D1266890

10TH EDITION

PHARMACOTHERAPY

A PATHOPHYSIOLOGIC APPROACH

Notice

Medicine is an ever-changing science. As new research and clinical experience broaden our knowledge, changes in treatment and drug therapy are required. The authors and the publisher of this work have checked with sources believed to be reliable in their efforts to provide information that is complete and generally in accord with the standards accepted at the time of publication. However, in view of the possibility of human error or changes in medical sciences, neither the authors nor the publisher nor any other party who has been involved in the preparation or publication of this work warrants that the information contained herein is in every respect accurate or complete, and they disclaim all responsibility for any errors or omissions or for the results obtained from use of the information contained in this work. Readers are encouraged to confirm the information contained herein with other sources. For example and in particular, readers are advised to check the product information sheet included in the package of each drug they plan to administer to be certain that the information contained in this work is accurate and that changes have not been made in the recommended dose or in the contraindications for administration. This recommendation is of particular importance in connection with new or infrequently used drugs.

10TH EDITION

PHARMACOTHERAPY

A PATHOPHYSIOLOGIC APPROACH

Editors

Joseph T. DiPiro, PharmD
Dean and Professor, Archie O. McCalley Chair
School of Pharmacy, Virginia Commonwealth University,
Richmond, Virginia

Robert L. Talbert, PharmD, FCCP, BCPS, FAHA
SmithKline Professor, College of Pharmacy, The University of Texas at Austin, Professor, School of Medicine, University of Texas Health Science Center at San Antonio, Texas

Gary C. Yee, PharmD, FCCP, BCOP
Professor and Associate Dean, Department of Pharmacy Practice, College of Pharmacy, University of Nebraska Medical Center, Omaha, Nebraska

Gary R. Matzke, PharmD, FCP, FCCP, FASN, FNAP
Professor and Founding Director, ACCP/ASHP/VCU Congressional Health Care Policy Fellow Program, Department of Pharmacotherapy and Outcome Sciences, School of Pharmacy, Virginia Commonwealth University, Richmond, Virginia

Barbara G. Wells, PharmD, FCCP, FASHP
Dean Emeritus and Professor Emeritus,
Department of Pharmacy Practice,
University of Mississippi, School of Pharmacy, Oxford, Mississippi

L. Michael Posey, BSPharm, MA
President, PENS Pharmacy Editorial & News Services,
Arlington, Virginia

Associate Editors

Vicki L. Ellingrod, PharmD, FCCP
Associate Dean for Research and John Gideon Searle Professor of Clinical and Translational Pharmacy, College of Pharmacy Professor of Psychiatry and Adjunct Professor of Psychology Associate Director, Michigan Institute for Clinical and Health Research (MICHR) and Director of the Education and Mentoring Group University of Michigan, Ann Arbor, Michigan

Stuart T. Haines, PharmD, BCPS, BCACP, BC-ADM
Professor, Department of Pharmacy Practice and Director, Division of Pharmacy Professional Development, University of Mississippi, School of Pharmacy, Jackson, Mississippi

Thomas D. Nolin, PharmD, PhD, FCCP, FCP, FASN
Associate Professor, Department of Pharmacy and Therapeutics, Center for Clinical Pharmaceutical Sciences, Department of Medicine, Renal-Electrolyte Division, University of Pittsburgh Schools of Pharmacy and Medicine, Pittsburgh, Pennsylvania

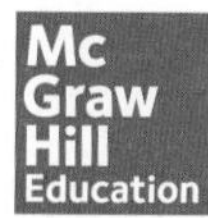

New York Chicago San Francisco Athens London Madrid Mexico City Milan New Delhi Singapore Sydney Toronto

Pharmacotherapy: A Pathophysiologic Approach, Tenth Edition

1 2 3 4 5 6 7 8 9 LWI 21 20 19 18 17 16

ISBN 978-1-259-58748-1
MHID 1-259-58748-7

This book was set in Minion Pro by Cenveo® Publishers Services.
The editors were Michael Weitz and Brian Kearns.
The production supervisor was Catherine H. Saggese.
Project management was provided by Rajinder Singh, Cenveo Publishers Services.
The interior designer was Alan Barnett.
The cover designer was Dreamit, Inc.
Cover Image: Shutterstock/Tsvetkov Maxim.
LSC Communications was printer and binder.

This book is printed on acid-free paper.

Library of Congress Cataloging-in-Publication Data

Names: DiPiro, Joseph T., editor.
Title: Pharmacotherapy : a pathophysiologic approach / [editors], Joseph T. DiPiro, Robert L. Talbert, Gary C. Yee, Gary R. Matzke, Barbara G. Wells, L. Michael Posey ; associate editors, Vicki L. Ellingrod, Stuart T. Haines, Thomas D. Nolin.
Other titles: Pharmacotherapy (New York)
Description: Tenth edition. | New York : McGraw-Hill Education, [2017] | Includes bibliographical references and index.
Identifiers: LCCN 2016035246| ISBN 9781259587481 (hardcover) | ISBN 1259587487
Subjects: | MESH: Drug Therapy
Classification: LCC RM263 | NLM WB 330 | DDC 615.5/8—dc23 LC record available at https://lccn.loc.gov/2016035246

Contents

SECTION 4 Gastrointestinal Disorders 433

Section Editor: *Joseph T. DiPiro*

SECTION 5 Renal Disorders 587

Section Editor: *Gary R. Matzke and Thomas D. Nolin*

SECTION 6 Neurologic Disorders 795

Section Editor: *Barbara G. Wells and Vicki L. Ellingrod*

SECTION 7 Psychiatric Disorders 943

Section Editor: *Barbara G. Wells and Vicki L. Ellingrod*

SECTION 14 Dermatologic Disorders 1535

Section Editor: *L. Michael Posey*

SECTION 15 Hematologic Disorders 1593

Section Editor: *Gary C. Yee*

SECTION 16 Infectious Diseases 1649

Section Editor: *Joseph T. DiPiro*

SECTION 17 Oncologic Disorders 2029

Section Editor: *Gary C. Yee*

SECTION 18 Nutritional Disorders 2323

Section Editor: *Gary R. Matzke*

SI Unit Conversions were produced by Dr. Ed Randell PhD DCC FCACB, Division Chief and Professor of Laboratory Medicine, Dept. of Lab. Medicine, Eastern Health Authority & Faculty of Medicine, Memorial University

Contributors

Val R. Adams, PharmD, FCCP, BCOP
Associate Professor
Department of Pharmacy Practice and Science
College of Pharmacy
University of Kentucky
Lexington, Kentucky
Chapter 129

Jeffrey R. Aeschlimann, PharmD
Associate Professor
Department of Pharmacy Practice
UConn School of Pharmacy
Storrs, Connecticut
Chapter e104

Aileen Ahiskali, PharmD
Antimicrobial Stewardship Pharmacist
Hennepin County Medical Center
Minneapolis, Minnesota
Chapter 129

Rondall E. Allen, BS, PharmD
Dean and Professor
School of Pharmacy and Health Professions
University of Maryland Eastern Shore
Princess Anne, Maryland
Chapter e38

Carlos A. Alvarez, PharmD, MSc, BCPS
Associate Professor
Texas Tech University Health Sciences
Center School of Pharmacy
University of Texas Southwestern
Dallas, Texas
Chapter 74

J. V. Anandan, PharmD
Consultant
Henry Ford Hospital
Detroit, Michigan
Chapter e115

Peter L. Anderson, PharmD
Professor
Department of Pharmaceutical Sciences
Skaggs School of Pharmacy and Pharmaceutical Sciences
University of Colorado Anschutz Medical Campus
Aurora, Colorado
Chapter 126

Jacqueline Argamany, PharmD
Pharmacotherapy Resident/MSc Candidate
College of Pharmacy
The University of Texas at Austin
Austin, TX
Adjoint Assistant Professor
Pharmacotherapy Education & Research Center
University of Texas Health Science Center at San Antonio
San Antonio, Texas
Chapter 117

Edward P. Armstrong, PharmD
Professor Emeritus
Department of Pharmacy Practice and Science
College of Pharmacy
University of Arizona
Tucson, Arizona
Chapter 118

Rebecca L. Attridge, PharmD, MSc, BCPS
Associate Professor
Department of Pharmacy Practice
University Incarnate Word Feik School of Pharmacy
Adjunct Assistant Professor
Division of Pulmonary Diseases and Critical Care Medicine
University of Texas Health Science Center
San Antonio, Texas
Chapter 28

Christine B. Baca, MD, MSHS
Assistant Professor
Department of Neurology
University of Colorado School of Medicine
Aurora, Colorado
Chapter 56

Jacquelyn L. Bainbridge, PharmD, FCCP
Professor
Department of Clinical Pharmacy and Neurology
University of Colorado
Anschutz Medical Campus
Skaggs School of Pharmacy and Pharmaceutical Sciences
Aurora, Colorado
Chapter 55

Jeffrey F. Barletta, PharmD, FCCM
Associate Professor and Vice Chair
Department of Pharmacy Practice
College of Pharmacy
Midwestern University
Glendale, Arizona
Chapter 12

Chad M. Barnett, PharmD, BCOP
Clinical Pharmacy Specialist-Breast Oncology
Division of Pharmacy
Clinical Pharmacy Services
University of Texas MD Anderson Cancer Center
Houston, Texas
Chapter 128

Brittany N. Bates, PharmD, BCPS
Clinical Assistant Professor and Clinical Pharmacist
Ohio Northern University
Lima Memorial Hospital
Lima, Ohio
Chapter 113

Marisa Battistella, BScPhm, PharmD, ACPR
Pharmacy Clinician Scientist
Assistant Professor
Leslie Dan Faculty of Pharmacy
University of Toronto
Clinical Pharmacist—Nephrology
University Health Network
Toronto, Ontario, Canada
Chapter 48

Larry A. Bauer, PharmD, FCP, FCCP
Professor
Department of Pharmacy
School of Pharmacy
Adjunct Professor
Department of Laboratory Medicine
School of Medicine
University of Washington
Seattle, Washington
Chapter e4

Steven J. Bauer, MD
Medical Director
Department of Psychiatry
Human Development Center
Duluth, Minnesota
Chapter e62

Jerry L. Bauman, PharmD, FCCP, FACC
Dean
College of Pharmacy
University of Illinois at Chicago
Professor
Departments of Pharmacy Practice and Medicine,
Section of Cardiology
Colleges of Pharmacy and Medicine
University of Illinois at Chicago
Chicago, Illinois
Chapter 18

Oralia V. Bazaldua, PharmD, FCCP, BCPS
Associate Professor
Department of Family and Community Medicine
University of Texas Health Science Center at San Antonio
San Antonio, Texas
Chapter e1

Donald Beam, MD
Pediatric Hematologist/Oncologist
Medical Director
Hemophilia and Bleeding Disorders Program
Cook Children's Medical Center
Fort Worth, Texas
Chapter 101

Nina Bemben, PharmD, BCPS
Assistant Professor
Department of Pharmacy Practice and Science
University of Maryland School of Pharmacy
Baltimore, Maryland
Chapter e8

Martha Blackford, PharmD, BCPS
Clinical Pharmacologist & Toxicologist
Clinical Pharmacology & Toxicology, Division of Critical Care
Department of Pediatrics
Akron Children's Hospital
Akron, Ohio
Chapter 107

Kathryn Blake, PharmD, BCPS, FCCP
Director, Center for Pharmacogenomics and Translational Research
Principal Research Scientist
Nemours Children's Specialty Care
Biomedical Research Department
Jacksonville, Florida
Chapter 26

Scott Bolesta, PharmD, BCPS, FCCM
Associate Professor
Department of Pharmacy Practice
Nesbitt College of Pharmacy
Wilkes University
Wilkes-Barre, Pennsylvania
AND
Visiting Investigator
Center for Pharmacy Innovation and Outcomes
Geisinger Health System
Danville, Pennsylvania
Chapter 39

Jill S. Borchert, PharmD, BCACP, BCPS, FCCP
Professor & Vice Chair
Pharmacy Practice
Director
PGY2 Ambulatory Care Residency Program
Midwestern University
Chicago College of Pharmacy
Chapter 92

Laura M. Borgelt, PharmD, FCCP, BCPS, NCMP
Associate Dean for Administration and Operations
Professor, Departments of Clinical Pharmacy and Family Medicine
Skaggs School of Pharmacy and Pharmaceutical Sciences
University of Colorado Anschutz Medical Campus
Aurora, Colorado
Chapter 82

Bonnie Lin Boster, PharmD, BCOP
Clinical Pharmacy Specialist
Division of Pharmacy
University of Texas MD Anderson Cancer Center
Houston, Texas
Chapter 128

Bradley A. Boucher, PharmD, FCCP, FCCM
Professor of Clinical Pharmacy
Associate Dean Strategic Initiatives and Operations
College of Pharmacy
University of Tennessee
Memphis, Tennessee
Chapter 58

Sharya Vaughan Bourdet, PharmD, BCPS
Critical Care Pharmacist/Clinical Inpatient Program Manager
Veterans Affairs Medical Center
Health Sciences Clinical Assistant Professor
School of Pharmacy
University of California
San Francisco, California
Chapter 27

Nancy C. Brahm, PharmD, MS, BCPP, CGP
Clinical Professor
College of Pharmacy
University of Oklahoma
Tulsa, Oklahoma
Chapter 73

Donald F. Brophy, PharmD, MSc, FCCP, BCPS
McFarlane Professor and Chairman
Department of Pharmacotherapy and Outcomes Sciences
School of Pharmacy
Virginia Commonwealth University
Richmond, Virginia
Chapter 51

Thomas ER Brown, PharmD
Associate Professor
Leslie Dan Faculty of Pharmacy
University of Toronto
Toronto, Ontario
Chapter 120

Peter F. Buckley, MD, MS
Dean
Professor of Psychiatry, Pharmacology, and Radiology
Medical College of Georgia
Augusta University
Augusta, Georgia
Chapter 67

David S. Burgess, PharmD, FCCP
Professor and Chair
University of Kentucky College of pharmacy
Department of Pharmacy Practice and Science
Lexington, Kentucky
Chapter 105

Karim Anton Calis, PharmD, MPH, FASHP, FCCP
Adjunct Senior Clinical Investigator
Office of the Clinical Director
Eunice Kennedy Shriver National Institute of Child Health and Human Development
National Institutes of Health
Bethesda, Maryland
Clinical Professor
University of Maryland
Baltimore, Maryland
Clinical Professor
Virginia Commonwealth University
Richmond, Virginia
Chapters e77, 82, and 144

Peggy L. Carver, PharmD, FCCP
Associate Professor of Pharmacy
Department of Clinical Pharmacy
University of Michigan College of Pharmacy
Ann Arbor, Michigan
Chapter 121

Larisa H. Cavallari, PharmD
Associate Professor
Department of Pharmacy Practice
University of Illinois at Chicago
Chicago, Illinois
Chapters e5 and 14

Alexandre Chan, PharmD, MPH, FCCP, BCPS, BCOP
Associate Professor and Assistant Head
Department of Pharmacy
Faculty of Science
National University of Singapore
Specialist Pharmacist (Oncology Pharmacy)
Department of Pharmacy
National Cancer Centre Singapore
Singapore
Chapter 132

C. Y. Jennifer Chan, PharmD, BCPPS
Clinical Assistant Professor of Pharmacy
Pharmacotherapy Education and Research Center
University of Texas at Austin—College of Pharmacy
Adjunct Associate Professor of Pediatrics
Department of Pediatrics
University of Texas Health Science Center
San Antonio, Texas
Chapter 102

Jack J. Chen, PharmD
Professor and Chair
Department of Pharmacy Practice
College of Pharmacy
Marshall B. Ketchum University
Fullerton, California
Department of Neurology
School of Medicine
Loma Linda University
Loma Linda, California
Chapters 56 and 59

Judy T. Chen, PharmD, BCPS, CDE, FNAP
Clinical Associate Professor
Department of Pharmacy Practice
Purdue University College of Pharmacy
Indianapolis, Indiana
Chapter 144

Katherine H. Chessman, PharmD, FCCP, BCPS, BCNSP
Professor
Department of Clinical Pharmacy and Outcomes Sciences
Medical University of South Carolina College of Pharmacy
Clinical Pharmacy Specialist, Pediatrics/Pediatric Surgery
Department of Pharmacy Services
Medical University of South Carolina Children's Hospital
Charleston, South Carolina
Chapters 49, 141, and 143

Sheryl L. Chow, PharmD, FCCP, FAHA, FHFSA, BCPS AQ-Cardiology
College of Pharmacy
Western University of Health Sciences
Pomona, California
Chapter e22

Mariann D. Churchwell, PharmD, BCPS, FCCP
Associate Professor
College of Pharmacy and Pharmaceutical Sciences
University of Toledo
Toledo, Ohio
Chapter 45

Peter A. Chyka, PharmD, FAACT, DABAT
Professor of Clinical Pharmacy and Associate Dean
College of Pharmacy
University of Tennessee Health Science Center
Knoxville, Tennessee
Chapter e9

Nathan P. Clark, PharmD, BCPS
Clinical Pharmacy Supervisor
Clinical Pharmacy, Anticoagulation and Anemia Service
Kaiser Permanente
Aurora, Colorado
Chapter 19

Jessica M. Clement, MD
Assistant Professor
Division of Hematology/Oncology
Department of Medicine
School of Medicine
UConn Health
Farmington, Connecticut
Chapter 130

Jennifer N. Clements, PharmD, BCPS, CDE, BCACP
Associate Professor
Department of Pharmacy Practice
Presbyterian College School of Pharmacy
Clinton, South Carolina
Chapter 37

Kristen Cook, PharmD, BCPS
Assistant Professor
Department of Pharmacy Practice
College of Pharmacy
University of Nebraska Medical Center
Omaha, Nebraska
Chapter 100

Lisa M. Cordes, PharmD, BCACP, BCOP
Oncology Clinical Pharmacy Specialist
Clinical Center Pharmacy Department
National Institutes of Health
Bethesda, Maryland
Chapter 127

Jason M. Cota, PharmD, MS
Vice Chair and Associate Professor
Department of Pharmacy Practice
University of the Incarnate Word Feik School of Pharmacy
San Antonio, Texas
Chapter e115

Elizabeth A. Coyle, PharmD, FCCM, BCPS
Assistant Dean of Assessment
Clinical Professor
University of Houston College of Pharmacy
Houston, Texas
Chapter 116

Catherine M. Crill, PharmD, BCPS, BCNSP
Associate Professor
Departments of Clinical Pharmacy and Pediatrics
University of Tennessee Health Science Center
Memphis, Tennessee
Chapter 142

M. Lynn Crismon, PharmD, FCCP, BCPP
Dean
James T. Doluisio Regents Chair and Behrens Centennial Professor
University of Texas at Austin—College of Pharmacy
Austin, Texas
Chapter 67

Daniel J. Crona, PharmD, PhD
Assistant Professor
Division of Pharmacotherapy and Experimental Therapeutics
University of North Carolina Eshelman School of Pharmacy
Chapel Hill, North Carolina
Chapter e138

Alix A. Dabb, PharmD
Pharmacy Specialist, Oncology Clinical Decision Support
Department of Pharmacy
Sidney Kimmel Comprehensive Cancer Center
Johns Hopkins Hospital
Baltimore, Maryland
Chapter 134

William E. Dager, PharmD, BCPS
Pharmacist Specialist
UC Davis Medical Center
Clinical Professor of Pharmacy
UC San Francisco School of Pharmacy
Clinical Professor of Medicine
UC Davis School of Medicine
Clinical Professor of Pharmacy
Touro School of Pharmacy
Sacramento, California
Chapter 43

Devra K. Dang, PharmD, BCPS, CDE
Associate Clinical Professor
School of Pharmacy
University of Connecticut
Storrs, Connecticut
Chapter 82

Khashayar Dashtipour, MD, PhD
Associate Professor Neurology and Basic Sciences
Director, Division of Movement Disorders
Department of Neurology/Movement Disorders
School of Medicine
Loma Linda University
Loma Linda, California
Chapter 59

Joseph F. Dasta, MSc, FCCM, FCCP
Adjunct Professor
University of Texas
Professor Emeritus
Ohio State University
Austin, Texas
Chapter 23

Dewayne A. Davidson, PharmD
Assistant Professor
Department of Family and Community Medicine
University of Texas Health Science Center at San Antonio
San Antonio, Texas
Chapter e1

Lisa E. Davis, PharmD, BCPS, BCOP
Professor
Department of Pharmacy Practice & Science
College of Pharmacy
University of Arizona
Tucson, Arizona
Chapter 130

Brian S. Decker, MD, PharmD, MS
Assistant Professor of Clinical Medicine
Nephrology Fellowship Training Program Director
Indiana University School of Medicine
Indianapolis, Indiana
Chapter 45

Simon de Denus, BPharm, MSC, PhD
Researcher Pharmacist
Montreal Heart Institute
Associate Professor
Faculty of Pharmacy Université de Montréal
Université de Montréal Beaulieu-Saucier Chair in Pharmacogenomics
Montreal, Quebec
Chapter 17

Paulina Deming, PharmD
Associate Professor
Department of Pharmacy Practice
College of Pharmacy-University of New Mexico Health Sciences Center
Albuquerque, New Mexico
Chapter 40

John W. Devlin, PharmD, FCCP, FCCM, BCPS
Professor
Department of Pharmacy and Health System Sciences
School of Pharmacy
Bouve College of Health Professions
Northeastern University
Boston, Massachusetts
Chapter 52

Joseph T. DiPiro, PharmD, BCPS
Dean and Professor
Archie O. McCalley Chair
School of Pharmacy
Virginia Commonwealth University
Richmond, Virginia
Chapter 114

Cecily DiPiro, PharmD
Consultant Pharmacist
Midlothian, Virginia
Chapter 35

Paul P. Dobesh, PharmD, FCCP, BCPS - AQ Cardiology
Professor of Pharmacy Practice
College of Pharmacy
University of Nebraska Medical Center
Omaha, Nebraska
Chapter 16

Paul L. Doering, MS
Distinguished Service Professor of Pharmacy Practice Emeritus
Department of Pharmacotherapy and Translational Research
College of Pharmacy
University of Florida
Gainesville, Florida
Chapters 65 and 66

Krista L. Donohoe, PharmD, BCPS, CGP
Assistant Professor
Department of Pharmacotherapy and Outcomes Science
Virginia Commonwealth University School of Pharmacy
Richmond, Virginia
Chapter 35

Julie A. Dopheide, PharmD, BCPP, FASHP
Professor of Clinical Pharmacy, Psychiatry, and the Behavioral Sciences
University of Southern California
School of Pharmacy and Keck School of Medicine
Director, Office of Continuing Professional Development
Director, PGY2 Psychiatric Pharmacy Residency
Los Angeles, California
Chapter 63

John M. Dopp, PharmD, MS
Associate Professor
School of Pharmacy
University of Wisconsin
Madison, Wisconsin
Chapter 72

Thomas C. Dowling, PharmD, PhD, FCCP, FCP
Professor,
Assistant Dean and Head
Pharmacy Practice Department
College of Pharmacy
Ferris State University
Grand Rapids, Michigan
Chapter e42

Shannon J. Drayton, PharmD
Associate Professor
Clinical Pharmacy and Outcomes Sciences
South Carolina College of Pharmacy
Medical University of South Carolina
Charleston, South Carolina
Chapter 69

Linda Dresser, PharmD, FCSHP
Assistant Professor
Leslie Dan Faculty of Pharmacy
University of Toronto
Pharmacotherapy Specialist - Antimicrobial Stewardship
University Health Network
Toronto, Ontario
Chapter 120

Bryson Duhon, PharmD, BCPS
Clinical Assistant Professor
The University of Texas College of Pharmacy
Austin, Texas
Chapter 117

Deepak P. Edward, MD
Jonas S Friedenwald Professor of Ophthalmology and Pathology
Department of Ophthalmology
Wilmer Eye Institute
Johns Hopkins University
Baltimore, Maryland
Chapter 94

Ramy Elshaboury, PharmD, BCPS AQ-ID
Clinical Pharmacy Coordinator - Infectious Diseases
Massachusetts General Hospital
Boston, Massachusetts
Chapter 106

Steven R. Erickson, PharmD
Associate Professor
Department of Clinical Pharmacy
College of Pharmacy
University of Michigan
Ann Arbor, Michigan
Chapter 73

Michael E. Ernst, PharmD
Professor (Clinical)
Department of Pharmacy Practice and Science
College of Pharmacy and Department of Family Medicine
Carver College of Medicine
University of Iowa
Iowa City, Iowa
Chapter 93

Brian L. Erstad, PharmD, FCCM, FCCP, FASHP
Professor
Department of Pharmacy Practice and Science
University of Arizona College of Pharmacy
Tucson, Arizona
Chapter 24

Patricia H. Fabel, PharmD, BCPS
Clinical Assistant Professor
Department of Clinical Pharmacy and Outcomes Sciences
South Carolina College of Pharmacy - University of South Carolina Campus
Columbia, South Carolina
Chapter 36

Susan C. Fagan, PharmD, BCPS, FCCP
Jowdy Professor, Assistant Dean
College of Pharmacy
University of Georgia
Athens, Georgia
Chapters 20 and e53

Christopher A. Fausel, PharmD, MHA, BCOP
Clinical Manager, Oncology Pharmacy
Department of Pharmacy
Indiana University Simon Cancer Center
Indianapolis, Indiana
Chapter 135

Christopher S. Fields, MD
Assistant Professor
Department of Psychiatry and Behavioral Sciences
Medical University of South Carolina
Charleston, South Carolina
Chapter 69

Shannon W. Finks, PharmD, FCCP, BCPS-AQ (Cardiology)
Associate Professor
College of Pharmacy
University of Tennessee
Memphis, Tennessee
Chapter 17

Richard G. Fiscella, PharmD, MPH
Clinical Professor Emeritus
Department of Pharmacy Practice
University of Illinois at Chicago
Chicago, Illinois
Chapter 94

Douglas N. Fish, PharmD, BCPS AQ-ID, FCCP, FCCM
Professor and Chair
Department of Clinical Pharmacy
Skaggs School of Pharmacy and Pharmaceutical Sciences
Aurora, Colorado
Chapters 110 and 122

Courtney V. Fletcher, PharmD
Dean and Professor
College of Pharmacy
University of Nebraska Medical Center
Omaha, Nebraska
Chapter 126

Rachel Flurie, PharmD, BCPS
Assistant Professor
Department of Pharmacotherapy and Outcomes Science
Virginia Commonwealth University School of Pharmacy
Richmond, Virginia
Chapter 51

Michelle Fravel, PharmD, BCPS
Clinical Assistant Professor
Clinical Pharmacy Specialist
Applied Clinical Science
Department of Pharmacy Practice and Science
University of Iowa College of Pharmacy
Iowa City, Iowa
Ambulatory Care Department of Pharmaceutical Care
University of Iowa Health Care
Iowa City, Iowa
Chapter 93

Bradi L. Frei, PharmD, MS, BCPS, BCOP
Associate Professor
Feik School of Pharmacy
University of the Incarnate Word
San Antonio, Texas
Chapter 108

Christopher R. Frei, PharmD, MS, FCCP, BCPS
Associate Professor and Division Head Pharmacotherapy Division
College of Pharmacy, The University of Texas at Austin
Center Director, Pharmacotherapy Education & Research Center,
School of Medicine, The University of Texas Health Science Center at San Antonio
San Antonio, Texas
Chapter 108

Melissa Frei-Jones, MD
Associate Professor
Department of Pediatrics
Division of Hematology/Oncology
School of Medicine
University of Texas Health Science Center
San Antonio, Texas
Chapter 102

Mark L. Glover, PharmD
Associate Consultant
Eli Lilly and Company
Indianapolis, Indiana
Chapter 107

Leigh Anne Hylton Gravatt, PharmD, BCPS
Assistant Professor
Department of Pharmacotherapy and Outcomes Science
Virginia Commonwealth University School of Pharmacy
Richmond, Virginia
Chapter 35

Shelly L. Gray, PharmD, MS
Professor and Vice Chair for Curriculum and Instruction
Department of Pharmacy
Director
Geriatric Pharmacy Program and PleinCertifi cate
School of Pharmacy
University of Washington
Seattle, Washington
Chapter e7

Elisa M. Greene, PharmD, BCACP
Assistant Professor
Department of Pharmacy Practice
Clinical Pharmacist—Siloam Family Health Center
College of Pharmacy
Belmont University
Nashville, Tennessee
Chapter 103

Alan E. Gross, PharmD, BCPS AQ-ID
Clinical Assistant Professor
Department of Pharmacy Practice
University of Illinois at Chicago College of Pharmacy
Chicago, Illinois
Chapter 114

Wayne P. Gulliver, MD, FRCPC
Professor of Dermatology and Medicine
Memorial University of Newfoundland
St. John's, Newfoundland and Labrador, Canada
Chapter 97

John G. Gums, PharmD, FCCP
Professor of Pharmacy and Translational Research
Department of Family Medicine
College of Pharmacy and Medicine
University of Florida
Gainesville, Florida
Chapter 76

Tracy M. Hagemann, PharmD, FCCP, FPPAG
Professor and Associate Dean
College of Pharmacy
University of Tennessee Health Sciences Center
Nashville, Tennessee
Chapters 101 and e103

Emily Hajjar, PharmD, BCPS, BCAP, CGP
Associate Professor
Department of Pharmacy Practice
Jefferson School of Pharmacy
Thomas Jefferson University
Philadelphia, Pennsylvania
Chapter e7

Jason S. Haney, PharmD, BCPS
Assistant Professor
Medical University of South Carolina
College of Pharmacy
Charleston, South Carolina
Chapter 49

Joseph T. Hanlon, PharmD, MS
Professor
Department of Medicine, Pharmacy and Therapeutics, and Epidemiology
University of Pittsburgh
Pittsburgh, Pennsylvania
Chapter e7

Michelle S. Harkins, MD
Associate Professor of Medicine
Department of Internal Medicine
University of New Mexico Health Sciences Center
Albuquerque, New Mexico
Chapter e30

T. Kristopher Harrell, PharmD, MA, FASHP
Associate Professor
Director of Experiential Affairs
Department of Pharmacy Practice
University of Mississippi
School of Pharmacy
Jackson, Mississippi
Chapter 61

Mary S. Hayney, PharmD, MPH, BCPS
Professor of Pharmacy
Division of Pharmacy Practice
University of Wisconsin --Madison School of Pharmacy
Madison, Wisconsin
Chapter 125

Brian A. Hemstreet, PharmD, FCCP, BCPS
Assistant Dean for Student Affairs
Professor of Pharmacy Practice
Regis University School of Pharmacy
Denver, Colorado
Chapter 34

Chris Herndon, PharmD
Associate Professor
School of Pharmacy
Southern Illinois University Edwardsville
Edwardsville, Illinois
Chapter 60

Lauren R. Hersh, MD
Instructor
Department of Family and Community Medicine
Thomas Jefferson University
Philadelphia, Pennsylvania
Chapter e7

David C. Hess, MD
Professor and Chairman
Department of Neurology
Medical College of Georgia
Augusta, Georgia
Chapter 20

Sarah E. Hobgood, MD
Assistant Professor
Geriatric Medicine
Department of Internal Medicine
School of Medicine
Virgina Commonwealth University
Richmond, Virginia
Chapter 54

Barbara J. Hoeben, Lt Col, USAF, PharmD, MSPharm, BCPS
Keesler Air Force Base
Biloxi, Mississippi
Chapter e10

Lisa M. Holle, PharmD, BCOP, FHOPA
Associate Clinical Professor
Department of Pharmacy Practice
School of Pharmacy
University of Connecticut
Storrs, Connecticut
Chapter 130

Jessica Holt, PharmD, BCPS (AQ-ID)
Infectious Diseases Pharmacy Coordinator
Department of Pharmacy
Abbott Northwestern Hospital, Part of Allina Health
Minneapolis, Minnesota
Chapter 106

Marcella N. Honkonen, PharmD, BCPS
Assistant Professor
Department of Pharmacy Practice and Science
University of Arizona College of Pharmacy
Tucson, Arizona
Chapter 118

Joanna Q. Hudson, PharmD, BCPS, FASN, FCCP, FNKF
Professor
Department of Clinical Pharmacy
Associate Professor
Department of Medicine (Nephrology)
University of Tennessee, Health Sciences Center
Memphis, Tennessee
Chapter 44

Andrew Y. Hwang, PharmD, BCPS
Postdoctoral Fellow, Family Medicine
University of Florida College of Pharmacy
Department of Pharmacotherapy and Translational Research
Gainesville, Florida
Chapter 76

Heather J. Johnson, PharmD, BCPS, FASN
Assistant Professor
Department of Pharmacy and Therapeutics
University of Pittsburgh School of Pharmacy
Clinical Specialist-Transplant, UPMC
Pittsburgh, Pennsylvania
Chapter 89

Jacqueline Jonklaas, MD, PhD
Associate Professor
Division of Endocrinology
Department of Medicine
Georgetown University
Washington, DC
Chapter 75

Joseph K. Jordan, PharmD, BCPS
Associate Professor
Department of Pharmacy Practice
Butler University College of Pharmacy and Health Sciences
Drug Information Specialist
Indiana University Health
Indianapolis, Indiana

Thomas Kakuda, PharmD
Scientific Director
Clinical Pharmacology
Alios BioPharma, Inc, part of the Janssen Pharmaceutical Companies of Johnson & Johnson
South San Francisco, California
Chapter 126

Sophia N. Kalantaridou, MD, PhD
Professor of Obstetrics and Gynecology
Department of Obstetrics and Gynecology
University of Ioannina Medical School
Ioannina, Greece
Chapter 82

Judith C. Kando, PharmD, BCPP
Shire Pharmaceuticals
Lead, U.S. Medical, BED
Lexington, Massachusetts
Chapter 68

Michael P. Kane, PharmD, FCCP, BCPS, BCACP
Professor
Department of Pharmacy Practice
School of Pharmacy and Pharmaceutical Sciences
Albany College of Pharmacy and Health Sciences
Clinical Pharmacy Specialist
Albany Medical Center Division of Community Endocrinology (formerly The Endocrine Group)
Albany, New York
Chapter 75

S. Lena Kang-Birken, PharmD, FCCP, AAHIVP
Associate Professor
Department of Pharmacy Practice
Thomas J Long School of Pharmacy and Health Sciences
University of the Pacific
Stockton, California
Chapter 119

Salmaan Kanji, PharmD
Clinical Pharmacy Specialist
The Ottawa Hospital
Associate Scientist
The Ottawa Hospital Research Institute
Ottawa, Ontario, Canada
Chapter 123

Rania S. Kattura, PharmD, MS, BCPP
Psychiatric Pharmacist
Austin State Hospital
Adjunct Assistant Professor
College of Pharmacy
University of Texas at Austin
Austin, Texas
Chapter 67

Patrick J. Kiel, PharmD, BCPS, BCOP
Clinical Pharmacy Specialist
Hematology/Oncology - Precision Genomics Program
Indiana University Simon Cancer Center
Indianapolis, Indiana
Chapter 135

Scott E. Kincaid, PharmD, BCPS
Director, Clinical Pharmacy Services
UK HealthCare
Adjunct Assistant Professor
Department of Pharmacy Practice and Science
University of Kentucky College of Pharmacy
Lexington, Kentucky
Chapter e124

William R. Kirchain, PharmD, CDE
Wilbur and Mildred Robichaux Endowed Professor
Division of Clinical and Administrative Sciences
Xavier University of Louisiana, College of Pharmacy
New Orleans, Louisiana
Chapter e38

Cynthia K. Kirkwood, PharmD, BCPP
Professor and Executive Associate Dean for Academic Affairs
School of Pharmacy
Virginia Commonwealth University
Richmond, Virginia
Chapters 70 and 71

Jacqueline M. Klootwyk, PharmD, BCPS, BCACP, TTS
Assistant Professor of Clinical, Social, and Administrative Sciences
Mylan School of Pharmacy
Duquesne University
Pittsburgh, Pennsylvania
Chapter 80

Leroy C. Knodel, PharmD
[DECEASED]
Associate Professor
Department of Surgery
University of Texas Health Science Center
San Antonio, Texas
Clinical Professor
University of Texas at Austin—College of Pharmacy
Austin, Texas
Chapter 117

Jill M. Kolesar, PharmD, MS, FCCP, BCPS
Professor
Department of Pharmacy Practice and Science
Department of Internal Medicine
Colleges of Pharmacy and Medicine
Director, Early Phase Clinical Trials Center
Markey Cancer Center
University of Kentucky
Lexington, Kentucky
Chapter 131

Lisa T Costanigro, PharmD
Clinical Pharmacist
Department of Pharmacy
Poudre Valley Hospital - University of Colorado Health
Fort Collins, Colorado
Chapter e10

Sunil Kripalani, MD, MSc
Associate Professor
Section of Hospital Medicine
Division of General Internal Medicine and Public Health
Department of Medicine
Vanderbilt University
Nashville, Tennessee
Chapter e1

Vanessa J. Kumpf, PharmD, BCNSP
Clinical Specialist, Nutrition Support
Center for Human Nutrition
Vanderbilt University Medical Center
Nashville, Tennessee
Chapters 141 and 143

Po Gin Kwa, MD, FRCPC
Clinical Assistant, Professor of Pediatrics
Faculty of Medicine
Memorial University of Newfoundland and Pediatrician
Eastern Health
St. John's, Newfoundland and Labrador, Canada
Chapter 98

Jeffrey A. Kyle, PharmD, BCPS
Associate Professor of Pharmacy Practice
Clinical Pharmacy Specialist, Shelby Baptist Medical Center
Department of Pharmacy Practice
McWhorter School of Pharmacy
Samford University
Birmingham, Alabama
Chapter 111

Y. W. Francis Lam, PharmD, FCCP
Professor
Department of Pharmacology (MSC 7764)
University of Texas Health Science Center at San Antonio
San Antonio, Texas
Chapter e5

Sum Lam, PharmD, CGP, BCPS, FASCP
Associate Clinical Professor
Department of Clinical Pharmacy Practice
St. John's University
Queens, New York
Chapter 85

Richard A. Lange, MD, MBA
President
Dean, Paul L. Foster School of Medicine
Rick and Ginger Francis Endowed Professor
El Paso, Texas
Chapter e11

Kerry L. Laplante, PharmD, BS
Infectious Diseases Pharmacotherapy Specialist
Providence Veterans Affairs Medical Center
Associate Professor of Pharmacy
College of Pharmacy
University of Rhode Island
Adjunct Associate Professor of Medicine
Warren Alpert School of Medicine
Brown University
Kingston, Rhode Island
Chapter e104

Alan H. Lau, PharmD, FCCP
Professor
Department of Pharmacy Practice
Director
International Clinical Pharmacy Education
College of Pharmacy
University of Illinois at Chicago
Chicago, Illinois
Chapter 47

Michael Lauzardo, MD, MSc
Chief
Division of Infectious Diseases and Global Medicine
Director
Southeastern National Tuberculosis Center
College of Medicine
University of Florida
Gainesville, Florida
Chapter 112

Rebecca Law, PharmD
School of Pharmacy and Discipline of Family Medicine
Faculty of Medicine
Memorial University of Newfoundland
St. John's Newfoundland, Canada
Chapter 98

David T. S. Law, BSc, MD, PhD, CCFP
Assistant Professor
Department of Family and Community Medicine
Faculty of Medicine
University of Toronto
Staff, Department of Family Practice
The Scarborough Hospital and Rouge Valley Health System
Scarborough, Ontario, Canada
Chapter e99

Rebecca Law, PharmD
School of Pharmacy and Discipline of Family Medicine
Faculty of Medicine
Memorial University of Newfoundland
St. John's Newfoundland, Canada
Chapters 97 and e99

Grace C. Lee, PharmD, PhD, BCPS
Assistant Professor
College of Pharmacy, The University of Texas at Austin
Austin, Texas
Pharmacotherapy Education and Research Center, School of Medicine, University of Texas Health Science Center at San Antonio
San Antonio, Texas
Chapter 105

Mary Lee, PharmD, BCPS, FCCP
Professor of Pharmacy Practice
Chicago College of Pharmacy
Midwestern University
Downers Grove, Illinois
Chapters 83 and 84

Timothy S. Lesar, PharmD
Director of Clinical Pharmacy Services
Patient Care Services Director
Department of Pharmacy
Albany Medical Center
Albany, New York
Chapter 94

Deborah J. Levine, MD, FCCP
Associate Professor of Medicine
Division of Pulmonary and Critical Care
University of Texas at San Antonio
San Antonio, Texas
Chapter 28

Stephanie M. Levine, MD
Professor of Medicine
Division of Pulmonary Diseases and Critical Care Medicine
University of Texas Health Science Center
San Antonio, Texas
Chapter e25

Robin Moorman Li, PharmD, BCACP, CPE
Assistant Director
Jacksonville Campus
Clinical Associate Professor
Department of Pharmacotherapy and Translational Research
College of Pharmacy
University of Florida
Gainesville, Florida
Chapters 65 and 66

Susanne Liewer, PharmD, BCOP
Clinical Pharmacy Coordinator, Stem Cell Transplant
Department of Pharmaceutical and Nutrition Care
Nebraska Medicine
Clinical Associate Professor
Department of Pharmacy Practice
College of Pharmacy
University of Nebraska Medical Center
Omaha, Nebraska
Chapter 140

Bryan L. Love, PharmD, BCPS-AQ ID
Associate Professor
Department of Clinical Pharmacy & Outcomes Sciences
South Carolina College of Pharmacy
University of South Carolina Campus
Columbia, South Carolina
Chapter 33

Amanda M. Loya
Clinical Associate Professor
University of Texas at El Paso
UT Austin Cooperative Pharmacy Program
University of Texas at El Paso College of Health Sciences
University of Texas at Austin—College of Pharmacy
Adjunct Clinical Assistant Professor
Department of Family and Community Medicine
Texas Tech University Health Sciences Center—El Paso
El Paso, Texas
Chapter e2

Robert MacLaren, BSc, PharmD, MPH, FCCM, FCCP
Professor
Department of Clinical Pharmacy
Skaggs School of Pharmacy and Pharmaceutical Sciences
University of Colorado Denver
Aurora, Colorado
Chapter 23

Eric J. MacLaughlin, PharmD, FCCP, BCPS
Professor and Head of Adult Medicine
Department of Pharmacy Practice
Professor
Departments of Family Medicine and Internal Medicine
Texas Tech University Health Sciences Center School of Pharmacy
Amarillo, Texas
Chapter 13

Jenana Halilovic Maker, PharmD, BCPS
Associate Professor
Department of Pharmacy Practice
Thomas J Long School of Pharmacy and Health Sciences
Stockton, California
Chapter 43

Robert A. Mangione, PharmD
Provost and Professor of Pharmacy
Office of the Provost
St. John's University
Queens, New York
Chapter 41

Steven J. Martin, PharmD, BCPS, FCCP, FCCM
Dean and Professor
Rudolph H. Raabe College of Pharmacy
Ohio Northern University
Ada, Ohio
Chapter 142

Gary R. Matzke, PharmD, FCP, FCCP, FASN, FNAP
Professor and Founding Director
ACCP/ASHP/VCU Congressional Health Care Policy
Fellow Program
Department of Pharmacotherapy and Outcome Sciences
School of Pharmacy
Virginia Commonwealth University
Richmond, Virginia
Chapters 48, 52

J. Russell May, PharmD
Clinical Professor
Department of Clinical and Administrative Pharmacy
University of Georgia College of Pharmacy
Augusta, Georgia
Chapter 95

Dianne May, PharmD, FCCP, BCPS
Clinical Professor
Department of Clinical and Administrative Pharmacy
Campus Director for Pharmacy Practice Experiences
Division of Experience Programs
University of Georgia College of Pharmacy
Augusta, Georgia
Chapter 32

Rachael McCaleb, PharmD
Assistant Professor
School of Pharmacy
University of Arkansas For Medical Sciences
Little Rock, Arkansas

Kristen B. McCullough, PharmD, BCPS, BCOP
Hematology/Oncology Clinical Pharmacy Specialist
Assistant Professor of Pharmacy
Mayo Clinic College of Medicine
Mayo Clinic
Rochester, Minnesota
Chapter e137

Kimberly McKeirnan, PharmD, BCACP
Clinical Assistant Professor
Department of Pharmacotherapy
Washington State University College of Pharmacy
Spokane, Washington
Chapter 10

Mary Lynn McPherson, PharmD, MA, BCPS, CPE
Professor
Executive Director, Advanced Post-Graduate Education in Palliative Care
Department of Pharmacy Practice and Science
University of Maryland School of Pharmacy
Baltimore, Maryland
Chapter 8

Sarah T. Melton, PharmD, BCPP, BCACP, FASCP
Professor of Pharmacy Practice
Department of Pharmacy Practice
Gatton College of Pharmacy at East Tennessee State University
Johnson City, Tennessee
Chapters 70 and 71

Julianna A. Merten, PharmD, BCPS, BCOP
Clinical Pharmacy Specialist - Hematology/Oncology
Assistant Professor of Pharmacy
Mayo Clinic College of Medicine
Mayo Clinic
Rochester, Minnesota
Chapter e137

Laura Boehnke Michaud, PharmD, FASHP, BCOP, CMQ
Manager, Clinical Pharmacy Services
Division of Pharmacy
Clinical Pharmacy Services
University of Texas MD Anderson Cancer Center
Houston, Texas
Chapter 128

Deborah S. Minor, PharmD
Professor
Department of Medicine
University of Mississippi
School of Medicine
Jackson, Mississippi
Chapter 61

Augusto Miravalle, MD
Associate Professor
Department of Neurology
University of Colorado School of Medicine
Associate Director
Neurology Residency Program
University of Colorado
Anschutz Medical Campus
Aurora, Colorado
Chapter 55

Phillip L. Mohorn, PharmD, BCPS, BCCCP
Clinical Pharmacy Specialist-Critical Care
Department of Pharmacy
Spartanburg Medical Center
Spartanburg Regional Healthcare System
Spartanburg, South Carolina
Chapter 33

Patricia A. Montgomery, PharmD, FCSHP
Clinical Pharmacy Specialist
Mercy General Hospital
Sacramento, CA
Adjunct Professor of Pharmacy
University of the Pacific
Stockton, California
Chapter 39

Rebecca Moote, PharmD, MSc, BCPS
Associate Professor
Department of Pharmacy Practice
Regis University School of Pharmacy
Denver, Colorado
Chapter 28

Scott W Mueller, PharmD, BCCCP
Assistant Professor
Department of Clinical Pharmacy
University of Colorado Skaggs School of Pharmacy and Pharmaceutical Sciences
Aurora, Colorado
Chapters 23 and 112

Milap Nahata, PharmD, MS, FCCP
Professor of Pharmacy
Pediatrics and Internal Medicine
Division Chair
Pharmacy Practice and Administration College of Pharmacy
Ohio State University
Associate Director of Pharmacy
Ohio State University Medical Center
Columbus, Ohio
Chapter e6

Rocsanna Namdar PharmD, BCPS, FCCP
Medical Science Liaison
Medical Affairs
Allergan, Inc.
Irvine, California
Chapter 112

Jennifer Greene Naples
Clinical Pharmacist, Pharmacovigilance
Pharmacovigilance Center, Office of The Surgeon General, Department of the Army
Falls Church, Virginia
Chapter e7

Jean Nappi, BS, PharmD, FCCP, BCPS
Professor of Clinical Pharmacy and Outcome Sciences
South Carolina College of Pharmacy—MUSC Campus Professor of Medicine, Medical University of South Carolina
Charleston, South Carolina
Chapter 14

Leigh Anne Nelson, PharmD, BCPP
Associate Professor
Division of Pharmacy Practice and Administration
University of Missouri–Kansas City School of Pharmacy
Kansas City, Missouri
Chapter e62

Viet-Huong V. Nguyen, PharmD, MPH, MS, BCPS
Assistant Professor
Department of Pharmacy Practice
Chapman University School of Pharmacy
Irvine, California
Chapter 56

Jessica Njoku, PharmD, MPH, BCPS
Clinical Director, Pharmacy Services/Antimicrobial Stewardship
Good Shepherd Health System
Longview, Texas
Chapter 109

Thomas D. Nolin, PharmD, PhD, FCCP, FCP, FASN
Associate Professor
Department of Pharmacy and Therapeutics
Center for Clinical Pharmaceutical Sciences
Department of Medicine, Renal-Electrolyte Division
University of Pittsburgh Schools of Pharmacy and Medicine
Pittsburgh, Pennsylvania
Chapter 46

LeAnn B. Norris, PharmD, BCPS, BCOP
Associate Professor
Department of Clinical Pharmacy and Outcomes Sciences
South Carolina College of Pharmacy
Columbia, South Carolina
Chapter 131

Elizabeth K. Nugent, MD
Assistant Professor
Department of Obstetrics, Gynecology and Reproductive Sciences
University of Texas Health Science Center McGovern Medical School
Houston, Texas
Chapter 133

Cindy L. O'Bryant, PharmD, BCOP, FCCP, FHOPA
Professor
Department of Clinical Pharmacy
Skaggs School of Pharmacy and Pharmaceutical Sciences
Clinical Specialist in Oncology
University of Colorado Anschutz Medical Campus
Aurora, Colorado
Chapter 139

Mary Beth O'Connell, PharmD, BCPS, FASHP, FCCP
Associate Professor
Department of Pharmacy Practice
Eugene Applebaum College of Pharmacy and Health Sciences
Wayne State University
Detroit, Michigan
Chapter 92

Brian Odle, PharmD
Associate Professor
Department of Pharmacy Practice
East Tennessee State University
Gatton College of Pharmacy
Johnson City, Tennessee
Chapter 111

Keith M. Olsen, PharmD, FCCP, FCCM
Dean and Professor
College of Pharmacy
University of Arkansas for Medical Sciences
Little Rock, Arkansas
Chapters e31 and 114

Oohed A. Owaidhah, MD
Glaucoma
King Khaled Eye Specialist Hospital
Riyadh, Saudi Arabia
Chapter 94

Amy Barton Pai, PharmD, BCPS, FASN, FCCP, FNKF
Associate Professor
Department of Clinical Pharmacy
College of Pharmacy
University of Michigan
Ann Arbor, Michigan
Chapter 50

Robert B. Parker, PharmD, FCCP
Professor
Department of Clinical Pharmacy
College of Pharmacy
University of Tennessee
Memphis, Tennessee
Chapter 14

Priti N. Patel, PharmD, BCPS
Clinical Associate Professor
Assistant Campus Director, St. Petersburg Campus
Department of Pharmacotherapy and Translational Science
University of Florida College of Pharmacy
St. Petersburg, Florida
Chapter 41

Charles Peloquin, PharmD, FCCP
Professor, and Director, Infectious Disease Pharmacokinetics Lab.
College of Pharmacy, and Emerging Pathogens Institute
University of Florida
Gainesville, Florida
Chapter 112

Janelle Perkins, PharmD, BCOP
Associate Professor
Department of Pharmacotherapeutics and Clinical Research
College of Pharmacy
University of South Florida
Tampa, Florida
Chapter 140

Emily P. Peron, PharmD, MS, BCPS, FASCP
Assistant Professor
Geriatric Pharmacotherapy Program
Department of Pharmacotherapy & Outcomes Science
School of Pharmacy
Virginia Commonwealth University
Richmond, Virginia
Chapter 54

Jay Peters, MD
Professor and Chief
Division of Pulmonary Critical Care
University of Texas Health Science Center
San Antonio, Texas
Chapter e25

Sarah Scarpace Peters, PharmD, MPH, BCOP
Associate Professor
Department of Pharmacy Practice
Albany College of Pharmacy and Health Sciences
Albany, New York
Chapter 129

Stephanie J. Phelps, PharmD
Associate Dean
Academic Affairs
Professor
Clinical Pharmacy and Pediatrics
College of Pharmacy
University of Tennessee Health Science Center
Memphis, Tennessee
Chapter 57

Bradley G. Phillips, PharmD, BCPS, FCCP
Milliken-Reeve Professor and Head
Department of Clinical and Administrative Pharmacy
University of Georgia College of Pharmacy
Athens, Georgia
Chapter 72

Amy M. Pick, PharmD, BCOP
Director of Faculty and Staff Development
Associate Professor
Department of Pharmacy Practice
School of Pharmacy and Health Professions
Creighton University
Omaha, Nebraska
Chapter 136

Nicole Weimert Pilch, PharmD, MSCR, BCPS, FAST
Quality and Outcomes Director, Transplant ICCE
Clinical Associate Professor
Department of Pharmacy and Clinical Sciences
South Carolina College of Pharmacy - MUSC Campus
Medical University of South Carolina
Charleston, South Carolina
Chapter 86

Kathleen J. Pincus, PharmD, BCPS
Assistant Professor
Department of Pharmacy Practice and Science
School of Pharmacy
University of Maryland
Baltimore, Maryland
Chapter 81

Steven R. Pliszka, MD
Division of Child and Adolescent Psychiatry
Dielmann Distinguished Professor and Chair
Department of Psychiatry
University of Texas Health Science Center at San Antonio
San Antonio, Texas
Chapter 63

Jamie C. Poust, PharmD, BCOP
Oncology & Palliative Care Pharmacy Specialist
Department of Pharmacy
University of Colorado Hospital
Anschutz Inpatient Pavilion
Aurora, Colorado
Chapter 139

Kacie E. Powers, PharmD, BCPS
Assistant Professor
Geriatric Pharmacotherapy Program
Department of Pharmacotherapy and Outcomes Science
School of Pharmacy
Virginia Commonwealth University
Richmond, Virginia
Chapter 54

Randall A. Prince, PharmD, FCCP, FCP, FIDSA
Professor
Department of Pharmacy Practice and Translational Research
University of Houston College of Pharmacy
Houston, Texas
Chapter 116

Kelly Ragucci, PharmD, FCCP, BCPS, CDE
Professor and Chair
Clinical Pharmacy and Outcomes Sciences
South Carolina College of Pharmacy
Medical University of South Carolina Campus
Charleston, South Carolina
Chapter 79

Hengameh H. Raissy, PharmD
Research Associate Professor of Pediatrics
Pulmonary Division
School of Medicine
University of New Mexico
Albuquerque, New Mexico
Chapter e30

Satish S. C. Rao, MD, PhD, FRCP
Georgia Health Sciences University
Medical College of Georgia
Professor of Medicine, Chief, Section of Gastroenterology/Hepatology
Director
Digestive Health Center
Augusta, Georgia
Chapter 32

Kamakshi V. Rao, PharmD, BCOP, CPP, FASHP
Clinical Pharmacist Practitioner, Bone Marrow Transplant
University of North Carolina Hospitals and Clinics
Associate Professor of Clinical Education
University of North Carolina Eshelman School of Pharmacy
Chapel Hill, North Carolina
Chapter 136

James B. Ray, PharmD, CPE
James A. Otterbeck OnePoint Patient Care
Clinical Associate Professor in Hospice and Palliative Care
Department of Pharmacy Practice and Science/Division of Applied Clinical Sciences
College of Pharmacy
University of Iowa
Iowa City, Iowa
Chapter 60

Brent N. Reed, PharmD, BCPS
Assistant Professor
Department of Pharmacy Practice and Science
School of Pharmacy
University of Maryland
Clinical Pharmacy Specialist
Department of Pharmacy
University of Maryland Medical Center
Baltimore, Maryland
Chapter 15

Michael D. Reed, PharmD, FCCP, FCP
Medical Writer
PPD
Wilmington, North Carolina
Chapter 107

Thomas Repas, DO, FACP, FACOI, FNLA, FACE, CDE
Clinical Associate Professor
Department of Internal Medicine
Sanford School of Medicine
University of South Dakota
Sioux Falls, South Dakota
Chapter 74

Beth H. Resman-Targoff, PharmD, FCCP
Clinical Professor
Department of Pharmacy
Clinical and Administrative Sciences
College of Pharmacy
University of Oklahoma
Oklahoma City, Oklahoma
Chapter 87

José O. Rivera, PharmD
Director and Clinical Professor
UT Austin Cooperative Pharmacy Program
College of Health Sciences
University of Texas at El Paso College of Health Sciences
Assistant Dean and Clinical Professor
University of Texas at Austin College of Pharmacy
El Paso, Texas
Chapter e2

Jo E. Rodgers, PharmD, FCCP, BCPS
Clinical Associate Professor
Department of Pharmacotherapy and Experimental Therapeutics
Eshelman School of Pharmacy
University of North Carolina at Chapel Hill
Chapel Hill, North Carolina
Chapter 15

Andrew M. Roecker, PharmD, BCPS
Professor and Chair
Department of Pharmacy Practice
Rudolph H. Raabe College of Pharmacy
Ohio Northern University
Ada, Ohio
Chapter 113

Kelly C. Rogers, PharmD, FCCP
Professor of Clinical Pharmacy
UTHSC Campus AED Program Coordinator
College of Pharmacy
University of Tennessee
Memphis, Tennessee
Chapter 17

Susan J. Rogers, PharmD
Assistant Clinical Professor (Retired)
University of Texas College of Pharmacy (Austin)
Clinical Pharmacy Specialist Neurology (Retired)
South Texas Healthcare System
Audie L. Murphy Memorial Veterans Hospital
San Antonio, Texas
Chapter 56

John C. Rotschafer, PharmD, FCCP
Professor
Experimental and Clinical Pharmacology
University of Minnesota
College of Pharmacy
Minneapolis, Minnesota
Chapter 106

Eric S. Rovner, MD
Professor of Urology
Department of Urology
Medical University of South Carolina
Charleston, South Carolina
Chapter 85

Valerie L. Ruehter, PharmD, BCPP
Clinical Associate Professor
Director of Experiential Learning
University of Missouri-Kansas City School of Pharmacy
Kansas City, Missouri
Chapter 64

Melody Ryan, PharmD, MPH, BCPS, CGP
Professor
College of Pharmacy
University of Kentucky
Lexington, Kentucky
Chapter e53

Stephen J. Ryan, MD, MS
Clinical Professor
College of Medicine
University of Kentucky
Lexington, Kentucky
Chapter e53

Michael J. Rybak, PharmD, MPH
Professor of Pharmacy & Medicine
Anti-Infective Research Laboratory
Department of Pharmacy Practice
Eugene Applebaum College of Pharmacy & Health Sciences
Wayne State University
Detroit, Michigan
Chapter e104

Cynthia A. Sanoski, PharmD, BCPS, FCCP
Chair and Associate Professor
Department of Pharmacy Practice
Jefferson School of Pharmacy
Thomas Jefferson University
Philadelphia, Pennsylvania
Chapter 18

Joseph J. Saseen, PharmD
Professor
Clinical Pharmacy and Family Medicine
Vice Chair
Department of Clinical Pharmacy
Anschutz Medical Campus
University of Colorado
Aurora, Colorado
Chapter 13

Mark E. Schneiderhan, PharmD, BCPP
Associate Professor
Human Development Center, Psychiatry Department
Mental Health Provider
University of Minnesota
College of Pharmacy—Duluth
Duluth, Minnesota
Chapter e62

Kristine S. Schonder, PharmD
Assistant Professor
Department of Pharmacy and Therapeutics
School of Pharmacy
University of Pittsburgh
Clinical Specialist-Transplantation, UPMC
Pittsburgh, Pennsylvania
Chapter 89

Arthur Schuna, MS, BCACP, FASHP
Clinical Professor
University of Wisconsin School of Pharmacy
Madison, Wisconsin
Chapter 91

Julie M. Sease, Pharm D, FCCP, BCPS, CDE, BCACP
Associate Dean for Academic Affairs and Professor of Pharmacy Practice
Presbyterian College School of Pharmacy
Clinton, South Carolina
Chapter 37

Jolynn Sessions, PharmD, BCOP
Clinical Pharmacist in Oncology
Mission Health System
Associate Professor of Clinical Education
University of North Carolina Eshelman School of Pharmacy
Asheville, North Carolina
Chapter 132

Amy Hatfield Seung, PharmD, BCOP
Senior Director, Clinical Initiatives
Physician Resource Management/Caret
Cary, North Carolina
Chapter 134

Roohollah Sharifi, MD, FACS
Professor of Surgery/Urology
University of Illinois at Chicago
College of Medicine
Chicago, Illinois
Chapters 83 and 84

Kayce Shealy, PharmD, BCPS, BCACP, CDE
Associate Professor
Department of Pharmacy Practice
Presbyterian College School of Pharmacy
Clinton, South Carolina
Chapter 36

Amy Heck Sheehan, PharmD
Associate Professor
Department of Pharmacy Practice
Purdue University College of Pharmacy
Indianapolis, Indiana
Chapters 77 and 144

Ziad Shehab, MD
Professor
Departments of Pediatrics and Pathology
University of Arizona College of Medicine
Tucson, Arizona
Chapter 118

Jessica M. Shenberger-Trujillo, PhD
Clinical Assistant Professor
Director of Assessment and Evaluation
University of Texas at El Paso
El Paso, Texas
Chapter e2

Stacy S. Shord, PharmD, FCCP, BCOP
Reviewer
Office of Clinical Pharmacology
Office of Translational Science
Center for Drug Evaluation and Research
U.S. Food and Drug Administration
Silver Spring, Maryland
Chapter 127

Sarah P. Shrader, PharmD, BCPS
Clinical Associate Professor
Department of Pharmacy Practice
University of Kansas School of Pharmacy
Lawrence, Kansas
Chapter 79

Jeri J. Sias, PharmD, MPH
Clinical Associate Professor
University of Texas at El Paso
UT Austin Cooperative Pharmacy Program
University of Texas at El Paso College of Health Sciences, University of Texas at Austin College of Pharmacy
Adjunct Clinical Assistant Professor
Department of Family and Community Medicine
Texas Tech University Health Sciences Center—El Paso
El Paso, Texas
Chapter e2

Debra Sibbald, BScPhm, RPh, ACPR, MA, PhD
Senior Lecturer
Division of Pharmacy Practice
Leslie Dan Faculty of Pharmacy
University of Toronto
Director
Department of Assessment Services
Centre for the Evaluation of Health Professionals Educated Abroad
Toronto, Ontario
Chapter 96

Tamara Simpson, MD
Clinical Associate Professor
Division of Pulmonary Diseases and Critical Care Medicine
University of Texas Health Science Center at San Antonio
San Antonio, Texas
Chapter e25

Douglas Slain, PharmD, BCPS, FCCP, FASHP
Professor
Infectious Diseases Clinical Specialist
West Virginia University
Health Sciences Center
Morgantown, West Virginia
Chapter e124

Patricia W. Slattum, PharmD, PhD, CGP
Director
Geriatric Pharmacotherapy Program
Department of Pharmacotherapy and Outcomes Science
School of Pharmacy
Virginia Commonwealth University
Richmond, Virginia
Chapters e7 and 54

Judith A. Smith, PharmD, BCOP, CPHQ, FCCP, FISOPP
Associate Professor
Director, Women's Health Integrative Medicine Research Program
Department of Obstetrics, Gynecology, and Reproductive Sciences
University of Texas Health Science Center McGovern Medical School
Houston, Texas
Chapter 133

Steven M. Smith, PharmD, MPH
Assistant Professor
Department of Clinical Pharmacy
Skaggs School of Pharmacy and Pharmaceutical Sciences
University of Colorado
Aurora, Colorado
Chapter 76

Christine A. Sorkness, PharmD
Professor of Pharmacy and Medicine
University of Wisconsin
Madison, Wisconsin
Chapter 26

Kevin M. Sowinski, PharmD, FCCP
Professor and Associate Head for Faculty Affairs
Department of Pharmacy Practice
Purdue University, College of Pharmacy
Adjunct Professor
Indiana University, School of Medicine
Indianapolis, Indiana
Chapter 45

Sarah A. Spinler, PharmD, FCCP, FAHA, FASHP, AACC, BCPS-AQ (Cardiology)
Professor of Clinical Pharmacy
Philadelphia College of Pharmacy
University of the Sciences in Philadelphia
Philadelphia, Pennsylvania
Chapter 17

Douglas W. Stewart, DO, MPH
Associate Professor
Department of Pediatrics
School of Community Medicine
University of Oklahoma
Tulsa, Oklahoma
Chapter 73

Steven C. Stoner, PharmD, BCPP
Chair and Clinical Professor
Division of Pharmacy Practice and Administration
UMKC School of Pharmacy
Kansas City, Missouri
Chapter 64

Jennifer M. Strickland, PharmD, BCPS
Millennium Health
Senior Vice President/General Manager, Medication Monitoring and Genetic Testing
Clinical Assistant Professor
University of Florida
College of Pharmacy
Lakeland, Florida
Chapter 60

Deborah A. Sturpe, PharmD, MA, BCPS
Associate Clinical Professor
College of Pharmacy
University of New England
Portland, Maine
Chapter 81

Lynne M. Sylvia, PharmD
Senior Clinical Pharmacy Specialist - Cardiology
Department of Pharmacy
Tufts Medical Center
Clinical Professor
School of Pharmacy
Northeastern University
Boston, Massachusetts
Chapter e88

Carol Taketomo, PharmD
Director of Pharmacy and Clinical Nutrition
Children's Hospital of Los Angeles
Adjunct Assistant Professor of Pharmacy Practice
School of Pharmacy
University of Southern California
Los Angeles, California
Chapter e6

Robert L. Talbert, PharmD, FCCP, BCPS, FAHA
SmithKline Professor
College of Pharmacy
The University of Texas at Austin
Professor
School of Medicine,
University of Texas Health Science Center
San Antonio, Texas
Chapter 21

Colleen M. Terriff, PharmD
Antimicrobial Stewardship Program Coordinator
Deaconess Hospital
Spokane, Washington
Chapter 10

Christian J. Teter, PharmD, BCPP
Associate Professor
Psychopharmacology
College of Pharmacy
Center for Excellence in the Neurosciences
University of New England
Portland, Maine
Chapter 68

Geoffrey M. Thiele, PhD
Professor
Division of Rheumatology and Immunology
Department of Medicine
College of Medicine
University of Nebraska Medical Center
Omaha, Nebraska
Chapter 86

Michael L. Thiman, PharmD, BCPS
Clinical Assistant Professor
Department of Clinical and Administrative Pharmacy
University of Georgia College of Pharmacy
Athens, Georgia
Chapter 32

Heidi Trinkman, PharmD
Pediatric Clinical Pharmacy Specialist
Hematology/Oncology and Stem Cell Transplantation
Cook Children's Medical Center
Fort Worth, Texas
Chapter 101

Curtis Triplitt, PharmD, CDE
Clinical Associate Professor
Department of Medicine
Division of Diabetes
University of Texas Health Science Center at San Antonio
Texas Diabetes Institute
University Health System
San Antonio, Texas
Chapter 74

Elena M. Umland, PharmD
Associate Dean for Academic Affairs
Professor of Pharmacy Practice
Jefferson College of Pharmacy
Thomas Jefferson University
Philadelphia, Pennsylvania
Chapter 80

Sara R. Vazquez, PharmD, BCPS
Clinical Pharmacist,
Department of Pharmacy Services, University of Utah Health Care,
Salt Lake City, Utah
Chapter 19

Yolanda Y. Vera, PharmD, BCPS
Pediatric Patient Care Pharmacist
Department of Pharmacy
The Children's Hospital at Scott & White
Temple, Texas
Chapter 29

Maria I. Velez
Assistant Professor of Medicine
Division of Pulmonary Diseases and Critical Care Medicine
University of Texas Health Science Center- San Antonio
San Antonio, Texas

Angie Veverka, PharmD, BCPS
Clinical Pharmacist Educator
RxPrep, Inc.
Manhattan Beach, California
Chapter 111

Kimberly Wahl, PharmD
Ambulatory Care Clinical Pharmacist
Department of Pharmacy
Ralph H. Johnson VA Medical Center
Myrtle Beach CBOC
Myrtle Beach, South Carolina
Chapter 91

Christine M. Walko, PharmD, FCCP, BCOP
Personalized Medicine Specialist
DeBartolo Family Personalized Medicine Institute
Moffitt Cancer Center
Tampa, Florida
Chapter 138

Kristina E. Ward, BS, PharmD, BCPS
Clinical Professor
Director
Drug Information Services
College of Pharmacy
University of Rhode Island
Kingston, Rhode Island
Chapter 78

Lori Wazny, BSc (Pharm), PharmD, EPPh
Clinical Pharmacist - Manitoba Renal Program
Clinical Assistant Professor - Colleges of Pharmacy, University of Manitoba and University of Florida Working Professional PharmD program
Department of Pharmaceutical Services
Health Sciences Centre
Winnipeg, Manitoba, Canada
Chapter 44

Robert J. Weber, PharmD, MS
Senior Director, Pharmaceutical Services
Department of Pharmacy
The Ohio State University Wexner Medical Center
Columbus, Ohio
Chapter e3

Barbara G. Wells, PharmD, FCCP, FASHP
Dean Emeritus and Professor Emeritus
University of Mississippi School of Pharmacy
Department of Pharmacy Practice
Oxford, Mississippi
Chapters 68 and 71

James W. Wheless, MD
Professor and Chief of Pediatric Neurology
LeBonheur Chair in Pediatric Neurology
University of Tennessee Health Science Center
Director
LeBonheur Comprehensive Epilepsy Program and Neuroscience Institute
LeBonheur Children's Hospital
Memphis, Tennessee
Chapter 57

Sara A. Wiedenfeld, PharmD, BCPS
Clinical Assistant Professor
Department of Pharmacy Practice and Science
Division of Applied Clinical Sciences
College of pharmacy
The University of Iowa
Iowa City, Iowa
Chapter 90

Dennis M. Williams, PharmD, BCPS
Associate Professor
Eshelman School of Pharmacy
University of North Carolina
Chapel Hill, North Carolina
Chapter 27

Daniel M. Witt, PharmD, FCCP, BCPS
Professor (Clinical) and Vice Chair
Department of Pharmacotherapy
University of Utah
College of Pharmacy
Salt Lake City, Utah
Chapter 19

Pei Shieen Wong, BSc (Pharm) (Hons), BCPS
Principal Pharmacist
Pharmacy Department
Singapore General Hospital
SingHealth
Singapore
Chapter 55

G. Christopher Wood, PharmD, FCCP, FCCM, BCPS (AQ-ID)
Associate Professor of Clinical Pharmacy
College of Pharmacy
University of Tennessee
Memphis, Tennessee
Chapter 58

Chanin Clark Wright, PharmD
Director of Pharmacy
McLane Children's Hospital
Assistant Professor
Department of Pediatrics
Texas A&M College of Medicine
Temple Texas
Adjunct Clinical Assistant Professor
University of Texas college of Pharmacy
Austin, Texas
Chapter 29

Jean Wyman, MN, PhD
Professor
Cora Meidl Siehl Chair in Nursing Research
Adult and Gerontological Health Cooperative
School of Nursing
University of Minnesota
Minneapolis, Minnesota
Chapter 85

Jack A. Yanovski, MD, PhD
Chief
Section on Growth and Obesity
Program in Developmental Endocrinology and Genetics
Eunice Kennedy Shriver National Institute of Child Health and Human Development
National Institutes of Health
Bethesda, Maryland
Chapter 144

Daniel A. Zlott, PharmD, BCOP
Clinical Pharmacy Specialist
Clinical Center Pharmacy Department
National Cancer Institute Surgery and Immunotherapy Programs
National Institutes of Health
Bethesda, Maryland
Chapter e86

Ashley M. Zurek, PharmD
Clinical Pharmacist, Internal Medicine Service
San Antonio Military Medical Center
Fort Sam Houston, Texas
Chapter e1

Foreword

Publication of the 10th edition of *Pharmacotherapy: A Pathophysiologic Approach* represents a milestone, in that almost 30 years have passed since publication of the 1st edition. Accordingly, this is a logical time to pause and reflect upon the mission and changes in *Pharmacotherapy*, health care delivery systems, and our profession. Hopefully, this reflection is not simply an academic exercise, but instead an opportunity to think about what the future may hold and how we might be able to lead the future such that clinical, humanistic, and economic outcomes of our patients are improved.

These are times of unprecedented change in health care. Since publication of the 1st edition, there has been growth and consolidation (through mergers) within health care systems, the pharmaceutical industry, and community pharmacy, especially within chain pharmacy.

Managed health care has become an increasingly stronger influence on how clinicians practice in an effort to ensure delivery of high-quality but cost conscious care. Patient-centered medical homes and accountable care organizations appear to be promising approaches to achieving higher-quality and cost-effective care while improving medication-related outcomes. Pharmacists will need to be integral members of the collaborative teams within patient-centered medical homes in order to maximize these improvements in patient outcomes.

In 2001, the National Academy of Medicine (NAM; formerly the Institute of Medicine) brought to the nation's attention the gap between the excellent care some patients received and the average care that most patients received. They also reported that our health care system is fragmented and uncoordinated, and that more than 43 million people at that time lacked health insurance. They called upon practitioners, health care organizations, and Congress to address these pressing deficiencies. Although some advances have been made, health care remains poorly coordinated, there are variations in quality, and limited progress has been made in integrating team based approaches. Additionally, medication adverse events continue to contribute to poor quality of care and high costs.

Passage of the Affordable Care Act in 2010 expanded access to health insurance coverage, including medications and medication therapy management. About 90% of Americans now have health insurance, but significant problems remain.

In 1985 spending for prescription drugs in the United States was just over $22 billion. IMS Health Holdings Inc. recently estimated that by 2020, that spending will climb to as high as $400 billion. These numbers do not include the ancillary costs of treatment failure, morbidity, and mortality associated with these drug therapies. Today the increasing cost of new drugs is garnering great media and even Congressional attention, as is the escalating costs of old drugs. Calls are being made for manufacturers to provide transparency in pricing and in some cases to justify pricing based on outcomes achieved.

Extensive efforts are now underway to enhance access to and coordinate electronic health records within and between hospitals, physicians' offices, and pharmacies.

As the health care environment has changed, so too has the pharmacy profession. When the 1st edition of *Pharmacotherapy* was published in 1988, the Board of Pharmacy Specialties (BPS; formerly called the Board of Pharmaceutical Specialties) had not yet approved Pharmacotherapy as a specialty within pharmacy, although they had acknowledged that the petition for approval of the specialty did document a specialist who did exist within the practice of pharmacy and whose expertise could be differentiated from the performance characteristics of those in general practice. BPS approval came later that year and signified that the pharmacotherapy specialist had taken unprecedented responsibilities in the collaborative management of patient-specific pharmacotherapy problems. That same year BPS recognized Nutrition Support as a specialty within pharmacy practice, bringing the number of recognized specialties to three. Since that time, five more specialties have been approved. Today more than 25,000 pharmacists worldwide are BPS certified.

The 2nd edition of *Pharmacotherapy* came in the early 1990s when pharmaceutical care emerged as the future mission for pharmacy practice. Pharmaceutical care emphasized the pharmacist's role to accept shared responsibility with other health care professionals for patients' drug therapy outcomes. Also of note, pharmacy practice and specialty practice residency programs were beginning to proliferate. The expansion of residencies in the 1990s and growth in demand for pharmacists in community and hospital settings resulted in substantial increases in pharmacist salaries and a pharmacist workforce shortage.

In 2003, President George W. Bush signed the Medicare Prescription Drug, Improvement, and Modernization Act which provided prescription drug benefits (Medicare Part D) to America's seniors starting in 2006.

In 2004, the Joint Commission of Pharmacy Practitioners and the 11 national pharmacy organizations that comprise its membership endorsed a future vision of pharmacy practice as follows:

> Pharmacists will be the health care professionals responsible for providing patient care that ensures optimal medication therapy outcomes.

Over the course of the last 30 years, pharmacy has matured into a clinical profession. Medication management is no longer provided only by pharmacists in tertiary care settings. Although the transformation is not complete, pharmacists provide evidence-based medication management and immunizations in many primary care and community pharmacy settings, and many pharmacists practice collaboratively with physicians and other health care professionals.

Today, the pace of entry of new drugs onto the market, limited efficacy, and potential toxicity create great complexity in selection and management of optimal medications for individual patients. Even when treatment guidelines are available for many specific diseases, far too many patients continue to receive suboptimal treatment. A 2000 NAM report documented that in the United States adverse drug effects are the sixth leading cause of death. Overuse of antibiotics and underuse of vaccines continue to challenge practitioners involved in delivery and oversight of drug therapy. These are only a few of the critical challenges that we must continue to address to improve the health of our nation. It is increasingly important that all patients have access to the expertise of a clinically trained pharmacist and that all pharmacists ensure that patients receive the most effective, safe, and economical pharmacotherapy. These contributions to patient care must be shared with other health care professionals and the resulting change in clinical outcomes documented to inform health policy decision makers of the value that pharmacists bring to patient care.

When the 1st edition of *Pharmacotherapy* was published in 1988, the PharmD was not the entry level degree, and 74 U.S. schools and colleges graduated only about 1000 PharmD graduates (in addition to approximately 5300 BS in pharmacy graduates). In 2015, 125 schools and colleges graduated approximately 14,000 first professional degree PharmD graduates, and 273 post-BS PharmD degrees were also conferred. The pharmacy education enterprise continues to grow, but at a slower pace than in the last decade of the 20th century and the first decade of the 21st century.

In the early 1990s, the American Association of Colleges of Pharmacy Commission to Implement Change in Pharmaceutical Education recommended a process to establish entry-level professional doctoral programs designed to produce graduates competent to provide pharmaceutical care upon entry into the pharmacy profession. The Commission also recommended curricular change to emphasize problem solving, communications, and improved practice skills. Responding to this, many colleges of pharmacy enhanced the practice component of the curriculum and are now delivering a significant portion of the curriculum using a problem-based, active learning format. Many schools and colleges are now experimenting with peer teaching and flipped classrooms. Curriculums continue to evolve to ensure that pharmacy students not only have a good grasp of the pharmaceutical sciences and pharmacotherapy, but that they can also think critically, communicate effectively, solve complex problems, and work effectively in teams.

Pharmacy educators recognize that information about prevention, diagnosis, and treatment is emerging more rapidly than ever before, largely due to our increasing knowledge of pharmacogenetics, pharmacogenomics, proteomics, and bioinformatics. This knowledge and information from other basic sciences will enable greater individualization of treatment and eventually precision medicine. It is very difficult to predict the pace of these advances, but relevant information from these disciplines is continuously being incorporated into the pharmacy curriculum.

The 1st edition of *Pharmacotherapy* included 111 chapters. In response to many of the advances and challenges noted above, the 10th edition includes 144 chapters. Chapters added to the Foundational Issues section include Medication Safety, Cultural Competency, Health Literacy, Pharmacogenetics, Palliative Care, and Clinical Management of Potential Bioterrorism-related Conditions. Several pedagogical features have also been added to facilitate learning. Recognizing a need to provide students and practitioners a mechanism to grow their clinical problem-solving skills, *Pharmacotherapy Casebook: A Patient Focused Approach* was introduced as a companion textbook in 1997.

Pharmacotherapy has evolved to provide much more information to support provision of medication management in ambulatory and community pharmacy settings, as pharmacy has evolved into a truly clinical profession. The selection of cases for the *Casebook*, the Clinical Controversies section, and other features in *Pharmacotherapy* have been critical in expanding this focus.

As stated in the Preface to the 1st edition, the book's purpose was to "provide a basis of principles and information that reflects the breadth and depth of knowledge appropriate for today's pharmacy student and practitioner. The Preface goes on to explain that "the sections on treatment attempt to place drug therapy in its proper perspective with other modalities" and also that "The pathophysiology sections are the key to imparting a way of thinking for the developing practitioner." Today, 30 years after those precepts were crafted, they are as true for the 10th edition as they were for the first. Each edition of the book provides the scientific knowledge foundation for the clinician who manages the drug therapy of patients. Building on this foundation, the clinician must stay abreast of new developments and advance his/her competence by interpretation and assimilation of new information in the primary literature.

We believe that over the last 30 years *Pharmacotherapy* has had a critical role in preparing pharmacy students and those already in practice to become medication managers and to define new clinical roles, thus helping to evolve our profession into a truly clinical one.

Pharmacy practitioners, students, teachers, and researchers must accept responsibility to help expand pharmacists' roles as providers of patient focused, comprehensive medication management. This includes providing the highest quality of care in our own practices and increasing awareness of pharmacists' roles and abilities by government, researchers, third-party payers, and the public. It is clear that we also have a responsibility to continue to define new and innovative models for the provision of medication management in all practice settings, including community pharmacies, community health clinics, managed care settings, and physician practices. Pharmacists will be key players in transformation of our medication use systems. Resources, including pharmacists, must be deployed more efficiently and effectively, taking advantage of their full scope of practice and breadth and depth of education and training. Strong leadership will be required to advance both generalist and specialty practices in pharmacy. Patient care of the future will be patient centered and will use a team based approach. Only when we optimize medication use will we be able to make meaningful improvements in the quality of care and decrease the costs of care. We are confident the evolution and maturation of our profession will not only continue, but that it will gain momentum in the years to come.

Barbara G. Wells
Robert L. Talbert
Gary R. Matzke

Foreword to the First Edition

Evidence of the maturity of a profession is not unlike that characterizing the maturity of an individual; a child's utterances and behavior typically reveal an unrealized potential for attainment, eventually, of those attributes characteristic of an appropriately confident, independently competent, socially responsible, sensitive, and productive member of society.

Within a period of perhaps 15 or 20 years, we have witnessed a profound maturation within the profession of pharmacy. The utterances of the profession, as projected in its literature, have evolved from mostly self-centered and self-serving issues of trade protection to a composite of expressed professional interests that prominently include responsible explorations of scientific/technological questions and ethical issues that promote the best interests of the clientele served by the profession. With the publication of *Pharmacotherapy: A Pathophysiologic Approach,* pharmacy's utterances bespeak a matured practitioner who is able to call upon unique knowledge and skills so as to function as an appropriately confident, independently competent pharmacotherapeutics expert.

In 1987, the Board of Pharmaceutical Specialties (BPS), in denying the petition filed by the American College of Clinical Pharmacy (ACCP) to recognize "clinical pharmacy" as a specialty, conceded nonetheless that the petitioning party had documented in its petition a specialist who does in fact exist within the practice of pharmacy and whose expertise clearly can be extricated from the performance characteristics of those in general practice. A refiled petition from ACCP requests recognition of "pharmacotherapy" as a Specialty Area of Pharmacy Practice. While the BPS had issued no decision when this book went to press, it is difficult to comprehend the basis for a rejection of the second petition.

Within this book one will find the scientific foundation for the essential knowledge required of one who may aspire to specialty practice as a pharmacotherapist. As is the case with any such publication, its usefulness to the practitioner or the future practitioner is limited to providing such a foundation. To be socially and professionally responsible in practice, the pharmacotherapist's foundation must be continually supplemented and complemented by the flow of information appearing in the primary literature. Of course this is not unique to the general or specialty practice of pharmacy; it is essential to the fulfillment of obligations to clients in any occupation operating under the code of professional ethics.

Because of the growing complexity of pharmacotherapeutic agents, their dosing regimens, and techniques for delivery, pharmacy is obligated to produce, recognize, and remunerate specialty practitioners who can fulfill the profession's responsibilities to society for service expertise where the competence required in a particular case exceeds that of the general practitioner. It simply is a component of our covenant with society and is as important as any other facet of that relationship existing between a profession and those it serves.

The recognition by BPS of pharmacotherapy as an area of specialty practice in pharmacy will serve as an important statement by the profession that we have matured sufficiently to be competent and willing to take unprecedented responsibilities in the collaborative, pharmacotherapeutic management of patient-specific problems. It commits pharmacy to an intention that will not be uniformly or rapidly accepted within the established health care community. Nonetheless, this formal action places us on the road to an avowed goal, and acceptance will be gained as the pharmacotherapists proliferate and establish their importance in the provision of optimal, costeffective drug therapy.

Suspecting that other professions in other times must have faced similar quests for recognition of their unique knowledge and skills I once searched the literature for an example that might parallel pharmacy's modern-day aspirations. Writing in the *Philadelphia Medical Journal*, May 27, 1899, D. H. Galloway, MD, reflected on the need for specialty training and practice in a field of medicine lacking such expertise at that time. In an article entitled "The Anesthetizer as a Speciality," Galloway commented:

> The anesthetizer will have to make his own place in medicine: the profession will not make a place for him, and not until he has demonstrated the value of his services will it concede him the position which the importance of his duties entitles him to occupy. He will be obliged to define his own rights, duties and privileges, and he must not expect that his own estimate of the importance of his position will be conceded without opposition. There are many surgeons who are unwilling to share either the credit or the emoluments of their work with anyone, and their opposition will be overcome only when they are shown that the importance of their work will not be lessened, but enhanced, by the increased safety and dispatch with which operations may be done. . . .

It has been my experience that, given the opportunity for one-on-one, collaborative practice with physicians and other health professionals, pharmacy practitioners who have been educated and trained to perform at the level of pharmacotherapeutics specialists almost invariably have convinced the former that "the importance of their work will not be lessened, but enhanced, by the increased safety and dispatch with which" individualized problems of drug therapy could be managed in collaboration with clinical pharmacy practitioners.

It is fortuitous—the coinciding of the release of *Pharmacotherapy: A Pathophysiologic Approach* with ACCP's petitioning of BPS for recognition of the pharmacotherapy specialist. The utterances of a maturing profession as revealed in the contents of this book, and the intraprofessional recognition and acceptance of a higher level of responsibility in the safe, effective, and economical use of drugs and drug products, bode well for the future of the profession and for the improvement of patient care with drugs.

Charles A. Walton, PhD
San Antonio, Texas

Preface

With publication of the 10th edition of *Pharmacotherapy: A Pathophysiologic Approach (PAPA)*, this textbook reaches a milestone that none of us on the original editorial team ever dreamed possible. It is thus appropriate that the changes with this edition are more focused on the team itself than on the specific elements readers have found useful over the past three decades.

With this edition of *PAPA*, readers will notice the addition of three Associate Editors to the editorial team. These individuals—Stuart T. Haines, Thomas D. Nolin, and Vicki L. Ellingrod, respectively—will replace three of our Editors beginning with the 11th edition: Robert L. Talbert (Founding Editor), Gary R. Matzke (Section Editor in the 1st edition and Editor beginning with the 2nd edition), and Barbara G. Wells (Author in the first two editions and Editor beginning with the 3rd edition). As the Editors transition to Editor Emeritus status, we thank them for the many hours spent identifying the best ways of conveying complicated disease pathophysiologic and pharmacotherapeutic concepts. The continuing Editors also welcome our new colleagues, all of whom are already contributing much to our editorial development and production processes.

As with the previous nine editions, the founding precepts for PAPA continue to guide our content decisions:

- Advance the quality of patient care through evidence-based medication therapy management based on sound pharmacotherapeutic principles.
- Enhance the health of our communities by incorporating contemporary health promotion and disease-prevention strategies in our practice environments.
- Motivate young practitioners to enhance the breadth, depth, and quality of care they provide to their patients.
- Challenge established pharmacists and other primary-care providers to learn new concepts and refine their understanding of the pathophysiologic tenets that undergird the development of individualized therapeutic regimens.
- Present the pharmacy and health care communities with innovative patient assessment, triage, and pharmacotherapy management skills.

Within these pages and in the online version of *PAPA* on the Access Pharmacy website (www.accesspharmacy.com), readers will find material that builds on and expands the foundation of previous editions. Key Concepts guide the student through each chapter, and material is always evidence based. When available, ratings of the level of evidence support the key therapeutic approaches. Personalized pharmacotherapy is emphasized in a special section, and disease-specific chapters have diagnostic flow diagrams, treatment algorithms, dosing guideline recommendations, and monitoring approaches with color codes to clearly distinguish treatment pathways. Drug dosing and monitoring tables provide both students and practitioners with a one-stop reference point in each chapter.

New in the 10th edition is a chapter on Travel Health (Chapter 124), added in recognition of the importance of emerging diseases and the travel vaccine services increasingly provided in pharmacies and alternative care settings. More content has been shifted from print to online presentation on our Access Pharmacy (www.accesspharmacy.com) digital home. Users of Access Pharmacy will find many features to enhance their learning and information retrieval. Thoughtful and provocative updates to *PAPA* chapters are added as new information mandates to keep our readers relevant in these times of rapid advancements. Also, the site has many new features such as education guides, Goodman & Gilman's animations, virtual cases, and many other textbooks. As in previous editions, the text coordinates well with *Pharmacotherapy: A Patient-Focused Approach*, which includes in-depth patient cases with questions and answers.

In closing, we acknowledge the many hours that *Pharmacotherapy's* more than 300 authors contributed to this labor of love. Without their devotion to the cause of improved pharmacotherapy and dedication in maintaining the accuracy, clarity, and relevance of their chapters, this text would unquestionably not be possible. In addition, we thank Michael Weitz, Brian Kearns, James Shanahan, and their colleagues at McGraw-Hill for their consistent support of the *Pharmacotherapy* family of resources, insights into trends in publishing and higher education, and the critical attention to detail so necessary in pharmacotherapy.

The Editors
December 2016

In Memoriam

Leroy C. Knodel (1954-2015), the author of "Sexually Transmitted Diseases" chapter in *Pharmacotherapy* since its first edition in 1989, received his BS and PharmD degrees from the University of Kentucky in 1977 and 1980, respectively. He served as a faculty member for The University of Texas at Austin and the University of Texas Health Science Center at San Antonio for more than 30 years. His chief academic responsibility was to coordinate experiential pharmacy education in the San Antonio region, a role he thoroughly embraced and enjoyed. He also directed the Drug Information Service for many years and held prominent service roles with state agencies, local health care institutions, and charitable organizations.

Leroy was an outstanding educator and tireless mentor who was universally loved by faculty, staff, students, and professional colleagues. He was a warm and caring person, known for his quick wit, great humor, and empathy. He was gifted in his ability to let those he encountered know they were important and appreciated. His contagious smile and laugh could brighten any room. Student pharmacists frequently cited him as one of the faculty members who made the biggest impact on their personal and professional development during their time in pharmacy school. Leroy touched many lives, and gave of himself unselfishly both professionally and personally. The thousands of students he helped educate and encourage during his academic career are his living legacy.

Health Literacy and Medication Use

e1

Oralia V. Bazaldua, DeWayne A. Davidson, Ashley Zurek, and Sunil Kripalani

KEY CONCEPTS

1. Limited health literacy is common and must be considered when providing medication management services.
2. Some groups of people are at higher risk for having limited literacy skills, but in general, you cannot tell by looking.
3. Patients with limited health literacy are more likely to misunderstand medication instructions and have difficulty demonstrating the correct dosing regimen.
4. Limited health literacy is associated with increased healthcare costs and worse health outcomes, including increased mortality.
5. Despite numerous efforts to improve safe medication practices, current strategies have been inadequate, and this may have a larger impact in patients with limited literacy.
6. Most printed materials are written at higher comprehension levels than most adults can read.
7. The United States Pharmacopeia has set new standards for prescription medication labeling to minimize patient confusion.
8. Several instruments exist to measure health literacy, but some experts advocate "universal precautions" under which all patients are assumed to benefit from plain language and clear communication.
9. Obtaining a complete medication history and providing medication counseling are vital components in the medication management of patients with limited health literacy.

INTRODUCTION

Every day, thousands of patients are not taking their medications correctly. Some take too much. Others take too little. Some use a tablespoon instead of a teaspoon. Parents pour an oral antibiotic suspension in their child's ear instead of giving it by mouth because it was prescribed for an ear infection. Others are in the emergency department because they did not know how to use their asthma inhaler. It is not a deliberate revolt against the doctor's orders but rather a likely and an unfortunate result of a hidden risk factor—limited health literacy.

1 *Literacy*, at the basic level, is simply the ability to read and write. When these skills are applied to a health context, it is called *health literacy*, but health literacy is more than just reading and writing. *Health literacy*, as defined by the Institute of Medicine (IOM), is "the degree to which individuals have the capacity to obtain, process, and understand basic health information and services needed to make appropriate health decisions." A growing body of evidence associates low health literacy with less understanding, worse outcomes, and increased cost. These poor outcomes have led this topic to receive national attention. Health literacy has been made "a priority area for national action" by the IOM[1,2] and Healthy People 2020.[3] As a result, federal policy initiatives promoting health literacy continue to be highlighted in Healthy People 2020, the Patient Protection and Affordable Care Act of 2010, and the Plain Writing Act of 2010.[4] A National Action Plan to Improve Health Literacy (Table e1-1) has also been developed by the Department of Health and Human Services (HHS).[5] Likewise, the Agency for Healthcare Research and Quality (AHRQ),[6,7] the National Institutes of Health (NIH),[8] and Centers for Disease Control and Prevention (CDC)[9] have each dedicated websites to this topic and have provided funding to support studies and interventions that are specifically relevant to health literacy. Additionally, state and private sector organizations, such as America's Health Insurance Plans (AHIP) and the American College of Physicians (ACP) Foundation, have led efforts to improve health literacy following the IOM's call to action.[10] Indeed, health literacy should be a national priority for the medical community as its consequences are far-reaching and cross-cutting.

More than one of every three American adults has difficulty understanding and acting on health information.[11] Patients with limited health literacy have less knowledge about how to manage their disease;[12] they misunderstand dosing instructions and warning labels on medication containers;[13,14] they are less likely to read or even look at medication guides;[15] their ability for medication management is limited as these persons are less able to identify or distinguish their medications from one another;[16,17] and they are less able to use a metered-dose inhaler (MDI) properly.[18] Limited health literacy skills have also been documented in caregivers of seniors[19] and in parents of children.[20] There is no question that limited health literacy is associated with adverse health outcomes[21] including an increased mortality rate[22] and increased healthcare costs.[23]

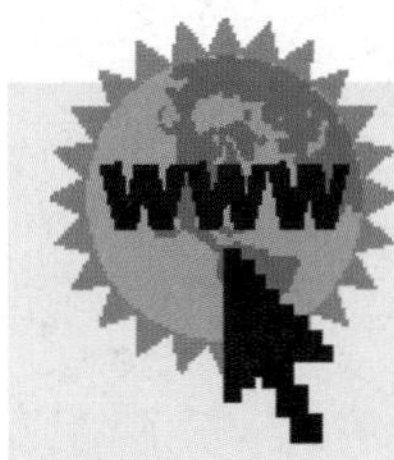

The complete chapter, learning objectives, and other resources can be found at **www.pharmacotherapyonline.com.**

Cultural Competency

e2

Jeri J. Sias, Amanda M. Loya, José O. Rivera, and Jessica M. Shenberger-Trujillo

KEY CONCEPTS

1. Healthcare providers should strive toward cultural competency to improve care and access unique resources for patients and communities from diverse cultures and backgrounds.
2. Changes in demographics in the United States, health disparities, and patient safety are among the reasons that cultural competency should be emphasized in healthcare.
3. A variety of models recognize cultural competency as a process, not an achievement.
4. Legal and regulatory issues surrounding cultural competency include understanding and interpreting accreditation standards for healthcare organizations and Title VI of the Civil Rights Act.
5. Patients may enter the healthcare setting with a different explanation of their illnesses than found in the Western biomedical model (WBM).
6. Cultural values and beliefs influence decisions and attitudes about healthcare, including race, ethnicity, age, gender, sexual orientation, and religious beliefs.
7. Developing communication skills to interact with diverse population involves recognizing personal styles and cultural values of communication as well as barriers to patient understanding.
8. Linguistic competency encompasses understanding the capacity of organizations and providers to communicate well with diverse populations such as patients with limited English proficiency (LEP), low literacy, or hearing impairments.
9. Before practitioners can understand other cultures, they should understand personal and organizational values and beliefs.
10. Skills for working with patients from diverse cultures include being able to listen to the patient's perception of health, acknowledging differences, being respectful, and negotiating treatment options.

CULTURE, COMMUNITY, AND SOCIAL DETERMINANTS OF HEALTH

Culture defines us.[1] Although our genetic makeup, which is largely nonmodifiable and affects our physical state of being, **social determinants of health** are also of great influence. Determinants of health describe the factors that affect the health of individuals. At the core of each person are their inherited traits as well as the choices that they make about their lifestyles (eg, diet, exercise, leisure activities). Their health is further marked by their exposure to healthy or risky behaviors based on the places where they live, work, worship, or go during the day and their built environment (eg, sidewalks, exposure to clean air, policies for healthy choices).[2] Basically, our socioeconomic status, race and ethnicity, gender, age, and communities (environments), as part of our cultures, shape us.[3]

Consider the following brief descriptions of three individuals and the determinants of health that influence them. Patient 1 is a 42-year-old bilingual Vietnamese American, Buddhist woman living on the West Coast whose family immigrated to the United States 35 years ago. Her lifestyle choices include a vegetarian diet, gardening, and daily meditation. She lives in a suburban community with her husband and three children, drives a hybrid electric/gas car to her work as a school teacher, and purchases food from a local farmer's market. She has health insurance and her city public policy includes no indoor smoking in public places and state policies include special low-emission requirements on vehicles. Weekend activities with the family include sports and dance for the kids along with others from the community center that serves a number of Asian-American families.

Patient 2 is a 27-year-old single African American, Muslim upper-middle-class man living in a major city in the Eastern Coast of the United States. Having just finished his graduate school degree, he lives in a high-rise apartment and walks or rides the subway to his work at a major corporation. In his leisure time, he enjoys reading and going to major sporting events with his college friends who come from diverse backgrounds. During the week, he also frequents the local mosque and community events that are supported by his neighborhood.

Patient 3 is a 55-year-old European American, Protestant middle class man living in the Midwest. His family moved from the rural South 2 years ago for a new full-time job. Due to recent economic changes in the community, he now has to work three part-time jobs (two in food industry and one in construction) so that he can help support his wife who is undergoing breast cancer treatment. As a result of his high work demands, he is not able to shop for groceries or exercise and so the couple often eats away from the home or they prepare quick and processed meals at home. He notices that he has gained about 10 pounds (4.5 kg) in the past 6 months and has difficulty sleeping. The family also has not had time to connect with their church or other friends due to his work and doctor appointments for his wife.

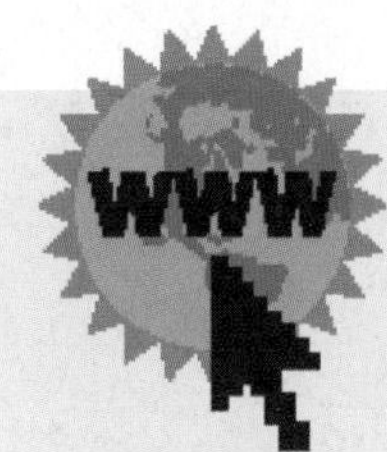

The complete chapter, learning objectives, and other resources can be found at **www.pharmacotherapyonline.com.**

Medication Safety Principles and Practices

e3

Robert J. Weber

KEY CONCEPTS

1. Medication errors (MEs) are defined as *any* mistake at *any* stage of the medication-use process; adverse drug events (ADEs) are the result of an injury as a result of an ME.
2. All MEs can be prevented, while ADEs can be categorized as preventable and potential.
3. MEs occur at an alarmingly high rate, with ADEs having fatal outcomes for patients.
4. MEs can occur at any step of the medication-use process: selection and procurement, storage, ordering and transcribing, preparing and dispensing, administration, or monitoring.
5. Determining the actual and potential root causes of MEs helps to correct future errors in the medication-use system.
6. Quality improvement methods that prevent MEs and thereby minimize ADEs include identifying the ME and/or ADE, understanding the reasons for the ME and/or ADE, designing and implementing changes to prevent an ADE or ME, and checking the outcome of that change.
7. Healthcare organizations have implemented various measures to reduce the incidence of MEs and ADEs, such as computerized physician order entry (CPOE), automated drug distribution systems, bar-code scanning, and "smart" infusion pumps with decision support and where information is passed in a bidirectional manner between the pump and the patient's electronic medical record (EMR).
8. Medication reconciliation or comparing a patient's current medication orders to *all* of the medications that the patient had been taking before any care transition (hospital admission, transfer, or discharge) is a vital process in preventing MEs and ADEs.
9. A "just culture" of medication safety cultivates trust in the workplace that makes personnel feel comfortable sharing safety information (eg, unsafe situations) and assuming personal responsibility and accountability for complying with safe medication practices.

INTRODUCTION

Medical errors are not a new phenomenon. Medical errors causing harm may lead to devastating effects on patients. In 1991, the Harvard Medical Practice Study showed that a significant number of people are victims of medication errors (MEs). This landmark study reviewed the incidence of adverse events and negligence in hospitalized patients in the state of New York showing that almost 4% of patients experienced an iatrogenic injury (one caused by healthcare practices or procedures), prolonging their hospital stays.[1] Importantly, nearly 14% of those mistakes were fatal. Examples of mistakes noted in the Harvard study included renal failure from angiographic dye and a missed diagnosis of colon cancer. Drug complications were the most common type of outcome attributed to negligence, accounting for 19% of these preventable adverse events.[1]

The goal of medication therapy is achieving defined therapeutic goals to improve a patient's quality of life while minimizing harm.[2] There are both known and unknown risks associated with the therapeutic use of prescription and nonprescription drugs and drug administration devices.[3] Mishaps related to medication therapy include both adverse drug events (ADEs) and MEs.[4]

Medication errors negatively affect patients' confidence in the healthcare system and increase healthcare costs. Research conducted by the American Society of Health-System Pharmacists (ASHP) showed that 61% of patients surveyed reported that they were "very concerned" about being given the wrong medicine during a hospital stay.[5] MEs are also very costly—to healthcare systems, patients and their families, and healthcare workers. The emotional cost of an ME is also significant, including the burden on the family for grieving loss or injury to the healthcare worker involved in an ME that caused harm.

Many MEs are not detected by standard reporting systems and often do not cause patient harm. According to the "Fourth Annual Report on Medication Errors in U.S. Hospitals" by the United States Pharmacopeia (USP), 49% of MEs never reach the patient.[6] Many MEs have little to no clinical importance or have minimal impact on patient care. According to the 2002 USP study of the anonymous Web-based reporting system MEDMARx, 98% of reported MEs (n = ~190,000) resulted in no harm to the patient. Tragically, however, MEs do sometimes result in serious patient morbidity and mortality.[7] In fact, preliminary data from the Centers for Disease Control and Prevention (CDC) list accidents (of which MEs are included) as the fifth leading cause of death in the United States in 2010.[8]

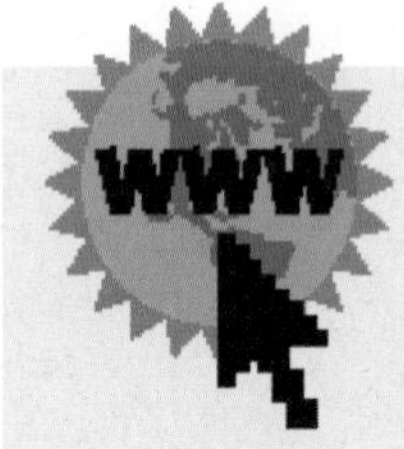

The complete chapter, learning objectives, and other resources can be found at **www.pharmacotherapyonline.com.**

Clinical Pharmacokinetics and Pharmacodynamics

e4

Larry A. Bauer

KEY CONCEPTS

1. Clinical pharmacokinetics is the discipline that describes the absorption, distribution, metabolism, and elimination of drugs in patients requiring drug therapy.
2. Clearance is the most important pharmacokinetic parameter because it determines the steady-state concentration for a given dosage rate. Physiologically, clearance is determined by blood flow to the organ that metabolizes or eliminates the drug and the efficiency of the organ in extracting the drug from the bloodstream.
3. The volume of distribution is a proportionality constant that relates the amount of drug in the body to the serum concentration. The volume of distribution is used to calculate the loading dose of a drug that will immediately achieve a desired steady-state concentration. The value of the volume of distribution is determined by the physiologic volume of blood and tissues and how the drug binds in blood and tissues.
4. Half-life is the time required for serum concentrations to decrease by one-half after absorption and distribution are complete. It is important because it determines the time required to reach steady state and the dosage interval. Half-life is a dependent kinetic variable because its value depends on the values of clearance and volume of distribution.
5. The fraction of drug absorbed into the systemic circulation after extravascular administration is defined as its *bioavailability*.
6. Most drugs follow linear pharmacokinetics, whereby steady-state serum drug concentrations change proportionally with long-term daily dosing.
7. Some drugs do not follow the rules of linear pharmacokinetics. Instead of steady-state drug concentration changing proportionally with the dose, serum concentration changes more or less than expected. These drugs follow nonlinear pharmacokinetics.
8. Pharmacokinetic models are useful to describe data sets, to predict serum concentrations after several doses or different routes of administration, and to calculate pharmacokinetic constants such as clearance, volume of distribution, and half-life. The simplest case uses a single compartment to represent the entire body.
9. Factors to be taken into consideration when deciding on the best drug dose for a patient include age, gender, weight, ethnic background, other concurrent disease states, and other drug therapy.
10. Cytochrome P450 is a generic name for the group of enzymes that are responsible for most drug metabolism oxidation reactions. Several P450 isozymes have been identified, including CYP1A2, CYP2C9, CYP2C19, CYP2D6, CYP2E1, and CYP3A4.
11. Membrane transporters are protein molecules concerned with the active transport of drugs across cell membranes. The importance of transport proteins in drug bioavailability, elimination, and distribution is continuing to evolve. A principal transport protein involved in the movement of drugs across biologic membranes is P-glycoprotein. P-glycoprotein is present in many organs, including the gastrointestinal (GI) tract, liver, and kidney. Other transport protein families include the organic cation transporters, the organic anion transporters, and the organic anion transporting polypeptides.
12. When deciding on initial doses for drugs that are renally eliminated, the patient's renal function should be assessed. A common, useful way to do this is to measure the patient's serum creatinine concentration and convert this value into an estimated creatinine clearance ($CL_{cr\ est}$). For drugs that are eliminated primarily by the kidney (more than or equal to 60% of the administered dose), some agents will need minor dosage adjustments for $CL_{cr\ est}$ between 30 and 60 mL/min (0.50 and 1.00 mL/s), moderate dosage adjustments for $CL_{cr\ est}$ between 15 and 30 mL/min (0.25 and 0.50 mL/s), and major dosage adjustments for $CL_{cr\ est}$ less than 15 mL/min (0.25 mL/s). For drugs approved after 2010, renal drug dosing adjustments may also include recommendations using estimated glomerular filtration rate (eGFR) in addition to $CL_{cr\ est}$. Supplemental doses of some medications also may be needed for patients receiving hemodialysis if the drug is removed by the artificial kidney or for patients receiving hemoperfusion if the drug is removed by the hemofilter.
13. When deciding on initial doses for drugs that are hepatically eliminated, the patient's liver function should be assessed. The Child-Pugh score can be used as an indicator of a patient's ability to metabolize drugs that are eliminated by the liver. In the absence of specific pharmacokinetic dosing guidelines for a medication, a Child-Pugh score equal to 8 or 9 is grounds for a moderate decrease (~25%) in the initial daily drug dose for agents that are metabolized primarily hepatically (more than or equal to 60%), and a score of 10 or greater indicates that a significant decrease in the initial daily dose (~50%) is required for drugs that are metabolized mostly hepatically.

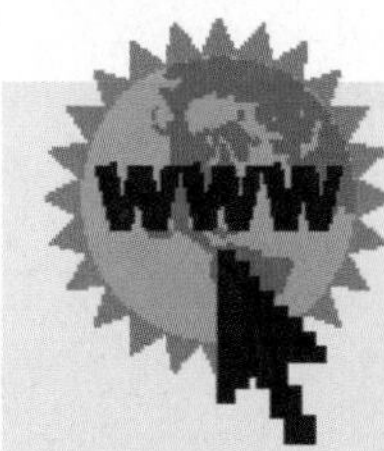

The complete chapter, learning objectives, and other resources can be found at **www.pharmacotherapyonline.com.**

Pharmacogenetics

e5

Larisa H. Cavallari and Y. W. Francis Lam

KEY CONCEPTS

1. Genetic variation contributes to pharmacokinetic and pharmacodynamic drug properties.
2. Genetic variation occurs for drug metabolism, drug transporter, and drug target proteins, as well as disease-associated proteins.
3. Single-nucleotide polymorphisms are the most common gene variations associated with drug response.
4. Genetic polymorphisms may influence drug effectiveness and risk for toxicity.
5. Pharmacogenetics is the study of the impact of genetic polymorphisms on drug response.
6. The goals of pharmacogenetics are to optimize drug efficacy and limit drug toxicity based on an individual's DNA.
7. Gene therapy aims to cure disease caused by genetic defects by changing gene expression.
8. Inadequate gene delivery and expression and serious adverse effects are obstacles to successful gene therapy.

PHARMACOGENETICS: INTRODUCTION

Great variability exists among individuals in response to drug therapy, and it is difficult to predict how effective or safe a medication will be for a particular patient. For example, when treating a patient with hypertension, it may be necessary to try several agents or a combination of agents before achieving adequate blood pressure control with acceptable tolerability. A number of clinical factors are known to influence drug response, including age, body size, renal and hepatic function, and concomitant drug use. However, considering these factors alone is often insufficient in predicting the likelihood of drug efficacy or safety for a given patient. For example, identical antihypertensive therapy in two patients of similar age, sex, race, and with similar medical histories and concomitant drug therapy may produce inadequate blood pressure reduction in one patient and symptomatic hypotension in the other.

1 2 The observed interpatient variability in drug response may result largely from genetically determined differences in drug metabolism, drug distribution, and drug target proteins. The influence of heredity on drug response was demonstrated as early as 1956 with the discovery that an inherited deficiency of glucose-6-phosphate dehydrogenase (G6PD) was responsible for hemolytic reactions to the antimalarial drug primaquine. Variations in genes encoding cytochrome P450 (CYP) and other drug-metabolizing enzymes are now well recognized as causes of interindividual differences in plasma concentrations of certain drugs. These variations may have serious implications for narrow-therapeutic-index drugs such as warfarin, phenytoin, and mercaptopurine. Other variations associated with drug response occur in genes for drug transporters such as the solute carrier organic anion transporter (OAT) family member 1B1 (SLCO1B1) and organic cation transporter 1 (OCT1), as well as drug targets such as receptors, enzymes, and proteins involved in intracellular signal transduction. Genetic variations for drug-metabolizing enzymes and drug transporter proteins may influence drug disposition, thus altering pharmacokinetic drug properties. Drug target genes may alter pharmacodynamic mechanisms by affecting sensitivity to a drug at its target site. Finally, genes associated with disease severity have been correlated with drug efficacy despite having no direct effect on pharmacokinetic or pharmacodynamic mechanisms.

PHARMACOGENETICS: A DEFINITION

3 4 Pharmacogenetics involves the search for genetic variations that lead to interindividual differences in drug response. The term *pharmacogenetics* often is used interchangeably with the term *pharmacogenomics*. However, pharmacogenetics generally refers to monogenetic variants that affect drug response, whereas pharmacogenomics refers to the entire spectrum of genes that interact to determine drug efficacy and safety. For example, a pharmacogenetic study would be one that examines the influence of the *CYP2C9* gene on warfarin dose requirements. A pharmacogenomic study might examine the interaction between the *CYP2C9*, vitamin K oxido reductase complex subunit 1 (*VKORC1*), and *CYP4F2* genes on warfarin dose requirements. Given that multiple proteins are involved in determining the ultimate response to most drugs, many investigators are taking a more pharmacogenomic approach to elucidating genetic contributions to drug response. For simplicity, this chapter treats pharmacogenetics and pharmacogenomics as synonymous.

5 The goals of pharmacogenetics are to optimize drug therapy and limit drug toxicity based on an individual's genetic profile. Thus, pharmacogenetics aims to use genetic information to choose a drug, drug dose, and treatment duration that will have the greatest likelihood for achieving therapeutic outcomes with the least potential for harm in a given patient. Pharmacogenetic discoveries have provided opportunities for clinicians to use genetic tests to predict individual responses to drug treatments and specifically select medications for patients based on DNA profiles. Genotype-guided therapy is already a reality for some diseases, such as cancer and cystic fibrosis, where novel drugs have been developed to target specific mutations. Clinical implementation of pharmacogenetics is beginning to emerge in other therapeutic areas, such as cardiology, neurology, pain management, and infectious disease.

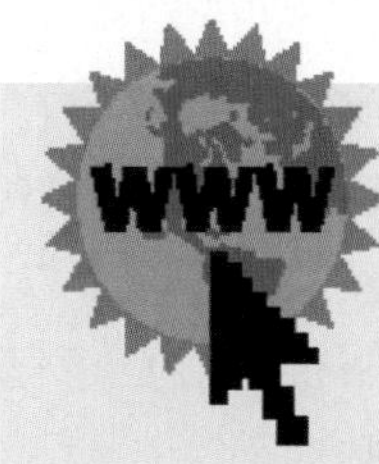

The complete chapter, learning objectives, and other resources can be found at **www.pharmacotherapyonline.com.**

Pediatrics

e6

Milap C. Nahata and Carol Taketomo

KEY CONCEPTS

1. Children are not just "little adults," and lack of data on important pharmacokinetic and pharmacodynamic differences has led to several disastrous situations in pediatric care.
2. Variations in absorption of medications from the gastrointestinal tract, intramuscular injection sites, and skin are important in pediatric patients, especially in premature and other newborn infants.
3. The rate and extent of organ function development and the distribution, metabolism, and elimination of drugs differ not only between pediatric versus adult patients but also among pediatric age groups.
4. The effectiveness and safety of drugs may vary among age groups and from one drug to another in pediatric versus adult patients.
5. Concomitant diseases may influence dosage requirements to achieve a targeted effect for a specific disease in children.
6. Use of weight-based dosing of medications for obese children may result in suboptimal drug therapy.
7. The myth that neonates and young infants do not experience pain has led to inadequate pain management in this pediatric population.
8. Special methods of drug administration are needed for infants and young children.
9. Many medicines needed for pediatric patients are not available in appropriate dosage forms; thus, the dosage forms of drugs marketed for adults may require modification for use in infants and children, necessitating assurance of potency and safety of drug use.
10. The pediatric medication-use process is complex and error prone because of the multiple steps required in calculating, verifying, preparing, and administering doses.

INTRODUCTION

Remarkable progress has been made in the clinical management of diseases in pediatric patients. This chapter highlights important principles of pediatric pharmacotherapy that must be considered when the diseases discussed in other chapters of this book occur in pediatric patients, defined as those younger than 18 years. Newborn infants born before 37 weeks of gestational age are termed *premature;* those between 1 day and 1 month of age are *neonates;* 1 month to 1 year are *infants;* 1 to 11 years are *children;* and 12 to 16 years are *adolescents.* This chapter covers notable examples of problems in pediatrics, pharmacokinetic differences in pediatric patients, drug efficacy and toxicity in this patient group, and various factors affecting pediatric pharmacotherapy. Specific examples of problems and special considerations in pediatric patients are cited to enhance understanding.

(1) Infant mortality up to 1 year of age has declined from 200 per 1,000 births in the 19th century to 75 per 1,000 births in 1925 and to 5.96 per 1,000 births in 2013.[1] This success has resulted largely from improvements in identification, prevention, and treatment of diseases once common during delivery and the infancy period. Although most marketed drugs are used in pediatric patients, only approximately one-fourth of the drugs approved by the US Food and Drug Administration (FDA) have indications specific for use in the pediatric population. Data on the pharmacokinetics, pharmacodynamics, efficacy, and safety of drugs in infants and children are scarce. Lack of this type of information led to disasters such as gray baby syndrome from chloramphenicol, phocomelia from thalidomide, and kernicterus from sulfonamide therapy. Gray baby syndrome was first reported in two neonates who died after excessive doses of chloramphenicol (100-300 mg/kg/day); the serum concentrations of chloramphenicol immediately before death were 75 and 100 mcg/mL (mg/L; 232 and 309 μmol/L). Patients with gray baby syndrome usually have abdominal distension, vomiting, diarrhea, a characteristic gray color, respiratory distress, hypotension, and progressive shock.

Thalidomide is well known for its teratogenic effects. Clearly implicated as the cause of multiple congenital fetal abnormalities (particularly limb deformities), thalidomide also can cause polyneuritis, nerve damage, and mental retardation. Isotretinoin (Accutane) is another teratogen, because it is used to treat severe acne vulgaris, which is common in teenage patients who may be sexually active but not willing to acknowledge that activity to healthcare professionals; isotretinoin has presented a difficult problem in patient education since its marketing in the 1980s.

Kernicterus was reported in neonates receiving sulfonamides, which displaced bilirubin from protein-binding sites in the blood to cause hyperbilirubinemia. This results in deposition of bilirubin in the brain and induces encephalopathy in infants.

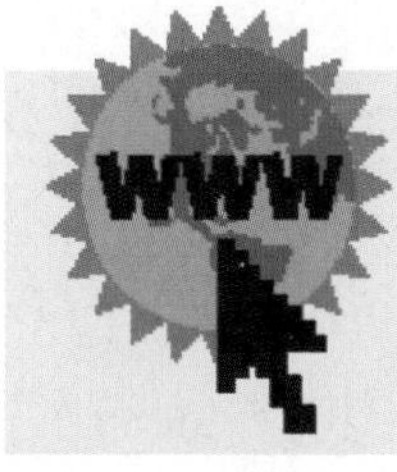

The complete chapter, learning objectives, and other resources can be found at **www.pharmacotherapyonline.com.**

Geriatrics

e7

Emily R. Hajjar, Shelly L. Gray, Patricia W. Slattum Jr, Lauren R. Hersh, Jennifer G. Naples, and Joseph T. Hanlon

KEY CONCEPTS

1. The population of persons age 65 years and older is increasing.
2. Age-related changes in physiology can affect the pharmacokinetics and pharmacodynamics of numerous drugs.
3. Improving and maintaining functional status is a cornerstone of care for older adults.
4. Drug-related problems in older adults are common and cause considerable morbidity.
5. Pharmacists can play a major role in optimizing drug therapy and preventing drug-related problems in older adults.

Pharmacotherapy for older adults can cure or palliate disease as well as enhance health-related quality of life (HRQOL). Health-related quality of life considerations for older adults include focusing on improvements in physical functioning (eg, activities of daily living), psychological functioning (eg, cognition, depression), social functioning (eg, social activities, support systems), and overall health (eg, general health perception).[1]

Despite the benefits of pharmacotherapy, HRQOL can be compromised by drug-related problems. Prevention of drug-related adverse consequences in older adults requires that health professionals become knowledgeable about a number of age-specific issues. To address these knowledge needs, this chapter discusses the epidemiology of aging; physiologic changes associated with aging, with emphasis on changes that can affect the pharmacokinetics and pharmacodynamics of drugs; clinical conditions commonly seen in older adult patients; epidemiology of drug-related problems in older adults; and an approach to reducing drug-related problems through the provision of comprehensive geriatric assessment.

EPIDEMIOLOGY OF AGING

1 The older American population is highly diverse and heterogeneous with respect to health status. The demographics and health characteristics of persons age 65 to 74 years differ from those of persons 85 years of age and older, as do those of persons who are institutionalized compared with those living in the community. Teasing apart the various threads of wellness and illness, independence and dependence, and function and dysfunction makes the available demographic and health status data relevant for clinical practice. Understanding the diversity and growth of older populations will allow society to plan for the training, research, and resources needed for future clinical practice and adequate healthcare.

The proportion of the population age 65 and older is increasing. In 2010, persons age 65 and older accounted for 13.0% (40 million) of the total US population, up from 12.4% in 2006. Among those older than 65 years, women accounted for 57% of this segment of the population. The gender gap widens with increasing age, with women accounting for 67% of the cohort 85 years and older.[2] In 2011, the first baby boomers turned 65 years old; this marked the beginning of a rapid increase in the older population. By 2030, this older population is projected to almost double in size; one in five Americans will be older than 65 years. This 20% projection will remain relatively stable through 2050. However, the proportion of the "oldest old" (greater than 85 years) will continue to grow; by 2050, almost one in four older adults will be 85 years or older.

The increase in the number of older persons is caused not only by the higher post-World War II birth rate but also by the declining mortality rate and overall improved health status among older adults.[3] The decline in early death and the better health of older adults arises from a variety of reasons: (a) public health measures affecting all age groups (eg, immunizations, prenatal care), (b) advances in medical technology, (c) promotion of a healthy lifestyle, and (d) improvements in living conditions.[4] More relevant to health professionals providing care to older Americans is the steadily increasing life expectancy at 65 and 85 years of age. In 2009, women 65 years of age could expect an average additional 20.30 years of life, and men could expect to live 17.6 additional years. Life expectancies are lower for black men and women.[2] Upon reaching 85 years of life, women may expect to live another 7.0 years and men another 5.9 years.[2] Nonetheless, the life expectancy at age 65 in the United States remains lower than that of many other industrialized countries. Interestingly, the number of centenarians (n = 53,364) increased by 5.8% between 2000 and 2010.

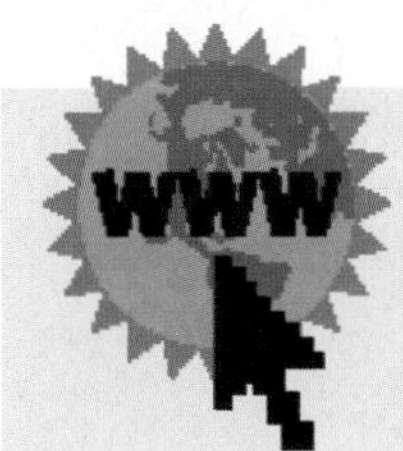

The complete chapter, learning objectives, and other resources can be found at **www.pharmacotherapyonline.com.**

e8

Palliative Care

Nina M. Bemben and Mary Lynn McPherson

KEY CONCEPTS

1. Palliative care may be provided to any patient with a serious illness, at any point in the course of the illness, including while a patient receives curative or disease-focused therapy.
2. Hospice is a form of palliative care, which has been defined by Medicare to encompass care solely focused on comfort and quality of life during the last 6 months of a patient's life.
3. Pain is a common symptom among patients receiving palliative care and may be managed safely and effectively using nonopioid, adjuvant, and/or opioid therapies.
4. Opioids are the drug of choice for the management of dyspnea.
5. Constipation, nausea, vomiting, anxiety, and delirium are common symptoms among patients receiving palliative care and may be managed effectively with drug and nondrug therapies.
6. End-of-life care can be provided to patients in the last days of their lives through palliative or hospice care, and provides management of common terminal symptoms.
7. Identifying a patient's goals and structuring care to achieve those goals is a key component of palliative care. Identifying a patient's goals of care involves communication with patients, their families and/or caregivers, as well as other healthcare professionals.
8. Addressing nonphysical needs, such as spirituality and faith, are key components of providing quality palliative care.

1 Palliative care, or palliative medicine, is specialized care provided to patients with serious illness with a goal of managing symptoms and helping patients to cope with their illnesses.[1] It is provided by an interdisciplinary team of healthcare professionals, including physicians, pharmacists, nurses, nurse practitioners, social workers, chaplains, and others.[2] Palliative care is appropriate for any patient with a serious or potentially life-limiting illness, at any point during the time course of that illness. Common diseases for which palliative care is appropriate include cancer, heart failure, advanced lung disease such as chronic obstructive pulmonary disease (COPD), organ failure such as liver or renal failure, and neurologic diseases such as dementia and Parkinson disease.[2] Patients may receive palliative care throughout the course of a serious illness, including while the patient receives treatment aimed at managing or curing the disease. If or when the serious illness progresses and disease-focused therapies are no longer helpful or desired, palliative care continues to be provided to manage symptoms and maximize quality of life.

Provision of palliative and hospice care to patients with limited prognoses has been shown to improve patient and caregiver satisfaction,[3-5] reduce healthcare utilization,[3,4] and decrease healthcare costs.[3,4,6] In addition to providing symptom management, improving patient and caregiver satisfaction, and reducing healthcare costs, early integration of palliative care has been shown to increase survival among patients with advanced cancer.[7,8]

Because of the evidence supporting the benefits of palliative care, clinical practice guidelines for serious illnesses incorporate palliative care into treatment recommendations. The American Society of Clinical Oncology and National Comprehensive Cancer Network both recommend palliative care as a component of oncology management.[9,10] In addition, the American College of Cardiology Foundation/American Heart Association practice guideline for the management of heart failure supports the incorporation of palliative care into the management of patients with advanced heart failure due to its effectiveness in increasing quality of life.[11]

WHAT IS HOSPICE?

2 In the United States, hospice care is a Medicare-defined benefit and is a form of palliative care that is focused on caring for patients with a life expectancy of 6 months or less.[12] While palliative care may be provided at any stage in the course of serious disease, including alongside curative, or disease-focused therapy, hospice care is generally provided when a patient is no longer pursuing disease-focused therapies and the decision has been made to focus solely on comfort and quality of life.[12,13] Although commonly associated with end-stage cancer, the frequency of noncancer diagnoses among hospice patients more than doubled between 1998 and 2008.[14] In 2014, the most recent year for which data are available, the most common hospice diagnoses were: non-cancer diagnoses (63.4% of hospice admissions) such as dementia (14.8%), heart disease (14.7%), and lung disease (9.3%). Cancer diagnoses accounted for 36.6% of hospice admissions.[14]

SYMPTOM MANAGEMENT IN PALLIATIVE CARE

Based on the diseases frequently encountered in hospice and palliative care, the most common symptoms managed by palliative care practitioners include pain, dyspnea, constipation, nausea and vomiting, anxiety, and delirium. The management of these symptoms is discussed below.

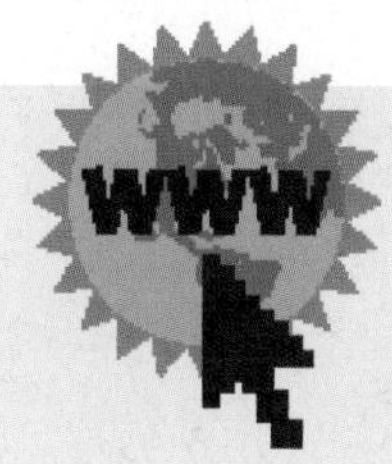

The complete chapter, learning objectives, and other resources can be found at **www.pharmacotherapyonline.com.**

e9

Clinical Toxicology

Peter A. Chyka

KEY CONCEPTS

1. Poisoning can result from exposure to excessive doses of any chemical, with medicines being responsible for most childhood and adult poisonings.
2. The total number and rate of poisonings have been increasing, but preventive measures, such as child-resistant containers, have reduced mortality in young children.
3. Immediate first aid may reduce the development of serious poisoning, and consultation with a poison control center may indicate the need for further therapy.
4. The use of ipecac syrup, gastric lavage, whole bowel irrigation, and cathartics has fallen out of favor as routine therapies, whereas activated charcoal remains useful for gastric decontamination of appropriate patients.
5. Antidotes can prevent or reduce the toxicity of certain poisons, but symptomatic and supportive care is essential for all patients.
6. Acute acetaminophen poisoning produces severe liver injury and occasionally kidney failure. A determination of serum acetaminophen concentration may indicate whether there is risk of hepatotoxicity and the need for acetylcysteine therapy.
7. Anticholinesterase insecticides may produce life-threatening respiratory distress and paralysis by all routes of exposure and can be treated with symptomatic care, atropine, and pralidoxime.
8. An overdose of calcium channel antagonists will produce severe hypotension and bradycardia and can be treated with supportive care, calcium, insulin with supplemental dextrose, and glucagon.
9. Poisoning with iron-containing drugs produces vomiting, gross gastrointestinal bleeding, shock, metabolic acidosis, and coma and can be treated with supportive care and deferoxamine.
10. Acute opioid poisoning and overdose can produce life-threatening respiratory depression that can be treated with assisted ventilation and naloxone.
11. Chemicals can be used for mass poisonings by acts of terrorism and warfare and typically produce life-threatening effects within minutes to hours, which warrant emergency preparedness at healthcare facilities and communities.

Poisoning is an adverse effect from a chemical that has been taken in excessive amounts. The body is able to tolerate and, in some cases, detoxify a certain dose of a chemical; however, toxicity ensues once a critical exposure threshold is exceeded. Poisoning can produce minor local effects that may be treated readily in the outpatient setting or systemic life-threatening effects that require intensive medical intervention. Virtually any chemical can become a poison when taken in sufficient quantity, but the potency of some compounds leads to serious toxicity with small quantities (Table e9-1). Poisoning by chemicals includes exposure to drugs, industrial chemicals, household products, plants, venomous animals, agrochemicals, and weapons for warfare and terrorism. This chapter describes some examples of the spectrum of toxicity, outlines means to recognize poisoning risk, and presents principles of treatment.

EPIDEMIOLOGY

Poisonings account for approximately 52,000 deaths, at least 2.3 million emergency department visits, and over 1.3 million nonfatal poisoning injuries each year in the United States.[1,2] Approximately 0.2% of poisoning deaths involve children younger than 5 years.[1] Of emergency department visits for drug-related poisoning, typically 1.1 million visits are made each year (3.5 per 100,000 population) with the highest rate observed for patients 20 to 34 years of age. One-fourth of emergency department visits for drug-related poisonings were hospitalized, which is twice the rate of other types of visits.[2] The age-adjusted death rates from poisonings from all circumstances have been increasing steadily, with a 224% increase from 2000 to 2014, representing 51,966 deaths in 2014 of which 91% were drug-related poisonings. This increasing mortality trend has placed poisoning since 2008 as the leading cause of injury death in the United States.[1]

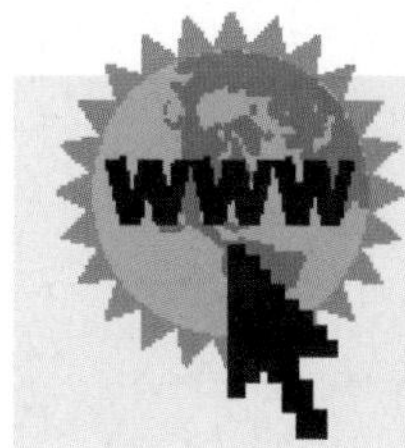

The complete chapter, learning objectives, and other resources can be found at **www.pharmacotherapyonline.com.**

Clinical Management of Potential Bioterrorism-related Conditions

e10

Colleen M. Terriff, Lisa T. Costanigro, Kimberly C. McKeirnan, and Barbara J. Hoeben

KEY CONCEPTS

1. The majority of emerging pathogens associated with public health outbreaks are zoonotic infections, passed from animals to humans.
2. Due to the high mortality rates with inhalation anthrax, postexposure prophylaxis may need to be rapidly offered to all people who were potentially exposed.
3. Pneumonic plague, one of the most lethal forms of plague, develops through primary (direct inhalation of infected droplets) or secondary exposure.
4. Rapid recognition of Ebola virus disease (EVD) is essential to initiate supportive care and infection control procedures.
5. While the incidence of measles-related deaths has, overall, significantly declined as the result of major global vaccination efforts, vigilance is still critical, since measles is extremely contagious and there are some gaps in vaccine coverage.
6. Middle Eastern Respiratory Syndrome (MERS) is an emerging viral respiratory illness, which can cause severe respiratory distress and has been fatal in one third of all patients who have contracted the disease.
7. A pertussis vaccination booster is recommended for all women during weeks 27 to 36 of gestation of each pregnancy to allow maximal maternal antibody response and passive in utero transfer of antibodies.
8. Infectious disease outbreaks following a natural disaster are common and usually attributable to critical infrastructure damage, limited access to quality healthcare, displacement, environmental and human condition changes, and vulnerability to pathogens.

Bioterrorism is characterized by an intentional exposure to animals or humans of an organism or toxin, which subsequently causes disease and/or death. Historically, these acts were planned and carried out against military personnel or directed towards select segments of the civilian population. Examples include diseased bodies flung over city walls, poisons added to drinking water, bacteria used to taint salad bars, and weaponized ricin and anthrax.[1,2] In general, while there is no catastrophic destruction of property associated with most acts of bioterrorism, there usually is fear, anxiety and confusion, some ensuing morbidity and mortality, economic disruption, and definite pressure on healthcare and public health systems.

After the intentional release of anthrax in 2001 public health officials, first responders, healthcare workers, employers, school officials, parents and community members incorporated the term bioterrorism in their emergency and disaster preparedness and response vocabulary. Subsequently, these groups wrote plans, conducted response exercises for potential scenarios, such as smallpox outbreaks and mass exposures of plague, that have, thankfully, not occurred. While these traditional bioterrorism agents are still threats, public health officials and healthcare professionals are starting to turn their focus on new or re-emerging concerns, many tied to Mother Nature or unintentional human acts.

(1) Similar to intentional acts of bioterrorism, disease outbreaks of Ebola and Middle Eastern Respiratory Syndrome Coronavirus (MERS) are a threat to global health security, associated with social unrest or instability and major economic disruption, in addition to significant morbidity and mortality.[3] The emergence and spread of these infectious diseases (ID) and the growing prevalence of drug resistance; ease of trade and travel; and rise of laboratories capable of creating dangerous microbes have heightened public concern.[3] Through a partnership of the Centers for Disease Control and Prevention (CDC), private and public stakeholders, and international organizations, The Global Health Security Agenda which focuses on efforts to prevent and reduce outbreaks, detect threats early to save lives, and rapidly and effectively respond to potential infectious disease threats has become a reality.[4] It is estimated that 75% of recently emerging infections are zoonotic, or passed between animals and humans.[5] The CDC recognizes the strong connection between humans, animals and the environment and has created the One Health Program to move forward an action agenda with both domestic and global activities. Initiatives of One Health are focused on improvements in research; detection or biosurveillance; clinical assessment, prevention and treatment; education and communication.[5] Many of these outbreaks, from pathogens like SARS and West Nile Virus, caused serious financial, political and public health ramifications, while eroding public confidence in the government's ability to anticipate and respond to these events.[5] Healthcare professionals are on the front lines of detection, clinical management and education related to these emerging zoonotic threats.

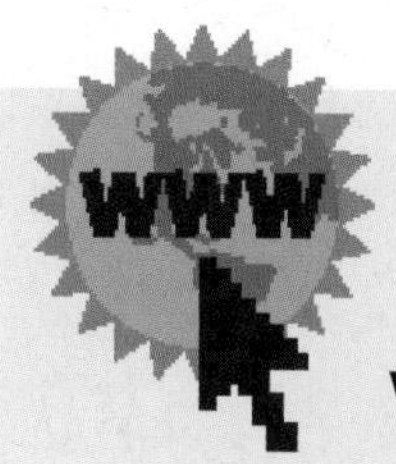

The complete chapter, learning objectives, and other resources can be found at **www.pharmacotherapyonline.com.**

Cardiovascular Testing

e11

Richard A. Lange

KEY CONCEPTS

1. A careful history and physical examination are extremely important in diagnosing cardiovascular disease; they should be performed before any testing.
2. Elevated jugular venous pressure (JVP) is an important sign of heart failure and may be used to assess its severity and the response to therapy.
3. Heart sounds and heart murmurs are important in identifying heart valve abnormalities and other structural cardiac defects.
4. Electrocardiography is useful for determining rhythm disturbances (tachy- or bradyarrhythmias).
5. Exercise stress testing provides important information concerning the presence and severity of coronary artery disease; changes in heart rate, blood pressure, and the electrocardiogram (ECG) are used to assess the response to exercise.
6. Echocardiography is used to assess valve structure and function as well as ventricular wall motion; transesophageal echocardiography is more sensitive than transthoracic echocardiography for detecting thrombus and vegetations.
7. Radionuclides, such as technetium-99m and thallium-201, are used to assess myocardial ischemia and myocardial viability in patients with suspected coronary artery disease.
8. When patients cannot exercise, pharmacologic stress testing is used to assess the likelihood of coronary artery disease.
9. Cardiac catheterization and angiography are used to assess coronary anatomy and ventricular performance.

INTRODUCTION

In the United States, cardiovascular disease (CVD) afflicts an estimated 85.6 million people (ie, greater than 1 in 3 adults) and accounts for 31% of all deaths. By 2030, 44% of the US population is projected to have some form of CVD. In 2011, the estimated direct and indirect cost of CVD—which includes hypertension, coronary heart disease, heart failure, and stroke—was $320.1 billion.[1]

Atherosclerosis, the cause of most CVD events, is typically present for decades before symptoms appear. With a thorough history, comprehensive physical examination, and appropriate testing, the individual with subclinical CVD usually can be identified, and the subject with symptomatic CVD can be assessed for the risk of an adverse event and can be managed appropriately.

THE HISTORY

The elements of a comprehensive history include the chief complaint, current symptoms, medical history, family history, social history, and review of systems.

The chief complaint is a brief statement describing the reason the patient is seeking medical attention. The patient is asked to describe his or her current symptoms, including their duration, quality, frequency, severity, progression, precipitating and relieving factors, associated symptoms, and impact on daily activities.

The medical history may reveal previous cardiovascular problems, conditions that predispose the patient to develop CVD (ie, hypertension, hyperlipidemia, or diabetes mellitus) (Table e11-1), or comorbid conditions that influence the identification or management of CVD. The patient should be asked about social habits that affect the cardiovascular system, including diet, amount of regular physical activity, tobacco use, alcohol intake, and illicit drug use. At present, family history of early onset CVD is the best available screening tool to identify patients with a genetic predisposition for CVD.

Cardiovascular History

1 Chest pain is a frequent symptom and may occur as a result of myocardial ischemia (angina pectoris) or infarction or a variety of noncardiac conditions, such as esophageal, pulmonary, or musculoskeletal disorders. The quality of chest pain, its location and duration, and the factors that provoke or relieve it are important in ascertaining its etiology.

Typically, patients with angina describe a sensation of heaviness or pressure in the retrosternal area that may radiate to the jaw, left shoulder, back, or left arm. It is precipitated by exertion, emotional stress, eating, smoking a cigarette, or exposure to cold, and it is usually relieved within minutes with rest or a sublingual nitroglycerin, although the latter also is effective in relieving chest pain due to esophageal spasm. Angina that is increasing in severity, longer in duration, or occurring at rest is called unstable angina; it should prompt the patient to seek medical attention expeditiously.

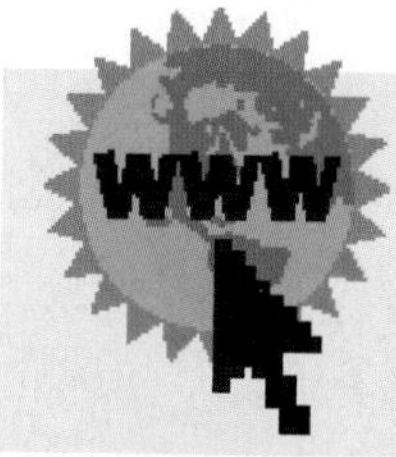

The complete chapter, learning objectives, and other resources can be found at **www.pharmacotherapyonline.com.**

12

Cardiac Arrest

Jeffrey F. Barletta

KEY CONCEPTS

1. High quality cardiopulmonary resuscitation (CPR) with minimal interruptions in chest compressions should be emphasized in all patients following cardiac arrest.
2. The AHA algorithm for basic life support following cardiac arrest emphasizes circulation, airway, and breathing forming the pneumonic "CAB" versus the historic pneumonic "ABC."
3. The purpose of using vasopressor therapy following cardiac arrest is to augment low coronary and cerebral perfusion pressures encountered during CPR.
4. Vasopressin appears to offer no benefit as a substitute over epinephrine.
5. Amiodarone remains the preferred antiarrhythmic during cardiac arrest with lidocaine considered as an alternative.
6. Successful treatment of both pulseless electrical activity (PEA) and asystole depends almost entirely on diagnosis of the underlying cause.
7. Intraosseous administration is the preferred alternative route for administration if IV access cannot be achieved.

CARDIAC ARREST

Cardiac arrest is defined as the cessation of cardiac mechanical activity as confirmed by the absence of signs of circulation (eg, a detectable pulse, unresponsiveness, and apnea).[1] While there is wide variation in the reported incidence of cardiac arrest, it is estimated that there are more than 320,000 people in the United States who experience emergency medical services (EMS)-assessed out-of-hospital cardiac arrest.[2] Survival to hospital discharge following out-of-hospital cardiac arrest is only 10.6% and survival with good neurologic function is only 8.3%.[2] While there has been minimal improvement in survival over the past 40 years, recent data have shown some progress from 2005 to 2012 (adjusted rate ratio = 1.47 [1.26-1.7]).[3] This improvement was attributed to both improved pre-hospital and in-hospital survival.

In-hospital cardiac arrests occur in roughly 200,000 patients in the United States annually and this rate may be increasing.[4] Similar to out-of-hospital arrests, some progress has been made over the past decade with survival rates to hospital discharge being 13.7% in 2000 and 22.3% in 2009.[5] Survival rates are substantially higher in victims with a shockable first documented rhythm as one study reported survival rates of 49% with ventricular fibrillation/pulseless ventricular tachycardia (VF/PVT) versus 11% with pulseless electrical activity (PEA)/asystole.[6]

EPIDEMIOLOGY

In adult patients, cardiac arrest usually results from the development of an arrhythmia.[7] Historically, VF and PVT have been the most common initial rhythm accounting for 40% to 60% of out-of-hospital arrests but their incidence now is estimated to be only about 24%.[8,9] In fact, data from the Cardiac Arrest Registry to Enhance Survival (CARES) project reported asystole to be the most common presenting rhythm (45%) which is similar to other registry data whereby nonshockable rhythms were more prevalent.[8,10,11] The reason for this change has not been firmly established. Possible explanations include the influence of noncardiac causes of arrest that typically present with apnea leading to bradycardia and then PEA or asystole. A second explanation is the increasing role of implantable pacemakers and defibrillators.[12] Finally, it has been suggested that beta-blockers and angiotensin-converting enzyme (ACE) inhibitors may shorten the duration of VF and the expanded use of these drug classes for ischemic heart disease and heart failure may account for the increased occurrence of non-VF/PVT rhythms.[9] Nonetheless, this declining incidence is particularly concerning as survival rates are substantially higher with shockable rhythms such as VF and PVT compared to nonshockable rhythms such as PEA and asystole. Survival rates with VF/PVT are roughly 27% versus 2% with asystole.[8]

A similar finding has been observed with in-hospital cardiac arrest. One study using the "Get with the Guidelines-Resuscitation" registry reported 79% of patients had an initial rhythm of asystole or PEA and 21% had VF or PVT.[5] Survival rates were 12.2% for asystole/PEA and 35% for VF/PVT. Similarly, a second study used the National Registry of CPR and noted the incidence of VF/PVT, PEA and asystole to be 24%, 37%, and 39%, respectively.[13] Survival rates were 37% for VF/PVT compared to 12% for PEA and 11% for asystole. Patients with VF/PVT were more likely to have myocardial infarction as the immediate factor pre-arrest while acute respiratory failure and hypotension were the immediate factors more commonly found in patients with PEA/asystole.

In pediatric patients, cardiac arrest typically results from respiratory failure and asphyxiation. As such, the initial rhythm most often encountered in out-of-hospital arrest is PEA or asystole.[14] Survival rates with out-of-hospital pediatric arrests range between 1% and 12% with lower rates in infants compared to children and adolescents.[15] Survival following in-hospital cardiac arrest appears higher with an overall rate of 34%.[16] Similar to the adult population, risk-adjusted survival rates have increased over the past decade from 14% in 2000 to 43% in 2009.[16]

ETIOLOGY

The most common clinical finding in adult patients who suffer cardiac arrest is coronary artery disease accounting for roughly 80% of sudden cardiac deaths.[7] Approximately 10% to 15% of sudden cardiac deaths occur in patients with cardiomyopathies (eg, hypertrophic cardiomyopathy, dilated cardiomyopathy) and the remaining 5% to 10% are composed of either structurally abnormal congenital cardiac conditions or patients with structurally normal but electrically abnormal heart. Unfortunately, in many patients (approximately two-thirds), cardiac arrest is the first clinical sign of coronary artery disease with no preceding signs or symptoms.[17]

In pediatric patients, cardiac arrest is often the terminal event of respiratory failure or progressive shock.[18] Out-of-hospital arrests frequently are associated with trauma, sudden infant death syndrome, drowning, poisoning, choking, severe asthma, and pneumonia. In-hospital arrests, on the other hand, are associated with sepsis, respiratory failure, drug toxicity, metabolic disorders, and arrhythmias.

PATHOPHYSIOLOGY OF CARDIAC ARREST

There are two distinctly different pathophysiologic conditions associated with cardiac arrest. The first is primary cardiac arrest whereby arterial blood is typically fully oxygenated at the time of arrest. The second is cardiac arrest secondary to respiratory failure in which lack of ventilation leads to severe hypoxemia, hypotension, and secondary cardiac arrest. It is important to understand the specific condition at hand as different treatment approaches are likely necessary.[19]

CLINICAL PRESENTATION

Cardiac arrest is characterized by the cessation of cardiac mechanical activity therefore signs and symptoms are consistent with those encountered when there is no circulation. In the setting of cardiac causes of arrest, anxiety, crushing chest pain, nausea, vomiting, and diaphoresis can precede the event. Following an arrest, individuals are unresponsive, apneic, hypotensive and do not have a detectable pulse. Extremities are cold and clammy and cyanosis is common.

TREATMENT

Cardiopulmonary resuscitation (CPR) is an attempt to restore spontaneous circulation by performing chest compressions (to restore threshold blood flows, particularly to the heart and brain) with or without ventilations. There are two proposed theories describing the mechanism of blood flow during CPR.[20] The original theory is known as the cardiac pump theory and is based on the active compression of the heart between the sternum and vertebrae thereby creating forward flow. Echocardiography, however, has revealed that left ventricular size does not always change with compressions and the mitral valve may in fact be open.[20] The second theory is the thoracic pump theory. This theory is based on intrathoracic pressure alterations induced by chest compressions and the differential compressibility of the arteries and veins. In this model, the heart merely acts as a passive conduit for flow. It is likely that both models contribute to the mechanism of blood flow with CPR.

High-quality CPR continues to be emphasized in the latest guidelines published by the American Heart Association. Clinicians must focus on proper technique, including adequate rate and depth of compressions, allowance of chest recoil after each compression, avoiding excessive ventilation, and minimizing interruptions.[21] One study, in patients suffering out-of-hospital VF, reported an increased chance of survival as chest compression fraction increased (eg, the proportion of resuscitation time without spontaneous circulation where chest compressions were administered).[22] Unfortunately, the provision of high-quality CPR is frequently suboptimal particularly when rescuers become fatigued.[23] There are several devices available that provide prompts and/or feedback in "real time"; however, data illustrating improvement in survival are lacking.[23] Additionally, mechanical devices designed to improve hemodynamics have been studied but inconsistent results limit their applicability in routine practice.[24]

Desired Outcome

The global goals of resuscitation are to preserve life, restore health, relieve suffering, limit disability, and respect the individual's decisions, rights, and privacy.[25] This can be accomplished via CPR by the return of spontaneous circulation (ROSC) with effective perfusion and ventilation as quickly as possible to minimize hypoxic damage to vital organs. Survival to hospital discharge with good neurologic function should be considered the primary treatment outcome sought by clinicians. Survival to hospital discharge in a vegetative or comatose state cannot be classified as a success and can impose a tremendous economic burden on the healthcare system. Additionally, most patients would choose not to continue living in a massively disabled state.[26]

The presence of a healthcare advanced directive allows patients to communicate their wishes and preferences regarding medical care and may lead to a "do not attempt resuscitation (DNAR)" order. As many cardiac arrests occur following terminal illnesses and end-of-life care, "allow natural death (AND)" has become a preferred term to replace DNAR.[27] These orders should explicitly state the resuscitation interventions that are to be performed and have clearly been communicated by the patient, their family or a surrogate decision maker.

General Approach to Treatment

Cardiopulmonary Resuscitation

Resuscitation techniques have been studied for many years. The first landmark article was published in 1960 and described the outcome of 20 patients who were given closed chest compressions at a rate of 60 per minute.[28] Artificial ventilation was used to augment the compressions, and three patients were given defibrillation for ventricular fibrillation. In this landmark article, all 20 patients had ROSC, and 14 lived for an extended period of time, with reported good neurologic status. Initial descriptions after this started to integrate the approach to cardiac arrest, including three phases.[29]

In 1966, the American Heart Association (AHA) first published guidelines for the treatment of cardiac arrest.[30] Since then, national conferences and organized committees have played a major role in encouraging widespread competency in CPR technique. There have been tremendous revisions of the guidelines over the years, and this is true of the most recent guidelines, published in 2015.[31] The 2015 guidelines represent a new era for the AHA Guidelines for CPR and Emergency Cardiovascular Care (ECC) because they will transition from a 5-year cycle of periodic revisions to a web-based format that is continuously updated. The intent is that this will allow for more rapid application of new research findings into daily patient care.

The 2015 guidelines continue to emphasize the "chain of survival" to highlight the treatment approach and illustrate the importance of a timely response. The updated guidelines however now includes two separate chains; one for out of hospital cardiac arrest and one for in-hospital cardiac arrest.[32] This has been done to reflect the differences in the steps needed to respond to a cardiac arrest in the in-patient and out-patient setting. The two chains converge in the hospital with post-cardiac arrest care as the last link. In summary, the five links in each chain of survival are as follows:

Out of hospital

1. Immediate recognition of cardiac arrest and activation of EMS.
2. Early CPR with an emphasis on chest compressions.
3. Rapid defibrillation.
4. Effective advanced life support.
5. Integrated postcardiac arrest care.

In-hospital

1. Appropriate surveillance and prevention of cardiac arrest.
2. Prompt notification and response by a multidisciplinary team of professional providers.
3. High-quality CPR.

4. Prompt defibrillation and advanced life support when appropriate.
5. Integrated postcardiac arrest care.

While all five links of the chain of survival are important, basic life support (BLS) is the foundation for saving lives after cardiac arrest (ie, immediate recognition, early CPR, and rapid defibrillation).[21] In fact, one large observational study compared the effects of BLS and advanced cardiac life support (ACLS) on outcomes following out-of-hospital cardiac arrest and survival to hospital discharge was greater among patients receiving BLS (13.1% vs 9.2%).[33] CPR provides critical blood flow to the heart and brain, prolongs the time VF is present (prior to the deterioration to asystole) and increases the likelihood that a shock will terminate VF resulting in a rhythm compatible with life.[21] For every minute that elapsed from collapse to successful defibrillation during witnessed VF arrests, survival rates decrease by 7 % to 10% if no CPR is provided.[34] If immediate CPR is added, the decrease in survival is more gradual (down to 3%-4% per minute post-collapse).[35] In effect, CPR can increase the likelihood of survival threefold from arrest to survival. Basic CPR alone, however, is not likely to terminate VF and lead to ROSC.

1 As in previous AHA guidelines for CPR and ECC, the AHA continues to emphasize the provision of high-quality CPR with minimal interruptions in chest compressions. In addition, algorithms continue to be more simplified, with emphasis on the use of end-tidal carbon dioxide ($ETCO_2$) to guide resuscitation.[36] Furthermore, there is growing importance of post-arrest care, reflecting that optimization of many organ systems may help improve outcomes.[37] The use of drug therapy and airway adjuncts, on the other hand, have continued to devolve to a minimal role as survival to hospital discharge does not appear to be impacted.

Basic Life Support The pneumonic for the CPR sequence is "CAB" which stands for circulation, airway, and breathing. 2 Historically, BLS and ACLS providers have been taught the pneumonic, "ABC." This change was made upon recognition of the importance of maintaining blood flow to the heart and brain and the consequences of delays or interruptions with chest compressions.

When first encountering a victim of cardiac arrest, the initial action is to determine responsiveness of the patient. If there is no response, the rescuer should immediately activate the emergency medical response team, and obtain (or call for) an automated external defibrillator (AED) (if one is available) and them immediately start CPR with chest compressions. A true cardiac arrest victim will be unresponsive, and agonal respirations can be confused with normal breathing. Thus, the "look, listen, and feel" for respirations is not recommended as part of the initial assessment.[21] Similarly, pulse recognition is often inaccurate, and it is recommended that lay rescuers not check for a pulse. Healthcare providers should assess for a pulse but take no more than 10 seconds to do so. If one is not detected within this short timeframe, then chest compressions should be initiated immediately.[21,38]

The prompt provision of chest compressions is thus of paramount importance, and rescuers should attempt them regardless of rescuer experience or skill level. The teaching of BLS now focuses on delivering high quality CPR with a rate of 100 to 120 beats/min, adequate depth (at least 2 inches in an adult), allowing full chest recoil, minimizing interruptions in compressions, and avoiding excessive ventilation.

While it is true that opening the airway has the potential to improve oxygenation and allow for better attempts at ventilation, this can be very challenging, especially if the rescuer is alone and is a novice. Thus, the simplified adult BLS algorithm calls for the initiation of CPR, with rhythm check every 2 minutes, shocking if indicated, with continued repetition.

Once chest compressions have been started, it is then appropriate for a trained rescuer to attempt to deliver rescue breaths, either by mouth-to-mouth, or preferentially by bag-mask ventilation. The current guidelines recommend delivering a breath over one second, use enough volume to elicit a visible chest rise, and to use a compression to ventilation ratio of 30 to 2 for one rescuer.[21]

The 2015 AHA guidelines for CPR and ECC continue to stress that there should be minimal interruptions in chest compressions. If there is no AED available, then cycles of compressions/breaths should continue, with pulse checks every 2 minutes until help arrives or the patient regains spontaneous circulation. If there is an AED available, then the rhythm should be checked to determine if defibrillation is advised. If so, then one shock should be delivered with the immediate resumption of chest compressions (and rescue breaths, if being provided). After 2 minutes (5 cycles of 30:2 compression to ventilation), the rhythm should be reevaluated to determine the need for defibrillation. This algorithm should be repeated until help arrives, or the rhythm is no longer "shockable." If the rhythm is not shockable, then chest compressions—rescue breath cycles should be continued until help arrives, or the victim recovers spontaneous circulation (Fig. 12-1).

Despite widespread dissemination of cardiac arrest guidelines and the ongoing education even of health care providers, there is ample evidence that chest compression quality remains poor in general. Furthermore, it have been reported that the rate of bystander CPR with out-of-hospital cardiac arrest in the United States is only 26%.[39] This has led to further educational interventions in an attempt to increase quality of CPR, and EMS dispatchers will often attempt to give instructions over the phone when EMS is activated.

There is now a push for hands-only CPR for lay persons, given data that show similar survival compared to the addition of rescue breaths. There has been reluctance on many bystanders to consider mouth-to-mouth, though one data set cites panic as a reason not to pursue bystander CPR rather than actual reluctance.[40]

Advanced Cardiac Life Support Once ACLS providers arrive, then further definitive therapy is given. An advanced airway (endotracheal tube, laryngeal mask airway, or even bag-valve mask) can be used to provide ventilation. When this occurs, the rescuers no longer need to provide the cycles of 30:2 compressions to ventilations. Instead, continuous chest compressions are recommended without pauses for ventilations, and the rescuer providing the ventilations needs to deliver a breath once every 6 to 8 seconds.

Monitoring during CPR has also evolved over time. Animal and human studies have shown that monitoring of $ETCO_2$, coronary perfusion pressure, and central venous oxygen saturation can provide valuable information as to the success of resuscitation.[36] Surprisingly, no study has ever shown the validity of checking a pulse during ongoing CPR. $ETCO_2$ is the concentration of carbon dioxide in exhaled air at the end of expiration. During cardiac arrest, the level of $ETCO_2$ decreases because there is no flow through the pulmonary circulation. Thus, a persistently low $ETCO_2$ (ie, less than 10 mm Hg) during CPR in intubated patients suggests that ROSC is unlikely.[36] In fact, one systematic review reported a mean $ETCO_2$ of 26 mm Hg in patients who achieved ROSC compared to 13 mm Hg in those who did not.[41] In patients without ROSC and persistently decreased $ETCO_2$, it is advised to evaluate the effectiveness of CPR, since good chest compressions can increase $ETCO_2$ somewhat. The latest guidelines recommend $ETCO_2$ monitoring during CPR if at all possible.[36]

Monitoring of coronary perfusion pressure and central venous oxygen saturation require more invasive monitoring and will not be covered.

If the cardiac rhythm is not deemed to be shockable, then it is likely to be either asystole or PEA (Fig. 12-2). For PEA, the rescuer must consider reversible causes. If the person is in VF or PVT, then one shock should be delivered (appropriate to the available electrical device), with the immediate resumption of chest compressions

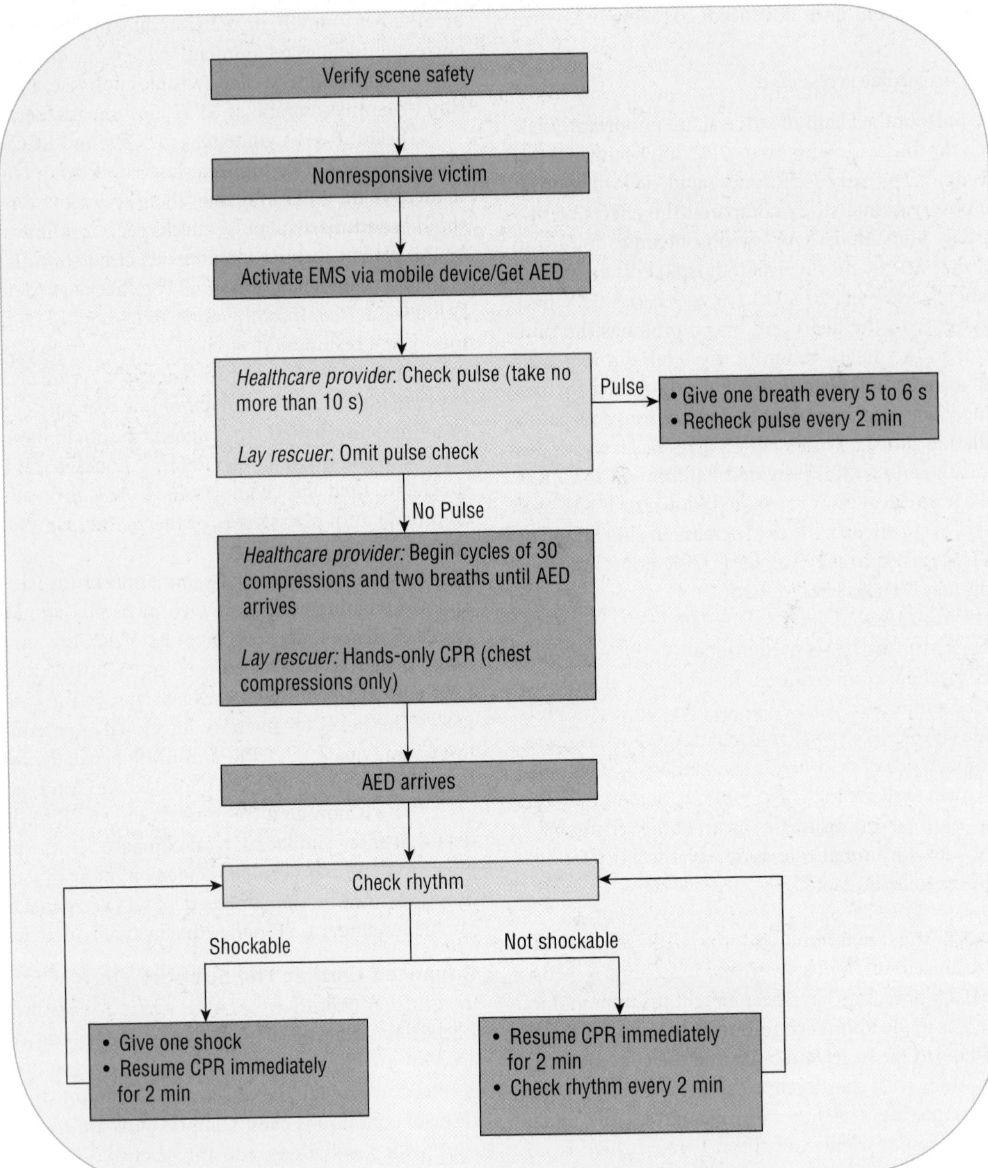

FIGURE 12-1 Treatment algorithm for adult cardiac arrest: Basic life support (BLS).

(using 30 compressions to 2 breaths for 5 cycles, or 2 minutes continuous compressions with assisted ventilations) prior to rechecking the rhythm or pulse. If there is still a shockable rhythm, then one shock should be delivered, and at this time pharmacologic intervention can be considered. Vasopressors are the initially recommended pharmacologic intervention at this point. After another unsuccessful shock, antiarrhythmics can be considered. Two minutes (five cycles of chest compressions: breaths) should be performed in between attempts at defibrillation. This algorithm will repeat until either a pulse is obtained with effective circulation, the rhythm changes, or the patient expires. For completeness, please refer to the guidelines published by the AHA.[36]

Cardiocerebral Resuscitation

In lieu of the relative lack of progress with survival rates following out-of-hospital cardiac arrest, an alternative approach for resuscitation was proposed called cardiocerebral resuscitation (CCR).[19] CCR has been embraced by the AHA guidelines, and is composed of three major components: a community component, an EMS component, and a hospital component.

The community component consists of prompt recognition (check), activation of EMS (call), and chest compression only CPR (compress). Chest compressions deliver a small but critical amount of oxygen to the brain and myocardium. Cerebral and coronary perfusion pressures, however, build up slowly once chest compressions are begun. These perfusion pressures are lost if chest compressions are stopped to deliver mouth-to-mouth ventilation. In fact, in earlier studies, approximately 16 seconds were required to deliver 2 breaths as recommended by earlier ECC guidelines.[42] The loss of perfusion during this time period has been shown to be extremely detrimental as ROSC is closely related to perfusion pressures generated during chest compressions.[43]

The EMS component of CCR consists of a revised ACLS algorithm. This protocol is based on the three-phase time-sensitive model of cardiac arrest.[44] The first phase is the electrical phase (0-5 minutes), where prompt defibrillation is the most important intervention. The second phase is the hemodynamic phase (5-15 minutes), where adequate coronary and cerebral perfusion pressures, before and after defibrillation, are crucial. In fact, defibrillation prior to CPR in this phase commonly leads asystole or PEA. This is likely due to the presence of global tissue ischemia and the need for blood flow (via chest compressions) to "flush out" deleterious metabolic factors that have accumulated during ischemia. The third phase is the metabolic phase (beyond 15 minutes) in which survival is very

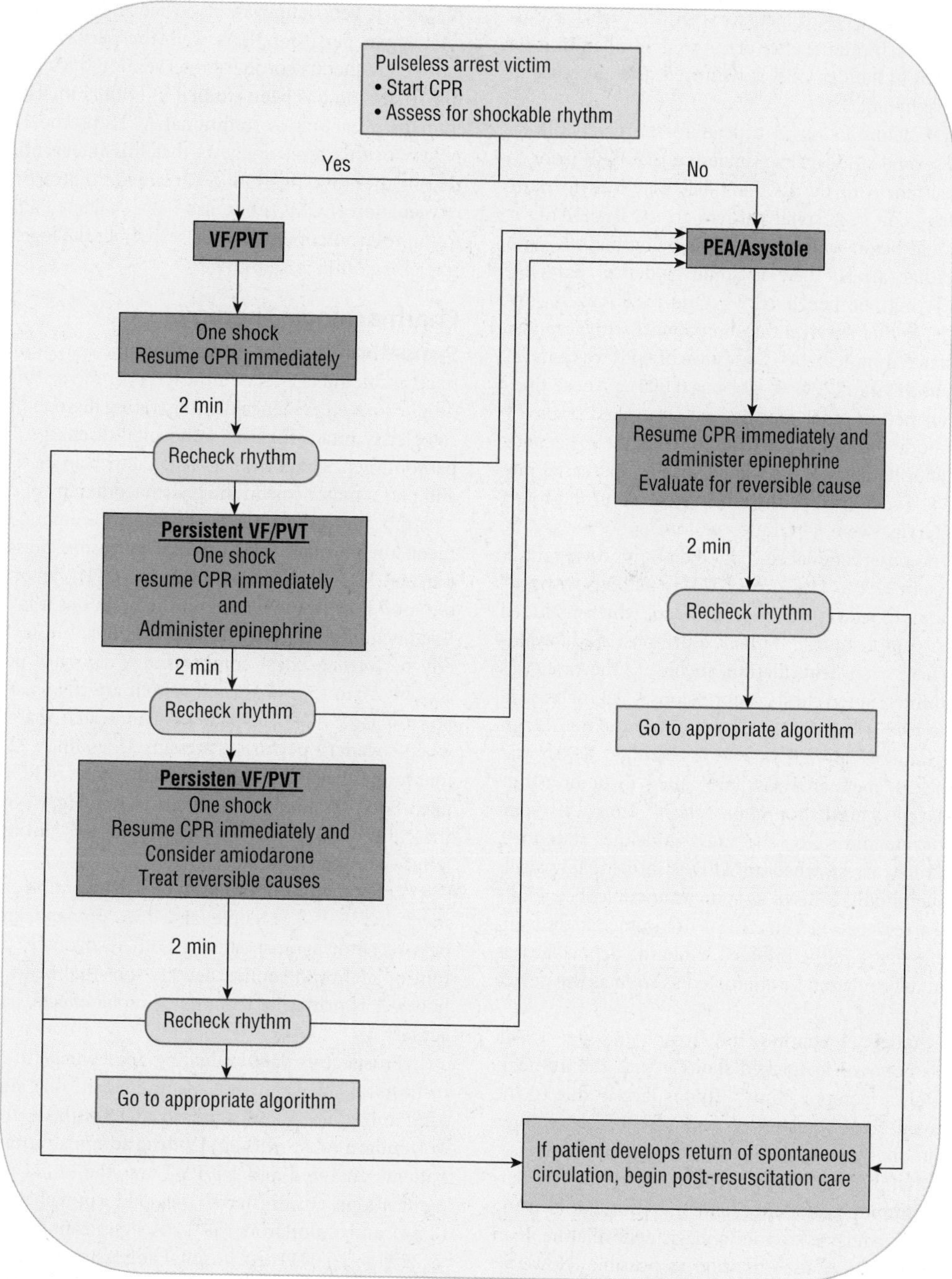

FIGURE 12-2 Treatment algorithm for adult cardiac arrest: Advanced cardiac life support (ACLS).

low and hypothermia may be the most beneficial approach. In situations where EMS personnel witness the arrest, immediate defibrillation is attempted.[45] Alternatively, the EMS protocol of CCR emphasizes prompt initiation of 2 minutes of continuous chest compressions before and immediately after a single indicated direct current shock.

The third component of CCR is the hospital which calls for aggressive postresuscitation care. This consists of the use of hypothermia for all comatose patients and emergent cardiac catheterization and percutaneous coronary intervention (PCI) for patients with myocardial ischemia as a potential cause of their arrest. This would entail the designation of cardiac receiving centers or hospitals with a commitment and expertise in postresuscitative care.

Since its conception in 2003, clinical studies evaluating CCR have demonstrated an improvement in survival of 250% to 300% compared to conventional CPR.[19] One systematic review compared CCR with CPR (as per the 2005 AHA Guidelines) and the odds ratio (OR) for survival was 2.26 (95% confidence interval [CI] 1.64-3.12).[46] A registry study demonstrated better survival with CCR which was observed across multiple age groups.[47] The greatest difference was noted in those who were younger than 40 years (OR 5.94; [95% CI] 1.82-19.26). Additionally, patients who received CCR had better neurologic outcomes.

Ventricular Fibrillation/Pulseless Ventricular Tachycardia

Nonpharmacologic Therapy

Electrical defibrillation is the only effective method of restoring a perfusing cardiac rhythm in either VF or PVT; therefore, it is a crucial link in the "chain of survival," especially for a witnessed arrest.[36] The probability of successful defibrillation is directly related to the time interval between the onset of VF and the delivery of the first shock.[35] In one study, a 23% relative improvement in survival was observed with each 1 minute reduction in the time to defibrillation

(OR 0.77; [95% CI] 0.73-0.81).[48] If fact, survival decreases an estimated 7% to 10% for each minute after arrest to defibrillation if no CPR is given.[34] When bystander CPR is delivered, this decrease in survival is cut almost in half.[35]

Although early defibrillation is crucial for survival following cardiac arrest, several studies have suggested that CPR prior to defibrillation (consistent with the CCR model) may lead to more successful outcomes. For in-hospital cardiac arrest, if an AED is available, CPR should begin while the AED is being placed. With out-of-hospital cardiac arrest, there is some evidence that CPR before defibrillation may be beneficial.[49-52] One randomized controlled trial revealed higher survival rates in patients with response intervals greater than 5 minutes when 3 minutes of CPR was administered prior to defibrillation (22% vs 4%; $p = 0.006$).[52] These findings were not confirmed in other randomized controlled trials.[53-56] An observational study found the provision of roughly 90 seconds of CPR prior to defibrillation was associated with an increased rate of hospital survival (compared with a historical control group) when response intervals were 4 minutes or longer (27% vs 17%; $p = 0.01$).[49] A second observational study noted an improvement in hospital survival (from 22% to 44%, $p = 0.0024$) in patients with witnessed VF using a modified resuscitation protocol which included 200 preshock chest compressions.[50] Finally, a pre-post study evaluated a protocol where each defibrillation, including the first, was preceded by 200 uninterrupted chest compressions.[51] An increase in total survival (57% [19/33] vs 20% [18/92], $p = 0.001$) and neurologically normal survival (48% [16/33] vs 15% [14/92], $p = 0.001$) was reported. Nevertheless, meta-analyses have failed to demonstrate benefit with a delayed defibrillation approach.[57-59] Thus, this is an issue of ongoing debate and study. The latest guidelines state for a witnessed adult cardiac arrest, when an AED is immediately available, the defibrillator should be used as soon as possible. For adults with unmonitored arrests or when an AED is not immediately available, it is reasonable that CPR be initiated while the defibrillator is being retrieved but defibrillation be attempted as soon as the device is ready for use.[21]

The current guidelines continue to recommend one shock for VF or PVT (as opposed to stacked shocks) with the immediate resumption of chest compressions.[36] This is largely due to the prolonged time noted (approximately 55 seconds) to deliver three stacked shocks without providing adequate chest compressions.[60] The defibrillation attempt should be with 120 to 200 J (biphasic defibrillator) or 360 J (monophasic defibrillator). Defibrillators using biphasic waveforms are preferred to monophasic defibrillators. If an AED is available, it should be used as soon as possible. However, CPR should be started immediately (after EMS activation) while the AED is being prepared.

After defibrillation is attempted, CPR should be immediately restarted and continued for 2 minutes without checking a pulse. The omission of the pulse check after defibrillation is related to myocardial stunning with resultant poor perfusion and diminished cardiac output immediately after electrical therapy.[36] After 2 minutes of chest compressions, the rhythm should be rechecked and if there is still evidence of VF or PVT, pharmacologic therapy with repeat attempts at single-discharge defibrillation should be attempted.

Endotracheal intubation and intravenous (IV) access should be obtained when feasible, but not at the expense of stopping chest compressions. The 2015 AHA guidelines for CPR and ECC continue to strongly stress the need for uninterrupted CPR.[21] Once an airway is achieved, patients should be ventilated with 100% oxygen. There are several airway adjuncts that are potentially available, such as laryngeal mask airways and esophageal-tracheal combination tubes. However, the definitive airway is an endotracheal tube placed with direct laryngoscopy.

Other interventions are also being evaluated as nonpharmacologic therapy. In a porcine model of VF arrest, a percutaneously placed left ventricular assist device (LVAD) was shown to sustain vital organ perfusion.[61] As well, the performance of angiography and percutaneous coronary intervention during suspected myocardial infarction has been studied in both animals and anecdotally in humans refractory to traditional ACLS protocol without ROSC. A review of this topic suggests that this intervention is feasible and that further investigation is warranted.[62] Extracorporeal membrane oxygenation (ECMO) has also been evaluated and has been shown to improve outcomes in some series, but the logistics of widespread implementation is daunting.[63]

Pharmacologic Therapy

Sympathomimetics Sympathomimetics continue to be the first pharmacologic agents administered in the setting of cardiac arrest despite limited evidence demonstrating their ability to increase neurologically intact survival to hospital discharge. Nevertheless sympathomimetics have been associated with an increased rate of ROSC and play a major role in the pharmacotherapy of cardiac arrest.

3 The primary goal of sympathomimetic therapy is to augment low coronary and cerebral perfusion pressures encountered during CPR. Chest compressions (via CPR) can provide some degree of blood flow to the heart and the brain but it is only about 25% of that encountered under basal conditions.[64] In fact, even with properly performed chest compressions, coronary perfusion pressures are only 10 to 15 mm Hg and systolic arterial pressure is rarely above 80 mm Hg.[65] Clinical data have indicated that ROSC is unlikely when coronary perfusion pressure is less than 15 mm Hg and animal studies have demonstrated higher rates of ROSC when coronary perfusion pressure was 31 versus 14 mm Hg.[66,67] Sympathomimetics therefore work to increase these pressures through their vasoconstrictive properties.

Epinephrine continues to be a drug of first choice for the treatment of VF, PVT, asystole, and PEA. Epinephrine is an alpha- and beta-receptor agonist causing both vasoconstriction and increased inotropic/chronotrophic activity on the heart. Its effectiveness however is primarily through its alpha effects, particularly alpha-2 activity.[68]

Prospective data evaluating epinephrine in the setting of out-of-hospital cardiac arrest are limited. In one study, patients were randomized to receive standard ACLS with IV drug administration or standard ACLS without IV drug administration.[69] There were 851 patients analyzed and VF/PVT was the initial rhythm in 34%. IV medications administered included epinephrine (79%), atropine (46%), and amiodarone (17%). A significant increase in ROSC (40% vs 25%, $p < 0.001$) and hospital admission (43% vs. 29%, $p < 0.001$) was noted in patients who received IV therapy. This difference was primarily observed in patients with initial rhythms other than VF/PVT. The role of epinephrine (vs other IV medications) in the contribution of these outcomes was not assessed. A second randomized, controlled trial compared epinephrine with placebo in 534 patients.[70] Ventricular fibrillation or PVT was the initial rhythm in 44% and 48% of patients in the epinephrine and placebo groups, respectively. Return of spontaneous circulation (23.5% vs 8.4%, $p < 0.001$) and survival to hospital admission (25.4% vs 13%, $p < 0.001$) was significantly higher with epinephrine but there was no difference in survival to hospital discharge (4% vs 1.9%, $p = 0.15$). While epinephrine was effective in achieving ROSC in both shockable (OR [95% CI] = 2.5 [1.2-4.5]) and nonshockable (OR [95% CI] = 6.9 [2.6-18.4]) rhythms, its effect was more pronounced in the latter cohort.

Several large observational studies have evaluated the impact of epinephrine on survival. One large registry study of over 400,000 patients failed to demonstrate a survival benefit with prehospital administration of epinephrine.[71] Despite a significant improvement in ROSC with epinephrine (adjusted OR [95% CI] = 2.36 [2.22-2.5]), 1-month survival (adjusted OR [95% CI] = 0.46 [0.42-0.51]) and survival with good neurologic function (adjusted OR [95% CI]

= 0.31 [0.26-0.36]) were both lower in patients who received epinephrine. A second study of evaluated outcomes of patients with witnessed out-of-hospital cardiac arrest.[72] After propensity matching, epinephrine was associated with improvements in survival at 1 month or discharge (17% vs 13.4%) in patients with VF/PVT but no difference in neurologically intact survival (6.6% vs 6.6%). The lack of agreement between these two studies may be related to the fact that epinephrine administration occurred earlier in the latter study (ie, within 10 minutes).

The influence of timing of epinephrine has been described in other analyses and earlier administration appears to be more beneficial than later.[73-78] One study though found an adverse association between epinephrine and intact survival which worsened as epinephrine administration was delayed.[79] These findings were replicated in a second study whereby a significant decrease in survival was noted with each minute increase in the time to epinephrine administration (adjusted OR [95% CI] = 0.95 [0.92-0.97]).[75] The time to epinephrine administration may therefore be a key factor associated with survival and future studies must consider this as a potential confounding variable.

Clinical **Controversy...**

The time to epinephrine administration may be an important confounding factor for the value of epinephrine during out-of-hospital cardiac arrest.

Given the disparate results with epinephrine in published research, it can be considered both a cure and a curse in cardiac arrest. One possible explanation for the negative effects of epinephrine is related to its mechanism of action. Epinephrine causes alpha-mediated vasoconstriction which increases coronary perfusion but can decrease perfusion to other vital organs. In fact, animal research has linked epinephrine to a decrease in cerebral microvascular blood flow and increase in brain tissue ischemia during and after CPR.[80] Epinephrine also stimulates beta-receptors which can increase myocardial oxygen demand, impair lactate clearance and advance the severity of post resuscitation myocardial dysfunction.[81] This has led some investigators to evaluate simultaneous adrenergic antagonist administration in conjunction with epinephrine therapy (thereby isolating the alpha-2 effects) using an animal model.[82] This approach has not been extensively studied in humans.

Several studies have compared epinephrine with other adrenergic agonists such as pure alpha-1 agonists (phenylephrine and methoxamine) and agents with more potent alpha-activity (norepinephrine).[83] When compared to pure alpha-1 agonists, no advantage in long-term survival could be reported. One potential reason could be the potent alpha-2 effects with epinephrine and the fact that these receptors lie extrajunctionally in the intima of the blood vessels making them more accessible to circulating catecholamines.[84] Furthermore, during ischemia, the number of postsynaptic alpha-1-receptors decreases which suggests a greater role for alpha-2 agonists during CPR.[85] Epinephrine has also been compared with norepinephrine, a potent alpha-agonist (both alpha-1 and alpha-2) with some beta-1 effects. In the only large-scale randomized, double-blind, prospective trial in out-of-hospital cardiac arrest, there were no significant differences in ROSC, hospital admission or discharge.[86] A second, smaller study demonstrated higher resuscitation rates with norepinephrine compared to epinephrine (64% vs 32%) but no significant difference in hospital discharge.[87] Since the use of epinephrine has been established for many decades in evidence-based guidelines, strong outcome-related data (eg, survival to hospital discharge) would be required for an alternative to replace it. Consequently, epinephrine remains the first-line sympathomimetic for CPR.

The recommended dose for epinephrine is 1 mg administered by IV or intraosseous (IO) injection every 3 to 5 minutes[36] (Table 12-1). The recommended dose for epinephrine was derived from animal studies (0.1 mg/kg in a 10-kg dog) and equates to approximately 0.015 mg/kg for a 70-kg human.[88] Both animal and human studies have demonstrated a positive dose-response relationship with epinephrine suggesting that higher doses might be necessary to improve hemodynamics and achieve successful resuscitation.[83] These results, however, have not been replicated in human studies. In fact, some studies have reported increased morbidity with high epinephrine doses, indicative of catecholamine toxicity, including decreased cardiac indices, left ventricular dysfunction, and decreased oxygen consumption and delivery. This discrepancy between animal and human studies could be related to most victims of cardiac arrest having coronary artery disease, which is not encountered in an animal model. Additionally, atherosclerotic plaques (in humans) can aggravate the balance between myocardial oxygen supply and demand and the interval from arrest to treatment is longer in human studies than that encountered in an animal model. High dose epinephrine is not recommended for routine use in cardiac arrest.

Vasopressin Vasopressin, also known as antidiuretic hormone, is a potent, nonadrenergic vasoconstrictor that increases blood pressure and systemic vascular resistance. Although it acts on various receptors throughout the body, its vasoconstrictive properties are due primarily to its effects on the V_1 receptor. Measurement of vasopressin levels in patients undergoing CPR has shown a high correlation between the levels of endogenous vasopressin released and the potential for ROSC.[89] In fact, in one study, plasma vasopressin concentrations were approximately three times as high in survivors compared with nonsurvivors, suggesting that vasopressin is released as an adjunct vasopressor to epinephrine in life-threatening events such as cardiac arrest.[90]

Vasopressin may have several advantages over epinephrine. First, the metabolic acidosis that frequently accompanies cardiac arrest can blunt the vasoconstrictive effect of adrenergic agents such as epinephrine. This effect does not occur with vasopressin. Second, the stimulation of beta-receptors caused by epinephrine can increase myocardial oxygen demand and complicate the postresuscitative phase of CPR. Because vasopressin does not act on beta-receptors, this effect does not occur with its use. Vasopressin also may have a beneficial effect on renal blood flow by stimulating V_2-receptors in the kidney, causing vasodilation and increased water reabsorption. With regard to splanchnic blood flow, however, vasopressin has a detrimental effect when compared to epinephrine.[89]

Despite these theoretical advantages with vasopressin, clinical trials have not consistently demonstrated superior results over that achieved with epinephrine (Table 12-2). In one large trial of out-of-hospital arrest, no significant differences were noted in ROSC, hospital admission rate or discharge rate.[91] Although, when patients were stratified according to their initial rhythm, patients with asystole had a significantly higher rate of hospital admission (29% vs 20%; $p = 0.02$) and discharge (4.7% vs 1.5%; $p = 0.04$) with vasopressin compared to epinephrine. In addition, a subgroup analysis of 732 patients who required additional epinephrine therapy despite the two doses of study drug revealed significant benefits in ROSC (37% vs 26%; $p = 0.002$), hospital admission rate (26% vs 16%; $p = 0.002$), and discharge rate (6.2% vs 1.7%; $p = 0.002$) with vasopressin. There was a trend, however, toward a poorer neurologic state or coma among the patients who survived to discharge and received vasopressin.

The favorable results observed in the subgroup analysis led to a prospective study evaluating the combination of vasopressin and epinephrine versus epinephrine alone.[92] In this study, patients were randomized to receive either 1 mg of epinephrine followed by 40 units of vasopressin (in less than 10 seconds) or 1 mg of epinephrine plus

TABLE 12-1 Evidence-Based Recommendations

Recommendations	Recommendation Grades[a]
Epinephrine	
Standard dose epinephrine (1 mg IV/IO every 3-5 minutes) may be reasonable for patients with cardiac arrest	Class IIb, LOE B-R
High dose epinephrine is not recommended for routine use in cardiac arrest	Class III: No benefit, LOE B-R
It may be reasonable to administer epinephrine as soon as feasible after the onset of cardiac arrest due to an initial nonshockable rhythm	Class IIb, LOE C-LD
Vasopressin	
Vasopressin offers no advantage as a substitute over epinephrine	Class III: No benefit, LOE B-R
Vasopressin in combination with epinephrine offers no advantage as a substitute for standard dose epinephrine	Class IIb, LOE B-R
For in-hospital cardiac arrest, the combination of intra-arrest vasopressin, epinephrine and methylprednisolone with post-arrest hydrocortisone may be considered	Class IIb, LOE C-LD
Amiodarone	
Amiodarone may be considered in patients with VF/PVT unresponsive to CPR, defibrillation, and a vasopressor.	Class IIb, LOE B-R
Lidocaine	
Lidocaine may be considered as alternative to amiodarone for VF/PVT that is unresponsive CPR, defibrillation, and a vasopressor.	Class IIb, LOE C-LD
Magnesium	
Magnesium is not routinely recommended for VF/PVT.	Class III: No benefit, LOE B-R
Thrombolysis	
Thrombolysis may be considered when cardiac arrest is suspected to be caused by pulmonary embolism.	Class IIb, LOE C-LD
Targeted Temperature Management	
Comatose adult patients with ROSC after cardiac arrest should have targeted temperature management.	Class I, LOE B-R (VF/PVT) Class I, LOE C-EO (non-VF/PVT and in-hospital arrests)
A constant temperature between 32°C and 36°C should be maintained.	Class I, LOE B-R
It is reasonable that targeted temperature management be maintained for at least 24 hours after achieving target temperature.	Class IIa, LOE C-EO
Routine prehospital cooling of patients after ROSC with rapid infusion of cold intravenous fluids is not recommended.	Class III: No benefit, LOE A
Miscellaneous	
Avoiding and immediately correcting hypotension (SBP <90 mm Hg or MAP <65 mm Hg) during postresuscitation care may be reasonable	Class IIb, LOE C-LD
The benefit of any specific target range of glucose management is uncertain	Class IIb, LOE B-R

CPR, cardiopulmonary resuscitation; IV, intravenous; IO, intraosseous, LOE, level of evidence; MAP, mean arterial pressure; PVT, pulseless ventricular tachycardia; ROSC, return of spontaneous circulation; SBP, systolic blood pressure; VF, ventricular fibrillation.

[a]Key for evidence-based classifications:

Class of recommendations:
Class I (Strong). Benefit >>> Risk
Class IIa (Moderate). Benefit >> Risk
Class IIb (Weak). Benefit ≥ Risk
Class III: No Benefit (Moderate). Benefit = Risk
Class III: Harm (Strong). Risk > Benefit

Levels of evidence (LOE):
Level A: High-quality evidence from more than 1 RCT, meta-analyses of high-quality RCTs, one or more RCT corroborated by high-quality registry studies.
Level B-R (Randomized): Moderate-quality evidence form 1 or more RCTs, meta-analyses of moderate-quality RCTs.
Level B-NR (Nonrandomized): Moderate-quality evidence from 1 or more well-designed nonrandomized studies, observational studies or registry studies, meta-analyses of such studies.
Level C-LD (Limited data): Randomized or nonrandomized observational or registry studies with limitations of design or execution, meta-analyses of such studies, physiological or mechanistic studies in human subjects.

Level C-EO (Expert opinion): Consensus of expert opinion based on clinical experience.

saline placebo. Unfortunately, there were no significant differences between the combination therapy group and epinephrine only group in any of the outcome measures studied (ROSC, survival to hospital admission, survival to hospital discharge, 1-year survival, and good neurologic recovery at discharge). In contrast, a post-hoc subgroup analysis revealed a lower rate of survival (0% vs 5.8%, $p = 0.02$) with combination therapy when the initial rhythm was PEA.

The utility of a multidrug regimen that also included corticosteroids has been evaluated in the setting of in-hospital cardiac arrest.[93,94] The rationale is based on the hemodynamic effects of steroids along with their potential to impact the intensity of the postresuscitation systemic inflammatory response and organ dysfunction. In a single-center trial, patients were randomized to receive either epinephrine alone or 20 units of vasopressin plus 1 mg of epinephrine and 40 mg of methylprednisolone (followed by hydrocortisone in the postresuscitative phase). Vasopressin 20 units plus epinephrine 1 mg were repeated during each of four subsequent CPR cycles. Significant benefits were observed in ROSC (81% vs 52%, $p = 0.003$) and

TABLE 12-2 Prospective, Randomized, Controlled Trials with Vasopressin in Cardiac Arrest

					Initial Resuscitation		Hospital Discharge	
Author	Setting	Initial rhythm	Intervention	N	Vasopressin	Epinephrine	Vasopressin	Epinephrine
Lindner et al[94a] (1997)	OOH	VF: 100%	Vasopressin 40 units vs epinephrine 1 mg for initial drug treatment	40	16/20 (80%)	11/20 (55%)	8/20 (40%)	3/20 (15%)
Stiell et al[94b] (2001)	IH	VF/PVT: 21% PEA: 48% Asystole: 31%	Vasopressin 40 units vs epinephrine 1 mg for initial drug treatment	200	62/104 (60%)	57/96 (59%)	12/104 (12%)	13/96 (14%)
Wenzel et al[91] (2004)	OOH	VF/PVT: 40% PEA: 16% Asystole: 45%	Vasopressin 40 units vs epinephrine 1 mg for two doses as initial drug treatment	1186	145/589 (25%)	167/597 (28%)	57/578 (10%)	58/588 (10%)
Callaway et al[94c] (2006)	OOH	VF: 15% PEA: 22% Asystole: 50%	Vasopressin 40 units or placebo as soon as possible after the first dose of epinephrine 1 mg	325	52/167 (31%)	48/158 (30%)	NR	NR
Gueugniaud et al[92] (2008)	OOH	VF: 9% PEA: 8% Asystole: 83%	Epinephrine 1 mg followed by vasopressin 40 units (<10 seconds apart) versus epinephrine alone for two doses	2894	413/1442 (29%)	428/1452 (30%)	24/1439 (1.7%)	33/1448 (2.3%)
Mentzelopoulos et al[93] (2009)	IH	VF/PVT: 14% PEA: 25% Asystole: 61%	Vasopressin 20 units + epinephrine 1 mg + methylprednisolone 40 mg (vasopressin + epinephrine were repeated during each of four subsequent CPR cycles vs epinephrine 1 mg) vs epinephrine 1 mg	100	39/48 (81%)[a]	27/52 (52%)	9/48 (19%)[a]	2/52 (4%)
Mukoyama et al[94d] (2009)	OOH	VF: 24% Asystole/ PEA: 76%	Vasopressin 40 units vs epinephrine 1 mg for a maximum of four doses	336	51/178 (29%)	42/158 (27%)	10/178(5.6%)	6/158 (3.8%)
Ong et al[94e] (2012)	OOH	VF/PVT: 8% PEA: 20% Asystole: 72%	Vasopressin 40 units vs epinephrine 1 mg	727	119/374 (32%)	106/353 (30%)	11/374 (2.9%)	8/353 (2.3%)
Mentzelopoulos et al[94] (2013)	IH	VF/PVT: 17% PEA: 16% Asystole: 67%	Vasopressin 20 units + epinephrine 1 mg + methylprednisolone 40 mg (vasopressin + epinephrine were repeated during each of four subsequent CPR cycles vs epinephrine 1 mg) vs epinephrine 1 mg	268	109/130 (84%)[a]	91/138 (66%)	18/130 (14%)[a]	7/138 (5.1%)

CPR, cardiopulmonary resuscitation; IH, in hospital; NR, not reported; OOH, out of hospital; PEA, pulseless electrical activity; PVT, pulseless ventricular tachycardia; VF, ventricular fibrillation.

[a] $p < 0.05$.

survival to hospital discharge (19% vs 4%, $p = 0.02$) with combination therapy including corticosteroids. These favorable results led to a multicenter trial conducted at three centers using the same drug regimen.[94] In this study, patients randomized to receive combination therapy had a higher probability for ROSC (84% vs 66%, $p = 0.005$) and a higher probability for survival to hospital discharge with good neurologic function (14% vs 5%, $p = 0.02$).

In lieu of the conflicting results with vasopressin therapy across randomized controlled trials, several meta-analyses have been performed.[95-99] The most recent study included 10 trials analyzing 6,120 patients (3 in-hospital arrest; 7 out-of-hospital arrest).[98] No significant improvements were noted with vasopressin therapy in ROSC (OR [95% CI] = 1.19 [0.93-1.52]), survival to hospital discharge (OR [95% CI] = 1.13 [0.89-1.43]) or favorable neurological outcome (OR [95% CI] = 1.02 [0.75-1.38]). Subgroup analyses revealed vasopressin may be associated with better outcomes in patients with in-hospital arrests or when used as repeated boluses of four or five times. These results may be confounded by the concomitant use of corticosteroids in some trials. A second meta-analysis included 4,745 patients from six studies (4 out-of-hospital arrest; 2 in-hospital arrest).[95] Similarly, no significant improvements were noted with vasopressin therapy in ROSC (OR [95% CI] = 1.25 [0.9-1.74]), long-term survival (OR [95% CI] = 1.13 [0.71-1.78]), or favorable neurologic outcome (OR [95% CI] = 0.87 [0.49-1.52]). When patients were stratified based on the presence of VF/PVT as their initial rhythm, the incidence of ROSC and long-term survival were similar with vasopressin but in patients with asystole, vasopressin was associated with superior long-term survival rates relative to control (OR [95% CI] = 1.8 [1.04-3.12]).

4 In summary, vasopressin appears to offer no benefit as a substitute over epinephrine. Additionally, vasopressin co-administered

with epinephrine offers no benefit compared to standard dose epinephrine alone. Vasopressin therefore has been removed from the 2015 cardiac arrest algorithm.[36] The combination of methylprednisolone, vasopressin and epinephrine can be considered as an alternative to epinephrine alone during CPR for in-hospital cardiac arrest. Future prospective trials are need to validate the role of vasopressin in certain sub-populations (eg, asystole).

Clinical **Controversy...**

The role of vasopressin continues to be debated due to lack of improvement in survival with good neurologic outcome. There are some sub-populations though where vasopressin may be beneficial. Future trials are needed in this area.

Antiarrhythmics The purpose of antiarrhythmic drug therapy following unsuccessful defibrillation and vasopressor administration is to prevent the development or recurrence of VF and PVT by raising the fibrillation threshold. Clinical evidence demonstrating improved survival to hospital discharge however is lacking.[100,101]

5 Amiodarone is the recommended antiarrhythmic in patients with VF or PVT, unresponsive to CPR, defibrillation, and vasopressor therapy. Amiodarone is classified as a class III antiarrhythmic but possesses electrophysiologic characteristics of all four Vaughn Williams classifications. A large, randomized, double-blind trial in patients with out-of-hospital cardiac arrest secondary to VF or PVT (referred to as the ARREST trial) randomized individuals to receive either amiodarone 300 mg or placebo.[102] Recipients of amiodarone were more likely to be resuscitated and survive to hospital admission (44% vs 34%, $p = 0.03$) but there was no difference in survival to hospital discharge (13.4% vs 13.2%, p = NS). This was the first trial to demonstrate the benefit of an antiarrhythmic agent over placebo in patients with out-of-hospital cardiac arrest. A subsequent trial (known as the ALIVE trial) compared amiodarone 5 mg/kg with lidocaine 1.5 mg/kg in patients with out-of-hospital cardiac arrest due to VF.[103] In this trial, amiodarone was associated with a relative improvement of 90% in survival to hospital admission compared with lidocaine (22.8% vs 12%; OR 2.17 [95% CI 1.21-3.83]; $p = 0.009$). Similar to the ARREST trial, there was no difference in survival to hospital discharge (amiodarone, 5% vs lidocaine, 3%; $p = 0.34$). A large, multicenter trial is currently underway comparing amiodarone, lidocaine or placebo in patients with out-of-hospital cardiac arrest.[104] The results of this trial will be pivotal in defining the role of antiarrhythmic drug use in cardiac arrest.

Adverse effects of amiodarone encountered in cardiac arrest include hypotension and bradycardia.[105] The effects however are largely due to the intravenous vehicle, polysorbate 80 and benzyl alcohol. A formulation of amiodarone exists that does not contain these solvents and adverse hemodynamic effects appear to be minimized. Nevertheless, administration of a vasoconstrictor prior to amiodarone can potentially prevent hypotension.

Lidocaine is currently recommended as an alternative to amiodarone, if amiodarone is not available.[36] Minimal evidence exists supporting lidocaine use for VF/PVT. In the only published case-control trial where patients were classified according to whether they received lidocaine, no significant difference was noted in ROSC, admission to the hospital, or survival to hospital discharge between groups.[106] Similarly, a prospective study comparing the effectiveness of lidocaine with that of standard-dose epinephrine showed not only a lack of benefit with lidocaine but also a higher tendency to promote asystole.[107] In contrast, a retrospective analysis in patients with VF indicated that lidocaine was associated with a higher rate of ROSC and hospitalization ($p < 0.01$) but not an increase in the hospital discharge rate.[108]

Magnesium Severe hypomagnesemia has been associated with VF/PVT but routine administration of magnesium during a cardiac arrest has not demonstrated any benefit in clinical outcome. Two observation trials though have noted an improvement in ROSC in patients with arrests associated with torsades de pointes.[36] Therefore, magnesium administration should only be administered to those patients.

Thrombolytics Since most cardiac arrests are related to either myocardial infarction or pulmonary embolism, several investigators have evaluated the role of thrombolytics during CPR. Earlier smaller studies have demonstrated some benefit with their use but in the two largest randomized controlled trials, no difference was noted.[105] In the first, 233 patients with PEA were randomized to receive either tissue plasminogen activator (tPA) or placebo.[109] The proportion of patients with ROSC was 21.4% and 23.3% for tPA and placebo treated patients, respectively. There was no significant difference in hemorrhage rates. The second study randomized patients with out-of-hospital cardiac arrest to receive either tenecteplase or placebo.[110] After a blinded review by the data and safety monitoring board, criteria for futility were met and enrollment was terminated. A total of 1,050 patients were analyzed and both ROSC (tenecteplase, 55% vs placebo, 55%; $p = 0.96$) and survival to hospital discharge (tenecteplase, 15.1% vs placebo, 17.5%, $p = 0.33$) were similar between groups. Furthermore, the incidence of intracranial hemorrhage was significantly greater with tenecteplase versus placebo (2.7% vs 0.4%, $p = 0.006$). Potential reasons for failure in this study include the omission of antiplatelet and antithrombin medication administration during CPR and decreased delivery of the thrombolytic to the coronary arteries (where the clots exist) due to impaired flow and perfusion. Given these results, fibrinolytic therapy should not be used routinely in cardiac arrest but when pulmonary embolism is suspected, their use is suggested.[111]

Pulseless Electrical Activity and Asystole

Nonpharmacologic Therapy

PEA is defined as the absence of a detectable pulse and the presence of some type of electrical activity other than VF or PVT. Several studies have documented that patients with PEA actually have mechanical cardiac contractions, but they are too weak to produce a palpable pulse or blood pressure. Although PEA is still classified as a "rhythm of survival," the success rate of treatment is much lower than the rates seen with VF/PVT.[112] PEA is often caused by treatable conditions, and the resuscitation team needs to identify and correct these conditions emergently if the resuscitation is to be successful (Table 12-3). Asystole is defined as the presence of a flat line of the electrocardiogram (ECG) monitor and often represents confirmation of death rather than a rhythm to be treated. Therefore, withdrawal of efforts must be strongly considered if there is not a rapid ROSC.[105] 6 Like PEA, successful treatment of asystole depends almost entirely on diagnosis of the underlying cause.

The algorithm for treatment of PEA is the same as the treatment of asystole. Both conditions require CPR, airway control, and IV access. Asystole should be reconfirmed by checking a second lead on the cardiac monitor. Defibrillation should be avoided in patients with asystole because the parasympathetic discharge that occurs with defibrillation may reduce the chance of ROSC and worsen the chance of survival. The emphasis in resuscitation is good quality CPR without interruption, and to try to identify a correctable cause. If available, transcutaneous pacing can be attempted.

Much like VF/PVT, there is an interest in hypothermia in these post-arrest patients. Metabolic parameters (eg, lactate and O_2 extraction) have been shown to be improved when post-arrest comatose adults survived their arrest and were treated with hypothermia.[113]

TABLE 12-3 Underlying Causes of Pulseless Electrical Activity and Asystole

Condition	Clues	Treatment
Hypovolemia	History, flat neck veins	Intravenous fluids
Hypoxia	Cyanosis, blood gases, airway problems	Ventilation, oxygen
Hydrogen ion (acidosis)	History of bicarbonate-responsive preexisting acidosis	Sodium bicarbonate, hyperventilation
Hyper (Hypo) kalemia	History of renal failure, diabetes, recent dialysis, dialysis fistulas, medications	Calcium chloride, insulin, glucose, sodium bicarbonate, sodium polystyrene sulfonate, dialysis
Hypothermia	History of exposure to cold, central body temperature	Rewarming, oxygen, intravenous fluids
Hypoglycemia	History of diabetes	Glucose infusion
Toxin (drug overdose)	Bradycardia, history of ingestion, empty bottles at the scene, pupils, neurologic examination	Drug screens, intubation, lavage, activated charcoal
Tamponade (cardiac)	History (trauma, renal failure, thoracic malignancy), no pulse with CPR, vein distention, impending tamponade-tachycardia, hypotension, low pulse pressure changing to sudden bradycardia as terminal event	Pericardiocentesis
Tension pneumothorax	History (asthma, ventilator, chronic obstructive pulmonary disease, trauma), no pulse with CPR, neck vein distention, tracheal deviation	Needle decompression
Thrombosis, coronary	History, ECG, enzymes	PCI, thrombolytics, oxygen, nitroglycerin, heparin, aspirin, morphine
Thrombosis, pulmonary	History, no pulse with CPR, distended neck veins	Pulmonary arteriogram, surgical embolectomy, thrombolytics
Trauma	History, examination	Volume infusion, intracranial pressure monitoring, bleeding control, surgical intervention

CPR, cardiopulmonary resuscitation; ECG, electrocardiogram.

Data from reference 36.

A meta-analysis though has failed to demonstrate any benefit in survival or neurologic outcome.[114] Further studies are warranted in this area.

Pharmacologic Therapy

The primary pharmacologic agent used in the treatment of asystole or PEA is epinephrine; vasopressin is no longer recommended. While data evaluating these therapies solely in patients with asystole or PEA are limited, these rhythms represent a majority of patients included in the published research. For example, in the largest observational trial evaluating the role of epinephrine in out-of-hospital arrest, 93% had either PEA or systole as the first documented rhythm.[71] In this study, epinephrine was associated with a significant improvement in ROSC but one-month survival and survival with good neurologic function were lower with epinephrine. A second study revealed similar findings but worse neurological outcomes were noted when epinephrine administration time exceeded 10 minutes.[76] In one study of more than 25,000 patients with in-hospital arrest and either asystole or PEA, a step-wise decrease in survival was observed with each incremental delay in epinephrine administration.[74] As with VF/PVT, time to epinephrine administration appears to be an important confounding factor.

Inconsistent results have also been reported with vasopressin. In a post-hoc subgroup analysis of patients with out-of-hospital arrest and asystole as the first identified rhythm, survival to hospital admission (29% vs 20%, $p = 0.02$) and discharge (4.7% vs 1.5%, $p = 0.04$) were significantly higher with vasopressin compared to epinephrine.[91] There was, however, a non-statistically significant increase in coma/vegetative state with vasopressin (40% vs 0%, $p = 0.14$). Similar findings were cited in a meta-analysis of randomized controlled trials comparing vasopressin with control.[95] Patients with asystole who had study drug administered within 20 minutes had higher rates of ROSC (OR [95% CI] = 1.7 [1.17-2.47]) and long-term survival (OR [95% CI] = 2.84 [1.19-6.79]). These results were largely influenced by the aforementioned trial which accounted for a majority of the weight in those statistics. In contrast to these findings, one randomized controlled trial, which evaluated combination therapy with vasopressin and epinephrine, did not report an advantage with vasopressin in patients with asystole.[92] In fact, a post-hoc subgroup analysis of patients with PEA as the initial rhythm, revealed a lower rate of survival (0% vs 5.8%, $p = 0.02$) with combination therapy compared to epinephrine alone.

Another agent that is no longer recommended in the setting of PEA or asystole is atropine.[36] Atropine is an antimuscarinic agent that blocks the depressant effect of acetylcholine on both heart rate and atrioventricular nodal conduction, thus decreasing parasympathetic tone. During asystole, parasympathetic tone may increase because of the vagal stimulation that occurs secondary to intubation, the effects of hypoxia and acidosis, or alterations in the balance of parasympathetic and sympathetic control.[115] Nevertheless, there are no prospective controlled trials showing benefit from atropine for the treatment of asystole or PEA and conflicting evidence exists across retrospective and observational reports. Therefore, atropine should not be routinely administered in this setting.

Acid-Base Management

Acidosis seen during cardiac arrest is the result of decreased blood flow (leading to anaerobic metabolism) or inadequate ventilation. Chest compressions generate only approximately 25% of normal cardiac output, leading to inadequate organ perfusion, tissue hypoxia, and metabolic acidosis. In addition, the lack of ventilation causes retention of carbon dioxide, leading to respiratory acidosis. This combined acidosis produces not only reduced myocardial contractility, but also the appearance of arrhythmias because of a lower fibrillation threshold. In early cardiac arrest, adequate alveolar ventilation has been considered the mainstay of control to limit the accumulation of carbon dioxide and control the acid-base imbalance.[105] With the evolution to CCR, however, there are experts arguing against ventilation because of the negative effects it can have on the effectiveness of CPR. This has led to evidence showing no negative effects if compression-only CPR is used for out-of-hospital cardiac arrest (exceptions being pediatric arrest, drowning, trauma, airway obstruction, non-cardiac etiology, or due to acute respiratory disease).[116] With arrests of long duration, buffer therapy is often considered, however few data support its use during cardiac arrest. In one randomized controlled trial, the early administration of bicarbonate (1 mEq/kg) had no effect on survival in pre-hospital cardiac arrest with only a trend toward improvement in prolonged arrest (more than 15 minutes).[117]

Although sodium bicarbonate was once given routinely to reduce the detrimental effects associated with acidosis (eg, reduced myocardial contractility), enhance the effect of epinephrine, and improve the rate of defibrillation, there are few clinical data supporting its use.[118] In fact, sodium bicarbonate may have some detrimental effects.[118,119] The effect of sodium bicarbonate can be described by the following reaction:

$$[HCO_3^-] + [H^+] \leftrightarrow [H_2O] + [CO_2]$$

When sodium bicarbonate is added to an acidic environment, this reaction will shift to the right, thereby increasing tissue and venous hypercarbia. The carbon dioxide generated by this reaction will diffuse into the cell and decrease intracellular pH. The accumulation of intracellular carbon dioxide, specifically within the myocardium, is inversely correlated with coronary perfusion pressure produced by CPR. Intracellular acidosis also will decrease myocardial contractility, further complicating the low-flow state associated with CPR.[118] Furthermore, treatment with sodium bicarbonate often overcorrects extracellular pH because sodium bicarbonate has a greater effect when the pH is closer to normal.[119] The induced alkalosis, causes an increase in the affinity of oxygen to hemoglobin ("left shift"), thus interfering with oxygen release into the tissues.

Sodium bicarbonate can be used in special circumstances (ie, underlying metabolic acidosis, hyperkalemia, salicylate overdose, or tricyclic antidepressant overdose), however, the dosage should be guided by laboratory analysis if possible. Tromethamine (THAM) is an alternative buffering agent which acts as a proton acceptor but there is a dearth of clinical experience with this agent in cardiac arrest and outcome studies are not currently available. [105]

Postresuscitative Care

Following the ROSC from a cardiac arrest, a complex phase of resuscitation begins which has been termed post-cardiac arrest syndrome.[120] There are four main components of post-cardiac arrest syndrome highlighting succinct pathophysiologic processes and potential areas for treatment. These are: post-cardiac arrest brain injury, myocardial dysfunction, systemic ischemia/reperfusion response, and persistent precipitating pathology. In general, many of the concepts within these four components surround the principles of basic ICU care (eg, early hemodynamic optimization, circulatory support, sedation, etc). Post-arrest care has the significant potential to reduce early mortality from altered hemodynamics and later morbidity and mortality from multiple organ dysfunction and central nervous system injury.[37,120,121]

After ROSC, it is imperative to ensure adequate airway and oxygenation. Securing the airway to prevent inadvertent loss is an important step. If there is any question of cervical spine injury, the patient should have a cervical collar placed, with subsequent appropriate evaluation. The head of the bed should be raised to 30 degrees (if this can be tolerated hemodynamically) to reduce the risk for aspiration, ventilator-associated pneumonia, and cerebral edema. Usually 100% oxygen is used during the initial resuscitation effort. If ROSC is obtained and the patient is placed on a mechanical ventilator, the health care team should titrate the oxygen fraction down as tolerated to avoid oxygen toxicity. Overventilation is common in the postresuscitation timeframe; the advent of widespread $ETCO_2$ usage can avoid this pitfall (ie, targeting an $ETCO_2$ of 40-45 mm Hg).

Because the most common cause of cardiac arrest is ischemia, a rapid search for electrocardiographic changes consistent with acute myocardial infarction should be undertaken as soon as possible in the post-arrest timeframe.[122] If there is an acute myocardial infarction present, urgent revascularization should be enacted immediately.

Therapeutic hypothermia or targeted temperature management is an integral component of postresuscitative care. Restoration of blood flow following cardiac arrest can lead to several chemical cascades and destructive enzymatic reactions that can result in cerebral injury. These reactions include free-radical production, excitatory amino acid release and calcium shifts, which ultimately lead to mitochondrial damage and apoptosis (programmed cell death).[123] Hypothermia can protect from cerebral injury by suppressing these chemical reactions, thereby reducing the production of free radicals. Additionally, therapeutic hypothermia can decrease cerebral metabolism and oxygen consumption as for each 1°C drop in temperature, cerebral metabolism can decrease by 6% to 10%.[124]

Early human success with hypothermia was described in two pivotal trials published in 2002.[125,126] The first was conducted in nine centers in five European countries.[125] In this trial, patients who had been resuscitated after cardiac arrest due to VF but remained comatose were assigned randomly to undergo therapeutic hypothermia, targeting a temperature of 32°C to 34°C, for 24 hours. The primary endpoint was favorable neurologic outcome which was achieved in 55% of patients in the hypothermia group as opposed to 39% in the normothermia group (p = 0.009). Additionally, mortality rates were improved significantly in the hypothermia group (41% vs 55%; p = 0.02). Based on this difference, seven patients would need to be treated with hypothermia to prevent one death. The second trial was conducted in four hospitals in Melbourne, Australia.[126] Entry criteria were similar to the previous trial, but the target temperature for hypothermia was 33°C, which was maintained for 12 hours. Forty-nine percent of patients in the hypothermia group had good neurologic function on discharge (to either home or a rehabilitation facility) compared with 26% of patients in the normothermia group (p = 0.046). Mortality rates were similar between the two groups (51% for the hypothermia group and 68% for the normothermia group; p = 0.145). Following these trials and widespread implementation across healthcare centers, there have been numerous observational studies describing the beneficial role of therapeutic hypothermia.[127] As a result, the utility of therapeutic hypothermia had markedly increased.[128]

Recently there have been 3 large-scale randomized controlled trials that have challenged the role of therapeutic hypothermia post-cardiac arrest.[129-131]

Clinical **Controversy...**

The role of therapeutic hypothermia has been challenged with the publication of recent studies. Some believe a temperature of 32°C to 34°C should be the target while others believe 36°C is the target with an emphasis on preventing hyperthermia.

The first was an international trial with 939 patients comparing targeted temperature management at 33°C versus 36°C.[131] The hypothermia intervention period was 36 hours. There was no significant differences noted in in all-cause, end of trial mortality (33°C, 50% vs 36°C, 48%, p = 0.51) or poor neurologic function (33°C, 54% vs 52°C, 48%, p = 0.78). The second trial assessed whether or not prehospital cooling improved survival in 1,364 patients.[129] Target temperature was less than 34°C which was reached approximately 1 hour sooner in the intervention group compared to controls. Prehospital cooling was not associated with increased survival to hospital discharge (63% vs 64%, p = 0.69) or improvement in neurological status (58% vs 62%, p = 0.69) in patients with VF. Similarly, prehospital cooling did not affect outcomes in patients without VF. Finally, the third study compared therapeutic hypothermia with therapeutic normothermia following out-of-hospital cardiac arrest in children.[130] In this study, the target temperature was 33°C (which was maintained for 48 hours) in the hypothermia groups and 36.8°C in the normothermia group. The primary outcome measure was survival with a good neurobehavioral outcome at 12 months using the Vineland Adaptive Behavior Scale, 2nd edition. No difference was noted between groups (20% vs 12%, $p = 0.14$).

Collectively, these studies raise the question of whether or not the benefits of hypothermia are related to hypothermia itself or avoidance of hyperthermia. In one of the earlier trials, that was pivotal to the widespread utilization of this intervention, there was no active temperature management in the control group. Mild fever, therefore occurred in some patients (average temperature was 37.8°C).[125] This is important because previous research has shown for each degree higher than 37°C, the risk of unfavorable neurologic recovery increases (OR ([95% CI] = 2.26 [1.24-4.12]).[132] Nevertheless, despite recent data showing no improvement in outcomes with hypothermia, the concept of targeted temperature management should not be abandoned. The most current guidelines recommend targeted temperature management (as opposed to no management) for all comatose adults patients after ROSC.[37] The target temperature should be between 32°C and 36°C and maintained for at least 24 hours. It is also reasonable to actively prevent fever following targeted temperature management. Further research is needed to discern the most appropriate temperature level, timing or subpopulations that may benefit from lower temperature targets.

Several methods exist to induce hypothermia which can be classified as surface cooling or invasive. Surface cooling devices are noninvasive and include simple ice packs, cooling blankets/gel pads, ice water immersion, and nasopharyngeal evaporative cooling devices.[133] Invasive cooling methods include ice cold intravenous fluids, endovascular cooling catheters, body cavity lavage, extracorporeal circuits, and selective brain cooling. While there is no consensus on the optimal method to induce hypothermia, target temperatures should be reached as quickly as possible (eg, the induction phase).[124] During the maintenance phase, core temperature should be tightly controlled with little or no fluctuations. The rewarming phase should consist of slow and controlled warming at a rate of 0.2°C to 0.5°C per hour.

Hypothermia must be used with caution, however, as there are several complications that can develop. Shivering occurs during the induction phase and can increase metabolic rate and myocardial oxygen demand. Several strategies exist to blunt the thermoregulatory response to hypothermia and these measures should be implemented accordingly.[134,135] Coagulopathy, dysrhythmias, cardiovascular changes, hyperglycemia, electrolyte disorders, and infectious risks have also been described.[134] In addition, hypothermia can have profound effects on drug distribution and clearance.[134] Although the duration of hypothermia is typically short, careful monitoring during this time period is necessary, particularly with vasoactive agents, sedatives, and opiates. Further research is required in this area.

Special Populations

Asthma

Asthma is a very common disorder, and despite modern therapies, there are still in excess of 2 million emergency room visits and 5,000 to 6,000 asthma-related deaths annually in the United States.[136] True cardiac arrest in asthma is infrequent, as the primary pathophysiology is respiratory compromise and the inability to ventilate.[137] Asthma exacerbations are a combination of bronchoconstriction, airway inflammation, and mucous plugging. This leads to severe air trapping, hyperinflation, and hemodynamic compromise. While wheezing is common in an asthma exacerbation, it does not correlate with the degree of airway obstruction. In contrast, as the airflow decreases with worsening disease, wheezing can disappear. In addition, several other disease states cause wheezing, including pulmonary edema, pneumonia, anaphylaxis, foreign bodies, and tumors.[136]

Patients with life-threatening asthma need to be treated aggressively with bronchodilators and corticosteroids. Adjunctive therapies include anticholinergics, magnesium sulfate, ketamine, helium/oxygen mixtures, or even inhaled anesthetics.[138-142] Noninvasive ventilation can be attempted if the patient is deteriorating and still awake for short-term support, and may prevent the need for mechanical ventilation.[143] The decision to intubate an asthmatic is a clinical judgment; the clinician needs to remain keenly aware that the endotracheal tube will not solve the airway problem, and that ongoing aggressive asthma management needs to continue after intubation. Mechanical ventilation in the asthmatic can be very difficult, and the intubation and positive pressure can trigger further bronchoconstriction or hemodynamic compromise.

The provision of BLS in asthma is unchanged. Similarly, standard advanced cardiac life support measures should be followed.[136] However, since the effect of auto-positive end expiratory pressure (PEEP), known as breath stacking, in an asthmatic with cardiac arrest is likely to be severe, a strategy of low respiratory rate and volume ventilation may be appropriate.[136] Similarly, for cardiac arrest in asthma, especially when ventilation is difficult, tension pneumothorax should be strongly considered.[136]

Anaphylaxis

Anaphylaxis is a severe allergic reaction involving most organs, and can lead to airway obstruction and cardiovascular collapse.[136] It still accounts for between 500 and 1,000 deaths annually in the United States.[144] The initial signs can be nonspecific, but with a severe reaction a "sense of impending doom" is common.[136] Rhinitis often leads to laryngeal edema with stridor in the upper airway, and bronchoconstriction often mimics an acute asthma attack as described earlier.

Cardiovascular collapse is common in severe reactions due to vasodilation and increased capillary permeability. This can rapidly lead to myocardial hypoperfusion and ischemia and to full cardiac arrest. There are no randomized trials of algorithms for arrest due to anaphylaxis.[136] Because of this lack of evidence, standard basic and advanced life support should be provided.

Early advanced airway management is recommended due to the potential for rapid edema development. Epinephrine has been the main-stay of treatment for years, and continues to be listed first.[136] The recommended dose is 0.2 to 0.5 mg and should be administered via intramuscular injection to all patients with signs of systemic allergy.[136] This can be repeated every 5 to 15 minutes in the absence of clinical improvement. Vasopressin has been used successfully in patients who did not respond to standard therapy.[145] Fluid resuscitation is usually required for restoration of circulation and has been evaluated in one study where hypotension did not respond immediately to vasoactive drugs.[146] There are no prospective trials evaluating other agents in anaphylactic shock or arrest. Antihistamines, inhaled beta-agonists, and intravenous corticosteroids have been used successfully in anaphylaxis and may be considered in cardiac arrest due to anaphylaxis.[136]

Pregnancy

Pregnancy is a unique situation in that survival of both the fetus and the mother depend on CPR. Despite the fact that pregnant patients are younger than the traditional cardiac arrest patient, the incidence of cardiac arrest in pregnancy seems to be on the rise, approximately 1 in 12,000 admissions for delivery in the United States.[111] In addition, the mortality rate of cardiac arrest with pregnancy seems to be higher, with one series reporting a survival rate of just 6.9%.[136,147]

The best hope for survival of the fetus is maternal survival. Because of the gravid uterus, resuscitation needs to be modified. Since the vena cava and aorta can be obstructed by a uterus of approximately 20 weeks gestation or later, manual lateral uterine displacement is suggested (ie, pulling the uterus to the side).[111] An alternative approach is to tilt the patient laterally (approximately 30 degrees), however, CPR quality is decreased. Thus, the current guidelines suggest that manual lateral uterine displacement in the supine position be attempted to optimize CPR quality.[111]

Airway control is important in the pregnant patient. The airway may be smaller because of the hormonal changes and edema which accompany pregnancy.[148] Similarly, because of increased intra-abdominal pressure exerted by the uterus, as well as hormonal changes that change the resting state of the gastroesophageal sphincter, clinicians need to be acutely aware of the increased risk of aspiration. Because of this, cricoid pressure needs to be maintained continuously during airway manipulation. The rescuer may need to give smaller tidal volumes than normal because of the diaphragm elevation that accompanies the later stages of pregnancy. Because of the increased ventilatory needs in pregnancy as well as the anatomic changes, some authors have suggested that it is important to perform early intubation during cardiac arrest in pregnancy and cite this rapid intubation as a difference from non-pregnant patients.[148] Similarly, circulatory support also has to be adjusted. In particular, chest compressions need to be administered slightly above the center of the sternum to adjust for the anatomic changes of the pregnant uterus.[136]

In an arrest situation during pregnancy the ACLS provider needs to follow the standard guidelines, including the same use of defibrillation and medications. While it is true that vasoactive agents, such as epinephrine, can diminish uterine blood flow, safer alternatives do not exist.[136] Available literature, though scant, suggests that the energy requirements for defibrillation do not change in pregnancy.[149]

While etiologies of arrest in pregnancy are often the same as in the non-pregnant patient, there are several unique situations that need to be considered in the differential diagnosis of a pregnancy arrest. These include excess magnesium sulfate administration (ie, iatrogenic from treating eclampsia) in which case the therapeutic administration of calcium gluconate can be lifesaving; amniotic embolism, which is associated with complete cardiovascular collapse during labor and delivery (cardiopulmonary bypass has been reportedly successful in salvaging this condition); pre-eclampsia/eclampsia developing after the 20th week of gestation producing hypertension and multiple organ dysfunction; as well as vascular events including acute coronary syndromes and acute pulmonary embolism.[148,150,151]

It is paramount to remember that unless circulation is restored to the mother, both the mother and the fetus will succumb, especially if standard therapy is not used correctly and promptly. Because of this, the resuscitation leader should consider the need for emergent cesarean delivery as soon as the arrest happens or if there is no immediate response after lateral uterine displacement and CPR.[111]

Hypothermia

Unintentional hypothermia (as opposed to the therapeutic hypothermia used post-arrest, described above) is defined by a body temperature less than 30°C (86°F), and is associated with marked derangements in body function. Because it can depress virtually every body system, including pulse and respiration, the patient may appear to be dead upon the initial evaluation. Hypothermia may lead to benefit on brain recovery after cardiac arrest (discussed earlier), thus aggressive intervention is clearly indicated when there is a hypothermic arrest victim.

If the patient still has a perfusing rhythm, therapy is mainly based upon rewarming techniques. For mild hypothermia (ie, more than 34°C [more than 93.2°F]), passive rewarming is recommended. For moderate hypothermia (ie, 30°C-34°C [86°F-93.2°F]), active external rewarming is recommended, and for severe hypothermia (ie, less than 30°C [less than 86°F]) active internal rewarming is recommended. These patients need to be manipulated very gently as VF is sometimes precipitated by movement.[152]

If the patient is in cardiac arrest, then the standard BLS algorithm should be followed. However, there are some modifications that the rescuer needs to consider. The rescuer should evaluate for pulse for a longer timeframe, since the heart rate may be slow or very difficult to palpate. If there is no pulse, then chest compressions and rescue breaths should ensue. If the patient is in VF or PVT then electrical therapy should be given in a standard manner. However, the hypothermic heart may be less responsive to medications or defibrillation, and thus there have been worries about the optimal temperature at which to start defibrillation attempts.[136] There are no published consensus guidelines regarding this, but animal data supports medications during CPR in cardiac arrest associated with hypothermia.[153] Immediately after defibrillation, CPR should resume as in the standard manner. During CPR, continued attempts at rewarming are of paramount importance. Included in this concept is preventing further heat loss (ie, removal of wet clothing, protection from the environment, etc). Patients often require significant volume challenges during the rewarming process. The use of steroids, antibiotics, and barbiturates has been proposed, but none of these agents have ever been shown to increase survival rates.[136]

It is debatable when to stop resuscitative efforts in the hypothermic patient. Many authors have proposed that a patient should not be pronounced dead until the core temperature has been restored to near normal.[136] Once the patient is in the hospital, it is still the judgment of the treating physician when efforts should be terminated.

Trauma

Cardiac resuscitation of the trauma arrest patient is basically performed with the same guidelines as any other arrest. There are some specific etiologies to rapidly consider however, since the survival of an out-of-hospital cardiac arrest due to trauma is rare.[136] The rescuer needs to consider airway obstruction, pneumothorax, tracheobronchial injury, cardiac or large arterial injury, cardiac tamponade, severe head injury with secondary cardiac collapse, and other injuries specific to the particular trauma.[136] The best survival seems to be in young patients with treatable penetrating injuries.

Trauma patients often suffer head or cervical injuries; thus cervical spine precautions should be used in these patients. A jaw thrust maneuver is the preferred way to open the airway, with in-line stabilization during attempts at advanced airway placement.[136] The rescuer must be vigilant for the development of tension pneumothorax during ventilation. Inadequate ventilation of one side is usually due to tube malposition, tension pneumothorax, or hemothorax. These conditions are usually treated by medical personnel at the hospital after transport.

Chest compressions should be performed in a standard manner. Any visible hemorrhage should be controlled with direct pressure. Fluid resuscitation is done with a goal of adequate blood pressure and organ perfusion. The specific details of fluid resuscitation are highly controversial however, and the optimal volume infusion for trauma resuscitation is a subject of ongoing debate.

Open thoracotomy for trauma-induced arrest has been performed in many instances. For penetrating chest trauma patients who arrest immediately before arrival or in the emergency department, open thoracotomy can allow relief of tamponade, control of major vessel hemorrhage, or direct repair of cardiac insult.[136] Furthermore, some have suggested that a physician-led, out-of-hospital thoracotomy for penetrating trauma may have a higher chance of survival.[154] In the case of blunt trauma, however, open thoracotomy has not been shown to definitively improve outcome.

A unique phenomenon of cardiac arrest (usually VF) caused by a blow of the anterior chest or sternum during the repolarization part of the cardiac cycle is called "Commotio Cordis."[155] These events are commonly seen in young athletes, and can be caused by a myriad of mechanisms, from falling directly on the sternum, to the strike of a baseball or hockey puck. Prompt recognition is of paramount importance, as rapid defibrillation is often lifesaving. Provision of basic life support, the use of an automatic external defibrillator, and standard advanced cardiac life support is appropriate for this type of arrest.

For definitive post-arrest care, trauma patients should be rapidly transferred to a facility with expertise in the provision of trauma care, and practitioners should consult guidelines for terminating efforts of cardiac arrest published by the National Association of EMS Physicians and the American College of Surgeons Committee on Trauma.[136,156]

Drowning

Drowning is a process resulting in primary respiratory impairment from immersion in a liquid. It is a common, preventable cause of morbidity and mortality. The most important inciting event is the hypoxia induced by submersion. The most powerful predictor of outcome therefore is duration of submersion. In fact, in one study the adjusted RR (95% CI) for a good outcome was only 0.02 (0.01-0.04) when the submersion duration exceeded 10 minutes.[157] With submersion durations that exceed 25 minutes, resuscitation efforts may be futile.

The presumed etiology of the arrest in a drowning patient is hypoxia thus the traditional A-B-C approach should be used instead of C-A-B. Early care consists of immediate rescue breathing, even before they are removed from the water. Once the victim is removed from the water, immediate chest compressions should be started if they are pulseless. Drowning victims can present with any of the pulseless rhythms; standard guidelines need to be followed for therapy of these rhythms. A Drowning Chain of Survival has been proposed to improve chances of survival and recovery from drowning.[158] The five links in the chain are: prevent drowning, recognize distress, provide flotation, remove from water, and provide care as needed.

Electrocution/Lightning

There are many etiologies of electrical shock injuries, from lightning strike (mortality estimated to be 30%, with 70% of survivors sustaining significant morbidity) to high-tension current, to household current.[136] The severity of injury depends on the site, type of current, duration of contact, pathway, and the magnitude of delivered electricity.

Cardiac arrest is common in electrical injury due to current passing through the heart during the "vulnerable period" of the cardiac cycle. In large-current events, such as lightning strike, the heart undergoes massive depolarization simultaneously.[159] Sometimes the intrinsic pacemaker can restore an organized cardiac electrical cycle, but because of injury to other muscles, specifically the thoracic musculature, the patient cannot retain or sustain viable circulation due to the lack of ventilation and oxygenation.[160]

When approaching a victim of electrocution, the rescuer must first be certain of his or her own safety. Thereafter, standard BLS, prompt CPR, and ACLS when available is indicated. Electric shock is often associated with multiple trauma, including spinal injury, multiple injuries to the skeletal muscles, as well as fractures. These factors need to be evaluated by the resuscitation team.

Airway control may be difficult due to the edema that often accompanies such injuries; thus an advanced airway early in the treatment process is recommended.[136] With soft tissue swelling, there is often a need for aggressive fluid resuscitation in these patients. The underlying tissue, or visceral organ damage, is often worse than the external appearance. It is usually recommended that these patients be transferred to centers with expertise in dealing with these types of injuries.

Drug Administration

The routes of administration available for drug delivery during CPR include IV (both central and peripheral access), IO, and endotracheal. The chosen route represents a compromise between the availability of access and their apparent efficacy in introducing the drug into the central circulation. When selecting a route for drug administration, it is of utmost importance to minimize any interruptions in chest compressions during CPR.

Central venous access will result in a faster and higher peak drug concentration than peripheral access but central line access is not needed in most resuscitation attempts. If a central line is already present, however, it should be the access site of choice. An appropriately trained provider may consider placing a central line if one is not present but CPR should not be interrupted. Central lines located above the diaphragm are preferable to those located below the diaphragm because of poor blood flow during CPR.[161] If IV access (either central or peripheral) has not been established a large peripheral venous catheter should be inserted. It has been suggested that only one attempt at peripheral IV insertion be allowed.[162] If this is not successful, an IO device should be inserted. Peripheral drug administration yields a peak concentration in the major systemic arteries in roughly 1.5 to 3 minutes but circulation time can be shortened by up to 40% if the drug is followed by a 20-mL fluid bolus with elevation of the extremity.[161]

7 IO administration is the preferred alternative route for administration if IV access cannot be achieved.[105] Several studies have documented the effectiveness and safety of this administration route in both adults and children.[163] Pharmacokinetic data have demonstrated similar areas under the curve and times to peak concentration for sternal IO and central IV administration.[164] There appears to be variability, though, based on the anatomic site for insertion as IO administration via the tibia delivered only 65% of the dose compared to the sternum. Potential anatomic sites for insertion for an IO needle are the distal tibia, the proximal tibia, the distal femur, the sternum, and the humerus.[163,164] There are several IO access devices that are commercially available allowing for rapid insertion and are easy to use. In fact, clinical trials have documented success rates of approximately 80% with placement times of roughly 1 to 2 minutes.[163] The high success rates for achieving vascular access (upon first attempt) allow for more rapid drug administration (versus IV therapy) and could offset the pharmacokinetic differences observed with this approach. Future pharmacokinetic studies are needed to identify the most optimal anatomic site for IO placement and if current dosing recommendations are appropriate.

In the event that neither IV nor IO access can be established, a few drugs can be administered through an endotracheal tube. These drugs are atropine, lidocaine, epinephrine, naloxone, and vasopressin.[105] There are no data with amiodarone. Medications administered through the endotracheal route, however, will have both a lower and delayed peak concentration than when they are administered by the IV or IO routes. In fact, animal studies have suggested that the lower epinephrine concentrations achieved with endotracheal administration may lead to vasodilation through beta-receptor activity. Clinical trials in humans have also failed to demonstrate any benefit with using the endotracheal route.[165,166] In one clinical trial, a lower rates of ROSC (15% vs 27%, $p \le 0.01$), hospital admission (9% vs 20%, $p \le 0.02$), and hospital discharge (0% vs 5%, $p \le 0.02$) was observed with endotracheal drug administration compared to IV.[166] If the endotracheal route is to be used, the recommended medication dose is 2 to 2.5 times larger than the IV/IO dose. Providers should dilute the medication in 5 to 10 mL of either sterile water or normal saline but better drug absorption may be achieved with sterile water.[105]

Personalized Pharmacotherapy

Several investigators have evaluated factors associated with good neurologic outcome following a cardiac arrest in an attempt to better predict prognosis, optimize resources, and decrease the percentage of patients who are left neurologically devastated. Many factors have been identified that are related to survival to hospital discharge. These include age, the occurrence of a witnessed arrest, rapid implementation of bystander CPR, presence of VF/PVT as the initial rhythm, early defibrillation therapy, achievement of ROSC in the field and time to ROSC.[167-171] In fact, one group developed a statistical prediction model whereby the probability for a good neurologic outcome was = exp(B)/1 + exp(B) where B = −0.02 (age in years) − 0.109 (time to ROSC in minutes) + 0.677 (ROSC prior to hospital arrival; 1 if yes, 0 if no) + 2.442 in patients with VF.[167] For patients with PEA/asystole, B = −0.037 (age in years) −0.076 (time to ROSC in minutes) + 1.735 (ROSC prior to hospital arrival; 1 if yes, 0 if no) + 1.462 (conversion to VF; 1 if yes, 0 if no) + 1.101. Areas under the receiver-operating characteristic curve were 0.867 for VF and 0.873 for PEA/asystole indicating a high predictive ability. A second study analyzed more than 390,000 cases of out-of-hospital cardiac arrest to develop a decision-tree prediction model for survival with good neurological outcome.[171] The single best predictor for survival with good neurological outcome was a shockable initial rhythm. Other identified predictors were age younger than 70 years, presence of a witnessed arrest or arrests witnessed by EMS personnel (Table 12-4). Other prediction models have been recommended which suggest a poor outcome is very likely if one or both of the following are present: bilateral absence of either pupillary and corneal reflexes and bilateral absence of the N20 wave of short-latency somatosensory evoked potentials, 72 hours post-ROSC.[37] A poor outcome is likely if two or more of the following are present: status myoclonus less than or equal to 48 hours post-ROSC, high neuron-specific enolase levels, unreactive burst-suppression, or status epilepticus on electroencephalogram (EEG) and diffuse anoxic injury on brain computed tomography/magnetic resonance imaging (CT/MRI). This prediction model does require a great deal of technical expertise which may not be available at every institution.

Other studies have evaluated prognostic indicators to identify scenarios whereby little or no chance of survival may be evident and prehospital termination of resuscitation would be appropriate.[172-174] From these data, two rules have been developed. The first rule, referred to as the BLS rule, has 3 criteria: (1) the event was not witnessed by EMS personnel, (2) no AED was used or manual shock applied, and (3) ROSC was not achieved in the out-of-hospital setting. The second rule, referred to as the advanced life support rule, consists of the BLS criteria plus (1) the arrest was not witnessed by a bystander and (2) no bystander CPR administered. In one validation study of 5,505 patients, these rules accurately identified patients who were unlikely to benefit from rapid transport to a hospital with a positive predictive value of 0.998 (BLS rule) and 1.000 (ALS rule) when all criteria were met, respectively.[175]

Prediction models have also been investigated for in-hospital cardiac arrest. One study queried the Get With the Guidelines-Resuscitation registry over a ten year period (January, 2000-October, 2009) to develop a score card with 11 variables that were identified in a multivariate analysis[176] (Table 12-5). This prediction tool was called the Cardiac Arrest Survival Postresuscitation In-hospital (CASPRI) score and was highly successful in predicting survival with favorable neurologic outcome ranging from 70% in the top decile and 2.8% in the bottom decile. A second prediction model also used the Get with the Guidelines-Resuscitation registry but limited their analysis to a three year period (2007-2009).[177] This model is referred to as the Good Outcome Following Attempted Resuscitation (GO-FAR) Score and was also successful in prediction survival with favorable neurologic outcome (see Table 12-5). While these scoring systems are not designed to identify scenarios where resuscitation may be futile, they can provide useful prognostic information for the medical team, patients, and families.

TABLE 12-4 Results from a Decision-Tree Model Identifying Prediction Groups for Out-of-Hospital Cardiac Arrest and Survival with Good Neurologic Outcome

Criteria				
Initial Rhythm	Age	Bystander Witnessed Arrest	EMS Witnessed Arrest	Survival with CPC Score 1 – 2
Shockable	<70	Yes	-	20.3%
Shockable	<70	No	-	8.1%
Shockable	≥70	-	Yes	23.2%
Shockable	≥70	-	No	6.9%
Unshockable	-	Yes	-	1.4%
Unshockable	-	No	-	0.3%

CPC, cerebral performance category; EMS, emergency medical services.

Dash mark indicates the respective variable was not identified as a predictor on multivariate decision-tree analysis.

Data from reference 171.

EVALUATION OF THERAPEUTIC OUTCOMES

To measure the success of resuscitation outcomes, therapeutic outcome monitoring should occur both during the resuscitation attempt and in the postresuscitation phase. The optimal outcome following CPR is an awake, responsive, spontaneously breathing patient. Patients must remain neurologically intact with minimal morbidity following the resuscitation if it is to be truly classified as a success.

Unfortunately, there are no reliable surrogate markers that can be used at the bedside to gauge the efficacy of CPR and a positive outcome. Nonetheless, heart rate, cardiac rhythm, and blood pressure should be assessed and documented throughout the resuscitation attempt and subsequent to each intervention. Determination of the presence or absence of a pulse is paramount to deciding which interventions may be appropriate. However, clinicians must be cautious to not exceed 10 seconds when checking for a pulse. Palpating a pulse to determine the efficacy of blood flow during CPR has not been shown to be useful.

A specific mean arterial pressure (MAP) that should be targeted remains unknown but avoiding and immediately correcting hypotension (MAP less than 65 mm Hg or systolic blood pressure [SBP] less than 90 mm Hg) is suggested.[37] Other hemodynamic measures remain undefined but coronary perfusion pressure (CPP = aortic diastolic pressure minus right atrial diastolic pressure) and central venous oxygen saturation (ScvO2) correlate with cardiac output and myocardial blood flow. Thresholds that have been identified which are associated with poor achievement of ROSC include less than 15 mm Hg for CPP and less than 30% for $ScvO_2$.[105] Because coronary perfusion pressures are not routinely available during CPR, arterial diastolic pressure can be used as a reasonable surrogate. Arterial diastolic pressure values less than 20 mm Hg are generally considered suboptimal.[105] $ETCO_2$ monitoring is another useful method to assess cardiac output during CPR and has been associated with ROSC. The main determinant for carbon dioxide excretion is the rate of

TABLE 12-5 Prediction Tools for Survival Following In-Hospital Cardiac Arrest

Cardiac Arrest Survival Postresuscitation In hospital (CASPRI) Scorecard

Predictor	Points
Age group (years)	
<50	0
50-59	0
60-69	1
70-79	2
≥80	4
Initial arrest rhythm	
VF/PVT time to defibrillation	
≤2 minutes	0
3 minutes	0
4-5 minutes	2
>5 minutes	3
PEA	6
Asystole	7
Prearrest CPC score	
1	0
2	2
3	9
≥4	9
Hospital location	
Telemetry unit	0
Intensive care unit	1
Nonmonitored unit	3
Duration of resuscitation (minutes)	
2	0
2-4	0
5-9	3
10-14	5
15-19	6
20-24	6
25-29	6
≥30	8
Mechanical ventilation	3
Renal insufficiency	2
Hepatic insufficiency	4
Sepsis	3
Malignant disease	4
Hypotension	3

INTERPRETATION

Score	Survival with CPC Score of 1-2
0-4	83%
5-9	67%
10-14	42%
15-19	23%
20-24	12%
25-29	5.2%
30-34	2.1%
35-39	0
≥40	0

Good Outcome Following Attempted Resuscitation (GO FAR) Scorecard[177]

SCORECARD

Predictor	Points
Neurologically intact or with minimal deficits at admission	−15
Major trauma	10
Acute stroke	8
Metastatic or hematologic cancer	7
Septicemia	7
Medical noncardiac diagnosis	7
Hepatic insufficiency	6
Admit from skilled nursing facility	6
Hypotension or hypoperfusion	5
Renal insufficiency or dialysis	4
Respiratory insufficiency	4
Pneumonia	1
Age group (years)	
70-74	2
75-79	5
80-84	6
≥85	11

INTERPRETATION

Score	Survival with CPC Score of 1
≥24	0.8%
14 to 23	2%
−5 to 13	9.2%
−15 to −6	27.8%

CPC, cerebral performance category; PVT, pulseless ventricular tachycardia; VF, ventricular fibrillation.

Data from references 176 and 177.

delivery from the peripheral sites (where it is produced) to the lungs. Increasing cardiac output (through effective CPR) will yield higher $ETCO_2$ levels as delivery of carbon dioxide to the lungs increases. Persistently low ETCO2 values (less than 10 mm Hg) during CPR in intubated patients suggest ROSC is unlikely.[36]

ABBREVIATIONS

ACLS	advanced cardiac life support
AED	automated external defibrillator
AHA	American Heart Association
AND	allow natural death
BLS	basic life support
CCR	cardiocerebral resuscitation
CI	confidence interval
CPP	coronary perfusion pressure
CPR	cardiopulmonary resuscitation
CT	computed tomography
DNAR	do not attempt resuscitation
ECC	emergency cardiovascular care
ECMO	extracorporeal membrane oxygenation
EEG	electroencephalogram
EMS	emergency medical services
$ETCO_2$	end-tidal carbon dioxide
IO	intraosseous
IV	intravenous
LVAD	left ventricular assist device
MI	myocardial infarction
MRI	magnetic resonance imaging
OR	odds ratio
PCI	percutaneous coronary intervention
PE	pulmonary embolism
PEA	pulseless electrical activity
PVT	pulseless ventricular tachycardia

ROSC return of spontaneous circulation
SBP systolic blood pressure
VF ventricular fibrillation

REFERENCES

1. Sandroni C, Nolan J, Cavallaro F, Antonelli M. In-hospital cardiac arrest: Incidence, prognosis and possible measures to improve survival. *Intensive Care Med* 2007;33:237-245.
2. Mozaffarian D, Benjamin EJ, Go AS, et al. Heart disease and stroke statistics–2015 update: A report from the American Heart Association. *Circulation* 2015;131:e29-322.
3. Chan PS, McNally B, Tang F, Kellermann A. Recent trends in survival from out-of-hospital cardiac arrest in the United States. *Circulation* 2014;130:1876-1882.
4. Merchant RM, Yang L, Becker LB, et al. Incidence of treated cardiac arrest in hospitalized patients in the United States. *Crit Care Med* 2011;39:2401-2406.
5. Girotra S, Nallamothu BK, Spertus JA, Li Y, Krumholz HM, Chan PS. Trends in survival after in-hospital cardiac arrest. *N Engl J Med* 2012;367:1912-1920.
6. Nolan JP, Soar J, Smith GB, et al. Incidence and outcome of in-hospital cardiac arrest in the United Kingdom National Cardiac Arrest Audit. *Resuscitation* 2014;85:987-992.
7. Chugh SS, Reinier K, Teodorescu C, et al. Epidemiology of sudden cardiac death: Clinical and research implications. *Prog Cardiovasc Dis* 2008;51:213-228.
8. McNally B, Robb R, Mehta M, et al. Out-of-hospital cardiac arrest surveillance—Cardiac Arrest Registry to Enhance Survival (CARES), United States, October 1, 2005–December 31, 2010. *MMWR Surveill Summ* 2011;60:1-19.
9. Weil MH, Tang W. Rhythms and outcomes of cardiac arrest. *Crit Care Med* 2010;38:310.
10. Andrew E, Nehme Z, Lijovic M, Bernard S, Smith K. Outcomes following out-of-hospital cardiac arrest with an initial cardiac rhythm of asystole or pulseless electrical activity in Victoria, Australia. *Resuscitation* 2014;85:1633-1639.
11. Thomas AJ, Newgard CD, Fu R, Zive DM, Daya MR. Survival in out-of-hospital cardiac arrests with initial asystole or pulseless electrical activity and subsequent shockable rhythms. *Resuscitation* 2013;84:1261-1266.
12. Weil MH, Fries M. In-hospital cardiac arrest. *Crit Care Med* 2005;33:2825-2830.
13. Meaney PA, Nadkarni VM, Kern KB, Indik JH, Halperin HR, Berg RA. Rhythms and outcomes of adult in-hospital cardiac arrest. *Crit Care Med* 2010;38:101-108.
14. Atkins DL, Everson-Stewart S, Sears GK, et al. Epidemiology and outcomes from out-of-hospital cardiac arrest in children: The Resuscitation Outcomes Consortium Epistry-Cardiac Arrest. *Circulation* 2009;119:1484-1491.
15. Atkins DL, Berger S. Improving outcomes from out-of-hospital cardiac arrest in young children and adolescents. *Pediatr Cardiol* 2012;33:474-483.
16. Girotra S, Spertus JA, Li Y, Berg RA, Nadkarni VM, Chan PS. Survival trends in pediatric in-hospital cardiac arrests: An analysis from Get With the Guidelines-Resuscitation. *Circ Cardiovasc Qual Outcomes* 2013;6:42-49.
17. Myerburg RJ, Castellanos A. Emerging paradigms of the epidemiology and demographics of sudden cardiac arrest. *Heart Rhythm* 2006;3:235-239.
18. Kleinman ME, Chameides L, Schexnayder SM, et al. Part 14: Pediatric advanced life support: 2010 American Heart Association Guidelines for Cardiopulmonary Resuscitation and Emergency Cardiovascular Care. *Circulation* 2010;122:S876-S908.
19. Ewy GA, Kern KB. Recent advances in cardiopulmonary resuscitation: Cardiocerebral resuscitation. *J Am Coll Cardiol* 2009;53:149-157.
20. Cooper JA, Cooper JD, Cooper JM. Cardiopulmonary resuscitation: History, current practice, and future direction. *Circulation* 2006;114:2839-2849.
21. Kleinman ME, Brennan EE, Goldberger ZD, et al. Part 5: Adult Basic Life Support and Cardiopulmonary Resuscitation Quality: 2015 American Heart Association Guidelines Update for Cardiopulmonary Resuscitation and Emergency Cardiovascular Care. *Circulation* 2015;132:S414-S435.
22. Christenson J, Andrusiek D, Everson-Stewart S, et al. Chest compression fraction determines survival in patients with out-of-hospital ventricular fibrillation. *Circulation* 2009;120:1241-1247.
23. Soar J, Edelson DP, Perkins GD. Delivering high-quality cardiopulmonary resuscitation in-hospital. *Curr Opin Crit Care* 2011;17:225-230.
24. Bottiger BW. Cardiopulmonary resuscitation and postresuscitation care 2015: Saving more than 200 000 additional lives per year worldwide. *Curr Opin Crit Care* 2015;21:179-182.
25. Mancini ME, Diekema DS, Hoadley TA, et al. Part 3: Ethical Issues: 2015 American Heart Association Guidelines Update for Cardiopulmonary Resuscitation and Emergency Cardiovascular Care. *Circulation* 2015;132:S383-S396.
26. Young GB. Clinical practice. Neurologic prognosis after cardiac arrest. *N Engl J Med* 2009;361:605-611.
27. Morrison LJ, Kierzek G, Diekema DS, et al. Part 3: Ethics: 2010 American Heart Association Guidelines for Cardiopulmonary Resuscitation and Emergency Cardiovascular Care. *Circulation* 2010;122:S665-S675.
28. Kouwenhoven WB, Jude JR, Knickerbocker GG. Closed-chest cardiac massage. *JAMA* 1960;173:1064-1067.
29. Safar P. Community-wide cardiopulmonary resuscitation. *J Iowa Med Soc* 1964;54:629-635.
30. Cardiopulmonary resuscitation. *JAMA* 1966;198:372-379.
31. Neumar RW, Shuster M, Callaway CW, et al. Part 1: Executive Summary: 2015 American Heart Association Guidelines Update for Cardiopulmonary Resuscitation and Emergency Cardiovascular Care. *Circulation* 2015;132:S315-S367.
32. Kronick SL, Kurz MC, Lin S, et al. Part 4: Systems of Care and Continuous Quality Improvement: 2015 American Heart Association Guidelines Update for Cardiopulmonary Resuscitation and Emergency Cardiovascular Care. *Circulation* 2015;132:S397-S413.
33. Sanghavi P, Jena AB, Newhouse JP, Zaslavsky AM. Outcomes after out-of-hospital cardiac arrest treated by basic vs advanced life support. *JAMA Intern Med* 2015;175:196-204.
34. Larsen MP, Eisenberg MS, Cummins RO, Hallstrom AP. Predicting survival from out-of-hospital cardiac arrest: A graphic model. *Ann Emerg Med* 1993;22:1652-1658.
35. Link MS, Atkins DL, Passman RS, et al. Part 6: Electrical therapies: automated external defibrillators, defibrillation, cardioversion, and pacing: 2010 American Heart Association Guidelines for Cardiopulmonary Resuscitation and Emergency Cardiovascular Care. *Circulation* 2010;122:S706-S719.
36. Link MS, Berkow LC, Kudenchuk PJ, et al. Part 7: Adult Advanced Cardiovascular Life Support: 2015 American Heart Association Guidelines Update for Cardiopulmonary Resuscitation and Emergency Cardiovascular Care. *Circulation* 2015;132:S444-S464.
37. Callaway CW, Donnino MW, Fink EL, et al. Part 8: Post-Cardiac Arrest Care: 2015 American Heart Association Guidelines Update for Cardiopulmonary Resuscitation and Emergency Cardiovascular Care. *Circulation* 2015;132:S465-S482.
38. Eberle B, Dick WF, Schneider T, Wisser G, Doetsch S, Tzanova I. Checking the carotid pulse check: Diagnostic accuracy of first responders in patients with and without a pulse. *Resuscitation* 1996;33:107-116.
39. Strategies to improve cardiac arrest survival: A time to act. Available at: http://ww.iom.edu/CardiacArrestSurvival. Accessed September 21, 2015.
40. Swor R, Khan I, Domeier R, Honeycutt L, Chu K, Compton S. CPR training and CPR performance: Do CPR-trained bystanders perform CPR? *Acad Emerg Med* 2006;13:596-601.
41. Hartmann SM, Farris RW, Di Gennaro JL, Roberts JS. Systematic review and meta-analysis of end-tidal carbon dioxide values associated with return of spontaneous circulation during cardiopulmonary resuscitation. *J Intensive Care Med* 2015;30:426-435.
42. Assar D, Chamberlain D, Colquhoun M, et al. Randomised controlled trials of staged teaching for basic life support. 1. Skill acquisition at bronze stage. *Resuscitation* 2000;45:7-15.
43. Ewy GA. Cardiocerebral resuscitation: The new cardiopulmonary resuscitation. *Circulation* 2005;111:2134-2142.
44. Weisfeldt ML, Becker LB. Resuscitation after cardiac arrest: a 3-phase time-sensitive model. *Jama* 2002;288:3035-3038.
45. Ewy GA, Bobrow BJ. Cardiocerebral resuscitation: An approach to improving survival of patients with primary cardiac arrest. *J Intensive Care Med* 2014.
46. Salmen M, Ewy GA, Sasson C. Use of cardiocerebral resuscitation or AHA/ERC 2005 Guidelines is associated with improved survival from out-of-hospital cardiac arrest: A systematic review and meta-analysis. *BMJ Open* 2012;2.
47. Mosier J, Itty A, Sanders A, et al. Cardiocerebral resuscitation is associated with improved survival and neurologic outcome

from out-of-hospital cardiac arrest in elders. *Acad Emerg Med* 2010;17:269-275.
48. De Maio VJ, Stiell IG, Wells GA, Spaite DW. Optimal defibrillation response intervals for maximum out-of-hospital cardiac arrest survival rates. *Ann Emerg Med* 2003;42:242-250.
49. Cobb LA, Fahrenbruch CE, Walsh TR, et al. Influence of cardiopulmonary resuscitation prior to defibrillation in patients with out-of-hospital ventricular fibrillation. *JAMA* 1999;281:1182-1188.
50. Garza AG, Gratton MC, Salomone JA, Lindholm D, McElroy J, Archer R. Improved patient survival using a modified resuscitation protocol for out-of-hospital cardiac arrest. *Circulation* 2009;119:2597-2605.
51. Kellum MJ, Kennedy KW, Ewy GA. Cardiocerebral resuscitation improves survival of patients with out-of-hospital cardiac arrest. *Am J Med* 2006;119:335-340.
52. Wik L, Hansen TB, Fylling F, et al. Delaying defibrillation to give basic cardiopulmonary resuscitation to patients with out-of-hospital ventricular fibrillation: A randomized trial. *JAMA* 2003;289:1389-1395.
53. Baker PW, Conway J, Cotton C, et al. Defibrillation or cardiopulmonary resuscitation first for patients with out-of-hospital cardiac arrests found by paramedics to be in ventricular fibrillation? A randomised control trial. *Resuscitation* 2008;79:424-431.
54. Jacobs IG, Finn JC, Oxer HF, Jelinek GA. CPR before defibrillation in out-of-hospital cardiac arrest: A randomized trial. *Emerg Med Australas* 2005;17:39-45.
55. Ma MH, Chiang WC, Ko PC, et al. A randomized trial of compression first or analyze first strategies in patients with out-of-hospital cardiac arrest: Results from an Asian community. *Resuscitation* 2012;83:806-812.
56. Stiell IG, Nichol G, Leroux BG, et al. Early versus later rhythm analysis in patients with out-of-hospital cardiac arrest. *N Engl J Med* 2011;365:787-797.
57. Huang Y, He Q, Yang LJ, Liu GJ, Jones A. Cardiopulmonary resuscitation (CPR) plus delayed defibrillation versus immediate defibrillation for out-of-hospital cardiac arrest. *Cochrane Database Syst Rev* 2014;9:CD009803.
58. Meier P, Baker P, Jost D, et al. Chest compressions before defibrillation for out-of-hospital cardiac arrest: a meta-analysis of randomized controlled clinical trials. *BMC Med* 2010;8:52.
59. Simpson PM, Goodger MS, Bendall JC. Delayed versus immediate defibrillation for out-of-hospital cardiac arrest due to ventricular fibrillation: A systematic review and meta-analysis of randomised controlled trials. *Resuscitation* 2010;81:925-931.
60. Valenzuela TD, Roe DJ, Nichol G, Clark LL, Spaite DW, Hardman RG. Outcomes of rapid defibrillation by security officers after cardiac arrest in casinos. *N Engl J Med* 2000;343:1206-1209.
61. Tuseth V, Salem M, Pettersen R, et al. Percutaneous left ventricular assist in ischemic cardiac arrest. *Crit Care Med* 2009;37: 1365-1372.
62. Sunde K. Experimental and clinical use of ongoing mechanical cardiopulmonary resuscitation during angiography and percutaneous coronary intervention. *Crit Care Med* 2008;36: S405-S408.
63. Varon J, Acosta P. Extracorporeal membrane oxygenation in cardiopulmonary resuscitation: Are we there yet? *Crit Care Med* 2008;36:2685-2686.
64. Chamberlain D, Frenneaux M, Fletcher D. The primacy of basics in advanced life support. *Curr Opin Crit Care* 2009;15:198-202.
65. Robinson LA, Brown CG, Jenkins J, et al. The effect of norepinephrine versus epinephrine on myocardial hemodynamics during CPR. *Ann Emerg Med* 1989;18:336-340.
66. Paradis NA, Martin GB, Rivers EP, et al. Coronary perfusion pressure and the return of spontaneous circulation in human cardiopulmonary resuscitation. *JAMA* 1990;263:1106-1113.
67. Reynolds JC, Salcido DD, Menegazzi JJ. Conceptual models of coronary perfusion pressure and their relationship to defibrillation success in a porcine model of prolonged out-of-hospital cardiac arrest. *Resuscitation* 2012;83:900-906.
68. Attaran RR, Ewy GA. Epinephrine in resuscitation: curse or cure? *Future Cardiol* 2010;6:473-482.
69. Olasveengen TM, Sunde K, Brunborg C, Thowsen J, Steen PA, Wik L. Intravenous drug administration during out-of-hospital cardiac arrest: A randomized trial. *JAMA* 2009;302:2222-2229.
70. Jacobs IG, Finn JC, Jelinek GA, Oxer HF, Thompson PL. Effect of adrenaline on survival in out-of-hospital cardiac arrest: A randomised double-blind placebo-controlled trial. *Resuscitation* 2011;82:1138-1143.
71. Hagihara A, Hasegawa M, Abe T, Nagata T, Wakata Y, Miyazaki S. Prehospital epinephrine use and survival among patients with out-of-hospital cardiac arrest. *JAMA* 2012;307:1161-1618.
72. Nakahara S, Tomio J, Takahashi H, et al. Evaluation of pre-hospital administration of adrenaline (epinephrine) by emergency medical services for patients with out of hospital cardiac arrest in Japan: Controlled propensity matched retrospective cohort study. *BMJ* 2013;347:f6829.
73. Andersen LW, Berg KM, Saindon BZ, et al. Time to epinephrine and survival after pediatric in-hospital cardiac arrest. *JAMA* 2015;314:802-810.
74. Donnino MW, Salciccioli JD, Howell MD, et al. Time to administration of epinephrine and outcome after in-hospital cardiac arrest with non-shockable rhythms: Retrospective analysis of large in-hospital data registry. *BMJ* 2014;348:g3028.
75. Ewy GA, Bobrow BJ, Chikani V, et al. The time dependent association of adrenaline administration and survival from out-of-hospital cardiac arrest. *Resuscitation* 2015;96:180-185.
76. Goto Y, Maeda T, Goto Y. Effects of prehospital epinephrine during out-of-hospital cardiac arrest with initial non-shockable rhythm: an observational cohort study. *Crit Care* 2013;17:R188.
77. Hayashi Y, Iwami T, Kitamura T, et al. Impact of early intravenous epinephrine administration on outcomes following out-of-hospital cardiac arrest. *Circ J* 2012;76:1639-1645.
78. Koscik C, Pinawin A, McGovern H, et al. Rapid epinephrine administration improves early outcomes in out-of-hospital cardiac arrest. *Resuscitation* 2013;84:915-920.
79. Dumas F, Bougouin W, Geri G, et al. Is epinephrine during cardiac arrest associated with worse outcomes in resuscitated patients? *J Am Coll Cardiol* 2014;64:2360-2367.
80. Ristagno G, Tang W, Huang L, et al. Epinephrine reduces cerebral perfusion during cardiopulmonary resuscitation. *Crit Care Med* 2009;37:1408-1415.
81. Rivers EP, Wortsman J, Rady MY, Blake HC, McGeorge FT, Buderer NM. The effect of the total cumulative epinephrine dose administered during human CPR on hemodynamic, oxygen transport, and utilization variables in the postresuscitation period. *Chest* 1994;106:1499-1507.
82. Huang L, Sun S, Fang X, Tang W, Weil MH. Simultaneous blockade of alpha1- and beta-actions of epinephrine during cardiopulmonary resuscitation. *Crit Care Med* 2006;34:S483-S485.
83. Larabee TM, Liu KY, Campbell JA, Little CM. Vasopressors in cardiac arrest: A systematic review. *Resuscitation* 2012;83: 932-939.
84. Ornato JP. Use of adrenergic agonists during CPR in adults. *Ann Emerg Med* 1993;22:411-416.
85. Brown C, Wiklund L, Bar-Joseph G, et al. Future directions for resuscitation research. IV. Innovative advanced life support pharmacology. *Resuscitation* 1996;33:163-177.
86. Callaham M, Madsen CD, Barton CW, Saunders CE, Pointer J. A randomized clinical trial of high-dose epinephrine and norepinephrine vs standard-dose epinephrine in prehospital cardiac arrest. *JAMA* 1992;268:2667-2672.
87. Lindner KH, Ahnefeld FW, Grunert A. Epinephrine versus norepinephrine in prehospital ventricular fibrillation. *Am J Cardiol* 1991;67:427-428.
88. Redding JS, Pearson JW. Evaluation of drugs for cardiac resuscitation. *Anesthesiology* 1963;24:203-207.
89. Wenzel V, Raab H, Dunser MW. Role of arginine vasopressin in the setting of cardiopulmonary resuscitation. *Best Pract Res Clin Anaesthesiol* 2008;22:287-297.
90. Lindner KH, Haak T, Keller A, Bothner U, Lurie KG. Release of endogenous vasopressors during and after cardiopulmonary resuscitation. *Heart* 1996;75:145-150.
91. Wenzel V, Krismer AC, Arntz HR, Sitter H, Stadlbauer KH, Lindner KH. A comparison of vasopressin and epinephrine for out-of-hospital cardiopulmonary resuscitation. *N Engl J Med* 2004;350:105-113.
92. Gueugniaud PY, David JS, Chanzy E, et al. Vasopressin and epinephrine vs. epinephrine alone in cardiopulmonary resuscitation. *N Engl J Med* 2008;359:21-30.
93. Mentzelopoulos SD, Zakynthinos SG, Tzoufi M, et al. Vasopressin, epinephrine, and corticosteroids for in-hospital cardiac arrest. *Arch Intern Med* 2009;169:15-24.
94. Mentzelopoulos SD, Malachias S, Chamos C, et al. Vasopressin, steroids, and epinephrine and neurologically favorable survival after in-hospital cardiac arrest: A randomized clinical trial. *JAMA* 2013;310:270-279.

94a. Lindner KH, Dirks B, Strohmenger HU, Prengel AW, Lindner IM, Lurie KG. Randomised comparison of epinephrine and vasopressin in patients with out-of-hospital ventricular fibrillation. *Lancet* 1997;349:535-537.

94b. Stiell IG, Hebert PC, Wells GA, et al. Vasopressin versus epinephrine for inhospital cardiac arrest: a randomised controlled trial. *Lancet* 2001;358:105-109.

94c. Callaway CW, Hostler D, Doshi AA, et al. Usefulness of vasopressin administered with epinephrine during out-of-hospital cardiac arrest. *Am J Cardiol* 2006;98:1316-1321.

94d. Mukoyama T, Kinoshita K, Nagao K, Tanjoh K. Reduced effectiveness of vasopressin in repeated doses for patients undergoing prolonged cardiopulmonary resuscitation. *Resuscitation* 2009;80:755-761.

94e. Ong ME, Tiah L, Leong BS, et al. A randomised, double-blind, multi-centre trial comparing vasopressin and adrenaline in patients with cardiac arrest presenting to or in the Emergency Department. *Resuscitation* 2012;83:953-960.

95. Mentzelopoulos SD, Zakynthinos SG, Siempos I, Malachias S, Ulmer H, Wenzel V. Vasopressin for cardiac arrest: Meta-analysis of randomized controlled trials. *Resuscitation* 2012;83:32-39.

96. Aung K, Htay T. Vasopressin for cardiac arrest: A systematic review and meta-analysis. *Arch Intern Med* 2005;165:17-24.

97. Biondi-Zoccai GG, Abbate A, Parisi Q, et al. Is vasopressin superior to adrenaline or placebo in the management of cardiac arrest? A meta-analysis. *Resuscitation* 2003;59:221-224.

98. Layek A, Maitra S, Pal S, Bhattacharjee S, Baidya DK. Efficacy of vasopressin during cardio-pulmonary resuscitation in adult patients: A meta-analysis. *Resuscitation* 2014;85:855-863.

99. Sillberg VA, Perry JJ, Stiell IG, Wells GA. Is the combination of vasopressin and epinephrine superior to repeated doses of epinephrine alone in the treatment of cardiac arrest-a systematic review. *Resuscitation* 2008;79:380-386.

100. Ong ME, Pellis T, Link MS. The use of antiarrhythmic drugs for adult cardiac arrest: A systematic review. *Resuscitation* 2011;82:665-670.

101. Huang Y, He Q, Yang M, Zhan L. Antiarrhythmia drugs for cardiac arrest: A systemic review and meta-analysis. *Crit Care* 2013;17:R173.

102. Kudenchuk PJ, Cobb LA, Copass MK, et al. Amiodarone for resuscitation after out-of-hospital cardiac arrest due to ventricular fibrillation. *N Engl J Med* 1999;341:871-878.

103. Dorian P, Cass D, Schwartz B, Cooper R, Gelaznikas R, Barr A. Amiodarone as compared with lidocaine for shock-resistant ventricular fibrillation. *N Engl J Med* 2002;346:884-890.

104. Kudenchuk PJ, Brown SP, Daya M, et al. Resuscitation Outcomes Consortium-Amiodarone, Lidocaine or Placebo Study (ROC-ALPS): Rationale and methodology behind an out-of-hospital cardiac arrest antiarrhythmic drug trial. *Am Heart J* 2014;167:653-9. e4.

105. Neumar RW, Otto CW, Link MS, et al. Part 8: Adult advanced cardiovascular life support: 2010 American Heart Association Guidelines for Cardiopulmonary Resuscitation and Emergency Cardiovascular Care. *Circulation* 2010;122:S729-S767.

106. Harrison EE. Lidocaine in prehospital countershock refractory ventricular fibrillation. *Ann Emerg Med* 1981;10:420-423.

107. Weaver WD, Fahrenbruch CE, Johnson DD, Hallstrom AP, Cobb LA, Copass MK. Effect of epinephrine and lidocaine therapy on outcome after cardiac arrest due to ventricular fibrillation. *Circulation* 1990;82:2027-2034.

108. Herlitz J, Ekstrom L, Wennerblom B, et al. Lidocaine in out-of-hospital ventricular fibrillation. Does it improve survival? *Resuscitation* 1997;33:199-205.

109. Abu-Laban RB, Christenson JM, Innes GD, et al. Tissue plasminogen activator in cardiac arrest with pulseless electrical activity. *N Engl J Med* 2002;346:1522-1528.

110. Bottiger BW, Arntz HR, Chamberlain DA, et al. Thrombolysis during resuscitation for out-of-hospital cardiac arrest. *N Engl J Med* 2008;359:2651-2662.

111. Lavonas EJ, Drennan IR, Gabrielli A, et al. Part 10: Special Circumstances of Resuscitation: 2015 American Heart Association Guidelines Update for Cardiopulmonary Resuscitation and Emergency Cardiovascular Care. *Circulation* 2015;132:S501-S518.

112. Mader TJ, Nathanson BH, Millay S, Coute RA, Clapp M, McNally B. Out-of-hospital cardiac arrest outcomes stratified by rhythm analysis. *Resuscitation* 2012;83:1358-1362.

113. Hachimi-Idrissi S, Corne L, Ebinger G, Michotte Y, Huyghens L. Mild hypothermia induced by a helmet device: A clinical feasibility study. *Resuscitation* 2001;51:275-81.

114. Kim YM, Yim HW, Jeong SH, Klem ML, Callaway CW. Does therapeutic hypothermia benefit adult cardiac arrest patients presenting with non-shockable initial rhythms?: A systematic review and meta-analysis of randomized and non-randomized studies. *Resuscitation* 2012;83:188-196.

115. Gonzalez ER. Pharmacologic controversies in CPR. *Ann Emerg Med* 1993;22:317-323.

116. Bohm K, Rosenqvist M, Herlitz J, Hollenberg J, Svensson L. Survival is similar after standard treatment and chest compression only in out-of-hospital bystander cardiopulmonary resuscitation. *Circulation* 2007;116:2908-2912.

117. Vukmir RB, Katz L, Sodium Bicarbonate Study G. Sodium bicarbonate improves outcome in prolonged prehospital cardiac arrest. *Am J Emerg Med* 2006;24:156-161.

118. Levy MM. An evidence-based evaluation of the use of sodium bicarbonate during cardiopulmonary resuscitation. *Crit Care Clin* 1998;14:457-483.

119. Bjerneroth G. Tribonat–a comprehensive summary of its properties. *Crit Care Med* 1999;27:1009-1013.

120. Neumar RW, Nolan JP, Adrie C, et al. Post-cardiac arrest syndrome: Epidemiology, pathophysiology, treatment, and prognostication. A consensus statement from the International Liaison Committee on Resuscitation (American Heart Association, Australian and New Zealand Council on Resuscitation, European Resuscitation Council, Heart and Stroke Foundation of Canada, InterAmerican Heart Foundation, Resuscitation Council of Asia, and the Resuscitation Council of Southern Africa); the American Heart Association Emergency Cardiovascular Care Committee; the Council on Cardiovascular Surgery and Anesthesia; the Council on Cardiopulmonary, Perioperative, and Critical Care; the Council on Clinical Cardiology; and the Stroke Council. *Circulation* 2008;118:2452-2483.

121. Safar P. Resuscitation from clinical death: Pathophysiologic limits and therapeutic potentials. *Crit Care Med* 1988;16:923-941.

122. Anyfantakis ZA, Baron G, Aubry P, et al. Acute coronary angiographic findings in survivors of out-of-hospital cardiac arrest. *Am Heart J* 2009;157:312-318.

123. Nolan JP, Morley PT, Vanden Hoek TL, et al. Therapeutic hypothermia after cardiac arrest: An advisory statement by the advanced life support task force of the International Liaison Committee on Resuscitation. *Circulation* 2003;108:118-121.

124. Polderman KH. Mechanisms of action, physiological effects, and complications of hypothermia. *Crit Care Med* 2009;37:S186-S202.

125. Mild therapeutic hypothermia to improve the neurologic outcome after cardiac arrest. *N Engl J Med* 2002;346:549-556.

126. Bernard SA, Gray TW, Buist MD, et al. Treatment of comatose survivors of out-of-hospital cardiac arrest with induced hypothermia. *N Engl J Med* 2002;346:557-563.

127. Polderman KH, Varon J. How low should we go? Hypothermia or strict normothermia after cardiac arrest? *Circulation* 2015;131: 669-675.

128. Dresden SM, O'Connor LM, Pearce CG, Courtney DM, Powell ES. National trends in the use of postcardiac arrest therapeutic hypothermia and hospital factors influencing its use. *Ther Hypothermia Temp Manag* 2015;5:48-54.

129. Kim F, Nichol G, Maynard C, et al. Effect of prehospital induction of mild hypothermia on survival and neurological status among adults with cardiac arrest: A randomized clinical trial. *JAMA* 2014;311:45-52.

130. Moler FW, Silverstein FS, Holubkov R, et al. Therapeutic hypothermia after out-of-hospital cardiac arrest in children. *N Engl J Med* 2015;372:1898-1908.

131. Nielsen N, Wetterslev J, Cronberg T, et al. Targeted temperature management at 33 degrees C versus 36 degrees C after cardiac arrest. *N Engl J Med* 2013;369:2197-2206.

132. Zeiner A, Holzer M, Sterz F, et al. Hyperthermia after cardiac arrest is associated with an unfavorable neurologic outcome. *Arch Intern Med* 2001;161:2007-2012.

133. Weng Y, Sun S. Therapeutic hypothermia after cardiac arrest in adults: mechanism of neuroprotection, phases of hypothermia, and methods of cooling. *Crit Care Clin* 2012;28:231-243.

134. Polderman KH, Herold I. Therapeutic hypothermia and controlled normothermia in the intensive care unit: practical considerations, side effects, and cooling methods. *Crit Care Med* 2009;37:1101-1020.

135. Sessler DI. Thermoregulatory defense mechanisms. *Crit Care Med* 2009;37:S203-S210.

136. Vanden Hoek TL, Morrison LJ, Shuster M, et al. Part 12: Cardiac arrest in special situations: 2010 American Heart Association Guidelines for Cardiopulmonary Resuscitation and Emergency Cardiovascular Care. *Circulation* 2010;122:S829-S861.

137. McFadden ER, Jr., Warren EL. Observations on asthma mortality. *Ann Intern Med* 1997;127:142-147.

138. Hess DR, Acosta FL, Ritz RH, Kacmarek RM, Camargo CA, Jr. The effect of heliox on nebulizer function using a beta-agonist bronchodilator. *Chest* 1999;115:184-189.
139. Petrillo TM, Fortenberry JD, Linzer JF, Simon HK. Emergency department use of ketamine in pediatric status asthmaticus. *J Asthma* 2001;38:657-664.
140. Rodrigo GJ, Castro-Rodriguez JA. Anticholinergics in the treatment of children and adults with acute asthma: A systematic review with meta-analysis. *Thorax* 2005;60:740-746.
141. Schultz TE. Sevoflurane administration in status asthmaticus: a case report. *AANA J* 2005;73:35-36.
142. Silverman RA, Osborn H, Runge J, et al. IV magnesium sulfate in the treatment of acute severe asthma: A multicenter randomized controlled trial. *Chest* 2002;122:489-497.
143. Soroksky A, Stav D, Shpirer I. A pilot prospective, randomized, placebo-controlled trial of bilevel positive airway pressure in acute asthmatic attack. *Chest* 2003;123:1018-1025.
144. Neugut AI, Ghatak AT, Miller RL. Anaphylaxis in the United States: An investigation into its epidemiology. *Arch Intern Med* 2001;161: 15-21.
145. Schummer C, Wirsing M, Schummer W. The pivotal role of vasopressin in refractory anaphylactic shock. *Anesth Analg* 2008;107:620-624.
146. Brown SG, Blackman KE, Stenlake V, Heddle RJ. Insect sting anaphylaxis; prospective evaluation of treatment with intravenous adrenaline and volume resuscitation. *Emerg Med J* 2004;21:149-154.
147. Dijkman A, Huisman CM, Smit M, et al. Cardiac arrest in pregnancy: increasing use of perimortem caesarean section due to emergency skills training? *BJOG* 2010;117:282-287.
148. Atta E, Gardner M. Cardiopulmonary resuscitation in pregnancy. *Obstet Gynecol Clin North Am* 2007;34:585-597.
149. Nanson J, Elcock D, Williams M, Deakin CD. Do physiological changes in pregnancy change defibrillation energy requirements? *Br J Anaesth* 2001;87:237-239.
150. Munro PT. Management of eclampsia in the accident and emergency department. *J Accid Emerg Med* 2000;17:7-11.
151. Stanten RD, Iverson LI, Daugharty TM, Lovett SM, Terry C, Blumenstock E. Amniotic fluid embolism causing catastrophic pulmonary vasoconstriction: Diagnosis by transesophageal echocardiogram and treatment by cardiopulmonary bypass. *Obstet Gynecol* 2003;102:496-498.
152. Hanania NA, Zimmerman JL. Accidental hypothermia. *Crit Care Clin* 1999;15:235-249.
153. Wira CR, Becker JU, Martin G, Donnino MW. Anti-arrhythmic and vasopressor medications for the treatment of ventricular fibrillation in severe hypothermia: a systematic review of the literature. *Resuscitation* 2008;78:21-29.
154. Lockey D, Crewdson K, Davies G. Traumatic cardiac arrest: Who are the survivors? *Ann Emerg Med* 2006;48:240-244.
155. Link MS, Maron BJ, Wang PJ, VanderBrink BA, Zhu W, Estes NA, 3rd. Upper and lower limits of vulnerability to sudden arrhythmic death with chest-wall impact (commotio cordis). *J Am Coll Cardiol* 2003;41:99-104.
156. Hopson LR, Hirsh E, Delgado J, et al. Guidelines for withholding or termination of resuscitation in prehospital traumatic cardiopulmonary arrest. *J Am Coll Surg* 2003;196:475-481.
157. Quan L, Mack CD, Schiff MA. Association of water temperature and submersion duration and drowning outcome. *Resuscitation* 2014;85:790-794.
158. Szpilman D, Webber J, Quan L, et al. Creating a drowning chain of survival. *Resuscitation* 2014;85:1149-1152.
159. Browne BJ, Gaasch WR. Electrical injuries and lightning. *Emerg Med Clin North Am* 1992;10:211-229.
160. Milzman DP, Moskowitz L, Hardel M. Lightning strikes at a mass gathering. *South Med J* 1999;92:708-710.
161. Vincent R. Drugs in modern resuscitation. *Br J Anaesth* 1997;79: 188-197.
162. Kellum MJ. Improving performance of emergency medical services personnel during resuscitation of cardiac arrest patients: The McMAID approach. *Curr Opin Crit Care* 2009;15:216-220.
163. Weiser G, Hoffmann Y, Galbraith R, Shavit I. Current advances in intraosseous infusion - A systematic review. *Resuscitation* 2012;83:20-26.
164. Hoskins SL, do Nascimento P, Jr., Lima RM, Espana-Tenorio JM, Kramer GC. Pharmacokinetics of intraosseous and central venous drug delivery during cardiopulmonary resuscitation. *Resuscitation* 2012;83:107-112.
165. Niemann JT, Stratton SJ. Endotracheal versus intravenous epinephrine and atropine in out-of-hospital "primary" and postcountershock asystole. *Crit Care Med* 2000;28:1815-1819.
166. Niemann JT, Stratton SJ, Cruz B, Lewis RJ. Endotracheal drug administration during out-of-hospital resuscitation: Where are the survivors? *Resuscitation* 2002;53:153-157.
167. Hayakawa K, Tasaki O, Hamasaki T, et al. Prognostic indicators and outcome prediction model for patients with return of spontaneous circulation from cardiopulmonary arrest: The Utstein Osaka Project. *Resuscitation* 2011;82:874-880.
168. Herlitz J, Engdahl J, Svensson L, Angquist KA, Young M, Holmberg S. Factors associated with an increased chance of survival among patients suffering from an out-of-hospital cardiac arrest in a national perspective in Sweden. *Am Heart J* 2005;149:61-66.
169. Sasson C, Rogers MA, Dahl J, Kellermann AL. Predictors of survival from out-of-hospital cardiac arrest: A systematic review and meta-analysis. *Circ Cardiovasc Qual Outcomes* 2010;3:63-81.
170. Stiell IG, Wells GA, Field B, et al. Advanced cardiac life support in out-of-hospital cardiac arrest. *N Engl J Med* 2004;351:647-656.
171. Goto Y, Maeda T, Goto Y. Decision-tree model for predicting outcomes after out-of-hospital cardiac arrest in the emergency department. *Crit Care* 2013;17:R133.
172. Morrison LJ, Verbeek PR, Vermeulen MJ, et al. Derivation and evaluation of a termination of resuscitation clinical prediction rule for advanced life support providers. *Resuscitation* 2007;74:266-275.
173. Morrison LJ, Visentin LM, Kiss A, et al. Validation of a rule for termination of resuscitation in out-of-hospital cardiac arrest. *N Engl J Med* 2006;355:478-487.
174. Verbeek PR, Vermeulen MJ, Ali FH, Messenger DW, Summers J, Morrison LJ. Derivation of a termination-of-resuscitation guideline for emergency medical technicians using automated external defibrillators. *Acad Emerg Med* 2002;9:671-678.
175. Sasson C, Hegg AJ, Macy M, et al. Prehospital termination of resuscitation in cases of refractory out-of-hospital cardiac arrest. *JAMA* 2008;300:1432-1438.
176. Chan PS, Spertus JA, Krumholz HM, et al. A Validated prediction tool for initial survivors of in-hospital cardiac arrestprediction tool for in-hospital cardiac arrest. *Arch Intern Med* 2012:1-7.
177. Ebell MH, Jang W, Shen Y, Geocadin RG. Development and validation of the Good Outcome Following Attempted Resuscitation (GO-FAR) score to predict neurologically intact survival after in-hospital cardiopulmonary resuscitation. *JAMA Intern Med* 2013;173:1872-1878.

Hypertension

13

Joseph J. Saseen and Eric J. MacLaughlin

KEY CONCEPTS

1. The risk of cardiovascular (CV) morbidity and mortality is directly correlated with blood pressure (BP).
2. Evidence from clinical trials has shown that antihypertensive drug therapy substantially reduces the risks of CV events and death in patients with high BP.
3. Essential hypertension is usually an asymptomatic disease. A diagnosis cannot be made based on only one elevated BP measurement. An elevated value from the average of two or more measurements, present during two or more clinical encounters, is needed to diagnose hypertension.
4. The overall goal of treating hypertension is to reduce associated morbidity and mortality from CV events. Antihypertensive drug therapy selection should be based on evidence demonstrating CV event reduction.
5. A goal BP of less than 140/90 mm Hg is appropriate for most patients with hypertension.
6. The magnitude of BP elevation should be used to guide the determination of the number of antihypertensive agents to start when implementing drug therapy. Most patients with stage 1 hypertension should be initially treated with one drug, with the option of starting treatment with two for some patients. However, most patients presenting with stage 2 hypertension should be initially treated with two drugs.
7. Lifestyle modifications should be prescribed to all patients, especially those with prehypertension and hypertension.
8. An Angiotensin-converting enzyme inhibitors (ACEi), angiotensin II receptor blocker (ARB), calcium channel blocker (CCB), and thiazide are first-line antihypertensive agents for most patients with hypertension. These first-line options are for patients with hypertension who do not a compelling indication(s) for a specific antihypertensive drug class.
9. For most patients with hypertension, treatment with a β-blockers does not reduce CV events as well as has been demonstrated with an ACEi, ARB, CCB, or thiazide.
10. Compelling indications are comorbid conditions where specific antihypertensive drug classes have been shown in clinical trials to reduce CV events in patients with the specific comorbidity.
11. Patients with diabetes and hypertension should ideally be treated with either an ACEi or an ARB, and often must be used in combination with one or more other antihypertensive agents to control BP.
12. Older patients are often at risk for orthostatic hypotension related to antihypertensive drug therapy. While antihypertensive drug therapy selection should be the same as in younger patients, low initial doses should be used to minimize the risk of orthostatic hypotension.
13. Alternative antihypertensive agents should only be used in combination with first-line antihypertensive agents to provide additional BP lowering because they do not have significant evidence demonstrating CV event reduction.
14. Initial therapy with the combination of two antihypertensive agents should be used in most patients presenting with stage 2 hypertension. This is also an option for patients presenting with stage 1 hypertension. Most patients require combination therapy to achieve goal BP.
15. Patients have resistant hypertension when they fail to achieve goal BP while adherent to a regimen that includes three antihypertensive agents at full doses (one of which includes a diuretic), or when four or more agents are needed to treat hypertension.
16. Hypertensive urgency is ideally managed by adjusting maintenance therapy, adding a new antihypertensive, and/or increasing the dose of a current antihypertensive medication. This provides a gradual reduction in BP, which is a safer treatment approach than rapid reductions in BP.

Hypertension is a common disease that is simply defined as persistently elevated arterial blood pressure (BP). Although elevated BP was perceived to be "essential" for adequate perfusion of vital organs during the early and middle 1900s, it is now identified as one of the most significant risk factors for cardiovascular (CV) disease. Increasing awareness and diagnosis of hypertension, and improving control of BP with appropriate treatment are considered critical public health initiatives to reduce CV morbidity and mortality.

The Joint National Committee (JNC) on Prevention, Detection, Evaluation, and Treatment of High Blood Pressure guidelines have been the most prominent evidence-based clinical guideline in the United States for the management of hypertension. The Seventh version of these guidelines, the Seventh Report of the Joint National Committee on Prevention, Detection, Evaluation, and Treatment of High Blood Pressure (JNC7), was published in 2003 and is the last version that was sponsored by the National Heart Lung and Blood Institute (NHLBI).[1] Other publications, particularly, the 2014 Report From the Panel Members Appointed to the Eighth Joint National Committee (JNC8), the 2014 Guidelines by the American Society of Hypertension/International Society of Hypertension (ASH/ISH), and the 2015 American Heart Association (AHA)/American College of Cardiology (ACC)/ASH Scientific Statement provide additional insight regarding pharmacotherapy for hypertension.[2-4] This chapter incorporates relevant components of these documents and additional evidence from clinical trials, with a focus on the pharmacotherapy of hypertension. However, when the ACC/AHA publishes their Guideline on the Management of Hypertension in late 2016, it will represent the most recent evidence-based guideline that should be used in clinical practice.

The National Health and Nutrition Examination Survey and the National Center for Health Statistics regularly assess hypertension in the United States.[5] Data from 2009 to 2012 indicate that approximately 80 million Americans aged 20 years and above have hypertension. Among these patients, 54.1% were at their goal BP, 76.5% were treated, and 82.7% were aware they had hypertension. While these statistics, particularly the control rate, are substantially higher than in the past, there remain many opportunities for clinicians to improve the care of patients with hypertension.

EPIDEMIOLOGY

Approximately one in three adult (age 20 years or older) Americans have elevated BP.[5] The overall incidence is similar between men and women, but varies depending on age. The percentage of men with high BP is higher than that of women before the age of 55 and is similar to that of women between the ages 55 and 64. However, after the age of 64, a much higher percentage of women have high BP than men.[5] Prevalence rates are highest in non-Hispanic blacks (46% in women, 45% in men), followed by non-Hispanic whites (30% in women, 33% in men), and Mexican Americans (30% in both women and men).[3] It is projected that by 2030, over 40% of American adults will have hypertension, which is an increase of 8.4% from 2012.[5]

BP values increase with age, and hypertension (persistently elevated BP values) is very common in the elderly. The lifetime risk of developing hypertension among those 55 years of age and older who are normotensive is 90%.[1] Most patients have prehypertension before they are diagnosed with hypertension, with most diagnoses occurring between the third and fifth decades of life.

ETIOLOGY

In most patients, hypertension results from unknown pathophysiologic etiology (*essential* or *primary hypertension*). This form of hypertension cannot be cured, but it can be controlled. A small percentage of patients have a specific cause of their hypertension (*secondary hypertension*). There are many potential secondary causes that either are concurrent medical conditions or are endogenously induced. If the cause can be identified, hypertension in these patients can be mitigated or potentially be cured.

Essential Hypertension

Over 90% of individuals with high BP have essential hypertension.[1] Numerous mechanisms have been identified that may contribute to the pathogenesis of this form of hypertension, so identifying the exact underlying abnormality is not possible. Genetic factors may play a role in the development of essential hypertension by affecting sodium balance, or other BP regulating pathways. In the future, genetic testing for these traits could lead to alternative approaches to preventing or treating hypertension. However, this is not currently recommended.

Secondary Hypertension

Fewer than 10% of patients have secondary hypertension where either a comorbid disease or a drug (or other product) is responsible for elevating BP (Table 13-1).[1,6] In most of these cases, renal dysfunction resulting from severe chronic kidney disease (CKD) or renovascular disease is the most common secondary cause. Certain drugs (or other products), either directly or indirectly, can cause hypertension or exacerbate hypertension by increasing BP. The most common agents are listed in Table 13-1. When a secondary cause is identified, removing the offending agent (when feasible) or treating/correcting the underlying comorbid condition should be the first step in management.

TABLE 13-1 Secondary Causes of Hypertension

Disease	Drugs and Other Products Associated with Hypertension[a]
Chronic kidney disease **Cushing's syndrome** **Coarctation of the aorta** **Obstructive sleep apnea** **Parathyroid disease** **Pheochromocytoma** **Primary aldosteronism** **Renovascular disease** **Thyroid disease**	**Prescription drugs** • Amphetamines (amphetamine, dexmethylphenidate, dextroamphetamine, lisdexamfetamine, methylphenidate, phendimetrazine, phentermine) • Antivascular endothelin growth factor agents (bevacizumab, sorafenib, sunitinib) • Corticosteroids (cortisone, dexamethasone, fludrocortisone, hydrocortisone, methylprednisolone, prednisolone, prednisone, triamcinolone) • Calcineurin inhibitors (cyclosporine, tacrolimus) • Decongestants (pseudoephedrine, phenylephrine) • Ergot alkaloids (bromocriptine, dihydroergotamine, methysergide) • Erythropoiesis-stimulating agents (erythropoietin, darbepoetin) • Estrogen-containing oral contraceptives • Nonsteroidal anti-inflammatory drugs—cyclooxygenase-2 selective (celecoxib) and nonselective (aspirin [at higher doses], choline magnesium trisalicylate, diclofenac, diflunisal, etodolac, fenoprofen, flurbiprofen, ibuprofen, indomethacin, ketoprofen, ketorolac, meclofenamate, mefenamic acid, meloxicam, nabumetone, naproxen, naproxen sodium, oxaprozin, piroxicam, salsalate, sulindac, tolmetin) • Others: desvenlafaxine, venlafaxine, bupropion Situations: β-blocker or centrally acting α-agonists (when abruptly discontinued); β-blocker without α-blocker first when treating pheochromocytoma; use of a monoamine oxidase inhibitor (isocarboxazid, phenelzine, tranylcypromine) with tyramine-containing foods or certain drugs **Street drugs and other products** • Cocaine and cocaine withdrawal • Ephedra alkaloids (eg, Ma huang), "herbal ecstasy," other analogues • Nicotine and withdrawal, anabolic steroids, narcotic withdrawal, ergot-containing herbal products, St. John's wort **Food substances** • Sodium • Ethanol • Licorice

[a]Agents of most clinical importance.

PATHOPHYSIOLOGY

Multiple factors that control BP are potential contributing components in the development of essential hypertension. These include malfunctions in either humoral (ie, the renin–angiotensin–aldosterone system [RAAS]) or vasodepressor mechanisms, abnormal neuronal mechanisms, defects in peripheral autoregulation, and disturbances in sodium, calcium, and natriuretic hormones. Many of these factors are cumulatively affected by the multifaceted RAAS, which ultimately regulates arterial BP. It is probable that no one factor is solely responsible for essential hypertension.

Arterial BP

Arterial BP is the pressure in the arterial wall measured in millimeters of mercury (mm Hg). The two identified arterial BP values are *systolic BP* (SBP) and *diastolic BP* (DBP). SBP represents the peak value, which is achieved during cardiac contraction. DBP is achieved after

TABLE 13-2 Potential Mechanisms of Pathogenesis

Blood pressure (BP) is the mathematical product of cardiac output and peripheral resistance. Elevated BP can result from increased cardiac output and/or increased total peripheral resistance.

Increased cardiac output	*Increased cardiac preload:* • Increased fluid volume from excess sodium intake or renal sodium retention *Venous constriction:* • Excess stimulation of the renin–angiotensin–aldosterone system (RAAS) • Sympathetic nervous system overactivity
Increased peripheral resistance	*Functional vascular constriction:* • Excess stimulation of the RAAS • Sympathetic nervous system overactivity • Genetic alterations of cell membranes • Endothelial-derived factors *Structural vascular hypertrophy:* • Excess stimulation of the RAAS • Sympathetic nervous system overactivity • Genetic alterations of cell membranes • Endothelial-derived factors • Hyperinsulinemia resulting from the metabolic syndrome

contraction when the cardiac chambers are filling, and represents the nadir value. The difference between SBP and DBP is called the *pulse pressure* and is a measure of arterial wall tension. Mean arterial pressure (MAP) is the average pressure throughout the cardiac cycle of contraction. It is sometimes used clinically to represent overall arterial BP, especially in hypertensive emergency. During a cardiac cycle, two-thirds of the time is spent in diastole and one third in systole. Therefore, the MAP is calculated by using the following equation:

$$\text{MAP} = \left(\text{SBP} \times \frac{1}{3}\right) + \left(\text{DBP} \times \frac{2}{3}\right)$$

Arterial BP is hemodynamically generated by the interplay between blood flow and the resistance to blood flow. It is mathematically defined as the product of cardiac output (CO) and total peripheral resistance (TPR) according to the following equation:

$$\text{BP} = \text{CO} \times \text{TPR}$$

CO is the major determinant of SBP, whereas TPR largely determines DBP. In turn, CO is a function of stroke volume, heart rate, and venous capacitance. Table 13-2 lists physiologic causes of increased CO and TPR and correlates them to potential mechanisms of pathogenesis.

Under normal physiologic conditions, arterial BP fluctuates throughout the day following a circadian rhythm. BP decreases to its lowest values during sleep followed by a sharp rise starting a few hours prior to awakening, with the highest values occurring mid-morning. BP is also increased acutely during physical activity or emotional stress.

Classification

The classification of BP in adults (age 18 years and older) is based on the average of two or more properly measured BP values from two or more clinical encounters (Table 13-3).[1] It includes four categories: normal, prehypertension, stage 1 hypertension, and stage 2 hypertension. Prehypertension is not a disease category, but identifies patients whose BP is likely to increase into the classification of hypertension in the future.

Hypertensive crises are clinical situations where there are extreme BP elevations, typically greater than 180/120 mm Hg. They are categorized as either *hypertensive emergency* or *hypertensive urgency.* Hypertensive emergencies are extreme BP elevations that are accompanied by acute or progressing end-organ damage.

TABLE 13-3 Classification of Blood Pressure in Adults (Age ≥18 Years)[a]

Classification	Systolic Blood Pressure (mm Hg)		Diastolic Blood Pressure (mm Hg)
Normal	<120	and	<80
Prehypertension[b]	120-139	or	80-89
Stage 1 hypertension	140-159	or	90-99
Stage 2 hypertension	≥160	or	≥100

[a]Classification determined based on the average of two or more properly measured seated BP values from two or more clinical encounters. If systolic and diastolic BP values yield different classifications, the highest category is used for the purpose of determining a classification.

[b]For certain patients, BP values within the prehypertension range are considered above goal (see Clinical Presentation "Desired Outcomes: Goal BP Values").

Hypertensive urgencies are extreme BP elevations without acute or progressing end-organ injury.

Cardiovascular Risk and Blood Pressure

1 Epidemiologic data demonstrate a strong correlation between BP and CV morbidity and mortality.[7] Risk of stroke, myocardial infarction (MI), angina, heart failure, kidney failure, or early death from a CV causes (all are hypertension-associated complications) is directly correlated with BP. Starting at a BP of 115/75 mm Hg, the risk of CV disease doubles with every 20/10 mm Hg increase.[1] Even patients with prehypertension have an increased risk of CV disease.

2 Treating patients with hypertension with antihypertensive drug therapy provides significant clinical benefits. Evidence from large-scale placebo-controlled clinical trials has shown that the increased risks of CV events and death associated with elevated BP are reduced substantially by antihypertensive therapy.[8-11] This is discussed in Treatment section of this chapter.

SBP is a stronger predictor of CV disease than DBP in adults aged 50 years and older; it is the most important clinical BP parameter for most patients.[1] Patients are considered to have *isolated systolic hypertension* when their SBP values are elevated (ie, greater than or equal to 140 mm Hg) and DBP values are not (ie, less than 90 mm Hg, but commonly less than 80 mm Hg). Isolated systolic hypertension is believed to result from pathophysiologic changes in the arterial vasculature consistent with aging. These changes decrease the compliance of the arterial wall and portend an increased risk of CV morbidity and mortality. The elevated pulse pressure (SBP minus DBP) is believed to reflect the extent of atherosclerotic disease in the elderly and is a measure of increased arterial stiffness. Higher pulse pressure values seen in those with isolated systolic hypertension are directly correlated with risk of CV mortality.

Humoral Mechanisms

Several humoral abnormalities involving the RAAS, natriuretic hormone, and hyperinsulinemia may be involved in the development of essential hypertension.

The Renin–Angiotensin–Aldosterone System

The RAAS is a complex endogenous system involved with most regulatory components of arterial BP. Activation and regulation is primarily governed by the kidney (Fig. 13-1). The RAAS regulates sodium, potassium, and blood volume. Therefore, this system significantly influences vascular tone and sympathetic nervous system activity, and is the most influential contributor to the homeostatic regulation of BP.

Renin is an enzyme that is stored in the juxtaglomerular cells, which are located in the afferent arterioles of the kidney. The release of renin is modulated by several factors: intrarenal factors (eg, renal perfusion pressure, catecholamines, angiotensin II) and extrarenal factors (eg, sodium, chloride, potassium).

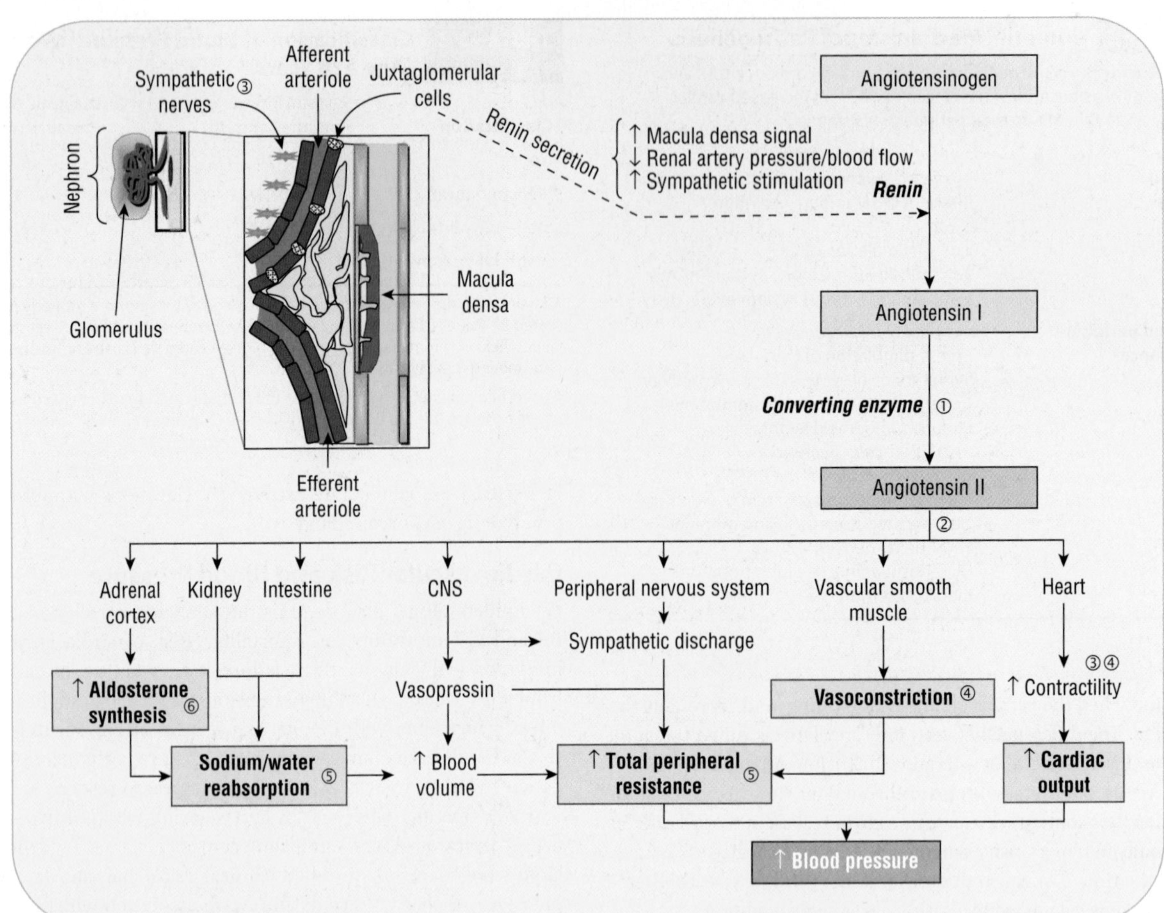

FIGURE 13-1 Diagram representing the renin–angiotensin–aldosterone system. The interrelationship between the kidney, angiotensin II, and regulation of blood pressure is depicted. Renin secretion from the juxtaglomerular cells in the afferent arterioles is regulated by three major factors to trigger conversion of angiotensinogen to angiotensin 1. The primary sites of action for major antihypertensive agents are included: 1 ACE inhibitor; 2 angiotensin II receptor blocker; 3 β-blocker; 4 calcium channel blocker; 5 thiazide; 6 aldosterone antagonist.

Juxtaglomerular cells function as a baroreceptor-sensing device. Decreased renal artery pressure and kidney blood flow is sensed by these cells and stimulates secretion of renin. The juxtaglomerular apparatus also includes a group of specialized distal tubule cells referred to collectively as the *macula densa*. A decrease in sodium and chloride delivered to the distal tubule stimulates renin release. Catecholamines increase renin release probably by directly stimulating sympathetic nerves on the afferent arterioles that in turn activate the juxtaglomerular cells.

Renin catalyzes the conversion of angiotensinogen to angiotensin I in the blood. Angiotensin I is then converted to angiotensin II by angiotensin-converting enzyme (ACE). After binding to specific receptors (classified as either angiotensin II type 1 [AT_1] or angiotensin II type 2 [AT_2] subtypes), angiotensin II exerts biologic effects in several tissues. The AT_1 receptor is located in brain, kidney, myocardium, peripheral vasculature, and the adrenal glands. These receptors mediate most responses that are critical to CV and kidney function. The AT_2 receptor is located in adrenal medullary tissue, uterus, and brain. Stimulation of the AT_2 receptor does not influence BP regulation.

Circulating angiotensin II can elevate BP through pressor and volume effects. Pressor effects include direct vasoconstriction, stimulation of catecholamine release from the adrenal medulla, and centrally mediated increases in sympathetic nervous system activity. Angiotensin II also stimulates aldosterone synthesis from the adrenal cortex. This leads to sodium and water reabsorption that increases plasma volume, TPR, and ultimately BP. Aldosterone also has a deleterious role in the pathophysiology of other CV diseases (eg, heart failure, MI, and kidney disease) by promoting tissue remodeling leading to myocardial fibrosis and vascular dysfunction. Clearly, any disturbance in the body that leads to activation of the RAAS could explain chronic hypertension.

The heart and brain contain a local RAAS. In the heart, angiotensin II is also generated by angiotensin I convertase (human chymase). This enzyme is not blocked by ACE inhibition. Activation of the myocardial RAAS increases cardiac contractility and stimulates cardiac hypertrophy. In the brain, angiotensin II modulates the production and release of hypothalamic and pituitary hormones, and enhances sympathetic outflow from the medulla oblongata.

Natriuretic Hormone

Natriuretic hormone inhibits sodium and potassium-ATPase and thus interferes with sodium transport across cell membranes. Inherited defects in the kidney's ability to eliminate sodium can cause increased blood volume. A compensatory increase in the concentration of circulating natriuretic hormone theoretically could increase urinary excretion of sodium and water. However, this hormone might block the active transport of sodium out of arteriolar smooth muscle cells. The increased intracellular sodium concentration ultimately would increase vascular tone and BP.

Neuronal Regulation

Central and autonomic nervous systems are intricately involved in the regulation of arterial BP. Many receptors that either enhance or inhibit norepinephrine release are located on the presynaptic surface of sympathetic terminals. The α and β presynaptic receptors play a role in negative and positive feedback to the norepinephrine—containing vesicles. Stimulation of presynaptic α-receptors (α_2) exerts a negative inhibition on norepinephrine release. Stimulation of presynaptic β-receptors facilitates norepinephrine release.

Sympathetic neuronal fibers located on the surface of effector cells innervate the α- and β-receptors. Stimulation of postsynaptic α-receptors (α_1) on arterioles and venules results in vasoconstriction. There are two types of postsynaptic β-receptors: β_1 and β_2. Both are present in all tissues innervated by the sympathetic nervous system. However, in some tissues β_1-receptors predominate (eg, heart), and in other tissues β_2-receptors predominate (eg, bronchioles). Stimulation of β_1-receptors in the heart results in an increase in heart rate (chronotropy) and force of contraction (ionotropy), whereas stimulation of β_2-receptors in the arterioles and venules causes vasodilation.

The baroreceptor reflex system is the major negative feedback mechanism that controls sympathetic activity. Baroreceptors are nerve endings lying in the walls of large arteries, especially in the carotid arteries and aortic arch. Changes in arterial BP rapidly activate baroreceptors that then transmit impulses to the brain stem through the ninth cranial nerve and vagus nerve. In this reflex system, a decrease in arterial BP stimulates baroreceptors, causing reflex vasoconstriction and increased heart rate and force of cardiac contraction. These baroreceptor reflex mechanisms may be less responsive in the elderly and those with diabetes.

Stimulation of certain areas within the central nervous system (eg, nucleus tractus solitarius, vagal nuclei, vasomotor center, and area postrema) can either increase or decrease BP. For example, α_2-adrenergic stimulation within the central nervous system decreases BP through an inhibitory effect on the vasomotor center. However, angiotensin II increases sympathetic outflow from the vasomotor center, which increases BP.

The purpose of these neuronal mechanisms is to regulate BP and maintain homeostasis. Pathologic disturbances in any of the four major components (autonomic nerve fibers, adrenergic receptors, baroreceptors, and central nervous system) could chronically elevate BP. These systems are physiologically interrelated. A defect in one component may alter normal function in another. Therefore, cumulative abnormalities may explain the development of essential hypertension.

Peripheral Autoregulatory Components

Abnormalities in renal or tissue autoregulatory systems could cause hypertension. It is possible that a renal defect in sodium excretion may develop, which can then cause resetting of tissue autoregulatory processes resulting in a higher BP. The kidney usually maintains a normal BP through a volume–pressure adaptive mechanism. When BP drops, the kidneys respond by increasing retention of sodium and water, which leads to plasma volume expansion that increases BP. Conversely, when BP rises above normal, renal sodium and water excretion are increased to reduce plasma volume and CO.

Local autoregulatory processes maintain adequate tissue oxygenation. When tissue oxygen demand is normal to low, the local arteriolar bed remains relatively vasoconstricted. However, increase in metabolic demand triggers arteriolar vasodilation that lowers peripheral vascular resistance (PVR) and increases blood flow and oxygen delivery.

Intrinsic defects in renal adaptive mechanisms could lead to plasma volume expansion and increased blood flow to peripheral tissues, even when BP is normal. Local tissue autoregulatory processes that vasoconstrict would then be activated to offset the increased blood flow. This effect would result in increased PVR and, if sustained, would also result in thickening of the arteriolar walls. This pathophysiologic component is plausible because increased TPR is a common underlying finding in patients with essential hypertension.

Vascular Endothelial Mechanisms

Vascular endothelium and smooth muscle play important roles in regulating blood vessel tone and BP. These regulating functions are mediated by vasoactive substances that are synthesized by endothelial cells. It has been postulated that a deficiency in local synthesis of vasodilating substances (eg, prostacyclin and bradykinin) or excess vasoconstricting substances (eg, angiotensin II and endothelin I) contributes to essential hypertension, atherosclerosis, and other CV diseases.

Nitric oxide is produced in the endothelium, relaxes the vascular epithelium, and is a very potent vasodilator. The nitric oxide system is an important regulator of arterial BP. Patients with hypertension may have an intrinsic nitric oxide deficiency, resulting in inadequate vasodilation.

Electrolytes

Epidemiologic and clinical data have associated excess sodium intake with hypertension. Population-based studies indicate that high-sodium diets are associated with a high prevalence of stroke and hypertension. Conversely, low-sodium diets are associated with a lower prevalence of hypertension. Clinical studies have shown that dietary sodium restriction lowers BP in many (but not all) patients with elevated BP. The exact mechanisms by which excess sodium leads to hypertension are not known.

Alterations in calcium and potassium may also play an important role in the pathogenesis of hypertension. A lack of dietary calcium hypothetically can disturb the balance between intracellular and extracellular calcium, resulting in an increased intracellular calcium concentration and alterations in vascular smooth muscle function. Potassium depletion may increase PVR, but the clinical significance of small serum potassium concentration changes is unclear. While altered calcium and potassium may play a role in the development of hypertension, data demonstrating reduced CV risk with supplementation are very limited.

CLINICAL PRESENTATION

The clinical presentation of hypertension is described in Clinical Presentation "Hypertension".

Diagnostic Considerations

3 Hypertension is called the *silent killer* because most patients do not have symptoms. The primary physical finding is elevated BP. The diagnosis of hypertension cannot be made based on only one elevated BP measurement. The average of two or more measurements taken during two or more clinical encounters is required to diagnose hypertension.[1] This BP average should be used to establish a diagnosis, and then classify the stage of hypertension using Table 13-3.

Measuring BP

The measurement of BP is a common routine medical screening tool that should be conducted at every healthcare encounter.[1]

Cuff Measurement The most common procedure to measure BP in clinical practice is the indirect measurement of BP using an oscillometric device or sphygmomanometry. The appropriate procedure to indirectly measure BP has been described by the AHA.[12] It is imperative that the measurement equipment (ie, inflation cuff, stethoscope, and manometer) meet national standards to ensure maximum quality and precision with measurement.

The AHA stepwise technique is recommended:

1. Patients should ideally refrain from nicotine and caffeine ingestion for 30 minutes and sit with lower back supported

CLINICAL PRESENTATION Hypertension

General: May Appear Healthy or May Have Additional CV Risk Factors:

- Age (greater than or equal to 55 years for men, greater than or equal to 65 years for women)
- Diabetes (type 1 or type 2)
- Dyslipidemia
- Albuminuria
- Family history of premature CV disease
- Overweight (body mass index [BMI] 27-29.9 kg/m^2) or Obesity (BMI greater than or equal to 30 kg/m^2)
- Physical inactivity
- Tobacco use

Symptoms: Usually none related to elevated BP.

Signs: Previously elevated BP values in the prehypertension or the hypertension category.

Routine laboratory tests: Blood urea nitrogen (BUN)/ serum creatinine, fasting lipid panel, fasting blood glucose, serum electrolytes (sodium, potassium), hemoglobin and hematocrit, and spot urine albumin-to-creatinine ratio. May have normal values and still have hypertension. However, some patients may have abnormal values consistent with either additional CV risk factors or hypertension-related damage.

Other tests: 12-Lead electrocardiogram, estimated GFR (using modification of diet in renal disease [MDRD] equation).

Hypertension-related complications: The patient may have a previous medical history or diagnostic findings that indicate the presence of hypertension-associated complications:

- **Brain** (stroke, transient ischemic attack, dementia)
- **Eyes** (retinopathy)
- **Heart** (left ventricular hypertrophy [LVH], angina, prior MI, prior coronary revascularization, heart failure)
- **Kidney** (chronic kidney disease [CKD])
- **Peripheral vasculature** (peripheral arterial disease [PAD])

in a chair. Their bare arm should be supported and resting near heart level. Feet should be flat on the floor (with legs not crossed). The measurement environment should be relatively quiet and ideally provide privacy. Measuring BP in a position other than seated (supine or standing position) may be required under special circumstances (eg, suspected orthostatic hypotension, dehydration).

2. Measurement should begin only after a 5-minute period of rest.
3. A properly sized cuff (pediatric, small, regular, large, or extra large) should be used. The inflatable rubber bladder should be at least 80% of arm circumference and a width that is at least 40% of arm circumference.
4. The palpatory method should be used to estimate the SBP:
   a. Place the cuff on the upper arm 2 to 3 cm above the antecubital fossa and attach it to the manometer.
   b. Close the inflation valve and inflate the cuff to 70 mm Hg. Palpate the radial pulse with the index and middle fingers of the opposite hand.
   c. Inflate further in increments of 10 mm Hg until the radial pulse can no longer be palpated.
   d. Note the pressure at which the radial pulse is no longer palpated. This is the estimated SBP.
   e. Release the pressure in the cuff by opening the valve.
5. The bell (use the diaphragm only if using the bell is not possible) of the stethoscope should be placed on the skin of the antecubital fossa, directly over where the brachial artery is palpated. The stethoscope earpieces should be inserted appropriately. The valve should be closed, with the cuff then inflated to 30 mm Hg above the estimated SBP from the palpatory method. The valve should then be slightly opened to slowly release pressure at a rate of approximately 2 mm Hg/s.
6. The clinician should listen for Korotkoff sounds with the stethoscope. The first phase of Korotkoff sounds is the initial presence of clear tapping sounds. Note the pressure at the first recognition of these sounds. This is the SBP. As pressure deflates, note the pressure when all sounds disappear, right at the last sound. This is the DBP.
7. Measurements should be rounded to the nearest 2 mm Hg.
8. A second measurement should be obtained after at least 1 minute. If these values differ by more than 5 mm Hg, additional measurements should be obtained.
9. Neither the patient nor the observer should talk during measurement.
10. When first establishing care with a patient, BP should be measured in both arms. If consistent inter-arm differences exist, the arm with the higher value should be used.

Inaccuracies with indirect measurements result from inherent biologic variability of BP, inaccuracies related to suboptimal technique, and the white coat effect.[12] Variations in BP occur with environmental temperature, the time of day and year, meals, physical activity, posture, alcohol, nicotine, and emotions. In the clinic setting, standard BP measurement procedures (eg, appropriate rest period, correct technique, wrong cuff size) are often not followed, which results in poor estimation of true BP. In addition, variations may occur between individuals measuring BP due to differences in hearing or technique. Due to various human factors related to manual measurements of BP, use of oscillometric devices is generally preferred.

Approximately 15% to 20% of patients have *white coat hypertension*, where BP values rise in a clinical setting but return to normal in nonclinical environments using home or ambulatory BP (ABP) measurements.[12] Interestingly, the rise in BP dissipates gradually after leaving the clinical setting. It may or may not be precipitated by other stresses in the patient's daily life. This is in contrast to *masked hypertension*, where a decrease in BP occurs in the clinical setting.[13] With masked hypertension, home BP is hypertensive, while the in-office BP is normotensive or substantially lower than that at home. This situation may lead to under treatment or lack of treatment for hypertension. Moreover, patients with either white coat or masked hypertension have a high risk of progressing to develop sustained hypertension, which can result in a higher risk of CV events compared with normotensive patients.[14]

Pseudohypertension is a falsely elevated BP measurement. It may be seen in the elderly, those with long-standing diabetes, or those with CKD due to rigid, calcified brachial arteries.[12] In these patients, the true arterial BP when measured directly with intra-arterial measurement (the most accurate measurement of BP) is much lower than that measured using the indirect cuff method. The Osler's maneuver can be used to test for pseudohypertension. In this maneuver, the BP cuff is inflated above peak SBP. If the radial artery remains palpable, the patient has a positive Osler's sign (rigid artery), which may indicate pseudohypertension.

Elderly patients with a wide pulse pressure may have an auscultatory gap that can lead to underestimated SBP or overestimated DBP measurements.[12] In this situation, as the cuff pressure falls from the true SBP value, the Korotkoff sound may disappear (indicating a false DBP measurement), reappear (a false SBP measurement), and then disappear again at the true DBP value. When an auscultatory gap is present, Korotkoff sounds are usually heard when pressure in the cuff first starts to decrease after inflation. This may be eliminated by raising the arm overhead by 30 seconds before bringing it to the proper position and inflating the cuff. This maneuver decreases the intravascular volume and improves inflow thereby allowing Korotkoff sounds to be heard.[12]

Ambulatory and Self-BP Monitoring Ambulatory BP (ABP) monitoring using an automated device can document BP at frequent time intervals (eg, every 15-30 minutes) throughout a 24-hour period.[12] ABP values are usually lower than clinic-measured values. The definition of hypertension for ABP is greater than or equal to 135/85 mm Hg during the day, greater than or equal to 120/75 mm Hg nighttime (or asleep), and greater than or equal to 130/80 mm Hg over 24 hours.[12] For self-BP monitoring, a BP greater than or equal to 135/85 mm Hg is considered hypertensive. Self-BP measurements are collected by patients, preferably in the morning, using home monitoring devices.

Neither ABP nor self-BP monitoring is required for the routine diagnosis of hypertension. However, these modalities can enhance the ability to identify patients with white coat and masked hypertension.[13] Recommendations from the United States Preventive Services Task Force recommend outside of clinical setting measurements for diagnostic confirmation before starting antihypertensive therapy.[15] ABP and self-BP measurements may also be useful in evaluating and optimizing BP control for patients on antihypertensive drug therapy. ABP monitoring may be helpful for patients with apparent drug resistance, hypotensive symptoms while on antihypertensive therapy, episodic hypertension (eg, white coat hypertension), autonomic dysfunction, and in identifying "nondippers" whose BP does not decrease by greater than 10% during sleep and who may portend increased risk of BP-related complications.[12]

Limitations of ABP and self-BP measurements may prohibit routine use in some patients. These include complexity of use, costs, and lack of prospective outcome data describing normal ranges for these measurements. Although self-monitoring of BP at home is less complicated and less costly than ambulatory monitoring, patients may omit or fabricate readings, or have poor technique (eg, not resting for adequate period of time, improper placement, wrong cuff size).

Clinical Evaluation

Frequently, the only sign of essential hypertension is elevated BP. The rest of the physical examination may be completely normal. However, a complete medical evaluation (a comprehensive medical history, physical examination, and laboratory and/or diagnostic tests) is recommended after diagnosis to (a) identify secondary causes, (b) identify other CV risk factors or comorbid conditions that may define prognosis and/or guide therapy, and (c) assess for the presence or absence of hypertension-associated complications. All patients with hypertension should have the tests described in Clinical Presentation "Hypertension" measured prior to initiating therapy.[1] For patients without a history of coronary artery disease, noncoronary atherosclerotic vascular disease (ASCVD), left ventricular dysfunction, or diabetes, it is also important to estimate future risk of CV disease and clinical ASCVD. The 10-year risk of clinical ASCVD (defined as coronary death or nonfatal myocardial infarction, or fatal or nonfatal stroke) based on the Pooled Cohort Equations and lifetime risk prediction tools can be found at: *http://tools.acc.org/ASCVD-Risk-Estimator/*

Secondary Causes

The most common secondary causes of hypertension are listed in Table 13-1. A complete medical evaluation should provide clues for identifying secondary hypertension.

Patients with secondary hypertension might have signs or symptoms suggestive of the underlying disorder. Patients with pheochromocytoma may have a history of paroxysmal headaches, sweating, tachycardia, and palpitations. Over half of these patients suffer from episodes of orthostatic hypotension. In primary hyperaldosteronism symptoms related to hypokalemia usually include muscle cramps and muscle weakness. Patients with Cushing's syndrome may complain of weight gain, polyuria, edema, menstrual irregularities, recurrent acne, or muscular weakness and have several classic physical features (eg, moon face, buffalo hump, hirsutism). Patients with coarctation of the aorta may have higher BP in the arms than in legs and diminished or even absent femoral pulses. Patients with renal artery stenosis may have an abdominal systolic–diastolic bruit.

Routine laboratory tests may also help identify secondary hypertension. Baseline hypokalemia may suggest mineralocorticoid-induced hypertension. Protein, red blood cells, and casts in the urine may indicate renovascular disease. Some laboratory tests are used specifically to diagnose secondary hypertension. These include plasma norepinephrine and urinary metanephrine for pheochromocytoma, plasma and urinary aldosterone concentrations for primary hyperaldosteronism, and plasma renin activity, captopril stimulation test, renal vein renin, and renal artery angiography for renovascular disease.

Certain drugs and other products can result in drug-induced hypertension (see Table 13-1). For some patients, the addition of these agents can be the cause of elevated BP or can exacerbate underlying hypertension. Identifying a temporal relationship between starting the suspected agent and developing elevated BP is most suggestive of drug-induced BP elevation.

Natural Course of Disease

Essential hypertension is usually preceded by elevated BP values that are in the prehypertension category. BP values may fluctuate between elevated and normal levels for a period. As the disease progresses, PVR increases, and BP elevation becomes chronic.

Hypertension-Associated Complications

There are several complications that can result as a consequence of high BP in patients with hypertension (see Clinical Presentation "Hypertension"). CV events (eg, MI, cerebrovascular events, kidney failure) are the primary causes of CV morbidity and mortality in patients with hypertension. The probability of CV events and CV morbidity and mortality in patients with hypertension is directly correlated with the severity of BP elevation.

Hypertension accelerates atherosclerosis and stimulates left ventricular and vascular dysfunction. These pathologic changes are thought to be secondary to both a chronic pressure overload and a variety of nonhemodynamic stimuli. Several nonhemodynamic disturbances have been implicated in these effects (eg, the adrenergic system, RAAS, increased synthesis and secretion of endothelin I, decreased production of prostacyclin and nitric oxide). Atherosclerosis in hypertension is accompanied by the proliferation of smooth muscle cells, lipid infiltration into the vascular endothelium, and enhancement of vascular calcium accumulation.

Cerebrovascular disease is a consequence of hypertension. A neurologic assessment can detect either gross neurologic deficits or a slight hemiparesis with some incoordination and hyperreflexia that are indicative of cerebrovascular disease. Stroke can result from lacunar infarcts caused by thrombotic occlusion of small vessels or intracerebral hemorrhage resulting from ruptured microaneurysms. Transient ischemic attacks secondary to atherosclerotic disease in the carotid arteries can also happen in patients with hypertension.

Retinopathies can occur in hypertension and may manifest as a variety of different findings. A funduscopic examination can detect hypertensive retinopathy, and the result can be categorized according to the Keith-Wagener-Barker retinopathy classification. Retinopathy manifests as arteriolar narrowing, focal arteriolar constrictions, arteriovenous crossing changes (nicking), retinal hemorrhages and exudates, and disk edema. Accelerated arteriosclerosis, a long-term consequence of essential hypertension, can cause nonspecific changes such as increased light reflex, increased tortuosity of vessels, and arteriovenous nicking. Focal arteriolar narrowing, retinal infarcts, and flame-shaped hemorrhages usually are suggestive of an accelerated or malignant phase of hypertension. Papilledema is swelling of the optic disk caused by a breakdown in autoregulation of capillary blood flow in the presence of high pressure. It is usually only present in hypertensive emergencies.

Heart disease is a commonly identified complication of hypertension. A thorough cardiac and pulmonary examination can identify cardiopulmonary abnormalities. Clinical manifestations include LVH, coronary heart disease (angina, prior MI, and prior coronary revascularization), and heart failure. These complications may lead to cardiac arrhythmias, angina, MI, and sudden death. Coronary disease (also called *coronary heart disease*) and associated CV events are the most common causes of death in patients with hypertension.

The kidney damage caused by hypertension is characterized pathologically by hyaline arteriosclerosis, hyperplastic arteriosclerosis, arteriolar hypertrophy, fibrinoid necrosis, and atheroma of the major renal arteries. Glomerular hyperfiltration and intraglomerular hypertension are early stages of hypertensive nephropathy. Albuminuria is followed by a gradual decline in renal function. The primary renal complication in hypertension is nephrosclerosis, which is secondary to arteriosclerosis. Atheromatous disease of a major renal artery may give rise to renal artery stenosis. Although overt kidney failure is an uncommon complication of essential hypertension, it is an important cause of end-stage kidney disease, especially in African Americans, Hispanics, and Native Americans.

The peripheral vasculature is a target organ. Physical examination of the vascular system can detect evidence of atherosclerosis, which may present as arterial bruits (aortic, abdominal, or peripheral), distended veins, diminished or absent peripheral arterial pulses, or lower extremity edema. Peripheral arterial disease (PAD) is a clinical condition that can result from atherosclerosis, which is accelerated in hypertension. Other CV risk factors (eg, smoking) can increase the likelihood of PAD as well as all other complications.

TREATMENT

Overall Goal of Treatment

4 The overall goal of treating hypertension is to reduce associated morbidity and mortality from CV events (eg, coronary events, cerebrovascular events, heart failure, kidney disease). Therefore, the specific selection of antihypertensive drug therapy should be based on evidence demonstrating CV event reduction.

Surrogate Targets—Blood Pressure Goals

5 Treating patients with hypertension to achieve a desired target BP value is a surrogate goal of therapy. Reducing BP to goal does not guarantee prevention of hypertension-associated complications, but is associated with a lower risk. Targeting a goal BP value is how clinicians evaluate response to therapy. It is the primary method used to determine the need for titration and regimen modification.

Most guidelines recommend a goal BP of less than 140/90 mm Hg for the management of hypertension in most patients (Clinical Presentation "Desired Outcomes: Goal BP Values").[1-4] The American Diabetes Association historically recommended lower BP goals for patients with diabetes, but now recommend a standard goal of less than 140/90 mm Hg for most patients with diabetes.[16] A lower BP goal of less than 130/80 mm Hg may be

CLINICAL PRESENTATION Desired Outcomes: Goal BP Values

Most patients, including diabetes and/or CKD and the elderly

- less than 140/90 mm Hg

Frail elderly at high risk for serious adverse effects

- less than 150/90 mm Hg

Certain Patients with lower goals as a therapeutic option (not a standard of care)

- Some patients with diabetes (eg, younger patients), less than 130/80 mm Hg may be an option if achieved without undue treatment burden
- Some patients with CKD (nondialysis) who have persistent urine albumin excretion of greater than 30 mg per 24 hours (or equivalent), less than 130/80 mm Hg may be an option if achieved without undue treatment burden
- Some patients greater than 50 years at increased risk of CV disease (one or more risk factors including clinical or subclinical CVD other than stroke, CKD with eGFR 20-60 mL/min/1.73m^2, 10-year risk of CVD greater than or equal to 15%, greater than or equal to 75 years) but without diabetes, may consider SBP goal less than 120 mm Hg

appropriate for certain patients (eg, younger patients) if achieved without undue treatment burden, but this is simply a therapeutic option. Similarly, the Kidney Disease Improving Global Outcomes (KDIGO) guidelines recommend a BP goal of 140/90 mm Hg for patients with hypertension and CKD (nondialysis), with a lower BP goal of less than 130/80 mm Hg only for those patients who have persistent albuminuria (greater than 30 mg urine albumin excretion per 24 hours or equivalent) as a therapeutic option.[17,18]

Until the new ACC/AHA guidelines are available, clinicians should follow the goals listed in Clinical Presentation "Desired Outcomes: Goal BP Values". Of note, the Systolic Blood Pressure Intervention Trial (SPRINT) was recently published that evaluated a BP goal of less than 120 mm Hg versus less than 140 mm Hg in certain high CV risk patients with hypertension, but without diabetes.[19] The study was stopped early after a median follow-up of 3.3 years due to significantly lower risk of the primary composite outcome (MI, other acute coronary syndromes, stroke, heart failure, or death from CV causes) and all-cause mortality in patients treated to the lower BP goal. Although SPRINT has demonstrated a benefit of a lower BP goal, clinicians should be cautious until details of this clinical trial have been fully interpreted and incorporated into evidence-based guidelines before broadly applying this lower BP goal. Treating patients to lower than normal BP goals may lead to harm. In SPRINT, there was increased risk of adverse events in the more intensive treatment group including hypotension, syncope, electrolyte abnormalities, and acute kidney injury or failure. However, this may be outweighed by the significant benefits. Therefore, waiting until full interpretation and application of SPRINT is recommended.

Evidence Supporting BP Goal of Less Than 140/90 mm Hg in Most Patients Lower goal DBP values have been evaluated prospectively in the Hypertension Optimal Treatment (HOT) study.[20] In this study, over 18,700 patients were randomized to DBP goals of less than equal to 90, less than equal to 85, less than equal to 80 mm Hg. Although actual DBP values achieved were 85.2, 83.2, and 81.1 mm Hg, respectively, there were no significant differences in risk of major CV events when the three DBP goal groups were compared with each other. Therefore, the HOT data did not demonstrate that lower DBP goals were better than the standard DBP goal of less than 90 mm Hg. However, when the relationship between actual BP values and risk of CV events was evaluated, there was a trend that lower DBP values were better.

A major limitation of the HOT study is the use of DBP goal values. SBP is more directly correlated to CV risk than DBP in most patients with hypertension, especially those above the age of 50. Therefore, data from the HOT study cannot determine the optimal SBP goal value. It is important to note that no J-curve relationship was seen. The *J-curve hypothesis* suggests that lowering BP too much might increase the risk of CV events.[21] This theoretical hypothesis was described many years ago and was originally suggested in observational studies. Therefore, it remains an unproven hypothesis, and may be viewed with particular skepticism considering the recent results of SPRINT.[19]

Additional data are available that suggest lower is better when SBP goal values are targeted. In a recent systematic review and meta-analysis of 19 trials involving 44,989 patients, CV events and renal outcomes were compared between intensive versus less intensive BP-lowering treatment. Compared to less intensive BP-lowering (mean BP 140/81 mm Hg), intensive treatment (mean BP 133/76 mm Hg) was associated with a reduced risk of major CV events, MI, stroke, albuminuria, and retinopathy progression. There was no significant reduction in heart failure, CV death, total mortality, or end-stage kidney disease. The risk of serious adverse events with intensive therapy was low and did not differ significantly compared to less-intensive treatment. However, severe hypotension was more frequent. Therefore, additional evidence is available supporting lower BP goals, particularly for patients at increased CV risk.[22]

Clinical **Controversy...**

HOW LOW TO GO IN MOST PATIENTS?

A standard BP goal of less than 140/90 mm Hg is recommended for most patients with hypertension. Lower goals were historically recommended in specific patient populations, but now are only a therapeutic option for select patients (eg, younger patients with diabetes, CKD patients that have persistent albuminuria). However, the SPRINT was a prospective randomized trial that compared a standard SBP goal of less than 140 mm Hg to a lower SBP goal of less than 120 mm Hg in high risk patients with hypertension. Patients with a history of diabetes or a history of stroke were excluded. The trial was stopped early due to a significant reduction in CVD events and mortality associated with the lower SBP goal. Until these data are fully interpreted and incorporated into evidence-based treatment guidelines, clinicians should use caution if applying the results of SPRINT widely and should consider using standard BP goals for most patients with hypertension.

Limited Evidence Supporting Lower BP Goals in Diabetes

A BP goal of less than 130/80 mm Hg was historically recommended for patients with diabetes for many years, by multiple organizations. The primary evidence supporting this recommendation was from the HOT study, where the only subgroup to show a lower risk of major CV events in the less than 80 mm Hg group versus the less than 90 mm Hg group was in patients with diabetes (n = 1,501).

The NHLBI-sponsored Action to Control Cardiovascular Risk in Diabetes Blood Pressure (ACCORD-BP) study evaluated the benefit of lower BP goals for patients with diabetes.[23] The ACCORD-BP was an open-label, factorial study that randomized 4,733 patients with type 2 diabetes to intensive therapy targeting a SBP of less than 120 mm Hg, or to standard therapy targeting a SBP less than 140 mm Hg for a mean follow-up of 4.7 years. After 1 year, an average of 3.4 medications was needed in the intensive therapy group to attain a mean SBP of 119.3 mm Hg, compared with an average of 2.1 medications in the standard therapy group to attain a mean SBP of 133.5 mm Hg. This difference was generally maintained throughout the study duration. However, there was no significant difference in the annual rate of the primary end point (nonfatal MI, nonfatal stroke, or CV death) between the two groups. The annual incidence of the secondary end point of stroke was lower with the intensive therapy group versus the standard therapy group, and this was the only prespecified end point that was different between the two groups. Reasons for discordant findings of ACCORD-BP compared to SPRINT could be due to study design and lack of power.

Despite consensus guidelines historically recommending a BP goal of less than 130/80 mm Hg for patients with diabetes, evidence supporting this approach over a standard goal of less than 140/90 mm Hg is marginal, and comes at the cost of increased side effects (eg, hypotension, hyperkalemia, bradycardia). While the ACCORD-BP provided additional evidence evaluating BP goals for patients with diabetes, these data do not provide all of the clinical answers that are needed. The ACCORD-BP was open label, and those in the standard group (SBP less than 140 mm Hg) actually had SBP values that were closer to 130 mm Hg than to 140 mm Hg. Based on these data, in 2015 the American Diabetes Association changed their recommendation to a goal BP of less than 140/90 mm Hg for most patients with hypertension and diabetes.[16] The KDIGO guidelines recommend a

BP goal of less than 140/90 mm Hg for patients with hypertension and CKD (nondialysis) and a BP goal of less than 130/80 mm Hg only for those patients who have persistently increased urine albumin excretion.[17]

Avoiding Clinical Inertia

Although hypertension is one of the most common medical conditions, BP control rates are poor. *Clinical inertia* in hypertension has been defined as an office visit at which no therapeutic move was made to lower BP in a patient with uncontrolled hypertension.[24] Clinical inertia is not the entire reason why many patients with hypertension do not achieve goal BP values. However, it is certainly a major reason that can be remedied simply through more aggressive treatment with drug therapy. This strategy can include initiating, titrating, or changing drug therapy.

General Approach to Treatment

Most patients should be placed on both lifestyle modifications and drug therapy concurrently after a diagnosis of hypertension. Lifestyle modification alone is appropriate for most patients with prehypertension. However, lifestyle modifications alone may not adequately lower BP in patients who have hypertension. Patients with additional CV risk factors or those with hypertension-associated complications will typically need antihypertensive drug therapy in addition to lifestyle modifications.

6 The choice of initial antihypertensive drug therapy depends on the degree of BP elevation and presence of compelling indications (discussed in the Pharmacotherapy section later). Most patients with stage 1 hypertension should be initially treated with a first-line antihypertensive drug or the combination of two. Combination drug therapy is recommended for patients with more severe BP elevation (stage 2 hypertension), using preferably two first-line antihypertensive drugs. This general approach is outlined in Fig. 13-2. There are six compelling indications where specific antihypertensive drug classes have evidence showing unique benefits in patients with hypertension and the listed compelling indication (Fig. 13-3).

Nonpharmacologic Therapy

7 All patients with prehypertension and hypertension should be prescribed lifestyle modifications. However, they should never be used as a replacement for antihypertensive drug therapy for patients with hypertension who are not at goal BP, especially in those with additional CV risk factors or hypertension-associated complications. Recommended modifications that have been shown to lower BP are listed in Table 13-4.[25] They can provide small to moderate reductions in SBP. Aside from lowering BP in patients with known hypertension, strict adherence with lifestyle modification can decrease the progression to hypertension in patients with prehypertension BP values.

A sensible dietary program is one that is designed to reduce weight gradually (for overweight and obese patients) and one that restricts sodium intake with only moderate alcohol consumption if one consumes alcohol. Successful implementation of dietary lifestyle modifications by clinicians requires aggressive promotion through patient education, encouragement, and continued reinforcement. The rationale for dietary intervention in hypertension can be explained to patients as follows:

1. Weight loss, as little as 5% to 10% of your body weight, can decrease BP significantly in overweight or obese patients.
2. Diets rich in fruits and vegetables and low in saturated fat have been shown to lower BP in patients with hypertension.
3. Most people experience some BP lowering with sodium restriction.

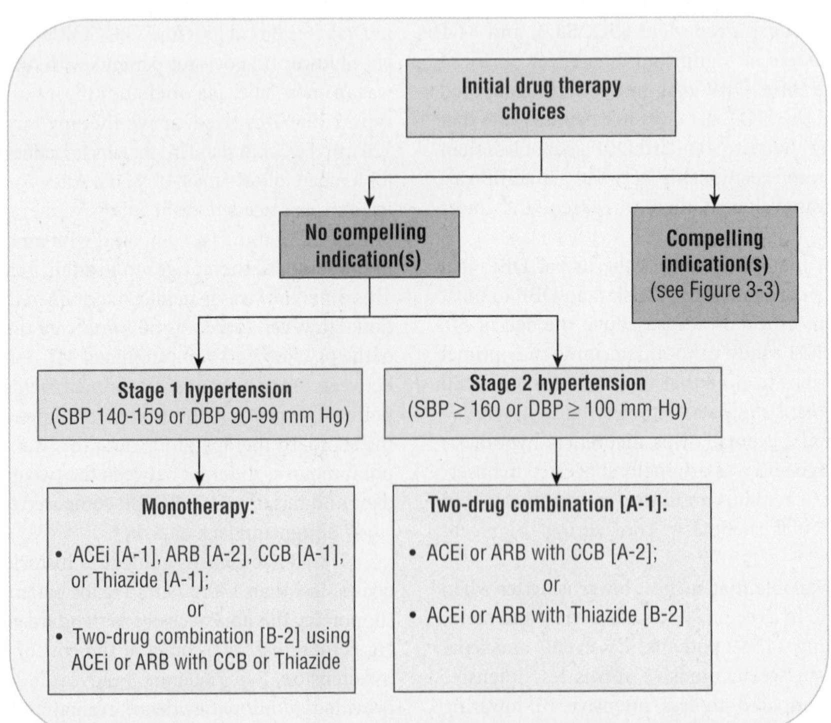

FIGURE 13-2 Algorithm for treatment of hypertension. Drug therapy recommendations are graded with strength of recommendation and quality of evidence in brackets. Strength of recommendations: A, B, and C are good, moderate, and poor evidence to support recommendation, respectively. Quality of evidence: (1) evidence from more than one properly randomized controlled trial; (2) evidence from at least one well-designed clinical trial with randomization, from cohort or case-controlled studies, or dramatic results from uncontrolled experiments or subgroup analyses; (3) evidence from opinions of respected authorities, based on clinical experience, descriptive studies, or reports of expert communities.

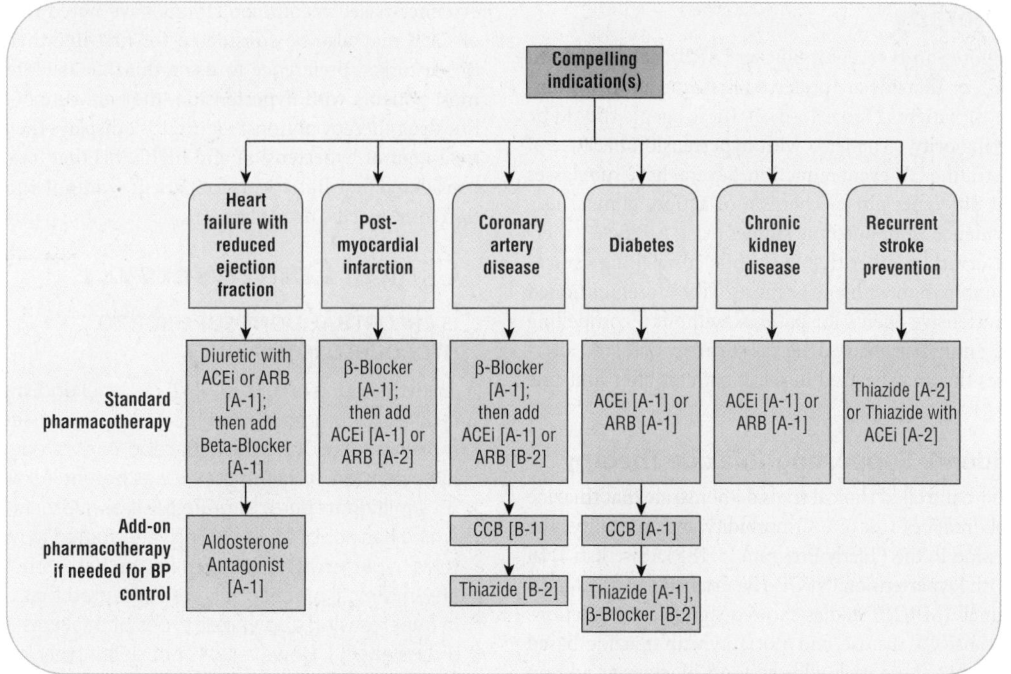

FIGURE 13-3 Compelling indications for individual drug classes. Compelling indications for specific drugs are evidenced-based recommendations from outcome studies or existing clinical guidelines. The order of drug therapies serves as a general guidance that should be balanced with clinical judgment and patient response. Add-on pharmacotherapy recommendations are when additional agents are needed to lower BP to goal values. Blood pressure control should be managed concurrently with the compelling indication. Drug therapy recommendations are graded with strength of recommendation and quality of evidence in brackets. Strength of recommendations: A, B, and C are good, moderate, and poor evidence to support recommendation, respectively. Quality of evidence: (1) evidence from more than one properly randomized controlled trial; (2) evidence from at least one well-designed clinical trial with randomization, from cohort or case-controlled analytic studies or multiple time series, or dramatic results from uncontrolled experiments or subgroup analyses; (3) evidence from opinions of respected authorities, based on clinical experience, descriptive studies, or reports of expert communities.

TABLE 13-4 Lifestyle Modifications to Prevent and Manage Hypertension[29]

Modification	Recommendation	Approximate Systolic Blood Pressure Reduction (mm Hg)[a]
Weight loss	Maintain normal body weight (body mass index, 18.5-24.9 kg/m^2)	5-20 per 10-kg weight loss
DASH-type dietary patterns	Consume a diet rich in fruits, vegetables, and low-fat dairy products with a reduced content of saturated and total fat	8-14
Reduced salt intake	Reduce daily dietary sodium intake as much as possible, ideally to ≈65 mmol/day (1.5 g/day sodium, or 3.8 g/day sodium chloride)	2-8
Aerobic physical activity	3 to 4 sessions/wk, lasting an average of 40 min/session, and involving moderate- to vigorous-intensity physical activity	4-9
Moderation of alcohol intake	Limit consumption to ≤2 drink equivalents per day in men and ≤1 drink equivalent per day in women and lighter-weight persons[b]	2-4

[a]Effects of implementing these modifications are time- and dose-dependent and could be greater for some patients.

[b]One drink equivalent is equal to 1.5 oz (approximately 45 mL) of 80-proof distilled spirits (eg, whiskey), a 5 oz (approximately 150 mL) glass of wine (12%), or 12 oz (approximately 350 mL) of beer.

The Dietary Approaches to Stop Hypertension (DASH) eating plan is a diet that is rich in fruits, vegetables, and low-fat dairy products with a reduced content of saturated and total fat. It is recommended as a reasonable and feasible diet that has proven to lower BP. Intake of sodium should be minimized as much as possible, ideally to 1.5 g/day, although an interim goal of less than 2.3 g/day may be reasonable considering the difficulty in achieving these low intakes. Patients should be aware of the multiple sources of dietary sodium (eg, processed foods, soups, and table salt) so that they may follow these recommendations. Potassium intake should be encouraged through fruits and vegetables with high content (ideally 4.7 g/day) in those with normal kidney function or without impaired potassium excretion. Excessive alcohol use can either cause or worsen hypertension. Patients with hypertension who drink alcoholic beverages should restrict their daily intake.

Aerobic physical activity consisting of 3 to 4 sessions per week, lasting on average 40 minutes per session, and involving moderate- to vigorous-intensity physical activity should be encouraged when possible. Studies have shown that aerobic physical activity can reduce BP, even in the absence of weight loss. Patients should consult their physicians before starting an exercise program, especially those with hypertension-associated complications.

Cigarette smoking is not a secondary cause of essential hypertension. Therefore, smoking cessation is not a recommended strategy to control BP. Smoking is a major, independent, modifiable risk factor for CV disease. Patients with hypertension who smoke should be counseled regarding the additional health risks that result from smoking. Moreover, the potential benefits that cessation can provide should be explained to encourage cessation.

Pharmacotherapy

8 An ACEi, angiotensin II receptor blocker (ARB), calcium channel blocker (CCB), or thiazide are preferred first-line antihypertensive agents for most patients (Table 13-5).[1-4] These agents should be used to treat the majority of patients with hypertension because of evidence demonstrating CV event reduction. Several have subclasses where significant differences in mechanism of action, clinical use, side effects, or evidence from outcome studies exist. β-Blocker therapy should be reserved to either treat a specific compelling indication or used in combination with one or more of the aforementioned first-line antihypertensive agents for patients without a compelling indication. Other antihypertensive drug classes are considered alternative drug classes that may be used in select patients after first-line agents (Table 13-6).

Historical Evidence Supporting Thiazide Therapy

Landmark placebo-controlled clinical trials demonstrate that thiazide therapy irrefutably reduces risk of CV morbidity and mortality. The Systolic Hypertension in the Elderly Program (SHEP),[8] Swedish Trial in Old Patients with Hypertension (STOP-Hypertension),[9] and Medical Research Council (MRC)[10] studies showed significant reductions in stroke, MI, all-cause CV disease, and mortality with thiazide-based therapy versus placebo. These trials allowed for β-blockers as add-on therapy for BP control. Agents such as an ACEi, ARB, and CCB were not available at the time of these studies. However, subsequent clinical trials have compared these antihypertensive agents with a thiazide and have demonstrated similar long-term benefits.[26-33]

The Antihypertensive and Lipid Lowering Treatment to Prevent Heart Attack Trial (ALLHAT) The results of the ALLHAT were the deciding evidence that the JNC7 used to justify thiazide therapy as first-line therapy.[29] It was designed to test the hypothesis that newer antihypertensive agents (an α-blocker, ACEi, or dihydropyridine CCB) would be superior to thiazide-based therapy. The primary objective was to compare the combined end point of fatal CHD and nonfatal MI. Other hypertension-related complications (eg, heart failure, stroke) were evaluated as secondary end points. This was the largest prospective hypertension trial ever conducted and included 42,418 patients aged 55 and older with hypertension and one additional CV risk factor. This double-blind trial randomized patients to chlorthalidone-, amlodipine-, doxazosin-, or lisinopril-based therapy for a mean of 4.9 years.

The doxazosin arm was terminated early when a significantly higher risk of heart failure versus chlorthalidone was observed.[34] The other arms were continued as scheduled and no significant differences in the primary end point was seen between the chlorthalidone and lisinopril or amlodipine treatment groups. However, chlorthalidone had statistically fewer secondary end points than amlodipine (heart failure) and lisinopril (combined CV disease, heart failure, and stroke). The study conclusions were that chlorthalidone-based therapy was superior in preventing one or more major forms of CV disease and was less expensive than amlodipine- or lisinopril-based therapy.

ALLHAT was designed as a superiority study with the hypothesis that amlodipine, doxazosin, and lisinopril would be better than chlorthalidone.[35] It did not prove this hypothesis because the primary end point was no different between chlorthalidone, amlodipine, and lisinopril. Many subgroup analyses of specific populations (eg, black patients, CKD, diabetes) from the ALLHAT have been conducted to assess response in certain unique patient populations.[36-38] Surprisingly, none of these analyses demonstrated superior CV event reductions with lisinopril or amlodipine versus chlorthalidone. Overall, thiazides remain unsurpassed in their ability to reduce CV morbidity and mortality in most patients.

The JNC7 guidelines (from 2003) recommend a thiazide as first-line therapy for most patients, and are consistent with the historical treatment of hypertension.[1] Subsequent guidelines and evidence-based recommendations have noted that an ACEi, ARB, or CCB may also be considered for first-line therapy. Contrary to the historical preference to use a thiazide as preferred for treating most patients with hypertension, they are simply one of four first-line drug therapy options. Figure 13-2 displays the algorithm for the treatment of hypertension and highlights that four drug classes are considered first-line agents for patients without a compelling indication for a specific drug class.

Clinical **Controversy...**

IS CHLORTHALIDONE SUPERIOR TO HYDROCHLOROTHIAZIDE?

Chlorthalidone (a thiazide-like diuretic) undisputedly reduces CV morbidity and mortality. It was used in the most landmark long-term placebo-controlled trials in hypertension. It is almost twice as potent in lowering BP on a milligram-per-milligram basis as hydrochlorothiazide, which has not been as extensively studied in major long-term hypertension clinical trials and has a much longer half-life. In clinical practice, it is well accepted that CV benefits in hypertension apply to all types of thiazides (considered a class effect). However, it is not definitively known if the clinical benefits of reducing CV morbidity and mortality that have been proven with chlorthalidone can be extrapolated to hydrochlorothiazide.

ACEi, ARB, and CCB as First-Line Agents

Clinical trial data cumulatively demonstrate that ACEi-, CCB-, or ARB-based antihypertensive therapy reduces CV events. These agents may be used for patients without compelling indications as a first-line therapy. The Blood Pressure Lowering Treatment Trialists' Collaboration has evaluated the incidence of major CV events and death among different antihypertensive drug classes from 29 major randomized trials in 162,341 patients.[39] In placebo-controlled trials, the incidences of major CV events were significantly lower with ACEi- and CCB-based regimens versus placebo. Although there were differences in the incidence of certain CV events in some comparisons (eg, stroke was lower with diuretic or CCB-based regiments vs ACEi-based regimens), there were no differences in total major CV events when an ACEi, CCB, or thiazide were compared with each other. In studies evaluating ARB-based therapy to control regimens, the incidence of major CV events was lower with ARB-based therapy. However, the control regimens used in these comparisons included both active antihypertensive drug therapies and placebo.

Data from meta-analyses may not be as influential as data from well-designed, prospective, randomized controlled trials (eg, the ALLHAT). However, they provide clinically useful data that support using ACEi-, CCB-, or ARB-based treatment for hypertension as first-line antihypertensive agents. Clinicians can use meta-analyses data as supporting evidence when selecting a first-line antihypertensive regimen for hypertension in most patients.

Other major consensus guidelines recommend multiple several first-line drug therapy options for treating hypertension in most patients. The 2013 European Society of Hypertension/European Society of Cardiology guidelines and the 2011 UK's National Institute for Health and the Clinical Excellence guidelines list more than one drug therapy option as an acceptable first-line treatment approach.[40,41] The European Society of Hypertension/European Society of Cardiology guidelines are founded on the principle that CV risk reduction is a function of BP control that is largely independent of specific antihypertensives.[40] The UK guidelines stratify patients based on age and race; they recommend an ACEi or ARB first-line for patients under the age of 55, and a CCB first-line for patients age 55 or older or for black patients.[41]

TABLE 13-5 First-Line and Other Common Antihypertensive Agents

Class	Subclass	Drug (Brand Name)	Usual Dose Range (mg/day)	Daily Frequency	Comments
ACEi		Benazepril (Lotensin)	10-40	1 or 2	May cause hyperkalemia in patients with CKD or in those receiving a potassium-sparing diuretic, aldosterone antagonist, ARB, or direct renin inhibitor; can cause acute kidney failure in patients with severe bilateral renal artery stenosis or severe stenosis in artery to solitary kidney; do not use in pregnancy or in patients with a history of angioedema; starting dose should be reduced 50% in patients who are on a thiazide, are volume depleted, or are very elderly due to risks of hypotension
		Captopril (Capoten)	12.5-150	2 or 3	
		Enalapril (Vasotec)	5-40	1 or 2	
		Fosinopril (Monopril)	10-40	1	
		Lisinopril (Prinivil, Zestril)	10-40	1	
		Moexipril (Univasc)	7.5-30	1 or 2	
		Perindopril (Aceon)	4-16	1	
		Quinapril (Accupril)	10-80	1 or 2	
		Ramipril (Altace)	2.5-10	1 or 2	
		Trandolapril (Mavik)	1-4	1	
ARB		Azilsartan (Edarbi)	40-80	1	May cause hyperkalemia in patients with CKD or in those receiving a potassium-sparing diuretic, aldosterone antagonist, ACEi, or direct renin inhibitor; can cause acute kidney failure in patients with severe bilateral renal artery stenosis or severe stenosis in artery to solitary kidney; do not cause a dry cough like an ACEi may; do not use in pregnancy; starting dose should be reduced 50% in patients who are on a thiazide, are volume depleted, or are very elderly due to risks of hypotension
		Candesartan (Atacand)	8-32	1 or 2	
		Eprosartan (Teveten)	600-800	1 or 2	
		Irbesartan (Avapro)	150-300	1	
		Losartan (Cozaar)	50-100	1 or 2	
		Olmesartan (Benicar)	20-40	1	
		Telmisartan (Micardis)	20-80	1	
		Valsartan (Diovan)	80-320	1	
Calcium channel blocker	Dihydropyridine	Amlodipine (Norvasc)	2.5-10	1	Short-acting dihydropyridines should be avoided, especially immediate-release nifedipine and nicardipine; dihydropyridines are more potent peripheral vasodilators than nondihydropyridines and may cause more reflex sympathetic discharge (tachycardia), dizziness, headache, flushing, and peripheral edema; have additional benefits in Raynaud's syndrome
		Felodipine (Plendil)	5-20	1	
		Isradipine (DynaCirc)	5-10	2	
		Isradipine SR (DynaCirc SR)	5-20	1	
		Nicardipine sustained release (Cardene SR)	60-120	2 1	
		Nifedipine long-acting (Adalat CC, Nifedical XL, Procardia XL)	30-90	1	
		Nisoldipine (Sular)	10-40		
	Nondihydropyridine	Diltiazem sustained release (Cardizem SR)	180-360	2 1	Extended-release products are preferred for hypertension; these agents reduce heart rate; may produce heart block, especially in combination with β-blockers; these products are not AB rated as interchangeable on an equipotent milligram-per-milligram basis due to different release mechanisms and different bioavailability parameters; Cardizem LA, Covera-HS, and Verelan PM have delayed drug release for several hours after dosing, when dosed in the evening can provide chronotherapeutic drug delivery starting shortly before patients awake from sleep; nondihydropyridines have additional benefits in patients with atrial tachyarrhythmia
		Diltiazem sustained release (Cardizem CD, Cartia XT, Dilacor XR, Diltia XT, Tiazac, Taztia XT)	120-480	1 (morning or evening) 1 or 2	
		Diltiazem extended release (Cardizem LA)	120-540	1 (in the evening)	
		Verapamil sustained release (Calan SR, Isoptin SR, Verelan)	180-480	1 (in the evening)	
		Verapamil controlled onset, extended release (Covera-HS)	180-420		
		Verapamil chronotherapeutic oral drug absorption system (Verelan PM)	100-400		
Diuretic	Thiazide	Chlorthalidone (Hygroton)	12.5-25	1	Hydrochlorothiazide is a "thiazide-type" agent; chlorthalidone, indapamide, and metolazone are "thiazide-like" agents. Dose in the morning to avoid nocturnal diuresis; thiazides are more effective antihypertensives than loop diuretics in most patients; use usual doses to avoid adverse metabolic effects; hydrochlorothiazide, chlorthalidone, and indapamide are preferred; chlorthalidone is approximately 1.5 times as potent as hydrochlorothiazide and has a much longer half-life; have additional benefits in osteoporosis; use with caution in patients with a history of gout
		Hydrochlorothiazide (Esidrix, HydroDiuril, Microzide, Oretic)	12.5-50	1 1	
		Indapamide (Lozol)	1.25-2.5	1	
		Metolazone (Zaroxolyn)	2.5-10		
	Loop	Bumetanide (Bumex)	0.5-4	2	Dose in the morning and late afternoon (when twice daily) to avoid nocturnal diuresis; higher doses may be needed for patients with severely decreased GFR or heart failure; preferred over thiazides in patient with concomitant renal dysfunction and resistant hypertension
		Furosemide (Lasix)	20-80	2	
		Torsemide (Demadex)	5-10	1	
	Potassium sparing	Amiloride (Midamor)	5-10	1 or 2	Weak diuretics that are generally used in combination with a thiazide to minimize hypokalemia; do not significantly lower BP unless used with a thiazide; should generally be reserved for patients experiencing diuretic-induced hypokalemia; avoid in patients with CKD (estimated creatinine clearance [CrCl] <30 mL/min [<0.5 mL/s]); may cause hyperkalemia, especially in combination with an ACEi, ARB, direct renin inhibitor, or potassium supplements
		Amiloride/hydrochlorothiazide (Moduretic)	5-10/50-100	1	
		Triamterene (Dyrenium)	50-100	1 or 2	
		Triamterene/hydrochlorothiazide (Dyazide)	37.5-75/25-50	1	

(continued)

TABLE 13-5 First-Line and Other Common Antihypertensive Agents (*Continued*)

Class	Subclass	Drug (Brand Name)	Usual Dose Range (mg/day)	Daily Frequency	Comments
	Aldosterone antagonist	Eplerenone (Inspra) Spironolactone (Aldactone) Spironolactone/hydrochlorothiazide (Aldactazide)	50-100 25-50 25-50/25-50	1 or 2 1 or 2 1	Dose in the morning and late afternoon (when twice daily) to avoid nocturnal diuresis; eplerenone contraindicated in patients with an estimated CrCl <50 mL/min (<0.83 mL/s), elevated serum creatinine (>1.8 mg/dL [159 μmol/L] in women, >2 mg/dL [177 μmol/L] in men), and type 2 diabetes with microalbuminuria; spironolactone often used as add-on therapy in resistant hypertension; avoid spironolactone in patients with CKD (estimated CrCl <30 mL/min [<0.5 mL/s]); may cause hyperkalemia, especially in combination with an ACEi, ARB, direct renin inhibitor, or potassium supplements
β-Blocker	Cardioselective	Atenolol (Tenormin) Betaxolol (Kerlone) Bisoprolol (Zebeta) Metoprolol tartrate (Lopressor) Metoprolol succinate extended release (Toprol XL)	25-100 5-20 2.5-10 100-400 50-200	1 1 1 2 1	Abrupt discontinuation may cause rebound hypertension; inhibit β_1-receptors at low to moderate dose, higher doses also block β_2-receptors; may exacerbate asthma when selectivity is lost; have additional benefits in patients with atrial tachyarrhythmia or preoperative hypertension
	Nonselective	Nadolol (Corgard) Propranolol (Inderal) Propranolol long acting (Inderal LA, Inderal XL, InnoPran XL) Timolol (Blocadren)	40-120 160-480 80-320 10-40	1 2 1 1	Abrupt discontinuation may cause rebound hypertension; inhibit β_1- and β_2-receptors at all doses; can exacerbate asthma; have additional benefits in patients with essential tremor, migraine headache, portal hypertension, thyrotoxicosis
	Intrinsic sympathomimetic activity	Acebutolol (Sectral) Carteolol (Cartrol) Pindolol (Visken)	200-800 2.5-10 10-60	2 1 2	Abrupt discontinuation may cause rebound hypertension; partially stimulate β-receptors while blocking against additional stimulation; no clear advantage for these agents; contraindicated in patients postmyocardial infarction
	Mixed α- and β-blockers	Carvedilol (Coreg) Carvedilol phosphate (Coreg CR) Labetalol (Normodyne, Trandate)	12.5-50 20-80 200-800	2 1 2	Abrupt discontinuation may cause rebound hypertension; additional α-blockade produces vasodilation and more orthostatic hypotension
	Cardioselective and vasodilatory	Nebivolol (Bystolic)	5-20	1	Abrupt discontinuation may cause rebound hypertension; additional vasodilation does not result in more orthostatic hypotension

(9) **β-Blocker Versus First-Line Agents** Clinical trial data cumulatively suggest that treatment with a β-blocker may not reduce CV events to the extent that an ACEi, ARB, CCB, or thiazide does. These data are from meta-analyses of clinical trials evaluating β-blocker-based therapy for hypertension.[42] Overall, these analyses demonstrated less CV event reduction benefits with β-blocker-based antihypertensive therapy compared mostly with ACEi- and CCB-based therapy. Although comparative data with ARB-based therapy are more limited, a similar trend was observed.

Meta-analyses data evaluating β-blockers and their ability to reduce CV events have limitations. Most studies that were included used atenolol as the β-blocker studied. Therefore, it is possible that

TABLE 13-6 Alternative Antihypertensive Agents

Class	Drug (Brand Name)	Usual Dose Range (mg/day)	Daily Frequency	Comments
α_1-Blocker	Doxazosin (Cardura) Prazosin (Minipress) Terazosin (Hytrin)	1-8 2-20 1-20	1 2 or 3 1 or 2	Give first dose at bedtime; patients should rise from sitting or laying down slowly to minimize risk of orthostatic hypotension; additional benefits in men with benign prostatic hyperplasia
Direct renin inhibitor	Aliskiren (Tekturna)	150-300	1	May cause hyperkalemia in patients with CKD and diabetes or in those receiving a potassium-sparing diuretic, aldosterone antagonist, ACEi, or ARB; may cause acute kidney failure in patients with severe bilateral renal artery stenosis or severe stenosis in artery to solitary kidney; do not use in pregnancy
Central α_2-agonist	Clonidine (Catapres) Clonidine patch (Catapres-TTS) Methyldopa (Aldomet)	0.1-0.8 0.1-0.3 250-1,000	2 1 weekly 2	Abrupt discontinuation may cause rebound hypertension; most effective if used with a thiazide to diminish fluid retention; clonidine patch is replaced once per week
Peripheral adrenergic antagonist	Reserpine (generic only)	0.05-0.25	1	Used in many of the landmark clinical trials; should be used with a thiazide to diminish fluid retention
Direct arterial vasodilator	Minoxidil (Loniten) Hydralazine (Apresoline)	10-40 20-100	1 or 2 2 to 4	Should be used with thiazide and β-blocker to diminish fluid retention and reflex tachycardia

atenolol is inferior and is the only β-blocker that reduces CV events less than the other first-line antihypertensive drug classes. However, consensus guidelines and expert recommendations do extrapolate these findings to the β-blocker drug class in general.[2-4] In the absence of a compelling indication, the 2011 UK guidelines recommend a β-blocker as fourth-line therapy, only after other first-line antihypertensive agents (ACEi or ARB, CCB, thiazide) have been used.[41] These findings also call in question the validity of results from prominent prospective, controlled clinical trials evaluating antihypertensive drug therapy that used β-blocker-based therapy, especially atenolol, as the primary comparator.[28,33] Of note, these studies used once-daily atenolol, which may be inadequate based on the short half-life of this agent.

β-Blocker therapy for patients without compelling indications still has a role in the management of hypertension. It is important for clinicians to remember that β-blocker-based antihypertensive therapy does not increase risk of CV events; β-blocker-based therapy reduces risk of CV events compared with no antihypertensive therapy. Using a β-blocker as a first-line antihypertensive agent is optimal when an ACEi, ARB, CCB, or thiazide cannot be used as the first-line agent. β-Blockers still have an important add-on role after first-line agents to reduce BP in patients with hypertension but without compelling indications.

Many of the clinical trials included in the meta-analyses that suggest β-blocker-based therapy may not reduce CV events as well as these other agents used atenolol dosed once daily.[42] Atenolol has a half-life of 6 to 7 hours and is nearly always dosed once daily, while immediate-release forms of carvedilol and metoprolol have half-lives of 6 to 10 and 3 to 7 hours, respectively, and are dosed at least twice daily.[42] Therefore, it is possible that these findings might only apply to atenolol and also that these findings may be a result of using atenolol once daily instead of twice daily. Based on available evidence, metoprolol succinate or carvedilol are preferred β-blocker if a β-blocker is to be used.

Patients with Compelling Indications

10 Compelling indications represent specific comorbid conditions where evidence from clinical trials supports using specific antihypertensive classes to treat both the compelling indication and hypertension. Drug therapy recommendations typically consist of combination drug therapy (see Fig. 13-3). Data from clinical trials have demonstrated reduction in CV morbidity and/or mortality that justify use for patients with hypertension and with such a compelling indication. Some compelling indications include recommendations that are provided by other national treatment guidelines, or from newer clinical trials, which are complementary to the hypertension guidelines.

Heart Failure with Reduced Ejection Fraction Five drug classes have compelling indications in heart failure with reduced ejection fraction (HF*r*EF), also known as systolic heart failure or left ventricular dysfunction.[43] The primary physiologic abnormality in this compelling indication is decreased CO resulting from a decrease left ventricular ejection fraction. An evidence-based pharmacotherapy regimen for HF*r*EF, sometimes called guideline-directed medical therapy, consists of three to four drugs: an ACEi or ARB plus diuretic therapy, followed by the addition of an evidence-based β-blocker (ie, bisoprolol, carvedilol, or metoprolol succinate) and possibly an aldosterone receptor antagonist.

Evidence from clinical trials shows that ACEi therapy significantly modifies disease progression by reducing morbidity and mortality. Although HF*r*EF was the primary disease in these studies, ACEi therapy will also control BP in these patients with concomitant hypertension. ARBs are acceptable as an alternative therapy for patients who cannot tolerate an ACEi. An ACEi or ARB should be started with low doses for patients with HF*r*EF, especially those with an acute exacerbation. Heart failure induces a compensatory high-renin condition, and starting an ACEi or ARB under these conditions can cause a pronounced first-dose effect and possible orthostatic hypotension.

Diuretics are also a part of standard pharmacotherapy primarily to control symptoms. They provide symptomatic relief of edema by inducing diuresis. Loop diuretics are often needed, especially for patients with more advanced heart failure and/or CKD. However, some patients with well-controlled heart failure and without significant CKD may be managed with a thiazide.

β-Blocker therapy is appropriate to further modify disease in HF*r*EF and is a component of standard therapy for these patients. For patients on an initial regimen of a thiazide and ACEi or ARB, β-blockers have been shown to reduce CV morbidity and mortality.[43] It is of paramount importance that β-blockers be dosed appropriately due to the risk of inducing an acute exacerbation of heart failure. They must be started in very low doses, doses much lower than that used to treat hypertension, and titrated slowly to high doses based on tolerability. Bisoprolol, carvedilol, and sustained-release metoprolol succinate are the only β-blockers proven to be beneficial in HF*r*EF.

After implementation of a standard three-drug regimen (diuretic, ACEi or ARB, and β-blocker), other agents may be added to further reduce CV morbidity and mortality, and reduce BP if needed. The addition of an aldosterone antagonist can reduce CV morbidity and mortality in HF*r*EF.[43] Spironolactone has been studied in severe HF*r*EF and has shown benefit in addition to diuretic and ACEi therapy. Eplerenone has been studied in patients with symptomatic HF*r*EF within 3 to 14 days after an acute MI in addition to a standard three-drug regimen and in patients with mild left ventricular dysfunction.[43] Spironolactone and eplerenone are similar in their ability to lower risk of CV events in HF*r*EF. For patients self-described as African Americans, the combination of a fixed dose of isosorbide dinitrate and hydralazine to standard three-drug regimen is recommended as an option to improve CV outcomes.[43]

Post-MI β-Blocker (those without intrinsic sympathomimetic activity [ISA]) and ACEi or ARB therapy are recommended in the AHA/American College of Cardiology Foundation and JNC7 guidelines.[1,4,44] β-Blockers decrease cardiac adrenergic stimulation and have been shown in clinical trials to reduce the risk of a subsequent MI or sudden cardiac death. ACEi treatment has been shown to improve cardiac remodeling and cardiac function and to reduce CV events post-MI. These two drug classes, with β-blockers first, are considered the first drugs of choice for patients who have experienced an MI.

Coronary Artery Disease Chronic stable angina and acute coronary syndrome (unstable angina and acute MI) are forms of coronary artery disease (aka ischemic heart disease).[44,45] These are the most common forms of hypertension-associated complications. This compelling indication is also referred to as high coronary and CV disease risk in the JNC7.[1] β-Blocker therapy has been considered a standard of care for treating patients with coronary artery disease and hypertension. β-Blockers are first-line therapy in chronic stable angina and have the ability to reduce BP and improve ischemic symptoms by decreasing myocardial oxygen consumption and demand. β-Blocker therapy seems to be most effective in reducing the risk of CV events in patients with recent MI and/or ischemic symptoms. However, evidence indicates that the long-term risk of CV events and mortality may not be reduced with β-blocker therapy in patients with very stable coronary artery disease (do not have ischemic symptoms or have a distant history of MI).[46]

Long-acting CCBs (the nondihydropyridine CCBs diltiazem and verapamil) may be considered alternatives to β-blockers or as add-on therapy (dihydropyridine CCBs) in chronic stable angina for patients with ischemic symptoms.[45] The International

Verapamil-Trandolapril Study (INVEST) demonstrated no difference in CV risk reduction when β-blocker-based therapy was compared with nondihydropyridine CCB-based therapy in this population.[47] Nonetheless, the preponderance of data is with β-blockers and they remain the therapy of choice.[1,44,45]

For acute coronary syndromes (ST-elevation MI and unstable angina/non-ST-segment MI), first-line therapy should consist of a β-blocker and ACEi.[48,49] An ARB is a reasonable alternative to an ACEi. This regimen will lower BP, control acute ischemia, and reduce CV risk.

CCBs (especially nondihydropyridine CCBs) and β-blockers provide anti-ischemic effects; they lower BP and reduce myocardial oxygen demand in patients with hypertension and coronary artery disease. However, cardiac stimulation may occur with dihydropyridine CCBs (particularly immediate release formulations) or β-blockers with ISA, making these agents less desirable. Therefore, β-blockers with ISA should be avoided. Nondihydropyridine CCBs should be used as alternatives to β-blockers, and dihydropyridines should be add-on therapy to β-blockers.

Once ischemic symptoms are controlled with β-blocker and/or CCB therapy, other antihypertensive drugs can be added to provide additional CV risk reduction. Clinical trials have demonstrated that the addition of an ACEi further reduces CV events in patients with chronic stable angina.[45] ARB therapy may provide similar benefits but have not been as extensively studied as ACEi therapy.[45] Therefore, in coronary artery disease, an ARB is generally considered an alternative to an ACEi. Thiazides can be added thereafter to provide additional BP lowering and to further reduce CV risk; they do not provide anti-ischemic effects.

Diabetes The primary cause of mortality in diabetes is CV disease, and hypertension management is a very important risk reduction strategy.[1,16] Five antihypertensive agents have evidence supporting their use in diabetes (see Fig. 13-3). All of these agents have been shown to reduce CV events in patients with diabetes. However, risk reduction may not be equal when comparing these agents.

11 Patients with diabetes and hypertension should ideally be treated with an ACEi or an ARB.[16] Pharmacologically, both of these agents should provide nephroprotection due to vasodilation in the efferent arteriole of the kidney. Moreover, ACEi therapy has overwhelming data demonstrating CV risk reduction in patients with established forms of heart disease. Evidence from clinical studies have demonstrated reductions in both CV risk (mostly with an ACEi) and reduction in risk of progressive kidney dysfunction (mostly with ARBs) in patients with diabetes.[16] There is debate surrounding which agent is better because data support both drug classes. Nonetheless, either drug class should ideally be used to control BP as one of the drugs in the antihypertensive regimen for patients with diabetes, because multiple agents are often needed to attain goal BP values. However, an ACEi should not be used in combination with an ARB as a treatment to control BP in patients with hypertension.

CCBs are the most appropriate add-on agents for BP control for patients with diabetes. Evidence demonstrates that these are the most optimal second agent added to either an ACEi or an ARB. Specifically, in the cohort of patients with diabetes from the Avoiding Cardiovascular Events Through Combination Therapy in Patients Living with Systolic Hypertension (ACCOMPLISH) trial, the combination of an ACEi with a CCB was better at reducing CV events than the combination of an ACEi with a thiazide.[50] The ACCOMPLISH trial is discussed later in this chapter.

A thiazide is recommended add-on therapy to lower BP and provide additional CV risk reduction. A subgroup analysis of patients with diabetes from the ALLHAT trial showed no difference in long-term risk of CV events in the chlorthalidone and lisinopril treatment groups.[37] Therefore, some argue that thiazides, used in low doses, are equally effective for patients with hypertension and diabetes. Nonetheless, the entire body of evidence evaluating pharmacotherapy for patients with hypertension and diabetes supports an ACEi or ARB first-line.[1,16,17]

A β-Blocker, similar to a CCB, is useful add-on therapy for BP control for patients with diabetes. These agents should also be used to treat another compelling indication (eg, post-MI). A β-Blocker (especially a nonselective agent) can possibly mask the signs and symptoms of hypoglycemia in patients with tightly controlled diabetes because most of the symptoms of hypoglycemia (eg, tremor, tachycardia, and palpitations) are mediated through the sympathetic nervous system. Sweating, a cholinergically mediated symptom of hypoglycemia, should still occur during a hypoglycemic episode despite β-blocker therapy. Patients may also have a delay in hypoglycemia recovery time because compensatory recovery mechanisms need the catecholamine inputs that are antagonized by β-blocker therapy. Finally, unopposed α-receptor stimulation during the acute hypoglycemic recovery phase (due to endogenous epinephrine release intended to reverse hypoglycemia) may result in acutely elevated BP due to vasoconstriction. Despite these potential problems, β-blockers can be safely used for patients with diabetes.

Based on the weight of all evidence, an ACEi or ARB are preferred first-line agents for controlling hypertension in diabetes. The need for combination therapy should be anticipated, and a CCB should be the second agent added. Thiazides, and even β-blockers, are useful evidence-based agents in this population, but are considered add-on therapies to the aforementioned agents.

Chronic Kidney Disease Patients with hypertension may develop damage to either the renal tissue (parenchyma) or the renal arteries.[18] CKD initially presents as moderately increased albuminuria (urine albumin-to-creatinine ratio 30 to 299 mg/g [3.4-33.8 mg/mmol] on a spot urine sample or greater than or equal to 30 mg albumin in a 24-hour urine collection) that can progress to overt kidney failure. The rate of kidney function deterioration is accelerated when both hypertension and diabetes are present. Once patients have an estimated glomerular filtration rate (GFR) less than 60 mL/min/1.73 m^2 or albuminuria, they have significant CKD and risk of CV disease and progression to severe CKD increases.[1] BP control can slow the decline in kidney function.

In addition to lowering BP, ACEi, and ARB therapy reduces intraglomerular pressure, which can theoretically provide additional benefits by further reducing the decline in kidney function. Using either an ACEi or ARB has been shown to slow progression of CKD in diabetes[16,17] and in those without diabetes.[18,51] It is difficult to differentiate whether the kidney protection benefits are from RAAS blockade versus BP lowering. A meta-analysis failed to demonstrate any unique long-term kidney protective effects of RAAS-blocking drugs compared with other antihypertensive drugs.[52] Moreover, a subgroup analysis of patients from the ALLHAT stratified by different baseline GFR values also did not show a difference in long-term outcomes with chlorthalidone versus lisinopril.[36] Patients may experience a rapid and profound drop in BP or acute kidney failure when given an ACEi or ARB. The potential to produce acute kidney failure is particularly problematic in patients with bilateral renal artery stenosis or a solitary functioning kidney with stenosis. Patients with renal artery stenosis are usually older, and the condition is more common in patients with diabetes or those who smoke. Patients with renal artery stenosis do not always have evidence of kidney disease unless sophisticated tests are performed. Starting with low dosages and evaluating serum creatinine soon after starting the drug can minimize this risk.

Recurrent Stroke Prevention Ischemic stroke (not hemorrhagic stroke) and transient ischemic attack are complications of hypertension.[52] Achieving goal BP values in patients who have experienced an ischemic stroke is considered a primary modality to reduce risk of a second stroke. A thiazide, either in combination with an ACEi or as monotherapy, is considered an evidence-based antihypertensive regimen for patients with a history of stroke or transient ischemic attack.[1,53,54] ARBs have also been studied in this population.[55,56] Antihypertensive drug therapy should only be implemented after patients have stabilized following an acute cerebrovascular event.

Alternative Drug Treatments

It is sometimes necessary to use other agents such as a direct renin inhibitor, α-blocker, central α_2-agonist, adrenergic inhibitor, and arterial vasodilator in some patients. Although these agents are effective in lowering BP, they either do not have compelling outcome data showing reduced morbidity and mortality in hypertension, or have poor tolerability and adverse effects that significantly limit their use. Alternative agents are generally reserved for patients with resistant hypertension or as add-on therapy with multiple other first-line antihypertensive agents.

Special Populations Selection of drug therapy should follow the recommendations provided by established guidelines, which are summarized in Figs. 13-2 and 13-3.[1] These should be maintained as the guiding principles of drug therapy. However, there are some patient populations where the approach to drug therapy may be slightly different, or utilize recommended agents using tailored dosing strategies. In some cases, this is because other agents have unique properties that benefit a coexisting condition, but may not be based on evidence from outcome studies in hypertension.

Hypertension in Older People Hypertension often presents as isolated systolic hypertension in the elderly.[57] Epidemiologic data indicate that CV morbidity and mortality are more directly correlated to SBP than to DBP for patients aged 50 and older. This population is at high risk for hypertension-associated complications.[1] Although several placebo-controlled trials have specifically demonstrated risk reduction in this form of hypertension, many older people with hypertension are either not treated, or treated but not controlled.

The SHEP was a landmark double-blind, placebo-controlled trial that evaluated chlorthalidone-based treatment (with atenolol or reserpine as add-on therapy) for isolated systolic hypertension.[8] A 36% reduction in total stroke, a 27% reduction in coronary artery disease, and 55% reduction in heart failure were demonstrated versus placebo. The Systolic Hypertension in Europe (Syst-Eur) trial was another placebo-controlled trial that evaluated treatment with a long-acting dihydropyridine CCB.[11] Treatment resulted in a 42% reduction in stroke, 26% reduction in coronary artery disease, and 29% reduction in heart failure. These data clearly demonstrate reductions in CV morbidity and mortality in older patients with isolated systolic hypertension, especially with thiazides and long-acting dihydropyridine CCBs.

The very elderly population (greater than or equal to 80 years of age) were underrepresented in the SHEP and Syst-Eur studies. Historically, this population often was not treated to goal either because of a fear of side effects or because of limited data demonstrating benefit. However, the Hypertension in the Very Elderly Trial (HYVET) provided definitive evidence that antihypertensive drug therapy provides significant clinical benefits in the very elderly.[58] The HYVET was a prospective controlled clinical trial that randomized patients 80 years and older with hypertension to placebo or antihypertensive drug therapy. It was stopped early after a median of only 1.8 years because the incidence of death was 21% higher in placebo-treated patients. Based on these results, hypertension should be treated in the very elderly.

Thiazide or β-blocker therapy has been compared with either an ACEi or CCB in elderly patients with either systolic hypertension, diastolic hypertension, or both in the Swedish Trial in Old Patients with Hypertension-2 (STOP-2) study.[59] In this trial, no significant differences were seen between conventional drugs and either an ACEi or CCB. However, there were significantly fewer MIs and cases of heart failure in the ACEi group compared with the CCB group. These data suggest that overall treatment may be more important than specific antihypertensive agents in this population.

Elderly patients are more sensitive to volume depletion and sympathetic inhibition than younger patients. This may lead to orthostatic hypotension (see next section). In the elderly, this can increase the risk of falls due to the associated dizziness. Centrally acting agents and α_1-blockers should generally be avoided or used with caution in the elderly because they are frequently associated with dizziness and orthostatic hypotension. A thiazide, ACEi, or ARB provides significant benefits and can safely be used in the elderly, but smaller-than-usual initial doses must be used for initial therapy.

The AHA expert consensus on hypertension in the elderly from 2011,[57] the ASH-ISH guidelines and JNC8 Report[2,3] all recommend higher than standard SBP goals in patients older than 80 years of age. The HYVET trial established that treating hypertension in patients aged 80 years or older with drug therapy to a SBP goal of less than 150 mm Hg was superior to placebo in reducing mortality.[58] However, a pre-specified subgroup analysis of SPRINT evaluated patients age 75 years and older. In this elderly group treatment to a SBP goal of less than 120 mm Hg reduced risk of CV events better than a SBP goal of less than 140 mm Hg. Although there was a slightly higher risk of adverse effects, these data indicated that lower BP goals were better than higher goals. When selecting BP goals in older patients clinicians should evaluate risk versus benefit. Using a higher SBP goal in older patients only seems reasonable when there is either concern for orthostatic hypotension or in frail patients. Absent these factors, standard SBP goals (less than 140 mm Hg) should be considered for elderly patients.

Treatment of hypertension in older patients should follow the same principles outlined for the general care of hypertension. However, lower initial drug doses, and dosage titrations over a longer period of time are usually needed to minimize risks.

12 **Patients at Risk for Orthostatic Hypotension** *Orthostatic hypotension* is a significant drop in BP when standing and can be associated with dizziness and/or fainting. It is defined as a SBP decrease of greater than 20 mm Hg or DBP decrease of greater than 10 mm Hg when changing from supine to standing.[1] The risk of orthostatic hypotension is increased in older patients (especially those with isolated systolic hypotension) and those with long-standing diabetes, severe volume depletion, baroreflex dysfunction, autonomic insufficiency (eg, diabetes), and on concomitant venodilators (α-blockers, mixed α-/β-blockers, nitrates, and phosphodiesterase inhibitors). For patients with these risks factors, antihypertensive agents should be started in low doses, especially a thiazide, ACEi or ARB.

Hypertension in Children and Adolescents Detecting hypertension in children requires special attention to BP measurement, which is defined as SBP and/or DBP that is greater than 95th percentile for sex, age, and height on at least three occasions.[61] BP between the 90th and 95th percentile, or greater than 120/80 mm Hg in adolescents, is considered prehypertension. Hypertensive children often have a family history of high BP, and many are overweight predisposing them to insulin resistance and associated CV disease. Unlike hypertension in adults, secondary hypertension is more common in children and adolescents. An appropriate workup for secondary causes is required if elevated BP is identified. Kidney disease (eg, pyelonephritis, glomerulonephritis) is the most common cause of secondary hypertension in children. Coarctation of the aorta can also produce secondary hypertension. Medical or surgical management of the underlying disorder usually normalizes BP.

Nonpharmacologic treatment, particularly weight loss in those overweight, is the cornerstone of therapy for essential hypertension in children.[61] The goal is to reduce the BP to less than 95th percentile for sex, age, and height, or less than 90th percentile if concurrent conditions such as CKD, diabetes, or hypertension-associated complications are present. An ACEi, ARB, β-blocker, CCB, and thiazide are all acceptable choices in children and have data supporting their use. An ACEi, ARB, or direct renin inhibitor should all be avoided in sexually active girls due to potential teratogenic effect. As with adults, selection of initial agents should be based on the presence of compelling indications or concurrent conditions that may warrant their use (eg, ACEi or ARB for those with diabetes or CKD).

Pregnancy Hypertension during pregnancy is a major cause of maternal and neonatal morbidity and mortality.[1] Hypertension during pregnancy is categorized as preeclampsia-eclampsia, chronic hypertension (of any cause), chronic hypertension superimposed preeclampsia, and gestational hypertension.[62] *Preeclampsia* is defined as hypertension (elevated BP greater than or equal to 140/90 mm Hg on more than two occasions at least 4 hours apart after 20 weeks' gestation or greater than or equal to 160/110 mm Hg confirmed within a short interval) in association with thrombocytopenia, impaired liver function, new development of renal insufficiency, pulmonary edema, or new-onset cerebral or visual disturbances. It can lead to life-threatening complications for both mother and fetus. Eclampsia, the onset of convulsions in preeclampsia, is a medical emergency. Chronic hypertension is hypertension that predates pregnancy; superimposed preeclampsia is chronic hypertension associated with preeclampsia. *Gestational hypertension* is defined as new-onset hypertension arising after 20 weeks of gestation in the absence of proteinuria or other systemic findings (eg, thrombocytopenia, renal insufficiency, pulmonary edema, cerebral, visual disturbances). It is controversial whether treating elevated BP for patients with chronic hypertension in pregnancy is beneficial. However, women with chronic hypertension prior to pregnancy are at increased risk of a number of complications including superimposed preeclampsia, preterm delivery, fetal growth restriction or demise, placental abruption, heart failure, and acute kidney failure. In a recent open, international, multicenter study of 987 women at 14 weeks 0 days to 33 weeks 6 days of gestation with nonproteinuric preexisiting or gestational hypertension, tighter DBP goals (less than 85 mm Hg) was not associated with decreased rates of the primary composite outcome of pregnancy loss or high-level neonatal care for more than 48 hours during the first 28 days. However, severe hypertension (greater than or equal to 160/110 mm Hg) developed less often in patients randomized to the tight control group compared to less-tight control (40.6% vs 27.5%).[63]

Definitive treatment of preeclampsia is delivery. Delivery is indicated if pending or frank eclampsia is present. Otherwise, management consists of restricting activity, bedrest, and close monitoring. Salt restriction, or any other measures that contract blood volume, should not be employed. Antihypertensive agents are used prior to induction of labor if DBP is greater than 105 mm Hg with a target DBP of 95 to 105 mm Hg. Intravenous (IV) hydralazine is most commonly used, and IV labetalol is also effective. Immediate-release oral nifedipine has been used in the past, but is not approved by the FDA for hypertension, and untoward fetal and maternal effects (hypotension with fetal distress) have been reported.

Many agents can be used to treat chronic hypertension in pregnancy (Table 13-7). Unfortunately, there are few data regarding the most appropriate therapy in pregnancy. Labetalol, long-acting nifedipine, or methyldopa is recommended as first-line agents due to favorable safety profile.[62] Other β-Blockers (other than atenolol) and CCBs are also reasonable alternatives. An ACEi, ARB, and direct renin inhibitor are known teratogens and are absolutely contraindicated.

TABLE 13-7 Treatment of Chronic Hypertension in Pregnancy

Drug/Class	Comments
Methyldopa	Long-term follow-up data supports safety; *considered a preferred agent*
β-Blocker	Generally safe, but intrauterine growth retardation reported (mostly with atenolol)
Labetalol	Increasingly used over methyldopa because of fewer side effects; *considered a first-line agent*
Clonidine	Limited data available; used mainly in third trimester
CCB	Limited data available; no increase in major teratogenicity with exposure (except immediate-release oral nifedipine should not be used); *long-acting nifedipine considered a preferred agent*
Thiazide	Not first-line agents but probably safe in low doses if started prior to conception for essential hypertension
ACEi, ARB, direct renin inhibitor	Contraindicated; major teratogenicity reported with exposure (fetal toxicity and death)

African Americans Hypertension affects African American patients at a disproportionately higher rate, and hypertension-associated complications are more prevalent than in other populations.[1,64] Reasons for these differences are not fully understood, but may be related to differences in electrolyte homeostasis, GFR, sodium excretion and transport mechanisms, plasma renin activity, and BP response to plasma volume expansion.

BP-lowering effects of antihypertensive classes vary in African Americans, primarily when used as monotherapy. CCBs and thiazides are most effective at lowering BP in African Americans. When either of these two classes (especially thiazides) are used in combination with a β-blocker, ACEi, or ARB (which are three classes known to be less effective at lowering BP in African Americans), antihypertensive response is significantly increased. This may be due to the low-renin pattern of hypertension in African Americans, which can result in less BP lowering with a β-blocker, ACEi, or ARB when used as monotherapy compared with white patients. Interestingly, African Americans have a higher risk of angioedema and cough from an ACEi compared with whites.[64]

Despite potential differences in antihypertensive effects, drug therapy selection should be based on evidence, no different from what is recommended for the hypertensive population in general. Drug therapies should be used if a compelling indication is present, even if the antihypertensive effect may not be as great as with another drug class (eg, a β-blocker is first-line for BP control in an African American patient who is post-MI).

Other Concomitant Conditions

Most patients with hypertension have some other coexisting conditions that may influence selection or utilization of drug therapy. The influence of concomitant conditions should only be complementary to, and never in replacement of, drug therapy choices indicated by compelling indications. Under some circumstances, these considerations are helpful in deciding on a particular antihypertensive agent when more than one antihypertensive class is recommended to treat a compelling indication. In some cases, an agent should be avoided because it may aggravate a concomitant disorder. In other cases, an antihypertensive can be used to treat hypertension, a compelling indication, and another concomitant condition. These are briefly summarized in Table 13-5.

Pulmonary Disease and Peripheral Arterial Disease β-Blockers, especially nonselective agents, have been generally avoided for patients with hypertension and reactive airway disease (asthma or chronic obstructive pulmonary disease [COPD] with a reversible obstructive component) due to a fear of inducing bronchospasm.[65] However, cardioselective β-blockers can safely be used in patients with asthma or COPD. Therefore, cardioselective

β-blockers should be used to treat a compelling indication (ie, post-MI, coronary disease, or heart failure) for patients with reactive airway disease.

PAD is considered a noncoronary form of ASCVD.[44,65] β-Blockers can theoretically be problematic for patients with PAD due to possible decreased peripheral blood flow secondary to unopposed stimulation of α_1-receptors that results in vasoconstriction. If problematic, this can be mitigated by using a β-blocker that also has α_1-blocking properties (eg, carvedilol). However, β-blockers are not contraindicated in PAD and have not been shown to adversely affect walking capacity.[65]

Metabolic Syndrome Metabolic syndrome is a cluster of multiple cardiometabolic risk factors.[66] It has been most recently defined as the presence of three of the following five criteria: abdominal obesity (based on waist circumference measurements), elevated triglycerides, low HDL cholesterol, elevated BP (greater than or equal to 130/greater than or equal to 85 mm Hg or receiving drug treatment for high BP), and elevated fasting blood glucose.[66]

Despite the debate regarding whether or not metabolic syndrome is a true "disease" or rather simply a cluster of risk factors, it is widely accepted that patients with metabolic syndrome have increased risk of developing CV disease and/or type 2 diabetes. Using an ACEi or ARB is associated with the lowest rate of developing new-onset diabetes in patients with hypertension.[67] However, studies specifically evaluating the most effective antihypertensive regimen for patients with metabolic syndrome have not been done. In addition, an ALLHAT subgroup analysis of patients with impaired fasting glucose showed that CV events were reduced more with chlorthalidone compared with lisinopril.[37] Thus, thiazides can be used first-line for patients with metabolic syndrome, similar to an ACEi, ARB, or CCB, but treated patients will have a higher risk of developing elevated fasting glucose.

Erectile Dysfunction Most antihypertensive agents have been associated with erectile dysfunction in men. However, it is not clear if erectile dysfunction associated with antihypertensive treatment is solely a result of drug therapy or rather a symptom of underlying vascular disease. β-Blockers have traditionally been labeled as agents that significantly cause sexual dysfunction, and many practitioners have avoided prescribing them as a result. However, data supporting this notion are limited. A systematic review of 15 studies involving 35,000 patients assessing β-blocker use for MI, heart failure, and hypertension found only a very slight increased risk for erectile dysfunction.[68] In addition, prospective long-term data from the Treatment of Mild Hypertension Study (TOMHS) and the Veterans Administration Cooperative trial show no difference in the incidence of erectile dysfunction between thiazide and β-blocker versus an ACEi and CCB.[69,70] Centrally acting agents are associated with higher rates of sexual dysfunction and should be avoided in men with erectile dysfunction.

Hypertensive men frequently have atherosclerotic vascular disease, which frequently results in erectile dysfunction. Therefore, erectile dysfunction is associated with chronic arterial changes resulting from elevated BP, and lack of control may increase the risk of erectile dysfunction. These changes are even more pronounced in hypertensive men with diabetes.

Individual Antihypertensive Agents

ACEi An ACEi is a first-line therapy option in most patients with hypertension.[1-4] The ALLHAT demonstrated less heart failure and stroke with chlorthalidone versus lisinopril.[28] However, another outcome study has demonstrated similar, if not better, outcomes with an ACEi versus hydrochlorothiazide.[31] It is possible that the different thiazides have different abilities to reduce CV events. Nonetheless, most clinicians will agree that if an ACEi is not the first agent used in most patients with hypertension, they should be the second agent used.

ACE facilitates production of angiotensin II that has a major role in arterial BP regulation as depicted in Fig. 13-1. ACE is distributed in many tissues and is present in several different cell types, but its principal location is in endothelial cells. Therefore, the major site for angiotensin II production is in the blood vessels, not the kidney. An ACEi blocks the ACE, thus inhibiting conversion of angiotensin I to angiotensin II. Angiotensin II is a potent vasoconstrictor that stimulates aldosterone secretion, causing an increase in sodium and water reabsorption with accompanying potassium loss. By blocking the ACE, vasodilation and a decrease in aldosterone occur.

An ACEi also blocks degradation of bradykinin and stimulates the synthesis of other vasodilating substances (prostaglandin E_2 and prostacyclin). The observation that an ACEi lowers BP in patients with normal plasma renin activity suggests that bradykinin and perhaps tissue production of ACE are important in the pathogenesis of hypertension. Increased bradykinin enhances the BP-lowering effects of an ACEi, but also is responsible for the side effect of a dry cough. An ACEi may effectively prevent or regress LVH by reducing direct stimulation by angiotensin II on myocardial cells.

There are many evidence-based uses for an ACEi (see Fig. 13-3). An ACEi reduces CV morbidity and mortality in patients with HF*r*EF and decrease progression of CKD. They should be first-line as disease-modifying therapy in all of these patients unless absolutely contraindicated. An ACEi (or ARB in certain patients) is first-line for patients with diabetes and hypertension because of demonstrated CV disease and kidney benefits. A regimen including an ACEi with a thiazide is considered first-line in recurrent stroke prevention based on benefits demonstrated from the PROGRESS trial showing reduced risk of secondary stroke.[30] In combination with β-blocker therapy, evidence shows that an ACEi further reduce CV risk in coronary disease and in patients post-MI.[44,45,48,49] These benefits of an ACEi occur in patients with atherosclerotic vascular disease even in the absence of left ventricular dysfunction and have the potential to reduce the development of new-onset type 2 diabetes.[71]

Most agents can be dosed once daily in hypertension (see Table 13-5). In some patients, especially when higher doses are used, twice-daily dosing is needed to maintain 24-hour effects with enalapril, benazepril, moexipril, quinapril, and ramipril.

ACEi therapy is generally well tolerated.[72] They decrease aldosterone and can increase potassium serum concentrations. While this increase is usually small, hyperkalemia is possible. Patients with CKD or those on concomitant potassium supplements, potassium-sparing diuretics, ARBs, or a direct renin inhibitor are at risk for hyperkalemia. Judicious monitoring of serum potassium and creatinine values within 4 weeks of starting or increasing the dose of an ACEi can often identify these abnormalities early before they evolve into serious adverse events.

The most worrisome adverse effect of ACEi therapy is acute kidney failure. This serious adverse effect is rare, occurring in less than 1% of patients. Preexisting kidney disease increases the risk of this side effect. Bilateral renal artery stenosis or unilateral stenosis of a solitary functioning kidney renders patients dependent on the vasoconstrictive effect of angiotensin II on the efferent arteriole of the kidney, thus explaining why these patients are particularly susceptible to acute kidney failure from an ACEi. Slow titration of the ACEi dose and judicious kidney function monitoring can minimize risk and allow for early detection of those with renal artery stenosis.

It is important to note that GFR does decrease somewhat in patients when started on an ACEi or ARB.[73] This is attributed to the inhibition of angiotensin II vasoconstriction on the efferent arteriole. This decrease in GFR often increases serum creatinine, and small increases should be anticipated when monitoring patients on an ACEi. Either modest elevations of less than or equal to 35% (for baseline creatinine values less than or equal to 3 mg/dL [265 μmol/L]) or absolute increases less than 1 mg/dL (88 μmol/L) do not warrant changes. If larger increases occur, ACEi therapy should be stopped or the dose reduced.

Angioedema is a serious potential complication of ACEi therapy. It occurs in less than 1% of the population, and it is more likely in African Americans and smokers. Symptoms include lip and tongue swelling and possibly difficulty breathing. Drug withdrawal is appropriate for treating patients with angioedema. However, angioedema associated with laryngeal edema and/or pulmonary symptoms occasionally occurs and requires additional treatment with icatibant, fresh frozen plasma, and/or emergent intubations to support respiration. A history of angioedema, even if not from an ACEi, precludes use of another ACEi (it is a contraindication). Cross-reactivity between an ACEi and an ARB does not appear to be a significant concern. The Telmisartan Randomized Assessment Study in ACE-Intolerant Subjects with Cardiovascular Disease (TRANSCEND) trial enrolled 75 patients with a history of ACEi–induced angioedema, and randomized these patients to either placebo or ARB therapy.[74] There were no cases of repeat angioedema among these patients. These data suggest the cross-reactivity is very low. Hence, an ARB can be used in a patient with a history of ACEi-induced angioedema when it is needed. However, clinicians should monitor for repeat occurrences, since idiopathic angioedema may still occur.

A persistent dry cough develops in up to 20% of patients treated with an ACEi. It is pharmacologically explained by the inhibition of bradykinin breakdown. This cough does not cause respiratory illness but is annoying to patients and can compromise adherence. It should be clearly differentiated from a wet cough due to pulmonary edema, which may be a sign of uncontrolled heart failure versus an ACEi-induced cough.

An ACEi, as well as an ARB or direct renin inhibitor, are absolutely contraindicated in pregnancy. Female patients of childbearing age should be counseled regarding effective forms of birth control as ACEi therapy has been associated with major congenital malformations when exposed in the first trimester and fetopathy (group of conditions that includes renal failure, renal dysplasia, hypotension, oligohydramnios, pulmonary hypotension, hypocalvaria, and death) has occurred when exposed in the second and third trimesters. Similar to a thiazide, an ACEi can increase lithium serum concentrations in patients on lithium therapy. Concurrent use of an ACEi with a potassium-sparing diuretic (including aldosterone antagonists), potassium supplements, an ARB, or a direct renin inhibitor may result in hyperkalemia.

Starting doses of an ACEi should be low, with even lower doses for patients at risk for orthostatic hypotension or severe renal dysfunction (eg, elderly, CKD). Acute hypotension may occur at the onset of ACEi therapy. Patients who are sodium or volume depleted, in a heart failure exacerbation, very elderly, or on concurrent vasodilators or thiazide therapy are at high risk for this effect. It is important to start with half the normal dose of an ACEi for all patients with these risk factors and to use slow dose titration.

ARB Angiotensin II is generated by two enzymatic pathways: the RAAS, which involves ACE, and an alternative pathway that uses other enzymes such as chymase (aka "tissue ACE"). An ACEi inhibits only the effects of angiotensin II produced through the RAAS, whereas ARBs inhibit angiotensin II from all pathways. It is unclear how these differences affect tissue concentrations of ACE. An ACEi only partially blocks the effects of angiotensin II, although the clinical significance of this is not known.

Angiotensin II receptor blocker therapy directly blocks the AT_1 receptor that mediates the known effects of angiotensin II in humans: vasoconstriction, aldosterone release, sympathetic activation, antidiuretic hormone release, and constriction of the efferent arterioles of the glomerulus. They do not block the AT_2 receptor. Therefore, beneficial effects of AT_2 receptor stimulation (vasodilation, tissue repair, and inhibition of cell growth) remain intact when ARBs are used. Unlike an ACEi, an ARB does not block the breakdown of bradykinin. Therefore, some of the beneficial effects of bradykinin, such as vasodilation, regression of myocyte hypertrophy and fibrosis, and increased levels of tissue plasminogen activator, are not present with ARB therapy.

An ARB is a first-line therapy option in most patients with hypertension.[1-4] ARB therapy has been directly compared with ACEi therapy in the management of hypertension.[75] The Ongoing Telmisartan Alone and in Combination with Ramipril Global End Point Trial (ON-TARGET) was a double-blind trial that randomized 25,620 patients with hypertension to ACEi-based therapy, ARB-based therapy, or the combination of an ACEi with an ARB. The primary end point was a composite end point of CV death or hospitalization for heart failure. After a median follow-up of 56 months, there was no difference in the primary end point between any of the three treatment groups. Therefore, these data establish that the CV event-lowering benefits of ARB therapy are similar to ACEi therapy in hypertension. Moreover, the combination of an ACEi with an ARB had no additional CV event lowering but was associated with a higher risk of side effects (renal dysfunction, hypotension). Therefore, there is no reason to use an ACEi with an ARB for the management of hypertension.

For patients with type 2 diabetes and nephropathy, progression of nephropathy has been shown to be significantly reduced with ARB therapy.[16] Some benefits appear to be independent of BP lowering, suggesting that the pharmacologic effects of ARBs on the efferent arteriole may result in attenuated progression of kidney disease. For patients with HF*r*EF, ARB therapy has been shown to reduce risk of hospitalization for heart failure when used as an alternative therapy in ACEi-intolerant patients.[43]

Angiotensin II receptor blockers have been compared head-to-head with CCBs. The Morbidity and Mortality After Stroke: Eprosartan Versus Nitrendipine in Secondary Prevention (MOSES) trial demonstrated that eprosartan reduced the risk of recurrent stroke greater than nitrendipine in patients with a past medical history of cerebrovascular disease.[55] Using nitrendipine was a reasonable comparator because the Syst-Eur had already demonstrated that nitrendipine reduces the occurrence of CV events, particularly stroke, in older patients with isolated systolic hypertension compared with placebo.[11] These data support the common notion that ARBs may have cerebroprotective effects that may explain CV event reductions. Another outcome study, the Valsartan Antihypertensive Long-Term Use Evaluation (VALUE) trial, showed that valsartan-based therapy is equivalent to amlodipine-based therapy for the primary composite outcome of first CV event in patients with hypertension and additional CV risk factors.[32] However, occurrence of certain components of the primary end point (stroke and MI) and new-onset type 2 diabetes was lower in the valsartan group. Although patients treated with amlodipine had slightly lower mean BP values than valsartan-treated patients, there was no difference in the primary end point.

The addition of a CCB or thiazide to an ARB significantly increases antihypertensive efficacy. Similar to an ACEi, most ARBs have long enough half-lives to allow for once-daily dosing. However, candesartan, eprosartan, losartan, and valsartan have the shortest half-lives and may require twice-daily dosing for sustained BP lowering.

Angiotensin II receptor blocker therapy has the lowest incidence of side effects compared with other antihypertensive agents.[72] Because ARBs do not affect bradykinin, they do not illicit a dry cough like an ACEi. While these drugs have been referred to as an "ACEi without the cough," pharmacologic differences highlight that they could have very different effects on vascular smooth muscle and myocardial tissue that can correlate to different effects when compared with an ACEi. Regardless, their first-line role for patients with hypertension is well established, and they are reasonable alternatives for patients requiring an ACEi but who experience an intolerable cough.

Like an ACEi, an ARB may cause renal insufficiency, hyperkalemia, and orthostatic hypotension. The same precautions that apply to ACEi therapy for patients with suspected bilateral renal artery stenosis, those on drugs that can raise potassium, and those on drugs that increase risk of hypotension apply to ARBs. As discussed in ACEi, ARB, or CCB as First-Line Agents above, patients with a history of ACEi angioedema can be treated with an ARB when needed.[74] An ARB should not be used in pregnancy.

CCB CCB therapy, including both dihydropyridine and nondihydropyridine types, are first-line therapy and are very effective antihypertensive agents.[1-4] They also have compelling indications in coronary artery disease and diabetes. However, with these compelling indications, they are in addition to, or instead of, other first-line antihypertensive drug classes.

Contraction of cardiac and smooth muscle cells requires an increase in free intracellular calcium concentrations from the extracellular fluid. When cardiac or vascular smooth muscle is stimulated, voltage-sensitive channels in the cell membrane are opened, allowing calcium to enter the cells. The influx of extracellular calcium into the cell releases stored calcium from the sarcoplasmic reticulum. As intracellular free calcium concentration increases, it binds to a protein, calmodulin, which then activates myosin kinase enabling myosin to interact with actin to induce contraction. CCBs work by inhibiting influx of calcium across the cell membrane. There are two types of voltage-gated calcium channels: a high-voltage channel (L-type) and a low-voltage channel (T-type). Currently available CCBs only block the L-type channel, which leads to coronary and peripheral vasodilation.

The two subclasses, dihydropyridines and nondihydropyridines (see Table 13-5), are pharmacologically very different from each other. Antihypertensive effectiveness is similar with both subclasses, but they differ somewhat in other pharmacodynamic effects. Nondihydropyridines (verapamil and diltiazem) decrease heart rate and slow atrioventricular nodal conduction. Similar to a β-blocker, these drugs may also treat supraventricular tachyarrhythmias (eg, atrial fibrillation). Verapamil produces negative inotropic and chronotropic effects that are responsible for its propensity to precipitate or cause systolic heart failure in high-risk patients. Diltiazem also has these effects but to a lesser extent than verapamil. All CCBs (except amlodipine and felodipine) have negative inotropic effects. Dihydropyridines may cause a baroreceptor-mediated reflex tachycardia because of their potent peripheral vasodilating effects. This effect appears to be more pronounced with the first-generation dihydropyridines (eg, nifedipine) and is significantly diminished with the newer agents (eg, amlodipine) and when given in sustained-release dosage forms. Dihydropyridines do not alter conduction through the atrioventricular node and thus are not effective agents in supraventricular tachyarrhythmias.

Dihydropyridine CCB The dihydropyridine CCBs have been extensively studied. In ALLHAT there was no difference in the primary outcome between chlorthalidone and amlodipine, and only the secondary outcome of heart failure was higher with amlodipine.[29] A subgroup analysis of ALLHAT directly compared amlodipine with lisinopril and demonstrated that there was no difference in the primary outcome.[76] However, amlodipine was superior to lisinopril for BP control in blacks, and for stroke reduction in blacks and in women. There was a lower risk of heart failure in the lisinopril group. As discussed previously, the VALUE study also showed no difference between valsartan and amlodipine in the primary outcome of first CV event in high-risk patients.[32]

Dihydropyridine CCBs are very effective in older patients with isolated systolic hypertension. The placebo-controlled Syst-Eur trial demonstrated that a long-acting dihydropyridine CCB reduced the risk of CV events markedly in isolated systolic hypertension.[11] A long-acting dihydropyridine CCB should be strongly considered as preferred add-on therapy when a thiazide is not controlling BP in a patient with isolated systolic hypertension and no other compelling indications.

Among dihydropyridines, short-acting nifedipine may rarely cause an increase in the frequency, intensity, and duration of angina in association with acute hypotension. This effect is most likely due to a reflex sympathetic stimulation and is likely obviated by using sustained-release formulations of nifedipine. For this reason, all other dihydropyridines have an intrinsically long half-life or are sustained-release formulations. Immediate-release nifedipine has been associated with an increased incidence of adverse CV effects, is not approved for treatment of hypertension, and should not be used to treat hypertension. Other side effects with dihydropyridines include dizziness, flushing, headache, gingival hyperplasia, peripheral edema, mood changes, and various GI complaints. Side effects due to vasodilation such as dizziness, flushing, headache, and peripheral edema occur more frequently with all dihydropyridines than with the nondihydropyridines (ie, verapamil, diltiazem) because they are less potent vasodilators.

Nondihydropyridine CCB Diltiazem and verapamil can cause cardiac conduction abnormalities such as bradycardia or atrioventricular block. These problems occur mostly with high doses or when used for patients with preexisting abnormalities in the cardiac conduction system. Heart failure has been reported in otherwise healthy patients due to negative inotropic effects. Both drugs can cause anorexia, nausea, peripheral edema, and hypotension. Verapamil causes constipation in about 7% of patients. This side effect also occurs with diltiazem, but to a lesser extent.

Verapamil and to a lesser extent diltiazem can cause drug interactions due to their ability to inhibit the cytochrome P450 3A4 isoenzyme system. This inhibition can increase serum concentrations of other drugs that are metabolized by this isoenzyme system (eg, cyclosporine, digoxin, lovastatin, simvastatin, tacrolimus, theophylline). Verapamil and diltiazem should be given very cautiously with a β-blocker because there is an increased risk of heart block with these combinations. When a CCB is needed in combination with a β-blocker for BP lowering, a dihydropyridine should be selected because it will not increase risk of heart block. The hepatic metabolism of CCBs, especially felodipine, nicardipine, nifedipine, and nisoldipine, may be inhibited by ingesting large quantities of grapefruit juice (eg, greater than or equal to 1 quart daily).

Many different formulations of verapamil and diltiazem are currently available (see Table 13-5). Although certain sustained-release verapamil and diltiazem products contain the same active drug (eg, Calan SR and Verelan), they are usually not AB rated by the FDA as interchangeable on a milligram-per-milligram basis due to different biopharmaceutical release mechanisms. However, the clinical significance of these differences is likely negligible.

Two sustained-release verapamil products (Covera-HS and Verelan PM) and one diltiazem product (Cardizem LA) are chronotherapeutically designed to target the circadian BP rhythm. These agents are primarily dosed in the evening (with the exception of Cardizem LA, which may be dosed in the morning or evening) so that drug is released during the early morning hours when BP first starts to increase. The rationale behind chronotherapy in hypertension is that blunting the early morning BP surge may result in greater reductions in CV events than conventional dosing of regular antihypertensive products in the morning. However, evidence from the Controlled Onset Verapamil Investigation of Cardiovascular End-Points (CONVINCE) trial showed that chronotherapeutic verapamil was similar to, but not better than, a thiazide-β-blocker-based regimen with respect to CV events.[27]

Thiazide and Other Diuretics There are four subclasses of diuretics that are used in the treatment of hypertension: thiazides, loops, potassium-sparing agents, and aldosterone antagonists (see Table 13-5).[77] A thiazide is the preferred type of diuretic for hypertension and is considered a first-line therapy option in most patients with hypertension.[1-4] The best available evidence justifying this recommendation is from the ALLHAT.[29] Moreover, when combination therapy is needed in hypertension to control BP, a thiazide as an add-on agent, but not necessarily the second agent, is very effective in lowering BP.

Loops are more potent agents for inducing diuresis, but they are not ideal antihypertensive agents unless relief of edema is also needed. In general, loops are sometimes needed over a thiazide for hypertension in patients with CKD when estimated GFR is less than 30 mL/min/1.73 m^2, especially when edema is present.[77] However, many patients with an estimated GFR of less than 30 mL/min/1.73 m^2 but not on dialysis will still have antihypertensive effects with thiazides. This is especially true with chlorthalidone.[77]

Potassium-sparing diuretics are very weak antihypertensive agents when used alone and provide minimal additive effect when used in combination with a thiazide or loop diuretic. Their primary use is in combination with another diuretic to counteract the potassium-wasting properties of the other diuretic agent. Aldosterone antagonists (spironolactone and eplerenone) may be technically considered potassium-sparing agents but are more potent as antihypertensives. However, they are viewed as an independent class due to evidence supporting compelling indications.

The exact hypotensive mechanism of action of diuretics is not known, but has been well hypothesized. The drop in BP seen when diuretics are first started is caused by an initial diuresis. Diuresis causes reductions in plasma and stroke volume, which decreases CO and BP. This initial drop in CO causes a compensatory increase in PVR. With chronic diuretic therapy, extracellular fluid and plasma volume return to near pretreatment values. However, PVR decreases to values that are lower than the pretreatment baseline. This reduction in PVR is responsible for chronic antihypertensive effects.

With thiazide therapy additional actions may further explain their antihypertensive effects. They mobilize sodium and water from arteriolar walls. This effect would lessen the amount of physical encroachment on the lumen of the vessel created by excessive accumulation of intracellular fluid. As the diameter of the lumen relaxes and increases, there is less resistance to the flow of blood and PVR further drops. High dietary sodium intake can blunt this effect and a low salt intake can enhance this effect. Thiazides are also postulated to cause direct relaxation of vascular smooth muscle.

Diuretics should ideally be dosed in the morning if given once daily and in the morning and late afternoon when dosed twice daily to minimize risk of nocturnal diuresis. However, with chronic use, thiazides, potassium-sparing diuretics, and aldosterone antagonists rarely cause a pronounced diuresis.

The major pharmacokinetic differences between the various thiazides are serum half-life and duration of diuretic effect. The clinical relevance of these differences is unknown because the serum half-life of most antihypertensive agents does not correlate with the hypotensive duration of action. Moreover, diuretics lower BP primarily through extrarenal mechanisms. Hydrochlorothiazide and particularly chlorthalidone are the two most frequently used thiazides in landmark clinical trials that have demonstrated reduced morbidity and mortality. Hydrochlorothiazide is considered a "thiazide-type" agent while chlorthalidone is a "thiazide-like" agent. These agents are not equipotent on a milligram-per-milligram basis; chlorthalidone is 1.5 to 2 times more potent than hydrochlorothiazide.[77] This has been attributed to a longer half-life (45-60 hours vs 8-15 hours) and longer duration of effect (48-72 hours vs 16-24 hours) with chlorthalidone.

A thiazide is very effective in lowering BP when used in combination with most other antihypertensives. This additive response is explained by two independent pharmacodynamic effects. First, when two drugs cause the same overall pharmacologic effect (BP lowering) through different mechanisms of action, their combination usually results in an additive or synergistic effect. This is especially relevant when a β-blocker or ACEi/ARB is indicated in an African American, but does not elicit sufficient antihypertensive effect. Adding a thiazide in this situation can often significantly lower BP. Second, a compensatory increase in sodium and fluid retention may be seen with antihypertensive agents. This problem is counteracted with the concurrent use of a thiazide.

Side effects of a thiazide include hypokalemia, hypomagnesemia, hypercalcemia, hyperuricemia, hyperglycemia, dyslipidemia, and sexual dysfunction. Many of these side effects were identified when high doses of thiazides were used in the past (eg, hydrochlorothiazide 100-200 mg/day). Current guidelines recommend dosing hydrochlorothiazide or chlorthalidone to 12.5 to 25 mg/day, which markedly reduces the risk for most metabolic side effects. However, the most effective antihypertensive dose of hydrochlorothiazide is 50 mg daily, although many clinicians are dissuaded from this higher dose due to potential higher risk of hypokalemia.[78] Loop diuretics may cause the same side effects. Although the effect on serum lipids and glucose is not as significant, hypokalemia is more pronounced, and hypocalcemia may occur.

Hypokalemia and hypomagnesemia may cause muscle fatigue or cramps. However, serious cardiac arrhythmias can occur in patients with severe hypokalemia and hypomagnesemia. Patients at greatest risk include those with LVH, coronary disease, post-MI, a history of arrhythmia, or concurrently receiving digoxin. Low-dose therapy (ie, 25 mg hydrochlorothiazide or 12.5 mg chlorthalidone daily) causes small electrolyte disturbances. However, the most effective doses of these two thiazides are hydrochlorothiazide 50 mg daily and chlorthalidone 25 mg daily. Efforts should be made to keep potassium in the therapeutic range by careful monitoring, especially if these higher doses are used.

Thiazide-induced hyperuricemia can precipitate gout. This side effect may be especially problematic for patients with a previous history of gout and is more common with thiazides. However, acute gout is unlikely in patients with no previous history of gout. If gout does occur in a patient who requires thiazide therapy, allopurinol can be given to prevent gout and will not compromise the antihypertensive effects of the thiazide. High doses of thiazide and loop diuretics may increase fasting glucose and serum cholesterol values. These effects, however, usually are transient and often inconsequential.[79]

Potassium-sparing diuretics can cause hyperkalemia, especially in patients with CKD or diabetes and in patients receiving concurrent treatment with an ACEi, ARB, direct renin inhibitor, or potassium supplements. Hyperkalemia is especially problematic for the newest aldosterone antagonist eplerenone. This agent is a very selective aldosterone antagonist, and its propensity to cause hyperkalemia is greater than with the other potassium-sparing agents and even spironolactone. Due to this increased risk of hyperkalemia, eplerenone is contraindicated for patients with impaired kidney function or type 2 diabetes with proteinuria (see Table 13-5). While spironolactone may cause gynecomastia in up to 10% of patients, this occurs rarely with eplerenone.

A thiazide can be used safely with most other agents. However, concurrent administration with lithium may result in increased lithium serum concentrations and can predispose patients to lithium toxicity.

β-Blocker A β-blocker has been used in several large outcome trials in hypertension. However, in most of these trials, a thiazide was the first-line agent with a β-blocker added for additional BP lowering. Moreover, as previously discussed, for patients with hypertension but without compelling indications, other first-line agents (ie, ACEi, ARB, CCB, thiazide) should be used as the initial first-line agent before a β-blocker. This recommendation is based on meta-analyses that suggest β-blocker-based therapy may not reduce CV events as well as these other agents when used as the initial drug to treat patients with hypertension and without a compelling indication for a β-blocker.[42]

A β-blocker is only considered an appropriate first-line agent to treat specific compelling indications (eg, post-MI, coronary artery disease, HF*r*EF). Numerous trials have shown a reduced risk of CV events when β-blockers are used following an MI, during an acute coronary syndrome, or in patients with chronic stable angina with ischemic symptoms. Although once contraindicated in heart failure, studies have shown that bisoprolol, carvedilol, and metoprolol succinate reduce mortality in patients with HF*r*EF who are treated with a diuretic and ACEi.

Several mechanisms of action have been proposed for β-blockers, but none of them alone has been shown to be consistently associated with a reduction in arterial BP. β-Blocker therapy has negative chronotropic and inotropic effects that reduce CO, which explains some of the antihypertensive effect. However, CO falls equally for patients treated with a β-blocker regardless of BP lowering. Additionally, β-blockers with ISA do not reduce CO, yet they lower BP and decrease peripheral resistance.

β-Adrenoceptors are also located on the surface membranes of juxtaglomerular cells, and a β-blocker inhibits these receptors and thus the release of renin. However, there is a weak association between plasma renin and antihypertensive efficacy of β-blocker therapy. Some patients with low plasma renin concentrations do respond to β-blocker therapy. Therefore, additional mechanisms likely also account for the antihypertensive effect of a β-blocker. However, the ability of a β-blocker to reduce plasma renin and thus angiotensin II concentrations may play a major role in their ability to reduce CV risk.

There are important pharmacodynamic and pharmacokinetic differences among β-blockers, but all agents provide a similar degree of BP lowering. There are three pharmacodynamic properties of β-blocker therapy that differentiate this class: cardioselectivity, ISA, and membrane-stabilizing effects. β-Blocker agents that possess a greater affinity for β_1-receptors than for β_2-receptors are *cardioselective*.

β_1-Adrenoceptors and β_2-adrenoceptors are distributed throughout the body, but they concentrate differently in certain organs and tissues. There is a preponderance of β_1-receptors in the heart and kidney, and a preponderance of β_2-receptors in the lungs, liver, pancreas, and arteriolar smooth muscle. β_1-Receptor stimulation increases heart rate, contractility, and renin release. β_2-Receptor stimulation results in bronchodilation and vasodilation. Cardioselective β-blocker therapy is not likely to provoke bronchospasm and vasoconstriction. Insulin secretion and glycogenolysis are mediated by β_2-receptors. Blocking β_2-receptors may reduce these processes and increase blood glucose or blunt recovery from hypoglycemia.

Cardioselective β-blockers (eg, atenolol, bisoprolol, metoprolol, and nebivolol) have clinically significant advantages over nonselective agents (eg, propranolol and nadolol), and are preferred when using a β-blocker to treat hypertension. Cardioselective agents are safer than nonselective agents for patients with asthma or diabetes who have a compelling indication for a β-blocker. However, cardioselectivity is a dose-dependent phenomenon; at higher doses, cardioselective agents lose their relative selectivity for β_1-receptors and block β_2-receptors as effectively as they block β_1-receptors. The dose at which cardioselectivity is lost varies from patient to patient.

Some β-blockers (eg, acebutolol, pindolol) have ISA and act as partial β-receptor agonists. When they bind to the β-receptor, they stimulate it, but far less than a pure β-agonist. If sympathetic tone is low, as it is during resting states, β-receptors are partially stimulated by ISA β-blockers. Therefore, resting heart rate, CO, and peripheral blood flow are not reduced when these types of β-blockers are used. Theoretically, ISA agents would appear to have advantages over a non-ISA β-blocker in certain patients with heart failure or sinus bradycardia. Unfortunately, they do not appear to reduce CV events as well as other β-blockers. In fact, they may increase CV risk post-MI or in those with coronary artery disease. Thus, agents with ISA are rarely needed.

All β-blockers exert a *membrane-stabilizing action* on cardiac cells when large doses are given. This activity is needed when β-blockers are used as an antiarrhythmic agent.

Pharmacokinetic differences among β-blockers relate to first-pass metabolism, route of elimination, degree of lipophilicity, and serum half-lives. Propranolol and metoprolol undergo extensive first-pass metabolism, so the dose needed to attain β-blockade with either drug varies from patient to patient. Atenolol and nadolol are renally excreted. The dose of these agents may need to be reduced for patients with moderate-to-severe CKD.

β-Blockers, especially those with high lipophilic properties, penetrate the central nervous system and may cause other effects. Propranolol is the most lipophilic drug and atenolol is the least lipophilic. Therefore, higher brain concentrations of propranolol compared with atenolol are seen after equivalent doses are given. It is thought that higher lipophilicity is associated with more central nervous system side effects (dizziness and drowsiness). However, the lipophilic properties can provide better effects for non-CV conditions such as migraine headache prevention, essential tremor, and thyrotoxicosis. BP lowering is equal among β-blockers regardless of lipophilicity.

Most side effects of β-blocker therapy are extensions of their ability to antagonize β-adrenoceptors. β-Blockade in the myocardium can be associated with bradycardia, atrioventricular conduction abnormalities (eg, second- or third-degree heart block), and the development of acute heart failure. The decrease in heart rate may benefit certain patients with atrial arrhythmias (atrial fibrillation and atrial flutter) and hypertension by both providing rate control and BP lowering. β-Blocker therapy usually only produce heart failure if used in high initial doses for patients with preexisting left ventricular dysfunction or if started in these patients during an acute heart failure exacerbation. Blocking β_2-receptors in arteriolar smooth muscle may cause cold extremities and may aggravate intermittent claudication or Raynaud's phenomenon as a result of decreased peripheral blood flow. In addition, there is an increase of sympathetic tone during periods of hypoglycemia in patients with diabetes that may result in a significant increase in BP because of unopposed α-receptor-mediated vasoconstriction.

Abrupt cessation of β-blocker therapy can produce unstable angina, MI, or even death in patients with coronary disease. Abrupt cessation may also lead to rebound hypertension (a sudden increase in BP to or above pretreatment values). To avoid this, β-blockers should always be tapered gradually over 1 to 2 weeks before eventually discontinuing the drug. This acute withdrawal syndrome is believed to be secondary to progression of underlying coronary disease, hypersensitivity of β-adrenergic receptors due to upregulation, and increased physical activity after withdrawal of a drug that decreases myocardial oxygen requirements. For patients without coronary disease, abrupt discontinuation may present as tachycardia, sweating, and generalized malaise in addition to increased BP.

Like a thiazide, β-blocker therapy has been shown to increase serum cholesterol and glucose values, but these effects are transient and of little clinical significance. For patients with diabetes, the reduction in CV events was as great with β-blocker therapy as with an ACEi in the United Kingdom Prospective Diabetes Study (UKPDS)[80] and far superior to placebo in the SHEP trial.[8] In the Glycemic Effects in Diabetes Mellitus: Carvedilol–Metoprolol Comparison in Hypertensives (GEMINI) trial, patients with diabetes and hypertension who were randomized to metoprolol tartrate had an increase in hemoglobin A1C values, while patients randomized to carvedilol did not.[81] This suggests that mixed α- and β-blocking effects of carvedilol may be preferential to metoprolol for patients with uncontrolled diabetes. However, differences in hemoglobin A1C values were small.

Nebivolol is considered a third-generation β-blocker. Similar to carvedilol and labetalol, this β-blocker results in vasodilation. However, carvedilol and labetalol cause vasodilation because of their ability to block α_1-receptors, while nebivolol causes vasodilation through release of nitric oxide. The long-term clinical benefits of the nitric oxide effects seen with nebivolol are currently unknown, but this might explain a lower risk of β-blocker-associated fatigue, erectile dysfunction, and metabolic side effects (eg, hyperglycemia) with this agent.

13 **Alternative Agents** The primary role of an alternative antihypertensive agent is to provide additional BP lowering in patients who are already treated with combination therapy consisting of first-line antihypertensive.

***α_1*-Blocker** Prazosin, terazosin, and doxazosin are selective α_1-receptor blockers. They work in the peripheral vasculature and inhibit the uptake of catecholamines in smooth muscle cells resulting in vasodilation and BP lowering.

Doxazosin was one of the original treatment arms of the ALLHAT. However, it was stopped prematurely when statistically more secondary end points of stroke, heart failure, and CV events were seen with doxazosin compared with chlorthalidone.[34] There were no differences in the primary end point of fatal coronary heart disease and nonfatal MI. These data suggest that thiazides are superior to α_1-blockers in preventing CV events in patients with hypertension. Therefore, α_1-blockers are alternative agents that should be used in combination with first-line antihypertensive agents.

An α_1-blocker can provide symptomatic benefits in men with benign prostatic hypertrophy. These agents block postsynaptic α_1-adrenergic receptors located on the prostate capsule, causing relaxation and decreased resistance to urinary outflow. However, when used to lower BP, they should only be in addition to other first-line antihypertensive agents.

A potentially severe side effect of an α_1-blocker is a "first-dose" phenomenon that is characterized by transient dizziness or faintness, palpitations, and even syncope within 1 to 3 hours of the first dose. This adverse reaction can also happen after dose increases. These episodes are accompanied by orthostatic hypotension and can be obviated by taking the first dose and subsequent first increased doses at bedtime. Because orthostatic hypotension and dizziness may persist with chronic administration, these agents should be used very cautiously in elderly patients, as they may increase the risk of falls. Even though antihypertensive effects are achieved through a peripheral α_1-receptor antagonism, these agents cross the blood–brain barrier and may cause central nervous system side effects such as lassitude, vivid dreams, and depression. α_1-Blocker therapy also may cause priapism. Sodium and water retention can occur with higher doses, and sometimes even with chronic administration of low doses. Therefore, these agents are most effective when given in combination with a thiazide to maintain antihypertensive efficacy and minimize potential edema.

Aliskiren Aliskiren is the only agent that is a direct renin inhibitor. This drug blocks the RAAS at its point of activation, which results in reduced plasma renin activity and BP lowering. It has a 24-hour half-life, is primarily eliminated through biliary excretion unchanged, and provides 24-hour antihypertensive effects with once-daily dosing.

The role of this drug class in the management of hypertension is very limited. Aliskiren is approved as monotherapy or in combination therapy. Since aliskiren is a RAAS blocker, it should not be used in combination with an ACEi or an ARB because of a higher risk of serious adverse effects without providing additional reduction in CV events.[82]

Many of the cautions and adverse effects seen with an ACEi or ARB applies to aliskiren. Aliskiren should never be used in pregnancy due to the known teratogenic effects of using other drugs that block the RAAS system. Angioedema has also been reported in patients treated with aliskiren. Increases in serum creatinine and serum potassium values have been observed. The mechanisms of these adverse effects are likely similar to those with an ACEi or ARB. It is reasonable to utilize similar monitoring strategies by measuring serum creatinine and serum potassium in patients treated with aliskiren.

Central α_2-Agonist Clonidine, guanabenz, guanfacine, and methyldopa lower BP primarily by stimulating α_2-adrenergic receptors in the brain. This stimulation reduces sympathetic outflow from the vasomotor center in the brain and increases vagal tone. It is also believed that peripheral stimulation of presynaptic α_2-receptors may further reduce sympathetic tone. Reduced sympathetic activity together with enhanced parasympathetic activity can decrease heart rate, CO, TPR, plasma renin activity, and baroreceptor reflexes. Clonidine is often used in resistant hypertension, and methyldopa is commonly used for pregnancy-induced hypertension.

Chronic use of a centrally acting α_2-agonist results in sodium and water retention, which is most prominent with methyldopa. Low doses of clonidine (and guanfacine or guanabenz) can be used to treat hypertension without the addition of a thiazide. However, methyldopa should be given in combination with a thiazide to avoid the blunting of antihypertensive effect that happens with prolonged use when used to treat chronic hypertension (not necessary in pregnancy-induced hypertension). Sedation and dry mouth are common anticholinergic side effects that typically improve with chronic use of low doses, but they are more troublesome in the elderly. As with other centrally acting antihypertensives, depression can occur, especially with high doses. The incidence of orthostatic hypotension and dizziness is higher than with other antihypertensive agents, so they should be used very cautiously in the elderly. Lastly, clonidine has a relatively high incidence of anticholinergic side effects (sedation, dry mouth, constipation, urinary retention, and blurred vision). Thus, it should generally be avoided for chronic antihypertensive therapy in the elderly.

Abrupt cessation of a central α_2-agonist may lead to rebound hypertension. This effect is thought to be secondary to a compensatory increase in norepinephrine release after abrupt discontinuation. In addition, other effects such as nervousness, agitation, headache, and tremor can also occur, which may be exacerbated by concomitant β-blocker use, particularly with clonidine. Thus, if clonidine is to be discontinued, it should be tapered. For patients who are receiving concomitant β-blocker therapy, the β-blocker should be gradually discontinued first several days before gradual discontinuation of clonidine.

Methyldopa can cause hepatitis or hemolytic anemia, although this is rare. Transient elevations in serum hepatic transaminases are occasionally seen with methyldopa therapy but are clinically irrelevant unless they are greater than three times the upper limit or normal. Methyldopa should be quickly discontinued if persistent increases in serum hepatic transaminases or alkaline phosphatase are detected because this may indicate the onset of fulminant life-threatening hepatitis. A Coombs-positive hemolytic anemia occurs in less than 1% of patients receiving methyldopa, although 20% exhibit a positive direct Coombs test without anemia. For these reasons, methyldopa has limited use in routine management of hypertension, except in pregnancy.

Reserpine Reserpine lowers BP by depleting norepinephrine from sympathetic nerve endings and blocking transport of norepinephrine into its storage granules. Norepinephrine release into the synapse following nerve stimulation is reduced and results in reduced sympathetic tone, PVR, and BP. Reserpine also depletes catecholamines in the brain and the myocardium, which may lead to sedation, depression, and decreased CO.

Reserpine can cause significant sodium and water retention; therefore, it should be given in combination with a thiazide. Reserpine's strong inhibition of sympathetic activity results in increased parasympathetic activity, which explains why side effects such as nasal stuffiness, increased gastric acid secretion, diarrhea, and bradycardia can occur. Depression, which is a consequence of central nervous system depletion of catecholamines and serotonin, has been reported with high dose therapy. However, when reserpine is dosed between 0.05 and 0.25 mg daily (recommended doses), the rate of depression is equal to that seen with a β-blocker, thiazide, or placebo.[8]

Reserpine was used as a third-line agent in many of the landmark clinical trials that have documented the benefit in treating hypertension, including the Veterans Administration Cooperative trials and the SHEP trial.[8] An analysis of the SHEP data found that reserpine was well tolerated and that the combination of a thiazide and reserpine is effective in reducing CV events.

Direct Arterial Vasodilator Hydralazine and minoxidil directly relax arteriolar smooth muscle resulting in vasodilation and BP lowering. They exert little to no venous vasodilation. Both agents cause potent reductions in perfusion pressure that activate baroreceptor reflexes. Activation of baroreceptors results in a compensatory increase in sympathetic outflow, which leads to an increase in heart rate, CO, and renin release. Consequently, tachyphylaxis can develop resulting in a loss of hypotensive effect with continued use. This compensatory baroreceptor response can be counteracted by concurrent use of a β-blocker.

All patients receiving hydralazine or minoxidil long-term for hypertension should first receive both a thiazide and a β-blocker. Direct arterial vasodilators can precipitate angina in patients with underlying coronary disease unless the baroreceptor reflex mechanism is blocked with a β-blocker. Nondihydropyridine CCBs (diltiazem and verapamil) can be used as an alternative to β-blockers in these patients, but a β-blocker is preferred. The side effect of sodium and water retention is significant but is minimized by using a thiazide concomitantly.

One side effect unique to hydralazine is a dose-dependent drug-induced lupus-like syndrome. Hydralazine is eliminated by hepatic *N*-acetyltransferase. This enzyme displays genetic polymorphism, and "slow acetylators" are especially prone to develop drug-induced lupus with hydralazine. This syndrome is more common in women and is reversible on discontinuation. Drug-induced lupus may be avoided by using less than 200 mg of hydralazine daily. Because of side effects, hydralazine has limited clinical use for chronic management of hypertension. However, it is especially useful for patients with severe CKD and in kidney failure on hemodialysis. Hydralazine, when used in combination with isosorbide dinitrate, has been shown to reduce the risk of CV events in black patients with HF*r*EF when added to a standard regimen of a thiazide, ACEi or ARB, and evidence-based β-blocker therapy.[43]

Minoxidil is a more potent vasodilator than hydralazine. Therefore, the compensatory increases in heart rate, CO, renin release, and sodium retention are even more dramatic. Due to significant water retention, a loop diuretic is often a more effective antihypertensive than a thiazide in patients treated with minoxidil. A troublesome side effect of minoxidil is hypertrichosis (hirsutism), presenting as increased hair growth on the face, arms, back, and chest. Hypertrichosis usually ceases when the drug is discontinued. Other minoxidil side effects include pericardial effusion and a nonspecific T-wave change on the electrocardiogram. Minoxidil is reserved for very difficult-to-control hypertension and for patients requiring hydralazine that experience drug-induced lupus.

Pharmacoeconomic Considerations

The cost of effectively treating hypertension is substantial. It is projected that the direct and indirect costs of treating hypertension will rise from \$4.64 billion in 2011 to \$274 billion in 2030.[5] However, these costs are offset by savings that would be realized by reducing CV morbidity and mortality. Cost related to treating CV events (eg, MI, end-stage kidney failure) can drastically increase healthcare costs.

Antihypertensive drug costs are a major portion of the total cost of hypertensive care. First-line drug classes (ie, ACEi, ARB, CCB, and thiazide) are predominantly generic. Using these agents to treat hypertension results in lower drug acquisition costs. There are even multiple generic fixed-dose combinations of these agents.

It is crucial to identify ways to control the cost of care without increasing the morbidity and mortality associated with uncontrolled hypertension. Using evidence-based pharmacotherapy will save costs. An ACEi, ARB, CCB, and thiazide are all first-line treatment options in most patients without compelling indications, and most are very inexpensive. Just utilizing generic agents, either as monotherapy or in combination, is appropriate under most circumstances in hypertension management. Brand name drugs may also be used when needed. However, considerations to implement once-daily options and fixed-dose combination options that are economical should be considered.

Team-Based Collaborative Care

Team-based care for patients with cardiovascular disease is highly recommended in the comprehensive care of patients.[83] A collaborative approach to management of hypertension is a proven strategy that improves goal BP attainment rates.[84,85] These patient care models are interprofessional and utilize physicians, pharmacists, nurses, and other healthcare professionals.

With the advent of healthcare reform, collaborative team-based approaches to chronic diseases are viewed as high-quality and cost-effective improvement modalities. Within these models, pharmacists have been proven to be an effective component of team-based models both in ambulatory clinic settings[84] and in community pharmacist settings.[86] In addition to optimizing selection and implementation of antihypertensive drug therapy, clinical interventions by pharmacists have been proven to reduce the risk of adverse drug events and medication errors in ambulatory patients with CV disease.[87] Clinical pharmacists have a substantial effect in a wide variety of roles in clinical settings, largely through optimization of drug use, avoidance of adverse drug events, and transitional care activities focusing on medication reconciliation and patient education.[88]

EVALUATION OF THERAPEUTIC OUTCOMES

Monitoring the Pharmacotherapy Plan

Routine ongoing monitoring to assess the desired effects of antihypertensive therapy (efficacy, including BP goal attainment), the undesired adverse side effects (toxicity), and disease progression is needed in all patients treated with antihypertensive drug therapy.

Efficacy

The most important strategy to prevent CV morbidity and mortality in hypertension is BP control to goal values (Clinical Presentation "Desired Outcomes: Goal BP Values"). Routine goal BP values should be attained in elderly patients and in those with isolated systolic hypertension, but actual BP lowering can occur at a gradual pace over a period of several months to avoid orthostatic hypotension. Modifying other CV risk factors (eg, smoking, dyslipidemia, diabetes) is also important.

Clinic-based BP monitoring remains the standard for managing hypertension. BP response should be evaluated 2 to 4 weeks after initiating or making changes in therapy. With some agents, monitoring BP 4 to 6 weeks later may better represent steady-state BP values (eg, thiazide, reserpine). Once goal BP values are attained, assuming no signs or symptoms of acute end-organ damage are present, BP monitoring can be done every 3 to 6 months. More frequent evaluations are required for patients with a history of poor control, nonadherence, progressive end-organ damage, or symptoms of adverse drug effects.

Self-measurements of BP or automated ABP monitoring can be useful clinically to establish effective 24-hour control. This type of monitoring may become the standard of care in the future because evolving data have demonstrated significant benefits of using these types of measurements to both diagnose hypertension[89,90] and optimize the use of antihypertensive drug therapy. Currently, ABP monitoring is used in select situations such as suspected white coat hypertension.[13] If patients are measuring their BP at home, it is important that they measure during the early morning hours for most days and then at different times of the day on alternative days of the week and use appropriate technique (e.g., proper cuff size, seated position, resting, etc.). It is also of paramount importance that clinicians remember self-BP and ABP measurements are lower than clinic BP measurements.[13] Goal BP values should be lowered accordingly when clinicians use self-BP or ABP measurements to monitor and/or adjust antihypertensive pharmacotherapy.

Toxicity

Patients should be monitored routinely for adverse drug effects. The most common side effects associated with each class of antihypertensive agents were discussed in Individual Antihypertensive Agents above, and laboratory parameters for first-line agents are listed in Table 13-8. Laboratory monitoring should typically occur 2 to 4 weeks after starting a new agent or dose increase, and then every 6 to 12 months in stable patients. Additional monitoring may be needed for other concomitant diseases if present (eg, diabetes, dyslipidemia, gout). Moreover, patients treated with an aldosterone antagonist (eplerenone or spironolactone) should have potassium concentrations and kidney function assessed within 3 days of initiation and again at 1 week to detect potential hyperkalemia. The occurrence of an adverse drug event may require dosage reduction or substitution with an alternative antihypertensive agent.

Disease Progression

Patients should be monitored for signs and symptoms of progressive hypertension-associated complications. A careful history for ischemic chest pain (or pressure), palpitations, dizziness, dyspnea, orthopnea, headache, sudden change in vision, one-sided weakness, slurred speech, and loss of balance should be taken to assess the presence of CV and cerebrovascular hypertensive complications. Other clinical monitoring parameters that may be used to assess hypertension-associated complications include funduscopic changes on eye examination, LVH on electrocardiogram, proteinuria, and changes in kidney function. These parameters should be monitored periodically because any sign of deterioration requires immediate assessment and follow-up.

TABLE 13-8 Select Monitoring for Antihypertensive Pharmacotherapy

Class	Parameters
Aldosterone antagonist	BP; BUN/serum creatinine; serum potassium
ACEi	BP; BUN/serum creatinine; serum potassium
ARB	BP; BUN/serum creatinine; serum potassium
Calcium channel blocker	BP; heart rate
Thiazide	BP; BUN/serum creatinine; serum electrolytes (potassium, magnesium, sodium); uric acid (for thiazides)
β-Blocker	BP; heart rate

Adherence and Persistence

Nonadherence and lack of persistence with hypertension treatment is a major problem in the United States and is associated with significant increases in costs due to development of complications. Since hypertension is a relatively asymptomatic disease, poor adherence is frequent, particularly in patients newly treated. It has been estimated that only 50% of patients with newly diagnosed hypertension are continuing treatment at 1 year.[91] It has also been demonstrated that long-term risk of CV events is significantly reduced when newly diagnosed patients are adherent with their antihypertensive drug therapy.[92] Therefore, it is imperative to assess patient adherence on a regular basis.

The American Society of Hypertension has outlined four global practical considerations and recommendations for adherence in patients with hypertension.[93] These include: (a) focus on clinical outcomes (eg, following national guidelines, simplifying drug regimens, encouraging self-monitoring of BP), (b) empowering informed, activated patients (eg, problem-solving and behavior change interventions, urge the use of pill boxes, help patients develop a system for refilling prescriptions), (c) implement a team approach (eg, implementing collaborative models of care, using office practice policies and procedures to improve BP control), and (d) advocating for health policy reform (eg, elevate medication adherence as a critical healthcare issue, structure/finance healthcare that stimulates behavioral aspects).

Identification of nonadherence should be followed up with appropriate patient education, counseling, and intervention. Once-daily regimens are preferred in most patients to improve adherence. Although some may believe that aggressive treatment may negatively impact quality of life and thus adherence, several studies have found that most patients actually feel better once their BP is controlled. Patients on antihypertensive therapy should be questioned periodically about changes in their general health perception, energy level, physical functioning, and overall satisfaction with treatment. Lifestyle modifications should always be recommended to provide additional BP lowering and other potential health benefits. Persistence with lifestyle modifications should be continually encouraged for patients engaging in such endeavors.

Combination Therapy

14 Initial therapy with a combination of two antihypertensive drugs is highly recommended for patients with stage 2 hypertension and is an option for treating patients with stage 1 hypertension.[94] Using a fixed-dose combination product is an option for these types of patients and has been shown to improve adherence.[95] Initial two-drug combination therapy may also be appropriate for patients with multiple compelling indications for different antihypertensive agents. Moreover, combination therapy is often needed to control BP in patients who are already treated with drug therapy because most patients require two or more agents.[1,40,94]

The Avoiding Cardiovascular Events Through Combination Therapy for Patients Living with Systolic Hypertension Trial

Long-term safety and efficacy of initial two-drug therapy for hypertension has been evaluated in the ACCOMPLISH trial.[96] This was a prospective, randomized, double-blind trial in 11,506 patients with hypertension and other CV risk factors. All of these patients either had stage 2 hypertension or were on antihypertensive drug therapy on enrollment. Patients were randomized to receive either benazepril with hydrochlorothiazide or benazepril with amlodipine as initial drug therapy. Treatment was titrated to a goal BP of less than 140/90 mm Hg for most patients and less than 130/80 mm Hg for patients with diabetes or CKD.

The trial was terminated early after a mean of 36 months because the incidence of CV events was 20% lower in the benazepril with amlodipine group compared with the benazepril with hydrochlorothiazide group. What is most important for clinical practice is that this trial established that initial two-drug therapy, as is recommended in JNC and AHA guidelines, was safe and highly effective in lowering BP. Mean BP measurements were 132/73 and 133/74 mm Hg in the benazepril with amlodipine and the benazepril with hydrochlorothiazide groups, respectively. However, rates of attaining a BP of less than 140/90 mm Hg were 75.4% and 72.4% (benazepril with amlodipine and benazepril with hydrochlorothiazide, respectively). These goal attainment rates are higher than in any other long-term prospective study and are higher than what is seen in clinical practice.

The ACCOMPLISH trial established initial two-drug antihypertensive therapy as an evidence-based strategy to treat hypertension. Clinicians should consider this study as justification for implementing initial two-drug therapy antihypertensive regimens in appropriate patients. Moreover, The ACCOMPLISH trial demonstrated that the combination of an ACEi with a dihydropyridine CCB was more effective in reducing risk of CV events than the combination of an ACEi with a thiazide. However, thiazides are very effective at lowering BP, especially when used in combination with other agents, and hydrochlorothiazide is available in many fixed-dose combination products.

Optimal Use of Combination Therapy

Clinicians should anticipate the need for combination drugs to control BP in most patients. Using low-dose combinations also provides greater reductions in BP compared with high doses of single agents, with fewer drug-related side effects.[72] Contrary to popular myth, appropriately increasing the number of antihypertensive medications to attain goal BP values does not increase the risk of adverse effects. The American Society of Hypertension has recommended three categories of combination therapy (see Clinical Presentation "Recommendations for Combination Therapy").[94] Preferred combinations are ideal for lowering BP, have complementary mechanisms of action, and use first-line drugs that have been shown to lower risk of CV events. Acceptable combinations may not provide all of the benefits that preferred combinations do, and may have additive side effect profiles. Less effective combinations are limited in their overall benefits, and should only be used when absolutely necessary.

Some combinations are not effective long-term in treating hypertension. As previously discussed, the ON-TARGET demonstrated that the use of an ACEi with an ARB in the management of hypertension resulted in no additional reduction in incidence of CV events.[75] Moreover, this combination resulted in a higher risk of adverse events which was also demonstrated in other trials. These same effects are seen when aliskiren is used in combination with an ARB.[82] These combinations (using two RAAS blockers together) should not be used for the purpose of managing hypertension. Other combinations such as a thiazide with a potassium-sparing diuretic, both of which appear to have overlapping mechanisms of action, should be implemented primarily to minimize side effects. The combination of two CCBs, a dihydropyridine with a nondihydropyridine, can provide additional BP lowering but has limited use in the routine management of most patients with hypertension.[97] Under no circumstance should two drugs from the exact same class of medications be used to treat hypertension.

Fixed-Dose Combination Products Many fixed-dose combination products are commercially available, and some are generic (Table 13-9). Most of these products contain a thiazide and have multiple dose strengths available. Individual dose titration is more complicated with fixed-dose combination products, but this strategy can reduce the number of daily tablets/capsules and can simplify regimens to improve adherence by decreasing pill burden.[94,95] This alone may increase the likelihood of achieving or maintaining goal BP values. Depending on the product, some may be less expensive to patients and to health systems. Nonadherence rates are 24% lower when fixed-dose combination products are used to treat hypertension compared with using free drug components (separate pills) to treat hypertension.[95]

Resistant Hypertension

15 Patients with resistant hypertension are those who fail to achieve goal BP with the use of three or more antihypertensive drugs.[98] This includes patients who are adhering to full doses of an appropriate three-drug regimen that includes a diuretic, but also includes patients who are controlled but require the use of four or more medications.[98] It has been estimated that 12% of patients with hypertension fall under this definition.[5] Patients with newly diagnosed hypertension or who are not treated with drug therapy should not be considered to have resistant hypertension. Difficult-to-control hypertension is persistently elevated BP despite treatment with two or three drugs that does not meet the criteria for resistant hypertension (eg, maximum doses that include a diuretic).

Several causes of resistant hypertension are listed in Table 13-10. Volume overload is a common cause, thus highlighting the importance of diuretic therapy in the management of hypertension.

CLINICAL PRESENTATION Recommendations for Combination Therapy

Preferred

- ACEi/CCB
- ARB/CCB
- ACEi/thiazide
- ARB/thiazide

Acceptable

- β-Blocker/thiazide
- CCB (dihydropyridine)/β-blocker
- CCB/thiazide
- Thiazide/potassium-sparing diuretic

Less Effective

- ACEi/β-blocker
- ARB/β-blocker
- CCB (nondihydropyridine)/β-blocker
- Centrally acting agent/β-blocker

TABLE 13-9 Fixed-Dose Combination Products

Combination	Drugs (Brand Name)	Strengths (mg/mg)	Daily Frequency
ACEi with CCB	Amlodipine/benazepril (Lotrel)	2.5/10, 5/10, 10/20	1
	Enalapril/felodipine (Lexxel)	5/5	1
	Trandolapril/verapamil (Tarka)	2/180, 1/240, 2/240, 4/240	1 or 2
ARB with CCB	Amlodipine/olmesartan (Azor)	5/20, 10/20, 5/40, 10/40	1
	Telmisartan/amlodipine (Twynsta)	40/5, 40/10, 80/5, 80/10	1
	Valsartan/amlodipine (Exforge)	5/160, 10/160, 5/320, 10/320	1
ACEi with a thiazide	Benazepril/hydrochlorothiazide (Lotensin HCT)	5/6.25, 10/12.5, 20/12.5, 20/25	1
	Captopril/hydrochlorothiazide (Capozide)	25/15, 25/25, 50/15, 50/25	1 to 3
	Enalapril/hydrochlorothiazide (Vaseretic)	5/12.5, 10/25	1
	Fosinopril/hydrochlorothiazide (Monopril HCT)	10/12.5, 20/25	1
	Lisinopril/hydrochlorothiazide (Prinizide, Zestoretic)	10/12.5, 20/12.5, 20/25	1
	Moexipril/hydrochlorothiazide (Uniretic)	7.5/12.5, 15/25	1 or 2
	Quinapril/hydrochlorothiazide (Accuretic)	10/12.5, 20/12.5, 20/25	1
ARB with a thiazide	Azilsartan/chlorthalidone (Edarbyclor)	40/12.5, 40/25	1
	Candesartan/hydrochlorothiazide (Atacand HCT)	16/12.5, 32/12.5	1
	Eprosartan/hydrochlorothiazide (Teveten HCT)	600/12.5, 600/25	1
	Irbesartan/hydrochlorothiazide (Avalide)	75/12.5, 150/12.5, 300/12.5	1
	Losartan/hydrochlorothiazide (Hyzaar)	50/12.5, 100/25	1
	Olmesartan/hydrochlorothiazide (Benicar HCT)	20/12.5, 40/12.5, 40/25	1
	Telmisartan/hydrochlorothiazide (Micardis HCT)	40/12.5, 80/12.5	1
	Valsartan/hydrochlorothiazide (Diovan HCT)	80/12.5, 160/12.5	1
β-Blocker with a thiazide	Atenolol/chlorthalidone (Tenoretic)	50/25, 100/25	1
	Bisoprolol/hydrochlorothiazide (Ziac)	2.5/6.25, 5/6.25, 10/6.25	1
	Metoprolol succinate/hydrochlorothiazide (Dutoprol)	25/12.5, 50/12.5, 100/12.5 mg	1
	Propranolol/hydrochlorothiazide (Inderide)	40/25, 80/25	2
	Propranolol LA/hydrochlorothiazide (Inderide LA)	80/50, 120/50, 160/50	1
	Metoprolol/hydrochlorothiazide (Lopressor HCT)	50/25, 100/25	1 or 2
	Nadolol/bendroflumethiazide (Corzide)	40/5, 80/5	1
	Timolol/hydrochlorothiazide (Timolide)	10/25	1 or 2
Direct renin inhibitor with thiazide	Aliskiren/hydrochlorothiazide (Tekturna HCT)	150/12.5, 150/25, 300/12.5, 300/25	1
Direct renin inhibitor with CCB	Aliskiren/amlodipine (Tekamlo)	100/5, 150/10, 300/5, 300/10	1
ARB with CCB with a thiazide	Amlodipine/valsartan/hydrochlorothiazide (Exforge HCT)	5/160/12.5, 5/160/25, 10/160/12.5, 10/160/25, 10/320/25	1
	Olmesartan/amlodipine/hydrochlorothiazide (Tribenzor)	20/5/12.5, 40/5/12.5, 40/5/25, 40/10/12.5, 40/10/25	1
Direct renin inhibitor with CCB with a thiazide	Aliskiren/amlodipine/hydrochlorothiazide (Amturnide)	150/5/12.5, 300/5/12.5, 300/5/25, 300/10/12.5, 300/10/25	1

Pseudoresistance should also be ruled out by assuring adherence with prescribed therapy and possibly use of home BP measurements (by using a self-monitoring device or 24-hour ABP monitor).[98] Patients should be closely evaluated to see if any of these causes can be reversed.

TABLE 13-10 Causes of Resistant Hypertension

Improper BP measurement

Volume overload:
- Excess sodium intake
- Volume retention from kidney disease
- Inadequate diuretic therapy

Drug induced or other causes:
- Nonadherence
- Inadequate antihypertensive doses
- Use of agents listed in Table 13-1

Associated conditions:
- Obesity, excess alcohol intake, obstructive sleep apnea
- Secondary hypertension

Treatment of patients with resistant hypertension should ultimately follow the principle of drug therapy selection from the JNC and AHA guidelines. Compelling indications, if present, should guide selection assuming these patients are on a thiazide or other type of diuretic. However, there are treatment philosophies that are germane to the management of resistant hypertension: (a) assuring adequate diuretic therapy, (b) appropriate use of combination therapies, and (c) using alternative antihypertensive agents when needed.

Assuring Appropriate Diuretic Therapy

Diuretics have a large role in the pharmacotherapy of resistant hypertension. Thiazides are the mainstay of treatment, but chlorthalidone (thiazide-like) should be preferentially used instead of hydrochlorothiazide, especially for patients with resistant hypertension, because it is more potent on a milligram-per-milligram basis.[77,98] Clinicians should identify that chlorthalidone therapy, like all thiazides, has dose-dependent metabolic side effects (hypokalemia and hyperglycemia) and that appropriate monitoring should be implemented. However, it does not seem as though side effects are more common with chlorthalidone versus hydrochlorothiazide. Though less commonly used, indapamide (similar to chlorthalidone as "thiazide like") is also a more potent antihypertensive agent than hydrochlorothiazide at commonly prescribed doses, and evidence does not demonstrate a higher risk of metabolic side effects.[99]

An aldosterone antagonist (eg, spironolactone) is highly effective as an add-on agent.[98] Data indicate that many patients with resistant hypertension have some degree of underlying hyperaldosteronism, emphasizing the role of adding an aldosterone antagonist. Spironolactone has been compared to an α-blocker and a β-blocker as add-on therapy in resistant hypertension in the Prevention And Treatment of Hypertension With Algorithm-based therapY-2 (PATHWAY-2) study.[100] Spironolactone was the most effective add-on drug for the treatment of resistant hypertension in this trial, reinforcing the important role of aldosterone antagonism in managing resistant hypertension.

Clinicians may consider using a loop diuretic, even in place of a thiazide, for patients with resistant hypertension who have very compromised kidney function (estimated GFR less than 30 mL/min/1.73m^2). Torsemide can be dosed once daily while furosemide must be dosed twice daily or three times daily.

Hypertensive Urgencies and Emergencies

Both hypertensive urgencies and emergencies are characterized by the presence of very elevated BP, typically greater than 180/120 mm Hg.[1] However, the need for urgent or emergent antihypertensive therapy must be determined based on the presence of acute or immediately progressing end-organ injury, not elevated BP alone. Urgencies are not associated with acute or immediately progressing end-organ injury, while emergencies are. Examples of acute end-organ injury include encephalopathy, intracranial hemorrhage, acute left ventricular failure with pulmonary edema, dissecting aortic aneurysm, unstable angina, and eclampsia or severe hypertension during pregnancy.

Hypertensive Urgency

16 A common error with hypertensive urgency is overly aggressive antihypertensive therapy. This treatment has likely been perpetrated by the classification terminology "urgency." Hypertensive urgencies are ideally managed by adjusting maintenance therapy, by adding a new antihypertensive, and/or by increasing the dose of a present medication. This is the preferred approach to these patients as it provides a more gradual reduction in BP. Very rapid reductions in BP to goal values should be discouraged due to potential risks. Because autoregulation of blood flow in patients with hypertension occurs at a much higher range of pressure than in normotensive persons, the inherent risks of reducing BP too precipitously include cerebrovascular accidents, MI, and acute kidney failure. Hypertensive urgency requires BP reductions with oral antihypertensive agents to stage 1 over a period of several hours to days. All patients with hypertensive urgency should be reevaluated within and no later than 7 days (preferably after 1 to 3 days).

Acute administration of a short-acting oral antihypertensive (eg, captopril, clonidine, labetalol) followed by careful observation for several hours to assure a gradual reduction in BP is an option for hypertensive urgency. However, there are no data supporting this approach as being absolutely needed. Oral captopril is one of the agents of choice and can be used in doses of 25 to 50 mg at 1- to 2-hour intervals. The onset of action of oral captopril is 15 to 30 minutes, and a marked fall in BP is unlikely to occur if no hypotensive response is observed within 30 to 60 minutes. For patients with hypertensive rebound following withdrawal of clonidine, 0.2 mg can be given initially, followed by 0.2 mg hourly until the DBP falls below 110 mm Hg or a total of 0.7 mg clonidine has been administered. A single dose may be all that is necessary. Labetalol can be given in a dose of 200 to 400 mg, followed by additional doses every 2 to 3 hours.

Oral or sublingual immediate-release nifedipine has been used for acute BP lowering in the past but is potentially dangerous. This approach produces a rapid reduction in BP. Immediate-release nifedipine should never be used for hypertensive urgencies due to risk of causing severe adverse events (eg, MI, stroke).

Hypertensive Emergency

Hypertensive emergencies are those rare situations that require immediate BP reduction to limit new or progressing end-organ damage (see Classification under Arterial BP above). Hypertensive emergencies require parenteral therapy, at least initially, with one of the agents listed in Table 13-11. The goal in hypertensive emergencies is not to lower BP to less than 140/90 mm Hg; rather, the initial target is a reduction in MAP of up to 25% within minutes to hours. If the patient is then stable, DBP can be reduced to 100 to 110 mm Hg within the next 2 to 6 hours. Precipitous drops in BP may lead to end-organ ischemia or infarction. If patients tolerate this reduction well, additional gradual reductions toward goal BP values can be attempted after 24 to 48 hours. The exception to this guideline is for patients with an acute ischemic stroke where maintaining an elevated BP is needed for a longer period of time.

The clinical situation should dictate which IV medication is used to treat hypertensive emergencies. Regardless, therapy should be provided in a hospital or emergency room setting with intraarticular BP monitoring. Table 13-11 lists special indications for agents that can be used.

Nitroprusside is widely considered the agent of choice for most cases, but it can be problematic for patients with CKD. It is a direct-acting vasodilator that decreases PVR but does not increase CO unless left ventricular failure is present. Nitroprusside can be given to treat most hypertensive emergencies, but in aortic dissection, propranolol should be given first to prevent reflex sympathetic activation. Nitroprusside is metabolized to cyanide and then to thiocyanate, which is eliminated by the kidneys. Therefore, serum thiocyanate levels should be monitored when infusions are continued longer than 72 hours. Nitroprusside should be discontinued if the concentration exceeds 12 mg/dL (approximately 2 mmol/L). The risk of thiocyanate accumulation and toxicity is increased for patients with impaired kidney function. The use of nitroprusside is limited by a recent and significant increase in the cost of this agent.

IV nitroglycerin dilates both arterioles and venous capacitance vessels, thereby reducing both cardiac afterload and cardiac preload, which can decrease myocardial oxygen demand. It also dilates collateral coronary blood vessels and improves perfusion to ischemic myocardium. These properties make IV nitroglycerin ideal for the management of hypertensive emergency in the presence of myocardial ischemia. IV nitroglycerin is associated with tolerance when used over 24 to 48 hours and can cause severe headache.

Fenoldopam, nicardipine, and clevidipine are newer and more expensive agents. Fenoldopam is a dopamine-1 agonist. It can improve renal blood flow and may be especially useful for patients with kidney insufficiency. Nicardipine and clevidipine are dihydropyridine CCBs that provide arterial vasodilation and can treat cardiac ischemia similar to nitroglycerin, but they may provide more predictable reductions in BP.

The hypotensive response of hydralazine is less predictable than with other parenteral agents. Therefore, its major role is in the treatment of eclampsia or hypertensive encephalopathy associated with renal insufficiency.

CONCLUSION

Hypertension is a very common medical condition in the United States. Treatment of patients with hypertension should include both lifestyle modifications and pharmacotherapy. Evidence from outcome-based clinical trials has definitively demonstrated that

TABLE 13-11 Parenteral Antihypertensive Agents for Hypertensive Emergency

Drug	Dose	Onset (minutes)	Duration (minutes)	Adverse Effects	Special Indications
Clevidipine	1-2 mg/h (32 mg/h maximum)	2-4	5-15	Headache, nausea, tachycardia, hypertriglyceridemia	Most hypertensive emergencies except acute heart failure; caution with coronary ischemia; contraindicated in soy or egg allergy, defective lipid metabolism, and severe aortic stenosis
Enalaprilat	1.25-5 mg IV every 6 hours	15-30	360-720	Precipitous fall in pressure in high-renin states; variable response	Acute left ventricular failure; avoid in acute myocardial infarction, eclampsia
Esmolol hydrochloride	250-500 mcg/kg/min IV bolus, and then 50-100 mcg/kg/min IV infusion; may repeat bolus after 5 minutes or increase infusion to 300 mcg/min	1-2	10-20	Hypotension, nausea, asthma, first-degree heart block, heart failure	Aortic dissection; perioperative; avoid in patients already on β-blocker, bradycardic, or decompensated heart failure
Fenoldopam mesylate	0.1-0.3 mcg/kg/min IV infusion	<5	30	Tachycardia, headache, nausea, flushing	Most hypertensive emergencies; caution with glaucoma
Hydralazine hydrochloride	12-20 mg IV 10-50 mg intramuscular	10-20 20-30	60-240 240-360	Tachycardia, flushing, headache vomiting, aggravation of angina	Eclampsia
Labetalol hydrochloride	20-80 mg IV bolus every 10 minutes; 0.5-2 mg/min IV infusion	5-10	180-360	Vomiting, scalp tingling, bronchoconstriction, dizziness, nausea, heart block, orthostatic hypotension	Most hypertensive emergencies except acute heart failure or heart block
Nicardipine hydrochloride	5-15 mg/h IV	5-10	15-30, may exceed 240	Tachycardia, headache, flushing, local phlebitis	Most hypertensive emergencies except acute heart failure; caution with coronary ischemia
Nitroglycerin	5-100 mcg/min IV infusion	2-5	5-10	Headache, vomiting, methemoglobinemia, tolerance with prolonged use	Coronary ischemia
Sodium nitroprusside	0.25-10 mcg/kg/min IV infusion (requires special delivery system)	Immediate	1-2	Nausea, vomiting, muscle twitching, sweating, thiocyanate and cyanide intoxication	Most hypertensive emergencies; caution with high intracranial pressure, azotemia, or in chronic kidney disease

treating hypertension reduces the risk of CV events and subsequently reduces morbidity and mortality. Moreover, evidence evaluating individual drug classes has resulted in an evidence-based approach to selecting pharmacotherapy in an individual patient. An ACEi, ARB, CCB, and thiazide are all first-line agents. Data suggest that using a β-blocker first-line to treat patients with hypertension, without the presence of a compelling indication, may not be as beneficial in reducing risk of CV events compared with ACEi-, ARB-, CCB-, or thiazide-based therapy. Therefore, they are not first-line therapy options unless an appropriate compelling indication is present.

Patients should be treated to a goal BP value. In addition to selecting the most appropriate agent, attaining a goal BP is also of paramount importance to ensure maximum reduction in risk for CV events is provided. A BP goal of less than 140/90 mm Hg is recommended for most patients with hypertension and some patients are candidates for lower goal values. Most patients with hypertension require more than one drug to attain goal BP values; therefore, combination therapy should be anticipated. Future evidence-based guidelines from the AHA (expected in 2016) will provide additional recommendations for the treatment of hypertension.

Optimizing hypertension management can be achieved many ways. Team-based approaches to implement care and attain goal BP values are effective. Judicious use of cost-effective treatments and fixed-dose combination products should always be considered to improve sustainability of treatment. Lastly, interventions to reinforce adherence and lifestyle modifications are needed for comprehensive management of hypertension.

ABBREVIATIONS

ABP	ambulatory blood pressure
ACCOMPLISH	Avoiding Cardiovascular Events Through Combination Therapy in Patients Living with Systolic Hypertension
ACCORD-BP	Action to Control Cardiovascular Risk in Diabetes Blood Pressure
ACE	angiotensin-converting enzyme
AHA	American Heart Association
ALLHAT	Antihypertensive and Lipid Lowering Treatment to Prevent Heart Attack Trial
ARB	angiotensin II receptor blocker
ASH	American Society of Hypertension
AT_1	angiotensin II type 1
AT_2	angiotensin II type 2
BP	blood pressure
BUN	blood urea nitrogen
CCB	calcium channel blocker
CKD	chronic kidney disease
CO	cardiac output
CONVINCE	Controlled Onset Verapamil Investigation of Cardiovascular End-Points
COPD	chronic obstructive pulmonary disease
CV	cardiovascular
DASH	Dietary Approaches to Stop Hypertension
DBP	diastolic blood pressure

GEMINI	Glycemic Effects in Diabetes Mellitus: Carvedilol–Metoprolol Comparison in Hypertensives
GFR	glomerular filtration rate
HOT	Hypertension Optimal Treatment
HFrEF	Heart Failure with reduced Ejection Fraction
HYVET	Hypertension in the Very Elderly Trial
INVEST	International Verapamil–Trandolapril Study
ISA	intrinsic sympathomimetic activity
ISH	International Society of Hypertension
JNC	Joint National Committee
KDIGO	Kidney Disease Improving Global Outcomes
LVH	left ventricular hypertrophy
MAP	mean arterial pressure
MDRD	modification of diet in renal disease
MI	myocardial infarction
MOSES	Morbidity and Mortality After Stroke: Eprosartan Versus Nitrendipine in Secondary Prevention
MRC	Medical Research Council
NHLBI	National Heart, Lung, and Blood Institute
ON-TARGET	Ongoing Telmisartan Alone and in Combination with Ramipril Global End Point Trial
PAD	Peripheral arterial disease
PATHWAY-2	Prevention And Treatment of Hypertension With Algorithm-based therapY-2
PVR	peripheral vascular resistance
RAAS	renin–angiotensin–aldosterone system
SBP	systolic blood pressure
SHEP	Systolic Hypertension in the Elderly Program
SPRINT	Systolic Pressure Intervention Trial
STOP-2	Swedish Trial in Old Patients with Hypertension-2
STOP-Hypertension	Swedish Trial in Old Patients with Hypertension
Syst-Eur	Systolic Hypertension in Europe
TOMHS	Treatment of Mild Hypertension Study
TPR	total peripheral resistance
TRANSCEND	Telmisartan Randomized Assessment Study in ACE-Intolerant Subjects with Cardiovascular Disease
UKPDS	United Kingdom Prospective Diabetes Study
VALUE	Valsartan Antihypertensive Long-Term Use Evaluation

REFERENCES

1. Chobanian AV, Bakris GL, Black HR, et al. Seventh report of the Joint National Committee on Prevention, Detection, Evaluation, and Treatment of High Blood Pressure. *Hypertension* 2003;42:1206-1252.
2. Weber MA, Schiffrin EL, White WB, et al. Clinical practice guidelines for the management of hypertension in the community: A statement by the American Society of Hypertension and the International Society of Hypertension. *J Clin Hypertens* 2014;16(1):14-26.
3. James PA, Oparil S, Carter BL, et al. 2014 evidence-Based Guideline for the Management of High Blood Pressure in Adults Report From the Panel Members Appointed to the Eighth Joint National Committee (JNC 8). *JAMA* 2014;311(5):507-520.
4. Rosendorff C, Lackland DT, Allison M, et al. Treatment of hypertension in patients with coronary artery disease a scientific statement from the American Heart Association, American College of Cardiology, and American Society of Hypertension. J Am Coll Cardiol 2015;65:1998-2038.
5. Mozaffarian D, Benjamin EJ, Go AS, et al. Heart disease and stroke statistics—2015 update: A report from the American Heart Association. *Circulation* 2015;131:e29-322.
6. Wilson L, Saseen JJ. Hypertension. In: Tisdale JE, Miller DA, eds. Drug-Induced Diseases: Prevention, Detection, and Management, 3rd ed. Bethesda: American Society of Health-Systems Pharmacists, Inc, 2016 [chapter 27].
7. MacMahon S, Peto R, Cutler J, et al. Blood pressure, stroke, and coronary heart disease. Part 1, prolonged differences in blood pressure: Prospective observational studies corrected for the regression dilution bias. *Lancet* 1990;335:765-774.
8. SHEP Cooperative Research Group. Prevention of stroke by antihypertensive drug treatment in older persons with isolated systolic hypertension. Final results of the Systolic Hypertension in the Elderly Program (SHEP). *JAMA* 1991;265:3255-3264.
9. Dahlof B, Lindholm LH, Hansson L, Schersten B, Ekbom T, Wester PO. Morbidity and mortality in the Swedish Trial in Old Patients with Hypertension (STOP-Hypertension). *Lancet* 1991;338:1281-1285.
10. MRC Working Party. Medical Research Council trial of treatment of hypertension in older adults: Principal results. *BMJ* 1992;304:405-412.
11. Staessen JA, Fagard R, Thijs L, et al. Randomised double-blind comparison of placebo and active treatment for older patients with isolated systolic hypertension. The Systolic Hypertension in Europe (Syst-Eur) Trial Investigators. *Lancet* 1997;350:757-764.
12. Pickering TG, Hall JE, Appel LJ, et al. Recommendations for blood pressure measurement in humans and experimental animals: Part 1: Blood pressure measurement in humans: A statement for professionals from the Subcommittee of Professional and Public Education of the American Heart Association Council on High Blood Pressure Research. *Circulation* 2005;111:697-716.
13. Pickering TG, White WB. ASH position paper: Home and ambulatory blood pressure monitoring. When and how to use self (home) and ambulatory blood pressure monitoring. *J Clin Hypertens* 2008;10:850-855.
14. Mancia G, Bombelli M, Facchetti R, et al. Long-term risk of sustained hypertension in white-coat or masked hypertension. *Hypertension* 2009;54:226-232.
15. U.S. Preventive Services Task Force. Screening for high blood pressure in adults: U.S. preventive services task force recommendation statement. *Ann Intern Med*. Published online 13 October 2015. doi:10.7326/M15-2223.
16. American Diabetes Association. Standards of medical care in diabetes—2015. *Diabetes Care* 2015;36(Suppl 1):s1-s93.
17. Kidney Disease Improving Global Outcomes. Chapter 4: Blood pressure management in CKD ND patients with diabetes mellitus. *Kidney Int Suppl* 2012;2:363-369.
18. Kidney Disease Improving Global Outcomes. Chapter 3: Blood pressure management in CKD ND patients without diabetes mellitus. *Kidney Int Suppl* 2012;2:357-362.
19. Wright JT, Williamson JD, Whelton PK, et al. A Randomized Trial of Intensive versus Standard Blood-Pressure Control. *New Engl J Med* 2015. doi: 10.1056/NEJMoa1511939.
20. Hansson L, Zanchetti A, Carruthers SG, et al. Effects of intensive blood-pressure lowering and low-dose aspirin in patients with hypertension: Principal results of the Hypertension Optimal Treatment (HOT) randomised trial. HOT Study Group. *Lancet* 1998;351:1755-1762.
21. Farnett L, Mulrow CD, Linn WD, Lucey CR, Tuley MR. The J-curve phenomenon and the treatment of hypertension. Is there a point beyond which pressure reduction is dangerous? *JAMA* 1991;265:489-495.
22. Xie X, Atkins E, Lv J, et al. Effects of intensive blood pressure lowering on cardiovascular and renal outcomes: updated systematic review and meta-analysis. Lancet. 2015;387(10017):435-443.
23. Cushman WC, Evans GW, Byington RP, et al. Effects of intensive blood-pressure control in type 2 diabetes mellitus. *N Engl J Med* 2010;362:1575-1585.
24. O'Connor PJ. Overcome clinical inertia to control systolic blood pressure. *Arch Intern Med* 2003;163:2677-2678.
25. Eckel RH, Jakicic JM, Ard JD, et al. 2013 AHA/ACC guideline on lifestyle management to reduce cardiovascular risk: A report of the American College of Cardiology/American Heart Association Task Force on Practice Guidelines. *Circulation* 2014;129:s76-s99.
26. Saseen JJ, MacLaughlin EJ, Westfall JM. Treatment of uncomplicated hypertension: Are ACE inhibitors and calcium channel blockers as effective as diuretics and beta-blockers? *J Am Board Fam Pract* 2003;16:156-164.
27. Black HR, Elliott WJ, Grandits G, et al. Principal results of the Controlled Onset Verapamil Investigation of Cardiovascular End Points (CONVINCE) trial. *JAMA* 2003;289:2073-2082.

28. Dahlof B, Devereux RB, Kjeldsen SE, et al. Cardiovascular morbidity and mortality in the Losartan Intervention For Endpoint reduction in hypertension study (LIFE): A randomised trial against atenolol. *Lancet* 2002;359:995-1003.
29. ALLHAT Officers and Coordinators for the ALLHAT Collaborative Research Group. Major outcomes in high-risk hypertensive patients randomized to angiotensin-converting enzyme inhibitor or calcium channel blocker vs diuretic: The Antihypertensive and Lipid-Lowering Treatment to Prevent Heart Attack Trial (ALLHAT). *JAMA* 2002;288:2981-2997.
30. PROGRESS Collaborative Group. Randomised trial of a perindopril-based blood-pressure-lowering regimen among 6,105 individuals with previous stroke or transient ischaemic attack. *Lancet* 2001;358:1033-1041.
31. Wing LM, Reid CM, Ryan P, et al. A comparison of outcomes with angiotensin-converting-enzyme inhibitors and diuretics for hypertension in the elderly. *N Engl J Med* 2003;348:583-592.
32. Julius S, Kjeldsen SE, Weber M, et al. Outcomes in hypertensive patients at high cardiovascular risk treated with regimens based on valsartan or amlodipine: The VALUE randomised trial. *Lancet* 2004;363:2022-2031.
33. Dahlof B, Sever PS, Poulter NR, et al. Prevention of cardiovascular events with an antihypertensive regimen of amlodipine adding perindopril as required versus atenolol adding bendroflumethiazide as required, in the Anglo-Scandinavian Cardiac Outcomes Trial-Blood Pressure Lowering Arm (ASCOT-BPLA): A multicentre randomised controlled trial. *Lancet* 2005;366:895-906.
34. Antihypertensive and Lipid-Lowering Treatment to Prevent Heart Attack Trial Collaborative Research Group. Diuretic versus alpha-blocker as first-step antihypertensive therapy: Final results from the Antihypertensive and Lipid-Lowering Treatment to Prevent Heart Attack Trial (ALLHAT). *Hypertension* 2003;42:239-246.
35. Davis BR, Cutler JA, Gordon DJ, et al. Rationale and design for the Antihypertensive and Lipid Lowering Treatment to Prevent Heart Attack Trial (ALLHAT). ALLHAT Research Group. *Am J Hypertens* 1996;9:342-360.
36. Rahman M, Pressel S, Davis BR, et al. Renal outcomes in high-risk hypertensive patients treated with an angiotensin-converting enzyme inhibitor or a calcium channel blocker vs a diuretic: A report from the Antihypertensive and Lipid-Lowering Treatment to Prevent Heart Attack Trial (ALLHAT). *Arch Intern Med* 2005;165:936-946.
37. Whelton PK, Barzilay J, Cushman WC, et al. Clinical outcomes in antihypertensive treatment of type 2 diabetes, impaired fasting glucose concentration, and normoglycemia: Antihypertensive and Lipid-Lowering Treatment to Prevent Heart Attack Trial (ALLHAT). *Arch Intern Med* 2005;165:1401-1409.
38. Wright JT Jr, Dunn JK, Cutler JA, et al. Outcomes in hypertensive black and nonblack patients treated with chlorthalidone, amlodipine, and lisinopril. *JAMA* 2005;293:1595-1608.
39. Turnbull F. Effects of different blood-pressure-lowering regimens on major cardiovascular events: Results of prospectively-designed overviews of randomised trials. *Lancet* 2003;362:1527-1535.
40. Mancia G, Fagard R, Narkiewicz K, et al. 2013 ESH/ESC Guidelines for the management of arterial hypertension: The Task Force for the management of arterial hypertension of the European Society of Hypertension (ESH) and of the European Society of Cardiology (ESC). *J Hypertens* 2013;31(7):1281-1357.
41. National Clinical Guideline Centre. Hypertension—The Clinical Management of Primary Hypertension in Adults. Clinical Guideline 127: Methods, Evidence, and Recommendations. London: The Royal College of Physicians; August 2011.
42. Ripley TL, Saseen JJ. β blockers: A review of their pharmacologic and physiologic diversity in hypertension. *Ann Pharmacother* 2014;48(6):723-733.
43. Yancy CW, Jessup M, Bozkurt B, et al. 2013 ACCF/AHA guideline for the management of heart failure: Executive Summary: A report of the American College of Cardiology Foundation/American Heart Association Task Force on Practice Guidelines. *Circulation* 2013;128:1810-1852.
44. Smith SC Jr, Benjamin EJ, Bonow RO, et al. AHA/ACCF secondary prevention and risk reduction therapy for patients with coronary and other atherosclerotic vascular disease: 2011 update: A guideline from the American Heart Association and American College of Cardiology Foundation. *Circulation* 2011;124:2458-2473.
45. Fihn SD, Blankenship JC, Alexander KP, et al. 2014 ACC/AHA/AATS/PCNA/SCAI/STS focused update of the guideline for the diagnosis and management of patients with stable ischemic heart disease: A report of the American College of Cardiology/American Heart Association Task Force on Practice Guidelines, and the American Association for Thoracic Surgery, Preventive Cardiovascular Nurses Association, Society for Cardiovascular Angiography and Interventions, and Society of Thoracic Surgeons. *Circulation* 2014;130:1749-1767.
46. Bangalore S, Steg G, Deedwania P, et al. Beta-blocker use and clinical outcomes in stable outpatients with and without coronary artery disease. *JAMA* 2012;308:1340-1349.
47. Pepine CJ, Handberg EM, Cooper-DeHoff RM, et al. A calcium antagonist vs a non-calcium antagonist hypertension treatment strategy for patients with coronary artery disease. The International Verapamil–Trandolapril Study (INVEST): A randomized controlled trial. *JAMA* 2003;290:2805-2816.
48. Jneid H, Anderson JL, Wright RS, et al. 2012 ACCF/AHA focused update of the guideline for the management of patients with unstable angina/non-ST-elevation myocardial infarction (updating the 2007 guideline and replacing the 2011 focused update): A report of the American College of Cardiology Foundation/American Heart Association Task Force on Practice Guidelines. *Circulation* 2012;126:875-910.
49. O'Gara PT, Kushner FG, Ascheim DD, et al. 2013 ACCF/AHA guideline for the management of ST-elevation myocardial infarction: A report of the American College of Cardiology Foundation/American Heart Association Task Force on Practice Guidelines. *J Am Coll Cardiol* 2013;61:e78-e140.
50. Weber MA, Bakris GL, Jamerson K, et al. Cardiovascular events during differing hypertension therapies in patients with diabetes. *J Am Coll Cardiol* 2010;56:77-85.
51. Wright JT Jr, Bakris G, Greene T, et al. Effect of blood pressure lowering and antihypertensive drug class on progression of hypertensive kidney disease: Results from the AASK trial. *JAMA* 2002;288:2421-2431.
52. Casas JP, Chua W, Loukogeorgakis S, et al. Effect of inhibitors of the renin–angiotensin system and other antihypertensive drugs on renal outcomes: Systematic review and meta-analysis. *Lancet* 2005;366:2026-2033.
53. Kernan WN, Ovbiagele B, Black HR, et al. Guidelines for the prevention of stroke in patients with stroke and transient ischemic attack: A guideline for healthcare professionals from the American Heart Association/American Stroke Association. *Stroke* 2014;45:2160-2236.
54. Rashid P, Leonardi-Bee J, Bath P. Blood pressure reduction and secondary prevention of stroke and other vascular events: A systematic review. *Stroke* 2003;34:2741-2748.
55. Schrader J, Luders S, Kulschewski A, et al. Morbidity and Mortality After Stroke, Eprosartan Compared with Nitrendipine for Secondary Prevention: Principal results of a prospective randomized controlled study (MOSES). *Stroke* 2005;36:1218-1226.
56. Yusuf S, Diener HC, Sacco RL, et al. Telmisartan to prevent recurrent stroke and cardiovascular events. *N Engl J Med* 2008;359:1225-1237.
57. Aronow WS, Fleg JL, Pepine CJ, et al. ACCF/AHA 2011 expert consensus document on hypertension in the elderly: A report of the American College of Cardiology Foundation Task Force on Clinical Expert Consensus Documents. *Circulation* 2011;123:2434-2506.
58. Beckett NS, Peters R, Fletcher AE, et al. Treatment of hypertension in patients 80 years of age or older. *N Engl J Med* 2008;358:1887-1898.
59. Hansson L, Lindholm LH, Ekbom T, et al. Randomised trial of old and new antihypertensive drugs in elderly patients: Cardiovascular mortality and morbidity the Swedish Trial in Old Patients with Hypertension-2 study. *Lancet* 1999;354:1751-1756.
60. Williamson JD, Supiano MA, Applegate WB, et al. Intensive vs standard blood pressure control and cardiovascular disease outcomes in adults aged ≥75 years. *JAMA* 2016;315(24):2673-2682.
61. National High Blood Pressure Education Program Working Group on High Blood Pressure in Children and Adolescents. The fourth report on the diagnosis, evaluation, and treatment of high blood pressure in children and adolescents. *Pediatrics* 2004;114:555-576.
62. American College of Obstetricians and Gynecologists, Task Force on Hypertension in Pregnancy. Hyperten-sion in pregnancy: report of the American College of Obstetricians and Gynecologists' Task Force on Hyper-tension in Pregnancy. *Obstet Gynecol* 2013;122:1122-1131.
63. Magee LA, von Dadelszen P, Rey E, et al. Less-tight versus tight control of hypertension in pregnancy. *N Engl J Med* 2015;372:407-417.
64. Flack JM, Sica DA, Bakris G, et al. Management of high blood pressure in blacks: An update of the International Society on Hypertension in Blacks consensus statement. *Hypertension* 2010;56:780-800.

65. Rooke TW, Hirsch AT, Misra S, et al. 2011 ACCF/AHA focused update of the guideline for the management of patients with peripheral artery disease (updating the 2005 guideline): A report of the American College of Cardiology Foundation/American Heart Association Task Force on Practice Guidelines. *Circulation* 2011;124:2020-2045.
66. Alberti KG, Eckel RH, Grundy SM, et al. Harmonizing the metabolic syndrome: A joint interim statement of the International Diabetes Federation Task Force on Epidemiology and Prevention; National Heart, Lung, and Blood Institute; American Heart Association; World Heart Federation; International Atherosclerosis Society; and Inter-national Association for the Study of Obesity. *Circulation* 2009;120:1640-1645.
67. Elliott WJ, Meyer PM. Incident diabetes in clinical trials of antihypertensive drugs: A network meta-analysis. *Lancet* 2007;369:201-207.
68. Ko DT, Hebert PR, Coffey CS, Sedrakyan A, Curtis JP, Krumholz HM. Beta-blocker therapy and symptoms of depression, fatigue, and sexual dysfunction. *JAMA* 2002;288:351-357.
69. Materson BJ, Reda DJ, Cushman WC, et al. Single-drug therapy for hypertension in men. A comparison of six antihypertensive agents with placebo. The Department of Veterans Affairs Cooperative Study Group on Antihypertensive Agents. *N Engl J Med* 1993;328:914-921.
70. Grimm RH Jr, Grandits GA, Prineas RJ, et al. Long-term effects on sexual function of five antihypertensive drugs and nutritional hygienic treatment in hypertensive men and women. Treatment of Mild Hypertension Study (TOMHS). *Hypertension* 1997;29:8-14.
71. Dagenais GR, Pogue J, Fox K, Simoons ML, Yusuf S. Angiotensin-converting-enzyme inhibitors in stable vascular disease without left ventricular systolic dysfunction or heart failure: A combined analysis of three trials. *Lancet* 2006;368:581-588.
72. Law MR, Wald NJ, Morris JK, Jordan RE. Value of low dose combination treatment with blood pressure lowering drugs: Analysis of 354 randomised trials. *BMJ* 2003;326:1427.
73. Bakris GL, Weir MR. Angiotensin-converting enzyme inhibitor-associated elevations in serum creatinine: Is this a cause for concern? *Arch Intern Med* 2000;160:685-693.
74. Yusuf S, Teo K, Anderson C, et al. Effects of the angiotensin-receptor blocker telmisartan on cardiovascular events in high-risk patients intolerant to angiotensin-converting enzyme inhibitors: A randomised controlled trial. *Lancet* 2008;372:1174-1183.
75. Yusuf S, Teo KK, Pogue J, et al. Telmisartan, ramipril, or both in patients at high risk for vascular events. *N Engl J Med* 2008;358:1547-1559.
76. Leenen FH, Nwachuku CE, Black HR, et al. Clinical events in high-risk hypertensive patients randomly assigned to calcium channel blocker versus angiotensin-converting enzyme inhibitor in the antihypertensive and lipid-lowering treatment to prevent heart attack trial. *Hypertension* 2006;48:374-384.
77. Ernst ME, Moser M. Use of diuretics in patients with hypertension. *N Engl J Med* 2009;361:2153-2164.
78. Messerli FH, Makani H, Benjo A, Romero J, Alviar C, Bangalore S. Antihypertensive efficacy of hydrochlorothiazide as evaluated by ambulatory blood pressure monitoring: A meta-analysis of randomized trials. *J Am Coll Cardiol* 2011;57:590-600.
79. Grimm RH Jr, Flack JM, Grandits GA, et al. Long-term effects on plasma lipids of diet and drugs to treat hypertension. Treatment of Mild Hypertension Study (TOMHS) Research Group. *JAMA* 1996;275:1549-1556.
80. UK Prospective Diabetes Study Group. Efficacy of atenolol and captopril in reducing risk of macrovascular and microvascular complications in type 2 diabetes: UKPDS 39. *BMJ* 1998;317:713-720.
81. Bakris GL, Fonseca V, Katholi RE, et al. Metabolic effects of carvedilol vs metoprolol in patients with type 2 diabetes mellitus and hypertension: A randomized controlled trial. *JAMA* 2004;292:2227-2236.
82. Parving HH, Brenner BM, McMurray JJ, et al. Cardiorenal end points in a trial of aliskiren for type 2 diabetes. *N Engl J Med* 2012;367:2204-2213.
83. Brush JE, Handberg EM, Biga C, et al. 2015 ACC health policy statement on cardiovascular team-based care and the role of advanced practice providers. *J Am Coll Cardiol* 2015;65(19):2118-2136.
84. Carter BL, Coffey CS, Ardery G, et al. Cluster-randomized trial of a physician/pharmacist collaborative model to improve blood pressure control. *Circ Cardiovasc Qual Outcomes*. 2015;8(3):235-243.
85. Carter BL, Rogers M, Daly J, Zheng S, James PA. The potency of team-based care interventions for hypertension: A meta-analysis. *Arch Intern Med* 2009;169:1748-1755.
86. Tsuyuki RT, Houle SKD, Charrois TL, et al. Randomized Trial of the Effect of Pharmacist Prescribing on Improving Blood Pressure in the Community The Alberta Clinical Trial in Optimizing Hypertension (RxACTION). *Circulation* 2015;132:93-100.
87. Murray MD, Ritchey ME, Wu J, Tu W. Effect of a pharmacist on adverse drug events and medication errors in outpatients with cardiovascular disease. *Arch Intern Med* 2009;169:757-763.
88. Dunn SP, Birtcher KK, Beavers CJ, et al. The role of the clinical pharmacist in the care of patients with cardiovascular disease. *J Am Coll Cardiol* 2015;66:2129-2139.
89. Lovibond K, Jowett S, Barton P, et al. Cost-effectiveness of options for the diagnosis of high blood pressure in primary care: A modelling study. *Lancet* 2011;378:1219-1230.
90. Hodgkinson J, Mant J, Martin U, et al. Relative effectiveness of clinic and home blood pressure monitoring compared with ambulatory blood pressure monitoring in diagnosis of hypertension: Systematic review. *BMJ* 2011;342:d3621.
91. Degli Esposti L, Valpiani G. Pharmacoeconomic burden of undertreating hypertension. *Pharmacoeconomics* 2004;22:907-928.
92. Mazzaglia G, Ambrosioni E, Alacqua M, et al. Adherence to antihypertensive medications and cardiovascular morbidity among newly diagnosed hypertensive patients. *Circulation* 2009;120:1598-1605.
93. Hill MN, Miller NH, Degeest S, et al. Adherence and persistence with taking medication to control high blood pressure. *J Am Soc Hypertens* 2011;5:56-63.
94. Gradman AH, Basile JN, Carter BL, Bakris GL. Combination therapy in hypertension. *J Am Soc Hypertens* 2010;4:42-50.
95. Bangalore S, Kamalakkannan G, Parkar S, Messerli FH. Fixed-dose combinations improve medication compliance: A meta-analysis. *Am J Med* 2007;120:713-719.
96. Jamerson K, Weber MA, Bakris GL, et al. Benazepril plus amlodipine or hydrochlorothiazide for hypertension in high-risk patients. *N Engl J Med* 2008;359:2417-2428.
97. Saseen JJ, Carter BL, Brown TE, Elliott WJ, Black HR. Comparison of nifedipine alone and with diltiazem or verapamil in hypertension. *Hypertension* 1996;28:109-114.
98. Calhoun DA, Jones D, Textor S, et al. Resistant hypertension: Diagnosis, evaluation, and treatment: A scientific statement from the American Heart Association Professional Education Committee of the Council for High Blood Pressure Research. *Circulation* 2008;117:e510-e526.
99. Roush GC, Ernst ME, Kostis JB, et al. Head-to-head comparisons of hydrochlorothiazide with indapamide and chlorthalidone antihypertensive and metabolic effects. *Hypertension* 2015;65:1041-1046.
100. Williams B, MacDonald TM, Morant S, et al. Spironolactone versus placebo, bisoprolol, and doxazosin to deter-mine the optimal treatment for drug-resistant hypertension (PATHWAY-2): a randomised, double-blind, crossover trial. Published Online Lancet September 21, 2015 (http://dx.doi.org/10.1016/S0140-6736(15)00257-3).

14

Chronic Heart Failure

Robert B. Parker, Jean M. Nappi, and Larisa H. Cavallari

KEY CONCEPTS

1 Heart failure (HF) is a progressive clinical syndrome that can result from any changes in cardiac structure or function that impair the ability of the ventricle to fill with or eject blood. HF may be caused by an abnormality in systolic function, diastolic function, or both. The leading causes of HF are coronary artery disease and hypertension. The primary manifestations of the syndrome are dyspnea, fatigue, and fluid retention.

2 In heart failure with reduced ejection fraction (HFrEF) there is a decrease in cardiac output, resulting in activation of a number of compensatory responses that attempt to maintain adequate cardiac output. These responses include activation of the sympathetic nervous system (SNS) and the renin–angiotensin–aldosterone system (RAAS), resulting in vasoconstriction and sodium and water retention as well as ventricular hypertrophy/remodeling. These compensatory mechanisms are responsible for the symptoms of HFrEF and contribute to disease progression.

3 Our current understanding of HFrEF pathophysiology is best described by the neurohormonal model. Activation of endogenous neurohormones including norepinephrine (NE), angiotensin II, aldosterone, vasopressin, and numerous proinflammatory cytokines plays an important role in ventricular remodeling and the subsequent progression of HF. Importantly, pharmacotherapy targeted at antagonizing this neurohormonal activation has slowed the progression of HFrEF and improved survival.

4 Most patients with HFrEF should be routinely treated with guideline directed medical therapy (GDMT) that includes an angiotensin-converting enzyme (ACE) inhibitor or angiotensin receptor blocker (ARB) and a β-blocker. Selected patients should also receive loop diuretics, hydralazine/nitrates, or aldosterone antagonists. The benefits of these medications on slowing HF progression, reducing morbidity and mortality, and/or improving symptoms are clearly established.

5 In patients with HFrEF, ACE inhibitors improve survival, slow disease progression, reduce hospitalizations, and improve quality of life. The doses for these agents should be targeted at those shown in clinical trials to improve survival. When ACE inhibitors are contraindicated or not tolerated, an ARB or the combination of hydralazine and isosorbide dinitrate is a reasonable alternative. Patients with asymptomatic left ventricular dysfunction and/or a previous myocardial infarction (MI) (Stage B of the American College of Cardiology [ACC]/American Heart Association [AHA] classification scheme) should also receive ACE inhibitors, with the goal of preventing symptomatic HF and reducing mortality.

6 The β-blockers carvedilol, metoprolol succinate, and bisoprolol have been shown to prolong survival, decrease hospitalizations and need for transplantation, and cause "reverse remodeling" of the left ventricle. These agents are recommended for all patients with HFrEF unless contraindicated. Therapy must be instituted at low doses, with slow upward titration to the target dose.

7 Although chronic loop diuretic therapy frequently is used in patients with either HFrEF or HFpEF, it is not mandatory. Diuretic therapy along with sodium restriction is required only in those patients with peripheral edema and/or pulmonary congestion. Many patients will need continued diuretic therapy to maintain euvolemia after fluid overload is resolved.

8 Aldosterone antagonists reduce mortality in patients with HFrEF and New York Heart Association (NYHA) class II to IV symptoms and thus should be strongly considered in these patients provided that potassium and renal function can be carefully monitored. Aldosterone antagonists should also be considered soon after MI in patients with left ventricular dysfunction and either HF or diabetes and may be considered to reduce the risk of hospitalization in patients with HFpEF.

9 The combination of hydralazine and nitrates improves the composite end point of mortality, hospitalizations for HF, and quality of life in African Americans receiving standard therapy for HFrEF. Current guidelines recommend the addition of hydralazine and nitrates to self-described African Americans with HFrEF and moderate to severe symptoms that are receiving GDMT with ACE inhibitors and β-blockers. Hydralazine and a nitrate might be reasonable in patients unable to tolerate either an ACE inhibitor or ARB because of renal insufficiency, hyperkalemia, or possibly hypotension.

10 Digoxin does not improve survival in patients with HFrEF but does provide symptomatic benefits. Digoxin doses should be adjusted to achieve plasma concentrations of 0.5 to 0.9 ng/mL (0.6-1.2 nmol/L); higher plasma concentrations are not associated with additional benefits but may be associated with increased risk of toxicity.

11 Treatment of heart failure with preserved ejection fraction (HFpEF) should be targeted at symptom reduction, causal clinical disease, and underlying basic mechanisms. Patients with HFpEF may be treated differently than those with HFrEF.

INTRODUCTION

1 2 Heart failure (HF) is a progressive clinical syndrome that can result from any abnormality in cardiac structure or function that impairs the ability of the ventricle to fill with or eject blood.[1] HF may be caused by an abnormality in systolic function,

diastolic function, or both. Making the distinction is important because the treatment of HF may be quite different depending on whether the predominant mechanism of the disorder is systolic or diastolic dysfunction. HF is the final common pathway for numerous cardiac disorders including those affecting the pericardium, heart valves, and myocardium. Diseases that adversely affect ventricular diastole (filling), ventricular systole (contraction), or both can lead to HF.

For many years it was believed that reduced myocardial contractility, or systolic dysfunction (ie, reduced left ventricular ejection fraction [LVEF]), now referred to as heart failure with reduced ejection fraction (HFrEF), was the sole disturbance in cardiac function responsible for HF. However, it is now recognized that large numbers of patients with the HF syndrome have relatively normal systolic function (ie, normal LVEF). This is now referred to as HF with preserved LVEF (HFpEF) and is believed to be primarily due to diastolic dysfunction of the heart.[1] Recent estimates suggest approximately 50% of patients with HF have preserved LVEF with disturbances in relaxation (lusitropic) properties of the heart, or diastolic dysfunction.[1,2] However, regardless of the etiology of HF, the underlying pathophysiologic process and principal clinical manifestations (fatigue, dyspnea, and often volume overload) are similar and appear to be independent of the initial cause. Historically, this disorder was commonly referred to as *congestive HF*; the preferred nomenclature is now *HF* since a patient may have the clinical syndrome of HF without having symptoms of congestion. This chapter will focus on treatment of patients with chronic HF from reduced as well as preserved LVEF. Chapter e5 will discuss the treatment of acute decompensated HF.

EPIDEMIOLOGY

Heart failure is an epidemic public health problem in the United States.[3] Nearly 6 million Americans have HF with over 800,000 new cases diagnosed each year.[3] Unlike most other cardiovascular diseases, the incidence and prevalence of HF are increasing and are expected to continue to increase over the next few decades as the population ages. A large majority of patients with HF are elderly, with multiple comorbid conditions that influence morbidity and mortality.[3] Improved survival after myocardial infarction (MI) is thought to be a likely contributor to the increased incidence and prevalence of HF.[4] Annual hospital discharges for HF now total over 1 million, and HF remains the most common hospital discharge diagnosis in individuals over age 65.[3] The disorder also has a tremendous economic impact, with this expected to increase markedly as the baby-boom generation ages. Current estimates suggest annual expenditures for HF of over $30 billion, with the majority of these costs spent on hospitalized patients.[3] Thus, HF is a major medical problem, with substantial economic impact that is expected to become even more significant as the population ages.

Despite prodigious advances in our understanding of the etiology, pathophysiology, and pharmacotherapy of HF, the prognosis for patients with this disorder remains grim. Although the mortality rates have declined over the last 50 years, the overall 5-year survival remains approximately 50% for all patients with a diagnosis of HF, with mortality increasing with symptom severity.[1,3] Death is classified as sudden in about 40% of patients, implicating serious ventricular arrhythmias as the underlying cause.[1] Factors affecting the prognosis of patients with HF include, but are not limited to, age, gender, LVEF, renal function, natriuretic peptide plasma concentrations, diabetes, metabolic syndrome, extent of underlying coronary artery disease, blood pressure (BP), HF etiology, and drug or device therapy. Recent models incorporating these and other factors enable clinicians to develop reliable estimates of an individual patient's prognosis.[1]

ETIOLOGY

1 2 Heart failure can result from any disorder that affects the ability of the heart to contract (systolic function) and/or relax (diastolic dysfunction); common causes of HF are shown in Table 14-1.[5] HF with reduced systolic function (ie, reduced LVEF) is the classic, more familiar form of the disorder and is now referred to as heart failure with reduced ejection fraction (HFrEF). Current estimates indicate up to 50% of patients with HF have preserved left ventricular systolic function with presumed diastolic dysfunction, now termed *heart failure with preserved ejection fraction* (HFpEF).[2,6] In contrast to HFrEF that is often caused by previous MI, patients with HFpEF typically are elderly, female, and obese, and have hypertension (HTN), atrial fibrillation, or diabetes.[2,6] Recent data indicate that survival is similar in patients with HFrEF or HFpEF.[1,2]

1 Coronary artery disease is the most common cause of HFrEF, accounting for nearly 70% of cases.[5] MI leads to reduction in muscle mass due to death of affected myocardial cells. The degree to which contractility is impaired depends on the size of the infarction. To attempt to maintain cardiac output (CO), the surviving myocardium undergoes a compensatory remodeling, thus beginning the maladaptive process that initiates the HF syndrome and leads to further injury to the heart. This is discussed in greater detail in Pathophysiology section of this chapter later. Myocardial ischemia and infarction also affect the diastolic properties of the heart by increasing ventricular stiffness and slowing ventricular relaxation. Thus, MI frequently results in systolic and diastolic dysfunction.

Impaired systolic function is a cardinal feature of dilated cardiomyopathies. Although the cause of reduced contractility frequently is unknown, abnormalities such as interstitial fibrosis, cellular infiltrates, cellular hypertrophy, and myocardial cell degeneration are seen commonly on histologic examination. Inherited forms of dilated as well as hypertrophic cardiomyopathies may also occur.[1,5]

Pressure or volume overload causes ventricular hypertrophy, which attempts to return contractility to a near-normal state. If the pressure or volume overload persists, the remodeling process results in alterations in the geometry of the hypertrophied myocardial cells and is accompanied by increased collagen deposition in the extracellular matrix. Thus, both systolic and diastolic functions may be impaired.[7] Examples of pressure overload include systemic or pulmonary HTN and aortic or pulmonic valve stenosis.

HTN remains an important cause and/or contributor to both HFrEF and HFpEF in many patients, particularly women, the elderly, and African Americans.[1,5] The role of HTN should not be underestimated because it is an important risk factor for ischemic

TABLE 14-1 Causes of Heart failure

Systolic dysfunction (decreased contractility)
- Reduction in muscle mass (eg, myocardial infarction)
- Dilated cardiomyopathies
- Ventricular hypertrophy
  - Pressure overload (eg, systemic or pulmonary hypertension, aortic or pulmonic valve stenosis)
  - Volume overload (eg, valvular regurgitation, shunts, high-output states)

Diastolic dysfunction (restriction in ventricular filling)
- Increased ventricular stiffness
  - Ventricular hypertrophy (eg, hypertrophic cardiomyopathy, other previous examples)
  - Infiltrative myocardial diseases (eg, amyloidosis, sarcoidosis, endomyocardial fibrosis)
  - Myocardial ischemia and infarction
- Mitral or tricuspid valve stenosis
- Pericardial disease (eg, pericarditis, pericardial tamponade)

Data from Mann DL. Management of patients with heart failure with reduced ejection fraction. In: Mann DL, Zipes DP, Libby P, Bonow RO, Braunwald E, eds. *Braunwald's Heart Disease: A Textbook of Cardiovascular Medicine*. 10th ed. Philadelphia, PA: Elsevier; 2015:512-546.

heart disease and thus is also present in a high percentage of the patients with coronary artery disease. HF is a largely preventable disorder such that appropriate management of lifestyle risk factors (eg, HTN, coronary heart disease, smoking, obesity, physical activity, diabetes, etc.) is key to minimize the risk of HF development.

PATHOPHYSIOLOGY

Normal Cardiac Function

To understand the pathophysiologic processes in HF, a basic understanding of normal cardiac function is necessary. CO is defined as the volume of blood ejected per unit time (L/min) and is the product of heart rate (HR) and stroke volume (SV):

$$\text{CO} = \text{HR} \times \text{SV}$$

The relationship between CO and mean arterial pressure (MAP) is given as follows:

$$\text{MAP} = \text{CO} \times \text{systemic vascular resistance (SVR)}$$

Heart rate is controlled by the autonomic nervous system. SV, or the volume of blood ejected during systole, depends on preload, afterload, and contractility.[7] As defined by the Frank–Starling mechanism, the ability of the heart to alter the force of contraction depends on changes in preload. As myocardial sarcomere length is stretched, the number of cross-bridges between thick and thin myofilaments increases, resulting in an increase in the force of contraction. The length of the sarcomere is determined primarily by the volume of blood in the ventricle; therefore, left ventricular end-diastolic volume (LVEDV) is the primary determinant of preload. In normal hearts, the preload response is the primary compensatory mechanism such that a small increase in end-diastolic volume results in a large increase in CO. Because of the relationship between pressure and volume in the heart, left ventricular end-diastolic pressure (LVEDP) is often used in the clinical setting to estimate preload. The hemodynamic measurement used to clinically estimate LVEDP is the pulmonary capillary wedge pressure (PCWP), also known as the pulmonary artery occlusion pressure (PAOP). Afterload is a more complex physiologic concept that can be viewed pragmatically as the sum of forces preventing active forward ejection of blood by the ventricle. Major components of afterload are ejection impedance, wall tension, and regional wall geometry. In patients with left ventricular systolic dysfunction, an inverse relationship exists between afterload (estimated clinically by SVR) and SV such that increasing afterload causes a decrease in SV (Fig. 14-1). Contractility is the intrinsic property of cardiac muscle describing fiber shortening and tension development.

Heart Failure with Preserved Ejection Fraction

Heart failure with preserved ejection fraction can be defined as a condition in which myocardial relaxation and filling are impaired and incomplete. The ventricle is unable to accept an adequate volume of blood from the venous system, does not fill at low pressure, and/or is unable to maintain normal SV. In its most severe form, HFpEF results in overt symptoms of HF. In modest HFpEF, symptoms of dyspnea and fatigue occur only during stress or activity, when HR and end-diastolic volume increase. In its mildest form, HFpEF can be manifested as a slow or delayed pattern of relaxation and filling with little or no elevation in diastolic pressure and few or no cardiac symptoms. The congestive symptoms that occur with HFpEF are a manifestation of increased pulmonary venous pressures. HFpEF is caused by impaired myocardial relaxation and/or increased diastolic stiffness. When HF is caused by a predominant abnormality in diastolic function, the ventricular chamber is not enlarged, and EF may be normal or even elevated.[2,8] Figure 14-2 shows the pressure–volume relationship in a patient with normal

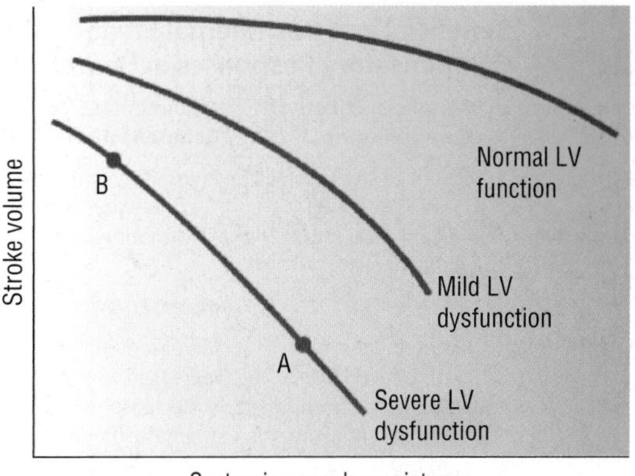

FIGURE 14-1 Relationship between stroke volume and systemic vascular resistance. In an individual with normal left ventricular (LV) function, increasing systemic vascular resistance has little effect on stroke volume. As the extent of LV dysfunction increases, the negative, inverse relationship between stroke volume and systemic vascular resistance becomes more important (B to A).

versus abnormal diastolic function. Changes in the myocardium are associated with a shift upward and to the left of the pressure–volume curve, so that for any increase in LV volume, diastolic pressure rises to a much greater level than normally would occur. Clinically, patients present with reduced exercise tolerance and dyspnea when they have elevated LV diastolic pressures. Patients with HFpEF have a predominant abnormality in diastolic function, whereas patients with HFrEF have a predominant abnormality in systolic function of the LV.

Recent data suggest that HFpEF may also be associated with abnormalities in endothelial and ventricular reserve function. During physical exertion, CO increases through integrated enhancements in venous return, contractility, HR, and peripheral vasodilation. The vasodilation that normally occurs during exercise is impaired in HFpEF. Pulmonary HTN is also a common finding. Abnormalities in each of these components of normal exercise reserve function have been identified in HFpEF and all may contribute to pathophysiology in individual patients.[2,8]

Compensatory Mechanisms in HFrEF

2 HFrEF is a progressive disorder initiated by any event that impairs the ability of the heart to contract and sometimes relax resulting in a decrease in CO. The index event may have an acute onset, as with MI, or the onset may be slow, as with long-standing HTN.

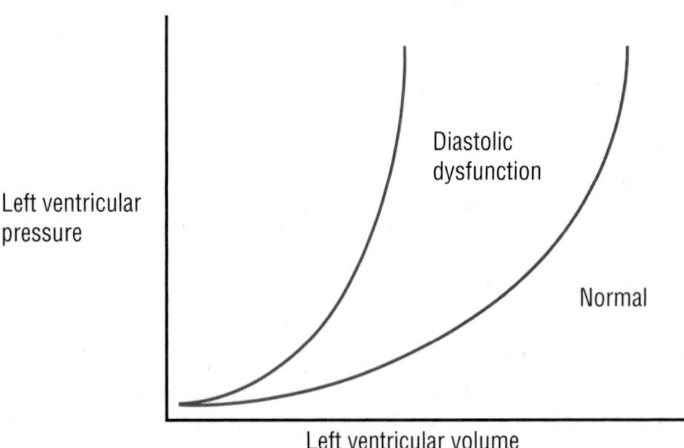

FIGURE 14-2 Diastolic pressure–volume relationship in a normal patient (*right trace*) and a patient with diastolic dysfunction (*left trace*).

TABLE 14-2 Beneficial and Detrimental Effects of the Compensatory Responses in Heart Failure

Compensatory Response	Beneficial Effects of Compensation	Detrimental Effects of Compensation
Increased preload (through Na^+ and retention)	Optimize stroke volume via Frank–Starling mechanism	Pulmonary and systemic congestion and edema formation Increased MVO_2
Vasoconstriction	Maintain BP in face of reduced CO Shunt blood from nonessential organs to brain and heart	Increased MVO_2 Increased afterload decreases stroke volume and further activates the compensatory responses
Tachycardia and increased contractility (due to SNS activation)	Helps maintain CO	Increased MVO_2 Shortened diastolic filling time β_1-receptor down-regulation, decreased receptor sensitivity Precipitation of ventricular arrhythmias Increased risk of myocardial cell death
Ventricular hypertrophy and remodeling	Helps maintain CO Reduces myocardial wall stress Decreases MVO_2	Diastolic dysfunction Systolic dysfunction Increased risk of myocardial cell death Increased risk of myocardial ischemia Increased arrhythmia risk Fibrosis

SNS, sympathetic nervous system; BP, blood pressure; MVO_2, myocardial oxygen demand; CO, cardiac output.

Regardless of the index event, a decrease in CO results in activation of compensatory responses to maintain the circulation.[7,9] These compensatory responses include: (a) tachycardia and increased contractility through sympathetic nervous system (SNS) activation, (b) the Frank–Starling mechanism, whereby an increase in preload results in an increase in SV, (c) vasoconstriction, and (d) ventricular hypertrophy and remodeling. Compensatory responses evolved to provide short-term support to maintain circulatory homeostasis after acute reductions in BP or renal perfusion. However, the persistent decline in CO in HF triggers long-term activation of these compensatory responses resulting in the complex functional, structural, biochemical, and molecular changes important for the development and progression of HF. The beneficial and detrimental effects of these compensatory responses are described later and are summarized in Table 14-2.

Tachycardia and Increased Contractility

The increase in HR and contractility that rapidly occurs in response to a drop in CO is primarily due to release of norepinephrine (NE) from adrenergic nerve terminals, although parasympathetic nervous system activity is also diminished.[9] Loss of atrial contribution to ventricular filling also can occur (atrial fibrillation, ventricular tachycardia), reducing ventricular performance even more. Because ionized calcium is sequestered into the sarcoplasmic reticulum and pumped out of the cell during diastole, the shortened diastolic time with increases in HR also results in a higher average intracellular calcium concentration during diastole, increasing actin–myosin interaction, augmenting the active resistance to fibril stretch, and reducing lusitropy. Conversely, the higher average calcium concentration translates into greater filament interaction during systole, generating more tension.[7] Increasing HR also increases myocardial oxygen demand. If ischemia is induced or worsened, both diastolic and systolic functions may become impaired, and SV can drop precipitously. In addition, polymorphisms in genes coding for adrenergic receptors (eg, β_1- and α_{2c}-receptors) and their signaling pathways may affect the risk for development of HF and alter the response to endogenous NE.[9,10]

Fluid Retention and Increased Preload

Augmentation of preload is another compensatory response that is rapidly activated in response to decreased CO. Renal perfusion in HF is reduced due to both depressed CO and redistribution of blood away from nonvital organs. The kidney interprets the reduced perfusion as an ineffective blood volume, resulting in activation of the renin–angiotensin–aldosterone system (RAAS) in an attempt to maintain BP and increase renal sodium and water retention. Reduced renal perfusion and increased sympathetic tone also stimulate renin release from juxtaglomerular cells in the kidney. As shown in Fig. 14-3, renin is responsible for conversion of angiotensinogen to angiotensin I. Angiotensin I is converted to angiotensin II by angiotensin-converting enzyme (ACE). Angiotensin II may also be generated via non-ACE-dependent pathways. Angiotensin II stimulates aldosterone release from the adrenal gland, thereby providing an additional mechanism for renal sodium and water retention. As intravascular volume increases secondary to sodium and water retention, left ventricular volume and pressure (preload) increase, sarcomeres are stretched, and the force of contraction is enhanced.[7] While the preload response is the primary compensatory mechanism in normal hearts, the chronically failing heart usually has exhausted its preload reserve.[7] As shown in Fig. 14-4, increases in preload will increase SV only to a certain point. Once the flat portion of the curve is reached, further increases in preload will only lead to pulmonary or systemic congestion, a detrimental result.[7] Figure 14-4 also shows that the curve is flatter in patients with left ventricular dysfunction. Consequently, a given increase in preload in a patient with HF will produce a smaller increment in SV than in an individual with normal ventricular function.

Vasoconstriction and Increased Afterload

Vasoconstriction occurs in patients with HFrEF to help redistribute blood flow away from nonessential organs to coronary and cerebral circulations to support BP, which may be reduced secondary to a decrease in CO (MAP = CO × SVR).[7] A number of neurohormones likely contribute to the vasoconstriction, including NE, angiotensin II, endothelin-1 (ET-1), neuropeptide Y, urotensin II, and arginine vasopressin (AVP).[7,9] Vasoconstriction impedes forward ejection of blood from the ventricle, further depressing CO and heightening the compensatory responses. The failing ventricle is exquisitely sensitive to changes in afterload (see Fig. 14-1). Thus, increases in afterload often potentiate a vicious cycle of continued worsening and downward spiraling of the HF state.

Ventricular Hypertrophy and Remodeling

3 While the signs and symptoms of HF are closely associated with the items described earlier, the progression of HF appears to be independent of the patient's hemodynamic status. It is now recognized that left ventricular hypertrophy and remodeling are key components in the pathogenesis of progressive myocardial failure.[7] *Ventricular hypertrophy* is a term used to describe an increase in ventricular muscle mass. *Cardiac or ventricular remodeling* is a broader term describing changes in both myocardial cells and extracellular matrix that result in changes in the size, shape, structure, and function of the heart.[11] These progressive changes in ventricular structure and function ultimately result in a change in shape of the left ventricle from an ellipse to a sphere. This change in ventricular size and shape serves to further depress the mechanical performance of the heart, increases regurgitant flow through the mitral valve, and, in turn, fuels the continued progression of remodeling. Ventricular hypertrophy and remodeling can occur in association with any condition

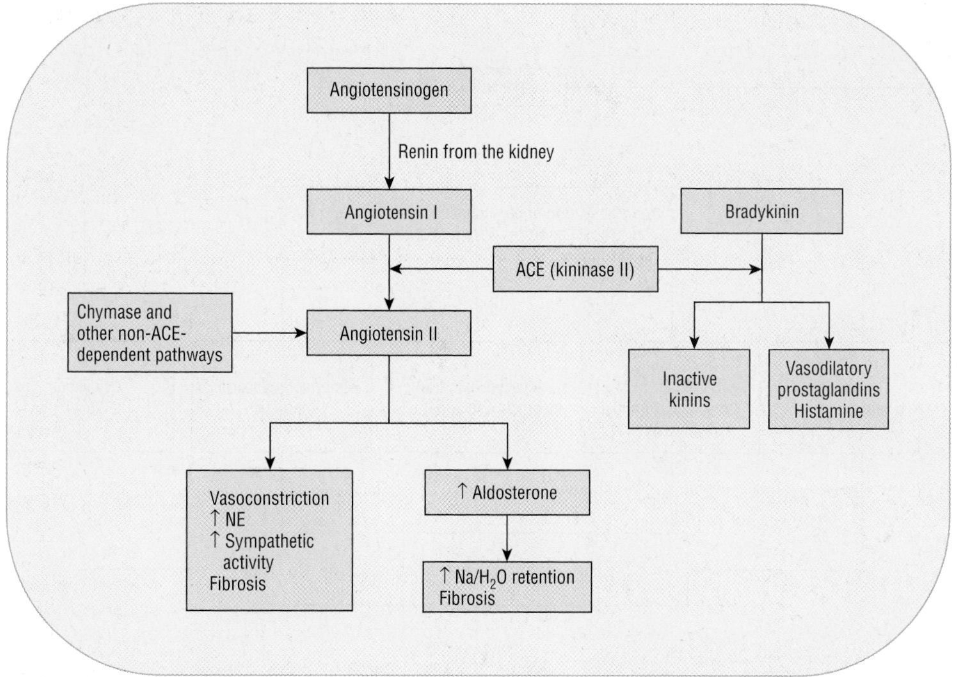

FIGURE 14-3 Physiology of the renin–angiotensin–aldosterone system. Renin produces angiotensin I from angiotensinogen. Angiotensin I is cleaved to angiotensin II by angiotensin-converting enzyme (ACE). Angiotensin II has a number of physiologic actions that are detrimental in heart failure. Note that angiotensin II can be produced in a number of tissues, including the heart, independent of ACE activity. ACE is also responsible for the breakdown of bradykinin. Inhibition of ACE results in accumulation of bradykinin that, in turn, enhances the production of vasodilatory prostaglandins.

that causes myocardial injury.[11] The onset of the remodeling process precedes the development of HF symptoms.

Cardiac remodeling is a complex process that affects the heart at the molecular and cellular levels.[7,11] Key elements in the process are shown in Fig. 14-5. Collectively, these events result in progressive changes in myocardial structure and function such as cardiac hypertrophy, myocyte loss, and alterations in the extracellular matrix. The progression of the remodeling process leads to reductions in myocardial systolic and/or diastolic function that, in turn, results in further myocardial injury, perpetuating the remodeling process and the decline in left ventricular performance. Angiotensin II, NE, ET, aldosterone, vasopressin, and numerous inflammatory cytokines, as well as substances under investigation, that are activated both systemically and locally in the heart and vasculature play an important role in initiating the signal transduction cascade responsible for ventricular remodeling. Although these mediators produce harmful effects on the heart, their increased circulating and tissue concentrations are also toxic to other organs and serve as an important reminder that HF is a systemic as well as a cardiac disorder.[7,9,11]

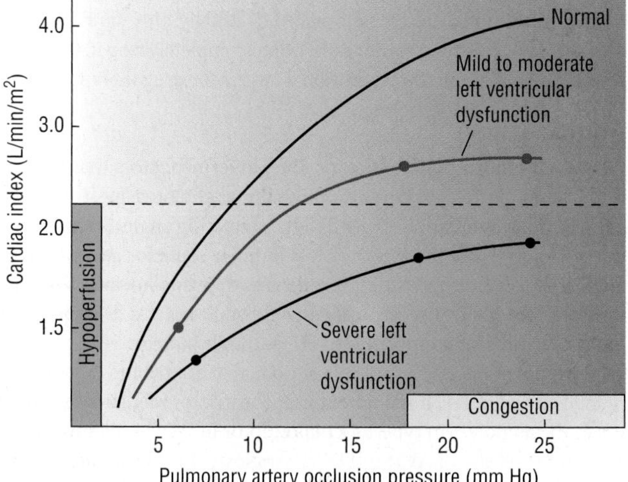

FIGURE 14-4 Relationship between cardiac output (shown as cardiac index which is CO/BSA) and preload (shown as pulmonary artery occlusion pressure).

Pressure overload (and probably hormonal activation) associated with HTN produces a concentric hypertrophy (increase in the ventricular wall thickness without chamber enlargement), that is often found in HFpEF.[8] Conversely, eccentric left ventricular hypertrophy (myocyte lengthening with increased chamber size with minimal increase in wall thickness) characterizes the hypertrophy seen in patients with systolic dysfunction or previous MI. As the myocytes undergo change, so do various components of the extracellular matrix. For example, collagen degradation may lead to myocyte slippage, fibroblast proliferation, and increased fibrillar collagen synthesis, resulting in fibrosis and stiffening of the entire myocardium. Thus, a number of important ventricular changes that occur with remodeling include alterations in the geometry of the heart from an elliptical to a spherical shape, increases in ventricular mass (from myocyte hypertrophy), and changes in ventricular composition (especially the extracellular matrix) and volumes, all of which contribute to the impaired cardiac function. If the event producing cardiac injury is acute (eg, MI), the ventricular remodeling process begins immediately. However, it is the progressive nature of this process that results in continual worsening of the HF state, and thus is now the major focus for identification of therapeutic targets. In fact, HF pharmacotherapy associated with decreased mortality, and/or slowing the progression of the disease, produces these effects largely by slowing or reversing ventricular remodeling, a process often referred to as *reverse remodeling*.

The Neurohormonal Model of Heart Failure and Therapeutic Insights It Provides

2 3 Over the years, several different paradigms have guided our understanding of the pathophysiology and treatment of HF.[7]

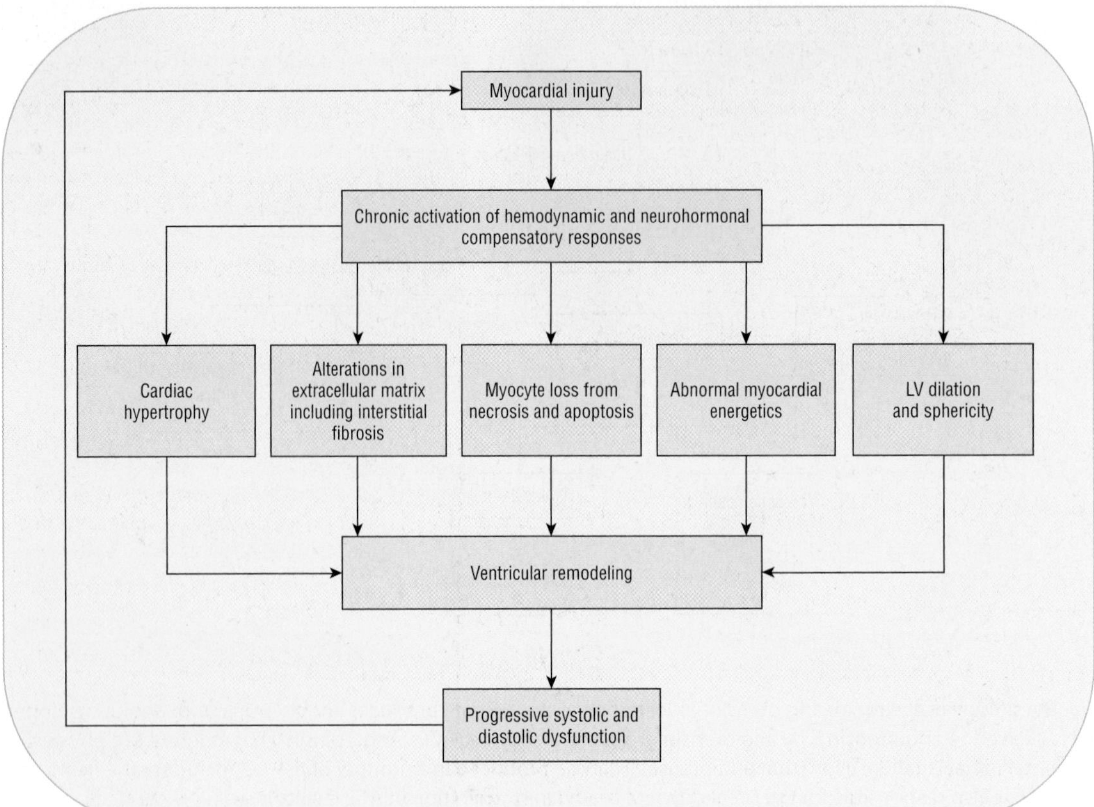

FIGURE 14-5 Key components of the pathophysiology of cardiac remodeling. Myocardial injury (eg, myocardial infarction) results in the activation of a number of hemodynamic and neurohormonal compensatory responses in an attempt to maintain circulatory homeostasis. Chronic activation of the neurohormonal systems results in a cascade of events that affect the myocardium at the molecular and cellular levels. These events lead to the changes in ventricular size, shape, structure, and function known as ventricular remodeling. The alterations in ventricular function result in further deterioration in cardiac systolic and diastolic functions that further promotes the remodeling process.

The early paradigm is often called the *cardiorenal model*, where the problem was viewed as excess sodium and water retention, and diuretic therapy was the main therapeutic approach. Next, the *cardiocirculatory model* focused on impaired CO (viewed as being due to both reduced pumping capacity of the heart and systemic vasoconstriction). Treatment strategies here focused on positive inotropes and, later, vasodilators, as the primary therapies to overcome reduced CO. While the therapeutic approaches associated with these paradigms provided some symptomatic benefits, they did little to slow progression of the disease. In fact, the detrimental effects of positive inotropic drugs on survival highlighted the inadequacy of the cardiocirculatory model to explain the progressive nature of HF.

Balanced (arterial and venous) vasodilation with ACE inhibitors was the basis for initial clinical trials with these agents. Subsequent discovery that ACE inhibitors provided benefits beyond their vasodilating effects, followed by the positive results with β-adrenergic receptor blockers and aldosterone antagonists, led to the current paradigm used to describe HF pathogenesis: the *neurohormonal model*.[7] This model recognizes an initiating event (eg, MI, long-standing HTN) that leads to decreased CO and begins the "HF state." The problem then moves beyond the heart, and it becomes a systemic disease whose progression is mediated largely by neurohormones and autocrine/paracrine factors that drive myocyte injury, oxidative stress, inflammation, and extracellular matrix remodeling. While the former paradigms still guide us to some extent in the symptomatic management of the disease (eg, diuretics and digoxin), it is the latter paradigm that helps us understand disease progression and, more important, the ways to slow disease progression. In the sections that follow, key neurohormones and autocrine/paracrine factors, sometimes now collectively termed *biomarkers*, are described with respect to their role in HF and its progression. The benefits of current and investigational drug therapies can be better understood through a solid understanding of the neurohormones they regulate/affect. Although the neurohormonal model provides a logical framework for our current understanding of HF progression and the role of various medications in attenuating this progression, it must be emphasized that this model does not completely explain HF progression. For example, drug therapies that target the neurohormonal perturbations in HF usually only slow the progressive nature of the disorder rather than completely stop it. Ongoing research will likely identify additional targets for drug therapy.

Angiotensin II

Of the neurohormones and autocrine/paracrine factors that play an important role in HFrEF pathophysiology, angiotensin II is probably the best understood.[7,12] Although circulating angiotensin II produced from ACE activity is the most familiar route for generation of angiotensin II, recent evidence indicates that this hormone is synthesized directly in the myocardium through non-ACE-dependent pathways and also contributes to HF pathophysiology.

Angiotensin II has multiple actions that contribute to its detrimental effects in HF. It is a potent vasoconstrictor mediated by binding to the angiotensin type 1 (AT1) receptor in the vasculature and it also causes release of AVP and ET-1. Angiotensin II facilitates release of NE from adrenergic nerve terminals, heightening SNS activation. It promotes sodium retention through direct effects on the renal tubules and by stimulating aldosterone release. Its vasoconstriction of the efferent glomerular arteriole helps to maintain renal perfusion pressure in patients with severe HF or impaired renal function. Finally, angiotensin II, and many of the neurohormones released in response to angiotensin II, plays a central role in stimulating ventricular hypertrophy, remodeling, myocyte apoptosis, oxidative stress, inflammation, and alterations in the myocardial extracellular matrix. Clinical data suggest that attenuating angiotensin II-mediated effects contributes substantially to the benefits of ACE inhibitor-treated and angiotensin receptor blocker (ARB)-treated patients with HFrEF.[12,13] The favorable effects of ACE inhibitors and ARBs on hemodynamics, symptoms, hospitalizations, and survival highlight the importance of angiotensin II in HF pathophysiology.

Norepinephrine

As described earlier in this chapter, NE plays a central role in the tachycardia, vasoconstriction, and increased contractility and plasma renin activity in HFrEF.[9] Plasma NE concentrations are elevated in correlation with the degree of HF, and patients with the highest plasma NE concentrations have the poorest prognosis.[14] Excessive SNS activation causes downregulation of β_1-receptors, with a subsequent loss of sensitivity to receptor stimulation. Excess catecholamines increase the risk of arrhythmias and can cause myocardial cell loss by stimulating both necrosis and apoptosis. Finally, NE contributes to ventricular hypertrophy and remodeling. The detrimental effects of SNS activation are further highlighted by the clinical trials of chronic therapy with β-agonists, phosphodiesterase inhibitors, or other drugs that cause SNS activation, since these agents are uniformly associated with increased mortality. Conversely, β-blockers, ACE inhibitors, and digoxin all help to decrease SNS activation, through various mechanisms, and are beneficial in HF. Thus, it is clear that NE plays a critical role in the pathophysiology of the HF state.

Aldosterone

Aldosterone-mediated sodium retention and its key role in volume overload and edema have long been recognized as important components of the HF syndrome.[15] Circulating aldosterone is increased in HF due to stimulation of its synthesis and release from the adrenal cortex by angiotensin II and due to decreased hepatic clearance from reduced hepatic perfusion. Recent studies demonstrate direct effects of aldosterone on the heart that may be even more important than sodium retention in HF pathophysiology. Chief among these is the ability of aldosterone to produce interstitial cardiac fibrosis through increased collagen deposition in the extracellular matrix of the heart. By increasing the stiffness of the myocardium, cardiac fibrosis may decrease systolic function and impair diastolic function. Current research shows that extra-adrenal production of aldosterone in the heart, kidneys, and vascular smooth muscle also contributes to the progressive nature of HF through target organ fibrosis and vascular remodeling. Induction of a systemic proinflammatory state, increased oxidative stress, wasting of soft tissues and bone, secondary hyperparathyroidism, and mineral/micronutrient dyshomeostasis are other important pathologic actions of aldosterone that directly contribute to ventricular remodeling and HF progression.[16] Aldosterone also may increase the risk of ventricular arrhythmias through a number of mechanisms, including creation of reentrant circuits as a result of fibrosis, inhibition of cardiac NE reuptake, depletion of intracellular potassium and magnesium, and impairment of parasympathetic traffic. Other detrimental effects of aldosterone include insulin resistance and endothelial and baroreceptor dysfunction. Clinical trials with the aldosterone antagonists spironolactone[17] and eplerenone[18,19] showing significant reductions in morbidity and mortality in patients with HFrEF provide compelling evidence of the important role of aldosterone in the initiation and progression of this syndrome. Although not studied as extensively as in HFrEF, aldosterone antagonists also show benefit in patients with HFpEF.[20,21]

Natriuretic Peptides

The natriuretic peptide family has three members, atrial natriuretic peptide (ANP), B-type natriuretic peptide (BNP), and C-type natriuretic peptide (CNP).[22] Of these, BNP is the most useful in the diagnosis and management of HF.[22] BNP and its related biologically inactive peptide, NT-proBNP, are synthesized and released from the ventricle in response to pressure or volume overload. BNP or NT-proBNP plasma concentrations are elevated in patients with HF functioning to increase natriuresis and diuresis and attenuate activation of the RAAS and SNS. The important role of these peptides in HF pathophysiology is supported by the recent clinical trial showing that neprilysin-mediated inhibition of natriuretic peptide breakdown improves outcomes in patients with HFrEF.[23]

The development of easily performed commercial assays for BNP and NT-proBNP, resulted in widespread interest in the role of these peptides as a biomarker for prognostic, diagnostic, and therapeutic use. In patients with chronic HFrEF, the degree of elevation in BNP concentrations is closely associated with increased mortality, risk of sudden death, symptoms, and hospital readmission.[22] Accurate diagnosis of acute decompensated HF in acute care settings is often difficult since many of the symptoms (eg, dyspnea) mimic those of other disorders such as pulmonary disease or obesity. The most well-established clinical application of BNP testing is in the urgent care setting where the BNP or NT-proBNP assay is useful when combined with clinical evaluation for differentiating dyspnea secondary to either HFrEF or HFpEF from other causes.[1]

Much interest has focused on the benefits of serial measurement of BNP as a target to guide drug therapy, primarily diuretics. Recent studies evaluating this approach have not shown consistent improvement in long-term outcomes compared with standard medical therapy, particularly in patients with HFpEF.[22,24-26] As a result, current guidelines reflect this uncertainty and do not support the routine use of serial measurement of BNP in the management of chronic HF.[1]

Arginine Vasopressin

AVP is a pituitary peptide hormone that regulates renal water excretion and plasma osmolality.[7] Plasma concentrations of AVP are elevated in patients with HF, supporting its role in the pathophysiology of this disorder. The physiologic effects of AVP are mediated through the V_{1a}, V_{1b}, and V_2 receptors. Stimulation of these receptors by increased circulating AVP results in several maladaptive responses including: (a) increased renal free water reabsorption in the face of plasma hypoosmolality resulting in volume overload and hyponatremia; (b) increased arterial vasoconstriction that contributes to reduced CO; and (c) stimulation of remodeling by cardiac hypertrophy and extracellular matrix collagen deposition.

Given the importance of AVP in HF, recent efforts have focused on the development of AVP antagonist drugs for treatment of acute and chronic HF. By blocking the AVP receptor, these agents primarily increase free water excretion (ie, an "aquaretic" effect). Although clinical trials with the AVP antagonists, tolvaptan, and conivaptain demonstrate improvements in acute symptoms and increases in serum sodium and urine output without affecting HR, BP, renal function, or other electrolytes, no improvements in morbidity and mortality were seen.[27]

Factors Precipitating/Exacerbating Heart Failure

Although significant advances have been made in treatment, symptom exacerbation, to the point that hospitalization is required, is a common and growing problem in patients with chronic HF. Hospitalization for HF exacerbation consumes large amounts of healthcare dollars and significantly impairs the patient's quality of life; thus, there is great interest in identifying and then remedying factors that increase the risk of decompensation. Appropriate therapy can often maintain patients in a "compensated" state, indicating that they are relatively symptom-free. However, there are many aggravating or precipitating factors that may cause a previously compensated patient to develop worsened symptoms necessitating hospitalization. Often, these precipitating factors are reversible or treatable, such that a thorough evaluation for their presence is imperative.

Cardiac events are a frequent cause of worsening HF.[1] Myocardial ischemia and infarction are potentially reversible causes that must be carefully considered since nearly 70% of patients with HF patients have coronary artery disease. Revascularization should be considered in appropriate patients. Atrial fibrillation occurs in up to 10% to 50% of patients with HF and is associated with increased morbidity and mortality.[28,29] It can exacerbate HF through rapid ventricular response and loss of atrial contribution to ventricular filling. Conversely, HF can precipitate atrial fibrillation by increasing atrial distension from ventricular volume overload. Control of ventricular response, maintenance of sinus rhythm in appropriate patients, and prevention of thromboembolism are important elements in the treatment of patients with concomitant HF and atrial fibrillation. Uncontrolled HTN is also an important contributing factor and should be treated according to current guidelines.[1]

Noncardiac events are also associated with HF decompensation. Pulmonary infections frequently cause worsening HF. Many of these events would be preventable with more widespread use of the pneumococcal and influenza vaccines. Pulmonary embolus, diabetes, worsening renal function, hypothyroidism, and hyperthyroidism should also be considered.

Nonadherence with prescribed HF medications or with dietary recommendations (eg, sodium intake and fluid restriction) is also a common cause of HF exacerbation.[1,30] Recent estimates indicate that nonadherence is an important contributor to poor outcomes and that socioeconomically disadvantaged patients appear to be disproportionately affected.

A number of drugs can precipitate or exacerbate HF by one or more of the following mechanisms: (a) negative inotropic effects; (b) direct cardiotoxicity; or (c) increased sodium and/or water retention (Table 14-3).[31,32] The resulting symptoms are typically those associated with volume overload, but in more severe cases hypoperfusion may also be present. Nonsteroidal antiinflammatory drugs (NSAIDs) are increasingly recognized for their ability to exacerbate HF and increase risk of hospitalization and mortality through volume retention, decreased renal function, and increased BP.[31,33]

What should be evident is that many of the precipitating factors are preventable, particularly through appropriate healthcare professional intervention. Specifically, patient education and counseling by a pharmacist should be able to identify and address inadequate HF therapy, detect medication nonadherence, and administration of drugs or the presence of drug–drug interactions that may worsen HF (see Table 14-3).[34,35] A careful medication history is an important aspect of evaluating the cause(s) of HF exacerbation. Discontinuation of medications known to exacerbate HF may help prevent hospitalizations. Use of medications such as antiarrhythmic agents, particularly disopyramide, dronedarone, and flecainide, and nondihydropyridine calcium channel blockers are important precipitants of exacerbations. The widespread use of NSAIDs, particularly the nonprescription agents that many patients perceive as having a low risk of adverse effects, is also problematic and should be discouraged. Thus, many of the factors precipitating HF exacerbations are amenable to pharmacist intervention. Attention to these factors may make important contributions to reducing the risk of adverse cardiovascular outcomes and improving the patient's quality of life.

TABLE 14-3 Drugs that May Precipitate or Exacerbate Heart Failure

Negative Inotropic Effect
Antiarrhythmics (eg, disopyramide, flecainide, propafenone)
Beta-blockers (eg, propranolol, metoprolol, carvedilol)
Calcium channel blockers (eg, verapamil, diltiazem)
Itraconazole
Cardiotoxic
Doxorubicin
Epirubicin
Daunomycin
Cyclophosphamide
Trastuzumab
Bevacizumab
Mitoxantrone
Ifosfamide
Mitomycin
Lapatinib
Sunitinib
Imatinib
Ethanol
Amphetamines (eg, cocaine, methamphetamine)
Sodium and Water Retention
NSAIDs
COX-2inhibitors
Rosiglitazone and pioglitazone
Glucocorticoids
Androgens and estrogens
Salicylates (high dose)
Sodium-containing drugs (eg, carbenicillin disodium, ticarcillin disodium)
Uncertain Mechanism
Adalimumab
Dronedarone
Etanercept
Infliximab

CLINICAL PRESENTATION

Signs and Symptoms

2 11 The primary manifestations of both HFrEF and HFpEF are dyspnea and fatigue, which lead to exercise intolerance, and fluid overload, which can result in peripheral edema and pulmonary congestion.[1,36] The presence of these signs and symptoms may vary considerably from patient to patient such that some patients have dyspnea but no signs of fluid retention, whereas others may have marked volume overload with few complaints of dyspnea or fatigue. However, many patients have both dyspnea and volume overload. Clinicians should remember that symptom severity often does not correlate with the degree of LV dysfunction. Patients with a low LVEF (less than 20%-25%) may be asymptomatic, whereas those with preserved LVEF may have significant symptoms. It is also important to note that symptoms can vary considerably over time in a given patient, even in the absence of changes in ventricular function or medications.

Systemic congestion is associated with a number of signs and symptoms. Jugular venous distension (JVD) is the simplest and most reliable sign of fluid overload. Examination of the right internal jugular vein with the patient at a 45 degree angle is the preferred method for assessing JVD. The presence of JVD more than 4 cm above the sternal angle suggests systemic venous congestion. In patients with mild systemic congestion, JVD may be absent at rest, but application of pressure to the abdomen will cause an elevation of JVD (hepatojugular reflux).

Peripheral edema is a cardinal finding in HF. Edema usually occurs in dependent parts of the body, and thus is seen as ankle or pedal edema in ambulatory patients, although it may be manifested as sacral edema in bedridden patients. Adults typically have a 10-lb (4.5-kg) fluid weight gain before trace peripheral edema is evident;

CLINICAL PRESENTATION Heart Failure

General

Patient presentation may range from asymptomatic to cardiogenic shock.

Symptoms

Dyspnea, particularly on exertion

Orthopnea

Paroxysmal nocturnal dyspnea

Exercise intolerance

Tachypnea

Cough

Fatigue

Nocturia

Hemoptysis

Abdominal pain

Anorexia

Nausea

Bloating

Poor appetite, early satiety

Ascites

Mental status changes

Weight gain or loss

Signs

Pulmonary rales

Pulmonary edema

S_3 gallop, mitral regurgitant murmur

Cool extremities

Pleural effusion

Cheyne-Stokes respiration

Tachycardia

Narrow pulse pressure

Cardiomegaly

Peripheral edema

Jugular venous distention

Hepatojugular reflux

Hepatomegaly

Venous stasis changes

Lateral displacement of apical impulse

Cachexia

Laboratory Tests

BNP > 100 pg/mL

NT-proBNP > 300 pg/mL

Electrocardiogram may be normal or it could show numerous abnormalities including acute ST-T wave changes from myocardial ischemia, atrial fibrillation, bradycardia, left ventricular hypertrophy

Serum creatinine: It may be increased due to hypoperfusion. Preexisting renal dysfunction can contribute to volume overload

Complete blood count useful to determine if heart failure due to reduced oxygen carrying capacity

Chest X-ray: Useful for detection of cardiac enlargement, pulmonary edema, and pleural effusions

Echocardiogram: Used to assess LV size, valve function, pericardial effusion, wall motion abnormalities, and ejection fraction

Hyponatremia: Serum sodium < 130 mEq/L is associated with reduced survival and may indicate worsening volume overload and/or disease progression

therefore, patients with acute decompensated HF may have no clinical evidence of systemic congestion except weight gain. Body weight is thus an excellent short-term end point for evaluating fluid status. Nonfluid weight gain and loss of muscle mass due to cardiac cachexia are potential confounders for long-term use of weight as a marker for fluid status. Hepatomegaly and ascites are other signs of systemic congestion.

Patients with HFrEF may exhibit signs and symptoms of low CO alone or in addition to volume overload. The primary complaint associated with hypoperfusion is fatigue. Poor appetite or early satiety may be due to limited perfusion of the GI tract. Conversely, patients with such GI complaints may simply be experiencing gut edema. Objective indicators of low CO include worsening renal function, cool extremities, altered mental status, resting tachycardia, and narrow pulse pressure.

Diagnosis

No single test is available to confirm the diagnosis of HF—it is a clinical syndrome associated with specific signs and symptoms.[1,36] Because HF can be caused or worsened by multiple cardiac and noncardiac disorders, some of which may be treatable or reversible, accurate diagnosis is essential for development of therapeutic strategies. HF is often initially suspected in a patient based on symptoms. However, signs and symptoms lack sensitivity for diagnosing HF since they are frequently found with many other disorders. Even in patients with known HF, there is poor correlation between the presence or severity of symptoms and the hemodynamic abnormality. With few exceptions, HFpEF cannot be distinguished from HFrEF on the basis of the history, physical examination, chest x-ray, and ECG alone.[37] Patients with HFpEF are often elderly, hypertensive women.[37]

A complete history and physical examination targeted at identifying cardiac or noncardiac disorders or behaviors that may cause or hasten HF development or progression are essential in the initial patient evaluation. However, the physical examination cannot distinguish between HFrEF and HFpEF. A careful medication history should also be obtained with a focus on use of ethanol, tobacco, illicit drugs (eg, cocaine or methamphetamine), vitamins and supplements (including herbal or "natural" supplements), NSAIDs, and antineoplastic agents (anthracyclines, cyclophosphamide, trastuzumab, and imatinib).

Particular attention should be paid to cardiovascular risk factors and to other disorders that can cause or exacerbate HF such as HTN, diabetes, atrial fibrillation, dyslipidemia, tobacco use, sleep-disordered breathing, and thyroid disease. Since coronary artery disease is the cause of HF in many patients, evaluation of the possibility of coronary disease is essential, especially in men. If coronary artery disease is detected, appropriate revascularization procedures may then be considered. The patient's volume status should be documented by assessing the body weight, JVD, and presence or absence of pulmonary congestion and peripheral edema. Laboratory testing may assist in identification of disorders that cause or worsen HF. The initial evaluation should include a complete blood count, serum electrolytes (including calcium and magnesium), assessment of renal and hepatic function, urinalysis, lipid profile, hemoglobin A1C, thyroid function tests, chest x-ray, and 12-lead ECG. There are no specific ECG abnormalities associated with HF, but findings may help detect coronary artery disease or conduction abnormalities that could affect prognosis and guide treatment decisions. Measurement of BNP or NT-proBNP may also assist in differentiating dyspnea caused by HF from other causes.

Although the history, physical examination, and laboratory tests provide important insight into the underlying cause of HF, the echocardiogram is the single most useful test in the evaluation of the patient. The echocardiogram is used to assess abnormalities in cardiac structure and function and should include evaluation of the pericardium, myocardium, and heart valves, and quantification of the LVEF to determine if systolic or diastolic dysfunction is present.

TREATMENT
Of Chronic Heart Failure

Desired Outcomes

The goals of therapy in management of chronic HF are to improve the patient's quality of life, relieve or reduce symptoms, prevent or minimize hospitalizations, slow progression of the disease, and prolong survival. Pharmacotherapy plays a key role in achieving these goals.[1] In addition, identification of risk factors for HF development and recognition of its progressive nature have led to increased emphasis on preventing the development of this disorder. With this in mind, the American College of Cardiology (ACC)/American Heart Association (AHA) guidelines for the evaluation and management of HF utilize a staging system that not only recognizes the evolution and progression of the disorder but also emphasizes risk factor modification and preventive treatment strategies (Fig. 14-6).[1] The four stages of this system differ from the NYHA functional classification (Table 14-4) with which most clinicians are familiar. The NYHA system is primarily intended to classify symptoms according to the clinician's subjective evaluation and does not recognize preventive measures or the progression of the disorder. A patient's symptoms can change frequently over a short period of time due to changes in medications, diet, intercurrent illnesses, etc. For example, a patient with ACC/AHA Stage C HF with NYHA class IV symptoms such as marked volume overload could rapidly improve to class I to II with aggressive diuretic therapy. Despite these limitations, this system can be useful for

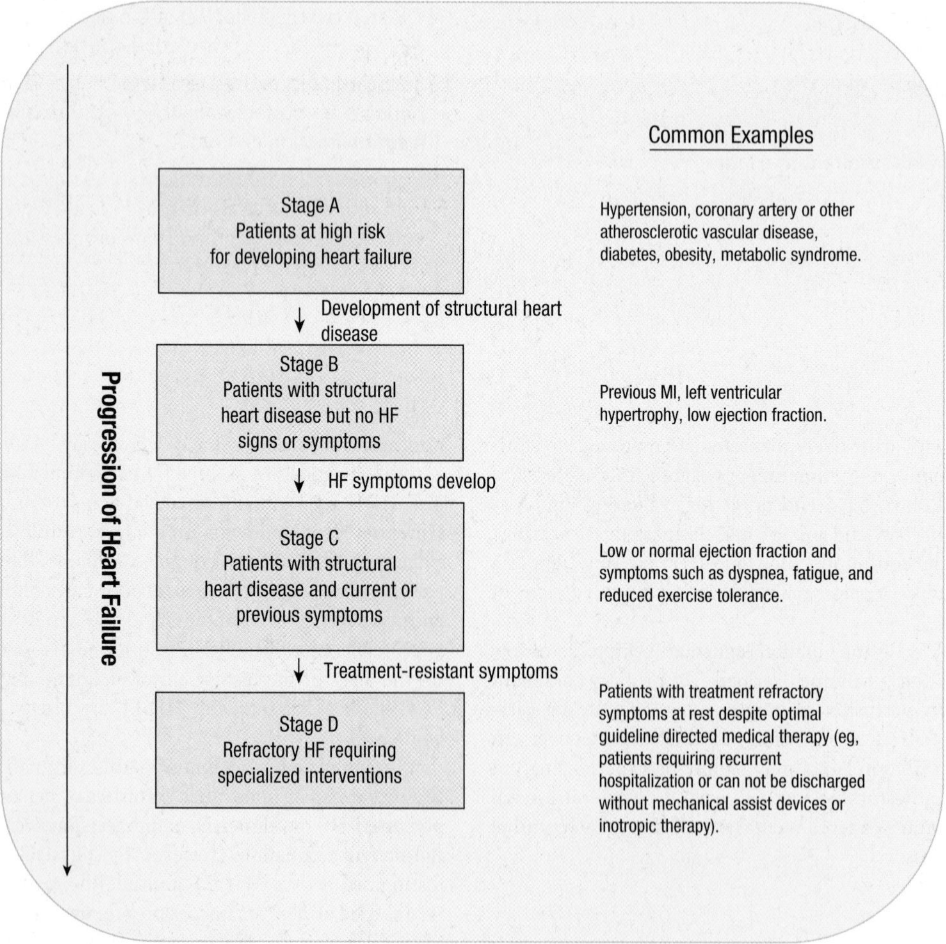

FIGURE 14-6 ACC/AHA heart failure staging system. (*Adapted from Yancy CW, Jessup M, Bozkurt B, et al. 2013 ACCF/AHA guideline for the management of heart failure: A report of the American College of Cardiology Foundation/American Heart Association Task Force on Practice Guidelines. J Am Coll Cardiol 2013;62:e147-239.*)

TABLE 14-4 New York Heart Association Functional Classification

Functional class

I. Patients with cardiac disease but without limitations of physical activity. Ordinary physical activity does not cause undue fatigue, dyspnea, or palpitation.

II. Patients with cardiac disease that results in slight limitations of physical activity. Ordinary physical activity results in fatigue, palpitation, dyspnea, or angina.

III. Patients with cardiac disease that results in marked limitation of physical activity. Although patients are comfortable at rest, less than ordinary activity will lead to symptoms.

IV. Patients with cardiac disease that results in an inability to carry on physical activity without discomfort. Symptoms of congestive heart failure are present even at rest. With any physical activity, increased discomfort is experienced.

monitoring patients and is widely used in HF studies. In contrast, and consistent with the progressive nature of HF, a patient's ACC/AHA HF stage could not improve (eg, go from Stage C to Stage B) even though the patient's symptoms could fluctuate from NYHA class IV to I.

The general principles used to guide the treatment of HFrEF are based on numerous large, randomized, double-blind, multicenter trials. Until recently, no such randomized trials had been performed in patients with HFpEF. Consequently, the guidelines for the management of HFpEF are based primarily on clinical investigations in relatively small groups of patients, clinical experience, and concepts based on the knowledge and understanding of the pathophysiology of the disease process. The treatment regimen outlined in Table 14-5 applies to patients with HFpEF who have clear manifestations of congestion either at rest or with exertion. Whether treatment of asymptomatic diastolic dysfunction confers any benefit has not been demonstrated.

TABLE 14-5 Targeted Approach to Treatment of HFpEF

Symptom-targeted treatment	Rationale	Agent
Decrease pulmonary venous pressure	Reduce left ventricular volume	Diuretics, nitrates, salt restriction
Decrease myocardial oxygen consumption	Reduce heart rate Control blood pressure	β-blockers, diltiazem, verapamil, ACE inhibitors, ARBs, calcium channel blockers
Maintain atrial contraction	Restore and/or maintain sinus rhythm	Cardioversion of atrial fibrillation
Improve exercise tolerance	As above	Use positive inotropic agents with caution
Disease-targeted treatment		
Prevent/treat myocardial ischemia		β-blockers, diltiazem, verapamil, nitrates
Prevent/regress ventricular hypertrophy		Antihypertensive therapy
Mechanism-targeted treatment		
Modify myocardial and extramyocardial mechanisms		Possibly ACE inhibitors or ARBs, diuretics, spironolactone
Modify intracellular and extracellular mechanisms		Possibly ACE inhibitors or ARBs, spironolactone

ACE, angiotensin-converting enzyme; ARB, angiotensin receptor blocker; HFpEF, heart failure with preserved ejection fraction.

General Measures

The complexity of the HF syndrome necessitates a comprehensive approach to management that includes accurate diagnosis, identification and treatment of risk factors, elimination or minimization of precipitating factors, appropriate pharmacologic and nonpharmacologic therapy, and close monitoring and followup.

The first step in management of chronic HF is to determine the etiology (see Table 14-1) and/or any precipitating factors. Appropriate treatment of underlying disorders (eg, hyperthyroidism, valvular heart disease) may obviate the need for specific HF treatment. Revascularization or anti-ischemic therapy in patients with coronary disease may reduce HF symptoms. Drugs that aggravate HF (see Table 14-3) should be discontinued if possible.

Restriction of physical activity reduces cardiac workload and is recommended for virtually all patients with acute congestive symptoms. However, once the patient's symptoms have stabilized and excess fluid is removed, restrictions on physical activity are discouraged. Exercise training may improve functional status, quality of life, and yield trends toward reduced hospitalizations and death from cardiovascular causes and is supported by current guidelines to improve functional status.[1,38]

Restriction of dietary sodium and fluid intake is an important lifestyle intervention for both HFrEF and HFpEF. Mild (less than 3 g/day) to moderate (less than 2 g/day) sodium restriction, in conjunction with daily measurement of weight, should be implemented to minimize volume retention and allow use of lower and safer diuretic doses. The typical American diet contains 8 to 10 g of sodium per day, so most patients would need to reduce their intake by over 50%. Patients should avoid adding salt to prepared foods and eliminate foods high in sodium (eg, salt-cured meats, salted snack foods, pickles, soups, delicatessen meats, and processed foods). In patients with hyponatremia (serum Na less than 130 mEq/L [less than 130 mmol/L]) or those with persistent volume retention despite high diuretic doses and sodium restriction, daily fluid intake should be limited to 2 L/day from all sources. However, both sodium and fluid restriction must be done with care in patients with HFpEF. Excessive restriction can lead to hypotension, low-output state, and/or renal insufficiency. Daily weights may help to assess volume status. Dietary and lifestyle factors that decrease the risk of development of CAD and HTN should be encouraged. Although guidelines indicate sodium restriction is reasonable to minimize congestion, proven benefits on clinical outcomes are lacking and some data suggest sodium restriction is associated with worse outcomes in patients with HFrEF.[39]

Other important general measures include patient and family counseling on the signs and symptoms of HF, detailed written instructions on the importance of appropriate medication use and compliance, activity level, diet, discharge medications, weight monitoring, continuity of care, and the need for close monitoring and followup to reinforce compliance and minimize the risk of HF exacerbations and subsequent hospitalization. These activities are now referred to as self-care and constitute an important means to improve such important outcomes as hospitalization and quality of life.[40]

General Approach to Treatment

4 The ACC/AHA treatment guidelines are organized around the four identified stages of HF, and the treatment recommendations are summarized in Figs. 14-7 and 14-8.[1] Clinicians are reminded that, in addition to the ACC/AHA, other cardiology professional societies publish guidelines for evaluation and treatment of HF including the Heart Failure Society of America (HFSA) and the European Society of Cardiology (ESC).[41,42] Although minor differences exist between the recommendations in these guidelines, they are in general agreement in their overall approach to evaluation and treatment of HF.

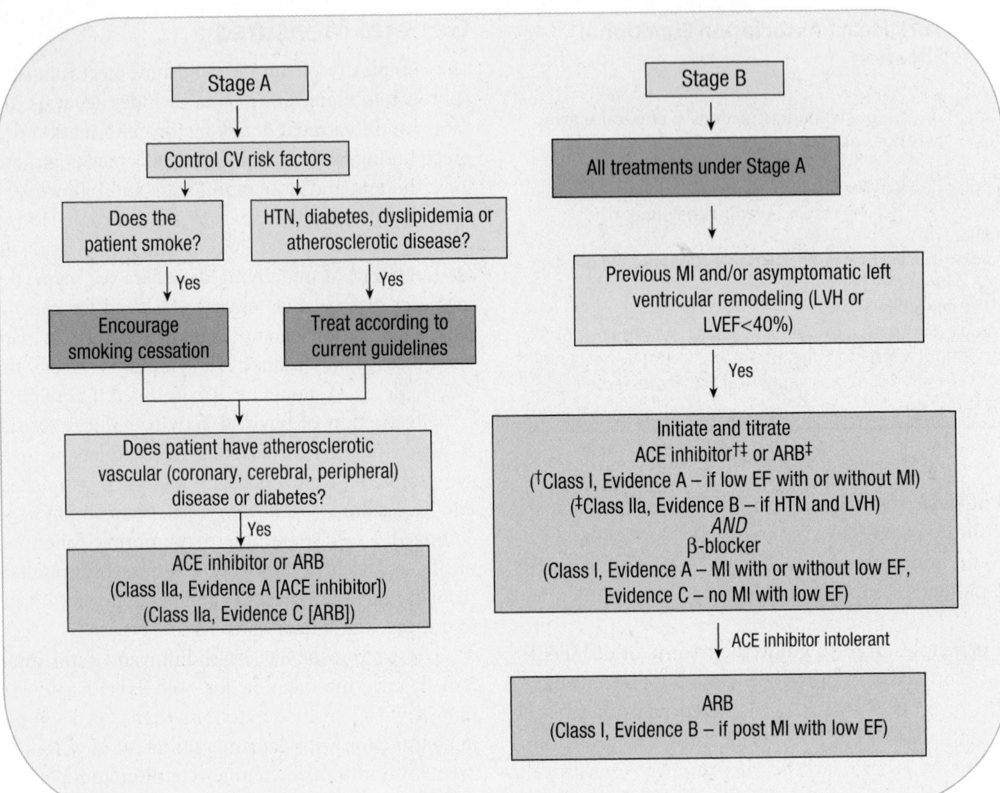

FIGURE 14-7 Treatment algorithm for patients with ACC/AHA Stage A and B heart failure. (*Adapted from Yancy CW, Jessup M, Bozkurt B, et al. 2013 ACCF/AHA guideline for the management of heart failure: A report of the American College of Cardiology Foundation/American Heart Association Task Force on Practice Guidelines. J Am Coll Cardiol 2013;62:e147-239.*)

In addition to chronic HFrEF, these guidelines now also provide thorough discussions of acute decompensated HF and management of patients with comorbid diseases often encountered in this population.

Heart Failure with Preserved Ejection Fraction

Less information on the treatment of HFpEF is available. This relative paucity of evidence is reflected in guidelines for the diagnosis and management of HFpEF published by the ACC/AHA, the ESC, and the HFSA.[1,41,42] In general, all three guidelines recommend treating comorbid conditions by controlling HR and BP, alleviating causes of myocardial ischemia, reducing volume, and restoring and maintaining sinus rhythm in patients with atrial fibrillation. Table 14-6 summarizes the therapeutic recommendations.

A recent study showing that use of guideline directed medical therapy (GDMT) improves mortality in patients with HFrEF reinforces the importance for clinicians to be familiar with these recommendations.[43] However, clinicians should also remember that these are only *guidelines* and that evaluation and treatment should be individualized for each patient.

As the management of HF has become increasingly complex, the development of disease management programs that use multidisciplinary teams has been studied extensively. These programs utilize several broad approaches including HF specialty clinics, home-based interventions, structured telephone support, and close patient followup. Most are multidisciplinary and may include physicians, advanced practice nurses, dieticians, and pharmacists. In general, the programs focus on optimization of drug and nondrug therapy, patient and family education and counseling, exercise and dietary advice, intense followup by telephone or home visits, improving adherence to medications and lifestyle recommendations, encouragement of self-care, and early recognition of and management of volume overload.[1] Such programs have typically focused on patients with more severe HF who are at high risk for hospital admission. In general, multidisciplinary disease management programs improve quality of life and reduce HF and all-cause hospitalizations and costs, although these benefits are not consistently demonstrated in all studies. Pharmacists can play an important role in the multidisciplinary team management of HF taking on such responsibilities as medication evaluation and therapeutic recommendations, improved use of GDMT, patient education, and followup telephone monitoring to reduce hospitalizations for HF, evaluation of adverse drug events, and medication errors.[34,44]

Treatment of Stage A Heart Failure

Patients in Stage A do not have structural heart disease or HF symptoms but are at high risk for developing HF because of the presence of risk factors (see Fig. 14-7). The emphasis here is on risk factor identification and modification to prevent the development of structural heart disease and subsequent HF. Commonly encountered risk factors include HTN, dyslipidemia, diabetes, obesity, metabolic syndrome, smoking, and coronary artery disease. Although each of these disorders individually increases risk, they frequently coexist in many patients and act synergistically to foster the development of both HFrEF and HFpEF.Effective blood pressure control reduces the risk of developing HF by approximately 50%; thus, current HTN treatment guidelines should be followed.[1] Obesity, diabetes, and metabolic syndrome also importantly contribute to the risk of developing HF although it remains unclear whether controlling these risk factors reduces the risk of developing HF.[45-47] Appropriate management of coronary disease and its associated risk factors is also important. Although treatment must be individualized, ACE inhibitors or ARBs and statins are recommended for HF prevention in patients with multiple vascular risk factors.[1]

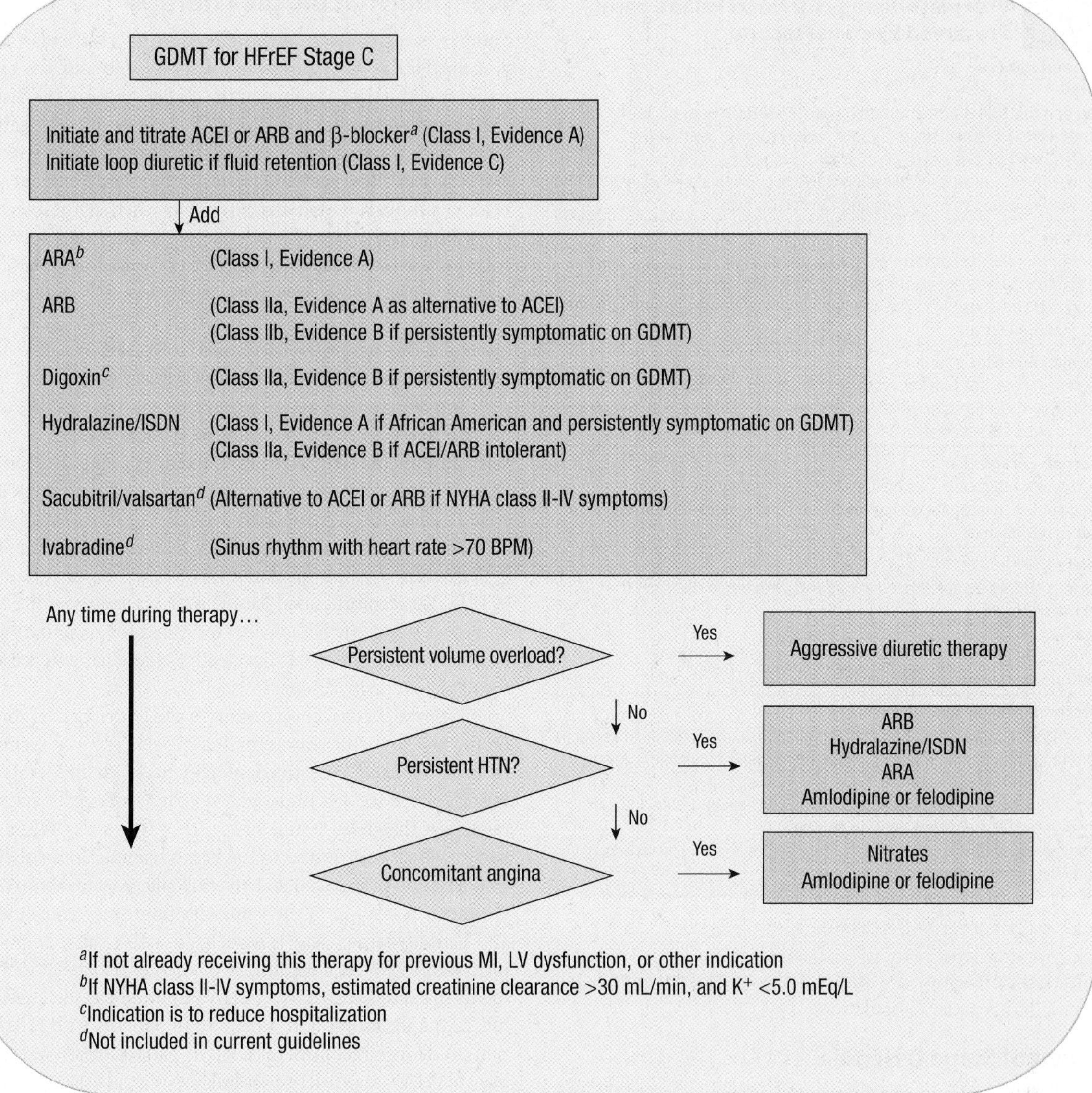

FIGURE 14-8 Guideline-directed treatment algorithm for patients with ACC/AHA Stage C heart failure with reduced ejection fraction. (*Adapted from Yancy CW, Jessup M, Bozkurt B, et al. 2013 ACCF/AHA guideline for the management of heart failure: A report of the American College of Cardiology Foundation/American Heart Association Task Force on Practice Guidelines. J Am Coll Cardiol 2013;62:e147-239.*)

Treatment of Stage B Heart Failure

Patients in Stage B have structural heart disease, but do not have HF symptoms (see Fig. 14-7). This group includes patients with left ventricular hypertrophy, recent or remote MI, valvular disease, or LVEF less than 40%. These individuals are at risk for developing HF, and treatment is targeted at minimizing additional injury and preventing or slowing the remodeling process. In addition to the treatment measures outlined in Stage A, ACE inhibitors or ARBs and β-blockers are important components of therapy. All patients with a reduced LVEF should receive an ACE inhibitor or ARB and a β-blocker to prevent development of HF, whether or not they have had an MI.[1] Patients with a previous MI and reduced LVEF should also receive an ACE inhibitor or ARB, evidence-based β-blockers, and a statin.[1]

Treatment of Stage C HF

4 5 6 7 8 9 10 11 Patients with structural heart disease and previous or current symptoms are classified in Stage C and include both HFrEF and HFpEF. In addition to treatments in Stages A and B, patients with HFrEF in Stage C should be routinely treated with GDMT that includes an ACE inhibitor or ARB and an evidence-based β-blocker (see Fig 14-8).[1] The benefits of these medications on slowing HF progression, reducing morbidity and mortality, and improving symptoms are clearly established. Loop diuretics, aldosterone antagonists, and hydralazine–isosorbide dinitrate (ISDN) are also routinely used in these patients. Digoxin can also be considered in selected patients, as can two newly approved medications, ivabradine and sacubitril/valsartan. Nonpharmacologic therapy with devices such as an implantable cardioverter-defibrillator (ICD) or cardiac resynchronization therapy (CRT) with a biventricular pacemaker is also indicated in certain patients with HFrEF in Stage C (see Nonpharmacologic Therapy). Other general measures noted earlier are also important as is careful followup and patient education to reinforce dietary and medication compliance to prevent clinical deterioration and reduce hospitalization.[1,48]

Dozens of trials evaluated pharmacotherapy in patients with HFrEF, but few focused on patients with HFpEF. In fact, most published HF studies specifically excluded patients with preserved EF. The results of some clinical trials for treatment of HFpEF as well as ongoing studies are summarized in Table 14-7. Phosphodiesterase inhibitors, ranolazine, interleukin-1 blockade, and cardiac

TABLE 14-6 Pharmacotherapy for Heart Failure with Preserved Ejection Fraction

Recommendations
Diuretics • A loop or a thiazide diuretic should be considered for patients with volume overload. However, with more severe volume overload or inadequate response to a thiazide, a loop diuretic should be implemented. Caution is warranted not to lower preload excessively, which may reduce stroke volume and cardiac output.
ACE inhibitors • ACE inhibitors may be considered in all patients. • ACE inhibitors should be considered in all patients who have symptomatic atherosclerotic cardiovascular disease or diabetes and one additional risk factor.
Angiotensin receptor blockers • Angiotensin receptor blockers may be considered in all patients. • In patients who are intolerant of ACE inhibitors, an angiotensin receptor blocker can be considered an alternative.
Aldosterone antagonists • Aldosterone antagonists can be considered to reduce the risk of hospitalization in patients that do not have contraindications or are at risk for hyperkalemia.
β-Blockers • β-blockers should be considered in patients with one or more of the following conditions: • Myocardial infarction • Hypertension • Atrial fibrillation requiring ventricular rate control
Calcium channel blockers • In patients with atrial fibrillation warranting ventricular rate control who either are intolerant to or have not responded to a β-blocker, diltiazem or verapamil should be considered. • A nondihydropyridine or dihydropyridine calcium channel blocker can be considered for symptom-limiting angina. • A nondihydropyridine or dihydropyridine calcium channel blocker can be considered for hypertension.

ACE, angiotensin-converting enzyme.

resynchronization therapy are some of the other strategies being investigated in this patient population.

Treatment of Stage D HFrEF

Stage D HF includes patients receiving maximally tolerated GDMT that have persistent symptoms. This is often referred to as advanced, refractory, or end-stage HF. These patients often undergo recurrent hospitalizations or cannot be discharged from the hospital without special interventions, have a poor quality of life, and are at high risk for morbidity and mortality. These individuals have the most advanced form of HF and should be referred to HF management programs so that specialized therapies including mechanical circulatory support, continuous IV positive inotropic therapy, and cardiac transplantation can be considered in addition to standard treatments outlined in Stages A to C.[1,49] Discussions with the patient and family members regarding prognosis, patient priorities for minimizing symptoms versus prolonging survival, options for additional treatments, and end-of-life and hospice care should be initiated. Several excellent resources are available that address these issues.[49-51]

Management of volume status can be challenging in these patients.[1,27] Restriction of sodium and fluid intake may be beneficial. High doses of diuretics, combination therapy with a loop and thiazide diuretic, or mechanical methods of fluid removal such as ultrafiltration may be required. Patients in Stage D may be less tolerant to ACE inhibitors (hypotension, worsening renal insufficiency) and β-blockers (worsening HF) as high levels of neurohormonal activation maintain circulatory homeostasis. Initiation of therapy with low doses, slow upward dose titration, and close monitoring for signs and symptoms of intolerance are essential in this group of patients. The approach to treatment of patients with Stage D HF is discussed in more detail in Chapter 15.

Nonpharmacologic Therapy

Sudden cardiac death, primarily due to ventricular tachycardia and fibrillation, is responsible for 40% to 50% of the mortality in patients with HFrF. Patients in the earlier stages of the disorder with milder symptoms are more likely to die from sudden death, whereas death from pump failure is more frequent in those with advanced HF. Many of these patients have complex and frequent ventricular ectopy, although it remains unknown whether these ectopic beats contribute to the risk of malignant arrhythmias or merely serve as markers for individuals at higher risk for sudden death. Although class I antiarrhythmic agents can suppress ventricular ectopy, empiric treatment with them adversely affects survival.[52] Drugs that attenuate disease progression such as β-blockers and aldosterone antagonists reduce the risk of sudden death.

Implantation of an ICD prevents sudden cardiac death and is an effective primary prevention to reduce the risk of mortality in selected patients with HFrEF.[1] Current guidelines recommend use of an ICD for primary prevention in patients receiving GDMT with NYHA class II–III symptoms with a LVEF less than or equal to 35% that are expected to live for at least one year.[1] In patients with NYHA class I symptoms and a LVEF less than or equal to 30%, an ICD is also recommended for primary prevention if life expectancy exceeds 1 year.[1] An ICD is also indicated for secondary prevention in survivors of sudden cardiac death as these patients are at high risk for recurrent arrhythmias.[1]

Delayed electrical activation of the left ventricle, characterized on the ECG by a QRS duration that exceeds 120 milliseconds, occurs in approximately one third of patients with moderate to severe HFrEF. Since the left and right ventricles normally activate simultaneously, this delay results in asynchronous contraction of the ventricles, which contributes to the hemodynamic abnormalities of HF. Implantation of a specialized biventricular pacemaker to restore synchronous activation of the ventricles improves ventricular function and hemodynamics and is associated with reverse remodeling and increased LVEF. As a result, use of CRT is associated with improvements in exercise capacity, NYHA symptom classification, quality of life, hospitalizations, and mortality in patients with HRrEF.[1,53] Current guidelines recommend CRT in patients receiving GDMT that have NYHA class II–III or ambulatory class IV symptoms and with a QRS duration greater than or equal to 150 milliseconds and LVEF less than or equal to 35%.[1] CRT can also be considered in selected patients with QRS durations of 120 to 149 milliseconds. Combined CRT and ICD devices are available and are frequently used if the patient meets the indications for both devices.

In patients with stage D HFrEF receiving GDMT, the use of mechanical circulatory support with a ventricular assist device (VAD) can be considered in certain patients.[1] Although the criteria for use of these devices continue to rapidly evolve, they are frequently used to bridge patients to cardiac transplant or as destination therapy in patients ineligible for transplant and their use in these settings is associated with better survival and improved functional capacity.[1,54]

Pharmacologic Therapy of HFpEF

11 With a few notable exceptions, many of the drugs used to treat HFrEF are the same as those for treatment of HFpEF. However, the rationale for their use, the pathophysiologic process that is being altered by the drug, and the dosing regimen may be entirely different depending on whether the patient has HFrEF or HFpEF. For example, β-blockers are recommended for the treatment of both HFrEF and HFpEF. In HFpEF, however, β-blockers are used to decrease HR, increase diastolic duration, and modify the hemodynamic response to exercise. In HFrEF, β-blockers are used in the long term to increase the inotropic state and modify LV remodeling. Diuretics also are used in the treatment of both HFrEF and HFpEF. However,

TABLE 14-7 Completed and Ongoing Large Clinical Trials for HFpEF

Trial (No. of Patients)	Treatment	Inclusion Criteria	Primary End Point	Results
DIG Ancillary Study (n = 988)[109]	Digoxin vs placebo for a mean of 37 months. Patients received ACE inhibitor (86%) and diuretics (85%)	EF >45%, NYHA II–IV, normal sinus rhythm	Composite of HF hospitalization or HF mortality	No significant difference was found in the primary end point between treatment groups (HR = 0.82, P = 0.136). Digoxin had no effect on all-cause mortality or cause-specific mortality or on all-cause or CV hospitalization. Compared with placebo, digoxin use was associated with a trend toward a reduction in HF hospitalizations (HR = 0.79, P = 0.094) and an increase in unstable angina admissions (HR = 1.37, P = 0.061).
CHARM-Preserved[68] (n = 3,023)	Candesartan vs placebo for a mean of 36.6 months. Patients continued their background HF medications: ACE inhibitor (19%), β-blocker (55%), diuretics (75%), spironolactone (11%)	EF >40%, NYHA II–IV, ≥1 hospitalization for CV reason	Composite of CV mortality or HF hospitalization	No significant difference was found in the primary end point between treatment groups (adjusted HR = 0.86, P = 0.051) or in CV deaths (adjusted HR = 0.95, P = 0.635). Compared with placebo, candesartan use was associated with fewer HF admissions (P = 0.047), lower incidence of new diabetes (HR = 0.60, P = 0.005), and a reduction in the composite of CV death, hospitalization for HF, MI, and stroke (adjusted HR = 0.86, P = 0.037).
PEP-CHF[159] (n = 850)	Perindopril vs placebo for a mean of 2.1 years	Clinical criteria for HF, EF ≥40%, age ≥70 years	Composite of total mortality and HF hospitalization	No significant difference was found in the primary end point between treatment groups (HR = 0.69, P = 0.055; HR = 0.70, P = 0.545). In a subgroup analysis, patients ≤75 years of age (HR = 0.29, P = 0.035) and with a history of MI (HR = 0.38, P = 0.004) showed a reduction in the primary end point. Compared with placebo, perindopril use at 1 year was associated with fewer unplanned hospital admissions (HR = 0.63, P = 0.033), greater improvements in exercise tolerance (P = 0.011), and improvement in NYHA class (P = 0.030).
I-Preserve[69] (n = 4,128)	Irbesartan vs placebo for 2 years. ACE inhibitor can be used for any indication other than HTN	Clinical criteria for HF or hospitalized within 6 months for HF, age ≥60 years, NYHA II–IV, EF ≥45%	Composite of all-cause mortality or CV hospitalization	No significant difference was found in the primary end point between treatment groups (HR = 0. 95, P = 0.35), overall death rates (HR = 1.00, P = 0.98), or CV hospitalization rate (HR = 0.95, P = 0.44).
SENIORS[160] (n = 2,111)	Nebivolol vs placebo for 21 months	Clinical criteria for HF with either documented heart failure hospitalization with 1 year or documented EF ≤35% within 6 months, age ≥70 years	All-cause mortality or cardiovascular hospitalization	In the study, 1,359 patients (64%) had an EF ≤35% (mean 28.7%), and 752 (36%) had an EF >35% (mean 49.2%). In patients with EF >35%, the HR for nebivolol vs placebo for the primary end point was 0.81 (P = 0.104). No significant difference existed between groups (EF ≤35% vs EF >35%, P = 0.720).
TOPCAT[21] (n = 3,345)	Spironolactone vs placebo for 2 years	Clinical criteria for HF, age ≥50 years, EF ≥45%, ≥1 hospitalization for HF, controlled SBP	CV mortality, aborted cardiac arrest, HF hospitalization	With a mean follow-up of 3.3 years, the primary outcome occurred in 18.6% of the spironolactone group and 20.4% in the placebo group (HR 0.89; P = 0.14).Only hospitalizations were significantly reduced by 17%. A posthoc analysis showed a significant benefit in the primary outcome in those patients enrolled in the Americas as compared to those enrolled in Russia and Georgia.
PARAGON-HF (n = 4,300)	Sacubitril/valsartan vs valsartan	NYHA class II–IV with EF >45%	Composite of CV death and total HF hospitalization	Estimated completion 2019. https://clinicaltrials.gov/ct2/show/NCT01920711

ACE, angiotensin-converting enzyme; CHARM, Candesartan in Heart Failure: Assessment of Reduction in Mortality and Morbidity; CV, cardiovascular; DIG, Digitalis Investigation Group.

the doses of diuretics used to treat HFpEF are, in general, much smaller than those used to treat HFrEF. Antagonists of the RAAS are useful in lowering BP and reducing LVH. Some drugs, however, are used to treat either HFrEF or HFpEF, but not both. Calcium channel blockers such as diltiazem, amlodipine, and verapamil have little utility in the treatment of HFrEF. In contrast, each of these drugs has been proposed as being useful in the treatment of HFpEF.

Drug Therapies for Routine Use in Guideline Directed Medical Therapy for Patients with Stage C HFrEF

4 5 6 7 8 9 10 A treatment algorithm for management of patients with Stage C HFrEF is shown in Fig. 14-8. In general, these patients should receive combined therapy with an ACE inhibitor or ARB and a β-blocker, plus a diuretic if there is evidence of fluid

retention. Other therapies including an aldosterone antagonist or the combination of hydralazine-nitrates should also be considered in selected patients.[1] Initiation of digoxin therapy can be considered to decrease hospitalizations in patients with HFrEF that remain symptomatic despite GDMT or added during intial treatment of patients with severe symptoms while GDMT is started.[1] Drug dosing and monitoring are summarized in Tables 14-8 and 14-9.

Diuretics 7 The compensatory mechanisms in HF stimulate excessive sodium and water retention, often leading to pulmonary and systemic congestion.[55,56] Diuretic therapy, in addition to sodium restriction, is recommended in all patients with clinical evidence of fluid retention. Once fluid overload has been resolved, many patients require chronic diuretic therapy to maintain euvolemia. Among the drugs used to manage HF, diuretics are the most rapid in producing symptomatic benefits. However, diuretics do not prolong survival or (with the possible exception of torsemide) alter disease progression, and therefore are not considered mandatory therapy. Thus, patients who do not have fluid retention would not require diuretic therapy.

The primary goal of diuretic therapy is to reduce symptoms associated with fluid retention, improve exercise tolerance and quality of life, and reduce hospitalizations from HF. Diuretics accomplish this by decreasing pulmonary and peripheral edema through reduction of preload. Although preload is a determinant of CO, the Frank–Starling curve (see Fig. 14-4) shows that patients with congestive symptoms have reached the flat portion of the curve. A reduction in preload improves symptoms but has little effect on the patient's SV or CO until the steep portion of the curve is reached. However, diuretic therapy must be used judiciously because overdiuresis can lead to a reduction in CO, renal perfusion, and symptoms of volume depletion.

Diuretic therapy is usually initiated in low doses in the outpatient setting, with dosage adjustments based on symptom assessment and daily body weight. Change in body weight is a sensitive marker of fluid retention or loss, and it is recommended that patients monitor their status by taking daily morning body weights. Patients who gain 1 lb/day for several consecutive days or 3 to 5 lb (1.4-2.3 kg) in a week should contact their healthcare provider for instructions (which often will be to increase the diuretic dose temporarily). Such action often will allow patients to prevent a decompensation that requires hospitalization. One study demonstrated a significant reduction in emergency department visits with a protocol that directed patients to self-adjust their diuretic dose based on changes in HF symptoms and daily body weight.[57] Hypotension or worsening renal function (eg, increases in serum creatinine) may be indicative of volume depletion and necessitates a reduction in the diuretic dose. Assessing volume status is particularly important before ACE inhibitor or β-blocker initiation or dose uptitration as overdiuresis may predispose patients to hypotension and other adverse effects with increases in ACE inhibitor or β-blocker doses.

11 In patients with HFpEF, diuretic treatment should be initiated at low doses in order to avoid hypotension and fatigue. Hypotension can be a significant problem in the treatment of HFpEF because these patients have a very steep LV diastolic pressure–volume curve such that a small change in volume causes a large change in filling pressure and CO. After the acute treatment of HFpEF has been completed, long-term treatment should include small to moderate oral doses of diuretics (furosemide 20-40 mg/day, chlorthalidone 25-100 mg, or hydrochlorothiazide 12.5-25 mg/day).

Thiazide Diuretics Thiazide diuretics such as hydrochlorothiazide block sodium reabsorption in the distal convoluted tubule (approximately 5%-8% of filtered sodium). The thiazides therefore are relatively weak diuretics and infrequently are used alone in HF. However, thiazides or the thiazide-like diuretic metolazone can be used in combination with loop diuretics to promote a very effective diuresis. In addition, thiazide diuretics may be preferred in patients with only mild fluid retention and elevated BP because of their more persistent antihypertensive effects compared with loop diuretics.

Loop Diuretics Loop diuretics are usually necessary to restore and maintain euvolemia in HF. They act by inhibiting a Na–K–2Cl transporter in the thick ascending limb of the loop of Henle, where 20% to 25% of filtered sodium normally is reabsorbed. Because loop diuretics are highly bound to plasma proteins, they are not highly filtered at the glomerulus. They reach the tubular lumen by active transport via the organic acid transport pathway. Competitors for this pathway (probenecid or organic by-products of uremia) can inhibit delivery of loop diuretics to their site of action and decrease effectiveness. Loop diuretics also induce a prostaglandin-mediated increase in renal blood flow, which contributes to their natriuretic effect. Coadministration of NSAIDs, including cyclooxygenase-2 (COX-2) inhibitors, blocks this prostaglandin-mediated effect and can diminish diuretic efficacy. Excessive dietary sodium intake may also reduce the efficacy of loop diuretics. Unlike thiazides, loop diuretics maintain their effectiveness in the presence of impaired renal function, although higher doses may be necessary to obtain adequate delivery of the drug to the site of action.

ACE Inhibitors 5 ACE inhibitors are a key component of the pharmacotherapy of patients with HFrEF.[1] By blocking the conversion of angiotensin I to angiotensin II by ACE, the production of angiotensin II and, in turn, aldosterone is decreased, but not completely eliminated.[13] This decrease in angiotensin II and aldosterone attenuates many of the deleterious effects of these neurohormones that drive HF progression including ventricular remodeling, myocardial fibrosis, myocyte apoptosis, cardiac hypertrophy, NE release, vasoconstriction, and sodium and water retention.[13] The endogenous vasodilator bradykinin, which is inactivated by ACE, is also increased by ACE inhibitors along with the release of vasodilatory prostaglandins and histamine.[16] The precise contribution of the effects of ACE inhibitors on bradykinin and vasodilatory prostaglandins is unclear. However, the persistence of clinical benefits with ACE inhibitors despite the fact that angiotensin II and aldosterone levels return to pretreatment levels in some patients suggests these are potentially important effects.[13]

Numerous placebo-controlled clinical trials in both symptomatic and asymptomatic patients with reduced LVEF have documented the favorable effects of ACE inhibitor therapy on symptoms, NYHA functional classification, clinical status, heart failure progression, hospitalizations, and quality of life.[13] Importantly, ACE inhibitors improve survival by 20% to 30% compared with placebo and these benefits are maintained with continued therapy.[13] The benefits of ACE inhibitor therapy are independent of the etiology of HF (ischemic vs nonischemic) and are greatest in patients with the most severe symptoms.[13] As efficacy has been demonstrated with numerous agents, the improved outcomes are likely a "class effect" of ACE inhibitors.[1,13]

The most common cause of HFrEF is ischemic heart disease, where MI results in loss of myocytes, followed by ventricular dilation and remodeling. Captopril, ramipril, and trandolapril all benefit post-MI patients whether therapy is initiated early or late after the infarct.[13] Collectively, these studies indicate that ACE inhibitors administered after MI improve overall survival, decrease development of severe HF, and reduce reinfarction and HF hospitalization rates.[13] The effects are most pronounced in higher-risk patients, such as those with symptomatic HF or reduced LVEF, with 20% to 30% reductions in mortality reported in these patients.[13] Post-MI patients without HF symptoms or reduced LVEF (Stage B) should also receive ACE inhibitors to prevent the development of HF and to reduce mortality.[1,13]

The use of ACE inhibitors in patients with chronic kidney disease is particularly relevant since it is a common co-morbidity in patients with HF and is associated with an increased risk of

TABLE 14-8 Drug Dosing Table

Drug	Brand Name	Initial Dose	Usual Range	Special Population Dose	Comments
Loop Diuretics					
Furosemide	Lasix®	20-40 mg once or twice daily	20-160 mg once or twice daily	Cl_{cr} 20-50 mL/min: 160 mg once or twice daily Cl_{cr}<20 mL/min: 400 mg daily	Single doses exceeding those listed are unlikely to elicit additional response
Bumetanide	Bumex®	0.5-1.0 mg once or twice daily	1-2 mg once or twice daily	Cl_{cr} 20-50 mL/min: 2 mg once or twice daily Cl_{cr}<20 mL/min: 8-10 mg daily	Single doses exceeding those listed are unlikely to elicit additional response
Torsemide	Demadex®	10-20 mg once daily	10-80 mg once daily	Cl_{cr} 20-50 mL/min: 40 mg once daily Cl_{cr}<20 mL/min: 200 mg daily	Single doses exceeding those listed are unlikely to elicit additional response
ACE Inhibitors					
Captopril	Capoten®	6.25 mg three times daily	50 mg three times daily*		
Enalapril	Vasotec®	2.5 mg twice daily	10-20 mg twice daily*		
Lisinopril	Zestril®, Prinivil®	2.5-5.0 mg once daily	20-40 mg once daily*		
Quinapril	Accupril®	5 mg twice daily	20-40 mg twice daily		
Ramipril	Altace®	1.25-2.5 mg	5 mg twice daily*		
Fosinopril	Monopril®	5-10 mg once daily	40 mg once daily		Undergoes both hepatic and renal elimination
Trandolapril	Mavik®	0.5-1.0 mg once daily	4 mg once daily*		Undergoes both hepatic and renal elimination
Perindopril	Aceon®	2 mg once daily	8-16 mg once daily		Undergoes both hepatic and renal elimination
Angiotensin Receptor Blockers					
Candesartan	Atacand®	4 mg once daily	32 mg once daily*		
Valsartan	Diovan®	20-40 mg twice daily	160 mg twice daily*		
Losartan	Cozaar®	25-50 mg once daily	150 mg once daily*		
Beta-Blockers					
Bisoprolol	Zebeta®	1.25 mg once daily	10 mg once daily*		
Carvedilol	Coreg®	3.125 mg twice daily	25 mg twice daily*	Target dose for patients weighing >85 kg is 50 mg twice daily	Should be taken with food
Carvedilol phosphate	Coreg CR®	10 mg once daily	80 mg once daily		Should be taken with food
Metoprolol succinate CR/XL	Toprol-XL®	12.5-25 mg once daily	200 mg once daily*		
Aldosterone Antagonists					
Spironolactone	Aldactone®	eGFR ≥50 mL/min/1.73m^2: 12.5-25 mg once daily	25-50 mg once daily*	eGFR 30-49 mL/min/1.73m^2: 12.5 mg once daily or every other day	The risk of hyperkalemia increases if serum creatinine is >1.6 mg/dL. Avoid if baseline potassium is ≥5 mEq/L
Eplerenone	Inspra®	eGFR ≥50 mL/min/1.73m^2: 25 mg once daily	50 mg once daily*	eGFR 30-49 mL/min/1.73m^2: 25 mg every other day	The risk of hyperkalemia increases if serum creatinine is >1.6 mg/dL. Avoid if baseline potassium is ≥5 mEq/L
Other					
Hydralazine-Isosorbide Dinitrate	Bidil®	Hydralazine 37.5 mg three times daily Isosorbide dinitrate 20 mg three times daily	Hydralazine 75 mg three times daily* Isosorbide dinitrate 40 mg three times daily*		Indicated in conjunction with standard heart failure therapy to improve survival and reduce hospitalizations in self-identified African-American patients
Digoxin	Lanoxin®	0.125-0.25 mg once daily	0.125-0.25 mg once daily	Reduce dose in elderly, patients with low lean body mass, and patients with impaired renal function	Target plasma concentration range is 0.5-0.9 ng/mL. Does not improve survival in patients with HFrEF

(continued)

TABLE 14-8 Drug Dosing Table (*Continued*)

Drug	Brand Name	Initial Dose	Usual Range	Special Population Dose	Comments
Ivabradine	Corlanor®	5 mg twice daily	5-7.5 mg twice daily	Avoid if resting heart rate <60 BPM before treatment	Indicated to reduce the risk of hospitalization in patients with HFrEF with a resting heart rate ≥70 BPM receiving maximally tolerated beta-blocker doses Take with meals
Sacubitril/valsartan	Entresto®	49/51 mg sacubitril/valsartan twice daily	97/103 mg sacubitril/valsartan twice daily*	For patients taking a low dose of or not taking an ACE inhibitor or ARB or if eGFR is <30 mL/min/1.73m^2, the starting dose is 24/26 mg sacubitril/valsartan twice daily	Discontinue ACE inhibitors at least 36 hours before initiating sacubitril/valsartn treatment

*Regimens proven in large clinical trials to reduce mortality.

Cl_{cr}, creatinine clearance; eGFR,estimated glomerular filtration rate; HFrEF, heart failure with reduced ejection fraction

Adapted from Brater DC. Pharmacology of diuretics *Am J Med Sci* 2000;319:38-50 and Yancy CW, Jessup M, Bozkurt B, et al. 2013 ACCF/AHA guideline for the management of heart failure: A report of the American College of Cardiology Foundation/American Heart Association Task Force on Practice Guidelines. *J Am Coll Cardiol* 2013;62:e147-e239.

TABLE 14-9 Drug Monitoring

Drug Class	Adverse Effect	Monitoring Parameters	Comments
ACE inhibitors	Angioedema, cough, hyperkalemia, hypotension, renal dysfunction	BP, electrolytes, BUN, and creatinine	Contraindicated in patients with bilateral renal artery stenosis, history of angioedema, or pregnancy. Assess BP, BUN, creatinine, and electrolytes at baseline and 1-2 weeks after initiation or increase in dose. Goal is target dose from clinical trials or highest tolerated.
ARBs	Hyperkalemia, hypotension, renal dysfunction	BP, electrolytes, BUN, and creatinine	Contraindicated in patients with bilateral renal artery stenosis or pregnancy. Assess BP, BUN, creatinine, and electrolytes at baseline and 1-2 weeks after initiation or increase in dose. Use with caution in patients with a history of ACE inhibitor-associated angioedema. Goal is target dose from clinical trials or highest tolerated.
Sacubitril/valsartan	Angioedema, hyperkalemia, hypotension, dizziness, renal dysfunction	BP, electrolytes, BUN, and creatinine	Contraindicated in patients with a history of angioedema associated with ACE inhibitor or ARB therapy or in pregnancy. Assess BP, BUN, creatinine, and electrolytes at baseline and 1-2 weeks after initiation or dose increase. Start with a low dose and double the dose every 2-4 weeks as tolerated based on BP, serum potassium, and renal function. Goal is target dose from clinical trials or highest tolerated.
Aldosterone antagonists	Gynecomastia/breast tenderness/menstrual irregularities (spironolactone), hyperkalemia, worsening renal function	BP, electrolytes, BUN, and creatinine	Assess BP, BUN, creatinine, and electrolytes at baseline. Check potassium 3 days and 1 week after initiation and then monthly for the first 3 months. Change to eplerenone if gynecomastia develops with spironolactone.
β-blockers	Bradycardia, heart block, bronchospasm, hypotension, worsening HF	BP, HR, ECG, signs and symptoms of worsening HF, blood glucose	Start with low dose and titrate upward no more often than every 2 weeks as tolerated based on BP, HR, and symptoms. Goal is target dose from clinical trials or highest tolerated. Patients may feel worse before they feel better.
Digoxin	GI and CNS adverse effects, brady- and tachyarrhythmias See table 11	electrolytes, BUN, creatinine, ECG, serum digoxin concentration	Target serum digoxin concentration 0.5-0.9 ng/mL.
Ivabradine	Bradycardia, hypertension, atrial fibrillation, luminous phenomena (phosphenes, transiently enhanced brightness in a portion of the visual field)	BP, HR, ECG	Start with 5 mg twice daily and after 2 weeks adjust dose to achieve a resting HR 50-60 BPM. Only use in patients in sinus rhythm.
Diuretics	Hypovolemia, hypotension, hyponatremia, hypokalemia, hypomagnesemia, hyperuricemia, renal dysfunction, thirst	BP, electrolytes, BUN, creatinine, glucose, uric acid, changes in weight, JVD	Dose should be adjusted based on volume status, renal function, electrolytes, and BP. Reassess these parameters 1-2 weeks after dose changes. Goal is lowest dose that maintains euvolemia.
Hydralazine	Hypotension, headache, rash, arthralgia, lupus, tachycardia	BP, HR	
Nitrates	Hypotension, headache, lightheadedness	BP, HR	

mortality.[58] In spite of the perceived risks, ACE inhibitors are effective in patients with chronic kidney disease and HFrEF.[59,60] Since many patients have concomitant disorders (eg, HTN, previous MI) that also may be favorably affected by ACE inhibitors, chronic kidney disease should not be an absolute contraindication to ACE inhibitor use in patients with reduced LVEF. However, these patients should be monitored carefully for the development of worsening renal function and/or hyperkalemia with special attention to risk factors associated with this complication of ACE inhibitor therapy.[1,60]

An important practical consideration is determining the proper dose of an ACE inhibitor. Despite the overwhelming benefit demonstrated with these agents, they remain underused and underdosed.[61] Also, for patients receiving an ACE inhibitor at hospital discharge, use significantly decreases over time and patients not prescribed ACE inhibitors at discharge were unlikely to have therapy initiated in the outpatient setting.[61] Common reasons cited for underuse or underdosing are concerns about safety and adverse reactions to ACE inhibitors, especially in patients with chronic kidney disease or low blood pressure. Clinical trials establishing the efficacy of these agents titrated drug doses to a predetermined target rather than according to therapeutic response. Although data on the dose-dependent effects of ACE inhibitors in patients with HF are limited, higher doses may reduce the risk of hospitalization, but not mortality, compared with lower doses.[62] In many positive trials of other HF therapies (eg, β-blockers, aldosterone antagonists), intermediate ACE inhibitor doses were generally used as background therapy. These results emphasize that clinicians should attempt to use ACE inhibitor doses proven beneficial in clinical trials, but if these doses are not tolerated, lower doses can be used with the knowledge that it is unlikely that there are differences in mortality between the high and low doses. Also, initiation of β-blocker therapy should not be delayed until target ACE inhibitor doses are achieved since the addition of a β-blocker is proven to reduce mortality, whereas that is not the case with increasing ACE inhibitor doses.

In summary, the evidence that ACE inhibitors improve symptoms, slow disease progression, and decrease mortality in patients with HFrEF is unequivocal. As a result, current guidelines recommend that all patients with HFrEF, regardless of whether or not symptoms are present, should receive ACE inhibitors, unless there are contraindications.[1] The clear benefit of ACE inhibitors is also evident by the selection of these agents as a key performance measure by the Joint Commission and Centers for Medicare and Medicaid Services (CMS). This measure states that patients with left ventricular systolic dysfunction discharged from the hospital should receive ACE inhibitors unless there is documentation in the medical record of an absolute contraindication or drug intolerance.

Angiotensin II Receptor Blockers 5 The crucial role of the RAAS in HF development and progression is well established as are the benefits of inhibiting this system with ACE inhibitors. ACE inhibitors decrease angiotensin II production in the short term, but these agents do not completely suppress generation of this hormone and angiotensin II can be formed in a number of tissues, including the heart, through non-ACE-dependent pathways (eg, chymase, cathepsin, and kallikrein).[7,13] By blocking the angiotensin II receptor subtype, AT1, ARBs attenuate the deleterious effects of angiotensin II on ventricular remodeling, regardless of the site of origin of the hormone. Since ARBs do not inhibit the ACE enzyme, these agents do not affect bradykinin, which is linked to ACE inhibitor cough and angioedema.

Although a number of ARBs are currently available, candesartan, losartan, or valsartan are recommended by the guidelines as the efficacy of these agents has been demonstrated in clinical trials.[1] In these studies, ARBs reduced mortality and hospitalizations and improved symptoms.[63]

A comparison of high-dose (150 mg) versus low-dose (50 mg) losartan treatment showed that higher doses slightly (~10%) reduced the primary end point of death or hospital admission for HF.[64] Significant increases in renal insufficiency, hyperkalemia, and hypotension were also associated with the higher dose. These findings point out the importance of titrating the doses of these medications to the targets achieved in clinical trials.

Combination therapy with an ACEI inhibitor and an ARB remains controversial. The addition of candesartan to ACE inhibitor and β-blocker therapy produced incremental reductions in cardiovascular death and hospitalizations for HF, but did not improve overall survival.[65] A meta-analysis showed that combination therapy is associated with increased risk of medication discontinuation due to adverse effects, hyperkalemia, renal insufficiency, and hypotension.[66] Collectively, these results suggest the addition of an ARB to optimal HF therapy (ACE inhibitors, β-blockers, diuretics, etc.) offers, at best, marginal benefits with increased risk of adverse effects. Current guidelines recommend the addition of an ARB can be considered in patients with HFrEF who remain symptomatic despite treatment with an ACE inhibitor and a β-blocker if an aldosterone antagonist cannot be used. Addition of an aldosterone antagonist is preferred over an ARB as this combination improves survival in patients with HFrEF.[17-19]

Although ACE inhibitors remain first-line therapy in patients with Stage C HFrEF, the current guidelines recommend the use of ARBs in patients who are unable to tolerate (usually due to cough) ACE inhibitors.[1] Caution should be exercised when ARBs are used in patients with angioedema from ACE inhibitors as some cross-reactivity is reported.[67] ARBs are not an alternative in patients with hypotension, hyperkalemia, or renal insufficiency secondary to ACE inhibitors because they are as likely to cause these adverse effects. Also, the combined use of ACE inhibitors, ARBs, and aldosterone antagonists is not recommended because of the increased risk of renal dysfunction and hyperkalemia.[1] The specific drugs and doses proven to be effective in clinical trials should be used (see Table 14-8).

11 The role of ARBs in the treatment of HFpEF is less clear. The CHARM-Preserved trial was the first large prospective study to demonstrate some benefit (reduction in hospitalizations for HF) of an ARB in patients with HFpEF receiving standard background treatment, although no improvement in cardiovascular death was observed.[68] Adverse effects of candesartan in this study were frequent; 22% of candesartan-treated patients discontinued therapy because of hypotension, increased serum creatinine, or hyperkalemia. In the Irbesartan in Heart Failure with Preserved EF (I-PRESERVE) trial, Irbesartan was compared with placebo in over 4,000 patients with symptoms of HF and a LVEF of at least 45%.[69] There was no significant difference between Irbesartan and placebo with regard to death or hospitalization for cardiovascular causes. No benefit was seen in quality-of-life measures. There was a high discontinuation rate of the study drug in this trial (33%), as well as a high rate of postrandomization initiation of ACE inhibitors (20%) and spironolactone (10%), which may have contributed to the outcome in this trial.

β-Blockers 6 There is overwhelming evidence from multiple randomized, placebo-controlled clinical trials that β-blockers reduce morbidity and mortality in patients with HFrEF. As such, the ACC/AHA guidelines on the management of HF recommend that β-blockers should be used in all stable patients with HF and a reduced left ventricular EF in the absence of contraindications or a clear history of β-blocker intolerance.[1] Patients should receive a β-blocker even if their symptoms are mild or well controlled with diuretic and ACE inhibitor therapy. Importantly, it is not essential that ACE inhibitor doses be optimized before a β-blocker is started because the addition of a β-blocker is likely to be of greater benefit than an increase in ACE inhibitor dose.[1] β-Blockers are also recommended for asymptomatic patients with a reduced left ventricular EF (Stage B) to decrease the risk of progression to HF.

β-Blockers have been studied in over 20,000 patients with HFrEF in placebo-controlled trials. Three β-blockers have been shown to significantly reduce mortality compared with placebo: carvedilol, metoprolol succinate (CR/XL), and bisoprolol. Each was studied in a large population with the primary end point of mortality. Carvedilol was the first β-blocker shown to improve survival in HF. In the United States Carvedilol Heart Failure Study, 1,094 patients were randomized to carvedilol or placebo in addition to standard therapy, including an ACE inhibitor, digoxin, and diuretic.[70] The study was stopped early because of a 65% reduction in the risk of death with carvedilol. Nearly 4,000 patients were randomized to metoprolol succinate (Toprol-XL®) or placebo in the Metoprolol CR/XL Randomised Intervention Trial in Congestive Heart Failure (MERIT-HF), the largest β-blocker mortality trial to date.[71] This trial was also stopped early because of a significant survival benefit with β-blockade. Specifically, metoprolol was associated with a 34% reduction in total mortality, a 41% reduction in sudden death, and a 49% reduction in death from worsening HF. Bisoprolol was studied in over 2,600 patients enrolled in the Cardiac Insufficiency Bisoprolol Study II (CIBIS II).[72] The study was also stopped prematurely because of a 34% reduction in total mortality with bisoprolol compared with placebo. Bisoprolol was also associated with a 44% reduction in sudden death and a 26% reduction in death due to worsening HF. Multiple posthoc subgroup analyses of data from the MERIT-HF and CIBIS II trials suggest that the benefits of β-blockade occur regardless of HF etiology or disease severity.

The majority of participants in MERIT-HF and CIBIS II had either NYHA class II or class III HFrEF. The efficacy and safety of β-blockers in patients with class IV HF were examined in the Carvedilol, Prospective, Randomized, Cumulative Survival (COPERNICUS) trial.[73] This trial randomized nearly 2,300 clinically stable patients who had symptoms at rest or with minimal exertion to carvedilol or placebo. Like the other studies, COPERNICUS was stopped prematurely after carvedilol produced a 35% relative reduction in mortality. Carvedilol was well tolerated in this population, with fewer participants receiving carvedilol compared with placebo requiring permanent discontinuation of study medication.

Data supporting the use of β-blockers in asymptomatic patients with left ventricular systolic dysfunction (Stage B) come from a study of carvedilol in post-MI patients with a decreased left ventricular EF.[74] While the primary end point of all-cause mortality or hospital admission for cardiovascular problems was similar in the carvedilol and placebo groups, carvedilol significantly reduced all-cause mortality alone compared with placebo. Cardiovascular mortality and nonfatal MI were also lower among carvedilol-treated patients.

In addition to improving survival, β-blockers have been shown to improve multiple other end points. All the large clinical trials demonstrated 15% to 20% reductions in all-cause hospitalization and 25% to 35% reductions in hospitalizations for worsening HF with β-blocker therapy.[72,75,76] Studies have also shown consistent improvements in left ventricular systolic function with β-blockers, with increases in LVEF of 5 to 10 units (eg, from an EF of 20%-25% or 30%) after several weeks to months of therapy. β-Blockers have also been shown to decrease ventricular mass, improve the sphericity of the ventricle, and reduce systolic and diastolic volumes (left ventricular end-systolic volume and LVEDV).[77] These effects are often collectively called *reverse remodeling*, referring to the fact that they return the heart toward more normal size, shape, and function.

The effects of β-blockers on symptoms and exercise tolerance varied among studies. Many studies showed improvements in NYHA functional class, patient symptom scores or quality-of-life assessments (such as the Minnesota Living with Heart Failure Questionnaire), and exercise performance, as assessed by the 6-minute walk test.[75,76] Other investigators found significant reductions in mortality with β-blockers but no significant improvement in symptoms.[78] As such, it is important to educate patients that β-blocker therapy is expected to positively influence disease progression and survival even if there is little to no symptomatic improvement.

Most participants in β-blocker trials were on ACE inhibitors at baseline since the benefits of ACE inhibitors were proven prior to β-blocker trials. Whether the strategy of starting a β-blocker prior to an ACE inhibitor is safe and effective was addressed in CIBIS III, in which patients with mild to moderate symptoms were randomized to initial therapy with either bisoprolol or enalapril.[79] Rates of death or hospitalization were similar with the two strategies. However, the trial failed to satisfy the prespecified statistical criterion for noninferiority of initial therapy with a β-blocker compared with an ACE inhibitor. In the absence of more compelling evidence, ACE inhibitors should be started first in most patients. Initiating a β-blocker first may be advantageous for patients with evidence of excessive SNS activity (eg, tachycardia) and may also be appropriate for patients whose renal function or potassium concentrations preclude starting an ACE inhibitor (or ARB) at that time. However, the risk for decompensation during β-blocker initiation may be greater in the absence of preexisting ACE inhibitor therapy, and careful monitoring is essential.

β-Blockers antagonize the detrimental effects of the SNS described earlier in the chapter. To this end, potential mechanisms to explain the favorable effects of β-blockers in HF include antiarrhythmic effects, attenuating or reversing ventricular remodeling, decreasing myocyte death from catecholamine-induced necrosis or apoptosis, preventing fetal gene expression, improving left ventricular systolic function, decreasing HR and ventricular wall stress thereby reducing myocardial oxygen demand, and inhibiting plasma renin release.[1]

Components that are critical for successful β-blocker therapy include appropriate patient selection, drug initiation and titration, and patient education. β-Blockers should be initiated in stable patients who have no or minimal evidence of fluid overload.[1] While β-blockers are typically started in the outpatient setting, there are data indicating that initiation of a β-blocker prior to discharge in patients who are hospitalized for decompensated HF increases β-blocker usage compared with outpatient initiation without increasing the risk of serious adverse effects.[76] However, β-blockers should not be started in patients who are hospitalized in the intensive care unit or recently required IV inotropic support. In unstable patients, other HF therapy should be optimized and then β-blocker therapy reevaluated once stability is achieved.

Initiation of a β-blocker at normal doses in patients with HF may lead to symptomatic worsening or acute decompensation owing to the drug's negative inotropic effect. For this reason, β-blockers are listed as drugs that may exacerbate or worsen HF (see Table 14-3). To minimize the likelihood for acute decompensation, β-blockers should be started in very low doses with slow upward dose titration and close monitoring. β-Blocker doses should be doubled no more often than every 2 weeks, as tolerated, until the target or maximally tolerated dose is reached. According to current guidelines, target doses are those associated with reductions in mortality in placebo-controlled clinical trials.[1] The starting and target doses achieved in clinical trials are described in Table 14-8. Data with both metoprolol and carvedilol suggest that HR may serve as a guide to the degree of β-blockade and that lower β-blocker doses might be considered reasonable if the reduction in HR indicates a good response to β-blocker therapy.[81] In fact, it remains uncertain whether β-blocker dose or the degree of HR reduction is the optimal end point to guide dose titration and predict survival.

A meta-analysis of 23 randomized trials involving over 19,000 patients receiving β-blockers for HF compared HR reduction and β-blocker dose as predictors of survival.[81] Overall, β-blocker treatment was associated with a 24% mortality reduction. However, trials with the largest decrease in HR (median 15 beats per minute) reported a 36% reduction in mortality, whereas trials with the smallest HR reduction (median 8 beats/min) showed only a 9% mortality reduction. Greater magnitude of HR reduction was significantly associated with greater improvement in survival. On the other hand, in contrast to findings from other investigators,[82] no relationship between β-blocker dose and magnitude of mortality decrease was found. The results from this study suggest that the degree of β-blocker-mediated reduction in resting HR, but not β-blocker dose, is associated with the magnitude of improved survival. However, the analysis is limited by its retrospective design, inability to account for other factors affecting HR (eg, vagal activity, β-receptor pharmacogenomics), and reliance on resting HR as a surrogate marker for extent of β-blockade. Although resting HR is routinely used clinically to evaluate extent of β-blockade, it is not as accurate as inhibition of exercise HR. Whether magnitude of resting HR reduction or achievement of clinical trial doses is the optimal surrogate marker for improved outcomes with β-blockers in HF remains uncertain and may only be definitively determined by prospective trials.

Of note, the smallest commercially available tablet of bisoprolol is a scored 5-mg tablet. Since the recommended starting dose of 1.25 mg/day is not readily available, bisoprolol is the least commonly used of the three agents and, in fact, is not approved by the FDA for use in HF. Thus, therapy is generally limited to either carvedilol or metoprolol succinate, and there is no compelling evidence that one drug is superior to the other. A controlled-release formulation of carvedilol (carvedilol CR) that allows once-daily dosing is available, and pharmacokinetic studies demonstrate similar degrees of drug exposure with the controlled- and immediate-release formations of the drug.[79]

Good communication between the patient and healthcare provider(s) is particularly important for successful therapy. Patients should understand that dose uptitration is a long, gradual process and that achieving the target dose is important to maximize the benefits of therapy. Patients should also be aware that response to therapy may be delayed and that HF symptoms may actually worsen during the initiation period. In the event of worsening symptoms, patients who understand the potential benefits of long-term β-blocker therapy may be more likely to continue treatment.

In summary, the data provide clear evidence that β-blockers slow disease progression, decrease hospitalizations, and improve survival in HFrEF. β-Blockers have also been shown to improve quality of life in many patients with HF, although this is not a universal finding. Based on these data, β-blockers are recommended as standard therapy for all patients with HFrEF, regardless of the severity of their symptoms. Clinical trial experience shows that target β-blocker doses can be achieved in the majority of patients provided that appropriate initiation, titration, and education are implemented.

11 In patients with HFpEF, β-blockers may help to lower and maintain low pulmonary venous pressures by decreasing HR and increasing the duration of diastole. Tachycardia is poorly tolerated in patients with HFpEF for several reasons. First, rapid HRs cause an increase in myocardial oxygen demand and a decrease in coronary perfusion time. This can promote ischemia even in the absence of epicardial CAD. Second, incomplete relaxation between cardiac cycles may result an increase in diastolic pressure relative to volume. Third, a rapid rate reduces diastolic filling time and ventricular filling. Thus, many clinicians use β-blockers (and nondihydropyridine calcium channel blockers) to prevent excessive tachycardia and produce a relative bradycardia in patients with diastolic dysfunction. However, excessive bradycardia can result in a fall of CO despite an increase in LV filling.[2] Such considerations underscore the need for individualizing therapeutic interventions that affect HR. In general, it is not necessary to start at an extremely low dose and titrate the β-blocker in a slow, progressive fashion in HFpEF as it is in HFrEF. However, because older patients have numerous comorbidities, and take many concomitant medications, it is prudent to start with a moderate dose of β-blockers. A meta-analysis examining the effects of β-blocker therapy on clinical outcomes in patients with HFpEF found lower all-cause mortality (relative risk 0.81, $p<0.001$) but no significant reduction for HF hospitalizations in observational studies.[84] These findings were not replicated in two small randomized trials; however those studies were underpowered and many patients were lost to followup.

Aldosterone Antagonists 8 Spironolactone and eplerenone are aldosterone antagonists that work by blocking the mineralocorticoid receptor, the target site for aldosterone, and, thus, they are also referred to as mineralocorticoid receptor antagonists. In the kidney, aldosterone antagonists inhibit sodium reabsorption and potassium excretion. While the diuretic effects with low doses of aldosterone antagonists are minimal, the potassium-sparing effects can have significant consequences as discussed later. In the heart, aldosterone antagonists inhibit cardiac extracellular matrix and collagen deposition, thereby attenuating cardiac fibrosis and ventricular remodeling.[81] Aldosterone antagonists also attenuate the systemic proinflammatory state, atherogenesis, and oxidative stress caused by aldosterone. In addition, there is evidence that aldosterone antagonists may attenuate aldosterone-induced calcium excretion and reductions in bone mineral density and protect against fractures in HF.[82] While spironolactone historically has been viewed as a diuretic, this is believed to contribute little to its benefits in HF, in part, because the doses used have minimal diuretic effect.[17] Thus, as with ACE inhibitors and β-blockers, the data on aldosterone antagonists also support the neurohormonal model of HF.

Three large, randomized controlled trials have evaluated low-dose aldosterone antagonism in patients with either HF or post-MI and left ventricular dysfunction. All three trials excluded patients with significant renal dysfunction (eg, serum creatinine above 2.5 mg/dL [221 μmol/L]) and elevated serum potassium (eg, above 5 mEq/L [5 mmol/L]) at baseline.

The RALES trial randomized over 1,600 patients with current or recent NYHA class IV HFrEF to aldosterone blockade with spironolactone 25 mg/day or placebo.[17] Patients were also treated with standard therapy, usually including an ACE inhibitor, loop diuretic, and digoxin. Those with a serum creatinine concentration above 2.5 mg/dL (221 μmol/L) or a serum potassium concentration above 5 mEq/L (5 mmol/L) was excluded. The study was stopped prematurely after an average followup of 24 months because of a significant 30% reduction in the primary end point of total mortality with spironolactone. Spironolactone reduced mortality due to both progressive HF and sudden cardiac death. It also produced a 35% reduction in hospitalizations for worsening HF and significant symptomatic improvement, as assessed by changes in NYHA functional class. The low dose of spironolactone was well tolerated in RALES. The most common adverse effect was gynecomastia, which occurred in 10% of men on spironolactone compared with 1% of men on placebo, and led to treatment discontinuation in 2% of patients. There were statistically (but not clinically) significant increases in serum creatinine (by 0.05-0.10 mg/dL) and potassium concentrations (by 0.30 mEq/L) with spironolactone. The incidence of serious hyperkalemia (greater than 6 mEq/L) was minimal and did not differ between spironolactone- and placebo-treated groups.

The EPHESUS trial evaluated the effect of selective antagonism of the mineralocorticoid receptor with eplerenone in patients with left ventricular dysfunction after MI.[18] To be eligible for study participation, patients had to have evidence of either HF or diabetes. Over 6,600 patients were randomized within 3 to 14 days of MI to eplerenone, titrated to 50 mg/day, or placebo in addition to standard therapy, which usually included an ACE inhibitor, β-blocker, aspirin, and diuretics. Treatment with eplerenone was associated with a significant 15% relative reduction in the risk for death from any cause and a 15% reduction in the risk of hospitalization from HF. Serious hyperkalemia occurred in 5.5% of eplerenone-treated patients and 3.9% of placebo-treated patients.

Most recently, the EMPHASIS-HF trial demonstrated significant improvements in clinical outcomes with aldosterone antagonism in mild HFrEF.[19] Over 2,700 patients with NYHA class II HF and a LVEF of 35% or less were randomized to eplerenone up to 50 mg/day (mean dose of 39 mg/day) or placebo, in addition to receiving treatment with an ACE inhibitor or ARB and β-blocker. Eligible patients were hospitalized for a cardiovascular reason within 6 months of study entry or had a plasma BNP of at least 250 pg/mL (72 pmol/L) or an N-terminal proBNP of at least 500 pg/mL (59 pmol/L) in men and 750 pg/mL (89 pmol/L) in women. The trial was stopped prematurely after a median followup of 21 months because of a significant benefit with eplerenone. Eplerenone treatment reduced the primary end point of cardiovascular death or HF hospitalization by 37%, all-cause and cardiovascular mortality by 24%, and hospitalization for HF by 42%. A posthoc analysis of the data also showed a reduction in the incidence of new-onset atrial fibrillation or flutter with eplerenone. The rate of serum potassium greater than 5.5 mEq/L (5.5 mmol/L) was 11.8% in the eplerenone group and 7.2% with placebo.

The TOPCAT trial examined the effect of spironolactone in patients with HFpEF.[21] TOPCAT randomized 3,445 patients with symptomatic heart failure and an ejection fraction of 45% or greater to spironolactone up to 45 mg/day (mean dose of 25 mg/day) or placebo. As an additional criterion for inclusion, patients had to either have a hospitalization within 1 year in which heart failure management was a major component or a BNP of at least 100 pg/mL (or N-terminal proBNP of at least 360 pg/mL) within 60 days of study entry. The primary outcome was the composite of death from cardiovascular causes, aborted cardiac arrest, or hospitalization for heart failure. After a mean follow-up of 3.3 years, there was no difference in the primary outcome or in the secondary outcomes of all-cause mortality, hospitalization for any reason, myocardial infarction, or stroke between groups. However, there was a significant 17% reduction in the risk for hospitalization for heart failure with spironolactone compared to placebo. There was a higher rate of hyperkalemia (serum potassium greater than or equal to 5.5 mEq/L) in the spironolactone group, but the incidence of serious side effects was similar between groups. Prespecified subgroup analysis showed a benefit with spironolactone among those enrolled on the basis of an elevated natriuretic peptide level, but not in those enrolled on the basis of the hospitalization criterion. There also appeared to be a difference in outcomes by region of enrollment. Approximately 51% of patients were enrolled from the Americans (United States, Canada, Argentina, and Brazil), and the remainder were enrolled from Eastern Europe (Russia and the Republic of Georgia). Posthoc analysis showed a greater reduction in the primary outcome with spironolactone among patients from the Americans, but not in those from Eastern Europe.[20] While the prespecified test for interaction between region and study arm was not significant, differences in baseline characteristics by region and the lower event rate overall in patients from Eastern Europe, confound the interpretation of the study results.

Current guidelines recommend adding a low-dose aldosterone antagonist to standard therapy to improve symptoms, reduce the risk of HF hospitalization, and increase survival in select patients provided that potassium and renal function can be carefully monitored.[1] Based on the clinical trial data low-dose aldosterone antagonists are appropriate for two groups of patients: those with mild to moderately severe HFrEF (NYHA class II-IV) who are receiving standard therapy and those with left ventricular dysfunction and either acute HF or diabetes early after MI.[1,85] Among patients with mild HFrEF (NYHA class II), aldosterone antagonists should be considered in those with a prior hospitalization for cardiovascular reasons or an elevated plasma BNP or N-terminal proBNP level. An aldosterone antagonist may be preferred over an ARB in patients with persisting symptoms despite ACE inhibitor and β-blocker therapy provided that serum potassium and renal function are acceptable.[1,85] Current guidelines were published prior to the completion of TOPCAT, and there are no clear guidelines on aldosterone antagonist use for patients with HFpEF or others who fall outside the populations studied in these clinical trials. On the basis of findings from TOPCAT, it may be reasonable to add an aldosterone antagonist to decrease risk for hospitalization for heart failure in patients with HFpEF, especially if plasma natriuretic peptide levels are elevated.

Despite the clear benefits of aldosterone antagonists in patients with mild to severe HFrEF, registry data show that only one third of patients meeting guideline criteria for an aldosterone antagonist actually receive one.[87] The low use of aldosterone antagonists is likely due in large part to safety concerns. The clinical trial data suggest that aldosterone antagonists in HF are associated with minimal risk when used appropriately (eg, in those with adequate renal function and with close laboratory monitoring). However, shortly after publication of RALES, an observational study of approximately 1.3 million elderly patients in the Ontario Drug Benefit Program found that the increase in the spironolactone prescription rate following the publication of RALES was accompanied by nearly threefold increases in the rate of hospital admissions and the rate of death related to hyperkalemia.[88] In addition, small case series showed that 25% to 35% of patients treated outside the controlled clinical trial setting developed hyperkalemia (greater than 5 mEq/L [greater than 5 mmol/L]) and that 10% to 12% developed serious hyperkalemia.[89]

Potential factors contributing to the high incidence of hyperkalemia in clinical practice include the initiation of aldosterone antagonists in patients with impaired renal function or high potassium concentrations and the failure to decrease or stop potassium supplements when starting aldosterone antagonists. Other risk factors for hyperkalemia include diabetes, inadequate laboratory monitoring, high potassium intake, and concomitant use of both ACE inhibitors and ARBs or NSAIDs. The ACC/AHA recommended strategies to minimize the risk for hyperkalemia with aldosterone antagonists in HF.[1] These strategies are summarized in Table 14-10. Chief among these recommendations is to avoid aldosterone antagonists in patients with renal dysfunction or elevated serum potassium. It is important to emphasize here that serum creatinine may overestimate renal function in the elderly and in patients with decreased muscle mass, in whom creatinine clearance should serve as a guide for the appropriateness of aldosterone antagonist therapy. The risk for hyperkalemia is dose dependent, and the morbidity and mortality reductions with aldosterone antagonists in clinical trials occurred at low doses (ie, spironolactone 25 mg/day and eplerenone 50 mg/day). Therefore, the doses of aldosterone antagonists should be limited to those associated with beneficial effects in order to decrease the risk for hyperkalemia. Initiation of every-other-day dosing is appropriate for patients with marginal renal function or who are otherwise at high risk for hyperkalemia. Spironolactone also interacts with androgen and progesterone receptors, which may lead to gynecomastia, impotence, and menstrual irregularities in some patients. Such adverse effects are less frequent with eplerenone owing to its low affinity for the progesterone and androgen receptors.

Only 10% of RALES participants were taking β-blockers at baseline since the benefits of β-blockers in HF were not appreciated fully at the time the trial began.[17] β-Blockers inhibit plasma renin

TABLE 14-10 Recommended Strategies for Reducing the Risk for Hyperkalemia with Aldosterone Antagonists

- Avoid starting aldosterone antagonists in patients with any of the following:
  - Serum creatinine concentration >2.0 in women or >2.5 mg/dL in men or a creatinine clearance <30 mL/min/1.73 m^2
  - Recent worsening of renal function
  - Serum potassium concentration >5.0 mEq/L
  - History of severe hyperkalemia
- Start with low doses (12.5 mg/day for spironolactone and 25 mg/day for eplerenone) especially in the elderly and in those with diabetes or a creatinine clearance <50 mL/min/1.73 m^2.
- Decrease or discontinue potassium supplements when starting an aldosterone antagonist.
- Avoid concomitant use of NSAIDs or COX-2 inhibitors.
- Avoid concomitant use of high-dose ACE inhibitors or ARBs.
- Avoid triple therapy with an ACE inhibitor, ARB, and aldosterone antagonist.
- Monitor serum potassium concentrations and renal function within 3 days and 1 week after the initiation or dose titration of an aldosterone antagonist or any other medication that could affect potassium homeostasis. Thereafter, potassium concentrations and renal function should be monitored monthly for the first 3 months, and then every 3 months.
- If potassium exceeds 5.5 mg/dL at any point during therapy, discontinue any potassium supplementation or, in the absence of potassium supplements, reduce or stop aldosterone antagonist therapy.
- Counsel patients to:
  - Limit intake of high potassium-containing foods and salt substitutes.
  - Avoid the use of over-the-counter NSAIDs.
  - Temporarily discontinue aldosterone antagonist therapy if diarrhea develops or diuretic therapy is interrupted.

Adapted from Yancy CW, Jessup M, Bozkurt B, et al. 2013 ACCF/AHA guideline for the management of heart failure: A report of the American College of Cardiology Foundation/American Heart Association Task Force on Practice Guidelines. J Am Coll Cardiol 2013;62:e147-239.

release and may provide additional suppression of the RAAS when used with ACE inhibitors. Thus, there has been some speculation about whether spironolactone will provide further benefit in patients receiving both ACE inhibitors and β-blockers. However, data from EPHESUS and EMPHASIS provide some clarity to this issue, since the majority of EPHESUS participants were on β-blockers at baseline, and the trial still demonstrated significant reductions in mortality with the addition of eplerenone.[18,19]

Drug Therapies to Consider for Selected Patients with HFrEF

Nitrates and Hydralazine 9 Nitrates and hydralazine were originally combined in the treatment of HFrEF because of their complementary hemodynamic actions. Nitrates, by serving as nitric oxide donors, activate guanylate cyclase to increase cyclic guanosine monophosphate (cGMP) in vascular smooth muscle resulting in venodilation and decreased preload. Hydralazine is a direct-acting arterial vasodilator causing a decrease in SVR and resultant increases in SV and CO (see Fig. 14-1). However, the beneficial effects of hydralazine and nitrates extend beyond their hemodynamic actions and are likely related to attenuating the biochemical processes driving HF progression.[90]

The efficacy of the combination of hydralazine and ISDN has been evaluated in three large, randomized clinical trials. The first trial predated the use of ACE inhibitors and β-blockers and found that the combination of hydralazine and isosorbide dinitrate reduced mortality compared with placebo in patients receiving diuretics and digoxin.[91] A subsequent study demonstrated that an ACE inhibitor improved survival compared to this combination.[92] Posthoc analysis of these trials suggested that the combination of hydralazine and ISDN was more effective in African Americans, and led to examining the efficacy of adding the combination to standard therapy in the African-American Heart Failure Trial (A-HeFT).[90] This study enrolled self-identified African Americans with NYHA class III or IV HFrEF receiving standard therapy and compared outcomes in patients randomized to the fixed-dose combination of hydralazine/Isosorbide dinitrate (BiDil®) or placebo.[93] The trial was terminated early because of a significant 43% reduction in all-cause mortality in patients receiving hydralazine/isosorbide compared with placebo. Based on these results, BiDil® was approved by the FDA to treat HFrEF in African Americans.

The mechanism for the beneficial effects of hydralazine/ISDN remains uncertain but is most likely related to normalization of the increased oxidative stress and reduced nitric oxide signaling that contributes to HF progression. By serving as a nitric oxide donor, nitrates increase nitric oxide bioavailability and hydralazine reduces oxidative stress.[90,91] Nitric oxide attenuates myocardial remodeling and may play a protective role in HF. African Americans may have less nitric oxide availability compared with non-African Americans, and, thus, may derive particular benefit from therapy that enhances nitric oxide bioavailability. Whether the benefits of adding hydralazine/ISDN to standard therapy extend to non-African Americans remains to be prospectively evaluated.

Guidelines recommend the addition of hydralazine/ISDN to self-described African Americans with HFrEF and NYHA class III–IV symptoms treated with ACE inhibitors and β-blockers.[1] Hydralazine/ISDN can also be useful in patients unable to tolerate either an ACE inhibitor or ARB because of renal insufficiency, hyperkalemia, or possibly hypotension.[1]

Several potential obstacles limit the use of hydralazine/ISDN.[90] The first is the need for frequent dosing, with the fixed-dose combination administered three times daily. Second, adverse effects are common with hydralazine/ISDN, with nearly 30% of patients reporting dizziness, as well as headache and GI distress, all occurring more frequently than with placebo.[91,93] A third potential obstacle is the high cost of the BiDil® fixed-dose combination product compared with that of the individual generic drugs purchased separately. Because of the high cost, many clinicians use generic hydralazine and ISDN as separate agents, rather than the combination product. Although the generic and brand name products are not bioequivalent as determined in healthy volunteer studies, it is unknown if these pharmacokinetic differences impact clinical outcomes.[90]

HFpEF In contrast to the beneficial effects of hydralazine/ISDN in patients with HFrEF, the effects in patients with HFpEF are less clear. Nitrates are frequently used in patients with HFpEF to improve exercise tolerance although their actual benefits are poorly understood. A recent study determined the effect of increasing doses of isosorbide mononitrate (30-120 mg daily) on exercise tolerance in 110 patients with HFpEF.[94] These investigators found that compared to placebo, a dose-dependent reduction in activity levels was found in patients receiving isosorbide mononitrate.[94] In addition, isosorbibe mononitrate did not improve quality of life or plasma NT-proBNP concentrations. Adverse events, including worsening HF and presyncope/syncope, were more frequent in the isosorbide mononitrate treatment arm. These findings suggest that in the absence of another indication for nitrate therapy (eg, angina), nitrates provide limited benefits to patients with HFpEF.

Angiotensin II Receptor Blocker/Neprilysin Inhibitor (ARNI) The first angiotensin receptor/neprilysin inhibitor approved for the treatment of patients with HFrEF is valsartan/sacubitril. It is a crystalline complex composed of the ARB valsartan and sacubitril, a neprilysin inhibitor prodrug. After ingestion, sacubitril dissociates from the complex and is cleaved into its active form LBQ657, which inhibits the action of neprilysin that degrades natriuretic peptides (NPs) and bradykinin.[95]

Natriuretic pepetides are beneficial because they cause vasodilation, increase glomerular filtration, natriuresis, and diuresis.

Neprilysin is a neutral endopeptidase, which is one of the enzymes that breaks down the body's endogenous NPs. By inhibiting neprilysin, LBQ657 promotes vasodilation through a different mechanism than the ARB.[95]

BNP and NT-proBNP plasma concentrations are elevated in the setting of worsening heart failure and have been used to evaluate and monitor the volume status of patients with HF. If patients are receiving sacubitril/valsartan, BNP concentrations will be "falsely elevated" and cannot be used in monitoring patients. However, NT-proBNP is not a substrate for neprilysin, therefore it may be used in monitoring.

The PARADIGM-HF study tested the hypothesis that treatment with an ARNI (sacubitril/valsartan) would be superior to ACE inhibition.[23] In this study, 8,442 patients with NYHA Class II–IV heart failure and an ejection fraction less than 40% were randomized to a target dose of sacubitril/valsartan 200 mg (97 mg/103 mg) twice daily or enalapril 10 mg twice daily. The primary outcome of the trial was a composite of death from cardiovascular causes or first hospitalization for heart failure. There was a statistically significant 20% relative risk reduction in the primary outcome for patients receiving sacubitril/valsartan (21.8%) compared to enalapril (26.5%). A similar reduction was seen in each component of the primary endpoint. Death from any cause was also significantly reduced in the sacubitril/valsartan treated patients. The trial was ended after a median of 27 months of follow-up. Twenty-one patients would need to treated for the duration of the study in order to prevent one primary event.[23]

The majority of patients in PARADIGM-HF were white (66%) males (78%) with NYHA class II symptoms (70%). At the time of randomization 80% of patients were taking diuretics, 93% β-blockers, 55% aldosterone antagonists, and 30% digitalis. A small number of patients in each group had an ICD (15%) or cardiac resynchronization therapy (7%). Hypotension occurred more frequently in patients randomized to sacubitril/valsartan compared to enalapril. However, more patients receiving enalapril experienced cough and hyperkalemia greater than 6.0 mEq/L. Angioedema was rare in either treatment group.

HFpEF Sacubitril/valsartan was studied in the phase II PARAMOUNT trial, where NT-proBNP levels were significantly reduced after 12 weeks of therapy when compared to valsartan alone.[96] This trial formed the basis of the larger phase III study PARAGON, which is intended to enroll over 4,000 patients with a preserved EF.

Ivabradine Ivabradine has been recently approved to reduce hospitalizations in patients with HFrEF. This agent has a unique pharmacology as it blocks the I_f current in the sinoatrial node that is responsible for controlling the heart rate.[97,98] By blocking this current, ivabradine slows the spontaneous depolarization of the sinus node resulting in a dose-dependent slowing of the heart rate. Ivabradine's effects are specific to the I_f current and this agent does not affect BP, myocardial contractility, or AV conduction.[97,98]

Elevated resting heart rate (greater than 70-80 BPM) is emerging as an important independent risk factor for adverse outcomes in patients with HF and is associated with increased hospital admissions, disease progression, and mortality.[99,100] Increased sympathetic nervous system activity is the likely cause of the heart rate increase but how this affects prognosis remains uncertain. Potential deleterious effects of elevated heart rate include increased myocardial oxygen demand, decreased oxygen supply, and tachycardia-induced cardiomyopathy.[97,100] The beneficial effects of β-blockers are more closely related to the degree of heart rate reduction than the dose of the β-blocker, further supporting the link between elevated heart rate and outcomes.[97,100] New approaches to address increased heart rate in these patients are needed because, for a variety of reasons, β-blockers are frequently underdosed in clinical practice.[97]

To determine the impact of heart rate lowering on clinical outcomes, the SHIFT trial examined the effect of ivabradine treatment in over 6,500 patients with an EF less than or equal to 35% and NYHA class II–III symptoms in sinus rhythm with a baseline heart rate greater than or equal to 70 BPM that were receiving standard background HF treatment (over 90% of the patients were taking β-blockers).[101] Patients were randomized to receive ivabradine 5 mg twice daily or placebo and the ivabradine dose could be increased to 7.5 twice daily if the patient's if the resting heart rate was greater than 60 BPM after 2 weeks of treatment with the lower dose. The primary composite endpoint of cardiovascular death or hospital admission for worsening HF was significantly reduced by 18% in the ivabradine treatment group compared to placebo (p<0.0001). The primary endpoint was largely driven by reduced hospitalizations for worsening HF and ivabradine did not affect overall or cardiovascular mortality. Ivabradine reduced resting heart rate by approximately 11 BPM compared to placebo. The most common adverse effects associated with ivabradine were bradycardia, atrial fibrillation, and visual disturbances.

Digoxin 10 In 1785, William Withering was the first to report extensively on the use of foxglove or *Digitalis purpurea* for the treatment of dropsy (ie, edema). Although digitalis glycosides have been in clinical use for more than 200 years, not until the 1920s were they clearly demonstrated to have a positive inotropic effect on the heart. Furthermore, it was not until the late 1980s that clinical trials were conducted to critically evaluate the role of digoxin in the therapy of chronic HF. The view of digoxin has also shifted over the past decade. While it was historically considered useful in HF because of its positive inotropic effects, it now seems clear that its real benefits in HF are related to its neurohormonal modulating activity.[102,103]

Clinical trials have shown that digoxin improves cardiac function, quality of life, exercise tolerance, and HF symptoms in patients with HFrEF.[104-106] However, these studies involved small numbers of patients followed for short time periods. Although these trials demonstrated hemodynamic and symptomatic improvement in HF patients receiving digoxin, an unresolved issue was the unknown effect of digoxin on mortality. This was of particular concern given the increased mortality seen with other positive inotropic drugs, and finally led to the Digitalis Investigation Group (DIG) trial to determine the effects of digoxin on survival in patients with HF in sinus rhythm.

The DIG trial was a double-blind, randomized, placebo-controlled trial with the primary end point of all-cause mortality.[107] Patients (n=6,800) with HF symptoms, a LVEF of 45% or less, and normal sinus rhythm were eligible for the main DIG trial and were randomized to receive digoxin or placebo for a mean followup period of 37 months. Most patients received background therapy with diuretics and ACE inhibitors. Digoxin serum concentrations of 0.5 to 2 ng/mL (0.6-2.6 nmol/L) were targeted, with a mean serum digoxin concentration (SDC) of 0.8 ng/mL (1 nmol/L) achieved at 12 months. No significant differences in all-cause mortality were found between patients receiving digoxin and placebo. A trend toward lower mortality due to worsening HF was observed in the digoxin group, although this was offset by a trend toward an increased mortality from other cardiovascular causes (presumably arrhythmias) in patients receiving digoxin. Importantly, digoxin reduced hospitalizations for worsening HF by 28% compared with placebo (P<0.001). Therefore, DIG is the first trial to show that a positive inotropic agent does not increase mortality and actually decreases morbidity in patients with HFrEF. On the other hand, among an additional 988 patients with a LVEF greater than 45% (HFpEF) who were enrolled in an ancillary DIG trial, there was no apparent benefit of digoxin on hospitalizations or mortality during the 37-month followup period.[108]

The PROVED and RADIANCE trials investigated the effect of digoxin withdrawal in patients with chronic HF and normal sinus rhythm and further defined the role of digoxin in this setting.[105,106] Both of these trials were short-term (12-week), prospective, randomized, and placebo-controlled and were conducted prior to the use of β-blockers. Together, data from these trials suggested that digoxin produces important symptomatic benefits and that digoxin withdrawal results in worsening HF, decreased exercise capacity, and a reduction in ejection fraction. A posthoc analysis of the DIG trial data supports findings that discontinuation of digoxin may be detrimental. Specifically, among patients treated with digoxin prior to enrollment in the DIG trial, those assigned to the placebo arm (ie, those discontinuing digoxin therapy) had an increased risk of all-cause hospitalization and HF-related hospitalization compared with patients assigned to the digoxin arm (ie, those continuing digoxin therapy).[106]

Retrospective analyses of the combined PROVED/RADIANCE database[110] and the DIG trial database[111] suggest that the clinical benefits of digoxin are achieved at lower SDCs, with no additional benefit with higher concentrations. In particular, analysis of digoxin-treated patients in the PROVED and RADIANCE trials showed similar clinical outcomes among those with a SDC between 0.5 and 0.9 ng/mL (between 0.6 and 1.2 nmol/L) as those with higher serum concentrations.[110] While the DIG trial showed no reduction in mortality in the study population overall, a comprehensive analysis of the DIG trial database found that lower SDCs were associated with decreased mortality, whereas higher concentrations were not.[111] Specifically, compared with placebo, SDCs of 0.5 to 0.9 ng/mL (0.6-1.2 nmol/L) 1 month after digoxin initiation were associated with lower mortality, all-cause hospitalizations, and HF hospitalizations. Serum concentrations greater than or equal to 1 ng/mL (1.3 nmol/L) were associated with lower HF hospitalizations with no effect on mortality. A digoxin dose of 0.125 mg daily or less was predictive of SDCs of 0.4 to 0.9 ng/mL (0.5-1.2 nmol/L). While an initial, well-publicized study suggested that digoxin might be harmful in women,[109] subsequent analyses show no increased risks with digoxin in women, particularly with SDCs less than 1 ng/mL (1.3 nmol/L).[111,113]

Based on the available data, for most patients, the target SDC should be 0.5 to 0.9 ng/mL (0.6-1.2 nmol/L). This more conservative target would also be expected to decrease the risk of adverse effects from digoxin toxicity and evidence indicates this is indeed the case[114] whereas other data show no change in ED admissions for digoxin toxicity.[115] In most patients with normal renal function, this serum concentration range can be achieved with a daily dose of 0.125 mg. Patients with decreased renal function or low body weight, the elderly, or those receiving interacting drugs (eg, amiodarone) should receive 0.125 mg daily or every other day. Routine measuring of SDCs is not necessary in the absence of suspected digoxin toxicity, worsening renal function, institution of an interacting drug, or other conditions that may significantly affect SDC. In patients with atrial fibrillation and a rapid ventricular response, the historic practice of increasing digoxin doses (and concentrations) until rate control is achieved is no longer recommended. Digoxin alone is often ineffective to control ventricular response in patients with atrial fibrillation and increasing the dose only increases the risk of toxicity. Digoxin combined with a β-blocker or amiodarone is superior to either agent alone for controlling ventricular response in patients with atrial fibrillation and HF.[1] Therefore, target SDCs are the same regardless of whether the patient is in sinus rhythm or atrial fibrillation. Several equations and nomograms have been proposed to estimate digoxin maintenance doses based on estimated renal function for a particular patient and population pharmacokinetic parameters. These methods are extensively reviewed elsewhere.[116] More recently, based on posthoc analyses from the DIG, PROVED, and RADIANCE trials, investigators developed a digoxin dosing nomogram that targets a lower digoxin plasma concentration.[117] In the absence of supraventricular tachyarrhythmias, a loading dose is not indicated because digoxin is a mild inotropic agent that will produce gradual effects over several hours, even after loading.

The DIG trial was conducted prior to the proven benefits and widespread use of β-blockers in HF, and, thus, recent observational studies have reexamined digoxin in the context of contemporary HF therapy and shown either neutral or detrimental effects of the drug on mortality.[118,119] Based on the totality of data, digoxin is not considered a first line agent in HF but a trial may be considered in conjunction with GDMT including ACE inhibitors, β-blockers, and diuretics in patients with symptomatic HFrEF to improve symptoms and reduce hospitalizations.[1] Digoxin may also be considered to help control ventricular response rate in patients with HFrEF and supraventricular arrhythmias, although β-blockers are generally more effective rate control agents, especially during exercise. In the absence of digoxin toxicity or serious adverse effects, digoxin should be continued in most patients. Digoxin withdrawal may be considered for asymptomatic patients who have significant improvement in systolic function with optimal ACE inhibitor and β-blocker treatment.[120]

There is no established role for digoxin in HFpEF when patients are in normal sinus rhythm. Digoxin may be of benefit in patients with concomitant HFpEF and atrial fibrillation.[121]

Calcium Channel Blockers 11 Calcium channel blockers can provide symptom-targeted treatment in patients with HFpEF by decreasing HR and increasing exercise tolerance. They can also provide disease-targeted therapy by treating HTN and coronary artery disease. However, the beneficial effect of these agents on exercise tolerance is not always paralleled by improved LV diastolic function or increased relaxation rate. Nonetheless, a number of small clinical trials have shown that the use of these agents results in both short- and long-term improvement in exercise capacity in patients with HFpEF.[41]

Of the calcium channel blockers, the nondihydropyridines (verapamil and diltiazem) are the most effective because they lower heart rate in addition to lowering BP. Nondihydropyridines are also frequently used to treat the co-morbidities of hypertension and atrial fibrillation in patients with HFpEF. Sustained-release nifedipine, because of its strong vasodilator properties, tends to cause hypotension, reflex tachycardia, and peripheral edema. These characteristics make it less useful in HFpEF. Amlodipine may be effective because it reduces BP. Initial daily doses are verapamil 120 to 240 mg, diltiazem 90 to 120 mg, and amlodipine 2.5 mg.

Heart block is a contraindication for the nondihydropyridines. The most common adverse effects are bradycardia and heart block (for the nondihydropyridines). Peripheral edema and headache also are common. Nondihydropyridines exacerbate the bradycardic effects of β-blockers, and verapamil raises digoxin serum concentrations by 70%. Diltiazem increases cyclosporine, tacrolimus, and sirolimus serum concentrations. Generic formulations, but not necessarily generic equivalents to the original brand names, are available for some of the calcium channel blockers.

Treatment of Concomitant Disorders

HF is often accompanied by other disorders whose natural history or therapy may affect morbidity, mortality, and treatment approach. Optimal management of these concomitant disorders in the context of the patient's HF is an important consideration in the overall careof the patient.

Hypertension Although ischemic heart disease has replaced HTN as the most common cause of HF, still nearly two thirds of patients with HF have current or a previous history of HTN.[1] HTN can contribute directly to the development of both HFrEF and HFpEF as well as indirectly by increasing the risk of coronary artery disease. Effective treatment of HTN reduces the risk of developing HF, especially in patients with diabetes.[1] Pharmacotherapy of HTN in patients with HFrEF should initially involve agents that can treat both disorders such as ACE inhibitors or ARBs, β-blockers, and diuretics. Target levels of BP should be consistent with current guidelines.[122] If control of HTN is not achieved after optimizing treatment with these agents, the addition of an ARB, aldosterone antagonist, ISDN/hydralazine, or a second-generation calcium channel blocker such as amlodipine (or possibly felodipine) should be considered. Medications that should be avoided in patients with HFrEF include the calcium channel blockers with negative inotropic effects (eg, verapamil, diltiazem) and direct-acting vasodilators (eg, minoxidil) that cause sodium retention.

In patients with HFpEF, both verapamil and diltiazem can be safely used. However, clinicians should remember that HFpEF is associated with HTN and aging, making it a common diagnosis in elderly women. Because these women often are frail and have low muscle mass, their creatinine clearance and renal function may be compromised. Special care must be taken when selecting and titrating doses of drugs such as diuretics, ACE inhibitors, and ARBs and close attention paid to monitoring serum creatinine and electrolytes.

Angina Coronary artery disease is the most common etiology of HFrEF. Appropriate management of coronary disease and its risk factors is thus an important strategy for the prevention and treatment of HF. Coronary revascularization should be strongly considered in patients with both HF and angina.[1] Pharmacotherapy of angina in patients with HF should utilize drugs that can effectively treat both disorders. Nitrates and β-blockers are effective antianginals and are the preferred agents for patients with both disorders since they may improve hemodynamics and clinical outcomes. It should be noted that the antianginal effectiveness of these agents may be significantly limited if fluid retention is not controlled with diuretics.

Similar to their use in HTN, both amlodipine and felodipine appear to be safe to use in this setting. Optimization of other treatments for secondary prevention of coronary and other atherosclerotic vascular disease should also be considered.[123] Statins have not been shown to improve outcomes in patients with HFrEF and are only recommended if other indications for their use are present (eg, post-MI).[1]

Atrial Fibrillation Atrial fibrillation is the most frequently encountered arrhythmia and it is commonly found in patients with HF (both HFrEF and HFpEF), affecting 5% to 50% of patients with the prevalence increasing in parallel to the severity of HF.[1,124] The high incidence of atrial fibrillation in these patients is not surprising since each disorder predisposes to the other and they share many risk factors including coronary artery disease, diabetes, obesity, and HTN. The presence of atrial fibrillation in patients with HF is associated with a worse long-term prognosis.[29,124] Detrimental effects of these disorders include increased risk of thromboembolism, a reduction in CO due to loss of the atrial contribution to ventricular filling, and hemodynamic compromise from the rapid ventricular response. Moreover, HF exacerbations and atrial fibrillation are closely linked and it is often difficult to determine which disorder caused the other. For example, worsening HF results in volume overload, which, in turn, causes atrial distension and increases the risk of atrial fibrillation. Similarly, atrial fibrillation with a rapid ventricular response can reduce CO and lead to HF exacerbation. Thus, optimal management according to established guidelines is required with careful attention paid to control of ventricular response, symptoms, and anticoagulation for stroke prevention.[121]

Digoxin is frequently used to slow ventricular response in patients with HF and atrial fibrillation. However, it is more effective at rest than with exercise and it does not affect the progression of HF. In addition, the potential for digoxin to increase mortality in patients with atrial fibrillation is a growing concern.[125,126] β-Blockers are more effective than digoxin and have the added benefits of improving morbidity and mortality in patients with HFrEF. Combination therapy with digoxin and a β-blocker may be more effective for rate control than either agent used alone. Calcium channel blockers with negative inotropic effects such as verapamil or diltiazem should be avoided in patients with HFrEF but are effective in patients with HFpEF.

There appear to be no differences in outcomes between the rhythm (restoration and maintenance of sinus rhythm) and rate control approaches to atrial fibrillation in patients with HF.[121,124] Rhythm control is often reserved for patients in whom the rate cannot be controlled or who remain symptomatic. In general, amiodarone is the preferred agent if the rhythm control approach is taken. Although it has many noncardiac toxicities, amiodarone does not have cardiodepressant or significant proarrhythmic effects and appears to be safe in HFrEF. Dofetilide also appears to be safe and effective in this population.[1,121] Class I antiarrhythmics should be avoided. Because of the limited efficacy and potential for serious adverse effects with antiarrhythmic drugs, there is growing interest in the use of catheter ablation for restoring sinus rhythm in these patients.[1]

Diabetes Diabetes is a common comorbid condition in patients with HF, present in 25% to 40% of patients with HF.[45] As an important risk factor for coronary artery disease, diabetes directly contributes to the development of HF. Importantly, diabetes is also a risk factor for developing HF, particularly in women, independent of coronary artery disease or HTN.[45] Diabetes is associated with more rapid HF progression and is a significant predictor of mortality and hospitalizations in patients with HF.[45]

Pharmacotherapy of diabetes in patients with HF should be targeted to control hyperglycemia according to current guidelines, although it remains uncertain if this approach reduces the risk of HF development.[1,46] The optimal approach to the treatment of diabetes in this population remains uncertain as many clinical trials of diabetes medications excluded patients with moderate to severe HF. Some medications used to treat diabetes can have important adverse effects in patients with HF. Because the thiazolidinediones (TZDs; pioglitazone and rosiglitazone) are associated with fluid retention, these medications should not be used in patients with NYHA class II–IV HF.[1] TZDs should be discontinued in patients developing symptoms related to volume overload. Use of metformin in patients with HF has been contraindicated because of the purported risk of lactic acidosis. However, a growing body of data demonstrates that not only is metformin safe in HF, but it is also associated with improved morbidity and mortality.[46,127] Nevertheless,careful monitoring of volume status and renal function is still needed when metformin is used in these patients. The use of the dipeptidylpeptidase-4 (DPP-4) inhibitors in patients with HF remains controversial with clinical trials showing association of some of these agents with increased risk of developing HF whereas other studies show no increased risk.[46,128]

Drug Class Information

Diuretics 7 Loop diuretics, as described earlier, represent the typical diuretic therapy for patients with HF due to their potency and, as such, are the only diuretics discussed here.[55,129] There are currently three loop diuretics available that are used routinely: furosemide, bumetanide, and torsemide. They share many similarities in their pharmacodynamics, with their differences being largely pharmacokinetic in nature. Relevant information on the loop diuretics is shown in Tables 14-8 and 14-9. Following oral administration, the peak effect with all the agents occurs in 30 to 90 minutes, with duration of 4 to 8 hours (longer for torsemide). Following IV administration, the diuretic effect begins within minutes. All three drugs are highly (greater than 95%) bound to serum albumin and enter the nephron by active secretion in the proximal tubule. The magnitude of effect is determined by the peak concentration achieved in the nephron, and there is a threshold concentration that must be achieved before any diuresis is seen.

The biggest difference between the agents is bioavailability. Bioavailability of bumetanide and torsemide is essentially complete (80%-100%), whereas furosemide bioavailability exhibits marked intrapatient and interpatient variability. Furosemide bioavailability ranges from 10% to 100%, with an average of 50%. Thus, if bioequivalent IV and oral doses are desired, oral furosemide doses should be approximately double that of the IV dose, whereas IV and oral doses are the same for torsemide and bumetanide. Coadministration of furosemide and bumetanide with food can decrease bioavailability significantly, whereas food has no effect on bioavailability of torsemide. The intra-abdominal congestion that can occur in HF also may slow the rate (and thus decrease the peak concentration) of furosemide, which can reduce the diuretic's efficacy. Thus, furosemide is most problematic with respect to rate and extent of absorption and the factors that influence it, whereas torsemide has the least variable bioavailability.

Data suggest that these differences in bioavailability and variability may have clinical implications. For example, several studies have suggested that torsemide is absorbed reliably and is associated with better outcomes than the more variably absorbed furosemide.[130] There is also some evidence that torsemide may modulate neurohormonal levels resulting in attenuation of cardiac remodeling.[131] Torsemide is preferred in patients with persistent fluid retention despite high doses of other loop diuretics. And while the costs of torsemide exceed those of furosemide, pharmacoeconomic analyses suggest that the costs of care are similar or less with torsemide.[132] These data require confirmation in controlled, double-blind clinical trials but provide preliminary evidence that the more reliably absorbed loop diuretics with potential neurohormonal modulating effects may be superior to furosemide.

Heart failure is one of the disease states in which the maximal response to loop diuretics is reduced. This is believed to result from a decrease in the rate of diuretic absorption and/or increased proximal or distal tubule reabsorption of sodium, possibly due to increased activity of the Na–K–2Cl transporter.[56] As a consequence, loop diuretics exhibit a ceiling effect in HF, meaning that once the ceiling dose is reached, no additional diuretic response is achieved by increasing the dose. Thus, when this dose is reached, additional diuresis can be achieved by giving the drug more often (twice daily or occasionally three times daily) or by giving combination diuretic therapy. Multiple daily dosing achieves a more sustained diuresis throughout the day. When dosed two or three times daily, the first dose is usually given first thing in the morning and the final dose in late afternoon/early evening. The appropriate chronic dose of a loop diuretic is that which maintains the patient at a stable dry weight without symptoms of dyspnea. Ranges of doses of loop diuretics and recommended ceiling doses are shown in Table 14-8.

Diuretics cause a variety of metabolic abnormalities, with severity related to the potency of the diuretic. The reader is referred to Chapter e3 for a detailed discussion on the adverse effects of diuretic therapy. Hypokalemia is the most common metabolic disturbance with thiazide and loop diuretics, which in HF patients may be exacerbated by hyperaldosteronism. Hypokalemia increases the risk for ventricular arrhythmias in HF and is especially worrisome in patients receiving digoxin. It is often accompanied by hypomagnesemia. Since adequate magnesium is necessary for entry of potassium into the cell, co-supplementation with both magnesium and potassium may be necessary to correct the hypokalemia. Concomitant ACE inhibitor (or ARB) and/or aldosterone antagonist therapy may help to minimize diuretic-induced hypokalemia because these drugs tend to increase serum potassium concentration through their inhibitory effect on aldosterone secretion. Nonetheless, the serum potassium concentration should be monitored closely in HF patients and supplemented appropriately when needed. In addition to metabolic abnormalities, a posthoc analysis of the DIG trial suggested that chronic diuretic use was associated with increased risk of mortality and hospitalization.[133] These findings must be interpreted with caution because this trial was not designed to evaluate outcomes associated with diuretic therapy. However, they do serve to remind clinicians of the importance of appropriate patient selection and monitoring when using diuretic therapy.

ACE Inhibitors 5 A number of ACE inhibitors are currently available; those commonly used in the treatment of patients with HF are summarized in Table 14-8. Although ACE inhibitors vary in their chemical structure (eg, sulfhydryl vs non-sulfhydryl-containing agents) and tissue affinity, the major differences in the ACE inhibitors are not in these pharmacologic properties but in their pharmacokinetic properties.[13] To date all ACE inhibitors studied improve symptoms and mortality in patients with HFrEF.[13] However, it seems most prudent to use those agents documented to reduce morbidity and mortality because the dose required for these end points has been determined.[1]

To minimize the risk of hypotension and renal insufficiency, ACE inhibitor therapy should be started with low doses followed by gradual titration as tolerated to the target doses.[1] Asymptomatic hypotension should not be considered a contraindication to starting therapy with an ACE inhibitor, although initiation or dose increases in patients with systolic blood pressures less than 90 to 100 mm Hg should be done cautiously. Renal function and serum potassium should be evaluated at baseline and within 1 to 2 weeks after therapy is started with subsequent periodic assessments. In the outpatient setting, clinicians should wait at least 2 weeks between dose increases and renal function and potassium should be checked 1 to 2 weeks after each increase. After titration of the drug to the target dose, most patients tolerate chronic therapy with few complications. Although symptoms may improve within a few days of initiating therapy, it may take weeks to months before the full benefits are apparent. Even if symptoms do not improve, long-term ACE inhibitor therapy should be continued to reduce the risk of mortality and hospitalization. Careful attention to appropriate doses of diuretics is important since fluid overload may blunt the beneficial effects of ACE inhibitors and overdiuresis increases the risk of hypotension and renal insufficiency.

Since ACE inhibitors were the first agents to show improvements in survival and were frequently used as background therapy in clinical trials of other medications, they are often used as the initial therapy in patients with HF. However, initiation of β-blocker therapy should not be delayed while the ACE inhibitor is titrated to the target dose since low-intermediate ACE inhibitor doses are equally effective as higher doses for improving symptoms and survival.[1,62] Also, in β-blocker clinical trials, most patients were receiving background therapy with low-intermediate ACE inhibitor doses. Thus, in most patients, ACE inhibitors should be the initial therapy but it is important to remember that even a small dose of ACE inhibitor is better than no ACE inhibitor and that the greatest benefit is seen when these agents are combined with a β-blocker.

Adverse Effects The primary adverse effects of ACE inhibitors are secondary to their major pharmacologic effects of suppressing angiotensin II and increasing bradykinin. The most common adverse effects with these agents are hypotension and functional renal insufficiency resulting from the drug-related reductions in angiotensin II. ACE inhibitors reduce BP in nearly all patients, with hypotension becoming problematic when symptoms such as dizziness, light-headedness, blurred vision, presyncope, or syncope are observed. Hypotension occurs most frequently soon after therapy is started or after an increase in dose, although it may occur at any time during treatment. Risk factors for hypotension include hyponatremia (serum sodium less than 130 mEq/L [less than 130 mmol/L]), hypovolemia, and overdiuresis. The risk of hypotension may be minimized by initiating therapy with lower ACE inhibitor doses and/or temporarily withholding or reducing the dose of diuretic, and liberalizing salt and fluid intake.[1] An often overlooked solution to hypotension is to space the administration times of vasoactive medications (eg, diuretics and β-blockers) throughout the day so that these medications are not all administered at or near the same time. Also, if the patient is receiving other vasodilating drugs (eg, nitrates, amlodipine), the need for these medications or at least the feasibility of dose reduction should be considered. Many patients who experience symptomatic hypotension early in therapy are still good candidates for long-term treatment if risk factors for low BP are addressed.

Functional renal insufficiency causes increases in serum creatinine and blood urea nitrogen (BUN). As CO and renal blood flow decline, renal perfusion is maintained by the vasoconstrictor effect of angiotensin II on the efferent arteriole. Patients most dependent on this system for maintenance of renal perfusion (and therefore most likely to develop functional renal insufficiency with ACE inhibitors) are those with severe HF, hypotension, hyponatremia, volume depletion, bilateral renal artery stenosis, and concomitant use of NSAIDs.[134] Sodium depletion, usually secondary to diuretic therapy, is the most important factor in the development of functional renal insufficiency with ACE inhibitor therapy. Renal insufficiency therefore can be minimized in some cases by reduction in diuretic dosage or liberalization of sodium intake. Increases in serum creatinine of 10% to 20% from baseline are commonly observed after initiation of ACE inhibitor therapy. In some patients, the serum creatinine will return to baseline levels without a reduction in ACE inhibitor dose.[134] Increases in serum creatinine of greater than 0.5 mg/dL if the baseline creatinine is less than 2 mg/dL or of greater than 1 mg/dL if the creatinine is greater than 2 mg/dL should prompt clinicians to reduce the dose of ACE inhibitors or reconsider ACE therapy and evaluate potential causes for the abrupt decline in renal function.[134] The safety and efficacy of ACE inhibitors in patients with baseline serum creatinine greater than 2.5 mg/dL (greater than 221 μmol/L) is uncertain as these patients were usually excluded from clinical trials. Caution should also be exercised when using ACE inhibitors in such patients. Since renal dysfunction with ACE inhibitors is secondary to alterations in renal hemodynamics, it is almost always reversible on discontinuation of the drug.[134]

Careful dose titration can minimize the risks of hypotension and transient worsening of renal function. Thus, usual initial doses should be about one fourth the final target dose with slow upward dose titration based on BP and serum creatinine. In certain patients, especially those hospitalized patients who seem at high risk for hypotension or worsening of renal function, it also may be advisable to initiate therapy with a short-acting agent such as captopril. This will help minimize the duration of these adverse effects should they occur. Once stabilized on captopril, the patient can then be switched to an agent given once daily.

Hyperkalemia with ACE inhibitor therapy can occur and is due to the reduced feedback of angiotensin II to stimulate aldosterone release. Hyperkalemia is most likely to occur in patients with renal insufficiency, in elderly patients, and in those taking concomitant potassium supplements, potassium-containing salt substitutes, or potassium-sparing diuretic therapy (including an aldosterone antagonist), especially if they have diabetes.[134] The more widespread use of aldosterone antagonists (eg, spironolactone) in patients with HF may increase the risk of hyperkalemia. Recent evidence shows that concomitant use of trimethoprim-sulfamethoxazole with either ACE inhibitors or ARBs increases the risk of hyperkalemia and sudden cardiac death.[135,136] The likely mechanism of this interaction is trimethoprim-induced reduction in renal potassium excretion as this agent is structurally similar to the potassium-sparing diuretic amiloride.[135]

ACE inhibitors are also associated with other important adverse effects. A dry, hacking cough is the most common reason for discontinuation of ACE inhibitors, and this adverse effect occurs with a similar frequency with all the agents.[1] Up to 15% to 20% of patients treated with ACE inhibitors will develop cough.[137] The cough is usually nonproductive, occurs within the first few months of therapy, resolves within 1 to 2 weeks of drug discontinuation, and reappears with rechallenge. Cough occurs in up to 40% of patients with HF, independent of ACE inhibitor use; therefore, it is important to rule out other potential causes of cough, such as pulmonary congestion. Because cough is a bradykinin-mediated effect, replacement of ACE inhibitor therapy with an ARB would be reasonable. Angioedema is a rare, occurring in less than 1% of patients receiving an ACE inhibitor, but potentially life-threatening complication that is also due to bradykinin accumulation. It occurs more frequently in African Americans, women, and patients with HF than in other populations.[138,139] Approximately 50% of patients develop angioedema within the first 90 days of therapy, but it can occur years after treatment was started.[139] Use of ACE inhibitors is contraindicated in patients with a history of angioedema. Extreme caution should be exercised if ARBs are used as an alternative therapy in patients with ACE inhibitor-induced angioedema, as cross-reactivity is reported.[1,138] ACE inhibitors are contraindicated during the second and third trimesters of pregnancy due to the increased risk of fetal renal failure, intrauterine growth retardation, and other congenital defects. An analysis of a Medicaid database of nearly 30,000 patients suggests that first-trimester use of ACE inhibitors should also be avoided as the risk of major congenital defects was increased 2.7-fold in infants exposed to these agents during the first trimester.[140]

Angiotensin II Receptor Blockers 5 Although ACE inhibitors remain the agents of first choice to treat HFrEF, ARBs are now the recommended alternatives in patients who are unable to tolerate an ACE inhibitor.[1] Although numerous ARBs are currently available, only three agents, candesartan, valsartan, and losartan, are recommended in the treatment guidelines.[1] The efficacy of these agents is supported by clinical trial data that document a target dose associated with improved survival and other important outcomes in patients with decreased EF.[1] ARBs are also alternatives to ACE inhibitors in patients with Stage A or B HF.[1]

The clinical use of ARBs is also similar to that of ACE inhibitors. Therapy should be initiated at low doses and then titrated to target doses (see Table 14-8).[1] Blood pressure, renal function, and serum potassium should be evaluated within 1 to 2 weeks after initiation of therapy and after increases in dose and these end points used to guide subsequent dose changes. It is not necessary to reach target doses before adding a β-blocker, although incremental benefits may be associated with higher doses of ARBs.[64]

Adverse Effects The ARBs have a low incidence of adverse effects. Since they do not affect bradykinin, they are not associated with cough and have a lower risk of angioedema than ACE inhibitors.[137] However, because of reports of recurrences of angioedema after ARB administration to patients with a history of ACE inhibitor-related angioedema, ARBs should be used with extreme caution in any patient with a history of angioedema as cross-reactivity may occur.[67]

The major adverse effects are related to suppression of the RAAS. The incidence and risk factors for developing hypotension, decreases in renal function, and hyperkalemia with the ARBs are similar to those with ACE inhibitors.[1] Thus, ARBs are not alternatives in patients who develop these complications from ACE inhibitors. Careful monitoring is required when an ARB is used with another inhibitor of the RAAS (eg, ACE inhibitor or aldosterone antagonist) as this combination increases the risk of these adverse effects. Similar to the ACE inhibitors, the ARBs are contraindicated in the second and third trimesters of pregnancy and should be avoided in the first trimester because of increased risk of fetal/neonatal morbidity and mortality. Neither candesartan nor valsartan is metabolized by the cytochrome P450 system, so no pharmacokinetic drug–drug interactions with these agents are expected.

Angiotensin II Receptor Blocker/Neprilysin Inhibitor (ARNI)

Deterimental effects of the activation of the SNS and RAAS are managed through the use of β-blockers, aldosterone antagonists, and either ACE inhibitors or ARBs. The combination of sacubitril/valsartan affects the RAAS and inhibits neprilysin. This two-pronged approach showed significant benefit in reducing mortality and hospitalizations in patients with HFrEF when compared to enalapril and is currently being studied in patients with HFpEF.[23]

The natriuretic peptides ANP and BNP cause vasodilation, natriuresis, and diuresis. In addition, they inhibit renin secretion, aldosterone production and attenuate ventricular hypertrophy and fibrosis.[141] When HF is present there are elevations in ANP, BNP and its inactive precursor NT-pro-BNP. Another structurally unrelated peptide called *adrenomedullin* (ADM) has similar vasodilatory and natriuretic properties. Neprilysin breaks down the natriuretic peptides ANP and BNP as well as ADM, bradykinin, and several other substances.[95,141] Inhibition of neprilysin as a therapeutic target has been of interest for several decades.

Omipatrilat was an ACE inhibitor neprilysin inhibitor that was abandoned due to an unacceptable rate of angioedema. Sacubitril/valsartan was designed to lessen the risk of angioedema by using an ARB instead of an ACE inhibitor and inhibiting only one of the enzymes that breaks down bradykinin. Neprilysin is also involved in the clearance of amyloid-β from the brain and CSF. Administration of sacubitril/valsartan is associated with increased levels of amyloid A β_{1-38};however the clinical relevance of this finding is unknown.

The half-lives of valsartan and LBQ657, the active component of sacubitril, are similar at 10 to 12 hours.[142] Both components are highly protein bound. The valsartan component of the combination product is 40% to 60% more bioavailable than conventional valsartan tablets. Thus, the 24 mg sacubitril/26 mg valsartan tablet is equivalent to 40 mg of valsartan.[142] The initial starting dose for most patients being treated for HFrEF is 49/51 mg sacubitril/valsartan twice daily and titrated to the target dose of 97/103 mg sacubitril/valsartan twice daily after 2 to 4 weeks. A reduced dose of 24/26 mg sacubitril/valsartan is available for patients taking a low dose of either an ACE inhibitor or an ARB prior to initiation, those with severe renal dysfunction (eGFR less than 30 mL/min/1.73 m^2) and those with moderate hepatic impairment (Child-Pugh B). Sacubitril/valsartan should be avoided in patients with severe hepatic impairment (Child-Pugh C).

Adverse Effects The most common adverse reactions and risk factors for their development are similar to those with ACE inhibitors or ARBs and include hypotension, dizziness, hyperkalemia, worsening renal function, and cough. Angioedema occurred more frequently with sacubitril/valsartan compared to enalapril (0.5% vs 0.2%, respectively).[23] The risk of angioedema is 4-fold higher in African-American patients.[142] Sacubitril/valsartan is contraindicated in patients with history of angioedema associated with an ACE inhibitor or ARB. Sacubitril/valsartan is also contraindicated in pregnancy and should not be used concurrently with ACE inhibitors or other ARBs. ACE inhibitors should be discontinued 36 hours prior to initiating sacubitril/valsartan. This agent should also be avoided with aliskiren in patients with diabetes.

β-Blockers 6 Metoprolol succinate, carvedilol, and bisoprolol are the only β-blockers shown to reduce mortality in large trials in patients with HFrEF. Metoprolol and bisoprolol selectively block the β_1-receptor, while carvedilol blocks the β_1-, β_2-, and α_1-receptors and also possesses antioxidant effects. While there is no clear evidence that these pharmacologic differences result in differences in efficacy among agents, they may aid in selection of a specific agent. For example, carvedilol is expected to have greater antihypertensive effects than the other agents because of its α-receptor blocking properties and may be preferred in patients with poorly controlled BP. Conversely, metoprolol or bisoprolol may be preferred in patients with low BP or dizziness and in patients with significant airway disease. Bisoprolol is eliminated approximately 50% by the kidneys, whereas metoprolol and carvedilol are essentially completely metabolized and undergo extensive hepatic first-pass metabolism.

There is fairly strong evidence that benefits of β-blockers in HFrEF are not a class effect. Specifically, in a study powered for mortality reduction, there was no difference in survival between the nonselective β-blocker bucindolol and placebo.[143] While there has been considerable debate over why bucindolol failed to provide a survival benefit, it may be related to the drug's ancillary properties or differences among β-blocker trials in the characteristics of study participants. Additional data suggest that bucindolol's effects on survival might be genotype specific, as described in Personalized Pharmacotherapy. In the absence of bucindolol's approval for HF, β-blocker use should be confined to one of the agents with proven survival benefits, especially given the diversity among β-blockers in their receptor sensitivities and ancillary properties.

There has been much debate over whether one β-blocker is superior to another. Specifically, it has been hypothesized that nonselective blockade with carvedilol might produce greater benefits than β_1-selective blockade. This hypothesis is based on observations that the β_1-receptor is downregulated, and the β_2- and α_1-receptors account for a larger proportion of total cardiac adrenergic receptors in the failing heart. Only one trial with a mortality end point has provided a head-to-head comparison of carvedilol and a β_1-selective blocker. The Carvedilol Or Metoprolol European Trial (COMET) compared carvedilol 25 mg twice daily and immediate-release metoprolol 50 mg twice daily and found a significant 17% lower mortality rate in patients treated with carvedilol.[144] However, concerns regarding the formulation and dose of metoprolol used in COMET limit the conclusions that can be drawn from these findings. Specifically, the study used the immediate-release formulation of metoprolol (metoprolol tartrate), not the sustained-release formation (metoprolol succinate) shown to reduce mortality. The efficacy of the immediate-release formulation in reducing mortality in HF has not been proven. Metoprolol succinate provides more consistent plasma concentrations over a 24-hour period and appears to provide more favorable effects on HR variability, autonomic balance, and BP, suggesting that this formulation might be superior to immediate-release metoprolol.[145] The target dose of metoprolol also differed between COMET and MERIT-HF. The target dose in COMET was 100 mg/day (50 mg twice daily), whereas the target dose of metoprolol in MERIT-HF was 200 mg/day. Many question whether the degree of β-blockade achieved in COMET with immediate-release metoprolol 50 mg twice daily is comparable to that achieved with metoprolol succinate 200 mg/day in MERIT-HF or carvedilol 25 mg twice daily in COMET. More recent data from heart failure registries suggest that metoprolol succinate and carvedilol are similarly effective.[146,147] While some clinicians may still argue the superiority of carvedilol, it seems clear that what is most important is that one of the three β-blockers proven to reduce mortality is used.

Adverse Effects Possible adverse effects with β-blocker use in HF include bradycardia or heart block, hypotension, fatigue, impaired glycemic control in diabetic patients, bronchospasm in patients with asthma, and worsening HF. Clinicians should monitor vital signs and carefully assess for signs and symptoms of worsening HF during β-blocker initiation and uptitration. Hypotension is more common with carvedilol due to its α_1-receptor blocking properties. Bradycardia and hypotension generally are asymptomatic and require no intervention; however, β-blocker dose reduction is warranted in symptomatic patients. Fatigue usually resolves after several weeks of therapy, but sometimes requires dose reduction. In diabetic patients, β-blockers may worsen glucose tolerance and can mask the tachycardia and tremor (but not sweating) that accompany hypoglycemia. In addition, nonselective agents such as carvedilol may prolong insulin-induced hypoglycemia and slow recovery from a hypoglycemic episode. Despite this, there is evidence that carvedilol produces better glycemic control in diabetic patients compared with immediate-release metoprolol and may improve insulin sensitivity.[147] Furthermore, posthoc analysis of HF trials shows that β-blockers are well tolerated and significantly reduce morbidity and mortality in patients with diabetes and HFrEF.[149] Thus, while β-blockers should be used cautiously in patients with recurrent hypoglycemia, concerns of masking symptoms of hypoglycemia or worsening glycemic control should not preclude β-blocker use in patients with diabetes. Patients with diabetes should be warned of these potential adverse effects, and blood glucose monitored with initiation, adjustment, and discontinuation of β-blocker therapy. Adjustment of hypoglycemic therapy may be necessary with concomitant β-blocker use in diabetics.

Uptitration should be avoided if the patient experiences signs of worsening HF, including volume overload and poor perfusion. Fluid overload may be asymptomatic and manifest solely as an increase in body weight. Mild fluid overload may be managed by intensifying diuretic therapy. Once the patient has been stabilized, dose titration may continue as tolerated until the target or highest tolerated dose is reached. Despite their negative inotropic effects, continuing β-blocker therapy during hospitalization for acute decompensated HF appears to neither worsen symptoms nor delay clinical improvement. In fact, β-blocker withdrawal may increase the risk for mortality after hospital discharge.[150] Further, stopping β-blocker therapy during acute decompensation may lead to lower chronic β-blocker use due to failure to reinstitute β-blocker therapy once the patient has stabilized.[151] Guidelines recommend continuing β-blocker therapy during hospitalization for HF whenever possible.[1]

Absolute contraindications to β-blocker use include uncontrolled bronchospastic disease, symptomatic bradycardia, advanced heart block without a pacemaker, and acute decompensated HF. However, β-blockers may be tried with caution in patients with asymptomatic bradycardia, COPD, or well-controlled asthma. Particular caution is warranted in patients with marked bradycardia (less than 55 beats/min) or hypotension (systolic BP less than 80 mm Hg).

Ivabradine Ivabradine reduces heart rate by selective inhibition of the I_f current responsible for controlling the depolarization rate of the sinus node.[97,98] Ivabradine does not affect AV conduction, blood pressure, or myocardial contractility.[97,98] Thus, ivabradine specifically targets the high resting heart rate that is associated with increased risk of adverse outcomes in this patient population.[99] This novel agent was recently approved for the treatment of patients with HFrEF in sinus rhythm with a heart rate greater than or equal to 70 beats/min that are receiving maximally tolerated treatment with β-blockers or have contraindications to β-blockers. Ivabradine is not included in current ACC/AHA HFrEF treatment guidelines as it was approved after publication of these guidelines.[1]

Ivabradine is extensively metabolized by intestinal and hepatic CYP3A4 resulting in an oral bioavailability of 40%.[98] The elimination half-life is approximately 6 hours and the drug's clearance is not affected by impaired renal function.[98] Ivabradine does not affect the metabolism of concomitantly administered medications. However, ivabradine pharmacokinetics are affected by other drugs that inhibit or induce CYP3A4.[98] Co-administration with strong CYP3A4 inhibitors (eg, itraconazole, macrolide antibiotics, HIV protease inhibitors) is contraindicated because of the large increase in exposure and potential for bradycardia or other conduction abnormalities. Moderate CYP3A4 inhibitors (eg, verapamil, diltiazem, grapefruit juice) and inducers (eg, St. John's wort, rifampin, phenytoin) should be avoided as well. Because QT interval prolongation can be increased by slower heart rates, ivabradine should be used cautiously, if at all, with other agents known to prolong the QT interval.

The starting dose of ivabradine in most patients is 5 mg twice daily with meals. After 2 weeks of treatment, resting heart rate should be evaluated and if between 50 and 60 beats/min, the dose should be continued. If the heart rate is greater than 60 beats/min, the dose can be increased to the maximum of 7.5 mg twice daily. If at any point, the heart rate is less than 50 beats/min or if the patient has symptomatic bradycardia, the dose should be reduced by 2.5 mg twice daily. In this case, if the patient is receiving only 2.5 mg twice daily, then ivabradine should be discontinued.

Adverse Effects Consistent with its mechanism of action, ivabradine's most common adverse effect is bradycardia, occurring in approximately 10% of patients, although it rarely leads to drug discontinuation.[101] Effects on vision are found in 3% of patients, primarily manifesting as phosphenes (transient brightness in portions of the visual field).[98,101] These often resolve with continued therapy. Also, atrial fibrillation occurred more frequently in patients receiving ivabradine.[98,101]

Digoxin 10 Digoxin exerts its positive inotropic effect by binding to sodium- and potassium-activated adenosine triphosphatase (Na,K-ATPase or sodium pump). Inhibition of Na,K-ATPase decreases outward transport of sodium and leads to increased intracellular sodium concentrations. Higher intracellular sodium concentrations favor calcium entry and reduce calcium extrusion from the cell through effects on the sodium–calcium exchanger. The result is increased storage of intracellular calcium in the sarcoplasmic reticulum and, with each action potential, a greater release of calcium to activate contractile elements. Digoxin also has beneficial neurohormonal actions. These effects occur at low plasma concentrations, where little inotropic effect is seen, and are independent of inotropic activity. Unlike other positive inotropes that increase intracellular cyclic adenosine monophosphate (cAMP), digoxin attenuates the excessive SNS activation present in HF patients. Although the precise mechanism is unknown, a digoxin-mediated reduction in central sympathetic outflow and improvement in impaired baroreceptor function appear to play an important role. Because mortality and progression of HF are linked to the extent of SNS activation, these sympatho inhibitory effects may be an important component of the clinical response to the drug. Chronic HF is also marked by autonomic dysfunction, most notably suppression of the parasympathetic (vagal) system. Digoxin increases parasympathetic activity in HF patients and leads to a decrease in HR, thus enhancing diastolic filling. The vagal effects also result in slowed conduction and prolongation of AV node refractoriness, thus slowing the ventricular response in patients with atrial fibrillation. Because atrial fibrillation is a common complication of HF, the combined positive inotropic, neurohormonal, and negative chronotropic effects of digoxin can be particularly beneficial for such patients. The overall response to digoxin is usually an increase in cardiac index and a decrease in PCWP with relatively little change in arterial BP.[103,120]

Pharmacokinetics Numerous studies of digoxin pharmacokinetics have been published and are summarized in Table 14-11. Digoxin has a large volume of distribution and is extensively bound to various tissues, most notably to Na,K-ATPase in skeletal and cardiac muscles. Because it does not distribute appreciably to body

TABLE 14-11 Clinical Pharmacokinetics of Digoxin

Oral bioavailability	
Tablets	0.5-0.9 (0.65)[a]
Elixir	0.75-0.85 (0.80)
Capsules	0.9-1.0 (0.95)
Onset of action	
Oral	1.5-6 h
Intravenous	15-30 min
Peak effect	
Oral	4-6 h
Intravenous	1.5-4 h
Terminal half-life	
Normal renal function	36 h
Anuric patients	5 d
Volume of distribution at steady state	7.3 L/kg
Fraction unbound in plasma	0.75-0.80
Fraction excreted unchanged in urine	0.65-0.70

[a]Range and mean value in parentheses.

Data from Schentag JJ, Bang AJ, Kozinski-Tober JL. In: Burton ME, Shaw LM, Schentag JJ, Evans WE, eds. *Applied Pharmacokinetics and Pharmacodynamics: Principles of Therapeutic Drug Monitoring*, 4th ed. Baltimore, MD: Lippincott Williams and Wilkins, 2006:410-439.

fat, loading doses of digoxin (when necessary) should be calculated based on estimates of lean body weight. There is a long "distribution phase" after administration of oral or IV digoxin, resulting in a lag time before maximum pharmacologic response is observed (see Table 14-11). Transiently elevated SDCs during the distribution phase are not associated with increased therapeutic or adverse effects, although they can mislead the clinician who is unaware of the timing of blood sampling relative to the previous digoxin dose. Consequently, blood samples for measurement of SDCs should be collected at least 6 hours and preferably 12 hours or more after the last dose.

In patients with normal renal function, 60% to 80% of a dose of digoxin is eliminated unchanged in urine via glomerular filtration and tubular secretion. The terminal half-life of digoxin is approximately 1.5 days in subjects with normal renal function but approximately 5 days in anuric patients (see Table 14-11). Recent evidence indicates that the drug efflux transporter P-glycoprotein (P-gp) plays an important role in the bioavailability, renal and nonrenal clearance, and drug interactions with digoxin. Clinically important pharmacokinetic/pharmacodynamic drug interactions are summarized in Table 14-12. An extensive review of the pharmacokinetics and pharmacodynamics of digoxin is available.[116]

Adverse Effects Digoxin can produce a variety of cardiac and noncardiac adverse effects, but it is usually well tolerated by most patients (Table 14-13).[103,120] Noncardiac adverse effects frequently involve the CNS or GI systems but also may be nonspecific

TABLE 14-12 Selected Digoxin Drug Interactions

Drugs	Mechanism/Effect	Suggested Clinical MGT
Amiodarone, dronedarone	Inhibits P-glycoprotein resulting in decrease in renal and nonrenal clearance; can increase SDC by 70%-100%	Monitor SDC and adverse effects; anticipate the need to reduce the dose by 30%-50%
Antacids	Concurrent administration may decrease digoxin bioavailability by 20%-35%	Space doses at least 2 h apart or avoid concurrent use if possible
Cholestyramine, colestipol	Bind digoxin in gut and decrease bioavailability 20%-35%; may also decrease enterohepatic recycling	Space doses at least 2 h apart or avoid concurrent use if possible
Cyclosporine	Inhibits P-glycoprotein resulting in decreased clearance	Monitor SDC and adverse effects; anticipate the need to reduce the dose
Diuretics	Thiazides or loop diuretics may cause hypokalemia and hypomagnesemia, thereby increasing the risk of digitalis toxicity	Monitor and replace electrolytes if necessary
Erythromycin, clarithromycin, tetracycline	Alter gut bacterial flora; bioavailability and SDC increase 40%-100% in about 10% of patients who extensively metabolize digoxin in the gut, may also be due to inhibition of P-glycoprotein by macrolides	Monitor SDC and anticipate the need to reduce the dose; avoid concurrent use if possible
Ketoconazole, itraconazole	Decrease in renal and nonrenal clearance by inhibition of P-glycoprotein; SDC may increase by 50%-100%	Monitor SDC and anticipate the need to reduce the dose by 50%
Kaolin-pectin	Large dose (30-60 mL) may decrease digoxin bioavailability by about 60%	Space doses at least 2 h apart or avoid concurrent use if possible
Metoclopramide	Increase in gut mobility may decrease bioavailability of slow dissolving tablets; unknown significance	Effect is minimized by administration of digoxin capsules
Neomycin, sulfasalazine	Decrease in bioavailability by 20%-25%	Space doses at least 2 h apart or avoid concurrent use if possible
Propafenone	Decrease in renal clearance; SDC may increase 30%-40%	Monitor SDC and anticipate the need to reduce the dose
Ranolazine	Inhibits P-glycoprotein; SDC may increase 50%	Monitor SDC
Ritonavir, telaprevir	Inhibits P-glycoprotein and may increase SDC	Monitor SDC and anticipate the need to reduce the dose
Quinidine	Inhibits P-glycoprotein resulting in decrease in renal and nonrenal clearance; also displacement of digoxin from tissue binding sites with decrease in the volume of distribution; SDC generally increases about twofold	Monitor SDC and adverse effects; anticipate the need to reduce dose by 50%
Spironolactone	Decrease in renal and nonrenal clearance; also interference with some digoxin assays thus increasing apparent SDC	Monitor SDC and anticipate the need to reduce dose; check assay for interference
Verapamil	Inhibits P-glycoprotein resulting in decrease in renal and nonrenal clearance, SDC may increase 70%-100%	Monitor SDC and anticipate the need to reduce the dose by 50%; consider using another calcium channel blocker

SDC, serum digoxin concentration.

TABLE 14-13 Signs and Symptoms of Digoxin Toxicity

Noncardiac (mostly CNS) adverse effects
Anorexia, nausea, vomiting, abdominal pain
Visual disturbances
Halos, photophobia, problems with color perception (ie, red-green or yellow-green vision), scotoma
Fatigue, weakness, dizziness, headache, neuralgia, confusion, delirium, psychosis
Cardiac adverse effects[a,b]
Ventricular arrhythmias
Premature ventricular depolarizations, bigeminy, trigeminy, ventricular tachycardia, ventricular fibrillation
Atrioventricular (A-V) block
First degree, second degree (Mobitz type I), third degree
A-V junctional escape rhythms, junctional tachycardia
Atrial arrhythmias with slowed A-V conduction or A-V block
Particularly paroxysmal atrial tachycardia with A-V block
Sinus bradycardia

[a]Some adverse effects may be difficult to distinguish from the signs/symptoms of heart failure.

[b]Digoxin toxicity has been associated with almost every known rhythm abnormality (only the more common manifestations are listed).

Data from Eichorn EJ, Gheorghiade M. *Prog Cardiovasc Dis* 2002;44:251-266.

(eg, fatigue or weakness). Cardiac manifestations include numerous different arrhythmias caused by the drug's multiple electrophysiologic effects (see Table 14-13). Cardiac arrhythmias may be the first evidence of toxicity in a patient (before any noncardiac symptoms occur). Rhythm disturbances are of particular concern because patients with chronic HF are already at increased risk for sudden cardiac death, presumably due to ventricular arrhythmias. Patients at increased risk of toxicity include those with impaired renal function, decreased lean body mass, the elderly, and those taking interacting drugs. Hypokalemia, hypomagnesemia, and hypercalcemia will predispose patients to cardiac manifestations of digoxin toxicity. Thus, concomitant therapy with diuretics may lead to electrolyte abnormalities and increase the likelihood of cardiac arrhythmias. Similarly, hypothyroidism, myocardial ischemia, and acidosis will also increase the risk of cardiac adverse effects. Although digoxin toxicity is commonly associated with plasma concentrations greater than 2 ng/mL (2.6 nmol/L), toxicity may occur at lower concentrations and clinicians should remember that digoxin toxicity is based on the presence of symptoms rather than a specific plasma concentration.[116] Usual treatment of digoxin toxicity includes drug withdrawal or dose reduction and treatment of cardiac arrhythmias and electrolyte abnormalities. In patients with life-threatening digoxin toxicity, purified digoxin-specific Fab antibody fragments should be administered. SDCs will not be reliable until the antidote has been eliminated from the body.[117]

Personalized Pharmacotherapy

Pharmacogenetics holds promise for future personalized HF therapy. Most HF pharmacogenetic research has focused on genetic association responses to β-blockers. For example, there is evidence that the β_1-adrenergic receptor (*ADRB1*) Arg389Gly polymorphism is associated with improvement in left ventricular EF with β-blockers.[152] Further, the Arg389Gly variant was associated with clinical outcomes with bucindolol, the only β-blocker among those studied in large, randomized, multicenter HF trials that did not significantly improve outcomes.[143] The trial with bucindolol was unique in that it included a large number of African American patients. A subgroup analysis showed survival improvement with bucindolol in whites, but not African Americans. African Americans have a higher frequency of the *ADRB1* 389Gly allele and the α_{2c}-adrenergic receptor (*ADRA2C*) Del322-325 variant, both of which are associated with a lack of improvement in HF outcomes with bucindolol.[153] In contrast, the nonvariant*ADRB1* and *ADRA2C* genotypes, which occur more often among whites, were associated with a reduced risk for hospitalization and death with bucindolol. The manufacturer of bucindolol sought FDA approval of the drug for patients with the more favorable response genotype; however, their efforts were unsuccessful.

Clinical **Controversy...**

Current treatment guidelines recommend that, in the absence of contraindications, all patients with HFrEF should receive an ACE inhibitor or ARB to improve survival and morbidity. Compared to enalapril, the recently approved combination product sacubitril/valsartan (neprilysin inhibitor/ARB) significantly reduced the risk of cardiovascular mortality and heart failure hospitalization in patients with HFrEF. Based on these new findings, the optimal initial approach to RAAS inhibition in these patients remains to be determined.

Both metoprolol and carvedilol are also substrates for the cytochrome P450 2D6 enzyme, which is known to be polymorphic. A total of 7% of the white population and 1% to 2% of the Asian-American and African-American populations who are CYP2D6 poor metabolizers would be expected to have higher plasma concentrations than anticipated at the usual doses of carvedilol and metoprolol. However, given that β-blockers have a wide therapeutic index, it is unclear whether CYP2D6 phenotype significantly impacts hemodynamic and clinical effects.

There is also preliminary evidence of genetic determinants of outcomes with hydralazine/ISDN. Specifically, the endothelial nitric oxide synthase-3 (NOS3) Glu298Asp polymorphism was associated with the effects of hydralazine/ISDN on the composite end point of survival, hospitalization, and quality of life, with greater improvement with the Glu298Glu genotype.[154] A separate analysis focused on the gene for corin, a protein expressed in cardiomyocytes that cleaves pro-ANP and proBNP into active natriuretic peptides. The corin Gln568Pro variant leads to a dysfunctional protein and was associated with an increased risk for death or HF hospitalization in the A-HeFT population.[155] However, no detrimental effect of the 568Pro variant was observed among patients treated with hydralazine/ISDN, suggesting that the drug combination attenuates the adverse consequences of the 568Pro allele. Both the NOS3 Glu-298Glu genotype and corin 568Pro variant occur predominately in persons of African descent, potentially explaining why hydralazine/ISDN is especially effective in African Americans.

Clinical **Controversy...**

Elevated resting heart rate in patients with HFrEF is associated with increased risk of adverse outcomes. The recently approved novel agent ivabradine reduces heart rate by selective inhibiton of the I_f current in the sinus node. This agent reduces the risk of hospitalization in patients with HFrEF in sinus rhythm that are receiving GDMT. Digoxin also decreases the risk of hospitalization in this patient population. In patients in sinus rhythm with a heart rate ≥70 BPM with persistent symptoms despite optimal GDMT, it remains uncertain whether adding ivabradine or digoxin is the best approach.

EVALUATION OF THERAPEUTIC OUTCOMES

Although mortality is an important end point, it does not give a complete measure of the overall impact of this disorder because many patients are hospitalized repeatedly for HF exacerbations and continue to survive, albeit with a significantly reduced quality of life. Thus, some of the more important therapeutic outcomes in HF management, such as prolonged survival or prevention or slowing of the progression of HF, cannot be quantified in an individual patient. However, after appropriate diagnostic evaluation to determine the etiology of HF, ongoing clinical assessment of patients typically focuses on evaluation of three general areas: (a) functional capacity, (b) volume status, and (c) laboratory monitoring.

The evaluation of functional capacity should focus on the presence and severity of symptoms the patient experiences during activities of daily living and how his or her symptoms affect these activities. Questions directed toward the patient's ability to perform specific activities may be more informative than general questions about what symptoms the patient may be experiencing. For example, patients should be asked if they could exercise, climb stairs, get dressed without stopping, check the mail, go shopping, or clean the house. Another important component of assessment of functional capacity is to ask patients what activities they would like to do but are now unable to perform.

Assessment of volume status is a vital component of the ongoing care of patients with HF. This evaluation provides the clinician important information about the adequacy of diuretic therapy. Since the cardinal signs and symptoms of HF are caused by excess fluid retention, the efficacy of diuretic treatment is readily evaluated by the disappearance of these signs and symptoms. The physical examination is the primary method for the evaluation of fluid retention, and specific attention should be focused on the patient's body weight, extent of JVD, presence of hepatojugular reflux, presence and severity of pulmonary congestion, and peripheral edema. Specifically, in a patient with pulmonary congestion, monitoring is indicated for resolution of rales and pulmonary edema and improvement or resolution of DOE, orthopnea, and PND. For patients with systemic congestion, a decrease or disappearance of peripheral edema, JVD, and hepatojugular reflux is sought. Other therapeutic outcomes include an improvement in exercise tolerance and fatigue, decreased nocturia, and a decrease in HR. Clinicians also will want to monitor BP and ensure that the patient does not develop symptomatic hypotension as a result of drug therapy. Body weight is a sensitive short-term marker of fluid loss or retention, and patients should be counseled to weigh themselves daily, reporting changes to their healthcare provider so that adjustments can be made in diuretic doses. Patients and healthcare providers should be aware that HF progression may be slowed even though symptoms have not resolved.

Routine monitoring of serum electrolytes and renal function is required in patients with HF. Assessment of serum potassium and magnesium is especially important because hypokalemia and hypomagnesemia are common adverse effects of diuretic therapy and are associated with an increased risk of arrhythmias and digoxin toxicity (hypokalemia). Serum potassium monitoring is also required because of the risk of hyperkalemia associated with ACE inhibitors, ARBs, and aldosterone antagonists. A serum potassium greater than or equal to 4mEq/L (greater than or equal to 4 mmol/L) should be maintained with some evidence suggesting it should be greater than or equal to 4.5 mEq/L (greater than or equal to 4.5 mmol/L).[156] Assessment of renal function (BUN and serum creatinine) is also an important end point for monitoring diuretic and ACE inhibitor therapy. Common causes of worsening renal function in patients with HF include overdiuresis, adverse effects of ACE inhibitor or ARB therapy, and hypoperfusion.

Most of these therapeutic end points are incorporated into the ACC/AHA performance measures outlined in Table 14-14.[157]

TABLE 14-14 ACC/AHA Clinical Performance Measures for Adults with HFrEF

Performance Measure	Recommendation
Inpatient Measures	
Evaluation of left ventricular systolic function[a]	Echocardiogram with Doppler flow studies is the most useful test as it enables clinicians to determine the presence of pericardial, myocardial, or valvular abnormalities. Patients with LVEF < 40% should be considered for specific therapy (eg, ACE inhibitors, β-blockers). *Class I recommendation, Level of Evidence C.*
ACE inhibitors or ARBs for patients with left ventricular systolic dysfunction[a]	Patients with a LVEF < 40% or moderate or severe systolic dysfunction should receive an ACE inhibitor or ARB unless contraindications are present or there is a history of intolerance to both drugs. ACE inhibitors: *Class I recommendation, Level of Evidence A.* ARBs: *Class 1, Level of Evidence A.*
Beta-blocker therapy for patients with left ventricular systolic dysfunction	All patients with stable heart failure and LVEF 40% should receive treatment with one of the three beta-blockers proven to reduce mortality unless contraindicated. *Class I recommendation, Level of Evidence A.*
Postdischarge follow-up appointment	At the time of hospital discharge, patients should receive an appointment for a follow-up visit to occur within 7-10 days of discharge.
Outpatient Measures	
Evaluation of left ventricular systolic function	Echocardiogram with Doppler flow studies is the most useful test as it enables clinicians to determine the presence of pericardial, myocardial, or valvular abnormalities. Patients with LVEF < 40% should be considered for specific therapy (eg, ACE inhibitors, β-blockers). *Class I recommendation, Level of Evidence C.*
Symptom and activity assessment	Both initial and ongoing quantitative assessment of symptom type, severity, duration, and their impact on the patient's functional capacity should be performed. This can be accomplished using the NYHA functional classification or other established evaluation instruments (eg, Minnesota Living with Heart Failure Questionnaire). *Class I recommendation, Level of Evidence C.*
Beta-blocker therapy for patients with left ventricular systolic dysfunction	All patients with stable heart failure and decreased LVEF should receive treatment with one of the three beta-blockers proven to reduce mortality unless contraindicated. *Class I recommendation, Level of Evidence A.*
ACE inhibitors or ARBs for patients with left ventricular systolic dysfunction	Patients with a LVEF < 40% or moderate or severe systolic dysfunction should receive an ACE inhibitor or ARB unless contraindications are present or there is a history of intolerance to both drugs. ACE inhibitors: *Class I recommendation, Level of Evidence A.* ARBs: *Class 1, Level of Evidence A.*

[a]Also Center for Medicare and Medicaid Services (CMS) and the Joint Commission Core Measures.

Adapted from Bonow RW, Ganiats TG, Beam CT, et al. ACCF/AHA/AMA-PCPI 2011 performance measures for adults with heart failure: A report of the American College of Cardiology Foundation/American Heart Association Task Force on Performance Measures and the American Medical Association-Physician Consortium for Performance Improvement. *J Am Coll Cardiol* 2012;59:1812-1832.

ABBREVIATIONS

ACC	American College of Cardiology
ACE	angiotensin converting enzyme
AHA	American Heart Association
ANP	atrial natriuretic peptide
ARB	angiotensin receptor blocker
AVP	arginine vasopressin
BNP	B-type natriuretic peptide
BP	blood pressure
BPM	beats per minute
BUN	blood urea nitrogen
cAMP	cyclic adenosine monophosphate
CNP	C-type natriuretic peptide
CO	cardiac output
COX-2	cyclooxygenase-2
CRT	cardiac resynchronization therapy
ET	endothelin
GDMT	guideline-directed medical therapy
HF	heart failure
HFpEF	heart failure with preserved ejection fraction
HFrEF	heart failure with reduced ejection fraction
HFSA	Heart Failure Society of America
HR	heart rate
HTN	hypertension
ICD	implantable cardioverter-defibrillator
JVD	jugular venous distension
LVAD	left ventricular assist device
LVEDV	left ventricular end diastolic volume
LVEDP	left ventricular end diastolic pressure
LVEF	left ventricular ejection fraction
MI	myocardial infarction
NE	norepinephrine
NSAID	non-steroidal anti-inflammatory drug
NYHA	New York Heart Association
PCWP	pulmonary capillary wedge pressure
P-gp	P-glycoprotein
RAAS	renin-angiotensin-aldosterone system
SDC	serum digoxin concentration
SNS	sympathetic nervous system
SVR	systemic vascular resistance
TZD	thiazolidinedione

REFERENCES

1. Yancy CW, Jessup M, Bozkurt B, et al. 2013 ACCF/AHA guideline for the management of heart failure: a report of the American College of Cardiology Foundation/American Heart Association Task Force on Practice Guidelines. J Am Coll Cardiol 2013;62:e147-e239.
2. Borlaug BA, Paulus WJ. Heart failure with preserved ejection fraction: pathophysiology, diagnosis, and treatment. Eur Heart J 2011;32:670-679.
3. Mozaffarian D, Benjamin EJ, Go AS, et al. Heart disease and stroke statistics–2015 update: a report from the American Heart Association. Circulation 2015;131:e29-e322.
4. Chen J, Normand SL, Wang Y, Krumholz HM. National and regional trends in heart failure hospitalization and mortality rates for Medicare beneficiaries, 1998-2008. JAMA 2011;306:1669-1678.
5. Mann DL. Management of patients with heart failure with reduced ejection fraction. In: DL Mann, DP Zipes, P Libby, RO Bonow, Braunwald E, eds. Braunwald's Heart Disease: A Textbook of Cardiovascular Medicine. 10th ed. Philadelphia, PA: Elsevier 2015:512-546.
6. Maeder MT, Kaye DM. Heart failure with normal left ventricular ejection fraction. J Am Coll Cardiol 2009;53:905-918.
7. Hasenfuss G, Mann DL. Pathophysiology of Heart Failure. In: DL Mann, DP Zipes, P Libby, RO Bonow, Braunwald E, eds. Braunwald's Heart Disease: A Textbook of Cardiovascular Medicine. 10th ed. Philadelphia, PA: Elsevier 2015:454-472.
8. Borlaug BA. The pathophysiology of heart failure with preserved ejection fraction. Nature reviews Cardiology 2014;11:507-515.
9. Lymperopoulos A, Rengo G, Koch WJ. Adrenergic nervous system in heart failure: pathophysiology and therapy. Circ Res 2013;113:739-753.
10. Johnson JA, Liggett SB. Cardiovascular pharmacogenomics of adrenergic receptor signaling: clinical implications and future directions. Clin Pharmacol Ther 2011;89:366-378.
11. Heusch G, Libby P, Gersh B, et al. Cardiovascular remodelling in coronary artery disease and heart failure. Lancet 2014;383:1933-1943.
12. McMurray JJ. CONSENSUS to EMPHASIS: the overwhelming evidence which makes blockade of the renin-angiotensin-aldosterone system the cornerstone of therapy for systolic heart failure. Eur J Heart Fail 2011;13:929-936.
13. Wong J, Patel RA, Kowey PR. The clinical use of angiotensin-converting enzyme inhibitors. Prog Cardiovasc Dis 2004;47:116-130.
14. Triposkiadis F, Karayannis G, Giamouzis G, Skoularigis J, Louridas G, Butler J. The sympathetic nervous system in heart failure physiology, pathophysiology, and clinical implications. J Am Coll Cardiol 2009;54:1747-1762.
15. Weber KT. The proinflammatory heart failure phenotype: a case of integrative physiology. Am J Med Sci 2005;330:219-226.
16. Weber KT, Weglicki WB, Simpson RU. Macro- and micronutrient dyshomeostasis in the adverse structural remodelling of myocardium. Cardiovasc Res 2009;81:500-508.
17. Pitt B, Zannad F, Remme WJ, et al. The effect of spironolactone on morbidity and mortality in patients with severe heart failure. Randomized Aldactone Evaluation Study Investigators. N Engl J Med 1999;341:709-717.
18. Pitt B, Remme W, Zannad F, et al. Eplerenone, a selective aldosterone blocker, in patients with left ventricular dysfunction after myocardial infarction. N Engl J Med 2003;348:1309-1321.
19. Zannad F, McMurray JJ, Krum H, et al. Eplerenone in patients with systolic heart failure and mild symptoms. N Engl J Med 2011;364:11-21.
20. Pfeffer MA, Claggett B, Assmann SF, et al. Regional variation in patients and outcomes in the Treatment of Preserved Cardiac Function Heart Failure With an Aldosterone Antagonist (TOPCAT) trial. Circulation 2015;131:34-42.
21. Pitt B, Pfeffer MA, Assmann SF, et al. Spironolactone for heart failure with preserved ejection fraction. N Engl J Med 2014;370:1383-1392.
22. Maisel AS, Choudhary R. Biomarkers in acute heart failure-state of the art. Nature reviews Cardiology 2012;9:478-490.
23. McMurray JJ, Packer M, Desai AS, et al. Angiotensin-neprilysin inhibition versus enalapril in heart failure. N Engl J Med 2014;371:993-1004.
24. Troughton RW, Frampton CM, Brunner-La Rocca HP, et al. Effect of B-type natriuretic peptide-guided treatment of chronic heart failure on total mortality and hospitalization: an individual patient meta-analysis. Eur Heart J 2014;35:1559-1567.
25. Savarese G, Trimarco B, Dellegrottaglie S, et al. Natriuretic peptide-guided therapy in chronic heart failure: a meta-analysis of 2,686 patients in 12 randomized trials. PloS one 2013;8:e582-e587.
26. Maeder MT, Rickenbacher P, Rickli H, et al. N-terminal pro brain natriuretic peptide-guided management in patients with heart failure and preserved ejection fraction: findings from the Trial of Intensified versus standard medical therapy in elderly patients with congestive heart failure (TIME-CHF). Eur J Heart Fail 2013;15:1148-1156.
27. Houston BA, Kalathiya RJ, Kim DA, Zakaria S. Volume Overload in Heart Failure: An Evidence-Based Review of Strategies for Treatment and Prevention. Mayo Clin Proc 2015;90:1247-1261.
28. Anter E, Jessup M, Callans DJ. Atrial fibrillation and heart failure: treatment considerations for a dual epidemic. Circulation 2009;119:2516-2525.
29. Mountantonakis SE, Grau-Sepulveda MV, Bhatt DL, Hernandez AF, Peterson ED, Fonarow GC. Presence of atrial fibrillation is independently associated with adverse outcomes in patients hospitalized with heart failure: an analysis of get with the guidelines-heart failure. Circulation Heart failure 2012;5:191-201.
30. Molloy GJ, O'Carroll RE, Witham MD, McMurdo ME. Interventions to enhance adherence to medications in patients with heart failure: a systematic review. Circulation Heart failure 2012;5:126-133.
31. Maxwell CB, Jenkins AT. Drug-induced heart failure. American journal of health-system pharmacy : AJHP : official journal of the American Society of Health-System Pharmacists 2011;68:1791-1804.
32. Yu AF, Steingart RM, Fuster V. Cardiomyopathy associated with cancer therapy. J Card Fail 2014;20:841-852.
33. Patrono C, Baigent C. Nonsteroidal anti-inflammatory drugs and the heart. Circulation 2014;129:907-916.

34. Milfred-LaForest SK, Chow SL, DiDomenico RJ, et al. Clinical pharmacy services in heart failure: an opinion paper from the Heart Failure Society of America and American College of Clinical Pharmacy Cardiology Practice and Research Network. Pharmacotherapy 2013;33:529-548.
35. Wiggins BS, Rodgers JE, DiDomenico RJ, Cook AM, Page RL, 2nd. Discharge counseling for patients with heart failure or myocardial infarction: a best practices model developed by members of the American College of Clinical Pharmacy's Cardiology Practice and Research Network based on the Hospital to Home (H2H) Initiative. Pharmacotherapy 2013;33:558-580.
36. Januzzi JL, Mann DL. Clinical assessment of heart failure. In: DL Mann, DP Zipes, P Libby, RO Bonow, Braunwald E, eds. Braunwald's Heart Disease: A Textbook of Cardiovascular Medicine. 10th ed. Philadelphia, PA: Elsevier; 2015:473-483.
37. Borlaug BA, Redfield MM. Diastolic and systolic heart failure are distinct phenotypes within the heart failure spectrum. Circulation 2011;123:2006-13.
38. Fleg JL, Cooper LS, Borlaug BA, et al. Exercise training as therapy for heart failure: current status and future directions. Circulation Heart failure 2015;8:209-220.
39. Gupta D, Georgiopoulou VV, Kalogeropoulos AP, et al. Dietary sodium intake in heart failure. Circulation 2012;126:479-485.
40. Riegel B, Lee CS, Dickson VV. Self care in patients with chronic heart failure. Nature reviews Cardiology 2011;8:644-654.
41. Lindenfeld J, Albert NM, Boehmer JP, et al. HFSA 2010 Comprehensive Heart Failure Practice Guideline. J Card Fail 2010;16:e1-e194.
42. McMurray JJ, Adamopoulos S, Anker SD, et al. ESC Guidelines for the diagnosis and treatment of acute and chronic heart failure 2012: The Task Force for the Diagnosis and Treatment of Acute and Chronic Heart Failure 2012 of the European Society of Cardiology. Developed in collaboration with the Heart Failure Association (HFA) of the ESC. Eur Heart J 2012;33:1787-1847.
43. Fonarow GC, Albert NM, Curtis AB, et al. Incremental Reduction in Risk of Death Associated With Use of Guideline-Recommended Therapies in Patients With Heart Failure: A Nested Case-Control Analysis of IMPROVE HF. J Am Heart Assoc 2012;1:16-26.
44. Dunn SP, Birtcher KK, Beavers CJ, et al. The Role of the Clinical Pharmacist in the Care of Patients With Cardiovascular Disease. J Am Coll Cardiol 2015;66:2129-2139.
45. Dei Cas A, Khan SS, Butler J, et al. Impact of diabetes on epidemiology, treatment, and outcomes of patients with heart failure. JACC Heart Fail 2015;3:136-145.
46. Gilbert RE, Krum H. Heart failure in diabetes: effects of anti-hyperglycaemic drug therapy. Lancet 2015;385:2107-2117.
47. Perrone-Filardi P, Paolillo S, Costanzo P, Savarese G, Trimarco B, Bonow RO. The role of metabolic syndrome in heart failure. Eur Heart J 2015;36:2630-2634.
48. Riegel B, Moser DK, Anker SD, et al. State of the science: promoting self-care in persons with heart failure: a scientific statement from the American Heart Association. Circulation 2009;120:1141-1163.
49. Fang JC, Ewald GA, Allen LA, et al. Advanced (stage D) heart failure: a statement from the Heart Failure Society of America Guidelines Committee. J Card Fail 2015;21:519-534.
50. Allen LA, Stevenson LW, Grady KL, et al. Decision making in advanced heart failure: a scientific statement from the American Heart Association. Circulation 2012;125:1928-1952.
51. Whellan DJ, Goodlin SJ, Dickinson MG, et al. End-of-life care in patients with heart failure. J Card Fail 2014;20:121-134.
52. Echt DS, Liebson PR, Mitchell LB, et al. Mortality and morbidity in patients receiving encainide, flecainide, or placebo. The Cardiac Arrhythmia Suppression Trial. N Engl J Med 1991;324:781-788.
53. Holzmeister J, Leclercq C. Implantable cardioverter defibrillators and cardiac resynchronisation therapy. Lancet 2011;378:722-730.
54. Mancini D, Colombo PC. Left Ventricular Assist Devices: A Rapidly Evolving Alternative to Transplant. J Am Coll Cardiol 2015;65:2542-2555.
55. Brater DC. Pharmacology of diuretics. Am J Med Sci 2000;319:38-50.
56. Shankar SS, Brater DC. Loop diuretics: from the Na-K-2Cl transporter to clinical use. Am J Physiol Renal Physiol 2003;284:F11-21.
57. Prasun MA, Kocheril AG, Klass PH, Dunlap SH, Piano MR. The effects of a sliding scale diuretic titration protocol in patients with heart failure. J Cardiovasc Nurs 2005;20:62-70.
58. Damman K, Valente MA, Voors AA, O'Connor CM, van Veldhuisen DJ, Hillege HL. Renal impairment, worsening renal function, and outcome in patients with heart failure: an updated meta-analysis. Eur Heart J 2014;35:455-469.
59. Ahmed A, Fonarow GC, Zhang Y, et al. Renin-angiotensin inhibition in systolic heart failure and chronic kidney disease. Am J Med 2012;125:399-410.
60. Damman K, Tang WH, Felker GM, et al. Current evidence on treatment of patients with chronic systolic heart failure and renal insufficiency: practical considerations from published data. J Am Coll Cardiol 2014;63:853-871.
61. Gheorghiade M, Albert NM, Curtis AB, et al. Medication dosing in outpatients with heart failure after implementation of a practice-based performance improvement intervention: findings from IMPROVE HF. Congest Heart Fail 2012;18:9-17.
62. Packer M, Poole-Wilson PA, Armstrong PW, et al. Comparative effects of low and high doses of the angiotensin-converting enzyme inhibitor, lisinopril, on morbidity and mortality in chronic heart failure. ATLAS Study Group. Circulation 1999;100:2312-2318.
63. Lee VC, Rhew DC, Dylan M, Badamgarav E, Braunstein GD, Weingarten SR. Meta-analysis: angiotensin-receptor blockers in chronic heart failure and high-risk acute myocardial infarction. Ann Intern Med 2004;141:693-704.
64. Konstam MA, Neaton JD, Dickstein K, et al. Effects of high-dose versus low-dose losartan on clinical outcomes in patients with heart failure (HEAAL study): a randomised, double-blind trial. Lancet 2009:1840-1848.
65. McMurray JJ, Ostergren J, Swedberg K, et al. Effects of candesartan in patients with chronic heart failure and reduced left-ventricular systolic function taking angiotensin-converting-enzyme inhibitors: the CHARM-Added trial. Lancet 2003;362:767-771.
66. Phillips CO, Kashani A, Ko DK, Francis G, Krumholz HM. Adverse effects of combination angiotensin II receptor blockers plus angiotensin-converting enzyme inhibitors for left ventricular dysfunction: a quantitative review of data from randomized clinical trials. Arch Intern Med 2007;167:1930-1936.
67. Haymore BR, DeZee KJ. Use of angiotensin receptor blockers after angioedema with an angiotensin-converting enzyme inhibitor. Ann Allergy Asthma Immunol 2009;103:83-84.
68. Yusuf S, Pfeffer MA, Swedberg K, et al. Effects of candesartan in patients with chronic heart failure and preserved left-ventricular ejection fraction: the CHARM-Preserved Trial. Lancet 2003;362:777-781.
69. Massie BM, Carson PE, McMurray JJ, et al. Irbesartan in patients with heart failure and preserved ejection fraction. N Engl J Med 2008;359:2456-2467.
70. Packer M, Bristow MR, Cohn JN, et al. The effect of carvedilol on morbidity and mortality in patients with chronic heart failure. U.S. Carvedilol Heart Failure Study Group. N Engl J Med 1996;334:1349-1355.
71. Effect of metoprolol CR/XL in chronic heart failure: Metoprolol CR/XL Randomised Intervention Trial in Congestive Heart Failure (MERIT-HF). Lancet 1999;353:2001-2007.
72. The Cardiac Insufficiency Bisoprolol Study II (CIBIS-II): a randomised trial. Lancet 1999;353:9-13.
73. Packer M, Coats AJ, Fowler MB, et al. Effect of carvedilol on survival in severe chronic heart failure. N Engl J Med 2001;344:1651-1658.
74. Dargie HJ. Effect of carvedilol on outcome after myocardial infarction in patients with left-ventricular dysfunction: the CAPRICORN randomised trial. Lancet 2001;357:1385-1390.
75. Hjalmarson A, Goldstein S, Fagerberg B, et al. Effects of controlled-release metoprolol on total mortality, hospitalizations, and well-being in patients with heart failure: the Metoprolol CR/XL Randomized Intervention Trial in congestive heart failure (MERIT-HF). MERIT-HF Study Group. JAMA 2000;283:1295-1302.
76. Packer M, Fowler MB, Roecker EB, et al. Effect of carvedilol on the morbidity of patients with severe chronic heart failure: results of the carvedilol prospective randomized cumulative survival (COPERNICUS) study. Circulation 2002;106:2194-2199.
77. Metra M, Nodari S, Parrinello G, et al. Marked improvement in left ventricular ejection fraction during long-term [beta]-blockade in patients with chronic heart failure: Clinical correlates and prognostic significance. Am Heart J 2003;145:292-299.
78. Bristow MR, Gilbert EM, Abraham WT, et al. Carvedilol produces dose-related improvements in left ventricular function and survival in subjects with chronic heart failure. MOCHA Investigators. Circulation 1996;94:2807-2816.
79. Willenheimer R, van Veldhuisen DJ, Silke B, et al. Effect on survival and hospitalization of initiating treatment for chronic heart failure with bisoprolol followed by enalapril, as compared with the opposite sequence: results of the randomized Cardiac Insufficiency Bisoprolol Study (CIBIS) III. Circulation 2005;112:2426-2435.

80. Gattis WA, O'Connor CM, Gallup DS, Hasselblad V, Gheorghiade M. Predischarge initiation of carvedilol in patients hospitalized for decompensated heart failure: results of the Initiation Management Predischarge: Process for Assessment of Carvedilol Therapy in Heart Failure (IMPACT-HF) trial. J Am Coll Cardiol 2004;43:1534-1541.
81. McAlister FA, Wiebe N, Ezekowitz JA, Leung AA, Armstrong PW. Meta-analysis: beta-blocker dose, heart rate reduction, and death in patients with heart failure. Ann Intern Med 2009;150:784-794.
82. Fiuzat M, Wojdyla D, Pina I, Adams K, Whellan D, O'Connor CM. Heart Rate or Beta-Blocker Dose? Association With Outcomes in Ambulatory Heart Failure Patients With Systolic Dysfunction: Results From the HF-ACTION Trial. JACC Heart Fail 2015.
83. Packer M. Controlled-release carvedilol: a concluding perspective. Am J Cardiol 2006;98:67-69.
84. Bavishi C, Chatterjee S, Ather S, Patel D, Messerli FH. Beta-blockers in heart failure with preserved ejection fraction: a meta-analysis. Heart Fail Rev 2015;20:193-201.
85. Butler J, Ezekowitz JA, Collins SP, et al. Update on aldosterone antagonists use in heart failure with reduced left ventricular ejection fraction Heart Failure Society of America guidelines committee. J Card Fail 2012;18:265-281.
86. Carbone LD, Cross JD, Raza SH, et al. Fracture risk in men with congestive heart failure risk reduction with spironolactone. J Am Coll Cardiol 2008;52:135-138.
87. Allen LA, Fonarow GC, Liang L, et al. Medication Initiation Burden Required to Comply With Heart Failure Guideline Recommendations and Hospital Quality Measures. Circulation 2015;132:1347-1353.
88. Juurlink DN, Mamdani MM, Lee DS, et al. Rates of hyperkalemia after publication of the Randomized Aldactone Evaluation Study. N Engl J Med 2004;351:543-551.
89. Svensson M, Gustafsson F, Galatius S, Hildebrandt PR, Atar D. How prevalent is hyperkalemia and renal dysfunction during treatment with spironolactone in patients with congestive heart failure? J Card Fail 2004;10:297-303.
90. Cole RT, Kalogeropoulos AP, Georgiopoulou VV, et al. Hydralazine and isosorbide dinitrate in heart failure: historical perspective, mechanisms, and future directions. Circulation 2011;123:2414-2422.
91. Cohn JN, Archibald DG, Ziesche S, et al. Effect of vasodilator therapy on mortality in chronic congestive heart failure: results of the Veterans Administration Cooperative Study. N Engl J Med 1986;316:1547-1552.
92. Cohn JN, Johnson G, Ziesche S, et al. A comparison of enalapril with hydralazine-isosorbide dinitrate in the treatment of chronic congestive heart failure. N Engl J Med 1991;325:303-310.
93. Taylor AL, Ziesche S, Yancy C, et al. Combination of isosorbide dinitrate and hydralazine in blacks with heart failure. N Engl J Med 2004;351:2049-2057.
94. Redfield MM, Anstrom KJ, Levine JA, et al. Isosorbide Mononitrate in Heart Failure with Preserved Ejection Fraction. N Engl J Med 2015;373:2314-2324.
95. Vardeny O, Miller R, Solomon SD. Combined neprilysin and renin-angiotensin system inhibition for the treatment of heart failure. JACC Heart Fail 2014;2:663-670.
96. Solomon SD, Zile M, Pieske B, et al. The angiotensin receptor neprilysin inhibitor LCZ696 in heart failure with preserved ejection fraction: a phase 2 double-blind randomised controlled trial. Lancet 2012;380:1387-1395.
97. Di Franco A, Sarullo FM, Salerno Y, et al. Beta-blockers and ivabradine in chronic heart failure: from clinical trials to clinical practice. Am J Cardiovasc Drugs 2014;14:101-110.
98. Perry CM. Ivabradine: in adults with chronic heart failure with reduced left ventricular ejection fraction. Am J Cardiovasc Drugs 2012;12:415-426.
99. Bohm M, Swedberg K, Komajda M, et al. Heart rate as a risk factor in chronic heart failure (SHIFT): the association between heart rate and outcomes in a randomised placebo-controlled trial. Lancet 2010;376:886-894.
100. Dobre D, Borer JS, Fox K, et al. Heart rate: a prognostic factor and therapeutic target in chronic heart failure. The distinct roles of drugs with heart rate-lowering properties. Eur J Heart Fail 2014;16:76-85.
101. Swedberg K, Komajda M, Bohm M, et al. Ivabradine and outcomes in chronic heart failure (SHIFT): a randomised placebo-controlled study. Lancet 2010;376:875-885.
102. Eichhorn EJ, Gheorghiade M. Digoxin. Prog Cardiovasc Dis 2002;44:251-266.
103. Ambrosy AP, Butler J, Ahmed A, et al. The use of digoxin in patients with worsening chronic heart failure: reconsidering an old drug to reduce hospital admissions. J Am Coll Cardiol 2014;63:1823-1832.
104. Gheorghiade M, Adams KF, Jr., Colucci WS. Digoxin in the management of cardiovascular disorders. Circulation 2004;109:2959-2964.
105. Packer M, Gheorghiade M, Young JB, et al. Withdrawal of digoxin from patients with chronic heart failure treated with angiotensin-converting-enzyme inhibitors. RADIANCE Study. N Engl J Med 1993;329:1-7.
106. Uretsky B, Young JB, Shahidi FE, al e. Randomized study assessing the effect of digoxin withdrawal in patients with mild to moderate chronic congestive heart failure: results of the PROVED trial. J Am Coll Cardiol 1993;22:955-962.
107. The Digitalis Investigation Group. The effect of digoxin on mortality and morbidity in patients with heart failure. N Engl J Med 1997;336:525-533.
108. Ahmed A, Rich MW, Fleg JL, et al. Effects of digoxin on morbidity and mortality in diastolic heart failure: the ancillary Digitalis Investigation Group trial. Circulation 2006;114:397-403.
109. Ahmed A, Gambassi G, Weaver MT, Young JB, Wehrmacher WH, Rich MW. Effects of discontinuation of digoxin versus continuation at low serum digoxin concentrations in chronic heart failure. Am J Cardiol 2007;100:280-284.
110. Adams KF, Gheorghiade M, Uretsky BF, et al. Clinical benefits of low serum digoxin concentrations in heart failure. J Am Coll Cardiol 2002;39:946-953.
111. Ahmed A, Rich MW, Love TE, et al. Digoxin and reduction in mortality and hospitalization in heart failure: a comprehensive post hoc analysis of the DIG trial. Eur Heart J 2006;27:178-186.
112. Rathore SS, Wang Y, Krumholz HM. Sex-based differences in the effect of digoxin for the treatment of heart failure. N Engl J Med 2002;347:1403-1411.
113. Adams KF, Jr., Patterson JH, Gattis WA, et al. Relationship of serum digoxin concentration to mortality and morbidity in women in the Digitalis Investigation Group trial: a retrospective analysis. J Am Coll Cardiol 2005;46:497-504.
114. Bauman JL, Didomenico RJ, Galanter WL. Mechanisms, manifestations, and management of digoxin toxicity in the modern era. Am J Cardiovasc Drugs 2006;6:77-86.
115. See I, Shehab N, Kegler SR, Laskar SR, Budnitz DS. Emergency department visits and hospitalizations for digoxin toxicity: United States, 2005 to 2010. Circulation Heart failure 2014;7:28-34.
116. Schentag J, Bang A, Kozinski-Tober J. Digoxin. In: Burton M, Shaw L, Schentag J, Evans W, eds. Applied Pharmacokinetics and Pharmacodynamics. 4th ed. Baltimore Lippincott Williams & Wilkins; 2006:411-439.
117. DiDomenico RJ, Bress AP, Na-Thalang K, et al. Use of a simplified nomogram to individualize digoxin dosing versus standard dosing practices in patients with heart failure. Pharmacotherapy 2014;34:1121-31.
118. Allen LA, Fonarow GC, Simon DN, et al. Digoxin Use and Subsequent Outcomes Among Patients in a Contemporary Atrial Fibrillation Cohort. J Am Coll Cardiol 2015;65:2691-2698.
119. Freeman JV, Yang J, Sung SH, Hlatky MA, Go AS. Effectiveness and safety of digoxin among contemporary adults with incident systolic heart failure. Circ Cardiovasc Qual Outcomes 2013;6:525-533.
120. Gheorghiade M, van Veldhuisen DJ, Colucci WS. Contemporary use of digoxin in the management of cardiovascular disorders. Circulation 2006;113:2556-2564.
121. January CT, Wann LS, Alpert JS, et al. 2014 AHA/ACC/HRS guideline for the management of patients with atrial fibrillation: a report of the American College of Cardiology/American Heart Association Task Force on practice guidelines and the Heart Rhythm Society. Circulation 2014;130:e199-e267.
122. James PA, Oparil S, Carter BL, et al. 2014 evidence-based guideline for the management of high blood pressure in adults: report from the panel members appointed to the Eighth Joint National Committee (JNC 8). JAMA 2014;311:507-520.
123. Smith SC, Jr., Benjamin EJ, Bonow RO, et al. AHA/ACCF Secondary Prevention and Risk Reduction Therapy for Patients with Coronary and other Atherosclerotic Vascular Disease: 2011 update: a guideline from the American Heart Association and American College of Cardiology Foundation. Circulation 2011;124:2458-2473.
124. Thihalolipavan S, Morin DP. Atrial Fibrillation and Heart Failure: Update 2015. Prog Cardiovasc Dis 2015;58:126-135.
125. Turakhia MP, Santangeli P, Winkelmayer WC, et al. Increased mortality associated with digoxin in contemporary patients with atrial fibrillation: findings from the TREAT-AF study. J Am Coll Cardiol 2014;64:660-668.
126. Vamos M, Erath JW, Hohnloser SH. Digoxin-associated mortality: a systematic review and meta-analysis of the literature. Eur Heart J 2015;36:1831-1838.

127. Eurich DT, Weir DL, Majumdar SR, et al. Comparative safety and effectiveness of metformin in patients with diabetes mellitus and heart failure: systematic review of observational studies involving 34,000 patients. Circulation Heart failure 2013;6:395-402.
128. Green JB, Bethel MA, Armstrong PW, et al. Effect of Sitagliptin on Cardiovascular Outcomes in Type 2 Diabetes. N Engl J Med 2015;373:232-242.
129. von Lueder TG, Atar D, Krum H. Diuretic use in heart failure and outcomes. Clin Pharmacol Ther 2013;94:490-498.
130. Murray MD, Deer MM, Ferguson JA, et al. Open-label randomized trial of torsemide compared with furosemide therapy for patients with heart failure. Am J Med 2001;111:513-520.
131. Lopez B, Gonzalez A, Beaumont J, Querejeta R, Larman M, Diez J. Identification of a potential cardiac antifibrotic mechanism of torasemide in patients with chronic heart failure. J Am Coll Cardiol 2007;50:859-867.
132. Young M, Plosker GL. Torasemide: a pharmacoeconomic review of its use in chronic heart failure. Pharmacoeconomics 2001;19:679-703.
133. Ahmed A, Husain A, Love TE, et al. Heart failure, chronic diuretic use, and increase in mortality and hospitalization: an observational study using propensity score methods. Eur Heart J 2006;27:1431-1439.
134. Schoolwerth AC, Sica DA, Ballermann BJ, Wilcox CS. Renal considerations in angiotensin converting enzyme inhibitor therapy: a statement for healthcare professionals from the Council on the Kidney in Cardiovascular Disease and the Council for High Blood Pressure Research of the American Heart Association. Circulation 2001;104:1985-1991.
135. Antoniou T, Gomes T, Juurlink DN, Loutfy MR, Glazier RH, Mamdani MM. Trimethoprim-sulfamethoxazole-induced hyperkalemia in patients receiving inhibitors of the renin-angiotensin system: a population-based study. Arch Intern Med 2010;170:1045-1049.
136. Fralick M, Macdonald EM, Gomes T, et al. Co-trimoxazole and sudden death in patients receiving inhibitors of renin-angiotensin system: population based study. BMJ 2014;349:g6196.
137. Bangalore S, Kumar S, Messerli FH. Angiotensin-converting enzyme inhibitor associated cough: deceptive information from the Physicians' Desk Reference. Am J Med 2010;123:1016-1030.
138. Makani H, Messerli FH, Romero J, et al. Meta-analysis of randomized trials of angioedema as an adverse event of Renin-Angiotensin system inhibitors. Am J Cardiol 2012;110:383-391.
139. Miller DR, Oliveria SA, Berlowitz DR, Fincke BG, Stang P, Lillienfeld DE. Angioedema incidence in US veterans initiating angiotensin-converting enzyme inhibitors. Hypertension 2008;51:1624-1630.
140. Cooper WO, Hernandez-Diaz S, Arbogast PG, et al. Major congenital malformations after first-trimester exposure to ACE inhibitors. N Engl J Med 2006;354:2443-2451.
141. Braunwald E. The path to an angiotensin receptor antagonist-neprilysin inhibitor in the treatment of heart failure. J Am Coll Cardiol 2015;65:1029-1041.
142. King JB, Bress AP, Reese AD, Munger MA. Neprilysin Inhibition in Heart Failure with Reduced Ejection Fraction: A Clinical Review. Pharmacotherapy 2015;35:823-837.
143. The Beta-Blocker Evaluation of Survival Trial Investigators. A trial of the beta-blocker bucindolol in patients with advanced chronic heart failure. N Engl J Med 2001;344:1659-1667.
144. Poole-Wilson PA, Swedberg K, Cleland JG, et al. Comparison of carvedilol and metoprolol on clinical outcomes in patients with chronic heart failure in the Carvedilol Or Metoprolol European Trial (COMET): randomised controlled trial. Lancet 2003;362:7-13.
145. Aquilante CL, Terra SG, Schofield RS, et al. Sustained restoration of autonomic balance with long- but not short-acting metoprolol in patients with heart failure. J Card Fail 2006;12:171-176.
146. Frohlich H, Zhao J, Tager T, et al. Carvedilol Compared With Metoprolol Succinate in the Treatment and Prognosis of Patients With Stable Chronic Heart Failure: Carvedilol or Metoprolol Evaluation Study. Circulation Heart failure 2015;8:887-896.
147. Pasternak B, Svanstrom H, Melbye M, Hviid A. Association of treatment with carvedilol vs metoprolol succinate and mortality in patients with heart failure. JAMA Intern Med 2014;174:1597-1604.
148. Bakris GL, Fonseca V, Katholi RE, et al. Metabolic effects of carvedilol vs metoprolol in patients with type 2 diabetes mellitus and hypertension: a randomized controlled trial. JAMA 2004;292:2227-2236.
149. Deedwania PC, Giles TD, Klibaner M, et al. Efficacy, safety and tolerability of metoprolol CR/XL in patients with diabetes and chronic heart failure: experiences from MERIT-HF. Am Heart J 2005;149:159-167.
150. Prins KW, Neill JM, Tyler JO, Eckman PM, Duval S. Effects of Beta-Blocker Withdrawal in Acute Decompensated Heart Failure: A Systematic Review and Meta-Analysis. JACC Heart Fail 2015;3:647-653.
151. Jondeau G, Neuder Y, Eicher JC, et al. B-CONVINCED: Beta-blocker CONtinuation Vs. INterruption in patients with Congestive heart failure hospitalizED for a decompensation episode. Eur Heart J 2009;30:2186-2192.
152. Davis HM, Johnson JA. Heart failure pharmacogenetics: past, present, and future. Current Cardiol Rep 2011;13:175-184.
153. Bristow MR, Murphy GA, Krause-Steinrauf H, et al. An alpha2C-adrenergic receptor polymorphism alters the norepinephrine-lowering effects and therapeutic response of the beta-blocker bucindolol in chronic heart failure. Circ Heart Fail 2010;3:21-28.
154. McNamara DM, Tam SW, Sabolinski ML, et al. Endothelial nitric oxide synthase (NOS3) polymorphisms in African Americans with heart failure: results from the A-HeFT trial. J Card Fail 2009;15:191-198.
155. Rame JE, Tam SW, McNamara D, et al. Dysfunctional corin i555(p568) allele is associated with impaired brain natriuretic peptide processing and adverse outcomes in blacks with systolic heart failure: results from the Genetic Risk Assessment in Heart Failure substudy. Circulation Heart failure 2009;2:541-548.
156. Macdonald JE, Struthers AD. What is the optimal serum potassium level in cardiovascular patients? J Am Coll Cardiol 2004;43:155-161.
157. Bonow RO, Ganiats TG, Beam CT, et al. ACCF/AHA/AMA-PCPI 2011 performance measures for adults with heart failure: a report of the American College of Cardiology Foundation/American Heart Association Task Force on Performance Measures and the American Medical Association-Physician Consortium for Performance Improvement. J Am Coll Cardiol 2012;59:1812-1832.
158. Cleland JG, Tendera M, Adamus J, Freemantle N, Polonski L, Taylor J. The perindopril in elderly people with chronic heart failure (PEP-CHF) study. Eur Heart J 2006;27:2338-2345.
159. van Veldhuisen DJ, Cohen-Solal A, Bohm M, et al. Beta-blockade with nebivolol in elderly heart failure patients with impaired and preserved left ventricular ejection fraction: Data From SENIORS (Study of Effects of Nebivolol Intervention on Outcomes and Rehospitalization in Seniors With Heart Failure). J Am Coll Cardiol 2009;53:2150-2158.

15

Acute Decompensated Heart Failure

Jo E. Rodgers and Brent N. Reed

KEY CONCEPTS

1. Patients presenting to the hospital with acute decompensated heart failure (ADHF) can be categorized into four hemodynamic subsets based on volume status (euvolemic or "dry" vs volume overloaded or "wet") and cardiac output (adequate cardiac output or "warm" vs hypoperfusion or "cold"). Patients may be warm and dry, warm and wet, cold and dry, or cold and wet.
2. While invasive hemodynamic monitoring using a pulmonary artery (PA) catheter does not alter outcomes in a broad population of ADHF patients, it may be considered in those who are refractory to initial therapy, whose volume status is unclear, or in those with clinically significant hypotension (ie, systolic blood pressure <80 mm Hg) or worsening renal function despite standard therapy.
3. Key hemodynamic parameters monitored with a PA catheter include pulmonary capillary wedge pressure (PCWP; reflecting fluid status or "preload"), cardiac output or cardiac index (CI; reflecting the innate contractility of the heart), and systemic vascular resistance (SVR; reflecting vascular tone or "afterload"). Although a normal PCWP (6-12 mm Hg) is desirable in healthy patients, higher ventricular filling pressures (15-18 mm Hg) are often necessary in patients with heart failure (HF).
4. Treatment goals for ADHF include relief of congestive symptoms, restoration of systemic tissue perfusion via improved cardiac output, and minimization of further cardiac damage and other adverse effects.
5. Optimizing oral chronic HF therapy in the setting of ADHF may assist with improving cardiac output, relieving congestion, and preventing hospital readmission.
6. Pharmacologic therapies used in the management of ADHF can be broadly classified according to whether they improve volume overload and/or low cardiac output. No therapy studied to date has conclusively been shown to reduce mortality and several may potentially worsen outcomes.
7. Intravenous (IV) loop diuretics are considered first-line therapy for the management of ADHF associated with volume overload refractory to orally administered diuretics. Administration as a bolus or continuous infusion appears to be equally efficacious and safe when selected as initial therapy, although high-dose loop diuretic therapy (ie, up to 2.5-times the oral regimen prior to admission) is associated with greater volume removal. The addition of a thiazide-type diuretic may be considered in patients with diuretic resistance. If patients continue to be refractory to, or experience worsening renal function with diuretic therapy, IV vasodilators and/or inotropes may be indicated. Placement of a PA catheter may be helpful in guiding therapy in such patients.
8. Intravenous vasodilators may be added to diuretics for rapid resolution of congestive symptoms, especially in patients with acute pulmonary edema or severe hypertension. Such therapy may also be considered in patients who fail to respond to aggressive treatment with diuretics. Vasodilators should be avoided in patients with symptomatic hypotension or reduced left ventricular filling pressure. Frequent blood pressure monitoring is necessary to ensure their safe use.
9. Vasopressin antagonists such as tolvaptan may be considered in patients with severe euvolemic or hypervolemic hyponatremia. Therapy should only be initiated in a hospital setting to allow for monitoring of volume status and serum sodium concentrations, as rapid correction of serum sodium may result in adverse neurological sequelae.
10. Ultrafiltration may be considered in patients with diuretic resistance or those with worsening renal impairment despite IV vasodilator and/or inotrope therapy.
11. In the absence of hypotension (systolic blood pressure <90 mm Hg or symptomatic hypotension), IV vasodilators should be considered prior to IV inotropes in patients with ADHF and evidence of low cardiac output.
12. Intravenous inotropes are recommended for maintaining systemic perfusion and end-organ function in hypotensive patients with evidence of severe left ventricular dysfunction and low cardiac output. Inotropic therapy may also be considered in patients who do not tolerate or respond to IV vasodilators or in patients with worsening renal function despite standard therapy, but should be avoided in patients with reduced left ventricular filling pressures. Patients receiving IV inotropes should be monitored continuously for arrhythmias.
13. Temporary mechanical circulatory support (MCS) is indicated in select patients with severe ADHF or those with advanced HF who are refractory to pharmacologic therapy. The intra-aortic balloon pump (IABP) is the most common type of temporary MCS but provides the least amount of hemodynamic support. Other types of temporary MCS include ventricular assist devices (VADs) and extracorporeal membrane oxygenation (ECMO).
14. Cardiac transplantation remains the only definitive therapy for advanced HF. Given the extended wait time for identifying suitable donors, implantation of a durable VAD may be considered for patients who are eligible for cardiac transplantation (ie, "bridge to transplant" or BTT) or in whom transplantation is not an option (ie, "destination therapy" or DT).

INTRODUCTION

An estimated 5.7 million American adults have heart failure (HF) and projections indicate another 3 million will develop HF by 2030, a 50% increase in prevalence from prior estimates.[1,2] Despite survival from HF having improved over time, 5-year mortality remains 50%.[1] In addition, the growing number of patients living with HF has led to substantial increases in hospitalization rates. Recent data indicate that over 1 million patients are hospitalized for HF annually, contributing to significant increases in morbidity and mortality and adding substantial burden to the healthcare system.[1,3] Hospitalization for HF has been independently associated with increases in subsequent hospitalization as well as decreased survival.[3,4] The cost of HF is projected to approach $70 billion by 2030, an increase thought to be driven primarily by the costs of acute care.[2]

The clinical course of HF manifests as periods of relative stability with increasingly frequent episodes of decompensation as the disease progresses.[5] Several terms have been used to characterize worsening HF requiring hospitalization. Patients with persistent symptoms or advanced HF requiring specialized interventions (eg, surgery) despite guideline-directed medical therapy (GDMT) are classified as Stage D according to the American College of Cardiology Foundation/American Heart Association (ACCF/AHA) system.[6] Due to the presence of HF symptoms with minimal activity or at rest, these patients are also typically classified as New York Heart Association (NYHA) class III or IV, respectively. The terms *acute decompensated heart failure* (ADHF) or *exacerbation of heart failure* refer to those patients with new or worsening signs or symptoms of HF (often as a result of volume overload and/or low cardiac output [CO]) requiring medical intervention such as an emergency department visit or hospitalization. The term *acute heart failure* may be misleading as it more often refers to patients with a sudden onset of HF signs or symptoms following previously normal cardiac function (eg, following myocardial infarction [MI]). This chapter focuses on the management of patients with ADHF, which may include those with heart failure with reduced ejection fraction (HFrEF) or heart failure with preserved ejection fraction (HFpEF).

Despite the considerable morbidity and mortality associated with ADHF, few randomized controlled trials have been conducted in this patient population. For those studies that have been published, the heterogeneity of patients enrolled often limits clinical application. Nonetheless, a comprehensive update to the clinical practice guidelines for HF was issued by ACCF/AHA in 2013, including sections specifically focused on the management of advanced HF and ADHF (Sections 7.4 and 8.1-8.9, respectively); these will be referenced where relevant throughout the remainder of this chapter.[6]

ETIOLOGY AND PATHOPHYSIOLOGY

The underlying etiology of ADHF varies and is often multifactorial. *De novo* HF may occur due to left ventricular dysfunction following a large MI or sudden elevation in blood pressure; such cases represent approximately 25% of admissions.[7] However, the majority of hospitalizations for ADHF (70%) are comprised of patients experiencing an acute worsening of chronic HF;[7] readers are referred to (Chapter 14) for a more detailed discussion of the pathophysiology of chronic HF. Patients can become refractory to oral therapies and decompensate after even a relatively mild insult (eg, dietary indiscretion, nonsteroidal anti-inflammatory drug use), medication nonadherence, or concurrent noncardiac illness (eg, infection). New or worsening cardiac processes, such as MI, atrial or ventricular arrhythmias, hypertensive crises, myocarditis, or acute valvular insufficiency, may also produce ADHF in an otherwise stable patient. Emerging evidence indicates that exacerbations of chronic HFrEF and HFpEF occur in approximately equal numbers.[6] A minority of patients (5%) present with progressive worsening of CO and refractoriness to therapy due to advanced left ventricular systolic dysfunction.[7]

Several studies have provided a better understanding of the prognostic factors associated with ADHF. Data from the Acute Decompensated Heart Failure National Registry (ADHERE) found blood urea nitrogen (BUN) greater than or equal to 43 mg/dL to be the best individual predictor of in-hospital mortality, followed by systolic blood pressure less than 115 mm Hg and serum creatinine greater than or equal to 2.75 mg/dL. Using these three parameters, patients may be classified as low, intermediate, high, and very high risk, with in-hospital mortalities of 2%, 6%, 13%, and 20%, respectively.[8] Hyponatremia, elevations in troponin I, ischemic etiology, and poor functional capacity are also negative prognostic factors.[3] In the Organized Program to Initiate Lifesaving Treatment in Hospitalized Patients with Heart Failure (OPTIMIZE-HF) Registry, low blood pressure and poor renal function were found to be negative prognostic markers for subsequent readmission or death.[9] Use of GDMT at discharge as well as coronary angiography or implantable cardioverter-defibrillator placement during hospitalization were associated with improved prognosis, suggesting that optimal management during hospitalization can yield beneficial effects on subsequent prognosis.[9]

CLINICAL PRESENTATION

A careful history and physical examination are key components of an ADHF diagnosis. The history should focus on potential etiologies of ADHF, the presence of precipitating factors, onset, duration, and severity of symptoms, and a careful medication history. Hemodynamic status should also be ascertained in order to guide initial therapy. (1) Patients presenting with ADHF may be categorized into one of four hemodynamic subsets based on volume status (euvolemic or "dry" vs volume overloaded or "wet") and CO (adequate CO or "warm" vs hypoperfusion or "cold"). The corresponding subsets are warm and dry (subset I), warm and wet (subset II), cold and dry (subset III), or cold and wet (subset IV) (Fig. 15-1). The term *cardiogenic shock* may also be used to describe patients in subsets III and IV who present with low blood pressure and evidence of tissue hypoperfusion. In addition to guiding therapeutic decision-making, these four hemodynamic profiles are also predictive of clinical outcomes. Compared to dry-warm patients, patients in the wet-warm and wet-cold subsets have a 2-fold and 2.5-fold greater risk of death at 1 year, respectively.[10]

Although hemodynamic status can be determined in a majority of patients based on signs and symptoms, a small subset of patients may require invasive hemodynamic monitoring to guide therapy. In this latter population, measurement of the pulmonary capillary wedge pressure (PCWP) and cardiac index (CI) may be used to categorize patients by volume status and CO, respectively. A PCWP greater than 18 mm Hg often reflects volume overload and is used to distinguish "wet" from "dry" subsets, whereas a CI less than 2.2 mL/min/m^2 is often used to distinguish "cold" from "warm" subsets; use of these invasive hemodynamic parameters will be discussed in further detail later in this chapter.

Hospitalization for ADHF should be considered based on the clinical findings listed in (Table 15-1). Most patients do not require admission to an intensive care unit and may be admitted to a monitored unit or general medical floor. If a patient experiences hemodynamic instability necessitating frequent monitoring of vital signs, invasive hemodynamic monitoring, or rapid titration of IV medications (with concurrent monitoring), admission to an intensive care unit may be required to ensure optimal outcomes.

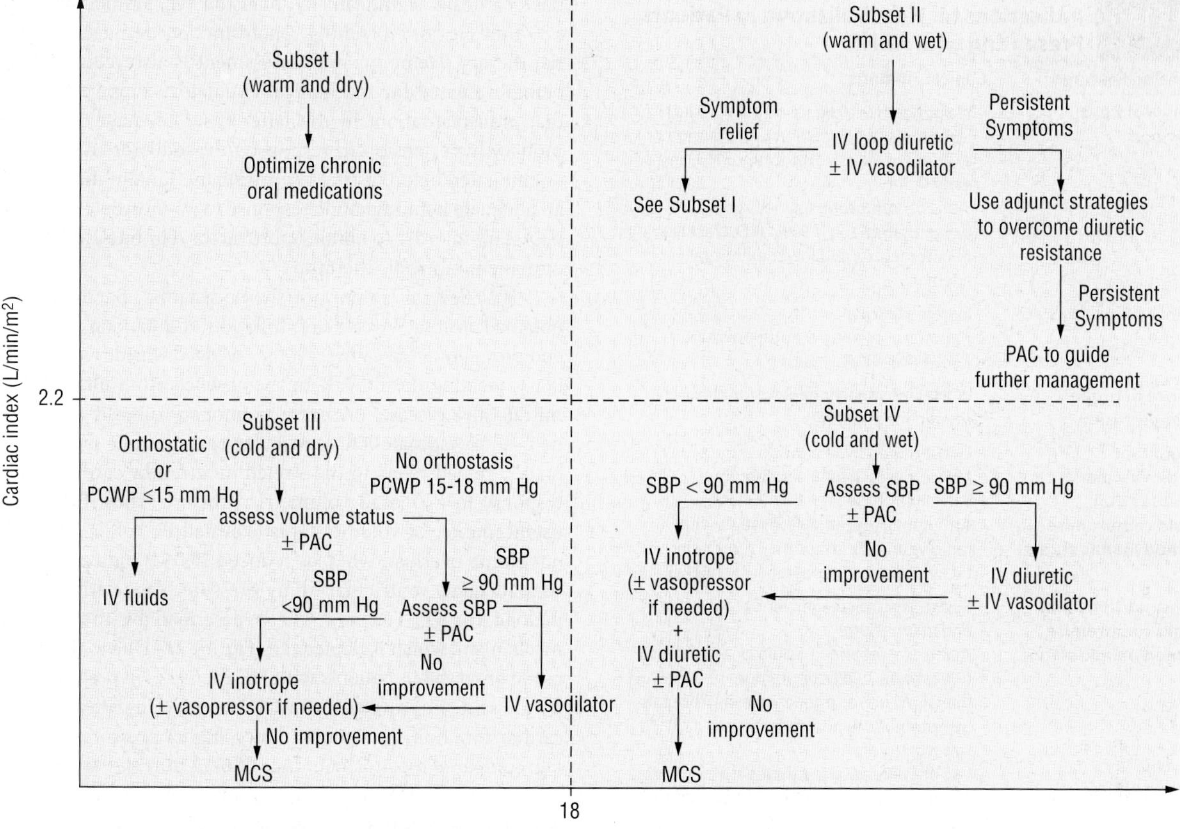

FIGURE 15-1 **General management algorithm for acute decompensated heart failure based on clinical presentation.** Patients may be categorized into a hemodynamic subset based on signs and symptoms or invasive hemodynamic monitoring. Adjunct strategies for overcoming diuretic resistance include increasing the dose of loop diuretic; switching to a continuous infusion; adding a diuretic with an alternative mechanism of action, an IV vasodilator, or an IV inotrope; and in select patients, ultrafiltration or a vasopressin antagonist. (IV, intravenous; MCS, mechanical circulatory support; PAC, pulmonary artery catheter; PCWP, pulmonary capillary wedge pressure; SBP, systolic blood pressure.)

Signs and Symptoms

Important elements of the physical examination include assessment of vital signs and weight, cardiac auscultation for heart sounds and murmurs, pulmonary auscultation for crackles, presence and severity of peripheral edema, and evidence of end-organ dysfunction. The most common presentation of ADHF is severe volume overload. Symptoms consistent with pulmonary congestion include orthopnea and dyspnea with minimal exertion, and those associated with systemic congestion include gastrointestinal (GI) discomfort, ascites, and peripheral edema. Orthopnea is the symptom that best correlates with elevated pulmonary pressure, whereas jugular venous pressure is the most reliable sign of volume status, warranting evaluation at admission as well as throughout the acute hospitalization as an indicator of diuretic efficacy.[10] An S3 gallop, suggestive of increased volume in the left ventricle, has high diagnostic specificity for ADHF.[10] Other physical findings, such as pulmonary crackles and lower extremity edema, have low specificity and sensitivity for the diagnosis of ADHF.

Signs and symptoms of low CO are often nonspecific and may include generalized fatigue, cool extremities, and pallor. Manifestations of impaired end-organ perfusion may also be present, such as altered mental status (decreased perfusion to the central nervous system) or decreased urine output (decreased renal perfusion). Hypotension and narrow pulse pressure may also suggest low CO. GI symptoms, such as poor appetite, nausea, and early satiety, may be a sign of poor perfusion to the GI tract, abdominal congestion, or both. Many patients will present with signs and symptoms of both wet and cold subsets; in these patients, symptoms of low CO may not be obvious until congestion has been optimally treated.

Laboratory Findings

Plasma B-type natriuretic peptide (BNP) and N-terminal pro-BNP concentrations are positively correlated with the degree of left ventricular dysfunction and HF, and are now frequently used to assist in the differential diagnosis of dyspnea (HF vs asthma, chronic obstructive pulmonary disease, or infection). A low BNP concentration, often defined as less than 100 pg/mL (ng/L; 29 pmol/L), has a 96% predictive value for excluding HF as an underlying etiology for dyspnea. In addition, an elevated BNP concentration prior to discharge is associated with an increased risk of poor long-term outcomes. However, some limitations exist. For example, any disease process that increases right heart pressures will elevate BNP, such as pulmonary emboli, chronic obstructive lung disease, and pulmonary arterial hypertension. In addition, BNP concentrations may be mildly increased with advanced age, female gender, and renal dysfunction, and lower in the setting of obesity.[10] Although the role of BNP in HF remains an area of ongoing research, guidelines currently recommend obtaining a BNP or NT-proBNP in order to assist with clinical decision-making when the diagnosis of ADHF is uncertain and for determining the prognosis or severity of disease.[6]

A number of other laboratory tests should also be obtained to identify precipitating factors for ADHF (eg, thyroid function tests,

TABLE 15-1 Indications for Hospitalization in Patients Presenting with ADHF

Presenting Features	Clinical Findings
Evidence of fluid overload	• Weight gain > 10 kg (consider if >5 kg) • Symptoms of congestion (eg, dyspnea on exertion or at rest, orthopnea, PND, and early satiety*) • Signs of congestion (eg, tachypnea + oxygen saturation < 90%, JVD, crackles, hepatomegaly, and lower extremity edema)
Evidence of low cardiac output	• Extreme fatigue • Hypotension, narrow pulse pressure • Cool extremities
Evidence of organ hypoperfusion	• Worsening renal or hepatic function • Altered mental status
Concomitant cardiovascular diseases that could compromise hemodynamic status	• Uncontrolled hypertension • Myocardial ischemia or infarction • Valvular disease • Arrhythmia (eg, atrial fibrillation with rapid ventricular response, ventricular tachycardia, and repeated ICD shocks)
Other conditions that could compromise hemodynamic status	• Severe electrolyte deficiency (potassium and magnesium) • Acute exacerbation of pulmonary disease (eg, asthma, COPD, or pulmonary embolus) • Infection such as pneumonia or urosepsis • Symptomatic hypothyroidism or hyperthyroidism • Use of medications with negative inotropic effects (eg, nondihydropyridine calcium antagonists) • Use of medications that promote fluid retention (eg, NSAIDs, steroids, thiazolidinediones, and pregabalin)

Abbreviations: COPD, chronic obstructive pulmonary disease; ICD, implantable cardioverter defibrillator; JVD, jugular venous distension; NSAIDs, nonsteroidal anti-inflammatory agents; PND, paroxysmal nocturnal dyspnea.

*Early satiety may also be a symptom of low cardiac output.

complete blood count to assess for infection). In particular, cardiac enzymes should be obtained to exclude the presence of myocardial ischemia. Routine serum chemistries (eg, serum creatinine, liver function tests) should also be obtained to assess end-organ perfusion. Profound volume overload may also contribute to aberrations in serum markers of end-organ function due to venous congestion. Other helpful laboratory tests include markers of peripheral tissue perfusion, such as venous oxygenation saturation and serum lactate concentrations.

Invasive Hemodynamic Monitoring

2 Invasive hemodynamic monitoring should be reserved for select patients with ADHF. Invasive hemodynamic monitoring is usually performed with a flow-directed pulmonary artery (PA) catheter (also known as Swan-Ganz catheter) placed percutaneously into a central vein and advanced through the right side of the heart and into the PA. This process may also be referred to as right heart catheterization (in contrast to left heart catheterization, which is often used to visualize the coronary arteries). In a clinical trial assessing routine PA catheter use in patients with ADHF, no impact on survival was observed, although those with a clear indication for its use (eg, titration of IV inotropes) were excluded.[11] Based on these results, the routine use of invasive hemodynamic monitoring in patients with ADHF is not currently recommended.[6] However, it often provides important information in patients whose clinical status is unclear or complicated, or as a guide for titrating rapidly acting medications (eg, IV vasodilators). As a consequence, invasive hemodynamic monitoring should be considered in patients who are refractory to initial therapy, those in whom volume status is unclear, or those who have clinically significant hypotension (eg, systolic blood pressure <80 mm Hg) or worsening renal function despite appropriate initial therapy. Hemodynamic assessment is also required in patients being evaluated for mechanical circulatory support (MCS) or cardiac transplantation; in the latter case, adequate reversal of pulmonary hypertension in response to vasodilator challenge must be documented before listing for transplant. Finally, documentation of an adequate hemodynamic response to IV inotropic therapy is often necessary in order to obtain approval for reimbursement for chronic outpatient inotropic therapy.[6]

3 Several important hemodynamic parameters can be obtained from a PA catheter. Inflation of a balloon proximal to the end port allows the catheter to be "wedged" inside a pulmonary capillary, yielding the PCWP. In the absence of an intracardiac shunt, mitral valve disease, or severe pulmonary disease, the PCWP may be used to estimate left ventricular end-diastolic pressure, or "preload." Preload refers to the stretch incurred by cardiac myocytes in response to increased volumetric pressure. Thus, PCWP can be a useful marker of volume status; elevated PCWP is often indicative of volume overload whereas reduced PCWP indicates dehydration or inadequate ventricular filling pressure. The relationship between preload (or PCWP) and CO is described by the Frank-Starling mechanism, which is depicted in Fig. 15-2A. Due to the much flatter curve observed in patients with HF, increases in preload do not confer the same improvements in CO observed in patients with normal cardiac function. As a consequence, higher pressures (ie, 15-18 mm Hg, compared to a normal range of 6-12 mm Hg) are often required in patients with HF in order to optimize CO. Excess preload (PCWP >18 mm Hg) manifests as signs and symptoms of congestion. Fortunately, PCWP can be lowered to 15 to 18 mm Hg with relatively little decrease in CO due to the flatter shape of the Frank-Starling curve in HF. Extreme elevations in PCWP (representing profound volume overload) are also thought to worsen cardiac function, although a mechanism for this phenomenon is not clearly understood.

A PA catheter may also be used to determine CO, or the volume of blood being pumped by the heart (particularly by the left ventricle) over a unit of time. CO is often normalized for body surface area to yield CI, which allows measurements to be made without regard to body size. Using parameters derived from the PA catheter, CO is calculated based on one of two methods. The thermodilution method for determining CO is performed by releasing cooled fluid from a proximal port on the PA catheter and measuring the resulting change in temperature at a downstream thermistor over a period of time. In the Fick method, blood flow is calculated using the difference between arterial and venous oxygen concentration, oxygen-carrying capacity of hemoglobin, and a population constant for oxygen consumption over time. The preferred method for determining CO varies by clinician, although the presence of certain comorbid conditions (eg, valvular abnormalities and pulmonary disease) may make one method more or less accurate in an individual patient.

The systemic vascular resistance (SVR) can also be calculated using parameters measured by the PA catheter, including CO, mean arterial pressure (MAP), and central venous pressure (CVP). Also referred to as total peripheral resistance or arterial impedance, SVR reflects "afterload," or the total sum of forces impeding ejection of blood from the left ventricle. Vasoconstriction (ie, decreased diameter of arterial vessel lumen) increases vascular resistance, whereas vasodilation decreases it. Although SVR is inversely related to CO, patients with normal left ventricular function can often withstand relatively high elevations in SVR, as shown in Fig. 15-2B. However, in patients with HF, even a moderately elevated SVR can compromise left ventricular performance. Elevated SVR is common in untreated HF and generally responsive to oral or IV vasodilators. Conversely, a reduction in resistance is consistent with vasodilatory shock (eg, sepsis) and is routinely managed with IV vasopressor therapy (see Chapter 23).

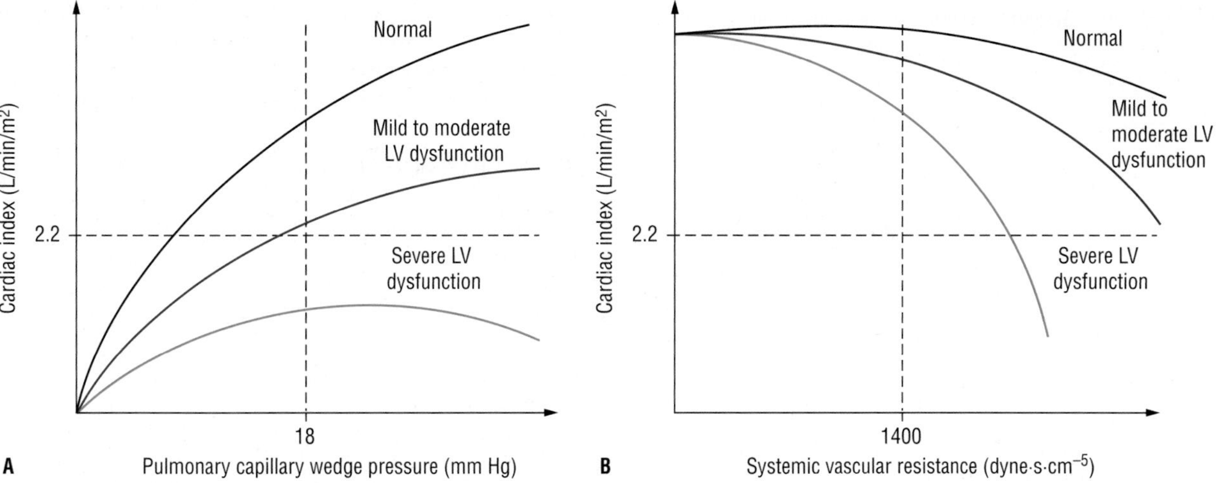

FIGURE 15-2 **Hemodynamic alterations in heart failure.** Figure A is an illustration of the relationship between cardiac output (displayed as cardiac index, which is cardiac output normalized for body surface area) and preload (displayed as pulmonary capillary wedge pressure) according to severity of left ventricular function. Figure B is an illustration of the corresponding relationship between cardiac output and afterload (displayed as systemic vascular resistance). (LV, left ventricular.)

A PA catheter can also be used to measure pulmonary vascular resistance (PVR), which represents the impedance of blood flow from the right ventricle to the pulmonary circulation. Pulmonary hypertension and pulmonary edema are two common causes of elevated PVR. As described previously, patients with elevated pulmonary pressure must have proven reversibility (in response to vasodilator challenge) prior to being listed for heart transplantation. Otherwise, if elevations in PVR are irreversible, isolated right ventricular failure is likely to occur immediately following heart transplantation. Just as SVR is calculated using MAP, PVR is calculated using the mean PA pressure, which incorporates the PA systolic and diastolic pressures. The PA diastolic pressure may also be useful if the PA catheter fails to wedge (making it impossible to obtain PCWP). If the PCWP and PA diastolic pressure have been correlated prior to the failure to wedge, then the PA diastolic pressure may be followed as a surrogate marker of volume status. Normal values for the aforementioned hemodynamic parameters are listed in Table 15-2.

TABLE 15-2 Normal Hemodynamic Values

Central Venous (Right Atrial) Pressure, mean, CVP	<5 mm Hg
Right Ventricular Pressure (Systolic/Diastolic)	25/0 mm Hg
Pulmonary Artery Pressure (Systolic/Diastolic), PAS/PAD	25/10 mm Hg
Pulmonary Arterial Pressure, mean, PAP	<18 mm Hg
Pulmonary Capillary Wedge Pressure, PCWP	<12 mm Hg
Systemic Arterial Pressure (Systolic/Diastolic), SBP/DBP	120/80 mm Hg
Mean Arterial Pressure, MAP = (DBP+[1/3 (SBP-DBP])	70-110 mm Hg
Cardiac Output, CO	4-6 L/min
Cardiac Index, CI = CO/BSA	2.8-4.2 L/min/m^2
Systemic Vascular Resistance, SVR = ([MAP–CVP]*80)/(CO)	900-1,400 dyne·sec·cm^{-5}
Pulmonary Vascular Resistance, PVR = ([PAP–CVP]*80)/(CO)	150-250 dyne·sec·cm^{-5}
Arterial Oxygen Saturation	90%-94%
Mixed Venous Oxygen Saturation	60%-80%

Abbreviation: BSA, body surface area.

TREATMENT

Desired Outcomes

4 The overall goals of therapy in ADHF are to provide symptomatic relief while optimizing volume status and CO so that a patient can be discharged in a stable compensated state on oral drug therapy. Although IV diuretic, vasodilator, and inotropic therapy can be very effective at achieving these goals, their efficacy must be balanced against the potential for serious adverse effects. All patients should also be evaluated for precipitating factors of ADHF, including arrhythmias, hypertension, myocardial ischemia or infarction, anemia, and thyroid disorders. Patients who may benefit from coronary revascularization should also be identified. Medications (including noncardiac medications) that may worsen cardiac function should also be evaluated. Prior to discharge, optimization of chronic oral therapy and patient education are critical to preventing rehospitalization. When available and appropriate, patients should be referred to an HF disease management program.[6]

General Approach to Treatment

An important step in the management of ADHF is to first assess medications being taken prior to admission and determine whether adjustment or discontinuation is required. If fluid retention is evident on physical examination, aggressive diuresis should be pursued. Although increasing the dose of oral diuretic therapy may be effective in some cases, the use of IV diuretics is often necessary. 5 In the absence of cardiogenic shock or symptomatic hypotension, every effort should be made to continue all GDMT for HF. β-blocker therapy may be temporarily held or dose-reduced if recent initiation or up-titration is responsible for acute decompensation. Otherwise, β-blocker discontinuation is discouraged as it has been associated with worse outcomes in patients with ADHF.[12,13] Appropriateness of initiating β-blockers prior to discharge will be discussed later in this chapter.

Select GDMT may also need to be temporarily held in the setting of renal dysfunction, especially if oliguria or hyperkalemia is present (eg, ACE inhibitors, angiotensin receptor blockers, neprilysin inhibitors, aldosterone antagonists). Therapies that may cause worsening renal function (eg, ACE inhibitor) should only be initiated or up-titrated cautiously during aggressive volume removal with IV diuretic therapy. Additionally, serum potassium concentrations should be monitored closely as IV diuretic therapy is transitioned

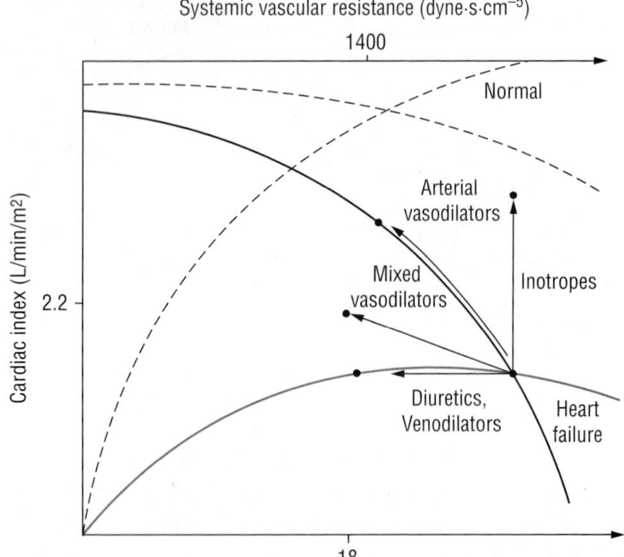

FIGURE 15-3 **Hemodynamic effects of pharmacologic therapy in acute decompensated heart failure.** Pharmacologic agents used in the management of acute decompensated heart failure exert important effects on cardiovascular hemodynamics. Although diuretics and venodilators reduce preload, this does not substantially reduce cardiac output in heart failure due to a flatter Frank-Starling curve. Arterial vasodilators reduce afterload, producing an increase in cardiac output as a consequence of improved left ventricular performance. Vasodilators with effects on both venous and arterial tissue may reduce both preload and afterload. Inotropes improve contractility directly, although some agents (eg, milrinone) may exert salutary effects on afterload via vasodilation.

to oral diuretic therapy, especially if an aldosterone antagonist has been initiated during the hospital stay; this ensures therapy can be tolerated on the intended oral diuretic dose prescribed at discharge. Most patients may continue to receive digoxin at doses targeting a trough serum concentration of 0.5 to 1 ng/mL.[6] Discontinuation of digoxin is generally discouraged as an association between withdrawal of therapy and worsening HF has been well-documented.[14,15] Digoxin should only be discontinued if serum concentrations cannot be safely maintained within the desirable range.

6 The acute management of ADHF is based primarily on hemodynamic status. The hemodynamic subsets described previously were first proposed for patients with left ventricular dysfunction following acute MI but are also applicable to patients with ADHF due to other causes.[16] Two general approaches exist for determining hemodynamic status. One is to use simple clinical parameters (eg, signs and symptoms, blood pressure, and organ function) and the other is to use these in conjunction with invasive hemodynamic monitoring. A management algorithm based on hemodynamic subset is depicted in Fig. 15-1. The hemodynamic effects exerted by pharmacologic therapies used in the management of ADHF are illustrated in Fig. 15-3.

Subset I (Warm and Dry)

Patients in subset I generally do not have signs and symptoms of volume overload or hypoperfusion and usually have CI and PCWP values within appropriate ranges. Patients in this subset have the lowest risk of mortality and do not require immediate intervention other than optimization of GDMT for HF. Patients with significant left ventricular dysfunction may still present in subset I because normal compensatory mechanisms and/or drug therapy may at least partially correct an otherwise abnormal hemodynamic profile.

Subset II (Warm and Wet)

Patients in subset II are likely to present with signs and symptoms of congestion (eg, orthopnea and peripheral edema) due to increased hydrostatic pressure in the pulmonary and systemic circulation, but without evidence of peripheral hypoperfusion. As a consequence, they often have adequate CO but a PCWP greater than 18 mm Hg. The primary goal of therapy in these patients is to relieve symptoms of congestion by lowering PCWP without reducing CO, increasing heart rate, or provoking neurohormonal activation.

Intravenous agents that reduce preload via diuresis and/or direct venodilation (eg, loop diuretics) are the most appropriate initial therapy for patients presenting in subset II. Despite a very rapid onset, the time required for significant improvement in oxygenation with IV loop diuretics may take several hours in select patients. Thus, IV vasodilators with effects on primarily the venous vasculature (eg, nitroglycerin) may be utilized for rapid venodilation (see Fig. 15-3), which can aid in acutely improving hypoxia. IV vasodilators should especially be considered in patients with acute pulmonary edema or severe hypertension but avoided in patients with symptomatic hypotension. Continuous blood pressure monitoring should be performed during IV vasodilator use. If symptomatic hypotension occurs with vasodilator therapy, the dose should be reduced or the agent discontinued. Resistance to loop diuretics may occur, requiring dose escalation or addition of thiazide-type diuretics. If patients fail to respond to the above therapies or experience worsening renal function, IV inotropic therapy (with or without PA catheter insertion) should be considered.

Patients in subset II should also be placed on a sodium restriction (<2 g daily). In patients with moderate hyponatremia (<130 mEq/L), fluid restriction (<2 L daily) should be considered, and in patients with worsening or severe hyponatremia (<125 mEq/L), stricter fluid restriction may be necessary.[6] Arginine vasopressin (AVP) antagonists may also be considered for severe euvolemic or hypervolemic hyponatremia, particularly if symptoms emerge. Finally, supplemental oxygen should be administered as needed for hypoxemia.

Subset III (Cold and Dry)

Patients in subset III present with evidence of peripheral hypoperfusion (eg, weakness, decreased urine output, and weak pulses) but no signs or symptoms of congestion. They often present with a CI of less than 2.2 L/min/m^2 but no abnormal elevation in PCWP. The mortality rate of patients in subset III is higher than that of patients with adequate perfusion.[16] Although the treatment goal is to alleviate signs and symptoms of hypoperfusion by increasing CI and perfusion to essential organs, therapy may differ based on initial presentation. If evidence of hypovolemia exists (eg, orthostatic hypotension) or PCWP is below 15 mm Hg, IV fluids should be administered to provide a more optimal left ventricular filling pressure (ie, 15-18 mm Hg), consequently improving CI (see Fig. 15-1). As this presentation most often occurs in the setting of overly aggressive diuresis, diuretic therapy should be withheld and fluid restriction liberalized; these interventions alone may obviate the need for IV fluids.

When only mild left ventricular dysfunction is present, IV fluid administration may be all that is necessary to achieve a CI above 2.2 L/min/m^2). However, in patients with more advanced HF, IV positive inotropic agents (eg, dobutamine and milrinone) and/or IV arterial vasodilators (eg, nitroprusside or nesiritide) may be necessary to achieve adequate CI (see Fig. 15-3). As with vasodilators,

IV inotrope administration requires frequent blood pressure monitoring as well as continuous monitoring for arrhythmias. If arrhythmias occur, dose reduction or discontinuation of inotropic therapy should be performed. IV inotropes should also be avoided in patients with low left ventricular filling pressure. In general, inotropic should be reserved for patients with evidence of severely low CO who are not candidates for IV vasodilators (ie, hypotension). They may also be used to "bridge" patients to MCS or heart transplantation, or as palliative therapy to improve functional status and quality of life in patients who are ineligible for definitive therapies.

Subset IV (Cold and Wet)

Patients in subset IV present with signs and symptoms of both volume overload and peripheral hypoperfusion, and often have a CI of less than 2.2 L/min/m^2 and a PCWP exceeding 18 mm Hg. This subset is characterized by the worst prognosis of all four and represents the most common hemodynamic profile for patients with end-stage HF. Given the severity of HF, patients in subset IV cannot maintain adequate CI despite elevated left ventricular filling pressure and increased myocardial fiber stretch. Treatment goals for these patients include alleviation of signs and symptoms associated with congestion and hypoperfusion by increasing CI to above 2.2 L/min/m^2 and reducing PCWP to 15 to 18 mm Hg while maintaining adequate MAP. Therapy often involves a combination of agents used in subsets II and III (ie, combination of IV diuretic plus vasodilator or inotrope). These targets may be difficult to achieve and often necessitate careful monitoring and individualization of drug therapy. In the presence of significant hypotension and low MAP, vasodilators should be avoided. In some cases, even the vasodilating effects of inotropic therapy may compromise MAP, requiring that combined inotrope and vasopressor therapy (eg, dobutamine plus norepinephrine) or an inotrope with vasopressor activity (eg, dopamine) be used to achieve adequate end-organ perfusion. Once peripheral perfusion has been restored, therapy can then be adjusted to obtain the desired clinical response (see Fig. 15-1).

PHARMACOLOGIC MANAGEMENT OF VOLUME OVERLOAD

Although IV loop diuretics are the mainstay of therapy for volume overload in ADHF, several additional therapies may be used in conjunction with loop diuretics in select patients. Until recently, an understanding of the appropriate management of volume overload had not substantially improved due to a dearth of clinical trial data in this population. However, several recent trials have expanded our understanding of both agent selection as well as method of administration, although many questions remain.

Diuretics

7 IV loop diuretics, including furosemide, bumetanide, and torsemide, are used commonly in the management of ADHF (Table 15-3), and furosemide remains the most widely studied and used in this setting. Current guidelines recommend the use of loop diuretics as first-line therapy for patients with ADHF and volume overload, and that they typically be administered IV.[6] Bolus administration reduces preload within 5 to 15 minutes by functional venodilation and later (>20 minutes) via sodium and water excretion, thereby improving pulmonary congestion. However, an acute reduction in venous return may severely compromise effective preload in patients with significant diastolic dysfunction, intravascular depletion, or those in whom CI is significantly dependent on adequate filling pressure (ie, preload-dependent). This reduction in preload may cause reflex neurohormonal activation (ie, elevation of renin, norepinephrine, and AVP), resulting in arteriolar and coronary vasoconstriction, tachycardia, and increased myocardial oxygen consumption. Unlike arterial vasodilators and positive inotropic agents, diuretics do not cause an upward shift in the Frank-Starling curve or significantly increase CO in most patients (see Table 15-3 and Fig. 15-3). In fact, excessive preload reduction (ie, PCWP of <15 mm Hg) can lead to a decline in CO (see Fig. 15-3). Although counterintuitive, patients with excessive fluid overload may initially present with compromised CO, which may improve with diuresis once PCWP approaches the normal range (see Fig. 15-3); this may explain why renal function occasionally improves in the setting of diuresis. Alternatively, the kidneys may simply be responsive to a reduction in venous congestion, similar to the improvement observed when an obstruction is removed in postrenal acute kidney injury.

Despite relative overload of total body fluid, intravascular volume depletion may occur in the setting of rapid diuresis due to a delay in the migration of fluid from the interstitial space back into the systemic vasculature. Most patients tolerate a two liter per day net negative diuresis. However, some patients with advanced HF will only tolerate a one liter per day net negative diuresis. Patients who are malnourished due to the early satiety commonly observed in advanced HF (as a consequence of abdominal edema and/or

TABLE 15-3 Diuretics Commonly Utilized for the Management of ADHF

	Furosemide	Bumetanide	Torsemide	Metolazone	Hydrochlorothiazide	Chlorothiazide
Mechanism	Loop diuretic	Loop diuretic	Loop diuretic	Thiazide-type diuretic	Thiazide-type diuretic	Thiazide-type diuretic
Oral Bioavailability	10%-100% (mean 50%)	80%-90%	80%-100%	40%-65%	65%-75%	N/A
Dose Equivalence (IV)	20-40 mg	0.5-1 mg	10-20 mg	N/A	N/A	N/A
Usual Intermittent Dose (maximum)	40-160 mg IV once to three times daily (200 mg/dose)	0.5-4 mg IV once to three times daily (5 mg/dose)	IV no longer available	2.5-5 mg PO once daily (20 mg/day)	25-50 mg PO once daily (100 mg/day)	500 mg-1 g IV once or twice daily (2 g/day)
Usual Continuous Infusion Dose (maximum)	5-20 mg/hr (40 mg/hr)	0.5-2 mg/hr (4 mg/hr)	IV no longer available	N/A	N/A	N/A
Onset of action (Peak effect)	30-60 min PO, 5 mins IV (2 hrs)	30-60 min PO, 2-3 mins IV (1-2 hrs)	1 hr PO (1-2 hrs)	2-3 hrs (6-8 hrs)	2 hrs (4 hrs)	2 hrs (3-6 hrs)
Duration of action	4-6 hrs	4-6 hrs	18-24 hrs	12-24 hrs	5-15 hrs	6-12 hrs

Abbreviations: CrCl, creatinine clearance; IV, intravenous; N/A, not applicable; PO, oral.

reduced perfusion to the GI tract) may be especially sensitive to rapid shifts in intravascular volume, as decreased oncotic pressure resulting from hypoalbuminemia decreases the rate at which fluid can effectively migrate from the interstitial space into the intravascular space. Due to these and other factors, diuretic therapy must be highly individualized in order to obtain the desired improvement in congestive symptoms while avoiding a reduction in CO, symptomatic hypotension, or worsening renal function. Electrolyte depletion should also be monitored closely, especially when high doses or combination diuretic therapy is utilized.

Adjunct Diuretics

Occasionally patients respond less optimally to escalating doses of loop diuretics, a phenomenon known as diuretic resistance. HF is the most common clinical setting in which this phenomenon is observed and multiple retrospective analyses suggest that diuretics, especially aggressive administration, may be associated with dose-dependent increases in mortality.[17] Evidence also suggests that high doses are associated with renal dysfunction in ADHF, which only further exacerbates diuretic resistance.[18,19] As a consequence, the need for increased exposure to diuretics in the setting of resistance warrants concern.

The mechanisms responsible for diuretic resistance in patients with HF are thought to be both pharmacokinetic and pharmacodynamic in nature.[20] The oral bioavailability of furosemide is relatively unchanged in patients with HF as long as GI perfusion has not been compromised, but the rate of absorption is prolonged by approximately twofold and peak concentrations are reduced by approximately half. Because loop diuretics have a sigmoidal-shaped concentration-response curve, prolonged absorption may result in concentrations that fail to reach the threshold necessary for producing effective diuresis. Resistance is also observed with IV administration, suggesting an equally important pharmacodynamic contribution to this phenomenon. The decreased responsiveness in patients with HF may be explained in part by compensatory reabsorption in the distal convoluted tubule in response to the high concentrations of sodium resulting from blocked reabsorption in the loop of Henle. Over time, the distal tubule may also undergo hypertrophy, thereby enhancing its ability to reabsorb sodium. Finally, neurohormonal activation, impaired CO, reduced renal perfusion, and decreased drug delivery to the kidney may also contribute to resistance.

Several strategies may be employed to overcome diuretic resistance. Current guidelines recommend one of two pharmacologic options in patients who do not initially respond to diuretic therapy: increased doses of loop diuretics or addition of an alternative diuretic with a different mechanism of action (eg, thiazide-type diuretics).[6] First, higher doses of loop diuretics are more likely to achieve concentrations near the top of the concentration-response curve. Although higher doses produce greater diuresis, these effects are not associated with improved long-term outcomes and must be weighed against the risk for transient worsening of renal function.[21] Importantly, guidelines emphasize higher doses may be administered as either an IV bolus or continuous infusion.[6] The use of continuous infusion loop diuretics has been considered another approach for overcoming diuretic resistance. Several small studies suggest a greater natriuretic effect with no difference in metabolic adverse effects when continuous infusion furosemide is compared to the same total daily dose given by IV bolus.[22,23] In contrast, a prospective randomized trial of 308 patients with ADHF compared low and high-dose furosemide administered as a continuous infusion or intermittent IV bolus every 12 hours; although differences were observed in the comparison of low and high-dose furosemide, no differences in relief of symptoms, urine output, weight loss, or long-term outcomes were observed between continuous infusion or intermittent IV bolus administration.[21] Importantly, the trial only evaluated the selection of initial diuretic therapy and did not specifically enroll patients with diuretic resistance, thus the role of continuous infusion diuretics in this population remains unknown.

A second strategy for overcoming diuretic resistance is to add a second diuretic with a different mechanism of action. Combining a loop diuretic with a distal tubule blocker such as oral metolazone, oral hydrochlorothiazide, or IV chlorothiazide (see Table 15-3) can produce a synergistic diuretic effect. Inhibition of sodium reabsorption in the loop of Henle increases sodium delivery to (and reabsorption in) the distal convoluted tubule, which can be subsequently blocked by a thiazide-type diuretic. The combination of a loop and thiazide-type diuretic should generally be reserved for hospitalized patients, as profound diuresis with severe electrolyte and intravascular volume depletion may occur. If used in the outpatient setting, very low doses or infrequent administration (eg, one to three times weekly) of a thiazide-type diuretic should be recommended. Patients should also receive close follow-up (eg, weight, vital signs, serum potassium, and assessment for orthostatic hypotension) to avoid serious adverse events.

Non-pharmacologic strategies for managing diuretic resistance include further limiting sodium and fluid beyond routinely recommended restrictions previously described (ie, less than 1 g and less than 1 L per day, respectively).

Vasodilators

8 IV vasodilators may also be helpful in select patients with refractory volume overload. The most commonly used IV vasodilators in ADHF are sodium nitroprusside, nitroglycerin, and nesiritide, and each can be classified according to its most prominent site of action (ie, arterial or venous circulation) (Table 15-4). As described in the section on patients in subset II, venodilators act as preload reducers by increasing venous capacitance, thus reducing symptoms of pulmonary congestion in patients with high ventricular filling pressures. Arterial vasodilators act as impedance-reducing agents, thereby reducing afterload and causing a reflexive increase in CO, which may promote diuresis via improved renal perfusion. Mixed vasodilators act on both resistance and capacitance vessels, reducing congestive symptoms while increasing CO. Nitroglycerin and nesiritide will be the focus of this section, as data to support their use for refractory congestive symptoms is the most robust. Because sodium nitroprusside demonstrates several unique properties that make it a reasonable consideration in patients with low CO, it will be discussed later in this chapter.

Nitroglycerin

Intravenous nitroglycerin is often preferred for preload reduction in patients with ADHF, especially those with evidence of pulmonary congestion. Because of its short half-life (1-3 minutes), IV nitroglycerin is administered by continuous infusion. Its major hemodynamic effects are reductions in preload and PCWP via functional venodilation and mild arterial vasodilation that is particularly evident in patients with HF and elevated SVR or when given in doses approaching 200 mcg/min (see Table 15-4). In higher doses, nitroglycerin displays potent coronary vasodilating properties, exerting beneficial effects on myocardial oxygen demand and supply and making it the vasodilator of choice for patients with severe HF and ischemic heart disease.

Nitroglycerin should be initiated at a dose of 5 to 10 mcg/min (0.1 mcg/kg/min) and increased every 5 to 10 minutes as tolerated. Hypotension and an excessive decrease in PCWP are important dose-limiting side effects. Maintenance doses usually vary from 35 to 200 mcg/min (0.5-3 mcg/kg/min). While tolerance to the hemodynamic effects of nitroglycerin may develop over 12 to 72 hours of continuous administration, some patients experience a sustained response. Like sodium nitroprusside, nitroglycerin should not be

TABLE 15-4 Vasodilators Commonly Utilized for the Management of ADHF[a]

Drug (Vasodilatory effect)	Onset, Half-life	Elimination	Dose	HR	MAP	PCWP	CO	SVR
Nitroglycerin (venous > arterial)	Immediate, <4 mins	Inactive metabolites in urine	10-20 mcg/min and titrate 10-20 mcg/min q10-20 mins, max 200 mcg/kg/min	0/↑	0/↓	↓	0/↑	0/↓
Nitroprusside (venous = arterial)	Immediate, 2 mins	Cyanide (hepatic), thiocyanate (renal)	0.1-0.2 mcg/ kg/min, titrate 0.1-0.2 mcg/kg/min q10-20 mins, max 3 mcg/kg/min	0/↑	0/↓	↓	↑	↓
Nesiritide (venous = arterial, natriuresis)	15 mins, 20 mins	Natriuretic peptide receptor C (no renal/ hepatic adjustment)	0.01 mcg/kg/min, titrate 0.005 mcg/kg/min q3 hrs, max 0.03 mcg/kg/min (IVB dose generally avoided)	0	0/↓	↓	↑	↓
Furosemide (venous only)	1 hr (PO)/ 5 mins (IV), 2 hrs	Urine	Variable[b]	0	0/↓	↓	0	0
Enalaprilat (arterial > venous)	N/A/11 hrs	Urine	1.25-2.5 mg q6-8h	0	0/↓	↓	↑	↓

Abbreviations: ↑, increase; ↓, decrease; 0, no change; HR, heart rate; MAP, mean arterial pressure; PCWP, pulmonary capillary wedge pressure; CI, continuous infusion; CO, cardiac output; IVB, intravenous bolus; SVR, systemic vascular resistance.

[a]See text for a more detailed description of the interpatient variability in response.

[b]Intravenous bolus administered <0.4 mg/min.

used in the presence of elevated intracranial pressure because it may worsen cerebral edema in this setting.

In contrast to sodium nitroprusside, one prospective randomized controlled trial has evaluated nitroglycerin in patients with ADHF. This study compared nitroglycerin to placebo as well as nesiritide and will be discussed in the following section.[24]

Nesiritide

Nesiritide is a recombinant form of BNP, which is secreted by the myocardium in response to volume overload. Exogenous administration of nesiritide mimics the vasodilatory and natriuretic actions of BNP by stimulating natriuretic peptide receptor A, leading to increased concentrations of cyclic guanosine monophosphate (cGMP) in target tissues. Nesiritide produces dose-dependent venous and arterial vasodilation; increases CO, natriuresis, and diuresis; decreases cardiac filling pressures; and impairs activation of the sympathetic nervous system and renin-angiotensin-aldosterone system. In contrast to nitroglycerin or dobutamine, tolerance does not develop to the pharmacologic actions of nesiritide. It also does not affect cyclic adenosine monophosphate (cAMP) or β-receptors, mechanisms thought to contribute to the myocardial toxicity associated with inotropes (eg, proarrhythmia). Nesiritide is eliminated by several metabolic pathways, including natriuretic peptide receptor C located on target tissues, proteolytic cleavage by neutral endopeptidase, and renal filtration. At 18 minutes, its elimination half-life is considerably longer than that of other IV vasoactive agents.

In a randomized, double-blind trial comparing nesiritide to nitroglycerin or placebo in patients with ADHF and dyspnea, nesiritide improved the incidence of dyspnea at 3 hours when compared to placebo but failed to demonstrate a significant difference compared to nitroglycerin.[24] In the subset of patients who received PA catheterization (permitted at the discretion of the investigators), nesiritide reduced PCWP at 3 hours when compared to both placebo and nitroglycerin. Two meta-analyses raised concern for an increased risk of adverse events with nesiritide, including an increased risk of worsening renal function and mortality.[25-27] In a large prospective randomized controlled trial designed to address these concerns, 7,141 patients hospitalized for ADHF were randomized to receive nesiritide at 0.01 mcg/kg/min (with an optional 2 mcg/kg IV bolus) or placebo for up to 7 days.[28] Nesiritide did not increase mortality nor worsen renal function. Rehospitalization for HF at 30 days was also not affected by the use of nesiritide, nor was patient self-assessment of dyspnea symptoms after 6 hours and 24 hours of treatment. In a more recent trial assessing the role of low-dose nesiritide (0.005 mcg/kg/min) added to IV loop diuretics in patients with ADHF and renal impairment, no improvements in urine output, congestive symptoms, or renal function were observed.[29] Despite the lower dose utilized in the trial, rates of hypotension were still higher in patients randomized to nesiritide.

Taken altogether, these trials indicate a limited role for nesiritide beyond the relief of congestive symptoms in patients with acute dyspnea. As a consequence, the use of nesiritide in the contemporary management of patients with ADHF has declined due to marginal improvements in clinical outcomes and its higher cost compared to other IV vasodilators.

Vasopressin Antagonists

Physiologic fluid balance depends on relative concentrations of sodium and water. An abnormally low serum sodium concentration, or *hyponatremia*, is commonly defined as less than 125 mmol/L and can be classified as hypovolemic, euvolemic (urine sodium <30 mmol/L), or hypervolemic (urine sodium >30 mmol/L) in nature. HF is most commonly associated with hypervolemic hyponatremia, although excess diuretic administration may result in hypovolemic hyponatremia. Other causes of hyponatremia include syndrome of inappropriate diuretic hormone (SIADH), cirrhosis with ascites, and medications.

Hyponatremia is often characterized by inappropriately elevated concentrations of AVP, or antidiuretic hormone. In the setting of HF, reduced CO leads to excess stimulation of arterial baroreceptors, which in turn enhances AVP secretion and consequently, net water retention. While the prevalence of hyponatremia in patients with HF varies by definition, as many as 1 in 5 patients hospitalized for acute HF present with serum sodium concentrations less than 136 mmol/L.[30] Furthermore, the presence of hyponatremia has been associated with increased mortality in this population.[31]

While many cases of hyponatremia are mild, asymptomatic, and self-limited, prompt diagnosis and management is critical for the less common but life-threatening presentation, which may include lethargy, confusion, respiratory arrest, cerebral edema, seizures, coma, or death. Treatment is specific to the underlying etiology, as well as duration and severity of symptoms. Strategies for managing hyponatremia include removal of the underlying cause, fluid restriction, isotonic or hypertonic saline administration, or administration of diuretics, vasopressin antagonists, or other therapies. Importantly, while neurological sequelae may occur if treatment is not initiated promptly, overly rapid correction of hyponatremia (>12 mmol/L per 24 hours) may be just as detrimental.

9 The two currently available vasopressin receptor antagonists, tolvaptan and conivaptan, inhibit one or two AVP receptors, V_{1A} or V_2. Stimulation of V_{1A} receptors, which are present in vascular smooth muscle and myocardium, results in vasoconstriction as well as myocyte hypertrophy, coronary vasoconstriction, and positive inotropic effects. V_2 receptors are located in the renal tubules where they regulate water reabsorption. Tolvaptan selectively binds to and inhibits the V_2 receptor, whereas conivaptan nonselectively inhibits both V_{1A} and V_2 receptors. Tolvaptan is orally bioavailable and indicated for the management of hypervolemic and euvolemic hyponatremia in patients with SIADH, cirrhosis, or HF. Tolvaptan is typically initiated at 15 mg daily and then titrated to 30 mg or 60 mg as needed for resolution of hyponatremia. Importantly, tolvaptan is a substrate of cytochrome P450 3A4 and is contraindicated with potent inhibitors of this enzyme. Conivaptan is an IV agent indicated for hypervolemic and euvolemic hyponatremia resulting from a variety of causes; however, because it is not indicated in patients with HF, conivaptan will not be discussed in further detail here. Patients receiving vasopressin antagonists must be monitored closely to avoid an overly rapid rise in serum sodium, which may result in hypotension or hypovolemia, requiring that therapy be discontinued. Therapy may be restarted at a lower dose if hyponatremia recurs or persists and/or adverse effects resolve.

The role of vasopressin antagonists in the long-term management of HF remains unclear at this time. In a trial comprised entirely of hospitalized patients with NYHA class III-IV HF, tolvaptan was associated with significant improvement in hyponatremia compared to placebo.[32,32] Additionally, patients receiving tolvaptan experienced an improvement in diuresis and symptoms of congestion. However, the study failed to demonstrate an improvement in global clinical status at discharge or a reduction in 2-year all-cause mortality, cardiovascular mortality, or HF rehospitalization.

Overall, tolvaptan is well tolerated; common side effects include dry mouth, thirst, urinary frequency, constipation, and hyperglycemia. While tolvaptan is orally available, therapy in clinical trials was initiated in the inpatient setting, where serum sodium and volume status could be closely monitored. Because of the adverse consequences of rapid changes in serum sodium concentrations or fluid balance, caution should be exerted when initiating therapy.

Ultrafiltration

Renal impairment is common among patients with ADHF, and advanced forms may warrant the use of renal replacement therapy (eg, hemodialysis). 10 Ultrafiltration has emerged as another strategy for rapid fluid removal, where salt and water may be eliminated at rates of up to 500 mL/h. Ultrafiltration reduces PCWP and increases diuresis without adversely affecting hemodynamics. Potential candidates for ultrafiltration include patients demonstrating diuretic resistance, renal impairment following diuretic administration, or continued renal impairment despite inotropic therapy. Complications of ultrafiltration include those associated with central venous access (eg, infection), rapid volume removal, and intravascular depletion, although electrolyte depletion is generally less significant compared to other modalities.

Small studies suggest that ultrafiltration represents an effective strategy for fluid removal in HF patients and that early initiation prior to IV diuretics reduces hospital length of stay and readmission rates. In a study comparing early ultrafiltration to IV diuretics in patients with ADHF and evidence of fluid overload, ultrafiltration resulted in greater weight loss at 48 hours (5 kg vs 3.1 kg) as well as net fluid loss (4.6 L vs 3.3 L), although no differences in dyspnea scores were observed.[33] Several additional endpoints were improved among patients in the ultrafiltration group, including the incidence and duration of rehospitalization and incidence of unscheduled office or emergency department visits at 90 days. Although these results were promising, a more recent study challenged these findings.[34] Patients with ADHF, worsened renal function, and persistent congestion were randomized to a strategy of stepped pharmacologic therapy or ultrafiltration. Ultrafiltration was inferior to pharmacologic therapy with respect to the bivariate endpoint of change from baseline in serum creatinine and body weight at 96 hours, primarily due worsening renal function in the ultrafiltration group. There was also no significant difference in weight loss and more patients in the ultrafiltration group experienced a serious adverse event. Subsequently, use of ultrafiltration has received greater scrutiny and ongoing trials are attempting to determine its role in managing volume overload.

Inotropes

Resistance to diuretic therapy may also result from worsening renal perfusion due to low CO. As a consequence, IV inotropes or arterial vasodilators may improve diuresis by improving central hemodynamics. However, given the adverse effect profile of IV inotropes, therapy should generally be reserved for patients not responding to other modalities or those with clear evidence of low CO (discussed in detail later in this chapter).

Administration of low doses of dopamine (ie, 2-5 mcg/kg/min) to enhance diuresis was once common practice, but evidence to support its use remains controversial, as most studies indicate minimal if any improvement in diuresis.[35] Despite an initial prospective randomized trial suggesting dopamine offered renal protection during aggressive diuresis, more recent investigations assessing low doses in conjunction with IV loop diuretics demonstrated no improvements in urine output, renal protection, or symptom relief, but with increased rates of tachycardia.[29,36,37] Given evidence of β-mediated effects at lower infusion rates, dopamine may not provide any advantages over a traditional inotrope when used in this setting.

MANAGEMENT OF LOW CARDIAC OUTPUT

Patients in subsets III and IV ("cold" subsets) require prompt correction of low CO in order to restore peripheral tissue perfusion and preserve end-organ function. The two most common pharmacologic strategies for improving CO in ADHF are the IV vasodilators and inotropes. Due to the risks associated with IV inotrope therapy, IV vasodilators are preferred although hypotension often precludes their use in many patients with advanced HF.

Importantly, these agents rarely, if ever, produce a single cardiovascular action. Even when intended for a specific purpose (eg, positive inotropic effects), other cardiovascular effects (tachycardia, vasodilation, or vasoconstriction) may either add to the therapeutic effect of the drug, or cause adverse effects that negate or even outweigh its intended therapeutic benefit. How an individual patient will respond to an intervention is often difficult to anticipate. For this reason, hemodynamic monitoring with a PA catheter may be useful.

Vasodilators

11 Current guidelines focus on the role of vasodilators in improving refractory congestive symptoms,[6] but they may also be helpful for

restoring CO in select patients. Activation of the sympathetic nervous system, renin–angiotensin–aldosterone system, and other neurohormonal mediators are characteristic features of both acute and chronic HF. Peripheral vasoconstriction and increased SVR often results, leading to a severe decline in stroke volume and thus CO. In these patients, IV vasodilators may be used to reduce arterial impedance, leading to improved left ventricular performance. However, for patients in whom SVR is already low, including those receiving GDMT with vasodilating effects (eg, ACE inhibitors) or those with advanced HF, hypotension may preclude the use of IV vasodilators. Additionally, their use has not been extensively studied in patients with HFpEF. Agents with venodilating effects should be used with caution in this latter population, as a sudden drop in preload may further compromise defects in ventricular filling.

As described previously, vasodilators are commonly classified according to their most prominent site of action (ie, arterial or venous circulation) (see Table 15-4; Fig. 15-3). Recall that in the setting of volume overload, agents with venodilatory effects are selected to reduce preload and filling pressures. However, in states of low CO, arterial vasodilators are selected to reduce afterload, resulting in a reflexive increase in CO. In the setting of both volume overload and low CO, mixed vasodilators (ie, sodium nitroprusside and nesiritide), which act on both resistance and capacitance vessels, may be selected to reduce congestive symptoms while simultaneously increasing CO. The following section will focus on the use of sodium nitroprusside, as other vasodilators have been discussed previously.

Sodium Nitroprusside

Sodium nitroprusside increases synthesis of nitric oxide in vascular smooth muscle, resulting in balanced arterial and venous vasodilation. As a result, it increases CI and decreases venous pressure to a similar degree as dobutamine and milrinone despite having no direct inotropic activity; however, greater decreases in PCWP, SVR, and blood pressure are generally observed. MAP may remain fairly constant due to reflexive improvements in stroke volume and CO but can decrease based on the extent of arterial smooth muscle relaxation. Patients with normal left ventricular function do not experience an increase in stroke volume when SVR falls because the normal ventricle is fairly insensitive to changes in afterload. Consequently, these patients may experience a significant decrease in blood pressure in response to arterial vasodilators. These differences explain why sodium nitroprusside is a potent antihypertensive agent in patients without HF but causes less hypotension and reflex tachycardia in the presence of left ventricular dysfunction (see Fig. 15-2B). Nonetheless, hypotension remains an important dose-limiting effect of sodium nitroprusside and its use should be primarily reserved for patients with elevated SVR. Close monitoring of therapy is warranted, as even modest increases in heart rate can have adverse consequences in patients with underlying ischemic heart disease and/or resting tachycardia.

Sodium nitroprusside is an effective strategy for short-term management of patients with severe HF across a variety of settings (eg, acute MI, valvular regurgitation, postcoronary bypass surgery, and ADHF). Generally, sodium nitroprusside does not worsen, and may even improve, the balance between myocardial oxygen demand and supply by lowering both left ventricular wall tension (thus reducing oxygen demand) and end-diastolic pressure (thereby increasing subendocardial blood flow). However, an excessive decrease in systemic arterial pressure may reduce coronary perfusion and worsen ischemia due to coronary steal.

Sodium nitroprusside has a rapid onset of action but its effects last less than 10 minutes, necessitating administration by continuous IV infusion. This method of administration also allows precise dose-titration based on clinical and hemodynamic response. As with other vasodilators used in ADHF, sodium nitroprusside should be initiated at low doses (0.1-0.2 mcg/kg/min) to avoid excessive hypotension and increased by small increments (0.1-0.2 mcg/kg/min) every 5 to 10 minutes as tolerated. Effective doses usually range from 0.5 to 3 mcg/kg/min. A rebound phenomenon, which may be due to reflex neurohormonal activation during sodium nitroprusside therapy, has been reported following abrupt withdrawal in patients with HF. Therefore, therapy should be tapered slowly when transitioning patients to oral medications. If renal perfusion pressure is compromised by sodium nitroprusside administration, salt and water retention may contribute to volume expansion and tachyphylaxis, although this is typically only observed in patients with chronic hypertension, baseline azotemia, or when augmentation of CO during therapy is minimal. Sodium nitroprusside should be avoided in the presence of elevated intracranial pressure as it may worsen cerebral edema in this setting. Given the potent pulmonary vasodilatory effects of sodium nitroprusside as well as its short half-life, it is frequently used to determine reversibility of pulmonary hypertension in patients being evaluated for heart transplantation.

Following IV administration, sodium nitroprusside interacts with hemoglobin to release cyanide, which undergoes hepatic conversion to thiocyanate before it is eliminated renally. As a consequence, sodium nitroprusside can cause cyanide and thiocyanate toxicity, but these effects are unlikely when doses less than 3 mcg/kg/min are administered for less than 3 days, except in patients with significant renal impairment (ie, serum creatinine concentration >3 mg/dL).

Unfortunately, no prospective randomized controlled trials have investigated the use of sodium nitroprusside in patients with ADHF. However, in one of the many retrospective studies in this population, patients with a reduced CI (ie, ≤2 L/min/m^2) treated with sodium nitroprusside (n = 78) experienced a reduction in all-cause mortality (P = 0.005) compared to patients who did not receive sodium nitroprusside (n = 97).[38] At baseline, patients receiving nitroprusside tended to have higher MAP, increased cardiac filling pressures, and lower CI, but the observed improvements in mortality remained even after including only those patients who had initial MAP less than or equal to 85 mm Hg (P = 0.0001).

Inotropes

12 Although IV inotropes can improve peripheral hypoperfusion by directly enhancing cardiac contractility, their association with adverse outcomes necessitates that they be reserved for select patients with refractory ADHF. Current guidelines recommend that inotrope therapy be considered only as a temporizing measure for maintaining end-organ perfusion in patients with cardiogenic shock or evidence of severely depressed CO and low systolic blood pressure (ie, ineligible for IV vasodilators) until definitive therapy can be initiated, as a "bridge" for those with advanced HF who are eligible for MCS or cardiac transplantation, or for palliation of symptoms in patients with advanced HF who are not eligible for MCS or cardiac transplantation.[6] Much of the concern regarding use of IV inotrope therapy in patients with ADHF is based on data from the ADHERE Registry (n = 15,230), which compared in-hospital mortality among patients receiving IV nitroglycerin, nesiritide, or the inotropes milrinone or dobutamine.[39] After adjusting for baseline parameters known to predict in-hospital mortality, both dobutamine- and milrinone-treated patients experienced higher in-hospital mortality compared to those receiving either nitroglycerin or nesiritide (P < 0.005). In-hospital mortality was higher among patients receiving dobutamine compared to milrinone (P = 0.027), and no difference in in-hospital mortality was observed between nitroglycerin- and nesiritide-treated patients (P = 0.58). Only one randomized controlled trial has prospectively evaluated the use of IV inotropic therapy as a strategy for improving clinical outcomes in patients with ADHF but no evidence of hypoperfusion. In 949 patients with ADHF randomized to a 48-hour infusion of milrinone or placebo,

no difference in length of stay was observed and adverse events were more common in the milrinone group, including sustained hypotension requiring intervention (10.7% vs 3.2%; $P < 0.001$) and new onset of atrial fibrillation or flutter (4.6% vs 1.5%; $P = 0.004$).[40]

Select populations with advanced HF may require placement of an indwelling IV catheter for continuous outpatient administration of inotropic therapy. This approach may be used to "bridge" patients awaiting durable MCS or cardiac transplantation, or as a palliative approach to facilitate discharge in patients who are not candidates for these advanced therapies but also cannot be weaned from inotropic support. Therapy in this latter group should only be considered after multiple unsuccessful attempts have been made to maximize oral therapy and discontinue IV inotropes. Although this strategy may be effective for symptom palliation, the risk of mortality is likely increased.

The two IV inotropic agents most commonly used for the management of ADHF are dobutamine and milrinone. Although both drugs increase intracellular concentrations of cAMP, they do so by different mechanisms. Dobutamine activates adenylate cyclase through direct stimulation of β-adrenergic receptors, thus catalyzing the conversion of adenosine triphosphate to cAMP, whereas milrinone reduces degradation of cAMP by inhibiting phosphodiesterase type 3. Increased intracellular cAMP enhances phospholipase (and subsequently phosphorylase) activity, increasing the rate and extent of calcium influx during systole and thus enhancing contractility. Additionally, cAMP enhances reuptake of calcium by the sarcoplasmic reticulum during diastole, improving active relaxation. Comparisons between dobutamine and milrinone indicate that the two agents generally produce similar hemodynamic effects, although dobutamine is usually associated with more pronounced increases in heart rate. Differences in the pharmacologic effects of the two agents may confer advantages or disadvantages in an individual patient; these and other clinical considerations for their use in the management of ADHF will be reviewed in the sections to follow.

Digoxin has a limited role in hemodynamically unstable patients due to its limited inotropic effects. In patients who take digoxin as chronic therapy, discontinuation or dose-adjustment during an acute decompensation is generally unnecessary unless changes in renal function increase the risk of toxicity. As discussed previously in this chapter, discontinuation should be discouraged in the absence of toxicity given the potential for digoxin withdrawal.[14,15]

Dobutamine

The receptor activities of dobutamine and other adrenergic agonists are summarized in Table 15-5. Dobutamine, a synthetic catecholamine, is a β_1- and β_2-receptor agonist with some α_1-agonist effects. Unlike dopamine, dobutamine does not result in the release of norepinephrine from nerve terminals. Consequently, the positive inotropic effects of dobutamine are attributed to its effects on β_1-receptors. Stimulation of cardiac β_1-receptors by dobutamine does not generally produce a significant change in heart rate, thus explaining its more modest chronotropic effects compared with dopamine. Modest peripheral β_2-receptor-mediated vasodilation tends to offset minor α_1-receptor-mediated vasoconstriction. In addition, the increase in CO often results in a reflexive decline in SVR. As a consequence, the net hemodynamic effect of dobutamine, particularly at low doses, is usually vasodilation.

The effects of dobutamine are observed within minutes but its peak effects may take up to 10 minutes to occur given an elimination half-life of 2 minutes. Initial doses of 2.5 to 5 mcg/kg/min may be increased progressively to 20 mcg/kg/min based on clinical and hemodynamic responses. CI is increased due to inotropic stimulation, arterial vasodilation, and a variable increase in heart rate. Because of offsetting changes in arteriolar resistance and CI, dobutamine usually causes relatively little change in MAP, unlike the more consistent increases observed with dopamine. The vasodilating action of dobutamine usually reduces PCWP, making it particularly useful in the presence of low CI and an elevated left ventricular filling pressure; conversely, these effects may be detrimental in the presence of a reduced filling pressure. Although its impact on heart rate is variable, the major adverse effects of dobutamine are tachycardia and ventricular arrhythmias. Potentially detrimental increases in oxygen consumption have also been observed. While concerns exist regarding the attenuation of its effects during prolonged administration, changes in receptor expression require that dobutamine be slowly tapered rather than abruptly discontinued.

Milrinone

Milrinone is a bipyridine derivative that inhibits phosphodiesterase III, an enzyme responsible for the breakdown of cAMP to adenosine monophosphate (AMP). Milrinone has supplanted the use of its prototype amrinone due to less frequent occurrence of thrombocytopenia. Because both inotropic and vasodilating effects contribute to its therapeutic effects in ADHF, milrinone is often referred to as an inodilator. The relative balance of these pharmacologic effects may vary with dose and underlying cardiovascular pathology.

During IV administration, milrinone produces an increase in stroke volume (and therefore CO) with minimal change in heart rate (see Table 15-5). Despite an increase in CI, MAP may remain constant due to a concomitant decrease in arteriolar resistance. However, the vasodilating effects of milrinone may predominate, leading to a decrease in blood pressure and reflex tachycardia. Like dobutamine, milrinone lowers PCWP by venodilation and thus is particularly useful in patients with a low CI and an elevated left ventricular

TABLE 15-5 Inotropes Commonly Utilized for the Management ADHF[a]

Drug	Onset, Half-life	Dose	Receptor Affinity ($\alpha_1/\beta_1/\beta_2/DA_1$)	HR	MAP	PCWP	CO	SVR
Dobutamine	<10 mins, 2 mins	1-2 mcg/kg/min, titrate 1-2 mcg/kg/min q10-20 mins, max 20 mcg/kg/min	↑/↑↑↑↑/↑↑/0	0/↑	0	↓	↑	↓
Milrinone	5-15 min, 1-4 hr, (prolonged if renal dysfunction)	0.1-0.2 mcg/kg/min, titrate 0.1 mcg/kg/min q4-16 hrs (titrate slowly in renal dysfunction), max 0.75 mcg/kg/min (IVB dose generally avoided)	Phosphodiesterase inhibition	0/↑	0/↓	↓	↑	↓
Dopamine	2 mins	0.5-3 mcg/kg/min	0/0/0/↑↑	0	0	0	0/↑	↓
		3-10 mcg/kg/min	0/↑↑↑↑/↑↑/↑↑	↑	↑	0	↑	0
		10-20 mcg/kg/min	↑↑↑↑/↑↑↑↑/↑↑/↑↑	↑	↑	↑	↑	↑

[a]See text for a more detailed description of the dose-dependent hemodynamic effects.

filling pressure. Such a reduction in preload, however, can be hazardous for patients without excessive filling pressure (especially those in subset III), thus blunting the improvement in CO produced by the positive inotropic and arterial dilating actions of milrinone. Furthermore, milrinone should be used cautiously in severely hypotensive patients because it does not increase, and may even decrease, arterial blood pressure.

Milrinone has a longer elimination half-life than other vasoactive agents. In healthy subjects, the half-life of milrinone is about 1 hour but may be as long as 3 to 6 hours in patients with renal dysfunction. The long elimination half-life of milrinone presents several disadvantages in this patient population, including the inability to perform minute-to-minute titrations based on hemodynamic changes and persistence of adverse effects (eg, arrhythmias or hypotension) following drug discontinuation. Although a loading dose is still listed in the product labeling for milrinone (50 mcg/kg administered over 10 minutes), this practice is uncommon due to an increased risk of hypotension. Most patients are started on a maintenance infusion of 0.1 to 0.3 mcg/kg/min (up to 0.75 mcg/kg/min), although lower initial doses may be considered. Milrinone is excreted unchanged in the urine, and thus, its infusion rate should be decreased by 50% to 70% in patients with significant renal impairment.

The most notable adverse effects associated with milrinone are arrhythmia, hypotension, and thrombocytopenia. Although the incidence of thrombocytopenia is rare, patients should still have platelet counts measured before and during therapy.

Inotrope Selection

Although inotrope selection is often clinician-dependent, certain characteristics may make one agent more ideal in an individual patient. Dobutamine should be considered when a significant decrease in MAP might further compromise hemodynamic function, as this is more common with the initiation of milrinone. Selection of an inotropic drug should also take into account whether patients are receiving chronic β-blocker therapy and whether a β_1-selective agent (eg, metoprolol succinate) or mixed α, β-blocking agent (eg, carvedilol) is used. Traditionally, milrinone has been advocated in patients who are receiving chronic β-blocker therapy because its inotropic effects do not involve β-receptor stimulation. However, this is not supported by evidence. In fact, the hemodynamic effects of dobutamine may persist in the presence of β-blocker therapy, particularly with β_1-selective agents as a result of β-receptor upregulation or selective activation of β_2-receptors by dobutamine.[41] Similar effects are not observed in the presence of carvedilol, which may inhibit the hemodynamic benefits of dobutamine entirely.[41] Concomitant β-blocker therapy may augment the hemodynamic effects of milrinone based on studies with a structurally similar phosphodiesterase inhibitor, enoximone.[41]

The combination of dobutamine and milrinone is likely to produce additive effects on CO and PCWP, suggesting that this regimen may be considered in patients who have dose-limiting adverse effects with either drug class. However, whether this combination provides a therapeutic advantage over the combined use of a positive inotrope and a traditional vasodilator (eg, sodium nitroprusside) is unclear.

Agents with Combined Inotropic and Vasopressor Activity

Although therapies that can increase SVR are generally avoided in ADHF, agents with combined inotropic and vasopressor activity, such as norepinephrine or dopamine, may be required in select scenarios where marked systemic hypotension may preclude the use of traditional IV inotropes (eg, septic shock, refractory cardiogenic shock). Alternatively, these agents may be used in combination with traditional inotropes so that adjustments can be made to each agent independently in order to achieve the desired hemodynamic response. Although these strategies are common in clinical practice, minimal data exist to support their use.

Norepinephrine is an endogenous catecholamine that exerts its hemodynamic effects via direct stimulation of α_1- and β_1-adrenergic receptors. Its effects on β_1-adrenergic receptors in myocardial tissue are thought to confer improvements in CO as a result of increases in heart rate and cardiac contractility. However, despite having similar affinity for α_1- and β_1-adrenergic receptors, enhanced vasoconstriction via activation of peripheral α_1-receptors appears to be the predominant hemodynamic effect observed clinically. The limited impact of norepinephrine on CO may be due to its lack of affinity for β_2-receptors, which would both enhance cardiac contractility as well as balance its effects on α_1-receptors in vascular smooth muscle. In contrast with dopamine, the affinity of norepinephrine for adrenergic receptors does not appreciably differ based on dose.

Dopamine is an endogenous precursor of norepinephrine and exerts its effects by directly stimulating adrenergic receptors as well as causing release of norepinephrine from adrenergic nerve terminals. Dopamine produces dose-dependent hemodynamic effects as a result of its relative affinity for α_1-, β_1-, β_2-, and D_1- (vascular dopaminergic) receptors (see Table 15-5).

The positive inotropic effects of dopamine are mediated primarily by β_1-receptors and become more prominent at doses of 2 to 5 mcg/kg/min. CI is increased because of an increase in stroke volume and a variable increase in heart rate, which is also partially dose-dependent. Minimal changes in SVR occur, presumably because neither vasodilation (D_1- and β_2-receptor-mediated) nor vasoconstriction (α_1-receptor-mediated) predominates. However, at doses between 5 and 10 mcg/kg/min, chronotropy and α_1-receptor-mediated vasoconstriction become more prominent. MAP is usually raised as a result of increases in both CI and SVR (see Table 15-5).

The vasoconstriction observed with higher doses of norepinephrine and dopamine may limit improvements in CI by concomitantly increasing afterload and preload. As a consequence, they should generally be reserved for patients with low CO and low systolic blood pressure despite adequate ventricular filling pressures, or as an adjunct to inotrope therapy when hypotension precludes the use of inotrope therapy alone. At higher doses, agents with vasopressor activity may alter several parameters that increase myocardial oxygen demand (eg, increased heart rate, contractility, and systolic pressure) and potentially decrease myocardial blood flow (eg, coronary vasoconstriction and increased wall tension), which may worsen ischemia in patients with coronary artery disease. As with dobutamine and milrinone, arrhythmogenesis is also more common at higher doses, although this risk appears to be greater with dopamine than with norepinephrine.[42]

Temporary Mechanical Circulatory Support

13 For patients with refractory ADHF, temporary MCS may be considered for hemodynamic stabilization until the underlying etiology of cardiac dysfunction resolves or has been corrected ("bridge to recovery") or until evaluation for definitive therapy (eg, durable MCS or cardiac transplantation) can be completed ("bridge to decision").[6] Due to the invasive nature of MCS and its potential complications, therapy should be reserved for patients who are refractory to maximally tolerated pharmacologic therapy. IV vasodilators and inotropic agents may also be used in conjunction with temporary MCS to maximize hemodynamic and clinical benefits or to facilitate device removal. Regardless of the modality selected, systemic anticoagulation is required to prevent device thrombosis. Temporary MCS should generally be avoided in patients with irreversible advanced HF and no plan for definitive management, those with contraindications to anticoagulation therapy, and those with comorbid conditions or anatomical abnormalities that preclude device implantation. The three most common modalities of temporary MCS are the

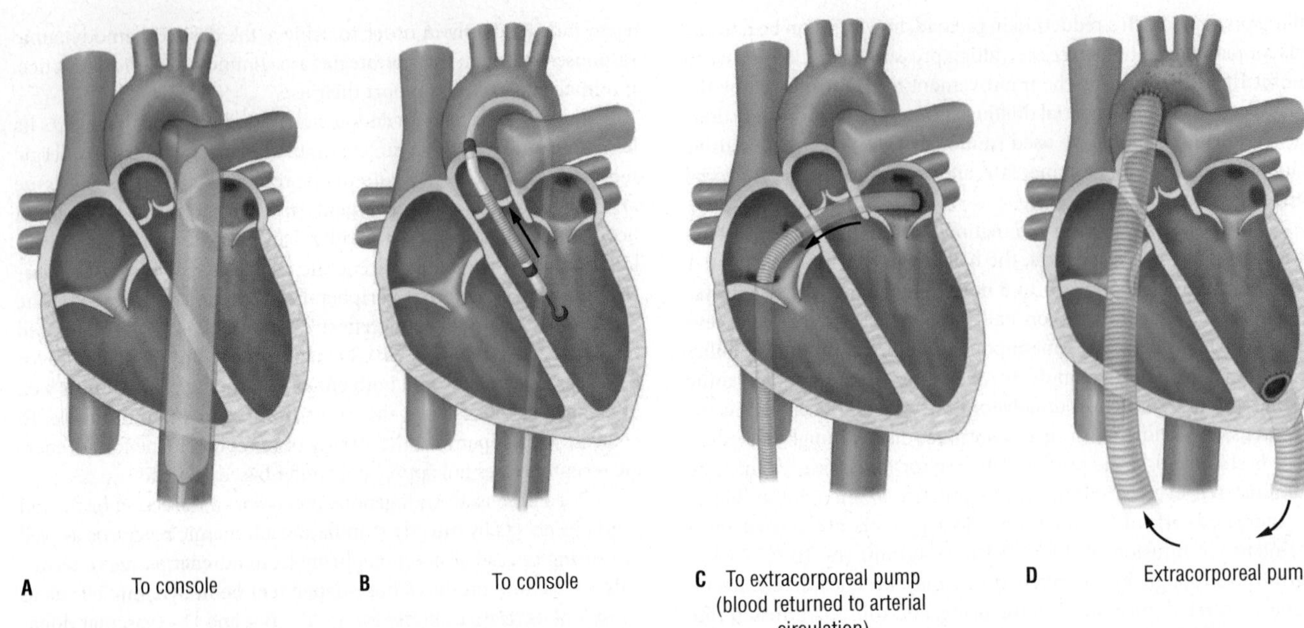

FIGURE 15-4 **Common types of temporary mechanical circulatory support.** As shown in Figure A, an intra-aortic balloon pump (IABP) is advanced into the descending aorta where it inflates during diastole (shown), displacing blood and improving coronary filling. During systole (not shown), the IABP deflates, producing a vacuum-like effect that reduces peripheral resistance. An example of an Impella percutaneous ventricular assist device (VAD) is illustrated in Figure B. An Impella device is advanced through the aortic valve, where blood is transferred from the left ventricle to the aorta by an axial flow pump. Figure C is an illustration of the TandemHeart device, which is inserted percutaneously into a large peripheral vein and advanced across the intra-atrial septum. Blood is removed from the left atrium and propelled by an extracorporeal centrifugal flow pump back into the systemic circulation (not shown). The cannulae of a CentriMag VAD are shown in Figure D. An inflow cannula is surgically inserted into the apex of the left ventricle, where blood is transferred to an extracorporeal centrifugal flow pump (not shown), where it is returned to the systemic circulation via an outflow cannula surgically inserted into the aorta. In extracorporeal membrane oxygenation (ECMO) (not shown), the inflow and outflow cannulae are inserted into peripheral vessels.

intra-aortic balloon pump (IABP), ventricular assist device (VAD), and extracorporeal membrane oxygenation (ECMO) (Fig. 15-4). Unique features, contraindications, and complications of each type of device will be discussed in the sections to follow.

Intra-aortic Balloon Pump

An IABP consists of a polyethylene balloon mounted on a catheter that is inserted percutaneously into the femoral artery and advanced into the descending thoracic aorta (see Fig. 15-4A). During counterpulsation, the balloon is synchronized with the electrocardiogram (or alternatively, changes in pressure) so that it inflates during diastole and displaces blood to the proximal aorta, thus increasing diastolic pressure and coronary perfusion. The balloon deflates just prior to the opening of the aortic valve during systole, which causes a sudden "vacuum-like" decrease in aortic pressure, allowing the left ventricle to pump against reduced arterial impedance. Although the IABP is the most commonly employed modality of temporary MCS due to its ease of use, it only provides an estimated 1.0 L/min of CO. As a consequence, the primary benefits of an IABP are enhanced coronary perfusion, increased myocardial oxygen supply, and reduced myocardial oxygen demand. It may be particularly useful for patients with myocardial ischemia complicated by cardiogenic shock, although it has not been shown to improve mortality in this setting.[43] Systemic anticoagulation is generally recommended although cases of IABP use without anticoagulation have been reported.[44] Complications of the IABP include vascular injury, thrombocytopenia, and renal impairment due to obstruction of the splanchnic circulation by balloon malposition. Use should be avoided in patients with severe peripheral vascular disease.

Ventricular Assist Devices

A VAD provides hemodynamic support by assisting and, in some cases, replacing the pumping functions of the right and/or left ventricles. Compared to an IABP, temporary VADs confer greater hemodynamic improvements but no differences in long-term survival.[45] A left ventricular assist device (LVAD) propels blood from the left ventricle or left atrium to the ascending aorta whereas a right VAD propels blood from the right ventricle or right atrium to the PA. A right VAD may be used alone or in conjunction with an LVAD; this latter configuration is known as a biventricular assist device. All VADs are preload-dependent, meaning that adequate intra-ventricular filling pressure (ie, volume) is required to optimize blood flow. As with the native ventricle in HF, VADs are also afterload-sensitive, meaning that excess peripheral resistance can impair blood flow. Complications of VAD implantation include bleeding, infections, and risks associated with the specific implantation technique. In addition, the devices can cause thrombosis, renal and hepatic dysfunction, and arrhythmias. Right ventricular failure is a unique complication of LVAD implantation as a result of increased venous return, persistently elevated pulmonary pressures, and changes in right ventricular geometry.

Percutaneous VADs include the Impella series (Abiomed, Danvers, MA) and TandemHeart (CardiacAssist, Pittsburgh, PA). Impella devices are inserted percutaneously into a large peripheral artery and advanced in a retrograde fashion across the aortic valve, where blood is advanced from the left ventricle to the ascending aorta via axial flow (see Fig. 15-4B). The amount of CO augmented by the Impella device depends on model; the Impella 2.5 and 5.0 models supply 2.5 L and 5.0 L/min of flow, respectively. Hemolysis is a common complication of Impella use due to the axial flow facilitated by the device. The TandemHeart device consists of an inflow cannula placed percutaneously into a large peripheral vein and advanced transseptally into the left atrium (see Fig. 15-4C). Blood is withdrawn from the left atrium by an extracorporeal pump and propelled via an outflow cannula placed percutaneously into a large artery. Up to 5.0 L/min of flow can be provided by the TandemHeart. Due to its placement across the intra-atrial septum, perforation and shunt formation are potential complications with this device.

The most common surgically implanted temporary VAD is the CentriMag (Thoractec Corp., Pleasanton, CA), which can provide right, left, or biventricular support and up to 10.0 L/min of CO. The CentriMag device consists of a centrifugal flow extracorporeal pump and surgically placed inflow and outflow cannulae supporting the affected ventricle (see Fig. 15-4D). Given the surgical technique required for placement of the CentriMag device, tissue injury is its most common complication.

Extracorporeal Membrane Oxygenation

Extracorporeal membrane oxygenation may be venoarterial or venovenous in nature. In venoarterial ECMO, deoxygenated blood is transported from the venous circulation to an extracorporeal oxygenator and centrifugal flow pump and returned as oxygenated blood to the arterial circulation. In contrast, venovenous ECMO consists of only extracorporeal oxygenation; hemodynamic support is provided by native cardiac function. As a consequence, venoarterial ECMO is more common in the management of refractory ADHF, where up to 8 L/min of cardiac support can be provided. Complications of ECMO include bleeding, infections, and organ dysfunction. Serum drug concentrations can also be significantly impacted as a result of increased volume of distribution, decreased elimination due to hepatic and/or renal impairment, and sequestration of drugs in the ECMO circuit.

ADVANCED THERAPIES

No consensus definition exists for advanced HF, or the stage at which patients should be considered for definitive therapies such as durable MCS and heart transplantation. Nonetheless, evaluation for these advanced therapies is commonly initiated during an admission for ADHF, particularly if hospitalization is accompanied by severe symptoms at rest, intolerance of GDMT, decline in organ function, refractory arrhythmias, or an inability to be successfully weaned from inotropic or temporary MCS support. Because of the complexity of care, potential risks, and resource implications of durable MCS and heart transplantation, patients with advanced HF must undergo a rigorous interdisciplinary evaluation before becoming eligible candidates. Components of this evaluation commonly include past medical, surgical, and psychosocial history, medication and adverse event history, adherence to medications and medical care, comorbid conditions, risks for postoperative complications, and health insurance coverage. Relative contraindications to the use of advanced therapies include excess perioperative risk, irreversible pulmonary hypertension, inability to manage postoperative care (eg, medication therapy, monitoring), and concurrent survival-limiting diseases (eg, malignancy).

Durable Mechanical Circulatory Support

The most common indications for durable MCS are temporary device implantation in patients awaiting heart transplantation who are unlikely to survive the duration of time required for identifying a suitable donor ("bridge to transplantation") and permanent device implantation in patients who are ineligible for heart transplantation due to advanced age or comorbid conditions ("destination therapy"). Although far less common than with temporary MCS, durable VADs may be implanted in patients who are likely to become eligible transplant candidates ("bridge to decision") but evaluation is incomplete or has been delayed until certain requirements can be satisfied (eg, smoking cessation). Durable MCS is almost exclusively comprised of LVAD implantation, although select patients may remain hospitalized with right VAD or biventricular support while awaiting transplantation.

Durable LVADs are implanted by inserting an inflow cannula into the apex of the left ventricle, which is connected to an intracorporeal pumping unit; blood is returned to the systemic circulation via an outflow cannula inserted into the aorta. Whereas previous devices provided hemodynamic support via pulsatile flow, newer-generation devices utilize a continuous flow mechanism, allowing them to be smaller in size, less subject to deterioration over time, and conferring an improvement in event-free survival.[46] Research suggests that prolonged unloading of the left ventricle with an LVAD in combination with drug therapy can produce sustained recovery in LV function, amelioration of symptoms, and in some cases, device explantation.[47] The two continuous flow LVADs currently approved for use in the United States are the axial flow HeartMate II LVAD (Thoratec Corp., Pleasanton, CA) and centrifugal flow HeartWare Ventricular Assist Device (HVAD) (HeartWare, Inc; Framingham, MA). Both devices are capable of providing up to 10 L/min of CO. For complete heart replacement therapy, total artificial heart systems continue to be investigated, although size and embolic complications limit widespread use.

Complications following durable LVAD placement are similar as those described for temporary devices. Device malfunction may occur with long-term use but has become rare with advances in technology. The most perplexing challenge in the care of LVAD patients remains identifying a chronic antithrombotic regimen that balances the risk of device thrombosis and bleeding. Antithrombotic regimens most often include a vitamin K antagonist and antiplatelet agent, although the goal international normalized ratio (INR) range and antiplatelet agents selected (eg, aspirin, dipyridamole, clopidogrel) may vary significantly by center. Suspected pump thrombosis should be promptly evaluated, although no consensus exists on an appropriate treatment strategy (eg, enhanced antiplatelet or anticoagulant therapy, thrombolysis, or pump exchange).[48]

Heart Transplantation

14 Orthotopic heart transplantation remains the optimal management strategy for patients with irreversible advanced HF, as 10-year survival rates approach 60% among patients transplanted after 2001.[49] Unfortunately, the shortage of acceptable donor hearts has prolonged waiting times and many patients succumb to their disease prior to transplantation. Another significant percentage of patients are deemed ineligible for heart transplantation because of age, concurrent illnesses, psychosocial factors, or other reasons. The shortage of donor hearts has prompted the development of new surgical strategies, including ventricular aneurysm resection, mitral valve repair, and myocardial cell transplantation, which have resulted in variable degrees of improvement. Further development of these and other techniques may offer additional options in patients who are not eligible for VAD implantation or heart transplantation. For a more detailed discussion of heart transplantation, see Chapter 89.

EVALUATION OF THERAPEUTIC OUTCOMES

Daily monitoring to assess the efficacy of drug therapy is critical to assuring optimal outcomes and should include weight, strict fluid intake and output, and HF signs and symptoms (Table 15-6). Foley catheter placement is not recommended unless close monitoring of urine output is not otherwise possible. As for safety endpoints,

TABLE 15-6 Monitoring Recommendations for Patients Hospitalized with ADHF

Parameter	Frequency	Notes
Weight	Daily	Assess after voiding in the morning Utilize same scale each day, if possible Account for increase or decrease in food intake
Fluid balance	Daily*	Strict intake and output
Vital Signs	More than daily	Blood pressure and heart rate including signs/symptoms of orthostatic hypotension, rhythm (continuous)
Signs of congestion and/or low output	Daily*	Jugular venous distension, crackles, hepatomegaly, splenomegaly, hepatojugular reflux, ascites, lower extremity edema, hypotension, narrow pulse pressures, cool extremities, altered mental status, worsening renal or hepatic function
Symptoms of congestion and/or low output	Daily*	Dyspnea on exertion or at rest, orthopnea, paroxysmal nocturnal dyspnea, nausea/vomiting, early satiety, fatigue, lightheadedness, chest pain, palpitations
Electrolytes	Daily*	Potassium, magnesium, sodium
Renal function	Daily*	Blood urea nitrogen and serum creatinine including ratio to assess volume status (ie, over-diuresis)
Hepatic function	Variable*	Alk Phos and GGT primarily for fluid overload, AST and ALT primarily for hypoperfusion
BNP, NT-proBNP	Admission, Discharge	Admission for diagnosis, discharge for prognosis
Other	Variable	Troponin and other cardiac enzymes if myocardial strain Arterial blood gas if hypoxic Lactate if hypoperfusion present

Alk Phos, alkaline phosphatase; AST, aspartate aminotransferase; ALT, alanine aminotransferase; GGT, gamma-glutamyltransferase.

*Daily unless change in clinical status warrants more frequent assessment.

monitoring for electrolyte depletion, symptomatic hypotension, and renal dysfunction should be assessed frequently. While many of the above parameters may be monitored daily, some will need to be monitored more frequently as dictated by patient clinical status. Vital signs should be assessed multiple times throughout the day at a frequency that is appropriate for the patient's degree of stability. Orthostatic blood pressure should be assessed at least once daily.

Patients with ADHF may have critically reduced CO, usually with low arterial blood pressure and systemic hypoperfusion resulting in organ system dysfunction (ie, cardiogenic shock). They may also have pulmonary edema with hypoxemia, respiratory acidosis, and markedly increased work of breathing. With cardiopulmonary support, response to interventions should be assessed promptly to allow for timely adjustments in treatment. Continuous monitoring of ECG, continuous pulse oximetry, urine flow, and automated blood pressure recordings are standards of care for critically ill patients with cardiopulmonary decompensation. Peripheral or femoral arterial catheters may be utilized for continuous and accurate assessment of arterial pressure.

Preparation for Discharge

Patients should not be discharged until optimal volume status is achieved and the patient is successfully transitioned from an IV to an oral diuretic regimen, GDMT is stable, and IV inotropes and vasodilators have been discontinued for at least 24 hours. If relevant, smoking cessation must be addressed to avoid delay in consideration for advanced therapies. The following should be documented in the medical record: left ventricular ejection fraction and ACE inhibitor and beta blocker use (for patients with reduced LVEF) or intolerance to such.[50]

Prior to discharge, patients and caregivers should be counseled on dietary sodium restriction as well as monitoring body weight daily and parameters for when to titrate diuretics or call a healthcare provider for further instruction (eg, two pound weight gain in 24 hours). Medication changes (initiation, discontinuation, dose change) should be clearly conveyed verbally and in writing and financial coverage for all medication assured. The importance of dietary and medication adherence should be emphasized. Appropriate follow-up should be scheduled including an appointment at 7-10 days post discharge including a nurse visit or phone call at 3 days for select patients. Pertinent follow-up labs (eg, potassium, serum creatinine) should also be scheduled including medication related labs (eg, INR for warfarin, serum digoxin concentration). All patients should be considered for referral to a formal disease management program.

Multidisciplinary disease management programs and other specialized interventions involving pharmacists have been associated with a wide range of benefits including reduced HF readmissions.[51] A recent systematic review of multidisciplinary teams involving a pharmacist showed reductions in all-cause and HF hospitalizations.[52] The American Heart Association recently published a statement describing transitional care interventions acknowledging that of the transition of care programs for patients with HF (n = 20), 75% used a collaborative, multidisciplinary team that included pharmacists.[53]

Clinical **Controversy...**

1. For patients with volume overload, administration of loop diuretic therapy as an IV bolus or continuous infusion appears to be similarly efficacious and safe when selected as initial therapy; however, the optimal strategy for facilitating volume removal in patients with diuretic resistance remains unknown. Higher doses (ie, 2.5-times the previous oral dose) of IV loop diuretic are more effective than lower doses (ie, equivalent to previous oral dose) but may also produce higher rates of transient renal dysfunction. The following controversies remain unaddressed: the role of adding a diuretic with an alternative mechanism of action (ie, thiazide-type diuretic), which alternative diuretic is most optimal (eg, metolazone, hydrochlorothiazide), and how adjunct diuretics compare to other treatment modalities, such as IV vasodilators or ultrafiltration.
2. For patients with low CO, appropriate selection of IV inotropes in the setting of chronic oral beta blockers is unclear. Theoretically milrinone should be the agent of choice for patients receiving beta blockade; however, many patients will not tolerate its potent vasodilatory effects. In addition, small studies suggest that the inotropic effects of dobutamine may be retained with select beta blockers. Furthermore, optimal dosing of beta blocker in the setting of low output (eg, maintain current dose vs dose reduction) has not been addressed, although complete discontinuation should generally be avoided. Additional investigation in this area is warranted.
3. In Chapter 14, several new therapies for the management of patients with stable chronic HF were discussed.

Unfortunately, trials evaluating these therapies enrolled very few patients with advanced HF and none with ADHF. As a consequence, it is currently unclear if these new therapies would exert beneficial effects in patients with ADHF or, perhaps more importantly, if they are safe. Additional research is warranted on the use of these agents in the ADHF population.

4. Evolving data continue to support the role of MCS as a bridge to transplantation or DT. However, additional research to define optimal candidates, determine timelines for implantation, and minimize complications is warranted. Another area lacking sufficient data is the appropriate management of medications in patients receiving ECMO.

CONCLUSION

Several recent clinical trials have addressed many controversies in the management of ADHF, including the appropriate dosing of diuretics and use of vasodilators and vasopressors (eg, dopamine) in patients with volume overload. Still, many unanswered questions remain, including inotrope selection in low CO and optimal use of GDMT in the setting of ADHF. Many advances in MCS have extended the lives of patients awaiting transplant; however, limited evidence exists to guide management of this patient population, including how to avoid and manage complications associated with these devices. Finally, ideal management of patients with ADHF includes optimization of GDMT, optimal communication with patients, caregivers, and other healthcare providers with each care transition, and outpatient follow-up with a collaborative, multidisciplinary team.

ABBREVIATIONS

ACCF	American College of Cardiology Foundation
ACE	angiotensin-converting enzyme
ADHERE	Acute Decompensated Heart Failure National Registry
ADHF	acute decompensated heart failure
AHA	American Heart Association
AMP	adenosine monophosphate
AVP	arginine vasopressin
BNP	B-type natriuretic peptide
BUN	blood urea nitrogen
cAMP	cyclic adenosine monophosphate
cGMP	cyclic guanosine monophosphate
CI	cardiac index
CO	cardiac output
CVP	central venous pressure
DT	destination therapy
ECMO	extracorporeal membrane oxygenation
GDMT	guideline-directed medical therapy
GI	gastrointestinal
HF	heart failure
HFpEF	heart failure with preserved ejection fraction
HFrEF	Heart failure with reduced ejection fraction
HVAD	HeartWare Ventricular Assist Device
IABP	intra-aortic balloon pump
INR	international normalized ratio
IV	intravenous
JVD	jugular venous distension
LVAD	left ventricular assist device
MAP	mean arterial pressure
MCS	mechanical circulatory support
MI	myocardial infarction
NYHA	New York Heart Association
OPTIMIZE-HF	Organized Program to Initiate Lifesaving Treatment in Hospitalized Patients with Heart Failure
PA	pulmonary artery
PCWP	pulmonary capillary wedge pressure
PVR	pulmonary vascular resistance
SIADH	syndrome of inappropriate diuretic hormone
SVR	systemic vascular resistance
VAD	ventricular assist device

REFERENCES

1. Mozaffarian D, Benjamin EJ, Go AS, et al. Heart disease and stroke statistics—2015 update: A report from the American Heart Association. *Circulation* 2015;131(4):e29-322.
2. Heidenreich PA, Albert NM, Allen LA, et al. Forecasting the impact of heart failure in the United States: A policy statement from the American Heart Association. *Circ Heart Fail* 2013;6(3):606-619.
3. Ambrosy AP, Fonarow GC, Butler J, et al. The global health and economic burden of hospitalizations for heart failure: Lessons learned from hospitalized heart failure registries. *J Am Coll Cardiol* 2014;63(12):1123-1133.
4. Weintraub NL, Collins SP, Pang PS, et al. Acute heart failure syndromes: Emergency department presentation, treatment, and disposition: Current approaches and future aims: A scientific statement from the American Heart Association. *Circulation* 2010;122(19):1975-1996.
5. Gheorghiade M, De Luca L, Fonarow GC, Filippatos G, Metra M, Francis GS. Pathophysiologic targets in the early phase of acute heart failure syndromes. *Am J Cardiol* 2005;96(6A):11G-17G.
6. Yancy CW, Jessup M, Bozkurt B, et al. 2013 ACCF/AHA guideline for the management of heart failure: A report of the American College of Cardiology Foundation/American Heart Association Task Force on Practice Guidelines. *J Am Coll Cardiol* 2013;62(16):e147-239.
7. Felker GM, Adams KF, Konstam MA, O'Connor CM, Gheorghiade M. The problem of decompensated heart failure: Nomenclature, classification, and risk stratification. *Am Heart J* 2003;145(2 Suppl): S18-25.
8. Fonarow GC, Adams KF, Abraham WT, et al. Risk stratification for in-hospital mortality in acutely decompensated heart failure: Classification and regression tree analysis. *JAMA* 2005;293(5):572-580.
9. O'Connor CM, Abraham WT, Albert NM, et al. Predictors of mortality after discharge in patients hospitalized with heart failure: An analysis from the Organized Program to Initiate Lifesaving Treatment in Hospitalized Patients with Heart Failure (OPTIMIZE-HF). *Am Heart J* 2008;156(4):662-673.
10. Nohria A, Mielniczuk LM, Stevenson LW. Evaluation and monitoring of patients with acute heart failure syndromes. *Am J Cardiol* 2005;96(6A):32G-40G.
11. Binanay C, Califf RM, Hasselblad V, et al. Evaluation study of congestive heart failure and pulmonary artery catheterization effectiveness: The ESCAPE trial. *JAMA* 2005;294(13):1625-1633.
12. Fonarow GC, Abraham WT, Albert NM, et al. Influence of beta-blocker continuation or withdrawal on outcomes in patients hospitalized with heart failure: Findings from the OPTIMIZE-HF program. *J Am Coll Cardiol* 2008;52(3):90-199.
13. Jondeau G, Neuder Y, Eicher J-C, et al. B-CONVINCED: Beta-blocker CONtinuation Vs. INterruption in patients with Congestive heart failure hospitalizED for a decompensation episode. *Eur Heart J* 2009;30(18):2186-2192.
14. Packer M, Gheorghiade M, Young JB, et al. Withdrawal of digoxin from patients with chronic heart failure treated with angiotensin-converting-enzyme inhibitors. RADIANCE Study. *N Engl J Med* 1993;329(1):1-7.
15. Uretsky BF, Young JB, Shahidi FE, Yellen LG, Harrison MC, Jolly MK. Randomized study assessing the effect of digoxin withdrawal in patients with mild to moderate chronic congestive heart failure: Results of the PROVED trial. PROVED Investigative Group. *J Am Coll Cardiol* 1993;22(4):955-962.
16. Forrester JS, Diamond G, Chatterjee K, Swan HJ. Medical therapy of acute myocardial infarction by application of hemodynamic subsets (first of two parts). *N Engl J Med* 1976;295(24):1356-1362.
17. Eshaghian S, Horwich TB, Fonarow GC. Relation of loop diuretic dose to mortality in advanced heart failure. *Am J Cardiol* 2006;97(12):1759-1764.

18. Butler J, Forman DE, Abraham WT, et al. Relationship between heart failure treatment and development of worsening renal function among hospitalized patients. *Am Heart J* 2004;147(2):331-338.
19. Stough WG, O'Connor CM, Gheorghiade M. Overview of current noninodilator therapies for acute heart failure syndromes. *Am J Cardiol* 2005;96(6A):41G-46G.
20. Cleland JGF, Coletta A, Witte K. Practical applications of intravenous diuretic therapy in decompensated heart failure. *Am J Med* 2006;119 (12 Suppl 1):S26-36.
21. Felker GM, Lee KL, Bull DA, et al. Diuretic strategies in patients with acute decompensated heart failure. *N Engl J Med* 2011;364(9):797-805.
22. Dormans TP, van Meyel JJ, Gerlag PG, Tan Y, Russel FG, Smits P. Diuretic efficacy of high dose furosemide in severe heart failure: Bolus injection versus continuous infusion. *J Am Coll Cardiol* 1996;28(2):376-382.
23. Thomson MR, Nappi JM, Dunn SP, Hollis IB, Rodgers JE, Van Bakel AB. Continuous versus intermittent infusion of furosemide in acute decompensated heart failure. *J Card Fail* 2010;16(3):88-193.
24. Publication Committee for the VMAC Investigators (Vasodilatation in the Management of Acute CHF). Intravenous nesiritide vs nitroglycerin for treatment of decompensated congestive heart failure: A randomized controlled trial. *JAMA* 2002;287(12):1531-1540.
25. Aaronson KD, Sackner-Bernstein J. Risk of death associated with nesiritide in patients with acutely decompensated heart failure. *JAMA* 2006;296(12):1465-1466.
26. Sackner-Bernstein JD, Kowalski M, Fox M, Aaronson K. Short-term risk of death after treatment with nesiritide for decompensated heart failure: A pooled analysis of randomized controlled trials. *JAMA* 2005;293(15):1900-1905.
27. Sackner-Bernstein JD, Skopicki HA, Aaronson KD. Risk of worsening renal function with nesiritide in patients with acutely decompensated heart failure. *Circulation* 2005;111(12):487-1491.
28. O'Connor CM, Starling RC, Hernandez AF, et al. Effect of nesiritide in patients with acute decompensated heart failure. *N Engl J Med* 2011;365(1):32-43.
29. Chen HH, Anstrom KJ, Givertz MM, et al. Low-dose dopamine or low-dose nesiritide in acute heart failure with renal dysfunction: The ROSE acute heart failure randomized trial. *JAMA* 2013;310(23):2533-2543.
30. Gheorghiade M, Gattis WA, O'Connor CM, et al. Effects of tolvaptan, a vasopressin antagonist, in patients hospitalized with worsening heart failure: A randomized controlled trial. *JAMA* 2004;291(16):1963-1971.
31. Lee WH, Packer M. Prognostic importance of serum sodium concentration and its modification by converting-enzyme inhibition in patients with severe chronic heart failure. *Circulation* 1986;73(2):257-267.
32. Gheorghiade M, Konstam MA, Burnett JC, et al. Short-term clinical effects of tolvaptan, an oral vasopressin antagonist, in patients hospitalized for heart failure: The EVEREST Clinical Status Trials. *JAMA* 2007;297(12):1332-1343.
33. Costanzo MR, Guglin ME, Saltzberg MT, et al. Ultrafiltration versus intravenous diuretics for patients hospitalized for acute decompensated heart failure. *J Am Coll Cardiol* 2007;49(6):675-683.
34. Bart BA, Goldsmith SR, Lee KL, et al. Ultrafiltration in decompensated heart failure with cardiorenal syndrome. *N Engl J Med* 2012;367(24): 2296-2304.
35. Vargo DL, Brater DC, Rudy DW, Swan SK. Dopamine does not enhance furosemide-induced natriuresis in patients with congestive heart failure. *J Am Soc Nephrol* 1996;7(7):1032-1037.
36. Giamouzis G, Butler J, Starling RC, et al. Impact of dopamine infusion on renal function in hospitalized heart failure patients: Results of the Dopamine in Acute Decompensated Heart Failure (DAD-HF) Trial. *J Card Fail* 2010;16(12):922-930.
37. Triposkiadis FK, Butler J, Karayannis G, et al. Efficacy and safety of high dose versus low dose furosemide with or without dopamine infusion: The Dopamine in Acute Decompensated Heart Failure II (DAD-HF II) Trial. *Int J Cardiol* 2014;172(1):15-121.
38. Mullens W, Abrahams Z, Francis GS, et al. Sodium nitroprusside for advanced low-output heart failure. *J Am Coll Cardiol* 2008;52(3):200-207.
39. Abraham WT, Adams KF, Fonarow GC, et al. In-hospital mortality in patients with acute decompensated heart failure requiring intravenous vasoactive medications: An analysis from the Acute Decompensated Heart Failure National Registry (ADHERE). *J Am Coll Cardiol* 2005;46(1):57-64.
40. Cuffe MS, Califf RM, Adams KF, et al. Short-term intravenous milrinone for acute exacerbation of chronic heart failure: A randomized controlled trial. *JAMA* 2002;287(12):1541-1547.
41. Metra M, Nodari S, D'Aloia A, et al. Beta-blocker therapy influences the hemodynamic response to inotropic agents in patients with heart failure: A randomized comparison of dobutamine and enoximone before and after chronic treatment with metoprolol or carvedilol. *J Am Coll Cardiol* 2002;40(7):1248-1258.
42. De Backer D, Biston P, Devriendt J, et al. Comparison of dopamine and norepinephrine in the treatment of shock. *N Engl J Med* 2010;362(9):779-789.
43. Thiele H, Zeymer U, Neumann F-J, et al. Intraaortic balloon support for myocardial infarction with cardiogenic shock. *N Engl J Med* 2012;367(14):1287-1296.
44. Pucher PH, Cummings IG, Shipolini AR, McCormack DJ. Is heparin needed for patients with an intra-aortic balloon pump? *Interact Cardiovasc Thorac Surg* 2012;15(1):36-139.
45. Cheng JM, den Uil CA, Hoeks SE, et al. Percutaneous left ventricular assist devices vs. intra-aortic balloon pump counterpulsation for treatment of cardiogenic shock: A meta-analysis of controlled trials. *Eur Heart J* 2009;30(17):2102-2108.
46. Slaughter MS, Rogers JG, Milano CA, et al. Advanced heart failure treated with continuous-flow left ventricular assist device. *N Engl J Med* 2009;361(23):2241-2251.
47. Birks EJ, Tansley PD, Hardy J, et al. Left ventricular assist device and drug therapy for the reversal of heart failure. *N Engl J Med* 2006;355(18):1873-1884.
48. Goldstein DJ, John R, Salerno C, et al. Algorithm for the diagnosis and management of suspected pump thrombus. *J Heart Lung Transplant Off Publ Int Soc Heart Transplant* 2013;32(7):667-670.
49. Lund LH, Edwards LB, Kucheryavaya AY, et al. The Registry of the International Society for Heart and Lung Transplantation: Thirty-second Official Adult Heart Transplantation Report-2015; Focus Theme: Early Graft Failure. *J Heart Lung Transplant Off Publ Int Soc Heart Transplant* 2015;34(10):1244-1254.
50. Wiggins BS, Rodgers JE, DiDomenico RJ, Cook AM, Page RL. Discharge counseling for patients with heart failure or myocardial infarction: A best practices model developed by members of the American College of Clinical Pharmacy's Cardiology Practice and Research Network based on the Hospital to Home (H2H) Initiative. *Pharmacotherapy* 2013;33(5):558-580.
51. Milfred-LaForest SK, Chow SL, DiDomenico RJ, et al. Clinical pharmacy services in heart failure: An opinion paper from the Heart Failure Society of America and American College of Clinical Pharmacy Cardiology Practice and Research Network. *Pharmacotherapy* 2013;33(5):529-548.
52. Koshman SL, Charrois TL, Simpson SH, McAlister FA, Tsuyuki RT. Pharmacist care of patients with heart failure: A systematic review of randomized trials. *Arch Intern Med* 2008;168(7):687-694.
53. Albert NM, Barnason S, Deswal A, et al. Transitions of care in heart failure: A scientific statement from the American Heart Association. *Circ Heart Fail* 2015;8(2):384-409.

Stable Ischemic Heart Disease

16

Paul P. Dobesh

KEY CONCEPTS

1. Stable ischemic heart disease (SIHD), if primary, is caused by an obstructive atherosclerotic plaque in one or more epicardial coronary vessels in which increases in myocardial demand in the setting of this fixed decrease in myocardial oxygen supply produces myocardial ischemia.
2. Some patients with SIHD also have a component of vasospasm that requires a slightly different pharmacologic approach.
3. Chest pain from exertion is the cardinal symptom of myocardial ischemia in patients with SIHD.
4. Assessment of successful treatment of angina includes not only reducing the number of episodes and increasing the amount of exertion needed to precipitate an episode, but also allowing patients to participate in activity that provides a high-level quality of life.
5. Revascularization can provide a survival advantage compared to medical therapy in patients with more extensive atherosclerotic disease.
6. In patients with less extensive atherosclerotic disease, percutaneous coronary intervention (PCI) has not demonstrated a clear advantage over guideline-directed medical therapy (GDMT) in patients with SIHD.
7. Aspirin and angiotensin converting enzyme (ACE) inhibitors play an important role preventing adverse cardiovascular events in patients with SIHD.
8. Management of modifiable atherosclerotic risk factors is key to improving the quantity of life in patients with SIHD.
9. β-blockers are typically regarded as first-line therapy in the management and control of episodes of angina in patients with SIHD
10. Calcium channel blockers (CCBs) and chronic long-acting nitrates are often used as additional therapy for the control of episodes of angina in patients with SIHD.
11. All patients with SIHD should receive sublingual nitroglycerin (SL NTG) for acute attacks, along with proper education of their use.
12. Ranolazine provides a reduction in episodes of angina by blocking excess accumulation of sodium, and consequentially calcium in the myocyte, without impacting heart rate (HR) or blood pressure (BP).

INTRODUCTION

Coronary artery disease (CAD) is the leading etiology of ischemic heart disease, and is typically the result atherosclerotic plaque in the epicardial vessels. The process of atherosclerosis begins early in life, with fatty steaks being present in many people in their teenage years or early twenties. These plaques grow over decades and start to become pathologic in a person's fifth decade of life and beyond. Besides CAD, atherosclerosis also manifest in other major vascular beds leading to cerebrovascular disease (stroke) and peripheral arterial disease. Ischemic heart disease may present as a medical emergency as an acute coronary syndrome (ACS), which includes unstable angina, non-ST-segment myocardial infarction (MI), or ST-segment elevation MI. It may also present as chronic stable exertional angina or ischemia without clinical symptoms (silent ischemia). Less common causes of stable IHD (SIHD) include microvascular angina, which is due to atherosclerosis in endocardial instead of epicardial vessels. Microvascular angina is more common in women and those with metabolic syndrome. Coronary vasospasm, also known as variant or Prinzmetal's angina, represents a form of SIHD that does not involve atherosclerotic plaque development. This chapter focuses on patients with SIHD. Inappropriate, insufficient, or untreated SIHD can not only lead to MI and cardiac death, but also the development of heart failure, arrhythmias, and valvular disease. Guidelines for the diagnosis and management of SIHD have been published by the American College of Cardiology (ACC) and American Heart Association (AHA), as well as the European Society of Cardiology.[1,2]

EPIDEMIOLOGY

According to AHA statistics in 2013, and estimated 85.6 million Americans had at least one form of cardiovascular disease (CVD), with more than 50% being 60 years of age or older.[3] Despite a reduction in mortality of slightly over 30% between 2001 and 2011, CVD remains the largest cause of death in men and women in the United States.[4] In 2011, CVD was listed as the main cause of death in 30.8% of the 2,596,993 deaths, or approximately 1 in every 3 deaths in the United States.[3] This calculates to approximately 2200 deaths per day or 1 death every 40 seconds. The overall death rate of CVD is 222.9 per 100,000 population, but varies based on gender and ethnicity. The death rate is 270.6 for white males, 356.7 for black males, 183.8 for white females, and 246.6 for black females. Estimated direct and indirect cost of CVD in 2012 was over $316 billion, with a projected direct medical cost of approximately $918 billion by 2030.[3] If all forms of CVD were eliminated, the predicted increase in life expectancy in the United States could rise by almost 7 years. CVD is not just a problem in the United Sates or "Western" cultures. Death due to CVD accounted for 17.3 million deaths per year (30%), making CVD the leading global cause of death, with numbers expecting to climb to almost 24 million deaths by 2030.[3] In 2010, the global cost of CVD was estimated at $863 billion, which is expected to climb to $1044 billion by 2030.

Among patients with CAD, the total number of patients with SIHD is difficult to determine. Statistics from the AHA estimate that approximately 8.2 million Americans have angina pectoris.[3] Stable angina pectoris is the initial manifestation of ischemic heart disease in approximately one-half of all patients who eventually have an MI. Using these numbers, along with estimates based on patients surviving MI, it is predicted that approximately 15.5 million Americans have coronary heart disease (CHD). These 15.5 million patients would receive treatment strategies that are similar to that for patients with SIHD as described in this chapter. In the United States, CHD is the underlying cause of death in approximately 1 in over 7 deaths, accounting for almost 400,000 deaths in 2013. The risk of mortality is greatest for black men, followed by white men, black females, and white females.[3] The 5 states with the lowest mortality from CHD are Minnesota, Hawaii, Utah, Oregon, and Colorado, with rates ranging from 65.6 to 72.8 per 100,000 populations.[3] The 5 states with the highest mortality from CHD are Oklahoma, Tennessee, New York, Arkansas, and Michigan, with rates being almost double those in the 5 states with the lowest mortality from CHD (130.8-149.8 per 100,000).[3] Estimated direct and indirect cost of CHD was $204 billion in 2010, with costs expected to double[This is a different figure that listed above] by 2030.[3] For countries reporting data, the United States ranks 10th for CHD death rates for males aged 35 to 74 years and 9th for females of the same age.[3] For both males and females, Ukraine, Russian Federation, Romania, and Hungary have the highest CHD death rates, with South Korea, Japan, and France having the lowest.[3]

Prognosis of patients with SIHD will be dependent on the extent of atherosclerotic disease, the presence of left ventricular (LV) dysfunction, as well as the presence of other comorbidities.[2] The severity of angina symptoms may also be used to determine prognosis as well.[5] In a study of 8,908 Veterans Administration patients with CAD, the risk of death increased with the self-reported degree of physical limitation due to angina.[6] It is thought that the degree of physical limitation may simply reflect the extent of underlying atherosclerotic disease. Besides the high mortality, morbidity is also considerable in patients with SIHD. Most of these patients will eventually need hospitalization for episodes of an ACS. These patients often have a reduced quality of life due to their inability to conduct activities of daily living without chest pain.[7,8] There is also a significant amount of lost time from work and lost productivity that can have a large indirect cost to patients and society. Data from the Bypass Angioplasty Revascularization Investigation (BARI) suggest that approximately 15% to 20% of patients rate their own health as fair or poor despite revascularization, and 30% of patients are never able to return to work.[9]

1 ETIOLOGY AND PATHOPHYSIOLOGY

Angina pectoris is typically a result of an imbalance between myocardial oxygen supply and myocardial oxygen demand (MVO_2). The process of maintaining adequate coronary blood flow to meet the metabolic demands of the myocytes is complex with multiple factors influencing both sides of the supply/demand equation.

The foundation pathophysiology of patients with SIHD is driven by an increase in myocardial oxygen demand (MVO_2) in the setting of a fixed decrease in myocardial oxygen supply.[10] The etiology of the fixed decrease in supply is long-standing, well developed atherosclerotic plaque. These plaques grow over several decades with the extensiveness and rate of growth determined by risk factors such as smoking, dyslipidemia, hypertension (HTN), diabetes mellitus (DM), and genetics (family history). The process and development of atherosclerosis is covered in detail in Chapter 17. The atherosclerotic plaques producing episodes of angina in patients with SIHD are not ones that rupture and produce rapid flow limiting thrombus as in the setting of an ACS.[11,12] In SIHD, the atherosclerotic plaques are more stable, have a reduced lipid core, and a firmer calcified covering. Since their geometry does not typically change acutely, they provide a relatively fixed decrease in myocardial oxygen supply.

Determinants of Myocardial Oxygen Demand

The major determinates of MVO_2 include heart rate (HR), myocardial contractility, and intramyocardial wall tension. A 2-fold increase in any of these individual determinates of MVO_2 requires an approximate 50% increase of coronary flow to maintain the myocardial supply—demand balance. Intramyocardial wall tension is the leading contributor to increased MVO_2 and is directly related to the radius or size of the ventricular cavity and blood pressure (BP), but indirectly related to the ventricular muscle mass. The larger the size of the ventricular cavity, the more energy or myocardial work is needed to begin myocardial contraction (systole). During early systole, myocardial work increases to a peak when the pressure in the LV becomes greater than the pressure outside the aortic valve. Once that occurs, the aortic valve is pushed open and blood is ejected into the systemic circulation. The higher the BP outside the aortic valve, the more MVO_2 needed per cardiac cycle. Increased ventricular muscle mass should make myocardial work easier and reduce MVO_2, for example as in an athlete's heart. Unfortunately, it is more common that the LV hypertrophy that occurs creates dysfunction myocytes that do not improve MVO_2. This type of LV hypertrophy also can worsen the supply/demand balance since blood vessel development (supply) is less than that of native myocardium.

The rate-pressure product, or double product, is a common noninvasive measure of MVO_2, which is the product of the HR and systolic BP. However, any change in contractility or volume loading of the LV is not considered by the double product. The increase in MVO_2 requirements commonly stems from release of norepinephrine by adrenergic nerve endings in the myocardium and vascular bed as part of the physiologic response to exertion, emotion, or mental stress. The rate of increase of MVO_2, or the rate at which a task is carried out, can be as important as the total amount of MVO_2. Hurrying is particularly likely to precipitate angina, as are efforts involving motion of the hands over the head. Mental and emotional stress may also precipitate angina, presumably by increasing adrenergic tone, and reduced vagal activity. Sexual activity may also precipitate angina due to the combination of physical exertion and emotional stimulation. Other precipitates of angina include physical exertion after a heavy meal and excessive metabolic demands imposed by chills, fever, thyrotoxicosis, tachycardia from any cause, exposure to cold, and hypoglycemia. Anger can also produce constriction of coronary arteries with preexisting narrowing, without necessarily directly affecting O_2 demand.

Determinates of Myocardial Oxygen Supply

Coronary Blood Flow

Meeting the metabolic demands of the myocardium is centered on the ability to maintain adequate coronary blood flow and coronary arterial pressure. Resting coronary blood flow under normal conditions averages 0.7 to 1.0 mL/min/g of myocardium.[13] The coronary vasculature is made up of larger epicardial vessels, also referred to as R_1 or conductance vessels, and smaller endocardial vessels, also referred to as R_2 or resistance vessels (Fig. 16-1).[14] Resistance to coronary blood flow is the sum of the resistance in the R_1 and R_2 vessels. The larger epicardial vessels typically offer little resistance to blood flow and are able to accommodate large increases in coronary flow without producing any significant drops in pressure. Therefore, these vessels mainly serve a conduit function. Most resistance to flow in normal coronary arteries is provided by the smaller endocardial (R_2) vessels. These vessels will contract and dilate to maintain blood flow based on the metabolic demands of the myocardium. When a person is at rest or not exerting themselves, and MVO_2 is low, the

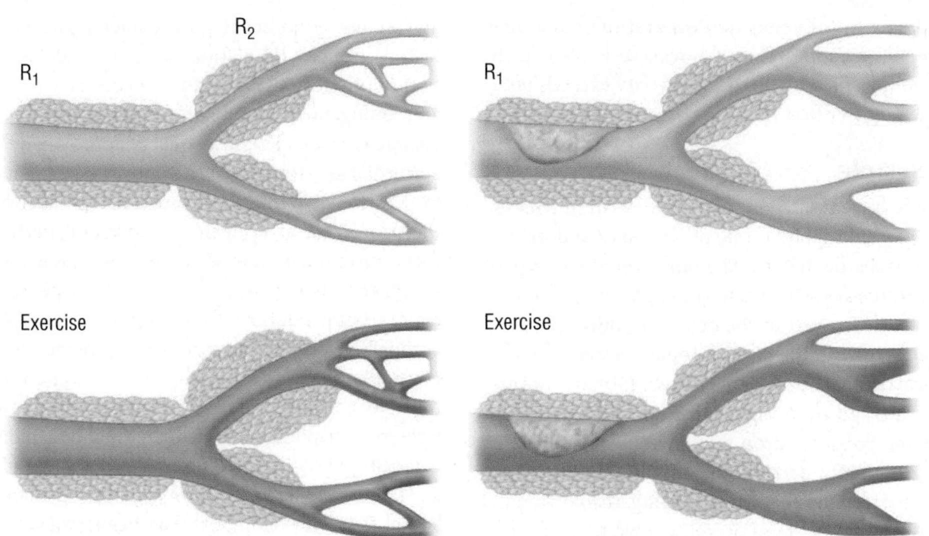

FIGURE 16-1 The coronary circulation with large epicardial conductance vessels (R_1) that offer little intrinsic resistance to myocardial blood flow and intramyocardial resistance arterioles (R_2). Resistance to flow equals $R_1 + R_2$ and R_2 resistance is normally much greater than R_1; hence flow is equal to the driving pressure across the coronary bed divided by the resistance in R_2. Dilation in R_2 normally occurs in response to exercise or increased myocardial oxygen demand. When an atherosclerotic lesion narrows the conductance vessel, the arterioles dilate under resting conditions to prevent ischemia. However, with stress, the vasodilator reserve becomes limited.

endocardial vessels with constrict since the need for blood flow is low. When this person undergoes physical exertion or emotional stress, the MVO_2 increases, and the endocardial vessels will dilate to increase myocardial oxygen supply in proportion to the increase in MVO_2 (see Fig. 16-1). This process in which the resistance vessels constrict and dilate based on MVO_2 is known as autoregulation.[13,14] Through autoregulation, coronary blood flow can increase 4- to 5-fold over that in normal resting conditions.[13] This increase in coronary flow above resting conditions is termed coronary flow reserve.

Coronary atherosclerotic plaque development typically occurs in the larger epicardial vessels. As these plaques continue to grow and cause luminal narrowing of the vessel, the vessel is transformed from one that originally provides minimal resistance into one that now provides considerable resistance to blood flow. This continues to a point where the epicardial artery resistance becomes dominate. Through autoregulation, this increase in resistance in the R_1 or conductance vessels is offset by vasodilation in the R_2 or resistance vessels to maintain flow.[14]

The amount of luminal diameter occupied by the atherosclerotic plaque is the major determine of the drop in pressure after the stenosis. The Bernoulli principle helps explain the fluid mechanics of a stenosis and the relationship between stenosis severity, pressure drop, and flow (Fig. 16-2).[15] The total pressure drop (and therefore flow) across a stenosis is governed by three hydrodynamic factors; viscous losses, separation losses, and turbulence, with turbulence representing a minor component of pressure loss. The most important determinant of stenosis resistance for any given level of flow is the minimum stenosis cross-sectional area.[16] Because resistance is inversely proportional to the square of the cross-sectional area, small dynamic changes in luminal area caused by atherosclerotic plaque size, thrombus creation, or vasospasm leads to major changes in the stenosis pressure-flow relation and reduce maximal perfusion during vasodilation.[16] Separation losses determine the steepness of the stenosis pressure-flow relation and become increasingly important as stenosis severity and/or flow rate increases. Stenosis length and changes in cross-sectional area distal to the stenosis are relatively minor determinates of resistance for most coronary lesions.

Coronary plaques that occupy less than 50% to 70% of the vessel luminal diameter rarely produce ischemia or angina.[14] As the intensity of exercise increases, the endocardial vessels dilate and resistance to flow decreases, leading to a proportional increase in myocardial blood flow so that there is not flow deficit or ischemia. Therefore, since these smaller plaques do not produce symptoms, the patient and clinician typically have no idea that they are there. Since small plaques have a rich lipid core and thin fibrous cap, they are more prone to rupture and acute thrombus production, making them quite dangerous and lethal (see Chapter 17).[11,12]

Once the epicardial vessel is significantly narrowed to 70% or more of the luminal diameter, the endocardial vessels dilate to maintain baseline coronary resistance at normal levels.[13,14] Therefore, much of the coronary flow reserve has been utilized and even low levels of exercise exhaust the remaining reserve. Further increments in exercise intensity can no longer be accompanied by further decreased in endocardial (R_2) resistance, and no further increments in flow can occur once autoregulation has reached its ceiling. This results in a flow deficit, causing myocardial ischemia and often angina. Therefore, the amount of exertion a patient can endure

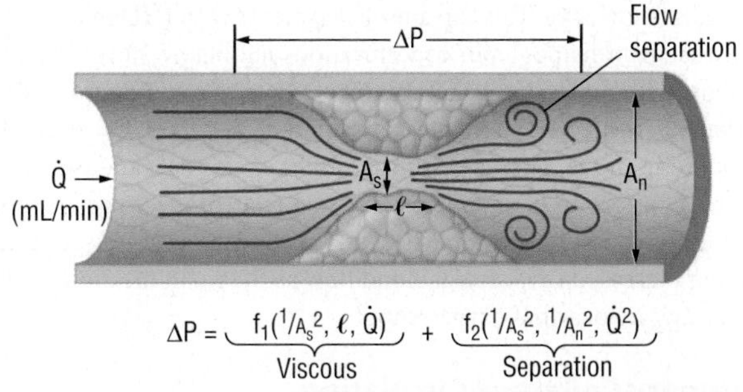

FIGURE 16-2 Fluid mechanics of a stenosis. The pressure drop across a stenosis can be predicted by the Bernouli equation. It is inversely related to the minimum stenosis cross-sectional area and varies with the square of the flow rate as stenosis severity increases. (A_n, area of the normal segment; A_s, area of the stenosis; f_1, viscous coefficient; f_2, separation coefficient; L, stenosis length; μ, viscosity of blood; ρ, density of blood; ΔP, pressure drop; Q, flow.)

is largely based on the extent of vessel stenosis and the remaining coronary flow reserve. The endocardial flow reserve is completely exhausted at rest when the epicardial stenosis severity exceeds 90%, which is also referred to as a critical stenosis.

Heart Rate and Systole

Increasing HR not only increases MVO_2, but also has an impact on reducing myocardial oxygen supply. While most tissues and organs are perfused during systole, the heart is the only organ that is perfused during diastole. There are two physiologic explanations for this difference.[17] First, pressure created in the ventricles during systole creates in increase in pressure in the distal coronary circulation well above that of the typical coronary perfusion pressure (50-60 mm Hg). Since coronary flow must go from higher to lower pressure, only during diastole does the pressures drop to allow downstream flow and myocardial oxygen supply. Second, the simple physical compression force of the myocardium that occurs during systole literally squeezes the downstream vessels closed preventing blood flow. During diastole, the myocytes relax and the downstream vessels open allowing coronary blood flow and myocardial oxygen delivery. During a typical cardiac cycle with a normal resting HR, the myocardial spends twice as much time in diastole compared to systole. When HR increases, time spend in diastole is reduced with little change in time spend in systole. During times of exertion and increased HR, the ratio to time spent in diastole to systole can be reduced from 2:1 to 1:1. This reduced time in diastole produces a reduced time for myocardial perfusion, and therefore, reduced total myocardial oxygen supply.[17]

Oxygen Extraction and Oxygen Carrying Capacity

Two additional determinants to myocardial oxygen supply are myocardial oxygen extraction and oxygen carrying capacity. Compared to most other vascular beds, myocardial oxygen extraction is near maximum at rest; nearly 60% to 80% of arterial oxygen content.[18] Coronary venous oxygen tension can only decrease from 25 mm Hg to a minimum of approximately 15 mm Hg. Therefore, during exertion, the ability to increase oxygen delivery to myocytes is limited through increasing the amount of oxygen extracted from the arterial blood.

Arterial oxygen content is equal to the product of the hemoglobin concentration and oxygen saturation. Small amounts of oxygen are also directly dissolved in plasma, but this does not contribute a measurable amount to myocardial oxygen supply. Consequently, patients with anemia (low hemoglobin) or hypoxia (low oxygen saturation) would have a reduction in their oxygen carrying capacity. The impact of anemia is thought to impact total oxygen carrying capacity to a greater degree than hypoxia unless the oxygen saturation falls below 50%. This explains why patients with IHD may receive transfusions if hemoglobin concentrations fall below 10 mg/dL, and patients without IHD are allowed to go as low as 6 to 8 mg/dL. Most patients have an arterial oxygen saturation of 95% to 100%, with little ability to improve. Therefore, during times of exertion and ischemia, there is little opportunity to improve myocardial oxygen supply through myocardial oxygen extraction or oxygen carrying capacity, leaving increased myocardial blood flow as the main mechanism for increasing myocardial oxygen supply.

Coronary Collateral Circulation

Most animals have some native collateral vessels from birth, though the extent can vary widely between species.[19] In the setting of SIHD, these native collateral vessels mature in a process termed arteriogenesis. As coronary stenosis exceeds 70%, resting distal pressure consistently falls due to maximized autoregulation. This extent of stenosis also contributes to episodes of exertion-induced ischemia. The ischemic episodes lead to the production of growth factors such as vascular endothelial growth factor and basic fibroblast growth factor through stimulation of nitric oxide synthase. The combination of physical forces of altered coronary pressure, growth factors, and endogenous vasodilators (eg, nitrous oxide and prostacyclin) change native collateral vessels of approximately 200 μm in existing epicardial anastomoses into mature vessels that can reach 1 to 2 mm in diameter.[20] While most functional collateral flow develops from the process of arteriogenesis, collateral perfusion can also occur from sprouting of new vessels in a process termed angiogenesis. The process of angiogenesis is also driven by physical forces and growth factors, but produces smaller, capillary-like vessels from preexisting coronary vessels. These vessels may provide collateral flow when they develop in the border between ischemic and nonischemic regions of the myocardium.[21] Capillary angiogenesis may also occur within the ischemic region and can reduce the intercapillary distance for oxygen delivery.

Investigation into pharmacologic mechanisms to improve collateral vessel development has been largely disappointing. While chronic nitrates may assist in development of collateral vessels, the use of growth factors and vasodilators have not produced the expected results. Due to the variability in collateral vessel development across different species, the use of animal models for study has significant limitations.[19]

Additional Factors Impacting Coronary Flow

While atherosclerotic coronary stenosis is the leading etiology in the development of SIHD and angina, there are a number of additional pathophysiologic mechanisms that are also occurring in these patients that contribute to disease onset and progression. These additional mechanisms include endothelial dysfunction, microvascular dysfunction, vasospasm, platelet activation and coagulation, as well as inflammation.[10,22] Endothelial dysfunction is manifested as a reduction in nitric oxide mediated vasodilation. This can be due to impairment in nitric oxide synthesis or availability. Reduced vasodilator response may lead to the development of ischemia at lower levels of exertion. There can also be impairment in how the microvascular response to endogenous vasodilators and vasoconstrictors, with reduced and exaggerated responses, respectively.[10] While atherosclerotic obstructive stenosis typically occurs in epicardial vessels, microvascular obstructions can also occasionally occur. Patients without epicardial stenosis, but presenting with demand driven ischemia, are classified as having cardiac syndrome X.[23]

Patients with an ACS event have ruptured atherosclerotic plaque with significant platelet accumulation and coagulation response producing an acute reduction in myocardial oxygen supply.[11,12] While this is not the pathophysiology of ischemia in patients with SIHD, there can be smaller plaques (30%-50% stenosis) that rupture that produce a fairly reserved platelet and coagulation response that does not produce an acute substantial reduction in myocardial oxygen supply. Instead, the process is arrested with an approximate 70% to 80% stenosis and reendothealialization.[11] Therefore, there is now a plaque that will lead to maximized flow reserve and exertion-driven ischemia that appears more sudden than the typically slowly accumulation plaque in most settings of SIHD. Finally, inflammation also plays a role in the pathophysiology of SIHD. In this setting, macrophages and T lymphocytes produce and secrete cytokines, chemokines, and growth factors that activate endothelial cells, increase vasoreactivity, and proliferation of vascular smooth muscle cells.[10,22] C-reactive protein, a marker of inflammation, has been shown to be elevated in patients with SIHD and correlates to adverse CV events. Statin therapy targeted at patients with elevated C-reactive protein and normal cholesterol levels has demonstrated a reduction in CV events.[24] While an obstructive atherosclerotic plaque contributes to ischemia and angina in patients with SIHD, the pathophysiology involves multiple mechanisms and the potential for multiple therapeutic targets.

2 Coronary Vasospasm and Prinzmetal's Angina

Most patients with SIHD have an obstructive coronary stenosis and exertion-induced ischemia. Since the size of the obstructive lesion does not change acutely, the amount of exertion needed to induce ischemia and angina is fairly predictable for an individual patient. For example, the patient knows when they work in the garden for 20 minutes or walk 5 blocks at a certain pace, before developing chest pain. Patients with this pattern of chest pain development are described as having a fixed angina threshold. Some patients can have what is described as having variable-threshold angina. In these patients the amount of exertion leading to chest pain may differ from day to day. An example would be the patient who could walk six blocks before experiencing angina yesterday, but today can only walk three blocks before becoming symptomatic. These patients also have an obstructing atherosclerotic plaque leading to a fixed decrease in supply, but they also have a reduction in myocardial oxygen supply due to transient vasospasm superimposed at the site of the obstructing plaque.[14,25] The vasospasm at or distal to the location of atherosclerotic plaque is typically induced by endothelial damage induced by the atherosclerotic plaque. Damaged endothelial cells produce less vasodilator substances such as endothelium-derived relaxing factor (EDRF), while also having an increased response to vasoconstrictors in response to exercise.[25] Patient symptoms will differ depending on the extent of the underlying fixed obstruction and the degree of dynamic change in coronary arterial tone. While the fixed obstruction is usually sufficient to produce symptoms with exertion, episodes of transient vasospasm superimposed on the obstruction significantly reduce myocardial blood flow leading to ischemia. The changing pattern of ischemia in these patients reflects a variable amount of vasospasm under certain conditions. Angina episodes are typically more common in the morning hours due to the circadian release of vasoconstrictors. Exposure to cold temperature, emotion, and mental stress has also been reported to lower the angina threshold in patients with variable threshold angina.

Patients may also have variant angina, also referred to as Prinzmetal's angina. Patients with variant angina typically have a different etiology of ischemia and angina compared to most patients with SIHD. Patients with variant angina usually do not have a coronary flow-obstructing atherosclerotic plaque, but instead have a significant reduction in myocardial oxygen supply due to substantial vasospasm in epicardial vessels.[25] The mechanism of this vasospasm is due to a reduced production of vasodilators, as well as an exaggerated response to endogenous vasoconstrictors. Patients with Prinzmetal's angina also have a different presentation compared to patients with SIHD and an obstructive coronary plaque. Patients with Prinzmetal's angina typically present with chest pain at rest, occur early in the morning, in younger patients, and have ST-segment elevation.[25]

CLINICAL PRESENTATION

A thorough patient history is key to the clinical assessment of a patient with SIHD. Exertional chest pain is the classical main presenting symptom of patients with SIHD. Since the differential diagnosis of "chest" pain is fairly broad (Table 16-1), it is important to determine if symptoms are due to a cardiac or noncardiac pathology. The description of a patient's chest pain also can be helpful in determining if a patient's pain is more likely to be due to SIHD or ACS. A commonly used method for incorporating the important aspects of the chest pain story is the PQRST mnemonic (Table 16-2).

3 The typical chest pain description of a patient with SIHD includes chest pain that is precipitated by exertion, such as walking, gardening, sexual activity, or some activities of daily living such as showering, cleaning house, or doing laundry. In this setting, the exertion produces an increase in MVO_2 that exceeds what can be provided by the fixed decrease in myocardial oxygen supply from the obstructive atherosclerotic plaque. Typically the most effective palliative measure is rest or the use of sublingual nitroglycerin (SL NTG). As the patient rests for a few minutes, the patient's HR and BP comes down to the level that can be met by the patient's reduced supply, reestablishing a balance between myocardial oxygen supply and demand, and the chest pain is relieved. Use of SL NTG also allows for relieve by acutely increasing myocardial oxygen supply through vasodilation of epicardial vessels and a reduction in preload.

The quality of cardiac chest pain is often described as squeezing, crushing, a heaviness, or tightness in the chest. It can also be more vague and described as a numbness or burning in the chest. Chest pain that is described as sharp in origin, pain that increases

TABLE 16-1 Differential Diagnosis of Episodic Chest Pain Resembling Angina Pectoris

	Duration	Quality	Provocation	Relief	Location	Comment
Effort angina	5-15 minutes	Visceral (pressure)	During effort or emotion	Rest, NTG	Substernal, radiates	First episode vivid
Rest angina	5-15 minutes	Visceral (pressure)	Spontaneous (with exercise?)	NTG	Substernal, radiates	Often nocturnal
Mitral prolapse	Minutes to hours	Superficial (rarely visceral)	Spontaneous (no pattern)	Time	Left anterior	No pattern, variable
Esophageal reflux	10 minutes to 1 hour	Visceral	Spontaneous, cold liquids, exercise, lying down	Foods, antacids, H_2 blockers, proton pump inhibitors, NTG	Substernal, radiates	Mimics angina
Peptic ulcer	Hours	Visceral, burning	Lack of food, "acid" foods	Foods, antacids, H_2 blockers, proton pump inhibitors	Epigastric, substernal	
Biliary disease	Hours	Visceral (wax and wane)	Spontaneous, food	Time, analgesia	Epigastric, radiates	Colic
Cervical disk	Variable (gradually subsides)	Superficial	Spontaneous, food	Time, analgesia	Arm, neck	Not relieved by rest
Hyperventilation	2-3 minutes	Visceral	Emotion, tachypnea	Stimulus removed	Substernal	Facial paraesthesia
Musculoskeletal	Variable	Superficial	Movement, palpation	Time, analgesia	Multiple	Tenderness
Pulmonary	30 minutes	Visceral (pressure)	Often spontaneous	Rest, time bronchodilator	Substernal	Dyspneic

NTG, nitroglycerin.

TABLE 16-2 PQRST Approach to Assessment of a Patient's Chest Pain

Factor	Presentation in Stable Ischemic Heart Disease
Precipitating factors	Typically brought on by some level of exercise or exertion
Palliative measures	Relieved by rest with or without a sublingual nitroglycerin in 5 to 10 minutes
Quality of the pain	Described as a squeezing, heaviness, or tightness
Region	Substernal
Radiation	Left or right arm, back, down into the abdomen, up into the neck
Severity	While pain is subjective, those who have pain report a 5 or higher on a 10-point scale
Temporal pattern (timing)	Pain last less than 20 minutes and usually relieved in 5 to 10 minutes

TABLE 16-3 Grading of Angina Pectoris by the Canadian Cardiovascular Society Classification System[26]

Class	Description of Stage
Class I	Ordinary physical activity does not cause angina such as walking and climbing stairs. Angina occurs with strenuous, rapid, or prolonged exertion at work or recreation
Class II	Slight limitation or ordinary activity. Angina occurs on walking or climbing stairs rapidly, on walking uphill, on walking or stair climbing after meals, in cold, in wind, under emotional stress, or only during the few hours after wakening. Walking more than two blocks on the level and climbing more than one flight of ordinary stairs at a normal pace and in normal condition
Class III	Marked limitations of ordinary physical activity. Angina occurs on walking one to two blocks on the level and climbing one flight of stairs in normal conditions and at a normal pace
Class IV	Inability to carry on any physical activity without discomfort—anginal symptoms may be present at rest

Used with permission from Campeau L. Grading of angina [letter]. Circulation 1976;54: 522-523, Copyright © 1976, Wolters Kluwer Health, Inc.

with inspiration or expiration, or a reproducible pain with palpation is usually not cardiac pain. The region of the pain is substernal and may radiate to the right or left shoulder, right or left arm (left more commonly than right), neck, back, or abdomen. Cardiac chest pain rarely radiates above the mandible or below the umbilicus. The severity of cardiac chest pain can be difficult to quantify since pain is a subjective measure, but the pain is usually considered severe and ranked a five or higher on a ten-point scale. The temporal pattern or duration of the chest pain in patients with SIHD is less than 20 minutes, but is usually around 5 to 10 minutes. Other symptoms that may also be present during times of ischemia include diaphoresis, nausea, vomiting, and dyspnea.

It is helpful to connect the pathophysiology with the clinical presentation. 1 In SIHD, ischemia is produced by an increase in MVO_2 in the setting of a fixed decrease in supply. 3 Exertion beyond the point in which autoregulation and coronary flow reserve are exhausted, the patient experiences chest pain. The patient then rest, or uses a SL NTG, and the MVO_2 comes down to a point in which myocardial supply and demand are back in balance, about 5 to 10 minutes, and the pain goes away and the patient feels better. [This sentence is covers concepts presented earlier and can be deleted] Relief of chest pain with the use of SL NTG can be a useful diagnostic tool for determining the origin of a patient's chest pain. However, esophageal pain also responds well to SL NTG. Esophageal pain is also relieved by food, antacids, milk, and occasionally warm liquids, while ischemic chest pain is not. The major differences between the pain with SIHD and the pain with an ACS would be the precipitating factors and the duration of the chest pain. The patient with an ACS typically has chest pain at rest that lasts longer than 20 minutes. The pathophysiology in a patient with an ACS is an abrupt decrease in myocardial oxygen supply from a plaque rupture, while increases in MVO_2 precipitate chest pain in patients with SIHD.

The severity of the angina and the impact of the disease on daily activity are often evaluated using the Canadian Cardiovascular Society (CCS) classification system (Table 16-3).[26] This system is a modification of the New York Heart Association functional classification used in patients with heart failure. Instead of determining the level of activity needed to produce dyspnea in patients with heart failure, the CSS system evaluates the level of activity needed to produce angina. There is also a scale developed by Goldman and associates that evaluates the metabolic cost to specific activities, and therefore, more specifically assesses the amount of MVO_2 a patient can achieve before producing angina.[27] Califf and associates developed an angina score that includes the tempo of angina along with ST and T wave changes on the electrocardiograph (ECG).[28] All of the current severity scores are limited by the subjective nature of a patient's pain as well as the reliability and reproducibility of patient observations.

Not all patients have a typical chest pain presentation.[1] "Typical" angina is comprised of three components: (1) substernal chest discomfort with a characteristic quality and duration that is (2) provoked by exertion or emotional stress and (3) relieved by rest or NTG. Patients with "atypical" angina meet two of the three criteria for typical angina. Patients meeting one or none of the typical angina characteristics are described as having noncardiac chest pain. Patient groups more likely to present with atypical angina include women and the elderly. Patients with DM may also have decreased sensation of pain due to complications of neuropathy.[29] Features of atypical angina or angina equivalents include symptoms such as midepigastric discomfort, effort intolerance, dyspnea, and excessive fatigue. To demonstrate the frequency of some of these symptoms, one study suggests that 65% of women with ischemia present with atypical symptoms.[30]

After a description of the chest pain has been obtained, a review of the patient's CAD risk factors should be performed. Non-modifiable risk factors include the patient's age and sex, and a family history of atherosclerotic disease in first-degree relatives (male onset before age 55 or female before age 65). The existence of the modifiable risk factors of HTN, DM, dyslipidemia, and cigarette smoking should also be evaluated. In addition to considering traditional risk factors, markers of inflammation, such as high sensitive C-reactive protein, have been investigated as risk factors for atherosclerosis. The value of C-reactive protein for primary prevention is growing, while the value for secondary prevention is less certain. Due to the systemic nature of atherosclerotic disease, patients with a history of cerebrovascular or peripheral arterial disease are also at high-risk for CAD. It is likely that patients having atherosclerosis in cerebral or peripheral arteries also have atherosclerosis in their coronary arteries even if it has not yet led to episodes of angina.

The physical examination of a patient with SIDH usually produces general and nonspecific findings. At the time of an ischemic episode, patients may present with tachycardia, diaphoresis, shortness of breath, and nausea. Other physical findings are related to the discovery of risk factors that may have led to the development of angina including an increased BP or a fourth heart sound reflecting long-standing HTN. Other positive findings may include pulmonary rales, displaced point of maximal impulse, or a third heart sound in patients with heart failure.

Diagnostic and Prognostic Testing

A number of noninvasive, as well as coronary angiography (invasive) testing can be done to assist in the diagnosis and evaluation of patients with SIHD. The most appropriate test based on available information and the clinical scenario for diagnosis is outlined in Figs. 16-3 and the use of testing for risk stratification is outlined in Fig. 16-4.[1] More information of how each test is preformed is available in Chapter 12.

Several tests can also provide prognostic information, which may help in determining the aggressiveness of pharmacotherapy and need for revascularization. All patients with symptoms suggestive of angina should receive a 12-lead ECG. In the resting state, the ECG will be normal in more than or equal to 50% of patients with SIHD. In patients with SIHD having a normal ECG at rest, about 50% will develop ischemic ST-T wave changes during an episode of angina. These changes can be observed on the ECG conducted during an exercise stress test. Exercise stress testing is a relatively easy and inexpensive method for detecting CAD. Since about 40% of patients who need a stress test cannot physically endure the test, the myocardium can also be stressed pharmacologically with adenosine, dipyridamole, or dobutamine. Stress testing can provide important diagnostic and prognostic information, especially when conducted with a nuclear imaging study to evaluate myocardial perfusion.

Coronary angiography is the most accurate test for the diagnosis and assessment of patients with CAD and is commonly considered the "gold standard." Unfortunately, coronary angiography is an invasive technique that requires arterial access. Findings in patients with SIHD routinely reveal that approximately 25% of patients have single-vessel disease, 25% have double-vessel disease, and 25% have triple-vessel disease, with 5% to 10% presenting with left main coronary disease and another 15% with no detectable critical vessel obstruction.

Coronary angiography is also useful in determining the fractional flow reserve (FFR) in patients with obstructive coronary stenosis. FFR is an indirect index determined by measuring the driving pressure of microcirculatory flow distal to the stenosis relative to the coronary driving pressure available in the absence of stenosis.[31] Although derived, the measurements are conceptually similar to those of relative coronary flow reserve because they only

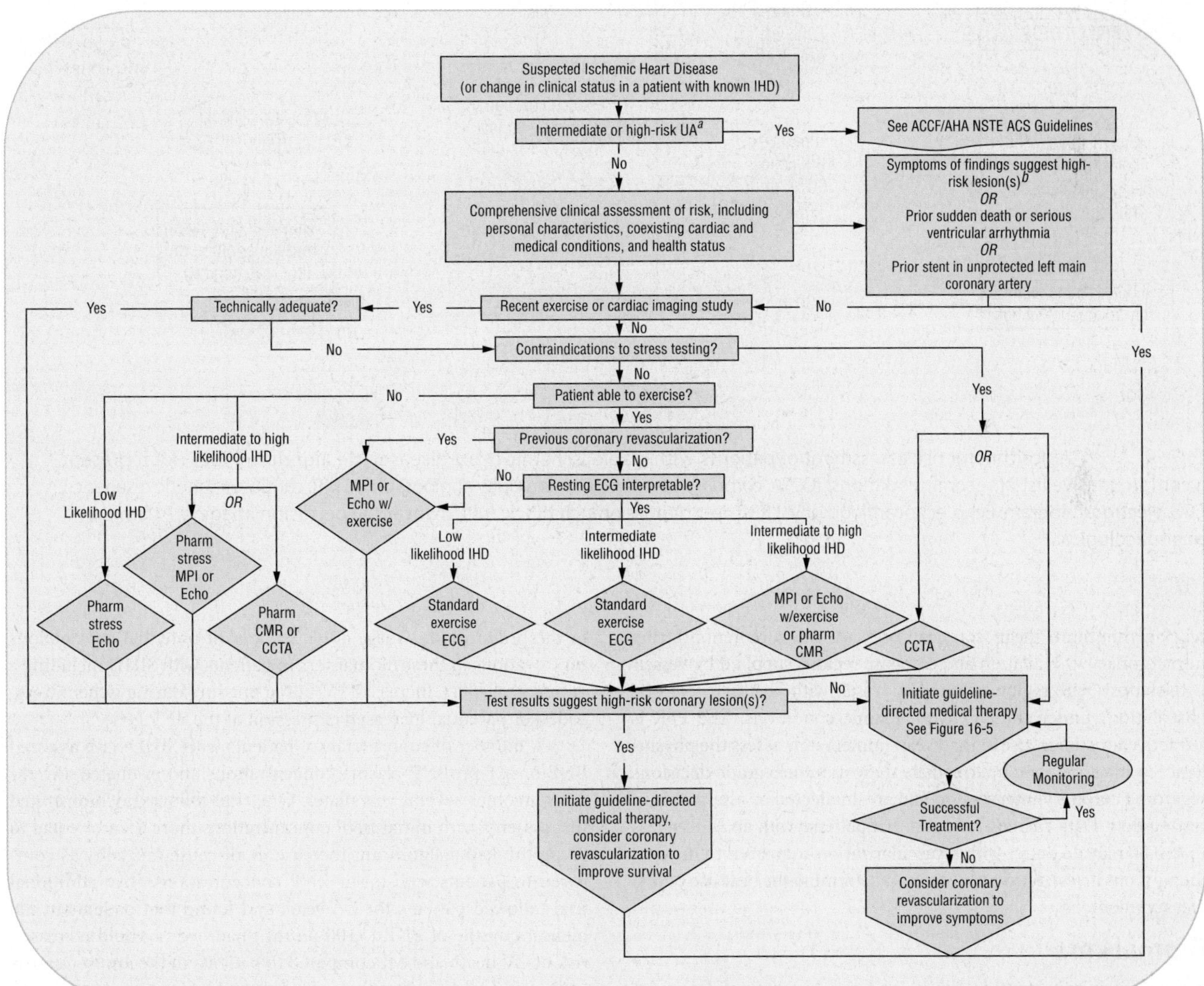

FIGURE 16-3 Diagnosis of patients with suspected ischemic heart disease. The algorithms do not represent a comprehensive list of recommendations (see ACC/AHA stable ischemic heart disease guidelines for all recommendations).
[a]See Table 16-2 in the ACC/AHA stable ischemic heart disease guidelines.
[b]CCTA is reasonable only for patients with intermediate probability of IHD.
(CCTA, computed coronary tomography angiography; CMR, cardiac magnetic resonance; ECG, electrocardiogram; Echo, echocardiography; IHD, ischemic heart disease; MI, myocardial infarction; MPI, myocardial perfusion imaging; Pharm, pharmacological; NSTE ACS, non-ST-segment elevation acute coronary syndrome; UA, unstable angina).

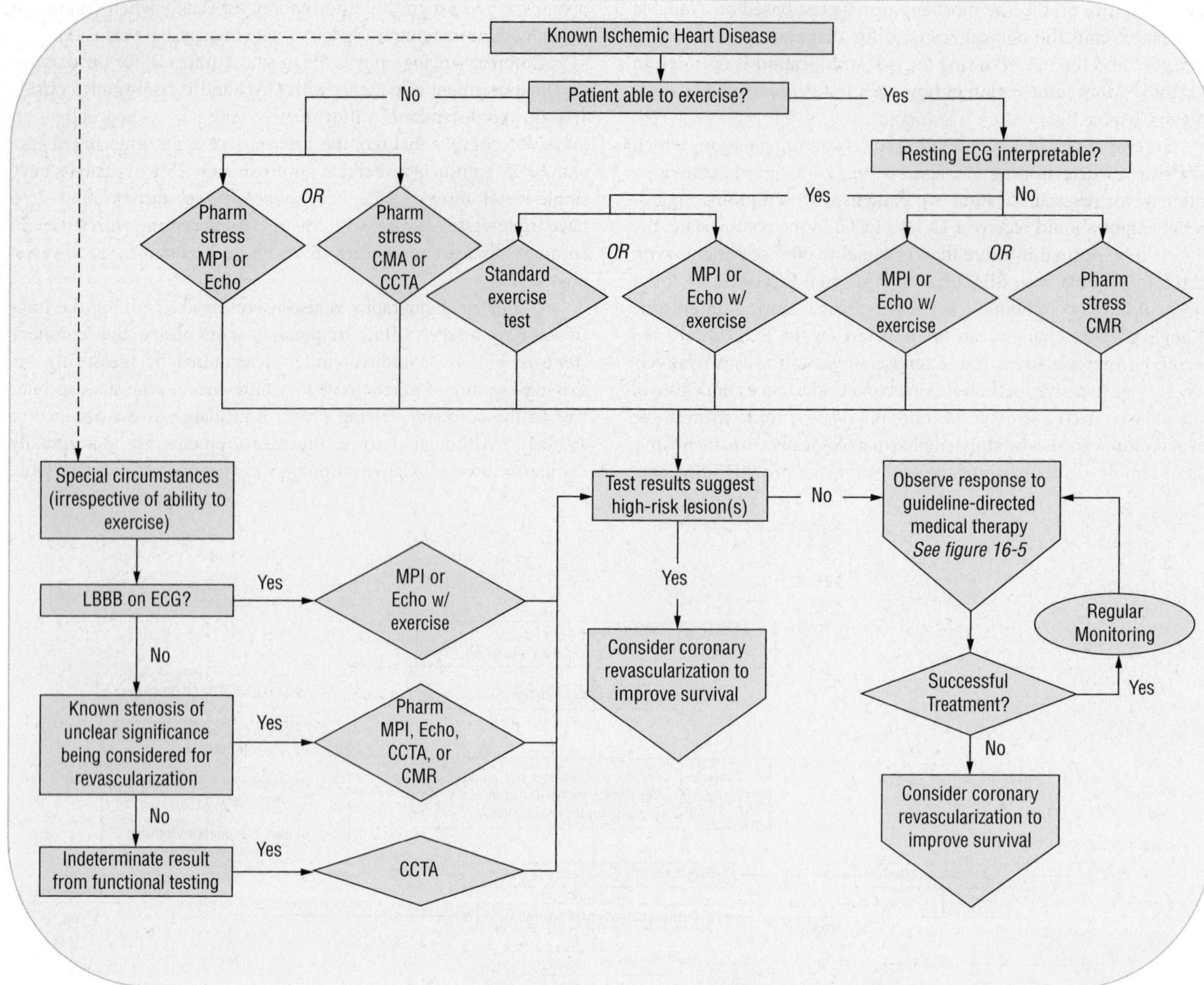

FIGURE 16-4 Algorithm for risk assessment of patients with stable ischemic heart disease. The algorithm does not represent a comprehensive list of recommendations. (CCTA, coronary computed tomography angiography; CMR, cardiac magnetic resonance; ECG, electrocardiogram; Echo, echocardiography; LBBB, left bundle branch block; MPI, myocardial perfusion imaging; Pharm, pharmacological.)

rely on minimum mean coronary pressure measurements during intracoronary vasodilation and compare regions supplied by vessels with stenosis with region supplied by vessels without atherosclerotic obstructions under similar hemodynamic conditions. The FFR is attractive for clinical use in that it can immediately assess the physiologic significance of an intermediate stenosis to help guide decisions regarding coronary intervention and are unaffected by alterations in resting flow. Data currently suggest that patients with an FFR of less than 0.80 may do better with revascularization compared to medical therapy, but investigation continues to determine the best use of this measurement.[31,32]

Biomarkers

B-type natriuretic peptide (BNP) and the N-terminal fragment (NT-proBNP) have been a useful biomarker in the diagnosis and prognosis of patients with heart failure and ACS for many years. Data on the prognostic implications of elevated natriuretic peptides in patients with SIHD have also been evaluated. BNP is a cardiac hormone that is mainly synthesized in the LV in response to increased ventricular volume and/or pressure creating ventricular wall stress.[33] The production of BNP begins as a prohormone (pro-BNP) that is enzymatically cleaved into the active hormone BNP and the NT-proBNP of the prohormone. There are a number of potential explanations for elevations in these biomarkers in patients with SIHD including a cumulative effect, increased LV filling pressure during ischemic episodes, or potential increased expression of the BNP gene.[33]

A number of cohort trials of patients with SIHD have assessed BNP or NT-proBNP plasma concentrations and evaluated adverse CV outcomes several years later. One trial followed demonstrated that patients with initial BNP concentrations more than or equal to 87 pg/mL had a significant increase in all-cause mortality as compared to patients with lower BNP concentrations.[34] An additional trial followed patients for 2.5 years and found that patients in the highest quartile of BNP (>100 pg/mL) had over a 4-fold increased risk of CV death and MI compared to patients in the lowest quartile (<12 pg/mL).[35] Based on these data, elevated plasma concentrations of BNP or NT-proBNP may be considered an emerging risk factor for SIHD.

Cardiac troponin concentrations are released when there is myocyte death (infarction), and hence are not typically elevated in patients with SIHD. In one study of patients undergoing percutaneous coronary intervention (PCI) for treatment of SIHD found that 6% of patients had an elevated troponin before PCI.[36] After adjusting for demographic, clinical, angiographic, and procedural factors, patients with an elevated pre-procedure troponin had a significant increase of inhospital death or MI compared to patients without an elevated troponin (13.4% vs 5.6%). The difference in these outcomes was still significant 1 year later.[36] Due to the fact there were multiple study sites, and therefore multiple reference ranges, no specific cut-off troponin value designating increased risk could be determined. The mechanism of the increase in troponin is not completely understood, but may be due to increased cardiac cell membrane permeability with repeated ischemia.

TREATMENT

Desired Outcomes

The management of patients with SIHD is typically divided into two parts (Fig. 16-5) that aim to improve the quantity and quality of life for the patient.[1] The first is directed toward slowing the progression of atherosclerosis and preventing complications of such as MI, heart failure, stroke, as well as death (either sudden cardiac death, or death secondary to progression of underlying CV conditions). Therapy in this approach generally is targeted at risk factor modification and other vasculoprotective therapies. While these therapies have demonstrated the ability to reduce mortality, and therefore, the quantity of life for the patient with SIHD, they typically have minimal impact on improving symptoms and limitations of angina, or the quality of life. 4 The other approach targets reducing the number of ischemic episodes as well as increasing the amount of exertion or exercise a patient can accomplish before inducing an ischemic episode. Therapies used in this approach rarely have demonstrated an improvement in improving the quantity of life, but do improve the quality of life through a reduction in symptoms. The ACC/AHA SIHD guidelines state that a goal of therapy should be the complete, or nearly complete, elimination of angina chest pain and return to normal activities and a functional capacity of CCS class I angina.[1] Recommendations from the ACC/AHA are organized in to a Class of Recommendation, which is an estimate of the size of the treatment effect, balancing efficacy and safety. Each recommendation is also based on a Level of Evidence (LOE), which describes the level of certainty or precision of the treatment effect and is based on the amount of evidence to support a recommendation. Table 16-4 describes the different classes of recommendation and the levels of evidence used to classify the ACC/AHA recommmendations.[1]

Guideline-Directed Medical Therapy

The primary method in which to improve mortality in patients with SIHD is providing guideline-directed medical therapy (GDMT), also referred to as optimal medical therapy.[1] 5 6 Besides certain settings of disease severity (Table 16-5), GDMT provides similar rates of death and MI compared to revascularization therapy. These are therapies that have demonstrated a reduction in mortality, and consequently improving the quantity of life for patients with SIHD. These therapies mainly include risk factor modifications (Table 16-6), but additionally medications such as aspirin and angiotensin converting enzyme (ACE) inhibition.

7 Antiplatelet Therapy

Aspirin provides its antiplatelet effect by providing nearly complete blockade of cyclooxygenase-1 (COX-1) activity (~ 95%) and subsequent thromboxane A_2 production. The reduction in thromboxane A_2 leads to reduced platelet activation and aggregation for the life of the platelet. Aspirin doses as small as 30 mg used chronically have been shown to provide the needed level of COX-1 inhibition. Therefore, further increases in aspirin doses above 75 to 100 mg would be expected to provide little additional antiplatelet potency of aspirin.[37] Aspirin is also thought to provide benefits through some nonplatelet mediated effects. Compared to higher doses of aspirin (≥325 mg daily), low-dose aspirin has demonstrated a lack of significant impairment of endothelial secretion of prostacyclin, which is a natural vasodilator. Even though there may be some inhibition of prostacyclin with the use of aspirin, the effects on the endothelium are reversible, compared to the effect on platelets.[38] After unbound aspirin has been removed from the circulation (half-life is about 30 minutes), prostacyclin secretion and its vasodilation effects are restored. Aspirin may also attenuate the synthesis of cytokines such as interleukin-2, interleukin-6, and interferon in leukocytes.[39] Aspirin may also prevent leukocyte rolling and macrophage-induced endothelial activation.[39,40]

Clinical evidence describing the effectiveness of aspirin in patients with SIHD first came from a subgroup analysis of the Physicians Health Study.[41] The original trial was a double-blind evaluation of the efficacy of low-dose aspirin (325 mg every other day) compared to placebo in the primary prevention of MI, stroke, or CV death. Of the 22,071 patients enrolled in the trial, 333 had a history of SIHD. After the 5-year follow-up period, the patients with SIHD had an 87% significant reduction in risk for first MI.[41] Similar to the overall trial results, this benefit came with a significant increase in hemorrhagic stroke, although none of the strokes were fatal. There was no difference in total or CV mortality, but there were too few patients with SIHD to provide a meaningful analysis of these endpoints.

These beneficial effects of aspirin were confirmed in the more robust SAPAT (Swedish Angina Pectoris Aspirin Trial).[42] The SAPAT trial randomized 2,035 patients with controlled angina on sotalol to 75 mg of aspirin daily or matching placebo. At the end of the 50 month follow-up, patients receiving aspirin had a 34% relative reduction in first MI or sudden death. There was no difference in major bleeding or stroke between the groups. These results support the ACC/AHA recommendation for the use of aspirin in patients with SIHD.[1]

Concern has been raised over the past decade about patients being nonresponsive to the antiplatelet effects of aspirin, and therefore, not receiving the clinical benefit. A recent meta-analysis reported the average rate of aspirin nonresponsiveness to be 24%, but the range of reported nonresponsiveness is wide (0%-57%).[43] If only studies that used light transmission aggregometry (the gold standard test) induced with arachidonic acid and/or measurement of serum thromboxane B_2 are used, the rate of aspirin nonresponsiveness is only 6%.[43] These results are similar to the findings of the ASPECT (Aspirin-Induced Platelet Effects) trial, in which aspirin nonresponsiveness defined by COX-1-nonspecific methods was 27%, compared to only 6% when COX-1-specific methods were used.[44] The ASPECT investigators also reported no difference in aspirin nonresponsiveness between patients receiving 81 mg, 162 mg, or 325 mg daily.[44] A lack of dose response to clinical outcomes is consistent with the findings of the Antithrombotic Trialists' Collaboration meta-analysis which found a similar protection against vascular events regardless if patients were receiving low dose (75-150 mg daily), moderate dose (160-325 mg daily), or high dose (500-1,500 mg daily) aspirin.[37]

Pharmacodynamic aspirin nonresponsiveness may occur because of changes to the COX-1 enzyme, such as changes to the enzyme structure, or the transient inaccessibility of the enzyme due to the blockade of the active site. Of particular concern is the potential for nonsteroidal anti-inflammatory drug therapy to inhibit the effect of aspirin on the COX-1 enzyme. Naproxen and ibuprofen have shown to interfere with aspirin's antiplatelet effect when coadministered due to competition for access to the site of action in the COX-1 enzyme.[45] Timing of coadministration appears to be an important factor in the extent of competition. The effect of aspirin on platelet aggregation is impaired when ibuprofen is given 2 hours before aspirin, but when aspirin is given first there is no effect on the ability of aspirin to inhibit platelet aggregation.

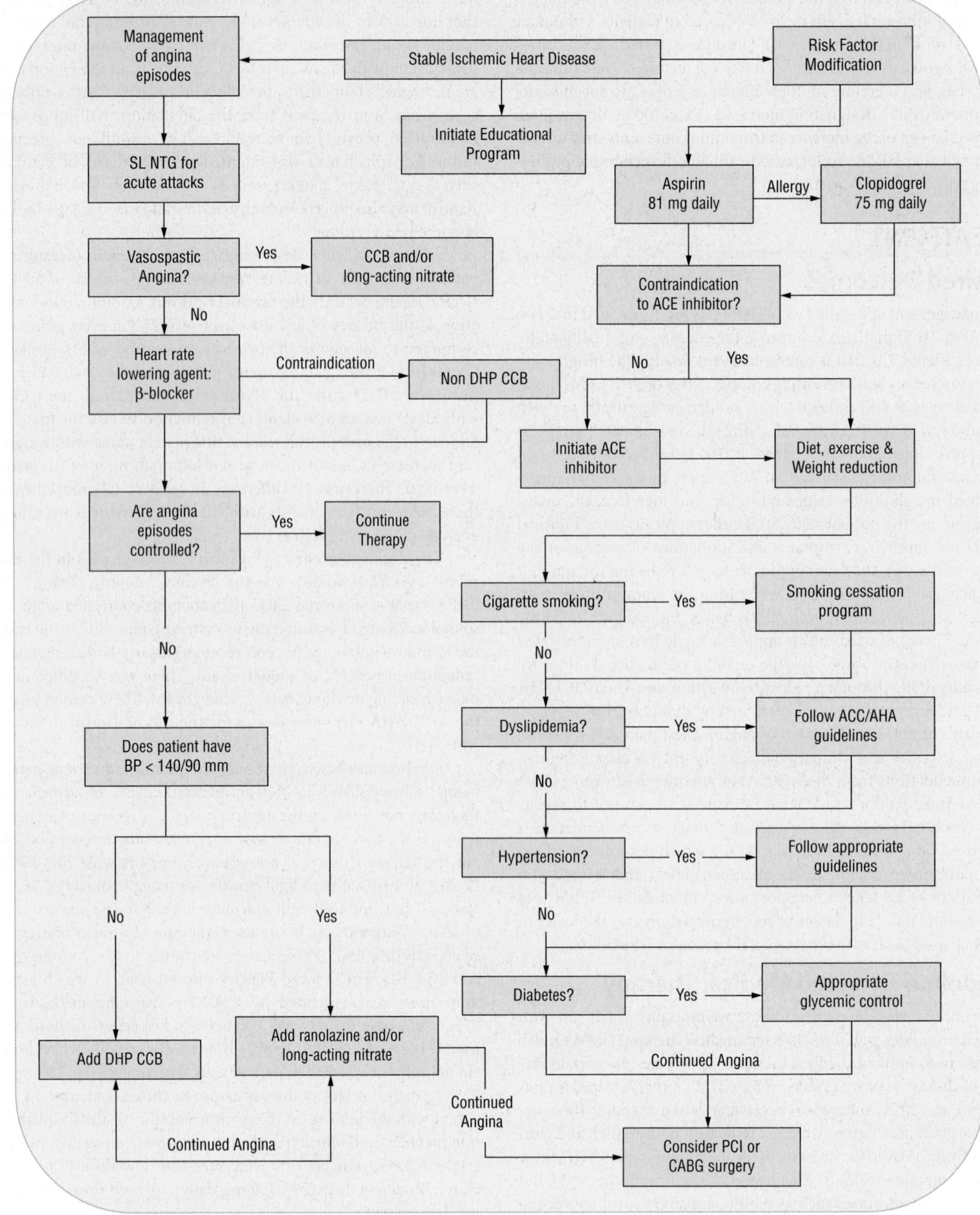

FIGURE 16-5 Algorithm for treatment of stable ischemic heart disease (Guideline-directed medical therapy).

A number of clinical trials have found a relationship between aspirin nonresponsiveness and increased risk of ischemic events. One commonly referenced trial of 325 patients with SIHD identified a lack of aspirin response in 5.2% of patients.[46] The incidence of death, MI, or stroke was significantly higher for nonresponders compared to responders (24% vs 10%).[46] Another trial of 468 patients with SIHD also found a 3-fold increase in risk of ischemic events associated with aspirin nonresponsiveness compared to responsive patients (15.6% vs 5.3%).[47] While aspirin nonresponsiveness does exist, the incidence is probably not as high as once thought. Even though patients with aspirin nonresponsiveness have demonstrated a higher rate of ischemic events, there are no recommendations for screening. Also, since increasing the dose of aspirin is unlikely to impact the incidence of nonresponsiveness or clinical outcomes, the only management strategy would be to change or add additional antiplatelet therapy.

TABLE 16-4 The American College of Cardiology and American Heart Association Evidence Grading System[1]

Recommendation Class	Level of Evidence
I Conditions for which there is evidence or general agreement that a given procedure or treatment is useful and effective II Conditions for which there is conflicting evidence or a divergence of opinion that the usefulness/efficacy of a given procedure or treatment is useful and effective IIa Weight of evidence/opinion is in favor or usefulness/efficacy IIb Usefulness/efficacy is less well established by evidence/opinion III Conditions for which there is evidence or general agreement that a given procedure or treatment is not useful/effective and in some cases may be harmful	A. Data derived from multiple randomized clinical trials with large numbers of patients B. Data derived from a limited number of randomized trials with small numbers of patients, careful analyses of nonrandomized studies, or observational registries C. Expert consensus was the primary basis for the recommendation

In patients unable to take aspirin due to allergy or intolerance, clopidogrel represents a suitable alternative antiplatelet agent to prevent MI and death in patients with CAD.[1] While clopidogrel significantly reduced the incidence of stroke, MI, or vascular death in patients with atherosclerotic vascular disease (previous MI, stroke, or peripheral arterial disease) compared to aspirin in the CAPRIE (The Clopidogrel versus Aspirin in Patients at Risk of Ischemic Events) trial (5.32% vs 5.83%; p = 0.043), the absolute difference in the primary outcome between the two strategies was quite small (0.5%, number need to treat = 200).[48] Only 22% of the patients in the CAPRIE trial

TABLE 16-5 Revascularization to Improve Survival: ACC/AHA Recommendations[1]

Left Main CAD Revascularization

Class I

1. CABG to improve survival is recommended for patients with significant (≥50% diameter stenosis) left main coronary artery stenosis. (LOE B)

Class IIa

1. PCI to improve survival is reasonable as an alternative to CABG in selected stable patients with significant (≥50% diameter stenosis) unprotected left main CAD with: (1) anatomic conditions associated with a low risk of PCI procedural complications and a high likelihood of good long-term (eg, a low SYNTAX score [≤22], ostial or trunk left main CAD); and (2) clinical characteristics that predict a significantly increased risk of adverse surgical outcomes (eg, STS-predicted risk of operative mortality ≥5%). (LOE B)
2. PCI to improve survival is reasonable in patients with UA/NSTEMI when an unprotected left main coronary artery is the culprit lesion and the patient is not a candidate for CABG. (LOE B)
3. PCI to improve survival is reasonable in patients with acute STEMI when an unprotected left main coronary artery is the culprit lesion, distal coronary flow is less than TIMI (Thrombolysis in Myocardial Infarction) grade 3, and PCI can be performed more rapidly and safely than CABG. (LOE C)

Class IIb

1. PCI to improve survival may be reasonable as an alternative to CABG in selected stable patients with significant (≥50% diameter stenosis) unprotected left main CAD with: (a) anatomic conditions associated with a low to intermediate risk of PCI procedural complications and an intermediate to high likelihood of good long-term outcome (eg, low-intermediate SYNTAX score of <33, bifurcation left main CAD); and (b) clinical characteristics that predict an increased risk of adverse surgical outcomes (eg, moderate-severe chronic obstructive pulmonary disease, disability from previous stroke, or previous cardiac surgery; STS-predicted risk of operative mortality >2%). (LOE B)

Class III: Harm

1. PCI to improve survival should not be performed in stable patients with significant (≥50% diameter stenosis) unprotected left main CAD who have unfavorable anatomy for PCI and who are good candidates for CABG. (LOE B)

Non-Left Main CAD Revascularization

Class I

1. CABG to improve survival in beneficial in patients with significant (≥70% diameter) stenosis in 3 major coronary arteries with or without involvement of the proximal LAD artery or in the proximal LAD artery plus 1 other major coronary artery. (LOE B)
2. CABG or PCI to improve survival is beneficial in survivors of sudden cardiac death with presumed ischemia-mediated ventricular tachycardia caused by significant (≥70% diameter) stenosis in a major coronary artery. (LOE C)

Class IIa

1. CABG to improve survival is reasonable in patients with significant (≥70% diameter) stenosis in 2 major coronary arteries with severe or extensive myocardial ischemia (eg, high-risk criteria on stress testing, abnormal intracoronary hemodynamic evaluation, or >20% perfusion defect by myocardial perfusion stress imaging) or target vessels supplying a large area of viable myocardium. (LOE B)
2. CABG to improve survival is reasonable in patients with mid-moderate LV systolic dysfunction (EF 35%-50%) and significant (≥70% diameter stenosis) multivessel CAD or proximal LAD coronary artery stenosis, when viable myocardium is present in the region of intended revascularization. (LOE B)
3. CABG with a left internal mammary artery (LIMA) graft to improve survival is reasonable in patients with significant (≥70% diameter) stenosis in the proximal LAD artery and evidence of extensive ischemia. (LOE B)
4. It is reasonable to choose CABG over PCI to improve survival in patients with complex 3-vessel CAD (eg, SYNTAX score >22), with or without involvement of the proximal LAD artery who are good candidates for CABG. (LOE B)
5. CABG is probably recommended in preference to PCI to improve survival in patients with multivessel CAD and diabetes mellitus, particularly if a LIMA graft can be anastomosed to the LAD artery. (LOE B)

Class IIb

1. The usefulness of CABG to improve survival is uncertain in patients with significant (70% diameter) stenoses in two major coronary arteries not involving the proximal LAD artery and without extensive ischemia. (LOE C)
2. The usefulness of PCI to improve survival is uncertain in patients with 2- or 3-vessel CAD (with or without involvement of the proximal LAD artery or 1-vessel proximal LAD disease. (LOE B)
3. CABG might be considered with the primary or sole intent of improving survival in patients with SIHD with severe LV systolic dysfunction (EF <35%) whether or not viable myocardium is present. (LOE B)
4. The usefulness of CABG or PCI to improve survival is uncertain in patient with CABG and extensive anterior wall ischemia on noninvasive testing. (LOE B)

Class III: Harm

1. CABG or PCI should not be performed with the primary or sole intent to improve survival in patients with SIHD with 1 or more coronary stenoses that are not anatomically or functionally significant (<70% diameter non-left main coronary artery stenosis, FFR >0.80, no or only mild ischemia on noninvasive testing), involve only the left circumflex or right coronary artery, or subtend only a small area of viable myocardium. (LOE B)

TABLE 16-6 Risk Factor Modification: ACC/AHA Recommendations[1]

Lipid Management

Class I

1. Lifestyle modifications, including daily physical activity and weight management, are strongly recommended for all patients with SIHD. (LOE B)
2. Dietary therapy for all patients should include reduced intake of saturated fats (to <7% of total calories), *trans* fatty acids (to <1% of total calories), and cholesterol (to <200 mg/day). (LOE B)
3. In addition to therapeutic lifestyle changes, a moderate or high dose of a statin therapy should be prescribed, in the absence of contraindications or documented adverse effects. (LOE A)

Class IIa

1. For patients who do not tolerate statins, LDL cholesterol-lowering therapy with bile acid sequestrates, niacin, or both is reasonable. (LOE B)

Blood Pressure Management

Class I

1. All patients should be counseled about the need for lifestyle modification: weight control; increased physical activity; alcohol moderation; sodium reduction; and emphasis on increased consumption of fresh fruits, vegetables, and low-fat dairy products. (LOE B)
2. In patients with SIHD with BP 140/90 mm Hg or higher, antihypertensive drug therapy should be instituted in addition to or after a trial of lifestyle modifications. (LOE A)
3. The specific medications used for treatment of high BP should be based on specific patient characteristics and may include ACE inhibitors and/or beta blockers, with addition of other drugs, such as thiazide diuretics or calcium channel blockers, if needed to achieve a goal BP of <140/90 mm Hg. (LOE B)

Diabetes Management

Class IIa

1. For selected individual patients, such as those with a short duration of diabetes mellitus and a long life expectancy, a goal HbA1c of 7% or less is reasonable. (LOE B)
2. A goal HbA1c between 7% and 9% is reasonable for certain patients according to age, history of hypoglycemia, presence of microvascular or macrovascular complications, or presence of coexisting medical conditions. (LOE C)

Class IIb

1. Initiation of pharmacotherapy interventions to achieve target HgA1c might be reasonable. (LOE A)

Class III: Harm

1. Therapy with rosiglitazone should not be initiated in patients with SIHD. (LOE C)

Physical Activity

Class I

1. For all patients, the clinician should encourage 30 to 60 minutes of moderate-intensity aerobic activity, such as brisk walking, at least 5 days and preferably 7 days per week, supplemented by an increase in daily lifestyle activities (eg, walking breaks at work, gardening, and household work) to improve cardiorespiratory fitness and move patients out of the least-fit, least-active, high-risk cohort (bottom 20%). (LOE B)
2. For all patients, risk assessment with a physical activity history and/or an exercise test is recommended to guide prognosis and prescription. (LOE B)
3. Medically supervised programs (cardiac rehabilitation) and physician-directed, home-based programs are recommended for at risk patients at first diagnosis. (LOE A)

Class IIa

1. It is reasonable for the clinician to recommend complementary resistance training at least 2 days per week. (LOE C)

Weight Management

Class I

1. BMI and/or waist circumference should be assessed at every visit, and the clinician should consistently encourage weight maintenance or reduction through an appropriate balance of lifestyle physical activity, structured exercise, caloric intake, and formal behavioral programs when indicated to maintain or achieve a BMI between 18.5 and 24.9 kg/m^2 and a waist circumference less than 102 cm (40 inches) in men and less than 88 cm (35 inches) in women (less for certain racial groups). (LOE B)
2. The initial goal of weight loss therapy should be to reduce body weight by approximately 5% to 10% from baseline. With success, further weight loss can be attempted if indicate. (LOE C)

Smoking Cessation Counseling

Class I

1. Smoking cessation and avoidance of exposure to environmental tobacco smoke at work and home should be encouraged for all patients with SIHD. Follow-up, referral to special programs, and pharmacotherapy are recommended, as is a stepwise strategy for smoking cessation (Ask, Advise, Assess, Assist, Arrange, Avoid). (LOE B)

Management of Psychological Factors

Class IIa

1. It is reasonable to consider screening SIHD patients for depression and to refer or treat when indicated. (LOE B)

Class IIb

1. Treatment of depression has not been shown to improve cardiovascular disease outcomes but might be reasonable for its other clinical benefits. (LOE C)

Alcohol Consumption

Class IIb

1. In patients with SIHD who use alcohol, it might be reasonable for nonpregnant women to have 1 drink (4 ounces of wine, 12 ounces of beer, or 1 ounce of spirits) a day and for men to have 1 or 2 drinks per day, unless alcohol is contraindicated (such as in patients with a history of alcohol abuse or dependence or with liver disease. (LOE C)

Avoiding Exposure to Air Pollution

Class IIa

1. It is reasonable for patients with SIHD to avoid exposure to increased air pollution to reduce the risk of cardiovascular events. (LOE C)

had documented SIHD and no specific subgroup analysis is available for those patients. Given the small magnitude of benefit along with significantly higher cost, clopidogrel has remained a second line choice behind aspirin in patients with CAD. When used in patients with SIHD, clopidogrel should be administered at a dose of 75 mg per day.

The role of dual antiplatelet therapy (DAPT) with aspirin and a $P2Y_{12}$ inhibitor, such as clopidogrel, has mainly been evaluated in patients receiving PCI with stents and in the post-ACS setting, and not in patients with SIHD. In a patient population similar to the CAPPRIE trial, the CHARISMA trial (Clopidogrel for High Atherothrombotic Risk and Ischemic Stabilization, Management, and Avoidance) evaluated aspirin compared to aspirin plus clopidogrel in patients (n=15,603) with documented vascular disease (CAD, cerebrovascular disease, peripheral arterial disease), or with no documented vascular disease but with multiple CV risk factors.[49]

The combination of aspirin plus clopidogrel for 28 months did not reduce the risk of death, MI, stroke, or coronary revascularization as compared to aspirin alone in the entire study population, although there was a significant reduction in the risk of death, MI and stroke in those patients receiving aspirin plus clopidogrel compared to aspirin alone (7.3% vs 8.8%, p = 0.01) in patients with established vascular disease at study entry (n = 12,319).[49,50] There was a significant increase in the risk of bleeding with the use of DAPT compared to aspirin alone. Therefore, there are limited data to support the use of DAPT in patients with SIHD who have not received PCI with stent placement or a recent ACS event.

A number of trials have demonstrated that there is extensive variability in patient response to clopidogrel, but for the most part, the antiplatelet activity follows a bell-shaped curve.[51] Due to the variety of tests evaluating clopidogrel activity, and the different definition of nonresponsiveness used, estimates reported in these trials range from 5% to 44%.[52,53] A number of different definitions have been evaluated for clopidogrel nonresponsiveness, and trials have correlated these definitions with clinical response.

There is currently significant confusion about what to do if a patient is found to have a lack of appropriate response to clopidogrel therapy. The most common cause of nonresponsiveness is noncompliance. If patients are even partially noncompliant with their clopidogrel therapy, the tests to evaluate clopidogrel therapy will demonstrate a lack of response. Data from the PREMIER (Prospective Registry Evaluating Myocardial Infarction: Events and Recovery) registry provides evidence that noncompliance is associated with increased ischemic events, as well as important insight into patient predictors of noncompliance.[54]

Conversion of clopidogrel to its active compound requires a two-step conversion process. While numerous cytochrome P450 (CYP) enzymes may play a role in conversion, the CYP2C19 enzyme seems to be the major contributor in both steps. This has led some to suggest a role for CYP2C19 genetic testing in patients receiving clopidogrel as a method to identify potential nonresponders to clopidogrel therapy.[55] Genetic polymorphisms to CYP2C19 may contribute to a lack of response to clopidogrel therapy, but do not fully explain a lack of response in most patients. Trials have demonstrated that identification of CYP2C19 status only explains 12% to 15% of the variability in clopidogrel response.[56,57] Therefore, many patients with "wild-type" CYP2C19 will still not achieve adequate antiplatelet response to clopidogrel. At this time genetic testing is not the answer to explaining poor antiplatelet response to clopidogrel therapy.

Another consideration when patients are found to have a lack of adequate response to clopidogrel is drug-drug interactions involving CYP 2C19. All proton pump inhibitors (PPIs) are metabolized by CYP 2C19 to varying degrees. These are the most widely prescribed medications worldwide and a number of trials evaluating the impact of PPIs on clopidogrel activity have been conducted. A number of pharmacodynamic and observational cohort trials have suggested that patients receiving a PPI (mainly omeprazole) and clopidogrel have reduced antiplatelet activity and more ischemic outcomes.[58,59] Other prospective data do not support that this drug interaction has significant clinical implications.[60]

Recommendations from the ACC/AHA for the use of antiplatelet agents in the management of SIHD include a Class I recommendation for the use of aspirin 75 to 162 mg daily, continued indefinitely in the absence of contraindications (LOE A).[1] Clopidogrel is considered a reasonable alternative when aspirin in contraindicated (LOE B). The guidelines state that treatment with aspirin (75-162 mg daily) and clopidogrel 75 mg daily might be reasonable in certain high-risk patients with SIHD as a Class IIb (LOE B) recommendation. The use of dipyridamole is a Class III recommendation (LOE B).

7 Angiotensin-Converting Enzyme Inhibitors

The use of ACE inhibitors has been shown to provide significant mortality benefit in patients with systolic heart failure or recent MI with reduced ejection fraction. They have also been shown to reduce the progression of nephropathy in patients with or without HTN. In the setting of atherosclerotic disease and SIHD, ACE inhibitors have demonstrated the ability to stabilize coronary plaque, provide restoration or improvement in endothelial function, inhibition of vascular smooth muscle cell growth, decreased macrophage migration, and possibly possess some antioxidant activities. They may also possess some antithrombotic properties through inhibition of platelet aggregation and augmentation of the endogenous fibrinolytic system. However, despite a reduction in silent ischemia on ambulatory ECG monitoring in a small number of trials, ACE inhibitors have not been shown to improve symptomatic ischemia.[61,62]

The role of ACE inhibitors in patients at high risk for CV events was evaluated in the HOPE (Heart Outcomes Prevention Evaluation) trial.[63] The HOPE trial investigators randomized patients to placebo or ramipril 10 mg daily. The HOPE trial evaluated patients with atherosclerotic disease (history of CAD, stroke, peripheral arterial disease, or DM with at least one additional risk factor), with approximately 80% of the patients having a history of CAD and approximately 55% had a history of SIHD.

After the 5-year follow-up period, ramipril patients had a significant reduction in the primary endpoint (CV death, MI, or stroke).[63] These impressive benefits were seen despite the minimal reduction in BP observed with the use of ramipril at 1 month (4/2 mm Hg), 2 years (3/2 mm Hg), and at the end of the 5-year period of the study (3/1 mm Hg). Benefits were consistent across all groups of patients enrolled, regardless of the location of atherosclerotic disease.

The results of the HOPE trial were confirmed in the EUROPA (European Trial on Reduction of Cardiac Events with Perindopril in Stable Coronary Artery Disease) trial.[64] The EUROPA trial evaluated only patients with SIHD, and not atherosclerotic disease in other vascular beds. In the EUROPA trial, perindopril 8 mg daily significantly reduced the incidence of CV death, MI, or cardiac arrest compared to placebo.[64] Data from the PEACE (Prevention of Events with Angiotensin Converting Enzyme Inhibitors) trial did not confirm the earlier results seen in the HOPE and EUROPA trials. In the PEACE trial, the addition of trandolapril 4 mg daily to standard therapy in patients with documented CAD did not significantly reduce the incidence of CV death, MI, or coronary revascularization.[65]

One possible explanation for the conflicting results in these three major trials may be related to the different agents and their relative dosing evaluated in the trials. Another explanation is the different patient populations and baseline therapy provided in the trials, with the patients enrolled in the PEACE trial appearing to be lower risk of ischemic event, and receiving better background therapy, such as statins and PCI, compared to the HOPE and EUROPA trials.

Regardless of whether there is a reasonable explanation for the discordant results of these trials, the PEACE trial does raise the issue of whether ACE inhibitors should be added to the pharmacotherapy regimen of all patients with SIHD. Based on existing well established benefits, it is appropriate to consider ACE inhibitors for patients with SIHD who have concomitant HTN, DM, HF, or who are post-MI.[1] Use of ACE inhibitors in all patients with SIHD would also be supported by a meta-analysis of seven trials with 33,960 patients that suggest a 14% significant reduction in morality ($p < 0.001$) when used in patients with CAD.[66]

Trials evaluating the role of angiotensin receptor blockers (ARBs) to determine if they provide a similar benefit as ACE inhibitors in the setting of CAD, and if the combination is better than either agent alone. In ONTARGET (ONgoing Telmisartan Alone and in combination with Ramipril Global Endpoint Trial), patients with existing CV disease and DM had similar benefit between the ACE inhibitor ramipril 10 mg daily and the ARB telmisartan 80 mg daily.[67] There was no added benefit of combination of the two agents, but there were significantly more adverse effects of hypotension, syncope, and renal dysfunction. In a second trial, there was no significant benefit of telmisartan over placebo in patients who were intolerant to ACE inhibitors.[68] Based on these conflicting data, an ARB would be used if the patient cannot tolerate ACE inhibitor therapy, and combination therapy is not justified.

Recommendations from the ACC/AHA for the use of ACE inhibition include a Class I recommendation for the use of ACE inhibitors in all patients with SIHD who also have HTN, DM, LV dysfunction, or chronic kidney disease, unless contraindicated (LOE A).[1] ARBs are recommended for the same patient populations if they are intolerant to ACE inhibitors (LOE A). It is a Class IIa recommendation to use ACE inhibitors in patients with both SIHD and other vascular diseases (LOE B), and ARBs in these patients if intolerant to ACE inhibitors (LOE B).

8 Risk Factor Modification

Lipid Management

Multiple studies have demonstrated a continuous, graded increase in coronary events with increasing low-density lipoprotein cholesterol (LDL-C) in men and women with or without initial SIHD. Multiple controlled clinical trials have demonstrated the ability of statin therapy to lower LDL-C and reduce CV events. The Cholesterol Treatment Trialist Collaborators published a meta-analysis of 26 trials of statin therapy, which demonstrated a 10% reduction in all-cause mortality for every 40 mg/dL reduction in LDL-C.[69] This same reduction in LDL-C was also associated with a 20% reduction in coronary mortality, with corresponding reductions in MI, stroke, and need for coronary revascularization. When comparing a higher dose to a lower dose statin regimen, there was a mean reduction of 20 mg/dL LDL-C more with the higher dose regimen. This resulted in a 15% lower rate of major vascular events, reflected by a 13% lower risk of MI, 16% lower risk of stroke, and a 19% lower risk of needing coronary revascularization, will a higher compared with a lower dose statin regimen.[69]

Until 2013, guidelines for the treatment of patients with dyslipidemia was centered around achieving particular LDL-C goals based on a patient's risk of CHD. Patients with existing CHD had a goal LDL-C of less than 100 mg/dL, and a goal of less than 70 mg/dL in patients considered to be at very high risk of coronary events. Unfortunately, the data to date do not support using statin therapy to achieve a specific target LDL-C to minimize CV events. The positive benefits demonstrated in most actively controlled trials support the use of a high dose or higher-intensity statin regimen. Therefore, the 2013 guidelines now recommend that all patients with known atherosclerotic CVD, such as SIHD, should receive high-intensity statin therapy.[70] Patients over the age of 75 years, or those who cannot tolerate high-intensity statin therapy, should receive moderate-intensity statin therapy. High-intensity statin options include atorvastatin 40 or 80 mg daily or rosuvastatin 20 or 40 mg daily. It should be noted that atorvastatin 80 mg is considered the preferred dose, and that the 40 mg dose was only used in one trial in patients who could not tolerate the 80 mg dose.[71] Also, rosuvastatin 20 mg daily is the preferred regimen based on the evidence, with the 40 mg daily dose being mentioned because it is also an approved dose. Moderate-intensity statin regimens include once daily atorvastatin 10 to 20 mg, rosuvastatin 5 to 10 mg, simvastatin 20 to 40 mg, pravastatin 40 mg, lovastatin 40 mg, pitavastatin 2 to 4 mg, and twice daily fluvastatin 40 mg.[70]

Other mechanisms for control of a patient's lipid profile, such as physical activity, weight management, management of psychological factors should also be implemented. Dietary approaches to lowering LDL-C include replacing saturated and *trans* fatty acids with dietary carbohydrates or unsaturated fatty acids and reducing dietary cholesterol. Although the response to dietary interventions is variable, a diet low in saturated fat and cholesterol typically lowers LDL-C by 10% to 15%. Other beneficial dietary interventions can include addition of plant stanols/sterols (2 g/day), which trials suggest lower LDL-C by 5% to 15%, and addition of viscous fiber (>10 g/day), which reduces LDL-C by 3% to 5%. A 10 lb weight loss reduces LDL-C by 5% to 8%. Regular physical exercise is key to therapeutic lifestyle modifications, but does not reliably lower LDL-C but facilitates weight loss and other beneficial effects on the lipid profile.

Blood Pressure Management

A number of observational trials have demonstrated a continuous and graded relationship between BP and risk of CV events. The risk of vascular death increases linearly over the BP range of 115/75 mm Hg to 185/115 mm Hg, with a doubling of risk for every 20 mm Hg increase in systolic BP or 10 mm Hg increase in diastolic BP.[72] Despite an abundance of trials evaluating when to initiate therapy and the target BP goal for patients with SIHD, the specific BP remains elusive. Current recommendations are to initiate pharmacotherapy, and treat to a BP goal of less than 140/90 mm Hg.[1,2,73] While observational trials suggest that patients with vascular disease might benefit from a lower target BP, other trials do not support this assumption. In the ACCORD (Action to Control Cardiovascular Risk in Diabetes) BP trial, patients with type 2 DM at high risk of CV events were randomized to a goal systolic BP of 120 mm Hg or 140 mm Hg.[74] There was no significant reduction in the incidence of CV death, MI, or stroke in patients randomized to a target systolic BP of 120 mm Hg compared to those treated to a target systolic BP of 140 mm Hg. Therefore, there was no benefit of a more aggressive BP reduction.

In contrast to the ACCORD trial, the SPRINT (Systolic Blood Pressure Intervention Trial) study found that patients with an initial baseline BP of 140/78 mm Hg treated to a target systolic BP of less than 120 mm Hg demonstrated a significant 25% reduction in CV events compared to those treated to a systolic BP of less than 140 mm Hg over a 3.26 year follow-up.[75] There was also a significant 27% reduction in all-cause mortality in patients in the more intense BP management group compared to the standard management group.[75] Some differences between the trials was the inclusion of patients with DM in the ACCORD trial and their exclusion in SPRINT, as well as the older patients being enrolled in SPRINT compared to the ACCORD trial (mean age 68 years vs 62 years). The most probable reason for the difference in the results is based on the size of the trials. While the ACCORD trial evaluates 4,733 patients, SPRINT had stronger statistical power by evaluating 9,361 patients. Based on the results of SPRINT, future guideline recommendations will likely be changing. Therefore, it seems reasonable to treat to a lower BP goal as long as adverse effects, such as hypotension, syncope, renal dysfunction, and electrolyte abnormalities, can be prevented or managed. Since approximately 30% of the patients in SPRINT were older than age 75, and they demonstrated a similar magnitude of benefit compared to younger patients, the current guideline recommendation to treat a goal systolic BP of less than 150 mm Hg in older patients needs to be reconsidered.[73]

Reduction of BP should consist of life style modifications as well as pharmacotherapy. This includes a diet rich in fruits, vegetables, and low-fat dairy products, regular physical exercise, a reduction in dietary sodium, and limited alcohol consumption. Many of these contribute to weight loss, where a 10-kg weight loss has contributed to a reduction in systolic BP of 5 to 20 mm Hg.

Several agents used to treat HTN have demonstrated the ability to reduce CV events. Drug selection in patients with SIHD includes a number of agents typically used to treat other aspects of the disease. Since β-blockers are usually the first agents selected for control of angina symptoms, they will also assist with lowering of BP. Patients may also be on ACE inhibitors based on the results of the HOPE trial or due to other comorbidities benefiting from ACE inhibitor therapy. Therefore, most patients with SIHD will typically get these two classes of agents for initial treatment of existing HTN. If additional therapy is needed, calcium channel blockers (CCBs) would be a good option since they could be used for the HTN, as well as help reduce angina episodes. Thiazide diuretics could also be an option based on their benefits in other populations and they would not be detrimental in patients with SIHD.

Smoking Cessation

Numerous observational studies have demonstrated that smoking significantly increases a patient's risk of having CV events.[76,77] Smoking increases risk by promoting atherosclerotic disease through a number of mechanism such as increasing platelet adhesion, increasing fibrinogen levels, causing endothelial dysfunction, decreasing high-density lipoprotein cholesterol (HDL-C) levels, and inducing vasoconstriction. While there have not been studies specifically in patients with SIHD, observational studies consistently demonstrate that smoking cessation is associated with a reduction in coronary events. A meta-analysis of 20 prospective cohort trials demonstrated a 30% relative risk reduction in mortality and MI for those who quit smoking compared to those who did not.[78] These benefits can occur within 2 to 3 years from initiation of smoking cessation.

One of the most important impacts of getting a patient to quit smoking is advice from their clinician recommending and discussing the importance of smoking cessation. Clinicians should approach smoking cessation by using the 6 A's framework:[1]

- Ask each patient about tobacco use at every visit;
- Advise each smoker to quit;
- Assess each smoker's wiliness to make a quit attempt;
- Assist each smoker in making a quit attempt by offering medication and referral for counseling;
- Arrange for follow-up; and
- Avoid exposure to environmental tobacco smoke.

Nonpharmacologic methods for smoking cessation are just as important as pharmacotherapy. Self-help programs, telephone counseling, behavioral therapy, and even exercise have had a beneficial effect at getting patients to quit smoking. Nicotine replacement therapy had demonstrated a nearly doubling of the rate of smoking cessation success.[79] There are a number of dosage forms available to fit the patient's lifestyle, such as patches, tablets, gum, lozenges, and a nasal spray. Sustained-release bupropion has also demonstrated a 2-fold increase in smoking cessation rates.[80] The partial agonist of the $\alpha_4\beta_2$ nicotinic receptor, varenicline, has demonstrated efficacy similar to that of buproprion.[81]

Diabetes Management

Diabetes mellitus is a significant risk factor of the development of CV disease in patients with type 1 and type 2 DM. Patients with type 1 DM have a 10-fold increase in risk of having a CV event compared to those without DM. Patients with type 2 DM have a 2- to 6-fold risk of CV death compared to those without DM. In fact, 80% of all deaths in patients with DM are associated with atherosclerotic disease.

The optimal goal HbA1c for patients with DM has not been determined. Studies have demonstrated that getting patients to an HbA1c of less than 7% is able to reduce microvascular complications of DM such as retinopathy, nephropathy, and neuropathy.[82] While subgroup analysis of larger trials have suggest a potential benefit, there have not been data from prospective trials to support reductions in macrovascular complications of DM, such as MI, stroke, and CV death.[83] In a trial that attempted to reduce these macrovascular complications by treating to a lower HbA1c (<6%), there was a failure to demonstrate any reductions in MI, stroke, or CV death, but did produce a 22% increase in all-cause mortality.[84]

Date from the EMPA-REG OUTCOME (Empagliflozin Cardiovascular Outcome Event Trial in Type 2 Diabetes Mellitus Patients) trial seems to be a breakthrough in the ability of glucose lowering agents to have a positive impact on CV events.[85] Patients with type 2 DM, with an HbA1c between 7% and 9% on glucose lowering therapy (up to 10% if treatment naïve) with established CV disease received 10 mg or 25 mg of empagliflozin once daily or placebo. Empagliflozin inhibits the sodium-glucose cotransporter 2, consequently inhibiting renal glucose resorption and thereby lowering plasma glucose levels. After approximately 3 years of follow-up patients receiving empagliflozin (n=4,687) had a significant relative reduction of 14% in CV events compared to placebo (10.5% vs 12.1%; p=0.04).[85] Interestingly, the 38% significantly lower rate of CV death was not due to lower rates of MI or stroke. There was a significant 35% relative reduction in hospitalizations for heart failure with the use of empagliflozin. There was no difference between the two doses of empagliflozin. It is unlikely the mechanism of the benefit of empagliflozin is due the magnitude of glucose lowering since there was only an approximate 0.5% reduction in HbA1c compared to placebo. Empagliflozin was more likely to cause genital infections compared to placebo, but otherwise adverse effects were similar between the groups. Based on these results, it would seem prudent that empagliflozin be part of the medication regimen for patients with DM and CVD. While studies are currently ongoing, it is unknown at this time of the other available sodium-glucose cotransporter inhibitors, canagliflozin or dapagliflozin, provide a similar benefit in patients with DM and CVD.

Metformin is typically the initial agent used in the treatment of DM in patients with SIHD. While sulfonylurea agents provide a similar reduction in HbA1c, their potentials to induce hypoglycemia and weight gain make metformin a more attractive option. Rosiglitazone should not be used in patients with SIHD due to an increase in CV events demonstrated with this agent. Pioglitazone has not been reported to carry this same risk of CV events, but is should not be used in patients with NYHA class III or IV heart failure due to risk of fluid retention.

Medical Therapy for Relief of Symptoms Recommendations[1]

Class I

1. β-blockers should be prescribed as initial therapy for relief of symptoms in patients with SIHD (LOE B).
2. Calcium channel blockers or long-acting nitrates should be prescribed for relief of symptoms when β-blockers are contraindicated or cause unacceptable side effects in patients with SIHD (LOE B).
3. Calcium channel blockers or long-acting nitrates, in combination with β-blockers, should be prescribed for relief of symptoms when initial treatment with β-blockers is unsuccessful in patients with SIHD (LOE B).
4. Sublingual nitroglycerin or nitroglycerin spray is recommended for immediate relief of angina in patients with SIHD (LOE B).

Class IIa

1. Treatment with a long-acting nondihydropyridine CCB (verapamil or diltiazem) instead of a β-blocker as initial therapy for relief of symptoms is reasonable in patients with SIHD (LOE B).

2. Ranolazine can be useful when prescribed as a substitute for β-blockers for relief of symptoms in patients with SIHD if initial treatment with β-blockers leads to unacceptable side effects or is ineffective or if initial treatment with β-blockers is contraindicated (LOE B).
3. Ranolazine in combination with β-blockers can be useful when prescribed for relief of symptoms when initial treatment with β-blockers is not successful in patients with SIHD (LOE A).

9 β-blockers

β-adrenergic blocking agents are commonly used in the management of patients with SIHD and are effective in reducing both symptomatic and silent episodes of myocardial ischemia. β-adrenergic blocking agents cause competitive inhibition of the effects of neuronally released and circulating catecholamines on β-adrenoceptors. The predominant adrenergic receptor type in the heart is the β_1-receptor, and competitive blockade minimizes the influence of endogenous catecholamines on the chronotropic and inotropic state of the myocardium. β-blockers also produce a moderate reduction in BP through competitive inhibition of β_1-receptors found in the kidney, leading to a reduction in renin release. By reducing HR, myocardial contractility, and intramyocardial wall tension (through BP reduction), β-blockers impact all of the major contributing factors of MVO_2.[86] HR reduction may also improve myocardial oxygen delivery by prolonging diastole filling time and increasing myocardial perfusion. Overall, β-blockers are effective agents for patients with effort-induced angina through their reduction in MVO_2.

β_1-selectivity does not influence the efficacy of β-blockers in the treatment of SIHD and all agents appear equally effective. β_1-selective agents would be preferred in patients with chronic obstructive pulmonary disease, peripheral arterial disease, DM, dyslipidemias, and sexual dysfunction, where blockage of the β_2-adrenergic receptor may be problematic. It should be noted that even β_1-selective agents lose their selectivity and provide additional β_2-blockage at higher doses. β-blockers with combined α_1 and β-blockade are also effective in the management of patients with angina. β-blockers with intrinsic sympathomimetic activity cause a slight to moderate activation of the β-receptor, in addition to preventing the binding of natural catecholamines. Due to this unique pharmacologic property, they provide little to no reduction in resting HR. There is a reduction in exercise HR when catecholamine concentrations are increased. While agents with intrinsic sympathomimetic activity can be useful for patients with peripheral arterial disease and dyslipidemia, they are not preferred in patients with CAD. In general, selection of a β-blocker in patients with SIHD usually depends on the presence of comorbid disease states, preferred dosing frequency, and cost.

Most side effects experienced with the use of β-blockers are typically an extension of their pharmacologic activity. Patients receiving β-blockers may experience bradycardia, hypotension, heart block, impaired glucose metabolism, and altered serum lipids. Changes in a patient's lipid profile are demonstrated as in increase in triglycerides, decrease in HDL-C, and no change in LDL-C. These change in a patient's lipid profile are more extensive with non-selective β-blockers and are usually transient. Central nervous system adverse effects, such as fatigue, depression, insomnia, and overall malaise, are somewhat less severe, but account for a significant number of β-blocker discontinuations. Impotence has been reported in approximately 1% of patients receiving β-blockers and inability to maintain an adequate erection has been reported in up to 25% of patients in some series. Patients with a history of airway disease may suffer from bronchospasm, and patients with LV systolic dysfunction may suffer from fluid overload. Patients without these preexisting disease states usually do not suffer from these adverse effects and it is important to note that even patients at risk for adverse effects receive significant benefit from the use of β-blockers. β-blockers are absolutely contraindicated in patients with existing bradycardia, hypotension, 2nd or 3rd degree atrioventricular (AV) block, a history of reactive airway disease (asthma), severe peripheral arterial disease, LV dysfunction with unstable fluid status, and difficult to control patients with DM who frequently have episodes of hypoglycemia. The highest risk post-MI patients should all receive β-blockers unless there is an absolute contraindication. A patient with SIHD who has never had an ACS, especially acute MI, with moderate chronic obstructive pulmonary disease could be treated adequately with an appropriate CCB or a β-blocker.

If β-blocker therapy needs to be discontinued, doses need to be tapered over 2 to 3 weeks to prevent abrupt withdrawal. During β-blocker therapy, there is a known up regulation of β-receptors on the myocardium. With abrupt withdrawal, these new receptors, along with all of the blocked receptors, are now exposed to be stimulated by endogenous catecholamines. This can produce a significant increase in MVO_2, induce ischemia, and even MI. If for some reason β-blockers cannot be tapered, patient should be instructed to avoid exertion as much as possible and manage angina episodes with SL NTG. Substitution with a non-dihydropyridine (DHP) CCB would be preferred if possible.

10 Calcium Channel Blockers

Calcium channel blockers are also effective agents in reducing angina episodes in patients with SIHD. All types of CCBs reduce MVO_2, as well as provide some increase in supply by inducing coronary vasodilation and preventing vasospasm. These effects are the result of CCB ability to modulate calcium entry into the myocardium and vascular smooth muscle, as well as a number of other tissues. This leads to a reduction in the cytosolic concentration of calcium responsible for activation of the actin-myosin complex leading to contraction of vascular smooth muscle and myocardium.

Calcium channel blockers should be considered as two separate classes of drugs. While they all inhibit influx of calcium ions, the location of the inhibition differs based on the chemical structure of the agents. The DHP CCBs, such as nifedipine, amlodipine, isradipine, and felodipine, provide their calcium channel blockade mainly in vascular smooth muscle cells, such as arterioles, with minimal effect on the myocardium. In contrast, the phenylalkylamine (verapamil) and benzothiazepine (diltiazem) agents, commonly referred to as non-DHP CCB, block calcium ion entry in mostly in the myocardium, with minimal effect on vascular smooth muscle. Verapamil is considered to have the most impact on myocardial calcium channels, with diltiazem having an effect intermediate between verapamil and a DHP CCB.

All CCBs reduce MVO_2 due to reduction in wall tension secondary to reduced arterial pressure and, to a minor extent, depressed contractility. While this is the main mechanism of benefit of DHP CCBs in patients with SIHD, non-DHPs are able to reduce all components of MVO2.

Like β-blockers, non-DHP CCBs also reduce HR and contractility through blockade of myocardial calcium channels. The DHP CCBs do produce a minimal reduction in contractility, and produce either a neural or increase in HR due to reflex tachycardia from direct arterial dilation. The effect on contractility and reflex tachycardia are not uniform across the class of DHP CCBs. Agents such as nifedipine produce more impairment of LV function than newer agents such as amlodipine and felopidine. Due to their propensity to cause reflex tachycardia, short acting DHP CCBs should not be used in the treatment of SIHD, as well as the treatment of chronic HTN, hypertensive crisis, or during an ACS event. If reflex tachycardia occurs with the use of longer acting DHP CCBs, it is typically less significant as than that seen with nitrate therapy, and can be prevented with β-blocker therapy.

Common side effects of CCBs vary between the classes. Patients taking non-DHP CCBs may experience bradycardia, hypotension,

AV block, and symptoms of LV depression. Non-DHP CCBs should not be used in patients who have contraindications or cannot tolerate β-blockers associated with these same effects. Non-DHP CCBs should be avoided in patients with concomitant systolic heart failure due to their negative inotropic effects, but can provide benefit to patients in atrial fibrillation with rapid ventricular response to due to their negative dromotropic effects. Verapamil also been reported to cause significant constipation in up 8% of patients. Patients taking DHP CCBs may experience reflex tachycardia, hypotension, headache, gingival hyperplasia, and peripheral edema. While most DHP CCBs are contraindicated in patients with systolic heart failure, amlodipine and felodipine are considered safe options in patients with systolic heart failure and concomitant SIHD and/or HTN.

Calcium channel blockers undergo hepatic oxidative biotransformation via the P450 isoenzyme 3A4 and other isoenzymes. Verapamil and diltiazem inhibit clearance of other substrates that utilize the 3A4 isoenzyme such as carbamazepine, cyclosporine, lovastatin, simvastatin, and benzodiazepines. The DHP CCBs generally do not have this same impact on these medications. Verapamil, and to a lesser extent diltiazem, also inhibit P-glycoprotein mediated drug transport. This interaction is partially responsible for increases in serum concentrations of agents such as digoxin and cyclosporine. Verapamil also decreases the clearance of digoxin, requiring close monitoring if these agents are used together. Agents that induce the P450 3A4 isoenzyme can reduce the effectiveness of all CCBs. Pharmacodynamic interactions also need to be monitored for in patients taking CCBs. Patients receiving verapamil or diltiazem concomitantly with other agents that reduce HR and AV nodal conduction (β-blockers, digoxin, and amiodarone) should be monitored for the development of bradycardia or heart block. Patients with LV dysfunction should not receive verapamil or diltiazem, especially if patients are treated with β-blockers.

10 Nitrates

Organic nitrates were found to have antianginal properties over 100 years ago when Murrell first reported in 1879 the ability of a 1% nitroglycerin solution administered orally relieved and prevented angina attacks. Organic nitrates are generally regarded as prodrugs that require biotransformation into the active compounds. This process leads to denitration of the nitrate and the release of nitric oxide, also known as EDRF. The EDRF works on the vascular endothelium to increase concentrations of cyclic guanosine monophosphate leading to a reduction in cytoplasmic calcium and vasodilation. Most of this vasodilation occurs on the venous side of the vascular system, leading to a reduction in preload, and subsequently a reduction in myocardial wall tension and MVO_2. As doses are increased, arterial vasodilation also occurs. This direct arterial vasodilatory effect can produce reflex tachycardia that can counter some of the antiangina benefits. Patients on adequate doses of β-blockers will not have reflex tachycardia, making this an effect combination for controlling a patient's angina symptoms.

Nitrates also provide vasodilation of stenotic vessels as well as the intracoronary collateral circulation. Due to the exponential reduction in flow with increasing stenosis, even small increases in vasodilation in these narrowed vessels can produce a significant increase in myocardial oxygen supply to ischemic portions of the myocardium. Nitrate-induced coronary vasodilation occurs predominately in epicardial vessels, with minimal effect on the coronary microcirculation. This explains why nitrates do not induce coronary steal similar to agents such as dipyridamole or sodium nitroprusside. Possible explanations for this lack of microcirculatory vasodilation include autoregulatory influences from the adjacent myocardium that counteract the vasodilatory effects of NTG, an absence of guanylate cyclase in these vessels, or an inability of the nitrate to undergo denitration in these vessels. Nitrates have been reported to have an antiaggregate effect on platelets, but the clinical relevance of this effect has not been documented.

Common side effects of nitrate therapy include headache, flushing, nausea, postural hypotension, and syncope. The hypotension is usually not severe but in volume depleted patients who rapidly try to stand, the hypotension can be accompanied with a paradoxical bradycardia. Headache will usually resolve after about 2 weeks of continued therapy. However, it is important to note that this does not necessarily represent tolerance or loss of antianginal effectiveness of the nitrate therapy. Acetaminophen has proven to be effective in managing nitrate-induced headache during the initial weeks of therapy. Patients utilizing transdermal nitroglycerin may experience skin erythema and inflammation. Initiating therapy with smaller doses and/or rotating the application site can manage adverse effects of transdermal NTG.

Several different formulations of nitrates are available for acute and chronic use (Table 16-7). 11 All patients with CAD should have access to SL NTG tables or spray for treatment of acute episodes of angina. Thorough patient education is critical for optimal benefit from SL NTG tablets and spray (Table 16-8). The SL route of administration is important to avoid the delay of gastrointestinal absorption and hepatic first pass metabolism. By going directly into the blood stream, SL NTG typically provides relief of angina within 5 minutes of administration. Despite the small tablet size of SL NTG, a dose of 300 to 400 mcg is substantial. Patients experience relief of symptoms due to the coronary artery vasodilation provided by this dose. This dose is also able to provide benefit, regardless if patients are already taking chronic long-acting nitrates. The side effects of flushing, headache, and postural hypotension can appear rapidly and the patient should be aware of this potential. Sublingual NTG can also be used for prophylaxis of acute episodes of angina. When patients want to involve themselves in a particular activity which they know leads to angina after a certain amount of exertion, they can take a SL NTG about 2 to 5 minutes before the activity. This prophylactic dose can provide up to 30 minutes of protection and allows the patient to take part in activities that they may otherwise be unable to because of angina episodes. Due to its longer half-life, sublingual isosorbide dinitrate could provide protection for up to 1 hour.

The use of chronic long-acting nitrate therapy for SIHD has been limited due to the phenomenon of nitrate tolerance. Several trials have shown that continuous nitrate therapy for more than 24 hours leads to a reduction or loss of the hemodynamic and antianginal effects of nitrates. In a trial of 562 patients receiving 24 hours

TABLE 16-7 Nitrate Products

Product	Onset (minutes)	Duration	Initial Dose
Nitroglycerin			
IV	1-2	3-5 minutes	5 mcg/min
Sublingual/lingual	1-3	30-60 minutes	0.3 mg
Oral	40	3-6 hours	2.5-9 mg three times a day
Ointment	20-60	2-8 hours	0.5-1 in
Patch	40-60	>8 hours	1 patch
Erythritol tetranitrate	5-30	4-6 hours	5-10 mg three times a day
Pentaerythritol tetranitrate	30	4-8 hours	10-20 mg three times a day
Isosorbide dinitrate			
Sublingual/chewable	2-5	1-2 hours	2.5-5 mg three times a day
Oral	20-40	4-6 hours	5-20 mg three times a day
Isosorbide mononitrate	30-60	6-8 hours	20 mg daily, twice a day[a]

[a]Product dependent.

TABLE 16-8 Education for Clinicians and Patients on Use of Sublingual Nitroglycerin

Education Point	Purpose
Keep in original dark glass container	SL NTG is degraded by sunlight and can lose potency.
Do not dump into a regular prescription bottle	SL NTG will interact with plastic and can lose potency. This is why it is packaged in a glass container.
Do not dispense in a larger plastic vial with safety cap	During an episode of angina you do not want the patient struggling to figure out how to open the safety cap.
Do not store in the bathroom	SL NTG will degrade in moisture and tablets will lose their integrity and potency.
Keep with them at all times, and may need multiple vials	SL NTG does not do the patient any good if they do not have it with them at the time of an episode of angina. Patient should consider having one at home, at work, in garage, etc.
Patient should be sitting down and resting with taking tablet	While the SL NTG tablets are small, the dose is not. It is likely the patient will have some flushing, may get a headache, and even become a little light headed. They need to know this can happen.
Describe how to use a SL tablet	The quick onset of a SL NTG is based on avoiding GI transite time and first-pass metabolism of the nitroglycerin. Therefore, the patient needs to know how to keep the tablet under the tongue until devolved and to try to attempt from swallowing the tablet.
Tablets need to be refilled every 6 months and spray every 3 years	Due to the instability of SL NTG tablets, they are typically only good for 6 months after they are opened.[a] Shelf-life of the spray is longer. Patients need to be advised to refill SL NTG even if they are not all gone once opened.
Remove cotton plug from the bottle	Larger quantity bottles commonly have a cotton plug. During an episode of angina you do not want the patient to be struggling with trying to get the cotton plug out of the bottle.
How to use prophylactically	SL NTG can be used to prevent episodes of angina if taken before partaking in an exertional event known to precipitate angina.
Contact 911 if first SL NTG does not relieve angina[b]	Most episodes of angina are relieved within 5 to10 minutes of rest and a single SL NTG. If pain persists, the episode may be an acute coronary syndrome, and not stable ischemic heart disease. This requires rapid medical attention.

SL NTG, sublingual nitroglycerin.

[a]product specific.

[b]may be patient specific base on their known experience with SL NTG and angina episodes.

of transdermal NTG, almost all of the patients lost control of their angina symptoms that could not be overcome with higher doses.

Nitrate tolerance is not necessarily an "all or none" phenomenon. Some patients may experience a reduction in the efficacy, while others may experience a total loss of efficacy. It is known that despite continued use of nitrates and a loss of antianginal effect, plasma volume remains expanded and some hemodynamic effects are maintained. Since the impact of continuous nitrate utilization varies from patient to patient and is unpredictable, the appropriate clinical strategy is to prescribe nitrates with a nitrate-free interval. Chronic administration of nitrates produces a state of oxidative stress leading to dysfunction of mitochondrial aldehyde dehydrogenase, the enzyme responsible for converting nitrates to the active agent NO.[87,88]

The mechanism of nitrate tolerance remains unknown, which has led to several pharmacologic approaches for its management and prevention. One thought is that tolerance is due to an exhausting of sulfhydryl groups needed for utilization of organic nitrates.[87] Based on this hypothesis, acetylcysteine has been investigated as a potential strategy for preventing nitrate tolerance because it supplies sulfhydryl groups. ACE inhibitors have also been investigated with mixed results. Agents such as captopril can supply sulfhydryl groups, but ACE inhibitors may prevent nitrate tolerance through other mechanisms. The inhibition of angiotensin II production can reduce superoxide anion production, leading to reduced nitrate degradation, as well as a reduction in protein kinase C and endothelin leading to a reduction in vasoconstriction. Unfortunately, none of these approaches have shown to be effective in maintaining the antianginal effects of continuous nitrate therapy despite their ability to maintain the hemodynamic effects of nitrates.

Despite multiple hypotheses for the mechanism of nitrate tolerance, the preferred management of nitrate tolerance for patients with CAD remains a 10- to 14-hour nitrate-free interval daily. This approach has been shown to maintain antianginal efficacy with the use of chronic nitrates. The rationale for this approach is based on the observation that although nitrate tolerance develops rapidly, it also is reversed rapidly. Unfortunately, this approach does not provide the patient anti-ischemic coverage during the nitrate-free interval and places the patient at risk for angina episodes. Usually the nitrate-free interval is provided during the nighttime hours when the patient is sleeping, and should have a reduced MVO_2. Several trials have utilized a nitrate-free interval and have demonstrated an increase in exercise time, a reduction in exercise induced ischemic events, and a reduction in the need for SL NTG. Despite these benefits, a nitrate-free interval would not provide protection to the 20% to 30% of patients with SIHD that also experience occasional nocturnal episodes of angina. The greatest concern with the use of chronic nitrates as the only antianginal therapy relates to the circadian timing of MI and other ischemic episodes. It is well documented that angina episodes and MI commonly occur in the morning hours, either right before or after awakening. Patients utilizing chronic nitrate therapy would generally not have taken or applied their nitrate therapy for the day during this critical time period. Nitrates should not be routinely used as monotherapy for SIHD because of the lack of coverage during the nitrate-free interval, lack of protection against circadian rhythm ischemic events, and potential for reflex tachycardia from vasodilatory properties. Trials have shown that patients taking intermittent transdermal NTG did not generally have rebound ischemia during the nitrate-free interval when concomitant β-blockers or diltiazem were also being administered.

10 While there are number of potential nitrate preparations that can be used for chronic long-term prevention of angina episodes, transdermal patches and isosorbide mononitrate (ISMN) are most commonly prescribed. Despite the fact that isosorbide dinitrate had proven to be effective, the three times a day dosing regimen would require that patients take a dose every 4 to 5 hours in order to provide an adequate nitrate-free interval. Two of the ISMN preparations are dosed twice daily. It is critical to be specific on the times of doses so patients do not take the dose 12 hours apart, and eliminate the nitrate-free interval. Dosing for these preparations should be dosed 7 hours apart, such as 7 am and 2 pm. One preparation is dosed once daily, which is designed as an extended-release preparation that provides 12 hours of nitrate exposure followed by a

12 hour nitrate-free interval. Transdermal NTG patches are typically prescribed as "on in the am and off in the pm." It would be best if instructions were clear to provide specific times for application and remove. Finally, third shift workers need to have the timing of their nitrate therapy altered to correlate with when they are active and resting during a day.

12 Ranolazine

Unlike other agents used for the management of episodes of angina, ranolazine does not provide its benefit by impacting hemodynamics such as HR, BP, the inotropic state, or increase coronary blood flow. Animal studies have demonstrated that ranolazine has little affinity for α_1, β_1, or β_2 adrenoreceptors and has minimal calcium channel blocking activity, but with no clinical significance. Ranolazine reduces ischemic episodes by selective inhibition of late sodium current (I_{Na}). Total sodium entry during an action potential in comprised of an early (fast) and late (slow) component. Under normal conditions, late I_{Na} constitutes only 1% of peak I_{Na}, or total I_{Na}. A number of preclinical studies have observed an increase in late I_{Na} that exceeds the duration of a typical action potential in ischemic and failing hearts.[89] It is not fully appreciated if this increase in late I_{Na} is due to an increase in density, or a dysfunction of these late Na^+ channels. The increase in intracellular Na^+ triggers an increase in the influx of Ca^{2+} through the reverse mode of the Na^+/Ca^{2+} exchanger, resulting in intracellular Ca^{2+} overload and eventually myocardial stunning.[90] It has also been demonstrated that intracellular Na^+ accumulation during ischemia is the substrate for reperfusion injury and that the Na^+ concentration kinetics during reperfusion, which is coupled with Ca^{2+} influx, also determines the degree of injury. Therefore, it is not the intracellular Na^+ concentration that produces ischemic damage, but its recognized role in Ca^{2+} accumulation via Na^+/Ca^{2+} exchange.[91] The rise in intracellular Ca^{2+} then directly contributes to lethal ischemic cell injury.[91] Increased intracellular Ca^{2+} also results in increased LV diastolic tension, increased myocardial oxygen consumption, depletion of adenosine triphosphate stores, and the potential for compression of the vascular space and further reduction of nutrient coronary blood flow to the ischemic territory. Through the mechanism of inhibiting late I_{Na}, ranolazine produces an overall reduction in intracellular Na^+. The reduction in intracellular Na^+ contributes to a reduction in the magnitude of ischemia-induced Ca^{2+} overload, and improves myocardial function as well as myocardial perfusion.[92]

Ranolazine is available as a sustained-release preparation with a half-life of approximately 7 hours and achieves steady state within 3 days of twice daily dosing. Ranolazine doses of 500 mg, 1,000 mg, and 1,500 mg, all twice daily, significantly increased total exercise duration, time to onset of angina, and time to 1 mm ST-segment depression compared to placebo.[93] While 1,000 mg twice daily was better than 500 mg twice daily, the difference between the 1,000 mg twice daily dose and the 1,500 mg twice daily dose was minimal. Due to the escalation of adverse events demonstrated with the 1,500 mg twice daily dose the 1,000 mg twice daily dose in the preferred regimen. When ranolazine 1,000 mg twice daily was added to existing therapy of atenolol (50 mg daily), diltiazem (180 mg daily), or amlodipine (5 mg daily), there was an increase in exercise duration, time to angina, time to 1 mm ST-depression, and a decrease in the number of angina episodes per week and number or SL NTG tablets used per week compared to the addition of placebo.[108] Ranolazine also demonstrated a significant reduction in weekly episodes of angina and SL NTG use when added to amlodipine 10 mg daily.[95]

In these trials, the average magnitude of increase in exercise duration over placebo was 29 to 50 seconds at peak and 24 to 34 seconds at trough. While these increases in exercise duration may seem of little clinical significance, this type of increase during an exercise tolerance test corresponds to a meaningful improvement in the ability of patients to carry on activities of daily living and take part in more minor types of exertion as compared to what is induced during testing. In one study, this magnitude of increase in exercise duration during testing was associated with a 25% reduction in the weekly number of angina episodes and SL NTG use over placebo and almost a 50% reduction from baseline.[94] These increases in exercise duration demonstrated with ranolazine is consistent with results produced in similar patients with β-blockers, CCBs, and chronic nitrates.[96,97]

Patients should be initiated on ranolazine 500 mg twice daily, with the dose increased to 1,000 mg twice daily within the next 1 to 2 weeks as long as there are not significant side effects. Clearance of ranolazine is reduced by renal insufficiency and moderate hepatic impairment. Ranolazine is primarily cleared by the liver metabolic enzyme cytochrome P450 (CYP) 3A4 (70%-85%) and CYP 2D6 (10%-15%), as well as being a substrate of P-glycoprotein. Ranolazine is contraindicated in patients with liver cirrhosis.

Due to the extensive hepatic metabolism of ranolazine there are a number of significant drug interactions to be considered. Potent inhibitors of CYP3A4 and P-glycoprotein (ketoconazole, itraconazole, protease inhibitors, clarithromycin and nefazodone) or potent inducers of CYP3A4 and P-glycoprotein (phenytoin, phenobarbital, carbamazepine, rifampin, rifabutin, rifapentine, or St. John's wort) are contraindicated with use with ranolazine due to significant increases and decreases in ranolazine drug concentrations, respectively. Moderate inhibitors of CYP3A4, such as diltiazem, verapamil, erythromycin, and fluconazole, can be used with ranolazine, but the maximum dose should not exceed 500 mg twice daily in these patients. Due to a weak inhibition of CYP3A4 by ranolazine, doses of simvastatin should not exceed 20 mg daily if coadministered. Ranolazine increases digoxin concentrations 1.4- to 1.6-fold at trough and approximately 2-fold at peak plasma concentrations, most likely through competition for intestinal and renal P-glycoprotein. Agents that are potent inhibitors of P-glycoprotein, such as cyclosporine, my increase ranolazine concentrations leading to increased side effects and a dose reduction of ranolazine.

Ranolazine and metformin compete for renal clearance through the organic cation transporter 2, which has to potential to increase metformin drug concentrations and increase the risk of lactic acidosis. The impact on metformin concentrations in only thought to be clinically meaningful when both full does ranolazine (1,000 mg twice daily) and full dose metformin (1,000 mg twice daily) are used together at the same time. In this setting, the metformin dose should be reduced to 850 mg twice daily. There is not expected to be any change in blood glucose control, as the metformin dose of 850 mg twice daily with ranolazine 1,000 mg twice daily produces similar metformin concentrations as 1,000 mg twice daily without the use of ranolazine. Patients on ranolazine 500 mg twice daily do not need to alter their metformin doses.

Clinical trials have identified adverse effects with ranolazine that range in incidence from 4% to 6% including constipation, nausea, dizziness, and headache. Ranolazine also has a linear relationship between QTc interval and ranolazine plasma concentration, with a 2.6 msec increase in QTc per 1,000 ng/mL. Clinical studies have reported QTc prolongation of 15 msec or less at therapeutic doses. However, an analysis of the electrophysiological data obtained from the MERLIN-TIMI 36 (Metabolic Efficiency With Ranolazine for Less Ischemia in Non ST-Elevation Acute Coronary Syndrome Thrombolysis in Myocardial Infarction 36) trial demonstrated that ranolazine was associated with a reduction in arrhythmias compared to placebo.[98] Patients should not receive doses of more than 1,000 mg twice daily and caution should be used in patients receiving concomitant QTc-prolonging agents. Ranolazine has also demonstrated the ability to produce reductions in HgA1C. One study found a statistically significant reduction in HgA1C of 0.70±0.18% with ranolazine 1,000 mg twice daily at 12 weeks.[94] Similarly, the MERLIN-TIMI 36 trial found a reduction in HgA1C of 0.64% from baseline.[98] These findings occurred in patients with or without diabetes. While ranolazine is not a treatment for DM, clinicians may find this property useful when targeting risk reduction goals.

While ranolazine has demonstrated efficacy and safety as monotherapy for patients with SIHD for treating angina episodes, it would only be an option in patient who cannot tolerate any of the traditional agents due to hemodynamic or other adverse effects. The number of patients fitting into this category would be expected to be relatively few. Ranolazine is recommended as add-on therapy to traditional anti-angina agents. Due to the lack of clinically meaningful impact on HR and BP, opportunities for ranolazine would be patients who achieve goal HR and BP and still have exertional angina symptoms, patients who cannot achieve these hemodynamic goals due to adverse effects, and patients who reach maximum dose of traditional agents, but still have angina symptoms.

NON-PHARMACOLOGIC THERAPY (REVASCULARIZATION)

Surgical revascularization plays an important and growing role in the treatment of SIHD. Revascularization options usually consist of coronary artery bypass grafting (CABG) surgery or PCI with or without stent placement. According to the AHA, approximately 492,000 PCI procedures are done in the United States annually, with about half being for management of SIHD.[3] Stents are used in over 90% of all patients undergoing PCI, with drug-eluting stents (DESs) accounting for 75% of all stent use compared to bare metal stent (BMS) use (25%). Approximately 219,000 patients undergo 397,000 CABG surgeries annually.[3] Other revascularization options are available and under development, but are less established.

The primary goal with revascularization is to prolong life, with the secondary goal being to eliminate or reduce symptoms. 5 Recommendations for revascularization over medical therapy as initial management to reduce mortality are described in Table 16-5, and recommendations for improvement in symptoms are described in Table 16-9.[1] 1 Whereas most of the pharmacologic approaches reduce MVO_2, revascularization increases myocardial oxygen supply in vessels with significant stenosis. This is accomplished by opening the vessel via PCI with or without stent placement, or using alternative transplanted vessels to bypass a critical stenosis in the setting of CABG surgery. While both of these therapies provide significant improvement in the care of patients with SIHD, and have advantages in certain groups of patients over a pharmacologic approach, both revascularization approaches have limitations.

Percutaneous Coronary Intervention

While the first use of balloon angioplasty was conducted on a femoral arterial stenosis by Dotter and Judkins in 1964, the first coronary balloon angioplasty was performed by Grüentizig in 1977. Initially, the procedure was done in a limited number of patients with symptomatic CAD who had single focal atherosclerotic plaque in a proximal coronary vessel. Since that time the use and techniques of the procedure have advanced several fold and is now performed in patients with multivessel CAD, total occlusions, diseased saphenous vein grafts (SVGs), and in patients with ST-elevation MI. The two major limitations of balloon angioplasty are abrupt vessel closure of the treated vessel, which occurred in 5% to 8% of cases and required emergency CABG surgery in 3% to 5%. The other main limitation is restenosis, which presents as recurrent symptoms and the need for repeat revascularization in approximately 30% to 50% of patients within the following year.[99] Today these complications have been dramatically reduced with the use of appropriate antithrombotic therapy and intracoronary stents, respectively. The term PCI encompasses the use of balloon angioplasty with stent placement, as well as other less commonly used intracoronary procedures such as rotational atherectomy and aspiration thrombectomy.

The PCI procedure requires arterial access. While the femoral approach is most commonly used, a brachial or radial artery approach is gaining in acceptance due to lower rates of bleeding compared to a femoral approach. A sheath is placed in the artery to maintain access during the procedure. A guide catheter is then introduced through the sheath and advanced to the ostium of the coronary arteries. A guide wire is then advanced through the guide catheter and across the stenosis in the coronary vessel. The deflated balloon is then slid along the guide wire and to the site of the coronary stenosis. The balloon is then inflated. The inflated balloon expands the coronary lumen by stretching and tearing the atherosclerotic plaque. Due to physical disruption of the plaque during this process, antithrombotic therapy is necessary to prevent acute thrombosis and abrupt vessel closure. After the balloon is deflated, elastic recoil of the stretched vessel wall generally leaves a 30% to 35% residual diameter stenosis. The balloon, guide wire, guide catheter, and sheath are then removed, with pressure and possibly a closure device used to prevent bleeding at the site of arterial access. Most elective PCI procedures are completed in 30 to 60 minutes, depending of the complexity of the patient's CAD.

Stents provide a stainless steel scaffold within coronary arterials that can treat acute vessels closure, but mainly reduce restenosis. The stent is placed over the deflated balloon and advanced to the area of coronary stenosis. When the balloon is inflated, the stent expands into the coronary vascular wall. The balloon is then deflated, leaving the expanded stent permanently in the diseased coronary vessel. While stents have had a dramatic effect of reducing restenosis, and therefore repeat revascularizations, they have not demonstrated an ability

TABLE 16-9 Revascularization to Improve Symptoms: ACC/AHA Recommendations[1]

Class I

1. CABG or PCI to improve symptoms is beneficial in patients with 1 or more significant (≥70% diameter) coronary artery stenoses amenable to revascularization and unacceptable angina despite GDMT. (LOE A)

Class IIa

1. CABG or PCI to improve symptoms is reasonable in patients with 1 or more significant (≥70% diameter) coronary artery stenoses and unacceptable angina for whom GDMT cannot be implemented because of medication contraindications, adverse effects, or patient preferences. (LOE C)
2. PCI to improve symptoms is reasonable in patients with previous CAGB, 1 or more significant (≥70% diameter) coronary artery stenoses associated with ischemia, and unacceptable angina despite GDMT. (LOE C)
3. It is reasonable to choose CABG over PCI to improve symptoms in patients with complex 3-vessel CAD (eg, SYNTAX score >22), with or without involvement of the proximal LAD artery, who are good candidates for CABG. (LOE B)

Class IIb

1. CABG to improve symptoms might be reasonable for patients with previous CABG, 1 or more significant (≥70% diameter) coronary artery stenoses not amenable to PCI, and unacceptable angina despite GDMT. (LOE C)
2. TMR performed as an adjunct to CABG to improve symptoms may be reasonable in patients with viable ischemic myocardium that is perfused by arteries that are not amenable to grafting. (LOE B)

Class III: Harm

1. CABG or PCI to improve symptoms should not be performed in patients who do not meet anatomic (≥50% diameter left main or ≥70% non-left main stenosis diameter) or physiological (eg, abnormal FFR) criteria for revascularization. (LOE C)

to prevent death or MI compared to stand alone balloon angioplasty. Currently, more than 90% of PCI procedures include the use of a stent.[3]

Restenosis is a phenomenon characterized by the loss of more than or equal to 50% diameter of the lumen at the site of prior successful intervention, and almost occurs within the first 3 to 6 months. The pathophysiology of restenosis involves a complex cascade of the effects of various growth factors and cytokines, as each contributes to the progressive loss of luminal diameter via smooth muscle cell proliferation.[100] Restenosis typically occurs by one of the following mechanisms: early vessel recoil, late constrictive ("negative") remodeling, or neointimal proliferation.[100]

Elastic recoil is a nearly instantaneous phenomenon, occurring during the first hour after successful dilation of the vessel. As the vessel is stretched during balloon angioplasty, the endothelium lining the vessel becomes damaged. In response to the balloon induced stretching of the elastic fibers, these fibers begin to recoil back to their previous size.[100] Late constrictive remodeling, also referred to as negative remodeling, is mediated by myofibroblasts of the adventitia layer of the coronary vessel. Balloon-induced injury often results in exposure of the adventitia to the lumen. Cell proliferation begins as activated fibroblasts contribute to the enlargement of the adventitia. In time, these activated fibroblasts differentiate into myofibroblasts that are involved in the profibrotic and remodeling effects of the vessel.[101] As the adventitia becomes thick and fibrotic, a decrease in arterial cross-sectional area results, contributing to the process of restenosis.

The scaffold-like properties of a BMS are effective at preventing restenosis by controlling elastic recoil and negative remodeling. Use of this technology has reduced restenosis rates from 30% to 50% with balloon angioplasty, to 15% to 30% with the use of BMS. However, stent-induced vessel injury and inflammatory reactions around stent struts trigger a set of events that ultimately lead to increased neointimal hyperplasia.[101] Neointimal proliferation, a normal response to vascular damage, is the target of the anti-proliferative effects of DES. Currently, DES are coated with sirolimus, paclitaxel, zotarolimus, or everolimus. These agents interrupt the cell cycle and prevent neointimal proliferation and reduce restenosis rates to approximately 5% to 10%.[102] This reduced need for repeat revascularization, along with the effectiveness of risk factor modification and better understanding of the patients who benefits from revascularization, has contributed to a slowing in the growth of the use of PCI over the last several years.

Despite the benefits in reducing restenosis demonstrated by the use of stents, the disadvantage is the risk of stent thrombosis due to exposed stent struts to circulating blood. Stent thrombosis is generally driven by the implantation of the stent into an atherosclerotic plaque, exposing platelet adhering proteins to the foreign stent surface. Patients are considered to be at risk of developing stent thrombosis until a thin layer of endothelial tissue can grow around the stent struts and prevent the exposure of the stent to the circulation. This process is called reendothelialization and typically occurs within 2 and 4 weeks after BMS deployment, with most adverse events occurring within the first 2 weeks after stent deployment. The process of reendotheliazation is significantly prolonged with the use of DES. The drugs used on these stents do not differentiate between a smooth muscle, neointimal, and an endothelial cell. Therefore, the mechanism of the benefit of reducing neointimal proliferation and restenosis also increases the duration of risk of stent thrombosis.

Stent thrombosis is a rare event (<5% of cases), but when it occurs it is usually catastrophic, with two-thirds of events associated with a large MI or death. The mortality rate alone from stent thrombosis ranges from 20% to 45%. Prevention of stent thrombosis is provided by the use of DAPT with aspirin and clopidogrel.

6 PCI vs Medical Therapy

Despite advancements in the technique of PCI and technology of stents, no study to date has demonstrated that PCI in patients with SIHD improves survival. This is most likely due the advancements in medical therapy and improved use of GDMT. A number of earlier studies demonstrated less recurrent angina in patients randomized to PCI compared to medical therapy, but PCI in these trials rarely included the use of stents, and medical therapy did not include the use of high-intensity statins or ACE inhibitors.[103]

The role of contemporary PCI and GDMT has been evaluated in two more recent clinical trials. In the COURAGE (Clinical Outcomes Utilizing Revascularization and Aggressive Drug Evaluation) trial, patients (n=2,287) with SIHD, and without elevated troponin or symptoms of heart failure, were randomized to GDMT alone or PCI with GDMT.[104] The components of GDMT in the COURAGE trial are defined in Table 16-10. Medication compliance was exceptional with more than 90% of patients being adherent to aspirin, β-blocker, and ACE inhibitor therapies. The LDL-C, systolic BP, and HgA1C goals were achieved in 70%, 65%, and 45% of patients, respectively. The primary outcome of death and MI was not different between the groups after a median follow-up of 4.6 years (19.0% in PCI group vs 18.5% in GDMT group). While more patients were angina-free in the PCI group compared to the GDMT group at 1 year (66% vs 58%), there was no difference at the 5-year follow-up time point (74% vs 72%). There was a reduction in the need for revascularization after 5 years for patients randomized to PCI with GDMT compared to GDMT alone (21.1% vs 32.6%; <0.001). This trial confirms that even in modern day practice, PCI with GDMT does not offer a reduction in death and MI compared to GDMT alone, and PCI should be reserved for management of medication refractory angina in patients with SIHD. A 12-year follow-up of 53% of the originally randomized patients from the COURGAE trial did not demonstrate any difference in mortality between these groups (25% vs 24%; p=0.76).[105] These data underscore the importance of aggressive, goal-oriented, pharmacotherapy use in patients with SIHD. Two limitations to consider when evaluating the COURAGE trial include the low use of DES (<1%) and the number of patients in the GDMT group who crossed over and received PCI (33%). Since DES placement reduces rates of restenosis, and not death or MI, there was unlikely an impact on the primary outcome of the COURAGE trial, but there would have probably been a larger difference in the need for revascularization. While one-third of patients in the GDMT group did need to receive PCI over the course of 5 years, two-thirds did not. Therefore, supporting the lack of a need for all patients with SIHD to be treated with PCI as an initial management strategy.

The BARI 2D trial (Bypass Angioplasty Revascularization Investigation 2 Diabetes) trial randomized patients similar to those in COURGE, but they all had to have type 2 DM.[106] Patients in the BARI 2D trial (n=2,368) were randomized to GDMT alone or GDMT and revascularization with PCI or CABG surgery. The primary endpoint of freedom from death, MI, or stroke was not different between the groups after 5 years of follow-up (77.2% revascularization group vs 75.0% GDMT group; p=0.70). While patients receiving CABG surgery did have a lower rate of the primary endpoint compared to GDMT alone, there was no difference between patients receiving PCI compared to GDMT therapy. Approximately 35% of patients undergoing PCI in the BARI 2D trial received a DES.

While the COURAGE and BARI 2D trials suggest that PCI in SIHD should be reserved for treatment of medication refractory disease instead of an initial treatment approach, the results remain controversial with strong opinions of both sides. The ISCHEMIA trial (International Study of Comparative Health Effectiveness with Medical and Invasive Approaches) is currently ongoing in an attempt to bring a final answer to this question. In an attempt to address limitation to the current data, the investigators will: (1) enroll patients before catheterization, so that anatomically high-risk patients are not excluded; (2) enrolling a higher-risk group with at least moderate ischemia; (3) minimizing crossovers; (4) using contemporary DES and physiologically guided decision making (FFR) to achieve

TABLE 16-10 Guideline-directed Medical Therapy in the COURAGE Trial[104]

Medication Class	Drug	Indication
Antiplatelet agents	Aspirin (clopidogrel if patients intolerant to aspirin)	Aspirin for all subjects; clopidogrel as part of dual antiplatelet therapy for at least 1 month after PCI with a BMS
ACE inhibitors	Lisinopril	Hypertension, heart failure, LVEF <40%; encouraged for all patients
Angiotensin receptor blocker	Losartan	Consider in individuals with hypertension, clinical evidence of heart failure, or LVEF <40% who are intolerant to ACE inhibitors
Beta-blockers	Long-acting metoprolol	Hypertension, angina, or postmyocardial infarction
Thiazide diuretic	Any	Hypertension
Statin	Simvastatin	All patients
Calcium channel blocker	Amlodipine	Hypertension or angina
Long-acting nitrates	Isosorbide mononitrate	Angina
Niacin	Extended-release niacin	LDL-C >85 mg/dL, HDL-C <40 mg/dL, or triglycerides >150 mg/dL despite statin
Cholesterol absorption inhibitor	Ezetimibe	LDL-C >85 mg/dL despite statin
Fibrate	Fenofibrate	Triglycerides >150 mgdL despite statin
Omega-3 fatty acids	Various formulations	Triglycerides >150 mg/dL despite statin
Risk factor	Goal	
Smoking	Cessation	
Total dietary fat/saturated fat	<30%/<7% of calories	
Dietary cholesterol	<200 mg/day	
Physical activity	30-45 minutes, moderate intensity 5 times per week	
Body weight by BMI	Initial BMI: 25-27.5 kg/m² Goal: <25 kg/m² Initial BMI: >27.5 kg/m² Goal: 10% relative weight loss	
Blood pressure	<130/85 mm Hg (<130/80 mm Hg if diabetes or renal disease present)	
LDL-C	60-85 mg/dL (goal became <70 mg/dL during the study)	
HDL-C	>40 mg/dL	
Triglycerides	<150 mg/dL	
Diabetes	HbAc <7.0%	

PCI, percutaneous coronary intervention; BMS, body mass index; ACE, angiotensin converting enzyme; LVEF, left ventricular ejection fraction; LDL-C, low-density lipoprotein cholesterol; HDL-C, high-density lipoprotein cholesterol; BMI, body mass index.

complete ischemic (rather than anatomic) revascularization; and (5) being adequately powered to demonstrate whether routine revascularization reduces CV death or MI in patients with SIHD and at least moderate ischemia. An important secondary outcome will be a quality of life assessment and evaluation of angina. An estimated 8,000 patients will be followed for an average of 4 years with enrollment projected to end in 2017.

Clinical **Controversy...**

Timing of PCI remains an issue of debate. One approach is to perform PCI once the diagnosis of SIHD is made. This approach has not demonstrated a reduction in hard outcomes such as death or MI. The most current data also do not support a reduction in episodes of angina. The ongoing ISHCEMIA trial should assist in settling this debate, but results are not due for several years.

Pharmacotherapy with PCI

The physical damage imposed on the atherosclerotic plaque during PCI with stent placement induces platelet recruitment and activation, leading to the potential for thrombus formation. Therefore, antithrombotic therapy with antiplatelet and anticoagulant therapy are necessary to produce a successful outcome. Antiplatelet therapy is also used after the procedure to reduce the risk of stent thrombosis.

All patients without a contraindication should receive aspirin before PCI and continued for life. Patients already on chronic aspirin therapy should take an additional 75 to 325 mg before PCI. Aspirin-naive patients should be given a dose of 325 mg at least 2 hours, and preferably 24 hours before PCI. Patients also receiving a stent (>90%) should also receive a $P2Y_{12}$ inhibitor before PCI.

A number of trials conducted in the 1990s demonstrated the benefit of glycoprotein (GP) IIb/IIIa inhibitors in patients undergoing elective PCI with stent placement. Abciximab demonstrated significant reduction in death and MI compared to placebo in the EPISTENT trial (Evaluation of Platelet IIb/IIIa Inhibition in Stenting).[107] There was also significant reduction in mortality with the use of abciximab at 1 year in the EPISTENT trial (1.0% vs 2.4%; p=0.037). In the ESPRIT trial (Enhanced Suppression of the Platelet IIb/IIIa Receptor with Integrilin Therapy) eptifibatide demonstrated a significant reduction in death and MI compared to placebo in patients undergoing PCI with stent placement.[108] The only head-to-head trial in these type of patients was TARGET (Do Tirofiban and ReoPro Give Similar Efficacy Trial), in which abciximab demonstrated a significant reduction in death, MI, or urgent revascularization compared to tirofiban (6.0% vs 7.6%; p=0.038).[109]

Despite the benefits demonstrated with GP IIb/IIIa inhibitors in patients undergoing PCI with stenting for SIHD, it is important to consider that these trials were conducted before pretreatment loading doses of clopidogrel 600 mg became part of standard of care. In the ISAR-REACT (Intracoronary Stenting and Antithrombotic Regimen-Rapid Early Action for Coronary Treatment) trial (n=2,159), patients received a clopidogrel 600 mg pretreatment dose at least 2 hours prior to elective PCI with stenting and were randomized to abciximab or placebo.[110] The incidence for the primary endpoints of death, MI, or revascularization between the abciximab and placebo groups at 30 days was similar (4% each). The ISAR-SWEET (Intracoronary Stenting and Antithrombotic Regimen: Is Abciximab a Superior Way to Eliminate Elevated Thrombotic Risk in Diabetics) trial (n=701) had a similar design as the ISAR-REACT trial, but included elective PCI patients with DM (excluded from ISAR-REACT).[111] The incidence of death and MI were similar between patients receiving abciximab and those not receiving abciximab (8.3% vs 8.6%). These data suggest that the addition of a GP IIb/IIIa inhibitor to patients undergoing elective PCI for refractory stable angina pretreated with clopidogrel 600 mg does not confer additional benefit in the prevention of adverse cardiovascular events. While prasugrel and ticagrelor are oral $P2Y_{12}$ inhibitors that provide faster and more potent antiplatelet effect compared to clopidogrel, they have not been prospectively evaluated in the setting of elective PCI. There use should be reserved to patients with ACS, where their benefits over clopidogrel have been clearly demonstrated.

After elective PCI, DAPT needs to be continued to reduce the risk of stent thrombosis. In patients receiving a BMS, 4 to 6 weeks of DAPT is needed. In patients at high risk of bleeding, a minimum of 2 weeks can be given, as most reendothelialization of the stent surface should have occurred. Patients receiving a DES should receive at least a year of DAPT due to the delay, and somewhat unknown duration of the reendothelialization process in this setting. A Class III (harm) recommendation from the ACC/AHA for patients to receive a stent if it is thought that they will not tolerate or comply with the recommended duration of DAPT.[1] While some evidence suggest that the second generation DES (everolimus and zotarolimus) may not need a full year of DAPT, these studies are limited by small sample size, low event rates, and poor patient enrollment. The theory for a shorter duration of DAPT is based mainly on stent design. Second generation DES have thinner and less stent struts compared to first generation stents, which exposes less "stent" to the blood, and theoretically should lower the risk of stent thrombosis. The trade-off is a slightly lower reduction in restenosis compared to first generation DES. The results of the DAPT trial not only suggest that there is not a difference between the type of DES received, but also that a longer duration of DAPT (up to 30 months) provides a better reduction in CV adverse events compared to 12 months.[112] Therefore, the optimal duration of DAPT is being debated, but at least 6 to 12 months of DAPT in patients receiving any DES seems prudent.

Clinical **Controversy...**

The duration of DAPT after DES placement has not been determined. A number of relatively poorly conducted trials suggest less than 1 year may be adequate, while the highest quality trial suggest more than a year is optimal.

Anticoagulant therapy during PCI has traditionally been provided with unfractionated heparin (UFH) 70 to 100 units/kg with additional bolus doses (2,000-5,000 units) sufficient to maintain the activated clotting time between 250 to 300 seconds with the HemoTec device and 300 to 350 seconds with the Hemochron device. When using UFH with a GP IIb/IIIa inhibitor, bolus doses of 50 to 70 units/kg should be used to maintain an activated clotting time between 200 and 300 seconds (regardless of the device) to reduce the risk of major bleeding.

Enoxaparin has been evaluated in the setting of elective PCI in the STEEPLE (SafeTy and Efficacy of Enoxaparin in PCI patients, an internationaL randomized Evaluation) trial. Immediately before PCI, patients (n=3,528) received either a single intravenous dose of 0.5 mg/kg enoxaparin, 0.75 mg/kg enoxaparin, or appropriately dosed UFH.[113] The primary endpoint of non-coronary artery bypass graft-related bleeding in the first 48 hours was significantly reduced with enoxaparin 0.5 mg/kg compared to UFH (5.9% vs 8.5%), but not with enoxaparin 0.75 mg/kg compared to UFH (6.5% vs 8.5%). Ischemic endpoints of death, MI, and revascularization were not different between the groups. Before the end of the trial, there was a significantly higher incidence of death in the patients receiving enoxaparin 0.5 mg/kg, and therefore, this arm of the trial was discontinued. At the end of the trial, and at the 1 year follow-up, this difference was not significant. It appears that either of these doses of enoxaparin are a possible alternative to UFH.

The direct thrombin inhibitor bivalirudin was evaluated in patients undergoing elective PCI in the REPLACE 2 (Randomized Evaluation in PCI Linking Angiomax to Reduced Clinical Events) trial.[114] Patients (n=6,010) in the REPLACE 2 trial were randomly assigned to receive bivalirudin with provisional GP IIb/IIIa inhibitor or UFH with planned GP IIb/IIIa inhibitor. The patient population involved both elective (about 75% of patients) and urgent PCI (about 25% of patients). Bivalirudin was administered as a 0.75 mg/kg bolus followed by a 1.75 mg/kg/h infusion for the duration of the procedure. The results of the REPLACE 2 trial demonstrated a significantly lower rate of bleeding with the use of bivalirudin compared to a GP IIb/IIIa inhibitor, with no significant difference in thrombotic events. Since GP IIb/IIIa inhibitors are typically reserved for high-risk patients with ACS, and rarely used in modern practice for patients undergoing PCI for SIHD, the utility of the REPLACE 2 data is difficult to determine.

Coronary Artery Bypass Graft Surgery

5 The majority of the data investigating the impact of CABG surgery on relieving angina symptoms and improving survival compared to initial medical therapy comes from three large multicenter randomized trials. These trials, the Veterans Administration Cooperative Study, the European Coronary Surgery Study and CASS (Coronary Artery Surgery Study), were initiated between 1972 and 1975.[115-117] All were powered to evaluate mortality benefit from CABG surgery compared to medical treatment. These trials have reported both short- and long-term outcomes and have provided the cardiology community valuable data on the role of CABG surgery in the treatment of SIHD.

There are several limitations to applying these data to current practice. As mentioned above, these trials were conducted three decades ago. Since that time cardiothoracic surgeons have gained significant experience in performing CABG surgery while newer techniques, such as off-pump and minimally invasive surgeries, have been utilized. Additionally, utilization of arterial grafts was limited to one trial in which only 14% of the patients received one vessel. These trials are also limited by the narrow spectrum of patients selected for enrollment. These trials primarily enrolled patients less than or equal to 65 years of age (>90%), very few women (<5%), and low to moderate risk patients who were clinically stable. Finally, the medical treatment in the comparative arm was clearly suboptimal by today's standard. Aspirin was not widely used, lipid lowering therapy and ACE inhibitors were not yet considered standard of care, and β-blockers were used in only about one-half of the patients.

5 Despite these issues, these trials along with a meta-analysis have provided us with valuable information about the role of an initial strategy of CABG surgery compared to medical management. Utilization of CABG surgery provides a mortality benefit in patients over medical management at 5 years (10.2% vs 15.8%; p=0.0001), 7 years (15.8% vs 21.7%; p<0.001) and at 10 years (26.4% vs 30.5%; p=0.03).[118]

5 Despite the survival benefit seen in the entire patient cohort, there were several subgroups of patients for which the survival benefit was even more profound. These patients included those at high risk of death without surgery (see Table 16-4). Patients with significant (>50% stenosis) left main CAD have a median survival of 13.3 years with CABG surgery compared to 6.6 years with medical treatment. Patients with left main equivalent disease (≥70% stenosis in both the proximal left anterior descending and proximal circumflex arteries) experience a similar survival advantage to CABG surgery.

Patients with three-vessel disease with reduced LV function, or two- or three-vessel disease with more than 75% stenosis in the proximal left anterior descending also have pronounced benefit from CABG surgery compared to medical therapy. Female and older patients have a higher risk of short-term mortality, but have a similar long-term prognosis compared to the general population.

There is an increase in the event rate in patients randomized to CABG surgery in the long-term follow-up period. This is related to the progressive atherosclerotic disease in native vessels as well as graft disease over time. Atherosclerotic obstruction of a native coronary vessel, leading to ischemic complications, usually takes five or more decades to accumulate, but the life span of a saphenous vein graft (SVG) is significantly shorter. Studies have shown occlusion rates of SVGs to be 20% to 25% at 5 years and almost 40% at 10 years, with one-half of all the remaining patent vessels showing atherosclerotic changes. This is due to the inability of SVG endothelium to withstand the increased BP seen on the arterial side compared to venous pressures. The endothelial damage and incorporation of LDL-C accelerates the atherosclerotic process significantly. The use of arterial grafts has provided promise in reducing occlusion of the coronary artery bypass grafts. The most commonly used arterial graft is the internal mammary artery (IMA), which has shown graft patency to be greater than 90% at 10 years. Due to similar endothelial and smooth muscle cell function, arterial grafts are better designed to accommodate arterial BP compared to SVGs. Limitations to the use of arterial grafts include vasospasm and long surgical times for harvest. Due to the increased time needed, arterial grafts are not ideal in the setting of emergency CABG surgery. There may also be an increase in wound infections in diabetic or obese patients receiving bilateral IMA grafts.

Despite the advancements in technique and patient care, CABG surgery still has some significant complications. One of the most feared and most common (~ 6%) complications is postoperative neurological impairment, which may be attributed to hypoxia, emboli, hemorrhage, or a metabolic abnormality during or shortly after the surgery. Neurological complications are divided into type 1 and type 2 deficits. A type 1 deficit is associated with major, focal neurological deficits, stupor, or coma. In a type 2 deficit, a reduction in intellectual function and memory is present. The incidence of neurologic deficits is equal between the two types, while mortality may be as high as 21% and 10% respectively. Many deficits are not clinically significant and resolve with time. Patients with advanced age and/or a history of HTN are at increased risk of a neurological complication after CABG surgery.

Other non-cardiac complications of CABG surgery include renal dysfunction and mediastinitis. Postoperative serum creatinine levels more than 2.0 mg/dL or an increase in baseline creatinine level of more than 0.7 mg/dL occurs in as many as 8% of CABG surgery patients. While most patients recover without problems, the mortality rate in these patients is 19%, and increases to almost 65% in the 1.5% of CABG surgery patients that require dialysis. Patients with advanced age, a history of heart failure, prior CABG surgery, DM type 1, and preexisiting renal impairment are at an increased risk of developing postoperative renal dysfunction. Patients with preoperative renal dysfunction (serum creatinine >2.5 mg/dL) are at an exceptionally high risk of needing postoperative hemodialysis (40%-50%). Despite the infrequent occurrence of mediastinitis (1%-4%), the mortality rate can be as high as 25%. Patients with obesity, reoperation, use of both IMAs, longer surgeries with increased complexity, and DM are at increased risk of developing postsurgical mediastinitis.

New approaches to CABG surgery have been developed in an attempt to minimize the morbidity related to the operation. One of these approaches is the off-pump bypass coronary surgery that is performed on a beating heart. This type of surgery currently accounts for about 20% of all CABG surgeries performed in the United States. Patients undergoing off-pump bypass experience the same relief from angina, vessel patency, and mortality benefit (evaluated out to 1 year) as traditional CABG surgery. Patients utilizing off-pump bypass with sternotomy can undergo multivessel bypass, but data on patients with left main disease and impaired LV function are limited. By reducing the need for cardiopulmonary bypass and preventing the need for clamping of the aorta, there is a significant reduction in adverse neurologic events, length of hospitalization, and cost. The cardiac motion is reduced by a number of pharmacological and mechanical devices. These include slowing the HR with β-blockers and non-DHP CCBs, creating a temporary cardiac arrest with adenosine, or vagal simulation.

The use of minimally invasive direct CABG is conducted without median sternotomy and without the use of cardiopulmonary bypass. In addition to the benefits of avoiding cardiopulmonary bypass, the prevention of sternotomy reduces the incidence of wound infections as well as patient recovery time. Due to the small incision and technical difficulty of the surgery, it is limited to patients with single vessel disease of either the LAD or right coronary artery. Both of these newer types of procedures are limited by the needed learning curve of the surgeon and lack of long-term follow-up for patency and mortality compared to standard CABG surgery.

Pharmacotherapy after CABG surgery includes aspirin and lipid-lowering therapy (ACC/AHA Class I recommendations). Aspirin in doses between 100 mg a day to 325 mg three times daily have been shown to be effective in reducing vein graft closure during the first year after the surgery. It is recommended that the first dose of aspirin be given within the first 24 hours of surgery. The efficacy of aspirin is lost if initiation is delayed more than 48 hours postoperatively. Aspirin is usually continued indefinitely due to its benefit in primary and secondary prevention of acute MI. If patients are truly aspirin allergic, clopidogrel is an acceptable alternative. Due to the accelerated atherosclerotic process in patients with SVGs, lipid-lowering therapy should be used aggressively to a target LDL-C of less than 100 mg/dL. The Cholesterol Lowering Atherosclerotic Study and the Post Coronary Artery Bypass Graft Trial have both shown angiographic evidence of significant reductions in SVG atherosclerosis. The need for long-term anti-angina therapy is significantly reduced with the use of CABG surgery. Only 30% of patients undergoing CABG surgery required chronic nitrate or β-blocker therapy compared with over 70% of medically treated patients. It would be reasonable to include a β-blocker and/or CCB for the treatment of preexisting HTN after surgery. Patients need to continue to have access to SL NTG after surgery. Smoking cessation (ACC/AHA Class 1 recommendation) and cardiac rehabilitation are also critical to successful postoperative outcomes.

CABG Surgery vs PCI

The decision to undergo PCI or CABG surgery as initial treatment is based on the severity of coronary stenoses, number of diseased vessels, location of stenosed vessels, as well as LV function. Several randomized clinical trials have compared revascularization strategies. Unfortunately, there are significant limitations to many of these trials. A number of the older trials compared CABG surgery with balloon angioplasty. Since less than 10% of patients who undergo PCI receive only balloon angioplasty without a stent, data from these trials are not reflective of modern practice. Most of the other trials compared CAGB surgery to PCI with a BMS, and only three trials comparing CABG surgery with PCI with a DES. Since 75% of stent use in modern practice is a DES, the seemingly large number of comparison trials does not offer as much information as would be expected. Even the more contemporary trials have limitations. Since CABG surgery was utilized for almost a decade before PCI, patient groups who had already demonstrated benefit from CABG surgery compared to medical treatment were not heavily included in these trials. Recruitment of patients in these trials proved to be difficult since patients with three-vessel disease seemed to be referred to CABG surgery, and patients with one- or two-vessel disease seemed to be referred to PCI prior to enrollment. Less than 10% of patients enrolled in these trials had an ejection fraction less than 50%. These trials enrolled patients with stable and unstable CAD, but the results did not appear to vary between the two types of patients.

One of the largest comparison study was the BARI trial, which randomized 1,792 patients to either PCI or CABG surgery to evaluate the primary endpoint of mortality at 5 years.[119] Most patients had normal LV function and had one- or two-vessel disease with a low utilization of stents. Survival at 5.4 years and freedom from MI was not different between the groups. There was a higher incidence of inhospital MI in patients receiving CABG surgery, but there was a significant increase in rehospitalization and need for repeat revascularization over the follow-up period for those randomized to PCI. Despite the initial increase in cost of CABG surgery, the cost of the two revascularization approaches became almost neutral, due to the higher need for repeat procedures in PCI patients. Despite the longer follow-up and larger number of patients compared to other trials, BARI is still limited due to the narrow scope of patients enrolled and the high crossover rate of PCI patient that received CABG surgery (31%).

The largest randomized clinical trial comparing CABG surgery to PCI with DES was the SYNTAX trial (Synergy between PCI with TAXUS and Cardiac Surgery).[120] In this trial 1,800 patients with left main or three-vessel disease were randomized to revascularization with PCI with DES or CABG surgery. At 3 years, the composite primary endpoint of death, stroke, MI, or repeat revascularization occurs significantly less often in the patients receiving CABG surgery compared to PCI with DES (20.2% vs 28.0%; $p<0.001$). While the rates of death and stroke were not different between the groups, the rates of MI (3.6% vs 7.1%) and repeat revascularizations (10.7% vs 19.7%) were higher with the use of PCI with DES compared to CABG surgery.

In the SYNTAX trial, the extent of CAD was assessed using the SYNTAX score. This scoring system is based on the location, severity, and extent of coronary stenoses, with a lower score indicating less complicated anatomic CAD. In a post-hoc analysis of the SYTNAX trial, a low score was defines as less than or equal to 22, an intermediate score was 23 to 32, and a high score was more than or equal to 33. The incidence of the primary endpoint correlated with the SYNTAX score for patients receiving PCI with DES, but not with those receiving CABG surgery. At 12 months, patients with a low SYNTAX score had a similar outcome regardless of the type of revascularization received, although those with intermediate or high scores did better if they received CABG surgery compared to PCI with DES. At the 3-year follow-up, the difference in the primary endpoint increased between PCI with DES and CABG surgery as the SYNTAX score increased. Therefore, patients with relatively uncomplicated and less extensive CAD could receive either revascularization approach, but those with more complex and diffuse disease would seem to benefit from CABG surgery.

MANAGEMENT OF EPISODES OF FIXED THRESHOLD ANGINA

Medical management of improving patient's quality of life through control of angina episodes follows a stepwise approach (see Fig. 16-5). 11 All patients should have access to SL NTG for treatment of a current episode of angina. Patients need to be sure to be adequately educated on appropriate use and storage, as well as being sure they have consistent access to the tablets or spray. This may require patients to have multiple vials or canisters that are in areas that they spend time (eg, home, work, car, and garage). While some patients may only need SL NTG for infrequent attacks, many patients will require chronic treatment for prevention of angina episodes. 4 Patients experiencing frequent angina episodes, or in whom angina is impacting quality of life, should receive chronic therapy. The goal of chronic therapy to provide complete or nearly complete elimination of angina episodes while having the patient take part in normal activities. The mechanism of chronic therapy is typically to prevent increases in MVO_2 that surpass the reduction in myocardial oxygen supply.

9 An initial goal in the reduction in MVO_2 is to lower the patient's resting HR to 50 to 60 beats per minute and an exercise HR of less than 100 beats per minutes. It should be noted that not all patients, especially elderly patients can tolerate an HR in this range, and therefore the goal HR would be as low as the patient can tolerate above 60 beats per minute. Reductions in HR also alter the cardiac cycle to increase diastolic filling time and an improvement in myocardial perfusion. Hence, initial chronic management of angina episodes to achieve this goal HR is either a β-blocker or a non-DHP CCB (verapamil or diltiazem). These agents not only reduce HR, but also contractility and myocardial wall tension (through BP reduction). Both agents are effective for increasing exercise duration and reducing the number of weekly angina episodes. While there have been a number of studies comparing β-blockers and CCBs in patients with SIHD, many of these trials demonstrating an advantage of β-blocker therapy were compared to DHP CCBs, and not HR lowering non-DHP CCBs. The APSIS trial (Angina Prognosis Study in Stockholm) did compare sustained-release metoprolol to sustained-release verapamil in patients with SIHD.[121] After the mean follow-up of 3.4 years, there was no significant difference in the occurrence of CV events (30.8% vs 29.3%) or mortality (5.4% vs 6.2%) between metoprolol and verapamil. These findings suggest that CV outcomes and mortality are similar regardless of whether a β-blocker or a non-DHP CCB is used as initial therapy in patients with SIHD.

9 β-blockers are currently recommended over CCBs as initial therapy for control of angina episodes in patients with SIHD.[1] This recommendation is mainly based on the improved survival demonstrated with the use of β-blockers in patients after MI. After the acute episode, these patients are often treated as those with SIHD. The mortality benefit in patients with LV dysfunction is also a contributing factor to this recommendation. It should be noted that only carvedilol, SR metoprolol, and bisoprolol should be used in patients with LV systolic dysfunction, starting with low doses and titrating up in a slow and set regimen. None of the non-DHP CCBs have demonstrated similar benefits in patients with MI or LV dysfunction. Patients with contraindications or intolerable side effects to β-blocker therapy, not related to HR lowering, should use verapamil or diltiazem as initial therapy. In patients without a history of MI or HF, the use of β-blocker therapy does not provide a survival advantage and is used purely for control of ischemic episodes and symptoms of angina.

If angina symptoms are controlled once the goal HR is achieved, then no further chronic therapy is necessary and patients are monitored for continued efficacy and side effects. Regardless of whether a β-blocker or non-DHP CCB are selected as initial therapy, many patients will require combination therapy to attain adequate control of their symptoms. 10 If additional therapy is required, control of BP helps decide the next step in therapy. Patients who continue to have a BP above the goal of 140/90 mm Hg should be prescribed a DHP CCB as their next agent. Since long-acting nitrates and ranolazine are not used to treat HTN, and DHP CCBs are effective agents for reducing MVO_2 and BP, they are a logical selection for use in these patients. The addition of a DHP CCP to a β-blocker has demonstrated efficacy in improving exercise duration and reducing weekly angina episodes.[122,123] While the addition of a DHP CCB to a non-DHP CCB is not often used, the different targets of calcium channel blockade do make this a rational regimen, so long as appropriate consideration is paid to the potential additive hemodynamic effects that may manifest in an individual patient.

10 12 Patients with continued angina episodes after achieving the goal HR, and having controlled BP, should receive a long-acting nitrate or ranolazine added to their regimen. Both agents have demonstrated efficacy when used in combination therapy. While long-acting nitrates are not optimal agents as monotherapy due to their ability to cause reflex tachycardia, this is avoided in patients who have already achieved HR control with a β-blocker or non-DHP CCB. The inability of ranolazine to reduce HR or BP make it an option in these patients who have already achieved their HR and BP goals, but still have exertional angina. The selection of one agent over the other is mainly based on patient preferences and tolerability. Long-acting nitrates do not provide 24-hour angina protection, but this may not be an issue for all patients. Ranolazine provides 24-hour protection, but is a more expensive agent compared to generic nitrates. Ranolazine has a more attractive side effect profile compared to long-acting nitrates, but the severity of these effects will be patient specific.

Clinical **Controversy...**

When to initiate ranolazine continues to be a point of controversy. While ranolazine has proven to be an effective and well tolerated agent for the management of episodes of angina, it is much more expensive. All other agents used for control of symptoms of angina are available in generic formulations, with many be only $4 a months.

Similar to the treatment of HTN, it is reasonable for patients to eventually end up on multiple agents in the attempt to achieve full control of angina symptoms and have patients fully participate in the activities that bring them joy in life. Patients who are unable to achieve this goal are defined as having refractory angina. Patients with refractory angina are those who continue to have symptoms, despite maximally tolerated therapy. Due to contraindications or intolerance to higher doses of medications, patients may end up with refractory angina with a smaller medication list than others, and not on full doses of anti-angina agents. Patients with refractory angina should be referred for revascularization therapy.

2 Management of Variable Threshold Angina and Prinzmetal's Angina

Patients with variable-threshold angina require pharmacotherapy that assists in management of vasospasm. While β-blockers are typically the agents of first choice in patients with fixed-threshold angina, they are not appropriate agents for patients with vasospasm. Although not all studies report increased painful episodes of angina with the addition of β-blockers in patients with vasospasm, they may induce coronary vasoconstriction and prolong ischemia, as documented by continuous ECG monitoring. The mechanism of worsening angina is most likely due to unopposed α^1-adrenergic receptor stimulation during β-blockade.

Both nitrates and CCBs are effective agents for reducing vasospasm. Most patients respond well to SL NTG for acute attacks. While long-acting nitrates can be used in the treatment of vasospasm, the high doses typically needed for adequate symptom control are not well tolerated. Therefore, nitrates are often given with CCBs. There is no preference to which agent is selected first, but CCBs are given less times a day and may allow for a single agent to be used to manage symptoms. Nifedipine, verapamil, and diltiazem are all equally effective as single agents for the initial management of coronary vasospasm. Dose titration is important to maximize the response with CCBs. Comparative trials are few in number and do not reveal significant differences among these three drugs for vasospasm. Patients unresponsive to calcium antagonists alone may have nitrates added.

EVALUATION OF THERAPEUTIC OUTCOMES

The two main therapeutic outcomes in the management of patients with SIHD are to prolong life and reduce symptoms of angina. Both of these should be accomplished while minimizing adverse effects to medications and improving the patient's quality of life. While "improved mortality" does not have a defined monitoring parameter, focus on surrogate endpoints, such as BP goal, use of high-intensity statin, HbA1c goal, smoking cessation, and weight loss from appropriate diet and exercise regimens, are targets that patients and clinicians can work on accomplishing. Patients may need to be evaluated every 1 to 2 months until goals are achieved. Follow-up then every 6 to 12 months would be appropriate.

4 Improvement in symptoms of angina should include reducing the number of angina episodes and weekly SL NTG use, as well as increasing their exercise capacity, or duration of exertion needed to induce angina. This should be accomplished while the patient is able to do the things in life that they want to do. It is not uncommon for patients to report reduced or no episodes of angina because they have given up on doing things that bring on angina. Once patients have been optimized on medical therapy, symptoms should improve over 2 to 4 weeks and remain stable until their disease progresses. There are several instruments such as the Seattle Angina Questionnaire and CCS, which can be used to improve the reproducibility of symptom assessment. If the patient is doing well, then no other assessment may be necessary. While objective assessment of control of ischemic episodes can be obtained by performing follow-up ETT with or without cardiac imaging, due to their expense they are rarely used unless patients are not responding to treatment. Patients receiving revascularization still require assessment of symptoms of angina at least every 6 to 12 months since a return of angina is not uncommon.

ABBREVIATIONS

ACC	American College of Cardiology
ACE	angiotensin converting enzyme
ACS	acute coronary syndrome
AHA	American Heart Association
ARB	angiotensin receptor blocker
ASPECT	aspirin-induced platelet effects
AV	atrioventricular
BARI	Bypass Angioplasty Revascularization Investigation
BMS	bare metal stent
BNP	B-type natriuretic peptide
BP	blood pressure
CAPRIE	The Clopidogrel versus Aspirin in Patients at Risk of Ischemic Events
CABG	coronary artery bypass grafting
CAD	coronary artery disease
CCS	Canadian Cardiovascular Society
CCB	calcium channel blocker
CHARISMA	Clopidogrel for High Atherothrombotic Risk and Ischemic Stabilization, Management, and Avoidance
CHD	coronary heart disease
COX	cyclooxygenase
CVD	cardiovascular disease
DAPT	dual antiplatelet therapy
DES	drug eluting stent
DHP	dihydropyridine
DM	diabetes mellitus
ECG	electrocardiogram

EDRF	endothelium-derived relaxing factor
FFR	fractional flow reserve
GDMT	guideline-directed medical therapy
GP	glycoprotein
HDL-C	high-density lipoprotein cholesterol
HR	heart rate
HTN	hypertension
IMA	internal mammary artery
ISMN	isosorbide mononitrate
LDL-C	low-density lipoprotein cholesterol
LOE	Level of Evidence
LV	left ventricular
MI	myocardial infarction
MVO_2	myocardial oxygen demand
NT-proBNP	N-terminal pro B-type natriuretic peptide
PCI	percutaneous coronary intervention
PPI	proton pump inhibitor
PREMIER	Prospective Registry Evaluating Myocardial Infarction: Events and Recovery
SIHD	stable ischemic heart disease
SL NTG	sublingual nitroglycerin
SVG	saphenous vein graft
UFH	unfractionated heparin

REFERENCES

1. Fihn SD, Gardin JM, Abrams, et al. 2012 ACCF/AHA/AATS/PCNA/SCAI/STS Guideline for the diagnosis and management of patients with stable ischemic heart disease. A report of the American College of Cardiology Foundation/American Heart Association task force on practice guidelines, and the American College of Physicians, American Association of Thoracic Surgery, Preventive Cardiovascular Nurses Association, Society for Cardiovascular Angiography and Interventions, and Society of Thoracic Surgeons. *J Am Coll Cardiol* 2012;60:e44-e164.
2. Motalescot G, Sechtem U, Achenbach S, et al. 2013 ESC guidelines on the management of stable coronary artery disease. The Task Force on the management of stable coronary artery disease by the European Society of Cardiology. *Eur Heart J* 2013;34:2949-3003.
3. Mozaffarian D, Benjamin EJ, Go AS, et al. Heart disease and stroke statistics—2016 update: A report from the American Heart Association. *Circulation* 2016;133:e38-e360.
4. Ford ES, Capewell S. Coronary heart disease mortality among young adults in the U.S. from 1980 through 2002: concealed leveling of mortality rates. *J Am Coll Cardiol* 2007;50:2128-2132.
5. Steg PG, Greenlaw N, Tendera M, et al. Prevalence of angina symptoms and myocardial ischemia and their effect on clinical outcomes in outpatients with stable coronary artery disease: Data from the International Observational CLARIFY Registry. *JAMA Intern Med* 2014;174:1651-1659.
6. Mozaffarian D, Bryson CL, Spertus JA, et al. Anginal symptoms consistently predict total mortality among outpatients with coronary artery disease. *Am Heart J* 2003;146:1015-1022.
7. Five-year clinical and functional outcome comparing bypass surgery and angioplasty in patients with multivessel coronary disease: A multicenter randomized trial. Writing Group for the Bypass Angioplasty Revascularization Investigation (BARI) Investigators. *JAMA* 1997;277:715-721.
8. Boini S, Briancon S, Guillemin F, Galan P, Hercberg S. Occurrence of coronary artery disease has an adverse impact on health-related quality of life: A longitudinal controlled study. *International Journal of Cardiology* 2006;113:215-222.
9. Hlatky MA, Rogers WJ, Johnstone I, et al. Medical care costs and quality of life after randomization to coronary angioplasty or coronary bypass surgery. Bypass Angioplasy Revascularization Investigation (BARI) Investigators. *N Engl J Med* 1997;336:92-99.
10. Marzilli M, Merz CNB, Boden WE, et al. Obstructive coronary atherosclerosis and ischemic heart disease: An elusive link! *J Am Coll Cardiol* 2012;60:951-956.
11. Fuster V, Badimon L, Badimon JJ, Chesebro JH. The pathogenesis of coronary heart disease and the acute coronary syndrome (first of two parts). *N Engl J Med* 1992;326:242-250.
12. Fuster V, Badimon L, Badimon JJ, Chesebro JH. The pathogenesis of coronary heart disease and the acute coronary syndrome (second of two parts). *N Engl J Med* 1992;326:310-318.
13. Klocke FJ. Coronary blood flow in man. *Prog Cardiovas Dis* 1976;19:117-166.
14. Epstein SE, Cannon RO III, Talbot TL. Hemodynamic principles in the control of coronary blood flow. *Am J Cardiol* 1985;56:4E-10E.
15. Canty JM Jr, Duncker. Coronary blood flow and myocardial ischemic. In: Mann DL, Zipes DP, Libby P, Bonow RO, eds. *Braunwald's Heart Disease: A Textbook of Cardiovascular Medicine.* 10th ed. Philadelphia PA: Elsevier Saunders; 2015:1029-1056.
16. Klocke FJ. Measurements of coronary blood flow and degree of stenosis: Current clinical implications and continues uncertainties. *J Am Coll Cardiol* 1983;1:31-41.
17. Hoffman JI, Spaan JA. Pressure-flow relations in coronary circulation. *Physiol Rev* 1990;70:331-390.
18. Laughlin MH, Davis MJ, Secher NH, et al. Peripheral circulation. *Compr Physiol* 2012;2:321-447.
19. Teunissen PFA, Horrevoets AJG, van Royen N. The coronary collateral circulation: genetic and environmental determinants in experimental models and humans. *J Mol Cell Cardiol* 2012;52:897-904.
20. Schaper W. Collateral circulation: Past and present. *Basic Res Cardiol* 2009;104:5-21.
21. Seiler C. The human coronary collateral circulation. *Eur J Clin Invest* 2010;40:465-476.
22. Pepine CJ, Douglas PS. Rethinking stable ischemic heart disease: Is this the beginning of a new era? *J Am Coll Cardiol* 2012;60:957-959.
23. Kaski JC, Russo G. Cardiac syndrome X: An overview. *Hospital Practice* 2000;35:75-91, 94.
24. Ridker PM, Danielson E, Fonseca FAH, et al., for the JUPITER Study Group. Rosuvastatin to prevent vascular events in men and women with elevated C-reactive protein. *N Engl J Med* 2008;359:2195-2207.
25. Hills LD, Braunwald E. Coronary-artery spasm. *N Engl J Med* 1978;299:695-702.
26. Campeau L. Grading of angina pectoris (letter). *Circulation* 1976;54:522-523.
27. Goldman L, Hashimoto B, Cook EF, Loscalzo A. Comparative reproducibility and validity of systems for assessing cardiovascular functional class: Advantages of a new specific activity scale. *Circulation* 1981;64:1227-1234.
28. Califf RM, Mark DB, Harell FE Jr, et al. Importance of clinical measures of ischemia in the prognosis of patients with documented coronary artery disease. *J Am Coll Cardiol* 1988;11:20-26.
29. Caracciolo EA, Chaitman BR, Forman SA, et al. Diabetics with coronary disease have a prevalence of asymptomatic ischemia during exercise treadmill testing and ambulatory ischemia monitoring similar to that of nondiabetic patients. An ACIP database study. *Circulation* 1996;93:2097-2105.
30. Pepine CJ, Balaban RS, Bonow RO, et al. Women's Ischemic Syndrome Evaluation: current status and future research directions: report of the National Heart, Lung and Blood Institute workshop: October 2-4, 2002; Section 1: diagnosis of stable ischemia and ischemic heart disease. *Circulation* 2004;109:e44-e46.
31. Gould KL, Johnson NP, Bateman TM, et al. Anatomic versus physiologic assessment of coronary artery disease: Role of coronary flow reserve, fractional flow reserve, and positron emission tomography imaging in revascularization decision-making. *J Am Coll Cardiol* 2013;62:1639-1653.
32. van de Hoef TP, Echavarría-Pinto M, van Lavieren MA, et al. Diagnostic and prognostic implications of coronary flow capacity: A comprehensive cross-modality physiological concept in ischemic heart disease. *J Am Coll Cardiol Intv* 2015;8:1670-1680.
33. Daniels LB, Maisel AS. Natriuretic peptides. *J Am Coll Cardiol* 2007;25:2357-2368.
34. Omland T, Richards AM, Wergeland R, Vik-Mo H. B-type natriuretic peptide and long-term survival in patients with stable coronary artery disease. *Am J Cardiol* 2005;95:24-28.
35. B-type natriuretic peptide and the risk of cardiovascular events and death in patients with stable angina: Results from the Athero*Gene* study. *J Am Cardiol Card* 2006;47:552-558.
36. Jeremias A, Kleiman NS, Nassif D, et al. Prevalence and prognostic significance of preprocedural cardiac troponin elevation among patients with stable coronary artery disease undergoing percutaneous coronary intervention: Results from the Evaluation of Drug Eluting Stents and Ischemic Events Registry. *Circulation* 2008;118:632-638.
37. Antithrombotic Trialists' Collaboration. Collaborative meta-analysis of randomised trials of antiplatelet therapy for prevention of death, myocardial infarction, and stroke in high risk patients. *BMJ* 2002;324:71-86.

38. Pairet M, Engelhardt G. Distinct isoforms (COX-1 and COX-2) of cyclooxygenase: Possible physiological and therapeutic implications. *Fundam Clin Pharmacol* 1996;10:1-17.
39. Awtry EH, Loscalzo J. Aspirin. *Circulation* 2000;101:1206-1218.
40. Lopez-Farre A, Caramelo C, Esteban A, et al. Effects of aspirin on platelet-neutrophil interactions. Role of nitric oxide and endothelin-1. *Circulation* 1995;91:2080-2088.
41. Ridker PM, Manson JE, Gaziano JM, Buring JE, Hennekens CH. Low-dose aspirin therapy for chronic stable angina: A randomized, placebo-controlled clinical trial. *Ann Intern Med* 1991;114:835-839.
42. Juul-Möller S, Edvardsson N, Jahnmatz B, et al. Double-blind trial of aspirin in primary prevention of myocardial infarction in patients with stable chronic angina pectoris. *Lancet* 1992;340:1421-1425.
43. Hovens MMC, Snoep JD, Eikenboom JCJ, van der Bom JG, Mertens BJA, Huisman MV. Prevalence of persistent platelet reactivity despite use of aspirin: A systematic review. *Am Heart J* 2007;153:175-181.
44. Gurbel PA, Bliden KP, DiChiara J, et al. Evaluation of dose-related effects of aspirin on platelet function: Results from the Aspirin-Induced Platelet Effect (ASPECT) study. *Circulation* 2007;115:3156-3164.
45. Catella-Lawson F, Reilly MP, Kapoor SC, et al. Cyclooxygenase inhibitors and the antiplatelet effects of aspirin. *N Engl J Med* 2001;345:1809-1817.
46. Gum PA, Kottke-Marchant K, Welsh PA, White J, Topol EJ. A prospective, blinded determination of the natural history of aspirin resistance among stable patients with cardiovascular disease. *J Am Coll Cardiol* 2003;41:961-965.
47. Chen W-H, Cheng X, Lee P-Y, et al. Aspirin resistance and adverse clinical events in patients with coronary artery disease. *Am J Med* 2007;120:631-635.
48. CAPRIE Steering Committee. A randomised, blinded trial of clopidogrel versus aspirin in patients at risk of ischaemic events (CAPRIE). *Lancet* 1996;348:1329-1339.
49. Bhatt DL, Fox KA, Hacke W, et al. Clopidogrel and aspirin versus aspirin alone for the prevention of atherothrombotic events. *N Engl J Med* 2006;354:1706-1717.
50. Bhatt DL, Flather MD, Hacke W, et al. Patients with prior myocardial infarction, stroke, or symptomatic peripheral arterial disease in the CHARISMA trial. *J Am Coll Cardiol* 2007;49:1982-1988.
51. Serebruany VL, Steinhubl SR, Berger PB, et al. Variability in platelet responsiveness to clopidogrel among 544 individuals. *J Am Coll Cardiol* 2005;45:246-251.
52. Wismann PP, Roest M, Asselbergs FW. Platelet-reactivity tests identify patients at secondary risk of secondary cardiovascular events: A systematic review and meta-analysis. *J Thromb Haemost* 2014;12:736-747.
53. Bonello L, Tantry US, Marcucci, R, et al. Consensus and future directions on the definition of high on-treatment platelet reactivity to adenosine diphosphate. *J Am Coll Cardiol* 2010;56:919-933.
54. Spertus JA, Kettelkamp R, Vance C, et al. Prevalence, predictors, and outcomes of premature discontinuation of thienopyridine therapy after drug-eluting stent placement: Results from the PREMIER registry. *Circulation* 2006;113:2803-2809.
55. Scott SA, Sangkuhl K, Stein CM, et al. Clinical pharmacogenetics implementation consortium guidelines for cytochrome P450-2C19 (CYP2C19) genotype and clopidogrel therapy: 2013 update. *Clin Pharmacol Ther* 2013;94:317-323.
56. Shuldiner AR, O'Connell JR, Bliden KP, et al. Association of cytochrome P450 2C19 genotype with the antiplatelet effect and clinical efficacy of clopidogrel therapy. *JAMA* 2009;302:849-857.
57. Hochholzer W, Trenk D, Fromm MF. Impact of cytochrome P450 2C19 loss-of-function polymorphism and of major demographic characteristics on residual platelet function after loading and maintenance treatment with clopidogrel in patients undergoing elective coronary stent placement. *J Am Coll Cardiol* 2010;55:2427-2434.
58. Gilard M, Arnaud B, Cornily J-C, et al. Influence of omeprazole on the antiplatelet action of clopidogrel associated with aspirin. The randomized, double-blind OCLA (Omeprazole CLopidogrel Aspirin) study. *J Am Coll Cardiol* 2008;51:256-260.
59. Norgard NB, Mathews KD, Wall GC. Drug-drug interaction between clopidogrel and the proton pump inhibitors. *Ann Pharmacother* 2009;43:1266-1274.
60. Bhatt DL, Cryer BL, Contant CF, et al. Clopidogrel with or without omeprazole in coronary artery disease. *N Engl J Med* 2010;363:1909-1917.
61. Klein WW, Khurmi MS, Eber B, Dusleag J. Effects of benazepril and metoprolol OROS alone and in combination on myocardial ischemia in patients with chronic stable angina. *J Am Coll Cardiol* 1990;16:948-956.
62. Ikram H, Low CJS, Shirlaw TM, et al. Angiotensin converting enzyme inhibition in chronic stable angina: Effects on myocardial ischaemia and comparison with nifedipine. *Br Heart J* 1994;71:30-33.
63. HOPE Investigators. Effects of an angiotensin-converting enzyme inhibitor, ramipril, on cardiovascular events in high risk patients. *N Engl J Med* 2000;342:145-153.
64. The European trial on reduction of cardiac events with perindopril in stable coronary artery disease investigators. Efficacy of perindopril in reduction of cardiovascular events among patients with stable coronary artery disease: Randomised, double-blind, placebo-controlled, multicenter trial (the EUROPA study). *Lancet* 2003;362:782-788.
65. PEACE Trial Investigators. Angiotensin-converting-enzyme inhibition in stable coronary artery disease. *N Engl J Med* 2004;351:2058-2068.
66. Danchin N, Cucherat M, Thuillez C, Durand E, Kadri Z, Steg PG. Angiotensin-converting enzyme inhibitors in patients with coronary artery disease and absence of heart failure or left ventricular systolic dysfunction: An overview of long-term randomized controlled trials. *Arch Intern Med* 2006;166:787-796.
67. The ONTARGET Investigators. Telmisartan, Ramipril, or both in patients at high risk for vascular events. *N Engl J Med* 2008;358:1547-1559.
68. The TRANSCEND Investigators. Effects of angiotensin-receptor blocker telmisartan on cardiovascular events in high-risk patients intolerant to angiotensin-converting enzyme inhibitors: A randomised controlled trial. *Lancet* 2008;372:1174-1183.
69. Baigent C, Blackwell L, Emberson J, et al. Efficacy and safety of more intensive lowering of LDL cholesterol: A meta-analysis of data from 170,000 participants in 26 randomised trials. *Lancet* 2010;376:1670-1681.
70. Stone NJ, Robinson JG, Lichtenstein AH, et al. 2013 ACC/AHA guideline on the treatment of blood cholesterol to reduce atherosclerotic cardiovascular risk in adults: A report of the American College of Cardiology/American Heart Association Task Force on practice guidelines. *Circulation* 2014;129(Suppl 2):S1-S45.
71. Pedersen TR, Faergeman O, Kastelein JJP, et al. High-dose atorvastatin vs usual-dose simvastatin for secondary prevention after myocardial infarction. The IDEAL study: A randomized controlled trial. *JAMA* 2005;294:2437-2445.
72. Lewington S, Clarke R, Qizilbash N, et al. Age-specific relevance of usual blood pressure to vascular mortality: A meta-analysis of individual data for one million adults in 61 prospective studies. *Lancet* 2002;360:1903-1913.
73. James PA, Oparil S, Carter BL, et al. 2014 evidence-based guideline for the management of high blood pressure in adults: Report from the panel members appointed to the Eighth Joint National Committee (JNC 8). *JAMA* 2014;311:507-520.
74. Ginsberg HN, Elam MB, Lovato LC, et al. Effects of combination lipid therapy in type 2 diabetes mellitus. *N Engl J Med* 2010;362:1563-1574.
75. The SPRINT Research Group. A randomized trial of intensive versus standard blood-pressure control. *N Engl J Med* 2015;373:2103-2116.
76. Doll R, Peto R. Mortality in relation to smoking: 20 years' observations on male British doctors. *Br Med J* 1976;2:1525-1536.
77. Willett WC, Green A, Stampfer MJ, et al. Relative and absolute excess risks of coronary heart disease among women who smoke cigarettes. *N Engl J Med* 1987;317:1303-1309.
78. Critchley J, Capewll S. Smoking cessation for the secondary prevention of coronary heart disease. *Cochrane Database Syst Rev* 2003;CD003041.
79. Silagy C, Lancaster T, Stead L, et al. Nicotine replacement therapy for smoking cessation. *Cochrane Database Syst Rev* 2004;CD000146.
80. Hughes J, Stead L, Lancaster T. Antidepressants for smoking cessation. *Cochrane Database Syst Rev* 2004;CD000031.
81. Jorenby DE, Hays JT, Rigotti NA, et al. Efficacy of varenicline, an alpha4beta2 nicotinic acetylcholine receptor partial agonist, vs placebo or sustained-release buproprion for smoking cessation: A randomized controlled trial. *JAMA* 2006;296:56-63.
82. The Diabetes Control and Complications Trial Research Group. The effect of intensive treatment of diabetes on the development and progression of long-term complications in insulin-dependent diabetes mellitus. *N Engl J Med* 1993;329:977-986.
83. McCormack J, Greenhalgh T. Seeing what you want to see in randomised controlled trials: Versions and perversions of UKPDS data. United Kingdom prospective diabetes study. *BMJ* 2000;320:1720-1723.
84. Gerstein HC, Miller ME, Byington RP, et al. Effects of intensive glucose lowering in type 2 diabetes. *N Engl J Med* 2008;358: 2545-2559.

85. Zinman B, Wanner C, Lachin JM, et al. Empagliflozin, cardiovascular outcomes, and mortality in type 2 diabetes. *N Engl J Med* 2015;373:2117-2128.
86. Messerli FH, Bangalore S, Yao SS, Steinberg JS. Cardioprotection with beta-blockers: Myths, facts and Pascal's wager. *J Intern Med* 2009;266:232-241.
87. Munzel T, Daiber A, Mulsch A. Explaining the phenomenon of nitrate tolerance. *Circ Res* 2005;97:618-628.
88. Daiber A, Oelze M, Wenzel P, et al. Nitrate tolerance as a model of vascular dysfunction: Roles for mitochondrial aldehyde dehydrogenase and mitochondrial oxidative stress. *Pharmacol Rep* 2009;61:33-48.
89. Undrovinas AI, Fleidervish IA, Makielski JC. Inward sodium current at resting potentials in single cardiac myocytes induced by the ischemic metabolite lysophosphatidylcholine. *Circ Res* 1992;71:1231-1241.
90. Kusuoka H, Hurtado MCC, Marban E. Role of sodium/calcium exchange in the mechanism of stunning: Protective effect of reperfusion with high sodium solution. *J Am Coll Cardiol* 1993;21:240-248.
91. Steenbergen C, Murphy E, Watts JA, London RE. Correlation between cytosolic free calcium, contracture, ATP, and irreversible ischemia injury in perfused rat heart. *Circ Res* 1990;66:135-146.
92. Belardinelli L, Antzelevitch C, Fraser H. Inhibition of late (sustained/persistent) sodium current: A potential drug target to reduce intracellular sodium-dependent calcium overload and its detrimental effects on cardiomyocyte function. *Eur Heart J Suppl* 2004;6(Suppl 1):13-17.
93. Chaitman BR, Skettino SL, Parker JO, et al. Anti-ischemic effects and long-term survival during ranolazine monotherapy in patients with chronic severe angina. *J Am Coll Cardiol* 2004;43:1375-1382.
94. Chaitman BR, Pepine CJ, Parker JO, et al. Effects of ranolazine with atenolol, amlodipine, or diltiazem on exercise tolerance and angina frequency in patients with severe chronic angina. A randomized controlled trial. *JAMA* 2004;291:309-316.
95. Stone PH, Gratsiansky NA, Blokhin A, Huang I-Z, Meng L. Antianginal efficacy of ranolazine when added to treatment with amlodipine. The ERICA (Efficacy of Ranolizine in Chronic Angina) Trial. *J Am Coll Cardiol* 2006;48:566-575.
96. Stone PH, Gibson RS, Glasser SP, et al. Comparison of propranolol, diltiazem, and nifedipine in the treatment of ambulatory ischemia in patients with stable angina. Differential effects on ambulatory ischemia, exercise performance, and anginal symptoms. *Circulation* 1990;82:1962-1972.
97. Davies RF, Habibi H, Klinke WP, et al, Effect of amlodipine, atenolol, and their combination on myocardial ischemia during treadmill exercise and ambulatory monitoring. *J Am Coll Cardiol* 1995;25:619-625.
98. Morrow DA, Scirica BM, Karwatowska-Prokopczuk E, et al. Effects of Ranolazine on recurrent cardiovascular events in patients with non-ST-elevatoin acute coronary syndromes: The MERLIN-TIMI 36 randomized trial. *JAMA* 2007;297:1775-1783.
99. Holmes DR Jr, Vlietstra RE, Smith HC, et al. Restenosis after percutaneous transluminal coronary angioplasty (PTCA): A report from the PTCA Registry of the National Heart, Lung, and Blood Institute. *Am J Cardiol* 1984;53:77C-81C.
100. Rajagopal V, Rockson SG. Coronary restenosis: A review of mechanisms and management. *Am J Med* 2003;115:547-553.
101. Mintz GS, Kent KM, Pichard AD, et al. Intravascular ultrasound insights into mechanisms of stenosis formation and restenosis. *Cardiol Clin* 1997;15:17-29.
102. Dobesh PP, Stacy ZA, Ansara AJ, Enders JM. Drug-eluting stents: A mechanical and pharmacologic approach to coronary artery disease. *Pharmacotherapy* 2004;24:1554-1577.
103. Stergiopoulos K, Boden WE, Hartigan P, et al. Percutaneous coronary intervention outcomes in patients with stable obstructive coronary artery disease and myocardial ischemia: A collaborative meta-analysis of contemporary randomized clinical trials. *JAMA Intern Med* 2014;174:232-240.
104. Boden WE, O'Rourke RA, Teo KK, et al. Optimal medical therapy with or without PCI for stable coronary disease. *N Engl J Med* 2007;356:1503-1516.
105. Sedlis SP, Hartigan PM, Teo KK, et al. Effects of PCI on long-term survival in patients with stable ischemic heart disease. *N Engl J Med* 2015;373:1937-1946.
106. The BARI 2D Study Group. A randomized trial of therapies for type 2 diabetes and coronary artery disease. *N Engl J Med* 2009;360:2503-2515.
107. Topol EJ, Mark DB, Lincoff AM, et al. Outcomes at 1 year and economic implications of platelet glycoprotein IIb/IIIa blockade in patients undergoing coronary stenting: Results from a multicenter randomised trial. *Lance* 1999;354:2019-2024.
108. O'Shea JC, Hafley GE, Greenberg S, et al. Platelet glycoprotein IIb/IIIa integrin blockade with eptifibatide in coronary stent intervention. The ESPRIT trial: A randomized controlled trial. *JAMA* 2001;285:2468-2473.
109. Topol EJ, Maliterno DJ, Herrmann HC, et al. Comparison of two platelet glycoprotein IIb/IIIa inhibitors, tirofiban and abciximab for the prevention of ischemic events with percutaneous coronary revascularization. *N Engl J Med* 2001;344:1888-1894.
110. Kastrati A, Mehilli J, Schühlen H, et al. A clinical trial of abciximab in elective percutaneous coronary intervention after pretreatment with clopidogrel. *N Engl J Med* 2004;350:232-238.
111. Mehilli J, Kastrati A, Schühlen H, et al. Randomized clinical trial of abciximab in diabetic patients undergoing elective percutaneous coronary interventions after treatment with a high loading dose of clopidogrel. *Circulation* 2004;110:3627-3635.
112. Mauri L, Kereiakes DJ, Yeh RW, et al. Twelve or 30 months of dual antiplatelet therapy after drug-eluting stents. *N Engl J Med* 2014;371:2155-2166.
113. Montalescot G, White HD, Gallo R, et al. Enoxaparin versus unfractionated heparin in elective percutaneous coronary intervention. *N Engl J Med* 2006;355:1006-1017.
114. Lincoff AM, Bittl JA, Harrington RA, et al. Bivalirudin and provisional glycoprotein IIb/IIIa blockade compared with heparin and planned glycoprotein IIb/IIIa blockade during percutaneous coronary intervention: REPLACE-2 randomized trial. *JAMA* 2003;289:853-863. [Erratum, *JAMA* 2003;289:1638.]
115. The Veterans Administration Coronary Artery Bypass Surgery Cooperative Study Group. Eighteen-year follow-up in the Veterans Affairs Cooperative Study of Coronary Artery Bypass Surgery for stable angina. *Circulation* 1992;86:121-130.
116. Varnauska E. Twelve-year follow-up of survival in the randomized European Coronary Surgery Study. *N Engl J Med* 1988;319:332-337.
117. Emond M, Mock MB, Davis KB, et al. Long-term survival of medically treated patients in the Coronary Artery Surgery Study (CASS) Registry. *Circulation* 1994;90:2645-2657.
118. Yusuf S, Zucker D, Peduzzi P, et al. Effect of coronary artery bypass graft surgery on survival: Overview of 10-year results from randomised trials by the Coronary Artery Bypass Graft Surgery Trialists Collaboration. *Lancet* 1994;344:563-570.
119. The Bypass Angioplasty Revascularization Investigation (BARI) Investigators. Comparison of coronary bypass surgery with angioplasty in patients with multivessel disease. *N Engl J Med* 1996;335:217-225. [Erratum, *N Engl J Med* 1997;336:147.]
120. Serruys PW, Morice M-C, Kappetein AP, et al. Percutaneous coronary intervention versus coronary-artery bypass grafting for severe coronary artery disease. *N Engl J Med* 2009;360:961-972.
121. Rehnqvist N, Hjemdahl P, Billing E, et al. Effects of metoprolol vs verapamil in patients with stable angina pectoris. The Angina Prognosis Study in Stockholm (APSIS). *Eur Heart J* 1996;17:76-81.
122. Kawanishi DT, Reid CL, Morrison EC, Rahimtoola SH. Response of angina and ischemia to long-term treatment in patients with chronic stable angina: A double-blind randomized individualized dosing trial of nifedipine, propranolol and their combination. *J Am Coll Cardiol* 1992;19:409-417.
123. Davies RF, Habibi H, Klinke WP, et al. Effect of amlodipine, atenolol and their combination on myocardial ischemia during treadmill exercise and ambulatory monitoring. *J Am Coll Cardiol* 1995;25:619-625.

17

Acute Coronary Syndromes

Kelly C. Rogers, Simon de Denus, Shannon W. Finks, and Sarah A. Spinler

KEY CONCEPTS

1. The cause of an acute coronary syndrome (ACS) is the rupture of an atherosclerotic plaque with subsequent platelet adherence, activation, and aggregation, and the activation of the clotting cascade. Ultimately, a clot forms composed of fibrin and platelets.
2. National guidelines exist for ACS patient care for ST-segment elevation (STE) myocardial infarction (MI) and non–ST-segment elevation (NSTE) ACS, including guidelines for patients undergoing percutaneous coronary intervention (PCI).
3. Patients with ischemic chest discomfort and suspected ACS are risk-stratified based on a 12-lead electrocardiogram (ECG), clinical presentation, past medical history, and results of the troponin assays. The diagnosis of MI is confirmed based on the results of the troponin biochemical marker tests.
4. Early reperfusion therapy with primary PCI of the infarct artery is recommended for patients presenting with STEMI within 12 hours of symptom onset.
5. The most recent PCI practice guidelines recommend coronary angiography with either PCI or coronary artery bypass graft (CABG) surgery revascularization as an early treatment (early invasive strategy) for patients with NSTE-ACS at an elevated risk for death or MI, including those with a high risk score or patients with refractory angina, acute heart failure, other symptoms of cardiogenic shock, or arrhythmias.
6. In addition to reperfusion therapy, other early pharmacotherapy that all patients with STEMI and without contraindications should receive within the first day of hospitalization, and preferably in the emergency department (ED), are intranasal oxygen (if oxygen saturation is low), sublingual (SL) nitroglycerin (NTG), aspirin, a $P2Y_{12}$ inhibitor (clopidogrel, prasugrel, or ticagrelor depending on reperfusion strategy), and anticoagulation with bivalirudin, unfractionated heparin (UFH), enoxaparin, or fondaparinux (Agent dependent on reperfusion strategy). A glycoprotein IIb/IIIa inhibitor (GPI) may be considered if UFH is selected as the anticoagulant for patients undergoing primary PCI. A high-intensity statin should be administered prior to PCI. Intravenous (IV) β-blockers and IV NTG should be administered cautiously in selected patients. Oral β-blockers should be initiated within the first day in patients without contraindications.
7. In the absence of contraindications, all patients with NSTE-ACS should be treated in the ED with intranasal oxygen (if oxygen saturation is low), SL NTG, aspirin, and an anticoagulant (UFH, enoxaparin, fondaparinux, or bivalirudin). High-risk patients should proceed to early angiography, and may receive a GPI. A $P2Y_{12}$ inhibitor (selection of agent and timing of indication dependent on interventional (PCI versus CABG surgery) versus conservative approach (medical managment/also referred to as "ischemia-guided approach")) and should be administered to all patients. A high-intensity statin should be administered prior to PCI. IV β-blockers and IV NTG should be administered cautiously in selected patients. Oral β-blockers should be initiated within the first day in patients without contraindications.
8. Secondary prevention guidelines suggest that following MI from either STEMI or NSTE-ACS, all patients, in the absence of contraindications, should receive indefinite treatment with aspirin, a β-blocker, a moderate to high-intensity statin, and an angiotensin-converting enzyme (ACE) inhibitor for secondary prevention of death, stroke, or recurrent infarction. A $P2Y_{12}$ inhibitor should be continued for at least 12 months for patients undergoing PCI and for patients treated medically (without PCI or thrombolytics). Clopidogrel should be continued for at least 14 days, and ideally 1 year, in patients with STEMI treated with fibrinolytics. An angiotensin II receptor blocker and an aldosterone antagonist should be given to selected patients. For all patients with ACS, treatment and control of modifiable risk factors such as hypertension (HTN), dyslipidemia, obesity, smoking, and diabetes mellitus (DM) are essential.
9. To determine the efficacy of nonpharmacologic treatments and pharmacotherapy, monitor patients for relief of ischemic discomfort, return of ECG changes to baseline, and absence or resolution of heart failure signs and symptoms. Patients should be monitored for adverse drug reactions that can be induced from pharmacotherapy of ACS.

INTRODUCTION

Cardiovascular disease (CVD) is the leading cause of death in the United States and one of the major causes of death worldwide. *Acute coronary syndrome* (ACS), including unstable angina (UA) and *myocardial infarction* (MI), is a form of coronary heart disease (CHD) that comprises the most common cause of CVD death.[1] (1) The cause of an ACS is primarily the rupture of an atherosclerotic plaque with subsequent platelet adherence, activation, and aggregation, and the activation of the clotting cascade. Ultimately, a clot forms composed of fibrin and platelets. (2) National guidelines recommend strategies for ACS patient care for *ST-segment elevation* (STE), *non–ST-segment elevation* (NSTE) ACS, and for *percutaneous coronary intervention* (PCI), including PCI in the setting of ACS.[2-4] These practice guidelines are based on a review of available clinical evidence, have graded recommendations based on evidence and expert opinion, and are updated periodically. These guidelines form the cornerstone for quality care of the ACS patient.

EPIDEMIOLOGY

One in seven deaths are secondary to CHD in America. It is estimated that every 42 seconds, an American will experience an MI.[1] Each year, more than 1.1 million persons are discharged from the hospital with a diagnosis of an ACS with 813,000 diagnosed with MI. Annually, approximately 660,000 Americans will have a new "coronary event" (a first hospitalization for an MI or CHD death), while 305,000 will have a recurrent event. It is estimated that 116,800 Americans die of an MI each year.[1] Moreover an estimated additional 160,000 Americans will have a "silent MI", which means that approximately more than 21% of individuals who experience a coronary event will not experience any, or only minimum symptoms. This nevertheless places these individuals at high-risk of subsequent additional events and death. Although the overall death rates from CHD has declined by 38% from 2003 to 2013, the estimated annual mortality in the first year following a new coronary event and MI remain high at 34% and 15%, respectively necessitating careful attention to secondary prevention measures.[1] Hospitals are required to report mortality rates and 30-day readmission rates following MI to the Centers for Medicare and Medicaid Services. These data are publically available and reported as better than, no different than, or worse than the national rate.[5]

Of patients presenting with suspected ACS, approximately 31% have STEMI, 32% NSTEMI, 26% UA, 8% another cardiac diagnosis, and 4% a noncardiac final diagnosis. The mean length of hospital stay is 3 days. An analysis of hospitalizations from the Healthcare Cost and Utilization Project's Nationwide Inpatient Sample reported unadjusted in-hospital mortality rates for STEMI of 3.52% in patients undergoing PCI and 14.91% for patients receiving no revascularization during hospitalization.[6] Analogous in-hospital mortality rates for NSTEMI were lower at 1.45% and 6.26%, respectively in 2011.[6] Nevertheless, data from Worcester, MA, indicate that at 1 year post-discharge mortality rates may be higher for NSTEMI than STEMI, with rates of 18.7% and 8.4%, respectively.[1] This suggests that more energy should be put in using disease-modifying therapies following hospital discharge in patients with NSTEMI. Other than persistent ST-segment changes and troponin, other predictors of in-hospital mortality include older age, elevated serum creatinine (SCr)/renal dysfunction, tachycardia, and heart failure (HF).

The cost of heart disease is high, with estimated direct and indirect costs of more than $207.3 billion in the United States.[1] These costs include MI and CHD, which at $11.5 and $10.4 billion respectively, represented 2 of the 10 most expensive hospital principal discharge diagnoses in 2011. The reported cost of hospitalization for STEMI or NSTEMI in the United States in 2011 was reported to be $19,000.[6]

ETIOLOGY

Endothelial dysfunction, inflammation, and the formation of fatty streaks contribute to the formation of atherosclerotic coronary artery plaques, the underlying cause of coronary artery disease (CAD).[7] 1 The predominant cause of ACS in more than 90% of patients is atheromatous plaque rupture, fissuring, or erosion of an unstable atherosclerotic plaque. This is called an MI type 1, which generally occurs in coronary arteries where the stenosis occludes less than 50% of the lumen prior to the event; rather than a more stable 70% to 90% stenosis of the coronary artery.[3,9,10]. MI type 2 is related to a reduction in myocardial oxygen supply or an increase in myocardial demand in the absence of a coronary artery process. MI type 3 is defined as MI resulting in death without the possibility of measuring biomarkers, while MI types 4 and 5 occur during revascularization procedures.[10] Stable plaques are characteristic of stable angina.

PATHOPHYSIOLOGY

Spectrum of ACS

Acute coronary syndrome includes all clinical syndromes compatible with acute MI resulting from an imbalance between myocardial oxygen demand and supply. In contrast to stable angina, an ACS results primarily from diminished myocardial blood flow secondary to an occlusive or partially occlusive coronary artery thrombus. ACS is classified according to electrocardiogram (ECG) changes into STEMI or NSTE-ACS (NSTEMI and UA) (Fig. 17-1).[3] A STEMI occurs when symptoms of myocardial ischemia occur in conjunction with new STE with subsequent release of biomarkers of myocardial necrosis, mainly *troponins T* or *I*.[2] 2 A STEMI typically results in an injury that transects the thickness of the myocardial wall. Following a STEMI, pathologic Q waves are frequently seen on the ECG, indicating transmural MI, whereas such an ECG manifestation is seen less commonly in patients with NSTEMI.[3] NSTEMI is limited to the subendocardial myocardium and is not as extensive as STEMI. NSTEMI differs from UA in that ischemia is severe enough to produce myocardial necrosis resulting in the release of a detectable amount of *troponins T* or *I*, from the necrotic myocytes in the bloodstream. The clinical significance of serum markers will be discussed in greater detail in later sections of this chapter.

Plaque Rupture and Clot Formation

Following plaque rupture, a clot (a partially or completely occlusive thrombus) forms on top of the ruptured plaque. The thrombogenic contents of the plaque are exposed to blood elements. Exposure of collagen and tissue factor induces platelet adhesion and activation, which promote the release of platelet-derived vasoactive substances including adenosine diphosphate (ADP) and thromboxane A_2 (TXA_2).[7] These produce vasoconstriction and potentiate platelet activation. Furthermore, during platelet activation, a change in the conformation in the glycoprotein (GP) IIb/IIIa surface receptors of platelets occurs that cross-links platelets to each other through fibrinogen bridges. This is considered the final common pathway of platelet aggregation. Inclusion of platelets gives the clot a white appearance. Simultaneously, the extrinsic coagulation cascade pathway is activated as a result of exposure of blood components to the thrombogenic lipid core and disrupted endothelium, which are rich in tissue factor. This leads to the production of thrombin (factor IIa), which converts fibrinogen to fibrin through enzymatic activity. Fibrin stabilizes the clot and traps red blood cells, which gives the clot a red appearance. Therefore, the clot is composed of cross-linked platelets and fibrin strands.[8]

Ventricular Remodeling Following an Acute MI

Ventricular remodeling is a process that occurs in several cardiovascular (CV) conditions including HF and following MI. It is characterized by left ventricular (LV) dilation and reduced pumping function of the LV, leading to HF.[11] Because HF represents one of the principal causes of morbidity and mortality following an MI, preventing ventricular remodeling is an important therapeutic goal.

Angiotensin-converting enzyme (ACE) inhibitors, angiotensin receptor blockers (ARBs), β-blockers, and aldosterone antagonists are all agents that slow down or reverse ventricular remodeling through inhibition of the renin–angiotensin–aldosterone system and/or through improvement in hemodynamics (decreasing preload, afterload or neurohormonal activation).[11] These agents also improve survival and will be discussed in more detail in subsequent sections of this chapter.

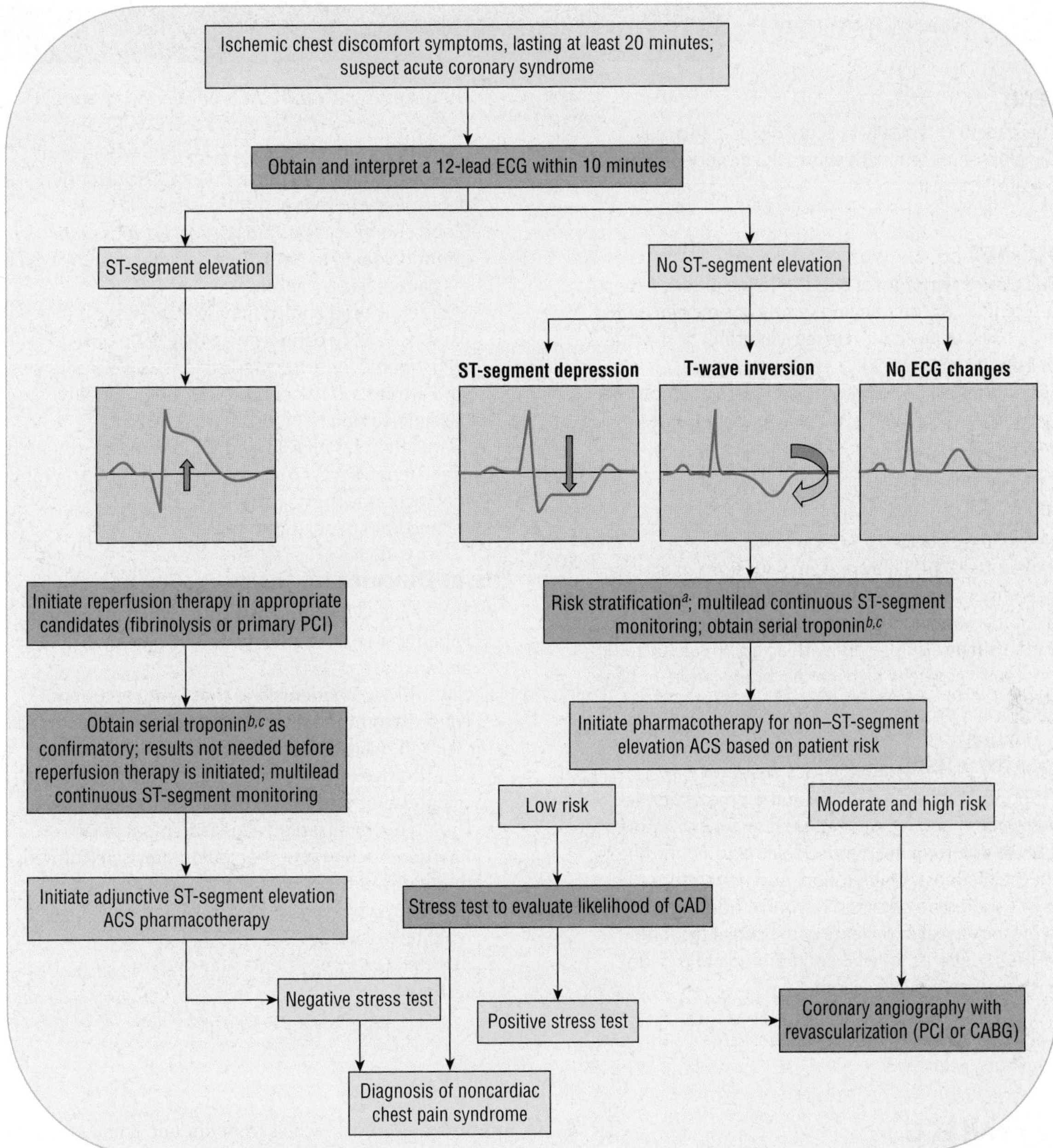

FIGURE 17-1 Evaluation of the acute coronary syndrome patient. [a]*As described in* Table 17-1. [b]"Positive": Above the myocardial infarction decision limit. [c]"Negative": Below the myocardial infarction decision limit. (ACS, acute coronary syndrome; CABG, coronary artery bypass graft; CAD, coronary artery disease; ECG, electrocardiogram; PCI, percutaneous coronary intervention.) *(Used with permission from Spinler SA. Evolution of antithrombotic therapy used in acute coronary syndromes. In: Richardson MM, Chant C, Cheng JWM, et al., eds. Pharmacotherapy Self-Assessment Program. Book 1: Cardiology, 7th ed. Lenexa, KS: American College of Clinical Pharmacy, 2010.)*

Complications

This chapter focuses on management of the uncomplicated ACS patient. However, it is important for clinicians to recognize complications of MI, because MI is associated with increased mortality. The most serious complication of MI is cardiogenic shock, occurring in approximately 5% to 10% of hospitalized patients presenting with STEMI.[12] Mortality of cardiogenic shock complicated by MI has been decreasing secondary to guideline-implemented therapies, yet remains high at approximately 34%.[12] Other complications that may result from MI are HF, valvular dysfunction, bradycardia, heart block, pericarditis, stroke secondary to LV thrombus embolization, venous thromboembolism, LV free wall or ventricular septal rupture, LV aneurysm formation, and ventricular and atrial tachyarrhythmias.[2]

Symptoms and Physical Examination Findings

The classic symptom of ACS is midline anterior anginal chest pain often described as crushing, burning, or a heavy pressure. It most often occurs when an individual is at rest, as a severe new onset, or as increasing angina that is at least 20 minutes in duration. The chest discomfort may radiate to the shoulder, down the left arm, and to the back or to the jaw. Associated symptoms that may accompany the chest discomfort include nausea, vomiting, diaphoresis, or shortness of breath. Although similar to stable angina, the duration may be longer and the intensity greater. All healthcare professionals should review these warning symptoms with patients at high risk for CHD. On physical examination, no specific features are indicative of ACS.[13]

CLINICAL PRESENTATION Diagnosis of ACS

General

- The patient is typically in acute distress and may develop or present with acute HF, cardiogenic shock, or cardiac arrest.

Symptoms

- The classic symptom of ACS is midline anterior chest discomfort. Accompanying symptoms may include arm, back, or jaw pain, nausea, vomiting, or shortness of breath.
- Patients less likely to present with classic symptoms include elderly patients, diabetic patients, and women.

Signs

- No signs are classic for ACS.
- Patients with ACS may present with signs of acute decompensated HF including jugular venous distention and an S_3 sound on auscultation.
- Patients may also present with arrhythmias, and therefore may have tachycardia, bradycardia, or heart block.

Laboratory Tests

- Troponin I or T are measured at the time of first assessment and repeated at least once, 3 to 6 hours later to ascertain heart muscle damage, confirmatory for the diagnosis of infarction. Additional troponin levels should be obtained beyond 6 hours after symptom onset in patients with normal troponin levels in patients for who an intermediate to high suspicion of ACS is present.
- For patients with NSTE-ACS, an elevated troponin is diagnostic for MI, defining a NSTEMI. Patients presenting with suspected NSTE-ACS who do not have an MI undergo further diagnostic testing to determine whether or not they have UA or ACS.
- Blood chemistry tests are performed with particular attention given to potassium and magnesium, which may affect heart rhythm.
- SCr is measured and creatinine clearance (CrCl) is used to identify patients who may need dosing adjustments for some medications as well as those who are at high risk of morbidity and mortality.
- Baseline complete blood count (CBC) and coagulation tests (aPTT and INR) should be obtained, as most patients will receive antithrombotic therapy that increases the risk for bleeding.
- Fasting lipid panel (optional).

Other Diagnostic Tests

- The 12-lead ECG is the first step in management. Patients are risk-stratified into two groups: STEMI and suspected NSTE-ACS.
- High-risk ACS patients and those with recurrent chest discomfort will undergo coronary angiography via a left heart catheterization and injection of contrast dye into the coronary arteries to determine the presence and extent of coronary artery stenosis.
- During hospitalization, a measurement of LV function, such as an echocardiogram, is performed to identify patients with low LV ejection fractions (EF) (≤40%) who are at high risk of death following hospital discharge.
- Selected low-risk patients may undergo early stress testing.

Twelve-Lead ECG

There are key features of a 12-lead ECG that identify and risk-stratify a patient with an ACS. Within 10 minutes of presentation to an ED with symptoms of ischemic chest discomfort, a 12-lead ECG should be obtained and interpreted. When possible, a 12-lead ECG should be performed by emergency medical system (EMS) providers in order to reduce the delay until myocardial reperfusion can be achieved. If available, a prior 12-lead ECG should be reviewed to identify whether or not the findings on the current ECG are new or old, with new findings being more indicative of ACS. Key findings on review of a 12-lead ECG that indicate myocardial ischemia or infarction are STE, ST-segment depression, and T-wave inversion (see Fig. 17-1).[2,13] ST-segment and/or T-wave changes in certain groupings of leads help to identify the location of the coronary artery that is the cause of the ischemia or infarction. In addition, the appearance of a new left bundle-branch block accompanied by chest discomfort is highly specific for acute MI. About one half of patients diagnosed with MI present with STE on their ECG, with the remainder having ST-segment depression, T-wave inversion, or, in some instances, no ECG changes. Some parts of the heart are more "electrically silent" than others, and myocardial ischemia may not be detected on a surface ECG. Therefore, it is important to review findings from the ECG in conjunction with biochemical markers of myocardial necrosis, such as troponin I or T, and other risk factors for CHD to determine the patient's risk for experiencing a new MI or having other complications.

Biochemical Markers/Cardiac Enzymes

Biochemical markers of myocardial cell death are important for confirming the diagnosis of MI. The diagnosis of acute MI is confirmed when the following conditions are met in a clinical setting consistent with myocardial ischemia: "Detection of a rise and/or fall of cardiac biomarkers with at least one value above the 99th percentile of the upper reference limit with at least one of the following: (a) symptoms of ischemia; (b) new or presumed new significant ST-segment–T wave changes or new left bundle-branch block; (c) development of pathologic Q waves; or (d) imaging evidence of new loss of viable myocardium or new regional wall motion abnormality."[10] Typically, a blood sample is obtained once in the ED, and then 3 to 6 hours after symptoms unset, and in patients at a high suspicion of MI but in whom previous measurements did not reveal elevations in biomarkers, further measurement can be performed beyond 6 hours after the onset of symptoms. A single measurement of troponin is not adequate to exclude a diagnosis of MI, as up to 15% of values that were initially below the level of detection (a "negative" test) rise to the level of detection (a "positive" test) in subsequent hours.

Troponins appear in the blood within 6 hours of infarction and stay elevated for up to 10 days.[10]

Risk Stratification

Patient symptoms, past medical history, ECG, and biomarkers are utilized to stratify patients into low, medium, or high risk of death, MI, or likelihood of failing pharmacotherapy and needing urgent coronary angiography and PCI (Table 17-1).[3,4] 3 Initial treatment according to risk stratification is depicted in Fig. 17-1.[2-4] Patients with STEMI are at the highest risk of death. Initial treatment of STEMI should proceed without evaluation of the troponins because these patients have a greater than 97% chance of having an MI subsequently diagnosed with biochemical markers. A target time to initiate reperfusion treatment within 30 minutes of hospital presentation for fibrinolytics (eg, streptokinase, alteplase, reteplase, and tenecteplase) and within 90 minutes or less from first medical contact for primary PCI is recommended.[2,4] The sooner the infarct-related coronary artery is opened for these patients, the lower their mortality and the greater the amount of myocardium that is preserved.[2] Although all patients should be evaluated for reperfusion therapy, not all patients may be eligible. Indications and contraindications for fibrinolytic therapy are described in the Treatment section of this chapter. Approximately 34% of hospitals in the United States are equipped to perform primary PCI.[14] Pharmacotherapy for STEMI patients should be initiated in the ED and the patient transferred to a coronary intensive care unit.[2]

Because NSTE-ACS is heterogeneous, risk stratification is more complex as patients with UA have a lower short-term mortality risk compared to NSTEMI. In-hospital outcomes for this group of patients vary with reported rates of death of 0% to 12%, reinfarction rates of 0% to 3%, and recurrent severe ischemia rates of 5% to 20%.[15,16] Not all patients presenting with suspected NSTE-ACS will even have CAD. Some will eventually be diagnosed with nonischemic chest discomfort. In general, among NSTE-ACS patients, those with ST-segment depression (see Fig. 17-1) and/or elevated biomarkers are at higher risk of death or recurrent infarction.[16]

TABLE 17-1 Risk Stratification for Acute Coronary Syndromes[3]

TIMI Risk Score for NSTE-ACS

One point is assigned for each of the seven medical history and clinical presentation findings. The point total is calculated, and the patient is assigned a risk for experiencing the composite endpoint of death, MI, or urgent need for revascularization as follows:

- Age 65 years or older
- Three or more CHD risk factors: smoking, hypercholesterolemia, hypertension, diabetes mellitus, family history of premature CHD death/events
- Known CAD (50% or greater stenosis of at least one major coronary artery on coronary angiogram)
- Aspirin use within the past 7 days
- Two or more episodes of chest discomfort within the past 24 hours
- ST-segment depression 0.5 mm or greater
- Positive biochemical marker for infarction

High-Risk	Medium-Risk	Low-Risk
TIMI Risk Score 5-7 points	TIMI Risk Score 3-4 points	TIMI Risk Score 0-2 points

TIMI Risk Score	Mortality, MI, or Severe Recurrent Ischemia Requiring Urgent Revascularization Through 14 Days
0/1	4.7%
2	8.3%
3	13.2%
4	19.9%
5	26.2%
6/7	40.9%

GRACE Risk Factors for Increased Mortality and the Composite of Death or MI in ACS

Signs and symptoms of heart failure
Low systolic blood pressure
Elevated heart rate
Older age
Elevated serum creatinine
Baseline risk factors on clinical evaluation: cardiac arrest at admission, ST-segment deviation, elevated troponin
A high-risk patient is defined as a GRACE Risk Score more than 140 points

ACS, acute coronary syndromes; CAD, coronary artery disease; CHD, coronary heart disease; GRACE, Global Registry of Acute Coronary Events; MI, myocardial infarction; NSTE, non-ST-segment elevation; TIMI, Thrombolysis in Myocardial Infarction.

An online calculator for the GRACE Risk Model is available at: http://www.outcomes-umassmed.org/GRACE/acs_risk/acs_risk_content.html. (Accessed January 25, 2016)

TREATMENT

Desired Outcomes

Short-term desired outcomes in a patient with ACS are: (a) early restoration of blood flow to the infarct-related artery to prevent infarct expansion (in the case of MI) or prevent complete occlusion and MI (in UA); (b) prevention of death and other MI complications; (c) prevention of coronary artery reocclusion; and as evidence of restoration of coronary artery blood flow; (d) relief of ischemic chest discomfort; and (e) resolution of ST-segment and T-wave changes on the ECG.

Long-term desired outcomes are control of CV risk factors, prevention of additional CV events, including reinfarction, stroke, and HF, and improvement in quality of life.

General Approach to Treatment

Selecting evidence-based therapies for patients without contraindications results in lower mortality.[17,18] General treatment measures for all STEMI and high- and intermediate-risk NSTE-ACS patients include admission to hospital, oxygen administration (if oxygen saturation is low, less than 90%), continuous multi-lead ST-segment monitoring for arrhythmias and ischemia, frequent measurement of vital signs, bed rest for 12 hours in hemodynamically stable patients, avoidance of the Valsalva maneuver (prescribe stool softeners routinely), and pain relief (Figs. 17-2 **and** 17-3).[2,3]

Because risk varies and resources are limited, it is important to triage and treat patients according to their risk category. Initial approaches to treatment of STEMI and NSTE-ACS patients are outlined in Figs. 17-2 and 17-3. Patients with STEMI are at high risk of death, and efforts to reestablish coronary perfusion, as well as adjunctive pharmacotherapy, should be initiated immediately.

Features identifying low-, moderate-, and high-risk NSTE-ACS patients are described in Table 17-1.[3,19,20]

Nonpharmacologic Therapy

Primary PCI for STEMIs

Early reperfusion therapy with primary PCI of the infarct artery within 90 minutes of first medical contact is the reperfusion treatment of choice for patients presenting with STEMI who present within 12 hours of symptom onset[2] 4 (see Fig. 17-2). EMS may be activated for a patient complaining of ischemic symptoms well in advance of hospital arrival. Paramedics can electronically transmit a 12-lead ECG where a physician can review and notify the cardiac catheterization medical team to alert them that a patient with STEMI is en route to the hospital for reperfusion. For primary PCI, the patient is taken

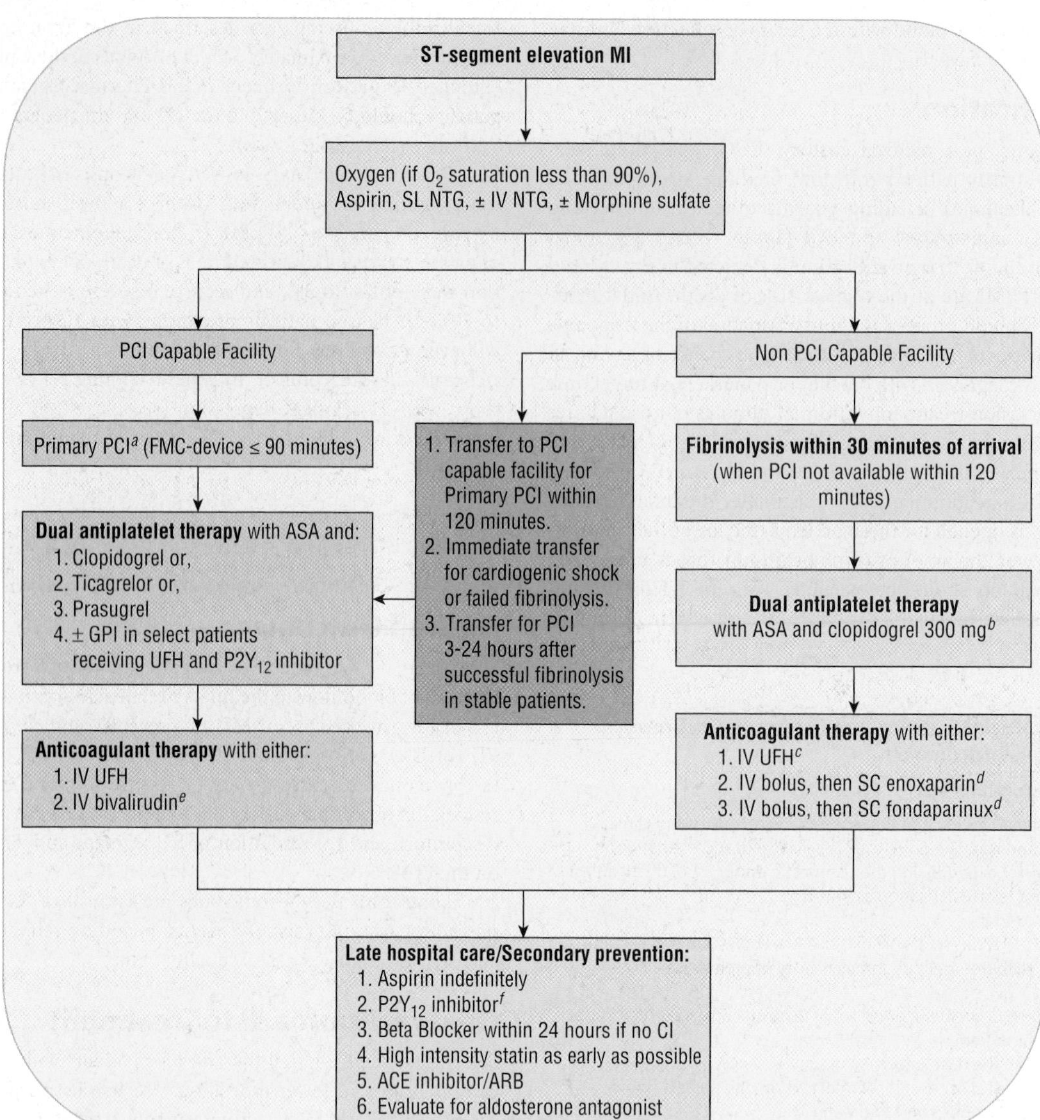

FIGURE 17-2 Initial pharmacotherapy for ST-segment elevation myocardial infarction. [a]Options after coronary angiography also include medical management alone or CABG surgery. [b]Clopidogrel preferred $P2Y^{12}$ inhibitor when fibrinolytic therapy is utilized. No loading dose recommended if age older than 75 years. [c]Given for up to 48 hours or until revascularization. [d]Given for the duration of hospitalization, up to 8 days or until revascularization. [e]If pretreated with UFH, stop UFH infusion for 30 minutes prior to administration of bivalirudin (bolus plus infusion). [f]In patients with STEMI receiving a fibrinolytic or who do not receive reperfusion therapy, administer clopidogrel for at least 14 days and ideally up to 1 year. (ACE, angiotensin-converting enzyme; ARB, angiotensin receptor blocker; ASA, aspirin; CI, contraindication; FMC, first medical contact; GPI, glycoprotein IIb/IIIa inhibitor; IV, intravenous; MI, myocardial infarction; NTG, nitroglycerin; PCI, percutaneous coronary intervention; SC, subcutaneous; SL, sublingual; UFH, unfractionated heparin.) *(Reproduced with permission from Rogers KC, de Denus S, Finks SW. Chapter 8. Acute Coronary Syndromes. In: Chisholm-Burns MA, Schwinghammer TL Wells BG, et al, eds. Pharmacotherapy: Principles and Practice. 4th ed. New York: McGraw-Hill Companies; 2016.)*

from the ED to the cardiac catheterization laboratory and undergoes coronary angiography with either balloon angioplasty or placement of a bare metal or drug-eluting intracoronary stent in the artery associated with the infarct. In order to meet the quality of care metric of less than 90 minutes from first medical contact to primary PCI, many transitions of care occur and care coordination between paramedics, ED staff, and cardiac catheterization is vital. Every minute delay results in additional myocardial cell damage that may be irreversible.

About 80% of patients with STEMI are treated with primary PCI; 11% are treated with fibrinolytics.[14,21] Results from a meta-analysis of trials comparing fibrinolysis with primary PCI indicate a lower mortality rate with primary PCI.[22] One reason for the superiority of primary PCI compared with fibrinolysis is that more than 90% of occluded infarct-related coronary arteries are opened with primary PCI compared with fewer than 60% of coronary arteries opened with currently available fibrinolytics.[2] In addition, intracranial hemorrhage (ICH) and major bleeding risks from primary PCI are lower than the risks of severe bleeding events following fibrinolysis. An invasive strategy of primary PCI is generally preferred in patients presenting to institutions with skilled interventional cardiologists and a catheterization laboratory immediately available, patients in cardiogenic shock, those with contraindications to fibrinolytics, and those with continuing symptoms 12 to 24 hours after symptom onset.[2]

Myocardial infarction performance measures are developed from practice guidelines and intended to permit the quality of patient care to be assessed, compared between institutions and ultimately,

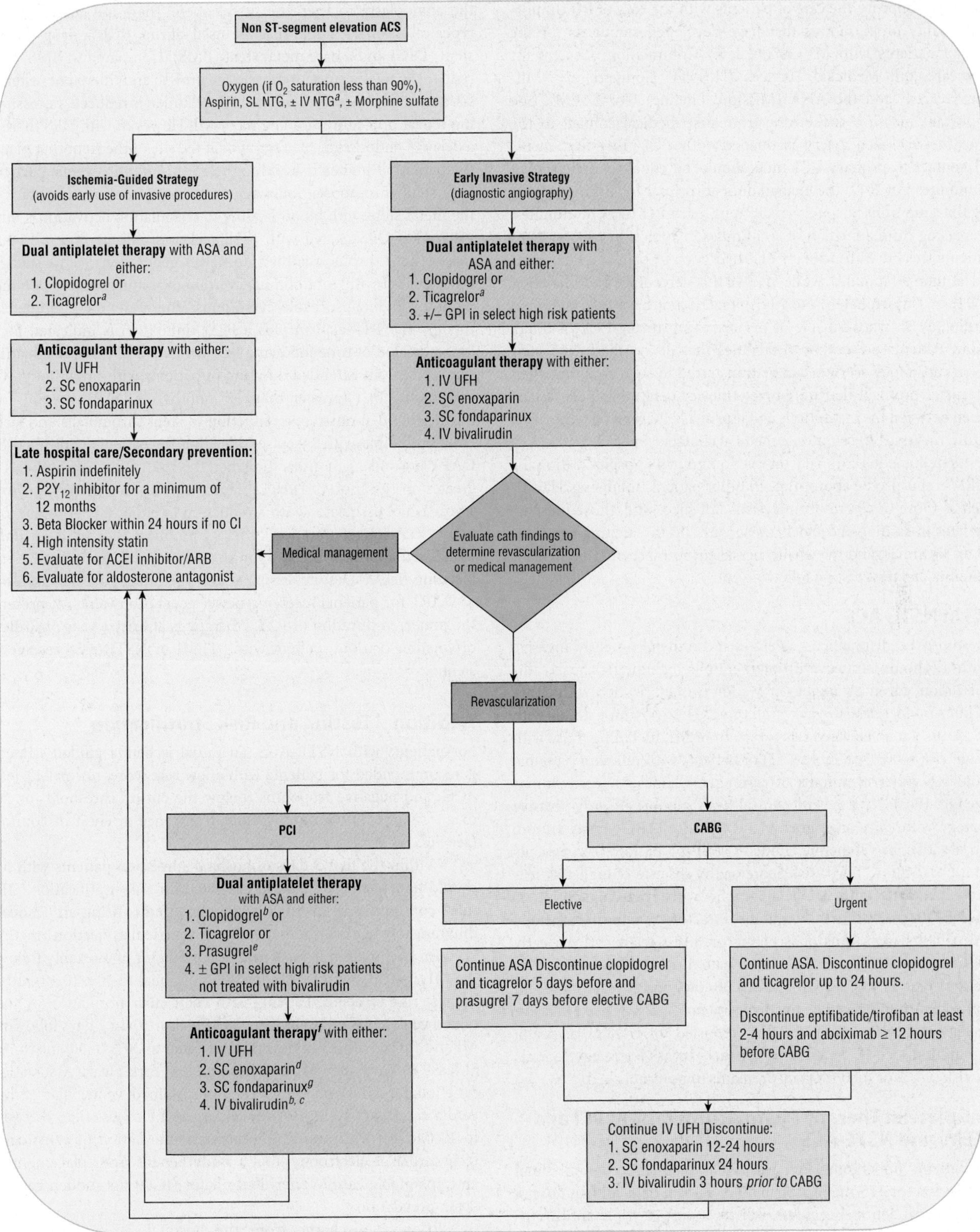

FIGURE 17-3 Initial pharmacotherapy for non–ST-segment elevation ACS. [a]For selected patients, see Table 17-2. [b]Preferred in patients at high risk for bleeding. [c]If pretreated with UFH, stop UFH infusion for 30 minutes prior to administration of bivalirudin bolus plus infusion. [d]May require IV supplemental dose of enoxaparin; see Table 17-2. [e]Do not use if prior history of stroke/transient ischemic attack (TIA), age older than 75 years, or body weight less than or equal to 60 kg. [f]Subcut enoxaparin or UFH can be continued at a lower dose for venous thromboembolism prophylaxis following PCI. [g]Requires an IV supplemental dose of UFH; see Table 17-2. (ACE, angiotensin-converting enzyme; ACS, acute coronary syndrome; ARB, angiotensin receptor blocker; CABG, coronary artery bypass graft; CAD, coronary artery disease; CHD, coronary heart disease; GP, glycoprotein; NTG, nitroglycerin; PCI, percutaneous coronary intervention; SC, subcutaneous; SL, sublingual; UFH, unfractionated heparin.) *(Reproduced with permission from Spinler SA, de Denus S. Acute coronary syndromes. In: Chisholm-Burns M, Wells BG, Schwinghammer TL, Malone PM, Kolesar JM, DiPiro JT, eds. Pharmacotherapy Principles and Practice. 3rd ed. New York: McGraw-Hill; 2013.)*

over time, improve the care of patients with the care of MI. Important quality organizations that have developed standards for the care of patients with MI are the Joint Commission, Centers for Medicare and Medicaid Services (Hospital Compare and Million Hearts), and the AHA (Mission: Lifeline). For STEMI, one important measure is the time from first medical contact to the time the occluded artery is opened with PCI. This first medical contact-to-primary PCI time should be equal to or less than 90 minutes.[2] In 2011, the median door-to-primary PCI time (meaning the time from hospital arrival to primary PCI) was 63 minutes, decreasing from a median of 96 minutes in 2005.[23] In 2005, 44% of patients treated with primary PCI had door-to-primary PCI times of less than 90 minutes, while in 2010 this percentage had increased to 94%.[23] Unfortunately, most hospitals do not have interventional cardiology services capable of performing primary PCI 24 hours a day. Patients presenting to facilities that do not have interventional cardiology services can be transferred to such facilities when a transfer protocol that minimizes transfer delays has been established between the institutions and if primary PCI can be performed within the first 120 minutes of medical contact.[2]

Percutaneous coronary intervention during hospitalization for STEMI may also be appropriate in other patients following STEMI, such as those in whom fibrinolysis is not successful, those presenting later in cardiogenic shock, those with life-threatening ventricular arrhythmias, and those with persistent rest ischemia or signs of ischemia on stress testing following MI.[2]

PCI in NSTE-ACS

The most recent practice guidelines recommend an early invasive (within 24 hours) strategy with interventions, including left heart catheterization, coronary angiography and revascularization with either PCI or *coronary artery bypass graft* (CABG) *surgery* for patients with NSTE-ACS at an elevated risk for death or MI, including those with a high risk score (see Table 17-1) or patients with refractory angina, acute HF, other symptoms of cardiogenic shock, or arrhythmias (see Fig. 17-3).[3,4] 5 Several clinical trials support an early invasive strategy with early angiography and PCI or CABG versus a more conservative or "ischemia guided" strategy in low-risk patients (those have a low TIMI Risk Score or the absence of high-risk features), whereby coronary angiography with revascularization is reserved for patients with symptoms refractory to pharmacotherapy and patients with signs of ischemia on stress testing.[4,24] An early invasive approach results in a lower rate of refractory angina over the first year as well as MI between 30 days and 5 years. A recent trial comparing immediate invasive strategy versus delayed invasive strategy in patients with NSTEMI reported lower rates of death, reinfarction, or MI.[24,25] Whether an early invasive strategy reduces the risk of CV or total mortality remains to be established.

Antiplatelet Therapy Pharmacotherapy in PCI and STEMI and NSTE-ACS

All patients undergoing PCI with ACS should receive an initial dose of 162- or 325-mg of aspirin followed by a daily aspirin dose of 81 mg/day indefinitely (unless aspirin is part of triple antithrombotic therapy [TT]—see Clinical Controversy 1) (Table 17-2).[2,4] A $P2Y_{12}$ inhibitor antiplatelet (clopidogrel, prasugrel, ticagrelor, or IV cangrelor) should be administered as early as possible concomitantly with aspirin and then an oral $P2Y_{12}$ agent should ideally be continued for at least 12 months following PCI (see Table 17-2).[2,4] Earlier discontinuation of the $P2Y^{12}$ inhibitor can be reasonable in patients at a high bleeding risk or with overt bleeding".[2,4,26] Either ticagrelor or prasugrel are preferred over clopidogrel secondary to improved efficacy with a reduction in the frequency of the composite endpoint of CV death, MI, or stroke.[3]

Stents are small, metal mesh tubes, which are inserted and expanded in the artery to prevent vessel closure during or following the angioplasty to keep the vessel open. There are currently two types of coronary stents that are used during PCI, a drug-eluting stent (DES) and a bare metal stent (BMS). Compared to BMS, DES reduce the rate of smooth muscle cell growth and thus stent restenosis, a gradual process whereby the stent lumen is reduced, necessitating repeat procedures for angina or MI. However, with DES there is a delay in endothelial cell regrowth at the site of the stent that places the patient at higher risk of long-term thrombotic events, particularly stent thrombosis, following PCI due to continued contact of the metal stent with blood leading to coagulation activation. Older generation DES coated with paclitaxel or sirolimus pose a higher risk of stent thrombosis than do newer generations stents such as those coated with zotarolimus, everolimus, biodegradable polymer biolimus or bioabsorbable everolimus. Therefore, dual antiplatelet therapy (DAPT—aspirin plus a $P2Y_{12}$ inhibitor) is indicated for a longer period of time following PCI with a DES.[26] Trials evaluating the need for an extended duration in patients with or without ACS undergoing PCI (greater than 12 months) of DAPT therapy following PCI demonstrate a reduction in stent thrombosis and ischemia endpoints with increased bleeding for patients continued on DAPT beyond 12 months.[27] Further, the risk of stent thrombosis is greater on cessation of DAPT.[27] However, continued DAPT beyond 1 year is not associated with a reduction in either CV or total mortality.[28,29] A longer duration of $P2Y_{12}$ inhibitor therapy is an individualized approach based upon the patient's risk for ischemic and bleeding risks.[29] Despite arising trials suggesting a shorter duration of DAPT for patients receiving newer generation stents, at present, the preferred duration of $P2Y_{12}$ therapy is at least 1 year regardless of whether or not a patient with STEMI or NSTE-ACS receives a stent.[2,4,26,30-32]

Additional Testing and Risk Stratification

For patients with NSTE-ACS, an initial ischemia guided strategy is recommended for patients with a low risk score, normal 12-lead ECG, and negative troponins (below the cut-off threshold for the diagnosis of MI) who are without recurrence of chest discomfort (see Fig. 17-3).[3]

Within the first 3 days of hospital admission patients with MI should have their LV function evaluated for risk stratification.[2] The most common way LV function is measured is using an echocardiogram to calculate the patient's left ventricular ejection fraction (LVEF). LV function is the single best predictor of mortality following MI. Patients with LVEFs less than or equal to 40% (0.40) are at highest risk of death. Patients with ventricular fibrillation or sustained ventricular tachycardia occurring more than 2 days following MI and those with LVEF less than or equal to 30% (0.30, measured at least 40 days after MI and have a New York Heart Association functional class I) or who have nonsustained ventricular tachycardia secondary to a prior MI and an LVEF of less than or equal to 40% (0.40) with inducible ventricular fibrillation or ventricular tachycardia at electrophysiology study benefit from placement of an implantable cardioverter-defibrillator (ICD) for sudden cardiac death prevention.[33]

Prior to discharge from the hospital, stress testing (see Fig. 17-3) is indicated in patients with NSTE-ACS where an initial ischemia guided strategy is selected and for patients with STEMI where coronary angiography was not performed and there has been no recurrent ischemia.[2,3] Following the stress test, patients deemed at higher risk should undergo left heart catheterization with coronary angiography and revascularization as indicated by the results.[3]

Early Pharmacotherapy for STEMI

Pharmacotherapy for early treatment of ACS is outlined in Fig. 17-2 and Table 17-2.[2-4] 6 According to the STEMI practice guidelines,

TABLE 17-2 Evidence-Based Pharmacotherapy for ST-Segment Elevation Myocardial Infarction and Non-ST-Segment Elevation Acute Coronary Syndrome[2-4,26]

Drug	Clinical Condition and Guideline Recommendations[a]	Contraindications[b]	Dose and Duration of Therapy
Aspirin	STEMI, class I recommendation for all patients. NSTE-ACS, class I recommendation for all patients.	Hypersensitivity, active bleeding, severe bleeding risk	160-325 mg orally once on hospital day 1. 81-162 mg once daily orally starting hospital day 2 and continued indefinitely in all patients. In STEMI, doses of up to 325 mg included in the guidelines, but a dose of 81 mg is preferred. In patients dual receiving dual antiplatelet therapy, a daily dose of 81 mg is recommended (Class I recommendation) Limit dose to <100 mg if using ticagrelor.
Clopidogrel	NSTE-ACS, class I recommendation added to aspirin. STEMI, class I recommendation added to aspirin. PCI in STE and NSTE-ACS, class I recommendation. In patients with aspirin allergy, class I recommendation.	Hypersensitivity, active bleeding, severe bleeding risk	300 mg-600 mg oral loading dose on hospital day 1 followed by a maintenance dose of 75 mg once daily starting on hospital day 2 in patients with NSTE-ACS. 300 mg oral loading dose followed by 75 mg orally daily in patients receiving a fibrinolytic or who do not receive reperfusion therapy with a STEMI, avoid loading dose in patients 75 years or older. 600 mg (class I recommendation) loading dose before or when PCI performed (unless within 24 hours of fibrinolytic therapy, a dose of 300 mg should be given). Discontinue at least 5 days before CABG surgery if bleeding risk outweighs benefit (class I recommendation). Administer indefinitely in patients with aspirin allergy (class I recommendation). Continue for at least 12 months (class I recommendation) and possibly beyond 12 months (class IIb recommendation) in patients with ACS managed with PCI/stent. In patients with NSTE-ACS treated medically, administer for up to 1 year (class I recommendation). In patients receiving a fibrinolytic or who do not receive reperfusion therapy, administer for at least 14 days (class I recommendation) and up to 1 year. In patients not at high-risk of bleeding and who have not add a bleeding complication, continuing dual antiplatelet therapy may be reasonable (class IIb recommendation). Genetic testing might be considered to identify patients at high risk of poor response (class IIb recommendation). In these patients, an alternative $P2Y_{12}$ inhibitor might be considered (class IIb recommendation). The routine use of genetic testing is not recommended (class III recommendation).
Prasugrel	PCI in STE and NSTE-ACS, added to aspirin, class I recommendation.	Active bleeding, prior stroke or TIA	Initiate in patients with known coronary artery anatomy only (so as to avoid use in patients needing CABG surgery; class I recommendation). Give no later than 1 hour after PCI. Patients who have history of prior stroke or TIA or are 75 years of age or more or weigh <60 kg (132 lb) have higher risk of bleeding and no added benefit compared with clopidogrel. 60 mg oral loading dose followed by 10 mg once daily for patients weighing 60 kg (132 lb) or more. Consider 5 mg once daily in patients weighing <60 kg (132 lb) (based on limited data). Discontinue at least 7 days prior to CABG surgery if bleeding risk outweighs benefit (class I recommendation). Continue for at least 12 months (class I recommendation) and possibly beyond 12 months (class IIb recommendation or treated with only medical therapy) in patients with ACS managed with PCI/stent.
Ticagrelor	PCI in STEMI and NSTE-ACS, added to aspirin, class I recommendation. Class IIa as preference over clopidogrel. Medically treated patients (without fibrinolytics or revascularization) STEMI and NSTE ACS added to aspirin, class I recommendation.	Active bleeding	180 mg (class I recommendation) oral loading dose in patients undergoing PCI or ischemia-guided management, followed by 90 mg twice daily for at least 12 months (class I recommendation) and possibly beyond 12 months (class IIb recommendation) in patients with ACS managed with PCI/stent. After 1 year, administer 60 mg twice daily. Current data are too limited to recommend use in patients with STEMI receiving fibrinolytics. Discontinue at least 5 days prior to CABG surgery if bleeding risk outweighs benefit (class I recommendation).
Cangrelor	PCI—adjunct in patients, not treated with oral $P2Y_{12}$ inhibitors or GPI. Newly FDA approved agent without guideline recommendations.	Active bleeding	30 mcg/kg IV bolus initiated prior to PCI followed by 4 mcg/kg/min IV infusion for duration of PCI or 2 hours, whichever is longer. To maintain platelet inhibition after infusion, initiate oral $P2Y_{12}$ agent as follows: ticagrelor 180 mg at any time during or immediately after infusion; clopidogrel 600 mg or prasugrel 60 mg immediately after discontinuation of infusion. Do not administer clopidogrel or prasugrel during infusion of cangrelor.

(*Continued*)

TABLE 17-2 Evidence-Based Pharmacotherapy for ST-Segment Elevation Myocardial Infarction and Non-ST-Segment Elevation Acute Coronary Syndrome[2-4] (*Continued*)

Drug	Clinical Condition and Guideline Recommendations[a]	Contraindications[b]	Dose and Duration of Therapy
Unfractionated heparin	STEMI, class I recommendation in patients undergoing PCI and for those patients treated with fibrinolytics; NSTE-ACS, class I recommendation in combination with antiplatelet therapy for ischemia-guided or early invasive approach PCI, class I recommendation (NSTE-ACS and STEMI).	Active bleeding, history of heparin-induced thrombocytopenia, severe bleeding risk, recent stroke	For STEMI with fibrinolytics, administer 60 Units/kg IV bolus (maximum 4,000 Units) heparin followed by a constant IV infusion at 12 Units/kg/h (maximum 1000 Units/h). For STEMI primary PCI, administer 50-70 Units/kg IV bolus if a GP IIb/IIIa inhibitor planned; 70-100 Units/kg IV bolus if no GP IIb/IIIa inhibitor planned and supplement with IV bolus doses to maintain target ACT. For NSTE-ACS, administer 60 Units/kg IV bolus (maximum 4,000 Units) followed by a constant IV infusion at 12 Units/kg/h (maximum 1,000 Units/h). Titrated to maintain an aPTT of 1.5-2.0 times control (approximately 50-70 seconds) for STEMI with fibrinolytics and for NSTE-ACS. Titrated to ACT of 250-350 seconds for primary PCI without a GP IIb/IIIa inhibitor and 200-250 seconds in patients given a concomitant GP IIb/IIIa inhibitor. The first aPTT should be measured at 4-6 hours for NSTE-ACS and STE ACS in patients not treated with fibrinolytics or undergoing primary PCI. The first aPTT should be measured at 3 hours in patients with STE ACS who are treated with fibrinolytics. Continue for 48 hours or until the end of PCI.
Enoxaparin	STEMI class I recommendation in patients receiving fibrinolytics and class IIa for patients not undergoing reperfusion therapy. NSTE-ACS, class I recommendation in combination with aspirin for conservative or invasive approach. For PCI, class IIa recommendation as an alternative to UFH in patients with NSTE-ACS. For primary PCI in STEMI, class IIb recommendation as an alternative to UFH.	Active bleeding, history of heparin-induced thrombocytopenia, severe bleeding risk, recent stroke, avoid enoxaparin if CrCl <15 mL/min (<0.25 mL/s), avoid if CABG surgery planned	Enoxaparin 1 mg/kg SC every 12 hours for patients with NSTE-ACS (CrCl ≥ to 30 mL/min [≥ to 0.50 mL/s]). Enoxaparin 1 mg/kg SC every 24 hours (CrCl 15-29 mL/min [0.25-0.49 mL/s]) for NSTE or STEMI. For all patients undergoing PCI following initiation of SC enoxaparin for NSTE-ACS, a supplemental 0.3 mg/kg IV dose of enoxaparin should be administered at the time of PCI if the last dose of SC enoxaparin was given 8-12 hours prior to PCI or who received less than two therapeutic SC doses. For patients with STEMI receiving fibrinolytics: • Age <75 years: Administer enoxaparin 30 mg IV bolus followed immediately by 1 mg/kg. • SC every 12 hours (first two doses administer maximum of 100 mg for patients weighing more than 100 kg). • Age ≥75 years: Administer enoxaparin 0.75 mg/kg SC every 12 hours (first two doses administer maximum of 75 mg for patients weighing more than 75 kg). Continue throughout hospitalization or up to 8 days for STEMI. Continue for 24-48 hours for NSTE-ACS or until the end of PCI for NSTEMI. Stop at least 12-24 hours after CABG surgery.
Bivalirudin	NSTE-ACS class I recommendation for invasive strategy. PCI in STEMI (class I recommendation).	Active bleeding, severe bleeding risk	For NSTE-ACS, administer 0.1 mg/kg IV bolus followed by 0.25 mg/kg/h infusion. For PCI in NSTE-ACS, administer a second bolus of 0.5 mg/kg IV and increase infusion rate to 1.75 mg/kg/h. For PCI in STEMI, administer 0.75 mg/kg IV bolus followed by 1.75 mg/kg/h infusion. If prior UFH given, discontinue UFH and wait 30 minutes before initiating bivalirudin. Dosage adjustment for severe renal failure and HD. Discontinue at end of PCI or continue at 0.25 mg/kg/h if prolonged anticoagulation necessary. Lower bleeding rates are mitigated when administered with a GPI inhibitor. Clopidogrel should be administered at least 6 hours before if a GPI inhibitor is not used. Discontinue at least 3 hours prior to CABG surgery.
Fondaparinux	STEMI class I recommendation receiving fibrinolytics and IIa for patients not undergoing reperfusion therapy. NSTE-ACS class I recommendation for invasive or conservative approach. Class III as sole agent in PCI.	Active bleeding, severe bleeding risk, SCr ≥3.0 mg/dL (≥265 μmol/L) or CrCl <30 mL/min (<0.50 mL/s)	For STEMI, 2.5 mg IV bolus followed by 2.5 mg SC once daily starting on hospital day 2. For NSTE-ACS, 2.5 mg SC once daily. Continue until hospital discharge or up to 8 days. For PCI, give additional 85 Units/kg IV UFH without and 60 Units/kg IV with GP IIb/IIIa inhibitor. Discontinue at least 24 hours prior to CABG surgery.

Fibrinolytic therapy	STEMI, class I recommendation for patients presenting within 12 hours following the onset of symptoms, class IIa in patients presenting between 12 and 24 hours following the onset of symptoms with continuing signs of ischemia. NSTE-ACS, class III recommendation.	Any prior intracranial hemorrhage, known structural cerebrovascular lesions, such as an arterial venous malformation, known intracranial malignant neoplasm, ischemic stroke within 3 months, active bleeding (excluding menses), significant closed head or facial trauma within 3 months	Streptokinase: 1.5 MU IV over 60 minutes. Alteplase: 15 mg IV bolus followed by 0.75 mg/kg IV over 30 minutes (maximum 50 mg) followed by 0.5 mg/kg (maximum 35 mg) over 60 minutes (maximum dose 100 mg). Reteplase: 10 Units IV × 2, 30 minutes apart. Tenecteplase: • <60 kg (<132 lb), 30 mg IV bolus • 60-69.9 kg (132-153 lb), 35 mg IV bolus • 70-80 kg (154-176 lb), 40 mg IV bolus
Glycoprotein IIb/IIIa receptor inhibitors (GPI)	NSTE-ACS PCI, class I recommendation for abciximab, high-bolus dose tirofiban or double-bolus eptifibatide at the time of PCI in high-risk patients already receiving aspirin and not adequately pretreated with a $P2Y_{12}$ inhibitor and not receiving bivalirudin as the anticoagulant; class IIa at the time of PCI for high-risk patients already receiving aspirin and pretreated with a $P2Y_{12}$ inhibitor; class IIb for upstream use in high-risk patients already receiving aspirin and pretreated with a $P2Y_{12}$ inhibitor and not receiving bivalirudin as the anticoagulant; class I for upstream use in addition to aspirin without $P2Y_{12}$ inhibitor pretreatment for moderate- to high-risk patients. NSTE-ACS for patients not undergoing PCI (ischemia guided management), class IIb recommendation (eptifibatide or tirofiban). STEMI primary PCI, class IIa recommendation for abciximab, high-bolus dose tirofiban or double-bolus eptifibatide.	Active bleeding, thrombocytopenia, prior stroke, renal dialysis (eptifibatide)	**Drug** / **Dose** / **Dosing adjustment for CKD** Abciximab / 0.25 mg/kg IV bolus followed by 0.125 mcg/kg/min(maximum 10 mcg/min) for 12 hours / None Eptifibatide / 180 mcg/kg IV bolus × 2, 10 minutes apart with an infusion of 2 mcg/kg/min for 18-24 hours after PCI / Reduce maintenance infusion to 1 mcg/kg/min for CrCl < 50 mL/min (<0.83 mL/s); contraindicated if patient dependent on dialysis. Patients weighing 121 kg (266 lb) or more should receive a maximum infusion rate of 22.6 mg per bolus and a maximum rate of 15 mg/h Tirofiban / 25mcg/kg IV bolus followed by an infusion of 0.15 mcg/kg/min for up to 18 hours / Reduce maintenance infusion to 0.075 mcg/kg/min for patients with CrCl ≤ 60 mL/min (<0.05 mL/s)
Nitroglycerin	STEMI and NSTE-ACS, class I recommendation in patients with ongoing ischemic discomfort, control of hypertension or management of HF.	Hypotension, sildenafil or vardenafil within 24 hours or tadalafil within 48 hours	0.4 mg SL, repeated every 5 minutes × 3 doses then assess need for IV infusion. 5-10 mcg/min IV infusion titrated up to 75-100 mcg/min until relief of symptoms or limiting side effects (headache) with a systolic blood pressure <90 mm Hg or more than 30% below starting mean arterial pressure levels if significant hypertension is present. Topical patches or oral nitrates are acceptable alternatives for patients without ongoing or refractory symptoms. Discontinue IV infusion after 24-48 hours.
β-Blockers[c]	STEMI and NSTE-ACS, class I recommendation for oral β-blockers in all patients without contraindications in the first 24 hours, class IIa for IV β-blockers STEMI patients with hypertension or those with ongoing ischemia. Class III for IV β-blockers in patients with risk factors for shock.	PR interval >0.24 seconds, second-degree or third-degree atrioventricular heart block, heart rate <60 beats/min, systolic blood pressure <90 mm Hg, shock, left ventricular failure with decompensated HF, severe reactive airway disease	Metoprolol 5 mg slow IV push (over 1-2 minutes), repeated every 5 minutes for a total of 15 mg followed in 1-2 hours by 25-50 mg orally every 6 hours; if a very conservative regimen is desired, initial doses can be reduced to 1-2 mg. Propranolol 0.5-1 mg IV dose followed in 1-2 hours by 40-80 mg orally every 6-8 hours. Atenolol 5 mg IV dose followed in 5 minutes by a second 5 mg IV dose for a total of 10 mg followed in 1-2 hours by 50-100 mg orally once daily. Alternatively, initial IV therapy can be omitted and treatment started with oral dosing. For dosing of carvedilol, metoprolol succinate and bisoprolol in patients with systolic HF, please refer to Chapter X. Continue oral β-blocker for 3 years and possibly indefinitely.
Calcium channel blockers	NSTE-ACS class I recommendation for patients with ongoing ischemia who are already taking adequate doses of nitrates and β-blockers or in patients with contraindications to or intolerance to β-blockers (diltiazem or verapamil preferred calcium channel blockers during initial presentation if EF > 40%). NSTE-ACS, class IIb recommendation for diltiazem for patients with AMI.	Pulmonary edema, evidence of left ventricular dysfunction, systolic blood pressure < 100 mm Hg, PR segment to >0.24 seconds second- or third-degree atrioventricular heart block for verapamil or diltiazem, pulse rate <60 beats/min for diltiazem or verapamil	Diltiazem 120-360 mg sustained release orally once daily. Verapamil 180-480 mg sustained release orally once daily. Amlodipine 5-10 mg orally once daily. Continue as indicated to manage angina, hypertension, or arrhythmias.

(*Continued*)

TABLE 17-2 Evidence-Based Pharmacotherapy for ST-Segment Elevation Myocardial Infarction and Non-ST-Segment Elevation Acute Coronary Syndrome[2-4] (*Continued*)

Drug	Clinical Condition and Guideline Recommendations[a]	Contraindications[b]	Dose and Duration of Therapy		
ACE inhibitors	NSTE-ACS and STEMI, class I recommendation for patients with HF left ventricular dysfunction and EF <40%, type 2 diabetes mellitus or CKD in the absence of contraindications. Consider in all patients with CAD (class I recommendation, class IIa in low-risk patients). Indicated indefinitely for all patients with EF <40% (class I recommendation).	Systolic blood pressure <100 mm Hg, history of intolerance to an ACE inhibitor, bilateral renal artery stenosis, serum potassium more than 5.5 mEq/L (>5.5 mmol/L), acute renal failure, pregnancy	**Drug**	**Initial Dose (mg)**	**Target Dose (mg)**
			Captopril	6.25-12.5	50 twice daily orally to 50 three times daily
			Enalapril	2.5-5.0	10 twice daily orally
			Lisinopril	2.5-5.0	10-20 once daily orally
			Ramipril	1.25-2.5	5 twice daily or 10 once daily orally
			Trandolapril	1.0	4 once daily orally
Angiotensin receptor blockers	NSTEMI and STEMI, class I recommendation in patients with HF or left ventricular EF <40% and intolerant of an ACE inhibitor, class IIa recommendation in patients with clinical signs of HF or EF <40% and no documentation of ACE inhibitor intolerance. Class I in other ACE inhibitor–intolerant patients with hypertension.	Systolic blood pressure <100 mm Hg, bilateral renal artery stenosis, serum potassium more than 5.5 mEq/L (>5.5 mmol/L), acute renal failure, pregnancy	**Drug**	**Initial Dose (mg)**	**Target Dose (mg)**
			Candesartan	4-8	32 once daily orally
			Valsartan	40	160 twice daily orally
			Losartan	12.5-25	150 daily
			Continue indefinitely		
Aldosterone antagonists	NSTEMI and STEMI class I recommendation in patients with EF <40% and either diabetes mellitus or HF who are already receiving an ACE inhibitor and *β*-blocker.	Hypotension, hyperkalemia, serum potassium >5.0 mEq/L (>5 mmol/L), SCr >2.5 mg/dL (221 μmol/L) for men and >2.0 mg/dL (177 μmol/L) for women and/or CrCl <30 mL/min (<0.50 mL/s)	**Drug**	**Initial Dose (mg)**	**Target Dose (mg)**
			Eplerenone	25	50 once daily orally
			Spironolactone	12.5	25-50 once daily orally
			Continue indefinitely		
Morphine sulfate	STEMI and NSTE-ACS (class IIb) recommendation for patients whose chest pain persists despite treatment with maximally tolerated anti-anginal drugs.	Hypotension, respiratory depression, confusion, obtundation	1-5 mg IV bolus dose May be repeated every 5-30 minutes as needed to relieve symptoms and maintain patient comfort		
Statins	NSTE-ACS and STEMI class I recommendation to initiate or continue high-intensity statin therapy during early hospital care. Consider moderate-intensity statin for patients >75.	Caution with use of fibrate and statin-specific drug interactions	High Intensity: Atorvastatin 40-80 mg daily; Rosuvastatin 20-40 mg daily Moderate Intensity: Atorvastatin 10-20 mg daily; Fluvastatin 80mg daily, Lovastatin 40 mg daily, Pitavastatin 2-4 mg daily, Pravastatin 40-80 mg daily, Rosuvastatin 5-10 mg daily, Simvastatin 20-40 mg daily.		

[a]Class I recommendations are conditions for which there is evidence and/or general agreement that a given procedure or treatment is useful and effective.

Class II recommendations are those conditions for which there is conflicting evidence and/or divergence of opinion about the usefulness/efficacy of a procedure or treatment. For Class IIa recommendations, the weight of the evidence/opinion is in favor of usefulness/efficacy. Class IIb recommendations are those for which usefulness/efficacy is less well established by evidence/opinion. Class III recommendations are those where the procedure or treatment is not useful and may be harmful.

[b]Allergy or prior intolerance contraindication for all categories of drugs listed in this chart.

[c]Choice of the specific agent is not as important as ensuring that appropriate candidates receive this therapy. If there are concerns about patient intolerance due to existing pulmonary disease, especially asthma, selection should favor a short-acting agent, such as metoprolol or the ultrashort-acting agent, esmolol. Mild wheezing or a history of chronic obstructive pulmonary disease should prompt a trial of a short-acting agent at a reduced dose (eg, 2.5 mg IV metoprolol, 12.5 mg oral metoprolol, or 25 mcg/kg/min esmolol as initial doses) rather than complete avoidance of *β*-blocker therapy.

ACE, angiotensin-converting enzyme inhibitor; ACS, acute coronary syndrome; ACT, activated clotting time; AMI, acute myocardial infarction; aPTT, activated partial thromboplastin time; CABG, coronary artery bypass graft; CAD, coronary artery disease; CKD, chronic kidney disease; CrCl, Creatinine clearance; ECG, electrocardiogram; EF, ejection fraction; GPI, glycoprotein IIb/IIIa inhibitor; HD, hemodialysis; HF, heart failure; IV, intravenous; MI, myocardial infarction; NSTEMI, non-ST-segment elevation myocardial infarction; PCI, percutaneous coronary intervention; SC, subcutaneous, SCAI, Society for Cardiac Angiography and Interventions; SCr, serum creatinine; SL, sublingual; STEMI, ST-segment elevation myocardial infarction; TIA, transient ischemic attack; UFH, unfractionated heparin.

in addition to reperfusion therapy, other early pharmacotherapy that all patients with STEMI and without contraindications should receive within the first day of hospitalization, and preferably in the ED, are intranasal oxygen (if oxygen saturation is low), sublingual (SL) nitroglycerin (NTG), aspirin, a $P2Y_{12}$ inhibitor (clopidogrel, prasugrel, or ticagrelor depending on reperfusion strategy), and anticoagulation with bivalirudin, unfractionated heparin (UFH), enoxaparin, or fondaparinux (agent dependent on reperfusion strategy; see Table 17-2). A GPI may be administered with UFH for patients undergoing primary PCI. Intravenous (IV) NTG should be given in selected patients (see Table 17-2). The use of IV β-blockers is reasonable at the time of presentation for patients with hypertension (HTN) and ongoing ischemia. Oral β-blockers are preferred to IV and should be initiated within the first day in patients without cardiogenic shock or other contraindications.[2-4] Morphine is administered to patients with refractory angina as an analgesic and a venodilator that lowers preload. However, morphine has been shown to slow the absorption of oral antiplatelet agents due to decreased gastric motility and its role in the contemporary management of ACS and contemporary trials suggest limiting morphine administration where possible.[34,35] These anti-ischemic agents are administered early while the patient is still in the ED. An ACE inhibitor is recommended to be administered within the first 24 hours in patients with STEMI who have either an anterior wall MI or an LVEF less than or equal to 40% (0.40) and no contraindications. Dosing and contraindications for SL and IV NTG, aspirin, clopidogrel, β-blockers, ACE inhibitors, anticoagulants, and fibrinolytics are described in Table 17-2.[2-4]

Fibrinolytic Therapy

Administration of a fibrinolytic agent is indicated in patients with STEMI who present within 12 hours of the onset of chest discomfort to a hospital not capable of primary PCI, have at least a 1 mm STE in two or more contiguous ECG leads, have no absolute contraindications to fibrinolytic therapy (Table 17-3) and are not able to be transferred and undergo primary PCI within 120 minutes of medical contact.[2] The mortality benefit of fibrinolysis is highest with early administration and diminishes after 12 hours.[2] The use of fibrinolytics between 12 and 24 hours after symptom onset should be limited to patients with ongoing ischemia. Fibrinolytic therapy is preferred over primary PCI where there is no cardiac catheterization laboratory or there would be a delay in "door-to-primary PCI" of more than 90 minutes (of first medical contact) within the institution or 120 minutes (of first medical contact) if the patient is transferred. Indications and contraindications for fibrinolysis are listed in Table 17-3.[2] It is not necessary to obtain the troponin result before initiating fibrinolytic therapy. Because administration of fibrinolytics results in clot lysis, patients or those who are at high risk of major bleeding (including a history of ICH) presenting with an absolute contraindication should not receive fibrinolytic therapy, and should be transferred to a hospital capable of performing PCI. In patients who have a contraindication to fibrinolytics and PCI, or who do not have access to a facility that can perform PCI, treatment with an anticoagulant (other than UFH) for up to 8 days can be administered.

The percentage of eligible patients who receive reperfusion therapy fibrinolytic therapy is a quality performance measure of care in patients with MI.[36] The primary reason for lack of reperfusion therapy is that most patients present more than 12 hours after the time of symptom onset. The door-to-needle time, the time from hospital presentation to start of fibrinolytic therapy, is another quality performance measure of timely and effective care. The guidelines recommend a door-to-needle time of less than 30 minutes from the time of hospital presentation until start of fibrinolytic therapy.[2] The median administration time in the United States in 2006 was 29 minutes, with only 50% of patients meeting the quality performance target of less than 30 minutes.[37] In the past 10 years, there has been little improvement in this quality measure with only 59% of patients receiving fibrinolytic reperfusion therapy having a door-to-needle time of less than 30 minutes in 2015. All hospitals should have protocols addressing fibrinolysis eligibility, dosing, and monitoring.[36]

A fibrin-specific agent, such as alteplase, reteplase, or tenecteplase, is preferred over a non–fibrin-specific agent such as streptokinase.[2] Fibrin-specific fibrinolytics open a greater percentage of infarcted arteries. Two trials compared alteplase with reteplase and alteplase with tenecteplase and found similar mortality between agents.[38,39] Therefore, alteplase, reteplase, and tenecteplase are acceptable as first-line agents. ICH and major bleeding are the most serious side effects of fibrinolytic agents. The risk of ICH is higher with fibrin-specific agents than with streptokinase.[2] However, the risk of systemic bleeding other than ICH is higher with streptokinase than with other more fibrin-specific agents and was higher with alteplase versus tenecteplase in one study.[2,38-40]

TABLE 17-3 Indications and Contraindications to Fibrinolytic Therapy for Management of ST-Segment Elevation Myocardial Infarction[2]

Indications

1. Ischemic chest discomfort at least 20 minutes in duration but 12 hours or less since symptom onset **and**

ST-segment elevation of at least two contiguous leads of ≥2 mm in men and ≥1.5 mm in women in leads V_2-V_3 and/or of ≥1 mm in other leads, or new or presumed new left bundle-branch block

2. Ongoing ischemic chest discomfort at least 20 minutes in duration 12-24 hours since symptom onset **and**

ST-segment elevation of at least 1 mm in height in two or more contiguous leads

Absolute Contraindications

- Active internal bleeding (not including menses)
- Previous intracranial hemorrhage at any time; ischemic stroke within 3 months (except acute ischemic stroke within 4.5 hours)
- Known intracranial neoplasm
- Known structural cerebral vascular lesion (eg, arteriovenous malformation)
- Suspected aortic dissection
- Significant closed head or facial trauma within 3 months
- Intracranial or intraspinal surgery within 2 months
- Severe uncontrolled hypertension (unresponsive to emergency therapy)
- For streptokinase, prior treatment within the previous 6 months

Aspirin

Aspirin is the preferred antiplatelet agent in the treatment of choice in all subsets of ACS.[2-4] Aspirin administration within 24 hours before or after hospital arrival to all patients without contraindications is recommended. The antiplatelet effects of aspirin are mediated by inhibiting the synthesis of TXA_2 through an irreversible inhibition of platelet cyclooxygenase-1. In patients undergoing PCI, aspirin prevents acute thrombotic occlusion during the procedure. In patients receiving fibrinolytics, aspirin reduces mortality, and its effects are additive to fibrinolysis alone.[2,4] Additionally, in patients undergoing PCI, aspirin, in addition to a $P2Y_{12}$ inhibitor, reduces the risk of stent thrombosis.[4]

In patients experiencing an ACS, an initial dose equal to or greater than 160 mg non-enteric aspirin is necessary to achieve a rapid platelet inhibition.[3] Current guidelines for STEMI recommend an initial aspirin dose of 162 to 325 mg (see Table 17-2).[2] This first dose can be chewed in order to achieve high blood concentrations and platelet inhibition rapidly. Preferably, patients undergoing PCI not previously taking aspirin should receive 325 mg non–enteric-coated aspirin.[4] Current data suggest that although an initial dose of 162 to 325 mg is required, long-term therapy with doses of 75 to 150 mg daily is as effective as higher doses, and therefore a daily maintenance dose of 75 to 162 mg is recommended in most patients to inhibit the 10% of the total platelet pool that is regenerated daily.[41] Most recent guidelines recommend a dose of 81 mg in patients receiving dual antiplatelet therapy.[26] In a large (n = 25,086) randomized trial, high-dose aspirin, 300 to 325 mg daily, had similar frequency of CV death, MI, or stroke as well as major bleeding compared with low-dose aspirin in the first 30 days following ACS presentation.[42,43] Minor bleeding and GI bleeding were less frequent with low-dose aspirin. In this trial, patients undergoing PCI during hospitalization had a lower frequency of death, MI, or stroke, but major bleeding was increased with high-dose aspirin.[44] Post-hoc analysis from the Harmonizing Outcomes with Revascularization and Stents in Acute Myocardial Infarction (HORIZONS-AMI) trial compared outcomes in patients treated with aspirin doses of less than or equal to 200 mg with doses of greater than 200 mg daily and found that higher doses were a predictor of major bleeding but demonstrated similar 3-year risk of CV events.[45] In the Study of Platelet Inhibition and Patient Outcomes (PLATO), a randomized, double-blind clinical trial comparing ticagrelor with clopidogrel in patients receiving aspirin, a post-hoc analysis suggested that maintenance doses of aspirin above 100 mg daily reduced the effectiveness of ticagrelor.[44] Because of increased bleeding risk in patients receiving aspirin plus a $P2Y_{12}$ inhibitor compared with aspirin alone, low-dose aspirin (81 mg daily) is preferred following PCI.[4,46] Low-dose aspirin should be continued indefinitely.[46]

Nonsteroidal anti-inflammatory agents other than aspirin, as well as cyclooxygenase-2 (COX-2) selective anti-inflammatory agents are contraindicated in STEMI and should be discontinued at the time of STEMI secondary to increased risk of death, reinfarction, HF, and myocardial rupture.[2]

The most frequent side effects of aspirin are dyspepsia and nausea. Patients should be counseled about the risk of bleeding, especially GI bleeding, with aspirin.

Platelet $P2Y_{12}$ Inhibitors

Clopidogrel, prasugrel, and ticagrelor are oral agents that block a subtype of the ADP receptor, the $P2Y_{12}$ receptor, on platelets, preventing the binding of ADP to the receptor and subsequent expression of platelet GP IIb/IIIa receptors, reducing platelet activation and aggregation. Both clopidogrel and prasugrel are thienopyridines and prodrugs that are converted to an active metabolite by a variety of cytochrome P450 (CYP) isoenzymes (Table 17-4).[47]

Both of these agents bind irreversibly to $P2Y_{12}$ receptor. Ticagrelor, which is not a thienopyridine, is a reversible, noncompetitive $P2Y_{12}$ receptor inhibitor. Ticagrelor's parent compound has antiplatelet effects and is also metabolized primarily by CYP3A to an active metabolite producing its antiplatelet effects.

A newer agent, cangrelor is an intravenous $P2Y_{12}$ inhibitor recently approved as an adjunct to PCI in patients not receiving prior oral $P2Y_{12}$ inhibitors or planned GPIs. Cangrelor is indicated to reduce periprocedural MI, repeat revascularization and stent thrombosis in patients undergoing PCI. In a randomized, double-blind study comparing cangrelor to clopidogrel in patients undergoing PCI (42% of patients with ACS), cangrelor reduced the rate of periprocedural complications of PCI without a statistically significant difference in risk of major bleeding.[48] At this time, there are no US guideline recommendations describing the role of cangrelor in ACS.

Both prasugrel and ticagrelor are more potent ADP inhibitors than clopidogrel. Prasugrel has the fewest significant drug–drug interactions of the oral $P2Y_{12}$ inhibitors. The production of clopidogrel's active metabolite and consequently its antiplatelet effect is reduced by moderate and strong inhibitors of CYP2C19, while ticagrelor's concentration is reduced by strong inhibitors of CYP3A. Labeled drug interactions are described in Table 17-4. A more detailed discussion of the interaction between clopidogrel and proton pump inhibitors may be found in Chapter 16. Both clopidogrel and prasugrel interact with cangrelor and cannot be administered until the end of the infusion as the patient would not have any antiplatelet effect of the oral agent until after the next administered dose. This does not appear to be the case with ticagrelor and it can be administered at any time during the active infusion of cangrelor.

Genetic variations in the gene coding for *CYP2C19* significantly modulate the antiplatelet effects of clopidogrel. Specifically, carriers of reduced-function allele (ie, *2 or *3) are not able to convert clopidogrel to its active metabolite in comparison to carriers of the wild-type allele (*1). This results in decreased antiplatelet effects, as well as higher rates of CV events, especially stent thrombosis and MI around the time of PCI.[49,50] Prasugrel and ticagrelor efficacy are not associated with *CYP2C19* genotype.[51] Hence, either ticagrelor or prasugrel are preferred in either intermediate metabolizers (*1/*2, *1/*3, *2/*17) or poor metabolizers (*2/*2, *2/*3, *3/*3) of *CYP2C19* reduced-function alleles if there is no contraindication.[52] Nevertheless, in the absence of a large randomized trial demonstrating the benefit of such genotype-based approach, the most recent practice guidelines have not endorsed routine genotyping to guide the prescription of $P2Y_{12}$ inhibitors.[2-4] Ongoing clinical trials should clarify the benefits of a genotype-guided use of these agents.

Administration of a $P2Y_{12}$ receptor inhibitor, in addition to aspirin, is recommended for all patients with STEMI.[2,26] For patients undergoing primary PCI, clopidogrel, prasugrel, ticagrelor, or IV cangrelor in addition to aspirin, should be administered to prevent subacute stent thrombosis and longer-term CV events (see Table 17-2).[2,4] Although not FDA approved, a clopidogrel loading dose of 600 mg is recommended over administration of 300 mg for patients undergoing PCI.[4] A systematic review and meta-analysis of randomized and nonrandomized trials in more than 25,000 patients demonstrated a reduction in CV ischemic events with a loading dose of 600 mg compared with 300 mg in patients undergoing PCI.[53] Although a modest benefit of using a 7-day course of clopidogrel 150 mg compared to 75 mg daily has been suggested, it is also associated with a higher risk of major bleeding. Thus, routine use of such dosing is not recommended in current practice guidelines.[2-4]

In the most recent PCI practice guidelines, no preference is given for one oral agent over the other.[4] Nevertheless, clinical trials comparing these agents have highlighted distinct clinical differences between these antiplatelet agents. Based on these evidences, the most recent NSTE-ACS guidelines nonetheless favor ticagrelor or prasugrel in selected patients and this will be discussed in a later section.[3]

A large randomized, double-blind study demonstrated that, compared with clopidogrel, the addition of prasugrel to aspirin for patients undergoing PCI in the setting of STEMI or NSTE-ACS significantly reduced risk of CV death or MI by 19% (9.9% vs 12.1%), as well as MI and stent thrombosis, but increased the risk of major bleeding (not ICH) by 32% (2.4% vs 1.8%).[54] Patients with a history of prior stroke or transient ischemic attack (TIA) had an increased risk of ICH and no net clinical benefit from prasugrel, therefore stroke or TIA is a contraindication to prasugrel.[54] Patients older than 75 years and those weighing less than 60 kg (132 lb) are at increased risk of bleeding with prasugrel compared with clopidogrel.[47] Two subgroups of patients do not have an increased bleeding risk with prasugrel compared with clopidogrel and have even greater benefit, namely, patients undergoing primary PCI for STEMI and patients with a history of diabetes mellitus (DM).[55,56]

Platelet Inhibition and Patient Outcomes compared ticagrelor with clopidogrel in patients receiving aspirin and presenting with either STEMI or NSTE-ACS and undergoing an intended interventional management strategy with PCI or conservative noninterventional management strategy with medical therapy alone. In this trial, ticagrelor significantly reduced the rate of the CV death, MI, stroke, and stent thrombosis compared with clopidogrel.[57] Although no increase in study-defined major bleeding was noted with ticagrelor, the frequency of non-CABG major bleeding was increased compared

TABLE 17-4 Clinical Considerations When Choosing a $P2Y_{12}$ Receptor Inhibitor[2-4,26,64,66,67,69]

	Clopidogrel	Prasugrel	Ticagrelor	Cangrelor
Pharmacologic class	Thienopyridine	Thienopyridine	Cyclopentyl triazolopyrimidine	Stabilized ATP analog
ADP receptor binding	Irreversible	Irreversible	Reversible	Reversible
Pharmacokinetics	Prodrug Converted twice to active metabolite primarily through CYP2C19	Prodrug Converted to active metabolite through CYP 3A4 and 2B6	Active moiety Converted to active metabolite through CYP 3A4/5	Active drug Independent of hepatic function; rapidly dephosphorylzed to inactive metabolite
	Elimination half-life of active metabolite is approximately 30 minutes after a 75-mg dose	Median elimination half-life of the active metabolite approximately 7.4 hours	Median elimination half-life of the parent compound is approximately 7 hours and active metabolite approximately 9 hours	Plasma half-life of 5-10 minutes; elimination half-life of 3-6 minutes
	Excretion is 50% urinary and 46% fecal	Excretion is primarily urinary (approximately 70%); fecal excretion <30%	Excretion is primarily metabolism (84%); fecal excretion 58%, urinary excretion (26%)	Excretion is 58% renal and 35% fecal (presumed biliary)
	No dose adjustment necessary in CKD	Not recommended when eGFR <15 mL/min/1.73 m^2	Not recommended when eGFR < 15 mL/min/1.73 m^2	No dose adjustment necessary in CKD
Dosing	300-600 mg Loading dose; 75 mg daily	60 mg loading dose; 10 mg daily	180 mg loading dose; 90 mg twice daily for 1 year, 60 mg twice daily thereafter	30 mcg/kg bolus; 4 mcg/kg/min IV infusion continued for at least 2 hours or the duration of PCI, whichever is longer
Onset of loading dose effect	Peak platelet inhibition occurs within 2 hours after 600 mg load and 6 hours after oral 300 mg load	Peak platelet inhibition reached within 1-1.5 hours after oral 60 mg load	Peak platelet inhibition within 1 hour after oral 180 mg load	Peak platelet inhibition within 2 minutes after 30 mcg/kg bolus
Duration of effect	3-10 days	7-10 days	3-5 days	1-2 hours
Drug and Disease considerations	Genetic polymorphisms may influence efficacy; Enhanced bleeding with NSAIDs; avoid use Enhanced bleeding with warfarin; monitor carefully for bleeding; target INR to 2.0-2.5 for most indications Avoid use with moderate or strong CYP2C19 inhibitors (omeprazole, esomeprazole, chloramphenicol, cimetidine, efavirenz, etravirine felbamate, fluoxetine, fluconazole, fluvoxamine, isoniazid, oxcarbazepine, ketoconazole, voriconazole); select alternative non-interacting $P2Y_{12}$ inhibitor or alternative non-interacting drug	Enhanced bleeding with warfarin and NSAIDs, avoid use	Enhanced bleeding with warfarin and NSAIDs Use aspirin doses <100 mg daily Avoid use with strong CYP3A inhibitors (atazanavir, clarithromycin, indinavir, itraconazole, nefazodone, nelfinavir, ketoconazole, ritonavir, saquinavir, telithromycin, voriconazole) Avoid use with potent CYP3A inducers (carbamazepine, dexamethasone, phenobarbital, phenytoin, rifampin) Avoid simvastatin and lovastatin doses more than 40 mg daily (ticagrelor inhibits CYP3A4 and increases statin concentration) Monitor digoxin serum concentrations with any change in ticagrelor dose (ticagrelor inhibits P-glycoprotein) Unique side-effects including dyspnea and bradycardia	Do not administer clopidogrel or prasugrel prior to the discontinuation of cangrelor infusion Ticagrelor may be given at any time during cangrelor infusion or immediately after the discontinuation of cangrelor infusion
Contraindications	Any active pathological bleeding	Any active pathological bleeding; any history of TIA/stroke	Any active pathological bleeding; ICH or severe hepatic disease	Significant active bleeding or hypersensitivity
Surgery hold time	5 days for elective surgery; 24 hours for urgent	7 days	5 days for elective surgery; 24 hours for urgent	1 hour
NSTE-ACS indication	May be used regardless of treatment strategy; additional non-ACS indications	Reasonable over clopidogrel in patients treated with PCI who are not at high risk for bleeding	Preferable to clopidogrel for NSTE ACS patients treated with early or invasive or ischemia-guided approach	No US guideline recommendation; May be considered in $P2Y_{12}$ inhibitor—naïve patients undergoing PCI

(*Continued*)

TABLE 17-4 Clinical Considerations When Choosing a $P2Y_{12}$ Receptor Inhibitor[2-4,26,64,66,67,69] **(*Continued*)**

	Clopidogrel	Prasugrel	Ticagrelor	Cangrelor
STEMI indication	Preferred when fibrinolytics used	Superior to clopidogrel in STEMI or in other high-risk patients like DM; Not studied in patients receiving fibrinolytic therapy	Superior to clopidogrel; Not studied in patients receiving fibrinolytic therapy	No US guideline recommendation; May be considered in $P2Y_{12}$ inhibitor—naïve patients undergoing PCI
Risk benefit considerations	Gold standard for reducing CV death and stent thrombosis compared to placebo Consider alternative if documented clopidogrel ineffectiveness (ie, poor metabolism, stent thrombosis during clopidogrel therapy)	Superior to clopidogrel with a significant increase in bleeding risk (driven mainly by reductions in MI and stent thrombosis); No clinical benefit when age ≥75 or weight <60 kg; Net harm in patients with history of TIA or stroke	Superior to clopidogrel with modest increase in major non-CABG related bleeding; Associated with an all-cause mortality reduction; Consider compliance with twice daily dosing	Demonstrated better efficacy than post PCI clopidogrel with minor increases in bleeding Has potential use as a bridge to CABG surgery in high-risk patients

ADP, adenosine diphosphate; CABG, coronary artery bypass grafting; CV, cardiovascular; CYP, cytochrome P450; DM, diabetes mellitus; ICH, intracranial hemorrhage; INR, international normalized ratio; NSAIDs, non-steroidal anti-inflammatory drugs; NSTE-ACS, Non-ST-segment elevation acute coronary syndrome; PCI, percutaneous coronary intervention; STEMI, ST-segment elevation myocardial infarction; TIA, transient ischemic attack.

with clopidogrel. As with the prasugrel trial described, several subgroups of patients enrolled in this trial had particular benefit with ticagrelor, including those with an intended invasive approach, those with an intended noninvasive approach, patients with STEMI primary PCI, and patients with DM.[58-61] Therefore, both of the more potent $P2Y_{12}$ inhibitors are more efficacious than clopidogrel but may also be associated with an increased risk of bleeding. No large randomized trial has directly compared ticagrelor and prasugrel.[62]

The recommended duration of $P2Y_{12}$ inhibitors for a patient undergoing PCI for ACS, either STEMI or NSTE-ACS, is at least 12 months for patients receiving either a BMS or DES.[2,4,26] The consequence of prolonging treatment beyond 12 months had been uncertain until recently.[2,4] Indeed, given the risk of late stent thrombosis, in particular with DES, it had been suggested that long-term use of DAPT could be beneficial, but the uncertainty related to the potential increased risk of bleeding associated with this approach translated in the need for clinical trials with long-term follow-up to properly assess the risk: benefit of such an approach. Many previous trials had suggested that indeed this approach was associated with a reduction in the risk of stent thrombosis with a higher risk of bleeding, and uncertain impact on mortality. The most definitive data comes from the PEGASUS-TIMI (Prevention of Cardiovascular Events in Patients with Prior Heart Attack Using Ticagrelor Compared to Placebo on a Background of Aspirin -Thrombolysis in Myocardial Infarction) 54 trial, which was published after the latest guidelines. In this trial, 21,162 patients who had a history of MI within the previous 1 to 3 years were randomly assigned in a double-blind fashion to receive, in addition to low-dose, aspirin: (1) ticagrelor (90 mg twice daily), (2) ticagrelor (60 mg twice daily), or (3) placebo. Eighty-three percent had a previous PCI. After a median follow-up of 33 months, both ticagrelor doses reduced the risk of the primary efficacy endpoint, which was a composite of CV death, MI, or stroke compared with placebo (ticagrelor 90 mg: 7.85%; ticagrelor 60 mg: 7.77%; placebo: 9.04%; $p < 0.01$ for each ticagrelor dose vs placebo). This benefit was at the expense of an increased risk of major bleeding (ticagrelor 90 mg: 2.60%; ticagrelor 60 mg: 2.30%; placebo: 1.06%); $p < 0.001$ for each dose vs placebo). CV mortality and all-cause mortality were not significantly reduced in any of the ticagrelor group compared to placebo. These results highlight a very fragile benefit: risk ratio of prolonging DAPT beyond 12 months and the necessity to carefully assess the CV and bleeding risk of a patient when contemplating the prolongation of DAPT beyond 12 months.[63] While there was no statistical comparison between doses reported in the PEGASUS-TIMI 54 publication, only the 60 mg dose is currently approved by the FDA for use beyond 1 year after an ACS.[64] The rates of dyspnea and bleeding were numerically lower with the 60 mg dose.[63]

Nonadherence to $P2Y_{12}$ inhibitors is a major risk factor for stent thrombosis, and hence the likelihood of adherence to DAPT (aspirin and a $P2Y_{12}$ inhibitor) should be assessed prior to angiography. The use of a BMS over a DES should be considered in patients who are anticipated to be nonadherent to 12 months of DAPT.[4]

To minimize the risk of CV events, elective noncardiac surgery should be delayed to more than 4 to 6 weeks after angioplasty or BMS implantation, or 12 months after DES implantation if the discontinuation of the $P2Y_{12}$ inhibitor is required. If CABG surgery is planned, clopidogrel and ticagrelor should be withheld preferably for 5 days, and prasugrel at least 7 days, to reduce the risk of postoperative bleeding, and restarted postoperatively, unless the need for immediate revascularization outweighs the bleeding risk. Low-dose aspirin should be continued.[2,4]

Although a variety of blood tests can assess functional platelet aggregation inhibition to $P2Y_{12}$ inhibitors, especially clopidogrel, there is no one gold standard test. Moreover, despite using a higher maintenance dose of clopidogrel (150 mg daily) in patients with a high level of on-treatment platelet aggregation (low platelet aggregation inhibition) that resulted in improved platelet aggregation inhibition, dosing of clopidogrel via platelet aggregation testing does not result in improved clinical outcomes.[65] Therefore, current practice guidelines do not recommend routine platelet aggregation testing to determine $P2Y_{12}$ inhibitor strategy.[2-4]

The most frequent side effects of clopidogrel and prasugrel are nausea, vomiting, and diarrhea, which occur in approximately 2% to 5% of patients.[66,67] Rarely, thrombotic thrombocytopenic purpura (TTP) has been reported with clopidogrel.[67] Clopidogrel hypersensitivity, most commonly presenting as rash develops in up to 6% of patients.[68] In addition to nausea (4%) and diarrhea (3%), use of ticagrelor is associated with dyspnea (up to 19% resulting in drug discontinuation in up to 7% of patients) and, rarely, ventricular pauses and bradyarrhythmias.[63] Patients at risk of bradycardia were excluded from PLATO and PEGASUS-TIMI 54.[57,63] Small non-clinically significant increases in SCr and serum uric acid have also been reported with ticagrelor.[64] A greater incidence of bleeding, hypersensitivity reactions, dyspnea, and worsening renal function has occurred with cangrelor compared to control.[69]

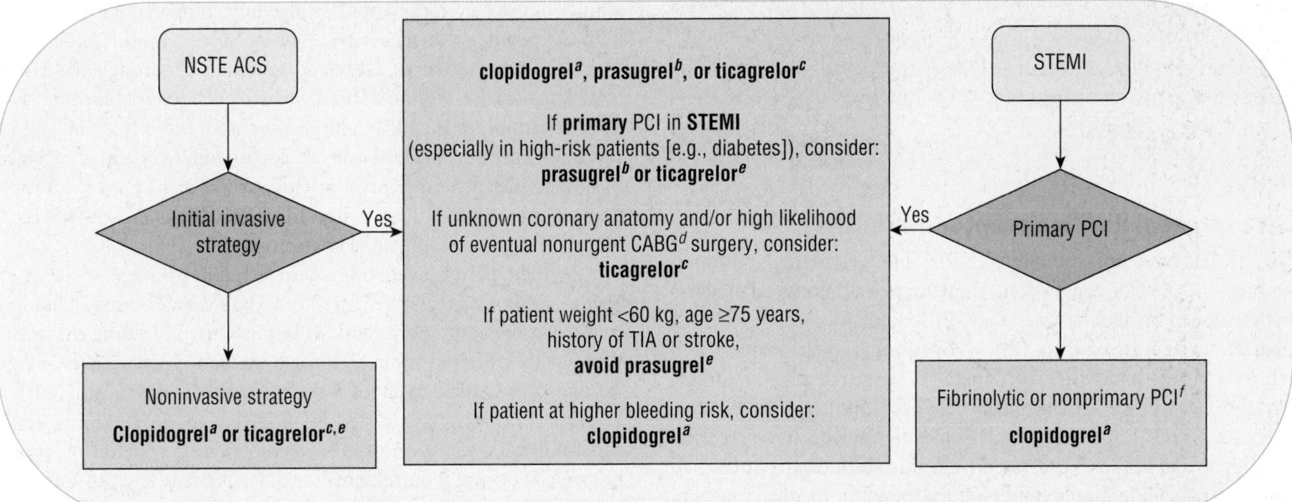

FIGURE 17-4 Proposed use of $P2Y_{12}$ inhibitors. [a]Do not use clopidogrel in patients with active pathologic bleeding; consider alternative $P2Y_{12}$ receptor inhibitor if documented clopidogrel ineffectiveness (eg, poor metabolism, stent thrombosis during clopidogrel therapy) or drug–drug interactions (eg, avoid moderate and strong CYP2C19 inhibitors); clopidogrel should be held for at least 5 days before CABG surgery, if the surgery can be delayed. [b]Do not use prasugrel in patients with active pathologic bleeding or a history of transient ischemic attack or stroke; if a patient subsequently goes on to receive CABG surgery, the drug should be held for at least 7 days if the surgery can be delayed. [c]Do not use ticagrelor in patients with active pathologic bleeding or a history of intracranial hemorrhage, or in patients planned to undergo urgent CABG surgery; concomitant maintenance aspirin dose above 100 mg should be avoided; dose of ticagrelor should be held for 5 days before CABG surgery, if the surgery can be delayed; when selecting this agent, consider patient compliance (dosed twice daily), unique adverse effects (e.g., dyspnea), and potential drug–drug interactions (e.g., avoid strong CYP3A inhibitors/inducers). [d]Prior to diagnostic angiography, it is difficult to determine the likelihood that an individual patient will receive CABG surgery; notable variables that predict this occurrence include previous CABG, male gender, previous heart failure, presence of diabetes, and previous percutaneous coronary intervention, among others. [e]Recommendation based on subgroup analysis. [f]At this time, there are insufficient data to support ticagrelor or prasugrel in the "fibrinolytic or nonprimary PCI" patient group. (ACS, acute coronary syndrome; CABG, coronary artery bypass graft; MI, myocardial infarction; NSTE, non–ST-segment elevation; PCI, percutaneous coronary intervention; STE, ST-segment elevation; TIA, transient ischemic attack.) *(Used with permission from Crouch MA, Colucci VJ, Howard PA, Spinler SA. P2Y12 receptor inhibitors: Integrating ticagrelor into management of acute coronary syndrome. Ann Pharmacother 2011;45:1151–1156. Reprinted by Permission of SAGE Publications.)*

In STEMI patients receiving fibrinolysis, early therapy with clopidogrel 75 mg once daily administered during hospitalization and up to 28 days (mean: 14 days) reduced mortality and reinfarction without increasing the risk of major bleeding.[2,70,71] In adult patients younger than 75 years of age receiving fibrinolytics, the first dose of clopidogrel can be a 300 mg loading dose.[2,71] Although prasugrel and ticagrelor have been studied in the setting of PCI, no studies have evaluated their use when added to both aspirin and a fibrinolytic.

Clopidogrel added to aspirin should be continued for at least 14 days (and up to 1 year) for patients presenting with STEMI who do not undergo reperfusion therapy with either primary PCI or fibrinolysis.[2,70] However, recent subgroup analysis from PLATO suggests that ticagrelor may also be an option in medically managed patients with ACS not receiving fibrinolysis because the frequency of CV death, MI, or stroke as well as mortality was lower in ticagrelor-treated patients compared with those receiving clopidogrel (Fig. 17-4). Ticagrelor use was not associated with a higher bleeding rate compared with clopidogrel.[58]

Clinical **Controversy...**

PERSONALIZED MEDICINE OF $P2Y_{12}$ INHIBITORS

In the last decade, a significant amount of information has been published with regard to the association of genetic factors with the antiplatelet response to clopidogrel.[47,50,72] Specifically, a great amount of evidence indicates that patients carrying a reduced or loss-of-function allele of the gene coding for *CYP2C19*, one of the isoenzymes implicated in the conversion of clopidogrel to its active metabolite, have a higher risk of CV events following an ACS, particularly those undergoing PCI. These data do not extend to other populations of patients receiving clopidogrel. Nevertheless, despite these extensive data, the most recent guidelines do not endorse routine genotyping in patients receiving an ADP $P2Y_{12}$ inhibitor, but favor a case-by-case approach in selected individuals.[2,3] On the other hand, guidelines from the Clinical Pharmacogenetics Implementation Consortium (CPIC) recommend the use of genetic information when it is available in patients with an ACS undergoing PCI for whom clopidogrel is being prescribed to personalize treatment.[73] The guidelines indicate that prasugrel or ticagrelor are preferred over clopidogrel in intermediate or poor metabolizers (for example, those carrying one or two *CYP2C19*2* alleles), when not contraindicated. These inconsistencies between two professional organizations reflect differences in their level of evidence to evaluate the data. The guidelines are primarily based on results from large, randomized controlled trials demonstrating a superiority of an approach before it can be strongly endorsed, whereas CPIC focused more on consistent results from well-designed clinical studies to give strong recommendations. Moreover, CPIC recommendations focus on "how to use" genetic information, rather than "when to genotype" patients.

Glycoprotein IIb/IIIa Receptor Inhibitors

GP IIb/IIIa receptor inhibitors (GPIs) block the final common pathway of platelet aggregation, namely, cross-linking of platelets by fibrinogen bridges between the GP IIb and IIIa receptors on the platelet surface. In patients with STEMI undergoing primary PCI who are treated with UFH, abciximab (IV or intracoronary administration), eptifibatide, or tirofiban may be administered.[2,4] Routine use of a GPI is not recommended in patients who have received fibrinolytics or in those receiving bivalirudin secondary to increased bleeding risk. GPIs should not be administered for medical management of the patient with STEMI who will not be undergoing PCI.[2] A meta-analysis of STEMI primary PCI trials demonstrated no reduction in mortality or 30-day reinfarction but increased risk of major bleeding with GPIs compared with control.[74] Although there are more clinical trial data with abciximab for primary PCI compared with the small-molecule GPIs eptifibatide and tirofiban, the small-molecule agents are used more commonly in clinical practice. A meta-analysis found no difference in efficacy and safety between abciximab and the small-molecule GPIs.[75]

Dosing and contraindications for GPIs are described in Table 17-2. Bleeding is the most significant adverse effect associated with administration of GPIs. GPIs should not be administered to patients with a prior history of hemorrhagic stroke or recent (less than 30 days) ischemic stroke. The risk of bleeding is increased in patients with chronic kidney disease.[76] The recommended dosing for tirofiban (high bolus dose) referenced in the STEMI guidelines is not an FDA-approved regimen but one that has been studied in more contemporary clinical trials.[77,78] This regimen is FDA-approved for patients with NSTE ACS. The dose of tirofiban should be halved in patients with CrCl less than 30 mL/min (0.50 mL/s).[79] No dosage adjustment for renal function is necessary for abciximab. An immune-mediated thrombocytopenia associated with both bleeding as well as thrombosis (when therapy is stopped) occurs in approximately 5% of patients with abciximab and less than 2% of patients receiving eptifibatide or tirofiban.[76,79,80]

Anticoagulants

Options for anticoagulant therapy for patients with STEMI are outlined in Fig. 17-2 and Table 17-2.[2,4] For patients undergoing primary PCI, either UFH or bivalirudin is preferred, whereas for fibrinolysis, UFH, enoxaparin, or fondaparinux may be administered. For patients undergoing PCI, anticoagulation is discontinued immediately following the PCI procedures. In patients receiving an anticoagulant plus a fibrinolytic, UFH is continued for a minimum of 48 hours and if either enoxaparin or fondaparinux is selected, those agents are continued for the duration of hospitalization, up to 8 days. In patients who do not undergo reperfusion therapy, it is reasonable to administer anticoagulant therapy for up to 48 hours for UFH or for the duration of hospitalization for enoxaparin or fondaparinux.[2,4]

Unfractionated heparin has been the traditional anticoagulant administered to patients with STEMI to prevent reocclusion of an infarct artery for more than 50 years. The results of a meta-analysis of more than 7,500 patients suggest that low-molecular-weight heparins (LMWHs) reduce both mortality and reinfarction compared with placebo in patients treated with fibrinolytics and aspirin.[81] Earlier trials favored bivalirudin, a direct thrombin inhibitor, over UFH plus a GPI (abciximab, eptifibatide, or tirofiban) due to bivalirudin's similar or greater efficacy but less bleeding compared with UFH.[82,83] Clinical practice patterns have evolved since time of these trials including a lower use of GPIs and greater PCI through the radial artery instead of the femoral artery which both reduce bleeding risk. Yet contemporary management also includes more frequent use of more potent $P2Y_{12}$ inhibitors than clopidogrel, which may increase bleeding risk. The superiority of either UFH or bivalirudin in primary PCI has been subject of recent trials, which demonstrate conflicting results (see Clinical Controversy).

While UFH or bivalirudin is preferred in primary PCI, enoxaparin, administered for a median of 7 days, has shown a reduction in the risk of death or nonfatal MI but increased bleeding risk compared with UFH (administered for a median of 2 days) in a large randomized clinical trial of patients treated with fibrinolytics.[84] Enoxaparin dosing is adjusted for body weight (mg/kg) and renal function, and when administered in combination with fibrinolysis, it has special dosing requirements for older patients and those weighing more than 100 kg (see Table 17-2).

Besides bleeding, the most serious adverse effect of UFH and enoxaparin is *heparin-induced thrombocytopenia*. ACS registry data indicate, however, that the frequency of heparin-induced thrombocytopenia is rare (less than 0.5%).[85] Bivalirudin would be a preferred anticoagulant for patients with a history of heparin-induced thrombocytopenia undergoing PCI.[2,4]

Clinical **Controversy...**

UFH or Bivalirudin in Primary PCI

Antiplatelet and anticoagulant regimens are used concomitantly during primary PCI to combat the physiological process of platelet aggregation and thrombin formation during STEMI as well as to reduce periprocedural complications. Both UFH and bivalirudin are recommended anticoagulants for patients with STEMI who are undergoing primary PCI.[2] Until recently, bivalirudin was preferred by practice guidelines to UFH as anticoagulant therapy in patients at high risk for bleeding because of data suggesting similar or greater efficacy but less bleeding compared with UFH plus GPI (abciximab, eptifibatide, or tirofiban).[82,83] Recently, data supporting the use of bivalirudin in preference to UFH have been criticized and the optimal anticoagulant for use in primary PCI has been debated. Earlier trials demonstrated reduced mortality and major bleeding favoring bivalirudin, a direct thrombin inhibitor, over UFH but the majority of data comparing the two anticoagulants in this setting is confounded by a high coadministration of GPIs with UFH but not with bivalirudin. Since then, clinical practice patterns have evolved including a more limited and selective use of GPIs, increased utilization of more potent $P2Y_{12}$ inhibitors, and percutaneous access through the radial instead of the femoral artery; all of which may influence safety and efficacy outcomes.

With current evidence, it is difficult to distinguish superiority of one agent over the other in terms of efficacy or safety because contemporary comparisons of UFH and bivalirudin during primary PCI have yielded differing results. Study design, definitions for primary and secondary endpoints including net or major adverse cardiac events, bleeding definitions, and clinical practice patterns (GPI use, $P2Y_{12}$ utilization, and access technique) have varied between the published studies. All trials to date have been open-label, for which potential bias cannot be ruled out. Very few trials have been powered to detect mortality differences.

Bleeding definitions were not standardized across the trials and thus differences between the anticoagulants cannot be easily compared. Studies with more liberal definitions of bleeding demonstrated results favoring bivalirudin.[83,86] Recent studies with more conservative definitions have mixed results overall and do not demonstrate the overwhelming benefit of bivalirudin over UFH in terms of bleeding outcomes.[87,88] Yet other variances such as concomitant antiplatelet use and access site of procedure can influence bleeding results, which have made comparisons of safety between the two anticoagulants difficult. Radial access, which is increasingly used in the United States for coronary angiography, reduces bleeding complications compared to femoral access.[89]

Importantly, recent concerns have been raised over increased risk for acute stent thrombosis with bivalirudin.[86,87] A post-intervention infusion of bivalirudin has been theorized to reduce the risk of stent thrombosis during the immediate post-procedure timeframe. Immediately after PCI, there may be a delay in the onset of full antiplatelet effect with a P2Y$_{12}$ inhibitor during the time that bivalirudin's anticoagulant effect is waning secondary to its short half-life and rapid clearance. Post-hoc and meta-analysis findings support the association between a full-dose post-PCI bivalirudin infusion and decreased stent thrombosis risk yet one prospective trial has not.[90]

At this point, there is no clearly superior agent and both UFH and bivalirudin remain as viable options for use in this setting, each with its own set of advantages and disadvantages when considering ischemic and bleeding complications as well as cost.

β-Blockers

In ACS, the benefit of β-blockers results mainly from the competitive blockade of β_1-adrenergic receptors located on the myocardium. β_1-Blockade produces a reduction in heart rate (HR), myocardial contractility, and blood pressure (BP), decreasing myocardial oxygen demand. In addition, the reduction in HR increases diastolic time, thus improving ventricular filling and coronary artery perfusion. As a result of these effects, β-blockers reduce the risk for recurrent ischemia, infarct size, risk of reinfarction, and occurrence of ventricular arrhythmias in the hours and days following MI.

Landmark clinical trials have established the role of early β-blocker therapy in reducing MI mortality. Most of these trials were performed in the 1970s and 1980s before routine use of early reperfusion therapy. However, data regarding the acute benefit of β-blockers in MI in the reperfusion era are derived mainly from a single large clinical trial that suggests that although initiating IV followed by oral β-blockers early in the course of STEMI was associated with a lower risk of reinfarction or ventricular fibrillation, there may be an early risk of cardiogenic shock, especially in patients presenting with pulmonary congestion or systolic BP less than 120 mm Hg.[91] Oral beta blockers are preferred over IV in the contemporary management of ACS. Initiation of β-blockers, particularly when administered IV, should be limited to patients who present with HTN and/or have ongoing signs of myocardial ischemia and do not demonstrate any signs or symptoms of acute HF.[2] Careful assessment for signs of hypotension and HF should be performed following β-blocker initiation and prior to any dose titration. Patients already taking β-blockers can continue taking them.[2]

The most serious side effects of β-blocker administration early in ACS are hypotension, acute HF, bradycardia, and heart block. Although initial acute administration of β-blockers is not appropriate for patients who present with acute HF, initiation of β-blockers may be attempted before hospital discharge in most patients following treatment of acute HF. β-Blockers should be continued for at least 3 years in patients with normal LV function and indefinitely in patients with LV systolic dysfunction and an LVEF less than or equal to 40% (0.40).[46]

Statins

A high-intensity statin (either atorvastatin 80 mg or rosuvastatin 40 mg) should be administered to all patients without contraindications prior to PCI (regardless of prior lipid-lowering therapy) to reduce the frequency of periprocedural MI (a Type IVa MI) following PCI.[4,10]

Nitrates

One SL NTG tablet should be administered every 5 minutes for up to three doses in order to relieve myocardial ischemia. If patients have been previously prescribed SL NTG and ischemic chest discomfort persists for more than 5 minutes after the first dose, the patient should be instructed to contact EMS before self-administering subsequent doses to activate EMS sooner. IV NTG should then be initiated in all patients with an ACS who have persistent ischemia, HF, or uncontrolled high BP in the absence of contraindications.[2] IV NTG should be continued for approximately 24 hours after ischemia is relieved (see Table 17-2). Nitrates promote the release of nitric oxide from the endothelium, which results in venous and arterial vasodilation. Venodilation lowers preload and myocardial oxygen demand. Arterial vasodilation may lower BP, thus reducing myocardial oxygen demand. Arterial vasodilation also relieves coronary artery vasospasm, dilating coronary arteries to improve myocardial blood flow and oxygenation. Although used to treat ACS, nitrates have been suggested to play a limited role in the treatment of ACS patients because randomized clinical trials failed to show a mortality benefit for IV nitrate therapy followed by oral nitrate therapy in acute MI. The most significant adverse effects of nitrates are tachycardia, flushing, headache, and hypotension. Nitrate administration is contraindicated in patients who have received oral phosphodiesterase-5 inhibitors, such as sildenafil and vardenafil, within the last 24 hours, and tadalafil within the last 48 hours.[2]

Calcium Channel Blockers

Calcium channel blockers in the setting of STEMI are used for relief of ischemic symptoms in patients who have certain contraindications to β-blockers. Current data suggest little benefit on clinical outcomes beyond symptom relief for calcium channel blockers in the setting of ACS.[2] Therefore, calcium channel blockers should be avoided in the acute management of all ACS unless there is a clear symptomatic need or a contraindication to β-blockers. Agent selection is based on presenting HR and LVF. Administration of an agent that lowers HR, either diltiazem or verapamil, is preferred unless the patient has LV systolic dysfunction, bradycardia, or heart block, and then either amlodipine or felodipine is preferred.[2] Nifedipine should be avoided because it has demonstrated reflex sympathetic activation, tachycardia, and worsened myocardial ischemia.[2] Dosing and contraindications are described in Table 17-2.

Early Pharmacotherapy for NSTE-ACS

In general, early pharmacotherapy of NSTE-ACS (see Fig. 17-3) is similar to that of STEMI. In the absence of contraindications, all patients with NSTE-ACS should be treated in the ED with intranasal oxygen (if oxygen saturation is low), SL NTG, aspirin, and an anticoagulant: UFH, enoxaparin, fondaparinux, or bivalirudin. High-risk patients should proceed to early angiography and may receive a GPI (optional with either UFH or enoxaparin but should be avoided with bivalirudin).[3] 7 A P2Y$_{12}$ inhibitor (choice of agent and timing of initiation dependent on selection of an interventional approach involving an early invasive strategy with either PCI or CABG surgery versus an ischemia-guided strategy with medical management alone) should be administered to all patients. IV β-blockers and IV NTG should be given in selected patients. Oral β-blockers should be initiated within the first 24 hours in patients without cardiogenic shock.[3] Morphine is also administered to patients with refractory angina as described previously. These agents should be administered early while the patient is still in the ED. Fibrinolytic therapy is never administered. Dosing and contraindications for SL and IV NTG (for selected patients), aspirin, $P2Y_{12}$ inhibitors, β-blockers, and anticoagulants are listed in Table 17-2.

Fibrinolytic Therapy

Fibrinolytic therapy is not indicated in any patient with NSTE-ACS because increased mortality has been reported with fibrinolytics compared with controls in clinical trials in which fibrinolytics have been administered to patients with NSTE-ACS (patients with normal or ST-segment depression ECGs).[3]

Aspirin

Aspirin reduces the risk of death or developing MI by about 50% (compared with no antiplatelet therapy) in patients with NSTE-ACS. Therefore, aspirin remains the cornerstone of early treatment for all patients with ACS. Dosing of aspirin for NSTE-ACS is the same as that for STEMI (see Table 17-2). Low-dose aspirin is continued indefinitely.[3,46]

Anticoagulants

The choice of anticoagulant for a patient with NSTE-ACS is guided by risk stratification and initial treatment strategy, either an early invasive approach with early coronary angiography and PCI or an early ischemic-guided with angiography in selected patients guided by relief of symptoms and stress testing (see Fig. 17-3). For patients treated by an early invasive strategy, UFH, enoxaparin, fondaparinux, or bivalirudin should be administered.[3,4] In a large open-label randomized clinical trial evaluating bivalirudin versus UFH or enoxaparin plus a GPI (abciximab, eptifibatide, or tirofiban) in moderate- and high-risk patients with NSTE-ACS undergoing an early invasive strategy, bivalirudin demonstrated similar efficacy in preventing CV ischemic events but a lower bleeding rate.[92] Similarly, in a smaller randomized trial specifically comparing abciximab plus UFH with bivalirudin for patients with NSTEMI undergoing PCI, bivalirudin demonstrated no differences in clinical outcomes but a lower bleeding risk.[93]

In patients in whom an initial ischemia-guided strategy is planned (ie, they are not anticipated to receive coronary angiography and revascularization), enoxaparin, UFH, or low-dose fondaparinux is recommended.[3] UFH and LMWH when added to aspirin reduce the frequency of death or MI in patients presenting with NSTE-ACS compared with control/placebo in patients primarily managed with a conservative strategy.[94,95] Compared with enoxaparin, fondaparinux showed similar ischemic outcomes with a lower bleeding rate in a large randomized trial of patients with NSTE-ACS primarily managed with a conservative strategy.[96] If fondaparinux is chosen for a patient initially receiving a conservative strategy who subsequently undergoes angiography and PCI, it should be administered in combination with UFH (and not as the sole anticoagulant) because the dose of fondaparinux studied appears too low to prevent thrombotic events during PCI.[4] Neither fondaparinux nor bivalirudin is FDA approved for NSTE-ACS despite being recommended by the NSTE-ACS guidelines. Bivalirudin has not been studied for initial therapy in patients intended to receive a conservative management strategy. Guideline-recommended dosing and contraindications are described in Table 17-2.

Therapy should be continued for up to at least 48 hours for UFH, until the patient is discharged from the hospital (or 8 days, whichever is shorter) for either enoxaparin or fondaparinux, or until the end of PCI or angiography procedure (or up to 72 hours following PCI for bivalirudin).[3,4] For patients undergoing CABG during the same hospitalization, UFH can be continued until a few hours before CABG and LMWH should be stopped 12 hours prior to the surgery.[97] Because enoxaparin is eliminated renally and patients with renal insufficiency generally have been excluded from clinical trials, some practice protocols recommend UFH for patients with CrCl rates of less than 30 mL/min (0.50 mL/s) based on total patient body weight using the Cockroft-Gault equation.[3] Although recommendations for dosing adjustment of enoxaparin in patients with CrCl between 10 and 30 mL/min (0.27 and 0.50 mL/s) are listed in the product manufacturer's label, the safety and efficacy of enoxaparin in this patient population remain vastly understudied.[98] Administration of enoxaparin should be avoided in dialysis patients with ACS. It is unclear whether or not bivalirudin requires dose adjustment for patients with significant renal dysfunction. Although bivalirudin is eliminated renally, the duration of infusion in recent trials has been short (several hours only), and therefore the actual need for dosing adjustment is unlikely. Practice guidelines recommend manufacturer's suggested dosing adjustment for patients with chronic kidney disease.[4] Patients with SCr greater than 3 mg/dL (265 μmol/L) were excluded from ACS trials with fondaparinux, and the product label states that fondaparinux is contraindicated in patients with CrCl less than 30 mL/min (0.50 mL/s) and in patients weighing less than 50 kg (110 lb).

Unfractionated heparin is monitored and the dose adjusted to a target activated partial thromboplastin time (aPTT) or anti-factor Xa levels, whereas enoxaparin is administered by a fixed actual body weight-based dose without routine monitoring of anti-factor Xa levels. Some experts recommend anti-factor Xa monitoring for LMWHs in patients with renal impairment during prolonged courses of administration of more than several days. No monitoring of coagulation is recommended for bivalirudin and fondaparinux.

$P2Y_{12}$ Inhibitors

Administration of $P2Y_{12}$ receptor inhibitors are recommended in addition to aspirin for most patients presenting with and following NSTE-ACS. Due to their effectiveness and potency following oral loading and maintenance therapy, the need for IV antiplatelets such as GPIs has diminished.

For patients with NSTE-ACS with an initial ischemia-guided approach, either clopidogrel (a 300 or 600-mg loading dose followed by 75 mg daily) or ticagrelor can be used in addition to low-dose aspirin. Ticagrelor is preferred by practice guidelines due to greater efficacy in this setting. If an invasive management strategy is selected, either clopidogrel or ticagrelor can be used either prehospital or in the ED. Following PCI, in patients not already treated with a $P2Y_{12}$ inhibitor, either clopidogrel, prasugrel or ticagrelor can be used (ticagrelor and prasugrel are preferred in patients not at high-risk of bleeding) and should be initiated at the time of or within 1 hour following PCI.[3,54] Specific dosing and contraindications of the $P2Y_{12}$ inhibitors are described in Table 17-2.

In a subgroup of patients undergoing PCI enrolled in a large clinical trial evaluating clopidogrel versus placebo added to aspirin in patients with NSTE-ACS, clopidogrel reduced the frequency of death or MI by 30%.[99] In the large pivotal trials of prasugrel versus clopidogrel (TRITON TIMI 38) and ticagrelor versus clopidogrel (PLATO), no added benefit of the newer $P2Y_{12}$ inhibitors was observed in the subgroup of patients with NSTE-ACS undergoing PCI.[54,57] Following PCI in ACS, for patients receiving either a BMS or a DES, oral DAPT (with aspirin plus clopidogrel, ticagrelor, or prasugrel) is continued for at least 12 months.[3] For patients receiving an initial ischemia-guided treatment strategy, either clopidogrel or ticagrelor in addition to aspirin should be given for up to 12 months.[3] After an NSTEMI, ticagrelor at a reduced dose of 60 mg/day may be continued beyond 12 months based on the results of the PEGASUS-TIMI 54 trial (results discussed previously).[63]

Glycoprotein IIb/IIIa Receptor Inhibitors

The role of GPIs in NSTE-ACS is diminishing as $P2Y_{12}$ inhibitors are used earlier in therapy, and bivalirudin is selected more commonly as the anticoagulant in patients receiving an early intervention approach. See $P2Y_{12}$ Inhibitors above, which includes the selection and timing of GPIs in patients with NSTE-ACS undergoing PCI.[3] Routine administration of eptifibatide (added to aspirin and clopidogrel) prior to angiography and PCI (ie, "upstream" use) in NSTE-ACS does not reduce ischemic events and increases bleeding risk compared to placebo.[100] Therefore, the two antiplatelet initial therapy options, described in the previous section, are preferred.[3,4]

For low-risk patients where a conservative management strategy is selected, there is no role for routine GPIs as the bleeding risk exceeds the benefit. For patients in whom an initial conservative strategy was selected but who experience recurrent ischemia (chest discomfort and ECG changes), HF, or arrhythmias after initial medical therapy necessitating a change in strategy to angiography and revascularization, a GPI may be added to aspirin and clopidogrel prior to the angiogram.[3]

Doses and contraindications to GPIs are described in Table 17-2.

Nitrates

Sublingual nitroglycerin followed by IV NTG should be administered to patients with NSTE-ACS and ongoing ischemia, HF, or uncontrolled high BP (see Table 17-2). The mechanism of action, dosing, contraindications, and adverse effects are the same as those described in Early Pharmacotherapy for STEMIs above. IV NTG is typically continued for approximately 24 hours following ischemia relief.

β-Blockers

The use of β-blockers in NSTE-ACS is similar to that in STEMI in that oral β-blockers should be initiated within 24 hours of hospital admission to all patients in the absence of contraindications. Benefits of β-blockers in this patient group are assumed to be similar to those seen in patients with STEMI. β-Blockers are continued indefinitely in patients with LVEF less than or equal to 40% (0.40) and for at least 3 years in patients with normal LV function.[3]

Calcium Channel Blockers

As described in the previous section, calcium channel blockers should not be administered to most patients with ACS. Their role is a second-line treatment for patients with certain contraindications to β-blockers and those with continued ischemia despite β-blocker and nitrate therapy. Agent selection for NSTE-ACS is identical to that for STEMI with either diltiazem or verapamil preferred unless the patient has LV systolic dysfunction, bradycardia, or heart block, and then either amlodipine or felodipine is preferred. Immediate-release nifedipine is contraindicated, especially in the absence of a β-blocker.[3]

Secondary Prevention Following MI

The long-term goals following MI are to (a) control modifiable CHD risk factors; (b) prevent the development of systolic HF; (c) prevent recurrent MI and stroke; (d) prevent death, including sudden cardiac death; and (e) prevent stent thrombosis following PCI. Pharmacotherapy, which has been proven to decrease mortality, HF, reinfarction or stroke, and stent thrombosis, should be initiated prior to hospital discharge for secondary prevention. Secondary prevention guidelines suggest that following an ACS all patients, in the absence of contraindications, should receive indefinite treatment with aspirin, an ACE inhibitor, and a "high-intensity" statin for secondary prevention of death, stroke, or recurrent infarction.[46,101] 8 A β-blocker should be continued for at least 3 years in patients with normal LV function and indefinitely in patients with LVEF of less than or equal to 40% (0.40) or HF symptoms.[46] It may be reasonable to continue a β-blocker indefinitely in patients without contraindications and with normal LVEF.[3] A $P2Y_{12}$ inhibitor should be continued for at least 12 months for patients undergoing PCI and for patients with NSTE-ACS receiving an ischemia-guided strategy of treatment.[3] Clopidogrel should be continued for at least 14 days in patients with STEMI not undergoing PCI.[2] An ARB and aldosterone antagonist should be given to selected patients as discussed in greater detail later in the chapter.[2,3,46] For all patients with ACS, treatment and control of modifiable risk factors, such as HTN, dyslipidemia, obesity, smoking, and DM, are essential.[46] Dosing and contraindications are described in detail in Table 17-2. Benefits and adverse effects of long-term treatment with these medications are discussed in more detail later. Use of ICDs for the prevention of sudden cardiac death following MI in patients with diminished LVF and nonsustained ventricular arrhythmias is discussed in more detail in Chapter 18.

Aspirin

Aspirin decreases the risk of death, recurrent infarction, and stroke following MI. All patients should receive aspirin indefinitely; those patients with a contraindication to aspirin should receive clopidogrel.[46] The risk of major bleeding from chronic aspirin therapy is approximately 2% and is dose related. Higher doses of aspirin, 160 to 325 mg, are not more effective than aspirin doses of 75 to 81 mg but have higher rates of bleeding.[102] Even in the setting of PCI, low-dose aspirin (75-100 mg daily) was found to be equally safe and efficacious compared with higher doses of aspirin (300-325 mg daily) in a prespecified subgroup analysis of 30-day outcomes in a large randomized, double-blind clinical trial of patients with ACS who underwent PCI.[45] Therefore, chronic doses of aspirin should not exceed 81 mg.[2,3,46]

$P2Y_{12}$ Inhibitors

For patients with either STEMI or NSTE-ACS, clopidogrel decreases the risk of CV events and stent thrombosis compared with placebo. Compared with clopidogrel, either prasugrel or ticagrelor lowers the risk of CV death, MI, or stroke by an additional 20% to 30% depending on the patient population studied. The frequency of stent thrombosis following PCI is also lower with prasugrel or ticagrelor compared with clopidogrel. However, the rate of non-CABG surgery-associated bleeding is higher with both prasugrel and ticagrelor compared with clopidogrel. For most patients with STEMI or NSTE-ACS, a $P2Y_{12}$ inhibitor should be continued for at least 1 year.[2-4,27,63] For patients with STEMI managed with fibrinolytics, clopidogrel should be continued for at least 14 days and ideally 1 year. For patients STEMI and NSTE-ACS patients who were medically treated, who received fibrinolytics or who had a PCI who are not at high-risk of bleeding and who have not had overt bleeding, new guidelines indicate it is reasonable to continue dual antiplatelet therapy after 12 months.

The combination of clopidogrel and aspirin increases the risk of major bleeding by approximately 50% and minor bleeding by approximately 40% but not fatal bleeding compared with single agent alone.[103] Compared with clopidogrel, ticagrelor increased the risk of major bleeding not related to CABG surgery by 18% in a large randomized comparative trial of patients presenting with ACS and undergoing either PCI or medical management while prasugrel increased major bleeding by 33% compared with clopidogrel in a pivotal trial of patients with ACS undergoing PCI.[54,57] Oral antiplatelet agents are the third leading cause of adverse drug reaction-associated hospital admissions after ED visits among senior citizens.[104] Therefore, patients should be counseled on the risks and sites of potential bleeding and should be told to seek medical care immediately if significant bleeding is noticed. Lower-weight patients (less than or equal to 60 kg) and elderly patients are at higher risk of bleeding with prasugrel or ticagrelor compared with clopidogrel.[105,106] Prasugrel is contraindicated in patients with a prior history of stroke as the risk of ICH is increased with prasugrel compared with clopidogrel.[54,66]

Clinical **Controversy...**

TRIPLE ORAL ANTITHROMBOTIC THERAPY

Patients with ACS undergoing PCI and intracoronary stent placement with either a BMS or a DES are managed with DAPT that reduces stent thrombosis risk and reinfarction risk.[4] But what antithrombotic therapy is best for patients with a chronic or new indication for longer-term anticoagulant therapy following hospital discharge such as atrial fibrillation, the presence of a mechanical heart valve, venous thromboembolism, or LV thrombus?

Which combination of antithrombotic agents is best to maximize efficacy while decreasing bleeding risk? Meta-analyses including mostly observational studies suggest a significant reduction in all-cause mortality at a cost of increased major bleeding with triple antithrombotic therapy (TT), such as aspirin, clopidogrel, and an oral vitamin K antagonist, compared with DAPT alone (aspirin plus clopidogrel).[107,108] Current practice guidelines recommend TT (warfarin, low-dose aspirin, and clopidogrel) for 1 to 6 months for patients following PCI with a BMS placement and between 6 and 12 months for patients following PCI with a DES placement, depending on bleeding risk. Thereafter, a single antiplatelet agent, either clopidogrel or low-dose aspirin, is recommended in addition to warfarin.[109]

Only one randomized trial, the *W*hat is the *O*ptimal Antiplatelet and Anticoagulant Therapy in Patients with Oral Anticoagulation and Coronary *S*tenting (WOEST) trial, has been published.[110] In this open-label study, patients undergoing PCI who were chronically treated with an oral vitamin K antagonist were randomized to receive clopidogrel alone or clopidogrel plus low-dose aspirin 80 to 100 mg/day. The target international normalized ratio (INR) of anticoagulation was that recommended based on the indication. At 1-year follow-up, the primary endpoint, any bleeding episode was increased more than twofold in patients randomized to TT compared with clopidogrel plus anticoagulation (44.4% vs 19.4%, $P < 0.0001$). GI bleeding was the most common type of bleeding and was increased threefold by aspirin (2.9% in patients receiving anticoagulation plus clopidogrel vs 8.8% in patients receiving triple therapy). In addition, there was no difference in the secondary endpoint of thromboembolic events. Therefore, consideration should be given to stopping aspirin in patients receiving TT as is an option in the practice guidelines recommended above.

The manufacturers of prasugrel and ticagrelor recommend against combining those $P2Y_{12}$ inhibitors with an oral anticoagulant due to a lack of data as well as clinical experience.[64,66] Therefore, when TT is needed, clopidogrel should be selected as the $P2Y_{12}$ inhibitor. Also, both rivaroxaban and apixaban have increased bleeding risk, including increased ICH risk when combined with aspirin plus clopidogrel in patients with ACS, and there is no information on long-term treatment with dabigatran, aspirin, and clopidogrel, and therefore warfarin should be selected as the anticoagulant of choice when TT is needed.[111,112] While guidelines suggest a tighter warfarin INR range goal of 2 to 2.5 in patients receiving TT, no clinical trial has prospectively tested this more stringent goal.[2,109,113]

In summary, TT, when needed, should consist of warfarin (INR target 2-2.5), low-dose aspirin 81 mg orally daily, and clopidogrel 75 mg orally daily. The anticoagulant should be discontinued if possible (such as in 3-6 months post-MI in patients at risk of LV thrombus but without actual thrombi present), and then either clopidogrel or preferably aspirin, discontinued after at least 1 month in a patient with a BMS and after at least 6 months in a patient with a DES. Concomitant use of a proton pump inhibitor is recommended in patients receiving TT undergoing PCI.[4,26,113]

β-Blockers, Nitrates, and Calcium Channel Blockers

Current treatment guidelines recommend that following an ACS, patients should receive a β-blocker for at least 3 years following MI in the absence of LV dysfunction and regardless of whether they have residual symptoms of angina or not. Patients with or without HF and LVEF less than or equal to 40% should receive a β-blocker indefinitely. Overwhelming data support the use of β-blockers in patients with a previous MI.[114] Currently, there are no data to support the superiority of one β-blocker over another in the absence of HF.

Although β-blockers should be avoided in patients with decompensated HF from LV systolic dysfunction complicating an MI, clinical trial data suggest it is safe to initiate β-blockers prior to hospital discharge in these patients once HF symptoms have resolved.[115] These patients may actually benefit more than those without LV dysfunction.[116] In patients who cannot tolerate or have a contraindication to a β-blocker, a calcium channel blocker can be used to prevent anginal symptoms but should not be used routinely in the absence of such symptoms.[2,3,117]

Finally, all patients should be prescribed short-acting, SL NTG or lingual NTG spray to relieve any anginal symptoms when necessary and instructed on its use.[117] Chronic long-acting nitrate therapy has not been shown to reduce CHD events following MI. Therefore, IV NTG is not routinely followed by chronic, long-acting oral nitrate therapy in ACS patients who have undergone revascularization, unless the patient has stable ischemic heart disease or significant coronary stenoses that were not revascularized.[117]

ACE Inhibitors and ARBs

Angiotensin-converting enzyme inhibitors should be initiated in all patients following MI to reduce mortality, decrease reinfarction, and prevent the development of HF.[2,4,46,118] The benefit of ACE inhibitors in patients with MI most likely comes from their ability to prevent cardiac remodeling. The largest reduction in mortality is observed in patients with LV dysfunction (low LVEF) or HF symptoms. Early initiation (within 24 hours) of an *oral* ACE inhibitor appears to be crucial during an acute MI because 40% of the 30-day survival benefit is observed during the first day, 45% from days 2 to 7, and approximately 15% from days 8 to 30.[119] However, current data do not support the early administration of IV ACE inhibitors in patients experiencing an MI because mortality may be increased.[120] Administration of ACE inhibitors should be continued indefinitely. Hypotension should be avoided because coronary artery filling may be compromised. Additional trials suggest that most patients with CAD, not just ACS or HF patients, benefit from ACE inhibitors. Therefore, ACE inhibitors should be considered in all patients following an ACS in the absence of a contraindication.

Many patients cannot tolerate chronic ACE inhibitor therapy secondary to adverse effects. The ARBs, candesartan, valsartan, and losartan, have been documented in trials to improve clinical outcomes in patients with HF.[121,122] Therefore, either an ACE inhibitor or candesartan, valsartan, or losartan is an acceptable choice for chronic therapy for patients who have a low LVEF and HF following MI. Besides hypotension, the most frequent adverse reaction to an ACE inhibitor is cough, which may occur in up to 30% of patients. Patients with an ACE inhibitor cough and either clinical signs of HF or LVEF less than or equal to 40% (0.40) may be prescribed an ARB.[46] Other, less common but more serious adverse effects to ACE inhibitors and ARBs include acute renal failure, hyperkalemia, and angioedema.

Aldosterone Antagonists

To reduce mortality, administration of an aldosterone antagonist, either eplerenone or spironolactone, should be considered within the first 7 days following MI in all patients who are already receiving an ACE inhibitor (or ARB) and a β-blocker and have an LVEF of less than or equal to 40% (0.40) and either HF symptoms or DM.[2,3,46] Aldosterone plays an important role in HF and in MI because it promotes vascular and myocardial fibrosis, endothelial dysfunction, HTN, LV hypertrophy, sodium retention, potassium and magnesium loss, and arrhythmias. Aldosterone antagonists have been shown in experimental and human studies to attenuate these adverse effects.[123] Spironolactone decreases all-cause mortality in patients with stable, severe HF.[124]

Eplerenone, like spironolactone, is an aldosterone antagonist that blocks the mineralocorticoid receptor. In contrast to spironolactone, eplerenone has no effect on the progesterone or androgen receptor, thereby minimizing the risk of gynecomastia, sexual dysfunction, and menstrual irregularities. In a large clinical trial, eplerenone significantly reduced mortality as well as hospitalization for HF in post-MI patients with an LVEF less than or equal to 40% (0.40) and symptoms of HF at any time during hospitalization.[125] Eplerenone has also been demonstrated to reduce mortality in patients with mild systolic HF.[126] The risk of hyperkalemia, however, was increased in both of these studies. Therefore, patients with serum potassium concentrations greater than 5 mmol/L (5 mEq/L) should not receive an aldosterone antagonist. Additional contraindications for spironolactone include a SCr greater than 2.5 mg/dL (221 μmol/L) for men, 2 mg/dL (177 μmol/L) for women, or CrCl less than 30 mL/min (0.5 mL/s). Specific contraindications for eplerenone include a SCr greater than or equal to 2 mg/dL (177 μmol/L) for men or 1.8 mg/dL (159 μmol/L) for women, or CrCl less than or equal to 50 mL/min (0.83 mL/s). Currently, there are no data to support that the more selective, more expensive eplerenone is superior to, or should be preferred to, the less expensive generic spironolactone unless a patient has experienced gynecomastia, breast pain, or impotence while receiving spironolactone.

Lipid-Lowering Agents

Following MI, statins reduce total mortality, CV mortality, and stroke. Results from landmark clinical trials have unequivocally demonstrated the value of statins in secondary prevention following MI. A meta-analysis of randomized controlled clinical trials in almost 18,000 patients with recent ACS (less than 14 days) found that statin therapy reduces mortality by 19%, with benefits observed after approximately 4 months of treatment.[127] In the 2013 ACC/AHA guidelines on managment of lipids, patients with clinical atherosclerotic vascular disease, such as MI, are one of the four groups of patients that benefit from moderate- or high-dose statins.[101] Therefore, all patients, regardless of low-density lipoprotein cholesterol level, should ideally be prescribed a high-intensity statin. Patients aged greater than 75 years may be prescribed a moderate-intensity statin as initial therapy because they are at higher risk of adverse drug effects and the data using high-dose statins in this patient subgroup are less robust. See Chapter 21 for a more detailed discussion. Use of other agents such as ezetimibe and proprotein convertase subtilisin kexin type 9 (PCSK9) inhibitors in patients already receiving statins for secondary prevention is supported by current guidelines with preference given to ezetimibe due to the benefit of ezetimibe-statin combination after ACS.[128]

Results of the Improved Reduction of Outcomes: Vytorin Efficacy International Trial Efficacy International Trial (IMPROVE-IT) study where ezetimibe added to moderate-dose simvastatin in patients with recent (within 10 days) ACS and an LDL level 50 mg/dL to 100 mg/dL reduced the frequency of a composite endpoint of CV events or stroke over a median follow-up of 6 years compared to simvastatin alone.[129] Patients on combined ezetimibe/simvastatin had a median LDL cholesterol level of 54 compared to 70 mg/dL in patients on simvastatin alone. Event rates were lower in patients with lower LDL cholesterols suggesting a direct relationship between LDL and benefit. Data with newer injectable PCSK9 inhibitors, such as alirocumab and evolocumab, added to high-intensity statins in patients with CHD or who are at high-risk for CHD are promising. However, current analyses indicate that they may not be cost-effective.[130] The results of ongoing clinical trials with prospective CV mortality endpoints are necessary before a more widespread use of PCSK9 inhibitors is employed.[128,131-134]

Other Modifiable Risk Factors

Smoking cessation, managing HTN, weight loss, exercise, and tight glucose control for patients with DM, in addition to treatment of dyslipidemia, are important treatments for secondary prevention of CHD events. Referral to a comprehensive CV risk reduction program for cardiac rehabilitation is recommended.[46] Behavioral therapy aided with nicotine replacement alone or combined with bupropion or varenicline, for smoking cessation should be absolutely considered in appropriate patients.[2,3,46] HTN should be strictly controlled according to published guidelines.[135] Patients who are overweight should be educated on the importance of regular exercise, healthy eating habits, and reaching and maintaining an ideal weight. Moderate-intensity aerobic exercise for at least 30 minutes, 7 days/wk (minimum 5 days/wk) is recommended.[46] The goal body mass index is less than 25 kg/m^2. Finally, because patients with DM have up to a fourfold increased mortality risk compared with patients without DM, the importance of blood glucose control, as well as other CHD risk factor modifications, cannot be overstated.[46]

OUTCOME EVALUATION

To determine the efficacy of nonpharmacologic therapy and pharmacotherapy for both STE and NSTE-ACS, monitor patients for: (a) relief of ischemic discomfort; (b) return of ECG changes to baseline; and (c) absence or resolution of HF signs and symptoms.

Monitoring parameters for recognition and prevention of adverse effects from ACS pharmacotherapy are described in Table 17-5. 9 In general, the most common adverse reactions from ACS therapies are hypotension and bleeding. To treat for bleeding and hypotension, discontinue the offending agent(s) until symptoms resolve. Severe bleeding resulting in hypotension secondary to hypovolemia may require blood transfusion.

Because poor medication adherence of secondary prevention medications following MI leads to worsened CV outcomes, patients should receive medication counseling (including counseling prior to hospital discharge) and be monitored for medication persistence.[2,3,136] Counseling should include assessment of health literacy level, assessment of barriers to adherence, assessment of access to medications, written and verbal instructions about the purpose of each medication, changes to previous medication regimen, optimal time to take each medication, new allergies or medication intolerances, need for timely prescription fill after discharge, anticipated duration

TABLE 17-5 Therapeutic Drug Monitoring of Pharmacotherapy for Acute Coronary Syndromes

Drug	Adverse Effects	Monitoring
Aspirin	Dyspepsia, bleeding, gastritis	Clinical signs of bleeding[a]; GI upset; baseline and every 6 months: Hgb, HCT, platelet count
Clopidogrel and prasugrel	Bleeding, diarrhea, rash, TTP (rare)	Clinical signs of bleeding[a]; baseline and every 6 months: Hgb, HCT, platelet count
Ticagrelor	Bleeding, dyspnea, diarrhea, rash, elevated SCr, elevated serum uric acid	Clinical signs of bleeding[a]; baseline and every 6 months: Hgb, HCT, platelet count
Unfractionated heparin	Bleeding, heparin-induced thrombocytopenia	Clinical signs of bleeding[a]; baseline aPTT, INR, Hgb, HCT, and platelet count; aPTT every 6 hours until target then every 24 hours; daily Hgb, HCT, and platelet
Enoxaparin	Bleeding, heparin-induced thrombocytopenia	Clinical signs of bleeding[a]; baseline SCr, aPTT, INR, Hgb, HCT, and platelet count; daily SCr, Hgb, HCT, and platelet count
Fondaparinux	Bleeding	Clinical signs of bleeding[a]; baseline SCr, aPTT, INR, Hgb, HCT, and platelet count; daily SCr, Hgb, HCT, and platelet count
Bivalirudin	Bleeding	Clinical signs of bleeding[a]; baseline SCr, aPTT, INR, Hgb, HCT, and platelet count
Fibrinolytics	Bleeding, especially intracranial hemorrhage	Clinical signs of bleeding[a]; baseline aPTT, INR, Hgb, HCT, and platelet count; mental status every 2 hours for signs of intracranial hemorrhage; daily Hgb, HCT, and platelet count
GPIs	Bleeding, acute profound thrombocytopenia	Clinical signs of bleeding[a]; baseline SCr (for eptifibatide and tirofiban), Hgb, HCT, and platelet count; platelet count at 4 hours after initiation; daily Hgb, HCT, and platelet count(and SCr for eptifibatide and tirofiban)
IV nitrates	Hypotension, flushing, headache, tachycardia	BP and HR every 2 hours
β-Blockers	Hypotension, bradycardia, heart block, bronchospasm, acute HF, fatigue, depression, sexual dysfunction	BP, RR, HR, 12-lead ECG, and clinical signs of HF every 5 minutes with bolus IV dosing; BP, RR, HR, and clinical signs of HF every shift with oral therapy, then BP and HR every 6 months following hospital discharge
Diltiazem and verapamil	Hypotension, bradycardia, heart block, HF, gingival hyperplasia	BP and HR every shift with oral therapy, then every 6 months following hospital discharge; dental examination and teeth cleaning every 6 months
Amlodipine	Hypotension, dependent peripheral edema, gingival hyperplasia	BP every shift with oral therapy, then every 6 months following hospital discharge; dental examination and teeth cleaning every 6 months
ACE inhibitors and ARBs	Hypotension, cough (with ACE inhibitors), hyperkalemia, prerenal azotemia, acute renal failure, angioedema (ACE inhibitors more so than ARBs)	BP every 4 hours × 3 for first dose, then every shift with oral therapy, then once every 6 months following hospital discharge; baseline SCr and potassium; daily SCr and potassium while hospitalized, then every 6 months (or 1–2 weeks after each outpatient dose titration); closer monitoring required in patients receiving spironolactone or eplerenone or if renal insufficiency; counsel patient on throat, tongue, and facial swelling
Aldosterone antagonists	Hypotension, hyperkalemia, increased SCr	BP and HR every shift with oral therapy, then once every 6 months; baseline SCr and serum potassium concentration then at 48 hours, at 7 days, monthly for 3 months, then every 3 months thereafter
Morphine	Hypotension, respiratory depression	BP and RR 5 minutes after each bolus dose
Statins	GI upset, myopathy, hepatotoxicity	Liver function tests at baseline. CK if indicated. Only repeat if patients present with sign/symptoms of liver failure or muscle symptoms; counsel patient on myalgia; baseline LDL cholesterol prior to treatment and at 4-6 weeks following initiation to determine adequate response and consideration of additional guideline-recommended lipid-lowering therapy

[a]Clinical signs of bleeding include bloody stools, melena, hematuria, hematemesis, bruising, and oozing from arterial or venous puncture sites.

ACE, angiotensin-converting enzyme; aPTT, activated partial thromboplastin time; ARB, angiotensin receptor blocker; BP, blood pressure; CK, creatine kinase; ECG, electrocardiogram; GI, gastrointestinal; GPI, glycoprotein IIb/IIIa inhibitor; Hgb, hemoglobin; HCT, hematocrit; HF, heart failure; HR, heart rate; INR, international normalized ratio; LDL, low-density lipoprotein RR, respiratory rate; SCr, serum creatinine, TTP, thrombotic thrombocytopenic purpura.

of therapy, consequences of nonadherence, common and/or serious adverse reactions that may develop, drug–drug and drug–food interactions, and an assessment of instruction understanding.

ABBREVIATIONS

ACE	angiotensin-converting enzyme
ACS	acute coronary syndrome
ADP	adenosine diphosphate
AMI	acute myocardial infarction
aPTT	activated partial thromboplastin time
ARB	angiotensin receptor blocker
BMS	bare metal stent
BP	blood pressure
CABG	coronary artery bypass graft
CAD	coronary artery disease
CBC	complete blood count
CHD	coronary heart disease
CPIC	clinical pharmacogenetics implementation consortium
CrCl	creatinine clearance
CV	cardiovascular
CVD	cardiovascular disease
CYP	cytochrome P450
DAPT	dual antiplatelet therapy
DES	drug-eluting stent
DM	diabetes mellitus
ECG	electrocardiogram
ED	emergency department
EF	ejection fraction
EMS	emergency medical system
GPI	glycoprotein IIb/IIIa inhibitor
HDL	high-density lipoprotein
HF	heart failure

HORIZONS-AMI	Harmonizing Outcomes with Revascularization and Stents in Acute Myocardial Infarction
HR	heart rate
HTN	hypertension
ICD	implantable cardioverter-defibrillator
ICH	intracranial hemorrhage
IMPROVE-IT	Improved Reduction of Outcomes: Vytorin Efficacy International Trial
INR	international normalized ratio
IV	intravenous
LDL	low-density lipoprotein
LMWH	low-molecular-weight heparin
LV	left ventricular
LVEF	left ventricular ejection fraction
MI	myocardial infarction
NSTEMI	non–ST-segment elevation myocardial infarction
NTG	nitroglycerin
PCI	percutaneous coronary intervention
PCSK9	proprotein convertase subtilisin kexin 9
PLATO	Platelet Inhibition and Patient Outcomes
SCr	serum creatinine
SL	Sublingual
STE	ST-segment elevation
STEMI	ST-segment elevation myocardial infarction
TIA	transient ischemic attack
TTP	thrombotic thrombocytopenic purpura
TXA_2	thromboxane A_2
UA	unstable angina
UFH	unfractionated heparin

REFERENCES

1. Mozaffarian D, Benjamin EJ, Go AS, et al. Heart Disease and Stroke Statistics-2016 Update: A Report From the American Heart Association. *Circulation* 2016;133(4):e38-e360.
2. O'Gara PT, Kushner FG, Ascheim DD, et al. 2013 ACCF/AHA guideline for the management of ST-elevation myocardial infarction: A report of the American College of Cardiology Foundation/ American Heart Association Task Force on Practice Guidelines. *J Am Coll Cardiol* 2013;61:e78-140.
3. Amsterdam EA, Wenger NK, Brindis RG, et al. 2014 AHA/ACC Guideline for the Management of Patients With Non-ST-Elevation Acute Coronary Syndromes: A Report of the American College of Cardiology/American Heart Association Task Force on Practice Guidelines. *J Am Coll Cardiol* 2014;64:e139-228.
4. Levine GN, Bates ER, Blankenship JC, et al. 2011 ACCF/AHA/ SCAI Guideline for Percutaneous Coronary Intervention. A report of the American College of Cardiology Foundation/American Heart Association Task Force on Practice Guidelines and the Society for Cardiovascular Angiography and Interventions. *J Am Coll Cardiol* 2011;58:e44-122.
5. Medicare.Gov: Hospital compare. Readmission & Deaths. Available at: https://www.medicare.gov/hospitalcompare/search.html. (Last accessed January 27, 2016)
6. Sugiyama T, Hasegawa K, Kobayashi Y, Takahashi O, Fukui T, Tsugawa Y. Differential time trends of outcomes and costs of care for acute myocardial infarction hospitalizations by ST elevation and type of intervention in the United States, 2001-2011. *J Am Heart Assoc* 2015;4:e001445.
7. Borissoff JI, Spronk HM, ten Cate H. The hemostatic system as a modulator of atherosclerosis. *N Engl J Med* 2011;364:1746-1760.
8. Antman EM. ST-segment myocardial infarction: Patholgy, pathophysiology, and clinical features. *Braunwald's Heart Disease: A Textbook of Cardiovascular Medicine*. 9th ed. Philiadelphia, PA: Elsevier/Saunders; 2012:1087-1110.
9. Bentzon JF, Otsuka F, Virmani R, Falk E. Mechanisms of plaque formation and rupture. *Circ Res* 2014;114:1852-1866.
10. Thygesen K, Alpert JS, Jaffe AS, et al. Third universal definition of myocardial infarction. *J Am Coll Cardiol* 2012;60:1581-1598.
11. Gajarsa JJ, Kloner RA. Left ventricular remodeling in the post-infarction heart: A review of cellular, molecular mechanisms, and therapeutic modalities. *Heart Fail Rev* 2011;16:13-21.
12. Kolte D, Khera S, Aronow WS, et al. Trends in incidence, management, and outcomes of cardiogenic shock complicating ST-elevation myocardial infarction in the United States. *J Am Heart Assoc* 2014;3:e000590.
13. Sabatine MS, Cannon, CP. Approach to the patient with chest pain. *Braunwald's Heart Disease: A Textbook of Cardiovascular Medicine*. 9th ed. Philiadelphia, PA: Elsevier/Saunders; 2012: 1076-1086.
14. Shah RU, Henry TD, Rutten-Ramos S, Garberich RF, Tighiouart M, Bairey Merz CN. Increasing percutaneous coronary interventions for ST-segment elevation myocardial infarction in the United States: Progress and opportunity. *JACC Cardiovasc Interv* 2015;8:139-146.
15. Brieger D, Fox KA, Fitzgerald G, et al. Predicting freedom from clinical events in non-ST-elevation acute coronary syndromes: The Global Registry of Acute Coronary Events. *Heart* 2009;95: 888-894.
16. Granger CB, Goldberg RJ, Dabbous O, et al. Predictors of hospital mortality in the global registry of acute coronary events. *Arch Int Med* 2003;163:2345-2353.
17. Heidenreich PA, Lewis WR, LaBresh KA, Schwamm LH, Fonarow GC. Hospital performance recognition with the Get With The Guidelines Program and mortality for acute myocardial infarction and heart failure. *Am Heart J* 2009;158:546-553.
18. Mehta RH, Chen AY, Alexander KP, Ohman EM, Roe MT, Peterson ED. Doing the right things and doing them the right way: Association between hospital guideline adherence, dosing safety, and outcomes among patients with acute coronary syndrome. *Circulation* 2015;131:980-987.
19. Antman EM, Cohen M, Bernink PJ, et al. The TIMI risk score for unstable angina/non-ST elevation MI: A method for prognostication and therapeutic decision making. *JAMA* 2000;284:835-842.
20. Pieper KS, Gore JM, FitzGerald G, et al. Validity of a risk-prediction tool for hospital mortality: The Global Registry of Acute Coronary Events. *Am Heart J* 2009;157:1097-1105.
21. Jortveit J, Govatsmark RE, Digre TA, et al. Myocardial infarction in Norway in 2013. *Tidsskr Nor Laegeforen* 2014;134:1841-1846.
22. Huynh T, Perron S, O'Loughlin J, et al. Comparison of primary percutaneous coronary intervention and fibrinolytic therapy in ST-segment-elevation myocardial infarction: Bayesian hierarchical meta-analyses of randomized controlled trials and observational studies. *Circulation* 2009;119:3101-109.
23. Krumholz HM, Herrin J, Miller LE, et al. Improvements in door-to-balloon time in the United States, 2005 to 2010. *Circulation* 2011;124:1038-1045.
24. Hoenig MR, Aroney CN, Scott IA. Early invasive versus conservative strategies for unstable angina and non-ST elevation myocardial infarction in the stent era. *Cochrane Database Syst Rev* 2010:Cd004815.
25. Milosevic A, Vasiljevic-Pokrajcic Z, Milasinovic D, et al. Immediate Versus Delayed Invasive Intervention for Non-ST-Segment Elevation Myocardial Infarction Patients: The RIDDLE-NSTEMI Study (Randomized study of ImmeDiate versus DeLayed invasivE intervention in patients with Non-ST-segment Elevation Myocardial Infarction). *JACC Cardiovasc Intervc* 2016;9(6):541-9.
26. Levine GN, Bates ER, Bittl JA, et al. 2016 ACC/AHA Guideline Focused Update on Duration of Dual Antiplatelet Therapy in Patients With Coronary Artery Disease: A Report of the American College of Cardiology/American Heart Association Task Force on Clinical Practice Guidelines. J Am Coll Cardiol. 2016; Sep 6;68(10):1082-1115. doi: 10.1016/j.jacc.2016.03.513. Epub 2016 Mar 29.
27. Mauri L, Kereiakes DJ, Yeh RW, et al. Twelve or 30 months of dual antiplatelet therapy after drug-eluting stents. *N Engl J Med* 2014;371:2155-2166.
28. Navarese EP, Andreotti F, Schulze V, et al. Optimal duration of dual antiplatelet therapy after percutaneous coronary intervention with drug eluting stents: Meta-analysis of randomised controlled trials. *BMJ* 2015;350:h1618.
29. Valgimigli M, Ariotti S, Costa F. Duration of dual antiplatelet therapy after drug-eluting stent implantation: Will we ever reach a consensus? *Eur Heart J* 2015;36:1219-1222.
30. Plavix (clopidogrel): FDA Drug Safety Communication—Long-term Treatment Does Not Change Risk of Death. Available at: http://www.fda.gov/Safety/MedWatch/SafetyInformation/ SafetyAlertsforHumanMedicalProducts/ucm471531.htm. (Last accessed, November 10, 2015)

31. Udell JA, Bonaca MP, Collet JP, et al. Long-term dual antiplatelet therapy for secondary prevention of cardiovascular events in the subgroup of patients with previous myocardial infarction: A collaborative meta-analysis of randomized trials. *Eur Heart J* 2016;37:390-399.
32. Elmariah S, Mauri L, Doros G, et al. Extended duration dual antiplatelet therapy and mortality: A systematic review and meta-analysis. *Lancet* 2015;385:792-798.
33. Epstein AE, DiMarco JP, Ellenbogen KA, et al. 2012 ACCF/AHA/HRS focused update incorporated into the ACCF/AHA/HRS 2008 guidelines for device-based therapy of cardiac rhythm abnormalities: A report of the American College of Cardiology Foundation/American Heart Association Task Force on Practice Guidelines and the Heart Rhythm Society. *J Am Coll Cardiol* 2013;61:e6-75.
34. Parodi G, Bellandi B, Xanthopoulou I, et al. Morphine is associated with a delayed activity of oral antiplatelet agents in patients with ST-elevation acute myocardial infarction undergoing primary percutaneous coronary intervention. *Circ Cardiovasc Interv* 2014;8(1). pii: e001593. doi:10.1161/CIRCINTERVENTIONS.114.001593.
35. Hobl EL, Stimpfl T, Ebner J, et al. Morphine decreases clopidogrel concentrations and effects: A randomized, double-blind, placebo-controlled trial. *J Am Coll Cardiol* 2014;63:630-635.
36. Medicare.Gov: Hospital compare. Timely and effective care. Available at: https://www.medicare.gov/hospitalcompare/about/timely-effective-care.html. (Last accessed, February 4, 2016)
37. Gibson CM, Pride YB, Frederick PD, et al. Trends in reperfusion strategies, door-to-needle and door-to-balloon times, and in-hospital mortality among patients with ST-segment elevation myocardial infarction enrolled in the National Registry of Myocardial Infarction from 1990 to 2006. *Am Heart J* 2008;156:1035-1044.
38. A comparison of reteplase with alteplase for acute myocardial infarction. The Global Use of Strategies to Open Occluded Coronary Arteries (GUSTO III) Investigators. *N Engl J Med* 1997;337:1118-1123.
39. Van De Werf F, Adgey J, Ardissino D, et al. Single-bolus tenecteplase compared with front-loaded alteplase in acute myocardial infarction: The ASSENT-2 double-blind randomised trial. *Lancet* 1999;354:716-722.
40. Effectiveness of intravenous thrombolytic treatment in acute myocardial infarction. Gruppo Italiano per lo Studio della Streptochinasi nell'Infarto Miocardico (GISSI). *Lancet* 1986;1:397-402.
41. Vandvik PO, Lincoff AM, Gore JM, et al. Primary and secondary prevention of cardiovascular disease: Antithrombotic Therapy and Prevention of Thrombosis, 9th ed: American College of Chest Physicians Evidence-Based Clinical Practice Guidelines. *Chest* 2012;141:e637S-668S.
42. Mehta SR, Bassand JP, Chrolavicius S, et al. Dose comparisons of clopidogrel and aspirin in acute coronary syndromes. *N Engl J Med* 2010;363:930-942.
43. Mehta SR, Tanguay JF, Eikelboom JW, et al. Double-dose versus standard-dose clopidogrel and high-dose versus low-dose aspirin in individuals undergoing percutaneous coronary intervention for acute coronary syndromes (CURRENT-OASIS 7): A randomised factorial trial. *Lancet* 2010;376:1233-1243.
44. Mahaffey KW, Wojdyla DM, Carroll K, et al. Ticagrelor compared with clopidogrel by geographic region in the Platelet Inhibition and Patient Outcomes (PLATO) trial. *Circulation* 2011;124:544-554.
45. Yu J, Mehran R, Dangas GD, et al. Safety and efficacy of high-versus low-dose aspirin after primary percutaneous coronary intervention in ST-segment elevation myocardial infarction: The HORIZONS-AMI (Harmonizing Outcomes With Revascularization and Stents in Acute Myocardial Infarction) trial. *JACC Cardiovasc Interv* 2012;5:1231-1238.
46. Smith SC Jr., Benjamin EJ, Bonow RO, et al. AHA/ACCF secondary prevention and risk reduction therapy for patients with coronary and other atherosclerotic vascular disease: 2011 update: A guideline from the American Heart Association and American College of Cardiology Foundation endorsed by the World Heart Federation and the Preventive Cardiovascular Nurses Association. *J Am Coll Cardiol* 2011;58:2432-2446.
47. Bhatt DL, Hulot JS, Moliterno DJ, Harrington RA. Antiplatelet and anticoagulation therapy for acute coronary syndromes. *Circ Res* 2014;114:1929-1943.
48. Bhatt DL, Stone GW, Mahaffey KW, et al. Effect of platelet inhibition with cangrelor during PCI on ischemic events. *N Engl J Med* 2013;368:1303-1313.
49. Sofi F, Giusti B, Marcucci R, Gori AM, Abbate R, Gensini GF. Cytochrome P450 2C19*2 polymorphism and cardiovascular recurrences in patients taking clopidogrel: A meta-analysis. *Pharmacogenomics J* 2011;11:199-206.
50. Mega JL, Close SL, Wiviott SD, et al. Cytochrome p-450 polymorphisms and response to clopidogrel. *N Engl J Med* 2009;360:354-362.
51. Mega JL, Close SL, Wiviott SD, et al. Cytochrome P450 genetic polymorphisms and the response to prasugrel: Relationship to pharmacokinetic, pharmacodynamic, and clinical outcomes. *Circulation* 2009;119:2553-2560.
52. Scott SA, Sangkuhl K, Stein CM, et al. Clinical Pharmacogenetics Implementation Consortium guidelines for CYP2C19 genotype and clopidogrel therapy: 2013 update. *Clin Pharmacol Therap* 2013;94:317-323.
53. Siller-Matula JM, Huber K, Christ G, et al. Impact of clopidogrel loading dose on clinical outcome in patients undergoing percutaneous coronary intervention: A systematic review and meta-analysis. *Heart* 2011;97:98-105.
54. Wiviott SD, Braunwald E, McCabe CH, et al. Prasugrel versus clopidogrel in patients with acute coronary syndromes. *N Engl J Med* 2007;357:2001-2015.
55. Montalescot G, Wiviott SD, Braunwald E, et al. Prasugrel compared with clopidogrel in patients undergoing percutaneous coronary intervention for ST-elevation myocardial infarction (TRITON-TIMI 38): Double-blind, randomised controlled trial. *Lancet* 2009;373:723-731.
56. Wiviott SD, Braunwald E, Angiolillo DJ, et al. Greater clinical benefit of more intensive oral antiplatelet therapy with prasugrel in patients with diabetes mellitus in the trial to assess improvement in therapeutic outcomes by optimizing platelet inhibition with prasugrel-Thrombolysis in Myocardial Infarction 38. *Circulation* 2008;118:1626-1636.
57. Wallentin L, Becker RC, Budaj A, et al. Ticagrelor versus clopidogrel in patients with acute coronary syndromes. *N Engl J Med* 2009;361:1045-1057.
58. James SK, Roe MT, Cannon CP, et al. Ticagrelor versus clopidogrel in patients with acute coronary syndromes intended for non-invasive management: Substudy from prospective randomised PLATelet inhibition and patient Outcomes (PLATO) trial. *BMJ* 2011;342:d3527.
59. James S, Angiolillo DJ, Cornel JH, et al. Ticagrelor vs. clopidogrel in patients with acute coronary syndromes and diabetes: A substudy from the PLATelet inhibition and patient Outcomes (PLATO) trial. *Eur Heart J* 2010;31:3006-3016.
60. Steg PG, James S, Harrington RA, et al. Ticagrelor versus clopidogrel in patients with ST-elevation acute coronary syndromes intended for reperfusion with primary percutaneous coronary intervention: A Platelet Inhibition and Patient Outcomes (PLATO) trial subgroup analysis. *Circulation* 2010;122:2131-2141.
61. Cannon CP, Harrington RA, James S, et al. Comparison of ticagrelor with clopidogrel in patients with a planned invasive strategy for acute coronary syndromes (PLATO): A randomised double-blind study. *Lancet* 2010;375:283-293.
62. Crouch MA, Colucci VJ, Howard PA, Spinler SA. $P2Y_{12}$ receptor inhibitors: integrating ticagrelor into the management of acute coronary syndrome. *Ann Pharmacother* 2011;45:1151-1156.
63. Bonaca MP, Bhatt DL, Cohen M, et al. Long-term use of ticagrelor in patients with prior myocardial infarction. *N Engl J Med* 2015;372:1791-1800.
64. Brilinta [package insert]. Wilmington, DE: AstraZeneca LP; 2015.
65. Price MJ, Berger PB, Teirstein PS, et al. Standard- vs high-dose clopidogrel based on platelet function testing after percutaneous coronary intervention: The GRAVITAS randomized trial. *JAMA* 2011;305:1097-1105.
66. Effient [package insert]. Indianapolis, IN: Eli Lilly and Company; 2015.
67. Plavix [package insert]. Bridgewater, NJ: Bristol-Myers Squibb/Sanofi Pharmaceuticals Partnership; July 2015.
68. Campbell KL, Cohn JR, Savage MP. Clopidogrel hypersensitivity: Clinical challenges and options for management. *Expert Rev Clin Pharmacol* 2010;3:553-561.
69. Kengreal [packge insert]. Parsippany, NJ: The Medicines Company; 2015.
70. Chen ZM, Jiang LX, Chen YP, et al. Addition of clopidogrel to aspirin in 45,852 patients with acute myocardial infarction: Randomised placebo-controlled trial. *Lancet* 2005;366:1607-1621.
71. Sabatine MS, Cannon CP, Gibson CM, et al. Addition of clopidogrel to aspirin and fibrinolytic therapy for myocardial infarction with ST-segment elevation. *N Engl J Med* 2005;352:1179-1189.

72. Roberts JD, Wells GA, Le May MR, et al. Point-of-care genetic testing for personalisation of antiplatelet treatment (RAPID GENE): A prospective, randomised, proof-of-concept trial. *Lancet* 2012;379:1705-1711.
73. Scott SA, Sangkuhl K, Stein CM, et al. Clinical Pharmacogenetics Implementation Consortium guidelines for CYP2C19 genotype and clopidogrel therapy: 2013 update. *Clin Pharmacol Therap* 2013;94:317-323.
74. De Luca G, Navarese E, Marino P. Risk profile and benefits from Gp IIb-IIIa inhibitors among patients with ST-segment elevation myocardial infarction treated with primary angioplasty: A meta-regression analysis of randomized trials. *Eur Heart J* 2009;30:2705-2713.
75. Gurm HS, Tamhane U, Meier P, Grossman PM, Chetcuti S, Bates ER. A comparison of abciximab and small-molecule glycoprotein IIb/IIIa inhibitors in patients undergoing primary percutaneous coronary intervention: A meta-analysis of contemporary randomized controlled trials. *Circ Cardiovasc Interv* 2009;2:230-236.
76. Integrilin [package insert]. Whitehouse Station, NJ: Merck & Co., Inc.; April 2014.
77. van 't Hof AW, Valgimigli M. Defining the role of platelet glycoprotein receptor inhibitors in STEMI: focus on tirofiban. *Drugs* 2009;69:85-100.
78. Valgimigli M, Campo G, Percoco G, et al. Comparison of angioplasty with infusion of tirofiban or abciximab and with implantation of sirolimus-eluting or uncoated stents for acute myocardial infarction: The MULTISTRATEGY randomized trial. *JAMA* 2008;299:1788-1799.
79. Aggrastat [package insert]. Somerset, NJ: Medicure Pharma, Inc.; April 2015.
80. Reopro [package insert]. Indianapolis, IN: Eli Lilly and Company; November 2013.
81. Eikelboom JW, Quinlan DJ, Mehta SR, Turpie AG, Menown IB, Yusuf S. Unfractionated and low-molecular-weight heparin as adjuncts to thrombolysis in aspirin-treated patients with ST-elevation acute myocardial infarction: a meta-analysis of the randomized trials. *Circulation* 2005;112:3855-3867.
82. Stone GW, Witzenbichler B, Guagliumi G, et al. Heparin plus a glycoprotein IIb/IIIa inhibitor versus bivalirudin monotherapy and paclitaxel-eluting stents versus bare-metal stents in acute myocardial infarction (HORIZONS-AMI): Final 3-year results from a multicentre, randomised controlled trial. *Lancet* 2011;377: 2193-2204.
83. Stone GW, Witzenbichler B, Guagliumi G, et al. Bivalirudin during primary PCI in acute myocardial infarction. *N Engl J Med* 2008;358: 2218-2230.
84. Antman EM, Morrow DA, McCabe CH, et al. Enoxaparin versus unfractionated heparin with fibrinolysis for ST-elevation myocardial infarction. *N Engl J Med* 2006;354:1477-1488.
85. Gore JM, Spencer FA, Gurfinkel EP, et al. Thrombocytopenia in patients with an acute coronary syndrome (from the Global Registry of Acute Coronary Events [GRACE]). *Am J Cardiol* 2009;103:175-180.
86. Steg PG, van 't Hof A, Hamm CW, et al. Bivalirudin started during emergency transport for primary PCI. *N Engl J Med* 2013;369:2207-2217.
87. Shahzad A, Kemp I, Mars C, et al. Unfractionated heparin versus bivalirudin in primary percutaneous coronary intervention (HEAT-PPCI): An open-label, single centre, randomised controlled trial. *Lancet* 2014;384:1849-1858.
88. Han Y, Guo J, Zheng Y, et al. Bivalirudin vs heparin with or without tirofiban during primary percutaneous coronary intervention in acute myocardial infarction: The BRIGHT randomized clinical trial. *JAMA* 2015;313:1336-1346.
89. Valgimigli M, Frigoli E, Leonardi S, et al. Bivalirudin or unfractionated Heparin in acute coronary syndromes. *N Engl J Med* 2015;373:997-1009.
90. Capodanno D, Gargiulo G, Capranzano P, Mehran R, Tamburino C, Stone GW. Bivalirudin versus heparin with or without glycoprotein IIb/IIIa inhibitors in patients with STEMI undergoing primary PCI: An updated meta-analysis of 10,350 patients from five randomized clinical trials. *Eur Heart J Acute Cardiovasc Care* 2016;5(3):253-262.
91. Chen ZM, Pan HC, Chen YP, et al. Early intravenous then oral metoprolol in 45,852 patients with acute myocardial infarction: Randomised placebo-controlled trial. *Lancet* 2005;366:1622-1632.
92. Stone GW, McLaurin BT, Cox DA, et al. Bivalirudin for patients with acute coronary syndromes. *N Engl J Med* 2006;355:2203-2216.
93. Kastrati A, Neumann FJ, Schulz S, et al. Abciximab and heparin versus bivalirudin for non-ST-elevation myocardial infarction. *N Engl J Med* 2011;365:1980-1989.
94. Oler A, Whooley MA, Oler J, Grady D. Adding heparin to aspirin reduces the incidence of myocardial infarction and death in patients with unstable angina. A meta-analysis. *JAMA* 1996;276:811-815.
95. Low-molecular-weight heparin during instability in coronary artery disease, Fragmin during Instability in Coronary Artery Disease (FRISC) study group. *Lancet* 1996;347:561-568.
96. Yusuf S, Mehta SR, Chrolavicius S, et al. Effects of fondaparinux on mortality and reinfarction in patients with acute ST-segment elevation myocardial infarction: The OASIS-6 randomized trial. *JAMA* 2006;295:1519-1530.
97. Hillis LD, Smith PK, Anderson JL, et al. 2011 ACCF/AHA Guideline for Coronary Artery Bypass Graft Surgery. A report of the American College of Cardiology Foundation/American Heart Association Task Force on Practice Guidelines. Developed in collaboration with the American Association for Thoracic Surgery, Society of Cardiovascular Anesthesiologists, and Society of Thoracic Surgeons. *J Am Coll Cardiol* 2011;58:e123-210.
98. Lovenox [package insert]. Bridgewater, NJ: Sanofi-Aventis U.S. LLC; October 2013.
99. Mehta SR, Yusuf S, Peters RJ, et al. Effects of pretreatment with clopidogrel and aspirin followed by long-term therapy in patients undergoing percutaneous coronary intervention: The PCI-CURE study. *Lancet* 2001;358:527-533.
100. Giugliano RP, White JA, Bode C, et al. Early versus delayed, provisional eptifibatide in acute coronary syndromes. *N Engl J Med* 2009;360:2176-2190.
101. Stone NJ, Robinson JG, Lichtenstein AH, et al. 2013 ACC/AHA guideline on the treatment of blood cholesterol to reduce atherosclerotic cardiovascular risk in adults: A report of the American College of Cardiology/American Heart Association Task Force on Practice Guidelines. *J Am Coll Cardiol* 2014;63: 2889-2934.
102. Serebruany VL, Malinin AI, Eisert RM, Sane DC. Risk of bleeding complications with antiplatelet agents: Meta-analysis of 338,191 patients enrolled in 50 randomized controlled trials. *Am J Hematol* 2004;75:40-47.
103. Serebruany VL, Malinin AI, Ferguson JJ, Vahabi J, Atar D, Hennekens CH. Bleeding risks of combination vs. single antiplatelet therapy: A meta-analysis of 18 randomized trials comprising 129,314 patients. *Fundam Clin Pharmacol* 2008;22:315-321.
104. Budnitz DS, Lovegrove MC, Shehab N, Richards CL. Emergency hospitalizations for adverse drug events in older Americans. *N Engl J Med* 2011;365:2002-2012.
105. Becker RC, Bassand JP, Budaj A, et al. Bleeding complications with the $P2Y_{12}$ receptor antagonists clopidogrel and ticagrelor in the PLATelet inhibition and patient Outcomes (PLATO) trial. *Eur Heart J* 2011;32:2933-2944.
106. Wiviott SD, Desai N, Murphy SA, et al. Efficacy and safety of intensive antiplatelet therapy with prasugrel from TRITON-TIMI 38 in a core clinical cohort defined by worldwide regulatory agencies. *Am J Cardiol* 2011;108:905-911.
107. Zhao HJ, Zheng ZT, Wang ZH, et al. "Triple therapy" rather than "triple threat": A meta-analysis of the two antithrombotic regimens after stent implantation in patients receiving long-term oral anticoagulant treatment. *Chest* 2011;139:260-270.
108. Liu J, Fan M, Zhao J, et al. Efficacy and safety of antithrombotic regimens after coronary intervention in patients on oral anticoagulation: Traditional and Bayesian meta-analysis of clinical trials. *Int J Cardiol* 2016;205:89-96.
109. Faxon DP, Eikelboom JW, Berger PB, et al. Antithrombotic therapy in patients with atrial fibrillation undergoing coronary stenting: A North American perspective: executive summary. *Circ Cardiovasc Interv* 2011;4:522-534.
110. Dewilde WJ, Oirbans T, Verheugt FW, et al. Use of clopidogrel with or without aspirin in patients taking oral anticoagulant therapy and undergoing percutaneous coronary intervention: An open-label, randomised, controlled trial. *Lancet* 2013;381:1107-1115.
111. Alexander JH, Lopes RD, James S, et al. Apixaban with antiplatelet therapy after acute coronary syndrome. *N Engl J Med* 2011;365: 699-708.
112. Mega JL, Braunwald E, Wiviott SD, et al. Rivaroxaban in patients with a recent acute coronary syndrome. *N Engl J Med* 2012;366:9-19.
113. Roffi M, Patrono C, Collet JP, et al. 2015 ESC Guidelines for the management of acute coronary syndromes in patients presenting without persistent ST-segment elevation: Task Force for the

Management of Acute Coronary Syndromes in Patients Presenting without Persistent ST-Segment Elevation of the European Society of Cardiology (ESC). *Eur Heart J* 2015.

114. Freemantle N, Cleland J, Young P, Mason J, Harrison J. beta Blockade after myocardial infarction: Systematic review and meta regression analysis. *BMJ* 1999;318:1730-1737.
115. Houghton T, Freemantle N, Cleland JG. Are beta-blockers effective in patients who develop heart failure soon after myocardial infarction? A meta-regression analysis of randomised trials. *Eur J Heart Fail* 2000;2:333-340.
116. Dargie HJ. Effect of carvedilol on outcome after myocardial infarction in patients with left-ventricular dysfunction: The CAPRICORN randomised trial. *Lancet* 2001;357:1385-1390.
117. Fihn SD, Gardin JM, Abrams J, et al. 2012 ACCF/AHA/ACP/AATS/PCNA/SCAI/STS Guideline for the diagnosis and management of patients with stable ischemic heart disease: A report of the American College of Cardiology Foundation/American Heart Association Task Force on Practice Guidelines, and the American College of Physicians, American Association for Thoracic Surgery, Preventive Cardiovascular Nurses Association, Society for Cardiovascular Angiography and Interventions, and Society of Thoracic Surgeons. *J Am Coll Cardiol* 2012;60:e44-e164.
118. Danchin N, Cucherat M, Thuillez C, Durand E, Kadri Z, Steg PG. Angiotensin-converting enzyme inhibitors in patients with coronary artery disease and absence of heart failure or left ventricular systolic dysfunction: An overview of long-term randomized controlled trials. *Arch Int Med* 2006;166:787-796.
119. Indications for ACE inhibitors in the early treatment of acute myocardial infarction: Systematic overview of individual data from 100,000 patients in randomized trials. ACE Inhibitor Myocardial Infarction Collaborative Group. *Circulation* 1998;97:2202-2212.
120. Swedberg K, Held P, Kjekshus J, Rasmussen K, Ryden L, Wedel H. Effects of the early administration of enalapril on mortality in patients with acute myocardial infarction. Results of the Cooperative New Scandinavian Enalapril Survival Study II (CONSENSUS II). *N Engl J Med* 1992;327:678-684.
121. Pfeffer MA, McMurray JJ, Velazquez EJ, et al. Valsartan, captopril, or both in myocardial infarction complicated by heart failure, left ventricular dysfunction, or both. *N Engl J Med* 2003;349:1893-1906.
122. Granger CB, McMurray JJ, Yusuf S, et al. Effects of candesartan in patients with chronic heart failure and reduced left-ventricular systolic function intolerant to angiotensin-converting-enzyme inhibitors: The CHARM-Alternative trial. *Lancet* 2003;362:772-776.
123. Makkar KM, Sanoski CA, Spinler SA. Role of angiotensin-converting enzyme inhibitors, angiotensin II receptor blockers, and aldosterone antagonists in the prevention of atrial and ventricular arrhythmias. *Pharmacotherapy* 2009;29:31-48.
124. Pitt B, Zannad F, Remme WJ, et al. The effect of spironolactone on morbidity and mortality in patients with severe heart failure. Randomized Aldactone Evaluation Study Investigators. *N Engl J Med* 1999;341:709-717.
125. Pitt B, Remme W, Zannad F, et al. Eplerenone, a selective aldosterone blocker, in patients with left ventricular dysfunction after myocardial infarction. *N Engl J Med* 2003;348:1309-1321.
126. Zannad F, McMurray JJ, Krum H, et al. Eplerenone in patients with systolic heart failure and mild symptoms. *N Engl J Med* 2011;364:11-21.
127. Hulten E, Jackson JL, Douglas K, George S, Villines TC. The effect of early, intensive statin therapy on acute coronary syndrome: A meta-analysis of randomized controlled trials. *Arch Int Med* 2006;166:1814-1821.
128. Lloyd-Jones DM, Morris PB, Ballantyne CM, et al. 2016 ACC Expert Consensus Decision Pathway on the Role of Non-statin Therapies for LDL-Cholesterol Lowering in the Management of Atherosclerotic Cardiovascular Disease Risk. J Am Coll Cardiol. 2016;68(1):92-125.
129. Cannon CP, Blazing MA, Giugliano RP, et al. Ezetimibe added to statin therapy after acute coronary syndromes. *N Engl J Med* 2015;372:2387-2397.
130. PCSK9 Inhibitors for Treatment of High Cholesterol: Effectiveness, Value, and Value-Based Price Benchmarks. November 2015. Available at: http://cepac.icer-review.org/wp-content/uploads/2015/04/Final-Report-for-Posting-11-24-15.pdf. (Last accessed, February 1, 2016)
131. Schwartz GG, Bessac L, Berdan LG, et al. Effect of alirocumab, a monoclonal antibody to PCSK9, on long-term cardiovascular outcomes following acute coronary syndromes: Rationale and design of the ODYSSEY outcomes trial. *Am Heart J* 2014;168:682-689.
132. Sabatine MS, Giugliano RP, Wiviott SD, et al. Efficacy and safety of evolocumab in reducing lipids and cardiovascular events. *N Engl J Med* 2015;372:1500-1509.
133. Robinson JG, Farnier M, Krempf M, et al. Efficacy and safety of alirocumab in reducing lipids and cardiovascular events. *N Engl J Med* 2015;372:1489-1499.
134. Kereiakes DJ, Robinson JG, Cannon CP, et al. Efficacy and safety of the proprotein convertase subtilisin/kexin type 9 inhibitor alirocumab among high cardiovascular risk patients on maximally tolerated statin therapy: The ODYSSEY COMBO I study. *Am Heart J* 2015;169:906-915. e13.
135. James PA, Oparil S, Carter BL, et al. 2014 evidence-based guideline for the management of high blood pressure in adults: Report from the panel members appointed to the Eighth Joint National Committee (JNC 8). *JAMA* 2014;311:507-520.
136. Ho PM, Spertus JA, Masoudi FA, et al. Impact of medication therapy discontinuation on mortality after myocardial infarction. *Arch Int Med* 2006;166:1842-1847.

18

The Arrhythmias

Cynthia A. Sanoski and Jerry L. Bauman

KEY CONCEPTS

1. The use of antiarrhythmic drugs (AADs) in the United States has declined because of major trials that show increased mortality with their use in several clinical situations, the realization of proarrhythmia as a significant side effect, and the advancing technology of nonpharmacologic therapies such as ablation and the implantable cardioverter-defibrillator (ICD).
2. AADs frequently cause side effects and are complex in their pharmacokinetic characteristics. Close monitoring is required of all of these drugs to assess for adverse effects as well as potential drug interactions.
3. The most commonly prescribed AAD is now amiodarone. This drug is effective in terminating and preventing a wide variety of symptomatic supraventricular and ventricular arrhythmias. However, because this AAD is plagued by frequent side effects, it requires close monitoring. The most concerning toxicity is pulmonary fibrosis; side effect profiles of the intravenous (IV) (acute, short-term) and oral (chronic, long-term) forms of amiodarone differ substantially.
4. In patients with atrial fibrillation (AF), therapy is traditionally aimed at controlling ventricular rate (digoxin, nondihydropyridine (non-DHP) calcium channel blockers (CCBs), β-blockers), preventing thromboembolic (TE) complications (warfarin, aspirin), and restoring and maintaining sinus rhythm (SR) (AADs, direct current cardioversion). Studies show there is no need to aggressively pursue strategies to maintain SR (ie, long-term AAD therapy); rate control alone (leaving the patient in AF) is often sufficient in patients who can tolerate it. Nonetheless, chronic AAD therapy may still be needed in patients who continue to have symptoms despite adequate ventricular rate control.
5. Paroxysmal supraventricular tachycardia (PSVT) is usually a result of reentry in or proximal to the atrioventricular (AV) node or AV reentry incorporating an extranodal pathway; common tachycardias can be terminated acutely with AV nodal blocking drugs such as adenosine, and recurrences can be prevented by ablation with radiofrequency current.
6. Patients with Wolff-Parkinson-White (WPW) syndrome may have several different tachycardias that are acutely treated by different strategies: orthodromic reentry (adenosine), antidromic reentry (adenosine or procainamide), and AF (procainamide or amiodarone). AV nodal blocking drugs are contraindicated in patients with WPW syndrome and AF.
7. Because of the results of the Cardiac Arrhythmia Suppression Trial (CAST) and other trials, AADs (with the exception of β-blockers) should not be routinely used in patients with prior myocardial infarction (MI) or left ventricular (LV) dysfunction and minor ventricular rhythm disturbances (eg, premature ventricular complexes [PVCs]).
8. Patients with hemodynamically significant ventricular tachycardia (VT) or ventricular fibrillation not associated with an acute MI who are successfully resuscitated (with electrical cardioversion, epinephrine, amiodarone) are at high risk for sudden cardiac death (SCD) and should receive an ICD ("secondary prevention").
9. Implantation of an ICD should be considered for the primary prevention of SCD in certain high-risk patient populations. High-risk patients include those with a history of MI and LV dysfunction (regardless of whether they have inducible sustained ventricular arrhythmias), as well as those with New York Heart Association (NYHA) class II or III heart failure (HF) as a result of either ischemic or nonischemic causes.
10. Life-threatening ventricular proarrhythmia generally takes two forms: sinusoidal or incessant monomorphic VT (class Ic AADs) and torsade de pointes (TdP) (class Ia or III AADs and many other noncardiac drugs).

The heart has two basic properties, namely, an electrical property and a mechanical property. The synchronous interaction between these two properties is complex, precise, and relatively enduring. The study of the electrical properties of the heart has grown at a steady rate, interrupted by periodic salvos of scientific breakthroughs. Einthoven's pioneering work allowed graphic electrical tracings of cardiac rhythm and probably represents the first of these breakthroughs. This discovery of the surface electrocardiogram (ECG) has remained the cornerstone of diagnostic tools for cardiac rhythm disturbances. Since then, intracardiac recordings and programmed cardiac stimulation have advanced our understanding of arrhythmias, and microelectrode, voltage clamping, and patch clamping techniques have allowed considerable insight into the electrophysiologic actions and mechanisms of AADs. Certainly, the new era of molecular biology and mapping of the human genome promises even greater insights into mechanisms (and potential therapies) of arrhythmias. Noteworthy in this regard is the discovery of genetic abnormalities in the ion channels that control electrical repolarization (heritable long QT syndrome) or depolarization (Brugada syndrome).

The clinical use of drug therapy started with the use of digitalis and then quinidine. A surge of new agents followed somewhat later in the 1980s. A theme of drug discovery during this decade was initially to find orally absorbed lidocaine congeners (such as mexiletine and tocainide); later, the emphasis was on drugs with extremely potent effects on conduction (ie, flecainide-like agents). The most recent focus of investigational AADs is the potassium channel blockers, with dronedarone being the most recently approved AAD in the United States in nearly a decade. Previously, there was some expectation that advances in AAD discovery would lead to a highly effective and nontoxic agent that would be effective for a majority of patients (ie, the so-called magic bullet). Instead, significant problems with drug toxicity and proarrhythmia have resulted in a decline in the overall volume of AAD usage in the United States since 1989. 1 The other phenomenon that has significantly contributed to the decline in AAD utilization is the development of extremely effective nonpharmacologic therapies. Technical advances have made it possible to permanently interrupt reentry circuits with radiofrequency ablation, which renders long-term AAD use unnecessary in certain arrhythmias. Furthermore, the impressive survival data associated with the use of ICDs for the primary and secondary prevention of SCD have led most clinicians to choose "device" therapy as the first-line treatment for patients who are at high risk for life-threatening ventricular arrhythmias. Both of these nonpharmacologic therapies have become increasingly popular for the management of arrhythmias so that the potential proarrhythmic effects and organ toxicities associated with AADs can be avoided.

This chapter reviews the principles involved in both normal and abnormal cardiac conduction and addresses the pathophysiology and treatment of the more commonly encountered arrhythmias. Certainly, many volumes of complete text could be (and have been) devoted to basic and clinical electrophysiology. Consequently, this chapter briefly addresses those principles necessary for clinicians.

ARRHYTHMOGENESIS

Normal Conduction

Electrical activity is initiated by the sinoatrial (SA) node and moves through cardiac tissue by a tree-like conduction network. The SA node initiates cardiac rhythm under normal circumstances because this tissue possesses the highest degree of automaticity or rate of spontaneous impulse generation. The degree of automaticity of the SA node is largely influenced by the autonomic nervous system in that both cholinergic and sympathetic innervations control the sinus rate. Most tissues within the conduction system also possess varying degrees of inherent automatic properties. However, the rates of spontaneous impulse generation of these tissues are less than that of the SA node. Thus, these latent automatic pacemakers are continuously overdriven by impulses arising from the SA node (primary pacemaker) and do not become clinically apparent.

From the SA node, electrical activity moves in a wave front through an atrial specialized conducting system and eventually gains entrance to the ventricle via the AV node and a large bundle of conducting tissue referred to as the bundle of His. The conducting tissues bridging the atria and ventricles are referred to as the junctional areas. Again, this area of tissue (junction) is largely influenced by autonomic input and possesses a relatively high degree of inherent automaticity (about 40 beats/min which is less than that of the SA node). From the bundle of His, the cardiac conduction system bifurcates into several (usually three) bundle branches: one right bundle and two left bundles. These bundle branches further arborize into a conduction network referred to as the Purkinje system. The conduction system as a whole innervates the mechanical myocardium and serves to initiate excitation-contraction coupling and the contractile process. After a cell or group of cells within the heart is electrically stimulated, a brief period of time follows in which those cells cannot again be excited. This time period is referred to as the refractory period. As the electrical wave front moves down the conduction system, the impulse eventually encounters tissue refractory to stimulation (recently excited) and subsequently dies out. The SA node subsequently recovers, fires spontaneously, and begins the process again.

Prior to cellular excitation, an electrical gradient exists between the inside and the outside of the cardiac cell membrane. At this time, the cell is polarized. In atrial and ventricular conducting tissues, the intracellular space is approximately −80 to −90 mV with respect to the extracellular environment. The electrical gradient just prior to excitation is referred to as the resting membrane potential (RMP) and is the result of differences in ion concentrations between the inside and the outside of the cell. At RMP, the cell is polarized primarily by the action of active membrane ion pumps, the most notable of these being the sodium-potassium pump. For example, this specific pump (in addition to other systems) attempts to maintain the intracellular sodium concentration at 5 to 15 mEq/L and the extracellular sodium concentration at 135 to 142 mEq/L, as well as the intracellular potassium concentration at 135 to 140 mEq/L and the extracellular potassium concentration at 3 to 5 mEq/L.

Electrical stimulation (or depolarization) of the cell will result in changes in membrane potential over time or a characteristic action potential curve (Fig. 18-1). The action potential curve results from the transmembrane movement of specific ions and is divided into different phases. Phase 0 or initial, rapid depolarization of atrial and ventricular tissues is caused by an abrupt increase in the permeability of the membrane to sodium influx. This rapid depolarization more than equilibrates (overshoots) the electrical potential, resulting in a brief initial repolarization or phase 1. Phase 1 (initial repolarization) is caused by a transient and active potassium efflux (ie, the I_{Kto} current). Calcium begins to move into the intracellular space at about −60 mV (during phase 0), causing a slower depolarization. Calcium influx continues throughout phase 2 of the action potential (plateau phase) and is balanced to some degree by potassium efflux. Calcium entrance (only through L channels in myocardial tissue) distinguishes cardiac conducting cells from nerve tissue and provides the critical ionic link to excitation-contraction coupling and the mechanical properties of the heart as a pump. The membrane remains permeable to potassium efflux during phase 3, resulting in cellular repolarization. Phase 4 of the action potential is the gradual depolarization of the cell and is related to a constant sodium leak into the intracellular space balanced by a decreasing (over time) efflux of potassium. The slope of phase 4 depolarization determines, in large part, the automatic properties of the cell. As the cell is slowly depolarized during phase 4, an abrupt increase in sodium permeability occurs, allowing the rapid cellular depolarization of phase 0. The juncture of phase 4 and phase 0 where rapid sodium influx is initiated is referred to as the threshold potential of the cell. The level of threshold potential also regulates the degree of cellular automaticity.

Not all cells in the cardiac conduction system rely on sodium influx for initial depolarization. Some tissues depolarize in response to a slower inward ionic current caused by calcium influx. These "calcium-dependent" tissues are found primarily in the SA and AV nodes (both L and T channels) and possess distinct conduction properties in comparison to "sodium-dependent" fibers. Calcium-dependent cells generally have a less negative RMP (−40 to −60 mV) and a slower conduction velocity. Furthermore, in calcium-dependent tissues, recovery of excitability outlasts full repolarization, whereas in sodium-dependent tissues, recovery is prompt after repolarization. These two types of electrical tissues also differ dramatically in how drugs modify their conduction properties.

Ion conductance across the lipid bilayer of the cell membrane occurs via the formation of membrane pores or "channels" (Fig. 18-2). Selective ion channels probably form in response to specific electrical potential differences between the inside and the outside of the cell (voltage dependence). The membrane itself is composed of both organized and disorganized lipids and phospholipids in a dynamic sol-gel matrix. During ion flux and electrical excitation, changes in this sol-gel equilibrium occur and permit the formation of activated ion channels. Besides channel formation and membrane composition, intrachannel proteins or phospholipids, referred to as gates, also regulate the transmembrane movement of ions. These gates are thought to be positioned strategically within the channel to modulate ion flow. Each ion channel conceptually

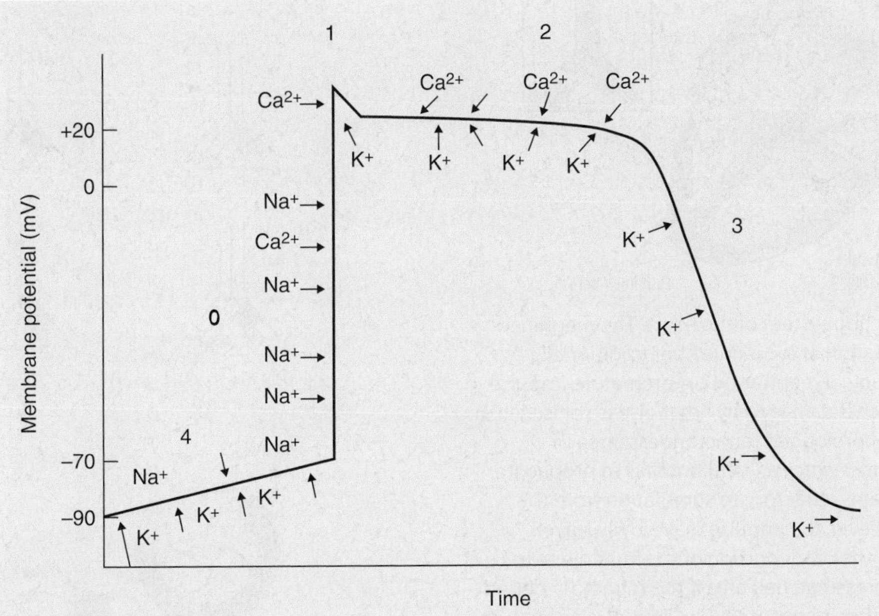

FIGURE 18-1 Purkinje fiber action potential showing specific ion flux responsible for the change in membrane potential. Ions outside of the line (eg, sodium) move from the extracellular space to the intracellular space and ions on the inside of the line (eg, potassium) move from the inside of the cell to the outside.

has two types of gates: an activation gate and an inactivation gate (see Fig. 18-2). The activation gate opens during depolarization to allow the ion current to enter or exit from the cell, and the inactivation gate later closes to stop ion movement. When the cell is in a rested state, the activation gates are closed and the inactivation gates are open. The activation gates then open to allow ion movement through the channel, and the inactivation gates later close to stop ion conductance. Thus, the cell cycles between three states: resting, activated or open, and inactivated or closed. Activation of SA and AV nodal tissue is dependent on a slow depolarizing current through calcium channels and gates, whereas the activation of atrial and ventricular tissues is dependent on a rapid depolarizing current through sodium channels and gates.

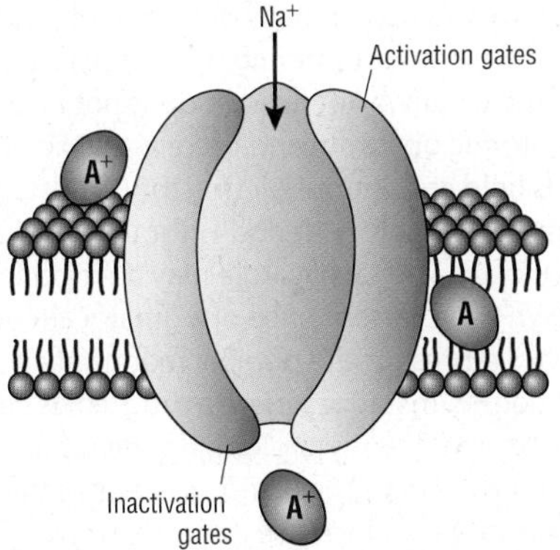

FIGURE 18-2 Lipid bilayer, sodium channel, and possible sites of action of the class I AADs (*A*). Class I AADs may theoretically inhibit sodium influx at an extracellular, intramembrane, or intracellular receptor site. However, all approved agents appear to block sodium conductance at a single receptor site by gaining entrance to the interior of the channel from an intracellular route. Active ionized drugs block the channel predominantly during the activated or inactivated state and bind and unbind with specific time constants (described as fast on-off, slow on-off, and intermediate). (AADs, antiarrhythmic drugs.)

Abnormal Conduction

The mechanisms of tachyarrhythmias have been classically divided into two general categories: those resulting from an abnormality in impulse generation or "automatic" tachycardias and those resulting from an abnormality in impulse conduction or "reentrant" tachycardias.

Automatic tachycardias depend on spontaneous impulse generation in latent pacemakers and may be a result of several different mechanisms. Drugs, such as digoxin or catecholamines, and conditions, such as hypoxia, electrolyte abnormalities (eg, hypokalemia), and fiber stretch (cardiac dilation), may lead to an increased slope of phase 4 depolarization in cardiac tissues other than the SA node. These factors that experimentally lead to abnormal automaticity are also known to be arrhythmogenic in clinical situations. The increased slope of phase 4 causes heightened automaticity of these tissues and competition with the SA node for dominance of cardiac rhythm. If the rate of spontaneous impulse generation of the abnormally automatic tissue exceeds that of the SA node, then an automatic tachycardia may result. Automatic tachycardias have the following characteristics: (a) the onset of the tachycardia is unrelated to an initiating event such as a premature beat; (b) the initiating beat is usually identical to subsequent beats of the tachycardia; (c) the tachycardia cannot be initiated by programmed cardiac stimulation; and (d) the onset of the tachycardia is usually preceded by a gradual acceleration in rate and termination is usually preceded by a gradual deceleration in rate. Clinical tachycardias resulting from the classic forms of enhanced automaticity already described are not as common as once thought. Examples are sinus tachycardia and junctional tachycardia.

Triggered automaticity is also a possible mechanism for abnormal impulse generation. Briefly, triggered automaticity refers to transient membrane depolarizations that occur during repolarization (early afterdepolarizations [EADs]) or after repolarization (late afterdepolarizations [LADs]) but prior to phase 4 of the action potential. Afterdepolarizations may be related to abnormal calcium and sodium influx during or just after full cellular repolarization. Experimentally, EADs may be precipitated by hypokalemia, class Ia AADs, or slow stimulation rates—any factor that blocks the ion channels (eg, potassium) responsible for cellular repolarization.

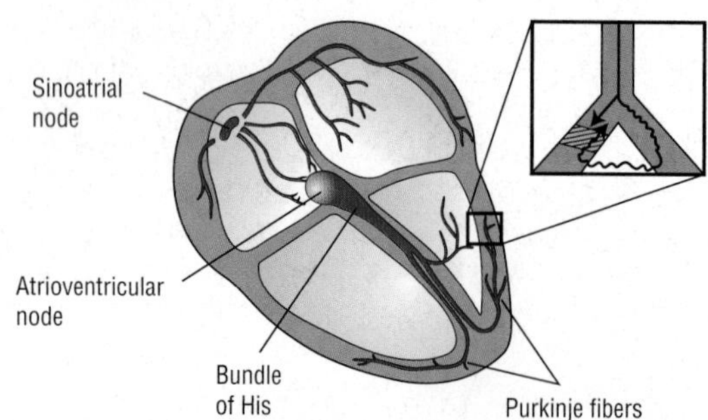

FIGURE 18-3 Conduction system of the heart. The magnified portion shows a bifurcation of a Purkinje fiber traditionally explained as the etiology of reentrant VT. A premature impulse travels to the fiber which is damaged by heart disease or ischemia. It encounters a zone of prolonged refractoriness (area of unidirectional block; *cross-hatched area*) but fails to propagate because the fiber remains refractory to stimulation from the previous impulse. However, the impulse may slowly travel (*squiggly line*) through the other portion of the Purkinje twig and will "reenter" the cross-hatched area if the refractory period is concluded and the fiber is now excitable. Thus, the premature impulse never meets refractory tissue; circus movement ensues. If this site stimulates the surrounding ventricle repetitively, clinical reentrant VT results. (VT, ventricular tachycardia.)

EADs provoked by drugs that block potassium conductance and delay repolarization are the underlying cause of TdP. LADs may be precipitated by digoxin or catecholamines and suppressed by CCBs, and have been suggested as the mechanism for multifocal atrial tachycardia, digoxin-induced tachycardias, and exercise-provoked VT. Triggered automatic rhythms possess some of the characteristics of automatic tachycardias and some of the characteristics of reentrant tachycardias (description follows).

Reentry is a concept that involves indefinite propagation of the impulse and continued activation of previously refractory tissue. There are three conduction requirements for the formation of a viable reentrant focus: (1) two pathways for impulse conduction, (2) an area of unidirectional block (prolonged refractoriness) in one of these pathways, and (3) slow conduction in the other pathway (Fig. 18-3). Usually, a critically timed premature beat initiates reentry. This premature impulse enters both conduction pathways but encounters refractory tissue in one of the pathways at the area of unidirectional block. The impulse dies out because the tissue is still refractory from the previous (sinus) impulse. Although it fails to propagate in one pathway, the impulse may still proceed in a forward direction (antegrade) through the other pathway because of this pathway's relatively shorter refractory period. The impulse may then proceed through a loop of tissue and "reenter" the area of unidirectional block in a backward direction (retrograde). Because the antegrade pathway has slow conduction characteristics, the area of unidirectional block has time to recover its excitability. The impulse can proceed in a retrograde fashion through this previously refractory tissue and continue around the loop of tissue in a circular fashion. Thus, the key to the formation of a reentrant focus is crucial conduction discrepancies in the electrophysiologic characteristics of the two pathways. The reentrant focus may excite surrounding tissue at a rate greater than that of the SA node, leading to formation of a clinical tachycardia. The above model is anatomically determined in that there is only one pathway for impulse conduction with a fixed circuit length. Another model of reentry, referred to as a functional reentrant loop or leading circle model, may also occur (Fig. 18-4).[1] In a functional reentrant focus, the length of the circuit may vary depending on the conduction velocity and recovery characteristics of the impulse. The area in the middle of the loop is continually kept refractory by the inwardly moving impulse. The length of the circuit is not fixed but is the smallest circle possible, such that the leading edge of the wave front is continuously exciting tissue just as it recovers. It differs from the anatomic model in that the leading edge of the

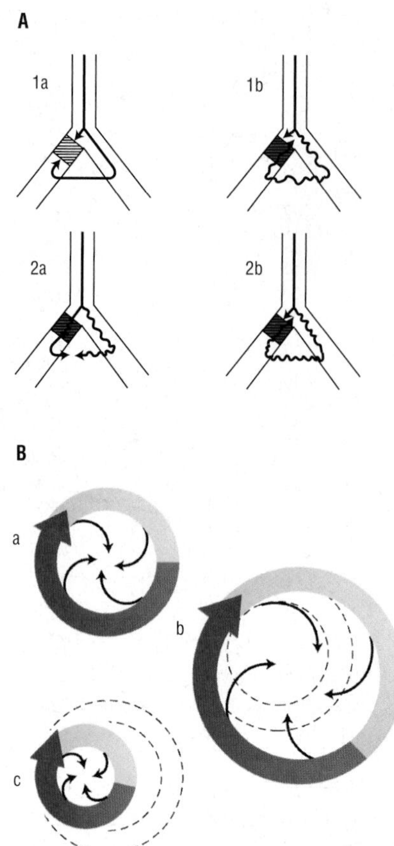

FIGURE 18-4 *A.* Possible mechanism of proarrhythmia in the anatomic model of reentry. *1a.* Nonviable reentrant loop due to bidirectional block (*shaded area*). *1b.* Instance where a drug slows conduction velocity without significantly prolonging the refractory period. The impulse is now able to reenter the area of unidirectional block (*shaded area*) because slowed conduction through the antegrade pathway allows recovery of the block. A new reentrant tachycardia may result. *2a.* Nonviable reentrant loop due to a lack of a unidirectional block. *2b.* Instance where a drug prolongs the refractory period without significantly slowing conduction velocity. The impulse moving antegrade meets refractory tissue (*shaded area*) allowing for unidirectional block. A new reentrant tachycardia may result. *B.* Mechanism of reentry and proarrhythmia. *a.* Functionally determined (*leading circle*) reentrant circuit. This model should be contrasted with anatomic reentry; here the circuit is not fixed (it does not necessarily move around an anatomic obstacle) and there is no excitable gap. All tissue inside is held continuously refractory. *b.* Instance where a drug prolongs the refractory period without significantly slowing conduction velocity. The tachycardia may terminate or slow in rate as shown as a consequence of a greater circuit length. The *dashed lines* represent the original reentrant circuit prior to drug treatment. *c.* Instance where a drug slows conduction velocity without significantly prolonging the refractory period (ie, class Ic *antiarrhythmic drugs*) and accelerates the tachycardia. The tachycardia rate may increase (proarrhythmia) as shown as a consequence of a shorter circuit length. The dashed lines represent the original reentrant circuit prior to drug treatment. *(Reproduced with permission from McCollam PL, Parker RB, Beckman KJ, et al. Proarrhythmia: A paradoxic response to antiarrhythmic agents.* Pharmacotherapy *1989;9:146.)*

impulse is not preceded by an excitable gap of tissue, and it does not have an obstacle in the middle or a fixed anatomic circuit. Clinically, many reentrant foci probably have both anatomic and functional characteristics. In the figure 8 model, a zone of unidirectional block is present, allowing for two impulse loops that join and reenter the area of block in a retrograde fashion to form a pretzel-shaped reentrant circuit. This model combines functional characteristics with an excitable gap. All of these theoretical models require a critical balance of refractoriness and conduction velocity within the circuit and as such have helped to explain the effects of drugs on terminating, modifying, and causing cardiac rhythm disturbances.

What causes reentry to become clinically manifest? Reentrant foci may occur at any level of the conduction system: within the branches of the specialized atrial conduction system, within the Purkinje network, and even within portions of the SA and AV nodes. The anatomy of the Purkinje system appears to provide a suitable substrate for the formation of microreentrant loops and is often used as a model to facilitate the understanding of reentry concepts. Of course, because reentry does not usually occur in normal, healthy conduction tissue, various forms of heart disease or conduction abnormalities must usually be present before reentry becomes manifest. In other words, the various forms of heart disease (eg, coronary artery disease [CAD], LV dysfunction) can result in changes in conduction in the pathways of a suitable reentrant substrate. An often-used example is reentry occurring as a consequence of ischemic or hypoxic damage; with inadequate cellular oxygen, cardiac tissue resorts to anaerobic glycolysis for adenosine triphosphate production. As high-energy phosphate concentrations diminish, the activity of the transmembrane ion pumps declines and RMP rises. This rise in RMP causes inactivation in the voltage-dependent sodium channel, and the tissue begins to assume slow conduction characteristics. If changes in conduction parameters occur in a discordant manner due to varying degrees of ischemia or hypoxia, then a reentry circuit may become manifest. Furthermore, an ischemic, dying cell liberates intracellular potassium, which also causes a rise in RMP. In other cases, reentry may occur as a consequence of anatomic or functional variants in the normal conduction system. For instance, patients may possess two (instead of one) conduction pathways near or within the AV node, or have an anomalous extranodal AV pathway that possesses different electrophysiologic characteristics from the normal AV nodal pathway. Reentry in these cases may occur within the AV node or encompass both atrial and ventricular tissues. Reentrant tachycardias have the following characteristics: (a) the onset of the tachycardia is usually related to an initiating event (ie, premature beat); (b) the initiating beat is usually different in morphology from subsequent beats of the tachycardia; (c) the initiation of the tachycardia can usually be incited with programmed cardiac stimulation; and (d) the initiation and termination of the tachycardia is usually abrupt without an acceleration or deceleration phase. There are many examples of reentrant tachycardias, including AF, atrial flutter (AFl), AV nodal or AV reentrant tachycardia, and recurrent VT.

ANTIARRHYTHMIC DRUGS

In a theoretical sense, drugs may have antiarrhythmic activity by directly altering conduction in several ways. First, a drug may depress the automatic properties of abnormal pacemaker cells. A drug may do this by decreasing the slope of phase 4 depolarization and/or by elevating threshold potential. If the rate of spontaneous impulse generation of the abnormally automatic foci becomes less than that of the SA node, normal cardiac rhythm can be restored. Second, drugs may alter the conduction characteristics of the pathways of a reentrant loop.[1,2] A drug may facilitate conduction (shorten refractoriness) in the area of unidirectional block, allowing antegrade conduction to proceed. On the other hand, a drug may further depress conduction (prolong refractoriness) either in the area of unidirectional block or in the pathway with slowed conduction and a relatively shorter refractory period. If refractoriness is prolonged in the area of unidirectional block, retrograde propagation of the impulse is not permitted, causing a "bidirectional" block. In the anatomic model, if refractoriness is prolonged in the pathway with slow conduction, antegrade conduction of the impulse is not permitted. In either case, drugs that reduce the discordance and cause uniformity in conduction properties of the two pathways may suppress the reentrant substrate. In the functionally determined model, if refractoriness is prolonged without significantly slowing conduction velocity, the tachycardia may terminate or slow in rate as a consequence of a greater circuit length (see Fig. 18-4). There are other theoretical ways to stop reentry: (a) a drug may eliminate the critically timed premature impulse that triggers reentry; (b) a drug may slow conduction velocity to such an extent that conduction is extinguished; or (c) a drug may reverse the underlying form of heart disease that was responsible for the conduction abnormalities that led to the arrhythmia (ie, "reverse remodeling").

AADs have specific electrophysiologic actions that alter cardiac conduction in patients with or without heart disease. These actions form the basis of grouping AADs into specific categories based on their electrophysiologic actions in vitro. Vaughan Williams proposed the most frequently used classification system (Table 18-1).[2] This classification has been criticized for the following reasons: (a) it is incomplete and does not allow for the classification of drugs such as digoxin or adenosine; (b) it is not pure, and many agents have properties of more than one class of drugs; (c) it does not incorporate drug characteristics such as mechanisms of tachycardia termination/prevention, clinical indications, or side effects; and (d) drugs become "labeled" within a class, although they may be distinct in many regards.[3] These criticisms formed the basis for an attempt to reclassify AADs based on a variety of basic and clinical characteristics (called the Sicilian Gambit[3]). Nonetheless, the Vaughan Williams classification remains the most frequently used despite many proposed modifications and alternative systems.

The class Ia AADs, quinidine, procainamide, and disopyramide, slow conduction velocity, prolong refractoriness, and decrease the automatic properties of sodium-dependent (normal and diseased) conduction tissue. Although class Ia AADs are primarily considered sodium channel blockers, their electrophysiologic actions can also be attributed to blockade of potassium channels. In reentrant tachycardias, these drugs generally depress conduction and prolong refractoriness, theoretically transforming the area of unidirectional block into a bidirectional block. Clinically, class Ia drugs are broad-spectrum AADs that are effective for both supraventricular and ventricular arrhythmias. Procainamide is only available in the IV formulation as all of its oral formulations have been discontinued. These AADs tend not to be used frequently in clinical practice for the management of either supraventricular or ventricular arrhythmias primarily because of their limited efficacy and significant toxicities.

The class Ib AADs, lidocaine, mexiletine, and phenytoin, were historically categorized separately from quinidine-like drugs. This was a result of early work demonstrating that lidocaine had distinctly different electrophysiologic actions. In normal tissue models, lidocaine generally facilitates actions on cardiac conduction by shortening refractoriness and having little effect on conduction velocity. Thus, it was postulated that these agents could improve antegrade conduction, eliminating the area of unidirectional block. Of course, arrhythmias do not usually arise from normal tissue, leading investigators to study the actions of lidocaine and phenytoin in ischemic and hypoxic tissue models. Interestingly, studies have shown these drugs to possess class Ia quinidine-like properties in diseased tissues. Therefore, it is probable that lidocaine acts in a similar fashion to the class Ia AADs (ie, prolongs refractoriness in diseased ischemic

TABLE 18-1 Classification of Antiarrhythmic Drugs

Class	Drug	Conduction Velocity[a]	Refractory Period	Automaticity	Ion Block
Ia	Quinidine Procainamide Disopyramide	↓	↑	↓	Sodium (intermediate) Potassium
Ib	Lidocaine Mexiletine	0/↓	↓	↓	Sodium (fast on–off)
Ic	Flecainide Propafenone[b]	↓↓	0	↓	Sodium (slow on–off)
II[c]	β-Blockers	↓	↑	↓	Calcium (indirect)
III	Amiodarone[d] Dofetilide Dronedarone[d] Sotalol[b] Ibutilide	0	↑↑	0	Potassium
IV[c]	Verapamil Diltiazem	↓	↑	↓	Calcium

[a]Variables for normal tissue models in ventricular tissue.

[b]Also has β-blocking actions.

[c]Variables for sinoatrial (SA) and atrioventricular (AV) nodal tissue only.

[d]Also has sodium, calcium, and β-blocking actions; see Table 18-2 (for amiodarone).

tissues leading to bidirectional block in a reentrant circuit). Lidocaine and similar agents have accentuated effects in ischemic tissue caused by the local acidosis and potassium shifts that occur during cellular hypoxia. Changes in pH alter the time that local anesthetics occupy the sodium channel receptor, thereby affecting the agent's electrophysiologic actions. In addition, the intracellular acidosis that ensues as a consequence of ischemia could cause lidocaine to become "trapped" within the cell, allowing increased access to the receptor. The class Ib AADs are considerably more effective in ventricular arrhythmias than supraventricular arrhythmias. As a group, these drugs are relatively weak sodium channel blockers (at normal stimulation rates).

The class Ic AADs, propafenone and flecainide, are extremely potent sodium channel blockers, profoundly slowing conduction velocity while leaving refractoriness relatively unaltered. The class Ic AADs theoretically eliminate reentry by slowing conduction to a point where the impulse is extinguished and cannot propagate further. Although the class Ic AADs are effective for both ventricular and supraventricular arrhythmias, their use for ventricular arrhythmias has been limited by the risk of proarrhythmia.

Class I AADs are grouped together because of their common action in blocking sodium conductance. The receptor site for these AADs is probably inside the sodium channel so that, in effect, the drug plugs the pore. The AAD may gain access to the receptor either via the intracellular space through the membrane lipid bilayer or directly through the channel. Several principles are inherent in antiarrhythmic sodium channel receptor theories[4]:

1. Class I AADs have predominant affinity for a particular state of the channel (eg, during activation or inactivation). For example, lidocaine and flecainide block sodium current primarily when the cell is in the inactivated state, whereas quinidine is predominantly an open (or activated)-channel blocker.
2. Class I AADs have specific binding and unbinding characteristics to the receptor. For example, lidocaine binds to and dissociates from the channel receptor quickly ("fast on-off") but flecainide has very "slow on-off" properties. This explains why flecainide has such potent effects on slowing ventricular conduction, whereas lidocaine has little effect on normal tissue (at normal heart rates). In general, the class Ic AADs are "slow on-off," the class Ib AADs are "fast on-off," and the class Ia AADs are intermediate in their binding kinetics.
3. Class I AADs possess rate dependence (ie, sodium channel blockade and slowed conduction are greatest at fast heart rates and least during bradycardia). For "slow on-off" drugs, sodium channel blockade is evident at normal rates (60-100 beats/min), but for "fast on-off" agents, slowed conduction is only apparent at fast heart rates.
4. Class I AADs (except phenytoin) are weak bases with a pK_a greater than 7 and block the sodium channel in their ionized form. Consequently, pH will alter these actions: acidosis accentuates and alkalosis diminishes sodium channel blockade.
5. Class I AADs appear to share a single receptor site in the sodium channel. It should be noted, however, that a number of class I AADs have other electrophysiologic properties. For instance, quinidine has potent potassium channel blocking activity (manifests predominantly at low concentrations) as does *N*-acetylprocainamide (manifests predominantly at high concentrations), the primary metabolite of procainamide. Additionally propafenone has β-blocking actions.

These principles are important in understanding additive drug combinations (eg, quinidine and mexiletine), antagonistic combinations (eg, flecainide and lidocaine), and potential antidotes to excess sodium channel blockade (sodium bicarbonate). They also explain a number of clinical observations, such as why lidocaine-like drugs are relatively ineffective for supraventricular arrhythmias. The class Ib AADs are "fast on-off," inactivated sodium channel blockers; atrial cells, however, have a very brief inactivated phase relative to ventricular tissue.

The β-blockers are classified as class II AADs. For the most part, the clinically relevant acute antiarrhythmic mechanisms of the β-blockers result from their antiadrenergic actions. Because the SA and AV nodes are heavily influenced by adrenergic innervation, β-blockers would be most useful in tachycardias in which these nodal tissues are abnormally automatic or are a portion of a reentrant loop. These drugs are also helpful in slowing ventricular response in atrial arrhythmias (eg, AF) by their effects on the AV node. Furthermore, some tachycardias are exercise-related or precipitated by states of high sympathetic tone (perhaps through triggered activity), and β-blockers may be useful in these instances. β-Adrenergic stimulation results in increased conduction velocity, shortened refractoriness, and increased automaticity of the nodal tissues; β-blockers will antagonize these effects. In the nodal tissues, β-blockers interfere with calcium entry into the cell by altering catecholamine-dependent channel integrity and gating kinetics. In sodium-dependent atrial and ventricular tissues, β-blockers shorten repolarization somewhat but otherwise have little direct effect. The antiarrhythmic properties of β-blockers observed with long-term, chronic therapy in patients with heart disease are less well understood. Although it is clear that β-blockers decrease the likelihood of SCD (presumably arrhythmic death) after MI, the mechanism for this benefit remains unclear but may relate to the complex interplay of changes in sympathetic tone, damaged myocardium, and ventricular conduction. In patients with HF, drugs such as β-blockers, angiotensin-converting enzyme inhibitors, and angiotensin II receptor blockers may prevent arrhythmias such as AF by attenuating the structural and/or electrical remodeling process in the myocardium.[5,6]

The class III AADs include those agents that specifically prolong refractoriness in atrial and ventricular tissues. This class includes amiodarone, dronedarone, sotalol, ibutilide, and dofetilide; these drugs share the common effect of delaying repolarization by blocking potassium channels. Amiodarone and sotalol are effective in most supraventricular and ventricular arrhythmias. Amiodarone displays electrophysiologic characteristics of all four Vaughan Williams classes; it is a sodium channel blocker with relatively "fast on-off" kinetics, has nonselective β-blocking actions, blocks potassium channels, and also has a small degree of calcium channel blocking activity (Table 18-2). At normal heart rates and with chronic use, its predominant effect is to prolong repolarization. With IV administration, its onset is relatively quick (unlike the oral form) and β-blockade predominates initially. Theoretically, amiodarone, like class I AADs, may interrupt the reentrant substrate by transforming an area of unidirectional block into an area of bidirectional block. However, electrophysiologic studies using programmed cardiac stimulation imply that amiodarone may leave the reentrant loop intact. The impressive effectiveness of amiodarone coupled with its low proarrhythmic potential has challenged the notion that selective ion channel blockade by AADs is preferable. Sotalol is a potent inhibitor of outward potassium movement during repolarization and also possesses nonselective β-blocking actions. Unlike amiodarone and sotalol, dronedarone, ibutilide, and dofetilide are only approved for the treatment of supraventricular arrhythmias. Both ibutilide (only available IV) and dofetilide (only available orally) can be used for the acute conversion of AF or AFl to SR. Dofetilide can also be used to maintain SR in patients with AF or AFl of longer than 1 week's duration who have been converted to SR. Dronedarone is approved to reduce the risk of cardiovascular (CV) hospitalization in patients with a history of paroxysmal or persistent AF who are currently in SR. Although structurally related to amiodarone, dronedarone's structure has been modified through the addition of a methylsulfonyl group and the removal of iodine. Dronedarone is also similar to amiodarone in exhibiting electrophysiologic characteristics of all four Vaughan Williams classes (sodium channel blocker with relatively "fast on-off" kinetics, nonselective β-blocker, potassium channel blocker, and calcium channel antagonist).

There are a number of different potassium channels that function during normal conduction; all approved class III AADs inhibit the delayed rectifier current (I_K) responsible for phase 2 and phase 3 repolarization. Subcurrents make up I_K: an ultrarapid component (I_{Kur}), a rapid component (I_{Kr}), and the slow component (I_{Ks}). Sotalol, ibutilide, and dofetilide selectively block I_{Kr}, whereas amiodarone and dronedarone block both I_{Kr} and I_{Ks}. New drugs that selectively block I_{Kur} (found predominantly in the atrium but not ventricle) are being investigated for supraventricular arrhythmias. The clinical relevance of selectively blocking components of the delayed rectifier current remains to be determined. Potassium channel blockers (particularly those with selective I_{Kr} blocking properties) display "reverse use dependence" (ie, their effects on repolarization are greatest at low heart rates). Sotalol and drugs like it also appear to be much more effective in preventing VF (in dog models) than the traditional sodium channel blockers. They also decrease defibrillation threshold in contrast to class I AADs which tend to increase this parameter. This feature could be important in patients with ICDs, as concurrent therapy with class I AADs may require more energy for successful cardioversion or may render the ICD ineffective in terminating the ventricular arrhythmia. The Achilles' heel of all class III AADs is an extension of their underlying ionic mechanism; that is, by blocking potassium channels and delaying repolarization, these medications may also cause proarrhythmia in the form of TdP by provoking EADs.

The non-DHP CCBs, verapamil and diltiazem, are categorized as class IV AADs. At least two types of calcium channels are operative in SA and AV nodal tissues: an L-type channel and a T-type channel. Both L-type channel blockers (verapamil and diltiazem) and selective T-type channel blockers (mibefradil was previously approved but withdrawn from the market) will slow conduction, prolong refractoriness, and decrease automaticity (eg, due to EADs or LADs) of the calcium-dependent tissue in the SA and AV nodes. Therefore, these agents are effective in automatic or reentrant tachycardias which arise from or use the SA or AV nodes. In supraventricular arrhythmias (eg, AF or AFl), these drugs can slow ventricular response by slowing AV nodal conduction. Furthermore, because calcium entry seems to be integral to exercise-related tachycardias and/or tachycardias caused by some forms of triggered automaticity, these agents may be effective in the treatment of these types of arrhythmias. The DHP CCBs (eg, nifedipine) do not have significant antiarrhythmic activity as they do not affect AV nodal conduction.

All AADs currently available have an impressive side effect profile (Table 18-3). A considerable percentage of patients cannot tolerate long-term therapy with these drugs and will have to discontinue therapy because of side effects. (2) Flecainide, propafenone, quinidine, procainamide, disopyramide, sotalol, and dronedarone

TABLE 18-2 Time Course and Electrophysiologic Effects of Amiodarone

				IV		Oral	
Class	Mechanism	EP	ECG	Minutes–Hours	Hours–Days	Days–Weeks	Weeks–Months
Class I	Na^+ block	↑HV	↑QRS	0	+	+	++
Class II	β-block	↑AH	↑PR ↓HR	++	++	++	++
Class III	K^+ block	↑VERP ↑AERP	↑QT	0	+	++	++++
Class IV	Ca^{2+} block[a]	↑AH	↑PR ↓HR	+	+	+	+

AERP, atrial effective refractory period; AH, atria–His interval; ECG, electrocardiographic effects; EP, electrophysiologic actions; HR, heart rate; HV, His–ventricle interval; IV, intravenous; VERP, ventricular effective refractory period.

[a]Rate-dependent.

TABLE 18-3 Side Effects of Antiarrhythmic Drugs

Disopyramide	Anticholinergic symptoms (dry mouth, urinary retention, constipation, blurred vision), nausea, anorexia, TdP, HF, conduction disturbances, ventricular arrhythmias
Procainamide[a]	Hypotension, TdP, worsening HF, conduction disturbances, ventricular arrhythmias
Quinidine	Cinchonism, diarrhea, abdominal cramps, nausea, vomiting, hypotension, TdP, worsening HF, conduction disturbances, ventricular arrhythmias, fever
Lidocaine	Dizziness, sedation, slurred speech, blurred vision, paresthesia, muscle twitching, confusion, nausea, vomiting, seizures, psychosis, sinus arrest, conduction disturbances
Mexiletine	Dizziness, sedation, anxiety, confusion, paresthesia, tremor, ataxia, blurred vision, nausea, vomiting, anorexia, conduction disturbances, ventricular arrhythmias
Flecainide	Blurred vision, dizziness, dyspnea, headache, tremor, nausea, worsening HF, conduction disturbances, ventricular arrhythmias
Propafenone	Dizziness, fatigue, blurred vision, bronchospasm, headache, taste disturbances, nausea, vomiting, bradycardia or AV block, worsening HF, ventricular arrhythmias
Amiodarone	Tremor, ataxia, paresthesia, insomnia, corneal microdeposits, optic neuropathy/neuritis, nausea, vomiting, anorexia, constipation, TdP (<1%), bradycardia or AV block (IV and oral use), pulmonary fi brosis, liver function test abnormalities, hypothyroidism, hyperthyroidism, photosensitivity, blue-gray skin discoloration, hypotension (IV use), phlebitis (IV use)
Dofetilide	Headache, dizziness, TdP
Dronedarone	Nausea, vomiting, diarrhea, serum creatinine elevations, bradycardia, worsening HF, hepatotoxicity, pulmonary fibrosis, acute renal failure, TdP (<1%)
Ibutilide	Headache, TdP, bradycardia or AV block, hypotension
Sotalol	Dizziness, weakness, fatigue, nausea, vomiting, diarrhea, bradycardia or AV block, TdP, bronchospasm, worsening HF

AV, atrioventricular; HF, heart failure; IV, intravenous; TdP, torsade de pointes.

[a]Side effects listed are for the IV formulation only; oral formulations are no longer available.

may precipitate worsening HF in a significant number of patients with underlying LV systolic dysfunction; consequently, these drugs should be avoided in patients with heart failure with reduced ejection fraction (HF*r*EF). The class Ib AAD, mexiletine, causes neurologic and/or gastrointestinal toxicity in a high percentage of patients. One of the most frightening side effects related to AADs is the aggravation of underlying ventricular arrhythmias or the precipitation of new (and life-threatening) ventricular arrhythmias.[7]

Amiodarone has assumed a prominent place in the treatment of both acute and chronic supraventricular and ventricular arrhythmias and is now the most commonly prescribed AAD.[8] Once considered a drug of last resort, it is now the first AAD considered for the treatment of many arrhythmias. Yet amiodarone is a peculiar and complex drug, displaying unusual pharmacologic effects, pharmacokinetics, dosing regimens, and multiorgan side effects. Amiodarone has an extremely long elimination half-life (approximately 60 days) and large volume of distribution; consequently, its onset of action with the oral form is delayed (days to weeks) despite the use of a loading regimen, and its effects persist for a long period (months) after discontinuation. Amiodarone is a substrate of the cytochrome P450 (CYP) 3A4 isoenzyme, a moderate inhibitor of many CYP isoenzymes (eg, CYP2C9, CYP2D6, CYP3A4), and a P-glycoprotein (P-gp) inhibitor, all of which can result in the potential for numerous drug interactions. Amiodarone interacts with digoxin and warfarin and can significantly increase plasma concentrations of both drugs. By inhibiting P-gp, amiodarone can increase digoxin concentrations by approximately 2-fold; therefore, the digoxin dose should be empirically reduced by 50% when amiodarone is initiated. By inhibiting CYP2C9 and CYP3A4, amiodarone can increase warfarin concentrations and the international normalized ratio (INR). Consequently, when amiodarone and warfarin are initiated concurrently, warfarin should be started at a dose of 2.5 mg daily. When amiodarone is initiated in a patient already receiving warfarin, the warfarin dose should be reduced by approximately 30%.[9] Through inhibition of P-gp, amiodarone can also increase concentrations of dabigatran, especially in patients with severe renal impairment (creatinine clearance [CrCl] 15-30 mL/min); consequently, the use of dabigatran should be avoided in these patients who are receiving amiodarone. Acute administration of amiodarone is usually well tolerated by patients; however, severe organ toxicities may result with chronic use. Severe bradycardia (sometimes requiring pacing to allow the patient to remain on amiodarone), hyperthyroidism, hypothyroidism, peripheral neuropathy, gastrointestinal discomfort, photosensitivity, and a blue-gray skin discoloration on exposed areas are common. Fulminant hepatitis (uncommon) and pulmonary fibrosis (5%-10% of patients) have caused death.[10,11] Although amiodarone can cause corneal microdeposits (usually do not affect vision) in virtually every patient, it has also been associated with the development of optic neuropathy/neuritis which can lead to blindness. Even though amiodarone markedly prolongs the QT interval, the risk of proarrhythmia (ie, TdP) is rare. All of these side effects mandate close and continued monitoring (liver enzymes, thyroid function tests, eye examinations, chest radiographs, pulmonary function tests) and have led to a proliferation of "amiodarone clinics" designed just for patients receiving this drug on a chronic basis (Table 18-4). 3 [12,13]

With the addition of a methylsulfonyl group and the deletion of the iodine moiety, dronedarone is less lipophilic than amiodarone; consequently, dronedarone is supposed to be less likely to accumulate in tissues and cause various organ toxicities. Dronedarone also has a considerably shorter half-life (approximately 24 hours) when compared with amiodarone, which allows for steady state to be achieved in 5 to 7 days without the need for loading doses. Like amiodarone, dronedarone is a substrate of the CYP3A4 isoenzyme and a moderate inhibitor of the CYP2D6 and CYP3A4 isoenzymes. Its use with potent CYP3A4 inhibitors or inducers should be avoided. Dronedarone may increase plasma concentrations of (*S*)-warfarin; therefore, the INR should be closely monitored with concurrent use of these drugs. Dronedarone also inhibits P-gp and can increase digoxin concentrations by about 2.5-fold. Consequently, when concomitantly using dronedarone and digoxin, the digoxin dose should be empirically reduced by 50%. Additionally, dronedarone can increase dabigatran and rivaroxaban concentrations in patients with renal impairment. To minimize the risk of bleeding when concomitantly using dronedarone and dabigatran in this patient population, the dose of dabigatran should be reduced to 75 mg twice daily in those with moderate renal impairment (CrCl 30-50 mL/min). The concomitant use of dronedarone and dabigatran should be avoided in patients with severe renal impairment (CrCl 15-30 mL/min). Rivaroxaban should only be used if the benefit outweighs the risk in patients receiving dronedarone who have a CrCl of 15 to 80 mL/min. While it was initially believed that dronedarone would cause fewer organ toxicities with the deletion of the iodine moiety, several postmarketing reports have suggested that this AAD may be associated with several significant organ toxicities, including severe hepatic injury, interstitial lung disease (ie, pulmonary fibrosis), and acute kidney injury.[14-16]

Table 18-5 summarizes the pharmacokinetics of the AADs and Table 18-6 lists recommended dosages of the oral dosage forms of the AADs. Table 18-7 lists the dosing recommendations for the IV forms of various AADs.

TABLE 18-4 Amiodarone Monitoring

Side Effect	Monitoring Recommendations	Management of Side Effect
Pulmonary fibrosis	Chest radiograph (baseline, and then every 12 months) Pulmonary function tests (baseline, and then if symptoms develop) High-resolution CT (if symptoms develop)	Discontinue amiodarone immediately; may consider corticosteroid therapy
Hypothyroidism	TFTs (baseline, and then every 6 months)	Thyroid hormone supplementation (eg, levothyroxine)
Hyperthyroidism	TFTs (baseline, and then every 6 months)	Antithyroid drugs (eg, methimazole, propylthiouracil) or corticosteroids; may need to discontinue amiodarone)
Optic neuritis/neuropathy	Ophthalmologic examination (baseline [only if visual impairment present], and then if symptoms develop)	Discontinue amiodarone immediately
Corneal microdeposits	Slit-lamp examination (routine monitoring not necessary)	No treatment necessary
Hepatotoxicity	LFTs (baseline, and then every 6 months)	Lower the dose or discontinue amiodarone if LFTs >2× the upper limit of normal
Bradycardia/heart block	ECG (baseline, and then every 3-6 months)	Lower the dose, if possible, or discontinue amiodarone if severe (or continue amiodarone and implant permanent pacemaker)
Tremor, ataxia, peripheral neuropathy	History/physical examination (each office visit)	Lower the dose, if possible, or discontinue amiodarone if severe
Photosensitivity/blue-gray skin discoloration	History/physical examination (each office visit)	Lower the dose; advise patients to wear sunblock while outdoors

ECG, electrocardiogram; LFTs, liver function tests, TFTs, thyroid function tests.

TABLE 18-5 Pharmacokinetics of Antiarrhythmic Drugs

Drug	Oral Bioavailability (%)	Primary Route of Elimination[a]	Substrate[b]	Inhibitor[b]	V_{Dss} (L/kg)	Protein Binding (%)	$t_{1/2}$[c]	Therapeutic Range (mg/L)
Disopyramide	70-95	H/R	CYP3A4 (M)	—	0.8-2	50-80	4-8 hours	2-6 (6-18 μmol/L)
Procainamide	—	H/R	NAT CYP2D6 (M)	—	1.5-3	10-20	5-6 hours (SAs) 2-3 hours (FAs)	4-15 (17-64 μmol/L)
Quinidine	70-80	H	CYP3A4 (M) CYP2C9	CYP2D6 (S) CYP3A4 (S) CYP2C9 P-gp	2-3.5	80-90	5-9 hours	2-6 (6-18 μmol/L)
Lidocaine	—	H	CYP3A4 (M) CYP2D6 (M) CYP1A2 CYP2C9	CYP1A2 (S) CYP2D6	1-2	65-75	1-3 hours	1.5-5 (6.4-21.3 μmol/L)
Mexiletine	80-95	H	CYP2D6 (M) CYP1A2 (M)	CYP1A2 (S)	5-12	60-75	12-20 hours (PMs) 7-11 hours (EMs)	0.8-2 (4.5-11.1 μmol/L)
Flecainide	90-95	H/R	CYP2D6 (M) CYP1A2	CYP2D6	8-10	35-45	14-20 hours (PMs) 10-14 hours (EMs)	0.2-1 (0.5-2.4 μmol/L)
Propafenone[d]	11-39	H	CYP2D6 (M) CYP1A2 CYP2D6	CYP1A2 CYP2D6	2.5-4	85-95	10-25 hours (PMs) 3-7 hours (EMs)	—
Amiodarone	22-88	H	CYP3A4 (M) CYP1A2 CYP2C19 CYP2D6	CYP2C9 CYP2D6 CYP3A4 CYP1A2 CYP2C19 P-gp	70-150	95-99	15-100 days	1-2.5 (1.6-3.9 μmol/L)
Dofetilide	85-95	R/H	CYP3A4	—	2.5-3.5	60-70	6-10 hours	—
Dronedarone	4 (fasting) 15 (with food)	H	CYP3A4	CYP2D6 CYP3A4	20	>98	13-19	—
Ibutilide	—	H	—	—	6-12	40-50	3-6 hours	—
Sotalol	90-95	R	—	—	1.2-2.4	30-40	10-20 hours	—
Diltiazem	35-50	H	CYP3A4 (M) CYP2C9 CYP2D6	CYP3A4 CYP2C9 CYP2D6 P-gp	3-5	70-85	4-10 hours	—
Verapamil	20-40	H	CYP3A4 (M) CYP1A2 CYP2C9	CYP3A4 CYP1A2 CYP2C9 CYP2D6 P-gp	1.5-5	95-99	4-12 hours	—

[a]H, hepatic; R, renal.

[b]CYP, cytochrome P450 isoenzyme; M, major; NAT, N -acetyltransferase; P-gp, P-glycoprotein; S, strong.

[c]EMs, extensive metabolizers; FAs, fast acetylators; PMs, poor metabolizers; SAs, slow acetylators.

[d]Variables for parent compound (not 5-OH-propafenone).

TABLE 18-6 Typical Maintenance Doses of Oral Antiarrhythmic Drugs

Drug	Dose	Dose Adjusted
Disopyramide	100-150 mg q 6 hours 200-300 mg q 12 hours (SR form)	HEP, REN
Quinidine	200-300 mg sulfate salt q 6 hours 324-648 gluconate salt q 8-12 hours	HEP
Mexiletine	200-300 mg q 8 hours	HEP
Flecainide	50-200 mg q 12 hours	HEP, REN
Propafenone	150-300 mg q 8 hours 225-425 mg q 12 hours (SR form)	HEP
Amiodarone	400 mg two to three times daily until 10 g total, and then 200-400 mg daily[a]	
Dofetilide	500 mcg q 12 hours	REN[b]
Dronedarone	400 mg twice daily (with meals)[c]	
Sotalol	80-160 mg q 12 hours	REN[d]

HEP, hepatic disease; REN, renal impairment; SR, sustained release.

[a]Usual maintenance dose for atrial fibrillation is 200 mg/day (may further decrease dose to 100 mg/day with long-term use if patient clinically stable in order to decrease risk of toxicity); usual maintenance dose for ventricular arrhythmias is 300-400 mg/day.

[b]Dose should be based on creatinine clearance; should not be used when creatinine clearance <20 mL/min.

[c]Should not be used in severe hepatic impairment.

[d]Should not be used for atrial fibrillation when creatinine clearance <40 mL/min.

TABLE 18-7 IV Antiarrhythmic Dosing

Drug	Clinical Situation	Dose
Amiodarone	Pulseless VT/VF	300 mg IV/IO push (can give additional 150 mg IV/IO push if persistent VT/VF or if VT/VF recurs), followed by infusion of 1 mg/min for 6 hours, and then 0.5 mg/min
	Stable VT (with a pulse)	150 mg IV over 10 minutes, followed by infusion of 1 mg/min for 6 hours, and then 0.5 mg/min
	AF (termination)	5 mg/kg IV over 30 minutes, followed by infusion of 1 mg/min for 6 hours, and then 0.5 mg/min
Diltiazem	PSVT; AF (rate control)	0.25 mg/kg IV over 2 minutes (may repeat with 0.35 mg/kg IV over 2 minutes), followed by infusion of 5-15 mg/h
Ibutilide	AF (termination)	1 mg IV over 10 minutes (may repeat if needed)
Lidocaine	Pulseless VT/VF	1-1.5 mg/kg IV/IO push (can give additional 0.5-0.75 mg/kg IV/IO push every 5-10 minutes if persistent VT/VF [maximum cumulative dose = 3 mg/kg]), followed by infusion of 1-4 mg/min (1-2 mg/min if liver disease or HF)
	Stable VT (with a pulse)	1-1.5 mg/kg IV push (can give additional 0.5-0.75 mg/kg IV push every 5-10 minutes if persistent VT [maximum cumulative dose = 3 mg/kg]), followed by infusion of 1-4 mg/min (1-2 mg/min if liver disease or HF)
Procainamide	AF (termination); stable VT (with a pulse)	15-18 mg/kg IV over 60 minutes, followed by infusion of 1-4 mg/min
Verapamil	PSVT; AF (rate control)	2.5-5 mg IV over 2 minutes (may repeat up to maximum cumulative dose of 20 mg); can follow with infusion of 2.5-10 mg/h

AF, atrial fibrillation; HF, heart failure; IO, intraosseous; IV, intravenous; PSVT, paroxysmal supraventricular tachycardia; VF, ventricular fibrillation; VT, ventricular tachycardia.

SUPRAVENTRICULAR ARRHYTHMIAS

The common supraventricular tachycardias that often require drug treatment are: (a) AF or AFl, (b) PSVT, and (c) automatic atrial tachycardias. Other common supraventricular arrhythmias that usually do not require drug therapy include premature atrial complexes, wandering atrial pacemaker, sinus arrhythmia, and sinus tachycardia. As an example, premature atrial complexes rarely cause symptoms and never cause hemodynamic compromise; therefore, drug therapy is usually not indicated. Likewise, sinus tachycardia is usually the result of underlying metabolic or hemodynamic disorders (eg, infection, dehydration, hypotension), and therapy should be directed at the underlying cause, not the tachycardia per se. Of course, there are exceptions to these suggestions. For example, sinus tachycardia may be deleterious in patients after cardiac surgery or MI. Therefore, AADs, such as β-blockers, may be indicated in these situations. Stated in another way, although many arrhythmias generally do not require therapy, clinical judgment and patient-specific variables play an important role in this decision. AF, AFl, and PSVT tend to be the most common supraventricular arrhythmias seen in clinical practice; therefore, this discussion will focus only on these arrhythmias.

Atrial Fibrillation and Atrial Flutter

Mechanisms and Background

AF continues to be the most common sustained arrhythmia encountered in clinical practice, affecting between 2.7 and 6.1 million Americans.[17] In the general population, the overall prevalence of AF is 0.4% to 1%, and this increases with age (eg, approximately an 8% prevalence in patients greater than 80 years old).[18,19] The prevalence of AF also appears to increase as patients develop more severe HF, increasing from 4% in asymptomatic NYHA class I patients to 50% in patients with NYHA class IV HF.[20] With the aging population, improved survival in patients with HF, CAD, and hypertension, and the increased frequency of surgical procedures being performed, it is expected that the prevalence of AF will dramatically increase to an estimated 12 to 15 million by the year 2050.[20] Based on data derived from the Framingham study cohort, the general lifetime risk for AF in men and women at least 40 years of age is estimated to be 1 in 4.[21]

AF and AFl may present as a chronic, established tachycardia, an acute tachycardia, or a self-terminating, paroxysmal form. The following semantics and definitions are sometimes used specifically for AF: acute AF (onset within 48 hours), paroxysmal AF (terminates spontaneously in less than 7 days), recurrent AF (two or more episodes), persistent AF (duration longer than 7 days and does not terminate spontaneously), and permanent AF (does not terminate with attempts at pharmacologic or electrical cardioversion).[22] AF is characterized by extremely rapid (atrial rate of 400 to 600 beats/min) and disorganized atrial activation. With this disorganized atrial activity, there is a loss of the contribution of synchronized atrial contraction (atrial kick) to forward cardiac output. Supraventricular

CLINICAL PRESENTATION Supraventricular Tachycardias

Atrial Fibrillation/Flutter

General

- These arrhythmias are usually not directly life-threatening and do not generally cause hemodynamic collapse or syncope; 1:1 AFl (ventricular response approximately 300 beats/min) is an exception. Also, patients with underlying forms of heart disease who are heavily reliant on atrial contraction to maintain adequate cardiac output (eg, mitral stenosis, obstructive cardiomyopathy) display more severe symptoms of AF or AFl.

Symptoms

- Most often, patients complain of rapid heart rate/palpitations and/or worsening symptoms of HF (dyspnea, fatigue). Medical emergencies are severe HF (ie, pulmonary edema, hypotension) or AF occurring in the setting of acute MI.

Diagnostic Tests/Signs (ECG)

- AF is an irregularly irregular supraventricular rhythm with no discernible, consistent atrial activity (P waves). Ventricular rate is usually 120 to 180 beats/min and the pulse is irregular. AFl is (usually) a regular supraventricular rhythm with characteristic flutter waves (or sawtooth pattern) reflecting more organized atrial activity. Commonly, the ventricular rate is in factors of 300 beats/min (eg, 150, 100, or 75 beats/min).

Paroxysmal Supraventricular Tachycardia Caused by Reentry

General

- This arrhythmia can be transient, resulting in little, if any, symptoms.

Symptoms

- Patients frequently complain of intermittent episodes of rapid heart rate/palpitations that abruptly start and stop, usually without provocation (but occasionally as a result of exercise). Severe symptoms include syncope. Often (in particular, those with AV nodal reentry), patients complain of a chest pressure or neck sensation. This is caused by simultaneous AV contraction with the right atrium contracting against a closed tricuspid valve. Life-threatening symptoms (syncope, hemodynamic collapse) are associated with an extremely rapid heart rate (eg, greater than 200 beats/min) and AF associated with an accessory AV pathway.

Diagnostic Tests/Signs (ECG)

- Most commonly, PSVT is a rapid, narrow QRS tachycardia (regular in rhythm) that starts and stops abruptly. Atrial activity, although present, is difficult to ascertain on surface ECG because P waves are "buried" in the QRS complex or T wave.

impulses penetrate the AV conduction system in variable degrees resulting in an irregular activation of the ventricles and an irregularly irregular pulse. The AV junction will not conduct most of the supraventricular impulses, causing the ventricular response to be considerably slower (120 to 180 beats/min) than the atrial rate. It is sometimes stated that "AF begets AF," that is, the arrhythmia tends to perpetuate itself. Long episodes are more difficult to terminate perhaps because of tachycardia-induced changes in atrial function (mechanical and/or electrical "remodeling").

AFl occurs less frequently than AF but is similar in its precipitating factors, consequences, and drug therapy approach. This arrhythmia is characterized by rapid (atrial rate of 270 to 330 beats/min) but regular atrial activation. The slower and regular electrical activity results in a regular ventricular response that is in approximate factors of 300 beats/min (ie, 1:1 AV conduction = ventricular rate of 300 beats/min; 2:1 AV conduction = ventricular rate of 150 beats/min; 3:1 AV conduction = ventricular rate of 100 beats/min). AFl may occur in two distinct forms (type I and type II). Type I flutter is the more common classic form with atrial rates of approximately 300 beats/min and the typical "sawtooth" pattern of atrial activation as shown by the surface ECG. Type II flutter tends to be faster, being somewhat of a hybrid between classic AFl and AF. Although the ventricular response usually has a regular pattern with this arrhythmia, AFl with varying degrees of AV block or that occur with episodes of AF ("fib-flutter") can cause an irregular ventricular rate.

It is generally accepted that the predominant mechanism of AF and AFl is reentry. AF appears to result from multiple atrial reentrant loops (or wavelets), whereas AFl is caused by a single, dominant, reentrant substrate (counterclockwise circus movement in the right atrium around the tricuspid annulus). AF or AFl usually occurs in association with various forms of structural heart disease (SHD) that cause left atrial distension, including myocardial ischemia or infarction, hypertensive heart disease, valvular disorders such as mitral stenosis or mitral insufficiency, congenital abnormalities such as septal defects, dilated or hypertrophic cardiomyopathy, and obesity. Disorders that cause right atrial stretch and are associated with AF or AFl include acute pulmonary embolism and chronic lung disease resulting in pulmonary hypertension and cor pulmonale. AF may also occur in association with states of high adrenergic tone such as thyrotoxicosis, surgery, alcohol withdrawal, sepsis, and excessive physical exertion. AF that develops in the absence of clinical, electrocardiographic, radiographic, and echocardiographic evidence of SHD is defined as lone AF. Other states in which patients are predisposed to episodes of AF are the presence of an anomalous AV pathway (ie, Kent's bundle) and sinus node dysfunction (ie, sick sinus syndrome).

Patients with AF or AFl may experience the entire range of symptoms associated with other supraventricular tachycardias, although syncope as a presenting symptom is uncommon. Because left atrial kick is lost with the onset of AF, patients with HF*r*EF or HF with preserved ejection fraction (HF*p*EF) may develop worsening signs and symptoms of HF as they often depend on the contribution of their atrial kick to maintain an adequate cardiac output. TE events, resulting from atrial stasis and poorly adherent mural thrombi, are an additional complication of AF. Of course, the most devastating complication in this regard is the occurrence of an embolic stroke. The average rate of ischemic stroke in patients with AF who are not receiving antithrombotic therapy is approximately 5% per year.[23] Stroke can precede the onset of documented AF, probably as a result of undetected paroxysms prior to the onset of established AF. The risk of stroke significantly increases with age, with the annual attributable risk increasing from 1.5% in individuals 50 to 59 years of age to almost 24% in those 80 to 89 years of age.[24] The risk of stroke in patients with only AFl has been traditionally believed to be low, prompting some to recommend only aspirin for prevention of thromboembolism in this particular patient population. However, because patients with AFl may also intermittently have episodes of AF, this patient population may also be at risk for a TE event. Although the role of antithrombotic therapy in patients with AFl has not been adequately studied in clinical trials, the most recent guidelines suggest that the same risk stratification scheme and antithrombotic recommendations used in patients with AF should also be applied to those with AFl.[22]

Management

The traditional approach to the treatment of AF can be organized into several sequential goals. First, evaluate the need for acute treatment (usually administering drugs that slow ventricular rate). Next, contemplate methods to restore SR, taking into consideration the risks (eg, thromboembolism). Lastly, consider ways to prevent the long-term complications of AF such as arrhythmia recurrence and thromboembolism. 4 One of the biggest controversies in the management of AF is whether restoring and maintaining SR is a desirable goal for all patients. A review of the management of AF and AFl, including a discussion of this controversy follows, organized according to the goals already outlined. Figure 18-5 shows an algorithm for the management of AF and AFl. In addition, Table 18-8 summarizes the recommendations for pharmacologically controlling ventricular rate and restoring and maintaining SR from the most recent AF guidelines developed by the American Heart Association (AHA)/American College of Cardiology (ACC)/Heart Rhythm Society (HRS).[22]

Acute Treatment First, consider the patient with new-onset, symptomatic AF or AFl. Although uncommon, patients may present with signs and/or symptoms of hemodynamic instability (eg, severe hypotension, angina, or pulmonary edema), which qualifies as a medical emergency. In these situations, direct current cardioversion (DCC) is indicated as first-line therapy in an attempt to immediately restore SR (without regard to the risk of thromboembolism). AFl often requires relatively low energy levels of countershock (ie, 50 joules [J]), whereas AF often requires higher energy levels (ie, greater than 200 J).

If patients are hemodynamically stable, there is no emergent need to restore SR. Instead, the focus should be directed toward controlling the patient's ventricular rate. Achieving adequate ventricular rate control should be a treatment goal for all patients with AF. To achieve this goal, drugs that slow conduction and increase refractoriness in the AV node (eg, β-blockers, non-DHP CCBs, or digoxin) should be used as initial therapy. Although loading doses of digoxin have been historically recommended as first-line treatment to slow ventricular rate, use of this drug for this purpose, especially in patients with normal LV systolic function (left ventricular ejection fraction [LVEF] greater than 40%), has declined.[8] Potential reasons for the declining use of digoxin in this patient population are its relatively slow onset and its inability to control the ventricular rate during exercise. Although an initial decrease in the ventricular rate can sometimes be observed within 1 hour of IV administration of digoxin, full control (heart rate less than 80 beats/min at rest and less than 100 beats/min during exercise) is usually not achieved for 24 to 48 hours. Digoxin also tends to be ineffective for controlling ventricular rate under conditions of increased sympathetic tone (ie, surgery, thyrotoxicosis) because it slows AV nodal conduction primarily through vagotonic mechanisms. Additionally, in several recent analyses, the use of digoxin in patients with AF has been associated with a significant increase in the risk of mortality.[25,26] In contrast, IV β-blockers and non-DHP CCBs have a relatively quick onset and can effectively control the ventricular rate at rest and during exercise. β-Blockers are also effective for controlling ventricular rate under conditions of increased sympathetic tone.

Based on the most recent AHA/ACC/HRS guidelines for the treatment of AF, the selection of a drug to control ventricular rate in the acute setting should be primarily based on the patient's LV function.[22] In patients with normal LV function (LVEF greater than 40%), an IV β-blocker (propranolol, metoprolol, esmolol) or non-DHP CCB (diltiazem or verapamil) is recommended as first-line therapy to control ventricular rate.[22] All of these drugs have proven efficacy in controlling the ventricular rate in patients with AF. Propranolol and metoprolol can be administered as intermittent IV boluses, whereas esmolol (because of its very short half-life of 5 to 10 minutes) must be administered as a series of loading doses followed by a continuous infusion. Likewise, because control of ventricular rate can be transient with a single bolus, verapamil or diltiazem can be given as an initial IV bolus followed by a continuous infusion.[27] These continuous infusions can be adjusted in monitored settings to the desired ventricular response (eg, acutely less than 100 beats/min). In situations where AF or AFl is precipitated by states of increased sympathetic tone (ie, surgery, thyrotoxicosis), IV β-blockers can be highly effective and should be considered as first-line therapy.

In patients with HF*r*EF (LVEF less than or equal to 40%), both IV diltiazem and verapamil should be avoided because of their potent negative inotropic effects.[22] IV β-blockers should be used with caution in this patient population and should be avoided if patients are in the midst of an episode of decompensated HF. In those patients who are having an exacerbation of HF symptoms, IV administration of either digoxin or amiodarone should be used as first-line therapy to achieve ventricular rate control. IV amiodarone can also be used in patients who are refractory to or have contraindications to β-blockers, non-DHP CCBs, and digoxin. However, clinicians should be aware that the use of amiodarone for controlling ventricular rate may also stimulate the conversion of AF to SR and place the patient at risk for a TE event, especially if the AF has persisted for at least 48 hours or is of unknown duration. In patients with stable HF*p*EF, either IV diltiazem or verapamil is recommended to acutely control ventricular rate; however, these agents should be avoided in these patients if they are experiencing decompensated HF.

Patients may present with a slow ventricular response (in the absence of AV nodal blocking drugs) and thus do not require therapy with β-blockers, non-DHP CCBs, or digoxin. This type of presentation should alert the clinician to the possibility of preexisting SA or AV nodal conduction disease such as sick sinus syndrome. In these patients, DCC should not be attempted without a temporary pacemaker in place.

Restoration of Sinus Rhythm After treatment with AV nodal blocking drugs and a subsequent decrease in the ventricular rate, the patient should be evaluated for the possibility of restoring SR if AF persists. Within the context of this evaluation, several factors should be considered. First, many patients spontaneously convert to SR without intervention, obviating the need for therapy to achieve this goal. For instance, AF occurs frequently as a complication of cardiac surgery and often spontaneously reverts to SR without therapy. Second, restoring SR is not a necessary or realistic goal in some patients. The results of six landmark clinical trials (Pharmacological Intervention in Atrial Fibrillation [PIAF], Rate Control versus Electrical Cardioversion for Persistent Atrial Fibrillation [RACE], Atrial Fibrillation Follow-Up Investigation of Rhythm Management [AFFIRM], Strategies of Treatment of Atrial Fibrillation [STAF],

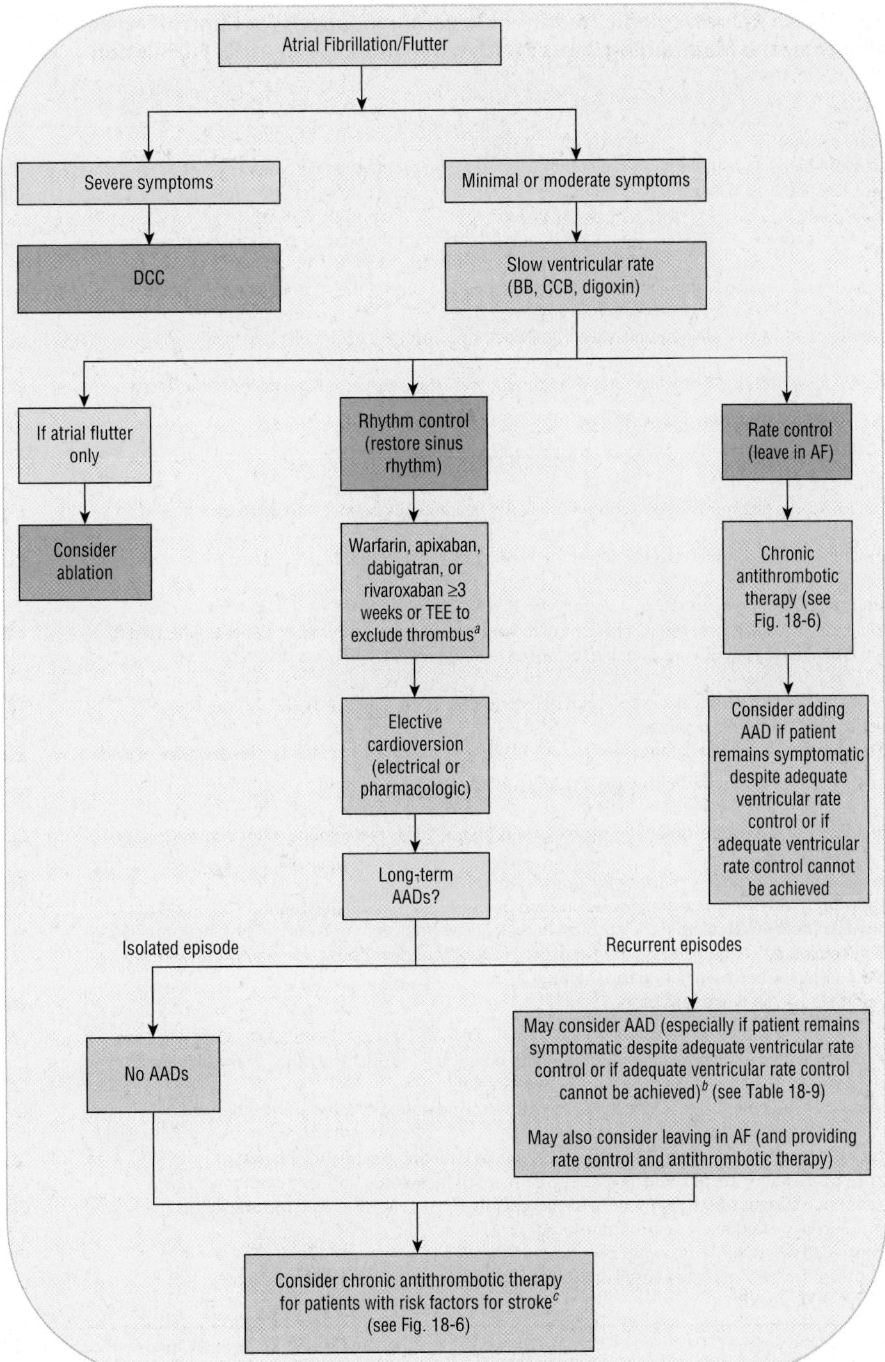

FIGURE 18-5 Algorithm for the treatment of AF and AFl. [a]If AF is less than 48 hours in duration, anticoagulation prior to cardioversion is unnecessary; initiate anticoagulation with unfractionated heparin, a low-molecular-weight heparin, apixaban, dabigatran, or rivaroxaban as soon as possible either before or after cardioversion for patients at high risk for stroke (this anticoagulant regimen or no antithrombotic therapy may be considered in low-risk patients). [b]Ablation may be considered for patients who fail or do not tolerate at least 1 AAD or as first-line therapy (before AAD therapy) for select patients with recurrent symptomatic paroxysmal AF. [c]Chronic antithrombotic therapy should be considered in all patients with AF and risk factors for stroke regardless of whether or not they remain in sinus rhythm. (AAD, antiarrhythmic drug; AF, atrial fibrillation; AFl, atrial flutter; BB, β-blocker; CCB, calcium channel blocker [ie, verapamil or diltiazem]; DCC, direct current cardioversion; TEE, transesophageal echocardiogram.)

How to Treat Chronic Atrial Fibrillation [HOT-CAFE], and Atrial Fibrillation and Congestive Heart Failure [AF-CHF]) have shed significant light on the comparative efficacy of rate-control (controlling ventricular rate; patient remains in AF) and rhythm-control (restoring and maintaining SR) treatment strategies in patients with AF.[28-33] The AFFIRM trial is the largest rate-control versus rhythm-control study to be conducted to date in patients with AF.[30] In this trial, patients with AF and at least one risk factor for stroke were randomized to either a rate-control or a rhythm-control group. Rate-control treatment involved AV nodal blocking drugs (digoxin, β-blockers, and/or non-DHP CCBs) first, and then nonpharmacologic treatment (AV nodal ablation with pacemaker implantation), if necessary. All patients in this group were anticoagulated with warfarin to achieve an INR of 2 to 3. In the rhythm-control group, class I

TABLE 18-8 Evidence-Based Pharmacologic Treatment Recommendations for Controlling Ventricular Rate, Restoring Sinus Rhythm, and Maintaining Sinus Rhythm in Patients with Atrial Fibrillation

Treatment Recommendations	ACC/AHA/ESC Guideline Recommendation
Ventricular rate control (acute setting)	
In the absence of an accessory pathway, an IV β-blocker or IV non-DHP CCB is recommended for patients without HF.	Class I
In the absence of an accessory pathway, IV digoxin or IV amiodarone is recommended to control the ventricular rate in patients with HF.	Class I
In the absence of an accessory pathway, an IV β-blocker is recommended to control the ventricular rate in patients with stable HF*r*EF.	Class I
In the absence of an accessory pathway, in IV non-DHP CCB is recommended to control the ventricular rate in patients with stable HF*p*EF.	Class I
In the absence of an accessory pathway, IV amiodarone is recommended to control the ventricular rate in critically ill patients.	Class IIa
IV amiodarone can be useful to control the ventricular rate when other measures are unsuccessful or contraindicated.	Class IIa
Digoxin, non-DHP CCBs, or IV amiodarone should not be used in patients with an accessory pathway.	Class III
IV β-blockers or IV non-DHP CCBs are not recommended in patients with decompensated HF.	Class III
Ventricular rate control (chronic setting)	
An oral β-blocker or non-DHP CCB is recommended to control the ventricular rate in patients with paroxysmal, persistent, or permanent AF.	Class I
An oral β-blocker or non-DHP CCB is recommended to control the ventricular rate in patients with persistent or permanent AF and compensated HF*p*EF.	Class I
Digoxin is effective for controlling resting heart rate in patients with HF*r*EF.	Class I
A combination of digoxin and a β-blocker is reasonable to control resting and exercise heart rate in patients with HF*r*EF.	Class IIa
A combination of digoxin and a non-DHP CCB is reasonable to control resting and exercise heart rate in patients with HF*p*EF.	Class IIa
Oral amiodarone can be used when the ventricular rate cannot be adequately controlled at rest and during exercise with an oral β-blocker, non-DHP CCB, and/or digoxin.	Class IIb
Oral non-DHP CCBs and dronedarone are not recommended to control the ventricular rate in patients with decompensated HF.	Class III
Dronedarone should not be used to control the ventricular rate in patients with permanent AF.	Class III
Restoration of SR	
In the absence of contraindications, flecainide, dofetilide, propafenone, or ibutilide is recommended for pharmacologic cardioversion of AF.	Class I
Oral amiodarone is a reasonable option for pharmacologic cardioversion of AF.	Class IIa
The "pill-in-the-pocket" approach with flecainide or propafenone can be used to terminate persistent AF on an outpatient basis once the treatment has been used safely in the hospital, in patients without sinus or AV node dysfunction, bundle-branch block, QT interval prolongation, Brugada syndrome, or SHD (*Note*: AV node must be adequately blocked with β-blocker or non-DHP CCB therapy before initiating this therapy).	Class IIa
Dofetilide should not be initiated on an outpatient basis.	Class III
Maintenance of SR	
The following AADs are recommended for maintaining SR, depending on underlying SHD and other comorbidities: amiodarone, dofetilide, dronedarone, flecainide, propafenone, and sotalol.	Class I
Because of its potential toxicities, amiodarone should only be used after consideration of its risks and when other agents have failed or are contraindicated.	Class I
The risk of the AAD, including proarrhythmia, should be considered before initiating treatment with that drug.	Class I
Antiarrhythmic therapy can be useful for maintaining SR for the treatment of tachycardia-induced cardiomyopathy.	Class IIa
It may be reasonable to continue current AAD therapy in the setting of infrequent, well-tolerated recurrences of AF when the drug has reduced the frequency or symptoms of AF.	Class IIb
An AAD should not be continued when the AF becomes permanent.	Class III
Dronedarone should not be used in patients with class III or IV HF or patients who have had an episode of decompensated HF in the last 4 weeks)	Class III

AAD, antiarrhythmic drug; ACC, American College of Cardiology; AF, atrial fibrillation; AHA, American Heart Association; AV, atrioventricular; CCB, calcium channel blocker; DCC, direct current cardioversion; DHP, dihydropyridine; HF, heart failure; HF*p*EF, heart failure with preserved ejection fraction; HF*r*EF, heart failure with reduced ejection fraction; HRS, Heart Rhythm Society; IV, intravenous; SHD, structural heart disease; SR, sinus rhythm.

Data from Fuster et al.[16] and Wann et al.

or III AADs were used to maintain SR. The choice of AAD therapy was left up to each patient's physician; however, by the end of the trial, more than 60% of patients had received at least one trial of amiodarone and approximately 40% of patients had received at least one trial of sotalol. In this group, anticoagulation was encouraged but could be discontinued if SR had been maintained for at least 4 weeks. After a mean follow-up period of 3.5 years, overall mortality was not statistically different between the two strategies but tended ($P = 0.08$) to be higher in the rhythm-control group. The results of the PIAF, RACE, STAF, and HOT-CAFE trials were consistent with those of the AFFIRM trial.[28,29,31,32] In addition, a meta-analysis of the data from all of these trials demonstrated no significant difference in overall mortality between rate-control and rhythm-control strategies, which persisted even when the results from the AFFIRM trial were excluded from this analysis.[34]

Even though the results of the PIAF, RACE, STAF, HOT-CAFE, and AFFIRM trials collectively demonstrate that a rate-control strategy is a viable alternative to a rhythm-control strategy in patients with persistent AF, a significant limitation of these results is that they cannot be applied to patients with HF because only a small proportion of patients enrolled in these trials had LV systolic dysfunction. The AF-CHF trial was conducted to specifically evaluate the safety and efficacy of rate-control and rhythm-control strategies in patients with HF*r*EF.[33] In this trial, patients with an LVEF less than or equal to 35%, a history of HF (defined as NYHA class II to IV HF within the last 6 months, NYHA class I HF with a hospitalization for HF during the previous 6 months, or an LVEF less than or equal to 25%), and a history of AF were randomized to either a rate-control or a rhythm-control group. Rate-control treatment involved concomitant therapy with a β-blocker and digoxin first, and then nonpharmacologic treatment (AV nodal ablation with pacemaker implantation), if necessary. In the rhythm-control group, amiodarone was the preferred AAD, whereas sotalol and dofetilide were considered alternatives (most of the patients ultimately received amiodarone). If patients in this group did not convert to SR within 6 weeks, electrical cardioversion was performed. Anticoagulation was recommended for all patients in both treatment groups. After a mean follow-up period of 37 months, no significant difference was observed between the treatment groups with regard to the primary end point of death from CV causes. Patients in the rhythm-control group tended to have more hospitalizations, primarily due to repeated cardioversions and adjustment of AAD therapy, compared with patients in the rate-control group; however, this difference was not statistically significant ($P = 0.06$). It is important to note that the results of this trial should not be applied to patients with HF*p*EF. Nevertheless, the results of this trial are generally consistent with those of the PIAF, RACE, AFFIRM, STAF, and HOT-CAFE trials and suggest that a rhythm-control strategy does not confer any advantage over a rate-control strategy in patients with AF and HF*r*EF.

Clearly, these important findings temper the old approach of aggressively attempting to maintain SR. Because a rhythm-control strategy does not offer any significant advantage over a rate-control strategy in the management of patients with persistent or recurrent AF (including those with concomitant HF*r*EF), it is acceptable to allow patients to remain in AF, while being chronically treated not only with AV nodal blocking drugs to achieve adequate ventricular rate control but also with appropriate antithrombotic therapy to prevent TE complications. 4 The important question with this rate-control approach is: What defines "adequate" ventricular rate control? While adequate ventricular rate control was previously considered to be achieving a heart rate less than 80 beats/min at rest and less than 100 beats/min during exercise, evidence from the RACE II trial has suggested that selecting a more lenient rate-control strategy (resting heart rate less than 110 beats/min) may be a reasonable approach for certain patients with AF.[35] In this trial, a lenient rate-control strategy (resting heart rate less than 110 beats/min) was considered to be noninferior to a strict heart rate-control strategy (resting heart rate less than 80 beats/min and heart rate during moderate exercise less than 110 beats/min) with regard to the primary end point of CV death, hospitalization for HF, stroke, systemic embolism, bleeding, and life-threatening arrhythmic events. According to the most recent AHA/ACC/HRS guidelines for AF, this lenient rate-control strategy is recommended for those patients with persistent AF provided that patients are asymptomatic and have preserved LV systolic function (LVEF >40%).[22] In patients who are symptomatic or have LV systolic dysfunction (LVEF less than or equal to 40%), a stricter rate-control approach (resting heart rate less than 80 beats/min) should be considered..

As in the acute setting, the selection of an AV nodal blocking drug to control ventricular rate in the chronic setting should be primarily based on the patient's LV function.[22] In patients with normal LV function (LVEF >40%) or in patients with stable HF*p*EF, an oral β-blocker or non-DHP CCB (diltiazem or verapamil) is preferred over digoxin because of their relatively quick onset and maintained efficacy during exercise. When adequate ventricular rate control cannot be achieved with one of these drugs, the addition of digoxin may result in an additive lowering of the heart rate. Verapamil and diltiazem should not be used in patients with HF*r*EF (LVEF ≤40%). Instead, β-blockers (ie, metoprolol succinate, carvedilol, or bisoprolol) and digoxin are preferred in these patients, as these drugs are also concomitantly used to treat chronic HF*r*EF. Specifically, in patients with NYHA class II or III HF, β-blockers should be considered over digoxin because of their survival benefits in patients with HF*r*EF. If patients are having an episode of decompensated HF (NYHA class IV), digoxin is preferred as first-line therapy to achieve ventricular rate control because of the potential for worsening HF symptoms with the initiation and subsequent titration of β-blocker therapy. If adequate ventricular rate control during rest and exercise cannot be achieved with β-blockers, non-DHP CCBs, and/or digoxin in patients with normal or depressed LV function, oral amiodarone can be used as alternative therapy to control the heart rate.

Because a rate-control strategy is now considered a reasonable initial approach for the chronic management of AF, the question that remains to be answered is, "In which patients should restoration of SR be considered?" Electrical or pharmacologic cardioversion should be considered for those patients with AF who remain symptomatic despite having adequate ventricular rate control or for those patients in whom adequate ventricular rate control cannot be achieved.[22] A rhythm-control strategy may also be considered in patients who are experiencing their first episode of AF if they are likely to convert to and remain in SR. Other factors that may lend themselves the use of a rhythm-control strategy include younger age, presence of tachycardia-induced cardiomyopathy, AF precipitated by acute illness, and patient preference.

In those patients in whom it is decided to restore SR, one must consider that this very act (regardless of whether an electrical or pharmacologic method is chosen) places the patient at risk for a TE event. The reason for this heightened risk is that the return of SR restores effective contraction in the atria, which may dislodge poorly adherent thrombi. Administering antithrombotic therapy prior to cardioversion not only prevents clot growth and the formation of new thrombi but also allows existing thrombi to become organized and well adherent to the atrial wall. It is a generally accepted principle that the risk of thrombus formation and a subsequent embolic event increases if the duration of the AF exceeds 48 hours. Therefore, it is vital for clinicians to estimate the duration of the patient's AF so that appropriate antithrombotic therapy can be administered prior to cardioversion if needed.

According to the most recent AHA/ACC/HRS guidelines for the treatment of AF, in patients undergoing elective cardioversion (electrical or pharmacologic) for AF lasting at least 48 hours or for an unknown duration, therapeutic anticoagulation with warfarin (INR target range 2 to 3), apixaban, dabigatran, or rivaroxaban should be given for at least 3 weeks before cardioversion is performed.[22] If 3 weeks of therapeutic oral anticoagulant therapy is not feasible in these patients, there is an alternative regimen whereby the patient can undergo a transesophageal echocardiogram (TEE) prior to cardioversion. If no thrombus is observed on TEE, the patient can undergo cardioversion. In these patients, anticoagulant therapy with either IV unfractionated heparin (UFH) (target activated partial thromboplastin time 60 seconds; acceptable range 50 to 70 seconds) or a low-molecular-weight heparin (LMWH) (subcutaneously at treatment doses) should be initiated at the time the TEE will be performed.[36] Cardioversion should then be performed within 24 hours of the TEE. Alternatively, warfarin therapy (INR target range 2 to 3) may be used for at least 5 days prior to the TEE and cardioversion. If cardioversion is successful, therapeutic anticoagulation with warfarin (INR target range 2 to 3), apixaban, dabigatran, or rivaroxaban should be continued for at least 4 weeks, regardless of the patient's baseline risk of stroke.[22] The reason for continuing anticoagulation for this additional 4-week time period is that after restoration of SR, full atrial contraction does not occur immediately. Rather, it returns gradually to a maximum contractile force over a 3- to 4-week period. Decisions regarding long-term antithrombotic therapy after this 4-week time period should be primarily based on the patient's risk for stroke and not on whether he/she is in SR.[22] If a thrombus is seen on TEE, cardioversion should not be performed and the patient should be anticoagulated indefinitely. If cardioversion is considered in these patients at a later time, a TEE should again be performed. Overall, the use of a TEE-guided approach to cardioversion in patients with AF has been compared with the conventional 3 weeks of anticoagulation before cardioversion in a large, multicenter, randomized trial.[37] In this trial, the incidence of TE events was not different between the two strategies, but bleeding episodes were higher in the group that received 3 weeks of warfarin therapy before cardioversion. Patients in the TEE strategy group had a higher success rate of achieving SR, probably because it is more difficult to terminate AF the longer a patient remains in this arrhythmia.

In patients with AF that is less than 48 hours in duration, anticoagulation prior to cardioversion is unnecessary because there has not been sufficient time to form atrial thrombi.[22] In those patients who are at high risk for stroke, IV UFH (target activated partial thromboplastin time 60 seconds; acceptable range 50 to 70 seconds), a LMWH (subcutaneously at treatment doses), apixaban, dabigatran, or rivaroxaban should be initiated as soon as possible either before or after cardioversion. If cardioversion is successful in these high-risk patients, therapeutic anticoagulation with warfarin (INR target range 2 to 3), apixaban, dabigatran, or rivaroxaban should be continued for at least 4 weeks. While the above anticoagulants can also be initiated immediately before or after cardioversion in patients at low risk for stroke, it is also reasonable to not initiate antithrombotic therapy in these patients. Decisions regarding long-term antithrombotic therapy in this low-risk population should be primarily based on the patient's risk for stroke and not on whether he/she is in SR.

After prior anticoagulation or TEE, the process of restoring SR can be considered. There are two methods of restoring SR in patients with AF or AFl: pharmacologic cardioversion and DCC. The decision to use either of these methods is generally a matter of clinical preference. The disadvantages of pharmacologic cardioversion are the risk of significant side effects (eg, drug-induced TdP), the potential for drug-drug interactions (eg, digoxin-amiodarone), and the lower efficacy of AADs when compared with DCC. The advantages of DCC are that it is quick and more often successful (80% to 90% success rate) compared to pharmacologic cardioversion. The disadvantages of DCC are the need for prior sedation/anesthesia and a risk (albeit small) of serious complications such as sinus arrest or ventricular arrhythmias.

Nonetheless, despite the relatively high success rate associated with DCC, clinicians often elect to use AADs first, and then resort to DCC in the event that these drugs fail. Pharmacologic cardioversion appears to be most effective when initiated within 7 days after the onset of AF.[22] According to the most recent treatment guidelines for AF, there is relatively strong evidence for efficacy of the class III pure I_K blockers (ibutilide and dofetilide), the class Ic AADs (flecainide and propafenone), and amiodarone (oral or IV) for cardioversion of AF.[22] Class Ia AADs have limited efficacy or have not been adequately studied in this setting. Sotalol is not effective for cardioversion of paroxysmal or persistent AF. Single, oral loading doses of propafenone (600 mg) and flecainide (300 mg) are effective compared with placebo for conversion of recent-onset AF and have been incorporated into the "pill-in-the-pocket" approach endorsed by the treatment guidelines.[22,38] With this method, outpatient, patient-controlled self-administration of a single, oral loading dose of either flecainide or propafenone can be a relatively safe and effective approach for the termination of recent-onset AF in a selected patient population that does not have sinus or AV node dysfunction, bundle-branch block, QT interval prolongation, Brugada syndrome, or SHD.[38] This treatment regimen should only be considered in patients who have previously been successfully cardioverted with these drugs on an inpatient basis.

Overall, when considering pharmacologic cardioversion, the selection of an AAD should be based on whether the patient has SHD (eg, LV dysfunction, CAD, valvular heart disease, LV hypertrophy).[22] In the absence of any type of SHD, the use of a single, oral loading dose of flecainide or propafenone is a reasonable approach for cardioversion. Ibutilide can also be used as an alternative in this patient population; however, use of this agent is restricted to a monitored setting in the hospital because it requires QT interval monitoring. In patients with underlying SHD, flecainide, propafenone, and ibutilide should be avoided because of the increased risk of proarrhythmia; amiodarone or dofetilide should be used instead. Although amiodarone can be administered safely on an outpatient basis because of its low proarrhythmic potential, dofetilide therapy can only be initiated in the hospital (for QT interval monitoring and assessment of renal function). Additionally, it should be remembered that a patient's ventricular rate should be adequately controlled with AV nodal blocking drugs prior to administering a class Ic AAD for cardioversion. The class Ic AADs may paradoxically increase ventricular response. The most likely mechanism for this effect is that by slowing atrial conduction, the class Ic AADs decrease the number of impulses reaching the AV node. Consequently, the AV node paradoxically allows more impulses to gain entrance to the ventricular conduction system, thereby increasing ventricular rate.

Long-Term Complications There are two forms of therapy that the clinician must consider in each patient with AF: long-term antithrombotic therapy to prevent stroke and long-term AADs to prevent recurrences of AF. Consider the issue of antithrombotic therapy first. Historically, warfarin has been the standard of care for stroke prevention in patients considered to be moderate or high risk for stroke. However, while warfarin is undoubtedly effective in preventing strokes in patients with AF, its use can be associated with a number of potential limitations, including a narrow therapeutic window, requirement for INR monitoring, food and drug interactions, and pharmacogenetic influences. Therefore, researchers have long been searching for an antithrombotic therapy that could be used as an alternative or even as a replacement for warfarin in patients with AF. Over the past few years, several oral antithrombotic therapies have been approved by the Food and Drug Administration for stroke prevention in patients with AF. These oral anticoagulant drugs, commonly referred to as target specific oral anticoagulants (TSOACs), include the direct thrombin inhibitor, dabigatran, and the factor Xa inhibitors, apixaban, edoxaban, and rivaroxaban.

When initiating chronic antithrombotic therapy in patients with AF, assessing the patient's risk for stroke becomes important for selecting the most appropriate regimen. Based on the most recent AHA/ACC/HRS guidelines for the treatment of AF, the CHA_2DS_2-VASc risk scoring system has been recommended for stroke risk stratification in patients with AF.[22] With this risk index, patients with AF are given 2 points each if they have a history of a previous stroke, transient ischemic attack, or thromboembolism, or if they are at least 75 years old. Patients are given one point each for being 65 to 74 years old, having hypertension, having diabetes, having congestive HF, having vascular disease (eg, MI, peripheral arterial disease, or aortic plaque), or being female. CHA_2DS_2-VASc is an acronym for each of these risk factors. The points are added up, and the total score is then used to determine the most appropriate antithrombotic therapy for the patient (Fig. 18-6). Patients with a CHA_2DS_2-VASc score of 2 or higher are considered to be at high risk for stroke. In these patients, oral anticoagulant therapy with warfarin (INR target range 2 to 3), apixaban, dabigatran, edoxaban, or rivaroxaban is preferred over aspirin. Patients with a CHA_2DS_2-VASc score of 1 are considered to be at intermediate risk for stroke. In these patients, oral anticoagulant therapy (warfarin [INR target range 2 to 3], apixaban, dabigatran, edoxaban, or rivaroxaban), aspirin 75 to 325 mg/day, or no antithrombotic therapy can be selected. Patients with a CHA_2DS_2-VASc score of 0 are considered to be at low risk for stroke. The guidelines state that it is reasonable to not give any antithrombotic therapy to this particular patient population.

The efficacy and safety of dabigatran were compared with those of warfarin in patients with AF in the Randomized Evaluation of

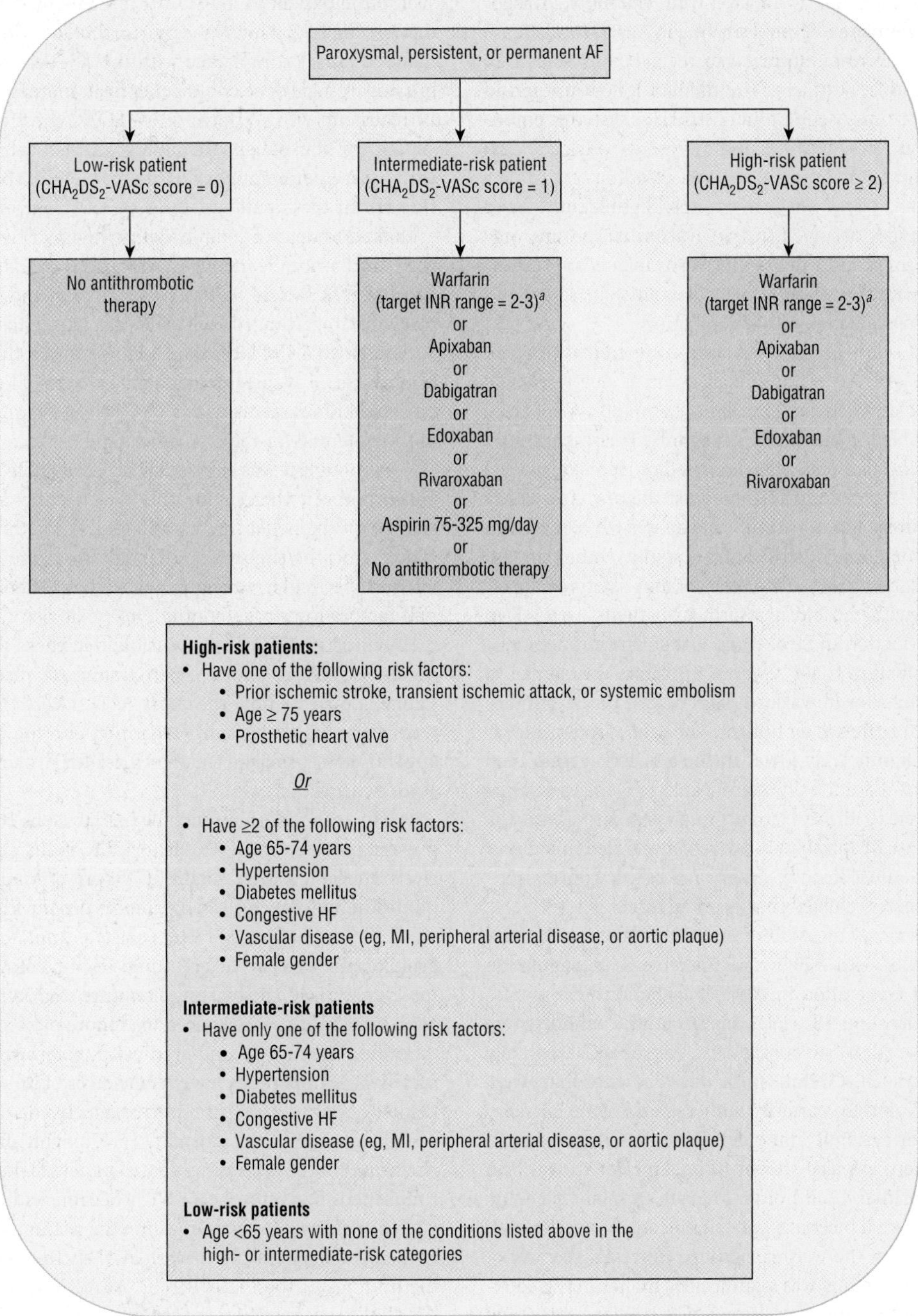

FIGURE 18-6 Algorithm for the prevention of thromboembolism in paroxysmal, persistent, or permanent AF. [a]The target INR for patients with prosthetic heart valves should be based on the type of valve that is present. (AF, atrial fibrillation; HF, heart failure; INR, international normalized ratio; MI, myocardial infarction.)

Long-Term Anticoagulation Therapy (RE-LY) trial.[39] In this study, patients were randomized to receive dabigatran 110 mg twice daily, dabigatran 150 mg twice daily or adjusted-dose warfarin. The median follow-up period was 2 years. For the primary end point of stroke or systemic embolism, both dabigatran groups were shown to be noninferior to warfarin. However, superiority was also assessed and the dabigatran 150-mg group was shown to be superior to warfarin in reducing this end point. The rate of major bleeding was similar between the dabigatran 150-mg and warfarin groups, while the rate of major bleeding was significantly lower in the dabigatran 110-mg group than in the warfarin group. The rate of intracranial hemorrhage was significantly lower in both dabigatran groups than in the warfarin group. Even though the 110- and 150-mg dosing regimens of dabigatran were evaluated in this trial, only the 150-mg dose was approved by the Food and Drug Administration for AF. A lower 75-mg dose was also approved for patients with a CrCl of 15 to 30 mL/min, even though this dose has not been evaluated in a randomized, prospective clinical trial in patients with AF; this dose has only pharmacokinetic data to support its use.[40] It is important to note that the RE-LY trial excluded patients with a CrCl less than 30 mL/min. Dabigatran is contraindicated in patients with mechanical heart valves because its use in this population has been associated with an increased risk of TE complications and bleeding.[41] The use of dabigatran is also not recommended in patients with bioprosthetic heart valves since the safety and efficacy of this antithrombotic have not been evaluated in this population. Patients with hemodynamically significant valvular disease or advanced liver disease are also not appropriate candidates for dabigatran therapy.

The efficacy and safety of rivaroxaban were compared with those of warfarin in patients with AF in the Rivaroxaban Once Daily

Oral Direct Factor Xa Inhibition Compared with Vitamin K Antagonism for Prevention of Stroke and Embolism Trial in Atrial Fibrillation.[42] In this study, patients were randomized to receive rivaroxaban 20 mg daily or adjusted-dose warfarin. The median follow-up period was 1.9 years. For the primary end point of stroke or systemic embolism, rivaroxaban was shown to be noninferior to warfarin. The rate of major and nonmajor clinically relevant bleeding was similar between the rivaroxaban and warfarin groups. Significantly fewer intracranial hemorrhages occurred in the rivaroxaban group compared with the warfarin group. The use of rivaroxaban is not recommended in patients with prosthetic heart valves since its safety and efficacy have not been evaluated in this population.

The efficacy and safety of apixaban were compared with those of aspirin in patients with AF in the Apixaban versus Acetylsalicylic Acid to Prevent Stroke in Atrial Fibrillation Patients Who Have Failed or Are Unsuitable for Vitamin K Antagonist Treatment trial.[43] This particular trial enrolled patients who failed or were considered unsuitable candidates for vitamin K antagonist therapy. This study was stopped prematurely when a significant benefit with regard to the primary efficacy outcome of stroke and systemic embolism was observed in the apixaban group. The efficacy and safety of apixaban were compared with those of warfarin in patients with AF in the Apixaban for Reduction in Stroke and Other Thromboembolic Events in Atrial Fibrillation trial.[44] Overall, apixaban was shown to be noninferior and superior to warfarin with regard to the primary end point of stroke or systemic embolism. The rate of major bleeding in this trial was significantly lower in the apixaban group than in the warfarin group. Additionally, significantly fewer intracranial hemorrhages occurred in the apixaban group compared with the warfarin group. The use of apixaban is not recommended in patients with prosthetic heart valves since the safety and efficacy of this anticoagulant have not been evaluated in this population.

The efficacy and safety of edoxaban were compared with those of warfarin in patients with AF in the Effective Anticoagulation with Factor Xa Next Generation in Atrial Fibrillation-Thrombolysis in Myocardial Infarction 48 trial.[45] In this study, patients were randomized to receive edoxaban 60 mg daily, edoxaban 30 mg daily or adjusted-dose warfarin. Overall, both doses of edoxaban were shown to be noninferior to warfarin with regard to the primary end point of stroke or systemic embolism. However, the edoxaban 60-mg dosing regimen was also shown to be superior to warfarin with regard to this primary end point. The rate of major bleeding and the risk of intracranial bleeding were significantly lower in both edoxaban groups than in the warfarin group. However, the risk of major gastrointestinal bleeding was significantly higher in the edoxaban 60-mg group but significantly lower in the edoxaban 30-mg group when compared to the warfarin group. The use of edoxaban is not recommended in patients with mechanical heart valves or moderate-to-severe mitral stenosis since the safety and efficacy of this anticoagulant have not been evaluated in this population.

The most recent AHA/ACC/HRS guidelines for the treatment of AF provide recommendations regarding the use of various anticoagulant agents for stroke prevention in patients with nonvalvular AF.[22] These recommendations state that warfarin, dabigatran, rivaroxaban and apixaban are all indicated for the prevention of initial and recurrent strokes in patients with nonvalvular AF. These guidelines were published prior to the Food and Drug Administration's approval of edoxaban, and consequently do not provide recommendations regarding the role of this oral anticoagulant for stroke prevention in patients with AF. Anticoagulant therapy should be individualized for each patient, with consideration given to stroke risk factors, drug cost, tolerability, patient preference and drug interaction potential. Additionally, if a patient has previously taken warfarin, the time that his/her INR has been within the therapeutic range should also be considered before making the decision to switch the patient to a TSOAC. If a patient is unable to maintain a therapeutic INR while on warfarin, therapy with a TSOAC is recommended. Strict compliance with the TSOACs is important because missing a single dose could result in an increased risk of TE events.[46] If treatment with warfarin or a TSOAC must be temporarily interrupted for the patient to undergo a medical procedure, coverage with a parenteral anticoagulant (eg, UFH, LMWH) should be considered. In these patients, the risks of stroke and bleeding must be evaluated to determine if bridging therapy is warranted. In patients with mechanical heart valves, warfarin is the anticoagulant of choice and the INR should be based on the type and location of the valve placed. Dabigatran, edoxaban, and rivaroxaban should be avoided in patients with a CrCl less than 15 mL/min. In this particular population, warfarin is the anticoagulant of choice. Edoxaban should also be avoided in patients with a CrCl greater than 95 mL/min because of the potential for reduced efficacy.

Although it was previously an acceptable practice to continue antithrombotic therapy for only 4 weeks after successful cardioversion (with the belief that a patient's risk for thromboembolism had abated since he/she was in SR), data from the RACE and AFFIRM trials, in particular, strongly suggest that patients with AF and other risk factors for stroke continue to be at risk for stroke even when maintained in SR.[29,30] It is possible that these patients may be having undetected episodes of paroxysmal AF, placing them at risk for stroke. Consequently, the most recent AHA/ACC/HRS guidelines recommend that decisions regarding chronic antithrombotic therapy should be based on a patient's risk for stroke using the CHA_2DS_2-VASc scoring system.[22]

The second form of chronic therapy to be considered is AADs to prevent recurrences of AF. Historically, many clinicians have aggressively attempted to maintain SR by prescribing oral AADs (usually quinidine) to prevent AF recurrences despite the fact that only small studies with conflicting results existed evaluating this approach. To evaluate the efficacy of quinidine in preventing AF, a well-known meta-analysis of the existing literature was completed.[47] This meta-analysis demonstrated that indeed more patients remain in SR with quinidine therapy (compared with placebo); however, approximately 50% of patients have recurrences of AF within a year despite the use of quinidine. This reported effectiveness was at the cost of an associated increase in mortality (presumably due, in part, to proarrhythmia) in the quinidine-treated patients. These disturbing results (published soon after the CAST[48]) became widely quoted and highly visible, making clinicians question the wisdom of long-term prevention of recurrences of AF with AADs. These results coupled with the findings of the PIAF, RACE, AFFIRM, STAF, HOT-CAFE, and AF-CHF trials question the need to use AADs to prevent AF recurrences.[28-33] In fact, based on the results of these landmark trials, the use of AADs to maintain SR may be more reasonable to consider in patients who remain symptomatic despite having adequate ventricular rate control or for those patients in whom adequate ventricular rate control cannot be achieved.

According to the most recent AHA/ACC/HRS treatment guidelines for AF, the class Ic or III AADs are reasonable to consider to maintain patients in SR (Table 18-9).[22] The role of the class Ia AADs for maintenance of SR has been deemphasized throughout these guidelines as they are considered less effective or incompletely studied compared with the class Ic and III AADs. Interestingly, a systematic review of AADs for the maintenance of SR after cardioversion in patients with AF demonstrated that AF recurrences were significantly reduced with the use of class Ia, Ic, and III AADs; however, mortality was significantly increased with the class Ia drugs, in particular.[49]

The class Ic AADs, flecainide and propafenone, are effective for maintaining SR. However, because of the increased risk for proarrhythmia, these drugs should be avoided in patients with SHD.

TABLE 18-9 Guidelines for Selecting Antiarrhythmic Drug Therapy for Maintenance of Sinus Rhythm in Patients with Recurrent Paroxysmal or Recurrent Persistent Atrial Fibrillation

No structural heart disease[a] (absence of heart failure, coronary artery disease, signifi cant LVH, and valvular disease) First line:[b] dofetilide, dronedarone, flecainide, propafenone, or sotalol Second line:[c] amiodarone
Heart failure[a] First line:[b] amiodarone or dofetilide Second line: catheter ablation
Coronary artery disease[a] First line:[b] dofetilide, dronedarone,[d] or sotalol[d] Second line:[c] amiodarone
Hypertension[a] Presence of signifi cant LVH: First line:[b] amiodarone or dronedarone Second line: catheter ablation Absence of signifi cant LVH: First line:[b] dofetilide, dronedarone, flecainide, propafenone, or sotalol Second line:[c] amiodarone

LVH, left ventricular hypertrophy.

[a]Drugs are listed alphabetically and not in order of suggested use.

[b]Catheter ablation may also be considered first-line therapy in select patients with paroxysmal atrial fibrillation.

[c]Catheter ablation may also be considered when patients are refractory or intolerant to at least 1 antiarrhythmic drug.

[d]Should only be used in this situation if the patient has normal left ventricular systolic function.

Although all of the oral class III AADs have demonstrated efficacy in preventing AF recurrences, amiodarone is clearly the most effective agent and is now the most frequently used AAD despite its potential for causing significant organ toxicity.[8] The superiority of amiodarone over other AADs for maintaining patients in SR has been demonstrated in a number of clinical trials. In the Canadian Trial of Atrial Fibrillation, amiodarone was significantly more effective than sotalol or propafenone in maintaining SR in patients with persistent or paroxysmal AF.[50] Furthermore, in a substudy of the AFFIRM trial, amiodarone appeared to be the most effective AAD in maintaining SR of those used in the study.[51] In the Sotalol Amiodarone Atrial Fibrillation Efficacy Trial, amiodarone and sotalol were equally effective at converting AF to SR.[52] However, amiodarone was significantly more effective than sotalol at maintaining SR in all patient subgroups, except for those with CAD where the efficacy of these two drugs was comparable.

Although sotalol is not effective for conversion of AF, it is an effective drug for maintaining SR. Sotalol appears to be at least as effective as quinidine or propafenone in preventing recurrences of AF.[50,53] However, treatment with either quinidine or sotalol is associated with a similar incidence of TdP. Because this form of proarrhythmia primarily occurs with higher doses of sotalol (quinidine usually causes TdP at low or therapeutic concentrations), it may be more easily predicted and therefore avoided. Nonetheless, sotalol may be similar to quinidine in increasing mortality in patients with AF; however, this finding requires further study.[54]

Dofetilide is effective in preventing recurrences of AF but has not been directly compared with either amiodarone or sotalol. In a large, multicenter trial, dofetilide was more effective than placebo in maintaining SR (approximately 35%-50% at 1 year).[55] The efficacy of dofetilide for the maintenance of SR has also specifically been demonstrated in patients with HF*r*EF.[56] Like sotalol and quinidine, dofetilide also has significant potential to cause TdP (in a dose-related fashion).

The safety and efficacy of dronedarone for the treatment of AF and AFl have been evaluated in several clinical trials. In the European Trial in Atrial Fibrillation or Flutter Patients Receiving Dronedarone for the Maintenance of Sinus Rhythm and the American-Australian-African Trial with Dronedarone in Atrial Fibrillation or Flutter Patients for the Maintenance of Sinus Rhythm, which were similar in design, dronedarone was more effective than placebo in maintaining SR in patients with paroxysmal or persistent AF or AFl.[57] In another trial, the use of dronedarone in patients with persistent or paroxysmal AF or AFl was associated with significantly fewer hospitalizations due to CV events or death when compared with placebo.[58] The safety and efficacy of dronedarone were also evaluated in a trial that included patients with NYHA class III or IV HF and an LVEF of 35% or less.[59] This trial was prematurely terminated because all-cause mortality (primarily due to worsening HF) was significantly higher in the dronedarone group when compared with the placebo group. Consequently, based on these findings, dronedarone is contraindicated in and has received a black box warning for patients with advanced HF (NYHA class IV or NYHA class II or III with a recent hospitalization for decompensated HF). The efficacy and safety of dronedarone in patients with AF have been compared with those of amiodarone.[60] In this trial, dronedarone was shown to be significantly less effective than amiodarone in reducing AF recurrences; however, tolerability was significantly better in the dronedarone group than in the amiodarone group as evidenced by higher rates of premature drug discontinuation and adverse events in the amiodarone group. Most recently, a trial that enrolled patients with permanent AF and risk factors for major vascular events was terminated prematurely after significantly more patients in the dronedarone group died (primarily from CV causes), were hospitalized for HF, and suffered a stroke when compared with the placebo group.[61] Based on the results of this trial, dronedarone is contraindicated in and has received a black box warning for patients with permanent AF.

Overall, the selection of an AAD to maintain SR should be primarily based on whether the patient has SHD.[22] However, other factors, including renal and hepatic function, concomitant disease states and drugs, and the AAD's side effect profile, also need to be considered. Based on the most recent AHA/ACC/HRS treatment guidelines for AF, dofetilide, dronedarone, flecainide, propafenone, or sotalol should be considered initially for those patients with no underlying SHD because these drugs have the most optimal long-term safety profile in this setting.[22] However, amiodarone could be used as alternative therapy if the patient fails or does not tolerate one of these initial AADs. In the presence of SHD, flecainide and propafenone should be avoided because of the risk of proarrhythmia. For those patients with HF*r*EF (LVEF ≤40%), amiodarone or dofetilide should be considered the AADs of choice. At this time, only amiodarone and dofetilide have been shown to be mortality-neutral in patients with AF and HF*r*EF. Both dronedarone and sotalol should be avoided in patients with HF*r*EF because of the risk for increased mortality (dronedarone) or worsening HF (dronedarone and sotalol). In patients with CAD, dofetilide, dronedarone, or sotalol can be used initially. Again, dronedarone and sotalol should not be used if patients have concomitant HF*r*EF. Amiodarone could be used as an alternative therapy if the patient fails or does not tolerate one of these initial AADs. The presence of LV hypertrophy may predispose the myocardium to proarrhythmic events. Because of their low proarrhythmic potential, amiodarone or dronedarone should be considered first-line AAD therapy in these patients.

Nonpharmacologic forms of therapy, designed to maintain SR, are becoming increasingly popular treatment options for patients with AF or AFl. For patients who have "pure" (ie, not associated with concurrent AF) type I AFl, ablation of the reentrant substrate with radiofrequency current is highly effective (approximately 90%) and can be considered first-line treatment of AFl to prevent recurrences.[62,63] Catheter ablation for patients with AF is much more technically difficult for a variety of reasons, including the lack of a single, identifiable, and ablatable reentrant focus (as in AFl). Nonetheless, progress has been made in this area. Patients with AF have been found to have arrhythmogenic foci that occur in atrial tissue near and within the pulmonary veins. During the ablation procedure, radiofrequency energy can be delivered to these areas in an attempt to abolish the foci. Historically, this procedure was often considered last-line therapy for patients who had failed all AADs, including amiodarone. However, in some of the recent trials, the use of catheter ablation in patients with AF has been associated with a significant reduction in recurrent episodes of AF and an improvement in quality of life when compared with AAD therapy.[64-66] There is also evidence to suggest that this procedure may be superior to AADs as first-line therapy of symptomatic AF.[67,68] According to the most recent AHA/ACC/HRS guidelines for AF, for those patients with symptomatic episodes of AF who fail or do not tolerate at least one class I or III AAD, catheter ablation is recommended for those with paroxysmal AF, reasonable for those with persistent AF, and may be considered for those with long-standing (more than 12 months) persistent AF.[22] For those patients with symptomatic episodes of AF who have not yet received treatment with a class I or III AAD, catheter ablation is reasonable for those with recurrent, paroxysmal AF and may be considered for persistent AF. This procedure is not without its risks, as major complications, such as pulmonary vein stenosis, TE events, cardiac tamponade, and new AFl, have been reported in 4.5% of patients.[69]

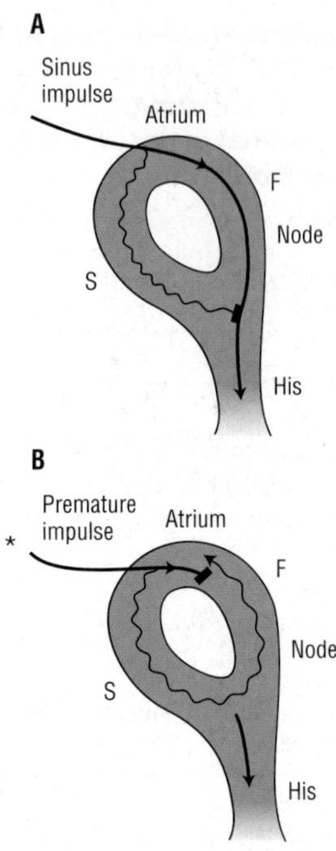

FIGURE 18-7 Reentry mechanism of dual AV nodal pathway PSVT. *A.* Sinus rhythm: the impulse travels from the atrium through the fast pathway (F) and then to the His-Purkinje system (His). The impulse also travels through the slow pathway (S) but is stopped when refractory tissue is encountered. *B.* Dual AV nodal reentry: a critically timed premature impulse (*) is stopped in the fast pathway (F) (because of prolonged refractoriness) but is able to travel antegrade down the slow pathway (S) and retrograde through the fast pathway. (AV, atrioventricular; PSVT, paroxysmal supraventricular tachycardia.)

Paroxysmal Supraventricular Tachycardia Caused By Reentry

PSVT arising by reentrant mechanisms includes those arrhythmias caused by AV nodal reentry, AV reentry incorporating an anomalous AV pathway, SA nodal reentry, and intraatrial reentry. AV nodal reentry and AV reentry are by far the most common of these tachycardias. 5

Mechanisms

The underlying substrate of AV nodal reentry is the functional division of the AV node into two (or more) longitudinal conduction pathways or "dual" AV nodal pathways.[70] It is now clear that there are not two distinct anatomic pathways inside the AV node itself; rather, it is likely that a fan-like network of perinodal fibers inserts into the AV node and represents the second pathway. The pathways possess key differences in conduction characteristics: one is a fast-conducting pathway with a relatively long refractory period (fast pathway) and the other is a slower-conducting pathway with a shorter refractory period (slow pathway). The presence of dual pathways does not necessarily imply that the patient will have clinical PSVT. In fact, it is estimated that between 10% and 50% of patients have discernible dual pathways, but the incidence of PSVT is considerably lower.[70] Sustenance of the tachycardia depends on the critical electrophysiologic discrepancies and the ability of one pathway (usually the slow) to allow repetitive antegrade conduction, and the ability of the other pathway (usually the fast) to allow repetitive retrograde conduction. During SR, a patient with dual pathways conducts supraventricular impulses antegrade through both pathways. Electrical activity reaches the distal common pathway at the level of or above the His bundle and continues to depolarize the ventricles in an antegrade direction. Conduction proceeds via the two pathways but reaches the distal common pathway first through the fast AV nodal route (Fig. 18-7). For this reason, a short PR interval is sometimes observed during SR.

PSVT caused by AV nodal reentry may occur by the following sequence of events. The occurrence of an appropriately timed premature impulse penetrates the AV node but is blocked in the fast pathway that is still refractory from the previous beat. However, the slow pathway, which has a shorter refractory period, permits antegrade conduction of the premature impulse. By the time the impulse has reached the distal common pathway, the fast pathway has recovered its excitability and now will permit retrograde conduction. The impulse reaches the common proximal pathway, preceded by an excitable gap of tissue, and reenters the slow pathway. A reentrant circuit that does not require atrial or ventricular tissue is completed within the AV node, and a tachycardia is thereby initiated. The common form of this tachycardia uses the slow pathway for antegrade conduction and the fast pathway for retrograde conduction; an uncommon form exists in which the reentrant impulse travels in the opposite direction.

AV reentrant tachycardia depends on the presence of an anomalous, or accessory, extranodal pathway that bypasses the normal AV conduction pathway. Several different types of accessory pathways have been described, depending on the specific anatomic areas they connect (eg, AV bundles or nodoventricular tracts); some are also referred to as eponyms, such as the Kent's bundle. A Kent's bundle is an extranodal AV connection that is associated with WPW syndrome. During SR (Fig. 18-8), patients with WPW syndrome depolarize the ventricles simultaneously through both AV pathways (AV nodal pathway and the Kent's bundle), creating a fusion pattern on the early portion of the QRS complex (delta wave). The degree of ventricular "preexcitation" depends on the contribution of antegrade ventricular activation through the accessory pathway. Patients may have an accessory pathway that is not evident on ECG, which is referred to as a "concealed" Kent's bundle. These concealed accessory pathways are often incapable of antegrade conduction and can only accept electrical stimulation in a retrograde fashion. The electrocardiographic expression of preexcitation (delta wave) depends on the location of the accessory pathway, the distance from the wave front of sinus activation, and the conduction characteristics

A

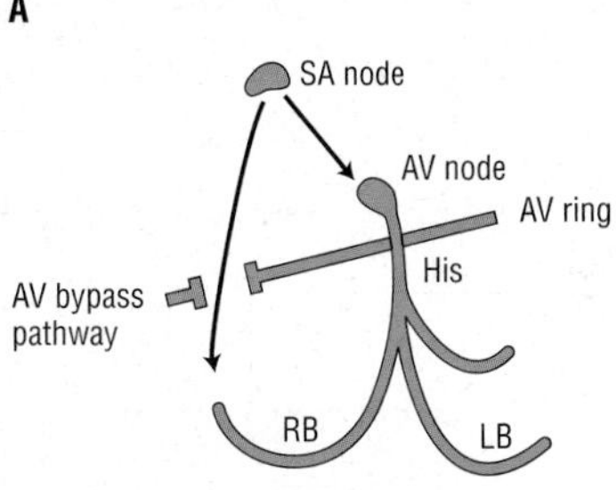

B

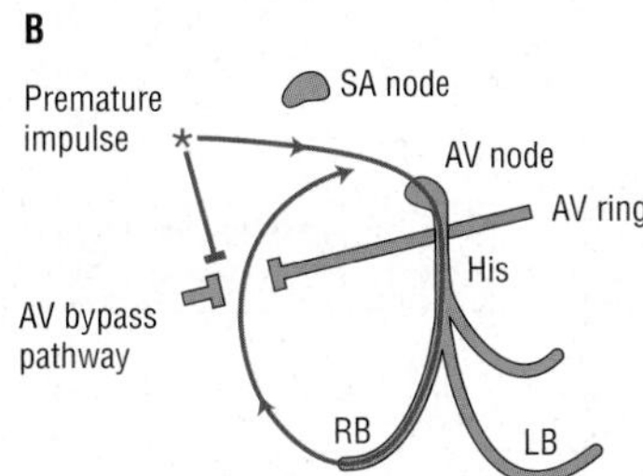

FIGURE 18-8 Reentry mechanism for AV accessory pathway PSVT in Wolff-Parkinson-White syndrome. *A.* Sinus rhythm: the impulse travels from the atrium to the ventricle by two pathways—the AV node and an accessory bypass pathway. *B.* AV reentry: a critically timed premature impulse (*) is stopped in the Kent's bundle (because of prolonged refractoriness) but travels antegrade through the AV node and retrograde through the Kent's bundle. (AV, atrioventricular; His, His-Purkinje system; LB, left bundle branch; PSVT, paroxysmal supraventricular tachycardia; RB, right bundle branch; SA, sinoatrial.)

of the various structures involved. It should be noted that (similar to patients with dual AV nodal pathways) not all patients with preexcitation with an accessory AV pathway are capable of having clinical PSVT.

Patients with an accessory AV pathway may have three forms of supraventricular tachycardia: (a) orthodromic reentry; (b) antidromic reentry; and/or (c) AF or AFl. AV reentrant PSVT usually occurs by the following sequence of events. Analogous to AV nodal reentry, two pathways (the normal AV nodal pathway and the accessory AV pathway) exist that have different electrophysiologic characteristics. The AV nodal pathway usually has a relatively slower conduction velocity and shorter refractory period, and the accessory pathway has a faster conduction velocity and a longer refractory period. A critically timed premature impulse may be blocked in the accessory pathway because this area is still refractory from the previous sinus beat. However, the AV nodal pathway, with a relatively shorter refractory period, may accept antegrade conduction of the premature impulse. Meanwhile, the accessory pathway may recover its excitability and now allow retrograde conduction. A macroreentrant tachycardia is thereby initiated in which the antegrade pathway is the AV nodal pathway, the distal common pathway is the ventricle, the retrograde pathway is the accessory pathway, and the proximal common pathway is the atrium (see Fig. 18-8). This sequence of events (down the AV node, up the Kent's bundle), termed *orthodromic PSVT*, is the common variety of reentry in patients with an accessory AV pathway, resulting in a narrow QRS tachycardia. In the uncommon variety, conduction proceeds in the opposite direction (down the Kent's bundle, up the AV node), resulting in a wide QRS tachycardia, which is termed *antidromic PSVT*. Patients with WPW syndrome can have a third type of tachycardia, namely, AF. The occurrence of AF in the setting of an accessory AV pathway (ie, WPW syndrome) can be extremely serious. As AF is an extremely rapid atrial tachycardia, conduction can proceed down the accessory AV pathway, resulting in a very fast ventricular response or even VF. Unlike the AV nodal pathway, the refractory period of the accessory bundle shortens in response to rapid stimulation rates.

Sinus node reentry and intraatrial reentry occur less commonly and are not as well described as AV nodal reentry and AV reentry. Aside from a characteristic abrupt onset and termination, coupled with subtle changes in P-wave morphology, these tachycardias can be difficult to diagnose. Electrophysiologic studies may be necessary to determine the ultimate mechanism of the PSVT.

Management

Both pharmacologic and nonpharmacologic methods have been used to treat patients with PSVT. Drugs used in the treatment of PSVT can be divided into three broad categories: (a) those that directly or indirectly increase vagal tone to the AV node (eg, digoxin); (b) those that depress conduction through slow, calcium-dependent tissue (eg, adenosine, β-blockers, and non-DHP CCBs); and (c) those that depress conduction through fast, sodium-dependent tissue (eg, quinidine, procainamide, disopyramide, and flecainide). Drugs within these categories alter the electrophysiologic characteristics of the reentrant substrate so that PSVT cannot be sustained. In PSVT caused by AV nodal reentry, class I AADs, such as flecainide, act primarily on the retrograde fast pathway. Digoxin and β-blockers may work on either the retrograde fast or the antegrade slow pathway. Verapamil, diltiazem, and adenosine prolong conduction time and increase refractoriness, primarily in the slow antegrade pathway of the reentrant loop. In PSVT caused by AV reentry incorporating an extranodal pathway, class I AADs increase refractoriness in the fast accessory pathway or within the His-Purkinje system. β-Blockers, digoxin, adenosine, and verapamil all act by their effects on the AV nodal (antegrade, slow) portion of the reentrant circuit. Regardless of the mechanism, treatment measures are directed first at terminating an acute episode of PSVT and then at preventing symptomatic recurrences of the arrhythmia.

For those patients with PSVT who present with severe symptoms (ie, syncope, near syncope, angina, or severe HF), synchronized DCC is the treatment of choice. Even at low energy levels (such as 25 J), DCC is almost always effective in quickly restoring SR and correcting symptomatic hypotension. Patients with only mild-to-moderate symptoms usually do not require DCC, and nonpharmacologic measures that increase vagal tone to the AV node can be used initially. Vagal techniques, such as unilateral carotid sinus massage, Valsalva maneuver, ice water facial immersion, or induced retching, are often successful in terminating PSVT, although carotid massage and Valsalva maneuver are the simplest, least obtrusive, and most frequently used of these techniques.

In the event that vagal maneuvers fail (approximately 80% of acute episodes) in those patients with tolerable symptoms, drug therapy is the next option. Figure 18-9 shows a therapeutic approach to the acute treatment of the different forms of reentrant PSVT. 6 This approach is based on analysis of the electrocardiographic characteristics of the rhythm because PSVT is not always discernible from other arrhythmias, and some forms of PSVT require different treatment. In patients with a narrow QRS, regular arrhythmia (AV nodal reentry or orthodromic AV reentry), IV verapamil (5-10 mg), IV diltiazem (15-25 mg), and adenosine (6-12 mg) are all equally efficacious. Approximately 80% to 90% of PSVT episodes will revert to SR within 5 minutes of these drug therapies.[71] The 2010 Guidelines for Cardiopulmonary Resuscitation (CPR) and Emergency Cardiovascular Care (ECC) from the AHA (no updated recommendations regarding treatment of PSVT in 2015 Guidelines Update for CPR and ECC), and the 2003 guidelines from the ACC/AHA/European Society of Cardiology,[63,72,73] promote adenosine as the drug of first choice in patients with PSVT.

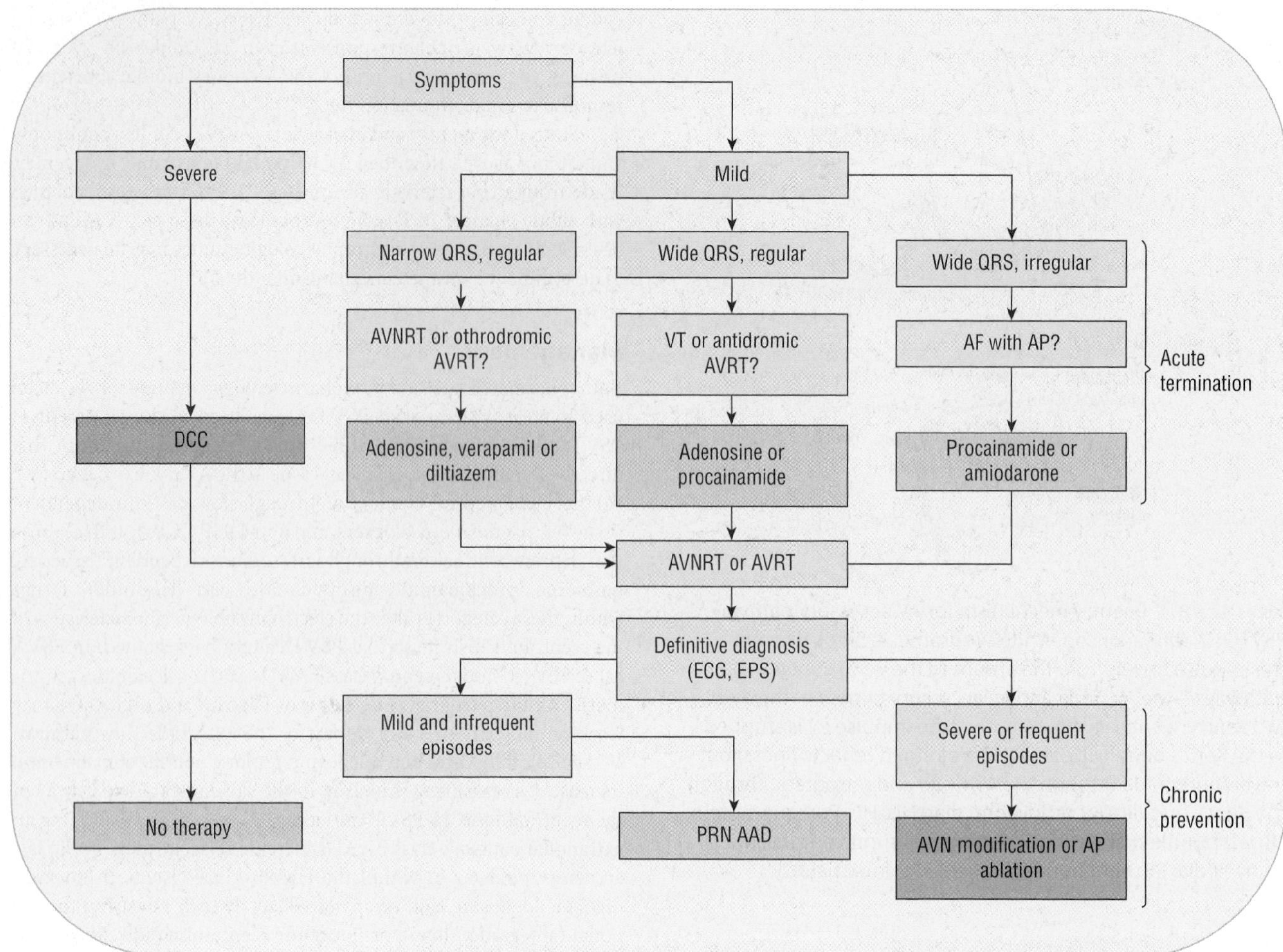

FIGURE 18-9 Algorithm for the treatment of acute (*top portion*) PSVT and chronic prevention of recurrences (*bottom portion*). *Note*: For empiric bridge therapy prior to ablation procedures, CCBs (or other AV nodal blockers) should not be used if the patient has AV reentry with an accessory pathway. (AAD, antiarrhythmic drug; AF, atrial fibrillation; AP, accessory pathway; AV, atrioventricular; AVN, atrioventricular nodal; AVNRT, atrioventricular nodal reentrant tachycardia; AVRT, atrioventricular reentrant tachycardia; CCBs, calcium channel blockers; DCC, direct current cardioversion; ECG, electrocardiogram; EPS, electrophysiologic studies; PRN, as needed; PSVT, paroxysmal supraventricular tachycardia; VT, ventricular tachycardia.)

5 These recommendations are particularly important when treating a patient who presents with a wide QRS, regular tachycardia that may be VT or PSVT (antidromic AV reentry or as a result of aberrancy). Because of its ultrashort duration of action (seconds), adenosine will not cause the severe and prolonged hemodynamic compromise seen in patients with VT who were mistakenly treated with verapamil and suffered from its negative inotropic effects and vasodilator properties.[74] If, in fact, the arrhythmia is PSVT, adenosine will likely terminate it. An alternative treatment for this type of patient is IV procainamide, which works on the fast, sodium-dependent extranodal pathway and is also effective for VT. Likewise, IV procainamide, or perhaps IV amiodarone (particularly in patients with LV dysfunction) should be used for the patient who presents with a wide QRS, irregular arrhythmia that is hemodynamically stable.[72] This rhythm could represent AF with rapid ventricular activation occurring primarily through an extranodal pathway. Administration of IV verapamil, diltiazem, digoxin, or adenosine to these patients may result in a paradoxical increase in ventricular response, causing severe symptoms requiring cardioversion. Consequently, these drugs are considered contraindicated in this specific setting.

Once the acute episode of PSVT is terminated, a decision on long-term preventive therapy must follow. Most patients require long-term therapy; preventive treatment is indicated if (a) frequent episodes occur that necessitate therapeutic intervention (ie, emergency department visits or interference with the patient's lifestyle) or (b) infrequent but severely symptomatic symptoms occur. For those patients in whom a preventive treatment is deemed necessary, two methods of management have been used: preventive drug therapy and catheter ablation.

AADs are no longer the treatment of choice to prevent recurrences of reentrant PSVT for the following reasons: (a) lifelong treatment is necessary in these generally young, but otherwise healthy, individuals; (b) there are few, if any, large controlled or comparative trials to assist the clinician in rationally choosing effective agents; and (c) most importantly, other nonpharmacologic treatments are clearly more effective. Nevertheless, drug therapy may occasionally be necessary in some patients, particularly those with mild symptoms and infrequent recurrences. A trial-and-error approach may be used, complemented by the use of ambulatory electrocardiographic recordings (Holter) or telephonic transmissions of cardiac rhythm (event monitors) to objectively document the efficacy or failure of the chosen drug regimen. Drugs known to be effective in preventing recurrences of PSVT are the AV nodal blocking drugs (digoxin, β-blockers, non-DHP CCBs, and combinations of these agents) and the class Ic AADs (flecainide, propafenone). Drugs such as quinidine, disopyramide, and amiodarone, although effective in some patients, should be discouraged because of the risk of toxicity with long-term treatment.

Catheter ablation using radiofrequency current on the PSVT substrate has dramatically altered the traditional treatment of these patients (Fig. 18-10). 5 Radiofrequency energy delivered through a transvenous or arterial catheter causes small, discrete lesions through thermal energy. During invasive electrophysiologic studies, portions of the reentrant circuit can be located (or mapped) by the use of a number of catheters. Once this is completed, radiofrequency energy is applied, creating thermal injury in the tissue necessary for reentry. In this way, the substrate for reentry is destroyed, "curing" the patient of recurrent episodes of PSVT and obviating the need for chronic drug therapy. Complications, although unusual, include cardiac tamponade, pericarditis, valvular insufficiency, and AV block. Radiofrequency ablation is highly effective, preventing the recurrences of PSVT in more than 90% of patients.[75,76] The procedure was originally used in patients with WPW syndrome.[75] In these patients, the extranodal pathway is most often located at the left lateral free wall of the left ventricle (see Fig. 18-10). After the pathway is located, the catheter is put as close to the site as possible, and radiofrequency current is applied to make small burns in the tissue. Ablation of the extranodal connection occurs promptly, and evidence of preexcitation (delta waves) disappears. Thereafter, a similar approach was developed for patients with AV nodal reentry, placing the catheter in the coronary sinus, proximal to the AV node.[76] The preferred method in these individuals is to apply small amounts of radiofrequency current to the slow pathway of the reentrant circuit in order to modify its properties enough so that PSVT cannot recur.

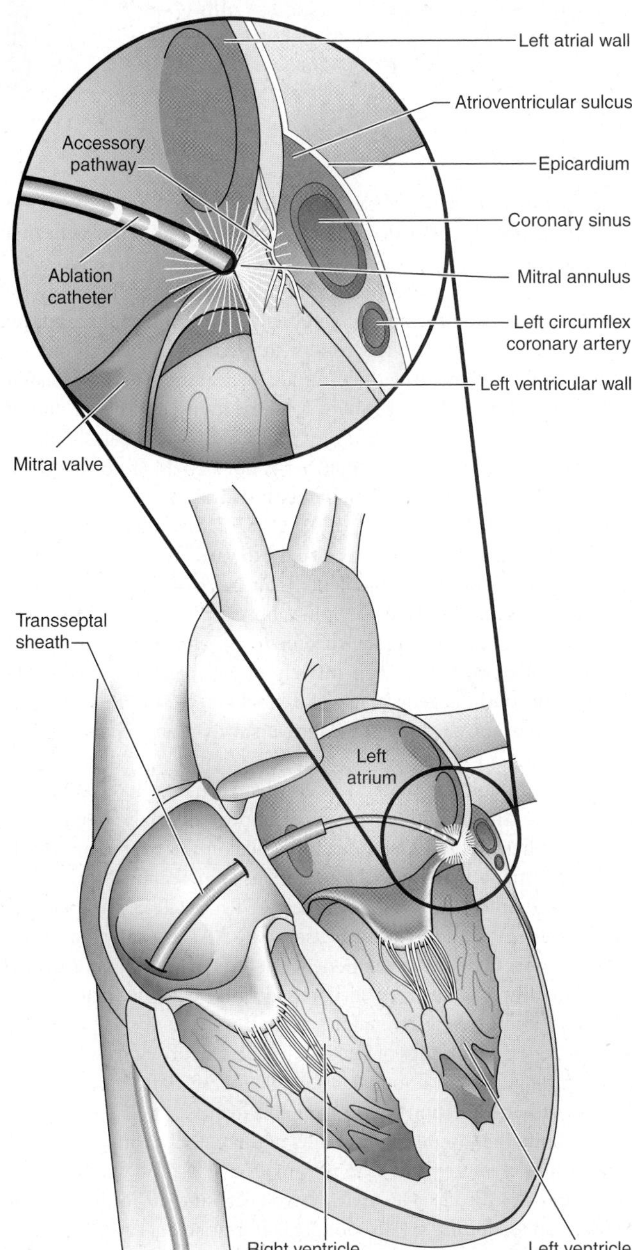

FIGURE 18-10 Drawing showing catheter placement for radiofrequency ablation of a left lateral free wall accessory pathway. Here, a venous (atrial) transseptal puncture to gain access to the Kent's bundle is shown; a retrograde arterial approach has also been used. *(Data from Lerman BB, Basson CT. High risk patients with ventricular preexcitation: A pendulum in motion.* N Engl J Med *2003;349:1787-1789. Copyright © 2003 Massachusetts Medical Society. All rights reserved.)*

Catheter ablation is now the preferred treatment strategy (over AADs) for patients with symptomatic PSVT because the procedure is highly effective and curative, rarely results in complications, and obviates the need for chronic AAD therapy.[63] Catheter ablation is also a cost-effective approach (in the long term) because, if effective, the costs of drugs and repeated hospital visits are avoided. In one cost-effectiveness analysis, radiofrequency ablation improved quality of life and reduced lifetime medical expenditures by nearly $30,000 compared with chronic drug treatment.[77]

VENTRICULAR ARRHYTHMIAS

The common ventricular arrhythmias include (a) PVCs, (b) VT, and (c) VF. These arrhythmias may result in a wide variety of symptoms. PVCs often cause no symptoms or only mild palpitations. VT may be a life-threatening situation associated with hemodynamic collapse or may be totally asymptomatic. VF, by definition, is an acute medical emergency necessitating CPR.

Premature Ventricular Complexes and Prevention of Sudden Cardiac Death

PVCs are very common ventricular rhythm disturbances that occur in patients with or without SHD. Experimental models show that PVCs may be elicited by abnormal automaticity, triggered activity, or reentrant mechanisms. It is well known that PVCs are commonly observed in apparently healthy individuals; in these patients, the PVCs seem to have little, if any, prognostic significance. PVCs occur more frequently and in more complex forms in patients with SHD than in healthy individuals. The prognostic meaning of PVCs has been well studied in patients with MI (acute or remote) with several consistent themes. Patients with some forms of PVCs are at higher risk for SCD than if they did not have these minor rhythm disturbances. SCD can be defined as unexpected death (without an obvious noncardiac cause) occurring in a patient within 1 hour of experiencing symptoms (witnessed episodes) or within 24 hours of last being observed in normal health (unwitnessed episodes).[78] Studies of patients who experienced SCD (and happened to be wearing an electrocardiographic monitor at the time) often demonstrate the cause to be VF preceded by a short run of VT and frequent PVCs.[79]

Significance

Historically, investigators promoted the concept that patients in the acute phase of MI may have types of PVCs that are predictive of VF and SCD. These types of PVCs were referred to as "warning arrhythmias" and included frequent ventricular ectopy (more than 5 beats/min), multiform configuration (different morphology), couplets (two in a row), and R-on-T phenomenon (PVCs occurring during the repolarization phase of the preceding sinus beat in the vulnerable period of ventricular recovery). However, as a result of using continuous electrocardiographic monitoring techniques, it has become apparent that almost all patients have warning arrhythmias

CLINICAL PRESENTATION Ventricular Arrhythmias

PVCs

- PVCs are non-life-threatening and usually asymptomatic. Occasionally, patients will complain of palpitations or uncomfortable heartbeats. Since the PVC, by definition, occurs early and the ventricle contracts when it is incompletely filled, patients do not feel the PVC. Rather, the next beat (after the PVC and a compensatory pause) is usually responsible for the patient's symptoms.

VT

- The symptoms of VT (monomorphic VT or TdP), if prolonged (ie, sustained), can vary from nearly completely asymptomatic to pulseless, hemodynamic collapse. Fast heart rates and underlying poor LV function will result in more severe symptoms. Symptoms of nonsustained, self-terminating VT also correlate with duration of episodes (eg, patients with 15-second episodes will be more symptomatic than those with three-beat episodes).

VF

- By definition, VF results in hemodynamic collapse, syncope, and cardiac arrest. Cardiac output and blood pressure are not recordable.

in the acute MI setting. In those patients who experience VF, warning arrhythmias are no more common than in those without VF. Consequently, warning arrhythmias observed during acute MI are neither sensitive nor specific for determining which patients will have VF. Thus, there is little need to direct drug therapy specifically at PVC suppression in these particular patients. Studies show that effective prevention of VF in the acute MI setting may be achieved without the abolition of PVCs.

Conversely, data strongly imply that PVCs documented in the convalescence period of MI do carry important long-term prognostic significance.[80] PVCs occurring after an MI seem to be a risk factor for patient death that is independent of the degree of LV dysfunction or the extent of coronary atherosclerosis. Ruberman et al. employed a simple classification of PVCs: simple or benign (infrequent and monomorphic) versus "complex" (≥5 PVCs/min, couplets, R-on-T beats, and multiform).[80] These investigators found that the presence of complex (but not simple) ventricular ectopy in the setting of CAD was associated with a higher incidence of overall mortality and cardiac death.

Because PVCs without associated SHD, in apparently healthy individuals, carry little or no risk, drug therapy is unnecessary. However, because of the prognostic significance of complex PVCs in patients with SHD, the use of AAD therapy to suppress them has been controversial. Historically, many supported the aggressive use of AAD therapy to suppress PVCs, based on the underlying premise of eliminating a risk factor for SCD in patients with CAD (namely, the presence of complex PVCs). However, others favored a more conservative approach and disregarded the use of AAD therapy in the absence of significant symptoms. An important study, the CAST, abruptly put an end to this debate in noteworthy fashion; its results are reviewed in the following section because of its great historical significance and lingering impact.[48]

The Cardiac Arrhythmia Suppression Trial

The CAST[48,81] was initiated by the National Institutes of Health in 1987 to determine if suppression of ventricular ectopy with encainide, flecainide, or moricizine could decrease the incidence of death from arrhythmia in patients who had suffered an MI. 7 Entrance criteria included documented MI between 6 days and 2 years prior to enrollment, and at least 6 PVCs/h (associated with no or minimal symptoms) without runs of VT greater than 15 beats in length. Also, patients were required to have an LVEF less than or equal to 55% if recruited within 90 days of the MI or an LVEF less than or equal to 40% if recruited at least 90 days after the MI. Patients with an LVEF less than 30% were randomized only to encainide or moricizine. Patients were randomized to receive AAD therapy or placebo after demonstrating PVC suppression with one of the agents.

In April 1989, a routine, preliminary review of the study by the Safety and Monitoring Board revealed alarming results, and the study was interrupted.[48] The results showed that when compared with placebo, treatment with encainide or flecainide was associated with a significantly higher rate of total mortality and death due to arrhythmia, presumably caused by proarrhythmia. Analysis of the moricizine arm indicated neither harm nor benefit from this therapy; therefore, only this portion of the study was allowed to continue as CAST II.[82] However, in July 1991, CAST II was also prematurely discontinued because there was a trend toward an increase in mortality in moricizine-treated patients. This increase in mortality was primarily observed during the initiation of moricizine (dose titration phase) but not during the chronic treatment phase. The overall results of the two CASTs conclusively prove that the use of AAD therapy (beyond the general use of β-blockers) to suppress PVCs in patients after an MI does not improve survival and is most likely detrimental.

Even though the CAST was conducted more than 2 decades ago, it is considered one of the most important trials ever undertaken and has had a tremendous influence on the overall approach to the treatment of arrhythmias, as well as a far-reaching impact on AAD development. The results of the CAST have clearly had a negative influence on the long-term use of all AADs, causing a broad skepticism in the risk-versus-benefit analysis of this class of drugs. Consequently, pharmaceutical companies have shifted their drug discovery and investigative efforts away from potent sodium channel blockers. The findings of the CAST have also provided additional fuel for the pursuit of nonpharmacologic therapies for arrhythmias, such as catheter ablation and implantable devices.

Despite the discouraging results of the CAST, post-MI patients with complex ventricular ectopy remain at risk for death. Other drugs, besides the class Ic AADs, have been studied in this patient population, including sotalol. Sotalol is comprised of a racemic mixture of D- and L- isomers: both isomers are class III potassium channel blockers but the L-isomer also has β-blocking actions. Chronic therapy with D-sotalol was studied in patients with a remote MI complicated by complex ectopy in the Survival with Oral D-Sotalol trial.[82] In this trial, D-sotalol treatment was not targeted at PVC suppression (unlike the CAST), yet (like the CAST) the trial was halted prematurely because of excessive mortality in the treatment arm. Again, the presumed reason for this observation was D-sotalol–related proarrhythmia. Currently, only two AADs have been shown *not* to increase mortality in post-MI patients with long-term use: amiodarone and dofetilide. A number of trials have shown amiodarone to decrease the incidence of sudden (or arrhythmic) death, but not total mortality, in post-MI patients with complex ventricular ectopy.[83,84] A meta-analysis of all trials (n = 6,553 patients) demonstrated a 13% reduction in total mortality with long-term amiodarone therapy.[85] It is unclear if these findings can be attributed to one of amiodarone's electrophysiologic properties (eg, β-blocking) or a combination of its complex pharmacologic effects on conduction. It is noteworthy to mention that in two major studies, patients treated with amiodarone and a β-blocker generally did better than when no β-blocker was used.[83,84] Clearly, because of its impressive side effect profile and its inability to improve survival, amiodarone should not routinely be recommended in patients with heart disease such as remote MI and complex PVCs. Two randomized controlled trials have also shown that chronic therapy with dofetilide has no effect on overall mortality in post-MI patients with LV dysfunction.[86,87]

How should the clinician approach the patient with documented asymptomatic PVCs? Clearly, attempts to suppress asymptomatic PVCs should *not* be made with any AAD. Indeed, those patients who are at risk for arrhythmic death (recent MI, LV dysfunction, complex PVCs) should also *not* be routinely given *any* class I or III AAD.[88] If these patients have symptomatic PVCs, chronic drug therapy should be limited to the use of β-blockers. The use of β-blockers in post-MI patients is associated with a reduction in the incidence of total mortality and SCD, especially in the presence of LV dysfunction. β-Blockers can also be used in patients without underlying SHD to suppress symptomatic PVCs. 7

Ventricular Tachycardia

Mechanisms and Types of VT

VT is a wide QRS tachycardia that may acutely occur as a result of metabolic abnormalities, ischemia, or drug toxicity, or chronically recur as a paroxysmal form. On ECG, VT may appear as repetitive monomorphic or polymorphic ventricular complexes. The definition of VT is three or more consecutive PVCs occurring at a rate greater than 100 beats/min. An acute episode of VT may be precipitated by severe electrolyte abnormalities (hypokalemia or hypomagnesemia), hypoxia, or digoxin toxicity, or (most commonly) may occur in patients presenting with acute MI or myocardial ischemia complicated by HF. In these cases, correction of the underlying precipitating factors will usually prevent further recurrences of VT. As an example, if VT occurs during the first 24 hours of an acute MI, it will probably not reappear on a chronic basis after the infarcted area has been reperfused or healed with scar formation. This form of acute VT may be caused by a transient reentrant mechanism within temporarily ischemic or dying ventricular tissue. In contrast, some patients have a chronic, recurrent form of VT that is almost always associated with some type of underlying SHD. Common examples are paroxysmal VT associated with idiopathic dilated cardiomyopathy or remote MI with an LV aneurysm. In chronic, recurrent VT, microreentry within the distal Purkinje network is presumed to be responsible for the underlying substrate in a large majority of patients (see Fig. 18-3). Theoretically, electrophysiologic discrepancies occur as a result of structural damage and heart disease within the ventricular conducting system. The reentrant circuit may possess both anatomically determined and functional properties coursing through normal tissue, damaged (but not dead) tissue, and islands of necrosed tissue. In a minority of patients, macroreentrant circuits may be responsible for recurrent VT, including reentry incorporating the bundle branches.

Patients with acute VT associated with a precipitating factor often suffer severe symptoms, requiring immediate treatment measures. Chronic, recurrent VT may also cause severe hemodynamic compromise but may also be associated with only mild symptoms that are generally well tolerated. Sustained VT is that which requires therapeutic intervention to restore a stable rhythm or persists for a relatively long time (usually more than 30 seconds). Nonsustained VT is that which self-terminates after a brief duration (usually less than 30 seconds). Patients who experience VT more frequently than SR (ie, VT is the dominant rhythm) are considered to have incessant VT. In monomorphic VT, the QRS complexes are similar in morphologic characteristics from beat to beat. In polymorphic VT, the QRS complexes vary in shape and/or size between beats. A characteristic type of polymorphic VT, in which the QRS complexes appear to undulate around a central axis and that is associated with evidence of delayed ventricular repolarization (long QT interval or prominent U waves), is referred to as TdP.

Most, but not all forms of recurrent VT occur in patients with extensive SHD. VT occurring in a patient without SHD is sometimes referred to as idiopathic VT and may take several forms, including fascicular VT and ventricular outflow tract VT.[89-91] Fascicular VT arises from a fascicle of the left bundle branch (usually posterior) and is usually not associated with severe underlying SHD. In distinct contrast to the common form of recurrent VT associated with extensive SHD, non-DHP CCBs (but not adenosine) are effective in terminating an acute episode of fascicular VT. Ventricular outflow tract VT (usually originating from the right ventricular outflow tract) originates from near the pulmonic valve (or uncommonly the aortic valve or LV outflow tract) and also occurs in patients with normal LV function without discernible SHD.[91] Unlike other forms of VT, right ventricular outflow tract VT often terminates with adenosine and may be prevented with β-blockers and/or non-DHP CCBs.

Some unusual forms of VT are congenital or heritable (Table 18-10). TdP can be associated with heritable defects in the flux of ions that govern ventricular repolarization. Although multiple syndromes and genetic mutations have been described, the more common examples are long QT syndrome 1 (depressed I_{Ks}), long QT syndrome 2 (depressed I_{Kr}), and long QT syndrome 3 (enhanced, inward sodium ion flux during repolarization).[92,93] Polymorphic VT (without a long QT interval) or VF may also occur as a result of a heritable defect in the sodium channel. This is the case in Brugada syndrome, which is described as a typical ECG pattern (ST-segment

TABLE 18-10 Heritable Polymorphic Ventricular Tachycardia

Syndrome	Channel Defect	Mutant Gene	Characteristics	Treatment
$LQTS_1$	$\downarrow I_{Ks}$	KVLQT1	SCD/TdP with exercise	BB/ICD
$LQTS_2$	$\downarrow I_{Kr}$	HERG	SCD/TdP with arousal	BB/ICD
$LQTS_3$	$\uparrow I_{Na}$ during plateau/ repolarization	SCN5A	SCD/TdP at rest/sleep	Flecainide/mexiletine/ICD
Brugada	$\downarrow I_{Na}$	SCN5A	SCD/PMVT or VF at rest/sleep in Asian males	ICD/quinidine

BB, β-blocker; ICD, implantable cardioverter-defibrillator; LQTS, long QT syndrome; PMVT, polymorphic ventricular tachycardia; SCD, sudden cardiac death; TdP, torsade de pointes; VF, ventricular fibrillation.

Note: LQTS can be provoked by potassium channel blockers (eg, quinidine, sotalol), and Brugada syndrome can be provoked by potent sodium channel blockers (eg, cocaine, flecainide). $LQTS_3$ and Brugada syndrome may coexist.

elevation in leads V_1 to V_3) in SR that is associated with SCD, and commonly occurs in males of Asian descent.[94]

Management

Consider the patient with the more common form of sustained monomorphic VT (ie, those with SHD, usually ischemic in nature). Like other rapid tachycardias, the initial management of an acute episode of VT (with a pulse) requires a quick assessment of the patient's signs and symptoms. If severe symptoms are present (ie, severe hypotension, angina, pulmonary edema), synchronized DCC should be delivered immediately to attempt to restore SR. An investigation should be made into possible precipitating factors, which should be corrected if possible. The diagnosis of acute MI should always be entertained. If the episode of VT is thought to be an isolated electrical event associated with a transient initiating factor (such as acute myocardial ischemia or digoxin toxicity), there is no need for long-term AAD therapy once the precipitating factors are corrected (eg, an MI has been reperfused and healed and the patient is stable). Nevertheless, the patient should be monitored closely for possible recurrences of VT.

Patients presenting with an acute episode of VT (with a pulse) associated with only mild symptoms can be initially treated with AADs. The reader is referred to the 2010 AHA Guidelines for CPR and ECC (no updated recommendations regarding treatment of VT [with a pulse] in 2015 Guidelines Update for CPR and ECC).[72] IV procainamide, amiodarone, or sotalol can be considered in this situation. Lidocaine can be considered as an alternative. In one small study, procainamide was shown to be superior to lidocaine in terminating VT.[95] Synchronized DCC should be delivered if the patient's status deteriorates, VT degenerates to VF (would be unsynchronized in this situation), or drug therapy fails.

Once an acute episode of sustained VT has been successfully terminated by electrical or pharmacologic means and an acute MI has been ruled out, the possibility of a patient having recurrent episodes of VT should be considered. Evidence for the possibility of VT recurrence can often be gleaned from invasive electrophysiologic studies using programmed ventricular stimulation. Because these patients are at extremely high risk for death, trial-and-error attempts to find effective therapy are unwarranted. To gain some objective evidence of a response to a specific AAD regimen, serial testing of these drugs using the following two surrogate end points has been used: (a) inability to induce sustained VT with programmed extrastimuli by invasive electrophysiologic studies and (b) suppression of ventricular ectopic beats by serial 24-hour continuous electrocardiographic (Holter) monitoring. These two strategies have been compared but largely abandoned for several reasons.[96,97] First, the yield for finding an effective AAD is low. For instance, sustained monomorphic VT can be rendered noninducible or nonsustained by programmed stimulation protocols in only 20% to 25% of patients. Therefore, the clinician frequently must search for other therapeutic options or settle for other treatment end points such as slower and more tolerable inducible VT. Second, amiodarone is the most effective (approximately 50% effective after 2 years) AAD in patients with recurrent VT; however, electrophysiologic drug testing does not necessarily predict the clinical efficacy of amiodarone. Patients may have continued inducibility of VT on amiodarone despite long-term success. Indeed, empiric amiodarone has been compared with therapy (with other AADs) guided by electrophysiologic testing in patients at high risk for recurrent VT.[98] In this trial, amiodarone therapy without invasive testing was superior in preventing SCD and recurrences of severe ventricular arrhythmias at all time points. Third, the recurrence rate of life-threatening VT is high (20%-50% per year depending on the AAD chosen), regardless of the method of acute drug testing. Fourth, as referred to previously, there is a substantial side effect profile of the class I and III AADs. Lastly, and perhaps most importantly, is the impressive demonstrated effectiveness of nonpharmacologic approaches to the treatment of recurrent VT/VF.[99] For instance, some forms of recurrent VT are amenable to catheter ablation therapy using radiofrequency current. This approach is highly effective (approximately 90%) in idiopathic VT (right ventricular outflow tract or fascicular VT), but less so in recurrent VT associated with a cardiomyopathic process or remote MI with LV aneurysm. In the latter patients, ablation is usually regarded as second-line therapy after other methods have failed. Additionally, numerous trials have established the ICD as a superior treatment over AAD therapy not only for the prevention of SCD in patients who have been resuscitated from an episode of cardiac arrest or had sustained VT ("secondary prevention") but also for the prevention of an initial episode of SCD in certain high-risk patient populations ("primary prevention").

The Implantable Cardioverter-Defibrillator The introduction of and advances in the ICD (Fig. 18-11) have obviated the need to rely solely on the use of AADs to prevent episodes of life-threatening ventricular arrhythmias.[100] (8) Numerous advancements in device technology have allowed the ICD to become smaller, less invasive to implant, and programmable with advanced functions. Early ICDs required a thoracotomy to place the generator in the abdomen, whereas with the newer, smaller models, the leads are implanted transvenously with the generator placed into the pectoral region in a manner similar to cardiac pacemakers. Modern ICDs now employ a "tiered-therapy approach," meaning that overdrive pacing (ie, antitachycardia pacing) can be attempted first to terminate the tachyarrhythmia (no painful shock delivered), followed by low-energy cardioversion, and, finally, by high-energy defibrillation shocks. In addition, backup antibradycardia pacing and extended battery lives have made these newer devices much more attractive. All models store recordings during delivery of pacing shocks, which is extremely important in discerning appropriate shocks (ie, delivers shock for serious ventricular arrhythmia) from inappropriate shocks (ie, delivers shock for AF with rapid ventricular rate) and in documenting true recurrences of the patient's tachycardia.

Although the ICD is a highly effective method for preventing SCD due to recurrent VT or VF, several problems remain. First, the

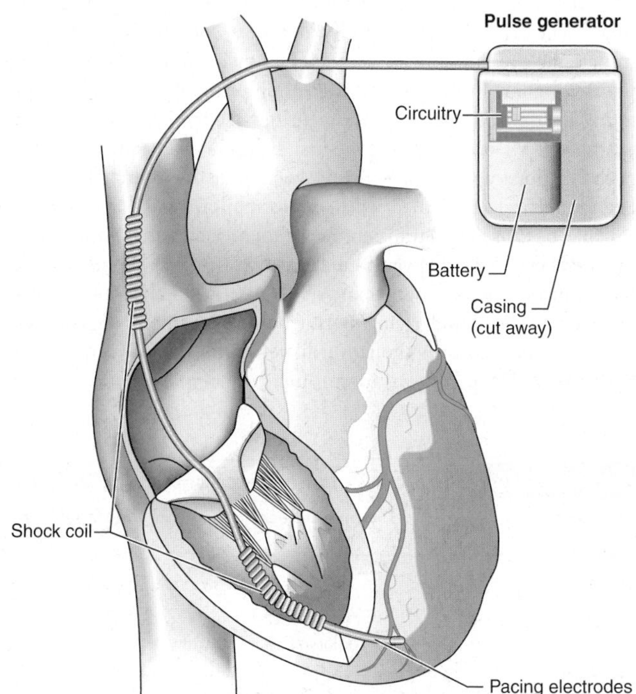

FIGURE 18-11 Drawing showing implantable cardioverter-defibrillator. *(Reproduced with permission from The Cascade Investigators. Randomized antiarrhythmic drug therapy in survivors of cardiac arrest (the CASCADE Study).* Am J Cardiol *1993;72:280-287.)*

device itself, the implantation procedure, electrophysiologic studies, hospitalization, and physician fees are costly. Given that the indications for receiving an ICD have significantly expanded over the past several years, the total cost associated with the implantation of this device is likely to place a great burden on the healthcare system. Second, many patients (as high as 70%) with ICDs end up receiving concomitant AAD therapy (usually amiodarone or sotalol).[101,102] AADs can be initiated in these patients for a number of reasons, including (a) decreasing the frequency of VT/VF episodes to subsequently reduce the frequency of appropriate shocks; (b) reducing the rate of VT so that it can be terminated with antitachycardia pacing; and (c) decreasing episodes of concomitant supraventricular arrhythmias (eg, AF, AFl) that may trigger inappropriate shocks. As a result of these potential benefits, the concomitant use of AADs can minimize patient discomfort and prolong the battery life of the ICD. The decision to initiate concomitant AAD therapy should be individualized, with treatment usually being reserved for those patients with frequent shocks because of VT or AF. If AADs are added to ICD therapy, one should note that many of these drugs alter defibrillation thresholds; consequently, the device may need to be reprogrammed to account for this alteration.[103]

Secondary Prevention of Sudden Cardiac Death The results of three trials, the Antiarrhythmics versus Implantable Defibrillators (AVID), Cardiac Arrest Study Hamburg (CASH), and Canadian Implantable Defibrillator Study (CIDS), definitively support the ICD as first-line therapy for the secondary prevention of SCD.[104-106] Of these, the AVID trial was the largest, randomizing more than 1,000 patients with resuscitated VF, sustained VT with syncope, or hemodynamically significant sustained VT (with LVEF ≤40%) to either an ICD or AADs (approximately 95% received amiodarone at discharge).[104] The trial was stopped early because of a demonstrated superiority of the ICD; patients in the ICD group had a better overall survival when compared with those in the AAD group (75% vs 64%, respectively, at 3 years). Although they were smaller trials, both CASH and CIDS demonstrated the efficacy of an ICD compared with amiodarone in patients with a history of sustained VT or VF, with the ICD reducing overall mortality by 20% to 25%.[105,106] Overall, the results of these three trials provide strong support for the aggressive use of the ICD in patients who are at high risk for recurrent, life-threatening ventricular arrhythmias.

Primary Prevention of Sudden Cardiac Death One of the patient populations that appears to be at high risk for a first episode of SCD includes those with a prior MI, LV dysfunction, and nonsustained VT. The use of AADs to prevent SCD in this high-risk group has been significantly limited by the results of the CAST and other similar trials that have collectively demonstrated that these drugs may actually increase the risk of mortality in these patients. As a result of these trials, clinicians have sought a more clearly defined strategy for risk stratification in these patients before initiating drug therapy.

Traditionally, there are three treatment strategies for patients with nonsustained VT: (a) conservative (ie, no AAD treatment beyond β-blockers); (b) empiric amiodarone; and (c) aggressive (ie, electrophysiologic studies with possible insertion of an ICD) (Fig. 18-12). 9 A number of early studies suggested that tests such as electrophysiologic studies could be used to determine long-term risk in patients with nonsustained VT.[107,108] For instance, Wilber et al. demonstrated that post-MI patients with nonsustained VT and inducible sustained VT after programmed stimulation were at increased risk for subsequent VT/VF or SCD compared with those in whom sustained VT could not be induced.[107] These data provided the basis for the Multicenter Automatic Defibrillator Implantation Trial (MADIT) and the Multicenter Unsustained Tachycardia Trial (MUSTT).[109,110] The MADIT was the first of these trials to be conducted to evaluate the efficacy of ICD therapy in this high-risk patient population. Specifically, this trial randomized patients with a previous MI, LVEF less than or equal to 35%, asymptomatic nonsustained VT, and inducible VT that was not suppressed with the use of IV procainamide to receive an ICD or conventional medical therapy (74% received amiodarone).[109] This trial was terminated prematurely after a significant survival benefit was detected in the ICD group. The findings of the MADIT were subsequently supported by those of the MUSTT. In the MUSTT, patients with a history of MI, LVEF less than or equal to 40%, asymptomatic nonsustained VT, and inducible sustained VT were randomized to a conservative approach (no AAD therapy beyond β-blockers) or electrophysiologically guided therapy (AADs and/or ICD).[110] The results showed that the conservative approach had a significantly higher event rate (cardiac arrest or death from arrhythmia). However, when the results of the electrophysiologically guided group were further stratified, those receiving only AADs (no ICD) were no different in terms of outcomes than those who received no treatment. In other words, only those treated with an ICD had a significantly lower event rate and greater survival. One problem with the MUSTT, however, is that, because the trial was initiated in 1989, nearly 50% of patients received class I AADs or drugs that are now known not to improve survival in patients with CAD, LV dysfunction, and ventricular arrhythmias; only 10% of patients received the most effective agent in this setting, amiodarone. Based on the results of the MADIT and MUSTT, it is reasonable for patients with CAD, LV dysfunction, and nonsustained VT to undergo electrophysiologic testing.[111] If these patients do not have inducible sustained VT/VF, chronic AAD therapy is unnecessary; however, if these patients do have inducible sustained VT/VF, implantation of an ICD is warranted.

Although the MADIT and MUSTT provide clinicians with important information regarding risk stratification, both of these trials targeted patients who had a history of nonsustained VT. The results of two landmark trials, the MADIT II and Sudden Cardiac Death in Heart Failure Trial (SCD-HeFT), have provided clinicians with additional information regarding the treatment of other groups of high-risk patients who have no prior history of ventricular arrhythmia (see Fig. 18-12).[112,113] In the MADIT II, patients with a prior MI and LVEF less than or equal to 30% were randomized to receive either an ICD or a conventional therapy (routine post-MI and HF therapy).[112] Neither a history of ventricular arrhythmia nor electrophysiologic testing was required for inclusion in this study. Patients in the ICD group experienced a significant reduction in mortality when compared with the conventional therapy group; the reduction in mortality in the ICD group was primarily due to a reduction in arrhythmic death. Whereas the MADIT, MUSTT, and MADIT II limited enrollment to patients with ischemic cardiomyopathy, the SCD-HeFT is the largest trial, to date, to evaluate the efficacy of an ICD in a nonischemic HF population. In this trial, patients with NYHA class II or III HF (of either ischemic or nonischemic etiology) and LVEF less than or equal to 35% were randomized to receive placebo, amiodarone, or an ICD.[113] All patients were treated with appropriate HF therapies, as indicated. Implantation of an ICD resulted in a significantly lower mortality rate compared with treatment with either placebo or amiodarone (there was no difference between placebo and amiodarone). The survival benefits of the ICD were observed regardless of the etiology of the HF.

Overall, as the ICD trials have evolved over the past decade, the indications for implanting these devices have significantly expanded (Table 18-11).[114] Based on the results of the MUSTT, MADIT, MADIT II, and SCD-HeFT, many patients will be eligible for an ICD. 9

Ventricular Proarrhythmia

All AADs have the potential to aggravate existing arrhythmias or to cause new arrhythmias. It is believed that AADs may cause proarrhythmia in nearly 30% of patients.[7] Many definitions for proarrhythmia have been proposed; however, in the simplest terms, it indicates the development of a significant new arrhythmia (such as VT, VF, or TdP) or worsening of an existing arrhythmia (episodes

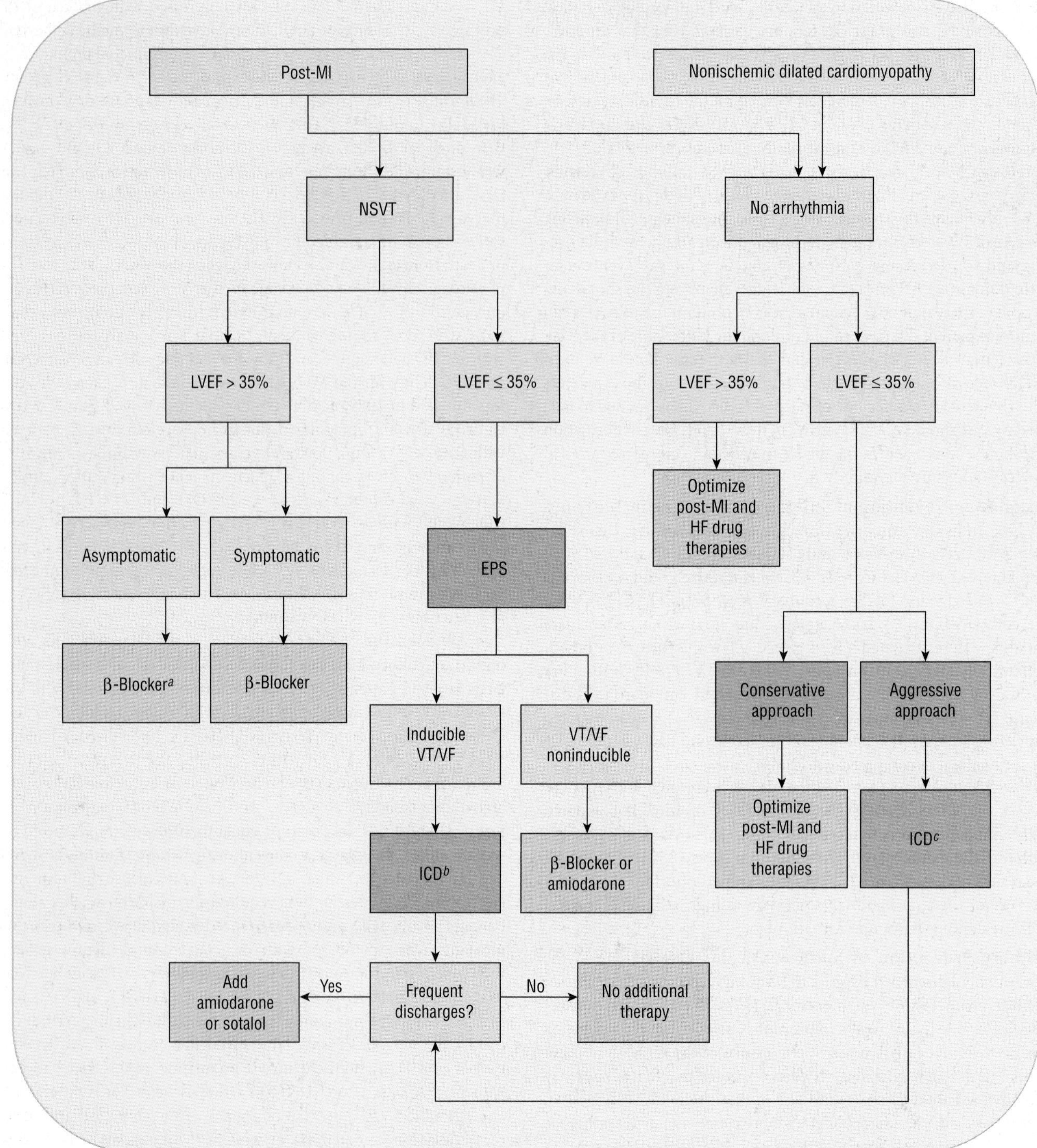

FIGURE 18-12 Algorithm for the primary prevention of SCD in patients with a history of MI or with a nonischemic dilated cardiomyopathy. [a]In these patients, the β-blocker is being used to reduce post-MI mortality. [b]Patients should be more than 40 days post-MI prior to insertion of the ICD. [c]Patients with an ischemic cardiomyopathy should be more than 40 days post-MI prior to insertion of the ICD. (EPS, electrophysiologic study; HF, heart failure; ICD, implantable cardioverter-defibrillator; LVEF, left ventricular ejection fraction; MI, myocardial infarction; NSVT, nonsustained VT; SCD, sudden cardiac death; VF, ventricular fibrillation; VT, ventricular tachycardia.)

are longer, faster, or more frequent). As with all arrhythmias, the consequences of proarrhythmia are varied. Some patients who develop proarrhythmia may be totally asymptomatic, others may notice a worsening of symptoms, and some may die suddenly. The development of proarrhythmia results from the same mechanisms that cause arrhythmias in general (eg, quinidine-induced TdP due to EADs) or from an alteration in the underlying substrate due to the AAD (eg, development of an accelerated tachycardia caused by flecainide, which decreases conduction velocity without significantly altering the refractory period).[7] The diagnosis of proarrhythmia is sometimes difficult to make because of the variable nature of the underlying arrhythmias. However, in all cases, the AAD should be discontinued if proarrhythmia is detected or suspected.

Incessant Monomorphic Ventricular Tachycardia

The prototypical form of proarrhythmia caused by the class Ic AADs is a rapid, sustained, monomorphic VT with a characteristic sinusoidal QRS pattern that is often resistant to resuscitation with

TABLE 18-11 Current Indications for Implantable Cardioverter-Defibrillator Implantation

Indications	ACC/AHA/HRS Guideline Recommendation
Secondary Prevention	
An ICD is *indicated* in the following individuals:	
Patients who survived an episode of cardiac arrest due to VF or have hemodynamically unstable sustained VT, not due to a reversible cause	Class I
Patients with structural heart disease who develop spontaneous sustained VT that is either hemodynamically stable or unstable	Class I
Patients with unexplained syncope who have hemodynamically unstable sustained VT or VF induced by EPS	Class I
An ICD is *considered reasonable* in the following individuals:	
Patients with unexplained syncope who have significant LV dysfunction and nonischemic dilated cardiomyopathy	Class IIa
Patients with sustained VT and normal or near-normal LV function	Class IIa
Primary Prevention	
An ICD is *indicated* in the following individuals:	
Patients with a prior MI (occurring >40 days before ICD implantation) and LVEF ≤30% who are in NYHA FC I	Class I
Patients with an LVEF ≤35% due to a prior MI (occurring >40 days before ICD implantation) who are in NYHA FC II or III	Class I
Patients with nonsustained VT due to prior MI, an LVEF ≤40%, and inducible, sustained VT or VF at EPS	Class I
Patients with nonischemic dilated cardiomyopathy and an LVEF ≤35% who are in NYHA FC II or III	Class I
An ICD is *considered reasonable* in patients who are not hospitalized and are awaiting cardiac transplantation	Class IIa
An ICD *may be considered* in patients with nonischemic dilated cardiomyopathy and an LVEF ≤35% who are in NYHA FC I	Class IIb

ACC, American College of Cardiology; AHA, American Heart Association; EPS, electrophysiologic study; FC, functional class; HRS, Heart Rhythm Society; ICD, implantable cardioverter-defibrillator; LV, left ventricular; LVEF, left ventricular ejection fraction; MI, myocardial infarction; NYHA, New York Heart Association; VF, ventricular fibrillation; VT, ventricular tachycardia.

cardioversion or overdrive pacing. 10 It is sometimes referred to as sinusoidal or incessant VT and is the result of excessive sodium channel blockade and slowed conduction. Sinusoidal VT caused by the class Ic AADs was thought to occur within the first several days of drug initiation; however, the results of the CAST indicate that the risk for this type of proarrhythmia may exist as long as the AAD is continued. Factors that can predispose a patient to this form of proarrhythmia include: (a) the presence of underlying ventricular arrhythmias; (b) CAD; and (c) LV dysfunction. Provocation of proarrhythmia by the class Ic AADs is sometimes reported during exercise, which is most likely a result of augmented slowed conduction at rapid heart rates (ie, rate-dependent sodium blockade). The incidence of proarrhythmia caused by class Ic AADs is greatest in patients with all three of the above risk factors (approximately 10% to 20%) and extremely uncommon in those without these risk factors, such as patients with supraventricular tachycardias and normal LV function. Other factors that have a less well-defined association with proarrhythmia are elevated AAD serum concentrations and rapid dosage escalation of the AAD. It has been proposed that the presence of underlying ventricular conduction delays may also pose a risk for proarrhythmia. As mentioned earlier, incessant monomorphic VT is often resistant to resuscitation; however, some have had success with lidocaine ("fast on-off" AAD, which successfully competes with a "slow on-off" agent such as flecainide for sodium channel receptor) or sodium bicarbonate (reverses the excessive sodium channel blockade).

Torsade de Pointes

As defined previously, TdP is a rapid form of polymorphic VT (Fig. 18-13) that is associated with evidence of delayed ventricular repolarization (long QT interval or prominent U waves) on ECG. It is important to note that most forms of polymorphic VT occurring in the setting of a normal QT interval are similar to monomorphic VT in terms of etiology and treatment strategies (thus, a long QT interval is crucial to the diagnosis of TdP). Much has been learned about the underlying etiology of TdP. Basic defects (genetic, drugs, or diseases) that delay repolarization by influencing ion movement (usually by blocking potassium efflux) provoke EADs preferentially in cells deep in the heart muscle, which, in turn, trigger reentry and TdP. Drugs that cause TdP usually delay ventricular repolarization in an inhomogeneous way (termed *dispersion of refractoriness*), which facilitates the formation of multiple reentrant loops in the ventricle.[115] TdP may occur in association with hereditary syndromes or as an acquired form (ie, a result of drugs or diseases). The underlying etiology in both cases is delayed ventricular repolarization due to blockade of potassium conductance. It is possible, however, that some individuals have a partially expressed form of these congenital syndromes but never suffer TdP unless some other external factor (eg, drugs, diseases, electrolyte disturbances, abrupt heart rate changes) further delays ventricular repolarization. Specifically, acquired forms of TdP are associated with electrolyte disturbances (hypokalemia or hypomagnesemia), subarachnoid hemorrhage, myocarditis, liquid protein diets, arsenic poisoning, severe hypothyroidism, or, most commonly, drug therapy (notably phenothiazines, antibiotics, antihistamines, antidepressants, and AADs) (Table 18-12). 10

The class Ia AADs (especially quinidine) and class III I_{Kr} blockers are most notorious for precipitating TdP; the class Ib and Ic AADs rarely, if ever, cause TdP as they do not appreciably delay repolarization. Most AADs with I_{Kr} blocking activity cause TdP in approximately 2% to 4% of patients, with the exceptions being amiodarone and dronedarone (<1%). Risk factors and associated features of drug-induced TdP have been identified and can be summarized as follow[116]: (a) high dosages or plasma concentrations of the offending drug ("dose-related") (except for quinidine-induced TdP, which tends to occur more frequently at low-to-therapeutic plasma concentrations); (b) concurrent SHD (eg, CAD, HF, and/or LV hypertrophy); (c) evidence of mild delayed repolarization (prolonged QT interval) at baseline; (d) evidence of a prolonged QT interval shortly

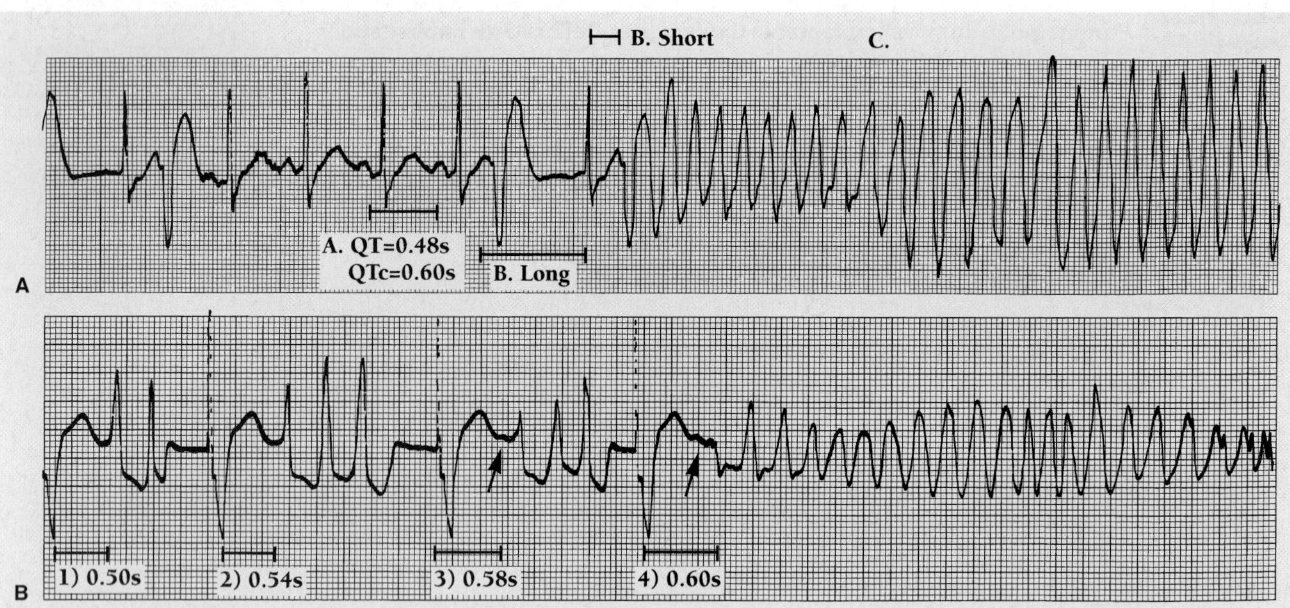

FIGURE 18-13 Torsade de pointes caused by quinidine. Note the presence of a couplet and two triplets following each extra systolic pause. The pause gets progressively longer until it is long enough to result in an episode of sustained torsade de pointes. Also, as the pause lengthens, discernible U waves (labeled ↑) (EADs?) begin to appear. The amplitude of the U wave is somewhat greater with the longest pause. *(Reproduced with permission from Bauman JL. Drug safety: Cardiac arrhythmias. Antihistamine update symposium.* Hosp Med *1995;31:24.)*

after initiation of the offending drug; (e) concomitant electrolyte disturbances such as hypokalemia or hypomagnesemia; (f) female gender; and (g) a characteristic long-short initiating sequence (so-called "pause dependence") of the TdP episode (see Fig. 18-13). However, none of these associations are absolute prerequisites to the development of drug-induced TdP. For instance, although TdP is usually documented early in the course of quinidine therapy, patients may develop this arrhythmia anytime during chronic treatment.[117] The reason for quinidine's relatively unique propensity for causing TdP at relatively low dosages and plasma concentrations requires explanation. Quinidine's ability to block I_{Kr} is clinically manifest at low plasma concentrations; at higher plasma concentrations, its sodium channel blocking properties predominate. Other drugs that block I_{Kr} usually do so in a concentration-dependent fashion. The observation that most patients who suffer drug-induced TdP have evidence of mildly delayed repolarization (long QT intervals) even before they are prescribed the offending drug has stimulated a search for a potential genetically linked risk. Indeed, it appears that at least some patients with acquired drug-induced TdP possess mutations of genes that encode for I_{Kr} or I_{Ks}.[116]

The common underlying electrophysiologic cause of TdP is a delay in ventricular repolarization (provoking EADs), which usually results from inhibition (drug-induced or genetic) of the I_K current and manifests as QT interval prolongation on the ECG. Therefore, the extent of QT interval prolongation has been used as a measurement of risk of TdP; however, considerable controversy exists regarding this practice. Amiodarone, for example, commonly causes significant QT prolongation but is a relatively infrequent cause of TdP. Nonetheless, the QT interval should be measured and monitored in all patients prescribed drugs that have a high potential for causing TdP (see Table 18-12). Patients with a baseline QT_c interval (QT interval corrected for heart rate, which can be calculated using Bazett's formula: $QT_c = QT\ measured/\sqrt{R-R\ Interval}$) greater than 450 milliseconds should not be given drugs that have a high potential for causing TdP; an increase in the QT_c interval to at least 560 milliseconds after the initiation of the drug is an indication to discontinue the agent or, at least, to reduce its dosage and carefully monitor.

Drug-induced TdP has become an extremely visible hazard plaguing new drugs, sometimes resulting in public health disasters. For instance, several drugs (cisapride, astemizole, levomethadyl, grepafloxacin, sparfloxacin, terfenadine, and high-dose [32 mg] IV ondansetron) have been withdrawn from the market in the United States because of their significant potential for causing TdP. One of the most visible and striking examples of drug withdrawal due to TdP occurred with the popular nonsedating antihistamine, terfenadine. Terfenadine is a potent I_{Kr} blocker but is rapidly metabolized by CYP3A4 to an active moiety (fexofenadine) that is not associated with delayed repolarization. Consequently, in the presence of drugs that block the CYP3A4 isoenzyme (eg, ketoconazole, erythromycin, diltiazem), accumulation of the parent compound, terfenadine, causes clinically significant blockade of I_{Kr} that could result in TdP and even death.[118] Because of experiences like this, all new drug entities under investigation are screened for their ability to block I_K and cause significant QT prolongation.

Acute treatment of TdP is different than treatment for the more common acute monomorphic VT. For an acute episode of TdP, most patients will require and respond to DCC. However, TdP tends to be paroxysmal in nature and often will rapidly recur after DCC. Therefore, after the initial restoration of a stable rhythm, therapy designed to prevent recurrences of TdP should be instituted. AADs that further prolong repolarization such as IV procainamide are absolutely contraindicated. Lidocaine is usually ineffective. Although there are no true efficacy trials, IV magnesium sulfate, by suppressing EADs, is considered the drug of choice in preventing recurrences of TdP.[119] If IV magnesium sulfate is ineffective, treatment strategies designed to increase heart rate, shorten ventricular repolarization, and prevent the pause dependency should be initiated. Either temporary transvenous pacing (105-120 beats/min) or pharmacologic pacing (isoproterenol or epinephrine continuous infusion) can be initiated for this purpose. All drugs that prolong the QT interval should be discontinued, and exacerbating factors (eg, hypokalemia or hypomagnesemia) should be corrected.

TABLE 18-12 Potential Causes of QT Interval Prolongation and Torsade de Pointes

Conditions
Congenital long QT syndromes
Heart failure
Hypokalemia
Hypomagnesemia
Myocardial ischemia/infarction
Myocarditis
Severe bradycardia (<50 beats/min)
Severe hypothermia
Severe starvation/liquid protein diets
Subarachnoid hemorrhage
Drugs
Antiarrhythmic drugs
Amiodarone (<1%)
Disopyramide
Dofetilide
Dronedarone (<1%)
Ibutilide
Procainamide (also *N*-acetylprocainamide)
Quinidine
Sotalol
Cancer chemotherapy or biologic agents
Ceritinib
Crizotinib
Dasatinib
Degarelix
Eribulin
Lapatinib
Leuprolide
Nilotinib
Oxaliplatin
Pazopanib
Sorafenib
Sunitinib
Toremifene
Vandetanib
Vemurafenib
Psychotropics
Atypical antipsychotics (eg, quetiapine, ziprasidone)
Droperidol
Haloperidol
Phenothiazines (eg, thioridazine, chlorpromazine)
Pimozide
Tricyclic and tetracyclic antidepressants
Toxins
Arsenic
Organophosphate insecticides
Antibiotics
Fluoroquinolones (levofloxacin, moxifloxacin, gemifloxacin)
Macrolides
Pentamidine
Trimethoprim-sulfamethoxazole
Voriconazole
Pain
Methadone
Miscellaneous
Chloroquine
Corticosteroids[a]
Diuretics[a]
Dolasetron
Liquid protein diets[a]
Ondansetron (IV)
Quinine
Tacrolimus

IV, intravenous

[a]More than likely a result of severe electrolyte imbalance.

Note: For a complete list, see *www.crediblemeds.org*.

Ventricular Fibrillation

Background and Prevention

VF is electrical anarchy of the ventricle resulting in no cardiac output and CV collapse. Death will ensue rapidly if effective treatment measures are not taken. Patients who die abruptly (within 1 hour of initial symptoms) and unexpectedly (ie, "sudden death") usually have VF recorded at the time of death.[120] SCD accounts for about 350,000 deaths per year in the United States.[17] It occurs most commonly in patients with CAD or LV dysfunction; it occurs less commonly in those with WPW syndrome or mitral valve prolapse, and occasionally in those without associated heart disease (eg, Brugada syndrome). Patients who have SCD (not associated with acute MI) but survive because of appropriate CPR and defibrillation (where warranted) often have inducible sustained VT and/or VF during electrophysiologic studies. These individuals are at high risk for the recurrence of VT and/or VF.

In contrast, patients who have VF associated with acute MI (ie, within the first 24 hours after symptoms) usually have little risk of recurrence. Of all patients who die as a result of an acute MI, approximately 50% die suddenly prior to hospitalization. VF associated with acute MI can be subdivided into two types: primary VF and complicated or secondary VF. Primary VF occurs in an uncomplicated MI not associated with HF; secondary VF occurs in an MI complicated by HF. The time course, incidence, mechanisms, treatment, and complications of these two forms of VF are different. For example, approximately 2% to 6% of patients with acute MI suffer primary VF within 24 hours of chest pain, but the risk of VF declines rapidly over time and is nearly zero after the initial 24-hour period. Complicated or secondary VF does not follow such a predictable time course and may occur in the late infarction period. The premise of prophylactic AADs administered to all patients with uncomplicated MI is based on (a) the inability to predict which patients are at risk for primary VF and (b) the predictable time course of primary VF (in contrast to complicated VF). Of the prophylactic therapies used, lidocaine has been the most widely debated and studied. Lie et al. performed the classic study showing the effectiveness of lidocaine in preventing primary VF.[121] Although lidocaine significantly reduced the incidence of VF compared with placebo, there was no significant difference in mortality due to VF between the groups. These results, along with the effectiveness of rapidly instituted defibrillation in modern coronary care units with sophisticated monitoring techniques, have caused most to reject the notion of prophylactic lidocaine administration for all patients with uncomplicated MI. In support of this, two meta-analyses concluded against the routine use of prophylactic lidocaine because of a possible increase in mortality in lidocaine-treated patients as well as the declining incidence of primary VF documented in recent years (probably a result of the more aggressive and rapid use of β-blockers, thrombolytics, and percutaneous intervention for the treatment of acute coronary syndromes).[122,123]

Acute Management

A patient with pulseless VT or VF should be managed according to the most recent AHA guidelines for CPR and ECC.[72,73] A detailed discussion regarding the acute management of pulseless VT/VF can be found in Chapter 12.

BRADYARRHYTHMIAS

The previous sections reviewed the pathophysiology and treatment of tachyarrhythmias, and this section serves to briefly consider the bradyarrhythmias. For the most part, the symptoms of bradyarrhythmias result from a decline in cardiac output. Because cardiac output decreases as heart rate decreases (to a point), patients with bradyarrhythmias may experience symptoms in association with hypotension, such as dizziness, syncope, fatigue, and confusion. If LV dysfunction exists, patients may experience worsening HF symptoms. Except in the case of recurrent syncope, symptoms associated with bradyarrhythmias are often subtle and nonspecific.

Sinus Bradycardia

Sinus bradyarrhythmias (heart rate <60 beats/min) are a common finding, especially in young, athletically active individuals, and usually are neither symptomatic nor in need of therapeutic intervention. On the other hand, some patients, particularly the elderly, have sinus node dysfunction. This may be the result of underlying SHD and the normal aging process that attenuate SA nodal function over time. Sick sinus syndrome refers to this process resulting in symptomatic sinus bradycardia and/or periods of sinus arrest.[124] Sinus node dysfunction is usually reflective of diffuse conduction disease, and accompanying AV block is relatively common. Furthermore, symptomatic bradyarrhythmias may be accompanied by alternating periods of paroxysmal tachycardias such as AF. In this instance, AF sometimes presents with a rather slow ventricular response (in the absence of AV nodal blocking drugs) because of diffuse conduction disease. The occurrence of alternating bradyarrhythmias and tachyarrhythmias is referred to as the tachy-brady syndrome. The occurrence of paroxysmal AF in a patient with sinus node dysfunction may be a result of underlying SHD with atrial dysfunction or atrial escape in response to reduced sinus node automaticity. In fact, because the rate of impulse generation by the sinus node is generally depressed or may fail altogether, other automatic pacemakers within the conduction system may "rescue" the sinus node. These rescue rhythms often present as paroxysmal atrial rhythms (eg, AF) or as a junctional escape rhythm.

The treatment of sinus node dysfunction involves the elimination of symptomatic bradycardia and potentially managing alternating tachycardias such as AF. In general, the long-term therapy of choice is a permanent ventricular pacemaker. Dual-chamber, rate-adaptive chronic pacing clearly improves symptoms and overall quality of life and decreases the incidence of paroxysmal AF and systemic embolism.[124] Drugs commonly employed to treat supraventricular tachycardias should be used with caution, if at all, in the absence of a functioning pacemaker. AADs prescribed to prevent AF recurrences may also suppress the escape or rescue rhythms that appear in severe sinus bradycardia or sinus arrest. Consequently, these drugs may transform an asymptomatic patient with bradycardia into a symptomatic one. The addition of class I AADs can also affect pacemaker threshold and result in loss of capture if the pacemaker is not appropriately interrogated and adjusted. Other drugs that depress SA or AV nodal function, such as β-blockers, non-DHP CCBs, and ivabradine, may also significantly exacerbate bradycardia. Even drugs with indirect sympatholytic actions, such as methyldopa and clonidine, may worsen sinus node dysfunction. The use of digoxin in these patients is controversial; however, in most cases, it can be used safely.

Other Causes

Another reason for paroxysmal bradycardia and sinus arrest that is not directly due to sinus node dysfunction is carotid sinus hypersensitivity.[125,126] Again, this syndrome occurs commonly in the elderly with underlying SHD, and may precipitate falls and hip fractures. Symptoms occur when the carotid sinus is stimulated, resulting in an accentuated baroreceptor reflex. Often, however, symptoms are not well correlated with the obvious physical manipulation of the carotid sinus (in the lateral neck region). Patients may experience intermittent episodes of dizziness or syncope because of sinus arrest caused by increased vagal tone and sympathetic withdrawal (the cardioinhibitory type), a drop in systemic blood pressure caused by sympathetic withdrawal (the vasodepressor type), or both (mixed cardioinhibitory and vasodepressor types). The diagnosis can be confirmed by performing carotid sinus massage with ECG and blood pressure monitoring in a controlled setting. Symptomatic carotid sinus hypersensitivity should also be treated with permanent pacemaker therapy.[125] However, some patients, particularly those with a significant vasodepressor component, still experience syncope or dizziness. The choice of definitive drug therapy in this situation is marred by the lack of controlled trials, although α-adrenergic stimulants such as midodrine are often tried in addition to the pacemaker.[126]

Vasovagal syndrome, by causing bradycardia, sinus arrest, and/or hypotension, is the cause of syncope in many patients who present with recurrent fainting of unknown origin.[127] By history, many individuals can recount rare instances of fainting spells at times of duress or fear. These episodes are most often caused by vasovagal syncope. However, some patients have extremely frequent, unexpected syncopal episodes that interfere with the patient's quality of life and cause physical danger (sometimes referred to as neurocardiogenic syncope syndrome or malignant vasovagal syndrome). Vasovagal syncope is presumed to be a neurally mediated, paradoxical reaction involving stimulation of cardiac mechanoreceptors (ie, Bezold-Jarisch reflex). Forceful contraction of the ventricle (eg, as with adrenergic stimulation) coupled with low ventricular volumes (eg, with upright posture or dehydration) provides a powerful stimulus for cardiac mechanoreceptors. Syncope results from the spontaneous development of transient hypotension (sympathetic withdrawal) and bradycardia (vagotonia). However, the true mechanism of vasovagal syncope remains to be definitively determined. For instance, patients with denervated hearts (eg, heart transplant recipients) can still experience this form of syncope. This observation has led some to question the ultimate role of the Bezold-Jarisch reflex in these patients. Regardless, patients believed to have frequent episodes of vasovagal syncope have been evaluated and diagnosed using the upright body-tilt test, a potent stimulus for the development of vasovagal symptoms.[128] Although commonly used, the sensitivity and reproducibility of this test have been questioned.[129]

Traditionally, β-blockers, such as metoprolol, were frequently chosen as the drugs of choice in preventing episodes of vasovagal syncope. Although these drugs may seem inappropriate to treat a syndrome resulting from vasodilation and bradycardia, the therapeutic approach is designed to block an inappropriate vasovagal reaction (ie, they inhibit the sympathetic surge that causes forceful ventricular contraction and precedes the onset of hypotension and bradycardia). To most clinicians' surprise, most controlled trials of the use of β-blockers in patients with severe vasovagal syncope have shown no effect compared with placebo in preventing syncopal episodes.[130] Some trials have suggested that β-blockers are more effective and should be used in older patients (older than 40 years of age) with vasovagal syncope rather than the relatively young.[131] Other drugs that have been used successfully (with or without β-blockers) include mineralocorticoids as volume expanders (fludrocortisone), anticholinergic drugs (scopolamine patches, disopyramide), α-adrenergic agonists (midodrine), adenosine analogs (theophylline, dipyridamole), and selective serotonin receptor antagonists (sertraline, paroxetine).[132] Permanent pacing has been used with some success but should be reserved for drug-refractory patients.[127] Because of the questionable effectiveness of β-blockers and the paucity of controlled or comparative trials, there is not a true drug of choice for severe vasovagal syncope, and clinicians are left with choosing agents and judging clinical effectiveness in individual patients on a case-by-case basis.

Atrioventricular Block

Conduction delay or block may occur in any area of the AV conduction system: the AV node, the His bundle, or the bundle branches. AV block is usually categorized into three different types based on ECG findings (Table 18-13). First-degree AV block is 1:1 AV conduction with a prolonged PR interval. Second-degree AV block is divided into two forms: Mobitz I AV block (Wenckebach periodicity) is less than 1:1 AV conduction with progressively lengthening PR intervals until a ventricular complex is dropped; Mobitz II AV block is intermittently dropped ventricular beats in a random fashion without progressive PR lengthening. Third-degree AV block is complete heart block where AV conduction is totally absent (AV dissociation). First-degree AV block usually represents prolonged conduction in the AV node. Mobitz I, second-degree AV block is also

TABLE 18-13 Forms of Atrioventricular Block

Type	Criteria	Site of Block
First-degree block	Prolonged PR interval (>0.2 second); 1:1 AV conduction	Usually AVN
Second-degree block		
Mobitz I	Progressive PR prolongation until QRS is dropped; <1:1 AV conduction	AVN
Mobitz II	Random nonconducted beats (absence of QRS); <1:1 AV conduction	Below AVN
Third-degree block	AV dissociation; absence of AV conduction	AVN or below

AV, atrioventricular; AVN, atrioventricular node.

usually caused by prolonged conduction in the AV node. In contrast, Mobitz II, second-degree AV block is usually caused by conduction disease below the AV node (ie, His bundle). Third-degree AV block may be caused by disease at any level of the AV conduction system: complete AV nodal block, His bundle block, or trifascicular block. In this situation, the ventricle beats independently of the atria (AV dissociation), and the rate of ventricular activation and QRS configuration are determined by the site of the AV block. The usual degree of automaticity of ventricular pacemakers progressively declines as the site of impulse generation moves down the ventricular conduction system. Therefore, the ventricular escape rate in cases of trifascicular block will be significantly less than complete AV nodal block. Consequently, trifascicular block is a much more dangerous form of AV block. For instance, complete AV block at the level of the AV node usually results in the ventricular rhythm being controlled by the stable AV junctional pacemaker (rate approximately 40 beats/min). In contrast, in complete AV block due to trifascicular or His bundle block, a much less reliable pacemaker with slower rates below the site of block controls ventricular rhythm.

AV block may be found in patients without underlying SHD such as trained athletes or during sleep when vagal tone is high. Also, AV block may be transient where the underlying etiology is reversible such as in myocarditis, myocardial ischemia, after CV surgery, or during drug therapy. β-Blockers, digoxin, or non-DHP CCBs may cause AV block, primarily in the AV nodal area. Class I AADs may exacerbate conduction delays below the level of the AV node (sodium-dependent tissue). In other cases, AV block may be irreversible, such as that caused by acute MI, rare degenerative diseases, primary myocardial disease, or congenital heart disease.

If patients with Mobitz II AV block or third-degree AV block develop signs or symptoms of poor perfusion (eg, altered mental status, chest pain, hypotension, shock), IV atropine (0.5 mg given every 3 to 5 minutes, up to 3 mg total dose) should be administered.[72] If these patients do not respond to atropine, transcutaneous pacing can be initiated. Sympathomimetic infusions such as epinephrine (2 to 10 mcg/min) or dopamine (2-10 mcg/kg/min) can also be used in the event of atropine failure and are particularly effective in sinus bradycardia/arrest and AV nodal block. An isoproterenol infusion (2-10 mcg/min) may be considered if the patient does not respond to dopamine or epinephrine; however, this drug should be used with caution because of its vasodilating properties and ability to increase myocardial oxygen consumption (particularly during active MI). As would be expected, these drugs usually do not help when the site of AV block is below the AV node (eg, Mobitz II or trifascicular AV block) because their primary mechanism is to accelerate conduction through the AV node. If patients with bradycardia or AV block present with signs and symptoms of adequate perfusion, no acute therapy other than close observation is recommended.

Patients with chronic symptomatic AV block should be treated with the insertion of a permanent pacemaker. Patients without symptoms can sometimes be followed closely without the need for a pacemaker. The reader is referred for more detail to the national consensus guidelines for pacemaker implantation.[114] Patients with acute MI and evidence of new AV block or conduction disturbances will often require the insertion of a temporary transvenous pacemaker. AV block more commonly occurs as a complication of inferior wall MIs because of high vagal innervation at this site, and the coronary blood flow to the nodal areas usually supplies the inferior wall. However, the AV block may only be transient, obviating the need for permanent pacing.

EVALUATION OF THERAPEUTIC AND ECONOMIC OUTCOMES

Generally, patients who suffer from tachyarrhythmias can be monitored for one or several possible therapeutic outcomes. Obviously, the presence or recurrence of any arrhythmia can be documented by electrocardiographic means (eg, surface ECG, Holter monitor, or event monitor). Furthermore, patients may experience a decrease in blood pressure that may result in symptoms ranging from lightheadedness to abrupt syncope, depending on the rate of the arrhythmia and the status of the underlying heart disease. For some patients, the potential alteration in hemodynamics may result in death if the arrhythmia is not detected and treated immediately. Besides these clinical outcomes, many patients with tachyarrhythmias experience alterations in quality of life as a result of recurrent symptoms of the arrhythmia or from side effects of therapy. And, finally, there are the economic considerations of medical or surgical intervention, continued medical care, and chronic drug or nonpharmacologic treatment.[133,134] Most of the studies are limited to the use of nonpharmacologic therapies such as the ICD or radiofrequency ablation.[77,135] Because that technology is rapidly evolving, what is not very cost-effective now may indeed be cost-effective in the next several years. For example, original cost-effectiveness analysis of the ICD showed it to be highly sensitive to the life of the generator, yet newer-generation devices have made significant advances not only in their size but also in their battery life. More recent data on the effect of the ICD on mortality coupled with the declining costs of an ICD imply that the device is indeed cost-effective in certain subsets of patients, which is similar to well-proven drug therapies used for other disorders.[135] Other nonpharmacologic treatments, such as catheter ablation for PSVT, not only improve quality of life but also save money on medical expenditures compared with chronic drug therapy.[76]

There are some therapeutic outcomes that are unique to certain arrhythmias. For instance, patients with AF or AFl need to be monitored for thromboembolism and for complications of antithrombotic therapy (bleeding, drug interactions). However, the most important monitoring parameters for most patients fall into the following categories: (a) mortality (total and arrhythmic); (b) arrhythmia recurrence (duration, frequency, symptoms); (c) hemodynamic consequences (heart rate, blood pressure, symptoms); and (d) treatment complications (side effects or need for alternative or additional drugs, devices, surgery) (Table 18-14). When evaluating the arrhythmia literature, care should be taken to consider real outcomes. For example, total mortality is more meaningful than SCD rates; it is possible an intervention prevents arrhythmic death but patients die from other causes, leaving all-cause mortality unaltered. Likewise, surrogate markers of drug efficacy (eg, noninducible tachycardia, suppression of minor arrhythmias) should be judged with a degree of skepticism. One should ask: Did the treatment make patients live longer (reduce mortality)? Did the treatment make them feel better (improve humanistic outcomes or quality of life)? Was the treatment economically worth it (cost-effective)?

TABLE 18-14 Arrhythmia Outcomes

Mortality
- Total, all-cause
- Arrhythmic death (ie, sudden cardiac death)

Recurrences documented by electrocardiogram
- Time to recurrence
- Frequency of recurrences

Tolerance
- Symptoms
- Blood pressure
- Rate of tachycardia

Surrogate markers of efficacy such as:
- Number of premature ventricular complexes per day
- Inducibility of tachycardia with programmed stimulation

Necessity of nondrug interventions (eg, ICD)

ICD shocks

Side effects of drugs/treatment complications

Quality of life

Economics

Outcomes specific to tachycardia (eg, systemic embolism in atrial fibrillation)

ICD, implantable cardioverter-defibrillator.

ABBREVIATIONS

AAD	antiarrhythmic drug
ACC	American College of Cardiology
AF	atrial fibrillation
AF-CHF	Atrial Fibrillation and Congestive Heart Failure
AFFIRM	Atrial Fibrillation Follow-Up Investigation of Rhythm Management
AFl	atrial flutter
AHA	American Heart Association
AV	atrioventricular
AVID	Antiarrhythmics versus Implantable Defibrillators
CAD	coronary artery disease
CASH	Cardiac Arrest Study Hamburg
CAST	Cardiac Arrhythmia Suppression Trial
CCB	calcium channel blocker
CIDS	Canadian Implantable Defibrillator Study
CPR	cardiopulmonary resuscitation
CrCl	creatinine clearance
CV	cardiovascular
CYP	cytochrome P450
DCC	direct current cardioversion
DHP	dihydropyridine
EAD	early afterdepolarization
ECC	emergency cardiovascular care
ECG	electrocardiogram
HF	heart failure
HF*p*EF	heart failure with preserved ejection fraction
HF*r*EF	heart failure with reduced ejection fraction
HOT-CAFE	How to Treat Chronic Atrial Fibrillation
HRS	Heart Rhythm Society
ICD	implantable cardioverter-defibrillator
INR	international normalized ratio
IV	intravenous
J	joules
LAD	late afterdepolarization
LMWH	low-molecular-weight heparin
LV	left ventricular
LVEF	left ventricular ejection fraction
MADIT	Multicenter Automatic Defibrillator Implantation Trial
MI	myocardial infarction
MUSTT	Multicenter Unsustained Tachycardia Trial
NYHA	New York Heart Association
P-gp	P-glycoprotein
PIAF	Pharmacological Intervention in Atrial Fibrillation
PSVT	paroxysmal supraventricular tachycardia
PVC	premature ventricular complex
RACE	Rate Control versus Electrical Cardioversion for Persistent Atrial Fibrillation
RE-LY	Randomized Evaluation of Long-Term Anticoagulation Therapy
RMP	resting membrane potential
SA	sinoatrial
SCD	sudden cardiac death
SCD-HeFT	Sudden Cardiac Death in Heart Failure Trial
SHD	structural heart disease
SR	sinus rhythm
STAF	Strategies of Treatment of Atrial Fibrillation
TdP	torsade de pointes
TE	thromboembolic
TEE	transesophageal echocardiography
TSOAC	target specific oral anticoagulant
UFH	unfractionated heparin
VF	ventricular fibrillation
VT	ventricular tachycardia
WPW	Wolff-Parkinson-White

REFERENCES

1. Alice MA, Bonke FIM, Schopman FJG. Circus movement in rabbit atrial muscle as a mechanism of tachycardia III. The "leading circle" concept: A new model of circus movement in cardiac tissue without the involvement of an anatomic obstacle. *Circ Res* 1977;41:9-18.
2. Vaughan Williams EM. A classification of antiarrhythmic actions reassessed after a decade of new drugs. *J Clin Pharmacol* 1984;24:129-147.
3. Working Group on Arrhythmias of the European Society of Cardiology. The Sicilian Gambit: A new approach to the classification of antiarrhythmic drugs based upon their actions on arrhythmogenic mechanisms. *Circulation* 1991;84:1831-1851.
4. Hondeghem LM, Katzung BG. Antiarrhythmic agents: The modulated receptor mechanism of action of sodium and calcium channel-blocking drugs. *Annu Rev Pharmacol Toxicol* 1984;24:387-423.
5. Nasr IR, Bouzamondo A, Hulot JS, et al. Prevention of atrial fibrillation onset by beta-blocker treatment in heart failure: A meta-analysis. *Eur Heart J* 2007;28:457-462.
6. Makkar KM, Sanoski CA, Spinler SA. Role of angiotensin-converting enzyme inhibitors, angiotensin II receptor blockers, and aldosterone antagonists in the prevention of atrial and ventricular arrhythmias. *Pharmacotherapy* 2009;29:31-48.
7. Podrid PJ. Proarrhythmia, a serious complication of antiarrhythmic drugs. *Curr Cardiol Rep* 1999;1:289-296.
8. Fang MC, Stafford RS, Ruskin JN, et al. National trends in antiarrhythmic and antithrombotic medication use in atrial fibrillation. *Arch Intern Med* 2004;164:55-60.
9. Sanoski CA, Bauman JL. Clinical observations with the amiodarone/warfarin interaction: Dosing relationships with long-term therapy. *Chest* 2002;121:19-23.
10. Camus P, Martin WJ, Rosenow EC. Amiodarone pulmonary toxicity. *Clin Chest Med* 2004;25:65-75.
11. Babatin M, Lee SS, Pollak PT. Amiodarone hepatotoxicity. *Curr Vasc Pharmacol* 2008;6:228-236.
12. Sanoski C, Schoen MD, Gonzalez RD, et al. Rationale, development and outcomes of a multidisciplinary clinic for patients receiving chronic oral amiodarone. *Pharmacotherapy* 1998;18:1465-1515.
13. Epstein AE, Olshansky B, Naccarelli GV, et al. Practical management guide for clinicians who treat patients with amiodarone. *Am J Med* 2016;129:468-475.
14. Jahn S, Zollner G, Lackner C, Stauber B. Severe toxic hepatitis associated with dronedarone. *Curr Drug Saf* 2013;8:201-202.
15. Siu CW, Wong MP, Ho CM, et al. Fatal lung toxic effects related to dronedarone use. *Arch Intern Med* 2012;172:516-517.

16. Young C, Maruthappu M, Wayne RP, Leaver L. Reversible acute kidney injury requiring haemodialysis five days after starting dronedarone in a stable 71-year-old man at risk of cardiovascular polypharmacy. *J R Coll Physicians Edinb* 2013;43:122-125.
17. Mozaffarian D, Benjamin EJ, Go AS, et al. Heart disease and stroke statistics—2016 update: A report from the American Heart Association. *Circulation* 2016;133:e38-e360.
18. Go AS, Hylek EM, Phillips KA, et al. Prevalence of diagnosed atrial fibrillation in adults: National implications for rhythm management and stroke prevention: The Anticoagulation and Risk Factors in Atrial Fibrillation (ATRIA) Study. *JAMA* 2001;285:2370-2375.
19. Feinberg WM, Blackshear JL, Laupacis A, et al. Prevalence, age distribution, and gender of patients with atrial fibrillation: Analysis and implications. *Arch Intern Med* 1995;155:469-473.
20. Miyasaka Y, Barnes ME, Gersh BJ, et al. Secular trends in incidence of atrial fibrillation in Olmsted County, Minnesota, 1980 to 2000, and implications on the projections for future prevalence. *Circulation* 2006;114:119-125.
21. Lloyd-Jones DM, Wang TJ, Leip EP, et al. Lifetime risk for developing atrial fibrillation: The Framingham Heart Study. *Circulation* 2004;110:1042-1046.
22. January CT, Wann LS, Alpert JS, et al. 2014 AHA/ACC/HRS guideline for the management of patients with atrial fibrillation: A report of the American College of Cardiology/American Heart Association Task Force on Practice Guidelines and the Heart Rhythm Society. *J Am Coll Cardiol*, 2014;64:e1-e76.
23. Atrial Fibrillation Investigators. Risk factors for stroke and efficacy of antithrombotic therapy in atrial fibrillation: Analysis of pooled data from five randomized controlled trials. *Arch Intern Med* 1994;154:1449-1457.
24. Wolf PA, Abbott RD, Kannel WB. Atrial fibrillation as an independent risk factor for stroke: the Framingham Study. *Stroke* 1991;22:983-988.
25. Turakjia MP, Santangeli P, Winkelmayer WC, et al. Increased mortality associated with digoxin in contemporary patients with atrial fibrillation: Findings from the TREAT-AF Study. *J Am Coll Cardiol* 2014;64:660-668.
26. Vamos M, Erath JW, Hohnloser SH. Digoxin-associated mortality: A systematic review and meta-analysis of the literature. *Eur Heart J* 2015;36:1831-1838.
27. Phillips BG, Gandhi AJ, Sanoski CA, et al. Comparison of intravenous diltiazem and verapamil for the acute treatment of atrial fibrillation and flutter. *Pharmacotherapy* 1997;17:1238-1245.
28. Hohnloser SH, Kuck KH, Lilienthal J. Rhythm or rate control in atrial fibrillation—Pharmacological Intervention in Atrial Fibrillation (PIAF): A randomised trial. *Lancet* 2000;356:1789-1794.
29. Van Gelder IC, Hagens VE, Bosker HA, et al. The Rate Control versus Electrical Cardioversion for Persistent Atrial Fibrillation Study Group. A comparison of rate control and rhythm control in patients with recurrent persistent atrial fibrillation. *N Engl J Med* 2002;347:1834-1840.
30. The Atrial Fibrillation Follow-Up Investigation of Rhythm Management (AFFIRM) Investigators. A comparison of rate control and rhythm control in patients with atrial fibrillation. *N Engl J Med* 2002;347:1825-1833.
31. Carlsson J, Miketic S, Windeler J, et al. Randomized trial of rate-control versus rhythm-control in persistent atrial fibrillation: The Strategies of Treatment of Atrial Fibrillation (STAF) study. *J Am Coll Cardiol* 2003;41:1690-1696.
32. Opolski G, Torbicki A, Kosior DA, et al. Rate control vs rhythm control in patients with nonvalvular persistent atrial fibrillation: The results of the Polish How to Treat Chronic Atrial Fibrillation (HOT CAFE) Study. *Chest* 2004;126:476-486.
33. Roy D, Talajic M, Nattel S, et al. Rhythm control versus rate control for atrial fibrillation and heart failure. *N Engl J Med* 2008;358: 2667-2677.
34. de Denus S, Sanoski CA, Carlsson J, Opolski G, Spinler SA. Rate vs rhythm control in patients with atrial fibrillation: A meta-analysis. *Arch Intern Med* 2005;165:258-262.
35. Van Gelder IC, Groenveld HF, Crijns HJ, et al. Lenient versus strict rate control in patients with atrial fibrillation. *N Engl J Med* 2010;362:1363-1373.
36. You JJ, Singer DE, Howard PA, et al. Antithrombotic therapy for atrial fibrillation: Antithrombotic Therapy and Prevention of Thrombosis, 9th ed: American College of Chest Physicians Evidence-Based Clinical Practice Guidelines. *Chest* 2012;141:e531S-e575S.
37. Klein AL, Grimm RA, Murray D, et al. Use of transesophageal echocardiography to guide cardioversion in patients with atrial fibrillation. *N Engl J Med* 2001;344:1411-1420.
38. Alboni P, Botto GL, Baldi N, et al. Outpatient treatment of recent-onset atrial fibrillation with the "pill-in-the-pocket" approach. *N Engl J Med* 2004;351:2384-2391.
39. Connolly SJ, Ezekowitz MD, Yusuf S, et al. Dabigatran versus warfarin in patients with atrial fibrillation. *N Engl J Med* 2009;361: 1139-1151.
40. Liesenfeld KH, Lehr T, Dansirikul C, et al. Population pharmacokinetic analysis of the oral thrombin inhibitor dabigatran etexilate in patients with non-valvular atrial fibrillation from the RE-LY trial. *J Thromb Haemost* 2011;9:2168-2175.
41. Eikelboom JW, Connolly SJ, Brueckmann M, et al. Dabigatran versus warfarin in patients with mechanical heart valves. *N Engl J Med* 2013;369:1206-1214.
42. Patel MR, Mahaffey KW, Garg J, et al. Rivaroxaban versus warfarin in nonvalvular atrial fibrillation. *N Engl J Med* 2011;365:883-891.
43. Connolly SJ, Eikelboom J, Joyner C, et al. Apixaban in patients with atrial fibrillation. *N Engl J Med* 2011;364:806-817.
44. Granger CB, Alexander JH, McMurray JJ, et al. Apixaban versus warfarin in patients with atrial fibrillation. *N Engl J Med* 2011;365: 981-992.
45. Giugliano RP, Ruff CT, Braunwald E, et al. Edoxaban versus warfarin in patients with atrial fibrillation. *N Engl J Med* 2013;369:2093-2104.
46. Patel MR, Hellkamp AS, Lokhnygina Y, et al. Outcomes of discontinuing rivaroxaban compared with warfarin in patients with nonvalvular atrial fibrillation: Analysis from the ROCKET AF trial (Rivaroxaban Once-Daily, Oral, Direct Factor Xa Inhibition Compared With Vitamin K Antagonism for Prevention of Stroke and Embolism Trial in Atrial Fibrillation). *J Am Coll Cardiol* 2013;61:651-658.
47. Coplen SE, Antman EM, Berlin JA, et al. Efficacy and safety of quinidine therapy for maintenance of sinus rhythm after cardioversion: A meta-analysis of randomized control trials. *Circulation* 1990;82:1106-1116.
48. Echt DS, Liebson PR, Mitchell B, et al. Mortality and morbidity in patients receiving encainide, flecainide, or placebo. The Cardiac Arrhythmia Suppression Trial. *N Engl J Med* 1991;324:781-788.
49. Lafuente-LaFuente C, Mouly S, Longás-Tejero MA, et al. Antiarrhythmic drugs for maintaining sinus rhythm after cardioversion of atrial fibrillation. *Arch Intern Med* 2006;166: 719-728.
50. Roy D, Talajic M, Dorian P, et al. Amiodarone to prevent recurrence of atrial fibrillation. Canadian Trial of Atrial Fibrillation Investigators. *N Engl J Med* 2000;324:913-920.
51. AFFIRM First Antiarrhythmic Drug Substudy Investigators. Maintenance of sinus rhythm in patients with atrial fibrillation: An AFFIRM substudy of the first antiarrhythmic drug. *J Am Coll Cardiol* 2003;42:20-29.
52. Singh BN, Singh SN, Reda DJ, et al. Amiodarone versus sotalol for atrial fibrillation. *N Engl J Med* 2005;352:1861-1872.
53. Juul-Moller S, Edvardsson N, Rehnqvist-Ahlberg N. Sotalol versus quinidine for the maintenance of sinus rhythm after direct current conversion of atrial fibrillation. *Circulation* 1990;82:1932-1939.
54. Southworth MR, Zarembski D, Viana M, Bauman JL. Comparison of sotalol versus quinidine for maintenance of normal sinus rhythm in patients with chronic atrial fibrillation. *Am J Cardiol* 1999;83:1629-1632.
55. Singh S, Zoble RG, Yellen L, et al. Efficacy and safety of oral dofetilide in converting and maintaining sinus rhythm in patients with chronic atrial fibrillation or atrial flutter. The Symptomatic Atrial Fibrillation Investigative Research on Dofetilide (SAFIRE-D) Study. *Circulation* 2000;102:2385-2390.
56. Pedersen OD, Bagger H, Keller N, et al. Efficacy of dofetilide in the treatment of atrial fibrillation-flutter in patients with reduced left ventricular function, a Danish Investigation of Arrhythmia and Mortality on Dofetilide (DIAMOND) Substudy. *Circulation* 2001;104:292-296.
57. Singh BN, Connolly SJ, Crijns HJGM, et al. Dronedarone for maintenance of sinus rhythm in atrial fibrillation or flutter. *N Engl J Med* 2007;357:987-999.
58. Hohnloser SH, Crijns HJGM, van Eickels M, et al. Effect of dronedarone on cardiovascular events in atrial fibrillation. *N Engl J Med* 2009;360:668-678.
59. Køber L, Torp-Pedersen C, McMurray JJV, et al. Increased mortality after dronedarone therapy for severe heart failure. *N Engl J Med* 2008;358:2678-2687.
60. Le Heuzey JY, De Ferrari GM, Radzik D, et al. A short-term, randomized, double-blind, parallel-group study to evaluate the efficacy and safety of dronedarone versus amiodarone in patients with persistent atrial fibrillation: The DIONYSOS study. *J Cardiovasc Electrophysiol* 2010;21:597-605.

61. Connolly SJ, Camm AJ, Halperin JL, et al. Dronedarone in high-risk permanent atrial fibrillation. *N Engl J Med* 2011;365:2268-2276.
62. Spector P, Reynolds MR, Calkins H, et al. Meta-analysis of ablation of atrial flutter and supraventricular tachycardia. *Am J Cardiol* 2009;104:671-677.
63. Blomstrom-Lundgrist C, Scheimanman MM, Aliot EM, et al. ACC/AHA/ESC guidelines for the management of patients with supraventricular arrhythmias. A report of the American College of Cardiology/American Heart Association Task Force and the European Society of Cardiology Committee for Practice Guidelines. *J Am Coll Cardiol* 2003;42:1493-1531.
64. Pappone C, Augello G, Sala S, et al. A randomized trial of circumferential pulmonary vein ablation versus antiarrhythmic drug therapy in paroxysmal atrial fibrillation: The APAF Study. *J Am Coll Cardiol* 2006;48:2340-2347.
65. Oral H, Pappone C, Chugh A, et al. Circumferential pulmonary-vein ablation for chronic atrial fibrillation. *N Engl J Med* 2006;354:934-941.
66. Wilber DJ, Pappone C, Neuzil P, et al. Comparison of antiarrhythmic drug therapy and radiofrequency catheter ablation in patients with paroxysmal atrial fibrillation: A randomized controlled trial. *JAMA* 2010;303:333-340.
67. Morillo C, Verma A, Kuck A, et al. Radiofrequency ablation vs antiarrhythmic drugs as first-line treatment of paroxysmal atrial fibrillation (RAAFT 2): A randomized trial. *JAMA* 2014;311: 692-700.
68. Cosedis NJ, Johannessen A, Raatkainen P, et al. Radiofrequency ablation as initial therapy in paroxysmal atrial fibrillation. *N Engl J Med* 2012;367:1587-1595.
69. Cappato R, Calkins H, Chen SA, et al. Updated worldwide survey on the methods, efficacy, and safety of catheter ablation for human atrial fibrillation. *Circ Arrhythm Electrophysiol* 2010;3:32-38.
70. Sung RJ, Lauer MR, Chun H. Atrioventricular node reentry: Current concepts and new perspectives. *Pacing Clin Electrophysiol* 1994;17:1413-1430.
71. DiMarco JP, Miles W, Akhtar M, et al. Adenosine for paroxysmal supraventricular tachycardia: Dose ranging and comparison with verapamil. Assessment in placebo-controlled, multicenter trials. *Ann Intern Med* 1990;1113:104-110.
72. 2010 American Heart Association guidelines for cardiopulmonary resuscitation and emergency cardiovascular care science. *Circulation* 2010;122:5640-5933.
73. Link MS, Berkow LC, Kudenchuk PJ, et al. Part 7: Adult advanced cardiovascular life support: 2015 American Heart Association guidelines update for cardiopulmonary resuscitation and emergency cardiovascular care. *Circulation* 2015;132:S444-S464.
74. Rankin AC, McGovern BA. Adenosine or verapamil for the acute treatment of supraventricular tachycardia? *Ann Intern Med* 1991;114: 513-515.
75. Jackman WM, Wang Z, Friday KJ, et al. Catheter ablation of accessory atrioventricular pathways (Wolff-Parkinson-White syndrome) by radiofrequency current. *N Engl J Med* 1991;324:1605-1611.
76. Jackman WM, Beckman KJ, McClelland JH, et al. Treatment of supraventricular tachycardia due to atrioventricular nodal reentry by radiofrequency catheter ablation of slow pathway conduction. *N Engl J Med* 1992;327:313-318.
77. Cheng CH, Sanders GD, Hlatky MA, et al. Cost effectiveness of radiofrequency ablation for supraventricular tachycardia. *Ann Intern Med* 2000;133:864-876.
78. Meyer L, Stubbs B, Fahrenbruch C, et al. Incidence, causes, and survival trends from cardiovascular related sudden cardiac arrest in children and young adults 0 to 35 years of age: A 30-year review. *Circulation* 2012;126:1363-1372.
79. Bayes deLuna A, Coumel P, LeClercq IF. Ambulatory sudden cardiac death: Mechanisms of production of fatal arrhythmia on the basis of data from 157 cases. *Am Heart J* 1989;117:151-159.
80. Ruberman W, Weinblatt E, Goldberg JD, et al. Ventricular premature beats and mortality after myocardial infarction. *N Engl J Med* 1977;297:750-757.
81. The Cardiac Arrhythmia Suppression Trial II Investigators. Effect of the antiarrhythmic agent moricizine on survival after myocardial infarction. *N Engl J Med* 1992;327:227-233.
82. Waldo AL, Camm AJ, deRuyter H, et al. Effect of *d*-sotalol on mortality in patients with left ventricular dysfunction and remote myocardial infarction. *Lancet* 1996;348:7-12.
83. Julian DG, Camm AJ, Frangin G, et al. Randomized trial of effect of amiodarone on mortality in patients with left ventricular dysfunction after recent myocardial infarction: EMIAT. *Lancet* 1997;349:667-674.
84. Cairns JA, Connolly SJ, Roberts R, et al. Randomized trial of outcome after myocardial infarction in patients with frequent or repetitive ventricular premature depolarizations: CAMIAT. *Lancet* 1997;349:675-682.
85. Amiodarone Trials Meta-Analysis Investigators. Effect of prophylactic amiodarone on mortality after acute myocardial infarction and in congestive heart failure: Meta-analysis of individual data from 6,500 patients in randomized trials. *Lancet* 1997;350:1417-1424.
86. Torp-Pederson C, Moller M, Bloch-Thomsen PE, et al. Dofetilide in patients with congestive heart failure and left ventricular dysfunction. *N Engl J Med* 1999;341:857-865.
87. Kober L, Block-Thomsen PE, Moller M, et al. Effect of dofetilide in patients with recent myocardial infarction and left ventricular dysfunction: A randomized trial. *Lancet* 2000;356:2052-2058.
88. Hilleman DE, Bauman JL. Role of antiarrhythmic therapy in patients at risk for sudden cardiac death: An evidence-based review. *Pharmacotherapy* 2001;21:556-575.
89. Edhouse J, Morris F. Broad complex tachycardia—Part I. *BMJ* 2002;312:719-722.
90. Edhouse J, Morris F. Broad complex tachycardia—Part II. *BMJ* 2002;324:776-779.
91. Cole CR, Marrouche NF, Natale A. Evaluation and management of ventricular outflow tract tachycardias. *Card Electrophysiol Rev* 2002;6:442-447.
92. Modell SM, Lehmann MH. The long QT syndrome family of cardiac ion channelopathies: A HuGE review. *Genet Med* 2006;8:143-155.
93. Keating MT, Sanguinetti MC. Molecular and cellular mechanisms of cardiac arrhythmias. *Cell* 2001;104:569-580.
94. Antzelevitch C, Brugada P, Brugada J, et al. Brugada syndrome: 1992–2002: A historical perspective. *J Am Coll Cardiol* 2003;41: 1665-1671.
95. Gorgels A, van den Dool A, Hofs A, et al. Comparison of procainamide and lidocaine in terminating sustained monomorphic ventricular tachycardia. *Am J Cardiol* 1996;78:43-46.
96. Mason JW; Electrophysiologic Study versus Electrocardiographic Monitoring Investigators. A comparison of electrophysiologic testing with Holter monitoring to predict antiarrhythmic drug efficacy for ventricular tachyarrhythmias. *N Engl J Med* 1993;329:445-451.
97. Mason JW; Electrophysiologic Study versus Electrocardiographic Monitoring Investigators. A comparison of seven antiarrhythmic drugs in patients with ventricular tachyarrhythmias. *N Engl J Med* 1993;329:452-458.
98. The Cascade Investigators. Randomized antiarrhythmic drug therapy in survivors of cardiac arrest (the CASCADE Study). *Am J Cardiol* 1993;72:280-287.
99. Aliot EM, Stevenson WG, Almendral-Garrote JM, et al. EHRA/HRS expert consensus on catheter ablation of ventricular arrhythmias: Developed in a partnership with the European Heart Rhythm Association (EHRA), a registered branch of the European Society of Cardiology (ESC), and the Heart Rhythm Society (HRS); in collaboration with the American College of Cardiology (ACC) and the American Heart Association (AHA). *Europace* 2009;11:771-817.
100. DiMarco JP. Implantable cardioverter-defibrillators. *N Engl J Med* 2003;349:1836-1847.
101. Pacifico A, Hohnloser SH, Williams JH, et al. Prevention of implantable-defibrillator shocks by treatment with sotalol. *N Engl J Med* 1999;340:1855-1862.
102. Connolly SJ, Dorian P, Roberts RS, et al. Comparison of beta-blockers, amiodarone plus beta-blockers, or sotalol for prevention of shocks from implantable cardioverter defibrillators: The OPTIC Study: A randomized trial. *JAMA* 2006;295:165-171.
103. Dopp AL, Miller JM, Tisdale JE. Effects of drugs on defibrillation capacity. *Drugs* 2008;68:607-630.
104. The AVID Investigators. A comparison of antiarrhythmic-drug therapy with implantable defibrillators in patients resuscitated from near-fatal ventricular arrhythmias. *N Engl J Med* 1997;337:1576-1583.
105. Connolly SJ, Gene M, Roberts TS, et al. Cardiac Implantable Defibrillator Study (CIDS): A randomized trial of the implantable cardioverter-defibrillator against amiodarone. *Circulation* 2000;101:1297-1302.
106. Kuck KH, Cappato R, Siebels J, et al. Randomized comparison of antiarrhythmic drug therapy with implantable defibrillators in patients resuscitated from cardiac arrest: The Cardiac Arrest Study Hamburg (CASH). *Circulation* 2000;102:748-754.
107. Wilber DJ, Olshansky B, Moran JF, et al. Electrophysiological testing and nonsustained VT. Use and limitations in patients with coronary artery disease and impaired ventricular function. *Circulation* 1990;82:350-358.

108. Buxton AE, Leek KL, DiCarlo L, et al. Electrophysiologic testing to identify patients with coronary artery disease who are at risk for sudden death. Multicenter Unsustained Tachycardia Trial. *N Engl J Med* 2000;342:1937-1945.
109. Moss AJ, Hall WJ, Cannom DS, et al. Improved survival with an implanted defibrillator in patients with coronary disease at high risk for ventricular arrhythmia. *N Engl J Med* 1996;335:1933-1940.
110. Buxton AE, Lee KL, Fisher JD, et al. A randomized study of the prevention of sudden death in patients with coronary artery disease. *N Engl J Med* 1999;341:1882-1890.
111. Pedersen CT, Kay GN, Kalman J, et al. EHRA/HRS/APHRS expert consensus on ventricular arrhythmias. *Heart Rhythm* 2014;11:e166-e196.
112. Moss AJ, Zareba W, Hall WJ, et al. Prophylactic implantation of a defibrillator in patients with myocardial infarction and reduced ejection fraction. *N Engl J Med* 2002;346:877-883.
113. Bardy GH, Lee KL, Mark DB, et al. Amiodarone or an implantable cardioverter-defibrillator for congestive heart failure. *N Engl J Med* 2005;352:225-237.
114. Epstein AE, DiMarco JP, Ellenbogen KA, et al. 2012 ACCF/AHA/HRS focused update incorporated into the ACCF/AHA/HRS 2008 guidelines for device-based therapy of cardiac rhythm abnormalities: A report of the American College of Cardiology/American Heart Association Task Force on Practice Guidelines and the Heart Rhythm Society. *J Am Coll Cardiol* 2013;61:e6-e75.
115. Antzelevitch C. Heterogeneity of cellular repolarization in LQTS: The role of M cells. *Eur Heart J* 2001;3:K2-K16.
116. Roden DM. Long QT syndrome: Reduced repolarization reserve and the genetic link. *J Intern Med* 2006;259:59-69.
117. Oberg KC, O'Toole MF, Gallastegui JL, Bauman JL. "Late" proarrhythmia due to quinidine. *Am J Cardiol* 1994;74:192-194.
118. Bauman JL. The role of pharmacokinetics, drug interactions and pharmacogenetics in the acquired long QT syndrome. *Eur Heart J* 2001;3:K93-K100.
119. Tzivoni D, Banai S, Schuger C, et al. Treatment of torsade de pointes with magnesium sulfate. *Circulation* 1987;77:392-397.
120. Koplan BA, Stevenson WG. Ventricular tachycardia and sudden cardiac death. *Mayo Clin Proc* 2009;84:289-297.
121. Lie KI, Wellens HJJ, Van Capelle FJ. Lidocaine in the prevention of primary ventricular fibrillation. *N Engl J Med* 1974;291:1324-1326.
122. MacMahon S, Collin R, Peto R, et al. Effects of prophylactic lidocaine in suspected acute myocardial infarction: An overview of results from the randomized controlled trials. *JAMA* 1988;260:1910-1916.
123. Antman EM, Berlin JA. Declining incidence of ventricular fibrillation in myocardial infarction: Implications for the prophylactic use of lidocaine. *Circulation* 1992;86:764-773.
124. Moya A, Sutton R, Ammirati F, et al. Guidelines for the diagnosis and management of syncope (version 2009). *Eur Heart J* 2009;30:2631-2671.
125. Sugrue DD, Gersh BJ, Holmes DR, et al. Symptomatic "isolated" carotid sinus hypersensitivity: Natural history and results of treatment with anticholinergic drugs or pacemaker. *J Am Coll Cardiol* 1986;7:158-162.
126. Seifer C. Carotid sinus syndrome. *Prog Cardiol Clin* 2013;31:111-121.
127. Grubb BP. Neurocardiogenic syncope. *N Engl J Med* 2005;352:1004-1010.
128. Milstein S, Reyes WJ, Benditt DG. Upright body tilt for evaluation of patients with recurrent, unexplained syncope. *Pacing Clin Electrophysiol* 1989;12:117-124.
129. Almquist A, Goldenberg I, Milstein S. Provocation of bradycardia and hypotension by isoproterenol and upright posture in patients with unexplained syncope. *N Engl J Med* 1990;320:346-351.
130. Brignole M. Randomized clinical trials of neurally mediated syncope. *J Cardiovasc Electrophysiol* 2003;14(Suppl):S64-S69.
131. Sheldon R, Connolly S, Rose S, for the POST Investigators. Prevention of Syncope Trial (POST). A randomized, placebo-controlled study of metoprolol in the prevention of vasovagal syncope. *Circulation* 2006;113:1164-1170.
132. Armaganijan L, Morillo CA. Treatment of vasovagal syncope: An update. *Curr Treat Options Cardiovasc Med* 2010;12:472-488.
133. Kupersmith J, Holmes-Novner M, Hogan A, et al. Cost-effectiveness analysis in heart disease, I: General principles. *Prog Cardiovasc Dis* 1994;37:161-184.
134. Kupersmith J, Holmes-Novner M, Hogan A, et al. Cost-effectiveness analysis in heart disease, III: Ischemia, congestive heart failure, and arrhythmias. *Prog Cardiovasc Dis* 1995;37:307-346.
135. Sanders GD, Hlatky MA, Owens DK. Cost-effectiveness of implantable cardioverter-defibrillators. *N Engl J Med* 2005;353:1471-1480.

19

Venous Thromboembolism

Daniel M. Witt, Nathan P. Clark, and Sara R. Vazquez

KEY CONCEPTS

1. Venous thromboembolism (VTE) is often associated with identifiable risk factors.
2. The diagnosis of VTE should be confirmed by objective testing.
3. During hospitalization, patients should receive prophylaxis against VTE corresponding to their degree and duration of risk.
4. Initial VTE treatment should include a rapid-acting anticoagulant.
5. During warfarin initiation injectable anticoagulants should be overlapped with warfarin for at least 5 days and until the patient's international normalized ratio is more than or equal to 2.0 for at least 24 hours.
6. Most patients with uncomplicated deep vein thrombosis (DVT) or pulmonary embolism (PE) can be safely treated as outpatients.
7. Most patients with VTE should receive 3 months of anticoagulation therapy; duration of anticoagulation therapy beyond 3 months should be based on risks for VTE recurrence and major bleeding as well as patient preferences.
8. Optimal anticoagulant management requires knowledge of pharmacologic and pharmacokinetic characteristics as well as systematic management and ongoing patient education.
9. Direct oral anticoagulants (DOACs), such as rivaroxaban, apixaban, dabigatran, and edoxaban, are a significant advancement in VTE treatment.

INTRODUCTION

Venous thromboembolism (VTE) is a potentially fatal disorder and significant health problem in our aging society.[1] VTE results from clot formation within the venous circulation and is manifested as deep vein thrombosis (DVT) and/or pulmonary embolism (PE) (Fig. 19-1).[1] DVT is rarely fatal, but PE can result in death within minutes of symptom onset, before effective treatment can be given. Beyond the symptoms produced by the acute event, VTE complications, such as the postthrombotic syndrome and chronic thromboembolic pulmonary hypertension (CTPH), also cause substantial disability and suffering.[1] Identifying VTE risk factors is important for targeting patients at high risk for VTE to guide prevention strategies.[2-4]

Rapid and accurate diagnosis is critical to making appropriate treatment decisions when VTE is suspected.[5] Optimal use of anticoagulant drugs for prevention and treatment of VTE requires an in-depth knowledge of their pharmacology and pharmacokinetic properties, and a comprehensive approach to patient management.[6] Bleeding is a common and serious complication of administering anticoagulant drugs.[2-4]

EPIDEMIOLOGY

Venous thromboembolism is associated with major global disease burden.[7] The incidence rate of symptomatic first VTE is estimated at 1.32 per 1,000 patient-years and occurs more frequently in women (55.6%).[8] When standardized by age, Asians appear to have the lowest VTE incidence (1.22 per 1,000 patient-years) followed by whites (1.91) and blacks (2.03).[8] The rate of recurrent VTE is highest in the 180 days following the initial event and declines slowly over the next 4 to 10 years to a relatively constant rate. The 10-year cumulative risk of recurrent VTE is approximately 25.0%.[8]

ETIOLOGY

1 A number of identifiable factors increase the risk of developing VTE (Table 19-1). Many risk factors fall into categories constituting what is known as Virchow's triad: blood stasis, vascular injury, and hypercoagulability.

Blood Stasis

Blood stasis favors clotting in part through reduced clearance of the elements responsible for blood clot formation.[9] Contraction of the calf and thigh muscles coupled with one-way valves in leg veins facilitate blood flow back to the heart and lungs; thus, damage to venous valves and periods of prolonged immobility result in venous stasis.[10] Blood stasis in the venous system partly explains why numerous medical conditions and surgical procedures are associated with an increased VTE risk (see Table 19-1).

Vascular Injury

Intact vascular endothelial cells separate flowing blood from vessel wall components responsible for preventing blood loss through clot formation (see detailed description in PATHOPHYSIOLOGY section). Vascular injury (eg, surgery and trauma) disrupts this protective barrier and initiates blood clot formation.[11]

Hypercoagulability

Inherited and acquired conditions and certain drugs have been linked to blood hypercoagulability (see Table 19-1). Inherited and acquired hypercoagulability disorders will be covered in detail later. Estrogen-containing contraception, estrogen replacement therapy, and selective estrogen receptor modulators are all linked to VTE risk.[12] Women with inherited hypercoagulability disorders are at particularly high risk of developing VTE during pregnancy and while taking estrogens.[12]

In many cases, VTE is the result of converging combinations of inherited and acquired thrombotic risk factors. Thus, many

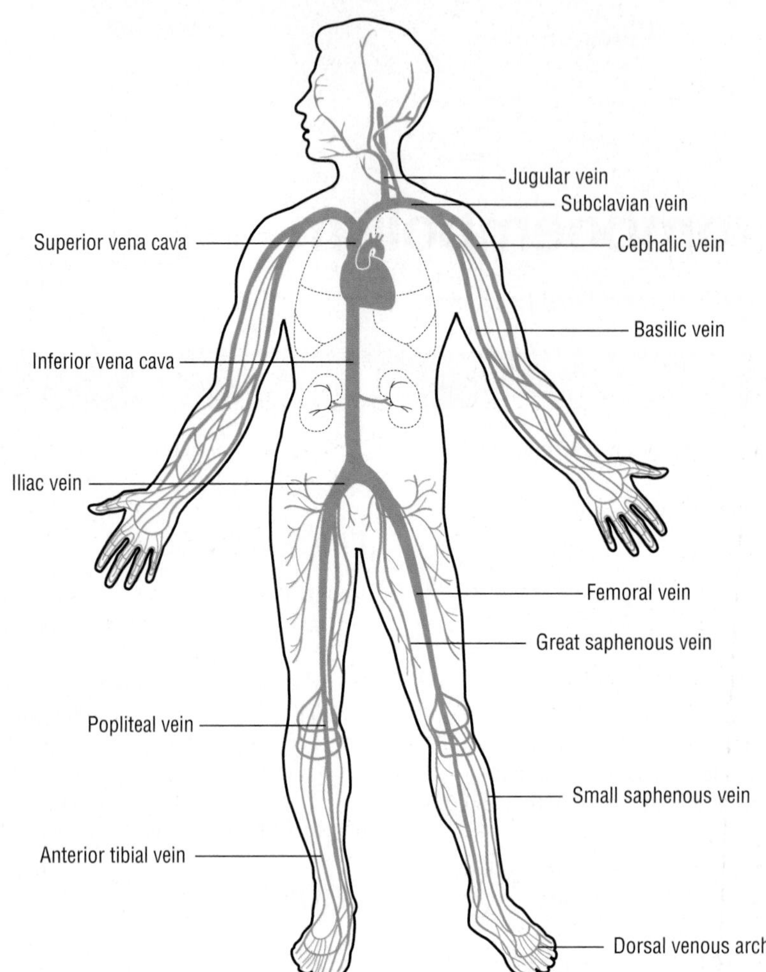

FIGURE 19-1 Venous circulation.

individuals with congenital hypercoagulable conditions experience VTE only after being placed in high-risk situations such as orthopedic surgery, immobilization, the use of estrogen-containing oral contraceptives, or pregnancy. Approximately 34.0% of VTEs are provoked by identifiable risk factors.[8]

PATHOPHYSIOLOGY

Hemostasis is the process responsible for maintaining the integrity of the circulatory system following blood vessel damage (Fig. 19-2).[11] Hemostatic clots remain localized to the vessel wall and do not greatly impair blood flow. In contrast, pathologic clots like those causing VTE result in blood flow impairment and often cause complete vessel occlusion.[11]

Collagen and tissue factor (TF) form a hemostatic barrier around blood vessels and organs. Under normal circumstances, endothelial cells lining the vessel wall physically separate collagen and TF from circulating platelets and clotting factors (namely, activated factor VII [VIIa]). Vessel injury results in platelet activation and TF-mediated initiation of the clotting factor cascade culminating in the formation of thrombin and ultimately fibrin clot, which seals the breach (see Fig. 19-2).[11] In contrast to physiologic hemostasis, pathologic VTE often occurs in the absence of gross vessel wall damage and may be triggered by TF brought to the clot formation site by circulating microparticles. Venous clots are mainly composed of fibrin with platelets and trapped red blood cells and often occur in areas of disturbed blood flow (eg, valve cusps in the deep leg veins).[11]

The activation of platelets and the coagulation cascade occur nearly simultaneously. Platelets become actively involved in thrombus formation after binding to various adhesion proteins (eg, von Willebrand factor, collagen) when blood is exposed to damaged vessel endothelium.[11] A platelet thrombus develops as activated platelets recruit additional platelets, some of which also become activated while others remain loosely associated without undergoing activation and ultimately break away from the growing thrombus. Activated platelets change shape and release components critical for sustaining further thrombus formation into the environment surrounding the developing clot.[11] Activated platelets accumulating in the thrombus also express P-selectin, an adhesion molecule that facilitates capture of blood-borne microparticles bearing TF triggering fibrin clot formation via the coagulation cascade (Fig. 19-3).[11] As described in the next section, important coagulation cascade reactions take place on the surfaces of activated platelets.[11]

The conceptual model for the coagulation cascade has evolved from the classic depiction of extrinsic, intrinsic, and common pathways (Fig. 19-4) to a more modern notion whereby highly regulated reactions take place on cell surfaces in three overlapping phases: initiation, amplification, and propagation. The cascade starts on TF-bearing cells, and continues on the surfaces of activated platelets (Fig. 19-5).[11]

The initiation phase takes place on TF-bearing cells exposed after vessel injury or captured via P-selectin (see Fig. 19-3). The TF/VIIa complex (known as extrinsic tenase) activates limited amounts of factors IX and X. The resulting factor Xa then associates with factor Va to form the prothrombinase complex, which cleaves prothrombin (factor II) to generate a small (picomolar) amount of thrombin (factor IIa) (see Fig. 19-5). Factor IXa moves from TF-bearing cells to the surface of activated platelets in the growing platelet thrombus.

TABLE 19-1 Risk Factors for Venous Thromboembolism

Risk Factor	Comments/Examples
Age	Annual incidence increases from 10 per 100,000 in adolescence to 1 per 100 in old age
History of VTE	Potent risk factor for recurrence, risk is highest during the first 180 days after VTE
Blood stasis	Acute medical illness requiring hospitalization Surgery (especially general anesthesia >30 minutes) Paralysis (eg, status post stroke, spinal cord injury) Immobility (eg, plaster casts, status post stroke or spinal cord injury) Polycythemia vera Obesity
Vascular injury	Major orthopedic surgery (eg, knee or hip replacement) Trauma (especially fractures of the pelvis, hip, or leg) Indwelling venous catheters
Hypercoagulability	Malignancy, diagnosed or occult Factor V Leiden (homozygous >>heterozygous) Prothrombin (G20210A) gene mutation Protein C deficiency Protein S deficiency Antithrombin deficiency Factor VIII excess (>90th percentile) Factor XI excess (>90th percentile) Antiphospholipid antibodies Lupus anticoagulant Anticardiolipin antibodies Anti-β_2-glycoprotein I antibodies Inflammatory bowel disease Nephrotic syndrome Paroxysmal nocturnal hemoglobinuria Pregnancy/postpartum Drug therapy (eg, estrogen-containing contraceptives, estrogen replacement therapy, tamoxifen, raloxifene, cancer therapy, heparin-induced thrombocytopenia)

VTE, venous thromboembolism.

Data from References 2, 3, 4, 12, 15.

Tissue factor pathway inhibitor (TFPI), an important regulator of TF/FVIIa-induced coagulation, rapidly terminates the initiation phase.[11]

In the amplification phase the small amount of thrombin produced during initiation activates factors V and VIII, which bind to platelet surfaces and support the large-scale thrombin generation occurring during the propagation phase. Platelet-bound factor XI is also activated by thrombin during this phase.[11]

A burst of thrombin generation occurs during the propagation phase as the VIIIa/IXa (known as "intrinsic tenase") and prothrombinase complexes assemble on the surface of activated platelets and accelerate the generation of factor Xa and thrombin, respectively. Thrombin generation is further supported by factor XIa bound to the platelet surface, which activates factor IX to form additional intrinsic tenase.[11]

Thrombin generated during the propagation phase converts fibrinogen to fibrin monomers that precipitate and polymerize to form fibrin strands. Factor XIIIa, which is also activated by the action of thrombin, covalently bonds these strands to one another (see Fig. 19-5) to form an extensive meshwork that surrounds and encases the aggregated platelet thrombus and red blood cells to form a stabilized fibrin clot.[11] Clot formation is eventually terminated when the expanding meshwork of platelets and fibrin "paves over" the initiation site and additional activated factors are unable to diffuse through the overlying layer of clot.

Normally, a number of tempering mechanisms control coagulation (see Fig. 19-2). Without effective self-regulation, thrombus formation would cause vascular occlusion. Intact endothelium adjacent to the damaged tissue actively secretes several antithrombotic substances.[9] Thrombomodulin modulates thrombin activity by converting protein C to its active form (aPC). When joined with its cofactor protein S, aPC inactivates factors Va and VIIIa regulating the functionality of the prothrombinase and tenase complexes, respectively.[9] aPC and protein S prevent coagulation reactions from spreading to healthy, uninjured vessel walls. Antithrombin is a circulating protein that inhibits thrombin and factor Xa. Heparan sulfate, a heparin-like compound secreted by endothelial cells, exponentially accelerates antithrombin activity.[9] As described previously, TFPI plays an important role by regulating the initiation of the coagulation cascade.[11] When these self-regulatory mechanisms are intact, fibrin clot is limited to the zone of vessel injury. However, disruptions in the system can result in hypercoagulability.[13]

The fibrinolytic system is responsible for blood clot dissolution.[14] Inactive plasminogen is converted by tissue plasminogen activator (tPA) to active plasmin, an enzyme that degrades fibrin mesh into soluble end products collectively known as fibrin degradation products including D-dimer.[14] The fibrinolytic system is also under the control of a series of stimulatory and inhibitory substances (see Fig. 19-2). Plasminogen activator inhibitor-1 inhibits tPA and α_2-antiplasmin inhibits plasmin activity. Impaired functioning of the fibrinolytic system has also been linked to hypercoagulability and thrombotic complications.[14]

Although a thrombus can form in any part of the venous circulation, most begin in the leg(s). Thrombus isolated in calf veins is unlikely to break loose (embolize), but thrombus involving the popliteal and larger veins above it are more likely to embolize and travel through the right side of the heart and lodge in the pulmonary artery or one of its branches, occluding blood flow to the lung and impairing gas exchange. Without treatment, the affected portion of the lung becomes necrotic and oxygen delivery to other vital organs decreases, potentially resulting in fatal circulatory collapse.[1]

Inherited and Acquired Hypercoagulability Disorders

Disturbances in hemostatic regulation processes may result in hypercoagulability. Disorders of hypercoagulability can be inherited or acquired.[13] aPC resistance increases the risk of VTE approximately threefold and is the most common inherited hypercoagulability disorder (prevalence rate in Caucasians 2.0%-7.0%).[13] Most aPC resistance results from a factor V gene mutation that renders it resistant to degradation by aPC. This mutation is known as factor V Leiden, named after the city of Leiden, Holland, where the defect was first described.[13]

The prothrombin G20210A mutation is the second most frequent inherited hypercoagulability disorder, occurring in about 2.0% to 4.0% of Caucasians and imparting about a threefold increased risk of VTE.[13] This mutation increases circulating prothrombin, and enhanced thrombin generation has been observed, but the mechanism whereby this disorder increases VTE risk is not completely understood.[15] Given the prevalence of factor V Leiden and prothrombin G20210A mutation in the general population, some patients inherit multiple genetic defects greatly increasing the lifetime VTE risk.[13]

Although an accurate quantification of the VTE risk associated with inherited protein C, protein S, and antithrombin deficiencies (present in less than 1% of the population) is not known, many experts believe the lifetime risk is high, perhaps sevenfold higher than patients without such disorders. Many patients with protein C, protein S, or antithrombin deficiency will suffer VTE prior to age 60.[15]

Acquired disorders of hypercoagulability may result from malignancy, the presence of antiphospholipid antibodies, or estrogen use. A strong link between cancer and thrombosis has long

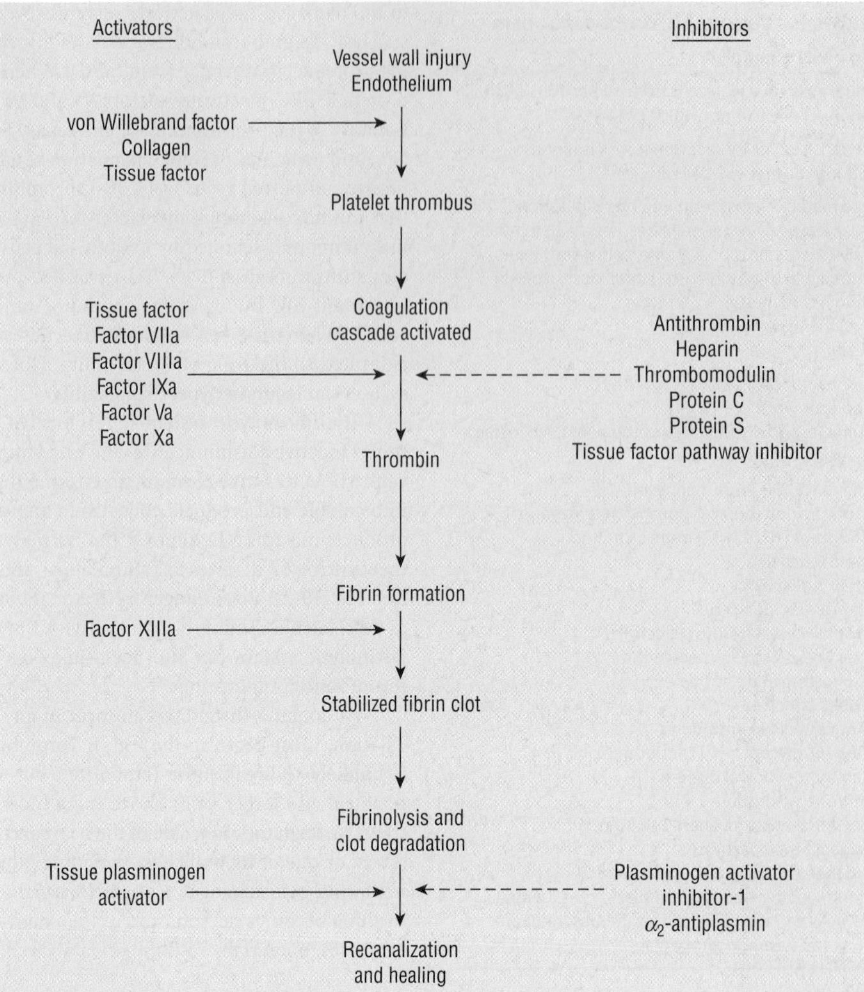

FIGURE 19-2 Overview of hemostasis.

been recognized.[16] Tumor cells secrete a number of procoagulant substances that activate the coagulation cascade, and patients with cancer often have suppressed levels of protein C, protein S, and antithrombin. Cancer cells may use thrombotic mechanisms to recruit a blood supply, metastasize, and create barriers against host defense mechanisms.[16]

Antiphospholipid antibodies are a heterogeneous group of antibodies targeting proteins that bind phospholipids.[15] These include antibodies that prolong phospholipid-based clotting assays, known as lupus anticoagulants, as well as anticardiolipin and β_2-glycoprotein (β_2-gp) I antibodies. Antiphospholipid antibodies are found in up to 5% of normal healthy populations but are more common in patients with autoimmune disorders such as systemic lupus erythematosus and inflammatory bowel disease. The precise mechanism by which antiphospholipid antibodies provoke thrombosis remains to be definitively determined. Contributing factors include complement activation, inhibition of protein C and fibrinolysis, platelet activation, and increased TF expression.[15]

CLINICAL PRESENTATION (INCLUDING DIAGNOSTIC CONSIDERATIONS)

2 The symptoms of DVT or PE are nonspecific and objective tests are required to confirm or exclude the diagnosis. Patients with DVT frequently present with unilateral leg pain and swelling.

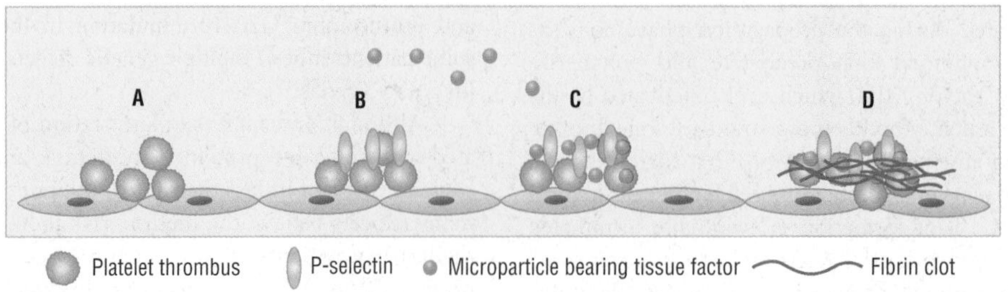

FIGURE 19-3 Model of pathologic thrombus formation: (*A*) activated platelets adhere to vascular endothelium; (*B*) activated platelets express P-selectin; (*C*) pathologic microparticles express active tissue factor and are present at a high concentration in the circulation—these microparticles accumulate, perhaps by binding to activated platelets expressing P-selectin; (*D*) tissue factor can lead to thrombin generation, and thrombin generation leads to fibrin clot formation. *(Adapted from reference 11.)*

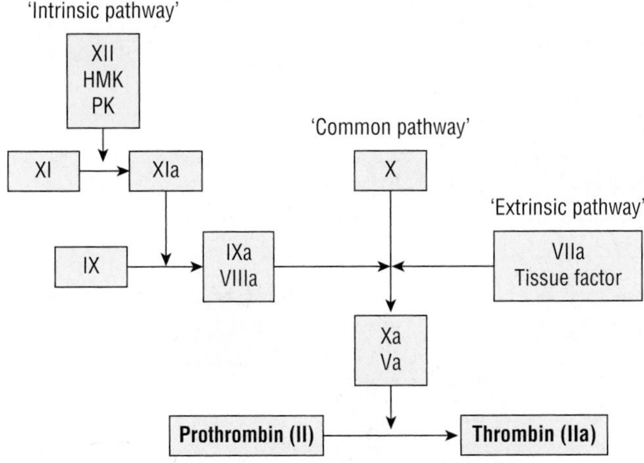

FIGURE 19-4 Classic depiction of the coagulation cascade.

Postthrombotic syndrome, a long-term complication of DVT caused by damage to the venous valves, may also result in chronic lower extremity swelling, pain, tenderness, skin discoloration, and, in the most severe cases, ulceration. PE typically presents with chest pain, shortness of breath, tachypnea, and tachycardia, which in some cases may result in cardiopulmonary collapse.[5,17]

Given that VTE can be debilitating or fatal, it is important to treat quickly and aggressively. Conversely, because major bleeding induced by anticoagulant drugs can be equally harmful, it is important to avoid treatment when the diagnosis is not a reasonable certainty. Assessment of the patient's status should focus on the search for risk factors in the patient's medical history (see Table 19-1). Even in the presence of mild, seemingly inconsequential symptoms, VTE should be strongly suspected in those with multiple risk factors.[17]

Radiographic contrast studies (venography and pulmonary angiography) are the most accurate VTE diagnostic methods, but are expensive invasive procedures technically difficult to perform and evaluate. Severely ill patients are often unable to tolerate these procedures, and many develop hypotension and cardiac arrhythmias. The contrast medium is also nephrotoxic and irritating to vessel walls and may paradoxically precipitate VTE.[18] For these reasons, less invasive tests, such as compression ultrasound (CUS) (either full leg or proximal segments only) and computed tomography pulmonary angiography (CTPA) are most used in clinical practice for the initial evaluation of patients with suspected VTE. In patients with allergy to contrast media, renal impairment, or high radiation exposure risk, the ventilation–perfusion (V/Q) scan is an alternative PE diagnostic test.[19]

D-dimer is a fibrin clot degradation product and levels are significantly elevated in patients with acute thrombosis. Although D-dimer is a very sensitive marker of clot formation, it is not sufficiently specific. A variety of conditions are associated with D-dimer elevations, including recent surgery or trauma, pregnancy, increasing age, and cancer; therefore, a positive D-dimer test is not conclusive evidence of VTE diagnosis. However, a *negative* D-dimer (for most assays defined as less than 500 ng/mL [mcg/L]) can be useful in ruling out the diagnosis of VTE.[19] As advanced age is known to elevate D-dimer levels, utilizing age-adjusted D-dimer cutoffs for ruling out VTE in patients over age 50 is being evaluated. The most promising strategy involves multiplying patient age by 10 to obtain an age-adjusted D-dimer threshold (eg, an 80-year-old patient's D-dimer threshold would be 800 ng/mL [mcg/L]). Appropriate use of D-dimer should include initial risk stratification using a validated clinical assessment tool.[19]

Clinical assessment significantly improves the diagnostic accuracy of noninvasive tests such as CUS, CTPA, and D-dimer. Simple clinical assessment checklists such as the Wells score can be used to determine if a patient is "likely" or "unlikely" to have DVT or PE (**Figs. 19-6 and 19-7**).[18] Patients with likely probability of VTE have more than 60% chance of VTE, compared with less than 10% chance for patient's with unlikely probability.[19] In general, patients with unlikely probability of VTE should first receive D-dimer testing. If the D-dimer result is below the defined cutoff point, VTE is ruled out; if above the cutoff point, the patient should receive appropriate diagnostic imaging (either CUS for suspected DVT or CTPA for suspected PE). All patients with likely probability of DVT should receive either proximal (popliteal, femoral, and iliac veins) or full leg CUS. A normal full leg ultrasound rules out DVT, whereas a normal proximal ultrasound requires additional testing with D-dimer, full leg ultrasound, or repeat proximal ultrasound surveillance in 1 week. Patients with CUS indicating proximal DVT should receive anticoagulant treatment. Evidence of distal vein DVT (anterior and posterior tibial, peroneal, gastrocnemius veins) after full leg ultrasound may be treated with anticoagulants or have further ultrasound surveillance to assess for propagation into the proximal deep veins of the leg (see Fig. 19-6). Patients with a likely probability of PE should receive imaging with either CTPA or V/Q scan. A negative imaging result rules out PE, whereas a positive imaging result indicates need for anticoagulant treatment (see Fig. 19-7).[5,17-19]

PREVENTION AND TREATMENT

Unfortunately, there is little public awareness of the life-threatening nature of DVT and PE. A global survey conducted by the International Society of Thrombosis and Hemostasis suggests that half of

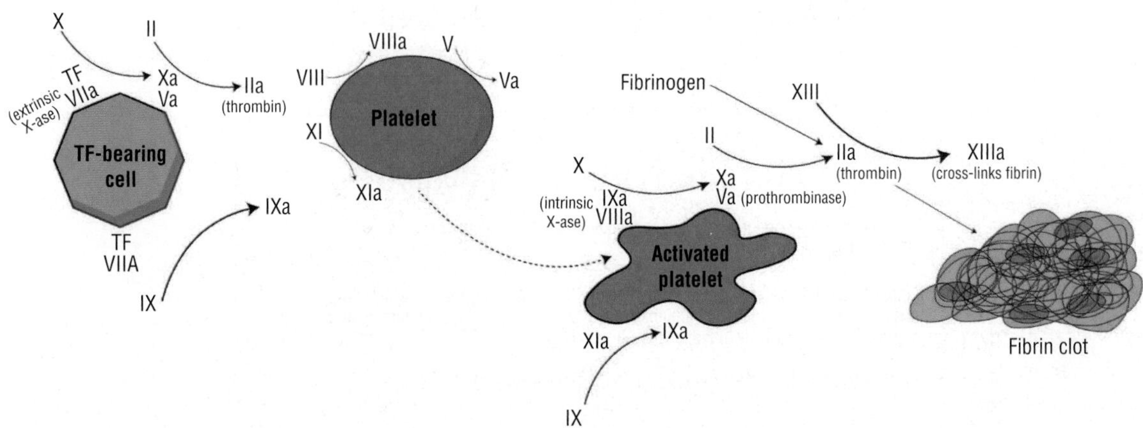

FIGURE 19-5 Cellular coagulation cascade model. *(Adapted from reference 11.)*

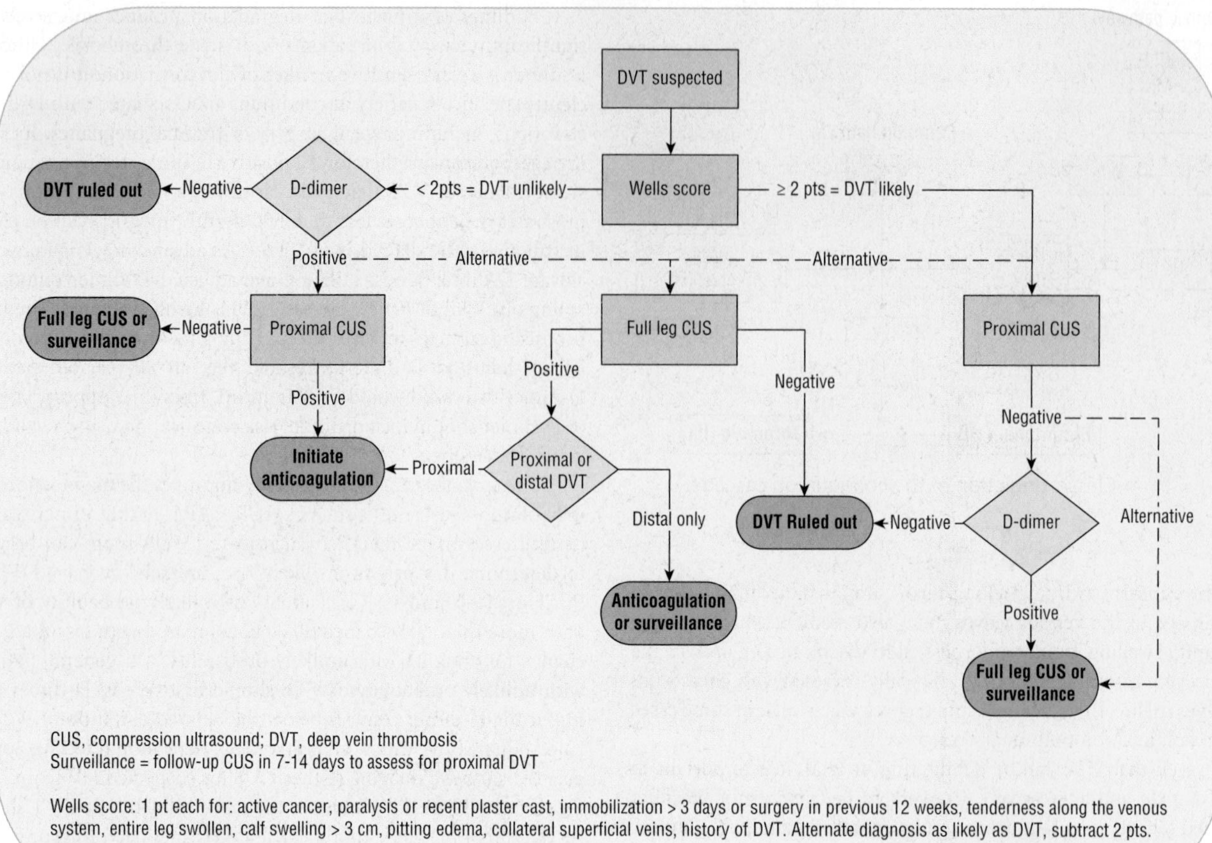

FIGURE 19-6 Deep vein thrombosis diagnostic algorithm.

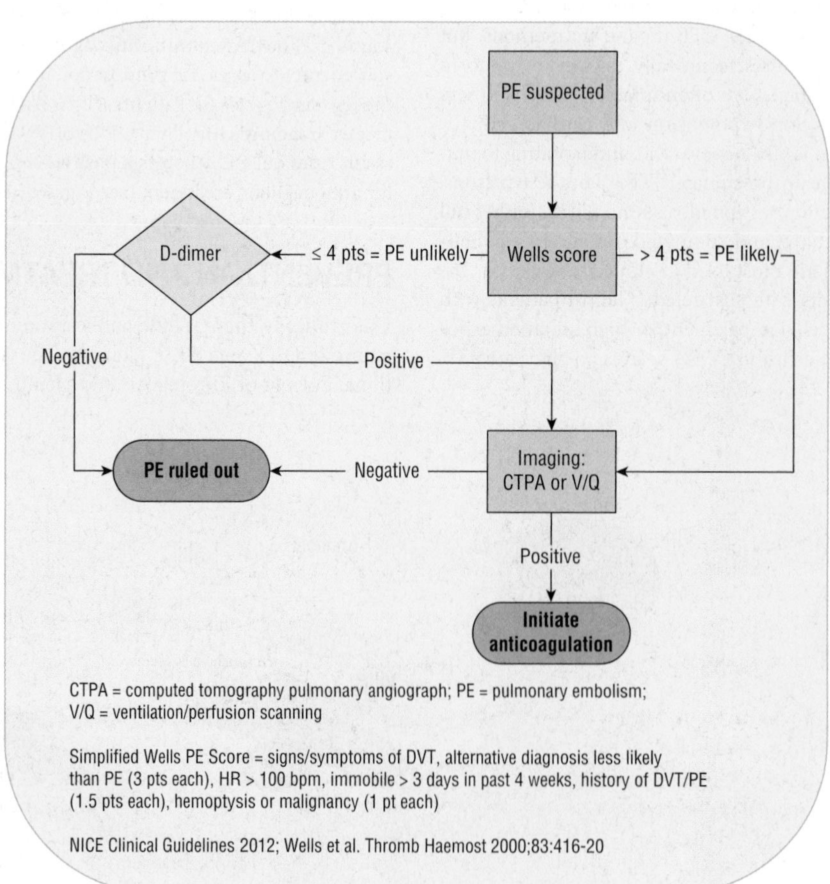

FIGURE 19-7 Pulmonary embolism diagnostic algorithm.

patients surveyed have little or no awareness of VTE, and less than half of respondents could identify VTE risk factors.[20] VTE awareness was substantially lower than for other disease states like stroke, heart attack, and breast cancer, each of which have major public awareness campaigns. This underscores the need to increase knowledge of the risks, signs, and symptoms of VTE through increased media visibility.

Desired Outcomes

Prevention strategies in at-risk populations positively impact patient outcomes because VTE is potentially fatal and costly to treat.[21] Treatment of VTE is aimed at preventing thrombus extension and embolization, reducing recurrence risk, and preventing long-term complications such as the postthrombotic syndrome and CTPH. Carefully managed use of anticoagulant drugs is important to reduce the risk of bleeding associated with these agents.

General Approach to the Prevention of Venous Thromboembolism

Effective prophylaxis can reduce the risk of fatal PE in high-risk surgical and medical populations, whereas early ambulation is often sufficient for those at low risk of VTE.[22] Educational programs and clinical decision support systems have been shown to improve the appropriate use of VTE prevention methods.[23]

3 Despite ongoing efforts to minimize hospital-acquired VTE, up to one-third of hospitalized patients at high VTE risk without contraindications to anticoagulant therapy still do not receive appropriate prophylaxis.[24] The American College of Chest Physicians' *Antithrombotic Therapy and Prevention of Thrombosis, 9th ed: Evidence-Based Clinical Practice Guidelines* (AT9) as well as the United Kingdom's National Institute for Health and Care Excellence (NICE) Guidelines provide evidence-based recommendations for VTE prevention and treatment.[17] A summary of AT9 VTE prophylaxis recommendations can be found in Table 19-2. Pharmacologic and mechanical methods are effective for preventing VTE and can be used alone or in combination.[2-4]

Nonpharmacologic Therapy

Compression stockings and intermittent pneumatic compression (IPC) devices prevent VTE by increasing the velocity of venous blood flow through graded pressure application. IPC devices utilize a series of cuffs wrapped around the patient's legs that inflate in continuous 1- to 2-minute cycles from the ankles to the thighs. IPC should be worn at least 18 hours/day for optimal effectiveness.

Graduated compression stockings do not reliably reduce VTE in medically ill patients.[2] However, they reduce the incidence of VTE (including asymptomatic and distal DVT) by approximately 65% when used after orthopedic surgery, cardiac surgery, gynecologic surgery, or neurosurgery.[3] IPC reduces the risk of VTE by more than 60% following general surgery, neurosurgery, and orthopedic surgery.[3] Both modalities can be used in combination with anticoagulation to maximize VTE prevention.[25]

Mechanical methods do not increase bleeding risk, which makes them attractive for postoperative VTE prophylaxis, especially in patients with contraindications to pharmacologic therapies. However, they are not risk-free, as discomfort, skin breakdown, and ulceration can occur.[2]

Inferior vena cava (IVC) filters can provide short-term protection against PE in very-high-risk patients by blocking embolization of thrombus formed below the filter.[27] Percutaneous insertion of an IVC filter is a minimally invasive procedure performed using fluoroscopic imaging to verify placement. Despite widespread IVC filter use, mortality benefit is unproven, and only limited nonrandomized data support effectiveness and long-term safety for VTE prevention. Frequently "retrievable" IVC filters are never retrieved; increasing risk for long-term complications such as DVT, filter migration, IVC occlusion, and insertion site thrombosis. As such, IVC filters should be reserved for patients at highest VTE risk in whom other prophylactic strategies cannot be used. IVC filters should be removed when VTE risk has passed or when anticoagulation is no longer contraindicated.[27]

Pharmacologic Therapy

Pharmacologic options for preventing VTE have been extensively evaluated in randomized clinical trials and significantly reduce the risk of VTE following hip and knee replacement, hip fracture repair, general surgery, myocardial infarction, ischemic stroke, and in selected hospitalized medical patients.[2-4] The optimal agent and dose for VTE prevention must be based on assessment of VTE and bleeding risk, as well as cost and availability.

Medical Patients

Several risk assessment models have been developed to identify hospitalized and critically ill patients at high VTE risk likely to benefit from thromboprophylaxis. The Padua Prediction Score is a prospectively validated VTE risk assessment tool for hospitalized medical patients.[2] Three points each are assigned for active cancer, previous VTE, reduced mobility, and thrombophilia; 2 points are assigned for trauma and/or surgery within the last month; and 1 point each is assigned for age older than or equal to 70 years, heart and/or respiratory failure, acute myocardial infarction or ischemic stroke, acute infection and/or rheumatologic disorder, body mass index more than or equal to 30 kg/m^2, or ongoing hormonal treatment. Among high-risk patients (score more than or equal to 4 points) not receiving prophylaxis, VTE occurred in 11.0% within 90 days compared with just 0.3% of low-risk patients.[2]

Recommendations for preventing VTE during medical illness are summarized in Table 19-2. Compared with placebo, low-dose unfractionated heparin (LDUH), low-molecular-weight heparin (LMWH), and fondaparinux all reduce symptomatic VTE and fatal PE among high-risk medical patients.[2] No direct oral anticoagulant (DOAC) is approved for use in this setting. Hospitalized and acutely ill medical patients at high VTE risk and low bleeding risk should receive pharmacologic prophylaxis with LDUH, LMWH, or fondaparinux during hospitalization or until fully ambulatory. Routine pharmacologic prophylaxis is not warranted in low-VTE-risk medical patients. Mechanical prophylaxis is preferred over anticoagulation therapy in medical patients at high bleeding risk (eg, active gastric or duodenal ulcer, history of bleeding within 90 days, or platelet count less than 50 × 10^9/L).[2] Mechanical prophylaxis should also be considered if more than one of the following are present: Age 85 years or more, hepatic failure, renal failure (creatinine clearance [CrCL] less than 30 mL/min [less than 0.5 mL/s]), admission to intensive care or cardiac care units, central venous catheter, rheumatic disease, active cancer, or male sex.[2] Patients with severe hepatic insufficiency are not adequately protected from VTE even if baseline INR is elevated. This population is particularly challenging as they are at risk for VTE without prophylaxis and bleeding with pharmacologic prophylaxis.[29,30]

Surgical Patients

General recommendations for reducing perioperative VTE risk includes stopping estrogen-containing medications 4 weeks prior to surgery and consideration for regional, rather than general anesthesia.[17] The Caprini score can be used to estimate VTE risk after general surgery by awarding 1, 2, 3, or 5 points to patient-specific risk factors (eg, age, body mass index, VTE history) and procedure-related risk factors including minor or major surgery, laparoscopic or open procedures, and elective arthroplasty. Summing risk factor

TABLE 19-2 Guidelines for the Prevention of Venous Thromboembolism

Medical illness

- For acutely ill hospitalized medical patients at increased risk of thrombosis, thromboprophylaxis with low-molecular-weight heparin (LMWH), low-dose unfractionated heparin (LDUH) twice or three times daily, or fondaparinux is recommended (Grade 1B)[a]
- For acutely ill hospitalized medical patients at low risk of thrombosis, use of pharmacologic prophylaxis or mechanical prophylaxis is not recommended (Grade 1B)
- For acutely ill hospitalized medical patients who are bleeding or at high risk for bleeding, anticoagulant thromboprophylaxis is not recommended (Grade 1B)
- For acutely ill hospitalized medical patients at increased risk of thrombosis who are bleeding or at high risk for major bleeding, optimal use of mechanical thromboprophylaxis with graduated compression stockings or intermittent pneumatic compression (IPC) is suggested (Grade 2C). When bleeding risk decreases, and if venous thromboembolism (VTE) risk persists, substitution of pharmacologic thromboprophylaxis for mechanical thromboprophylaxis is suggested (Grade 2B)
- For critically ill patients, thromboprophylaxis with LMWH or LDUH is suggested over no prophylaxis (Grade 2C)
- For critically ill patients who are bleeding, or are at high risk for major bleeding, mechanical thromboprophylaxis with graduated compression stockings or IPC is suggested (Grade 2C). When bleeding risk decreases, substitution of pharmacologic thromboprophylaxis for mechanical thromboprophylaxis is suggested (Grade 2C)
- In outpatients with cancer who have no additional risk factors for VTE, routine prophylaxis is not recommended with LMWH or LDUH (Grade 2B) or warfarin (Grade 1B)
- Routine thromboprophylaxis is not recommended for chronically immobilized persons residing at home or at a nursing home (Grade 2C)
- For long-distance travelers at increased risk of VTE (including previous VTE, recent surgery or trauma, active malignancy, pregnancy, estrogen use, advanced age, limited mobility, severe obesity, or known thrombophilia disorder), frequent ambulation, calf muscle exercise, sitting in an aisle seat or below-the-knee graduated compression stockings providing 15-30 mm Hg (2-4 kPa) pressure at the ankle are suggested (Grade 2C)
- In persons with thrombophilia but no previous history of VTE, the long-term daily use of mechanical or pharmacologic thromboprophylaxis to prevent VTE is not recommended (Grade 1C)

Surgical populations excluding orthopedics

- For general and abdominal–pelvic surgery patients at very low risk for VTE, no specific pharmacologic (Grade 1B) or mechanical (Grade 2C) prophylaxis other than early ambulation is recommended
- For patients at low risk of VTE after abdominal–pelvic surgery or cardiac surgery with an uncomplicated course, mechanical prophylaxis, preferably with IPC, over no prophylaxis is suggested (Grade 2C)
- For patients at moderate VTE risk after general, abdominal–pelvic, or thoracic surgery, or cardiac surgery with a prolonged course not at high risk for major bleeding complications, LMWH or LDUH (Grade 2B), or mechanical prophylaxis, preferably with IPC (Grade 2C), is suggested over no prophylaxis
- For patients at moderate risk for VTE after general, abdominal–pelvic surgery, thoracic surgery, or cardiac surgery who are at high risk for major bleeding complications or those in whom the consequences of bleeding are thought to be particularly severe, mechanical prophylaxis, preferably with IPC, is suggested over no prophylaxis (Grade 2C)
- For patients at high risk for VTE after general, abdominal–pelvic, and thoracic surgery who are not at high risk for major bleeding complications, pharmacologic prophylaxis with LMWH (Grade 1B) or LDUH (Grade 1B) is suggested over no prophylaxis. Combination with graduated compression stockings or IPC is also suggested (Grade 2C)
- For high-VTE-risk general, abdominal–pelvic, and thoracic surgery patients who are at high risk for major bleeding complications or those in whom the consequences of bleeding are thought to be particularly severe, the use of mechanical prophylaxis, preferably with IPC, is suggested over no prophylaxis until the risk of bleeding diminishes and pharmacologic prophylaxis may be initiated (Grade 2C)
- For high-VTE-risk patients undergoing abdominal or pelvic surgery for cancer who are not otherwise at high risk for major bleeding complications, extended-duration pharmacologic prophylaxis (4 weeks) with LMWH is recommended over shorter-duration prophylaxis (Grade 1B)
- For general and abdominal–pelvic surgery patients at high risk for VTE in whom both LMWH and LDUH are contraindicated or unavailable and who are not at high risk for major bleeding complications, low-dose aspirin (Grade 2C), fondaparinux (Grade 2C), or mechanical prophylaxis, preferably with IPC (Grade 2C), is suggested over no prophylaxis
- For general and abdominal–pelvic surgery patients, an inferior vena cava (IVC) filter is not recommended for primary VTE prevention (Grade 2C)

Orthopedic surgery

- In patients undergoing total hip arthroplasty (THA) or total knee arthroplasty (TKA), use of one of the following for a minimum of 10-14 days is recommended: LMWH, fondaparinux, apixaban, dabigatran, rivaroxaban, LDUH, adjusted-dose warfarin, aspirin (all Grade 1B), or IPC (Grade 1C)
- In patients undergoing hip fracture surgery (HFS), use of one of the following is recommended: antithrombotic prophylaxis for a minimum of 10-14 days, LMWH, fondaparinux, LDUH, adjusted-dose warfarin, aspirin (all Grade 1B), or IPC (Grade 1C)
- For patients undergoing major orthopedic surgery (THA, TKA, HFS) and receiving LMWH as thromboprophylaxis, starting either 12 hours or more preoperatively or 12 hours or more postoperatively is recommended over starting within 4 hours or less preoperatively or 4 hours or less postoperatively (Grade 1B)
- In patients undergoing THA, TKA, or HFS, irrespective of the concomitant use of IPC or length of treatment, the use of LMWH is suggested over other recommended alternatives, including fondaparinux, apixaban, dabigatran, rivaroxaban, LDUH (all Grade 2B), adjusted-dose warfarin, or aspirin (all Grade 2C)
- For patients undergoing major orthopedic surgery, extending thromboprophylaxis in the outpatient period for up to 35 days from the day of surgery is suggested (Grade 2B)
- In patients undergoing major orthopedic surgery, dual prophylaxis with an antithrombotic agent and IPC is suggested during the hospital stay (Grade 2C)
- In patients undergoing major orthopedic surgery who decline injections or IPC, apixaban or dabigatran (alternatively rivaroxaban or adjusted-dose warfarin) is recommended over alternative forms of prophylaxis (all Grade 1B)
- For primary prevention of VTE after major orthopedic surgery, no thromboprophylaxis is suggested over placement of an IVC filter in patients with an increased bleeding risk or contraindications to both pharmacologic and mechanical thromboprophylaxis (Grade 2C)
- The use of screening compression ultrasound in asymptomatic patients following major orthopedic surgery is not recommended (Grade 1B)
- No prophylaxis is suggested rather than pharmacologic thromboprophylaxis in patients with isolated lower leg injuries requiring leg immobilization (Grade 2C)
- For patients undergoing knee arthroscopy without a history of prior VTE, no thromboprophylaxis is suggested (Grade 2B)

[a]Recommendations are graded as strong (Grade 1) or weak (Grade 2) based on high-quality (Grade A), moderate-quality (Grade B), or weak-quality (Grade C) evidence.

Data from references 2, 3 and 4.

points yields VTE risk categorized as very low (0 to 1 point), low (2 points), moderate (3 to 4 points), or high (more than or equal to 5 points).[3] Estimating surgical bleeding risk is challenging due to the wide variety of surgery types, the effect of surgical technique, and the lack of a validated bleeding predication rule. Table 19-2 summarizes the AT9 recommendation for preventing VTE following nonorthopedic surgery. In general, patients at high VTE risk but low bleeding risk should receive LDUH or LMWH prophylaxis in addition to graduated compression stockings or IPC. Patients at high bleeding risk should receive IPC if VTE risk is moderate or high. Low risk patients able to ambulate early after surgery do not routinely require VTE prophylaxis.[3]

Total joint arthroplasty is associated with very high postoperative VTE risk. Recommended pharmacologic agents for VTE

CLINICAL PRESENTATION Deep Vein Thrombosis

General

- Deep vein thrombosis (DVT) most commonly develops in patients with identifiable risk factors (see Table 19-1) during or following a period of acute illness or hospitalization. Many have asymptomatic disease.

Symptoms

- The patient may complain of leg swelling, pain, or warmth. Symptoms are nonspecific and objective testing must be performed to establish the diagnosis.

Signs

- The patient's superficial veins may be dilated and a "palpable cord" may be felt in the affected leg.
- The patient may experience pain in back of the knee when the examiner dorsiflexes the foot of the affected leg (Homan's sign).

Laboratory tests

- Serum concentration of D-dimer, a by-product of fibrin degradation, is nearly always elevated. D-dimer values less than 500 ng/mL (mcg/L) combined with clinical decision rules are useful in ruling out the diagnosis of DVT.

Diagnostic tests

- Compression ultrasound is the most commonly used test to diagnose DVT. It is a noninvasive test that can visualize clot formation in veins of the legs. It cannot reliably detect small blood clots in calf veins. Coupled with a careful clinical assessment, it can rule in or out the diagnosis in the majority of cases.
- Venography is the gold standard for the diagnosis of DVT. However, it is an invasive test that involves injection of radiopaque contrast dye into a foot vein. It is expensive and can cause anaphylaxis and nephrotoxicity.

prevention following joint replacement surgery include aspirin, adjusted-dose warfarin, UFH, LMWH, fondaparinux, dabigatran, apixaban, and rivaroxaban for 10 days postsurgery, minimum.[4] Head-to-head trials fail to reliably demonstrate differences in clinically relevant outcomes such as symptomatic VTE, fatal PE, major hemorrhage, and surgical site complications between agents.[4]

AT9 suggests using LMWHs preferentially over other agents after total joint arthroplasty based on favorable pharmacologic

CLINICAL PRESENTATION Pulmonary Embolism

General

- Pulmonary embolism (PE) most commonly develops in patients with risk factors for venous thromboembolism (see Table 19-1) during or following a hospitalization. Although many patients develop a symptomatic deep vein thrombosis prior to developing a PE, some do not. Patients may die suddenly from cardiogenic shock and circulatory collapse before effective treatment can be initiated.

Symptoms

- The patient may complain of cough, chest pain, chest tightness, shortness of breath, or palpitation. The patient may spit or cough up blood (hemoptysis). When PE is massive, the patient may complain of dizziness or light-headedness. Symptoms may be confused with myocardial infarction, requiring objective testing to establish the diagnosis.

Signs

- The patient may have tachypnea, tachycardia, and appear diaphoretic. The patient's neck veins may be distended. In massive PE, the patient may appear cyanotic and become hypotensive. In such cases, oxygen saturation by pulse oximetry or arterial blood gas will likely indicate that the patient is hypoxic. In the worse cases, the patient may go into cardiogenic shock and die within minutes.

Laboratory tests

- Serum concentration of D-dimer, a by-product of fibrin degradation, is nearly always elevated. D-dimer values less than 500 ng/mL (mcg/L) combined with clinical decision rules are useful in ruling out the diagnosis of PE.

Diagnostic tests

- Computerized tomography pulmonary angiography (CTPA) is the most commonly used test to diagnose PE, but some centers still use the ventilation–perfusion (V/Q) scan. A V/Q scan measures the distribution of blood and airflow in the lungs. When there is a large mismatch between blood and airflow in one area of the lung, there is a high probability that the patient has a PE.
- Pulmonary angiography is the gold standard for the diagnosis of PE. However, it is an invasive test that involves injection of radiopaque contrast dye into the pulmonary artery. The test is expensive and associated with a significant risk of mortality.

properties and extensive clinical use.[4] LMWH bleeding risk following orthopedic surgery relates closely to thromboprophylaxis initiation timing. LMWH administration within 2 hours preoperatively or postoperatively increases bleeding risk up to fivefold compared with starting 12 hours after surgery.[4]

Warfarin remains a commonly prescribed agent for VTE prevention after total joint arthroplasty due to low acquisition cost and oral administration.[31] Warfarin's delayed onset of anticoagulant effect confers both a potential advantage (reduced immediate risk of postoperative bleeding) and disadvantage (increased risk of early VTE). Many orthopedic surgeons prefer low-intensity warfarin (eg, international normalized ratio [INR] 1.5 to 2.5) due to perceived lower postoperative bleeding risk.[31] AT9 now simply recommends "dose-adjusted warfarin" without specific guidance on target INR, and American Academy of Orthopaedic Surgery guidelines also no longer recommend a specific INR target.[4,32] Warfarin use following orthopedic surgery requires a well-coordinated monitoring system and timely INR testing.[33] Arranging INR testing following joint replacement surgery can be challenging due to limited patient mobility and often requires home phlebotomy services or point-of-care INR monitoring devices; this increases complexity and erodes warfarin's cost advantage.

Direct oral anticoagulants offer convenient oral administration and fixed dosing without need for routine coagulation testing. Clinical trials have demonstrated safety and efficacy similar to enoxaparin after total joint replacement, but studies after hip fracture surgery are lacking.[4] AT9 expresses a preference for apixaban, dabigatran, or warfarin in patients unwilling to use LMWH injections.[4]

Duration of Therapy

Optimal VTE prophylaxis duration following surgery is not well established. Prophylaxis should be given throughout the period of increased VTE risk. For general surgical procedures once patients are able to ambulate regularly and other risk factors are no longer present, prophylaxis can be discontinued.[2,3] Because of relatively high VTE incidence in the month following hospital discharge among patients undergoing lower extremity orthopedic procedures, extended prophylaxis appears to be beneficial.[4] Most clinical trials support the use of antithrombotic prophylaxis for 21 to 35 days following total hip replacement and hip fracture repair surgeries.[4]

General Approach to the Treatment of Venous Thromboembolism

4 Anticoagulation therapies remain the mainstay of VTE treatment. DVT and PE are manifestations of the same disease process and are treated similarly (Figs. 19-8 **and** 19-9, Table 19-3). Before prescribing anticoagulation therapy for VTE treatment, establishing an accurate diagnosis is imperative in preventing unnecessary bleeding risk and expense to the patient.[5] Patients with likely VTE probability may need rapid-onset anticoagulation therapy while awaiting diagnostic testing results, whereas patients with unlikely probability but positive D-dimer may need rapid-onset anticoagulation only if diagnostic testing will be delayed more than 4 hours.[17]

Strict bedrest was traditionally recommended following acute DVT based on the assumption that leg movement would dislodge

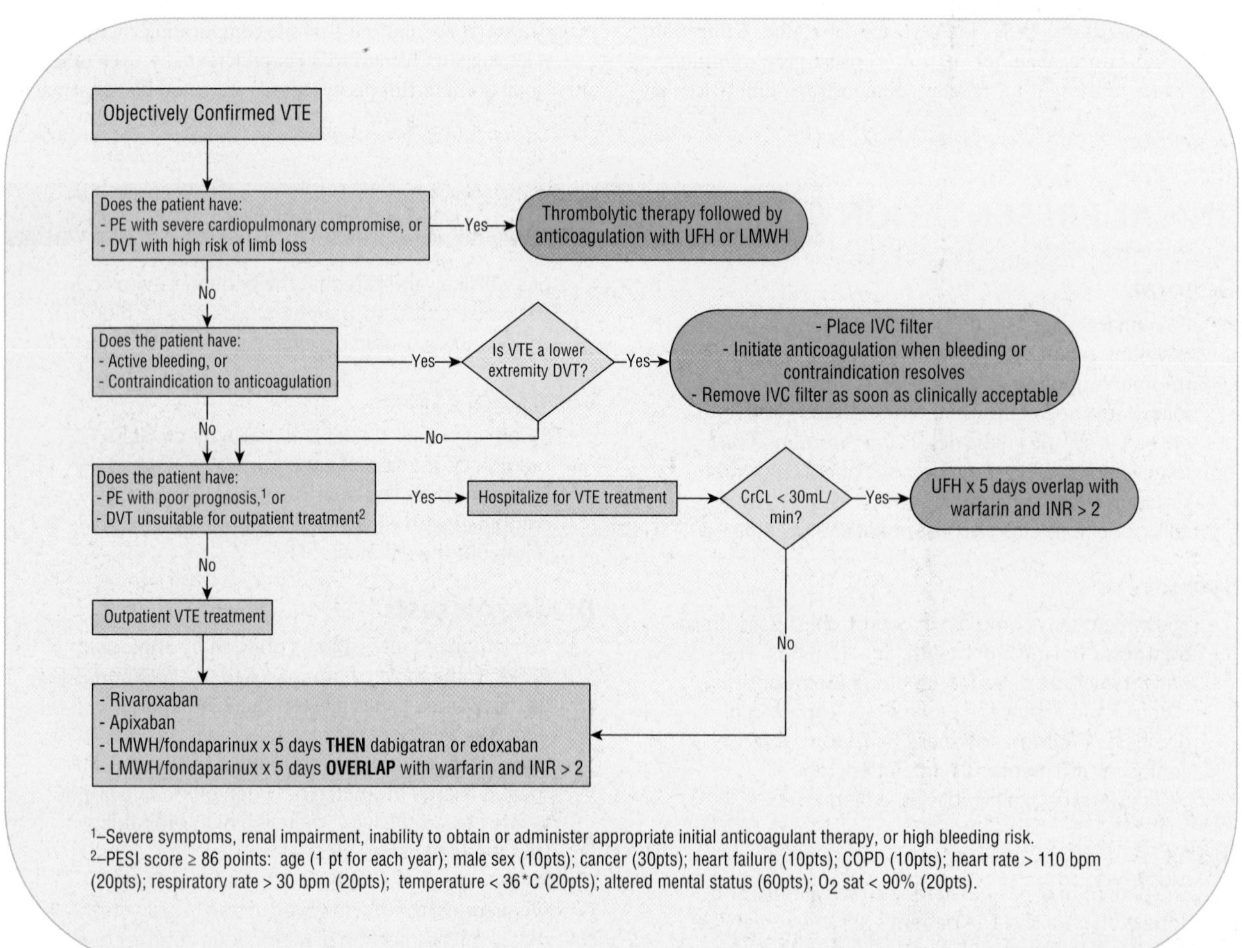

FIGURE 19-8 Treatment of venous thromboembolism (VTE). CrCl, creatinine clearance; DVT, deep vein thrombosis; IV, intravenous; LMWH, low-molecular-weight heparin; PE, pulmonary embolism; PESI, pulmonary embolism severity index; SC, subcutaneous; UFH, unfractionated heparin. (*Data from references 34 and 35.*)

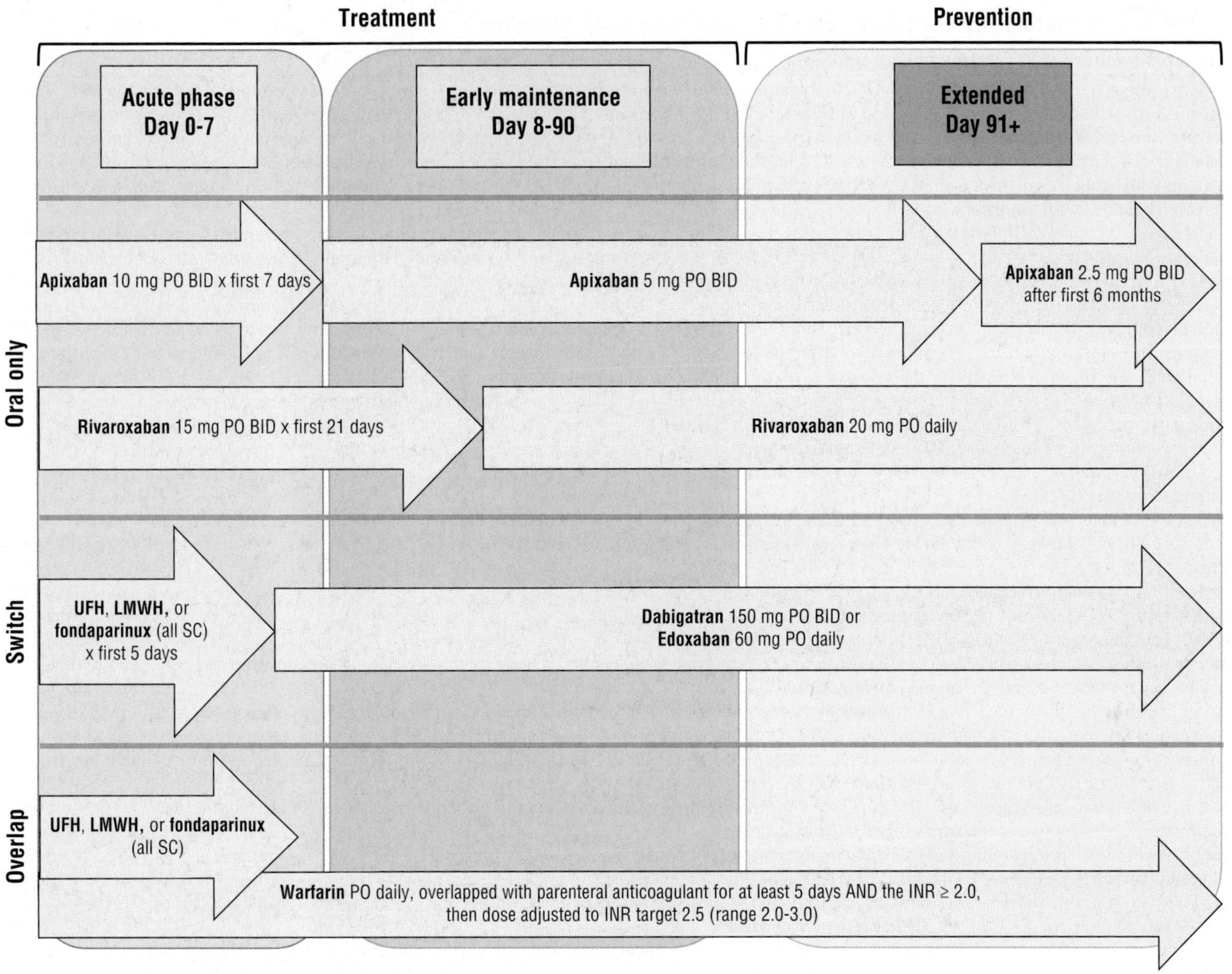

FIGURE 19-9 Overview of VTE treatment strategies.

the clot, resulting in PE. However, ambulation in conjunction with graduated compression stockings results in faster reduction in pain and swelling with no apparent increase in embolization rate. Patients should be encouraged to ambulate as much as symptoms permit. If ambulation increases pain and swelling, the patient should be instructed to lie down and elevate the affected leg until symptoms subside.

Inferior vena cava filters also have a limited role in the management of acute VTE, and should only be used when anticoagulants are contraindicated due to active bleeding.[28] As soon as the bleeding risk resolves, patients should receive a conventional course of anticoagulant therapy and have the filter removed within 90 to 120 days of implantation.[5,17,27] In life- or limb-threatening circumstances, elimination of the obstructing thrombus may be warranted and the use of thrombolysis or thrombectomy considered.[5,34] Removable IVC filter insertion is an option in patients with contraindications to anticoagulation therapy or when anticoagulant therapy has failed.[5,34]

Once the diagnosis of VTE has been objectively confirmed (see Clinical Presentation and Diagnosis discussed earlier), anticoagulant therapy with a rapid-acting anticoagulant should be instituted as soon as possible (see Fig. 19-8). 6 Available anticoagulants can be administered in the outpatient setting in most patients with DVT and in carefully selected hemodynamically stable patients with PE. The decision to initiate outpatient therapy should be based on institutional resources and patient-specific variables (Table 19-4).[34,35]

7 The appropriate initial duration of anticoagulation therapy to effectively treat an acute first episode of VTE for all patients is 3 months, as this reduces recurrent VTE risk to as low as can be achieved by a time-limited therapy duration.[28] To prevent new VTE episodes not directly related to the preceding episode, continuing anticoagulation therapy is required.[1] Individually tailoring anticoagulation therapy duration therapy past 3 months requires careful consideration of the circumstances surrounding the initial thromboembolic event, the presence of ongoing thromboembolic risk factors, bleeding risk, and patient preference.[28]

The most important considerations in determining recurrent VTE risk are whether the initial thrombotic event was associated with a major transient or reversible risk factor (eg, surgery, plaster cast leg immobilization, or hospitalization in the month prior to VTE) and the presence of active cancer.[28] The estimated cumulative risk of recurrent VTE after stopping anticoagulant therapy for VTE provoked by surgery is 1% after 1 year and 3% after 5 years, and that for VTE provoked by a nonsurgical reversible risk factor is 5% after 1 year and 15% after 5 years. Three months of anticoagulation therapy is recommended in these situations.[5] Patients with a first unprovoked (idiopathic) VTE have approximately 10% recurrence risk in the first year and approximately 30% and 50% over 5 and 10 years, respectively. These patients should be considered for extended anticoagulation therapy when feasible.[28] Extended therapy refers to continuing anticoagulation beyond 3 months without a scheduled stop date, but stopping therapy if there is a subsequent increase in bleeding risk or change in patient preference for anticoagulation.[28] For patients with a second idiopathic VTE episode, extended anticoagulation is recommended.[28] Anticoagulation is rarely stopped in patients with VTE and active cancer because of high recurrence risk.[28] Factors that may lead to the decision to stop warfarin therapy after 3 months include noncompliance with therapy, initial clot isolated in calf veins (even if idiopathic), or moderate to high bleeding risk.[28]

TABLE 19-3 Guidelines for the Treatment of Venous Thromboembolism

Deep vein thrombosis (DVT) and pulmonary embolism (PE)

In patients with acute DVT of the leg or PE, a DOAC (dabigatran, rivaroxaban, apixaban, or edoxaban) is suggested over warfarin therapy (Grade 2B)[a]

In patients with acute DVT of the leg or PE treated with warfarin therapy, initial treatment with LMWH, fondaparinux, IV UFH, or SC UFH is recommended (Grade 1B)

In patients with acute DVT of the leg or PE, early initiation of warfarin (eg, same day as parenteral therapy is started) over delayed initiation, and continuation of parenteral anticoagulation for a minimum of 5 days and until the international normalized ratio (INR) is 2 or above for at least 24 hours are recommended (Grade 1B)

In patients with acute DVT of the leg or PE, LMWH or fondaparinux is suggested over IV UFH (Grade 2C [2B for fondaparinux in PE]) and over SC UFH (Grade 2B for LMWH; Grade 2C for fondaparinux)

In patients with proximal DVT of the leg or PE provoked by surgery, treatment with anticoagulation for 3 months is recommended over treatment of a shorter period (Grade 1B), treatment of a longer time-limited period (eg, 6 or 12 months) (Grade 1B), or extended therapy (Grade 1B regardless of bleeding risk)

In patients with proximal DVT of the leg or PE provoked by a nonsurgical transient risk factor, treatment with anticoagulation for 3 months is recommended over treatment of a shorter period (Grade 1B), treatment of a longer time-limited period (eg, 6 or 12 months) (Grade 1B), and extended therapy if there is a high bleeding risk (Grade 1B); anticoagulation for 3 months is suggested over extended therapy if there is a low or moderate bleeding risk (Grade 2B)

In patients with a first unprovoked DVT of the leg or PE, treatment with anticoagulation for at least 3 months is recommended over treatment of a shorter duration (Grade 1B); after 3 months of treatment, the risk-to-benefit ratio of extended therapy should be evaluated; for patients with low or moderate bleeding risk, extended anticoagulant therapy is suggested over 3 months of therapy (Grade 2B); for patients with high bleeding risk, 3 months of anticoagulant therapy is recommended over extended therapy (Grade 1B)

In patients with recurrent unprovoked VTE, extended anticoagulant therapy is recommended over 3 months of therapy in those with low bleeding risk (Grade 1B), and suggested in those with moderate bleeding risk (Grade 2B); in patients with high bleeding risk, 3 months of therapy is suggested over extended therapy (Grade 2B)

In all patients who receive extended anticoagulant therapy, the continuing use of treatment should be reassessed at periodic intervals (eg, annually)

In patients with DVT of the leg or PE who are treated with warfarin, a therapeutic INR range of 2-3 (target INR of 2.5) is recommended for all treatment durations (Grade 1B)

In patients with DVT of the leg or PE and no cancer and not treated with a DOAC, warfarin therapy is suggested over LMWH for long-term therapy (Grade 2C)

In patients with DVT of the leg or PE and cancer, LMWH is suggested over warfarin therapy or a DOAC (Grade 2C for all); in patients with DVT or PE and cancer who are not treated with LMWH, either warfarin or a DOAC may be used

In patients with DVT of the leg or PE who receive extended therapy, there is no need to change the choice of anticoagulant after the first 3 months unless patient circumstances dictate a change in therapy (Grade 2C)

In patients with acute DVT of the leg or PE, the use of an inferior vena cava (IVC) filter in addition to anticoagulants is not recommended (Grade 1B) unless anticoagulation therapy is contraindicated (Grade 1B); a conventional course of anticoagulant therapy is suggested if the risk of bleeding resolves (Grade 2B)

In patients who are incidentally found to have asymptomatic DVT of the leg or PE, the same initial and long-term anticoagulation as for comparable patients with symptomatic DVT of PE is suggested (Grade 2B)

In patients with unprovoked proximal DVT of the leg or PE who are stopping anticoagulant therapy and do not have a contraindication to aspirin, aspirin is suggested over no aspirin to prevent recurrent VTE (Grade 2C)

In patients with subsegmental PE (no involvement of more proximal pulmonary arteries) and no proximal DVT in the legs who have a low risk for recurrent VTE, clinical surveillance is suggested over anticoagulation (Grade 2C); if high risk for recurrent VTE anticoagulation is suggested over clinical surveillance (Grade 2C)

In patients with recurrent VTE while on warfarin therapy (in the therapeutic range) or on DOAC (and believed to be compliant), switching to treatment with LMWH at least temporarily is suggested (Grade 2C)

In patients who have recurrent VTE while on long-term LMWH (and are believed to be compliant), increasing the LMWH dose by about one-quarter to one-third is suggested (Grade 2C)

DVT specific

In patients with acute DVT of the leg and whose home circumstances are adequate, initial treatment at home is recommended over treatment in hospital (Grade 1B)

In patients with acute DVT of the leg, early ambulation is suggested over initial bedrest (Grade 2C)

In patients with acute proximal DVT of the leg, anticoagulant therapy alone is suggested over catheter-directed thrombolysis (Grade 2C)

In patients with acute symptomatic DVT of the leg, suggest against the routine use of graduated compression stockings for the purpose of preventing postthrombotic syndrome (Grade 2B)

PE specific

In patients with low-risk PE and whose home circumstances are adequate, treatment at home or early discharge is suggested over standard discharge (eg, after first 5 days of treatment) (Grade 2B)

In patients with acute PE associated with hypotension (eg, systolic BP <90 mm Hg) who do not have a high bleeding risk, systemically administered thrombolytic therapy is suggested (Grade 2B)

In most patients with acute PE not associated with hypotension, systemically administered thrombolytic therapy is not recommended (Grade 1B)

In selected patients with acute PE who deteriorate after starting anticoagulant therapy but have yet to develop hypotension and who have a low bleeding risk, systemically administered thrombolytic t herapy is suggested over no therapy (Grade 2C)

In patients with acute PE who are treated with a thrombolytic agent, systemically administered thrombolytic therapy is suggested over catheter directed thrombolysis (Grade 2C) In patients with acute PE, when a thrombolytic agent is used, short infusion times (eg, a 2-hour infusion) are suggested over prolonged infusion times (eg, a 24-hour infusion) (Grade 2C); thrombolytic administration through a peripheral vein is suggested over a pulmonary artery catheter (Grade 2C)

In patients with acute PE associated with hypotension and who have high bleeding risk, failed systemic thrombolysis, or shock that is likely to cause death before systemic thrombolysis can take effect (eg, within hours), catheter-assisted thrombus removal is suggested over no such intervention if appropriate expertise and resources are available (Grade 2C); In patients with chronic thromboembolic pulmonary hypertension (CTPH), extended anticoagulation is recommended over stopping therapy (Grade 1B); in selected patients with CTPH who are identified by an experienced thromboendarterectomy team, pulmonary thromboendarterectomy is suggested (Grade 2C)

Upper extremity DVT

In patients with acute upper extremity DVT (UEDVT) involving the axillary or more proximal veins, acute treatment with parenteral anticoagulation (LMWH, fondaparinux, IV UFH, or SC UFH) is recommended over no such acute treatment (Grade 1B); LMWH or fondaparinux is suggested over IV UFH (Grade 2C) and over SC UFH (Grade 2B); anticoagulant therapy alone is suggested over thrombolysis (Grade 2C)

In patients with UEDVT who undergo thrombolysis, the same intensity and duration of anticoagulant therapy as in similar patients who do not undergo thrombolysis is recommended (Grade 1B)

In most patients with UEDVT associated with a central venous catheter, not removing the catheter is suggested if it is functional and there is an ongoing need for the catheter (Grade 2C)

In patients with UEDVT involving the axillary or more proximal veins, a minimum duration of anticoagulation of 3 months is suggested over a shorter period (Grade 2B); in patients who have UEDVT that is not associated with a central venous catheter or with cancer, 3 months of anticoagulation is recommended over a longer duration of therapy (Grade 1B); in patients who have UEDVT that is associated with a central venous catheter that is not removed, anticoagulation that continues as long as the central venous catheter remains is recommended over stopping after 3 months of treatment in patients with cancer (Grade 1C), and is suggested in patients with no cancer (Grade 2C)

[a]Recommendations are graded as strong (Grade 1) or weak (Grade 2) based on high-quality (Grade A), moderate-quality (Grade B), or weak-quality (Grade C) evidence.

Data from references 5 and 28.

TABLE 19-4 Outpatient Treatment Suggestions for Deep Venous Thrombosis and Pulmonary Embolism

Inclusion	Patients with objectively diagnosed VTE
Relative exclusion	Patients who are hemodynamically unstable
Exclusion	Arterial thromboembolism or patients who are currently receiving dialysis, actively bleeding, have had recent (within 2 weeks) major surgery/trauma, or have other severe uncompensated comorbid conditions

Suggested procedure: may vary depending on the patient's clinical condition
Confirm diagnosis of VTE by objective testing
Day 1
Baseline laboratory evaluation
  International normalized ratio (INR)—if use of warfarin anticipated
  Serum creatinine (Scr)
  Complete blood count (CBC) with platelets
Medication—see Fig. 19-7
Patient education
  Clinical pharmacy/nursing
- Educate patient regarding the importance of proper monitoring of anticoagulation therapy (if applicable) and warning signs that should prompt additional medical evaluation; document activities in the medical record
- If applicable, teach patient how to self-administer LMWH/fondaparinux (if patient or family member unwilling or unable to self-administer injection, visiting nurse services should be arranged or consider single oral anticoagulant approach); initial injection should be administered in the medical office or hospital
- Instruct patient regarding local therapy: elevation of affected extremity, localized heat, antiembolic exercises (flexion–extension of ankle for lower extremity VTE, or hand squeezing–relaxation for upper extremity VTE)

  Pharmacy operations
- Reinforce patient education regarding indication, use, monitoring, side effects, and drug interactions with antithrombotic therapy
- Screen patient's pharmacy profile for potential drug–drug interactions with anticoagulation therapy
- Dispense anticoagulant therapy
- Anticoagulation service enrollment

Days 3-4
Laboratory evaluation if on warfarin: check INR
Assess for symptoms of pulmonary embolism
Medications: continue anticoagulant medication(s) as directed
Anticoagulation service
  If on warfarin interpret results of INR and adjust dose of warfarin to achieve a target INR of 2.5
  Patient activity: continue reduced activity as long as pain persists (when possible, elevate extremity); increase activity as tolerated
  Document activities in medical record
Day 5
Laboratory evaluation if on warfarin: check INR
Assess for symptoms of pulmonary embolism
Medications: continue anticoagulant medication(s) as directed
Anticoagulation service
  If on warfarin interpret results of INR and adjust dose of warfarin to achieve a target INR of 2.5 (stop LMWH if INR ≥2.0)
  Patient activity: no restriction; if pain increases, contact primary care provider
  Document activities in medical record
Day 6 (Dabigatran or Edoxaban)
Medications: transition from parenteral to oral medication
Assess for symptoms of pulmonary embolism
Anticoagulation service
  Verify adherence, affordability, and tolerability of oral medication
  Patient activity: no restriction; if pain increases, contact primary care provider
  Review key education points (eg, keep in original container [dabigatran])
  Document activities in medical record
Day 7 (Apixaban)
Medications: Decrease apixaban dose
Anticoagulation service
  Patient activity: no restrictions; if pain increases contact primary care provider
  Verify adherence, affordability, and tolerability of oral medication
  Document activities in medical record
Day 21 (Rivaroxaban)
Medications: Decrease riaroxaban dose
Anticoagulation service
  Verify adherence, affordability, and tolerability of oral medication
  Patient activity: no restriction; if pain increases, contact primary care provider
  Review key education points (eg, take with food [rivaroxaban])
  Document activities in medical record

Clinically important bleeding risk factors include age more than 75 years, previous noncardioembolic stroke, history of gastrointestinal bleeding, renal or hepatic impairment, anemia, thrombocytopenia, concurrent antiplatelet use (avoid if possible), noncompliance, poor anticoagulant control (for patients on warfarin), serious acute or chronic illness, and the presence of structural lesions (eg, tumor, recent surgery) that could bleed. One to two bleeding risk factors suggest moderate bleeding risk while three or more suggest high bleeding risk.[5]

Various secondary strategies aimed at identifying patients with very low recurrence risk after a first idiopathic VTE have evaluated whether safe withdrawal of anticoagulation therapy may be possible if reliable identification of these patients proves possible. Some factors that may predict lower recurrence risk include female gender, low D-dimer levels 1 month after stopping anticoagulation therapy, absence of residual clot on ultrasound, absence of hereditary and acquired thrombophilia, and absence of the postthrombotic syndrome. Risk assessment derived from combining several independent recurrence risk factors has also been investigated.[5] Further validation is needed before any one factor or prediction rule using a combination of factors can justify stopping anticoagulation. The decision to continue extended warfarin therapy should be reassessed periodically. Patients should be involved in any decision to continue anticoagulation therapy with consideration given to long-term prognosis, risk of bleeding, ability to adhere to anticoagulation therapy instructions, financial resources, lifestyle, and quality of life.[5] When anticoagulation therapy is stopped, there is a similar risk of recurrence whether patients have been treated for 3 months or longer.[28]

Patients with VTE are often tested for hereditary and acquired hypercoagulable states (thrombophilia). The available evidence does not support a strong association between genetically transmitted thrombophilia (especially factor V Leiden and prothrombin G20210A) and higher recurrent VTE rates.[15] Routine testing for thrombophilia is not recommended.[17]

For patients with proximal DVT, wearing graduated compression stockings does not reduce the risk of developing the postthrombotic syndrome.[26] However, for patients with persistent leg pain and swelling, graduated compression stockings can be suggested for symptomatic relief.

PREVENTION OF VTE

- Conduct an accurate assessment of VTE and bleeding risks to weigh the competing hazards of symptomatic VTE and bleeding and appropriately target prevention strategies.
- An effective VTE prophylaxis program should not only quantify patients' risks, but also assist providers in selecting prophylaxis regimens that optimally balance these risks in a cost-effective manner.

TREATMENT OF VTE

- Establish an accurate diagnosis of VTE.
- Prevent thrombus extension and embolization with rapidly acting anticoagulants (acute phase of VTE treatment [~7 days]).
- Reduce the risk of long-term sequelae such as the postthrombotic syndrome and CTPH by allowing formed clot to be slowly dissolved by endogenous thrombolytic processes (early maintenance phase [7 days to 3 months]).
- Prevent recurrent VTE (long-term anticoagulation therapy extending beyond 3 months).

Pharmacologic Therapy

The anticoagulant drugs used to treat VTE are the same as those used for VTE prevention; however, there are important differences in the approach to VTE treatment in terms of the doses used and duration of therapy.

Direct Oral Anticoagulants

9 Clinical trials have demonstrated that single-drug therapy with rivaroxaban or apixaban is noninferior to warfarin overlapped with enoxaparin at initiation (traditional therapy) for both acute DVT and PE with similar rates of recurrent VTE.[36-38] Major bleeding was lower with rivaroxaban in the PE trial,[37] but not in the DVT trial.[38] Apixaban caused significantly less major bleeding than traditional therapy.[36] Both drugs are initiated with a higher dose with eventual transition to maintenance dosing (see Fig. 19-9). Neither drug requires routine coagulation monitoring. Patients with CrCL less than 25-30 mL/min (less than 0.42-0.5 mL/s), active cancer, and those requiring thrombolytic therapy were excluded from clinical trials.[36-38] Until further data are available, traditional anticoagulation therapy should be utilized in these patient populations. Replacing the effective but cumbersome combination of injectable anticoagulants and warfarin with a single-drug regimen simplifies VTE treatment; however, the higher acquisition cost of rivaroxaban and apixaban and lack of an effective reversal agent is concerning to some patients and clinicians.

Clinical **Controversy...**

Even though the treatment of acute VTE using apixaban and rivaroxaban is less complex than traditional therapy with warfarin overlapped with LMWH, most patients do not receive therapy with these agents. Clinical inertia may be the primary reason why clinicians continue to use traditional therapy in light of the relative simplicity of apixaban or rivaroxaban therapy compared to daily injections of LMWH coupled with the need for frequent INR monitoring. Therapy with apixaban or rivaroxaban should be the default anticoagulant for acute VTE treatment with other therapies reserved for those situations where DOAC therapy is less desirable (eg, renal dysfunction, cancer-associated VTE, VTE associated with antiphospholipid antibody syndrome).

Oral dabigatran 150 mg twice daily and oral edoxaban 60 mg once daily have each been compared with traditional therapy in randomized, double-blind, noninferiority trials involving patients with acute VTE.[39,40] In these trials, all patients were initially given at least 5 days of parenteral anticoagulation therapy (unfractionated heparin [UFH] or LMWH) and then randomized to study treatment. Both dabigatran and edoxaban were noninferior to warfarin following the parenteral anticoagulant lead-in for the outcome of recurrent VTE. Dabigatran caused similar major bleeding[39] and edoxaban significantly less bleeding than warfarin.[40] Similar to the other DOACs, patients with hemodynamically unstable PE or at high bleeding risk were excluded and should not receive treatment with dabigatran or edoxaban until further data are available. Patients with CrCL less than 30 mL/min (less than 0.5 mL/s) should not receive dabigatran, but for patients with a CrCL 15-50 mL/min (0.25-0.83 mL/s), edoxaban with dose reduced from 60 mg once daily to 30 mg once daily can be prescribed.[40] The requirement for parenteral anticoagulation prior to initiation of dabigatran or edoxaban therapy is a disadvantage compared with single-drug approaches to VTE treatment (see Fig. 19-9). DOACs are preferred over conventional anticoagulation for management of VTE in the American College of Chest Physician 10th edition guidelines.[28]

Low-Molecular-Weight Heparin

Low-molecular-weight heparin has largely replaced UFH for initial VTE treatment due to improved pharmacokinetic and pharmacodynamic profiles and ease of use. LMWH given subcutaneously in fixed, weight-based doses (Table 19-5) is at least as effective as UFH given intravenously for the treatment of VTE.[6] Given the predictable response and reduced need for laboratory monitoring with LMWH, stable patients with DVT or PE who have normal vital signs, low bleeding risk, and no other uncontrolled comorbid conditions requiring hospitalization can be discharged early or treated entirely on an outpatient basis (see Table 19-4).[28] Not all patients are appropriate candidates for outpatient VTE treatment. At a minimum, patients must be reliable or have adequate caregiver support and be willing and active participants in outpatient VTE management. Important patient education aspects for outpatient VTE treatment are summarized in Table 19-6. Hemodynamically unstable patients with PE should generally be admitted for anticoagulation therapy initiation. Rapidly reversible UFH is preferred if thrombolytic therapy or embolectomy is anticipated.[41] In patients without cancer,

TABLE 19-5 FDA-Approved Venous Thromboembolism Indications and Doses for Low-Molecular-Weight Heparins

Indications	Enoxaparin	Dalteparin
Hip replacement surgery (prophylaxis)	30 mg SC q 12 h initiated 12-24 hours after surgery *Or* 40 mg SC q 24 h initiated 12 hours prior to surgery Extended prophylaxis may be given for up to 3 weeks	Postoperative start: 2,500 units SC given 4-8 hours after surgery, and then 5,000 units SC q 24 h *Or* Preoperative start (evening before surgery): 5,000 units SC 10-14 hours before surgery, then 5,000 units given 4-8 hours after surgery, and then 5,000 units SC q 24 h *Or* Preoperative start (day of surgery): 2,500 units SC within 2 hours of surgery, then 2,500 units given 4-8 hours after surgery, and then 5,000 units SC q 24 h
Knee replacement surgery (prophylaxis)	30 mg SC q 12 h initiated 12-24 hours after surgery	
Abdominal surgery (prophylaxis)	40 mg SC q 24 h initiated 2 hours prior to surgery	2,500 units SC q 24 h initiated 1-2 hours prior to surgery Patients with malignancy: 5,000 units SC the evening prior to surgery, and then 5,000 units SC q 24 h *Or* 2,500 units SC 1-2 hours prior to surgery, and then 2,500 units 12 hours after surgery followed by 5,000 units SC q 24 h
Acute medical illness (prophylaxis)	40 mg SC q 24 h	5,000 units SC q 24 h
Deep vein thrombosis treatment (with or without pulmonary embolism)	1 mg/kg SC q 12 h *Or* 1.5 mg/kg SC q 24 h	
Venous thromboembolism treatment in patients with cancer		200 units/kg SC q 24 h for 30 days, followed by 150 units SC q 24 h (total daily dose should not exceed 18,000 units)

acute treatment with LMWH is generally transitioned to long-term warfarin therapy after about 5 to 10 days.

Clinical **Controversy...**

Despite recommendations from AT9, the American Society of Clinical Oncology, and the National Comprehensive Cancer Network that patients with cancer should be given LMWH monotherapy for the long-term treatment of VTE, most patients with cancer-related VTE continue to receive warfarin-based therapy. Moreover, a survey of clinicians indicated that 82% of respondents indicated LMWH was their first choice for treating VTE in patients with cancer.[89,90] Possible explanations for this observation might be patient preference for oral therapy over daily injections, and/or the higher cost of LMWH. In addition, pooled analysis of clinical trials demonstrates no survival advantage of LMWH monotherapy compared with traditional therapy with warfarin.[5]

Fondaparinux

Fondaparinux has been shown to be a safe and effective alternative to LMWH for acute VTE treatment.[5] It is dosed once daily via weight-based SC injection as follows: 5 mg if less than 50 kg, 7.5 mg if 50 to 100 kg, and 10 mg if more than 100 kg.[42] Compared with weight-based LMWH dosing, this flexible dosing scheme may be particularly useful with obese patients. Careful attention should be paid to renal function as fondaparinux is contraindicated if CrCL is less than 30 mL/min (less than 0.5 mL/s).[42]

Unfractionated Heparin

Unfractionated heparin may be administered subcutaneously or by continuous intravenous infusion (Table 19-7). Because the anticoagulant response to UFH is highly variable, it is standard practice to adjust the dose based on coagulation test results. The activated partial thromboplastin time (aPTT) is generally used to monitor UFH anticoagulant effect. The therapeutic aPTT range at each institution should be adapted to the responsiveness of the reagent and instrument used.[6] Either weight-based (see Table 19-7) or fixed UFH dosing (eg, 5,000 unit bolus followed by 1,000 units/h continuous infusion) produces similar clinical outcomes.[33] However, failure to give a sufficient intravenous UFH dose has been shown to increase VTE recurrence risk during initial treatment and long-term therapy.[6] Intravenous UFH requires hospitalization with frequent aPTT monitoring and dose adjustment and some patients still fail to achieve an adequate response to UFH therapy.[6] Consequently, traditional intravenous UFH in the acute treatment of VTE has largely been replaced by LMWH or fondaparinux. However, as clearance of LMWH, fondaparinux, and DOACs is dependent in some degree on renal function, UFH will continue to have a role for acute VTE treatment in patients with CrCL less than 30 mL/min (less than 0.5 mL/s).[5,28,43]

If a sufficient dose of UFH is administered subcutaneously (initial dose 333 units/kg followed by 250 units/kg twice daily), aPTT-guided dose titration may be unnecessary.[6] UFH administered in this manner might be a less costly option for treatment of acute VTE in appropriately selected patients. For patients weighing more than 80 kg, injection volume may be problematic.

Warfarin

Warfarin monotherapy is unacceptable for acute VTE treatment because the slow onset of effect is associated with high incidence of recurrent thromboembolism. However, warfarin is effective in the long-term VTE management provided it is started concurrently with rapid-acting injectable anticoagulant therapy.[5] 5 Injectable anticoagulation should overlap with warfarin therapy for at least 5 days and until an INR more than or equal to 2 has been achieved for at least 24 hours.[5] The initial dose of warfarin should be 5 to 10 mg for most patients and periodically adjusted to achieve and maintain an INR between 2 and 3 (Fig. 19-10).

Alternative Treatment

Most VTE cases require only anticoagulation therapy. In rare cases removing the occluding thrombus by pharmacologic or

TABLE 19-6 Patient Education for Outpatient Venous Thromboembolism Therapy

General information regarding VTE and the goals of treatment

- Anticoagulant medications (injections and warfarin tablets, injections and dabigatran or edoxaban, or rivaroxaban or apixaban) have been prescribed to prevent your blood clot from growing larger so that the body can begin to dissolve the clot
- Your body may be able to completely dissolve the clot, but in some cases the clot never goes completely away; even with adequate anticoagulation therapy, some people will have chronic pain and swelling in the affected limb; people who have had one clot are at increased risk of having future clots
- Warfarin tablets take several days to begin to work, so at first LMWH or fondaparinux injections and warfarin tablets are used together
- When the warfarin has become effective, you will be able to stop the LMWH or fondaparinux injections; you will continue to take warfarin tablets for 3 months or longer to prevent blood clots from returning
- It is important for you to administer your LMWH or fondaparinux and warfarin exactly as directed
- It is important not to use LMWH at the same time as dabigatran or edoxaban—first use LMWH then switch to dabigatran or edoxaban

Subcutaneous injection technique (if needed)

- You must learn to give yourself an injection of LMWH or fondaparinux under the skin; alternatively, you may have a family member or visiting nurse give it to you
- If your LMWH or fondaparinux syringes were filled by the manufacturer, they can be stored at room temperature; if your syringes were filled by the pharmacy, they should be stored in the refrigerator; if you were instructed to fill your own syringes, you should prepare the syringe immediately prior to injecting its contents
- If you see a bubble in the syringe, do not try to get it out; you may accidentally squirt out part of your dose
- Choose an injection site on your abdomen; clean the area with alcohol, and then position an uncapped syringe at a 90° angle; pinch the skin, stick the needle in as far as it will go, and gently but firmly push the plunger down; this will inject the medicine into the skin; when all the medication has been injected, remove the needle and dispose of it in an appropriate container
- You will likely experience a burning sensation when the medication is injected; this will go away after a few minutes
- Rotate injection sites from side to side; do not inject into the same site more than once; avoid the area around your navel; do not inject into any bruises

Blood test monitoring

- If you are taking warfarin, regular blood tests are required to make sure your medication is working properly
- The prothrombin time tells how quickly your blood forms a clot; it is used to tell how well warfarin is working
- The INR is a way to standardize the prothrombin time between laboratories; your goal INR range is between 2 and 3; if your INR is < 2, you are at higher risk for clotting; if your INR is > 3, you are at higher risk for bleeding; your dose of warfarin will be adjusted based on the results of this test
- You need to have a complete blood count test before you begin therapy
- If you are taking LMWH, fondaparinux, dabigatran, edoxaban, rivaroxaban, or apixaban you need to have a blood test to determine how well your kidneys are working

Warfarin information

- Each strength of warfarin has a unique color; each time you refill your prescription, make sure your new tablets are the same color as the ones you have been taking; if not, ask your pharmacist why
- Warfarin should be taken at approximately the same time each day
- The most common and serious side effect of warfarin is bleeding; you should be careful to avoid situations or activities that increase your risk of injury; apply direct pressure to control bleeding from superficial cuts
- Warfarin has many drug interactions; always check with your provider before taking any new medications (including nonprescription medications and dietary supplements)
- Foods rich in vitamin K (green leafy vegetables, etc.) may interfere with warfarin; do not avoid foods rich in vitamin K, but try to maintain consistent dietary habits
- Alcohol can increase your risk for bleeding and interfere with warfarin therapy; drink alcohol in moderation (one to two drinks per day); avoid binge drinking

Dabigatran, edoxaban, rivaroxaban, apixaban information

- Take rivaroxaban 15- or 20-mg doses with food to make sure the medication is well absorbed from your stomach
- It is very important that you take each dose of your medication. These medications leave your body in a few hours; so missing a dose of medication may place you at a higher risk of blood clots
- If you need to have a surgery or procedure, talk to your provider to make a plan for how to take your medication before and after the procedure. Do not stop taking your medication without first talking to your provider
- There are a few drug interactions with dabigatran, edoxaban, rivaroxaban, and apixaban; always check with your provider before taking any new medications (including nonprescription medications and dietary supplements)

Contact your provider if you experience

- Persistent bleeding from a cut or scrape
- Blood in your urine
- Blood in your stool
- Persistent nose bleeding
- Increased swelling or pain in your affected extremity

Go to the emergency department if you experience

- Shortness of breath
- Chest pain
- Coughing up blood
- Black tarry-appearing stool
- Severe headache of sudden onset
- Slurred speech

INR, international normalized ratio; LMWH, low-molecular-weight heparin.

surgical means may be warranted. Consensus panel recommendations regarding thrombolysis or thrombectomy in VTE management are based on low-quality evidence, and more study is needed to clarify their precise role.[5,44]

Thrombolytic agents are proteolytic enzymes that enhance conversion of plasminogen to plasmin.[5] Thrombolytic therapy for DVT improves early venous patency, but this does not necessarily translate into improved long-term outcomes.[28] If thrombolytic therapy is pursued, systemic administration via peripheral vein is preferred to catheter-directed thrombolysis.[28] Patients with extensive proximal DVT presenting within 14 days of symptom onset, with good functional status, low bleeding risk, and a life expectancy of a year or more are thrombolysis candidates (Table 19-8). Catheter-directed DVT thrombolysis is preferred provided appropriate expertise and

TABLE 19-7 Weight-Based[a] Dosing for Unfractionated Heparin Administered by Continuous IV Infusion

Indication	Initial Loading Dose	Initial Infusion Rate
Deep venous thrombosis/ pulmonary embolism	80-100 units/kg Maximum = 10,000 units	17-20 units/kg/h Maximum = 2,300 units/h
Activated Partial Thromboplastin Time (seconds)	**Maintenance Infusion Rate** ***Dose Adjustment***	
<37 (or anti–factor Xa <0.20 unit/mL [kU/L])	80 units/kg bolus, and then increase infusion by 4 units/kg/h	
37-47 (or anti–factor Xa 0.20-0.29 unit/mL [kU/L])	40 units/kg bolus, and then increase infusion by 2 units/kg/h	
48-71 (or anti–factor Xa 0.30-0.70 unit/mL [kU/L])	No change	
72-93 (or anti–factor Xa 0.71-1 unit/mL [kU/L])	Decrease infusion by 1-2 units/kg/h	
>93 (or anti–factor Xa >1 unit/mL [kU/L])	Hold infusion for 1 hour, and then decrease by 3 units/kg/h	

[a]Use actual body weight for all calculations. Adjusted body weight may be used for obese patients (>130% of ideal body weight).

Data from reference 6.

resources are available. Catheter-based thrombus fragmentation, with or without thrombus fragment aspiration, can be combined with catheter-directed thrombolysis and is associated with shorter treatment times and reduced cost. The same anticoagulation therapy duration and intensity is recommended as for patients with DVT not receiving thrombolysis.[5] Patients with DVT involving the iliac and common femoral veins are at highest risk for postthrombotic syndrome and may have the greatest potential to benefit from thrombus removal strategies. In patients with impending venous gangrene despite optimal anticoagulant therapy, thrombus removal is indicated; for all other patients with acute DVT, AT9 suggests anticoagulation therapy alone over either catheter-directed or systemic thrombolysis.[5]

In acute PE management successful clot dissolution with thrombolytic therapy reduces elevated pulmonary artery pressure and normalizes right ventricular dysfunction. However, the risk of death from PE should outweigh the risk of serious bleeding associated with thrombolytic therapy. Patients being considered for thrombolytic therapy should be screened carefully for contraindications relating to bleeding risk (see Table 19-8).[5,45] Thrombolytic therapy is considered necessary in addition to aggressive interventions such as volume expansion, vasopressor therapy, intubation, and mechanical ventilation for patients with massive PE accompanied by shock and cardiovascular collapse (about 5% of patients with PE).[5,45] Thrombolytic therapy in these patients should be administered without delay to reduce risk of progression to multisystem organ failure and death. While lifesaving in the acute phase of massive PE with hypotension, the hemodynamic benefit of thrombolysis is comparable to that of UFH after a few days.[46]

The benefit of thrombolytic therapy in patients with PE without hemodynamic compromise is less clear and rapid risk stratification is required to determine whether patients may benefit from thrombolysis or embolectomy in addition to anticoagulation therapy.[41] Risk stratification helps inform the initial treatment intensity, low-risk patients being discharged early or managed as outpatients and high-risk patients receiving surveillance in the intensive care unit and/or advanced therapies such as thrombolysis.[47] Key components of risk stratification are clinical evaluation, determination of cardiac biomarker levels such as troponin, and assessment of right ventricular size and function.[5] The Pulmonary Embolism Severity Index (PESI) is a prognostic tool utilizing 11 routinely available clinical parameters: demographics (age and gender), comorbid illnesses (cancer, heart failure, and chronic lung disease), and clinical findings (pulse, systolic blood pressure, respiratory rate, temperature, mental status, and arterial oxygen saturation). PESI stratifies patients into five risk classes with classes I and II considered low risk.[47] AT9 suggests that patients with acute PE presenting without hypotension be risk stratified predominantly by signs that indicate clinical instability including decrease in systolic blood pressure but still more than 90 mm Hg, tachycardia, elevated jugular venous pressure, clinical evidence of poor tissue perfusion, hypoxemia, and failure to improve on anticoagulant therapy.[5] Patients with one or more of these clinical features are at high risk for PE-related morbidity and mortality and may benefit from thrombolytic therapy, provided bleeding risk is acceptable, even in the absence of hemodynamic compromise (see Table 19-8).[5] The optimal role of thrombolysis in the management of PE requires further study.

In rare circumstances surgical thrombectomy for extensive ileofemoral DVT may be necessary, but catheter-directed thrombolysis is preferred if bleeding risk is acceptable.[28] For acute PE treatment, catheter-based embolectomy might be suitable in settings where expertise and resources are available for patients who have contraindications to thrombolytic therapy, have failed thrombolytic therapy, or in whom death is likely before thrombolytic onset.[28] In the absence of contraindications, catheter-based PE embolectomy is usually combined with thrombolytic therapy unless bleeding risk is high.[5] Surgical embolectomy is reserved for massive PE and hemodynamic instability when thrombolysis is contraindicated, and for when thrombolysis has failed clinically or will not have sufficient time to take effect.[5] In chronic PE cases—where persistent emboli produce CTPH, hypoxemia, and right-sided heart failure—surgical pulmonary thromboendarterectomy offers greater benefit than anticoagulants and may be the treatment of choice if performed by an experienced surgical team. A permanent IVC filter is usually inserted before or during the procedure and long-term warfarin therapy targeted to an INR of 2 to 3 is needed.[5]

Special Populations

Some patient populations with VTE require special consideration due to increased risk for recurrence, adverse events, or altered anticoagulant pharmacokinetics.

Pregnancy

Anticoagulation therapy is commonly used for the prevention and treatment of VTE during pregnancy.[12] UFH and LMWH do not cross the placenta and are preferred during pregnancy (Table 19-9).[12] Warfarin crosses the placenta and can result in fetal bleeding, central nervous system abnormalities, and embryopathy and should not be used for VTE treatment during pregnancy.[12] Women of childbearing age taking warfarin must be counseled regarding fetal risks and need for effective contraception. DOACs should be avoided in pregnancy until more information regarding safety is available.[48-51] Fondaparinux has not been extensively studied in pregnancy and may cross the placenta.[42] However, fondaparinux may be a viable option in pregnant patients intolerant to LMWH or those with a history of heparin-induced thrombocytopenia (HIT).[52]

Pregnant women with a history of VTE should receive VTE prophylaxis for 6 to 12 weeks after delivery.[53] Antenatal prophylaxis may also be indicated depending on other risk factors, such as history of multiple VTE, VTE associated with pregnancy or estrogen therapy, or known thrombophilia. Anticoagulation for acute VTE during pregnancy should continue for at least 6 weeks postpartum and a minimum total duration of 3 months.[12] Warfarin, UFH, and LMWH are safe during breast-feeding.[6,54] It is not

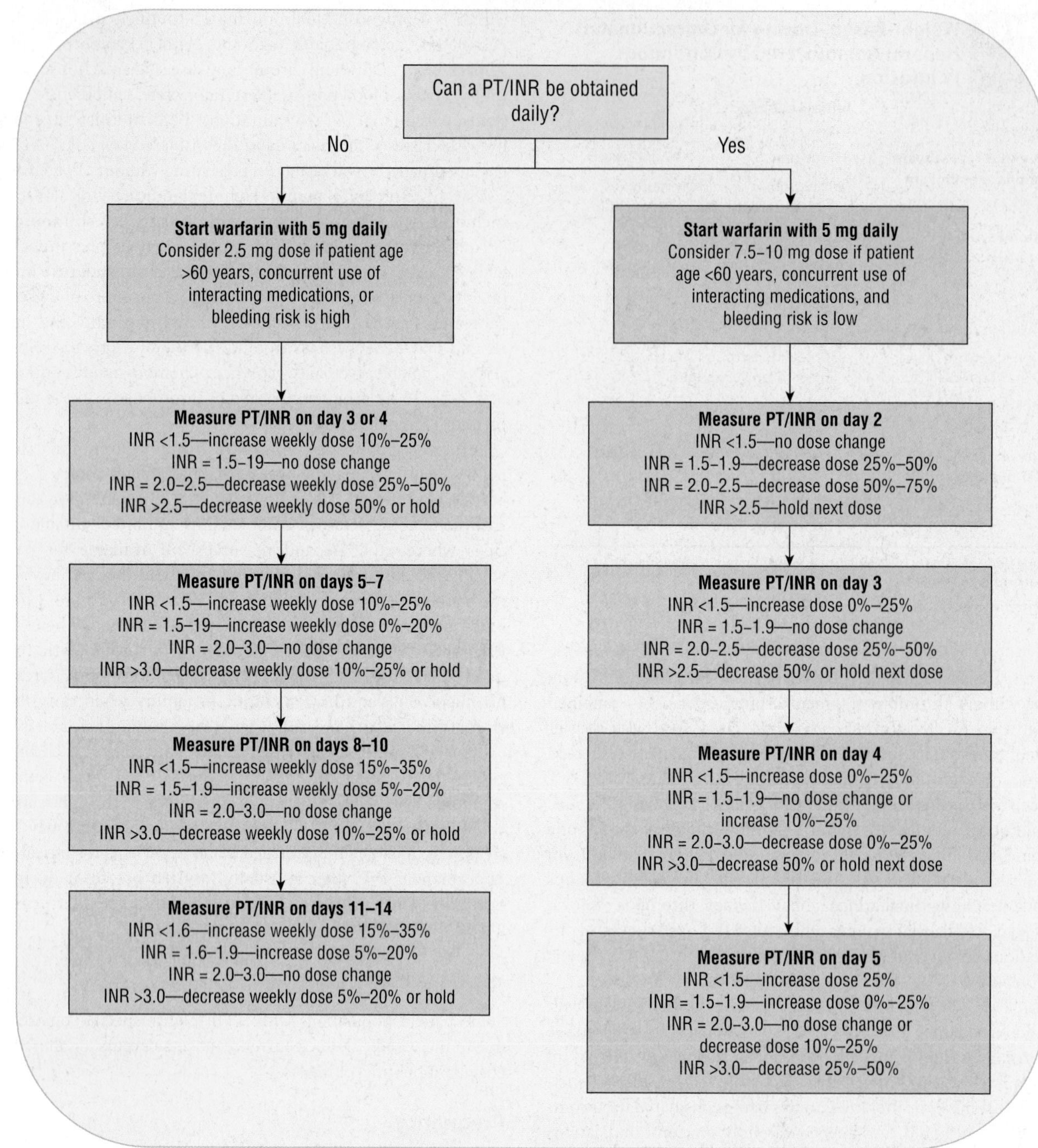

FIGURE 19-10 Initiation of warfarin therapy. INR, international normalized ratio; PT, prothrombin time.

known if DOACs are excreted in human milk and breast-feeding is not recommended.[48-51]

Pediatric Patients

Venous thromboembolism in pediatric patients is increasing secondary to prematurity, cancer, trauma, surgery, congenital heart disease, and systemic lupus erythematosus. Pediatric patients rarely experience unprovoked VTE, but often develop DVTs associated with indwelling central venous catheters.[55] Recommendations for anticoagulant therapy in pediatric patients are largely extrapolated from adults; however, there are important pharmacokinetic and pharmacodynamic differences that should be taken into consideration. The majority of literature supporting pediatric recommendations is derived from uncontrolled studies, case reports, or in vitro experiments. When possible, a pediatric hematologist with experience managing VTE should manage pediatric patients.[55]

Anticoagulation with UFH and warfarin remains the most frequently used approach for VTE treatment in pediatric patients and the recommended target aPTT and INR ranges as well as the duration of therapy are extrapolated from adults.[55] The recommended initial bolus dose of UFH is 75 to 100 units/kg given intravenously over 10 minutes followed by a maintenance infusion of 28 units/kg/h for infants 2 to 12 months of age and 20 units/kg/h for children aged 1 year or older.[55] Subsequent infusion rate adjustments should be made every 4 to 6 hours to maintain the aPTT within the institution-specific therapeutic range. The usual warfarin starting dose is 0.2 mg/kg with a maximum of 10 mg. Infants require higher warfarin doses per kilogram to maintain a target INR of 2 to 3 compared with teenagers and adults (mean dose 0.33 mg/kg, 0.09 mg/g, and 0.04 to 0.08 mg/kg, respectively).[55] The INR target range for VTE treatment in children is 2.0 to 3.0. Frequent INR monitoring and warfarin dose adjustments are typically required. When compared with adults,

TABLE 19-8 Thrombolysis for the Treatment of Venous Thromboembolism

- The majority of patients with VTE do not require thrombolytic therapy
- Thrombolytic therapy for DVT should be reserved for patients who present with extensive proximal DVT (eg, ileofemoral) within 14 days of symptom onset, have good functional status, and are at low risk of bleeding
- Thrombolytic therapy should be administered to patients with massive PE with evidence of hemodynamic compromise (hypotension or shock) unless contraindicated by bleeding risk
- Thrombolytic therapy should be considered for selected high-risk patients without hypotension provided the risk of bleeding is acceptable
- Factors associated with high risk for adverse PE outcomes include:
  - Ill-appearing patients with marked dyspnea, anxiety, and low oxygen saturation
  - Elevated troponin levels
  - Right ventricular dysfunction on echocardiography
  - Right ventricular enlargement on chest CT
- Factors that increase the risk of bleeding must be evaluated before thrombolytic therapy is initiated (ie, recent surgery, trauma or internal bleeding, uncontrolled hypertension, recent stroke or intracranial hemorrhage)
- Baseline labs should include CBC and blood typing in case transfusion is needed
- Alteplase 100 mg infused via peripheral vein over 2 hours is the most commonly used thrombolytic for patients with PE
- Before thrombolytic therapy for PE, IV UFH should be administered in full therapeutic doses
- During thrombolytic therapy it is acceptable to either continue or suspend IV UFH (suspending UFH is the most common practice in the United States)
- aPTT should be measured following the completion of thrombolytic therapy
  - If aPTT is <80 seconds, UFH infusion should be started and adjusted to maintain aPTT in therapeutic range
  - If aPTT is >80 seconds, measure every 2-4 hours and start UFH infusion when aPTT is <80 seconds
- Avoid phlebotomy, arterial puncture, and other invasive procedures during thrombolytic therapy to minimize the risk of bleeding

aPTT, activated partial thromboplastin time; CBC, complete blood cell count; DVT, deep vein thrombosis; PE, pulmonary embolism; UFH, unfractionated heparin.

Data from references 1 and 28.

only 10% to 20% of pediatric patients can be safely monitored with once monthly INRs.[55] Obtaining blood for coagulation monitoring tests in pediatric patients is problematic because many have poor venous access; many clinicians recommend using finger-stick blood samples with portable point-of-care INR monitors.[55] Despite need for daily injections, LMWH is an attractive alternative for pediatric patients due to low drug interaction potential and less frequent laboratory testing. Most experts recommend anti-Xa activity monitoring with goal anti–factor Xa levels between 0.5 and 1.0 unit/mL (kU/L) 4 to 6 hours following subcutaneous injection. Compared with adults, children younger than 3 months or weighing less than 5 kg have higher per-kilogram dose requirements to achieve a "therapeutic" anti-Xa response. The LMWH dose for older children is generally similar to weight-adjusted doses used in adults.[55] Warfarin can be initiated concurrently with UFH or LMWH therapy. Therapy should be overlapped for a minimum of 5 days and until the INR is therapeutic. Warfarin should be continued for at least 3 months for provoked VTE and 6 months for unprovoked VTE.[55] DOACs are attractive alternatives in pediatric patients due to oral administration and no need for routine coagulation monitoring; however, safety and effectiveness in this population have not been established.[48-51] Thrombolysis and thrombectomy have been successfully employed in pediatric patients, but published data are very limited—routine use is not recommended.[55]

Patients with Cancer

Cancer-related VTE is associated with threefold higher rates of recurrent VTE, 2.5 to 6-fold higher rates of bleeding, and more resistance to standard warfarin-based therapy compared to patients without cancer.[56] Warfarin therapy in cancer patients is often complicated by drug interactions (eg, chemotherapy and antibiotics) and the need to interrupt therapy for invasive procedures. Maintaining stable INR control is also more difficult in this patient population because of nausea, anorexia, and vomiting.[5]

Randomized trials provide evidence that long-term LMWH monotherapy for cancer-related VTE significantly decreases recurrent VTE rates without increasing bleeding risks compared with warfarin-based therapy; most consensus guideline panels therefore recommend LMWH monotherapy for VTE treatment in patients

TABLE 19-9 Unfractionated and Low-Molecular-Weight Heparin Use During Pregnancy

Acute treatment[a]	LMWH • Enoxaparin 1 mg/kg SC q 12 h or 1.5 mg/kg q 24 h *Or* • Dalteparin 100 units/kg SC q 12 h *Or* UFH • Initiate using weight-based IV therapy and adjust dose to achieve therapeutic anti-Xa level for at least 5 days • Transition to SC adjusted-dose UFH administered q 8-12 h with mid-interval anti-Xa activity in the therapeutic range[b]
Long-term treatment[c]	LMWH Maintain initial LMWH dose regimen throughout pregnancy *Or* Alter LMWH dose in proportion to any weight change (usually gain) *Or* Obtain monthly anti-Xa level measurements 4-6 hours after morning dose and adjust LMWH dose based on anti-Xa level (target = 0.5-1.2 units/mL [kU/L] if twice-daily dosing; 1-2 units/mL [kU/L] if once-daily dosing) *Or* UFH Obtain anti-Xa level at the midpoint of the dosing interval and adjust UFH dose to achieve an anti-Xa level of 0.3-0.7 unit/mL [kU/L]
Issues at time of delivery	Elective induction of labor • Discontinue UFH or LMWH 24 hours prior to induction • Initiate therapeutic doses of UFH by IV infusion and discontinue 4-6 hours prior to expected time of delivery if risk of recurrent VTE is deemed high Spontaneous labor • For LMWH, if there is a reasonable expectation that significant anticoagulant effect will be present at time of delivery: (a) epidural should be avoided and (b) reversal with protamine sulfate may be considered • For UFH, monitor the aPTT and reverse with protamine sulfate if aPTT is prolonged near the time of delivery Postpartum • Commence UFH or LMWH as soon as safely possible (usually 12 hours following delivery) • Concurrently initiate warfarin therapy and discontinue UFH or LMWH when the INR is 2 or greater • Continue anticoagulants for at least 6 weeks following delivery • Warfarin can be safely used by women who are breast-feeding

aPTT, activated partial thromboplastin time; INR, international normalized ratio; LMWH, low-molecular-weight heparin; SC, subcutaneously; UFH, unfractionated heparin; VTE, venous thromboembolism.

[a]Twice-daily LMWH preferred during pregnancy due to increased clearance.

[b]Anti-Xa monitoring preferred as the relationship between aPTT and heparin levels differs in pregnant compared with nonpregnant patients.

[c]As pregnancy progresses the volume of distribution of LMWH changes, glomerular filtration rate increases, and most women gain weight.

Data from reference 12.

with cancer.[5,16,57,58] Advantages of LMWH over warfarin for VTE treatment in cancer are expected to be greatest in those with one or more of the following: metastatic disease, treatment with aggressive chemotherapy, extensive VTE at presentation, liver dysfunction, poor or unstable nutritional status, or desire to avoid frequent blood draws for coagulation monitoring.[5]

For patients with cancer and VTE receiving LMWH, therapy should continue for at least the first 3 to 6 months of long-term treatment, at which time LMWH can be continued or warfarin therapy substituted. Anticoagulation therapy should continue for as long as the cancer is "active" and while the patient is receiving antitumor therapy.[5] A risk-to-benefit assessment should be performed on a regular basis considering overall clinical status, bleeding risk, quality of life, and life expectancy.[5] For patients with cancer who have VTE recurrence despite receiving anticoagulant therapy, LMWH appears to be more effective than warfarin-based therapy in preventing further recurrences and increasing the anticoagulant intensity may not be necessary in this situation.[56] A meta-analysis evaluated the outcomes of the subset of patients with cancer within the phase three VTE treatment trials comparing DOACs and conventional therapy with LMWH followed by warfarin.[59] There were similar recurrent VTE and major bleeding rates in the two groups suggesting DOACs are not inferior to conventional warfarin therapy for cancer-associated VTE management.[59] However, until DOACs are compared to LMWH monotherapy they cannot be recommended as first-line agents for cancer-related VTE.

Patients with Renal Insufficiency

Patients with acute or chronic kidney disease often require anticoagulation for VTE prevention or treatment. With the exception of warfarin, most anticoagulants have at least some dependency on renal elimination. Accumulation of drug is possible during treatment with LMWH, fondaparinux, and DOACs.[6,54] In addition, patients with chronic kidney disease are at increased risk of bleeding, independent of drug clearance.[60]

Low-molecular-weight heparins are renally eliminated and should be used with caution in patients with severe renal impairment.[61] Enoxaparin has specific labeling for patients with CrCL less than 30 mL/min (less than 0.5 mL/s), but supporting evidence is limited to pharmacokinetic modeling analyses.[62] Bleeding and recurrent VTE outcomes for patients with CrCL less than 30 mL/min (less than 0.5 mL/s) receiving enoxaparin 1 mg/kg once daily for acute VTE treatment were observed to be comparable to patients with normal renal function in one retrospective study.[43] However, UFH remains preferred for acute VTE treatment in this setting until further evidence becomes available.[5]

Direct oral anticoagulants rely to varying degrees on renal elimination and require dose adjustment for renal impairment.[48-51] Use of these anticoagulants in patients with CrCL less than 30 mL/min (less than 25 mL/min for apixaban) (or less than 0.5 mL/s and less than 0.42 mL/s for apixaban) should be avoided.

Patients Undergoing Invasive Procedures

Patients scheduled to undergo invasive procedures often require temporary discontinuation of anticoagulation therapy.[63] The decision to withhold anticoagulation therapy should be based on the type of surgical procedure being performed and the patient's bleeding and thromboembolic risk. Anticoagulation therapy should generally not be discontinued in patients undergoing minimally invasive procedures such as dental work, cataract surgery, or minor dermatologic procedures.[64] If the bleeding risk from the procedure is considerable, near-normal hemostasis should be achieved prior to the procedure. For DOACs, the time required for restoration of normal hemostasis after interrupting therapy is dependent on renal function. Stopping DOACs 2 days prior to invasive procedures is usually sufficient to restore near normal hemostasis for patients with normal renal function. Additional days off therapy may be required for patients with impaired renal function.[48-51] The anticoagulant effect of dabigatran can be rapidly reversed with idarucizumab for patients requiring urgent surgical interventions.[65] Up to 5 days may be required for restoration of normal hemostasis after warfarin discontinuation. Patients at high thromboembolic risk (ie, DVT or PE in the previous month) can be considered for so-called bridge therapy with UFH or an LMWH before and/or after the procedure.[64] Bridge therapy has been associated with increased major bleeding without offering additional recurrent VTE risk reduction; therefore, most patients with VTE can safely interrupt warfarin for invasive procedures without using bridge therapy.[63]

DRUG CLASS INFORMATION

8 Optimal use of anticoagulant therapies requires knowledge of pharmacologic and pharmacokinetic characteristics as well as systematic management and ongoing patient education to reduce the risks of bleeding and therapeutic failure (Tables 19-10 and 19-11).

Direct Oral Anticoagulants

Shortcomings with warfarin, LMWH, fondaparinux, and UFH have driven the search for replacements with rapid anticoagulant onset and oral administration without the need for monitoring. The DOACs represent a major advance in VTE prevention and treatment (see Fig. 19-9).

Pharmacology/Mechanism of Action

Rivaroxaban, apixaban, and edoxaban are potent and selective inhibitors of both free and clot-bound factor Xa and do not require antithrombin to exert their anticoagulant effect.[48,50,51] Dabigatran is a selective, reversible, direct factor IIa inhibitor.[49]

Pharmacokinetics

All Factor Xa inhibitors have good oral bioavailability (80%, 60%, and 62% for rivaroxaban, apixaban, and edoxaban, respectively) whereas dabigatran is formulated as a prodrug (dabigatran etexilate) to overcome poor oral bioavailability.[48-51] All DOACs reach peak plasma concentrations in about 2 hours. Each drug is renally eliminated to some degree (33%, 27%, 50%, and 80% for rivaroxaban, apixaban, edoxaban, and dabigatran, respectively) with terminal half-lives of 9 to 12 hours for the Factor Xa inhibitors, and 14 to 17 hours for dabigatran.[48-51] DOACs should be used with caution in patients with renal dysfunction.[66] Rivaroxaban and apixaban are substrates of cytochrome p450 (CYP) 3A4, and the P-glycoprotein (P-gp) transporter.[48,50] Neither edoxaban nor dabigatran undergo significant CYP 3A4 metabolism, but both are P-gp substrates.[49,51] Inhibitors and inducers of CYP 3A4 enzymes or P-gp may cause changes in DOAC exposure and increase risk of bleeding or VTE events.[48-51]

Efficacy

Direct oral anticoagulants are noninferior to warfarin therapy overlapped with LMWH during initiation for reducing recurrence during VTE treatment.[48-51] Similarly, compared to LMWH, the Xa inhibitors are noninferior for preventing VTE following hip or knee replacement surgery.[48-51] Approved DOAC indications for prevention and treatment of VTE are summarized in Table 19-12.

Adverse Effects

The most common adverse effect associated with DOAC therapy is bleeding.[48-51] The International Society for Thrombosis and Haemostasis defines major bleeding as fatal bleeding, any bleeding into a critical anatomic space (eg, intracranial bleeding, hemarthrosis, pericardial bleeding, or intraocular bleeding), bleeding that requires transfusion of 2 or more units of whole blood or red cells,

TABLE 19-10 Comparison of the Chemical and Pharmacokinetic Properties of Antithrombotic Drugs Used for Venous Thrombosis

Agent	FDA Approved	Method of Preparation	Mean Molecular Weight (d)	Plasma Half-Life	Anti-Xa: Anti-IIa Activity	Bioavailability
Unfractionated heparin	Yes	Extracted from porcine gut mucosa or beef lung	≈15,000	30-90 minutes (dose dependent)	1:1	SC: 30%-70% (dose dependent)
Low-molecular-weight heparins						
Dalteparin (Fragmin)	Yes	Nitrous acid depolymerization	≈6,000	119-139 minutes	2.7:1	SC: 87%
Enoxaparin (Lovenox)	Yes	Benzoylation and alkaline depolymerization	≈4,200	129-180 minutes	3.8:1	SC: 92%
Anti–factor Xa inhibitors						
Fondaparinux (Arixtra)	Yes	Synthetic	1,728	15-18 hours	100% anti-Xa	SC: 100%
Rivaroxaban (Xarelto)	Yes	Synthetic	436	7-11 hours	100% anti-Xa	Oral: 80%-100%
Apixaban (Eliquis)	Yes	Synthetic	459	9-14 hours	100% anti-Xa	Oral: 50%
Edoxaban (Savaysa)	Yes	Synthetic	548	10-14 hours	100% anti-Xa	Oral: 62%
Direct thrombin inhibitors						
Dabigatran (Pradaxa)	Yes	Synthetic	471	14 hours	100% anti-IIa	Oral: 7%
Vitamin K antagonists						
Warfarin (Coumadin)	Yes	Synthetic	330	40 hours	1:1	Oral: 90%-100%

SC, subcutaneous.

TABLE 19-11 Risk Factors for Major Bleeding While Taking Anticoagulation Therapy

Anticoagulation intensity
Initiation of therapy (first few days and weeks)
Unstable anti-coagulation response
Age >65 years
Concurrent antiplatelet therapy
Concurrent nonsteroidal anti-inflammatory drug use
History of GI bleeding
Recent surgery or trauma
High risk for fall/trauma
Heavy alcohol use
Renal failure
Cerebrovascular disease
Malignancy

Data from reference 60.

or bleeding that leads to a greater than 2 g/dL (20 g/L; 1.24 mmol/L) drop in hemoglobin concentration. Bleeding that does not meet the major bleeding criteria but requires medical intervention or alteration of therapy is sometimes termed clinically relevant non-major bleeding. All other bleeding is considered minor and is common during anticoagulation therapy even in the most expertly managed patients. Patients presenting with significant bleeding during DOAC therapy should receive routine supportive care (fluid resuscitation, blood transfusion, maintenance of renal function, bleeding source identification, and surgical intervention if needed), and discontinuation of anticoagulation therapy.[67] Because DOACs have relatively short half-lives, these measures may control bleeding in many patients, especially those with normal renal function.[67] Activated charcoal may provide some benefits if drug intake occurred within a couple of hours of presentation, and hemodialysis may be of benefit for reversal of dabigatran.[67] Idarucizumab rapidly reverses the dabigatran anticoagulant effect following IV administration.[65] Idarucizumab can be used during emergency situations such as life-threatening bleeding and when there is need for urgent surgical intervention. Specific reversal agents for apixaban, edoxaban, and rivaroxaban are not available at this time, although several

TABLE 19-12 Approved Indications and Dosing for the Direct Oral Anticoagulants

	VTE prophylaxis following Orthopedic Surgery	Acute VTE Treatment	Extended VTE Treatment (after the first 6 months of anticoagulant therapy)
Dabigatran	Not approved for use	150 mg PO twice daily with or without food FOLLOWING at least 5 days of parenteral anticoagulant therapy	150 mg PO twice daily with or without food
Rivaroxaban	10 mg PO once daily with or without food beginning 6-10 hours after surgery as soon as hemostasis is achieved and continuing for 12-35 days postoperatively	15 mg PO twice daily with food for Days 1-21, then 20 mg PO once daily with food beginning on Day 22	20 mg PO once daily with food
Apixaban	2.5 mg PO twice daily with or without food beginning 12-24 hours after surgery and continuing for 12-35 days postoperatively	10 mg PO twice daily with or without food for Days 1-7, then 5 mg PO twice daily with or without food beginning on Day 8	2.5 mg PO twice daily with or without food
Edoxaban	Not approved for use	60 mg PO once daily with or without food FOLLOWING at least 5 days of parenteral anticoagulant therapy	Not approved for use

PO, by mouth; VTE, venous thromboembolism.

Data from references 48-51.

TABLE 19-13 Reversal Agents for the Direct Oral Anticoagulants

Reversal Agent	Target	Outcomes and Current Status
Idarucizumab (monoclonal antibody fragment)	Dabigatran	Reversed anticoagulant effect of dabigatran in patients with serious bleeding or needing urgent reversal for a procedure Approved by FDA October 2015
Andexanet (modified recombinant Factor Xa)	Rivaroxaban, Apixaban, LMWH	Reversed anticoagulant effect of rivaroxaban and apixaban in healthy volunteers Phase III clinical trial underway
Ciraparantag (synthetic molecule)	UFH, LMWH, Rivaroxaban, Apixaban, Edoxaban, Dabigatran	Reversed anticoagulant effect of Rivaroxaban, Apixaban, Edoxaban, and Dabigatran in animal studies Reversed anticoagulant effect of Rivaroxaban, Apixaban, and Edoxaban in human in vitro studies Reversed anticoagulant effect of Edoxaban in healthy volunteers Phase III trials not yet begun

Data from references 65, 86, and 87.

are in development: andexanet alfa for rivaroxaban, apixaban, and LMWH and ciraparantag for UFH, LMWH, and each of the DOACs (Table 19-13). If traditional hemostatic measures fail in a life-threatening bleeding situation in patients receiving Xa inhibitors, it may be reasonable to consider the use of prothrombin complex concentrates (PCCs) (3-factor, 4-factor, or activated PCCs) or recombinant Factor VIIa, while weighing the associated risk for thrombotic events. Animal, in vitro, and healthy volunteer studies have shown that these agents reverse coagulation laboratory parameters, but controlled studies of these agents in bleeding patients taking DOACs are not available. Fresh-frozen plasma (FFP) is unlikely to provide clinical benefit.[67] The most frequent nonbleeding adverse events in clinical trials of DOACs were gastrointestinal complaints.[48-51]

Drug–drug and Drug–food Interactions

Adding aspirin to DOAC therapy nearly doubles bleeding rates and should be avoided in most patients with VTE. All DOACs are P-gp substrates and subject to changes in anticoagulant effect when coadministered with P-gp inhibitors or inducers. Rivaroxaban and apixaban are subject to interactions involving inhibitors or inducers of CYP 3A4.[48-51] During DOAC therapy, concurrent use of interacting drugs should be avoided because the anticoagulant effect cannot be easily monitored. When interacting drugs cannot be avoided it may be best to switch to warfarin for dose adjustment guided by INR monitoring.

Clinical **Controversy...**

Should aspirin be used for VTE prevention after major surgery? For more than a decade, the ACCP recommended against the use of aspirin as a sole agent for prophylaxis after high VTE risk, such as major orthopedic sugery. The rationale provided for this recommendation was not that aspirin was ineffective but rather that anticoagulants were substantially more effective. The evidence supporting the superiority of anticoagulants relied heavily on trials including a primary outcome of asymptomatic DVT found on screening ultrasound or venography. AT9 focused on symptomatic VTE and bleeding events in their comparison of pharmacologic agents. As a result, aspirin was included as an option for VTE prophylaxis in AT9 and added to the list of approved VTE prophylaxis strategies in the Surgical Care Improvement Project (SCIP) guidelines in 2014. However, NICE guidelines do not include aspirin or other antiplatelet agents as an approved option for VTE prophylaxis in high-risk medical or surgical populations.

Dosing and Administration

Rivaroxaban and apixaban utilize a single-drug approach for acute VTE treatment, whereas at least 5 days of parenteral anticoagulant therapy is required prior to edoxaban or dabigatran initiation for acute VTE (see Fig. 19-9). The 15- and 20-mg doses of rivaroxaban should be taken with food to enhance oral absorption, but all other DOACs can be taken irrespective of food.[48-51] Dosing information for VTE prevention and treatment is summarized in Table 19-12.

Low-Molecular-Weight Heparin

Low-molecular-weight heparin fragments produced by either chemical or enzymatic depolymerization of UFH (see Table 19-10) are heterogeneous mixtures of sulfated glycosaminoglycans with approximately one-third the mean UFH molecular weight.[6] Advantages of LMWH over UFH include predictable anticoagulation dose response, improved subcutaneous bioavailability, dose-independent clearance, longer biologic half-life, lower incidence of thrombocytopenia, and reduced need for routine laboratory monitoring.[6]

Pharmacology/Mechanism of Action

Low-molecular-weight heparin prevents thrombus growth and propagation by enhancing and accelerating the activity of antithrombin similar to UFH.[6] The principal difference in the pharmacologic activity of LMWH and UFH is their relative inhibition of factor Xa and thrombin. Because of smaller chain lengths, LMWH has limited activity against thrombin (Fig. 19-11). The ratio of anti–factor Xa:IIa activity varies between 4:1 and 2:1. By comparison, UFH has an anti–factor Xa:IIa activity ratio of 1:1.[6]

Pharmacokinetics

Compared with UFH, LMWH has a more predictable anticoagulation response. The improved pharmacokinetic profile of LMWH is the result of reduced binding to proteins and cells.[6] The bioavailability of LMWH is about 90% when administered subcutaneously. The peak anticoagulation effect is seen in 3 to 5 hours.[6] The predominant mode of elimination for LMWH is renal. Consequently, biologic half-life may be prolonged in patients with renal impairment.[6] The plasma half-life of LMWH preparations is 3 to 6 hours. The clearance of LMWH is independent of dose.[6]

Efficacy

The efficacy of LMWH for prevention of VTE was established in clinical trials in comparison to LDUH and placebo. For treatment of VTE, the efficacy of fixed weight-based LMWH was compared to aPTT-adjusted intravenous UFH; all patients were transitioned to warfarin for long-term therapy.[62,68]

Adverse Effects

As with other anticoagulants, bleeding is the most common LMWH adverse effect.[60] The frequency of major bleeding is purported to be less with LMWH than with UFH, but this has not been consistently demonstrated in clinical trials.[60] Although there is no proven method for reversing LMWH anticoagulation if major bleeding occurs, IV protamine sulfate can be administered. However, because of limited binding to the shorter LMWH chains, protamine sulfate neutralizes

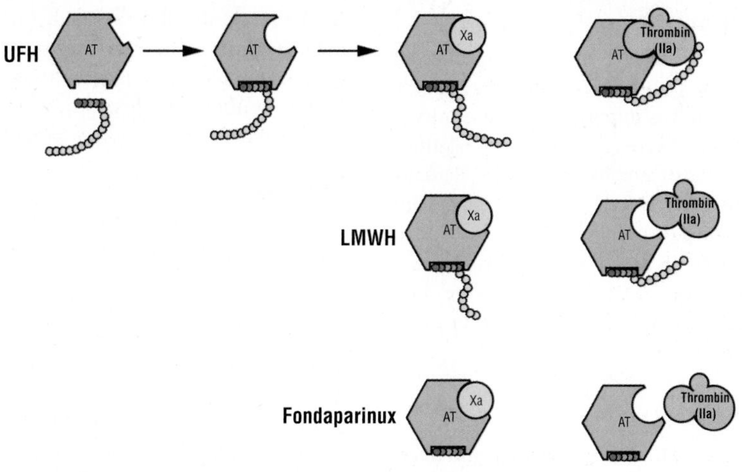

FIGURE 19-11 Pharmacologic activity of unfractionated heparin, low-molecular-weight heparins (LMWHs), and fondaparinux.

only around 60% to 75% of LMWH anticoagulant activity.[6] The recommended dose of protamine sulfate is 1 mg/1 mg of enoxaparin or 1 mg/100 anti–factor Xa units of dalteparin administered in the previous 8 hours. A second protamine sulfate dose of 0.5 mg/1 mg or 100 anti–factor Xa units can be given if bleeding continues. Smaller doses of protamine sulfate can be used if the LMWH dose was given in the previous 8 to 12 hours. The use of protamine sulfate is not recommended if LMWH was administered more than 12 hours earlier.[6] Two additional agents are in development that may have an important role in the future of management of LMWH-related bleeding. Andexanet alfa is a recombinant modified Factor Xa molecule that lacks enzymatic activity while binding to anticoagulant medications and ciraparantag (also known as PER977) may have utility in rapidly reversing LMWH.[69]

Although thrombocytopenia can occur with LMWH use, the incidence of HIT is three times lower than that observed with UFH, perhaps due to the reduced propensity of LMWH to bind to platelets.[6] Because LMWH exhibits nearly 100% cross-reactivity with heparin antibodies in vitro, LMWH should be avoided in patients with an established diagnosis or history of HIT.[6] The risk of osteoporosis appears to be lower with LMWH than with UFH, but both agents have been associated with osteopenia.[6]

Drug–drug Interactions

Drugs enhancing bleeding risk should be avoided during LMWH therapy, if possible. This includes aspirin, non-steroidal anti-inflammatory drugs, dipyridamole, or sulfinpyrazone.[62,68]

Dosing and Administration

Low-molecular-weight heparin is given in fixed or weight-based doses based on the product and indication (see Table 19-5). Doses should be based on actual body weight and dose capping is not recommended.[61] The dose for enoxaparin is expressed in milligrams, whereas dalteparin doses are expressed in units of anti–factor Xa activity. LMWH is given by subcutaneous injection as described in Table 19-6.

Significant LMWH accumulation is possible in patients with severe renal impairment.[6] The enoxaparin dose should be reduced or the dosing interval extended to once daily in patients with CrCL less than 30 mL/min (less than 0.5 mL/s).[62] Dalteparin pharmacokinetics are less well characterized in renal insufficiency.[70] LMWH use in patients with end-stage renal disease receiving hemodialysis is poorly understood; thus, UFH is preferred for these patients.[6] Some experts recommend measuring anti–factor Xa activity if LMWH therapy is continued for more than a few days in patients with severe renal disease.[6] For patients with CrCL less than 30 mL/min (less than 0.5 mL/s) who require VTE prophylaxis, enoxaparin 30 mg once daily is recommended.[6]

Fondaparinux

Fondaparinux is a synthetic molecule consisting of the five critical saccharide units that bind specifically, but reversibly, to antithrombin. Unlike UFH or LMWH, fondaparinux inhibits only factor Xa activity.[6]

Pharmacology/Mechanism of Action

Fondaparinux prevents thrombus generation and clot formation by indirectly inhibiting factor Xa activity through its interaction with antithrombin (see Fig. 19-11). Fondaparinux is not destroyed during this process and is released to bind other antithrombin molecules.[6]

Pharmacokinetics

Fondaparinux is rapidly and completely absorbed following subcutaneous administration achieving peak plasma concentrations approximately 2 hours after a single dose and 3 hours with repeated once-daily dosing. At therapeutic concentrations fondaparinux does not bind to red blood cells or other plasma proteins.[6] Fondaparinux is primarily eliminated unchanged in the urine. The terminal elimination half-life is 17 to 21 hours.[6] The anticoagulant effect of fondaparinux persists for 2 to 4 days following discontinuation of the drug in patients with normal renal function.

Efficacy

The efficacy of fondaparinux for prevention of VTE was established in clinical trials in comparison to LMWH. For treatment of VTE, the efficacy of fixed weight-based fondaparinux was compared to fixed weight-based LMWH; all patients were transitioned to warfarin for long-term therapy.[42]

Adverse Effects

The primary adverse effect associated with fondaparinux therapy is bleeding.[42] Fondaparinux should be used with extreme caution with neuraxial anesthesia or following spinal puncture because of the risk for spinal or epidural hematoma formation.[42] Some case reports have implicated fondaparinux as a cause of HIT, while others have documented successful HIT treatment with fondaparinux.[71] A specific antidote to reverse the antithrombotic activity of fondaparinux is not currently available.[6]

Drug–drug Interactions

Fondaparinux has no known pharmacokinetic drug interactions; other drugs with anticoagulant, fibrinolytic, or antiplatelet activity increase the risk of bleeding.[42]

Dosing and Administration

The dose of fondaparinux for VTE prevention is 2.5 mg injected subcutaneously once daily starting 6 to 8 hours following surgery if hemostasis has been established. It is important to avoid initiating fondaparinux too soon because there is a significant relationship between first dose timing and major bleeding risk.[6] Patients weighing less than 50 kg should not receive VTE prophylaxis with fondaparinux.[42] The usual duration of prophylaxis is 5 to 9 days, but extended prophylaxis for up to 35 days following hospital discharge may be used.[4] For the treatment of DVT or PE, the dose of fondaparinux is 5 mg for patients up to 50 kg, 7.5 mg for 50 to 100 kg, and 10 mg for more than 100 kg.[42]

Unfractionated Heparin

Unfractionated heparin has been used for VTE prevention and treatment for decades. Commercially available UFH preparations are derived from bovine lung or porcine intestinal mucosa. Although some differences exist between the two sources, no differences in antithrombotic activity have been demonstrated.[6]

Pharmacology/Mechanism of Action

Unfractionated heparin is a heterogeneous mixture of sulfated mucopolysaccharides of variable lengths and pharmacologic properties (see Table 19-10).[6] The anticoagulant profile and clearance of each UFH molecule varies based on its length. Smaller chains are cleared less rapidly than their longer counterparts.[6]

The anticoagulant effect of UFH is mediated through a specific pentasaccharide sequence that binds to antithrombin, provoking a conformational change (see Fig. 19-11). Only one-third of the UFH molecules possess the unique pentasaccharide sequence with affinity for antithrombin. The UFH–antithrombin complex is 100 to 1,000 times more potent as an anticoagulant compared with antithrombin alone. Antithrombin inhibits factor IXa, Xa, XIIa, and IIa activity. UFH prevents thrombus growth and propagation allowing endogenous thrombolytic systems to lyse the clot.[6]

Thrombin and Xa are most sensitive to UFH–antithrombin complex inhibition. To inactivate thrombin, the heparin molecule must form a ternary complex bridging between antithrombin and thrombin (see Fig. 19-11).[6] Only molecules containing more than 18 saccharides are able to bind to both antithrombin and thrombin simultaneously. Smaller heparin molecules cannot facilitate the interaction between antithrombin and thrombin. In contrast, the inactivation of factor Xa does not require UFH to form a bridge with antithrombin, but requires only UFH binding to antithrombin via the specific pentasaccharide sequence. UFH molecules with as few as five saccharide units are able to catalyze the inhibition of factor Xa. After it has produced its effect UFH uncouples from antithrombin and quickly recouples with another antithrombin molecule.[6]

Pharmacokinetics

Unfractionated heparin is not reliably orally absorbed as a result of its large molecular size and anionic structure. The bioavailability and biologic activity of UFH is limited by a propensity to bind plasma proteins, platelet factor-4, macrophages, fibrinogen, lipoproteins, and endothelial cells. This may explain the substantial interpatient and intrapatient variability observed in the anticoagulation response to UFH.[6]

The onset of anticoagulant effect after subcutaneous injection is 1 to 2 hours, peaking at 3 hours.[6] Continuous infusion is preferred for intravenous UFH administration.[5] Intramuscular administration is discouraged because of the risk of large hematoma formation.

Unfractionated heparin has a dose-dependent half-life of approximately 30 to 90 minutes.[6] There are two primary mechanisms for UFH elimination, a rapid, but saturable zero-order process involving enzymatic inactivation of heparin molecules bound to endothelial cells and macrophages, and renal elimination via a slower, nonsaturable first-order process. With typical therapeutic UFH regimens the zero-order process predominates.[6]

Efficacy

The clinical effectiveness of UFH for prevention and treatment of VTE has been determined through many years of clinical use.

Adverse Effects

Low-dose subcutaneous UFH is associated with a minimal major bleeding risk, while rates for patients receiving therapeutic UFH doses range from 0% to 2%.[60] Close monitoring for bleeding signs and symptoms during UFH therapy is crucial.[6,60] When major bleeding occurs, UFH should be discontinued and the underlying bleeding source identified and treated. Protamine sulfate in a dose of 1 mg per 100 units of UFH (maximum of 50 mg) can be administered via slow intravenous infusion to reverse the anticoagulant effects of UFH.[6] Protamine sulfate neutralizes UFH in 5 minutes, and persists for 2 hours. Multiple doses or prolonged infusion of protamine sulfate may be necessary if bleeding continues.[6]

Heparin-induced thrombocytopenia is a rare drug-induced immunologic reaction requiring immediate intervention.[72] The most common complication of HIT is VTE; arterial thromboembolic events occur less frequently. Approximately 5% to 10% of patients with HIT die, usually from thrombotic complications.[72] Thrombocytopenia (defined as a platelet count less than $150 \times 10^3/mm^3$ [less than $150 \times 10^9/L$]) is the most common clinical HIT manifestation. Thrombocytopenia occurs in up to 95% of patients with confirmed HIT if platelet counts that decrease by 30% to 50% but remain above $150 \times 10^3/mm^3$ ($150 \times 10^9/L$) are included in the definition.[72] The characteristic onset of falling platelet count in HIT is 5 to 10 days after initiation of UFH (day 0 being the first day of UFH), particularly when administered perioperatively.[72] Thrombocytopenia alone is not sufficient for diagnosing HIT; serologic confirmation of heparin antibodies using an assay available only in a few specialty laboratories is required.[72] Falsely diagnosing HIT can have serious consequences including unnecessary anxiety, unnecessary UFH withdrawal, and the use of alternative anticoagulants with higher bleeding risk. One decision analysis found that strict adherence to platelet monitoring for HIT could, at best, prevent one thrombosis per 1,000 patients screened at the cost of one major bleeding event.[72] For these reasons, AT9 suggests monitoring platelet counts every 2 to 3 days from day 4 to 14 of UFH only in populations where the expected HIT risk exceeds 1%.[72] The use of a clinical prediction rule, such as the four Ts score (*T*hrombocytopenia, *T*iming of platelet count fall or thrombosis, *T*hrombosis, o*T*her explanation for thrombocytopenia), can improve the predictive value of platelet count monitoring and heparin antibody testing.[72,73] A four Ts score should be calculated when HIT is suspected in patients receiving heparin (UFH or LMWH). If the four Ts score is low, no further workup is needed, whereas, further HIT workup including serologic testing should be undertaken if the four Ts score is moderate or high.[74] In the setting of new thrombosis occurring in conjunction with falling platelets and a moderate or high four Ts score all sources of heparin should be discontinued. Alternative anticoagulation with a direct thrombin inhibitor should then be initiated. If warfarin therapy is being used, it should be discontinued and reversed with vitamin K; once platelet counts have recovered warfarin can be carefully resumed with direct thrombin inhibitor overlap until the INR is more than or equal to 2.0.[72]

Using UFH in doses more than or equal to 20,000 units/day for more than 6 months, especially during pregnancy, is associated with significant bone loss and may lead to osteoporosis.[6]

Drug–drug and Drug–food Interactions

Few drug interactions are reported with UFH, but concurrent use with other anticoagulant, thrombolytic, and antiplatelet agents increases bleeding risk.[6]

Dosing and Administration

Unfractionated heparin dose is expressed in units of activity. For VTE prevention, UFH is given by subcutaneous injection in the abdominal fat layer. The typical prophylaxis dose is 5,000 units every 8 to 12 hours. When immediate and full anticoagulation is required, an intravenous bolus dose followed by a continuous infusion is preferred (see Table 19-7).[6] Subcutaneous UFH (initial dose of 333 units/kg followed by 250 units/kg every 12 hours) also provides adequate therapeutic anticoagulation for the treatment of acute VTE.[6]

Warfarin

Because of its narrow therapeutic index, predisposition to drug and food interactions, and propensity to exacerbate bleeding, warfarin requires continuous patient monitoring and education to achieve optimal outcomes.[54]

Pharmacology/Mechanism of Action

Warfarin exerts its anticoagulation effect by inhibiting the enzymes responsible for the cyclic vitamin K interconversion in the liver.[54] Vitamin K in its reduced form is a required cofactor for vitamin K-dependent carboxylation of factors II, VII, IX, and X, as well as the endogenous anticoagulant proteins C and S. Hepatic carboxylation of the N-terminal region of these proteins is required for biologic activity. By inhibiting the reduced vitamin K supply used in the production of these proteins, warfarin therapy produces partially carboxylated and decarboxylated coagulation proteins with reduced activity.[54] Warfarin has no direct effect on previously circulating clotting factors or previously formed thrombus. The time required for warfarin to achieve its pharmacologic effect is dependent on coagulation protein elimination half-lives (6 hours for factor VII and 72 hours for prothrombin).[54] Full antithrombotic effect is not achieved for at least 6 days after warfarin therapy initiation. By suppressing fully functional clotting factor production, warfarin prevents initial thrombus formation and propagation.[54]

Pharmacokinetics

Warfarin is a racemic mixture of *R* and *S* isomers, with *S*-warfarin being 2.7 to 3.8 times more potent than *R*-warfarin.[54] Warfarin is rapidly and extensively absorbed from the GI tract (bioavailability more than 90%) and reaches peak plasma concentration within 4 hours of oral administration. Warfarin is 99% bound to plasma proteins and undergoes stereoselective metabolism via CYP 1A2, 2C9, 2C19, 2C8, 2C18, and 3A4 isoenzymes in the liver, with 2C9 being the main enzyme to modulate in vivo anticoagulant activity.[75] Warfarin pharmacokinetics varies substantially between individuals leading to large interpatient differences in dose requirements. Genetic variations in the 2C9 isoenzyme and vitamin K epoxide reductase (VKOR) have been shown to correlate with warfarin dose requirements.[54] Given the greater potency of *S*-warfarin, coadministration of drugs that induce or inhibit the CYP 2C9 isoenzyme is more likely to cause clinically significant interactions.[54]

Efficacy

The clinical effectiveness of warfarin for prevention and treatment of VTE has been determined through many years of clinical use.

Adverse Effects

Warfarin's primary adverse effect is bleeding that can range from mild to life threatening.[54] Although warfarin does not cause bleeding per se, it exacerbates bleeding from existing lesions and enables massive bleeding from ordinarily minor sources.[54] Anticoagulation therapy intensity is an important bleeding risk factor; the likelihood of bleeding rises with increasing INR values.[54] Therefore, correcting high INR values is important to reduce bleeding risk. For INR more than 4.5 without evidence of bleeding, AT9 suggests withholding warfarin, decreasing the warfarin dose, and/or providing a small dose of vitamin K to shorten the time required to return to normal INR.[33] Vitamin K can be administered parenterally or orally; the oral route is preferred in the absence of serious bleeding. AT9 suggests against routine vitamin K use if the INR is between 4.5 and 10 and no bleeding is present as it has not been shown to affect the risk of developing subsequent bleeding or thromboembolism compared with simply withholding warfarin alone. For INRs more than 10 without evidence of bleeding, oral vitamin K 2.5 mg is suggested.[33] Vitamin K should be used cautiously in patients at high thromboembolism risk due to the possibility of INR overcorrection. Conversely, simply withholding warfarin therapy may not lower high INRs quickly enough in patients at high bleeding risk. Most patients with asymptomatic INR elevations can be safely managed by withholding warfarin alone.

Patients with warfarin-associated major bleeding require supportive care, and in addition AT9 suggests rapid reversal of anticoagulation with four-factor PCCs (rather than FFP) and 5 to 10 mg of vitamin K administered via slow intravenous injection.[33]

Other adverse effects associated with warfarin are uncommon, but can be serious.[54] The etiology of the "purple toe syndrome" is unknown, but is thought to be the result of cholesterol microembolization into the arterial circulation of the toes.[54] Warfarin-induced skin necrosis is a serious dermatologic reaction usually manifesting in the first week of therapy as a painful maculopapular rash and ecchymosis or purpura that subsequently progresses to necrotic gangrene. Areas of the body rich in subcutaneous fat, such as the breasts, thighs, buttocks, and abdomen are most commonly affected.[54] If skin necrosis is suspected, warfarin therapy should be discontinued immediately and reversed with FFP or PCC and vitamin K, and full-dose UFH or LMWH therapy initiated. Patients with a history of skin necrosis should restart warfarin with extreme caution, if at all, using small doses and gradual titration under full-dose UFH or LMWH coverage until a therapeutic INR is achieved.[54]

Drug–drug and Drug–food Interactions

The pharmacokinetic and pharmacodynamic properties of warfarin predispose to numerous clinically important food and drug interactions.[76] Vitamin K can reverse warfarin's pharmacologic activity, and many foods contain sufficient vitamin K to reduce the anticoagulation effect if consumed in large portions or repetitively within a short period of time.[54] Patients should be instructed to maintain a relatively consistent intake of vitamin K-rich foods (Table 19-14). It is important to stress consistency rather than abstinence.

Pharmacokinetic drug interactions with warfarin primarily result from alterations in hepatic metabolism. Drugs inhibiting or inducing CYP 2C9, 1A2, and 3A4 isoenzymes have the greatest potential to significantly alter warfarin therapy response.[54] Drugs altering hemostasis or platelet function (eg, aspirin, clopidogrel) can increase bleeding risk without altering warfarin metabolism.[54] Clinicians should advise patients on warfarin to seek information about potential interactions whenever a drug product, dietary supplement, or herbal product is initiated or stopped, whether prescribed or available over the counter. If there is a known drug interaction or doubt about potential to alter the response to warfarin, more frequent INR testing is recommended with warfarin dose adjustments as needed to maintain INRs in the target range.[76]

TABLE 19-14 Vitamin K Content of Select Foods[a]

Very High (>200 mcg)	High (100-200 mcg)	Medium (50-100 mcg)	Low (<50 mcg)
Brussel sprouts	Basil	Apple, green	Apple, red
Chickpea	Broccoli	Asparagus	Avocado
Collard greens	Chive	Cabbage	Beans
Coriander	Coleslaw	Cauliflower	Breads, grains
Endive	Cucumber (with peel)	Mayonnaise	Carrot
Kale	Canola oil	Nuts, pistachio	Cereal
Lettuce, red leaf	Green onion/scallion	Squash, summer	Celery
Parsley	Lettuce, butterhead		Coffee
Spinach	Mustard greens		Corn
Swiss chard	Soybean oil		Cucumber (without peel)
Tea (green)			Dairy products
Tea (black)			Eggs
Turnip greens			Fruit (varies)
Watercress			Lettuce, iceberg
			Meats, fish, poultry
			Pasta
			Peanuts
			Peas
			Potato
			Rice
			Tomato

[a]Approximate amount of vitamin K per 100 g (3.5 oz) serving.

Data from reference 88.

Dosing and Administration

The dose of warfarin is individualized based on the desired target INR range and anticoagulant response.[54] The pharmacodynamic response and pharmacokinetic disposition of warfarin between and within patients are highly variable. Therefore, the dose of warfarin must be individualized based on continual clinical and laboratory monitoring.[54]

The average weekly warfarin dose is between 25 and 55 mg, but some patient-related variables are associated with lower than usual dose requirement including advanced age (more than 65 years), elevated baseline INR, poor nutritional status, liver disease, genetic polymorphisms in CYP 2C9 and VKOR, and concurrent use of medications known to enhance the effect of warfarin.[54] It is important to collect a complete medication history, including use of herbal and nutritional products as these can influence warfarin's metabolism and/or increase the risk of bleeding.[54]

Initiating warfarin therapy with 5 to 10 mg daily and adjusting the dose based on the INR response will produce therapeutic INRs in 4 to 5 days for most patients (see Fig. 19-10). Lower starting doses may be acceptable based on patient-related factors such as advanced age, malnutrition, liver disease, or heart failure. Starting doses more than 10 mg should be avoided.[54] When warfarin therapy is initiated in the outpatient setting the INR should be measured every 1 to 3 days until stabilized. For patients with acute VTE, UFH, LMWH, or fondaparinux should be overlapped with warfarin therapy for at least 5 days regardless of whether the target INR has been achieved earlier.[5,54]

It is important to allow sufficient time for changes in the INR to occur when adjusting the dose of warfarin. In general, maintenance dose changes should not be made more frequently than every 3 days. When adjusting maintenance warfarin doses the weekly dose should be reduced or increased by 5% to 25%; the full effect of dose changes may not become evident for 5 to 7 days or longer.[54]

Personalized Pharmacotherapy

To personalize anticoagulation therapy for the prevention or treatment of VTE several factors should be considered.

Prevention vs Treatment of VTE

Lower doses of LMWH and DOACs are used for VTE prevention than during VTE treatment. Warfarin may be targeted to traditional INR (ie, 2.0 to 3.0) or reduced intensity (INR 1.5 to 2.5) for VTE prophylaxis. Orthopedic surgeons frequently prefer the lower INR range due to perceived lower bleeding risk. VTE prophylaxis in high-risk hospitalized patients is typically discontinued at discharge. In contrast, after major orthopedic surgery VTE prophylaxis continues following discharge for up to 35 days.

Venous thromboembolism treatment requires full therapeutic anticoagulant doses. Patients unwilling to self-administer LMWH or fondaparinux injections may prefer apixaban or rivaroxaban. Duration of anticoagulant therapy after acute VTE is principally determined by whether the clot was provoked or recurrent. Three months of therapeutic anticoagulation is sufficient following a first episode of VTE provoked by major transient risk factors such as surgery, pregnancy, or trauma. Appropriately selected patients with unprovoked or recurrent VTE should receive long-term anticoagulation for secondary VTE prevention. Patients selected for long-term secondary anticoagulation traditionally receive standard therapeutic doses of anticoagulant agents with one exception. Prophylactic dose apixaban (2.5 mg twice daily) may be used for long-term secondary VTE prevention after 6 months of therapeutic intensity has been completed. Switching to aspirin for long-term secondary VTE prevention is also an option, but is less effective than continuing anticoagulation therapy.[77,78]

Renal Function

Periodic renal function assessment is important during long-term DOAC therapy, especially for patients with CrCL less than 50 mL/min (less than 0.83 mL/s). DOACs should not be used in patients with CrCL less than 25 mL/min (less than 0.42 mL/s) (apixaban) or 30 mL/min (0.5 mL/s) (rivaroxaban and dabigatran). Edoxaban dosing is reduced to 30 mg once daily in patients with CrCL 15 to 50 mL/min (0.25 to 0.83 mL/s).[48-51] LMWHs also rely upon renal elimination and UFH remains preferred in patients with severe renal compromise (eg, CrCL less than 30 mL/min [less than 0.5 mL/s]).[28]

Weight

Patients at extremes of body weight were underrepresented in DOAC VTE treatment trials. There is speculation regarding whether very obese or very small patients receive equivalent on-treatment DOAC exposure compared to other patients. DOACs should be used with caution in very obese or very small patients until additional information substantiating equivalent outcomes becomes available.

Low-molecular-weight heparin dosing in obesity frequently causes concern. Patients weighing more than 90 kg would exceed the maximum dose specified in approved labeling for dalteparin (18,000 units). However, evidence supports similar anti-Xa exposure to LMWH and no increase in bleeding risk compared to non-obese patients when doses based on actual body weight without capping are administered.[79] Fondaparinux is a convenient option for obese patients as the 10 mg dose is suitable for acute VTE treatment in patients more than 100 kg.[42] Obese patients requiring VTE prophylaxis may need higher than normal LMWH doses. For example enoxaparin 40 mg subcutaneously twice daily may be more effective than usual VTE prophylaxis doses for patients undergoing bariatric surgery.[80]

Response to Previous Therapy

Other than bleeding, anticoagulants are generally well tolerated. However, adverse reactions, treatment failure, or allergies during previous therapy may necessitate preferential use of one anticoagulant over another.

Warfarin allergy is rare and often related to dyes or tablet excipients rather than the active ingredient. Warfarin 10 mg tablets contain no dye and can be considered when allergy is suspected. Patients experiencing dabigatran-related dyspepsia can try taking the dose with a full glass of water or food. Transitioning to another DOAC or warfarin may be necessary.

Cost is an important aspect of personalizing anticoagulant therapy for VTE prevention and treatment. For patients unable to afford DOACs, warfarin may remain the lone cost-effective option.

Patient having recurrent VTE during anticoagulant therapy should be assessed for nonadherence and have imaging compared to historical data to ensure the clot is in fact new. Determining and correcting the causes of nonadherence to anticoagulation therapy should occur before pursuing alternate anticoagulant therapy. Investigation for malignancy should be considered when nonadherence is ruled out. Switching to LMWH is recommended for management of breakthrough VTE during oral anticoagulation therapy.[28] Patients having breakthrough VTE during LMWH should be switched to twice daily injections (if receiving once daily LMWH) and considered for dose escalation of 25% to 33%.[28] Switching between oral anticoagulants in response to a breakthrough VTE is less desirable since DOACs and warfarin showed similar efficacy in preventing VTE recurrence when compared head-to-head. Patients with cancer experiencing recurrent VTE during warfarin therapy should be switched to LMWH.[28]

Pharmacogenomics

CYP2C9 is the hepatic microsomal enzyme responsible for metabolism of the more potent S-enantionmer of warfarin. Polymorphisms in CYP2C9 and the gene coding for VKOR (known as Vitamin K Epoxide Reductase Complex 1) explain a substantial proportion of warfarin dose variability between patients. Dosing algorithms using CYP2C9 and VKOR pharmacogenomics, as well as clinical and drug interaction information, have been developed to assist providers more accurately select initial warfarin doses based upon a predicted maintenance warfarin dose for an individual patient (see www.warfarindosing.org). The FDA updated the warfarin package label to include use of pharmacogenetic testing in 2007.[75]

There are several barriers to the widespread application of pharmacogenomic testing for warfarin. First, and most important, is the INR. The ability to rapidly assess a patient's physiologic response to warfarin using an inexpensive and widely available test limits the need for pharmacogenomic information. Second is the timeliness of receiving pharmacogenomic test results. Pharmacogenomic information is most valuable when selecting the first 3 or 4 warfarin doses. However, pharmagenomic testing outside of clinical trials may require several days or longer before results become available. Delaying warfarin initiation is rarely a safe alternative, thus pharmacogenomic test results are only meaningfully if they available in the first 2 to 3 days after treatment initiation. Although poor metabolizing CYP2C9 subtypes have been associated with increased risk of bleeding compared to wild-type, clinical trials have not demonstrated improved bleeding or thromboembolic outcomes with the application of pharmacogenomic warfarin information compared to usual care.[81,82] As a result, the clinical utility and cost-effectiveness of warfarin pharmacogenomics is poorly defined and AT9 suggests against routine use.[33]

Evaluation of Therapeutic Outcomes

Warfarin dose titration based on INR monitoring and UFH dose titration based on aPTT monitoring allows a degree of personalized therapy not available with other anticoagulants. The intensity of warfarin or UFH therapy can be easily titrated in high-risk situations such as invasive procedures, accidental or intentional overdose, suspected nonadherence, or concomitant therapy with interacting drugs. Titrating DOAC therapy in similar situations cannot be accomplished due to lack of readily available quantitative coagulation assays.[83]

While laboratory coagulation monitoring is unnecessary during DOAC therapy, clinical surveillance may be beneficial. In clinical trials comparing DOACs to warfarin, patients receiving DOAC therapy had healthcare provider contact at least every 4 weeks where screenings for bleeding, changes in renal or hepatic function, drug adherence, potential drug interactions, and planning for invasive procedures occurred. A recent study performed in patients with atrial fibrillation taking dabigatran found that pharmacist involvement in appropriate initial drug selection, education, and follow-up contacts improved drug adherence.[84] Adherence is essential to preventing recurrent VTE during DOAC therapy due to their short half-lives. Pharmacist involvement during DOAC initiation may be especially important to ensure proper transitions from LMWH to dabigatran or edoxaban or from initiation to maintenance dosing with rivaroxaban or apixaban. An ABCDEF checklist may be helpful for DOAC therapy clinical surveillance: A—Adherence with DOAC therapy, B—Bleeding risk assessment, C—Creatinine clearance/renal function monitoring, D—Drug interaction evaluation, E—Examination for adverse events and therapeutic effectiveness, and F—Final assessment and recommendations regarding the need for ongoing DOAC therapy.[85] What remains unclear is how frequently DOAC clinical surveillance should be performed, and whether it should be performed for all patients taking DOACs or only those at highest-risk.

Because LMWH anticoagulant response is predictable when given subcutaneously, routine laboratory monitoring is unnecessary.[6] Prior to LMWH initiation, baseline complete blood cell counts with platelets, and serum creatinine should be obtained. The complete blood cell count can be checked every 5 to 10 days during the first 2 weeks of LMWH therapy and every 2 to 4 weeks thereafter to monitor for occult bleeding. If neuraxial anesthesia has been used, patients should be closely monitored for signs and symptoms of neurologic impairment.[62]

Anti–factor Xa activity is the most widely used test to monitor the anticoagulant effect of LMWH in clinical practice. Routine anti–factor Xa activity measurement is unnecessary in uncomplicated patients in stable condition.[6] Measuring anti–factor Xa activity may be helpful in patients who have significant renal impairment (eg, CrCL less than 30 mL/min [less than 0.5 mL/s]), weigh less than 50 kg, are morbidly obese, and require prolonged therapy (eg, longer than 14 days). Periodic anti–factor Xa activity monitoring may also be useful in women treated with LMWH during pregnancy due to changing volume of distribution and renal function.[6]

When anti–factor Xa activity is used to monitor LMWH therapy, the sample should be drawn during the peak anti–factor Xa activity—once steady state has been achieved (after the second or third dose) and approximately 4 hours after the subcutaneous injection.[6] The anti–factor Xa activity therapeutic range is not well defined and has not been clearly correlated with efficacy or the risk of bleeding. For the treatment of VTE, an acceptable target range for the peak anti-Xa level for twice-daily enoxaparin dosing is 0.6 to 1 unit/mL (kU/L). For once daily dosing likely peak targets are more than 1 unit/mL (kU/L) for enoxaparin and 1.05 units/mL (kU/L) for dalteparin.[6] The suggested target range for peak anti-Xa concentrations during cancer-associated VTE treatment with dalteparin is 0.5 to 1.5 units/mL (kU/L).[68]

Prior to initiating fondaparinux baseline kidney function should be determined as fondaparinux is contraindicated when CrCL is less than 30 mL/min (less than 0.5 mL/s).[42] Signs and symptoms of bleeding should be monitored daily, particularly in patients with a baseline CrCL between 30 and 50 mL/min (0.5 and 0.83 mL/s). If neuraxial anesthesia has been used, patients should be closely monitored for signs and symptoms of neurologic impairment.[42] Fondaparinux does not alter coagulation tests such as the aPTT and PT. The role of anti–factor Xa monitoring during fondaparinux is not well defined, but routine coagulation testing is not required.[42]

Administration of UFH requires close monitoring because of the unpredictable anticoagulant patient response.[6] Although the aPTT has several limitations, most experts advocate using the aPTT to monitor UFH provided that institution-specific therapeutic ranges are defined.[6] The aPTT should be measured prior to the initiation of therapy to determine the patient's baseline. With intravenous infusion, the aPTT response to UFH therapy should be measured 6 hours after initiation or dose changes. UFH doses should be adjusted based on patient response and the institution-specific aPTT therapeutic range (see Table 19-7).[6]

The prothrombin time (PT) measures the biologic activity of factors II, VII, and X and has been used for decades to monitor the anticoagulation effects of warfarin. The PT is performed by measuring the time required for clot formation after adding calcium and thromboplastin to citrated plasma.[54] Interpreting the PT is problematic because thromboplastins of differing sensitivity produce substantially different results, some of which could lead to inappropriate dosing decisions. The World Health Organization (WHO) addressed the need for standardization in the late 1970s by developing a reference thromboplastin and recommending the use of the INR to monitor warfarin therapy.[54] The INR attempts to correct for differences in thromboplastin reagents through the following formula:

$$\text{INR} = \left(\frac{\text{PT}^{\text{patient}}}{\text{PT}^{\text{control}}}\right)^{\text{ISI}}$$

The International Sensitivity Index (ISI) is a measure of thromboplastin responsiveness compared with the WHO reference standard.[54] The ISI for each thromboplastin reagent should be used to calculate the INR, and although the INR system has a number of potential problems, it remains the preferred method for monitoring warfarin therapy.[54]

The recommended target INR for treatment of VTE is 2.5 with an acceptable range of 2.0 to 3.0.[54] A baseline INR and complete blood cell count should be obtained prior to initiating warfarin therapy. In patients with an acute thromboembolic event, an INR should be measured minimally every 3 days during the first week of therapy (daily INRs are common in hospitalized patients). Once the patient's dose–response is established, an INR should be determined every 7 to 14 days until it stabilizes and optimally every 4 to 12 weeks thereafter.[33]

At each encounter and especially when the INR is not in range, patients on warfarin therapy should be questioned regarding adherence to prior dosing instructions, other medication use, changes in health status, and symptoms related to bleeding and thromboembolic complications. Any changes in medications, including changes in dose as well as nonprescription drug and dietary supplement use, should be carefully explored. Dietary intake of vitamin K–rich foods should also be evaluated.[54]

Anticoagulation therapy management services can optimize the care of patients who take warfarin therapy by providing structured care, comprehensive patient education, and evaluation of outcomes. When anticoagulation management services are not available, individual clinicians should strive to implement similar structured care processes.[33]

Portable finger-stick INR devices are available for monitoring warfarin therapy. These devices permit clinicians to do "real-time" therapeutic INR monitoring, and enable patients to engage in self-testing and/or management at home.[33] Patients who engage in INR self-monitoring and warfarin self-management report high levels of satisfaction with care and maintain INRs within the therapeutic range slightly more frequently than those managed by "usual care." However, home INR testing and self-management is not for everyone and requires careful patient selection and considerable patient education.[33] Finger-stick INR devices are relatively expensive, but some patients qualify for limited coverage of the monitor and testing supplies.

CONCLUSION

Venous thromboembolism is a significant public health issue, yet there is little public awareness of the life-threatening nature of this commonly occurring condition. Given the number and variety of clinical conditions or circumstances that place individuals at VTE risk, improvements in VTE prevention and care have the potential to benefit many patients. Over the past decade, the focus on quality healthcare has included systematic measures to improve the use of effective VTE prophylaxis and evidence-based VTE treatments. The concerted efforts of government and accrediting agencies working with hospitals and other healthcare institutions will hopefully reduce VTE rates. Systematic approaches to this problem are needed at every level, starting with increased public and health practitioner awareness, continuing with the uniform use of effective prophylactic strategies in patients at risk, and concluding with greater accountability for quality VTE treatment strategies using expanding anticoagulant drug options.

ABBREVIATIONS

aPC	activated protein C
aPTT	activated partial thromboplastin time
AT9	*Antithrombotic Therapy and Prevention of Thrombosis, 9th ed: Evidence-Based Clinical Practice Guidelines* published by the American College of Chest Physicians
β_2-gp	β_2-glycoprotein
CrCL	creatinine clearance
CTPA	computed tomography pulmonary angiography
CTPH	chronic thromboembolic pulmonary hypertension
CUS	compression ultrasound
CYP	cytochrome p450
DOAC	direct oral anticoagulant
DVT	deep vein thrombosis
FFP	fresh-frozen plasma
HIT	heparin-induced thrombocytopenia
INR	international normalized ratio
IPC	intermittent pneumatic compression
ISI	International Sensitivity Index
IVC	inferior vena cava
LDUH	low-dose unfractionated heparin
LMWH	low-molecular-weight heparin
NICE	National Institute for Health and Care Excellence
PCCs	prothrombin complex concentrates
PE	pulmonary embolism
PESI	Pulmonary Embolism Severity Index
P-gp	P-glycoprotein
PT	prothrombin time
TF	tissue factor
TFPI	tissue factor pathway inhibitor
tPA	tissue plasminogen activator
UFH	unfractionated heparin
V/Q	ventilation–perfusion
VKOR	vitamin K epoxide reductase
VTE	venous thromboembolism
WHO	World Health Organization

REFERENCES

1. Goldhaber SZ, Bounameaux H. Pulmonary embolism and deep vein thrombosis. *Lancet* 2012;379:1835-1846.
2. Kahn SR, Lim W, Dunn AS, et al. Prevention of VTE in nonsurgical patients: Antithrombotic Therapy and Prevention of Thrombosis. 9th ed. American College of Chest Physicians Evidence-Based Clinical Practice Guidelines. *Chest* 2012;141:e195S-226S.
3. Gould MK, Garcia DA, Wren SM, et al. Prevention of VTE in nonorthopedic surgical patients: Antithrombotic Therapy and Prevention of Thrombosis. 9th ed. American College of Chest Physicians Evidence-Based Clinical Practice Guidelines. *Chest* 2012;141:e227S-277S.
4. Falck-Ytter Y, Francis CW, Johanson NA, et al. Prevention of VTE in orthopedic surgery patients: Antithrombotic Therapy and Prevention of Thrombosis. 9th ed. American College of Chest Physicians Evidence-Based Clinical Practice Guidelines. *Chest* 2012;141:e278S-325S.
5. Kearon C, Akl EA, Comerota AJ, et al. Antithrombotic therapy for VTE disease: Antithrombotic Therapy and Prevention of Thrombosis. 9th ed. American College of Chest Physicians Evidence-Based Clinical Practice Guidelines. *Chest* 2012;141: e419S-494S.
6. Garcia DA, Baglin TP, Weitz JI, Samama MM, American College of Chest P. Parenteral anticoagulants: Antithrombotic Therapy and Prevention of Thrombosis. 9th ed. American College of Chest Physicians Evidence-Based Clinical Practice Guidelines. *Chest* 2012;141:e24S-43S.
7. ISTH Steering Committee for World Thrombosis Day. Thrombosis: A major contributor to the global disease burden. *J Thromb Haemost* 2014;12:1580-1590.
8. Martinez C, Cohen AT, Bamber L, Rietbrock S. Epidemiology of first and recurrent venous thromboembolism: A population-based cohort study in patients without active cancer. *Thromb Haemost* 2014;112:255-263.
9. Turpie AG, Esmon C. Venous and arterial thrombosis—pathogenesis and the rationale for anticoagulation. *Thromb Haemost* 2011;105: 586-596.
10. Reitsma PH, Versteeg HH, Middeldorp S. Mechanistic view of risk factors for venous thromboembolism. *Arterioscler Thromb Vasc Biol* 2012;32:563-568.
11. De Caterina R, Husted S, Wallentin L, et al. General mechanisms of coagulation and targets of anticoagulants (Section I). Position Paper of the ESC Working Group on Thrombosis—Task Force on Anticoagulants in Heart Disease. *Thromb Haemost* 2013;109:569-579.
12. Bates SM, Greer IA, Middeldorp S, et al. VTE, thrombophilia, antithrombotic therapy, and pregnancy: Antithrombotic Therapy and Prevention of Thrombosis. 9th ed. American College of Chest Physicians Evidence-Based Clinical Practice Guidelines. *Chest* 2012;141:e691S-736S.
13. Margaglione M, Grandone E. Population genetics of venous thromboembolism. A narrative review. *Thromb Haemost* 2011;105:221-231.
14. Rijken DC, Lijnen HR. New insights into the molecular mechanisms of the fibrinolytic system. *J Thromb Haemost* 2009;7:4-13.
15. Anderson JA, Weitz JI. Hypercoagulable states. *Crit Care Clin* 2011;27:933-952, vii.
16. Khorana AA. Cancer and coagulation. *Am J Hematol* 2012; 87(Suppl 1):S82-87.
17. Chong LY, Fenu E, Stansby G, Hodgkinson S, Guideline Development G. Management of venous thromboembolic diseases and the role of thrombophilia testing: Summary of NICE guidance. *BMJ* 2012;344:e3979.
18. Bates SM, Jaeschke R, Stevens SM, et al. Diagnosis of DVT: Antithrombotic Therapy and Prevention of Thrombosis. 9th ed. American College of Chest Physicians Evidence-Based Clinical Practice Guidelines. *Chest* 2012;141:e351S-418S.
19. Le Gal G, Righini M. Controversies in the diagnosis of venous thromboembolism. *J Thromb Haemost* 2015;13(Suppl 1):S259-265.
20. Wendelboe AM, McCumber M, Hylek EM, et al. Global public awareness of venous thromboembolism. *J Thromb Haemost* 2015;13:1365-1371.
21. Mahan CE, Holdsworth MT, Welch SM, Borrego M, Spyropoulos AC. Deep-vein thrombosis: A United States cost model for a preventable and costly adverse event. *Thromb Haemost* 2011;106:405-415.
22. Guyatt GH, Eikelboom JW, Gould MK, et al. Approach to outcome measurement in the prevention of thrombosis in surgical and medical patients: Antithrombotic Therapy and Prevention of Thrombosis. 9th ed. American College of Chest Physicians Evidence-Based Clinical Practice Guidelines. *Chest* 2012;141:e185S-194S.
23. Gray J, Razmus I. Improving venous thromboembolism prevention processes and outcomes at a community hospital. *Jt Comm J Qual Patient Saf* 2012;38:61-66.
24. Schiro TA, Sakowski J, Romanelli RJ, et al. Improving adherence to best-practice guidelines for venous thromboembolism risk assessment and prevention. *Am J Health Syst Pharm* 2011;68:2184-2189.
25. Zareba P, Wu C, Agzarian J, Rodriguez D, Kearon C. Meta-analysis of randomized trials comparing combined compression and anticoagulation with either modality alone for prevention of venous thromboembolism after surgery. *Br J Surg* 2014;101:1053-1062.
26. Kahn SR, Shapiro S, Wells PS, et al. Compression stockings to prevent post-thrombotic syndrome: A randomised placebo-controlled trial. *Lancet* 2014;383:880-888.
27. Rajasekhar A, Streiff MB. Vena cava filters for management of venous thromboembolism: A clinical review. *Blood Rev* 2013;27:225-241.
28. Kearon C, Akl EA, Ornelas J, et al. Antithrombotic therapy for VTE disease: CHEST guideline and Expert Panel Report. *Chest* 2016;149(2):315-352.
29. Reichert JA, Hlavinka PF, Stolzfus JC. Risk of hemorrhage in patients with chronic liver disease and coagulopathy receiving pharmacologic venous thromboembolism prophylaxis. *Pharmacotherapy* 2014;34:1043-1049.
30. Ali M, Ananthakrishnan AN, McGinley EL, Saeian K. Deep vein thrombosis and pulmonary embolism in hospitalized patients with cirrhosis: A nationwide analysis. *Dig Dis Sci* 2011;56:2152-2159.
31. Anderson FA Jr, Huang W, Friedman RJ, et al. Prevention of venous thromboembolism after hip or knee arthroplasty: Findings from a 2008 survey of US orthopedic surgeons. *J Arthroplasty* 2012;27:659-666.e5.
32. Mont MA, Jacobs JJ, Boggio LN, et al. Preventing venous thromboembolic disease in patients undergoing elective hip and knee arthroplasty. *J Am Acad Orthop Surg* 2011;19:768-776.
33. Holbrook A, Schulman S, Witt DM, et al. Evidence-based management of anticoagulant therapy: Antithrombotic Therapy and Prevention of Thrombosis. 9th ed. American College of Chest Physicians Evidence-Based Clinical Practice Guidelines. *Chest* 2012;141:e152S-184S.
34. Wells PS, Forgie MA, Rodger MA. Treatment of venous thromboembolism. *JAMA* 2014;311:717-728.
35. Meyer G, Planquette B, Sanchez O. Pulmonary embolism: Whom to discharge and whom to thrombolyze? *J Thromb Haemost* 2015;13(Suppl 1): S252-258.
36. Agnelli G, Buller HR, Cohen A, et al. Oral apixaban for the treatment of acute venous thromboembolism. *N Engl J Med* 2013;369:799-808.
37. Investigators E-P, Buller HR, Prins MH, et al. Oral rivaroxaban for the treatment of symptomatic pulmonary embolism. *N Engl J Med* 2012;366:1287-1297.
38. Investigators E, Bauersachs R, Berkowitz SD, et al. Oral rivaroxaban for symptomatic venous thromboembolism. *N Engl J Med* 2010;363: 2499-2510.
39. Schulman S, Kakkar AK, Goldhaber SZ, et al. Treatment of acute venous thromboembolism with dabigatran or warfarin and pooled analysis. *Circulation* 2014;129:764-772.
40. Hokusai VTEI, Buller HR, Decousus H, et al. Edoxaban versus warfarin for the treatment of symptomatic venous thromboembolism. *N Engl J Med* 2013;369:1406-1415.
41. Goldhaber SZ. Advanced treatment strategies for acute pulmonary embolism, including thrombolysis and embolectomy. *J Thromb Haemost* 2009;7(Suppl 1):322-327.
42. GlaxoSmithKline. Arixtra Prescribing Information 2015.
43. Martinez K, Kosirog E, Billups SJ, Clark NP, Delate T, Witt DM. Clinical outcomes and adherence to guideline recommendations during the initial treatment of acute venous thromboembolism. *Ann Pharmacother* 2015;49:869-875.
44. Bashir R, Zack CJ, Zhao H, Comerota AJ, Bove AA. Comparative outcomes of catheter-directed thrombolysis plus anticoagulation vs anticoagulation alone to treat lower-extremity proximal deep vein thrombosis. *JAMA Intern Med* 2014;174:1494-1501.
45. Wang TF, Squizzato A, Dentali F, Ageno W. The role of thrombolytic therapy in pulmonary embolism. *Blood* 2015;125:2191-2199.
46. Baglin T. What happens after venous thromboembolism? *J Thromb Haemost* 2009;7(Suppl 1):287-290.
47. Aujesky D, Hughes R, Jimenez D. Short-term prognosis of pulmonary embolism. *J Thromb Haemost* 2009;7(Suppl 1):318-321.
48. Bristol Myers Squibb C. Eliquis Prescribing Information: 2015. Available at: http://packageinserts.bms.com/pi/pi_eliquis.pdf. (Accessed August 30, 2015)
49. Boehringer-Ingelheim. Pradaxa Prescribing Information; 2015. Available at: http://bidocs.boehringer-ingelheim.com/BIWebAccess/ViewServlet.ser?docBase=renetnt&folderPath=/Prescribing Information/PIs/Pradaxa/Pradaxa.pdf. (Accessed August 30, 2015.)

50. Janssen Pharmaceuticals I. Xarelto Prescribing Information: 2015. Available at: https://www.xareltohcp.com/shared/product/xarelto/prescribing-information.pdf. (Accessed August 30, 2015.)
51. Daiichi Sankyo I. Savaysa Prescribing Information: 2015. Available at: http://dsi.com/prescribing-information-portlet/getPIContent?productName=Savaysa&inline=true. (Accessed August 30, 2015.)
52. Knol HM, Schultinge L, Erwich JJ, Meijer K. Fondaparinux as an alternative anticoagulant therapy during pregnancy. *J Thromb Haemost* 2010;8:1876-1879.
53. Kamel H, Navi BB, Sriram N, Hovsepian DA, Devereux RB, Elkind MS. Risk of a thrombotic event after the 6-week postpartum period. *N Engl J Med* 2014;370:1307-1315.
54. Ageno W, Gallus AS, Wittkowsky A, et al. Oral anticoagulant therapy: Antithrombotic Therapy and Prevention of Thrombosis. 9th ed. American College of Chest Physicians Evidence-Based Clinical Practice Guidelines. *Chest* 2012;141:e44S-88S.
55. Monagle P, Chan AK, Goldenberg NA, et al. Antithrombotic therapy in neonates and children: Antithrombotic Therapy and Prevention of Thrombosis. 9th ed. American College of Chest Physicians Evidence-Based Clinical Practice Guidelines. *Chest* 2012;141:e737S-801S.
56. Schulman S, Zondag M, Linkins L, et al. Recurrent venous thromboembolism in anticoagulated patients with cancer: Management and short-term prognosis. *J Thromb Haemost* 2015;13:1010-1018.
57. Easaw JC, Shea-Budgell MA, Wu CM, et al. Canadian consensus recommendations on the management of venous thromboembolism in patients with cancer. Part 2: treatment. *Curr Oncol* 2015;22:144-155.
58. Farge D, Debourdeau P, Beckers M, et al. International clinical practice guidelines for the treatment and prophylaxis of venous thromboembolism in patients with cancer. *J Thromb Haemost* 2013;11:56-70.
59. Vedovati MC, Germini F, Agnelli G, Becattini C. Direct oral anticoagulants in patients with VTE and cancer: A systematic review and meta-analysis. *Chest* 2015;147:475-483.
60. Schulman S, Beyth RJ, Kearon C, Levine MN, American College of Chest P. Hemorrhagic complications of anticoagulant and thrombolytic treatment: American College of Chest Physicians Evidence-Based Clinical Practice Guidelines (8th ed.). *Chest* 2008;133:257S-298S.
61. Clark NP. Low-molecular-weight heparin use in the obese, elderly, and in renal insufficiency. *Thromb Res* 2008;123(Suppl 1):S58-61.
62. Sanofi-Aventis. Lovenox Prescribing Information: 2015. Available at: http://products.sanofi.us/lovenox/lovenox.html. (Accessed August 30, 2015)
63. Clark NP, Witt DM, Davies LE, et al. Bleeding, Recurrent Venous Thromboembolism, and Mortality Risks During Warfarin Interruption for Invasive Procedures. *JAMA Intern Med* 2015;175:1163-1168.
64. Douketis JD, Spyropoulos AC, Spencer FA, et al. Perioperative management of antithrombotic therapy: Antithrombotic Therapy and Prevention of Thrombosis. 9th ed. American College of Chest Physicians Evidence-Based Clinical Practice Guidelines. *Chest* 2012;141:e326S-350S.
65. Pollack CV Jr, Reilly PA, Eikelboom J, et al. Idarucizumab for Dabigatran Reversal. *N Engl J Med* 2015;373:511-520.
66. Yeh CH, Gross PL, Weitz JI. Evolving use of new oral anticoagulants for treatment of venous thromboembolism. *Blood* 2014;124:1020-1028.
67. Weitz JI, Pollack CV Jr. Practical management of bleeding in patients receiving non-vitamin K antagonist oral anticoagulants. *Thromb Haemost* 2015;114(6):1113-1126.
68. Labs P. Fragmin Prescribing Information: 2015. Available at: http://labeling.pfizer.com/ShowLabeling.aspx?id=2293. (Accessed September 1, 2015)
69. Crowther M, Crowther MA. Antidotes for novel oral anticoagulants: Current status and future potential. *Arterioscler Thromb Vasc Biol* 2015;35:1736-1745.
70. Park D, Southern W, Calvo M, et al. Treatment with Dalteparin is Associated with a Lower Risk of Bleeding Compared to Treatment with Unfractionated Heparin in Patients with Renal Insufficiency. *J Gen Intern Med* 2016;31(2):182-187.
71. Blackmer AB, Oertel MD, Valgus JM. Fondaparinux and the management of heparin-induced thrombocytopenia: The journey continues. *Ann Pharmacother* 2009;43:1636-1646.
72. Linkins LA, Dans AL, Moores LK, et al. Treatment and prevention of heparin-induced thrombocytopenia: Antithrombotic Therapy and Prevention of Thrombosis. 9th ed. American College of Chest Physicians Evidence-Based Clinical Practice Guidelines. *Chest* 2012;141:e495S-530S.
73. Crowther MA, Cook DJ, Albert M, et al. The 4Ts scoring system for heparin-induced thrombocytopenia in medical-surgical intensive care unit patients. *J Crit Care* 2010;25:287-293.
74. Cuker A, Gimotty PA, Crowther MA, Warkentin TE. Predictive value of the 4Ts scoring system for heparin-induced thrombocytopenia: A systematic review and meta-analysis. *Blood* 2012;120:4160-4167.
75. Bristol Myers Squibb C. Coumadin Prescribing Information: 2015. Available at: http://packageinserts.bms.com/pi/pi_coumadin.pdf. (Accessed September 4, 2015)
76. Clark NP, Delate T, Riggs CS, et al. Warfarin interactions with antibiotics in the ambulatory care setting. *JAMA Intern Med* 2014;174:409-416.
77. Becattini C, Agnelli G, Schenone A, et al. Aspirin for preventing the recurrence of venous thromboembolism. *N Engl J Med* 2012;366:1959-1967.
78. Brighton TA, Eikelboom JW, Mann K, et al. Low-dose aspirin for preventing recurrent venous thromboembolism. *N Engl J Med* 2012;367:1979-1987.
79. Al-Yaseen E, Wells PS, Anderson J, Martin J, Kovacs MJ. The safety of dosing dalteparin based on actual body weight for the treatment of acute venous thromboembolism in obese patients. *J Thromb Haemost* 2005;3:100-102.
80. Parker SG, McGlone ER, Knight WR, Sufi P, Khan OA. Enoxaparin venous thromboembolism prophylaxis in bariatric surgery: A best evidence topic. *Int J Surg* 2015;23:52-56.
81. Pirmohamed M, Burnside G, Eriksson N, et al. A randomized trial of genotype-guided dosing of warfarin. *N Engl J Med* 2013;369:2294-2303.
82. Kimmel SE, French B, Kasner SE, et al. A pharmacogenetic versus a clinical algorithm for warfarin dosing. *N Engl J Med* 2013;369:2283-2293.
83. Cuker A, Siegal DM, Crowther MA, Garcia DA. Laboratory measurement of the anticoagulant activity of the non-vitamin K oral anticoagulants. *J Am Coll Cardiol* 2014;64:1128-1139.
84. Shore S, Ho PM, Lambert-Kerzner A, et al. Site-level variation in and practices associated with dabigatran adherence. *JAMA* 2015;313:1443-1450.
85. Gladstone DJ, Geerts WH, Douketis J, Ivers N, Healey JS, Leblanc K. How to Monitor Patients Receiving Direct Oral Anticoagulants for Stroke Prevention in Atrial Fibrillation: A Practice Tool Endorsed by Thrombosis Canada, the Canadian Stroke Consortium, the Canadian Cardiovascular Pharmacists Network, and the Canadian Cardiovascular Society. *Ann Intern Med* 2015;163:382-385.
86. Greinacher A, Thiele T, Selleng K. Reversal of anticoagulants: An overview of current developments. *Thromb Haemost* 2015;113:931-942.
87. Ansell JE, Bakhru SH, Laulicht BE, et al. Use of PER977 to reverse the anticoagulant effect of edoxaban. *N Engl J Med* 2014;371:2141-2142.
88. Booth SL, Centurelli MA. Vitamin K: A practical guide to the dietary management of patients on warfarin. *Nutr Rev* 1999;57:288-296.
89. Delate T, Witt DM, Ritzwoller D, et al. Outpatient use of low molecular weight heparin monotherapy for first-line treatment of venous thromboembolism in advanced cancer. *Oncologist* 2012;17:419-427.
90. Kleinjan A, Aggarwal A, Van de Geer A, et al. A worldwide survey to assess the current approach to the treatment of patients with cancer and venous thromboembolism. *Thromb Haemost* 2013;110:959-965.

20

Stroke

Susan C. Fagan and David C. Hess

KEY CONCEPTS

1. Stroke can be either ischemic (87%) or hemorrhagic (13%) and the two types are treated differently.
2. Transient ischemic attacks (TIAs) require urgent intervention to reduce the risk of stroke, which is known to be highest in the first few days after TIA.
3. Carotid endarterectomy should be performed in ischemic stroke patients with 70% to 99% stenosis of the ipsilateral carotid artery, provided that it is done in an experienced center.
4. Carotid stenting is an option for stroke patients eligible for carotid endarterectomy, especially in patients younger than 70 years.
5. Early reperfusion (less than 4.5 hours from onset) with tissue plasminogen activator (tPA) has been shown to reduce the ultimate disability due to ischemic stroke.
6. Endovascular thrombectomy with a stent retriever (within 6 hours) improves stroke outcomes in selected patients with proximal large artery occlusion and preservable penumbral tissue.
7. Antiplatelet therapy is the cornerstone of antithrombotic therapy for the secondary prevention of noncardioembolic ischemic stroke.
8. Oral anticoagulation is recommended for the secondary prevention of cardioembolic stroke in patients with atrial fibrillation.
9. Blood pressure lowering is effective in both the primary and secondary prevention of both ischemic and hemorrhagic stroke.
10. Blood pressure lowering in the acute ischemic stroke period (first 7 days) may result in decreased cerebral blood flow and worsened symptoms.

(1) Stroke is the leading cause of disability among adults and the fifth leading cause of death in the United States, behind cardiovascular disease, cancer, chronic lower respiratory diseases, and accidental death.[1] Despite a 35% reduction in stroke mortality between 2001 and 2011, stroke occurs in the United States at a rate of almost 800,000 per year and resulted in 128,932 deaths in 2011.[1,2] Aggressive efforts to organize stroke care at the local and regional levels and increased utilization of evidence-based recommendations and national guidelines may have contributed to the improved outcomes.

EPIDEMIOLOGY

There are currently 6.6 million stroke survivors in the United States, and stroke is the leading cause of adult disability.[2] Of those free of the diagnosis of stroke or transient ischemic attack (TIA), however, almost 20% of individuals older than 45 years reported at least one stroke symptom,[3] suggesting rampant underdiagnosing. Owing in part to the need for expensive posthospitalization rehabilitation and nursing home care, the annual cost of stroke in the United States is estimated to be $33.6 billion.[2]

Not all groups have benefitted equally from advances in care and prevention of stroke. African Americans have stroke rates that are twice those of whites, and the difference is exaggerated at younger ages.[2] In addition, geographic disparity in stroke incidence exists, such that many states in the southeastern United States have stroke mortality rates 40% higher than the national average.[2] Lastly, case fatality due to hemorrhagic stroke has not declined in the past decade, with 30-day rates remaining around 40%.

Etiology

(2) Stroke can be either ischemic or hemorrhagic (87% and 13%, respectively, of all strokes in the 2015 American Heart Association [AHA] report).[2] Hemorrhagic strokes include subarachnoid hemorrhage (SAH) and intracerebral hemorrhage (ICH). SAH occurs when blood enters the subarachnoid space (where cerebrospinal fluid is housed) owing to trauma, rupture of an intracranial aneurysm, or rupture of an arteriovenous malformation (AVM). By contrast, ICH occurs when a blood vessel ruptures within the brain parenchyma itself, resulting in the formation of a hematoma. These types of hemorrhages very often are associated with uncontrolled high blood pressure and sometimes antithrombotic or thrombolytic therapy. Hemorrhagic stroke, although less common, is significantly more lethal than ischemic stroke, with 30-day case-fatality rates of 46.5% compared to 9% to 23% in ischemic stroke.[4]

Ischemic strokes are caused either by local thrombus formation or by embolic phenomena, resulting in occlusion of a cerebral artery. Atherosclerosis, particularly of the cerebral vasculature, is a causative factor in most cases of ischemic stroke, although 30% are cryptogenic. Emboli can arise from either intracranial or extracranial arteries (including the aortic arch) or, as is the case in 20% of all ischemic strokes, the heart. Cardiogenic embolism is presumed to have occurred if the patient has concomitant atrial fibrillation, valvular heart disease, or any other condition of the heart that can lead to clot formation.[2] Distinguishing between cardiogenic embolism and other causes of ischemic stroke is important in determining long-term pharmacotherapy in a given patient.

Risk Factors

Risk factors for stroke can be subdivided into nonmodifiable, modifiable, and potentially modifiable. In addition, risk factors can be either well documented or less well documented.[5] The main risk factors of stroke are listed in Table 20-1. Recommendations for risk factor reduction aggressively target the modifiable, well-documented risk factors, even in individuals with nonmodifiable risk.[5] The nonmodifiable risk factors are age, race, sex, low birth weight, and

TABLE 20-1 Risk Factors for Ischemic Stroke

Nonmodifiable risk factors or risk markers
Age
Low birth weight
Race
Genetic factors
Modifiable, well documented
Cigarette smoking
Hypertension
Diabetes
Asymptomatic carotid stenosis
Dyslipidemia
Atrial fibrillation
Sickle cell disease
Poor diet
Obesity
Physical inactivity
Other cardiac diseases (coronary heart disease, heart failure, PAD)
Potentially modifiable, less well documented
Migraine
Metabolic syndrome
Drug and alcohol abuse
Inflammation and Infection
Elevated Lp(a)
Homocysteinemia
Sleep-disordered breathing

Lp(a); lipoprotein(a); PAD, peripheral arterial disease.

Data from reference 5.

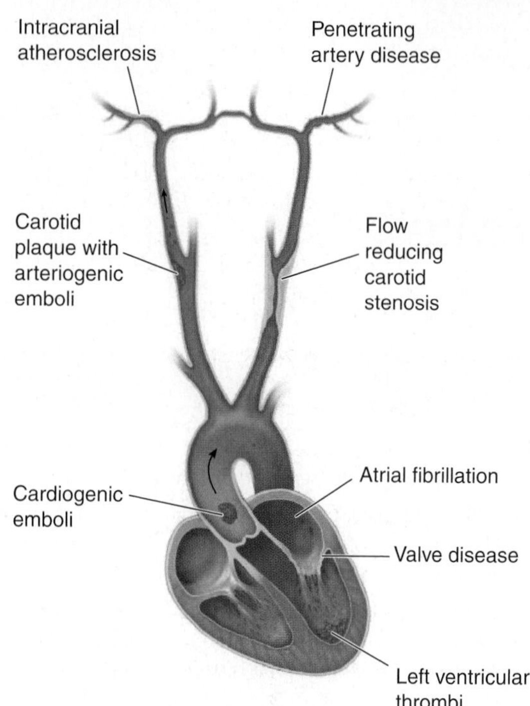

FIGURE 20-1 Pathophysiology of ischemic stroke. Diagram illustrating the three major mechanisms underlying ischemic stroke including occlusion of an intracranial vessel by an embolus that arises from a distant site (eg, cardiogenic embolus), in situ thrombosis of an intracranial vessel, typically affecting the small penetrating arteries, and hypoperfusion caused by flow-limiting stenosis of a major extracranial artery. *(Reproduced with permission from Chapter 370. Cerebrovascular Diseases. In: Longo DL, Fauci AS, Kasper DL, et al.* Harrison's Principals and Practice of Internal Medicine, *18th ed. New York: McGraw-Hill, 2012.)*

genetic factors. An individual's risk of having a stroke increases substantially as he or she ages, with a doubling of risk for each decade older than 55 years. African Americans, Asian-Pacific Islanders, and Hispanics experience higher death rates than their white counterparts.[2] Men are at a higher risk of stroke than women at younger ages, but women who suffer from a stroke are more likely to die from it.[2]

The most common modifiable, well-documented risk factors for stroke include hypertension, cigarette smoking, diabetes, atrial fibrillation, and dyslipidemia. Hypertension is the most common of all, affecting almost one in three adults in the United States. A second very important risk factor for stroke is cardiac disease. Patients with coronary artery disease, congestive heart failure, left ventricular hypertrophy, and especially atrial fibrillation are at increased risk of stroke.[5] In fact, the presence of atrial fibrillation is one of the most potent risk factors for ischemic stroke, with stroke rates from 5% to 20% per year depending on the patient's comorbid conditions.[5] Other known risk factors for atherosclerosis are also known to place patients at risk of stroke. Diabetes mellitus, dyslipidemia, and cigarette smoking are known atherogenic states that lead to cerebrovascular disease and ischemic stroke.[5]

PATHOPHYSIOLOGY

Ischemic Stroke

Ischemic stroke results from an occlusion of a cerebral artery, leading to a reduction in cerebral blood flow. The pathophysiologic mechanisms of ischemic stroke are given in Fig. 20-1. Normal cerebral blood flow averages 50 mL/100 g per minute, and this is maintained over a wide range of blood pressures (mean arterial pressures of 50-150 mm Hg) by a process called *cerebral autoregulation*. Cerebral blood vessels dilate and constrict in response to changes in blood pressure, but this process can be impaired by atherosclerosis, chronic hypertension, and acute injury, such as stroke. Arterial occlusion leads to severe reductions in cerebral blood flow leading to *infarction*. Tissue that is ischemic but maintains membrane integrity is referred to as the *ischemic penumbra* because it usually surrounds the infarct core.[6] This penumbra is potentially salvageable through therapeutic intervention and is assessed urgently prior to endovascular intervention with a stent retriever.

Reduction in the provision of nutrients to the ischemic cell eventually leads to depletion of the high-energy phosphates (eg, adenosine triphosphate [ATP]) and accumulation of extracellular potassium, intracellular sodium, and water, leading to cell swelling and eventual lysis. The increase in intracellular calcium that follows results in the activation of lipases, proteases, and endonucleases and the release of free fatty acids from membrane phospholipids. In addition, there is a release of excitatory amino acids, such as glutamate and aspartate, which perpetuate the neuronal damage and the accumulation of free fatty acids, including arachidonic acid, and result in the formation of prostaglandins, leukotrienes, and free radicals. In ischemia, the magnitude of free radical production overwhelms normal scavenging systems, leaving these reactive molecules to attack cell membranes and contribute to the mounting intracellular acidosis. All these events occur within 2 to 3 hours of the onset of ischemia and contribute to the ultimate cell death.[6]

Later targets for intervention in the pathophysiologic process involved after cerebral ischemia include inflammation and apoptosis, or programmed cell death, occurring many hours after the acute insult and can interfere with recovery and repair of brain tissue.[6]

Hemorrhagic Stroke

Intensive worldwide interest and attention has led to recent advances in the diagnosis and management of ICH. Urgent imaging of ICH patients has revealed that up to 38% expand dramatically more than 3 hours after the onset of symptoms and expansion is associated with worsened outcomes. Ultimately, clot volume is a very important predictor of outcome, and the ICH score has been shown to reliably predict 30-day mortality rates.[7] The highest mortality is seen in patients with low Glasgow Coma Score (GCS; 3-4), ICH volumes greater than 30 cc, intraventricular extension, brain stem involvement and age older than 80 years.[4] The presence of blood in the brain parenchyma causes mechanical compression of vulnerable tissue and subsequent activation of inflammation and neurotoxins. The molecular mediators of secondary brain injury and perihematomal edema are being investigated for potential therapeutic targets but no clinically proven pharmacologic intervention exists.[4]

CLINICAL PRESENTATION (INCLUDING DIAGNOSTIC CONSIDERATIONS)

Stroke is a term used to describe an abrupt-onset focal neurologic deficit that lasts at least 24 hours and is of presumed vascular origin. A TIA is the same but lasts less than 24 hours and usually less than 30 minutes. The abrupt onset and the duration of the symptoms are determined through the history. The use of sensitive imaging techniques (magnetic resonance imaging [MRI] with diffusion-weighted imaging [DWI]) has revealed that symptoms lasting more than 1 hour and less than 24 hours are associated with infarction, making TIA and minor stroke clinically indistinguishable. The location of the central nervous system (CNS) injury and its reference to a specific arterial distribution in the brain are determined through the neurologic examination and confirmed by imaging studies such as computed tomography (CT) scanning and MRI. The main arterial supply to the cerebral hemispheres is illustrated in Fig. 20-2. Further diagnostic tests are performed to identify the cause of the patient's stroke and to design appropriate therapeutic strategies to prevent further events.[8]

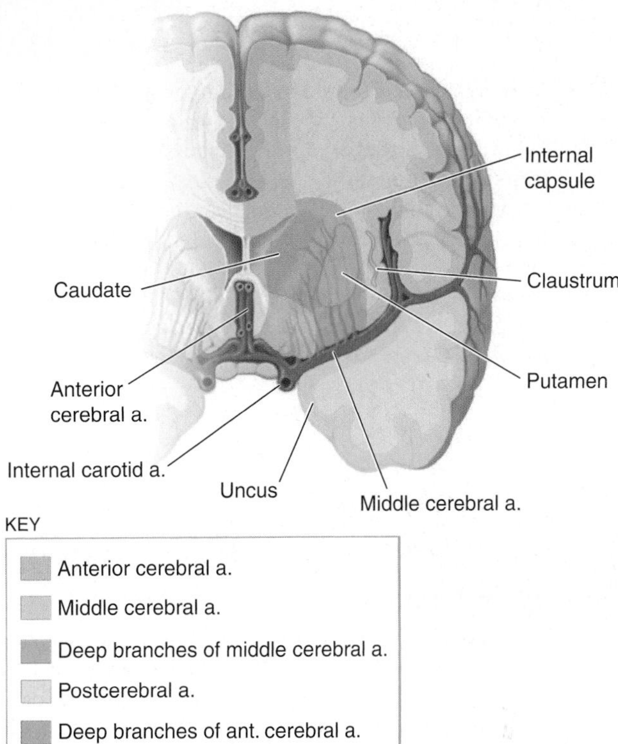

FIGURE 20-2 Diagram of a cerebral hemisphere in coronal section showing the territories of the major cerebral vessels branching from the internal carotid arteries. *(Reproduced with permission from Chapter 370. Cerebrovascular Diseases. In: Longo DL, Fauci AS, Kasper DL, et al.* Harrison's Principals and Practice of Internal Medicine, *18th ed. New York: McGraw-Hill, 2012.)*

CLINICAL PRESENTATION Stroke

General

- The patient may not be able to reliably report the history owing to cognitive or language deficits. A reliable history may have to come from a family member or another witness.

Symptoms

- The patient may complain of weakness on one side of the body, inability to speak, loss of vision, vertigo, or falling. Ischemic stroke is not usually painful, but patients may complain of headache, and with hemorrhagic stroke, it can be very severe.

Signs

- Patients usually have multiple signs of neurologic dysfunction, and the specific deficits are determined by the area of the brain involved.
- Hemiparesis or monoparesis occurs commonly, as does a hemisensory deficit.
- Patients with vertigo and double vision are likely to have posterior circulation involvement.
- Aphasia is seen commonly in patients with anterior circulation strokes.
- Patients may also suffer from dysarthria, visual field defects, and altered levels of consciousness.

Laboratory Tests

- Tests for hypercoagulable states (protein C deficiency, antiphospholipid antibody) should be done only when the cause of the stroke cannot be determined based on the presence of well-known risk factors for stroke. Protein C, protein S, and antithrombin III are best measured in the "steady state," not in the acute stage. Antiphospholipid antibodies as measured by anticardiolipin antibodies, β_2-glycoprotein I, and lupus anticoagulant screen are of higher yield than protein C, protein S, and antithrombin III but should be reserved for patients who are young (less than 50 years), have had multiple venous/arterial thrombotic events, or have livedo reticularis (a skin rash).

Other Diagnostic Tests

- CT scan of the head will reveal an area of hyperintensity (white) in the area of hemorrhage and will be normal or hypointense (dark) in the area of infarction. The CT scan may take 24 hours (and rarely longer) to reveal the area of infarction.
- MRI of the head will reveal areas of ischemia with higher resolution and earlier than the CT scan. DWI will reveal an evolving infarct within minutes.

(Continued)

CLINICAL PRESENTATION Stroke (*Continued*)

- Carotid Doppler (CD) studies will determine whether the patient has a high degree of stenosis in the carotid arteries supplying blood to the brain (extracranial disease).
- An electrocardiogram (ECG) will determine whether the patient has atrial fibrillation, a potent etiologic factor for stroke.
- Transthoracic echocardiography (TTE) will determine whether valve abnormalities or wall-motion abnormalities are sources of emboli to the brain. A "bubble test" can be done to look for an intra-atrial shunt indicating an atrial septal defect or a patent foramen ovale.
- Transesophageal echocardiography (TEE) is a more sensitive test for thrombus in the left atrium. It is effective at examining the aortic arch for atheroma, a potential source of emboli.
- Transcranial Doppler (TCD) will determine whether the patient is likely to have intracranial stenosis (eg, middle cerebral artery stenosis).

TREATMENT

Desired Outcomes

The goals of treatment of acute stroke are to (a) reduce the ongoing neurologic injury and decrease mortality and long-term disability, (b) prevent complications secondary to immobility and neurologic dysfunction, and (c) prevent stroke recurrence.[9] Primary prevention of stroke is reviewed elsewhere.[5]

General Approach to Treatment

The initial approach to the patient with a presumed acute stroke is to ensure that the patient is supported from a respiratory and cardiac standpoint and to quickly determine whether the lesion is ischemic or hemorrhagic, based on a CT scan. Ischemic stroke patients presenting within hours of the onset of their symptoms should be evaluated for reperfusion therapy. 3 TIAs also require urgent intervention to reduce the risk of stroke, which is known to be highest in the first few days after TIA.[10] According to the American Stroke Association guidelines, patients with elevated blood pressure should remain untreated unless their blood pressure exceeds 220/120 mm Hg, or they have evidence of aortic dissection, acute myocardial infarction (AMI), pulmonary edema, or hypertensive encephalopathy. If blood pressure is treated, short-acting parenteral agents, such as labetalol and nicardipine, are favored. Current recommendations regarding management of arterial hypertension in ischemic stroke patients are given in Table 20-2.[9] In ICH patients with blood pressure between 150 and 220 mm Hg systolic, early treatment designed to achieve a pressure of less than 140 mm Hg systolic has been shown to be safe and improve functional outcome.[7] Once the patient is out of the hyperacute phase, attention is placed on preventing worsening, minimizing complications, and instituting appropriate secondary prevention strategies. The acute phase of the stroke includes the first week after the event.[9]

TABLE 20-2 Blood Pressure Treatment Guidelines in Acute Ischemic Stroke Patients Treated with tPA

Treatment	Received tPA
None	<180/105
Labetalol IV[a] or nicardipine IV[b]	180-230/105-120
Nitroprusside[c]	Diastolic >120

tPA, tissue plasminogen activator.

[a]Labetalol IV: 10 mg, followed by an infusion of 2-8 mg/min.

[b]Nicardipine IV: infusion starting at 5 mg/h up to 15 mg/h.

[c]Nitroprusside IV: infusion starting at 0.5 mcg/kg/min, with continuous arterial blood pressure monitoring.

Data from reference 9.

Nonpharmacologic Therapy

Ischemic Stroke In 2015, AHA/ASA performed a focused update of the acute ischemic stroke guidelines to consider the evidence from eight clinical trials of endovascular intervention to reperfuse the ischemic brain.[11] Although early thrombectomy trials were disappointing, later investigations with more sophisticated devices called "stent retrievers" and careful selection of patients with proximal artery occlusions and salvageable tissue (on imaging), were universally positive. If administered within 6 hours of symptom onset (after intravenous [IV] tissue plasminogen activator [tPA]) in these patients, stent retrievers double the likelihood of recanalization, compared to tPA alone, and significantly increased the proportion of patients independent at 90 days (53%-70% vs 29.3%-40%). These findings dramatically changed the way in which stroke patients with large artery occlusion are managed in comprehensive stroke centers and increased the need for interventionalists in ischemic stroke care.

In less than 10% of patients with a large infarction in the middle cerebral artery territory, decompressive surgery to reduce intracranial pressure has been shown to significantly reduce mortality. However, the surgery must be performed within 48 hours of stroke onset in patients younger than 60 years to significantly improve functional outcome and this is at the cost of an increased number of surviving patients with severe disability.[12] In cases of significant swelling associated with a cerebellar infarction, surgical decompression can be lifesaving. Beyond surgical intervention, however, the use of an organized, multidisciplinary approach to stroke care that includes early rehabilitation has been shown to be very effective in reducing the ultimate disability owing to ischemic stroke. In fact, the use of "stroke units" has been associated with outcomes similar to those achieved with early thrombolysis when compared with usual care.[9]

4 In secondary prevention, carotid endarterectomy of an ulcerated and/or stenotic carotid artery is a very effective way to reduce stroke incidence and recurrence in appropriate patients and in centers where the operative morbidity and mortality are low. In fact, in ischemic stroke patients with 70% to 99% stenosis of an ipsilateral internal carotid artery, recurrent stroke risk can be reduced by up to 48% compared with medical therapy alone when combined with aspirin 325 mg daily.[13] In patients younger than 70 years, carotid stenting is a less invasive alternative and can be effective in reducing recurrent stroke risk.[14] However, in patients with intracranial stenosis, aggressive medical management was shown to be superior to stenting in reducing recurrent stroke.[15]

Hemorrhagic Stroke In patients with SAH owing to a ruptured intracranial aneurysm or AVM, surgical intervention to either clip or ablate the offending vascular abnormality substantially reduces mortality owing to rebleeding.[16] In the case of primary ICH, surgical evacuation may be of benefit in patients with intermediate hemorrhage volumes (20-50 mL) but this remains under investigation.[17] Insertion of an external ventricular drain (EVD) for hydrocephalus and subsequent monitoring of intracranial pressure are done commonly and are the least invasive of the procedures done in these patients.

Pharmacologic Therapy

Ischemic Stroke

Drug Treatments of First Choice: Published Guidelines The Stroke Council of the American Stroke Association have created and published guidelines that address the management of acute ischemic stroke.[9] For acute treatment, the only two pharmacologic agents with class I recommendations are IV tPA within 4.5 hours of onset and aspirin within 48 hours of onset.[9]

5 Early reperfusion (less than 4.5 hours from onset) with IV tPA has been shown to reduce the ultimate disability caused by ischemic stroke.[18,19] Caution must be exercised when using this therapy, and adherence to a strict protocol is essential to achieving positive outcomes.[9] The essentials of the treatment protocol can be summarized as (a) stroke team activation, (b) treatment as early as possible within 4.5 hours of onset, (c) CT scan to rule out hemorrhage, (d) meeting inclusion and exclusion criteria (Table 20-3), (e) administration of tPA 0.9 mg/kg over 1 hour, with 10% given as initial bolus over 1 minute, (f) avoidance of antithrombotic (anticoagulant or antiplatelet) therapy for 24 hours, and (g) close patient monitoring for elevated blood pressure, response, and hemorrhage.[9] 6 Endovascular thrombectomy with a stent retriever is indicated after tPA but within 6 hours, for patients with proximal vessel occlusion and a small core injury on imaging.[11]

Early aspirin therapy has also been shown to reduce long-term death and disability[20,21] but should never be given within 24 hours of the administration of tPA because it can increase the risk of bleeding in such patients.[9]

Antiplatelet therapy is the cornerstone of antithrombotic therapy for the secondary prevention of ischemic stroke and should be used in noncardioembolic strokes. Acetylsalicylic acid (ASA), extended-release dipyridamole plus aspirin (ERDP-ASA) and clopidogrel are all recommended for secondary stroke prevention.[10] In patients with atrial fibrillation and a presumed cardiac source of embolism, oral anticoagulation with either vitamin K antagonism (warfarin), apixaban, dabigatran, or rivaroxaban is recommended for secondary stroke prevention.[10] Other pharmacotherapy recommended for secondary prevention of stroke includes blood pressure lowering and statin therapy. Current recommendations regarding the acute treatment and secondary prevention of stroke are given in Table 20-4.

TABLE 20-3 Inclusion and Exclusion Criteria for tPA Use in Acute Ischemic Stroke[9]

Inclusion criteria
- Age 18 years or older
- Clinical diagnosis of ischemic stroke causing a measurable neurologic deficit
- Time of symptom onset well established to be <4.5 hours before treatment would begin

Exclusion criteria
- History of previous intracranial hemorrhage
- Symptoms suggestive of SAH
- Active internal bleeding
- Acute bleeding diathesis, including but not limited to a platelet count <100,000/mm³ (<100 × 10¹²/L)
- Patient has received heparin within 48 hours, resulting in an elevated APTT
- Recent anticoagulant use and elevated INR (>1.7) or PT (>15 seconds)
- Current use of direct thrombin inhibitors or direct factor Xa inhibitors with elevated sensitive laboratory tests (such as aPTT, INR, platelet count, and ECT; TT; or appropriate factor Xa activity assays)
- Significant head trauma or previous stroke within 3 months
- Arterial puncture at noncompressible site within 7 days
- Intracranial neoplasm, arteriovenous malformation, or aneurysm
- SBP >185 mm Hg or DBP >110 mm Hg
- Blood glucose <50 mg/dL (2.7 mmol/L)
- CT demonstrates multilobar infarction (hypodensity >1/3 cerebral hemisphere)

Relative exclusion criteria (considering risk to benefit in individual patients, may be wise to administer tPA despite 1 or more of the following:)
- Only minor or rapidly improving symptoms
- Pregnancy
- Seizure at onset with postictal residual impairments
- Major surgery or serious trauma within 14 days
- Gastrointestinal or urinary tract hemorrhage within 21 days
- Acute myocardial infarction within 3 months

Additional exclusion criteria if within 3–4.5 hours of onset:
- Age greater than 80 years
- Current treatment with oral anticoagulants
- NIH Stroke Scale Score >25 (severe stroke)
- Imaging evidence of large infarct (>1/3 MCA territory)
- History of both stroke and diabetes

APTT, activated partial thromboplastin time; CT, computed tomography; DBP, diastolic blood pressure; ECT, Ecarin clotting time; INR, international normalized ratio; MCA, middle cerebral artery; PT, prothrombin time; SBP, systolic blood pressure; SAH, subarachnoid hemorrhage; TT, thrombin time.

General Information Regarding Safety and Efficacy (Including Pivotal Clinical Trials)

tPA The effectiveness of IV tPA in the treatment of ischemic stroke was first demonstrated in the National Institute of Neurologic Disorders and Stroke (NINDS) Recombinant Tissue-Type Plasminogen Activator (rtPA) Stroke Trial, published in 1995.[18] In 624 patients treated in equal numbers with either tPA 0.9 mg/kg IV or placebo

TABLE 20-4 Recommendations for Pharmacotherapy of Ischemic Stroke

	Recommendation	Evidence[a]
Acute treatment	tPA 0.9 mg/kg IV[9] (maximum 90 mg) over 1 hour in selected patients within 3 hours of onset	IA
	tPA 0.9 mg/kg IV[9] (maximum 90 mg) over 1 hour between 3 and 4.5 hours of onset	IB
	ASA 160-325 mg daily[9] started within 48 hours of onset	IA
Secondary prevention		
Noncardioembolic	Antiplatelet therapy	IA
	Aspirin 50-325 mg daily[10]	IB
	Aspirin 25 mg + extended-release dipyridamole	IB
	200 mg twice daily[10]	
	Clopidogrel 75 mg daily[10]	IIaB
Cardioembolic (especially atrial fibrillation)	VKA (INR = 2.5)[10]	IA
	Apixaban 5 mg twice daily[10]	IA
	Dabigatran 150 mg twice daily[10]	IB
	Rivaroxaban 20 mg daily[10]	IIaB
Atherosclerosis + LDL > 100 mg/dL	High intensity statin therapy[10]	IB
BP > 140/90	BP reduction[10]	IB

ASA, acetylsalicylic acid; INR, international normalized ratio; IV, intravenous; LDL, low-density lipoprotein; tPA, tissue plasminogen activator; VKA, vitamin K antagonist.

[a]Classes: I, evidence or general agreement about usefulness and effectiveness; II, conflicting evidence about the usefulness; IIa, weight of evidence in favor of the treatment; IIb, usefulness less well established; III, not useful and maybe harmful. Levels of evidence: A, multiple randomized clinical trials; B, a single randomized trial or nonrandomized studies; C, expert opinion or case studies.[10]

Data from references 9 and 10.

within 3 hours of the onset of their neurologic symptoms, 39% of the treated patients achieved an "excellent outcome" at 3 months compared with 26% of the placebo patients. An "excellent outcome" was defined as minimal or no disability by several different neurologic scales. This beneficial effect was reported despite a 10-fold increase in the risk of symptomatic ICH in the tPA-treated patients (0.6% vs 6.4%). Overall mortality was not significantly different between the two groups (17% with tPA and 21% with placebo). Patients with very severe symptoms at baseline (National Institutes of Health Stroke Scale [NIHSS] greater than 20) and early ischemic changes on CT scan were shown to be at highest risk for the development of symptomatic intracranial hemorrhage. Even in patients at highest risk for bleeding, however, those receiving tPA had better outcomes at 90 days than those who received placebo.[18]

Thirteen years after the NINDS trial, the European Cooperative Acute Stroke Study (ECASS) III demonstrated that, even when administered between 3 and 4.5 hours after the onset of symptoms, ischemic stroke patients benefit from tPA when compared with placebo (52.4% vs 45.2% excellent outcome; $P = 0.04$).[19] The benefit was less than that reported with earlier treatment but the rate of excess hemorrhage was similar, leading to a change in AHA guidelines to recommend extension of the window.[9] An important caveat was that the exclusion criteria for later treatment are more strict and are given in Table 20-3. The International Stroke Trial (IST)-3 reported subsequently, in a large group of 3,035 patients treated within 6 hours of ischemic stroke onset, that even patients outside the rigid criteria set forth by both the NINDS and ECASS III trials may experience improved functional outcome.[22] These investigators advocate that patients over the age of 80, presenting outside the 3-hour treatment window, may benefit from a personalized assessment of risk and benefit prior to excluding them from thrombolytic therapy.

ASA The use of early ASA to reduce long-term death and disability owing to ischemic stroke is supported by two large randomized clinical trials. In the IST,[21] aspirin 300 mg/day significantly reduced stroke recurrence within the first 2 weeks without effect on early mortality, resulting in a significant decrease in death and dependency at 6 months. In the Chinese Acute Stroke Trial (CAST),[20] aspirin 160 mg/day reduced the risk of recurrence and death in the first 28 days, but long-term death and disability were not different than with placebo. In both trials, a small but significant increase in hemorrhagic transformation of the infarction was demonstrated. Overall, the beneficial effects of early aspirin have been embraced and adopted into clinical guidelines.

Antiplatelet Agents All patients who have had an acute ischemic stroke or TIA should receive long-term antithrombotic therapy for secondary prevention.[10] 7 In patients with noncardioembolic stroke, this will be some form of antiplatelet therapy. In a comprehensive meta-analysis, the overall benefit of antiplatelet therapy in patients with atherothrombotic disorders was estimated to be 22%.[23] ASA is the best studied of the available agents but published literature has supported the use of the combination product ERDP-ASA and clopidogrel as additional first-line agents in secondary stroke prevention.[10]

In the European Stroke Prevention Study 2 (ESPS-2), ASA 25 mg and ERDP 200 mg twice daily were compared alone and in combination with placebo for their ability to reduce recurrent stroke over a 2-year period.[24] In a total of more than 6,600 patients, all three treatment groups were shown to be superior to placebo—ASA alone (18% relative risk reduction [RRR]), ERDP alone (16% RRR), and the combination (37% RRR). In addition, the combination demonstrated a significant advantage over the ASA-alone group (23% RRR; $P = 0.006$) and the ERDP-alone group (24% RRR; $P = 0.002$). Headache resulting in discontinuation occurred in approximately 15% of the ERDP groups (four times more common than in the placebo group), and the ASA-treated patients, even at the low dose of 50 mg/day, experienced significantly more bleeding than the other groups. In a large, multinational trial (Prevention Regimen for Effectively Avoiding Second Strokes [PRoFESS]) comparing ERDP-ASA with clopidogrel, the risk of recurrent stroke was similar for the two antiplatelet agents, but clopidogrel was better tolerated with less bleeding and headache.[25]

The efficacy of clopidogrel as an antiplatelet agent in atherothrombotic disorders was demonstrated in the Clopidogrel versus Aspirin in Patients at Risk of Ischemic Events (CAPRIE) trial.[26] In this study of more than 19,000 patients with a history of myocardial infarction (MI), stroke, or peripheral arterial disease (PAD), clopidogrel 75 mg/day was compared with ASA 325 mg/day for its ability to decrease MI, stroke, or cardiovascular death. In the final analysis, clopidogrel was slightly (8% RRR) more effective than ASA ($P = 0.043$) and had a similar incidence of adverse effects. It is not associated with the blood dyscrasias (neutropenia) common with its congener, ticlopidine, and is used widely in patients with atherosclerosis.

Oral Anticoagulants 8 Oral anticoagulation is the treatment of choice for the prevention of stroke in patients with atrial fibrillation.[5,10] In patients with atrial fibrillation and a recent history of stroke or TIA, the risk of recurrence places these patients in one of the highest risk categories known. In the European Atrial Fibrillation Trial (EAFT), 669 patients with nonvalvular atrial fibrillation (NVAF) and a prior stroke or TIA were randomized to warfarin (international normalized ratio [INR] = 2.5-4), ASA 300 mg/day, or placebo. Patients in the placebo group experienced stroke, MI, or vascular death at a rate of 17% per year compared with 8% per year in the warfarin group and 15% per year in the ASA group. This represents a 53% reduction in risk with anticoagulation.[27] Subsequent studies in the primary prevention of stroke in patients with NVAF have demonstrated that targeting an INR of 2.5 prevents stroke with the lowest bleeding risk (Stroke Prevention in Atrial Fibrillation [SPAF III]); therefore, a target INR of 2.5 is recommended in the secondary prevention of stroke.[5,10] Newer oral anticoagulants including dabigatran (direct thrombin inhibitor), rivaroxaban, and apixaban (direct factor Xa inhibitors) have significant advantages over warfarin in terms of ease of dosing and less food and drug interactions. In addition, in the prevention of stroke in selected patients with atrial fibrillation, all three agents have been shown to be as effective as, and in some cases, superior to, warfarin in reducing recurrent events and intracranial hemorrhage.[28-30]

Blood Pressure Lowering 9 Elevated blood pressure is very common in ischemic stroke patients, and treatment of hypertension in these patients is associated with a decreased risk of stroke recurrence.[38] In the Perindopril pROtection aGainst REcurrent Stroke Study (PROGRESS), a multinational stroke population (40% Asian) was randomized to receive either blood pressure lowering with the angiotensin-converting enzyme (ACE) inhibitor perindopril (with or without the thiazide diuretic indapamide) or placebo.[31] Treated patients achieved an overall 9 mm Hg systolic and 4 mm Hg diastolic blood pressure reduction, and this was associated with a 28% reduction in stroke recurrence. In the patients who received the combination treatment (clinician's discretion), the average blood pressure lowering achieved was 12 mm Hg systolic and 5 mm Hg diastolic, and this was associated with an even larger reduction in stroke recurrence (43%). Similar results were achieved in patients with and without hypertension. AHA/ASA guidelines recommend reduction of blood pressure greater than 140/90 in patients with stroke or TIA.[10] 10 Early blood pressure lowering can worsen symptoms; however, therefore, recommendations are limited to patients outside of the acute stroke period (first 7 days).[10]

Statins The statins have been shown to reduce the risk of stroke by approximately 30% in patients with coronary artery disease and elevated plasma lipids.[32] The Stroke Prevention by Aggressive

Reduction in Cholesterol (SPARCL) study demonstrated that atorvastatin 80 mg daily reduced the risk of recurrent stroke by 16% and coronary events by 42% in patients with no cardiac history. Although the high-dose statin caused an increase in liver enzymes, there was no increase in myopathy.[33] It is now recommended that patients experiencing ischemic stroke of presumed atherosclerotic origin, with low-density lipoprotein (LDL) greater than 100 mg/dL, be treated with high-intensity statin therapy for secondary stroke prevention.[10]

Heparin for Prophylaxis of Deep Vein Thrombosis (DVT) The use of low-molecular-weight heparins or low-dose subcutaneous unfractionated heparin (5,000 units three times daily) can be recommended for the prevention of DVT in hospitalized patients with decreased mobility owing to their stroke and should be used in all but the most minor strokes.[9] In ICH patients, intermittent pneumatic compression (IPC) devices in combination with thigh high elastic stockings should be employed for DVT prophylaxis until the risk of further expansion of the hematoma is thought to be low.[7]

Alternative Drug Treatments

ASA Plus Clopidogrel In the Management of AТherothrombosis with Clopidogrel in High-risk patients (MATCH) study, clopidogrel in combination with ASA 75 mg daily was no better than clopidogrel alone in secondary stroke prevention.[34] Also, when clopidogrel was used with ASA, the risk of life-threatening bleeding increased from 1.3% to 2.6%.[34] Again, in the Stroke Prevention in Subcortical Stroke (SPS)-3 trial of patients with recent minor strokes, the arm of the trial studying the combination of clopidogrel and ASA was stopped early because of excess mortality due to bleeding in this group.[35] However, the combination has been studied in patients with TIA or minor stroke, and short-term (3-month) use of the combination of clopidogrel and ASA was associated with improved outcomes.[36]

Heparins The use of full-dose unfractionated heparin in the acute stroke period has never been proven to positively affect stroke outcome, and it significantly increases the risk of ICH. Trials of low-molecular-weight heparins or heparinoids have been largely negative and do not support their routine use in stroke patients.[37-39] Other potential but unproven uses for treatment doses of either unfractionated or low-molecular-weight heparins include bridge therapy in patients being initiated on warfarin, carotid dissection, or continuous worsening of ischemia despite adequate antiplatelet therapy.[40]

Drug Class Information

ASA ASA exerts its antiplatelet effect by irreversibly inhibiting cyclooxygenase, which, in platelets, prevents conversion of arachidonic acid to thromboxane A_2 (TXA_2), which is a powerful vasoconstrictor and stimulator of platelet aggregation. Platelets remain impaired for their life span (5-7 days) after exposure to aspirin. ASA also inhibits prostacyclin (PGI_2) activity in the smooth muscle of vascular walls. PGI_2 inhibits platelet aggregation, and the vascular endothelium can synthesize PGI_2 such that the platelet antiaggregating effect is maintained.[40] There is probably a point at which lower doses of ASA do not completely block TXA_2, and recent studies indicate that the lowest effective dose may be in the range of 50 mg/day.[41] Upper gastrointestinal (GI) discomfort and bleeding are the most common adverse effects of ASA and have been shown to be dose related. The highest rates of GI bleeding (5%) have been reported in patients receiving 1,200 mg/day as compared with rates of 2% in patients taking the more commonly prescribed 300 mg/day. Upper GI symptoms are much more common than frank bleeding; however, with 40% of patients affected at 1,200 mg/day and 25% at 300 mg/day.[42] In the ESPS-2 study, even 50 mg/day of ASA was associated with a twofold increase in bleeding over the placebo group.[24]

The onset of the antiplatelet effect of ASA is less than 60 minutes.[43] It has been reported, however, that some patients either have or develop "aspirin resistance" and can require higher doses to achieve the desired antiplatelet effect.[44] Despite this, routine testing for ASA resistance is not recommended. It was observed that administration of ibuprofen prior to the administration of a daily aspirin dose inhibits the ASA from binding irreversibly to the cyclooxygenase and can decrease its antiplatelet effect.[45] Current recommendations are to administer ASA at least 2 hours before ibuprofen or to wait at least 4 hours after an ibuprofen dose.

Clopidogrel Clopidogrel has a unique platelet antiaggregatory effect in that it is an inhibitor of the adenosine diphosphate (ADP) pathway of platelet aggregation and inhibits known stimuli to platelet aggregation.[26,40] This effect causes an alteration of the platelet membrane and interference with the membrane–fibrinogenic interaction leading to a blocking of the platelet glycoprotein IIb/IIIa receptor. A time lag of 3 to 7 days before the antiplatelet effect is maximal should be expected. The tolerability of clopidogrel 75 mg/day is at least as good as medium-dose (325 mg/day) ASA, and there is less GI bleeding.[26] Clopidogrel is associated with an increased risk of diarrhea and rash, but discontinuation rates owing to adverse effects are similar to those with ASA 325 mg/day (5.3% and 6%, respectively).[26] There is no excess neutropenia in patients taking clopidogrel, and rates of thrombotic thrombocytopenic purpura probably are no greater than background rate.

Extended-Release Dipyridamole Plus ASA Early studies of the role of dipyridamole in stroke prevention failed to show a benefit over that realized by ASA alone. Dipyridamole in high doses is thought to inhibit platelet aggregation by inhibiting phosphodiesterase, leading to accumulation of cyclic adenosine monophosphate (cAMP) and cyclic guanosine monophosphate (cGMP) intracellularly, which prevent platelet activation. In addition, dipyridamole also enhances the antithrombotic potential of the vascular wall.[46] The ESPS-2 demonstrated the efficacy of high-dose ERDP alone and in combination with ASA in secondary stroke prevention.[24] The extended-release formulation of dipyridamole is important in that it allows twice-daily administration and higher doses to be tolerated in patients. The use of immediate-release generic dipyridamole in combination with regular ASA, in order to reduce costs, is unproven and should be discouraged.

In the ESPS-2, 25% of the patients who received combination dipyridamole and ASA discontinued the therapy early, and the rate of discontinuation owing to headache was more than three times as common (10%) as in the aspirin-alone group (3%).[24] Even when patients were carefully educated and coached in the PRoFESS trial, discontinuation due to headache was six times higher in the ERDP-ASA group (5.9% vs 0.9%).[25]

Investigational Strategies

Neuroprotection and Neurorestoration Although many different neuroprotective agents have been studied in clinical trials of acute ischemic stroke, all have been unsuccessful[47] and the drug development pipeline for acute neuroprotection is essentially nonexistent. However, hope exists that clinicians will be able to enhance the reparative process of the brain (neurorestoration) through targeted neurorehabilitation, growth factor enhancement, and the use of neural and cell transplantation.[48]

Hemorrhagic Stroke

There are currently no standard pharmacologic strategies for treating ICH.[7] Medical guidelines for the management of blood pressure, raised intracranial pressure, and other medical complications of ICH are those required for the management of any acutely ill patient in a neurointensive care unit.[7] When ICH occurs in a patient on oral anticoagulants, reversal of anticoagulation to prevent expansion and allow surgical intervention is recommended. The methods recommended to achieve reversal include IV vitamin K, fresh-frozen plasma (FFP), and hemostatic agents (factor VIIa and prothrombin complex concentrate [PCC]).[7] All patients with warfarin-associated ICH should receive IV vitamin K and therapy to replace the affected clotting factors. PCC has advantages over FFP alone in this regard in that it results in a faster normalization of the INR and less chance of fluid overload. In a large clinical trial, 4-factor PCC was noninferior to FFP alone in warfarin reversal with no excess in thromboembolic events: 7.4% versus 6.4%, respectively.[49]

SAH owing to aneurysm rupture is associated with a high incidence of delayed cerebral ischemia (DCI) in the 2 weeks following the bleeding episode. Vasospasm of the cerebral vasculature is thought to be responsible for DCI and occurs between 4 and 21 days after the bleed, peaking at days 5 to 9.[16] The calcium channel blocker nimodipine (60 mg every 4 hours for 21 days), along with maintenance of intravascular volume with pressor therapy, is recommended to reduce the incidence and severity of neurologic deficits owing to DCI.[16]

PERSONALIZED PHARMACOTHERAPY

Clopidogrel is a thienopyridine prodrug and needs to be biotransformed by the liver to an active metabolite. Evidence suggests that the antiplatelet effects of clopidogrel can be diminished in patients with reduced-function cytochrome P450 2C19 (CYP2C19)[50] or in those receiving agents that inhibit hepatic metabolism.[51] In patients receiving clopidogrel after stent placement, reduced-function CYP2C19 is associated with an increase in recurrent vascular events.[51] Although high doses of the lipophilic statins atorvastatin and simvastatin can diminish the effectiveness of clopidogrel to inhibit platelet aggregation in vitro, there does not appear to be any adverse effect on atherothrombotic event rates.[52] In contrast, in a retrospective analysis of 8,205 patients, concomitant proton pump inhibitor and clopidogrel treatment was associated with increased adverse vascular outcomes after acute coronary syndromes.[50] Careful consideration should be given to using clopidogrel in patients with reduced ability to biotransform the agent to its active metabolite.

The availability of genetic testing to identify patients with altered sensitivity to warfarin has led to questions regarding the ability of the tests to improve patient care. Polymorphisms in CYP2C9 and vitamin K epoxide reductase complex subunit 1 (VKORC1) contribute to the variability in warfarin response, but it is unclear whether knowledge of these genetic variations will improve dosing accuracy and reduce adverse events.[53] Clinical trial evidence is needed prior to instituting these tests in stroke patients who are candidates for warfarin therapy.

EVALUATION OF THERAPEUTIC OUTCOMES

Monitoring of the Pharmaceutical Care Plan

Patients with acute stroke should be monitored intensely for the development of neurologic worsening (recurrence or extension), complications (thromboembolism or infection), or adverse effects from pharmacologic or nonpharmacologic interventions. The most common reasons for deterioration in a stroke patient are (a) extension of the original lesion—ischemic or hemorrhagic—in the brain, (b) development of cerebral edema and raised intracranial pressure, (c) hypertensive emergency, (d) infection (urinary and respiratory most common), (e) venous thromboembolism (DVT and pulmonary embolism), (f) electrolyte abnormalities and cardiac rhythm disturbances (can be associated with brain injury), and (g) recurrent stroke.

The approach to monitoring drug therapy in the hospitalized stroke patient is summarized in Table 20-5. The plan should be customized for individual patients based on their comorbidities and ongoing disease processes.

TABLE 20-5 Monitoring Stroke Therapy

Drug	Adverse Effect	Monitoring Parameters	Comments
tPA	Bleeding	Neurologic examination	Every 15 minutes × 1 hour; every 0.5 hour × 6 hours; every 1 hour × 17 hours; every shift after
ASA	Bleeding		Daily
Clopidogrel	Bleeding		Daily
ERDP-ASA	Headache, bleeding		Daily
Warfarin	Bleeding	INR, Hb/Hct	Daily
Oral anticoagulants	Bleeding		Daily

ERDP-ASA, extended-release dipyridamole plus aspirin; Hb/Hct, hemoglobin/hematocrit; INR, international normalized ratio; tPA, tissue plasminogen activator.

Clinical Controversy...

It is unclear when it is safe to start oral anticoagulation with one of the newer agents (apixaban, dabigatran, or rivaroxaban) in a stroke patient with atrial fibrillation and a large infarction.

In patients requiring rapid reversal of warfarin anticoagulation in the setting of ICH, it is unclear whether to target an INR of less than 1.3 or less than 1.5.

ABBREVIATIONS

ACE	angiotensin-converting enzyme
ADP	adenosine diphosphate
AHA	American Heart Association
AMI	acute myocardial infarction
ASA	acetylsalicylic acid
ATP	adenosine triphosphate
AVM	arteriovenous malformation
cAMP	cyclic adenosine monophosphate
CAPRIE	Clopidogrel versus Aspirin in Patients at Risk of Ischemic Events
CAST	Chinese Acute Stroke Trial
CD	carotid Doppler
cGMP	cyclic guanosine monophosphate
CNS	central nervous system
CT scan	computed tomographic scan
CYP2C19	cytochrome P450 2C19
DCI	delayed cerebral ischemia
DVT	deep vein thrombosis
DWI	diffusion-weighted imaging
EAFT	European Atrial Fibrillation Trial
ECASS	European Cooperative Acute Stroke Study
ECG	electrocardiogram
ERDP	extended-release dipyridamole
ESPS-2	European Stroke Prevention Study 2
EVD	external ventricular drainage
FFP	fresh-frozen plasma
GCS	Glasgow Coma Score

GI	gastrointestinal
ICH	intracerebral hemorrhage
INR	international normalized ratio
IPC	intermittent pneumatic compression
IST	International Stroke Trial
LDL	low-density lipoprotein
MATCH	Management of ATherothrombosis with Clopidogrel in High-risk patients
MI	myocardial infarction
MRI	magnetic resonance imaging
NIHSS	National Institutes of Health Stroke Scale
NINDS	National Institute of Neurologic Disorders and Stroke
NVAF	nonvalvular atrial fibrillation
PAD	peripheral arterial disease
PCC	prothrombin complex concentrate
PGI_2	prostacyclin
PRoFESS	Prevention Regimen for Effectively Avoiding Second Strokes
PROGRESS	Perindopril pROtection aGainst REcurrent Stroke Study
RRR	relative risk reduction
rtPA	recombinant tissue-type plasminogen activator
SAH	subarachnoid hemorrhage
SPAF III	Stroke Prevention in Atrial Fibrillation
SPARCL	Stroke Prevention by Aggressive Reduction in Cholesterol
SPS	Stroke Prevention in Subcortical Stroke
TCD	transcranial Doppler
TEE	transesophageal echocardiography
TIA	transient ischemic attack
tPA	tissue plasminogen activator
TTE	transthoracic echocardiography
TXA_2	thromboxane A_2
VKORC1	vitamin K epoxide reductase complex subunit 1

REFERENCES

1. Kochanek KD, Murphy SL, Xu J, Arias E. Mortality in the United States, 2013. National Center for Health Statistics. Centers for Disease Control and Prevention. US Department of Health and Human Services, No. 178, December, 2014.
2. Mozaffarian D, Benjamin EJ, Go AS, et al. Heart disease and stroke statistics—2015 update: A report from the American Heart Association. *Circulation* 2015:131, January 27, 2015.
3. Howard VJ, McClure LA, Meschia JF, Pulley L, Orr SC, Friday GH. High prevalence of stroke symptoms among persons without a diagnosis of stroke or transient ischemic attack in a general population: The Reasons for Geographic and Racial Differences in Stroke (REGARDS) Study. *Arch Int Med* 2006;166:1952-1958.
4. Godoy DA, Pinero GR, Koller P, Masotti L, Napoli M. Steps to consider in the approach and management of critically ill patient with spontaneous intracerebral hemorrhage. *World J Crit Care Med* 2015;4:213-229.
5. Meschia JF, Bushnell C, Boden-Albala B, et al. Guidelines for the primary prevention of ischemic stroke. A guideline for healthcare professionals from the American Heart Association/American Stroke Association. *Stroke* 2014;45(12):3754-3832.
6. Xing C, Arai K, Lo EH, Hommel M. Pathophysiologic cascades in ischemic stroke. *Int J Stroke* 2012;7:378-385.
7. Hemphill JC, Greenberg SM, Anderson CS, et al. Guidelines for the management of spontaneous intracerebral hemorrhage. A guideline for healthcare professionals from the American Heart Association/American Stroke Association. *Stroke* 2015;46:2032-2060.
8. Smith WS, English JD, Johnston SC. Cerebrovascular diseases. In: Longo DL, Fauci AS, Kasper DL, et al., eds. *Harrison's Principles of Internal Medicine*, 18th ed. New York: McGraw-Hill, 2012:3270-3299.
9. Jauch EC, Saver JL, Adams HP, et al. Guidelines for the early management of patients with ischemic stroke: A guideline for healthcare professionals from the American Heart Association/American Stroke Association. Stroke 2013;44:870-947.
10. Kernan WN, Ovbiogele B, Black HR, et al. Guidelines for the prevention of stroke in patients with stroke and transient ischemic attack: A guidelines for healthcare professionals from the American Heart Association/American Stroke Association. *Stroke* 2014;45:2160-2236.
11. Powers WJ, Derdeyn CP, Biller J, et al. 2015 AHA/ASA Focused update of the 2013 guidelines for the early management of patients with acute ischemic stroke regarding endovascular treatment. A guideline for health professionals from the American Heart Association/American Stroke Association. *Stroke* 2015;46, June 29 [Stroke 2015;46(10):3020-3035].
12. Wijdicks EFM, Sheth K, Carter BS, et al. Recommendations for the management of cerebral and cerebellar infarction with swelling: A statement for healthcare professionals from the American Heart Association/American Stroke Association. 2014;45:1222-1238.
13. Cina CA, Clase CM, Haynes RB. Carotid endarterectomy for symptomatic carotid stenosis [Cochrane review on CD-ROM]. In: The Cochrane Library, Issue 1. Oxford: Update Software, 2001.
14. Brott TG, Hobson RW, Howard G, et al. Stenting versus endarterectomy for treatment of carotid artery stenosis. *N Engl J Med* 2010;363:11-23.
15. Chimowitz MI, Lynn MJ, Derdeyn CP, et al. Stenting versus aggressive medical therapy for intracranial arterial stenosis. *N Engl J Med* 2011;365:993-1003.
16. Connolly ES, Rabinstein AA, Carhuapoma JR, et al. Guidelines for the management of aneurysmal subarachnoid hemorrhage. A guideline for healthcare professionals from the American Heart Association/American Stroke Association. *Stroke* 2012;43:1711-1717.
17. Gregson BA, Broderick JP, Auer LM, et al. Individual patient data subgroup meta analysis of surgery for spontaneous supratentorial intracerebral hemorrhage. *Stroke* 2012;43:1496-1504.
18. The National Institute of Neurological Disorders and Stroke rt-PA Stroke Study Group. Tissue plasminogen activator for acute ischemic stroke. *N Engl J Med* 1995;333:1581-1587.
19. Hacke W, Kaste M, Bluhmki E, et al. Thrombolysis with alteplase 3 to 4.5 hours after acute ischemic stroke. *N Engl J Med* 2008;359:1317-1329.
20. Chinese Acute Stroke Trial (CAST) Collaborative Group. CAST: A randomized, placebo-controlled trial of early aspirin use in 20,000 patients with acute ischemic stroke. *Lancet* 1997;349:1641-1649.
21. International Stroke Trial Collaborative Group. The International Stroke Trial (IST): A randomized trial of aspirin, subcutaneous heparin, both, or neither among 19,435 patients with acute ischemic stroke. *Lancet* 1997;349:1560-1581.
22. The IST-3 Collaborative Group. The benefits and harms of intravenous thrombolysis with recombinant tissue plasminogen activator within 6 h of acute ischaemic stroke (the third international stroke trial [IST-3]): A randomized controlled trial. *Lancet* 2012;379:2352-2363 [Epub ahead of print]. doi:10.1016/50140-6736(12)60768-5.
23. Antithrombotic Trialists' Collaboration. Collaborative meta analysis of randomized trials of antiplatelet therapy for prevention of death, myocardial infarction, and stroke in high risk patients. *BMJ* 2002;324:71-86.
24. Diener HC, Cunha L, Forbes C, et al. European Stroke Prevention Study 2: Dipyridamole and acetylsalicylic acid in the secondary prevention of stroke. *J Neurol Sci* 1996;143:1-13.
25. Sacco RL, Diener HC, Yusuf S, et al. Aspirin and extended-release dipyridamole versus clopidogrel for recurrent stroke. *N Engl J Med* 2008;359:1238-1251.
26. CAPRIE Steering Committee. A randomized, blinded trial of clopidogrel versus aspirin in patients at risk of ischaemic events (CAPRIE). *Lancet* 1995;348:1329-1339.
27. European Atrial Fibrillation Trial Study Group. Secondary prevention in nonrheumatic atrial fibrillation after transient ischaemic attack or minor stroke. *Lancet* 1993;342:1255-1262.
28. Connolly SJ, Ezekowitz MD, Yusuf S, et al. Dabigatran versus warfarin in patients with atrial fibrillation. *N Engl J Med* 2009;361(12):1139-1151.
29. Granger CB, Alexander JH, McMurray JJV, et al. Apixaban versus warfarin in patients with atrial fibrillation. *N Engl J Med* 2011;August 28; 365(11):981-992.
30. Patel MR, Mahaffey KW, Garg J, et al. Rivaroxaban versus warfarin in nonvalvular atrial fibrillation. *N Engl J Med* 2011; August 10; 365(10):883-891.
31. PROGRESS Collaborative Group. Randomized trial of perindopril-based blood-pressure-lowering regimen among 6105 individuals with previous stroke or transient ischaemic attack. *Lancet* 2001;358:1033-1041.
32. Hebert PR, Gaziano JM, Chan KS, Hennekens CH. Cholesterol lowering with statin drugs, risk of stroke, and total mortality: An overview of randomized trials. *JAMA* 1997;278:313-321.
33. The Stroke Prevention by Aggressive Reduction in Cholesterol Levels (SPARCL) Investigators. High-dose atorvastatin after stroke or transient ischemic attack. *N Engl J Med* 2006;355:549-559.

34. Diener HC, Bogousslavsky J, Brass LM, et al. Aspirin and clopidogrel compared with clopidogrel alone after recent ischemic stroke or transient ischaemic attack in high-risk patients (MATCH): Randomized, double-blind, placebo-controlled trial. *Lancet* 2004;364:331-337.
35. The SPS3 Investigators. Effects of clopidogrel added to aspirin in patients with recent lacunar stroke. *N Engl J Med* 2012;367:817-825.
36. Wang Y, Wang Y, Zhou X, et al. Clopidogrel with aspirin in acute minor stroke or transient ischemic attack. *N Engl J Med* 2013;June 26; 369(1): 11-19.
37. The Publications Committee for the Trial of ORG 10172 in Acute Stroke Treatment (TOAST) Investigators. Low-molecular-weight heparinoid, ORG 10172 (danaparoid), and outcome after acute ischemic stroke: A randomized, controlled trial. *JAMA* 1998;279:1265-1272.
38. Bath PM, Lidenstrom E, Boysen G, et al. Tinzaparin in acute ischaemic stroke (TAIST): A randomized, aspirin-controlled trial. *Lancet* 2001;358:702-710.
39. Berge E, Abdelnoor M, Nakstad PH, et al. Low-molecular-weight heparin versus aspirin in patients with acute ischaemic stroke and atrial fibrillation: A double-blind, randomised study. HAEST Study Group. Heparin in Acute Embolic Stroke Trial. *Lancet* 2000;355:1205-1210.
40. Lansberg MG, O'Donnell MJ, Khatri P, et al. Antithrombotic and thrombolytic therapy for ischemic stroke: Antithrombotic therapy and prevention of thrombosis, 9th ed: American College of Chest Physicians evidence-based clinical practice guidelines. *Chest* 2012;141:e601S-e636S.
41. Food and Drug Administration. FDA Approves New Prescribed Uses for Aspirin. FDA Talk Paper T98-76. 1998, *www.fda.gov/bbs/topics/ANSWERS/ANS00919.html.*
42. Farrell B, Godwin J, Richards S, Warlow C. The United Kingdom transient ischaemic attack (UK-TIA) aspirin trial: Final results. *J Neurol Neurosurg Psychiatry* 1991;54:1044-1054.
43. Serebruany VL, Malinin AI, Sane DC. Rapid platelet inhibition after a single capsule of Aggrenox: Challenging a conventional full-dose aspirin antiplatelet advantage? *Am J Hematol* 2003;72:280-281.
44. Eikelboom JW, Hankey GJ. Aspirin resistance: A new independent predictor of vascular events? *J Am Coll Cardiol* 2003;41:966-968.
45. Catella-Lawson F, Reilly MP, Kapoor SC, et al. Cyclooxygenase inhibitors and the antiplatelet effects of aspirin. *N Engl J Med* 2001;345:1809-1817.
46. Eisert WG. Near-field amplification of antithrombotic effects of dipyridamole through vessel wall cells. *Neurology* 2001;57(Suppl 2): S20-S23.
47. Grupke S, Hall J, Dobbs M, Bix GJ, Fraser JF. Understanding history, and not repeating it. Neuroprotection for acute ischemic stroke: From review to preview. *Clin Neurol Neurosurg* 2015;129:1-9.
48. George PM, Steinberg GK. Novel stroke therapeutics: Unraveling stroke pathophysiology and its impact on clinical treatments. *Neuron* 2015;July 15; 87(2):297-309.
49. Sarode R, Milling TJ, Refaai MA, Mangione A, Schneider A, Durn BL, Goldstein JN. Efficacy and safety of a 4-Factor Prothrombin Complex concentrate in patients on vitamin K antagonists presenting with major bleeding. *Circulation* 2013;128:1234-1243.
50. Ho PM, Maddox TM, Wang L, et al. Risk of adverse outcomes associated with concomitant use of clopidogrel and proton pump inhibitors following acute coronary syndrome. *JAMA* 2009;301:937-944.
51. Mega JL, Close SL, Wiviott SD, et al. Cytochrome P-450 polymorphisms and response to clopidogrel. *N Engl J Med* 2009;360:354-362.
52. Saw J, Steinhubl SR, Berger PB, et al. Lack of adverse clopidogrel atorvastatin clinical interaction from secondary analysis of a randomized, placebo-controlled clopidogrel trial. *Circulation* 2003;108:921-924.
53. Johnson JA, Cavallari LH. Pharmacogenetics and cardiovascular disease—Implications for personalized medicine. *Pharmacol Rev* 2013;65:987-1009.

Dyslipidemia

Robert L. Talbert

21

KEY CONCEPTS

1. Hypercholesterolemia, elevated low density lipoprotein, and low high density lipoprotein are unequivocally linked to increased risk for coronary heart disease (CHD) and cerebrovascular morbidity and mortality; LDL is the primary target.
2. Multiple genetic abnormalities and environmental factors are involved in clinical lipid abnormalities and routinely used clinical laboratory measurements do not define the underlying abnormalities.
3. Initial therapy for any lipoprotein disorder is therapeutic life-style changes with restricted intake of total and saturated fat and cholesterol and a modest increase in polyunsaturated fat intake along with a program of regular exercise and weight reduction if needed.
4. If pharmacologic therapy is insufficient after therapeutic lifestyle changes (TLC), lipid-lowering agents should be chosen based on the specific lipoprotein disorder presentation and the severity of the lipid abnormality.
5. Considering compliance, adverse effects and effectiveness, statins are the drugs of choice for patients with hypercholesterolemia because they are the most potent form of monotherapy and are cost-effective in patients with known coronary artery disease (CAD) or multiple risk factors and in high-risk primary prevention patients.
6. Patients not responding to statin monotherapy may be treated with combination therapy for hypercholesterolemia, but should be monitored closely because of an increased risk for adverse effects and drug interactions.
7. Hypertriglyceridemia usually responds well to niacin, gemfibrozil, and fenofibrate; high dose niacin should be used cautiously in diabetics because of worsening glycemic control. Statins lower triglycerides to a variable extent depending on baseline triglyceride concentration and statin potency.
8. Low HDL-C is addressed with life-style modifications such as smoking cessation and increased exercise; niacin and gemfibrozil and fenofibrate can significantly increase HDL-C as well.
9. Reductions in elevated total cholesterol and LDL-C reduce CHD mortality and total mortality; increasing HDL reduces CHD events as well. Aggressive treatment of hypercholesterolemia results in fewer patients progressing to myocardial infarction, angina, and stroke, and reduces the need for interventions such as coronary artery bypass graft and percutaneous transluminal coronary angioplasty.
10. Lipid lowering therapy is generally considered to be cost effective, particularly in secondary intervention and high risk patients.
11. Lomitapide, mipomersen, alirocumab, and evolocumab have been recently approved for the treatment of homozygous familial hypercholesterolemia. All have novel mechanisms of action to lower total and LDL cholesterol and are used as adjuncts to statin therapy or in lieu of statins if patients are statin intolerant.

Cholesterol, triglycerides, and phospholipids are the major lipids in the body and they are transported as complexes of lipid and proteins known as lipoproteins. Plasma lipoproteins are spherical particles with surfaces that consist largely of phospholipid, free cholesterol, and protein, and cores that consist mostly of triglyceride and cholesterol ester (Fig. 21-1). The three major classes of lipoproteins found in serum are low density lipoproteins (LDL),[1] high density lipoproteins (HDL),[2] and very low density lipoproteins,[3] VLDL is carried in the circulation as triglyceride and VLDL can be estimated by dividing the triglyceride concentration by five if the triglyceride concentration is below 250 mg/dL (2.83 mmol/L). Intermediate density lipoprotein resides between VLDL and LDL and is included in the LDL measurement in routine clinical measurement. Abnormalities of plasma lipoproteins can result in a predisposition to coronary, cerebrovascular, and peripheral vascular arterial disease and constitutes one of the major risk factors for coronary heart disease (CHD). Accumulating evidence over the last decades had linked elevated total and LDL cholesterol and reduced HDL to the development of CHD. Premature coronary atherosclerosis, leading to the manifestations of ischemic heart disease (IHD) (see Chapter 16), is the most common and significant consequence of dyslipidemia. In 2014 the American Heart Association (AHA) and the American College of Cardiology published revised guidelines on the treatment of blood cholesterol to reduce atherosclerotic risk in adults. This report supersedes the National Cholesterol Education Program[4] Adult Treatment Panel III (ATP III) published more than a decade ago.[5,6,170] The 2014 guidelines did not find sufficient evidence to recommend specific targets for any lipid, but rather, it identifies four groups of patients who qualify for treatment with statins. The other substantive change is the method used for risk assessment resulting in identifying significantly more patients who would qualify for therapy. The AHA also provides guidelines for primary and secondary prevention of CHD.[7-9]

Total cholesterol and LDL-C increase throughout life in men and women, representing an atherogenic pattern characteristic of Westernized society diets.[10] Based on estimates from the AHA, 42.8% or 100,100,000 million American adults over age 20 years have total cholesterol levels of 200 mg/dL (5.17 mmol/L) or higher.[11] More than half of individuals at borderline-high risk remain unaware that they have hypercholesterolemia and fewer than half of highest risk persons (those with symptomatic CHD) are receiving lipid-lowering treatment. About one third of treated patients are achieving their LDL goal; fewer than 20% of CHD patients are at their LDL goal.

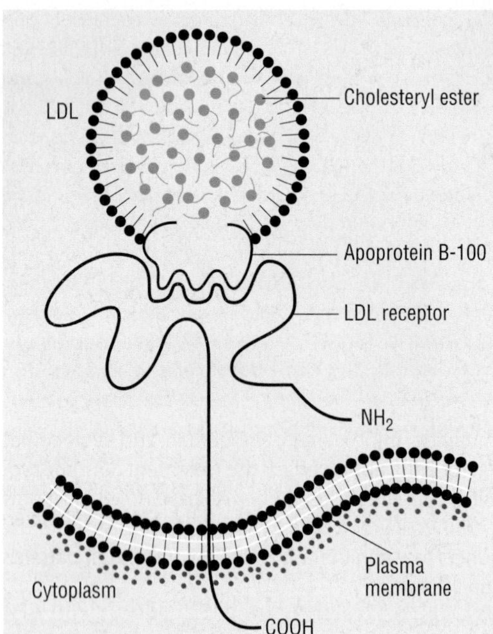

FIGURE 21-1 Diagrammatic representation of the structure of lowdensity lipoprotein (LDL), the LDL receptor, and the binding of LDL to the receptor via apolipoprotein B-100. *(Reproduced with permission from Chapter 17. Energy Balance, Metabolism, and Nutrition. In: Ganong WF. Review of Medical Physiology, 22nd ed. New York: McGraw-Hill, 2005.)*

Changes in the NCEP guidelines have increased the number of persons eligible for therapeutic life style changes (TLC) or lipid-lowering therapy by millions.[171,172] NCEP estimates that only 26% of patients have an optimal LDL-C (less than 100 mg/dL [less than 2.59 mmol/L]) and that large numbers of patients are either untreated or under-treated.[5] Unfortunately, those patients at highest risk are less likely to be treated to desirable levels of LDL.[12] Although these numbers seem staggering in their enormity, substantial progress has been made, and the number of Americans with a desirable blood cholesterol level (less than 200 mg/dL [less than 5.17 mmol/L]) has risen to 49% from 45% from the earlier survey (1976-1980), while the average total cholesterol in this country has fallen from 220 mg/dL (5.69 mmol/L) in 1960 to 195 mg/dL for men and 201 mg/dL for women.[13] Patients who are at risk but who have not yet experienced their first cardiovascular or cerebrovascular event (eg, myocardial infarction [MI]) are termed primary prevention, whereas those with manifest vascular disease are termed secondary intervention.

1 Data from the Framingham study and from other studies demonstrate that the risk for developing cardiovascular disease is related to the degree of total cholesterol and LDL elevation in a graded, continuous fashion.[14] Hypercholesterolemia is additive to the other non-lipid risk factors for CHD, including cigarette smoking, hypertension, diabetes, low HDL levels, and electrocardiographic abnormalities. The presence of established CHD or prior MI increases the risk of MI five to seven times that seen in men or women without CHD, and LDL is a significant predictor of subsequent morbidity and mortality. About 50% of all myocardial infarctions and at least 70% of CHD deaths occur in patients with known CHD, and these patients should therefore be a target for screening, identification, and treatment. Unfortunately, the identification of patients at high risk because of hypercholesterolemia or other lipid disorders is too frequently overlooked, because blood lipid levels are not always evaluated in this population even after an event such as MI.

A comparison of the United States to other countries shows similar relationships between total cholesterol, LDL, and an inverse relationship with HDL to coronary artery disease (CAD) mortality.[14] On a positive note, the U.S. mortality rate is midway among the countries studied, and this country has had the greatest decline in CAD mortality (35%-40%) in men and women over the last 10 years as compared to other countries. A decline in the prevalence of hypercholesterolemia in certain segments of the U.S. population parallels these trends in mortality.[5] LDL and the ratio of LDL to HDL have also been used to assess risk, but their use adds little information to total cholesterol alone unless HDL is abnormally high or low. McQueen et al. found that the ratio of apolipoprotein (Apo) B to ApoA1 was more predictive and consistent across gender and ethnic groups.[15] HDL transports cholesterol from lipid-laden foam cells to the liver. HDL has been shown to be protective for the occurrence of CHD, and an inverse relationship exists between CHD and HDL levels.[16] Recent clinical trials attempting to raise HDL have failed to demonstrate clinically meaningful reductions in cardiovascular endpoints challenging the importance of increasing HDL fractions and ApoA1.[17]

Very low density lipoproteins, the major lipoprotein associated with triglycerides is enriched with cholesterol esters, is smaller, denser, and more atherogenic than less-dense VLDL. Routine measurement of triglycerides cannot distinguish between the types of VLDL present in plasma. Elevation of triglyceride-rich lipoproteins is associated with low HDL, and this ratio predicts increased risk. The 8-year follow-up of the Copenhagen male study found a clear gradient of risk of IHD with increasing triglyceride levels within each level of HDL cholesterol. When compared to the lowest tertile of triglyceride concentrations; the highest tertile had 2.2 relative risk for IHD and the relationship extended across all concentrations of HDL.[18] The Helsinki Heart Study shows that hypertriglyceridemia and low HDL are associated with obesity (body mass index [BMI] greater than 26 kg/m^2), smoking, sedentary life-style, blood pressure of greater than or equal to 140/90 mm Hg, and blood glucose above 79 mg/dL (4.4 mmol/L), and that the benefit of gemfibrozil (risk reduction 68%, $P < 0.03$) was largely confined to overweight subjects.[19] Hypertriglyceridemia in certain instances—for example, diabetes mellitus, nephrotic syndrome, and chronic renal disease, and perhaps in women—is associated with increased cardiovascular risk. This is thought to be a consequence of the presence of atherogenic lipoproteins and of hypertriglyceridemia being a marker for them, as triglycerides are usually not independently predictive for CHD.[20]

LIPOPROTEIN METABOLISM AND TRANSPORT

Cholesterol and triglycerides, as the major plasma lipids, are essential substrates for cell membrane formation and hormone synthesis, and provide a source of free fatty acids.[21] Dyslipidemia may be defined as an elevation total cholesterol, elevation in LDL cholesterol, elevation in triglycerides or low HDL cholesterol concentration or some combination of these abnormalities. Lipids, being water immiscible, are not present in free form in the plasma, but rather circulate as lipoproteins. Hyperlipoproteinemia describes an increased concentration of the lipoprotein macromolecules that transport lipids in the plasma. The density of plasma lipoproteins is determined by their relative content of protein and lipid. Density, composition, size, and electrophoretic mobility divide lipoproteins into four classes (Table 21-1).

Low density lipoproteins has been further divided into LDL_1, or IDL (density 1.006-1.019 g/mL), and LDL_2 (1.019-1.063 g/mL). LDL_2 is the major LDL component in plasma and it carries 60% to 70% of the total serum cholesterol. HDL has been subfractionated into HDL_2 (density 1.063-1.125 g/mL) and HDL_3 (1.125-1.21 g/mL). Fluctuations in HDL are usually caused by alterations in the levels of HDL_2. HDL normally carries about 20% to 30% of the total cholesterol. VLDL has also been subdivided into three classes, and it carries about 10% to 15% of serum cholesterol and most of the triglyceride in the fasting state. VLDL is the precursor for LDL, and

TABLE 21-1 Composition of Lipoprotein Isolated from Normal Subjects

			Composition (Weight %)				
					Cholesterol		
Lipoprotein Class*	Density Range (g/mL)	Diameter (nm)	Protein	Triglyceride	Free	Ester	Phospholipid
Chylomicrons	<0.94	75-1,200	1-2	80-95	1-3	2-4	3-9
VLDL	0.94-1.006	30-80	6-10	55-80	4-8	16-22	10-20
LDL	1.006-1.063	18-25	18-22	5-15	6-8	45-50	18-24
HDL	1.063-1.21	5-12	45-55	5-10	3-5	15-20	20-30

*VLDL, very-low-density lipoprotein; LDL, low-density lipoprotein; HDL, density lipoprotein.

VLDL remnants may also be atherogenic. Table 21-2 shows the characteristics of the protein constituent of lipoproteins known as apolipoproteins. The structure of LDL, the LDL receptor, and the binding of the LDL to the receptor via apolipoprotein (Apo) B-100 is shown in Fig. 21-1.

Chylomicrons, large triglyceride-rich particles containing apolipoprotein B-48, B-100, and E, are formed from dietary fat solubilized by bile salts in intestinal mucosal cells. Chylomicrons are normally not present in the plasma after a fast of 12 to 14 hours and are catabolized by lipoprotein lipase (LPL), which is activated by apolipoprotein C-II and in the vascular endothelium and hepatic lipase to form chylomicron remnants. The remnants that contain apolipoprotein E (Fig. 21-2) are taken up by the "remnant receptor," which may be an LDL receptor-related protein, in the liver. Free cholesterol is liberated intracellularly after attachment to the remnant receptor. Chylomicrons also function to deliver dietary triglyceride to skeletal muscle and adipose tissue. During the catabolism of nascent chylomicrons to remnants, triglyceride is converted to free fatty acids and apolipoproteins A-I, A-II, A-IV (free in plasma), C-I, C-II, and C-III, and phospholipids are transferred to HDL. Apolipoprotein E and apolipoprotein C-II are transferred to chylomicrons from HDL and eventually back through these metabolic events. Hepatic VLDL synthesis is regulated in part by diet and hormones, and is inhibited by uptake of chylomicron remnants in the liver. VLDL is secreted from the liver and serially converted via LPL to intermediate-density lipoprotein (IDL), and, finally, to LDL. VLDL receptors are found in adipose tissue and muscle, and bear close homology to the structure of LDL receptors.

Low density lipoproteins, the major cholesterol transport lipoprotein and having virtually only apolipoprotein B-100, is mostly derived from VLDL catabolism and cellular synthesis. When fasting and on low-fat intake in normal subjects, most cholesterol is synthesized and used in the extrahepatic organs, while most of the cholesterol carried by LDL is taken up by the liver for catabolism. In patients with homozygous familial hypercholesterolemia, enhanced synthesis of LDL may occur, because LDL clearance is reduced as a consequence of the lack of LDL receptors. LDL is catabolized through interaction of cell surface receptors found on liver, adrenal, and peripheral cells (including fibroblasts and smooth-muscle cells). These cells recognize apolipoprotein B-100 on LDL, and after binding to a receptor on the cell membrane, LDL is internalized and degraded. In the normal fasting state, approximately 70% of LDL is cleared through receptor-dependent mechanism, although this is highly dependent on the availability and type of saturated and

TABLE 21-2 Characteristics and Functions of Apolipoproteins

Apolipoprotein	Lipoprotein Density Class	Approximate Plasma Concentration, mg/dL (g/L)	Approximate Molecular Weight (kDa)	Reported Functions	Major Site of Synthesis
A-I	Chylomicrons, HDL	120 (1.2)	28	Cofactor with LCAT, structural protein on HDL, ligand for HDL receptor	Liver, intestine
A-II	Chylomicrons, HDL	35 (0.35)	17	Structural protein for HDL, ligand for HDL receptor	Liver
A-IV	Chylomicrons, 1.21B	15 (0.15)	46	Possibly facilitates transfer of other apos between HDL and chylomicrons	Intestine
ApoLp(a)	LDL, HDL	10 (0.10)	500±	Bound to B-100, high homology with plasminogen, may prevent LDL uptake by B, E receptor	Liver
B-100	VLDL, LDL, IDL	100 (1.0 g/L)	540	Necessary for assembly and secretion of VLDL from the liver, structural protein of VLDL, IDL, LDL, ligand for LDL receptor	Liver
B-48	Chylomicrons	Trace	264	Necessary for assembly and secretion of chylomicrons from the small intestine	Intestine
C-I	Chylomicrons, VLDL, HDL	7 (0.07)	6.6	Cofactor with LCAT; may inhibit hepatic uptake of chylomicron and VLDL remnants	Liver
C-II	Chylomicrons, VLDL, HDL	4 (0.04)	8.9	Activator of LPL	Liver
C-III	Chylomicrons, VLDL, HDL	13 (0.13)	8.8	Inhibitor with LPL; may inhibit hepatic uptake of chylomicron and VLDL remnants	Liver
D	HDL	6 (0.06)	32	?	?
E2-E4	Chylomicrons, VLDL, HDL	5 (0.05)	34	Ligand for several lipoproteins to LDL receptor, LRP and possibly to a separate hepatic apo E receptor	Liver

LCAT, lecithin-cholesterol acyltransferase; HL, hepatic lipase; IDL, intermediate density lipoprotein; LRP, LDL receptor related protein. Other abbreviations are in Table 19.1.

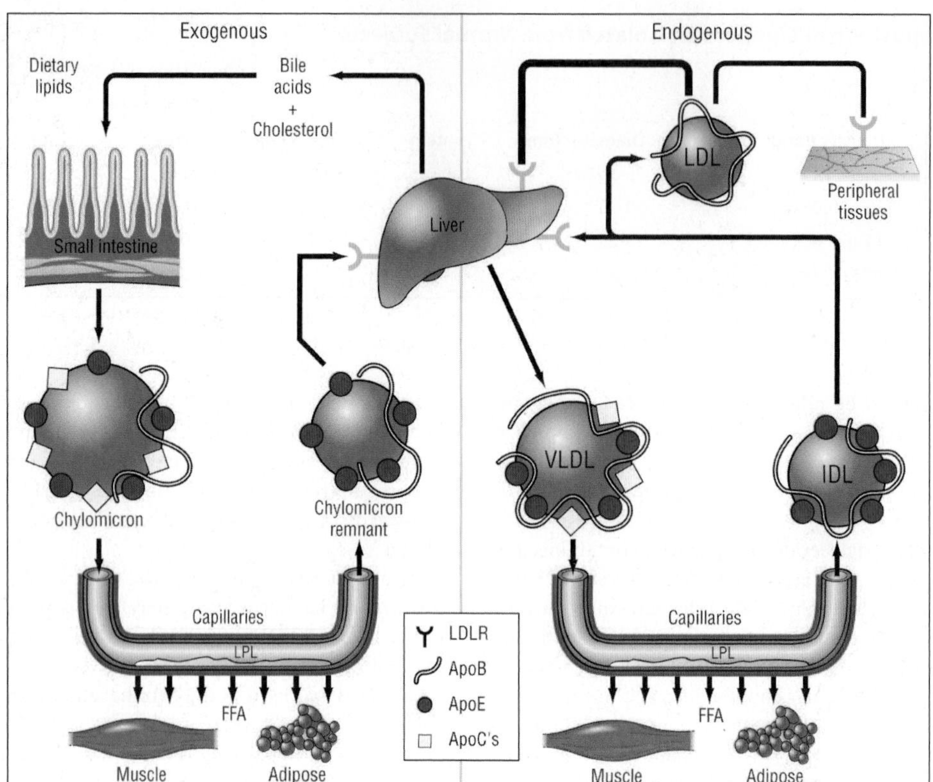

FIGURE 21-2 Simplified diagram of lipoprotein systems for transporting lipids in humans. In the exogenous system, chylomicrons rich in triglycerides of dietary origin are converted to chylomicron remnants rich in cholesteryl esters by the action of lipoprotein lipase (LPL). In the endogenous system, very-low-density lipoproteins (VLDL) rich in triglycerides are secreted by the liver and converted to intermediate density lipoproteins (IDL) and then to low-density lipoproteins (LDL) rich in cholesteryl esters. Some of the LDLs enter the subendothelial space of arteries, are oxidized, and then are taken up by macrophages, which become foam cells. The letters on the chylomicrons, chylomicron remnants, VLDL, IDL, and LDL identify the primary apoproteins (ApoB, ApoC, ApoE) found in them. (LDLR, low-density lipoprotein receptor.) *(Reproduced with permission from Kasper DL, Braunwald E, Fauci AS, et al., eds. Harrison's Principles of Internal Medicine, 16th ed. New York, McGraw-Hill, 2005, p. 2289.)*

mono- or polyunsaturated fat from dietary sources. Ingestion of cholesterol and saturated fatty acids such as C12:0, C14:0, and C16:0 is associated with reduction in LDL receptor activity, increased LDL production rate, and elevation in LDL plasma concentration. Receptor-independent mechanisms are also involved to a lesser extent in the catabolism of LDL, and these receptors are present in many tissues but are most active in animals in the adrenals and ovary. Increased intracellular cholesterol resulting from LDL catabolism inhibits the activity of 3-hydroxy-3-methylglutaryl coenzyme A reductase (HMG-CoA reductase), the rate-limiting enzyme for intracellular cholesterol biosynthesis (Fig. 21-3). Additional consequences of increased intracellular cholesterol include reduced synthesis of LDL receptors, which limits subsequent cholesterol uptake from the plasma, and accelerated activity of acyl coenzyme-A: cholesterol acyltransferase to facilitate cholesterol storage within cells. LDL cholesterol may also be excreted into bile and become part of the enterohepatic pool or may be lost in the stool. Lp(a) is a cholesterol-rich lipoprotein similar to LDL in composition and density and with close homology to fibrinogen; it is reported to be an important independent risk factor for the development of premature cardiovascular disease.

Nascent HDL is derived from liver and gut synthesis primarily in the form of apolipoprotein A-I phospholipid discs.[16] Esterification of free cholesterol in nascent HDL and from peripheral tissues to cholesteryl esters by lecithin-cholesterol acyltransferase (LCAT) results in the production of HDL_3. Further addition of tissue cholesterol to HDL_3 results in the formation of HDL_2. HDL_2 can also be formed from remodeling of chylomicrons and VLDL catabolism. HDL_2 may be converted back to HDL_3 by the action of hepatic lipase and by the transfer of cholesteryl esters to the liver, LDL, and VLDL. Apolipoprotein A-I production is increased by estrogens, leading to higher HDL levels in women and in individuals receiving estrogen. Transfer of excess cholesterol from peripheral tissues by HDL is called *reverse cholesterol transport.* Putative HDL receptors in peripheral cells facilitate the uptake of cholesterol by HDL, which transfers cholesterol to either VLDL and LDL or to the liver for secretion into bile or conversion into bile acids. These processes serve to rid peripheral tissue (eg, coronary arteries) of excessive amounts of cholesterol, and account for some of the protective effects noted with increasing HDL in women and other factors that elevate HDL levels. Variants of the cholesterol ester transfer protein (CETP) have been demonstrated in humans, and the B1B1 genotype is associated with lower HDL and progression of coronary atherosclerosis. Inhibition of CETP leads to elevations in HDL, unfortunately when CETP inhibitors have been tested in clinical trials they did not induce regression of atherosclerotic plaque and were associated with higher blood pressure and CHD events.[22-25] The effect of CETP inhibition on blood pressure and HDL is disconcordant with some of these agents and several compounds continue to be investigated.[26,27]

The "response-to-injury" hypothesis states that risk factors such as oxidized LDL, mechanical injury to the endothelium (eg, percutaneous transluminal angioplasty), excessive homocysteine, immunologic attack, or infection-induced (eg, *Chlamydia,* herpes simplex virus-1) changes in endothelial and intimal function lead to endothelial dysfunction and a series of cellular interactions that culminate in atherosclerosis. C-reactive protein (CRP) is an acute phase reactant and a marker for inflammation; it may be useful in identifying patients at risk for developing CAD.[28] The transcription factor

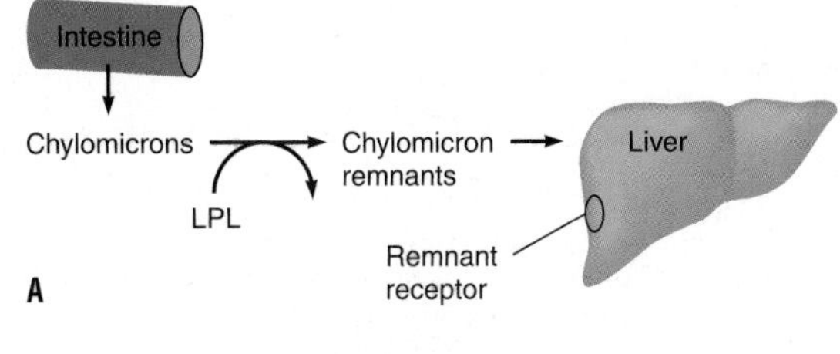

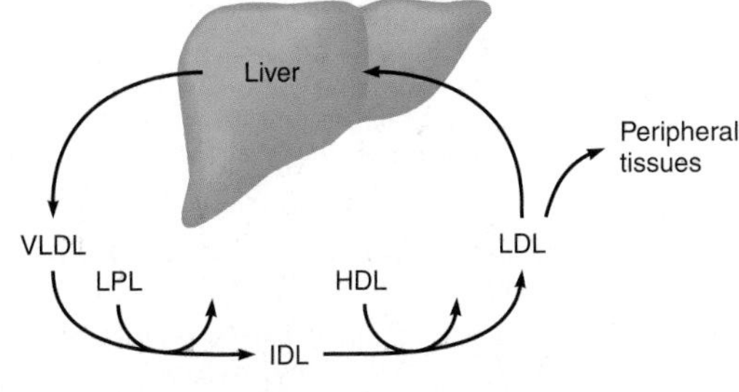

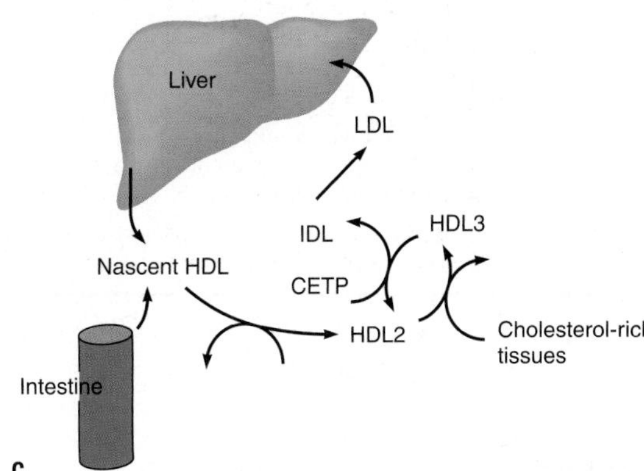

FIGURE 21-3 Biosynthetic pathway for cholesterol. The rate-limiting enzyme in this pathway is 3-hydroxy-3-methylglutaryl coenzyme A reductase (HMG-CoA reductase). (CETP, cholesterolester transfer protein; HDL, high-density lipoprotein; IDL, intermediate-density lipoprotein; LDL, low-density lipoprotein; LPL, lipoprotein lipase; VLDL, very-low-density lipoprotein.) *A.* Exogenous pathway; *B.* Endogenous pathway; C. Reverse cholesterol transport. *(Adapted from Breslow JL. Genetic basis of lipoprotein disorders. J Clin Invest 1989;84:373.)*

Kruppel-like factor 2 (KLF2) may be induced by statins in liver sinusoidal endothelial cells (SEC), orchestrating an efficient vasoprotective response. Upregulation of hepatic endothelial KLF2-derived transcriptional programs by statins confers vasoprotection and stellate cells deactivation, reinforcing the therapeutic potential of these drugs for liver diseases that course with endothelial dysfunction.

The eventual outcomes of this atherogenic cascade are clinical events such as angina, MI, arrhythmias, stroke, peripheral arterial disease, abdominal aortic aneurysm, and sudden death. Atherosclerotic lesions are thought to arise from transport and retention of plasma LDL-cholesterol through the endothelial cell layer into the extracellular matrix of the subendothelial space. Once in the artery wall, LDL is chemically modified through oxidation and non-enzymatic glycation. Mildly oxidized LDL then recruits monocytes into the artery wall, which become transformed into macrophages. Macrophages have tremendous potential for accelerating LDL oxidation and apolipoprotein B accumulation, and altering the receptor-mediated uptake of LDL into the artery wall from the usual LDL-receptor to a "scavenger receptor" not regulated by cell content of cholesterol. Oxidized LDL increases plasminogen inhibitor levels (promotion of coagulation), induces the expression of endothelin (vasoconstrictive substance), inhibits the expression of nitric oxide (a vasodilator and platelet inhibitor), and is toxic to macrophages if highly oxidized. As oxidation of biologically active lipids proceeds, other lipids such as lysophosphatidylcholine, hydroperoxides, aldehydic breakdown products of fatty acids and oxysterol are formed, which continue the reaction within the tissue. These events lead to a massive accumulation of cholesterol. The cholesterol-laden macrophages become foam cells; foam cells are the earliest recognized cells of the arterial fatty streak.

Oxidized LDL provokes an inflammatory response, which is mediated by a number of chemoattractants and cytokines. Examples of each that appear to be involved at different stages of lesion development include monocyte chemoattractant protein 1 (MCP-1); monocyte colony stimulating factor (M-CSF); *gro;* vascular cell adhesion molecule (VCAM-1); E-selectin (ELAM-1); intercellular adhesion molecule (ICAM-1); platelet-derived growth factor (PDGF); vascular endothelial growth factor (VEGF); transforming growth factors (TGFα and TGFβ); interleukin-1 and interleukin-6 (IL-1, IL-6); and the ratio of interleukin-10 and interleukin-12 (IL-10, IL-12). It appears that some of these factors (eg, MCP-1 and M-CSF) participate early in the process of monocyte-macrophage attachment and transmigration across the endothelium, whereas others (PDGF and VCAM-1) promote later lesion growth.[29] The extent of oxidation and the inflammatory response is under genetic control of a major gene termed *Ath*-1 based on murine model studies. The process of aging may lead to lipoproteins that are more susceptible to oxidation and have longer resident time in the vascular compartment. Two proteins associated with HDL—apolipoprotein J (apoJ) and paraxonase (PON)—appear to play an important role to minimize the oxidation of LDL-C.[30] Increased recognition of the role of these growth-regulatory molecules provides the possibility of future directions for antagonists to regulatory molecules such as PDGF, TGFβ, and the interleukins. Repeated injury and repair within an atherosclerotic plaque eventually leads to a fibrous cap protecting the underlying core of lipids, collagen, calcium, and inflammatory cells such as T-lymphocytes. Maintenance of the fibrous plaque is critical to prevent plaque rupture and subsequent coronary thrombosis.[31] An imbalance between plaque synthesis and degradation may lead to a weakened or vulnerable plaque prone to rupture. The fibrous cap may become weakened through decreased synthesis of the extracellular matrix or increased degradation of the matrix. The cytokine interferon-γ, produced by T-lymphocytes, inhibits the ability of smooth-muscle cells to synthesize collagen, a structurally important component of the fibrous cap. A family of enzymes known as matrix metalloproteinases can degrade all major constituents of the vascular extracellular matrix: collagen, elastin, and proteoglycans.[32]

Lipoprotein disorders are classified into six categories, which are commonly used for phenotypical description of dyslipidemia (Table 21-3). Specific genetic defects with disrupted protein, cell, and organ function give rise to several disorders within each family of lipoproteins (Table 21-4). In other words, an elevated cholesterol

TABLE 21-3 Fredrickson-Levy-Lees Classification of Hyperlipoproteinemia

Type	Lipoprotein Elevation
I	Chylomicrons
IIa	LDL
IIb	LDL + VLDL
III	IDL (LDL1)
IV	VLDL
V	VLDL + Chylomicrons

IDL, intermediate-density lipoprotein; LDL, low-density lipoprotein; VLDL, very low-density lipoprotein.

TABLE 21-4 Lipoprotein Disorders

		Lipoproteins		
Lipid Phenotype	Plasma Lipid Levels, mg/dL (mmol/L)	Elevated	Phenotype	Clinical Signs
Isolated Hypercholesterolemia				
Familial hypercholesterolemia	Heterozygotes TC = 275-500 (7.1-12.9)	LDL	IIa	Usually develop xanthomas in adulthood and vascular disease at 30-50 years
	Homozygotes TC > 500 (>12.9)	LDL	IIa	Usually develop xanthomas in adulthood and vascular disease in childhood
Familial defective apo B100	Heterozygotes TC = 275-500 (7.1-12.9)	LDL	IIa	
Polygenic hypercholesterolemia	TC = 250-350 (6.5-9.0)	LDL	IIa	Usually asymptomatic until vascular disease develops; no xanthomas
Isolated Hypertriglyceridemia				
Familial hypertriglyceridemia	TG = 250-750 (2.8-8.5)	VLDL	IV	Asymptomatic; maybe associated with increased risk of vascular disease
Familial LPL deficiency	TG > 750 (>8.5)	Chylomicrons, VLDL	I, V	May be asymptomatic; may be associated with pancreatitits, abdominal pain, hepatosplenomegaly
Familial apo CII deficiency	TG > 750 (>8.5)	Chylomicrons, VLDL	I, V	As above
Hypertriglyceridemia and Hypercholesterolemia				
Combined hyperlipidemia	TG = (250-750 (2.8-8.5); TC = 250-500 (6.5-12.9)	VLDL, LDL	IIb	Usually asymptomatic until vascular disease develops; familial form may also present as isolated high TG or an isolated high LDL cholesterol
Dysbetalipoproteinemia	TG = 250-750 (2.8-8.5); TC = 250-500 (6.5-12.9)	VLDL, IDL; LDL normal	III	Usually asymptomatic until vascular disease develops; may have palmar or tuboeruptive xanthomas

LPL, lipoprotein lipase. Other abbreviations as in Table 23.1; TC, total cholesterol; TG, triglycerides.

level does not necessarily equate with familial hypercholesterolemia or type IIa, as cholesterol may also be elevated in other lipoprotein disorders and the lipoprotein pattern does not describe the underlying genetic defect. The preceding discussion has focused on primary or genetic dyslipoproteinemia; it should be remembered that secondary forms exist and that several drugs may also elevate lipid levels (Table 21-5). These secondary forms of hyperlipidemia should be initially managed by correcting the underlying abnormality, including modification of drug therapy when appropriate.

Familial hypercholesterolemia is characterized by (a) a selective elevation in the plasma level of LDL; (b) deposition of LDL-derived cholesterol in tendons (xanthomas) and arteries (atheromas); and (c) inheritance as an autosomal dominant trait with homozygotes more severely affected than heterozygotes. Homozygotes (prevalence 1 in 1,000,000) have severe hypercholesterolemia (650-1,000 mg/dL [16.8-25.9 mmol/L]), with the early appearance of cutaneous xanthomas and fatal CHD generally before the age of 20. The primary defect in familial hypercholesterolemia is the inability to bind LDL to the LDL receptor (LDL-R) or, rarely, a defect of internalizing the LDL-R complex into the cell after normal binding. Homozygotes have essentially no functional LDL receptors. This leads to lack of LDL degradation by cells and unregulated biosynthesis of cholesterol, with total cholesterol and LDL-C being inversely proportional to the deficit in LDL receptors. Heterozygotes have only about one-half of the normal number of LDL receptors, total cholesterol levels in the range of 300-600 mg/dL (7.76-15.52 mmol/L) and cardiovascular events beginning in the third and fourth decades of life.

Familial LPL deficiency is a rare, autosomal recessive trait characterized by a massive accumulation of chylomicrons and corresponding increase in plasma triglycerides or a type I lipoprotein pattern. VLDL concentration is normal. The presenting manifestations include repeated attacks of pancreatitis and abdominal pain, eruptive cutaneous xanthomatosis, and hepatosplenomegaly beginning in childhood. Symptom severity is proportional to dietary fat

TABLE 21-5 Secondary Causes of Lipoprotein Abnormalities

Hypercholesterolemia	Hypothyroidism Obstructive liver disease Nephrotic syndrome Anorexia nervosa Acute intermittent porphyria Drugs: progestins, thiazide diuretics, glucocorticoids, beta-blockers, isotretinoin, protease inhibitors, cyclosporine, mirtazapine, sirolimus
Hypertriglyceridemia	Obesity Diabetes mellitus Lipodystrophy Glycogen storage disease Ileal bypass surgery Sepsis Pregnancy Acute hepatitis Systemic lupus erythematous Monoclonal gammopathy: multiple myeloma, lymphoma Drugs: Alcohol, estrogens, isotretinoin, beta blockers, glucocorticoids, bile-acid resins, thiazides; asparaginase, interferons, azole antifungals, mirtazapine, anabolic steroids, sirolimus, bexarotene
Hypocholesterolemia	Malnutrition Malabsorption Myeloproliferative diseases Chronic infectious diseases: AIDS, tuberculosis Monoclonal gammopathy Chronic liver disease
Low HDL	Malnutrition Obesity Drugs: non-ISA beta blockers, anabolic steroids, probucol, isotretinoin, progestins

CLINICAL PRESENTATION

General

- Most patients are asymptomatic for many years prior to clinically evident disease.
- Patients with the metabolic syndrome may have 3 or more of the following: abdominal obesity, atherogenic dyslipidemia, raised blood pressure, insulin resistance ± glucose intolerance, prothrombotic state or proinflammatory state.

Symptoms

- None to chest pain, palpitations, sweating, anxiety, shortness of breath, loss of consciousness or difficulty with speech or movement, abdominal pain, and sudden death.

Signs

- None to abdominal pain, pancreatitis, eruptive xanthomas, peripheral polyneuropathy, high blood pressure, BMI greater than 30 kg/m^2 or waist size greater than 40 inches (102 cm) in men (35 inches [89 cm] in women).

Laboratory Tests

- Elevations in total cholesterol, LDL, triglycerides, apolipoprotein B, and high sensitivity C-reactive protein (hsCRP).
- Low HDL

Other diagnostic Tests

- Lipoprotein (a), and small, dense LDL (pattern B), HDL subclassification, apolipoprotein E isoforms, apolipoprotein A-1, fibrinogen, folate, lipoprotein-associated phospholipase A_2.
- Various screening tests for manifestations of vascular disease (ankle-brachial index, exercise testing, and magnetic resonance imaging) and diabetes (fasting glucose, oral glucose tolerance test, and hemoglobin A_{1c}).

intake, and consequently to the elevation of chylomicrons. LPL is normally released from vascular endothelium or by heparin and hydrolyzes chylomicrons and VLDL (see Fig. 21-2). Diagnosis is based on low or absent enzyme activity with normal human plasma or apolipoprotein C-II, a cofactor of the enzyme. Accelerated atherosclerosis is not associated with this disease. Abdominal pain, pancreatitis, eruptive xanthomas, and peripheral polyneuropathy characterize type V (VLDL and chylomicrons). Symptoms may occur in childhood, but usually the disorder is expressed at a later age. The risk of atherosclerosis is increased with this disorder. These patients are commonly obese, hyperuricemic, and diabetic, and alcohol intake, exogenous estrogens, and renal insufficiency tend to be exacerbating factors.

Patients with familial type III hyperlipoproteinemia (also called dysbetalipoproteinemia, broad-band or β-VLDL) develop these clinical features after 20 years of age: xanthoma striata palmaris (yellow discolorations of the palmar and digital creases); tuberous or tuberoeruptive xanthomas (bulbous cutaneous xanthomas); and severe atherosclerosis involving the coronary arteries, internal carotids, and abdominal aorta. A defective structure of apolipoprotein E does not allow normal hepatic surface receptor binding of remnant particles derived from chylomicrons and VLDL (known as IDL); aggravating factors such as obesity, diabetes, or pregnancy may promote overproduction of apo-B-containing lipoproteins. Although homozygosity for the defective allele (E_2/E_2) is common (1 in 100), only 1 in 10,000 express the full-blown picture, and interaction with other genetic or environmental factors, or both, is needed to produce clinical disease.

Familial combined hyperlipidemia is characterized by elevations in total cholesterol, triglycerides, decreased HDL, increased apolipoprotein B and small, dense LDL.[33] It is associated with premature CHD and may be difficult to diagnose since the lipid levels do not consistently display the same pattern.

Type IV hyperlipoproteinemia is common and occurs in adulthood primarily in patients who are obese, diabetic, and hyperuricemic and do not have xanthomas. It may be secondary to alcohol ingestion and can be aggravated by stress, progestins, oral contraceptives, thiazides, or β-blockers. Two genetic patterns occur in type IV hyperlipoproteinemia: familial hypertriglyceridemia, which does not carry a great risk for premature CAD, and familial combined hyperlipidemia, which is associated with increased risk of cardiovascular disease.

Rare forms of lipoprotein disorders may include hypobetalipoproteinemia, abetalipoproteinemia, Tangier disease, LCAT deficiency (fish-eye disease), cerebrotendinous xanthomatosis, and sitosterolemia. Most of these rare lipoprotein disorders do not result in premature atherosclerosis, with the exceptions of familial LCAT deficiency, cerebrotendinous xanthomatosis (CTX), and sitosterolemia with xanthomatosis. Their treatment consists of dietary restriction of plant sterols (sitosterolemia with xanthomatosis), chenodeoxycholic acid (CTX), or, potentially, blood transfusion (LCAT deficiency).

PATIENT EVALUATION

A fasting (preferred) lipoprotein profile including total cholesterol, LDL-C, HDL-C, and triglycerides should be measured in all adults 20 years of age or older at least once every 5 years.[5] If the profile is obtained in the nonfasted state, only total cholesterol and HDL-C will be usable because LDL-C is usually a calculated value; if total cholesterol is greater than or equal to 200 mg/dL (greater than or equal to 5.17 mmol/L), or if HDL-C is less than 40 mg/dL (less than 1.03 mmol/L), a follow-up fasting lipoprotein profile should be obtained. After a lipid abnormality is confirmed (Table 21-6), major components of the evaluation are the history (including age, gender, and, if female, menstrual and hormone replacement status), physical examination, and laboratory investigations. A complete history and physical exam should assess (a) presence or absence of cardiovascular risk factors or definite cardiovascular disease in the individual; (b) family history of premature cardiovascular disease or lipid disorders; (c) presence or absence of secondary causes of lipid abnormalities, including concurrent medications (see Table 21-5); and (d) presence or absence of xanthomas or abdominal pain, or history of pancreatitis, renal or liver disease, peripheral vascular disease, abdominal aortic aneurysm, or cerebral vascular disease (carotid bruits, stroke, or transient ischemic attack). Diabetes mellitus is regarded as a CHD risk equivalent.[5] The presence of diabetes in patients without known CHD is associated with the same level

TABLE 21-6 Classification of Total-, Ldl-, Hdl-Cholesterol and Triglycerides

Total Cholesterol	
<200 mg/dL (<5.17 mmol/L)	Desirable
200-239 mg/dL (5.17-6.20 mmol/L)	Borderline high
≥240 mg/dL (≥6.21 mmol/L)	High
LDL Cholesterol	
<100 mg/dL (<2.59 mmol/L)	Optimal
100-129 mg/dL (2.59-3.35 mmol/L)	Near or above optimal
130-159 mg/dL (3.36-4.13 mmol/L)	Borderline high
160-189 mg/dL (4.14-4.90 mmol/L)	High
≥190 mg/dL (≥4.91 mmol/L)	Very high
HDL Cholesterol	
<40 mg/dL (<1.03 mmol/L)	Low
≥60 mg/dL (≥1.55 mmol/L)	High
Triglycerides	
<150 mg/dL (<1.70 mmol/L)	Normal
150-199 mg/dL (1.70-2.25 mmol/L)	Borderline high
200-499 mg/dL (2.26-5.64 mmol/L)	High
≥500 mg/dL (≥5.65 mmol/L)	Very high

HDL, high-density lipoproteins; LDL, low-density lipoproteins.

of risk as patients without diabetes but having confirmed CHD.[34,35] ATP III identified four categories of risk that modify the goals and modalities of LDL-lowering therapy (Table 21-8).[6] However in the current guidelines, pooled cohort equations are currently recommended. The components of the estimator include gender, age, race, total cholesterol, HDL, systolic blood pressure, hypertension that is being treated, presence of diabetes, and smoking status. Cohort Equations and lifetime risk prediction tools can be found at: http://tools.acc.org/ASCVD-Risk-Estimator/. The expert panel was unable to find sufficient evidence from randomized clinical trials to support the use of specific LDL or non-LDL treatment targets (no recommendation).[36] Rather than specific treatment targets, the panel identified four groups most likely to benefit from treatment with statins to reduce the 10-year risk of atherosclerotic cardiovascular disease in secondary and primary intervention.

Heart-healthy lifestyle and habits should be encouraged for all individuals (I/A). Table 21-7 outlines the key recommendations for treatment of blood cholesterol to reduce ASCVD risk in adults. Other recommendations not appearing in Table 21-7 address adherence, lipid panel testing, screening for comorbidities and monitoring. The Expert Panel established categories of statin intensity including High-, Moderate-, and Low-intensity statin therapy (see Table 21-8) based on evidence from randomized clinical trials and package insert information. Figure 21-4 further outlines the process for statin initiation for the treatment of blood cholesterol to reduce ASCVD risk in adults.

Measurement of plasma cholesterol (which is about 3% lower than serum determinations), triglyceride, and HDL-C levels after a 12-hour or longer fast is important, as triglycerides may be elevated in non-fasted individuals; total cholesterol is only modestly affected by fasting. Analytic and biologic variability can have a major impact on the measurement and interpretation of cholesterol (or any other laboratory test). Analytic variability can be minimized through the use of adequate quality-control procedures, including internal training, routine calibration and monitoring, and external proficiency testing. Even with these measures, the coefficient of variability in the best procedures can acceptably be up to 5%, and when combined with average biologic variability, total variability may be as high as about 22%. Analytic variability with desktop equipment generally is greater in the fingerstick capillary blood methods, usually yielding measurements less than those from a clinical laboratory, and this technology should be considered for use only as a screening method. Reliance on desktop methods can result in misclassification of 7% to 14% of

TABLE 21-7 Key Recommendations to Reduce the Risk of ASCVD in Adults

Recommendations	ACC/AHA COR	ACC/AHA LOE
Heart healthy lifestyle for everyone		
Appropriate intensity of statin therapy should be initiated or continued		
1. Clinical ASCVD*		
a. Age <75 y and no safety concerns: High-intensity statin therapy	I	A
b. Age >65 y or safety concerns: Moderate-intensity statin therapy	I	A
2. Primary prevention—Primary LDL ≥190 mg/dL		
a. Rule out secondary causes of dyslipidemia	I	B
b. Age ≥21 y: High-intensity statin therapy	I	B
c. Achieve at least a 50% reduction in LDL	IIa	B
d. LDL lowering nonstatin therapy may be considered to further reduce LDL	IIb	C
3. Primary prevention—Diabetes 40-75 years of age and LDL 70-189 mg/dL		
a. Moderate-intensity statin therapy	I	A
b. Consider high-intensity statin when ≥7.5% 10-y ASCVD risk using the Pooled Cohort Equations	II	B
4. Primary prevention—no diabetes, 40-75 years of age and LDL 70-189 mg/dL		
a. Estimate 10-y ASCVD risk based on Pooled Cohort Equations in those not receiving a statin; estimate risk every 4-6 y	I	B
b. To determine if statin should be initiated, engage in a clinical-patient discussion concerning risk adverse reactions, drug interactions and patient preferences	IIa	C
c. Re-emphasize heart-healthy lifestyle and address other risk factors	I	A
i. ≥7.5% 10-y ASCVD risk: Moderate or high-intensity statin therapy	I	A
ii. 5%-7.5% 10-y ASCVD risk: Consider moderate-intensity statin therapy	IIb	C
iii. Other risk factors may be considered: LDL ≥160 mg/dL, family history of premature ASCVD, hs-CRP ≥2 mg/dL, CAC score ≥300 Agaston units, ABI <0.9 or lifetime risk	IIb	C
5. Primary prevention when LDL <190 mg/dL and age <40 or >75 y, or <5% 10-y ASCVD risk		
a. Statin therapy may be considered in selected individuals	IIb	C
6. Statin therapy is not routinely recommended for individuals with NYHA Class 11-IV heart failure or who are receiving maintenance hemodialysis		

ABI, ankle brachial index; ACC/AHA, American College of Cardiology/American Heart Association; ASCVD, Atherosclerotic cardiovascular disease; y, years; CAC, coronary artery calcium; COR, Class of recommendation; hsCRP, high-sensitivity C reactive protein; LDL-, low density lipoprotein; LOE, Level of evidence; NYHA, New York Heart Association.

*Clinical ASCVD includes nonfatal MI, CHD death, and nonfatal and fatal stroke, TIA or peripheral arterial disease presumed to be of atherosclerotic origin.

TABLE 21-8 Intensity of Statin Therapy by Drug and Dose

High-intensity Statin Therapy	Moderate-intensity Statin Therapy	Low-intensity Statin Therapy
Daily dose lowers LDL on average by ≥50%	Daily dose lowers LDL on average by 30 to <50%	Daily dose lowers LDL on average by <30%
Atorvastatin (40)-80 mg	**Atorvastatin 10 (20) mg**	Simvastatin 10 mg
Rosuvstatin (20)-40 mg	**Rosuvastatin (5)-20 mg**	**Pravastatin 10-20 mg**
	Simvastatin 20-40 mg[*]	**Lovastatin 20 mg**
	Pravastatin 40-(80) mg	Fluvastatin 20-40 mg
	Lovastatin 40 mg	Pitavastin 1 mg
	Fluvastin XL 80 mg	
	Fluvastatin 40 mg BID	
	Pitavastatin 2-4 mg	

[*]Simvastatin is not recommended by the FDA to be started at 80 mg/day due to increased risk of myopathy and rarely rhabdomyolysis .

Boldface type indicates specific states that have been tested in RCT.

Legend: FDA, Food and Drug Administration; RCT, Randomized clinical trials.

patients if capillary blood is used. Two determinations, 1 to 8 weeks apart, with the patient on a stable diet and weight, and in the absence of acute illness, are recommended to minimize variability and to obtain a reliable baseline.[5,36] If the total cholesterol is greater than 200 mg/dL (5.17 mmol/L), a second determination is recommended, and if the values are more than 30 mg/dL (0.78 mmol/L) apart, the average of three values should be used. Familiarity with the method and quality control procedures employed by local laboratories is essential for interpretation of reported values. If the physical examination and history are insufficient to diagnose a familial disorder, then agarose-gel lipoprotein electrophoresis is useful to determine which class of lipoproteins is affected. If the triglyceride levels are below 400 mg/dL (4.52 mmol/L) and neither type III hyperlipidemia nor chylomicrons are detected by electrophoresis, then one can calculate VLDL and LDL concentrations: VLDL = triglyceride/5; LDL = total cholesterol – (VLDL + HDL).

Because total cholesterol is comprised of cholesterol derived from LDL, VLDL, and HDL, determination of HDL is useful when total plasma cholesterol is elevated. HDL may be elevated by moderate alcohol ingestion (less than two drinks per day), physical exercise, smoking cessation, weight loss, oral contraceptives, phenytoin, and terbutaline. Smoking, obesity, a sedentary lifestyle and drugs such as β-blockers lower HDL. Only exercise and smoking cessation could be recommended as interventions for low HDL concentrations. Niacin and gemfibrozil also increase HDL concentrations.

The range of lipid concentrations represents a population mean plus or minus two standard deviations and does not define the risk of disease. Reference values for plasma total, LDL, and HDL cholesterol concentrations for men and women, as well as various ethnic groups, are available from the NHANES III.[10] Cholesterol and triglycerides increase throughout life until about the fifth decade for men and the sixth decade for women. Past these ages, total cholesterol and LDL plateau and fall slightly. HDL tends to fall slightly with time and more rapidly after menopause in women. Institution of a population-based approach for cholesterol reduction should shift the entire curve to the left, and the potential reduction in cardiovascular mortality would be proportional to mean reductions at any cholesterol concentration.

Based on a careful review of the experimental pathologic, genetic, and epidemiologic evidence relating to the relationship between blood cholesterol levels and CHD, the ATP III of the NCEP recommends that a fasting lipoprotein profile and risk factor assessment be used in the initial classification of adults.[5,37] If total cholesterol is less than 200 mg/dL (5.17 mmol/L), then the patient has a *desirable blood cholesterol level* (see Table 21-6). Cholesterol levels between 200 and 239 mg/dL (5.17 and 6.18 mmol/L) are classified as *borderline-high blood cholesterol levels,* and assessment of risk factors (see Table 21-7) is needed to more clearly define disease risk. Blood cholesterol levels of 240 mg/dL (6.21 mmol/L) and above are classified as *high blood cholesterol levels.* If the total cholesterol is below 200 mg/dL (5.17 mmol/L) and the HDL is above 40 mg/dL (1.03 mmol/L), no further follow-up is recommended for patients without known CHD and who have fewer than two risk factors. An increasing number of persons have the metabolic syndrome that is characterized by abdominal obesity, atherogenic dyslipidemia (elevated triglycerides, small LDL particles, and low HDL-C), raised blood pressure, insulin resistance (with or without glucose intolerance), and prothrombotic and proinflammatory states. Non-HDL is calculated by subtracting HDL from total cholesterol and the targets are 30 mg/dL (0.78 mmol/L) greater than LDL for each risk stratum. Non-HDL takes into consideration atherogenic particles such as remnant lipoproteins and IDL that are not measured in routine clinical laboratory testing.[38] HDL-raising has potential benefit but no specific goals are set in the current guidelines and the evidence is modest to support aggressively increasing HDL levels.[39]

The Expert Panel on Children and Adolescents of the NCEP recommends screening in higher-risk children (positive family history or parental high blood cholesterol, greater than or equal to 240 mg/dL [greater than or equal to 6.21 mmol/L]).[40] The American Academy of Pediatrics categorizes total and LDL cholesterol into Acceptable (less than 75th percentile; total cholesterol less than 170 mg/dL [less than 4.40 mmol/L]), Borderline (75th-95th percentile; total cholesterol 170-199 mg/dL [4.40-5.15 mmol/L], LDL cholesterol 110-129 mg/dL [2.84-3.34 mmol/L]) and Elevated (greater than 95th percentile; total cholesterol greater than 200 mg/dL [greater than 5.17 mmol/L], LDL cholesterol greater than 130 mg/dL [greater than 3.36 mmol/L]).[40] The rationale, in part, for this approach is based on the recognition that atherosclerosis begins in the childhood and adolescent years as documented in the pathobiologic determinants of atherosclerosis in youth (PDAY) and the Bogalusa studies.[41] Similarly, if children with high blood lipids or lipoprotein levels are identified, and the levels in the parents are unknown, the parents should be screened as well, as they are likely to be at high risk. Racial and gender differences do exist in the determination of lipoprotein fractions, and these factors should be considered in screening. Use of the serum cholesterol level alone may be of insufficient specificity or sensitivity, depending on the cut points used in screening, and other discretionary factors, such as hypertension, smoking, obesity, high-fat diet, and use of cholesterol-raising medication, may be needed to correctly identify children at risk. Presently, children over the age of 10 years are candidates for drug therapy if a trial of diet (6 months-1 year) proves to be inadequate and LDL-C remains above 190 mg/dL (4.91 mmol/L), or above 160 mg/dL (4.14 mmol/L) if two or more risk factors or CHD are present in the child or adolescent, or if there is a history of premature CHD. In children with diabetes mellitus, pharmacologic treatment should be considered when LDL cholesterol is greater than or equal to 130 mg/dL (greater than or equal to 3.36 mmol/L).[40] The Dietary Intervention Study in Children (DISC) in pubertal children found that a fat restricted diet modestly lowered LDL-C and maintained psychologic well-being and dietary changes are acceptable to children.[42,43] Although bile acid sequestrants have been the recommended drugs for this population, clinical trials demonstrate that statin therapy is effective and well tolerated in pediatric populations.[44,45] The long-term consequences of drug therapy in this population are unknown. In special instances, familial hypercholesterolemia (particularly the homozygous form), or the existence of CHD or two or more risk factors in the child, would prompt the earlier institution of drug therapy after a trial of dietary intervention.

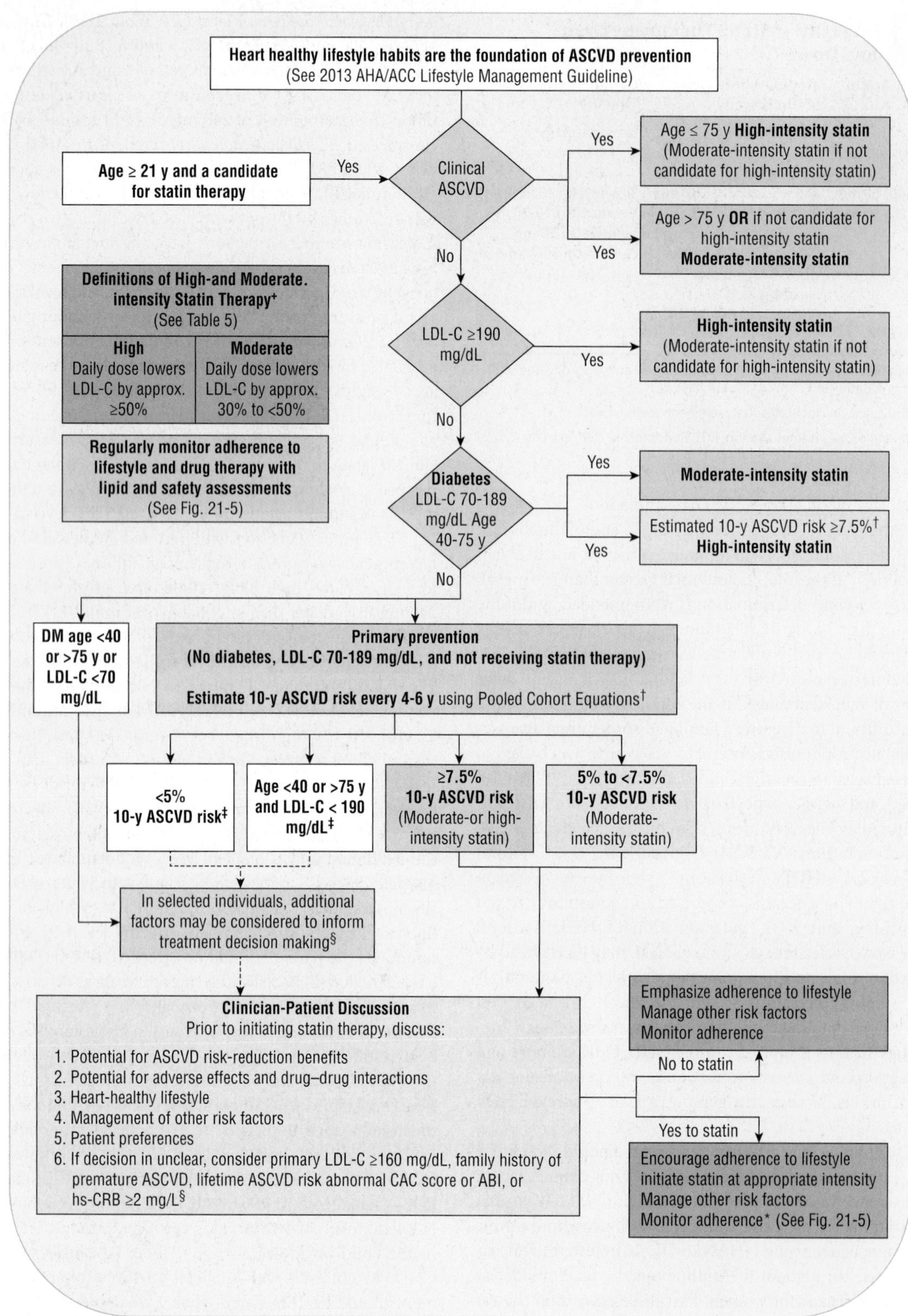

FIGURE 21-4 Statin Initation.

TREATMENT

Desired Outcomes

The goals of therapy expressed as LDL-C levels and the level of initiation of TLC and drug therapy are provided in Tables 21-7 and **21-9** for adults and children, respectively. While these goals are surrogate endpoints, the primary reason to institute TLC and drug therapy is reduce the risk first or recurrent events such as MI, angina, heart failure, ischemic stroke, or other forms of peripheral arterial disease such as carotid stenosis or abdominal aortic aneurysm.

General Approach[1]

Establishing targeted changes and outcomes with consistent reinforcement of goals and measures at follow up visits to attain goals are important to reduce barriers for optimizing TLC and pharmacologic

TABLE 21-9 Cut Points for Total Cholesterol and LDL Concentrations in Children and Adolescents

Category	Percentile	Total Cholesterol, mg/dL (mmol/L)	LDL Cholesterol, mg/dL (mmol/L)
Acceptable	<75th	<170 (<4.40)	<110 (<2.84)
Borderline	75th-95th	170-199 (4.40-5.16)	110-129 (2.84-3.35)
Elevated	>95th	>200 (>5.17)	>130 (>3.36)

Adapted from American Academy of Pediatrics. National Cholesterol Education Program: report of the expert panel on blood cholesterol levels in children and adolescents. Pediatrics. 1992;89(3 pt 2): 525 -584.

TABLE 21-10 Macronutrient Recommendations for the TLC Diet

Component*	Recommended Intake
Total fat	25%-35% of total calories
Saturated fat	Less than 7% of total calories
Polyunsaturated fat	Up to 10% of total calories
Monounsaturated fat	Up to 20% of total calories
Carbohydrates#	50%-60% of total calories
Cholesterol	<200 mg/day
Dietary Fiber	20-30 grams/d
Plant sterols	2 grams/d
Protein	Approximately 15% of total calories
Total calories	To achieve and maintain desirable body weight

*Calories from alcohol not included.

#Carbohydrates should derive from foods rich in complex carbohydrates such as whole grains, fruits, and vegetables.

therapy. 3 TLC should be implemented in all patients prior to considering drug therapy. The components of TLC include reduced intakes of saturated fats and cholesterol, dietary options to reduce LDL such as plant stanols and sterols and increased soluble fiber intake, weight reduction, and increased physical activity. In general, physical activity of moderate intensity 30 minutes per day for most days of the week should be encouraged.[46,47] Patients with known CAD or at high risk should be evaluated before undertaking vigorous exercise. Weight and BMI should be determined at each visit and lifestyle patterns to induce a weight loss of 10% should be discussed in persons who are overweight. All patients should also be counseled to stop smoking and to meet the Joint National Committee VII guidelines for control of hypertension.

Nonpharmacologic Therapy

Individualized diet counseling that provides acceptable substitutions for unhealthy foods and ongoing reinforcement by a registered dietitian are necessary for maximal effect. The objectives of dietary therapy are to progressively decrease the intake of total fat, saturated fatty acids (ie, saturated fat), and cholesterol, and to achieve a desirable body weight. Typical American diets now include 13% to 20% of total calories from saturated fat and a cholesterol intake of 350 to 450 mg/day, both in excess of a "heart healthy" diet for normal Americans, let alone patients with a lipid disorder. Excessive dietary intake of cholesterol and saturated fatty acids leads to decreased hepatic clearance of LDL and deposition of LDL and oxidized LDL in peripheral tissues. The targeted saturated fatty acids have carbon chain lengths of 12 (lauric acid), 14 (myristic acid), and 16 (palmitic acid). The rationale for using a nutritionally balanced low-fat, low-cholesterol diet for the treatment of hypercholesterolemia is based on these principles: (a) it represents a reasonable extension of the diet recommended for the general public; (b) it progressively decreases the major cholesterol-raising constituent of the diet; (c) it precludes large intakes of polyunsaturated fats; and (d) it facilitates weight reduction by removing foods of high caloric density.[48-51]

Dietary expertise in providing a wide range of options and suggestions in preparation of food can make the difference between a good or an inadequate response to diet. Information concerning eating out in a healthy fashion and advice for shopping are also important factors for success in diet therapy. An example is being aware of products with misleading labels such as coffee creamers that state they contain "no cholesterol," when they may contain hydrogenated (saturated) fats or oils (eg, palmitic acid, palm kernel oil, or coconut oil), which makes them undesirable because of their saturated fat content. Variations in polyunsaturated and saturated fat and cholesterol intake influence the LDL concentration, but the amount of cholesterol has been found to have a greater effect than the proportion of polyunsaturated or saturated fat. There were also racial differences in elevation of LDL with high saturated fat diets being greater in whites than in other racial groups. The isomeric form of fatty acids is also important.[48] Fatty acids with the *cis* configuration are the preferred substrate for the ACAT reaction and significantly increase hepatic LDL receptor clearance while reducing LDL cholesterol production rate. The *trans* isomeric form cannot be used by ACAT and is biologically inactive with no effect on LDL concentration.

Ideally, therapeutic TLC including reduced intake of saturated fats and cholesterol, increased stanol/sterol and fiber intake, weight reduction, and increased physical activity should be used to attain lower LDL-C and to achieve reductions in CHD risk (Table 21-10). TLC may obviate the need for drug therapy, augment LDL-lowering drug therapy, and allow for lower doses. Weight control plus increased physical activity reduces risk beyond LDL-cholesterol lowering, is the primary management approach for the metabolic syndrome, raises HDL and reduces non-HDL cholesterol.[52,53] Many persons should be given a three-month trial (two visits spaced 6 weeks apart) of dietary therapy and TLC before advancing to drug therapy unless patients are at very high risk (severe hypercholesterolemia, known CHD, CHD risk equivalents, multiple risk factors, and strong family history). Although changes in blood lipid levels may change before three months, adoption of a different eating pattern may require a longer period of time. It is important to involve all family members, especially if the patient is not the primary person preparing food. The NCEP and AHA both have excellent internet based resources to aid patients in altering their diet in a culturally sensitive manner (http://www.americanheart.org/presenter.jhtml?identifier=1200009; http://www.nhlbi.nih.gov/health/index.htm). If all of the recommended dietary changes from NCEP, the estimated reduction, on average, in LDL would range from 20% to 30%.[5] Adherence to diet and inter-individual variability in macronutrient intake would obviously influence the eventual LDL level achieved. Based on the NHANES data, less than one-half of the patients who should be instructed on heart healthy diet receive any dietary instructions.

Other dietary interventions or diet supplements may be useful in certain patients with lipid disorders. Increased intake of soluble fiber in the form of oat bran, pectins, certain gums, and psyllium products can result in useful adjunctive reductions in total and LDL cholesterol, but these dietary alterations or supplements should not be substituted for more active forms of treatment. Total daily fiber intake should be about 20 to 30 g/d, with about 25% or 6 g/d, being soluble fiber.[5] Studies with psyllium seed in doses of 10 to 15 g/d show reductions in total and LDL cholesterol ranging from about 5% to 20%.[54,55] They have little or no effect on HDL-C or triglyceride concentrations. These products may also be useful in managing constipation associated with the bile acid sequestrants. Psyllium binds cholesterol in the gut but also reduces hepatic production and clearance. Fish oil supplementation provides an increased amount of the omega-3 polyunsaturated fatty acids such as eicosapentaenoic acid and docosahexaenoic acid. In epidemiologic studies, ingestion of large amounts of cold water, oily fish is associated with a reduction in CHD risk, but it is unclear whether the same advantage is conferred with commercially prepared fish oil products. Each 20 gm per day ingestion of fish lowers CHD risk by 7% and eating fish once weekly or more should reduce CHD mortality.[56] Fish oil supplementation has a fairly large effect in reducing triglycerides and VLDL-C, but it either has no effect on total and LDL cholesterol or may cause elevations in these fractions. Other actions of fish oil may account for their protective effects. These effects include quantitative and qualitative alterations in the synthesis of prostanoid substances, changes in immune function and cellular proliferation, and potential antioxidative actions.[57] Responses noted with fish oil are further discussed under drug therapy.[58]

Fat substitutes such as Olestra (Olean, sucrose polyester, Procter and Gamble), a mixture of hexa-, hepta-, and octa-esters formed from the reaction of sucrose with long-chain fatty acids, are approved by the FDA as a nondigestible, nonabsorable, and noncaloric fat substitute for snack foods. Olestra is heat stable, an advantage over several other fat substitutes, enabling it to be used in the preparation of fried and baked foods. It is similar in composition to triglycerides, but Olestra is not hydrolyzed in the gastrointestinal tract by pancreatic lipase, and, consequently, is not taken up by the intestinal mucosa. The principal adverse effects associated with Olestra use are bloating, flatulence, diarrhea, and "anal leakage." Because of the ability of Olestra to solubilize lipophilic substances, there has been concern over potential drug interactions in which lipophilic drugs (eg, cyclosporin, or colchicine) or vitamins (vitamins A, D, E, and K) are solubilized in Olestra and excreted in the feces.

Recent studies have demonstrated the LDL-lowering effect of plant sterols, which are isolated from soybean and tall pine-tree oils. Ingestion of 2 to 3 grams per day will reduce LDL by 6% to 15%.[5] Plant sterols can be esterified to unsaturated fatty acids (creating sterol esters) to increase lipid solubility. Hydrogenating sterols produces plant stanols and, with esterification, stanol esters. The efficacy of plant sterols and plant stanols is considered to be comparable. Because lipids are needed to solubilize stanol/sterol esters, they are usually available in commercial margarines. The presence of plant stanols/sterols is listed on the food label. When margarine products are used, persons must be advised to adjust caloric intake to account for the calories contained in the products. Benecol® (McNeil), as an example, is a butter-like spread that contains a plant stanol ester, an ingredient that can lower cholesterol and which is derived from plant stanols found naturally in small amounts in foods like wheat, rye, and corn.[59] In August 2007, the Food and Drug Administration issued a warning about the consumption of red yeast rice and red yeast rice/policosonal containing products. These products contained lovastatin that could interact with other drugs and would have the same toxicity of statins but would not be recognized by the consumer and the reduction in LDL is minimal.[60]

Drug therapy is indicated following an adequate trial of TLC changes as outlined in Tables 21-8 and 21-9.

Pharmacologic Therapy

There are now numerous randomized, double-blinded clinical trials demonstrating that reduction of LDL reduces CHD event rates in primary prevention, secondary intervention, and in angiographic trials.[61] Generally speaking, for every 1% reduction in LDL, there is a 1% reduction in CHD event rates.[5] However, if treatment extends beyond the typical duration of a clinical trial (2-5 years), the accumulated benefit could be greater. Elevations of HDL of 1% result in approximately 2% reduction in CHD events.[16,62] Of interest, angiographic trials, which typically cause small changes in luminal diameter (eg, about a 0.04-mm difference in change between placebo and active treatment), result in fewer clinical events such as MI or the need for revascularization. This unexpected finding suggests that plaque size and luminal encroachment by plaque may be less important than the effects that cholesterol lowering may have on the activity in the plaque and endothelial dysfunction. These studies provide a strong rationale for attempting to lower plasma cholesterol and LDL in patients with hypercholesterolemia.

4 Although many efficacious lipid-lowering drugs exist, none is effective in all lipoprotein disorders, and all such agents are associated with some adverse effects.[63] Lipid-lowering drugs can be broadly divided into agents that decrease the synthesis of VLDL and LDL, agents that enhance VLDL clearance, agents that enhance LDL catabolism, agents that decrease cholesterol absorption, agents that elevate HDL, or some combination of these characteristics (Table 21-11). Table 21-12 lists recommended drugs of choice for each lipoprotein phenotype and alternate agents. Table 21-13 lists available products and their doses.

Treatment of type I hyperlipoproteinemia is directed toward reduction of chylomicrons derived from dietary fat with the subsequent reduction in plasma triglycerides. Total daily fat intake should be no more than 10 to 25 g/d, or approximately 15% of total calories. Secondary causes of hypertriglyceridemia (see Table 21-5) should be excluded or, if present, the underlying disorder should be treated appropriately. Type V hyperlipoproteinemia also requires a stringent restriction of the fat component of dietary intake; in addition, drug therapy is indicated, as outlined in Table 21-12, if the response to diet alone is inadequate. Medium-chain triglycerides, which are absorbed without chylomicron formation, may be used as a dietary supplement for caloric intake if needed for types I and V. Hepatic fibrosis has been reported with medium-chain triglycerides. Omega-3 fatty acids may be useful in LPL deficiency in some patients. In patients with apolipoprotein C-II deficiency, infusion of plasma may normalize plasma triglyceride levels.

Primary hypercholesterolemia (familial hypercholesterolemia, familial combined hyperlipidemia, and type IIa hyperlipoproteinemia) is treated with the bile acid resins or sequestrants (BAR, colestipol, cholestyramine, and colesevelam), HMG Co-A reductase inhibitors (statins), niacin or eztimibe. 5 Of these choices, statins are first choice because they are the most potent LDL lowering agents. Statins interrupt the conversion of HMG-CoA to mevalonate, the rate-limiting step in de novo cholesterol biosynthesis, by inhibiting HMG-CoA reductase (see Fig. 21-3). Currently available products include lovastatin, pravastatin, simvastatin, fluvastatin, atorvastatin, and pitvastatin.[64] Rosuvastatin is the most potent statin currently on the market. Table 21-14 lists the pharmacokinetic properties of the statins.[65] The plasma half-lives for all the statins are reported to be short except for atorvastatin and rosuvastatin, and this may account for their potency. In CURVES, the largest head-to-head comparison of statins, atorvastatin was found to be the most potent drug for lowering total cholesterol and LDL-C, with reductions in LDL-C of 38%, 46%, 51%, and 54% for the 10-, 20-, 40-, and 80-mg doses, respectively.[66] Metabolic studies with statins in normal volunteers and patients with hypercholesterolemia suggest reduced synthesis of LDL-C, as well as enhanced catabolism of LDL mediated through LDL receptors, as the principal mechanisms for lipid-lowering effects. Total and LDL cholesterol are reduced in a dose-related fashion by 30% or more on average when added to dietary therapy, with the effects being more pronounced in nonfamilial than in familial hypercholesterolemia. 6 Combination therapy with bile acid sequestrants and lovastatin is rational as LDL receptor numbers are increased, leading to greater degradation of LDL-C; intracellular synthesis of cholesterol is inhibited, and enterohepatic recycling of bile acids is interrupted. Combination therapy with a statin plus eztimibe is also so rational since eztimibe inhibits cholesterol absorption across the gut border and adds 12% to 20% further reduction when combined to a statin or other drugs.[67] However, the combination of a statin and eztimibe has not been shown to affect surrogate endpoints such as carotid intimal medial

TABLE 21-11 Effects of Drug Therapy on Lipids and Lipoproteins

Drug	Mechanism of Action	Effects on Lipids	Effects on Lipoproteins	Comment
Cholestyramine, colestipol and colesevelam	↑ LDL catabolism Cholesterol ↓ absorption	↓ Cholesterol	↓ LDL ↑ VLDL	Problem with compliance; binds many co-administered acidic drugs
Niacin	↓ LDL and VLDL ↓ synthesis	↓ Triglyceride and ↓ cholesterol	↓ VLDL, ↓ LDL, ↑ HDL	Problems with patient acceptance; good in combination with bile acid resins; extended release niacin causes less flushing and is less hepatotoxic than sustained release
Gemfibrozil, fenofibrate, clofibrate	↑ VLDL clearance ↓ VLDL synthesis	↓ Triglyceride and cholesterol	↓ VLDL, ↓ LDL, ↑ HDL	Clofibrate causes cholesterol gall stones; modest LDL lowering; raises HDL; gemfibrozil inhibits glucuronidation of simvastatin, lovastatin and atorvastatin
Lovastatin, Pravastatin, Simvastatin, Fluvastatin, Atorvastatin Rosuvastatin	↑ LDL catabolism; inhibit LDL synthesis	↓ Cholesterol	↓ LDL	Highly effective in heterozygous familial hypercholesterolemia and in combination with other agents
Ezetimibe	Blocks cholesterol absorption across the intestinal border	↓ Cholesterol	↓ LDL	Few adverse effects; effects additive to other drugs
Mipomerson	Inhibitor of Apolipoprotein B-100	↓ Cholesterol, LDL, non-HDL	↓ LDL, non-HDL	Increase in transaminases, risk of hepatosteatosis and hepatotoxicity; must be given by SQ injection. Only indicated for familial hypercholesterolemia. To be used along with other lipid lowering therapies (statins)
Lomitapide	Microsomal triglyceride transfer protein inhibitor	↓ Cholesterol	↓ LDL, non-HDL	Hepatotoxicity must be monitored via Juxtapid Risk Evaluation and Mitigation Strategy program. Only indicated for familial hypercholesterolemia. To be used along with other lipid lowering therapies (statins)
Alirocumab	PCSK9 inhibitor	↓ Cholesterol, ↓ Lpa	↓ Cholesterol and LDL	Given by SQ injection, injection site pain, low risk of hepatoxicity
Evolocumab	PCSK9 inhibitor	↓ Cholesterol, ↓ Lpa	↓ Cholesterol and LDL	Given by SQ injection, injection site pain, low risk of hepatoxicity

thickness (CIMT) even with further reduction in LDL cholesterol.[68] Elevation of serum transaminase levels (primarily alanine aminotransferase) to greater than three times the upper limit of normal occurs in approximately 1.3% of patients on moderate to high doses of statins and serious muscle toxicity occurs in less than 0.6% of patients.[69] Meta-analysis of placebo controlled studies with statins demonstrate a low risk of abnormal ALT or CK and a low risk of myopathy without or with rhadomyolysis.[70] Lens opacities have been reported with lovastatin; however, in the age groups studied, these abnormalities are common and tend to wax and wane with time irrespective of drug therapy, and no statistical association is known to exist. As a category of monotherapy, the HMG-CoA reductase inhibitors are the most potent total and LDL cholesterol-lowering agents and among the best tolerated.[69,70] In an analysis of more than 75,000 patients allocated to statins in clinical trials, Alsheikh-Ali et al. found that risk of statin-associated elevated liver enzymes or rhabdomyolysis is not related to the magnitude of LDL-C lowering. A highly significant inverse relationship between achieved LDL-C levels and rates of newly diagnosed cancer was observed ($R^2 = 0.43$, $p = 0.009$).[71] The WHO Foundation Collaborating Centre for International Drug Monitoring has issued a report suggesting that a rare relationship may exist between statin use and the onset of upper motor neuron diseases such as amyotrophic lateral sclerosis but this association remains uncertain.[72] Statin use is associated with a small risk of diabetes (9%).[73] There are numerous pharmacokinetic and pharmacodynamic differences among statins and patients that give rise to variable response to therapy.[74]

TABLE 21-12 Lipoprotein Phenotype and Recommended Drug Treatment

Lipoprotein Type	Drug of Choice	Combination Therapy
I	Not indicated	—
II[a]	Statins Cholestyramine or colestipol Niacin	Niacin or BAR Statins or niacin Statins or BAR Ezetimibe Mipomersen, lomitapide[b]
II[b]	Statins Fibrates Niacin	BAR or Fibrates or niacin Statins or niacin or BAR[a] Statins or Fibrates Ezetimibe
III	Fibrates Niacin	Statins or niacin Statins or Fibrates Ezetimibe
IV	Fibrates Niacin	Niacin Fibrates
V	Fibrates Niacin	Niacin Fish oils

BAR, bile acid resins; fibrates includes gemfibrozil or fenofibrate.

[a]BAR are not used as first-line therapy if triglycerides are elevated at baseline since hypertriglyceridemia may be worsen with BAR alone.

[b]Mipomersen and lomitapide are used in combinations with other lipid lowering therapy, in particular, statins for patients with familial hypercholestermia (homozygotes or heterzygotes) and in patient who cannot be managed adequately with maximally tolerated statin therapy.

The primary action of BAR is to bind bile acids in the intestinal lumen, with a concurrent interruption of enterohepatic circulation of bile acids and a markedly increased excretion of acidic steroids in the feces. This decreases the bile acid pool size and stimulates hepatic synthesis of bile acids from cholesterol. Depletion of the hepatic pool of cholesterol results in an increase in cholesterol biosynthesis and an increase in the number of LDL receptors on the hepatocyte membrane. The increased number of receptors stimulates an enhanced rate of catabolism from plasma and lowers LDL levels. CETP, which is correlated with total and LDL cholesterol concentrations, is also reduced by BAR, perhaps by interfering with hepatic microsomal cholesterol content but this effect is not as great as with statins.[75] Patients with homozygous familial hypercholesterolemia genetically lack the ability to increase synthesis of LDL receptors and bile acid

TABLE 21-13 Comparison of Drugs Used in the Treatment of Hyperlipidemia

Drug	Manufacturer	Dosage Forms	Usual Daily Dose	Maximum Daily Dose
Cholestyramine (Questran)	BMS	Bulk powder/4-g packets	8 g tid	32 g
Cholestyramine (Questran Light)	BMS	Bulk powder/4-g packets		
Cholestyramine (Cholybar)	Parke-Davis	4-g resin per bar		
Colestipol hydrochloride (Colestid)	Upjohn	Bulk powder/5-g packets	10 g bid	30 g
Colesevelam (Welchol)	Sankyo	625 mg tablets	1,875 mg bid	4,375 mg
Niacin	Various	50-, 100-, 250-, and 500-mg tablets; 125-, 250-, and 500-mg capsules	2 g tid	9 g
Extended release niacin (Niaspan)	Kos	500, 750 and 1,000 mg tablets	500 mg	2,000 mg
Extended release niacin + lovastatin (Advicor)*	Kos	Niacin/lovastatin 500 mg/20 mg tablets Niacin/lovastatin 750 mg/20 mg tablets Niacin/lovastatin 1,000 mg/20 mg tablets	Niacin/lovastatin 500 mg/20 mg	Niacin/lovastatin 1,000 mg/20 mg
Fenofibrate (Tricor and others)	Abbott, various	67, 134 and 200 mg capsules (micronized); 54 and160 mg tablets; 40, 120 mg tablets; 50, 160 mg tablets	54 mg or 67 mg	201 mg
Gemfibrozil (Lopid)	Parke-Davis	300-mg capsules	600 mg bid	1.5 g
Lovastatin (Mevacor)	MSD	20- and 40-mg tablets	20-40 mg	80 mg
Pravastatin (Pravachol)	Bristol-Myers Squibb	10- and 20-mg tablets	10-20 mg	40 mg
Simvastatin (Zocor)	MSD	5, 10, 20, 40, and 80-mg tablets	10-20 mg	80 mg
Atorvastatin (Lipitor)	Pfizer	10 mg tablets	10 mg	80 mg
Rosuvastatin (Crestor)	Astra-Zeneca	5- and 10-mg tablets	5 mg	40 mg
Pitavastatin (Livalo)	Kowa	1, 2, and 4 mg tablets	2 mg	4 mg
Ezetimibe (Zetia)	MSD	10 mg tablet	10 mg	10 mg
Atorvastatin/amlodipine (Caduet)	Pfizer	Atorvastatin/amlodipine 10 mg/5 mg Atorvastatin/amlodipine 20 mg/5 mg Atorvastatin/amlodipine 40 mg/5 mg Atorvastatin/amlodipine 80 mg/5 mg Atorvastatin/amlodipine 10 mg/10 mg Atorvastatin/amlodipine 20 mg/10 mg Atorvastatin/amlodipine 40 mg/10 mg Atorvastatin/amlodipine 80 mg/10 mg	Atovastatin/amlodipine 10 mg/5 mg	Atovastatin/amlodipine 80 mg/10 mg
Pravastatin/aspirin (Pravigard PAC)	BMS	Pravastatin/aspirin 20 mg/81 mg Pravastatin/aspirin 20 mg/325 mg Pravastatin/aspirin 40 mg/81 mg Pravastatin/aspirin 40 mg/325 mg Pravastatin/aspirin 80 mg/81 mg Pravastatin/aspirin 80 mg/325 mg		
Simvastatin/ezetimibe (Vytorin)	Merck/Schering-Plough	Simvastatin/ezetimibe 10 mg/ 10 mg Simvastatin/ezetimibe 20 mg/ 10 mg Simvastatin/ezetimibe 40 mg/ 10 mg	Simvastatin/ezetimibe 20 mg/10 mg	Simvastatin/ezetimibe 40 mg/10 mg
Omega-3 acid ethyl esters (Lovaza)	Reliant	Eicosapentaenoic acid (EPA) 465 mg, docosahexaenoic acid (DHA) 375 mg	41 gram capsules QD or 21 gram capsules BID	41 gram capsules QD or 21 gram capsules BID
Lomitapide	Aegerion	5, 10, 20 mg capsules	5 mg QD increasing at 2 week intervals to response or maximum dose; dose 2 hours after evening meal	60 mg QD
Mipomersen	Genzyme	200 mg/ml for SQ injection	200 mg SQ once weekly	200 mg SQ once weekly
Alirocumab		75 or 150 mg	SQ every two weeks	150 mg
Evolocumab		140 mg or 420 mg	SQ 140 mg every 2 weeks or 420 mg once a month	420 mg

BID, twice daily; probucol is no longer on the market in the US; gemfibrozil, fenofibrate, and lovastatin are available as generic products. BMS, Bristol-Myers Squibb; MSD, Merck Sharp & Dohme; SQ, subcutaneously.

*The manufacturer does not recommend use of the fixed combination as initial therapy of primary hypercholesterolemia or mixed dyslipidemia. It is specifically indicated in patients receiving lovastatin alone plus diet who require an additional reduction in triglyceride levels or increase in HDL-cholesterol levels; it is also indicated in those treated with niacin alone who require additional decreases in LDL cholesterol. Lomitapide and mipomersen can be hepatotoxic and close monitoring is recommended for both.

TABLE 21-14 Pharmacokinetics of the Statins

Parameter	Lovastatin	Simvastatin	Pravastatin	Fluvastatin	Atorvastatin	Rosuvastatin	Pitavastatin
Isoenzyme	3A4	3A4	None	2C9	3A4	2C9/2C19	UGT1A3/UGT2B7
Lipophilic	Yes	Yes	No	Yes	Yes	No	Yes
Protein binding (%)	>95	95-98	~50	>90	96	88	99
Active metabolites	Yes	Yes	No	No	Yes	Yes	No
Elimination half-life (h)	3	2	1.8	1.2	7-14	13-20	12

Isoenzyme refers to the specific isoenzyme in the cytochrome P450 system which is responsible for the metabolism of each drug. Pharmacokinetic parameters in this table are based on studies and reviews presented in the literature.

resins are generally ineffective. The increase in hepatic cholesterol biosynthesis may be paralleled by increased hepatic VLDL production and, consequently, bile acid resins may aggravate hypertriglyceridemia in patients with combined hyperlipidemia. Gastrointestinal complaints of constipation, bloating, epigastric fullness, nausea, and flatulence are most commonly reported.[5] With intensive education, patients can learn to tolerate resins on a long-term basis as evidenced by adherence in clinical trials to active drug regimens but in routine clinical practice 40% or more of patients will discontinue therapy within 1 year but with pharmacists interventions, adherence rates can be improved.[76,77] These adverse effects can be managed by increasing the fluid intake, modifying the diet to increase bulk, and using stool softeners. The other major limiting complaint is the gritty texture and bulk; these problems may be minimized by mixing the powder with orange drink or juice. Tablet forms of bile acid sequestrants should help in improving compliance with this form of therapy, whereas the bar does not improve compliance.[78] Other potential adverse effects include impaired absorption of fat-soluble vitamins A, D, E, and K; hypernatremia and hyperchloremia; gastrointestinal obstruction; and reduced bioavailability of acidic drugs such as coumarin anticoagulants, nicotinic acid, thyroxine, acetaminophen, hydrocortisone, hydrochlorothiazide, loperamide, and possibly iron. Hyperchloremic metabolic acidosis, hypernatremia, and gastrointestinal obstruction have been reported almost exclusively in children, and malabsorption of fat-soluble vitamins is probably most common with high doses (eg, 30 g/d of cholestyramine) of the bile acid resins. Drug interactions may be avoided by alternating administration times with an interval of 6 hours or greater between the bile acid resin and other drugs. Colestipol and cholestyramine have comparable side effects; however, colestipol may have better palatability because it is odorless and tasteless. Colesevelam is the newest BAR and total and LDL-C reduction is dose related. The adverse effects are qualitatively similar to the older BAR but may occur less often. Because of adverse effects occurring commonly with BAR at higher doses, BARs are increasingly used in combination with other drugs, as low doses are tolerated well and they work in a complementary fashion with other agents.

Niacin (nicotinic acid) may also be used in primary hypercholesterolemia in combination with bile acid sequestrants or as monotherapy for this disorder and others (see Table 21-12). Niacin reduces the hepatic synthesis of VLDL, which, in turn, leads to a reduction in the synthesis of LDL. Factors responsible for decreased production of VLDL include inhibition of lipolysis with a decrease in free fatty acids in plasma, decreased hepatic esterification of triglycerides, and a possible direct effect on the hepatic production of apolipoprotein B.[79] The complementary action of niacin and bile acid sequestrants to increase catabolism and decrease synthesis of LDL may account for the additive effects of this combination in hyperlipidemia. Niacin also increases HDL by reducing its catabolism. Niacin selectively decreases hepatic removal of HDL apoA-I but not removal of cholesterol esters, thereby increasing the capacity of retained apoA-I to augment reverse cholesterol transport in isolated hepatic cells. The principal use of niacin is for mixed hyperlipemia or as a second-line agent in combination therapy for hypercholesterolemia. It is also considered to be the first-line agent or an alternative for the treatment of hypertriglyceridemia and diabetic dyslipidemia.[80,81] There are numerous smaller trials suggesting that lower doses of niacin may be combined with statins or gemfibrozil to minimize adverse effects and maximize response. One meta-analysis showed that combination therapy was no more effective than high dose statin therapy.[82] These combinations require careful monitoring because interactions do occur.

Niacin has many adverse drug reactions that occur commonly; fortunately, most of the symptoms and biochemical abnormalities seen do not require discontinuation of therapy. Cutaneous flushing and itching appear to be prostaglandin mediated and can be reduced by aspirin 325 mg given shortly before niacin ingestion.[5,83] Flushing seems to be related to rising plasma concentrations of niacin; taking the dose with meals and slowly titrating the dose upward may minimize these effects. Laropiprant is a selective antagonist of the prostaglandin D[84] receptor subtype 1 (DP1), which may mediate niacin-induced vasodilation. Coadministration of laropiprant 30, 100, and 300 mg with extended-release (ER) niacin significantly lowered flushing symptom scores (by approximately 50% or more) and also significantly reduced malar skin blood flow measured by laser Doppler perfusion imaging.[85,86] Gastrointestinal intolerance and flushing are common problems. Acanthosis nigricans, a darkening of the skin in skinfold areas and an external marker of insulin resistance, may be seen with high doses of niacin. Sustained-release products may minimize these complaints in some patients, but controlled trials with regular-release products do not demonstrate much of a difference between sustained- and regular-release products. The only legend form of niacin, Niaspan® (Abbott), is an extended release form of niacin with pharmacokinetics intermediate between instant and sustained-release products which are sold as food supplements rather than legend products. In controlled trials, Niaspan® is reported to have fewer dermatologic reactions and has a low risk for hepatoxicity. When combined with statins, this combination produces large reductions in LDL and increases in HDL.[87] Potentially important laboratory abnormalities occurring with niacin therapy include elevated liver function tests, hyperuricemia, and hyperglycemia. Recent experience with niacin in diabetes suggests that some diabetic patients do not have worsened glycemic control with dose-titration and sustained-release products.[88] BMI and fasting plasma glucose predict loss of blood glucose control.[89] With less than 3 grams per day, the degree of liver function test elevation is generally not marked and often transient, and a temporary reduction in dosage frequently corrects the problem. Niacin-associated hepatitis is more common with sustained-release preparations, and their use should be restricted to patients intolerant of regular-release products.[88,90] Sustained-release products are often more expensive and given the lack of data for reduced adverse effects and increased incidence of hepatitis, regular-release products should always be used first. Preexisting gout and diabetes may be exacerbated by niacin; these patients should be monitored more closely and their medication titrated appropriately. Patients with well controlled Type 2 diabetes mellitus do not have significant changes in glycemic control with niacin at doses of 2 grams per day or less.[90] Niacin is contraindicated in patients with active liver disease. Dry eyes and other ophthalmologic complaints are also occasionally noted. Concomitant alcohol and hot drinks may magnify flushing and pruritus with niacin and they should be avoided at the time of ingestion. Nicotinamide should not be used in the treatment of hyperlipidemia, as it does not effectively leads to lower cholesterol or triglyceride levels.

Combined hyperlipoproteinemia (type IIb) may be treated with statins, niacin, or gemfibrozil combinations to lower LDL cholesterol without elevating VLDL and triglycerides. Niacin is the most effective agent and may be combined with a bile acid sequestrant. Bile acid resins alone in this disorder may elevate VLDL and triglycerides, and their use as single agents for treating combined hyperlipoproteinemia should be avoided. Fibric acid (gemfibrozil, fenofibrate) monotherapy is effective in reducing VLDL, but a reciprocal rise in LDL may occur, and total cholesterol values may remain relatively unchanged. Gemfibrozil reduces the synthesis of VLDL and, to a lesser extent, apolipoprotein B, with a concurrent increase in the rate of removal of triglyceride-rich lipoproteins from plasma. Plasma HDL concentrations may rise 10% to 15% or more with fibrates. Fenofibrate may have fewer drug interactions than gemfibrozil but fenofibrate has been reported to worsen renal function.[91] Ezetimibe could also be used in combination therapy in Type IIb. Gastrointestinal complaints with fibric acid derivatives occur in 3% to 5% of patients; rash in 2% of patients; dizziness in 2.4% of patients; and transient elevations in transaminase levels and alkaline phosphatase in 4.5% and 1.3% of patients, respectively.[92] Gemfibrozil and probably fenofibrate may enhance the formation of gallstones associated with an increase in the lithogenic index; however, the rate is low (0.5%-7%) and similar to that seen with placebo in the Helsinki heart study.[92] Fibric acid derivatives may potentiate the effects of oral anticoagulants and international normalized ratio (INR) should be monitored very closely with this combination.

Type III hyperlipoproteinemia may be treated with fibric acid derivatives or niacin. Although fibric acid derivatives have been suggested as the drugs of choice for this disorder, given the lack of data supporting its efficacy in altering cardiovascular mortality in the major studies on hypercholesterolemia, and numerous, well-documented, and serious adverse effects, it is reasonable to consider niacin. Gemfibrozil increases the activity of LPL and reduces to a lesser extent the synthesis or secretion of VLDL from the liver into the plasma. A myositis syndrome of myalgia, weakness, stiffness, malaise, and elevations in creatinine phosphokinase and aspartate aminotransaminase is seen with the fibric acid derivatives, and it seems to be more common in patients with renal insufficiency.[92] Enhanced hypoglycemic effects are reported to occur when fibric acid derivative is given to patients on sulfonylurea compounds, but the mechanisms for these interactions are not well understood.

Three fibric acid derivatives (gemfibrozil and fenofibrate) are approved in the United States. Both reduce LDL-C by 20% to 25% in heterozygous familial hypercholesterolemia. The response of LDL-C, HDL-C, and triglycerides to this category of drug is very dependent on the specific lipoprotein type (eg, type IIa vs IIb) and the baseline triglyceride concentration.[93]

As a potential alternative therapy, for this phenotype, numerous epidemiologic and normal volunteer studies have found that diets high in omega-3 polyunsaturated fatty acids (from fish oil), mostly commonly eicosapentaenoic acid, reduce cholesterol, triglycerides, LDL-C, and VLDL-C, and may elevate HDL-C.[58] The effects of fish oil on lipoprotein metabolism are mediated through a reduction in VLDL production and suppression of VLDL apolipoprotein B. In patients with hypertriglyceridemia, either phenotypes type IIb or type V, a diet high in omega-3 fatty acids given for 4 weeks reduced cholesterol 27% and 45%, and triglyceride 64% and 79%, in the type IIb and type V patients, respectively.[56] A diet high in eicosapentaenoic acid given to hyperlipidemic hemodialysis patients resulted in significant decreases in cholesterol and triglycerides for as long as 13 weeks. Fish oil supplementation may be most useful in patients with hypertriglyceridemia; however, its role in treatment is not well defined. Potential complications of fish oil supplementation, such as thrombocytopenia and bleeding disorders, have been noted, especially with high doses (eicosapentaenoic acid 15 to 30 g/d); and well-controlled trials are needed to determine if fish oils are safe and effective before their use may be broadly recommended. Based on a recent meta-analysis, fish consumption lowers the risk of CHD but nutraceuticals have not been adequately tested.[56] Recently, a prescription form of concentrated fish oil, Lovaza®, has become available.[58] This product lowers triglycerides by 14% to 30% and raises HDL by about 10% depending on baseline values. Another fish oil derivative product being considered by the FDA, Epanova contains EPA and DHA in their free fatty acid form at a total concentration of 50% to 60% EPA and 15% to 25% DHA along with other potentially active omega-3 fatty acids stored in a patent—protected capsule with a patent—protected coating, designed to maximize bioavailability and tolerability™. There is no convincing evidence that fish supplementation in any form reduces the risk of ASCVD.

Combination drug therapy may be considered after adequate trials of monotherapy and for patients documented compliant to the prescribed regimen. Two or three lipoprotein profiles at 6-week intervals should confirm lack of response prior to initiation of combination therapy. Cholestyramine may be added in patients with fasting hypertriglyceridemia, but it should not be used as the initial drug, because triglycerides are likely to increase. Contraindications to and drug interactions with combined therapy should be carefully screened, as well as consideration of the extra cost of drug product and monitoring that may be required. In general, a statin and a BAR or niacin with a BAR provide the greatest reduction in total and LDL cholesterol. Regimens intended to increase HDL levels should include either gemfibrozil or niacin, and it should be remembered that statins combined with either of these drugs may result in a greater incidence of hepatotoxicity or myositis. This is particularly important for statins that are eliminated via cytochrome 3A4 or through glucuronidation.[65] Familial combined hyperlipidemia may respond better to a fibric acid and a statin than to a fibric acid and a BAR.[94]

Severe forms of hypercholesterolemia—such as familial hypercholesterolemia, familial defective apolipoprotein B-100, severe polygenic hypercholesterolemia, familial combined hyperlipidemia, and familial dysbetalipoproteinemia (type III)—may require more intensive therapy. In particular, familial hypercholesterolemia patients often require combination therapy (two or three drugs) and are managed with surgical therapy (partial ileal bypass), plasmapheresis (LDL-apheresis), and liver transplantation (to replace LDL receptors).

HYPERTRIGLYCERIDEMIA

It is important to remember that lipoprotein pattern types I, III, IV, and V are associated with hypertriglyceridemia, and that these primary lipoprotein disorders and underlying diseases should be excluded prior to implementing therapy (see Table 21-5). In a national survey, approximately one third of participants tested had a triglyceride concentration exceeding 150 mg/dL (1.70 mmol/L).[95] A positive family history of CHD is important in identifying patients at risk for premature atherosclerosis.[20,96] If a patient with CHD has elevated triglycerides, the associated abnormality is probably a contributing factor to CHD and should be treated.[37]

High serum triglycerides (see Tables 21-6 and 21-12) should be treated by achieving desirable body weight, consumption of a low saturated fat and cholesterol diet, regular exercise, smoking cessation, and restriction of alcohol (in selected patients). ATP III identifies the sum of LDL + VLDL (termed *non-HDC* [total cholesterol − HDL]) as a secondary target of therapy in persons with high triglycerides (greater than or equal to 200 mg/dL [greater than or equal to 2.26 mmol/L]).[5,37] This approach is used when triglycerides exceed 200 mg/dL (2.26 mmol/L) and accounts for atherogenic particles carried in VLDL and remnant particles. The goal for non-HDL in persons with high serum triglycerides can be set at 30 mg/dL (0.78 mmol/L) higher than that for LDL on the premise that a VLDL level less than or equal to 30 mg/dL (less than or equal to 0.78 mmol/L) is normal. 7 In patients with borderline-high triglycerides but with accompanying risk factors of established CHD disease, family history of premature CHD, concomitant LDL elevation or low HDL, and genetic forms of hypertriglyceridemia associated with CHD (familial dysbetalipoproteinemia, familial combined hyperlipidemia), drug therapy with niacin should be considered. Niacin may be used cautiously in diabetics based on the results of the ADMIT trial, which found triglycerides were reduced by 23%, HDL-C increased by 29%, only a slight increase in glucose (mean 8.7 mg/dL [0.5 mmol/L]), and no change in hemoglobin A_{1c}.[97] Elevated BMI and plasma glucose predict loss of glycemic control.[89] Alternative therapies include gemfibrozil or fenofibrate, statins, and fish oil.[20,98,99] Fibrates may increase LDL, and their use in borderline-high triglyceridemia requires careful monitoring to detect this deleterious change in lipid profile. Statins may also be used, because they provide modest reductions in triglycerides and modest elevations in HDL. Higher doses of statins may reduce HDL as well as LDL and triglycerides with amount of reduction related to the baseline concentration and dose.[20,99] The goal of therapy in this situation is to lower triglycerides and VLDL particles that may be atherogenic, increase HDL, and reduce LDL.

Very high triglycerides are associated with pancreatitis and other consequences of the chylomicron syndrome. At this level of elevation of triglycerides, a genetic form of hypertriglyceridemia often coexists with other causes of elevated triglycerides such as diabetes. Dietary fat restriction (10%-20% of calories as fat), weight loss, alcohol restriction, and treatment of the coexisting disorder are the basic elements of management. Drugs useful in hypertriglyceridemia include gemfibrozil or fenofibrate, niacin, and higher potency statins (atorvastatin, rosuvastatin, pitvastatin, and simvastatin). Gemfibrozil or fenofibrate are the preferred drugs in diabetics because of the effect of niacin on glycemic control unless the newer ER forms are used. Fenofibrate may be preferred in combination with statin therapy since it does not impair glucuronidation and minimizes potential drug interactions. Success in treatment is defined as a reduction in triglycerides below 500 mg/dL (5.65 mmol/L).[5]

LOW HDL CHOLESTEROL

Low HDL is a strong independent risk predictor of CHD. ATP III redefined low HDL-C as less than 40 mg/dL (less than 1.03 mmol/L), but specified no goal for HDL-C raising.[5] Low HDL may be a consequence of insulin resistance, physical inactivity, Type 2 diabetes, cigarette smoking, very high carbohydrate intake, and certain drugs (see Table 21-5). 8 In low HDL the primary target remains LDL according to ATP III, but emphasis shifts to weight reduction, increased physical activity, and smoking cessation, and if drug therapy is required, to fibric acid derivatives and niacin. Niacin has the potential for the greatest increase in HDL and the effect is more pronounced with regular or immediate-release forms than with sustained-release forms; however, no randomized clinical trial data have shown a reduction in ASCVD risk by raising HDL.[100]

DIABETIC DYSLIPIDEMIA

Diabetic dyslipidemia is characterized by hypertriglyceridemia, low HDL, and LDL that is minimally elevated. Small, dense LDL (pattern B) in diabetes is more atherogenic than larger, more buoyant forms of LDL (pattern A); routine lipoprotein profiles do not differentiate between pattern A and pattern B.[101-103] Diabetes in ATP III is a CHD risk equivalent and the primary target is LDL with a goal of treatment being to lower LDL-C less than 100 mg/dL (less than 2.59 mmol/L).[5] When LDL is greater than 130 mg/dL (greater than 3.36 mmol/L), most patients will require simultaneous therapeutic life-style changes and drug therapy. When LDL-C is between 100 and 129 mg/dL (2.59 and 3.34 mmol/L), intensifying glycemic control, adding drugs for the atherogenic dyslipidemia (fibric acid derivatives, niacin) and intensifying LDL-C-lowering therapy are options. Because the primary target is LDL-C in diabetic dyslipidemia, statins are considered by many to be initial drugs of choice.[5,37] The relative risk reduction for CHD in diabetics versus nondiabetics is greater in the West of Scotland, (37% vs 20%)[104] AFCAPS/TexCAPS (43% vs 36%),[105] CARE (25% vs 23%),[106] and 4S (55% vs 32%) trials.[107] All statins are fairly comparable in triglyceride lowering and because statins differ in potency for LDL reduction, a ratio of LDL reduction to triglyceride reduction can be applied. Statin therapy may protect against the development of diabetes.[34] The most recent trial LDL lowering in Type 2 diabetes mellitus is the Collaborative Atorvastatin Diabetes Study (CARDS).[108] This was a randomized, double-blind placebo comparison of atorvastatin 10 mg per day versus placebo in 2838 diabetes to reduce first CHD events. Baseline LDL was 118 mg/dL (3.05 mmol/L) and with atorvastatin LDL fell by 46 mg/dL (1.19 mmol/L). The primary end point, a composite of acute CHD death, nonfatal MI, hospitalized unstable angina, resuscitated cardiac arrest, coronary revascularization or stroke, was reduced by 37%. This study suggests that all diabetics should have a LDL much lower than 100 mg/dL (2.59 mmol/L) and these results are consistent with the Heart Protection Study analysis of diabetic patients.[109]

Fenofibrate, according to the DIAS trial, reduced the angiographic progression of CAD in Type 2 diabetes.[110] Fewer CHD events were seen with fenofibrate compared with placebo but the difference was not significant. Fibric acids principally lower VLDL and triglycerides while increasing HDL with only modest lowering of total and LDL cholesterol; on occasion, fibric acid derivatives may increase LDL levels. Fibric acid derivatives tend to improve glucose tolerance, in contrast to niacin; the greatest effect has been seen with bezafibrate. The Helsinki Heart Study found gemfibrozil to be most effective in diabetic dyslipidemia.[111] Although the effect of statins on triglycerides and HDL abnormalities commonly seen in diabetes is less than with fibric acids, the subgroup analyses cited earlier suggest that they reduce CHD risk significantly. In the Action to Control Cardiovascular Risk in Diabetes (ACCORD) the combination of a statin and fenofibrate in patients with Type 2 diabetes did not reduce the rate of fatal cardiovascular events, nonfatal myocardial infarction, or nonfatal stroke compared to simvastatin alone.[112] Cholestyramine in diabetic patients may result in lower LDL levels, but VLDL and triglyceride levels, which are commonly elevated in diabetes, may be further increased in this population. Resins may aggravate constipation, which is common in diabetics. As demonstrated in the ADMIT and ADVENT trials, immediate-release and ER niacin are very effective in raising HDL and lowering triglycerides and LDL.[97,113]

SPECIAL CONSIDERATIONS

Elderly

Hypercholesterolemia is an independent risk factor for CHD in the elderly (greater than 65 years old), as it is in the younger patient. The attributable risk, which is the difference in absolute rates of CHD between segments of the population with higher or lower serum cholesterol levels, increases with age. Older patients potentially benefit to a greater extent from cholesterol lowering than younger populations. Data from studies of elderly men in a variety of settings are consistent with a relative risk of at least 1.5 in the highest compared to the lowest quartile of cholesterol levels and a relative risk reduction of 22% for heart-related mortality.[114-116] Treatment of hypercholesterolemia in the elderly may bring about a comparable reduction in absolute risk to that obtained in younger persons.[5] Subgroup analyses of the West of Scotland (primary) and 4S (secondary) intervention studies show that elderly patients have lower CHD risk reduction (relative risk reduction of 27% and 29%, respectively) as compared to younger patients (relative risk reduction of 40% and 39%, respectively).[104,117] The Framingham study suggests that elderly women are at higher risk because of high blood cholesterol levels, but no other large studies included women; and their risks or benefits from cholesterol reduction are not well defined. Primary prevention in younger patients requires about 2 years before reduction in CHD risk is apparent, and this lag time should be taken into consideration in patient selection for therapy. Non-lipid CHD risk factors do not decline in relative risk with aging, and aggressive management of the modifiable non-lipid risk factors is important in the older patient. High-risk elderly patients are less likely to be prescribed statins and their potent benefits are not realized.[118] Because most women with CHD are elderly and also at risk for osteoporosis, they are logical candidates for diet therapy with consideration of calcium intake consistent with osteoporosis prevention, exercise, and perhaps estrogen replacement therapy. Recent evidence suggests that statins may reduce the risk of osteoporosis; however, there are conflicting data from various studies.[119]

Drug therapy in principle differs little from younger patients, and older patients respond to lipid-lowering drugs as well as younger patients.[120,121] Based on the Heart Protection Study with more elderly patients than any other trial, simvastatin 40 mg per day produced the CHD event rate reduction in patients over 70 years of age as in younger patients.[122] The gain in life expectancy may be small depending on the age at the start of treatment and the magnitude of cholesterol reduction. Changes in body composition, renal function, and other physiologic changes of aging may make older patients more susceptible to adverse effects of lipid-lowering drug therapy. In particular, older patients are more likely to have constipation (bile acid resins), skin and eye changes (niacin), gout (niacin), gallstones (fibric acid derivatives), and bone/joint disorders (fibric acid derivatives, statins). Therapy should be started with lower doses and titrated up slowly to minimize adverse effects.

Women

Cholesterol is an important determinant of CHD in women, but the relationship is not as strong as that seen in men. HDL may be a more important predictor of disease in women.[8] LDL and HDL genetic regulation in women and men does not appear to be different. Based on the Nurses' Health Study, obesity is an important determinant of CHD in women, with the relative risk being 3.3 in the highest Quetelet index (weight in kilograms divided by the square of the height in meters) as compared to the lowest category (ie, less than 21 vs greater than or equal to 29); low HDL levels usually accompany obesity.[123] No major differences exist in the influence of exercise, alcohol ingestion, and smoking on lipid levels between men and women. Women in the highest tertile of cholesterol appear to be more responsive to dietary therapy than those in the lower tertiles, and more responsive than formulas based on men predict.

Based on the HERS[124] and WHI trials,[125-127] published national guidelines recommended similar types of lifestyle and risk factor goals and interventions as recommended by NCEP for the entire population.[8] Hormone therapy may continue to have a role for postmenopausal symptoms; however, a notable exception is hormone replacement therapy and heart protection. Combined estrogen plus progestin hormone therapy should not be initiated to prevent CVD in postmenopausal women. Combined estrogen plus progestin hormone therapy should not be continued to prevent CVD in postmenopausal women. Other forms of menopausal hormone therapy (eg, unopposed estrogen) should not be initiated or continued to prevent CVD in postmenopausal women pending the results of ongoing trials. Results of the WISDOM trial confirm lack of benefit as seen in HERS and WHI.[128] In a recent, post-hoc analysis of the WHI, women who initiated hormone therapy closer to menopause tended to have reduced CHD risk compared with the increase in CHD risk among women more distant from menopause, but this trend did not meet statistical signifance.[125] Based on the Justification for the Use of Statins in Prevention: An Intervention Trial Evaluating Rosuvastatin (JUPITER) trial, women experience the same benefit of LDL cholesterol lowering as men with rosuvastatin.[129]

Cholesterol and triglyceride levels rise progressively throughout pregnancy, with an average increment in cholesterol of 30 to 40 mg/dL (0.78-1.03 mmol/L) occurring around the 36th to 39th weeks. Triglyceride levels may go up by as much as 150 mg/dL (1.70 mmol/L). Drug therapy is not instituted nor is it usually continued during pregnancy. If the patient is very high risk, a bile acid resin may considered since there is no systemic drug exposure.[5] Statins are category X and are contraindicated. Ezetimibe might be an alternative since it is a Category C drug (animal studies have shown that the drug exerts teratogenic or embryocidal effects, and there are no adequate, well-controlled studies in pregnant women, or no studies are available in either animals or pregnant women) but no data are available in humans. Dietary therapy is the mainstay of treatment, with emphasis on maintaining a nutritionally balanced diet as per the needs of pregnancy.

Children

Drug therapy in children is not recommended until the age of 8 years or older, and the guidelines for institution of therapy and the goals of therapy are different from those in adults (see Table 21-9).[130] Younger children are generally managed with therapeutic life-style changes until after the age of 2 years.[5,51] Although bile acid sequestrants have been recommended in the past as first line therapy, there is now evidence that statins are safe and effective in children and provide greater lipid lowering than BAR.[131-134] Severe forms of hypercholesterolemia (eg, familial hypercholesterolemia) may require more aggressive treatment.

Concurrent Disease States

Nephrotic syndrome, end-stage renal disease and nephrotic syndrome, and hypertension compound the risk of dyslipidemia and may present difficult-to-treat lipid abnormalities. Abnormalities of lipoprotein metabolism in the nephrotic syndrome include elevated total and LDL cholesterol, Lp(a), VLDL, and triglycerides. The apolipoprotein C-III to C-II ratio is elevated, consistent with greater LPL inhibitor activity, and the extent of hypoalbuminemia is correlated with dyslipidemia. The basic abnormality appears to be one of overproduction of LDL-apoB from VLDL, rather than reduced clearance of LDL-C and related proteins. Protein restriction and a "vegan" diet corrects lipid abnormalities to some extent. Statins have been shown to be effective in reducing elevated total and LDL cholesterol in the nephrotic syndrome, although the levels do not usually return to normal.[135] Fibric acid derivatives and statins reduce small, dense LDL-C by different mechanisms, suggesting a potential role for combination therapy to optimize lowering of small, dense LDL-C and remnant lipoproteins. Statins appear to be safe and effective for lowering LDL cholesterol in renal insufficiency but they may not affect CHD endpoints.[136,137]

Renal insufficiency without proteinuria leads to hypertriglyceridemia, slightly elevated total and LDL cholesterol (particularly with chronic ambulatory peritoneal dialysis), and low HDL levels (especially during hemodialysis). These abnormalities are thought to be caused by a deficiency in apolipoprotein C-II, perhaps as a result of sustained use of heparin during hemodialysis and depletion of LPL, carbohydrate-induced obesity and hypertriglyceridemia, loss of carnitine during hemodialysis, use of acetate buffer (acetate is a precursor to fatty acid synthesis) during hemodialysis, and decreased LCAT activity during hemodialysis. Dialysis does not correct the lipid abnormalities. Renal transplantation may correct lipid abnormalities in some patients; however, in others, the use of transplantation-related medications, such as corticosteroids, cyclosporine, and certain antihypertensive agents, may aggravate the lipid abnormalities. Cyclosporine interferes with the metabolism of statins metabolized by cytochrome P450 3A4 (see Table 21-14), and patients need to be observed closely for myositis and worsening renal function. Of interest, correction of lipid abnormalities may improve renal hemodynamics. Pravastatin and fluvastatin may be safer than other statins, but this needs to be validated in larger, long-term trials. Diet will modify lipoprotein levels and polyunsaturated fatty acids may have a role in impeding the progression of renal disease as well as the cardiovascular complications. Bile acid sequestrants do not correct the lipid abnormalities seen in renal insufficiency. Lovastatin or its active metabolite may accumulate in renal insufficiency, and lower doses of reductase inhibitors should be used to avoid adverse effects. Gemfibrozil may be used with caution as its pharmacokinetics are unchanged and it lowers triglycerides and increases HDL.[138] Statins (simvastatin, lovastatin, and atorvastatin) and fibric acid derivatives may increase the risk of severe myopathy, and attention to symptoms of myositis is needed. Niacin may also be useful in nondiabetic patients with renal insufficiency.

Hypertensive patients have a greater-than-expected prevalence of high blood-cholesterol levels and, conversely, patients with hypercholesterolemia have a higher than expected prevalence of hypertension caused by the metabolic syndrome. Recommendations for the management of hypertension in patients with hypercholesterolemia include avoiding the use of drugs that elevate cholesterol such as diuretics and β-blockers and using agents that are either lipid-neutral or that may reduce cholesterol slightly.[5] Bile acid sequestrants may bind to thiazide diuretics and some β-blockers, and may interfere with their absorption; reaction may be avoided by giving the antihypertensive 1 hour before or 4 hours after the resin. Niacin may magnify the hypotensive effects of vasodilators.

PHARMACOECONOMIC CONSIDERATIONS

The clinical benefits of lipid-lowering therapy for primary and secondary intervention are now well established based on the results of studies showing a reduction in CHD morbidity and mortality.[139-141] The balance of benefits and costs has been examined in a few studies. The cost per year of life saved has been estimated to range from less than \$10,000 to over \$1 million dollars depending on the presence or absence of CHD, age of the patient, baseline total or LDL-C level and reduction in cholesterol, and number of risk factors present. In general, intervention in patients with known CHD, those who have CHD risk equivalents or those with a 10-year risk of 10% to 20% are cost-effective with statin therapy, while other types of therapy may be cost-effective if certain assumptions concerning compliance, efficacy, and so forth, are met. The range for secondary intervention based on the 4S study is \$3,800 for a 70-year-old man with a high cholesterol level to \$27,400 per year of life gained for a middle-aged woman with an average cholesterol level.[142] In contrast, primary prevention in men based on the West of Scotland trial averages about \$35,000 per year of life gained.[143] These studies demonstrate that primary and secondary interventions are well within the accepted boundary of less than \$50,000 for a medical intervention to be considered cost-effective. Based on the specific lipoprotein phenotype, fibric acid derivatives, niacin, or combination therapy of statins plus BAR may be cost-effective. Cost-effectiveness is maximized by treating high-risk patients and those with established CHD.

Specialty lipid clinics have become increasingly popular and many use pharmacists to provide direct patient care in this setting. An interesting recent analysis shows that a specialty clinic may be more expensive (\$659 ± \$43 vs \$477 ± \$42 per patient, $P < 0.001$) than usual care. However, the overall cost-effectiveness is improved when expressed as program costs per unit (mmol/L) reduction in the LDL-C, a measure of cost-effectiveness that was significantly lower for specialized care (\$758 ± \$58 vs \$1,058 ± \$70, $P = 0.002$) because more patients achieve their targeted goal.[144] Project ImPACT demonstrated that pharmacists, working collaborative with patients and physicians, can improve persistence and compliance and that nearly two thirds of patients achieved their NCEP lipid goal.[145] Other programs show similar trends.[77,146,147]

OTHER THERAPIES

Partial ileal bypass has been used in severe heterozygous and homozygous familial hypercholesterolemia; however, it is ineffective in the latter case. Ileal bypass removes the site of bile acid reabsorption, depleting the bile acid pool and increasing the catabolism of cholesterol. A randomized trial of diet versus surgery, program on the surgical control of the hyperlipidemias (POSCH), reported that total and LDL cholesterol were decreased (23.3% and 37.7%, respectively) and HDL increased (4.3%) in patients who had undergone ileal bypass for hypercholesterolemia.[148] Overall death was delayed by nearly 3 years ($P = 0.032$) and CHD mortality was delayed by nearly 4 years ($P = 0.046$) by surgery, as compared to the control group. Revascularization procedures were delayed by an average of 7 years ($P < 0.001$). Post-surgery diarrhea was more common in the surgical group, as was the rate of kidney stones (4% vs 0.4%), gallstones (10% vs 2%), and bowel obstruction (13.5% vs 3.6%).

Portacaval shunts have been used to decrease the formation of LDL-C and reductions of 10% to 20% have been reported. Plasma exchange combined with niacin was found to reduce plasma cholesterol levels by about 50% in homozygous familial hypercholesterolemia over 5 years, and coronary atherosclerosis did not progress as documented by angiography. LDL-apheresis, selective removal of LDL-C via a filtering system, plus statin therapy is effective in LDL-C and appears to affect the progression of vascular disease. LDL-apheresis may be combined with statin therapy for greater effect. Combined liver and heart transplantation in homozygous familial hypercholesterolemia reduces total and LDL cholesterol concentrations from about 1,100 and 900 mg/dL (28.45 and 23.27 mmol/L) to about 300 and 185 mg/dL (7.76 and 4.78 mmol/L), prior to and after surgery, respectively. Liver transplantation replaced the missing LDL receptors, enhanced catabolism, and reduced lipoprotein synthesis in this patient.

SUMMARY OF MAJOR STUDIES

9 Primary and secondary prevention diet and drug trials have been performed to determine whether lowering of cholesterol will prevent CHD; **Tables 21-15** and **21-16** summarize these trials. A number of earlier angiographic studies demonstrated that cholesterol reduction leads to regression of atherosclerosis and plaque stabilization. Most of the primary and secondary studies were double blinded, randomized, and placebo controlled, lasting for 5 years or longer, and most had sufficient patient numbers to be meaningful. Exceptions to these qualifications were seen in the early studies such as the Newcastle and Edinburgh trials, which were small and generally did not show much benefit; and the Coronary Drug Project (CDP) using dextrothyroxine, which was terminated early due to adverse effects on CHD mortality. The Helsinki heart study, using gemfibrozil, resulted in a reduction in nonfatal MI, which was the primary contributor to reduced CHD incidence (see Table 21-15).[19]

Total and LDL cholesterol were reduced to an average of 13.4% and 20.3%, respectively, by cholestyramine in the LRC-CPPT, and the reduction of lipid levels was related to the amount of drug ingested (eg, 1 to 2 packets, 5.4% reduction in total cholesterol, versus 5 or more packets, 19.0% reduction).[149] The prescribed dose of cholestyramine was 24 g, or 6 packets, per day. The cholestyramine group experienced a 19% reduction in risk ($P < 0.05$) of the primary end point—definite CHD death and/or definite nonfatal MI—reflecting a 24% reduction in definite CHD death and a 19% reduction in nonfatal MI. Other end points were reduced by 25%, 20%, and 21% for new positive exercise tests, angina, and coronary bypass surgery, respectively. Death from all causes was not significantly reduced by cholestyramine secondary to more accidents and violence in this group. The mean falls in total and LDL cholesterol in the cholestyramine group were 8% and 12% relative to levels in placebo-treated men, providing evidence that for every 1% reduction in cholesterol, a 2% decline in CHD mortality can be realized.

AFCAPS/TexCAPS, a primary prevention trial conducted in 6,605 men and women aged 57 to 63 years with average total cholesterol and LDL (less than 221 mg/dL and less than 150 mg/dL [less than 5.72 and less than 3.88 mmol/L], respectively) who were treated with lovastatin 20 to 40 mg/d for 5.2 years, a 37% reduction

TABLE 21-15 Primary Prevention Trials with Lipid Lowering Drugs

Trial	F/U (yr)	*N*	Treatment	Control Events (%)	Treatment Events (%)	*p* Value	RRR	ARR (%)	NNT
AFCAPS/TexCAPS	5	6,605	Lovastatin 20-40 mg	5.5	3.5	<0.001	36.4%	2.0	50
Helsinki	5	4,081	Gemfibrozil 1,200 mg	4.1	2.7	<0.02	34.0%	1.4	71
LRC-CPPT	7.4	3,806	Cholestyramine 24 g	9.8	8.1	<0.05	17.3%	1.7	59
Oslo	5	1,232	Diet + Smoking Cessation	4.2	2.5	0.03	40.5%	1.7	59
WOSCOPS	4.9	6,595	Pravastatin 40 mg	7.8	5.5	<0.001	29.5%	2.3	43
ALLHAT	4.8	10,355	Usual care Pravastatin 40 mg	10.4	9.3	0.16	9%	1.1	91
WHI	5.2	16,608	Usual care Diet, CEE 0.625 mg + MPA 2.5 mg	1.5	1.9	0.05	1.29*	0.4	200**
WHI	5.2	16,608	Usual care Diet, CEE 0.625 mg	3.7	3.3	NA	9%	0.4	250
CARDS	4	2,838	Atorvastatin 10 mg	9.0	5.8	0.001	37%	3.2	32
JUPITER	1.9	17,802	Rosuvastatin 20 mg	2.82	1.59	0.00001	44%	1.2	82

AFCAPS/TexCAPS, Air Force/Texas Coronary Atherosclerosis Prevention Study (Downs et al., 1998); ALLHAT, Antihypertensive and Lipid-Lowering Treatment to Prevent Heart Attack Trial; approximately 13%-15% of patients had a history of coronary heart disease (CHD); events are CHD events only; ARR, Absolute Risk Reduction; CARDS, Collaborative Atorvastatin Diabetes Study (presented at the 2004 American Diabetes Association meeting); CEE, conjugated equine estrogen; Helsinki, The Helsinki Heart Study (Frick et al., 1987); *HR, hazard ratio. The risk of CHD was increased by 29%; JUPITER, Justification for the Use of Statins in Prevention (Ridker, 2008); LRC-CPPT, The Lipid Research Clinics Coronary Primary Prevention Trial (Insull et al., 1984); MPA, medtroxyprogesterone acetate; NA, Not available; NNT, Number Needed to Treat; Oslo, The Oslo Study (Hjermann et al., 1988); RRR, Relative Risk Reduction; WHI, Women's Health Initiative; WOSCOPS, The West of Scotland Coronary Prevention Study (Shepherd et al., 1995).

**Number needed to harm since CEE + MPA was worse than placebo.

TABLE 21-16 Secondary Prevention Trials with Lipid Lowering Drugs

Trial	F/U (yr)	*N*	Treatment	Control Events	Treatment Events	*p* Value	RRR	ARR	NNT
VA-HIT	5.1	2,531	Gemfibrozil 1,200 mg	23.7%	17.3%	0.006	22%	4.4%	23
AVERT	1.5	341	Atorvastatin 80 mg	21%	13%	0.048	38%	8%	12
CARE	5	4,159	Pravastatin 40 mg	13.2%	10.2%	0.003	22.7%	3.0%	33
CDP	5	8,341	Niacin 3 g + Clofibrate 1.8 g	20.9%	20.6%	NS	1.4%	0.3%	333
HERS	4.1	2,673	Estrogen 0.625 mg + Progestin 2.5 mg	12.7%	12.5%	0.91	1.6%	0.2%	500
LIPID	7.4	3,806	Pravastatin 40 mg	9.8%	8.1%	<0.05	17.3%	1.7%	59
4S	5	4,444	Simvastatin 20 mg	11.5%	8.2%	0.0003	28.7%	3.3%	30
WHO	5.3	15,745	Clofibrate 1.6 g	3.9%	3.1%	<0.005	20.5%	0.8%	125
BIP	6.2	3,090	Placebo Bezafibrate 400 mg	15.0%	13.6%	0.26	9.3%	1.4%	72
TIMI-22	2	4,162	Pravastatin 40 mg Atorvastatin 80 mg	26.3% (P)	22.4% (A)	0.005	16%	3.9%	26
HPS	5	20,536	Simvastatin 40 mg	14.7%	12.9%	0.003	13%	1.8%	56
MIRACL		3,086	Atorvastatin 80 mg	17.4%	14.8%	0.048	16%	2.6%	39
PROSPER	3	5,804	Pravastatin 40 mg	16.2%	14.1%	0.014	24%	2.1%	48
SPARCL	4.0	4,731	Atorvastatin 80 mg	13.1	11.2	0.03	16%	2.2	46
TNT	4.9	10,001	Atorvastatin 10 mg vs 80 mg	10.9	8.7	<0.001	22%	2.2	46
ACCORD	4.7	5,518	Fenofibrate 160 mg	2.4%	2.2%	0.32	8%	0.2%	500
AIM-HIGH	2	3,414	Niacin 1,500-2,000 mg + simvastatin	16.2%	16.4	0.80	−0.2%	+1.2%	NA
HPS 2-THRIVE	3.9	25,673	Niacin 2 gm + laropripant	13.7%	13.2%	0.29	4.9%	0.5%	200
IMPROVE-IT	7	18,144	Simvastatin ± ezetimibe	34.7	32.7	0.016	6.4	2.0	50

ACCORD, Action to Control Cardiovascular Risk in Diabetes (Accord Study Group, 2010); AIM-HIGH, Low HDL/High Triglycerides: Impact on Global Health Outcomes (AIM-HIGH Investigators); ARR, Absolute Risk Reduction; AVERT, The Atorvastatin Versus Revascularization Treatments; BIP, Bezafibrate Infarction Prevention; CARE, Cholesterol and Recurrent Events (Melendez et al., 1996); CDP, Coronary Drug Project (Berge et al., 1975); HERS, Heart and Estrogen Replacement Study (Hulley et al., 1998); HPS, Heart Protection Study; results expressed as all cause mortality (HPS Collaborative Group, 2002); HPS2-THRIVE, Heart Protection Study—Treatment of HDL to Reduce the Incidence of Vascular Events; IMPROVE-IT, Improved Reduction in Outcomes: Vytorin Efficacy International Trial; LIPID, Long-Term Intervention with Pravastatin in Ischaemic Disease Study (MacMahon et al., 1995); MIRACL, Myocardial Ischemia Reduction with Aggressive Cholesterol Lowering (Schwartz et al., 2001); NNT, Number Needed to Treat; PROSPER, PROspective Study of Pravastatin in the Elderly at Risk (Shepher, 2002); RRR, Relative Risk Reduction; SPARCL, Stroke Prevention by Aggressive Reduction in Cholesterol Levels (SPARCL investigators, 2006); 4S, Scandinavian Simvastatin Survival Study (Pederson et al., 1994); TIMI-22, Thrombolysis in Myocardial Infarction study 22; also known as the PROVE-IT trial (Cannon et al., 2004); TNT, Treatment to New Targets (LaRosa, 2005); VA-HIT, Veterans Administration-High-Density Lipoprotein Cholesterol (HDL-C) Intervention Trial; WHO, World Health Organization (Committee of Principal Investigators, 1978).

($P < 0.001$) was shown in the risk for first acute major coronary event (fatal or nonfatal MI, unstable angina, or sudden cardiac death).[105] The need for revascularization procedures was also reduced by 33% ($P < 0.001$). The implications of this trial are enormous; potentially millions of "normal" people could benefit from lipid-lowering with statins based on these results. The number of patients that need to be treated (NNT, see Table 21-15) for primary prevention ranges from 43 in the West of Scotland trial to 71 in the Helsinki Heart Study. This range is within the typical boundary used for treatment decisions and described previously; cost-effectiveness is achieved routinely in patients with moderate to high risk. The Antihypertensive and Lipid-Lowering Treatment to Prevent Heart Attack Trial (ALLHAT-LLT) tested pravastatin 40 mg per day versus placebo in hypertensive patients with at least one CHD risk factor. Pravastatin did not reduce either all-cause mortality or CHD significantly when compared with usual care in older participants with well-controlled hypertension and moderately elevated LDL-C. The results may be due to the modest differential in total cholesterol (9.6%) and LDL-C (16.7%) between pravastatin and usual care compared with prior statin trials supporting cardiovascular disease prevention.[150] The Women's Health Initiative trial proved to be disappointing with no beneficial effects on CHD event reduction in the hormone replacement arm (conjugated equine estrogens [CEE] + medroxgprogesterone) or the CEE alone arm compared to placebo.[124,126] Women did experience greater risk for thromboembolism and a slight increase in breast cancer and a reduced risk of hip fracture. Consequently, hormone replacement therapy can no longer be recommended for cardiovascular protection.[8] Publication of the recent WISDOM trial found that when combined hormone therapy ($n = 2196$) was compared with placebo ($n = 2189$), there was a significant increase in the number of major cardiovascular events (7 vs 0, $P = 0.016$) and venous thromboembolism (22 vs 3, hazard ratio 7.36 [95% CI 2.20-24.60]) confirming the findings of HERS and WHI. There were no statistically significant differences in numbers of breast or other cancers cerebrovascular events, fractures, and overall death.[128]

Niacin in the CDP significantly reduced definite, nonfatal MI as compared to placebo (10.1% vs 13.9%), whereas clofibrate did not reduce death from any cause or nonfatal or fatal MI at the 5-year followup period.[151]

One of the most important studies published in the last few years is the 4S trial, a secondary intervention trial in a large number of patients.[152] Simvastatin, 20 to 40 mg/d, reduced LDL cholesterol by 35% and reduced the risk of death from any cause by 30%. Coronary deaths were also reduced with simvastatin (relative risk, 0.58; confidence interval, 0.46-0.73). Therapy was also shown to be effective in women (18%-19% of patients enrolled) and in the elderly (greater than or equal to 60 years). Indeed, the relative risk of death or major coronary event was reduced to a greater extent in the elderly than in younger patients. Death from noncardiovascular causes was similar for simvastatin and placebo (2.1% and 2.2%, respectively). The survival curves for simvastatin and placebo began to separate at 1 year and became more divergent with additional follow-up. The 4S study clearly demonstrates the benefit in cholesterol lowering and placates long-held fears of death from non-CHD causes. The long-term intervention with pravastatin in ischemic disease (LIPID) study ($N = 7,498$ men and 1,516 women) has investigated the effect of pravastatin on CHD mortality in patients with prior MI or unstable angina and mean cholesterol level of 219 mg/dL (5.66 mmol/L) over 6 years.[153] Pravastatin reduced the risk of CHD mortality by 24% (8.3% vs 6.4%, $P = 0.0004$) and total mortality by 23% (14.1% vs 11.0%, $P = 0.00002$); stroke was also reduced by 20% (4.3% vs 3.5%, $P = 0.22$) as well as reduction in the need for coronary artery bypass graft (11.3% vs 8.9%, $P = 0.0001$) or percutaneous transluminal coronary angioplasty (5.3% vs 4.4%, $P = 0.04$).

The Veterans Administration High-Density Lipoprotein intervention trial [154] was a double-blind trial that compared gemfibrozil (1,200 mg/day) with placebo in 2,531 men with CHD, an HDL cholesterol level of less than or equal to 40 mg/dL (less than or equal to 1.03 mmol/L), and an LDL cholesterol level of less than or equal to 140 mg/dL (less than or equal to 3.62 mmol/L).[155] The primary study outcome was nonfatal MI or death from coronary causes. The median follow-up was 5.1 years. At 1 year, the mean HDL cholesterol level was 6% higher, the mean triglyceride level was 31% lower, and the mean total cholesterol level was 4% lower in the gemfibrozil group than in the placebo group. LDL cholesterol levels did not differ significantly between the groups. A primary event occurred in 21.7% of the patients assigned to placebo and in 17.3% of the patients assigned to gemfibrozil. The overall reduction in the risk of an event was 4.4 percentage points, and the reduction in relative risk was 22% ($P = 0.006$). This trial presents the strongest evidence to date that raising HDL-C and lowering triglycerides reduces risk for CHD.

The Atorvastatin Versus Revascularization Treatments[156] study compared atorvastatin 80 mg/day with percutaneous transluminal coronary angioplasty.[157] The follow-up period was 18 months. Of the patients who received aggressive lipid-lowering treatment with atorvastatin, 13% had ischemic events, as compared to 21% of the patients who underwent angioplasty. The incidence of ischemic events was thus 36% lower in the atorvastatin group over an 18-month period ($P = 0.048$, which was not statistically significant after adjustment for interim analyses). This reduction in events was because of a smaller number of angioplasty procedures, coronary-artery bypass operations, and hospitalizations for worsening angina (the most common end point). As compared to the patients who were treated with angioplasty and usual care, the patients who received atorvastatin had a significantly longer time to the first ischemic event ($P = 0.03$). In low-risk patients with stable CAD, aggressive lipid-lowering therapy is at least as effective as angioplasty and usual care in reducing the incidence of ischemic events.

Pravastatin in the elderly individuals at risk for vascular disease[158] studied men and women in the age range of 70 to 82 years and found that pravastatin 40 mg per day reduced CHD events by 24% with no effect on cognitive function.[158] A more recent trial, TIMI-22 (also known as PROVE-IT, Pravastatin or Atorvastatin Evaluation and Infection Therapy) enrolled 4162 patients who had been hospitalized for an acute coronary syndrome within the preceding 10 days and compared 40 mg of pravastatin daily (standard therapy) with 80 mg of atorvastatin daily (intensive therapy).[159] An intensive lipid lowering statin regimen with atorvastatin 80 mg per day provided greater protection against death or major cardiovascular events than does a standard regimen. This study clearly points to 'lower is better' for LDL concentration and will likely lead to revision in guideline goals to lower LDL levels. The Treatment to New Targets (TNT) assessed the efficacy and safety of lowering LDL cholesterol levels below 100 mg per deciliter (2.6 mmol per liter) in patients with stable CHD.[160,161] Intensive lipid-lowering therapy with 80 mg of atorvastatin per day in patients with stable CHD provides significant clinical benefit beyond that afforded by treatment with 10 mg of atorvastatin per day providing further evidence that intensive lipid lowering brings greater benefits.

Statins reduce the incidence of strokes among patients at increased risk for cardiovascular disease; whether they reduce the risk of stroke after a recent stroke or transient ischemic attack (TIA) was addressed by Stroke Prevention by Aggressive Reduction in Cholesterol Levels[162]. During a median follow-up of 4.9 years, 265 patients (11.2 percent) receiving atorvastatin 80 mg/day and 311 patients (13.1 percent) receiving placebo had a fatal or nonfatal stroke (5-year absolute reduction in risk, 2.2%; adjusted hazard ratio, 0.84; 95% confidence interval, 0.71-0.99; $P = 0.03$; unadjusted $P = 0.05$).[163] JUPITER randomized healthy patients to rosuvastatin on placebo the basis of elevated CRP found a 55% reduction in vascular events (event rate 1.11 vs 0.51 per 100 person-years; hazard ratio 0.45, $p < 0.0001$).[28]

Recent clinical trials attempting to increase HDL-C have been disappointing and one was stopped early due to futility.[164] Neither the AIM-HIGH or HPS2-THRIVE trial demonstrated a reduction in cardiovascular endpoints.[17] Both trials included background therapy with statins ± ezetimibe and the changes in HDL-C was somewhat smaller than expected. Some have suggested that extensive prior treatment may have depleted the lipid core making plaque less susceptible to rupture leading to clinical events.

Clinical **Controversy...**

The CETP inhibitor torcetrapib was associated with a substantial increase in HDL cholesterol and decrease in LDL cholesterol. It was also associated with an increase in blood pressure, and there was no significant decrease in the progression of coronary atherosclerosis. The lack of efficacy may be related to the mechanism of action of this drug class or to molecule-specific adverse effects. Other means of raising HDL cholesterol (HDL mimetics, which include ApoA1 mutants and peptide mimetics of ApoA1 and HDL Milano A, a synthetic form of HDL) still hold hope of HDL modification leading a reduction in clinical events.

The enzyme acyl-coenzyme A: cholesterol acyltransferase[165] esterifies cholesterol in a variety of tissues. In some animal models, ACAT inhibitors have antiatherosclerotic effects. Unfortunately, when tested in clinical trials, ACAT inhibition is not an effective strategy for limiting atherosclerosis and may promote atherogenesis.[165]

With the failure of AIM-HIGH and HPS2-THRIVE, the HDL hypothesis, raising HDL-C lowers cardiovascular risk, may called into question. Others argue that trial design limited the outcome in these studies and a true test of the HDL-C hypothesis remains to be completed.

Statins differ in their pharmacokinetic properties and in pleotropic effects (ie, non-lipid lowering). The contribution of lipid lowering alone (a class effect) versus other effects (anti-inflammatory, antithombotic, etc.) continues to create controversy.

Proteinuria has been associated with high dose rosuvastatin therapy (40 mg/day) but a review of a clinical trial database revealed that an increase in eGFR for rosuvastatin-treated patients was consistent across all major demographic and clinical subgroups of interest, including patients with baseline proteinuria, baseline eGFR less than 60 mL/min/1.73 m^2 (less than 0.58 mL/s/m^2), and in patients with hypertension and/or diabetes.[166]

Mipomersen is an oligonucleotide inhibitor of apolipprotein B-100 synthesis indicated as an adjunct to lipid lowering medications and diet to reduce LDL-cholesterol, apolipoprotein B, total cholesterol and non-high density lipoprotein cholesterol in patients with homozygous familial hypercholesterolemia. The average reduction in LDL-cholesterol is ~25% with the most common adverse events being injection site pain (~10%).[167] Lomitapide oral capsule is a microsomal triglyceride transfer protein (MTP) inhibitor. Inhibiting MTP reduces the level of cholesterol that the liver and intestines assemble and secrete into the circulation.[168] The average decrease in LDL-cholesterol beyond baseline is ~40%. Hepatic steatosis associated with lomitapide may be a risk factor for progressive liver disease including steatohepatitis and cirrhosis. Gastrointestinal complaints and mild to moderate elevations in liver enzymes have been reported with both drugs.

A new category of LDL lowering therapy was approved by the Food and Drug Administration in 2015. Currently, there are two agents in this category including alirocumab and evolcumab. Their mechanism of action is to inhibit proprotein convertase subtilisin/kexin type 9 (PCKS9). PCSK9 promotes intracellular degradation of hepatic LDL, prevents LDL recycling to the cell surface, and reduces LDL clearance from the circulation. Therefore, inhibiting PCSK9 will lower LDL concentrations significantly. Alirocumab and evolocumb are given by subcutaneous injection. Alirocumb is given every 2 weeks at either 75 or 150 mg dose per injection. Evolocumab is given every 140 mg every 2 weeks or 420 mg every month as 3 × 140 mg subcutaneous injections. The typical LDL reduction ranges from about 40% to over 60% with both drugs. The most common adverse effect reported in clinical trials is injection site pain.

Cholesterol ester transport inhibitors (CETP) are currently being studied but early trials with torcetrapib were disappointing with increased CV events that were attributed to increases in blood pressure. Other analogs (eg, anacetrapib and evacetrapib) are continuing under development. Both reduce LDL by approximately 40% to 50% and raise HDL by 80% to 130%. Randomized trials with hard CVD outcomes are needed before large-scale use is possible.

The role of non-traditional risk factors (hsCRP, homocysteine, etc.) is continuing to be clarified and may lead to recommendations for the use of these tests in patient evaluation.

EVALUATION OF THERAPEUTIC OUTCOMES

Short-term evaluation of therapy for hyperlipidemia is based on response to diet and drug treatment as measured in the clinical laboratory by total cholesterol, LDL cholesterol, HDL cholesterol, and triglycerides for patients being treated for primary intervention, as well as on response to secondary intervention. The interval for follow-up is dependent on the severity of illness, and patients with known CAD or multiple risk factors should be monitored more closely. Less commonly used laboratory measurements include CRP, homocysteine, apolipoprotein B, and Lp(a) levels. Because many patients being treated for primary hyperlipidemia have no symptoms and may not have any clinical manifestations of a genetic lipid disorder such as xanthomas or eruptions, monitoring and outcome are solely laboratory based. In patients treated for secondary intervention, symptoms of atherosclerotic cardiovascular disease, such as angina or intermittent claudication, may improve over months to years. If patients have xanthomas or other external manifestations of hyperlipidemia, these lesions should regress with therapy. Lipid measurements should be obtained in the fasted state to minimize interference from chylomicrons, and once the patient is stable, monitoring is needed at intervals of 6 months to 1 year.

Patients with multiple risk factors and established CHD should also be monitored and evaluated for progress in managing their other risk factors such as hypertension, smoking cessation, exercise and weight control, and glycemic control if diabetic. The goals are to maintain a blood pressure of below 140/80 mm Hg or less (presence of diabetes or renal insufficiency), stop smoking, maintain an ideal body weight, exercise for at least 20 minutes three or more times per week, and keep plasma glucose below 100 mg/dL (5.6 mmol/L) (threshold for glucose intolerance). Invasive evaluation, such as cardiac catheterization, is useful in patients with established CHD and is typically used for planning revascularization rather than monitoring of lipid-lowering therapy.

Evaluation of dietary therapy is part of the outcome evaluation for treating hyperlipidemia and the assistance of a dietitian is recommended. Use of diet diaries and recall survey instruments enable information about diet to be collected in a systematic fashion and may improve patient adherence to dietary recommendations. Patients on resin therapy should have a FLP panel checked every 4 to 8 weeks until a stable dose; triglycerides should be checked at stable dose to insure they have not increased. Niacin requires baseline liver function tests, uric acid and glucose; repeat tests are appropriate at doses of 1,000 to 1,500 mg per day. Symptoms myopathy or diabetes-like symptoms should be investigated and may require CK or glucose determinations; more frequent monitoring in diabetics may be necessary. A FLP 4 to 8 weeks after the initial dose or dose changes with statins is appropriate. Liver function tests should be obtained at baseline and periodically thereafter based on package insert information; recognized experts believe that monitoring for hepatotoxicity and myopathy should be symptom-triggered.[63,70] Ezetimibe requires little specific monitoring however, with the publication of the SEAS trial, there is concern over the increased risk of cancer.[169] More recent meta-analyses have not noted a relationship nor were any signal see in the IMPROVE-IT trial. IMPROVE-IT also demonstrated a small reduction in overall cardiovascular events (32.7 vs 34.7%, $p = 0.016$, relative risk reduction of 6.4%.[173]

ABBREVIATIONS

ACCORD	Action to Control Cardiovascular Risk in Diabetes
AHA	American Heart Association
ATP III	Adult Treatment Panel III
BMI	Body mass index
CAD	Coronary artery disease
CARDS	Collaborative Atorvastatin Diabetes Study
CDP	Coronary Drug Project
CETP	Cholesterol ester transfer protein
CHD	Coronary heart disease
CIMT	Carotid intimal medial thickness
CRP	C-reactive protein
DISC	Dietary Intervention Study in Children
ER	Extended-release
hsCRP	High sensitivity C-reactive protein
IDL	Intermediate-density lipoprotein
IHD	Ischemic heart disease
INR	International normalized ratio
KLF2	Kruppel-like factor 2
LCAT	Lecithin-cholesterol acyltransferase
LIPID	Long-term intervention with pravastatin in ischemic disease
LPL	Lipoprotein lipase
MCP-1	Monocyte chemoattractant protein 1
PDAY	Pathobiologic determinants of atherosclerosis in youth
POSCH	Program on the surgical control of the hyperlipidemias
SEC	Sinusoidal endothelial cells
TIA	Transient ischemic attack
TLC	Therapeutic life style changes
TNT	Treatment to New Targets

REFERENCES

1. Svahn JC, Feldl F, Raiha NC, Koletzko B, Axelsson IE. Fatty acid content of plasma lipid fractions, blood lipids, and apolipoproteins in children fed milk products containing different quantity and quality of fat. *J Pediatr Gastroenterol Nutr* 2000;31:152-161.
2. Abbasi F, McLaughlin T, Lamendola C, et al. High carbohydrate diets, triglyceride-rich lipoproteins, and coronary heart disease risk. *Am J Cardiol* 2000;85:45-48.
3. Abbott RD, Levy D, Kannel WB, et al. Cardiovascular risk factors and graded treadmill exercise endurance in healthy adults: The Framingham Offspring Study. *Am J Cardiol* 1989;63:342-346.
4. Gotto AM, Ncep ATP III. NCEP ATP III guidelines incorporate global risk assessment. *Am J Manag Care Suppl* 2003;1-3.
5. Expert Panel on Detection E, and Treatment of High Blood Cholesterol in Adults. Executive summary of the third report of the National Cholesterol Education Program (NCEP) Expert Panel on Detection, Evaluation and Treatment of High Blood Cholesterol in Adults (Adult Treatment Panel III). *JAMA* 2001;285:2486-2497.
6. Grundy SM, Cleeman JI, Merz CN, et al. Implications of recent clinical trials for the National Cholesterol Education Program Adult Treatment Panel III guidelines. [erratum appears in Circulation. 2004 Aug 10;110(6):763]. *Circulation* 2004;110:227-239.
7. Smith SC Jr, Allen J, Blair SN, et al. AHA/ACC guidelines for secondary prevention for patients with coronary and other atherosclerotic vascular disease: 2006 update: Endorsed by the National Heart, Lung, and Blood Institute. [erratum appears in Circulation. 2006 Jun 6;113(22):e847]. *Circulation* 2006;113:2363-2372.
8. Mosca L, Banka CL, Benjamin EJ, et al. Evidence-based guidelines for cardiovascular disease prevention in women: 2007 update. *Circulation* 2007;115:1481-1501.
9. Fletcher B, Berra K, Ades P, et al. Managing abnormal blood lipids: A collaborative approach. *Circulation* 2005;112:3184-3209.
10. Ford ES, Mokdad AH, Giles WH, Mensah GA. Serum total cholesterol concentrations and awareness, treatment, and control of hypercholesterolemia among US adults: Findings from the National Health and Nutrition Examination Survey, 1999 to 2000. *Circulation* 2003;107:2185-2189.
11. Mozaffarian D, Benjamin EJ, Go AS, et al. Executive Summary: Heart Disease and Stroke Statistics—2015 Update: A Report From the American Heart Association. *Circulation* 2015;131:434-441.
12. Foley KA, Denke MA, Kamal-Bahl S, et al. The impact of physician attitudes and beliefs on treatment decisions: Lipid therapy in high-risk patients. *Med Care* 2006;44:421-428.
13. Go AS, Mozaffarian D, Roger VL, et al. Heart disease and stroke statistics—2013 update: A report from the American Heart Association. *Circulation* 2013;127:e6-e245.
14. Menotti A, Lanti M, Nedeljkovic S, Nissinen A, Kafatos A, Kromhout D. The relationship of age, blood pressure, serum cholesterol and smoking habits with the risk of typical and atypical coronary heart disease death in the European cohorts of the Seven Countries Study. *Int J Cardiol* 2006;106:157-163.
15. McQueen MJ, Hawken S, Wang X, et al. Lipids, lipoproteins, and apolipoproteins as risk markers of myocardial infarction in 52 countries (the INTERHEART study): A case-control study. *Lancet* 2008;372: 224-233.
16. Rader DJ. Mechanisms of disease: HDL metabolism as a target for novel therapies. *Nat Clin Pract Cardiovasc Med* 2007;4:102-109.
17. Investigators A-H, Boden WE, Probstfield JL, et al. Niacin in patients with low HDL cholesterol levels receiving intensive statin therapy. *N Engl J Med* 2011;365:2255-2267.
18. Jeppesen J, Hein HO, Suadicani P, Gyntelberg F. Triglyceride concentration and ischemic heart disease: An eight-year follow-up in the Copenhagen Male Study. *Circulation* 1998;97:1029-1036.
19. Huttunen JK, Manninen V, Manttari M, et al. The Helsinki Heart Study: Central findings and clinical implications. *Ann Med* 1991;23: 155-159.
20. Yuan G, Al-Shali KZ, Hegele RA. Hypertriglyceridemia: Its etiology, effects and treatment. *CMAJ Can Med Assoc J* 2007;176: 1113-1120.
21. Ganong WF. *Pathophysiology of Disease: An Introduction to Clinical Medicine*. 5th ed. New York: McGraw Hill; 2006.
22. Nissen SE, Tardif JC, Nicholls SJ, et al. Effect of torcetrapib on the progression of coronary atherosclerosis. *N Engl J Med* 2007;356:1304-1316.
23. Libby P, Aikawa M, Jain MK. Vascular endothelium and atherosclerosis. *Handbook of Experimental Pharmacology* 2006;176:285-306.
24. Miller DT, Ridker PM, Libby P, Kwiatkowski DJ. Atherosclerosis: the path from genomics to therapeutics. *J Am Coll Cardiol* 2007;49:1589-1599.
25. Schwartz GG, Olsson AG, Abt M, et al. Effects of dalcetrapib in patients with a recent acute coronary syndrome. *N Engl J Med* 2012;367:2089-2099.
26. Sofat R, Hingorani AD, Smeeth L, et al. Separating the mechanism-based and off-target actions of cholesteryl ester transfer protein inhibitors with CETP gene polymorphisms. *Circulation* 2010;121: 52-62.
27. Raal FJ, Blom DJ. Anacetrapib in familial hypercholesterolaemia: Pros and cons. *Lancet* 2015;385:2124-2126.
28. Ridker PM, Danielson E, Fonseca FA, et al. Reduction in C-reactive protein and LDL cholesterol and cardiovascular event rates after initiation of rosuvastatin: A prospective study of the JUPITER trial. *Lancet* 2009;373:1175-1182.
29. Eagle KA, Ginsburg GS, Musunuru K, et al. Identifying patients at high risk of a cardiovascular event in the near future: Current status and future directions: Report of a national heart, lung, and blood institute working group. *Circulation* 2010;121:1447-1454.
30. Kujiraoka T, Hattori H, Miwa Y, et al. Serum apolipoprotein j in health, coronary heart disease and type 2 diabetes mellitus. *J Atheroscler Thromb* 2006;13:314-322.

31. Libby P. How our growing understanding of inflammation has reshaped the way we think of disease and drug development. *Clin Pharmacol Ther* 2010;87:389-391.
32. Huang CY, Wu TC, Lin WT, et al. Effects of simvastatin withdrawal on serum matrix metalloproteinases in hypercholesterolaemic patients. *Eur J Clin Invest* 2006;36:76-84.
33. Suviolahti E, Lilja HE, Pajukanta P. Unraveling the complex genetics of familial combined hyperlipidemia. *Ann Med* 2006;38:337-351.
34. Buse JB, Ginsberg HN, Bakris GL, et al. Primary prevention of cardiovascular diseases in people with diabetes mellitus: A scientific statement from the American Heart Association and the American Diabetes Association. *Diabetes Care* 2007;30:162-172.
35. Grundy SM, Cleeman JI, Daniels SR, et al. Diagnosis and management of the metabolic syndrome: An American Heart Association/National Heart, Lung, and Blood Institute Scientific Statement. [erratum appears in Circulation. 2005 Oct 25;112(17):e297]. *Circulation* 2005;112:2735-2752.
36. Stone NJ, Robinson JG, Lichtenstein AH, et al. 2013 ACC/AHA guideline on the treatment of blood cholesterol to reduce atherosclerotic cardiovascular risk in adults: A report of the American College of Cardiology/American Heart Association Task Force on Practice Guidelines. *Circulation* 2014;129:S1-S45.
37. Grundy SM, Cleeman JI, Merz CN, et al. A summary of implications of recent clinical trials for the National Cholesterol Education Program Adult Treatment Panel III guidelines. *Arterioscler Thromb Vasc Biol* 2004;24:1329-1330.
38. Grundy SM, Cleeman JI, Merz CN, et al. Implications of recent clinical trials for the National Cholesterol Education Program Adult Treatment Panel III Guidelines. *J Am Coll Cardiol* 2004;44:720-732.
39. Singh IM, Shishehbor MH, Ansell BJ. High density lipoprotein as a therapeutic target. A systematic review. *JAMA* 2007;298:786-798.
40. Daniels SR, Greer FR. Lipid screening and cardiovascular health in childhood. *Pediatrics* 2008;122:198-208.
41. Strong JP, Malcom GT, Oalmann MC, Wissler RW. The PDAY Study: Natural history, risk factors, and pathobiology. Pathobiological Determinants of Atherosclerosis in Youth. *Ann N Y Acad Sci* 1997;811:226-235; discussion 35-37.
42. Lauer RM, Obarzanek E, Hunsberger SA, et al. Efficacy and safety of lowering dietary intake of total fat, saturated fat, and cholesterol in children with elevated LDL cholesterol: The Dietary Intervention Study in Children. *Am J Clin Nutr* 2000;72:1332S-1342S.
43. Van Horn L, Obarzanek E, Friedman LA, Gernhofer N, Barton B. Children's adaptations to a fat-reduced diet: The Dietary Intervention Study in Children (DISC). *Pediatrics* 2005;115:1723-1733.
44. Iughetti L, Predieri B, Balli F, Calandra S. Rational approach to the treatment for heterozygous familial hypercholesterolemia in childhood and adolescence: A review. *J Endocrinol Invest* 2007;30:700-719.
45. Wierzbicki AS, Viljoen A. Hyperlipidaemia in paediatric patients: The role of lipid-lowering therapy in clinical practice. *Drug Saf* 2010;33:115-125.
46. Trejo-Gutierrez JF, Fletcher G. Impact of exercise on blood lipids and lipoproteins. *J Clin Lipidol* 2007;1:175-181.
47. Williams MA, Haskell WL, Ades PA, et al. Resistance exercise in individuals with and without cardiovascular disease: 2007 update: A scientific statement from the American Heart Association Council on Clinical Cardiology and Council on Nutrition, Physical Activity, and Metabolism. *Circulation* 2007;116:572-584.
48. Eckel RH, Borra S, Lichtenstein AH, Yin-Piazza SY; Trans Fat Conference Planning G. Understanding the complexity of trans fatty acid reduction in the American diet: American Heart Association Trans Fat Conference 2006: Report of the Trans Fat Conference Planning Group. *Circulation* 2007;115:2231-2246.
49. American Heart Association Nutrition C, Lichtenstein AH, Appel LJ, et al. Diet and lifestyle recommendations revision 2006: A scientific statement from the American Heart Association Nutrition Committee. [erratum appears in Circulation. 2006 Jul 4;114(1):e27]. *Circulation* 2006;114:82-96.
50. Sacks FM, Lichtenstein A, Van Horn L, et al. Soy protein, isoflavones, and cardiovascular health: An American Heart Association Science Advisory for professionals from the Nutrition Committee. *Circulation* 2006;113:1034-1044.
51. Gidding SS, Dennison BA, Birch LL, et al. Dietary recommendations for children and adolescents: A guide for practitioners: Consensus statement from the American Heart Association. [erratum appears in Circulation. 2005 Oct 11;112(15):2375]. *Circulation* 2005;112:2061-2075.
52. Grundy SM, Cleeman JI, Daniels SR, et al. Diagnosis and management of the metabolic syndrome: An American Heart Association/National Heart, Lung, and Blood Institute scientific statement. *Curr Opin Cardiol* 2006;21:1-6.
53. Assmann G, Guerra R, Fox G, et al. Harmonizing the definition of the metabolic syndrome: Comparison of the criteria of the Adult Treatment Panel III and the International Diabetes Federation in United States American and European populations. *Am J Cardiol* 2007;99:541-548.
54. Shrestha S, Volek JS, Udani J, et al. A combination therapy including psyllium and plant sterols lowers LDL cholesterol by modifying lipoprotein metabolism in hypercholesterolemic individuals. *J Nutr* 2006;136:2492-2497.
55. Petchetti L, Frishman WH, Petrillo R, Raju K. Nutriceuticals in cardiovascular disease: Psyllium. *Cardiol Rev* 2007;15:116-122.
56. He K, Song Y, Davigius ML, et al. Accumulated evidence on fish consumption and coronary heart disease mortality: A meta-analysis of cohort studies. *Circulation* 2004;109:2705-2711.
57. von Schacky C, Harris WS. Cardiovascular benefits of omega-3 fatty acids. *Cardiovas Res* 2007;73:310-315.
58. McKenney JM, Sica D. Role of prescription omega-3 fatty acids in the treatment of hypertriglyceridemia. *Pharmacotherapy* 2007;27:715-728.
59. Bhattacharya S. Therapy and clinical trials: Plant sterols and stanols in management of hypercholesterolemia: Where are we now? *Curr Opin Lipidol* 2006;17:98-100.
60. Berthold HK, Unverdorben S, Degenhardt R, Bulitta M, Gouni-Berthold I. Effect of policosanol on lipid levels among patients with hypercholesterolemia or combined hyperlipidemia: A randomized controlled trial. *JAMA* 2006;295:2262-2269.
61. Baigent C, Keech A, Kearney PM, et al. Efficacy and safety of cholesterol-lowering treatment: Prospective meta-analysis of data from 90,056 participants in 14 randomised trials of statins. *Lancet* 2005;366:1267-1278.
62. Link JJ, Rohatgi A, de Lemos JA. HDL cholesterol: Physiology, pathophysiology, and management. *Curr Probl Cardiol* 2007;32:268-314.
63. McKenney JM. Introduction. Report of the National Lipid Association's Safety Task Force: The nonstatins. *Am J Cardiol* 2007;99:1C-58C.
64. Wensel TM, Waldrop BA, Wensel B. Pitavastatin: A new HMG-CoA reductase inhibitor. *Ann Pharmacother* 2010;44:507-514.
65. Shitara Y, Sugiyama Y. Pharmacokinetic and pharmacodynamic alterations of 3-hydroxy-3-methylglutaryl coenzyme A (HMG-CoA) reductase inhibitors: Drug-drug interactions and interindividual differences in transporter and metabolic enzyme functions. *Pharmacol Ther* 2006;112:71-105.
66. Jones P, Kafonek S, Laurora I, Hunninghake D, Investigators C. Comparative dose efficacy study of atorvastatin versus simvastatin, pravastatin, lovastatin, and fluvastatin in patients with hypercholesterolemia (the CURVES study). *Am J Cardiol* 1998;81:582-587.
67. Robinson JG, Davidson MH. Combination therapy with ezetimibe and simvastatin to achieve aggressive LDL reduction. *Expert Rev Cardiovasc Therapy* 2006;4:461-476.
68. Nissen SE. ENHANCE and ACCORD: Controversy over surrogate end points. *Curr Cardiol Rep* 2008;10:159-161.
69. Davidson MH, Robinson JG. Safety of aggressive lipid management. *J Am Coll Cardiol* 2007;49:1753-1762.
70. McKenney JM, Davidson MH, Jacobson TA, Guyton JR; National Lipid Association Statin Safety Assessment Task F. Final conclusions and recommendations of the National Lipid Association Statin Safety Assessment Task Force. *Am J Cardiol* 2006;97:17.
71. Alsheikh-Ali AA, Maddukuri PV, Han H, Karas RH. Effect of the magnitude of lipid lowering on risk of elevated liver enzymes, rhabdomyolysis, and cancer: Insights from large randomized statin trials. *J Am Coll Cardiol* 2007;50:409-418.
72. Edwards IR, Star K, Kiuru A. Statins, neuromuscular degenerative disease and an amyotrophic lateral sclerosis-like syndrome: An analysis of individual case safety reports from vigibase. *Drug Saf* 2007;30:515-525.
73. Sattar N, Preiss D, Murray HM, et al. Statins and risk of incident diabetes: A collaborative meta-analysis of randomised statin trials. *Lancet* 2010;375:735-742.
74. Mangravite LM, Thorn CF, Krauss RM. Clinical implications of pharmacogenomics of statin treatment. *Pharmacogenomics J* 2006;6:360-374.

75. McPherson R. Comparative effects of simvastatin and cholestyramine on plasma lipoproteins and CETP in humans. *Can J Clin Pharmacol* 1999;6:85-90.
76. Tsuyuki RT, Bungard RJ. Poor adherence with hypolipidemic drugs: A lost opportunity. *Pharmacotherapy* 2001;21:576-582.
77. Tsuyuki RT, Olson KL, Dubyk AM, Schindel TJ, Johnson JA. Effect of community pharmacist intervention on cholesterol levels in patients at high risk of cardiovascular events: The Second Study of Cardiovascular Risk Intervention by Pharmacists (SCRIP-plus). *Am J Med* 2004;116:130-133.
78. McCrindle BW, O'Neill MB, Cullen-Dean G, Helden E. Acceptability and compliance with two forms of cholestyramine in the treatment of hypercholesterolemia in children: A randomized, crossover trial. *J Pediatr* 1997;130:266-273.
79. Zhang Y, Schmidt RJ, Foxworthy P, et al. Niacin mediates lipolysis in adipose tissue through its G-protein coupled receptor HM74A. *Biochem Biophys Res Commun* 2005;334:729-732.
80. Carlson LA. Nicotinic acid: the broad-spectrum lipid drug. A 50th anniversary review. *J Intern Med* 2005;258:94-114.
81. Shepherd J, Betteridge J, Van Gaal L, European Consensus P. Nicotinic acid in the management of dyslipidaemia associated with diabetes and metabolic syndrome: A position paper developed by a European Consensus Panel. *Curr Med Res Opin* 2005;21:665-682.
82. Sharma M, Ansari MT, Abou-Setta AM, et al. Systematic review: Comparative effectiveness and harms of combination therapy and monotherapy for dyslipidemia. *Ann Intern Med* 2009;151: 622-630.
83. Stern RH. The role of nicotinic acid metabolites in flushing and hepatoxicity. *J Clin Lipidol* 2007;1:191-193.
84. Recto CS 2nd, Acosta S, Dobs A. Comparison of the efficacy and tolerability of simvastatin and atorvastatin in the treatment of hypercholesterolemia. *Clin Cardiol* 2000;23:682-688.
85. Lai E, De Lepeleire I, Crumley TM, et al. Suppression of niacin-induced vasodilation with an antagonist to prostaglandin D2 receptor subtype 1. *Clin Pharmacol Ther* 2007;81:849-857.
86. Maccubbin D, Koren MJ, Davidson M, et al. Flushing profile of extended-release niacin/laropiprant versus gradually titrated niacin extended-release in patients with dyslipidemia with and without ischemic cardiovascular disease. *Am J Cardiol* 2009;104:74-81.
87. McKenney JM, Jones PH, Bays HE, et al. Comparative effects on lipid levels of combination therapy with a statin and extended-release niacin or ezetimibe versus a statin alone (the COMPELL study). *Atherosclerosis* 2007;192:432-437.
88. McKenney J. Niacin for dyslipidemia: Considerations in product selection. *Am J Health Syst Pharm* 2003;60:995-1005.
89. Libby A, Meier J, Lopez J, Swislocki AL, Siegel D. The effect of body mass index on fasting blood glucose and development of diabetes mellitus after initiation of extended-release niacin. *Metab Syndr Relat Disord* 2010;8:79-84.
90. Guyton JR, Bays HE. Safety considerations with niacin therapy. *Am J Cardiol* 2007;99:19.
91. Forsblom C, Hiukka A, Leinonen ES, Sundvall J, Groop PH, Taskinen MR. Effects of long-term fenofibrate treatment on markers of renal function in type 2 diabetes: The FIELD Helsinki substudy. *Diabetes Care* 2010;33:215-220.
92. Davidson MH, Armani A, McKenney JM, Jacobson TA. Safety considerations with fibrate therapy. *Am J Cardiol* 2007;99:19.
93. Sveger T, Flodmark CE, Nordborg K, Nilsson-Ehle P, Borgfors N. Hereditary dyslipidaemias and combined risk factors in children with a family history of premature coronary artery disease. *Arch Dis Child* 2000;82:292-296.
94. Grundy SM, Vega GL, Yuan Z, Battisti WP, Brady WE, Palmisano J. Effectiveness and tolerability of simvastatin plus fenofibrate for combined hyperlipidemia (the SAFARI trial). [erratum appears in Am J Cardiol. 2006 Aug 1;98(3):427-8]. *Am J Cardiol* 2005;95:462-468.
95. Ford ES, Li C, Zhao G, Pearson WS, Mokdad AH. Hypertriglyceridemia and its pharmacologic treatment among US adults. *Arch Intern Med* 2009;169:572-578.
96. Capell WH, Eckel RH. Treatment of hypertriglyceridemia. *Curr Diabetes Rep* 2006;6:230-240.
97. Elam MB, Hunninghake DB, Davis KB, et al. Effect of niacin on lipid and lipoprotein levels and glycemic control in patients with diabetes and peripheral arterial disease: The ADMIT study: A randomized trial. Arterial Disease Multiple Intervention Trial. *JAMA* 2000;284:1263-1270.
98. McKenney JM, Sica D. Prescription omega-3 fatty acids for the treatment of hypertriglyceridemia. *Am J Health Syst Pharm* 2007;64:595-605.
99. Oh RC, Lanier JB. Management of hypertriglyceridemia. *Am Fam Physician* 2007;75:1365-1371.
100. McKenney J. New perspectives on the use of niacin in the treatment of lipid disorders. *Arch Intern Med* 2004;164:697-705.
101. Gadi R, Samaha FF. Dyslipidemia in type 2 diabetes mellitus. *Curr Diabetes Rep* 2007;7:228-234.
102. Tan KC. Management of dyslipidemia in the metabolic syndrome. *Cardiovasc Hematol Disord Drug Targets* 2007;7:99-108.
103. Garg A, Simha V. Update on dyslipidemia. *J Clin Endocrinol Metab* 2007;92:1581-1589.
104. Shepherd J, Cobbe SM, Ford I, et al. Prevention of coronary heart disease with pravastatin in men with hypercholesterolemia. West of Scotland Coronary Prevention Study Group. *N Engl J Med* 1995;333:1301-1307.
105. Downs JRMD, Clearfield MDO, Weis SDO, et al. Primary Prevention of Acute Coronary Events With Lovastatin in Men and Women With Average Cholesterol Levels: Results of AFCAPS/TexCAPS. *JAMA* 1998;279:1615-1622.
106. Sacks FM, Pfeffer MA, Moye LA, et al. The effect of pravastatin on coronary events after myocardial infarction in patients with average cholesterol levels. *N Engl J Med* 1996;335:1001-1009.
107. Anonymous. Design and baseline results of the Scandinavian Simvastatin Survival Study of patients with stable angina and/or previous myocardial infarction. *Am J Cardiol* 1993;71:393-400.
108. Colhoun HM, Betteridge DJ, Durrington PN, et al. Primary prevention of cardiovascular disease with atorvastatin in type 2 diabetes in the Collaborative Atorvastatin Diabetes Study (CARDS): Multicentre randomised placebo-controlled trial. *Lancet* 2004;364:685-696.
109. Collins R, Armitage J, Parish S, Sleight P, Peto R; Heart Protection Study Collaborative G. Effects of cholesterol-lowering with simvastatin on stroke and other major vascular events in 20536 people with cerebrovascular disease or other high-risk conditions. *Lancet* 2004;363:757-767.
110. Anonymous. Effect of fenofibrate on progression of coronary-artery disease in type 2 diabetes: The Diabetes Atherosclerosis Intervention Study, a randomised study. *Lancet* 2001;357:905-910.
111. Backes JM, Gibson CA, Ruisinger JF, Moriarty PM. Fibrates: What have we learned in the past 40 years? *Pharmacotherapy* 2007;27:412-424.
112. Effects of combination lipid therapy in Type 2 diabetes mellitus. *N Engl J Med* 2010;362:1563-1574.
113. Grundy SM, Vega GL, McGovern ME, et al. Efficacy, safety, and tolerability of once-daily niacin for the treatment of dyslipidemia associated with type 2 diabetes: Results of the assessment of diabetes control and evaluation of the efficacy of niaspan trial. *Arch Intern Med* 2002;162:1568-1576.
114. Davidson MH, Kurlandsky SB, Kleinpell RM, Maki KC. Lipid management and the elderly. *Prev Cardiol* 2003;6:128-133.
115. Mazza A, Tikhonoff V, Schiavon L, Casiglia E. Triglycerides + high-density-lipoprotein-cholesterol dyslipidaemia, a coronary risk factor in elderly women: The CArdiovascular STudy in the ELderly. *Intern Med J* 2005;35:604-610.
116. Afilalo J, Duque G, Steele R, Jukema JW, de Craen AJ, Eisenberg MJ. Statins for secondary prevention in elderly patients: A hierarchical bayesian meta-analysis. *J Am Coll Cardiol* 2008;51:37-45.
117. Anonymous. Randomised trial of cholesterol lowering in 4444 patients with coronary heart disease: The Scandinavian Simvastatin Survival Study (4S). *Lancet* 1994;344:1383-1389.
118. Berger AK, Duval SJ, Armstrong C, Jacobs DR Jr, Luepker RV. Contemporary diagnosis and management of hypercholesterolemia in elderly acute myocardial infarction patients: A population-based study. *Am J Geriatr Cardiol* 2007;16:15-23.
119. Hatzigeorgiou C, Jackson JL. Hydroxymethylglutaryl-coenzyme A reductase inhibitors and osteoporosis: A meta-analysis. *Osteoporos Int* 2005;16:990-998.
120. Blue Cross Blue Shield A, Technology Evaluation C. Special report: The efficacy and safety of statins in the elderly. *Technol Eval Cent Assess Program Exec Summ* 2007;21:1-3.
121. Anonymous. Pravastatin benefits elderly patients: Results of PROSPER study. *Cardiovasc J S Afr* 2003;14.
122. Heart Protection Study Collaborative G. MRC/BHF Heart Protection Study of cholesterol lowering with simvastatin in 20,536 high-risk individuals: A randomised placebo-controlled trial. [summary for patients in Curr Cardiol Rep. 2002 Nov;4(6):486-7; PMID: 12379169]. *Lancet* 2002;360:7-22.

123. Abate N. Obesity and cardiovascular disease. Pathogenetic role of the metabolic syndrome and therapeutic implications. *J Diabetes Complicat* 2000;14:154-174.
124. Hulley S, Grady D, Bush T, et al. Randomized trial of estrogen plus progestin for secondary prevention of coronary heart disease in postmenopausal women. Heart and Estrogen/progestin Replacement Study (HERS) Research Group. *JAMA* 1998;280:605-613.
125. Rossouw JE, Prentice RL, Manson JE, et al. Postmenopausal hormone therapy and risk of cardiovascular disease by age and years since menopause. *JAMA* 2007;297:1465-1477.
126. Anderson GL, Limacher M, Assaf AR, et al. Effects of conjugated equine estrogen in postmenopausal women with hysterectomy: The Women's Health Initiative randomized controlled trial. *JAMA* 2004;291:1701-1712.
127. Wassertheil-Smoller S, Hendrix SL, Limacher M, et al. Effect of estrogen plus progestin on stroke in postmenopausal women: The Women's Health Initiative: A randomized trial. *JAMA* 2003;289:2673-2684.
128. Vickers MR, MacLennan AH, Lawton B, et al. Main morbidities recorded in the women's international study of long duration oestrogen after menopause (WISDOM): A randomised controlled trial of hormone replacement therapy in postmenopausal women. *BMJ* 2007;335:doi:10.1136/bmj.39266.425069.AD.
129. Mora S, Glynn RJ, Hsia J, MacFadyen JG, Genest J, Ridker PM. Statins for the primary prevention of cardiovascular events in women with elevated high-sensitivity C-reactive protein or dyslipidemia: Results from the Justification for the Use of Statins in Prevention: An Intervention Trial Evaluating Rosuvastatin (JUPITER) and meta-analysis of women from primary prevention trials. *Circulation* 2010;121:1069-1077.
130. Davis V, Schatz D, Winter W. Pediatric lipid disorders in clinical practice. *eMedicine* 2006; http://www.emedicine.com/ped/topic2787.htm#section~pictures.
131. Clauss SB, Holmes KW, Hopkins P, et al. Efficacy and safety of lovastatin therapy in adolescent girls with heterozygous familial hypercholesterolemia. *Pediatrics* 2005;116:682-688.
132. Wiegman A, Hutten BA, de Groot E, et al. Efficacy and safety of statin therapy in children with familial hypercholesterolemia: A randomized controlled trial. *JAMA* 2004;292:331-337.
133. de Jongh S, Ose L, Szamosi T, et al. Efficacy and safety of statin therapy in children with familial hypercholesterolemia: A randomized, double-blind, placebo-controlled trial with simvastatin. *Circulation* 2002;106:2231-2237.
134. O'Gorman CS, Higgins MF, O'Neill MB. Systematic review and metaanalysis of statins for heterozygous familial hypercholesterolemia in children: Evaluation of cholesterol changes and side effects. *Pediatr Cardiol* 2009;30:482-489.
135. Toto RD, Grundy SM, Vega GL. Pravastatin treatment of very low density, intermediate density and low density lipoproteins in hypercholesterolemia and combined hyperlipidemia secondary to the nephrotic syndrome. *Am J Nephrol* 2000;20:12-17.
136. Fellstrom BC, Jardine AG, Schmieder RE, et al. Rosuvastatin and cardiovascular events in patients undergoing hemodialysis. *N Engl J Med* 2009;360:1395-1407.
137. Baber U, Toto RD, de Lemos JA. Statins and cardiovascular risk reduction in patients with chronic kidney disease and end-stage renal failure. *Am Heart J* 2007;153:471-477.
138. Samuelsson O, Attman PO, Knight-Gibson C, et al. Effect of gemfibrozil on lipoprotein abnormalities in chronic renal insufficiency: A controlled study in human chronic renal disease. *Nephron* 1997;75:286-294.
139. Peterson AM, McGhan WF. Pharmacoeconomic impact of non-compliance with statins. *Pharmacoeconomics* 2005;23:13-25.
140. Tarraga-Lopez PJ, Celada-Rodriguez A, Cerdan-Oliver M, et al. A pharmacoeconomic evaluation of statins in the treatment of hypercholesterolaemia in the primary care setting in Spain. [erratum appears in Pharmacoeconomics. 2006;24(1):106]. *Pharmacoeconomics* 2005;23:275-287.
141. Cziraky MJ, Watson KE, Talbert RL. Targeting low HDL-cholesterol to decrease residual cardiovascular risk in the managed care setting. *J Manag Care Pharm* 2009;14:S3-S28.
142. Johannesson M, Jonsson B, Kjekshus J, Olsson AG, Pedersen TR, Wedel H. Cost effectiveness of simvastatin treatment to lower cholesterol levels in patients with coronary heart disease. Scandinavian Simvastatin Survival Study Group. *N Engl J Med* 1997;336:332-336.
143. Caro J, Klittich W, McGuire A, et al. The West of Scotland coronary prevention study: Economic benefit analysis of primary prevention with pravastatin. *BMJ* 1997;315:1577-1582.
144. Schectman G, Wolff N, Byrd JC, Hiatt JG, Hartz A. Physician extenders for cost-effective management of hypercholesterolemia. *J Gen Intern Med* 1996;11:277-286.
145. Bluml BM, McKenney JM, Cziraky MJ. Pharmaceutical care services and results in project ImPACT: Hyperlipidemia. *J Am Pharm Assoc* 2000;40:157-165.
146. Charrois TL, Johnson JA, Blitz S, Tsuyuki RT. Relationship between number, timing, and type of pharmacist interventions and patient outcomes. *Am J Health Syst Pharm* 2005;62:1798-1801.
147. Yamada C, Johnson JA, Robertson P, Pearson G, Tsuyuki RT. Long-term impact of a community pharmacist intervention on cholesterol levels in patients at high risk for cardiovascular events: Extended follow-up of the second study of cardiovascular risk intervention by pharmacists (SCRIP-plus). *Pharmacotherapy* 2005;25:110-115.
148. Buchwald H, Campos CT, Boen JR, Nguyen PA, Williams SE. Disease-free intervals after partial ileal bypass in patients with coronary heart disease and hypercholesterolemia: Report from the Program on the Surgical Control of the Hyperlipidemias (POSCH). *J Am Coll Cardiol* 1995;26:351-357.
149. Anonymous. The lipid research clinics coronary primary prevention trial results. I. Reduction in incidence of coronary heart disease. *JAMA* 1984;251:351-364.
150. Officers A, Coordinators for the ACRGTA, Lipid-Lowering Treatment to Prevent Heart Attack T. Major outcomes in moderately hypercholesterolemic, hypertensive patients randomized to pravastatin vs usual care: The Antihypertensive and Lipid-Lowering Treatment to Prevent Heart Attack Trial (ALLHAT-LLT). *JAMA* 2002;288:2998-3007.
151. Canner PL, Berge KG, Wenger NK, et al. Fifteen year mortality in Coronary Drug Project patients: Long-term benefit with niacin. *J Am Coll Cardiol* 1986;8:1245-1255.
152. Strandberg TE, Pyorala K, Cook TJ, et al. Mortality and incidence of cancer during 10-year follow-up of the Scandinavian Simvastatin Survival Study (4S). *Lancet* 2004;364:771-777.
153. Tonkin AM, Colquhoun D, Emberson J, et al. Effects of pravastatin in 3260 patients with unstable angina: Results from the LIPID study. *Lancet* 2000;356:1871-1875.
154. Robins SJ, Collins D, Wittes JT, et al. Relation of gemfibrozil treatment and lipid levels with major coronary events: VA-HIT: A randomized controlled trial. *JAMA* 2001;285:1585-1591.
155. Rubins HB, Robins SJ, Collins D. The Veterans Affairs High-Density Lipoprotein Intervention Trial: Baseline characteristics of normocholesterolemic men with coronary artery disease and low levels of high-density lipoprotein cholesterol. Veterans Affairs Cooperative Studies Program High-Density Lipoprotein Intervention Trial Study Group. *Am J Cardiol* 1996;78:572-575.
156. Leaverton PE, Sorlie PD, Kleinman JC, et al. Representativeness of the Framingham risk model for coronary heart disease mortality: A comparison with a national cohort study. *J Chronic Dis* 1987;40:775-784.
157. Pitt B, Waters D, Brown WV, et al. Aggressive lipid-lowering therapy compared with angioplasty in stable coronary artery disease. Atorvastatin versus Revascularization Treatment Investigators. *N Engl J Med* 1999;341:70-76.
158. Shepherd J, Blauw GJ, Murphy MB, et al. Pravastatin in elderly individuals at risk of vascular disease (PROSPER): A randomised controlled trial. *Lancet* 2002;360:1623-1630.
159. Cannon CP, Braunwald E, McCabe CH, et al. Intensive versus moderate lipid lowering with statins after acute coronary syndromes. [erratum appears in N Engl J Med. 2006 Feb 16;354(7):778]. *N Engl J Med* 2004;350:1495-1504.
160. LaRosa JC, Grundy SM, Waters DD, et al. Intensive lipid lowering with atorvastatin in patients with stable coronary disease. *N Engl J Med* 2005;352:1425-1435.
161. Waters DD, LaRosa JC, Barter P, et al. Effects of high-dose atorvastatin on cerebrovascular events in patients with stable coronary disease in the TNT (treating to new targets) study. *J Am Coll Cardiol* 2006;48:1793-1799.
162. Amarenco P, Bogousslavsky J, Callahan AS, et al. Design and baseline characteristics of the stroke prevention by aggressive reduction in cholesterol levels (SPARCL) study. [erratum appears in Cerebrovasc Dis. 2004;17(1):91-2]. *Cerebrovasc Dis* 2003;16:389-395.
163. Amarenco P, Bogousslavsky J, Callahan A 3rd, et al. High-dose atorvastatin after stroke or transient ischemic attack. *N Engl J Med* 2006;355:549-359.
164. Group HTC. HPS2-THRIVE randomized placebo-controlled trial in 25 673 high-risk patients of ER niacin/laropiprant: Trial design, pre-specified muscle and liver outcomes, and reasons for stopping study treatment. *Eur Heart J* 2013;34:1279-1291.

165. Nissen SE, Tuzcu EM, Brewer HB, et al. Effect of ACAT inhibition on the progression of coronary atherosclerosis. [erratum appears in N Engl J Med. 2006 Aug 10;355(6):638]. *N Engl J Med* 2006;354:1253-1263.
166. Vidt DG, Harris S, McTaggart F, Ditmarsch M, Sager PT, Sorof JM. Effect of short-term rosuvastatin treatment on estimated glomerular filtration rate. *Am J Cardiol* 2006;97:1602-1606.
167. Raal FJ, Santos RD, Blom DJ, et al. Mipomersen, an apolipoprotein B synthesis inhibitor, for lowering of LDL cholesterol concentrations in patients with homozygous familial hypercholesterolaemia: A randomised, double-blind, placebo-controlled trial. *Lancet* 2010;375: 998-1006.
168. Cuchel M, Meagher EA, du Toit Theron H, et al. Efficacy and safety of a microsomal triglyceride transfer protein inhibitor in patients with homozygous familial hypercholesterolaemia: A single-arm, open-label, phase 3 study. *Lancet* 2013;381:40-46.
169. Pedersen TR. Lipid-lowering drugs and risk for cancer. *Curr Atheroscler Rep* 2009;11:350-357.
170. Stone, N. J., Robinson, J. G., Lichtenstein, A. H., et al. 2013 ACC/AHA guideline on the treatment of blood cholesterol to reduce atherosclerotic cardiovascular risk in adults: a report of the American College of Cardiology/American Heart Association Task Force on Practice Guidelines Circulation 2014;129:S1-45.
171. Arnett, D. K. Jacobs, D. R., Jr. Luepker, R. V., el al. Twenty-year trends in serum cholesterol, hypercholesterolemia, and cholesterol medication use: the Minnesota Heart Survey, 1980-1982 to 2000-2002. *Circulation* 2005;112:3884-91.
172. Lloyd-Jones, D. Adams, R. J. Brown, T. M., et al. Executive Summary: Heart Disease and Stroke Statistics-2010 Update A Report From the American Heart Association. *Circulation* 010;121:948-54.
173. Cannon, C. P., Blazing, M. A., Giugliano, R. P., et al. Ezetimibe Added to Statin Therapy after Acute Coronary Syndromes. *N Eng J Med* 2015;372:2387-97.

e22

Peripheral Arterial Disease

Sheryl L. Chow and Barbara J. Hoeben

KEY CONCEPTS

1. The prevalence of peripheral arterial disease (PAD) is dependent on age and the presence of traditional risk factors for cardiovascular disease (CVD) and many patients are undiagnosed; undiagnosed patients have substantial risk for coronary and cerebrovascular events.
2. The clinical presentation of PAD is variable and includes a range of symptoms. The two most common characteristics of PAD are intermittent claudication (IC) and pain at rest in the lower extremities.
3. The ankle-brachial index (ABI) is a simple, noninvasive, quantitative test that has been proven to be a highly sensitive and specific tool in the diagnosis of PAD.
4. As with any atherosclerotic condition, several risk factors play an important role in the morbidity and mortality of peripheral vascular disease. Many of these risk factors are modifiable with the help of various nonpharmacologic and pharmacologic interventions.
5. Nonpharmacologic interventions such as smoking cessation and walking exercise programs have the ability to positively impact several of the pathophysiologic abnormalities present in patients with PAD.[1]
6. Data proving that antiplatelet therapies can prevent or delay the progression of PAD are currently unavailable. However, aspirin therapy has repeatedly been proven to significantly reduce serious vascular events in these "high-risk" patients and, in the absence of contraindications, is highly recommended.
7. After appropriate exercise therapy and therapeutic lifestyle changes (TLC) have been implemented, patients who continue to experience severe IC may benefit from additional pharmacologic therapy with cilostazol.

Peripheral arterial disease (PAD), the most common form of peripheral vascular disease, is a manifestation of progressive narrowing of arteries due to atherosclerosis.[1] PAD is associated with elevated risk of cardiovascular disease (CVD) morbidity and mortality, even in the absence of history of acute myocardial infarction (AMI), stroke, or other manifestations of CVD.[2] Patients with PAD have approximately the same relative risk of death from CVD as do patients with a history of coronary or cerebrovascular disease, and PAD should be considered a surrogate marker of subclinical coronary artery disease (CAD) and other vascular territories. The treatment of PAD focuses on decreasing the functional impairment caused by symptoms of intermittent claudication (IC) through nonpharmacologic and pharmacologic therapy and by minimizing the impact of other cardiovascular risk factors.[3]

EPIDEMIOLOGY

1 PAD affects approximately 8.5 million with an estimated prevalence of 2.76% of adults aged 40 years and older in the United States.[1] The prevalence of PAD is highly dependent on age, being infrequent in younger individuals and common in older individuals (Fig. e22-1). In age- and gender-adjusted logistic regression analyses, black race/ethnicity (odds ratio [OR] 2.83), current smoking (OR 4.46), diabetes (OR 2.71), hypertension (HTN; OR 1.75), hypercholesterolemia (OR 1.68), and impaired renal function (estimated glomerular filtration rate less than 60 mL/min/1.73 m^2) (OR 2) were associated with more prevalent PAD.[4] Individuals with PAD are also more likely to have a self-reported history of any CAD or CVD but, interestingly, no association with elevated body mass index. The reported relative risk of death from CVD in patients with PAD is reported to range from 2 to 5.1 in patients with or without CVD and 2.9 to 5.7 in patients with known CVD.[5] CVD accounts for 75% of all deaths in patients with PAD.[6] The risk of death is approximately the same in men and women and is elevated even in asymptomatic patients. Annual mortality is 25% in patients with critical leg ischemia who have the lowest ankle-brachial index (ABI).[7]

The complete chapter, learning objectives, and other resources can be found at **www.pharmacotherapyonline.com.**

Use of Vasopressors and Inotropes in the Pharmacotherapy of Shock

23

Robert Maclaren, Scott W. Mueller, and Joseph F. Dasta

KEY CONCEPTS

1. Continuous hemodynamic monitoring with an arterial catheter and/or a central venous catheter should be used early and throughout the course of septic shock to assess mean arterial pressure (MAP), intravascular fluid status and arterial and venous oxygenation and monitor response to therapies. They can be used for monitoring the response to drug therapy and guiding dosage titration.

2. Lactate production is increased under anaerobic conditions. Mixed venous oxygen saturation (Svo_2) or central venous oxygen saturation ($Scvo_2$) are indicative of tissue perfusion. Elevated serum lactate concentrations or low Svo_2/$Scvo_2$ represent global perfusion abnormalities. Lactate clearance or Svo_2/$Scvo_2$ may be used to assess repayment of oxygen to the tissues. Gastrointestinal tonometry and sublingual capnometry represent methods of assessing regional perfusion but are used infrequently.

3. Early goal-directed therapy with aggressive fluid resuscitation within the first 6 hours of presentation improves survival of patients with sepsis and septic shock.

4. Goals of therapy with vasopressors and inotropes in septic shock should be predetermined and should optimize global and regional perfusion parameters (eg, cardiac, renal, mesenteric, and periphery) to normalize cellular metabolism. This can be accomplished by continuous or intermittent measurements. Targeted goals should be central venous pressure (CVP) of 8 to 12 mm Hg (up to 15 mm Hg in mechanically ventilated patients, patients with preexisting left ventricular dysfunction, or patients with abdominal distension), MAP more than or equal to 65 mm Hg, urine production more than or equal to 0.5, mL/kg/h, and either lactate clearance of more than or equal to 20% or Svo_2 more than or equal to 65% or $Scvo_2$ more than or equal to 70%.

5. Derangements in adrenergic receptor sensitivity or activity frequently result in resistance to catecholamine vasopressor and inotropic therapy in critically ill patients. These changes may be a function of endogenous catecholamine concentrations, dosage/duration of exposure to and type of exogenously administered vasopressors, stage of septic shock, preexisting illness, and other factors.

6. In refractory septic shock, rational use of vasopressor or inotropic agents should be guided by receptor activity, pharmacologic and pharmacokinetic characteristics, and regional and systemic hemodynamic effects of the drug and should be tailored to the patient's physiologic needs. Pharmacologically sound combinations of vasopressor and/or inotrope agents should be initiated early to optimize and facilitate rapid response.

7. Dose titration and monitoring of vasopressor and inotropic therapy should be guided by the "best clinical response" while observing for and minimizing evidence of myocardial ischemia (eg, tachydysrhythmias, electrocardiographic changes, troponin elevation), renal (decreased glomerular filtration rate and/or urine production), splanchnic/gastric (low intramucosal pH, bowel ischemia), or peripheral (cold extremities) hypoperfusion, and worsening of partial pressure of arterial oxygen (PaO_2), pulmonary artery occlusive pressure, and other hemodynamic variables.

8. Much higher dosages of all vasopressors and inotropes than traditionally recommended are required to improve hemodynamic and oxygen-transport variables in patients with septic shock. Arbitrarily targeting vasopressor and inotrope therapy to supranormal values of global oxygen-transport variables cannot be recommended because of the lack of clear benefit and possible increased morbidity.

9. First-line therapy of septic shock is aggressive volume resuscitation with crystalloid or colloid types of fluids. Norepinephrine is the preferred initial vasopressor agent for hemodynamic support. Norepinephrine achieves greater hemodynamic response than dopamine and is less likely to cause tachydysrhythmias and a decrease in splanchnic oxygen utilization. Dopamine is also limited by its inability to adequately increase CO and complications of increased pulmonary artery occlusive pressure and decreased splanchnic oxygen use. Low-dose dopamine should not be used to prevent renal failure.

10. Phenylephrine may be a particularly useful alternative in patients who cannot tolerate tachycardia or tachydysrhythmia associated with the use of other agents. Its effects on cardiac performance and splanchnic oxygen utilization are variable.

11. Epinephrine is an effective initial agent and as an add-on agent. It is particularly useful in the young, in patients with otherwise healthy myocardium, and potentially in patients when used early in the course of treatment. However, because epinephrine causes a significant increase in lactate and worsening of splanchnic oxygen utilization, it is not the agent of first choice in patients with septic shock and is reserved as adjunctive therapy when other vasopressors do not adequately increase MAP. It should be used cautiously in patients with a history of coronary artery disease or underlying cardiac disturbances.

12. Dobutamine may be used as adjunctive therapy for its inotropic effect. It enhances CO and may increase global perfusion. Concurrent vasopressor therapy is needed because dobutamine causes vasodilation. Dobutamine therapy may be limited by tachycardia and dysrhythmias.

13 Therapy with vasopressors and inotropes is continued until the myocardial depression and vascular hyporesponsiveness of septic shock improve, usually measured in hours to days. Discontinuation of vasopressor or inotropic therapy should be executed slowly; therapy should be "weaned" to avoid a precipitous worsening in regional and systemic hemodynamics.

14 Vasopressin produces vasoconstriction independent of adrenergic receptors and reduces the dosages of catecholamine vasopressors. Physiologic replacement dosages of vasopressin (0.01-0.04 units/min) can be considered in patients with septic shock refractory to catecholamine vasopressors despite adequate fluid resuscitation. Dosage rates should not be titrated upward. Vasopressin may enhance urine production but it may worsen splanchnic and peripheral perfusion. Given the current data, corticosteroids can be administered to patients with septic shock refractory to vasopressors or when adrenal insufficiency is suspected. Side effects of short-term corticosteroids are minimal.

Shock is an acute, generalized state of inadequate perfusion of critical organs that can produce serious pathophysiologic consequences, including death, when therapy is not optimal. Shock is defined as systolic blood pressure less than 90 mm Hg or reduction of at least 40 mm Hg from baseline with perfusion abnormalities despite adequate fluid resuscitation.[1] Previously, mortality from septic or cardiogenic shock exceeded 70% but now ranges between 20% and 40%.[1-5] This chapter reviews the theory and current status of hemodynamic monitoring and presents an update on the optimal use of inotropes and vasopressor drugs in shock states, specifically septic shock.[1,2,4-9]

The general goal of therapy during resuscitation from shock is to achieve and maintain mean arterial pressure (MAP) consistently above 65 mm Hg while ensuring adequate perfusion to the critical organs.[1,2,4-9] Hemodynamic and perfusion monitoring can be categorized into two broad areas: global versus regional monitoring. Global parameters, such as systemic blood pressure, oxygen tension, and lactate, assess perfusion and oxygen utilization of the entire body. Regional monitoring techniques focus on tissue-specific oxygen delivery and subsequent changes in functional indices of individual organs.[1,2,4-16] These measurements include coagulation abnormalities (disseminated intravascular coagulation), altered renal and/or hepatic function, altered gastrointestinal perfusion, cool extremities, cardiac ischemia, and altered sensorium. Although none of these indices alone is a reliable indicator of adequate resuscitation, they offer immediate detection and may be prognostic of recovery when combined and defined at the level of organ function. As a result, these indices are frequently used as surrogate end points for the goals of resuscitation.[1,2,4-16] While it is assumed that normalization of these parameters infers benefit, the clinician must first treat the patient clinically rather than relying solely on data from continuous monitoring to guide therapy.[1,2,4-16]

Patients in shock generally have several modes of monitoring so therapies are based on all gathered information and correlated with the patient's dynamic clinical response. Normal values for commonly monitored parameters are listed in Table 23-1. Evidence-based goals of therapy are listed in Table 23-2.[2,4-16]

TABLE 23-1 Hemodynamic and Oxygen-Transport Monitoring Parameters

Parameter	Normal Value^a
Blood pressure (systolic/diastolic)	100-130/70-85 mm Hg
Mean arterial pressure (MAP)	80-100 mm Hg
Pulmonary artery pressure (PAP)	25/10 mm Hg
Mean pulmonary artery pressure (MPAP)	12-15 mm Hg
Central venous pressure (CVP)	8-12 mm Hg
Pulmonary artery occlusion pressure (PAOP)	12-15 mm Hg
Heart rate (HR)	60-80 beats/min
Cardiac output (CO)	4-7 L/min
Cardiac index (CI)	2.8-3.6 L/min/m^2
Stroke volume index (SVI)	30-50 mL/m^2
Systemic vascular resistance index (SVRI)	1,300-2,100 dyne • s/m^2 • cm^5
Pulmonary vascular resistance index (PVRI)	45-225 dyne • s/m^2 • cm^5
Arterial oxygen saturation (Sao_2)	97% (range, 95%-100%)
Mixed venous oxygen saturation (Svo_2)	70%-75%
Arterial oxygen content (Cao_2)	20.1 vol% (range, 19-21)
Venous oxygen content (Cvo_2)	15.5 vol% (range, 11.5-16.5)
Oxygen content difference ($C[a-v]O_2$)	5 vol% (range, 4-6)
Oxygen consumption index (VO_2)	131 mL/min/m^2 (range, 100-180)
Oxygen delivery index (Do_2)	578 mL/min/m^2 (range, 370-730)
Oxygen extraction ratio (O_2ER)	25% (range, 22-30)
Intramucosal pH (pHi)	7.40 (range, 7.35-7.45)
Index (I)	Parameter indexed to body surface area

^{a}Normal values may not be the same as values needed to optimize the management of a critically ill patient.

GLOBAL PERFUSION MONITORING

Arterial Blood Pressure Measurement

Mean arterial pressure is the product of cardiac output (CO) and systemic vascular resistance (SVR). Conditions that may lower blood pressure through diminished CO in critically ill patients include cardiac failure (etiology may be myocardial infarction, arrhythmia, acute heart failure, or valvular disease), cardiac obstruction to reduce blood flow into or out of the heart (etiology may be cardiac tamponade, cardiac tumors, massive pulmonary embolism, or tension pneumothorax) and hypovolemia (etiology may be hemorrhage, intractable diarrhea, or heat stroke).[1] Vasodilatory conditions, such as sepsis, anaphylaxis, pancreatitis, acute hepatic failure, or neurotrauma, lower blood pressure by reducing SVR.[1] Arterial blood pressure is the commonly used end point of therapy; however, restoration of adequate perfusion pressure is the primary criterion of effectiveness.[1-16] Profound hypotension (MAP less than 60 mm Hg) is associated with pressure-dependent decreases in coronary, cerebral, and renal blood flow and may rapidly produce myocardial, cerebral, and renal ischemia. Therefore, a goal MAP of 65 mm Hg is often targeted for shock to maintain perfusion; however, patient specific characteristics must be considered in establishing a MAP goal and determining an adequate perfusion response to resuscitation.

Arterial blood pressure can be determined by noninvasive and invasive methods. All noninvasive blood pressure monitoring techniques depend on the use of an occluding cuff. Systolic and diastolic blood pressures are further determined by oscillometry, auscultation, palpation (systolic pressure only), or Doppler technique (systolic pressures are most reliable). Oscillometry is the only noninvasive method used in the intensive care unit (ICU) to measure MAP because the data are valid during low-flow states and the method provides automatic cycling and serial measurements (every 1-3 minutes) that do not require operator intervention. The oscillometry method

TABLE 23-2 Evidence-Based Treatment Recommendations for Management of Severe Sepsis or Septic Shock

Recommendations	Grade
Crystalloids are the initial fluid resuscitation of severe sepsis.	1B
Albumin is additional therapy after substantial amounts of crystalloid have been used in the initial resuscitation regimen of severe sepsis and septic shock.	2C
Hydroxyethyl starches with molecular weights exceeding 200 Da or molar substitution exceeding 0.4 should not be used.	1B
An incremental fluid challenge technique of fluid boluses should be applied wherein fluid administration is continued until hemodynamic improvement, either based on dynamic (eg, pulse pressure and stroke volume variation) or static (arterial pressure and heart rate) variables.	1C
The following therapies should be completed within THREE hours of presentation: measure lactate, obtain cultures and administer antibiotics, administer 30 mL/kg of crystalloid for hypotension or lactate blood lactate more than or equal to 4 mmol/L.	Ungraded
The following therapies should be completed within SIX hours of presentation: apply vasopressors to maintain MAP more than or equal to 65 mm Hg, reassess volume status, remeasure blood lactate if the initial lactate was elevated.	Ungraded
Resuscitation of patients with sepsis-induced shock, defined as tissue hypoperfusion (hypotension persisting after fluid challenge or blood lactate more than or equal to 4 mmol/L) should be protocolized. This protocol should be initiated as soon as hypoperfusion is recognized and should not be delayed pending ICU admission. The goal of initial resuscitation of sepsis-induced hypotension during the initial 6 hours should include all of the following: (1) CVP 8-12 mm Hg,[a] (2) MAP more than or equal to 65 mm Hg, (3) urine production more than or equal to 0.5 mL/kg/h, and (4) lactate clearance or Svo_2 more than or equal to 65% or $Scvo_2$ more than or equal to 70%.	1C
Resuscitation should target normal lactate concentrations in patients with elevated lactate levels as a marker of tissue hypoperfusion.	2C
Use vasopressors to initially target MAP more than or equal to 65 mm Hg.	1C
Norepinephrine is the initial vasopressor of choice.	1B
Epinephrine (added or substituted) should be used when an additional agent is needed to maintain adequate blood pressure.	2B
Dopamine should be used as an alternative vasopressor agent to norepinephrine in highly select patients with low CO and/or low heart rate and at very low risk of arrhythmias.	2C
A trial of dobutamine infusion should be administered or added to vasopressor therapy in the presence of (1) myocardial dysfunction as suggested by elevated filling pressures, low CO, or left ventricular dysfunction or (2) ongoing signs of hypoperfusion despite achieving adequate intravascular volume and adequate MAP.	1C
Vasopressin 0.03 U/min may be added to norepinephrine with the intent of raising MAP or decreasing norepinephrine dosage.	Ungraded
Do not use corticosteroid in adult septic shock patients if adequate fluid resuscitation and vasopressor therapy are able to restore hemodynamic stability. If hemodynamic stability is not achieved, hydrocortisone at daily doses of 200 mg by continuous intravenous infusion may be administered.	2C
ACTH stimulation test should not be used to identify the subset of adult patients with septic shock who should receive hydrocortisone.	2B
Corticosteroid therapy may be weaned once vasopressors are no longer required.	2D
Do not use corticosteroids to treat sepsis in the absence of shock unless the patient's endocrine or corticosteroid history warrants it.	1D

ACTH, adrenocorticotropic hormone; CO, cardiac output; CVP, central venous pressure; MAP, mean arterial pressure; $Scvo_2$, central-venous oxygen saturation; Svo_2, mixed venous oxygen saturation. Level of recommendations: 1, a strong recommendation indicating that the intervention's desirable effects clearly outweigh its undesirable effects; 2, a suggestion indicating that the tradeoff between desirable and undesirable effects is less clear. Quality of evidence: A, supported by a randomized control trial; B, supported by a downgraded randomized control trial or upgraded observational studies; C, supported by observational studies; D, supported by case series or expert opinion.

[a]A higher target CVP of 12-15 mm Hg may be required in the presence of mechanical ventilation or preexisting left ventricular dysfunction or abdominal distension.

Data from references 2 and 4-12.

operates by sensing arterial blood pressure changes, or oscillation amplitudes, against an inflated cuff. Unexpected high or low readings should be investigated as the use of improperly fitting cuffs can result in erroneous values. Fingertip devices offer another avenue for continuous indirect blood pressure measurement, but their accuracy in ICU patients may be significantly diminished by concurrent administration of vasoactive drugs.

1 The use of invasive arterial catheters makes possible the continuous measurement of MAP as well as procurement of blood samples for laboratory testing. The radial artery is the most commonly used vessel, but the dorsalis pedis, femoral, brachial, and axillary arteries and the umbilical artery in the newborn also can be accessed. This method of blood pressure monitoring is the standard technique used in the ICU against which all other methods are compared. Major complications of peripheral artery catheterization include infection and distal ischemia. Acute distal ischemia and catheter-related bacteremia occur in less than 1% of catheter insertions. This translates to 2.3 to 2.9 bloodstream infections per 1,000 catheter-days.[2] Ischemia is most common in patients with multiple or prolonged arterial cannulations, hypertension, or vasopressor therapy.[2] Invasive techniques are labor intensive, require aseptic techniques, and offer potential sources of equipment errors, such as length and quality of tubing, air bubbles, stopcocks, thrombus formation, tube kinking, and transducer placement. Hypertension, advanced age, and atherosclerosis also may affect the accuracy of invasive blood pressure readings.

Central Venous Catheter

1 2 The central venous catheter is used to measure the central venous pressure (CVP), to obtain venous samples for laboratory testing, and to administer drugs or fluids directly to the central circulation. A triple-lumen catheter frequently is used, whereby drugs with known incompatibility can be administered. Blood volume, venous wall compliance, right-sided cardiac function, intra-abdominal and intrathoracic pressures, and vasopressor therapy affect CVP. The CVP is not a reliable estimate of blood volume but can be used to qualitatively assess blood volume changes in patients during the early phases of fluid resuscitation.[2,17,18] The goal of fluid administration is to maintain the CVP at 8 to 12 mm Hg, but values of 15 mm Hg may be targeted in mechanically ventilated patients or patients with abdominal distension or preexisting ventricular dysfunction.[2,6,17,18] Sustained elevated pressures may be indicative of fluid overloading. While the results of early studies showed CVP monitoring of fluid therapy during resuscitation of septic shock was

associated with reduced mortality,[19,20] recent trials suggest the uniform use of central catheters for CVP monitoring is not associated with reduced mortality and is unlikely to be cost-effective.[21-24] Therefore, resuscitative therapies should not be delayed in the absence of CVP monitoring or while a central venous catheter is being inserted.

Pulmonary Artery Catheter

1 Pulmonary artery catheterization provides multiple cardiovascular parameters, including CVP, pulmonary artery pressure, pulmonary artery occlusion pressures (PAOP, commonly called the "wedge pressure"), CO, SVR, and the mixed-venous oxygen saturation (Svo_2).[25] Ideally, the pulmonary artery catheter should be positioned fluoroscopically; however, satisfactory placement also may be obtained by observing pulmonary artery pressure readings and electrocardiographic waveforms during catheter advancement. Proper positioning, or wedging, in the lower lung (zone 3) is essential to measure PAOP and to prevent distal pulmonary artery collapse. Inflation of the balloon at the catheter tip occludes the pulmonary artery, isolates the distal catheter tip from the right side of the heart, and allows the user to measure the PAOP, an approximate measure of the left ventricular end-diastolic volume and a major determinant of left ventricular preload. Poor wedging may be caused by catheter migration, patient movement, mechanical ventilation, or eccentric balloon inflation. Pulmonary artery catheters equipped with a distal thermistor also allow measurement of CO by thermodilution. Rapid injection of cold saline or dextrose solutions via the right atrial port allows complete mixing of blood with the injectate, and the resulting change in blood temperature is measured in the pulmonary artery. From the temperature change, the patient's CO can be calculated. Some pulmonary artery catheters contain a temperature coil or filament that intermittently warms the blood in the right ventricle for near-continuous CO measurement. Significant tricuspid regurgitation, an intracardiac shunt, the respiratory phase, and significant positive end-expiratory pressure decrease the accuracy of CO measurements. The most common complications of pulmonary artery catheterization include mural thrombus formation (14%-91%), transient ventricular tachydysrhythmias (11%-63%), pulmonary infarction (1%-7%), pulmonary artery rupture (0.06%-2.0%), and sepsis (0.3%-0.5%).[25,26] Most pulmonary artery catheters are heparin bonded which requires consideration in patients with unexplained thrombocytopenia. The relative risk (RR) of infection is 2.6 per 1,000 patient-days, similar to the risk with central venous catheters.[25,26] Controversy surrounds the utility and safety of the pulmonary artery catheter, including issues of correct placement and impact of the device on patient outcome as studies have failed to demonstrate beneficial outcomes with the use of the pulmonary artery catheter.[2,6,26] Careful evaluation of the indications and the risk of placing a pulmonary artery catheter for resuscitation of critically ill patients is warranted.[2,6,26,27]

1 The optimal PAOP needs to be individualized for each patient. Administering a fluid bolus followed by simultaneous PAOP and CO measurements with the goal of increasing the PAOP until CO does not change can be accomplished and is based on Starling's law of the heart. However, clinical experience suggests that most patients have an optimal response to PAOP values in the range from 12 to 15 mm Hg. CVP and PAOP guided therapies are equivalent in terms of clinical outcomes, including mortality.[27] Therefore, a pulmonary artery catheter should only be inserted when hemodynamic data are needed that cannot be obtained from a central venous catheter or when the validity of measurements from the central venous catheter or other assessments of perfusion are questionable.

1 Other methods used to assess CO include carbon dioxide (CO_2) partial rebreathing, esophageal Doppler, transpulmonary (ultrasound) indicator dilution, and the passive leg raise test.[1,2,7,13-16] The CO_2 partial rebreathing technique compares end-tidal CO_2 partial pressure obtained during a nonrebreathing period with that obtained during a subsequent rebreathing period. The ratio of change in end-tidal CO_2 and CO_2 elimination estimates CO but must be corrected for blood shunting. Poor to acceptable agreement exists between this method and the thermodilution method of assessing CO in critically ill patients. Also, low minute ventilation, a high shunt fraction, or a high CO produces inaccurate results. The esophageal Doppler technique measures flow velocity in the descending aorta by means of a Doppler transducer. CO is calculated based on the diameter of the aorta, the distribution of CO to the aorta, and the flow velocity of blood in the aorta. The CO reported by this method correlates with therapeutic interventions and demonstrates excellent agreement with the pulmonary artery catheter. Unfortunately, this method is technologically difficult and may not produce reliable measurements over time. The transpulmonary (ultrasound) indicator dilution method is functionally similar to the pulmonary artery catheter in that it employs thermodilution to calculate CO but it uses a central venous catheter rather than introducing a catheter into the pulmonary artery. This method of measuring CO correlates well with the values obtained from the pulmonary artery catheter and may display less respiratory phase variations. It also may estimate global end diastolic volume but other hemodynamic variables are not readily obtained. Passively lifting a leg 45° for 60 to 90 seconds when a patient is fully supine provides a 250 to 500 mL bolus of fluid as pooled venous blood is mobilized to the heart and increases stroke volume. A dynamic increase in blood pressure of 10% reflects increased CO and is highly sensitive and specific that the patient requires fluid resuscitation.[6] Special hemodynamic monitors are available that specifically assess changes in stroke volume and CO in response to a passive leg raise but they are rarely used in practice due to cost and technical requirements.

Oxygen Tension and Saturation Monitoring

Partial pressure of arterial oxygen (PaO_2) and arterial oxygen saturation (SaO_2) can be assessed subjectively by assessing capillary refill or invasively by obtaining an arterial blood sample. Arterial blood gases measured by conventional arterial sampling are considered standard, but their accuracy and usefulness are affected by poor sampling techniques, transportation and analysis delays, analyzer accuracy, sample cellular metabolism, and inability to trend results. Indwelling fiberoptic and electrochemical systems that allow continuous monitoring and trend analyses of blood pH, Pao_2, and partial pressure of arterial carbon dioxide ($Paco_2$) while decreasing patient blood loss from less frequent sampling are available but rarely employed due to cost. Svo_2 and central-venous oxygen saturation ($Scvo_2$) reflect oxygen delivery (Do_2, or Do_2I, indexed to body surface area) with low values indicative of inadequate tissue perfusion that may occur during the early stages of septic shock, cardiogenic shock, or hypovolemic shock. Both measurements depend on CO, oxygen demand, hemoglobin, and Sao_2.

2 Mixed-venous oxygen saturation is measured in patients using a pulmonary artery catheter. Initially, critically ill septic patients may present with a low Svo_2 value (less than 65%), indicating high extraction of oxygen by tissues or lack of adequate Do_2 to tissues. In patients with sepsis and other conditions who present with low Svo_2 values, rapid intervention should be undertaken to increase Do_2 to tissues, with the goal of obtaining Svo_2 more than or equal to 65%.[17,19,28,29] The length of time Svo_2 is less than 65% is associated with mortality.[17] As sepsis worsens, however, Svo_2 may be more than or equal to 65%. This occurs because extraction of oxygen in the arteriolar beds is hampered and is indicative of poor outcome.

1 2 3 Central-venous oxygen saturation is a less invasive measure of venous oxygen saturation because the catheter is placed at the junction of the inferior and superior venae cavae rather than at the pulmonary artery.[13-16,28,29] It is as accurate as Svo_2 but provides slightly higher normal values. Concentrations of $Scvo_2$ less than

70% reliably indicate inadequate oxygenation in shock states and detect subclinical ("cryptic") shock much earlier than hypotension. Targeting fluid and hemodynamic resuscitation to achieve $Scvo_2$ more than or equal to 70% is a sensitive indicator and measure of the extent of global tissue hypoxia and a determinant of the adequacy of hemodynamic resuscitation. While the results of early studies showed $Scvo_2$ monitoring as a determinant of resuscitation was associated with improved survival in patients with sepsis and septic shock,[19,20] recent studies failed to show a reduction in mortality.[21-24] This likely reflects practice changes over time to provide more aggressive early resuscitation with response measured by clinical outcomes rather than laboratory parameters.[20,24] As a result, $Scvo_2$ (or Svo_2) monitoring to guide resuscitation should not be used routinely and should be reserved for cases when clinical monitoring parameters are conflicting or difficult to measure. Resuscitative therapies should not be delayed in the absence of $Scvo_2$ (or Svo_2) measurements or while a catheter is being inserted.

Oxygen Delivery and Consumption

1 2 Tissue oxygen debt is indicative of organ damage in critical illness. In normal individuals, oxygen consumption (Vo_2 or Vo_2I, indexed to body surface area) depends on Do_2 (or Do_2I) up to a certain critical level (Vo_2 flow dependency). At this point, tissue oxygen requirements apparently are satisfied and further increases in Do_2 will not alter Vo_2 (Vo_2 flow independency). The point that Vo_2 becomes dependent on Do_2 represents a pathologic transition from aerobic to anaerobic cellular metabolism and lactate production.[16,17,28-31] Although animal models of sepsis substantiate this relationship, studies in critically ill humans show a continuous, pathologic dependence relationship of Vo_2 with Do_2.[16,17,28-31] The Vo_2/Do_2 ratio, or oxygen extraction ratio (O_2ER), can be used to assess adequacy of perfusion and metabolic response.[16,17,28-31] Maintaining the O_2ER at less than 25% without decreasing Vo_2 may be helpful in maintaining or improving the body's reserve in meeting the oxygen demands. Low Vo_2 and O_2ER values are indicative of poor oxygen utilization and greater mortality. Patients who are able to increase Vo_2 when Do_2 is increased show improved survival. This finding became the basis for targeting supranormal Do_2 and Vo_2 values in the treatment of ICU patients in the 1970s and 1980s but this practice is no longer favored as the results of studies failed to show improved regional organ blood flow or oxygenation and survival with the achievement of supranormal Do_2 and Vo_2.[16,28,29]

The apparent linear relationship between Do_2 and Vo_2 has been questioned because both share variables, and this *mathematical coupling* can produce artifactual relationships between variables.[16,17] Inconsistent relationships between Do_2 and Vo_2 are observed when Vo_2 is measured independently by indirect calorimetry. While the systematic assessments of Do_2 and Vo_2 and their dependence are rarely practiced, the concepts of enhancing Do_2 are frequently applied. The Do_2 and Vo_2 indexed parameters are calculated as follows:

$$Do_2 = CI \times Cao_2$$
$$Vo_2 = CI \times (Cao_2 - Cvo_2)$$

where CI = cardiac index, Cao_2 = arterial oxygen content determined by hemoglobin concentration and Sao_2, and Cvo_2 = mixed venous oxygen content determined by hemoglobin concentration and Svo_2.

2 3 4 The rapid initiation of therapy to optimize the components of Do_2 (CO, hemoglobin, and Sao_2) improves survival. In a prospective, randomized controlled trial, Rivers et al. demonstrated a significant reduction in hospital mortality (30.5% vs 46.5%; $P < 0.001$) in patients with severe sepsis and septic shock randomized to receive therapy based on goal-directed hemodynamic end points that were achieved within 6 hours of hospital presentation.[19] They used a systematic strategy to optimize Do_2 of serially administering (1) fluids rapidly to achieve CVP 8 to 12 mm Hg, (2) vasopressor agents to achieve MAP at least 65 mm Hg, (3) red blood cell transfusion to maintain hematocrit more than or equal to 30%, and (4) dobutamine to achieve $Scvo_2$ more than or equal to 70%. During the 6-hour window, the goal-directed therapy group received substantially more fluid, blood transfusions, and dobutamine administration but required less vasopressor and ventilator support later. While this approach demonstrates the benefits of initiating therapy early in the course of sepsis, the benefit of directing therapies toward clearly defined goals for the purpose of optimizing Do_2 has been challenged by the results of three multicenter studies.[21-23] Nearly 3,800 patients with severe sepsis and septic shock were randomized across three multicenter trials to receive therapies based on the same goal-directed hemodynamic end points as the Rivers et al. trial or receive usual care of practice as directed by the clinician. In general, subjects randomized to goal-directed therapies were more likely to receive vasopressors, blood transfusions, and dobutamine administration but 60-day and 90-day mortality rates were comparable to the usual care groups (18.2%-29.5% vs 18.8%-29.2%). Unlike the Rivers et al. trial, the volume of fluid during the initial periods of resuscitation did not differ between study regimens suggesting that usual care practices have changed over time to encourage aggressive early fluid administration. Another study demonstrated no benefit of administering blood transfusions to maintain hematocrit more than or equal to 30% for the purpose of increasing Do_2 and achieving $Scvo_2$ more than or equal to 70%.[32] While current guidelines endorse the application of defined goals for optimizing Do_2 (eg, $Scvo_2$ more than or equal to 70%),[6] many clinicians only apply clinical monitoring parameters or use other measurements of tissue oxygen debt (eg, serum lactate concentration) or indicators of Do_2 optimization. Experts generally agree on the importance of aggressive early resuscitation regardless of whether components of Do_2 are systematically measured.

Blood Lactate

2 Lactate is a metabolic product of pyruvate. Its production is increased under anaerobic conditions when Vo_2 exceeds Do_2, such as may occur during shock.[16,28,33-35] Blood lactate concentrations are used as a diagnostic and prognostic tool in sepsis; they also are used to measure the repayment of oxygen debt to tissues.[16,28,33-35] Several studies have demonstrated risk stratification of mortality rates based on initial lactate concentrations.[33-36] Serial lactate concentrations may show better correlation with outcome than oxygen transport parameters and may be superior to hemodynamic markers in determining adequacy of restoration of systemic oxygenation. Continuously elevated concentrations are predictive of morbidity and mortality. Lactate elimination (commonly termed "clearance") of 10% for 6 hours during initial resuscitation produces similar survival outcomes as achieving $Scvo_2$ more than or equal to 70%.[37] The utility of blood lactate measurements in guiding therapy was demonstrated in a study of 348 septic patients that showed targeting a 20% lactate reduction during the first 2 hours of resuscitation reduced hospital mortality compared to conventional assessment methods (hazard ratio [HR], 0.61; 95% CI, 0.43-0.87; $P = 0.006$).[38] The results of a meta-analysis of four trials of septic patients (N = 547) showed reduced mortality with therapies directed toward early lactate clearance (RR, 0.65; 95% CI, 0.49-0.85; $P = 0.002$). Therefore, lactate clearance (or normalization) should be targeted as a goal of resuscitation in patients with evidence of tissue hypoperfusion and is preferred to $Scvo_2$ (or Svo_2).[6]

Several caveats guide the use of lactate concentrations in septic patients. First, lactate may accumulate in patients with other conditions, such as significant hepatic dysfunction or acute respiratory distress syndrome, who are not in shock. Second, both well-perfused and poorly perfused tissues contribute to arterial and mixed venous lactate concentrations and therefore are not reflective of regional perfusion. Third, elevated lactate concentrations may result from cellular metabolic failure or medications rather than global hypoperfusion in shock. Fourth, evidence of organ perfusion and function should always be considered in conjunction with lactate clearance.[6]

REGIONAL PERFUSION MONITORING

4 Blood pressures, CO, blood lactate, and global oxygen homeostasis parameters do not offer information about perfusion to individual organs. Organ-specific hypoxia may be evident by coagulopathy as indicated by thrombocytopenia (platelet count less than 100,000/L) and/or prolonged clotting times (international normalized ratio greater than 1.5 or activated partial thromboplastin time at least 1.5-fold the upper limit of normal), impaired renal function with urine production less than 0.5 mL/kg/h and/or increased serum concentrations of blood urea nitrogen and creatinine, altered hepatic function with substantially increased serum concentrations of transaminases and bilirubin, altered gastrointestinal perfusion manifested by ileus and diminished bowel sounds, cool extremities, cardiac ischemia with elevated troponin levels and electrocardiogram or echocardiography changes, pulmonary ischemia with worsening PaO_2, and altered sensorium.[1,2,5,6] The success of resuscitation should be based on the combination of blood pressure, organ-specific parameters of regional perfusion, and global perfusion measurements. For example, early resuscitation goals in septic shock may include CVP, MAP, urine production, echocardiography sensorium, and lactate (or possibly $Scvo_2$ or Svo_2).

Gastrointestinal Tonometry

2 Other measurements of regional perfusion to detect inadequate tissue oxygenation have focused on the mesenteric/splanchnic circulation, which is sensitive to changes in blood flow and oxygenation for several reasons.[13-15,29-31] Normally, most blood flow to the gut mucosa is redistributed toward the serosa and muscularis. Second, the gut may have a higher critical Do_2 threshold than other organs. Third, the tip of the villus has a countercurrent oxygen-exchange mechanism, rendering it highly sensitive to alterations in regional blood flow and oxygenation.

Gastric tonometry measures gut luminal partial pressure of carbon dioxide (Pco_2) at equilibrium by placing a saline- or air-filled gas-permeable balloon in the gastric lumen. Assuming that CO_2 permeates freely among tissues and that the arterial bicarbonate (HCO_3^-) concentration is equal to that of the gut mucosa, the intramucosal pH (pHi) may be calculated using the Henderson-Hasselbalch equation:

$$pHi = 6.1 \log (HCO_3^-)\ 0.03 \times Pco_2$$

Increases in mucosal Pco_2 and calculated decreases in pHi are associated with mucosal hypoperfusion.[13-15,29-31] Calculation of pHi can be confounded by increases in luminal Pco_2, such as may occur when buffering antacids are used. Histamine$_2$-receptor antagonists or proton pump inhibitors can be used instead. The presence of respiratory acid-base disorders; systemic bicarbonate administration; arterial blood gas measurement errors; or enteral feeding products, blood, or stool in the gut may confound pHi determinations. As a result, the change in gastric mucosal Pco_2 may be more accurate than pHi. Furthermore, because mucosal Pco_2 is influenced by arterial Pco_2, the mucosal-arterial Pco_2 difference (Pco_2 gap) likely is the optimal measurement.[13-15,29-31] The clinical utility of gastric tonometry is minimal as clinical trials of pHi-directed therapy do not show that it aids resuscitation when other goals are concomitantly targeted. Gastric tonometry, in general, inconsistently predicts mortality but has provided insight into perfusion differences of vasopressor activity.

2 Evidence suggests that the most proximal part of the gastrointestinal tract, the sublingual mucosa, may be an acceptable location for monitoring regional perfusion and Pco_2.[13-15,29-31] Unlike gastrointestinal circulation, limited intra- and interpatient variability exists in the microvasculature and only few arterioles are available for assessment. Sublingual capnometry is noninvasive, is not technically complex, and provides results within minutes. Small studies of critically ill patients with and without sepsis and septic shock show that the sublingual carbon dioxide pressure ($Pslco_2$) and the sublingual-to-arterial Pco_2 gap correlate better with the enhancement of Do_2 with dobutamine than the mucosal Pco_2 and the mucosal-to-arterial Pco_2 gap.[13-15,29-31] The initial sublingual-to-arterial Pco_2 gap is a better predictor of mortality. These pilot studies must be expanded before this technology becomes part of routine practice, but it offers the possibility of noninvasive measurement of regional perfusion.

Myocardial Dysfunction

1 4 Although loss of vascular tone is the hallmark of septic shock, myocardial dysfunction characterized by transient impairment of contractility is a recognized complication.[39] The range of left ventricular ejection fraction (LVEF) upon presentation is wide, but approximately 35% of patients with septic shock have left ventricular hypokinesis (mean ejection fraction 38% ± 17%) and low CO.[39] Because LVEF also is affected by preload and afterload, the low SVR of septic shock may mask depressed myocardial contractility that may be revealed upon restoration of MAP by administration of fluid and vasopressors. Therefore, CO may not reflect the extent of myocardial dysfunction. While it requires technical and interpretive training, echocardiography is a relatively simple method of assessing cardiac function and ventricular response to therapies.[40] It can assess chamber size, ventricular contractility, valve function, blood flow, and CO. Patients with tissue hypoxia or a hypercontractile left ventricle may benefit from fluid administration or vasopressor therapy; whereas, patients with poor left ventricular function may require inotropic intervention.

Cardiac troponin release in septic patients occurs in the absence of flow-limiting disease, likely due to a loss in membrane integrity with subsequent leakage or microvascular thrombosis. Elevation of cardiac troponin concentrations in patients with sepsis indicates left ventricular dysfunction and portends a poor prognosis.[39-41] Troponin concentrations also correlate with the duration of hypotension and the intensity of vasopressor therapy. Early recognition of myocardial dysfunction is crucial for administration of appropriate therapy. In the absence of other mechanisms for assessing cardiac function, echocardiographic findings and troponin concentrations may help guide and monitor therapy. Whereas cardiac troponins may be integrated into the monitoring of myocardial dysfunction to identify patients requiring aggressive therapy, natriuretic peptides show variable correlation with LVEF and should not be routinely monitored.[39-41]

VASOPRESSORS AND INOTROPES

6 Vasopressors and inotropes in patients with septic shock are required when volume resuscitation fails to maintain adequate blood pressure (MAP more than or equal to 65 mm Hg) and organs and tissues remain hypoperfused.[5-12] In addition, vasopressors may be needed temporarily to treat life-threatening hypotension when filling pressures are inadequate despite aggressive fluid resuscitation. Inotropes are frequently used to optimize Do_2 in cases of septic shock and cardiac function in cases of cardiogenic shock.[2-6] The clinician must decide on the choice of agent, therapeutic end points, and safe and effective doses of vasopressors and inotropes to be used. This section reviews adrenergic receptor pharmacology, exogenous

catecholamine use, and alterations in receptor function in critically ill patients. It also provides guidance for the clinical use of adrenergic agents, optimization of pharmacotherapeutic outcomes, and minimization of adverse effects in critically ill patients with septic shock.

Vasopressin and corticosteroids, as they relate to septic shock, also are emphasized because they have pharmacologic interactions with catecholamine vasopressors, possess hemodynamic effects, and are frequently used. Other agents such as phosphodiesterase III inhibitors, naloxone, nitric oxide (NO) synthase (NOS) inhibitors, and calcium sensitizers have been used as inotropes and vasopressors in shock states. These therapies are not discussed below as they are rarely used for septic shock and pharmacologic principles of other shock etiologies are discussed in other chapters.

Catecholamine Receptor Pharmacology

5 Comparative receptor activities of endogenous and exogenously administered catecholamines is summarized in Table 23-3.[6-12,42,43] Endogenous catecholamines are responsible for regulation of vascular and bronchiolar smooth muscle tone and myocardial contractility. These effects are mediated by sympathetic adrenergic receptors of the autonomic nervous system located in the vasculature, myocardium, and bronchioles. Postsynaptic adrenoceptors are located at or near the synaptic junction. These receptors can be activated by naturally circulating or exogenous catecholamines (eg, norepinephrine, epinephrine, and phenylephrine), whereas presynaptic adrenoceptors are stimulated by locally released neurotransmitters (eg, norepinephrine) and are controlled by a negative feedback mechanism.

The signal transduction pathways associated with catecholamine and vasopressin-induced effects in the heart and blood vessels are illustrated in Fig. 23-1.[6-12,42,43] Agonists of β-adrenoceptors and dopamine (D_1) receptors stimulate adenylate cyclase by a G-protein (G_s)-dependent mechanism (see Fig. 23-1, top). Adenylate cyclase generates cyclic adenosine monophosphate (cAMP) from adenosine triphosphate (ATP). cAMP-dependent protein kinase A, which is activated by elevations in intracellular cAMP, phosphorylates target proteins to modify cellular function. Through these mechanisms, β_1-adrenoceptor activation exerts positive inotropic and chronotropic effects in the heart, and β_2-adrenoceptor and D_1-receptor activation induces vascular smooth muscle relaxation. Agonists of α_1-adrenoceptors stimulate phospholipase C-β (PLC-β) through a G-protein (G_q)-dependent process (see Fig. 23-1, bottom). PLC-β produces inositol trisphosphate and diacylglycerol from cell membrane phosphatidylinositol bisphosphate. Diacylglycerol activates protein kinase C, an enzyme that phosphorylates several key proteins (eg, extracellular signal-regulated kinases, c-Jun NH2-terminal kinases, and mitogen-activated protein kinases) that modify cellular function (eg, hypertrophy). Inositol trisphosphate elicits the release of calcium from intracellular stores, such as the sarcoplasmic reticulum. Calcium forms a complex with calmodulin, which then activates calcium–calmodulin-dependent protein kinases (CaMK). CaMKs phosphorylate target proteins to alter cellular function. Myosin light-chain kinase is an example of a CaMK. Its action of phosphorylating myosin light chain leads to vascular smooth muscle contraction.

The normal heart contains primarily postsynaptic β_1-receptors, which when stimulated cause increased rate and force of contraction. This effect is mediated by activation of adenylate cyclase and subsequent generation and accumulation of cAMP. Stimulation of postsynaptic cardiac α_1-receptors causes a significant increase in contractility without an increase in rate, an effect mediated by PLC rather than adenylate cyclase. The increased contractility is more pronounced at lower heart rates and has a slower onset and longer duration in comparison with β_1-mediated inotropic response. Presynaptic α_2-adrenoceptors also are found in the heart and appear to be activated by norepinephrine released by the sympathetic nerve itself. Their activation inhibits further norepinephrine release from the nerve terminal.

TABLE 23-3 Adrenergic, Dopaminergic, and Vasopressin Receptor Pharmacology and Organ Distribution

Effector Organ	Receptor Subtype	Physiologic Response
Heart		
Sinoatrial node	β_1, β_2	Increased heart rate
Atria	β_1, β_2	Increased contractility
		Increased conduction velocity
Atrioventricular node	β_1, β_2	Increased automaticity
		Increased conduction velocity
His-Purkinje system	β_1, β_2	Increased automaticity
		Increased conduction velocity
Ventricles	β_1, β_2	Increased contractility
		Increased conduction velocity
		Increased automaticity
		Increased rate idioventricular pacemaker cells
Arterioles		
Coronary	$\alpha_1, \alpha_2, V_1; \beta_2, D_1, V_2$ (via NO)	Constriction; dilation
Skin and mucosa	α_1, α_2, V_1	Constriction
Skeletal muscle	$\alpha_1, V_1; \beta_2$	Constriction; dilation
Cerebral	$\alpha_1, V_1; V_2$ (via NO)	Constriction (slight); dilation
Pulmonary	$\alpha_1; \beta_2, V_2$ (via NO)	Constriction; dilation
Abdominal viscera (mesentery)	$\alpha_1, V_1; \beta_2, D_1$	Constriction; dilation
Renal	$\alpha_1, \alpha_2, V_1; \beta_1, \beta_2, D_1$	Constriction; dilation
Veins (systemic)	$\alpha_1, \alpha_2; \beta_2$	Constriction; dilation
Lungs		
Tracheal/bronchial smooth muscle	β_2	Relaxation
Bronchial glands	$\alpha_1; \beta_2$	Decreased; increased secretion
Stomach		
Motility and tone	$\alpha_1, \alpha_2, \beta_1, \beta_2$	Decreased (usually)
Sphincter	α_1	Contraction (usually)
Secretions	α_2	Inhibition
Intestine		
Motility and tone	$\alpha_1, \alpha_2, \beta_1, \beta_2; V_1$	Decreased (usually); increased?
Sphincters	α_1	Contraction
Secretions	α_2	Inhibition
Kidney		
Renin secretion	$\alpha_1; \beta_1$	Decreased; increased
Reabsorption of water	V_2	Increased
Skeletal muscle	β_2	Increased contractility, glyconeogenesis, K^+ uptake
Liver	α_1, β_2	Glycogenolysis and gluconeogenesis
Fat cells	$\alpha_1, \beta_1, \beta_2$	Lipolysis (thermogenesis)

D, dopamine; NO, nitric oxide; V, vasopressin.

Data from references 6-12, 42 and 43.

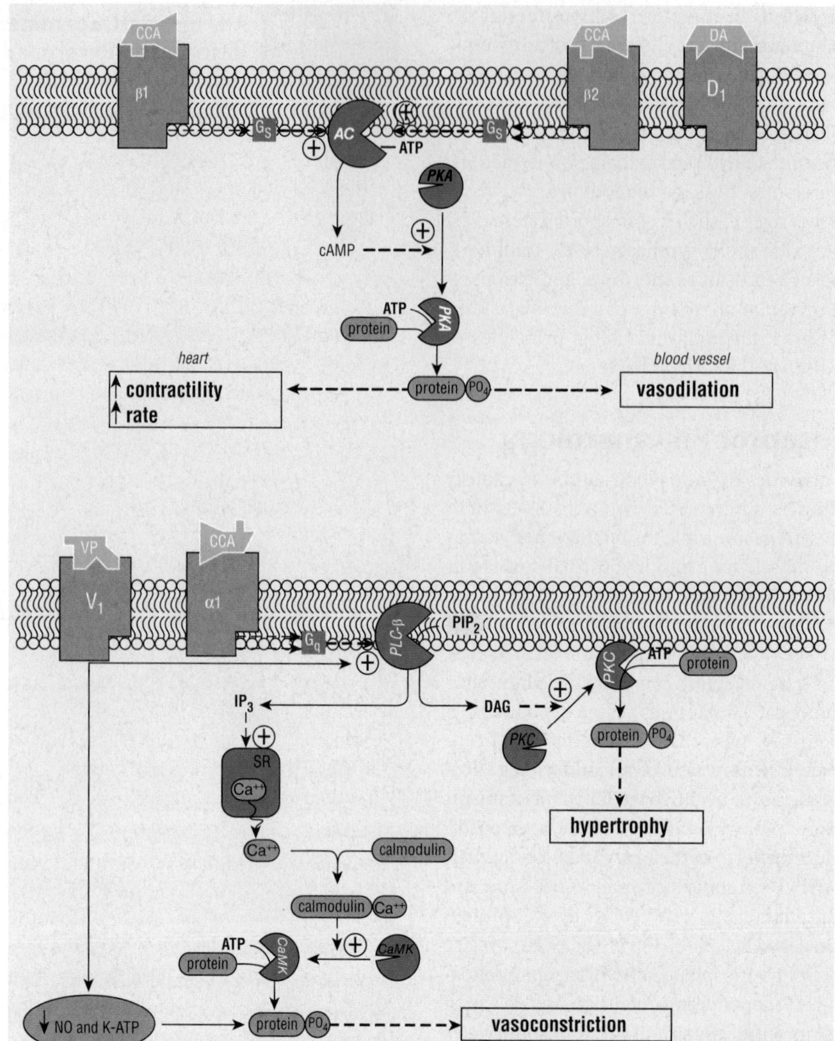

FIGURE 23-1 Signal transduction pathways in heart and blood vessels. *Top:* Catecholamine (CCA)-induced effects mediated in heart (β_1) or vascular smooth muscle (β_2, D_1). (Abbreviations: AC, adenylate cyclase; ATP, adenosine triphosphate; cAMP, cyclic adenosine monophosphate; PKA, cAMP-dependent protein kinase; +, stimulation.) *Bottom:* CCA (α_1) and vasopressin (VP)-induced actions in vascular smooth muscle. (Abbreviations: Ca^{++}, calcium ion; CaMK, calcium/calmodulin-dependent protein kinase; DAG, diacylglycerol; IP3, inositol trisphosphate; NO, nitric oxide; PIP2, phosphatidylinositol bisphosphate; PKC, protein kinase C; PLC-β, phospholipase C-β; SR, sarcoplasmic reticulum.) These pathways have been extensively simplified, and denoted cellular effects represent one of many produced. *(Data from references 6-12, 42, 43.)*

Both presynaptic and postsynaptic adrenoceptors are present in the vasculature. Postsynaptic α_1- and α_2-receptors mediate vasoconstriction, whereas postsynaptic β_2-receptors induce vasodilation. Presynaptic α_2-receptors inhibit norepinephrine release in the vasculature, also promoting vasodilation. Presynaptic β_1-adrenoceptors promote neurotransmitter release. Stimulation of peripheral D_1-receptors produces renal, coronary, and mesenteric vasodilation and a natriuretic response. Stimulation of D_2-receptors inhibits norepinephrine release from sympathetic nerve endings, sequesters prolactin and aldosterone, and may induce nausea and vomiting. D_1- and D_2-receptor stimulation also suppresses peristalsis and may precipitate ileus.

5 Vasopressin-induced vasoconstriction occurs through a variety of direct and indirect mechanisms.[12,42,43] Stimulation of vascular vasopressin (V_1) receptors causes vasoconstriction by receptor-coupled activation of PLC and calcium release from intracellular stores via secondary messengers similar to α_1-adrenergic stimulation (see Fig. 23-1, bottom). Vasopressin also directly inhibits vascular potassium-sensitive ATP channels to produce vasoconstriction (see Fig. 23-1, bottom). V_1-receptor stimulation inhibits the actions of interleukin (IL)-1β and thereby facilitates vasoconstriction. Vasopressin also increases the activity of adrenergic receptors. The greatest vasoconstriction occurs in the skin and soft tissue, skeletal muscle, fat tissue, pancreas, and thyroid gland. In contrast, vasopressin causes vasodilation in the cerebral, pulmonary, coronary, and selected renal vascular beds by enhancing endothelial NO release through V_1-receptor stimulation in these tissues.[12,42,43] Vasopressin has minimal to no inotropic or chronotropic effects.

V_2 receptors located in the kidneys are responsible for the antidiuretic properties of vasopressin.[12,42,43] Stimulation of V_2 receptors facilitates integration of aquaporins into the luminal cell membrane of distal tubules and collecting duct capillaries to increase permeability and thus retain intravascular volume. However, vasopressin stimulation of V_1 receptors causes vasoconstriction of efferent arterioles and relative vasodilation of afferent arterioles to increase glomerular perfusion pressure and filtration rate to enhance urine production.

Vasopressin rapidly increases serum cortisol concentration by stimulating V_3 receptors in the pituitary gland to enhance the release of adrenocorticotropic hormone (ACTH).[12,42,43] Cortisol helps regulate the proinflammatory state associated with sepsis and increases blood pressure through several mechanisms, including inhibition of inducible NOS (iNOS) to reduce NO production, reversal of adrenergic receptor desensitization, and increased intravascular volume through retention of sodium and water.

Altered Adrenoceptor Function: Implications for Critically Ill Patients

5 Most of the work describing receptor function and associated clinical pharmacology has been performed in either animal models or human volunteers. In critically ill septic patients, derangements in adrenergic receptor activity may result in resistance to exogenously administered catecholamine.[6-12,42,43] This "desensitization" frequently is characterized by myocardial and vascular hyporesponsiveness to high dosages of inotropes and vasopressor agents. Prolonged exposure of vascular endothelial tissue to vasopressor drugs (α-adrenergic agonists) or endogenous catecholamines may promote additional receptor downregulation. Increased endogenous catecholamine concentrations have been reported in endotoxemic and other critically ill patients, suggesting an acquired adrenergic receptor defect and desensitization of adrenergic receptors and alteration in voltage-sensitive calcium channels. The problem in critically ill patients may be related to decreased receptor activity or density. However, in patients with septic shock, catecholamine concentrations are even higher, so abnormalities in adrenergic receptor function are greater, with associated reductions in the concentrations of intracellular signal transduction mediators. The worsened receptor abnormality may be explained by defects distal to the receptor site, such as uncoupling of adrenergic receptors from adenylate cyclase or PLC, or dysfunction in the regulatory G-protein unit of signal transduction pathways.

In addition to catecholamines, circulating inflammatory cytokines may be partly responsible for distal alterations.[12,42,43] Macrophage-derived IL-1 and tumor necrosis factor (TNF)-α produce impaired coupling of β-adrenoceptors to adenylate cyclase. Patients with septic shock exhibit impaired β-adrenergic receptor stimulation of cAMP associated with myocardial hyporesponsiveness to various vasopressors and inotropes. However, increased chronotropic sensitivity to β-adrenergic stimulation with hypersensitivity of the adenylate cyclase system to isoproterenol stimulation also has been reported in animal models of bacteremia and endotoxemia. In the presence of intrinsic myocardial dysfunction and increased metabolic demands, this dysfunctional adrenergic system is incapable of mobilizing functional cardiac reserve to maintain adequate myocardial performance.[39,42,43]

IL-1 and TNF-α suppress gene expression of α_1-adrenoceptors, resulting in fewer receptor proteins. Overproduction of NO by iNOS directly contributes to vasodilation by cyclic guanosine monophosphate-mediated smooth muscle relaxation. NO indirectly produces vasodilation by combining with superoxide to form peroxynitrite, a highly toxic reactive species that causes endothelial dysfunction, uncoupling of α_1-adrenoceptors to PLC, and deactivation of catecholamines. The result of sepsis-induced inflammation is a system that promotes adrenergic receptor dysfunction to accentuate vasodilation and shock.[39,42,43]

5 Functional α_1-adrenergic receptor changes occur at various stages of sepsis; thus, adrenoceptor sensitivity may be time dependent during progression of sepsis to septic shock. The findings are not always consistent in various animal models of sepsis and in critically ill septic patients. Time-dependent alterations in the production of NO, a potent vasodilator, may explain the apparent differences in vascular reactivity to phenylephrine during the phases of endotoxemia. Furthermore, β-adrenergic receptor changes are present within 24 to 48 hours of septic shock. These findings suggest that the clinical response to vasopressors and possibly inotropic agents is variable during the stages of hemodynamic, myocardial, and peripheral vascular derangements of septic shock. In summary, α- and β-adrenergic receptor derangements may vary among patients and during each bacteremic insult; therefore, dose responsiveness of catecholamines vary among patients and during the insult.[6-12,39,42,43] For these reasons, these drugs should be dosed to clinical end points and not to arbitrary maximal dosages. High dosages are frequently required.

Relative Deficiencies of Vasopressin and Cortisol

14 Endogenous arginine vasopressin, a peptide hormone also known as antidiuretic hormone, is important for osmoregulation under normal physiologic conditions. Vasopressin is produced in the hypothalamus, stored in the posterior pituitary, and released from magnocellular neurons of the hypothalamus.[12,43] Increased serum osmolality and hypovolemia are the major stimuli for vasopressin release.[43] Other stimuli commonly associated with shock are dopamine, histamine, angiotensin II, prostaglandins, pain, hypoxia, acidosis, hypotension, hypercarbia, and α_1-adrenergic receptor stimulation. Vasopressin release is inhibited by NO, natriuretic peptides, γ-aminobutyric acid, β-adrenergic receptor stimulation, and α_2-adrenergic receptor stimulation.[43]

Normal serum vasopressin concentrations are less than 4 pg/mL.[43] Serum vasopressin concentrations are elevated with hypotension. Vasopressin response in septic shock is biphasic. During the first 8 hours of septic shock requiring catecholamine adrenergic therapy, serum concentrations of vasopressin are appropriately high to help maintain blood pressure and organ perfusion. Thereafter, serum vasopressin concentrations decline dramatically over the next 96 hours to physiologically normal but inappropriately low values, resulting in a state of "relative deficiency." In contrast, serum vasopressin concentrations remain elevated in patients with cardiogenic shock. Administration of vasopressin at 0.01 to 0.06 units/min produces concentrations similar to those observed in early septic shock and other hypotensive states; however, vasopressin concentrations do not correlate with blood pressure.[43] Administration of vasopressin augments the decline of inflammatory mediators and improves arterial pressure while minimizing the dosage of catecholamine vasopressors.[43,44]

The mechanism of vasopressin insufficiency in septic shock is not well understood. Neurohypophyseal stores in the posterior lobe of the pituitary gland are depleted during septic shock, likely as a result of excessive and continuous baroreceptor stimulation that eventually exhausts the limited vasopressin secretory stores. In addition, secretion of vasopressin is inhibited by enhanced endothelial production of NO, high circulating concentrations of adrenergic agonists (both endogenous and exogenous), and tonic inhibition by stretch receptors in response to volume replacement and mechanical ventilation.[43]

14 As with vasopressin, during sepsis a state of "relative adrenal insufficiency" is produced by continuous activation of the hypothalamic-pituitary-adrenal axis by IL-1, IL-6, and TNF-α that causes depletion of cortisol in the adrenal glands.[45,46] Administration of corticosteroids improves arterial pressure while minimizing the dosage of catecholamine vasopressors. Current proposed mechanisms of the vasoconstrictor effect of corticosteroids include increasing the number and stimulating the function of α_1- and β-adrenergic receptors and attenuating the production of inflammatory mediators responsible for vasodilation.

The use of corticosteroids for treatment of septic shock has been a topic of controversy for many years. Early studies of steroids in patients with sepsis demonstrated a lack of benefit and potential harm in sepsis and septic shock. Interest in corticosteroid use is driven by the awareness of adrenocortical insufficiency in critically ill patients with septic shock.[45] Relative adrenal insufficiency has been defined as a random cortisol concentration less than 10 mcg/dL (278 nmol/L) or an increase of less than 9 mcg/dL (250 nmol/L) following a dose of synthetic ACTH irrespective of the initial serum cortisol concentration.[46] Although absolute insufficiency is rare, relative adrenocortical insufficiency is present in 50% to 70% of patients with septic shock and is associated with a poor outcome.[46-49]

Conversely, an elevated random cortisol concentration (more than 34 mcg/dL) is also a predictor of mortality.[46] Mortality is further increased if ACTH response is less than 9 mcg/dL, suggesting that the risk of mortality is greatest in situations of adrenal gland "fatigue" (ie, degree of stress is not matched by sufficient cortisol production by the adrenal glands despite operating at maximal functional capacity).

Clinical Pharmacology of Vasopressors and Inotropes

5 14 The receptor selectivity of clinically used, catecholamine-based vasopressors and inotropes and hemodynamic effects are listed in Table 23-4.[5-12,42,43,50-52] In general, these drugs are fast acting, with short durations of action. As such, these drugs are given as continuous infusions and titrated rapidly to predetermined effects with the exception of vasopressin which is administered as a replacement dosage of 0.01 to 0.04 units/min and should not be titrated.[6,43] Careful monitoring and calculation of infusion rates are advised for all vasopressors because dosing adjustments are made frequently, and varying admixtures and concentrations are used.

9 Norepinephrine is a combined α- and β-agonist that produces vasoconstriction primarily via its more prominent α-effects on all vascular beds, thus increasing SVR. Norepinephrine administration generally produces either no change or some increase in CO. Norepinephrine is considered the first-line option for initial vasopressor therapy of septic shock.[2,6,50-52]

10 Phenylephrine is a pure α_1-agonist and increases blood pressure through vasoconstriction.[6-12,42,50-52] Given the presence of cardiac α_1-receptors, phenylephrine also may increase contractility and CO although no change or a slight reduction in CO is often observed. It is a therapeutic option in hypotensive patients experiencing a tachyarrhythmia when a vasopressor with minimal to no β_1-agonist activity is indicated.[2,6]

11 Epinephrine exerts combined α- and β-agonist effects.[6-12,42,51,52] At the high epinephrine infusion rates used for patients with septic shock, predominantly α-adrenergic effects are observed, and SVR and MAP are increased. While epinephrine traditionally has been reserved as the vasopressor of last resort due to peripheral vasoconstriction, particularly in the splanchnic and renal beds, it is considered second-line therapy in septic shock according to the current guidelines.[6] It is commonly used in other countries where other agents may not be readily available or are relatively expensive.

9 Dopamine has been described as having dose-related receptor activity at D_1-, D_2-, β_1-, and α_1-receptors (see Table 23-4).[5-12,42,43,50-52] This dose-response relationship has not been confirmed in critically ill patients. In patients with septic shock, great overlap of hemodynamic effects occur, even at dosages as low as 3 mcg/kg/min. Tachydysrhythmias are common and it is no longer considered a first-line therapy for septic shock.[6] Dopamine may increase PAOP through pulmonary vasoconstriction. It may depress ventilation and worsen hypoxemia in patients dependent on the hypoxic ventilatory drive.

12 Dobutamine, a synthetic catecholamine, is primarily a selective β_1-agonist with mild β_2- and vascular α_1-activity, resulting in strong positive inotropic activity without concomitant vasoconstriction.[6-12,42,51,52] In comparison with dopamine, dobutamine produces a larger increase in CO and is less arrhythmogenic. α_1-Adrenoceptors in the heart are directly stimulated by the (−) isomer of dobutamine, but β_1 and β_2 activity resides in the (+) isomer. The strong inotropic action of dobutamine is a function of its structure, the additive effect of cardiac α_1- and β_1-agonist activity, and a relatively weak chronotropic effect limited to the (+) isomer action on the β-receptors. Clinically, β_2-induced vasodilation and the increased myocardial contractility with subsequent reflex reduction in sympathetic tone lead to a decrease in SVR. Optimal uses of dobutamine in septic shock are for patients with low CO and high filling pressures (eg, low CI, left ventricular dysfunction demonstrated with echogardiography) or ongoing signs of global or regional hypoperfusion despite adequate resuscitation; however, vasopressors may be needed to counteract arterial vasodilation.[6]

TABLE 23-4 Receptor Pharmacology and Adverse Events of Selected Inotropic and Vasopressor Agents Used in Septic Shock[a]

Agent (Adverse Events)	α_1	α_2	β_1	β_2	D	V_1	V_2
Dobutamine (0.5-4 mg/mL D_5W or NS)	Tachycardia, dysrhythmias, hypotension						
2-10 mcg/kg/min	+	0	++++	++	0	0	0
>10-20 mcg/kg/min	++	0	++++	+++	0	0	0
Dopamine (0.8-3.2 mg/mL D_5W or NS)	Tachycardia, dysrhythmias, decreased PaO_2, mesenteric hypoperfusion, gastrointestinal motility inhibition, T-cell inhibition						
1-3 mcg/kg/min	0	0	+	0	++++	0	0
3-10 mcg/kg/min	0/+	0	++++	+	++++	0	0
>10-20 mcg/kg/min	+++	0	++++	+	0	0	0
Epinephrine (0.008-0.016 mg/mL D_5W or NS)	Tachycardia, dysrhythmias, decreased PaO_2, mesenteric hypoperfusion, increased lactate, hyperglycemia, immunomodulation						
0.01-0.05 mcg/kg/min	++	++	++++	+++	0	0	0
0.05-3 mcg/kg/min	++++	++++	+++	+	0	0	0
Norepinephrine (0.016-0.064 mg/mL D_5W)	Mixed effects on myocardial performance and mesenteric perfusion, peripheral ischemia						
0.02-3 mcg/kg/min	+++	+++	+++	+/++	0	0	0
Phenylephrine (0.1-0.4 mg/mL D_5W or NS)	Mixed effects on myocardial performance, peripheral ischemia						
0.5-9 mcg/kg/min	+++	+	+	0	0	0	0
Vasopressin (0.8 units/mL D_5W or NS)	Mixed effects on myocardial performance, mesenteric hypoperfusion, peripheral ischemia, hyponatremia, thrombocytopenia						
0.01-0.04 units/min	0	0	0	0	0	+++	+++

D, dopamine; D_5W, dextrose 5% in water; NS, normal saline; PaO_2, partial pressure of arterial oxygen; V, vasopressin.

Data from references 5-12, 42, 43 and 50-52.

[a]Activity ranges from no activity (0) to maximal (++++) activity.

Clinical **Controversy...**

DOBUTAMINE THERAPY

Increasing Do_2 by enhancing cardiac output with dobutamine is based on obtaining Svo_2 or $Scvo_2$ more than or equal to 70% or more than or equal to 65%, respectively in the original study of early goal directed therapy.[19] In the absence of measuring Svo_2 or $Scvo_2$, current guidelines suggest considering dobutamine if cardiac output is low or left ventricular dysfunction is present.[6] The assessment of either of these, however, requires technical methods such as echocardiography that may not be readily available to the bedside clinician. Instead, dobutamine may be tried if regional hypoperfusion is indicated by organ-specific dysfunction despite adequate arterial pressure and fluid resuscitation. This warrants caution as dobutamine may lower systemic vascular resistance and cause hypotension.

14 Unlike adrenergic receptor agonists, the vasoconstrictive effects of vasopressin are preserved during hypoxia and severe acidosis. Initiating vasopressin at less than or equal to 0.04 units/min in patients with septic shock increases SVR and arterial blood pressure to reduce the dosage requirements of catecholamine adrenergic agents.[43,52-54] These effects are rapid and sustained. Organ-specific vasodilation reduces pulmonary artery pressure and may preserve cardiac and renal function. It may enhance urine production, likely due to increased glomerular filtration rate.[43,55] At dosages exceeding 0.04 units/min, however, vasopressin is associated with ischemia of the mesenteric mucosa, skin, and myocardium. Limiting the dosage to a maximum of 0.04 units/min may minimize the development of these adverse effects. At present, vasopressin is not recommended as a replacement for norepinephrine in patients with septic shock but may be considered as adjunctive therapy in patients who are refractory to catecholamine vasopressors despite adequate fluid resuscitation.[6] If used for septic shock, vasopressin should be administered at a dosage of 0.03 or 0.04 units/min to not exceed 0.04 units/min.[6,43,52,53]

Desired Outcomes and Clinical Application

Resuscitation Goals of Septic Shock

4 7 9 Initial hemodynamic therapy for septic shock is the administration of intravenous fluid (30 mL/kg of crystalloid fluid), with the aim of using the least amount of fluid and lowest CVP to achieve end organ perfusion. If assessed, the recommended goal CVP is 8 to 12 mm Hg or 15 mm Hg in mechanically ventilated patients or patients with abdominal distension or preexisting ventricular dysfunction.[2,5-12] Greater than 30 mL/kg of crystalloid fluids may be needed to obtain goal MAP, reverse global hypoperfusion (lactate clearance, $Scvo_2$ more than or equal to 70%), or achieve clinical indication of regional organ-specific perfusion (eg, urine production). Therefore dynamic fluid response and clinical assessment should occur frequently following each fluid challenge.[5,6] Current recommendations are to measure serum lactate and administer 30 mL/kg of crystalloid for hypotension within three hours of presentation and obtain MAP more than or equal to 65 mm Hg with vasopressors, reassess volume status, and remeasure serum lactate if the initial lactate was elevated within 6 hours of presentation.[6]

6 9 Crystalloid fluids (eg, normal saline and Ringer lactate) and colloid fluids (eg, albumin, gelatins, dextrans, and blood products) are arguably considered equivalent for shock resuscitation.[6,56-62] The Saline vs Albumin Fluid Evaluation (SAFE) study randomly assigned 6,997 patients requiring resuscitation to albumin 4% or normal saline (sodium chloride 0.9% solution) and found similar 28-day mortality rates (20.9% vs 21.1%; $P = 0.87$).[56] Secondary outcomes also did not differ although a trend toward lower mortality was apparent in the albumin group in patients with sepsis (30.7% vs 35.3%; $P = 0.09$). A pragmatic multicenter trial of 1,857 patients with hypovolemic shock (including sepsis) also found similar 28-day mortality rates with colloid and crystalloid resuscitation strategies (25.4% vs 27%; $P = 0.26$) but secondary outcomes including 90-day mortality (30.7% vs 34.2%, RR, -0.92; 95% CI, 0.86-0.99; $P = 0.03$) and days alive without mechanical ventilation or vasopressor therapy were improved with colloid therapy.[57] These outcomes were not reported for the subgroup of patients with sepsis. In contrast, exogenous replacement with albumin 20% to target a serum albumin concentration of 3 g/dL found no difference in 28-day mortality (31.8% vs 32%; $P = 0.94$) or 90-day mortality (41.1% vs 43.6%; $P = 0.29$) when compared to crystalloid resuscitation in 1,818 patients with severe sepsis and septic shock.[58] The results of meta-analyses are conflicting with regard to a survival benefit associated with colloid administration; however, they are in agreement that resuscitation with albumin achieves higher values of CVP and MAP more rapidly than crystalloid fluids with a lower overall fluid balance.[59-61] Crystalloid fluids are generally preferred as they are readily available at a lower cost unless patients are at risk for adverse events from redistribution of intravenous fluids to extravascular tissues and/or are fluid restricted (eg, patients with renal dysfunction, decompensated heart failure, ascites compromising diaphragmatic function).[2,6,59-62] In contrast, hydroxyethyl starch (a colloid) is associated with increased risks of acute kidney injury in a dose-dependent manner and mortality.[63,64] The use of hydroxyethyl starch warrants extreme caution and consideration of a dosage threshold if not avoided altogether.

Clinical **Controversy...**

CHOICE OF FLUID FOR RESUSCITATION

Crystalloid fluids (eg, normal saline and Ringer lactate) and colloid fluids (eg, albumin) are arguably considered equivalent for shock resuscitation. Studies are conflicting with respect to mortality differences between normal saline and albumin as this outcome was either similar between groups or favored albumin. Current guidelines recommend normal saline as the initial fluid of choice for resuscitation and reserving albumin for refractory cases or in situations of clinical evidence of hypervolemia.[6] Many clinicians prefer albumin as this fluid achieves higher values of arterial pressure more rapidly with lower overall fluid balance. Also, the large quantities of chloride in normal saline may contribute to metabolic acidosis. For this reason, some experts suggest the preferred crystalloid is Ringer lactate.

6 8 Norepinephrine is the preferred initial vasopressor agent in septic shock patients not responding to fluid administration.[2,6,50-52] Other agents include phenylephrine, epinephrine, dopamine, and the inotrope, dobutamine. Optimizing MAP to 65 mm Hg as the goal of vasopressor therapy does not uniformly correlate with decreased mortality in patients with septic shock but global perfusion may be improved.[13-16,65] A randomized trial of 776 patients with septic shock failed to show reduced mortality when targeting a higher MAP of 80 to 85 mm Hg compared to 65 to 70 mm Hg (36.6% vs 34%; $P = 0.57$).[66] Therefore, the goal of resuscitation is a MAP more than or equal to 65 mm Hg, reversal of global hypoperfusion (eg, lactate clearance or $Scvo_2$ more than or equal to 70%), and evidence of regional organ-specific perfusion (eg, urine production).[6-12] Initial resuscitation of septic shock should be protocolized with quantitative goals achieved within 3 to 6 hours.[6]

6 7 9 10 11 12 13 Dosage titration and monitoring of vasopressor and inotropic therapy should be guided by the "best clinical response," the goals of early goal-directed therapy,

and lactate clearance.[2,5-12] Norepinephrine is considered the agent of choice as initial vasopressor therapy.[5,6] Epinephrine may be added to (or substituted for) norepinephrine when suboptimal hemodynamic response is obtained from norepinephrine alone.[6] Phenylephrine may be tried in cases of severe tachydysrhythmias, when CO is known to be high, or as salvage therapy when combination vasopressors including low dose vasopressin fail to achieve goals.[6] Dobutamine is used in states of low CO despite adequate fluid resuscitation pressures (eg, CI less than 3 L/min/m^2, left ventricular dysfunction demonstrated with echocardiography) or ongoing signs of global or regional hypoperfusion despite adequate resuscitation. Low dosage rates of these medications are initiated and titrated rapidly (usually every 5-15 minutes) to clinical response. Clinically effective dosing of vasopressors and inotropes in septic shock often requires dosages much higher than recommended by most references.[2,5-12] These large infusion rates must be tempered with the development of adverse effects. The goal is to use the lowest effective infusion rate while minimizing evidence of global hypoperfusion (lactate, $Scvo_2$) and regional hypoperfusion such as myocardial ischemia (eg, tachydysrhythmias, electrocardiographic changes, and troponin elevations), renal (decreased glomerular filtration rate and/or urine output), splanchnic/gastric (low pHi, bowel ischemia, and elevated transaminases), pulmonary (worsening Pao_2), or peripheral (cold extremities).

14 Vasopressin 0.03 units/min may be considered as adjunctive therapy in patients who are refractory to catecholamine vasopressors despite adequate fluid resuscitation.[5,6] Dosages of less than or equal to 0.04 units/min increases SVR and arterial blood pressure to reduce the dose requirements of catecholamine adrenergic agents.[43,53]

13 Therapy with catecholamine vasopressors and inotropes is continued until myocardial depression and vascular hyporesponsiveness (ie, blood pressure) of septic shock improve, usually measured in hours to days.[6] Discontinuation of vasopressor or inotropic therapy should be executed slowly; therapy should be "weaned" to avoid a precipitous worsening in regional and systemic hemodynamics. Careful monitoring of global and regional end points also should be geared toward discontinuation of vasopressors and inotropes as soon as the patient is hemodynamically stable. This requires constant observation. Because vasopressors and inotropes often are started while the patient is not yet optimally volume resuscitated, clinicians should reevaluate intravascular volume status continuously so that the patient can be weaned from the vasopressor as soon as possible. Dosage rates should be titrated downward approximately every 10 minutes to determine if the patient can tolerate gradual withdrawal and eventual discontinuation of the vasopressor and/or inotrope. Discontinuation of agents may occur only minutes to hours after their initiation, or it may take days to weeks. Septic shock requiring vasopressor and/or inotropic support usually resolves within several days to 1 week.

Comparative Studies of Catecholamine Vasopressors

7 9 The results of several observational and randomized studies support norepinephrine as the first-line vasopressor for septic shock.[6] A meta-analysis of 11 trials (N = 1,718) showed norepinephrine was associated with survival compared to dopamine with an absolute risk reduction of 11% (RR, 0.89; 95% CI, 0.81-0.98; $P = 0.02$).[52] Tachydysrhythmias were less common with norepinephrine (RR, 0.48; 95% CI, 0.40-0.58; $P < 0.001$). The results of two studies contribute to the majority of data. The first randomized 1,679 patients with shock unresponsive to volume resuscitation to norepinephrine or dopamine and found similar 28-day mortality rates (48.5% vs 52.5% of patients; $P = 0.10$) although death from refractory shock tended to occur less frequently with norepinephrine (41% vs 46%; $P = 0.05$).[67] Mortality rate was significantly lower in the subgroup of 280 patients with cardiogenic shock that received norepinephrine ($P = 0.03$). Overall, patients receiving norepinephrine had fewer arrhythmic events (12.4% vs 24.2%; $P < 0.001$) despite using dobutamine more frequently, had more vasopressor-free days, and were less likely to require open-label vasopressor support (20% vs 26%; $P < 0.001$). Limitations of this landmark study include combining heterogeneous shock etiologies (cardiogenic, septic, hypovolemic, and other), the use of a relatively conservative definition of "shock unresponsive to fluid administration" (only 1 L of crystalloid or 0.5 L of colloid), the use of open-label norepinephrine in patients with inadequate hemodynamic response to study drug regimens, and the lack of standardization of other shock therapies that affect hemodynamic variables (eg, corticosteroids, vasopressin, dobutamine, additional fluid administration). Another prospective study of 252 septic shock patients found statistically similar 28-day mortality rates between norepinephrine and dopamine (43% vs 50%; $P = 0.282$).[68] Similar to the aforementioned study, arrhythmic events were less likely to occur with norepinephrine (5.3% vs 23.3%; $P < 0.0001$).

7 9 11 Two randomized, double blind studies compared epinephrine with norepinephrine in 330 and 280 patients with septic shock, respectively.[69,70] Both studies found similar 28-day mortality rates with epinephrine and norepinephrine (40% vs 31%; $P = 0.31$; and 22.5% vs 26.1%; $P = 0.48$). Time to hemodynamic recovery and vasopressor withdrawal were also similar between agents in both studies. One study found more events of tachydysrhythmias with epinephrine leading to study discontinuation.[69] Both studies also showed that epinephrine was associated with lower arterial pH values and higher serum lactate concentrations over the first days of therapy, possibly demonstrating deleterious circulation, exaggerated glycogenolysis and glycolysis, or mobilization of lactate with epinephrine. These findings support the use of epinephrine in septic shock but it is considered second-line therapy due to its association with impaired lactate clearance.[6]

Vasopressin

14 Small studies of septic shock patients demonstrate that initial therapy with vasopressin achieves blood pressure control as effectively as traditional catecholamine vasopressors but the response is delayed.[43] Therefore, vasopressin therapy should not be initiated as first-line therapy. Several small studies showed that adjunctive vasopressin therapy reduces the dose requirements of catecholamine vasopressors and maintains blood pressure to expedite the discontinuation of catecholamine vasopressors with some documenting enhanced urine production.[43,55] A meta-analysis of 10 trials (N = 1,134) confirmed a negative correlation between vasopressin and norepinephrine dosages.[54] The results of a randomized, double-blind study of 776 patients with septic shock requiring catecholamine vasopressors showed that 28-day mortality rates were similar when vasopressin 0.01 to 0.03 units/min or norepinephrine 5 to 15 mcg/min was added to traditional catecholamine therapy (35.4% vs 39.3%; $P = 0.26$).[53] A trend toward reduced 28-day mortality favored vasopressin in the subset of patients categorized as having less severe septic shock defined by a baseline norepinephrine requirement of less than 15 mcg/min (26.5% vs 35.7%; $P = 0.05$). This trend was evident when sepsis severity was defined by lactate quartiles or number of organ failures, suggesting that adjunctive vasopressin may be most beneficial when it is started prior to escalation of therapy with catecholamine vasopressors. Posthoc analyses demonstrated greatest benefit with early vasopressin treatment relative to the onset of shock. The adverse event profiles were similar between groups. Of note, vasopressin therapy expedited the discontinuation of catecholamine vasopressors in all patients and helped preserve renal function in patients with acutely declining urine production as defined by the injury (doubling of serum creatinine concentration, glomerular

filtration rate reduced by half, or urine production less than 0.5 mL/kg/h) category of Risk, Injury, Failure, Loss, End-stage renal disease (RIFLE) criteria.[55] Whereas V_2 stimulation promotes water retention from the distal tubules and collecting ducts, V_1 receptors cause vasoconstriction of efferent arterioles and relative vasodilation of afferent arterioles to increase glomerular perfusion pressure and filtration rate, enhancing urine production. Adjunctive use of fixed dosage vasopressin for preventing dose escalation of adrenergic or reducing their dosages should be considered, but the risks must be weighed prior to initiating therapy. At present, vasopressin should not be used for the sole purpose of improving or maintaining renal function nor should dosages exceed 0.04 units/min.[6]

Clinical **Controversy...**

EPINEPHRINE OR VASOPRESSIN

Current guidelines suggest epinephrine or vasopressin may be added to norepinephrine but do not delineate which agent is preferred or when this should occur with respect to resuscitation goals.[6] Adding epinephrine may worsen lactate clearance while adding vasopressin may enhance the occurrence of ischemic events to digits. Both agents may worsen splanchnic circulation.

Corticosteroids

14 Several randomized controlled trials of low-dose corticosteroids in vasopressor-dependent septic shock patients have been published.[46-48] In general, studies demonstrating a survival benefit with corticosteroids administer lower total doses (hydrocortisone equivalents: 1,209 mg vs 23,975 mg; $P = 0.01$) starting later in septic shock (23 hours vs less than 2 hours; $P = 0.02$) for longer courses (6 days vs 1 day; $P = 0.01$) to patients with higher control group mortality rates (mean, 57% vs 34%; $P = 0.06$) who were more likely to be vasopressor dependent (100% vs 65%; $P = 0.03$). The results of meta-analyses are conflicting with regard to a survival benefit associated with corticosteroid administration; however, they are in agreement that corticosteroid use improves hemodynamics with more rapid shock reversal and shorter durations of vasopressor support.[47,71-73] Corticosteroids do not alter the rates of gastrointestinal bleeding, super infections, and neuromuscular weakness.

14 Two, somewhat discordant, studies contribute to the majority of data surrounding corticosteroid use in septic shock.[48,49] The first randomized 300 patients with septic shock within 8 hours of hypotension to placebo or a daily combination of hydrocortisone 50 mg IV every 6 hours and fludrocortisone 0.05 mg enterally for 7 days and found reduced 28-day mortality with corticosteroid therapy (OR, 0.65; 95% CI, 0.39-1.07; $P = 0.09$)[48] The placebo group was more likely to continually require vasopressor therapy (HR, 1.54; 95% CI, 1.10-12.16; $P = 0.01$). These beneficial outcomes were exhibited only in the 77% of patients with adrenal insufficiency as defined by the lack of cortisol response to ACTH administration. The second study randomized 499 of 800 intended subjects with severe sepsis or shock within 72 hours of presentation to placebo or hydrocortisone 50 mg IV every 6 hours for 5 days followed by a 6-day taper.[49] Mortality rates were similar between groups (32% vs 34%), irrespective of adrenal function. Median time to shock reversal was shorter in patients receiving corticosteroid therapy (3.3 vs 5.8 days; $P < 0.001$), again irrespective of adrenal function. Reversal of organ dysfunction was also expedited with corticosteroid therapy. Unlike the previous study, however, only 47% of patients demonstrated adrenal insufficiency likely reflective of the entry criteria and lower overall mortality rate of the study population.

Clinical **Controversy...**

CORTICOSTEROID THERAPY

Current guidelines do not suggest assessing adrenal function to determine the need for corticosteroid therapy.[6] Instead, they recommend initiating corticosteroids when hemodynamic goals are not achieved with fluid resuscitation or vasopressor therapy. This is controversial given the limitations and differences between studies and the difficulty of determining the adequate achievement of hemodynamic goals in patients requiring vasopressor therapy.

14 A post hoc analysis of the large vasopressin study revealed a significant interaction between vasopressin and corticosteroids.[74] In patients receiving vasopressin therapy, concurrent corticosteroid administration increased vasopressin concentrations by 33% to 67% over the initial 24 hours compared with patients only receiving vasopressin. The addition of corticosteroids to vasopressin was associated with reduced mortality compared with concurrent administration of corticosteroids and norepinephrine (35.9% vs 44.7%; $P = 0.03$). In the absence of corticosteroid therapy, however, mortality was greater with vasopressin therapy compared with norepinephrine (33.7% vs 21.3%; $P = 0.06$). Similar results have been reported in cohort studies but have not been validated in a prospective trial.

Hemodynamic Considerations and Adverse Effects

5 7 9 10 11 Catecholamine vasopressors may result in adverse peripheral vasoconstrictive, metabolic, and dysrhythmogenic effects that limit or outweigh their positive effects on the central circulation.[6-12,42,43] Table 23-4 lists potential adverse effects of commonly used vasopressors and inotropes.[5-12,42,43,50-52] Excessive peripheral vasoconstriction may cause ischemia or necrosis of already poorly perfused tissues such as the skin and the mesenteric and splanchnic circulations. Some of these profound vasoconstrictive effects may be compounded by under resuscitation with fluid administration prior to initiating the vasopressor or the concurrent use of other vasopressor agents. When these agents are used in the context of late septic shock, where hypotension is refractory to less selective vasoconstrictors (eg, dopamine), large doses of norepinephrine, epinephrine, or phenylephrine are required but provide little or no benefit. Myocardial ischemia and dysrhythmias may occur in patients with coronary artery disease, atherosclerosis, cardiomyopathies, left ventricular hypertrophy, congestive heart failure, or underlying dysrhythmias because of their inability to tolerate β_1 cardiac stimulation that mediates increases in CO. However, in young patients with healthy myocardium, β_1 cardiac stimulation is usually well tolerated, leading to decreased ventricular filling pressures and increased CO and Do_2, with a resulting increase in peripheral perfusion. The dysrhythmogenic potential of catecholamine vasopressors includes a variety of atrial and ventricular arrhythmias. Norepinephrine, phenylephrine, and especially epinephrine can produce lactic acidosis secondary to excessive constriction in peripheral arterioles or enhanced glycogenolysis, or as a result of mobilization of lactate from peripheral tissues as a result of improved oxygenation. Catecholamine vasopressors also have been found to possess immunomodulatory actions, primarily mediated by β_2-adrenergic actions (eg, epinephrine) because almost all immune cells express this receptor. In general, catecholamines inhibit the production of inflammatory cytokines (eg, IL-6 and TNF-α), may enhance anti-inflammatory cytokines (eg, IL-4 and IL-10), suppress oxygen-free radical production from neutrophils, and direct proapoptotic effects. Dopamine suppresses prolactin secretion from the anterior pituitary gland, which may lead to reduced T-cell responsiveness. These

anti-inflammatory effects may be either beneficial or deleterious by dampening harmful effects of oxygen-free radical–mediated tissue injury or by reducing neutrophilic defense against bacteria. The clinical significance of these actions on overall mortality in sepsis remains unknown.

Vasopressor catecholamines have the potential to cause extravasation-associated tissue damage if infusions infiltrate during peripheral administration. In the event of infiltration, an α-receptor antagonist such as phentolamine (10 mg in 10 mL saline) should be injected intradermally to reverse local vasoconstriction, with administration of vasopressor drugs into a large central vein.

Norepinephrine

7 8 9 13 Norepinephrine is the first-line therapy for septic shock as it effectively increases MAP.[2,6-12] It has combined strong α_1-activity and less potent β_1-agonist effects while maintaining weak vasodilatory effects of β_2-receptor stimulation.[5-12,50] Several studies have demonstrated improved MAP and mortality in ICU patients with severe hypotension treated with norepinephrine either as first-line therapy or after therapeutic failure with fluid resuscitation treatment.[50-52]

Norepinephrine infusions are initiated at 0.05 to 0.1 mcg/kg/min and rapidly titrated to preset goals of MAP (usually more than or equal to 65 mm Hg), improvement in global and regional peripheral perfusion (eg, restore urine production, decrease blood lactate), and/or achievement of desired oxygen-transport variables while not compromising the cardiac index. Norepinephrine 0.01 to 2 mcg/kg/min reliably and predictably improves hemodynamic parameters to "normal" values in most patients with septic shock. As with other vasopressors, norepinephrine dosages exceeding those recommended by most references frequently are needed in critically ill patients with septic shock to achieve predetermined goals. A significant increase in MAP generally is caused by an increase in SVR. Heart rate generally does not increase significantly with norepinephrine because of diminished stimulation of cardiac β_1-receptors in septic shock and reflex bradycardia from increased SVR.[5-12,50-52] Increasing norepinephrine doses to maintain higher MAPs may increase heart rates, cardiac index, Do_2, and cutaneous blood flow but these results are inconsistent. Older patients may benefit from the combined α- and β-adrenergic effects of norepinephrine given the higher incidence of coronary disease and compromised ventricles in this patient population. By virtue of restored MAP and hence coronary perfusion, cardiac index is increased in older patients, whereas in younger patients with less coronary artery disease and a higher cardiac index at baseline, norepinephrine acts primarily as a vasoconstrictor. Norepinephrine does not influence PAOP.

The effect of norepinephrine on oxygen transport parameters is variable and depends on baseline values and concurrently administered vasoactive agents. In most studies of norepinephrine alone, either an increase or no change in Do_2 is seen with no change in O_2ER, particularly when Do_2 values were "supranormal" prior to therapy. Norepinephrine demonstrates either no effect or improvement in Pco_2 gap, pHi, or serum lactate concentrations. Splanchnic blood flow and fractional blood flow are higher with norepinephrine than either dopamine or epinephrine despite higher CO with the two latter agents.

Taken together, these data suggest that norepinephrine is the primary vasopressor of choice in patients in septic shock because of its multiple benefits: (1) norepinephrine may decrease mortality in septic shock; (2) it reverses inappropriate vasodilation and low global oxygen extraction; (3) it attenuates myocardial depression at unchanged or increased CO and increased coronary blood flow; (4) it improves renal perfusion pressure and renal filtration; (5) it enhances splanchnic perfusion; and (6) it is less likely than other vasopressors to cause tachydysrhythmias.[5-12,50-53] The primary limitation to use is that norepinephrine is not commercially available as premixed ready-to-use solutions so use requires preparation time. Institutions may stock compounded admixtures in preparation for administration, but they must follow sterile compounding and storage regulations.

Phenylephrine

7 8 10 13 Despite its purported use in refractory septic shock, little information is available regarding the clinical efficacy of phenylephrine. Nevertheless, it is an attractive agent for use in sepsis because of its selective α-agonism with primarily vascular effects.[5-12,51,52] As with other vasopressors, phenylephrine dosages required to achieve goals of therapy are significantly higher than dosages traditionally recommended for use.

Phenylephrine 0.5 to 9 mcg/kg/min, used alone or in combination with dobutamine or low dosages of dopamine, improves blood pressure and myocardial performance in fluid-resuscitated septic patients. Incremental doses of phenylephrine result in linear dose-related increases in SVR and MAP when administered alone as a single agent in stable, nonhypotensive but hyperdynamic, volume-resuscitated surgical ICU patients. In septic shock, phenylephrine does not significantly impair the cardiac index, PAOP, or peripheral perfusion. In sepsis, phenylephrine improves MAP by increasing SVR and stroke index through enhanced venous return to the heart. It improves myocardial performance in hyperdynamic, normotensive septic patients but worsens myocardial performance in cardiac controls. In cardiac patients, myocardial performance worsens as a result of a decrease in the cardiac index and an increase in SVR. Therefore, phenylephrine use warrants caution and should not be used as an initial vasopressor in septic shock patients with impaired myocardial performance.

In septic shock, phenylephrine appears to increase global tissue oxygen use, although data regarding the relationship of the oxygen-transport variables with increases in MAP and cardiac index are conflicting. Increases in Vo_2 appear to be dissociated from Do_2, representing an increase in O_2ER as the cardiac index remains unchanged. Increases in Vo_2 may result from redistribution of blood flow to previously underperfused areas, improving oxygen use as a result of changes in MAP and SVR. Evidence of globally improved peripheral tissue perfusion is observed as lactic acid concentration declines or remains unchanged and urine production increases significantly at increased or maximal Vo_2. An increased O_2ER may contribute to improved tissue response.

Few data regarding the effect of phenylephrine on regional hemodynamics and oxygen-transport variables are available. When phenylephrine replaced norepinephrine in patients with septic shock, phenylephrine selectively reduced splanchnic blood flow and thus splanchnic Do_2 and splanchnic lactate uptake rate without changing the overall splanchnic Vo_2. Concomitantly, pHi decreased and arterial lactate concentrations increased. Because all of these parameters normalized when norepinephrine was reinstated, these data suggest that exogenous β-adrenergic stimulation (norepinephrine) may determine hepatosplanchnic perfusion and oxygen availability but not utilization in septic shock. Phenylephrine and norepinephrine demonstrate similar short-term hemodynamic profiles and indices of global and regional perfusion when used as an initial vasopressor in septic shock.[6-12]

The available data on hemodynamics, oxygen-transport variables, and mortality with phenylephrine in septic shock patients may not be generalizable because of the small numbers of patients evaluated. Adverse effects, such as tachydysrhythmias, are notably infrequent with phenylephrine, particularly when it is used as a single agent or at higher doses, because phenylephrine does not exert any activity on β_1-adrenergic receptors. Whether the beneficial effects can be sustained with longer administrations of phenylephrine is unclear. Phenylephrine may be a particularly useful alternative in patients who cannot tolerate tachycardia or tachydysrhythmias with use of dopamine or norepinephrine and in patients who are refractory to dopamine or norepinephrine (because of β-adrenergic receptor desensitization).[6,51,52] Its use in patients with myocardial dysfunction warrants caution. Like norepinephrine, it is not commercially available as premixed ready-to-use solutions. Institutions may stock compounded admixtures in preparation for administration but they must follow sterile compounding and storage regulations.

Epinephrine

7 8 11 13 Epinephrine is an acceptable choice for hemodynamic support of septic shock because of its combined vasoconstrictor and inotropic effects but it is associated with tachydysrhythmias and lactate elevation.[5-12,51,52,69,70] As a result, it is considered second line or as adjunctive therapy to norepinephrine.[6] It is as effective as norepinephrine for blood pressure control. Epinephrine infusion rates of 0.04 to 1 mcg/kg/min alone increase hemodynamic and oxygen-transport variables to "supranormal" values without adverse effects in septic patients without coronary artery disease. Large dosages (0.5-3 mcg/kg/min) often are required. Smaller dosages (0.10-0.50 mcg/kg/min) are effective when epinephrine is added to other vasopressors and inotropes. In addition, younger patients appear to respond better to epinephrine, possibly due to greater β-adrenergic reactivity.

Despite a linear dose-response curve with rapid improvement of hemodynamic variables and Do_2, epinephrine has deleterious effects on regional hemodynamics and oxygen utilization. Although Do_2 increases mainly as a function of increases in the cardiac index and a more variable increase in SVR, Vo_2 may not increase, and O_2ER may fall. A decrease in pHi may be seen during epinephrine administration but the impairment in gastric mucosal perfusion can be counteracted in part by dobutamine. This may be explained by the vasodilatory effect of dobutamine on gastric mucosal microcirculation resulting in a redistribution of blood flow toward the mucosa. In contrast to other vasopressors, lactate concentrations frequently rise during epinephrine therapy resulting in variable arterial pH values. When compared with a combination of norepinephrine and dobutamine, epinephrine preferentially decreases splanchnic Do_2, worsens pHi, and increases systemic lactate concentration without increasing Vo_2. The effects of epinephrine on absolute and fractional splanchnic blood flow are more pronounced during severe shock. The increase in lactate may be a result of worsened Do_2 to the liver (and subsequent anaerobic metabolism) or to the hepatosplanchnic circulation, direct increase in calorigenesis and breakdown of glycogen (enhanced aerobic lactate production via β_2-adrenergic receptor stimulation), or lactate mobilization. However, evidence suggests that epinephrine, in contrast to dopamine, increases the proportion of total CO delivered to the splanchnic circulation, although Vo_2 is not increased sufficiently. As a result, O_2ER values are usually lower with epinephrine than with other vasopressors but the concomitant administration of dobutamine helps maintain O_2ER. Of all the vasopressors, epinephrine exhibits the most pronounced capacity to induce hyperglycemia by increased gluconeogenesis and glycogenolysis with α-mediated suppression of insulin secretion.[42]

Despite the administration of high doses, epinephrine-associated clinically important dysrhythmias or cardiac ischemia occur at variable rates irrespective of age or underlying cardiac status.[5-12,51,52,69,70] Nevertheless, caution must be exercised before considering epinephrine for managing hypoperfusion in hypodynamic patients with coronary artery disease, in whom ischemia, chest pain, or myocardial infarction may result. Based on the current evidence, epinephrine may be used as a second-line vasopressor or added on to norepinephrine in patients with septic shock refractory to fluid administration.[6] Although it effectively increases CO and Do_2, it has deleterious effects on the splanchnic circulation. If it is used, factors that may influence successful therapy with epinephrine include the time from onset of septic shock to effective therapy, the age of the population, and the selection of concurrent vasopressors and inotropes. Like norepinephrine and phenylephrine, it is not commercially available as premixed ready-to-use solutions. Institutions may stock compounded admixtures in preparation for administration but they must follow sterile compounding and storage regulations.

Dopamine

7 8 9 13 Dopamine is a natural precursor to norepinephrine and epinephrine and generally not as effective as these two agents for achieving goal MAP in patients with septic shock.[5-12,42,50-52] Most studies of patients with septic shock have shown that dopamine at dosages of 5 to 10 mcg/kg/min increase the cardiac index by improving contractility and heart rate, primarily from its β_1 effects. It increases MAP and SVR as a result of both increased CO and, at higher doses (more than 10 mcg/kg/min), its α_1 effects.

The clinical utility of dopamine as a vasopressor in the setting of septic shock is limited because large dosages are frequently necessary to maintain CO and MAP. At dosages exceeding 20 mcg/kg/min, further improvement in cardiac performance and regional hemodynamics is limited. Its clinical use frequently is hampered by tachycardia and tachydysrhythmias, which may lead to myocardial ischemia. Although tachydysrhythmias theoretically should not be expected to occur until administration of dopamine 5 to 10 mcg/kg/min, these β_1 effects are observed with dosages as low as 3 mcg/kg/min. They seem to be more prevalent in patients who are inadequately resuscitated (hypovolemic), in the elderly, in those with preexisting or concurrent cardiac ischemia or dysrhythmias, and in patients currently receiving other dysrhythmogenic agents, including vasopressors and inotropes.

Dopamine increases PAOP and pulmonary shunting to decrease Pao_2. The increase in PAOP may be due to changes in diastolic volumes from decreased cardiac compliance or increased venous return to the heart by α-adrenergic receptor-mediated venoconstriction. This may affect gas exchange and decrease Pao_2. The increase in pulmonary shunting also may result from acute enhancement of pulmonary blood flow to nonhomogeneous lung regions. Thus, dopamine should be used with caution in patients with elevated preload because the drug may worsen pulmonary edema. In the instance of high filling pressures, tachycardia, or tachydysrhythmias, dopamine should be replaced by another vasopressor and/or inotrope such as norepinephrine, dobutamine, phenylephrine, or epinephrine, depending on the desired effect.

The effect of dopamine on global oxygen-transport variables parallels the hemodynamic effects. Although dopamine improves global Do_2 in septic patients, it may compromise O_2ER in the splanchnic and mesenteric circulations by α_1-mediated vasoconstriction. Splanchnic blood flow and Do_2 increase with dopamine, but with no preferential increase in splanchnic perfusion as a fraction of CO and systemic increases in Do_2. Large doses of dopamine worsen pHi and the Pco_2 gap. This is reflected by a decrease or lack of change in regional Vo_2 and a decrease in tissue O_2ER. Dopamine at low or vasopressor dosages directly impedes gastric motility in critical illness and may aggravate gut ischemia in septic shock. Similar to high-dose administration, low-dose dopamine increases splanchnic blood flow but lowers splanchnic Vo_2 in sepsis. Therefore, dopamine at all dosages impairs hepatosplanchnic metabolism despite an increase in regional perfusion. Low dosages increase renal blood flow and glomerular filtration rate in studies of animals and healthy volunteers but did not demonstrate improved renal function in a randomized, placebo-controlled study of 328 critically ill patients with early renal dysfunction.[75] A meta-analysis of 61 trials (N = 3,359) confirmed that low-dose dopamine fails to enhance renal function or survival in critically ill patients.[76]

While dopamine may improve hemodynamic function, the use of dopamine for septic shock is questionable because regional hemodynamics, oxygen-transport variables, and functional parameters of improved organ perfusion are not consistently enhanced in a sustained manner and may be negatively impaired.[6] The negative findings of low-dose dopamine use and the deleterious effects of inotropic and vasopressor dosages of dopamine on regional hemodynamics, oxygen transport, and functional performance of organ perfusion raise concern over whether dopamine should even be considered in patients with severe sepsis or septic shock.[6,75] Unlike other vasopressor agents, however, dopamine is commercially available as premixed ready-to-use solutions of various concentrations that can be stored in automated dispensing systems for rapid initiation.

Dobutamine

6 7 12 13 Dobutamine is an inotrope with vasodilatory properties (an "inodilator").[5-12,42] It is used for treatment of septic and cardiogenic shock to increase the cardiac index, typically by 25% to 50%.[6] In septic shock, LVEF and right ventricular function are depressed despite a high cardiac index, whereas ventricular volumes and compliance are increased. Stroke index is maintained by an increased heart rate and ventricular dilation. In survivors, myocardial depression is reversible and normalizes 5 to 10 days after the onset of sepsis. Dobutamine increases stroke index, left ventricular stroke work index, and thus cardiac index and Do_2 without increasing PAOP.[6-12] It also enhances chronotropy effect. However, dosage increments of dobutamine beyond 20 mcg/kg/min are limited by complications of tachycardia, ischemic changes on electrocardiogram, hypertension, and tachydysrhythmias despite the absence of preexisting cardiac abnormalities. The combination of dobutamine and norepinephrine results in a lower increase in heart rate compared with use of epinephrine alone.

Increased cardiac performance measures in response to adjunctive dobutamine therapy are predictive of survival during sepsis. However, the achievement of supranormal oxygen transport values with dobutamine is of little value compared with treatment to normal values. In addition, administration of dobutamine to achieve these high values may increase mortality rate and/or the incidence of adverse effects. Dobutamine increases Do_2 without affecting Vo_2, resulting in decreased O_2ER. Arterial lactate concentrations decrease significantly with norepinephrine and dobutamine compared with dopamine and epinephrine infusions.

Studies have focused on the effects of dobutamine on gastric mucosal flow and the splanchnic circulation. The addition of dobutamine to other vasopressors improves gastric mucosal perfusion without increasing the cardiac index. This is consistent with findings that dobutamine may improve pHi and mucosal perfusion in septic patients. The addition of dobutamine to norepinephrine or epinephrine treatment improves gastric mucosal perfusion as measured by improvements in pHi and Pco_2 gap. This effect may relate to blood flow redistribution toward gastric mucosa, due to either an increase in the fraction of CO distributed to the global hepatosplanchnic blood flow and/or a redistribution of blood flow within gastric wall layers toward the mucosa by "stealing" blood away from the muscularis potentially as a result of greater β_2-mediated vasodilation. Sublingual microcirculation improves after dobutamine is added to vasopressor-dependent septic shock patients in a manner unrelated to arterial pressure or cardiac index, suggesting that enhanced perfusion is the result of the "steal" phenomenon. Of note, gastric mucosal perfusion and tissue oxygen utilization are most improved with concurrent norepinephrine and dobutamine therapies compared with other vasopressor combinations at the same level of MAP.

Dobutamine should be started at dosages ranging from 2.5 to 5 mcg/kg/min. In the studies of early goal-directed therapy, dobutamine was administered to 13.7% to 18.1% of patients within 6 hours of resuscitation to achieve $Scvo_2$ more than or equal to 70%.[19-24] While dobutamine was only administered to 0.8% to 7.5% of subjects in the groups receiving usual aggressive care which did not include $Scvo_2$ monitoring, overall mortality rates across all studies did not differ.[24] Therefore, dobutamine administration purely to achieve a $Scvo_2$ more than or equal to 70% is not best clinical practice. Current guidelines recommend a trial of dobutamine infusion up to 20 mcg/kg/min in the presence of myocardial dysfunction (elevated cardiac filling pressures, low CO, and echocardiography displaying left ventricular dysfunction) or continued signs of global or regional hypoperfusion despite meeting volume and MAP goals.[6] Although a dose response may be seen, evidence suggests that dosages more than 5 mcg/kg/min may provide limited beneficial effects on oxygen transport values and hemodynamics and may increase adverse cardiac effects. If given to patients who are intravascularly depleted, dobutamine will result in hypotension and a reflexive tachycardia. Pathophysiologic factors influence dosing requirements and pharmacokinetic parameters over the time course of the illness and the duration of the infusion. Decreases in PaO_2, as well as myocardial adverse effects such as tachycardia, ischemic changes on electrocardiogram, tachydysrhythmias, and hypotension are seen. Thus, infusion rates should be guided by clinical end points, echocardiography, and global perfusion goals. Dobutamine, like other inotropes, usually is given until improvement in myocardial function with resolution of the septic episode or dose-limiting side effects are observed. Dobutamine is commercially available as premixed ready-to-use solutions.

Vasopressin

14 Studies involving vasopressin infusion for management of septic shock show rapid and sustained improvement in hemodynamic parameters.[43,53-55] These effects are evident with administration of dosages not exceeding 0.04 units/min. Administration of dosages more than 0.04 units/min are associated with negative changes in CO and mesenteric mucosal perfusion. The reduction in CO likely is the result of lowered stroke volume.[43] The studies that reported cardiac function indicate patients had adequate CO prior to initiating vasopressin therapy. Cardiac ischemia appears to be a rare occurrence when low dosage rates are used. Therefore, higher dosages of vasopressin in septic shock patients with cardiac dysfunction warrant extreme caution.

Mesenteric ischemia associated with vasopressin may be clinically relevant. Increased hepatic transaminases and total bilirubin concentrations may occur with vasopressin therapy, suggesting impaired hepatic blood flow or a direct effect on excretory hepatic function.[43] While mesenteric vasoconstriction occurs at vasopressin serum concentrations as low as 10 pg/dL, the results of studies indicate that vasopressin dosages exceeding 0.04 units/min worsen pHi or PCO_2 gap when it is added to low or high doses of catecholamine vasopressors.[43] The effect is additive with norepinephrine despite substantially reduced dosages of norepinephrine when vasopressin is initiated.

Vasopressin's strongest vasoconstrictive action occurs in the skin and soft tissues, skeletal muscles, and fat tissues.[43] As a result, ischemic skin lesions have been observed in several studies, with an occurrence rate as high as 30% after vasopressin was added to norepinephrine-resistant shock.[43] Although vasopressin may have deleterious effects on mesenteric and skin perfusion, studies report vasodilation of cerebral, pulmonary, coronary, and some renal vasculature beds. The clinical outcomes associated with selective vasodilation are not yet known except for the possibility of enhanced urine production in patients not anuric at baseline.[55]

In order to minimize the potential for adverse events and maximize the beneficial effects, vasopressin should be used as add-on therapy to catecholamine adrenergic agents rather than as first-line therapy or salvage therapy and dosages should be limited to 0.04 units/min (generally fixed dose of 0.03-0.04 units/min).[5,6,43] The results of studies showed that vasopressin markedly reduced the requirements for adrenergic agents, but few studies demonstrated complete discontinuation of these therapies.[43,53,54] Therefore, vasopressin should be used when response to one or two adrenergic agents is inadequate or as a method for reducing the dosage of these therapies.[6] Increased arterial pressure should be evident within the first hour of vasopressin therapy, at which time the dose(s) of adrenergic agent(s) should be reduced while maintaining goal MAP. This method should help limit the degree of ischemia.

Most studies evaluated vasopressin use for less than 48 hours, and several studies reported difficulty discontinuing vasopressin therapy. Whether additional benefits, deleterious effects, or tolerance is observed with longer infusions remains unclear. Long-term administration of vasopressin is associated with hyponatremia and thrombocytopenia. Because vasopressin is being used to replace a physiologic deficiency, it stands to reason that the requirement for vasopressin will subside with reversal of the septic process. Attempts to discontinue vasopressin should occur when the dosage(s) of adrenergic agent(s) has been minimized (eg, dopamine less than or equal to 5 mcg/kg/min, norepinephrine less than or equal to 0.1 mcg/kg/min, phenylephrine less than or equal to 1 mcg/kg/min, and epinephrine less than or equal to 0.15 mcg/kg/min). Vasopressin is not available as premixed ready-to-use solutions.

Corticosteroids

14 Corticosteroids can be initiated in cases of septic shock when adrenal insufficiency is suspected (eg, patients receiving long-term corticosteroid therapy for other indications prior to the onset of shock), when vasopressor dosages are escalating, or when weaning of vasopressor therapy proves futile.[5,6,45-48,72,73] Assessment of adrenal function to guide therapy is not recommended.[6] Adverse events are few because corticosteroids are administered for a finite period of time, usually 7 days. Acutely, elevated serum concentrations of blood urea nitrogen, white blood cell count, glucose, and sodium occur. Although long-term administration of corticosteroids is associated with several chronic disease states, meta-analyses do not show an increase in major adverse events, including gastrointestinal hemorrhage, superinfections, and neuromuscular weakness.[46,47,72,73] Therefore, therapy of septic shock with corticosteroids improves hemodynamic variables and lowers catecholamine vasopressor dosages with minimal to no effect on patient safety.[6]

EXPERIMENTAL THERAPIES

Nitric Oxide Inhibitors

Nitric oxide is a short-acting, potent vasodilator derived from enzymatic oxidation of arginine. Its production is under control of NOS. This enzyme is present (expressed) in two forms: (1) a constitutive form (ecNOS) and (2) an inducible form (iNOS). Small amounts of NO normally are produced by the vascular endothelium under the control of ecNOS for physiologic control of vascular tone and blood flow distribution. Under pathophysiologic conditions such as stimulation by lipopolysaccharide or cytokines, iNOS becomes diffusely expressed, producing large amounts of NO. The latter has been implicated in the cardiovascular failure of septic shock.

Pharmacologic inhibition of NO production has been investigated as an adjunct to standard therapies of septic shock.[77,78] L-Arginine analogs, such as monomethyl-L-arginine (L-NMMA) and L-arginine-methylester (L-NAME), are competitive inhibitors of NOS and have been shown to increase blood pressure, partially restore vascular reactivity, and reduce vasopressor use. However, because these arginine analogs nonselectively block ecNOS and iNOS, their use has been associated with extensive vasoconstriction, decreased CO, and regional hypoperfusion, thus promoting organ failure and mortality.[78,79] Some *S*-substituted thiourea derivatives have demonstrated, both in vitro and in vivo (rodent), dose-dependent selectivity for iNOS inhibition, but the clinical application must be evaluated. Several phase I/IIa clinical trials of septic shock patients are underway.

Pyridoxalated hemoglobin polyoxyethylene is a scavenger of NO. A phase II study of 62 patients with vasodilatory shock requiring vasopressors showed that an infusion of 20 mg/kg/h for up to 100 hours rapidly increased blood pressure and shortened the duration of vasopressor therapy.[80] However, a Phase III study was terminated early due to a signal of increased mortality in more severely ill patients with pyridoxalated hemoglobin polyoxyethylene despite favorable vasopressor-free survival time.[81]

Methylene Blue

Methylene blue counteracts ecNOS, iNOS, and soluble guanylate cyclase to reduce serum concentrations of NO and cyclic guanosine monophosphate.[82] Despite these effects, methylene blue does not alter the expression of inflammatory cytokines. Clinically, methylene blue at dosages of 0.25 to 3 mg/kg/h increases SVR, MAP, myocardial contractility, and Do_2 in septic shock patients refractory to vasopressors while improving Pco_2 gap.[82] Dosages exceeding 3 mg/kg/h worsen splanchnic perfusion. It may increase pulmonary vascular resistance, potentially worsening oxygenation. Additional studies are needed before methylene blue can be recommended; at present, it has been used only for salvage therapy.

Terlipressin

Terlipressin, a prodrug that is converted into lysine vasopressin, has been used in septic shock patients and is available in other countries.[12] This drug has a half-life of 6 hours and acts via vascular V_1 receptors and renal tubular V_2 receptors. Terlipressin increases MAP to a greater extent than norepinephrine when it is used as the initial vasopressor in septic shock. Despite a decrease in CO, heart rate, and Do_2I, terlipressin increases gastric mesenteric perfusion, urine production, and creatinine clearance while reducing lactate concentration. Both terlipressin and vasopressin increase blood pressure and decrease heart rate to the same extent but terlipressin is associated with less supplemental norepinephrine usage and improved mesenteric perfusion.[12] These preliminary findings suggest that a clinical trial evaluating mortality as well as hemodynamic effects should be conducted with terlipressin.

Levosimendan

Levosimendan is a novel inotropic and vasodilator calcium-sensitizing drug.[83] In acute decompensated heart failure, it improves cardiac contractility by sensitizing troponin C to calcium. In septic shock patients with and without left ventricular dysfunction, levosimendan 0.1 to 0.2 mcg/kg/min decreases PAOP, increases LVEF and cardiac index, improves mesenteric and sublingual perfusion, and enhances urine production.[83] Levosimendan improves $Scvo_2$ to the same extent as dobutamine when it is used in early goal-directed therapy. Levosimendan is associated with declining serum lactate concentrations. The results of a meta-analysis of seven studies (N = 246) suggest it is associated with reduced mortality compared to traditional inotropes when used in severe sepsis.[84] While additional clinical trials of levosimendan in septic shock are needed, increased mortality was demonstrated in studies of acute decompensated heart failure.

Esmolol

High sympathetic stress and excessive adrenergic tone may, in part, lead to many sequelae seen in late septic shock including myocardial dysfunction.[85] Contrasting the proposed benefits of stimulating β-adrenergic activity in septic shock, a study of 154 hemodynamically "optimized" patients (PAOP more than or equal to 12 mm Hg,

CVP more than or equal to 8 mm Hg, Svo_2 more than 65% and MAP more than or equal to 65 mm Hg) with septic shock requiring norepinephrine with a heart rate more than 94 beats per minute were randomized to receive esmolol to a goal heart rate of 80 to 94 beats per minute or standard of care.[86] Patients were excluded if they had cardiac dysfunction or significant valvular heart disease. The esmolol group had significantly lower heart rate and higher stroke volume while maintaining similar MAP values despite lower SVR and norepinephrine requirements. Do_2, Vo_2, fluid requirements, acidosis, serum lactate, and markers of myocardial injury were decreased in the esmolol group. Mortality at day 28 was lower in the esmolol group (49.4% vs 80.5%; $P < 0.001$), although this was a secondary outcome. The concept of targeted heart rate control requires additional study before application occurs in practice.

Other Therapies

As with vasopressin and cortisol, critical illness impairs hypothalamic-pituitary function, producing relative deficiencies of triiodothyronine (T_3) and thyroxine (T_4). This condition, referred to as *euthyroid sick syndrome*, may contribute to hypotension and mortality.[87] Concentrations of thyrotropin-releasing hormone and thyroid-stimulating hormone are inappropriately low. Measured concentrations of free T_3 and T_4 may be low or normal, but synthesis is consistently impaired. Only scant data regarding the replacement of these hormones in critically ill patients are available, and the results are variable, depending on the extent of additional hormone replacement (growth hormone, gonadotropin-releasing hormone, leptin, insulin, thyrotropin-releasing hormone, and thyroid-stimulating hormone). Given the data for replacing vasopressin and cortisol in septic shock, it is reasonable to assume that one day a "thyroid replacement" regimen will be offered as an adjunctive treatment to vasopressors.

GENERAL CONCLUSION AND RECOMMENDATIONS

Norepinephrine is the recommended first-line vasopressor for septic shock.[6] The choice of additional vasopressor or inotropic agents should be made according to the clinical needs of the patient and the data obtained from hemodynamic and global and regional perfusion monitoring.[2,5-15] Figure 23-2 presents an algorithm for the management of septic shock.[2,5,6-12] This algorithm suggests a stepwise approach of early goal-directed therapy to optimize MAP, first with fluid resuscitation and using norepinephrine. Dobutamine may be added for states low CO or left ventricular dysfunction or to optimize lactate clearance or Svo_2/$Scvo_2$. Occasionally, epinephrine and phenylephrine are used when necessary. Although this approach is empirical, it is used broadly in clinical practice and has been justified by the desire to avoid the adverse events associated with strong vasoconstriction. Developing a strategy to rapidly titrate therapy early in the course of illness to predetermined values reduces mortality. Goals of initial resuscitation should include fluids to achieve CVP of 8 to 12 mm Hg, vasopressor agents to achieve MAP at least 65 mm Hg, and frequent clinical assessments to meet global and regional perfusion goals (eg, additional fluid challenge or inotropic therapy to achieve lactate clearance more than or equal to 20% or $Scvo_2$ more than or equal to 70% or urine production output to more than or equal to 0.5mL/kg/h).[2,5,6] For all catecholamine vasopressors, doses higher than recommended traditionally are required for goal-directed therapy to achieve goal MAP and for normalization of oxygen-transport variables. Patients who develop supranormal Do_2 and Vo_2 values have lower mortality, but targeting these with exogenous administration of vasopressors/inotropes is not beneficial and cannot be recommended. Further work is required to better elucidate the differential effects of vasopressors on regional hemodynamic and oxygen-transport values as measures of local tissue perfusion.

Clinical **Controversy...**

PERFUSION GOALS OF EARLY GOAL-DIRECTED THERAPY

The goal of resuscitation is to reverse tissue hypoxia by facilitating Do_2. Both Svo_2 and $Scvo_2$ measure global tissue perfusion. Current guidelines recommend targeting Svo_2 or $Scvo_2$ more than or equal to 70% or more than or equal to 65%, respectively, based on the original study of early goal directed therapy.[6,19] In contrast, the results of three large multicenter studies conducted after the guidelines were published found usual care without the assessment of Svo_2 or $Scvo_2$ resulted in similar survival outcomes as strategies of early goal directed therapy that incorporated these as goals of global perfusion.[21-23] Lactate clearance reliably assesses tissue perfusion and predicts survival. The decision to use Svo_2 or $Scvo_2$ as a goal of early goal directed therapy will depend on clinician's preference and patient's characteristics but the guidelines will be revised to include lactate clearance. Many clinicians already apply lactate clearance as a goal of global perfusion in addition to organ-specific indicators of regional perfusion as end points of early goal directed therapy that should be achieved within 3 to 6 hours of sepsis presentation.

This algorithmic approach (see Fig. 23-2) is consistent with the recommendations made in the Surviving Sepsis Campaign[6] and the American College of Critical Care Medicine's guidelines to the hemodynamic support of adult patients with sepsis (see Table 23-2).[2,4-16] Personalized pharmacotherapy (Table 23-5) for hemodynamic support of shock may be rationale in certain situations (such as long standing baseline hypertension, or home corticosteroid use) but may be difficult to achieve because patient response is variable and the acute nature of emergent resuscitation often necessitates treatment before pharmacotherapy can be personalized. In the future, vasopressor therapies may be directed to pharmacogenomic profiles as recent research indicates effectiveness and safety may be influenced by gene polymorphisms.

Although difficult to demonstrate, true differences in clinical outcomes as a result of differences in the pharmacologic activity of vasopressors and inotropes may exist. For example, evidence suggests that norepinephrine, when used appropriately with fluid replenishment, is safe and effective in treating septic shock; it decreases mortality, particularly when started early in the course of septic shock. It is effective in optimizing hemodynamic variables and improving systemic and regional (eg, renal, gastric mucosal, and splanchnic) perfusion. Epinephrine causes a greater increase in the cardiac index and Do_2 and increases gastric mucosal flow but may not preserve splanchnic circulation adequately. It may cause increases in lactic acid. Epinephrine, however, may be particularly useful when used earlier in the course of septic shock in young patients. Unlike epinephrine, dopamine does not increase the proportion of CO that preferentially goes to the splanchnic circulation. The ability of dopamine to increase CO by no more than 35% accompanied by a tachycardia or tachydysrhythmias limits its utility. Dopamine, as opposed to norepinephrine, has been shown to worsen splanchnic Vo_2 and O_2ER and is of limited value in improving urine production. Low-dose dopamine has not been shown consistently to increase the glomerular filtration rate, does not prevent renal failure, and actually worsens splanchnic tissue oxygen utilization and therefore should not be used. Phenylephrine may be used when a pure vasoconstrictor

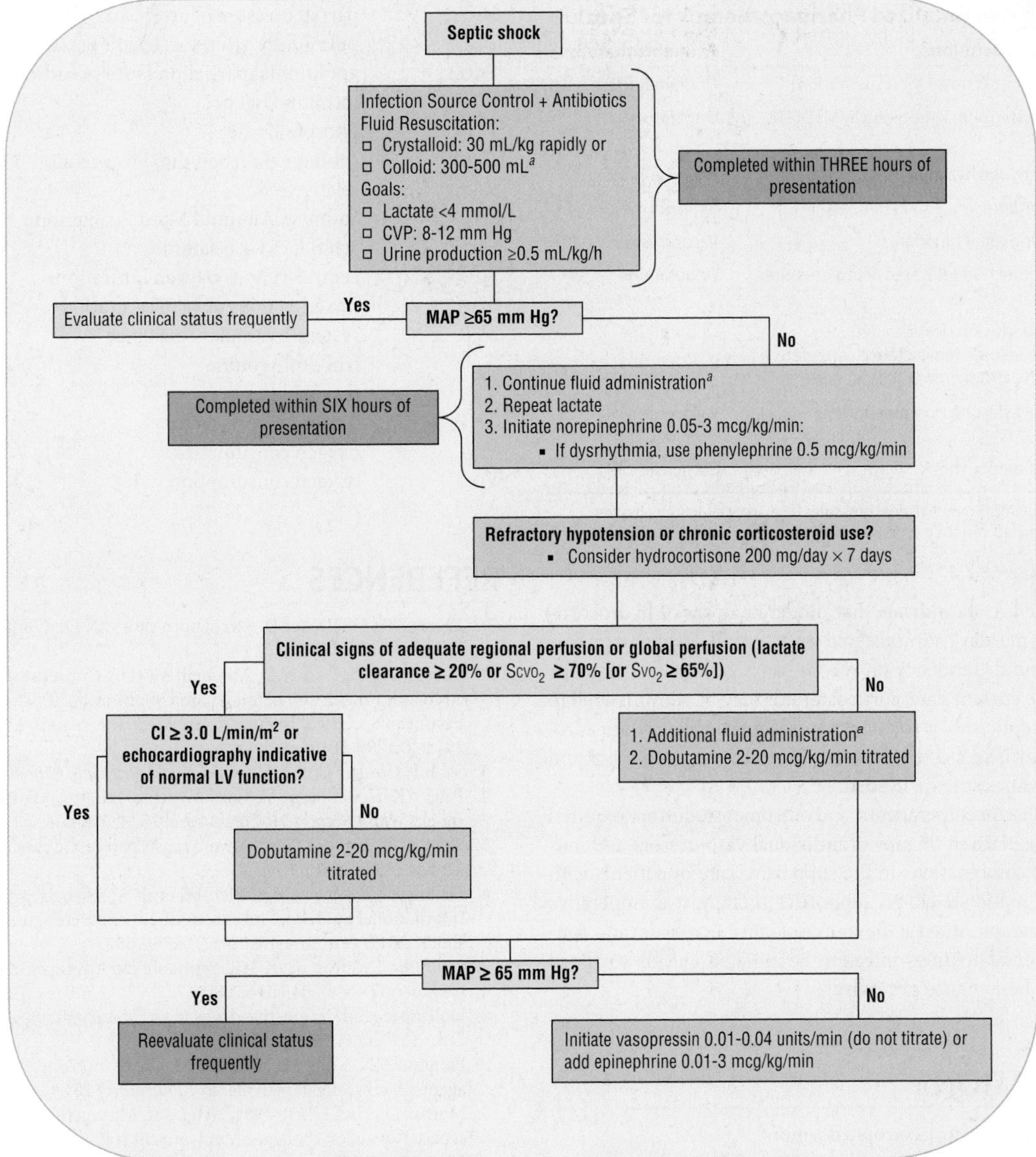

FIGURE 23-2 Algorithmic approach to resuscitative management of septic shock. Algorithmic approach is intended to be used in conjunction with clinical judgment, hemodynamic monitoring parameters, global and regional perfusion goals, and therapy end points, as discussed in the text. [a]Colloid (albumin) may be initiated in patients at risk for adverse events from redistribution of intravenous fluids to extravascular tissues (eg, patients with renal dysfunction, decompensated heart failure, ascites compromising diaphragmatic function), those that are fluid restricted, or those not responding to crystalloid therapy. (Abbreviations: CI, cardiac index; CVP, central venous pressure; echo, echocardiography; Hct, hematocrit; MAP, mean arterial pressure; $Scvo_2$, central venous oxygen saturation; Svo_2, mixed venous oxygen saturation.) (*Data from references 2, 5-12.*)

is desired in patients who may not require or cannot tolerate the β-effects of other vasopressors or inotropes. In patients with a high filling pressure and hypotension, the combination of phenylephrine and dobutamine may be useful.

Shortcomings of study methodology prevent the establishment of definitive conclusions regarding catecholamines. As a consequence, published guidelines for the management of severe sepsis and septic shock have many inconclusive recommendations (see Table 23-2). Short infusions during studies may show differences that are not clinically significant after 24 hours, as demonstrated for epinephrine and dobutamine. Most studies comparatively evaluated vasopressors once patients were hemodynamically stable as the process of obtaining consent and randomization precluded the initiation of study drug during early resuscitation. Clinically, vasopressors and inotropes are used for hours to days. Possible confounding factors are the variable times at which studies are initiated with respect to the stage of sepsis or septic shock, the inherent differences in circulating catecholamine concentrations, changes in receptor activity, as well as differences in prestudy duration and type of exogenous catecholamine administration.

Initial studies with vasopressin suggest a potential role in the management of vasopressor-dependent septic shock patients. Vasopressin reduces the requirements of adrenergic agents while maintaining hemodynamic function. While it may enhance urine production, it is associated with mesenteric and peripheral ischemia. Therefore, fixed dose vasopressin should be used if response to one or two adrenergic agents is inadequate or as a method for reducing the dosage of these therapies. Close monitoring of ischemic

TABLE 23-5 Personalized Pharmacotherapy for Shock

Situational Considerations	Pharmacotherapy
Initial vasopressor of choice for resuscitation	Norepinephrine
Rapidly progressing shock requiring IMMEDIATE therapy	Dopamine
Presence of tachydysrhythmia	Phenylephrine
Healthy myocardium (eg, young patients)	Epinephrine
Acutely declining renal function	Vasopressin
Myocardial dysfunction (elevated filling pressures and low CO)	Dobutamine
Regional hypoperfusion despite adequate intravascular volume (eg, lactate clearance <20% or Sc_VO_2 <70% or SvO_2 <65%)	Dobutamine
MAP <65 mm Hg despite norepinephrine	Vasopressin or epinephrine
Vasopressor refractory shock	Corticosteroid

CO, cardiac output; MAP, mean arterial pressure; $Scvo_2$, central-venous oxygen saturation; Svo_2, mixed venous oxygen saturation.

events is needed. Data indicate that moderate doses of hydrocortisone (200-300 mg/day) administered over several days may reverse septic shock and dependency on vasopressor agents. Given the discrepancy of the current data, corticosteroids may be administered to patients with septic shock refractory to vasopressors or when adrenal insufficiency is suspected. Data on optimal dosage regimens and definitive outcomes still are needed.

Further pharmacotherapeutic and outcomes studies are required to elucidate the place in therapy of individual vasopressors and inotropes or their combinations in the supportive care of patients with bacteremia or septic shock. As supportive therapy, it is imperative that primary therapy aimed at the source of (antimicrobials) and consequences of (anticytokines) infection be initiated quickly to afford the patient the best chance of survival.

ABBREVIATIONS

ACTH	adrenocorticotropic hormone
ATP	adenosine triphosphate
CaMK	calcium–calmodulin-dependent protein kinase
cAMP	cyclic adenosine monophosphate
CaO_2	arterial oxygen content
CI	cardiac index
CO	cardiac output
CO_2	carbon dioxide
Cvo_2	venous oxygen content
CVP	central venous pressure
Do_2	oxygen delivery
Do_2I	oxygen delivery index
ecNOS	constitutive nitric oxide synthase
HR	hazard ratio
ICU	intensive care unit
IL	interleukin
iNOS	inducible nitric oxide synthase
L-NAME	L-arginine-methylester
L-NMMA	monomethyl-L-arginine
LVEF	left ventricular ejection fraction
MAP	mean arterial pressure
NO	nitric oxide
NOS	nitric oxide synthase
O_2ER	oxygen extraction ratio
OR	odds ratio
$Paco_2$	partial pressure of arterial carbon dioxide pressure (tension)
Pao_2	partial pressure of arterial oxygen (tension)
PAOP	pulmonary artery occlusion pressure
Pco_2	gut luminal partial pressure of carbon dioxide
pHi	intramucosal pH
PLC	phospholipase
$Pslco_2$	sublingual carbon dioxide pressure
RR	relative risk
SAFE	Saline vs Albumin Fluid Evaluation
Sao_2	arterial oxygen saturation
$Scvo_2$	central-venous oxygen saturation
Svo_2	mixed-venous oxygen saturation
SVR	systemic vascular resistance
T_3	triiodothyronine
T_4	thyroxine
TNF	tumor necrosis factor
Vo_2	oxygen consumption
Vo_2I	oxygen consumption index

REFERENCES

1. Vincent JL, De Backer D. Circulatory shock. *N Engl J Med* 2013;369:1726-1734.
2. Cecconi M, De Backer D, Antonelli M, et al. Consensus on circulatory shock and hemodynamic monitoring. Task force of the European Society of Intensive Care Medicine. *Intensive Care Med* 2014;40:1795-1815.
3. Shah P, Cowger JA. Cardiogenic shock. *Crit Care Clin* 2014;30:391-412.
4. Patel AK, Hollenberg SM. Cardiovascular failure and cardiogenic shock. *Semin Respir Crit Care Med* 2011;32:598-606.
5. Angus DC, van der Poll T. Severe sepsis and septic shock. *New Engl J Med* 2013;369:840-851.
6. Dellinger RP, Levy MM, Carlet JM, et al. Surviving sepsis campaign: International guidelines for management of severe sepsis and septic shock: 2012. *Crit Care Med* 2013;41:580-637.
7. Seymour CW, Rosengart MR. Septic shock. Advances in diagnosis and treatment. *JAMA* 2015;314:708-717.
8. Hollenberg SM. Vasoactive drugs in circulatory shock. *Am J Respir Crit Care Med* 2011;183:847-855.
9. Bangash MN, Kong ML, Pearse RM. Use of inotropes and vasopressor agents in critically ill patients. *Br J Pharmacol* 2012;165:2015-2033.
10. Martin-Loeches I, Levy MM, Artigas A. Management of severe sepsis: Advances, challenges, and current status. *Drug Des Devel Ther* 2015;9:2079-2088.
11. Marik PE. Early management of severe sepsis. Concepts and controversies. *Chest* 2014;145:1407-1418.
12. Jentzer JC, Coons JC, Link CB, Schmidhofer M. Pharmacotherapy update on the use of vasopressors and inotropes in the intensive care unit. *J Cardiovasc Pharmacol Ther* 2015;20:249-260.
13. Vincent JL, Rhodes A, Perel A, et al. Clinical review: Update on hemodynamic monitoring—a consensus of 16. *Crit Care* 2011;15:229.
14. Holley A, Lukin W, Paratz J, Hawkins T, Boots R, Lipman J. Review article: Part one: Goal-directed resuscitation—which goals? Haemodynamic targets. *Emerg Med Australas* 2012;24:14-22.
15. Holley A, Lukin W, Paratz J, Hawkins T, Boots R, Lipman J. Review article: Part two: Goal-directed resuscitation—which goals? Perfusion targets. *Emerg Med Australas* 2012;24:127-135.
16. Nichols D, Nielsen ND. Oxygen delivery and consumption: A macrocirculatory perspective. *Crit Care Clin* 2010;26:239-253.
17. Maddirala S, Khan A. Optimizing hemodynamic support in septic shock using central and mixed venous oxygen saturation. *Crit Care Clin* 2010;26:323-333.
18. Walley KR. Use of central venous oxygen saturation to guide therapy. *Am J Respir Crit Care Med* 2011;184:514-520.
19. Rivers E, Nguyen B, Havstad S, et al. Early goal-directed therapy in the treatment of severe sepsis and septic shock. *N Engl J Med* 2001;345:1368-1377.
20. Gupta RG, Hartigan SM, Kashiouris MG, Sessler CN, Bearman GM. Early goal-directed resuscitation of patients with septic shock: Current evidence and future directions. *Crit Care* 2015;19:286.
21. Yealy DM, Kellum JA, Huang DT, et al. A randomized trial of protocol-based care for early septic shock. *New Engl J Med* 2014;370:1683-1693.
22. Peake SL, Delaney A, Bailey M, et al. Goal-directed resuscitation for patients with early septic shock. *New Engl J Med* 2014;371:1496-1506.

23. Mouncey PR, Osborn TM, Power GS, et al. Trial of early, goal-directed resuscitation for septic shock. *New Engl J Med* 2015;372:1301-1311.
24. Gu WJ, Wang F, Bakker J, Tang L, Liu JC. The effect of goal-directed therapy on mortality in patients with sepsis—earlier is better: A meta-analysis of randomized controlled trials. *Crit Care* 2014;18:570.
25. Greenberg SB, Murphy GS, Vender JS. Current use of the pulmonary artery catheter. *Curr Opin Crit Care* 2009;15:249-253.
26. Evans DC, Doraiswamy VA, Prosciak MP, et al. Complications associated with pulmonary artery catheters: A comprehensive clinical review. *Scand J Surg* 2009;98:199-208.
27. Practice guidelines for pulmonary artery catheterization: An updated report by the American Society of Anesthesiologists Task Force on Pulmonary Artery Catheterization. *Anesthesiology* 2003;99:988-1014.
28. Joshi R, de Witt B, Mosier JM. Optimizing oxygen delivery in the critically ill: The utility of lactate and central venous oxygen saturation ($ScvO_2$) as a roadmap of resuscitation in shock. *J Emerg Med* 2014;47:493-500.
29. Saugel B, Trepte CJ, Heckel K, Wagner JY, Reuter DA. Hemodynamic management of septic shock: Is it time for "individualized goal-directed hemodynamic therapy" and for specifically targeting the microcirculation? *Shock* 2015;43:522-529.
30. Loiacono LA, Shapiro DS. Detection of hypoxia at the cellular level. *Crit Care Clin* 2010;26:409-421.
31. De Backer D, Ospina-Tascon G, Salgado D, Favory R, Creteur J, Vincent JL. Monitoring the microcirculation in the critically ill patients: Current methods and future approaches. *Intensive Care Med* 2010;36:1813-1825.
32. Holst LB, Haase N, Wetterslev J. Lower versus higher hemoglobin threshold for transfusion in septic shock. *N Engl J Med* 20149;371:1381-1391.
33. Garcia-Alvarez M, Marik P, Bellomo R. Sepsis-associated hyperlactemia. *Crit Care* 2014;18:503.
34. Walley KR, Suetrong B. Lactic acidosis in sepsis: It's not all anaerobic. Implications for diagnosis and management. *Chest* 2015;149(1):252-261.
35. Gu W, Zhang Z, Bakker J. Early lactate clearance-guided therapy in patients with sepsis: A meta-analysis with trial sequential analysis of randomized controlled trials. *Intensive Care Med* 2015;41:1862-1863.
36. Fuller BM, Dellinger RP. Lactate as a hemodynamic marker in the critically ill. *Curr Opin Crit Care* 2012;18:267-272.
37. Jones AE, Shapiro NI, Trzeciak S, et al. Lactate clearance vs. central venous oxygen saturation as goals on early sepsis therapy. A randomized clinical trial. *JAMA* 2010;303:739-746.
38. Jansen TC, van Bommel J, Schoonderbeek J, et al. Early lactate-guided therapy in intensive care unit patients. A multicenter, open-label, randomised controlled trial. *Am J Respir Crit Care Med* 2010;182:752-761.
39. Zanotti-Cavazzoni SL, Hollenberg SM. Cardiac dysfunction in severe sepsis and septic shock. *Curr Opin Crit Care* 2009;15:392-397.
40. Griffee MJ, Merkel MJ, Wei KS. The role of echocardiography in hemodynamic assessment of septic shock. *Crit Care Clin* 2010;26:365-382.
41. Ventetuolo CE, Levy MM. Cardiac biomarkers in critically ill. *Crit Care Clin* 2011;27:327-343.
42. Boerma EC, Ince C. The role of vasoactive agents in the resuscitation of microvascular perfusion and tissue oxygenation in critically ill patients. *Intensive Care Med* 2010;36:2004-2018.
43. Russell JA. Bench-to-bedside review: Vasopressin in the management of septic shock. *Crit Care* 2011;15:226.
44. Russell JA, Fjell C, Hsu JL, et al. Vasopressin compared with norepinephrine augments the decline of plasma cytokine levels in septic shock. *Am J Respir Crit Care Med* 2013;188:356-364.
45. Marik PE, Pastores SM, Annane D, et al. Recommendations for the diagnosis and management of corticosteroid insufficiency in critically ill adult patients: Consensus statements from an international task force by the American College of Critical Care Medicine. *Crit Care Med* 2008;36:1937-1949.
46. Annane D, Sebille V, Troche G, et al. A 3-level prognostic classification in septic shock based on cortisol levels and cortisol response to corticotropin. *JAMA* 2000;283:1038-1045.
47. Annane D, Bellissant E, Bollaert PE, et al. Corticosteroids in the treatment of severe sepsis and septic shock in adults. *JAMA* 2009;301:2362-2375.
48. Annane D, Sébille V, Charpentier C, et al. Effect of treatment with low doses of hydrocortisone and fludrocortisone on mortality in patients with septic shock. *JAMA* 2002;288:862-871.
49. Sprung CL, Annane D, Keh D, et al. Hydrocortisone therapy for patients with septic shock. *N Engl J Med* 2008;358:111-124.
50. De Backer D, Aldecoa C, Nimi H, Vincent JL. Dopamine versus norepinephrine in the treatment of septic shock: A meta-analysis. *Crit Care Med* 2012;40:725-730.
51. Zhou F, Mao Z, Zeng X, et al. Vasopressors in septic shock: A systematic review and network meta-analysis. *Ther Clin Risk Manag* 2015;11:1047-1059.
52. Avni T, Lador A, Lev S, Leibovici L, Paul M, Grossman A. Vasopressors for the treatment of septic shock: Systematic review and meta-analysis. *PLoS One* 2015;10:e0129305.
53. Russell JA, Walley KR, Singer J, et al. Vasopressin versus norepinephrine in patients with septic shock. *N Engl J Med* 2008;358:877-887.
54. Polito A, Parisini E, Ricci Z, Picardo S, Annane D. Vasopressin for treatment of vasodilatory shock: An ESICM systematic review and meta-analysis. *Intensive Care Med* 2012;38:9-19.
55. Gordon AC, Russell JA, Walley KR, et al. The effects of vasopressin on acute kidney injury in septic shock. *Intensive Care Med* 2010;36:83-91.
56. Finfer S, Bellomo R, McEvoy S, et al. A comparison of albumin and saline for fluid resuscitation in the intensive care unit. *N Engl J Med* 2004;350:2247-2256.
57. Annane D, Siami S, Jaber S, et al. Effects of fluid resuscitation with colloids vs crystalloids on mortality in critically ill patients presenting with hypovolemic shock: The CRISTAL randomized trial. *JAMA* 2013;310:1806-1817.
58. Caironi P, Tognoni G, Masson S, et al. Albumin replacement in patients with severe sepsis or septic shock. *N Engl J Med* 2014;370:1412-1421.
59. Xu JY, Chen QH, Xie JF, et al. Comparison of the effects of albumin and crystalloid on mortality in adult patients with severe sepsis and septic shock: A meta-analysis of randomized clinical trials. *Crit Care* 2014;18:702.
60. Rochwerg B, Alhazzani W, Gibson A, et al. Fluid type and the use of renal replacement therapy in sepsis: A systematic review and network meta-analysis. *Intensive Care Med* 2015;41:1561-1571.
61. Patel A, Laffan MA, Waheed U, Brett SJ. Randomised trials of human albumin for adults with sepsis: Systematic review and meta-analysis with trial sequential analysis of all-cause mortality. *BMJ* 2014;349:g4561.
62. Douglas JJ, Walley KR. Fluid choices impact outcome in septic shock. *Curr Opin Crit Care* 2014;20:378-384.
63. Brunkhorst FM, Engel C, Bloos F, et al. Intensive insulin therapy and pentastarch resuscitation in severe sepsis. *N Engl J Med* 2008;358:125-139.
64. Perner A, Hasse N, Guttormsen AB, et al. Hydroxyethyl starch 130/0.42 versus Ringer's acetate in severe sepsis. *N Engl J Med* 2012;367:124-134.
65. Leone M, Asfar P, Radermacher P, Vincent JL, Martin C. Optimizing mean arterial pressure in septic shock: A critical reappraisal of the literature. *Crit Care* 2015;19:101.
66. Asfar P, Meziani F, Hamel JF, et al. High versus low blood-pressure target in patients with septic shock. *N Engl J Med* 2014;370:1583-1593.
67. De Backer D, Biston P, Devriendt J, et al. Comparison of dopamine and norepinephrine in the treatment of shock. *N Engl J Med* 2010;362:779-789.
68. Patel GP, Grahe JS, Sperry M, et al. Efficacy and safety of dopamine versus norepinephrine in the management of septic shock. *Shock* 2010;33:375-380.
69. Myburgh JA, Higgins A, Jovanovska A, et al. A comparison of epinephrine and norepinephrine in critically ill patients. *Intensive Care Med* 2008;34:2226-2234.
70. Annane D, Vignon P, Renault A, et al. Norepinephrine plus dobutamine versus epinephrine alone for the management of septic shock: A randomised trial. *Lancet* 2007;370:678-684.
71. Minneci PC, Deans KJ, Banks SM, et al. Meta-analysis: The effect of steroids on survival and shock during sepsis depends on the dose. *Ann Intern Med* 2004;141:47-56.
72. Volbeda M, Wetterslev J, Gluud C, Zijlstra JG, van der Horst IC, Keus F. Glucocorticosteroids for sepsis: Systematic review with meta-analysis and trial sequential analysis. *Intensive Care Med* 2015;41:1220-1234.
73. Wang C, Sun J, Zheng J, et al. Low-dose hydrocortisone therapy attenuates septic shock in adult patients but does not reduce 28-day mortality: A meta-analysis of randomized controlled trials. *Anesth Analg* 2014;118:346-357.
74. Russell JA, Walley KR, Gordon AC, et al. Interaction of vasopressin infusion, corticosteroid treatment, and mortality of septic shock. *Crit Care Med* 2009;37:811-818.
75. Bellomo R, Chapman M, Finfer S, et al. Low-dose dopamine in patients with early renal dysfunction: A placebo-controlled randomized trial. Australian and New Zealand Intensive Care Society (ANZICS) Clinical Trials Group. *Lancet* 2000;356:2139-2143.

76. Friedrich JO, Adhikari N, Herridge MS, et al. Meta-analysis: Low-dose dopamine increases urine output but does not prevent renal dysfunction or death. *Ann Intern Med* 2005;142:510-524.
77. Suffredini AF, Munford RS. Novel therapies for septic shock over the past 4 decades. *JAMA* 2011;306:194-199.
78. Sharawy N, Lehmann C. New directions for sepsis and septic shock. *J Surg Res* 2015;194:520-527.
79. Lopez A, Lorente JA, Steingrub J, et al. Multiple-center, randomized, placebo-controlled, double-blind study of the nitric oxide synthase inhibitor 546C88: Effect on survival in patients with septic shock. *Crit Care Med* 2004;32:21-30.
80. Kinasewitz GT. Privalle CT, Imm A, et al. Multicenter, randomized, placebo-controlled study of the nitric oxide scavenger pyridoxalated hemoglobin polyoxyethylene in distributive shock. *Crit Care Med* 2008;36:1999-2007.
81. Vincent JL, Marshall JC, Dellinger RP, et al. Talactoferrin in Severe Sepsis: Results From the Phase II/III Oral tAlactoferrin in Severe sepsIS Trial. *Crit Care Med* 2015;43:1832-1838.
82. Paciullo CA, McMahon Horner D, Hatton KW, Flynn JD. Methylene blue for the treatment of septic shock. *Pharmacotherapy* 2010;30:702-715.
83. Pierrakos C, Velissaris D, Franchi F, Muzzi L, Karanikolas M, Scolletta S. Levosimendan in critical illness: A literature review. *Clin Med Res* 2014;6:75-85.
84. Zangrillo A, Putzu A, Monaco F, et al. Levosimendan reduces mortality in patients with severe sepsis and septic shock: A meta-analysis of randomized trials. *J Crit Care* 2015;30(5):908-913.
85. Sanfilippo F, Santonocito C, Morelli A, Foex P. Beta-blocker use in severe sepsis and septic shock: A systematic review. *Curr Med Res Opin* 2015;31:1817-1825.
86. Morelli A, Ertmer C, Westphal M, et al. Effect of heart rate control with esmolol on hemodynamic and clinical outcomes in patients with septic shock: A randomized clinical trial. *JAMA* 2013;310:1683-1691.
87. Angelousi AG, Karageorgopoulos DE, Kapaskelis AM, Falagas ME. Association between thyroid function tests at baseline and the outcome of patients with sepsis or septic shock: A systematic review. *Eur J Endocrinol* 2011;164:147-155.

24

Hypovolemic Shock

Brian L. Erstad

KEY CONCEPTS

1. Plasma does not have to be lost from the body for hypovolemic shock to occur.
2. Patients may die of hypovolemic shock despite having normal serum electrolyte concentrations.
3. Although the Starling's equation of fluid transport is useful for understanding the factors involved in fluid shifting between compartments, it is not a practical tool for use in the clinical setting.
4. Patients may have complications and death as a result of reperfusion injury as well as the initial insult.
5. The clinical presentation of patients with hypovolemic shock can vary substantially, depending on concomitant disease states, medications, and cause of hypovolemia.
6. The initial monitoring of a patient with suspected intravascular depletion always should include vital signs, urine output, mental status, and physical examination.
7. The need for intravenous (IV) (vs oral) rehydration in children often is overestimated.
8. Crystalloid (sodium-containing) solutions should be used for most forms of circulatory insufficiency that are associated with hemodynamic instability.
9. Neither crystalloids nor colloids have the oxygen-carrying properties of red blood cells.
10. Vasoactive medications should not be considered for hypovolemic shock until fluid resuscitation has been optimized.

INTRODUCTION

This chapter discusses the assessment and management of hypovolemic shock. Other forms of shock such as obstructive (eg, cardiac tamponade), distributive (eg, spinal cord injury, septic or anaphylactic shock), and left ventricular dysfunction (eg, myocardial infarction, arrhythmia) often are considered separately from hypovolemic shock because fluid loss from the body is not necessary for their occurrence. Although these forms of shock are not discussed in detail, it is important to note that intravenous (IV) fluid administration (in conjunction with vasoactive medications) is a mainstay of therapy because circulating volume is decreased. In this regard, adequate fluid resuscitation to maintain circulating blood volume is a common principle in managing all forms of shock.

EPIDEMIOLOGY

Because shock is not a reportable category by state and federal agencies that track causes of death, the incidence is unknown. Estimates of deaths due to shock are complicated by differences in definitions and classification systems. Part of the problem is defining when progressive circulatory insufficiency results in the loss of normal compensatory responses by the body, which could reverse the processes leading to irreversible organ dysfunction. This loss of appropriate compensation varies from patient to patient and is not always readily apparent during the initial patient presentation. Therefore, forms of hypovolemic shock, such as hemorrhagic shock, are subsumed by more readily identifiable categories of death, such as accidental injuries and homicides. Crude and conservative estimates of death due to hypovolemic shock are available for some of its forms. More than 39 deaths per 100,000 standard population occur each year in the United States due to unintentional injuries that frequently involve bleeding,[1] and more than 600 deaths each year are due to natural heat-related illness.[2] The figures are much higher when considered on a global basis. For example, electrolyte depletion and dehydration due to diarrheal disease result in approximately 2 million deaths each year in children younger than 5 years.[3] The most liberal estimates of death include all causes of circulatory failure (ie, the last stage of shock).

ETIOLOGY

1 Hypovolemic shock is extracellular volume depletion that may result from blood loss (plasma and red blood cells) due to trauma, surgery, or internal hemorrhage or from plasma loss due to fluid sequestered within the body or lost from the body (Table 24-1). In some cases, such as in postoperative patients, a number of these problems occur at the same time. For example, a patient may have blood loss secondary to trauma or surgery, with additional fluid being third spaced (eg, as tissue edema in the gastrointestinal [GI] tract with a concomitant ileus) and lost through a high-output GI fistula postoperatively. As this example of third-spaced fluid indicates, fluid (ie, plasma) does not have to be lost from the body for a person to develop hypovolemic shock, although the fistula output would clearly aggravate the situation. Approximately 10 L of fluid is secreted and reabsorbed daily in the GI tract; so, it is not surprising that volume loss could be substantial depending on the location of the fistula and function of the tract preceding the fistula.

The term dehydration implies primary intracellular water depletion, in contrast to volume depletion, which implies extracellular, and particularly intravascular, sodium and water loss. However, there is substantial overlap in the definitions and use of terms such as dehydration and volume depletion in the medical literature, so the reader must be cognizant of the intended meaning. Dehydration may result from primary water deficiency, usually because of decreased intake, but in some instances (eg, diabetes insipidus) it may result from increased losses of water. With most forms of dehydration, such as those caused by diarrheal disease and heat-related illness, a combination of inadequate intake and higher than normal losses occurs. Initially with intracellular water depletion, the patient may be thirsty and possibly have some mental status changes, such as confusion. If cellular dehydration occurs slowly, intracellular substances, referred

TABLE 24-1 Causes of Hypovolemic Shock[a]

Decreased blood (plasma + red blood cells) volume
- External: Surgery or trauma
- Internal (eg, cerebral, chest, GI and other abdominal sources, long bone fractures, and retroperitoneum)

Decreased plasma volume
- External: Losses from urine, GI tract (eg, vomiting, nasogastric suctioning, fistula, and diarrhea), lungs, or skin (including thermal injury)
- Internal (decreased oncotic pressure or increased capillary permeability): fluid accumulation in bowel, peritoneal or pleural cavities

GI, gastrointestinal.

[a]Shock may result from various combinations of blood and plasma volume losses listed (ie, causes are not mutually exclusive).

to as *idiogenic osmoles,* develop that limit progressive complications (eg, cerebral edema or coma). Death due to primary water deficit, if it occurs, is usually a result of delayed circulatory failure. With combined water and salt deficiencies, such as might occur with GI (eg, diarrhea) and skin losses (eg, heat stroke), interstitial and intravascular depletion is an early occurrence. Fortunately, dehydration is relatively easy to prevent with routine vigilance and water replacement compared with some of the other causes of shock.

PATHOPHYSIOLOGY

2 Hypovolemic shock often is described in terms of monitoring parameters such as lowered blood pressure, but patients with shock may die despite normal surrogate markers of circulatory insufficiency. Therefore, an appropriate definition should mention the underlying problem, which is inadequate tissue perfusion resulting from circulatory failure. In the case of hypovolemic shock, the cause of the altered perfusion is fluid (or volume) depletion resulting from trauma, surgery, thermal injury, or some form of dehydration. Figure 24-1 provides a simplified view of the pathophysiology of circulatory insufficiency assuming the acute insult causing the plasma volume depletion did not result in immediate patient death. Cell damage and death may occur from the primary insult or from reperfusion injury. The latter problem is associated most frequently with trauma and blood loss that cause a systemic inflammatory response syndrome (SIRS) with the release of a multitude of mediators of inflammation and injury that have complex interactions. Cells have varying responses to hypoxia, ranging from astrocytes that quit functioning almost immediately to other cells that may tolerate more prolonged periods of hypoperfusion. Left unmitigated, cell death occurs with prolonged injury and is usually heralded by acidosis, hypothermia, and coagulopathy—referred to as the *lethal triad.*

The body attempts to compensate for volume depletion beginning with autoregulatory changes involving smaller blood vessels. When the cause of circulatory insufficiency continues unabated, local mechanisms eventually fail to provide adequate compensation, and macrocirculatory changes ensue. The majority of blood volume is contained in venous capacitance vessels, with gravity being the major impedance to flow back to the heart. With increasing volume depletion, blood flow to the heart (preload) is decreased, with subsequent activation of baroreceptors and chemoreceptors leading to sympathetic discharge. Also, fluid shifting from the interstitial space

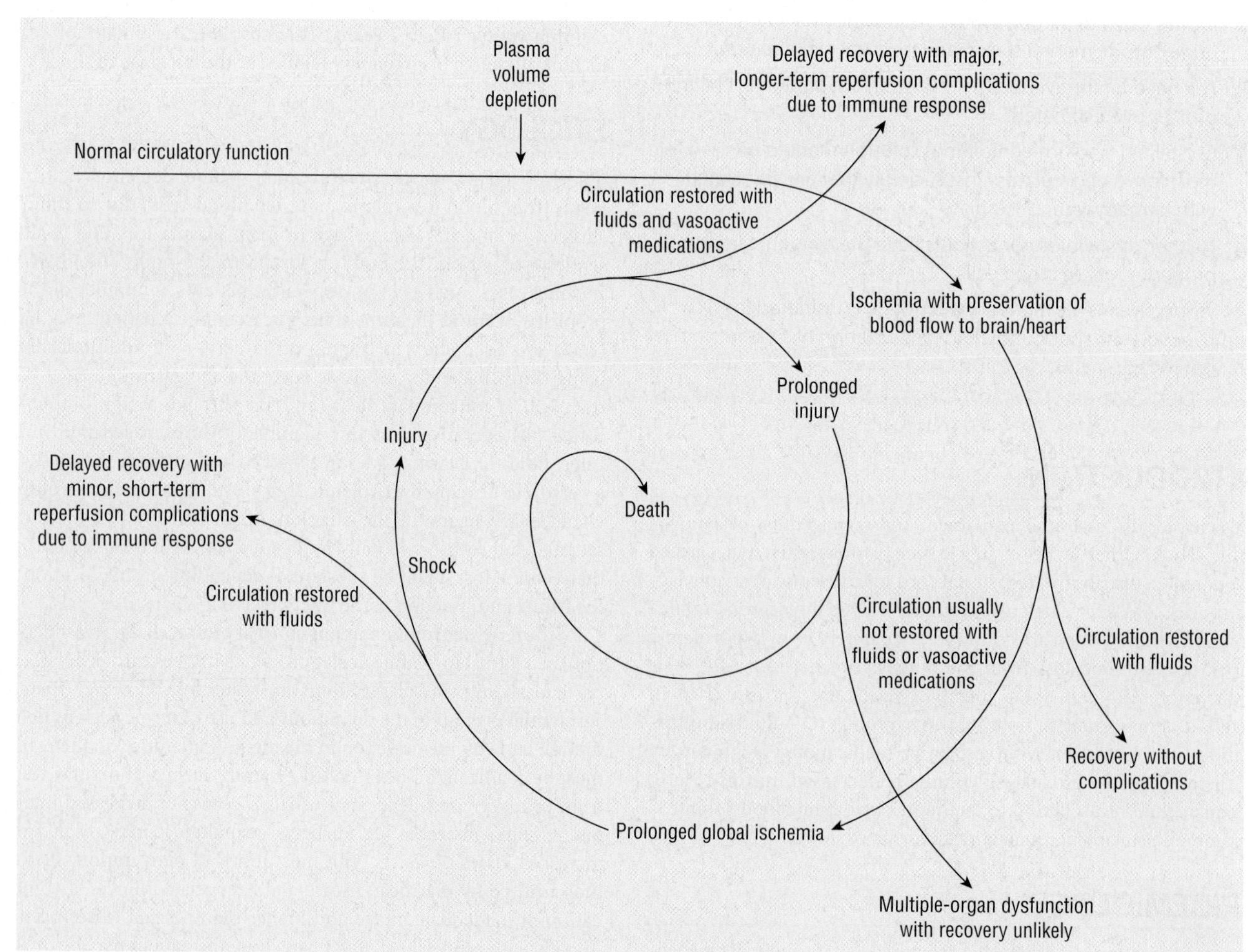

FIGURE 24-1 Pathophysiology of circulatory insufficiency and failure (shock).

to the intravascular space occurs through a phenomenon known as *transcapillary refill*, and hormones (eg, adrenocorticotropic hormone, angiotensin, catecholamines, and vasopressin) that cause sodium and water retention by the kidneys are released. The phenomenon of transcapillary refill means that the body can have fluid losses exceeding normal plasma volume. These responses cause alterations in stroke volume, heart rate, and peripheral vascular resistance so that blood pressure and hence tissue perfusion can be maintained.

The microcirculatory changes associated with shock are complex and difficult to study. Although some mediators such as catecholamines, angiotensin II, arginine vasopressin, and endothelin-1 cause vasoconstriction, other mediators, such as adenosine and nitric oxide, yield vasodilation. These changes result in hypoperfusion or hyperperfusion, depending on the organs involved. As these microcirculatory changes fail to maintain adequate organ perfusion, more widespread sympathetic nervous system activation and vasoconstriction ensue. Even assuming general circulation is restored, capillaries may not function properly due to ongoing edema and ischemia. Failure to respond to sympathetic stimulation and fluid administration is indicative of the vasodilation that occurs in the final phase of circulatory failure leading to death.

The factors involved in fluid shifting between the intravascular and interstitial spaces are described by the modified Starling's equation:

$$J_v = K_{f,c}[(P_c - P_t) - [\sigma(\pi_{esl} - \pi_t)]]$$

where J_V is the net transvascular flow rate (cannot be measured in the clinical setting), $K_{f,c}$ is the capillary filtration coefficient for fluids (cannot be measured in the clinical setting), P_c is the capillary hydrostatic pressure (indirectly estimated in the clinical setting, eg, pulmonary artery occlusive pressure), P_t is the tissue or interstitial hydrostatic pressure (cannot be measured in the clinical setting), σ is the reflection coefficient for proteins (cannot be measured in the clinical setting), π_{esl} is the oncotic pressure in the endothelial surface layer (not usually measured in the clinical setting, but technology is available), and π_t is the oncotic pressure below the endothelial surface layer that determines the tissue or interstitial oncotic pressure (cannot be measured in the clinical setting).

Proteins act as oncotic agents in each of these spaces to attract fluid, whereas hydrostatic forces push fluid into or out of the vessels. The equation has distinct permeability values for water and protein because each crosses the vascular membrane at a different rate. The values for the variables listed in the equation are not the same for capillaries in all parts of the body. For example, on a scale from 0 to 1 with 0 being free passage of protein and 1 being impermeable to protein, the typical value for the reflection coefficient in most capillaries is more than 0.9. Capillaries in the central nervous system and glomeruli have coefficients near 1 so in the absence of disease states minimal protein transport occurs. However, in the pulmonary capillaries the value is closer to 0.7 and approaches 0 in inflammatory states associated with increased capillary permeability.[4] As the value approaches 0, the capillaries are freely permeable not only to the usual fluid and electrolytes but also to plasma proteins such as albumin. Because albumin accounts for approximately 80% of the plasma oncotic pressure, its free passage into the interstitial space effectively negates its intravascular oncotic benefit. 3 Although the Starling's equation is useful to practitioners in terms of understanding the factors involved in fluid shifting between compartments, the rate and direction of transvascular flow cannot be calculated accurately in the clinical setting because most factors cannot be measured directly and the values for the factors vary in different capillaries in the body.

The body's compensatory mechanisms may have beneficial and harmful consequences. For example, cardiac output can be increased substantially by increases in stroke volume or heart rate. Although this may be useful for providing blood flow to inadequately perfused tissues, it may cause large increases in oxygen consumption by the heart that could aggravate preexisting ischemia in patients with underlying coronary artery disease (CAD). Another example is the sympathetic nervous system–mediated vasoconstriction that causes blood to shift from the skin, skeletal muscle, and some internal organs such as the kidneys and GI tract to organs (eg, heart and brain) that are less tolerant of inadequate flow. If the vasoconstriction continues unabated, the hypoperfused organs eventually become damaged. Figure 24-2 provides an overview of the compensatory changes that occur with a loss of circulating blood volume.

4 In addition to the more acute implications of hypovolemia and attendant complications, reperfusion damage is likely to occur, particularly after prolonged resuscitation attempts. In addition to edematous obstruction of capillaries and oxygen-free radical damage of cell membranes, a number of cellular (eg, white blood cells and platelets) and humoral (eg, procoagulants, anticoagulants, complement, and kinins) components are activated, causing the release of other inflammatory mediators. The resulting reperfusion injury may range from readily reversible organ dysfunction to multiple-organ failure and death. The lungs are frequently the first system affected either by excessive fluid resuscitation or by the mediators of secondary reperfusion injury. The latter form of injury often results in the acute respiratory distress syndrome that is defined by an arterial oxygen tension-to-fraction of inspired oxygen ratio of less than or equal to 300 (with additional subdivisions of mild, moderate, and severe) with bilateral lung opacities in the absence of hypervolemia.

Although the basic pathophysiology is similar for the various causes of hypovolemic shock, there are unique considerations relative to each. For example, whereas isolated head injuries associated with trauma typically do not result in substantial blood loss or shock, long bone or pelvic fractures may sequester several liters of blood. Patients with traumatic or thermal injuries, as well as postoperative patients, may have substantial fluid accumulation in sites where the fluid cannot be readily transferred back into blood vessels (ie, third-spaced fluid) for maintaining pressure. With these types of injuries, prompt control of compressible bleeding sources with rapid patient transfer to the hospital for definitive treatment may preclude the cascade of events leading to shock. Indeed, with trauma patients, a "scoop and run" approach that places a priority on rapid transport to a hospital is used by most urban hospitals.

In the case of hemorrhagic shock, prompt attention must be given to cellular as well as plasma losses. Red blood cells lost during the bleeding episode may lead to ischemic damage in vital organs. Packed red blood cell transfusions may be needed to increase the oxygen-carrying capacity of the blood because oxygen transport is a function not only of cardiac output but also of hemoglobin concentration and saturation and of hemoglobin affinity for oxygen. Once hemostasis has been achieved, a more restrictive transfusion strategy (ie, transfusion if hemoglobin less than 7 g/dL [less than 70 g/L; 4.34 mmol/L]) is indicated for the majority of patients without severe cardiovascular disease (see Trauma/Perioperative Patients below).

Clotting factors and platelets are also lost in hemorrhage. The resulting bleeding problems may be aggravated by the dilutional effect of fluid resuscitation on clotting factor activity. Fresh-frozen plasma that contains necessary clotting factors and platelets is needed in massive blood loss to restore adequate coagulation. On the other hand, trauma patients are at increased risk for deep vein thrombosis and pulmonary embolism caused by multiple factors, including vessel damage, abnormal blood flow patterns,

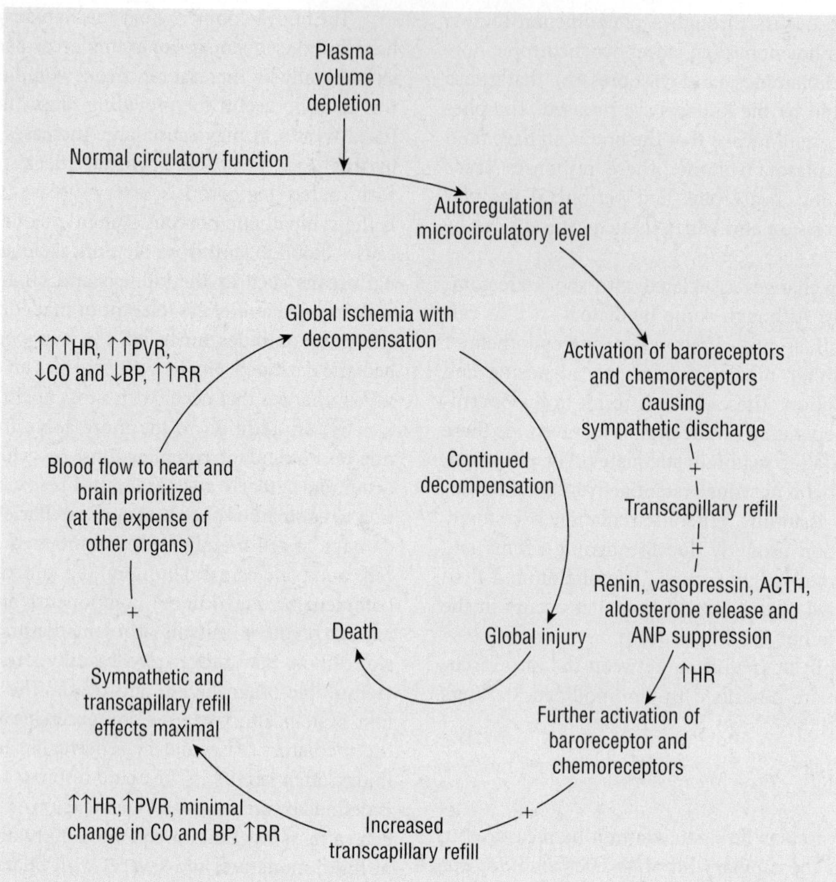

FIGURE 24-2 Activation of compensatory mechanisms with loss of circulatory volume. Certain stages may be absent, depending on a number of factors, such as age, preexisting disease states, and cause of circulatory insufficiency. (ACTH, adrenocorticotropin; ANP, atrial natriuretic peptide; BP, blood pressure; CO, cardiac output; HR, heart rate; PVR, peripheral vascular resistance; RR, respiratory rate.)

and the hypercoagulable state associated with injury. Therefore, some form of venous thromboembolism prophylaxis usually is indicated in multiple-trauma patients or patients with severe single-system injuries (eg, spinal cord damage) once hemostasis of major injury-related bleeding has been achieved.

The pathophysiology becomes more complicated if the severity of shock is sufficient to require patient admission to the intensive care unit (ICU) after initial resuscitation or surgery. Most patients admitted to the ICU have SIRS, which is the body's response to injury. This syndrome is defined by a number of hypermetabolic changes reflected in the patient's temperature, white blood cell count and differential, and respiratory and heart rates. The stress response involves complex interactions between the nervous system and immunomodulating substances and has similar (if not the same) harmful and helpful consequences described with reperfusion following shock. If the underlying problems are left untreated, the patient with SIRS may develop multiple-organ dysfunction syndrome (MODS) during the final stages of illness.

CLINICAL PRESENTATION

5 The initial presentation of patients with suspected volume depletion can vary markedly, depending on factors such as age, concomitant disease states and medications, and the etiology and rapidity of depletion (see Clinical Presentation of Hypovolemic Shock box). Intravascular depletion as a consequence of blood loss is signified by postural vital sign changes (ie, changes in pulse and blood pressure between supine, sitting, and standing measurements), and such measurements should be performed unless the diagnosis is obvious, as in the case of bleeding associated with trauma. Early signs and symptoms of dehydration and intravascular depletion caused by GI or urinary losses often are relatively nonspecific. Plasma volume losses of less than 10 mL/kg of body weight usually are associated with minor signs and symptoms of distress. Larger losses are not likely to be well tolerated (Table 24-2), particularly in patients older than 65 years. An 18-year-old athlete and a 65-year-old sedentary individual are likely to have much different responses to a similar amount of fluid loss. The young patient may lose one-fourth of his or her circulating blood volume with minimal changes in arterial blood pressure and a relatively low heart rate. However, the elderly patient may have orthostatic changes in blood pressure that are not well tolerated by organs such as the kidneys. Unfortunately, this same elderly patient may not have common signs and symptoms of volume depletion, such as skin turgor changes or thirst, but instead may have more subtle changes (eg, mental status alterations).

The diagnosis of dehydration and intravascular depletion in children is complicated by difficulties in obtaining an accurate history. However, some excellent resources are available for healthcare providers, such as the Centers for Disease Control and Prevention (CDC) guidelines (*www.cdc.gov*), which discuss the evaluation and management of diarrhea in patients of all ages. In younger children, parental observations are important for estimating fluid deficits and deciding whether hospitalization is necessary. Fortunately, prospective data suggest that parental histories are predictive of acidosis and the need for hospitalization.[5] 6 Regardless of patient age or preexisting conditions, the initial monitoring of a patient with suspected volume depletion should include the following noninvasive

TABLE 24-2 Acute Circulatory Insufficiency: Initial Presentation and Therapy[a]

	Mild	Severe
Plasma/blood loss	Adult: 10 mL/kg Child: 20 mL/kg	Adult: 30 mL/kg Child: 35 mL/kg
Mental status/level of consciousness	None to small changes (eg, anxious, irritable)	Marked changes (eg, confusion to unconsciousness)
Vital signs/orthostatic changes	Minor changes	Marked changes
Therapy	20 mL/kg lactated Ringer or normal saline IV[a] over 10-15 minutes Unlikely to need blood cell replacement even if hemorrhagic loss	Lactated Ringer or normal saline IV as rapidly as possible until response in adult, and then decrease rate of infusion 20 mL/kg lactated Ringer or normal saline IV in child (repeat quickly if minimal response); likely to need blood cell replacement and surgery if hemorrhagic

[a]Patients may have intermediate degrees of volume loss in addition to those listed, but the amount of loss often is difficult to quantify. The presentations may also vary greatly in patients with similar amounts of loss (young athlete vs sedentary, elderly person). In patients particularly prone to complications associated with fluid overload, the fluid can be administered in multiple smaller boluses titrated to clinical response. See text for a more in-depth discussion of some of the guidelines in this table.

parameters: vital signs, urine output, mental status, and physical examination (Fig. 24-3). An increase in blood pressure with passive leg raising may also be useful for the assessment of suspected hypovolemia, but should not be used to guide responsiveness to fluid administration.

Although the presenting signs and symptoms of circulatory insufficiency are variable, patients usually have decreased blood pressure, increased heart and respiratory rates, and a normal or low–normal temperature (eg, 36°C-37°C [96.8°F-98.6°F]) in the absence of infection, exposure to extremes of temperature, and medications that impair thermoregulation. As mentioned earlier, recordings of vital signs must be interpreted in light of known or suspected baseline conditions. For example, alcohol, β-blockers, diuretics, and medications with anticholinergic effects may impair thermoregulation. Medications such as β-blockers and calcium channel blockers may alter resting blood pressure and heart rate, as well as the subsequent response to therapeutic interventions.

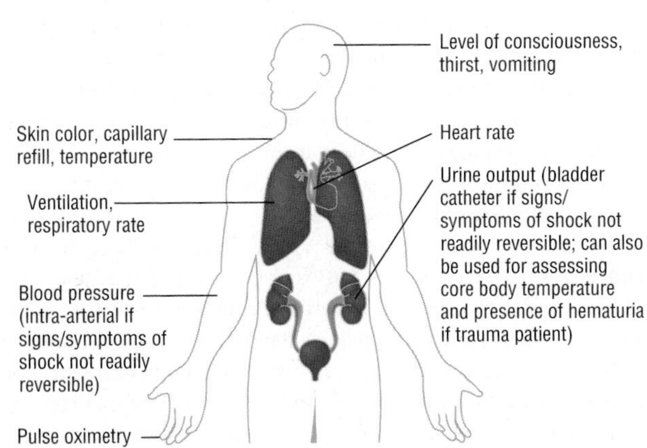

FIGURE 24-3 Noninvasive assessment of circulatory insufficiency.

Although a blood pressure reading of 110/70 mm Hg (systolic/diastolic) may be acceptable in many patients, it may be inadequate in a patient with preexisting hypertension who normally has a blood pressure of 170/105 mm Hg. At the other extreme, patients with very low blood pressure may have inaudible or inaccurate determinations with cuff (sphygmomanometric) measurements. Chapters e11 and 13 detail blood pressure measurement (eg, cuff size, position). In this case, intra-arterial monitoring is indicated. The respiratory rate may be elevated because of anxiety or as a compensatory mechanism for the metabolic acidosis caused by lactic acidosis associated with poor tissue perfusion.

Although the kidneys continually produce urine, the bladder stores the urine for intermittent elimination. For the initial diagnosis and management of acute circulatory insufficiency, a catheter can be inserted into the bladder for measuring urine output. In contrast to thirst, which is a relatively insensitive indicator of volume depletion, urine output is generally diminished with inadequate fluid administration and increases with appropriate resuscitation. This presumes, of course, that acute renal failure or medications such as diuretics are not altering the expected response. Adults should produce at least 0.5 to 1 mL/kg/h of urine, whereas children up to 12 years should produce at least 1 mL/kg/h (2 mL/kg/h if younger than 1 year).

Mental status changes associated with volume depletion, if present, may range from subtle fluctuations in mood to unconsciousness. Although the latter finding typically is indicative of more severe depletion, less dramatic findings should not be interpreted as indicating mild fluid deficits. Losses of 3 to 4 L of plasma volume may be associated only with lassitude in an otherwise healthy adult patient. Similar interpretation difficulties must be considered when performing the initial physical examination. An orderly progression from warm, reddish skin with appropriate capillary refill (rapid return of blood flow to the extremity after removal of compression) to cold, cyanotic discoloration with impaired refill may not occur. Also, dry mucous membranes in elderly patients may be caused by mouth breathing or medications and not by fluid depletion.

TREATMENT

Milder forms of volume depletion may be managed in outpatient settings. For example, supplemental fluids can be added to the usual estimated daily requirements of 30 to 35 mL/kg in patients older than 12 years with dehydration. Commercially available carbohydrate/electrolyte drinks generally are more palatable than water and may promote earlier recovery. The rationale for combining carbohydrates with sodium is based on the cotransport absorption mechanism in the intestinal tract. With diarrheal states in particular, sodium absorption is impaired. Because water follows sodium, the diarrhea is likely to continue despite oral crystalloid fluid administration until the intestinal pathology resolves. However, when dextrose and sodium are combined in 1:1 equimolar amounts, both are absorbed via the cotransport mechanism, which also allows for absorption of water. This concept forms the basis for the World Health Organization's (WHO) oral rehydration solution, which contains 75 mmol/L of dextrose, 75 mmol/L of sodium, 20 mmol/L of potassium, 65 mmol/L of chloride, and 10 mmol/L of citrate for a total osmolarity of 245 mOsm/L.[3] Commercially available nonprescription rehydration drinks for children in the United States also have an osmolarity of approximately 250 mOsm/L but typically contain 50 mmol/L or less of sodium, and the dextrose-to-sodium ratio often is 3:1. How these differences between commercially available formulations and the WHO rehydration formula might affect hospitalization rates is unclear, but ad hoc attempts to alter the commercially available products to make them more consistent with the WHO formula may be dangerous and are not recommended.

CLINICAL PRESENTATION Hypovolemic Shock

General

- The initial presentation of adult patients with suspected volume depletion could vary markedly, depending on factors such as age, concomitant disease states and medications, and the etiology and rapidity of depletion.
- Plasma volume losses of less than 10 mL/kg of body weight usually are associated with minor signs and symptoms of distress.

Symptoms

- Patients may present with thirst, nausea, anxiousness, weakness, light-headedness, and dizziness.
- Patients may report scanty urine output and dark yellow urine.

Signs

With more severe volume loss:

- Patients would have marked increases in heart rate (eg, greater than 120 beats/min) and respiratory rate (eg, greater than 30 breaths/min).
- Blood pressure would be decreased (eg, systolic blood pressure less than 90 mm Hg).
- Mental status changes or unconsciousness may occur.
- Agitation may be present if the patient is conscious.
- Body temperature would be low or normal (eg, 36°C-37°C [96.8°F-98.6°F]) in the absence of concomitant infection with cold extremities and decreased capillary refill on physical examination.

Laboratory Tests

- Sodium and chloride concentrations usually are high with acute depletion but may be low or normal depending on type of fluid intake.
- The ratio of blood urea nitrogen (BUN) to creatinine is likely to be elevated initially, but the creatinine level would increase as renal dysfunction occurs.
- Elevated base deficit and lactate concentrations in conjunction with decreased bicarbonate concentrations and pH due to metabolic acidosis.
- The complete blood count should be normal in the absence of concomitant disease states such as infection; in hemorrhagic shock, the red cell count, hemoglobin, and hematocrit would decrease over time, while the prothrombin time (PT) and international normalized ratio would increase.
- With more severe volume depletion, other organs may become dysfunctional, which may be reflected in laboratory testing (eg, elevated transaminase levels with hepatic dysfunction).

Other Diagnostic Tests

- Urine output would be decreased to less than 0.5 to 1 mL/h.

Outpatient rehydration of children usually is recommended for those with uncomplicated (eg, vomiting less than 48 hours) acute gastroenteritis and relatively mild dehydration after the exclusion of more severe illnesses such as bowel obstruction. (7) The need for IV rehydration often is overestimated. Randomized studies conducted in pediatric emergency departments have found oral or nasogastric rehydration to be at least as effective as IV rehydration using end points such as length of stay and need for hospital admission.[6,7] While dehydration is primarily a problem of intracellular fluid depletion, ongoing losses will result in extracellular fluid depletion as well. The remainder of this chapter will focus on more severe forms of volume depletion (ie, hypovolemic shock) that are not amenable to oral rehydration.

Desired Outcome

Reduce morbidity and mortality by preventing disease progression with subsequent organ damage.

To the extent possible, reverse organ dysfunction that has already taken place.

General Approach to Treatment

Hospitalization is indicated for more severe forms of circulatory insufficiency. If access to the circulatory system for administration of fluids and medication is not obtained prior to hospitalization, this should be a priority. Venous access generally is obtained during the preliminary examination process that includes the ABCs of life support (ie, airway, breathing, and circulation), assessment of vital signs and mental status, and determination of urine output after catheterization. Whenever large-volume fluid resuscitation is expected, as in hemorrhagic shock, at least two IV catheters are desirable. Because flow is a function of tubing length and catheter diameter, large-bore peripheral IV lines are preferred over longer central lines. Unfortunately, vascular access in some patients may be problematic, and other routes such as intraosseous infusion may be necessary. Prior to the past decade, use of intraosseous fluid and drug administration in the United States was mostly restricted to children with IV access issues, but it is increasingly being used in adult patients as well. One interesting method of fluid administration that has been investigated in elderly patients is subcutaneous infusion, or hypodermoclysis. With hypodermoclysis, common dextrose- and sodium-containing fluids typically given by the IV route are given by subcutaneous infusion at sites such as the upper arm, chest, abdomen, or thigh, depending on factors such as patient or provider preference. Hyaluronidase has been used as a spreading agent to facilitate fluid absorption by this route, but its benefit versus risk profile has yet to be clearly elucidated; in particular, allergic reactions with this agent have been a concern, although a recombinant form is now available that has the potential for fewer reactions compared with the older bovine-derived products. Hypodermoclysis is not used commonly in the United States, probably because of concerns of adverse effects that were found in early studies that used excessively hypotonic or hypertonic solutions, as well as issues related to reimbursement when considered in ambulatory, home, or palliative care settings. Although relatively high fluid administration rates have been achieved in some studies involving hypodermoclysis, this method of infusion should not be used in patients with more severe forms of dehydration or hypovolemia until additional supportive information from clinical trials is available. Although alternative methods of fluid administration, such as hypodermoclysis, are desirable, well-conducted trials are needed before such methods can be recommended for routine use.

After the immediate postresuscitation phase of the treatment of hypovolemic shock, proper attention must be paid to general supportive care measures that include appropriate assessment and management of pain, anxiety/agitation, and delirium. This is particularly true for patients who develop shock after trauma, surgery, or thermal injury and require admission to an ICU.

Nonpharmacologic Therapy

Nonpharmacologic therapy for shock is dependent on the inciting event, although the basic life support measures such as a secure airway with appropriate oxygenation apply to all patients. For patients with more severe traumatic injury, additional measures would include surgery, stabilization of fractures, control of blood loss by physical compression or surgical control, and prevention of heat loss since hypothermia may aggravate other problems such as bleeding. For patients with heat exposure, cooling measures are indicated. Patients with thermal injuries should have the wound sites covered with cool, moist sterile dressings until more definitive care can take place.

Pharmacologic Therapy

Since IV fluids are the primary therapy for hypovolemic shock, they will be considered pharmacologic agents for this discussion.

Drug Treatments of First Choice

8 Dextrose-in-water solutions may be appropriate for uncomplicated dehydration caused by water deprivation, but isotonic crystalloid (sodium-containing) solutions should be used for forms of circulatory insufficiency that are associated with hemodynamic instability. In the latter situation, IV solutions with sodium concentrations approximating normal serum sodium values usually are indicated because they cause more expansion of the intravascular and interstitial spaces compared with dextrose solutions (Table 24-3). Lactated Ringer and normal saline solutions are examples of such crystalloid solutions that frequently need to be administered in large volumes when given to patients with more severe forms of hypovolemia. A "large" amount of fluid does not mean a single bolus volume typically used as fluid challenge in a critically ill patient. An isolated bolus (eg, 250-500 mL) in a young adult trauma patient is unlikely to cause a substantial change in blood pressure or acid–base balance.[8] Therefore, multiple fluid boluses usually are often needed in such patients to achieve hemodynamic stability in the perioperative period. On the other hand, overly aggressive fluid administration should be avoided, especially in patients with heart failure or impending pulmonary edema. In a randomized trial involving patients with acute lung injury and radiographic presence of pulmonary edema, a more conservative fluid management strategy beginning postresuscitation (~40 hours after admission in the study) led to significantly fewer ventilator-free days and days not spent in an ICU (P less than 0.001).[9]

Published Guidelines or Treatment Protocols Recommendations for shock associated with trauma have been published as part of the Advanced Trauma Life Support (ATLS) course (http://www.facs.org/trauma/atls/).[10] In the past, the ATLS guidelines were derived more from consensus of expert participants than evidence, but this has changed in more recent revisions. Guidelines for prehospital fluid administration in patients with trauma have been published by the Eastern Association for the Surgery of Trauma (EAST).[11] Other evidence relative to fluid choice for resuscitation is available from systematic reviews,[12-14] a guideline for perioperative fluid resuscitation,[15] and a guideline pertaining to burn shock resuscitation.[16] Taken as a whole, the recommendations from all of these sources are consistent in that isotonic (or near isotonic) crystalloid solutions are the initial fluid of choice for resuscitation in hypovolemic shock (Table 24-4).

General Information Reporting Efficacy and Safety The choice between normal saline and lactated Ringer solutions for hypovolemia is largely based on clinician preference and adverse effect concerns (Table 24-5). Lactated Ringer solution has been recommended for patients with hemorrhage because it is unlikely to cause the hyperchloremic metabolic acidosis and possibly acute kidney injury due to excess chloride administration that is seen with infusions of large volumes of normal saline. But concerns have been raised relative to the proinflammatory effects (eg, neutrophil activation) of the D-isomer form of lactate that is contained along with the L-isomer in commercially available racemic isomer solutions. There are advocates for the use of lactated Ringer solution containing only L-isomer lactate, particularly for more severe forms of hemorrhagic shock, since it avoids the proinflammatory effects of the racemic solution, while avoiding the hyperchloremia associated with normal saline.[17] Additionally, other substitutes for racemic lactate such as ketone or pyruvate have shown beneficial effects on neutrophil activation and gene expression in vitro and are the subject of ongoing studies.

TABLE 24-3 Fluid Distribution and Major Indications[a]

Fluid	Intracellular	Interstitial	Intravascular	Major Indication
Normal saline or lactated Ringer	None	750 mL	250 mL	Intravascular repletion in symptomatic patients
3% sodium chloride	→	750 mL+	250 mL+	Small amounts (eg, 250 mL) by intermittent infusion have been used in conjunction with normal saline or lactated Ringer for intravascular depletion in patients with head trauma
5% dextrose/0.45% sodium chloride	333 mL	500 mL	167 mL	Maintenance fluid in euvolemic or dehydrated (sodium and water loss) patients with mild signs/symptoms of volume depletion
5% dextrose	667 mL	250 mL	83 mL	Dehydration (primarily water loss) in patients with mild signs/symptoms of volume depletion
5% albumin	None	None	1,000 mL[b]	Intravascular repletion in symptomatic patients
25% albumin	→	→	1,000 mL+++[b]	Usually given by intermittent infusion of small volumes (eg, 50-100 mL) or by continuous infusion titrated to response in hypovolemic patients with excess interstitial fluid accumulation

[a]Based on administration of 1 L of each solution *for comparative purposes only*. This amount of fluid, particularly for 3% saline and 25% albumin, would be inappropriate and likely harmful if given over a short period of time. Numbers are approximations and are likely not reflective of actual fluid distribution in critically ill patients; arrows indicate direction of fluid shift and plus signs indicate fluid pulled from other compartments.

[b]After distribution and attainment of steady-state conditions, 60% of albumin (and associated fluid) is in interstitial compartment and 40% is in intravascular compartment.

TABLE 24-4 Summary of Evidence for Choice of Plasma Expander for Hypovolemic Shock

Source	Type of Evidence	Recommendation/Conclusion
ATLS recommendations[10]	Evidence-based consensus recommendations of fluids in trauma patients with shock	Warmed isotonic crystalloid solutions such as normal saline or lactated Ringer should be used (LOE3); hypertonic sodium chloride is an alternative with no mortality advantage (LOE4)
EAST guideline[11]	Evidence-based consensus recommendations for prehospital fluids in trauma patients	Insufficient data to recommend one fluid over another when comparing normal saline, lactated Ringer, 3% sodium chloride, or 7.5% sodium chloride (level I)
Cochrane Collaboration[12]	Systematic review of colloids versus crystalloids in critically ill patients	No evidence that colloids reduce mortality compared with crystalloids in patients with trauma or burns, or after surgery; hydroxyethyl starch products may increase mortality
Cochrane Collaboration[13]	Systematic review of different colloids for fluid resuscitation	No evidence that one colloid is more effective than another in terms of efficacy or safety; could not exclude clinically important differences due to wide confidence intervals; did not include trials after December 1, 2011
Cochrane Collaboration[14]	Systematic review of albumin solutions versus no albumin or crystalloids for fluid resuscitation in critically ill patients	No evidence that albumin reduces mortality when compared with crystalloid solutions such as normal saline but cannot exclude benefit in specific subsets of critically ill patients
British consensus guidelines[15]	Guidelines for perioperative fluid prescribing	Balanced salt solutions such as lactated Ringer's are preferred over normal saline for crystalloid resuscitation unless hypochloremia is present (level 1b); balanced salt solutions or colloids until packed red blood cells are available for hypovolemia with blood loss (level 1b)
American Burn Association[16]	Guidelines for burn shock resuscitation that include fluid recommendations	Near isotonic crystalloid recommended for initial resuscitation (grade C); hypertonic sodium chloride reserved for clinicians experienced with use (grade B); addition of colloid after 12-24 hours postburn may decrease fluid requirements (grade A)

ATLS, Advanced Trauma Life Support; EAST, Eastern Association for the Surgery of Trauma; grade A, at least one large prospective trial with clear-cut results; grade B, several small prospective trials with similar results; grade C, single small prospective trial, retrospective studies, or expert opinion; level 1b, randomized controlled trial with narrow confidence interval, or quality cohort studies (specific definitions); level I, convincingly justifiable; LOE3, level of evidence based on case–control or retrospective cohort studies, or a systematic review with at least three studies; LOE4, level of evidence based on case series.

Although lactated Ringer solution does contain lactate, it does not cause substantial elevations in circulating lactate concentrations when used as a resuscitation solution.[18] Once adequate plasma volume has been restored by fluid administration, the body can readily clear the blood of the excess lactate that has accumulated from both anaerobic metabolism and lactated Ringer solution. However, blood samples for lactate determinations drawn through catheters (arterial and venous) that have not been cleared appropriately may have spurious increases or decreases in lactate concentrations because of retained lactated Ringer and nonlactated solutions (eg, varying concentrations of dextrose-in-water or sodium chloride), respectively.[19] Therefore, blood samples for lactate concentration determinations should be drawn from a catheter that has been cleared adequately (eg, 5 mL) of infusate after temporarily stopping the fluid infusion.

TABLE 24-5 Adverse Effects of Plasma Expanders: Crystalloids

Normal saline
- Primarily extensions of pharmacologic actions (eg, fluid overload, dilutional coagulopathy)
- Hyperchloremic metabolic acidosis (has 154 mEq/L [154 mmol/L] of chloride)
- Hypernatremia (has 154 mEq/L [154 mmol/L] of sodium)

Lactated Ringer
- Primarily extensions of pharmacologic actions (eg, fluid overload, dilutional coagulopathy)
- Hyponatremia (has 130 mEq/L [130 mmol/L] of sodium)
- Aggravation of preexisting hyperkalemia (has 4 mEq/L [4 mmol/L] of potassium)

Hypertonic saline
- Primarily extensions of pharmacologic actions (eg, fluid overload, dilutional coagulopathy; intracellular volume depletion)
- Hypernatremia (has 513 mEq/L [513 mmol/L] of sodium)
- Hyperchloremia (has 513 mEq/L [513 mmol/L] of chloride)

Alternative Drug Treatments

A number of pharmacologic therapies show promise in animal models of shock, but few demonstrate success in subsequent trials involving patients with shock. In large part this is a result of the lack of acceptable animal models of shock that mimic the pathophysiology of patients. In cases in which a relevant animal model is available, care must be taken when extrapolating the information to forms of shock other than the one under study. This may be the problem with naloxone, which has been shown to raise blood pressure in some studies of shock but not in others.

While research continues on medications that improve oxygen transport, optimize oxygen utilization, and reduce reactive oxygen species and reperfusion injuries, fluids remain the mainstay of therapy for shock. Hypertonic sodium chloride solutions have been studied as alternatives to isotonic crystalloid solutions for hypovolemic shock, particularly in patients with traumatic brain injuries. By causing redistribution (ie, pulling fluid) from the intracellular space, hypertonic solutions cause rapid expansion of the intravascular compartment, which is essential for vital organ perfusion. In head-injured patients, it has been postulated that this redistribution should decrease intracranial pressure because the vessels of the brain are more impermeable to sodium ions than are vessels in other areas of the body. Additionally, hypertonic sodium chloride solutions have beneficial immunomodulating actions when compared with more isotonic solutions in experiments with animals. Unfortunately, the theoretical benefits associated with hypertonic sodium chloride solutions have not translated into improved outcomes when used for the initial resuscitation of patients with hypovolemic shock.

From a safety standpoint, hypertonic sodium chloride is considered to be a high-risk concentrated electrolyte solution. Potential dosing and administration errors and related adverse events can occur when hypertonic sodium solution is ordered and administered by clinicians relatively unfamiliar with its use. Potential adverse events include cellular crenation and damage caused by the dramatic fluid shifts associated with hypernatremia, hyperchloremic metabolic acidosis from hyperchloremia, and peripheral vein destruction from high osmolality. The osmolarity of 3% sodium chloride is 1,026 mOsm/L. Although there are some notable exceptions (eg, peripheral parenteral nutrition solutions often approach 1,000 mOsm/L), IV solutions with osmolarity values above 600 mOsm/L are usually recommended for administration by central lines. In the limited number of studies conducted in humans to date, adverse effects related to hypertonic sodium solutions have been uncommon and apparently of little clinical importance.

Larger-molecular-weight solutions (ie, greater than 30,000 Da) known as *colloids* have been recommended in conjunction with or as replacements for crystalloid solutions, although their use is controversial. The major theoretical advantage of these compounds is their prolonged intravascular retention time compared with crystalloid solutions. In contrast to isotonic crystalloid solutions that have substantial interstitial distribution within minutes of IV administration, colloids remain in the intravascular space for hours or days, depending on factors such as the size of the colloid molecules and capillary permeability. Examples of colloids used as plasma expanders in the United States include albumin, hydroxyethyl starch, and much less commonly, dextran. Albumin is known as a *monodisperse colloid* because all its molecules are of the same molecular size and weight (~67,000 Da), whereas hydroxyethyl starch and dextran solutions are *polydisperse compounds* with molecules of varying molecular size that are roughly proportional to molecular weight (weight-*averaged* molecular weights of 600,000 Da [range 450,000-800,000 Da] for 6% hetastarch in normal saline 450/0.75, 670,000 Da [range 450,000-800,000 Da] for 6% hetastarch in lactated electrolyte 670/0.75, 130,000 Da [range 110,000-150,000 Da] for 6% tetrastarch in normal saline 130/0.4, 40,000 Da [range 10,000-90,000 Da] for dextran 40, or 70,000 to 75,000 Da [range 20,000-200,000 Da] for dextran 70 or dextran 75, respectively). In light of these differences, colloid comparisons are based on weight-averaged ([number of molecules at each weight × particle weight]/total weight of all molecules) or number-averaged (arithmetic mean of all particles' weights) molecular weight.[20] The size and weight differences of the colloids have important implications for the distribution of the products because lower-molecular-weight substances are retained in the intravascular space for a shorter period of time as a result of more rapid leakage across the vessel membrane. The theoretical benefit common to all colloids is based on their increased molecular weight (average molecular weight in the case of hydroxyethyl starch and dextran) that corresponds to increased intravascular retention time in the absence of increased capillary permeability compared with crystalloids. Even in patients with intact capillary permeability, small and intermediate size colloid molecules such as albumin eventually will leak through capillary membranes with a few notable exceptions (eg, those in the central nervous system and glomeruli). In the case of albumin with a distribution half-life of 15 hours in normal subjects, approximately 60% of administered albumin molecules (and associated fluid) would be shifted to the interstitial space within 3 to 5 days of exogenous administration. In patients with altered permeability (eg, acute respiratory distress syndrome), the leakage of albumin from the intravascular to the interstitial space may occur within hours, not days. The primary adverse effect concern of all colloids is fluid overload, which is an extension of their pharmacologic action. Another adverse effect of increasing concern is renal dysfunction that seems to be related to hyperoncotic (eg, 25%) albumin and other starch and dextran products. The mechanism of this adverse effect may be related to alteration of normal glomerular oncotic pressure differences or formation of lesions in the kidney.[21]

Clinical **Controversy...**

There is no widespread agreement on the upper limit of osmolarity for hypertonic sodium solutions that are given by peripheral vein infusion under emergent conditions, but 600 or 900 mOsm/L is the usual recommended upper limit for prolonged IV infusions.

Albumin is available in 5% and 25% concentrations. Plasma protein fraction has oncotic actions similar to a 5% albumin solution, which is not surprising because albumin is the predominant protein in this product. When given in equipotent amounts, albumin is much more costly than crystalloid solutions. Additionally, the 5% and 25% albumin solutions typically are priced such that no cost saving is associated with dilution of the 25% product to make a 5% concentration. In general, dilution should be avoided because of the possibility of preparation errors; cases of hemolysis and death have occurred when 25% albumin was inappropriately diluted with sterile water for injection, causing a dramatic lowering of effective osmolarity. The 5% albumin solution is relatively *iso-oncotic*, which means that it does not pull fluid into the compartment in which it is contained. In contrast, 25% albumin is referred to as *hyperoncotic* albumin because it tends to pull fluid into the compartment containing the albumin molecules. In general, the 5% albumin solution is used for hypovolemic states. The 25% solution should not be used for acute circulatory insufficiency unless it is used in combination with other fluids or it is being used in patients with excess total body water but intravascular depletion as a means of pulling fluid into the intravascular space. An example of the latter condition is cirrhosis with ascites in which total body water is substantially increased, but the patient is hypotensive as a consequence of lack of intravascular volume. To justify this use of hyperoncotic albumin from a cost-effectiveness standpoint presumes that there is evidence of adverse effects associated with the excess water (eg, interstitial fluid accumulation in the lungs) and that the albumin remains in the intravascular space long enough to be of benefit. Albumin has a variety of functions beyond plasma expansion, such as binding properties, inflammatory gene modification, and antioxidant and free radical scavenging effects, which have been used to justify its administration instead of less expensive crystalloid or other colloid products. Although appealing theoretically, improved patient outcomes related to these properties have not been documented in adequately powered, randomized controlled trials. Additionally, the clinician must realize that the properties of commercially available albumin products are not biologically identical to those of native albumin. For example, denaturation of the products may lead to inefficient binding and decreased oncotic activity.

Hydroxyethyl starch products have been developed as synthetic alternatives to albumin that is derived through the fractionation of donated human blood. The various products are differentiated by two numbers, one for the average mean molecular weight and one for the degree of hydroxyethyl substitution of glucose. For example, hetastarch is expressed as 450/0.7 based on weight and substitution, respectively. Most of the trials comparing albumin with hydroxyethyl starch products for volume expansion were inadequately powered and found no significant differences in clinically important outcomes (eg, mortality). Two large randomized trials have directly compared hydroxyethyl starch products with crystalloid solutions for intravascular expansion. Although these trials used newer, low-molecular-weight (140), low-substitution (0.4 or 0.42) starch products, hemostasis and renal function problems noted in older trials involving high-molecular-weight, high-substitution starch products were found, suggesting these are class adverse effects. One of these large trials (Scandinavian Starch for Severe Sepsis/Septic Shock, also known as the 6S trial) found significantly higher rates of renal replacement therapy, red blood cell transfusions, and 90-day mortality in patients receiving hydroxyethyl starch versus a Ringer acetate solution.[22] The second trial (Crystalloid versus Hydroxyethyl Starch Trial referred to as the CHEST trial) involved 7,000 general ICU patients, making it the largest randomized study to date involving a starch product. As in the other large trial, patients in the hydroxyethyl starch group required significantly more renal replacement therapy versus patients receiving normal saline, but the 90-day mortality rates were similar.[23] Possible explanations for the lack of a mortality difference include the relatively low overall mortality that might be related to the exclusion criteria (eg, patients unlikely to survive), or to the use of normal saline as a control solution since saline has a high concentration of chloride ion and a low strong ion difference compared to plasma.

Hydroxyethyl starch may aggravate bleeding through mechanisms specific to this colloid (eg, decreased factor VIII/von Willebrand factor). These mechanisms have not been well elucidated and often are difficult to distinguish from the dilutional effects on clotting factors caused by all plasma expanders; however, the risk of coagulopathy appears to be related to increasing doses and durations of administration.[22] Renal dysfunction associated with hydroxyethyl starch products may also be a function of dose and duration of administration. Regardless of potential mechanisms, the Food and Drug Administration (FDA) considers the serious adverse effects of the hydroxyethyl starch products to be class effects that warrant changes to product labeling. The changes include a boxed warning that states these products are contraindicated in critically ill patients. Additional warnings have also been added about excessive bleeding when used in patients undergoing cardiopulmonary bypass. Hydroxyethyl starch may cause elevations in serum amylase concentrations but does not cause pancreatitis.

Clinical **Controversy...**

The mechanisms by which hydroxyethyl starch products cause bleeding and acute kidney injury have yet to be fully elucidated, but these problems are of sufficient concern to question the use of such products outside the confines of well-controlled trials.

Dextran 40, dextran 70, and dextran 75 are available for use as plasma expanders in the United States. The numbers refer to the average molecular weight of the solutions. In general, dextran solutions are not used as often as albumin for plasma expansion because of a lack of adequately powered randomized trials, and because of concerns related to aggravation of bleeding (ie, anticoagulant actions related to inhibiting stasis of microcirculation), acute kidney injury, and anaphylaxis that is more likely to occur with the higher-molecular-weight solutions. There are few comparative trials involving the dextran solutions, but the intravascular expansion within hours after infusion is approximately equal to the amount of dextran infused. Apart from the acute kidney injury and bleeding associated with starch and dextran products, adverse effects associated with colloids generally are extensions of their pharmacologic activity (Table 24-6).

From a historical perspective, the so-called crystalloid versus colloid debate was intensified when a meta-analysis by the well-respected Cochrane group found an overall increase in mortality associated with albumin using pooled results of randomized investigations.[24] The meta-analysis involved 30 randomized trials with 1,419 patients (relative risk of death with albumin vs no administration or crystalloid administration, 1.68; 95% confidence interval [CI], 1.26-2.23). For hypovolemia (caused by blood loss in the majority of studies), the risk of death associated with albumin administration was not quite statistically significant (relative risk, 1.46; 95% CI, 0.97-2.22). With the notable exception of trauma patients, a subsequent and more comprehensive systematic review did not find increased mortality attributable to albumin.[25] Furthermore, a landmark investigation involving almost 7,000 critically ill patients (conducted after the previously mentioned meta-analyses) did not find statistically significant differences in 28-day mortality between patients resuscitated with either normal saline or 4% albumin.[26] As in the previous meta-analysis, there was a trend toward increased mortality in patients with trauma, which became statistically significant ($P = 0.003$) when analyzed at 24 months in a subset of patients with traumatic brain injury.[27] This multicenter, randomized, double-blind investigation, referred to as the *Saline versus Albumin Fluid Evaluation* (SAFE) study, involved a heterogeneous group of ICU patients and was not sufficiently powered to look at various subsets, so clinicians must be cautious when extrapolating the results to more specific patient populations.

The colloids are expensive solutions. Therefore, it is difficult to justify the additional cost of colloidal products unless the benefit-to-risk ratio is substantially greater than that associated with inexpensive crystalloid solutions. This does not appear to be the case based on randomized controlled studies and meta-analyses comparing colloid and crystalloid solutions for acute circulatory insufficiency. While the use of albumin in specific patient populations (eg, septic shock) is still debated, the documented adverse effect profile of hydroxyethyl starch products and the lack of adequately powered trials for dextran products renders them all unsuitable for use in critically ill patients including those with shock.

In contrast to other forms of shock such as anaphylactic or septic, medications are a distant alternative to the primary therapy

TABLE 24-6 Adverse Effects of Plasma Expanders: Colloids

Albumin
- Primarily extensions of pharmacologic actions (eg, fluid overload; dilutional coagulopathy)
- Amino acid profile and catabolism alterations (clinical significance?); potential protein overload if given with exogenous protein (eg, parenteral nutrition)
- Anaphylactoid/anaphylaxis reactions (life-threatening reactions rare; higher in patients with immunoglobulin A deficiency)
- Infectious complications (all reported cases have been associated with improper handling by manufacturer or institution; no reported cases of human immunodeficiency virus or hepatitis transmission)
- Interactions with medications and nutrients (clinical significance varies)
- Metal loading, particularly aluminum (long-term administration in patients with renal failure)
- Negative inotropic effect; reductions in ionized calcium concentrations (not well documented)
- Pyrogenic reactions (not well documented)
- Renal dysfunction with hyperoncotic albumin

Hydroxyethyl starch
- Primarily extensions of pharmacologic actions (eg, fluid overload, dilutional coagulopathy)
- Bleeding; not recommended in critically ill patients or in patients with bleeding conditions such as subarachnoid hemorrhage
- Macroamylase formation may cause elevation in blood amylase that leads to inaccurate diagnosis of pancreatitis
- Anaphylactoid/anaphylaxis reactions
- Pruritus (particularly when large amounts are given; may take months to resolve)
- Renal dysfunction; not recommended in critically ill patients, patients at risk for renal dysfunction or patients with preexisting renal dysfunction

Dextrans
- Primarily extensions of pharmacologic actions (eg, fluid overload, dilutional coagulopathy)
- Anaphylactoid/anaphylaxis reactions (increased incidence of anaphylaxis with increased molecular weight)
- Bleeding (sometimes used for anticoagulant activity, so not recommended for patients with or at risk for bleeding)
- Renal dysfunction

for hypovolemic shock, fluids. In hypovolemic shock, peripheral resistance is high due to compensatory mechanisms aimed at maintaining tissue perfusion. Early or overzealous use of vasopressors in lieu of fluids may exacerbate this resistance to the point that flow is stopped. Therefore, vasoactive agents that dilate the peripheral vasculature such as dobutamine are preferred if the blood pressure is stable and high enough to tolerate the vasodilation. Vasopressors are only used as a temporizing measure or as a last resort when all other measures to maintain perfusion have been exhausted.[28] Because vasopressors have such a limited role in hypovolemic shock, there are very few studies that compare various agents. In one of the few studies that included patients with hypovolemic shock, norepinephrine and dopamine had similar effects on mortality, but dopamine was associated with more adverse effects, particularly atrial fibrillation.[29]

Special Populations

Trauma/Perioperative Patients

The need for immediate treatment of hemorrhagic circulatory insufficiency with plasma expanders (ie, crystalloids or colloids) seems obvious, but no large, well-controlled trials conducted in humans have supported this practice. To the contrary, evidence suggests that fluid resuscitation beyond minimal levels (ie, mean arterial pressure greater than 60 mm Hg) is harmful in patients with penetrating abdominal trauma due to hemodilution and clot destabilization. One prospective study involving 598 adult patients with gunshot or stab wound injuries to the torso and systolic blood pressure measurements of 90 mm Hg or less found that delayed fluid resuscitation until operation was associated with increased survival and discharge from the hospital ($P = 0.04$).[30] Since concerns were expressed about the comparability of the immediate and delayed resuscitation groups, particularly because true randomization did not take place, a follow-up randomized trial was conducted to verify the findings. There were no differences in survival (four deaths in each group) in the second trial regardless of whether systolic blood pressure was titrated to greater than 100 mm Hg or to 70 mm Hg.[31] Both studies were conducted in populated urban areas with approximately 2 hours from the time of injury to operation. Therefore, the results may not be applicable to rural areas with extended transport times. There also is a concern in applying the results of these investigations to patients with certain kinds of single-system injuries, particularly head trauma, where cerebral perfusion pressure is of primary importance. Although the applicability of these studies to other populations and settings is debatable, the *presumption* of benefits from immediate plasma expansion in all preoperative patients with circulatory insufficiency caused by hemorrhage is no longer valid. Instead, the initial priority should be surgical control of the bleeding source; until this is possible, fluids should be given in small aliquots to yield a palpable pulse and to maintain mean arterial pressures no more than 60 mm Hg and systolic pressures no more than 90 mm Hg based on accurate measurements (eg, arterial monitoring).

Beneficial outcome data attributable to hypertonic sodium chloride solutions are lacking. Most of these studies were conducted in prehospital and emergency department settings using 250 mL of 7.5% sodium chloride with or without 6% dextran 70. For example, a double-blind, randomized controlled trial involving 229 patients with hypotension and severe brain injury demonstrated no significant differences in neurologic function at 6 months when 250 mL of 7.5% saline or lactated Ringer solution was administered as part of a prehospital resuscitation regimen.[32] Part of the explanation for this finding may be related to supplemental crystalloid fluids that were given routinely to patients in both the treatment and control groups, which probably would increase the number of patients needed to demonstrate a statistically significant difference in mortality.

In order to address ongoing questions of efficacy, the National Heart, Lung, and Blood Institute evaluated hypertonic sodium chloride solutions with or without a colloid (ie, 7.5% sodium chloride or 7.5% sodium chloride in 6% dextran 70) for prehospitalized trauma patients with shock and severe traumatic brain injury in two trials conducted by a network of sites known as the Resuscitation Outcomes Consortium (ROC). Both the parallel trials were stopped when it was determined that the hypertonic sodium chloride solutions were no better than normal saline and further enrollment would not change the 33 outcomes.[33,34] Therefore, normal saline is the fluid of choice since it is equal in efficacy with a lower risk of adverse effects compared with hypertonic solutions that are high-risk electrolyte solutions. Given their relatively poor intravascular expansion and association with poor outcome in animal models of closed head injury, hypotonic solutions should be avoided in this population.

In addition to crystalloid solutions, colloids have been used for plasma expansion in trauma patients with perioperative circulatory insufficiency. No large randomized studies have compared crystalloids and colloids for circulatory insufficiency in trauma patients. Until such studies are performed, there is no compelling reason to suspect that colloids have any substantial clinical benefits beyond crystalloids in these patients given the results of previous trials and systematic reviews performed in more general critical care populations. Further, bleeding and renal injury concerns for both starch and dextran products precludes their use in critically ill trauma patients.

The preceding discussion dealt primarily with acute circulatory insufficiency, but there are other considerations with regard to fluid replacement in other patients undergoing surgical procedures. Preoperative fluid deficits in patients undergoing minor procedures may be associated with increased perioperative morbidity, some of which (eg, drowsiness, dizziness) may be reduced by appropriate fluid administration prior to surgery. However, care must be taken to avoid overhydration in the perioperative period because excess fluid will lead to weight gain and decreased pulmonary function. Some evidence suggests that fluid restriction on the day of surgery may reduce postoperative morbidity in patients undergoing major surgical procedures. In one randomized, multicenter trial, use of a restricted intraoperative and postoperative IV fluid protocol led to significantly fewer cardiopulmonary (7% vs 24%; $P = 0.007$) and wound (16% vs 31%; $P = 0.04$) complications.[35] As the preceding discussion indicates, the benefits and risks of fluid administration in the perioperative period are not just a function of too little or too much fluid but involve other patient- and procedure-related issues.

Another consideration in the patient with penetrating injuries or surgery is the potential need for blood product administration (Table 24-7) to replace oxygen-carrying and clotting functions.

TABLE 24-7 General Indications for Blood Products in Acute Circulatory Insufficiency due to Hemorrhage

Packed red blood cells
Increase oxygen-carrying capacity of blood: Usually indicated in patients with continued deterioration after volume replacement or obvious exsanguination; must be warmed, particularly when used in children
Fresh-frozen plasma
Replacement of clotting factors: Generally overused; indicated if ongoing hemorrhage in patients with PT/PTT >1.5 times normal, severe hepatic disease, or other bleeding diathesis
Platelets
Used for bleeding due to severe thrombocytopenia (ie, platelet count <10,000/μL [$<10 \times 10^9$/L]) or rapidly dropping platelet counts as would occur with massive bleeding
Other products
With the exception of recombinant activated factor VII, which is currently undergoing trials for use in life-threatening hemorrhage unresponsive to traditional blood product administration, components such as cryoprecipitate and factor VIII are generally not indicated in acute hemorrhage but rather are used after specific deficiencies are identified

PT, prothrombin time; PTT, partial thromboplastin time.

[a]Although whole blood can be used for large-volume blood loss, most hospitals use component therapy, and use crystalloids or colloids for plasma expansion.

Although a small group of trauma patients respond to the initial fluid bolus and remain stable, most patients respond initially and then deteriorate. The latter patients, as well as patients undergoing blood loss associated with surgery, frequently need blood components such as packed red blood cells. 9 In the case of the latter component, red blood cells contain hemoglobin that delivers oxygen to tissues. Neither crystalloids nor colloids perform this function.

Administration of excessive blood products may be counterproductive. In the case of red blood cells, attempts to raise the hematocrit to high–normal or supranormal concentrations may decrease oxygen delivery by increasing blood viscosity. Additionally, there are immunomodulatory concerns with red blood cell administration. Although there is no optimal hematocrit value for all patients, a minimum hematocrit of 30% (0.30) (equivalent to a hemoglobin concentration of 10 g/dL [100 g/L; 6.21 mmol/L]) traditionally has been used as the threshold for transfusion, particularly in patients at risk for ischemia, such as those with CAD. Use of a more liberal transfusion strategy has been curtailed in many institutions with the publication of a randomized, multicenter trial involving critically ill patients that found 30-day mortality to be similar whether patients were transfused at a hemoglobin concentration less than 7 or 10 g/dL (70-100 g/L; 4.34-6.21 mmol/L) (18.7% vs 23.3%, respectively; $P = 0.11$).[36] The mortality during hospitalization was significantly lower in the restrictive group (22.2% vs 28.1%; $P = 0.05$). Although the investigators were cautious about extrapolating the results of this investigation to patients with myocardial ischemia, a subsequent study performed in patients undergoing cardiac surgery found similar results.[37] With the exception of the critically ill or perioperative patient with acute exsanguination, there is little justification for a liberal transfusion strategy based solely on hemoglobin concentrations.

Blood products have risks beyond immunomodulation. There is the rare but important risk of virus transmission (eg, human immunodeficiency virus [HIV], hepatitis). Citrate that is added to stored blood to prevent coagulation may bind to calcium, resulting in hypocalcemia, although potassium and phosphate concentrations often are elevated in stored blood, particularly when hemolysis has occurred during storage. In patients receiving large amounts of blood, prophylactic calcium administration may be warranted until levels are available. Other issues that must be considered with blood product administration include monitoring for transfusion-related reactions and attention to appropriate warming, particularly when large volumes are given to pediatric patients, because hypothermia is associated with increased fluid requirements and mortality.

Since its commercial release in the United States, recombinant factor VIIa has been used for a variety of off-label uses related to trauma and bleeding. For example, in patients with massive blood loss a cocktail of cryoprecipitate, platelets, and recombinant factor VIIa has been suggested to rapidly attain hemostasis. These more severe forms of blood loss are a function of not only the type of injury but also factors such as medications (eg, aspirin, Coumadin, clopidogrel, enoxaparin, newer oral anticoagulants) and disease states that impair normal coagulation. Large well-controlled trials are needed to define the role of recombinant factor VIIa in clinical practice given its high cost and potential thromboembolic complications. Concerns with its use in trauma patients are issues related to appropriate dose, timing, and diminished effectiveness in patients with acidosis and severe hypothermia. Evidence of efficacy in a general trauma population that would offset these concerns is lacking. In the largest randomized controlled trial conducted to date that enrolled patients with penetrating and blunt trauma, factor VIIa did not decrease mortality compared with placebo when the trial was prematurely terminated due to futility.[38]

The periodic shortages, high costs, and adverse effect concerns related to blood products have prompted investigations of alternative "bloodless" strategies. In addition to the use of more restrictive transfusion thresholds, as mentioned previously, these strategies have included hemoglobin-based oxygen carriers and perfluorocarbon compounds to deliver oxygen to tissues. Other strategies have aimed at reducing blood loss through the use of improved procedural and surgical techniques, as well as the administration of hemostatic medications. The only hemostatic medication with a proven mortality benefit is the antifibrinolytic agent, tranexamic acid. The best evidence for efficacy was data from a multicenter trial involving more than 20,000 adult trauma patients with significant bleeding (or risk for significant bleeding) who were randomized to IV tranexamic acid (1 g over 10 minutes followed by 1 g over 8 hours by infusion) or matching placebo within 8 hours of injury.[39] There was a significant reduction in all-cause mortality with tranexamic acid compared with placebo (14.5% vs 16%, $P = 0.0035$) with no increase in vascular or other adverse events. A more in-depth review of the results of this trial suggests that the beneficial effects are most likely to occur if tranexamic acid is given within the first 3 hours of injury. While additional data are still needed in specific subpopulations such as patients with traumatic brain injuries, this study is relatively unique in that an intervention apart from surgery and blood product administration was demonstrated to reduce mortality.

Patients with Thermal Injuries

There are a number of formulas for estimating fluid requirements in thermally injured patients, but there is little reason to choose one over another based on well-controlled studies. In general, the amount of loss corresponds to the size of the thermal injury. Guidelines recommend approximately 2 to 4 mL/kg of isotonic fluid (lactated Ringer solution) for each percent burn can be used for calculating the expected fluid requirements for the first 24 hours after the burn.[16] For example, a 60-kg person with 30% body surface area (BSA) burns is expected to require 5,400 to 7,200 mL of fluid over the initial 24 hours. Regardless of the calculated deficit, fluids should be administered until adequate tissue perfusion has been documented (eg, maintenance of urine output of 0.5-1 mL/kg in adults) or adverse effects (eg, pulmonary edema) occur. Crystalloids are preferred as initial therapy for burn victims because there is no substantial evidence that colloids mobilize edematous fluid, and there is a theoretical concern that extravascular fluid accumulation might be prolonged by the oncotic actions of albumin and other colloid products that have leaked through vessel walls. Additionally, there is no evidence that colloids reduce mortality in patients with thermal injuries and there is a concern that hydroxyethyl starch and dextran products might even increase mortality through deleterious effects on coagulation and renal function. Some novel therapies for thermal resuscitation have been studied, although larger confirmatory trials are needed prior to use apart from research protocols. For example, in a prospective study involving patients with more than 30% BSA burns, antioxidant therapy with extremely high doses of IV vitamin C (66 mg/kg/h for 24 hours) reduced resuscitation fluid requirements and wound edema.[40] The proposed mechanism is reduction in free radical–induced increases in capillary permeability.

Personalized Pharmacotherapy

At this time there is little genetic/genomic information that is available to guide personalized pharmacotherapy in patients with hypovolemic shock. Further, as stressed throughout this chapter, fluids are by far the first choice of therapy in conjunction with other definitive interventions such as surgery for traumatic injuries. Nevertheless, there are individual factors that may influence the specific fluid being administered. For example, the lower chloride concentration in lactated Ringer would usually make it preferred over normal saline in patients with a hyperchloremic metabolic acidosis, while the increased osmolarity of normal saline would usually make it preferred over lactated Ringer in a patient with increased intracranial pressure.

Clinical **Controversy...**

Some clinicians believe that hypertonic sodium-containing solutions should be the intervention of choice to lower intracranial pressure in patients with head injuries.

The appropriate use of invasive hemodynamic monitoring tools, such as right-sided heart catheterization in patients with hypovolemic shock, is controversial.

Some clinicians believe that more balanced crystalloid solutions are preferred over normal saline for IV fluid resuscitation given the association between high-chloride-containing solutions and acute kidney injury.

EVALUATION OF THERAPEUTIC OUTCOMES

Monitoring of the Pharmaceutical Care Plan

One form of monitoring that may take place in the emergency and operating rooms, as well as in the ICU, requires placement of a central venous pressure (CVP) line. Monitoring of CVP provides the clinician with a somewhat insensitive yet useful estimate of the relationship between increased right atrial pressure and cardiac output. A protocol that used a particular type of central catheter to perform continuous monitoring of central venous oxygen saturation in conjunction with so-called early goal-directed therapy (EGDT) in the first 6 hours of patient arrival in an urban emergency department resulted in decreased mortality compared with standard monitoring (30.5% vs 46.5%; $P = 0.009$).[41] However, the results of this landmark study that used continuous central venous oxygen saturation monitoring as part of an EGDT protocol have been called into question by two more recent studies (Protocolized Care for Early Septic Shock [ProCESS] and Australasian Resuscitation in Sepsis Evaluation [ARISE]).[42,43] In ProCESS and ARISE, no significant differences were found in mortality (or a variety of other secondary endpoints) between groups that received the continuous invasive monitoring versus groups receiving usual, less invasive monitoring. These follow-up investigations suggest it may have been the protocols of care and not the invasive catheter that was responsible for the mortality benefit noted in the original landmark study. Also of note is that patients in all of these studies had severe sepsis and septic shock, so the results might not be applicable to other forms of shock with different pathophysiologic considerations. For example, in hemorrhagic shock due to trauma, the most important intervention is surgical control of bleeding, and anything that delays this control is likely to increase, not decrease, mortality. In fact, so-called "upstream" measurements of perfusion such as CVP are not a useful guide for fluid management in hospitalized patients, and are being replaced by "downstream" markers such as urine output and lactate levels that are more likely to reflect end-organ dysfunction.[44] A more complete discussion of invasive and noninvasive hemodynamic monitoring is given in Chapter e11.

Clinical **Controversy...**

The most appropriate, cost-effective, and practical parameter(s) for monitoring adequacy of fluid resuscitation in shock is unresolved.

A number of laboratory tests are indicated for subacute monitoring of shock in the ICU setting. These include a renal battery for assessing possible electrolyte alterations and kidney perfusion (eg, BUN and creatinine). Among other things, a complete blood count will enable assessment of possible infection (white blood cell count), oxygen-carrying capacity of the blood (hemoglobin, hematocrit), and ongoing bleeding (hemoglobin, hematocrit, and platelet count). The PT or international normalized ratio and partial thromboplastin time (PTT) will give an indication of the ability of the blood to clot because, in the case of hemorrhagic shock, clotting factors are lost and diluted. An increasing lactate concentration (arterial, mixed venous, or central venous), an increasing arterial base deficit, or a decreasing bicarbonate concentration are global markers indicative of inadequate perfusion leading to anaerobic metabolism with accumulation of lactic acid. Although the value of these surrogate markers for improving patient outcomes is more controversial, they are considered traditional end points of resuscitation in certain populations such as trauma patients. Other tests may be indicated if organ dysfunction is likely. For example, when blood flow to the liver is interrupted because of sustained hypotension, a condition known as *shock liver* may occur. In this condition, the levels of transaminases on a liver panel may be markedly elevated in the first couple of days after marked hypotension, although the concentrations should decrease over time. Along with laboratory testing, a more extensive history can be obtained during the subacute monitoring period.

The value of pulmonary artery catheters (also known as *right-sided heart* or *Swan-Ganz catheters*) has been debated hotly since their introduction. Such catheters are placed to obtain various oxygen-transport variables, some of which cannot be determined reliably from peripheral or other central vessels. The debate was intensified when early studies suggested improved outcomes when cardiac output and other oxygen-transport variables were raised to supranormal levels, the monitoring of which required placement of a pulmonary artery catheter. The controversy led to consensus conferences and workshops, the development of organizational guidelines, and the publication of a meta-analysis (which found a statistically significant reduction in *morbidity* using pulmonary artery catheters to guide therapy).[45] Ultimately, a large randomized controlled trial involving pulmonary artery catheters was conducted in high-risk surgical patients.[46] The trial involved 1,994 patients. The mortality was almost identical for the catheter and control groups (7.8% vs 7.7%; 95% CI, 2.3-2.5). There were no episodes of pulmonary embolism in the catheter group and eight episodes in the control group ($P = 0.004$). This trial is important not only because of the implications for high-risk surgical patients but also because it allows for the conduct of future trials in other patient populations without some of the ethical issues raised about such trials in the past.

Part of the concern regarding pulmonary artery catheterization relates to interpretation of its results by inexperienced practitioners. Studies in Europe and the United States found that one of two physicians incorrectly interpreted a tracing from a pulmonary artery catheter.[47] This could explain some of the results of studies finding no benefits to pulmonary artery catheterization or, in some cases, worse outcomes in the pulmonary artery catheterization group by actions taken as a result of inaccurate measurements or misinterpretation of information obtained from the monitoring process.

Complications related to pulmonary artery catheter insertion, maintenance, and removal include damage to vessels and organs during insertion, arrhythmias, infections, and thromboembolic damage. To avoid the complications associated with pulmonary artery catheterization, other less invasive tools were developed to obtain similar information. For example, cardiac output determinations have been made by Doppler, bioimpedance, dye, and ionic dilution techniques, although such measurements would not provide other data that are obtained routinely with pulmonary artery catheters (eg, left-sided heart filling pressure). Additionally, advances in pulmonary artery catheter technology that expand the information obtained from such monitoring (eg, mixed venous oxyhemoglobin) are under investigation. However, given the lack of well-defined outcome data associated with pulmonary artery catheterization, its use is best reserved for complicated cases of shock not responding to conventional fluid and medication therapies.

Commonly measured and calculated hemodynamic and oxygen-transport indices associated with invasive monitoring are primarily global indicators of tissue perfusion. Attempts have been made to find regional and local indicators of hypoperfusion so that circulatory insufficiency could be treated before overt shock occurs. One focus of recent research has been monitoring modalities involving the GI tract. Although the literature is fairly consistent concerning low gastric intramucosal pH (pHi) values being predictive of death, pHi-guided therapy to decrease mortality has not been demonstrated.[48] Additionally, a number of technical considerations remain to be resolved when using pHi or, more recently, capnometry (luminal PCO_2 tonometry) for monitoring and therapy. Despite these concerns, measures of regional tissue oxygenation continue to be investigated through a variety of novel monitoring techniques.

In addition to regional monitoring of tissue perfusion, local methods of monitoring are being studied. For example, subcutaneous measurement of tissue oxygen pressure shows promise in preliminary investigations. Regional and local measurements likely will not replace more global indicators of perfusion; rather, the methods will complement each other.

Monitoring of the Pharmaceutical Care Plan after Initial Fluid Resuscitation

Proper attention to monitoring of plasma volume must be continued into the intraoperative and postoperative periods. A number of neurohormonal changes take place that affect urine output, and patients may have substantial third spacing of fluid depending on the operation and preexisting conditions. Furthermore, postoperative patients are prone to hyponatremia from renal generation of electrolyte-free water and from antidiuretic hormone release. As in acute resuscitation, the administration of hypotonic solutions in the perioperative period does not prevent the decrease in extracellular volume that often occurs. Therefore, although excess fluid administration is to be avoided in the perioperative setting, isotonic crystalloid solutions should be used when fluids are indicated to prevent intravascular depletion and circulatory insufficiency.

Of the randomized studies comparing albumin with crystalloid solutions in the perioperative period, the majority found no statistically significant differences between groups. Any significant differences found involved isolated hemodynamic or respiratory variables with no obvious clinical correlates (eg, duration of mechanical ventilation). Therefore, albumin cannot be recommended for the prevention or initial treatment of circulatory insufficiency, although its use may be appropriate in patients who are not responding to crystalloids and are developing problems such as interstitial fluid accumulation.

There is no evidence that vasoactive medications improve outcome in patients with hypovolemic shock assuming that fluid therapy is adequate. (10) In a multicenter cohort study of blunt-injured patients with hemorrhagic shock, the use of vasopressors within 12 hours of injury was associated with significantly higher mortality at 24 hours ($P = 0.001$).[49] Therefore, pressor agents such as norepinephrine and high-dose dopamine are to be avoided, if possible, because they may increase blood pressure at the expense of peripheral tissue ischemia. Some sources use stronger language and state that vasopressors are contraindicated in certain forms of shock (eg, hemorrhagic). This does not help the clinician who is treating a patient with unstable blood pressure despite massive fluid replacement and increasing interstitial fluid accumulation. Although the search for a cryptogenic source (eg, intra-abdominal bleeding in a trauma patient) should continue, the clinician may need to administer vasoactive medications to improve perfusion. In such situations, inotropic agents such as dobutamine are preferred if blood pressure is adequate (eg, systolic blood pressure ≥80-90 mm Hg) because they should not aggravate the existing vasoconstriction. The inotropic agents are justified by presumed inadequate cardiac output for the specific situation, although the measured values may be in the normal range.

When pressure cannot be maintained with inotropic agents or when inotropic agents with vasodilatory properties cannot be used because of inadequate blood pressure concerns, pressors may be required as a last resort. In general, the need for pressors is predictive of the development of MODS and increased length of hospital stay. Although the response to pressor agents may be variable in hypovolemic shock, there does not appear to be resistance as a consequence of altered receptor response, as is sometimes seen in patients with septic shock. Potent vasoconstrictors such as norepinephrine and phenylephrine should be given through central veins because of the possibility of extravasation and necrosis with peripheral administration.

In managing patients with hypovolemic shock, the clinician must be aware of potential adverse effects of medications being used for supportive care purposes. For example, some patients are particularly susceptible to the histamine release associated with morphine and may have substantial decreases in blood pressure. Sodium bicarbonate would seem to be a logical therapy in patients with shock who typically have a metabolic acidosis, but bicarbonate administration has not been shown to improve surrogate hemodynamic markers or patient outcomes and has known disadvantages such as the associated increase in arterial carbon dioxide levels and decrease in serum ionized calcium levels.[50] Agents such as propofol and dexmedetomidine are commonly used for sedation in the ICU, but they may cause substantial decreases in blood pressure. The initial doses of such agents should be substantially reduced or preferably the agents should be avoided in patients with hemorrhagic shock who may not be fully resuscitated.

A number of interesting treatments for shock are under investigation, including autotransfusion for removing harmful cytokines from the body. Various alternatives to conventional blood components also are being studied, such as stroma-free hemoglobin and perfluorocarbon compounds, as virus-free alternatives to red blood cell transfusion. Hopefully, these methods will be useful adjuncts to adequate volume replacement, which is the primary therapeutic intervention in managing acute circulatory insufficiency as a result of volume depletion.

CLINICAL BOTTOM LINE

Figure 24-4 is an algorithm that summarizes many of the treatment principles discussed in this chapter. The algorithm is an example of one approach to the adult patient presenting with hypovolemic shock. It presumes that initial rehydration attempts (ie, outpatient or prehospital) were unsuccessful in restoring circulation. Obviously, modifications may be needed for patient-specific forms of hypovolemic shock. For example, in patients with severe traumatic brain injury albumin would be contraindicated as a plasma expander, while hypertonic sodium solution might be considered for its ability to lower elevated intracranial pressure without causing the diuresis associated with mannitol administration. Other limitations of the algorithm should be recognized, particularly the decisions to add or to substitute medication therapies when crystalloid solutions are not yielding desired results and when to perform pulmonary artery catheterization for more invasive monitoring. Medications become more important for the ongoing management of hypovolemic shock, but only when the patient is unresponsive to fluids (Fig. 24-5). Medications for more complicated cases of hemorrhagic shock should not

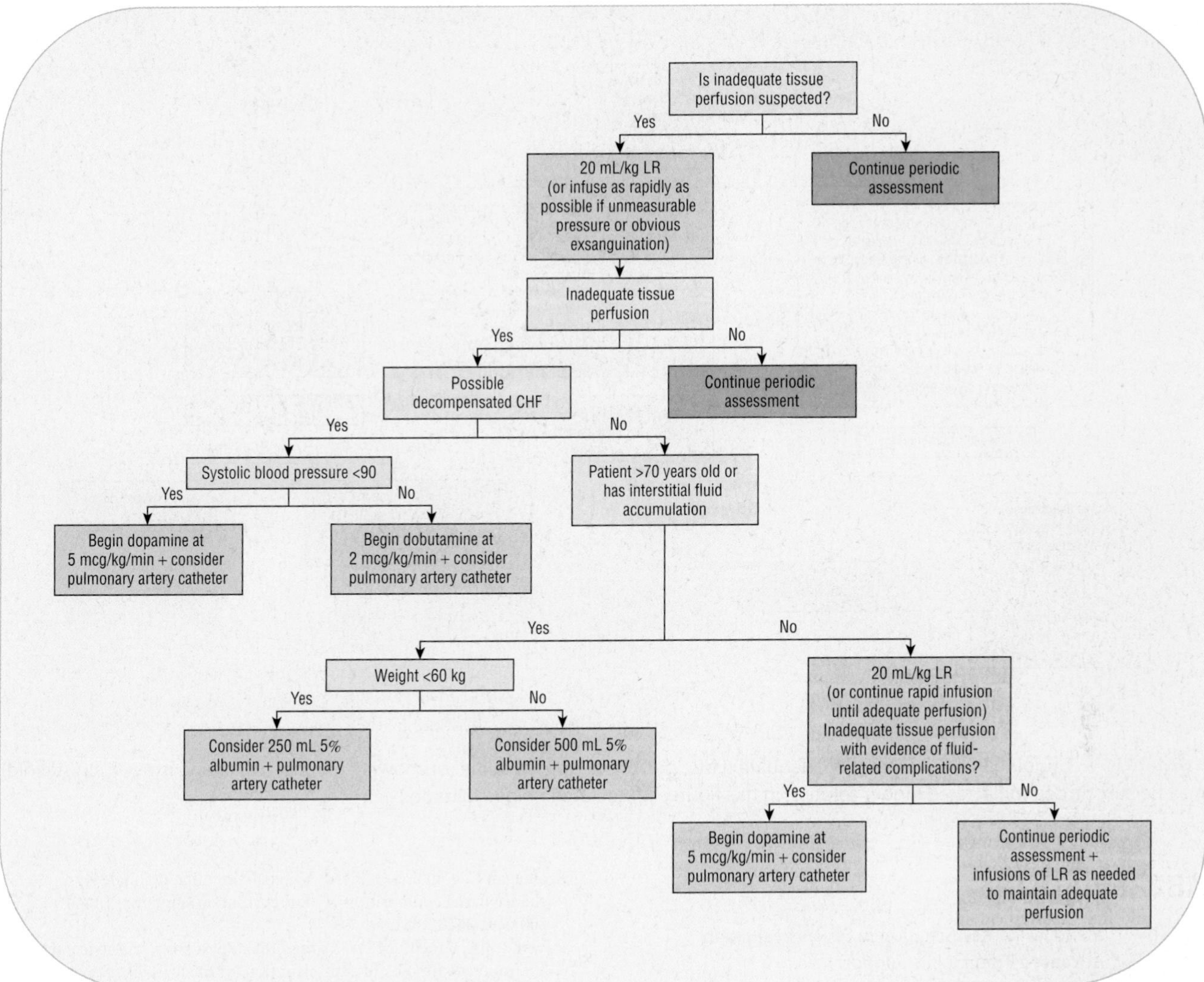

FIGURE 24-4 Hypovolemia protocol for adults. Normal saline (or a lower chloride-containing isotonic crystalloid) may be used instead of lactated Ringer solution. This protocol is not intended to replace or delay therapies such as surgical intervention or blood products for restoring oxygen-carrying capacity or hemostasis. For the resuscitation of patients with trauma prior to bleeding control, usually no more than 1 L of crystalloid should be given initially in an attempt to use the minimal amount of fluid necessary to maintain perfusion and not exacerbate bleeding. If available, some measurements can be used in addition to those listed in the algorithm, such as mean arterial pressure or pulmonary artery catheter recordings. The latter can be used to assist in medication choices (eg, agents with primary pressor effects may be desirable in patients with normal cardiac outputs, whereas dopamine or dobutamine may be indicated in patients with suboptimal cardiac outputs). Lower maximal doses of the medications in this algorithm should be considered when pulmonary artery catheterization is not available. See text for an in-depth discussion of these and other issues involved in this protocol. (CHF, congestive heart failure; LR, lactated Ringer solution.)

detract from the primary effective resuscitative measure—surgical stabilization of bleeding.

The algorithm in Fig. 24-4 attempts to incorporate economic considerations and potential fluid shortages. The institutional cost of 1 L of most crystalloid solutions is less than $1. Assuming that such fluids are used, the associated costs of personnel and equipment then become the primary economic considerations in the resuscitation of patients with hypovolemic shock. However, as mentioned, many clinicians recommend that colloid plasma expanders (eg, albumin, hydroxyethyl starch, or dextrans) be used to replace some or all of the standard crystalloid solutions. Although the costs of these solutions vary, depending on contractual arrangements, in general, albumin solutions are more expensive than older hydroxyethyl starch and dextran products. All these solutions are markedly more costly than crystalloid solutions; in some cases, the differences are 50- to 100-fold, even when used in equipotent amounts. It is important to note that these cost minimization statements assume no differences in efficacy or toxicity between colloids and crystalloids when given in equipotent amounts. This is almost certainly not the case with respect to adverse effects of hydroxyethyl starch and dextran products. A cost-effectiveness analysis that takes into account adverse effects would be needed for the latter products and such an analysis would likely demonstrate they are not cost-effective versus crystalloids even if equipotent efficacy is presumed.

Because medications are not simply alternatives to crystalloids but rather are used when crystalloid therapy has been optimized, there is little reason to compare medication and fluid therapies from an economic perspective. Furthermore, there are no economic comparisons of the various inotropic and vasopressor medications used in the treatment of hypovolemic shock.

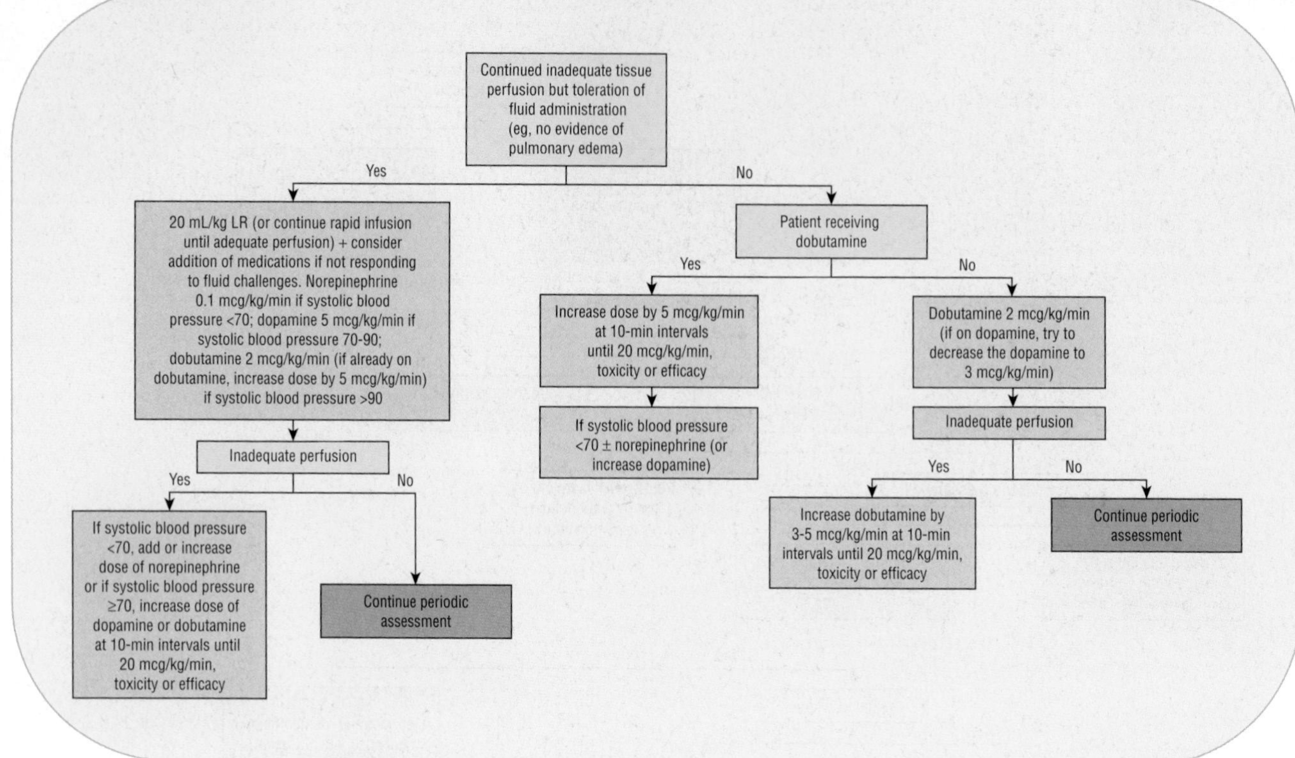

FIGURE 24-5 Ongoing management of inadequate tissue perfusion. Normal saline (or a lower chloride-containing isotonic crystalloid) may be substituted for lactated Ringer solution in this figure. (LR, lactated Ringer solution.)

ABBREVIATIONS

ARISE	Australasian Resuscitation in Sepsis Evaluation
ATLS	Advanced Trauma Life Support
BSA	body surface area
BUN	blood urea nitrogen
CAD	coronary artery disease
CDC	Centers for Disease Control and Prevention
CI	confidence interval
CVP	central venous pressure
EAST	Eastern Association for the Surgery of Trauma
EGDT	early goal directed therapy
FDA	Food and Drug Administration
GI	gastrointestinal
HIV	human immunodeficiency virus
ICU	intensive care unit
IV	intravenous
MODS	multiple-organ dysfunction syndrome
pHi	gastric intramucosal pH
ProCESS	Protocolized Care for Early Septic Shock
PT	prothrombin time
PTT	partial thromboplastin time
ROC	Resuscitation Outcomes Consortium
SAFE	Saline versus Albumin Fluid Evaluation
SIRS	systemic inflammatory response syndrome
WHO	World Health Organization

REFERENCES

1. Kochanek KD, Murphy SL, Xu J, Arias E. Mortality in the United States, 2013. NCHS data brief, no. 178. Hyattsville, MD: National Center for Health Statistics, 2014.
2. Anonymous. QuickStats: Number of Heat-Related Deaths,* by Sex—National Vital Statistics System, United States, 1999–2010. *MMWR Morb Mortal Wkly Rep* 2012;61(36):729.
3. Duggan C, Fontaine O, Pierce NF, et al. Scientific rationale for a change in the composition of oral rehydration solution. *JAMA* 2004;291:2628-2631.
4. Vercueil A, Grocott MPW, Mythen MG. Physiology, pharmacology, and rationale for colloid administration for the maintenance of effective hemodynamic stability in critically ill patients. *Trans Med Rev* 2005;19:93-109.
5. Porter SC, Fleisher GR, Kohane IS, Mandl KD. The value of parental report for diagnosis and management of dehydration in the emergency department. *Ann Emerg Med* 2003;41:196-205.
6. Spandorfer PR, Alessandrini EA, Joffe MD, et al. Oral versus intravenous rehydration of moderately dehydrated children: A randomized, controlled trial. *Pediatrics* 2005;115:295-301.
7. Atherly-John YC, Cunningham SJ, Crain EF. A randomized trial of oral vs intravenous rehydration in a pediatric emergency department. *Arch Pediatr Adolesc Med* 2002;156:1240-1243.
8. Axler OA, Tousiganant C, Thompson CR, et al. Small hemodynamic effect of typical rapid volume infusions in critically ill patients. *Crit Care Med* 1997;25:965-970.
9. The National Heart, Lung, and Blood Institute Acute Respiratory Distress Syndrome (ARDS) Clinical Trials Network. Comparison of two fluid-management strategies in acute lung injury. *N Engl J Med* 2006;354:2564-2575.
10. The ATLS Subcommittee, American College of Surgeons' Committee on Trauma, and the International ATLS working group. Advanced trauma life support (ATLS®): The ninth edition. *J Trauma Acute Care Surg* 2013;74:1363-1366.
11. Cotton BA, Jerome R, Collier BR, et al. Guidelines for prehospital fluid resuscitation in the injured patient. *J Trauma* 2009;67:389-402.
12. Perel P, Roberts I, Ker K. Colloids versus crystalloids for fluid resuscitation in critically ill patients. Cochrane Database Syst Rev 2013, Issue 2. Art. No.: CD000567. DOI: 10.1002/14651858.CD000567.pub6.
13. Bunn F, Trivedi D. Colloid solutions for fluid resuscitation. Cochrane Database Syst Rev 2012, Issue 7. Art. No.: CD001319. DOI: 10.1002/14651858. CD001319.pub5.
14. Roberts I, Blackhall K, Alderson P, Bunn F, Schierhout G. Human albumin solution for resuscitation and volume expansion in critically ill patients. Cochrane Database Syst Rev 2011, Issue 11. Art. No.: CD001208. DOI: 10.1002/14651858.CD001208.pub4.
15. Soni N. British consensus guidelines on intravenous fluid therapy for adult surgical patients—Cassandra's view. *Anesthesia* 2009;64:235-238.

16. Pham TN, Cancio LC, Gibran NS. American Burn Association practice guidelines burn shock resuscitation. *J Burn Care Res* 2008;29:257-266.
17. Alam HB, Rhee P. New developments in fluid resuscitation. *Surg Clin North Am* 2007;87:55-72.
18. Didwania A, Miller J, Kassel D, et al. Effect of intravenous lactated Ringer's solution infusion on the circulating lactate concentration: Results of a prospective, randomized, double-blind, placebo-controlled trial. *Crit Care Med* 1997;25:1851-1854.
19. Jackson EV, Wiese J, Sigal B, et al. Effects of crystalloid solutions on circulating lactate concentrations: 1. Implications for the proper handling of blood specimens obtained in critically ill patients. *Crit Care Med* 1996;24:1840-1846.
20. Grocott MPW, Mythen MG, Gan TJ. Perioperative fluid management and clinical outcomes in adults. *Anesth Analg* 2005;100:1093-1106.
21. Schortgen F, Giron E, Deye N, Brochard L. The risk associated with hyperoncotic colloids in patients with shock. *Intensive Care Med* 2008;34:2157-2168.
22. Perner A, Haase N, Guttormsen AB, et al. Hydroxyethyl starch 130/0.42 versus Ringer's acetate in severe sepsis. *N Engl J Med* 2012;367:124-134.
23. Myburgh JA, Finfer S, Bellomo R, et al. Hydroxyethyl starch or saline for fluid resuscitation in intensive care. *N Engl J Med* 2012;367:1901-1911.
24. Cochrane Injuries Group Albumin Reviewers. Human albumin administration in critically ill patients: Systematic review of randomized controlled trials. *BMJ* 1998;317:235-240.
25. Choi PTL, Yip G, Quinonez LG, Cook DJ. Crystalloids vs. colloids in fluid resuscitation: A systematic review. *Crit Care Med* 1999;27:200-210.
26. The SAFE Study Investigators. A comparison of albumin and saline for fluid resuscitation in the intensive care unit. *N Engl J Med* 2004;350:2247-2256.
27. The SAFE Study Investigators. Saline or albumin for fluid resuscitation in patients with traumatic brain injury. *N Engl J Med* 2007;357:874-884.
28. Hollenberg SM. Vasoactive drugs in circulatory shock. *Am J Respir Crit Care Med* 2011;183:847-855.
29. De Backer D, Biston P, Devriendt J, et al. Comparison of dopamine and norepinephrine in the treatment of shock. *N Engl J Med* 2010;362:779-789.
30. Bickell WH, Wall MJ, Pepe PE, et al. Immediate versus delayed fluid resuscitation for hypotensive patients with penetrating torso injuries. *N Engl J Med* 1994;331:1105-1109.
31. Dutton RP, Mackenzie CF, Scalea TM. Hypotensive resuscitation during active hemorrhage: Impact on in-hospital mortality. *J Trauma* 2002;52:1141-1146.
32. Cooper DJ, Myles PS, McDermott FT, et al. Prehospital hypertonic saline resuscitation of patients with hypotension and severe traumatic brain injury. *JAMA* 2004;291:1350-1357.
33. Bulger EM, May S, Brasel KJ, et al. Out-of-hospital hypertonic resuscitation following severe traumatic brain injury: a randomized controlled trial. *JAMA* 2010;304:1455-1464.
34. Bulger EM, May S, Kirby JD, et al. Out-of-hospital hypertonic resuscitation after traumatic hypovolemic shock: A randomized, placebo controlled trial. *Ann Surg* 2011;253:431-441.
35. Brandstrup B, Tonnesen H, Beier-Holgersen R, et al. Effects of intravenous fluid restriction on postoperative complications: Comparison of two perioperative fluid regimens. *Ann Surg* 2003;238:641-648.
36. Hebert PC, Wells G, Blajchman MA, et al. A multicenter, randomized, controlled clinical trial of transfusion requirements in critical care. *N Engl J Med* 1999;340:409-417.
37. Hajjar LA, Vincent JL, Galas FRBG, et al. Transfusion requirements after cardiac surgery: The TRACS randomized controlled trial. *JAMA* 2010;304:1559-1567.
38. Hauser CJ, Boffard K, Dutton R, et al. Results of the CONTROL trial: Efficacy and safety of recombinant activated factor VII in the management of refractory traumatic hemorrhage. *J Trauma* 2010;69:489-500.
39. CRASH-2 Trial Collaborators. Effects of tranexamic acid on death, vascular occlusive events, and blood transfusion in trauma patients with significant hemorrhage (CRASH-2): A randomised, placebo-controlled trial. *Lancet* 2010;376:23-32.
40. Tanaka J, Matsuda T, Miyagantani Y, et al. Reduction of resuscitation fluid volumes in severely burned patients using ascorbic acid administration. *Arch Surg* 2000;135:326-331.
41. Rivers E, Nguyen B, Havstad S, et al. Early goal-directed therapy in the treatment of severe sepsis and septic-shock. *N Engl J Med* 2001;345:1368-1377.
42. The ProCESS Investigators. A randomized trial of protocol-based care for early septic shock. *N Engl J Med* 2014;370:1683-1693.
43. The ARISE Investigators and the ANZICS Clinical Trials Group. Goal-directed resuscitation for patients with early septic shock. *N Engl J Med* 2014;371:1496-1506.
44. Marik PE, Baram M, Vahid B. Does central venous pressure predict fluid responsiveness? *Chest* 2008;134:172-178.
45. Ivanov R, Allen J, Calvin JE. The incidence of major morbidity in critically ill patients managed with pulmonary artery catheters: A meta-analysis. *Crit Care Med* 2000;28:615-619.
46. Sandham JD, Hull RD, Brant RF, et al. A randomized, controlled trial of the use of pulmonary-artery catheters in high-risk surgical patients. *N Engl J Med* 2003;348:5-14.
47. Ginosar Y, Thijs LG, Sprung CL. Raising the standard of hemodynamic monitoring: Targeting the practice or the practitioner? *Crit Care Med* 1997;25:209-211.
48. Gomersall CD, Joynt GM, Freebairn RC, et al. Resuscitation of critically ill patients based on the results of gastric tonometry: A prospective, randomized, controlled trial. *Crit Care Med* 2000;28:607-614.
49. Sperry JL, Minei JP, Frankel HL, et al. Early use of vasopressors after injury: Caution before constriction. *J Trauma* 2008;64:9-14.
50. Boyd JH, Walley KR. Is there a role for sodium bicarbonate in treating lactic acidosis from shock? *Curr Opin Crit Care* 2008;14:379-383.

Introduction to Pulmonary Function Testing

e25

Maria I. Velez, Tamara D. Simpson, Stephanie M. Levine, and Jay I. Peters

KEY CONCEPTS

1. Normal ventilation–perfusion ratio. The function of the lungs is to maintain arterial partial pressure of oxygen (PaO_2) and arterial partial pressure of carbon dioxide ($PaCO_2$) within normal ranges. This goal is accomplished by matching 1 mL mixed venous blood with 1 mL fresh air ($\dot{V}/\dot{Q} = 1$). Normally, ventilation ($\dot{V}$) is less than perfusion ($\dot{Q}$, and $\dot{V}/\dot{Q}$ ratio is 0.8.
2. The air in the lung is divided into four compartments: tidal volume—air exhaled during quiet breathing; inspiratory reserve volume (IRV)—maximal air inhaled above tidal volume; expiratory reserve volume (ERV)—maximum air exhaled below tidal volume; and residual volume (RV)—air remaining in the lung after maximal exhalation. The sum of all four components is the total lung capacity (TLC).
3. Obstructive lung disease is defined as an inability to get air out of the lung. It is identified on spirometry when forced expiratory volume in the first second of expiration (FEV_1)/forced vital capacity (FVC) (total amount of air that can be exhaled during a forced exhalation) (FEV_1/FVC) is less than 70% to 75% (or below the lower limit of normal (LLN) based on population studies).
4. Reversible airway obstruction is common in asthma and is sometimes seen in chronic obstructive pulmonary disease (COPD). An increase in FEV_1 of 12% (and greater than 0.2 L in adults) after an inhaled β-agonist suggests an acute bronchodilator response.
5. Restrictive lung disease is defined as an inability to get air into the lung and is best defined as a reduction in TLC (usually less than 80% predicted). It is suspected when FVC is low (less than 80% predicted) and FEV_1/FVC is normal.
6. Restrictive lung disease can be produced by a number of defects, such as increased elastic recoil (interstitial lung disease), respiratory muscle weakness (myasthenia gravis), mechanical restrictions (pleural effusion or kyphoscoliosis), and poor effort.

INTRODUCTION

The primary function of the respiratory system is to maintain normality of arterial blood gases, that is, arterial partial pressure of oxygen (PaO_2) and arterial partial pressure of carbon dioxide ($PaCO_2$). To achieve this goal, several processes must be accomplished, including alveolar ventilation, pulmonary perfusion, ventilation–perfusion matching, and gas transfer across the alveolar–capillary membrane. Alveolar ventilation is achieved by the cyclic process of air movement in and out of the lung. During inspiration, the inspiratory muscle contracts and generates negative pressure in the pleural space. This pressure gradient between the mouth and the alveoli draws fresh air (tidal volume [V_T]) into the lung. Approximately one third of the inspired gas stays in the conducting airways (dead space), and two third reaches the alveoli.

1 The human lung contains a series of branching, progressively tapering airways that originate at the glottis and terminate in a matrix of thin-walled alveoli. Coursing through this matrix of alveoli is a rich network of capillaries that originates from the pulmonary arterioles and terminates in the pulmonary venules. The adequacy of respiration in each gas exchange unit depends on the apposition of a thin film of mixed venous blood with just the right amount of fresh alveolar gas. During "ideal" gas exchange, blood flow and ventilation are uniform; accordingly, there is no alveolar–arterial difference (or gradient) in the partial pressure of oxygen ($P[A–a]O_2$, sometimes called the A–a gradient). However, gas exchange is not perfect, even in the normal lung. Normally, alveolar ventilation is less than pulmonary blood flow, and the overall ventilation–perfusion ratio is 0.8 (not 1.0).

Normal expiration is a passive process, and when the inspiratory muscles end their contraction, the elastic recoil of the lung pulls the lung back to its original size and shape. This process makes the alveolar pressure positive relative to the pressure at the mouth, and air flows out of the lung. During inspiration, the respiratory muscles must overcome the elastic properties of the lung (elastic recoil) and the resistance to air flow by the airways. During expiration, the flow of air is determined primarily by the elastic recoil and airway resistance.

Different pulmonary function tests (PFTs) are used to evaluate the physiologic processes of the respiratory system. Physiologic abnormalities that can be measured by pulmonary function testing include obstruction to airflow, restriction of lung size, and decrease in transfer of gas across the alveolar–capillary membrane. Simple spirometry is frequently used to screen patients for evidence of obstruction or restrictive lung disease when they present with pulmonary complaints. Abnormal values on PFTs are outside the range of values obtained from a group of normal individuals matched according to age, height, sex, and race. A PFT is labeled abnormal when the results fall outside the range in which 95% of people of same age, height, and sex would be found (95% confidence interval). This definition is arbitrary and may misclassify a small percentage of normal individuals as having lung dysfunction; it also may miss patients with mild pulmonary disease. Therefore, clinical correlation and serial pulmonary function testing may be necessary for optimal interpretation of PFTs.

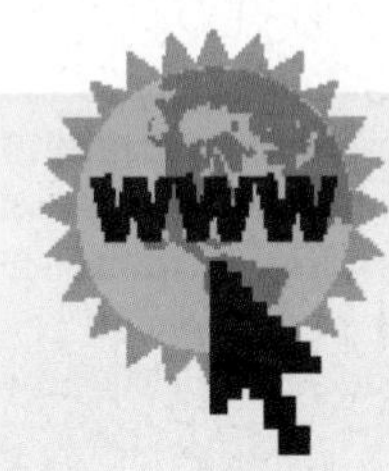

The complete chapter, learning objectives, and other resources can be found at **www.pharmacotherapyonline.com.**

26 Asthma

Christine A. Sorkness and Kathryn V. Blake

KEY CONCEPTS

1. Asthma is a disease of increasing prevalence that is a result of genetic predisposition and environmental interactions; it is one of the most common chronic diseases of childhood.
2. Asthma is primarily a chronic inflammatory disease of the airways of the lung for which there is no known cure or primary prevention; the immunohistopathologic features include cell infiltration by neutrophils, eosinophils, T-helper type 2 lymphocytes, mast cells, and epithelial cells.
3. Asthma is characterized by either the intermittent or persistent presence of highly variable degrees of airflow obstruction from airway wall inflammation and bronchial smooth muscle constriction; in some patients, persistent changes in airway structure occur.
4. The inflammatory process in asthma is treated most effectively with corticosteroids, with the inhaled corticosteroids (ICSs) having the greatest efficacy and safety profile for long-term management.
5. Bronchial smooth muscle constriction is prevented or treated most effectively with inhaled β_2-adrenergic receptor agonists.
6. Variability in response to medications requires individualization of therapy within existing evidence-based guidelines for management. This is most evident in patients with severe asthma phenotypes.
7. Ongoing patient education, for a partnership in asthma care, is essential for optimal patient outcomes and includes trigger avoidance and self-management techniques.

Asthma has been known since antiquity, yet it is a disease that still defies precise definition. The word *asthma* is of Greek origin and means "panting." More than 2,000 years ago, Hippocrates used the word *asthma* to describe episodic shortness of breath; however, the first detailed clinical description of the asthmatic patient was made by Aretaeus in the second century.[1] The National Institutes of Health, National Asthma Education and Prevention Program (NAEPP) Expert Panel Report 3 (EPR3), has provided the following working definition of asthma[2]:

> "Asthma is a chronic inflammatory disorder of the airways in which many cells and cellular elements play a role: in particular, mast cells, eosinophils, T-lymphocytes, macrophages, neutrophils, and epithelial cells. In susceptible individuals, this inflammation causes recurrent episodes of wheezing, breathlessness, chest tightness, and coughing, particularly at night or in the early morning. These episodes are usually associated with widespread but variable airflow obstruction that is often reversible either spontaneously or with treatment. The inflammation also causes an associated increase in the existing bronchial hyper-responsiveness (BHR) to a variety of stimuli. Reversibility of airflow limitation may be incomplete in some patients with asthma."
>
> The Global Initiative for Asthma (GINA) provides a new practical asthma definition[3]:
>
> "Asthma is a *heterogeneous* disease, usually characterized by chronic airway inflammation. It is defined by the history of respiratory symptoms such as wheeze, shortness of breath, chest tightness, and cough that vary over time and in intensity, together with variable expiratory airflow limitation."

These definitions encompass the important heterogeneity of the clinical presentation of asthma by describing the scientific and clinically accepted characteristics of asthma.

EPIDEMIOLOGY

1 An estimated 25.7 million persons in the United States have asthma (about 8.4% of the population).[4] Asthma is the most common chronic disease among children in the United States, with approximately 7 million children affected. The prevalence rate is highest in children 0 to 17 years of age at 9.5%.[4] In the United States, as in other industrialized countries, the prevalence of asthma has increased from 7.3% in 2001. Asthma prevalence is higher in persons with incomes below 100% of poverty level at 11.2% and in blacks 11.2% and multiple races 14.1%. Asthma accounts for 1.6% of all ambulatory care visits (10.6 million physician office visits and 1.2 million hospital outpatient visits) and resulted in 479,000 hospitalizations and 2.1 million emergency department (ED) visits in 2009 (both declined from peaks in the 1990s).[5] It is still a leading cause of preventable hospitalization in the United States; however, hospitalizations decreased 24% between 2003 and 2010. Asthma accounts for more than 14.4 million lost school days per year.[5] In young children (0-10 years of age), the risk of asthma is greater in boys than in girls, becomes about equal during puberty, and then is greater in women than in men.[5]

Ethnic minorities continue to share the burden of asthma disproportionately. African Americans are two times as likely to be hospitalized and approximately two times more likely to die from asthma than whites.[4] Hispanics in general, with the exception of Puerto Ricans, have lower disease and hospitalization rates than African Americans or whites.

The estimated direct healthcare costs of asthma in the United States from 2002 to 2007 was $50.1 billion.[5] The societal burden of asthma (indirect medical expenditures: loss of productivity and death) in the United States was $5.9 billion. Prescription drugs were the largest single direct medical expenditure.[5]

The natural history of asthma is still not well defined. Although asthma can occur at any time, it is principally a pediatric disease, with most patients being diagnosed by 5 years of age and up to 50% of children having symptoms by 2 years of age.[2] Between 30% and 70% of children with asthma will improve markedly or become symptom-free by early adulthood; chronic disease persists in about 30% to 40% of patients, and generally 20% or less develop severe chronic disease.[2] Predictors of persistent adult asthma include atopy, onset during school age, and presence of bronchial hyperresponsiveness (BHR).[2] Diminished lung growth may occur in some children (approximately 10%) with asthma.[2]

In adults, most longitudinal studies have suggested a more rapid rate of decline in lung function in asthmatics than in nonasthmatic normals, primarily reflected in forced expiratory volume in 1 second (FEV_1).[2] However, the annual decline in FEV_1 is less than in smokers or in patients with a diagnosis of emphysema. In general, individuals with less frequent asthma attacks and normal lung function on initial assessment have higher remission rates, whereas smokers have the lowest remission and highest relapse rates.[2] The level of BHR tends to predict the rate of decline in FEV_1, with a greater decline with high levels of BHR.[2] Thus, airway obstruction in asthma may become irreversible and also worsen over time owing to airway remodeling (see below).[2] However, most patients do not die from long-term progression of their disease and their life span is not different from the general population.[2]

As with prevalence and morbidity, mortality from acute exacerbations of asthma has been decreasing over the past 10 years, with a death rate of 0.14 per 1,000 persons with asthma reported in 2009.[3] Despite the relatively low number of asthma deaths, 80% to 90% are preventable.[2] Most deaths from asthma occur outside the hospital, and death is rare after hospitalization. The most common cause of death from asthma is inadequate assessment of the severity of airway obstruction by the patient or healthcare professional and inadequate therapy. The most common cause of death in hospitalized patients is also inadequate or inappropriate therapy. Thus, the key to prevention of death from asthma, as advocated by both US NAEPP and GINA, is education.[2,3]

ETIOLOGY

1 Epidemiologic studies strongly support the concept of a genetic predisposition plus environmental interaction to the development of asthma, yet the picture remains complex and incomplete.[6] Genetic factors account for 60% to 80% of the susceptibility. Asthma represents a complex genetic disorder in that the asthma phenotype is likely a result of polygenic inheritance or different combinations of genes. Initial searches focused on establishing links between atopy (genetically determined state of hypersensitivity to environmental allergens) and asthma, but genome-wide searches have also found linkages with genes for metalloproteinases involved in the airway remodeling process (eg, *ADAM33*) and those associated with asthma development and disease deterioration (*CHI3L1*).[6] Although genetic predisposition to atopy is a significant risk factor for developing asthma, not all atopic individuals develop asthma, nor do all patients with asthma exhibit atopy. Disparate phenotypes of asthma (progressive or remodeled vs non-progressive) are likely genetically determined.[6]

1 Environmental risk factors for the development of asthma include socioeconomic status, family size, exposure to secondhand tobacco smoke in infancy and in utero, allergen exposure, ambient air pollution, urbanization, viral respiratory infections including respiratory syncytial virus (RSV) and rhinovirus, and decreased exposure to common childhood infectious agents.[7,8] The "hygiene hypothesis" proposes that genetically susceptible individuals develop allergies and asthma by allowing the allergic immunologic system (T-helper cell type 2 [Th_2] lymphocytes) to develop instead of the system to fight infections (T-helper type 1 [Th_1] lymphocytes) and may explain the increase of asthma in developed countries.[7,8] The first 2 years of life appear to be most important for the exposures to produce an alteration in the immune response system.[7] The hygiene hypothesis is supported by studies demonstrating a lower risk for asthma in children who are exposed to high levels of bacteria or endotoxin, in those with a large number of older siblings, in those with early enrollment into child care, in those with exposure to cats, dogs, and farm animals early in life, or in those with exposure to fewer antibiotics.[6-9]

Risk factors for early (less than 3 years of age) recurrent wheezing associated with viral infections include low birth weight, male gender, and parental smoking. However, this early pattern is due to smaller airways, and these risk factors are not necessarily risk factors for asthma in later life.[7] Atopy is the predominant risk factor for children to have continued asthma.[7,8] Asthma can begin in adults later in life. Occupational asthma in previously healthy individuals emphasizes the effect of environment on the development of asthma.[10] The heterogeneity of the asthma phenotype appears most obvious when listing the diverse triggers of bronchospasm[2,7] (Table 26-1). The various triggers have relative degrees of importance from patient to patient. Environmental exposures are the most important precipitants of severe asthma exacerbations (see Table 26-1). Epidemics of severe asthma in cities have followed exposures to high concentrations of aeroallergens. Viral respiratory tract infections remain the single most significant precipitant of severe asthma in children and are an important trigger in adults as well.[11] Other possible factors include air pollution, sinusitis, and drugs.

TABLE 26-1 List of Agents and Events Triggering or Increasing Susceptibility to Asthma

Respiratory infection
Respiratory syncytial virus (RSV), rhinovirus, influenza, parainfluenza, *Mycoplasma pneumonia*, *Chlamydia*
Allergens
Airborne pollens (grass, trees, weeds), house dust mites, animal dander, rodents, cockroaches, fungal spores
Environment
Cold air, fog, ozone, sulfur dioxide, nitrogen dioxide, tobacco smoke (including 2nd and 3rd hand), wood smoke, energy efficient buildings (increase indoor air pollution), meteorological conditions related to climate change, scented home products, cleaners, and perfumes
Emotions
Anxiety, stress, laughter
Exercise
Particularly in cold, dry climate
Drugs/preservatives
Acetaminophen, Aspirin, NSAIDs (cyclooxygenase inhibitors), sulfites, benzalkonium chloride, nonselective β-blockers
Occupational stimuli
Bakers (flour dust); farmers (hay mold); spice and enzyme workers; occupational cleaners, printers (arabic gum); chemical workers (azo dyes, anthraquinone, ethylenediamine, toluene diisocyanates, polyvinyl chloride); plastics, rubber, and wood workers (formaldehyde, western cedar, dimethylethanolamine, anhydrides)
Host factors: obesity, African American race, Hispanic ethnicity, low socioeconomic status

PATHOPHYSIOLOGY

2 Major characteristics of asthma include a variable degree of airflow obstruction (related to bronchospasm, edema, and mucous hypersecretion), BHR, and airway inflammation (Fig. 26-1). To understand the pathogenetic mechanisms that underlie the many phenotypes of asthma, it is critical to identify factors that initiate, intensify, and modulate the inflammatory response of the airways

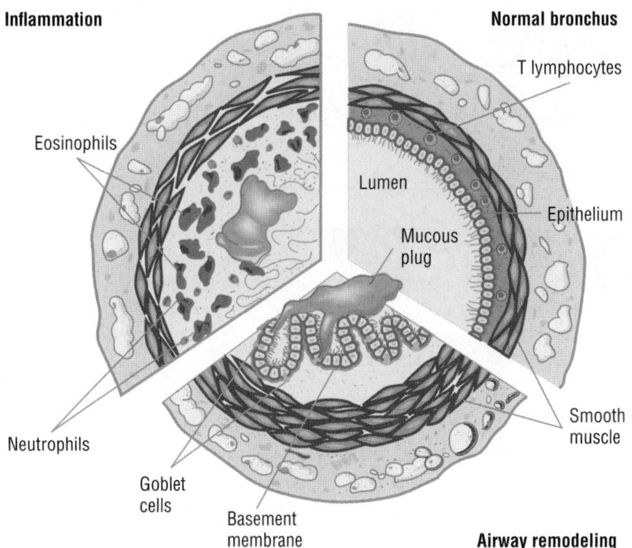

FIGURE 26-1 Representative illustration of the pathology found in the asthmatic bronchus compared with a normal bronchus (*upper right*). Each section demonstrates how the lumen is narrowed. Hypertrophy of the basement membrane, mucus plugging, smooth muscle hypertrophy, and constriction contribute (*lower section*). Inflammatory cells infiltrate, producing submucosal edema, and epithelial desquamation fills the airway lumen with cellular debris and exposes the airway smooth muscle to other mediators (*upper left*).

and to determine how these processes produce the characteristic airway abnormalities.

Acute Inflammation

Inhaled allergen challenge models contribute most to our understanding of acute inflammation in asthma.[8] Inhaled allergen challenge in allergic patients leads to an early phase reaction that, in some cases, may be followed by a late-phase reaction. The activation of cells bearing allergen-specific immunoglobulin E (IgE) initiates the early phase reaction. It is characterized by the rapid activation of airway mast cells and macrophages leading to the rapid release of pro-inflammatory mediators such as histamine, eicosanoids, and reactive oxygen (O_2) species that induce contraction of airway smooth muscle, mucous secretion, and vasodilation.[8] The bronchial microcirculation has an essential role in this inflammatory process. Inflammatory mediators induce microvascular leakage with exudation of plasma in the airways.[8] Acute plasma protein leakage induces a thickened, engorged, and edematous airway wall and a consequent narrowing of the airway lumen. Plasma exudation may compromise epithelial integrity, and the presence of plasma in the lumen may reduce mucus clearance.[8] Plasma proteins also may promote the formation of exudative plugs mixed with mucus and inflammatory and epithelial cells. Together these effects contribute to airflow obstruction (see Fig. 26-1).

The late-phase inflammatory reaction occurs 6 to 9 hours after allergen provocation and involves the recruitment and activation of eosinophils, CD4$^+$ thymically derived lymphocytes (T cells), basophils, neutrophils, and macrophages.[8] There is selective retention of airway T cells, the expression of adhesion molecules, and the release of selected pro-inflammatory mediators and cytokines involved in the recruitment and activation of inflammatory cells.[8] The activation of T cells after allergen challenge leads to the release of Th_2-like cytokines that may modulate the late-phase response.[8] The release of preformed cytokines by mast cells is the likely initial trigger for the early recruitment of inflammatory cells that then recruit and induce the more persistent involvement by T cells.[8] The enhancement of nonspecific BHR usually can be demonstrated after the late-phase reaction but not after the early phase reaction following allergen or occupational challenge.

Chronic Inflammation

Airway inflammation has been demonstrated in all forms of asthma, and an association between the extent of inflammation and the clinical severity of asthma has been demonstrated in selected studies.[8] It is accepted that both central and peripheral airways are inflamed.

In asthma, all cells of the airways are involved and become activated (Fig. 26-2). Included are eosinophils, neutrophils, T cells, mast cells, alveolar macrophages and dendritic cells, epithelial cells, fibroblasts, and bronchial smooth muscle cells. These cells also regulate airway inflammation and initiate the process of remodeling by the release of cytokines and growth factors.[8,12]

Epithelial Cells

Bronchial epithelial cells participate in mucociliary clearance and removal of noxious agents; however, they also enhance inflammation by releasing eicosanoids, peptidases, matrix proteins, cytokines, chemokines, and nitric oxide (NO).[8] Epithelial cells can be activated by IgE-dependent mechanisms, viruses, pollutants, or histamine. In asthma, especially fatal asthma, extensive epithelial shedding occurs. The functional consequences of epithelial shedding may include heightened BHR, release of the chemokine eotaxin that attracts eosinophils, altered permeability of the airway mucosa, depletion of epithelial-derived relaxant factors, and loss of enzymes responsible for degrading pro-inflammatory neuropeptides. The integrity of airway epithelium may influence the sensitivity of the airways to various provocative stimuli. Epithelial cells also may be important in the regulation of airway remodeling and fibrosis.[8,12]

Eosinophils

Eosinophils play an effector role in asthma by releasing pro-inflammatory mediators, cytotoxic mediators, and cytokines.[8] Circulating eosinophils migrate to the airways by cell rolling, through interactions with selectins, and eventually adhere to the endothelium through the binding of integrins to adhesion proteins (vascular cell adhesion molecule 1 [VCAM-1] and intercellular adhesion molecule 1 [ICAM-1]). As eosinophils enter the matrix of the membrane, their survival is prolonged by interleukin 5 (IL-5) and granulocyte-macrophage colony-stimulating factor (GM-CSF). On activation, eosinophils release inflammatory mediators such as leukotrienes (LTs) and granule proteins to injure airway tissue.[8]

Lymphocytes

Mucosal biopsy specimens from patients with asthma contain lymphocytes, many of which express surface markers of inflammation. There are two types of T-helper CD4$^+$ cells. Th_1 cells produce IL-2 and interferon-γ (IFN-γ), both essential for cellular defense mechanisms. Th_2 cells produce cytokines (IL-4, 5, and 13) that mediate allergic inflammation. It is known that Th_1 cytokines inhibit the production of Th_2 cytokines, and vice versa. It is hypothesized that allergic asthmatic inflammation results from a Th_2-mediated mechanism (an imbalance between Th_1 and Th_2 cells).[8] However, it has also been observed that there exists a low Th_2 cytokine phenotype of asthma in adults that appears more resistant to usual therapies for asthma.[13]

Th_1 and Th_2 Cell Imbalance

The T-cell population in the cord blood of newborn infants is skewed toward a Th_2 phenotype.[7,8] The extent of the imbalance between Th_1 and Th_2 cells (as indicated by diminished IFN-γ production) during the neonatal phase may predict the subsequent development of allergic disease, asthma, or both. It has been suggested that infants at

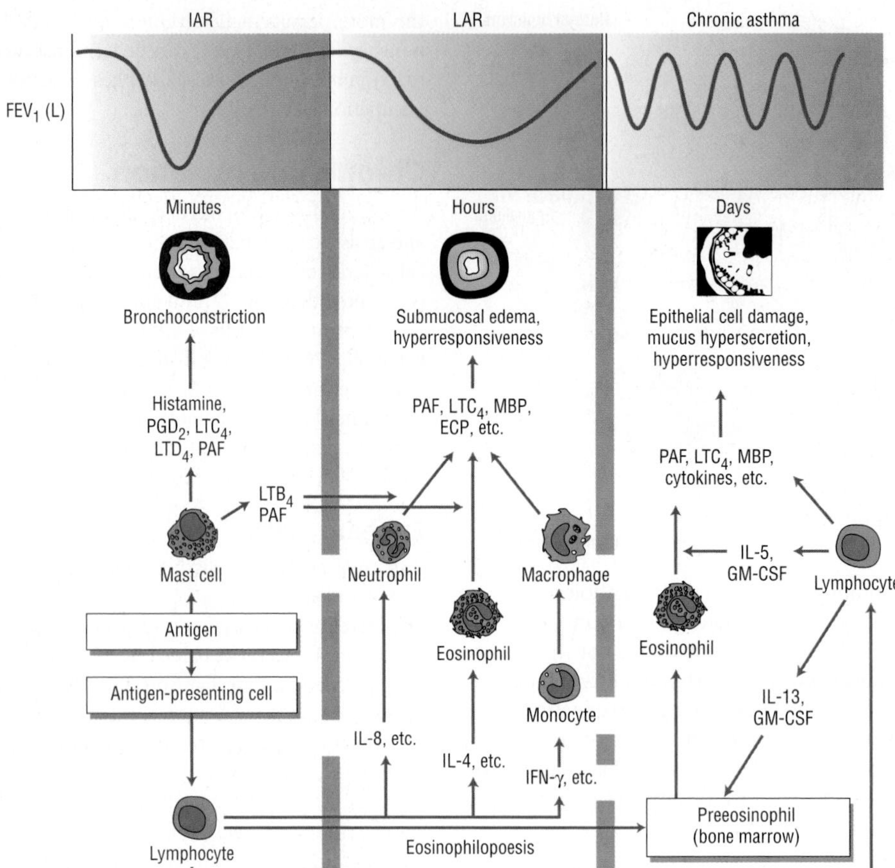

FIGURE 26-2 Diagrammatic presentation of the relationship between inflammatory cells, lipid and preformed mediators, inflammatory cytokines, and proposed pathogenesis and clinical presentation in asthma. See text for details. (GM-CSF, granulocyte-macrophage colony-stimulating factor; IL, interleukin; LT, leukotriene; MBP, major basic protein; PAF, platelet-activating factor; PG, prostaglandin.)

high risk of asthma and allergies should be exposed to stimuli that upregulate Th_1-mediated responses in order to restore the balance during a critical time in the development of the immune system and the lungs.[7]

The basic premise of the hygiene hypothesis is that the newborn's immune system needs timely and appropriate environmental stimuli to create a balanced immune response. Factors that enhance Th_1-mediated responses include infection with *Mycobacterium tuberculosis*, measles virus, and hepatitis A virus; endotoxin exposure; increased exposure to infections through contact with older siblings; and daycare attendance during the first 6 months of life. Restoration of the balance between Th_1 and Th_2 cells may be impeded by frequent administration of oral antibiotics, with concomitant alterations in GI flora. Other factors favoring the Th_2 phenotype include residence in an industrialized country, urban environment exposure, diet, and sensitization to house dust mites and cockroaches.[7] Immune "imprinting" may begin in utero by transplacental transfer of allergens and cytokines.

Mast Cells

Mast cell degranulation is important in the initiation of immediate responses following exposure to allergens.[2] Mast cells reside throughout the walls of the respiratory tract, and increased numbers of these cells (threefold to fivefold) have been described in the airways of allergic asthmatics.[8] Once binding of allergen to cell-bound IgE occurs, mediators such as histamine; eosinophil and neutrophil chemotactic factors; LTs C_4, D_4, and E_4; prostaglandins; platelet-activating factor (PAF); and others are released from mast cells (see Fig. 26-2). Histologic examination has revealed decreased numbers of granulated mast cells in the airways of patients who have died from acute asthma attacks, suggesting that mast cell degranulation is a contributing factor. Sensitized mast cells are also activated by osmotic stimuli to account for exercise-induced bronchospasm (EIB).[14]

Alveolar Macrophages

The primary function of alveolar macrophages in the normal airway is to serve as "scavengers," engulfing and digesting bacteria and other foreign materials. Macrophages are found in large and small airways, ideally located for affecting the asthmatic response. A number of mediators produced and released by macrophages have been identified, including proinflammatory and anti-inflammatory cytokines, reactive oxygen species, and eicosanoids.[7] In addition, alveolar macrophages are able to produce neutrophil chemotactic factor and eosinophil chemotactic factor, which in turn amplify the inflammatory process.

Neutrophils

The role of neutrophils in the pathogenesis of asthma remains somewhat unclear because they normally may be present in the airways and usually do not infiltrate tissues showing chronic allergic inflammation despite the potential to participate in late-phase inflammatory reactions. However, high numbers of neutrophils have been observed in the airways of patients who died from sudden-onset fatal asthma and in those with severe disease.[15] This suggests that neutrophils may play a pivotal role in the disease process, at least in some patients with long-standing or corticosteroid-resistant asthma.[13,15] The neutrophil also can be a source for a variety of mediators, including PAF, prostaglandins, thromboxanes, and LTs, that contribute to BHR and airway inflammation.[15]

Fibroblasts and Myofibroblasts

Fibroblasts are found frequently in connective tissue. Human lung fibroblasts may behave as inflammatory cells on activation by IL-4 and IL-13. The myofibroblast may contribute to the regulation of inflammation via the release of cytokines and to tissue remodeling. In asthma, myofibroblasts are increased in numbers beneath the reticular basement membrane, and there is an association between their numbers and the thickness of the reticular basement membrane.[8,12]

Inflammatory Mediators

Associated with asthma for many years, histamine is capable of inducing smooth muscle constriction and bronchospasm and is thought to play a role in mucosal edema and mucous secretion.[2] Lung mast cells are an important source of histamine. The release of histamine can be stimulated by exposure of the airways to a variety of factors, including physical stimuli (airway drying with exercise) and relevant allergens.[8] Histamine is involved in acute bronchospasm following allergen exposure; however, other mediators such as LTs are also involved.

Besides histamine release, mast cell degranulation releases ILs, proteases, and other enzymes that activate the production of other mediators of inflammation. Several classes of important mediators, including arachidonic acid and its metabolites (ie, prostaglandins, LTs, and PAF), are derived from cell membrane phospholipids.

Once arachidonic acid is released, it can be metabolized by the enzyme cyclooxygenase to form prostaglandins. Prostaglandin D_2 is a potent bronchoconstricting agent; however, it is unlikely to produce sustained effects and its role in asthma remains to be determined. Similarly, prostaglandin $F_2\alpha$ is a potent bronchoconstrictor in patients with asthma and can enhance the effects of histamine.[2,8] However, its pathophysiologic role in asthma is unclear. Another cyclooxygenase product, prostacyclin (prostaglandin I_2), is known to be produced in the lung and may contribute to inflammation and edema owing to its effects as a vasodilator.

Thromboxane A_2 is produced by alveolar macrophages, fibroblasts, epithelial cells, neutrophils, and platelets within the lung.[8] It may have several effects, including bronchoconstriction, involvement in the late asthmatic response, and involvement in the development of airway inflammation and BHR.

The 5-lipoxygenase pathway of arachidonic acid metabolism is responsible for the production of the *cysteinyl LTs*.[8] LTC_4, LTD_4, and LTE_4 are released during inflammatory processes in the lung. LTs D_4 and E_4 share a common receptor (LTD_4 receptor) that, when stimulated, produces bronchospasm, mucous secretion, microvascular permeability, and airway edema, whereas LTB_4 is involved with granulocyte chemotaxis.

Thought to be produced by macrophages, eosinophils, and neutrophils within the lung, PAF is involved in the mediation of bronchospasm, sustained induction of BHR, edema formation, and chemotaxis of eosinophils.[8]

Adhesion Molecules

Adhesion molecules are glycoproteins that facilitate infiltration and migration of inflammatory cells to the site of inflammation. They have additional functions involved in the inflammatory process aside from promoting cell adhesion, including activation of cells and cell–cell communication, and promoting cellular migration and infiltration.[2] Many adhesion molecules are divided into families on the basis of their chemical structure. These families are the integrins, cadherins, immunoglobulin supergene family, selectins, vascular adressins, and carbohydrate ligands.[8] Those thought to be important in inflammation include the integrins, immunoglobulin supergene family, selectins, and carbohydrate ligands, including ICAM-1 and VCAM-1.[8] Adhesion molecules are found on a variety of cells, such as neutrophils, monocytes, lymphocytes, basophils, eosinophils, granulocytes, platelets, endothelial cells, and epithelial cells, and can be expressed or activated by the many inflammatory mediators present in asthma.[8]

Clinical Consequences of Chronic Inflammation

Chronic inflammation is associated with nonspecific BHR and increases the risk of asthma exacerbations. Exacerbations are characterized by increased symptoms and worsening airway obstruction over a period of days or even weeks, and rarely hours. Hyper-responsiveness of the airways to physical, chemical, and pharmacologic stimuli is a hallmark of asthma.[2] BHR also occurs in some patients with chronic bronchitis and allergic rhinitis.[2] Normal healthy subjects also may develop a transient BHR after viral respiratory infections or ozone exposure. However, the degree of BHR in patients with asthma is quantitatively greater than in other populations. Bronchial responsiveness of the general population fits a unimodal distribution that is skewed toward increased reactivity; individuals with clinical asthma represent the extreme end of this distribution. The degree of BHR within asthma correlates with its clinical course and medication requirement necessary to control symptoms.[2] Patients with mild symptoms or in remission demonstrate lower levels of BHR.

The current understanding is that the BHR seen in asthma is at least in part due to and correlative with the extent of airway inflammation.[2] Airway remodeling also correlates somewhat with BHR.[12]

Remodeling of the Airways

Acute inflammation is a beneficial, nonspecific response of tissues to injury and generally leads to repair and restoration of the normal structure and function. In contrast, asthma represents a chronic inflammatory process of the airways followed by healing that in some may result in altered structure referred to as *remodeling*.[12] Repair involves replacement of injured tissue by parenchymal cells of the same type and replacement by connective tissue and its maturation into scar tissue. In asthma, remodeling presents as extracellular matrix fibrosis, an increase in smooth muscle and mucous gland mass, and angiogenesis.[12]

The precise mechanisms of remodeling of the airways are under intense study. Airway remodeling is of concern because it may represent an irreversible process that can have more serious sequelae such as the development of chronic obstructive pulmonary disease (COPD).[2,12] Observations in children with asthma indicate that some loss of lung function may occur during the first 5 years of life.[7] Importantly, no current therapies have been shown to alter either early decreased lung growth or later progressive loss of lung function.

Mucus Production

The mucociliary system is the lung's primary defense mechanism against irritants and infectious agents. Mucus, composed of 95% water and 5% glycoproteins, is produced by bronchial epithelial glands and goblet cells.[8] The lining of the airways consists of a continuous aqueous layer controlled by active ion transport across the epithelium in which water moves toward the lumen along the concentration gradient. Catecholamines and vagal stimulation enhance the ion transport and fluid movement. Mucus transport depends on its viscoelastic properties. Mucus that is either too watery or too viscous will not be transported optimally. The exudative inflammatory process and sloughing of epithelial cells into the airway lumen impair mucociliary transport. The bronchial glands are increased in size and the goblet cells are increased in size and number in asthma. Expectorated mucus from patients with asthma tends to have a high viscosity. The mucous plugs in the airways of patients who died in status asthmaticus are tenacious and tend to be connected by mucous strands to the goblet cells. Asthmatic airways also may become plugged with casts consisting of epithelial and inflammatory cells. Although it is tempting to speculate that death from asthma attacks is a result of the mucous plugging resulting in irreversible obstruction, there is no direct evidence for this. Autopsies of asthmatics who died from other causes have shown similar pathology. In addition, some patients who have died of sudden severe asthma did not show the characteristic mucous plugging on necropsy.[8]

Airway Smooth Muscle

The airway smooth muscle extends from the trachea through the respiratory bronchioles. When expressed as a percentage of wall thickness, the smooth muscle represents 5% of the large central airways and up to 20% of the wall thickness in the bronchioles. Total smooth muscle mass decreases rapidly past the terminal bronchioles to the alveoli, so the contribution of smooth muscle tone to airway diameter in this region is relatively small. In the large airways of asthmatics, smooth muscle may account for 11% of the wall thickness. It is possible that the increased smooth muscle mass of the asthmatic airways is important in magnifying and maintaining BHR in persistent disease. However, it appears that the hypertrophy and hyperplasia are secondary processes caused by chronic inflammation and are not the primary cause of BHR.[16]

Neural Control/Neurogenic Inflammation

The airway is innervated by parasympathetic, sympathetic, and non-adrenergic inhibitory nerves.[2] Parasympathetic innervation of the smooth muscle consists of efferent motor fibers in the vagus nerves and sensory afferent fibers in the vagus and other nerves.[16] Normal resting tone of human airway smooth muscle is maintained by vagal efferent activity. Maximum bronchoconstriction mediated by vagal stimulation occurs in the small bronchi and is absent in the small bronchioles. The non-myelinated C fibers of the afferent system lie immediately beneath the tight junctions between epithelial cells lining the airway lumen.[16] These nerve endings probably represent the irritant receptors of the airways. Stimulation of these irritant receptors by mechanical stimulation, chemical and particulate irritants, and pharmacologic agents such as histamine produces reflex bronchoconstriction.[8]

The non-adrenergic, non-cholinergic (NANC) nervous system has been described in the trachea and bronchi. Substance P, neurokinin A, neurokinin B, and vasoactive intestinal peptide (VIP) are the best characterized neurotransmitters in the NANC nervous system.[8] VIP is an inhibitory neurotransmitter. Inflammatory cells in asthma can release peptidases that can degrade VIP, producing exaggerated reflex cholinergic bronchoconstriction. NANC excitatory neuropeptides such as substance P and neurokinin A are released by stimulation of C-fiber sensory nerve endings. The NANC system may play an important role in amplifying inflammation in asthma by releasing NO.

Nitric Oxide

NO is produced by cells within the respiratory tract. It has been thought to be a neurotransmitter of the NANC nervous system.[17] Endogenous NO is generated from the amino acid L-arginine (L-Arg) by the enzyme NO synthase.[17] Three isoforms of NO synthase exist. One isoform is induced in response to pro-inflammatory cytokines, inducible NO synthase (iNOS), in airway epithelial cells and inflammatory cells of asthmatic airways.[17] NO produces smooth muscle relaxation in the vasculature and bronchials; however, it appears to amplify the inflammatory process and is unlikely to be of therapeutic benefit. Investigations measuring the fraction of exhaled NO (FeNO) concentrations have suggested that it may be a useful measure of ongoing lower airway inflammation in patients with asthma and for guiding asthma therapy.[17]

CLINICAL PRESENTATION Chronic Ambulatory Asthma

General

- Asthma is a disease of exacerbation and remission, so the patient may not have any signs or symptoms at the time of examination.

Symptoms

- The patient may complain of episodes of shortness of breath, chest tightness, coughing (particularly at night), wheezing, or a whistling sound when breathing. These often occur in association with exercise, but also occur spontaneously or in association with known allergens.

Signs

- Expiratory wheezing (rhonchi) on auscultation, dry hacking cough, or signs of atopy (allergic rhinitis and/or atopic dermatitis) may occur.

Laboratory

- Spirometry demonstrates obstruction (reduced FEV_1/forced vital capacity [FVC]) with reversibility following inhaled β_2-agonist administration (FEV_1 increases by more than 12% and 200 mL). The FEV_1/FVC ratio is normally more than 0.75 to 0.80 in adults, and more than 0.90 in children.

Other Diagnostic Tests

- Excessive variability in twice daily peak expiratory flow (PEF) over 2 weeks (greater than 10% in adults and greater than 13% in children). A fall in FEV_1 of at least 10% following 6 minutes of near maximal exercise. Elevated eosinophil count and IgE concentration in blood. Elevated FeNO (greater than 20 ppb in children younger than 12 years of age and greater than 25 ppb in adults). Positive methacholine challenge (PC_{20} FEV_1 less than 12.5 mg/mL) or mannitol challenge (FEV_1 decrease of at least 15% from baseline after 635 mg or less).

CLINICAL PRESENTATION

Chronic Asthma

3 Classic asthma is characterized by episodic and variable respiratory symptoms; however, the clinical presentation of asthma is as diverse as the number of triggering events (see Clinical Presentation: Chronic Ambulatory Asthma above). Although wheezing is the characteristic symptom of asthma, the medical literature is replete with the warning that "not all that wheezes is asthma." A wheeze is a high-pitched, whistling sound created by turbulent airflow through an obstructed airway, so any condition that produces significant obstruction can result in wheezing as a symptom. In addition, "all of asthma does not wheeze" is an equally justifiable warning. Patients may present with a chronic persistent cough (cough variant asthma) as their only symptom.[2,3]

There is no single diagnostic test for asthma. The diagnosis is based primarily on a good history.[2,3] The patient may have a family history of allergy or asthma or have symptoms of allergic rhinitis, or atopic dermatitis.[2,3] Reversibility of airway obstruction following administration of a short-acting inhaled β_2-agonist provides confirmation but is not by itself diagnostic. GINA adds excessive variability in twice daily PEF over 2 weeks as an alternative diagnostic test.[3] Patients with normal values of spirometry can be challenged by exercise or substances that produce bronchoconstriction, such as methacholine or mannitol, to determine if they have BHR, but, again, positive challenges are not diagnostic. Newer tests of inflammation in the airways such as induced sputum eosinophil and/or neutrophil counts and FeNO measurements are consistent with but not diagnostic of asthma.

GINA recommends confirmation of the diagnosis of asthma in patients already taking controller treatment using objective testing. The process depends on the patient's symptoms and lung function, and may include a trial of either a lower or a higher dose of controller treatment.[3]

Asthma has a widely variable presentation from chronic daily symptoms to only intermittent symptoms. The intervals between symptoms can be days, weeks, months, or years. Asthma also can vary as to its severity, the intrinsic intensity of the disease process. Severity is most easily and directly measured in a patient who is not currently receiving asthma treatment. The NAEPP has provided a means of classifying asthma severity that is divided into two domains: impairment and risk.[2] This classification system is individualized for three age groups (0-4, 5-11, and greater than or equal to 12 years) and summarized in Table 26-2. GINA has provided a means of determining chronic therapy for children and adults aged 6 years and older based on symptom control and future risk of adverse outcomes, described later in this chapter.

TABLE 26-2 Classifying Asthma Severity for Patients Who Are Not Currently Taking Long-Term Control Medications

			Children 0-4 and 5-11 Years of Age		
			Persistent		
	Components	**Intermittent**	**Mild**	**Moderate**	**Severe**
Impairment	Symptoms	≤2 days/wk	>2 days/wk but not daily	Daily	Throughout the day
	Nighttime awakenings (0-4 years)	0	1-2 × month	3-4 × month	>1 × week
	5-11 years	≤2 × month	3-4 × month	>1 × week, but not nightly	Often 7 × week
	SABA use for Sx control	≤2 days/wk	>2 days/wk but not daily	Daily	Several times per day
	Interference with normal activity	None	Minor limitation	Some limitation	Extremely limited
	Lung function	FEV_1 > 80%	FEV_1 > 80%	FEV_1 60%-80%	FEV_1 < 60%
	5-11 years	FEV_1/FVC >85% (>0.85)	FEV_1/FVC >80% (>0.80)	FEV_1/FVC 75%-80% (0.75-0.80)	FEV_1/FVC <75% (<0.75)
	Exacerbations	**Intermittent**	**Persistent**		
Risk	0-4 years	0-1/y	≥2 in 6 months or ≥4 wheezing episodes/1 year lasting >1 day		
	5-11 years	0-2/y	>2 in 1 year →		
	Recommended step for initiating treatment	Step 1	Step 2	Step 3 and consider short course of oral corticosteroids	
			Youths ≥ 12 Years of Age and Adults		
			Persistent		
	Components	**Intermittent**	**Mild**	**Moderate**	**Severe**
Impairment	Symptoms	≤2 days/wk	>2 days/wk but not daily	Daily	Throughout the day
	Nighttime awakenings	≤2 × month	3-4 × month	>1 × week, but not nightly	Often 7 × week
	SABA use for Sx control	≤2 days/wk	>2 days/wk, but not >1 × day	Daily	Several times per day
	Interference with normal activity	None	Minor limitation	Some limitation	Extremely limited
	Lung function[a]	FEV_1 > 80%	FEV_1 > 80%	FEV_1 60%-80%	FEV_1 < 60%
		FEV_1/FVC normal	FEV_1/FVC normal	FEV_1/FVC reduced 5% (0.05)	FEV_1/FVC reduced >5% (> 0.05)
	Exacerbations	**Intermittent**	**Persistent**		
Risk		0-2/y	>2 in 1 year →		
	Recommended step for initiating treatment	Step 1	Step 2	Step 3 and consider short course of oral corticosteroids	Step 4 or 5 and consider course of oral corticosteroid

SABA, short-acting β-agonist.

[a]Normal FEV_1/FVC: 8-19 years 85% (0.85); 20-39 years 80% (0.80); 40-59 years 75% (0.75); 60-80 years 70% (0.70).

CLINICAL PRESENTATION Acute Severe Asthma

General

- An episode can progress over several days or hours (usual scenario) or progresses rapidly over 1 to 2 hours.

Symptoms

- The patient is anxious in acute distress and complains of severe dyspnea, shortness of breath, chest tightness, or burning. The patient is only able to say a few words with each breath. Symptoms are unresponsive to usual measures (short-acting inhaled β_2-agonist administration).

Signs

- Signs include expiratory and inspiratory wheezing on auscultation (breath sounds may be diminished with very severe obstruction), dry hacking cough, tachypnea, tachycardia, pale or cyanotic skin, hyperinflated chest with intercostal and supraclavicular retractions, and hypoxic seizures if very severe.

Laboratory

- Peak expiratory flow and/or FEV_1 less than 40% of normal predicted values. Decreased arterial O_2 (PaO_2), and O_2 saturations by pulse oximetry (SaO_2 less than 90% [0.90] on room air is severe). Decreased arterial or capillary CO_2 if mild, but in the normal range or increased in moderate to severe obstruction.

Other Diagnostic Tests

- Blood gases to assess metabolic acidosis (lactic acidosis) in severe obstruction. Complete blood count if there are signs of infection (fever and purulent sputum). Serum electrolytes as therapy with β_2-agonist and corticosteroids can lower serum potassium, magnesium, and phosphate, and increase glucose. Chest radiograph if signs of consolidation on auscultation.

The intermittent and/or chronic nature of symptoms does not necessarily determine the severity of symptoms during exacerbations. Asthma severity is determined by lung function, symptoms, nighttime awakenings, and interference with normal activity prior to therapy. Patients can present with a range from intermittent symptoms that require no medications or only occasional use of short-acting inhaled β_2-agonists to severe persistent asthma symptoms despite treatment with multiple medications.

Acute Severe Asthma

Uncontrolled asthma, with its inherent variability, can progress to an acute state where inflammation, airway edema, excessive mucus accumulation, and severe bronchospasm result in a profound airway narrowing that is poorly responsive to usual bronchodilator therapy[2,3] (see Clinical Presentation: Acute Severe Asthma above). Although this progression is the most common scenario, some patients experience rapid-onset or hyper-acute attacks.[2,3] Hyperacute attacks are associated with neutrophilic as opposed to eosinophilic infiltration and resolve rapidly with bronchodilator therapy, suggesting that smooth muscle spasm is the major pathogenic mechanism.[15] In most cases, ED visits for acute severe asthma represent the failure of an adequate therapeutic regimen to control persistent asthma. Underutilization of anti-inflammatory drugs and excessive reliance on short-acting inhaled β_2-agonists are the major risk factors for severe exacerbations.[2,3] However, frequent exacerbations may represent a specific phenotype of asthma. A blunted perception of airway obstruction may predispose certain individuals to fatal asthma attacks.[2]

Exercise-Induced Bronchospasm

During vigorous exercise, pulmonary function measurements (FEV_1 and PEF) in patients with asthma increase during the first few minutes but then begin to decrease after 6 to 8 minutes (Fig. 26-3).[2] EIB is defined as a drop in FEV_1 of 10% or greater from baseline (pre-exercise value).[14] Most studies suggest that many patients with persistent asthma experience EIB.[2] The exact pathogenesis of EIB is unknown, but heat loss and/or water loss from the central airways appears to play an important role.[14] EIB is provoked more easily in cold, dry air, ambient ozone, and airborne particulate matter; alternatively, warm, humid air can blunt or block it.[14] Studies have demonstrated increased plasma histamine, cysteinyl leukotrienes, prostaglandins, and tryptase concentrations during EIB, suggesting a role for mast cell degranulation.[14] These findings led to the development of inhaled mannitol, an osmotic agent, as an indirect pharmacologic bronchoprovocation test to assist in the diagnosis of asthma.[18]

A refractory period following EIB lasts up to 4 hours after exercise in some patients. During this period, repeat exercise of the same intensity produces either no decrease in pulmonary function or a drop of less than 50% of the initial response.[14] The refractory period is thought to be caused by an acute depletion of mast cell mediators and time required for their repletion.

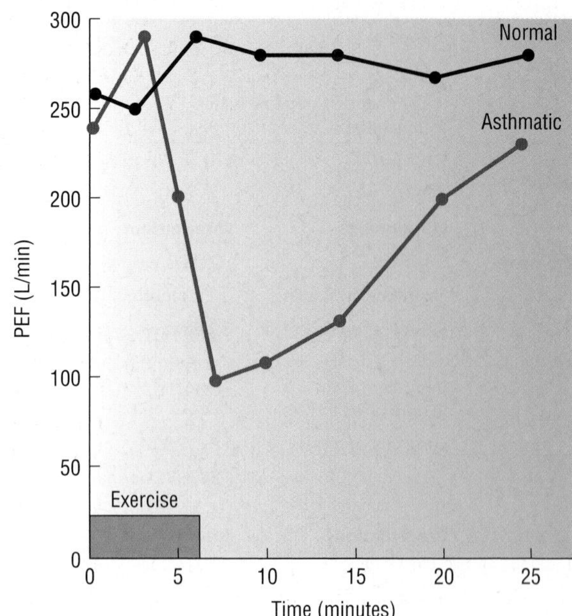

FIGURE 26-3 Typical responses to exercise in a normal subject and an asthmatic subject. Note the initial bronchodilation. (PEF, peak expiratory flow.)

Exercise-induced bronchospasm is believed to be a reflection of increased BHR associated with asthma. A correlation, though not perfect, exists between EIB and reactivity to histamine, methacholine, and mannitol.[14] Other patient groups with BHR (eg, after viral infection, cystic fibrosis, or allergic rhinitis) show bronchoconstriction after exercise to a lesser degree (5%-10% drops) than patients with asthma (15%-40% drops).[14] Patients will not always demonstrate the same sensitivity. During periods of remission, a decreased sensitivity to the same degree of exercise is often observed. Finally, a number of children and adults with EIB are otherwise normal, without symptoms or abnormal pulmonary function except in association with exercise.[2] Elite athletes have a higher prevalence of EIB than the general population.[14]

Nocturnal Asthma

3 Worsening of asthma during sleep is referred to as *nocturnal asthma*. Patients with nocturnal asthma exhibit significant falls in pulmonary function between bedtime and awakening.[2] Typically, their lung function reaches a nadir at 3 to 4 AM. Although the pathogenesis of this phenomenon is unknown, it has been associated with diurnal patterns of endogenous cortisol secretion and circulating epinephrine.[2] Direct evidence for an inflammatory component to nocturnal asthma includes increased circulating histamine and activated eosinophils and LT excretion at night associated with increased BHR to methacholine.[2]

Numerous other factors that may affect nocturnal worsening of asthma, including allergies and improper environmental control, gastroesophageal reflux, obstructive sleep apnea, and sinusitis, also must be considered when evaluating these patients.[2] Experts consider nocturnal symptoms to be a sign of inadequately treated persistent asthma.[2] Awakening from nocturnal asthma is a sensitive indicator of both severity and inadequate control.[2]

FACTORS CONTRIBUTING TO ASTHMA SEVERITY

Viral Respiratory Infections

Viral respiratory infections are primarily responsible for exacerbations of asthma, particularly in children under age 10.[11] Children aged 5 or younger may have wheezing (which may or may not be asthma) associated with upper respiratory tract infections up to 6 to 8 times per year.[3] Infants are particularly susceptible to airway obstruction and wheezing with viral infections because of their small airways. Approximately 50% of infants who have severe RSV bronchiolitis will subsequently be diagnosed with asthma. The most common cause of exacerbations in both children and adults is the rhinovirus, which is the most frequent virus associated with the common cold and distributed worldwide.[11] Other viruses isolated include RSV, parainfluenza virus, adenoviruses, coronavirus, and influenza viruses. Certain viruses (RSV and parainfluenza virus) are capable of inducing specific IgE antibodies, and rhinovirus can activate eosinophils directly in asthmatics.[11] The increase in asthma symptoms and BHR that occurs may last for days or weeks following resolution of the symptoms of the viral infection. Evidence does not support a beneficial effect of influenza vaccine for preventing asthma exacerbations from subsequent influenza infections.[2] However, patients with moderate-severe asthma should be vaccinated against influenza annually.[3]

Environmental and Occupational Factors

The development and heterogeneity of persistent asthma is driven by complex gene-environment interactions. Agents and events that are known to trigger asthma are listed in Table 26-1. The mechanisms for inducing symptoms are as varied as the exposure factor and include both IgE and cell-mediated reactions.[3] The World Allergy Organization predicts an increase in the incidence and prevalence of asthma due to environmental exposures from climate change. Greater temperature variability, industrial pollution, more frequent forest fires, higher concentration of ground level ozone, increased trans-boundary movement of respiratory infectious agents, and changes in aeroallergen distribution are all cited factors. Exposure to 0.2 ppm ozone for 2 to 3 hours can induce bronchoconstriction and increase BHR in asthmatics.[2,10] Sulfur dioxide in the ambient atmosphere is highly irritating and presumably induces bronchoconstriction through mast cell or irritant-receptor involvement.[2] Asthma produced by repeated prolonged exposure to industrial inhalants is a significant health problem. It has been estimated that occupational asthma accounts for 15% of all asthmatic persons.[3] An estimated 5% to 20% of new cases of adult-onset asthma can be attributed to occupational exposure.[3] Occupational asthma can be difficult to diagnose as the latency between exposure and symptom development can extend from months to years.[3] Persons with occupational asthma have the typical symptoms of asthma with cough, dyspnea, and wheeze. Typically, the symptoms are related to workplace exposure and improve on days off and during vacations.[10] Once occupational asthma has developed, the symptoms persist in most patients even after exposure is no longer present. [GINA Appendix 2015][3]

Stress, Depression, and Psychosocial Factors in Asthma

Observational studies demonstrate an association between increased stress and worsening asthma, but the role is not clearly defined.[2] Bronchoconstriction from psychological factors appears to be mediated primarily through excess parasympathetic input. Atropine has been shown to block experimental psychogenic bronchoconstriction. Persons with asthma are more likely to have depression than those without asthma. The episodic nature of both diseases may be related to abnormal expression of Th2 cytokines which have effects in the brain as well as the airway. It is most important to emphasize to both patients and parents that asthma is not an emotional disease; however, coping skills may benefit the patient who becomes emotionally distraught during an asthma attack.

Chronic Rhinosinusitis

Disorders of the upper respiratory tract, particularly rhinitis and sinusitis, have been linked with asthma for many years. As many as 40% to 50% of asthmatics have abnormal sinus radiographs.[2] The prevalence of allergic sensitization increases with asthma severity; nasal polyposis is often seen in those with allergic rhinitis. It has been postulated that transport of mucus chemotactic factors and inflammatory mediators from nasal passages during allergic rhinitis into the lungs may accentuate BHR. However, chronic sinusitis may just represent a nonbacterial coexisting condition with allergic asthmatics because the histologic changes in the paranasal sinuses are similar to those seen in the lung and nose.[2] Thus, it would seem that treatment of upper airway disease could optimize overall asthma control. However, a large study of children and adults found that treatment of chronic sinonasal disease with intranasal corticosteroids for six months did not improve asthma control nor improve BHR, suggesting that the treatment of sinus disease and asthma be managed separately.[19]

Gastroesophageal Reflux Disease

Symptoms of gastroesophageal reflux disease (GERD) as well as asymptomatic reflux are common in both children and adults who have asthma.[2] Nocturnal asthma may be associated with nighttime reflux.[2] Reflux of acidic gastric contents into the esophagus is thought to initiate a vagally mediated reflex bronchoconstriction.[2] Also of concern is that most medications that decrease airway smooth muscle tone may have a relaxant effect on gastroesophageal sphincter tone. There is no benefit from treating asymptomatic reflux in asthma.[3,20] Treatment with proton pump inhibitors does not improve asthma control even in those with documented reflux.[20] Symptomatic reflux should be treated for its general health benefits.[3]

Female Hormones and Asthma

Asthma symptoms may vary significantly during different stages of the menstrual cycle. Premenstrual worsening of asthma has been reported in as many as 30% to 40% of women in some studies, whereas worsening of pulmonary functions has been reported even in women not aware of worsening symptoms.[21] The pathophysiology is uncertain because estrogen replacement in postmenopausal women has been shown to worsen asthma, whereas estradiol and progesterone administration has been variably reported to improve or have no effect on asthma in women with premenstrual asthma.[21,22] The clinical significance of menstruation-related asthma is still unclear because some studies have reported that up to 50% of ED visits by women were premenstrual, whereas others have reported no association with menstrual phase.[21,22] Pregnancy may cause worsening, improvement or no change in asthma symptoms and the changes seem to occur with equal frequency. These changes are suspected to be related to altered sex hormones, stress, and fetal antigens.[22]

Foods, Drugs, Additives and Vitamins

Documentation in the literature of food allergens as triggers for asthma is not available.[2] However, additives, specifically sulfites used as preservatives, can trigger life-threatening asthma exacerbations. Beer, wine, dried fruit, and open salad bars, in particular, have high concentrations of metabisulfites.[2] Severe oral corticosteroid-dependent patients should be warned about ingesting foods processed with sulfites.

Aspirin and other nonsteroidal anti-inflammatory drugs can cause severe asthma exacerbations (aspirin-exacerbated respiratory disease).[3] The mechanism is related to cyclooxygenase-1 (COX-1) inhibition, and inhaled corticosteroids (ICSs) are the primary preventive treatment although oral corticosteroids may be required; leukotriene receptor antagonists (LTRAs) may be useful.[3] The prevalence increases with age and severity of asthma.[2] The greatest frequency occurs in severe corticosteroid-resistant asthmatics in their fourth and fifth decades who also have perennial rhinitis and nasal polyposis (presence of several polyps).[2] Other drugs that do not precipitate bronchospasm but that prevent its reversal are the nonselective β-blocking agents.[2,3]

Children with vitamin D insufficiency have been considered at greater risk of uncontrolled asthma (increased hospitalizations, BHR, and eosinophil counts).[25] Vitamin D helps regulate T cells and improves their secretion of anti-inflammatory cytokines in response to corticosteroids.[25] In adults with asthma, Vitamin D supplementation in those with levels below 30 ng/mL does not provide protection against exacerbations compared with placebo.[26] There are no published data evaluating Vitamin D treatment in children with asthma.

Obesity

Epidemiologic data suggest that obesity increases the prevalence of asthma and may reduce asthma control, although it may be difficult to distinguish obesity-induced respiratory symptoms from true asthma symptoms particularly because obesity often precedes the onset of asthma.[23] Lung volume and tidal volume are reduced in obesity, promoting airway narrowing. Obesity also produces low-grade systemic inflammation that may act on the lung to worsen asthma.[23] The mechanism may be the release of adipose-derived pro-inflammatory mediators such as IL-6, IL-10, eotaxin, tumor necrosis factor-α, transforming growth factors-β_1, C-reactive protein, leptin, and adiponectin or a result of common predisposing dietary factors. Although not all studies find relationship between body mass index and asthma control, management of asthma in obese patients should include weight loss measures.[24] Additional co-morbidities of obesity that may independently contribute to asthma symptoms include obstructive sleep apnea, GERD, and metabolic syndrome.[3]

Smoking History

During performance of a history that considers age, respiratory symptoms (onset, exacerbations, progression, variability, seasonality or periodicity, and persistence), past history, and previous diagnoses and treatment and response to treatment, the query of social and occupational risk factors may identify a smoking history of importance. The clinician is then faced with distinguishing asthma from COPD. Some patients have clinical features of both, now termed asthma COPD Overlap Syndrome (ACOS).[27] Physical examination findings, lung function measures, and radiology data are then combined with the history, to confirm this syndromic diagnosis. GINA and the Global Initiative for Chronic Obstructive Lung Disease provide recommendations for initial therapy of ACOS, if the differential diagnosis is equally balanced between asthma and COPD.[27] Referral for expert advice and further diagnostic evaluation may be necessary. A recent literature review has been published to characterize the prevalence of ACOS and the effect of different disease definitions on these estimates, to help guide decision making for both refining the ACOS definition and trial design aimed at effective treatment.[28]

TREATMENT

Asthma

Aerosol Therapy for Asthma

4 5 Aerosol delivery of drugs for asthma has the advantage of being site specific and thus enhancing the therapeutic ratio.[2,29] Inhalation of short-acting β_2-agonists provides more rapid bronchodilation than either parenteral or oral administration, as well as the greatest degree of protection against EIB and other challenges.[2] ICSs have been developed with rapid oral and systemic clearance to enhance lung activity and reduce systemic activity. Specific agents (eg, formoterol, salmeterol, and ipratropium bromide) are only effective by inhalation.[2] Therefore, an understanding of aerosol drug delivery is essential to optimal asthma therapy. Table 26-3 lists the factors determining lung deposition of therapeutic aerosols.

Device Determinants of Delivery

Devices used to generate therapeutic aerosols include jet nebulizers, ultrasonic nebulizers, metered-dose inhalers (MDIs), and dry powder inhalers (DPIs). The single most important device factor determining the site of aerosol deposition is particle size.[29] Devices for delivering therapeutic aerosols generate particles with mass median aerodynamic diameters (MMAD) from 0.5 to 35 μm.[29] Particles larger than 10 μm deposit in the oropharynx, particles between 5 and 10 μm deposit in the trachea and large bronchi, particles 1 to 5 μm in size reach the lower airways, and particles smaller than 0.5 μm act as a gas and are exhaled. As a result of the Montreal Protocol of 1987, chlorofluorocarbon (CFC) propellants in MDIs were phased out and replaced with hydrofluoroalkane (HFA) propellants that do not have ozone depleting properties.[29] The resultant MDIs, particularly for corticosteroid inhalers, are solution aerosols (vs suspensions) with extra-fine particle size distributions (MMAD of 1.1 μm) and high lung deposition. It has been suggested, but not robustly proven in clinical trials, that ICS HFA MDIs may improve asthma outcomes in patients due to greater penetration into the peripheral airways.

TABLE 26-3 Factors Determining Lung Deposition of Aerosols

Device	Device Factors	Patient Factors
Metered-dose inhaler (MDI)	Canister held inverted Formulation (solution or suspension) Actuator cleanliness Addition of a spacer device	Inspiratory flow (slow, deep) Breath-holding Tilting head back Coordinating actuation with inhalation Priming and shaking the device
Dry powder inhaler (DPI)	Device cleanliness Resistance to inhalation Humidity	Inspiratory flow (deep, forceful) Tilting head back Maintaining parallel to ground once activated
Jet nebulizer (small volume)	Volume fill (3-6 mL) Gas flow (6-12 L/min) Dead space volume Open vs closed system Thumb-activating valve Mouthpiece vs face mask	Inspiratory flow (slow, deep) Breath-holding Tapping nebulizer
Ultrasonic nebulizer	Volume fill Not effective for suspensions Mouthpiece vs face mask	Inspiratory flow (slow, deep) Breath-holding Tapping nebulizer
Spacer device	Volume (≥650 mL) One-way valves Holding chamber vs open-ended Antistatic lining Mouthpiece vs face mask	Inspiratory flow (slow, deep) Time between actuation and inhalation (<5 seconds) Cleaning with detergent to reduce static Multiple actuations (all at once) decrease delivery Coordination of actuation and inhalation for the simple open-tube spacers

In asthma, the airways, not the alveoli, are the target for delivery. Respirable particles are deposited in the airways by three mechanisms: (a) inertial impaction, (b) gravitational sedimentation, and (c) Brownian diffusion.[29] The first two mechanisms are the most important for therapeutic aerosols and probably are the only factors that can be manipulated by patients.

Each delivery device within a classification generates specific aerosol characteristics, so extrapolation of delivery data from one device cannot be applied to the other devices in the class. For instance, MDIs can deliver 15% to 50% of the actuated dose; DPIs, 10% to 30% of the labeled dose; and nebulizers, 2% to 15% of the starting dose.[29] MDIs and DPIs are portable and convenient, unlike jet nebulizers. Small portable ultrasonic nebulizers have also been developed.

Metered-dose inhalers consist of a pressurized canister with a metering valve; the canister contains active drug, low-vapor-pressure propellants such as HFA, co-solvents, and/or surfactants.[29] With any change in the components of an MDI, the FDA considers it to be a new drug that requires stability, safety, and efficacy studies prior to approval. The MDI drug is either in solution or a suspended micronized powder. In order to disperse the suspension for accurate delivery, the canister must be shaken. The metering chamber measures a liquid volume, and, therefore, the device must be held with the valve stem downward so that the chamber is covered with liquid[29] (Fig. 26-4). If not used for a period of time the drug in the chamber evaporates which could lead to an inadequate therapeutic dose. Inhalers have to be primed before first use to fill the chamber and after an interval of nonuse.[29] When the canister is actuated, the device releases the propellant and drug in a forceful spray whose particles are large (MMAD = 45 μm)[29] (see Fig. 26-4). As evaporation occurs, the particle size is reduced to a final MMAD of 0.5 to 5.5 μm depending on the MDI. The aerosol cloud extends about 6 inches beyond the

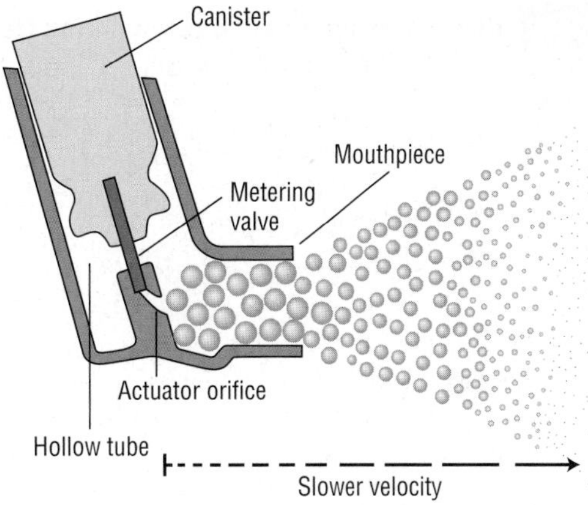

FIGURE 26-4 Illustration of a metered-dose inhaler demonstrating the particle size difference as the aerosol cloud extends outward.

MDI at the lowest MMAD.[29] Each MDI has different conditions for storage, priming, and durations to expiration, so the clinician must become familiar with and counsel the patient on these factors.

Spacer devices are used frequently with an MDI to decrease oropharyngeal deposition and enhance lung delivery.[2,3] However, not all spacer devices produce similar effects. The design of spacers varies from simple open-ended tubes that separate the MDI from the mouth to valved holding chambers (VHCs) with one-way valves that open during inhalation (the preferred system); some VHCs have a face mask to accommodate drug delivery in children 5 years or younger.[3] A VHC allows evaporation of the propellant prior to inhalation permitting a greater number of drug particles to achieve a respirable droplet size. VHC use also allows inhalation after actuation of the MDI, obviating the need for good hand–lung coordination.[29] Additionally, the large particles that normally would deposit in the oropharynx "rain out" in the spacer.[29] Spacer size may affect the amount of drug available for inhalation; a lower volume spacer (less than 350 mL) is advantageous in very young children.[3]

All the available spacers significantly reduce oropharyngeal deposition from MDIs, with the VHCs being superior to the open-ended tubes.[29] This reduction in oropharyngeal deposition is an important factor in reducing local adverse effects (eg, hoarseness and thrush) from ICSs.[29] The change in lung delivery depends on both the MDI and the drug, where one spacer device may enhance delivery with one MDI preparation and decrease delivery with others.[29] Therefore, once a patient is stabilized on a drug and chamber combination, the chamber should not be substituted in order to avoid changes in the dose delivered to the lungs. Finally, over time, holding chambers (eg, plastic) can build up static electricity that attracts small particles to the sides of the chamber, significantly reducing aerosol availability. Some spacers should be washed weekly with household detergent with a single rinse and allowed to drip dry.[2] Other VHCs have been developed with antistatic materials.

Dry micronized powders can be inhaled directly into the lungs. A number of DPIs are now available for use in the United States.[29] Currently, there are no generic DPIs as each drug plus device has its own patent. Each DPI has unique characteristics with advantages and disadvantages (Table 26-4). The primary advantage of DPIs is that they are breath actuated and require minimal hand–lung coordination, and it is thus easier to teach patients proper technique.[29] Some DPIs are more flow dependent than others.[29] Thus, similar to MDIs and spacers, delivery data from one DPI cannot be extrapolated to another.

Nebulizers come in two basic types, the jet nebulizer and the ultrasonic nebulizer. Jet nebulizers produce an aerosol from a liquid solution or suspension placed in a cup. A tube connected to a

TABLE 26-4 Characteristics of Various Inhalation Devices

Device	Drugs	Breath Activated	Dose Counter	Other Excipients	Disadvantages
MDI	All classes	No	No/yes	Propellants, surfactants, cosolvents	Requires coordination of actuation and inhalation. Large pharyngeal deposition. Difficult to teach
Pressair	aclidinium	Yes	Yes	Lactose filler	Requires rapid inhalation to activate
Respiclick	albuterol	Yes	Yes	Lactose filler	Requires rapid inhalation to activate
MDI plus valved holding chamber	All classes	No	No		More expensive than MDI alone; less portable; some payers will not pay; inconsistent effect on delivery; nonstatic preferred
Jet nebulizers	All classes	No	—	Preservatives in some solutions	Significant interbrand variability; expensive and time consuming; less efficient than MDIs; contamination possible; preparations may be light and temperature sensitive (short shelf life)
Ulrasonic nebulizer	Cromolyn solution, short-acting β_2-agonist solutions	No	—	Preservatives in some solutions	Same as for jet nebulizers plus cannot be used for suspensions; battery operated are portable
Flexhaler	Budesonide	Yes	Yes	Lactose filler	Requires high inspiratory flow (60 L/min) Pharyngeal deposition Not approved for <6 years of age
Diskus	Fluticasone; salmeterol; fluticasone/salmeterol	Yes	Yes	Lactose filler	Not approved for <4 years of age Requires inspiratory flow of 30-60 L/min
Ellipta	Fluticasone furoate Fluticasone/vilanterol	Yes	Yes	Lactose filler	Not approved for <12 years of age (18 years for fluticasone/vilanterol) Requires inspiratory flow of 60 L/min
Aerolizer	Formoterol	Yes	—	Lactose filler	Single-dose capsules. Not approved for <5 years of age Requires flow of 30-60 L/min
Neohaler	Indacaterol	Yes	—	Lactose filler	Single-dose capsules. Not approved for children Requires flow of 60 L/min
Handihaler	Tiotropium	Yes	—	Lactose filler	Single-dose capsule. Not approved for children Requires flow of 20 L/min
Twisthaler	Mometasone	Yes	Yes	Lactose filler	Not approved for <4 years of age
Respimat	Tiotropium Albuterol/Ipratropium Olodaterol	No	Yes	Preservative	Requires slow deep breath. Not approved for <12 years of age

stream of compressed air or O_2 flows up through the bottom and draws the liquid up an adjacent open-ended tube.[29] The air and liquid strike a baffle, creating a droplet cloud that is then inhaled.[29] Ultrasonic nebulizers produce an aerosol by vibrating liquid lying above a transducer at speeds of about 1 mHz.[29] Both produce similar degrees of lung deposition, with the exception that ultrasonic nebulizers are ineffective for nebulizing currently available micronized suspensions.[29] The aerosol output and lung delivery vary significantly among the commercially available jet nebulizers even when operated in the same manner.[29] Increasing fill volume will increase the total amount of drug delivered; however, it also will take longer for the patient to nebulize the dose.[29] The MMAD of the droplets is related directly to the gas flow, with flows of 5 to 12 L/min providing an aerosol cloud with an MMAD of 4 to 8 μm for most jet nebulizers.[29] Each jet nebulizer comes with its optimal operating and cleaning instructions.

Patient Determinants of Delivery

6 7 The most important patient factor determining aerosol deposition is inspiratory flow (see Table 26-3).[2,29] High inspiratory flows with MDIs increase the degree of deposition owing to impaction of particles of any size, thereby increasing deposition centrally (ie, throat and large airways) and decreasing peripheral deposition. Optimal inspiratory flow for most MDIs is slow and deep (approximately 30 L/min or 5 seconds for a full inhalation).[2,3] In general, DPIs require higher inspiratory flows (greater than or equal to 60 L/min) and a change in inhalation technique (ie, deep, forceful inspiration) for optimal dispersion of the powder, which, in turn, increases the amount of drug delivered to the larger central airways.[29] However, this difference in delivery may not produce clinically significant differences.[29] Patients should be cautioned not to exhale into DPIs because this causes loss of dose and moistens the dry powder, causing aggregation into larger particles. Patient factors that cannot be controlled include interpatient variability in airway geometry (particularly the differences between children and adults)[29] and the effects of bronchospasm, edema, and mucus hypersecretion. Mild obstruction increases aerosol deposition; however, severe obstruction probably leads to increased central deposition from impaction.[29] The absolute delivery to the lung is not as important as consistency of delivery, assuming that a sufficient dose to produce the desired therapeutic effect is achieved. No single inhalation device is the best for all patients. Table 26-4 lists the differing characteristics of inhalation devices.

Appropriate inhalation technique is essential to achieve optimal drug delivery and therapeutic effect.[2,3] The components are illustrated in Fig. 26-5. Approximately 50% to 80% of a dose from MDIs and DPIs impacts on the oropharynx and is then swallowed; the rest is either left in the device or exhaled.[29] It is important that MDI actuation occurs during inhalation, although the time during inspiration is unimportant.[2,29] Although radiolabeled studies with MDIs indicate improved delivery by holding the actuator 2 to 3 cm in front of an open mouth to allow more evaporation and less impaction, physiologic studies with bronchodilators have failed to document an advantage for this method.[2,29] Many patients do not use their MDIs optimally, and patient instruction with demonstration is the most effective means of improving inhaler technique.[2,3] Even with instruction, up to 30% of patients, particularly young

Steps For Using Your Inhaler

Please demonstrate your inhaler technique at every visit.

1. Remove the cap and hold inhaler upright.
2. Shake the inhaler.
3. Tilt your head back slightly and breathe out slowly.
4. Position the inhaler in one of the following ways (B is acceptable for those who have difficulty with A or C: C is required for breath-activated inhalers):

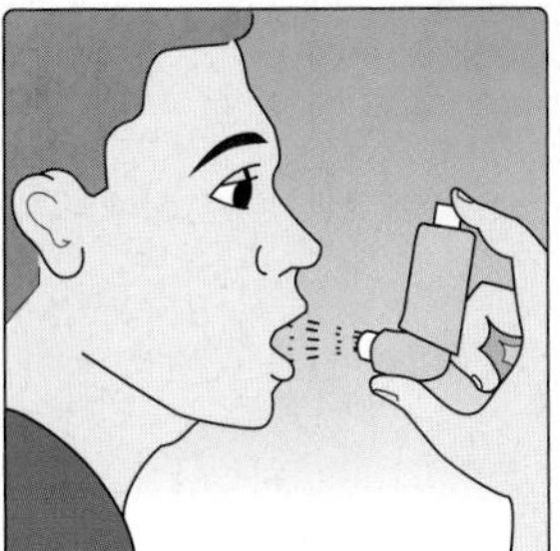

A Open mouth with inhaler 1-2 in away.

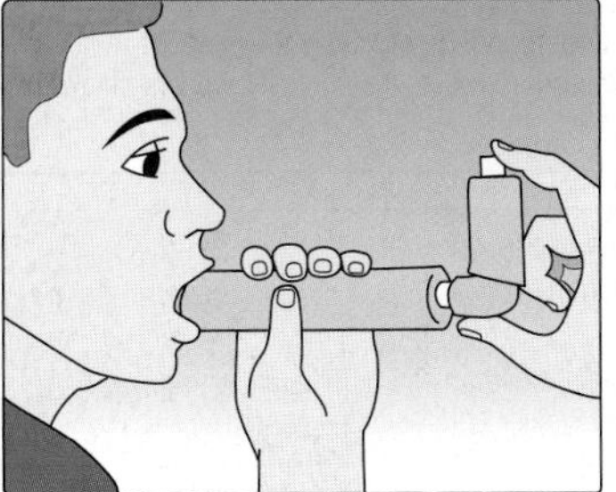

B Use spacer/holding chamber (which is recommended especially for young children and for people using corticosteroids).

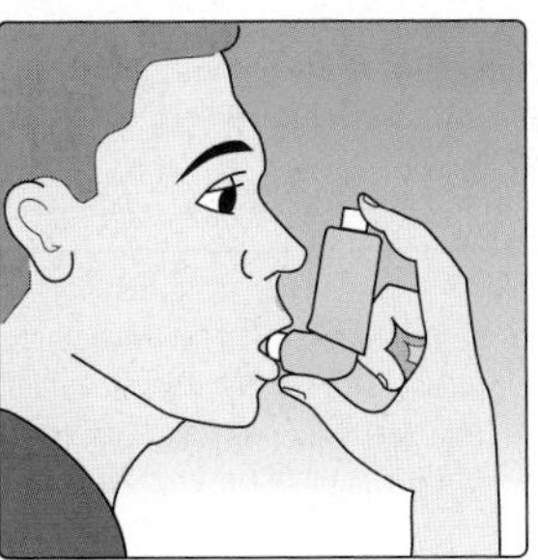

C In the mouth.

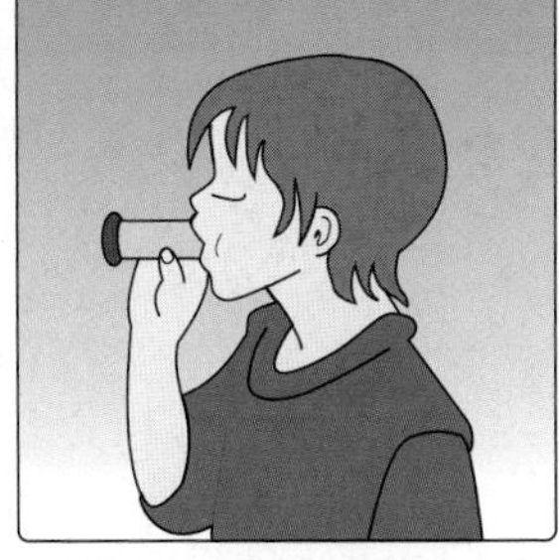

D NOTE: Inhaled dry powder capsules require a different inhalation technique. To use a dry powder inhaler, it is important to close the mouth tightly around the mouthpiece of the inhaler and to inhale rapidly.

5. Press down on the inhaler to release medication as you start to breathe in slowly.
6. Breathe in slowly (3-5 seconds).
7. Hold your breath for 10 seconds to allow the medicine to reach deeply into your lungs.
8. Repeat puff as directed. Waiting 1 minute between puffs may permit second puff to penetrate your lungs better.
9. Spacers/holding chambers are useful for all patients. They are particularly recommended for young children and older adults and for use with corticosteroids.

Avoid common inhaler mistakes. Follow these inhaler tips:

- Breathe out *before* pressing your inhaler.
- Inhale *slowly*.
- Breathe in through your mouth, not your nose.
- Press down on your inhaler at the *start* of inhalation (or within the first second of inhalation).
- Keep inhaling as you press down on inhaler.
- Press your inhaler only *once* while you are inhaling (one breath for each puff).
- Make sure you breathe in evenly and deeply.

NOTE: Other inhalers are becoming available in addition to those illustrated above. Different types of inhalers require different techniques.

FIGURE 26-5 Instructions for inhaler use from the adapted NAEPP Expert Panel Report 2. *http://www.nhlbi.nih.gov/guidelines/archives/epr-2/index.htm. (Data from reference 3.)*

children and the elderly, cannot master the use of an MDI. For these patients, attachment of a VHC to the MDI can improve efficacy significantly.[2,29] However, addition of a VHC offers no advantage in patients who can use an MDI optimally alone.[29] Mouth rinsing following treatment with MDI- and DPI-ICSs is important to minimize local adverse effects and oral absorption.[2,29]

Delivery from high-resistance DPIs is more flow dependent than from low-resistance DPIs. Thus, younger children and possibly elderly adults will have more variability in delivery from high-resistance devices.[29] Most children younger than 4 years of age cannot generate a sufficient inspiratory flow to use DPIs. Young children (younger than 4 years) and infants generally require the use of a face mask attached to either an MDI plus VHC or nebulizer. The use of a face mask results in a reduction in lung delivery due to the portion of the aerosol inhaled nasally, so the doses of drugs used in these patients are often not decreased.

TREATMENT

Acute Severe Asthma in the Emergency Department

The primary goal is prevention of life-threatening asthma by early recognition of signs of deterioration and early intervention. Initial assessment includes history, physical examination, and objective assessments. It is important that therapy not be delayed, so the history and physical examination should be obtained while initial therapy is being provided. The brief history will assess for: onset and causes of the exacerbation; severity of symptoms and if associated with anaphylaxis; medication use, adherence, and response to current therapy; and risk factors for asthma-related death. The asthma-related risk factors for death include: a history of near-fatal asthma requiring intubation and mechanical ventilation; hospitalization or emergency care in the past year; current or recent use of oral corticosteroids; no current use of ICSs; over use of short-acting β_2-agonist therapy (more than one canister per month); history of psychiatric disease or psychosocial problems; poor medication adherence; lack of a written asthma action plan; and food allergy.[3]

The physical exam will assess vital signs and any complicating factors such as pneumonia or anaphylaxis as well as other comorbid conditions that could be causing acute shortness of breath such as inhaled foreign body, congestive heart failure, pulmonary infection, and pulmonary embolism.[3]

Objective assessments are keys to monitoring response to therapy and should be made before initiation of oxygen or drug treatment. Lung function testing by PEF or FEV_1 should be measured before treatment if possible and thereafter at one hour after start of treatment and then periodically until response is achieved or no further improvement is evident.[3] Oxygen saturation is also monitored closely preferably by pulse oximetry and is a key parameter in young children who may not be able to perform lung function. Arterial blood gases are typically reserved for patients who are poorly responsive to initial treatment or deteriorating. A chest X-ray is

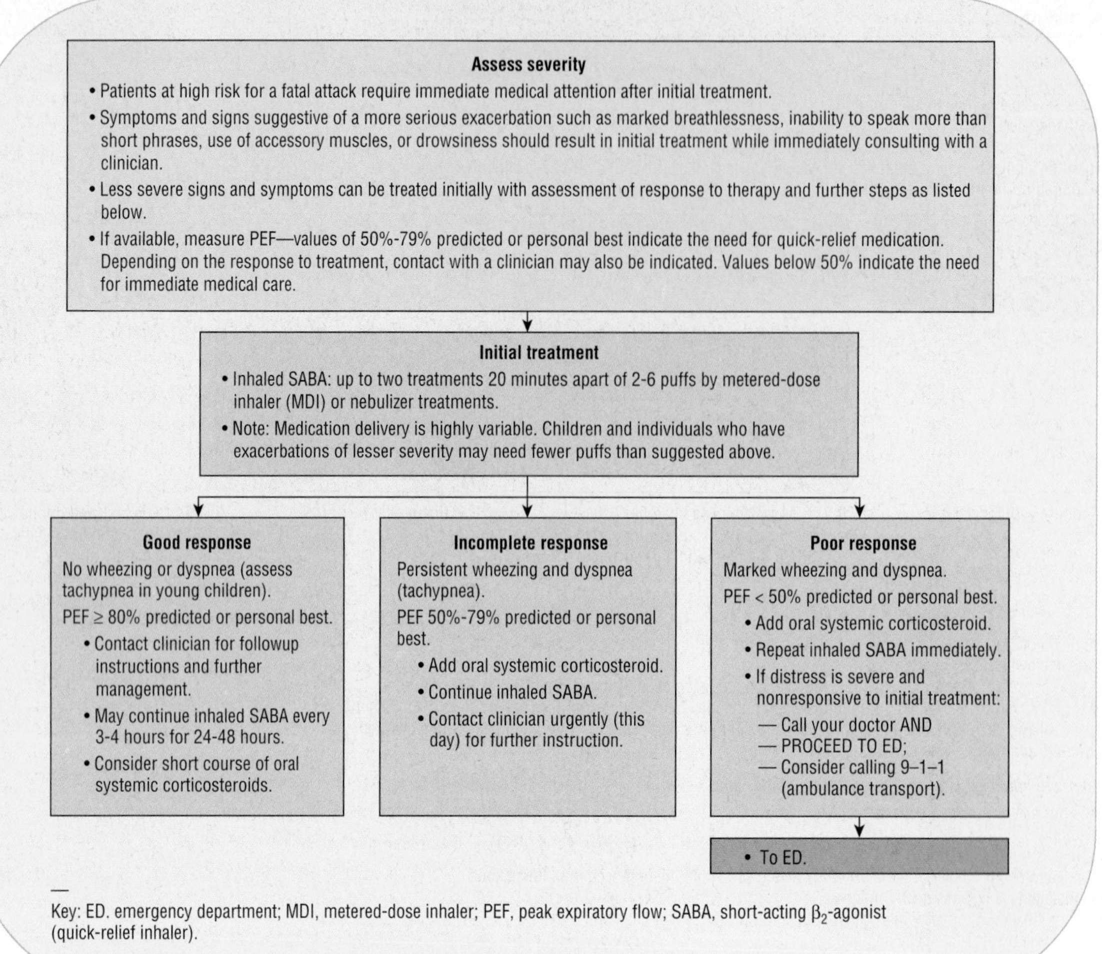

Assess severity
• Patients at high risk for a fatal attack require immediate medical attention after initial treatment.
• Symptoms and signs suggestive of a more serious exacerbation such as marked breathlessness, inability to speak more than short phrases, use of accessory muscles, or drowsiness should result in initial treatment while immediately consulting with a clinician.
• Less severe signs and symptoms can be treated initially with assessment of response to therapy and further steps as listed below.
• If available, measure PEF—values of 50%-79% predicted or personal best indicate the need for quick-relief medication. Depending on the response to treatment, contact with a clinician may also be indicated. Values below 50% indicate the need for immediate medical care.
Initial treatment
• Inhaled SABA: up to two treatments 20 minutes apart of 2-6 puffs by metered-dose inhaler (MDI) or nebulizer treatments.
• Note: Medication delivery is highly variable. Children and individuals who have exacerbations of lesser severity may need fewer puffs than suggested above.
Good response
No wheezing or dyspnea (assess tachypnea in young children).
PEF ≥ 80% predicted or personal best.
• Contact clinician for followup instructions and further management.
• May continue inhaled SABA every 3-4 hours for 24-48 hours.
• Consider short course of oral systemic corticosteroids.
Incomplete response
Persistent wheezing and dyspnea (tachypnea).
PEF 50%-79% predicted or personal best.
• Add oral systemic corticosteroid.
• Continue inhaled SABA.
• Contact clinician urgently (this day) for further instruction.
Poor response
Marked wheezing and dyspnea.
PEF < 50% predicted or personal best.
• Add oral systemic corticosteroid.
• Repeat inhaled SABA immediately.
• If distress is severe and nonresponsive to initial treatment:
— Call your doctor AND
— PROCEED TO ED;
— Consider calling 9–1–1 (ambulance transport).
• To ED.
Key: ED. emergency department; MDI, metered-dose inhaler; PEF, peak expiratory flow; SABA, short-acting β2-agonist (quick-relief inhaler).

FIGURE 26-6 Self-management of worsening asthma in adults and adolescents with a written asthma action plan. *(Used with permission from Global Initiative for Asthma. Global strategy for asthma management and prevention, 2015. Available from: www.ginasthma.org)*

rarely indicated unless there are physical signs of other or additional complicating features such as foreign body aspiration.

Oxygen therapy is initiated to achieve an arterial oxygen saturation of 93% to 95% in adolescents and adults and 94% to 98% in school-aged children and pregnant women or those with cardiac disease.[2,3] Oxygen therapy is continued until the patient has stabilized with continued use of pulse oximetry to monitor further oxygen need and response to medications.

The primary therapy of acute exacerbations is pharmacologic, which includes short-acting inhaled β_2-agonists and, depending on the severity, systemic corticosteroids, inhaled ipratropium, and O_2. Treatments are typically administered concurrently to facilitate rapid improvement (Figs. 26-6 and 26-7).[2] New evidence supports the use of heliox versus oxygen for nebulized β_2-agonist administration in patients with moderate to severe exacerbations who do not respond to standard therapy.[3,30] Heliox is a combination of helium and oxygen (often 70:30) that has a lower density than air which reduces resistance to flow and increases ventilation by converting turbulent flow to more efficient laminar flow.[31] Limited data suggest that the benefits with heliox therapy are apparent in those with severe exacerbations by improving PEF and reducing the risk of hospitalizations in both children and adults.[30]

A complete blood count may be appropriate for patients with fever or purulent sputum, but modest leukocytosis is common in asthma exacerbations due to viral infection or secondary to corticosteroid administration. Leukocytosis associated with corticosteroid administration does not cause a shift to the left as is seen in bacterial infections. Serum electrolytes should be monitored in patients who take diuretics regularly and in patients with coexistent cardiovascular disease as short-acting inhaled β_2-agonists can produce transient decreases in potassium, magnesium, and phosphate.[2] The combination of high-dose β_2-agonists and systemic corticosteroids occasionally may result in excessive elevations of glucose and lactic acid.[31]

Initial response is measured one hour after the first three inhaled bronchodilator treatments are administered and provides the best indicator for the need for hospitaliztion.[3] Indicators for hospitalization include an initial FEV_1 less than 25% predicted or PEF that is less than 40% of their personal best, and post-treatment FEV_1 or PEF that is 40% to 60%.[3] Other indicators of severe asthma include monosyllabic speech, inaudible breath sounds, sitting hunched forward, and use of accessory muscles.[3] Patients with lung function that is 40% to 60% predicted *may* be considered for discharge after assessment of risk factors for death from asthma and the likelihood for follow up care. Those with higher lung function can be discharged after risk factor and follow-up care assessment.[3]

Discharge planning after an ED visit or hospitalization includes arrangement for follow-up care within one week as well as review of strategies to improve asthma management. Referral to a specialist is suggested for those who have been hospitalized or frequently seek care in the ED despite having regular primary care. Strategies for preventing future urgent care visits includes ensuring the patient understands the cause of the exacerbation, how to modify risk factors, how to use medications correctly and for what purpose, and has a written asthma action plan that includes self-assessment of worsening symptoms and home PEF values.[3]

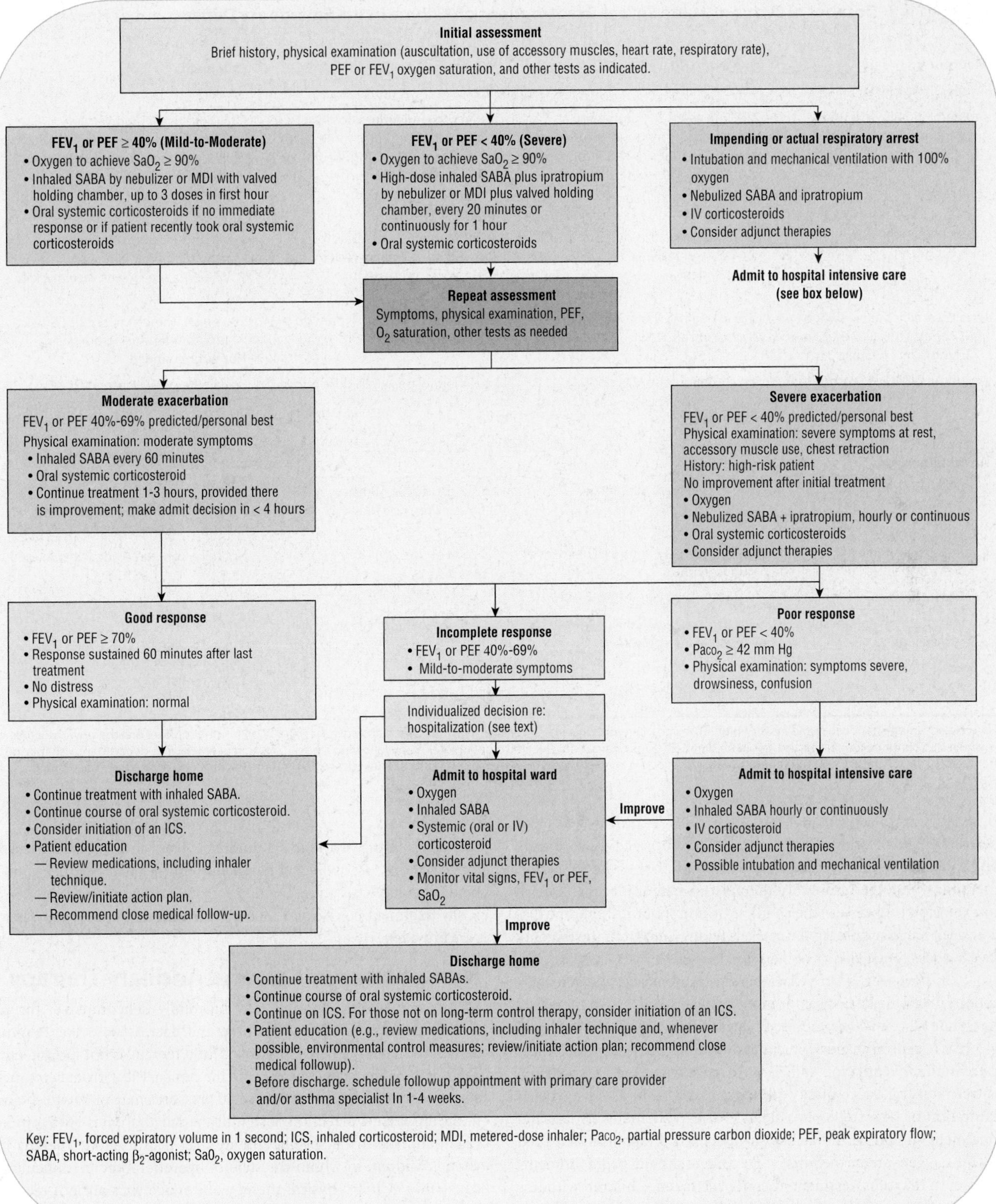

FIGURE 26-7 Management of asthma exacerbations in acute care facility, For example, emergency department. *(Used with permission from Global Initiative for Asthma. Global strategy for asthma management and prevention, 2015. Available from: www.ginasthma.org.)*

Figures 26-6 and 26-7 illustrate the recommended therapies for the treatment of acute asthma exacerbations in home and ED/hospital settings, respectively.[2] The dosages of the drugs for acute severe exacerbations are provided in Table 26-5.[2] Institutions should strongly consider developing critical pathways/treatment algorithms for their EDs because their implementation has been shown to improve outcomes and decrease the cost of care.[32]

Acute Severe Asthma in Children 5-Years and Younger

Infants and children younger than 5 years of age may be at greater risk of respiratory failure than older children and adults. Although treated with the same drugs, these younger children require the use of a face mask as opposed to a mouthpiece for delivery of

TABLE 26-5 Dosages of Drugs of Acute Severe Exacerbations of Asthma in the Emergency Department or Hospital

	Dosages		
Medications	**≥12 Years Old**	**<12 Years Old**	**Comments**
Inhaled β-Agonists			
Albuterol nebulizer solution (5 mg/mL, 0.63 mg/3 mL, 1.25 mg/3 mL, 2.5 mg/3 mL)	2.5-5 mg every 20 minutes for three doses, and then 2.5-10 mg every 1-4 hours as needed, or 10-15 mg/h continuously	0.15 mg/kg (minimum dose 2.5 mg) every 20 minutes for three doses, and then 0.15-0.3 mg/kg up to 10 mg every 1-4 hours as needed, or 0.5 mg/kg/h by continuous nebulization	Only selective β_2-agonists are recommended. For optimal delivery, dilute aerosols to minimum of 4 mL at gas flow of 6-8 L/min. Use face mask if <4 years
Albuterol MDI (90 mcg/puff)	4-8 puffs every 30 minutes up to 4 hours, and then every 1-4 hours as needed	4-8 puffs every 20 minutes for three doses, and then every 1-4 hours as needed	In patients in severe distress, nebulization is preferred; use VHC-type spacer with face mask if <4 years old
Levalbuterol nebulizer solution (0.31 mg/3 mL, 0.63 mg/3 mL, 2.5 mg/1 mL, 1.25 mg/3 mL)	Give at one half the milligram dose of albuterol above	Give at one half the milligram dose of albuterol above	The single isomer of albuterol is twice as potent on a milligram basis Not recommended
Levalbuterol MDI (45 mcg/puff)	See albuterol dose MDI dose	See albuterol dose MDI dose above	See albuterol MDI dose one half as potent as albuterol on a microgram basis Not recommended
Anticholinergics			
Ipratropium bromide nebulizer solution (0.25 mg/mL)	500 mcg every 30 minutes for three doses, and then every 2-4 hours as needed	250 mcg every 20 minutes for three doses, and then 250 mcg every 2-4 hours	May mix in same nebulizer with albuterol; only add to β_2-agonist therapy
Ipratropium bromide MDI (18 mcg/puff)	8 puffs every 20 minutes as needed for up to 3 hours	4-8 puffs as needed every 2-4 hours	Not to be continued once hospitalized
Corticosteroids			
Prednisone, methylprednisolone, prednisolone	50 mg in one or two divided doses (prednisone equivalent)	1 mg/kg (maximum 40 mg/day) in two divided doses (prednisone equivalent)	For outpatient "burst" use 1-2 mg/kg/day, maximum 60 mg, for 3-5 days in children and 40-60 mg/day in one or two divided doses for 5-7 days in adults

Note: No advantage has been found for very-high-dose corticosteroids in acute severe asthma, nor is there any advantage for IV administration over oral therapy. The usual regimen is to continue the oral corticosteroid for duration of hospitalization. The final duration of therapy following a hospitalization or emergency department visit may be from 3 to 10 days. If patients are then started on ICSs, there is no need to taper the systemic corticosteroid dose. ICSs can be started at any time during the exacerbation.

Data from reference 3.

aerosolized medication. The face mask should be sized appropriately and should fit snugly over the nose and mouth. Use of the "blow-by" method, where the respiratory therapist or parent places the mask or extension tubing near the child's nose and mouth, should be discouraged because holding the mask as few as 2 cm from the patient's face reduces lung delivery of the aerosol by 80%.[2,29]

Children with severe exacerbations present with oxygen saturation of 92% or less, speak in monosyllabic words, have increased heart rate (above 200 beats/min if 0-3 years or above 180 beats/min if 4-5 years), central cyanosis, and inaudible breath sounds which indicate minimal ventilation sufficient to cause wheezing.[3] Hypoxemia is treated using a face mask with oxygen at 24% to achieve oxygen saturation of 94% to 98%. Avoidance of hypoxemia is critical and treatment should be initiated with nebulized β_2-agonists delivered by an oxygen-driven nebulizer. Treatment should begin immediately even if a full assessment has not been taken. Children with less severe symptoms can be treated with 2.5 mg of albuterol by nebulizer or 2 to 6 inhalations of albuterol with a spacer/facemask every 20 minutes for 3 doses with re-assessment at the end of this treatment. Subsequent doses by nebulizer or 2 to 3 inhalations by spacer/facemask can be given every hour, but if symptoms do not resolve after 10 inhalations administered over 3 to 4 hours then a hospital admission is required.[3] As in older children and adults, oral corticosteroids are administered at the time of inhaled β_2-agonists or systemically in children unable to swallow. Inhaled ipratropium bromide can be administered with β_2-agonist treatment but should not be continued for more than 3 doses in an hour. There is no evidence for continuing inhaled anticholinergics added to β_2-agonists in hospitalized children.[33] Nebulized magnesium sulfate may be administered as 3 doses in the first hour in children 2 years and older with severe exacerbations.[3] As in older children and adults, young children should be discharged with a prescription for oral corticosteroids for a 3 to 5 day treatment course and followed up within 7 days by a primary care provider.

Non-pharmacologic and Ancillary Therapy

Infants and young children may be mildly dehydrated owing to increased insensible loss, vomiting, and decreased intake.[2] Unless dehydration has occurred, increased fluid therapy is not indicated in acute asthma management because the capillary leak from cytokines and increased negative intrathoracic pressures may promote edema in the airways.[2] Correction of significant dehydration is always indicated, and the urine specific gravity may help to guide therapy in young children, in whom the state of hydration may be difficult to determine.[2] Chest physical therapy and mucolytics are not recommended in the therapy of acute asthma.[2] Sedatives should not be given because anxiety may be a sign of hypoxemia, which could be worsened by central nervous system depressants. Antibiotics also are not indicated routinely because viral respiratory tract infections are the primary cause of asthma exacerbations.[2] Antibiotics should be reserved for patients who have signs and symptoms of pneumonia (eg, fever, pulmonary consolidation, and purulent sputum from polymorphonuclear leukocytes). *Mycoplasma* and *Chlamydia* are infrequent causes of severe asthma exacerbations but should be considered in patients with high O_2 requirements.[2,34]

Respiratory failure or impending respiratory failure as measured by rising $PaCO_2$ (greater than or equal to 45 mm Hg [greater than or equal to 6 kPa]) or failure to correct hypoxemia with supplemental O_2 therapy is treated with intubation and mechanical ventilation.[3]

Pharmacotherapy

β_2-Agonists

4 The short-acting inhaled β_2-agonists are the most effective bronchodilators and the treatment of first choice for the management of acute severe asthma.[3] In adults, administration as either continuous or intermittent (every 20 minutes for 3 doses) over 1 hour results in equivalent improvement.[2] In the subset of more severely obstructed patients, continuous nebulization decreases the hospital admission rate, provides greater improvement in the FEV_1 and PEF, and reduces duration of hospitalization when compared with intermittent (hourly) nebulized albuterol in the same total dose.[2] Thus, continuous nebulization is recommended for patients having an unsatisfactory response (achieving less than 50% of normal FEV_1 or PEF) following the initial three doses (every 20 minutes) of aerosolized β_2-agonists and potentially for patients presenting initially with PEF or FEV_1 values of less than 30% of predicted normal.[2] Intravenous β_2-agonists do not have a role in the routine management of patients with severe exacerbations.[3] Effective doses of aerosolized β_2-agonists can be delivered successfully through mechanical ventilator circuits to infants, children, and adults in respiratory failure secondary to severe airway obstruction.[29]

The doses of inhaled β_2-agonists for acute severe asthma exacerbations (see Table 26-5) have been derived empirically. The β_2-agonists follow a log-linear dose–response curve. In addition, the dose–response curve is shifted to the right by more severe bronchospasm or by increased concentrations of bronchospastic mediators, which is characteristic of functional antagonists.[35] The ability to increase the dose of the short-acting aerosolized β_2-agonists by as much as 5- to 10-fold over doses producing adequate bronchodilation in chronic stable asthma is what contributes to their efficacy in reversing the bronchospasm of acute severe exacerbations. The nebulizer dose of inhaled β_2-agonists for children often is listed on a weight basis (milligrams per kilogram). However, a fixed minimal dose (2.5 mg albuterol or equivalent), as opposed to a weight-adjusted dose, is more appropriate in younger children because children younger than 5 years of age receive a lower lung dose.[2] Adults dosed on a weight basis demonstrate excessive cardiac stimulation, so they have fixed maximal doses[2] (see Table 26-5). Initial doses of inhaled β_2-agonists can produce vasodilation, worsening ventilation–perfusion mismatch, slightly lowering O_2 saturation or PaO_2.[32] High doses of inhaled β_2-agonists can produce a decrease in serum potassium concentration, an increase in heart rate, and an increase in serum glucose and lactic acid concentration.[3] Electrolyte monitoring may be needed in patients with preexisting heart disease who receive frequent doses for an acute exacerbation.[3] Hyperlactatemia is common but is not accompanied by metabolic acidosis and does not increase the risk of hospitalization.[31] Both children and adults receiving continuously nebulized β_2-agonists have demonstrated decreased heart rate as their lung function improves.[2] Thus, an elevated heart rate is not an indication to use lower doses or to avoid using inhaled β_2-agonists.

There is no evidence to support the use of levalbuterol over albuterol for the treatment of acute severe exacerbations in either children or adults with respect to efficacy or adverse effects.[35] A meta-analysis which showed a lower risk for hospitalization in the levalbuterol treated patients was driven by one study only.[35]

The inhaled β_2-agonists produce similar efficacy whether delivered by MDI plus VHC or nebulization in treating acute severe exacerbations in the ED and hospital; thus, the choice depends on the experience and comfort of the treating clinicians.[3] The DPIs are currently not indicated for the treatment of acute severe asthma exacerbations due to the higher inspiratory flows required for adequate drug delivery.[2]

Corticosteroids

Systemic corticosteroids are indicated in all patients with acute severe asthma exacerbations not responding completely to initial inhaled β_2-agonist administration (every 20 minutes for three doses) and should be administered within one hour of presentation.[2,3] Clinical improvement is noted after approximately 4-hours. IV therapy offers no therapeutic advantage over oral administration except in patients who are too dyspneic to swallow, vomiting, or intubated.[2,3] This therapy usually is continued until hospital discharge. Tapering the systemic corticosteroid dose following discharge from the hospital appears unnecessary, provided that patients are prescribed ICSs for outpatient therapy.[3] Adults are effectively treated with a 5 to 7 day course of therapy but children typically require only 3 to 5 days.[3] It is recommended that a full dose of the corticosteroid be continued until the patient's PEF reaches 70% of predicted normal or personal best.[2] Dexamethasone as 1 or 2 doses versus a 5-day course of prednisone/prednisolone may be an option for children and has the benefit of causing less vomiting.[36]

Multiple daily dosing of systemic corticosteroids for the initial therapy of acute asthma exacerbations appears warranted because receptor binding affinities of lung corticosteroid receptors are decreased in the face of airway inflammation.[37] However, patients with less severe exacerbations may be treated adequately with once-daily administration. High-dose and very-high-pulse-dose corticosteroid regimens have not been shown to enhance the outcomes in severe acute asthma but are associated with a higher likelihood of side effects.[37]

Inhaled corticosteroids initiated within one hour of presentation to the ED reduce hospitalization rate in those not treated with systemic corticosteroids.[3] However, current evidence suggests there is no rationale for combining inhaled and systemic therapy nor for replacing systemic with inhaled therapy.[3]

Anticholinergics

Inhaled ipratropium bromide produces a further improvement in lung function of 10% to 15% over inhaled β_2-agonists alone. In children and adults, multiple-dose ipratropium bromide added to initial therapy reduces hospitalization rate in the subset of patients with moderate to severe asthma exacerbations.[3] However, there is no benefit to continuing combined anticholinergic and β_2-agonist therapy during hospitalization on duration of stay or clinical outcomes.[33] Ipratropium bromide, a quaternary amine, is poorly absorbed and produces minimal or no systemic effects.[38] Care should be taken when administering ipratropium bromide by nebulizer. If a tight mask or mouthpiece is not used, the ipratropium bromide that deposits in the eyes may produce pupillary dilation and difficulty in accommodation.[2]

Magnesium Sulfate

Intravenous and nebulized magnesium sulfate have been used in addition to standard therapies (β_2-agonists, systemic corticosteroids, anticholinergics, and oxygen) in children and adults with severe or life-threatening asthma. Magnesium sulfate is a moderately potent bronchodilator, producing relaxation of smooth muscle by blocking calcium ion influx into smooth muscles and it may have anti-inflammatory effects.[39] A meta-analysis found strong evidence that single infusion of 1.2 or 2 g magnesium sulfate administered to adults with moderate, severe, or life-threatening asthma who had not sufficiently responded to β_2-agonists, systemic corticosteroids, and oxygen reduced hospital admission rate (7 fewer admissions per 100 treated) and improved lung function.[40] Previous meta-analyses have shown inconsistent effects in adults on respiratory function and hospitalization rate when administered by the intravenous or nebulized route but it was not clear if magnesium sulfate was given concurrently with standard therapy or after failure to respond to standard therapy.[41,42] There are fewer studies in children with severe or life-threatening asthma though one meta-analysis found intravenous use improved respiratory function and reduced hospitalizations but again it was not clear exactly when in the course of care magnesium was administered.[42] For patients with severe asthma exacerbations, current guidelines suggest that a single 2 g intravenous infusion can be helpful in reducing hospital admissions in adults who have a FEV_1 less than 25% to 30% predicted upon arrival in the ED, children and adults who have persistent hypoxemia after standard treatment, and children whose FEV_1 remains below 60% predicted after 1 hour of standard treatment.[3] The adverse effects of magnesium sulfate include hypotension, facial flushing, sweating, depressed deep tendon reflexes, hypothermia, cardiac, CNS and respiratory depression.

Alternative Therapies

The inhalational anesthetics halothane, isoflurane, and enflurane all have been reported to have a positive effect in children and adults with acute severe asthma on mechanical ventilation that is unresponsive to standard medical therapy.[43] The proposed mechanisms for inhalational anesthetics include β_2-adrenergic receptor stimulation, direct relaxation on bronchial smooth muscle, inhibition of airway reflexes, attenuation of histamine-induced bronchospasm, and alteration of the nitric oxide pathway in epithelial cells.[43] Well-controlled trials with these agents have not been completed.[43] Potential adverse effects include myocardial depression, vasodilation, arrhythmias, and depression of mucociliary function.[43] In addition, the practical problem of delivery and scavenging these agents in the intensive care environment as opposed to the operating room and the avoidance of environmental pollution to treating caregivers is a concern. The use of volatile anesthetics cannot be recommended based on insufficient evidence of efficacy.

Ketamine has been recommended for rapid induction of anesthesia in patients with asthma who require intubation and mechanical ventilation.[44,45] In addition, intravenous ketamine has been used as a bolus followed by continuous infusion in both intubated and nonintubated patients with severe asthma exacerbations but controlled trials have not provided evidence of efficacy.[2] Purported mechanisms for beneficial effects in asthma include inhibition of histamine and acetylcholine-induced bronchoconstriction and acting as a sympathomimetic agent.[2] Ketamine has several significant adverse effects, including the anesthesia emergence reaction, which can alter mood and cause delirium. These emergence phenomena occur in at least 25% of patients over 16 years of age; the incidence seems to be much lower in younger patients.[2] Other adverse effects include hypertension and sinus tachycardia or hypotension and sinus bradycardia

Drug Class Information for Management of Acute Asthma

Short-Acting β_2-Agonists

5 6 The β_2-agonists are the most effective bronchodilators available. The β_2-adrenergic receptors are transmembrane proteins consisting of clusters of seven helices of amino acids that form the ligand-binding core.[46] The human β_2-adrenergic receptors are polymorphic in structure, with the most common polymorphisms in the amino terminus of the receptor at amino acid positions 16 (encoding either arginine [Arg] or glycine [Gly]) and 27 (encoding either glutamine [Gln] or glutamic acid [Glu]).[47] This activation, in turn, decreases unbound intracellular calcium, producing smooth muscle relaxation, mast cell membrane stabilization, and skeletal muscle stimulation.[46] Despite the fact that β_2-agonists are potent inhibitors of mast cell degranulation in vitro, they do not inhibit the late asthmatic response to allergen challenge or the subsequent BHR.[2,46] Long-term administration of β_2-agonists does not reduce BHR, confirming a lack of significant anti-inflammatory activity. β_2-Adrenergic stimulation also activates Na^+-K^+-ATPase, produces gluconeogenesis, and enhances insulin secretion, resulting in a mild to moderate decrease in serum potassium concentration by driving potassium intracellularly.[32] The chronotropic response to β_2-agonists is mediated in part by baroreceptor reflex mechanisms as a result of the drop in blood pressure from vascular smooth muscle relaxation, as well as by direct stimulation of cardiac β_2-receptors and some β_1 stimulation at high concentrations.[32] Table 26-6 lists the pharmacologic effects of adrenergic receptor stimulation. Because β_1-receptor stimulation produces excessive cardiac stimulation, resulting in cardiac arrhythmias, and because the inotropic effect enhancing myocardial O_2 consumption leads to myocardial necrosis, there is no rationale for using non-β_2-selective agonists in the treatment of asthma.[2]

TABLE 26-6 Pharmacologic Responses to Sympathomimetic Agonists

Tissue	Receptor Type	Response
Airways	β_2	Smooth muscle relaxation (bronchodilation), increased ciliary beat, increased serous secretion, and inhibition of mast cell degranulation
	α	Smooth muscle contraction (bronchoconstriction?)
Heart	β_1	Inotropic and chronotropic
	β_2	Chronotropic
Vasculature	β_2	Vasodilation, decreased microvascular leakage
	α	Vasoconstriction
Skeletal	β_2	Increased neuromuscular transmission (tremor and increased strength of contraction)
Uterus	β_2	Relaxation (tocolysis)
Metabolic	α, β_1	Glycogenolysis, lipolysis
	β_2	Gluconeogenesis, hypokalemia, increased lactate production

Table 26-7 compares the various short-, long-, and ultra-long-acting β-adrenergic agonists used in asthma in terms of selectivity, potency, and onset and duration of action.[75] The β_2-agonists are functional or physiologic antagonists in that they relax airway smooth muscle regardless of the mechanism for constriction.[46] When administered in equipotent doses, all the short-acting drugs produce the same intensity of response; the only differences are in duration of action and cardiac toxicity.[2,46] The catecholamine derivatives all have the disadvantage of rapid inactivation of their 3,4-hydroxyl catechol group from catechol-*O*-methyltransferase located in the GI tract, rendering them orally inactive. In addition, catecholamines are taken up rapidly into tissues by secondary uptake mechanisms that limit their receptor occupancy and thus have a shorter duration of action.[46] All the β_2-agonists are more bronchoselective when administered by the aerosol route. Aerosol administration of the short-acting β_2-agonists provides more rapid response and greater protection against provocations that induce bronchospasm such as exercise and allergen challenges than does systemic administration.[2,46] Differences in myocardial effects are discernible between selective and nonselective agents even when administered as aerosols, particularly at the higher doses used for acute severe asthma. The β_2-agonists also differ in efficacy or ability to activate the β_2-adrenergic receptors. Full agonists include the catecholamines while the synthetic β_2-agonists all exhibit various levels of partial agonism (see Table 26-7).[46] Although partial agonists by definition cannot produce maximum dilation or protection as full agonists and can potentially block the effect of a full agonist, these differences have not been proven to be clinically significant.

TABLE 26-7 Relative Selectivity, Potency, Onset and Duration of Action of the β-Adrenergic Agonists

	β_2 Activity			Onset and Duration of Action[a]		
Agent	β_2 Intrinsic Efficacy	β_2 Selectivity over β_1	Agonist at β_2 (full/partial)	Bronchodilation (hours)	Protection (hours)[a]	Onset of bronchodilation
Isoproterenol	1	0.24	Full	0.5-2	0.5-1	1-2 minutes
Albuterol/levalbuterol	Not done	27	Partial	4-8	2-4	1-2 minutes
Formoterol	0.95	150	Full	≥12	≥12	1-2 minutes
Salmeterol	0.41	3000	Partial	≥12	≥12	10 minutes
Indacaterol	0.86	16	Nearly full	≥24	≥24	1-2 minutes
Olodaterol	Not done	Not done	Nearly full	≥24	≥24	1-2 minutes
Vilanterol	0.70	2400	Nearly full	≥24	Not studied	1-2 minutes

[a]Protection refers to the prevention of bronchoconstriction induced by exercise or nonspecific bronchial challenges.

The majority of synthetic β_2-agonists are 1:1 racemic mixtures of two mirror images (enantiomers) owing to an asymmetric or chiral carbon.[46] Since most physiologic functions (receptor occupancy and activation and enzymatic metabolism) are stereoselective, the (*R*)-enantiomers of the β_2-agonists are the most pharmacologically active isomer.[46] While it was felt initially that the (*S*)-enantiomers were essentially inactive owing to the 100- to 1,000-fold potency difference between the enantiomers, studies in animal models and isolated in vitro tissue preparations have suggested that the (*S*)-enantiomer of albuterol may be pro-inflammatory and could induce BHR.[46] However, evidence that this occurs consistently in humans or is clinically relevant is lacking.[46] The pharmacokinetics are stereoselective as well, although not predictable. (*R*)-Albuterol is metabolized more rapidly than (*S*)-albuterol, which could lead to accumulation of (*S*)-albuterol with continued dosing.[46] Levalbuterol tartrate is the (*R*)-enantiomer of albuterol, and is a comparable selective beta$_2$-adrenergic receptor agonist.

Both the intensity and duration of response are dose dependent, and, more important, the dose–response relationship is dynamic.[46] At increasing levels of baseline bronchoconstriction (irrespective of the stimulus), the dose–response curve is shifted to the right, and the duration of bronchodilation is decreased.[46] This shift is reflected in the need for higher, more frequent doses in acute asthma exacerbations; the duration of protection against significant provocation is much less than the duration of bronchodilation in chronic stable asthma for short-acting B$_2$-agonists (see Table 26-7).[46]

Chronic administration of β_2-agonists leads to downregulation (decreased number of β_2-receptors) and a decreased binding affinity (desensitization) for these receptors.[46] Systemic corticosteroid therapy can both prevent and partially reverse this phenomenon.[2,46] However, the use of ICSs appears to have minimal ability to prevent tolerance to β_2-agonists.[46] Tolerance primarily reduces duration of bronchodilation as opposed to peak response, although the latter can occur as well. A significantly greater tolerance develops in other tissues (eg, lymphocytes and cardiac and skeletal muscle) compared with the lung, primarily as a result of the surplus β_2-receptors found in respiratory smooth muscle.[46] Tolerance to the extra-pulmonary effects (cardiac stimulation and hypokalemia) may account for a lack of significant cardiac effects with retention of the bronchodilator response despite chronic inhaled β_2-agonist therapy, whereas tolerance to mast cell stabilization may be a drawback to chronic use.[46] Thus, chronic β_2-agonist administration produces a tolerance of minimal clinical significance that is overcome easily by increasing the dose or by administering corticosteroids.[2,46] Most of the tolerance occurs within a week of regular administration and does not worsen with continued administration. As would be expected from a receptor phenomenon, tolerance is a cross-tolerance to all β_2-agonists.[46] Regular treatment (four times daily) does not improve symptom control over as-needed use and is not indicated.[2,3] Regular treatment with the long-acting inhaled β_2-agonists (LABAs) is discussed in Chronic Asthma below.

In conclusion, the short-acting inhaled selective β_2-agonists are indicated for the as-needed treatment of intermittent episodes of bronchospasm. They are the first treatment of choice for acute severe asthma and EIB.[2,3,14] They inhibit EIB in a dose-dependent fashion and provide complete protection for a 2-hour period following inhalation with varying levels of patient-dependent protection over 4 hours.[14] Although the regular administration of β_2-agonists slightly decreases the protective effect, two inhalations prior to exercise still essentially block EIB completely (1% vs 5% drop in FEV$_1$).[14,46]

Systemic Corticosteroids

4 The corticosteroids are the most effective anti-inflammatories available to treat asthma.[2,3] Actions useful in treating asthma include (a) increasing the number of β_2-adrenergic receptors and improving the receptor responsiveness to β_2-adrenergic stimulation, (b) reducing mucus production and hypersecretion, (c) reducing BHR, and (d) reducing airway edema and exudation.[2,47] The glucocorticoid receptor is found in the cytoplasm of most body cells, explaining the multiple effects of systemic corticosteroids. There is no difference between glucocorticoid receptors found throughout the body; however, genetic differences between glucocorticoid receptors from different individuals may determine some of the variations in response.[47] The corticosteroids are lipophilic, readily cross the cell membrane, and combine with the glucocorticoid receptor. The activated complex then enters the nucleus, where it acts as a transcription factor leading to gene activation or suppression.[48] This leads to specific mRNA production, resulting in increased production of anti-inflammatory mediators; suppression of several pro-inflammatory cytokines such as IL-1, GM-CSF, IL-4, IL-5, IL-6, and IL-8, reducing inflammatory cell activation, recruitment, and infiltration; and decreasing vascular permeability.[48] In addition, the activated glucocorticoid receptor complex can act directly with cytoplasmic transcription factors, nuclear factor-κB, and activating protein 1 to prevent the action of pro-inflammatory cytokines on the cell.[48]

Owing to the mechanism that modifies gene expression, the time required to see a particular effect depends on the time required for new protein synthesis, decreased formation of the particular mediator, and resolution of the inflammatory response.[48] Generally, the cellular and biochemical effects are immediate, but varying amounts of time are required to produce a clinical response. β_2-Receptor density increases within 4 hours of corticosteroid administration.[48] Improved responsiveness to β_2-agonists occurs within 2 hours.[48] In acute severe asthma, 4 to 12 hours may be required before any clinical response is noted.[38,48] Reversal of seasonally increased BHR requires at least 1 week of therapy.[48] The chronic use of corticosteroids does not induce a state of corticosteroid dependence, there is no evidence of tolerance produced by chronic administration.

TABLE 26-8 Pharmacodynamic/Pharmacokinetic Comparison of the Corticosteroids

Systemic	Antiinflammatory Potency	Mineralocorticoid Potency	Duration of Biologic Activity (hours)	Elimination Half-Life (hours)
Hydrocortisone	1	1	8-12	1.5-2
Prednisone	4	0.8	12-36	2.5-3.5
Methylprednisolone	5	0.5	12-36	3.3
Dexamethasone	25	0	36-72	3.4-4
ICS	**Receptor Binding Affinity**	**Oral Bioavailability (%)**	**Systemic Clearance (L/h)**	**Half-Life (hours) (IV/Inhaled)**
BDP/BMP[a]	0.4/13.5	20/40	150/120	(0.5/2.7)/(UK/2.7)
BUD	9.4	11	84	2.8/2
CIC/des-CIC[a]	0.12/12	<1/<1	152/228	(0.36/3.4)/(0.5/4.8)
FLU	1.8	20	58	1.6/1.6
FP	18	≤1	66	7.8/14.4
MF	23[b]	<1	53	5.8/UK

Note: Receptor binding affinities are relative to dexamethasone equal to 1. BDP, beclomethasone dipropionate; BMP, beclomethasone 17-monopropionate; BUD, budesonide; CIC, ciclesonide; des-CIC, des-ciclesonide; FLU, flunisolide; FP, fluticasone propionate; MF, mometasone furoate; UK, unknown.

[a]BDP and CIC are prodrugs that are activated in the lung to their active metabolites BMP and des-CIC, respectively.

[b]MF studied in a different receptor system. Value estimated from relative values of BDP and FP in that system.

The corticosteroids used in asthma are compared in Table 26-8.[48,49] Besides acute severe asthma, systemic corticosteroids are also recommended for the treatment of impending episodes of severe asthma unresponsive to bronchodilator therapy.[2,3] The effects of corticosteroids in asthma are dose and duration dependent. This pattern is true for the adverse effects as well (Table 26-9). The clinician must continually balance the toxicity of chronic systemic corticosteroid therapy with control of asthma symptoms. Because short-term (1-2 weeks) high-dose corticosteroids (1-2 mg/kg/day of prednisone) do not produce serious toxicities, the ideal use is to administer the systemic corticosteroids in a short "burst" and then to maintain the patient on appropriate long-term control therapy with ICSs (discussed below).[2] In general, therapy for more than 5 days at doses that exceed the usual physiologic endogenous cortisol production will cause temporary aberration in adrenal cortisol release.[48] However, this hypothalamic–pituitary–adrenal (HPA) axis suppression is short-lived (1-3 days) and readily reversible following short bursts (less than or equal to 10 days) of pharmacologic doses.[48] A maximum number of short bursts that a patient can receive probably exists, after which chronic corticosteroid side effects occur. Adult patients receiving at least eight bursts (more than or equal to 10 days each) have a similar decrease in trabecular bone density as patients on daily or alternate-day corticosteroids over 1 year.[47] Children who received four or more bursts per year of prednisone exhibited a subnormal response to hypoglycemic stress or adrenocorticotropic hormone (ACTH) administration.[48] Very short courses (3-5 days) have been effective in reducing hospitalization from acute exacerbations.[2,3] Use of the shorter-acting corticosteroids such as prednisone will produce less adrenal suppression than the longer-acting dexamethasone.[48]

TABLE 26-9 Adverse Effects of Chronic Systemic Glucocorticoid Administration

Hypothalamic–pituitary–adrenal suppression	Hypertension
Growth retardation	Skin striae
Skeletal muscle myopathy	Impaired wound healing
Osteoporosis/fractures	Inhibition of leukocyte and monocyte function
Aseptic necrosis of bone	Subcutaneous tissue atrophy
Pancreatitis	Glaucoma
Pseudotumor cerebri	Posterior subcapsular cataracts
Psychiatric disturbances	Moon facies
Sodium and water retention	Central redistribution of fat
Hypokalemia/hyperglycemia	

Anticholinergics

The anticholinergic agents have a long history of use for asthma, with an evolving role in the management of asthma.[2,3,50] Anticholinergics are competitive inhibitors of muscarinic receptors.[50] Unlike β_2-agonists, they are not functional antagonists; they only reverse cholinergic-mediated bronchoconstriction. Normal bronchial tone is maintained through parasympathetic innervation of the airways via the vagus nerve.[50] A number of the triggers and mediators of asthma (ie, histamine, prostaglandins, sulfur dioxide, exercise, and allergens) produce bronchoconstriction in part through vagal reflex mechanisms.[50] Studies consistently demonstrate that anticholinergics are effective bronchodilators in asthma. Anticholinergics attenuate but do not block allergen-induced asthma in a dose-dependent fashion and have no effect on BHR.[50] Anticholinergics attenuate but do not block EIB.[14] Five muscarinic receptor subtypes (M_1 through M_5), all inhibited by atropine, have been identified; M_1, M_2, and M_3 are the principal receptors in the airway.[50]

Ipratropium bromide is a nonselective antagonist of M_1, M_2, and M_3 receptors. Although ipratropium produces net bronchodilation, blockade of M_2 receptors allows further release of presynaptic acetylcholine, and may antagonize the bronchodilatory effect of blocking M_3, a possible basis of paradoxical bronchoconstriction.[50] Only the quaternary ammonium derivatives such as ipratropium bromide and tiotropium should be used because they have the advantage of little absorption across respiratory mucosa and do not penetrate the blood–brain barrier. This attribute contributes to negligible systemic effects with a prolonged local effect (ie, bronchodilation). In addition, the quaternary compounds do not appear to significantly alter mucociliary clearance or respiratory secretions.[50] Ipratropium bromide has duration of action of 4 to 8 hours. Both intensity and duration of action are dose dependent. Tiotropium bromide, a long-acting inhaled anticholinergic with duration of 24 hours, has a higher affinity for muscarinic receptors than ipratropium; it dissociates from muscarinic receptors more slowly than ipratropium.[50] Time to reach maximum bronchodilation for ipratropium is considerably slower than for aerosolized short-acting β_2-agonists (30-60 minutes vs 5-10 minutes). However, this difference is of little clinical consequence because some bronchodilation is seen within 30 seconds; 50% of maximum response occurs within 3 minutes.[50] Ipratropium bromide is only indicated as adjunctive therapy in acute severe asthma not completely responsive to β_2-agonists alone.[2,3] Recent trials of tiotropium bromide in chronic asthma suggest that it may be as effective as LABAs added to ICSs and add additional control in severe asthma when added to ICS/LABA combinations.[50-52]

EVALUATION OF THERAPEUTIC OUTCOMES

General Principles, Long-Term Management Goals, and Treatment of Chronic Asthma

Whereas, the NAEPP[2] and GINA[3] have outlined sound strategies for management and treatment of chronic asthma, the following chapter sections rely on the GINA document.[3] GINA is more current (updated in 2015), and describes levels of evidence used in their report.[3] Evidence level A provides a rich body of data consisting of randomized controlled trials (RCTs) and meta-analyses; Evidence level B has a more limited body of data, but still relies on RCTs and meta-analyses. Evidence C includes outcomes of nonrandomized trials or observational studies, and evidence D relies on panel consensus judgment.

Global Initiative for Asthma's long-term goals of asthma management are: (1) to achieve good control of symptoms and maintain normal activity levels and (2) to minimize future risk of exacerbations, fixed airflow limitation, and side effects.[3] The importance of eliciting the patient's own goals is emphasized, as is the development of a patient-healthcare provider partnership. Key components are strategies to both facilitate good communication and reduce the impact of impaired health literacy.[3] Self-management education reduces asthma morbidity in both adults and children (Evidence A).[3] GINA recommends control-based asthma management, adjusting pharmacological and non-pharmacological treatment in a continuous cycle of assessment, treatment, and review. Assessment includes symptom control, risk factors, inhaler technique and adherence, and patient preferences. Response review includes symptoms, exacerbations, medication side effects, patient satisfaction, and lung function.[3] GINA does not recommend neither sputum-guided treatment nor FeNO-guided treatment for the general asthma population.[3]

Global Initiative for Asthma discriminates between preferred treatment options at a population level (based on efficacy, effectiveness, safety, and availability/cost at this level) versus choosing between asthma controller options for individual patients. A shared-decision making approach is recommended for the latter, to include preferred treatment, patient characteristics or phenotype,[3] patient/parent preference, and practical issues (inhaler technique, adherence, and cost).[3]

Non-pharmacologic Therapy

Although the mainstay of the management of asthma is pharmacologic therapy, it is likely to fail without concurrent attention to relevant environmental control and management of comorbidities that may contribute to respiratory symptoms and poor quality of life. Non-pharmacologic therapies are incorporated into GINA's recommendations for initiation of regular daily controller treatment, as well as the stepwise approach for adjusting treatment in adults, adolescents, and children.[3] The guidelines were designed to give healthcare providers a framework with which to develop the proper approach to the individualized therapy of patients. The heterogeneity of asthma demands an individualized approach to therapy with the basic goals of therapy as primary outcome measures.[3] The focus of controller therapy is the reduction of airway inflammation, control of symptoms, and reduction of future risks. Thus, current therapeutic options in asthma consist of acute reliever (rescue) medications for as-needed relief of breakthrough symptoms and exacerbations, and long-term control medications used for the prevention of symptoms and exacerbations and the suppression of inflammation and reduction of BHR.[3] GINA emphasizes the importance of concurrently identifying and treating modifiable risk factors, such as active smoking and exposure to tobacco smoke, obesity, major psychological problems, major socioeconomic problems, confirmed food allergy, and allergen exposure if sensitized.[3] Avoidance of occupational exposures, indoor allergens, and medications that may make asthma worse should be considered when relevant.

7 The development of a patient-healthcare provider partnership in care through patient education and the teaching of patient self-management skills should be the cornerstone of any treatment program.[3] There are a number of published self-management programs for children and adults available through local American Lung Association chapters, as well as asthma treatment centers, and nationally through the NAEPP, GINA, and the Asthma and Allergy Foundation of America.[2,3] Asthma self-management programs have been shown to improve patient adherence to medication regimens, improve self-management skills, and improve use of healthcare services.[53,54]

Self-management programs instruct patients in the pathogenesis of asthma and the appropriate use of their medications but focus principally on teaching patients to recognize triggers for their asthma, how to recognize early signs of deterioration and how to keep track of symptoms (with or without a diary), and take action.[2,3,53] Home PEF monitoring is part of some programs, however, routine PEF monitoring in and of itself does not improve patient outcomes.[2] Short-term PEF monitoring may be useful: following an exacerbation, to monitor recovery; following a change in treatment to assess response; if symptoms appear excessive; and to assist in trigger identification. Long-term PEF monitoring may be useful for earlier detection of exacerbations, especially in patients with poor perception of airflow limitation; for patients with a history of sudden severe exacerbations; and for patients with difficult-to-control or severe asthma.[3]

The NAEPP has recommended a PEF monitoring system based on a traffic light scenario (based on percentage of normal predicted values or personal best values): the green zone is equal to 80% to 100%, the yellow zone is equal to 50% to 79%, and the red zone is less than 50%. The yellow zone is cautionary and requires increasing as-needed bronchodilator use and possibly beginning prednisone if not improved, whereas the red zone warrants contacting the patient's healthcare provider.[2]

Patient education is essential before monitoring can be effective. It proved successful regardless of the healthcare provider who provides it. The NAEPP and GINA advocate significant involvement of all points of patient care in the educational process.[2,3] The provision of written action plans enhances the success of education and is considered an essential component of care.[2,3] Samples of clinically tested written action plans are available from NAEPP and GINA guidelines and other sources.[2,3]

In patients with known allergic triggers for their asthma, allergen avoidance has resulted in an improvement in symptoms, a reduction in medication use, and a decrease in BHR.[2] A comprehensive approach to environmental control is advocated. For example, for patients with house dust mite allergy removing carpeting from bedrooms, washing sheets in hot water (greater than 54.4°C [greater than 130°F]) and using special dust-proof pillow and mattress covers can reduce symptoms and need for medications.[2] Obvious environmental triggers (eg, animal dander and cockroaches), if the patient is sensitive, should be avoided. Evidence for home air-filtering systems and chemicals for killing house dust mites is limited.[2] Immunotherapy (allergy shots) with single antigens particularly has been beneficial and may be considered in patients with persistent asthma with documented sensitivity.[2] Immunotherapy with multiple antigens has been less effective.

Pharmacologic Therapy

The current GINA recommendations for initial controller treatment in adults and adolescents with persistent asthma are summarized in Table 26-10.[3] Regardless of the long-term therapy, all patients need

TABLE 26-10 GINA Recommendations for Initial Controller Treatment in Adults and Adolescents

Symptom Presentation	Preferred Treatment (Evidence Level)
Symptoms or need for SABA lt; 2x/mo; no waking due to asthma in last month; and no risk factors for exacerbations, including in prior year	No controller (D)
Infrequent symptoms, but patient has ≥ risk factor for exacerbation, eg, low lung function, use of OCS in prior year, intensive care treatment for asthma ever	Low dose ICS (D)
Symptoms or need for SABA between 2x/mo and 2x/week, or patient wakes due to asthma ≥ (x) mo.	Low dose ICS (B)
Symptoms or need for SABA > 2x/week	Low dose ICS* (A)
Troublesome symptoms most days or waking ≥ 1x/week, esp. if any risk factors exist	Medium/high dose ICS(A) or Low dose ICS/LABA** (A)
Symptoms consistent with severely uncontrolled asthma, or with an acute exacerbation	OCS short course AND start of high-dose ICS(A) or moderate-dose ICS/LABA** (D)

*Less effective options are LTRA or theophylline.

**Not recommended for initial controller treatment in children 6-11 years.

ICS, inhaled corticosteroids; LABA, long-acting beta$_2$-agonist; LTRA, leukotriene receptor antagonist; OCS, oral corticosteroids; SABA, short-acting beta$_2$-agonist.

to have quick-relief medication in the form of short-acting inhaled β_2-agonists available for acute symptoms. Ensure that the patient can use both the reliever and controller delivery devices correctly. Schedule an appointment for a healthcare provider visit after 2 to 3 months, or earlier depending on clinical urgency. Step down treatment once good control is maintained for 3 months.[3]

The GINA stepwise approach for control-based management is outlined in Table 26-11.[3] This GINA approach emphasizes three components[3]:

> ASSESS—documentation of symptom control and risk factors, and if these are uncontrolled, check inhaler technique and adherence, and consider whether symptoms are due to a co-morbid condition such as allergic rhinitis, GERD, or obesity rather than asthma.
>
> ADJUST therapy (up or down)—both drug therapy and non-pharmacological strategies; treat modifiable risk factors.
>
> REVIEW RESPONSE—assess and optimize asthma control about every 3 months.

Global Initiative for Asthma provides general principles for step-down of controller treatment.[3] Consideration is warranted if symptoms have been well controlled and lung function stable for more than or equal to 3 months (D). An appropriate time should be chosen (no respiratory infection, not travelling, not pregnant). Engage the patient in this therapeutic trial, monitor with symptoms and/or PEF, and schedule follow-up (D). Stepping down ICS doses by 25% to 50% at 3 month intervals is considered feasible and safe for most patients (B).

The ICSs are considered the preferred long-term control therapy for persistent asthma in all patients due to their potency and consistent effectiveness.[3] Low- to medium-dose ICSs reduce BHR, improve lung function, and reduce severe exacerbations leading to ED visits and hospitalizations. They are more effective than theophylline or the LTRAs.[3,55] In addition, the ICS is the only therapy that reduces the risk of dying from asthma.[2,3] In the low to medium doses recommended by GINA (Table 26-12), ICSs are safe for long-term administration (see below).[3,55] They do not appear to reduce airway remodeling and loss of lung function found in some patients with persistent asthma. The ICSs do not enhance lung growth in children with asthma, prevent the development of asthma in high-risk infants, or induce remission of asthma as BHR and other measures of inflammation return to pretreatment levels on discontinuation of therapy.[57] The sensitivity and consequent clinical response to ICSs can vary among patients.[2,3]

Although studies of the alternative long-term control therapies (eg, LTRAs and theophylline) demonstrate improvement in symptoms, lung function, and as-needed, short-acting inhaled β_2-agonist use, they do not reduce BHR, suggesting minimal anti-inflammatory activity.[2,3] The evidence suggests minimal to no differences in efficacy between these alternatives.

For those patients inadequately controlled on low-dose ICSs either an increased dose of the ICS or the combination of ICS and LABA is recommended Step 3 to gain control of more moderate persistent asthma.[3] Alternatives could be the addition of LTRAs or theophylline to ICSs.[3] The addition of theophylline or LTRAs to ICSs is no more effective than doubling the dose of the ICS.[2] The combination of ICS/LABA is more effective at reducing severe asthma exacerbations than doubling the dose of ICS in moderate persistent asthma; increasing the dose of ICSs fourfold also will result in

TABLE 26-11 GINA Stepwise Approach to Control Symptoms and Minimize Future Risk[7]

Step	Preferred Option (Evidence Level)	Other Recommended Options (Evidence Level)
1	As-needed SABA (A)	Consider low dose ICS, in addition to as-needed SABA, for patients at risk for exacerbations (B)
2	Low dose ICS, plus as-needed SABA (A)	LTRA (A) Low-dose ICS/LABA (A) ICS started with symptoms of allergic asthma, for seasonal treatment only (D)
3	Low dose ICS/LABA, plus as-needed SABA for adults/adolescents (A) OR low dose ICS/formoterol as both maintenance and reliever (A) For children 6-11 years, mod. dose ICS, plus as-needed SABA	Medium dose ICS, for adults/adolescents (A) Low dose ICS plus LTRA (A) or low dose, sustained release theophylline (B)
4	Medium dose ICS/LABA, plus as-needed SABA for adults/adolescents (B) OR medium dose ICS/formoterol as both maintenance and reliever (A) For children 6-11 years, refer child to asthma specialist	Add-on therapy with tiotropium for adults with exacerbation history (B)
5	Referral to specialist and consideration of add-on treatment	Tiotropium if < 18 years (B) Omalizumab for moderate-severe allergic asthma (A) Sputum-guided treatment adjusted by eosinophilia >3% (A) Bronchial thermoplasty in some adults with severe asthma (B) Add-on low dose OCS (≤7.5 mg/day prednisone equivalent) (B)

ICS, inhaled corticosteroids; LABA, long-acting beta$_2$-agonist; LTRA, leukotriene receptor antagonist; OCS, oral corticosteroids; SABA, short-acting beta$_2$-agonist.

TABLE 26-12 Available Inhaled Corticosteroid Products, Lung Delivery, and Comparative Daily Dosages

ICS	Product		Lung Delivery[a]
Beclomethasone dipropionate (BDP)	40 and 80 mcg/actuation HFA MDI		50%-60%
Budesonide (BUD)	90 or 180 mcg/dose DPI, Flexhaler		15%-30%
	200 and 500 mcg ampules, 1 mg		5%-8%
Ciclesonide (CIC)	80 or 160 mcg/actuation HFA MDI		50%
Flunisolide (FLU)	80 mcg/actuation HFA MDI		68%
Fluticasone furoate (FF)	100, 200 mcg/actuation DPI, Ellipta		80%-85%
Fluticasone propionate (FP)	44, 110, and 220 mcg/actuation HFA MDI		20%
	50, 100, and 250 mcg/dose DPI, Diskus		15%
Mometasone furoate (MF)	110 and 220 mcg/dose DPI, Twisthaler; 100 mcg and 200 mcg/actuation HFA MDI		11%
	Comparative Daily Dosages (mcg) of Inhaled Corticosteroids		
	Low Daily Dose Child[a]/Adult	**Medium Daily Dose Child[a]/Adult**	**High Daily Dose Child[a]/Adult**
BDP			
HFA MDI	80-160/80-240	>160-320/>240-480	>320/>480
BUD			
DPI	180-360/180-540	>360-720/>540-1,080	>720/>1,080
Nebules	500/UK	1,000/UK	2,000/UK
CIC HFA MDI	80-160/160-320	>160-320/>320-640	>320/>640
FLU			
HFA MDI	160/320	320/320-640	≥640/>640
FFDPI		UK/100	UK/200
FP			
HFA MDI	88-176/88-264	176-352/264-440	>352/>440
DPIs	100-200/100-300	200-400/300-500	>400/>500
MF, DPI	110/110-220	220-440/>220-440	>440/>440

[a]5-11 years of age, except for BUD Nebules, which is 2-11 years of age.

a significant reduction in exacerbations.[58,59] However, doses of ICSs in the high range significantly enhance the risk of toxicity.[56] Thus, high doses of ICSs plus LABA are reserved for patients with severe persistent asthma.[2,3]

Although the addition of a third controller medication is often used clinically in patients with severe persistent asthma uncontrolled on high-dose ICS/LABA, there are limited studies evaluating this practice.[3] LTRAs or theophylline added to high-dose combination ICS/LABA do not improve outcomes.[3] Omalizumab, a recombinant anti-IgE, has demonstrated significant activity in these severe uncontrolled atopic patients.[60] More recently tiotropium bromide has shown promise as add-on to ICS or ICS/LABA combination for use in asthma.[61-63] Studies also point to a beneficial role of tiotropium in the treatment of difficult-to-control asthma and a potential function in ACOS treatment.[64]

Special Populations

6 The management of asthma in children younger than 5 years of age follows the same stepwise approach as in older children and adults but many treatments have not been studied adequately. Thus, many of the recommendations in this age group are extrapolated from older children and adults.[3] The primary differences in management are that no controller treatment is necessarily indicated for Step 1 and the recommended treatment in Step 3 is doubling the dose of ICS rather than adding LABA as is recommended for older children and adults; LABA are not recommended for this age group at any step unless there is evaluation and a clear indication from a specialist.[3] Due to the risk of LABA contributing to asthma exacerbation risk, the FDA required manufacturers of LABA containing products to conduct safety studies in children and adults and there is an ongoing study specifically in children 4 to 11 years of age. Most of the available ICS have been studied in young children but not all have marketing approval from the FDA in this age group. Lack of an approved indication in children under 5 years of age could affect insurance coverage for specific products. ICSs are available as MDI, DPI, and nebulized formulations but the preferred method of delivery is by MDI with a valved spacer and facemask, if needed.[3] Smaller spacers (less than 350 mL) are preferred because 5 to 10 breaths after actuation are required to inhale the complete dose. It is also recommended to not change the spacer type once a child is stable on a specific dose of ICS due to large differences in delivery between devices.[3] ICS use, even with low doses, causes reductions in growth velocity in children that are clinically important.[65,66] Thus, the lowest effective should be used and height should be regularly measured during treatment.[65,66] Treatment of moderate to severe asthma exacerbations may require use of oral corticosteroids but high-dose nebulized budesonide administered intermittently (1 mg twice a day for 7 days) at early signs of upper respiratory tract infections was as effective at preventing severe episodes of wheezing in infants 12 to 53 months of age with recurrent wheezing as low-dose (0.5 mg daily) continuous therapy.[67]

The FDA approval for montelukast (a leukotriene receptor antagonist) in children younger than age 6 was based on safety and pharmacokinetic studies establishing doses but not on efficacy, although improvement in symptoms and as-needed bronchodilators was noted.[2] Based on data from older children, a small minority of children may respond better to montelukast than ICS.[2] ICSs are recommended as first line therapy but the initial choice between a trial of ICS or montelukast should be based on shared decision making between the provider and caregiver.

The elderly are at highest risk from dying of asthma and there are multiple contributing factors.[3] As in very young children, there have been few prospective studies evaluating drug therapies.[3] In addition, the elderly have a high co-morbidity burden which may impact response to therapies differently than with younger patients, and which contributes to the difficultly with adherence when multiple medications for different diseases are given daily. Control of co-morbid conditions (obesity, smoking, depression, and rhinosinusitis) may be required to improve treatment outcomes.[68] Arthritis, vision impairment, and muscle weakness which may affect inspiratory flow, should be considered when selecting inhaler devices.[3] In addition, the elderly may have difficulty distinguishing breathlessness due to ageing or cardiovascular disease from symptoms of asthma.[3] Owing to the increased risk of osteoporosis and cataracts in the elderly, patients requiring high doses of ICSs should have routine height measurements, bone mineral density determinations, and ophthalmic examinations.[2,69] Appropriate therapies for prevention of osteoporosis should be instituted.[2,69] ICS use may contribute to skin bruising which is already common in the elderly.

Asthma affects 8% of pregnant women, making it potentially the most common serious medical condition to complicate pregnancy.[70] Maternal asthma has been reported to increase the risk of perinatal mortality, preeclampsia, preterm birth, and low-birth-weight infants.[70] More severe asthma is associated with increased risks, whereas better-controlled asthma is associated with decreased risks. A systematic review of the evidence on the safety of asthma medications has concluded that it is safer for pregnant women with asthma to be treated with effective medications than for them to have exacerbations.[70] Proper monitoring and control of asthma should enable a woman with asthma to maintain a normal pregnancy with little or no risk to mother or her fetus. Patients should be monitored monthly as exacerbations are more common in the second trimester and should include objective assessment of lung function and validated assessment of symptoms.[3,70]

A stepwise approach to managing asthma during pregnancy and lactation has been published, with low-dose ICSs recommended as preferred treatment for mild persistent asthma with the addition of a LABA if not adequately controlled.[22,70] Budesonide is considered the preferred ICS to initiate because it has the greatest amount of safety data, and the data are reassuring; however, patients who are well-controlled on a particular ICS should remain on current treatment as changing doses could jeopardize asthma control.[22,70] Stepping down treatment should not be initiated during pregnancy due to a risk of perturbations in asthma control.[3] Albuterol is considered the preferred rescue therapy.[70] Conditions that may aggravate asthma such as allergic rhinitis, sinusitis, and GERD should be aggressively treated.[71] Pregnant women are particularly susceptible to viral infections which may lead to exacerbations and worsening asthma symptoms, and should be aggressively treated to avoid fetal hypoxia.[3] Moderate to severe exacerbations should be treated per usual treatment guidelines with a target oxygen saturation of 95%.[3] Hyperventilation during labor may induce bronchoconstriction and should be treated with short-acting inhaled β_2-agonist.[3] Fentanyl, rather than morphine, should be used for pain control as morphine may induce histamine release and respiratory depression.[71]

Drug Class Information for Management of Chronic Asthma

Inhaled Corticosteroids

The mechanism of action of the corticosteroids has been reviewed (see above). The principal advantage of the ICSs is their high topical potency to reduce inflammation in the lung and low systemic activity.[49] The ICSs have high anti-inflammatory potency, approximately 1,000-fold greater than endogenous cortisol, and differ from each other by as much as fourfold to sixfold.[49] However, potency differences, which are simply a measure of binding affinity to the receptor, can be overcome simply by giving different microgram dosages of drug. Aerosol delivery of the preparations is remarkably variable, ranging from 10% to 60% of the nominal dose (ie, that dose which leaves an actuator for an MDI or, in the case of a DPI, that which is released on actuation of the inhaler).[49] Different devices for the same chemical entity may result in twofold differences in delivery, so that delivery method can make a significant difference in the relative comparable dose or therapeutic index.[2,49]

The ICSs, beclomethasone dipropionate, budesonide, ciclesonide, flunisolide, fluticasone propionate, fluticasone furoate, and mometasone furoate, that are currently available for use are compared and listed in Table 26-12. The ICSs have pharmacokinetic differences that result in different topical/systemic activity.[49] Most evidence is consistent with log-linear dose–response curves for both indirect and direct responses. The log-linear nature of the dose–response curve for ICS activity raises the issue of how much of a difference in dose (or lung delivery) or potency is detectable. The measures used to assess efficacy (lung function, BHR, symptoms, and as-needed short-acting inhaled β_2-agonist use) are downstream events from the anti-inflammatory activity. It takes a fourfold difference in potency or dose to detect clinically significant differences in efficacy.[59] The table of comparable ICS doses (see Table 26-12) is based on extensive clinical trial data.[3,49] Clinically comparable doses take into consideration drug potency differences as well as device delivery differences but not the potential for systemic activity.

Since the glucocorticoid receptors within the various tissues are the same, differences in the pharmacokinetic profile are required to produce differences in the topical/systemic effect ratio (therapeutic index).[49] Pharmacokinetic properties that enhance topical selectivity include rapid systemic clearance, poor oral bioavailability, and prolonged residence time in the lung.[49] Owing to their high lipophilicity, systemic clearance of the available ICSs is very rapid, approaching the rate of liver blood flow with the exception of ciclesonide, which is inactivated by blood esterases as well.[49] However, the ICSs differ markedly in their oral bioavailability, although they all undergo rather extensive first-pass metabolism to less active substances when absorbed[49] (see Table 26-8). The ICSs produce dose-dependent systemic effects, contributed by the orally absorbed fraction and the fraction absorbed from the lung[2,49] (Table 26-13). Essentially all the drug that reaches the lung is absorbed systemically; thus, a slow absorption from the lung results in an apparent long elimination half-life and enhances topical selectivity by lowering the systemic concentration.[49] Ciclesonide and beclomethasone dipropionate differ from the other ICSs in that the parent compounds are prodrugs that are metabolized in the lung to the active compounds desciclesonide and beclomethasone monopropionate.[49] The potential advantage of the drugs with low oral bioavailability is obviated by using a spacer device with the MDI for the drugs with higher oral bioavailability because appropriate spacers reduce the oral amount delivered by 80%.[49] The use of VHCs also can increase systemic activity by increasing lung delivery of drugs not absorbed significantly orally.[49] If this increase in lung deposition is twofold or less,

TABLE 26-13 Effects of Inhaled Corticosteroids

Beneficial Effects	Potential Adverse Effects
Decrease eosinophil numbers Decrease mast cell numbers Decrease T-lymphocyte cytokine production Inhibit transcription of inflammatory genes in airway epithelium Reduce endothelial cell leak Upregulate β_2-receptor production Reduce airway epithelial subbasement membrane thickening	Hoarseness, dysphonia, thrush Growth retardation, skeletal muscle myopathy Osteoporosis, fractures and aseptic necrosis of hip Posterior subcapsular cataract formation and glaucoma Adrenal axis suppression, immunosuppression Impaired wound healing, easy bruising, skin striaeHyperglycemia/ hypokalemia, hypertension Psychiatric disturbances

it will increase systemic activity without producing a clinically important increase in efficacy, thus decreasing the therapeutic index.[49] Mouth rinsing and spitting will also reduce the oral availability and are particularly useful for DPI devices.[2,49] Although ciclesonide and its active metabolite have rapid systemic clearance suggesting an improved therapeutic index, it has not yet been clearly established in clinical trials.[49]

The response to ICSs is somewhat delayed. Most patients' symptoms will improve in the first 1 to 2 weeks of therapy and will reach maximum improvement in 4 to 8 weeks.[2] Improvement in baseline FEV_1 and PEF may require 3 to 6 weeks for maximum improvement, whereas improvement in BHR requires 2 to 3 weeks and approaches maximum in 1 to 3 months but may continue to improve over 1 year.[2] Most of the improvement in these parameters occurs at low to medium doses, and there is a large variability in response, with 10% of patients not demonstrating an improvement in either parameter.[2] Whether these nonresponders also show no improvement in rates of exacerbations is unknown. Significant decreases in FeNO occur within 1 to 2 days with maximum effect in 2 to 3 weeks. Sensitivity to exercise challenge decreases after 4 weeks of therapy.[14] Although single doses do not inhibit the immediate asthmatic response to antigen challenge or exercise, continued therapy for 1 week partially suppresses the response. The two latter effects are likely due to a reduction in mucosal mast cells.[2]

Local adverse effects from ICSs include oropharyngeal candidiasis and dysphonia that are dose dependent. The dysphonia (reported in 5%-20% of patients) appears to be due to a local corticosteroid-induced myopathy of the vocal cords.[2] The use of a spacer device with MDIs can decrease oropharyngeal deposition and thus decrease the incidence and severity of local side effects.[2] In infants who require ICS delivery through a face mask, the parent should clean the nasal–perioral area with a damp cloth following each treatment to prevent topical candidiasis.

Systemic adverse effects can occur with any of the ICSs given in a sufficiently high dose.[2,3] Long-term adverse effects of greatest concern include growth suppression in children, osteoporosis, cataracts, dermal thinning, and adrenal insufficiency and crisis.[2,49] Of these, only growth retardation occurs in low to medium doses. However, the growth reduction appears to be transient in that growth velocity is reduced in the first 6 months to 2 years of therapy and then returns to normal.[2,49] The effect is small (1-2 cm total) and not cumulative, but does persist into adulthood.[72] The suppression of the HPA axis and decreased bone mineralization are dose dependent and do not appear to be significant clinically except at high doses.[56] The risks therefore depend on the therapeutic index of each ICS and its delivery device. The effect of delivery device is illustrated by fluticasone propionate, which has both the greatest therapeutic index when administered by DPI and the lowest therapeutic index when administered by MDI plus VHC.[49] Many of the ICSs, including fluticasone propionate, budesonide, ciclesonide, and mometasone furoate, are metabolized in the GI tract and liver by CYP3A4 isoenzymes. Potent inhibitors of CYP3A4 such as ritonavir and ketoconazole have the potential for increasing systemic concentrations of these ICSs by increasing oral availability and decreasing systemic clearance.[49] Some cases of clinically significant Cushing's syndrome and secondary adrenal insufficiency have been reported.[49]

Most patients with moderate disease can be controlled with twice-daily dosing of most ICSs.[2,3,49] Twice-daily dosing produces less thrush than three- to four-times-daily dosing regimens. In milder asthma, once-daily dosing is often sufficient to maintain control.[49] Some of the newer products have gained once-daily dosing indications, particularly in mild asthma once initial control is established.[49] There is no specific pharmacologic or pharmacokinetic aspect of the current ICSs that allows for once-daily dosing because all the agents studied (both the older low-potency ICSs and newer high-potency ICSs) have been effective, provided that patients had relatively mild-to-moderate asthma.[49] More severe patients require multiple daily dosing. The inflammatory response of asthma has been shown to inhibit corticosteroid-receptor binding.[49] Once asthma is controlled, many patients are able to reduce the ICS dose and maintain control.[49] There has been interest in using ICSs as needed or intermittently in patients with mild persistent asthma; however, the as-needed use has shown inconsistent results with better overall control from regular use.[73,74]

Long-Acting Inhaled β_2-Agonists

The two LABAs, formoterol and salmeterol, provide long-lasting bronchodilation (greater than or equal to 12 hours)[75] (see Table 26-7). Unlike the more water-soluble short-acting β_2-agonists, the long-acting agents are lipid soluble, readily partitioning into the outer phospholipid layer of the cell membrane.[75] In addition, ultra-LABA (indacaterol, vilanterol, and olodaterol), are now available and have a 24-hour bronchodilator duration of effect. Vilanterol in combination with fluticasone furoate is available for once daily dosing for asthma in adults aged 18 and older in the United States and for children and adults aged 12 and older in European countries. Currently, products containing indacterol and olodaterol are only indicated for COPD, but are being evaluated for asthma.

The LABAs and ultra-LABAs are more β_2-selective than albuterol and more bronchoselective by virtue of their property of remaining in the lung tissue cell membrane, which produces its longer duration.[75] The LABAs have a duration of bronchodilator effect of about 12 hours and are dosed twice daily whereas the ultra-LABAs have extended bronchodilator characteristics and last up to 24 hours permitting once daily dosing.[75] The onset of action (time required to increase FEV_1 by 12% over baseline) is similar to that of albuterol for LABAs and ultra-LABAs with the exception of salmeterol which has an onset of approximately 10 minutes. However, this difference is of little consequence as salmeterol, formoterol, and vilanterol are recommended for chronic therapy only in combination with ICSs in the United States (in European countries combination ICS with formoterol are also used on-demand for acute relief of symptoms).[3] LABAs are available as single entity and as fixed-dose combinations with ICSs (see below) though single entity LABA products are FDA approved for use only with ICS. Patients need to be counseled to continue to use their short-acting inhaled β_2-agonists for acute exacerbations while receiving the LABA/ICS combination products.

The LABAs are preferred adjunctive therapy to ICSs in children 12 years and older and adults for step 3 and children 6 to 11 years of age for steps 4 and 5.[3] Combination treatment with ICS/LABA provides greater asthma control than increasing the dose of ICS alone, while at the same time reducing the frequency of mild and severe exacerbations.[3]

As with short-acting β_2-agonists, tolerance can occur with chronic administration of LABAs and seems to plateau after about 1 week of regular therapy but response recovers rapidly after only 3 days of non-use.[75] Long-term trials have shown no diminution in bronchodilator response but a partial loss of the bronchoprotective effect against methacholine, histamine, and exercise challenge.[75] These effects do not seem to have a significant impact on the quality of asthma control with chronic daily use.

Concern for risks with long-acting β_2-agonist use began shortly after approval of the first available LABA, salmeterol, with reports of respiratory deaths in salmeterol users.[76] Two large studies of over 25,000 adult patients found an increased risk of death in patients using salmeterol which was observed to be greater in African Americans than whites in one study.[77,78] An FDA review of data revealed similar increases in exacerbation rates with both salmeterol and formoterol including effects in children.[79] However, whether concomitant use of ICS mitigated the risk was unclear. Therefore, FDA has required manufacturers of long-acting β_2-agonists to conduct large (over 40,000 participants) clinical trials separately in adults and children (4-11 years) to evaluate effects on asthma control.[80] The results of the first large study in adults found no increased risk for serious asthma-related events nor asthma-related deaths with LABA/ICS treatment compared to ICS treatment alone; other studies are ongoing.

Methylxanthines

Methylxanthines have been used for asthma therapy for more than 50 years, but their use has declined markedly owing to the high risk of severe life-threatening toxicity and numerous drug interactions, as well as decreased efficacy compared with ICSs and LABAs. Theophylline, the primary methylxanthine of interest, is a moderately potent bronchodilator with mild anti-inflammatory properties.[2] Like the β_2-agonists, the methylxanthines are functional antagonists of bronchospasm; however, their clinical utility is limited by their low therapeutic index.[2] Theophylline as a sustained-release product is the preferred oral preparation, whereas its complex with ethylenediamine (aminophylline) is the preferred injectable product owing to increased solubility.[2]

The mechanism by which theophylline produces bronchodilation appears to be through nonselective phosphodiesterase (PDE) inhibition—producing increased cAMP and cyclic guanosine monophosphate (cGMP) concentrations.[2] The PDE isoenzymes currently thought to be important for theophylline's clinical effects are isoenzymes III, predominant in airway smooth muscle, and IV, important in inflammatory cell regulation such as mast cells, neutrophils, eosinophils, and T lymphocytes.[2] Selective PDE isoenzyme IV inhibitors, however, have no significant effects in clinical asthma. Theophylline also activates histone deacetylase that is involved in the corticosteroid-induced decrease in pro-inflammatory gene expression.[81] It is a competitive antagonist of adenosine and stimulates endogenous catecholamine release, which are important determinants of toxic symptoms of excess theophylline.[2]

Theophylline has a log-linear dose–response curve.[82] Most chronic stable patients with asthma will obtain significant bronchodilation when the serum theophylline concentration reaches 5 mcg/mL (28 μmol/L), and most patients will have no toxic symptoms with serum concentrations of less than 15 mcg/mL (83 μmol/L).[2,82] The percentage of patients experiencing adverse effects increases sharply as concentrations exceed 15 mcg/mL (83 μmol/L). As with the β_2-agonists, the dose–response curves for smooth muscle relaxation by theophylline are dynamic and shifted to the right in the face of increasing contractile stimuli.[82] This property probably explains theophylline's relative lack of bronchodilatory effect in acute severe asthma.[2,82] The severity of theophylline's toxicity precludes even doubling the usual dosage. Toxicities include caffeine-like effects of nausea, vomiting, tachycardia, jitteriness, and difficulty sleeping to more severe toxicities such as cardiac tachyarrhythmias and seizures. Death has occurred in children receiving their usual doses of theophylline during acute systemic viral illnesses due to a reduction in clearance.[82]

Routine monitoring of serum concentrations is essential for the safe and effective use of theophylline.[2] Theophylline is eliminated primarily by metabolism via the hepatic cytochrome P450 (CYP) mixed-function oxidase microsomal enzymes (primarily the CYP1A2 and CYP3A3 isozymes), with 10% or less excreted unchanged in the kidney.[2] Theophylline clearance is age dependent, with 1- to 9-year-olds having the highest systemic clearances and therefore requiring the largest dosages (on a weight basis). However, even within the same age groups, theophylline clearance can vary twofold to threefold.[2] Figure 26-8 outlines a dosing and monitoring schedule for theophylline. Factors affecting theophylline's hepatic metabolism are listed in Table 26-14.[2] Only drugs or diseases that produce a greater than or equal to 20% inhibition or a greater than or equal to 50% induction of theophylline metabolism are likely to result in clinically significant interactions.[82]

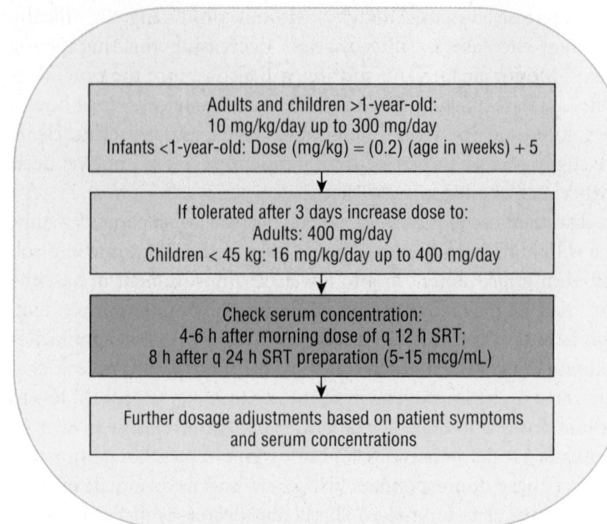

FIGURE 26-8 Algorithm for slow titration of theophylline dosage and guide for final dosage adjustment based on serum theophylline concentration measurement. For infants younger than 1 year of age, the initial daily dosage can be calculated by the following regression equation: Dose (mg/kg) = (0.2) (age in weeks) + 5. Whenever side effects occur, dosage should be reduced to a previously tolerated lower dose.

Sustained-release theophylline is less effective than ICSs and no more effective than oral sustained-release β_2-agonists or LT antagonists.[2,3] The addition of theophylline to ICSs is similar to doubling the dose of the ICS and is overall less effective than the LABAs as adjunctive therapy.[2] The addition of theophylline to patients with poorly controlled asthma receiving ICS/LABA combination does not improve outcomes.[83]

Leukotriene Modifiers

Two cysteinyl LT receptor antagonists (zafirlukast and montelukast) and one 5-lipoxygenase inhibitor (zileuton) are available in the United States.[84] In challenge studies, they reduce allergen-, exercise-, cold-air hyperventilation-, irritant-, and aspirin-induced asthma.[84] Clinical use of zileuton is limited due to the potential for elevated liver enzymes (especially in the first 3 months of therapy),

TABLE 26-14 Factors Affecting Theophylline Clearance

Decreased Clearance	% Decrease	Increased Clearance	% Increase
Cimetidine	−25 to −60	Rifampin	+53
Macrolides: erythromycin, TAO, clarithromycin	−25 to −50	Carbamazepine Phenobarbital Phenytoin	+50 +34 +70
Allopurinol	−20	Charcoal-broiled meat	+30
Propranolol	−30		
Quinolones ciprofloxacin, enoxacin, perfloxacin	−20 to −50	High-protein diet Smoking	+25 +40
Interferon	−50	Sulfinpyrazone	+22
Thiabendazole	−65	Moricizine	+50
Ticlopidine	−25	Aminoglutethimide	+50
Zileuton	−35		
Systemic viral illness	−10 to −50		

and the potential inhibition of drugs metabolized by the CYP3A4 isoenzymes.[84] They are not preferred alternatives in mild persistent asthma nor as alternative add-on therapy for moderate persistent asthma (see Tables 26-10 and 26-11).[3]

These drugs improve pulmonary function tests (FEV_1 and PEF), decrease nocturnal awakenings and β_2-agonist use, and improve asthma symptoms.[84] A major advantage is that they are effective orally, and can be administered once or twice a day.[84] However, they are less effective in asthma than low doses of ICSs.[2,3,55] Although montelukast is approved for EIB in adults, it is significantly less effective than short-acting inhaled β_2-agonists.[14] In adults with severe uncontrolled asthma they do not improve outcomes.[84] They are not as effective as LABAs when added to ICSs for moderate persistent asthma.[84] It is not yet possible to predict which patients respond best to LT modifiers, although there is some evidence that patients with aspirin-sensitive asthma do well, as predicted by studies showing increased cysteinyl LT production in these patients.[84] It is possible that genetic polymorphisms in the 5-lipoxygenase or LTC_4 synthase pathways or in cys-LT_1 receptors might predict better responders in the future.[84] LTRAs also have modest efficacy in allergic rhinitis.

In general, the LTD_4 receptor antagonists are well tolerated and do not appear to have serious class-specific effects.[2] An idiosyncratic syndrome similar to the Churg-Strauss syndrome, with marked circulating eosinophilia, heart failure, and associated eosinophilic vasculitis, has been reported in a small number of patients treated with zafirlukast and montelukast.[82] The majority of these patients had been receiving high-dose ICS or oral corticosteroids and were able to reduce the dose as a consequence of the LTD_4 receptor antagonists. It is unclear whether the increased reports are due to increased case findings among patients with asthma prescribed a new drug or whether the syndrome is related to corticosteroid dose reduction or an idiosyncratic effect of LTRAs in general. Whatever the cause, it appears to be a rare syndrome, with an estimated incidence of less than 1 case per 15,000 to 20,000 patient-years of treatment.[82]

Reports of adverse neuropsychiatric events have caused the manufacturers of the LT inhibitors to revise their labeling. However, evidence for causality of suicidal thoughts and suicide is lacking.[85] Reports of fatal hepatic failure associated with zafirlukast have prompted a warning for patients to be made aware of signs and symptoms of hepatic dysfunction.[2]

Zileuton can be administered twice daily as controlled-release tablets.[2] Efficacy data are more limited, liver function monitoring is recommended, and drug interactions are reported with warfarin and theophylline.

Anti-IgE (Omalizumab)

Omalizumab is a recombinant anti-IgE antibody approved for the treatment of allergic asthma not well controlled on oral corticosteroids or ICSs.[86] It is a composite of 95% human and 5% antihuman murine IgE sequences. Omalizumab binds to the Fc portion of the IgE antibody preventing the binding of IgE to its high-affinity receptor (FcεRI) on mast cells and basophils. The decreased binding of IgE on the surface of mast cells leads to a decrease in the release of mediators in response to allergen exposure. Omalizumab also decreases FcεRI expression on basophils and airway submucosal mast cells over 8 to 12 weeks.[86]

Omalizumab is administered subcutaneously and has a slow absorption rate; peak serum concentration is achieved in 3 to 14 days.[86] Omalizumab is eliminated primarily through the reticuloendothelial system and has an elimination half-life of 17 to 22 days; serum free IgE levels return to previous level in about 3 weeks.[86] Omalizumab should be administered under medical observation with drugs for treating anaphylaxis available.

The dosage of omalizumab is determined by the patient's baseline total serum IgE level (international units per milliliter) and body weight (kilograms).[86] Doses range from 150 to 375 mg and are given at either 2- or 4-week intervals. No further adjustments for variations in total serum IgE are required, and patients receive a consistent dose for the duration of treatment.[86] Omalizumab is approved for patients greater than 6 years with allergic asthma.[86] Due to its significant cost, it is only indicated as step 5 or 6 care for patients who have allergies and severe persistent asthma that are inadequately controlled with the combination of high-dose ICS/LABA and at risk for severe exacerbations.[2,3] It is the only adjunctive therapy that has demonstrated improved outcomes in patients uncontrolled on ICS/LABA and has allowed oral corticosteroid reduction in a number of studies.[2,3,86] Omalizumab therapy is associated with a 0.2% rate of anaphylaxis prompting an FDA warning that patients should remain in the healthcare provider's office for a reasonable period of time past the injection as 70% of reactions occur within 2 hours. In addition, patients should be counseled on the signs and symptoms of anaphylaxis because some reactions have occurred up to 24 hours following an injection.[2,86]

EVALUATION OF ASTHMA CONTROL

The two domains of asthma control are "symptom control" and "future risk of adverse outcomes."[3] Symptom control is assessed from the frequency of daytime and night-time asthma symptoms, reliever medication use, and activity limitations; poor symptom control is an indicator of future risk for exacerbations.[3] However, even when perceived symptom control is good, assessments of future risk of exacerbations, airflow limitation (which may be under-perceived by patients), and medication adverse effects need to be assessed.[3] Factors contributing to asthma severity and future risk of exacerbations and are discussed previously in this chapter.

Future risk of adverse outcomes includes assessment of risks for: future exacerbations, fixed airflow limitation (and thus diminished response to therapy), and medication adverse effects.[3] To assess the risk for future exacerbations (with exacerbation defined as a worsening of asthma requiring the use of systemic corticosteroids or an increase in the use of systemic corticosteroids for patients on a stable maintenance dose to prevent a serious outcome), lung function should be measured before the start of treatment and then 2 months later when maximum response to controller medications is likely attained.[3,87,88] This benchmark of "personal best" can then be used for ongoing risk assessment. Other factors that affect future risk of exacerbations and are to be evaluated include exacerbation history in the previous year (one or more exacerbations requiring systemic corticosteroids is a risk factor) or intubation or intensive care unit stay for asthma as well as ED visits for urgent care.[3,88] Fixed airflow limitation can be affected by lack of ICS treatment, smoking exposure, and low lung function. During ongoing care, spirometry should be measured yearly but long-term PEF monitoring is typically reserved for those with severe asthma.[3] Adverse effect risks are influenced by oral and ICS dose and potential drug interactions with cytochrome P450 inhibitors.[3] In addition, poor inhaler technique (such as not rinsing and spitting after ICS use) can lead to oral candidiasis or an increase in the swallowed fraction of the dose that could influence linear growth in children.

There are several simple screening questionnaires that can be used to assess asthma symptom control quickly in a clinic setting. The Asthma Control Test is a validated simple 5-question survey for patients 12 years and older that yields a numerical score; a score of 19 or less indicates poor asthma control and several institutions have incorporated the survey into the electronic health record in order to evaluate changes over time.[89,90] There is a companion Childhood Asthma Control Test survey for children 4 to 11 years.[89,90] A number of other validated questionnaires exist such as the Asthma Therapy Assessment Questionnaire (ATAQ) and the Asthma Control Questionnaire (ACQ).[89,90]

Patients should also be asked about exercise tolerance as perceived good exercise tolerance may be biased by a sedentary lifestyle adapted to the frequency of bothersome symptoms. All patients on inhaled drugs should have their inhalation delivery technique evaluated periodically—monthly initially and then every 3 to 6 months. Before stepping up therapy, adherence, environmental control, and comorbid conditions should be reviewed.[3]

Following initiation of anti-inflammatory therapy or an increase in dosage, most patients should begin experiencing a decrease in symptoms in 1 to 2 weeks and achieve maximum symptomatic improvement within 4 to 8 weeks. The use of higher ICS doses or more potent agents may accelerate the process. Improvement in FEV_1 and PEF should follow a similar time frame; however, a decrease in BHR, as measured by morning PEF, PEF variability, and exercise tolerance, may take longer and improve over 1 to 3 months.[3] Patients should be informed that following a viral respiratory infection, they may experience decreased exercise tolerance for up to 4 weeks.

Initial visits with the patient should focus on the patient's concerns, expectations, and goals of treatment. Basic education should focus on asthma as a chronic lung disease, the types of medications, and how they are to be used. Inhaler technique is taught, as is when to seek medical advice. Written action plans should be provided. Both peak flow-based or symptom-based self-monitoring can be effective, if taught and followed correctly.[3] The first follow-up visit should include repetition of the educational messages from the first visit, as well as review of the patient's current medications, adherence, and any difficulties related to the therapy.

FUTURE THERAPIES: BIOLOGIC AGENTS IN ASTHMA

Since asthma represents a heterogeneous disease with multiple phenotypes and different pathobiologies, natural histories, symptom burden, and therapeutic responses, approaches to management can no longer be "one-size-fits all." Whereas, the investigation of long-acting muscarinic antagonists (LAMAs) as alternatives to LABAs is a first step, the development of targeted biologic agents is close behind, especially for patients defined as severe asthma.[91]

The World Health Organization (WHO) includes 3 groups of patients who would meet criteria for the diagnosis of severe asthma:[92] (1) untreated severe asthma; (2) difficult-to-treat severe asthma; and (3) treatment-resistant severe asthma. This latter group includes both those individuals for whom control is not achieved despite the highest level of recommended treatment (refractory asthma and corticosteroid-resistant asthma) *and* those individuals for which control can be maintained only with the highest level of recommended treatment.

Alternative definitions of severe asthma have been provided by the American Thoracic Society (ATS).[93] The ATS defines refractory or severe asthma on the basis of 2 major and 7 minor criteria.[93] To meet the ATS definition, patients must have 1 of the 2 major criteria (OCS for greater than 50% of past year or continuous high-dose ICS) and 2 of the 7 minor criteria (concurrent use of greater than or equal to 1 other controller, daily symptoms requiring SABA, FEV_1 less than 80% predicted, greater than or equal to 1 urgent care visits in past year, greater than or equal to 3 OCS bursts in past year, deterioration with decrease in corticosteroid dose of 25%, and history of near-fatal event). This definition of severe asthma may include patients with good disease control and focuses on the need of high doses of corticosteroids; the NLHBI Severe Asthma Research Program uses these criteria as do many of the pharmaceutical manufacturers developing drugs to meet the unmet need of the severe disease phenotype.[91] Gaps still remain about the determinants of severe asthma in children, and trials of novel therapeutic strategies for severe asthma in childhood populations are essential to guide therapy rather than reliance of extrapolation of results from trials conducted in adults.[94]

Table 26-15 outlines the current biologic agents either FDA approved or in trials, as well as the biomarkers predicting therapeutic responses and the biomarkers modulated by therapy.[91,95,96] These agents are targeting the IgE pathway (relevant to allergic asthma) or IL-4, IL-13, and IL-5 pathways (relevant to eosinophilic disorders).

Omalizumab (described earlier) is currently recommended for the treatment of patients greater than 6 years of age with moderate-to-severe asthma, which is not adequately controlled by ICS, ICS/LABA, and is some cases, OCS. Clinical trials that have included children less than 12 years with allergic asthma and poor disease control demonstrate nearly complete elimination of the spring and fall exacerbations.[97]

Eosinophils drive asthmatic inflammation and contribute to airway dysfunction secondary to release of their pro-inflammatory cytokines, chemokines, lipid mediators, and cytotoxic granules from these cells.[96] Reduced sputum eosinophils by ICS reduced asthma exacerbations and contributes to disease control. IL-5 (produced by lymphocytes, mast cells, and maybe eosinophils) contributes to terminal differential, survival, migration, and activation of eosinophils.[96] Thus, this cytokine has been a primary target in asthma treatment.

Mepolizumab (Nucala®) is the first anti-IL5 agent approved in the U.S. for use in combination with other medications for maintenance treatment of severe asthma in patients aged 12 years or older

TABLE 26-15 Targeted Biologic Therapies for Asthma and Potential Biomarkers

Pathway	Biologic Agents Approved/in Trials	Biomarkers Predicting Therapeutic Response	Biomarkers Modulated by Therapy
IgE	Omalizumab (Xolair®)	FeNO Blood eosinophils Periostin	FeNO Sputum eosinophils
IL-4/IL-13	Pitrakinra (competitive antagonist) Dupilumab (receptor antibody)	FeNO Sputum eosinophils Blood eosinophils	FeNO
IL-13	Tralokinomab	Periostin FeNO Eosinophils Sputum IL-13 (periostin surrogate)	
IL-15	Mepolizumab (Nucala®) Reslizumab (Cinqair) (blocks IL-5 alpha receptor) Benralizumab	Sputum eosinophils Blood eosinophils	Sputum eosinophils Blood eosinophils

FeNO, functional exhaled nitric oxide.

with an eosinophic phenotype.[91] It is administered as a 100 mg fixed dose subcutaneous injection every 4 weeks. Those individuals who were shown to benefit from mepolizumab in the Phase III clinical trials had blood eosinophil levels of 150 cells/mcl or greater just prior to treatment. Patients treated with mepolizumab experienced fewer exacerbations; the medication was well-tolerated. Adverse effects most commonly reported included headache, injection-site reactions, back pain, and fatigue.[91]

CONCLUSION

Asthma is a complex disease with a multitude of clinical presentations. The exact defect in asthma has not been defined, and it may be that asthma is a common presentation of a heterogeneous group of diseases. Asthma is defined and characterized by excessive reactivity of the bronchial tree to a wide variety of noxious stimuli. The reaction is characterized by bronchospasm, excessive mucus production, and inflammation. The central role of inflammation in inducing and maintaining BHR is now becoming widely appreciated. The goal of asthma therapy is to normalize, as much as possible, the patient's life and prevent chronic irreversible lung changes. Drugs are the mainstay of asthma management. The goal of drug therapy is to use the minimum amount of medications possible to completely control the disease. In persistent asthma, therapy should be aimed at both bronchospasm and inflammation in order to produce the best results. Patients should be followed and monitored diligently for toxicities. Although death from asthma is an uncommon event, the most common cause of death is underassessment of the severity of obstruction either by the patient or by the clinician; the next common cause is under-treatment. A cornerstone of any therapy is education and the realization that most asthma deaths are avoidable.

ABBREVIATIONS

ACOS	Asthma COPD Overlap Syndrome
ACQ	Asthma Control Questionnaire
ACT	Asthma Control Test
ACTH	adrenocorticotropic hormone
Arg	arginine
ATAQ	Asthma Therapy Assessment Questionnaire
BHR	bronchial hyperresponsiveness
cAMP	cyclic adenosine monophosphate
CFC	chlorofluorocarbon
cGMP	cyclic guanosine monophosphate
COPD	chronic obstructive pulmonary disease
CYP	cytochrome P450
DPI	dry powder inhaler
ED	emergency department
EIB	exercise-induced bronchospasm
EPR3	Expert Panel Report 3
FeNO	fraction of exhaled nitric oxide
FEV_1	forced expiratory volume in 1 second
FVC	forced vital capacity
GERD	gastroesophageal reflux disease
GINA	Global Initiative for Asthma
Gln	glutamine
Glu	glutamic acid
Gly	glycine
GM-CSF	granulocyte-macrophage colony-stimulating factor
HFA	hydrofluoroalkane
HPA	hypothalamic–pituitary–adrenal
ICAM-1	intercellular adhesion molecule 1
ICS	inhaled corticosteroid
IFN-γ	interferon-γ
IgE	immunoglobulin E
IL	interleukin
iNOS	inducible nitric oxide synthase
LABA	long-acting inhaled β_2-agonist
LAMA	long-acting muscarinic antagonist
LT	leukotriene
MDI	metered-dose inhaler
MMAD	mass median aerodynamic diameter
NAEPP	National Asthma Education and Prevention Program
NANC	nonadrenergic, noncholinergic
NO	nitric oxide
O_2	oxygen
PAF	platelet-activating factor
PDE	phosphodiesterase
PEF	peak expiratory flow
PKA	protein kinase A
RCT	randomized controlled trial
RSV	respiratory syncytial virus
SABA	short-acting beta-agonist
T cells	thymically derived lymphocytes
Th_1	type 1 T-helper
Th_2	T-helper cell type 2
VCAM-1	vascular cell adhesion molecule 1
VHC	valved holding chamber
VIP	vasoactive intestinal peptide
WHO	World Health Organization

REFERENCES

1. Rosenblatt MB. History of bronchial asthma. In: Weiss EB, Segal MS, Stein M, eds. *Bronchial Asthma: Mechanisms and Therapeutics*, 2nd ed. Boston: Little, Brown, 1976:5-17.
2. National Institutes of Health, National Heart, Lung, and Blood Institute. National Asthma Education and Prevention Program. Full Report of the Expert Panel: Guidelines for the Diagnosis and Management of Asthma (EPR-3). July 2007. Available at: http://www.nhlbi.nih.gov/guidelines/asthma. Accessed November 2, 2015.
3. Global Initiative for Asthma. Global strategy for asthma management and prevention, 2015. Available at: www.ginasthma.org.
4. Akinbami LJ, Moorman JE, Bailey C, et al. Trends in asthma prevalence, health care use, and mortality in the United States, 2001-2010. *NCHS Data Brief* 2012;94:1-8.
5. American Lung Association. Trends in Asthma Morbidity and Mortality. American Lung Association Epidemiology & Statistics Unit, Research and Health Education Division. September 2012. Available at: http://www.lungusa.org. Accessed November 2, 2015.
6. Melén E, Pershagen G. Pathophysiology of asthma: Lessons from genetic research with particular focus on severe asthma. *J Intern Med* 2012;272:108-120.
7. Gelfand EW. Pediatric asthma: A different disease. *Proc Am Thorac Soc* 2009;6:278-282.
8. Busse WW, Lemanske RF Jr. Asthma. *N Engl J Med* 2001;344:350-362.
9. Fall T, Lundholm C, Ortqvist AK, et al. Early exposure to dogs and farm animals and the risk of childhood asthma. *JAMA Pediatr* 2015;169(11):e153219.
10. Dykewicz MS. Occupational asthma: Current concepts in pathogenesis, diagnosis, and management. *J Allergy Clin Immunol* 2009;123:519-528.
11. Busse WW, Lemanske RF Jr, Gern JE. Role of viral respiratory infections in asthma and asthma exacerbations. *Lancet* 2010;376(9743): 826-834.
12. Murdoch JR and Lloyd CM. Chronic inflammation and asthma. *Mutat Res* 2010;690(1-2):24-39.
13. Gauthier M, Ray A, and Wenzel SE. Evolving concepts of asthma. *Am J Respir Crit Care Med* 2015;192(6):660-668.
14. Parsons JP, Hallstrand TS, Mastronarde JG, et al. An official American Thoracic Society clinical practice guideline: Exercise-induced bronchoconstriction. *Am J Respir Crit Care Med* 2013;187(9):1016-1027.
15. Fahy JV. Eosinophilic and neutrophilic inflammation in asthma: Insights from clinical studies. *Proc Am Thorac Soc* 2009;6:256-259.
16. An SS, Bai TR, Bates JHT, et al. Airway smooth muscle dynamics: A common pathway of airway obstruction in asthma. *Eur Respir J* 2007;29:834-860.

17. Haccuria A, Michils A, Michiels S, et al. Exhaled nitric oxide: A biomarker integrating both lung function and airway inflammation changes. *J Allergy Clin Immunol* 2014;134:554-559.
18. Anderson SD, Charlton B, Weiler JM, et al. Comparison of mannitol and methacholine to predict exercise-induced bronchoconstriction and a clinical diagnosis of asthma. *Respir Res* 2009;10:4.
19. American Lung Association – Asthma Clinical Research Centers' Writing Committee. Effect of nasal mometasone for the treatment of chronic sinonasal disease in patients with inadequately controlled asthma. *J Allergy Clin Immunol* 2015;135(3):701-709.
20. The American Lung Association Clinical Research Centers. Efficacy of esomeprazole for treatment of poorly controlled asthma. *N Engl J Med* 2009;360(15):1487-1499.
21. Brenner BE, Holmes TM, Mazal B, Camargo CA Jr. Relation between phase of the menstrual cycle and asthma presentations in the emergency department. *Thorax* 2005;60:806-809.
22. National Institutes of Health, National Heart, Lung and Blood Institute. *NAEPP Expert Panel Report Managing Asthma During Pregnancy: Recommendations for Pharmacologic Treatment—Update 2004*. NIH Publication No. 04-5246. Bethesda, MD: National Heart, Lung and Blood Institute, National Institutes of Health, March; 2004.
23. Dixon AE, Holguin F, Sood A, et al. An official American Thoracic Society workshop report: Obesity and asthma. *Proc Am Thorac Soc* 2010;7(5):325-335.
24. Marcon A, Corsico A, Cazzoletti L, et al. Body mass index, weight gain, and other determinants of lung function decline in adult asthma. *J Allergy Clin Immunol* 2009;123:1069-1074.
25. Brehm JM, Schuemann B, Fuhlbrigge AL, et al. Serum vitamin D levels and severe asthma exacerbations in the Childhood Asthma Management Program study. *J Allergy Clin Immunol* 2010;126:52-58.
26. Castro M, King TS, Kunselman SJ, et al. Effect of vitamin D3 on asthma treatment failures in adults with symptomatic asthma and lower vitamin D levels: the VIDA randomized clinical trial. *JAMA* 2014;311(20):2083-2091.
27. Diagnosis of Diseases of Chronic Airflow Limitation: Asthma, COPD, and Asthma – COPD Overlap Syndrome (ACOS), 2015. Available at: www.ginasthma.org. Accessed November 2, 2015.
28. Wurst KE, Kelly-Reif K, Bushnell GA, Pascoe S, Barnes N. Understanding asthma-chronic obstructive pulmonary disease overlap syndrome. *Resp Med* 2016;110:1-11.
29. Dolovich MB, Dhand R. Aerosol drug delivery: Developments in device design and clinical use. *Lancet* 2011;377(9770):1032-1045.
30. Rodrigo GJ, Castro-Rodriguez JA. Heliox-driven beta2-agonists nebulization for children and adults with acute asthma: a systematic review with meta-analysis. *Ann Allergy Asthma Immunol* 2014;112: 29-34.
31. Rodrigo GJ. Advances in acute asthma. *Curr Opin Pulm Med* 2015;21: 22-26.
32. Schatz M, Kazzi AAN, Brenner B, et al. American Thoracic Society documents: Joint task force report: Supplemental recommendations for the management and follow-up of asthma exacerbations. *Proc Am Thorac Soc* 2009;6:353-393.
33. Vezina K, Chauhan BF, Ducharme FM. Inhaled anticholinergics and short-acting beta(2)-agonists versus short-acting beta2-agonists alone for children with acute asthma in hospital. *Cochrane Database Syst Rev* 2014;7:CD010283.
34. Guilbert TW, Denlinger LC. Role of infection in the development and exacerbation of asthma. *Expert Rev Respir Med* 2010;4:71-83.
35. Jat KR, Khairwa A. Levalbuterol versus albuterol for acute asthma: A systematic review and meta-analysis. *Pulm Pharmacol Ther* 2013;26: 239-248.
36. Keeney GE, Gray MP, Morrison AK, et al. Dexamethasone for acute asthma exacerbations in children: A meta-analysis. *Pediatrics* 2014;133:493-499.
37. Rowe BH, Edmonds ML, Spooner CH, Diner B, Camargo CA, Jr. Corticosteroid therapy for acute asthma. *Respir Med* 2004;98:275-284.
38. Lazarus SC. Clinical practice. Emergency treatment of asthma. *N Engl J Med* 2010;363:755-764.
39. Powell CV. The role of magnesium sulfate in acute asthma: Does route of administration make a difference? *Curr Opin Pulm Med* 2014;20:103-108.
40. Kew KM, Kirtchuk L, Michell CI. Intravenous magnesium sulfate for treating adults with acute asthma in the emergency department. *Cochrane Database Syst Rev* 2014;5:CD010909.
41. Powell C, Dwan K, Milan SJ, et al. Inhaled magnesium sulfate in the treatment of acute asthma. *Cochrane Database Syst Rev* 2012;12: CD003898.
42. Shan Z, Rong Y, Yang W, et al. Intravenous and nebulized magnesium sulfate for treating acute asthma in adults and children: A systematic review and meta-analysis. *Respir Med* 2013;107:321-330.
43. Tobias JD. Inhalational anesthesia: Basic pharmacology, end organ effects, and applications in the treatment of status asthmaticus. *J Intensive Care Med* 2009;24:361-371.
44. Jat KR, Chawla D. Ketamine for management of acute exacerbations of asthma in children. *Cochrane Database Syst Rev* 2012;11:CD009293.
45. D'Souza DC, Ahn K, Bhakta S, et al. Nicotine fails to attenuate ketamine-induced cognitive deficits and negative and positive symptoms in humans: Implications for schizophrenia. *Biol Psychiatry* 2012;72:785-794.
46. Kelly HW. Risk versus benefit considerations for the beta(2)-agonists. *Pharmacotherapy* 2006;26:164S-174S.
47. Tse SM, Tantisira K, Weiss ST. The pharmacogenetics and pharmacogenomics of asthma therapy. *Pharmacogenomics J* 2011;11:383-392.
48. Green RH, Wardlaw AJ. Systemic corticosteroids in asthma. In: Li JT, ed. *Pharmacotherapy of Asthma*. New York, NY: Taylor and Francis; 2006;233-262.
49. Raissy HH, Kelly HW, Harkins M et al. Inhaled corticosteroids in lung diseases. *Am J Respir Crit Care Med* 2013;187(8):798-803.
50. Peters SP and Dykewicz MS. Anticholinergic therapies. *Middleton's Allergy Principles and Practice*, Volume 2. Philadelphia, PA: Elsevier Saunders; 2014;1552-1566.
51. Peters SP, Kunselman SJ, Icitovic N, et al. Tiotropium bromide step-up therapy for adults with uncontrolled asthma. *N Engl J Med* 2010;363:1715-1726.
52. Kerstjens HA, Disse B, Schröder-Babo W, et al. Tiotropium improves lung function in patients with severe uncontrolled asthma: A randomized controlled trial. *J Allergy Clin Immunol* 2011;128:308-314.
53. Boyd M, Lasserson TJ, McKean MC, Gibson PG, Ducharme FM, Haby M. Interventions for educating children who are at risk of asthma-related emergency department attendance. *Cochrane Database Syst Rev* 2009;(2):CD001290.
54. Janson SL, McGrath KW, Covington JK, Cheng SC, Boushey HA. Individualized asthma self-management improves medication adherence and markers of asthma control. *J Allergy Clin Immunol* 2009;123:840-846.
55. Chauhan BF, Ducharme FM. Anti-leukotriene agents compared to inhaled corticosteroids in the management of recurrent and/or chronic asthma in adults and children. *Cochrane Database Syst Rev* 2012;5:CD002314.
56. Pedersen S. Clinical safety of inhaled corticosteroids for asthma in children: An update of long-term trials. *Drug Saf* 2006;29:599-612.
57. Strunk RC, Sternberg AL, Szefler SJ, et al. Long-term budesonide or nedocromil treatment, once discontinued, does not alter the course of mild to moderate asthma in children and adolescents. *J Pediatr* 2009;154:682-687.
58. Ducharme F, Ni Chroinin M, Greenstone I, Lasserson TJ. Addition of long-acting beta2-agonists to inhaled corticosteroids versus same dose inhaled corticosteroids for chronic asthma in adults and children. *Cochrane Database Syst Rev* 2010;(5):CD005535.
59. Kelly HW. Inhaled corticosteroid dosing: Double for nothing? *J Allergy Clin Immunol* 2011;128:278-281.
60. Casale TB, Stokes JR. Immunomodulators for allergic respiratory disorders. *J Allergy Clin Immunol* 2008;121:288-296.
61. Anderson DE, Kew KM, Boyter AC. Long-acting muscarinic antagonists (LAMA) added to inhaled corticosteroids (ICS) versus the same dose of ICS alone for adults with asthma. *Cochrane Database Rev* 2015;8:CD011397.
62. Evans DJW, Kew KM, Anderson DE, Boyter AC. Long-acting muscarinic antagonists (LAMA) added to inhaled corticosteroids (ICS) versus higher dose ICS for adults with asthma. *Cochrane Database Rev* 2015;7:CD011437.
63. Kerstjens HA, Engel M, Dahl R, et al. Tiotropium in asthma poorly controlled with standard combination therapy. *N Engl J Med* 2012;367: 1198-1207 [Epub ahead of print].
64. Alvarado-Gonzalez A and Arce I. Tiotropium bromide in chronic obstructive pulmonary disease and bronchial asthma. *J Clin Med Res* 2015;7(11):831-839.
65. Zhang L, Prietsch SO, Ducharme FM. Inhaled corticosteroids in children with persistent asthma: Effects on growth. *Evid Based Child Health* 2014;9:829-930.
66. Pruteanu AI, Chauhan BF, Zhang L, Prietsch SO, Ducharme FM. Inhaled corticosteroids in children with persistent asthma: Dose-response effects on growth. *Evid Based Child Health* 2014;9:931-1046.

67. Zeiger RS, Mauger D, Bacharier LB, et al. Continuous or intermittent budesonide in preschool children with recurrent wheezing. *N Engl J Med* 2011;365:1990-2001.
68. Song WJ, Cho SH. Challenges in the Management of Asthma in the Elderly. *Allergy Asthma Immunol Res* 2015;7:431-439.
69. Weldon D. The effects of corticosteroids on bone growth and bone density. *Ann Allergy Asthma Immunol* 2009;103:3-11.
70. Namazy JA, Schatz M. The safety of asthma medications during pregnancy: An update for clinicians. *Ther Adv Respir Dis* 2014;8: 103-110.
71. Maselli DJ, Adams SG, Peters JI, Levine SM. Management of asthma during pregnancy. *Ther Adv Respir Dis* 2013;7:87-100.
72. Kelly HW, Sternberg AL, Lescher R, et al. Effect of inhaled glucocorticoids in childhood on adult height. *N Engl J Med* 2012;367:904-912.
73. Papi A, Canonica GW, Maestrelli P, et al. Rescue use of beclomethasone and albuterol in a single inhaler for mild asthma. *N Engl J Med* 2007;356(20):2040-2052.
74. Martinez FD, Chinchilli VM, Morgan WJ, et al. Use of beclomethasone dipropionate as rescue treatment for children with mild persistent asthma (TREXA): A randomised, double-blind, placebo-controlled trial. *Lancet* 2011;377(9766):650-657.
75. Cazzola M, Page CP, Calzetta L, Matera MG. Pharmacology and therapeutics of bronchodilators. *Pharmacol Rev* 2012;64:450-504.
76. Finkelstein FN. Risks of salmeterol? *N Engl J Med* 1994;331:1314.
77. Castle W, Fuller R, Hall J, Palmer J. Serevent nationwide surveillance study: Comparison of salmeterol with salbutamol in asthmatic patients who require regular bronchodilator treatment. *BMJ* 1993;306:1034-1037.
78. Nelson HS, Weiss ST, Bleecker ER, Yancey SW, Dorinsky PM. The Salmeterol Multicenter Asthma Research Trial: A comparison of usual pharmacotherapy for asthma or usual pharmacotherapy plus salmeterol. *Chest* 2006;129:15-26.
79. McMahon AW, Levenson MS, McEvoy BW, Mosholder AD, Murphy D. Age and risks of FDA-approved long-acting beta(2)-adrenergic receptor agonists. *Pediatrics* 2011;128:e1147-1154.
80. Sears MR. The FDA-mandated trial of safety of long-acting beta-agonists in asthma: Finality or futility? *Thorax* 2013;68:195-198.
81. Adcock IM, Barnes PJ. Molecular mechanisms of corticosteroid resistance. *Chest* 2008;134:394-401.
82. Kelly HW. Non-corticosteroid therapy for the long-term control of asthma. *Expert Opin Pharmacother* 2007;8:2077-2087.
83. The American Lung Association Asthma Clinical Research Centers. Clinical trial of low-dose theophylline and montelukast in patients with poorly controlled asthma. *Am J Respir Crit Care Med* 2007;175:235-242.
84. O'Byrne PM, Gauvreau GM, Murphy DM. Efficacy of leukotriene receptor antagonists and synthesis inhibitors in asthma. *J Allergy Clin Immunol* 2009;124:397-403.
85. Manalai P, Woo JM, Postolache TT. Suicidality and montelukast. *Expert Opin Drug Saf* 2009;8:273-282.
86. Ledford DK. Omalizumab: Overview of pharmacology and efficacy in asthma. *Expert Opin Biol Ther* 2009;9:933-943.
87. Reddel HK, Taylor DR, Bateman ED, et al. An official American Thoracic Society/European Respiratory Society statement: Asthma control and exacerbations: Standardizing endpoints for clinical asthma trials and clinical practice. *Am J Respir Crit Care Med* 2009;180:59-99.
88. Fuhlbrigge A, Peden D, Aptar AJ, et al. Asthma outcomes: Exacerbations. *J Allergy Clin Immunol* 2012;129(3 Suppl):S34-S48.
89. Bime C, Nguyen J, Wise RA. Measures of asthma control. *Curr Opin Pulm Med* 2012;18:48-56.
90. Cloutier MM, Schatz M, Castro M, et al. Asthma outcomes: Composite scores of asthma control. *J Allergy Clin Immunol* 2012;129(3 Suppl): S24-S33.
91. Bell MC and Busse WW. Severe asthma: An expanding and mounting clinical challenge. *J Allergy Clin Immunol: In Practice* 2013;1(2):110-121.
92. Bousquet J, Mantzouranis E, Cruz AA, et al. Uniform definition of asthma severity, control, and exacerbations: Document presented for the World Health Organization Consultation on Severe Asthma. *J Allergy Clin Immunol* 2010;126:926-938.
93. American Thoracic Society. Proceedings of the ATS workshop on refractory asthma: Current understanding, recommendations, and unanswered questions. *Am J Resp Crit Care Med* 2000;162:2341-2351.
94. Guilbert TW, Bacharier LB, and Fitzpatrick AM. Severe asthma in children. *J Allergy Clin Immunol: In Practice* 2014;2(5):489-500.
95. Darveaux J and Busse WW. Biologics in asthma—The next step toward personalized treatment. *J Allergy Clin Immunol* 2015;3(2):152-166.
96. Legrand F and Klion D. Biologic therapies targeting eosinophils: Current status and future prospects. *J Allergy Clin Immunol* 2015;3(2): 167-174.
97. Busse WW, Morgan WJ, Gergen PJ, et al. Randomized trial of omalizumab (anti-IgE) for asthma in inner-city children. *N Engl J Med* 2011;364:1005-1015.

Chronic Obstructive Pulmonary Disease

27

Sharya V. Bourdet and Dennis M. Williams

KEY CONCEPTS

1. Chronic obstructive pulmonary disease (COPD) is a treatable and preventable disease characterized by progressive airflow limitation that is not fully reversible and is associated with an abnormal inflammatory response of the lungs to noxious particles or gases.
2. Chronic obstructive pulmonary disease is historically described as either *chronic bronchitis* or *emphysema*. Chronic bronchitis is defined in clinical terms, whereas emphysema is defined in terms of anatomic pathology. Because most patients exhibit some features of each phenotype, the appropriate emphasis of COPD pathophysiology is on small airway disease and parenchymal damage that contributes to chronic airflow limitation.
3. Mortality from COPD has increased steadily over the past 3 decades; it currently is the third leading cause of death in the United States.
4. The primary cause of COPD is cigarette smoking, implicated in 85% of diagnosed cases. Other risks include a genetic predisposition, environmental exposures (including occupational dusts and chemicals), and air pollution.
5. Smoking cessation and avoidance of other known toxins are the only management strategies proven to slow the progression of COPD.
6. Oxygen therapy has been shown to reduce mortality in selected patients with COPD. Oxygen therapy is indicated for patients with a resting PaO_2 of less than 55 mm Hg or a PaO_2 of less than 60 mm Hg and evidence of right-sided heart failure, polycythemia, or impaired neurologic function.
7. Bronchodilators represent the mainstay of drug therapy for COPD. Pharmacotherapy is used to relieve patient symptoms, improve quality of life, and reduce exacerbation risks. Guidelines recommend short-acting bronchodilators as initial therapy for patients with mild or intermittent symptoms.
8. For the patient who experiences chronic symptoms, long-acting bronchodilators are appropriate. Either a β_2-agonist or an anticholinergic offers significant benefits. Combining long-acting bronchodilators is recommended if necessary.
9. The role of inhaled corticosteroid (IC) therapy in COPD is controversial. International guidelines suggest that patients with severe COPD and frequent exacerbations may benefit from ICs.
10. Acute exacerbations of COPD have a significant impact on disease progression and mortality. Treatment of acute exacerbations includes intensification of bronchodilator therapy and a short course of systemic corticosteroids.
11. Antimicrobial therapy should be used during acute exacerbations of COPD if the patient exhibits at least two of the following: increased dyspnea, increased sputum volume, and increased sputum purulence.

1 Chronic obstructive pulmonary disease (COPD) is a common lung disease characterized by airflow limitation that is not fully reversible and is both chronic and progressive.[1] COPD is preventable and treatable and causes significant extrapulmonary effects that contribute to disease severity in a subset of patients. The prevalence and mortality of COPD have increased substantially over the past 2 decades. In the United States, approximately 24 million Americans are estimated to have COPD, and it accounts for 120,000 deaths annually which is the 3rd leading cause of death.[2] Among the top 5 leading causes of death, only COPD increased in incidence between 2007 and 2010.[3]

In order to standardize the care of patients with COPD and present evidence-based recommendations, the National Heart, Lung, and Blood Institute (NHLBI) and the World Health Organization (WHO) launched the Global Initiative for Chronic Obstructive Lung Disease (GOLD) in 2001. This report was most recently revised in January 2016.[1] The goals of the GOLD organization are to increase awareness of COPD and reduce morbidity and mortality associated with the disease. International guidelines have also been developed through a collaborative effort of the American College of Physicians (ACP), the American College of Chest Physicians (ACCP), the American Thoracic Society (ATS), and the European Respiratory Society (ERS) and are widely available.[4] In addition, the British guidelines were updated in 2010.[5] All of these guidelines are generally concordant in their recommendations. Finally, ACCP and the Canadian Thoracic Society collaborated on a guideline focusing on the prevention of COPD exacerbations which was published in 2015.[6]

Chronic obstructive pulmonary disease is differentiated from asthma in that the airflow limitation present is not fully reversible. Within a patient, the degree of reversibility is typically small; however, between patients, there can be substantial differences in the extent of variability. For some patients airflow obstruction is fixed with minimal improvement in response to a bronchodilator or with optimal treatment. Other patients can demonstrate a significant improvement with pharmacotherapy. The chronic and progressive nature of COPD is associated with an abnormal inflammatory response of the lungs to noxious particles or gases.[1,4,5] Nonetheless, COPD is preventable and treatable. In recent years, there has been an increased appreciation for the impact of the systemic consequences of chronic inflammatory diseases, including COPD, and for the impact of comorbidities in individual patients that can complicate COPD management.

Historically, clinicians and researchers have exhibited a nihilistic attitude toward the value of treatments for COPD. This was based on the paucity of effective therapies, the destructive nature of the condition, and the fact that the common etiology is cigarette smoking, a modifiable health risk. There is now a renewed interest in evaluating the value of treatments and prevention based on the availability of new therapeutic options for pharmacotherapy and guidelines based on evidence. Additionally, a variety of new agents are available for treatment. The international guidelines emphasize the terms *preventable* and *treatable* to support a positive approach to managing the patient with COPD. Support is also reflected in the availability of research funding to improve understanding about this disease and its management. This includes NHLBI funding of Specialized Centers of Clinically Oriented Research (SCCOR) programs in COPD that have an objective to promote multidisciplinary research on clinically relevant questions enabling basic science findings to be more rapidly applied to clinical problems.[7]

2 The term *COPD* has historically been used to describe various pulmonary diseases with a fixed component of airflow limitation. The two principal conditions are chronic bronchitis and emphysema, which are referred to as phenotypes. Chronic bronchitis is associated with chronic or recurrent excessive mucus secretion into the bronchial tree with cough that is present on most days for at least 3 months of the year for at least 2 consecutive years in a patient in whom other causes of chronic cough have been excluded.[1,5] While chronic bronchitis is defined in clinical terms, emphysema is defined in terms of anatomic pathology. Emphysema historically was defined on histologic examination at autopsy. Because this histologic definition is of limited clinical value, emphysema also has been defined as abnormal permanent enlargement of the airspaces distal to the terminal bronchioles accompanied by destruction of their walls, yet without obvious fibrosis.[1]

Differentiating COPD as either chronic bronchitis or emphysema as descriptive subsets of COPD is no longer considered relevant. This is based on the observation that the majority of COPD is caused by a common risk factor (cigarette smoking) and most patients exhibit features of both chronic bronchitis and emphysema. Currently, emphasis is placed on the pathophysiologic features of small airways disease and parenchymal destruction as contributors to chronic airflow limitation. Chronic inflammation affects the integrity of the airways and causes damage and promotes destruction of the parenchymal structures. The underlying problem is persistent exposure to noxious particles or gases that sustain the inflammatory response. The airways of both the lung and the parenchyma are susceptible to inflammation, and the result is the chronic airflow limitation that characterizes COPD (Fig. 27-1).

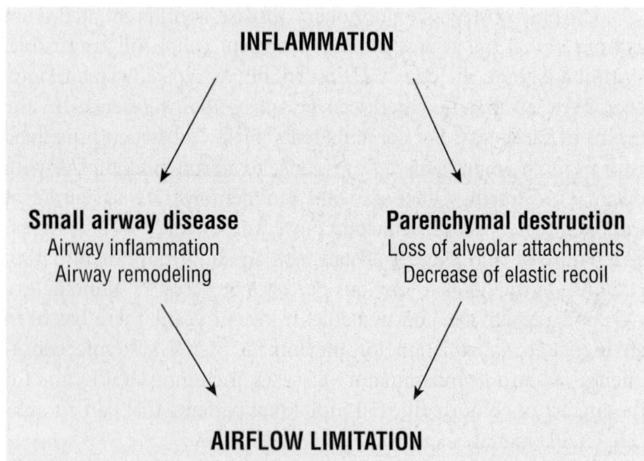

FIGURE 27-1 Mechanisms for developing chronic airflow limitation in COPD. *Data from reference 1.*

EPIDEMIOLOGY

The true prevalence of COPD is likely underreported in the United States. According to national surveys, the true prevalence of people with chronic airflow obstruction as measured by spirometry may exceed 28 million, although more than half are not diagnosed.[8] Surveys indicate that women are twice as likely to be diagnosed with COPD compared to men.[8]

3 Chronic obstructive pulmonary disease is the third leading cause of death in the United States, exceeded only by cancer and heart disease.[2,9] Overall, the mortality rate is six times higher in males; however, the female death rate has doubled over the past 25 years, and the number of female deaths exceeded male deaths in each year since 2000. The mortality rate is higher in whites compared with that in blacks.[9]

Cigarette smoking is the primary cause of COPD and, although the prevalence of cigarette smoking has declined compared with 1965, approximately 23% of individuals in the United States currently smoke.[1] The trend of increasing COPD mortality likely reflects the long latency period between smoking exposure and complications associated with COPD.

The mortality of COPD is significant; however, morbidity associated with the disease also has a significant impact on patients, their families, and the healthcare system. Patients with COPD accounted for over 15 million physician office visits and over 700,000 hospitalizations. A survey by the American Lung Association revealed that among COPD patients, 51% reported that their condition limits their ability to work, 70% were limited in normal physical activity, 56% were limited in performing household chores, and 50% reported that sleep was affected adversely.[9]

The economic impact of COPD continues to increase as well. In the United States, the direct costs of COPD are $29.5 billion with indirect costs of $20.4 billion.[1] These costs are nearly twice that for patients without the disease, and are directly related to the severity of COPD and exacerbation frequency.[2]

ETIOLOGY

4 Cigarette smoking is the most common risk factor and accounts for 85% to 90% of cases of COPD.[1,4,5] Components of tobacco smoke activate inflammatory cells, which produce and release the inflammatory mediators characteristic of COPD. Smokers are 12 to 13 times more likely to die from COPD than nonsmokers.[10] Although the risk is lower in pipe and cigar smokers, it is still higher than in nonsmokers. Age of starting, total pack-years, and current smoking status are predictive of COPD mortality.

However, only 15% to 20% of all smokers go on to develop COPD, and not all smokers who have equivalent smoking histories develop the same degree of pulmonary impairment, suggesting that other host and environmental factors contribute to the degree of lung dysfunction. Nevertheless, the rate of loss of lung function is determined primarily by smoking status and history.[1,5] Children and spouses of smokers have increased risk of developing significant pulmonary dysfunction through passive smoking, also known as *environmental tobacco smoke* or *secondhand smoke.*

In addition to cigarette smoking, COPD is attributed to a combination of risk factors that results in lung injury and tissue destruction. Risk factors can be divided into host factors and environmental factors (Table 27-1), and, commonly, the interaction between these risks leads to expression of the disease. Host factors, such as genetic predisposition, may not be modifiable but are important for identifying patients at high risk of developing the disease.

Environmental factors, such as tobacco smoke, occupational dust, and chemicals are modifiable factors that, if avoided, may reduce the risk of disease development. Environmental exposures associated with COPD are particles that are inhaled by the

TABLE 27-1 Risk Factors for Development of Chronic Obstructive Pulmonary Disease (COPD)

Exposures	Host Factors
Environmental tobacco smoke	Genetic predisposition (AAT deficiency)
Occupational dusts and chemicals	Airway hyperresponsiveness
Air pollution	Impaired lung growth

individual, which result in inflammation and cell injury. Exposure to multiple environmental toxins increases the risk of COPD. Thus, the total burden of inhaled particles (eg, cigarette smoke as well as occupational and environmental particles and pollutants) can play a significant role in the development of COPD. In such cases, it is helpful to assess an individual's total burden of inhaled particles. For example, an individual who smokes and works in a textile factory has a higher total burden of inhaled particles than an individual who smokes and has no occupational exposure.

In nonindustrialized countries, occupational exposures may be a more common risk than cigarette smoking. These exposures include dust and chemicals such as vapors, irritants, and fumes. Reduced lung function and deaths from COPD are higher for individuals who work in gold and coal mining, in the glass or ceramic industries with exposure to silica dust, and in jobs that expose them to cotton dust or grain dust, toluene diisocyanate, or asbestos. Other occupational risk factors include chronic exposure to open cooking or heating fires.

It is unclear whether air pollution alone is a significant risk factor for the development of COPD in smokers and nonsmokers with normal lung function. However, in individuals with existing pulmonary dysfunction, significant air pollution worsens symptoms. As evidence for this, emergency department visits are increased during higher-intensity periods of air pollution.

Individuals exposed to the same environmental risk factors do not have the same chance of developing COPD, suggesting that host factors play an important role in pathogenesis.[1,5] While many not-yet-identified genes may influence the risk of developing COPD, the best documented genetic factor is a hereditary deficiency of α_1-antitrypsin (AAT). AAT-associated emphysema is an example of a pure genetic disorder inherited in an autosomal recessive pattern. Inheritance is sometimes described as autosomal codominant by some researchers, because heterozygotes can also have decreased concentrations of AAT enzyme.[1,4] The consequences of AAT deficiency are discussed in the following section as the protease–antiprotease imbalance. True AAT deficiency accounts for less than 1% of COPD cases.[4]

AAT is a 42 kDa plasma protein that is synthesized in hepatocytes. A primary role of AAT is to protect cells, especially those in the lung, from destruction by elastase released by neutrophils. In fact, AAT may be responsible for 90% of the inhibition of this destructive enzyme.[11] In individuals with the most common allele (M), plasma levels of AAT are approximately 20 to 50 μmol (100-350 mg/dL). The protective effect of AAT in the lungs is significantly diminished when plasma levels are less than 11 μmol (80 mg/dL).[1] AAT is an acute-phase reactant, and the serum concentration can be quite variable.

Several types of AAT deficiency have been identified and are due to mutations in the AAT gene. Two main gene variants, S and Z, have been identified. For patients who are homozygous with the S variant, AAT levels are at least 60% of those of normal individuals. These patients usually do not have an increased risk of COPD compared with normal individuals. Patients with homozygous Z deficiency (ZZ) represent 95% of clinical cases[11] and have AAT levels that are 10% of those of normal individuals, while patients with heterozygous Z variant (SZ) have levels closer to 40% of those of normal individuals. Homozygous Z patients have a higher risk of developing COPD compared with heterozygous Z patients. A history of cigarette smoking increases this risk. A small number of patients have a null phenotype and are at high risk for developing emphysema because they produce virtually no AAT.

Patients with AAT deficiency develop COPD at an early age (20-50 years) primarily owing to an accelerated decline in lung function. Compared with an average annual decline in forced expiratory volume in 1 second (FEV_1) of 25 mL/y in healthy nonsmokers, patients with homozygous Z deficiency have been reported to have declines of 54 mL/y for nonsmokers and 108 mL/y for current smokers. Effective diagnosis is dependent on clinical suspicion, diagnostic testing of serum concentrations, and genotype confirmation.[11] Patients developing COPD at an early age or those with a strong family history of COPD should be screened for AAT deficiency. If the concentration is low, genotype testing (DNA) should be performed.

Other genes have been implicated with increased risk of developing COPD, including chromosome 2q, transforming growth factor β_1, microsomal epoxide hydrolase 1, and tumor necrosis factor-α (TNF-α). However, there are no definite conclusions about an association other than AAT. One genetic factor that may reduce the risk of developing COPD is a polymorphism in the gene encoding for matrix metalloproteinase 12 (MMP12). A cohort of smokers with the polymorphism exhibited a lower risk for developing COPD (relative risk of 0.63).[12]

Two additional host factors that may influence the risk of COPD include airway hyperresponsiveness and lung growth. Individuals with airway hyperresponsiveness to various inhaled particles may have an accelerated decline in lung function compared with those without airway hyperresponsiveness. Additionally, individuals who do not attain maximal lung growth owing to low-birth-weight, prematurity at birth, or childhood illnesses may be at risk for COPD in the future.[1]

PATHOPHYSIOLOGY

Chronic obstructive pulmonary disease is characterized by chronic inflammatory changes that lead to destructive changes and the development of chronic airflow limitation. The inflammatory process is widespread and not only involves the airways but also extends to the pulmonary vasculature and lung parenchyma. The inflammation of COPD is often referred to as *neutrophilic* in nature, but macrophages and CD8+ lymphocytes also play major roles.[1,4,13] The inflammatory cells release a variety of chemical mediators, of which TNF-α, interleukin 8 (IL-8), and leukotriene B_4 (LTB_4) play major roles.[1,13] The actions of these cells and mediators are complementary and redundant, leading to the widespread destructive changes. The stimulus for activation of inflammatory cells and mediators is an exposure to noxious particles and gas through inhalation. The most common etiologic factor is exposure to environmental tobacco smoke, although other chronic inhalational exposures can lead to similar inflammatory changes.

Other processes that have been proposed to play a major role in the pathogenesis of COPD include oxidative stress and an imbalance between aggressive and protective defense systems in the lungs (proteases and antiproteases).[1,13] These processes may be the result of ongoing inflammation or occur as a result of environmental pressures and exposures (Fig. 27-2).

An altered interaction between oxidants and antioxidants present in the airways is responsible for the increased oxidative stress present in COPD. Increases in markers (eg, hydrogen peroxide and nitric oxide) of oxidants are seen in the epithelial lining fluid.[1] The increased oxidants generated by cigarette smoke react with and damage various proteins and lipids, leading to cell and tissue damage. Oxidants also promote inflammation directly and exacerbate

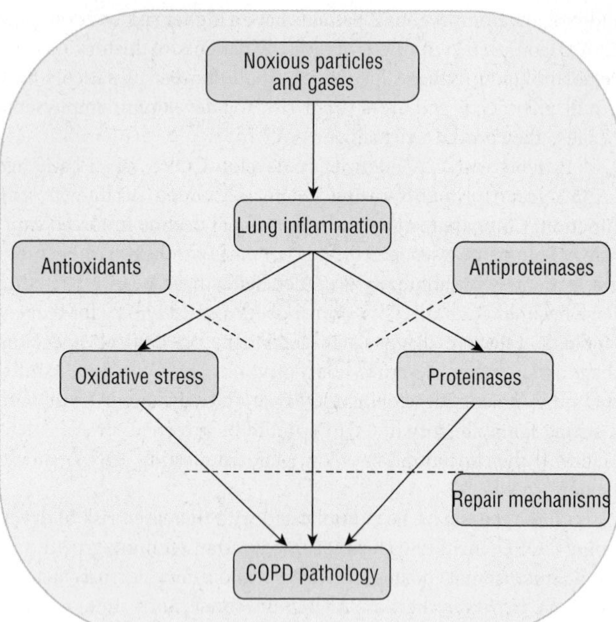

FIGURE 27-2 Pathogenesis of COPD.

the protease–antiprotease imbalance by inhibiting antiprotease activity.[13]

The consequences of an imbalance between proteases and antiproteases in the lungs were described over 40 years ago when the hereditary deficiency of the protective antiprotease AAT was discovered to result in an increased risk of developing emphysema prematurely. As discussed earlier, the enzyme (AAT) is responsible for inhibiting several protease enzymes, including neutrophil elastase. In the presence of unopposed activity, elastase attacks elastin, a major component of alveolar walls.[1]

In the inherited form of emphysema, there is an absolute deficiency of AAT. In cigarette smoking-associated emphysema, the imbalance is likely associated with increased protease activity or reduced activity of antiproteases. Activated inflammatory cells release several proteases other than AAT, including cathepsins and metalloproteinases (MMPs). In addition, oxidative stress reduces antiprotease (or protective) activity.

It is helpful to differentiate inflammation occurring in COPD from that present in asthma because the response to antiinflammatory therapy differs. The inflammatory cells that predominate differ between the two conditions, with neutrophils playing a major role in COPD and eosinophils and mast cells in asthma. Mediators of inflammation also differ leukotriene B_4 (LTB_4), interleukin 8 (IL-8), and tumor necrosis factor alpha (TNF-α) predominating in COPD, compared with leukotriene D_4 (LTD_4), interleukin 4 (IL-4), and interleukin 5 (IL-5) among the numerous mediators modulating inflammation in asthma.[1,13] Characteristics of inflammation for the two diseases are summarized in Table 27-2.

Pathologic changes of COPD are widespread, affecting large and small airways, lung parenchyma, and the pulmonary vasculature.[1] An inflammatory exudate is often present that leads to an increase in the number and size of goblet cells and mucus glands. Mucus secretion is increased, and ciliary motility is impaired. There is also a thickening of smooth muscle and connective tissue in the airways. Inflammation is present in central and peripheral airways. The chronic inflammation results in a repeated injury and repair process that leads to scarring and fibrosis. Diffuse airway narrowing is present and is more prominent in smaller peripheral airways. The decrease in FEV_1 is attributed to the presence of inflammation in the

TABLE 27-2 Features of Inflammation in COPD Compared with Asthma

	COPD	Asthma
Cells	Neutrophils Large increase in macrophages Increase in CD8+ T lymphocytes	Eosinophils Small increase in macrophages Increase in CD4+ Th2 lymphocytes Activation of mast cells
Mediators	LTB_4 IL-8 TNF-α	LTD_4 IL-4, IL-5 (Plus many others)
Consequences	Squamous metaplasia of epithelium Parenchymal destruction Mucus metaplasia Glandular enlargement	Fragile epithelium Thickening of basement membrane Mucus metaplasia Glandular enlargement
Response to treatment	Glucocorticosteroids have variable effect	Glucocorticosteroids inhibit inflammation

airways, while the blood gas abnormalities result from impaired gas transfer due to parenchymal damage and loss of alveolar-capillary networks.

Parenchymal changes affect the gas-exchanging units of the lungs, including the alveoli and pulmonary capillaries. The distribution of destructive changes varies depending on the etiology. Most commonly, smoking-related disease results in centrilobular emphysema that primarily affects respiratory bronchioles. Panlobular emphysema is seen in AAT deficiency and extends to the alveolar ducts and sacs.

The vascular changes of COPD include a thickening of pulmonary vessels and often are present early in the disease.[1,13] Increased pulmonary pressures early in the disease are due to hypoxic vasoconstriction of pulmonary arteries. If persistent, the presence of chronic inflammation may lead to endothelial dysfunction of the pulmonary arteries. Later, structural changes lead to an increase in pulmonary pressures, especially during exercise. In severe COPD, secondary pulmonary hypertension leads to the development of right-sided heart failure.

Mucus hypersecretion is present early in the course of the disease and is associated with an increased number and size of mucus-producing cells. The presence of chronic inflammation perpetuates the process, although the resulting airflow obstruction and chronic airflow limitation may be reversible or irreversible. The various causes of airflow obstruction are summarized in Table 27-3.

Thoracic overinflation is a relevant feature in the pathophysiology of COPD, because it is a central factor in causing dyspnea. Chronic airflow obstruction leads to air trapping, resulting in thoracic hyperinflation that can be detected on chest radiograph. This problem results in several dynamic changes in the chest, including flattening of diaphragmatic muscles. Under normal circumstances, the diaphragms are dome-shaped muscles tethered at the base of

TABLE 27-3 Etiology of Airflow Limitation in COPD

Etiology
Reversible
Presence of mucus and inflammatory cells and mediators in bronchial secretions
Bronchial smooth muscle contraction in peripheral and central airways
Dynamic hyperinflation during exercise
Irreversible
Fibrosis and narrowing of airways
Reduced elastic recoil with loss of alveolar surface area
Destruction of alveolar support with reduced patency of small airways

the lungs. When the diaphragm contracts, the muscle becomes shorter and flatter, which creates the negative inspiratory force through which air flows into the lung during inspiration. In the presence of thoracic hyperinflation, the diaphragmatic muscle is placed at a disadvantage and is a less efficient muscle of ventilation. The increased work required by diaphragmatic contractions predisposes the patient to muscle fatigue, especially during periods of exacerbations.

The other consequence of thoracic hyperinflation is a change in lung volumes. For patients with COPD who exhibit thoracic hyperinflation, there is an increase in the functional residual capacity (FRC), which is the amount of air left in the lung after exhalation at rest. Therefore, these patients are breathing at higher lung volumes that perturb gas exchange. In addition, the increased FRC limits the inspiratory reserve capacity, which is the amount of air that the patient can inhale to fill the lungs. The increased FRC also limits the duration of inhalation time, and this has been associated with an increase in dyspnea complaints by patients.[1,2,5] Drug therapy for COPD, especially bronchodilators, can reduce thoracic hyperinflation by reducing airflow obstruction and air trapping. This explains the improvement in symptoms reported by patients with COPD despite minimal improvements in expiratory lung function with drug therapy.

Airflow limitation is assessed through spirometry, which represents the "gold standard" for diagnosing and monitoring COPD. The hallmark of COPD is a reduction in the ratio of FEV_1 to forced vital capacity (FVC) to less than 70%.[1,5] The FEV_1 generally is reduced, except in very mild disease, and the rate of FEV_1 decline is greater in COPD patients compared with that in normal subjects.

The impact of the numerous pathologic changes in the lung perturbs the normal gas-exchange and protective functions of the lung. Ultimately, these are exhibited through the common symptoms of COPD, including dyspnea and a chronic cough productive of sputum. As the disease progresses, abnormalities in gas exchange lead to hypoxemia and/or hypercapnia, although there often is not a strong relationship between pulmonary function and arterial blood gas (ABG) results.

Significant changes in ABGs usually are not present until the FEV_1 is less than 1 L.[1] In these patients, hypoxemia and hypercapnia can become chronic problems. Initially, when hypoxemia is present, it usually is associated with exertion. However, as the disease progresses, hypoxemia at rest develops. Patients with severe COPD can have a low arterial oxygen tension (pressure exerted by oxygen gas in arterial blood [PaO_2] = 45-60 mm Hg) and an elevated arterial carbon dioxide tension (pressure exerted by carbon dioxide gas in arterial blood [$PaCO_2$] = 50-60 mm Hg). The hypoxemia is attributed to hypoventilation ($\dot{V}$) of lung tissue relative to perfusion ($\dot{Q}$) of the area. This low ($\dot{V}/\dot{Q}$) ratio will progress over a period of several years, resulting in a consistent decline in the PaO_2. Some COPD patients lose the ability to increase the rate or depth of respiration in response to persistent hypoxemia. In addition as COPD progresses and lung function and gas exchange worsens, some patients exhibit chronic hypercapnia, and are referred to as carbon dioxide retainers. In these patients, the central respiratory response to a chronically increased $PaCO_2$ can be blunted. These changes in PaO_2 and $PaCO_2$ are subtle and progress over a period of many years. As a result, the pH usually is nearly normal because the kidneys compensate by retaining bicarbonate. If acute respiratory distress develops, such as might be seen in pneumonia or a COPD exacerbation with impending respiratory failure, the $PaCO_2$ may rise sharply, and the patient presents with a worsening respiratory acidosis.

The consequences of long-standing COPD and chronic hypoxemia include the development of secondary pulmonary hypertension that progresses slowly if appropriate treatment of COPD is not initiated. Pulmonary hypertension is the most common cardiovascular complication of COPD and can result in cor pulmonale, or right-sided heart failure.[14]

The elevated pulmonary artery pressures are attributed to vasoconstriction (in response to chronic hypoxemia), vascular remodeling, and loss of pulmonary capillary beds. When elevated pulmonary pressures are sustained, cor pulmonale develops, characterized by hypertrophy of the right ventricle in response to increases in pulmonary vascular resistance. The risks of cor pulmonale include venous stasis with the potential for thrombosis and pulmonary embolism.

Another important systemic consequence of COPD is a loss of skeletal muscle mass and general decline in the overall health status. These changes are partially attributed to systemic inflammation which is a characteristic of COPD.[15] A consequence is widespread skeletal muscle dysfunction, especially in the leg muscles involved with ambulation.[15] The systemic manifestations can have devastating effects on overall health status and comorbidities. These include cardiovascular events associated with ischemia, cachexia, osteoporosis, anemia, and muscle wasting. There is some interest in the role of measuring C-reactive protein as a parameter to assess systemic inflammation and its impact on COPD severity; however, it is premature to recommend this strategy currently.[16]

CLINICAL PRESENTATION

Symptoms

- Chronic cough
- Sputum production
- Dyspnea

Exposure to Risk Factors

- Tobacco smoke
- α_1-Antitrypsin deficiency
- Occupational hazards

Physical Examination

- Cyanosis of mucosal membranes
- Barrel chest
- Increased resting respiratory rate
- Shallow breathing
- Pursed lips during expiration
- Use of accessory respiratory muscles

Diagnostic Tests

- Spirometry with reversibility testing
- Radiograph of chest
- Arterial blood gas (not routinely assessed in chronic management; has utility in acute decompensation)

PATHOPHYSIOLOGY OF EXACERBATION

The natural history of COPD is characterized by recurrent exacerbations associated with increased symptoms and a decline in overall health status. An exacerbation is defined as a change in the patient's baseline symptoms (dyspnea, cough, or sputum production) beyond day-to-day variability sufficient to warrant a change in management.[1,6,17] Exacerbations have a significant impact on the natural course of COPD and occur more frequently for patients with more severe chronic disease. Because many patients experience chronic symptoms, the diagnosis of an exacerbation is based, in part, on subjective measures and clinical judgment; thus, it can be considered a syndrome. Exacerbations are significant events in that if they hasten disease progress. Additionally, exacerbations, especially those requiring hospitalization, are associated with an increased mortality risk.[17]

There are limited data about pathology during exacerbations owing to the nature of the disease and the condition of patients. However, inflammatory mediators including neutrophils and eosinophils are increased in the sputum. Chronic airflow limitation is a feature of COPD and may not change remarkably even during an exacerbation.[1] The lung hyperinflation present in chronic COPD is worsened during an exacerbation, which contributes to worsening dyspnea and poor gas exchange.

The primary physiologic change is often a worsening of ABG results due to poor gas exchange and increased muscle fatigue. For a patient experiencing a severe exacerbation, profound hypoxemia and hypercapnia can be accompanied by respiratory acidosis and respiratory failure.

CLINICAL PRESENTATION

The diagnosis of COPD is made based on the patient's symptoms, including cough, sputum production, and dyspnea, and a history of exposure to risk factors such as tobacco smoke and occupational exposures. Patients may experience cough for several years before dyspnea develops and often will not seek medical attention until dyspnea is significant. A diagnosis of COPD should be considered for any patient, age 40 years or older, with persistent or progressive dyspnea, with chronic cough productive of sputum, and who exhibits an unusual or abnormal decline in activity, especially in the presence of exposure to environmental tobacco smoke. In addition, the presence of genetic factors, including AAT deficiency, and occupational exposures should be evaluated because approximately 15% of patients with COPD do not have a history of cigarette smoking.

The presence of airflow limitation should be confirmed with spirometry. Spirometry represents a comprehensive assessment of lung volumes and capacities. The hallmark of COPD is an FEV_1:FVC ratio of less than 70%, which indicates airway obstruction.[1] A fixed ratio of less than 70% may be problematic because normal aging may affect this result; however, it continues to be the current standard. Previous criteria for the diagnosis of COPD included measuring the degree of airflow limitation before and after inhaled bronchodilator challenge. It is no longer recommended to obtain pre-bronchodilator values or to calculate the degree of reversibility in order to diagnose COPD (Table 27-4).[1] Post-bronchodilator spirometry results should be used in assessing lung function in patients with COPD. The use of peak expiratory flow measurements as a diagnostic tool is not adequate for COPD due to low specificity and the high degree of effort dependence; however, a low peak expiratory flow is consistent with the clinical presentation of COPD. A comprehensive discussion about spirometry can be found in Chapter 26.

Spirometry combined with a physical examination improves the diagnostic accuracy of COPD.[1,4] Spirometry also is useful to determine the severity of airflow limitation. Patients with all levels of severity of COPD exhibit the hallmark finding of airflow obstruction, specifically, a reduction in the FEV_1/FVC ratio to less than 70%. FVC is the total amount of air exhaled after a maximal inhalation. Currently, the GOLD consensus guidelines suggest a four-grade classification of airflow limitation (Table 27-5). Patients in GOLD 3 or 4 have the most significant airflow limitation and are at the highest risk for future exacerbations, while patients in GOLD 1 and 2 have less airflow limitation and are at lower risk for exacerbations.

Dyspnea is typically the most troublesome complaint for the patient with COPD and often is the stimulus for the patient seeking medical attention. It can impair exercise performance and functional capacity and is frequently associated with depression and anxiety. Together, these have a significant effect on health-related quality of life.[1,4,5] As a subjective symptom, dyspnea is often difficult for the clinician to assess. Various tools are available to evaluate the severity of dyspnea. The modified Medical Research Council (mMRC) scale is commonly employed and categorizes dyspnea grades from 0 to 4.[1,3] In recent years, the impact of COPD on other measures of health status has been recognized and newer patient assessment tools, such as COPD assessment Test (CAT) and Clinical COPD Questionnaire (CCQ), include more items related to overall symptoms and activities.[18,19] Currently, there are three patient assessment questionnaires that are amenable to use in routine clinical practice and are recommended by international guidelines (Table 27-6).[1]

Previously, guidelines have defined disease severity solely by spirometry. Observations that patients with similar spirometric parameters exhibit variations in symptom severity and risk of adverse health events, such as exacerbations, have led to a revision in severity classification. In order to incorporate multiple factors that contribute to disease risk, the revised GOLD consensus guidelines

TABLE 27-4 Procedures for Postbronchodilator Testing

Preparation
Tests should be performed when patients are clinically stable and free from respiratory infection.
Patient must be able to participate with maximal effort during test.
Spirometry
Bronchodilators can be given by either metered-dose inhaler or nebulization.
Usual doses are 400 mcg of β-agonist, 160 mcg of anticholinergic, or the two combined.
FEV_1 should be measured 10-15 minutes after a short-acting β-agonist or 30-45 minutes after a short-acting anticholinergic or combination.
Results
Airflow limitation is confirmed by a postbronchodilator FEV_1/FVC <0.70.

Data from reference 1.

TABLE 27-5 Classification of Severity of Airflow Obstruction (Based on Postbronchodilator FEV_1)

GOLD 1: mild
FEV_1/FVC < 70%
FEV_1 ≥ 80%
With or without symptoms
GOLD 2: moderate
FEV_1/FVC <70%
50% ≤ FEV_1 <80%
With or without symptoms
GOLD 3: severe
FEV_1/FVC <70%
30% ≤ FEV_1 <50%
With or without symptoms
GOLD 4: very severe
FEV_1/FVC <70%
FEV_1 <30%

Data from reference 1.

TABLE 27-6 Comparison of Patient Assessment Questionnaires Used in COPD

Name	Description of Scoring System	Link to Assessment Tool
COPD Assessment Test (CAT)	• Includes 8 items related to health status and impact of COPD on daily activities • Each item scored 0-5 with additive total score of 40 • Score of <10 means less symptoms • Score of ≥10 means more symptoms	http://catestonline.org
Modified Medical Research Council Dyspnea Questionnaire (mMRC)	• Includes 5 descriptive statements related to dyspnea only • Patient chooses most appropriate statement • Each statement corresponds to score of 0-4 • Score of <2 means less symptoms • Score of ≥2 means more symptoms	http://www.goldcopd.org
Clinical COPD Questionnaire (CCQ)	• Includes 10 items in 3 domains related to symptoms, functional state, mental state • Assesses clinical control of disease in past week • Score weighted for each domain • Score <1 means less symptoms[a] • Score ≥1 means more symptoms[a]	http://www.ccq.nl

[a]Exact cut point values have not yet been established for this assessment questionnaire.

recommend that three separate parameters be assessed when classifying disease severity. Parameters include an assessment of airflow limitation by spirometry, measurement of symptom severity, and an assessment of exacerbation frequency. Symptom assessment should be measured at baseline and then during routine visits using CAT, mMRC or CCQ. Defined cut points for patients exhibiting "more symptoms" and "less symptoms" have been established for CAT and mMRC but are not as well defined for CCQ. Until further evaluated, it is reasonable to define "more symptoms" as a CCQ score greater than 1 to 1.5.[1] Frequency of exacerbations can be assessed either by predicted risk of future exacerbations based on classification of airflow limitation or through a review of exacerbation history for the past 12 months. Patients with at least two exacerbations in the last 12 months, or one exacerbation requiring hospitalization, would be considered high risk for future exacerbations. If both methods of exacerbation risk are assessed, the method with the highest risk result should be used to classify the patient (Table 27-7).

While a physical examination is appropriate in the diagnosis and assessment of COPD, most patients who present in the milder stages of COPD will have a normal physical examination. In later stages of the disease, when airflow limitation is severe, patients may have cyanosis of mucosal membranes, development of "barrel chest" due to hyperinflation of the lungs, an increased respiratory rate and shallow breathing, and changes in breathing mechanics such as pursing of the lips to help with expiration or use of accessory respiratory muscles.

Classification Based on Severity

In 2011, the GOLD guidelines included a modified system for classifying COPD based on severity. As discussed above, the new system is based on numerous factors that have a significant impact on the patient, including the degree of airflow obstruction, the frequency and severity of symptoms, and the frequency of exacerbations (see Table 27-7). A patient can first be classified according to the severity of airflow obstruction into grades ranging from 1 to 4 (see Table 27-5). Then the patient is placed into a group (Patient Category A, B, C, or D) based on the impact of symptoms and the risk for future exacerbations. The extent of symptoms is assessed using a validated symptom assessment tool (eg, mMRC, CAT or CCQ). Finally, the risk for an exacerbation is based on previous exacerbations. A patient is categorized based on a history of less than two annual exacerbations, or two or more. A history of at least one exacerbation requiring hospitalization in the past 12 months automatically places the patient in Patient Category C or D. This new classification system by group provides an appropriate emphasis for each of the parameters included (see Table 27-7). Another advantage is that classifying patients according to these groups informs treatment decisions.

Prognosis

For the patient with COPD, the combination of impaired lung function and recurrent exacerbations promotes a clinical scenario characterized by dyspnea, reduced exercise tolerance and physical activity, and deconditioning. These factors lead to disease progression, poor quality of life, possible disability, and premature mortality. COPD is ultimately a fatal disease if it progresses and advanced directives and end-of-life care options are appropriate to consider. The primary causes of death of patients with COPD include respiratory failure, cardiovascular events or diseases, and lung cancer.[1]

Patients with COPD are a heterogeneous group and multiple factors, such as airflow limitation, age, frequency and severity of exacerbations, and comorbidities, have been implicated in rate of disease progression and prognosis.[20] The mortality rate of patients with COPD increases with worsening airflow limitation. In the Towards a Revolution in COPD Health (TORCH) and Understanding Potential Long-Term Impacts on Function with Tiotropium (UPLIFT) trials, 3-year mortality in patients with COPD was reported to be 11% for GOLD 2 (moderate airflow limitation),

TABLE 27-7 Combined Assessment of COPD Severity

Patient Category	Description	Spirometry	Exacerbations in Last Year[a]	CAT	mMRC	CCQ
A	Less symptoms; low risk	FEV_1 ≥ 50% of predicted	0-1	<10	0-1	0-1
B	More symptoms; low risk	FEV_1 ≥ 50% of predicted	0-1	≥10	≥2	≥1
C	Less symptoms; high risk	FEV_1 < 50% of predicted	≥2	<10	0-1	0-1
D	More symptoms; high risk	FEV_1 < 50% of predicted	≥2	≥10	≥2	≥1

[a]> exacerbation, or one requiring hospitalization equals high risk (e.g. Patient Category C or D)

Data from reference 1.

15% for GOLD 3 (severe airflow limitation), and 24% for GOLD 4 (very severe airflow limitation).[21,22]

The average rate of decline of FEV_1 is a useful objective measure to assess the course of COPD over time. However, patients with similar FEV_1 values may differ in the frequency and severity of symptoms and exacerbation history, thus emphasizing the need for a combined assessment for all patients. The average rate of decline in FEV_1 for healthy, nonsmoking patients owing to age alone is 25-30 mL/y. The rate of decline for smokers is steeper, especially for heavy smokers compared with light smokers. The decline in pulmonary function is a steady curvilinear path. The more severely diminished the FEV_1 at diagnosis, the steeper is the rate of decline. Greater numbers of years of smoking and number of cigarettes smoked also correlate with a steeper decline in pulmonary function.[1,5,13] Patients with COPD should have spirometry performed at least annually to assess disease progression. At each clinic visit, patients should be assessed for smoking cessation readiness, if applicable, symptoms and impact on daily activities, and exacerbation history.[1]

Pulmonary gas exchange, affecting both oxygenation and expiration of carbon dioxide, can be impaired in severe disease. Pulse oximetry measures oxygen saturation in the blood and is useful to assess need for supplemental oxygen therapy. It is recommended for all stable patients with FEV_1 less than 35% of predicted and for unstable patients who have signs of respiratory failure, severe exacerbation, or right heart failure.[1] For patients with an oxygen saturation less than 92%, an ABG should be obtained to assess the pO_2 more precisely and to evaluate for hypercapnia.

Asthma is usually differentiated from COPD based on the patient's medical history, risk factors, and improvements on postbronchodilator spirometry; however, in some cases, asthma patients exhibit COPD-like features and COPD patients exhibit asthma-like features. It is also possible for the two conditions to coexist. This coexistence of conditions has been termed "asthma and COPD overlap syndrome" (ACOS) and has been included in the most recent update of the international COPD guidelines.[1] Phenotypes of patients who may meet the ACOS features include those with partially reversible airflow obstruction, an atopic symptoms, and minimal smoking history. Optimal management strategies for a patient with ACOS is not clear; however, there is evidence that this condition is associated with substantially greater treatment costs compared to asthma alone.[23]

CLINICAL PRESENTATION OF COPD EXACERBATION

Because of the subjective nature of defining an exacerbation of COPD, the criteria used among clinicians vary widely; however, most rely on a change in one or more of the following clinical findings: worsening symptoms of dyspnea, increase in sputum volume, or increase in sputum purulence. Acute exacerbations have a significant impact of the economics of treating COPD as well, estimated at 35% to 45% of the total costs of the disease in some settings.[2,13,17]

A widely accepted definition of an exacerbation is that it is an event in the natural course of COPD that is characterized by a worsening in baseline dyspnea, cough, and/or sputum that is beyond the normal day-to-day variation, is acute in onset, and may warrant a change in regular medication. With an exacerbation, patients using rapid-acting bronchodilators may report an increase in the frequency of use. Exacerbations are commonly staged as mild, moderate, or severe according to the criteria summarized in Table 27-8.[1]

TABLE 27-8 Staging Acute Exacerbations of COPD[a]

Mild (type 1)	One cardinal symptom[a] plus at least one of the following: URTI[b] within 5 days, fever without other explanation, increased wheezing, increased cough, increase in respiratory or heart rate >20% above baseline
Moderate (type 2)	Two cardinal symptoms[a]
Severe (type 3)	Three cardinal symptoms[a]

[a]Cardinal symptoms include worsening of dyspnea, increase in sputum volume, and increase in sputum purulence.

[b]URTI, upper respiratory tract infection.

An important complication of a severe exacerbation is acute respiratory failure. In the emergency department or hospital, an ABG usually is obtained to assess the severity of an exacerbation. The diagnosis of acute respiratory failure in COPD is made based on an acute change in the ABGs. Defining acute respiratory failure as a PaO_2 of less than 50 mm Hg or a $PaCO_2$ of greater than 50 mm Hg often may be incorrect and inadequate because these values may not represent a significant change from a patient's baseline values. A more precise definition is an acute drop in PaO_2 of 10 to 15 mm Hg or any acute increase in $PaCO_2$ that decreases the serum pH to 7.3 or less. Additional acute clinical manifestations of respiratory failure include restlessness, confusion, tachycardia, diaphoresis, cyanosis, hypotension, irregular breathing, miosis, and unconsciousness.

Prognosis

Chronic obstructive pulmonary disease exacerbations are associated with significant morbidity and mortality. While mild exacerbations may be managed at home, mortality rates are higher for patients admitted to the hospital. COPD exacerbations contribute to in hospital mortality and deaths after discharge, in addition to hastening the decline of lung function. Many patients experiencing an exacerbation do not have a return to their baseline clinical status for several weeks, significantly affecting their quality of life. Additionally, as many as half the patients originally hospitalized for an exacerbation are readmitted within 6 months.[2,6,17]

There is good evidence that acute exacerbations of COPD have a tremendous impact on disease progression and ultimate mortality. For exacerbations requiring hospitalizations, mortality rates range from 22% to 43% after 1 year, and 36% to 49% in 2 years.[24,25]

TREATMENT
Chronic Obstructive Pulmonary Disease

Desired Outcome

Given the nature of COPD, a major focus in healthcare should be on prevention. However, for patients with a diagnosis of COPD, the primary goal is to prevent or minimize progression. Specific goals of management are listed in Table 27-9. The primary goal of pharmacotherapy has been relief of symptoms, including dyspnea. However, more recently there has been increased interest in the value of therapeutic interventions that reduce exacerbation frequency and severity, as well as reduce mortality. In fact, a reduction in exacerbation frequency is an important outcome measure to consider when evaluating the role and benefit of individual chronic therapies used in COPD management.

Optimally, these goals can be accomplished with minimal risks or side effects. The therapy of the patient with COPD is multifaceted and includes pharmacologic and nonpharmacologic strategies. Appropriate measures of effectiveness of the management plan include continued smoking cessation, symptom improvement, reduction in FEV_1 decline, reduction in the number of exacerbations, improvements in physical and psychological well-being, and reduction in mortality, hospitalizations, and days lost from work.

CLINICAL PRESENTATION Features of COPD Exacerbation

Symptoms

- Increased sputum volume
- Acutely worsening dyspnea
- Chest tightness
- Presence of purulent sputum
- Increased need for bronchodilators
- Malaise, fatigue
- Decreased exercise tolerance

Physical Examination

- Fever
- Wheezing, decreased breath sounds

Diagnostic Tests

- Sputum sample for Gram stain and culture
- Chest radiograph to evaluate for new infiltrates

Unfortunately, most treatments for COPD have not been shown to improve survival or to slow the progressive decline in lung function. However, many therapies do improve pulmonary function and quality of life and reduce exacerbations and duration of hospitalization. Several disease-specific quality-of-life measures are available to assess the overall efficacies of therapies for COPD, including the CAT, CCQ, Chronic Respiratory Questionnaire (CRQ), and the St. George's Respiratory Questionnaire (SGRQ). These questionnaires measure the impact of various therapies on such disease variables as severity of dyspnea and level of activity. They do not measure impact of therapies on survival. While earlier studies of COPD therapies focused primarily on improvements in pulmonary function measurements such as FEV_1, there is a trend towards greater use of these disease-specific quality-of-life measures to evaluate the benefits of therapy on larger clinical outcomes.

General Approach to Treatment

To be effective, the clinician should address four primary components of management: assess and monitor the condition, avoid or reduce exposure to risk factors, manage stable disease, and treat exacerbations. These components are addressed through a variety of nonpharmacologic and pharmacologic approaches.

Nonpharmacologic Therapy

Patients with COPD should receive education about their disease, treatment plans, and strategies to slow progression and prevent complications.[1,5] Advice and counseling about smoking cessation are essential, if applicable, and should be addressed for patients in all stages of the disease. Because the natural course of the disease leads to respiratory failure, the clinician should address end-of-life decisions and advanced directives prospectively with the patient and family. Increasingly, palliative care services, which include both end-of-life and hospice care for patients with all types of life-threatening acute and chronic illnesses, have been utilized for patients with severe COPD.[26]

Smoking Cessation

5 Smoking cessation represents the single most important intervention in preventing the development, as well as the progression, of COPD. A primary component of COPD management is avoidance of or reduced exposure to risk factors. Exposure to environmental tobacco smoke is a major risk factor, and smoking cessation is the most effective strategy to reduce the risk of developing COPD and to slow or stop disease progression. The cost-effectiveness of smoking-cessation interventions compares favorably with interventions made for other major chronic diseases.[1,4,5] The importance of smoking cessation cannot be overemphasized. Smoking cessation leads to decreased symptomatology and slows the rate of decline of pulmonary function even after significant abnormalities in pulmonary function tests have been detected. As confirmed by the Lung Health Study, smoking cessation is the only intervention proven to affect long-term decline in FEV_1 and slow the progression of COPD.[27] In this 5-year prospective trial, smokers with early COPD were randomly assigned to one of the following three groups: smoking-cessation intervention plus inhaled ipratropium three times a day, smoking-cessation intervention alone, or no intervention. During an 11-year followup, the rate of decline in FEV_1 among subjects who continued to smoke was more than twice the rate in sustained quitters. Smokers who underwent smoking-cessation intervention had fewer respiratory symptoms and a smaller annual decline in FEV_1 compared with smokers who had no intervention. However, this study also demonstrated the difficulty in achieving and sustaining successful smoking cessation.

Tobacco cessation has mortality benefits beyond those related to COPD. A follow-up analysis of the Lung Health Study data conducted more than 14 years later demonstrated an 18% reduction in all-cause mortality in patients who received the intervention compared with usual care.[47] Intervention patients had lower death rates due to coronary artery disease (the leading cause of mortality), cardiovascular diseases, and lung cancer, although all categories did not reach clinical significance.

Every clinician has a responsibility to assist smokers in smoking-cessation efforts. A clinical practice guideline for treating tobacco dependence from the US Public Health Service (PHS) was last updated in 2008.[28] The major findings and recommendations of that report are summarized in Table 27-10. A more recent review of tobacco cessation strategies, including the potential role of electronic nicotine dispensing systems (eg, e-cigarettes), was published in 2015.[29] Since 2004, reports from the Surgeon General on the health consequences of smoking have emphasized the detrimental effects of cigarette smoking on the general health of smokers and individuals exposed to secondhand smoke. It is estimated that over 20 million Americans have died prematurely from exposure to cigarette smoking since 1964.

All clinicians should take an active role in assisting patients with tobacco dependence in order to reduce the burden on the individual, his or her family, and the healthcare system. It is estimated that over 75% of smokers want to quit and that one-third have made a serious effort. Yet complete and permanent tobacco cessation is difficult.[28,29] Counseling that is provided by clinicians is associated with greater success rates than self-initiated efforts.

TABLE 27-9 Goals of COPD Management

Goals of COPD Management
Prevent disease progression
Relieve symptoms
Improve exercise tolerance
Improve overall health status
Prevent and treat exacerbations
Prevent and treat complications
Reduce morbidity and mortality

TABLE 27-10 Key Guideline Recommendations Regarding Tobacco Use and Dependence

Tobacco dependence is a chronic disease that often requires repeated intervention and multiple attempts to quit. Effective treatments are available that can significantly improve rates of long-term abstinence.

Clinicians and healthcare delivery systems should consistently identify and document tobacco use status and treat every tobacco user.

Tobacco-dependence treatments are effective over a broad range of populations. Clinicians should encourage every patient willing to make a quit attempt to use counseling treatments and medications recommended in the guideline.

Brief tobacco-dependence treatments are effective. Clinicians should offer every patient who uses tobacco at least these brief treatments.

Individual, group, and telephone counseling are effective, and their effectiveness increases with treatment intensity. Practical counseling (problem-solving and/or skills training) and social support are especially effective and should be employed as a part of treatment.

There are numerous effective medications for tobacco dependence, and clinicians should encourage their use by patients during a quit attempt, except when medically contraindicated or with populations in which the evidence of effectiveness is insufficient (pregnancy, smokeless tobacco users, light smokers, and adolescents). Seven first-line medications (5 nicotine and 2 non-nicotine) consistently increase long-term abstinence rates. Clinicians should also consider the use of combinations as identified in the guideline.

Counseling and medication are effective when used by themselves for treating tobacco dependence. The combination of the two is more effective than either alone. Patients should be encouraged to use both counseling and medication.

Telephone quitline counseling is effective for diverse populations and offers the advantage of broad reach. Clinicians should ensure patient access to quitlines and promote quitline use.

For a tobacco user who is currently unwilling to make a quit attempt, clinicians should use motivational treatments that have been shown to be effective in increasing future quit attempts.

Tobacco-dependence treatments are both clinically effective and highly cost-effective relative to interventions for other clinical disorders. Providing coverage for these treatments increases quit rates. Insurers and purchasers should ensure that all insurance plans include the counseling and medications identified as effective in the guideline as covered benefits.

Data from reference 28.

The PHS guidelines recommend that clinicians take a comprehensive approach to smoking-cessation counseling. Advice should be given to smokers even if they have no symptoms of smoking-related disease or if they are receiving care for reasons unrelated to smoking. Clinicians should be persistent in their efforts because relapse is common among smokers owing to the chronic nature of dependence. Brief interventions (3 minutes) of counseling are proven effective. However, it must be recognized that the patient must be ready to stop smoking because there are several stages of decision making. Based on this, a five-step intervention program is proposed (Table 27-11).

There is strong evidence to support the use of pharmacotherapy to assist in smoking cessation. In fact, it should be offered to most patients as part of a cessation attempt. In general, available therapies will double the effectiveness of a cessation effort. Agents that are considered first line are listed in Table 27-12. The usual duration of therapy is 8 to 12 weeks, although some individuals may require longer courses of treatment. Precautions to consider before using bupropion include a history of seizures or an eating disorder. Nicotine replacement therapies are contraindicated for patients with unstable coronary artery disease, active peptic ulcers, or recent myocardial infarction or stroke. Nicotine patch, bupropion, and the combination of bupropion and the nicotine patch were compared with placebo in a controlled trial.[30] The treatment groups that received bupropion had higher rates of smoking cessation than the groups that received placebo or the nicotine patch. The addition of the nicotine patch to bupropion slightly improved the smoking-cessation rate compared with bupropion monotherapy. Varenicline, a nicotine acetylcholine receptor partial agonist, relieves physical withdrawal symptoms and reduces the rewarding properties of nicotine. Nausea and headache are the most frequent complaints associated with varenicline. Currently, varenicline has not been studied in combination with other tobacco cessation therapies. Second-line agents are less effective or associated with greater side effects; however, they may be useful in selected clinical situations. These therapies include clonidine and nortriptyline, a tricyclic antidepressant. Given the significant increase in use of e-cigarettes and other electronic nicotine delivery systems (ENDS), there is interest in the potential role of these agents as a smoking cessation strategy. It is not clear that substituting ENDS for traditional smoking aids with tobacco cessation.[29] These agents should not be recommended as part of a smoking related strategy until additional evidence is available.

TABLE 27-11 Five-Step Strategy for Smoking-Cessation Program (5 A's)

Ask	Use systematic approach to identify all tobacco users.
Advise	Urge all tobacco users to quit.
Assess	Determine willingness to make a cessation attempt.
Assist	Provide support for the patient to quit smoking.
Arrange	Schedule follow-up and monitor for continued abstinence.

Behavioral modification techniques or other forms of psychotherapy also may be helpful in assisting in smoking cessation. Programs that address the many issues associated with smoking (ie, learned behaviors, environmental influences, and chemical dependence) using a team approach are more likely to be successful. The role of alternative medicine therapies in smoking cessation is controversial. Hypnosis may aid in improving abstinence rates when added to a smoking-cessation program but appears to give little benefit when used alone.

Other Environmental Triggers

Although cigarette smoke represents the overwhelming majority of risk for developing COPD, exposure to other environmental toxins also confers risks.[1] Exposures to occupational dusts and fumes have been implicated as a cause of COPD in 19% of smokers and 31% of nonsmokers with COPD in the United States. In the case of known environmental hazards, primary prevention is appropriate. Policies to limit airborne exposures in the workplace and outdoors, as well as education efforts of workers and policy makers, are recommended.

Pulmonary Rehabilitation

Exercise training is beneficial in the treatment of COPD to improve exercise tolerance and to reduce symptoms of dyspnea and fatigue.[1,3,5] Pulmonary rehabilitation programs are an integral component in the management of COPD and should include exercise training along with smoking cessation, breathing exercises, optimal medical treatment, psychosocial support, and health education. Pulmonary rehabilitation has no direct effect on lung function or gas exchange. Instead, it optimizes other body systems so that the impact of poor lung function is minimized. Exercise training reduces the CNS response to dyspnea, ameliorates anxiety and depression, reduces thoracic hyperinflation, and improves skeletal muscle function.[15] High-intensity training (70% maximal workload) is possible even in advanced COPD patients, and the level of intensity improves peripheral muscle and ventilatory function. Studies have demonstrated that pulmonary rehabilitation with exercise three to seven times per week can produce long-term

TABLE 27-12 First-Line Pharmacotherapies for Smoking Cessation

Agent	Usual Dose	Duration	Common Complaints
Bupropion SR	150 mg orally daily for 3 days, then twice daily	12 weeks, up to 6 months	Insomnia, dry mouth
Nicotine gum	2-4 mg gum prn, up to 24 pieces daily	12 weeks	Sore mouth, dyspepsia
Nicotine inhaler	6-16 cartridges daily	Up to 6 months	Sore mouth and throat
Nicotine nasal spray	8-40 doses daily	3-6 months	Nasal irritation
Nicotine patches	Various, 7-21 mg every 24 hours	Up to 8 weeks	Skin reaction, insomnia
Varenicline	0.5 mg daily orally for 3 days, then 0.5 mg twice daily for 4 days, then 1 mg twice daily	12 weeks	Nausea, sleep disturbances

improvement in activities of daily living, quality of life, exercise tolerance, and dyspnea for patients with moderate-to-severe COPD.[31] Improvements in dyspnea can be achieved without concomitant improvements in spirometry. While rehabilitation programs vary based on length of program, and exercise frequency and intensity, those with longer length and more frequent sessions have demonstrated the best clinical benefit.

Immunizations

Vaccines can be considered as pharmacologic agents; however, their role is described here in reducing risk factors for COPD exacerbations. Because influenza is a common complication in COPD that can lead to exacerbations and respiratory failure, an annual vaccination with the inactivated intramuscular influenza vaccine is recommended. Immunization against influenza can reduce serious illness and death by 50% in COPD patients.[32] Influenza vaccine should be administered annually during each influenza season. Vaccination against influenza can begin as early as August, with most patients being vaccinated during regular medical visits or at vaccination clinics in October and November. COPD patients should receive an inactivated form of the influenza virus vaccine. An oral antiinfluenza agent (oseltamivir) can be considered for patients with COPD during an outbreak for patients who have not been immunized; however, this therapy is less effective and causes more side effects.[33]

The Centers for Disease Control and Prevention (CDC) and the American Lung Association recommend the 23-valent pneumococcal polysaccharide vaccine (PPSV23) for people from 2 to 64 years of age who have chronic lung disease and for all people older than 65 years.[33] In 2009, the CDC added smokers over the age of 18 years to the recommendations. Although evidence for the benefit of the polysaccharide pneumococcal vaccine in COPD is not strong, the argument for continued use is that the current vaccine provides coverage for 85% of pneumococcal strains causing invasive disease and the increasing rate of resistance of pneumococcus to selected antibiotics.[34] Currently, administering the vaccine remains the standard of practice and is recommended by the CDC and the American Lung Association. The GOLD guidelines recommend immunization with pneumococcal polysaccharide vaccine for all COPD patients who are 65 years and older and for patients less than 65 years only if the FEV_1 is less than 40% predicted.[1] Repeated vaccination with the 23-valent product is not recommended for patients aged 2 to 64 years with chronic lung disease; however, revaccination is recommended for patients over 65 years of age if the first vaccination was more than 5 years earlier and the patient was younger than age 65. In 2014, the Advisory Committee on Immunization Practices (ACIP) recommended vaccination with the 13-valent pneumococcal conjugate vaccine (PCV13) for all adults aged 65 years or older. This recommendation will impact the immunization strategies for patients with COPD. At age 65, it is recommended to administer PCV13 followed in 1 year with PPSV23, as long as at least 5 years have passed since the previous PPSV23.

Long-Term Oxygen Therapy

6 The use of supplemental oxygen therapy increases survival in COPD patients with chronic hypoxemia. Although long-term oxygen has been used for many years for patients with advanced COPD, it was not until 1980 that data became available documenting its benefits. At that time, the Nocturnal Oxygen Therapy Trial Group published its data comparing nocturnal oxygen therapy (NOT), 12 h/day, with continuous oxygen therapy (COT), average of 20 h/day.[35] Among patients who were followed for at least 12 months, the results revealed a mortality rate in the NOT group that was nearly double that of the COT group (51% vs 26%). Statistical estimates of the COT group suggest that COT may have added 3.25 years to a COPD patient's life. Additional data from the Nocturnal Oxygen Therapy Trial Group revealed that COT patients had fewer (but statistically insignificant) hospitalizations, improved quality of life and neuropsychological function, reduced hematocrit, and decreased pulmonary vascular resistance.[35]

The decline in mortality with oxygen therapy is proven with 15 h/day of oxygen versus no supplemental oxygen in COPD patients. Patients receiving oxygen therapy for at least part of the day have lower rates of mortality than those not receiving oxygen. Long-term oxygen therapy provides even more benefit in terms of survival after at least 5 years of use, and it improves the quality of life of these patients by increasing walking distance and neuropsychological condition and reducing time spent in the hospital.[1,4,5] Before patients are considered for long-term oxygen therapy, they should be stabilized in the outpatient setting, and pharmacotherapy should be optimized. Once this is accomplished, long-term oxygen therapy should be instituted if either of the following two conditions is observed and documented twice in a 3-week period:

1. A resting PaO_2 of less than 55 mm Hg or SaO_2 less than 88% with or without hypercapnia.
2. A resting PaO_2 between 55 and 60 mm Hg or SaO_2 less than 88% with evidence of right-sided heart failure, polycythemia, or pulmonary hypertension.

The most practical means of administering long-term oxygen is with the nasal cannula, at 1 to 2 L/min, which provides 24% to 28% oxygen. The goal is to raise the PaO_2 above 60 mm Hg. Patient education about flow rates and avoidance of flames (ie, smoking) is of the utmost importance.

There are three different ways to deliver oxygen, including (a) in liquid reservoirs, (b) compressed into a cylinder, and (c) via an oxygen concentrator. Although conventional liquid oxygen and compressed oxygen are quite bulky, smaller, portable tanks are available to permit greater patient mobility. Oxygen concentrator devices separate nitrogen from room air and concentrate oxygen. These are the most convenient and the least expensive method of oxygen delivery. Oxygen-conservation devices are available that allow oxygen to flow only during inspiration, making the supply last longer. These may be particularly useful to prolong the oxygen supply for mobile patients using portable cylinders. However, the devices are bulky and subject to failure.

Adjunctive Therapies

In addition to supplemental oxygen, adjunctive therapies to consider as part of a pulmonary rehabilitation program are psychoeducational care and nutritional support. Psychoeducational care (such as relaxation) has been associated with improvement in the functioning and well-being of adults with COPD.[1,4] The role of nutritional support for patients with COPD is controversial. Several studies have shown an association among malnutrition, low body mass index (BMI), and impaired pulmonary status among patients with COPD. However, results from multiple studies suggest that the effect of nutritional support on physical and functional outcomes in COPD is small and may be most beneficial for malnourished patients.[36]

Pharmacologic Therapy

Results from numerous clinical trials have improved insight and understanding about the respective roles of various medications used in chronic COPD management. Yet, some controversies still exist related to both effectiveness and safety. In contrast to the survival benefit conferred by supplemental oxygen therapy, there is no medication available for the treatment of COPD that has been conclusively shown to modify the progressive decline in lung function or prolong survival.[1,4,5] There is limited evidence that chronic treatment with pharmacotherapy can reduce the rate of decline in spirometry in a subset of patients with more severe disease. Currently, the primary goal of pharmacotherapy is to control patient symptoms and reduce complications, including the frequency and severity of exacerbations, and improving the overall health status and exercise tolerance of the patient.

Currently available inhalational therapies for COPD are summarized in Tables 27-13 and 27-14. International guidelines recommend a stepwise approach to the use of pharmacotherapy based on disease severity, which is determined by the results of spirometry, nature of symptoms, and exacerbation rates.[1,5] The impact of recurrent exacerbations on accelerating disease progression is increasingly recognized as an important factor to be considered. The primary goals of pharmacotherapy are to control symptoms (including dyspnea), reduce exacerbations, and improve exercise tolerance and health status. Currently, there is inadequate evidence to support the use of more aggressive pharmacotherapy early in the course of disease because of the lack of a disease-modifying benefit. Because of the progressive nature of COPD, pharmacotherapy tends to be chronic and cumulative and step-down approaches in stable patients are not successful, although recent evidence suggests that this practice requires further evaluation. Patients exhibit variable responses to available therapies and the treatment approach should be individualized.

Pharmacotherapy of COPD typically involves the use of inhaled medications, requiring patient knowledge, understanding, and skills using the various inhalation devices. Several delivery devices are available (eg, metered-dose inhalers [MDIs], dry powder inhalers [DPIs], soft-mist inhalers [SMIs], nebulizers, and ancillary devices such as holding chambers), and the instructions about proper use vary. Comorbidities that are common for patients with COPD, including physical and mental conditions, can have a significant effect on the patient's ability to use the devices. Periodic and frequent reinforcement and observation by the clinician is required for the patient's benefit.

7 Pharmacotherapy focuses on the use of bronchodilators to control symptoms. Bronchodilators relax bronchial smooth muscle, improve lung emptying, reduce thoracic hyperinflation at rest and during exercise, and improve exercise tolerance.[1] These effects can be seen in the absence of objective improvements on spirometry. There are several classes of bronchodilators to choose from, and classes differ with respect to onset and duration of action, and adverse events. The initial and subsequent choice of medications should be based on the specific clinical situation and patient characteristics. Short-acting medications can be used as needed or on a scheduled basis depending on the clinical situation, and additional therapies should be added in a stepwise manner depending on the response and severity of disease. Considerations should be given to individual patient response, tolerability, adherence, and economic factors. Recommendations for management of COPD have been proposed based on a combined assessment of airflow limitation, symptoms, and risk of exacerbations, according to the new classification system for disease severity (see Table 27-13). This schema provides clearer guidance on management compared with previous recommendations, and also allows for the individualization of pharmacotherapy based on patient-specific factors of lung function, symptom frequency and severity, and exacerbation risk.

According to the guidelines, patients with intermittent symptoms and low risk for exacerbations (Group A) should be treated with short-acting bronchodilators as needed. When symptoms become more persistent (Group B), long-acting bronchodilators should be initiated. For patients at high risk for exacerbations (Groups C and D), ICS combined with long-acting bronchodilators should be considered. Short-acting bronchodilators relieve symptoms and increase exercise tolerance. Long-acting bronchodilators relieve symptoms, reduce exacerbation frequency, and improve quality of life and health status. Patients have a variety of choices in using inhalational therapies, including MDIs, DPIs, SMIs or nebulizers. There is no clear advantage of one delivery method over another, and it is recommended that patient-specific factors and preferences should be considered in selecting the device.[1]

The benefit of individual therapies in reducing the severity and frequency of exacerbations has been a major focus for the past several years. With the exception of short-acting bronchodilators,

TABLE 27-13 Recommended Pharmacologic Therapy for Stable COPD

Patient Category	First Choice	Second Choice	Alternate Therapy
A (less symptoms, less risk)	SABA prn or SAMA prn	LAMA or LABA or SAMA and SABA	Theophylline
B (more symptoms, less risk)	LAMA or LABA	LAMA and LABA	SABA and/or SAMA theophylline
C (less symptoms, more risk)	ICS and LABA or LAMA	LAMA and LABA or LAMA and PDE4I or LABA and PDE4I	SABA and/or SAMA theophylline
D (more symptoms, more risk)	ICS and LABA and/or LAMA	ICS and LABA and LAMA or ICS and LABA and PDE4I or LAMA and LABA or LAMA and PDE4I	SABA and/or SAMA Theophylline

ICS, inhaled corticosteroids; LABA, long acting beta agonist; LAMA, long-acting muscarinic antagonists; PDE4I, phosphodiesterase type 4 inhibitor (roflumilast); SABA, short acting beta-agonist; SAMA, short-acting muscarinic antagonists.

TABLE 27-14 COPD Medication Chart

Brand Name	Device	SABA	SAMA	ICS	LABA	LAMA	Other	Dosing
Proair, Ventolin, Proventil		Albuterol						
	MDI	90 mcg						1-2 puffs q4-6h prn
Xopenex		Levalbuterol						
	MDI	45 mcg						1-2 puffs q4-6h prn
Combivent		Albuterol	Ipratropium					
	Respimat	100 mcg	20 mcg					1 puff q6h
Atrovent			Ipratropium					
	MDI		17 mcg					2 puffs q6h
Advair				Fluticasone	Salmeterol			
	MDI			45, 115, 230 mcg	21 mcg			2 puffs BID
	Diskus			100 mcg	50 mcg			1 puff BID
				250 mcg	50 mcg			1 puff BID
				500 mcg	50 mcg			1 puff BID
Symbicort				Budesonide	Formoterol			
	MDI			80 mcg	4.5 mcg			2 puffs BID
				160 mcg	4.5 mcg			2 puffs BID
Breo	Ellipta			Fluticasone	Vilanterol			
				100 mcg	25 mcg			1 puff once daily
				200 mcg	25 mcg			1 puff once daily
Serevent	Diskus				Salmeterol			
					50 mcg			1 puff BID
Foradil	Aerolizer				Formoterol			
					12 mcg			1 puff BID
Striverdi	Respimat				Olodaterol			
					2.5 mcg			2 puffs once daily
Arcapta	Neohaler				Indacaterol			
					75 mcg			1 puff once daily
Anoro	Ellipta				Vilanterol	Umeclidinium		
					25 mcg	62.5 mcg		1 puff once daily
Stiolto	Respimat				Olodaterol	Tiotropium		
					2.5 mcg	2.5 mcg		2 puffs once daily
Spiriva	Handihaler					Tiotropium		
	Respimat					18 mcg		1 puff once daily
						2.5 mcg		2 puffs once daily
Tudorza	Pressair					Aclidinium		
						400 mcg		1 puff BID
Incruse	Ellipta					Umeclidinium		
						62.5 mcg		1 puff once daily
Utibron	Neohaler				Indacaterol	Glycopyrrolate		
					27.5 mcg	15.6 mcg		1 puff twice daily
Seebri	Neohaler					Glycopyrrolate		
						15.6 mcg		1 puff twice daily
Daliresp	(Oral)						Roflumilast (PDE-4 Inhibitor)	500 mcg orally daily
Theophylline	Oral						PDE inhibitor; Adenosine Antagonist	Variable dosing in Patients

each of the agents typically used in the long-term treatment of COPD has been shown to reduce exacerbation frequency, and each does so to a similar degree. In a meta-analysis that included many clinical trials, it was reported that exacerbations were reduced by long-acting inhaled β_2-agonists (LABAs) (23%), tiotropium (29%), ICs (22%), and ICs plus LABAs (28%).[37] There were no significant differences between the agents, with regards to exacerbation frequency. These exacerbation reduction rates are consistent with those seen in the large clinical trials for tiotropium (UPLIFT and TORCH [ICs plus LABAs]).[21,22]

Bronchodilators

Bronchodilator classes available for the treatment of COPD include β_2-agonists, anticholinergics, and methylxanthines. Bronchodilators generally work by reducing the tone of airway smooth muscle (relaxation), thus minimizing airflow limitation. For patients with COPD, the clinical benefits of bronchodilators include increased exercise capacity, decreased air trapping in the lungs, and relief of symptoms such as dyspnea. However, use of bronchodilators may not be associated with significant improvements in pulmonary function measurements of expiratory airflow such as FEV_1. In general, side effects of bronchodilator medications are related to their pharmacologic effects and are dose dependent. Because COPD patients are older and more likely to have comorbid conditions, the risk for side effects and drug interactions is higher compared with patients with asthma.

There is no clear benefit to one bronchodilator agent or class over others, although inhaled therapy generally is preferred. In general, it can be more difficult for patients with COPD to use inhalation devices effectively compared with other populations owing to advanced age and the presence of other comorbidities. Clinicians should advise, counsel, and observe patient technique with the devices frequently and consistently.

Short-Acting Bronchodilators The initial therapy for COPD patients who experience symptoms intermittently is short-acting bronchodilators. Among these agents, the choices are a short-acting β_2-agonist or an anticholinergic. Either class of agents has a relatively rapid onset of action, relieves symptoms, and improves exercise tolerance and lung function. In general, both classes are equally effective.

Short-Acting Sympathomimetics (β_2-Agonists) β_2-agonists cause bronchodilation by stimulating the enzyme adenyl cyclase to increase the formation of cyclic adenosine monophosphate (cAMP). cAMP is responsible for mediating relaxation of bronchial smooth muscle, leading to bronchodilation. In addition, β_2-agonists may improve mucociliary clearance. Older agents with less selectivity are no longer available and the choices for short-acting, selective β_2-agonists are albuterol and levalbuterol. Racemic epinephrine is available as an over the counter therapy but is not appropriate for chronic treatment.

The preferred route of administration for short-acting, selective β_2-agonists is by inhalation. The use of oral and parenteral β-agonists in COPD is discouraged because they are no more effective than a properly used inhalation device, and the incidence of systemic adverse effects such as tachycardia and hand tremor is greater. Administration of β_2-agonists in the outpatient and emergency room settings via inhalers (MDIs or DPIs) is at least as effective as nebulization therapy and usually favored for reasons of cost and convenience.[1,3,5] Chapter 26 includes a complete description of the devices used for delivering aerosolized medication and a comparison of β_2-agonist therapies.

Albuterol is the most frequently used β_2-agonist. It is available as an oral and inhaled preparation. Albuterol is a racemic mixture of (*R*)-albuterol, which is responsible for the bronchodilator effect, and (*S*)-albuterol, which has no therapeutic effect. (*S*)-Albuterol is considered by some clinicians to be inert, whereas others believe that it may be implicated in worsening airway inflammation and antagonizing the response to (*R*)-albuterol. Levalbuterol is a single-isomer formulation of (*R*)-albuterol. Despite years of clinical use, there is not compelling evidence to suggest that levalbuterol offers consistent advantages in terms of clinical effectiveness or safety, and it is more expensive than albuterol.[38]

In COPD patients, β_2-agonists exert a rapid onset of effect, although the response generally is less than that seen in asthma. Short-acting inhaled β_2-agonists cause only a small improvement in FEV_1 acutely but may improve respiratory symptoms and exercise tolerance despite the small improvement in spirometric measurements.[1,13] Patients with COPD can use quick-onset β_2-agonists as needed for relief of symptoms or on a scheduled basis to prevent or reduce symptoms. The duration of action of short-acting β_2-agonists is 4 to 6 hours.

Inhaled β_2-agonists are generally well tolerated. They can cause sinus tachycardia and rhythm disturbances in predisposed patients, but these are rarely reported. Skeletal muscle tremors can occur initially but subside as tolerance develops.

Short-Acting Anticholinergics When given by inhalation, anticholinergics produce bronchodilation by competitively inhibiting cholinergic receptors in bronchial smooth muscle. This activity blocks acetylcholine, with the net effect being a reduction in cyclic guanosine monophosphate (cGMP), which normally acts to constrict bronchial smooth muscle. Muscarinic receptors on airway smooth muscle include M_1, M_2, and M_3 subtypes. Activation of M_1 and M_3 receptors by acetylcholine results in bronchoconstriction; however, activation of M_2 receptors inhibits further acetylcholine release.

Ipratropium is the primary short-acting anticholinergic agent used for COPD in the United States. The lack of systemic absorption of ipratropium greatly diminishes the anticholinergic side effects such as blurred vision, urinary retention, nausea, and tachycardia associated with atropine. Ipratropium is also available as a MDI and SMI in combination with albuterol and as a solution for nebulization at 200 mcg/mL. The soft-mist inhaler (available as Respimat®) is a new type of inhalation device and requires specific patient education to ensure proper use. Ipratropium has a peak effect in 1.5 to 2 hours and has a duration of effect of up to 8 hours. Compared with standard β_2-agonists, ipratropium has a slower onset of action and a more prolonged bronchodilator effect. Because of the slower onset of effect (15-20 minutes compared with 5 minutes for albuterol), it may be less suitable for as-needed use; however, it is often prescribed in that manner.

The role of inhaled anticholinergics in COPD is well established.[1,3,4] However, results from the Lung Health Study showed that treatment with ipratropium did not affect the progressive decline in lung function.[27] Studies comparing ipratropium with inhaled β_2-agonists have generally reported similar improvements in pulmonary function. Others report a modest benefit with ipratropium, including a lower incidence of side effects such as tachycardia.[1,4] Although the recommended dose of ipratropium is 2 puffs four times a day, there is evidence for a dose–response, so the dose can be titrated upward often to 24 puffs a day. Ipratropium has been shown to increase maximum exercise performance in stable COPD patients with doses of 8 to 12 puffs prior to exercise but not with doses of 4 puffs or less.[39] Ipratropium is well tolerated. The most frequent patient complaints are dry mouth, nausea, and an occasional metallic taste.

Clinicians differ about preference in choosing the initial short-acting bronchodilator therapy for the patient with COPD. Both a short-acting β_2-agonist and ipratropium represent reasonable choices for initial therapy. When a patient does not achieve adequate control of symptoms with one agent, the combination of a short-acting β_2-agonist and ipratropium is a reasonable alternative.

8 **Long-Acting Bronchodilators** For patients with moderate-to-severe COPD who experience symptoms on a regular and consistent basis, or in whom short-acting therapies do not provide adequate relief (category B and D), long-acting bronchodilator therapies are the recommended treatment. Long-acting agents are also recommended for patients at high risk for exacerbation (category C and D). Long-acting inhaled bronchodilator therapy can be administered as an inhaled β_2-agonist (LABA) or an anticholinergic (LAMA). Long-acting, inhaled bronchodilator therapy is more

convenient and effective, compared with short-acting agents, for patients with chronic symptoms. There are superior outcomes in lung function as measured by spirometry, symptoms including dyspnea, and, importantly, reductions in exacerbation frequency and improved quality of life.

Long-Acting Inhaled β_2-Agonists LABAs offer the convenience and benefit of a long duration of action for patients with persistent symptoms. Some LABAs (eg, salmeterol, formoterol, and arformoterol) are dosed every 12 hours and provide sustained bronchodilation. Two ultra-long-acting agents, indacaterol (approved 2011) and olodaterol (approved 2014), require only once-daily dosing. Another ultra-long-acting agent, vilanterol, is also administered once daily but is currently available in the United States only as a combination product with an inhaled corticosteroid (IC) (fluticasone) or long-acting anticholinergic (umeclidinium). Arformoterol, formoterol, indacaterol and olodaterol have an onset of action similar to albuterol (less than 5 minutes), whereas salmeterol has a slower onset (15-20 minutes); however, none of these agents are recommended for acute relief of symptoms. There is no dose titration for any of these agents; the starting dose is the effective and recommended dose for all patients. The clinical benefits of LABAs compared with short-acting therapies include similar or superior improvements in lung function and symptoms, as well as reduced exacerbation rates and need for hospitalization.[40] The use of the long-acting agents should be considered for patients with frequent and persistent symptoms and those at higher risk for exacerbation (see Table 27-13). When patients require short-acting β_2-agonists on a scheduled basis, LABAs are more convenient based on dosing frequency but may be more expensive. Salmeterol and indacaterol are available in dry powder inhalation devices. Formoterol and arformoterol are available as solutions for nebulization, and olodaterol is formulated as a soft-mist inhaler (Respimat). In addition to decreasing frequency of exacerbations, LABAs are also useful to reduce nocturnal symptoms and improve quality of life. When compared with short-acting bronchodilators or theophylline, both salmeterol and formoterol improve lung function, symptoms, exacerbation frequency, and quality of life.[3,13,17] These benefits are apparent even for patients with poorly reversible lung function and are related to improvements in inspiratory capacity. Similar to salmeterol and formoterol, indacaterol has been shown to have beneficial effects on health care status, frequency of exacerbations and bronchodilation.[41] In direct comparison trials, indacaterol has greater effect on bronchodilation than salmeterol and formoterol. Comparative data for olodaterol and other bronchodilators are limited. Available studies have demonstrated similar effects with olodaterol on FEV_1 and symptoms compared with other long-acting bronchodilators; however, the effect on other outcomes such as exacerbation frequency has not been evaluated.

Long-Acting Anticholinergics Tiotropium bromide, a long-acting quaternary anticholinergic agent, has been available in the United States since 2004. Additional long-acting anticholinergic agents, aclidinium and umeclidinium, were approved in 2012 and 2014. Inhaled anticholinergics block the effects of acetylcholine by binding to muscarinic receptors in airway smooth muscle and mucus glands, inhibiting the cholinergic effects of bronchoconstriction and mucus secretion. Long-acting anticholinergic agents, such as tiotropium, are more selective than ipratropium at blocking important muscarinic receptors. They dissociate slowly from M_3 receptors, resulting in prolonged bronchodilation with once or twice a day dosing.[42] There is no dose titration for any of these agents. Aclidinium has a faster onset of action (30 minutes) compared to tiotropium (80 minutes); however, none of these agents are recommended for acute relief of symptoms. In the United States, tiotropium, is available as a dry-powder and soft-mist inhaler. Aclindium and umeclidinium are available as dry-powder inhalers. Because it acts locally, tiotropium is well tolerated, with the most common complaint being a dry mouth. Other anticholinergic side effects that are reported include constipation, urinary retention, tachycardia, blurred vision, and precipitation of narrow-angle glaucoma symptoms.

The benefits of tiotropium have been evaluated in numerous trials of patients with COPD. Compared to placebo and ipratropium, treatment with tiotropium results in significantly greater improvements in lung function, quality of life and reduces the frequency of exacerbation and need for hospitalization.[43] For outcomes such as bronchodilation, quality of life and frequency of exacerbations, tiotropium therapy has equal or superior efficacy compared with LABAs in various studies.[44,45]

The most notable study involving the use of tiotropium in recent years for patients with COPD was the UPLIFT trial.[22] This was a randomized, double-blind study over 4 years. A total of 5,993 subjects received either tiotropium 18 mcg daily inhaled via a handihaler dry-powder device or a matching placebo. All other COPD therapies were allowed except for other anticholinergic therapies (eg, ipratropium). The mean postbronchodilator FEV_1 among subjects was 1.32 L, and the primary outcome was the rate of decline in FEV_1 on spirometry. The results showed that tiotropium treatment resulted in a significant improvement in FEV_1 from baseline. However, the rate of decline in the mean FEV_1 result was not statistically significant between the groups. Tiotropium-treated subjects benefited from treatment as reflected in improved quality-of-life scores, reduced exacerbation rates, fewer hospitalizations, and instances of respiratory failure. Tiotropium was associated with a lower overall risk of mortality, including deaths from respiratory and cardiac causes.

Previously, retrospective analyses have reported an increased risk of cardiovascular events associated with ipratropium and tiotropium use.[46] However, the UPLIFT study, which was a prospective trial over 4 years, did not report an increased cardiovascular risk associated with tiotropium use when administered from both devices.[22] Additionally, a prospective, noninferiority trial (TIOSPIR) was published in 2013 which compared the effects of tiotropium delivered via Handihaler or Respimat devices among 17,000 patients with COPD over a median 2.3 year period.[47] The primary outcomes in this trial were risk of death and risk of first COPD exacerbation. Secondary outcomes included cardiovascular safety. No significant differences were seen in any of the primary or secondary outcomes when comparing tiotropium delivery devices. Further studies are needed to evaluate the cardiovascular safety of ipratropium.

In clinical trials, aclidinium has been shown to have similar improvements in spirometry and symptom scores compared to tiotropium.[48] However, reduction in exacerbation frequency has not been observed in trials to date. While available as both a single-drug and combination inhaler (with vilanterol), umeclidinium has primarily been evaluated as part of a combination bronchodilator regimen.

Combination Anticholinergics and β-Agonists Combination regimens of bronchodilators are used often in the treatment of COPD, especially as the disease progresses and symptoms worsen over time. Combining bronchodilators with different mechanisms of action allows the lowest possible effective doses to be used and reduces potential adverse effects from individual agents.[1] Combinations of both short- and long-acting β_2-agonists with ipratropium provide added symptomatic relief and improvements in pulmonary function. A combination of albuterol and ipratropium (Combivent Respimat) is available as a soft-mist inhaler in the United States for chronic maintenance therapy of COPD. This product offers the obvious convenience of two classes of bronchodilators in a single inhaler.

Although clinical practice guidelines have recommended that combinations of long-acting bronchodilators are appropriate for patients who do not receive adequate benefit from a single agent, data to support the use of these combinations have been lacking. These approaches have been the focus of more recent research. A recent Cochrane review evaluated five trials comparing combination long-acting bronchodilators (LABA plus tiotropium) versus tiotropium alone. Combination therapy resulted in significant improvement in FEV_1 and quality-of-life measures compared with tiotropium alone, although no difference was shown for frequency of exacerbations or symptom scores.[49]

In 2013, the first LABA-LAMA combination inhaler (umeclidinium/vilanterol—DPI) was approved in the United States and another combination inhaler was approved in 2015 (tiotropium/olodaterol—SMI). As a result of this drug development process, there is now more evidence for the efficacy and safety of using long-acting bronchodilators in combination.[50-52] To date, efficacy has been demonstrated for improvements in lung function and symptoms scores with combination long-acting bronchodilators compared to single-therapy; however, additional benefit in exacerbation reduction needs to be evaluated.

Methylxanthines Methylxanthines, including theophylline and aminophylline, have been available for the treatment of COPD for at least 5 decades and at one time were considered first-line therapy. However, with the availability of LABAs and inhaled anticholinergics, the role of methylxanthine therapy is significantly limited. Inhaled bronchodilator therapy is preferred for COPD. Because of the risk for drug interactions and the significant intrapatient and interpatient variability in dosage requirements, theophylline therapy generally is considered for patients who are intolerant or unable to use an inhaled bronchodilator. Theophylline is still an alternative to commonly used inhaled therapies partially due to the potential for multiple mechanisms (bronchodilation and antiinflammatory) and the possible benefit that systemic administration may exert on peripheral airways.[1,5]

The methylxanthines may produce bronchodilation through numerous mechanisms, including (a) inhibition of phosphodiesterase, thereby increasing cAMP levels, (b) inhibition of calcium ion influx into smooth muscle, (c) prostaglandin antagonism, (d) stimulation of endogenous catecholamines, (e) adenosine receptor antagonism, and (f) inhibition of release of mediators from mast cells and leukocytes.[1]

Chronic theophylline use for patients with COPD may offer improvements in lung function, including vital capacity (VC), FEV_1, minute ventilation, and gas exchange. Subjectively, theophylline has been shown to reduce dyspnea, increase exercise tolerance, and improve respiratory drive in COPD patients.[1] Other nonpulmonary effects of theophylline that may contribute to improved overall functional capacity for patients with COPD include improved cardiac function and decreased pulmonary artery pressure.

Regular use of methylxanthines has not been shown to have either a beneficial or a detrimental effect on the progression of COPD. However, methylxanthines may be added to the treatment plan of patients who have not achieved an optimal clinical response to inhaled bronchodilators. The efficacy of combination therapy with salmeterol and theophylline for patients with COPD can improve pulmonary function and reduce dyspnea better than either treatment alone.[1] Combination treatment has also been associated with a reduced number of exacerbations only when compared with the theophylline group, suggesting that the salmeterol component was responsible for this beneficial effect.

As is the case with other bronchodilator therapy, parameters other than objective measurements, such as FEV_1, should be monitored to assess efficacy of theophylline in COPD. Subjective parameters, such as perceived improvements in symptoms of dyspnea and exercise tolerance, become increasingly important in assessing the acceptability of methylxanthines for COPD patients. Although objective improvement may be minimal, patients may experience an improvement in clinical symptoms, and thus benefit to the individual may be meaningful.

Although theophylline is available in a variety of oral dosage forms, sustained-release preparations are most appropriate for the long-term management of COPD. These products have the advantages of improving patient compliance and achieving more consistent serum concentrations over rapid-release theophylline and aminophylline preparations. However, caution must be used in switching from one sustained-release preparation to another because there are considerable variations in sustained-release characteristics.[53] Aside from IV aminophylline, there is no need to use any of the various salt forms of theophylline.

Therapy can be initiated at 200 mg twice daily and titrated upward every 3 to 5 days to the target dose. Most patients require daily doses of 400 to 900 mg. Dosage adjustments generally should be made based on serum concentration results. Traditionally, the therapeutic range of theophylline was identified as 10 to 20 mcg/mL; however, because of the frequency of dose-related side effects and the relatively minor benefit of higher concentrations, a more conservative therapeutic range of 8 to 15 mcg/mL often is targeted. This is especially preferable for the elderly. When concentrations are measured, trough measurements are most appropriate.

Once a dose is established, serum concentrations should be monitored once or twice a year unless the patient's disease worsens, medications that interfere with theophylline metabolism are added to therapy, or toxicity is suspected. The most common side effects of theophylline therapy are related to the GI system, the cardiovascular system, and the CNS. Side effects are dose related; however, there is overlap in side effects between the therapeutic and toxic ranges. Minor side effects include dyspepsia, nausea, vomiting, diarrhea, headache, dizziness, and tachycardia. More serious toxicities, especially at toxic concentrations, include arrhythmias and seizures.

Factors that decrease theophylline clearance and lead to reduced maintenance dose requirements include advanced age, bacterial or viral pneumonia, left or right ventricular failure, liver dysfunction, hypoxemia from acute decompensation, and use of drugs such as cimetidine, macrolides, and fluoroquinolone antibiotics. Factors that may enhance theophylline clearance and result in the need for higher maintenance doses include tobacco and marijuana smoking, hyperthyroidism, and the use of such drugs as phenytoin, phenobarbital, and rifampin.

In summary, there are decades of experience with theophylline and other methylxanthine products in the management of patients with COPD. However, inhalation therapy is currently preferred based on superior efficacy and safety, as well as ease of use by the clinician. Theophylline is a challenging medication to dose, monitor, and manage due to the significant intrapatient and interpatient variability in pharmacokinetics and the potential for drug interactions and toxicities.

Corticosteroids

9 Corticosteroid therapy has been studied and debated in COPD therapy for half a century; however, owing to the poor risk-to-benefit ratio, chronic systemic corticosteroid therapy should be avoided if possible.[1] Because of the potential role of inflammation in the pathogenesis of the disease, clinicians hoped that corticosteroids would be promising agents in COPD management. However, their use continues to be debated, especially in the management of stable COPD.

The antiinflammatory mechanisms whereby corticosteroids exert their beneficial effect in COPD include (a) reduction in capillary permeability to decrease mucus, (b) inhibition of release of proteolytic enzymes from leukocytes, and (c) inhibition of prostaglandins. Unfortunately, the clinical benefits of systemic corticosteroid therapy in the chronic management of COPD are often not evident, and the risk of toxicity is extensive and far-reaching. Currently, the appropriate situations to consider corticosteroids in COPD include (a) short-term systemic use for acute exacerbations and (b) inhalation therapy for chronic stable COPD in selected patients.

Chronic therapy with oral steroids is not warranted. Only a small fraction (10%) of COPD patients treated with steroids show clinically significant improvement in baseline FEV_1 (increase of 20%) compared with those treated with placebo. While a small number of COPD patients are considered responders to oral steroids, many of these patients actually may have an asthmatic, or reversible, component to their disease. Previously, a common clinical practice was to administer a short course (2 weeks) of oral corticosteroids as a trial to predict which patients would benefit from chronic oral or ICS. There is now sufficient evidence suggesting that this practice is not effective in predicting a long-term response to ICS and should not be recommended.

Long-term adverse effects associated with systemic corticosteroid therapy include osteoporosis, muscular atrophy, thinning of the skin, development of cataracts, and adrenal suppression and insufficiency. The risks associated with long-term steroid therapy are much greater than the clinical benefits. If a decision to treat with long-term systemic corticosteroids is made, the lowest possible effective dose should be given once per day in the morning to minimize the risk of adrenal suppression. If therapy with oral agents is required, an alternate-day schedule should be used.

Initially, it was postulated that ICS might be beneficial in COPD to slow disease progression. Unfortunately, the results of major clinical trials have failed to demonstrate any benefit from chronic treatment with ICS in modifying long-term decline in lung function that is characteristic of COPD.[1,4,5,13,17] However, ICS have been associated with other important benefits in some patients, including a decrease in exacerbation frequency and improvements in overall health status.[1,54] Patients with severe to very severe COPD (FEV_1 less than 60% predicted) and those at high risk of exacerbation receive the most benefit from ICS.

Although a dose–response relationship for ICS has not been demonstrated in COPD, the major clinical trials employed moderate to high doses for treatment. At these doses, adverse effects are a consideration with long-term therapy. Recent trials have reported that treatment with ICS increases the risk of pneumonia for patients with COPD.[21,54,55] Other adverse effects include hoarseness, sore throat, oral candidiasis, and skin bruising. Severe adverse effects, such as adrenal suppression, osteoporosis, and cataract formation, have been reported less frequently than with systemic corticosteroids, but clinicians should monitor patients who are receiving high-dose chronic therapy.

There is conflicting evidence supporting a dose relationship between ICS use and the risk of fractures. In a cohort of over 1,600 subjects with a diagnosis of asthma or COPD (mean age 80 years), the risk of a fracture was 2.53 times higher (CI, 1.65-3.89) in those receiving a mean daily dose of ICS of 601 mcg or greater.[56] A meta-analysis found no evidence supporting an increased risk of fractures or decreased bone mineral density with chronic ICS use.[57] It appears prudent to suggest that, to minimize the risk of fracture, patients should be treated with the lowest effective dose of ICS. It may also be helpful to recommend adequate intake of calcium and vitamin D and possibly periodic bone mineral density testing.

Currently, the recommended role of ICS therapy is for patients with severe or very severe COPD and at high risk of exacerbation (Groups C and D) who are not controlled with inhaled bronchodilators. Given the risks associated with long-term ICS therapy, clinicians should appropriately identify patients who will receive the best benefit, such as reduction in exacerbations. Evaluations of current practice has shown that many patients with COPD may be inappropriately prescribed an IC (eg, not high risk for exacerbations); thus, exposing them to unnecessary adverse effects.[58]

Two recent trials have evaluated the effects of withdrawing ICS from therapy in patients with moderate and severe COPD.[59,60] In the INSTEAD trial, patients with moderate COPD and low risk of exacerbations (eg, no exacerbation in the previous 12 months) were transitioned from salmeterol/fluticasone combination therapy to indacaterol alone. At 12 weeks, there was no difference in lung function, symptoms or health status between treatment groups. Effect of therapy change on long-term risk of exacerbation was not evaluated.[59] In another trial, patients with severe COPD receiving "triple therapy" (eg, LAMA-LABA-ICS) had their ICS tapered over 12 weeks and then discontinued. Discontinuation of ICS therapy did not result in a significant increase in exacerbations. However, some patients experienced a decrease in FEV_1 or return of symptoms with ICS withdrawal.[60] These trials provide more information to clinicians who may wish to scale back ICS therapy due to observed adverse effects, such as recurrent pneumonia, or in patients who are not at high risk for exacerbations and can be maintained on long-acting bronchodilators alone.

Combination Therapy: Bronchodilators and Inhaled Corticosteroids

Following the disappointing results of chronic ICS studies and the progressive decline in lung function, investigators became interested in the combination of potent antiinflammatory therapies and long-acting bronchodilators. In various studies, combination therapy with LABA and ICS was associated with greater improvements in clinical outcomes such as FEV_1, health status, and frequency of exacerbations compared with ICS or long-acting bronchodilators alone.[61] The availability of combination inhalers (eg, salmeterol plus fluticasone, budesonide plus formoterol, and mometasone plus formoterol) makes administration of both ICS and long-acting bronchodilators more convenient for patients and decreases the total number of inhalations needed daily.

One of the largest prospective studies evaluating combination therapy to date is referred to as the TORCH study.[21] This trial included 6,112 patients who received one of four treatments for 3 years. Treatment groups were placebo, salmeterol 50 mcg twice daily, fluticasone 500 mcg twice daily, or the combination of salmeterol and fluticasone in a single inhaler. The primary outcome was death from any cause and secondary outcomes were exacerbation rates, lung function, and health status. None of the active treatments differed significantly from placebo, although the combination of salmeterol and fluticasone trended toward fewer deaths ($P = 0.052$). The combination also reduced exacerbation rates, and improved lung function and health status compared with the other treatments. Exacerbation rates were also significantly reduced with combination therapy compared with either single agent alone. Both treatment groups that included fluticasone had higher rates of pneumonia. Although this study did not reflect a mortality benefit, the authors indicated that the relative risk of death was reduced by 17.5% with the combination therapy.

In a posthoc analysis of this trial, both individual agents and the combination decreased the rate of spirometry decline in patients with an FEV_1 of less than 60% predicted.[62] While this observation is interesting, it is in contrast to previous randomized controlled studies that have not demonstrated an effect of pharmacotherapy on rate of disease progression.

In a head-to-head trial, a large study comparing a combination of salmeterol and fluticasone with tiotropium alone showed no difference in the exacerbation rates between the groups, although the combination therapy was associated with a higher study completion rate.[63]

Combinations of Long-Acting Bronchodilators Compared with Long-Acting Bronchodilators Plus Inhaled Corticosteroids

Given that COPD is a progressive disease, common practice is to add therapies over time to achieve symptom control and prevent exacerbations. Ultimately, many patients may receive combination therapy with multiple agents, despite a lack of strong evidence for efficacy. For patients with more symptoms and at high risk of exacerbation (category D), triple therapy (LABA-LAMA-IC) may be considered as a first or second choice.

The benefit of triple therapy was evaluated in a 1-year randomized, double-blind, placebo-controlled study involving 449 subjects with moderate-to-severe COPD. Treatment consisted of tiotropium, tiotropium plus salmeterol, or tiotropium, salmeterol, and fluticasone.[64] There was no difference between treatments for the primary outcome of percentage of patients experiencing an exacerbation requiring systemic corticosteroids or antibiotics. The triple-drug regimen improved lung function, quality of life, and reduced hospitalization compared with tiotropium alone, while two-drug therapy did not offer any benefit in lung function improvement or hospitalization rates compared with the single agent.

These data involving combinations of long-acting bronchodilators and ICS are limited and preliminary.[65,66] More research is required and should include other outcome parameters including relief of symptoms, exacerbation rates, and quality of life. Larger sample sizes and longer durations will provide insight into the value of combinations.

Phosphodiesterase Inhibitors

Phosphodiesterase 4 (PDE4) is the major phosphodiesterase found in airway smooth muscle cells and inflammatory cells and is responsible for degrading cAMP. Inhibition of PDE4 results in relaxation of airway smooth muscle cells and decreased activity of inflammatory cells and mediators such as TNF-α and IL-8. One PDE4 inhibitor, roflumilast, was approved in 2011 to reduce the risk of exacerbations in patients with severe COPD. When either used as monotherapy or added to a maintenance regimen with other inhaled bronchodilators, roflumilast was associated with a modest increase in FEV_1 and reduction in rate of exacerbation by approximately 15%.[67] Of note, patients in phase III trials evaluating roflumilast were not allowed to receive ICS as part of their maintenance regimen.

A more recent study evaluated the addition of roflumilast to combination therapy with IC and LABA.[68] Patients with severe COPD were randomized to receive placebo or roflumilast in addition to an IC and LABA for 1 year. Open-label LAMA was also allowed, and approximately 70% of patients in both groups were receiving a LAMA as part of their therapy prior to randomization. The primary outcome was frequency of moderate to severe exacerbations, and secondary outcomes of lung function, symptoms and health status were also measured. Treatment with roflumilast was associated with a significant decrease in exacerbation rate and need for hospitalization compared to placebo. No significant improvements were seen in symptom scores or health status with roflumilast therapy.

Roflumilast is dosed at 500 mcg orally once a day. Major adverse effects include weight loss and neuropsychiatric effects such as suicidal thoughts, insomnia, anxiety, and new or worsened depression. Weight loss may be of concern in patients with low BMI and drug discontinuation may be necessary if significant weight loss is observed. Both patients and family members should be counseled regarding the potential for mood and behavior changes and to alert healthcare providers if they occur.

Roflumilast is metabolized by CYP3A4 and 1A2 and coadministration with strong inducers of cytochrome P450 is not recommended due to potential for subtherapeutic plasma concentrations. Although there are no recommended dose adjustments, caution should also be used when administering roflumilast with strong inhibitors of cytochrome P450 due to potential for adverse effects.

Given the limited evidence demonstrating long-term clinical benefit, the role of roflumilast in the management of COPD is not entirely clear. Current consensus guidelines recommend roflumilast for patients with severe or very severe COPD who are at high risk of exacerbation (Groups C and D) and are not controlled by inhaled bronchodilators (see Table 27-13). Roflumilast may also be considered for patients who are intolerant or unable to use inhaled bronchodilators or corticosteroids. Given that both theophylline and roflumilast have similar mechanisms of action through inhibition of phosphodiesterases, it is not recommended to use both together for the management of COPD.

α_1-Antitrypsin Replacement Therapy

For patients with inherited AAT deficiency-associated emphysema, treatment focuses on reduction of risk factors such as smoking, symptomatic treatment with bronchodilators, and augmentation therapy with replacement AAT. Based on knowledge about the relationship between serum concentrations of AAT and the risk of developing emphysema, the rationale for augmentation therapy is to maintain serum concentrations above the protective threshold throughout the dosing interval.[1,5] Indirect evidence of AAT activity in the interstitium of the lung has been demonstrated by measuring concentrations of the enzyme in epithelial lining fluid obtained during bronchoalveolar lavage. Augmentation therapy consists of weekly infusions of pooled human AAT to maintain AAT plasma levels over 10 μmol/L. Much of the data supporting the use of AAT replacement are based on evidence of biochemical efficacy (eg, administering the product and demonstrating protective serum concentrations of AAT).

Clinical evidence for slowing lung function decline or improving outcomes with augmentation therapy is sparse. Stated challenges to performing randomized clinical trials include the large sample size and long duration of follow-up required, and the expense of conducting such a trial. One observational study followed patients in the National Registry of Severe AAT Deficiency over a period of several years and documented clinical outcomes. In this study, patients who received weekly augmentation therapy with purified AAT had slower declines in FEV_1 and decreased mortality compared with patients who never received augmentation therapy.[69] However, this was an observational study of patients, not a randomized, placebo-controlled trial, and so direct cause-and-effect relationships cannot be concluded. One randomized, placebo-controlled study of patients with severe AAT deficiency (ZZ phenotype) did show a significant reduction in lung tissue loss and destruction as measured by computed tomographic (CT) scan for patients receiving augmentation therapy.[70] Other measures of lung function and mortality were not recorded.

The recommended dosing regimen for replacement AAT is 60 mg/kg administered IV once a week at a rate of 0.08 mL/kg/min, adjusted to patient tolerance. This form of augmentation therapy will cost over $54,000 annually. In the absence of alternative treatments, it is difficult to assess the cost-effectiveness using conventional criteria. There have been repeated problems with supply of this biologic replacement therapy (derived from pooled blood donors) related to production difficulty and contamination issues. Currently, there are four products available (Prolastin-C [Talecris], Aralast and Aralast-NP [Baxter], Zemaira [CSL Behring]), that should minimize this problem in the future. Drug development research continues in the area of recombinant products and inhalational therapy.

TREATMENT
COPD Exacerbation

Desired Outcomes

10 The goals of therapy for patients experiencing exacerbations of COPD are (a) prevention of hospitalization or reduction in hospital stay, (b) prevention of acute respiratory failure and death, and (c) resolution of exacerbation symptoms and a return to baseline clinical status and quality of life.[1,6,17] Acute exacerbations can range from mild to severe. Factors that influence the severity, and subsequently the level of care required, include the severity of airflow limitation, presence of comorbidities, and the history of previous exacerbations. Table 27-15 includes factors that warrant treatment in the hospital.

Various therapeutic options for exacerbation management are summarized in Table 27-16. Pharmacotherapy consists of intensification of bronchodilator therapy and a short course of systemic corticosteroids. Antimicrobial therapy is indicated in the presence of selected symptoms. Since the frequency and severity of exacerbations are closely related to each patient's overall health status, all patients should receive optimal chronic treatment, including smoking cessation, appropriate pharmacologic therapy, and preventative therapy such as vaccinations.

Nonpharmacologic Therapy

Controlled Oxygen Therapy

Oxygen therapy should be provided for patients with significant hypoxemia during an exacerbation (eg, oxygen saturation less than 90%). Caution must be used, however, because many patients with COPD rely on mild hypoxemia to trigger their drive to breathe. In normal, healthy individuals, the drive to breathe is triggered by carbon dioxide accumulation. For patients with COPD who retain carbon dioxide as a result of their disease progression, hypoxemia rather than hypercapnia becomes the main trigger for their respiratory drive. Overly aggressive administration of oxygen to patients with chronic hypercapnia may result in respiratory depression and respiratory failure. Oxygen therapy should be used to achieve a PaO_2 of greater than 60 mm Hg or oxygen saturation of greater than 90%. However, an ABG should be obtained after oxygen initiation to monitor carbon dioxide retention owing to hypoventilation.

Noninvasive Mechanical Ventilation

Noninvasive positive-pressure ventilation (NPPV) provides ventilatory support with oxygen and pressurized airflow using a face or nasal mask with a tight seal but without endotracheal intubation. There have been numerous trials reporting the benefits of NPPV for patients with acute respiratory failure due to COPD exacerbations. NPPV has been associated with lower mortality, lower intubation rates, and shorter hospital stays for COPD exacerbations. A recent analysis regarding NPPV in patients with respiratory failure in general included a subset of patients with COPD and reported that the risk of hospital-based mortality and long-term mortality was reduced by 56%.[71] The benefits seen with NPPV generally can be attributed to a reduction in the complications that often arise with invasive mechanical ventilation. Not all patients with COPD exacerbations are appropriate candidates for NPPV. Patients with altered mental status may not be able to protect their airway and thus may be at increased risk for aspiration. Patients with severe acidosis (pH <7.25), respiratory arrest, or cardiovascular instability should be not considered for NPPV. Patients failing a trial of NPPV or those considered poor candidates might be considered for intubation and mechanical ventilation.

TABLE 27-15 Factors Favoring Hospitalization for Treatment of COPD Exacerbation

Presence of high risk comorbidity (eg, pneumonia, arrhythmia, CHF, diabetes, renal or hepatic failure)
Suboptimal response to outpatient management
Marked worsening of dyspnea
Inability to eat or sleep due to symptoms
Worsening hypoxemia or hypercapnia
Mental status changes
Lack of home support for care
Uncertain diagnosis

TABLE 27-16 Therapeutic Options for Acute Exacerbations of COPD

Therapy	Comments
Antibiotics	Recommended if two or more of the following are present: Increased dyspnea Increased sputum production Increased sputum purulence
Corticosteroids	Oral or IV therapy may be used. If IV is used, it should be changed to oral after improvement in pulmonary status. If continued longer than 14 days, then the dose should be tapered to avoid HPA Axis suppression.
Bronchodilators	MDIs and DPIs equal in efficacy to nebulization. β-Agonists also may increase mucociliary clearance. Long-acting β-agonists or long-acting antimuscarinics should not be used for quick relief of symptoms or on an as-needed basis.
Controlled oxygen therapy	Titrate oxygen to desired oxygen saturation (>90%). Monitor arterial blood gas for development of hypercapnia.
Noninvasive mechanical ventilation	Consider for patients with acute respiratory failure. Not appropriate for patients with altered mental status, severe acidosis, respiratory arrest, or cardiovascular instability.

Pharmacologic Therapy

Bronchodilators

During exacerbations, intensification of bronchodilator regimens is used commonly. The doses and frequency of bronchodilators are increased to provide symptomatic relief. Short-acting β_2-agonists are preferred owing to rapid onset of action. Anticholinergic agents may be added if symptoms persist despite increased doses of β_2-agonists. In fact, combinations of these agents are employed often, although data are lacking about the benefit versus higher doses of one agent. Bronchodilators may be administered via MDIs or nebulization with equal efficacy. Nebulization may be considered for patients with severe dyspnea who are unable to hold their breath after actuation of an MDI. Clinical evidence supporting the use of theophylline during exacerbations is lacking, and thus theophylline generally should be avoided. However, addition of theophylline may be considered for patients not responding to other therapies. The risk of adverse effects such as cardiac arrhythmias should be considered and serum levels monitored closely.

Corticosteroids

The role of systemic corticosteroids for COPD exacerbations is well established based on several studies that document the value of systemic corticosteroids in exacerbations of COPD.[17,72-74] The Systemic Corticosteroids in COPD Exacerbations (SCCOPE) trial evaluated three groups of patients hospitalized for exacerbations of COPD.[72] The first group received an 8-week course of corticosteroids given as methylprednisolone 125 mg IV every 6 hours for 72 hours, followed by once-daily oral prednisone (60 mg on days 4-7, 40 mg on days 8-11,

20 mg on days 12-43, 10 mg on days 44-50, and 5 mg on days 51-57). The second group received a 2-week course given as methylprednisolone 125 mg IV every 6 hours for 72 hours, followed by oral prednisone (60 mg on days 5-7, 40 mg on days 8-11, and 20 mg on days 12-15) and placebo on days 16 to 57. The third group received placebo for all 57 days of study. Rates of treatment failure and hospital stay were significantly higher in the placebo group than in either treatment group at 30 and 90 days. Groups randomized to corticosteroid treatment also had a significantly shorter length of hospital stay compared with the placebo group. The 8-week regimen was not found to be superior to the 2-week regimen. Significant treatment benefits were no longer evident at 6 months.

Davies et al.[73] evaluated the oral use of corticosteroids in hospitalized patients with acute exacerbations of COPD. Patients received either 30 mg/day oral prednisolone or placebo for 14 days. Patients who were treated with corticosteroids had a significantly more rapid improvement in FEV_1 and a shorter hospital stay than did patients who received placebo. There was no significant difference between groups at 6-week follow-up.

In total, results from these trials suggest that patients with acute exacerbations of COPD should receive a short course of IV or oral corticosteroids. However, because of the large variability in dosage ranges, the optimal dose and duration of corticosteroid treatment are not known. Several trials used high initial doses of steroids before tapering to a lower maintenance dose. Adverse effects such as hyperglycemia, insomnia, and hallucinations may occur at higher doses. Depending on the clinical status of the patient, treatment may be initiated at a lower dose or tapered more quickly if these effects occur. It appears that a regimen of prednisone 40 mg orally daily (or equivalent) for 10 to 14 days can be effective for most patients. If steroid treatment is continued for greater than 2 weeks, a tapering oral schedule should be employed to avoid hypothalamic–pituitary–adrenal (HPA) axis suppression.

A recent systematic review reported benefits from either oral or parenteral corticosteroids in reducing treatment failures (OR 0.48 with CI of 0.35-0.67), risk of relapse (HR 0.78 with CI of 0.63-0.97), but no beneficial effect on mortality.[75] There was also an increase in the risk for adverse effects with the use of corticosteroids (OR 2.33 with CI of 1.59-3.43).

It may be possible to limit adverse effects without compromising the effectiveness of systemic corticosteroids.[76] The REDUCE trial evaluated a 5 day course of prednisone 40 mg versus 14 days in a non-inferiority study.[76] For the primary outcome which was time to the next exacerbation in 6 months, the shorter treatment duration was non-inferior with a hazard ratio of 0.95%. Shorter courses of corticosteroids may be as effective as longer courses and have a lower risk of associated adverse effects owing to less time of exposure.

Antimicrobial Therapy

11 It is thought that most acute exacerbations of COPD are caused by viral or bacterial infections. However, as many as 30% of exacerbations are caused by unknown factors.[1] The data supporting the need and the efficacy of antibiotics for COPD exacerbations are remarkably sparse. It is suggested that antibiotics are of most benefit and should be initiated if at least two of the following three symptoms are present: increased dyspnea, increased sputum volume, and increased sputum purulence.[77] The utility of sputum Gram stain and culture is questionable because some patients have chronic bacterial colonization of the bronchial tree between exacerbations.

The emergence of drug-resistant organisms has mandated that antibiotic regimens be chosen judiciously. Selection of empirical antimicrobial therapy should be based on the most likely organism(s) thought to be responsible for the infection based on the individual patient profile and site-specific sensitivities. The most common organisms for any acute exacerbation of COPD are *Haemophilus influenzae*, *Moraxella catarrhalis*, *Streptococcus pneumoniae*, and *Haemophilus parainfluenzae*. More virulent bacteria may be present for patients with more complicated acute exacerbations of COPD, including drug-resistant pneumococci, β-lactamase–producing *H. influenzae* and *M. catarrhalis*, and enteric gram-negative organisms, including *Pseudomonas aeruginosa*. Table 27-17 summarizes recommended antimicrobial therapy for exacerbations of COPD and the most common organisms based on patient presentation.[78]

The benefits of antimicrobial therapy are unclear; however, they continue to be recommended as part of standard therapy, especially in more severe exacerbations. Therapy with antibiotics generally should be continued for at least 7 to 10 days. Studies evaluating shorter treatment courses (usually 5 days) with the fluoroquinolones, second- and third-generation cephalosporins, and macrolide antimicrobials have demonstrated comparable efficacy with the longer treatment regimens.[79] If the patient deteriorates or does not improve as anticipated, hospitalization may be necessary, and more aggressive attempts should be made to identify potential pathogens responsible for the exacerbation.

Other Management Considerations

Chronic obstructive pulmonary disease patients are at increased risk for pulmonary embolism during severe exacerbations requiring hospitalizations. An increased awareness of this risk and appropriate preventative measures are warranted.[80]

TABLE 27-17 Recommended Antimicrobial Therapy in Acute Exacerbations of COPD

Patient Characteristics	Likely Pathogens	Recommended Therapy
Uncomplicated exacerbations <4 exacerbations per year No comorbid illness FEV_1 >50% of predicted	*S. pneumoniae* *H. influenzae* *M. catarrhalis* *H. parainfluenzae* Resistance uncommon	Macrolide (azithromycin, clarithromycin) Second- or third-generation cephalosporin Doxycycline Therapies not recommended[a]: TMP/SMX, amoxicillin, first-generation cephalosporins, and erythromycin
Complicated exacerbations: Age ≥65 and >4 exacerbations per year FEV_1 <50% but >35% of predicted	As above plus drug-resistant pneumococci, β-lactamase–producing *H. influenzae* and *M. catarrhalis*	Amoxicillin/clavulanate Fluoroquinolone with enhanced pneumococcal activity (levofloxacin, gemifloxacin, and moxifloxacin)
Complicated exacerbations with risk of *P. aeruginosa* Chronic bronchial sepsis[b] Need for chronic corticosteroid therapy Resident of nursing home with <4 exacerbations per year FEV_1 <35% of predicted	Some enteric gram-negatives As above plus *P. aeruginosa*	Fluoroquinolone with enhanced pneumococcal and *P. aeruginosa* activity (levofloxacin) IV therapy if required: β-lactamase resistant penicillin with antipseudomonal activity 3rd- or 4th-generation cephalosporin with antipseudomonal activity

[a]TMP/SMX should not be used due to increasing pneumococcal resistance; amoxicillin and first-generation cephalosporins are not recommended due to β-lactamase susceptibility; and erythromycin is not recommended due to insufficient activity against *H. influenzae*.

[b]In sepsis, double antipseudomonal coverage should be considered (eg, addition of aminoglycoside).

Complications

Cor Pulmonale

Cor pulmonale is right-sided heart failure secondary to pulmonary hypertension. Long-term oxygen therapy and diuretics have been the mainstays of therapy for cor pulmonale. Increasing the PaO_2 above 60 mm Hg with supplemental oxygen therapy decreases pulmonary hypertension and thus decreases the force against which the right ventricle has to work. While diuretics may help decrease fluid overload, caution should be used because patients with significant right-sided heart failure are highly dependent on preload for cardiac output. Therefore, the decision to use diuretics must be based on a risk-to-benefit ratio. Digitalis glycosides have no role in the treatment of cor pulmonale.

Beta blocker therapy is indicated to treat systolic heart failure including patients who have experienced a myocardial infarction. Beta blocker therapy can present unique challenges for patients with airway disease but are generally well tolerated by patients with COPD who do not exhibit bronchial hyperreactivity. Patients with COPD should be treated with $beta_1$ selective agents when appropriate. The use of beta blocker therapy for patients with COPD and cardiac disease has been associated with improved overall survival.[81,82]

Polycythemia

Polycythemia secondary to chronic hypoxemia in COPD patients can be improved by either oxygen therapy or periodic phlebotomy if oxygen therapy alone is not sufficient. COT was shown by the Nocturnal Oxygen Therapy Trial Group to reduce hematocrit values in treated patients. Acute phlebotomy is indicated if the hematocrit is above 55% to 60% and the patient is experiencing CNS effects suggestive of sludging from high blood viscosity. Long-term oxygen then can be used to maintain a lower hematocrit.

Other Pharmacologic Considerations

A number of other treatments have been explored over the years. Among these therapies, either there is insufficient evidence to warrant recommending their use or they have been proven to not be beneficial in the management of COPD. A brief summary is provided because the clinician likely will encounter patients who are receiving or inquire about these treatments.

Suppressive Antimicrobial Agents

Because COPD patients often are colonized with bacteria and experience recurrent exacerbations of their condition, a common practice employed in the past has been the use of low-dose antimicrobial therapy as preventative or prophylaxis against these acute exacerbations. However, clinical studies over the past 40 years have failed to demonstrate any significant benefit from this practice.[1]

In certain pulmonary conditions such as cystic fibrosis and bronchiectasis, chronic therapy with macrolide antibiotics, specifically azithromycin, has shown clinical benefit based on its proposed antiinflammatory properties and is used in clinical practice. In a study evaluating chronic azithromycin in patients with COPD, patients were randomized to azithromycin (250 mg orally daily) or placebo in addition to maintenance therapy for COPD and were followed for 1 year.[83] Chronic azithromycin was associated with a lower rate of exacerbations and improved quality-of-life scores; however, more patients in the azithromycin group reported hearing deficits (25% vs 20% in the placebo group). Therapy with azithromycin was also associated with a higher rate of colonization with macrolide-resistant bacteria during the study period. Of note, patients were carefully screened for hearing impairment and risk factors for QT prolongation prior to entering the study and were excluded if either was present.

In 2012, a retrospective, observational study reported an increase in cardiac events with short courses of azithromycin and the FDA has since updated the product labeling to include a precaution about QT prolongation.[84] Given the limited evidence for long-term treatment (beyond 1 year) with azithromycin, it would be prudent to wait for more long-term safety data before routinely recommending this therapy for patients with COPD who are at risk for exacerbations. Other therapies that reduce exacerbation risk (IC, LABA, LAMA, and roflumilast) should be considered first. Clinicians may choose to consider azithromycin for individual patients at high risk for exacerbations after weighing the risks and benefits of therapy.

Expectorants and Mucolytics

Adequate water intake generally is acceptable to maintain hydration and assist in the removal of airway sections. Mucolytics and expectorants such as compounded saturated solutions of potassium iodide, ammonium chloride, N-acetylcysteine, and guaifenesin have been evaluated as adjunctive therapy for patients with COPD. In one recent trial, patients with moderate to severe COPD were randomized to either placebo or oral N-acetylcysteine 600 mg twice daily for 1 year. Patients were not required to be on ICs prior to randomization. N-acetylcysteine was associated with a significant decrease in exacerbation rate among patients with moderate disease only (GOLD 2).[85] Strong evidence of clinical benefit is lacking for the routine use of mucolytics in the treatment of COPD.[86]

In 2011, the FDA announced its intention to remove various unapproved cough and cold preparations (including several containing guaifenesin) from the market due to safety and efficacy concerns. Two extended release tablet formulations are currently approved by the FDA. Other approved formulations of guaifenesin contain dextromethorphan or pseudoephedrine and should not be used for COPD maintenance therapy.

Opioids

Systemic (oral and parenteral) opioids, especially morphine, can relieve dyspnea for patients with end-stage COPD. Nebulized therapy is sometimes used in clinical practice, although data about clinical benefit are lacking. Opioids should be used carefully, if at all, to avoid adverse effects on ventilatory drive.

Respiratory Stimulants

There is no role for respiratory stimulants in the long-term management of COPD.[1] Agents that have shown some utility in the acute setting include almitrine and doxapram. However, almitrine is available only in Europe, and its usefulness is limited by neurotoxicity. Doxapram is available for IV use only and may be no better than intermittent NPPV.

Targeted Therapy for Pulmonary Hypertension

Secondary pulmonary hypertension is a feature of severe COPD. This has prompted interest about the potential role of agents used to treat pulmonary arterial hypertension. However, the use of an endothelin receptor antagonist (bosentan) failed to improve exercise tolerance and worsened hypoxemia in one trial.[87] Investigations with sildenafil, a phosphodiesterase type 5 (PDE5) inhibitor, have been conflicting in uncontrolled clinical trials. Due to concerns that PDE5 inhibitors may worsen gas exchange in patients with COPD, they are not recommended outside of clinical trials.[88]

Surgical Intervention

Various surgical options have been employed in the management of COPD. These include bullectomy, lung volume reduction surgery (LVRS), and lung transplantation. Bullectomy has been performed for many years and may be useful when large bullae (more than 1 cm) are noted on computerized axial tomography (CT or CAT) scan. The presence of bullae may contribute to complaints of dyspnea, and their removal can improve lung function and reduce symptoms, although there is no evidence of a mortality benefit.

Because of the prevalence of COPD, it is the most frequent indication for lung transplantation. Transplantation is considered when predicted survival is less than 2 years, FEV_1 is less than 25% predicted, and hypoxemia, hypercapnia, and pulmonary hypertension exist despite medical management.[5] Experience to date shows 2-year survival of 65% to 90%, and 5-year survival of 41% to 53%.

Short-term trials comparing the effects of pulmonary rehabilitation plus LVRS with pulmonary rehabilitation alone reported that the combination of treatments resulted in greater improvements in lung function, gas exchange, and quality of life at 3 months. The National Emphysema Treatment Trial (NETT), a prospective, randomized trial evaluating the long-term effects of LVRS plus pulmonary rehabilitation compared with pulmonary rehabilitation alone, followed 1,218 patients for 3 years.[89] The primary end points for the study were mortality and maximal exercise capacity 2 years after randomization. Secondary end points included pulmonary function, distance walked in 6 minutes, and quality-of-life measurements. At an interim analysis, patients with an FEV_1 of less than 20% of predicted or a carbon monoxide diffusing capacity of less than 20% of predicted were noted to be at high risk of death after surgery and subsequently were excluded from the study. Results of the study showed no mortality benefit with LVRS compared with pulmonary rehabilitation alone. Patients undergoing surgery had improved exercise capacity, lung function, and quality of life at 2 years, but these patients also had a higher risk of short-term morbidity and mortality associated with the surgery. A subgroup analysis of the study noted that patients with predominately upper-lobe emphysema and low exercise capacity undergoing surgery had lower mortality rates at 2 years compared with patients treated with medical therapy alone. Because of the costs and risks associated with LVRS, more studies are needed to better determine the ideal surgical candidates and identify subgroups of patients that would benefit most from surgery. The long-term benefits of LVRS are exhibited as improved oxygenation and decreased requirements for supplemental oxygen during treadmill walking as well as self-reported oxygen requirements for up to 24 months after the procedure.[90]

Dietary Supplements

There has been increasing interest in the role of antioxidants, including vitamins E and C and β-carotene, in reducing the frequency of exacerbations. It is postulated that they may be beneficial in COPD as a result of an imbalance between oxidants and antioxidants that has been considered in the pathogenesis of smoking-induced lung disease. However, there is no good evidence that antioxidant therapies improve COPD symptoms or slow disease progression. Nutritional supplements, including creatine, have not proven beneficial to improve the benefit of pulmonary rehabilitation programs.[91]

Investigational Therapies

Much of the recent progress concerning pharmacotherapies has focused on long-acting bronchodilators and corticosteroid agents. In addition, based on the knowledge about the importance of neutrophilic inflammation in COPD and potential therapeutic benefit of inhibition of neutrophil activity, a number of antiinflammatory compounds are being explored. Specifically, agents inhibiting LTB_4, neutrophil elastase, and phosphodiesterases have being evaluated. Studies of these strategies have been disappointing. As noted above, therapies targeting oxidative stress have not borne promising results, although vitamin D continues to be an area of exploration.[92]

Manipulation of various cytokines have been evaluated despite earlier studies involving infliximab, a TNFα-blocker, which failed to demonstrate any benefits on quality of life or secondary end points including lung function, exercise capacity, or exacerbation rates. The discontinuation rate due to adverse events was high (20%-27%) in the active treatment group.[93] Other current areas of investigation include p38 mitogen activated protein kinase inhibitors (MAPK), inhibitors of interleukin 1 and interleukin 5, epithelial growth factor receptor inhibitors, and neutrophil elasatase inhibitors.[92,94]

The role of HMG-CoA reductase inhibitors for patients with COPD has continued to garner interest because of the systemic inflammation that is present. A recent meta-analysis reported a hazard ratio of 0.62 for all-cause mortality, 0.48 for COPD mortality, and 0.93 for cardiovascular mortality.[95] The risk for COPD exacerbations was also reduced (HR 0.64). These results suggest the need for a prospective trial. In the meantime, patients receiving statin therapy for other reasons likely derive benefits related to their COPD.

PHARMACOECONOMIC CONSIDERATIONS

The overall cost of therapy is an important consideration in contemporary medical practice. Meaningful cost analysis goes beyond the cost of the medication itself and incorporates the impact of a given therapeutic agent on overall healthcare cost. Because of the relative lack of benefit among objective outcome measures in COPD clinical trials, pharmacoeconomic studies can be useful in decision making about pharmacotherapy options. Although there appears to be substantial interest in describing the pharmacoeconomic impact of COPD, much of the current literature appears to address modeling and predicting costs.[96,97]

A recent database study evaluating 8,554 patients with a mean age of 70.1 years reported the economic impact of exacerbations.[98] The population was predominantly insured by Medicare and, during a 2 year period, 49.8% of the patients had experienced an exacerbation. The COPD-related mean annual costs were $4,069 overall and $6,381 for patients with two or more exacerbations. All-cause health care costs were $18,976 overall and $23,901 for patients with two or more exacerbations. The authors concluded that exacerbations add significantly to the annual costs.

Another systematic review reported that direct health costs increased 38% between 1987 and 2007, and continued to rise 5% annually through 2009.[99] The annual healthcare costs were 10 fold higher in patients who experienced an exacerbation and two studies suggested that long-acting bronchodilator therapy reduced the risk of exacerbations by 16% to 17%, with a resultant lowering in costs.

Few data are available about the cost-effectiveness of educational programs for patients with COPD. In an outpatient clinic, patients attending one 4-hour group session, followed by one to two individual sessions with a clinician, reported improved outcomes, and costs were reduced in an evaluation 12 months later.[100] Additional research is needed regarding the best model for education and also the specific self-management strategies to teach. One modeling study evaluated the cost effectiveness of improving adherence to therapy and inhalation technique among patients.[101] The study reported a 10% reduction in annual costs mostly related to a reduced risk of hospitalization.

One literature review focused on the cost-effectiveness of pharmacotherapy in ambulatory care settings.[102] The author concluded (without providing quantitative assessments) that pharmacotherapeutic strategies for managing ambulatory COPD patients are cost effective, with particular benefit for more severe patients.

Clinical **Controversy...**

In the United States, all products containing a LABA agent, either alone or in combination with ICs, include a black box warning about an increased risk of severe asthma attacks or death associated with their use. This caution applies to patients with asthma, and it is strongly recommended that LABAs use should always be in conjunction with another controller therapy (eg, ICs) and that use should be limited in duration. This concern only applies to patients with asthma and is not relevant concerning the use of LABA therapy for COPD patients.

Combination products of a long-acting inhaled β-agonist and an IC agent are the most commonly prescribed medications for lung disease, including COPD. However, in expert guidelines, ICs are indicated only for patients with more severe disease who experience frequent exacerbations. Many patients now receiving therapy with the combination inhaler may be candidates for bronchodilator therapy alone, although the benefit of ICs continues to be a focus of clinical research, including the potential for a mortality benefit.

The role of systemic corticosteroids for acute exacerbations of COPD has been clarified in recent years. However, the appropriate dosage regimen is not well established. Regimens range from initial high doses (methylprednisolone 125 mg every 6 hours) to more conservative dosing (prednisone 40-60 mg/day). Consensus guidelines indicate that bronchodilator therapy is the focus of pharmacotherapy for COPD. However, there is no clear choice for the initial agent. For patients with daily but not persistent symptoms, either ipratropium or albuterol offers advantages as initial therapy. Both also have limitations if chosen as the initial therapy.

International guidelines recommend long-acting bronchodilator therapy for patients with moderate to very severe disease or when symptoms are not adequately managed with short-acting agents or as-needed therapy. When response to a single long-acting bronchodilator is not optimal, guidelines recommend the use of combinations. However, data are lacking presently about the therapeutic benefit of combinations of long-acting bronchodilators, and this approach is associated with substantial costs.

EVALUATION OF THERAPEUTIC OUTCOMES

To evaluate therapeutic outcomes of COPD effectively, the practitioner must first delineate between chronic stable COPD and acute exacerbations. In chronic stable COPD, pulmonary function tests should be assessed periodically and with any therapy addition, change in dose, or deletion of therapy. Because objective improvements often are minimal, subjective assessments are important. Other outcome parameters are commonly evaluated, including dyspnea score, quality-of-life assessments, and exacerbation rates, including visits to the emergency department or hospitalization. In acute exacerbations of COPD, white blood cell count, vital signs, chest x-ray, and changes in frequency of dyspnea, sputum volume, and sputum purulence should be assessed at the onset and throughout treatment of an exacerbation. In more severe exacerbations, ABGs and oxygen saturation also should be monitored. As with any drug therapy, patient adherence to therapeutic regimens, side effects, potential drug interactions, and subjective measures of quality of life also must be evaluated.

To date, there is no evidence that any of the available pharmacotherapies for COPD impact disease progression. Removal of the primary causative factor for COPD (eg, cessation of cigarette smoking) does improve survival, as does supplemental oxygen therapy in a subset of patients with COPD. The most pertinent clinical outcomes that have emerged from clinical trials over the past decade are symptom improvement and reductions in exacerbation frequency. While it is important to continue to explore strategies to improve survival, consideration should be given to these two relevant and important outcome measures when initiating, continuing, and monitoring therapy. Because of the tremendous impact of exacerbations on disease progression, a reduction in exacerbation frequency may be predicted to show a benefit; however, this has not been proven.

END-OF-LIFE CARE

Based on the natural course of COPD, characterized by the progressive decline in lung function and development of complications, consideration should be given to end-of-life decisions and advanced directives.[1] Factors associated with expected mortality within 1 year have been identified. These include older age, diagnosis of depression, declining overall health status, hypercapnia, an FEV_1 of less than 30% predicted, ability to walk only a few steps without resting, more than one emergent hospitalization in the past year, and the presence of comorbidities, including congestive heart failure. An effective strategy to discuss end-of-life care involves the patient's participation in identifying advanced directives. Patients should be assured that symptoms, including pain, will be managed and their dignity will be preserved. Specific issues that should be addressed include location and provider for terminal care, desires to use or withhold mechanical ventilation, and involvement of other family members in decisions on behalf of the patient.

ABBREVIATIONS

AAT	α_1-antitrypsin
ABG	arterial blood gas
ACCP	American College of Chest Physicians
ACIP	Advisory Committee on Immunization Practices
ACOS	asthma and COPD overlap syndrome
ACP	American College of Physicians
ATS	American Thoracic Society
BMI	body mass index
cAMP	cyclic adenosine monophosphate
CAT	COPD Assessment Test
CCQ	Clinical COPD Questionnaire
CDC	Centers for Disease Control and Prevention
cGMP	cyclic guanosine monophosphate
COPD	chronic obstructive pulmonary disease
COT	continuous oxygen therapy
CRQ	Chronic Respiratory Questionnaire
CT	computed tomographic
DPI	dry powder inhaler
ENDS	electronic nicotine delivery systems
ERS	European Respiratory Society
FEV_1	forced expiratory volume in 1 second
FRC	functional residual capacity
FVC	forced vital capacity
GOLD	Global Initiative for Chronic Obstructive Lung Disease
HPA	hypothalamic–pituitary–adrenal
ICS	inhaled corticosteroid
IL	interleukin
LABA	long-acting inhaled β_2-agonist

LTB_4	leukotriene B_4
LVRS	lung volume reduction surgery
MDI	metered-dose inhaler
MMP12	matrix metalloproteinase 12
mMRC	modified Medical Research Council
NETT	National Emphysema Treatment Trial
NHLBI	National Heart, Lung, and Blood Institute
NOT	nocturnal oxygen therapy
NPPV	noninvasive positive-pressure ventilation
$PaCO_2$	pressure exerted by carbon dioxide gas in arterial blood
PaO_2	pressure exerted by oxygen gas in arterial blood
PDE4	phosphodiesterase 4
PDE5	phosphodiesterase type 5
PHS	Public Health Service
SCCOPE	Systemic Corticosteroids in Chronic Obstructive Pulmonary Disease Exacerbations
SCCOR	Specialized Centers of Clinically Oriented Research
SGRQ	St. George's Respiratory Questionnaire
TNF-α	tumor necrosis factor-α
TORCH	Towards a Revolution in COPD Health
UPLIFT	Understanding Potential Long-Term Impacts on Function with Tiotropium
VC	vital capacity
WHO	World Health Organization

REFERENCES

1. Global Initiative for Chronic Obstructive Lung Disease. Global Strategy for the Diagnosis, Management, and Prevention of Chronic Obstructive Pulmonary Disease (GOLD). 2016. Available at: http://www.goldcopd.
2. Qureshi H, Sharafkhaneh A, Hanania NA. Chronic obstructive pulmonary disease exacerbations: Latest evidence and clinical implications. *Ther Adv Chronic Dis* 2014;5(5):212-227.
3. Hatipoglu U, Aboussquan L. Chronic obstructive pulmonary disease: An update for the primary physician. *Clev Clin J Med* 2014;81(6):373-383.
4. Qaseem A, Wilt TJ, Weinberger SE, et al. Diagnosis and management of stable COPD: A clinical practice guideline update from the American College of Physicians, the American College of Chest Physicians, the American Thoracic Society, and the European Respiratory Society. *Ann Intern Med* 2011;155:179-191.
5. National Clinical Guideline Centre. Chronic obstructive pulmonary disease: Management of chronic obstructive pulmonary disease in adults in primary and secondary care. London: National Clinical Guideline Centre. 2010. Available at: http://guidance.nice.org.uk/CG101/Guidance/pdf/English.
6. Criner GJ, Bourbeau J, Diekemper RL, et al. Prevention of acute exacerbations of COPD. *Chest* 2015;147(4):894-942.
7. Postow L, Punturieri A, Croxton TL, Weinmann GG, Kiley JP. A decade of National Heart, Lung, and Blood Institute programs supporting COPD research and education. *J COPD F* 2014;1(1):64-72. http://journal.copdfoundation.org.
8. Ford ES, Mannino DM, Wheaton AG, Giles WH, Presley-Cantrell LR, Croft JB. Trends in the prevalence of obstructive and restrictive lung function among adults in the United States: Findings from the National Health and Nutrition Examination Survey from 1988-1994 to 2007-2010. *Chest* 2013;143(5):1395-1406.
9. Chronic Obstructive Pulmonary Disease (COPD) Fact Sheet. Washington, DC: American Lung Association, February 2010. Available at: www.lungusa.org/lung-disease/COPD/resources/fact-figures/COPD-Fact-Sheet.html.
10. U.S. Department of Health and Human Services. The Health Consequences of Smoking—50 Years of Progress: A Report of the Surgeon General. Atlanta, GA: U.S. Department of Health and Human Services, Centers for Disease Control and Prevention, National Center for Chronic Disease Prevention and Health Promotion, Office on Smoking and Health, 2014.
11. Sandford AJ, Silverman EK. Chronic obstructive pulmonary disease. 1: Susceptibility factors for COPD the genotype—environment interaction. *Thorax* 2002;57:736-741.
12. Hunninghake GM, Cho MH, Tesfaigzi Y, et al. MMP12, lung function, and COPD in high-risk populations. *N Engl J Med* 2009;361:2599-2608.
13. Gladysheva ES, Malhotra A, Owens RL. Influencing the decline of lung function in COPD: Use of pharmacotherapy. *Int J Chron Obstruct Pulmon Dis* 2010;5:153-164. PubMed PMID: 20631815; PubMed Central PMCID: PMC2898088.
14. Shujaat A, Minkin R, Eden E. Pulmonary hypertension and chronic cor pulmonale in COPD. *Int J Chron Obstruct Pulmon Dis* 2007;2(3):273-282.
15. McCarthy B, Casey D, Devane D, Murphy K, Murphy E, Lacasse Y. Pulmonary rehabilitation for chronic obstructive pulmonary disease. *Cochrane Database Syst Rev* 2015;2:CD003793.
16. Patel N, Belcher J, Thorpe G, Forsyth NR, Spiteri MA. Measurement of C-reactive protein, procalcitonin and neutrophil elastase in saliva of COPD patients and healthy controls: Correlation to self-reported wellbeing parameters. *Respir Res* 2015;16:62-69.
17. Hurst JR, Wedzicha JA. Management and prevention of chronic obstructive pulmonary disease exacerbations: A state of the art review. *BMC Med* 2009;7:40. doi: 10.1186/1741-7015-7-40. PubMed PMID: 19664218; PubMedCentral PMCID: PMC2734841.
18. Jones PW, Harding G, Berry P, Wiklund L, Chen W-H, Kline Leidy N. Development and first validation of the COPD Assessment Test. *Eur Respir J* 2009;34:648-665.
19. van der Molen T, Willemse BW, Schokker S, ten Hacken NH, Postma DS, Juniper EF. Development, validity and responsiveness of the Clinical COPD Questionnaire. *Health Qual Life Outcomes* 2003;1:13.
20. Agusti A, Calverley PM, Celli B, et al. Characterisation of COPD heterogeneity in the ECLIPSE cohort. *Respir Res* 2010;11:122.
21. Calverley PMA, Anderson JA, Celli B, et al. Salmeterol and fluticasone propionate and survival in chronic obstructive pulmonary disease (TORCH). *N Engl J Med* 2007;356:775-789.
22. Tashkin DP, Celli B, Senn S, et al. A 4 year trial of tiotropium in chronic obstructive pulmonary disease. *N Engl J Med* 2008;359:1543-1554.
23. Gerhardsson de Verdier M, Andersson M, Kern DW, Zhou S, Tunceli O. Asthma and chronic obstructive pulmonary disease overlap syndrome: Doubled costs compared with patients with asthma alone. *Value Health* 2015;18:759-766.
24. Eriksen N, Vestbo J. Management and survival of patients admitted with an exacerbation of COPD: Comparison of two Danish cohorts. Clin Respir J 2010;4(4):208-214.
25. Gudmundsson G, Ulrik CS, Gislason T, el al. Long-term survival in patients hospitalized for chronic obstructive pulmonary disease: A prospective observational study in the Nordic countries. *Int J Chron Obstruct Pulmon Dis* 2012;7:571-576.
26. Vermylen JH, Szmuilowicz E, Kalhan R. Palliative care in COPD: An unmet area for quality improvement. *Int J Chron Obstruct Pulmon Dis* 2015;10:1543-1551.
27. Anthonisen NR, Connett JE, Kiley JP, et al. Effects of smoking intervention and the use of an inhaled anticholinergic bronchodilator on the rate of decline in FEV_1: The Lung Health Study. *JAMA* 1994;272:1497-1505.
28. Fiore MC, Jaén CR, Baker TB, et al. Treating Tobacco Use and Dependence: 2008 Update. *Clinical Practice Guideline. Public Health Service*. Rockville, MD: U.S. Department of Health and Human Services. May 2008. Available at: www.surgeongeneral.gov/tobacco.
29. Patnode CD, Henderson JT, Thompson JH, Senger CA, Fortmann SP, Whitlock EP. Behavioral counseling and pharmacotherapy interventions for tobacco cessation in adults, including pregnant women: A review of reviews for the U.S. Preventive Services Task Force. *Ann Intern Med* 2015;163(8):608-621.
30. Jorenby DE, Leischow SJ, Nides MA, et al. A controlled trial of sustained-release bupropion, a nicotine patch, or both for smoking cessation. *N Engl J Med* 1999;340:685-691.
31. Spruit MA, Singh SJ, Garvey C, et al. An official American Thoracic Society/European Respiratory Society statement: Key concepts and advances in pulmonary rehabilitation. *Am J Respir Crit Care Med* 2013;188(8):e13-e64.
32. Poole PJ, Chacko E, Wood-Baker RW, Cates CJ. Influenza vaccine for patients with chronic obstructive pulmonary disease. *Cochrane Database Syst Rev* 2006;25(1):CD002733.
33. Centers for Disease Control and Prevention (CDC). Advisory Committee on Immunization Practices (ACIP) Adult Immunization Work Group. Advisory committee on immunization practices recommended immunization schedule for adults aged 19 years or older—United States 2015. *MMWR Morb Mortal Wkly Rep* 2015;64(4):91-92.

34. Walters JA, Smith S, Poole P, Granger RH, Wood-Baker R. Injectable vaccines for preventing pneumococcal infection in patients with chronic obstructive pulmonary disease. *Cochrane Database Syst Rev* 201010;(11):CD001390.
35. Nocturnal Oxygen Therapy Trial Group. Continuous or nocturnal oxygen therapy in hypoxemic chronic obstructive lung disease. *Ann Intern Med* 1980;93:391-398.
36. Ferreira IMI, Brooks D, White J, Goldstein R. Nutritional supplementation for stable chronic obstructive pulmonary disease. *Cochrane Database Syst Rev* 2012;12:CD000998.
37. Puhan MA, Bachmann LM, Kleijnen J, ter Riet G, Kessels AG. Inhaled drugs to reduce exacerbations in patients with chronic obstructive pulmonary disease: A network meta-analysis. *BMC Med* 2009;7:2.
38. Asmus MJ, Hendeles L. Levalbuterol nebulizer solution: Is it worth five times the cost of albuterol? *Pharmacotherapy* 2000;20:123-129.
39. Ikeda A, Nishimura K, Koyama H, et al. Dose–response study of ipratropium bromide aerosol on maximum exercise performance in stable patients with chronic obstructive pulmonary disease. *Thorax* 1996;51:48-53.
40. Kew KM, Mavergames C, Walters JA. Long-acting beta2- agonists for chronic obstructive pulmonary disease. *Cochrane Database Syst Rev* 2013;10:CD010177.
41. Dahl R, Chung KF, Buhl R, et al. Once-daily indacaterol versus twice-daily salmeterol for COPD: A placebo-controlled comparison. *Eur Respir J* 2011;37(2):273-279.
42. Melani AS. Long-acting muscarinic antagonists. *Expert Rev Clin Pharmacol* 2015;8(4):479-501.
43. Cheyne L, Irvin-Sellers MJ, White J. Tiotropium versus ipratropium bromide for chronic obstructive pulmonary disease. *Cochrane Database Syst Rev* 2015;9:CD009552. [Epub ahead of print]
44. Chong J, Karner C, Poole P. Tiotropium versus long-acting beta-agonists for stable chronic obstructive pulmonary disease. *Cochrane Database Syst Rev* 2012;9:CD009157.
45. Kim JS, Park J, Lim SY, et al. Comparison of clinical efficacy and safety between indacaterol and tiotropium in COPD: Meta-analysis of randomized controlled trials. *PLoS One* 2015;10(3):e0119948.
46. Celli B, Decramer M, Leimer I, Vogel U, Kesten S, Tashkin DP. Cardiovascular safety of tiotropium in patients with COPD. *Chest* 2010;137:2-30.
47. Wise RA, Anzueto A, Cotton D, Dahl R, Devins T, Disse B, et al. for the TIOSPIR Investigators. Tiotripium Respimat Inhaler and the Risk of Death in COPD. *N Engl J Med* 2013;369(16):1491-1501.
48. Ni H, Soe Z, Moe S. Aclidinium bromide for stable chronic obstructive pulmonary disease. *Cochrane Database Syst Rev* 2014;9:CD010509.
49. Karner C, Cates CJ. Long-acting beta$_2$-agonist in addition to tiotropium versus either tiotropium alone or long-acting beta$_2$-agonist alone for chronic obstructive pulmonary disease. *Cochrane Database Syst Rev* 2012;4:CD008989.
50. Huisman EL, Cockle SM, Ismaila AS, Karabis A, Punekar YS. Comparative efficacy of combination bronchodilator therapies in COPD: A network meta-analysis. *Int J Chron Obstruct Pulmon Dis* 2015;10:1863-1881.
51. D'Urzo T, Donohue JF, Price D, Miravitlles M, Kerwin E. Dual bronchodilator therapy with aclidinium bromide/formoterol fumarate for chronic obstructive pulmonary disease. *Expert Rev Respir Med* 2015;9(5):519-532.
52. Rodrigo GJ, Neffen H. A systematic review of the efficacy and safety of a fixed-dose combination of umeclidinium and vilanterol for the treatment of COPD. *Chest* 2015;148(2):397-407.
53. Barnes PJ. Theophylline: New perspectives for an old drug. *Am J Respir Crit Care Med* 2003;167:813-818.
54. Yang IA, Clarke MS, Sim EH, Fong KM. Inhaled corticosteroids for stable chronic obstructive pulmonary disease. *Cochrane Database Syst Rev* 2012;7:CD002991.
55. Kew KM, Seniukovich A. Inhaled steroids and risk of pneumonia for chronic obstructive pulmonary disease. *Cochrane Database Syst Rev* 2014;3:CD010115.
56. Hubbard R, Tatterfield A, Smith C, et al. Use of inhaled corticosteroids and the risk of fracture. *Chest* 2006;130:1082-1088.
57. Jones A, Fay JK, Burr M, Stone M, Hood K, Roberts G. Inhaled corticosteroid effects on bone metabolism in asthma and mild chronic obstructive pulmonary disease. *Cochrane Database Syst Rev* 2002;(1):CD003537.
58. Franssen FM, Spruit MA, Wouters EF. Determinants of polypharmacy and compliance with GOLD guidelines in patients with chronic obstructive pulmonary disease. *Int J Chron Obstruct Pulmon Dis* 2011;6:493-501.
59. Rossi A, van der Molen T, del Olmo R, et al. INSTEAD: A randomised switch trial of indacaterol versus salmeterol/fluticasone in moderate COPD. *Eur Respir J* 2014;44(6):1548-1556.
60. Magnussen H, Disse B, Rodriguez-Rosin R, et al. Withdrawal of inhaled glucocorticoids and exacerbations of COPD (WISDOM). *N Engl J Med* 2014;371:1285-1294.
61. Nannini LJ, Poole P, Milan SJ, Holmes R, Normansell R. Combined corticosteroid and long-acting beta$_2$-agonist in one inhaler versus placebo for chronic obstructive pulmonary disease. *Cochrane Database Syst Rev* 2013;11:CD003794.
62. Celli BR, Thomas NE, Anderson JA, et al. Effect of pharmacotherapy on rate of decline of lung function in chronic obstructive pulmonary disease: Results from the TORCH study. *Am J Respir Crit Care Med* 2008;178:332-338.
63. Wedzicha JA, Calverley PM, Seemungal TA, et al. The prevention of chronic obstructive pulmonary disease exacerbations by salmeterol/fluticasone propionate or tiotropium bromide. *Am J Respir Crit Care Med* 2008;177:19-26.
64. Aaron SD, Vandemheen KL, Fergusson D, et al. Tiotropium in combination with placebo, salmeterol or fluticasone–salmeterol for treatment of chronic obstructive pulmonary disease. *Ann Intern Med* 2007;146:545-555.
65. Karner C, Cates CJ. Combination inhaled steroid and long-acting beta(2)-agonist in addition to tiotropium versus tiotropium or combination alone for chronic obstructive pulmonary disease. *Cochrane Database Syst Rev* 2011;3:CD008532.
66. Siler TM, Kerwin E, Sousa AR, Donald A, Ali R, Church A. Efficacy and safety of umeclidinium added to fluticasone furoate/vilanterol in chronic obstructive pulmonary disease: Results of two randomized studies. *Respir Med* 2015;109(9):1155-1163.
67. Calverley PM, Rabe KF, Goehring UM, et al. Roflumilast in symptomatic chronic obstructive pulmonary disease: Two randomised clinical trials. *Lancet* 2009;374(9691):685-694.
68. Martinez FJ, Calverley PM, Goehring UM, et al. Effect of roflumilast on exacerbations inpatients with severe chronic obstructive pulmonary disease uncontrolled by combination therapy (REACT): A multicentre randomised controlled trial. *Lancet* 2015;385(9971):857-866.
69. Alpha-1-Antitrypsin Deficiency Registry Study Group. Survival and FEV_1 decline in individuals with severe deficiency of alpha-1-antitrypsin. *Am J Respir Crit Care Med* 1998;158:49-59.
70. Dirksen A, Dijkman JH, Madsen F, et al. A randomized clinical trial of alpha-1-antitrypsin augmentation therapy. *Am J Respir Crit Care Med* 1999;160:1468-1472.
71. Cabrini L, Landoni G, Oriani A, et al. Noninvasive ventilation and survival in acute care settings: A comprehensive systematic review and meta-analysis of randomized controlled trials. *Crit Care Med* 2014;43(4):880-888.
72. Niewoehner DE, Erbland ML, Deupree RH, et al. Effect of systemic glucocorticoids on exacerbations of chronic obstructive pulmonary disease. Department of Veterans Affairs Cooperative Study Group. *N Engl J Med* 1999;340:1941-1947.
73. Davies L, Angus RM, Calverley PMA. Oral corticosteroids in patients admitted to hospital with exacerbations of chronic obstructive pulmonary disease: A prospective, randomised, controlled trial. *Lancet* 1999;354:456-460.
74. Aaron SD, Vandemheen KL, Hebert P, et al. Outpatient oral prednisone after emergency treatment of chronic obstructive pulmonary disease. *N Engl J Med* 2003;348:2618-2625.
75. Hernandez JM, Edmonds M. Do systemic corticosteroids improve outcomes in chronic obstructive pulmonary disease exacerbations? *Ann Emerg Med* 2015 doi.org/10.1016/j.annemergmed.2015.07.009.
76. Leuppi JD, Schuetz P, Bingisser R, et al. Short-term vs convential glucocorticoid therapy in acute exacerbations of chronic obstructive pulmonary disease. *JAMA* 2013;309(21):2223-2231.
77. Wilson R, Sethi S, Anzueto A, Miravittles M. Antibiotics for treatment and prevention of exacerbations of chronic obstructive pulmonary disease. *J Infect* 2013;67:497-515.
78. Niederman MS. Antibiotic therapy for exacerbations of chronic bronchitis. *Semin Respir Infect* 2000;15:59-70.
79. Chodosh S, DeAbate C, Haverstock D, Aneiro L, Church D. Short-course moxifloxacin therapy for treatment of acute bacterial exacerbations of chronic bronchitis. *Respir Med* 2000;94:18-27.
80. Rizkallah J, Man SF, Sin DD. Prevalence of pulmonary embolism in acute exacerbations of COPD: A systematic review and metaanalysis. *Chest* 2009;135:786-793.

81. Quint JK, Herrett E, Bhaskaran K, et al. Effect of beta blockers on mortality after myocardial infarction in adults with COPD: Population-based cohort study of UK electronic healthcare records. *BMJ* 2013;347:16650.
82. Etminan M, Jafari S, Carleton B, Fitzgerald JM. Beta-blocker use and COPD mortality: A systematic review and meta-analysis. *BMC Pulm Med* 2012;12:48-54.
83. Albert RK, Connett J, Bailey WD, et al. Azithromycin for prevention of exacerbation in COPD. *N Engl J Med* 2011;365:689-698.
84. Ray WA, Murray KT, Hall K, et al. Azithromycin and the risk of cardiovascular death. *N Engl J Med* 2012;366:1881-1890.
85. Zheng JP, Wen FQ, Bai CX, et al. PANTHEON study group. Twice daily N-acetylcysteine 600 mg for exacerbations of chronic obstructive pulmonary disease (PANTHEON): A randomised, double- blind placebo-controlled trial. *Lancet Respir Med* 2014;2(3):187-194.
86. Poole P, Black PN, Cates CJ. Mucolytic agents for chronic bronchitis or chronic obstructive pulmonary disease. *Cochrane Database Syst Rev* 2012;8:CD001287.
87. Stolz D, Linka A, Di Valentino M, Meyer A, Brutsche M, Tamm M. A randomized, controlled trial of bosentan in severe COPD. *Eur Respir J* 2008;32:619-628.
88. Galie N, Hoeper MM, Humbert M, et al. Guidelines for the diagnosis and treatment of pulmonary hypertension. *Eur Respir J* 2009;34:1219-1263.
89. Fishman A, Martinez F, Naunheim K, et al. A randomized trial comparing lung-volume-reduction surgery with medical therapy for severe emphysema. *N Engl J Med* 2003;348:2059-2073.
90. Snyder ML, Goss CH, Neradilek B, et al. National Emphysema Treatment Trial Research Group. Changes in arterial oxygenation and self-reported oxygen use after lung volume reduction surgery. *Am J Respir Crit Care Med* 2008;178:339-345.
91. Deacon SJ, Vincent EE, Greenhaff PL, et al. Randomized controlled trial of dietary creatine as an adjunct therapy to physical training in chronic obstructive pulmonary disease. *Am J Respir Crit Care Med* 2008;178:233-239.
92. Matera MG, Cazzola M. Treatment of COPD: No longer nihilism, but there is still an urgent need for new therapies. *Curr Opin Pharmacol* 2012;12:225-228.
93. Rennard SI, Fogarty C, Kelsen S, et al. The safety and efficacy of infliximab in moderate to severe chronic obstructive pulmonary disease. *Am J Respir Crit Care Med* 2007;175:926-934.
94. Babu KS, Morjaria JB. Emerging therapeutic strategies in COPD. *Drug Discov Today* 2015;20(3):371-379.
95. Cao C, Wu Y, Lv D, et al. The effect of statins on chronic obstructive pulmonary disease and mortality: A systematic review and meta-analysis of observational research. *Nat Sci Rep* 2015;5:16461 doi: 10.1038/srep16461.
96. van Boven JF, Roman-Rodriguez M, Kocks JW, Soriano JB, Postma MJ, van der Molen T. Predictors of cost-effectiveness of selected COPD treatments in primary care: UNLOCK study protocol. *NPJ Prim Care Respir Med* 2015;25:15051.
97. Srivastava S, Thakur D, Sharma S, Punekar KS. Systematic review of humanistic and economic burden of symptomatic chronic obstructive pulmonary disease. *Pharmacoeconomics* 2015;33(5):467-88.
98. Pasquale MK, Sun SX, Song f, Hartnett HJ, Sternkowski SA. Impact of exacerbations on health care costs and resource utilization in chronic obstructive pulmonary disease patients with chronic bronchitis from a predominately Medicare population. *Int J COPD* 2012;7:757-764.
99. Blanchette CM, Gross NJ, Altman P. Rising costs of COPD and the potential for maintenance therapy to slow the trend. *Am Health Drug Benefits* 2014;7(2):98-106.
100. Gallefoss F. The effects of patient education in COPD in a 1-year follow-up randomized, controlled trial. Patient Educ Couns 2004;52: 259-266.
101. van Boven JF, Tommelein E, Bossery K, et al. Improving inhaler adherence in patients with chronic obstructive pulmonary disease: A cost-effectiveness analysis. *Respir Res* 2014;15:66.
102. Simoens S. Cost-effectiveness of pharmacotherapy for COPD in ambulatory care:A review. *J Eval Clin Pract* 2013;19:1004-1011.

Pulmonary Arterial Hypertension

28

Rebecca Moote, Rebecca L. Attridge, and Deborah J. Levine

KEY CONCEPTS

1. Pulmonary arterial hypertension (PAH) is defined as a mean pulmonary artery pressure (mPAP) more than or equal to 25 mm Hg at rest with a pulmonary wedge pressure or left ventricular end-diastolic pressure (LVEDP) less than or equal to 15 mm Hg and a pulmonary vascular resistance (PVR) more than 3 Wood units (WU) measured by right cardiac catheterization.
2. Diagnosis of PAH is growing because of increased awareness and knowledge of the disease state, leading to earlier and improved evaluation and identification.
3. Regardless of the etiology, be it unknown or related to an associated medical condition, subgroups of PAH are based on similar clinical and pathologic physiology.
4. The underlying cause of PAH is a complicated amalgam of endothelial cell dysfunction, a procoagulant state, platelet activation, vasoconstriction, loss of relaxing factors, cellular proliferation, hypertrophy, fibrosis, and inflammation.
5. Patients with PAH present with exertional dyspnea, fatigue, weakness, and exertion intolerance. As the disease progresses, symptoms of right heart dysfunction and failure, such as dyspnea at rest, lower extremity edema, chest pain, and syncope, are seen.
6. The only way to make a definitive diagnosis of PAH is by right heart catheterization. The right heart catheterization provides important prognostic information and can be used to assess pulmonary vasoreactivity prior to initiating therapy.
7. The goals of treatment are to alleviate symptoms, improve the quality of life, slow the progression of the disease, and improve survival.
8. A general goal of PAH treatment is to correct the imbalance between vasoconstriction and vasodilation and prevent adverse thrombotic events to improve oxygenation, functional class, exercise capacity, and quality of life.
9. Nonpharmacologic therapy is frequently used to address comorbid conditions that often accompany PAH.
10. Conventional therapy of PAH includes oral anticoagulants, diuretics, oxygen, and digoxin.
11. Prostacyclin analogs such as epoprostenol, treprostinil, and iloprost induce potent vasodilation of pulmonary vascular beds. Only epoprostenol has demonstrated improved survival.
12. Endothelin receptor antagonists, bosentan, ambrisentan and macitentan, improve exercise capacity, hemodynamics, and functional class in PAH. Macitentan also significantly decreases the composite end point of events related to PAH or death.
13. Phosphodiesterase-5 inhibitors, including sildenafil and tadalafil, are potent and highly specific drugs that have been shown to reduce mPAP and improve functional class.
14. Riociguat is a novel soluble guanylate cyclase stimulator shown to improve exercise capacity, hemodynamic parameters, and functional class.
15. Calcium channel blockers may be considered in a small number of patients who have a positive response on acute vasoreactivity testing.
16. Combination therapy in PAH may address more than one mechanism causing this disease. Combination therapy may be initiated sequentially or as the initial regimen in patients with worse functional classes. Recent evidence demonstrated that initial combination therapy was associated with a significant reduction in time to clinical failure and PAH hospitalizations.

Pulmonary hypertension is a term describing a group of conditions relating to elevated blood pressure measured within the pulmonary artery. Pulmonary hypertension is not a specific diagnosis; rather it is a complex group of disorders relating to the pulmonary circulation. Pulmonary hypertension is classified into five groups according to the World Health Organization (WHO; Table 28-1).[1] Pulmonary arterial hypertension (PAH) or Group 1 pulmonary hypertension is a progressive disease characterized by an elevation in pulmonary arterial pressure and pulmonary vascular resistance (PVR). 1 PAH may be defined as a mean pulmonary artery pressure (mPAP) more than or equal to 25 mm Hg at rest, with a pulmonary capillary wedge pressure or left ventricular end-diastolic pressure (LVEDP) less than or equal to 15 mm Hg and a PVR more than 3 Wood units (WU) measured by cardiac catheterization.[2,3,4]

PAH may occur in the setting of underlying medical conditions or as an idiopathic disease (idiopathic PAH [IPAH]). Historically, medical treatment of PAH has been limited because of lack of effective, targeted therapy. Without medical therapy, IPAH portends a poor prognosis (median survival 2.8 years) after diagnosis.[5] Prior to the availability of disease-specific therapy for IPAH, survival rates for 1, 3, and 5 years were 68%, 48%, and 34%, respectively.[6] Since the approval of epoprostenol in 1995, a number of new therapeutic options have been developed. A recent epidemiologic study demonstrated survival rates at 1 and 3 years were 85% and 68%, respectively, in patients with PAH, and 91% and 74%, respectively, in patients with IPAH.[7]

EPIDEMIOLOGY

The prevalence of PAH is estimated to be 15 to 26 patients per million individuals.[8] Unfortunately, only 15,000 to 20,000 of the afflicted patients worldwide have an established diagnosis of PAH and are currently receiving treatment. In a French registry study of more than 600 patients with PAH, Humbert found that the most common cause of PAH was IPAH (approximately 40%), followed by PAH

TABLE 28-1 World Health Organization Classification of Pulmonary Hypertension

Group 1—PAH
1.1. IPAH
1.2. Heritable
1.2.1. BMPR2
1.2.2. Other mutations: ALK-1, ENG, SMAD9, CAV1, KCNK3
1.3. Drugs and toxins induced
1.4. APAH
1.4.1. Connective tissue diseases
1.4.2. HIV infection
1.4.3. Portal hypertension
1.4.4. Congenital heart diseases
1.4.5. Schistosomiasis
1.5. Pulmonary venoocclusive disease and/or pulmonary capillary hemoangiomatosis
1.5.1. Idiopathic
1.5.2. Heritable
1.5.2.1. EIF2AK4 mutation
1.5.2.2. Other mutations
1.5.3. Drugs, toxins, and radiation induced
1.5.4. Associated with:
1.5.4.1. Connective tissue disease
1.5.4.2. HIV infection
1.6. Persistent pulmonary hypertension of the newborn
Group 2—Pulmonary Hypertension due to Left Heart Disease
2.1. Left ventricular systolic dysfunction
2.2. Left ventricular diastolic dysfunction
2.3. Valvular disease
2.4. Congenital/acquired left heart inflow/outflow tract obstruction and congenital cardiomyopathies
2.5. Congenital/acquired pulmonary veins stenosis
Group 3—Pulmonary Hypertension due to Lung Diseases and/or Hypoxia
3.1. Chronic obstructive pulmonary disease
3.2. Interstitial lung disease
3.3. Other pulmonary diseases with mixed restrictive and obstructive pattern
3.4. Sleep-disordered breathing
3.5. Alveolar hypoventilation disorders
3.6. Chronic exposure to high altitude
3.7. Developmental abnormalities
Group 4—CTEPH
4.1. Chronic thromboembolic pulmonary hypertension
4.2. Other pulmonary artery obstructions
4.2.1. Angiosarcoma
4.2.2. Other intravascular tumors
4.2.3. Arteritis
4.2.4. Congenital pulmonary arteries stenosis
4.2.5. Parasites (hydatidosis)
Group 5—Pulmonary Hypertension with Unclear and/or Multifactorial Mechanisms
5.1. Hematological disorders: chronic hemolytic anemia, myeloproliferative disorders, splenectomy
5.2. Systemic disorders: sarcoidosis, pulmonary Langerhans' cell histiocytosis, lymphangioleiomyomatosis
5.3. Metabolic disorders: glycogen storage disease, Gaucher disease, thyroid disorders
5.4. Others: pulmonary tumoral thrombotic microangiopathy, fibrosing mediastinitis, chronic renal failure (with/without dialysis), segmental pulmonary hypertension

ALK-1, activin receptor-like kinase type-1; APAH, associated pulmonary hypertension; BMPR2, bone morphogenetic protein receptor 2; CAV1, caveolin-1; CTPH, chronic thromboembolic pulmonary hypertension; EIF2AK4, eukaryotic translation initiation factor 2 alpha kinase 4; ENG, endoglin; HIV, human immunodeficiency virus; IPAH, idiopathic pulmonary arterial hypertension; PAH, pulmonary arterial hypertension.

Data from Galiè N, Humbert M, Vachiery J-L, et al. 2015 ESC/ERS Guidelines for the diagnosis and treatment of pulmonary hypertension. Eur Heart J. *August 2015:ehv317.*

associated with connective tissue diseases (15.3%), congenital heart disease (11.3%), portal hypertension (10.4%), and familial PAH (FPAH) (3.9%).[9] The US based REVEAL registry (Registry to Evaluate Early and Long-Term Pulmonary Arterial Hypertension Disease Management) also provides helpful insight in to the epidemiology of PAH. The registry includes over 3,500 patients and found that 46% of PAH was idiopathic while 25% was associated with connective tissue diseases and 10% was associated with congenital heart diseases.[10] 2 However, diagnosis of PAH is growing because of increased awareness and knowledge of the disease state, leading to earlier and improved evaluation and identification.

ETIOLOGY

PAH most often originates with a predisposing state and one or more inciting factors that could be genetic or environmental exposures.[11] Once a permissive environment exists, multiple mechanisms can be activated leading to vascular constriction, cellular proliferation, and a prothrombotic state resulting in PAH and its sequelae.[12] PAH can be associated with numerous conditions as well as being an idiopathic condition (IPAH). The incidence of IPAH is estimated to be 2.0 to 7.6 per 1 million in North America and Europe, with a marked female predominance (male-to-female ratio, 1:1.7), and mean age at time of recognition is approximately 37 years, although there is considerable variation.[1,2,3] Based on recent registry data, PAH overall is now being diagnosed more commonly in older patients, with a mean age at diagnosis ranging from 50 to 65 years.[1,2,4] Although uncommon in the United States, the most common form of PAH worldwide is schistosomiasis followed by congenital heart disease and pulmonary hypertension of early childhood.[3] Rheumatologic diseases such as scleroderma, systemic lupus erythematosus, rheumatoid arthritis, and myositis are also associated with development of PAH. Patients with scleroderma who develop PAH, estimated between 7% and 12% of patients, have markedly worse outcomes in comparison to other PAH subgroups. Patients with human immunodeficiency virus (HIV) infection can develop PAH with a prevalence of 0.5%. In patients with liver disease, portal hypertension may cause concurrent pulmonary hypertension in an estimated 2% to 6% of patients.[3] Multiple drugs and toxins have been associated with PAH but those that definitively precipitate PAH include anorexigens such as aminorex, fenfluramine, benfluorex, and dexfenfluramine.[1,3,4] Other definite precipitants include toxic rapeseed oil and selective serotonin reuptake inhibitors (SSRIs), specifically in pregnant patients exposed to SSRIs after 20 weeks of gestation.[3,4] Other drugs considered to be likely or possible causative agents for PAH include amphetamines, L-tryptophan, cocaine, interferon α and β, dasatinib and certain chemotherapeutic agents (mitomycin C, carmustine, etoposide, cyclophosphamide, bleomycin).[34] Heritable PAH (HPAH) includes both IPAH with germline mutations and familial cases without an identified mutation. Germline mutations seen in PAH include bone morphogenetic protein receptor 2 (BMPR2) and activin receptor-like kinase 1 (ALK-1). About 75% of patients with HPAH have BMPR2 mutations.[2] Genetic testing for these mutations may be offered and professional genetic counseling should be provided at expert centers.[3]

PATHOPHYSIOLOGY

PAH is a disease progressive vasoconstriction of the small pulmonary arteries that eventually leads to right ventricular hypertrophy and failure. The right ventricle is thin-walled and used to the much lower pressures of the pulmonary system and therefore does not have the reserve that the LV does.[14] 3 Regardless of etiology, all subgroups of PAH are based on similar clinical and pathologic physiology. 4 The pathobiology of PAH involves several key biologic events, including endothelial cell dysfunction, thrombotic lesions, platelet activation, gain of constricting factors, loss of relaxing factors, intimal proliferation, medial hypertrophy, fibrosis, and inflammation—all combining to produce progressive and deleterious vascular remodeling (Fig. 28-1).[15,16] Multiple genetic mutations are known to contribute

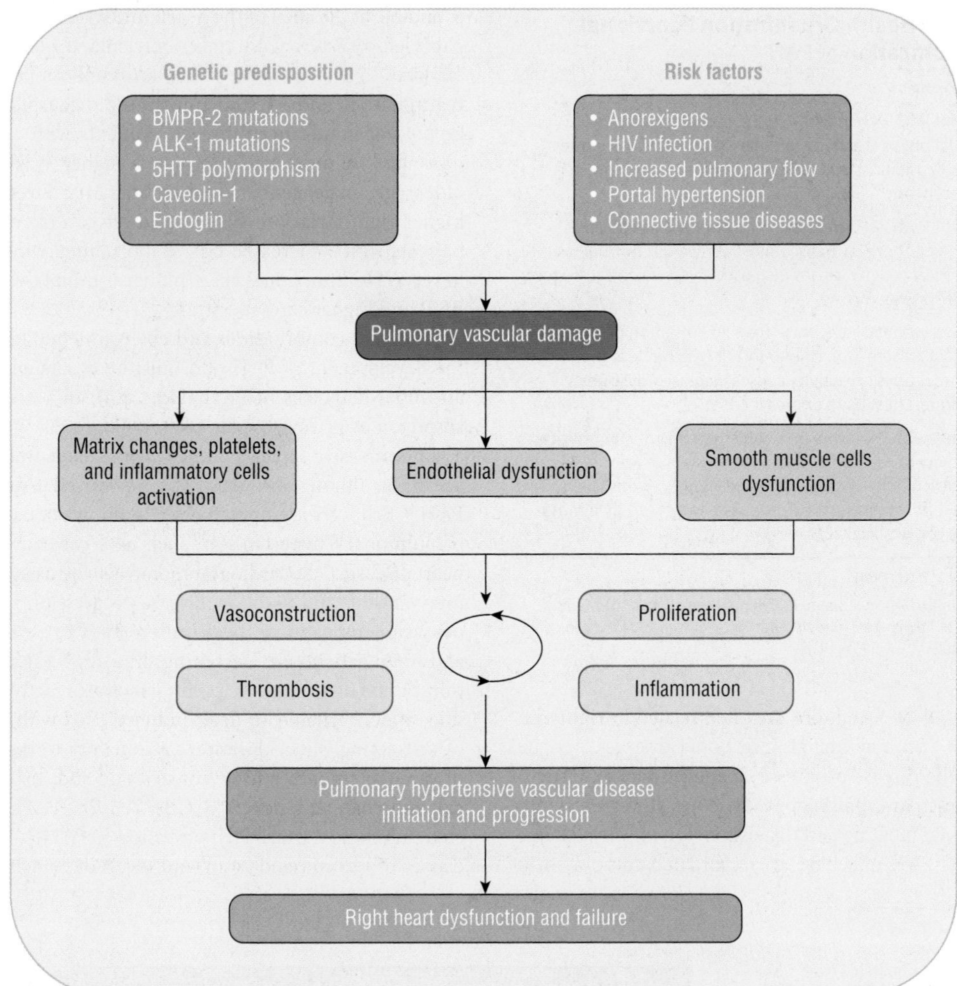

FIGURE 28-1 Pulmonary arterial hypertension; potential pathogenetic and pathobiologic mechanisms. (5-HTT, serotonin transporter gene; ALK-1, activin receptor-like kinase 1 gene; BMPR-2, bone morphogenetic receptor 2 gene; HIV, human immunodeficiency virus.) *(Reproduced with permission from Galie N, Torbicki A, Barst R. Guidelines on diagnosis and treatment of pulmonary arterial hypertension.* Eur Heart J *2004;25:2243-2278.)*

to the pathophysiology of PAH, including BMPR2, ALK-1, Caveolin-1, KCNK3, nitric oxide synthase (ec-NOS), 5-hydroxytryptamine (serotonin [5-HT]) transporter (5-HTT), and others.[3,15,17] A mutation of BMPR2 receptor is an aberration of signal transduction in the pulmonary vascular smooth muscle cell that is postulated to alter apoptosis favoring cellular proliferation. ALK-1 is part of the transforming growth factor-β superfamily and is seen in hereditary hemorrhagic telangiectasia and PAH.[18] 5-HTT is associated with pulmonary artery smooth muscle proliferation and is present in IPAH in the homozygous form in 65% of patients.[19] Dysregulation of 5-HT synthesis mediated via tryptophan hydroxylases is closely linked to the hypoxic PAH phenotype in mice and may contribute to PAH development.[20]

Molecular, cellular, and genetic mechanisms are mediated by a variety of biologically active compounds, including prostacyclin (PGI_2), endothelin-1 (ET-1), nitric oxide (NO), and 5-HT. PGI_2 is a vasodilatory and antiproliferative substance that is produced by the endothelial cells, and the synthesis of PGI_2 and its circulating levels are reduced in PAH. Furthermore, thromboxane, a vasoconstrictor, is increased in PAH. ET-1 is produced in the endothelium, and it possesses potent vasoconstrictor and mitogenic effects. ET-1 levels are increased in PAH and clearance is reduced. ET-1 acts via the endothelin receptors (ET_A and ET_B) to promote vascular smooth muscle proliferation and vasoconstriction.[16,21] Plasma levels of ET-1 are correlated with severity of PAH and prognosis.[22] NO is produced in the endothelium via NO synthase and leads to vasodilation and opening of cell membrane potassium channels to allow potassium ion efflux, membrane depolarization, and calcium channel inhibition. Voltage-dependent potassium channels are inhibited by a number of stimuli that promote PAH, including hypoxia and fenfluramine, resulting in downregulated potassium channels in patients with PAH. Entering calcium is a signal for release of sarcoplasmic calcium and activation of the contractile apparatus. NO promotes vasodilation through calcium channel inhibition. In PAH there is evidence of decreased NO synthase expression, leading to vasoconstriction and cellular proliferation.[23] Elevated 5-HT has been observed and vasoconstriction mediated via the increased expression of the 5-HT_{1B} receptor is seen in PAH.[3]

Autoantibodies, proinflammatory cytokines, and inflammatory infiltrates may also participate in the pathogenesis of PAH. Coagulation is disordered in PAH as evidenced by increased levels of von Willebrand factor, plasma fibrinopeptide A, plasminogen activator inhibitor-1, 5-HT, and thromboxane. Furthermore, tissue plasminogen activator, thrombomodulin, NO, and PGI_2 are decreased, leading to an imbalance favoring thrombosis. Endothelial dysfunction is the common denominator of mechanisms for PAH, and a variety of injuries, such as shear stress, inflammation, toxins, and hypoxia, are thought to be involved.[3,15]

5 The signs and symptoms of PAH are highly variable depending on the stage of the disease and comorbidities. The impact of these signs and symptoms on functional capacity can be generally described using the World Health Organization functional

TABLE 28-2 World Health Organization Functional Classification of PAH

Class	Description
I	Patients with PAH in whom there is no limitation of usual physical activity; ordinary physical activity does not cause increased dyspnea, fatigue, chest pain, or presyncope.
II	Patients with PAH who have mild limitation of physical activity. There is no discomfort at rest, but normal physical activity causes increased dyspnea, fatigue, chest pain, or presyncope.
III	Patients with PAH who have marked limitation of physical activity. There is no discomfort at rest, but less than normal physical activity causes increased dyspnea, fatigue, chest pain, or presyncope.
IV	Patients with PAH who are unable to perform any physical activity at rest and who may have signs of right ventricular failure. Dyspnea and/or fatigue may be present at rest, and symptoms are increased by almost any physical activity.

PAH, pulmonary arterial hypertension.

Data from Badesch DB, Abman SH, Simonneau G, Rubin LJ, McLaughlin VV. Medical therapy for pulmonary arterial hypertension: Updated ACCP evidence-based clinical practice guidelines. Chest *2007;131:1917-1928.*

classification (Table 28-2). Symptoms are often related to right ventricular dysfunction and may include exertional dyspnea, fatigue, and weakness.[4] As the disease progresses, patients may experience dyspnea at rest, chest pain, presyncope, syncope, lower extremity edema, and abdominal bloating and distension. On physical examination, patients with PAH may have an accentuated component of S_2 audible at the apex of the heart, midsystolic ejection murmur, palpable left parasternal lift, right ventricular S_4 gallop, and a prominent "a" wave.[3] Hepatojugular reflux, a diastolic murmur of pulmonary regurgitation, and a systolic murmur of tricuspid regurgitation may be present in advanced disease.[3] Patients with an increased risk of mortality are more likely to have a higher WHO functional class, older age, male gender, higher brain natriuretic peptide (BNP), higher right atrial pressure and lower cardiac output. In contrast, patients with a decreased risk of mortality are more likely to have a lower WHO functional class, higher 6-minute walk distance, lower BNP, and higher cardiac output.[24]

Several comorbidities and environmental factors play a role in the development of PAH and must be evaluated when establishing an initial diagnosis of PAH (Fig. 28.2). In patients with a clinical suspicion of PAH, Doppler echocardiography should be performed as a noninvasive screening test that can detect increased pulmonary pressures, although this study cannot be used to definitively diagnose PAH.[25] Echocardiography is also useful in evaluating specific causes of pulmonary hypertension, such as a cardiac shunt or left-sided heart disease. Echocardiography can also be used to assess treatment interventions and to follow disease progression.[3] 6 However, right heart catheterization is the definitive study to use in diagnosis of PAH and when patients are worsening clinically.[17] Right heart catheterization can be used to assess pulmonary vasoreactivity in patients with idiopathic, heritable, or drug-induced PAH with the administration of fast-acting, short-duration vasodilators to determine the extent of vascular smooth muscle constriction and vasodilator response to calcium channel blockers (CCBs; I-C for IPAH; IIIb-C for associated pulmonary arterial hypertension [APAH]).[1] Table 28-3 lists the classes of recommendations and levels of evidence, and Table 28-4

CLINICAL PRESENTATION Pulmonary Arterial Hypertension

Symptoms

- Exertional dyspnea
- Fatigue
- Weakness
- Exertional chest pain
- Complaints of general exertion intolerance
- Dyspnea at rest as disease progresses
- Syncope
- Lower extremity edema

Symptoms of Related Conditions

- Paroxysmal nocturnal dyspnea as a result of left-sided heart disease
- Raynaud phenomenon, arthralgia, or swollen hands and other symptoms of connective tissue disease
- Orthopnea

Symptoms of Disease Progression

- Leg swelling
- Abdominal bloating and distension
- Anorexia
- Profound fatigue
- May develop as right ventricular dysfunction and tricuspid valve regurgitation evolve

Signs

- Accentuated component of S_2 audible at the apex of the heart
- Early systolic ejection click
- Midsystolic ejection murmur
- Palpable left parasternal lift
- Right ventricular S_4 gallop
- Prominent "a" wave due to increased right ventricular stiffness

Signs of Advanced Disease

- Diastolic murmur of pulmonary regurgitation
- Pansystolic murmur of tricuspid regurgitation
- Hepatojugular reflux
- A pulsatile liver
- Right ventricular S_3 gallop
- Marked distension of jugular veins
- Peripheral edema
- Hypotension
- Cool extremities suggesting markedly reduced cardiac output and peripheral vasoconstriction
- Diminished pulse pressure
- Cyanosis (suggests right-to-left shunting)
- Digital clubbing
- Rales
- Dullness
- Decreased breath sounds
- Accessory muscle use
- Prolonged exhalation
- Peripheral venous insufficiency (suggests venous thrombosis or pulmonary thrombotic disease)

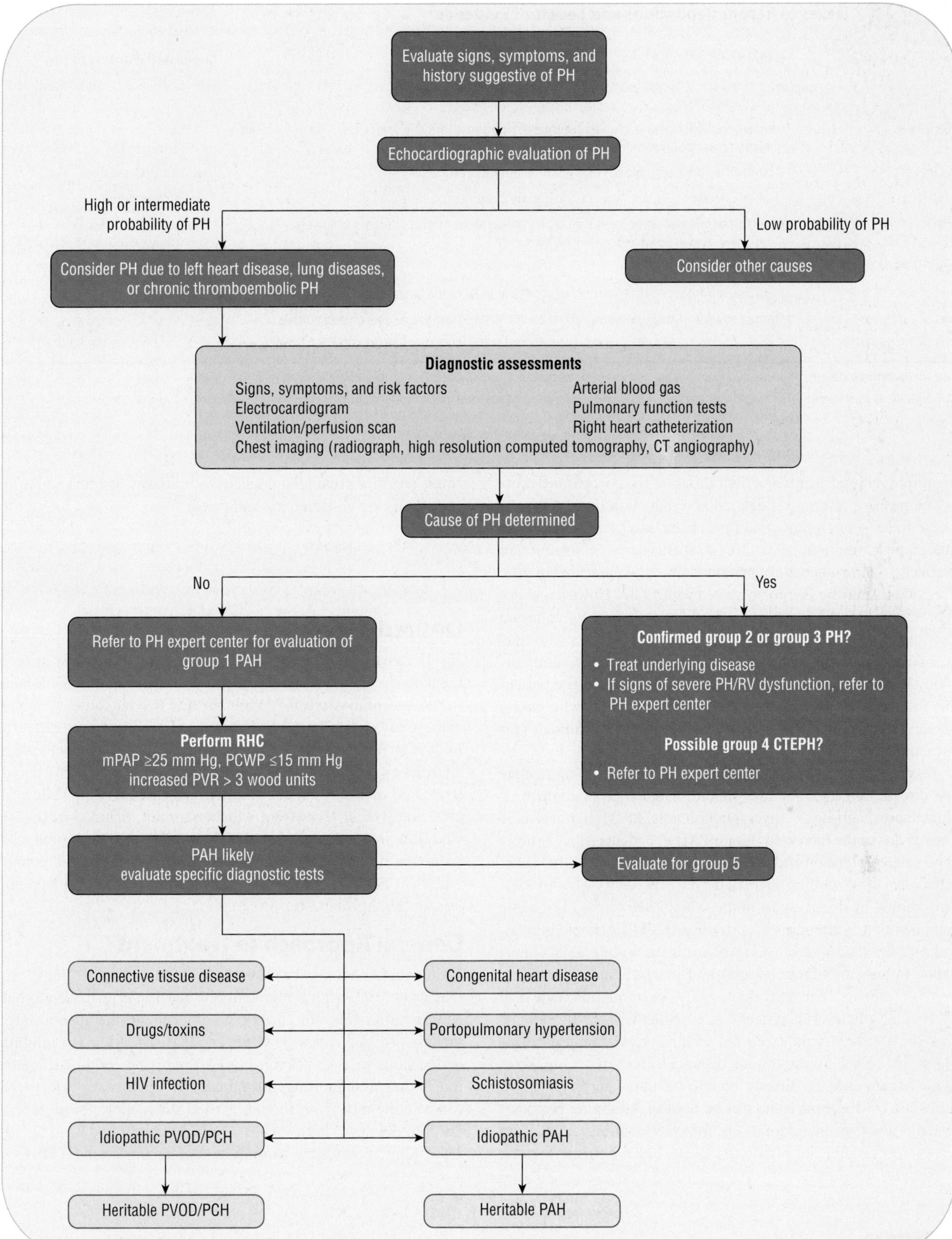

FIGURE 28-2 Diagnostic algorithm of PAH. (CTEPH, chronic thromboembolic pulmonary hypertension; HIV, human immunodeficiency virus; PVOD/PCH, pulmonary venoocclusive disease or pulmonary capillary hemangiomatosis; RHC, right heart catheterization.) *(Data from Galie N, Humbert M, Vachiery JL, et al. 2015 ESC/ERA Guidelines for the diagnosis and treatment of pulmonary hypertension. Eur Respir J 2015.)*

TABLE 28-3 Classes of Recommendations and Levels of Evidence[a]

Classes of Recommendations	Definition	Suggested Wording to Use
Class I	Evidence and/or general agreement that a given treatment or procedure is beneficial, useful, effective.	Is recommended/Is indicated.
Class II	Conflicting evidence and/or a divergence of opinion about the usefulness/efficacy of the given treatment or procedure.	
Class IIa	Weight of evidence/opinion is in favor of usefulness/efficacy.	Should be considered.
Class IIb	Usefulness/efficacy is less well established by evidence/opinion.	May be considered.
Class III	Evidence or general agreement that a given treatment or procedures is not useful/effective, and in some cases may be harmful.	Is not recommended.
Levels of Evidence	**Definition**	
Level of evidence A	Data derived from multiple randomized clinical trials or meta-analyses.	
Level of evidence B	Data derived from a single randomized clinical trial or large nonrandomized studies.	
Level of evidence C	Consensus of opinion of the experts and/or small studies, retrospective studies, registries.	

[a]Classes of Recommendations and Levels of Evidence are consistent between the ESC/ERS Guidelines and the WHO Guidelines.

Data from Galiè N, Humbert M, Vachiery J-L, et al. 2015 ESC/ERS Guidelines for the diagnosis and treatment of pulmonary hypertension. Eur Heart J. *August 2015:ehv317.*

lists commonly used agents and their dosages. The consensus definition of a positive response is defined as a reduction of mPAP by at least 10 mm Hg to a value of 40 mm Hg or less.[26] Patients with an acute response (approximately 13% of patients on initial testing) are most likely to have a beneficial hemodynamic and clinical response. These patients may be able to be treated with CCBs. However, about half of these patients lose an acute vasodilator response when tested 1 year later.[27] Therefore, even this small group of patients who may be treated with CCBs must be followed closely for safety and efficacy. If the patient loses the acute vasodilator response, the patient needs to be switched to different PAH therapy. Patients who have a negative response on initial vasodilator testing are not candidates for treatment with CCBs.[3,28]

Because PAH commonly occurs in the setting of connective tissue disease, serologic markers should be obtained to confirm or exclude these diagnoses.[3,29] Liver function tests (LFTs) should also be evaluated due to the increased risk for PAH in patients with cirrhosis and portal hypertension and as a baseline for certain PAH therapies. HIV is associated with an increased prevalence of PAH, and HIV testing should be done as part of the initial PAH workup.[3] Chronic thromboembolic pulmonary hypertension (CTEPH) should be evaluated with ventilation–perfusion lung scans and/or pulmonary angiography. Pulmonary function testing and arterial blood oxygenation should be evaluated. The diffusing capacity of carbon monoxide may be particularly helpful in systemic sclerosis and PAH.[3] In patients with PAH, serial determinations of functional class, exercise capacity (assessed by the 6-minute walk distance), and serial biomarkers provide benchmarks for disease severity, response to therapy, and progression.[3,29] These variables can be used to determine risk level in patients and may aid in prognosis. Table 28-5 outlines calculation of low, intermediate, and high-risk patients based on these factors. Table 28-6 also provides guidelines for initial assessment and timing and when each assessment is indicated.

TREATMENT

Desired Outcomes

7 The goals of treatment are alleviation of symptoms, improvement in the quality of life, prevention of disease progression, and improvement in survival.[13] While the first two outcomes are obtainable based on data from randomized trials, controversy exists over improvement in survival with current treatment regimens. Meta-analyses are conflicting; a 2007 meta-analysis of 16 trials demonstrated no mortality benefit in functional classes III/IV while a later 2009 study of 21 trials (6 of which were not included in the 2007 study) in predominately functional class III patients showed a 43% reduction in mortality.[30] Unfortunately, overall mortality remained high.[31] In addition, individual trials also show survival benefit, at least in the short term (ie, 3 years).[32]

General Approach to Treatment

Treatment of PAH may be categorized into nonpharmacologic, pharmacologic, and surgical interventions. 8 The principal endothelial abnormalities that are current pharmacologic therapeutic targets include (a) supplementing endogenous vasodilators, (b) inhibiting endogenous vasoconstrictors, and (c) reducing endothelial platelet interaction and limiting thrombosis. Nonpharmacologic therapy can be quite broad and should be used when clinically appropriate. Surgical therapy is indicated in certain situations and includes atrial septostomy, pulmonary thromboendarterectomy for CTEPH, and

TABLE 28-4 Agents for Vasodilator Testing in PAH

	NO	Epoprostenol	Adenosine
Route	Inhaled	IV	IV
Dose range	10-80 ppm	2-10 ng/kg/min	50-250 mcg/kg/min
Dosing increments	10-80 ppm for 5 min	2 ng/kg/min every 15 min	50 mcg/kg/min every 2 min
Common side effects	None	Headache, flushing, nausea	Chest tightness, dyspnea

NO, nitric oxide; PAH, pulmonary arterial hypertension.

Data from reference 33.

TABLE 28-5 Risk Assessment in PAH

Determinants of Prognosis[a] (Estimated 1-year Mortality)	Low Risk <5%	Intermediate Risk 5%-10%	High Risk >10%
Clinical signs of right heart failure	Absent	Absent	Present
Progression of symptoms	No	Slow	Rapid
Syncope	No	Occasional syncope[b]	Repeated syncope[c]
WHO functional class	I, II	III	IV
6MWD	>440 m	165-440 m	<165 m
Cardiopulmonary exercise testing	Peak VO_2 >15 mL/min/kg (>65% pred.) Ve/VCO_2 slope <36	Peak VO_2 11-15 mL/min/kg (35%-65% pred.) Ve/VCO_2 slope 36-44.9	Peak VO_2 <11 mL/min/kg (<35% pred.) Ve/VCO_2 slope ≥45
NT-proBNP plasma levels	BNP <50 ng/L NT-proBNP <300 ng/mL	BNP 50-300 ng/L NT-proBNP 300-1400 ng/mL	BNP >300 ng/L NT-proBNP >1400 ng/mL
Imaging (echocardiography, CMR imaging)	RA area <18 cm^2 No pericardial effusion	RA area 18-26 cm^2 No or minimal, pericardial effusion	RA area >26 cm^2 Pericardial effusion
Hemodynamics	RAP <8 mm Hg CI ≥2.5 L/min/m^2 SvO_2 >65%	RAP 8-14 mm Hg CI 2.0-2.4 L/min/m^2 SvO_2 60%-65%	RAP >14 mm Hg CI ≤2.0 L/min/m^2 SvO_2 <60%

6MWD, 6-minute walking distance; NT-proBNP, N-terminal pro-brain natriuretic peptide; RA, right atrium; RAP, right atrial pressure; SvO2, mixed venous oxygen saturation; VCO2, ventilatory equivalents for carbon dioxide; VO2, oxygen consumption.

[a]Most of the proposed variables and cut-off values are based on expert opinion. They may provide prognostic information and may be used to guide therapeutic decisions, but applications to individual patients must be done carefully. One must also note that most of these variables have been validated mostly for IPAH and the cut-off values used above may not necessarily apply to other forms of PAH. Futhermore, the use of approved therapies and their influence on the variables should be considered in the evaluation of the risk.

[b]Occasional syncope during brisk or heavy exercise, or occasional orthostatic syncope in the otherwise stable patient.

[c]Repeated episodes of syncope, even with little or regular physical activity.

Data from N. Galie et al. 2015ESC/ERS Guidelines for the diagnosis and treatment of pulmonary hypertension. Eur Respir J 2015.

lung or heart–lung transplantation (for disease that is not responsive to medical therapy). Bilateral lung and lung-heart transplantation has been shown to improve survival rates in patients with PAH.[1]

Nonpharmacologic Therapy

9 Nonpharmacologic therapy is frequently used to address comorbid conditions that often accompany PAH. Patients with PAH should be counseled on several important points. Pregnancy should be avoided due to high morbidity and mortality rates in females with PAH during pregnancy and in the postpartum course (I-C).[5] Immunization against influenza and pneumococcal disease should be provided (I-C).[3] Hypoxemia may aggravate vasoconstriction in patients with PAH; therefore, PAH patients may require supplemental oxygen (I-C), particularly when using air travel due to a reduction in ambient air concentration of oxygen.[33] Patients should adhere to a low-sodium diet to avoid fluid retention predisposing to right heart failure.[34] Cardiopulmonary rehabilitation improves functional status, exercise capacity, and quality of life in patients with PAH (I-A).[1]

TABLE 28-6 Suggested Assessment and Timing for the Follow-up of Patients with PAH

	At Baseline	Every 3-6 Months[a]	Every 6-12 Months[a]	3-6 Months after Changes in Therapy[a]	In Case of Clinical Worsening
Medical assessment and determination of functional class	+	+	+	+	+
ECG	+	+	+	+	+
6MWT/Borg dyspnea score	+	+	+	+	+
CPET	+		+		+[a]
Echo	+		+	+	+
Basic laboratories[b]	+	+	+	+	+
Extended lab[c]	+		+		+
Blood gas analysis[d]	+		+	+	+
Right heart catheterization	+		+[e]	+[f]	+[f]

6MWT, 6-minute walking test; ALT, alanine aminotransferase; AST, aspartate aminotransferase; BGA, blood gas analysis; BNP, brain natriuretic peptide; CPET, cardiopulmonary exercise testing; ECG, electrocardiogram; Echo, echocardiography; ERAs, endothelin receptor antagonists; FC, functional class; INR, international normalized ratio; lab, laboratory assessment; NT-proBNP, N-terminal pro-brain natriuretic peptide; PAH, pulmonary arterial hypertension; RHC, right heart catheterization; TSH, thyroid stimulating hormone.

[a]Intervals to be adjusted according to patient needs.

[b]Basic lab includes blood count, INR (in patients receiving vitamin K antagonists), serum creatinine, sodium, potassium, AST/ALT (in patients receiving ERAs), bilirubin and BNP/NT-proBNP.

[c]Extended lab includes TSH, troponin, uric acid, iron status (iron, ferritin, soluble transferrin receptor) and other variables according to individual patient need.

[d]From arterial or arterialized capillary blood; may be replaced by peripheral oxygen saturation in stable patients or if BGA is not available.

[e]Some centers perform RHCs at regular intervals during follow-up.

[f]Should be considered.

Data from Galiè N, Humbert M, Vachiery J-L, et al. 2015 ESC/ERS Guidelines for the diagnosis and treatment of pulmonary hypertension. Eur Heart J. *August 2015:ehv317.*

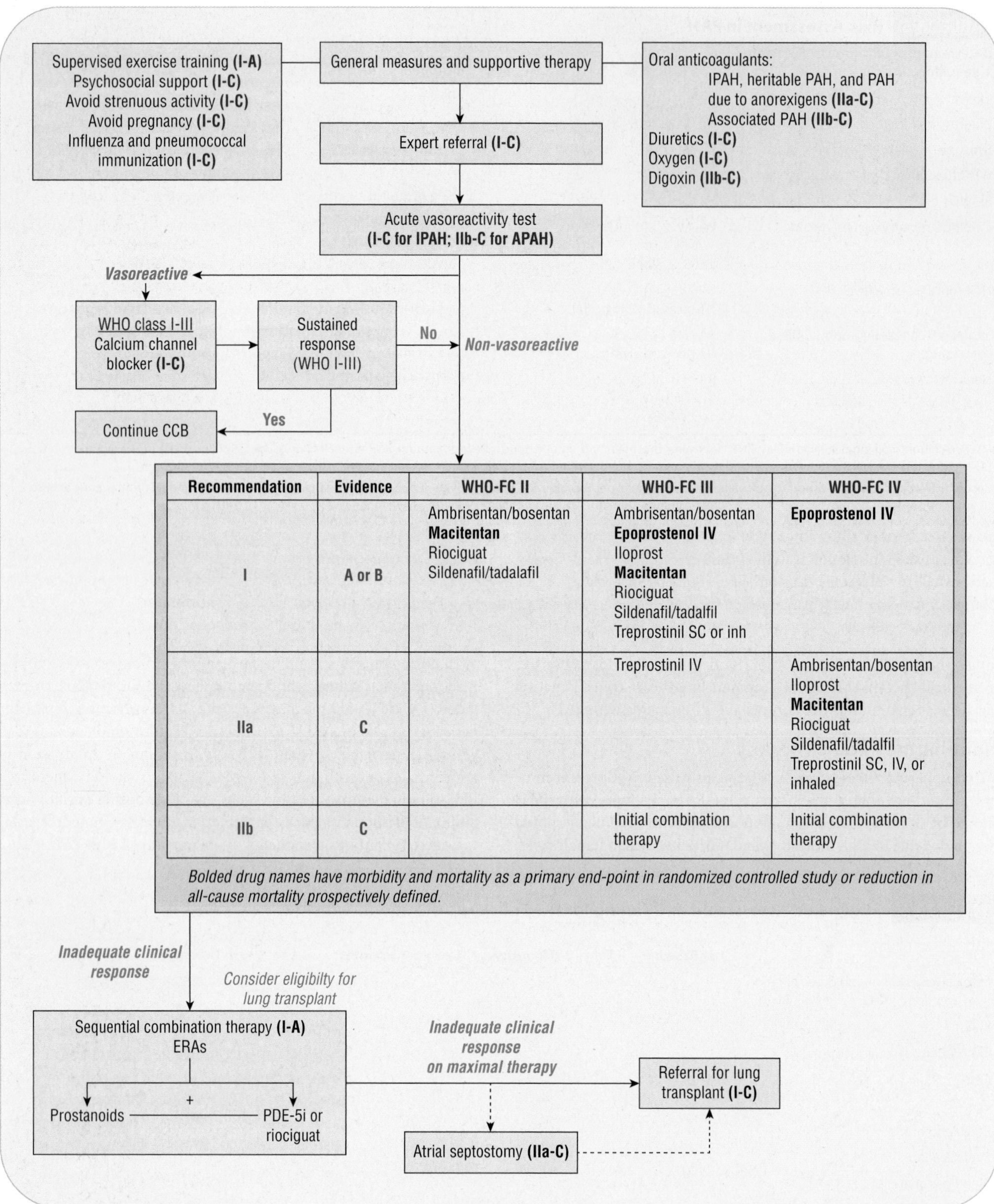

Recommendation	Evidence	WHO-FC II	WHO-FC III	WHO-FC IV
I	A or B	Ambrisentan/bosentan **Macitentan** Riociguat Sildenafil/tadalafil	Ambrisentan/bosentan **Epoprostenol IV** Iloprost **Macitentan** Riociguat Sildenafil/tadalfil Treprostinil SC or inh	**Epoprostenol IV**
IIa	C		Treprostinil IV	Ambrisentan/bosentan Iloprost **Macitentan** Riociguat Sildenafil/tadalfil Treprostinil SC, IV, or inhaled
IIb	C		Initial combination therapy	Initial combination therapy

FIGURE 28-3 Treatment algorithm for pulmonary arterial hypertension (PAH). Levels of evidence and strength of recommendation are defined in Table 28-3. (APAH, associated pulmonary arterial hypertension; CCBs, calcium channel blocker; ERA, endothelin receptor antagonist; IPAH, idiopathic pulmonary arterial hypertension; PDE-5i, phosphodiesterase type-5 inhibitor, WHO-FC, World Health Organization functional class.) *(Adapted from Galie N, Corris PA, Frost A, et al. Updated treatment algorithm of pulmonary arterial hypertension.* J Am Coll Cardiol *2013;62:D60-72.)*

Pharmacologic Therapy

The number of potential therapies for PAH has expanded dramatically in the last decade. In addition to adjunctive background therapy, multiple drugs have been developed specifically for treatment of PAH. Figure 28-3 illustrates the current recommended treatment algorithm based on the most recent guidelines.[15]

Conventional Pharmacologic Treatment 10 Conventional therapy includes oral anticoagulants, diuretics, oxygen, and digoxin.[29]

Anticoagulation with warfarin may be considered in patients with PAH, particularly if they have IPAH. The rationale for oral anticoagulants is based on the presence of traditional risk factors for venous thromboembolism, such as heart failure and sedentary lifestyle, as well as on the demonstration of thrombotic predisposition and thrombotic changes in the pulmonary microcirculation. Small retrospective and prospective studies support a survival benefit with anticoagulation.[35-38] The target international normalized ratio (INR) in most centers is 1.5 to 2.5.[3,26] Anticoagulation is recommended for patients with IPAH, HPAH, and PAH due to anorexigens (IIb-C) as well as in associated PAH (IIb-C).[1] It may also be recommended in patients on long-term intravenous prostaglandin therapy as these patients are at risk for catheter-associated thrombosis.[4]

Loop diuretics such as furosemide are helpful adjunctive therapy in patients with decompensated right heart failure and associated findings of increased central venous pressure, abdominal organ congestion, peripheral edema, and ascites.[3] Appropriate diuretic therapy in right heart failure provides symptomatic and clinical benefits in patients with PAH (I-C).[1] Patients should be maintained at as close to a euvolemic state as possible.

Oxygen therapy with a goal oxygen saturation greater than 90% (0.90) may be beneficial in some patients, although there are no data regarding the long-term effects of oxygen treatment in PAH (I-C).[1] Oxygen treatment is controversial in patients with PAH associated with shunts (ie, Eisenmenger syndrome).

Digoxin may be used for patients with PAH with right heart failure as adjunctive therapy along with diuretics to control symptoms as well as in patients with atrial arrhythmias (I-C).[1] There are no long-term trials and benefit is uncertain. Optimal plasma concentrations are unknown; however, in light of recent trials of digoxin in left systolic dysfunction, the typical target concentration is between 0.5 and 0.8 ng/mL (0.64 and 1 nmol/L). Patients on digoxin should receive periodic monitoring of potassium.

Specific Pharmacologic Therapy In recent years, there has been a surge in availability of drug therapy for the treatment of PAH. Figure 28-4 illustrates the timeline of drug approval over the past few decades.

Synthetic Prostacyclin and Prostacyclin Analogs 11 PGI_2 is produced predominantly by endothelial cells, and it induces potent vasodilation of all vascular beds. It is also a potent inhibitor of platelet aggregation and possesses cytoprotective and antiproliferative activities. PGI_2 synthase expression is reduced in pulmonary arteries, and urinary excretion of PGI_2 metabolites is reduced in PAH. Epoprostenol is a synthetic analog of PGI_2 and has a short half-life of 3 to 5 minutes; consequently, it must be given by continuous IV infusion. Initiation of epoprostenol should be done in a hospital setting at low doses ranging from 2 to 4 ng/kg/min and increased at a rate limited by side effects (flushing, headache, diarrhea, jaw pain, backache, abdominal cramping, extremity pain, and hypotension). The two available products, Flolan® (now available generic) and Veletri®, have unique stability and reconstitution parameters; both pharmacists and patients should be aware of the differences and follow the manufacturer recommendations. Due to the short half-life of the drug, it is recommended that the patient have a backup supply of the drug and infusion pump as interruption of epoprostenol may lead to life-threatening pulmonary vasoconstriction.[39] Because the drug must be administered by continuous infusion with a central venous catheter and pump, infection, catheter obstruction, and sepsis are potential complications. A Centers for Disease Control and Prevention study found that bloodstream infections occurred with epoprostenol and treprostinil in the range of 0.3 to 2.1 per 1,000 medicine days (approximately 1 infection every 3 years) when these drugs are given by the IV route.[40] The target dose for the first 2 to 4 weeks is around 10 to 15 ng/kg/min, and periodic dose increases are then required to maximize efficacy. Optimal doses are variable but are in the range of 25 to 40 ng/kg/min.[33,41] Multiple observational series have documented an improvement in survival in patients with IPAH compared with either historical control or predicted survival based on the National Institutes of Health Registry equation.[41-43] Based on current guidelines, epoprostenol is indicated for WHO functional class III and IV (I-A).[1]

Treprostinil (Remodulin) is a stable analog of PGI_2 given for subcutaneous (SC) or IV infusion approved for functional classes II, III, and IV.[41] The major advantages of treprostinil over epoprostenol include ease of use and increased safety due to a longer half-life, lowering the risk of rebound effects that may happen with drug interruption.[21] Treprostinil has been shown to improve 6-minute walk distance and hemodynamics with outcomes that are similar to epoprostenol.[44,45] In clinical trials, the greatest exercise improvement was observed in patients who were more compromised at baseline and in patients who could tolerate doses in the upper quartile (≥13.8 ng/kg/min). The initial dose for treprostinil is 1.25 ng/kg/min by either the SC or the IV route. If not tolerated, the dose should be reduced

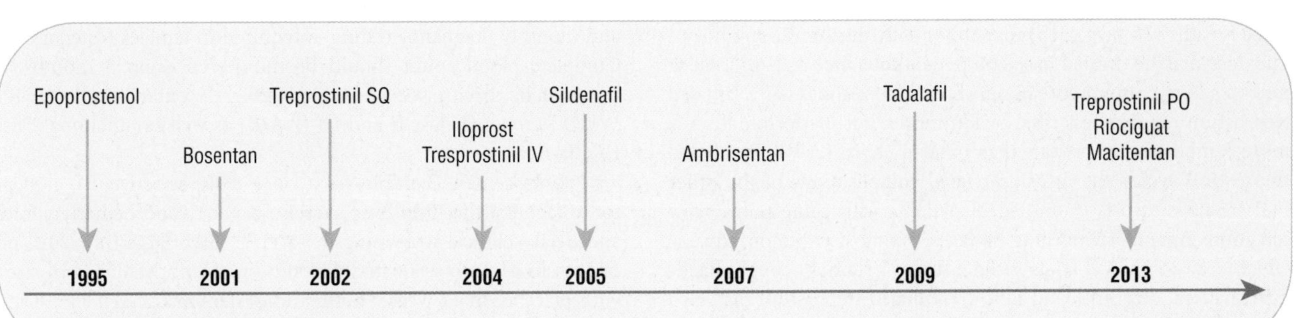

Epoprostenol: 1995
Treprostnil: SQ 2002, IV 2004, PO 2013
Iloprost: 2004
Bosentan: 2001
Ambrisentan: 2007
Sildenafil: 2005
Tadalafil: 2009
Riociguat: 2013
Macitentan: 2013

FIGURE 28-4 Timeline of pulmonary arterial hypertension (PAH) medication approvals.

to 0.625 ng/kg/min and retitration attempted at 4 weeks. Infusion site pain is common with the SC route and can occur in up to 85% of patients, leading to discontinuation of treatment in 8% of patients and limiting upward dose titration.[33] Patients unable to tolerate SC can be transitioned to IV treprostinil.[26] Transitions between prostacyclin agents or routes should be performed in an inpatient setting at an expert referral center. Bloodstream infections, primarily due to gram-negative pathogens, are more likely with IV treprostinil than with IV epoprostenol.[46] Recent data demonstrate that use of the diluent used for epoprostenol, which has a more basic pH, to reconstitute IV treprostinil may decrease rates of bloodstream infections to a rate similar to that seen with epoprostenol.[47] Other side effects are similar to epoprostenol. Based on international guidelines, treprostinil is recommended for functional class III (SC administration—I-A/B; IV administration—IIa-C), and functional class IV (SC and IV administration—IIa-C).[1]

In an effort to prevent complications and use of pumps and central venous catheters for PGI_2 analog administration, aerosolized formulations were developed. The first approved formulation, iloprost (Ventavis), is a PGI_2 analog that is given by inhalation using a dosing system provided by the manufacturer (ADD system) with the initial inhaled dose being 2.5 mcg six to nine times per day up to every 2 hours during waking hours. The dose should be titrated and maintained at 5 mcg/dose if tolerated. In a 3-month, randomized, double-blind, placebo-controlled trial, iloprost via inhalation provided at least a 10% improvement in 6-minute walking distance and improvement in functional class.[48] Inhaled iloprost can be cumbersome to use as each inhalation dose can take 4 to 10 minutes to administer and multiple inhalations are required for a full dose. Patients should also be instructed to have a backup supply as iloprost has a short half-life, similar to epoprostenol.[26] Adverse effects are similar to other PGI_2 analogs, including cough, headache, flushing, and jaw pain. Inhaled iloprost is indicated for functional class III (I-A/B) and functional class IV (IIa-C), although many clinicians prefer using the IV or SC route in patients with more severe disease.[1]

The second aerosolized formulation, inhaled treprostinil (Tyvaso), was approved by the FDA in July 2009 to improve exercise capacity in functional class III patients. In a randomized, double-blind, 12-week trial, patients receiving inhaled treprostinil experienced a 20-m improvement in 6-minute walk distance compared with those on placebo ($P < 0.0006$). All patients included in the trial were concurrently receiving bosentan or sildenafil for at least 3 months.[49] An open-label extension of the trial found that inhaled treprostinil provided sustained benefit and was safe and efficacious over a 2-year period.[50] The approved dosing of inhaled treprostinil is three breaths (18 mcg each) four times daily during waking hours. The dose may be titrated based on patient tolerance at 1- to 2-week intervals to maximum dose of nine breaths four times daily. Inhaled treprostinil requires less time to administer, but the formulation is more complicated to prepare than inhaled iloprost.[26] While inhaled treprostinil avoids the infusion-related complications of the other PGI_2 analogs, use is cautioned in patients with acute pulmonary infections or underlying lung disease. The most common adverse effects seen in clinical trials include throat irritation, cough, headache, nausea, dizziness, and flushing. Inhaled treprostinil may also cause systemic hypotension, and patients should be monitored carefully if they are concurrently on diuretics, antihypertensives, or other vasodilators. Inhaled treprostinil is indicated for patients with functional class III (I-A/B) and IV (IIa-C).[1]

Finally, the first oral prostacyclin analog, sustained-release trepostinil (Orenitram), was approved by the FDA in December 2013 for patients with functional class II and III PAH. Oral treprostinil was studied as monotherapy in a 12-week study of 349 patients with PAH and was associated with a significant increase of 23 meters in 6-minute walk distance.[51] No differences were observed between treprostinil and placebo in time to clinical worsening or WHO functional class. Two randomized controlled trials followed evaluating use of oral treprostinil in addition to endothelin receptor antagonists and/or phosphodiesterase-5 inhibitors. Both studies used change in 6-minute walk distance as the primary endpoint and neither study demonstrated a significant improvement with oral treprostinil therapy.[52,53] The average increase in 6-minute walk distance did correspond to treprostinil dose, with patients receiving higher doses demonstrating more improvement in exercise capacity as measured by 6-minute walk distance. Adverse events in studies included headache, nausea, diarrhea, and jaw pain. Like other prostacyclin analogs, oral treprostinil inhibits platelet aggregation and may increase risk of bleeding, especially in patients treated with anticoagulants. Of note, oral trepostinil must be taken with food to improve absorption and cannot be crushed due to the osmotic release formulation. Oral treprostinil was not available at the time of recent guidelines publication and current data do not support use of oral treprostinil in combinations with endothelin receptor antagonists or PDE-5 inhibitors therefore.

Endothelin Receptor Antagonists (ERAs) 12 ET-1, a peptide produced primarily by the vascular endothelial cells, is characterized as a powerful vasoconstrictor and mitogen for smooth muscle. Activation of the ET-1 system has been shown in both plasma and lung tissue of PAH patients. Bosentan (Tracleer) is an orally active dual ET_A and ET_B receptor antagonist that improves exercise capacity, functional class, hemodynamics, echocardiographic and Doppler variables, and time to clinical worsening.[54,55] In one of the larger studies with bosentan, patients were started on 62.5 mg twice daily for 4 weeks followed by 125 or 250 mg twice daily for a minimum of 12 weeks. Both doses were better than placebo, and the higher dose provided greater improvement in 6-minute walking distance. Increases in hepatic aminotransferases occurred in 11% of patients and were dose-dependent.[55] The mechanism of increased liver enzymes is thought to be competition by bosentan and its metabolites with the biliary excretion of bile salts, resulting in retention of bile salts that can be cytotoxic to hepatocytes. Because of this toxicity, bosentan is only available through a distribution program, the Tracleer Access Program.[26] Bosentan should be started at 62.5 mg twice daily in adults and adolescents for 4 weeks. After 4 weeks of therapy, the dose should be increased to 125 mg twice daily. If LFTs are confirmed to be in the range of three to five times the upper limit of normal, reduce the daily dose or interrupt treatment. If LFTs return to pretreatment levels, bosentan may be continued or reintroduced if indicated. LFTs should be monitored at baseline and monthly thereafter, and monthly pregnancy testing is required in females (category X). Complete blood count should be monitored every 3 months as bosentan has been associated with anemia. Bosentan is indicated for WHO functional class II and III (I-A/B) as well as functional class IV (IIa-C).[1]

Ambrisentan (Letairis) is a once-daily selective ET_A receptor antagonist that improves exercise capacity and hemodynamics and delays clinical worsening in PAH.[56,57] Two large (n = 202 and 192) trials recently evaluated the efficacy of ambrisentan compared with placebo. In 12 weeks, both studies demonstrated a significant improvement in functional capacity at doses of 2.5, 5, and 10 mg daily (range of 31-59 m). However, greater response was seen with increased doses. All doses were well tolerated, with no patients on therapy experiencing an increase in LFTs >3 times the upper limit of normal. Similar to bosentan, ambrisentan is category X for pregnancy; the distribution program for ambrisentan is referred to as Letairis Education and Access Program (LEAP).[26] Unlike bosentan, liver toxicity occurs very rarely with ambrisentan (0.8% in 12-week trials and 2.8% for up to 1 year).[42] Common side effects include peripheral edema, nasal congestion, flushing, anemia, and palpitations. Treatment should be initiated with 5 mg once daily and increased to 10 mg once daily if required. Ambrisentan is recommended for WHO functional class II and III (I-A/B) as well as functional class IV (IIa-C).[3]

Macitentan (Opsumit) was FDA approved in 2013 as a once-daily dual ERA. Macitentan was approved based on the results of the Study with an Endothelin Receptor Antagonist in Pulmonary Arterial Hypertension to Improve Clinical Outcome (SERAPHIN) trial.[58] In this phase 3 multicenter, placebo-controlled study, patients (n = 742) were randomized to placebo, macitentan 3 mg orally daily, or macitentan 10 mg orally daily. Patients from WHO functional class II, III, and IV were included. Patients could be on concomitant therapy, if at stable doses for 3 months, with oral or inhaled prostanoids, calcium channel blockers, or oral phosphodiesterase inhibitors. Patients on intravenous or subcutaneous prostacyclins were excluded. The majority of patients (more than 80%) were functional class II or III. The most common diagnosis was IPAH. Over a treatment period of about 3 months, both doses demonstrated statistically significant decreases in the composite end point of events related to PAH or death compared to placebo. Worsening of PAH was the most common event (defined as a decrease in 6-minute walk distance, worsening symptoms, and need for additional treatment). Increase in LFTs was similar across all groups, about 3.5% to 4.5%. More patients in the macitentan groups experienced nasopharyngitis, headache, and anemia than with placebo. The FDA-approved dose is 10 mg by mouth daily. Macitentan is considered category X for pregnancy and female patients must go through a Risk Evaluation and Mitigation Strategy (REMS) program to receive the drug. Macitentan is recommended for WHO functional class II and III (I-A/B) as well as functional class IV (IIa-C).[1]

Phosphodiesterase Inhibitors There are two phosphodiesterase-5 inhibitors available for the treatment of PAH—sildenafil (Revatio) and tadalafil (Adcirca). 13 Sildenafil is a potent and highly specific phosphodiesterase-5 inhibitor that is approved for erectile dysfunction but also has been shown to reduce mPAP and improve functional class. Sildenafil exerts its pharmacologic effect by increasing the intracellular concentration of cyclic guanosine monophosphate, leading to vasorelaxation and antiproliferative effects on vascular smooth muscle cells. In a double-blind, placebo-controlled trial, sildenafil with conventional therapy significantly improved 6MWD and hemodynamic parameters at 12 weeks compared with placebo. A 1-year extension study showed a continued improvement in 6MWD of 51 m (95% CI 41-60).[59] The FDA-approved dose is 20 mg by mouth three times (TID) per day; however, much higher doses are routinely used clinically. Common adverse effects include headaches, flushing, epistaxis, dyspepsia, and diarrhea. Sildenafil may also cause systemic hypotension. Changes in vision have been reported, including blue-tinted vision and sudden loss of vision. In the event of sudden loss of vision, the drug should be stopped. Concurrent administration of sildenafil and bosentan leads to a 50% decrease in sildenafil concentrations through cytochrome P450 3A4 induction, requiring dose adjustment of sildenafil. Nitrate therapy may lead to excessive blood pressure reduction should be avoided with sildenafil. Based on the current guidelines, sildenafil is recommended for functional class II and III patients with PAH (I-A/B) in addition to functional class IV patients (IIa-C).[1]

Another phosphodiesterase-5 inhibitor, tadalafil (Adcirca), was approved by the FDA in 2009 for the treatment of PAH. In a 16-week study, tadalafil 40 mg daily significantly improved exercise capacity (an average of +33 m; $P < 0.01$) and quality of life measures. Tadalafil 40 mg also improved the time to clinical worsening (P = 0.041), which has not been demonstrated with sildenafil. Fifty-three percent of patients in this study were also on background bosentan therapy. Treatment-naïve patients demonstrated not only greater improvement in exercise capacity than those on bosentan therapy (+44 m vs 23 m) but also greater improvement on all secondary outcomes. One possible explanation is decreased tadalafil levels as bosentan is a potent CYP450 3A4 inducer. Higher doses of tadalafil may be required in patients on concurrent bosentan therapy.[60] The most commonly reported adverse events were headache, myalgia, and flushing. The recommended dose is 40 mg by mouth once a day.[61] Concurrent use with nitrate therapy should also be avoided with tadalafil. Current guidelines indicate tadalafil for functional class II and III (I-A/B) and functional class IV (IIa-C).[1]

Guanylate Cyclase Stimulator 14 A new class of medication recently became available in the treatment of PAH, soluble guanylate cyclase stimulators. Riociguat (Adempas®) was approved by the FDA in 2013. Riociguat works synergistically with nitric oxide and directly stimulates soluble guanylate cyclase. In the phase 3 study Pulmonary Arterial Hypertension Soluble Guanylate Cyclase-Stimulator Trial 1 (PATENT-1), riociguat 2.5 mg by mouth TID daily improved 6MWD over 12 weeks compared to placebo ($P < 0.001$).[62] Hemodynamic parameters and WHO functional class were also statistically significantly improved. Syncope occurred in 1% of riociguat patients compared to 4% in the placebo group. Of note, patients were continued on baseline therapy of endothelin-receptor antagonists or nonintravenous prostacyclin analogs. However, use of riociguat with phosphodiesterase-5 inhibitors is contraindicated due to the additive risk of hypotension. The recommended starting dose is 1 mg by mouth TID daily, titrated by 0.5 mg TID every 2 weeks to a maximum dose of 2.5 mg by mouth TID. Riociguat is considered category X for pregnancy and female patients must go through a REMS program to receive the drug. Riociguat is recommended for WHO functional class II and III (I-A/B) as well as functional class IV (IIa-C).

Calcium Channel Blockers 15 Since such a small number of patients with IPAH, HPAH, or PAH induced by drugs or toxins have a positive response to acute vasodilator testing, CCBs are infrequently used in the management of PAH in these subgroups. Approximately 13% of patients with IPAH will demonstrate an acute vasodilator response and may be initiated on CCB therapy; however, the number responding to long-term therapy is low (7%).[27] CCBs should not be used in the absence of demonstrated acute vasoreactivity.[1] If used in patients without acute vasoreactivity, CCBs are associated with systemic hypotension leading to reflex tachycardia, sympathetic stimulation, and right ventricular ischemia, ultimately increasing patient morbidity.[5] The preferred drugs are dihydropyridine CCBs as they lack the negative inotropic effects seen with verapamil. Diltiazem may be used in patients with tachycardia to slow heart rate through atrioventricular node blockade. If left ventricular systolic dysfunction is present, diltiazem and verapamil should not be used because of their negative inotropic effects. Assessment of CCB therapy should occur soon after initiation, and if improvement in functional class to class I or II is not seen, additional or alternative PAH therapy must be initiated. In acute responders, CCBs may be used in WHO functional classes I to IV (I-C).[1] The doses of these drugs are relatively high—that is, up to 20 to 30 mg/day for amlodipine, 120 to 240 mg/day for nifedipine, and 240 to 720 mg/day for diltiazem—however, initial doses should be much lower and titrated upward to response.[5] The most common adverse effect is peripheral edema. More specific information concerning individual drugs used for PAH is shown in Tables 28-7 to 28-9.

Combination Therapy 16 Combination therapy is an attractive option to address the multiple pathophysiologic mechanisms in PAH, resulting in improvement in hemodynamics, symptoms, and exercise capacity. Combination therapy can be pursued by the simultaneous initiation of two (or more) treatments or by the addition of a second (or third) agent if previous treatment has been insufficient. The goal with combination therapy is for the patient to achieve

TABLE 28-7 Drug Dosing Table

Drug	Brand Name	Initial Dose	Usual Range	Other
Epoprostenol	Flolan®	Starting dose 2-4 ng/kg/min IV	Titrate up to 20-40 ng/kg/min	
Treprostinil (IV or SC)	Remodulin®	Initially 1.25 ng/kg/min continuous subcutaneous or IV infusion	Decrease to 0.625 ng/kg/min if not tolerated Increase by no more than 1.25 ng/kg/min weekly for the first 4 wk of therapy and no more than 2.5 ng/kg/min weekly for the duration of therapy	
Treprostinil (inhaled)	Tyvaso®	Initially three breaths (18 mcg) via oral inhalation four times daily during waking hours (approximately 4 h apart)	Reduce to one to two breaths if three breaths not tolerated; increase to three breaths when tolerance improves Goal maintenance dose is nine breaths (54 mcg) per treatment four times daily; titrate by increasing three breaths at 1- to 2-wk intervals as tolerated	
Treprostinil (Oral)	Orenitram®	0.25 mg every 12 hours or 0.125 mg every 8 hours	Titrate dose in increments of 0.25-0.5 mg every 12 h or 0.125 mg every 8 h every 3-4 days Maximum dose is determined by tolerability Avoid abrupt discontinuation; if not tolerated, decrease dose stepwise in 0.25-0.5 mg increments	If unable to continue oral therapy temporarily while inpatient, consider initiation of IV or SC treprostinil; 1/5 of total daily dose is estimate of total daily parenteral dose
Iloprost	Ventavis®	Initially 2.5 mcg inhaled six to nine times daily (dosing at ≥2-h intervals while awake)	Titrate to 5 mcg per dose with a maximum daily dose of 45 mcg	
Bosentan	Tracleer®	Initially 62.5 mg orally twice daily for 4 wk	Increase to 125 mg orally twice daily	Available through Tracleer Access Program
Ambrisentan	Letairis®	Initial dose 5 mg orally daily	Titrate to maximum dose of 10 mg daily	Available through Letairis Education and Access Program
Macitentan	Opsumit®	Initial dose 10 mg orally daily	Maximum dose of 10 mg orally daily	Available through Opsumit Risk Evaluation and Mitigation Strategy Program
Sildenafil	Revatio®	Initial dose 20 mg orally three times daily, taken at least 4-6 h apart	Maximum FDA-approved dose is 20 mg orally three times a day; higher doses frequently used clinically	
Tadalafil	Adcirca®	40 mg orally once daily, with or without food	40 mg orally once daily	Not recommended to divide the dose
Riociguat	Adempas®	Initial dose 0.5-1 mg orally three times daily	Maximum dose is 2.5 mg orally three times daily Titrate every 2 wk to maximum tolerated dose; dose limited by hypotension	Use is contraindicated with PDE-5 inhibitors due to additive risk of hypotension Available through Adempas Risk Evaluation and Mitigation Program

TABLE 28-8 Drug Monitoring Information

Drug	ADR	Monitoring Parameter	Comments
Synthetic Prostacyclin and Prostacyclin Analogs			
Epoprostenol	Pain (chest and jaw), flushing, headache	Titrate to balance efficacy and adverse effect	Occurs with dose titration
	GI (nausea, vomiting, diarrhea, anorexia)		
	Hypotension	Blood pressure	Occurs with dose titration; additive hypotensive effects with other anithypertensives, vasodilators, and diuretics
	Thrombocytopenia	Platelets; signs and symptoms of bleeding	Monitor with concurrent anticoagulant and antiplatelet agents
Treprostinil (IV or SC)	SC site pain	Local pain at SC administration site	Frequent site rotation may improve; may also use cool compresses, lidocaine-based creams or patches, or PLO to relieve pain
	See epoprostenol		
Treprostinil (inhaled)	Cough and throat irritation		
Treprostinil (oral)			
Iloprost	Throat irritation		
	Cough		
Endothelin Receptor Antagonists			
Bosentan	Hepatotoxicity	Baseline and monthly liver function tests required	Black box warning for liver injury
	Anemia	Hemoglobin	Usually resolves after the first 3 mo of therapy
	Edema	Edema on physical examination	May require dose increase of diuretic therapy
Ambrisentan and Macitentan	Anemia	Hemoglobin	Usually resolves after the first 3 mo of therapy
	Edema	Edema on physical examination	May require dose increase of diuretic therapy

(Continued)

TABLE 28-8 Drug Monitoring Information (*Continued*)

Drug	ADR	Monitoring Parameter	Comments
Phosphodiesterase-5 Inhibitors			
Sildenafil and Tadalafil	Headache	Self-report by patient; occurs due to vasodilation	
	Nasal congestion		
	Hypotension	Blood pressure	Concurrent use with nitrates potentiates effects
	Visual changes	Consider baseline examination; repeat examination if visual changes occur	
Soluble Guanylate Cyclase Stimulator			
Riociguat	Headache		
	Hypotension	Blood pressure	
	Peripheral edema	Edema on physical examination	
	Major bleeding	Hemoglobin and hematocrit Signs and symptoms of bleeding	
	GERD		

GERD, gastroesophageal reflux disease; IV, intravenous; PLO, pluronic lecithin organogel; SC, subcutaneous.

TABLE 28-9 Potentially Signficant Drug Interactions with Pulmonary Arterial Hypertension Drugs

PAH drug	Mechanism of interaction	Interacting drug	Interaction
Ambrisentan	?	Cydosporine Ketoconazole	Caution is required in the co-administration of ambrisentan with ketoconazole and cyclosporine.
Bosentan	CYP3A4 inducer	Sildenafil	Sildenafil levels fall 50%; bosentan levels increase 50%. May not require dose adjustments of either drug.
	CYP3A4 substrate	Cydosporine	Cyclosporine levels fall 50%; bosentan levels 4-fold. Combination contraindicated.
	CYP3A4 substrate	Erythromycin	Bosentan levels increase. May not require dose adjustement of bosentan during a short course.
	CYP3A4 substrate	Ketoconazole	Bosentan levels increase twofold.
	CYP3A4 substrate + bile salt pump inhibitor	Glibenclamide	Increase incidence of elevated aminotransferases. Potential decrease of hypoglycaemic effect of glibendamide. Combination contraindicated.
	CYP2C9 and CYP3A4 substrate	Fluconazole, amlodarone	Bosentan levels increase considerably. Combination contraindicated.
	CYP2C9 and CYP3A4 inducers	Rifampicin, phenytoin	Bosentan levels decrease by 58%. Need for dose adjustment uncertain.
	CYP2C9 inducer	HMG CoA reductase inhibitors	Simvastatin levels reduce 50%; similar effects likely with atorvastatin. Cholesterol level should be monitored.
	CYP2C9 inducer	Warfarin	Increases warfarin metabolism, may need to adjust warfarin dose. Intensified monitoring of warfarin recommended following initiation but dose adjustment usually unnecessary.
	CYP2C9 and CYP3A4 inducers	Hormonal contraceptives	Hormone levels decrease. Contraception unreliable.
Macitentan			To be determined.
Selexipag			To be determined.
Sildenafil[43]	CYP3A4 substrate	Bosentan	Sildenafil levels fall 50%; bosentan levels increase 50%. May not require dose adjustments of either drug.
	CYP3A4 substrate	HMG CoA reductase inhibitors	May increase simvastatin/atorvastatin levels through competition for metabolism. Sildenafil levels may increase. Possible increased risk or rhabdomyolysis.
	CYP3A4 substrate	HIV protease inhibitors	Ritonavir and saquinovir increase sildenafil levels markedly.
	CYP3A4 Inducer	Phenytoin	Sildenafil level may fall.
	CYP3A4 substrate	Erythromycin	Sildenafil levels increase. May not require dose adjustment for a short course.
	CYP3A4 substrate	Ketoconaczole	Sildenafil levels increase. May not require dose adjustment.
	CYP3A4 substrate	Cimetidine	Sildenafil levels increase. May not require dose adjustment.
	cGMP	Nitrates, Nicorandil Molsidomine	Profound systemic hypotension, combination contraindicated.
Tadalafil[44]	CYP3A4 substrate	Bosentan	Tadalafil exposure decreases by 42%, no significant changes in bosentan levels.(44) May not require dose adjustment.
	cGMP	Nitrates, Nicorandil	Profound systemic hypotension, combination contraindicated.
Rioclguat[18]	cGMP	Sildenafil, other PDE-5 inhibitors	Hypotension, servere side effects, combination contraindicated.
	cGMP	Nitrates, Nicorandil	Profound systemic hypotension, combination contraindicated.

cGMP, cyclic guanosine monophosphate; HMG CoA, 3-hydroxy-3-methylglutaryl-CoA reductase; PDE-5, phosphodiesterase type 5.

Data from N. Galie et al. 2015 ESC/ERS Guidelines for the diagnosis and treatment of pulmonary hypertension. Eur Respir J 2015.

TABLE 28-10 Recommendations for Efficacy of Initial Drug Combination Therapy for PAH (Group 1) according to World Health Organization Functional Class. Sequence Is by Rating

	Class[a]-Level[b]					
Measure/Treatment	**WHO-FC II**		**WHO-FC III**		**WHO-FC IV**	
Ambrisentan + tadalafil[d]	I	B	I	B	IIb	C
Other ERA + PDE-5i	IIa	C	IIa	C	IIb	C
Bosentan + sildenafil + IV epoprostenol	-	-	IIa	C	IIa	C
Bosentan + IV epoprostenol	-	-	IIa	C	IIa	C
Other ERA or PDE-5i + SC treprostinil			IIb	C	IIb	C
Other ERA or PDE-5i + other IV prostacyclin analogues			IIb	C	IIb	C

ERA, endothelin receptor antagonist; IV, intravenous; PAH, pulmonary arterial hypertension; PDE-5i, phosphodiesterase type 5 inhibitor; RCT, randomized controlled trial; SC, subcutaneous; WHO-FC, World Health Organization functional class.

[a]Class of recommendation.

[b]Level of evidence.

[c]Reference(s) supporting recommendations.

[d]Time to clinical failure as primary endpoint in RCTs or drugs with demonstrated reduction in all-cause mortality (prospectively defined).

WHO functional class I or II along with normalization of the cardiac index and BNP.[1] Combination therapy may be started as initial therapy or added sequentially throughout treatment. Table 28-10 and Table 28-11 show current treatment recommendations for initial combination and sequential combination therapy, respectively.

ERAs plus PDE-5 inhibitors, PDE-5 inhibitors with PGI_2 analogs, ERAs with PGI_2 analogs, and all three classes used in combination have all shown improved functional outcomes.[54,55,60,63,64] Sequential combination therapy is recommended for patients with inadequate clinical response to monotherapy; combinations of prostanoids, phosphodiesterase-5 inhibitors, and endothelin antagonists may be used (I-A).[1] Certain combinations, such as riociguat and phosphodiesterase-5 inhibitors, should be avoided due to unsafe adverse effects.

Recent results of the AMBITION trial comparing ambrisentan and tadalafil together versus either alone suggest that initial combination therapy was associated with a significant reduction in time to clinical failure and PAH hospitalizations. Adverse effects such as peripheral edema, headache, nasal congestion, and anemia were more common in the combination group than either monotherapy group. However, there was no difference in drug discontinuation due to adverse events.[65] Based on the results of this trial, the FDA approved combination use of ambrisentan and tadalafil as first line therapy for patients with WHO Class II or II PAH in October 2015.

Evaluation of Therapeutic Outcomes

Response to treatment in PAH can be objectively measured by the 6-minute walk distance, echocardiography to assess pulmonary pressures, and right heart catheterization as the gold standard to assess ventricular function and pulmonary pressures (see Table 28-6). The WHO functional classification system is clinically useful, but

TABLE 28-11 Recommendations for Efficacy of Sequential Drug Combination Therapy for PAH (Group 1) according to World Health Organization Functional Class. Sequence Is by Rating and by Alphabetical Order

	Class[a]-Level[b]					
Measure/Treatment	**WHO-FC II**		**WHO-FC III**		**WHO-FC IV**	
Macitentan added to sildenafil[d]	I	B	I	B	IIa	C
Riociguat added to bosentan	I	B	I	B	IIa	C
Selexipag[e] added to ERA and/or PDE-5i[d]	I	B	I	B	IIa	C
Sildenafil added to epoprostenol	-	-	I	B	IIa	B
Treprostinil inhaled added to sildenafil or bosentan	IIa	B	IIa	B	IIa	C
Iloprost inhaled added to bosentan	IIb	B	IIb	B	IIb	C
Tadalafil added to bosentan	IIa	C	IIa	C	IIa	C
Ambrisentan added to sildenafil	IIb	C	IIb	C	IIb	C
Bosentan added to epoprostenol	-	-	IIb	C	IIb	C
Bosentan added to sildenafil	IIb	C	IIb	C	IIb	C
Sildenafil added to bosentan	IIb	C	IIb	C	IIb	C
Other double combinations	IIb	C	IIb	C	IIb	C
Other triple combinations	IIb	C	IIb	C	IIb	C
Riociguat added to sildenafil or other PDE-5i	III	B	III	B	III	B

EMA, European Medicines Agendy; ERA, endothelin receptor antagonist; PAH, pulmonary arterial hypertension; PDE-5i, phosphodiesterase type 5 inhibitor; RCT, randomized controlled trial; WHO-FC, World Health Organization functional class.

[a]Class of recommendation.

[b]Level of evidence.

[c]Reference(s) supporting recommendations.

[d]Time to clinical failure as primary endpoint in RCTs or drugs with demonstrated reduction in all-cause mortality (prospectively defined).

[e]This drug was not approved by the EMA at the time of publication of these guidelines.

correlations to hemodynamics may be imprecise. Other outcomes that are useful in clinical trials include hospitalization for exacerbations of PAH and the development of complications and death. Table 28-6 provides recommendations regarding specific baseline and follow-up assessments and when they are indicated.

CONCLUSION

Significant advances have been made in elucidating the pathogenesis of PAH as well as in the evaluation and treatment of these patients over the past 3 decades. With approved targeted therapies such as ERAs, phosphodiesterase-5 inhibitors, and PGI_2 analogs, clinical improvement is possible in most patients, leading to a better quality of life and delay of disease progression. Patient education is important to improve acceptance of this disease and referral to specialty care centers may provide the best outcomes.

ABBREVIATIONS

ALK-1	activin receptor-like kinase 1
APAH	associated pulmonary arterial hypertension
BMPR2	bone morphogenetic protein receptor 2
BNP	brain natriuretic peptide
CCB	calcium channel blocker
CTEPH	chronic thromboembolic pulmonary hypertension
ec-NOS	nitric oxide synthase
ERA	endothelin receptor antagonist
ET-1	endothelin-1
FPAH	familial pulmonary arterial hypertension
5-HT	serotonin
5-HTT	5-hydroxytryptamine transporter
HIV	human immunodeficiency virus
HPAH	heritable pulmonary arterial hypertension
INR	international normalized ratio
IPAH	idiopathic pulmonary arterial hypertension
LEAP	Letairis Education and Access Program
LFT	liver function test
LVEDP	left ventricular end-diastolic pressure
mPAP	mean pulmonary artery pressure
NO	nitric oxide
PAH	pulmonary arterial hypertension
PGI_2	prostacyclin
SC	subcutaneous
WHO	World Health Organization

REFERENCES

1. Galiè N, Corris PA, Frost A, et al. Updated treatment algorithm of pulmonary arterial hypertension. *J Am Coll Cardiol* 2013;62(25):D60-D72. doi:10.1016/j.jacc.2013.10.031.
2. Hoeper MM, Bogaard HJ, Condliffe R, et al. Definitions and diagnosis of pulmonary hypertension. *J Am Coll Cardiol* 2013;62(25):D42-D50. doi:10.1016/j.jacc.2013.10.032.
3. McLaughlin V V, Shah SJ, Souza R, Humbert M. Management of pulmonary arterial hypertension. *J Am Coll Cardiol* 2015;65(18):1976-1997. doi:10.1016/j.jacc.2015.03.540.
4. Galiè N, Humbert M, Vachiery J-L, et al. 2015 ESC/ERS Guidelines for the diagnosis and treatment of pulmonary hypertension. *Eur Heart J* August 2015:ehv317.
5. Taichman DB, Ornelas J, Chung L, et al. Pharmacological therapy for pulmonary arterial hypertension in adults: CHEST Guideline. *Chest* 2014;146(2):449-475. doi:10.1378/chest.14-0793.
6. D'Alonzo GE. Survival in patients with primary pulmonary hypertension. *Ann Intern Med* 1991;115(5):343. doi:10.7326/0003-4819-115-5-343.
7. Benza RL, Miller DP, Gomberg-Maitland M, et al. Predicting survival in pulmonary arterial hypertension: insights from the Registry to Evaluate Early and Long-Term Pulmonary Arterial Hypertension Disease Management (REVEAL). *Circulation* 2010;122(2):164-172. doi:10.1161/CIRCULATIONAHA.109.898122.
8. McGoon MD, Benza RL, Escribano-Subias P, et al. Pulmonary Arterial hypertension. *J Am Coll Cardiol* 2013;62(25):D51-D59. doi:10.1016/j.jacc.2013.10.023.
9. Humbert M, Sitbon O, Chaouat A, et al. Pulmonary arterial hypertension in France: Results from a national registry. *Am J Respir Crit Care Med* 2006;173(9):1023-1030. doi:10.1164/rccm.200510-1668OC.
10. Badesch DB, Raskob GE, Elliott CG, et al. Pulmonary arterial hypertension: Baseline characteristics from the REVEAL Registry. *Chest* 2010;137(2):376-387. doi:10.1378/chest.09-1140.
11. Yuan JX-J. Pathogenesis of pulmonary arterial hypertension: The need for multiple hits. *Circulation* 2005;111(5):534-538. doi:10.1161/01.CIR.0000156326.48823.55.
12. McGoon MD, Benza RL, Escribano-Subias P, et al. Pulmonary arterial hypertension: epidemiology and registries. *J Am Coll Cardiol* 2013;62(25 Suppl):D51-D59. doi:10.1016/j.jacc.2013.10.023.
13. Simonneau G, Gatzoulis MA, Adatia I, et al. Updated clinical classification of pulmonary hypertension. *J Am Coll Cardiol* 2013;62(25):D34-D41. doi:10.1016/j.jacc.2013.10.029.
14. Shah SJ. Pulmonary hypertension. *JAMA* 2012;308(13):1366. doi:10.1001/jama.2012.12347.
15. Schermuly RT, Ghofrani HA, Wilkins MR, Grimminger F. Mechanisms of disease: Pulmonary arterial hypertension. *Nat Rev Cardiol* 2011; 8(8):443-455. doi:10.1038/nrcardio.2011.87.
16. Olsson KM, Hoeper MM. Novel approaches to the pharmacotherapy of pulmonary arterial hypertension. *Drug Discov Today* 2009;14(5-6):284-290.
17. Humbert M. Update in Pulmonary hypertension 2008. *Am J Respir Crit Care Med* 2009;179(8):650-656. doi:10.1164/rccm.200901-0136UP.
18. Trembath RC, Thomson JR, Machado RD, et al. Clinical and molecular genetic features of pulmonary hypertension in patients with hereditary hemorrhagic telangiectasia. *N Engl J Med* 2001;345(5):325-334.
19. Eddahibi S, Humbert M, Fadel E, et al. Serotonin transporter overexpression is responsible for pulmonary artery smooth muscle hyperplasia in primary pulmonary hypertension. *J Clin Invest* 2001;108(8):1141-1150.
20. Izikki M, Hanoun N, Marcos E, et al. Tryptophan hydroxylase 1 knockout and tryptophan hydroxylase 2 polymorphism: effects on hypoxic pulmonary hypertension in mice. *Am J Physiol Lung Cell Mol Physiol* 2007;293(4):L1045-L1052.
21. Park MH. Advances in diagnosis and treatment in patients with pulmonary arterial hypertension. *Catheter Cardiovasc Interv* 2008;71(2):205-213. doi:10.1002/ccd.21389.
22. Rubens C, Ewert R, Halank M, et al. Big endothelin-1 and endothelin-1 plasma levels are correlated with the severity of primary pulmonary hypertension. *Chest* 2001;120(5):1562-1569.
23. Giaid A, Saleh D. Reduced expression of endothelial nitric oxide synthase in the lungs of patients with pulmonary hypertension. *N Engl J Med* 1995;333(4):214-221.
24. McGoon MD, Benza RL, Escribano-Subias P, et al. Pulmonary arterial hypertension: Epidemiology and registries. *J Am Coll Cardiol* 2013;62(25 Suppl):D51-D59.
25. Janda S, Shahidi N, Gin K, Swiston J. Diagnostic accuracy of echocardiography for pulmonary hypertension: a systematic review and meta-analysis. *Heart* 2011;97(8):612-622. doi:10.1136/hrt.2010.212084.
26. Bishop BM, Mauro VF, Khouri SJ. Practical considerations for the pharmacotherapy of pulmonary arterial hypertension. *Pharmacotherapy* 2012;32(9):838-855. doi:10.1002/j.1875-9114.2012.01114.x.
27. Sitbon O. Long-term response to calcium channel blockers in idiopathic pulmonary arterial hypertension. *Circulation* 2005;111(23):3105-3111. doi:10.1161/CIRCULATIONAHA.104.488486.
28. O'Callaghan DS, Savale L, Montani D, et al. Treatment of pulmonary arterial hypertension with targeted therapies. *Nat Rev Cardiol* 2011;8(9):526-538. doi:10.1038/nrcardio.2011.104.
29. Agarwal R, Gomberg-Maitland M. Current therapeutics and practical management strategies for pulmonary arterial hypertension. *Am Heart J* 2011;162(2):201-213. doi:10.1016/j.ahj.2011.05.012.
30. Macchia A, Marchioli R, Marfisi R, et al. A meta-analysis of trials of pulmonary hypertension: A clinical condition looking for drugs and research methodology. *Am Heart J* 2007;153(6):1037-1047. doi:10.1016/j.ahj.2007.02.037.
31. Galie N, Manes A, Negro L, Palazzini M, Bacchi-Reggiani ML, Branzi A. A meta-analysis of randomized controlled trials in pulmonary arterial hypertension. *Eur Heart J* 2008;30(4):394-403. doi:10.1093/eurheartj/ehp022.

32. McLaughlin V V, Presberg KW, Doyle RL, et al. Prognosis of pulmonary arterial hypertension: ACCP evidence-based clinical practice guidelines. *Chest* 2004;126(1 Suppl):78S - 92S. doi:10.1378/chest.126.1_suppl.78S.
33. Galiè N, Torbicki A, Barst R, et al. Guidelines on diagnosis and treatment of pulmonary arterial hypertension. The Task Force on Diagnosis and Treatment of Pulmonary Arterial Hypertension of the European Society of Cardiology. *Eur Heart J* 2004;25(24):2243-2278.
34. McGoon M, Gutterman D, Steen V, et al. Screening, early detection, and diagnosis of pulmonary arterial hypertension: ACCP evidence-based clinical practice guidelines. *Chest* 2004;126(1 Suppl):14S-34S.
35. Frank H, Mlczoch J, Huber K, Schuster E, Gurtner HP, Kneussl M. The effect of anticoagulant therapy in primary and anorectic drug-induced pulmonary hypertension. *Chest* 1997;112(3):714-721. doi:10.1378/chest.112.3.714.
36. Fuster V, Steele PM, Edwards WD, Gersh BJ, McGoon MD, Frye RL. Primary pulmonary hypertension: Natural history and the importance of thrombosis. *Circulation* 1984;70(4):580-587. doi:10.1161/01.CIR.70.4.580.
37. Olsson KM, Delcroix M, Ghofrani HA, et al. Anticoagulation and survival in pulmonary arterial hypertension: Results From the Comparative, Prospective Registry of Newly Initiated Therapies for Pulmonary Hypertension (COMPERA). *Circulation* 2014;129(1):57-65. doi:10.1161/CIRCULATIONAHA.113.004526.
38. Caldeira D, Loureiro MJ, Costa J, Pinto FJ, Ferreira JJ. Oral anticoagulation for pulmonary arterial hypertension: Systematic Review and Meta-analysis. *Can J Cardiol* 2014;30(8):879-887. doi:10.1016/j.cjca.2014.04.016.
39. Coons JC, Clarke M, Wanek MR, Bauer A, Bream-Rouwenhorst HR. Safe and effective use of prostacyclins to treat pulmonary arterial hypertension. *Am J Heal Pharm* 2013;70(19):1716-1723. doi:10.2146/ajhp130005.
40. Kallen AJ, Lederman E, Balaji A, et al. Bloodstream infections in patients given treatment with intravenous prostanoids. *Infect Control Hosp Epidemiol* 2008;29(4):342-349. doi:10.1086/529552.
41. McLaughlin V V, Archer SL, Badesch DB, et al. ACCF/AHA 2009 expert consensus document on pulmonary hypertension: A report of the American College of Cardiology Foundation Task Force on Expert Consensus Documents and the American Heart Association developed in collaboration with the American College of. *J Am Coll Cardiol* 2009;53(17):1573-1619.
42. Badesch DB, Tapson VF, McGoon MD, et al. Continuous intravenous epoprostenol for pulmonary hypertension due to the scleroderma spectrum of disease. A randomized, controlled trial. *Ann Intern Med* 2000;132(6):425-434.
43. Sitbon O, Humbert M, Nunes H, et al. Long-term intravenous epoprostenol infusion in primary pulmonary hypertension: Prognostic factors and survival. *J Am Coll Cardiol* 2002;40(4):780-788.
44. Simonneau G, Barst RJ, Galie N, et al. Continuous subcutaneous infusion of treprostinil, a prostacyclin analogue, in patients with pulmonary arterial hypertension: A double-blind, randomized, placebo-controlled trial. *Am J Respir Crit Care Med* 2002;165(6):800-804.
45. Gomberg-Maitland M, Tapson VF, Benza RL, et al. Transition from intravenous epoprostenol to intravenous treprostinil in pulmonary hypertension. *Am J Respir Crit Care Med* 2005;172(12):1586-1589. doi:10.1164/rccm.200505-766OC.
46. Kitterman N, Poms A, Miller DP, Lombardi S, Farber HW, Barst RJ. Bloodstream infections in patients with pulmonary arterial hypertension treated with intravenous prostanoids: Insights From the REVEAL REGISTRY®. *Mayo Clin Proc* 2012;87(9):825-834. doi:10.1016/j.mayocp.2012.05.014.
47. Rich JD. The Effect of diluent pH on bloodstream infection rates in patients receiving iv treprostinil for pulmonary arterial hypertension. *Chest J* 2012;141(1):36. doi:10.1378/chest.11-0245.
48. Olschewski H, Simonneau G, Galiè N, et al. Inhaled iloprost for severe pulmonary hypertension. *N Engl J Med* 2002;347(5):322-329.
49. McLaughlin V V, Benza RL, Rubin LJ, et al. Addition of inhaled treprostinil to oral therapy for pulmonary arterial hypertension: A randomized controlled clinical trial. *J Am Coll Cardiol* 2010;55(18):1915-1922. doi:10.1016/j.jacc.2010.01.027.
50. Benza RL, Seeger W, McLaughlin V V, et al. Long-term effects of inhaled treprostinil in patients with pulmonary arterial hypertension: The Treprostinil Sodium Inhalation Used in the Management of Pulmonary Arterial Hypertension (TRIUMPH) study open-label extension. *J Heart Lung Transplant* 2011;30(12):1327-1333. doi:10.1016/j.healun.2011.08.019.
51. Jing Z-C, Parikh K, Pulido T, et al. Efficacy and safety of oral treprostinil monotherapy for the treatment of pulmonary arterial hypertension: A Randomized, controlled trial. *Circulation* 2013;127(5):624-633. doi:10.1161/CIRCULATIONAHA.112.124388.
52. Tapson VF. Oral Treprostinil for the treatment of pulmonary arterial hypertension in patients on background endothelin receptor antagonist and/or phosphodiesterase type 5 inhibitor therapy (The FREEDOM-C Study). *Chest J* 2012;142(6):1383. doi:10.1378/chest.11-2212.
53. Tapson VF. Oral treprostinil for the treatment of pulmonary arterial hypertension in patients receiving background endothelin receptor antagonist and phosphodiesterase type 5 inhibitor therapy (The FREEDOM-C2 Study). *Chest J* 2013;144(3):952. doi:10.1378/chest.12-2875.
54. Hoeper MM. Combining inhaled iloprost with bosentan in patients with idiopathic pulmonary arterial hypertension. *Eur Respir J* 2006;28(4):691-694. doi:10.1183/09031936.06.00057906.
55. Humbert M. Combination of bosentan with epoprostenol in pulmonary arterial hypertension: BREATHE-2. *Eur Respir J* 2004;24(3):353-359. doi:10.1183/09031936.04.00028404.
56. Galié N, Badesch D, Oudiz R, et al. Ambrisentan therapy for pulmonary arterial hypertension. *J Am Coll Cardiol* 2005;46(3):529-535.
57. Barst RJ. A review of pulmonary arterial hypertension: Role of ambrisentan. *Vasc Health Risk Manag* 2007;3(1):11-22.
58. Pulido T, Adzerikho I, Channick RN, et al. Macitentan and morbidity and mortality in pulmonary arterial hypertension. *N Engl J Med* 2013;369(9):809-818.
59. Galiè N, Ghofrani HA, Torbicki A, et al. Sildenafil citrate therapy for pulmonary arterial hypertension. *N Engl J Med* 2005;353(20):2148-2157.
60. Abraham T, Wu G, Vastey F, Rapp J, Saad N, Balmir E. Role of combination therapy in the treatment of pulmonary arterial hypertension. *Pharmacotherapy* 2010;30(4):390-404.
61. Galiè N, Brundage BH, Ghofrani HA, et al. Tadalafil therapy for pulmonary arterial hypertension. *Circulation* 2009;119(22):2894-2903.
62. Ghofrani H-A, Galiè N, Grimminger F, et al. Riociguat for the treatment of pulmonary arterial hypertension. *N Engl J Med* 2013;369(4):330-340. doi:10.1056/NEJMoa1209655.
63. Ghofrani HA, Wiedemann R, Rose F, et al. Combination therapy with oral sildenafil and inhaled iloprost for severe pulmonary hypertension. *Ann Intern Med* 2002;136(7):515-522.
64. Simonneau G, Rubin LJ, Galiè N, et al. Addition of sildenafil to long-term intravenous epoprostenol therapy in patients with pulmonary arterial hypertension: A randomized trial. *Ann Intern Med* 2008;149(8):521-530.
65. Galiè N, Barberà JA, Frost AE, et al. Initial use of ambrisentan plus tadalafil in pulmonary arterial hypertension. *N Engl J Med* 2015;373(9):834-844.

29

Cystic Fibrosis

Chanin C. Wright and Yolanda Y. Vera

KEY CONCEPTS

1. Good nutrition with appropriate pancreatic enzyme and vitamin supplementation are essential in the management of cystic fibrosis (CF).
2. Airway clearance and anti-inflammatory therapies are key components to improve pulmonary health in CF patients.
3. Antipseudomonal agents are the cornerstone of antibiotic therapy for chronic lung infections in the CF patient.
4. Altered pharmacokinetics of CF patients can impact the dosing and clearance of pharmacologic therapy.

"Woe to that child which when kissed on the forehead tastes salty. He is bewitched and soon must die." This European adage accurately describes the fate of an individual diagnosed with cystic fibrosis (CF) during ancient times.[1]

CF is a disease state resulting from a dysfunction in the cystic fibrosis transmembrane conductance regulator (CFTR). It is the most common life-limiting genetic disorder in the Caucasian population, with an incidence of 1 in 2,000 to 4,000 live births and a prevalence of 30,000 affected individuals in the United States.[2-7]

Currently with care, affected individuals have an expected life span of 41 years. Multiple organ systems are affected in CF individuals, especially, the lungs, the digestive system, and the reproductive organs. Mortality is most commonly due to chronic organ damage or resistant pulmonary infections.[8]

The pharmacist plays an essential role in the development and management of a pharmacotherapeutic care plan for the CF patient.

EPIDEMIOLOGY

CF occurs in approximately 1 in 3,500 Caucasian newborns. In the 1970s, patients only survived into their teen years. By 2013, progress in care had extended survival to 41 years. Institution of care at a young age impacts long-term survival; hence, timing of diagnosis and recognition of signs and symptoms are crucial.[2-7]

Although CF occurs in all ethnicities, other ethnicities besides the Caucasian population display lower frequencies: 1 in 13,500 Hispanic-Americans, 1 in 15,000 African Americans, and 1 in 31,000 to 100,000 Asians, Native Hawaiian, and Pacific Islanders. The carrier frequency is 1 in 28 North American white populations, 1 in 29 Ashkenazi Jews, and 1 in 84 African Americans.[6]

Etiology

The cause of CF is due to a mutation of the *CFTR* gene. Extensive genetic studies have increased awareness regarding the large spectrum of mutations in the CF population. Over 1,800 mutations have been identified due to the extensive collaboration of the CF Foundation with international researchers. The most common mutation identified in CF patients is *ΔF508*.[3]

CF is an autosomal recessive disease, in which one mutation present on each allele of the *CFTR* gene results in presentation of the disease. The presentation of a mutation on only one allele of the *CFTR* gene will prevent the full expression of CF. Genetic studies have increased the understanding of genotype–phenotype relationships. Various mutations on the *CFTR* gene can result in various pathologies such as primary lung disease to minor gastrointestinal (GI) involvement.[3]

PATHOPHYSIOLOGY

In order to successfully treat CF, a good understanding of the disease's underlying mechanism of action is crucial. It is well established that gene mutations cause an abnormality in the CFTR. This initiates the sequence of events responsible for the manifestations of CF. Mucosal obstruction occurs in the distal airways of the lung and submucosal glands, which express the CFTR. The CFTR also performs numerous cellular functions, including the regulation of chloride transport across the cell membrane. Studies in genotype–phenotype relationships have shown that an abnormality on the CFTR contributes to the expression of other gene proteins involved with inflammatory responses, ion transport, and cell signaling. These various expressions result in differences in clinical severity among patients with the same mutations on the CFTR.[3,9-11]

Under normal conditions, the CFTR helps regulate ion transport and salt homeostasis in the sweat glands. Typically, the sodium ion is followed by the chloride ion, and is reabsorbed from the lumen by the CFTR and apical sodium channels. As a result of the CFTR's malfunction in CF patients, chloride fails to be reabsorbed, which impacts the sodium ion reabsorption as well. This failed process produces sweat that contains high levels of salt. The endpoint of this process is a highly negatively charged lumen, which leads to an increased salt content in the sweat gland. This is known as the transepithelial potential difference, which is two to three times greater in CF patients than in patients without CF. These processes can lead to organ damage in the CF patient (Fig. 29-1).

There are several theories as to how mucosal obstruction occurs in the airways. One of these theories, known as the "low-volume model," explains that the pulmonary surface epithelium behaves the opposite of a sweat gland in CF patients. There is an increased absorption of sodium, chloride, and fluid, which causes dehydration of the airway surfaces and defective mucociliary transport. An alternative theory known as the "high-salt model" indicates that the pulmonary surface epithelium behaves similarly to the sweat gland. A high salt content predisposes the CF patient to bacterial infections. Both theories agree that CF airways lack the ability to transport chloride through the CFTR.[9,12,13]

One of the common causes of morbidity and mortality in CF patients is mucosal obstruction of the exocrine glands. Mucosal obstruction causes the ducts to dilate, which results in the coating of lung surfaces by thick, viscous, neutrophil-dominated debris. These

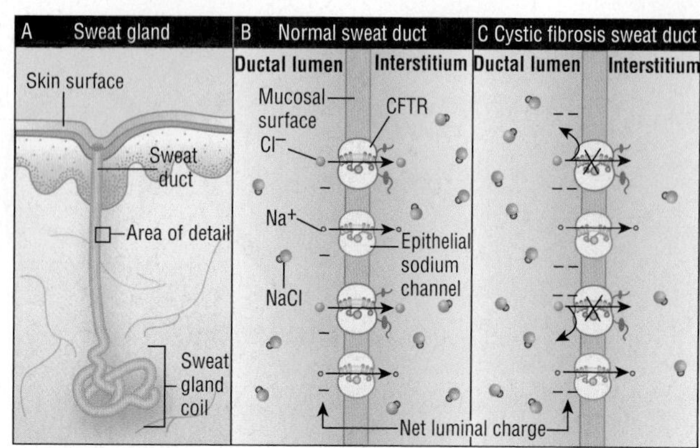

FIGURE 29-1 Mechanism of underlying elevated sodium chloride levels in the sweat of patients with cystic fibrosis (CF). Sweat ducts (Panel *A*) in patients with CF differ from those in people without the disease in the ability to reabsorb chloride before the emergence of sweat on the surface of the skin. A major pathway for Cl^- absorption is through CFTR, situated within luminal plasma membranes of cells lining the duct (ie, on the apical, or mucosal, cell surface) (Panel *B*). Diminished chloride reabsorption in the setting of continued sodium uptake leads to an elevated transepithelial potential difference across the wall of the sweat duct, and the lumen becomes more negatively charged because of a failure to reabsorb chloride (Panel *C*). The result is that total sodium chloride flux is markedly decreased, leading to increased salt content. The thickness of the arrows corresponds to the degree of movement of ions. *(Used with permission from Rowe SM, Miller S, Sorscher EJ. Cystic fibrosis. N Engl J Med 2005;352(19):1992–2001. Copyright © 2005 Massachusetts Medical Society. All rights reserved.)*

secretions initiate a cascade of events that lead to inflammation and formation of scar tissue in the lungs[14] (Fig. 29-2).

Other organ systems are impacted by the absence of CFTR activity as well. Ten percent of CF patients are born with meconium ileus, which is an intestinal obstruction that may be fatal if left untreated. Blockage of the pancreatic duct leads to complications such as chronic fibrosis and fatty replacement of the pancreatic gland. Bile duct obstruction causes cirrhosis of the liver, and male CF patients can experience infertility due to obstruction of the vas deferens in utero.[9]

Sinus and Pulmonary Presentation

CF patients will usually experience chronic infections and frequently develop polyps in the sinus cavity. Daily symptomatology includes shortness of breath and cough, with sputum production. A common finding in radiology chest films is a flat diaphragm with an increased chest diameter and air trapping. Pulmonary function tests will reflect a decrease in forced expiratory volume at 1 second (FEV_1). Older patients will experience digital clubbing, a deformity of the fingers and fingernails often associated with chronic hypoxia.

Bacterial growth in the lungs will often drive CF patients to a state of exacerbation, resulting in increased cough, a reduction in pulmonary function, and increased sputum production with a change in color.

Gastrointestinal System Presentation

Most patients with nonclassic CF will maintain adequate pancreatic function. However in classic CF patients, steatorrhea, or greasy stools, is typically present that can lead to a failure to thrive, resulting in malnutrition. Infants and small children will show an increase in frequency of small stools. Newborns may present with meconium ileus, which is considered diagnostic of CF. Older patients may experience constipation, abdominal cramping, and flatulence. This presentation is due to the obstruction of the pancreatic ducts and intestinal tract and their inability to digest essential nutrients.

Pancreatic malfunction can also lead to an insulin deficiency, which is often a later finding detected by a loss in weight, an increase in blood glucose levels, and a failed oral glucose tolerance test (OGTT).

Reproductive Presentation

As patients reach adolescent and adult ages, tests may show azoospermia due to blockage of or the congenital bilateral absence of the vas deferens. Females may experience reduced fertility as cervical fluids have lower water content and decreased thinning during ovulation.[9,15,16]

CLINICAL PRESENTATION

In the classic presentation of CF, there are two mutations present (Table 29-1). The patients show signs and symptoms of chronic sinus and pulmonary infections, pancreatic insufficiency, and elevated sweat chloride levels. Patients with nonclassic CF have one mutation present, therefore retaining partial function of the CFTR and maintaining appropriate pancreatic function (Fig. 29-3).

DIAGNOSIS

All states are required to perform CF newborn screening.[17] The screening test checks for immunoreactive trypsinogen (IRT), a chemical produced by the pancreas. The IRT tends to be high in babies with CF. A second test may be done with a follow-up IRT test or a DNA test to look for a genetic mutation that causes CF. The CF newborn screening consists of a test called the quantitative pilocarpine iontophoresis sweat test (QPIT). The QPIT came about due to the risk of hyperpyrexia associated with older methods that utilized plastic body bags to make patients sweat. QPIT uses only a small area on the forearm, which is then stimulated to secrete sweat through the skin by iontophoresis of pilocarpine. Sweat from the stimulated area is then collected and analyzed for chloride content. Chloride concentrations are quantified as: normal: ≤39 mmol/L; intermediate: 40 to 59 mmol/L; and abnormal: ≥60 mmol/L. Values more than or equal to 60 mmol/L are consistently diagnostic of CF. It is suggested that samples from two sites will increase the reliability of the diagnosis[3-5] (Fig. 29-4).

Desired Outcomes

Pharmacists play a vital role in assisting patients to reach the following long- and short-term goals. Since CF affects multiple organ systems, there are several therapeutic goals that must be addressed for each system.[8]

Sinopulmonary

1. Prevent and treat sinusitis.
2. Increase FEV_1 and promote optimal pulmonary function tests and prevent pulmonary exacerbations.
   a. Promote effective airway clearance by providing counseling on the use of appropriate medications and chest physiotherapy.
   b. Prevent and treat colonization of the lungs with pathogens.
   c. Prevent and treat acute exacerbations.

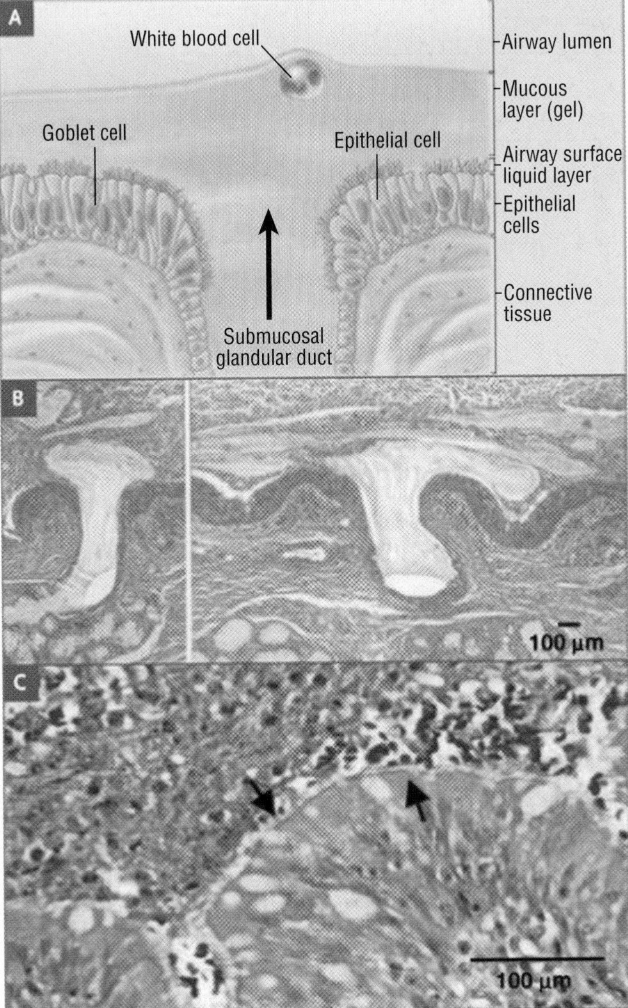

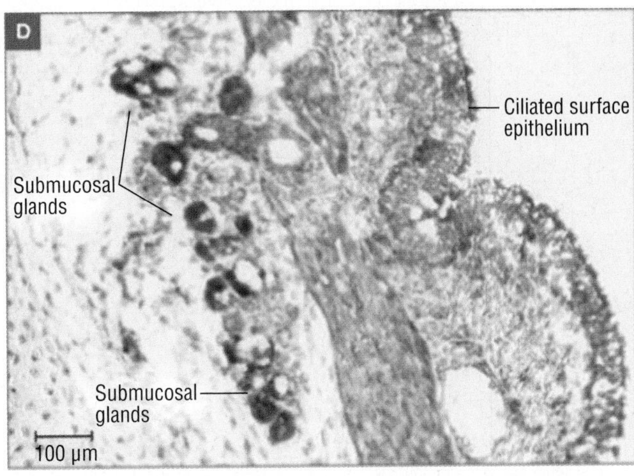

FIGURE 29-2 Extrusion of mucus secretion onto the epithelial surface of airways in cystic fibrosis (CF). Panel *A* shows a schematic of the surface epithelium and supporting glandular structure of the human airway. In Panel *B*, the submucosal glands of a patient with CF are filled with mucus, and mucopurulent debris overlies the airway surfaces, essentially burying the epithelium. Panel *C* is a higher-magnification view of a mucus plug tightly adhering to the airway surface, with arrows indicating the interface between infected and inflamed secretions and the underlying epithelium to which the secretions adhere. (Both Panels *B* and *C* were stained with hematoxylin and eosin, with the colors modified to highlight structures.) Infected secretions obstruct airways and, over time, dramatically disrupt the normal architecture of the lung. In Panel *D*, CFTR is expressed in surface epithelium and serous cells at the base of submucosal glands in a porcine lung sample, as shown by the dark staining, signifying binding by CFTR antibodies to epithelial structures (aminoethylcarbazole detection of horseradish peroxidase with hematoxylin counterstain). *(Used with permission from Rowe SM, Miller S, Sorscher EJ. Cystic fibrosis. N Engl J Med 2005;352(19):1992–2001. Copyright © 2005 Massachusetts Medical Society. All rights reserved.)*

Gastrointestinal

1. Control pancreatic insufficiency by providing adequate enzyme supplementation.
2. Optimize growth and nutritional status.
3. Promote healthy bowel habits.
4. Maintain normal fat-soluble vitamin levels.

Reproduction

1. Provide mutation analysis with appropriate genetic counseling at the time of diagnosis and periodically thereafter.

TABLE 29-1 Cystic Fibrosis Foundation Diagnosis Criteria and Clinical Presentation

A. Meets one or more of the following clinical features associated with the CF phenotype plus:
  a. Two CF mutations
  b. Two positive QPIT results
  c. An abnormal transepithelial potential difference value

B. The following are typical phenotypes associated with CF:
  a. Chronic sinopulmonary disease
    i. Persistent colonization/infection with pathogens typical of CF lung disease
    ii. Endobronchial disease manifested by
      1. Cough and sputum production
      2. Wheeze and air trapping
      3. Radiographic abnormalities
      4. Evidence of obstruction on pulmonary function test
      5. Digital clubbing
    iii. Chronic sinus disease
      1. Nasal polyps
      2. Radiographic changes
  b. GI/nutritional abnormalities
    i. Intestinal abnormalities
      1. Meconium ileus
      2. Exocrine pancreatic insufficiency
      3. Distal intestinal obstruction syndrome
      4. Rectal prolapse
      5. Recurrent pancreatitis
    ii. Chronic hepatobiliary disease manifested by clinical and/or laboratory evidence of
      1. Focal biliary cirrhosis
      2. Multilobar cirrhosis
    iii. Failure to thrive
    iv. Hypoproteinemia–edema
    v. Fat-soluble vitamin deficiencies
  c. Obstructive azoospermia in males
  d. Salt-loss syndromes
    i. Acute salt depletion
    ii. Chronic metabolic alkalosis
  e. CF in a first-degree relative

CF, cystic fibrosis; GI, gastrointestinal; QPIT, quantitative pilocarpine iontophoresis test.

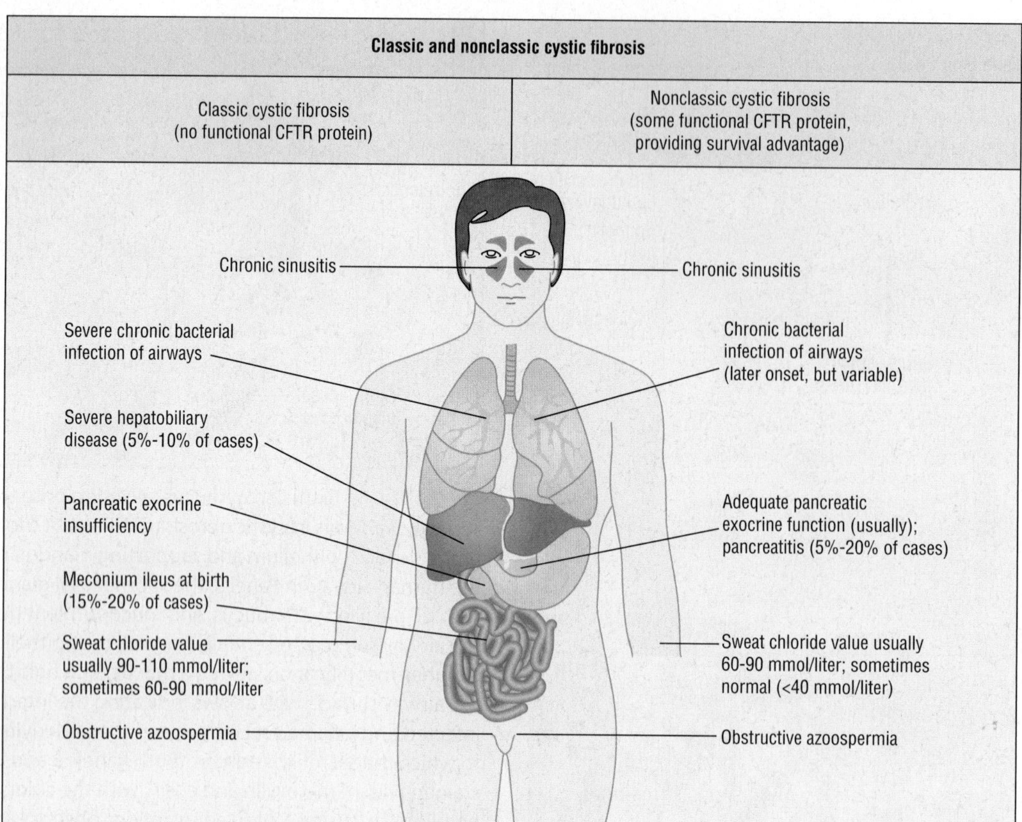

FIGURE 29-3 Classic and nonclassic cystic fibrosis (CF). The findings in classic CF are shown on the left-hand side, and those of nonclassic CF on the right-hand side. Patients with nonclassic CF have better nutritional status and better overall survival. Although the lung disease is variable, patients with nonclassic CF usually have late-onset or more slowly progressive lung disease. Sweat-gland function, as evidenced by the sweat chloride test, is abnormal but not to the extent noted in classic CF. Pancreatitis may occur in patients with nonclassic disease. However, chronic sinusitis and obstructive azoospermia occur in both groups of patients. On the basis of these findings, one can infer that mutations in *CTFR*, perhaps coupled with other genetic or environmental factors, may confer a predisposition to sinusitis, pancreatitis, or congenital bilateral absence of the vas deferens (azoospermia) in the general population. *(Used with permission from Knowles MR, Durie PR. What is cystic fibrosis? N Engl J Med 2002;347(6):439–442. Copyright © 2002 Massachusetts Medical Society. All rights reserved.)*

Psychosocial

1. Keep these patients living essentially normal lives by being active in school and the workplace.
2. Encourage adherence with pharmacological and nonpharmacological therapies in order to help prolong CF patient's lives.

NUTRITION

1 In healthy individuals, the pancreas is vital to the absorption and digestion of essential nutrients for the body's growth and function. In pancreatic-insufficient CF individuals, the resulting inability to absorb these nutrients may lead to malnourishment. The focus of treatment lies in achieving and maintaining normal weight for adults and normal growth patterns for children. This is mostly achieved by managing GI and pulmonary symptoms, monitoring nutrient and energy intakes, and addressing psychosocial and financial issues. The CF Foundation recommends that both children and adults optimize nutritional status, due to its association with healthy pulmonary function, including better FEV_1, and an increase in survival.

To help meet this desired outcome, the CF Foundation recommends energy intakes greater than the standard for the general population to support weight gain and maintenance in children over 2 years and in adults. Trial evidence gathered from population-based studies has shown that energy intakes of 110% to 200% compared to the general health population intakes yield improved nutritional status in CF individuals. The CF Foundation has also established consensus-based assessment parameters to monitor nutritional status in CF individuals. These parameters and goals are listed in Table 29-2. In order to achieve these goals, pancreatic enzyme replacement therapy (PERT) is used to improve fat absorption due to pancreatic insufficiency. For patients who consistently fail to meet weight requirements, the clinician must consider the use of nutritional supplements that may be given orally or enterally via a percutaneous endoscopic gastrostomy (PEG) tube.

PERT has been proven both safe and efficacious in improving nutritional status in CF patients and is recommended in addition to adequate dietary intake. Consensus-based guidelines have established a dose of 500 to 2,500 lipase units per kilogram (kg) of body weight per meal; or 10,000 units per kg per day; or 4,000 units per gram of dietary fat per day. Generic enzyme supplements are not bioequivalent; therefore, the CF Foundation does not recommend their use.

Historically, pancreatic enzymes were considered nutritional supplements, and were not under the Food and Drug Administration (FDA) jurisdiction. New regulations now require all pancreatic enzyme supplements to obtain FDA approval. Table 29-3 shows currently used enzyme preparations.[18-39]

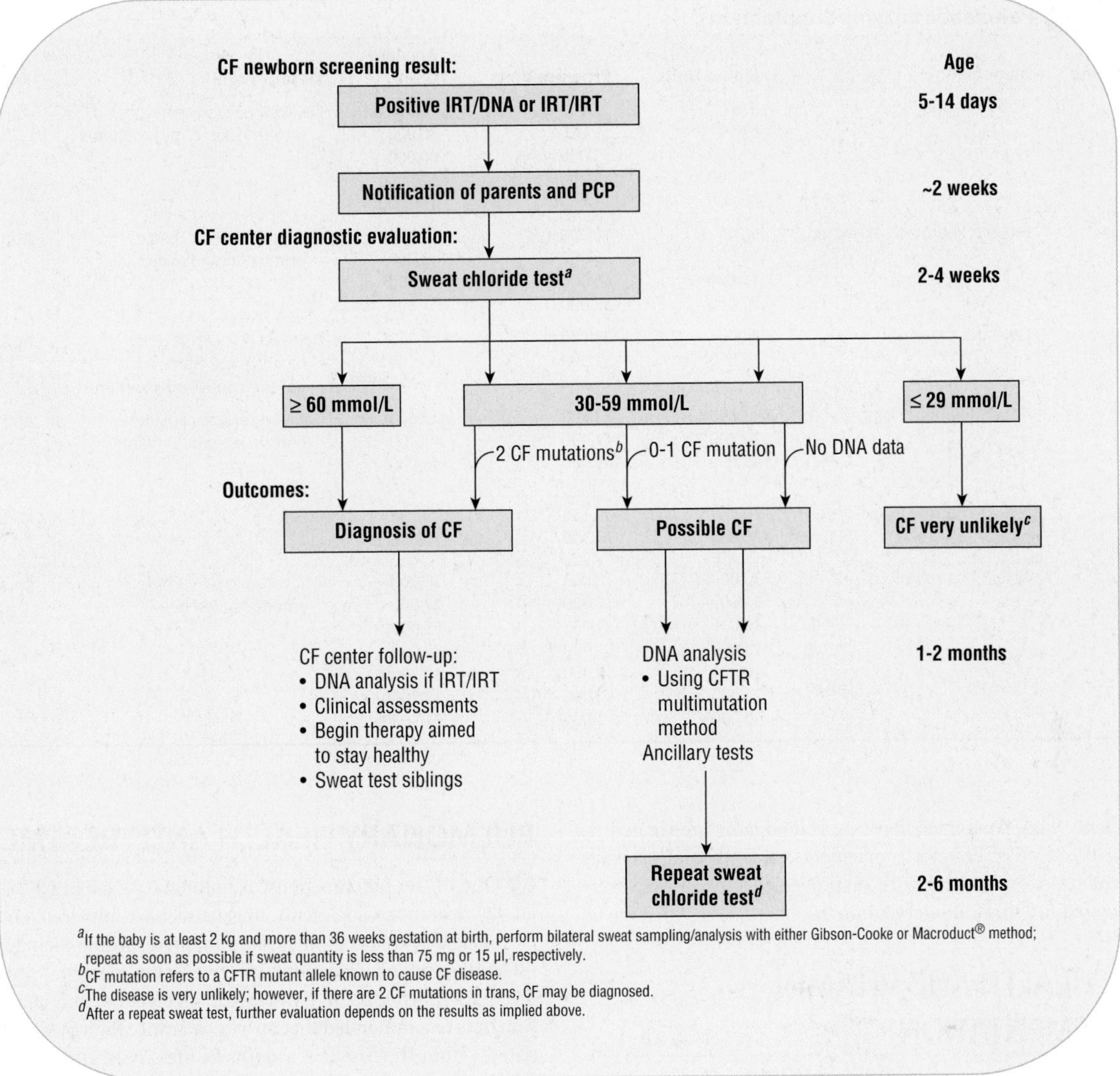

FIGURE 29-4 The cystic fibrosis (CF) diagnostic process for screened newborns. *(Used with permission from Farrell PM, Rosenstein BJ, White TB, et al. Guidelines for the diagnosis of cystic fibrosis in newborns through older adults: Cystic Fibrosis Foundation Consensus Report.* J Pediatr *2008;153(2):S4-S14.)*

TABLE 29-2 Cystic Fibrosis Foundation Nutritional Assessment Parameters and Recommendations

- Age-appropriate BMI method should be utilized to assess weight and height.
- Better FEV_1 status at about 80% (0.80) predicted or above was associated with BMI % at 50th percentile or higher.
- For children and adolescents aged 2-20 years, the CF Foundation recommends that weight-for-stature assessment uses the BMI percentile method and those children and adolescents maintain a BMI at or above the 50th percentile.
- For children diagnosed <2 years, the CF Foundation recommends that children reach a weight-for-length status of 50th percentile by 2 years.
- For adults 20 years and older, the CF Foundation recommends that weight-for-stature assessment use the BMI method and that women maintain a BMI ≥22, and men maintain a BMI ≥23.
- For adults 20 years and older, the CF Foundation recommends that unintentional weight loss be avoided. When encountered in patient care, unintentional weight loss should be evaluated in the context of the patient's usual weight and health status.

BMI, body mass index; CF, cystic fibrosis; FEV_1, forced expiratory volume at 1 second.

Most preparations are capsules containing enteric-coated microspheres or enteric-coated tablets designed to withstand the acidic environment in the stomach allowing for absorption in the small intestine. Frequently CF patients require the addition of histamine receptor antagonists or proton-pump inhibitors in order to create an alkaline environment in the intestine. Enteric-coated capsules should not be crushed but may be opened and mixed with nonalkaline food. However, if allowed to sit in food for a prolonged amount of time, the enteric coating will be lost and enzymes inactivated. Enzymes are administered prior to meals, snacks, and fat-soluble vitamins.[40]

Patients dosed beyond the recommended guidelines may develop fibrosing colonopathy, which leads to colonic strictures. This condition should be considered in individuals who have evidence of obstruction, bloody diarrhea, or ascites, as well as in patients who have a combination of abdominal pain, ongoing diarrhea, and/or poor weight gain. Risk factors for fibrosing colonopathy include: age less than 12 years; enzyme dosages more than 6,000 lipase units/kg/meal for more than 6 months; history of meconium ileus or distal intestinal obstruction syndrome (DIOS); history of any intestinal surgery; and inflammatory bowel disease.

TABLE 29-3 Pancreatic Enzyme Supplements

Trade Name	Manufacturer	Lipase Units	Protease Units	Amylase Units	Dosage Form	FDA Approval
Creon®	Abbott Laboratories	3,000 6,000 12,000 24,000 36,000	9,500 19,000 38,000 76,000 114,000	15,000 30,000 60,000 120,000 180,000	Delayed release capsule, enteric-coated microspheres	Approved
Pancreaze®	Janssen Pharmaceuticals, Inc.	4,200 10,500 16,800 21,000	10,000 25,000 40,000 37,000	17,500 43,750 70,000 61,000	Delayed release capsule, enteric-coated microtablets	Approved
Pertzye®	Digestive Care, Inc.	8,000 16,000	28,750 57,500	30,250 60,500	Delayed-release capsule, bicarbonate-buffered enteric-coated microspheres	Approved
Ultresa®	Aptalis Pharma US, Inc.	13,800 20,700 23,000	27,600 41,400 46,000	27,600 41,400 46,000	Delayed-release capsule, enteric-coated minitablets	Approved
Viokace	Aptalis Pharma US, Inc.	10,440 20,880	39,150 78,300	39,150 78,300	Tablet	Approved
Zenpep®	Aptalis Pharma US, Inc.	3,000 5,000 10,000 15,000 20,000 25,000 40,000	10,000 17,000 34,000 51,000 68,000 85,000 136,000	16,000 27,000 55,000 82,000 109,000 136,000 218,000	Delayed-release capsule, enteric-coated beads	Approved

Patients who experience fibrosing colonopathy are treated by reducing the dose of enzyme supplements, or with oral laxatives and/or enemas, all of which have been proven effective. More severe cases may require surgical intervention.[41]

BONE HEALTH AND VITAMIN SUPPLEMENTATION

Increased longevity in CF patients has revealed bone disease as an emerging complication. Many studies have observed that 50% to 75% of CF adults have low bone density and increased rates of fractures. CF patients are especially at risk as a result of several contributing factors: malabsorption of vitamin D, poor nutritional status, physical inactivity, glucocorticoid therapy, delayed pubertal maturation, and early hypogonadism. Increased bone resorption and decreased bone formation are likely stimulated by elevated serum cytokine levels triggered by chronic pulmonary inflammation. Additionally, chronic infections lead to bone loss in patients regardless of pancreatic sufficiency. Pancreatic-insufficient CF patients lack the ability to absorb fat-soluble vitamins A, D, E, and K (ADEK). Decreased calcium absorption and intake can also compound this problem. As bone disease progresses, this can lead to exclusion from lung transplantation, which is often a life-saving operation for individuals with CF.

Appropriate bone density monitoring for CF patients requires obtaining levels of fat-soluble vitamins yearly, as well as treatment with daily supplementation. Special multivitamin formulations contain high amounts of fat-soluble vitamins designed to deliver the appropriate doses required. Recommended vitamin D levels are a minimum of 30 ng/mL (75 nmol/L). Even with these precautions, adequate vitamin D levels may be difficult to maintain due to altered absorption, reduced fat mass, and minimal exposure to sun light. Medical management of CF patients can also contribute to bone disease by the administration of glucocorticoids, posttransplant immunosuppressant therapies, and antibiotic therapies that require protection from sunlight exposure.[42-51]

PULMONARY HEALTH AND TREATMENT

2 One of the fundamentals of pulmonary care in CF patients is airway clearance. CF patients, in general, have impaired mucociliary clearance that results in thick sputum, predisposing them to chronic infections and inflammation. Effective airway clearance involves the use of a bronchodilator, a mucolytic medication, and chest percussion. It is recommended that airway clearance therapy (ACT) be initiated within the first few months of life. Table 29-4 shows typical medications used in airway clearance.

Choosing a particular ACT routine for a patient is based on the patient's needs. There is no consensus on the optimal method of ACT. The regimen including duration or number of treatments per day may be changed in response to acute illness or exacerbations.

Chest percussion was originally performed with a cupped hand pounding on the chest that generated percussion or vibration. Currently, the most convenient method is the use of a percussion vest. Aerobic exercise is also effective and recommended for improved airway clearance.[52]

The recommended sequence of clearance therapy or "pulmonary toilet" regimen is as follows (note that these therapies are recommended for individuals ≥6 years and are administered concurrently with percussion therapy):

1. Bronchodilator: Albuterol is commonly used for this indication. It helps open up the airways and prevents bronchospasm.
2. Hypertonic saline (HyperSal®): It hydrates the airway mucus secretions and facilitates mucociliary function.

TABLE 29-4 Airway Clearance Therapies

	Dose
Albuterol	2 puffs prior to therapy 2-4 times a day
HyperSal® (hypertonic saline)	4 mL delivered via a nebulizer 2-4 times a day
Pulmozyme® (dornase alfa)	2.5 mg delivered via a nebulizer 1-2 times a day

3. Dornase alfa (Pulmozyme®): Enzyme that cleaves extracellular DNA, which results in decreased viscosity of mucus.
4. Aerosolized antibiotics (ie, Aztreonam [Cayston], tobramycin [TOBI®]): If this therapy is indicated based on severity of lung disease and sputum cultures, it is administered after the CF patient completes percussion therapy.

Bronchodilator therapy is recommended for patients 6 years or older who demonstrate bronchiole hyperresponsiveness or a bronchodilator response. Chronic use of bronchodilator therapy is recommended to improve lung function by enhancing mucociliary action.[53,54]

Inhaled hypertonic saline is a novel agent used for the treatment of CF. Based on the "low-volume model" theory, the use of hypertonic saline would restore airway hydration and enhance mucociliary function.[55] Hypertonic saline is recommended for patients 6 years or older. A study conducted in Australia showed that CF patients who surfed had better pulmonary outcomes than other patients who did not surf.[56] Researchers believed that the inhalation of ocean water helped improve FEV_1 in CF patients who surfed. In this study, 24 patients were randomly assigned to receive a daily treatment of 7% hypertonic saline with or without pretreatment of a control. Clearance and pulmonary function were measured during a 14-day period. Results showed significant improvement in FEV_1 and forced vital capacity (FVC), as well as improvement of respiratory symptoms in hypertonic saline patients. The study also demonstrated that these patients were able to sustain mucus clearance for more than 8 hours. Other studies assessing the use of hypertonic saline have supported this study, showing an improvement in lung function and a 56% reduction in exacerbations. Known side effects during administration include irritation to the airways, which may lead to a drop in FEV_1, increased cough, sore throat, and chest tightness. In an attempt to ameliorate these symptoms, providers may use a lower concentration of 3% hypertonic saline.[53-57]

Dornase alfa (Pulmozyme®) is also recommended in all patients 6 years or older, and is strongly recommended in patients with moderate-to-severe lung disease, to improve lung function and reduce exacerbations. Three randomized controlled trials and a crossover trial involving 520 patients were conducted. Study results showed improvement in FEV_1 by 3.2% and a reduction in exacerbations.[53,58,59]

Anti-inflammatory Therapies

Pulmonary inflammation begins early in life, as shown by the predominance of proinflammatory mediators that can be seen on bronchiolar lavage. A normal inflammatory response to bacteria becomes pathologic in CF patients who have both a prolonged and exaggerated reaction. Treatment of this inflammatory response is crucial to treating the CF patient.

Anti-inflammatory therapies must address the neutrophil response and inhaled therapies will target the endobronchial location, which is the site of inflammation. Using medications that terminate the inflammatory process may be effective. Airway clearance and antibiotics will help control the inflammatory stimulation. Steroids and nonsteroidal anti-inflammatory drugs (NSAIDs) are not widely used because of long-term safety concerns. High-dose ibuprofen (20-30 mg/kg of body weight twice daily) has proven efficacious in a study where patients showed less decline in pulmonary function when compared with patients given placebo. Patients on high dose ibuprofen were able to maintain weight and had less hospital admissions. The benefits of this regimen exceed the risks of GI complications and nephrotoxicity. Despite these outcomes, less than 5% of CF patients in the United States are on this regimen. The low number of patients using this proven therapy may be related to the requirement to obtain a specific therapeutic level of ibuprofen, which in turn requires frequent blood draws for pharmacokinetic monitoring.[7,53,60-63]

Studies with macrolides have shown an inhibition of the neutrophil migration and a decrease in production of proinflammatory mediators. It is unclear at this point if the anti-inflammatory effects of macrolides are a combination of antimicrobial and/or immunomodulatory mechanisms of action. A study conducted in Japan first demonstrated the benefit of macrolides against *Pseudomonas aeruginosa*. Four randomized controlled trials have since demonstrated this effect with azithromycin (250-500 mg) given three times weekly, which has led to increased nutritional status and decreased pulmonary infections. Other treatments are under investigation, but larger studies are needed before they become recommended therapies.[53,60,64,65]

Infectious Disease

3 Antibiotic therapy plays two integral roles in the treatment of CF patients: improving pulmonary function and preventing pulmonary failure. Oral, IV, and aerosolized antibiotic formulations are indicated and used in patients who experience acute pulmonary exacerbations, are chronically infected with *P. aeruginosa*, or require prevention of chronic *P. aeruginosa* infection. A major disadvantage of treatment in CF patients is that pathogens are not fully eradicated from the airways and will often develop resistance. Unfortunately, this limits antimicrobial selection, and can contribute to deterioration of pulmonary function (Table 29-5).

Early in life, patients will routinely be colonized with *Staphylococcus aureus* and then later with *P. aeruginosa*. A 5- to 7-year study of cephalexin prophylaxis in young CF children showed decreased *S. aureus* colonization; however, there was an increase in frequency of *P. aeruginosa* infections. Ultimately, this study showed no significant improvement in health outcomes, therefore, prophylaxis for *S. aureus* colonization is not recommended.[66,67]

The finding of *P. aeruginosa* on sputum culture is a predictor of morbidity and mortality. There are relatively few antibiotics available for the treatment of *P. aeruginosa*. Antibiotics available include extended-spectrum penicillins, select cephalosporins, select carbapenems, aztreonam, quinolones, colistimethate, and aminoglycosides. The only two mechanisms of action represented in this group are cell wall destruction and inhibited cell wall synthesis by ribosomal attachment. Standard practice is to combine these two mechanisms for the best bactericidal results. It is not unusual for patients to have multiple organisms growing in their sputum. The clinician can review the quantitative sputum culture for both the organisms present and the amount or colony forming units grown. By targeting the organisms with the most numerous organisms present and reviewing the susceptibility panels, the clinician can choose the most appropriate regimen. After years of drug exposure, older CF patients will exhibit multidrug-resistant *P. aeruginosa*. At this point, sputum cultures can be sent to specialized laboratories that will test combinations of antibiotics and report out any synergy results. Aerosolized antibiotics are directly deposited into the lung, providing concentrations that may overcome the standard measures of resistance.[68]

Other organisms that may be seen are *Alcaligenes*, *Stenotrophomonas*, *Mycobacteria*, *Aspergillus*, and *Burkholderia*. The importance of *Alcaligenes* as a pathogen is not well described. Originally only thought to have a prevalence of 2.7%, better lab testing and more studies have found infection rates closer to 8% in CF patients older than 6 years.[69-72] *Stenotrophomonas* is intrinsically multidrug resistant and pathogenic. A risk factor for acquiring this organism may be broad-spectrum antibiotic use (carbapenems and cephalosporins).[73,74] Quite often this bacteria is misidentified and confirmatory testing may show *Burkholderia*. Prevalence in American CF patients is reported to be 8.4%; however, some centers report incidence to be as high as 25%.[75-77] Treatment choice is trimethoprim–sulfamethoxazole or doxycycline. *Mycobacteria* have been reported with more frequency in the past 10 years. Species include *M. tuberculosis*, nontuberculosis *M. chelonei, M. fortuitum*, and *M. avium-intracellulare* (MAI). The impact of *Mycobacteria* in the CF patient is unclear. Caseating granulomas have been found in some patients with clinical disease while other patients with

TABLE 29-5 Antimicrobial Agents Used in Cystic Fibrosis

Antibiotic Oral	Pediatric Dose (mg/kg/day)	Adult Dose	Frequency Range	Pathogens
Ciprofloxacin	40	750 mg	Q 12 H	*Pseudomonas, Alcaligenes*
Sulfamethoxazole/ Trimethoprim	15-20 mg of TMP	15-20 mg of TMP/kg/day	Q 6-8 H	*Staphylococcus* (MRSA, MSSA), *Burkholderia Stenotrophomonas, Alcaligenes*
Doxycycline	2-4	Max 200 mg/day	Q 12-24 H	*Stenotrophomonas, Staphylococcus*
IV				
Amikacin	30	15 mg/kg/day	Q 8 H	*Pseudomonas*
Aztreonam	200-300	2 g	Q 6-8 H	*Pseudomonas*
Cefepime	150-200	2 g	Q 8 H	*Pseudomonas*
Ceftazidime	150-200	2 g	Q 8 H	*Pseudomonas, Burkholderia, Alcaligenes*
Ciprofloxacin	30	400 mg	Q 8 H	*Pseudomonas, Alcaligenes*
Colistimethate	5-8	5-8 mg/kg/day	Q 8 H	*Pseudomonas*
Doxycycline	4	Max 200 mg/day	Q 12-24 H	*Stenotrophomonas, Staphylococcus*
Gentamicin	10-12	7.5-10 mg/kg/day	Q 6-8 H	*Pseudomonas*
Imipenem	60-100	2-4 g	Q 6 H	*Pseudomonas, Burkholderia, Alcaligenes*
Meropenem	120	1-2 g	Q 8 H	*Pseudomonas, Burkholderia, Alcaligenes*
Piperacillin–Tazobactam	300-400 (piperacillin component)	4.5 g	Q 4-6 H	*Pseudomonas, Alcaligenes, Staphylococcus* MSSA
Ticarcillin–Clavulanate	300-400 (ticarcillin component)	3.1 g	Q 4 H	*Pseudomonas, Alcaligenes Staphylococcus* (MSSA)
Tobramycin	10-12	7.5-10 mg/kg/day	Q 6-8H	*Pseudomonas*
Vancomycin	60	15 mg/kg	Q 6-12 H	*Staphylococcus* (MRSA, MSSA)
Inhalation				
Tobramycin (Tobi®, Bethkis®)	60-600 mg/day	60-600 mg/day	Q 12 H	*Pseudomonas*
Tobramycin (TOBI Podhaler®)	224 mg/day	224 mg/day	Q 12 H	
Colistimethate	75 mg/day	75 mg/day	Q 12 H	*Pseudomonas*
Aztreonam (Cayston®)	225 mg/day	225 mg/day	Q 8 H	*Pseudomonas*

nontuberculous mycobacteria (NTM) have shown no adverse consequences.[78-81] *Aspergillus* species has a prevalence of 10% to 25% in American CF patients. During the TOBI® trials, patients treated with aerosolized tobramycin appeared to be more at risk for colonization with *Aspergillus* than the placebo group. Although *Aspergillus* does not directly inhibit lung function, it may cause allergic bronchopulmonary aspergillosis which is an immunologic-mediated response to the presence of *Aspergillus* in the lungs.[82,83] *B. cepacia* is now known to be a bacterial species called "genomovars." Currently, up to nine species have been identified.

The two typical antimicrobial choices to treat *B. cepacia* are ceftazidime and trimethoprim-sulfamethoxazole®. It is important to recognize the transmission of *B. cepacia* from patient to patient has been shown via droplet route and therefore proper infection control precautions should be taken.[84-86]

Although CF patients are not more susceptible to respiratory viral infections, the outcome of such illnesses may be more severe. Decline in pulmonary function can be directly related to the number of annual viral infections. Newborns diagnosed with CF should be evaluated to receive respiratory syncytial virus (RSV) prevention with Synagis® (palivizumab), a monoclonal antibody for the first 2 years of life. Synagis® is usually dosed at 15 mg/kg intramuscularly once a month during the RSV season. All CF patients who are 6 months of age or older should receive the annual influenza vaccine.[87-93]

The CF Foundation recommends inhaled tobramycin (TOBI®) to CF patients 6 years or older, with mild to severe lung disease with persistent *Pseudomonas* present in sputum cultures. Aerosolized antibiotics deliver drug locally to the lung while decreasing the risk of systemic side effects. In 1998, the FDA approved TOBI® for treating bacterial lung infections in patients with CF. Routine monitoring of serum aminoglycoside levels is unnecessary in patients with normal renal function using approved doses. It is recommended that CF patients use a preservative-free formulation of aerosolized antibiotics to prevent occurrence of bronchospasm.[94]

Geller et al. describes the pharmacokinetics of inhaled TOBI®, specifically looking at sputum concentrations in CF patients receiving three cycles of routine TOBI® (ie, 28 days on, 28 days off), 300 mg twice daily. The study followed 258 patients for 24 weeks, and showed that approximately 95% of patients achieved sputum concentrations of more than 25 times the minimum inhibitory concentration (MIC) of *Pseudomonas* isolates. This confirmed that inhaled TOBI® can be efficacious in helping prevent the progression of lung disease. At 25 times the MIC, tobramycin has a bactericidal effect.[95]

In 2010, the FDA approved an inhaled formulation of aztreonam, known as, Cayston®, for the treatment of *Pseudomonas*. Cayston® is approved for CF patients older than 6 years with mild to severe lung disease and persistent *Pseudomonas* present in sputum cultures. This inhaled formulation of aztreonam has demonstrated improvement in respiratory symptoms and lung function in patients older than 6 years. Cayston® has been compared with TOBI® in a head-to-head trial and met noninferiority and superiority endpoints. It requires an Altera nebulizer that can deliver the medication in 3 minutes. This in itself increases compliance and has a positive impact on the quality of life in CF patients.[96]

Pharmacokinetics

4 CF patients are unique in respect to a larger volume of distribution and a faster rate of clearance. With a larger volume of distribution, patients may require larger antibiotic doses. Dosing intervals become shorter because drugs are eliminated faster. Critically ill patients may vary from their baseline function and require closer monitoring. However, as patients age, they tend to approach normal population parameters. Therapeutic drug monitoring and necessary dosage and regimen adjustments are critical to the successful treatment of CF patients.

Once daily dosing of intravenous aminoglycosides is preferred for ease of home care administration, and may actually work well in this setting. However, given the possibility of a shortened half-life, each patient's unique pharmacokinetic parameters must be calculated to determine if once daily dosing is appropriate.[97,98]

Reproduction

Fertility discussions with older CF patients may arise during clinic visits, and these conversations should include genetic counseling and options for contraception. Drug–drug interactions between oral contraceptive pills (OCPs) and antibiotics should be monitored. Studies have shown that OCP use in CF patients is safe and effective in comparison to other contraception methods. Patches may not reliably adhere to the skin as a result of increased sweat on the surface of the skin.

The issues surrounding the use of contraception among CF men are similar to those among the normal population. CF men should not assume they are infertile, and should adhere to using protective measures in order to prevent unwanted pregnancy and the spread of sexually transmitted diseases. Should a CF male with a nonfunctioning vas deferens desire to become a biological parent, microsurgical epididymal aspiration of spermatozoa with intracytoplasmic sperm injection into the oocyte can be performed.[16]

Diabetes

As CF patients live longer, glucose intolerance and cystic fibrosis related diabetes (CFRD) are common complications. Even though it shares features of type 1 and type 2 diabetes, CFRD is unique because it is influenced by factors specific to CF, including insulin deficiency, undernutrition, chronic and acute infection, elevated energy expenditure, glucagon deficiency, malabsorption, abnormal intestinal transit time, and liver dysfunction.[99] In comparison to the general CF population, patients with CFRD show a higher mortality rate. In a study of 448 patients, 60% of non-CFRD population and 25% of the CFRD were alive at age 30. The average onset of CFRD is between 18 and 21 years, with a slight female predominance and is more commonly seen in CF gene mutation *ΔF508*.[99-104]

It is recommended that at age 10 years and every year thereafter, CF patients be screened for CFRD. The OGTT should be used as the HbA1c is not a reliable indicator of diabetes in this population. In stable outpatients, fasting glucose levels of more than or equal to 126 mg/dL (7.0 mmol/L) are diagnostic of CFRD. A 2-hour OGTT plasma glucose level of more than or equal to 200 mg/dL (greater than 11.1 mmol/L) repeated on two separate days may also be diagnostic of CFRD.[105]

A desired goal in this population is to control hyperglycemia and prevent hypoglycemia in order to reduce acute and chronic diabetes complications. Because insulin deficiency is the hallmark of CFRD, insulin is the recommended medical treatment. Insulin regimens are individualized based on the patient's lifestyle and circumstances. Exercise is encouraged because it can improve peripheral insulin sensitivity and have beneficial effects in overall health, pulmonary function, and well-being.[100-103]

Oral antidiabetic agents have inconsistent results in the literature; therefore, support for their use in therapy for CFRD patients is not recommended. Medications that help improve insulin sensitivity do not address the primary problem of insulin deficiency in CF. Metformin's mechanism of action is to improve hepatic and peripheral insulin sensitivity; however, it is contraindicated in patients with hypoxia due to the risk of fatal lactic acidosis. Additionally, metformin's multiple GI effects include anorexia, diarrhea, flatulence, and abdominal discomfort. Thiazolidinediones help enhance peripheral insulin sensitivity, but there is serious potential for hepatic toxicity due to the underlying liver problems in CF patients. The use of acarbose is also discouraged due to its mechanism of action, which reduces postprandial glucose and insulin excursion by limiting intestinal absorption of glucose. This inhibits the energy absorption in malnourished individuals while causing diarrhea, anorexia, and abdominal discomfort. Sulfonylureas are being considered due to their ability to enhance insulin secretion by acting on a specific islet beta-cell receptor; however, evidence has also shown that these agents bind and inhibit the CFTR. Use of sulfonylureas is not recommended at this time.[100,104] Newer antidiabetic agents effective for treatment of Type 1 and Type 2 diabetes are currently being studied for treatment of CFRD. One current focus is in glucagon-like-peptide (GLP)1, which is an incretin hormone the body releases in response to eating. At least one study has found that CF patients may have a deficiency of this hormone. This deficiency was found in both CF patients with diagnosed diabetes and those without diabetes. It is not yet known how this plays into the future determination of diabetes in CF patients. There are ongoing studies evaluating the results of supplementation with GLP-1 in CF patients. A disadvantage of utilizing these new agents in CFRD is that these therapies target weight loss as well as glycemic control. Weight loss in CF patients may be detrimental to overall health, as the goal is to optimize nutrition status which contributes to optimal pulmonary health and survival.[100-104]

SPECIAL POPULATIONS

Pregnancy

As women with CF live longer, more choose to become pregnant. CF women considering pregnancy and their partners should both undergo genetic counseling. CF women who become pregnant are considered a high-risk pregnancy; therefore, several considerations should be addressed at the onset of and during pregnancy. At the beginning, both current medications and medications that might be used to treat exacerbations need to be considered. Several of these medications are classified as category C and may pose a potential harm to the fetus. These patients should also be screened and treated accordingly for CFRD.

Several complications that will arise during CF pregnancy include increases in minute ventilation, increased oxygen uptake, increased blood volume, and cardiac output. In a woman with severe lung disease, these changes can cause right-sided heart failure.

Other pharmacotherapy issues that are seen in this population are altered pharmacokinetics and increased maintenance of nutritional and pulmonary health.

The addition of the fetus impacts the CF woman's health by placing a strain on a precariously balanced state of being. The CF woman who chooses to breastfeed must take into account the additional nutritional requirement of approximately 500 kcal/day (2,093 kJ/day).[16]

Pediatrics

Education of the parents is emphasized in this population, concerning administration of pancreatic enzymes and infant formula. Parents are also counseled to encourage their child to adhere with pulmonary health and nutritional health practices. As the child grows into adolescence, compliance becomes an issue. Peer pressure and social restraints may interfere with CF compliance and may influence the patients to disregard their personal well-being.

Transplant Patients

Lung transplantation has become an option with a 5-year survival rate of approximately 50%. Criteria for selection of transplant candidates include not only an FEV_1 of less than 30% (less than 0.30), but also gender, nutritional status, diabetic status, sputum microbiology, and number of pulmonary exacerbations. Factors affecting compliance to CF care and to immunosuppressant therapy may also be taken under consideration for candidacy.[16]

NEW THERAPIES

Bronchitol, an inhaled dry powder form of mannitol, is a new agent to help restore normal airway hydration by drawing water to the airway surface, which hydrates secretions to help improve airway clearance. Bronchitol completed two large multinational phase 3 trials, has been approved for CF treatment in Australia, and was submitted to the FDA in 2012. The FDA rejected the new drug application (NDA), due to failure to prove safety and efficacy.[111]

An exciting breakthrough in CF treatment focuses on treating the basic defect of the disease: CFTR dysfunction. Kalydeco® (ivacaftor) was approved on January 31, 2012, for patients 6 years or older with the *G551D* mutation. Ivacaftor works by potentiating the activity of the CFTR protein so that the channels stay open longer on the cell surface. As a result, mucus is thinned by fluid movement into the airways making airway clearance easier for the patient.

In a randomized, double-blind, placebo-controlled trial evaluating ivacaftor in patients 12 years or older, ivacaftor met effectiveness endpoints. Researchers saw significant improvements in lung function, risk of pulmonary exacerbations, respiratory symptoms, and weight and sweat chloride concentrations. The change in baseline FEV_1 was greater than 10.6 percentage points (0.106) in comparison with placebo (*P* less than 0.001) with an improvement in pulmonary function noted by 2 weeks and sustained through week 48. An average weight increase of 2.7 kg was seen in the ivacaftor group versus placebo at the end of 48 weeks. No significant safety issues were noted in the study. Currently, 87.5% of eligible patients are taking ivacaftor.[112,113]

Orkambi® is a combination of ivacaftor and lumacaftor, a CFTR potentiator and CFTR corrector. It was approved by FDA in 2015 for patients 12 years or older with the *ΔF508* mutation. In 2 phase 3 placebo controlled, randomized control trials, Orkambi® showed improvement in percentage of predicted FEV_1, as well as reduction in pulmonary exacerbations in comparison to placebo.[112,113]

Clinical **Controversy...**

CF is a worldwide problem, with a variety of approaches toward treatment. Discussions regarding controversial methods are constantly being held while new therapies are tried. Due to the relatively small population of CF patients, any studies that are conducted are frequently small in number or do not accurately reflect this population. This makes it difficult to extrapolate and come to a consensus regarding therapy. Some of these controversies will be discussed.

Contraceptive use in CF women continues to be a difficult issue to manage due to limited studies and recommendations. According to these studies, majority of CF women are sexually active, and use a variety of contraceptive methods. The most common method reported was the OCP. Although without further research, providers must consider several compounding factors regarding the use of OCPs. Several pharmacokinetic factors are altered in this population, including decreased absorption, increased rate of metabolism, and increased clearance. Drug interactions should also be considered, as CF women will be on antibiotics that may compromise the efficacy of the pill. Emerging therapy modalities such as the CFTR modulators (ie, ivacaftor) need more studies to confirm lack of drug interactions that may compromise contraception. Other risks associated with OCP use include thromboembolic events that may be potentiated in the CF patient with an indwelling central vascular device.

Other contraceptive methods should be considered, such as estrogen patches, intrauterine devices, vaginal rings, and hormone implants. These methods may be beneficial by avoiding first pass metabolism, reducing the risk of drug interactions. Medroxyprogesterone acetate may be beneficial in improving nutritional status, however, contributes to bone mineral density (BMD) loss, leading to early osteoporosis.

In light of this interesting, but sparse data, there is an encouraging possibility that exogenous hormone therapy has a potential benefit to prolong the life span of CF women. In comparison to CF men, women have a worsened disease severity and shorter life span. It is possible that fluctuating estradiol levels are associated with increased pulmonary exacerbations. However, studies in this area are limited and need to be substantiated as hormone therapy is not without risk.

SOCIAL

The social worker is an integral part of the CF team, due to the complex social issues that surround CF patients. Maintaining health insurance is a lifelong problem for CF patients. The inability to pay for CF medications may often influence compliance. Employment is difficult to maintain because some employers may penalize for frequent hospitalizations. Thus, many CF patients have low-paying jobs without insurance coverage.

Building relationships and confiding in others about personal health issues can be intimidating and difficult for CF patients. Due to infection control guidelines, group settings are limited. The use of new technology now allows support groups via video conferencing and online discussion. The decision to marry and/or have children is complicated by an awareness of their abbreviated life span.[16]

SUMMARY

Multidisciplinary care for CF patients should involve pulmonologists, gastroenterologists, pharmacists, social workers, respiratory therapists, and dieticians. Complexity of care requires good communication within the CF team. Although intravenous (IV) antibiotics have historically been a mainstay of therapy, recent focus has shifted to optimizing nutrition status and promoting effective pulmonary clearance. New treatment modalities such as CFTR modulators will necessitate greater involvement by pharmacists. As patients live longer, more social issues arise and medical issues become more complex.

ABBREVIATIONS

ACT	airway clearance therapy
ADEK	fat-soluble vitamins A, D, E, K
BMD	bone mineral density
CF	cystic fibrosis
CFRD	cystic fibrosis related diabetes
CFTR	cystic fibrosis transmembrane conductance regulator
DIOS	distal intestinal obstruction syndrome
FDA	Food and Drug Administration
FEV_1	forced expiratory volume at 1 second
FVC	forced vital capacity
GI	gastrointestinal
IRT	immunoreactive trypsinogen
IV	intravenous
MAI	*Mycobacterium avium-intracellulare*
MIC	minimum inhibitory concentration
NDA	new drug application
NSAIDs	nonsteroidal anti-inflammatory drugs
NTM	nontuberculous mycobacteria
OGTT	oral glucose tolerance test
OCPs	oral contraceptive pills
PEG	percutaneous endoscopic gastrostomy
PERT	pancreatic enzyme replacement therapy
QPIT	quantitative pilocarpine iontophoresis test
RSV	respiratory syncytial virus

REFERENCES

1. Quinton PM. Cystic fibrosis: Lessons from the sweat gland. *Physiology* 2007;22:212-225.
2. American Lung Association. State of Lung Disease in Diverse Communities 2010: Cystic Fibrosis. www.lungusa.org 31August2015.
3. Farrell PM, Rosenstein BJ, White TB, et al. Guidelines for the diagnosis of cystic fibrosis in newborns through older adults: Cystic Fibrosis Foundation Consensus Report. *J Pediatr* 2008;153(2):S4-S14.
4. Sontag MK, Hammond KB, Zielenski J, et al. Two-tiered immunoreactive trypsinogen (IRT/IRT)-based newborn screening for cystic fibrosis in Colorado: Screening efficacy and diagnostic outcomes. *J Pediatr* 2005;147(3 Suppl):S83-S88.
5. Parad RB, Corneau AM. Newborn screening for cystic fibrosis. *Pediatr Ann* 2003;32:528-535.
6. Rohlfs, E, Zhou Z, Heim RA, et al. Cystic fibrosis carrier testing in an ethnically diverse US population. *Clin Chem* 2011;57(6):841-848.
7. Cystic Fibrosis Foundation. Cystic Fibrosis Foundation Patient Registry, 2013 Annual Data Report to the Center Directors. Bethesda, MD: Cystic Fibrosis Foundation, 2014.
8. Cystic Fibrosis Foundation. Clinical Practice Guidelines for Cystic Fibrosis: Preventive and maintenance care for the patient with cystic fibrosis. May 2006;1-24. https://www.portcf.org/Resources/Consensus%20&%20Guidelines/Chapter%201.pdf.
9. Rowe SM, Miller S, Sorscher EJ. Cystic fibrosis. *N Engl J Med* 2005;352(19):1992-2001.
10. Groman JD, Karczeski B, Sheridan M, et al. Phenotypic and genetic characterization of patients with features of "nonclassic" forms of cystic fibrosis. *J Pediatr* 2005;146:675-680.
11. Mickle JE, Cutting GR. Genotype–phenotype relationships in cystic fibrosis. *Med Clin North Am* 2000;84:597-607.
12. Mall M, Grubb BR, Harkema JR, et al. Increased airway epithelial Na+ absorption produces cystic fibrosis-like lung disease in mice. *Nat Med* 2004;10:487-493.
13. Smith JJ, Travis SM, Greenberg EP, et al. Cystic fibrosis airway epithelia fail to kill bacteria because of abnormal airway surface fluid. *Cell* 1996;85:229-236.
14. Engelhardt JF, Yankaskas JR, Ernst SA, et al. Submucosal glands are the predominant site of CFTR expression in the human bronchus. *Nat Genet* 1992;2:240-248.
15. Knowles MR, Durie PR. What is cystic fibrosis? *N Engl J Med* 2002;347(6):439-442.
16. Yankaskas JR, Marshall BC, Sufian B, et al. Cystic fibrosis adult care. *Chest* 2004;125:1S-39S.
17. Kerr M. Cystic fibrosis screening legislated for all newborns by 2010. Medscape Medical News. 2009 Medscape, LLC. July 15, 2009. *http://www.medscape.com/viewarticle/705589_print.*
18. Stallings VA, Stark LJ, Robinson KA, et al. Evidence-based practice recommendations for nutrition-related management of children and adults with cystic fibrosis and pancreatic insufficiency: Results of a systematic review. *J Am Diet Assoc* 2008;108(5):832-839.
19. Steinkamp G, Demmelmair H, Ruhl-Bagheri I, et al. Energy supplements rich in linoleic acid improve body weight and essential fatty acid status of cystic fibrosis patients. *J Pediatr Gastroenterol Nutr* 2000;31:418-423.
20. Richardson I, Nyulasi I, Cameron K, et al. Nutritional status of an adult cystic fibrosis population. *Nutrition* 2000;16:255-259.
21. Stark LJ, Bowen AM, Tyc VL, et al. A behavioral approach to increasing calorie consumption in children with cystic fibrosis. *J Pediatr Psychol* 1990;15:309-326.
22. Stark LJ, Knapp LG, Bowen AM, et al. Increasing calorie consumption in children with cystic-fibrosis—Replication with 2-year follow-up. *J Appl Behav Anal* 1993;26:435-450.
23. Lloyd-Still JD, Smith AE, Wessel HU. Fat intake is low in cystic fibrosis despite unrestricted dietary practices. *JPEN J Parenter Enteral Nutr* 1989;13:296-298.
24. Luder E, Kattan M, Thornton JC, et al. Efficacy of a nonrestricted fat diet in patients with cystic fibrosis. *Am J Dis Child* 1989;143:458-464.
25. Shepherd RW, Holt TL, Cleghorn G, et al. Short-term nutritional supplementation during management of pulmonary exacerbations in cystic fibrosis: A controlled study, including effects of protein turnover. *Am J Clin Nutr* 1988;48:235-239.
26. Hanning RM, Blimkie CJR, Baror O, et al. Relationships among nutritional status and skeletal and respiratory muscle function in cystic fibrosis: Does early dietary supplementation make a difference? *Am J Clin Nutr* 1993;57:580-587.
27. Bentur L, Kalnins D, Levison H, et al. Dietary intakes of young children with cystic fibrosis: Is there a difference? *J Pediatr Gastroenterol Nutr* 1996;22:254-258.
28. Vaisman N, Clarke R, Pencharz PB. Nutritional rehabilitation increases resting energy expenditure without affecting protein turnover in patients with cystic fibrosis. *J Pediatr Gastroenterol Nutr* 1991;13:383-390.
29. Van Biervliet S, De Waele K, Van Winekel M, et al. Percutaneous endoscopic gastrostomy in cystic fibrosis: Patient acceptance and effect of overnight tube feeding on nutritional status. *Acta Gastroenterol Belg* 2004;67:241-244.
30. Peterson ML, Jacobs DR Jr, Mills CE. Longitudinal changes in growth parameters are correlated with changes in pulmonary function in children with cystic fibrosis. *Pediatrics* 2003;112(3 Pt 1):588-592.
31. Konstan MW, Butler SM, Wohl ME, et al. Growth and nutritional indexes in early life predict pulmonary function in cystic fibrosis. *J Pediatr* 2003;142:624-630.
32. Thomson MA, Quirk P, Swanson CE, et al. Nutritional growth-retardation is associated with defective lung growth in cystic-fibrosis: A preventable determinant of progressive pulmonary dysfunction. *Nutrition* 1995;11:350-354.
33. Walker SA, Gozal D. Pulmonary function correlates in the prediction of long-term weight gain in cystic fibrosis patients with gastrostomy tube feedings. *J Pediatr Gastroenterol Nutr* 1998;27:53-56.
34. Navarro J, Rainisio M, Harms HK, et al. Factors associated with poor pulmonary function: Cross-sectional analysis of data from the ERCF. European Epidemiologic Registry of Cystic Fibrosis. *Eur Respir J* 2001;18:298-305.
35. Oliver MR, Heine RG, Ng CH, et al. Factors affecting clinical outcomes in gastrostomy-fed children with cystic fibrosis. *Pediatr Pulmonol* 2004;37:324-329.
36. Smith DL, Clarke JM, Stableforth DE. A nocturnal nasogastric feeding programme in cystic fibrosis adults. *J Hum Nutr Diet* 1994;7:257-262.
37. Williams SG, Ashworth F, McAlweenie A, et al. Percutaneous endoscopic gastrostomy feeding in patients with cystic fibrosis. *Gut* 1999;44:87-90.
38. Steinkamp G, von der Hardt H. Improvement of nutritional status and lung function after long-term nocturnal gastrostomy feedings in cystic fibrosis. *J Pediatr* 1994;124:244-249.
39. FDA approves pancreatic enzyme replacement product for marketing in United States: Creon designed to help those with cystic fibrosis, others with exocrine pancreatic insufficiency. U.S. Food and Drug Administration. U.S. Department of Health & Human Services, 2009.
40. Cystic Fibrosis Foundation. Concepts in CF Care, Vol X, Section 1. Consensus Conferences. Bethesda, MD: Cystic Fibrosis Foundation, 2001.
41. Houwen RH, van der Doef HP, Sermer I, et al. Defining DIOS and constipation in cystic fibrosis with a multicentre study on the incidence, characteristics, and treatment of DIOS. *J Pediatr Gastroenterol Nutr* 2009;49(1):54-58.
42. Aris RM, Merkel PA, Bachrach LK, et al. Consensus statement: Guide to bone health and disease in cystic fibrosis. *J Clin Endocrinol Metab* 2005;90(3):1888-1896.
43. Elkin SL, Fairney A, Burnett S, et al. Vertebral deformities and low bone mineral density in adults with cystic fibrosis: A cross-sectional study. *Osteoporos Int* 2001;12:366-372.
44. Aris RM, Renner JB, Winders AD, et al. Increased rate of fractures and severe kyphosis: Sequelae of living to adulthood with cystic fibrosis. *Ann Intern Med* 1998;128:186-193.
45. Conway SP, Morton AM, Oldroyd B, et al. Osteoporosis and osteopenia in adults and adolescents with cystic fibrosis: Prevalence and associated factors. *Thorax* 2000;55:798-804.
46. Borowitz D, Baker RD, Stallings V. Consensus report on nutrition for pediatric patients with cystic fibrosis. *J Pediatr Gastroenterol Nutr* 2002;35:246-259.
47. Wilson DC, Rashid M, Durie PR, et al. Treatment of vitamin K deficiency in cystic fibrosis: Effectiveness of a daily fat-soluble vitamin combination. *J Pediatr* 2001;138:851-855.
48. Ontjes DA, Lark RK, Lester GE, et al. Vitamin D depletion and replacement in patients with cystic fibrosis. In: Norman A, Bouillon R, eds. *Vitamin D Endocrine System: Structural, Biological, Genetic and Clinical Aspects.* Riverside, CA: Thomasset, University of California, 2000:893-896.
49. Haworth CS, Selby PL, Adams JE, et al. Effect of intravenous pamidronate on bone mineral density in adults with cystic fibrosis. *Thorax* 2001;56:314-316.
50. Haworth CS, Selby PL, Webb AK, et al. Severe bone pain after intravenous pamidronate in adult patients with cystic fibrosis. *Lancet* 1998;86:1753-1754.
51. Tangpricha V, Kelly A, Stephenson A, et al. An update on the screening, diagnosis, management, and treatment of vitamin D deficiency in individuals with cystic fibrosis: Evidence-based recommendations

from the Cystic Fibrosis Foundation. *J Clin Endocrinol Metab* 2012;2011-3050.

52. Flume PA, Robinson KA, O'Sullivan BP, et al. Cystic fibrosis pulmonary guidelines: Airway clearance therapies. *Respir Care* 2009;54(4):522-537.
53. Mogayzel, PJ, Naureckas, ET, Robinson KA, et al. Cystic fibrosis pulmonary guidelines: Chronic medications for maintenance of lung health. *Am J Respir Crit Care Med* 2013;187:680-689.
54. Halfhide C, Evans HJ, Couriel J. Inhaled bronchodilators for cystic fibrosis. *Cochrane Database Syst Rev* 2008;4:CD003428.
55. Ratjen F. Restoring airway surface liquid in cystic fibrosis. *N Engl J Med* 2006;354(3):291-293.
56. Robinson M, Rose BR, et al. A controlled trial of long-term inhaled hypertonic saline in patients with cystic fibrosis. *N Engl J Med* 2006;354(3):229-240.
57. Ballmann M, von der Hart H. Hypertonic saline and recombinant human DNase: A randomised cross-over pilot study in patients with cystic fibrosis. *J Cyst Fibros* 2002;1:35-37.
58. Quan JM, Tiddens HA, Sy JP, et al. A two-year randomized, placebo-controlled trial of dornase alfa in young patients with cystic fibrosis with mild lung function abnormalities. *J Pediatr* 2001;139(6):813-820.
59. Nasr SZ, Kuhns LR, Brown RW, et al. Use of computerized tomography and chest x-rays in evaluating efficacy of aerosolized recombinant human DNase in cystic fibrosis patients younger than age 5 years: A preliminary study. *Pediatr Pulmonol* 2001;31(5):377-382.
60. Nichols DP, Konstan MW, Chmiel JF. Anti-inflammatory therapies for cystic fibrosis-related lung disease. *Clin Rev Allerg Immunol* 2008;35(3):135-153.
61. Lands LC, Milner R, Cantin AM, et al. High-dose ibuprofen in cystic fibrosis: Canadian safety and effectiveness trial. *J Pediatr* 2007;151(3):249-254.
62. Konstan MW, Schluchter MD, Xue W, et al. Clinical use of ibuprofen is associated with slower FEV1 decline in children with cystic fibrosis. *Am J Respir Crit Care Med* 2007;176(11):1084-1089.
63. Konstan MW, Byard PJ, Hoppel CL, et al. Effect of high-dose ibuprofen in patients with cystic fibrosis. *N Engl J Med* 1995;332(13):848-854.
64. Saiman L, Marshall BC, Mayer-Hamblett N, et al. Azithromycin in patients with cystic fibrosis chronically infected with *Pseudomonas aeruginosa*: A randomized controlled trial. *JAMA* 2003;290(13):1749-1756.
65. Wolter J, Seeney S, Bell S, et al. Effect of long term treatment with azithromycin on disease parameters in cystic fibrosis: A randomised trial. *Thorax* 2002;57(3):212-216.
66. Saiman L, Siegel J. Infection control recommendations for patients with cystic fibrosis: Microbiology, important pathogens, and infection control practices to prevent patient-to-patient transmissions. *Infect Control Hosp Epidemiol* 2003;24(5):S6-S52.
67. Stutman HR, Lieberman JM, Nussbaum E, et al. Antibiotic prophylaxis in infants and young children with cystic fibrosis: A randomized controlled trial. *J Pediatr* 2002;140:299-305.
68. Saiman L, Mehar F, Niu WW, et al. Antibiotic susceptibility of multiply resistant *Pseudomonas aeruginosa* isolated from patients with cystic fibrosis, including candidates for transplantation. *Clin Infect Dis* 1996;23:532-537.
69. Cystic Fibrosis Foundation. Patient Registry 1996. In: *Annual Report*. Bethesda, MD: Cystic Fibrosis Foundation, 1997.
70. Cystic Fibrosis Foundation. Patient Registry 1997. In: *Annual Report*. Bethesda, MD: Cystic Fibrosis Foundation, 1998.
71. Burns JL, Emerson J, Stapp JR, et al. Microbiology of sputum from patients at cystic fibrosis centers in the United States. *Clin Infect Dis* 1998;27:158-163.
72. Saiman L, Chen Y, Tabibi S, et al. Identification and antimicrobial susceptibility of *Alcaligenes xylosoxidans* isolated from patients with cystic fibrosis. *J Clin Microbiol* 2001;39:3942-3945.
73. Sattler C, Mason EJ, Kaplan S. Nonrespiratory *Stenotrophomonas maltophilia* infection at a children's hospital. *Clin Infect Dis* 2000;31:1321-1330.
74. Elting LS, Khardori N, Bodey GP, et al. Nosocomial infection caused by *Xanthomonas maltophilia*: A case–control study of predisposing factors. *Infect Control Hosp Epidemiol* 1990;11:134-138.
75. Burde DR, Noble MA, Campbell ME, et al. *Xanthomonas maltophilia* misidentified as *Pseudomonas cepacia* in cultures of sputum from patients with cystic fibrosis: A diagnostic pitfall with major clinical implications. *Clin Infect Dis* 1995;20:445-448.
76. Demko CA, Stern RC, Doershuk CF. *Stenotrophomonas maltophilia* in cystic fibrosis: Incidence and prevalence. *Pediatr Pulmonol* 1998;25:304-308.
77. Denton M, Todd NJ, Kerr KG, et al. Molecular epidemiology of *Stenotrophomonas maltophilia* isolated from clinical specimens from patients with cystic fibrosis and associated environmental samples. *J Clin Microbiol* 1998;36:1953-1958.
78. Kilby JM, Gilligan PH, Yankaskas JR, et al. Nontuberculous mycobacteria in adult patients with cystic fibrosis. *Chest* 1992;102:70-75.
79. Torrens JK, Dawkins P, Conway SP, et al. Non-tuberculous mycobacteria in cystic fibrosis. *Thorax* 1998;53:182-185.
80. Tomashefski JF Jr, Stern RC, Demko CA, et al. Nontuberculous mycobacteria in cystic fibrosis. An autopsy study. *Am J Respir Crit Care Med* 1996;154:523-528.
81. Cullen AR, Cannon CL, Mark EJ, et al. *Mycobacterium abscessus* infection in cystic fibrosis. Colonization or infection? *Am J Respir Crit Care Med* 2003;167:828-834.
82. Equi A, Balfour-Lynn IM, Bush A, et al. Long term azithromycin in children with cystic fibrosis: A randomised, placebo-controlled crossover trial. *Lancet* 2002;360(9338)978-980.
83. Bargon J, Dauletbaev N, Kohler B, et al. Prophylactic antibiotic therapy is associated with an increased prevalence of *Aspergillus* colonization in adult cystic fibrosis patients. *Respir Med* 1999;93:835-838.
84. Coenye T, Vandamme P, Govan JRW, et al. Taxonomy and identification of the *Burkholderia cepacia* complex. *J Clin Microbiol* 2001:3427-3436.
85. Humphreys H, Peckham D, Patel P, et al. Airborne dissemination of *Burkholderia* (*Pseudomonas*) *cepacia* from adult patients with cystic fibrosis. *Thorax* 1994;49:1157-1159.
86. McMeamin JD, Zaccone TM, Coenye T, et al. Misidentification of *Burkholderia cepacia* in US cystic fibrosis treatment centers: An analysis of 1,051 recent sputum isolates. *Chest* 2000;117:1661-1665.
87. Ramsey BW, Gore EJ, Smith AL, et al. The effect of respiratory viral infections on patients with cystic fibrosis. *Am J Dis Child* 1989;143:662-668.
88. Hiatt PW, Grace SC, Kozinetz CA, et al. Effects of viral lower respiratory tract infection on lung function in infants with cystic fibrosis. *Pediatr* 1999;103:619-626.
89. Abman SH, Ogle JW, Harbeck RJ, et al. Early bacteriologic, immunologic, and clinical courses of young infants with cystic fibrosis identified by neonatal screening. *J Pediatr* 1991;119:211-217.
90. Synagis (Palivizumab) package insert. MedImmune Incorporated. July 2008.
91. Gruber WC, Campbell PW, Thompson JM, et al. Comparison of live attenuated and inactivated influenza vaccines in cystic fibrosis patients and their families: Results of a 3-year study. *J Infect Dis* 1994;169:241-247.
92. Gross PA, Denning CR, Gaerlan PF, et al. Annual influenza vaccination: Immune response in patients over 10 years. *Vaccine* 1996;14:1280-1284.
93. Grohskopf L, Uyeki T, Bresee J, et al. Prevention and control of influenza with vaccines: Recommendations of the Advisory Committee on Immunization Practices (ACIP)—United States, 2012-2013 Influenza Season. *MMWR* 2012;61:613-618.
94. Fiel SB. Aerosolized antibiotics in cystic fibrosis: Current and future trends. Expert Rev Respir Med 2009 Medscape, LLC. July 15, 2009. *http://www.medscape.com/viewarticle/579507_print.*
95. Geller, DE, Pitlick WH, Nardella PA. "Pharmacokinetics and bioavailability of aerosolized tobramycin in cystic fibrosis." *Chest* 2002:22(1):219-226.
96. Assael BM, Pressler T, Bilton D, et al. Inhaled aztreonam lysine vs. inhaled tobramycin in cystic fibrosis: A comparative efficacy trial. *J Cyst Fibros* 2012;12(2):130-140. doi:10.1016/j.jcf.2012.07.006.
97. Yaffe S, Gerbracht LM, Mosovich LL, et al. Pharmacokinetics of methicillin in patients with cystic fibrosis. *J Infect Dis* 1977;135(5):828-831.
98. Powell SH, Thompson WL, Luthe MA, et al. Once-daily vs. continuous aminoglycoside dosing: Efficacy and toxicity in animal and clinical studies of gentamicin, netilmicin and tobramycin. *J Infect Dis* 1983;5:918-932.
99. Cystic Fibrosis Foundation. Clinical Care Guidelines for Cystic Fibrosis- Related Diabetes. American Diabetes Association, 2010.
100. Rosenecker J, Eichler I, Kuhn L, et al. Genetic determination of diabetes mellitus in patients with cystic fibrosis. *J Pediatr* 1995;127:441-443.
101. Lanng S, Thorsteinsson B, Lund-Andersen C, et al. Diabetes mellitus in Danish CF patients: Prevalence and late diabetic complications. *Acta Paediatr* 1994;83:72-77.
102. Finkelstein SM, Wielinski CL, Elliott GR, et al. Diabetes mellitus associated with cystic fibrosis. *J Pediatr* 1988;112:373-377.

103. Geffner ME, Lippe BM, Maclaren NK, et al. Role of autoimmunity in insulinopenia and carbohydrate derangements with cystic fibrosis. *J Pediatr* 1988;112:419-421.
104. Sheppard DJ, Welsh MJ. Effect on ATP-sensitive K^+ channel regulators on cystic fibrosis transmembrance conductance regulator chloride currents. *J Gen Physiol* 1992;100:573-591.
105. Moran A, Brunzell C, Cohen RC, et al. Clinical care guidelines for cystic fibrosis-related diabetes. *Diabetes Care* 2010;33(12): 2697-2708.
106. Trouvanziam R, Conrad CK, Bottiglieri T, et al. High-dose oral *N*-acetylcysteine, a glutathione prodrug, modulates inflammation in cystic fibrosis. *Proc Natl Acad Sci USA* 2006;103:4628-4633.
107. Aris RM, Lester GE, Camaniti M, et al. Alendronate for cystic fibrosis adults with low bone density: Results of a randomized, controlled trial. *Am J Respir Crit Care Med* 2006;169:77-82.
108. Rebelo K. ATS 2009: Inhalation powder tobramycin safe, effective to treat *Pseudomonas aeruginosa* in cystic fibrosis patients. *Medscape Medical News*. 2009 Medscape, LLC. July 15, 2009. *http://www.medscape.com/viewarticle/702973_print.*
109. PARI's Altera Delivers Gilead's Cayston, approved by European Commission to treat cystic fibrosis. 2009 PARI Pharma. Sept 23, 2009. http://www.paripharma.com.
110. Cystic Fibrosis Foundation Website, 2013. Cystic Fibrosis Drug Pipeline: Arikace. http://www.cff.org/research/DrugDevelopmentPipeline/.
111. Cystic Fibrosis Foundation Website, 2013. Cystic Fibrosis Drug Pipeline: Bronchitol. http://www.cff.org/research/DrugDevelopmentPipeline/.
112. Ramsey BW, Davies J, McElvaney NG et al. A CFTR potentiator in patients with cystic fibrosis and the G551D mutation. *N Eng J Med* 2011;365:1663-1672.
113. Wainwright CE, Elborn JS, Ramsey BW, et al. Lumacaftor-Ivacaftor in patients with cystic fibrosis homozygous for Phe508del CFTR. *N Eng J Med* 2015;373:220-231.

Drug-Induced Pulmonary Diseases

e30

Hengameh H. Raissy and Michelle Harkins

KEY CONCEPTS

1. Select populations may be more susceptible to toxicities associated with specific agents.
2. Primary treatment is discontinuation of the offending agent and supportive care.

The manifestations of drug-induced pulmonary diseases span the entire spectrum of pathophysiologic conditions of the respiratory tract. As with most drug-induced diseases, the pathological changes are nonspecific. Therefore, the diagnosis is often difficult and, in most cases, is based on exclusion of all other possible causes. In addition, the true incidence of drug-induced pulmonary disease is difficult to assess as a result of the pathological nonspecificity and the interaction between the underlying disease state and the drugs.

Considering the physiologic and metabolic capacity of the lung, it is surprising that drug-induced pulmonary disease is not more common. The lung is the only organ of the body that receives the entire circulation. In addition, the lung contains a heterogeneous population of cells capable of various metabolic functions, including *N*-alkylation, *N*-dealkylation, *N*-oxidation, reduction of *N*-oxides, and *C*-hydroxylation.

In Unites States, more than 2 million cases of adverse drug reactions occur every year with 100,000 reported deaths;[1] 0.3% of hospital deaths are drug-related.[2] Evaluation of epidemiologic studies on adverse drug reactions provides a perspective on the importance of drug-induced pulmonary disease. In a 2-year prospective survey of a community-based general practice, 41% of 817 patients experienced adverse drug reactions.[3] Four patients, or 0.5% of the total respondents, experienced adverse respiratory symptoms. Respiratory symptoms occurred in 1.2% of patients experiencing adverse drug reactions. In a recent retrospective analysis of clinical case series in France, 898 patients had reported drug allergy, with a bronchospasm incidence of 6.9%. When these patients were rechallenged with the suspected drug, only 241 (17.6%) tested positive. The incidence of bronchospasm in patients with positive provocation test was 7.9%.[4]

Adverse pulmonary reactions are uncommon in the general population but are among the most serious reactions, often requiring intervention. In a study of 270 adverse reactions leading to hospitalization from two populations, 3.0% were respiratory in nature.[5] Of the reactions considered to be life threatening, 12.3% were respiratory. An early report on death caused by drug reactions from the Boston Collaborative Drug Surveillance Program indicated that 7 of 27 drug-induced deaths were respiratory in nature.[6] This was confirmed in a follow-up study in which 6 of 24 drug-induced deaths were respiratory in nature.[7]

DRUG-INDUCED APNEA

Apnea may be induced by central nervous system depression or respiratory neuromuscular blockade (Table e30-1). Patients with chronic obstructive airway disease, alveolar hypoventilation, and chronic carbon dioxide retention have an exaggerated respiratory depressant response to narcotic analgesics and sedatives. In addition, the injudicious administration of oxygen in patients with carbon dioxide retention can worsen ventilation-perfusion mismatching, further elevating pCO_2 and thus producing apnea.[8] Although the benzodiazepines are touted as causing less respiratory depression than barbiturates, they may produce a profound additive or synergistic effect when taken in combination with other respiratory depressants. Combining intravenous diazepam with phenobarbital to stop seizures in an emergency department frequently results in admissions to an intensive care unit for a short period of assisted mechanical ventilation, regardless of the drug administration rate. Too rapid intravenous administration of any of the benzodiazepines, even without coadministration of other respiratory depressants, will result in apnea. The risk appears to be the same for the various available agents (diazepam, lorazepam, and midazolam). Respiratory depression and arrests resulting in death and hypoxic encephalopathy have occurred following rapid intravenous administration of midazolam for conscious sedation prior to medical procedures. (1) This has been reported more commonly in the elderly and the chronically debilitated or in combination with opioid analgesics. Concurrent use of inhibitors of cytochrome P450 3A4 with benzodiazepines is likely to lead to greater risk of respiratory depression.

(1) Prolonged apnea may follow administration of any of the neuromuscular blocking agents used for surgery, particularly in patients with hepatic or renal dysfunction. In addition, persistent neuromuscular blockade and muscle weakness have been reported in critically ill patients who are receiving neuromuscular blockers continuously for more than 2 days to facilitate mechanical ventilation.[9,10] This has resulted in delayed weaning from mechanical ventilation and prolonged intensive care unit stays. The prolonged neuromuscular blockade has been confined principally to pancuronium and vecuronium in patients with renal disease. Both agents have pharmacologic active metabolites that are excreted renally. The persistent muscular weakness is less well defined but appears to represent an acute myopathy.[9,11-13] High-dose corticosteroids appear to produce a synergistic effect, supported by animal studies showing that corticosteroids at dosages greater than or equal to 2 mg/kg per day of prednisone produce atrophy in denervated muscle.[14] The fluorinated corticosteroids (eg, triamcinolone) appear to be more myopathic.[15] Dose-dependent respiratory muscle weakness has been reported in chronic obstructive pulmonary disease (COPD) and asthma patients receiving repeated short courses of oral prednisone in the previous 6 months,[16,17] as well as patients with steroid-dependent asthma.

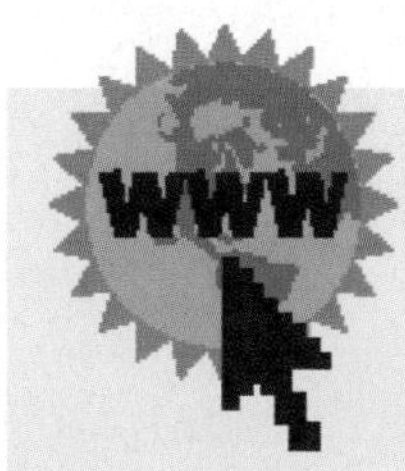

The complete chapter, learning objectives, and other resources can be found at **www.pharmacotherapyonline.com.**

e31 Evaluation of the Gastrointestinal Tract

Keith M. Olsen and Rachael V. McCaleb

KEY CONCEPTS

1. The patient history is key to evaluating gastrointestinal (GI) tract disorders and should include the problem onset, the setting in which it developed, and its presentation. Patient warning signs and alarm symptoms should be identified quickly and referral for further evaluation should be obtained in a prompt manner.
2. A complete physical examination should be performed, the severity and location of symptoms directing the focus of the examination.
3. Contrast agents, barium sulfate and Gastrograffin® (diatrizoate meglumine and diatrizoate sodium solution), have gradually been replaced by endoscopy, but allow evaluation of the hollow organs of the digestive tract for mucosally based lesions as well as narrowing or strictures involving the GI tract.
4. The upper GI series involves radiographic visualization of the esophagus, stomach, and duodenum; whereas, the lower GI series involves visualization of the colon and rectum.
5. Enteroclysis is used to evaluate the small bowel by introducing contrast agents by tube through the nose or mouth directly into the small intestine.
6. Transabdominal ultrasound, computed tomography, and magnetic resonance imaging provide images of the gallbladder, liver, pancreas, and abdominal wall.
7. Radionuclide imaging is sometimes useful to visualize and evaluate the liver, spleen, bile ducts, and gallbladder.
8. The endoscope, an illuminated optical instrument, remains the cornerstone of GI diagnosis and most importantly therapy. Common examples of endoscopic procedures include esophagogastroduodenoscopy, colonoscopy, enteroscopy, endoscopic retrograde cholangiopancreatography, and endoscopic ultrasound.
9. Capsule endoscopy, a newer less invasive endoscopic technique, takes pictures of the GI tract in the assessment of the small bowel in particular.
10. Ambulatory esophageal pH measurement is an important diagnostic test for gastroesophageal reflux disease and is often performed in conjunction with upper endoscopy. Most systems today are completely wireless and patient friendly.
11. Multichannel intraluminal impedance and pH monitoring combines acid exposure with impedance changes in resistant flow to aid the diagnosis of reflux in patients receiving a proton pump inhibitor and other antisecretory medications.

The gastrointestinal (GI) tract is an organ system responsible for nutrient absorption, waste excretion, and immunity. It is composed of the upper GI tract (oral cavity, esophagus, and duodenum), lower GI tract (small intestine, cecum, colon, rectum, and anus), and associated glandular organs (gallbladder, pancreas, and liver). A variety of symptoms can arise from GI tract dysfunction, including heartburn, dyspepsia, abdominal pain, nausea, vomiting, diarrhea, constipation, and GI bleeding. Signs and symptoms of malabsorption, hepatitis, and GI infection are also commonly seen. All clinicians must recognize warning symptoms that include weight loss, intractable vomiting, anemia, dysphagia, odynophagia, and bleeding; and a patient presenting with any of these symptoms should be immediately referred for further diagnostic interventions.

Despite the rapid proliferation of technology for the diagnosis of digestive diseases, the patient history and physical examination remain important for initial assessment, triage, and guidance of further diagnostic interventions. When combined with a thorough patient history and physical examination, diagnostic procedures are essential in the evaluation of GI disorders. This chapter describes the most commonly used clinical tools to evaluate patients with GI tract-related diseases.

The complete chapter, learning objectives, and other resources can be found at **www.pharmacotherapyonline.com.**

Gastroesophageal Reflux Disease

32

Dianne May, Michael Thiman, and Satish S.C. Rao

KEY CONCEPTS

1. Gastroesophageal reflux disease (GERD) can be described on the basis of either esophageal symptoms or esophageal tissue injury. The common symptoms include heartburn, acid brash, regurgitation, chest pain, and dysphagia.
2. Endoscopy is commonly used to evaluate mucosal injury from GERD and to assess for the presence of Barrett's esophagus or other complications such as strictures.
3. Whereas ambulatory reflux monitoring only measures acid reflux, combined impedance–pH monitoring measures both acid and nonacid reflux.
4. The goals of GERD treatment are to alleviate symptoms, decrease the frequency of recurrent disease, promote healing of mucosal injury, and prevent complications.
5. GERD treatment is determined by disease severity and includes lifestyle changes and patient-directed therapy, pharmacologic treatment, and antireflux surgery.
6. Patients with typical GERD symptoms should be treated with lifestyle modifications as appropriate and a trial of empiric acid suppression therapy. Those who do not respond to empiric therapy or who present with alarm symptoms such as dysphagia, weight loss, or GI bleeding should undergo endoscopy.
7. Surgical intervention is a viable alternative treatment for select patients when long-term pharmacologic management is undesirable or when patients have complications.
8. Acid suppression is the mainstay of GERD treatment. Proton pump inhibitors provide the greatest symptom relief and the highest healing rates, especially for patients with erosive disease or moderate to severe symptoms or with complications.
9. Many patients with GERD will relapse if medication is withdrawn; so long-term maintenance treatment may be required. A proton pump inhibitor is the drug of choice for maintenance of patients with moderate to severe GERD.
10. Patient medication profiles should be reviewed for drugs that may aggravate GERD. Patients should be monitored for adverse drug reactions and potential drug–drug interactions.

Gastroesophageal reflux disease (GERD) is a common medical disorder. A consensus definition of GERD is "symptoms or complications resulting from refluxed stomach contents into the esophagus or beyond, into the oral cavity (including the larynx) or lung."[1] The key is that these troublesome symptoms adversely affect the well-being of the patient. Episodic heartburn that is not frequent enough or painful enough to be considered bothersome by the patient is not included in this definition of GERD.

Gastroesophageal reflux disease can be further classified as either symptom-based or tissue injury-based depending on how the patient presents.[1] Symptom-based GERD may exist with or without esophageal injury and most commonly presents as heartburn, regurgitation, or dysphagia. Less commonly, odynophagia (painful swallowing) or hypersalivation may occur. The absence of tissue injury or erosions is commonly termed nonerosive reflux disease (NERD). Tissue injury-based GERD may exist with or without symptoms. The spectrum of injury includes esophagitis (inflammation of the lining of the esophagus), Barrett's esophagus (when tissue lining the esophagus is replaced by tissue similar to the lining of the intestine), strictures, and esophageal adenocarcinoma.[1] Esophagitis occurs when the esophagus is repeatedly exposed to refluxed gastric contents for prolonged periods of time. This can progress to erosion of the squamous epithelium of the esophagus (erosive esophagitis). Complications of long-term reflux may include the development of strictures, Barrett's esophagus, or possibly adenocarcinoma of the esophagus.

Gastroesophageal reflux symptoms associated with disease processes in organs other than the esophagus are referred to as extraesophageal reflux syndromes. Patients with extraesophageal reflux syndromes may present with chest pain, hoarseness of voice, chronic cough/throat clearing, or asthma. An association between these syndromes and GERD should only be considered when they occur along with esophageal GERD syndrome because these extraesophageal symptoms are nonspecific and have many other causes.[1]

Many patients suffering from mild GERD do not go on to develop erosive esophagitis and are often managed with lifestyle changes, antacids, and nonprescription histamine-2 (H_2)-receptor antagonists or nonprescription proton pump inhibitors. Those with more severe symptoms (with or without tissue injury) predictably follow a course of relapsing disease, requiring more intensive treatment with acid suppression therapy followed by long-term maintenance therapy. Antireflux surgery offers an alternative for select patients in whom prolonged medical management is undesirable or who have complications. Bariatric surgery may be an option in obese patients.

EPIDEMIOLOGY

GERD occurs in people of all ages but is most common in those older than age 40 years. Although mortality is rare, GERD symptoms may have a significant economic impact and impact on quality of life. The true prevalence of GERD is difficult to assess because many patients do not seek medical treatment, symptoms do not always correlate well with the severity of the disease, and there is no standardized definition or universal gold standard method for diagnosing the disease. However, the prevalence has risen significantly over the last 20 years with approximately 20% of adults in North America suffering from GERD symptoms on a weekly basis.[2,3] The prevalence of GERD varies depending on the geographic region but appears highest in Western countries and is on the rise.[2,3]

Except during pregnancy, there does not appear to be a major difference in incidence between men and women. Although gender does not generally play a major role in the development of GERD, it is an important factor in the development of Barrett's esophagus and esophageal adenocarcinoma, which are both more common in men. Adenocarcinoma of the esophagus is five-fold more common in those with chronic GERD symptoms than those who do not have GERD.[2] The relationship of adenocarcinoma to Barrett's esophagus, or even just long-standing GERD, which may be an independent risk factor for esophageal adenocarcinoma, remains to be clearly defined.

Other risk factors and comorbidities that may contribute to the development or worsening of GERD symptoms include family history, obesity, smoking, alcohol consumption, certain medications and foods, respiratory diseases, and reflux chest pain syndrome. Obese patients are 2.5 times more likely to experience GERD symptoms.[4] An increased prevalence of GERD was noted in patients with major depressive disorder in a population-based study conducted in a Taiwanese patient population. The exact mechanism of this association cannot be determined at this time.[5]

PATHOPHYSIOLOGY

The key factor in the development of GERD is the abnormal reflux of gastric contents from the stomach into the esophagus, oral cavity, and/or the lung.[1] In some cases, gastroesophageal reflux is associated with defective lower esophageal sphincter (LES) pressure or function (Fig. 32-1). Patients may have decreased gastroesophageal sphincter pressures related to (a) spontaneous transient LES relaxations, (b) transient increases in intra-abdominal pressure, or (c) an atonic LES, all of which may lead to the development of gastroesophageal reflux. Problems with other normal mucosal defense mechanisms, such as abnormal esophageal anatomy, improper esophageal clearance of gastric fluids, reduced mucosal resistance to acid, delayed or ineffective gastric emptying, inadequate production of epidermal growth factor, and reduced salivary buffering of acid, may also contribute to the development of GERD. Substances that may promote esophageal damage on reflux into the esophagus include gastric acid, pepsin, bile acids, and pancreatic enzymes. Thus, the composition and volume of the refluxate, as well as duration of exposure, are important aggressive factors in determining the consequences of gastroesophageal reflux.

The presence of an "acid pocket" has gained attention as a potential explanation for postprandial reflux symptoms and may represent a target for treatment of reflux disease. While gastric acidity is buffered by food, pH monitoring has shown that this buffering effect may vary in different parts of the stomach and esophagus. The acid pocket is thought to be an area of unbuffered acid in the proximal stomach that accumulates after a meal and may contribute to GERD symptoms postprandially.[6] It is thought to occur due to meal-stimulated acid not mixing well with the chyme in the proximal stomach. Gastric secretions form a distinct layer above the chyme.[6] GERD patients are predisposed to upward migration of acid from the acid pocket. In addition, the acid pocket may also be positioned above the diaphragm in patients, especially in those with hiatal hernia, which increases the risk for acid reflux.

Lower Esophageal Sphincter Pressure

The LES is a specialized thickening of the smooth muscle lining of the distal esophagus with an elevated basal resting pressure. The sphincter is normally in a tonic, contracted state, preventing the reflux of gastric material from the stomach, but relaxes on swallowing to permit the passage of food into the stomach. There are three mechanisms by which defective LES pressure may cause gastroesophageal reflux. First, and probably most importantly, reflux may occur following spontaneous transient LES relaxations that are not associated with swallowing. Although the exact mechanism is unknown, esophageal distension, vomiting, belching, and retching cause relaxation of the LES. While not thought to contribute significantly to erosive esophagitis, these transient relaxations, which are normal postprandially, may play an important role in symptom-based esophageal reflux syndromes. Transient decreases in sphincter pressure are responsible for more than half of the reflux episodes in patients with GERD. The propensity to develop gastroesophageal reflux secondary to transient decreases in LES pressure is probably dependent on numerous factors, including the degree of sphincter relaxation, efficacy of esophageal clearance, patient position (more common in recumbent position), gastric volume, and intragastric pressure. Secondly, reflux may occur following transient increases in intra-abdominal pressure (stress reflux). An increase in intra-abdominal pressure such as that occurring during straining, bending over, coughing, eating, or a Valsalva maneuver may overcome a weak LES, and thus may lead to reflux. Thirdly, the LES may be atonic, thus permitting free reflux as seen in patients with scleroderma.

Various foods and medications may aggravate esophageal reflux by decreasing LES pressure or by precipitating symptomatic reflux by direct mucosal irritation (Table 32-1). Pregnancy is a condition in which reflux is common. There are many postulated reasons for the increased incidence of heartburn during pregnancy, including hormonal effects on esophageal muscle, LES tone, and physical factors (increased intra-abdominal pressure) resulting from an enlarging

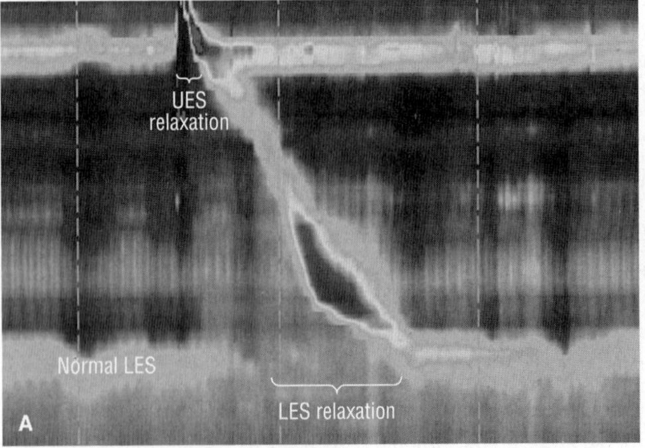

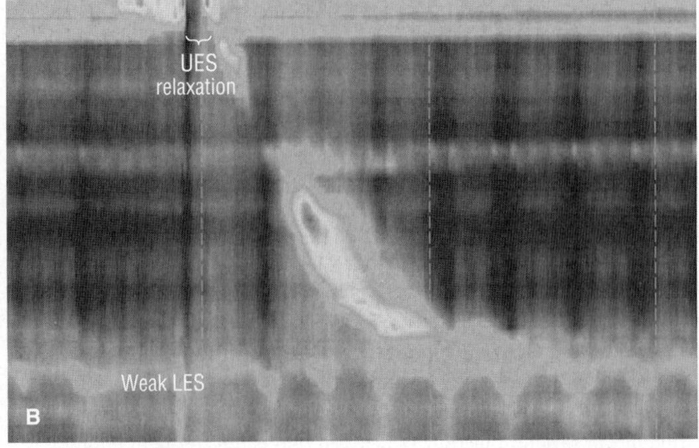

FIGURE 32-1 Comparison of a normal esophageal high-resolution manometry showing normal upper esophageal sphincter and lower esophageal sphincter (LES) resting pressure and relaxations with a water bolus (*A*), compared with that seen in a patient with GERD and a weak resting LES (*B*).

TABLE 32-1 Foods and Medications That May Worsen GERD Symptoms

Foods/Beverages	Medications
Decreased Lower Esophageal Sphincter Pressure	
Fatty meal	Anticholinergics
Carminatives (peppermint, spearmint)	Barbiturates
Chocolate	Caffeine
Coffee, cola, tea	Dihydropyridine calcium channel blockers
Garlic	Dopamine
Onions	Estrogen
Chili peppers	Nicotine
Alcohol (wine)	Nitrates
	Progesterone
	Tetracycline
	Theophylline
Direct Irritants to the Esophageal Mucosa	
Spicy foods	Aspirin
Orange juice	Bisphosphonates
Tomato juice	Nonsteroidal anti-inflammatory drugs (NSAIDs)
Coffee	Iron
Tobacco	Quinidine
	Potassium chloride

uterus. A decrease in LES pressure resulting from any of the previously mentioned causes is not always associated with gastroesophageal reflux. Likewise, individuals who experience decreases in sphincter pressures and subsequently reflux do not always develop GERD. The other natural defense mechanisms (anatomic factors, esophageal clearance, mucosal resistance, and other gastric factors) must be evoked to explain this phenomenon.

Anatomic Factors

Disruption of the normal anatomic barriers by a hiatal hernia (when a portion of the stomach protrudes through the diaphragm into the chest) was once thought to be a primary etiology of gastroesophageal reflux and esophagitis. Now it appears that a more important factor related to the presence or absence of symptoms in patients with hiatal hernia is the LES pressure. Patients with hypotensive LES pressures and large hiatal hernias are more likely to experience gastroesophageal reflux following abrupt increases in intra-abdominal pressure compared with patients with a hypotensive LES and no hiatal hernia. Although anatomic factors are still considered significant by some, the diagnosis of hiatal hernia is currently considered a separate entity with which gastroesophageal reflux may simultaneously occur.

Esophageal Clearance

In many patients with GERD, the problem is not that they produce too much acid but that the acid spends too much time in contact with the esophageal mucosa. Contact time is dependent on the rate at which the esophagus clears the noxious material, as well as the frequency of reflux. Swallowing contributes to esophageal clearance by increasing salivary flow. Saliva contains bicarbonate that buffers the residual gastric material on the surface of the esophagus. The production of saliva decreases with increasing age, making it more difficult to maintain a neutral intraesophageal pH. In addition, swallowing is decreased during sleep, making nocturnal GERD a problem in many patients.

Mucosal Resistance

Within the esophageal mucosa and submucosa there are mucus-secreting glands that may contribute to the protection of the esophagus. Bicarbonate moving from the blood to the lumen can neutralize acidic refluxate in the esophagus. When the mucosa is repeatedly exposed to the refluxate in GERD, or if there is a defect in the normal mucosal defenses, hydrogen ions diffuse into the mucosa, leading to the cellular acidification and necrosis that ultimately cause esophagitis. In theory, mucosal resistance may be related not only to esophageal mucus but also to tight epithelial junctions, epithelial cell turnover, nitrogen balance, mucosal blood flow, tissue prostaglandins, and the acid–base status of the tissue. Saliva is also rich in epidermal growth factor, stimulating cell renewal.

Gastric Emptying/Increased Intra-abdominal Pressure

Delayed gastric emptying can contribute to gastroesophageal reflux. An increase in gastric volume may increase both the frequency of reflux and the amount of gastric fluid available to be refluxed. Gastric volume is related to the volume of material ingested, rate of gastric secretion, rate of gastric emptying, and amount and frequency of duodenal reflux into the stomach. Factors that increase gastric volume and/or decrease gastric emptying, such as smoking and high-fat meals, are often associated with gastroesophageal reflux. This partially explains the prevalence of postprandial gastroesophageal reflux. Fatty foods may increase postprandial gastroesophageal reflux by increasing gastric volume, delaying the gastric emptying rate, and decreasing the LES pressure. Patients with gastroesophageal reflux, particularly infants, may have a defect in gastric antral motility. The delay in emptying may promote regurgitation of feedings, which might, in turn, contribute to two common complications of GERD in infants (eg, failure to thrive and pulmonary aspiration).[7]

Increased GERD symptoms and complications have been seen in obese patients. Obesity is considered an independent risk factor for GERD due to increased intra-abdominal pressure. Interestingly, even weight gain in a non-obese patient has been associated with increased new-onset GERD symptoms. Transient LES relaxations, incompetent LES and impaired esophageal motility have all been attributed to obesity.[8]

Composition of Refluxate

The composition, pH, and volume of the refluxate are important aggressive factors in determining the consequences of gastroesophageal reflux. If the pH of the refluxate is less than 2, esophagitis may develop secondary to protein denaturation. In addition, pepsinogen is activated to pepsin at this pH and may also cause esophagitis. Duodenogastric reflux esophagitis, or "alkaline esophagitis," refers to esophagitis induced by the reflux of bilious and pancreatic fluid. The term alkaline esophagitis may be a misnomer in that the refluxate may be either weakly alkaline or acidic in nature. Although bile acids have both a direct irritant effect on the esophageal mucosa and an indirect effect of increasing hydrogen ion permeability of the mucosa, symptoms are more often related to acid reflux than to bile reflux. Specifically, the percentage of time that the esophageal pH is less than 4 is greater for patients with severe disease as compared with that for patients with mild disease. Nevertheless, the combination of acid, pepsin, and/or bile is a potent refluxate in producing esophageal damage.

Complications

Several complications may occur with gastroesophageal reflux, including esophagitis, esophageal strictures, Barrett's esophagus, and esophageal adenocarcinoma. Strictures are common in the distal esophagus and are generally 1 to 2 cm in length. The use of nonsteroidal anti-inflammatory drugs or aspirin is an additional risk factor that may contribute to the development or worsening of GERD complications. Although GERD may lead to esophageal bleeding, the blood loss is usually chronic and low grade in nature, but anemia may occur. In some patients, the reparative process leads to the replacement of the squamous epithelial lining of the esophagus by specialized columnar-type epithelium (Barrett's esophagus), which increases the incidence of esophageal strictures by as much as 30%. Barrett's esophagus is most prevalent in white males in Western countries. The risk of esophageal adenocarcinoma may be higher for patients with Barrett's esophagus as compared with that for the general population, although not as high as previously thought. The absolute annual risk of esophageal adenocarcinoma was 0.12% in those with Barrett's esophagus.[9]

The pathophysiology of gastroesophageal reflux is a complex cyclic process. It is difficult, if not impossible, to determine which occurs first: gastroesophageal reflux leading to defective peristalsis with delayed clearing or an incompetent LES pressure leading to gastroesophageal reflux. Understanding the factors associated with the development of GERD provides insight into the treatment modalities currently used to manage patients suffering from this disease.

CLINICAL PRESENTATION

1 GERD can be described on the basis of either esophageal symptoms or esophageal tissue injury. The severity of the symptoms of gastroesophageal reflux does not always correlate with the degree of esophageal tissue injury, but it does correlate with the duration of reflux. Similar frequency and severity of both heartburn and regurgitation have been found in patients with NERD compared with those with erosive esophagitis with some differences noted based on gender.[10] It is important to distinguish GERD symptoms from those of other diseases, especially when chest pain or pulmonary symptoms are present.

Diagnostic Tests

The most useful tool in the diagnosis of gastroesophageal reflux is the clinical history, including presenting symptoms and associated risk factors. Patients presenting with typical symptoms of reflux, such as heartburn or regurgitation, do not usually require invasive esophageal evaluation. These patients generally benefit from an initial empiric trial of acid-suppression therapy. A clinical diagnosis of GERD can be assumed in patients who respond to appropriate therapy.[1] Further diagnostic evaluation is useful to prevent misdiagnosis, identify complications, and assess treatment failures.[11] Diagnostic tests should be performed in those patients who do not respond to therapy and in those who present with alarm symptoms (eg, dysphagia, odynophagia, and weight loss), which may be more indicative of complicated disease.

Useful tests in diagnosing GERD include upper endoscopy, ambulatory reflux monitoring, combined impedance–pH monitoring, manometry/high-resolution esophageal pressure topography, and impedance manometry. 2 Endoscopy is commonly used to evaluate mucosal injury from GERD and to assess other complications, such as strictures, Barrett's esophagus or adenocarcinoma. It should be performed in patients not responding to twice daily proton pump inhibitor therapy, and those with dysphagia or unexplained weight loss. Currently endoscopic screening is only recommended in patients with chronic GERD and at least one additional risk factor for esophageal adenocarcinoma.[12]

A camera-containing capsule swallowed by the patient offers the newest technology for visualizing the esophageal mucosa via endoscopy. The PillCam ESO is less invasive than traditional endoscopy and takes less than 15 minutes to perform in the clinician's office. Images of the esophagus are downloaded through sensors placed on the patient's chest that are connected to a data collector.

CLINICAL PRESENTATION GERD[1,11]

Symptom-based GERD Syndromes (With or Without Esophageal Tissue Injury)

Typical symptoms (may be aggravated by activities that worsen gastroesophageal reflux such as recumbent position, bending over, or eating a meal high in fat):

- Heartburn (hallmark symptom described as a substernal sensation of warmth or burning rising up from the abdomen that may radiate to the neck; may be waxing and waning in character)
- Regurgitation/belching
- Reflux chest pain

Alarm symptoms (these symptoms may be indicative of complications of GERD such as Barrett's esophagus, esophageal strictures, or esophageal adenocarcinoma and require further diagnostic evaluation):

- Dysphagia (common)
- Odynophagia
- Bleeding
- Weight loss

Tissue Injury-based GERD Syndromes (With or Without Esophageal Symptoms)

Symptoms (may present with alarm symptoms such as dysphagia, odynophagia, or unexplained weight loss):

- Esophagitis
- Strictures
- Barrett's esophagus
- Esophageal adenocarcinoma

Extraesophageal GERD Syndromes

- Symptoms (these symptoms have an association with GERD, but causality should only be considered if a concomitant esophageal GERD syndrome is also present):
- Chronic cough
- Laryngitis
- Wheezing
- Asthma (~50% with asthma have GERD)

Diagnostic Tests For GERD

Clinical History:

- Generally sufficient to diagnose GERD in patients with typical symptoms

Endoscopy:

- Preferred for assessing for mucosal injury and to assess for complications, such as strictures. Biopsies needed to identify Barrett's esophagus, adenocarcinoma, and eosinophilic esophagitis (a nonacid-related esophageal disorder that generally does not respond well to proton pump inhibitor therapy).

(continued)

CLINICAL PRESENTATION GERD[1,11] (*continued*)

- Non-inflammatory GERD and major motor disorders may be missed by endoscopy.

Ambulatory Reflux Monitoring:

- Identifies patients with excessive esophageal acid exposure and helps determine if symptoms are acid-related
- Useful for patients not responding to acid-suppression therapy
- Documents the percentage of time the intraesophageal pH is <4 and determines the frequency and severity of reflux
- Measures only acid reflux (not nonacid reflux)

Combined Impedance–pH Monitoring:

- Measures both acid and nonacid reflux

Manometry/High-Resolution Esophageal Pressure Topography (HREPT):

- Useful in those who have failed twice-daily proton pump inhibitor therapy with normal endoscopic findings to identify motor disorders, to evaluate peristaltic function in those who are candidates for antireflux surgery, and to assure proper placement of pH probes (the recent advancement of the tubeless pH monitoring system using endoscopic landmarks for placement may negate the need for manometry for ensuring proper placement of esophageal pH probes)

Impedance Manometry:

- Evaluates bolus transit esophageal clearance/retention
- Evaluates LES and upper esophageal sphincter pressures and peristalsis

Empiric Proton Pump Inhibitor as a Diagnostic Test for GERD:

- Less expensive and more convenient than ambulatory pH monitoring but lacks standardized dosing regimen and duration of the diagnostic trial

Barium Radiography:

- Not routinely used to diagnose GERD because it lacks sensitivity and specificity; cannot identify Barrett's esophagus. Can detect hiatal hernia.

The camera-containing capsule is later eliminated in the stool. The main disadvantage of the PillCam is that biopsies cannot be obtained.

Unfortunately, the presence or absence of mucosal damage does not prove the patient's symptoms are reflux related; for that, ambulatory reflux monitoring is useful. 3 Whereas ambulatory reflux monitoring only measures acid reflux, combined impedance–pH monitoring measures both acid and nonacid reflux.

Ambulatory reflux monitoring can be performed by passing a small pH probe transnasally and placing it approximately 5 cm above the LES. Patients are asked to keep a diary of symptoms that later are correlated with the pH measurement corresponding to the time the symptom was reported (Fig. 32-2). Approximately 24 hours of data can be obtained using this method. The wireless pH monitoring involves attaching a radiotelemetry capsule to the esophageal mucosa. The advantages of this method are that a longer period of monitoring is possible (48 hours), it may demonstrate superior recording accuracy compared with some catheter designs, and it is more comfortable for the patient because a nasogastric tube is unnecessary.[1] Proton pump inhibitor therapy should be withheld for 7 days prior to performing ambulatory catheter pH, impedance–pH, or wireless pH monitoring when evaluating patients who have failed an initial empiric therapy and who have normal findings on endoscopy and manometry. However, when testing for nonacid reflux, only impedance–pH monitoring should be performed and testing should be done while patient is still on a proton pump inhibitor.[1] Early referral for ambulatory pH monitoring reduced cost compared to long duration trials of proton pump inhibitors.[13]

Manometry can be performed before ambulatory reflux/impedance testing. Manometry is useful for patients who are candidates for antireflux surgery and for ensuring proper placement of pH probes.

TREATMENT

Therapeutic modalities used in the treatment of gastroesophageal reflux are targeted at reversing the various pathophysiologic abnormalities.

Desired Outcomes

4 The goals of treatment are to (a) alleviate or eliminate the patient's symptoms, (b) decrease the frequency or recurrence and duration of gastroesophageal reflux, (c) promote healing of the injured mucosa, and (d) prevent the development of complications. Therapy is directed at augmenting defense mechanisms that prevent reflux and/or decrease the aggressive factors that worsen reflux or mucosal damage. Therapy is directed at (a) decreasing the acidity of the refluxate, (b) decreasing the gastric volume available to be refluxed, (c) improving gastric emptying, (d) increasing LES pressure, (e) enhancing esophageal acid clearance, and (f) protecting the esophageal mucosa.

General Approach to Treatment

5 GERD treatment is determined by disease severity and includes: (a) lifestyle changes and patient-directed therapy with antacids, nonprescription H_2-receptor antagonists, and/or nonprescription proton pump inhibitors; (b) pharmacologic treatment with prescription-strength acid suppression therapy; (c) and antireflux surgery (Table 32-2).[1,14] The initial therapeutic modality used is in part dependent on the patient's condition (frequency of symptoms, degree of esophagitis, and presence of complications) (Table 32-3). A step-down approach, starting with a proton pump inhibitor, instead of an H_2-receptor antagonist, and then stepping down to the lowest dose of acid suppression (either an H_2-receptor antagonist or proton pump inhibitor) needed to control symptoms, is most often advocated. The clinician should determine the most appropriate approach for the individual patient. Every attempt should be made to aggressively control symptoms and to prevent relapses early in the course of the patient's disease in order to prevent the complications. For patients with moderate to severe GERD, especially those with erosive disease, starting with a proton pump inhibitor as initial therapy is advocated because of its superior efficacy over H_2-receptor antagonists.

While weight loss in obese patients and elevation of the head end of the bed are beneficial for most GERD patients, recommending all lifestyle modifications to all patients is not recommended.[1]

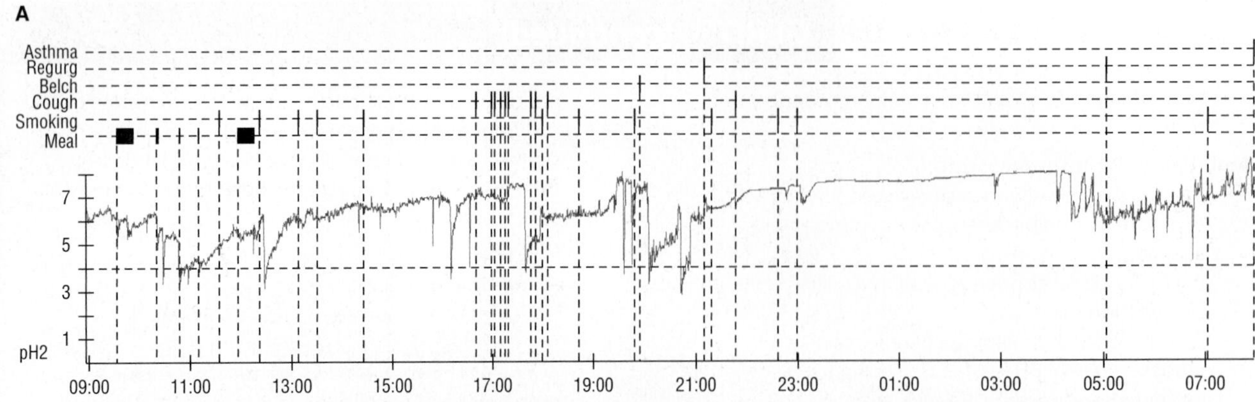

Normal 24 hour ambulatory esophageal pH test						
	Total	Normal	Upright	Normal	Supine	Normal
• Fraction time pH <4 (%)	1.9	<4.2	1.9	<6.3	0%	<1.2
• Number of refluxes	81		81		0	
• Number of long refluxes (>5 min)	0		0		0	
• Duration of longest reflux (min)	2.3		2.3		0	
• Time pH <4 (min)	25.9		25.9		0	

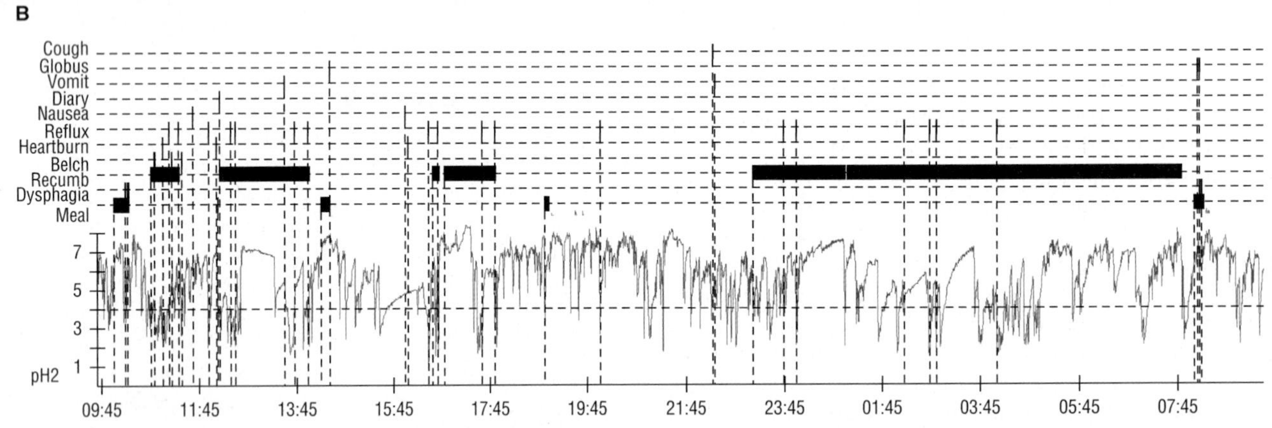

Abnormal 24-hour ambulatory esophageal pH test						
	Total	Normal	Upright	Normal	Supine	Normal
• Fraction time pH <4 (%)	16	<4.2	10.6	<6.3	20.6	<1.2
• Number of refluxes	332		143		189	
• Number of long refluxes (>5 min)	10		6		4	
• Duration of longest reflux (min)	7.9		7.1		7.9	
• Time pH <4 (min)	220.5		66.8		153.7	

FIGURE 32-2 Graphical representation of a normal 24-hour ambulatory esophageal pH test profile in a healthy subject and a table summarizing key results (*A*) compared with an abnormal 24-hour ambulatory esophageal pH test (*B*) showing significant acid reflux (multiple events of pH drop below 4) and abnormal 24-hour profile in the table.

Instead, education on lifestyle modifications should be tailored to the individual needs of the patient. Table 32-4 lists some of the lifestyle modifications that can be recommended on an individualized basis.[11]

6 Initially, patients with typical GERD symptoms should be treated with lifestyle modifications and patient-directed therapy. Patients who do not respond to lifestyle modifications and patient-directed therapy after 2 weeks or those with alarm symptoms, such as dysphagia, should seek medical attention and are generally started on empiric therapy consisting of an acid suppression agent. Those who do not respond to empiric therapy or who present with alarm symptoms should undergo endoscopy. Acid suppression therapy with proton pump inhibitors or H_2-receptor antagonists is the mainstay of GERD treatment. Patients presenting with moderate to severe symptoms (with or without esophageal erosions) should be started on a proton pump inhibitor as initial therapy because it provides the most rapid symptomatic relief and healing in the highest percentage of patients.[1] H_2-receptor antagonists in divided doses are effective for patients with milder GERD symptoms. However, when standard doses of H_2-receptor antagonist therapy are not effective at relieving symptoms, it is considered more cost-effective and efficacious to switch to a proton pump inhibitor.

TABLE 32-2 Evidence-Based Treatment Recommendations for GERD in Adults[1,14]

Recommendation	Level of Evidence and Strength of Evidence[a]
Lifestyle Modifications	
• Weight loss in overweight GERD patients or those who have recently gained weight.	Moderate, Conditional
• Elevation of the head end of the bed and avoidance of food 2-3 hours before bedtime if nocturnal GERD symptoms present.	Low, Conditional
• Routine elimination of foods that can trigger reflux is not recommended in the treatment of GERD.	Low, Conditional
Acid Suppression Therapy	
• Therapy of choice for symptom relief and healing of erosive esophagitis is an 8-week proton pump inhibitor course. There is similar efficacy among all proton pump inhibitors.	High, Strong
• For maximal pH control, delayed-release proton pump inhibitors should be administered 30-60 minutes before meals.	Moderate, Strong
• Proton pump inhibitors should be started at once daily dosing prior to the first meal each day.	Moderate, Strong
• Patients with Barrett's esophagus can be treated similarly to those with GERD who do not have Barrett's esophagus.	Moderate, Strong
• Flexibility with meal time administration may be seen with newer proton pump inhibitors (eg, dexlansoprazole).	Moderate, Conditional
• When clinically indicated, proton pump inhibitors are considered safe in pregnancy.	Moderate, Conditional
• Adjustments of dose timing and/or twice daily dosing may be beneficial in patients with night-time symptoms, variable schedules, and/or sleep disturbances who are partial responders to proton pump inhibitor therapy.	Low, Strong
• In patients with typical GERD symptoms who also have extraesophageal symptoms, a proton pump inhibitor trial is recommended.	Low, Strong
• Optimization of proton pump inhibitor therapy should be assessed in anyone with refractory GERD symptoms.	Low, Strong
• Increasing to twice daily dosing or switching proton pump inhibitor may be beneficial in partial responders to proton pump inhibitor therapy.	Low, Conditional
• Further evaluation is recommended for nonresponders to proton pump inhibitor therapy.	Low, Conditional
• If adverse effects occur with proton pump inhibitor, may consider switching to an alternative proton pump inhibitor.	Low, Conditional
• Patients with osteoporosis can use a proton pump inhibitor.	Moderate, Conditional
• Concern for hip fracture with proton pump inhibitor should be considered in those with osteoporosis AND other risk factors for hip fracture.	Moderate, Conditional
• Proton pump inhibitors are a risk factor for development of *Clostridium difficile.*	Moderate, Moderate
• Proton pump inhibitors are a risk factor for development of Community-Acquired Pneumonia with short-term use (but not long-term use).	Moderate, Conditional
• Proton pump inhibitors can be used in patients on clopidogrel and there is not an increased risk for adverse cardiovascular events.	High, Strong
Promotility Therapy and Other Nonacid Suppression Therapies	
• Prokinetic medications and/or baclofen should not be used to manage GERD without diagnostic evaluation.	Moderate, Conditional
• Sulcralfate is not generally recommended in nonpregnant GERD patients.	Moderate, Conditional
Maintenance Therapy	
• Maintenance therapy is recommended for (1) patients with continued symptoms after proton pump inhibitor discontinuation; (2) patients with complications including erosive esophagitis and Barrett's esophagus.	Moderate, Strong
• The lowest effective dose should be used when long-term proton pump inhibitor therapy is indicated for maintenance. Strategies such as on-demand and intermittent therapy may be beneficial.	Low, Conditional
• H_2-receptor antagonists may be used as maintenance therapy in patients without erosive disease when the goal is heartburn relief.	Moderate, Conditional
Surgery	
• Surgery is a long-term treatment option in GERD patients.	High, Strong
• Surgery is not generally recommended in proton pump inhibitor nonresponders.	High, Strong
• Surgery is not generally recommended in patients with extraesophageal symptoms not responding to proton pump inhibitor therapy.	Moderate, Strong
• Endoscopic therapy or transoral incisionless fundoplication not recommended as alternative to medical or traditional surgical procedures.	Moderate, Strong
• Bariatric surgery (Gastric bypass) should be considered in obese patients contemplating surgical therapy.	Moderate, Conditional

[a]Level of evidence per Grades of Recommendation, Assessment, Development, and Evaluation (GRADE) system: High = further research not likely to change authors' confidence in the estimate of effect; Moderate = further research would likely have an impact on the confidence in the estimate of effect; Low = further research would be expected to have an important impact on the confidence in the estimate of the effect and would be likely to change the evidence.

Strength of evidence per GRADE system: Strong = desired effects of an intervention clearly outweigh the undesireable effects; Conditional = there is uncertainty about the trade-offs between desirable effects and undesirable effects.[1,14]

Promotility agents (such as metoclopramide) are not as effective as acid suppression agents. Combining a promotility agent with acid suppression medications offer only modest improvements in symptoms over standard doses of H_2-receptor antagonists and should not be routinely recommended. In addition, the availability of a promotility agent that has an acceptable adverse effect profile is lacking. Mucosal protectants, such as sucralfate, have a limited role in the treatment of GERD.

Maintenance therapy is generally necessary to control symptoms and to prevent complications. For patients with more severe symptoms (with or without esophageal erosions) or for patients with other complications, maintenance therapy with a proton pump

TABLE 32-3 Therapeutic Approach to GERD in Adults

Recommended Treatment Regimen	Brand Name	Oral Dose	Comments
Intermittent, mild heartburn (individualized lifestyle modifications + patient-directed therapy with antacids and/or nonprescription H_2-receptor antagonists *or* nonprescription proton pump inhibitor)			
Individualized lifestyle modifications			Lifestyle modifications should be individualized for each patient
Patient-directed therapy with antacids (≥12 years old)			
Magnesium hydroxide/aluminum hydroxide with simethicone	Maalox®	10-20 mL as needed or after meals and at bedtime	If symptoms are unrelieved with lifestyle modifications and nonprescription medications after 2 weeks, patient should seek medical attention; do not exceed 16 teaspoonfuls per 24 hours
Antacid/alginic acid	Gaviscon®	2-4 tablets or 10-20 mL after meals and at bedtime	Note: Content of alginic acid varies greatly among products; the higher the alginic acid the better
Calcium carbonate	Tums®	500 mg, 2-4 tablets as needed	
Patient-directed therapy with nonprescription H_2-receptor antagonists (up to twice daily) (≥12 years old)			
Cimetidine	Tagamet HB®	200 mg	If symptoms are unrelieved with lifestyle modifications and nonprescription medications after 2 weeks, patient should seek medical attention
Famotidine	Pepcid AC®	10-20 mg	
Nizatidine	Axid AR®	75 mg	
Ranitidine	Zantac®	75-150 mg	
Patient-directed therapy (>18 years old) with nonprescription proton pump inhibitors (taken once daily)			
Esomeprazole	Nexium® 24HR	20 mg	If symptoms are unrelieved with lifestyle modifications and nonprescription medications after 2 weeks, patient should seek medical attention
Lansoprazole	Prevacid® 24HR	15 mg	
Omeprazole	Prilosec OTC®	20 mg	
Omeprazole/sodium bicarbonate	Zegerid OTC®	20 mg/1,100 mg	
Symptomatic relief of GERD (individualized lifestyle modifications + prescription-strength H_2-receptor antagonists *or* prescription-strength proton pump inhibitors)			
Individualized lifestyle modifications			Lifestyle modifications should be individualized for each patient
Prescription-strength H_2-receptor antagonists (for 6-12 weeks)			
Cimetidine (off-label use)	Tagamet®	400 mg four times daily or 800 mg twice daily	• For typical symptoms, treat empirically with prescription-strength acid suppression therapy • If symptoms recur, consider maintenance therapy. Note: Most patients will require standard doses for maintenance therapy
Famotidine	Pepcid®	20 mg twice daily	
Nizatidine	Axid®	150 mg twice daily	
Ranitidine	Zantac®	150 mg twice daily	
Prescription-strength proton pump inhibitors (for 4-8 weeks)			
Dexlansoprazole	Dexilant®	30 mg once daily for 4 weeks	• For typical symptoms, treat empirically with prescription-strength acid suppression therapy • Patients with moderate to severe symptoms should receive a proton pump inhibitor as initial therapy • If symptoms recur, consider maintenance therapy
Esomeprazole	Nexium®	20-40 mg once daily	
Lansoprazole	Prevacid®	15mg once daily	
Omeprazole	Prilosec®	20 mg once daily	
Omeprazole/sodium bicarbonate	Zegerid®	20 mg once daily	
Pantoprazole (Off-label use)	Protonix®	40 mg once daily	
Rabeprazole	Aciphex®	20 mg once daily	
Healing of erosive esophagitis or treatment of patients with moderate to severe symptoms or complications (individualized lifestyle modifications + high-dose H_2-receptor antagonists *or* proton pump inhibitors *or* antireflux surgery)			
Individualized lifestyle modifications			Lifestyle modifications should be individualized for each patient.
Proton pump inhibitors (up to twice daily for up to 8 weeks)			
Dexlansoprazole	Dexilant®	60 mg daily	• For extraesophageal or alarm symptoms, obtain endoscopy with biopsy to evaluate mucosa • If symptoms are relieved, consider maintenance therapy. Proton pump inhibitors are the most effective maintenance therapy for patients with extraesophageal symptoms, complications, and erosive disease. Start with twice-daily proton pump inhibitor therapy if reflux chest syndrome present • Patients not responding to pharmacologic therapy, including those with persistent extraesophageal symptoms, should be evaluated via manometry and/or ambulatory reflux monitoring • Twice daily dosing of proton pump inhibitors is considered off-label use
Esomeprazole	Nexium®	20-40 mg daily	
Lansoprazole	Prevacid®	30 mg once or twice daily	
Omeprazole	Prilosec®	20 mg once or twice daily	
Rabeprazole	Aciphex®	20 mg once or twice daily	
Pantoprazole	Protonix®	40 mg once or twice daily	

(Continued)

TABLE 32-3 Therapeutic Approach to GERD in Adults (*Continued*)

Recommended Treatment Regimen	Brand Name	Oral Dose	Comments
High-dose H_2-receptor antagonists (for 8-12 weeks)			
Cimetidine	Tagamet®	400 mg four times daily or 800 mg twice daily	Note: If high-dose H_2-receptor antagonist needed, may consider using proton pump inhibitor to lower cost, increase convenience, and increase tolerability Note: Four times daily H_2-receptor antagonist is considered off-label use for Nizatidine
Famotidine	Pepcid®	20-40 mg twice daily	
Nizatidine	Aciphex®	150 mg two-four times daily	
Ranitidine	Zantac®	150 mg four times daily	
Interventional therapy			
Antireflux surgery			

inhibitor is most effective. Routine use of combination therapy has no role in GERD maintenance therapy. In cases of refractory GERD, the diagnosis should be confirmed through further diagnostic tests before long-term, high-dose therapy is considered.[1]

Nonpharmacologic Therapy

Nonpharmacologic treatment of GERD includes lifestyle modifications and antireflux surgery, which may be viable maintenance modalities in select patients. Endoscopic therapies, such as endoscopic sewing devices and endoluminal application of radiofrequency heat energy, have fallen out of favor and are not routinely recommended.

Lifestyle Modifications

The most common lifestyle modifications that a patient should be educated about include weight loss in obese patients and elevation of the head end of the bed, especially for those patients who have symptoms while in a recumbent position. Other lifestyle modifications should be individualized based on the patient's specific situation. These include consumption of smaller meals and not sleeping for at least 3 hours after eating, avoidance of foods or medications that exacerbate GERD, smoking cessation, avoidance of tight-fitting clothes, and avoidance of alcohol (see Table 32-4).[15]

Obesity increases the risk of GERD symptoms and complications including Barrett's esophagus. A clear association has been shown between body mass index (BMI), waist circumference and weight gain.[1] Surprisingly, weight gain in those considered to have a normal BMI has also been associated with new onset GERD symptoms.[1] Even more alarming is the potential association between BMI and cancer in the esophagus and gastric cardia.[1]

TABLE 32-4 Nonpharmacologic Treatment of GERD with Lifestyle Modifications[15]

- Elevate the head end of the bed (increases esophageal clearance). Use 6- to 8-in. (15-20 cm) blocks under the head side of the bed
- Weight reduction (reduces symptoms) in obese patients
- Avoid foods that may decrease lower esophageal sphincter pressure or increase transient lower esophageal sphincter relaxation (TLESR) (fats, chocolate, alcohol, peppermint, and spearmint)
- Include protein-rich meals in diet (augments lower esophageal sphincter pressure)
- Avoid foods that have a direct irritant effect on the esophageal mucosa (spicy foods, orange juice, tomato juice, and coffee)
- Behaviors that may reduce esophageal acid exposure:
  - Eat small meals and avoid sleeping immediately after meals (sleep after 3 hours if possible; decreases gastric volume)
  - Stop smoking (decreases spontaneous esophageal sphincter relaxation)
  - Avoid alcohol (increases amplitude of the lower esophageal sphincter, peristaltic waves, and frequency of contraction)
  - Avoid tight-fitting clothes
  - Always take drugs in the sitting upright or standing position and with plenty of liquid, especially for those that have a direct irritant effect on the esophageal mucosa (eg, bisphosphonates, tetracyclines, quinidine, potassium chloride, iron salts, aspirin, nonsteroidal anti-inflammatory drugs)

A high-fat meal will decrease LES pressure for 2 hours or more postprandially. In contrast, a high-protein, low-fat meal will elevate LES pressure. Consequently, weight loss and a low-fat diet may help to improve GERD symptoms.

Elevating the head end of the bed by approximately 6″ to 8″ (15-20 cm) with a foam wedge under the mattress (not just elevating the head with pillows) decreases nocturnal esophageal acid contact time and should be recommended. Many foods may worsen the symptoms of GERD. Some foods decrease LES pressure (eg, fats and chocolates), while other foods can act as direct contact irritants to the esophageal mucosa (citrus juice, tomato juice, coffee, and pepper) (see Table 32-1).

Patient profiles should be evaluated to identify potential medications that may exacerbate GERD symptoms. Some medications decrease LES pressure, while other medications can act as direct contact irritants to the esophageal mucosa. Proper patient education can help prevent dysphagia or esophageal ulceration. Patients should be closely monitored for worsening symptoms when any of these medications are started. If symptoms worsen, alternative therapies may be warranted. The clinician must weigh the risks and benefits of continuing a medication known to worsen GERD and esophagitis.

Smoking can cause aerophagia (ie, air swallowing), which leads to increased belching and regurgitation. Smoking cessation has historically been recommended as an important lifestyle modification in the management of GERD patients; however, data are lacking to show that symptoms improve for patients who quit smoking and the current guidelines do not recommend this as an effective nonpharmacologic option for GERD. Nevertheless, patients with GERD should be encouraged to quit smoking. Alcohol, although not thought to play a role in severe disease, decreases LES pressure and may exacerbate symptoms such as heartburn.

Many patients are noncompliant with lifestyle modifications, and even those who do comply generally continue to have symptoms that require acid suppression therapy. Nonetheless, it is important to regularly stress the potential benefits of lifestyle modifications that would benefit each individual patient.

Interventional Approaches

Interventional approaches include antireflux surgery and endoscopic therapies. These are discussed in more detail below.

Antireflux Surgery 7 Surgical intervention is a viable alternative treatment for select patients when long-term pharmacologic management is undesirable or when patients have complications. The goal of antireflux surgery is to re-establish the antireflux barrier, to position the LES within the abdomen where it is under positive (intra-abdominal) pressure, and to close any associated defect in the diaphragmatic hiatus by reinforcing the crural muscles. Antireflux surgery should be considered for patients (a) who opt for surgery despite successful treatment because of lifestyle considerations, including age, time, or expense of medications, or (b) who have complications of GERD (eg, Barrett's esophagus and strictures). Current guidelines do not generally recommend surgery for patients who do not respond to proton pump inhibitor therapy.[1] The antireflux surgical procedure chosen depends on the surgeon's expertise and preference, as well as on anatomic considerations. In general, 90% of patients have symptom resolution following successful Nissen fundoplication. The major complications with antireflux surgery include gas bloat syndrome (inability to belch or vomit), dysphagia, vagal denervation, and splenic trauma. Antireflux surgery is superior to medical management with an H_2-receptor antagonist or a promotility agent. A meta-analysis comparing fundoplication and medical management favored fundoplication at multiple quality of life endpoints; however a substantial number of patients remained on acid suppression medication following surgical intervention.[16] Long-term effectiveness of antireflux surgery is uncertain.

Bariatric surgery, specifically Roux-en-Y gastric bypass surgery, should be considered in obese patients contemplating surgery.[1] The consideration of bariatric surgery in obese patients for improvement of GERD symptoms is a result of the proposed difference in pathophysiology in this patient population. Abdominal pressure may play a greater role in the development of GERD in obese patients. Gastric banding may improve GERD through weight loss however, it may also precipitate acid reflux through other mechanisms. Studies evaluating the effect of gastric banding procedures on GERD have shown mixed results, while studies have more consistently demonstrated the benefits of gastric bypass in the management of GERD in obese patients.[17]

Endoscopic Therapies Endoscopic approaches for the management of GERD have included endoscopic sewing devices and endoluminal application of radiofrequency heat energy resulting in tissue injury or nerve ablation (the Stretta procedure). Unfortunately, results from these endoscopic therapies have proven disappointing and are not routinely recommended. Currently in their infancy stages, natural orifice transluminal surgery and surgical techniques have been tested and may offer an option in the future. Endoscopic stapling has demonstrated improvement in quality of life scores but several limitations were noted in comparison to laparoscopic fundoplication.[18]

Other Therapies Radiofrequency ablation is an endoscopic therapy used for the management of Barrett's esophagus primarily when dysplasia is present. Radiofrequency ablation is recommended in patients with Barrett's esophagus with high-grade dysplasia and current guidance additionally acknowledges radiofrequency ablation as a treatment option in low-grade dysplasia.[19] Radiofrequency ablation prompts reversal to normal squamous epithelium and reduces development of esophageal cancer in those with high-grade dysplasia.[19]

The FDA approved a device for magnetic sphincter augmentation to improve lower esophageal resistance and reduce symptoms of GERD. A study comparing magnetic sphincter augmentation with traditional laparoscopic fundoplication found similar improvement in symptoms and quality of life, with 67% of participants who underwent magnetic sphincter augmentation retaining the ability to belch in comparison to no patients who underwent fundoplication.[20] Postmarketing results have also demonstrated that a majority of patients can discontinue their proton pump inhibitor and have GERD-health-related quality of life (HRQL) scores similar to patients without GERD.[21] However concerns related to long-term safety of this approach have been raised.[22]

Pharmacologic Therapy

Pharmacologic treatment consists of (a) patient-directed therapy with nonprescription antacids, H_2-receptor antagonists, or proton pump inhibitors and (b) prescription-strength acid-suppression therapy or promotility medications.

Patient-Directed Therapy

Patient-directed therapy, where patients self-treat themselves with nonprescription medications, is appropriate for mild, intermittent symptoms. Patients with continuous symptoms lasting longer than 2 weeks should seek medical attention.

Antacids and Antacid–Alginic Acid Products Patients should be educated that antacids are an appropriate component of treating milder GERD symptoms, even though documentation of their efficacy in placebo-controlled clinical trials is lacking. Antacids may offer immediate symptomatic relief and help maintain the intragastric pH greater than 4, which decreases the activation of pepsinogen to pepsin, a proteolytic enzyme. The neutralization of gastric fluid may also lead to increased LES pressure. Patients who require frequent use of antacids for chronic symptoms should be treated with prescription-strength acid suppression therapy.

Some antacid products are combined with alginic acid, which is not a potent neutralizing agent and does not enhance LES pressure; however, it does form a highly viscous solution or "raft" that floats on the surface of the gastric contents. This viscous solution is thought to serve as a protective barrier for the esophagus against reflux of gastric contents. It also reduces the frequency of the reflux episodes. The combination product may be superior to antacids alone in relieving the symptoms of GERD.[23] The alginic acid "raft" can adapt to the acid pocket, continuously floating above newly secreted acid near the esophagogastric junction. Weakly acidic or nonacidic reflux has been associated with refractory GERD symptoms. There are many Gaviscon® products with varying amounts of alginic acid. Products with a higher alginic acid component are preferred (eg, 500 mg). Patients should be encouraged to check medication labels for ingredients. Some of the Gaviscon® products contain lower amounts of alginic acid or list alginic acid under inactive ingredients with no amounts specified. Efficacy data indicating endoscopic healing are lacking.

Antacid or antacid combination products interact with a variety of medications by altering gastric pH, increasing urinary pH, adsorbing medications to their surfaces, providing a physical barrier to absorption, or forming insoluble complexes with other medications. Antacids have clinically significant drug interactions with tetracycline, ferrous sulfate, isoniazid, sulfonylureas, and quinolone antibiotics. Antacid–drug interactions are influenced by composition, dose, dosage schedule, and formulation of the antacid. They may also cause constipation or diarrhea depending on the magnesium or aluminum content.

Dosage recommendations for antacids in the management of GERD are somewhat difficult to derive from the literature. Doses range from hourly to an as-needed basis (see Table 32-3). In general, antacids have a short duration of action, which necessitates frequent administration throughout the day to provide continuous neutralization of acid. Taking antacids after meals can increase the duration of action from about 1 to 3 hours; however, nighttime acid suppression cannot be maintained with bedtime doses.

Nonprescription H_2-Receptor Antagonists and Proton Pump Inhibitors Nonprescription H_2-receptor antagonists (cimetidine, famotidine, nizatidine, and ranitidine) are effective in diminishing gastric acid secretion when taken prior to meals and decrease GERD symptoms associated with exercise. Antacids may have a slightly faster onset of action, while the H_2-receptor antagonists have a much longer duration of action compared with antacids.

The proton pump inhibitors esomeprazole, omeprazole (alone or combined with sodium bicarbonate) and lansoprazole are available without a prescription for the short-term treatment of heartburn. Patients who do not respond to lifestyle modifications and patient-directed therapy after 2 weeks should be seen by their clinician.

Acid Suppression Therapy

8 Acid suppression is the mainstay of GERD treatment. Proton pump inhibitors provide the greatest symptom relief and the highest healing rates, especially for patients with erosive disease, moderate to severe symptoms, or complications.

Proton Pump Inhibitors (Dexlansoprazole, Esomeprazole, Lansoprazole, Omeprazole [with or without Sodium Bicarbonate], Pantoprazole, and Rabeprazole) Proton pump inhibitors are superior to H_2-receptor antagonists in treating patients with moderate to severe GERD and should be given empirically to those with troublesome symptoms. This includes not only patients with esophageal tissue injury (eg, Barrett's esophagus, strictures, or esophagitis) but also patients with symptom-based GERD syndromes. Twice-daily proton pump inhibitor use is indicated in those not responding to a standard once-daily course of therapy. Before increasing the frequency to twice daily, optimization of proton pump therapy should be assessed (eg, taken 30-60 minutes prior to largest meal each day, etc.). In patients who are partial responders to initial proton pump inhibitor therapy, a trial of an alternative proton pump inhibitor may also be considered. Patients with Barrett's esophagus should be treated similarly to patients without Barrett's esophagus.[1] Further diagnostic evaluation is indicated for patients not responding to twice-daily proton pump inhibitor therapy.

Proton pump inhibitors block gastric acid secretion by inhibiting gastric H^+/K^+-adenosine triphosphatase in gastric parietal cells. This produces a profound, long-lasting antisecretory effect capable of maintaining the gastric pH greater than 4, even during postprandial acid surges. A correlation exists between the percentage of time the gastric pH remains greater than 4 during the 24-hour period and healing erosive esophagitis.

In general, healing rates at 4 and 8 weeks are similar among proton pump inhibitors. Symptomatic relief is seen in approximately 83% of patients with endoscopic evidence of injury after 8 weeks treated with a proton pump inhibitor, whereas the endoscopic healing rate at 8 weeks is 78%.[1] Symptom response to NERD has been found to be less robust with approximately 60% of patients experiencing complete relief with proton pump inhibitor therapy.[1]

Clinical **Controversy...**

With continued increased recognition of potential adverse effects associated with proton pump inhibitor therapy, there is a focus on ensuring de-escalation of therapy in appropriate patients. Appropriate patients for de-escalation of therapy are not well-defined.

The most cost common adverse effects associated with proton pump inhibitors include headache, diarrhea, constipation and abdominal pain. Community-acquired pneumonia has occurred with short-term use in GERD patients.[1] Enteric infections, vitamin B_{12} deficiency, hypomagnesemia, and bone fractures are potential long-term adverse effects associated with proton pump inhibitors (Table 32-5).[24-29] In one study, dysmotility and proton pump

TABLE 32-5 Drug Monitoring[23-28]

Drug	Adverse Drug Reaction	Monitoring Parameter	Comments
Antacids			
• Magnesium hydroxide/aluminum hydroxide • Antacid/alginic acid • Calcium carbonate	• Diarrhea or constipation (depending on product) • Alterations in mineral metabolism • Acid–base disturbances	• Periodic calcium and phosphate levels in patients on chronic therapy	• Use caution with aluminum- and calcium-containing antacids in patients with renal impairment • Aluminum-containing antacids may bind to phosphate in the gut and lead to bone demineralization
H_2-Receptor Antagonists			
• Cimetidine • Famotidine • Nizatidine • Ranitidine	• Headache, somnolence, fatigue, dizziness, and either constipation or diarrhea	• Monitor for CNS effects, especially in the elderly • Monitor vitamin B_{12} serum concentrations in those on chronic, long-term therapy or in those on higher doses	• May see increased CNS effects (rare) in those over 50 years of age or in those with renal or hepatic dysfunction • May be associated with vitamin B_{12} deficiency with longer duration therapy and in higher doses
Proton Pump Inhibitors			
• Dexlansoprazole • Esomeprazole • Lansoprazole • Omeprazole • Omeprazole/sodium bicarbonate • Pantoprazole • Rabeprazole	*Most common adverse effects:* • Headache, dizziness, somnolence, diarrhea, constipation, flatulence, abdominal pain, and nausea *Other important adverse effects:* • Enteric infections (*C. difficile* infections) • Increased risk of pneumonia *Long-term adverse effects:* • Hypomagnesemia • Bone fractures • Vitamin B_{12} deficiency	• Number and type of diarrhea episodes • Periodic magnesium levels warranted in those on higher doses or who are on therapy for greater than 1 year • Routine bone density studies or calcium supplementation should only be considered if other risk factors for osteoporosis or bone fractures are present • Respiratory symptoms within first 30 days of therapy • Periodic vitamin B_{12} serum concentration with long-term use	• Acid suppression may result in loss of host defense against ingested spores and bacteria permitting a higher burden of exposure. Recent meta-analysis showed 65% increase in *Clostridium difficile*–associated diarrhea among those on proton pump inhibitors[23] • Hypomagnesemia is uncommon but can be life-threatening; has been seen as soon as 3 months after starting therapy but more likely in those on proton pump inhibitors >1 year • May increase risk for osteoporosis-related fractures of the hip, wrist or spine; Most common with high-dose (eg, multiple daily doses) and long-term use (eg, ≥1 year) Patients with known osteoporosis can remain on proton pump inhibitor • Proton pump inhibitors may inhibit secretion of intrinsic factor, which potentially can lead to vitamin B_{12} deficiency; this is not common and usually associated with use for >3 years • May increase risk of community-acquired pneumonia, particularly within the first 30 days of therapy

inhibitor use were found to be independent risk factors for not only for small intestinal bacterial overgrowth, but also small intestinal fungal overgrowth.[30] Overuse of proton pump inhibitors should be minimized as the clinical implications of chronic therapy are better elucidated.

Drug interactions with the proton pump inhibitors vary slightly with each agent. All proton pump inhibitors can decrease the absorption of medications such as ketoconazole or itraconazole, which require an acidic environment to be absorbed. While no drug interactions with lansoprazole, pantoprazole, or rabeprazole have been seen with CYP2C19 substrates such as diazepam, warfarin, and phenytoin, concerns have been raised regarding the concomitant use of proton pump inhibitors, particularly omeprazole, with clopidogrel since it is the strongest inhibitor of CYP2C19.[31,32] Clopidogrel, a prodrug, is converted to its active metabolite via the CYP2C19 and CYP3A4 enzymes. Inhibition of CYP2C19 by proton pump inhibitors, specifically omeprazole, may decrease the effectiveness of clopidogrel. Careful review of the risk-to-benefit profile regarding the use of proton pump inhibitors for patients on clopidogrel should be considered. Selection of a proton pump inhibitor with less inhibition of CYP2C19 may limit the risk of interaction with clopidogrel.

Patients with upper GI bleeding or those with multiple risk factors for GI bleeding who require antiplatelet therapy would benefit from proton pump inhibitor therapy. Risk factors for GI bleeding include advanced age, use of anticoagulants, steroids or nonsteroidal anti-inflammatory drugs, presence of *Helicobacter pylori*, or previous history of bleeding or peptic ulcer disease complications.[33] Otherwise, using an alternative agent, such as an H_2-receptor antagonist, may be prudent in this patient population.

Esomeprazole does not appear to interact with warfarin or phenytoin, and an interaction with diazepam is generally not considered clinically relevant. Although generally not a problem, omeprazole has the potential to inhibit the metabolism of warfarin, diazepam, and phenytoin, and lansoprazole may decrease theophylline concentrations. Patients on potentially interacting medications, such as warfarin, should be monitored closely for potential problems.

The proton pump inhibitors degrade in acidic environments and are therefore formulated in a delayed-release capsule or tablet formulation. Dexlansoprazole, esomeprazole, lansoprazole, and omeprazole contain enteric-coated (pH-sensitive) granules in a capsule form. Dexlansoprazole is unique in that the capsule is a dual delayed-release formulation, with the first release occurring 1 to 2 hours after the dose and the second release occurring 4 to 5 hours after the dose. The clinical significance of this dual release is to allow the medication to have a longer lasting benefit, at least 16 to 18 hours. Patients taking pantoprazole or rabeprazole should be instructed not to crush, chew, or split the delayed-release tablets.

For patients who are unable to swallow the capsule or for pediatric patients, there are several alternative administration methods available. The contents of the delayed-release capsules can be mixed in applesauce or placed in orange juice. If a patient has a nasogastric tube, the contents of an omeprazole capsule can be mixed in 8.4% sodium bicarbonate solution. Esomeprazole granules can be dispersed in water. Esomeprazole, omeprazole, and pantoprazole are also available in a delayed-release oral suspension powder packet, and lansoprazole is available as a delayed-release, orally disintegrating tablet. Esomeprazole and pantoprazole are available in an IV formulation, which offers an alternative route of administration for patients who are unable to take an oral proton pump inhibitor. Importantly, the IV product is not more efficacious than oral proton pump inhibitors and is significantly more expensive. Careful patient selection is necessary to avoid the increased cost from the use of the IV product.

The newest dosage form of omeprazole is in a delayed-release tablet; it is also available in a combination product with sodium bicarbonate in an immediate-release capsule and oral suspension (Zegerid®). This is the first immediate-release proton pump inhibitor and it should be taken on an empty stomach at least 1 hour before a meal. Zegerid® powder for oral suspension offers an alternative to the delayed-release capsules, powder for suspension, or IV formulation in adult patients with a nasogastric tube. The Zegerid® capsule should be swallowed whole and not opened, sprinkled on food, or administered via nasogastric tube. The 20 mg and 40 mg Zegerid® capsules have the same amount of sodium bicarbonate so two 20 mg capsules cannot be substituted for a 40 mg capsule.

Patients should be instructed to take their proton pump inhibitor in the morning, 30 to 60 minutes before breakfast or before their biggest meal of the day, to maximize efficacy, because these agents inhibit only actively secreting proton pumps. Dexlansoprazole can be taken without regards to meals. Patients with nocturnal symptoms may benefit from taking their proton pump inhibitor prior to the evening meal. If dosed twice daily, the second dose should be administered approximately 10 to 12 hours after the morning dose and prior to a meal or snack.

H_2-Receptor Antagonists (Cimetidine, Famotidine, Nizatidine, and Ranitidine) H_2-receptor antagonists in divided doses are effective in treating patients with mild to moderate GERD.[15] The majority of the trials assessing the efficacy of standard doses of H_2-receptor antagonists indicate that symptomatic improvement is achieved in an average of 60% of patients after 12 weeks of therapy.[15] However, endoscopic healing rates tend to be lower, an average of 50% of patients at 12 weeks.[15]

The efficacy of H_2-receptor antagonists in the management of GERD is extremely variable and is frequently lower than desired. Response to the H_2-receptor antagonists is dependent on the (a) severity of disease, (b) dosage regimen used, and (c) duration of therapy. These factors are important to keep in mind when comparing clinical trials and/or assessing a patient's response to therapy. The severity of esophagitis at baseline has a profound impact on the patient's response to H_2-receptor antagonists. For symptomatic relief of mild GERD, low-dose, nonprescription H_2-receptor antagonists or standard doses given twice daily may be beneficial. Patients who do not respond to standard doses may be hypersecreters of gastric acid and will require higher doses. Although higher doses of H_2-receptor antagonists may provide higher symptomatic and endoscopic healing rates, limited information exists regarding the safety of these regimens, and they can be less effective and more costly than once-daily proton pump inhibitors. Unlike duodenal ulcer disease, in which the duration of therapy is relatively short (eg, 4-6 weeks), prolonged courses of H_2-receptor antagonists are frequently required in the treatment of GERD.

Because all of the H_2-receptor antagonists have similar efficacy, selection of the specific agent to use in the management of GERD should be based on factors such as differences in pharmacokinetics, safety profile, and cost. Patients should be monitored for the presence of adverse effects as well as potential drug interactions, especially when on cimetidine. Cimetidine may inhibit the metabolism of theophylline, warfarin, phenytoin, nifedipine, and propranolol, among others. An alternate H_2-receptor antagonist should be selected if the patient is on any of these medications. Headache, fatigue, dizziness, and constipation/diarrhea are the most common adverse effects associated with the use of H_2-receptor antagonists.

Promotility Agents

Promotility agents may be useful as an adjunct to acid suppression therapy for patients with a known motility defect (eg, LES incompetence, decreased esophageal clearance, and delayed gastric emptying). Unfortunately, all available promotility agents are fraught with undesirable adverse effects and are not generally as effective as acid suppression therapy.

Metoclopramide Metoclopramide, a dopamine antagonist, increases LES pressure in a dose-related manner and accelerates gastric emptying in gastroesophageal reflux patients. However, it does not improve esophageal clearance. Metoclopramide provides symptomatic improvement for some patients with GERD; however, substantial data supporting endoscopic healing are lacking. In addition, metoclopramide's adverse effect profile, including extrapyramidal effects, tardive dyskinesia, and other CNS effects, limits its usefulness in treating many patients with GERD. The risk of adverse effects is much greater for elderly patients and for patients with renal dysfunction because the drug is primarily eliminated by the kidneys. Contraindications include Parkinson's disease, mechanical obstruction, concomitant use of other dopamine antagonists or anticholinergic agents, and pheochromocytoma.

Bethanechol Bethanechol, a promotility drug, has limited value in the treatment of GERD because of unwanted adverse effects, such as urinary retention, abdominal discomfort, nausea, and flushing. It is not routinely recommended for the treatment of GERD.

Other Promotility Drugs Under Investigation Other promotility drugs under investigation include itopride and baclofen. Because domperidone does not cross the blood–brain barrier, it does not cause the CNS effects seen with metoclopramide. However, it is not currently available in the United States. Baclofen, a gamma aminobutyric acid (GABA) receptor type B agonist, may decrease esophageal acid exposure and the number of reflux episodes by decreasing the number of transient relaxations of the LES. However, this agent has many adverse effects, limiting its usefulness in GERD. Other GABA type B agonists, as well as metabotropic glutamate type 5 (mGluR5) receptor antagonists are under development as potential prokinetic agents; however their effectiveness has not been promising to date.[34]

Mucosal Protectants

Sucralfate, a nonabsorbable aluminum salt of sucrose octasulfate, has limited value in the treatment of GERD. It may not be useful in the routine treatment of acid reflux but may useful in the management of radiation esophagitis and bile or nonacid reflux GERD.

Combination Therapy

Combination therapy with an acid suppression agent and a promotility agent or a mucosal protectant agent would seem logical given the multifactorial nature of the disease, particularly in light of the disappointing results seen with many monotherapy regimens. However, data to support combination therapy are limited, and this approach should not routinely be recommended unless a patient has GERD plus motor dysfunction occurring. The effectiveness of the addition of an H_2-receptor antagonist at bedtime to proton pump inhibitor therapy for the treatment of nocturnal symptoms may decrease over time due to tachyphylaxis with H_2-receptor antagonists. In light of this, "as needed" use of bedtime H_2-receptor antagonist may be a more appropriate approach if combination with a proton pump inhibitor is deemed necessary. Using the omeprazole–sodium bicarbonate immediate-release product in addition to once-daily proton pump inhibitors may offer an alternative for nocturnal GERD symptoms.

Clinical **Controversy...**

The use of a bedtime H_2-receptor antagonist in addition to daytime proton-pump inhibitor therapy is sometimes encountered in clinical practice to manage nocturnal GERD symptoms; however the long-term efficacy of this regimen is not well-established and a low-level of evidence exists.

Maintenance Therapy

9 Many patients with GERD will relapse if medication is withdrawn; so long-term maintenance treatment may be required. A proton pump inhibitor is the drug of choice for maintenance of patients with moderate to severe GERD, erosive disease, or other complication.

Although healing and/or symptomatic improvement may be achieved via many different therapeutic modalities, a large percentage of patients with gastroesophageal reflux will relapse following discontinuation of proton pump inhibitor or H_2-receptor antagonist therapy, especially those with more severe disease. Patients who have symptomatic relapse following discontinuation of therapy or lowering of medication doses, including patients with complications such as Barrett's esophagus, strictures, or erosive esophagitis, should be considered for long-term maintenance therapy to prevent complications or worsening of esophageal function.[15] The goal of maintenance therapy is to improve quality of life by controlling the patient's symptoms and preventing complications. Patients should be counseled on the importance of complying with lifestyle changes and long-term maintenance therapy in order to prevent recurrence or worsening of disease.[15]

Clinical **Controversy...**

While trials exist supporting the efficacy of "on-demand" use of proton pump inhibitors as maintenance therapy—reliable methods for identifying most appropriate patients for this approach are not available.

H_2-receptor antagonists may be effective maintenance therapy for patients with mild disease.[1] Proton pump inhibitors are the drugs of choice for maintenance treatment of moderate to severe esophagitis or symptoms. Low doses of a proton pump inhibitor or alternate-day dosing may be effective in some patients with mild symptoms, thereby allowing dose reduction in some cases. "On-demand" maintenance therapy, by which patients take their proton pump inhibitor only when they have symptoms, may be effective for patients with endoscopy-negative GERD.[1] Although not well studied, many patients with only mild to moderate symptoms may decide on their own to use "on-demand" for the financial benefit. However, patients with persistent symptoms and/or complications generally require standard doses of proton pump inhibitors.

Long-term chronic use of proton pump inhibitor doses, higher than standard treatment doses, is not indicated unless the patient has complicated symptoms, has erosive esophagitis per endoscopy, or has had further diagnostic evaluation to determine the level of acid exposure. Metoclopramide is not approved for maintenance therapy, and its use is limited by adverse effect profile. Antireflux surgery may also be considered a viable alternative to long-term drug therapy for maintenance of healing for patients who are candidates.

Maintenance Therapy with H_2-Receptor Antagonist The studies evaluating the efficacy of the H_2-receptor antagonists in maintaining GERD patients in remission have been disappointing. Currently, ranitidine 150 mg twice daily is the only H_2-receptor antagonist regimen that is FDA approved for maintenance of healing of erosive esophagitis.

Maintenance Therapy with Proton Pump Inhibitors Long-term use of the proton pump inhibitors is associated with adverse effects such as hypomagnesemia, enteric infections, and risk for bone fractures; however, there is no evidence of carcinoid tumors directly linked to their use. Prolonged hypergastrinemia leading to the development of colonic polyps, and potentially adenocarcinoma, was also a concern that has proven unfounded with long-term use.

However, the role of *H. pylori* status for patients with GERD has been questioned. As a consequence of the controversy surrounding *H. pylori* and GERD, specific guidelines on how to handle patients who are *H. pylori* positive are lacking. Most clinicians would probably opt to eradicate *H. pylori* infections once detected. However, routine screening for *H. pylori* is not recommended as part of the diagnosis and management of GERD. Further studies are needed to determine the role of *H. pylori* for patients with GERD.

Special Populations

There are several special populations that should be considered when discussing GERD, such as patients with extraesophageal symptoms, pediatric patients, elderly patients, and patients with refractory symptoms.

Patients with Extraesophageal GERD

Extraesophageal symptoms (such as asthma, laryngitis, or chest pain) should prompt investigation for other possible causes outside of GERD. Patients presenting with extraesophageal symptoms, with concomitant typical GERD symptoms, should receive a trial of proton pump inhibitor therapy. Patients with extraesophageal symptoms without the presence of typical GERD symptoms should undergo esophageal reflux monitoring prior to initiation of proton pump inhibitor therapy. If symptoms continue, patients should be evaluated with manometry, ambulatory reflux monitoring, or impedance–pH monitoring to rule out dysmotility or refractory symptoms.[1] Because there are many causes of asthma and laryngeal symptoms, a concomitant esophageal GERD syndrome must also be present to associate these symptoms with GERD. A trial of proton pump inhibitor therapy is recommended for those with extraesophageal symptoms with concurrent typical GERD symptoms. The optimal dose of proton pump inhibition is not well-defined. For patients not responding to empiric therapy, ambulatory reflux monitoring may be beneficial in determining acid exposure as it relates to symptoms. Maintenance therapy is generally indicated for patients who respond to the therapeutic trial or have endoscopic evidence of reflux. Antireflux surgery may be an option in select patients but is generally not recommended for management of extraesophageal symptoms that persist despite proton pump inhibitor therapy.

Pediatric Patients with GERD

Many infants have physiologic reflux with little or no clinical consequence. Uncomplicated gastroesophageal reflux usually manifests as regurgitation or "spitting up" and resolves without incident by about 12 months of life.[7] It usually responds to supportive therapy, including dietary adjustments, postural management, and reassurance for the parents. Thickened feedings may be useful in milder cases. While this does not decrease reflux episodes, it may decrease the incidence of regurgitation.[7] This strategy of thickening feedings may be appropriate for full-term infants, however may be associated with necrotizing enterocolitis in preterm infants. Chronic vomiting associated with gastroesophageal reflux must be distinguished from other causes, such as neurologic, metabolic, eating, and rumination disorders. Smaller, more frequent feedings may be beneficial. In formula-fed infants, an extensively hydrolyzed protein may help identify milk protein sensitivity as the cause of unexplained GERD-like symptoms, likewise, exclusion of milk and eggs in the maternal diet for breastfeeding infants may be appropriate.[7]

Developmental immaturity of the LES is one suspected cause of gastroesophageal reflux in infants. Like adults, transient LES relaxations seem to be the most common cause of gastroesophageal reflux in children. Other causes include impaired luminal clearance of gastric acid, neurologic impairment, and type of infant formula. Complications, although rare, include distal esophagitis, failure to thrive, esophageal peptic strictures, Barrett's esophagus, and pulmonary disease. Further diagnostic evaluation is indicated in all who experience apnea or an apparent life-threatening event.

The benefits of using promotility medications, such as metoclopramide, erythromycin, bethanechol, and baclofen, are outweighed by the potential adverse effects that may occur and, therefore, cannot be routinely recommended.[7] Careful consideration should be made before medication is recommended, especially in children younger than 1 year of age. Overprescribing of acid suppression therapy may lead to increased risk of infection and other adverse effects in premature infants.[35,36] When medication is deemed necessary, ranitidine is commonly used at a dose of 5 to 10 mg/kg/day in 2 to 3 divided doses in pediatric patients aged 1 month to 16 years.[7] Tachyphylaxis may develop making the effectiveness of H_2-receptor antagonists less than optimal.

Proton pump inhibitor use in children is increasing, especially in those with esophagitis. Most patients will respond to once-daily proton pump inhibitor dosing. Lansoprazole and omeprazole are indicated for treating symptomatic and erosive GERD for pediatric patients older than age 1 year, while esomeprazole is indicated in patients older than 1 month of age. Omeprazole has been used off-label for children younger than 1 year of age at a dose of 1 mg/kg/day. Rabeprazole is indicated for short-term treatment of symptomatic GERD in adolescents 12 years and older and for treatment of GERD in pediatric patients 1 to 11 years of age.

Table 32-6 details indications and dosing of proton pump inhibitors in pediatric patients. Dexlansoprazole and pantoprazole have not been adequately studied in pediatric patients. A review of the current evidence for use of proton pump inhibitor therapy in infants and children found little efficacy in infants with better evidence in children and adolescents particularly with omeprazole, rabeprazole, and lansoprazole.[37] When examining adverse effect data from currently available trial data the authors noted that overall proton pump inhibitor therapy was well tolerated with mostly mild to moderate adverse effects in the short-term. Adverse effects with individual agents included diarrhea, abdominal pain, and vomiting with headache noted in older age groups and upper and lower respiratory tract infections noted in infants. It was stated that additional long-term data is needed in this population and that overall data was limited in infants younger than 1 year of age.[37] Long-term use of a proton pump inhibitor without a clear diagnosis of GERD is not recommended.[7]

Elderly Patients with GERD

Many elderly patients have decreased host defense mechanisms, such as saliva production. In addition, they have more comorbidities, medications, and physiologic changes that put them at higher risk. Often these patients do not seek medical attention because they feel their symptoms are part of the normal aging process. They may also present with atypical symptoms such as chest pain, asthma, poor dentition, or jaw pain. Decreased GI motility is a common problem in elderly patients. Unfortunately, there are no good promotility agents available to these patients. Elderly patients are especially sensitive to the CNS effects of metoclopramide. They may also be sensitive to the CNS effects of H_2-receptor antagonists. Proton pump inhibitors appear to be the most useful treatment modality because they have superior efficacy and are dosed once daily, which is beneficial in all patients, but is especially beneficial in the elderly. Long-term risk of bone fractures may be of concern in this population. Patients at risk for bone fractures should be monitored appropriately.

Patients with Refractory GERD

What constitutes refractory GERD is not well-defined. Prior to increasing the dose to twice daily, adherence and proper timing of proton pump inhibitor therapy should be optimized. Refractory GERD should be considered in patients who have not responded to

TABLE 32-6 Oral Proton Pump Inhibitor Therapy in Pediatric Patients

	Indication	Recommended Oral Dose (daily)		
Lansoprazole	GERD, erosive esophagitis	1-11 years	≤30 kg	15 mg
			>30 kg	30 mg
	Erosive esophagitis	12-17 years		30 mg
	Nonerosive GERD	12-17 years		15 mg
Esomeprazole	Erosive esophagitis	1 month-1 year	3-5 kg	2.5 mg
			>5 to 7.5 kg	5 mg
			>7.5 to 12 kg	10 mg
		1-11 years	<20 kg	10 mg
			≥20 kg	10-20 mg
		12-17 years		20-40 mg
	Symptomatic GERD	1-11 years		10 mg
		12-17 years		20 mg
Omeprazole	GERD, maintenance of healing of erosive esophagitis	1-16 years	5 to <10 kg	5 mg
			10 to <20 kg	10 mg
			≥20 kg	20 mg
Pantoprazole	Short-term treatment of erosive esophagitis	≥5 years	≥15 to <40 kg	20 mg
			≥40 kg	40 mg
Rabeprazole	GERD	1-11 years	<15 kg	5-10 mg
			≥15 kg	10 mg
		≥12 years		20 mg

a standard course of twice-daily proton pump inhibitor therapy. In this case, other causes for the patient's symptoms should be evaluated. The majority of patients with refractory symptoms experience nocturnal acid breakthrough. Other reasons for refractory symptoms may be related to compliance, timing of proton pump inhibitor, and drug metabolism differences in certain patients. Switching to another proton pump inhibitor may be effective for refractory symptoms in some patients. Manometry or ambulatory esophageal reflux monitoring is useful for patients who are not responding to therapy with normal endoscopic findings. If tests are negative, ISERT the patient is unlikely to have GERD and proton pump inhibitor therapy should be discontinued.[1] The addition of an H_2-receptor antagonist at bedtime for nocturnal symptoms has been suggested; however, the effect may be short-lived due to tachyphylaxis. Eosinophilic esophagitis or dysmotility syndromes may be causes of nonacid-related esophageal symptoms.[38]

PERSONALIZED PHARMACOTHERAPY

Significant liver impairment may result in a seven-fold to nine-fold increase in area under the serum concentration versus time curve and increase serum half-life of proton pump inhibitors. While clear recommendations are not available, it may be prudent to consider a lower dose in this population.

The hepatic enzyme CYP2C19 is involved in the metabolism of many medications, including proton pump inhibitors, particularly omeprazole. Further evaluation is needed to determine the role of polymorphic gene variation in the hepatic activity of CYP2C19.

Drug interactions with omeprazole are of particular concern for patients who are considered "slow metabolizers" of omeprazole, which is more common in the Asian population but also found in approximately 3% of the white population. Unfortunately, it is unclear which patients have the polymorphic gene variation that makes them slow metabolizers. Like omeprazole, the metabolism of esomeprazole may also be altered for patients with this polymorphic gene variation.

EVALUATION OF THERAPEUTIC OUTCOMES

The long-term benefits of treatment are difficult to assess because of the limited information known about the epidemiology and natural history of GERD. Consequently, successful outcomes are generally measured in terms of three separate end points: (a) relieving symptoms, (b) healing the injured mucosa, and (c) preventing complications.

The short-term goal of therapy is to relieve symptoms such as heartburn and regurgitation to the point at which they do not impair the patient's quality of life. Patients should be educated regarding specific lifestyle modifications that are applicable to their individual situation including weight loss and raising the head end of the bed. 10 In addition, patient medication profiles should be reviewed for medications that may aggravate GERD. Patients should be monitored for adverse drug reactions. Table 32-5 reviews common adverse drug reactions and monitoring of medications used in GERD. Drug-drug interactions should also be assessed and these agents should be avoided if possible. Table 32-7 lists recommendations for providing pharmaceutical care to patients with GERD.

The frequency and severity of symptoms should be monitored, and patients should be counseled on symptoms that suggest the presence of complications requiring immediate medical attention, such as dysphagia. Patients should also be monitored for the presence of extraesophageal symptoms, such as laryngitis asthma or chest pain. These symptoms require further diagnostic evaluation. Long-term maintenance treatment is indicated for patients who have strictures because the strictures commonly recur if reflux esophagitis is not treated.

The second goal is to heal the injured mucosa. Again, individualized lifestyle modifications and the importance of complying with the therapeutic regimen chosen to heal the mucosa should be stressed. Patients should be educated about the risk of relapse and the need for long-term maintenance therapy to prevent recurrence or complications.

TABLE 32-7 Recommendations for Providing Pharmaceutical Care to Patients with GERD

1. Assess the patient's symptoms to determine if patient-directed therapy is appropriate or whether patient should be evaluated by a clinician. Determine the type of symptoms, frequency, and exacerbating factors. Refer any patient with alarm or atypical symptoms to a clinician for further diagnostic workup
2. Obtain a thorough history of prescription, nonprescription, and natural drug product use
3. Counsel the patient on lifestyle modifications that will improve symptoms
4. Recommend appropriate drug therapy based on patient presentation
5. Develop a plan to assess effectiveness of acid-suppression therapy after an appropriate amount of time (8-16 weeks). Recommend alternative therapy if necessary
6. Assess improvement in quality-of-life measures such as physical, psychological, and social functioning and well-being
7. Evaluate patient for the presence of adverse drug reactions, allergies, and drug interactions
8. Stress the importance of compliance with the therapeutic regimen, including lifestyle modifications. Recommend a therapeutic regimen that is easy for the patient to accomplish
9. Provide patient education with regard to disease state, lifestyle modifications, and drug therapy. Patients should be counseled on:
   - What causes GERD and what things to avoid
   - When to take their medications
   - What potential adverse effects or drug interactions may occur
   - What alarm signs they should report to their clinician

The final, long-term goal of therapy is to decrease the risk of complications (esophagitis, strictures, Barrett's esophagus, and esophageal adenocarcinoma). A small subset of patients may continue to fail treatment despite therapy with high doses of H_2-receptor antagonists or a proton pump inhibitor. Patients should be monitored for the presence of continual pain, dysphagia, or odynophagia.

ABBREVIATIONS

BMI	body mass index
CYP	cytochrome P450
GABA	gamma aminobutyric acid
GERD	gastroesophageal reflux disease
H_2	histamine-2
HREPT	high-resolution esophageal pressure topography
HRQL	health-related quality of life
LES	lower esophageal sphincter
mGluR5	metabotropic glutamate type 5
NERD	nonerosive reflux disease
TLESR	transient lower esophageal sphincter relaxation

REFERENCES

1. Katz PO, Gerson LB, Vela MF. Guidelines for the diagnosis and management of gastroesophageal reflux disease. *Am J Gastroenterol* 2013;108:308-328. doi:10.1038/ajg.2012.444.
2. Rubenstein JH, Chen JW. Epidemiology of gastroesophageal reflux disease. *Gastroenterol Clin North Am* 2014;43(1):1-14.
3. El-Serag HB, Sweet S, Winchester CC, Dent J. Update on the epidemiology of gastro-oesophageal reflux disease: A systematic review. *Gut* 2014;63(6):871-880.
4. Nwokediuko SC. Current trends in the management of gastroesophageal reflux disease: A review. *ISRN Gastroenterol* 2012; Article 391631:1-11. doi:10.5402/2012/391631.
5. Chou PH, Lin CC, Lin CH, et al. Prevalence of gastroesophageal reflux disease in major depressive disorder: A population-based study. *Psychosomatics* 2014;55(2):155-162.
6. Kahrilas PJ, McColl K, Fox M, et al. The acid pocket: A target for treatment in reflux disease? *Am J Gastroenterol* 2013;108:1058-1064. doi:10.1038/ajg.2013.132.
7. Lightdale JR, Gremse DA, and Section on Gastroenterology, Hepatology, and Nutrition. Gastroesophageal reflux: Management guidance for the pediatrician. *Pediatrics* 2013;131:e1684-e1695. doi: 10.1542/peds.2013-0421.
8. Herbella FA, Patti MG. Gastroesophageal reflux disease: From pathophysiology to treatment. *World J Gastroenterol* 2010;16(30):3745-3749.
9. Hvid-Jensen F, Pedersen L, Drewes AM, et al. Incidence of adenocarcinoma among patients with Barrett's esophagus. *N Engl J Med* 2011;365:1375-1383.
10. Lee SW, Lee TY, Lien HC, Yang SS, Yeh HZ, Chang CS. Characteristics of symptom presentation and risk factors in patients with erosive esophagitis and nonerosive reflux disease. *Med Prin Pract* 2014;23(5):460-464.
11. Kahrilas PJ. Gastroesophageal reflux disease. *N Engl J Med* 2008;359:1700-1707.
12. Dunbar KB, Spechler SJ. Controversies in Barrett esophagus. *Mayo Clin Proc* 2014;89(7):973-984.
13. Kleiman DA, Beninato T, Bosworth BP, et al. Early referral for esophageal pH monitoring is more cost-effective than prolonged empiric trials of proton-pump inhibitors for suspected gastroesophageal reflux disease. *J Gastrointest Surg* 2014;18(1):26-33.
14. GRADE Working Group. Grading quality of evidence and strength of recommendations. *BMJ* 2004;328:1490-1494.
15. DeVault KR, Castell DO. Updated guidelines for the diagnosis and treatment of gastroesophageal reflux disease. *Am J Gastroenterol* 2005;100:190-200.
16. Rickenbacher N, Kötter T, Kochen MM, et al. Fundoplication versus medical management of gastroesophageal reflux disease: Systematic review and meta-analysis. *Surg Endosc* 2014;28:143-155.
17. Nadaleto BF, Herbella FA, Patti MG. Gastroesophageal reflux disease in the obese: Pathophysiology and treatment [published online ahead of print June 5 2015]. *Surgery* 2015;159:475-486. doi:10.1016/j.surg.2015.04.034.
18. Danalioglu A, Cipe G, Toydemir T, Kocaman O, Ince AT, et al. Endoscopic stapling in comparison to laparoscopic fundoplication for the treatment of gastroesophageal reflux disease. *Dig Endosc* 2014;26(1):37-42.
19. Spechler SJ, Sharma P, Souza RF, et al. American Gastroenterological Association medical position statement on the management of Barrett's esophagus. *Gastroenterology* 2011;140:1084-1091.
20. Louie BE, Farivar AS, Shultz D, et al. Short-term outcomes using magnetic sphincter augmentation versus Nissen fundoplication for medically resistant gastroesophageal reflux disease. *Ann Thorac Surg* 2014;98(2):498-504.
21. Smith CD, DeVault KR, Buchanan M. Introduction of mechanical sphincter augmentation for gastroesophageal reflux disease into practice: Early clinical outcomes and keys to successful adoption. *J Am Coll Surg* 2014;218(4):776-781.
22. Bortolotti M. The "magnetic collar": The ultimate solution for gastroesophageal reflux? *Scand J Astroenterol* 2014;49(4):511-512.
23. Sweis R, Kaufman E, Anggiansah A, et al. Post-prandial reflux suppression by a raft-forming alginate (Gaviscon Advance) compared to a simple antacid documented by magnetic resonance imaging and pH-impedance monitoring: Mechanistic assessment in healthy volunteers and randomized, controlled, double-blind study in reflux patients. *Aliment Pharmacol Ther* 2013;37:1093-1102.
24. Janarthanan S, Ditah I, Phil M, et al. *Clostridium difficile*-associated diarrhea and proton pump inhibitor therapy: A meta-analysis. *Am J Gastroenterol* 2012;107:1001-1010.
25. Thomson ABR, Sauve MD, Kassam N, Kamitakahara H. Safety of the long-term use of proton pump inhibitors. *World J Gastroenterol* 2010;16(19):2323-2330.
26. FDA Drug Safety Communication: Possible Increased Risk of Fractures of the Hip, Wrist, and Spine with the Use of Proton Pump Inhibitors. 2010. Available at: www.fda.gov.
27. FDA Drug Safety Communication: Possible Increased Risk of Fractures of the Hip, Wrist, and Spine with the Use of Proton Pump Inhibitors. Update. 2011. Available at: www.fda.gov.
28. Ngamruengphong S, Leontiadis GI, Radhi S, et al. Proton pump inhibitors and risk of fracture: A systematic review and meta-analysis of observational studies. *Am J Gastroenterol* 2011;106:1209-1218.
29. Corley DA, Kubo A, Zhao W, Quesenberry C. Proton pump inhibitors and histamine-2 receptor antagonists are associated with hip fractures among at-risk patients. *Gastroenterology* 2010;139:93-101.
30. Jacobs C, Coss Adame E, Attaluri A, et al. Dysmotility and proton pump inhibitor use are independent risk factors for small intestinal bacterial and/or fungal overgrowth. *Aliment Pharmacol Ther* 2013;37:1103-1111.
31. Ho MP, Maddox TM, Wang L, et al. Risk of adverse outcomes associated with concomitant use of clopidogrel and proton pump inhibitors following acute coronary syndrome. *JAMA* 2009;301:937-944.

32. Laine L, Henneken SC. Proton pump inhibitor and clopidogrel interaction: Fact or fiction? *Am J Gastroenterol* 2010;105:34-41.
33. Abraham NS, Hlatky MA, Antman EM, et al. ACCF/ACG/AHA 2010 expert consensus document on the concomitant use of proton pump inhibitors and thienopyridines: A focused update of the ACCF/ACG/AHA 2008 expert consensus document on reducing the gastrointestinal risks of antiplatelet therapy and NSAID use: A report of the American College of Cardiology Foundation Task Force on Expert Consensus Documents. *Circulation* 2010;122:2619-2633.
34. Kuo P, Holloway RH. Beyond acid suppression: New pharmacologic approaches for treatment of GERD. *Curr Gastroenterol Rep* 2010;12:175-180.
35. Hassall E. Over-prescription of acid-suppressing medications in infants: How it came about, why it's wrong, and what to do about it. *J Pediatr* 2012;160(2):193-198.
36. Terrin G, Passariello A, De Curtis M, et al. Ranitidine is associated with infections, necrotizing enterocolitis, and fatal outcome in newborns. *Pediatrics* 2012;129:e40-e45.
37. Kierkus J, Oracz G, Dorczowski B, et al. Comparative safety and efficacy of proton pump inhibitors in pediatric gastroesophageal reflux disease. *Drug Safety* 2014;37(5):309-316.
38. Dellon ES, Shaheen NJ. Persistent reflux symptoms in the proton pump inhibitor era: The changing face of gastroesophageal reflux disease. *Gastroenterology* 2010;139:7-13.

Peptic Ulcer Disease and Related Disorders

33

Bryan L. Love and Phillip L. Mohorn

KEY CONCEPTS

1. Psychological stress, cigarette smoking, nonsteroidal anti-inflammatory drug (NSAID) use and certain foods/beverages can exacerbate ulcer symptoms and should be avoided.
2. Eradication of *Helicobacter pylori* is recommended in all patients who test positive, especially in those patients with an active ulcer, a documented history of a prior ulcer, or a history of ulcer-related complications.
3. The selection of an *H. pylori* eradication regimen should be based on several factors, including: efficacy, safety, antibiotic resistance, cost, and the likelihood of medication adherence. The preferred initial treatment is a proton pump inhibitor (PPI)–based three-drug regimen. Subsequent salvage treatment for *H. pylori* should contain different antibiotics due to potential resistance.
4. PPI co-therapy reduces the risk of NSAID-related gastric and duodenal ulcers and is at least as effective as recommended dosages of misoprostol and superior to the histamine-2 receptor antagonists (H2RAs).
5. Standard PPI dosages and a nonselective NSAID are as effective as a selective cyclooxygenase-2 (COX-2) inhibitor in reducing the risk of NSAID-induced ulcers and upper gastrointestinal (GI) complications.
6. Patients with peptic ulcer disease (PUD), especially those receiving *H. pylori* eradication or misoprostol cotherapy, require patient education regarding their disease and drug treatment to successfully achieve a positive therapeutic outcome.
7. Treatment for severe peptic ulcer bleeding after appropriate endoscopic treatment includes IV administration of a PPI loading dose followed by a 72-hour continuous infusion.
8. Coagulopathy and respiratory failure requiring mechanical ventilation are two of the highest risk factors for developing stress-related mucosal bleeding (SRMB). Prophylactic drug therapy should be administered to critically ill patients with one of these complications.
9. Since there are limited data to support the selection of a PPI over an IV H2RA for SRMB prophylaxis, agent selection should be based on appropriate individual patient characteristics (eg, nothing by mouth, presence of nasogastric tube, thrombocytopenia, renal failure).

PEPTIC ULCER DISEASE

Gastric-acid is a critical component of upper gastrointestinal (GI) tract complications including gastritis, erosions, and peptic ulcer.[1-3] Peptic ulcer disease (PUD) differs from gastritis and erosions in that ulcers are larger (greater than or equal to 5 mm) and extend deeper into the muscularis mucosa.[1] The three common forms of peptic ulcers can be grouped according to their etiology: *Helicobacter pylori*-positive, nonsteroidal anti-inflammatory drug (NSAID)-induced, and stress-related mucosal damage (SRMD) (Table 33-1).

H. pylori-positive and NSAID-induced ulcers are chronic peptic ulcers that differ in etiology, clinical presentation, and tendency to recur (see Table 33-1). These ulcers develop most often in the stomach and duodenum of ambulatory patients (Fig. 33-1). Occasionally, ulcers develop in the esophagus, jejunum, ileum, or colon. The natural course of chronic PUD is characterized by frequent ulcer recurrence. The cause of ulcer recurrence is often multifactorial, although *H. pylori* infection and NSAID use are commonly associated. In addition, cigarette smoking, alcohol use, gastric acid hypersecretion, and medication nonadherence are frequently related.

Other conditions such as Zollinger-Ellison syndrome (ZES), radiation, chemotherapy, vascular insufficiency, and other chronic diseases (Table 33-2) are associated with development and recurrence of peptic ulcers.[1,2] Although a strong association exists between chronic pulmonary diseases, chronic renal failure including hemodialysis, and cirrhosis, the pathophysiologic mechanisms of these associations remain unclear.[1] In contrast, SRMD occurs primarily in the stomach of critically ill patients (see Table 33-1).[1]

This chapter focuses on issues surrounding chronic PUD due to *H. pylori* and NSAIDs. A brief discussion of other PUD-related disorders (ZES, upper GI bleeding, and SRMD) is also included.

EPIDEMIOLOGY

The epidemiology of PUD is complicated and the prevalence is difficult to estimate given the variability in *H. pylori* infection, NSAID use, and cigarette smoking. In addition, endoscopy, radiology, symptoms, or other methods have different sensitivity and specificity to detect ulcers.[1,4] The prevalence and incidence of PUD in the United States also reflects improvements in drug therapy, the dramatic shift to ambulatory management, and changes in the criteria and coding system for mortality and hospitalization data reflected by continued declines in mortality, hospitalization, and age-adjusted ambulatory care visits. Mortality rates are higher among those older than or 65 years and in males compared to females.[4] Despite continued improvements, PUD remains one of the most common GI diseases, resulting in impaired quality of life, work loss, and high-cost medical care.

Helicobacter pylori

The prevalence of *H. pylori* varies by geographic location, socioeconomic conditions, ethnicity, and age. In industrialized countries, *H . pylori* prevalence is less common than in developing countries and correlates with socioeconomic levels.[2,5,6] The prevalence of *H. pylori* in the United States is 30% to 40% but is much higher in individuals older than 60 years (50%-60%) than in children younger than 12 years (10%-15%).[2,5] Although most individuals in the United States

TABLE 33-1 Comparison of Common Forms of Peptic Ulcer

Characteristic	*H. pylori*-Induced	NSAID-Induced	SRMD
Condition	Chronic	Chronic	Acute
Site of damage	Duodenum > stomach	Stomach > duodenum	Stomach > duodenum
Intragastric pH	More dependent	Less dependent	Less dependent
Symptoms	Usually epigastric pain	Often asymptomatic	Asymptomatic
Ulcer depth	Superficial	Deep	Most superficial
GI bleeding	Less severe, single vessel	More severe, single vessel	More severe, superficial mucosal capillaries

GI, gastrointestinal; NSAID, nonsteroidal anti-inflammatory drug; SRMD, stress-related mucosal damage.

acquire *H. pylori* in childhood, the rate of acquisition in children is declining and most likely will continue to fall as a consequence of improved socioeconomic conditions.[2] Whites are infected with *H. pylori* less frequently than African Americans and Hispanic persons, but this is thought to be related to lower socioeconomic status and living conditions. Infection rates do not differ with gender or smoking status.

Nonsteroidal Anti-Inflammatory Drugs

Gastroduodenal ulcers develop in up to 15% to 30% of chronic NSAID users with continued use.[7] Gastric ulcers are most common, occur primarily in the antrum, and are of greater concern because of their potential to cause ulcer-related upper GI complications. Between 2% and 4% of patients with an NSAID ulcer will bleed or perforate.[7] In the United States at least 100,000 hospitalizations and between 7,000 and 10,000 deaths are directly attributed to NSAIDs each year.[7-9] Ulcer-related complications and death among regular NSAID users are 3 to 10 times higher compared with nonusers.

ETIOLOGY

H. pylori infection and NSAID use are the most common risk factors for PUD. Less common factors including ZES with hypersecretion of acid (see Table 33-2) can also be involved.[1] Disruptions in normal mucosal defense and healing mechanisms allow acid and pepsin to reach the gastric epithelium.[1] Benign gastric ulcers, erosions, and gastritis can occur anywhere in the stomach, although the antrum and lesser curvature represent the most common locations (see Fig. 33-1). Most duodenal ulcers occur in the first part of the duodenum (duodenal bulb).

H. pylori

H. pylori is a gram-negative, microaerophilic, urease producing bacteria most commonly found in the stomach or duodenum. Bacterial urease production, to alkalinize the microenvironment, and flagella that allows for motility enable the bacterium to survive in the acidic environment of the stomach. *H. pylori* is primarily transmitted via person to person routes by either gastro–oral (vomitus) or fecal–oral (diarrhea) contact. Risk factors for acquiring *H. pylori* include close contact within households, low socioeconomic status, and country of origin.[2]

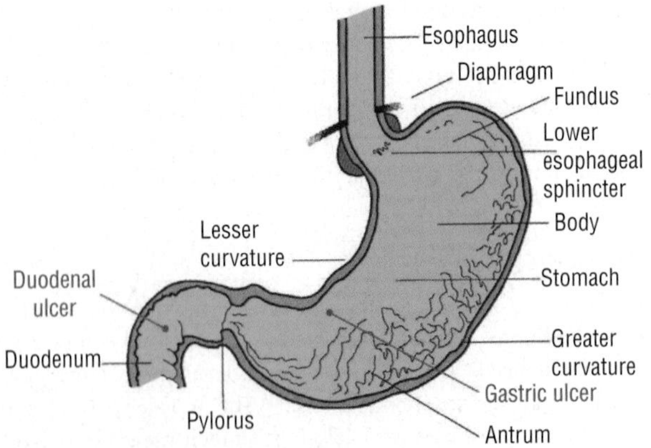

H. pylori infection can cause both acute and chronic gastritis in infected individuals and is associated with multiple GI complications. PUD, mucosa-associated lymphoid tissue (MALT) lymphoma, and gastric cancer (Fig. 33-2) have all been linked to *H. pylori* infection.[1,2,5,6,10,11] Most infected individuals remain asymptomatic, but 10% to 20% will develop PUD during their lifetime and about 1% will develop gastric cancer.[1,2] Environmental factors, host genetics and *H. pylori* strain virulence factors play an important role in the pathogenesis of PUD and gastric cancer.[2] *H. pylori* infection increases the risk of GI bleeding and peptic ulcers by threefold to sevenfold.[5] No specific link has been established between *H. pylori* and dyspepsia, nonulcer dyspepsia (NUD), or gastroesophageal reflux disease (GERD).[5,10,12] However, some patients with dyspepsia and NUD may have symptom improvement from *H. pylori* eradication.[5] Conversely, eradication of *H. pylori* may worsen GERD symptoms in some patients, but eradication should be attempted due to the known gastric cancer risk.[5,10] *H. pylori* is also associated with iron deficiency anemia, although the benefit of eradication remains unknown.[5,12]

Nonsteroidal Anti-Inflammatory Drugs

Prescription and nonprescription NSAIDs (Table 33-3), are widely used in the United States, and have been linked to PUD. There is overwhelming evidence linking chronic NSAID (including low-dose aspirin) use to upper GI tract injury, PUD, gastritis, and

FIGURE 33-1 Anatomic structure of the stomach and duodenum and most common locations of gastric and duodenal ulcers.

TABLE 33-2 Potential Causes of Peptic Ulcer

Common causes
Helicobacter pylori infection
NSAIDs
Critical illness (stress-related mucosal damage)
Uncommon causes of chronic peptic ulcer
Idiopathic (non–*H. pylori*, non-NSAID peptic ulcer)
Hypersecretion of gastric acid (eg, Zollinger-Ellison syndrome)
Viral infections (eg, cytomegalovirus)
Vascular insufficiency (eg, crack cocaine associated)
Radiation therapy
Chemotherapy (eg, hepatic artery infusions)
Infiltrating disease (eg, Crohn disease)
Diseases and medical conditions associated with chronic peptic ulcer
Cirrhosis
Chronic renal failure
Chronic obstructive pulmonary disease
Cardiovascular disease
Organ transplantation

NSAIDs, nonsteroidal anti-inflammatory drugs.

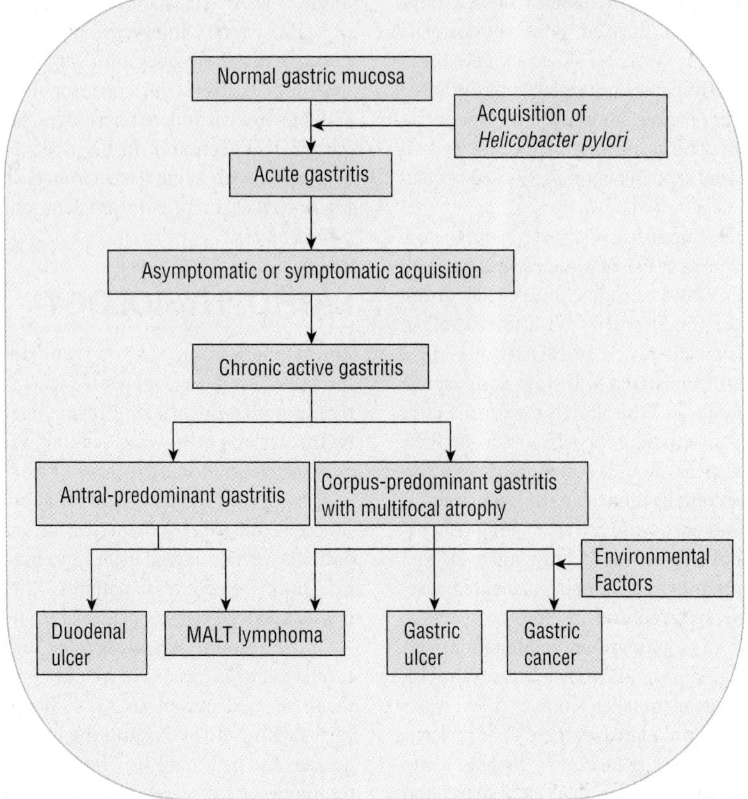

FIGURE 33-2 The natural history of Helicobacter pylori infection in the pathogenesis of gastric ulcer and duodenal ulcer, mucosaassociated lymphoid tissue (MALT) lymphoma, and gastric cancer.

superficial erosion.[1,7,13-17] In susceptible individuals, NSAIDs cause superficial mucosal damage consisting of petechiae (intramucosal hemorrhages) within minutes of ingestion, and progress to erosions with continued use.[1] These lesions typically heal within a few days and rarely cause ulcers or acute upper GI bleeding. NSAID-induced ulcers occur less frequently in the esophagus, small bowel, and colon.[17,18] The mechanisms by which NSAIDs damage the lower GI tract is not clear, but the enteropathy is associated with lower GI bleeding.

Table 33-4 lists the risk factors associated with NSAID-induced ulcers and upper GI complications. Combinations of factors confer an additive risk.[7,14-17,19] Advanced age is an independent risk factor, and the incidence of NSAID-induced ulcers increases linearly with the age of the patient.[1] The high incidence of ulcer complications in older individuals may be explained by age-related changes in gastric mucosal defense. The relative risk of NSAID complications is increased for patients with a previous peptic ulcer and may be as high as 14-fold in those with a history of an ulcer-related complication.[1,17] Although the risk of ulcer complications is greatest during the first few months after initiating continuous NSAID therapy, it does not vanish with long-term treatment.[7]

NSAID ulcers and related complications are dependent upon the dose, duration of use, and type of NSAID. Although dose is important, low doses of nonprescription NSAIDs and low cardioprotective dosages of aspirin (81-325 mg/day) can also be attributed to increased risk of ulcer formation.[1,7,14-17] Factors such as NSAID potency, longer duration of effect, and a greater propensity to inhibit cyclooxygenase-1 (COX-1) versus cyclooxygenase-2

TABLE 33-3 Selected NSAIDs and COX-2 Inhibitors

Nonsalicylates[a]
Nonselective (traditional) NSAIDs: indomethacin, piroxicam, ibuprofen, naproxen, sulindac, ketoprofen, ketorolac, flurbiprofen
Partially selective NSAIDs: etodolac, nabumetone, meloxicam, diclofenac, celecoxib
Selective COX-2 inhibitors: rofecoxib,[b] valdecoxib[b]
Salicylates
Acetylated: aspirin
Nonacetylated: salsalate, trisalicylate

COX-2, cyclooxygenase-2; NSAIDs, nonsteroidal anti-inflammatory drugs.

[a]Based on COX-1-to-COX-2 selectivity ratio.

[b]Withdrawn from US market.

TABLE 33-4 Risk Factors Associated with INSAID–Induced Ulcers and Upper GI Complications[a]

Age > 65
Previous peptic ulcer
Previous ulcer-related upper GI complication
High-dose NSAIDs
Multiple NSAID use
Selection of NSAID (eg, COX-1 vs COX-2 inhibition)
NSAID-related dyspepsia
Aspirin (including cardioprotective dosages)
Concomitant use of
NSAID plus low-dose aspirin
Oral bisphosphonates (eg, alendronate)
Corticosteroids
Anticoagulant or coagulopathy
Antiplatelet drugs (eg, clopidogrel)
Selective serotonin reuptake inhibitor
Chronic debilitating disorders (eg, cardiovascular disease, rheumatoid arthritis)
Helicobacter pylori infection
Cigarette smoking
Alcohol consumption

COX-2, cyclooxygenase-2; GI, gastrointestinal; NSAIDs, nonsteroidal anti-inflammatory drugs.

[a]Combinations of risk factors are additive.

Data from references 1, 7, 8, and 13 to 16.

(COX-2) isoenzymes are associated with increased risk (see Table 33-3).[1,17,19,20] NSAID-related dyspepsia, in itself, does not correlate directly with mucosal injury or clinical events. However, new-onset dyspepsia, changes in severity, or dyspepsia not relieved by antiulcer medications may suggest an ulcer or ulcer complication.[1] Nonacetylated salicylates (eg, salsalate) may be associated with decreased GI toxicity.[1] Buffered or enteric-coated aspirin confers no added protection from upper GI events.[14]

NSAID ulcer and GI complication risk are increased with the use of multiple NSAIDs or the concomitant use of low-dose aspirin, oral bisphosphonates, corticosteroids, anticoagulants, antiplatelet drugs, and selective serotonin reuptake inhibitors.[1,7,14-17,21] The risk of an ulcer-related GI complication is greater when an NSAID or COX-2 inhibitor (see Table 33-3) is coadministered with low-dose aspirin than when either drug is taken alone.[1,14,17] The NSAID may also reduce the antiplatelet effects of aspirin, although NSAIDs vary in their effects on platelet function.[14-16] Corticosteroids, when used alone, do not potentiate the risk of ulcer or complications, but the relative risk is increased twofold in corticosteroid users who are also taking concurrent NSAIDs.[1,17] The relative risk of GI bleeding increases up to 20-fold when NSAIDs are taken concomitantly with anticoagulants (eg, warfarin) and up to sixfold with the concurrent use of serotonin reuptake inhibitors.[17,18] Coadiministration of clopidogrel in combination with aspirin, an NSAID, or an anticoagulant significantly increases the risk of GI bleeding compared with either agent taken alone.[14,17] Even when prescribed as monotherapy, clopidogrel increases the risk of rebleeding for patients with a history of a bleeding ulcer.[14,15,17] Prasugrel and ticagrelor have more potent platelet inhibition than clopidogrel and are associated with a greater risk of bleeding.[14,22]

H. pylori and NSAIDs act independently to increase ulcer risk and ulcer-related bleeding and appear to have additive effects.[5,17] Thus, the incidence of peptic ulcer is higher in *H. pylori*–positive NSAID users. Whether *H. pylori* infection is actually a risk factor for NSAID ulcers remains controversial.[1,5,17] However, eradication is reported to reduce the incidence of peptic ulcer if undertaken prior to starting the NSAID but does not reduce the risk for patients who were previously taking an NSAID.[1,5,17]

Cigarette Smoking

Cigarette smoking has been linked to PUD, but it is uncertain whether smoking causes peptic ulcers.[1] The prevalence of ulcer disease is nearly double in current and former smokers (11.43% and 11.52%) compared to those who never smoked (6%). The risk of peptic ulcers in smokers with a large daily use, but ulcer risk is modest when fewer than 10 cigarettes are smoked per day.[23] Cigarette smoking impairs ulcer healing, promotes ulcer recurrence, and increases ulcer risk.[1] However, the underlying mechanisms by which cigarette smoking exerts these adverse effects remains unclear. Possible mechanisms include mucosal ischemia, inhibition of pancreatic bicarbonate secretion, and increases in gastric acid and mucous secretion, but these effects are inconsistent.[24]

Psychological Stress

The importance of psychological factors in the pathogenesis of PUD remains controversial.[1] Clinical observation suggests that ulcer patients are adversely affected by stressful life events. However, results from controlled trials are conflicting and have failed to document a cause-and-effect relationship.[1] Emotional stress may induce behavioral risks such as smoking and the use of NSAIDs or alter the inflammatory response or resistance to *H. pylori* infection. The role of stress and how it affects PUD is complex and probably multifactorial.

Dietary Factors

The effects of diet and nutrition on the pathophysiology PUD is uncertain. Carbonated beverages, coffee, tea, beer, milk, and spices often cause dyspepsia, but they do not appear to increase the risk of PUD.[1] Dietary interventions such as bland or restricted diets do not alter the frequency of ulcer recurrence. Although caffeine is a gastric acid stimulant, constituents in decaffeinated coffee or tea, caffeine-free carbonated beverages, beer, and wine may also increase gastric acid secretion. In high concentrations, alcohol ingestion is associated with acute gastric mucosal damage and upper GI bleeding; however, there is insufficient evidence to confirm that alcohol causes ulcers.[1]

PATHOPHYSIOLOGY

The pathophysiology of gastric and duodenal ulcers is determined by the balance between aggressive (gastric acid and pepsin) and protective (mucosal defense and repair) factors.[1,3] Gastric acid is secreted by the parietal cells, which contain receptors for histamine, gastrin, and acetylcholine.[1] Acid (as well as *H. pylori* infection and NSAID use) is an independent factor that contributes to the disruption of mucosal integrity.[1] Increased acid secretion has been observed for patients with duodenal ulcers and may be a consequence of *H. pylori* infection.[2,25] In contrast, patients with gastric ulcer usually have normal or reduced rates of acid secretion (hypochlorhydria).

The amount of acid secreted under basal or fasting conditions is referred to as basal acid output (BAO); after maximal stimulation, maximal acid output (MAO).[1] Basal and maximal acid secretion varies with time of day and the individual's psychological state, age, gender, and health status. The BAO follows a circadian rhythm, with the highest acid secretion occurring at night and the lowest in the morning. An increase in the BAO:MAO ratio suggests a basal hypersecretory state such as ZES.

Pepsin is an important enzyme cofactor in the proteolytic activity involved in ulcer formation.[21] Pepsinogen, the inactive precursor of pepsin, is secreted by the chief cells in the gastric fundus (see Fig. 33-1). Pepsin activity is determined by pH as it is activated by acid pH (optimal pH of 1.8-3.5), reversibly inactivated at pH 4, and irreversibly destroyed at pH 7.

Mucus and bicarbonate secretion, intrinsic epithelial cell defense, and mucosal blood flow protect the gastroduodenal mucosa from noxious endogenous and exogenous substances.[1,21] The viscous nature and near-neutral pH of the mucus–bicarbonate barrier protect the stomach from the acidic contents in the gastric lumen. Mucosal repair after injury is related to epithelial cell restitution, growth, and regeneration. Endogenous prostaglandins' (PGs) production facilitate mucosal integrity and repair. The term *cytoprotection* is often used to describe this process, but *mucosal defense* and *mucosal protection* are more accurate terms, as PGs prevent deep mucosal injury and not superficial damage to individual cells. Gastric hyperemia and increased PG synthesis characterize adaptive cytoprotection, the short-term adaptation of mucosal cells to mild topical irritants that enables the stomach to initially withstand the damaging effects of irritants. Alterations in mucosal defense that are induced by *H. pylori* or NSAIDs are the most important cofactors in the formation of peptic ulcers.

Helicobacter pylori

In infected people, *H. pylori* resides between the gastric mucus layer and surface epithelial cells, or any location where gastric-type epithelium is found.[2,25] Its spiral shape and flagellum permits it to move from the lumen of the stomach, where the pH is low, to the mucus layer, where the local pH is neutral. *H. pylori* produces large amounts of urease, which hydrolyzes urea in the gastric juice and converts it to ammonia and carbon dioxide.[2] The local buffering effect of ammonia creates a neutral microenvironment within and surrounding the bacterium, protecting it from the lethal effect of gastric acid. *H. pylori* also produces acid-inhibitory proteins, which allow it to adapt to the low-pH environment of the stomach.[2]

H. pylori binds to gastric-type epithelium by adherence pedestals, which prevent the organism from being shed during cell turnover and mucus secretion.[2] Colonization of the antrum and corpus (body) of the stomach is associated with gastric ulcer and cancer.[1,25] Antral organisms colonize gastric tissue that develops in the duodenum secondary to changes in gastric acid or bicarbonate secretion leading to duodenal ulcer (see Fig. 33-2).[1,2] Although *H. pylori* causes chronic gastric mucosal inflammation in all infected individuals, only a minority actually develop an ulcer or gastric cancer.[1] The difference in the diverse clinical outcomes is related to variations in bacterial pathogenicity and host susceptibility.[2,25]

Bacterial enzymes (urease, lipases, and proteases), bacterial adherence, and *H. pylori* virulence factors produce gastric mucosal injury.[2,25] Lipases and proteases degrade gastric mucus, ammonia produced by urease may be toxic to gastric epithelial cells, and bacterial adherence enhances the uptake of toxins into gastric epithelial cells. *H. pylori* induces gastric inflammation by altering the host inflammatory response and damaging epithelial cells directly by cell-mediated immune mechanisms or indirectly by activated neutrophils or macrophages attempting to phagocytose bacteria or bacterial products.[2,25] However, *H. pylori* strains are genetically diverse and account for differences in adaptation within the human host. Two of the most important are cytotoxin-associated gene protein (CagA) and vacuolating cytotoxin (VacA). About 60% of *H. pylori* strains in the United States possess CagA, but CagA-positive strains increase the risk for severe PUD, gastritis, and gastric cancer compared with CagA-negative strains.[2,26] The VacA gene codes for the VacA cytotoxin, a vacuolating toxin. Although VacA is present in most *H. pylori* strains, strains vary in cytotoxicity and increased risk for peptic ulcer and gastric cancer.[2] Host polymorphisms are important markers of disease susceptibility and may identify high-risk patients.[2,25]

Nonsteroidal Anti-Inflammatory Drugs

NSAIDs, including aspirin (see Table 33-3), cause gastric mucosal damage by direct or topical irritation of the gastric epithelium and systemic inhibition of endogenous mucosal PG synthesis.[1,13] The onset of injury is initiated by the acidic properties of many of the NSAIDs while systemic inhibition of the protective PGs limits the ability of the mucosa to defend against injury and thus plays the predominant role in the development of gastric ulcer.[1,13]

Acidic NSAIDs (eg, aspirin) have topical irritant properties and they decrease the hydrophobicity of the mucous gel layer in the gastric mucosa. Most nonaspirin NSAIDs have topical irritant effects, but aspirin is the most damaging. Although NSAID prodrugs, enteric-coated aspirin tablets, salicylate derivatives, and parenteral or rectal preparations are associated with less acute gastric mucosal injury, they can cause ulcers and related GI complications as a result of systemic inhibition of endogenous PGs.[1]

COX is the rate-limiting enzyme in the conversion of arachidonic acid to PGs and is inhibited by NSAIDs (Fig. 33-3). Two similar COX isoforms have been identified: COX-1 is found in most body tissue, including the stomach, kidney, intestine, and platelets; COX-2 is undetectable in most tissues under normal physiologic conditions, but its expression can be induced during acute inflammation and arthritis (Fig. 33-4).[1,13] COX-1 produces protective PGs that regulate physiologic processes such as GI mucosal integrity, platelet homeostasis, and renal function. COX-2 is induced (unregulated) by inflammatory stimuli such as cytokines and produces PGs involved with inflammation, fever, and pain. It is also constitutionally expressed in organs such as the brain, kidney, and reproductive tract. Adverse effects (eg, GI or renal toxicity) of NSAIDs are primarily associated with the inhibition of COX-1, whereas anti-inflammatory actions result primarily from NSAID inhibition of COX-2.[1,13]

The COX-1-to-COX-2 inhibitory ratio determines the relative GI toxicity of a specific NSAID. Nonselective NSAIDs, including aspirin (see Table 33-3), inhibit both COX-1 and COX-2 to varying degrees and are associated with an increased propensity to cause gastric ulcers.[1,13] In contrast, the selective COX-2 inhibitors have a reduced risk of ulcers and related GI complications, but the benefit of celecoxib is less than that of rofecoxib and valdecoxib (see Table 33-3). The addition of aspirin to a selective COX-2 inhibitor reduces its ulcer-sparing benefit and increases ulcer risk.[1,13] Aspirin and nonaspirin NSAIDs irreversibly inhibit platelet COX-1, resulting in decreased platelet aggregation and prolonged bleeding times, thereby increasing the potential for upper and lower GI bleeding.[1,13,15] Coadministration of NSAIDs may reduce the antiplatelet effects of aspirin.[13,15,16] Clopidogrel and other medications

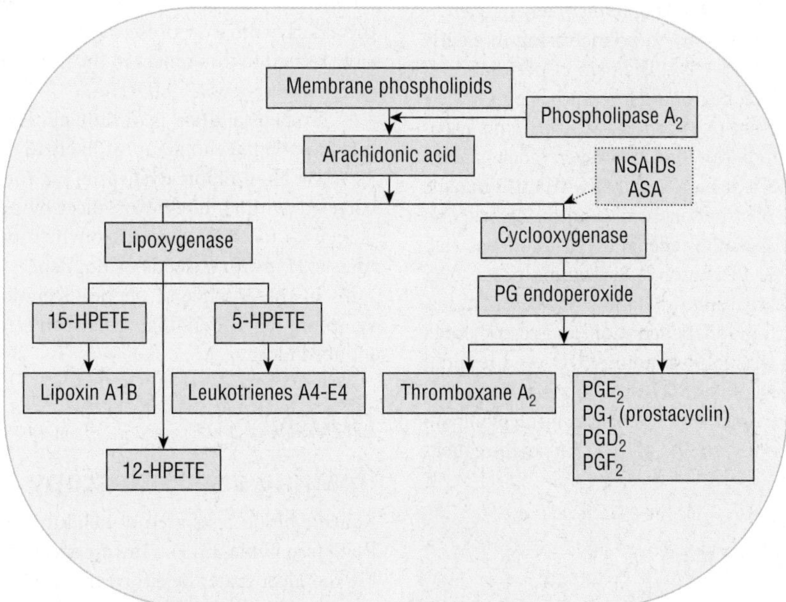

FIGURE 33-3 Metabolism of arachidonic acid after its release from membrane phospholipids. Broken arrow indicates inhibitory effects. (ASA, aspirin; HPETE, hydroperoxyeicosatetraenoic acid; NSAIDs, nonsteroidal antiinflammatory drugs; PG, prostaglandin.)

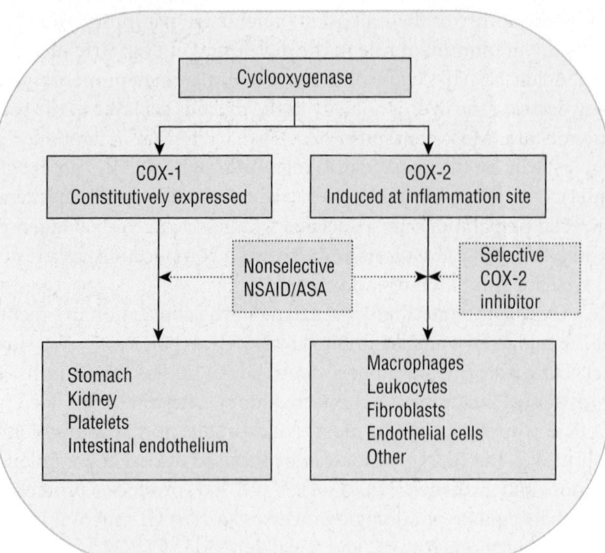

FIGURE 33-4 Tissue distribution and actions of cyclooxygenase (COX) isoenzymes. Nonselective nonsteroidal antiinflamatory drugs (NSAIDs) including aspirin (ASA) inhibit COX-1 and COX-2 to varying degrees; COX-2 inhibitors inhibit only COX-2. Broken arrow indicates inhibitory effects.

that impair angiogenesis do not cause ulcers, per se, but may impair healing of gastric erosions leading to ulceration.[13,15]

Complications

The most serious, life-threatening complications of chronic PUD are upper GI bleeding, perforation, and obstruction.[1,27] Bleeding is caused by the erosion of an ulcer into an artery. It may be occult (hidden) and insidious or may present as melena (black-colored stools) or hematemesis (vomiting of blood). NSAID use (especially in older adults) is the most important risk factor for upper GI bleeding. Deaths occur primarily in patients who continue to bleed or in those patients who rebleed after the initial bleeding has stopped (see section "Upper GI Bleeding" below).

Gastric perforation into the peritoneal cavity is the second most common ulcer-related complication, occurring in up to 7% of patients with PUD.[1,27] The ulcer may penetrate into an adjacent structure (pancreas, biliary tract, or liver) rather than opening freely into a cavity. The incidence of perforation appears to be increasing in elderly possibly due to increased use of NSAIDs. The pain of perforation is usually sudden, sharp, and severe, beginning first in the epigastrium, but quickly spreading over the entire abdomen. Most patients experience ulcer symptoms prior to perforation. However, older patients who experience perforation in association with NSAID use may be asymptomatic. Gastric outlet obstruction is mechanical obstruction caused by scarring, muscular spasm, or edema of the duodenal bulb usually resulting from chronic ulceration.[23] Symptoms occur over several months and include early satiety, bloating, anorexia, nausea, vomiting, and weight loss. Perforation, penetration, and gastric outlet obstruction occur most often with long-standing PUD. As a result of improvements in PUD treatment, rates of obstruction have decreased significantly, occurring in fewer than 2% of patients.[1] Intractability to drug therapy is an infrequent manifestation of PUD and an infrequent indication for surgery.

CLINICAL PRESENTATION

There is significant variability in the clinical presentation of PUD depending on the severity of epigastric pain and the presence of complications (Table 33-5).[1] Pain related to duodenal ulcer often occurs 1 to 3 hours after meals and is usually relieved by food, but this is variable. Food may precipitate or accentuate gastric ulcer pain. Antacids usually provide immediate pain relief in most ulcer patients. Pain usually diminishes or disappears during treatment; however, recurrence of epigastric pain after healing often suggests an unhealed or recurrent ulcer.

The presence or absence of epigastric pain does not define an ulcer[1] and ulcer healing does not necessarily render the patient asymptomatic. Symptoms may remain because of sensitization of afferent nerves in response to mucosal injury.[1] Conversely, the absence of pain does not preclude an ulcer diagnosis especially in the elderly who may present with a "silent" ulcer complication possibly related to differences in the way the elderly perceive pain or the analgesic effect of NSAIDs.

Dyspepsia alone is of little clinical value when assessing subsets of patients who are most likely to have an ulcer. Patients taking NSAIDs often report dyspepsia, but these symptoms do not always correlate with an ulcer. Non-ulcer dyspepsia, or NUD, refers to the lack of an ulcer upon endoscopy in a patient with ulcer-like symptoms.[28] *H. pylori* gastritis or duodenitis may cause ulcer-like symptoms in the absence of peptic ulceration. There is no one sign or symptom that differentiates between *H. pylori*–positive and NSAID-induced ulcer.

TABLE 33-5 Clinical Presentation of PUD

General
• Mild epigastric pain or acute life-threatening upper GI complications
Symptoms
• Abdominal pain that is often epigastric and described as burning but may present as vague discomfort, abdominal fullness, or cramping
• A typical nocturnal pain that awakens the patient from sleep (especially between 12 and 3 AM)
• The severity of ulcer pain varies from patient to patient and may be seasonal, occurring more frequently in the spring or fall; episodes of discomfort usually occur in clusters, lasting up to a few weeks and followed by a pain-free period or remission lasting from weeks to years
• Changes in the character of the pain may suggest the presence of complications
• Heartburn, belching, and bloating often accompany the pain
• Nausea, vomiting, and anorexia are more common for patients with gastric ulcer than with duodenal ulcer but may also be signs of an ulcer-related complication
Signs
• Weight loss associated with nausea, vomiting, and anorexia
• Complications including ulcer bleeding, perforation, penetration, or obstruction
Laboratory tests
• Gastric acid secretory studies
• The hematocrit and hemoglobin are low with bleeding, and stool hemoccult tests are positive
• Tests for *Helicobacter pylori* (see Table 33-6)
Diagnostic tests
• Fiber-optic upper endoscopy (esophagogastroduodenoscopy) detects more than 90% of peptic ulcers and permits direct inspection, biopsy, visualization of superficial erosions, and sites of active bleeding
• Upper GI radiography with barium has been replaced with upper endoscopy as the diagnostic procedure of choice for suspected peptic ulcer

GI, gastrointestinal; PUD, peptic ulcer disease.

DIAGNOSIS

Imaging and Endoscopy

Routine blood tests are not helpful in establishing the diagnosis of PUD (see Table 33-5).[1] The diagnosis of PUD depends on visualizing the ulcer crater by either upper GI radiography or upper endoscopy (see Table 33-5).[1] Upper endoscopy has replaced radiography as the diagnostic procedure of choice because it provides a more accurate diagnosis and permits direct visualization of the ulcer and

TABLE 33-6 Tests for Detection of *Helicobacter pylori*

Test	Description	Comments
Endoscopic tests		
Histology	Microbiologic examination using various stains	Gold standard; greater than 95% sensitive and specific; permits classification of gastritis; results are not immediate; not recommended for initial diagnosis; tests for active *H. pylori* infection
Culture	Culture of biopsy	Enables sensitivity testing to determine appropriate treatment or antibiotic resistance; 100% specific; results are not immediate; not recommended for initial diagnosis; used after failure of second-line treatment; tests for active *H. pylori* infection
Biopsy (rapid) urease	*H. pylori* urease generates ammonia, which causes a color change	Test of choice at endoscopy; greater than 90% sensitive and specific; easily performed; rapid results (usually within 24 hours); tests for active *H. pylori* infection
Polymerase chain reaction	*H. pylori* DNA detected in gastric tissue	Test is highly specific and sensitive; high rate of false-positives and false-negatives; positive DNA does not directly equate to presence of the organism; considered a research technique
Nonendoscopic tests		
Antibody detection (laboratory-based)	Detects antibodies to *H. pylori* in serum using laboratory-based ELISA tests and latex agglutination techniques	Quantitative; less sensitive and specific than endoscopic tests; more accurate than in office; unable to determine if antibody is related to active or cured infection; antibody titers vary markedly among individuals and take 6 months to 1 year to return to the uninfected range; not affected by PPIs or bismuth; antibiotics given for unrelated indications may cure the infection, but antibody test will remain positive
Antibody detection (can be performed in office or near patient)	Detects IgG antibodies to *H. pylori* in whole blood or finger stick	Qualitative; quick (within 15 minutes); unable to determine if antibody is related to active or cured infection; most patients remain seropositive for at least 6 months to 1 year after *H. pylori* eradication; not affected by PPIs, bismuth, or antibiotics
Urea breath test	*H. pylori* urease breaks down ingested labeled C-urea, patient exhales labeled CO_2	Tests for active *H. pylori* infection; 95% sensitive and specific; results take about 2 days; antibiotics, bismuth, PPIs, and H2RAs may cause false-negative results; withhold PPIs or H2RAs (1-2 weeks) and bismuth or antibiotics (4 weeks) prior to testing; recommended test to confirm posttreatment eradication of *H. pylori*
Fecal antigen	Identifies *H. pylori* antigen in stool by enzyme immunoassay using polyclonal anti–*H. pylori* antibody	Tests for active *H. pylori* infection; sensitivity and specificity comparable to urea breath test when used for initial diagnosis; antibiotics, bismuth, and PPIs may cause false-negative results, but to a lesser extent than with the urea breath test; may be used posttreatment to confirm eradication, but patients may have a reluctance to obtain stool samples

ELISA, enzyme-linked immunosorbent assay; H2RA, H_2-receptor antagonist; PPIs, proton pump inhibitors.

Data from references 2, 5, and 35.

implementation of therapeutic maneuvers such as injection of epinephrine or deployment of hemostatic clips to control bleeding.

Tests for *Helicobacter pylori*

The diagnosis of *H. pylori* infection can be made using endoscopic or nonendoscopic tests (Table 33-6).[2,5,29] Testing that requires upper endoscopy is invasive, more expensive, and usually requires a mucosal biopsy for histology, culture, or detection of urease activity. The updated Sydney system recommends taking five tissue samples from different sites within the stomach, as patchy distribution of *H. pylori* infection can lead to false-negative results.[30] Because antibiotics and bismuth salts may decrease the sensitivity of rapid urease test, they should be withheld for 4 weeks and proton pump inhibitors (PPIs) for 2 weeks prior to endoscopic testing.[2,5,29,31] If the patient has been taking these medications, then a gastric biopsy for histology should be performed.[5]

Nonendoscopic tests may identify active infection or detect antibodies (see Table 33-6) and are less invasive, more convenient, and less expensive than the endoscopic tests.[2,5,29] Antibody tests do not differentiate between active infection and previously eradicated *H. pylori*. The nonendoscopic tests include the urea breath test (UBT), serologic antibody detection tests, and the fecal antigen test.

The UBT is the most accurate noninvasive test and is based on *H. pylori* urease activity.[30] The ^{13}Carbon (nonradioactive isotope) and ^{14}Carbon (radioactive isotope) tests require that the patient ingest radiolabeled urea, which is then hydrolyzed by *H. pylori* (if present in the stomach) to ammonia and radiolabeled bicarbonate. The radiolabeled bicarbonate is absorbed in the blood and excreted in the breath. In addition to being noninvasive, another advantage of UBT over biopsy is that it overcomes the possible sampling error associated with endoscopic biopsy secondary to irregular distribution of *H. pylori*.[30] The fecal antigen test is less expensive and easier to perform than the UBT, and may be useful in children.

Serologic tests are a cost-effective alternative for the initial diagnosis of *H. pylori* infection in the untreated patient.[25] Antibodies to *H. pylori* usually develop about 3 weeks after infection and remain present after successful eradication.[5] Therefore, serology should not be used to confirm *H. pylori* eradication.[25] Office-based tests are less expensive, widely available, and provide rapid results, but the results are less accurate and more variable than the laboratory-based tests. Salivary and urine antibody tests are under investigation.

Testing for *H. pylori* is only recommended if eradication therapy is planned. Serologic antibody testing is a reasonable choice if endoscopy is not planned. The diagnostic accuracy of *H. pylori* tests for patients with an active bleeding ulcer has been questioned because of the potential for false-negative results. However, endoscopic biopsy-based tests such as the rapid urease test have a high degree of specificity in these patients (see "Peptic Ulcer–Related Bleeding").[5]

Confirmation of eradication is indicated post-treatment of active ulcers, previous ulcers, MALT lymphoma, endoscopic resection of gastric cancer, and uninvestigated dyspepsia. Routine testing for all patients is not recommended, and the cost-effectiveness needs to be further studied.[5] However, as resistance and treatment failures increase, the decision to confirm post-treatment eradication will also increase. The decision to test post-treatment should be patient-specific and take into consideration the patient's diagnosis, age, and ulcer history. The UBT and fecal antigen are the preferred nonendoscopic tests to confirm *H. pylori* eradication but must be delayed at least 4 weeks after the completion of treatment to avoid confusing bacterial suppression with eradication. The term *eradication* or *cure* is used when post-treatment tests conducted 4 weeks after the end of treatment do not detect the organism. Quantitative antibody tests are impractical for post-treatment confirmation as antibody titers remain elevated for long periods of time. A negative post-treatment antibody test, however, is considered reliable.

CLINICAL COURSE AND PROGNOSIS

PUD is characterized by periods of exacerbations and remissions.[1] Ulcer pain is usually recognizable and episodic, but symptoms are variable, especially in older adults and for patients taking NSAIDs. Antiulcer medications, including the histamine-2 receptor antagonists (H2RAs), PPIs, and sucralfate, relieve symptoms, accelerate ulcer healing, and reduce the risk of ulcer recurrence, but they do not cure the disease. Both duodenal and gastric ulcers recur unless the underlying cause (*H. pylori* or NSAID) is removed. Successful *H. pylori* eradication markedly decreases ulcer recurrence and complications. Prophylactic co-therapy or a COX-2 inhibitor decreases the risk of upper GI events for patients who are taking NSAIDs. GI bleeding, perforation, and obstruction remain troublesome complications of chronic PUD. Mortality for patients with gastric ulcer is slightly higher than in duodenal ulcer and the general population. The development of gastric cancer in *H. pylori*–infected individuals is a slow process that occurs over 20 to 40 years and is associated with a lifetime risk of less than 1%.[11]

TREATMENT

Desired Outcome

The goal of therapy for *H. pylori*–positive patients with an active ulcer, a previously documented ulcer, or a history of an ulcer-related complication is to eradicate *H. pylori*, heal the ulcer, and cure the disease. Successful eradication heals ulcers and reduces the risk of recurrence for most patients. The goal of therapy for a patient with an NSAID-induced ulcer is to heal the ulcer as rapidly as possible. Patients who are at high risk of developing NSAID ulcers should receive prophylactic co-therapy or be switched to a selective COX-2 inhibitor NSAID when possible to reduce ulcer risk and related complications.

General Approach to Treatment

The treatment of chronic PUD varies depending on the etiology of the ulcer (*H. pylori* or NSAID), whether the ulcer is initial or recurrent, and whether complications have occurred (Fig. 33-5). Treatment is aimed at relieving ulcer pain, healing the ulcer, preventing ulcer recurrence, and reducing ulcer-related complications. Antimicrobials such as clarithromycin, metronidazole, amoxicillin, bismuth salts, and antisecretory drugs (PPIs or H2RAs) eradicate *H. pylori* infection healing the ulcer and relieving ulcer symptoms. PPIs are preferred to H2RAs or sucralfate for healing *H. pylori*-negative NSAID-induced ulcers because they accelerate ulcer healing and provide more effective relief of symptoms.

Dietary modifications are important for patients who are unable to tolerate certain foods and beverages. Lifestyle modifications such as reducing stress and smoking cessation are encouraged. Surgery is reserved for patients with ulcer-related complications.

Nonpharmacologic Therapy

1 Patients with PUD should eliminate or reduce psychological stress, cigarette smoking, and the use of NSAIDs (including aspirin). Although there is no "antiulcer diet," the patient should avoid foods and beverages (eg, spicy foods, caffeine, and alcohol) that cause dyspepsia or that exacerbate ulcer symptoms. If possible, alternative agents such as acetaminophen or nonacetylated salicylate (eg, salsalate) should be used for relief of pain. Elective surgery for PUD is rarely performed today because of highly effective medical management. A subset of patients, however, may require emergency surgery for bleeding, perforation, or obstruction. In the past, surgical procedures were performed for medical treatment failures and included vagotomy with pyloroplasty or vagotomy with antrectomy.[1] Vagotomy (truncal, selective, or parietal cell) inhibits vagal stimulation of gastric acid. A truncal or selective vagotomy frequently results in postoperative gastric dysfunction and requires a pyloroplasty or antrectomy to facilitate gastric drainage. When an antrectomy is performed, the remaining stomach is anastomosed with the duodenum (Billroth I) or with the jejunum (Billroth II). A vagotomy is unnecessary when an antrectomy is performed for gastric ulcer. Postoperative consequences include postvagotomy diarrhea, dumping syndrome, anemia, and recurrent ulceration.

Pharmacologic Therapy

Recommendations

2 Table 33-7 presents guidelines for the eradication of infection in *H. pylori*–positive individuals. Table 33-8 lists regimens used to eradicate *H. pylori* infection.

3 The most cost-effective drug regimen should be used whenever feasible. First-line therapy is usually initiated with a PPI-based three-drug regimen for 14 days. If a second course of treatment is required, the salvage regimen should contain different antibiotics or a four-drug regimen with a bismuth salt, metronidazole, tetracycline, and a PPI should be used.

Patients with NSAID-induced ulcers should be tested to determine their *H. pylori* status. If *H. pylori*-positive, treatment should be initiated with a PPI-based three-drug regimen. If *H. pylori*-negative, the NSAID should be discontinued, and the patient treated with a PPI, H2RA, or sucralfate (see Table 33-9). If the NSAID is continued, treatment should be initiated with a PPI (if *H. pylori*-negative) or with a PPI-based three-drug regimen (if *H. pylori*-positive). Co-therapy with a PPI or misoprostol or switching to a selective COX-2 inhibitor (if available) is recommended for patients at risk of developing an ulcer-related complication.

Maintenance therapy with a PPI or H2RA should be limited to high-risk patients with ulcer complications, patients who fail eradication, and those with *H. pylori*-negative ulcers. Treatment failure is associated with poor medication adherence, antimicrobial resistance, NSAID use, cigarette smoking, acid hypersecretion, or tolerance to the antisecretory effects of an H2RA.

Treatment of *Helicobacter pylori*–Positive Ulcers

This chapter focuses on the eradication of *H. pylori* in adults. A discussion of the treatment of *H. pylori* infection in children is found elsewhere.[32]

The treatment of *H. pylori*–positive PUD should be effective, well tolerated, easy to adhere to, and cost-effective. Historically, none of these factors have been addressed in a systematic way making it difficult to identify the best evidence-based treatment regimens.[1] Successful eradication depends on the drug regimen, resistance to the antibiotics used, duration of therapy, medication adherence, and genetic polymorphism.[33,34] *H. pylori* regimens should have eradication (cure) rates of at least 80% based on intention-to-treat analysis or at least 90% based on per-protocol analysis, and they should minimize the potential for antimicrobial resistance.[1,8,35] Not one antibiotic, bismuth salt, or antiulcer drug achieves this goal, but clarithromycin has been considered the single most effective antibiotic. Two-drug regimens that combine a PPI and either amoxicillin or clarithromycin have yielded marginal and variable eradication rates in the United States and are not recommended.[1,5] In addition, the use of only one antibiotic is associated with a higher rate of antimicrobial resistance and is therefore not recommended.

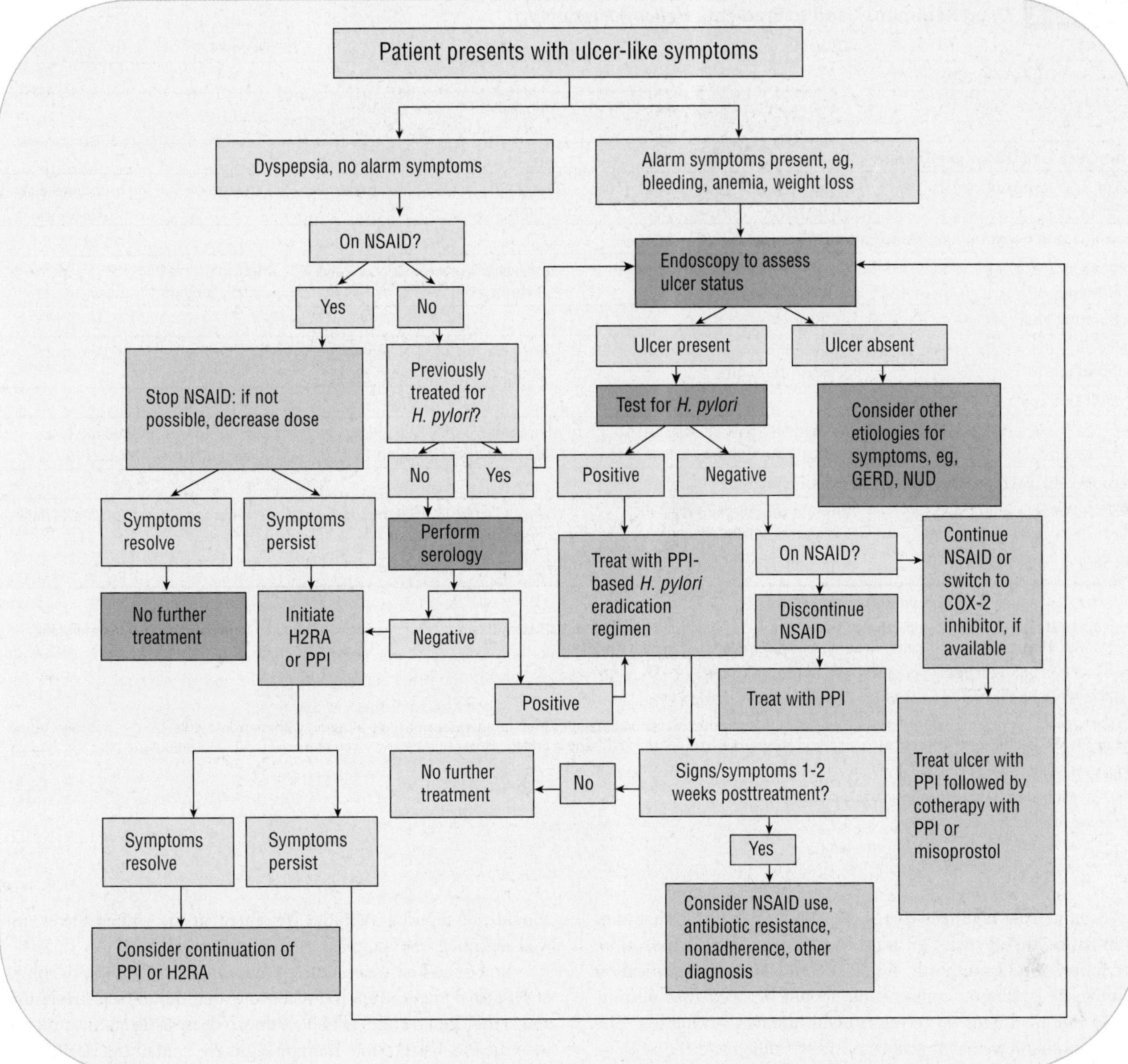

FIGURE 33-5 Algorithm. Guidelines for the evaluation and management of a patient who presents with dyspeptic or ulcer-like symptoms. (COX-2, cyclooxygenase-2; GERD, gastroesophageal reflux disease; H_2 RA, H_2-receptor antagonist; NSAID, nonsteroidal antiinflammatory drug; NUD, nonulcer dyspepsia; PPI, proton pump inhibitor.)

TABLE 33-7 Guidelines for the Eradication of *Helicobacter pylori* Infection

Indications for treatment of *H. pylori* infection
- Established indications for the treatment of *H. pylori* include gastric or duodenal ulcer, MALT lymphoma, after endoscopic resection of gastric cancer, and uninvestigated dyspepsia
- Controversial indications for the treatment of *H. pylori* infection include nonulcer dyspepsia, gastroesophageal reflux disease, individuals taking NSAIDs, individuals at high risk for gastric cancer, and unexplained iron deficiency anemia

Initial treatment of *H. pylori* infection
- Use only those eradication regimens that are of proven effectiveness in the United States
- In the United States, first-line treatment should include a PPI, clarithromycin, and either amoxicillin or metronidazole (PPI-based triple therapy) for 10-14 days
- The PPI-based triple-therapy amoxicillin-containing regimen is preferred initially because bacterial resistance to amoxicillin is almost absent, it has fewer adverse effects, and it leaves metronidazole as a backup agent for second-line therapy
- In penicillin-allergic patients, metronidazole should be substituted for amoxicillin in the PPI-based triple-therapy regimen and yields similar results when combined with clarithromycin
- An alternate initial strategy includes a PPI or H2RA, bismuth salt, tetracycline, and metronidazole (bismuth-based quadruple therapy) for 10-14 days
- Sequential therapy consisting of a PPI and amoxicillin for 5 days followed by a PPI, clarithromycin, and metronidazole for 5 days is an alternative to PPI-based triple therapy or PPI-based quadruple therapy, but requires further validation before it can be recommended as first-line therapy in the United States

Eradication of *H. pylori* after initial treatment failure
- Avoid antibiotics that have been used in previous eradication regimens
- Bismuth-based quadruple therapy with a bismuth salt, tetracycline, metronidazole, and a PPI or H2RA for 10–14 days is an acceptable treatment regimen for persistent *H. pylori* infections
- PPI-based triple therapy with levofloxacin and amoxicillin for 10 days may be more effective and better tolerated than PPI-based quadruple therapy with a bismuth salt, tetracycline, and metronidazole, but it requires further validation in the United States

MALT, mucosa-associated lymphoid tissue; NSAIDs, nonsteroidal anti-inflammatory drugs, PPI, proton pump inhibitor.
Data from references 5, 8, 35, 37 to 39.

TABLE 33-8 Drug Regimens Used to Eradicate *Helicobacter pylori*

Drug #1	Drug #2	Drug #3	Drug #4
PPI-Based Triple Therapy[a]			
PPI once or twice daily[b]	Clarithromycin 500 mg twice daily	Amoxicillin 1 g twice daily *or* metronidazole 500 mg twice daily	
Bismuth-Based Quadruple Therapy[a]			
PPI or H2RA once or twice daily[b,c]	Bismuth subsalicylate[d] 525 mg four times daily	Metronidazole 250-500 mg four times daily	Tetracycline 500 mg four times daily
Non-Bismuth Quadruple or "Concomitant" Therapy[e]			
PPI once or twice daily on days 1 through 10[b]	Clarithromycin 250-500 mg twice daily on days 1-10	Amoxicillin 1 g twice daily on days 1 through 10	Metronidazole 250-500 mg twice daily on days 1 through 10
Sequential Therapy[e]			
PPI once or twice daily on days 1 through 10[b]	Amoxicillin 1 g twice daily on days 1 through 5	Metronidazole 250-500 mg twice daily on days 6 through 10	Clarithromycin 250-500 mg twice daily on days 6 through 10
Hybrid Therapy[e]			
PPI once or twice daily on days 1 through 14[b]	Amoxicillin 1 g twice daily on days 1 through 14	Metronidazole 250-500 mg twice daily on days 7 through 14	Clarithromycin 250-500 mg twice daily on days 7 through 14
Second-Line (Salvage) Therapy for Persistent Infections			
PPI or H2RA once or twice daily[b,c]	Bismuth subsalicylate[d] 525 mg four times daily	Metronidazole 250-500 mg four times daily	Tetracycline 500 mg four times daily
PPI once or twice daily[b,f]	Amoxicillin 1 g twice daily	Levofloxacin 250 mg twice daily	

H2RA, H_2-receptor antagonist; PPI, proton pump inhibitor.

[a]Although treatment is minimally effective if used for 7 days, 10-14 days is recommended. The antisecretory drug may be continued beyond antimicrobial treatment for patients with a history of a complicated ulcer, for example, bleeding, or in heavy smokers.

[b]Standard PPI peptic ulcer healing dosages given once or twice daily.

[c]Standard H2RA peptic ulcer healing dosages may be used in place of a PPI.

[d]Bismuth subcitrate potassium (biskalcitrate) 140 mg, as the bismuth salt, is contained in a prepackaged capsule (Pylera), along with metronidazole 125 mg and tetracycline 125 mg; three capsules are taken with each meal and at bedtime; a standard PPI dosage is added to the regimen and taken twice daily. All medications are taken for 10 days.

[e]Requires validation as first-line therapy in the United States.

[f]Requires validation as rescue therapy in the United States.

Data from references 5, 8, 35, 37 to 39.

Several drug regimens (see Table 33-8) are available that offer combination therapy with an antisecretory drug, with two or more antibiotics, or a bismuth salt. When selecting an initial eradication regimen, an antibiotic combination should be used that permits second-line treatment (if necessary) with different antibiotics. The antibiotics that have been most extensively studied and found to be effective in various combinations include clarithromycin, amoxicillin, metronidazole, and tetracycline.[1] Because of insufficient data, ampicillin should not be substituted for amoxicillin, doxycycline should not be substituted for tetracycline, and azithromycin or erythromycin should not be substituted for clarithromycin.[36] Antisecretory drugs enhance antibiotic activity and stability by increasing intragastric pH and by decreasing intragastric volume thereby enhancing the topical antibiotic concentration.[37]

Proton Pump Inhibitor–Based Three-Drug Regimens

PPI-based triple therapy (see Table 33-8) is the initial treatment of choice for eradicating *H. pylori* (see Table 33-7).[5,8,35,37-39] The regimens that combine either clarithromycin and amoxicillin or clarithromycin and metronidazole are more effective than the amoxicillin–metronidazole regimen. In most cases, increasing the antibiotic dosage does not improve eradication rates. The clarithromycin–amoxicillin regimen is preferred initially (see Table 33-7), but metronidazole should be substituted for amoxicillin for penicillin-allergic patients unless alcohol is consumed.[5,35,37-39] Unfortunately, eradication rates for PPI-based triple therapy have declined substantially in recent years in North America and Europe due primarily to an increase in clarithromycin-resistant *H. pylori* strains (see "Factors that Predict *H. pylori* Eradication Outcomes" below).[5,8,35,37-39] Other antibiotics and antibiotic combinations have been investigated, but these regimens should not be used as initial treatment in the United States until well-designed trials confirm their effectiveness.[5,37]

Since the first treatment regimen offers the highest likelihood of *H. pylori* eradication, the recommended duration of triple-therapy in the United States is 14 days due to decreasing eradication rates with the PPI-based triple-therapy regimens containing clarithromycin, particularly with shorter durations.[5] Although a 7-day course has been approved by the FDA and is used in Europe, higher eradication and lower resistance rates are generally associated with longer treatment durations.[5,8,35,37-39]

The PPI is an integral part of the three-drug regimen and should be taken 30 to 60 minutes before a meal (see Table 33-8).[5] Prolonged PPI treatment beyond 2 weeks after eradication is usually not necessary for ulcer healing. A single daily dose of a PPI may be less effective than a twice-daily dose.[40,41] Substitution of one PPI for another is acceptable and does not enhance or diminish *H . pylori* eradication.[41] An H2RA should not be substituted for a PPI unless there are significant tolerability issues, as H2RA is associated with lower eradication rates.[42,43] Pretreatment with a PPI does not influence *H. pylori* eradication regardless of the pretreatment duration.[44]

Bismuth-Containing Quadruple Therapy

Bismuth-based quadruple therapy (see Table 33-8) is recommended as an alternative first-line eradication therapy (see Table 33-7) for those allergic to penicillin.[5,35,37-39] Although this regimen may be used initially, it is often reserved as a second-line therapy after treatment failure with the PPI-based clarithromycin–amoxicillin regimen (see "Eradication of *H. pylori* After Initial Treatment Failure" below). Eradication rates for bismuth-based quadruple therapy (bismuth salicylate, metronidazole, tetracycline, and either a PPI

TABLE 33-9 Drug Dosing Table

Drug	Brand Name	Initial Dose	Usual Range	Special Population Dose	Other
Proton Pump Inhibitors					
Omeprazole, sodium bicarbonate	Prilosec, Zegerid	40 mg daily	20-40 mg/day	Consider adjustment for hepatic disease	Pregnancy Category C
Lansoprazole	Prevacid, various	30 mg daily	15-30 mg/day	Consider adjustment for hepatic disease	Pregnancy Category B
Rabeprazole	Aciphex	20 mg daily	20-40 mg/day	Use with caution in severe hepatic disease	Pregnancy Category B
Pantoprazole	Pantoprazole, various	40 mg daily	40-80 mg/day	Consider adjustment for severe hepatic disease	Pregnancy Category B
Esomeprazole	Nexium	40 mg daily	20-40 mg/day	Limit dose to 20 mg/day in severe hepatic disease	Pregnancy Category B
Dexlansoprazole	Dexilant	30-60 mg daily	30-60 mg/day	Consider dose limit of 30 mg/day in moderate hepatic impairment, dose not established in severe hepatic disease	Pregnancy Category B
H_2-Receptor Antagonists					
Cimetidine	Tagamet, various	300 mg four times daily, 400 mg twice daily, or 800 mg at bedtime	800-1,600 mg/day in divided doses	Adjust dose for renal and severe hepatic impairment	Pregnancy Category B
Famotidine	Pepcid, various	20 mg twice daily, or 40 mg at bedtime	20-40 mg/day	Adjust dose for renal impairment	Pregnancy Category B
Nizatidine	Axid, various	150 mg twice daily, or 300 mg at bedtime	150-300 mg/day	Adjust dose for renal impairment	Pregnancy Category B
Ranitidine	Zantac, various	150 mg twice daily, or 300 mg at bedtime	150-300 mg/day	Adjust dose for renal impairment	Pregnancy Category B
Mucosal Protectants					
Sucralfate	Carafate, various	1 g four times daily, or 2 g twice daily	2-4 g/day		Aluminum may accumulate in renal failure, Pregnancy Category B
Misoprostol	Cytotec	100-200 mcg four times daily	400-800 mcg/day		Pregnancy Category X

Data from references 79, 81, and 82.

or H2RA) are similar to those achieved with PPI-based triple therapy.[5,37,45] Eradication rates are comparable when bismuth subcitrate potassium (biskalcitrate) is substituted for bismuth subsalicylate (see Table 33-8).[46] Bismuth salts have a topical antimicrobial effect.[1] The antisecretory drug hastens ulcer healing and relieves pain in patients with an active ulcer. All medications except the PPI should be taken with meals and at bedtime.

The original bismuth-based regimens contained an H2RA but have largely been replaced by PPI as the antisecretory agent due to greater efficacy. Although shorter treatment durations have been studied, a 10- to 14-day duration is recommended in the United States as it generally provides higher eradication rates.[5,47] When treating an active ulcer, the antisecretory drug is usually continued for 2 (PPI) to 4 (H2RA) weeks after stopping bismuth and antibiotics. Bismuth-based quadruple therapy is the treatment of choice when medication costs are of overriding importance. However, major concerns include a four-times-a-day dosing regimen (see Table 33-8), poor medication adherence, and frequent adverse effects. A simplified twice-daily quadruple regimen has been piloted with high eradication rates (90%) and improved adherence.[48] Adverse effects are similar compared to those reported for the PPI-based triple therapy.[47]

Sequential Therapy Sequential therapy is a form of eradication therapy in which the antibiotics are administered in a sequence rather than together.[5,8,38] The basis for sequential therapy is to initially treat with antibiotics that rarely promote resistance (eg, amoxicillin) to reduce the bacterial load and any preexisting resistant organisms that are susceptible. The second sequence follows with different antibiotics (eg, clarithromycin and metronidazole) to kill any remaining organisms. Treatment typically consists of a PPI and amoxicillin for 5 days followed by a PPI, clarithromycin, and tinidazole (or metronidazole) for an additional 5 days (see Table 33-8).[5,38,49] Although this regimen has achieved eradication rates that are superior to the PPI-based three-drug regimens containing clarithromycin,[49] the regimen requires a change in medication midtreatment, which may contribute to nonadherence.[50] Though promising, the advantages of sequential therapy have yet to be fully validated in the United States, and has yet to be incorporated into guidelines as a first-line *H. pylori* eradication therapy (see Table 33-7).[5,37,38]

Clinical **Controversy...**

Although sequential, hybrid, and non-bismuth quadruple therapies have higher overall eradication rates than traditional triple-therapy regimens, current guidelines do not recommend these as first-line therapy. Although these treatment strategies need to be validated in North American populations before they can be recommended as first-line therapy, they are more likely to be beneficial in situations where antibiotic (particularly clarithromycin) resistance is high.

Non-Bismuth Quadruple "Concomitant" Therapy and Hybrid Therapy

Non-bismuth quadruple therapy, also called "concomitant" therapy, is a regimen with a PPI, amoxicillin, clarithromycin, and metronidazole taken together at standard doses for 10 days. Hybrid therapy combines the strategies of concomitant and sequential therapy. Patients take 7 days of dual therapy (PPI and amoxicillin) followed by 7 days of quadruple therapy (PPI, amoxicillin, clarithromycin, and metronidazole). Both hybrid and non-bismuth quadruple therapies have demonstrated higher eradication rates when compared with traditional triple-therapy,[51,52] although similar eradication rates are likely in areas of low antimicrobial resistance.[34,49,53]

Eradication of *Helicobacter pylori* After Initial Treatment Failure

H. pylori eradication is often more difficult after initial treatment fails and successful eradication after retreatment is extremely variable.[5,54] Treatment failures should be referred to a gastroenterologist for further diagnostic evaluation. Second-line (salvage) treatment should (a) use antibiotics that were not previously used during initial therapy; (b) use antibiotics that are not associated with resistance; (c) use a drug that has a topical effect such as bismuth; and (d) extend the duration of treatment to 14 days.[5,55] The most commonly used second-line therapy, after unsuccessful initial treatment with a PPI–amoxicillin–clarithromycin regimen, is a 14-day course of the PPI-based bismuth-containing quadruple therapy (see Table 33-8).[5,37,38,55] A levofloxacin-based triple therapy regimen (see Table 33-8) containing amoxicillin and a PPI may be an alternative second-line eradication regimen and may be better tolerated than PPI-based bismuth-containing quadruple therapy (see Table 33-7).[56] A 10-day therapy containing PPI, bismuth, tetracycline, and levofloxacin achieved a high eradication rate after failure of first-line treatment with sequential therapy.[57] However, concerns about using fluoroquinolones to treat *H. pylori* include development of resistance and adverse effects (eg, tendonitis and hepatotoxicity).[38] Other salvage regimens that include rifabutin and furazolidone are also effective, but these are discussed in more detail elsewhere.[5,38] European guidelines recommend obtaining antimicrobial sensitivity information following the second failed attempt to eradicate *H. pylori* when available.

Factors that Predict *Helicobacter pylori* Eradication Outcomes

Factors that predict *H. pylori* eradication outcomes include antibiotic resistance, poor medication adherence, short duration of therapy, CagA status, high bacterial load, low intragastric pH, and genetic polymorphism.[5,26,55,58] Medication adherence decreases with multiple medications, increased frequency of administration, intolerable adverse effects, and costly drug regimens. Tolerability varies with different regimens, but common adverse effects include nausea, vomiting, abdominal pain, diarrhea, and taste disturbances (metronidazole and clarithromycin). Adverse effects with metronidazole are dose-related (especially when more than 1 g/day) and include a disulfiram-like reaction with alcohol. Tetracycline may cause photosensitivity and should not be used in children because of possible tooth discoloration. Bismuth salts may cause darkening of the stool and tongue. Antibiotic-associated diarrhea and *Clostridium difficile*–associated disease can occur. Oral thrush and vaginal candidiasis may also occur.[1,5]

An important predictor of *H. pylori* eradication is the presence or absence of resistant microorganisms.[5,34,59] A worldwide meta-analysis including North American data from 2000 to 2008 reveal resistance rates among *H. pylori* strains (n = 818 isolates) for clarithromycin (30.8%), metronidazole (30.5%), amoxicillin (2%), tetracycline (0%), and levofloxacin (14.2%).[59] While amoxicillin and tetracycline resistance remains low, these data represent notable increases in resistance for metronidazole (25%) and clarithromycin (13%) compared to prior studies.[60,61] It is possible that the increased rate of clarithromycin resistance partially explains the decrease in efficacy of triple therapy clarithromycin-containing regimens. Prior antibiotic exposure is likely a factor in the development of resistance as was seen in one study where the proportion of clarithromycin resistance increased from 7% resistance with no prior macrolide exposure to 80% resistance with more than or equal to five courses.[62] Therefore, prior antibiotic use should prompt consider for possible *H. pylori* resistance. The clinical importance of metronidazole resistance remains uncertain, as resistance can be overcome by using higher dosages and by combining metronidazole with other antibiotics.[5] Resistance to tetracycline and amoxicillin is uncommon.[5] Resistance to bismuth has not been reported. Although the role of antibiotic sensitivity testing prior to initiating *H. pylori* treatment has not been formally established, newly developed molecular-based tests may offer quick and easy determination of *H. pylori* resistance to macrolides and fluoroquinolones which allows for optimal regimen selection.[63]

Probiotics

Probiotics (eg, strains of *Lactobacillus* and *Bifidobacterium*) and foodstuffs (eg, cranberry juice and some milk proteins) with bioactive components have been used proactively to control *H. pylori* colonization in at-risk individuals. Although the quality of the data in this area is not optimal, probiotics taken as a supplement to antibiotic therapy, increases eradication rates compared to placebo and may reduce the adverse effects of PPI-based triple therapy.[64-66] However, the administration of probiotics alone does not eradicate *H. pylori* infection. In the future, the regular intake of probiotics may constitute a low-cost alternative for individuals who are at risk for *H. pylori* infection and, in combination with antibiotics, augment eradication rates. These preliminary data are encouraging and warrant more research in this area.

Treatment of Nonsteroidal Anti-Inflammatory Drug-Induced Ulcers

Nonselective NSAIDs should be discontinued (when possible) on confirmation of an active ulcer. If the NSAID is stopped, most uncomplicated ulcers heal with standard 4-week regimens of an H2RA, PPI, or sucralfate (see Table 33-9).[1,8,13,14] However, PPIs are usually preferred because they provide more rapid symptom relief and ulcer healing. If the NSAID is continued despite ulceration, consideration should be given to reducing the NSAID dose, switching to acetaminophen or a nonacetylated salicylate, or using a more selective COX-2 inhibitor (see Table 33-3). PPI treatment duration should be extended from 4 to 8-12 weeks if the NSAID must be continued. PPIs are the drugs of choice when the NSAID is continued, as potent acid suppression is required to accelerate ulcer healing.[1,8,13,14] If the ulcer is *H. pylori*-positive, eradication should be initiated with a regimen that contains a PPI.[1,8,13,14]

Strategies to Reduce the Risk of NSAID Ulcer and GI Complications There are three therapeutic approaches to reducing the risk of NSAID ulcers and related upper GI complications (see Table 33-10). Medical co-therapy with either a PPI or misoprostol decreases ulcer risk and GI complications in high-risk pat ients.[7,8,13,14,16,17] The use of a selective COX-2 inhibitor instead of a nonselective NSAID also decreases risk of ulcers and upper GI events.[7,8,13,14,16,17] Unfortunately, these strategies do not completely eliminate ulcers and complications for patients at the "highest risk." When selecting a gastroprotective strategy, the GI benefits must be balanced against the cardiovascular risks associated with selective COX-2 inhibitor NSAIDs, nonselective NSAIDs, and concomitant antiplatelet therapy.[7,13-17] Strategies aimed at reducing the topical

TABLE 33-10 Drug Monitoring Table

Drug	Adverse Drug Reaction	Monitoring Parameter	Comments
PPIs	Headache, N/V/D, flatulence Less common: thrombocytopenia, neutropenia, hypomagnesemia, hypocalcemia, liver function abnormalities, renal impairment	Baseline and periodic CBC, serum electrolytes, renal/liver function	Well tolerated; may be associated with increased risk of fractures, pneumonia, *Clostridium difficile* infection
H_2RA	Headache, dizziness, diarrhea, somnolence, gynecomastia (cimetidine) Less common: thrombocytopenia, neutropenia, liver function abnormalities, renal impairment, pancreatitis	Baseline and periodic CBC, serum electrolytes, renal/liver function	
Sucralfate	Constipation		
Misoprostol	Diarrhea, abdominal pain, headache, nausea/vomiting, flatulence, dysmenorrhea, hypophosphatemia	Pregnancy test Serum phosphate	Avoid in pregnancy

CBC, complete blood count; H_2RA, H_2-receptor antagonists; PPIs, proton pump inhibitors.

Data from references 79, 81, 82, 95 to 102.

irritant effects of nonselective NSAIDs, for example, prodrugs, slow-release formulations, and enteric-coated products, do not prevent ulcers or GI complications.

Misoprostol Cotherapy Misoprostol, 200 mcg orally four times per day, reduces the risk of NSAID-induced gastric and duodenal ulcer, and related upper GI complications, but diarrhea and abdominal cramping limit its use.[7,17,67] Because a dosage of 200 mcg three times per day is comparable in efficacy to 800 mcg/day, the lower dosage should be considered for patients unable to tolerate the higher dose.[7,17] Reducing the misoprostol dosage to 400 mcg/day or less to minimize diarrhea compromises its gastroprotective effects. A fixed combination of misoprostol 200 mcg and diclofenac (50 or 75 mg) may enhance compliance, but the flexibility to individualize drug dosage is lost. A large clinical trial in rheumatoid arthritis patients provided the most compelling evidence that misoprostol reduces the risk of upper GI complications for high-risk patients.[68]

Proton Pump Inhibitor Cotherapy 4 PPI cotherapy reduces NSAID-related gastric and duodenal ulcer risk and is better tolerated than misoprostol.[7,13,14,16,67] All PPIs are effective when used in standard dosages (see Table 33-9). Although head-to-head comparative trials are lacking, observational data indicate that PPIs are superior to H2RA at standard dosages.[7,14,17] When lansoprazole (15 or 30 mg/day) was compared with misoprostol 800 mcg/day or placebo, both dosages of lansoprazole and misoprostol effectively reduced ulcer recurrence, although the PPI was better tolerated.[69] A greater proportion of those in the misoprostol group reported treatment-related adverse events and withdrew early from the study. Results from observational studies and meta-analyses indicate the PPIs reduce the risk of NSAID-related ulcer bleeding.[7,17,70,71]

H_2-Receptor Antagonist Cotherapy Standard H2RA dosages (eg, famotidine 40 mg/day) are effective in reducing NSAID-related duodenal ulcer but not gastric ulcer (the most frequent type of ulcer associated with NSAIDs).[7,14,17] Higher dosages (eg, famotidine 40 mg twice daily, ranitidine 300 mg twice daily) may reduce the risk of gastric and duodenal ulcer, but studies comparing double dosages with PPIs or misoprostol are not available.[7,14] One study suggests that famotidine 20 mg twice daily may be an alternative to PPIs for patients taking low cardioprotective dosages of aspirin, but additional studies are required to confirm these findings.[72] The H2RAs are not recommended as prophylactic co-therapy because it is likely that they are not as effective as the PPIs or misoprostol in preventing NSAID-induced gastric ulcer and related GI complications.[17] An H2RA, however, may be used to relieve NSAID-related dyspepsia.

Cyclooxygenase-2 Inhibitors Two large outcome trials have compared celecoxib[73] and rofecoxib with nonselective NSAIDs. Patients in the Celecoxib Long-Term Arthritis Safety Study (CLASS) trial who were taking celecoxib and required cardioprotection (antiplatelet effects of aspirin) were permitted to take low-dose aspirin. Although a 6-month analysis found a non-significant reduction in ulcer complications with celecoxib when compared with ibuprofen and diclofenac, results after 1 year found no difference between the groups.[73] Today, celecoxib is not considered a selective COX-2 inhibitor (Table 33-3) by the FDA as it contains the same GI warnings as the nonselective and partially selective NSAIDs.[74] Gastroprotective benefits of celecoxib were negated in aspirin users. Similar effects have been observed with rofecoxib. Additionally, an increased number of nonfatal myocardial infarctions and thrombotic stroke were observed in studies of rofecoxib leading to its withdrawal from the market.[75] Subsequently, valdecoxib was withdrawn from the market amid concerns about cardiovascular risk.[76]

Cardiovascular safety was also evaluated in the CLASS trial, but serious cardiovascular thromboembolic events were no different between celecoxib and the comparative nonselective NSAIDs. In contrast, the results of a meta-analysis of randomized trials of COX-2 inhibitor NSAIDs reported a dose-dependent increase in cardiovascular events with all COX-2 inhibitor NSAIDs, including celecoxib.[65] Increased cardiovascular risk appears to be dependent on a number of factors including increased COX-2 selectivity, higher dosages, and a longer duration of treatment.[7,19,20] Thus, the lowest effective celecoxib dose should be used for the shortest duration of time. Dyspepsia and abdominal pain, fluid retention, hypertension, and renal toxicity are associated with the COX-2 inhibitors and nonselective NSAIDs.[1]

COX-2 Inhibitor versus NSAID Plus PPI 5 For high-risk, *H. pylori*-negative patients, a COX-2 inhibitor NSAID may be as beneficial as a nonselective NSAID plus a PPI in reducing NSAID-related ulcer complications.[7,19,20] However, neither the COX-2 inhibitor NSAID nor the NSAID plus a PPI will eliminate upper GI events for these patients. Combining a COX-2 inhibitor NSAID with a PPI may be considered for very high-risk patients, but this regimen is likely to be of modest benefit.[7,19]

Gastrointestinal and Cardiovascular Safety Issues

There is no difference in cardiovascular risk between the selective COX-2 inhibitor NSAIDs and the nonselective or partially selective NSAIDs, with the exception of naproxen.[7,19] Thus, individual patient risk factors for NSAID-related GI bleeding and cardiovascular events must be weighed when determining treatment (see Table 33-11). Naproxen is preferred compared with other nonselective NSAIDs and COX-2 inhibitors because of its comparative cardiovascular safety and not because of its GI safety profile. There is insufficient evidence regarding the preferred NSAID for patients

TABLE 33-11 Guidelines for Reducing GI Risk for Patients Receiving Chronic NSAID Therapy

Cardiovascular Risk	No or Low GI Risk (No Risk Factors)	Moderate GI Risk (1-2 Risk Factors)	High GI Risk (Greater than 2 Risk Factors or Prior Ulcer or Ulcer-Related Complication)
GI Risk Factors (see Table 33-4)			
	Age < 65 years	Age ≥ 65 years High-dose NSAIDs Concomitant use of aspirin, corticosteroids, or anticoagulants	Age ≥ 65 years Concomitant use of aspirin corticosteroids, or anticoagulants Dual antiplatelet therapy
No or low CV risk (patient does not require low-dose aspirin)	Nonselective NSAID or partially selective NSAID (see Table 33-3)	Nonselective NSAID or partially selective NSAID + PPI or misoprostol Selective COX-2 inhibitor NSAID (if available)	Avoid NSAID or selective COX-2 inhibitor, if possible; use alternative therapy Nonselective NSAID or partially selective NSAID + PPI or misoprostol Selective COX-2 inhibitor NSAID (if available) + PPI or misoprostol
High CV risk (patient requires low-dose aspirin), no NSAID	No prophylaxis required	PPI or misoprostol	PPI or misoprostol
High CV risk (patient requires low-dose aspirin) and NSAID	Naproxen + PPI or misoprostol	Naproxen + PPI or misoprostol	Avoid NSAID or selective COX-2 inhibitor If antiinflammatory drug is needed and CV risk is >GI risk, use naproxen and aspirin + PPI or misoprostol If antiinflammatory drug and aspirin are needed and GI risk is >CV risk, use selective COX-2 inhibitor + PPI or misoprostol

COX-2, cyclooxygenase-2 inhibitor; CV, cardiovascular; GI, gastrointestinal; NSAID, nonsteroidal anti-inflammatory drug; PPI, proton pump inhibitor.

Data from references 7, 13 to 16, 19, 20, and 71.

also taking low-dose aspirin.[19] Clopidogrel should not be substituted for low-dose aspirin in order to reduce recurrent GI bleeding as it is inferior to a PPI plus low-dose aspirin.[14] Despite limited evidence to suggest an interaction via the hepatic cytochrome P450 (CYP450) pathway, combining a PPI and clopidogrel with or without low-dose aspirin results in less GI bleeding.[14] Ongoing studies for patients with cardiovascular disease should provide the necessary information to help resolve these issues. The lowest possible daily dose of a COX-2 inhibitor should be used as the cardiovascular risk may be dose dependent. However, no studies, to date, have evaluated the safety of low-dose COX-2 inhibitor NSAIDs for patients with or at risk for cardiovascular disease. In the future, there will be new formulations and classes of NSAIDs and COX-2 inhibitors with an improved GI and cardiovascular safety profile.[77] Until then patients who take NSAIDs or COX-2 inhibitors should be counseled about the signs and symptoms of upper GI bleeding and major cardiovascular events and what they should do if they occur.

Treatment of Non–*Helicobacter pylori*, Non-Nonsteroidal Anti-Inflammatory Drug Ulcers

Few individuals have non–*H. pylori*, non-NSAID (idiopathic) ulcers.[8,78] Patients should be double-checked to verify that they are *H. pylori*-negative and that they are not taking ulcerogenic medications. Possible explanations for *non–H. pylori*, non-NSAID ulcers include gastric hypersecretion, gastric outlet obstruction, genetic predisposition, concomitant diseases (see Table 33-2), and heavy tobacco use. Treatment should be initiated with conventional ulcer healing therapy (see Table 33-9). Although standard H2RA or sucralfate dosage regimens heal the majority of gastric and duodenal ulcers in 6 to 8 weeks, PPIs provide comparable ulcer healing rates in 4 weeks.[79] A higher daily dose or a longer treatment duration is sometimes needed to heal larger gastric ulcers. Antacids are not used as single agents to heal ulcers because of the high volume and frequent doses required. When conventional antiulcer therapy is discontinued after ulcer healing, most patients develop a recurrent ulcer within 1 year.[79] Maintenance therapy may be required to prevent ulcer recurrence.

Long-Term Maintenance of Ulcer Healing

Long-term maintenance of ulcer healing and the prevention of ulcer-related complications may be necessary in some patients. Because *H. pylori* eradication dramatically decreases ulcer recurrence, continuous maintenance therapy is primarily used to treat high-risk patients who failed *H. pylori* eradication, have a history of ulcer-related complications, have frequent recurrences of *H. pylori*-negative ulcers, and are heavy smokers or NSAID users. For most patients, standard maintenance dosages (see Table 33-9) are effective.[79]

Treatment of Refractory Ulcers

Ulcers are considered refractory to therapy when symptoms, ulcers, or both persist beyond 8 to 12 weeks despite conventional treatment or when several courses of *H. pylori* eradication fail.[1,55] Poor patient compliance, antimicrobial resistance, cigarette smoking, NSAID use, gastric acid hypersecretion, or tolerance to the antisecretory effects of an H2RA (see "Antiulcer Agents" below) may contribute to refractory PUD. Patients with refractory ulcers should undergo upper endoscopy to confirm a nonhealing ulcer, exclude malignancy, and assess *H. pylori* status. *H. pylori*-positive patients should receive eradication therapy (see "Treatment of *H. pylori*–Positive Ulcers" above). In *H. pylori*-negative patients, higher PPI dosages (eg, omeprazole 40 mg/day) heal the majority of ulcers. Continuous treatment with a PPI is often necessary to maintain healing, as refractory ulcers recur when therapy is discontinued or the dose is reduced. Switching from one PPI to another is not beneficial. Patients with refractory gastric ulcer may require surgery because of the possibility of malignancy.

Antiulcer Agents

Proton Pump Inhibitors PPIs (omeprazole, esomeprazole, lansoprazole, dexlansoprazole, rabeprazole, and pantoprazole) dose-dependently inhibit basal and stimulated gastric acid secretion.[79] The duration of acid suppression is a function of binding to the H^+/K^+-adenosine triphosphatase (ATPase) enzyme.[79] When PPI therapy is initiated, the degree of acid suppression increases over the first 3 to 4 days of therapy, as more proton pumps are inhibited.[79] PPIs inhibit only those proton pumps that are actively secreting acid, thus they are most effective when taken 30 to 60 minutes before meals.[79] Symptomatic acid rebound on withdrawal of a PPI has been reported in healthy volunteers after 8 weeks of treatment.[80]

PPIs are formulated as delayed-release enteric-coated dosage forms that have pH-sensitive granules contained in gelatin capsules

TABLE 33-12 PPI Formulations and Options for Administration

	Omeprazole	Esomeprazole	Lansoprazole	Pantoprazole	Rabeprazole	Dexlansoprazole
Commercially available oral formulations						
Capsule	X[a]	X	X			X[b]
Tablet	X[c]			X	X	
Oral disintegrating tablet			X			
Packet for oral suspension	X[d]	X[d]				
Extemporaneous oral preparations						
Pellets from capsule in water		X				
Pellets from capsule in applesauce	X		X			X
Pellets from capsule in juice	X	X[e]	X			
Extemporaneous preparation of delayed-release PPI in bicarbonate (omeprazole-sodium bicarbonate)	X		X	X		
Parenteral formulations						
IV	Not available in the United States	X		X		

PPI, proton pump inhibitor; X, product is available.

[a]Omeprazole is available as delayed-release enteric-coated pellets in a capsule or as immediate-release capsule that contains 20 or 40 mg of omeprazole with 1,100 mg sodium bicarbonate (equivalent to 304 mg of sodium). Because 20 and 40 mg dosages contain the same amount of bicarbonate, two 20 mg capsules should not be substituted for the 40 mg immediate-release omeprazole-sodium bicarbonate capsule.

[b]Dexlansoprazole is available as a dual delayed-release formulation in capsules for oral administration. The capsule contains dexlansoprazole in a mixture of two types of enteric-coated granules with different pH-dependent dissolution profiles.

[c]Omeprazole oral tablets are available as 20 mg delayed-release nonprescription tablets.

[d]Omeprazole oral suspension is available as 20 or 40 mg omeprazole with 1,680 mg sodium bicarbonate (equivalent to 460 mg of sodium). Because 20 and 40 mg dosages contain the same amount of bicarbonate, two 20 mg packets should not be substituted for the 40 mg immediate-release omeprazole-bicarbonate packet.

[e]No published information; based on omeprazole data.

Data from references 79, 81, and 82.

(omeprazole, esomeprazole, prescription and nonprescription lansoprazole, and dexlansoprazole), rapidly disintegrating tablets (lansoprazole), and delayed-release enteric-coated tablets (rabeprazole, pantoprazole, and nonprescription omeprazole) (see Table 33-12).[79] The pH-sensitive enteric coating prevents degradation and premature protonation of the drug in stomach allowing the drug to be dissolved then absorbed in the duodenum at a higher pH. Dexlansoprazole is formulated with a dual-release mechanism that provides inhibition of proton pumps that become activated after initial release of the medication while omeprazole is also available as an immediate-release formulation (oral suspension, oral capsule) containing sodium bicarbonate, which can control intragastric pH in the absence of food.[81,82] IV products available in the United States include pantoprazole and esomeprazole.

Five of the PPIs provide similar rates of ulcer healing (omeprazole, esomeprazole, lansoprazole, rabeprazole, and pantoprazole), maintenance of ulcer healing, and symptom relief when used in recommended dosages (see Table 33-9). Higher than indicated daily doses should be divided in order to obtain better 24-hour control of intragastric pH. Older adults and patients with renal impairment do not require dosage reductions, but dosage reductions should be considered in patients with severe hepatic disease.[79] Short-term adverse effects of the PPIs are similar to those observed with the H2RAs (headache, nausea, and abdominal pain).[79] Immediate-release formulations contain sodium bicarbonate, and thus are contraindicated for patients with metabolic alkalosis and hypokalemia. Sodium content in these immediate-release products should also be taken into consideration for patients who are on sodium-restricted diets (eg, congestive heart failure patients, chronic kidney disease patients).

Drug Interactions Since PPIs increase intragastric pH, they may alter the bioavailability of orally administered drugs that are weak bases (eg, ketoconazole), digoxin, or pH-dependent dosage forms.[79,83] This interaction is especially important with atazanavir, a protease inhibitor used for treatment of HIV. Concomitant use with a PPI can significantly reduce the oral bioavailability of atazanavir leading to therapeutic failure and viral resistance in patients infected with HIV.[84] Omeprazole and esomeprazole selectively inhibit the hepatic CYP2C19 pathway and may decrease the elimination of several drugs (eg, phenytoin, warfarin, diazepam, and carbamazepine).[79] PPIs may increase the metabolic clearance and decrease the GI absorption of levothyroxine resulting in increased thyroid-stimulating hormone levels and a corresponding increase in the levothyroxine dose.[85] Clinically significant drug interactions with PPIs are rare and usually do not constitute a major clinical risk.[86,87]

Clinical **Controversy...**

PPIs have been linked with various enteric infections, but the most convincing data are with *C. difficile*. PPIs provide elevations in intragastric pH which facilitate the survival of *C. difficile* spores. Even though a possible association exists, the magnitude of risk varies and causality is difficult to establish prompting the need for large prospective studies.

A controversial PPI drug interaction involves the antiplatelet drug clopidogrel. Clopidogrel is converted to its active form through CYP2C19. PPIs may attenuate the antiplatelet effect of clopidogrel by inhibiting or competing for this metabolic pathway. FDA safety guidelines recommend that the coadministration of omeprazole, omeprazole/sodium bicarbonate, or esomeprazole with clopidogrel be avoided because they reduce the effectiveness of clopidogrel.[88] Warnings regarding omeprazole, esomeprazole, and other interacting drugs (eg, cimetidine), are contained in the clopidogrel package insert as well.[89] A reduced antiplatelet effect of clopidogrel may also result from genetic polymorphisms of the CYP2C19 pathway leading to decreased biotransformation of the drug to its active form which complicates the drug interaction.[90,91] Whether the use of other PPIs such as pantoprazole, lansoprazole, dexlansoprazole, and rabeprazole interacts with clopidogrel remains uncertain as the capacity to inhibit CYP2C19 varies among these PPIs.[92,93] Some reports suggest a "class effect" among the different PPIs. Other pharmacodynamic studies suggest an interaction with omeprazole and esomeprazole but not with pantoprazole.[92,93] The only randomized double-blind trial comparing clopidogrel with or without omeprazole yielded no apparent increase in cardiovascular events due to clopidogrel and omeprazole cotherapy; however, there was a significant reduction in the rate of upper GI bleeding.[94] This trial has been criticized for the low number of cardiovascular events, formulation of omeprazole used, and premature termination of the study due to loss of funding by the sponsor. Patients should have an acceptable indication for a PPI recognizing that risk versus benefit must be weighed on an individual basis. If a PPI is absolutely necessary with clopidogrel, avoiding the use of omeprazole or esomeprazole may be warranted.

Potential Risks and Long-Term Safety Issues Prolonged hypergastrinemia and chronic hypochlorhydria from long-term PPI use has been associated with numerous potential risks and safety issues (see Table 33-13).[79,95-98] In most cases, causality is difficult to ascertain because of the study design, confounding variables, and subject selection. All of the PPIs dose-dependently increase serum gastrin concentrations twofold to fourfold as a function of their potent acid-inhibitory effect.[79,95] Fasting gastrin elevations are usually within the normal range and return to baseline within 1 month of discontinuing the drug. In humans, PPIs may lead to enterochromaffin-like (ECL) hyperplasia, but there is no evidence that these changes result in dysplasia, carcinoid tumors, or gastric adenocarcinoma.[95,96] Long-term PPI therapy in *H. pylori*–positive individuals is associated with progressive atrophic gastritis, but there are insufficient data to link chronic PPI use with gastric cancer in *H. pylori*–positive patients.[95,96] There is also no evidence to support an association between PPIs and colonic polyps or colorectal cancer.[95,96] Bacterial overgrowth can occur in the stomach as a consequence of hypochlorhydria, but the full biological significance of this change in quantity and diversity of bacteria in the stomach and small intestine of PPI users remains unclear.[95,98]

Chronic PPI therapy may be associated with an increased risk of infection and nutritional deficiences.[95-97] Gastric acid plays an important role in the defense against bacterial colonization of the stomach and in nutrient absorption. Acid suppression has been implicated as a risk factor for community-acquired pneumonia (CAP) and enteric infections (*C. difficile, Salmonella, Campylobacter*).[96] Several studies, including one meta-analysis, demonstrate a higher adjusted relative risk of CAP for patients currently using PPIs compared with controls particularly in patients receiving higher doses or within the first 30 days of therapy.[99-101] The results of these retrospectively designed studies, however, need to be interpreted cautiously because of the variability in the length of therapy for current PPI users and the inclusion of older (older than 60 years) patients with concomitant comorbidities. A systematic review of the literature has linked PPIs with various enteric infections, but the most convincing data were with *C. difficile*.[102] It is likely that sustained elevations in intragastric pH facilitate the survival of *C. difficile* spores. However, the magnitude of risk varies and causality is difficult to establish. The risk of various infections associated with PPI therapy cannot be firmly established until the results of large prospective studies are made available.

The absorption of vitamin B_{12}, dietary iron, and calcium requires an acidic environment and may be adversely affected by long-term use of PPIs (see Table 33-10).[96] Although this adverse effect has been investigated, the clinical importance of their effect on absorption has not been established, and routine monitoring of B_{12} and iron levels cannot be recommended.[96] Adequate supplementation and monitoring should be considered in high-risk populations (eg, older patients, vegetarians, alcoholism) who may be already depleted.[95,96] High PPI dosage and long-term therapy have been associated with an increased risk of hip, wrist, and spine fractures related to reduction in calcium absorption.[38,103] The FDA has revised the warnings and precautions of prescription and nonprescription PPIs to reflect this potential risk.[103] Routine bone density tests for osteoporosis screening, calcium supplementation, or other precautions cannot be recommended solely based on chronic PPI therapy.[87] However, it is appropriate to screen and treat older patients for osteoporosis regardless of whether they are receiving long-term PPI therapy.

Hypomagnesemia, both symptomatic and asymptomatic, has been reported with PPI use with serious adverse events including tetany, arrhythmias, and seizures (see Table 33-10). In most cases it occurs in patients taking PPIs more than 1 year, but can occur with as little as 3 months of therapy. The FDA has revised the warnings and precautions of prescription and nonprescription PPIs.

H_2-Receptor Antagonists Ulcer healing is comparable among H2RAs (cimetidine, famotidine, nizatidine, and ranitidine) with equipotent multiple daily doses or a single full dose given after dinner or at bedtime (see Table 33-9), but tolerance to their antisecretory effect may occur.[104] Twice-daily administration may be beneficial in patients with daytime ulcer pain while cigarette smokers may require higher doses or a longer duration of treatment. H2RAs are renally eliminated thus a dosage reduction is recommended for patients with moderate-to-severe renal failure.[3] The short- and long-term safety of all four H2RAs is similar. Thrombocytopenia is a common yet likely overestimated hematologic adverse effect that occurs with all H2RAs and is reversible (see Table 33-10). The H2RAs decrease acid secretion and may alter the bioavailability of orally administered drugs, similar to that seen with the PPIs. Cimetidine inhibits several CYP450 isoenzymes, resulting in numerous drug interactions (eg, theophylline, lidocaine, phenytoin, warfarin, and clopidogrel). Ranitidine has less potential for hepatic CYP450 drug interactions, while famotidine and nizatidine do not interact with drugs metabolized by the hepatic CYP450 pathway.[3]

Sucralfate Sucralfate heals peptic ulcers, but is not widely used today for this indication.[1] Deterrents to its use include the requirement for multiple doses per day, large tablet size, and the need to separate the drug from meals and potentially interacting medications. Drug interactions can be minimized by giving the interacting drug at least 2 hours before sucralfate. Alternative therapy is warranted for patients taking oral fluoroquinolones.

TABLE 33-13 Potential Risks and Safety Issues Associated with the PPIs

Gastric cancers or malignancy
Carcinoid tumors
Atrophic gastritis
Adenocarcinoma
Bacterial overgrowth
Increase in *N*-nitroso compounds from ingested nitrates (carcinogenic)
Enteric infections (*Clostridium difficile, Salmonella typhimurium*, and *Campylobacter jejuni*)
Community-acquired pneumonia
Decreased nutrient absorption:
Iron
Calcium
Cyanocobalamin (vitamin B_{12})
Magnesium
Osteoporosis and related fractures

PPI, proton pump inhibitor.

Data from references 79, 95 to 98.

Constipation may be troublesome especially in older individuals. Seizures may occur in dialysis patients taking aluminum-containing antacids. Hypophosphatemia may develop with long-term treatment. Gastric bezoar formation has also been reported (see Table 33-10).

Prostaglandins Misoprostol, a synthetic PGE_1 analogue, moderately inhibits acid secretion and enhances mucosal defense.[1,3] Antisecretory effects are dose dependent over the range of 50 to 200 mcg, and cytoprotective effects occur in humans at doses of greater than 200 mcg. Because protective effects occur at higher doses, it is difficult to establish the protective effect independent of the antisecretory action. A dose of 200 mcg four times daily or 400 mcg twice daily (although not recommended in the United States) heals duodenal ulcers and gastric ulcers comparable to standard H2RA or sucralfate regimens. The most troublesome adverse effect is diarrhea which is dose-dependent; develops in 10% to 30% of patients; and is accompanied by abdominal cramping, nausea, flatulence, and headache.[1,3] Taking the drug with or after meals and at bedtime may and avoidance of magnesium containing antacids minimize the diarrhea (see Table 33-10). Misoprostol is contraindicated in pregnant women because it produces uterine contractions that may endanger pregnancy. If misoprostol is prescribed to women in their childbearing years, contraceptive measures must be confirmed and a negative serum pregnancy test should be documented within 2 weeks of initiating treatment (see Table 33-10).[3]

Bismuth Preparations Bismuth subsalicylate and bismuth subcitrate potassium (biskalcitrate) are the only available bismuth salts in the United States.[1] Possible ulcer healing mechanisms include an antibacterial effect, a local gastroprotective effect, and stimulation of endogenous PGs. Bismuth salts do not inhibit or neutralize acid. Bismuth subsalicylate is regarded as safe and has few adverse effects when taken in recommended dosages. Bismuth salts should be used with caution in older patients and in renal failure as renal insufficiency may decrease bismuth elimination. Bismuth subsalicylate may cause salicylate sensitivity or bleeding disorders and should be used with caution for patients receiving concurrent salicylate therapy. Bismuth salts impart a black color to stool and possibly the tongue with liquid preparations. Long-term use of bismuth salts is not recommended due to the potential for bismuth toxicity.

Antacids Antacids neutralize gastric acid, inactivate pepsin, and bind bile salts.[1] Aluminum-containing antacids also suppress *H. pylori* and enhance mucosal defense. The GI adverse effects are most common and are dose dependent: Aluminum-containing antacids cause constipation, and magnesium salts can cause an osmotic diarrhea. Aluminum-containing antacids (except aluminum phosphate) form insoluble salts with dietary phosphorus and interfere with phosphorus absorption. Hypophosphatemia occurs most often for patients with low dietary phosphate intake (eg, malnutrition or alcoholism). Combined treatment with sucralfate may amplify the hypophosphatemia and aluminum toxicity.

Magnesium excretion is impaired in patients with a creatinine clearance of less than 30 mL/min (0.5 mL/s) which may lead to toxicity; thus, magnesium-containing antacids should be avoided in these patients. Hypercalcemia may occur for patients with normal renal function taking more than 20 g/day of calcium carbonate and for patients with renal failure who are taking more than 4 g/day. The milk-alkali syndrome (ie, hypercalcemia, alkalosis, renal stones, increased blood urea nitrogen, and increased serum creatinine concentration) occurs with high calcium intake for patients with systemic alkalosis produced by either ingestion of absorbable antacids (sodium bicarbonate) or prolonged vomiting. Antacids may alter the absorption and excretion of drugs when administered concomitantly (eg, iron, warfarin, tetracycline, digoxin, quinidine, isoniazid, ketoconazole, or the fluoroquinolones).[1] Most interactions can be avoided by separating the antacid from the oral drug by at least 2 hours.

PERSONALIZED PHARMACOTHERAPY

The metabolism of PPIs occurs primarily through CYP2C19 and polymorphisms of CPY2C19 result in significant differences in enzymatic activity (poor, intermediate, or rapid metabolizers). For example, approximately 85% of white and nearly 100% of Asian populations have polymorphisms resulting in poor metabolism of substrates for CYP2C19. Eradication response rates of *H. pylori* are influenced by pharmacogenomics, with poor metabolizers achieving 100% eradication, intermediate metabolizers achieving 60%, and rapid metabolizers achieving 30% eradication.[105] Prior knowledge of CYP2C19 genotype may help to optimize the PPI dose and interval to minimize therapeutic failure. Rapid metabolizers may need more frequent PPI dosing, up to four times daily, to ensure an optimal gastric pH. Further studies are required to determine if increased AUC achieved in poor metabolizers translates to an additional risk of adverse effects.[106] Pharmacologic properties such as bioavailability and plasma concentrations of individual PPIs differ between individuals, but it remains unclear whether these differences impact the efficacy of *H. pylori* eradication.

Patients with high body-mass index have reduced antibiotic concentration at the gastric mucosal level and may result in higher risk of treatment failure. Likewise, prior allergy information and history of antimicrobial use is important in tailoring a regimen for *H. pylori* eradication. Tailoring eradication therapy based on *H. pylori* clarithromycin sensitivities is gaining popularity as molecular diagnostic testing improves. In one study, eradication rates improved from 70% in the control group to 94.3% in the treatment arm by tailoring eradication therapy from detection of clarithromycin-resistant *H. pylori* in feces.[107]

Smoking is a risk factor for treatment failure or ulcer recurrence; therefore, patients should be encouraged to quit smoking.

EVALUATION OF THERAPEUTIC OUTCOMES

6 Table 33-14 lists the recommendations for treating and monitoring patients with PUD. Relief of epigastric pain should be monitored throughout the course of treatment for patients with either *H. pylori*- or NSAID-related ulcers. Ulcer pain typically resolves in a few days when NSAIDs are discontinued and within 7 days upon initiation of antiulcer therapy. Patients with uncomplicated PUD are usually symptom free after treatment with any of the recommended antiulcer regimens. Persistent or recurrent symptoms within 14 days following treatment completion suggests failure of ulcer healing or *H. pylori* eradication or presence of an alternate diagnosis such as GERD. Most patients with uncomplicated *H. pylori*-positive ulcers do not require confirmation of ulcer healing or *H. pylori* eradication. However, eradication should be confirmed after treatment in individuals who are at risk for complications, for example, individuals who had a prior bleeding ulcer. The UBT and fecal antigen are the preferred methods to confirm *H. pylori* eradication when endoscopy is not indicated. Medication adherence should be assessed for patients who fail therapy. Many at-risk patients treated with NSAIDs do not receive adequate prophylaxis for GI complications; however, therapeutic outcomes can be improved by advocating preventive strategies. Any signs or symptoms of bleeding, obstruction, penetration, or perforation require prompt investigation to avoid complications. A follow-up endoscopy is justified for patients with frequent symptomatic recurrence, refractory disease, complications, or suspected hypersecretory states.

TABLE 33-14 Recommendations for Treating and Monitoring Patients with *Helicobacter pylori*–Associated and NSAID-Induced Ulcers

***H. pylori*-associated ulcer**

1. Recommend drug treatment as presented in the chapter text. See Tables 33-7 and 33-8
2. Assess patient allergies to determine if allergic to penicillin (or other antibiotics) so that drug regimens that contain penicillin (or other antibiotics) can be avoided. Avoid regimens that contain tetracycline in children
3. Assess patient use of alcohol or alcohol-containing products with metronidazole and oral birth control medications with antibiotics and counsel appropriately
4. Assess likelihood of nonadherence to the drug regimen as a cause of treatment failure
5. Recommend a different antibiotic combination if *H. pylori* eradication fails and a second treatment is planned
6. Inform the patient of change in stool color when bismuth salicylate is included in an *H. pylori* eradication regimen
7. Assess and monitor patients for potential adverse effects, especially those associated with metronidazole, clarithromycin, and amoxicillin
8. Assess and monitor patients for potential drug interactions, especially those receiving metronidazole, clarithromycin, or cimetidine
9. Monitor patients for salicylate toxicity, especially patients receiving cotherapy with other salicylates and anticoagulants and patients with renal failure
10. Monitor patients for persistent or recurrent symptoms within 14 days after completion of a course of *H. pylori* eradication therapy
11. Provide patient education to patients who are receiving *H. pylori* eradication therapy and include why antibiotic and antiulcer combinations are used; when and how to take medications; adverse effects; alarm symptoms; the importance of adherence to the entire course of drug treatment; and contact their healthcare provider if alarm symptoms develop (eg, blood in the stools, black tarry stools, vomiting, severe abdominal pain), or if symptoms persist or return after *H. pylori* eradication

NSAID-induced ulcer

1. Recommend drug treatment as presented in the chapter text
2. Assess risk factors for NSAID-induced ulcers and ulcer-related complications and recommend appropriate strategies for reducing ulcer risk (see Table 33-11)
3. Weigh patient risk factors for NSAID-related GI bleeding and cardiovascular events when selecting a strategy to reduce ulcer risk
4. Recommend eradication treatment for *H. pylori*-positive patients taking NSAIDs
5. Monitor patients for signs and symptoms of NSAID-related upper GI complications
6. Assess and monitor patients for potential drug interactions and adverse effects (especially misoprostol)
7. Provide patient education to patients who are at risk of NSAID-induced ulcers or GI-related complications and include why cotherapy is used with nonselective NSAIDs, when and how to take medications, adverse effects, alarm symptoms, when to contact their healthcare provider, and the importance of adherence to drug treatment

RELATED DISORDERS

Upper Gastrointestinal Bleeding

Upper GI bleeding is one of the most common GI emergencies with more than 300,000 hospital admissions annually. There are about 48 to 160 cases of upper GI bleeding per 100,000 adults annually in the United States, and the mortality rate associated with acute hemorrhage remains relatively high between 6% and 14% despite a decreased incidence of PUD and improvements in the management of upper GI bleeding. Upper GI bleeding is categorized as variceal or nonvariceal bleeding. A complete discussion of variceal bleeding is found elsewhere (Chapter 37). Two common types of nonvariceal bleeding are bleeding from chronic peptic ulcers and bleeding from stress-related mucosal damage (SRMD).[108] Upper GI bleeding associated with chronic PUD usually precedes hospital admission. Bleeding associated with SRMD develops in severely ill patients during hospitalization.[108-111] The underlying pathophysiology of bleeding from a peptic ulcer or from SRMD is similar in that impaired mucosal defense in the presence of gastric acid and pepsin leads to mucosal damage. In chronic PUD, *H. pylori* infection and NSAID use are the most important etiologic factors. The primary pathogenic factor of SRMD in critically ill patients is thought to be mucosal ischemia, which is a result of reduced gastric blood flow resulting from splanchnic hypoperfusion.[108-111] Stress-related mucosal lesions are characteristically asymptomatic, numerous, located in the proximal stomach, and unlikely to perforate. Bleeding from SRMD occurs from superficial mucosal capillaries, whereas bleeding associated with chronic PUD usually results from a single vessel.[108-111] The mortality rate associated with clinically important stress-related mucosal bleeding (SRMB) is approximately 50% and is related to disease severity and comorbidities in this patient population. The mortality associated with chronic PUD-related bleeding is approximately 10% but can increase dramatically in select patient populations.[108-111] Initial management of acute upper GI bleeding focuses on aggressive resuscitation and hemodynamic stability.

Peptic Ulcer-Related Bleeding

Clinical Presentation and Diagnosis

Hematemesis (vomiting up blood), melena (dark, tarry stools), or both are most common presenting signs and symptoms of PUD-related bleeding. Risk for adverse outcomes must be rapidly assessed in order to determine if the patient's condition constitutes a medical emergency.[112,113] Two risk stratification tools exist for early assessment and triage. The Blatchford score is used to evaluate the need for urgent endoscopic intervention for patients presenting with PUD-related bleeding. The scale values range from 0 to 23, with higher scores indicating higher risk. The Rockall Score is composed of two assessments: the clinical score, which is performed prior to endoscopy, and the endoscopic score. The use of these risk stratification tools can reduce the requirement of endoscopic procedures and lead to early discharge for low-risk patients while ensuring rapid intervention for patients at higher risk.[112,113] When considering the risk of death due to PUD bleeding, the following patients generally have poorer prognoses and usually require more aggressive intervention including admission to an intensive care unit (ICU): age older than 65 years, shock, poor overall health, comorbid conditions, low initial hemoglobin/hematocrit, active bleeding (red blood per rectum or hematemesis), sepsis, and elevated serum creatinine or serum transaminases.[109] Diagnostic endoscopy is usually performed within 24 hours of presentation to identify the source of the bleeding, assess the potential risk for rebleeding using the Forrest classification of lesions, and, if appropriate, employ therapeutic interventions to promote hemostasis.[108,109,112,113]

The appearance of the ulcer at the time of endoscopy is a prognostic indicator for the risk of rebleeding. Clean-based (Forrest type III) and flat spot (pigmented; Forrest type IIc) ulcers are most commonly seen and are associated with a low risk of rebleeding (5% and 10%, respectively). In most cases, patients with clean-based ulcers can be treated as an outpatient after endoscopy on antiulcer therapy, while patients with flat spot ulcers may be admitted to the general hospital ward for brief observation.[108,112] Patients with an adherent clot overlying the ulcer base (Forrest type IIb) are at intermediate risk of rebleeding (22%-33%), and controversy exists as to the appropriate management of these patients. Patients with a visible vessel (Forrest type IIa) or active bleeding (Forrest type Ia or Ib) are at the highest risk of rebleeding (43%-50% and 55%-90%, respectively) and should receive ICU care for at least 24 hours followed by monitoring on a general medical/surgical service for an additional 48 hours as rebleeding significantly increases mortality.[108,112]

Treatment

Initial therapy for patients with defined hemostatic instability should focus on correcting fluid volume loss though appropriate volume resuscitative measures. This is usually accomplished with a continuous 0.9% sodium chloride infusion or blood products if clinically indicated.[112,113] The use of nasogastric (NG) tubes remains controversial but may aid in early assessment and gastric lavage.[109,113] Several endoscopic treatment approaches (eg, thermocoagulation, argon plasma coagulation therapy, injection sclerotherapy, hemoclipping, and ligation) can be used. To maximize the likelihood of positive outcomes, patients should be treated with a combination of at least two endoscopic modalities, such as thermocoagulation and injection of lesions with epinephrine.[108,109,112,113]

Antisecretory agents are often used as adjuvant therapy to endoscopic procedures to prevent PUD rebleeding in high-risk patients because acid impairs clot stability. PPIs reduce the incidence of rebleeding and need for surgery but have no significant impact on overall mortality.[109,112,114] Historically, practice guidelines recommended that high-dose continuous-infusion PPI therapy (equivalent to omeprazole 80 mg given IV as a loading dose, followed by 8 mg/h continuous infusion for 72 hours) be used to reduce the risk of rebleeding in high risk patients who have undergone endoscopy hemostasis. A Cochrane Review comparing different regimens of PPIs and a meta-analysis comparing intermittent and continuous PPI therapy for high-risk bleeding ulcers showed no benefit in high dose or continuous therapy respectively.[114,115] Thus intermittent IV dosing of PPIs (at cumulative daily doses of 80-160 mg) may be a therapeutic option that provides a greater ease of administration. PPI therapy is not a replacement for interventional endoscopy in patients with a high risk of rebleeding, as data demonstrate that the combination of a PPI with therapeutic endoscopy is superior to either strategy alone.[109,112,113] The risk of rebleeding is greatest within the first 72 hours, and thus antisecretory therapy to prevent rebleeding in high-risk patients should be employed in this time frame. Patients should be transitioned to an oral PPI on completion of IV therapy.[109,112,113]

Patients with upper GI bleeding should be tested for *H. pylori* at the time of endoscopy (see "Tests for *H. pylori*" above). However, the tests are associated with an increased rate of false-negatives when obtained during acute bleeding episodes. If the initial results of the rapid urease test and/or histology are negative, a confirmatory test should be performed following the acute bleeding episode.[109] Ulcer treatment, including *H. pylori* eradication, if appropriate, should be initiated after the acute bleeding episode has resolved (see "Treatment of *H. pylori*–Positive Ulcers and Treatment of NSAID-Induced Ulcers" above).

Stress-Related Mucosal Bleeding

Epidemiology and Risk Factors

Clinically important bleeding increases ICU length of stay, results in excessive healthcare costs, and is associated with increased mortality. Thus, attempts to prevent SRMB are warranted in high-risk patients. Prophylactic therapy to prevent bleeding is most effective if initiated early in the patient's course.[111] Majority (75%-100%) of critically ill patients develop SRMD within the first 1 to 3 days of admission to an ICU, but the incidence of clinically important SRMB (defined as overt bleeding with concomitant hemodynamic instability and likely requirement for blood products) is 1% to 6%.[111]

Patients who are at risk for SRMB include those with respiratory failure (need for mechanical ventilation for longer than 48 hours), coagulopathy (INR greater than 1.5, platelet count less than 50,000 mm^3[less than 50×10^9 /L]), hypotension, sepsis, hepatic failure, acute renal failure, high-dose corticosteroid therapy (more than 250 mg/day hydrocortisone or equivalent), multiple trauma, severe burns (more than 35% of body surface area), head injury, traumatic spinal cord injury, major surgery, prolonged ICU admission (more than 7 days), or history of GI bleeding.[116] The relative importance of the various risk factors remains controversial, but most clinicians concur that patients with respiratory failure or coagulopathy should receive prophylaxis, as these two factors are independent risk factors for SRMB.[117]

Prevention and Treatment

Prevention of SRMB includes resuscitative measures that restore mucosal blood and pharmacotherapy that either maintains an intragastric pH of greater than 4 or provides gastric mucosal protection.[111,116] Although the benefits of enteral nutrition to patient outcome (eg, improved nutritional status enhances mucosal integrity) are of overall clinical importance, its precise role as a sole modality to prevent SRMB remains controversial. Two meta-analyses suggest that patients receiving enteral nutrition may not require SRMB prophylaxis and that such therapies may increase the risk of adverse complications of these therapies.[118,119] Therapeutic options for the prevention of SRMB include antacids (which are no longer used because of cumbersome dosage schedules and side effects), antisecretory drugs (H2RAs and PPIs), and sucralfate.[111,116]

Sucralfate is an evidence-based option but requires multiple daily dosage administration (up to four times daily), which may occlude nasogastric (NG) tubes, cause constipation, interact with several medications, or increase the potential for aluminum toxicity in patients with renal dysfunction and is thus not used very frequently for SRMB prophylaxis.[116] Antisecretory therapy is generally preferred for SRMB prophylaxis. The PPIs are more potent than H2RAs in inhibiting acid secretion and, unlike H2RAs, tolerance does not develop. PPIs have become the most widely used therapy despite conflicting evidence of their superiority over H2RAs for SRMB prophylaxis.[111,120-123] In addition, adverse events that have been described when the PPIs are used for SRMB prophylaxis include an increased risk of enteric infections, including *C. difficile*–associated diarrhea and nosocomial pneumonia thus potentially increasing hospital-associated costs and providing an argument against their routine use for SRMB prophylaxis.[111,116,121-123] Based on available evidence, several PPI dosing regimens for SRMB prophylaxis exist (see Table 33-15).[111,116]

Even though PPIs have become the most widely used prevention therapy, numerous studies and years of experience support the use of H2RAs, and they remain a recommended option for the prevention of SRMB.[111,116,121,122] Parenteral H2RAs may be administered as either continuous infusions or intermittent bolus doses (see Table 33-15). Cimetidine, given as a continuous IV infusion, is the only FDA-labeled H2RA for the prevention of SRMB. Drug interactions are more common with cimetidine, thus the other H2RAs (famotidine, ranitidine) are used more frequently.[111,116] Adverse events associated with the use of H2RAs for the critically ill patient include thrombocytopenia, mental status changes (more common in older patients or individuals with renal or hepatic compromise), and tachyphylaxis (especially with parenteral or high-dose therapy). Given that the H2RAs are renally eliminated, dosage reductions are recommended for patients with renal dysfunction.[116]

When deciding on the most appropriate pharmacotherapy plan for the prevention of SRMB for a specific patient, the clinical presentation of the patient and medication costs should be used as a guide. Patients who can take oral medication or have a working NG tube in place may be placed on an oral H2RA or PPI suspension as a cost-effective measure. For most patients who are not able to utilize one of these routes, an IV H2RA is appropriate. However, if the patient has any relative or absolute contraindications to an H2RA, then an IV PPI may be the most appropriate prophylaxis option.

TABLE 33-15 Pharmacotherapy Options for Prophylaxis of Stress-Related Mucosal Bleeding

Drug and Route	Dosage
Parenteral H2RAs	
Cimetidine	300 mg IV loading dose followed by 50 mg/h as a continuous infusion[a] or 300 mg IV every 6-8 hours
Ranitidine	6.25 mg/h as a continuous infusion or 50 mg IV every 6-8 hours
Famotidine	1.7 mg/h as a continuous infusion or 20 mg IV every 12 hours
Oral/NG Tube PPIs	
Omeprazole	20-40 mg orally/NG tube[b] every 12-24 hours
Omeprazole/bicarbonate powder for oral suspension	40 mg orally/NG tube to start, then followed by an additional 40 mg in 6-8 hours as a loading dose, and then 40 mg every 24 hours
Lansoprazole	30 mg orally/NG tube[b,c] every 12-24 hours
Pantoprazole	40 mg orally/NG tube[b] every 12-24 hours
Parenteral PPIs	
Pantoprazole	40-80 mg IV every 12-24 hours
Esomeprazole	40 mg IV every 12-24 hours

H_2RA, histamine-2 receptor antagonist; NG, nasogastric; PPI, proton pump inhibitor.

[a]Product is FDA approved for the prevention of stress-related mucosal bleeding.

[b]Administered as an extemporaneously compounded suspension made with sodium bicarbonate.

[c]Administered as a rapidly disintegrating tablet given orally or by NG tube dissolved in 10 mL of water.

Improvement in the patient's overall medical condition (resolution of risk factors, discharge from the ICU, extubation, and oral intake) suggests that prophylactic therapy can be discontinued. Often patients are continued on SRMB prophylaxis on transition to the general medical/surgical unit and are often discharged on oral PPI therapy without an appropriate indication. This results in unnecessary costs for the patient and the healthcare system.[122,123] Patients in whom SRMB prophylaxis is no longer indicated should be identified. If a patient develops clinically important bleeding, endoscopic evaluation of the GI tract is indicated along with aggressive antisecretory therapy (see "Peptic Ulcer–Related Bleeding" above).

Clinical **Controversy...**

The precise role of enteral nutrition as a sole modality to prevent SRMB remains controversial. Two meta-analyses suggest that patients receiving enteral nutrition may not require SRMB prophylaxis thus preventing adverse complications of these therapies. However, more randomized-controlled trials are needed to confirm benefit.

Zollinger-Ellison Syndrome

ZES, characterized by hypersecretion of gastric acid and severe gastroesophageal PUD, is caused by a neuroendocrine tumor (gastrinoma) that is present in the duodenum or pancreas.[124-127] Gastrinoma has a yearly incidence of approximately one to three cases per million in the United States with ZES being the underlying cause of PUD in 0.1% to 1% of patients.[126] ZES occurs spontaneously in 75% to 80% of patients, but 20% to 25% of patients have the familial form associated with multiple endocrine neoplasia type 1 (MEN1), an autosomal-dominant syndrome due to defects in the *MEN1* gene.[125,126] MEN1 patients commonly develop hyperparathyroidism, pituitary adenomas, and neuroendocrine tumors. Half (50%) of patients with MEN1 have ZES making gastrinoma and ZES the most common functional neuroendocrine tumor and syndrome in MEN1.[125,126] Gastrinomas are usually slow growing, but approximately 60% to 90% are malignant with metastases to regional lymph nodes, liver, and other distant sites at time of diagnosis.[126]

Pathophysiology

Gastrinomas are derived from the enteroendocrine cells, form tumors mainly in the pancreas and proximal small intestine, and are generally classified under the larger term of neuroendocrine tumors. Most gastrinomas arise in the duodenum. Gastrinomas located in the pancreas carry a greater malignant potential.[127] ZES pathophysiology is related to the trophic action of gastrin on parietal cells of the gastric antrum and the resulting hypersecretion of gastric acid. A majority of patients consequently develop large peptic ulcers frequently in the distal duodenum and even proximal jejunum which is an uncommon location for ulcers resulting from *H. pylori* or the use of NSAIDs.[127]

Clinical Presentation and Diagnosis

Historically, patients with ZES presented with refractory PUD or complications of acid hypersecretion (perforation, penetration, bleeding, and esophageal stricture). Due to the widespread use of PPIs and H2RAs, this form of presentation has decreased drastically.[125] Currently, patients commonly present with severe refractory heartburn, epigastric pain, and profound diarrhea. Diarrhea maybe the only symptom in 10% to 20% of patients and is due to the osmotic load of high gastric acid, inhibition of sodium and water reabsorption by the intestinal brush border of high gastric acid secretion, and a malabsorptive component from inactivation of pancreatic digestive enzymes by gastric acid.[125,127]

ZES diagnosis is established when the serum gastrin is greater than 1,000 pg/mL (ng/L; greater than 481 pmol/L) and the basal acid output (BAO) is more than or equal to 15 mEq/h (more than or equal to 15 mmol/h) for patients with an intact stomach (BAO more than or equal to 5 mEq/h [greater than or equal to 5 mmol/h] for patients with previous gastric surgery) or when hypergastrinemia is associated with a gastric pH value of more than or equal to 2.[126,127] In situations in which the serum gastrin is between 100 and 1,000 pg/mL (ng/L; 48 and 481 pmol/L) and gastric pH is less than or equal to 2, a secretin or calcium proactive test is used to aid the diagnosis. Identification of the location of the tumor with imaging techniques is essential, as early surgical resection prior to liver metastases is often curative.[124-127] The widespread use of PPIs, although effective in reducing symptoms, may mask the clinical presentation and PPI-related hypergastrinemia may further complicate the diagnosis.[124,125]

Treatment

Historically, only total gastrectomy was effective at controlling gastric acid hypersecretion. With the development of H2RAs and PPIs, medical management of ZES is now feasible in almost all patients. Because of their long duration of action and potency, PPIs are now the drugs of choice for treating gastric acid hypersecretion in patients with ZES.[124-126] Many of the PPIs (omperazole, esomeprazole, lansoprazole, esomeprazole, rabeprazole, and pantoprazole) are effective in ZES. Initial doses of 80 mg/day for pantoprazole (or an equivalent dose of other available PPIs) given every 8 to 12 hours is most effective at controlling gastric acid hypersecretion and reliving symptoms. IV PPIs can be used for those patients who do not tolerate oral therapy. PPIs must be dose adjusted in patients with ZES to normalize BAO levels to less than 15 mEq/h (less than 15 mmol/h) or less than 5 mEq/h (5 mmol/h) in patients with reflux esophagitis or prior operations to reduce acid secretion, such as subtotal gastrectomy. PPI therapy can be gradually decreased after adequate control of hypersecretion is achieved.[124-126] Since 60% to 90% of gastrinomas are malignant, management of advanced disease may include surgical resection of primary and metastatic gastrinomas. Nonsurgical therapy may include treatment with chemotherapy, somatostatin analogues such as octreotide, interferon, and targeted-molecular therapies such as a mTor inhibitor (everolimus) or a tyrosine-kinase inhibitor (sunitinib).[124-126]

ACKNOWLEDGMENT

This chapter is a revision of the chapter on Peptic Ulcer Disease in the 8th edition written by Rosemary R. Berardi and Randolph V. Fugit.

ABBREVIATIONS

ATPase	adenosine triphosphatase
BAO	basal acid output
CAP	community-acquired pneumonia
CLASS	Celecoxib Long-Term Arthritis Safety Study
COX	cyclooxygenase
COX-1	cyclooxygenase-1
COX-2	cyclooxygenase-2
CYP450	cytochrome P450
ECL	enterochromaffin-like
GERD	gastroesophageal reflux disease
H_2RA	histamine-2 receptor antagonist
ICU	intensive care unit
IL	interleukin
INR	international normalized ratio
MALT	mucosa-associated lymphoid tissue
MAO	maximal acid output
MEN 1	multiple endocrine neoplasia type 1
NG	nasogastric
NSAID	nonsteroidal anti-inflammatory drug
NUD	nonulcer dyspepsia
PG	prostaglandin
PPI	proton pump inhibitor
PUD	peptic ulcer disease
SRMB	stress-related mucosal bleeding
SRMD	stress-related mucosal damage
TNF-α	tumor necrosis factor-α
UBT	urea breath test
ZES	Zollinger-Ellison syndrome

REFERENCES

1. Del Valle J. Peptic Ulcer Disease and Related Disorders. In: Kasper D, Fauci A, Hauser S, Longo D, Jameson J, Loscalzo J. eds. Harrison's Principles of Internal Medicine, 19e. New York, NY: McGraw-Hill; 2015. http://accessmedicine.mhmedical.com Accessed August 03, 2016.
2. Lew E. Peptic ulcer disease. In: Greenberger NJ, Blumberg RS, Burakoff R, eds. *Current Diagnosis & Treatment: Gastroenterology, Hepatology, & Endoscopy*. 2nd ed. New York, NY: McGraw-Hill Medical; 2012.
3. Love BL, Meade LT. Upper gastrointestinal disorders. In: SS S, ed. *NAPLEX Review Guide*. New York, NY: McGraw-Hill Medical; 2015.
4. Everhart JE, Ruhl CE. Burden of digestive diseases in the United States part I: Overall and upper gastrointestinal diseases. *Gastroenterology* 2009;136(2):376-386.
5. Chey WD, Wong BC. Practice Parameters Committee of the American College of G. American College of Gastroenterology guideline on the management of *Helicobacter pylori* infection. *Am J Gastroenterol* 2007;102(8):1808-1825.
6. Azevedo NF, Huntington J, Goodman KJ. The epidemiology of *Helicobacter pylori* and public health implications. *Helicobacter* 2009;14 (Suppl 1):1-7.
7. Lanza FL, Chan FK, Quigley EM. Practice Parameters Committee of the American College of G. Guidelines for prevention of NSAID-related ulcer complications. *Am J Gastroenterol* 2009;104(3):728-738.
8. Malfertheiner P, Chan FK, McColl KE. Peptic ulcer disease. *Lancet* 2009;374(9699):1449-1461.
9. Laine L, Curtis SP, Cryer B, Kaur A, Cannon CP. Risk factors for NSAID-associated upper GI clinical events in a long-term prospective study of 34 701 arthritis patients. *Aliment Pharmacol Ther* 2010;32(10):1240-1248.
10. Furuta T, Delchier JC. *Helicobacter pylori* and non-malignant diseases. *Helicobacter* 2009;14 (Suppl 1):29-35.
11. Talley NJ, Fock KM, Moayyedi P. Gastric Cancer Consensus conference recommends *Helicobacter pylori* screening and treatment in asymptomatic persons from high-risk populations to prevent gastric cancer. *Am J Gastroenterol* 2008;103(3):510-514.
12. Pellicano R, Franceschi F, Saracco G, Fagoonee S, Roccarina D, Gasbarrini A. Helicobacters and extragastric diseases. *Helicobacter* 2009;14 (Suppl 1):58-68.
13. Bhatt DL, Scheiman J, Abraham NS, et al. ACCF/ACG/AHA 2008 expert consensus document on reducing the gastrointestinal risks of antiplatelet therapy and NSAID use. *Am J Gastroentero.* 2008;103(11):2890-2907.
14. Abraham NS, Hlatky MA, Antman EM, et al. ACCF/ACG/AHA 2010 expert consensus document on the concomitant use of proton pump inhibitors and thienopyridines: A focused update of the ACCF/ACG/AHA 2008 expert consensus document on reducing the gastrointestinal risks of antiplatelet therapy and NSAID use. *Am J Gastroenterol* 2010;105(12):2533-2549.
15. Cryer B. Management of patients with high gastrointestinal risk on antiplatelet therapy. *Gastroenterol Clin North Am* 2009;38(2):289-303.
16. Chan FK, Abraham NS, Scheiman JM, et al. Management of patients on nonsteroidal anti-inflammatory drugs: a clinical practice recommendation from the First International Working Party on Gastrointestinal and Cardiovascular Effects of Nonsteroidal Anti-inflammatory Drugs and Anti-platelet Agents. *Am J Gastroenterol* 2008;103(11):2908-2918.
17. Rostom A, Moayyedi P. Hunt R, Canadian Association of Gastroenterology Consensus G. Canadian consensus guidelines on long-term nonsteroidal anti-inflammatory drug therapy and the need for gastroprotection: benefits versus risks. *Aliment Pharmacol Ther* 2009;29(5):481-496.
18. Lanas A, Sopena F. Nonsteroidal anti-inflammatory drugs and lower gastrointestinal complications. *Gastroenterol Clin North Am* 2009;38(2):333-352.
19. Chan FK. The David Y. Graham lecture: use of nonsteroidal antiinflammatory drugs in a COX-2 restricted environment. *Am J Gastroenterol* 2008;103(1):221-227.
20. Scheiman JM. Balancing risks and benefits of cyclooxygenase-2 selective nonsteroidal anti-inflammatory drugs. *Gastroenterol Clin North Am* 2009;38(2):305-314.
21. Jiang HY, Chen HZ, Hu XJ, et al. Use of selective serotonin reuptake inhibitors and risk of upper gastrointestinal bleeding: a systematic review and meta-analysis. *Clin Gastroenterol Hepatol* 2015;13(1):42-50 e43.
22. Amsterdam EA, Wenger NK, Brindis RG, et al. 2014 AHA/ACC guideline for the management of patients with non-ST-elevation acute coronary syndromes: A report of the American College of Cardiology/American Heart Association Task Force on Practice Guidelines. *Circulation* 2014;130(25):e344-426.
23. Li LF, Chan RL, Lu L, et al. Cigarette smoking and gastrointestinal diseases: the causal relationship and underlying molecular mechanisms (review). *Int J Mol Med* 2014;34(2):372-380.
24. Zhang L, Ren JW, Wong CC, et al. Effects of cigarette smoke and its active components on ulcer formation and healing in the gastrointestinal mucosa. *Curr Med Chem* 2012;19(1):63-69.
25. Costa AC, Figueiredo C, Touati E. Pathogenesis of *Helicobacter pylori* infection. *Helicobacter* 2009;14 (Suppl 1):15-20.
26. Amieva M, Peek RM, Jr. Pathobiology of *Helicobacter pylori*-induced gastric cancer. *Gastroenterology*; 2015.
27. Hernandez-Diaz S, Martin-Merino E, Garcia Rodriguez LA. Risk of complications after a peptic ulcer diagnosis: Effectiveness of proton pump inhibitors. *Dig Dis Sci* 2013;58(6):1653-1662.
28. Talley NJ. Functional (non-ulcer) dyspepsia and gastroesophageal reflux disease: One not two diseases? *Am J Gastroenterol* 2013;108(5):775-777.
29. Calvet X. Diagnosis of *Helicobacter pylori* Infection in the proton pump inhibitor era. *Gastroenterol Clin North Am* 2015;44(3):507-518.
30. Ferwana M, Abdulmajeed I, Alhajiahmed A, et al. Accuracy of urea breath test in *Helicobacter pylori* infection: meta-analysis. *World J Gastroenterol* 2015;21(4):1305-1314.
31. Kilincalp S, Ustun Y, Akinci H, Coban S, Yuksel I. Letter: effect of proton pump inhibitor use on invasive detection of *Helicobacter pylori* gastritis. *Aliment Pharmacol Ther* 2015;41(6):599.
32. Roma E, Miele E. *Helicobacter pylori* infection in pediatrics. *Helicobacter* 2015;20 (Suppl 1):47-53.

33. Dos Santos AA, Carvalho AA. Pharmacological therapy used in the elimination of *Helicobacter pylori* infection: A review. *World J Gastroentero.* 2015;21(1):139-154.
34. Heo J, Jeon SW. Optimal treatment strategy for *Helicobacter pylori*: Era of antibiotic resistance. *World J Gastroenterol* 2014;20(19):5654-5659.
35. Malfertheiner P, Megraud F, O'Morain C, et al. Management of *Helicobacter pylori* infection–the Maastricht IV/Florence Consensus Report. *Gut* 2012;61(5):646-664.
36. Almeida N, Romaozinho JM, Donato MM, et al. Triple therapy with high-dose proton-pump inhibitor, amoxicillin, and doxycycline is useless for *Helicobacter pylori* eradication: A proof-of-concept study. *Helicobacter* 2014;19(2):90-97.
37. Vakil N. H. pylori treatment: New wine in old bottles? *Am J Gastroenterol* 2009;104(1):26-30.
38. O'Connor A, Gisbert J, O'Morain C. Treatment of *Helicobacter pylori* infection. *Helicobacter* 2009;14 (Suppl 1):46-51.
39. Rokkas T, Sechopoulos P, Robotis I, Margantinis G, Pistiolas D. Cumulative *H. pylori* eradication rates in clinical practice by adopting first and second-line regimens proposed by the Maastricht III consensus and a third-line empirical regimen. *Am J Gastroenterol* 2009;104(1):21-25.
40. Sugimoto M, Graham DY. High-dose versus standard-dose PPI in triple therapy for *Helicobacter pylori* eradication. *Nat Clin Pract Gastroenterol Hepatol* 2009;6(3):138-139.
41. Nagaraja V, Eslick GD. Evidence-based assessment of proton-pump inhibitors in *Helicobacter pylori* eradication: A systematic review. *World J Gastroenterol* 2014;20(40):14527-14536.
42. Gisbert JP, Khorrami S, Calvet X, Gabriel R, Carballo F, Pajares JM. Meta-analysis: Proton pump inhibitors vs. H_2-receptor antagonists—their efficacy with antibiotics in *Helicobacter pylori* eradication. *Aliment Pharmacol Ther* 2003;18(8):757-766.
43. Graham DY, Hammoud F, El-Zimaity HM, Kim JG, Osato MS, El-Serag HB. Meta-analysis: proton pump inhibitor or H2-receptor antagonist for *Helicobacter pylori* eradication. *Aliment Pharmacol Ther* 2003;17(10):1229-1236.
44. Yoon SB, Park JM, Lee JY, et al. Long-term pretreatment with proton pump inhibitor and *Helicobacter pylori* eradication rates. *World J Gastroenterol* 2014;20(4):1061-1066.
45. Luther J, Higgins PD, Schoenfeld PS, Moayyedi P, Vakil N, Chey WD. Empiric quadruple vs. triple therapy for primary treatment of *Helicobacter pylori* infection: Systematic review and meta-analysis of efficacy and tolerability. *Am J Gastroenterol* 2010;105(1):65-73.
46. Laine L, Hunt R, El-Zimaity H, Nguyen B, Osato M, Spenard J. Bismuth-based quadruple therapy using a single capsule of bismuth biskalcitrate, metronidazole, and tetracycline given with omeprazole versus omeprazole, amoxicillin, and clarithromycin for eradication of *Helicobacter pylori* in duodenal ulcer patients: A prospective, randomized, multicenter, North American trial. *Am J Gastroenterol* 2003;98(3):562-567.
47. Venerito M, Krieger T, Ecker T, Leandro G, Malfertheiner P. Meta-analysis of bismuth quadruple therapy versus clarithromycin triple therapy for empiric primary treatment of *Helicobacter pylori* infection. *Digestion* 2013;88(1):33-45.
48. Graham DY, Belson G, Abudayyeh S, Osato MS, Dore MP, El-Zimaity HM. Twice daily (mid-day and evening) quadruple therapy for *H. pylori* infection in the United States. *Dig Liver Dis* 2004;36(6):384-387.
49. He L, Deng T, Luo H. Meta-analysis of sequential, concomitant and hybrid therapy for *Helicobacter pylori* eradication. *Intern Med* 2015;54(7):703-710.
50. O'Morain CA, O'Connor JP. Is sequential therapy superior to standard triple therapy for the treatment of *Helicobacter pylori* infection? *Nat Clin Pract Gastroenterol Hepatol* 2009;6(1):8-9.
51. Oh DH, Lee DH, Kang KK, et al. Efficacy of hybrid therapy as first-line regimen for *Helicobacter pylori* infection compared with sequential therapy. *J Gastroenterol Hepatol* 2014;29(6):1171-1176.
52. Yanai A, Sakamoto K, Akanuma M, Ogura K, Maeda S. Non-bismuth quadruple therapy for first-line *Helicobacter pylori* eradication: A randomized study in Japan. *World J Gastrointest Pharmacol Ther* 2012;3(1):1-6.
53. Papastergiou V, Georgopoulos SD, Karatapanis S. Treatment of *Helicobacter pylori* infection: Meeting the challenge of antimicrobial resistance. *World J Gastroenterol* 2014;20(29):9898-9911.
54. Luther J, Chey WD, Saad RJ. A clinician's guide to salvage therapy for persistent *Helicobacter pylori* infection. *Hosp Pract (1995)* 2011;39(1):133-140.
55. Napolitano L. Refractory peptic ulcer disease. *Gastroenterol Clin North Am* 2009;38(2):267-288.
56. Di Caro S, Fini L, Daoud Y, et al. Levofloxacin/amoxicillin-based schemes vs quadruple therapy for *Helicobacter pylori* eradication in second-line. *World J Gastroenterol* 2012;18(40):5669-5678.
57. Hsu PI, Chen WC, Tsay FW, et al. Ten-day Quadruple therapy comprising proton-pump inhibitor, bismuth, tetracycline, and levofloxacin achieves a high eradication rate for *Helicobacter pylori* infection after failure of sequential therapy. *Helicobacter* 2014;19(1):74-79.
58. Kang JM, Kim N, Lee DH, et al. Effect of the CYP2C19 polymorphism on the eradication rate of *Helicobacter pylori* infection by 7-day triple therapy with regular proton pump inhibitor dosage. *J Gastroenterol Hepatol* 2008;23(8 Pt 1):1287-1291.
59. Ghotaslou R, Leylabadlo HE, Asl YM. Prevalence of antibiotic resistance in *Helicobacter pylori*: A recent literature review. *World J Methodol* 2015;5(3):164-174.
60. Duck WM, Sobel J, Pruckler JM, et al. Antimicrobial resistance incidence and risk factors among *Helicobacter pylori*-infected persons, United States. *Emerg Infect Dis* 2004;10(6):1088-1094.
61. Meyer JM, Silliman NP, Wang W, et al. Risk factors for *Helicobacter pylori* resistance in the United States: the surveillance of *H. pylori* antimicrobial resistance partnership (SHARP) study, 1993-1999. *Ann Intern Med* 2002;136(1):13-24.
62. McMahon BJ, Hennessy TW, Bensler JM, et al. The relationship among previous antimicrobial use, antimicrobial resistance, and treatment outcomes for *Helicobacter pylori* infections. *Ann Intern Med* 2003;139(6):463-469.
63. Megraud F, Benejat L, Ontsira Ngoyi EN, Lehours P. Molecular approaches to identify *Helicobacter pylori* antimicrobial resistance. *Gastroenterol Clin North Am* 2015;44(3):577-596.
64. Dang Y, Reinhardt JD, Zhou X, Zhang G. The effect of probiotics supplementation on *Helicobacter pylori* eradication rates and side effects during eradication therapy: A meta-analysis. *PLoS One* 2014;9(11):e111030.
65. Wang ZH, Gao QY, Fang JY. Meta-analysis of the efficacy and safety of Lactobacillus-containing and Bifidobacterium-containing probiotic compound preparation in *Helicobacter pylori* eradication therapy. *J Clin Gastroenterol* 2013;47(1):25-32.
66. Zhu R, Chen K, Zheng YY, et al. Meta-analysis of the efficacy of probiotics in *Helicobacter pylori* eradication therapy. *World J Gastroenterol* 2014;20(47):18013-18021.
67. Targownik LE, Metge CJ, Leung S, Chateau DG. The relative efficacies of gastroprotective strategies in chronic users of nonsteroidal anti-inflammatory drugs. *Gastroenterology* 2008;134(4):937-944.
68. Silverstein FE, Graham DY, Senior JR, et al. Misoprostol reduces serious gastrointestinal complications in patients with rheumatoid arthritis receiving nonsteroidal anti-inflammatory drugs. A randomized, double-blind, placebo-controlled trial. *Ann Intern Med* 1995;123(4):241-249.
69. Graham DY, Agrawal NM, Campbell DR, et al. Ulcer prevention in long-term users of nonsteroidal anti-inflammatory drugs: results of a double-blind, randomized, multicenter, active- and placebo-controlled study of misoprostol vs lansoprazole. *Arch Intern Med* 2002;162(2):169-175.
70. Scheiman JM. The use of proton pump inhibitors in treating and preventing NSAID-induced mucosal damage. *Arthritis Res Ther* 2013;15 (Suppl 3):S5.
71. Arora G, Singh G, Triadafilopoulos G. Proton pump inhibitors for gastroduodenal damage related to nonsteroidal anti-inflammatory drugs or aspirin: Twelve important questions for clinical practice. *Clin Gastroenterol Hepatol* 2009;7(7):725-735.
72. Taha AS, McCloskey C, Prasad R, Bezlyak V. Famotidine for the prevention of peptic ulcers and oesophagitis in patients taking low-dose aspirin (FAMOUS): A phase III, randomised, double-blind, placebo-controlled trial. *Lancet* 2009;374(9684):119-125.
73. Silverstein FE, Faich G, Goldstein JL, et al. Gastrointestinal toxicity with celecoxib vs nonsteroidal anti-inflammatory drugs for osteoarthritis and rheumatoid arthritis: the CLASS study: A randomized controlled trial. Celecoxib Long-term Arthritis Safety Study. *JAMA* 2000;284(10):1247-1255.
74. US Food and Drug Administration. FDA Drug Safety Communication: COX-2 Selective and non-selective non-steroidal anti-inflammatory drugs (NSAIDs). Available at: http://www.fda.gov/cder/drug/infopage/cox2/default.htm. Accessed: 8/3/2016
75. Bresalier RS, Sandler RS, Quan H, et al. Cardiovascular events associated with rofecoxib in a colorectal adenoma chemoprevention trial. *N Engl J Med* 2005;352(11):1092-1102.
76. Becker MC, Wang TH, Wisniewski L, et al. Rationale, design, and governance of Prospective Randomized Evaluation of Celecoxib Integrated Safety versus Ibuprofen Or Naproxen (PRECISION), a cardiovascular end point trial of nonsteroidal antiinflammatory agents in patients with arthritis. *Am Heart J* 2009;157(4):606-612.

77. Fiorucci S. Prevention of nonsteroidal anti-inflammatory drug-induced ulcer: Looking to the future. *Gastroenterol Clin North Am* 2009;38(2):315-332.
78. Gisbert JP, Calvet X. Review article: *Helicobacter pylori*-negative duodenal ulcer disease. *Aliment Pharmacol Ther* 2009;30(8):791-815.
79. Boparai V, Rajagopalan J, Triadafilopoulos G. Guide to the use of proton pump inhibitors in adult patients. *Drugs* 2008;68(7):925-947.
80. Reimer C, Sondergaard B, Hilsted L, Bytzer P. Proton-pump inhibitor therapy induces acid-related symptoms in healthy volunteers after withdrawal of therapy. *Gastroenterology* 2009;137(1):80-87, 87 e1.
81. Metz DC, Vakily M, Dixit T, Mulford D. Review article: Dual delayed release formulation of dexlansoprazole MR, a novel approach to overcome the limitations of conventional single release proton pump inhibitor therapy. *Aliment Pharmacol Ther* 2009;29(9):928-937.
82. Orbelo DM, Enders FT, Romero Y, et al. Once-daily omeprazole/sodium bicarbonate heals severe refractory reflux esophagitis with morning or nighttime dosing. *Dig Dis Sci* 2015;60(1):146-162.
83. Lahner E, Annibale B, Delle Fave G. Systematic review: Impaired drug absorption related to the co-administration of antisecretory therapy. *Aliment Pharmacol Ther* 2009;29(12):1219-1229.
84. Beique L, Giguere P, la Porte C, Angel J. Interactions between protease inhibitors and acid-reducing agents: A systematic review. *HIV Med* 2007;8(6):335-345.
85. Sachmechi I, Reich DM, Aninyei M, Wibowo F, Gupta G, Kim PJ. Effect of proton pump inhibitors on serum thyroid-stimulating hormone level in euthyroid patients treated with levothyroxine for hypothyroidism. *Endocr Pract* 2007;13(4):345-349.
86. Parikh N, Howden CW. The safety of drugs used in acid-related disorders and functional gastrointestinal disorders. *Gastroenterol Clin North Am* 2010;39(3):529-542.
87. Kahrilas PJ, Shaheen NJ, Vaezi MF, et al. American Gastroenterological Association Medical Position Statement on the management of gastroesophageal reflux disease. *Gastroenterology* 2008;135(4):1383-1391, 1391 e1381-1385.
88. US Food and Drug Administration. Reminder to avoid concomitant use of Plavix (clopidogrel) and omeprazole. Available at: http://www.fda.gov/drugs/drugsafety/ucm231161.htm. Accessed: 8/3/2016
89. Plavix (clopidogrel bisulfate tablets). Bridgewater, NJ: Mristol-Myers Squibb/Sanofi Pharmaceuticals Partnership. Revised 7/2015. Available at: http://packageinserts.bms.com/pi/pi_plavix.pdf. Accessed: 8/3/2016
90. Mega JL, Close SL, Wiviott SD, et al. Cytochrome p-450 polymorphisms and response to clopidogrel. *N Engl J Med* 2009;360(4):354-362.
91. Freedman JE, Hylek EM. Clopidogrel, genetics, and drug responsiveness. *N Engl J Med* 2009;360(4):411-413.
92. Last EJ, Sheehan AH. Review of recent evidence: potential interaction between clopidogrel and proton pump inhibitors. *Am J Health Syst Pharm* 2009;66(23):2117-2122.
93. Norgard NB, Mathews KD, Wall GC. Drug-drug interaction between clopidogrel and the proton pump inhibitors. *Ann Pharmacother* 2009;43(7):1266-1274.
94. Bhatt DL, Cryer BL, Contant CF, et al. Clopidogrel with or without omeprazole in coronary artery disease. *N Engl J Med* 2010;363(20):1909-1917.
95. Sheen E, Triadafilopoulos G. Adverse effects of long-term proton pump inhibitor therapy. *Dig Dis Sci* 2011;56(4):931-950.
96. Ali T, Roberts DN, Tierney WM. Long-term safety concerns with proton pump inhibitors. *Am J Med* 2009;122(10):896-903.
97. Heidelbaugh JJ, Goldberg KL, Inadomi JM. Overutilization of proton pump inhibitors: a review of cost-effectiveness and risk. *Am J Gastroenterol* 2009;104 (Suppl 2):S27-32.
98. Tsuda A, Suda W, Morita H, et al. Influence of proton-pump inhibitors on the luminal microbiota in the gastrointestinal tract. *Clin Transl Gastroenterol* 2015;6:e89.
99. Lambert AA, Lam JO, Paik JJ, Ugarte-Gil C, Drummond MB, Crowell TA. Risk of community-acquired pneumonia with outpatient proton-pump inhibitor therapy: A systematic review and meta-analysis. *PLoS One* 2015;10(6):e0128004.
100. de Jager CP, Wever PC, Gemen EF, et al. Proton pump inhibitor therapy predisposes to community-acquired Streptococcus pneumoniae pneumonia. *Aliment Pharmacol Ther* 2012;36(10):941-949.
101. Giuliano C, Wilhelm SM, Kale-Pradhan PB. Are proton pump inhibitors associated with the development of community-acquired pneumonia? A meta-analysis. *Expert Rev Clin Pharmacol* 2012;5(3):337-344.
102. Leonard J, Marshall JK, Moayyedi P. Systematic review of the risk of enteric infection in patients taking acid suppression. *Am J Gastroenterol* 2007;102(9):2047-2056; quiz 2057.
103. US Food and Drug Administration. FDA Drug Safety Communication: Possible increased risk of fractures of the hip, wrist, and spine with the use of proton pump inhibitors. Available at: http://www.fda.gov/drugs/drugsafety/postmarketdrugsafetyinformationforpatientsandproviders/ucm213206.htm Accessed: 8/3/2016.
104. Furuta K, Adachi K, Komazawa Y, et al. Tolerance to H2 receptor antagonist correlates well with the decline in efficacy against gastroesophageal reflux in patients with gastroesophageal reflux disease. *J Gastroenterol Hepatol* 2006;21(10):1581-1585.
105. Kuo CH, Lu CY, Shih HY, et al. CYP2C19 polymorphism influences *Helicobacter pylori* eradication. *World J Gastroenterol* 2014;20(43):16029-16036.
106. Ma Q, Lu AY. Pharmacogenetics, pharmacogenomics, and individualized medicine. *Pharmacol Rev* 2011;63(2):437-459.
107. Kawai T, Yamagishi T, Yagi K, et al. Tailored eradication therapy based on fecal *Helicobacter pylori* clarithromycin sensitivities. *J Gastroenterol Hepatol* 2008;23 (Suppl 2):S171-174.
108. Rotondano G. Epidemiology and diagnosis of acute nonvariceal upper gastrointestinal bleeding. *Gastroenterol Clin North Am* 2014;43(4):643-663.
109. Trawick EP, Yachimski PS. Management of non-variceal upper gastrointestinal tract hemorrhage: controversies and areas of uncertainty. *World J Gastroenterol* 2012;18(11):1159-1165.
110. Wollenman CS, Chason R, Reisch JS, Rockey DC. Impact of ethnicity in upper gastrointestinal hemorrhage. *J Clin Gastroenterol* 2014;48(4):343-350.
111. Bardou M, Quenot JP, Barkun A. Stress-related mucosal disease in the critically ill patient. *Nat Rev Gastroenterol Hepatol* 2015;12(2):98-107.
112. Klein A, Gralnek IM. Acute, nonvariceal upper gastrointestinal bleeding. *Curr Opin Crit Care* 2015;21(2):154-162.
113. Khamaysi I, Gralnek IM. Acute upper gastrointestinal bleeding (UGIB) - initial evaluation and management. *Best Pract Res Clin Gastroenterol* 2013;27(5):633-638.
114. Neumann I, Letelier LM, Rada G, et al. Comparison of different regimens of proton pump inhibitors for acute peptic ulcer bleeding. *Cochrane Database Syst Rev* 2013;6:CD007999.
115. Sachar H, Vaidya K, Laine L. Intermittent vs continuous proton pump inhibitor therapy for high-risk bleeding ulcers: A systematic review and meta-analysis. *JAMA Intern Med* 2014;174(11):1755-1762.
116. ASHP Therapeutic Guidelines on Stress Ulcer Prophylaxis. ASHP Commission on Therapeutics and approved by the ASHP Board of Directors on November 14, 1998. *Am J Health Syst Pharm* 1999;56(4):347-379.
117. Cook DJ, Fuller HD, Guyatt GH, et al. Risk factors for gastrointestinal bleeding in critically ill patients. Canadian Critical Care Trials Group. *N Engl J Med* 1994;330(6):377-381.
118. Marik PE, Vasu T, Hirani A, Pachinburavan M. Stress ulcer prophylaxis in the new millennium: a systematic review and meta-analysis. *Crit Care Med* 2010;38(11):2222-2228.
119. Chanpura T, Yende S. Weighing risks and benefits of stress ulcer prophylaxis in critically ill patients. *Crit Care* 2012;16(5):322.
120. Alhazzani W, Alenezi F, Jaeschke RZ, Moayyedi P, Cook DJ. Proton pump inhibitors versus histamine 2 receptor antagonists for stress ulcer prophylaxis in critically ill patients: a systematic review and meta-analysis. *Crit Care Med* 2013;41(3):693-705.
121. Krag M, Perner A, Wetterslev J, Moller MH. Stress ulcer prophylaxis in the intensive care unit: is it indicated? A topical systematic review. *Acta Anaesthesiol Scand* 2013;57(7):835-847.
122. Frandah W, Colmer-Hamood J, Nugent K, Raj R. Patterns of use of prophylaxis for stress-related mucosal disease in patients admitted to the intensive care unit. *J Intensive Care Med* 2014;29(2):96-103.
123. Barletta JF, Sclar DA. Use of proton pump inhibitors for the provision of stress ulcer prophylaxis: clinical and economic consequences. *Pharmacoeconomics* 2014;32(1):5-13.
124. Ito T, Igarashi H, Uehara H, Jensen RT. Pharmacotherapy of Zollinger-Ellison syndrome. *Expert Opin Pharmacother* 2013;14(3):307-321.
125. Ito T, Igarashi H, Jensen RT. Zollinger-Ellison syndrome: Recent advances and controversies. *Curr Opin Gastroenterol* 2013;29(6):650-661.
126. Krampitz GW, Norton JA. Current management of the Zollinger-Ellison syndrome. *Adv Surg* 2013;47:59-79.
127. Epelboym I, Mazeh H. Zollinger-Ellison syndrome: Classical considerations and current controversies. *Oncologist* 2014;19(1):44-50.

34

Inflammatory Bowel Disease

Brian A. Hemstreet

KEY CONCEPTS

1. The exact cause of inflammatory bowel disease (IBD) is unknown. Proposed causes include infectious, genetic, and environmental factors, as well as immune dysregulation.
2. Ulcerative colitis (UC) is confined to the rectum and colon, causes continuous lesions, and affects primarily the mucosa and the submucosa. Crohn's disease (CD) can involve any part of the GI tract, often causes discontinuous (skip) lesions, and is a transmural process that can result in fistulas, perforations, or strictures.
3. Common GI complications of IBD include rectal fissures, fistulas (CD), perirectal abscess (UC), toxic megacolon (UC), and colon cancer. Extraintestinal manifestations include hepatobiliary complications, arthritis, uveitis, skin lesions (including erythema nodosum and pyoderma gangrenosum), osteoporosis, anemia, and aphthous ulcerations of the mouth.
4. The severity of UC may be assessed by stool frequency, presence of blood in stool, fever, pulse, hemoglobin, erythrocyte sedimentation rate (ESR), C-reactive protein (CRP), abdominal tenderness, and radiologic or endoscopic findings. The severity of CD can be assessed using similar parameters, in addition to the CD Activity Index, which includes stool frequency, presence of blood in stool, endoscopic appearance, and physician's global assessment.
5. The goals of IBD treatment are resolution of acute inflammation and complications, alleviation of systemic manifestations, maintenance of remission, and improvement in quality of life (QOL).
6. The first line of treatment for mild to moderate extensive UC consists of oral aminosalicylates (ASAs) with oral controlled release budesonide as an alternative. Mesalamine or corticosteroid enemas or suppositories may be used for distal disease. Mesalamine is less effective for CD; however, certain delayed-release oral formulations of mesalamine may be used for Crohn's ileitis. Controlled-release budesonide is preferred as a first-line agent for CD confined to the terminal ileum and/or ascending colon.
7. Systemic corticosteroids are often required for acute UC or CD. The duration of steroid use should be minimized and the dose tapered gradually over 3 to 4 weeks.
8. Infliximab, adalimumab, and golimumab are treatment options for patients with moderate to severe active UC and for those patients with UC who are corticosteroid dependent. Azathioprine or mercaptopurine may be used for maintenance of remission in UC as an alternative to or in combination with tumor necrosis factor-alpha (TNF-*α*) inhibitors, and in patients failing ASAs or with corticosteroid dependency. Vedolizumab may be used for patients failing TNF-*α* inhibitors.
9. IV continuous infusion of cyclosporine may be effective in treating severe colitis that is refractory to corticosteroids as an option to delay or prevent the need for surgery.
10. Aminosalicylates may prevent recurrence of acute UC in many patients, while corticosteroids are ineffective for this purpose.
11. Treatments for CD include infliximab, adalimumab, and certolizumab (for moderate to severe or fistulizing disease as both induction and maintenance therapies); methotrexate, azathioprine, or mercaptopurine (for inadequate response or to reduce steroid dosage and in combination with TNF-*α* inhibitors); metronidazole (for perineal or colonic disease); natalizumab or vedolizumab (for patients failing TNF-*α* antagonists); and cyclosporine (for refractory disease).

There are two forms of idiopathic inflammatory bowel disease (IBD): (a) ulcerative colitis (UC), a mucosal inflammatory condition confined to the rectum and colon, and (b) Crohn's disease (CD), a transmural inflammation of the GI tract that can affect any part, from the mouth to the anus.

EPIDEMIOLOGY

Inflammatory bowel disease is most prevalent in Western countries and in areas of northern latitude.[1] Rates of IBD are highest in North America, Northern Europe, and Great Britain.[1,2] The incidence of IBD is increasing worldwide.[2,3] CD has an incidence of 6 to 15.5 cases per 100,000 persons per year and a prevalence of 3.6 to 214 per 100,000 people per year.[1,2] The incidence of UC ranges from 1.2 to 20 cases per 100,000 persons per year with a prevalence of 7.6 to 246 per 100,000 persons per year.[1] Although most epidemiologic studies combine ulcerative proctitis with UC, 17% to 49% of cases are classified as proctitis.

Both sexes are affected somewhat equally with IBD, although 20% to 30% more women are affected with CD and slightly more males (60%) are affected with UC.[2] Both UC and CD have bimodal distributions in age of initial presentation. The peak incidence generally occurs in the second (CD) or third (UC) decade of life, with a second peak occurring between 60 and 70 years of age.[1-3] A higher incidence of IBD occurs in the Jewish population, while black and Asian populations have a relatively similar, and possibly lower, incidence of IBD.[2]

ETIOLOGY

1 The exact etiology of UC and CD is unknown; however, there are similar factors believed responsible for both conditions. The major theories behind the cause of IBD involve a combination of infectious, genetic, environmental, and immunologic factors. This may

involve abnormal regulation of the innate immune response or a reaction to various antigens.[4-6] The microflora of the GI tract may provide an environmental trigger to activate inflammation and are highly implicated in the development of IBD.[5,6]

Infectious Factors

Microorganisms are proposed to be a major factor in the initiation of inflammation in IBD. In general, there is thought to be shift toward the presence of more proinflammatory bacteria in the GI tract, often referred to as dysbiosis.[4,7] However, no one definitive infectious cause of IBD has been found. Patients with IBD have an increased density of intestinal microbiotica compared with those without IBD, including increased numbers of mucus, mucosal, and intraepithelial bacteria.[1,4] The development and composition of the intestinal microbiotica may be influenced by dietary factors.[5] The pathogenesis of IBD may involve a loss of tolerance toward normal GI bacterial flora.[1] Other supporting evidence for an infectious etiology are that colitis does not appear to occur in genetically altered germ-free animals, intestinal lesions in IBD predominate in areas of highest bacterial exposure, and differences are observed in the makeup of the resident luminal and mucosal bacterial flora in healthy subjects versus those with IBD.[7,8]

Microorganisms may play a key role in the development of IBD. Suspect infectious agents include viruses, protozoans, mycobacteria such as *Mycobacterium paratuberculosis* or *avium*, and other bacteria such as *Ruminococcus gnavus*, *Ruminococcus torques*, *Listeria monocytogenes*, *Chlamydia trachomatis*, and *Escherichia coli*.[4-9] Patients with CD typically have circulating antibodies to *Saccharomyces cerevisiae*, which demonstrates some immunologic response to intestinal organisms.[4] Bacterial gene products may promote alteration of the intestinal barrier while bacterial antigens or ligands may include and propagate the inflammatory response.[4,5,10]

Genetic Factors

Genetic factors play a significant role in the predisposition to IBD. Studies of monozygotic twins demonstrate a high concordance rate of IBD in both individuals (particularly CD).[1,11] First-degree relatives of patients with IBD may have up to a 20-fold increase in the risk of disease and risk is extended to second and third degree relatives.[4,12] Several genetic markers and loci have been identified that occur more frequently in patients with IBD. Genes may not act independently, but rather function in an integrated manner. This is referred to as the "limited pathway model."[4] The nucleotide-binding oligomerization domain protein 2 (NOD2), a key component involved in pathogen recognition in the innate immune system, is the major contributor of genetic predisposition to CD.[11,12] Other genes involved in the innate immune system autophagy, such as ATG16L1 and IRGM, as well as genes involved in the interleukin (IL) biologic pathway such as polymorphisms of the IL-23 receptor IL-23R, and IL-12B, STAT3, and CCR6, are strongly associated with CD and possibly UC (IL-23R).[1,10-12] The major genetic region for UC is on chromosome 6p21, in the major histocompatibility region, near human leukocyte antigen (HLA) class II genes.[11] Alterations in the genes encoding for IL-10 and the IL-10 receptor have been implicated in UC.[11,12] Other possible high-risk loci involved in epithelial barrier function, such as ECM1, HNF4A, CDH1, and LAMB1, and Th1 and Th17, involved with helper T-cell types, are implicated in the pathophysiology of UC.[1] Lastly, an emerging area of interest in IBD pathogenesis is in the role of microRNAs, which are small noncoding RNAs that regulate gene expression.[15]

Immunologic Mechanisms

The immune system plays a critical role in the pathogenesis of IBD. Potential immunologic mechanisms include both autoimmune and nonautoimmune phenomena. The innate immune system largely involves the intestinal wall epithelial barrier and its associated secretions in response to contact with organisms.[4] NOD proteins (for recognition of organisms) and toll-like membrane receptors (TLRs) are involved in intestinal surveillance and can lead to release of antibacterial peptides such as defensins, among other functions.[4] Reduction in defensin secretion by Paneth cells is thought to be one contributing factor in the loss of effective barrier function.[4,10] Consequently, the bowel wall in CD is infiltrated with lymphocytes, plasma cells, mast cells, macrophages, and neutrophils, often leading to formation of granulomas. Similar infiltration has been observed in the colonic mucosal layer in patients with UC. Given that inflammation is limited to the colon in UC, dysfunction of colonocytes is highly implicated.[1] The colonic mucosal layer in UC may be thinner and less effective in protecting the epithelial cells. This may be due to reduced mucin secretion secondary to defective goblet cell differentiation.[4,10,14] Autoimmune features may be directed against mucosal epithelial cells or against neutrophil cytoplasmic elements.

Antineutrophil cytoplasmic antibodies are found in a high percentage of patients with UC (70%) and less frequently in CD.[6,14] Circulating antibodies to goblet cells and anti-tropomyosin are present in UC, although their contribution to the disease process is not fully elucidated.[10] Overproduction of circulating IgG1 antibodies in UC may react with epithelium in the eyes, skin, joints, and biliary tract.[1] Dysfunction or reduced expression of the peroxisome proliferator–activated receptor γ in colonocytes may play a role in this process.[1]

Dysregulation of cytokines is a key component of IBD. Specifically, Th1 cytokine activity is excessive in CD and increased expression of interferon-γ in the intestinal mucosa and production of IL-12 production are features of the immune response in CD.[6,10] In contrast, Th2 cytokine activity is excessive with UC.[1,14,16] This is mediated by excess production of IL-13, which contributes to epithelial cell dysfunction by enhancing natural killer T-cell cytotoxicity, and IL-5, which is involved with eosinophil recruitment and activation.[1,10,14] Upregulation of the IL-13 receptor-2α occurs as well.[1,10,14,16] Activated epithelial cells secrete a variety of substances involved in the recruitment of inflammatory cells. These include IL-1β, epithelial neutrophil-activating peptide 78, IL-8, and monocyte chemoattractant protein 1.[1] Neutrophils produce proteolytic enzymes, such as matrix metalloproteinase-8 and neutrophil elastase, which further contribute to epithelial damage.[14]

Lastly, tumor necrosis factor-alpha (TNF-α) is a pivotal proinflammatory cytokine that is increased in the mucosa and intestinal lumen of patients with CD and UC. TNF-α can recruit inflammatory cells to inflamed tissues, activate coagulation, promote the formation of granulomas in patients with CD, and possibly modify epithelial cell apoptosis.[1,14,16]

Psychological Factors

Mental health changes, particularly stress, appear to possibly correlate with disease flares in IBD, but whether psychological factors are true etiologic factors in the pathophysiologic process is unclear.[17-19] Given the complex nature of the disease process and lack of standard measurement processes, documenting the effects of stress in IBD is difficult.[18] Some studies demonstrate that perceived stress and negative mood is significantly different between patients in remission and those experiencing a disease flare.[18,19] Mood-related components, such as anxiety and depression, may contribute to exacerbations of CD.[20] Approximately 50% of patients with IBD reported some type of significant stress during any 3-month period.[21] Additionally, subjects with IBD matched by sex, age, and geographic region to control subjects reported significantly worse psychological well-being and more distress compared with controls.[22] Stress-related interventions in another study did not appear to alter disease course for patients with IBD, but may result in improved quality of life (QOL).[23] While stress and psychological factors may not be a direct cause of IBD, they may significantly affect QOL. This is compounded by the fact that many patients are young at the time of diagnosis, and may require surgical intervention and temporary or permanent ostomy placement.[24]

Lifestyle, Dietary, and Drug-Related Causes

Several theories regarding dietary influence on the development of IBD have been proposed. Intake of refined sugars has been associated with development of CD, while increased protein intake has been associated with a higher risk of developing IBD.[13] Diet composition may directly influence the makeup of the gut microbiotica, possibly triggering IBD.[25,26] The "hygiene hypothesis" proposes that cleaner conditions in more industrialized countries expose patients to fewer microorganisms at an early age. The immune response to these organisms is altered when encountered later in life.[13,26] Diets low in fruits and vegetables and high in ω-6 polyunsaturated fats have been suggested to increase the risk of CD.[25] Changes in expression of the aryl hydrocarbon receptor, a transcription factor activated by dietary ligands and involved in the maintenance of the innate immune response, may increase development of IBD.[27] Recent interest has arisen in vitamin D deficiency as a possible cause of IBD given that vitamin D is involved with NOD2 gene induction.[28]

Smoking plays an important but contrasting role in UC and CD. It appears to be protective for UC and is associated with fewer disease flare-ups and reduced disease severity. The risk of developing UC is increased for 2 to 3 years after smoking cessation in patients without IBD.[24] In contrast, smoking is associated with increased frequency and severity of CD, and appears to worsen ileal disease more than colonic.[25] Patients with CD who stop smoking have a disease severity that is similar to nonsmokers. Smoking cessation should be offered to all patients. There are data to support transdermal nicotine replacement as an adjunctive therapy in UC.[29]

Use of nonsteroidal anti-inflammatory drugs (NSAIDs) may trigger disease occurrence or lead to disease flares.[25,30,31] Inhibition of prostaglandin production through cyclooxygenase inhibition may impair mucosal barrier protective mechanisms. Alteration in platelet function, release of inflammatory mediators, and alteration in the microvascular response to stress are other potential mechanisms of worsening of IBD. Cyclooxygenase-2 inhibitors and cyclooxygenase-1 inhibitors increase risk; however, it is unclear whether cyclooxygenase-2 inhibitors may be safer in select patients with IBD.[2] A large cohort study in U.S. women revealed an increase in risk of developing IBD with NSAID use; however, no association was found with use of aspirin.[30] Use of NSAIDs may be warranted in some patients with IBD, particularly those with arthritic symptoms, if the benefit outweighs the potential risk of disease flare.

An association with development of IBD following use of antibiotics has been found, but a direct causal relationship remains unclear.[25,31] Since antibiotics alter the intestinal flora, this appears to be a viable mechanism; however, delineating antibiotics as a causative factor is difficult given that symptoms may not manifest for several weeks to years following a treatment course. Furthermore, antibiotics may induce *Clostridium difficile* infection, which is a cause of colitis.[25,31] Patients presenting with severe diarrhea for whom a diagnosis of IBD is being entertained should be asked about recent antibiotic use.

Oral contraceptives and isotretinoin have been implicated in the development of IBD as well.[25,32]

PATHOPHYSIOLOGY

Ulcerative colitis and CD differ in two general respects: the extent and distribution of inflammation within the GI tract and depth of involvement within the bowel wall. A small fraction of patients have features of both diseases. Confusion can occur, particularly when the inflammation is limited to the colon. For patients in whom it cannot be determined whether they have UC or CD, they are often classified as indeterminate colitis.[1] Table 34-1 compares pathologic and clinical findings of the two diseases.

TABLE 34-1 Comparison of the Clinical and Pathologic Features of Crohn's Disease and Ulcerative Colitis

Feature	Crohn's Disease	Ulcerative Colitis
Clinical		
Malaise, fever	Common	Uncommon
Rectal bleeding	Common	Common
Abdominal tenderness	Common	May be present
Abdominal mass	Common	Absent
Abdominal pain	Common	Unusual
Abdominal wall and internal fistulas	Common	Absent
Distribution	Discontinuous	Continuous
Aphthous or linear ulcers	Common	Rare
Pathologic		
Rectal involvement	Rare	Common
Ileal involvement	Very common	Rare
Strictures	Common	Rare
Fistulas	Common	Rare
Transmural involvement	Common	Rare
Crypt abscesses	Rare	Very common
Granulomas	Common	Rare
Linear clefts	Common	Rare
Cobblestone appearance	Common	Absent

Ulcerative Colitis

2 Ulcerative colitis is confined to the rectum and colon and affects the mucosal and the submucosal layers. In some instances, a short segment of terminal ileum may be inflamed; this is referred to as *backwash ileitis*. Unlike CD, the deeper longitudinal muscular layers, serosa, and regional lymph nodes are not usually involved.[1] Fistula, perforation, or obstruction is uncommon because this is a superficial inflammation.

In UC, abscess formation in the crypts of the mucosa occurs (crypts of Lieberkuhn) secondary to infiltration of lymphocytes, plasma cells, and granulocytes.[1] Crypt abscesses are usually visible only with microscopy but may be visible when coalescence results in ulceration. Reduced crypt density, distorted crypt architecture and atrophy, and depletion of goblet cells are typical findings.[1,33] Extension and coalescence of ulcers may surround areas of uninvolved mucosa, causing *pseudopolyp* formation. Mucosal damage and friability in UC can result in significant diarrhea and bleeding, although a small percentage of patients experience constipation.

3 Complications of UC may be local, including hemorrhoids, anal fissures, or perirectal abscesses, and are more likely to be present during active colitis. Extraintestinal manifestations (not directly associated with the colon) may occur and are discussed later.

A major complication is toxic megacolon, which is a segmental or total colonic distension of greater than 6 cm with acute colitis and signs of systemic toxicity.[1,34] It occurs in up to 7.9% of UC patients admitted to hospitals and results in death rates of up to 50%. With toxic megacolon, ulceration extends below the submucosa, sometimes reaching the serosa. Vasculitis, swelling of the vascular endothelium, and thrombosis of small arteries occur. Involvement of the muscularis propria causes loss of colonic tone, leading to dilation and potential perforation. Patients typically have a high fever, tachycardia, distended abdomen, elevated white blood cell count, and a dilated colon observed on x-ray.[7,34] Colonic perforation may occur with or without toxic megacolon and is a greater risk with the first episode. Another infrequent major complication is massive colonic hemorrhage. Colonic stricture, sometimes with clinical obstruction, may also complicate long-standing UC.

The risk of colonic dysplasia with transition to colorectal carcinoma (CRC) is fivefold greater for patients with chronic UC with colonic involvement compared with the general population.[35] Patients with ulcerative proctitis or proctosigmoiditis are generally not considered to be at increased risk.[35,36] The cumulative risk of developing CRC in patients with chronic UC may be as high as 20% to 30% at 30 years.[1] Risk factors for CRC include young age at onset (<50 years), severe inflammation, a positive family history, and presence of primary sclerosing cholangitis (PSC) or inflammatory polyps.[1,35,36] Screening colonoscopy with multiple biopsies should be performed at 8 years after onset of symptoms in patients with left-sided or extensive colitis, with subsequent screenings at 1 to 2 years if negative.[36] Patients with PSC should undergo yearly colonoscopy.[36]

Crohn's Disease

Crohn's disease is characterized as a transmural inflammatory process. The terminal ileum is the most common site of the disorder, but it may occur in any part of the GI tract from mouth to anus.[37,38] Patients often have normal bowel separating segments of diseased bowel resulting in discontinuous disease. The mesentery first becomes thickened and edematous, and then fibrotic. Ulcers are typically deep and elongated and extend along the longitudinal axis of the bowel, at least into the submucosa. The "cobblestone" appearance of the bowel wall results from deep mucosal ulceration intermingled with nodular submucosal thickening.

Bowel wall injury is generally extensive, and the intestinal lumen is often narrowed. Small bowel stricture and subsequent obstruction is a complication that may require surgery. Fistula formation is also common, occurring much more frequently than with UC, and is reported as a 20% to 40% lifetime risk in CD.[37] Fistulas often occur in highly inflamed areas, where loops of bowel become matted together by fibrous adhesions. Fistulas may connect a segment of the GI tract to skin (enterocutaneous), two segments of the GI tract (enteroenteric), or the intestinal tract with the bladder (enterovesicular) or vagina. Fistulae associated with CD frequently require surgical treatment.

Bleeding with CD is usually not as severe as with UC, although patients with CD may develop hypochromic anemia. The risk of carcinoma is increased but not as greatly as with UC.[36]

Nutritional deficiencies are common with CD.[39,40] Reported deficiencies include folate, vitamin B_{12}, vitamins A-D, calcium, magnesium, iron, and zinc.[40] Major contributing factors include decreased food intake, intestinal loss, malabsorption, hypermetabolic state, drug-nutrient interactions, and those receiving long-term total parenteral nutrition.[40]

Extraintestinal Manifestations of IBD

Both forms of IBD are associated with development of symptoms and organ involvement outside of the GI tract referred to as extraintestinal manifestations.

Hepatobiliary Complications

Approximately 11% of patients with UC are reported to have hepatobiliary complications with overall frequencies ranging from 5% to 95% for patients with IBD.[1,41,42] Hepatic complications include fatty liver, pericholangitis, autoimmune hepatitis, and cirrhosis. Biliary complications include PSC, cholangiocarcinoma, and cholelithiasis.[1,41]

Fatty infiltration of the liver may result from malabsorption, protein-losing enteropathy, or corticosteroid use. Pericholangitis (acute inflammation surrounding the intrahepatic portal venules, bile ducts, and lymphatics) occurs in up to one third of UC patients. PSC is associated with progressive fibrosis of intrahepatic and extrahepatic bile ducts in 3% to 7% of patients with UC.[41] Cirrhosis may result from cholangitis or chronic active hepatitis. Often the severity of hepatic disease does not correlate with GI disease activity. Gallstones occur in 13% to 34% of patients with CD (particularly with terminal ileal disease) and are related to bile salt malabsorption.[41]

Joint Complications

Arthritis in IBD is typically asymmetric (unlike rheumatoid arthritis) and migratory, involving one or a few usually large joints. The severity parallels IBD disease activity.[1,42] Arthritis may be peripheral or axial in nature and includes sacroiliitis, ankylosing spondylitis, and IBD-associated spondyloarthropathy. Patients positive for HLA-B27 often exhibit axial arthropathy, such as ankylosing spondylitis. Rheumatoid factors are generally not detected and the arthritis is nondeforming and nondestructive. Patients may exhibit enthesopathy, tenosynovitis, or dactylitis.[42]

Ocular Complications

Ocular complications including iritis, uveitis, episcleritis, and conjunctivitis occur in up to 2% to 29% of patients with IBD.[1,42] Commonly reported symptoms with iritis and uveitis include blurred vision, eye pain, and photophobia. Episcleritis is associated with scleral injection, burning, and increased secretions. These complications may parallel the severity of intestinal disease, and recurrence after colectomy with UC is uncommon.

Dermatologic and Mucocutaneous Complications

Skin and mucosal lesions associated with IBD include erythema nodosum, pyoderma gangrenosum, aphthous ulceration, and Sweet's syndrome.[42] Raised, red, tender nodules on the tibial surfaces of the legs and arms that vary in size from 1 cm to several centimeters are manifestations of erythema nodosum, and may occur in 2% to 20% of patients with IBD.[42] These lesions are more commonly observed in CD patients and often correlate with disease severity.

Pyoderma gangrenosum occurs in 0.5% to 2% of patients with IBD and is characterized by discrete skin ulcerations that have a necrotic center and a violaceous color of the surrounding skin.[1,42] They can be seen on any part of the body but commonly occur on the lower extremities.

Oral lesions are found in 4% to 20% of patients with IBD.[37,42] The most common lesion seen with CD is aphthous stomatitis. The severity of these lesions tends to parallel the disease course. Sweet's syndrome, also known as acute febrile neutrophilic dermatosis, is characterized by tender erythematous skin lesions secondary to dermal neutrophil infiltration, and is often associated with fever and a distribution on the upper trunk, face, neck, and arms.[42]

Hematologic, Coagulation, and Metabolic Abnormalities

Patients with IBD may develop anemia, with a prevalence reported up to 74%.[1,40,42] The anemia may present as iron deficiency related to chronic blood loss, ongoing inflammation, malnutrition, hemolysis, or bone marrow suppression from drug treatment.[40,42] Alternatively, it may be more characteristic of anemia of chronic disease secondary to chronic inflammation and overproduction of cytokines. Patients with IBD are at a 1.5 to 3.6 times higher risk of venous thromboembolism (VTE) compared with the general population.[43] This is secondary to activation of the clotting cascade and platelet activation secondary to inflammation.[42,43] Occurrence of VTE is higher during disease flares and occurs more often in peripheral veins.[1,43] Patients should be considered for pharmacologic VTE prophylaxis when admitted to the hospital for a disease flare. Patients with IBD may be at increased risk for metabolic bone disease and development of osteoporosis. Osteomalacia is less common in IBD.[42,44]

Bone disease may be related to a combination of nutritional deficiencies, especially calcium and vitamin D, chronic cytokine-related inflammatory effects on bone, disease-associated hypogonadism, and use of corticosteroids.[42,44]

CLINICAL PRESENTATION

The patterns of clinical presentation of IBD can vary widely. Patients may have a single acute episode that resolves and does not recur, but most patients experience acute flares with alternating periods of remission.

Ulcerative Colitis

There is a wide range of presentation in UC, ranging from mild abdominal cramping with frequent small-volume bowel movements to profuse diarrhea (Table 34-2). Most patients with UC experience intermittent bouts of illness after varying intervals of remission with symptoms. A small percentage of patients have continuous unremitting symptoms or a single acute attack with no subsequent symptoms.

4 While various disease classifications are available for UC, a standard disease severity scoring system is not universally accepted.[45] The arbitrary distinctions of mild, moderate, severe, and fulminant disease activity are generally used in treatment guideline recommendations, and are determined largely by clinical signs and symptoms:[1,33,45]

1. Mild: Fewer than four stools daily, with or without blood, with no systemic disturbance and a normal erythrocyte sedimentation rate (ESR)
2. Moderate: More than four stools per day but with minimal systemic disturbance
3. Severe: More than six stools per day with blood, with evidence of systemic disturbance as shown by fever, tachycardia, anemia, or ESR of greater than 30 mm/h (8.3 μm/s)
4. Fulminant: More than 10 bowel movements per day with continuous bleeding, toxicity, abdominal tenderness, requirement for transfusion, and colonic dilation

With severe disease, the patient typically has profuse bloody diarrhea with a high fever, leukocytosis, and hypoalbuminemia. The patient may be dehydrated with tachycardia and hypotension. This presentation may have a sudden onset with rapid progression.

Determining disease extent, that is, which sections of the colon are involved, is important. This is accomplished via endoscopy. Patients with "distal" disease have inflammation limited to areas distal to the splenic flexure (also referred to as *left-sided* disease), while those with "extensive disease" have inflammation extending proximal to the splenic flexure.[1,33] Inflammation confined to the rectal area is referred to as *proctitis*, while disease involving the rectum and sigmoid colon is referred to as *proctosigmoiditis*. Inflammation of the majority of the colon is called *extensive disease*, sometimes referred to as *pancolitis*.

The diagnosis of UC is made on clinical suspicion and confirmed by biopsy, stool examinations, sigmoidoscopy or colonoscopy, or barium radiographic contrast studies. The presence of extracolonic manifestations may also aid in establishing the diagnosis.[1,33,42]

TABLE 34-2 Clinical Presentation of Ulcerative Colitis

Signs and symptoms
- Abdominal cramping
- Frequent bowel movements, often with blood in the stool
- Weight loss
- Fever and tachycardia in severe disease
- Blurred vision, eye pain, and photophobia with ocular involvement
- Arthritis
- Raised, red, tender nodules that vary in size from 1 cm to several centimeters

Physical examination
- Hemorrhoids, anal fissures, or perirectal abscesses may be present
- Iritis, uveitis, episcleritis, and conjunctivitis with ocular involvement
- Dermatologic findings with erythema nodosum, pyoderma gangrenosum, or aphthous ulceration

Laboratory tests
- Decreased hematocrit/hemoglobin
- Increased ESR or CRP
- Leukocytosis and hypoalbuminemia with severe disease
- (+) perinuclear antineutrophil cytoplasmic antibodies

Crohn's Disease

As with UC, the presentation of CD is highly variable. The time between the onset of complaints and the initial diagnosis may be as long as 3 years. The patient typically presents with diarrhea and abdominal pain. Hematochezia occurs in about one half of patients with colonic involvement and much less frequently when there is no colonic involvement. A patient may first present with a perirectal or perianal lesion (Table 34-3). The diagnosis should also be suspected in children with growth retardation, especially with abdominal complaints.

Much like UC, global classification guidelines for scoring severity of active CD are not available. For patients with luminal nonfistulizing CD, the Crohn's Disease Activity Index (CDAI) is used most often to gauge response to therapy and determine remission and is employed mostly in the research setting.[46] This score system ranges from 0 to 600, with score great than 150 defined as active disease. The Harvey-Bradshaw Index (HBI) is another scoring system that is also used for CD, and tends to correlate well with the CDAI.[46] A decrease of 3 points in the HBI is defined as a clinical response with complete remission defined as a score of less than 4. Treatment guidelines use the presence of signs and symptoms as their marker for disease activity and severity.[37] Patients with mild to moderate CD are typically ambulatory and have no evidence of dehydration, systemic toxicity, loss of body weight, or abdominal tenderness, mass, or obstruction. Moderate to severe disease is considered in patients who fail to respond to treatment for mild to moderate disease or those with fever, weight loss, abdominal pain or tenderness, vomiting, intestinal obstruction, or significant anemia. Severe to fulminant CD is classified as the presence of persistent symptoms or evidence of systemic toxicity despite corticosteroid or biologic treatment or presence of cachexia, rebound tenderness, intestinal obstruction, or abscess. Disease activity may be assessed and correlated by evaluation of serum C-reactive protein (CRP) concentrations.

The course of CD is characterized by periods of remission and exacerbation. Patients may be symptom-free for years, while others experience chronic symptoms in spite of medical therapy. As with UC, the diagnosis of CD involves a thorough evaluation using laboratory, endoscopic, and radiologic testing to detect the extent

TABLE 34-3 Clinical Presentation of Crohn Disease

Signs and symptoms
- Malaise and fever
- Abdominal pain
- Frequent bowel movements
- Hematochezia
- Fistula
- Weight loss and malnutrition
- Arthritis

Physical examination
- Abdominal mass and tenderness
- Perianal fissure or fistula

Laboratory tests
- Increased white blood cell count, ESR, and CRP
- (+) anti-*Saccharomyces cerevisiae* antibodies

and characteristic features of the disease. Small bowel involvement, strictures detected on radiographs, and presence of fistulae are characteristic of CD. A clinical decision support tool which contains recommendations and algorithms for initial laboratory, radiologic, and physical assessment of CD, has been published by the American Gastroenterological Association and is available for use on their website.[47]

TREATMENT

Desired Outcomes

5 The clinician must have a clear concept of realistic therapeutic goals for each patient with IBD. Goals may relate to resolution of acute inflammatory processes, resolution of complications (eg, fistulae and abscesses), alleviation of extraintestinal manifestations, maintenance of remission, or surgical palliation or cure.

When determining goals of therapy and selecting therapeutic regimens, it is important to understand the natural history of IBD.[1,13,33,37] Some cases of acute UC are self-limited. With mild to moderate acute colitis without systemic symptoms, 20% of patients may experience spontaneous improvement in their disease within a few weeks; however, a small percentage of patients may go on to experience more serious disease. With severe colitis, improvement without treatment cannot be expected. The response to medical management of toxic megacolon is variable and emergent colectomy may be required. When remission of UC is achieved, it is likely to last at least 1 year with medical therapy; however, long-term sustained remission rates are typically less than 50%.[45] In the absence of medical therapy, one half to two-thirds of patients relapse within 9 months.[33]

Approximately 20% of patients with CD will experience a relapse annually.[37] Sustained remission is impacted by response to treatment. Patients remaining in remission for 1 year have an 80% chance of remaining in remission the subsequent year, while 70% of patients will continue to have active disease in the year following a 12-month period in which they had active disease.[37] Thus, inducing and maintaining remission is an important aspect of treatment to improve outcomes and QOL and reduce complications. There has been recent interest in mucosal healing as a more objective end point or goal for the treatment of IBD.[48,49] Mucosal healing is accessed via endoscopy; however, there is not a universal scoring system that has been adopted for either CD or UC. The natural course of the disease may be altered and outcomes improved, such as sustained remission and reduced hospitalization, if mucosal healing is achieved.[48,49] Mucosal healing is directly related to the efficacy of drug therapies used in the treatment of IBD and may be used to determine the need for escalation or de-escalation of drug therapy.[48,49] At this time mucosal healing is a promising end point; however, as more studies incorporate this end point, it can be better determined if this is achievable in all patients, particularly those with CD whose disease typically penetrates below the mucosal layer.

General Approach To Treatment

6 Treatment of IBD centers on agents used to relieve the inflammatory process and induce disease remission. Aminosalicylates (ASAs), corticosteroids, antimicrobials, immunosuppressive, and biologic agents are commonly used to treat active disease and for some agents to maintain disease remission. The severity and extent of the disease should be taken into account, as this will often dictate the dose, route, frequency, and formulation of drug therapy that will be most effective. Patient preference for different drug formulations and cost of therapies should also be taken into account.

Surgical procedures are sometimes performed when active disease is inadequately controlled with drugs or when the required drug dosages pose an unacceptable risk of adverse effects. Nutritional considerations are also important because many patients may develop malnutrition. A variety of adjunctive therapies may be used to address complications or symptoms of IBD.

Nonpharmacologic Therapy

Nutritional Support

Proper nutritional support is an important aspect of the treatment of patients with IBD. Specific types of diets are not useful in alleviating the inflammatory conditions; however, patients with moderate to severe disease are often malnourished.[39,40,50] Malabsorption or maldigestion may occur secondary to the catabolic effects of the disease process. Elevated activity of IL-6 and TNF-α increases protein turnover, resulting in protein loss and muscle wasting.[40] Malabsorption and malnutrition may occur more often in the patient with CD with involvement of the small bowel, as this is where many nutrients are absorbed.[50] Protein–energy malnutrition and suboptimal weight is reported in up to 85% of patients with CD.[50] Patients who have undergone multiple small bowel resections may have reduction in the absorptive surface of the intestine (ie, "short gut"). Maldigestion with accompanying diarrhea can also occur if there is a bile salt deficiency in the gut.

Many specific diets have been tried to improve nutritional status and symptoms in IBD, but none has gained widespread acceptance. On an individual patient basis, elimination of specific foods that appear to exacerbate symptoms can be tried; however, exclusion diets are generally not endorsed, even in the setting of severe disease.[51] If attempted, the elimination process must be conducted cautiously, as patients may exclude a wide range of nutritious products without adequate justification. Some patients with IBD may have lactase deficiency as well; therefore, diarrhea may be associated with intake of dairy products. For these patients, avoidance of dairy products or supplementation with lactase generally improves the patient's symptoms.[51] Patients with small bowel strictures due to CD should avoid excessive high-residue foods, such as citrus fruits and nuts, in order to prevent obstruction.

The nutritional needs of patients with IBD may be adequately addressed with oral supplementation or use of enteral supplementation in acute or chronic situations.[39,40,50] Use of enteral nutrition has favorable effects on reducing inflammation and intestinal cytokine production.[50] This may lead to a greater chance of induction and maintenance of remission as well as facilitation of mucosal healing, particularly in patients with CD.[50] No specific enteral formula is recommended, so initiation of polymeric feeds may be tried first.[50] Monitoring for efficacy of the enteral feeding is similar to other patient populations receiving enteral nutrition.

Parenteral nutrition has a more limited role in CD or UC. It is generally reserved for patients with severe malnutrition or those who fail enteral therapy or have a contraindication to receiving enteral therapy, such as perforation, protracted vomiting, short-bowel syndrome, or severe intestinal stenosis.[50] Parenteral therapy is not preferred as primary therapy for IBD even in the setting of acute disease flares in hospitalized patients.[51] Home parenteral nutrition may be necessary for patients requiring long-term therapy, particularly those with short-bowel syndrome. Parenteral nutrition is more costly and is associated with more complications, such as serious infections, compared with enteral nutrition.

Given that the intestinal microbiotica may play a key role in IBD pathogenesis, probiotic administration as an adjunctive treatment of IBD has been explored. Postulated mechanisms for using probiotics in IBD include reestablishment of normal bacterial flora within the gut, reduction in bacterial adhesion and competition for nutrients with pathogenic bacteria, production of antibacterial substances, and promotion of favorable effects on the host immune response.[52-54] Probiotic preparations often contain various organisms such as nonpathogenic *E. coli Nissle*, bifidobacteria, lactobacilli,

Streptococcus thermophilus, or Saccharomyces boulardii. Probiotics have demonstrated some effectiveness in inducing and maintaining remission in some trials for patients with UC; however, differences in methodology, probiotics used, and underlying treatments for IBD make comparison of trials difficult.[52-57] A formulation of *Bifidobacterium*, lactobacilli, and streptococci (VSL #3) is marketed specifically for use in UC as an adjunctive therapy and for patients who have a surgically constructed ileal pouch anal anastomosis (IPAA) to prevent or treat pouchitis.[33,52-54] Use of probiotics as adjunctive agents to avoid stepping up drug therapy to potentially more toxic agents is another potential use.[52] Evidence of probiotic use in the induction and maintenance of CD is less compelling and has led to recommendations not supporting widespread use, but rather further investigation.[52-57] While probiotics are considered to be generally safe in patients with IBD, the added cost and requirement to often take multiple doses per day, coupled with the lack of quality data to support their use, should also weigh into the decision to use them in IBD.

Surgery

Despite the availability of medications to treat IBD, many patients will often require surgery. Surgical procedures may involve resection of segments of intestine that are affected, as well as correction of complications (eg, fistulas) or drainage of abscesses.

Rates of colectomy for UC are 5% to 30%.[1,33,58,59] Colectomy may be necessary when the patient has disease uncontrolled by maximum medical therapy or when there are complications of the disease such as colonic perforation, toxic megacolon, uncontrolled colonic hemorrhage, or colonic strictures.[1,33,59] Colectomy may be indicated for patients with long-standing disease (greater than 8-10 years), as a prophylactic measure against the development of CRC, and for patients with premalignant changes (severe dysplasia) on surveillance mucosal biopsies.[35,36,59] Proctocolectomy, after which the patient is left with a permanent ileostomy, is generally considered curative for UC; however, the decision to perform this should take into account the effects on the patient's QOL. Restorative proctocolectomy with construction of an IPAA is the most common surgical procedure performed in UC and is typically well tolerated with a reported failure rate of less than 10%.[59] Patients may develop inflammation of the IPAA, often referred to as pouchitis.[56]

Indications for surgery with CD are not as well established as for UC. Surgery is usually reserved for patients with complications of the disease. A recognized problem with intestinal resection for CD is the high rate of recurrence. Surgery may be appropriate in well-selected patients who have severe or incapacitating disease or obstruction in spite of aggressive medical management. The surgical procedures performed most often include resections of the major intestinal areas of involvement. Patients who undergo multiple resections of the small intestine may develop malabsorption related to short-bowel syndrome. For some patients with severe rectal or perianal disease, particularly abscesses, diversion of the fecal stream is performed with a colostomy. Other indications for surgery include resection of strictures or performance of stricturoplasty, or presence of colon cancer, an inflammatory mass, intestinal perforation, or fistulas.[37]

Pharmacologic Therapy

Drug therapy plays an integral role in the treatment of IBD. None of the drugs used for IBD are curative; therefore, reasonable goals of drug therapy are resolution of acute disease symptoms and induction and maintenance of remission. The major types of drug therapy used in IBD include ASAs, corticosteroids, immunosuppressive agents (azathioprine, mercaptopurine, cyclosporine, and methotrexate), antimicrobials (metronidazole and ciprofloxacin), and agents to inhibit TNF-α (anti–TNF-α antibodies) or leukocyte adhesion and migration (natalizumab and vedolizumab).[58]

Sulfasalazine is the prototypical ASA, and is composed of a sulfonamide moiety (sulfapyridine) and mesalamine (5-aminosalicylate acid [5-ASA]) joined by a diazo bond in the same molecule.[60] Sulfasalazine has been used for years to treat IBD but was originally intended to treat arthritis. It is cleaved by gut bacteria in the colon to sulfapyridine (which is mostly absorbed and excreted in the urine) and mesalamine (which mostly remains in the colon and is excreted in stool).[60-63]

The active component of sulfasalazine is mesalamine, which exerts its effects locally in the GI tract; however, the mechanism of action is not completely understood. Beneficial effects of mesalamine may include scavenging of free radicals, inhibition of leukocyte motility, interference with TNF-α, transforming growth factor-β (TGF-β) and nuclear factor κ B (NF-κ β), suppression of IL-1 production, and inhibition of leukotriene and prostaglandin production.[60-63]

Because the effectiveness of sulfasalazine is not related to the sulfapyridine component and since sulfapyridine is believed to be responsible for many of the adverse reactions to sulfasalazine, mesalamine can be administered alone. Given that mesalamine is rapidly and completely absorbed in the small intestine but poorly absorbed in the colon, drug formulations must be designed to deliver mesalamine to the affected areas in the GI while preventing premature absorption.[58-64] Mesalamine can be used topically as an enema, to treat left-sided disease, or as a suppository for treatment of proctitis (Fig. 34-1). In general, the use of topical mesalamine preparations, such as enemas and suppositories, is more effective than oral preparations.[64,65] Likewise, these therapies may be used concomitantly with the oral mesalamine preparations, which may result in additive efficacy in patients with UC.[65] Oral slow-release formulations will deliver mesalamine to the small intestine and/or colon based on the product design (Table 34-4). Slow-release oral formulations of mesalamine, such as Pentasa, release mesalamine from the duodenum to the ileum, with up to 59% of the drug passing into the colon.[60,61] Some dose forms (Asacol, Asacol HD, Delzicol) utilize a pH-dependent coating that releases in response to intestinal pH.[62] Another tablet formulation of mesalamine (Lialda) uses a pH-dependent coating that releases at a pH of 7, in combination with a polymeric matrix core, referred to as the Multi-MatriX (MMX) system, and releases drug evenly throughout the colon also allowing for once-daily dosing.[63] A capsule formulation of mesalamine (Apriso) utilizes enteric-coated mesalamine granules in a polymer matrix for delayed and extended delivery of mesalamine to the colon and also allows for once-daily dosing.[61,62] Use of once-daily oral mesalamine preparations may enhance adherence, which may help to prevent relapse.[61,62] Olsalazine is a dimer of two 5-ASA molecules linked by an azo bond. Mesalamine is released in the colon after colonic bacteria cleave the azo bond.[60] Balsalazide is a mesalamine prodrug that couples mesalamine with the inert carrier molecule 4-aminobenzoyl-β-alanine and

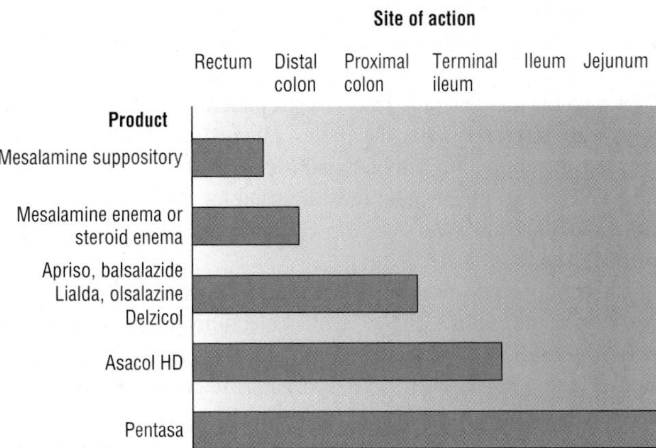

FIGURE 34-1 Site of activity of various agents used to treat inflammatory bowel disease.

TABLE 34-4 Agents for the Treatment of Inflammatory Bowel Disease

Drug	Brand Name	Initial Dose (g)	Usual Range
Sulfasalazine	Azulfidine Azulfidine EN	500 mg-1 g 500 mg-1 g	4-6 g/day 4-6 g/day
Mesalamine suppository	Rowasa	1 g	1 g daily to three times weekly
Mesalamine enema	Canasa	4 g	4 g daily to three times weekly
Mesalamine (oral)	Asacol HD Apriso Lialda Pentasa Delzicol	1.6 g/day 1.5 g/day 1.2-2.4 g/day 2 g/day 1.2 g/day	2.8-4.8 g/day 1.5 g/day once daily 1.2-4.8 g/day once daily 2-4 g/day 2.4-4.8 g/day
Olsalazine	Dipentum	1.5 g/day	1.5-3 g/day
Balsalazide	Colazal	2.25 g/day	2.25-6.75 g/day
Azathioprine	Imuran, Azasan	50-100 mg	1-2.5 mg/kg/day
Cyclosporine	Gengraf Neoral, Sandimmune	2-4 mg/kg/day IV 2-8 mg/kg/day oral	2-4 mg/kg/day IV
Mercaptopurine	Purinethol	50-100 mg	1-2.5 mg/kg/day
Methotrexate	No branded IM injection	15-25 mg IM weekly	15-25 mg IM weekly
Adalimumab	Humira	160 mg SC day 1	80 mg SC 2 (day 15), and then 40 mg every 2 weeks
Certolizumab	Cimzia	400 mg SC	400 mg SC weeks 2 and 4, and then 400 mg SC monthly
Infliximab	Remicade	5 mg/kg IV	5 mg/kg weeks 2 and 6, 5-10 mg/kg every 8 weeks
Natalizumab	Tysabri	300 mg IV	300 mg IV every 4 weeks
Budesonide	Enterocort EC, Uceris	9 mg	6-9 mg daily
Vedolizumab	Entyvio	300 mg IV	300 mg IV weeks 2 and 6 and then every 8 weeks
Golimumab	Simponi	200 mg SC	100 mg SC weeks 2 and 4

SC, subcutaneous; IM, intramuscular.

is also enzymatically cleaved in the colon to release mesalamine.[60] The recommended daily doses of the oral mesalamine derivatives are intended to approximate the molar equivalent of mesalamine present in 4 g of sulfasalazine. Because the oral mesalamine formulations are delayed-release coated tablets or granules, they should not be crushed or chewed. Unlike sulfasalazine, all of these agents are safe to use for patients with sulfonamide allergies.

7 Corticosteroids are used to suppress acute inflammation in the treatment of IBD, and may be given parenterally, orally, or rectally.[66] They modulate the immune system and inhibit production of cytokines and mediators. It is not clear whether the most important steroid effects are systemic or local (mucosal). Budesonide is a corticosteroid that is administered orally in a controlled-release formulation designed to release in the terminal ileum or the colon depending on the product. The drug undergoes extensive first-pass metabolism; so systemic exposure is thought to be minimized.[38,66]

Immunosuppressive agents such as azathioprine, mercaptopurine, methotrexate, or cyclosporine are also used for the treatment of IBD (see Table 34-4). Azathioprine and mercaptopurine are effectively used in long-term treatment of both CD and UC.[1,33,37,67-69] These agents are generally reserved for patients who fail ASA therapy or are refractory to or dependent on corticosteroids. They may be used in conjunction with mesalamine derivatives, corticosteroids, and TNF-α antagonists, and must be used for extended periods of time, ranging from a few weeks up to 12 months, before benefits may be observed.[58,67-69]

Cyclosporine has a short-term benefit in the treatment of acute, severe UC to avoid colectomy in patients failing corticosteroids.[1,13,33,51,70] It is used initially as a continuous IV infusion of 2 to 4 mg/kg daily.[51,58,71] Cyclosporine poses a risk of nephrotoxicity and neurotoxicity. Studies evaluating tacrolimus for the treatment of IBD suggest a potential role for use for patients with luminal or perianal CD; however, results have been variable with few data to support its routine use.[72] Methotrexate 15 to 25 mg given intramuscularly or subcutaneously once weekly may useful for maintenance therapy of CD and may result in steroid-sparing effects, while data supporting use in UC are lacking.[13,37,64,58,67]

Clinical **Controversy...**

Treatment with thiopurines remains a viable option for maintenance of remission in patients with IBD either as monotherapy or in combination with anti–TNF-α inhibitors. While effective in many patients, the optimal duration of thiopurine use is unknown. Long-term use may be associated with development of significant adverse effects such as infection and lymphoma. The benefit of maintaining remission must be weighed against the potential for adverse effects and risk for relapse if therapy is discontinued. Relapse rates after thiopurine discontinuation are reported in up to 23% of patients with CD and 12% of patients with UC at 12 months.[73]

Antimicrobial agents, particularly metronidazole and ciprofloxacin, are frequently used as adjunctive therapies in IBD. Metronidazole and ciprofloxacin, often given in combination, have demonstrated some value in both induction of remission and decrease in relapse rates in CD with some data supporting use in UC as well.[13,38,46,58,74] Antibiotics are often used in patients with perineal CD or when fistulas or abscesses are present or for pouchitis.[5,58] Rifamycin antibiotics have demonstrated some efficacy in treatment of both UC and CD.[58,74] Risks of long-term antibiotic use include the development of antibiotic resistance, predisposition to *C. difficile* infection, and adverse effects such as neurotoxicity secondary to metronidazole use.

Biologic agents that target TNF-α have become a key class of agents in the treatment and maintenance of IBD.[58,75-77]

Infliximab is an IgG1 chimeric monoclonal antibody that is administered IV and binds TNF-α and inhibits its inflammatory effects. In addition, it lyses activated T cells and macrophages and induces T-cell apoptosis.[58,76,77] Infliximab is useful for moderate to severe active CD and UC disease, as well as steroid-dependent or fistulizing disease, as both an induction and a maintenance therapy. Adalimumab is also an IgG1 antibody to TNF-α; however, this agent, unlike infliximab, is fully humanized and contains no murine sequences. Theoretically, the lack of a murine component in adalimumab reduces antibody development seen with use of infliximab. This agent is administered subcutaneously and is a treatment option for patients with moderate to severe active UC and CD and those previously treated with infliximab who have lost response. Certolizumab pegol is a humanized pegylated Fab fragment directed against TNF-α that is also administered subcutaneously. Golimumab is similar in structure to adalimumab and offers similar efficacy to the currently approved agents. Lastly, natalizumab and vedolizumab are a novel biologic agent that inhibits leukocyte adhesion and migration by targeting the α_4 subunit of integrin.[76,77] Vedolizumab works similar to natalizumab but is more specific for the $\alpha_4\beta_7$ subunit of integrin, which targets leukocyte trafficking in the gut.[58,77]

Clinical **Controversy...**

The optimal management of corticosteroid refractory patients with acute severe UC remains unclear. The sequential use of TNF-α inhibitors, cyclosporine or tacrolimus in this patient population has traditionally yielded conflicting results, and may have more risk than benefit. However, if effective these agents may prevent the need for colectomy. Recent data suggest report the risk of severe adverse effects 23.0% (95% CI, 17.7%-28.3%) with these therapies versus remission rates of 39.9% (95% CI, 33.5%-44.3%).[78] Based on these data use of TNF-α inhibitors, cyclosporine or tacrolimus should be considered prior to colectomy.

Treatment of Ulcerative Colitis

Mild to Moderate Active Disease Most patients with mild to moderate active UC can be managed on an outpatient basis with oral and/or topical ASAs (Fig. 34-2; Table 34-5). For patients with extensive disease, oral sulfasalazine or an oral mesalamine derivative is preferred, with rates of induction of remission reported as 36% to 60% in 2 to 4 weeks after initiating therapy.[1,33,64,65,79,80] Topical mesalamine in an enema or suppository formulation is more effective than oral mesalamine or topical steroids for distal disease.[64,65] The combination of oral and topical mesalamine is more effective than either alone for patients with left-sided or extensive disease; however, patients may be less willing to use these formulations.[64,65] Usually 4 to 6 g/day of sulfasalazine given in four divided doses is required to suppress active inflammation.[33] There does not appear to be an increased rate of response with dosages over 6 g/day, although adverse effects typically increase.

Oral mesalamine derivatives (see Table 34-2) are alternatives to sulfasalazine for treatment of mild to moderate UC with similar rates of efficacy. Mesalamine preparations are typically better tolerated than sulfasalazine and thus are often chosen preferentially as first-line therapies. Mesalamine suppositories will only reach to approximately 10 to 20 cm within the lower GI tract and thus are reserved for patients with proctitis.[1] Enemas will reach to the splenic flexure and can be used for left-sided disease.[64] The various oral mesalamine products generally have similar rates of efficacy and the effective daily dose range is 2.4 to 4.8 g/day. Doses greater than 2.4 g/day generally do not demonstrate significant additional benefit; however, patients with moderate disease may respond better to higher doses.[1,13,58,71,79] The choice of oral formulations may be dictated by patient-specific factors, such as use of a once-daily formulation to help improve patient adherence and reduce pill burden, or use of a generically available product in patients with limited financial resources.[60-63,81] Controlled release budesonide (Uceris) is an alternative for mild-moderate UC. Oral corticosteroids in doses of 40 to 60 mg/day prednisone equivalent can be used for patients with moderate extensive disease who are refractory to oral ASAs or require more rapid control of symptoms.[33,66] Topical corticosteroids, given as foams, enemas, and suppositories, while effective for patients with distal disease, are generally less effective than mesalamine but can be used for patients with tenesmus.[33]

Moderate to Severe Active Disease Patients with moderate to severe active disease require prompt initiation of therapies to quickly suppress inflammation. Systemic corticosteroids are used in the treatment of moderate to severe active UC regardless of disease location or in those patients who are unresponsive to maximal doses of oral and/or topical mesalamine derivatives.[22,33] Oral doses of 40 to 60 mg prednisone equivalent daily are recommended.[33]

Use of TNF-α inhibitors is an option for patients with moderate to severe disease who are unresponsive to ASAs, corticosteroids, or other immunosuppressive agents and is generally the next step in therapy. In general infliximab, adalimumab, and golimumab have similar rates of efficacy when used as monotherapy in UC.[58,77] Certolizumab is not approved for use in UC in the United States. Some data demonstrate that combining infliximab and azathioprine is more effective in inducing corticosteroid-free remission in patients with acute severe colitis.[69,77] Vedolizumab can be used for patients who fail immunosuppressive and TNF-α inhibitors, or for as an alternative those patients with contraindications to TNF-α inhibitors.[77] Vedolizumab should not be used in combination with any immunosuppressive agents or TNF-α inhibitors.

Severe or Fulminant Disease Patients with uncontrolled severe colitis or those with incapacitating symptoms require hospitalization for effective management. Under these conditions, patients generally receive nothing by mouth to promote bowel rest. Medications are given by the parenteral route and oral sulfasalazine or mesalamine derivatives are not typically beneficial in this setting because of rapid elimination of these agents from the colon with diarrhea.

Systemic corticosteroids are used in the treatment of severe disease and may allow some patients to avoid colectomy. IV hydrocortisone 300 mg daily in three divided doses or methylprednisolone 60 mg once daily is considered a first-line agent.[33,71] Methylprednisolone is typically preferred due to its lesser mineralocorticoid effects. A trial of corticosteroids is warranted in most patients before proceeding to colectomy, unless the condition is grave or rapidly deteriorating. The length of corticosteroid therapy before consideration of surgery is open to debate, with recommendations ranging from 3 to 7 days.[1,33,51] Steroids do increase surgical risk, particularly infectious, if an operation is required later.

8 Patients, who are unresponsive to parenteral corticosteroids after 3 to 7 days, have the option of receiving higher-potency agents such as cyclosporine or infliximab. Seventy-six percent to 85% of hospitalized patients who are unresponsive to corticosteroids will typically respond to IV cyclosporine.[70] A continuous IV infusion of cyclosporine 2 to 4 mg/kg/day is the typical dose range utilized and may delay the need for colectomy.[1,33,51,70,71] Persistent fever, tachycardia, elevated CRP, hypoalbuminemia, and deep colonic ulcerations may be predictors of failure to respond to cyclosporine.[33,70] Patients who are controlled on IV cyclosporine can then be switched to an oral cyclosporine (4-8 mg/kg/day) tapered regimen with transition to azathioprine or MP.[1,33,51,71,82] Infliximab is an alternative to cyclosporine at a dose of 5 mg/kg and has demonstrated similar results regarding delaying the need for colectomy for patients with severe disease unresponsive to steroids.[1,51,71] Patients who respond

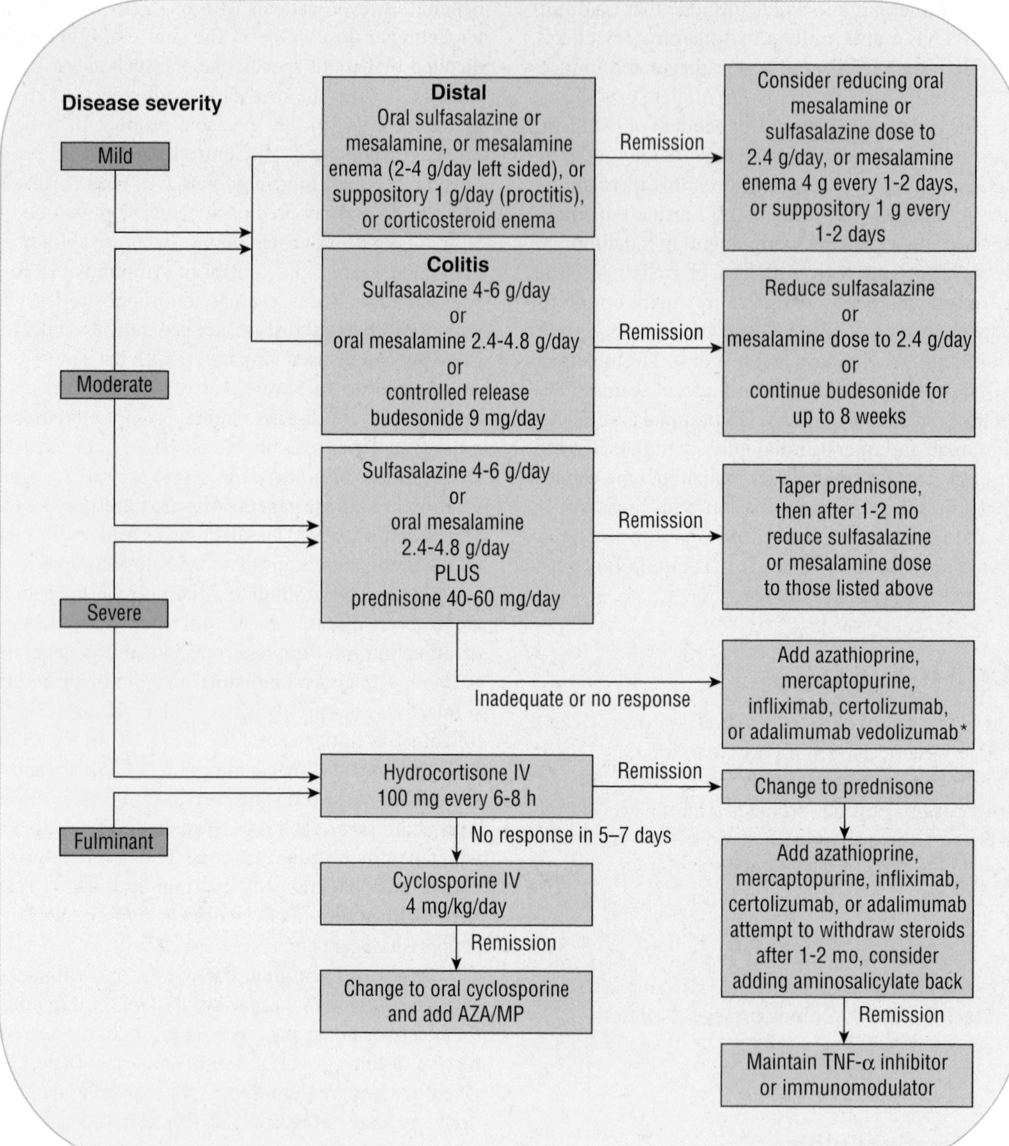

FIGURE 34-2 Treatment approaches for ulcerative colitis.
*Can be considered as an alternative to TNF-alpha inhibitors.

to infliximab should be considered for additional doses at 2 and 6 weeks later.[51] The sequential use of cyclosporine and infliximab, or the drugs given in reverse order, is not generally recommended.[51] The adverse effects of both cyclosporine and infliximab are potentially serious and should be taken into consideration when using either therapy for patients with severe disease.[70,71]

Clinical **Controversy...**

Patients with IBD manifesting arthritic symptoms may benefit from the use of anti-inflammatory agents such as NSAIDs or corticosteroids. However, NSAIDs may exacerbate IBD symptoms by compromising the intestinal barrier. The ability of COX-2 specific NSAIDs, such as celecoxib, to exacerbate IBD compared to traditional NSAIDs is unclear. Few studies of COX-2 inhibitors have been conducted in patients with IBD. A recent Cochrane analysis reveals risk may be low with the use of COX-2 inhibitors; however, the ability to draw clinically relevant conclusions is hampered by the low number of patients and studies included. Both NSAIDs and COX-2 inhibitors should be used with caution in patients with IBD.[83]

Maintenance of Remission

9 After remission from active disease is achieved, the goal of therapy is to maintain remission. The major agents used for maintenance of remission are sulfasalazine and the newer mesalamine derivatives, infliximab, adalimumab, golimumab, and azathioprine or MP.

Oral agents, including sulfasalazine, mesalamine, and balsalazide, are all effective options for maintenance therapy. The optimal dose to prevent relapse is 2 to 2.4 g/day of mesalamine equivalent, with rates of relapse over 6 to 12 months reported as 40%.[13,33,76,79,80] The newer mesalamine derivatives are generally better tolerated than sulfasalazine and are associated with fewer adverse effects often making them a preferred choice.[33,79] For patients with left-sided disease or proctitis, mesalamine enemas or suppositories are preferred.[64] The frequency of administration of topical agents may possibly be lessened to every third night over time.[31,64,65] The combination of topical and oral mesalamine is superior to either regimen alone for maintenance therapy.[65]

Corticosteroids do not have a role in the maintenance of remission with UC because they are ineffective and are associated with serious adverse effects with long-term use.[1,33] Steroids should be gradually withdrawn after 2 to 4 weeks after induction of remission. For patients who require chronic steroid use and are steroid dependent,

TABLE 34-5 Levels of Evidence for Therapeutic Interventions in Inflammatory Bowel Disease

Interventions	Evidence Grades[a]
Ulcerative Colitis	
Mild to moderate active distal disease may be treated with oral aminosalicylates, topical mesalamine, or topical steroids	A
Combined oral and topical aminosalicylates are more effective than either is alone for mild to moderate active distal disease	A
Oral prednisone in doses of 40-60 mg/day or 1 mg/kg/day may be used in patients with mild to moderate distal disease unresponsive to oral or topical aminosalicylates	B
Sulfasalazine in doses of 4-6 g/day or an alternate aminosalicylate in doses of up to 4.8 g/day of the active 5-aminosalicylate moiety is effective for induction of mild to moderate extensive colitis	A
Infliximab, adalimumab, and golimumab are effective for moderate to severe disease in those patients not responding to corticosteroids or an immunosuppressive agent	A
Systemic corticosteroids are effective in moderate to severe active disease	A
Hospitalization for parenteral steroids is indicated for patients with severe disease or those failing to respond to oral steroids	A
Failure to demonstrate improvement following 3 days of parenteral steroids in patients with severe disease is an indication for cyclosporine or colectomy	1B
Sulfasalazine, mesalamine, or balsalazide is effective in maintenance of remission of distal disease; combining oral and topical mesalamine is more effective than is either alone	A
Sulfasalazine, olsalazine, mesalamine, and balsalazide are effective in preventing relapses in patients with mild to moderate extensive disease	A
Corticosteroids are not effective as maintenance treatment	A
Azathioprine, mercaptopurine, infliximab, and adalimumab are effective in lowering or eliminating corticosteroid use in corticosteroid-dependent patients	A
Azathioprine, mercaptopurine, or infliximab may be effective in patients with severe disease flares or those requiring retreatment with corticosteroids within 1 year	C
Oral cyclosporine is effective for patients with corticosteroid refractory disease but requires concomitant administration of azathioprine or mercaptopurine	C
Infliximab, adalimumab, and golimumab therapy is effective for maintenance if there is an initial response	A
Infliximab combined with azathioprine are effective for induction therapy in active moderately severe disease	B
Budesonide is effective for induction in mild-moderate active colonic disease	A
Vedolizumab is effective in moderate to severe disease in patients failing other therapies	B
Crohn's Disease	
Oral aminosalicylates are effective for mild to moderate ileal, ileocolonic, or colonic active disease	D
Metronidazole may be effective in patients not responding to sulfasalazine	D
Ileal release budesonide is effective for mild to moderate ileal or right-sided colonic disease	A
Topical hydrocortisone is effective for distal colonic inflammation	A
Systemic corticosteroids are effective in moderate to severe active disease	A
Systemic corticosteroids are not effective for patients with perianal fistulas	C
Hospitalization for parenteral steroids is indicated for patients with severe disease or those failing to respond to oral steroids	A
Parenteral methotrexate is effective for induction of remission in patients with active disease and for reducing corticosteroid dependency	B
Infliximab, adalimumab, and certolizumab are effective for moderate to severe disease in those patients not responding to corticosteroids or an immunosuppressive agent	A
Infliximab, adalimumab, and certolizimab are effective for those patients with fistulas who have not responded to antibiotics, immunosuppressive agents, or surgical drainage	A
High-dose oral cyclosporine (7.6 mg/kg) has short-term efficacy in patients with active disease	B
IV cyclosporine is effective for the treatment of fistulizing disease	B
Corticosteroids are not effective as maintenance treatment	A
Budesonide is effective as short-term maintenance therapy (3 months) but not long term	A
Azathioprine, mercaptopurine, infliximab, adalimumab, and certolizumab are effective in lowering or eliminating corticosteroid use in corticosteroid-dependent patients	A
Azathioprine or mercaptopurine is effective for maintenance of remission regardless of disease distribution	A
Azathioprine or mercaptopurine may be effective for treating perianal or enteric fistulae	C
Methotrexate maintenance therapy (15-25 mg IM weekly) is effective for patients whose active disease has responded to IM methotrexate	A
Methotrexate 25 mg IM for up to 16 weeks followed by 15 mg IM weekly is effective for patients with chronic active disease	A
Infliximab, adalimumab, and certolizumab therapy is effective for maintenance if there is an initial response	A
Natalizumab is effective in moderate to severe disease in patients failing other therapies	B
Vedolizumab is effective in moderate to severe disease in patients failing other therapies	B
Infliximab combined with azathioprine are effective for induction therapy in active moderately severe disease	A

[a]A, homogenous evidence from multiple well-designed, randomized (therapeutic) or cohort (descriptive) controlled trials, each involving a number of participants to be of sufficient statistical power; B, evidence from at least one large well-designed clinical trial with or without randomization from cohort or case-control analytic studies or well-designed meta analysis; C, evidence based on clinical experience, descriptive studies, or reports of expert committees; D, not rated.

Data from references 33, 37, 48, 77, 87, 88, 89, 91.

there is a strong justification for use of alternative therapies. Azathioprine is effective in preventing relapse of UC for patients who fail ASAs or who are steroid dependent.[1,13,67,68,69] Approximately one third of patients will maintain remission on azathioprine; however, the onset of action is slow and 3 to 6 months may be required before beneficial effects are noted.[58,68] As mentioned earlier, azathioprine is also recommended for patients with severe UC who are transitioned to oral cyclosporine.[1,13,33,51,68,70,82]

The TNF-α inhibitors are options for maintenance in patients with moderate to severe UC following induction, and in those who are steroid dependent or have failed azathioprine. Clinically up to one third of patients may not respond and those that do may lose effectiveness over time due to antibody development.[58,77]

Crohn's Disease

Management of CD often proves more difficult than management of UC because of the greater complexity of presentation (Fig. 34-3; see Table 34-3). There is a greater potential for reliance on drug therapy with CD because resection of involved areas of the GI tract may not be possible. Recurrence of CD is common following surgery with reported rates of endoscopic recurrence reported as up to 75% at 1 year.[84]

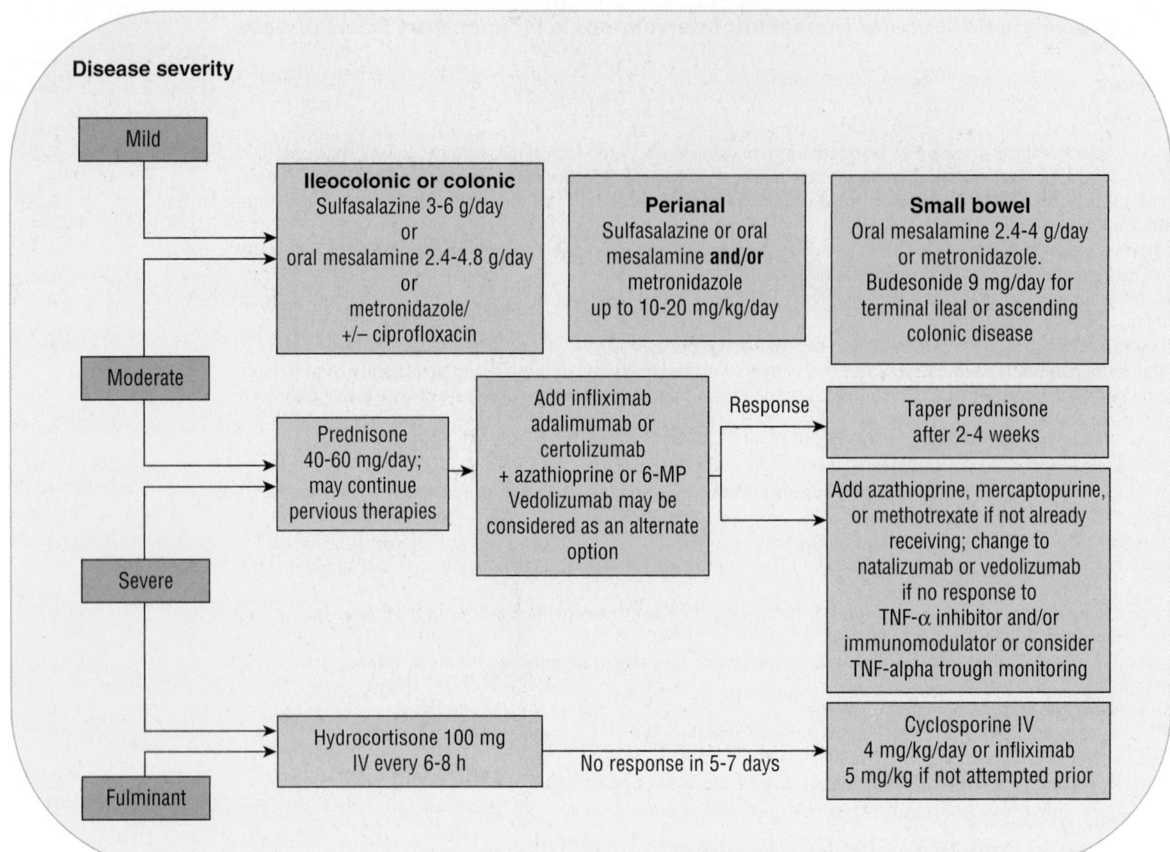

FIGURE 34-3 Treatment approaches for Crohn's disease.

The drug treatment of CD involves many of the same agents used for UC. While the treatment strategy for CD has often followed a similar "step-up" pattern as seen with UC, which involves initiating therapy with ASAs first, there has been interest in using higher-potency agents first, such as TNF-α inhibitors in a "top-down" approach in patients with severe disease.[38]

Mild to Moderate Active Crohn's Disease

While effective in UC, ASAs have not demonstrated significant efficacy in CD. Sulfasalazine is reported to have marginal efficacy when compared with placebo for patients with mild to moderate CD, while the newer mesalamine derivatives are generally considered to have minimal efficacy.[13,37,38,46,76,85] Despite limited and variable effectiveness, the mesalamine derivatives are often tried as an initial therapy for mild to moderate CD given their favorable adverse effect profile. Since CD often involves the small intestine, formulations such as Pentasa, which release in the small intestine, may be used.

Systemic corticosteroids are frequently used for the treatment of moderate to severe active CD; however, controlled-release budesonide (Entocort) at a dose of 9 mg daily is a viable first-line option for patients with mild to moderate ileal or right-sided (ascending colonic) disease.[13,37,38,46,66] This agent is superior to placebo and has demonstrated superiority to mesalamine and is preferred for patients with ileal disease.[13,46,76,86]

Antibiotics may have some roles in the treatment of CD. Metronidazole, given orally as 10 to 20 mg/kg/day in divided doses, has demonstrated variable efficacy but may possibly be useful in some patients with CD, particularly for patients with colonic or ileocolonic involvement, those with perineal disease, or those who are unresponsive to sulfasalazine.[13,37,38,74] For patients with colonic or perineal disease, metronidazole can be added to a mesalamine product or steroids as adjunctive therapy when satisfactory control of CD is not gained with first-line agents, or in attempts to reduce steroid dosage.[38] Ciprofloxacin 1 g/day is another antibiotic used in CD, often in combination with metronidazole for patients with perianal disease or pouchitis; however, results have been variable due to differences in study design and patient numbers.[37,43,46,58,74,87] Other antibiotics, such as rifaximin and clofazimine, have also been studied with variable efficacy reported.[46,74] While there has been some demonstrated efficacy with antibiotics in mild to moderate CD, they are generally not recommended as a first-line therapy.[37,38,46,58,74]

Moderate to Severe Active Crohn's Disease

Patients with moderate to severe active CD require rapid suppression of inflammation for symptom improvement and prevention of complications. Oral corticosteroids, such as prednisone 40 to 60 mg/day, are generally considered first-line therapies for moderate to severe active CD who are unresponsive to ASAs and are effective in inducing remission for up to 70% of patients.[13,38,66] Traditional oral systemic steroids have greater efficacy in inducing remission compared with budesonide in patients with moderate disease; however, the potential for adverse effects is greater.[66,76] Hospitalized patients with moderate to severe disease who are unable to tolerate oral therapy are candidates for administration of parenteral steroids, with methylprednisolone or hydrocortisone being first-line options.[38,51] Systemic steroids do not appear to be effective for treatment of perianal fistulas.[38,76]

10 Immunomodulators (azathioprine and MP) are not recommended to induce remission in moderate to severe CD; however, they are effective in maintaining steroid-induced remission, in patients not achieving adequate response to standard medical therapy or those with steroid dependency, or in combination with TNF-α inhibitors.[13,38,67,88] Clinical response to azathioprine and mercaptopurine may be related to whole-blood concentrations of the metabolite 6-thioguanine (TGN). Concentrations of TGN greater than 230 to 260 pmol/8 × 10^8 erythrocytes have been demonstrated to have beneficial effects, but monitoring is not routinely performed or may not be available at some sites.[68]

11 Although mostly used in the setting of maintenance therapy as an alternative to azathioprine, methotrexate given weekly intramuscularly or subcutaneously in doses of 15 to 25 mg has demonstrated some efficacy in induction of remission in CD and corticosteroid-sparing effects; however, its use as a first line agent for induction is not recommended.[58,88]

The TNF-α inhibitors are the most effective and thus the preferred agents in the management of moderate to severe CD.[88,89] All agents in this class, with the exception of golimumab, which is not approved for use in CD in the United States, have similar rates of efficacy. The choice of agent depends on patient preference, route of administration, and cost. Adalimumab and certolizumab have the advantage of subcutaneous administration and may be considered alternates to infliximab as initial therapy or in those patients losing response to infliximab. Collectively these agents have demonstrated higher likelihood of induction of remission compared to placebo: RR 1.6 (95% CI 1.17-2.36).[89]

The use of TNF-α inhibitors in combination with thiopurines has quickly become the preferred approach to treatment of moderate to severe CD. Combination therapy results in added efficacy and reduction in antibody formation to the TNF-α inhibitor, which extends the duration of efficacy. Studies comparing infliximab with azathioprine and the combination of infliximab and azathioprine demonstrated significantly greater rates of remission of 57% at week 26 with the combination and infliximab alone (44%) compared with azathioprine alone (30%) in immunomodulator and biologic naive patients with CD.[88-91] For this reason the combination of TNF-α inhibitors and thiopurines is the recommended treatment approach.[88]

The integrin antagonists are options for patients who do not respond to steroids or TNF-α inhibitors (vedolizumab may as an alternative to TNF-alpha inhibitors for moderate to sever disease).[58,77,92] Vedolizumab is preferred over natalizumab due to the reduced risk of adverse effects, particularly progressive multifocal leukoencephalopathy (PML). These agents should not be used in combination with other immunosuppressants or biologic agents.

Severe/Fulminant Active Disease

Patients with severe or fulminant disease require prompt management in the inpatient setting and are often considered for surgical intervention. Parenteral corticosteroids at a dose equivalent of 40 to 60 mg prednisone should be instituted once the presence of abscess has been excluded.[38] Unresponsive cyclosporine has been tried at doses of 2 to 4 mg/h via IV infusion with reported in-hospital colectomy rates of 12.5%; however, despite these findings, there are few data to support its use in this setting.[13,93] It may also be effective as a last-line option for patients with severe fistulizing disease.[93]

Maintenance of Remission

Maintaining remission is typically more difficult with CD than with UC. There is minimal evidence that sulfasalazine and oral mesalamine derivatives are effective therapies for maintenance of CD following medically induced remission.[37,80,84,85] Despite these findings, an attempt to maintain remission with sulfasalazine or oral mesalamine following a medically induced remission may be carried out given the favorable side-effect profile and cost of these drugs compared with those of immunosuppressive and biologic agents. Mesalamine appears to have some efficacy in preventing postsurgical relapse following resection, with absolute risk reductions of approximately 14% for relapse in some studies, and can be considered in patients who do not qualify for or have a contraindication to immunosuppressive therapy.[84]

Systemic corticosteroids have no place in the prevention of recurrence of CD. These agents do not alter the long-term course of the disease and predispose patients to serious adverse effects with long-term use.[38] Budesonide has been studied at maintenance doses of 6 mg/day for up to 52 weeks with minimal efficacy in maintaining remission.[13,80,86] Despite this recommendation, use of budesonide as maintenance therapy for up to 1 year can be considered, particularly in patients who have become corticosteroid dependent, for whom switching to budesonide is an option.[13]

Azathioprine and mercaptopurine are most effective in maintaining corticosteroid induced remission in CD.[58,68,80,82] Patients who may also benefit from these agents include those with quiescent disease who are steroid dependent or refractory, postsurgical patients to prevent recurrence, those with frequent flares requiring steroid bursts, and those with perianal or enteric fistulas.[13,68,80] Methotrexate may be considered as an alternative to thiopurines to maintain corticosteroid induced remission; however, the evidence for its use is weak.[58,88]

All of the TNF-α inhibitors currently approved for use in CD are viable options for maintenance of remission.[87,91] If induction of remission was obtained via combination therapy with a thiopurine, the decision will need to be made as to whether both drugs should be continued, or one of the two agents discontinued to promote use of monotherapy given the risk of adverse effects increases with continued use of both agents.[88]

Selected Complications

Toxic Megacolon

The treatment required for toxic megacolon includes general supportive, consideration for early surgical intervention, and drug therapy.[34,38] Perforation is reported in up to 36% of patients and can significantly worsen outcomes.[51] Aggressive fluid and electrolyte management is required for dehydration. Transfusion may be necessary if significant blood loss has occurred. Opiates and medications with anticholinergic properties should be discontinued because these agents enhance colonic dilation, thereby increasing the risk of bowel perforation.[51] Broad-spectrum antimicrobials that include coverage for gram-negative bacilli and intestinal anaerobes should be used as preemptive therapy in the event that perforation occurs.[34] If the patient is not receiving corticosteroids, then high-dose IV therapy should be administered to reduce acute inflammation. Emergent surgical intervention, mainly an abdominal colectomy with formation of an ileostomy, is an important consideration for patients with toxic megacolon and prevents death in some patients.[51]

Extraintestinal Manifestations

For some extraintestinal manifestations of IBD, specific therapies can be instituted, whereas for others the treatment that is used for the GI inflammatory process also addresses the systemic manifestations.

Anemia secondary to blood loss from the GI tract can be treated with oral ferrous sulfate. If the patient is unable to take oral medication and the patient's hematocrit is sufficiently low, blood transfusions or IV iron infusions may be required.[42] Anemia may also be related to malabsorption of vitamin B_{12} or folic acid, particularly for patients who have had ileal resection, so supplementation may be required. Screening for osteoporosis via dual x-ray absorptiometry is recommended for patients using steroids for more than 3 months, in postmenopausal females, patients of age over 60, and those who have sustained a low-stress fracture.[44] If the patient is deemed high risk for osteoporosis or exhibits a reduced serum vitamin D concentration, vitamin D and calcium should be instituted. If osteoporosis is present, then calcium, vitamin D, and a bisphosphonate or possibly teriparatide are recommended.[42,44] Corticosteroid use should be avoided or limited, and weight-bearing exercise initiated if possible.

There are no consistently recommended therapies for aphthous ulcers; however, topical viscous lidocaine may provide symptom relief while topical corticosteroids may promote healing.[42] Episcleritis or uveitis is often worse during exacerbations of the intestinal disease, and measures improving intestinal disease will improve these systemic manifestations. Cool compresses and topical corticosteroids may provide symptomatic relief, while TNF-α inhibitors when in use may also provide benefit.[42] For arthritis associated with IBD, aspirin or another NSAID may be beneficial, as are corticosteroids. However, NSAID use may exacerbate the underlying IBD and predispose patients to GI bleeding. Intraarticular corticosteroids may be tried to limit the adverse effects of systemically administered agents.[42] Skin manifestations often require local wound care and use of topical or systemic corticosteroids.[42] Anti–TNF-α therapies may also improve severe dermatologic manifestations. Although ursodiol may improve liver enzymes in patients with IBD-associated PSC, it has not been demonstrated to have favorable effects on outcomes.[41,42] Liver transplantation is being used more frequently for definitive treatment of PSC.

Special Considerations

Pregnancy and Breastfeeding

The occurrence or consideration of pregnancy may cause significant concerns for the patient with IBD. Patients with IBD have similar infertility rates as the general female population. The rate of normal childbirth is similar to that for healthy populations.[94,95] Some studies have noted a greater risk of spontaneous abortion, low birth weight, caesarian section, congenital abnormalities, low Apgar scores, preterm rupture of membranes, and preeclampsia.[94-96] However, most patients can conceive normally and have a normal pregnancy.[94-99] There is a small risk of preterm labor or low-gestational-weight infants.[94,98,99] Preconception counseling is key for female patients with IBD who are considering becoming pregnant. This includes improving prepregnancy nutrition, implementing supplementation with folate, calcium, and vitamin D, ceasing alcohol and tobacco use, and inducing disease remission if possible.[94] Overall, pregnancy appears to have minimal effects on the course of IBD.[93-98] Likewise, IBD appears to have little effect on the course of pregnancy, particularly if the IBD is quiescent at the time of conception.[94,95,98] Patients who are pregnant experience IBD recurrence rates similar to those of nonpregnant females.[98] Patients are recommended to wait until their disease is in remission for 3 months prior to conceiving if possible.[93] Patients requiring colectomy for UC should preferentially receive rectal-sparing surgery if they are considering conceiving, followed by IPAA after delivery.[94]

Most classes of medications used in IBD are relatively safe in pregnancy. Sulfasalazine is generally well tolerated; however, it does interfere with folate absorption, so supplementation with folic acid 1 mg twice daily should be used during the pregnancy.[94,95] Sulfasalazine causes decreased sperm counts and reduced fertility in males and corticosteroids may adversely affect fertility as well.[100] This effect is reversible on discontinuation of the drug, and it is not reported with mesalamine. Other ASAs can be used as well; however, there are concerns regarding the presence of dibutyl phthalate in the coating of Asacol.[94] Mesalamine preparations not containing dibutyl phthalate should be preferentially used. Steroids given systemically do not appear to be detrimental to the fetus, with the exception of dexamethasone, and should be limited in duration.[94,98,100] Maternal cortisol is generally inactivated by placental 11β-hydroxysteroid dehydrogenase type 2; however, dexamethasone is not inactivated by this enzyme and may accumulate in fetal tissue. Therefore, dexamethasone should be avoided in pregnancy.[94] Immunosuppressive drugs (azathioprine and mercaptopurine) may be associated with fetal deformities in humans and are classified as pregnancy category D; however, they have been used commonly in IBD without detriment for most patients.[94,98] Infliximab, adalimumab, and certolizumab appear to be relatively safe for use in pregnant patients.[94-99] Use of infliximab should be restricted to the first and second trimesters if possible due to placental transfer of infliximab and the potential for neonatal adverse effects.[99] There is a similar concern with adalimumab, although this agent is more difficult to detect in the neonatal bloodstream. Consideration can be given to stopping it 8 to 10 weeks prior to delivery.[99] Natalizumab was formerly pregnancy category C drug and not much is known about its safety in pregnancy, and thus may be used if benefit is thought to outweigh risk.[91] Vedolizumab was a pregnancy category B drug and pregnancies occurring while receiving this agent should be reported to the manufacturers pregnancy exposure registry. Metronidazole may be used for short courses for treatment of trichomoniasis, but prolonged use should be avoided due to potential mutagenic effects.[98] Methotrexate should not be used during pregnancy, as it is a known abortifacient (former category X).[94-99] Cyclosporine has been used in pregnant patients with success and therefore is an option for patients with severe disease.[94,98]

Use of agents in breastfeeding women is also a consideration. Sulfasalazine does pose a small risk of kernicterus, as levels of sulfapyridine in breast milk are low or undetectable, and thus monitoring for this symptom should be implemented.[94] Other mesalamine derivatives are considered safe in breastfeeding.[94,98] Corticosteroids can be detected in breast milk, with fetal levels approximately 10% to 12% of maternal levels.[95] However, breastfeeding is believed to be safe for the infant when doses of prednisone less than 40 mg are used.[95] Optimally mothers should wait at least 4 hours after an oral dose of systemic corticosteroids before breastfeeding to limit exposure to the child.[94,98] The anti–TNF-α agents are generally considered safe for use in breastfeeding and carry minimal risk of adverse effects.[95,99] Metronidazole and cyclosporine should not be given to nursing mothers because these agents are excreted into breast milk and may cause adverse effects.[94-98]

Adverse Drug Effects

Drug intolerance often limits the usefulness of agents used to treat IBD. In some cases, adverse effects can be significant and require discontinuation of the therapy. Knowledge of the common or important adverse reactions will assist in avoiding or minimizing their effects.

Compared with mesalamine, sulfasalazine is more often associated with adverse drug effects, and these effects may be classified as either dose related or idiosyncratic (Table 34-6).[58,101] The sulfapyridine portion of the sulfasalazine molecule is believed to be responsible for much of the sulfasalazine toxicity.[33] Dose-related side effects usually include GI disturbances such as nausea, vomiting, diarrhea, or anorexia but may also include headache and arthralgia. These adverse reactions tend to occur more commonly on initiation of therapy and decrease in frequency as therapy is continued. Approaches to the management of these adverse effects include discontinuing the agent for a short period and then reinstituting therapy at a reduced dosage with subsequent slower dose escalation, administration with food, or substituting another enteric-coated 5-ASA product. Folic acid absorption is impaired by sulfasalazine, which may lead to anemia, so oral folic acid supplementation should be administered.

Idiosyncratic effects commonly include rash, fever, or hepatotoxicity, as well as relatively uncommon but serious reactions such as bone marrow suppression, thrombocytopenia, pancreatitis, pneumonitis, interstitial nephritis, and hepatitis. For most patients with idiosyncratic reactions, sulfasalazine must be discontinued. In some patients who have experienced allergic reactions to sulfasalazine, a desensitization procedure can be instituted. By gradually increasing sulfasalazine dosage over weeks to months, patient tolerance has been improved.[33]

Oral mesalamine derivatives may impose a lower frequency of adverse effects as compared with sulfasalazine.[33,78] Up to 80% of patients who are intolerant to sulfasalazine will tolerate oral mesalamine derivatives.[33] The most commonly encountered adverse effects are nausea, vomiting, and headache.[79] However, olsalazine may cause watery diarrhea in up to 25% of patients, often requiring drug discontinuation.

TABLE 34-6 Drug Monitoring Guidelines

Drug(s)	Adverse Drug Reaction	Monitoring Parameters	Comments
Sulfasalazine	Nausea, vomiting, headache Rash, anemia, pneumonitis Hepatotoxicity, nephritis Thrombocytopenia, lymphoma	Folate, complete blood count Liver function tests, Scr, BUN	Increase the dose slowly, over 1-2 weeks
Mesalamine	Nausea, vomiting, headache	GI disturbances	
Corticosteroids	Hyperglycemia, dyslipidemia	Blood pressure, fasting lipid panel	Avoid long-term use if possible or consider budesonide
	Osteoporosis, hypertension, acne	Glucose, vitamin D, bone density	
	Edema, infection, myopathy, psychosis		
Azathioprine/ mercaptopurine	Bone marrow suppression, pancreatitis	Complete blood count	Check TPMT activity
	Liver dysfunction, rash, arthralgia	Scr, BUN, liver function tests, genotype/phenotype	May monitor TGN
Methotrexate	Bone marrow suppression, pancreatitis	Complete blood count, Scr, BUN	Check baseline pregnancy test
	Pneumonitis, pulmonary fibrosis, hepatitis	Liver function tests	Chest x-ray
Infliximab	Infusion-related reactions (infliximab), infection	Blood pressure/heart rate (infliximab)	Need negative PPD and viral serologies
Adalimumab	Heart failure, optic neuritis, demyelination, injection site reaction, signs of infection	Neurologic exam, mental status	
Certolizumab	Lymphoma	Trough concentrations (infliximab)	
Golimumab		Antidrug antibodies (all agents)	
Natalizumab Vedolizumab	Infusion-related reactions	Brain MRI, mental status, progressive multifocal leukoencephalopathy	Vedolizumab not associated with PML

There is a greater potential for adverse effects from corticosteroids when used for the treatment of IBD because there is often a requirement for use of high doses for extended periods of time. Adverse effects of corticosteroids include hyperglycemia, hypertension, osteoporosis, acne, fluid retention, electrolyte disturbances, myopathies, muscle wasting, increased appetite, psychosis, infection, and adrenocortical suppression.[33,66] To minimize corticosteroid effects, clinicians have used alternate-day steroid therapy; however, some patients do not do well clinically on the days when no steroid is given. For most patients a single daily corticosteroid dose suffices, and divided daily doses are unnecessary. Adrenal insufficiency after abrupt steroid withdrawal often necessitates gradual tapering of steroid therapy for patients using these agents daily for more than 2 to 3 weeks. Due to its lower bioavailability and lower potential for adverse effects, budesonide may be used as alternate steroid therapy in CD involving the ileum or right colon, or in UC, or may be substituted for prednisone in CD patients who are steroid dependent or require long-term therapy.[37,38,66]

Azathioprine and mercaptopurine may be associated with serious adverse effects such as lymphomas, pancreatitis, or nephrotoxicity.[33,38,68,69] Adverse events to thiopurines are typically divided into two groups: type A and type B.[68,101,102] Type A are dose related and include malaise, nausea, infectious complications, hepatitis, and myelosuppression. Complete blood counts with differential should be monitored every 2 weeks while doses are being titrated. Type B reactions are considered idiosyncratic and include fever, rash, arthralgia, and pancreatitis (3%-15% of patients).[100,101] Predisposition to development of these adverse effects may be related to polymorphisms in the enzyme thiopurine methyltransferase (TPMT), which is partially responsible for activation and metabolism of these drugs. Determination of TPMT activity is recommended prior to initiation of therapy to determine which patients require lower doses of these agents.[38,68,102] Alternatively, evaluating TPMT genotype or phenotype can also assist in assessing a patient's risk for toxicity.[67-69,102] Doses may need to be reduced by 30% to 70% if low TPMT activity is present.[102] Adjusting azathioprine and MP doses by measuring concentrations of metabolites, particularly TGN, may be useful, with higher levels associated with greater remission rates.[67-69,101,102]

With the advent of coadministration of azathioprine with infliximab, development of hepatosplenic T-cell lymphoma (HSTCL) has become a concern. The overall impact of using both drugs together, the contribution of drug classes to the development of lymphoma, and the risk and effects of both drugs are unclear. Those most at risk appear to be younger male patients and most of the risk is thought to be conferred by the thiopurine component.[67,103-105] Methotrexate is associated with the development of nausea, vomiting, pulmonary fibrosis, pneumonitis, hepatotoxicity, anemia, and renal dysfunction, and is a known abortifacient. Patients should have baseline liver function tests, serum creatinine, BUN, complete blood count, and chest x-ray prior to use. Female patients should have a negative pregnancy test prior to use. Some patients may require supplementation with folic acid.

Most patients receiving metronidazole for CD tolerate the agent fairly well; however, mild adverse effects occur frequently. They commonly include nausea, metallic taste, urticaria, and glossitis.[34,37] More serious effects that occur with long-term use include development of paresthesias and reversible peripheral neuropathy. Other effects include a disulfiram-like reaction if alcohol is ingested in conjunction.

The TNF-α inhibitors may be associated with development of serious adverse effects and carry similar adverse effect profiles for the available agents. Patients who receive infliximab often develop antibodies to infliximab (ATIs), also referred to as antidrug antibodies (ADAs). These ADAs can develop in response to administration of the other TNF-α inhibitors as well. Overall up to 50% of patients may lose efficacy after 1 year of treatment due to ADA development.[106] The development of ADAs also results in increases in the occurrence of serious infusion-related reactions and loss of response to the drug.

Up to 10% of patients per year require discontinuation of infliximab due to adverse effects and loss of efficacy related to development of ATIs.[76,88,106]

Strategies to reduce ATI formation include administration of a second dose within 8 weeks of the first dose, concurrent administration of steroids (hydrocortisone 200 mg IV on the day of the infusion or oral prednisone the day prior), and use of concomitant immunosuppressive agents such as thiopurines.[76,97,106] Loss of efficacy may be managed by a dose escalation to 10 mg/kg, reducing the dosing interval, or switching to another TNF-α inhibitor.[87,88,106] Delayed hypersensitivity reactions may also occur up to 14 days after administration, with 5 to 7 days being the most common time frame.[87,104] Autoimmune phenomena, such as lupus and hemolytic anemia, may also occur during infliximab therapy but are uncommon, as are adverse neurologic events such as optic neuritis and demyelinating syndrome.[77,86,104] For these reasons patients with a history of demyelinating disease, optic neuritis, or lymphoma should avoid use of TNF-α antagonists.[104] Infliximab may also cause worsening of heart failure and thus is contraindicated for patients with New York Heart Association Class III or IV heart failure.[91] While the mechanism is unclear, it may relate in part to the cytoprotective effects of TNF on ischemic cardiac tissue, increases in production of nitric oxide and increased peripheral perfusion secondary to TNF, or TNF's role in cardiac remodeling and repair. Due to administration via the subcutaneous route, adalimumab, certolizumab, and golimumab may be more associated with injection site reactions versus infusion-related reactions.

All TNF-α inhibitors predispose patients to development of serious infections, including fungal, bacterial, and viral. Patients with clinically significant active infections should not receive TNF-α inhibitors. While the overall risk of hospitalization for serious infections may be less than previously suspected, development of infection remains a serious concern.[107] Reactivation of latent mycobacterial infections may occur because of the inhibition of TNF-protective mechanisms; therefore, patients should receive a tuberculin skin test (purified protein derivative [PPD] test) and a chest x-ray prior to initiating therapy to rule out undiagnosed tuberculosis.[93,107] Reactivation of hepatitis B may occur; thus, patients should also be screened for hepatitis B virus infection prior to initiating therapy. Patients should also be screened for hepatitis C infection, although it does not appear that use of TNF-α inhibitors is unsafe or significantly alters the disease course. Lastly, use of natalizumab is associated with development of PML and is only available via the manufacturer's TOUCH prescribing program.[95] Patients receiving natalizumab should be monitored for development of adverse neurologic events and undergo MRI of the brain should development of PML be suspected. Vedolizumab has not been associated with development of PML to date.

PERSONALIZED PHARMACOTHERAPY

The approach to treatment of IBD should consider all aspects of each individual patient in order to maximize therapy, improve patient symptoms and QOL, and prevent complications. To ensure optimal drug therapy, an assessment of each patient's health literacy and potential barriers to understanding and adherence should be performed. Involving the patient in the care process will help to keep him or her engaged. For the drug classes that are used in the management of IBD, there are several aspects of individualization that may improve efficacy and safety. Since patients with IBD are often seen by GI specialists or surgeons, ensuring that each provider has a current, accurate, and complete medication list will help to prevent potential medication errors. Female patients of childbearing age should discuss with their providers their goals for becoming pregnant, as this may dictate the choice of drugs used.

For the ASAs, picking the appropriate formulation and dose of drug for the disease severity and extent is key. Enemas and suppositories, while generally more effective than oral preparations, may not be as acceptable for use, particularly by younger patients. Therefore, individuating the patient's preference for a specific formulation should be taken into account when choosing ASA preparations.[57] Consideration can be given to the use of once-daily products if there is evidence that multiple-daily dosing is affecting patient adherence.[61-63] This must be weighed against the higher cost of these preparations. If expense is an issue, use of generically available agents may be preferred.

Patients receiving systemic corticosteroids for extended periods of time should be assessed for risk of bone loss and fracture and the need for vitamin D and calcium supplementation. In addition, a review of the patient's medical history should be performed to identify other conditions that may be worsened by corticosteroids, such as diabetes or hypertension. Adjustment of medications for these types of conditions may need to be made based on the dose and duration of corticosteroid use.

Patients in whom azathioprine or mercaptopurine is being considered should undergo TPMT activity testing or have a genotype or phenotype test performed to determine if dose adjustments are required. Since the initial dosing of these agents is weight based, obtaining a current accurate weight for the patient is necessary as well. Obtaining a family history regarding lymphoproliferative disorders or lymphoma is important for determining if the potential risks outweigh the benefits of long-term use. For female patients in whom methotrexate is being considered, a pregnancy test should be obtained and the potential desire to become pregnant in the future should be discussed. Female patients of childbearing age opting to use methotrexate should have a safe and effective method of birth control available that is based on their preference.

For patients receiving TNF-α inhibitors, baseline screening for latent infections should be performed. Obtaining an accurate weight will assist in the dosing of infliximab. Likewise use of infliximab requires administration in an observed infusion center or clinic. If patients are unable to afford to get to their appointment, use of a self-administered agent, such as adalimumab or certolizumab, may be preferred. If patients appear to be losing response to infliximab, evaluating for ADAs, if assays are available, in addition to evaluating serum trough concentrations may assist the clinician in determining if dose and frequency need to be altered. Trough concentrations of 3 to 7 mcg/mL (mg/L) are considered optimal, while ADA concentrations specific for infliximab are considered high if greater than 9.1 U/mL (kU/L).[106]

From a health maintenance standpoint, patients should be evaluated for use of recommended vaccines; however, if patients are receiving immunosuppressants or biologic agents, the use of live or attenuated vaccines may be contraindicated. Patients who currently use tobacco should be encouraged to undergo tobacco cessation, as tobacco use will worsen CD. Since nicotine often improves symptoms in UC, it may be more difficult to cease tobacco use in this patient population. Choice of tobacco cessation products should also be based on current amount and patient preference. Nutritional status of patients should also be routinely assessed and patient-specific diets or delivery, such as enteral or parenteral nutrition, should be implemented.

EVALUATION OF THERAPEUTIC OUTCOMES

The success of therapeutic regimens to treat IBD can be measured by patient-reported complaints, signs, and symptoms; by direct clinician examination (including endoscopy); by history and physical examination; by selected laboratory tests; and by QOL measures.

Evaluation of IBD severity is difficult because much of the assessment is subjective. Disease rating scales, such as the CDAI or other indices, have been created to try and make disease assessment more objective. The CDAI is a commonly used scale for patients with nonfistulizing disease and for evaluation of patients during clinical trials.[46] The scale incorporates eight elements: (a) number of stools in the past 7 days, (b) sum of abdominal pain ratings from the past 7 days, (c) rating of general well-being in the past 7 days, (d) use of antidiarrheals, (e) body weight, (f) hematocrit, (g) finding of abdominal mass, and (h) a sum of extraintestinal symptoms present in the past week. Elements of this index provide a guide for those measures that may be useful in assessing the effectiveness of treatment regimens. A decrease in CDAI of 100 points is considered a clinically significant response, with a score of less than 150 considered to be disease remission.[46] A subsequent scale was developed specifically for perianal CD, known as the *Perianal Crohn's Disease Activity Index* (PDAI).[46] The PDAI includes five items: presence of discharge, pain, restriction of sexual activity, type of perianal disease, and degree of induration. The HBI may also be used in place of the CDAI.

Standardized assessment tools have also been constructed for UC.[45] Elements in these scales vary and include (a) stool frequency, (b) presence of blood in the stool, (c) mucosal appearance (from endoscopy), and (d) physician's global assessment based on physical examination, endoscopy, and laboratory data. While these tools are often used for assessment of patients in clinical trials, they are sometimes used in the clinical setting as well.

Additional studies that are often useful include direct endoscopic examination of affected areas and/or radiocontrast studies. As mentioned earlier, mucosal healing is being explored as a major end point for patients with luminal disease.[48] For patients with acute disease, assessment of fluid and electrolyte status is important, because these may be lost during diarrheal episodes. Other laboratory tests, such as serum albumin, transferrin, or other markers of visceral protein status as well as markers of inflammation such as ESR or CRP, may be used to monitor disease and drug therapy. Lastly assessing for both trough concentrations of infliximab and presence of ADAs can help guide therapy in patients who are not responding to normal doses.

Assessment of the IBD patient must include consideration of adverse drug effects. Because many of the agents used have a relatively high probability of causing adverse effects, particularly corticosteroids and other immunosuppressive agents, patient assessment should include collection of history and physical and laboratory data that are necessary to prevent or recognize adverse drug effects.

Finally, a patient QOL assessment should be performed regularly.[45,46] Inquiry should be made regarding patient's general well-being, emotional function, and social function. Social function may include assessment of the ability to perform routine daily functions and to maintain occupational activities, sexual function, and recreation. The most common tool used to assess QOL is the Inflammatory Bowel Disease Questionnaire (IBDQ), a 32-item questionnaire that covers four disease dimensions: bowel function, emotional status, systemic symptoms, and social function. The IBDQ has shown good correlation with the CDAI.[46] The standard short form-36 is often used as a measure of QOL in IBD intervention trials.[45,46]

ABBREVIATIONS

ADA	antidrug antibody
ASA	aminosalicylate
ATI	antibody to infliximab
CD	Crohn's disease
CDAI	Crohn's Disease Activity Index
CRC	colorectal carcinoma
CRP	C-reactive protein
ESR	erythrocyte sedimentation rate
HBI	Harvey-Bradshaw Index
HLA	human leukocyte antigen
HSTCL	hepatosplenic T-cell lymphoma
IBD	inflammatory bowel disease
IBDQ	Inflammatory Bowel Disease Questionnaire
IL	interleukin
IPAA	ileal pouch anal anastomosis
MMX	Multi-MatriX
MP	mercaptopurine
NF-κ B	nuclear factor κ B
NOD2	nucleotide-binding oligomerization domain protein 2
NSAID	nonsteroidal anti-inflammatory drug
PDAI	Perianal Crohn's Disease Activity Index
PML	progressive multifocal leukoencephalopathy
PPD	purified protein derivative
PSC	primary sclerosing cholangitis
QOL	quality of life
TGF-β	transforming growth factor-β
TGN	thioguanine
TLR	toll-like membrane receptor
TNF-α	tumor necrosis factor-α
TPMT	thiopurine methyltransferase
UC	ulcerative colitis
VTE	venous thromboembolism

REFERENCES

1. Danese S, Fiocchi C. Ulcerative colitis. *N Engl J Med* 2011;356(18): 1713-1725.
2. Cosnes J, Gower-Rousseau C, Seksik P, Cortot A. Epidemiology and natural history of inflammatory bowel diseases. *Gastroenterology* 2011;140:1786-1795.
3. Molodecky NA, Soon IS, Rabi DM, et al. Increasing incidence and prevalence of the inflammatory bowel diseases with time, based on systematic review. *Gastroenterology* 2012;142:46-54.
4. Gerseman M, Wehkamp J, Strange EF. Innate immune dysfunction in inflammatory bowel disease. *J Intern Med* 2012;271:421-428.
5. Scharl M, Rogler G. Inflammatory bowel disease pathogenesis: What is new? *Curr Opin Gastroenterol* 2012;28:301-309.
6. Nanau R, Neuman MG. Metabolome and inflammasome in inflammatory bowel disease. *Transl Res* 2012;160:1-28.
7. Norman JM, Handley SA, Baldridge MT, et al. Disease specific alterations in the enteric virome in inflammatory bowel disease. *Cell* 2015;160:447-460.
8. Gentschew L, Ferguson LR. Role of nutrition and microbiota in susceptibility to inflammatory bowel diseases. *Mol Nutr Food Res* 2012;56:524-535.
9. Guo AY, Stevens BW, Wilson RG, et al. Early life environment and natural history of inflammatory bowel disease. *BMC Gastroenterol* 2014;14:216.
10. Murphy SF, Kwon JH, Boone DL. Novel players in inflammatory bowel disease pathogenesis. *Curr Gastroenterol Rep* 2012;14:146-152.
11. Cho JH, Brant SR. Recent insights into the genetics of inflammatory bowel disease. *Gastroenterology* 2011;140:1704-1712.
12. Moller FT, AndersenV, Wohlfahrt J, et al. Familial risk if inflammatory bowel disease: A population-based cohort study 1977-2011. *Am J Gastroenterol* 2015;110:564-571.
13. Neuman MG, Nanau R. Single nucleotide polymorphisms in inflammatory bowel disease. *Transl Res* 2012;160:45-64.

13a. Talley NJ, Abreu MT, Achkar JP, et al. An evidence-based systematic review on medical therapies for inflammatory bowel disease. *Am J Gastroenterol* 2011;106:S2-S25.

14. Di Sabatino A, Biacnheri P, Rovedatti L, MacDonald TT, Corazza GR. Recent advances in understanding ulcerative colitis. *Intern Emerg Med* 2012;7:103-111.
15. Chapman CG, Pekow J. The emerging role of miRNAs in inflammatory bowel disease: A review. *Ther Adv Gastroenterol* 2015;8(1):4-22.

16. Hamilton MJ, Snapper SB, Blumberg RS. Update on biologic pathways in inflammatory bowel disease and their therapeutic relevance. *J Gastroenterol* 2012;47:1-8.
17. Andrews JM, Holtmann G. Stress causes flares of IBD—Much evidence is enough? *Nat Rev Gastroenterol Hepatol* 2011;8:13-14.
18. Rampton DS. The influence of stress on the development and severity of immune mediated diseases. *J Rheumatol* 2011;38(Suppl 88):43-47.
19. Rampton DS. Does stress influence inflammatory bowel disease? The clinical data. *Dig Dis* 2009;27(Suppl 1):76-79.
20. Camara RJ, Schoepfer AM, Pittet V, Begre S, von Kanel R, Swiss Inflammatory Bowel Disease Cohort Study (SIBDCS) Group. Mood and nonmood components of perceived stress and exacerbation of Crohn's disease. *Inflamm Bowel Dis* 2011;17(11):2358-2365.
21. Singh S, Blanchard A, Walker JR, Graff LA, Miller N, Bernstein CN. Common symptoms and stressors among individuals with inflammatory bowel diseases. *Clin Gastroenterol Hepatol* 2011;9(9): 769-775.
22. Graff LA, Walker JR, Clara I, Lix L, Miller N, Rogala L. Stress coping, distress, and health perceptions in inflammatory bowel disease and community controls. *Am J Gastroenterol* 2009;104(12):2959-2969.
23. Boye B, Lundin KE, Jantschek G, et al. INSPIRE study: Does stress management improve the course of inflammatory bowel disease and disease-specific quality of life in distressed patients with ulcerative colitis or Crohn's disease? A randomized controlled trial. *Inflamm Bowel Dis* 2011;17(9):1863-1873.
24. Savard J, Woodgate R. Young peoples' experience of living with ulcerative colitis and an ostomy. *Gastroenterol Nurs* 2009;32(1): 33-41.
25. Neuman MG, Nanau RM. Inflammatory bowel disease: Role of diet, microbiota, life style. *Transl Res* 2012;160:29-44.
26. Albenberg LG, Lewis JD, Wu GD. Food and gut microbiotica in inflammatory bowel disease: A critical connection. *Curr Opin Gastroenterol* 2012;28:314-320.
27. Monteleone I, MacDonald TT, Pallone F, Monteleone G. The aryl hydrocarbon receptor in inflammatory bowel disease: Linking environment to disease pathogenesis. *Curr Opin Gastroenterol* 2012;28:310-313.
28. Palmer MT, Weaver CT. Linking vitamin D deficiency to inflammatory bowel disease. *Inflamm Bowel Dis* 2013;19:2245-2256.
29. McGrath J, McDonald JWD, MacDonald JK. Transdermal nicotine for induction of remission in ulcerative colitis. *Cochrane Database Syst Rev* 2004;(4):CD004722. doi:10.1002/14651858.CD004722.pub2.
30. Ananthakrishnan AN, Higuchi LM, Huang ES, et al. Aspirin, nonsteroidal anti-inflammatory drug use, and risk for Crohn disease and ulcerative colitis. *Ann Intern Med* 2012;156:350-359.
31. Singh S, Graff LA, Bernstein CN. Do NSAIDs, antibiotics, infections, or stress trigger flares in IBD? *Am J Gastroenterol* 2009;104: 1298-1313.
32. Crockett SD, Porter CQ, Martin CF, Sandler RS, Kappelman MD. Isotretinoin use and the risk of inflammatory bowel disease: A case-control study. *Am J Gastroenterol* 2010;105(9):1986-1993.
33. Kornbluth A, Sachar DB. Ulcerative practice guidelines in adults: American College of Gastroenterology, Practice Parameters Committee. *Am J Gastroenterol* 2010;105:501-523.
34. Auten DM, Baumgart DC. Toxic Megacolon. *Inflamm Bowel Dis* 2012;18:584-591.
35. Velayos F. Managing risks of neoplasia in inflammatory bowel disease. *Curr Gastroenterol Rep* 2012;14:174-180.
36. Farraye FA, Odze RD, Eaden J, Itzkowitz SH. AGA technical review on the diagnosis and management of colorectal neoplasia in inflammatory bowel disease. *Gastroenterology* 2010;138(2):746-774.
37. Lichtenstein GR, Hanauer SB, Sandborn WJ, The Practice Parameters Committee of the American College of Gastroenterology. Management of Crohn's disease in adults. *Am J Gastroenterol* 2009;104:465-483.
38. Buchner AM, Blonski W, Lichtenstein GR. Update on the management of Crohn's disease. *Curr Gastroenterol Rep* 2011;3: 465-474.
39. Hartman C, Eliakim R, Shamir R. Nutritional status and nutritional therapy in inflammatory bowel diseases. *World J Gastroenterol* 2009;15:2570-2578.
40. Hwang C, Ross V, Mahadevan U. Micronutrient deficiencies in inflammatory bowel disease: From A to zinc. *Inflamm Bowel Dis* 2012;18:1961-1981.
41. Navaneethan U, Shen B. Hepatopancreatobiliary manifestations and complications associated with inflammatory bowel disease. *Inflamm Bowel Dis* 2010;16(9):1598-1619.
42. Larsen S, Bendtzen K, Nielsen OH. Extraintestinal manifestations of inflammatory bowel disease: Epidemiology, diagnosis, and management. *Ann Med* 2010;42(2):97-114.
43. Murthy SK, Nguyen CG. Venous thromboembolism in inflammatory bowel disease: An epidemiological review. *Am J Gastroenterol* 2011;106:713-718.
44. American Gastroenterological Association medical position statement: Guidelines on osteoporosis in gastrointestinal diseases. *Gastroenterology* 2003;124:791-794.
45. Travis SPL, Higgins PDR, Orchard T, et al. Review article: Defining remission in ulcerative colitis. *Aliment Pharmacol Ther* 2011;34: 113-124.
46. Cottone M, Renna S, Orlando A, Mocciaro F. Medical management of Crohn's disease. *Expert Opin Pharmacother* 2011;12(16): 2505-2525.
47. AGA Institute Guidelines for the Identification, Assessment and Initial Medical Treatment in Crohn's Disease Clinical Decision Support Tool. Available at: http://campaigns.gastro.org/algorithms/IBDCarePathway/. (Accessed October 12, 2015)
48. Pineton de Chambrun G, Lemann M, Peyrin-Biroule L. Clinical implications of mucosal healing for the management of IBD. *Nat Rev Gastroenterol Hepatol* 2010;7:15-29.
49. Flynn A, Kane S. Mucosal healing in Crohn's disease and ulcerative colitis: What does it tell us? *Curr Opin Gastroenterol* 2011;27: 342-345.
50. Forbes A, Goldesgeyme E, Paulon E. Nutrition in inflammatory bowel disease. *J Parenter Enteral Nutr* 2011;35:571-580.
51. Bitton A, Buie D, Enns R, et al. Treatment of hospitalized adult patients with severe ulcerative colitis: Toronto consensus statements. *Am J Gastroenterol* 2012;107:179-194.
52. Meijer BJ, Dieleman LA. Probiotics in the treatment of human inflammatory bowel diseases update 2011. *J Clin Gastroenterol* 2011;45:S139-S144.
53. Cain AM, Dowhower Karpa K. Clinical utility of probiotics in inflammatory bowel disease. *Altern Ther Health Med* 2011;17(l): 72-79.
54. Jonkers D, Penders J, Masclee A, Pierik M. Probiotics in the management of inflammatory bowel disease: A systematic review of intervention studies in adult patients. *Drugs* 2012;72(6):803-823.
55. Shen J, Zuo Z, Mao A. Effect of Probiotics on Inducing Remission and Maintaining Therapy in Ulcerative Colitis, Crohn's Disease, and Pouchitis: Meta-analysis of Randomized Controlled Trials. *Inflamm Bowel Dis* 2014;20:21-35.
56. Prantera C, Scribano ML. Antibiotics and probiotics in inflammatory bowel disease: Why, when, and how. *Curr Opin Gastroenterol* 2009;25:329-333.
57. Beneficial effects of Probiotics, prebiotics, synbiotics, and psychobiotics in inflammatory bowel disease. *Inflamm Bowel Dis* 2015;21;1674-1682.
58. Bernstein CN. Treatment of IBD: Where we are and where we are going. *Am J Gastroenterol* 2015;110:114-126.
59. Biondi A, Zoccali M, Costa S, Troci A, Contessini-Avesani E, Fichera A. Surgical treatment of ulcerative colitis in the biologic therapy era. *World J Gastroenterol* 2012;18(16):1861-1870.
60. Campregher C, Gasche C. Aminosalicylates. *Best Pract Res Clin Gastroenterol* 2011;25:535-546.
61. Tindall WN. New approaches to adherence issues when dosing oral aminosalicylates in ulcerative colitis. *Am J Health Syst Pharm* 2009;66:451-457.
62. Oliveira L, Cohen RD. Maintaining remission in ulcerative colitis—Role of once daily extended-release mesalamine. *Drug Des Dev Ther* 2011;5:111-116.
63. Yang LPH, McCormack PL. MMX mesalamine: A review of its use in the management of mild to moderate ulcerative colitis. *Drugs* 2011;71(2):221-235.
64. Cohen RD, Dalal SR. Systematic review: Rectal therapies for the treatment of distal forms of ulcerative colitis. *Inflamm Bowel Dis* 2015;21:1719-1736.
65. Ford AC, Khan KJ, Achkar JP, Moayyedi P. Efficacy of oral vs. topical, or combined oral and topical 5-aminosalicylates, in ulcerative colitis: Systematic review and meta-analysis. *Am J Gastroenterol* 2012;107:167-176.
66. Ford AC, Bernstein CN, Khan KJ, et al. Glucocorticosteroid therapy in inflammatory bowel disease: Systematic review and meta-analysis. *Am J Gastroenterol* 2011;106:590-599.
67. Khan KJ, Dubinsky MC, Ford AC, Ullman TA, Talley NJ, Moayyedi P. Efficacy of immunosuppressive therapy for inflammatory bowel

disease: A systematic review and meta-analysis. *Am J Gastroenterol* 2011;106:630-642.

68. Louis E, Irving P, Beaugerie L. Use of azathioprine in IBD: Modern aspects of an old drug. *Gut* 2014;63(11):1695-1699.
69. Cohen BL, Torres J, Colombel JF. Immunosuppression in inflammatory bowel disease: How much is too much? *Curr Opin Gastroenterol* 2012;28:341-348.
70. Burger DC, Travis S. Colon salvage therapy for acute severe colitis: Cyclosporine or infliximab? *Curr Opin Gastroenterol* 2011;27:358-362.
71. Hoentjen F, Sakuraba A, Hanauer S. Update on the management of ulcerative colitis. *Curr Gastroenterol Rep* 2011;13:475-485.
72. McSharry K, Dalzell AM, Leiper K, El-Matary W. Systematic review: The role of tacrolimus in the management of Crohn's disease. *Aliment Pharmacol Ther* 2011;34:1282-1294.
73. Kennedy NA, Kalla R, Warner B, et al. Thiopurine withdrawal during sustained clinical remission in inflammatory bowel disease: Relapse and recapture rates, with predictive factors in 237 patients. *Aliment Pharmacol Ther* 2014;40:1313-1323.
74. Khan KJ, Ullman TA, Ford AC, et al. Antibiotic therapy in inflammatory bowel disease: A systematic review and meta-analysis. *Am J Gastroenterol* 2011;106:661-673.
75. Ford AC, Sandborn WJ, Khan KJ, Hanauer SB, Talley NJ, Moayyedi P. Efficacy of biological therapies in inflammatory bowel disease: Systematic review and meta-analysis. *Am J Gastroenterol* 2011;106:644-659.
76. Blonski W, Buchner AM, Lichtenstein GR. Inflammatory bowel disease therapy: Current state-of-the-art. *Curr Opin Gastroenterol* 2011;27:346-357.
77. Cote-Daigneault J, Bouin M, Lahaie R, et al. Biologics in inflammatory bowel disease: what are the data? *Un Eur Gastroenterol J* 2015;0(0):1-10.
78. Narula N, Fine M, Colombe JF, et al. Systematic review: Sequential rescue therapy in severe ulcerative colitis: Do the benefits outweigh the risks? *Inflamm Bowel Dis* 2015;21:1683-1694.
79. Ford AC, Ackhar AC, Khan KJ, et al. Efficacy of 5-aminosalicylates in ulcerative colitis: Systematic review and meta-analysis. *Am J Gastroenterol* 2011;106:601-616.
80. Peyrin-Biroulet L, Lémann M. Review article: Remission rates achievable by current therapies for inflammatory bowel disease. *Aliment Pharmacol Ther* 2011;33:870-879.
81. Zhu Y, Tang R, Zhao P, Zhu S, Li Y, Li J. Can oral 5-aminosalicylic acid be administered once daily in the treatment of mild-to-moderate ulcerative colitis? A meta-analysis of randomized-controlled trials. *Eur J Gastroenterol Hepatol* 2012;24:487-494.
82. Cheifetz AS, Stern J, Garud S, et al. Cyclosporine is safe and effective in patients with severe ulcerative colitis. *J Clin Gastroenterol* 2011;45:107-112.
83. Miao XP, Li JS, Ouyang Q, Hu RW, Zhang Y, Li HY. Tolerability of selective cyclooxygenase 2 inhibitors used for the treatment of rheumatological manifestations of inflammatory bowel disease. *Cochrane Database of Syst Rev* 2014;(10):CD007744. doi: 10.1002/14651858.CD007744.pub2.
84. Ford AC, Khan KK, Talley NJ, Moayyedi P. 5-Aminosalicylates prevent relapse of Crohn's disease after surgically induced remission: Systematic review and meta-analysis. *Am J Gastroenterol* 2011;106:413-420.
85. Ford AC, Kane SV, Khan KJ, Achkar AJ, Talley NJ, Marshall JK. Efficacy of 5-aminosalicylates in Crohn's disease: Systematic review and meta-analysis. *Am J Gastroenterol* 2011;106:617-629.
86. Moja L, Danese S, Fiorino C, et al. Systematic review with network meta-analysis: comparative efficacy and safety of budesonide and mesalazine (mesalamine) for Crohn's disease. *Aliment Pharmacol Ther* 2015;41:1055-1065.
87. Gecse KB, Bemelman W, Kamm MA, et al. A global consensus on the classification, diagnosis and multidisciplinary treatment of perianal fistulising Crohn's disease. *Gut* 2014;63:1381-1392.
88. Terdiman JP, Gruss CB, Heidelbaugh JJ, et al. American Gastroenterological Association Institute guideline on the use of thiopurines, methotrexate, and anti-TNF-α biologic drugs for the induction and maintenance of remission in Crohn's disease. *Gastroenterology* 2013;145:1459-63.
89. Stidham RW, Lee THC, Higgens PDR, et al. Systematic review with network meta-analysis: The efficacy of anti-TNF agents for the treatment of Crohn's disease. *Aliment Pharmacol Ther* 2014;39:1349-1362.
90. Colombel J-F, Sandborn WJ, Reinisch W, et al. Infliximab, azathioprine, or combination therapy for Crohn's disease. *N Engl J Med* 2010;362:1383-1395.
91. Akobeng AA, Sandborn WJ, Bickston SJ, et al. Tumor necrosis factor-alpha antagonists twenty years later: What do cochrane reviews tell us? *Inflamm Bowel Dis* 2014;20:2132-2141.
92. Beniwal-Patel P, Saha S. The role of integrin antagonists in the treatment of inflammatory bowel disease. *Expert Opin Biol Ther* 2014;14:1815-1823.
93. Nakase H, Yoshino T, Matsuura M. Role in calcineurin inhibitors for inflammatory bowel disease in the biologics era: When and how to use. *Inflamm Bowel Dis* 2014;20:2151-2156.
94. Dubinsky M, Abraham B, Mahadevan U. Management of the pregnant IBD patient. *Inflamm Bowel Dis* 2008;14:1736-1750.
95. Habal FM, Huang VW. Review article: A decision-making algorithm for the management of pregnancy in the inflammatory bowel disease patient. *Aliment Pharmacol Ther* 2012;35:501-515.
96. Boyd HA, Basit S, Harpsoe MC, et al. Inflammatory bowel disease and risk of adverse pregnancy outcomes. *PLoS One* 2015;10(6): e0129567. doi:10.1371/journal.pone.0129567.
97. Nasef NA, Ferguson LR. Inflammatory bowel disease and pregnancy: Overlapping pathways. *Transl Res* 2012;160:65-83.
98. Beaulieu DB, Kane S. Inflammatory bowel disease in pregnancy. *Gastroenterol Clin North Am* 2011;40:399-413.
99. van Mahade U, Cucchiara S, Hyams JS, et al. The London Position Statement of the World Congress of Gastroenterology on Biological Therapy for IBD with the European Crohn's and Colitis Organization: Pregnancy and pediatrics. *Am J Gastroenterol* 2011;106:214-223.
100. Sands K, Jansen R, Zaslau, et al. Review article: The safety of therapeutic drugs in male inflammatory bowel disease patients wishing to conceive. *Aliment Pharmacol Ther* 2015;41:821-834.
101. Thomas A, Lohida N. Advanced Therapy for Inflammatory Bowel Disease: A Guide for the Primary Care Physician. *J Am Board Fam Med* 2014;27:411-420.
102. Relling MV, Gardner EE, Sandborn WJ, et al. Clinical pharmacogenetics implementation consortium guidelines for thiopurine methyltransferase genotype and thiopurine dosing: 2013 update. *Clin Pharmacol Ther* 2013;93(4):324-325.
103. Kotlyar DS, Osterman MT, Diamond RH, et al. A systematic review of factors that contribute to hepatosplenic T-cell lymphoma in patients with inflammatory bowel disease. *Clin Gastroenterol Hepatol* 2011;9:36-41.e1.
104. Andersen NN, Pasternak B, Basit S, et al. Association between tumor necrosis factor-α antagonists and risk of cancer in patients with inflammatory bowel disease. *JAMA* 2014;311(23):2406-2413.
105. Connor V. Anti-TNF therapies: A comprehensive analysis of adverse effects associated with immunosuppression. *Rheumatol Int* 2011;31:327-337.
106. Yarur AJ, Rubin DT. Therapeutic drug monitoring of anti-tumor necrosis factor agents in patients with inflammatory bowel disease. *Inflamm Bowel Dis* 2015;21:1709-1718.
107. Grijalva CG, Chen L, Delzell E, et al. Initiation of tumor necrosis factor antagonists and the risk of hospitalization for infection in patients with autoimmune diseases. *JAMA* 2011;306(21):2331-2339.

35

Nausea and Vomiting

Leigh Anne Hylton Gravatt, Krista L. Donohoe, and Cecily V. DiPiro

KEY CONCEPTS

1. Nausea and/or vomiting is often a part of the symptom complex for a variety of gastrointestinal (GI), cardiovascular, infectious, neurologic, metabolic, or psychogenic processes.
2. Nausea or vomiting is caused by a variety of medications or other noxious agents.
3. The overall goal of treatment should be to prevent or eliminate nausea and vomiting regardless of etiology.
4. Treatment options for nausea and vomiting include drug and non-drug modalities such as relaxation, biofeedback, and self-hypnosis.
5. The primary goal with chemotherapy-induced nausea and vomiting (CINV) is to prevent nausea and/or vomiting and the emetic risk of the chemotherapeutic regimen is a major factor to consider when selecting a prophylactic regimen.
6. Patients at high risk of vomiting should receive prophylactic antiemetics for postoperative nausea and vomiting (PONV).
7. Patients undergoing radiation therapy (RT) to the upper abdomen or receiving total or hemibody irradiation should receive prophylactic antiemetics for radiation-induced nausea and vomiting (RINV).
8. Beneficial therapy for patients with balance disorders can most reliably be found among the antihistaminic–anticholinergic agents.

Nausea and vomiting are common complaints from individuals of all ages. Management can be simple or detailed and complex, depending on the etiology. This chapter provides an overview of nausea and vomiting, two multifaceted problems.

Nausea is defined as the inclination to vomit or as a feeling in the throat or epigastric region alerting an individual that vomiting is imminent. Vomiting is the ejection or expulsion of gastric contents through the mouth and is often a forceful event. Either condition may occur transiently with no other associated signs or symptoms; however, these conditions also may be only part of a more complex clinical presentation.

ETIOLOGY

(1) Nausea and vomiting may be associated with a variety of conditions, including gastrointestinal (GI), cardiovascular, infectious, neurologic, or metabolic disease processes. Nausea and vomiting may be a feature of such conditions as pregnancy, or may follow operative procedures or administration of certain medications, such as those used in cancer chemotherapy. Psychogenic etiologies of these symptoms may be present. Anticipatory etiologies may be involved, such as in patients who have previously received cytotoxic chemotherapy. Table 35-1 lists specific etiologies associated with nausea and vomiting.[1]

The etiology of nausea and vomiting may vary with the age of the patient. For example, vomiting in the newborn during the first day of life suggests upper digestive tract obstruction or an increase in intracranial pressure. (2) Drug-induced nausea and vomiting are of particular concern, especially with the increasing number of patients receiving cytotoxic treatment. A four-level classification system defines the risk for emesis with agents used in oncology (Table 35-2).[2] Although some agents may have greater emetic risk than others, combinations of agents, high doses, clinical settings, psychological conditions, prior treatment experiences, and unusual stimulus of sight, smell, or taste may alter a patient's response to drug treatment. In this setting, nausea and vomiting may be unavoidable and some patients experience these problems so intensely that chemotherapy is postponed or discontinued.

PATHOPHYSIOLOGY

The three consecutive phases of emesis include nausea, retching, and vomiting. Nausea, the imminent need to vomit, may be considered a separate and singular symptom. Retching is the labored movement of abdominal and thoracic muscles before vomiting. The final phase of emesis is vomiting, the forceful expulsion of gastric contents caused by GI retroperistalsis. The act of vomiting requires the coordinated contractions of the abdominal muscles, pylorus, and antrum, a raised gastric cardia, diminished lower esophageal sphincter pressure, and esophageal dilation.[1] Vomiting should not be confused with regurgitation, an act in which the gastric or esophageal contents rise to the pharynx but is not usually associated with forceful ejection seen with vomiting. Accompanying autonomic symptoms of pallor, tachycardia, and diaphoresis account for many of the distressing feelings associated with emesis.

Vomiting is triggered by afferent impulses to the vomiting center (VC), a nucleus of cells in the medulla. Impulses are received from sensory centers, which include the chemoreceptor trigger zone (CTZ), cerebral cortex, and visceral afferents from the pharynx and GI tract. The VC integrates the afferent impulses, resulting in efferent impulses to the salivation center, respiratory center, and the pharyngeal, GI, and abdominal muscles, leading to vomiting.

The CTZ, located in the area postrema of the fourth ventricle of the brain, is a major chemosensory organ for emesis and is usually associated with chemically induced vomiting. Because of its location, bloodborne and cerebrospinal fluid toxins have easy access to the CTZ. Cytotoxic agents primarily stimulate this area rather than the cerebral cortex and visceral afferents. Similarly, pregnancy-associated vomiting probably occurs through stimulation of the CTZ.

Numerous neurotransmitter receptors are located in the VC, CTZ, and GI tract, including cholinergic, histaminic, dopaminergic, opiate, serotonergic, neurokinin (NK), and benzodiazepine receptors. Chemotherapeutic agents, their metabolites, or other emetic compounds theoretically trigger the process of emesis through stimulation of one or more of these receptors. Antiemetics have been developed to antagonize or block these emetogenic receptors.

TABLE 35-1 Specific Etiologies of Nausea and Vomiting

GI mechanisms
Mechanical obstruction
Gastric outlet obstruction
Small bowel obstruction
Functional GI disorders
Gastroparesis
Nonulcer dyspepsia
Chronic intestinal pseudoobstruction
Irritable bowel syndrome
Organic GI disorders
Peptic ulcer disease
Pancreatitis
Pyelonephritis
Cholecystitis
Cholangitis
Hepatitis
Acute gastroenteritis
Viral
Bacterial
Cardiovascular diseases
Acute myocardial infarction
Congestive heart failure
Radio-frequency ablation
Neurologic processes
Increased intracranial pressure
Migraine headache
Vestibular disorders
Metabolic disorders
Diabetes mellitus (diabetic ketoacidosis)
Addison's disease
Renal disease (uremia)
Psychiatric causes
Psychogenic vomiting
Anxiety disorders
Anorexia nervosa
Therapy-induced causes
Cytotoxic chemotherapy
Radiation therapy
Theophylline preparations
Anticonvulsant preparations
Digitalis preparations
Opiates
Antibiotics
Volatile general anesthetics
Drug withdrawal
Opiates
Benzodiazepines
Miscellaneous causes
Pregnancy
Noxious odors
Operative procedures

Adapted from reference 1.

CLINICAL PRESENTATION

Nausea and vomiting are commonly seen in many clinical situations. Patients may present in varying degrees of distress summarized in Table 35-3 as *simple* or *complex* in presentation.

TREATMENT

Desired Outcomes

3 The overall goal of antiemetic therapy is to prevent or eliminate nausea and vomiting. This should be accomplished without adverse effects or with clinically acceptable adverse effects. In addition to these clinical goals, appropriate cost issues should be considered, particularly in the management of chemotherapy-induced nausea and vomiting (CINV) and postoperative nausea and vomiting (PONV).

General Approach to Treatment

4 Treatment options include drug and non-drug modalities such as relaxation, biofeedback, and self-hypnosis. Initially patients may choose to not treat or to self-medicate with nonprescription drugs. As symptoms become worse or are associated with more serious medical problems, patients are more likely to utilize prescription antiemetic drugs. When prescribed and used appropriately, these agents can provide relief; however, some patients will never be totally free of symptoms. This lack of relief is most disabling when it is associated with an unresolved medical problem or when the necessary therapy for this condition is the cause of the nausea or vomiting, as in the case of patients who are receiving chemotherapy of moderate or high emetic risk.

Nonpharmacologic Management

Nonpharmacologic management of nausea and vomiting involves dietary, physical, or psychological strategies that are consistent with the etiology of nausea and vomiting. For patients who are suffering due to excessive or disagreeable food or beverage consumption, avoidance or moderation in dietary intake may be lead to symptom resolution. Patients suffering symptoms of systemic illness may quickly improve as their underlying condition resolves. Finally, patients in whom these symptoms result from labyrinthine changes produced by motion may benefit quickly by assuming a stable physical position.

Nonpharmacologic interventions are classified as behavioral interventions and include relaxation, biofeedback, hypnosis, cognitive distraction, optimism, guided imagery, acupuncture, yoga, and systematic desensitization.[3,4] Some of these modalities, such as with P6 acupuncture bands, have shown to be effective at preventing nausea and vomiting in the surgical population.[5] Other therapies, such as ginger and pyridoxine, are beneficial in specific situations as with chemotherapy-induced nausea and vomiting (CINV) and nausea and vomiting related to pregnancy.

Pharmacologic Therapy

Although many approaches to the treatment of nausea and vomiting have been suggested, antiemetic drugs (nonprescription and prescription) are most often recommended. These agents work in various ways that may be used singularly or in conjunction with each other and represent a number of delivery mechanisms.

Factors that enable the clinician to choose the appropriate regimen include: (a) the suspected etiology of the symptoms; (b) the frequency, duration, and severity of the episodes; (c) the ability of the patient to use oral, rectal, injectable, or transdermal medications; and (d) the success of previous antiemetic medications. Please see Table 35-4 for dosing information of commonly available antiemetic preparations.

The treatment of simple nausea and vomiting often involves self-care from a list of nonprescription products. Both nonprescription and prescription drugs are useful in the treatment of simple nausea and vomiting in small, infrequently administered doses and are associated with minimal side effects. Changes in diet such as restricting oral intake, eating smaller meals, avoiding spicy or fried foods and instead eating bland foods such as with the BRAT diet (Bananas, Rice, Applesauce and Toast) can help alleviate symptoms. As the symptoms persist or become worse, prescription medications may be chosen, either as single-agent therapy or in combination.

The management of complex nausea and vomiting, such as in patients who are receiving cytotoxic chemotherapy, may require initial combination therapy. In combination regimens, the goal is to achieve symptomatic control through administration of agents with different pharmacologic mechanisms of action.

TABLE 35-2 Emetic Risk of Agents Used in Oncology

Emetic Risk (If No Prophylactic Medication Is Administered)	Cytotoxic Agent (in Alphabetical Order)
High (>90%)	Combination of either doxorubicin or epirubicin + cyclophosphamide
	Carmustine
	Cisplatin (>50 mg/m^2)
	Cyclophosphamide (≥1,500 mg/m^2)
	Dacarbazine
	Ifosfamide (>10 g/m^2)
	Mechlorethamine
	Streptozotocin
Moderate (30%-90%)	Aldesleukin (>12-15 million units/m^2)
	Amifostine (>300 mg/m^2)
	Arsenic trioxide
	Azacitidine
	Bendamustine
	Busulfan
	Carboplatin
	Cisplatin (<50 mg/m^2)
	Clofarabine
	Cytarabine (>200 mg/m^2)
	Cyclophosphamide (<1,500 mg/m^2)
	Daunorubicin
	Dactinomycin
	Doxorubicin
	Epirubicin
	Idarubicin
	Ifosfamide
	Interferon alfa (10 million units/m^2)
	Irinotecan
	Melphalan
	Methotrexate (>250 mg/m^2)
	Oxaliplatin
	Procarbazine
	Temozolomide
Low (10%-30%)	Cabazitaxel
	Capecitabine
	Cetuximab
	Cytarabine (≤200 mg/m^2)
	Docetaxel
	Eribulin
	Erlotinib
	Etoposide
	Floxuridine
Low (10%-30%) (Continued)	Fluorouracil
	Gemcitabine
	Interferon alfa (<10 million units/m^2)
	Ixabepilone
	Lapatinib
	Methotrexate (<250 mg/m^2)
	Mitomycin
	Mitoxantrone
	Paclitaxel
	Paclitaxel albumin
	Pemetrexed
	Pentostatin
	Romidepsin
	Sorafenib
	Sunitinib
	Thiotepa
	Topotecan
	Trastuzumab
Minimal (<10%)	Alemtuzumab
	Asparaginase
	Bevacizumab
	Bleomycin
	Bortezomib
	Cladribine
	Cytarabine (<200 mg/m^2)
	Decitabine
	Denileukin diftitox
	Dexrazoxane
	Fludarabine
	Ipilimumab
	Nelarabine
	Ofatumumab
	Panitumumab
	PEG-asparaginase
	Rituximab
	Temsirolimus
	Trastuzumab
	Valrubicin
	Vinblastine
	Vincristine
	Vinorelbine

Data from references 2 and 30.

TABLE 35-3 Clinical Presentation of Nausea and Vomiting

General

Depending on severity of symptoms, patients may present in mild to severe distress

Symptoms

Simple: Self-limiting, resolves spontaneously, and requires only symptomatic therapy

Complex: Not relieved after administration of antiemetics; progressive deterioration of patient secondary to fluid-electrolyte imbalances; usually associated with noxious agents or psychogenic events

Signs

Simple: Patient complaint of queasiness or discomfort

Complex: Weight loss; fever; abdominal pain

Laboratory tests

Simple: None

Complex: Serum electrolyte concentrations; upper/lower GI evaluation

Other information

Fluid input and output

Medication history

Recent history of behavioral or visual changes, headache, pain, or stress

Family history positive for psychogenic vomiting

Antacids

Patients who are experiencing simple nausea and vomiting may initially use antacids, as many of these products are readily available without a prescription. In this setting, single or combination products, especially those containing magnesium hydroxide, aluminum hydroxide, and/or calcium carbonate, may provide rapid relief, primarily through gastric acid neutralization. These agents are most effective for those with symptoms related to acid reflux or heartburn and must be used with caution in those who experience acute or chronic kidney disease due to the risk of accumulation. These agents may exacerbate other GI complaints that accompany nausea and vomiting, such as diarrhea or constipation, so attention must be paid to which of these agents may worsen these other conditions.

Antihistamine–Anticholinergic Drugs

Antiemetic drugs from the antihistaminic–anticholinergic category work on muscarinic and histamine receptors in the VC and the vestibular system that stimulates nausea and vomiting. As such, these agents are frequently initiated as self-care to prevent nausea and vomiting associated with motion disturbances such as vertigo and motion sickness.

TABLE 35-4 Common Antiemetic Preparations and Adult Dosage Regimens

Drug	Adult Dosage Regimen	Dosage Form/ Route	Availability	Adverse Drug Reactions	Monitoring Parameters	Comments
Antacids						
Antacids (various)	15-30 mL every 2-4 hours prn	Liquid/oral	OTC	Magnesium products: diarrhea Aluminum or calcium products: constipation	Assess for symptom relief	Useful with simple nausea/vomiting
Antihistaminic–Anticholinergic Agents						
Dimenhydrinate (Dramamine)	50-100 mg every 4-6 hours prn	Tab, chew tab, cap	OTC	Drowsiness, confusion, blurred vision, dry mouth, urinary retention	Assess for episodic relief of motion sickness or nausea/ vomiting	Especially problematic in the elderly Increased risk of complications in patients with BPH, narrow angle glaucoma, or asthma
Diphenhydramine (Benadryl)	25-50 mg every 4-6 hours prn 10-50 mg every 2-4 hours prn	Tab, cap, liquid IM, IV	Rx/OTC			
Hydroxyzine (Vistaril, Atarax)	25-100 mg every 4-6 hours prn	IM (unlabeled use)	Rx			
Meclizine (Bonine, Antivert)	12.5-25 mg 1 hour before travel; repeat every 12-24 hours prn	Tab, chew tab	Rx/OTC			
Scopolamine (Transderm Scop)	1.5 mg every 72 hours	Transdermal patch	Rx			
Trimethobenzamide (Tigan)	300 mg three to four times daily 200 mg three to four times daily	Cap IM	Rx			
Benzodiazepines						
Alprazolam (Xanax)	0.5-2 mg three times daily prior to chemotherapy	Tab	Rx (C-IV)	Dizziness, sedation, appetite changes, memory impairment	Assess for episodes of ANV	Place in therapy: ANV
Lorazepam (Ativan)	0.5-2 mg on night before and morning of chemotherapy	Tab	Rx (C-IV)			
Butyrophenones						
Haloperidol (Haldol)	1-5 mg every 12 hours prn	Tab, liquid, IM, IV	Rx	Sedation, constipation, hypotension	Observe for additive sedation especially if used with narcotic analgesics	Place in therapy: palliative care
Droperidol (Inapsine)[a]	2.5 mg; additional 1.25 mg may be given	IM, IV	Rx	QT prolongation and/or torsade de pointes	12-Lead electrocardiogram prior to administration, followed by cardiac monitoring for 2-3 hours after administration	Limited use outside of clinical trials
Cannabinoids						
Dronabinol (Marinol)	5-15 mg/m² every 2-4 hours prn	Cap	Rx (C-III)	Euphoria, somnolence, xerostomia	Assess for symptom relief	May be useful with refractory CINV
Nabilone (Cesamet)	1-2 mg twice daily	Cap	Rx (C-II)	Somnolence, vertigo, xerostomia		
Corticosteroids						
Dexamethasone	See Table 35-6 for CINV dosing and Table 35-8 for PONV dosing	Tab, IV	Rx	Insomnia, GI symptoms, agitation, appetite stimulation	Assess for efficacy as prophylactic agent: episodes of nausea/ vomiting and hydration status	Useful as single-agent or combination therapy for prophylaxis of CINV and PONV

(Continued)

TABLE 35-4 Common Antiemetic Preparations and Adult Dosage Regimens (*Continued*)

Drug	Adult Dosage Regimen	Dosage Form/ Route	Availability	Adverse Drug Reactions	Monitoring Parameters	Comments
Histamine (H2) Antagonists						
Cimetidine (Tagamet HB)	200 mg twice daily prn	Tab	OTC	Headache	Assess for symptom relief	Useful when nausea due to heartburn or GERD
Famotidine (Pepcid AC)	10 mg twice daily prn	Tab	OTC	Constipation, diarrhea		
Nizatidine (Axid AR)	75 mg twice daily prn	Tab	OTC	Diarrhea, headache		
Ranitidine (Zantac 75)	75 mg twice daily prn	Tab	OTC	Constipation, diarrhea		
5-Hydroxytryptamine-3 Receptor Antagonists						
	See Table 35-6 for CINV dosing and Table 35-8 for PONV dosing	Tab, IV	Rx	Asthenia, constipation, headache	Assess for efficacy as prophylactic agent: episodes of nausea/ vomiting and hydration status	Useful as single-agent or combination therapy for prophylaxis of CINV and PONV
Miscellaneous Agents						
Metoclopramide (Reglan)	10 mg four times daily	Tab	Rx	Asthenia, headache, somnolence	Assess for symptom relief	Prokinetic activity useful in diabetic gastroparesis
Olanzapine (Zyprexa)	2.5-5 mg twice daily	Tab	Rx	Sedation	Assess for decrease in episodes of nausea/ vomiting	Use with caution in elderly. May be useful in breakthrough CINV
Phenothiazines						
Chlorpromazine (Thorazine)	10-25 mg every 4-6 hours prn	Tab, liquid	Rx	Constipation, dizziness, tachycardia, tardive dyskinesia	Assess for decrease in episodes of nausea/ vomiting	Useful with simple nausea/vomiting
	25-50 mg every 4-6 hours prn	IM, IV		See above		
Prochlorperazine (Compazine)	5-10 mg three to four times daily prn	Tab, liquid	Rx	Prolonged QT interval, sedation, tardive dyskinesia	Assess for decrease in episodes of nausea/ vomiting	Useful with simple nausea/ vomiting and for breakthrough CINV
	5-10 mg every 3-4 hours prn	IM				
	2.5-10 mg every 3-4 hours prn	IV	Rx			
	25 mg twice daily prn	Supp	Rx			
Promethazine (Phenergan)	12.5-25 mg every 4-6 hours prn	Tab, liquid, IM, IV, supp	Rx	Drowsiness, sedation	Assess for decreased nausea/vomiting episodes and improvement in hydration status	
Substance P/Neurokinin 1 Receptor Antagonist						
Aprepitant	See Table 35-6 for CINV dosing and Table 35-8 for PONV dosing	Cap, IV	Rx	Constipation, diarrhea, headache, hiccups	Assess for efficacy as prophylactic agent: episodes of nausea/ vomiting and hydration status	Useful in combination therapy for prophylaxis of CINV and PONV
Fosaprepitant		IV	Rx			
Netupitant/ palonosetron		Cap	Rx	Same as above plus dyspepsia and fatigue		
Rolapitant		Cap	Rx			Long half-life and no drug interactions

ANV, anticipatory nausea and vomiting; C-II, C-III, and C-IV, controlled substance schedule 2, 3, and 4, respectively; cap, capsule; chew tab, chewable tablet; CINV, chemotherapy-induced nausea and vomiting; GERD, gastroesophageal reflux disease; liquid, oral syrup, concentrate, or suspension; OTC, nonprescription; PONV, postoperative nausea and vomiting; Rx, prescription; supp, rectal suppository; tab, tablet.

[a]See text for current warnings.

Benzodiazepines

Benzodiazepines are relatively weak antiemetics and are primarily used for their anxiolytic activity to prevent anxiety or anticipatory nausea and vomiting (ANV) that is common in patients receiving highly emetogenic chemotherapy. Either agent, alprazolam, or lorazepam, may be used as adjuncts to other antiemetics in patients treated with cisplatin-containing regimens. Both agents may be used orally, with alprazolam and the sublingual formulation of lorazepam having an onset of action of 60 minutes.

Butyrophenones

Haloperidol and droperidol work to block dopaminergic stimulation of the CTZ, which in turn decreases the incidence of nausea and vomiting. Although each agent is effective in relieving nausea and vomiting, these agents are limited due to their propensity to cause extra-pyramidal symptoms and risk of QTc prolongation. For these reasons, haloperidol is not considered first-line therapy for uncomplicated nausea and vomiting but has been used in palliative care situations.[6] The labeling of droperidol recommends that all patients should undergo a 12-lead electrocardiogram prior to administration, followed by cardiac monitoring for 2 to 3 hours after administration because of the possibility of the development of potentially fatal QT prolongation and/or torsade de pointes.[7] The clinical use of droperidol has effectively ceased outside of clinical trials in anesthesia.

Cannabinoids

Cannabinoids have complex effects on the CNS and their effects at receptors in neural tissues may explain efficacy in CINV. Oral dronabinol and nabilone are therapeutic options when CINV is refractory to other antiemetics. These agents are limited by their route of administration and slow onset of action; however, a newer agent, nabiximol, which is available as a oromucosal spray, is currently being investigated in the prevention of CINV and resolves some of the key limitations of the currently available products.[8] Cannabinoids have the advantage of being effective for other cancer related side effects such as serving as a treatment of cancer related pain and an appetite stimulant.[9-11] Despite these advantages, cannabinoids are not indicated as first-line agents.

Corticosteroids

Corticosteroids have demonstrated antiemetic efficacy since the initial recognition that patients who received prednisone as part of their Hodgkin's disease protocol appeared to develop less nausea and vomiting than did those patients who were treated with protocols that excluded this agent. Methylprednisolone has also been used as a component of an antiemetic regimen, but the majority of trials have studied dexamethasone. The site and mechanism of action of corticosteroids for CINV and PONV is unknown.

Dexamethasone is the most commonly used corticosteroid in the management of CINV and PONV, either as a single agent or in combination with 5-hydroxytryptamine-3 receptor antagonists (5-HT3-RA). Dexamethasone is effective in the prevention of both CINV acute emesis and delayed nausea and vomiting when used alone or in combination.[12,13] Given the risk of corticosteroids such as hyperglycemia, fluid retention and even psychosis, steroids are not indicated for the treatment of simple nausea and vomiting.

H2-Receptor Antagonists (H2RA)

Histamine2-receptor antagonists work by decreasing gastric acid production and are used to manage simple nausea and vomiting associated with heartburn or gastroesophageal reflux. Except for potential drug interactions with cimetidine, these agents cause few side effects when used for episodic relief.

5-Hydroxytryptamine-3 Receptor Antagonists

5-Hydroxytryptamine-3 receptor antagonists block serotonin receptors on sensory vagal fibers in the gut wall, thus blocking the acute phase of CINV. These agents do not completely block the acute phase of CINV and are less efficacious in preventing the delayed phase, but they are considered the standard of care in the management of CINV, PONV, and radiation-induced nausea and vomiting (RINV). Issues involved in the use of dolasetron, granisetron, ondansetron, and palonosetron are reviewed in detail in the sections that follow.

Metoclopramide

Metoclopramide works by blocking dopaminergic receptors centrally in the CTZ. It also increases lower esophageal sphincter tone, aids gastric emptying, and accelerates transit through the small bowel, possibly through the release of acetylcholine. The prokinetic activity of metoclopramide makes it useful in patients with nausea and vomiting associated with diabetic gastroparesis.

Olanzapine

Olanzapine is an antipsychotic that blocks several neurotransmitters including dopamine, serotonin, adrenergic, histamine (H1) and 5-HT3-RA. Use of olanzapine, in combination with palonosetron and dexamethasone, effectively controlled acute and delayed CINV in patients receiving highly emetogenic chemotherapy as compared with aprepitant, palonosetron, and dexamethasone in a randomized, phase 3 clinical trial.[14] It has also been studied as an option for those who have failed their initial antiemetic prophylactic therapy. When compared to metoclopramide, olanzapine had significantly lower nausea or vomiting rates in this population.[15] The National Comprehensive Cancer Network (NCCN) antiemesis practice guideline includes olanzapine as one of many options in patients who experience breakthrough nausea and/or vomiting following prophylaxis for CINV.[16] Sedation, constipation, and restlessness are the most common side effects with olanzapine; it should be used with caution in the elderly.

Phenothiazines

Phenothiazines have been the most widely prescribed antiemetic agents and appear to block dopamine receptors, most likely in the CTZ. They are marketed in an array of dosage forms, none of which appears to be more efficacious than another. These agents may be most practical for long-term treatment and are inexpensive in comparison with newer drugs. Rectal administration is a reasonable alternative in patients in whom oral or parenteral administration is not feasible.

Phenothiazines are most useful in adult patients with simple nausea and vomiting. Intravenously administered prochlorperazine provided quicker and more complete relief with less drowsiness than IV promethazine in adult patients treated in an emergency department for nausea and vomiting associated with uncomplicated gastritis or gastroenteritis.[17]

Neurokinin 1 Receptor Antagonists

Substance P is a peptide neurotransmitter in the NK family whose preferred receptor is the NK1 receptor. The acute phase of CINV is believed to be mediated by both serotonin and substance P, where substance P is believed to be the primary mediator of the delayed phase. Aprepitant and fosaprepitant are the first NK1 receptor antagonists in clinical use; however, newer agents are available such as the new combination NK1 receptor antagonist/5-HT3-RA product, netupitant/palonosetron (NEPA) and the NK1 receptor antagonist, rolapitant.[18]

Agents, such as rolapitant, aprepitant, or fosaprepitant, are used in patients receiving moderate to highly emetogenic chemotherapy as part of a three drug combination consisting of an NK1 receptor antagonist, dexamethasone, and a 5-HT3-RA. This combination is now considered the standard of care for CINV and has shown improved protection from vomiting for up to 5 days after chemotherapy administration as compared with dual therapy of dexamethasone and a 5-HT3-RA inhibitor.[16]

Aprepitant has the potential for numerous drug interactions because it is a substrate, moderate inhibitor, and an inducer of cytochrome isoenzyme CYP3A4 as well as an inducer of CYP2C9. It can increase serum concentrations of many drugs, including many chemotherapeutic agents, metabolized by CYP3A4, including docetaxel, paclitaxel, etoposide, irinotecan, ifosfamide, imatinib, vinorelbine, vincristine, and vinblastine. Other significant drug interactions include decreased effectiveness of oral contraceptives, and a decrease in the international normalized ratio when used with warfarin.[19] The dose of oral dexamethasone should be reduced 50% when coadministered with aprepitant, because of the 2.2-fold increase in observed area under the plasma-concentration-versus-time curve.[20]

Fosaprepitant, an injectable form of aprepitant, has been approved by the FDA as an IV substitute for oral aprepitant on day 1 of the standard 3-day CINV prevention regimen, with oral aprepitant administered on days 2 and 3.[21]

Rolapitant is the newest NK1 receptor antagonist and has the unique advantage over other NK1 receptor antagonist in that it has a significantly longer half-life in comparison with aprepitant, 7 days versus 9 hours. This allows less frequent administration with this drug only being administered in one dose prior to chemotherapy in combination with a 5-HT3-RA and dexamethasone.[18] Another unique advantage of rolapitant is that it has no effects on CYP3A4, which could be useful in those regimens that would otherwise have significant drug interactions with aprepitant.[22]

Netupitant/palonosetron (NEPA) is an oral, coformulated product that when given in just one dose combination with dexamethasone, was superior to a combination regimen of aprepitant, oral palonosetron, and dexamethasone regimen in individuals receiving highly emetogenic chemotherapy. NEPA prevented both acute and delayed nausea and vomiting; this effect was sustained up to 5 days from chemotherapy administration.[23,24] As with aprepitant, it is also a moderate inhibitor of CYP3A4, and also requires a significant decrease in the dexamethasone dose when used together. The most common side effects of NEPA were headache, asthenia, fatigue, and dyspepsia.[25]

CHEMOTHERAPY-INDUCED NAUSEA AND VOMITING

There are five categories of CINV: acute, delayed, anticipatory, breakthrough, and refractory. Nausea and vomiting that occurs within 24 hours of chemotherapy administration is defined as acute CINV, whereas when it starts more than 24 hours after chemotherapy administration, it is defined as delayed CINV.

Nausea or vomiting that occurs prior to receiving chemotherapy is termed anticipatory nausea and vomiting (ANV). ANV is believed to be a learned, conditioned, or psychological response that occurs in about 25% of patients by the fourth cycle of chemotherapy.[26] ANV triggers include tastes, odors, sights, or thoughts associated with chemotherapy. Risk factors associated with ANV include age under 50, nausea and/or vomiting after the previous chemotherapy session, anxiety, sweating and a feeling of warmth after the last chemotherapy cycle, and susceptibility to motion sickness.[27]

In the setting of optimal antiemetic prophylaxis and no prior history of emesis, reported chemotherapy-induced ANV is rare. Use of newer antiemetic regimens appears to have resulted in a decreased rate of ANV.[28]

TABLE 35-5 Non-Chemotherapy Etiologies of Nausea and Vomiting in Cancer Patients

Fluid and electrolyte abnormalities
Hypercalcemia
Volume depletion
Water intoxication
Adrenocortical insufficiency
Drug induced
Opiates
Antibiotics
Antifungals
GI obstruction
Increased intracranial pressure
Peritonitis
Metastases
Brain
Meninges
Hepatic
Uremia
Infections (septicemia, local)
Radiation therapy

Data from reference 26.

Breakthrough nausea and vomiting is defined as emesis occurring despite prophylactic administration of antiemetics and requiring the use of rescue antiemetics. Breakthrough emesis occurs in 10% to 40% treated with modern-day antiemetics.[29]

Refractory nausea and vomiting is evident when there is a poor response to multiple antiemetic regimens. It is also important to rule out other potential causes of nausea and vomiting in the cancer population such as with brain metastases, electrolytes imbalances, infections, uremia, treatment with opioids, anxiety or bowel obstruction.[16]

5 The primary goal with CINV is to prevent nausea and/or vomiting and the emetic risk of the chemotherapeutic regimen is a major factor to consider when selecting a prophylactic regimen.[16]

Clinical practice guidelines for the use of antiemetics in CINV have been published by the NCCN,[16] the Multinational Association of Supportive Care in Cancer/European Society of Oncology (MASCC/ESMO),[30] and the American Society of Clinical Oncology (ASCO).[31] The NCCN guidelines are updated annually, while the ASCO and ESMO guidelines are updated less frequently. Despite the demonstrated improvement in outcomes with the use of these practice guidelines, they are underutilized by a high percentage of practitioners.[30] Furthermore, product availability and recommended doses are often institution-specific and may vary considerably from the doses listed in Table 35-6.

Principles of Antiemetic Use for CINV

The ASCO, MASCC, and NCCN consensus groups share several of the principles listed below that appear to be important for the effective prevention of CINV in adults:[32,33]

1. The primary goal of emesis prevention is no nausea and/or vomiting throughout the period of emetic risk.
2. The duration of emetic risk is 2 days for patients receiving moderately emetogenic chemotherapy and 3 days for highly emetogenic chemotherapy. Emetic prophylaxis should be provided through the entire period of risk.
3. The selection of the antiemetic regimen should be based on the chemotherapy drug with highest emetogenicity (see Table 35-2). Prior emetic experience and patient-specific factors should also be considered.
4. When given in equipotent doses, oral and IV 5-HT3-RAs are equivalent in efficacy.
5. The toxicities of antiemetics should be considered and managed appropriately.

Prophylaxis of Acute CINV

Each of the practice guidelines states that the most effective classes of drugs for the prevention of acute emesis are the 5-HT3-RAs, NK1 receptor antagonists, olanzapine and glucocorticoids (especially dexamethasone). Treatment recommendations for the different categories of emesis are outlined in Table 35-6.

High Emetogenic Chemotherapy

Patients receiving high emetogenic chemotherapy (HEC) have three different options that may be used. The first option includes an initial three drug antiemetic regimen that is initiated prior to the administration moderate/low emetogenic chemotherapy, day 1, which includes a 5-HT3-RA agent, dexamethasone, and an NK1 receptor antagonist. Due to the CYP3A4 interactions, lower doses of dexamethasone are used for aprepitant or fosaprepitant versus a standard dose of dexamethasone with a rolapitant regimen; steroids may be continued for days 2 to 4 as outlined in Table 35-6.

The second option includes a two drug regimen containing the NK1 receptor antagonist/5-HT3 antagonist combination of NEPA, in addition to reduced dose dexamethasone due to the drug interactions with CYP3A4, similar to the dose used with aprepitant. As with the first option, dexamethasone is continued on days 1 to 3.

The third option includes an olanzapine based therapy in combination with a 5-HT3-RA, specifically palonosetron, along with dexamethasone. This regimen is unique in that it is steroid sparing and only the olanzapine is continued through days 2 to 4 as outlined in Table 35-6.

Any of the 5-HT3-RAs may be used on day 1; however, the ASCO and NCCN guidelines prefer IV palonosetron.[30,31] In regards to dolasetron, in 2010 the FDA released a statement that IV dolasetron should not be used for treatment of CINV due to an increased risk of QTc prolongation and other cardiac conduction abnormalities. Only the oral formulation of dolasetron should be used for CINV.[34] Non-oral/IV options do exist such as the granisetron transdermal patch, which should be applied 24 to 48 hours prior to chemotherapy. This patch continues to work for up to 7 days. The final choice of 5-HT3-RA should be based on route of administration, potential side effects and cost concerns.

Clinical **Controversy...**

Is QT prolongation a concern for 5-HT3-RAs? 5-HT3-RAs are widely used antiemetics in oncology; however, QT prolongation has been observed. Only a few studies have addressed ECG changes in cancer patients treated for CINV. Further studies are needed in this population as patients are often older, have a higher incidence of comorbidities and polypharmacy, as well as the potential for more drug-drug interactions than those who have previously been included in clinical trials for PONV. The incidence of cardiac adverse effects in cancer patients who have known heart disease needs to be addressed in those who may receive a 5-HT3-RA for the prophylaxis of CINV.[35]

Moderate Emetogenic Chemotherapy

Patients receiving moderate emetogenic chemotherapy (MEC) also have three options of antiemetic regimens. The first is a two-drug regimen 5-HT3-RA on day 1 with dexamethasone and either a 5-HT3-RA or dexamethasone continued through day 3. Both ASCO and NCCN guidelines recommend IV palonosetron as the preferred 5-HT3-RA for MEC.[30,31] The exception to this recommendation is in patients who are receiving combination chemotherapy with the following therapies: carboplatin, cisplatin, doxorubicin, epirubicin, ifosfamide, irinotecan, or methotrexate. It is recommended that these patients be given an NK1 receptor antagonist in addition the 5-HT3-RA and dexamethasone.[16]

The second option is the combination of an NK1 receptor antagonist/5-HT3 receptor antagonist, NEPA plus dexamethasone on day 1 of therapy, with dexamethasone continued through days 2 to 3. The third and final option is the same as with the HEC based olanzapine therapy in combination with palonosetron and dexamethasone, with only olanzapine continued for days 2 to 3.[16]

For chemotherapy regimens that are of low emetic risk, dexamethasone or any of the following may be used: prochlorperazine, metoclopramide, or a 5-HT3-RA such as dolasetron, granisetron or ondansetron alone.[16]

Prophylaxis of Delayed CINV

The best strategy for preventing delayed CINV, nausea and/or vomiting occurring 24 or more hours after chemotherapy, is to control acute CINV and provide adequate prophylaxis for delayed CINV. As with prevention of acute CINV, the agent used is highly dependent on the emetogenic potential of the regimen. It is also imperative to realize that the regimen used in the prevention of acute CINV in each patient will often dictate the regimen to be used for delayed nausea and vomiting. These regimens frequently include continuing dexamethasone or olanzapine for up to 3 days for those receiving HEC.[16,30,31] For those who use aprepitant for prevention of acute CINV, aprepitant must be continued for 3 days in addition to dexamethasone. This is the only NK1 antagonist that is recommended for continued dosing for prevention of CINV, and other NK1 antagonists do not require repeated dosing administrations.[16] Those receiving MEC can often continue with just a single drug therapy with options with 5-HT3-RAs, dexamethasone, olanzapine, or potentially use a combination of these agents. Further details including agents and days of therapy are outlined in Table 35-6.

Any of the above regimens, whether it be HEC, MEC, or low risk, may be used in combination with an acid suppressing agent such as an H2RA or a proton pump inhibitor. These patients may also use lorazepam 0.5-2 mg PO/IV every 6 hours as needed for additional nausea relief.[16,30,31]

Prophylaxis and Treatment of Anticipatory Nausea and Vomiting

All three guidelines, MASCC, ASCO, as well as the NCCN, are all in agreement that prevention of CINV from the beginning of chemotherapy is essential in preventing ANV.[16,30,31] There are some nonpharmacologic options, such as use of behavioral therapy, hypnosis, acupuncture/acupressure or music therapy, may be of use for ANV. Benzodiazepine therapy may be used the decrease the occurrence of ANV; however, these therapies may become less effective over time.[28] If ANV occurs, options such as oral alprazolam 0.5-1 mg or oral lorazepam 0.5-2 mg starting the evening prior to chemotherapy and then an addition dose 1 to 2 hours prior to chemotherapy administration may be used.[16]

Treatment of Breakthrough CINV

A general principle in all patients receiving chemotherapy is to prescribe an antiemetic from a different pharmacologic class for rescue of breakthrough nausea and vomiting. Rescue medications used in adult patients include prochlorperazine, promethazine, lorazepam, metoclopramide, haloperidol, 5-HT3-RAs, dexamethasone, cannabinoids, or olanzapine.[16,31,36]

Around-the-clock dosing of rescue antiemetics should be considered rather than as-needed administration. If the rescue antiemetics are useful, there should be consideration of changing the current antiemetic therapy to a higher level of primary treatment for the subsequent cycles.[16,31] The choice of agent should be based on patient-specific factors, including potential adverse drug reactions and cost. Chlorpromazine, lorazepam, and dexamethasone are recommended for pediatric patients.[37]

Treatment of Refractory Nausea and Vomiting

The general approach to the management of refractory CINV is to upgrade the antiemetic strategy to the next level of prophylaxis or to add breakthrough antiemetics to the regimen.[16] Some patients will experience nausea and vomiting despite optimal acute and delayed prophylaxis and failure of rescue antiemetics. Addition of another agent from a different pharmacologic class is recommended and routes other than the oral route may be required.

Treatment of Multiday Chemotherapy

Chemotherapy regimens are occasionally administered over multiple days. The MASCC guidelines state that the combination of a 5-HT3-RA plus daily dexamethasone is the standard of care.[30] For HEC or MEC, it is recommended that dexamethasone be administered either IV or PO and be continued for up to 2 to 3 days after the chemotherapy has ended and that 5-HT3-RA administration should be started prior to start of chemotherapy.[16] When using NK1 antagonist for HEC regimens, there is some data supporting the use of aprepitant for up to 4 to 5 days; there is another trial that suggests that for 5-day cisplatin therapy, initiate aprepitant on day 3 and continue a lower dose of aprepitant through day 7 along with a 5-HT3-RA on days 1 to 5 along with dexamethasone on days 1 to 2.[38] Dexamethasone should not be prescribed for patients receiving a corticosteroid in their chemotherapy regimen or with regimens containing interferon alpha or interleukin-2.[33]

POSTOPERATIVE NAUSEA AND VOMITING

Postoperative nausea and vomiting in adults occurs in 30% of patients and usually within 24 hours of undergoing anesthesia.[39] Patients with multiple risk factors are at highest risk for PONV (Table 35-7). Patients with zero or one of the four risk factors present in Table 35-7 are at lowest risk (10%-20%) and those with three to five risk factors are at highest risk for PONV (50%-80%). Moderate risk is defined by this model as the presence of two to three risk factors and high risk is defined as greater than three risk factors. The use of a risk assessment tool can help identify patients most likely to benefit from prophylaxis.[40-42]

In addition to using prophylactic antiemetics in moderate and high-risk patients, other strategies to prevent PONV include using regional rather than systemic anesthesia, propofol, and hydration, as well as avoiding the use of nitrous oxide, volatile anesthetics, or opioids.[41]

Prophylaxis of PONV

Adherence to consensus guidelines for prophylaxis and treatment of PONV decreases emetic episodes.[41] 6 Patients at highest risk of vomiting should receive two or more prophylactic antiemetics from different pharmacologic classes, while those at moderate risk should receive one or two drugs.[41] Timing the administration of the antiemetic is dependent on the agent used. Scopolamine patches must be initiated the evening before the surgery or at least 2 hours prior, whereas NK1 antagonists should be given during the induction of anesthesia; all other agents are recommended to be given at the end of the surgery. Pharmacological options for the prevention of PONV include 5-HT3-RAs, NK1 antagonist, corticosteroids, droperidol, haloperidol, antihistamines, and anticholinergics.

Of the available 5-HT3-RAs available, ondansetron is still considered the "gold standard" agent and has the most data supporting its use at the end of surgical procedures. Ondansetron has greater anti-vomiting activity versus anti-nausea activity and is as effective as dexamethasone, droperidol, and IV haloperidol. It was however found to be less effective than the NK1 antagonist, aprepitant, in decreasing emesis and less effective than fellow 5-HT3-RA, palonosetron for decreasing the incidence of PONV.[41,43,44] Palonosetron is a second generation 5-HT3-RA, which is unique with a prolonged half-life of 40 hours and it is one of the only 5-HT3-RAs that does not affect the QT interval. Granisetron is as effective as other first generation 5-HT3-RAs, but this agent may not be as effective in those who are ultra-metabolizers of CYP2D6 pathway.[45]

Steroids, such as dexamethasone and methylprednisolone are useful low cost agents used in preventing PONV. Utilizing higher doses of dexamethasone (more than 0.1 mg/kg) has been associated with a decrease in nausea and vomiting, and improvement in other important postoperative complications such as decreasing pain, need for opiates, and improvement in sleep. Dexamethasone should be administered after the induction of anesthesia, and due to its effects on glycemic control, its use should be avoided in patients with uncontrolled diabetes.[41,46,47]

When the different combinations of antiemetics were compared, no differences were found between 5-HT3-RA plus droperidol, 5-HT3-RA plus dexamethasone, and droperidol plus dexamethasone.[48] However, QT prolongation and/or torsade de pointes has been reported in some cases, with some fatalities in patients receiving droperidol at doses at or below recommended doses. Droperidol should be avoided in patients who have a history of QT prolongation, are over 65 years old, or have a history of alcohol abuse, or when used concomitantly with benzodiazepines, volatile anesthetics, and IV opiates.[7] Low-dose haloperidol has also been studied as a potential alternative to droperidol therapy and is beneficial in PONV. This agent also carries a risk for potential QTc prolongation and should be used with caution in individuals at high risk for this complication.[41]

Monotherapy with perphenazine, metoclopramide, scopolamine are as effective as placebo for the prophylaxis of PONV.[41] The guidelines advocate the use of combination therapy versus monotherapy; however, an optimal combination of antiemetics for PONV has not been established. The agents with the most data supporting their use includes dexamethasone plus either a 5-HT3-RA or droperidol or a 5-HT3-RA plus droperidol.[41] The choice should be based on use of different mechanisms of action, agents with different adverse effects along with cost considerations. Table 35-8 summarizes the doses for prophylactic antiemetics from the consensus guidelines.[41]

Aprepitant, an NK1 antagonist, was approved for the prevention of PONV when given orally within 3 hours prior to induction of anesthesia.[19] Aprepitant is equivalent to ondansetron 4 mg IV in reducing the incidence of nausea and the need for rescue in the 24 hours after surgery, but was significantly better than ondansetron for preventing vomiting in the 24 and 48 hours after surgery.[49] It has also been studied in combination with dexamethasone in comparison with an ondansetron plus dexamethasone combination and the aprepitant combination was more effective than the ondansetron combination group.[50] The newest and longest acting NK1-antagonist, rolapitant, is currently being investigated for prophylaxis of PONV and was found to be more effective than placebo in a small trial, but currently only has an indication for CINV.[51]

Treatment of PONV

Patients who experience PONV after receiving prophylactic treatment with a combination of 5-HT3-RA plus dexamethasone should be given rescue therapy from a different drug class such as a phenothiazine, metoclopramide, or droperidol.[41] Repeating the agent given for PONV prophylaxis within 6 hours of surgery offers no additional benefit.[52] Furthermore, a repeated dose of a 5-HT3-RA is not effective in treatment of PONV.[53,54] An emetic episode occurring more than 6 hours postoperatively can be treated with any of the drugs used for prophylaxis except dexamethasone and transdermal scopolamine.[41]

If no prophylaxis was given initially, the recommended treatment is low-dose 5-HT3-RA such as ondansetron 1 mg. Alternative

TABLE 35-6 Dosage Recommendations for CINV for Adult Patients

Emetogenic Risk	Acute NV Prevention (Day 1)—Prior to Chemotherapy			Delayed NV Prevention (Days 2-4)		
High[b,c,g]	***Option 1—NK1 + 5-HT3 + Steroid***					
	NK1 Antagonist	*5-HT3 Antagonist*	*Steroid*	*Day 2*	*Day 3*	*Day 4*
	Aprepitant 125 mg PO × 1	Dolasetron 100 mg PO × 1	Dexamethasone 12 mg PO/IV × 1[a]	Aprepitant 80 mg PO + Dexamethasone 8 mg IV/PO	Aprepitant 80 mg PO + Dexamethasone 8 mg IV/PO	Dexamethasone 8 mg IV/PO
	Fosaprepitant 150 mg IV × 1	Granisetron 2 mg PO × 1 OR 1 mg PO twice daily OR 0.01 mg/kg (Max 1 mg) IV OR 3.1 mg/h transdermal patch applied 24-48 hours prior to chemo		Dexamethasone 8 mg IV/PO	Dexamethasone 8 mg IV/PO twice daily	Dexamethasone 8 mg IV/PO twice daily
	Rolapitant 180 mg PO × 1	Ondansetron 16-24 mg PO × 1 OR 8-16 mg IV × 1	Dexamethasone 20 mg PO/IV × 1	Dexamethasone 8 mg IV/PO twice daily	Dexamethasone 8 mg IV/PO twice daily	Dexamethasone 8 mg IV/PO twice daily
		Palonosetron 0.25 mg IV × 1				
	Option 2—NK1/5-HT3 + Steroid			*Day 2*	*Day 3*	*Day 4*
	Netupitant 300 mg PO/Palonosetron 0.5 mg PO × 1 + Dexamethasone 12 mg PO/IV × 1			Dexamethasone 8 mg IV/PO	Dexamethasone 8 mg IV/PO	Dexamethasone 8 mg IV/PO
	Option 3—Olanzapine + 5-HT3 + Steroid			*Day 2*	*Day 3*	*Day 4*
	Olanzapine 10 mg PO × 1+ Palonosetron 0.25 mg IV + Dexamethasone 20 mg IV × 1			Olanzapine 10 mg PO	*Olanzapine 10 mg PO*	*Olanzapine 10 mg PO*
Moderate[b,c]	***Option 1-5—HT3 (Palonosetron Preferred) + Steroid (Same doses as listed above) ± NK1***			***Option 1-5—HT3 Monotherapy, Days 2-3***		
				Dolasetron 100 mg PO daily		
				Granisetron 1-2 mg PO daily OR 1 mg PO twice daily OR 0.01 mg/kg (Max 1 mg) IV		
				Ondansetron 8 mg PO twice daily OR 16 mg PO daily OR 8-16 mg IV daily		
				Option 2—Steroid Monotherapy, Days 2-3		
				Dexamethasone 8 mg IV/PO daily		
				Option 3—NK1 + Steroid, as listed with High-Risk Delayed Regimen		
	Option 2—NK1/5-HT3 + Steroid at Doses listed above			± Dexamethasone 8 mg IV/PO daily, Days 2-3		
	Option 3—Olanzapine +5-HT3 + Steroid at Doses listed above			Olanzapine 10 mg PO daily, Days 2-3		
Low[b,c]	Dexamethasone 12 mg IV/PO IV daily			None		
	Metoclopramide 10-40 mg IV/PO, then every 4-6 hours prn					
	Prochlorperazine 10 mg IV/PO, then every 6 hour prn (max 40 mg/day)					
	5-HT3 Antagonist Dolasetron 100 mg PO daily Granisetron 1-2 mg PO daily Ondansetron 8-16 mg PO daily					
Minimal	None			None		

[a]Use a lower dose of Dexamethasone if Aprepitant or Fosaprepitant is used

[b]± Use of H2RA or Proton Pump Inhibitor See References 16, 24, and 27 for the above information.

[c]± Use of Lorazepam 0.5-2 mg PO/IV/SL every 6 hours prn on Days 1-4

treatments for established PONV include dexamethasone 2 to 4 mg IV, droperidol 0.625 mg IV, or promethazine 6.25 to 12.5 mg IV.[55]

RADIATION-INDUCED NAUSEA AND VOMITING

Nausea and vomiting associated with radiation therapy (RT) is not well understood and often underestimated by radiation oncologists.[56] RINV is neither as predictable nor as severe as CINV, and many patients receiving RT will not experience nausea or vomiting. The incidence of RINV ranges from 50% to 80%, is site dependent, and can have a substantial impact on a patient's quality of life. Risk factors associated with the development of RINV include combination chemoradiotherapy, prior CINV, upper abdomen RT, and field size.[57]

Four radiotherapy-induced emesis risk groups have been defined by the Antiemetic Subcommittee of the MASCC and the ASCO antiemetic practice guidelines:[30,31]

1. Highest risk: Total-body or nodal irradiation (TBI/TNI)
2. Moderate risk: Upper body or abdomen and hemibody RT
3. Low risk: Cranial, craniospinal, head and neck, lower thorax, and pelvic RT
4. Minimal risk: Extremity or breast RT

TABLE 35-7 Risk Factors for Postoperative Nausea and Vomiting (PONV)

Patient-related factors
Age less than 50 years old
Female gender (two to three times greater incidence of PONV vs males)
Nonsmoker
History of PONV or motion sickness (threefold increase in incidence of PONV)
Hydration status
Factors related to anesthesia
Use of general anesthesia
Use of volatile anesthetics
Nitrous oxide
Use of opioids (intraoperative or postoperative)
Factors related to surgery
Type of surgical procedure (laparoscopic, gynecological, cholecystectomy)
Duration of surgery

Data from references 45 and 47.

Prophylaxis of RINV

7 Patients undergoing RT to the upper abdomen or receiving total or hemibody irradiation should receive prophylactic antiemetics for RINV. Several randomized trials have demonstrated that the combination of prophylactic 5-HT3-RA plus dexamethasone is more effective than placebo,[57] which was confirmed by a meta-analysis.[57] In addition, 5-HT3-RAs were more effective than placebo or non-5-HT3-RAs (prochlorperazine or metoclopramide), even in patients undergoing TBI.[57,58]

The ASCO, ESMO/MASCC, and NCCN recommend preventive therapy with a 5-HT3-RA throughout RT and dexamethasone on fractions 1 through 5 in patients who are receiving TBI (high emetic risk).[16,30,31] Patients undergoing RT procedures with moderate emetic risk should receive a 5-HT3-RA prior to each fraction and dexamethasone on fractions 1 through 5. Those receiving low emetic risk radiotherapy may be given a 5-HT3-RA either throughout RT or only as needed for rescue. For minimal emetic risk, a 5-HT3-RA, metoclopramide, or prochlorperazine may be offered.[16,30,31]

There has not a study of prophylactic NK1 antagonists, palonosetron, or transdermal granisetron in the setting of RINV.

DISORDERS OF BALANCE

Disorders of balance include vertigo, dizziness, and motion sickness. The etiology of these complaints may include diseases that are infectious, postinfectious, demyelinative, vascular, neoplastic, degenerative, traumatic, toxic, psychogenic, or idiopathic. Symptoms of imbalance perceived by the patient present a particular clinical challenge.

8 Beneficial therapy for patients with balance disorders can most reliably be found among the antihistaminic–anticholinergic agents. However, the precise mechanisms of action of these agents are currently unknown. Oral regimens of antihistaminic–anticholinergic agents given one to several times each day may be effective, especially when the first dose is administered prior to motion.

Motion sickness may be associated with nausea and vomiting. A Cochrane review of 14 randomized controlled trials showed that scopolamine is effective for the prevention of motion sickness and is considered first-line for this indication.[59] The usefulness of scopolamine in preventing motion sickness was enhanced with the development of the transdermal system (patch) that increased patient satisfaction and decreased untoward side effects. The patch should be placed several hours before the anticipated motion exposure. First-generation sedating antihistamines are also effective. However, second-generation non-sedating antihistamines, ondansetron, and ginger root are not effective in the prevention and treatment of motion sickness.[60]

ANTIEMETIC USE DURING PREGNANCY

As many as 75% of pregnant women experience nausea and vomiting to some degree during the first trimester of pregnancy. The severity of the symptoms varies considerably, from mild nausea to incapacitating nausea and vomiting. The etiology of nausea and vomiting of pregnancy (NVP) is not well understood. Symptoms are self-limited for a majority of women, although approximately 1% develop hyperemesis gravidarum, a serious condition marked by severe physical symptoms and/or medical complications requiring hospitalization. In its most severe state, hyperemesis gravidarum may result in volume contraction, starvation, and electrolyte abnormalities.

Initial management of NVP often involves dietary changes and/or lifestyle modifications, such as eating smaller, more frequent meals and avoiding foods or odors that trigger symptoms. Ginger has also

TABLE 35-8 Recommended Prophylactic Doses of Selected Antiemetics for Postoperative Nausea and Vomiting in Adults and Postoperative Vomiting in Children

Drug	Adult Dose	Pediatric Dose (IV)	Timing of Dose[a]
Aprepitant[b]	40 mg orally	Not labeled for use in pediatrics	Within 3 hours prior to induction
Dexamethasone	4-5 mg IV	150 mcg/kg up to 5 mg	At induction
Dimenhydrinate	1 mg/kg IV	0.5 mg/kg up to 25 mg	Not specified
Dolasetron	12.5 mg IV	350 mcg/kg up to 12.5 mg	At end of surgery
Droperidol[c]	0.625-1.25 mg IV	10-15 mcg/kg up to 1.25 mg	At end of surgery
Granisetron	0.35-3 mg IV	40 mcg/kg up to 0.6 mg	At end of surgery
Haloperidol	0.5-2 mg (IM or IV)	*d*	Not specified
Methylprednisolone	40 mg IV	*d*	At induction
Ondansetron	4 mg IV, 8 mg ODT	50-100 mcg/kg up to 4 mg	At end of surgery
Palonosetron[b]	0.075 mg IV	*d*	At induction
Promethazine[c]	6.25-12.5 mg IV	*d*	At induction
Scopolamine	Transdermal patch	*d*	Prior evening or 4 hours before surgery

[a]Based on recommendations from consensus guidelines.

[b]Labeled for use in PONV but not included in consensus guidelines.

[c]See FDA "black box" warning.

[d]Pediatric dosing not included in consensus guidelines.

Data from reference 47.

been shown to be beneficial in reducing nausea.[61,62] Persistent nausea and/or vomiting leads to the consideration of drug therapy at a time when teratogenic potential of each agent must be considered.

Treatment recommendations for the management of NVP are available from the American College of Obstetricians and Gynecologists (ACOG).[62] Pyridoxine, with or without doxylamine is recommended as first-line therapy.[62,63] The U.S. Food and Drug Administration approved a delayed-release formulation of doxylamine and pyridoxine hydrochloride (Diclegis[R]) in April 2013.[64]

Patients with persistent NVP or who show signs of dehydration should receive IV fluid replacement with thiamine. Ondansetron, promethazine, and metoclopramide have similar effectiveness for hyperemesis gravidarum, although ondansetron may be better tolerated due to less adverse effects.[63,65,66] Metoclopramide should not be used for more than 12 weeks due to the risk of tardive dyskinesia. Glucocorticoids may be used in patients with severe NVP or hyperemesis gravidarum, but should be used only after 10 weeks of gestation due to the increased risk of cleft lip.[63]

Clinical **Controversy...**

Which antiemetic is best to use during breastfeeding? There is a paucity of clinical trials to determine the most effective, safest medication to use for nausea and/or vomiting in breastfeeding. More studies are needed to look at the extent antiemetics are excreted into breast milk and the adverse effects to infants if the drugs are excreted. An important clinical consideration is to try to minimize exposure to medications and use them for the shortest duration possible. LactMed provides information on individual antiemetics in breastfeeding.[67]

ANTIEMETIC USE IN SPECIAL POPULATIONS

Chemotherapy-Induced Nausea and Vomiting in Children

Updated practice guidelines recommend that a corticosteroid (such as dexamethasone) plus a 5-HT3-RA be administered as prophylaxis of acute CINV to children receiving chemotherapy of high or moderate emetic risk.[68] Consensus guidelines suggest that there are no differences between 5-HT3-RAs in safety or efficacy. 5-HT3-RAs are more efficacious and have less adverse effects than metoclopramide, phenothiazines, and cannabinoids in children for the prevention of CINV.[68]

One small study has evaluated the safety and efficacy of aprepitant in adolescents. Patients were randomized to dexamethasone and ondansetron with or without aprepitant, using the recommended oral adult 3-day regimen. The emetogenicity of the chemotherapy administered was not discussed. Patients in the aprepitant arm had higher complete response rates and a parallel pharmacokinetic study suggests that the adult dose regimen was appropriate for adolescents.[69]

Gastroenteritis in Children

Nausea and vomiting associated with pediatric gastroenteritis is usually self-limited and improves with correction of dehydration. The majority of patients can be successfully treated with oral rehydration therapy. Pediatric practitioners may prescribe antiemetics for intractable vomiting due to gastroenteritis. The use of promethazine is contraindicated in patients less than 2 years old and should be used in caution in older children due to the potential risk of fatal respiratory depression.[70] Administration of ondansetron is associated with deceased vomiting and a reduced need for intravenous therapy and hospital admissions.[71-73]

Antiemetic Use in Geriatric Patients

Many of the commonly used antiemetics are on the Beers Criteria list, which are considered medications that may be considered potentially inappropriate in the older adults due to the risks outweighing the benefits.[74] These include first-generation antihistamines and scopolamine due to their highly anticholinergic side effects. Metoclopramide is also a Beers Criteria medication that may cause extrapyramidal effects including tardive dyskinesia especially in frail older adults. Ondansetron may be considered a preferred antiemetic in older adults; however, consider drug–drug interactions and potential side effects before prescribing.[75]

PERSONALIZED PHARMACOTHERAPY

Antiemetics are 70% to 80% effective in the prevention of CINV. One potential factor that might explain a less than optimal response is the variability in genetic enzymes responsible for the metabolism, transport, and receptor affinity of antiemetics.[76] The literature on the pharmacogenetics of antiemetic drugs is limited regarding the impact of the polymorphic variability in the drug transport mechanisms such as the ABCB1 or multidrug resistance gene (MDR1), or polymorphisms of metabolism with either CYP2D6 genes, which all may impact the efficacy of the 5-HT3-RAs. Individuals who are either rapid or ultra-metabolizers of the CYP2D6 enzymes generally respond poorly to 5-HT3-RAs and dopamine D2 receptor antagonists (prochlorperazine and metoclopramide).[77] Those patients with specific polymorphisms of the ABCB1 transporter, which is found in 5-HT3-RAs such as ondansetron, and are found to have the 3435T variant had a better response of short-term nausea and vomiting control versus those with the 3435C variant.[78] There are many limitations given the relatively small number of individuals studied in these trials, typically less than 300 patients, studied in limited ethnic populations and the fact that there are no tests readily available to test for these genetic polymorphisms. Given that granisetron is the only 5-HT3-RA available that does not require metabolism via CYP2D6, this agent should be used as an alternative if a patient is less responsive to initial 5-HT3-RA therapy with other agents.[77] Until there are confirmatory studies of these results, it is premature to utilize genomic analysis for personalized clinical decision-making for use of 5-HT3-RAs.

EVALUATION OF EMETIC OUTCOMES

In assessing emetic outcomes, standardized monitoring criteria should include a subjective assessment and objectives parameters including:

1. Severity of nausea
2. Change in patient weight
3. Number of vomiting episodes each day
4. Estimated fluid loss
5. Acid-base balance
6. Serum sodium, potassium, and chloride concentrations
7. Serum BUN and creatinine concentrations
8. Daily urine volume and urine-specific gravity

Physical assessment should include evaluation of mucous membranes and skin turgor. For patients on chemotherapy, evaluation of emetic outcomes should occur after the administration of each chemotherapy cycle. Adherence to outpatient antiemetic regimens occurs in only about 65% of patients. Patients receiving high-risk regimens are most likely to report symptoms of nausea and vomiting on day 3 after chemotherapy.[79] Documentation of nausea and/or vomiting events will assist the clinician in modifying the antiemetic regimen for the next cycle of chemotherapy.

ABBREVIATIONS

ACOG	American College of Obstetricians and Gynecologists
ANV	anticipatory nausea and vomiting
ASCO	American Society of Clinical Oncology
BRAT	Bananas, rice, applesauce or toast
CINV	chemotherapy-induced nausea and vomiting
CTZ	chemoreceptor trigger zone
GI	gastrointestinal
ESMO	European Society of Oncology
HEC	high emetogenic chemotherapy
5-HT3-RA	5-hydroxytryptamine-3 receptor antagonist
MASCC	Multinational Association of Supportive Care in Cancer
MDR1	multidrug resistance gene
MEC	moderate emetogenic chemotherapy
NCCN	National Comprehensive Cancer Network
NEPA	netupitant/palonosetron
NK1	neurokinin 1
NVP	nausea and vomiting of pregnancy
ORT	oral rehydration therapy
PONV	postoperative nausea and vomiting
RINV	radiation-induced nausea and vomiting
RT	radiation therapy
TBI	total-body irradiation
TNI	total nodal irradiation
VC	vomiting center

REFERENCES

1. Malagelada JR, Malagelada C. Nausea and vomiting. In: Feldman M, ed. *Sleisenger and Fordtran's Gastrointestinal and Liver Disease: Pathophysiology/Diagnosis/Management*. St. Louis, MO: Elsevier; 2010:197-209.
2. Grunberg SM, Osoba D, Hesketh PJ, et al. Evaluation of new antiemetic agents and definition of antineoplastic agent emetogenicity—An update. *Support Care Cancer* 2011;19(Suppl 10): S43-S47.
3. Kamen C, Tejani MA, Chandwani K, et al. Anticipatory nausea and vomiting due to chemotherapy. *Eur J Pharmacol* 2014;722:172-179.
4. Roscoe JA, Morrow GR, Aapro MS, et al. Anticipatory nausea and vomiting. *Support Care Cancer* 2011;19(10):1533-1538.
5. Cheong KB, Chang JP, Huang, Y, Zhang ZJ. The effectiveness of acupuncture in the prevention and treatment of postoperative nausea and vomiting—A systematic review and meta-analysis. *PLoS One* 2013;8(12):e82474.
6. Perkins P, Dorman S. Haloperidol for the treatment of nausea and vomiting in palliative care patients. *Cochrane Database Syst Rev* 2009;(2):CD006271.
7. Inapsine (Droperidol). 2012.
8. Kramer JL. Medicinal marijuana for cancer. *CA Cancer J Clin* 2015;65(2):109-122.
9. Whiting PF, Wolff RF, Deshpande S, et al. Cannabinoids for medicinal use: A systematic review and meta-analysis. *JAMA* 2015;313(24):2456-2473.
10. Todaro B. Cannabinoids in the treatment of chemotherapy-induced nausea and vomiting. *J Natl Compr Canc Netw* 2012;10:487-492.
11. Meda Pharmaceuticals Inc. Cesamet [package insert]. Somerset, NJ: Meda Pharmaceuticals Inc; 2011. Available at: cesamet.com/pdf/Cesamet_PI_5-_count.pdf. (Accessed August 31st, 2015)
12. Italian Group for Antiemetic Research. Double-blind, dose-finding study of four intravenous doses of dexamethasone in the prevention of cisplatin-induced acute emesis. *J Clin Oncol* 1998;16:2937-2942.
13. Gan TJ, Diemunsch P, Habib AS, et al. Consensus Guidelines for the management of postoperative nausea and vomiting. *Anesth Analg* 2014;118:85-113.
14. Navari RM, Gray SE, Kerr AC. Olanzapine versus aprepitant for the prevention of chemotherapy-induced nausea and vomiting: A randomized phase III trial. *J Support Oncol* 2011;9:188-195.
15. Navari RM, Nagy CK, Gray SE. The use of olanzapine versus metoclopramide for the treatment of breakthrough chemotherapy-induced nausea and vomiting in patients receiving highly emetogenic chemotherapy. *Support Care Cancer* 2013;21:1655-1663.
16. National Comprehensive Cancer Network. Clinical Practice Guidelines in Oncology. Antiemesis. Version 2. 2015. Available at: http://www.nccn.org/professionals/physician_gls/pdf/antiemesis.pdf Accessed June 28, 2016.
17. Ernst A, Weiss SJ, Park S, et al. Prochlorperazine versus promethazine for uncomplicated nausea and vomiting in the emergency department: A randomized, double-blind clinical trial. *Ann Emerg Med* 2000;36:89-94.
18. Schnadig ID, Modiano MR, Poma A, et al. Phase 3 trial results for rolapitant, a novel NK-1 receptor antagonist, in prevention of chemotherapy induced nausea and vomiting (CINV) in subjects receiving moderately emetogenic chemotherapy (MEC). *J Clin Oncol* 2014;32(5s suppl):abstr 9633.
19. Merck & Co Inc. Prescribing Information. Emend (Aprepitant) Capsules. 2011.
20. McCrea JB, Majumdar AK, Goldberg MR, et al. Effects of the neurokinin-1 receptor antagonist aprepitant on the pharmacokinetics of dexamethasone and methylprednisolone. *Clin Pharmacol Ther* 2003;74:17-24.
21. Van Belle S, Cocquyt V. Fosaprepitant dimeglumine (MK-0517 or L-785,298), an intravenous neurokinin-1 antagonist for the prevention of chemotherapy induced nausea and vomiting. *Expert Opin Pharmacother* 2008;9:3261-3270.
22. Poma A, Christensen JC, Pentkls HP, et al. Rolapitant and its major metabolite do not affect the pharmacokinetics of midazolam, a sensitive cytochrome P450 3A4 substrate. *Support Care Cancer* 2013;21:S154;Abstr 441.
23. Aapro M, Rugo H, Rossi G, et al. A randomized phase III study evaluating the safety and efficacy of NEPA, a fixed-dose combination of netupitant and palonosetron, for prevention of chemotherapy-induced nausea and vomiting following moderately emetogenic chemotherapy. *Ann Oncol* 2014;25:1328-1333.
24. Gralla RJ, Bosnjak SM, Hontsa A, et al. A phase III study evaluating the safety and efficacy of NEPA, a fixed-dose combination of netupitant and palonosetron, for prevention of chemotherapy-induced nausea and vomiting over repeated cycles of chemotherapy. *Ann Oncol* 2014;25:1333-1339.
25. Akynzeo. Package Insert:(Netupitant and Palonosetron) Capsules, for Oral Use [Prescribing Information]. Woodcliff Lake, NY: Easai, Inc.; 2014.
26. Roscoe JA, Morrow GR, Aapro MS, et al. Anticipatory nausea and vomiting. *Support Care Cancer* 2011;19:1533-1538.
27. Kamen C, Tejani MA, Chandwani K, et al. Anticipatory nausea and vomiting due to chemotherapy. *Eur J Pharmacol* 2014;722: 172-179.
28. Roila F, Herrstedt J, Aapro M, et al. Guideline update for MASCC and ESMO in the prevention of chemotherapy- and radiotherapy-induced nausea and vomiting: Results of the third Perugia consensus conference. *Ann Oncol* 2010;21(Suppl 5):v232-v243.
29. Navari RM. Treatment of Breakthrough and Refractory Chemotherapy-Induced Nausea and Vomiting. BioMed Research International 2015;2015:1-6.
30. Jordan K, Gralla R, Jahn F, Molassiotts A. International antiemetic guidelines on chemotherapy induced nausea and vomiting (CINV): Content and implementation in daily practice. *European Journal of Pharmacology* 2014;722:197-222.
31. Basch E, Prestrud AA, Hesketh PJ, et al. Antiemetics: American Society of Clinical Oncology clinic practice guideline update. *J Clin Oncol* 2011;29:4189-4198.
32. Wickham R. Best practice management of CINV in oncology patients II. Antiemesis guidelines and rational for use. *J Support Oncol* 2010;8(2 Suppl 1):10-15.
33. Ettinger DS, Armstrong DK, Barbour S, et al. Antiemesis. Clinical practice guidelines in oncology. *J Natl Compr Canc Netw* 2012;10: 456-485.
34. FDA. FDA Drug Safety Communication: Abnormal Heart Rhythms Associated with Use of Anzemet (Dolasetron Mesylate) [Safety Communication]. Available at: http://www.fda.gov/Drugs/DrugSafety/ucm237081.htm|~http://www.fda.gov/Drugs/DrugSafety/ucm237081.htm. (Accessed September 1, 2015)
35. Brygger L, Herrstedt J, on behalf of the Academy of Geriatric Cancer Research (AgeCare). 5-Hydroxytryptamine3 receptor antagonists and cardiac side effects. *Expert Opin Drug Saf* 2014;13(10):1407-1422.

36. Hawkins R, Grunberg S. Chemotherapy-induced nausea and vomiting: Challenges and opportunities for improved outcomes. *Clin J Oncol Nurs* 2009;13:54-64.
37. Dupuis LL, Nathan PC. Optimizing emetic control in children receiving antineoplastic therapy: Beyond the Guidelines. *Pediatr Drugs* 2010;12(1):51-61.
38. Albancy C, Brames MJ, Fausel C, et al. Randomized, double blind, placebo controlled, phase III crossover study evaluating the oral neurokinin-1 antagonist aprepitant in combination with a 5HT3 receptor antagonist and dexamethasone in patients with germ cell tumors receiving 5 day Cisplatin combination chemotherapy regimens: A Hoosier Oncology Group Study. *J Clin Oncol* 2012;20:3998-4003.
39. Wiesmann T, Kranke P, Eberhart L. Postoperative nausea and vomiting–A narrative review of pathophysiology, pharmacotherapy and clinical management strategies. *Expert Opin Pharmacother* 2015;16(7):1069-1077.
40. Apfel CC, Philip BK, Cakmakkaya OS, et al. Who is at risk for postdischarge nausea and vomiting after ambulatory surgery? *Anesthesiology* 2012;117:475-486.
41. Gan TJ, Diemunsch P, Habib AS, et al. Consensus Guidelines for the management of postoperative nausea and vomiting. *Anesth Analg* 2014;118:85-113.
42. Apfel CA, Korttila K, Abdalla M, et al. A factorial trial of six interventions for the prevention of postoperative nausea and vomiting. *N Engl J Med* 2004;350:2441-2451.
43. Diemunsch P, Gan TJ, Philip BK, et al. Single-dose aprepitant vs ondansetron for the prevention of postoperative nausea and vomiting: A randomized, double-blind phase III trial in patients undergoing open abdominal surgery. *Br J Anaesth* 2007;99:202-211.
44. Park SK, Cho EJ. A randomized, double-blind trial of palonosetron compared with ondansetron in preventing postoperative nausea and vomiting after gynaecological laparoscopic surgery. *J Int Med Res* 2011;39:399-407.
45. Janicki PK, Schuler HG, Jarzembowski TM, Rossi M 2nd. Prevention of postoperative nausea and vomiting with granisetron and dolasetron in relation to CYP2D6 genotype. *Anesth Analg* 2006;102:1127-1133.
46. De Oliveira GS Jr, Ahmad S, Fitzgerald PC, et al. Dose ranging study on the effect on preoperative dexamethasone on postoperative quality of recovery and opioid consumption after ambulatory gynaecological surgery. *Br J Anaesth* 2011;107:362-367.
47. Waldron NH, Jones CA, Gan TJ, et al. Impact of perioperative dexamethasone on postoperative analgesia and side-effects: Systematic review and meta-analysis. *Br J Anaesth* 2013;110:191-200.
48. Habib AS, El-Moalem HE, Gan TJ. The efficacy of the 5-HT3 receptor antagonists combined with droperidol for PONV prophylaxis is similar to their combination with dexamethasone. A meta-analysis of randomized controlled trials. *Can J Anaesth* 2004;51:311-319.
49. Gan TJ, Apfel C, Kovac A, et al. A randomized, double-blind comparison of the NK1 antagonist, aprepitant versus ondansetron for the prevention of postoperative nausea and vomiting. *Anesth Analg* 2007;104:1082-1089.
50. Habib AS, Keifer JC, Borel CO, White WD, Gan TJ. A comparison of the combination of aprepitant and dexamethasone versus the combination of ondansetron and dexamethasone for the prevention of postoperative nausea and vomiting in patients undergoing craniotomy. *Anesth Analg* 2011;112:813-818.
51. Gan TJ, Gu J, Singla N, et al. Rolapitant for the prevention of postoperative nausea and vomiting: A prospective, double-blinded, placebo-controlled randomized trial. *Anesth Analg* 2011;112:804-812.
52. Kovac AL, O'Connor TA, Pearman MH, et al. Efficacy of repeat intravenous dosing of ondansetron in controlling postoperative nausea and vomiting: A randomized, double-blind, placebo-controlled multicenter trial. *J Clin Anesth* 1999;11:453-459.
53. Kreisler NS, Spiekermann BF, Ascari CM, et al. Small-dose droperidol effectively reduces nausea in a general surgical adult patient population. *Anesth Analg* 2000;91:1256-1261.
54. Candiotti KA, Nhuch F, Kamat A, et al. Granisetron versus ondansetron treatment for breakthrough postoperative nausea and vomiting after prophylactic ondansetron failure: A pilot study. *Anesth Analg* 2007;104:1370-1373.
55. Habib AS, Gan TJ. The effectiveness of rescue antiemetics after failure of prophylaxis with ondansetron or droperidol: A preliminary report. *J Clin Anesth* 2005;17:62-65.
56. Fever P, Maranzano E, Molassiotis A, et al. Radiotherapy-induced nausea and vomiting (RINV): MASCC/ESMO guideline for antiemetics in radiotherapy: Update 2009. *Support Care Cancer* 2011;19(Suppl 1):S5-S14.
57. Maranzano E, De Angelis V, Pergolizzi S, et al. A prospective observational trial on emesis in radiotherapy: Analysis of 1020 patients recruited in 45 Italian radiation oncology centres. *Radiother Oncol* 2010;94:36-41.
58. Salvo N, Doble B, Khan L, et al. Prophylaxis of radiation-induced nausea and vomiting using 5-hydroxytryptamine-3 serotonin receptor antagonists: A systematic review of randomized trials. *Int J Radiat Oncol Biol Phys* 2012;82:408-417.
59. Spinks AB, Wasiak J, Villaneuva EV, Bernath V. Scopolamine (hyoscine) for preventing and treating motion sickness. *Cochrane Database Syst Rev* 2011;(6):CD002851.
60. Brainard A, Gresham C. Prevention and treatment of motion sickness. *Am Fam Physician* 2014;90(1):41-46.
61. Matthews A, Dowswell T, Haas DM, et al. Interventions for nausea and vomiting in early pregnancy. *Cochrane Database Syst Rev* 2010;(9):CD007575.
62. Nausea and vomiting of pregnancy. Practice Bulletin No. 153. American College of Obstetricians and Gynecologists. *Obstet Gynecol* 2015;126:e12-24.
63. Herrell HE. Nausea and vomiting of pregnancy. *Am Fam Physician* 2014;89(12):965-970.
64. Koren G, Clark S, Hankins GD, et al. Maternal safety of the delayed-release doxylamine and pyridoxine combination for nausea and vomiting of pregnancy; a randomized placebo controlled trial. *BMC Pregnancy Childbirth* 2015;15:59.
65. Abas MN, Tan PC, Azmi N, Omar SZ. Ondansetron compared with metoclopramide for hyperemesis gravidarum: A randomized controlled trial. *Obstet Gynecol* 2014;123(6):1272-1279.
66. Tan PC, Khine PP, Vallikkannu N, Omar SZ. Promethazine compared with metoclopramide for hyperemesis gravidarum: A randomized controlled trial. *Obstet Gynecol* 2010;115(5):975-981.
67. LactMed: A Toxnet database. National Library Medicine. "Antiemetics." Available at: http://toxnet.nlm.nih.gov/newtoxnet/lactmed.htm. Updated September 2015. (Accessed September 24, 2015)
68. Jordan K, Roila F, Molassiotis A, et al. Antiemetics in children receiving chemotherapy. MASCC/ESMO guideline update 2009. *Support Care Cancer* 2011;19(Suppl 1):S37-S42.
69. Gore L, Chawla S, Petrilli A, et al. Aprepitant in adolescent patients for prevention of chemotherapy-induced nausea and vomiting: A randomized, double-blind, placebo-controlled study of efficacy and tolerability. *Pediatr Blood Cancer* 2009;52:242-247.
70. Buck ML. Promethazine: Recommendations for safe use in children. *Pediatr Pharm* 2010;16(3). Available at: http://www.medscape.com/viewarticle/720608_8. Accessed June 28, 2016.
71. Hervás D, Armero C, Carrión T, Utrera JF, Hervás JA. Clinical and economic impact of oral ondansetron for vomiting in a pediatric emergency department. *Pediatr Emerg Care* 2012;28(11):1166-1168.
72. Levine DA. Oral ondansetron decreases vomiting, as well as the need for intravenous fluids and hospital admission, in children with acute gastroenteritis. *Evid Based Med* 2012;17(4):112-113.
73. Fedorowicz Z, Jagannath VA, Carter B. Antiemetics for reducing vomiting related to acute gastroenteritis in children and adolescents. *Cochrane Database Syst Rev* 2011;(9):CD005506.
74. American Geriatrics Society 2012 Beers Criteria Update Expert Panel. American Geriatrics Society updated Beers Criteria for potentially inappropriate medication use in older adults. *J Am Geriatr Soc* 2012;60(4):616-631.
75. Reuben DB, Herr KA, Pacala JT, et al. *Geriatrics At Your Fingertips: 2015*, 17th ed. New York, NY: The American Geriatrics Society; 2015.
76. Perwitasari DA, Gelderblom H, Atthobari J, et al. Anti-emetic drugs in oncology: Pharmacology and individualization by pharmacogenetics. *Int J Clin Pharm* 2011;33:33-43.
77. Trammel M, Roedere M, Patel J, McLeod H. Does pharmacogenomics account for variability in the control of acute chemotherapy induced nausea and vomiting with 5-hydroxytryptamine type 3 antagonist? *Curr Oncol Rep* 2013;15(3):276-285.
78. Perwitasari DA, Wessles J, van der Straaten R, et al. Association of ABCB1, 5-HT3B Receptor and CYP2D6 Genetic Polymorphisms with Ondansetron and Metoclopramide Antiemetic Response in Indonesian Cancer Patients Treated with Highly Emetogenic Chemotherapy. *Jpn J Clin Oncol* 2011;41(10):1168-1176.
79. Shih V, Wan HS, Chan A. Clinical predictors of chemotherapy-induced nausea and vomiting in breast cancer patients receiving adjuvant doxorubicin and cyclophosphamide. *Ann Pharmacother* 2009;43:444-452.

Diarrhea, Constipation, and Irritable Bowel Syndrome

36

Patricia H. Fabel and Kayce M. Shealy

KEY CONCEPTS

1 Diarrhea is caused by many viral and bacterial organisms. It is most often a minor discomfort, not life-threatening, and usually self-limited.

2 The four pathophysiologic mechanisms of diarrhea have been linked to the four broad diarrheal groups, which are secretory, osmotic, exudative, and altered intestinal transit. The three mechanisms by which absorption occurs from the intestines are active transport, diffusion, and solvent drag.

3 Management of diarrhea focuses on preventing excessive water and electrolyte losses, dietary care, relieving symptoms, treating curable causes, and treating secondary disorders.

4 Bismuth subsalicylate is marketed for indigestion, relieving abdominal cramps, and controlling diarrhea, including traveler's diarrhea, but may cause interactions with several components if given excessively.

5 Constipation is defined as difficult or infrequent passage of stool, at times associated with straining or a feeling of incomplete defecation.

6 Underlying causes of constipation should be identified when possible and corrective measures taken (eg, alteration of diet or treatment of diseases such as hypothyroidism).

7 The foundation of treatment of constipation is dietary fiber or bulk-forming laxatives that provide 20 to 25 g/day of raw fiber.

8 Irritable bowel syndrome (IBS) is one of the most common GI disorders characterized by lower abdominal pain, disturbed defecation, and bloating. Many non-GI manifestations also exist with IBS. Visceral hypersensitivity is a major culprit in the pathophysiology of the disease.

9 Diarrhea-predominant IBS should be managed by dietary modification and drugs such as loperamide when diet changes alone are insufficient to promote control of symptoms.

10 Several drug classes are involved in the treatment of the pain associated with IBS including tricyclic compounds and the gut-selective calcium channel blockers.

DIARRHEA

Diarrhea is a troublesome discomfort that affects most individuals in the United States at some point in their lives and can be thought of as both a symptom and a sign. Usually diarrheal episodes begin abruptly and subside within 1 or 2 days without treatment. This chapter focuses primarily on noninfectious diarrhea, with only minor reference to infectious diarrhea (see Chapter 113 for a discussion of gastrointestinal infections). Diarrhea is often a symptom of a systemic disease, and not all possible causes of diarrhea are discussed in this chapter. Acute diarrhea is commonly defined as less than 14 days' duration, persistent diarrhea as more than 14 days' duration, and chronic diarrhea as more than 30 days' duration.

To understand diarrhea, one must have a reasonable definition of the condition; unfortunately, the literature is extremely variable on this. Simply put, diarrhea is an increased frequency and decreased consistency of fecal discharge as compared with an individual's normal bowel pattern. Frequency and consistency are variable within and between individuals. For example, some individuals defecate as often as three times per day, whereas others defecate only two or three times per week. A Western diet usually produces a daily stool weighing between 100 and 300 g, depending on the amount of nonabsorbable materials (mainly carbohydrates) consumed. Patients with serious diarrhea may have a daily stool weight in excess of 300 g; however, a subset of patients experience frequent small, watery passages. Additionally, vegetable fiber-rich diets, such as those consumed in some Eastern cultures (eg, those in Africa), produce stools weighing more than 300 g/day.

Diarrhea may be associated with a specific disease of the intestines or secondary to a disease outside the intestines. For instance, bacillary dysentery directly affects the gut, whereas diabetes mellitus causes neuropathic diarrheal episodes. Furthermore, diarrhea can be considered as acute or chronic disease. Infectious diarrhea is often acute; diabetic diarrhea is chronic. Congenital disorders in GI ion transport mechanisms are another cause of chronic diarrhea.[1] Whether acute or chronic, diarrhea has the same pathophysiologic causes that help in identification of specific treatments.

Epidemiology

The epidemiology of diarrhea varies in developed versus developing countries.[2] In the United States, diarrheal illnesses are usually not reported to the Centers for Disease Control and Prevention (CDC) unless associated with an outbreak or an unusual organism or condition. For example, the acquired immune deficiency syndrome (AIDS) has been identified with protracted diarrheal illness. Diarrhea is a major problem in daycare centers and nursing homes, probably because early childhood and senescence plus environmental conditions are risk factors. Although an exact epidemiologic profile in the United States is not available through the CDC or published literature, chronic diarrhea affects approximately 5% of the adult population and ranges from 3% to 20% in children worldwide.[2-4] In developing countries, diarrhea is a leading cause of illness and death in children, creating a tremendous economic strain on health care costs.

1 Most cases of acute diarrhea are caused by infections with viruses, bacteria, or protozoa and are generally self-limited.[5] Although viruses are more commonly associated with acute gastroenteritis, bacteria are responsible for more cases of acute diarrhea.

Evaluation of a noninfectious cause is considered if diarrhea persists and no infectious organism can be identified, or if the patient falls into a high-risk category for metabolic complications with persistent diarrhea. Common causative bacterial organisms include *Shigella*, *Salmonella*, *Campylobacter*, *Staphylococcus*, and *Escherichia coli*. Foodborne bacterial infection is a major concern, as several major food poisoning episodes have occurred that were traced to poor sanitary conditions in meat processing plants. Acute viral infections are attributed mostly to the Norwalk and rotavirus groups.

Physiology

In the fasting state, 9 L of fluid enters the proximal small intestine each day. Of this fluid, 2 L is ingested through diet, while the remainder consists of internal secretions. Because of meal content, duodenal chyme is usually hypertonic. When chyme reaches the ileum, the osmolality adjusts to that of plasma, with most dietary fat, carbohydrate, and protein being absorbed. The volume of ileal chyme decreases to about 1 L/day on entering the colon, which is further reduced by colonic absorption to 100 mL daily. If the small intestine water absorption capacity is exceeded, chyme overloads the colon, resulting in diarrhea. In humans, the colon absorptive capacity is about 5 L daily. Colonic fluid transport is critical to water and electrolyte balance.

Absorption from the intestines back into the blood occurs by three mechanisms: active transport, diffusion, and solvent drag. Active transport and diffusion are the mechanisms of sodium transport. Because of the high luminal sodium concentration (142 mEq/L [mmol/L]), sodium diffuses from the sodium-rich gut into epithelial cells, where it is actively pumped into the blood and exchanged with chloride to maintain an isoelectric condition across the epithelial membrane.

Hydrogen ions are transported by an indirect mechanism in the upper small intestine. As sodium is absorbed, hydrogen ions are secreted into the gut. Hydrogen ions then combine with bicarbonate ions to form carbonic acid, which then dissociates into carbon dioxide and water. Carbon dioxide readily diffuses into the blood for expiration through the lung. The water remains in the chyme.

Paracellular pathways are major routes of ion movement. As ions, monosaccharides, and amino acids are actively transported, an osmotic pressure is created, drawing water and electrolytes across the intestinal wall. This pathway accounts for significant amounts of ion transport, especially sodium. Sodium plays an important role in stimulating glucose absorption. Glucose and amino acids are actively transported into the blood via a sodium-dependent cotransport mechanism. Cotransport absorption mechanisms of glucose–sodium and amino acid–sodium are extremely important for treating diarrhea.

Gut motility influences absorption and secretion. The amount of time in which luminal content is in contact with the epithelium is under neural and hormonal control. Neurohormonal substances, such as angiotensin, vasopressin, glucocorticoid, aldosterone, and neurotransmitters, also regulate ion transport.

Pathophysiology

2 Four general pathophysiologic mechanisms disrupt water and electrolyte balance, leading to diarrhea, and are the basis of diagnosis and therapy. These are (a) a change in active ion transport by either decreased sodium absorption or increased chloride secretion; (b) change in intestinal motility; (c) increase in luminal osmolarity; and (d) increase in tissue hydrostatic pressure. These mechanisms have been related to four broad clinical diarrheal groups: secretory, osmotic, exudative, and altered intestinal transit.

Secretory diarrhea occurs when a stimulating substance either increases secretion or decreases absorption of large amounts of water and electrolytes. Substances that cause excess secretion include vasoactive intestinal peptide (VIP) from a pancreatic tumor, unabsorbed dietary fat in steatorrhea, laxatives, hormones (such as secretion), bacterial toxins, and excessive bile salts. Many of these agents stimulate intracellular cyclic adenosine monophosphate and inhibit Na^+/K^+-adenosine triphosphatase (ATPase), leading to increased secretion. Also, many of these mediators inhibit ion absorption simultaneously. Secretory diarrhea is recognized by large stool volumes (more than 1 L/day) with normal ionic contents and osmolality approximately equal to plasma. Fasting does not alter the stool volume in these patients.

Poorly absorbed substances retain intestinal fluids, resulting in osmotic diarrhea. This process occurs with malabsorption syndromes, lactose intolerance, administration of divalent ions (eg, magnesium-containing antacids), or consumption of poorly soluble carbohydrate (eg, lactulose). As a poorly soluble solute is transported, the gut adjusts the osmolality to that of plasma; in so doing, water and electrolytes flux into the lumen. Clinically, osmotic diarrhea is distinguishable from other types, as it ceases if the patient resorts to a fasting state.

Inflammatory diseases of the GI tract discharge mucus, serum proteins, and blood into the gut. Sometimes bowel movements consist only of mucus, exudate, and blood. Exudative diarrhea affects other absorptive, secretory, or motility functions to account for the large stool volume associated with this disorder.

Altered intestinal motility produces diarrhea by three mechanisms: (1) reduction of contact time in the small intestine, (2) premature emptying of the colon, and (3) bacterial overgrowth. Chyme must be exposed to intestinal epithelium for a sufficient time period to enable normal absorption and secretion processes to occur. If this contact time decreases, diarrhea results. Intestinal resection or bypass surgery and drugs (such as metoclopramide) cause this type of diarrhea. On the other hand, an increased time of exposure allows fecal bacteria overgrowth. A characteristic small intestine diarrheal pattern is rapid, small, coupling bursts of waves. These waves are inefficient, do not allow absorption, and rapidly dump chyme into the colon. Once in the colon, chyme exceeds the colonic capability to absorb water.

Etiologic Examination of the Stool

Stool characteristics are important in assessing the etiology of diarrhea. A description of the frequency, volume, consistency, and color provides diagnostic clues. For instance, diarrhea starting in the small intestine produces a copious, watery or fatty (greasy), and foul-smelling stool; contains undigested food particles; and is usually free from gross blood. Colonic diarrhea appears as small, pasty, and sometimes bloody or mucoid movements. Rectal tenesmus with flatus accompanies large intestinal diarrhea.

Clinical Presentation

Table 36-1 outlines the clinical presentation of diarrhea, and Table 36-2 shows common drug-induced causes of diarrhea. A medication history is extremely important in identifying drug-induced diarrhea. Many agents, including antibiotics and other drugs, cause diarrhea or, less commonly, pseudomembranous colitis. Self-inflicted laxative abuse for weight loss is popular.

Most acute diarrhea is self-limiting, subsiding within 72 hours. However, infants, young children, the elderly, and debilitated persons are at risk for morbid and mortal events in prolonged or voluminous diarrhea. These groups are at risk for water, electrolyte, and acid–base disturbances, and potentially cardiovascular collapse and death. The prognosis for chronic diarrhea depends on the cause; for example, diarrhea secondary to diabetes mellitus waxes and wanes throughout life.

TABLE 36-1 Clinical Presentation of Diarrhea

General
- Usually, acute diarrheal episodes subside within 72 hours of onset, whereas chronic diarrhea involves frequent attacks over extended time periods

Signs and symptoms
- Abrupt onset of nausea, vomiting, abdominal pain, headache, fever, chills, and malaise
- Bowel movements are frequent and never bloody, and diarrhea lasts 12-60 hours
- Intermittent periumbilical or lower right quadrant pain with cramps and audible bowel sounds is characteristic of small intestinal disease
- When pain is present in large intestinal diarrhea, it is a gripping, aching sensation with tenesmus (straining, ineffective, and painful stooling). Pain localizes to the hypogastric region, right or left lower quadrant, or sacral region
- In chronic diarrhea, a history of previous bouts, weight loss, anorexia, and chronic weakness are important findings

Physical examination
- Typically demonstrates hyperperistalsis with borborygmi and generalized or local tenderness

Laboratory tests
- Stool analysis studies include examination for microorganisms, blood, mucus, fat, osmolality, pH, electrolyte and mineral concentration, and cultures
- Stool test kits are useful for detecting GI viruses, particularly rotavirus
- Antibody serologic testing shows rising titers over a 3- to 6-day period, but this test is not practical and is nonspecific
- Occasionally, total daily stool volume is also determined
- Direct endoscopic visualization and biopsy of the colon may be undertaken to assess for the presence of conditions such as colitis or cancer
- Radiographic studies are helpful in neoplastic and inflammatory conditions

TREATMENT

Prevention

Acute viral diarrheal illness often occurs in daycare centers and nursing homes. Because person-to-person contact is the mechanism by which viral disease spreads, isolation techniques must be initiated. For bacterial, parasitic, and protozoal infections, strict food handling, sanitation, water, and other environmental hygiene practices can prevent transmission. If diarrhea is secondary to another illness, controlling the primary condition is necessary. Antibiotics and bismuth subsalicylate are advocated to prevent traveler's diarrhea, in conjunction with treatment of drinking water and caution with consumption of fresh vegetables.[6,7]

TABLE 36-2 Drugs Causing Diarrhea

- Laxatives
- Antacids containing magnesium
- Antineoplastics
- Auranofin (gold salt)
- Antibiotics
  - Clindamycin
  - Tetracyclines
  - Sulfonamides
  - Any broad-spectrum antibiotic
- Antihypertensives
  - Reserpine
  - Guanethidine
  - Methyldopa
  - Guanabenz
  - Guanadrel
  - Angiotensin-converting enzyme inhibitors
- Cholinergics
  - Bethanechol
  - Neostigmine
- Cardiac agents
  - Quinidine
  - Digitalis
  - Digoxin
- Nonsteroidal antiinflammatory drugs
- Misoprostol
- Colchicine
- Proton pump inhibitors
- H_2-receptor blockers

Desired Outcome

3 If prevention is unsuccessful and diarrhea occurs, therapeutic goals are to (a) manage the diet; (b) prevent excessive water, electrolyte, and acid–base disturbances; (c) provide symptomatic relief; (d) treat curable causes; and (e) manage secondary disorders causing diarrhea (Figs. 36-1 and 36-2).

Clinicians must clearly understand that diarrhea, like a cough, may be a body defense mechanism for ridding itself of harmful substances or pathogens. The correct therapeutic response is not necessarily to stop diarrhea at all costs.

Nonpharmacologic Management

Dietary management is a first priority in the treatment of diarrhea. Feeding should continue in children with acute bacterial diarrhea. Fed children have less morbidity and mortality, whether or not they receive oral rehydration fluids. Studies are not available in the elderly or in other high-risk groups to determine the value of continued feeding in bacterial diarrhea.

Clinical Controversy...

Most clinicians recommend discontinuing consumption of solid foods and dairy products for 24 hours in patients with acute diarrhea. However, withholding food is considered inappropriate in patients with no signs of severe dehydration. In osmotic diarrhea, it may control the problem. If the mechanism is secretory, diarrhea persists. For patients who are experiencing nausea and/or vomiting, a mild, digestible, low-residue diet should be administered for 24 hours. If vomiting is present and uncontrollable with antiemetics (see Chapter 35), nothing is taken by mouth. As bowel movements decrease, a bland diet is begun.

Water and Electrolytes

Rehydration and maintenance of water and electrolytes are primary treatment goals until the diarrheal episode ends. If the patient is volume depleted, rehydration should be directed at replacing water and electrolytes to normal body composition. Then water and electrolyte composition are maintained by replacing losses. Many patients will not develop volume depletion and therefore will only require maintenance fluid and electrolyte therapy. Parenteral and enteral routes may be used for supplying water and electrolytes. If vomiting and dehydration are not severe, enteral feeding is the less costly and preferred method. In the United States, many commercial oral rehydration preparations are available (Table 36-3).

Because of concerns about hypernatremia, physicians continue to hospitalize patients and use IV fluids to correct fluid and electrolyte deficits in severe dehydration. Oral solutions are strongly recommended.[8-10] In developing countries, the World Health Organization oral rehydration solution (WHO-ORS) saves the lives of millions of children annually.

During diarrhea, the small intestine retains its ability to actively transport monosaccharides such as glucose. Glucose actively carries sodium with water and other electrolytes. The WHO now recommends an ORS with a lower osmolarity, sodium content, and glucose load (see Table 36-3).[11] A separate oral supplement of zinc 20 mg daily for 10 days in addition to ORS significantly reduces the severity and duration of acute diarrhea in developing countries.[2] ORS is

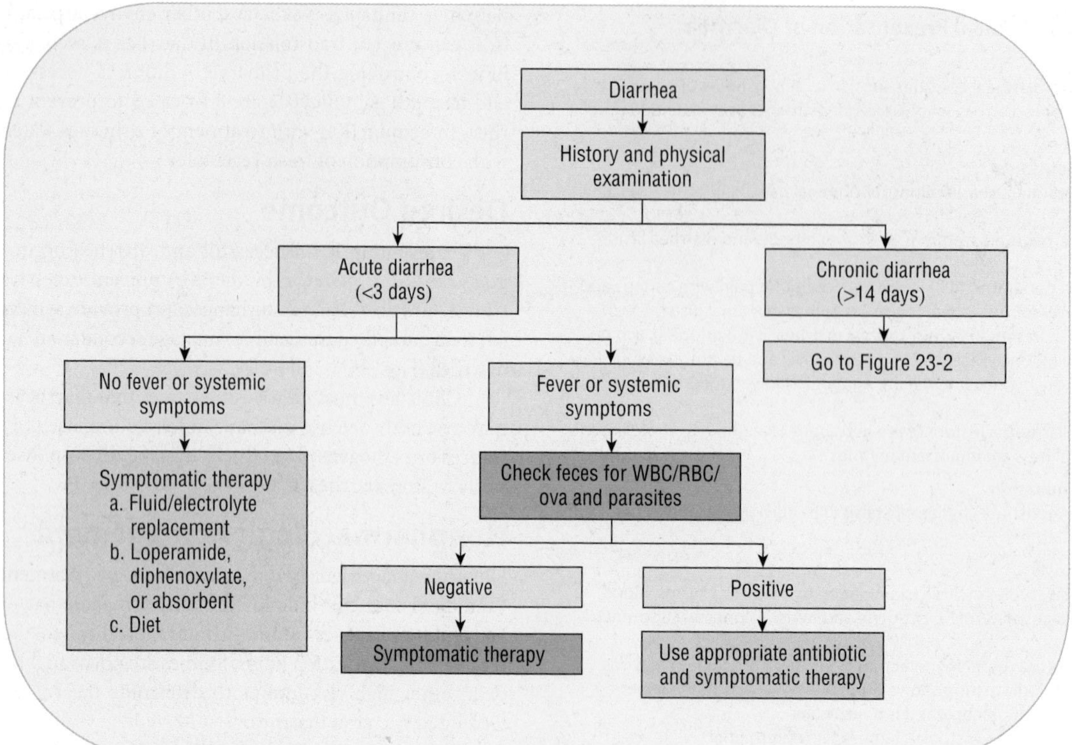

FIGURE 36-1 Recommendations for treating acute diarrhea. Follow the following steps: (a) Perform a complete history and physical examination. (b) Is the diarrhea acute or chronic? If chronic diarrhea, go to Fig. 36-2. (c) If acute diarrhea, check for fever and/or systemic signs and symptoms (ie, toxic patient). If systemic illness (fever, anorexia, or volume depletion), check for an infectious source. If positive for infectious diarrhea, use appropriate antibiotic/anthelmintic drug and symptomatic therapy. If negative for infectious cause, use only symptomatic treatment. (d) If no systemic findings, then use symptomatic therapy based on severity of volume depletion, oral or parenteral fluid/electrolytes, antidiarrheal agents (see Table 36-4), and diet (RBC, red blood cells; WBC, white blood cells).

a lifesaving treatment for millions afflicted in developing countries. Acceptance in developed countries is less enthusiastic; however, the advantage of this product in reducing hospitalizations may prove its use as a cost-effective alternative, saving millions of dollars in health care expenditures.

Pharmacologic Therapy

Various drugs have been used to treat diarrheal attacks (Table 36-4), including antimotility agents, adsorbents, antisecretory compounds, antibiotics, enzymes, and intestinal microflora. Usually these drugs are not curative but palliative.

Opiates and Their Derivatives

Opiates and opioid derivatives (a) delay the transit of intraluminal contents or (b) increase gut capacity, prolonging contact and absorption. Enkephalins, which are endogenous opioid substances, regulate fluid movement across the mucosa by stimulating absorptive processes. Limitations to the use of opiates include an addiction potential (a real concern with long-term use) and worsening of diarrhea in selected infectious diarrhea.

Most opiates act through peripheral and central mechanisms with the exception of loperamide, which acts only peripherally. Loperamide is antisecretory; it inhibits the calcium-binding protein calmodulin, controlling chloride secretion. Loperamide, available as 2 mg capsules or 1 mg/5 mL solution (both are nonprescription products), is suggested for managing acute and chronic diarrhea. The usual adult dose is initially 4 mg orally, followed by 2 mg after each loose stool, up to 16 mg/day. Used correctly, this agent has rare side effects, such as dizziness and constipation. If the diarrhea is concurrent with a high fever or bloody stool, the patient should be referred to a physician. Also, diarrhea lasting 48 hours beyond initiating loperamide warrants medical attention. Loperamide can also be used in traveler's diarrhea. It is comparable to bismuth subsalicylate for treatment of this disorder.[6]

Diphenoxylate is available as a 2.5 mg tablet and as a 2.5 mg/5 mL solution. A small amount of atropine (0.025 mg) is included in the product to discourage abuse. In adults, when taken as 2.5 to 5 mg three or four times daily, not to exceed a 20 mg total daily dose, diphenoxylate is rarely toxic. Some patients may complain of atropinism (blurred vision, dry mouth, and urinary hesitancy). Like loperamide, it should not be used in patients who are at risk of bacterial enteritis with *E. coli*, *Shigella*, or *Salmonella*.

Difenoxin, a diphenoxylate derivative also chemically related to meperidine, is also combined with atropine and has the same uses, precautions, and side effects. Marketed as a 1 mg tablet, the adult dosage is 2 mg initially, followed by 1 mg after each loose stool, not to exceed 8 mg/day.

Paregoric, camphorated tincture of opium, is marketed as a 2 mg/5 mL solution and is indicated for managing both acute and chronic diarrhea. It is not widely prescribed today because of its abuse potential.

Adsorbents

Adsorbents are used for symptomatic relief. These products, many not requiring a prescription, are nontoxic, but their effectiveness remains unproven. Adsorbents are nonspecific in their action; they adsorb nutrients, toxins, drugs, and digestive juices. Polycarbophil absorbs 60 times its weight in water and can be used to treat both diarrhea and constipation. It is a nonprescription product and is sold as a 500 mg chewable tablet. This hydrophilic, nonabsorbable

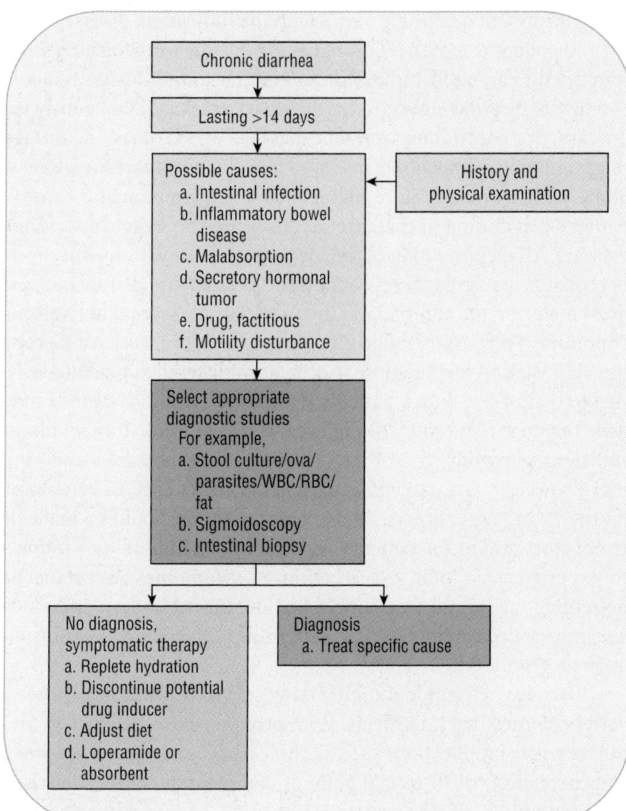

FIGURE 36-2 Recommendations for treating chronic diarrhea. Follow the following steps: (a) Perform a careful history and physical examination. (b) The possible causes of chronic diarrhea are many. These can be classified into intestinal infections (bacterial or protozoal), inflammatory disease (Crohn's disease or ulcerative colitis), malabsorption (lactose intolerance), secretory hormonal tumor (intestinal carcinoid tumor or vasoactive intestinal peptide-secreting tumor [VIPoma]), drug (antacid), factitious (laxative abuse), or motility disturbance (diabetes mellitus, irritable bowel syndrome, or hyperthyroidism). (c) If the diagnosis is uncertain, selected appropriate diagnostic studies should be ordered. (d) Once diagnosed, treatment is planned for the underlying cause with symptomatic antidiarrheal therapy. (e) If no specific cause can be identified, symptomatic therapy is prescribed (RBC, red blood cells; WBC, white blood cells).

product is safe and may be taken four times daily, up to 6 g/day in adults. See Table 36-4 for selected antidiarrheal preparations.

Antisecretory Agents

Bismuth subsalicylate appears to have antisecretory, antiinflammatory, and antibacterial effects. As a nonprescription product, it is marketed for indigestion, relieving abdominal cramps, and controlling diarrhea, including traveler's diarrhea. Bismuth subsalicylate dosage strengths are a 262 mg chewable tablet, 262 mg/5 mL liquid, and 524 mg/15 mL liquid. The usual adult dose is two tablets or 30 mL every 30 minutes to 1 hour up to eight doses per day.

4 Bismuth subsalicylate contains multiple components that might be toxic if given excessively to prevent or treat diarrhea. For instance, an active ingredient is salicylate, which may interact with anticoagulants or may produce salicylism (tinnitus, nausea, and vomiting). Bismuth reduces tetracycline absorption and may interfere with select GI radiographic studies. Patients may complain of a darkening of the tongue and stools with repeat administration. Salicylate can induce gout attacks in susceptible individuals.

Bismuth subsalicylate suspension has been evaluated in the treatment of secretory diarrhea of infectious etiology as well. In a dose of 30 mL every 30 minutes for eight doses, unformed stools decrease in the first 24 hours. Bismuth subsalicylate may also be effective in preventing traveler's diarrhea.

Octreotide, a synthetic octapeptide analog of endogenous somatostatin, is effective for the symptomatic treatment of carcinoid tumors and other peptide-secreting tumors, dumping syndrome, and chemotherapy-induced diarrhea.[12] It has had limited success in patients with AIDS-associated diarrhea and short-bowel syndrome, does not appear to have an advantage over various opiate derivatives in the treatment of chronic idiopathic diarrhea, and has the disadvantage of being administered by injection.[13] Metastatic intestinal carcinoid tumors secrete excessive amounts of vasoactive substances, including histamine, bradykinin, serotonin (5-hydroxytryptamine, 5-HT), and prostaglandins. Primary carcinoid tumors occur throughout the GI tract, with most in the ileum. Predominant signs and symptoms experienced by patients with these tumors are attributable to excessive concentrations of 5-hydroxytryptophan and 5-HT. The totality of their clinical effects is termed the carcinoid syndrome. Some patients have a violent, watery diarrhea with abdominal cramping. Initially, diarrhea might be managed with various agents such as codeine, diphenoxylate, cyproheptadine, methysergide, phenoxybenzamine, or methyldopa. But octreotide is now considered first-line therapy for carcinoid syndrome.

TABLE 36-3 Oral Rehydration Solutions

	WHO-ORS[a]	Pedialyte[b] (Ross)	CeraLyte (Cera Products)	Enfalyte (Mead Johnson)
Osmolality (mOsm/kg or mmol/kg)	245	250	220	167
Carbohydrates[b] (g/L)	13.5	25	40[c]	30[c]
Calories (cal/L [J/L])	65 (272)	100 (418)	160 (670)	126 (527)
Electrolytes (mEq/L; mmol/L)				
Sodium	75	45	50-90	50
Potassium	20	20	20	25
Chloride	65	35	40-80	45
Citrate	—	30	30	34
Bicarbonate	30	—	—	—
Calcium	—	—	—	—
Magnesium	—	—	—	—
Sulfate	—	—	—	—
Phosphate	—	—	—	—

[a]World Health Organization reduced osmolarity oral rehydration solution.
[b]Carbohydrate is glucose.
[c]Rice syrup solids are carbohydrate source.

TABLE 36-4 Selected Antidiarrheal Preparations

	Dose Form	Adult Dose
Antimotility		
Diphenoxylate	2.5 mg/tablet	5 mg four times daily; do not exceed 20 mg/day
	2.5 mg/5 mL	
Loperamide	2 mg/capsule	Initially 4 mg, and then 2 mg after each loose stool; do not exceed 16 mg/day
	2 mg/capsule	
Paregoric	2 mg/5 mL (morphine)	5-10 mL one to four times daily
Opium tincture	10 mg/mL (morphine)	0.6 mL four times daily
Difenoxin	1 mg/tablet	Two tablets, and then one tablet after each loose stool; up to eight tablets per day
Adsorbents		
Kaolin-pectin mixture	5.7 g kaolin + 130.2 mg pectin/30 mL	30-120 mL after each loose stool
Polycarbophil	500 mg/tablet	Chew 2 tablets four times daily or after each loose stool; do not exceed 12 tablets per day
Attapulgite	750 mg/15 mL 300 mg/7.5 mL 750 mg/tablet 600 mg/tablet 300 mg/tablet	1,200-1,500 mg after each loose bowel movement or every 2 hours; up to 9,000 mg/day
Antisecretory		
Bismuth subsalicylate	1,050 mg/30 mL 262 mg/15 mL 524 mg/15 mL 262 mg/tablet	Two tablets or 30 mL every 30 minutes to 1 hour as needed up to eight doses per day
Enzymes (lactase)	1,250 neutral lactase units/4 drops 3,300 FCC lactase units per tablet	Three to four drops taken with milk or dairy product
Bacterial replacement (*Lactobacillus acidophilus, Lactobacillus bulgaricus*)		Two tablets or one granule packet three to four times daily; give with milk, juice, or water
Octreotide	0.05 mg/mL 0.1 mg/mL 0.5 mg/mL	Initial: 50 mcg subcutaneously One to two times per day and titrate dose based on indication up to 600 mcg/day in two to four divided doses

Octreotide blocks the release of 5-HT and many other active peptides and has been effective in controlling diarrhea and flushing. It is reported to have direct inhibitory effects on intestinal secretion and stimulatory effects on intestinal absorption. Non-gastrin-secreting adenomas of the pancreas are tumors associated with profuse watery diarrhea. This condition has been referred to as Verner–Morrison syndrome, WDHA (watery diarrhea, hypokalemia, and achlorhydria) syndrome, pancreatic cholera, watery diarrhea syndrome, and vasoactive intestinal peptide-secreting tumor (VIPoma). Excessive secretion of VIP from a retroperitoneal or pancreatic tumor produces most of the clinical features. Surgical tumor dissection is the treatment of choice. In nonsurgical candidates, the profuse watery diarrhea and other symptoms commonly encountered are managed with octreotide.

The dose of octreotide varies with the indication, disease severity, and patient response.[12] For managing diarrhea and flushing associated with carcinoid tumors in adults, the initial dosage range is 100 to 600 mcg/day in two to four divided doses subcutaneously for 2 weeks. For controlling secretory diarrhea of VIPomas, the dosage range is 200 to 300 mcg/day in two to four divided doses for 2 weeks. Some patients may require higher doses for symptomatic control. Patients responding to these initial doses may be switched to Sandostatin LAR Depot, a long-acting octreotide formulation. This product consists of microspheres containing the drug. Initial doses consist of 20 mg given intramuscularly intragluteally at 4-week intervals for 2 months. It is recommended that during the first 2 weeks of therapy the short-acting formulation also be administered subcutaneously. At the end of 2 months, patients with good symptom control may have the dose reduced to 10 mg every 4 weeks, while those without sufficient symptom control may have the dose increased to 30 mg every 4 weeks. For patients experiencing recurrence of symptoms on the 10 mg dose, dosage adjustment to 20 mg should be made. It is not uncommon for patients with carcinoid tumors or VIPomas to experience periodic exacerbation of symptoms. Subcutaneous octreotide for several days should be reinstituted in these individuals. In so-called carcinoid crisis, octreotide is given as an IV infusion at 50 mcg/h for 8 to 24 hours.

Because octreotide inhibits many other GI hormones, it has a variety of intestinal side effects. With prolonged use, gallbladder and biliary tract complications such as cholelithiasis have been reported. Approximately 5% to 10% of patients complain of nausea, diarrhea, and abdominal pain. Local injection pain occurs with about an 8% incidence. With high doses, octreotide may reduce dietary fat absorption, leading to steatorrhea.

Two other somatostatin analogs, lanreotide and vapreotide, have been studied.[13,14] Lanreotide is approved for use in the United States for acromegaly. The starting dose is 90 mg subcutaneously every 4 weeks for 3 months, and then the dose is adjusted based on growth hormone and insulin-like growth factor levels.[15] Vapreotide is an orphan drug that is indicated for pancreatic and GI fistulas as well as esophageal variceal bleeding.

Miscellaneous Products

Probiotics are microorganisms that have been used for many years to replace colonic microflora. This supposedly restores normal intestinal function and suppresses the growth of pathogenic microorganisms. *Saccharomyces boulardii*, *Lactobacillus* GG, and *Lactobacillus acidophilus* decrease the duration of infectious and antibiotic-induced diarrhea in adults and children.[16] A meta-analysis suggests that probiotics may prevent antibiotic-associated diarrhea (AAD).[17] However, a randomized control trial in hospitalized patients over the age of 65 years found no difference in cases of AAD between a probiotic preparation (two strains of lactobacillus acidophilus and Bifidobacterium) and placebo.[18] The dosage of probiotic preparations varies depending on the brand used. Intestinal flatus is the primary patient complaint experienced with this modality.

Anticholinergic drugs such as atropine block vagal tone and prolong gut transit time. Drugs with anticholinergic properties are present in many nonprescription products. Their value in controlling diarrhea is questionable and limited because of side effects. Angle-closure glaucoma, selected heart diseases, and obstructive uropathies are relative contraindications to the use of anticholinergic agents.

Lactase enzyme products are helpful for patients who are experiencing diarrhea secondary to lactose intolerance. Lactase is required for carbohydrate digestion. When a patient lacks this enzyme, eating dairy products causes an osmotic diarrhea. Several products are available for use each time a dairy product, especially milk or ice cream, is consumed.

Clinical **Controversy...**

The use of probiotics to treat and prevent AAD is controversial. A meta-analysis published in 2012 concluded that adjunctive probiotics significantly reduce the risk of acquiring AAD, but individual studies, including a well-designed randomized control trial published in 2013, have been unable to show a difference when compared with placebo. Additional studies are needed to compare different probiotic formulations, determine optimal dosing, and evaluate whether efficacy differs based on the antibiotic used. Additional safety data are also required before probiotics can be recommended routinely for this purpose.

Vaccines

Vaccines are a new therapeutic frontier in controlling infectious diarrheas, especially in developing countries.[19,20] An oral vaccine for cholera is licensed and available in other countries (Dukoral from SBL Vaccines) and appears to provide somewhat better immunity and has fewer adverse effects than the previously available parenteral vaccine. However, the CDC does not recommend cholera vaccines for most travelers, nor is the vaccine available in the United States.

Oral *Shigella* vaccine, although effective under field conditions, requires five weekly oral doses and repeat booster doses, thereby limiting its practicality for use in developing nations. With about 1,500 serotypes for *Salmonella*, a vaccine is not currently available for humans. There are two newer typhoid vaccine formulations, one a parenteral inactivated whole-cell vaccine and the other an oral live-attenuated (Ty21a) vaccine that is administered in four doses on days 1, 3, 5, and 7, to be completed at least 1 week before exposure. Two rotavirus vaccines have been shown to prevent gastroenteritis due to rotavirus infection in infants and children.[21] The pentavalent human-bovine reassortant vaccine (RotaTeq from Merck) is administered as a three-oral-dose sequence, and the monovalent human vaccine (Rotarix from GlaxoSmithKline) is administered as a two-oral-dose sequence. A rotavirus vaccine program has been formed to reduce child morbidity and mortality from diarrheal disease by accelerating the availability of rotavirus vaccines appropriate for use in developing countries.

Evaluation of Therapeutic Outcomes

Therapeutic outcomes are directed toward key symptoms, signs, and laboratory studies. Constitutional symptoms usually improve within 24 to 72 hours. Monitoring for changes in the frequency and character of bowel movements on a daily basis in conjunction with vital signs and improvement in appetite are of utmost importance. Also, the clinician needs to monitor body weight, serum osmolality, serum electrolytes, complete blood cell counts, urinalysis, and culture results (if appropriate).

Acute Diarrhea

Most patients with acute diarrhea experience mild to moderate distress. In the absence of moderate to severe dehydration, high fever, and blood or mucus in the stool, this illness is usually self-limiting within 3 to 7 days. Mild to moderate acute diarrhea is usually managed on an outpatient basis with oral rehydration, symptomatic treatment, and diet. Elderly persons with chronic illness as well as infants may require hospitalization for parenteral rehydration and close monitoring.

Severe Diarrhea

In the urgent/emergent situation, restoration of the patient's volume status is the most important outcome. Toxic patients (fever dehydration, hematochezia, or hypotension) require hospitalization, IV fluids and electrolyte administration, and empiric antibiotic therapy while awaiting culture and sensitivity results. With timely management, these patients usually recover within a few days.

CONSTIPATION

5 Constipation is a common complaint among the general population and accounts for many medical visits each year in the United States.[22] It is generally defined by the American Gastroenterology Association (AGA) as difficult or infrequent passage of stool, at times associated with straining or a feeling of incomplete defecation.[23]

Constipation may be further defined by quantitative or qualitative measures. For instance, physicians often use stool frequency to define constipation (most commonly fewer than three bowel movements per week); however, the "normal" frequency of bowel movement is not well established and can vary from person to person. Patients more often describe constipation in terms of symptoms or a combination of quantitative and qualitative descriptors that are difficult to quantify: bowel movement frequency, stool size or consistency (hard or lumpy stools), straining on defecation, inability to defecate at will, and symptoms such as sensation of incomplete evacuation. The condition is considered chronic if symptoms last for at least 3 months. Many people believe that daily bowel movements are required for normal health or that accumulation of toxic substances will occur with infrequent defecation. Inappropriate laxative use by the general public may result from these misconceptions.

Though often considered more of a minor uncomfortable or unpleasant problem, constipation can have serious consequences and be costly to the health care system. Costs for medical evaluation of constipation alone have been estimated at more than $2,500 per patient, and patients spend more than $800 million each year on nonprescription laxatives.[22,24]

Epidemiology

The prevalence of constipation depends on the definition used and whether the condition is self-reported or provider-diagnosed. A systematic review of 45 studies reported the prevalence of chronic constipation in adults (elder than or equal to 15 years old) worldwide to be 14%.[23] The highest incidence was found in South America (16%) and the lowest incidence in Southeast Asia. A review of the epidemiology of constipation in North America found a prevalence up to 27%, with most reported estimates ranging from 12% to 19%.[25] Similarly, in a multinational survey of 13,879 adults from seven countries, the rate of self-reported constipation was 12.3% overall (range 5%-18%).[25,26]

Constipation is more common in women (2.4-fold more likely) and the elderly.[23] Other factors associated with constipation in some reports include inactivity, lower socioeconomic class, lower income, non-white race, symptoms of depression, and history of physical or sexual abuse.

Pathophysiology

Constipation may be primary or secondary. Primary, or idiopathic, constipation occurs without an identifiable underlying cause, whereas secondary constipation may be the result of constipating drugs, lifestyle factors, or medical disorders (Table 36-5).[27] Primary constipation can be further divided into three categories—normal transit, slow transit, and pelvic floor dysfunction, or disordered defecation.[28] Normal transit constipation, often referred to as functional, is the most common type. These patients have normal GI motility and stool frequency but may experience difficulty evacuating, passage of hard stools, or bloating and abdominal discomfort. Slow transit constipation represents an abnormality of GI transit time that leads to infrequent defecation. Dysfunction of the pelvic floor muscles and/or anal sphincter is the most frequently encountered

TABLE 36-5 Possible Causes of Constipation

Conditions	Possible Causes
GI disorders	Irritable bowel syndrome
	Diverticulitis
	Upper GI tract diseases
	Anal and rectal diseases
	Hemorrhoids
	Anal fissures
	Ulcerative proctitis
	Tumors
	Hernia
	Volvulus of the bowel
	Syphilis
	Tuberculosis
	Helminthic infections
	Lymphogranuloma venereum
	Hirschsprung's disease
Metabolic and endocrine disorders	Diabetes mellitus with neuropathy
	Hypothyroidism
	Panhypopituitarism
	Pheochromocytoma
	Hypercalcemia
	Enteric glucagon excess
Cardiac disorders	Heart failure
Pregnancy	Depressed gut motility
	Increased fluid absorption from colon
	Use of iron salts
Lifestyle factors	Dietary changes
	Inadequate fluid intake
	Low dietary fiber
	Decreased physical activity
Neurogenic causes	CNS diseases
	Trauma to the brain (particularly the medulla)
	Spinal cord injury
	CNS tumors
	Cerebrovascular accidents
	Parkinson's disease
Psychogenic causes	Ignoring or postponing urge to defecate
	Psychiatric diseases
Drug induced	See Table 36-6

TABLE 36-6 Drugs Causing Constipation

Analgesics
Inhibitors of prostaglandin synthesis
Opiates
Anticholinergics
Antihistamines
Antiparkinsonian agents (eg, benztropine or trihexyphenidyl)
Phenothiazines
Tricyclic antidepressants
Antacids containing calcium carbonate or aluminum hydroxide
Barium sulfate
Calcium channel antagonists
Clonidine
Diuretics (non–potassium-sparing)
Ganglionic blockers
Iron preparations
Muscle blockers (D-tubocurarine, succinylcholine)
Nonsteroidal antiinflammatory agents
Polystyrene sodium sulfonate

reason for disordered defecation. In patients with defecatory disorders, these muscles or sphincter contract during defecation instead of relax and impede evacuation of stool. It is common for patients to have and present with more than one type of constipation.

Factors associated with the increased prevalence of constipation in the elderly include a higher number of daily medications, particularly anticholinergic agents, increased incidence of chronic comorbidities, and changes in mobility status.[24] Changes in diet such as decreased fluid and/or fiber intake, diminished physical activity, and institutionalization can lead to constipation. Physiologic changes such as mesenteric dysfunction and changes in anorectal function, including loss of rectal wall elasticity, are also thought to predispose elderly patients to constipation.

Drug-Induced Constipation

Use of drugs that inhibit the neurologic or muscular function of the GI tract, particularly the colon, may result in secondary constipation.[27] Medications that are commonly associated with causing constipation include opiates, anticholinergic agents, and certain antacids.[24] With most of the agents listed in Table 36-6, the inhibitory effects on bowel function may be dose dependent, with larger doses causing constipation more frequently.

Opiates have effects on all segments of the bowel, but effects are most pronounced on the colon.[23] The major mechanism by which opiates produce constipation has been proposed to be prolongation of intestinal transit time by causing spastic, nonpropulsive contractions. Additionally, anal sphincter tone may be increased with an accompanying decrease in reflex relaxation leading to difficult rectal evacuation.[29]

While all opiate derivatives are associated with constipation, the degree of intestinal inhibitory effects seems to differ between agents. Orally administered opiates appear to have greater inhibitory effects than parenterally administered products. In some reports, transdermal fentanyl has been associated with less constipation than oral sustained-release morphine.[30]

Other medications may increase the risk of constipation by a variety of mechanisms. Anticholinergic agents decrease contractility of intestinal muscle while calcium channel blockers are thought to cause rectosigmoid dysfunction, leading to constipation. Nonsteroidal antiinflammatory drugs (NSAIDs) may lead to constipation due to their inhibition of prostaglandin synthesis.[24]

Clinical Presentation

A symptom-based system for classifying functional constipation (and other functional GI disorders) is often used to define constipation in clinical trials. The Rome criteria encompass both quantitative (frequency) and qualitative (stool consistency, etc.) symptoms associated with constipation.[31] Table 36-7 outlines general clinical presentation of patients with constipation. According to the Rome III criteria, patients should have at least two of the signs and symptoms listed in Table 36-7 apply to a minimum of 25% of bowel movements.

Evaluation of constipation should attempt to clarify the patient's specific symptoms (ie, exactly what the patient means by constipation).[31] A complete and thorough history should be obtained from the patient, including frequency of bowel movements and duration of symptoms. Constipation occurring abruptly in an adult may indicate significant colon pathology such as malignancy. Constipation present since early infancy may be indicative of neurologic disorders. The patient should also be carefully questioned about usual diet and laxative regimens. Does the patient have a diet consistently deficient in high-fiber items and containing mainly high refined foods? What laxatives or cathartics has the patient used to attempt relief of constipation? The patient should be questioned about other concurrent medications, with interest focused on agents that might cause constipation.

Evaluation should also include perianal and anal examinations to identify fecal impaction or other anatomical obstructions that may be contributing to or causing constipation. General health status, signs of underlying medical illness (ie, hypothyroidism), and psychological status (eg, depression or other psychological illness)

TABLE 36-7 Clinical Presentation of Constipation

Signs and symptoms
- Infrequent bowel movements (<3 per week)
- Stools that are hard, small, or dry
- Difficulty or pain of defecation
- Feeling of abdominal discomfort or bloating, incomplete evacuation, etc.

Alarm signs and symptoms
- Hematochezia
- Melena
- Family history of colon cancer
- Family history of inflammatory bowel disease
- Anemia
- Weight loss
- Anorexia
- Nausea and vomiting
- Severe, persistent constipation that is refractory to treatment
- New-onset or worsening constipation in elderly without evidence of primary cause

Physical examination
- Perform rectal exam for presence of anatomical abnormalities (such as fistulas, fissures, hemorrhoids, rectal prolapse) or abnormalities of perianal descent
- Digital examination of rectum to check for fecal impaction, anal stricture, or rectal mass

Laboratory and other diagnostic tests
- No routine recommendations for lab testing—as indicated by clinical discretion
- In patients with signs and symptoms suggestive of organic disorder, specific testing may be performed (ie, thyroid function tests, electrolytes, glucose, complete blood count) based on clinical presentation
- In patients with alarm signs and symptoms or when structural disease is a possibility, select appropriate diagnostic studies:
  1. Protoscopy
  2. Sigmoidoscopy
  3. Colonoscopy
  4. Barium enema

should also be assessed. Laboratory tests may be performed, particularly if the patient is presumed to suffer from secondary causes and is still experiencing symptoms after a trial of fiber supplementation or other nonprescription therapies.[28]

Specific attention should be given to identify any "alarm symptoms" that would warrant further diagnostic workup (see Table 36-7).[32] Patients with alarm symptoms, a family history of colon cancer, or those more than 50 years old with new symptoms may need further diagnostic evaluation.

TREATMENT

Desired Outcome

The major goals of treatment are to (a) relieve symptoms; (b) reestablish normal bowel habits; and (c) improve quality of life by minimizing adverse effects of treatment.

General Approach to Treatment

Table 36-8 presents a general treatment algorithm for the management of constipation.

6 Approaches to the treatment of constipation should begin with attempts to determine its cause. If an underlying disease is recognized as the cause of constipation, attempts should be made to correct it. GI malignancies may be removed via surgical resection. Endocrine and metabolic derangements should be corrected by the appropriate methods. For example, when hypothyroidism is the cause of constipation, cautious institution of thyroid replacement therapy is the most important treatment measure. If a patient is consuming medications known to cause constipation, consideration should be given to alternative agents. If a patient must remain on constipating medications, then more attention must be given to general measures for prevention of constipation, as discussed in the next section. Also, patients with opioid-induced constipation (OIC) may require the routine use of pharmacologic agents, also discussed below.

TABLE 36-8 Constipation Treatment Algorithm

Diagnosis
1. Treat specific cause
2. No underlying diagnosis, then choose symptomatic therapy
   A. Dietary modification to increase fiber ± supplementation (bulk agents)
   B. Add Osmotic laxative (ie, PEG) if no relief; trial 2-4 weeks
   C. Add stimulant laxative (ie, bisacodyl) if no relief or no BM in 2 days
   D. Lubiprostone or linaclotide trial
   E. Opioid-receptor antagonists if opioid-induced constipation

The proper management of constipation will require a combination of nonpharmacologic and pharmacologic therapies. Osmotic laxative therapy is considered the preferred first line for the treatment of constipation, in addition to increasing dietary fiber or using fiber supplementation.[28] Patients are often encouraged to increase daily fluid intake and physical activity as well dedicate time to respond to the urge to defecate, although efficacy data are conflicting for these measures.[33]

Nonpharmacologic Therapy

Dietary Modification

The most important aspect of therapy for constipation for the majority of patients is dietary modification to increase the amount of fiber consumed. Fiber, the portion of vegetable matter not digested in the human GI tract, increases stool bulk, retention of stool water, and rate of transit of stool through the intestine. The result of fiber therapy is an increased frequency of defecation. Also, fiber decreases intraluminal pressures in the colon and rectum, which is thought to be beneficial for diverticular disease and for irritable bowel syndrome (IBS).

7 The specific physiologic effects of fiber are not well understood. Patients should be advised to gradually increase daily fiber intake to 20 to 25 g, through either dietary changes or fiber supplement products (see Bulk-Forming Agents below), a grade B recommendation from the American College of Gastroenterology.[34] Fruits, vegetables, and cereals typically have the highest fiber content. Bran, a by-product of milling of wheat, is often added to foods to increase fiber content and contains a high amount of soluble fiber, which may be extremely constipating in larger doses. Raw bran is generally 40% fiber. A small randomized controlled trial revealed that adding prunes (approximately 6 g fiber/day), or dried plums, to daily diet was more effective than adding psyllium (6 g fiber/day) in treating mild to moderate constipation.[35]

A trial of dietary modification with high-fiber content should be continued for at least 1 month before effects on bowel function are determined. Most patients begin to notice effects on bowel function 3 to 5 days after beginning a high-fiber diet, but some patients may require a considerably longer period of time. Patients should be cautioned that abdominal distension and flatulence may be particularly troublesome in the first few weeks of fiber therapy, especially with high bran consumption. Gradually increasing dietary fiber over a few weeks to the goal of 20 to 25 g may help reduce some of the adverse abdominal effects, as well as ensuring adequate fluid intake. In most cases these problems resolve with continued use.

Surgery

In a small percentage of patients who present with complaints of constipation, surgical procedures are necessary because of the presence of colonic malignancies or GI obstruction from a number of other causes. Patients who have slow-transit-type primary constipation that is refractory to treatment are also surgical candidates.[33] Surgery may be required in some endocrine disorders that cause constipation, such as pheochromocytoma, which requires removal of a tumor. In each case, the involved segment of intestine may be resected or revised.

Biofeedback

Patients with constipation due to pelvic floor dysfunction/disordered defecation may have a less favorable response to fiber therapy than other constipation subtypes.[34] Many adult patients with functional defecatory disorders appear to benefit from pelvic floor retraining with biofeedback therapy. The goals of biofeedback are to improve pelvic floor relaxation to facilitate the passage of stool and the procedure is typically performed over 4- to 6-hour-long sessions. Success rates of 65% to 80% have been reported in controlled and uncontrolled studies, and improvement has been sustained for up to 1 year. The value of biofeedback in children with chronic constipation has not been well demonstrated.

Electrical Stimulation

Sacral nerve stimulation is a minimally invasive technique that has been used for treatment of fecal incontinence and there are some reports of its use in severe refractory chronic constipation.[36] However, clinical data supporting the use of electrical stimulation for this purpose are limited and there are currently no recommendations for general practice.

Pharmacologic Therapy

Three general classes of laxatives are discussed in this section: (a) those causing softening of feces in 1 to 3 days; (b) those that result in soft or semifluid stool in 6 to 12 hours; and (c) those causing watery evacuation in 1 to 6 hours (Table 36-9). Other pharmacologic agents available for the treatment of constipation include a calcium channel activator, guanylate cyclase C agonist, and serotonergic agents.

TABLE 36-9 Dosage Recommendations for Laxatives and Cathartics

Agent	Recommended Dose
Agents that Cause Softening of Feces in 1-3 Days	
Bulk-forming agents/osmotic laxatives	
Methylcellulose	4-6 g/day
Polycarbophil	4-6 g/day
Psyllium	Varies with product
Emollients	
Docusate sodium	50-360 mg/day
Docusate calcium	50-360 mg/day
Docusate potassium	100-300 mg/day
Polyethylene glycol 3350	17 g/dose
Lactulose	15-30 mL orally
Sorbitol	30-50 g/day orally
Agents that Result in Soft or Semifluid Stool in 6-12 Hours	
Bisacodyl (oral)	5-15 mg orally
Senna	Dose varies with formulation
Magnesium sulfate (low dose)	<10 g orally
Agents that Cause Watery Evacuation in 1-6 Hours	
Magnesium citrate	18 g 300 mL water
Magnesium hydroxide	2.4-4.8 g orally
Magnesium sulfate (high dose)	10-30 g orally
Sodium phosphates	Varies with salt used
Bisacodyl	10 mg rectally
Polyethylene glycol-electrolyte preparations	4 L

Bulk-Forming Agents

Medicinal products, often called "bulk-forming agents," such as psyllium hydrophilic colloids, methylcellulose, or polycarbophil, have properties similar to those of dietary fiber and may be taken as tablets, powders, or granules.[24] These agents increase the water content of stool to increase stool bulk and weight and relieve the symptoms of constipation within 3 days of initiating therapy.

Bulk-forming laxatives have few adverse effects. The most common effects include flatulence, abdominal bloating, and distention. Rarely, these agents may lead to bowel obstruction. Patients should also be cautioned to consume sufficient fluid while supplementing with bulk-forming agents to avoid obstruction of the esophagus, stomach, small intestine, and colon.

Emollient Laxatives

Emollient laxatives, including docusate in its various salts, are surfactant agents that work by facilitating mixing of aqueous and fatty materials within the intestinal tract; these are commonly referred to as stool softeners.[37] They may increase water and electrolyte secretion in the small and large bowel. Increased stool moisture content should lead to a softer, easier-to-pass stool. These products are generally given orally, although docusate potassium has also been used rectally. With these products, softening of stools occurs within 1 to 3 days of therapy.

Emollient laxatives are ineffective in treating constipation but are used mainly to prevent this condition. They may be helpful in situations in which straining at stool should be avoided, such as after recovery from myocardial infarction (MI), with acute perianal disease, or after rectal surgery. It is unlikely that these agents would be effective in preventing constipation if major causative factors (eg, heavy opiate use, uncorrected pathology, or inadequate dietary fiber) are not concurrently addressed. The use of mineral oil is generally not recommended due to safety concerns.

Although docusates are generally safe, a few adverse effects have been noted. They may increase the intestinal absorption of agents administered concurrently and alter toxic potential. Reports of increased fecal soiling associated with docusate use in elderly patients may limit their use in this population.[37]

Hyperosmolar Agents

Lactulose and Sorbitol Lactulose is a nonabsorbable disaccharide that is metabolized by colonic bacteria to low-molecular-weight acids, resulting in an osmotic effect whereby fluid is retained in the colon.[37] The fluid retained in the colon lowers the pH and increases colonic peristalsis within 2 to 3 days of use. Lactulose increases stool frequency and consistency in patients with chronic constipation (vs placebo) and may be more effective than fiber alone. In comparison to polyethylene glycol (PEG), lactulose is slightly less effective in increasing stool frequency per week and patients are more likely to need additional products for constipation relief.[38] The most common adverse effects include flatulence, nausea, and abdominal discomfort or bloating—although lactulose can be useful in some patients. It may be justified as an alternative for acute constipation or in patients with an inadequate response to increased dietary fiber and bulking agents. In some patients with more complex disease or nonmodifiable risk factors for constipation (such as bedridden, elderly patients with chronic or debilitating illnesses and constipating medications), lactulose may be required on a more regular basis.[37] In addition to the adverse abdominal effects associated with lactulose, diarrhea and electrolyte imbalances can occasionally occur. Sorbitol, a monosaccharide, also exerts its effect by osmotic action and has been recommended as a cost-effective alternative to lactulose. It is as effective as lactulose but may cause less nausea and is much less expensive.

Polyethylene Glycol PEG is FDA-approved for treatment of constipation at low doses and is expected to produce a bowel movement in 1 to 3 days.[37,38] For this indication, PEG is administered in smaller volumes (10-30 or 17-34 g per 120-240 mL) usually once (or twice) daily. PEG is not absorbed systemically or metabolized by colonic bacteria, and therefore has a lower incidence of adverse effects compared with other osmotic laxatives. Daily use in low dose (17 g) may be safe and effective for up to 6 months.[39] PEG has a grade A recommendation from the American College of Gastroenterology for the treatment of chronic constipation and is available as a nonprescription drug.[31] It is also preferred by the American Gastroenterology Association if fiber supplementation is insufficient due to high efficacy based on high quality of evidence available.[28] The most common adverse effects are GI-related and include nausea, vomiting, flatulence, and abdominal cramping.[37] PEG solutions with electrolytes are used as bowl cleansing regimens prior to GI-related procedures, and should not be used routinely for treatment of constipation.

Magnesium Salts Magnesium salts, including hydroxide, phosphate, and citrate, and sodium phosphate are categorized as saline cathartics.[37] These agents are frequently used as bowel preparations prior to diagnostic procedures such as colonoscopy.[27] Milk of magnesia (an 8% suspension of magnesium hydroxide), though, may be used occasionally to treat constipation in otherwise healthy adults, but efficacy data are limited. Saline cathartics should not be used on a routine basis. These agents may cause fluid and electrolyte depletion. Also, magnesium or sodium accumulation may occur in patients with renal dysfunction or congestive heart failure. These risks increase with long-term use.

Glycerin Glycerin is usually administered as a suppository and exerts its effect by osmotic action in the rectum. As with most agents given as suppositories, the onset of action is usually less than 30 minutes. Glycerin is considered a safe laxative, although it may occasionally cause rectal irritation. Its use is acceptable on an intermittent basis for constipation or fecal impaction, particularly in children.[40]

Stimulant Laxatives

Stimulant laxatives such as diphenylmethane (bisacodyl) and anthraquinone (senna and others) derivates primarily affect the colon.[37] These agents stimulate the mucosal nerve plexus of the colon and may also affect intestinal fluid secretion by altering fluid and electrolyte transport, and are expected to cause a bowel movement within 8 to 12 hours of administration. Stimulant laxatives may cause severe abdominal cramping and electrolyte imbalances, particularly with chronic use. Compared with placebo, bisacodyl is effective in treatment of constipation;[40] however, stimulant laxatives are not recommended as first-line treatment. These agents are typically reserved for intermittent use or in patients who fail to respond adequately to bulking and osmotic laxatives. Some patients, though, with severe chronic constipation and nonmodifiable risk factors may use these agents on a more regular basis.[28,41]

Clinical **Controversy...**

The long-term use of stimulant laxatives is controversial. Newer studies do not report damage to the enteric nervous system like earlier studies. Nerve damage may actually be the cause of the constipation rather than the result of using laxatives. Patients requiring regular use of laxatives, though, may still need to be monitored for these effects.

Intestinal Secretagogues

Lubiprostone

Lubiprostone (Amitiza) is a chloride channel activator that acts locally in the gut to open chloride channels on the GI luminal epithelium, which, in turn, stimulates chloride-rich fluid secretion into the intestinal lumen. Increased intraluminal fluid secretion helps to soften stool and accelerate GI transit time.[23] Lubiprostone is FDA-approved for adults with chronic idiopathic constipation as well as treatment of patients with constipation-predominant irritable bowel syndrome (IBS-C) at a recommended dose of one 24 mg capsule twice daily with food. Patients treated with lubiprostone have a significant increase in spontaneous bowel movements versus placebo as well as improvement in straining, stool consistency, and overall constipation severity.[42] Lubiprostone appears safe and effective for long-term treatment (up to 48 weeks). For most patients, bowel movements occur within 24 to 48 hours of lubiprostone administration. Common adverse effects include nausea, headache, and diarrhea and may be dose dependent.[27] Because of its high cost (especially relative to other available laxative agents) and lack of comparative data with other laxative therapies, lubiprostone is reserved for patients with chronic constipation who fail conventional first-line agents such as osmotic laxatives and fiber supplementation, or for those with OIC.

Linaclotide

Linaclotide (Linzess) is approved for the treatment of constipation and IBS-C.[43] It is a synthetic 14-amino-acid peptide that binds to and activates the guanylate cyclase C receptor found on the intestinal epithelium. This increases intestinal fluid secretion and quickens intestinal motility. In two randomized controlled trials involving approximately 1,276 patients, linaclotide 145 and 290 mcg daily was more effective than placebo at increasing spontaneous bowel movements in patients with chronic constipation at 12 weeks.[44] Only the 145 mcg dose is approved for treatment of constipation due to the lack of improved efficacy with the higher dosing. Diarrhea was the most commonly reported adverse event in clinical trials, followed by flatulence and abdominal pain. Linaclotide should not be used in patients under the age of 18.[43]

Opioid Receptor Antagonists

Alvimopan (Entereg) is an oral GI-specific μ-opioid antagonist approved for short-term use in hospitalized patients to accelerate recovery of bowel function after large or small bowel resection.[45] It antagonizes the GI (peripheral) effects of opioids without affecting analgesia because it does not cross the blood–brain barrier. Alvimopan is only available through a special use program (ENTEREG access support and education [EASE]), which requires hospitals to register and meet all requirements before the drug can be administered. Additionally, alvimopan is contraindicated in patients receiving therapeutic doses of opioids for more than 7 consecutive days prior to surgery as they may be more sensitive to the drug's effects. Dosing for alvimopan is as follows: 12 mg capsule administered 30 minutes to 5 hours before surgery and then 12 mg twice daily for up to 7 days or until discharge (maximum of 15 doses).

Methylnaltrexone (Relistor) is μ-receptor antagonist approved for OIC in patients with advanced disease receiving palliative care or when response to laxative therapy has been insufficient.[45] This agent does not cross the blood–brain barrier or antagonize analgesia; it acts on peripheral μ-receptors to block unwanted opioid side effects such as constipation. It is administered at a weight-based dose as a subcutaneous injection, usually every other day (no more than once daily), and is contraindicated in patients with known or suspected GI obstruction.

Naloxegol (Movantik) was approved by the FDA in September 2014 for the treatment of OIC in adult patients with noncancer pain.[46]

It is an oral pegylated naloxone molecule and antagonizes the μ-receptor. Pegylation reduces naloxegol's passive permeability of the blood–brain barrier. The recommended dose is 25 mg by mouth once daily, 1 hour before or 2 hours after a meal. The dose should be reduced by half in patients with diminished renal function (CrCl <60 mL/min [<1.0 mL/s]) or in those unable to tolerate 25 mg. The most common side effects are abdominal pain, diarrhea, and nausea. In clinical trials, naloxegol significantly increased the number and frequency of bowel movements compared to placebo at 12 weeks.[29]

Other Agents

Prucalopride is a selective 5-hydroxytryptamine-4 (5-HT_4) receptor agonist approved for treatment of chronic constipation in Europe.[47] It demonstrates proenterokinetic effects (increased colonic motility and transit), specifically in the GI tract. Prucalopride, however, is more selective than the previously available serotonergic agonists cisapride and tegaserod with higher affinity for the 5-HT_4 receptor. Receptor selectivity is thought to improve the safety profile of prucalopride over cisapride and tegaserod, which were removed from the market due to concerns for adverse cardiovascular events. In clinical trials, prucalopride significantly increased the number of complete, spontaneous bowel movements in adults with chronic constipation. Constipation symptoms and quality of life were also improved with prucalopride. This agent has been safely tolerated in clinical trials with no adverse cardiovascular effects versus placebo (although data are limited). Prucalopride has not yet been approved by the FDA.

Probiotics may be useful in the treatment of constipation. Five randomized controlled trials conducted in children and adults revealed that certain strains of probiotics increased weekly stool frequency.[48] However, these trials were small (370 patients total) and only slight improvement was realized (one additional stool per week). More studies are needed to strengthen evidence involving probiotics, but these may be an option for patients seeking alternative treatment.

Prevention

For patients recovering from MI or rectal surgery, straining at defecation should be avoided. The basis of preventive therapy in these patients should be bulk-forming laxatives. Additionally, the use of docusate is popular, although its effectiveness is debated. In pregnant patients, constipation may result because of alterations in hormones or iron supplementation. As described earlier, bulk-forming laxatives and docusates should be the first line of prevention.

Evaluation of Therapeutic Outcomes

The ultimate goal of treatment for constipation is to prevent further episodes of constipation. Short-term goals include alleviation of acute constipation with relief from symptoms. For patients with chronic constipation, the goals include use of proper diet and decreased reliance on laxatives in addition to relief of symptoms for the patient so that quality of life is not diminished. Effective treatment of constipation requires the patient to become more knowledgeable about the causes of constipation, proper diet, and appropriate use of laxatives.

IRRITABLE BOWEL SYNDROME

Irritable bowel syndrome is a GI syndrome characterized by chronic abdominal pain and altered bowel habits in the absence of any organic cause. It is the most commonly diagnosed GI condition.

Epidemiology

The prevalence of IBS is approximately 5% to 15% based on North American and European population-based studies; however, there is a wide variation in prevalence by individual country.[49-51] IBS affects men and women, young patients, and the elderly with an overall 2:1 female predominance in North America.[52] However, younger patients and women are more likely to be diagnosed with IBS. Although only 15% of those affected actually seek medical attention, IBS is the cause of between 25% and 50% of all referrals to gastroenterologists.[49]

Pathophysiology

Although the exact pathophysiologic abnormalities with IBS are still being actively investigated, IBS likely results from altered somatovisceral and motor dysfunction of the intestine from a variety of causes. Abnormal CNS processing of afferent signals may lead to visceral hypersensitivity, with the specific nerve pathway affected determining the exact symptomatology expressed. This visceral hypersensitivity is a neuroenteric phenomenon that is independent of motility and psychological disturbances.[51] Factors known to contribute to these alterations include genetics, motility factors, inflammation, colonic infections, mechanical irritation to local nerves, stress, and other psychological factors.

The enteric nervous system contains a significant percentage of the body's 5-HT receptors.[53] Two types of 5-HT receptors exist within the gut: serotonin type 3 (HT_3) and serotonin type 4 (HT_4), which are responsible for secretion, sensitization, and motility. There is an increase in the postprandial levels of 5-HT in the GI tract in those who suffer from diarrhea-predominant IBS when compared with nonsufferers.[53] Therefore, stimulation and antagonism of these 5-HT receptors have become a focused area for research on new drug therapies for both diarrhea- and constipation-predominant diseases.

Clinical Presentation

(8) Irritable bowel syndrome presents as either diarrhea- or constipation-predominant disease and can be defined as lower abdominal pain, disturbed defecation (constipation, diarrhea, or an alternating pattern of both), and bloating in the absence of structural or biochemical factors that might explain these symptoms (Table 36-10). Because IBS can have variable signs and symptoms, two diagnostic criteria "checklists" are commonly used to aid in the workup of a patient suspected of having IBS.[54] The Manning criteria were first proposed in 1978, whereas the Rome criteria were initially proposed in 1999 and revised as recently as 2006 by an international working group in an effort to help standardize the diagnostic criteria used in clinical research protocols. Table 36-11 shows the symptom criteria for both of the Manning[55] and Rome III[31] symptom-based criteria.

TABLE 36-10 Clinical Presentation of Irritable Bowel Syndrome

Signs and symptoms
- Lower abdominal pain
- Abdominal bloating and distension
- Diarrhea symptoms, >3 stools/day
- Extreme urgency
- Passage of mucus
- Constipation symptoms, <3 stools/wk, straining, incomplete evacuation
- Psychological symptoms such as depression and anxiety

Non-GI symptoms
- Urinary symptoms
- Fatigue
- Dyspareunia

Other concurrent conditions
- Fibromyalgia
- Functional dyspepsia
- Chronic fatigue syndrome

Reduced health-related quality of life

TABLE 36-11 Symptom-Based Criteria for Irritable Bowel Syndrome

The Manning criteria[56]

Chronic or recurrent abdominal pain for at least 6 months and two or more of the following:

1. Abdominal pain relieved with defecation
2. Abdominal pain associated with more frequent stools
3. Abdominal pain associated with looser stools
4. Abdominal distension
5. Feeling of incomplete evacuation after defecation
6. Mucus in stools

Rome III diagnostic criteria for irritable bowel syndrome[33]

Recurrent abdominal pain or discomfort at least 3 days per month in the last 3 months associated with two or more of the following:

1. Relieved with defecation
2. Onset associated with a change in frequency of stool
3. Onset associated with a change in form (appearance) of stool

Additional diagnostic steps that can be taken include sigmoidoscopy or colonoscopy, examination of the stool for occult blood and ova and parasites, complete blood cell count, erythrocyte sedimentation rate, and serum electrolytes. In some cases, radiographic imaging studies, such as computed tomography scans or barium swallows or enemas, may also be necessary if the findings of the foregoing assessment are not typical for IBS.[49]

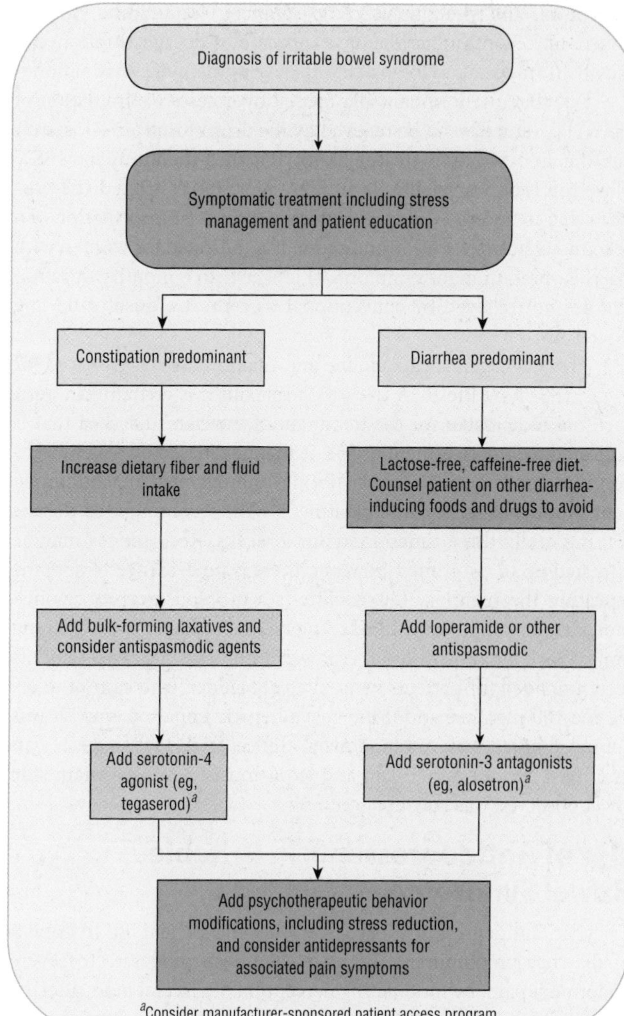

FIGURE 36-3 A general stepwise approach to the management of both constipation- and diarrhea-predominant irritable bowel syndrome.

TREATMENT

General Approach to Treatment

The treatment approach to IBS is based on the predominant symptoms and their severity (Fig. 36-3). Milder, less frequent episodes can be managed with lifestyle changes such as dietary restrictions, a higher-fiber diet, physical activity, and relaxation techniques.[56] More persistent disease may require as-needed uses of various antispasmodic or antidiarrheal agents such as loperamide. Lastly, the most severe forms of this disease may call for pharmacologic agents directed specifically at the underlying neurohormonal imbalance, such as the 5-HT_4 agonists (eg, tegaserod), or the 5-HT_3 receptor antagonists (eg, alosetron).

Alosetron, a 5-HT_3 receptor antagonist, was withdrawn from the U.S. market in 2000 as a result of serious adverse effects, including severe constipation and ischemic colitis that did not appear in the initial clinical trials. It was reintroduced in 2002 and is now limited to an FDA-approved restricted-use program in lower initial doses, and requires extensive postmarketing surveillance. Results of these trials are necessary to definitively determine alosetron's true safety profile, especially with regard to its association with or causation of fatal ischemic colitis.

Constipation-Predominant Disease

In the constipation-predominant patient, dietary fiber may be beneficial. Patients should be instructed to begin with one tablespoonful of fiber with one meal daily and gradually increase the dose to include fiber with two and three meals a day until the desired outcome is achieved. End points that the patient should aim for include bulkier and more easily passed stools. For patients unable to tolerate dietary bran, bulking agents such as psyllium may be substituted.[56] PEG laxatives may be used; however, other laxatives should only be used in the smallest dose for the least amount of time. When lifestyle modifications alone do not control symptoms, linaclotide should be recommended.[52]

The 5-HT_4 partial agonist tegaserod was the first therapy approved by the FDA specifically for short-term, intermittent treatment of IBS-C in women.[57-59] Tegaserod is available in the United States through a restricted-access program due to a small, yet significant, increase in ischemia events (MI, cerebrovascular accident [CVA], and unstable angina) in patients with preexisting cardiovascular disease and/or cardiovascular risk factors. It is given as 2 or 6 mg doses given twice daily 30 minutes prior to a meal with water for up to 12 weeks.[58] Stimulation of the 5-HT_4 receptors by tegaserod increases gastric secretions and promotes motility, with improvement in symptoms generally occurring within the first week of therapy. Diarrhea was the most common adverse effect, resulting in drug discontinuation in 1.6% of study subjects.

Diarrhea-Predominant Disease

9 For patients in whom diarrhea is the primary complaint, avoidance of certain food products may be necessary. Caffeine, alcohol, and artificial sweeteners (sorbitol, fructose, and mannitol) are known to irritate the gut and produce a laxative effect. Lactose intolerance should be considered in certain patients; however, the prevalence of this condition may be exaggerated.

Herbal medicines or teas often contain senna, which may produce diarrhea. In patients with disease persistence following dietary modification, loperamide may be used for episodic management of urgent diarrhea, or in situations in which the patient wishes to avoid the possibility of an acute onset of symptoms.[52] Loperamide decreases intestinal transit, enhances water and electrolyte absorption, and strengthens rectal sphincter tone. Some patients may require continuous therapy, and careful dosage titration can usually be undertaken to prevent the development of constipation.

Diarrhea-predominant IBS caused by excessive stimulation of the 5-HT_3 receptor can be relieved by the drug alosetron. Alosetron was the first effective treatment for diarrhea-predominant IBS.[52] Alosetron is only available via an FDA-approved restricted-use program due to severe GI adverse effects. Additional information can be found at http://www.lotronex.com. It is indicated for women with diarrhea-predominant symptoms of longer than 6 months' duration that are not relieved by conventional therapy at a dose of 0.5 mg twice daily.

Two new agents, eluxadoline and rifaximin, were approved for use in IBS-D by the FDA in 2015.[60] Rifaximin is a rifamycin antibacterial indicidated for the treatment of travelers' diarrhea that is indicated for the treatment of IBS-D in adults based on several randomized control trials demonstrating improvement in abdominal pain, stool consistency, and bloating.[52,61] The recommended dose is 550 mg orally three times a day for 2 weeks. Recurrences may be retreated up to two times; however, there is no evidence to support repeating the regimen. Eluxadoline is a μ-opiod receptor agonist indicated for adults with IBS-D. The recommended dose is 100 mg orally twice a day with food. A lower dose of 75 mg twice daily is recommended for patients without a gallbladder, who cannot tolerate the 100 mg dose and if they have hepatic impairement.[62] It was approved based on two randomized clinical trials that suggested an improved in abdominal pain and stool consistency. The main side effect observed was constipation.

Use of Antidepressants in Irritable Bowel Syndrome

Tricyclic antidepressants have shown some benefit in treatment of diarrhea-predominant IBS associated with moderate to severe abdominal pain, by modulating perception of visceral pain, altering GI transit time, and treating underlying comorbidities.[63,64] Selective 5-HT reuptake inhibitors are less well studied, with only one report with paroxetine showing some improvement in stool passage and "well-being" but no decrease in abdominal pain.[65-67]

Figure 36-3 shows a general stepwise approach to the management of both constipation and diarrhea-predominant IBS.

Pain in Irritable Bowel Syndrome

10 Some patients with IBS suffer significant pain associated with their disease. Data supporting the use of antispasmodic agents in these patients are conflicting.[49] A trial of low-dose antidepressant therapy is indicated, especially if pain is associated with eating. Both tricyclic antidepressants and 5-HT reuptake inhibitors produce analgesia and may relieve depressive symptoms if present. Preprandial doses of drugs containing anticholinergic properties may suppress pain (and/or diarrhea) associated with an overactive postprandial gastrocolonic response. Tricyclic antidepressants should be avoided in patients with pain and constipation. In addition, psychotherapy, including cognitive behavioral therapy, relaxation therapy, and hypnotherapy, has been shown to decrease IBS symptoms.[68]

Evaluation of Therapeutic Outcomes

Irritable bowel syndrome is usually classified as constipation-predominant, diarrhea-predominant, or IBS with abdominal pain and bloating. Therapeutic goals in IBS should focus on the patient's primary complaint. Dietary and drug therapy goals should focus on end-organ treatment to relieve abdominal pain (antispasmodic drugs) or disturbed bowel habits (antidiarrheals and bulk-forming agents). Additionally, severe symptoms from CNS dysregulation should be treated with antidepressants, psychotherapy, relaxation/stress management, cognitive behavior treatment, and/or hypnosis aimed at specific affective disorders.[49] Lastly, the 5-HT receptor agonists and antagonists can be used in carefully selected patients whose symptoms are not adequately controlled with other agents. The AGA recommends that patients with severe IBS consider psychological treatments such as psychotherapy, relaxation/stress management, and/or cognitive behavior treatment.

ABBREVIATIONS

AAD	antibiotic-associated diarrhea
AGA	American Gastroenterology Association
AIDS	acquired immune deficiency syndrome
ATPase	adenosine triphosphatase
CDC	Centers for Disease Control and Prevention
CVA	cerebrovascular accident
EASE	ENTEREG access support and education
5-HT	serotonin
HT_3	serotonin type 3
HT_4	serotonin type 4
5-HT_4	5-hydroxytryptamine-4
IBS	irritable bowel syndrome
IBS-C	constipation-predominant irritable bowel syndrome
MI	myocardial infarction
NSAID	nonsteroidal antiinflammatory drug
OIC	opioid-induced constipation
ORS	oral rehydration solution
PEG	polyethylene glycol
VIP	vasoactive intestinal peptide
VIPoma	vasoactive intestinal peptide-secreting tumor
WDHA	watery diarrhea, hypokalemia, and achlorhydria
WHO	World Health Organization
WHO-ORS	World Health Organization oral rehydration solution

REFERENCES

1. Sandle GI. Infective and inflammatory diarrhea: Mechanisms and opportunities for novel therapies. *Curr Opin Pharmacol* 2011;11(6):634-639.
2. Farthing M, Salam M, Lindberg G, et al. Acute diarrhea in adults and children: A global perspective. World Gastsroenterology Organization Guidelines. 2012. Available at: *http://www.worldgastroenterology.org/acute-diarrhea-in-adults.html.* Accessed date, July 14, 2016.
3. Scallan E, Majowicz S, Hall G, et al. Prevalence of diarrhoea in the community in Australia, Canada, Ireland, and the United States. *Int J Epidemiol* 2005;34:454-460.
4. Jones T, McMillian M, Scallan E, et al. A population-based estimate of the substantial burden of diarrhoeal disease in the United States; FoodNet, 1996-2003. *Epidemiol Infect* 2007;135:293-301.
5. Musher DM, Musher BL. Contagious acute gastrointestinal infections. *N Engl J Med* 2004;351(23):2417-2427.
6. DuPont HL, Ericsson CD, Farthing MJG, et al. Expert review of the evidence base for self-therapy of travelers' diarrhea. *J Travel Med* 2009;16(3):161-171.
7. Steffen R, Hill DR, Dupont HL. Traveler's diarrhea: A clinical review. *JAMA* 2015;313(1):71-80.
8. Bhatnagar S, Bhandari N, Mouli U, Bhan M. Consensus statement of IAP National Task Force: Status report on management of acute diarrhea. *Indian Pediatr* 2004;41:335-348.
9. Atia AN, Buchman AL. Oral rehydration solutions in non-cholera diarrhea: A review. *Am J Gastroenterol* 2009;104(10):2596-2604.
10. Fine KD, Schiller LR. AGA technical review on the evaluation and management of chronic diarrhea. *Gastroenterology* 1999;116(6):1464-1486.
11. World Health Organization. WHO/UNICEF Joint Statement: Clinical Management of Acute Diarrhea (WHO/FCH/CAH/04.7). Geneva, Switzerland: World Health Organization, 2004.
12. Harris AG, Odorisio TM, Woltering EA, et al. Consensus statement—Octreotide dose titration in secretory diarrhea—Diarrhea Management Consensus Development Panel. *Dig Dis Sci* 1995;40(7):1464-1473.

13. Schiller LR. Review article: Anti-diarrhoeal pharmacology and therapeutics. *Aliment Pharmacol Ther* 1995;9(2):87-106.
14. Ruszniewski P, Ducreux M, Chayvialle JA, et al. Treatment of the carcinoid syndrome with the longacting somatostatin analogue lanreotide: A prospective study in 39 patients. *Gut* 1996;39(2):279-283.
15. Lombardi G, Minuto F, Tamburrano G, et al. Efficacy of the new long-acting formulation of lanreotide (lanreotide Autogel) in somastatin analogue-naive patients with acromegaly. *J Endocrinol Invest* 2009;32(3):202-209.
16. Floch MH, Walker WA, Guandalini S, et al. Recommendations for probiotic use—2008. *J Clin Gastroenterol* 2008;42:S104-S108.
17. Hempel S, Newberry SJ, Maher AR, et al. Probiotics for the prevention and treatment of antibiotic-associated diarrhea. A systematic review and meta-analysis. *JAMA* 2012;307(18):1959-1969.
18. Allen SJ, Wareham K, Wang D, et al. A high-dose preparation of lactobacilli and bifidobacteria in the prevention of antibiotic-associated and Clostridium difficile diarrhoea in older people admitted to hospital: A multicentre, randomised, double-blind, placebo-controlled, parallel arm trial (PLACIDE). *Health Technol Assess* 2013;17(57):1-140.
19. Thompson RF, Bass DM, Hoffman SL. Travel vaccines. *Infect Dis Clin North Am* 1999;13(1):149-167.
20. Tacket CO, Kotloff KL, Losonsky G, et al. Volunteer studies investigating the safety and efficacy of live oral El Tor *Vibrio cholerae* 01 vaccine strain CVD 111. *Am J Trop Med Hyg* 1997;56(5):533-537.
21. CDC. Prevention of rotavirus gastroenteritis among infants and children: Recommendations of the Advisory Committee on Immunization Practices (ACIP). *MMWR* 2009;58(RR-2):1-26.
22. Choung RS, Locke GR, Rey E, et al. Factors associated with persistent and nonpersistent chronic constipation, over 20 years. *Clin Gastroenterol Hepatol* 2012;10:494-500.
23. Suares NC, Ford AC. Prevalence of, and risk factors for, chronic idiopathic constipation in the community: Systematic review and meta-analysis. *Am J Gastroenterol* 2011;106:1582-1591.
24. Gallegos-Orozco JF, Foxx-Orenstein AE, Sterler SM, Stoa JM. Chronic constipation in the elderly. *Am J Gastroenterol* 2012;107:18-25.
25. Higgins P, Johanson J. Epidemiology of constipation in North America: A systematic review. *Am J Gastroenterol* 2004;99(4):750-759.
26. Wald A, Scarpignato C, Mueller-Lissner S, et al. A multinational survey of prevalence and patterns of laxative use among adults with self-defined constipation. *Aliment Pharmacol Ther* 2008;28(7):917-930.
27. Foxx-Orenstein AE, McNally MA, Odunsi ST. Update on constipation: One treatment does not fit all. *Cleve Clin J Med* 2008;75(11):813-824.
28. Bharucha AE, Pemberton JH, Locke GR III. American Gastroenterological Association technical review on constipation. *Gastroenterology* 2013;144:218-238.
29. Siemens W, Gaertner J, Becker G. Advances in pharmacotherapy for opioid-induced constipation—A systematic review. *Expert Opin Pharmacother* 2015;16(4):515-535.
30. Allan L, Richarz U, Simpson K, Slappendel R. Transdermal fentanyl versus sustained release oral morphine in strong-opioid naive patients with chronic low back pain. *Spine* 2005;30(22):2484-2490.
31. Longstreth G, Thompson W, Chey W, Houghton L, Mearin F, Spiller R. Functional bowel disorders. *Gastroenterology* 2006;130(5):1480-1491.
32. Brandt L, Prather C, Quigley E, Schiller L, Schoenfeld P, Talley N. Systematic review on the management of chronic constipation in North America. *Am J Gastroenterol* 2005;100:S5-S21.
33. Ternent CA, Bastawrous AL, Morin NA, et al. Practice parameters for the evaluation and management of constipation. *Dis Colon Rectum* 2007;50:2013-2022.
34. Schey R, Cromwell J, Rao SSC. Medical and surgical management of pelvic floor disorders affecting defecation. *Am J Gastroenterol* 2012;107:1624-1633. doi:10.1038/ajg.2012.247.
35. Attaluri A, Donahoe R, Valestin J, Brown K, Rao SSC. Randomised clinical trial: Dried plums (prunes) vs psyllium for constipation. *Aliment Pharmacol Ther* 2011;33:822-828.
36. Ortiz H, de Miguel M, Rinaldi M, Oteiza F, Altomare DE. Functional outcome of sacral nerve stimulation in patients with severe constipation. *Dis Colon Rectum* 2012;55:876-880.
37. Gallagher PF, O'Mahony D, Quigley EM. Management of chronic constipation in the elderly. *Drugs Aging* 2008;25(10):807-821.
38. Lee-Robichaud H, Thomas K, Morgan J, Nelson RL. Lactulose versus polyethylene glycol for chronic constipation. *Cochrane Database Syst Rev* 2010;(7):CD007570. doi:10.1002/14651858.CD007570.pub2.
39. DiPalma JA, Cleveland MV, McGowan J, Herrar JL. A randomized, multicenter, placebo-controlled trial of polyethylene glycol laxative for chronic treatment of chronic constipation. *Am J Gastroenterol* 2007;102:1436-1441.
40. North American Society for Pediatric Gastroenterology, Hepatology, and Nutrition. Evaluation and treatment of constipation in infants and children: Recommendations from the North American Society of Pediatric Gastroenterology, Hepatology, and Nutrition. *J Pediatr Gastroenterol Nutr* 2006;43(3):e1-e13.
41. Ford AC, Suares NC. Effect of laxatives and pharmacological therapies in chronic idiopathic constipation: Systematic review and meta-analysis. *Gut* 2011;60:209-218.
42. Lembo AJ, Johanson JF, Parkman HP, Rao SS, Miner PB Jr, Ueno R. Long-term safety and effectiveness of lubiprostone, a calcium channel (ClC-2) activator, in patients with chronic idiopathic constipation. *Dig Dis Sci* 2011;56:2639-2645.
43. Food and Drug Administration (FDA). FDA approves Linzess to treat certain cases of irritable bowel syndrome and constipation [news release]. Silver Spring, MD: FDA; August 30, 2012.
44. Lembo AJ, Schneier AH, Shiff SJ, et al. Two randomized trials of linaclotide for chronic constipation. *N Engl J Med* 2011;365:527-536.
45. Camilleri M. Opioid-induced constipation: Challenges and therapeutic opportunities. *Am J Gastroenterol* 2011;106:835-842.
46. Leonard J, Baker DE. Naloxegol: Treatment for opioid-induced constipation in chronic non-cancer pain. *Ann Pharmocother* 2015;49(3):360-365.
47. Shin A, Camilleri M, Kolar G, Erwin P, West CP, Murad MH. Systematic review with meta analysis: Highly selective 5-HT4 agonists (prucalopride, velusetrag, or naronapride) in chronic constipation. *Aliment Pharmacol Ther* 2014;39:239-253.
48. Chmielewska A, Szajewska H. Systematic review of randomized controlled trials: Probiotics for functional constipation. *World J Gastroenterol* 2010;16(7):69-75.
49. Brandt L, Chey W, Foxx-Orenstein A, et al. An evidence-based position statement on the management of irritable bowel syndrome. *Am J Gastroenterol* 2009;104(S1):S1-S35.
50. Chang FY. Irritable bowel syndrome: The evolution of multi-dimensional looking and multidisciplinary treatments. *World J Gastroenterol.* 2014;20(10):2499-2514.
51. Hungin A, Chang L, Locke G, Dennis E, Barghout V. Irritable bowel syndrome in the United States: Prevalence, symptom patterns and impact. *Aliment Pharmacol Ther* 2005;21(11):1365-1375.
52. Weinberg DS, Smalley W, Heidelbaugh JJ, Sultan S. American Gastroenterological Association Institute Guideline on the pharmacological management of irritable bowel syndrome. *Gastroenterology* 2014;147(5):1146-1148.
53. Ford AC, Brandt LJ, Young C, et al. Efficacy of 5-Ht3 antagonists and 5-HT5 agonists in irritable bowel syndrome: A systematic review and meta-analysis. *Am J Gastroenterol* 2009;104:1831-1843.
54. Dang J, Ardila-hani A, Amichai MM, Chua K, Pimentel M. Systematic review of diagnostic criteria for IBS demonstrates poor validity and utilization of Rome III. *Neurogastroenterol Motil* 2012;24(9):853-e397.
55. Manning A, Thompson W, Heaton K, Morris A. Towards positive diagnosis of the irritable bowel. *Br Med J* 1978;2(6138):653-654.
56. National Institute for Health and Care Excellence. Addendum to Guideline CG61. Irritable bowel syndrome in adults: Diagnosis and management of irritable bowel syndrome in primary care. 2015. Available at: *http://www.nice.org.uk/guidance/cg61/chapter/ 1-recommendations#clinical-management-of-ibs*. Accessed date, July 14, 2016.
57. Camilleri M. Review article: Tegaserod. *Aliment Pharmacol Ther* 2001;15(3):277-289.
58. Tougas G, Snape WJ, Otten MH, et al. Long-term safety of tegaserod in patients with constipation-predominant irritable bowel syndrome. *Aliment Pharmacol Ther* 2002;16(10):1701-1708.
59. Muller-Lissner SA, Fumagalli I, Bardhan KD, et al. Tegaserod, a 5-HT4 receptor partial agonist, relieves symptoms in irritable bowel syndrome patients with abdominal pain, bloating and constipation. *Aliment Pharmacol Ther* 2001;15(10):1655-1666.
60. Food and Drug Administration. FDA approves two therapies to treat IBS-D [news release]. Silver Spring, MD: FDA; May 27, 2015.
61. Xifaxan® [package insert]. Raleigh, NC: Salix Pharmaceuticals Inc; 2015.
62. Viberzi® [package insert]. Cincinnati, OH: Patheon Pharmaceuticals Inc; 2015.
63. Rahimi R, Nikfar S, Rezaie A, Abdollahi M. Efficacy of tricyclic antidepressants in irritable bowel syndrome: A meta-analysis. *World J Gastroenterol* 2009;15(13):1548-1553.
64. Abdul-Baki S, El Hajj I, ElZahabi L, et al. A randomized controlled trial of imipramine in patients with irritable bowel syndrome. *World J Gastroenterol* 2009;15(29):3636-3642.

65. Tabas G, Beaves M, Wang J, Friday P, Mardini H, Arnold G. Paroxetine to treat irritable bowel syndrome not responding to high-fiber diet: A double-blind, placebo-controlled trial. *Am J Gastroenterol* 2004;99(5):914-920.
66. Han C, Masand PS, Krulewicz S, et al. Childhood abuse and treatment response in patients with irritable bowel syndrome: A post-hoc analysis of a 12-week, randomized, double-blind, placebo-controlled trial of paroxetine controlled release. *J Clin Pharm Ther* 2009;34(1):79-88.
67. Masand PS, Pae C-U, Krulewicz S, et al. A double-blind, randomized, placebo-controlled trial of paroxetine controlled-release in irritable bowel syndrome. *Psychosomatics* 2009;50(1):78-86.
68. Heymann-Monnikes I, Arnold R, Florin I, Herda C, Melfsen S, Monnikes H. The combination of medical treatment plus multicomponent behavioral therapy is superior to medical treatment alone in the therapy of irritable bowel syndrome. *Am J Gastroenterol* 2000;95(4):981-994.

Portal Hypertension and Cirrhosis

37

Julie M. Sease and Jennifer N. Clements

KEY CONCEPTS

1. Cirrhosis is a severe, chronic, irreversible disease associated with significant morbidity and mortality. However, the progression of cirrhosis secondary to alcohol abuse can be interrupted by abstinence. It is therefore imperative for the clinician to educate and support abstinence from alcohol as part of the overall treatment strategy of the underlying liver disease.
2. Patients with cirrhosis should receive endoscopic screening for varices, and certain patients with varices should receive primary prophylaxis with nonselective β-adrenergic blockade therapy to prevent variceal hemorrhage.
3. When nonselective β-adrenergic blocker therapy is used to prevent rebleeding, therapy can be titrated to achieve a goal heart rate of 55 to 60 beats/min or the maximal tolerated dose.
4. Octreotide is the preferred vasoactive agent for the medical management of variceal bleeding. Endoscopic band ligation is the primary therapeutic tool for the management of acute variceal bleeding.
5. The combination of spironolactone and furosemide is the recommended initial diuretic therapy for patients with ascites.
6. All patients who have survived an episode of spontaneous bacterial peritonitis (SBP) should receive long-term antibiotic prophylaxis.
7. The mainstay of therapy of hepatic encephalopathy (HE) involves therapy to lower blood ammonia concentrations and includes diet therapy, lactulose, and antibiotics alone or in combination with lactulose.

Chronic liver injury causes damage to normal liver tissue resulting in the development of regenerative nodules surrounded by fibrous bands.[1] Cirrhosis is an advanced stage of liver fibrosis that leads to shunting of the portal and arterial blood supply directly into hepatic outflow through the central veins with compromised exchange between hepatic sinusoids and hepatocytes. Clinical consequences of cirrhosis include impaired hepatocyte function, the increased intrahepatic resistance of portal hypertension, and hepatocellular carcinoma. Circulatory irregularities, such as splanchnic vasodilation, vasoconstriction and hypoperfusion of the kidneys, water and salt retention, and increased cardiac output, also occur. The word *cirrhosis* is derived from the Greek *kirrhos*, meaning orange-yellow, and refers to the color of the cirrhotic liver as seen on autopsy or during surgery.[2]

1 While cirrhosis has many causes (Table 37-1), in the Western world, excessive alcohol intake and hepatitis C are the most common causes.[1,3] Nonalcoholic steatohepatitis is also an important cause of cirrhosis in the end diagnosis of cirrhosis without an apparent cause occurs infrequently today.[1] This chapter elucidates the pathophysiology of cirrhosis and the resultant effects on human anatomy and physiology. Treatment strategies for managing the most commonly encountered clinical complications of cirrhosis are discussed.

EPIDEMIOLOGY

The exact prevalence of cirrhosis is unknown, but a reasonable estimate is that 1% of populations have histologically diagnosable cirrhosis.[1] Chronic liver disease and cirrhosis were responsible for nearly 35,000 deaths in America in 2012 making it the 11th leading cause of death among whites, 15th leading cause of death among blacks, 5th leading cause of death among American Indians and Alaska Natives and 13th leading cause of death among Asians and Pacific Islanders.[4] Acute variceal bleeding and spontaneous bacterial peritonitis (SBP) are among the immediately life-threatening complications of cirrhosis. Associated conditions causing significant morbidity include ascites and hepatic encephalopathy (HE). Approximately 50% of patients with cirrhosis develop ascites during 10 years of observation and, within 2 years, nearly half of patients who develop ascites will die.[5]

PATHOPHYSIOLOGY OF CIRRHOSIS

Any discussion of cirrhosis must be based on a firm understanding of hepatic anatomy and vascular supply. Conceptually, the liver can be thought of as an elaborate blood filtration system receiving blood from the hepatic artery and the portal vein (Fig. 37-1), with portal blood originating from the small intestines.[6] Blood enters the liver via the portal triad, which contains branches of the portal vein, hepatic artery, and bile ducts. It then drains through the sinusoidal spaces (also known as the space of Disse) of the hepatic lobule (Fig. 37-2), which are lined by the workhorses of the liver, the hepatocytes. Individual hepatocytes are arranged in plates that are one cell thick and organized around individual central veins. The six or more surfaces of each individual hepatocyte make contact with adjacent hepatocytes, border the bile canaliculi, or are exposed to the sinusoidal space. Filtered blood travels into the terminal hepatic venules, also called central veins, and then empties into larger hepatic veins and eventually into the inferior vena cava. Functional gradients of hepatocytes based on oxygen saturation have been reported. Hepatocytes closest to the portal triad, which contains the hepatic artery, have greater oxygen saturation than those hepatocytes nearer to the terminal hepatic venule. Blood flows past hepatocytes in zone one, then zone two, and finally zone three before entering the central vein. Hepatocytes in zone one are involved in gluconeogenesis, urea synthesis, and oxidative energy metabolism while those in zone three carry out the functions of glycolysis and lipogenesis.

TABLE 37-1 Etiology of Cirrhosis

Chronic alcohol consumption
Chronic viral hepatitis (types B and C)
Metabolic liver disease
Hemochromatosis
Wilson's disease
α_1-antitrypsin deficiency
Nonalcoholic steatohepatitis ("fatty liver")
Immunologic disease
Autoimmune hepatitis
Primary biliary cirrhosis
Vascular disease
Budd–Chiari
Cardiac failure
Drugs
Isoniazid, methyldopa, amiodarone, amoxicillin-clavulanate, nitrofurantoin, diclofenac, methotrexate, nevirapine, propylthiouracil, valproate

Data from references 1 and 3.

Normally, hepatic stellate cells function to store vitamin A and help to maintain the normal matrix in the sinusoidal space.[7] During chronic liver disease, however, hepatic stellate cells undergo an "activation" process, which is the central event in the development of hepatic fibrosis. Activation causes stellate cells to lose vitamin A, become highly proliferative, and synthesize fibrotic scar tissue, which accumulates in the sinusoidal space. This leads to loss of hepatocyte microvilli, loss of sinusoidal endothelial fenestrae, deterioration of hepatocyte function, and, if fibrosis progresses, eventual cirrhosis.

Cirrhosis causes changes to the splanchnic vascular bed as well as the systemic circulation.[8] Splanchnic vasodilation, decreased responsiveness to vasoconstrictors, and the formation of new blood vessels contribute to an increased splanchnic blood flow, formation of gastroesophageal varices, and variceal bleeding. All of these components are part of the portal hypertensive syndrome. Portal hypertension is characterized by hypervolemia, increased cardiac index, hypotension, and decreased systemic vascular resistance. This is so-called hyperkinetic syndrome that leads to a marked activation of neurohumoral vasoactive factors, a response that occurs in an effort to maintain the arterial blood pressure within normal limits. Activation of neurohumoral vasoactive factors is a main component in the pathophysiology of the ascites and renal dysfunction that often accompany chronic liver disease. Portal-systemic shunting may also occur and is involved in HE and other complications.

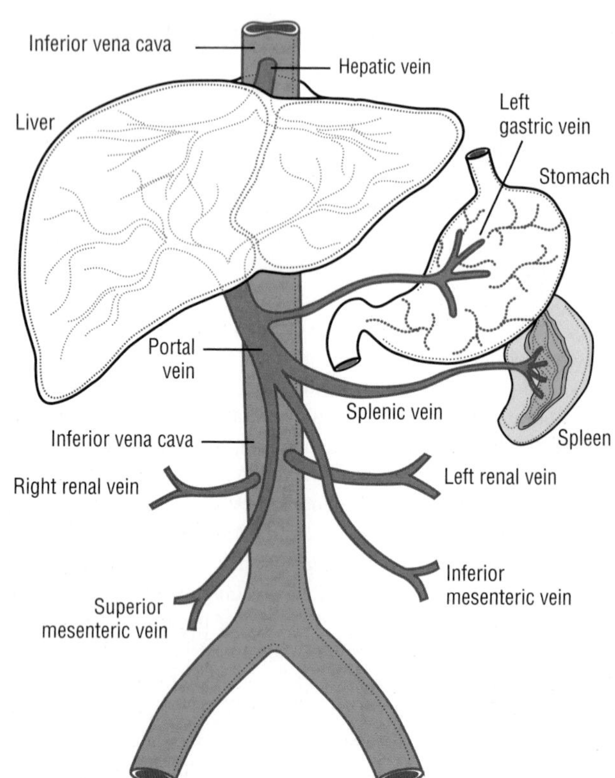

FIGURE 37-1 The portal venous system.

ANATOMIC AND PHYSIOLOGIC EFFECTS OF CIRRHOSIS

Cirrhosis and the pathophysiologic abnormalities that cause it result in the commonly encountered problems of ascites, portal hypertension, esophageal varices, HE, and coagulation disorders. Other less commonly seen problems in patients with cirrhosis include hepatorenal syndrome, hepatopulmonary syndrome, and endocrine dysfunction. These are discussed under heads Management of Portal Hypertension and Variceal Bleeding.

Ascites

Ascites is the accumulation of an excessive amount of fluid within the peritoneal cavity.[9] It is the most commonly occurring major complication of cirrhosis.[5] Approximately half of all cirrhotic patients develop ascites within 10 years of diagnosis. Several hypotheses have been offered to explain the mechanism for the development of ascites in decompensated cirrhosis.[9] Most acceptable theories state that ascites formation begins as a result of the development of sinusoidal hypertension and portal hypertension. Portal hypertension activates vasodilatory mechanisms that are mediated mostly by nitric oxide overproduction. This leads to splanchnic and peripheral arteriolar vasodilation and, in advanced disease, a drop in arterial pressure. Baroreceptor-mediated activation of the renin–angiotensin–aldosterone system, activation of the sympathetic nervous system, and release of antidiuretic hormone occur in response to the resulting arterial hypotension in an effort to restore normal blood pressure (Fig. 37-3). These changes cause renal sodium and water retention. Additionally, ongoing splanchnic vasodilation increases splanchnic lymph production beyond the capacity of the lymph transportation system. Leakage of lymphatic fluid into the peritoneal cavity occurs. Persistent renal sodium and water retention, increased splanchnic vascular permeability, and lymphatic leakage into the peritoneal cavity combine to create the sustained ascites formation of end-stage liver disease.

Portal Hypertension and Varices

Sinusoidal portal hypertension is most often caused by cirrhosis.[10] It is associated with acute variceal bleeding, a medical emergency which is among the most severe complications of cirrhosis.[11] Portal hypertension is defined by the presence of a gradient of greater than 5 mm Hg (0.7 kPa) between the portal and central venous pressures (see Fig. 37-1).[10] This gradient is called the hepatic venous pressure gradient (HVPG). Esophageal and gastric varices and variceal bleeding may arise after an HVPG pressure gradient of 10 mm Hg (1.3 kPa) is reached.

Progression to bleeding can be predicted by Child-Pugh score, size of varices, and the presence of red wale markings on the varices. First variceal hemorrhage occurs at an annual rate of about 15% and carries a mortality of 7% to 15%. Rebleeding is common following initial hemorrhage with a median rate of 60% and carries a mortality rate as high as 33%. Prevention of bleeding is a major goal in the therapy of portal hypertension, and strategies include both pharmacologic and surgical approaches.

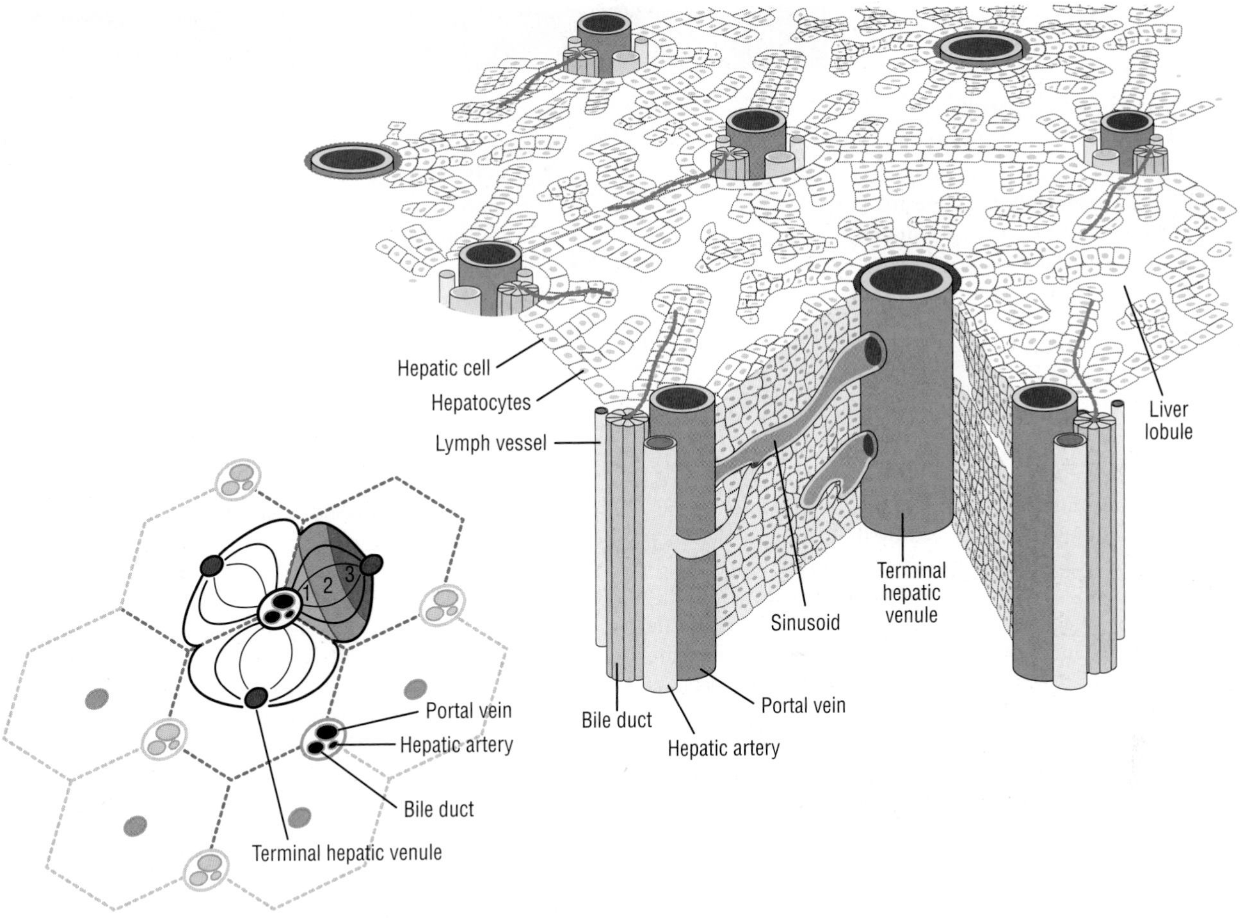

FIGURE 37-2 The hepatic lobule.

Hepatic Encephalopathy

Hepatic encephalopathy is a metabolically induced functional disturbance of the brain that is potentially reversible.[12] Symptoms of HE are thought to result from an accumulation of gut-derived nitrogenous substances in the systemic circulation as a consequence of decreased hepatic functioning and shunting through portosystemic collaterals bypassing the liver.[13] Once these substances enter the CNS, they cause alterations of neurotransmission that affect consciousness and behavior. Ammonia is the most commonly cited culprit in the pathogenesis of HE, but glutamine, benzodiazepine receptor agonists, aromatic amino acids, and manganese are also potential causes.[12,13] Arterial ammonia levels are increased commonly in both acute and chronic liver diseases, but an established correlation between blood ammonia levels and mental status does not exist.[13] Despite this, interventions to lower blood ammonia levels remain the mainstay of treatment for HE.

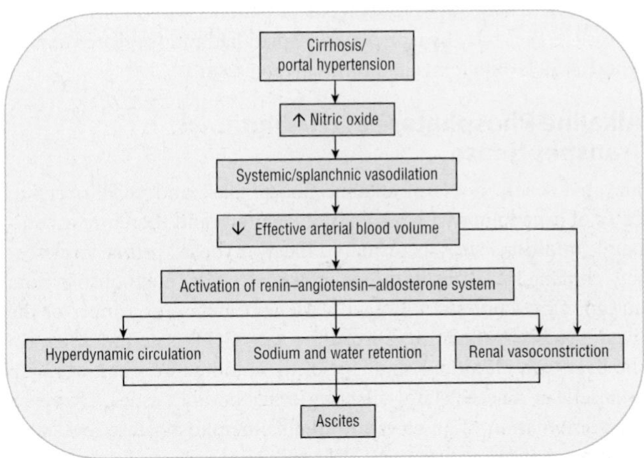

FIGURE 37-3 Pathogenesis of ascites.

Hepatic encephalopathy is categorized as type A, B, or C based on nomenclature developed by the 11th World Congress of Gastroenterology.[12] Type A is HE induced by acute liver failure, type B is due to portal-systemic bypass without associated intrinsic liver disease, and type C is HE that occurs in patients with cirrhosis. Minimal HE refers to cirrhotic patients who do not suffer clinically overt cognitive dysfunction but who are found to have cognitive impairment on psychological studies. The onset of HE in a patient with liver failure may be related to the presence of several known precipitating factors. In cases of HE associated with a precipitant, if that precipitant can be cured or discontinued, it may also be possible to discontinue treatment for HE. In many cases, no precipitant is found and, therefore, long-term treatment of HE may be required.

Coagulation Defects

End stage chronic liver disease is associated with decreased synthetic capability of the liver leading to decreased levels of most procoagulant factors as well as the naturally occurring anticoagulants, antithrombin and protein C.[14] However; two procoagulant factors, factor VIII, and von Willebrand factor, are actually elevated in chronic liver disease. Traditionally, it was thought that chronic liver disease induced an "autoanticoagulation" owing to the decrease in most procoagulant factors, but it is now believed that, thanks to the increased levels of factor VIII and von Willbrand factor and the decreased levels of antithrombin and protein C, these patients actually live in a tenuous state of hemostatic homeostasis. The rebalanced homeostasis seen in chronic liver disease can be tipped toward either

CLINICAL PRESENTATION Cirrhosis

Signs and Symptoms

- Asymptomatic
- Hepatomegaly and splenomegaly
- Pruritus, jaundice, palmar erythema, spider angiomata, and hyperpigmentation
- Gynecomastia and reduced libido
- Ascites, edema, pleural effusion, and respiratory difficulties
- Malaise, anorexia, and weight loss
- Encephalopathy

Laboratory Tests

- Hypoalbuminemia
- Elevated prothrombin time (PT)
- Thrombocytopenia
- Elevated alkaline phosphatase
- Elevated aspartate transaminase (AST), alanine transaminase (ALT), and γ-glutamyl transpeptidase (GGT)

thrombosis or clinically significant bleeding at any time depending on the circumstances experienced by the patient at the time. The prothrombin time (PT) is a standard component of the Child-Pugh scoring system and the international normalized ratio (INR) is utilized in the Model for End-Stage Liver Disease, a prognostic evaluation tool. The ability of the PT and INR to accurately measure bleeding risk and assist with estimation of the severity of a patient's liver disease has been called into question.

Both platelet number and function may be affected in cirrhosis. Thrombocytopenia, a common finding in cirrhosis, could promote bleeding. However, given the relatively high levels of von Willebrand factor present in cirrhosis, platelet function is actually increased. Cirrhotic patients with platelet counts as low as 60×10^9 per liter are able to preserve thrombin formation similar to the lower end of the normal range for healthy persons. Fibrinolysis is another process that is likely rebalanced in cirrhosis. While it has been observed that hyperfibrinolysis occurs in chronic liver disease owing to increased levels of tissue plasminogen activator and thrombin-activatable fibrinolysis inhibitor, reduced levels of plasminogen and increased levels of plasminogen activator inhibitor are also observed, both of which promote a hypofibrinolytic state.

CLINICAL PRESENTATION

Cirrhotic patients may present in a variety of ways, from asymptomatic with abnormal radiographic or laboratory studies to decompensated with ascites, SBP, HE, or variceal bleeding.[15]

The approach to a patient with suspected liver disease begins with a thorough history and physical examination. Some presenting characteristics of patients with cirrhosis include anorexia, weight loss, weakness, fatigue, jaundice, pruritus, GI bleeding, coagulopathy, increasing abdominal girth with shifting flank dullness, mental status changes, and vascular spiders. Osteoporosis, as a result of vitamin D malabsorption and resultant calcium deficiency, can also occur.

A thorough history including risk factors that predispose patients to cirrhosis should be taken. Quantity and duration of alcohol intake should be determined. Risk factors for hepatitis B and C transmission should be inquired about. These include birthplace in endemic areas, sexual history, intranasal or IV drug use, body piercing or tattooing, and accidental contamination of body tissues or blood. Information concerning any history of transfusions, as well as any personal history of autoimmune or hepatic diseases, should be gathered. A family history should also be taken, looking especially for any family member with a prior history of autoimmune or hepatic diseases.

Laboratory Abnormalities

There are no laboratory or radiographic tests of hepatic function that can accurately diagnose cirrhosis. Despite this, liver function tests, a complete blood count with platelets, and a PT test should be performed if liver disease is suspected. Tests that measure the level of serum liver enzymes are usually referred to as liver function tests.[16] However, these tests actually reflect hepatocyte integrity or cholestasis, not liver function.

Routine liver tests include alkaline phosphatase, bilirubin, AST, ALT, and GGT. Additional markers of hepatic synthetic activity include albumin and PT. Liver function tests are often the first step in the evaluation of patients who present with symptoms or signs suggestive of cirrhosis.[15] The use of liver function tests in the diagnosis and management of cirrhosis is discussed in the following sections. It may be useful to group the tests into two broad categories: (1) markers of hepatocyte integrity such as the transaminases and (2) markers of liver function mass such as PT and albumin.[16]

Aminotransferases

The aminotransferases, AST and ALT, are enzymes that are highly concentrated in the liver. Liver injury, whether acute or chronic, results, at some point in the course of the disease, in increases in the serum concentrations of the aminotransferase enzymes. The degree of elevation, rate of rise, and nature of the course of alteration in aminotransferase serum levels are helpful in suggesting possible etiologies. Liver function tests will typically be elevated to the highest levels in acute viral, ischemic, or toxic liver injury. Chronic hepatitis and cirrhosis patients may present with elevated aminotransferase levels, but they may also present with aminotransferase levels within the normal reference range. The degree of aminotransferase level elevation is dependent on the course of the hepatic injury being experienced by the patients and also depends on when the enzyme levels are tested. In a landmark study by Cohen and Kaplan, alcoholic liver disease resulted in AST elevations of only six to seven times the upper limit of normal in 98% of patients.[17] The ratio of AST to ALT also provides information in patients with suspected alcoholic liver disease. Seventy percent of patients with alcoholic liver disease in the study by Cohen and Kaplan had ratios greater than 2, whereas 92% of patients had ratios greater than 1.

Alkaline Phosphatase and γ-Glutamyl Transpeptidase

Elevated serum levels of alkaline phosphatase and GGT occur in cases of liver injury with a cholestatic pattern and therefore accompany conditions such as primary biliary cirrhosis, primary sclerosing cholangitis, drug-induced cholestasis, bile duct obstruction, autoimmune cholestatic liver disease, and metastatic cancer of the liver.[16] Neither alkaline phosphatase nor GGT is found solely in the liver, and elevations in either of these biomarkers can occur in a variety of disease states affecting other bodily tissues. However, the combination of an elevation in alkaline phosphatase level with a concomitant elevation in GGT level increases clinical suspicion of hepatic etiology.

TABLE 37-2 Criteria and Scoring for the Child–Pugh Grading of Chronic Liver Disease

Score	1	2	3
Total bilirubin (mg/dL)	<2 (<34.2 μmol/L)	2-3 (34.2-51.3 μmol/L)	>3 (>51.3 μmol/L)
Albumin (g/dL)	>3.5 (>35 g/L)	2.8-3.5 (28-35 g/L)	<2.8 (<28 g/L)
Ascites	None	Mild	Moderate
Encephalopathy (grade)	None	1 and 2	3 and 4
Prothrombin time (seconds prolonged)	<4	4-6	>6

Grade A, <7 points; grade B, 7-9 points; grade C, 10-15 points.

Data from reference 18.

Child-Pugh Classification and Model for End-Stage Liver Disease Score

The Child-Pugh classification system has gained widespread acceptance as a means of quantifying the myriad effects of the cirrhotic process on the laboratory and clinical manifestations of this disease.[18] Recommended drug dosing adjustments for patients in liver failure, when available, are normally based on the Child-Pugh score. The newer MELD scoring system is now the accepted classification scheme used by the United Network for Organ Sharing in the allocation livers for transplantation.[19] The Child-Pugh classification system employs a combination of physical and laboratory findings (Table 37-2), whereas the MELD score calculation takes into account a patient's serum creatinine, bilirubin, INR, and etiology of liver disease, omitting the more subjective reports of ascites and encephalopathy used in the Child-Pugh system.

The MELD scoring calculation* is as follows:[20]

$$\begin{aligned}\text{MELD score} &= 0.957 \times \log_e(\text{creatinine [mg/dL]}) \\ &+ 0.378 \times \log_e(\text{bilirubin [mg/dL]}) \\ &+ 1.120 \times \log_e(\text{INR}) + 0.643\end{aligned}$$

or using SI units:*

$$\begin{aligned}\text{MELD score} &= 0.957 \times \log_e(\text{creatinine [}\mu\text{mol/L]} \times 0.01131) \\ &+ 0.378 \times \log_e(\text{bilirubin [}\mu\text{mol/L]} \times 0.05848) \\ &+ 1.120 \times \log_e(\text{INR}) + 0.643\end{aligned}$$

These classification systems are important because they are used to assess and define the severity of the cirrhosis, and as a predictor for patient survival, surgical outcome, and risk of variceal bleeding.

Bilirubin

Bilirubin is the product of the breakdown of hemoglobin molecules in the reticuloendothelial system.[16] Elevations in serum conjugated bilirubin indicate that the liver has lost at least half of its excretory capacity and are usually a sign of liver disease. When found in conjunction with markedly elevated AST and ALT, conjugated hyperbilirubinemia indicates the possible presence of acute viral hepatitis, autoimmune hepatitis, toxic liver injury, or ischemic liver injury. Elevated conjugated bilirubin levels with concomitant increases in alkaline phosphatase and normal aminotransferase levels are a sign of cholestatic disease and possible cholestatic drug reactions. Causes of elevations in unconjugated bilirubin include hemolysis, Gilbert's syndrome, hematoma reabsorption, and ineffective erythropoiesis.

*Multiply the score by 10 and round to the nearest whole number. (Laboratory values <1 are rounded up to 1 for the purposes of the MELD calculation.)

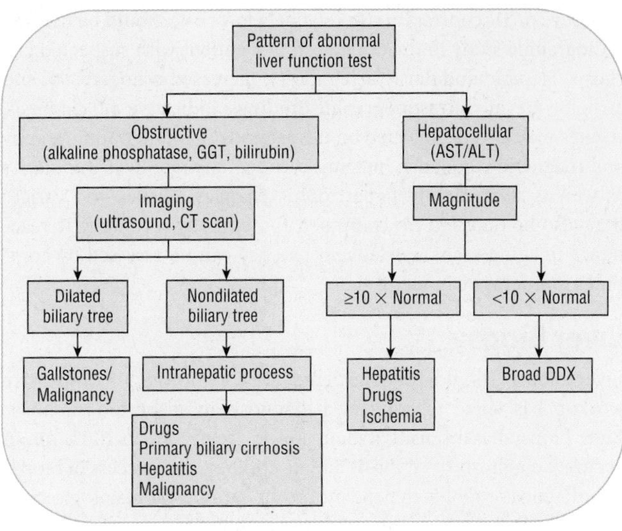

FIGURE 37-4 Interpretation of liver function tests. (DDX, differential diagnosis)

Causes of conjugated hyperbilirubinemia include bile duct obstruction, hepatitis, cirrhosis, primary sclerosing cholangitis, primary biliary cirrhosis, total parenteral nutrition, drug toxins, and vanishing bile duct syndrome. When cirrhosis has been established, the degree of bilirubin elevation has prognostic significance and is used as a component of the Child-Pugh and MELD scoring systems for quantifying the degree of cirrhosis.[18,20]

Figure 37-4 describes a general algorithm for the interpretation of liver function tests. The algorithm first separates the tests into two categories based on the underlying pathology (pattern of elevations): obstructive (alkaline phosphatase, GGT, and bilirubin) versus hepatocellular (AST and ALT). If a hepatocellular pattern predominates, the magnitude of elevation provides diagnostic assistance. If the degree of elevation is greater than 10 times normal, the etiology is likely a result of drugs or other toxins, ischemia, or acute viral hepatitis.[16] Elevations less than 10 times normal have a broad differential. Unfortunately, most liver enzyme abnormalities will fall into a mixed pattern providing limited diagnostic assistance.

Albumin and Coagulation Factors

Albumin and coagulation proteins are markers of hepatic synthetic activity and are therefore used to estimate the level of hepatic functioning in cirrhosis. Albumin and PT are used in the Child-Pugh system for quantifying liver disease, and the INR is used in the MELD scoring system as a marker of coagulation.[18,20] Albumin levels can be affected by a number of factors, including malnutrition, malabsorption, and protein losses from renal and intestinal sources.[16]

Thrombocytopenia

Thrombocytopenia is a common feature of chronic liver disease.[14] A platelet count below 160,000 per mm^3 (160 × 10^9/L) is indicative of cirrhosis in patients with hepatitis C with a sensitivity of 80%.[15] When liver abnormality is suspected, a complete blood cell count with platelets should be evaluated. Platelet count should also be evaluated prior to liver biopsy.

Endoscopic and Radiographic Abnormalities

While no radiographic test is considered a diagnostic standard for cirrhosis, radiographic studies may be used to detect ascites, hepatosplenomegaly, hepatic or portal vein thromboses, and hepatocellular carcinoma. Ultrasonography, because it does not require radiation exposure or IV contrast and is relatively low cost, should be the first radiographic study in the evaluation of a patient with suspected cirrhosis. Hepatic nodularity, irregularity, increased echogenicity, and atrophy are all ultrasonographic findings indicative of cirrhosis. Ascites may also be detected on ultrasound. Computed tomography and magnetic resonance imaging can demonstrate liver nodularity as well as atrophic and hypertrophic changes. Ascites and varices may also be detected on computed tomography or magnetic resonance imaging scans. Portal vein patency can be assessed by computer tomography imaging.

Liver Biopsy

Liver biopsy should be considered after a thorough noninvasive workup has failed to confirm a diagnosis in suspected cirrhosis. Liver biopsy has a sensitivity and specificity of 80% to 100% for an accurate diagnosis of cirrhosis and its etiology. The success of biopsy as a diagnostic tool is dependent on the number of histologic samples retrieved as well as the sampling method used.

TREATMENT

General Approaches to Treatment

General approaches to therapy in cirrhosis should include the following:

1. Identify and eliminate, where possible, the causes of cirrhosis (eg, alcohol abuse).
2. Assess the risk for variceal bleeding and begin pharmacologic prophylaxis when indicated. Prophylactic endoscopic therapy can be used for patients with high-risk medium and large varices as well as in patients with contraindications or intolerance to nonselective β-adrenergic blockers. Endoscopic therapy is also appropriate for patients suffering acute bleeding episodes. Variceal obliteration with endoscopic techniques in conjunction with pharmacologic intervention is the recommended treatment of choice in patients with acute bleeding.
3. Evaluate the patient for clinical signs of ascites and manage with pharmacologic therapy (eg, diuretics) and paracentesis. Careful monitoring for SBP should be used in patients with ascites who undergo acute deterioration.
4. HE is a common complication of cirrhosis and requires clinical vigilance and treatment with dietary restriction, elimination of precipitating factors, and therapy to lower ammonia levels.
5. Frequent monitoring for signs of hepatorenal syndrome, pulmonary insufficiency, and endocrine dysfunction is necessary.

Desired Outcomes

The desired therapeutic outcomes can be viewed in two categories: *resolution of acute complications* such as tamponade of bleeding and resolution of hemodynamic instability for an episode of acute variceal hemorrhage and *prevention of complications* through lowering of portal pressure with medical therapy using non-selective β-adrenergic blocker therapy or supporting abstinence from alcohol. Treatment end points and desired therapeutic outcomes are presented for each of the recommended therapies discussed.

Management of Portal Hypertension and Variceal Bleeding

The management of varices involves three strategies: (a) primary prophylaxis (prevention of the first bleeding episode); (b) treatment of acute variceal hemorrhage; and (c) secondary prophylaxis (prevention of rebleeding in patients who have previously bled).[11]

Primary Prophylaxis

β-Adrenergic Blockade The mainstay of primary prophylaxis is the use of nonselective β-adrenergic blocking agents such as propranolol, nadolol, or carvedilol.[10,11,21] These agents reduce portal pressure by reducing portal venous inflow via two mechanisms: a decrease in cardiac output through β_1-adrenergic blockade and a decrease in splanchnic blood flow through β_2-adrenergic blockade.[10]

Endoscopic Variceal Ligation (EVL) EVL is an endoscopic therapy that consists of placing rubber bands around varices until the varices are obliterated.[21]

Treatment Recommendations: Variceal Bleeding—Primary Prophylaxis

2 All patients with cirrhosis should be screened for varices on diagnosis.[10,11,21] Transient elastography that shows liver stiffness below 20 kPa in patients with platelets over 150,000/mm^3 (150 × 10^9/L) do not require screening endoscopy.[10] Others should undergo screening endoscopy to identify and evaluate varices. β-Adrenergic blocker therapy is not indicated in patients without varices to prevent the formation of varices.[10,11,21] Patients with small varices plus risk factors for variceal hemorrhage including red wale marks or Child-Pugh grade C should receive prophylaxis therapy with a nonselective β-adrenergic blocker. β-Adrenergic blocker therapy is recommended preferentially to EVL in this situation due to the technical difficulty of EVL in the treatment of small varices. β-Adrenergic blocker therapy is not recommended for patients with small varices in the absence of risk factors as there is insufficient evidence to support this therapy to slow the growth of varices in this scenario. All patients found to have medium to large varices that have not bled should receive primary prophylaxis therapy with a nonselective β-adrenergic blocker or EVL. The choice of treatment should be based on a consideration of resources and expertise as well as patient preferences and characteristics with a particular emphasis on side effects and contraindications.[11] If β-adrenergic blocker therapy is chosen, initiate therapy with oral propranolol 20 mg twice daily, nadolol 20 to 40 mg once daily, or carvedilol 6.25 mg daily and titrate every 2 to 3 days to maximal tolerated dose to heart rates of 55 to 60 beats/min.[10,21,22] Once a patient is started on nonselective β-adrenergic blocker therapy, it should be continued indefinitely or until the occurrence of end-stage liver disease when the risks may outweigh the benefits.[11] Following initiation and appropriate titration of the β-adrenergic blocker, further endoscopic surveillance is not needed.[10,21,23] If EVL is chosen, it will be performed every 1 to 2 weeks until the obliteration of varices.[21] Follow-up surveillance will occur at 1 to 3 months and again every 6 to 12 months thereafter.

Patients with contraindications to therapy with nonselective β-adrenergic blockers (ie, those with asthma, insulin-dependent diabetes with episodes of hypoglycemia, and peripheral vascular disease) or intolerance to β-adrenergic blockers should be considered for alternative prophylactic therapy with EVL.[23] Also, EVL may be considered as a possible first option for primary prophylaxis in patients with high-risk medium to large varices. Nitrates are no longer recommended as alternative therapy for primary prophylaxis against variceal bleeding in patients with intolerance to nonselective β-adrenergic blocker due to a potential for higher mortality with this therapy.[21] At this time, there is also insufficient evidence to support the use of other therapies and procedures (such as combination nonselective β-adrenergic blocker therapy with isosorbide mononitrate, combination nonselective β-adrenergic blocker therapy with spironolactone, combination nonselective β-adrenergic blocker therapy with EVL, shunt surgery, and endoscopic sclerotherapy) for primary prevention of variceal hemorrhage.

Acute Variceal Hemorrhage

Variceal hemorrhage is a medical emergency that carries a mortality rate of 15% to 20%, requires admission to an intensive care unit, and is one of the most feared complications of cirrhosis.[10,21] Treatment of acute variceal bleeding includes general stabilizing and assessment measures as well as specific measures to control the acute hemorrhage and prevent complications.

Initial treatment goals include (a) adequate blood volume resuscitation, (b) protection of airway from aspiration of blood, (c) correction of significant coagulopathy and/or thrombocytopenia with fresh-frozen plasma and platelets, (d) prophylaxis against SBP and other infections, (e) control of bleeding, (f) prevention of rebleeding, and (g) preservation of liver function.[23] Prompt stabilization of blood volume with a goal of maintaining hemodynamic stability and a hemoglobin of 8 g/dL (80 g/L; 4.97 mmol/L) should be undertaken. Volume should be expanded to maintain a systolic blood pressure of 90 to 100 mm Hg and a heart rate of less than 100 beats/min, but vigorous resuscitation with saline solution should generally be avoided because this may lead to recurrent variceal hemorrhage or accumulation of ascites and/or fluid at other anatomic sites.[21,23] Use of recombinant factor VIIa therapy is not recommended in cirrhotic patients with GI hemorrhage at this time. Airway management is critical in patients with variceal hemorrhage, especially those with concomitant HE or severe bleeding.[23] Elective or more emergent intubation may be required prior to diagnostic endoscopy. Combination pharmacologic therapy plus endoscopic therapy with preferably EVL, or sclerotherapy if EVL is not technically feasible, is considered the most rational approach to the treatment of acute variceal bleeding.[10,21]

Vasoactive drug therapy (usually octreotide) is routinely used early to stop or slow bleeding for patient management as soon as a diagnosis of variceal bleeding is suspected, and potentially even before endoscopy. Antibiotic therapy to prevent SBP and other infections, as well as to prevent rebleeding and decrease mortality, should be implemented. Figure 37-5 presents an algorithm for the management of variceal hemorrhage.

Drugs employed to manage acute variceal bleeding in the United States include (a) the somatostatin analogue octreotide and (b) vasopressin. These agents work as splanchnic vasoconstrictors, thus decreasing portal blood flow and pressure.[21] Agents available in other countries also include terlipressin, which is an analogue of vasopressin, and another somatostatin analogue, vapreotide.

Somatostatin and Octreotide

Somatostatin is a naturally occurring tetradecapeptide hormone, and octreotide is a synthetic octapeptide that shares a four amino acid segment with somatostatin and has similar pharmacologic activity with greater potency and longer duration of action as compared with somatostatin.[24] Somatostatin and octreotide cause a reduction in portal pressure and port-collateral blood flow through inducing splanchnic vasoconstriction without causing the systemic effects associated with vasopressin.[23,24] The splanchnic vasoconstriction found with somatostatin and octreotide therapy is due to inhibition of the release of vasodilatory peptides such as glucagon; however, octreotide has a local vasoconstrictive effect confined to the splanchnic vasculature.[23] Somatostatin and somatostatin analogues are associated with fewer side effects as compared with vasopressin. The side effects of somatostatin therapy may include sinus bradycardia, hypertension, arrhythmia, and abdominal pain.[10] The recommended dosing of octreotide for variceal bleeding consists of an initial IV bolus of 50 mcg followed by a continuous IV infusion of 50 mcg/h. Because octreotide is safe for continuation for multiple days and because around half of early recurrent bleeding occurs within the first 3 to 5 days, guidelines suggest continuation of octreotide for 5 days after acute variceal bleeding.[11,21]

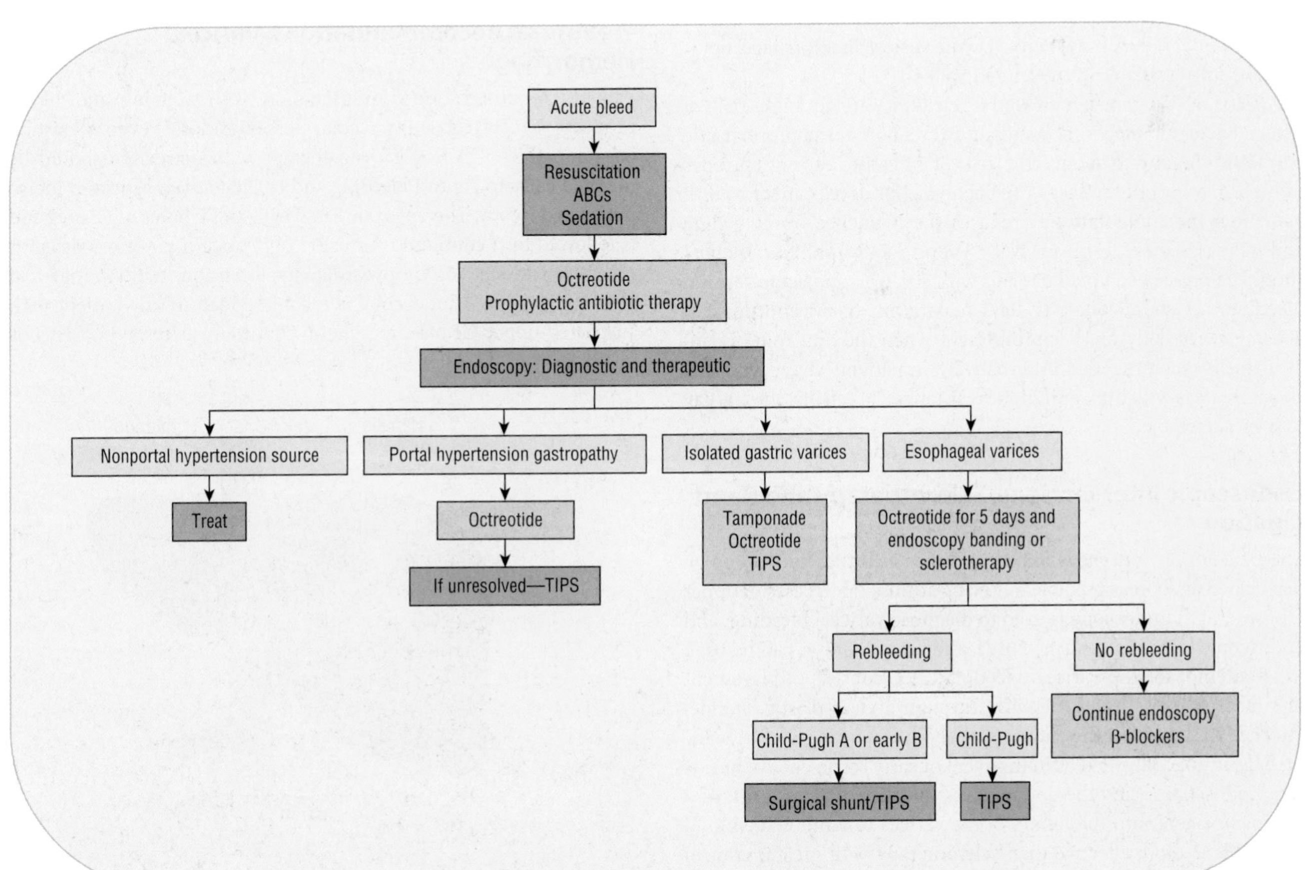

FIGURE 37-5 Management of acute variceal hemorrhage. TIPS, transjugular intrahepatic portosystemic shunt.

Vasopressin

Vasopressin (also known as antidiuretic hormone) is a potent, nonselective vasoconstrictor that reduces portal pressure by causing splanchnic vasoconstriction, which reduces splanchnic blood flow.[24] Unfortunately, the vasoconstrictive effects of vasopressin are nonselective—the vasoconstriction is not restricted to the splanchnic vascular bed. Potent systemic vasoconstriction induces peripheral resistance, which reduces cardiac output, heart rate, and coronary blood flow. These effects on cardiac hemodynamics can lead to myocardial ischemia or infarction, arrhythmias, mesenteric ischemia, ischemia of the limbs, and cerebrovascular accidents. A meta-analysis comparing vasopressin and somatostatin in the management of acute esophageal variceal hemorrhage found somatostatin more efficacious for controlling acute hemorrhage from esophageal varices with significantly less adverse effects.[25] Only four patients must be treated with somatostatin over vasopressin for one to derive additional benefit in terms of initial control of bleeding, and only nine patients need to be treated with somatostatin instead of vasopressin in order for one to experience benefit in terms of avoidance of rebleeding. Although somatostatin is not available in the United States today, its analogue octreotide is commonly used instead of vasopressin for acute variceal hemorrhage.

A recommended dosing strategy for vasopressin is a continuous IV infusion of 0.2 to 0.4 units/min, which can be increased to a maximal dose of 0.8 units/min.[23] Vasopressin should only be used at the highest effective dose continuously for a maximum of 24 hours and should always be administered with IV nitroglycerin at a starting dose of 40 mcg/min (which can be increased to a maximum of 400 mcg/min and adjusted to maintain systolic blood pressure over 90 mm Hg) in order to minimize the risk of serious adverse events. With the addition of safer and equally effective treatment alternatives, vasopressin, alone or combined with nitroglycerin, can no longer be recommended as first-line therapy for the management of variceal hemorrhage.[10,23] Terlipressin, a synthetic analogue of vasopressin, has fewer side effects and a longer duration of action than vasopressin. It reduces mortality in acute variceal hemorrhage, but is not currently available in the United States.[10]

Cirrhotic patients with active bleeding are at high risk of severe bacterial infections such as SBP.[23] Short-term prophylactic antibiotic therapy to reduce the risk of infection during episodes of bleeding not only reduces the likelihood of development of SBP and other infections but also reduces the incidence of rebleeding and increases short-term survival.[21] Prophylactic antibiotic therapy should be prescribed for all patients with cirrhosis and acute variceal bleeding.[23] A short course (7 days maximum) of oral norfloxacin 400 mg twice daily or IV ciprofloxacin when the oral route is not available is recommended. Alternatively, in patients with severe cirrhosis in areas with high quinolone resistance, IV ceftriaxone 1 g/day may be preferable.[11]

Endoscopic Interventions: Sclerotherapy and Band Ligation

The Baveno VI Consensus Report recommends that endoscopy be performed as soon as possible following admission in cases of upper GI bleeding.[11] Endoscopy is used to diagnose variceal bleeding, and endoscopic techniques, such as EVL and sclerotherapy, can be used in an attempt to stop variceal bleeding. EVL consists of placement of rubber bands around the varix through a clear plastic channel attached to the end of the endoscope.[21] EVL can be repeated if hemorrhage is not controlled or in the event of early recurrence of bleeding. Endoscopic sclerotherapy involves injection of 1 to 4 mL of a sclerosing agent into the lumen of the varices to tamponade blood flow. EVL is more effective than sclerotherapy with greater control of hemorrhage, less risk for rebleeding, lower likelihood of adverse events, and lower mortality.[10] Therefore, consensus recommendation calls for EVL (in conjunction with pharmacologic therapy) as the recommended form of endoscopic therapy for acute variceal bleeding.[11] Endoscopic injection of the tissue adhesive *N*-butyl cyanoacrylate is recommended to control acute *gastric* variceal bleeding from isolated gastric varices and gastroesophageal varices type 2 that extend beyond the cardia. EVL or tissue adhesive can be used for bleeding from gastroesophageal varices type 1. A pre-endoscopy infusion of erythromycin 250 mg IV, 30 to 120 minutes prior to the procedure, is recommended in the absence of QT interval prolongation.

Interventional and Surgical Treatment Approaches

Standard therapy fails to control initial bleeding or early rebleeding in 10% to 20% of patients with acute variceal hemorrhage.[21] In these cases, a salvage procedure, such as balloon tamponade or transjugular intrahepatic portosystemic shunt (TIPS), is necessary. Balloon tamponade is effective in controlling variceal bleeding temporarily; however, rebleeding is common after balloon deflation, and complications result in mortality rates of up to 20% with balloon tamponade. Sengstaken-Blakemore tubes are recommended for use in esophageal variceal bleeding. Linton tubes are preferred for bleeding from fundal gastric varices. Balloon tamponade should be reserved as a temporizing measure until a more definitive treatment, such as TIPS, can be performed.

The TIPS procedure involves the placement of one or more stents between the hepatic vein and the portal vein (Fig. 37-6). TIPS (preferably with polytetrafluoroethylene-covered stents) is recommended for patients who fail to achieve hemostasis despite combined endoscopic and pharmacologic therapy.[11] TIPS provides an effective decompressive shunt without laparotomy and can be employed regardless of Child-Pugh score, unlike shunt surgery, which is restricted to Child-Pugh grade A patients.[23] TIPS decreases the incidence of variceal rebleeding and decreases the incidence of deaths due to rebleeding.[26] There is a significantly increased rate of posttreatment encephalopathy found in TIPS-treated patients.

Treatment Recommendations: Variceal Hemorrhage

Patients require cautious resuscitation with colloids and blood products to correct intravascular losses and to reverse existing coagulopathies.[10,11,21,23] 4 Drug therapy with octreotide should be initiated early to control bleeding and facilitate diagnostic and therapeutic endoscopy. Therapy is initiated with an IV bolus of 50 mcg and is followed by a continuous infusion of 50 mcg/h for 3 to 5 days.[21,23] Monitor patients for bradycardia, hypertension, arrhythmia, and abdominal pain.[10] Endoscopy is recommended in any patient with suspected upper GI bleeding due to ruptured varices.[10,11,21,23] EVL is

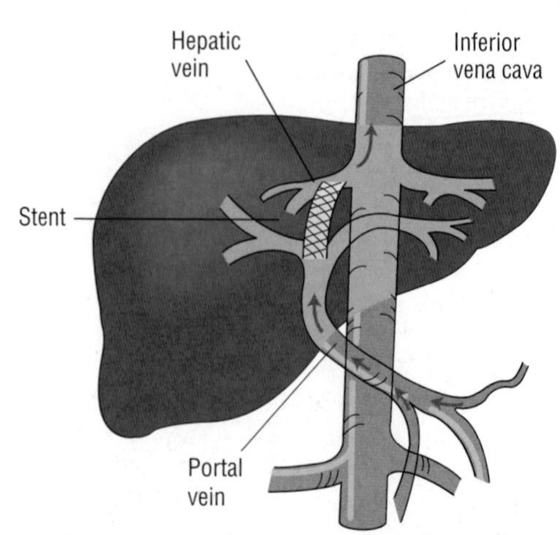

FIGURE 37-6 Transjugular intrahepatic portosystemic shunt (TIPS).

the recommended form of endoscopic therapy, but endoscopic sclerotherapy may be employed if EVL is technically difficult. An additional endoscopic therapy option is injection of the tissue adhesive *N*-butyl cyanoacrylate for gastric varices.[11] Short-term antibiotic prophylaxis (maximum 7 days) is recommended.[11,23] Appropriate choices include norfloxacin 400 mg twice daily or IV ciprofloxacin if the oral route is unavailable.[5,23] In patients with advanced cirrhosis in areas of high quinolone resistance, IV ceftriaxone 1 g daily may be preferred. Surgical shunts and TIPS are employed as salvage therapy in patients who have failed repeated endoscopy and vasoactive drug therapy.[11]

Secondary Prophylaxis

Because rebleeding after initial control of variceal hemorrhage occurs in a median of 60% of patients and because rebleeding carries a mortality rate of 33%, it is inappropriate to simply observe patients for evidence of further bleeding.[10,23] Only patients who underwent shunt surgery or TIPS to control their initial acute bleeding require no further intervention as secondary prophylaxis. Patients who underwent one of these procedures to treat their initial bleeding should be referred for transplantation if they are a candidate. Candidates include those with a Child-Pugh score greater than or equal to 7 or MELD score greater than or equal to 15.[23] Combination therapy with β-adrenergic blockers and chronic EVL to eradicate varices is the best treatment option for secondary prophylaxis of variceal bleeding.[10,11,21,23] Secondary prophylaxis should be started once vasoactive drug therapy is discontinued and as soon as possible (as early as day 6) following the acute bleeding event.[10]

Clinical **Controversy...**

While carvedilol is now an accepted alternative β-adrenergic blocker for primary prophylaxis against variceal bleeding in patients with portal hypertension, it is not recommended for secondary prophylaxis against variceal bleeding in patients with a history of prior bleed.[11] Propranolol or nadolol should be chosen as the non-selective β-adrenergic blocker therapy in secondary prophylaxis since carvedilol has not been adequately studied in comparison to the current standard of care in this population.

Drug Therapy

The combination of EVL and a nonselective β-adrenergic blocking agent provides the most rational approach for secondary prophylaxis because nonselective β-adrenergic blocking agents can protect against variceal rebleeding before variceal obliteration can be accomplished through EVL, and β-adrenergic blocking agents will also delay variceal recurrence.[21,23] The addition of isosorbide mononitrate to nonselective β-adrenergic blocker therapy reduces portal pressure more than β-adrenergic blocker alone, but there is no difference in the overall rate of rebleeding with this combination and side effects are more likely than with β-adrenergic blocker monotherapy (namely, headache and light-headedness).[27] Pharmacologic therapy (either isosorbide mononitrate plus nonselective β-adrenergic blocker therapy or β-adrenergic blocker therapy alone) plus EVL is associated with lower rebleeding rates than either pharmacologic or EVL therapy alone.[28,29]

The lowest rate of variceal rebleeding occurs in patients when pharmacologic therapy leads to a reduction in HVPG of at least 10% of baseline or to a measurement less than or equal to 12 mm Hg (1.6 kPa).[11] Ideally, portal pressure monitoring would be used to assess the response to nonselective β-adrenergic blocker therapy and identify responders from nonresponders earlier in the treatment course. Nonselective β-blocker therapy should be utilized regardless of the possibility of HVPG monitoring.

Treatment Recommendations: Variceal Bleeding—Secondary Prophylaxis

The combination of EVL plus pharmacologic therapy to prevent rebleeding is currently considered the most rational therapeutic approach.[21,23] Pharmacologic therapy should be initiated with a nonselective β-blocker such as propranolol 20 mg twice daily or nadolol at a dose of 20 to 40 mg once daily.[21] (3) β-Blocker therapy can be titrated to achieve a goal heart rate of 55 to 60 beats/min or the maximal tolerated dose. Monitor patients for evidence of heart failure, bronchospasm, and glucose intolerance, particularly hypoglycemia in patients with insulin-dependent diabetes. EVL should be conducted every 1 to 2 weeks until variceal obliteration, and then the patient should be followed by surveillance endoscopy in 1 to 3 months and then every 6 to 12 months. Patients who cannot tolerate or who fail pharmacologic and endoscopic interventions can be considered for TIPS or surgical shunting to prevent bleeding.[11] A summary of evidence-based treatment recommendations regarding portal hypertension and variceal bleeding is found in Table 37-3.

Management of Ascites and Spontaneous Bacterial Peritonitis

Patients with cirrhosis experience overt fluid retention and ascites as liver disease progresses.[9] The classic physical examination findings of ascites are a bulging abdomen with shifting flank dullness.[5] The development of ascites in patients with cirrhosis is an indication of advanced liver disease and is a poor prognostic sign.[5,9] The principle therapeutic goals for patients with ascites are to control the ascites; to prevent or relieve ascites-related symptoms such as

TABLE 37-3 Evidence-Based Table of Selected Treatment Recommendations: Variceal Bleeding in Portal Hypertension

Recommendation	Grade
Prevention of variceal bleeding	
Nonselective β-blocker therapy should be initiated in:	
Patients with small varices and criteria for increased risk of hemorrhage	IIaC
Patients with medium/large varices without high risk of hemorrhage	IA
Endoscopic variceal ligation (EVL) should be offered to patients who have contraindications or intolerance to nonselective β-blockers	IA
EVL may be recommended for prevention in patients with medium/large varices at high risk of hemorrhage instead of nonselective β-blocker therapy	IA
Treatment of variceal bleeding	
Short-term antibiotic prophylaxis should be instituted on admission	IA
Vasoactive drugs should be started as soon as possible, prior to endoscopy, and maintained for 3-5 days	IA
Endoscopy should be performed within 12 hours to diagnose variceal bleeding and treat bleeding with either sclerotherapy or EVL	IA
Secondary prophylaxis of variceal bleeding	
Nonselective β-blocker therapy plus EVL is the best therapeutic option for prevention of recurrent variceal bleeding	IA

Recommendation grading:
Class I—Conditions for which there is evidence and/or general agreement
Class II—Conditions for which there is conflicting evidence and/or a divergence of opinion
Class IIa—Weight of evidence/opinion is in favor of efficacy
Class IIb—Efficacy less well established
Class III—Conditions for which there is evidence and/or general agreement that treatment is not effective and/or potentially harmful
Level A—Data from multiple randomized trials or meta-analyses
Level B—Data derived from single randomized trial or nonrandomized studies
Level C—Only consensus opinion, case studies, or standard of care

Data from reference 23.

dyspnea, abdominal pain, and abdominal distention; and to prevent life-threatening complications such as SBP and the hepatorenal syndrome.[9] Treatment of ascites is expected to have little effect on survival, however.[21] Workup includes a history and physical examination, abdominal paracentesis and/or ultrasound, and ascitic fluid analysis.[5] The treatment of ascites is based on oral diuretics and is carried out in a slow, stepwise fashion.[21] Treatment of ascites should be initiated only in stable patients (eg, those without ongoing variceal hemorrhage, bacterial infection, or renal dysfunction).

Spontaneous bacterial peritonitis is an infection of ascitic fluid that occurs in the absence of any evidence of an intraabdominal, surgically treatable source of infection.[5] It is a common complication that develops in 10% to 20% of patients hospitalized with severe liver disease, cirrhosis, and ascites.[21] The key mechanism behind the development of SBP is thought to be bacterial translocation.[30] Decreased motility of the GI tract with disturbances of the gut flora, changes in the structure of the GI tract, and reduced local and humoral immunity combine to lead to the free flow of microorganisms and endotoxins to the mesenteric lymph nodes. Most episodes of SBP are caused by *Escherichia coli*, *Klebsiella pneumonia*, and pneumococci.[5] Symptoms and signs of SBP include fever, abdominal pain, abdominal tenderness, rebound, encephalopathy, renal failure, acidosis, peripheral leukocytosis, and altered mental status.[5,30] Paralytic ileus, hypotension, and hypothermia are poor prognostic indicators.[30] Thirteen percent of patients with SBP present with no symptoms. For this reason, a diagnostic paracentesis with analysis of ascitic fluid should be performed in all patients admitted with ascites.[5] SBP is diagnosed when there is possible ascitic fluid bacterial culture and ascitic fluid cell counts show an absolute polymorphonuclear (PMN) leukocyte count of greater than or equal to 250 cells/mm^3 (0.25×10^9/L).

The following treatment guidelines for the management of adult patients with ascites and SBP were updated and approved by the Practice Guidelines Committee of the American Association for the Study of Liver Diseases (AASLD).

Ascites

In adult patients with new-onset ascites as determined by physical examination or radiographic studies, abdominal paracentesis should be performed, and ascitic fluid analysis should include a cell count with differential, ascitic fluid total protein, and a serum-ascites albumin gradient (SAAG). If infection is suspected, ascitic fluid cultures should be obtained at the time of the paracentesis. The SAAG can accurately determine whether ascites is a result of portal hypertension or another process. If the SAAG is greater than or equal to 1.1 g/dL (11 g/L), the patient almost certainly has portal hypertension. The treatment of ascites secondary to portal hypertension is relatively straightforward and includes abstinence from alcohol, sodium restriction, and diuretics.

1 Abstinence from alcohol is an essential element of the overall treatment strategy. Abstinence from alcohol can result in improvement of the reversible component of alcoholic liver disease, resolution of ascites, or improved responsiveness of ascites to medical therapy. Patients with cirrhosis not caused by alcohol have less reversible liver disease, and, by the time ascites is present, these patients may be best managed with liver transplantation rather than protracted medical therapy.

Beyond avoidance of alcohol, the primary treatment of ascites due to portal hypertension and cirrhosis is salt restriction and oral diuretic therapy. Fluid loss and weight change depend directly on sodium balance in these patients. A goal of therapy is to increase urinary excretion of sodium to greater than 78 mmol/day. Evaluation of urinary sodium excretion, preferably utilizing a 24-hour urine[5] collection, may be helpful, although this collection can be difficult. A random spot urine sodium concentration that is greater than the potassium concentration correlates very well with a 24-hour urinary sodium excretion over 78 mmol/day and is an easier test to complete. Severe hyponatremia, defined as serum sodium less than a threshold of 120 to 125 mEq/L (mmol/L), does warrant fluid restriction.[5] However, hyponatremia of this severity is rare among patients with cirrhosis and ascites and, for this reason, rarely requires specific treatment.

Diuretic Therapy The AASLD practice guidelines recommend that diuretic therapy be initiated with the combination of spironolactone and furosemide or spironolactone alone.[5] Due to the likelihood for development of drug-induced hyperkalemia with spironolactone when used as monotherapy, it is best to use spironolactone as a lone diuretic agent only in patients with minimal fluid overload. Furosemide as lone diuretic therapy is inferior to spironolactone in the treatment of ascites and is not recommended. If tense ascites is present, paracentesis should be performed prior to institution of diuretic therapy and salt restriction. For patients who respond to diuretic therapy, this approach is preferred over the use of serial paracenteses. In patients with refractory ascites, serial paracenteses may be employed. Albumin infusion postparacentesis is reasonable for extraction volumes exceeding 5 L.[5] Laboratory tests for renal function and electrolytes need to be monitored during therapy. Referral for liver transplantation should be made in patients with refractory ascites. TIPS is a therapeutic modality for the treatment of refractory ascites that may be considered in appropriately selected patients. Peritoneovenous shunting may be considered in treatment refractory patients who are not candidates for paracenteses, transplant, or TIPS.

Clinical **Controversy...**

Patients with cirrhosis and ascites should avoid nonsteroidal anti-inflammatory drugs, angiotensin converting enzyme inhibitors, and angiotensin receptor blockers except under special circumstances.[5] Angiotensin converting enzyme inhibitors and angiotensin receptor blockers should not be used in patients with refractory ascites. While these therapies are not part of the standard therapies of the complications of cirrhosis, non-selective β-adrenergic blocker therapy is indicated for primary and secondary prophylaxis against variceal bleeding in portal hypertension. Unfortunately, non-selective β-adrenergic blocker therapy can cause hypotension in patients with refractory ascites making the condition worse. For this reason, the risks versus benefits of non-selective β-adrenergic blocker therapy in refractory ascites must be carefully weighed and non-selective β-adrenergic blockers avoided or not started in this population unless the benefit of bleeding prophylaxis is considered to outweigh the risk of worsening ascites.

Spontaneous Bacterial Peritonitis

Relatively broad-spectrum antibiotic therapy that adequately covers the three most commonly encountered pathogens (*E. coli*, *K. pneumoniae*, and pneumococci) is warranted in patients with documented or suspected SBP.[5,21,30] Empiric therapy should not be delayed while awaiting culture results. In some patients, signs and symptoms of infection are present such as fever, abdominal pain, and unexplained encephalopathy at the bacterascites stage (ie, signs and symptoms are present before the PMN count in the ascitic fluid is elevated).[5] In these patients, signs and symptoms of infection justify empiric antibiotic therapy until culture results are known, regardless of the PMN count in the ascitic fluid.

Cefotaxime 2 g every 8 hours, or a similar third-generation cephalosporin, is considered the drug of choice for SBP. A 5-day course of antibiotic therapy is as efficacious as 10 days of therapy. Ofloxacin 400 mg every 12 hours administered orally for an average of 8 days is an alternative for patients without vomiting, shock, significant HE, or serum creatinine over 3 mg/dL (265 μmol/L). IV ciprofloxacin offers another potential treatment alternative. Patients with SBP who previously received quinolone therapy as prophylaxis should be treated with an alternative agent since patients who have received quinolone therapy may become infected with quinolone-resistant flora.

Secondary bacterial peritonitis, ascitic fluid infection caused by a surgically treatable intraabdominal source, can masquerade as SBP. Free perforation should be considered when multiple or atypical organisms are cultured, a very high ascitic fluid PMN count is seen, or at least two of the following are seen on ascitic fluid analysis: total protein greater than 1 g/dL (10 g/L), lactate dehydrogenase greater than the upper limit of normal for serum, and glucose less than 50 mg/dL (2.8 mmol/L). A 48-hour follow-up PMN count that rises above pretreatment levels despite antibiotic treatment is indicative of secondary nonperforation peritonitis. Patients with free perforation or nonperforation secondary peritonitis should receive a third-generation cephalosporin plus anaerobic coverage in addition to undergoing laparotomy.

Treatment Recommendations: Ascites and Spontaneous Bacterial Peritonitis

Adult patients admitted to the hospital with new-onset ascites should have an abdominal paracentesis performed to establish the SAAG, the ascitic fluid cell count and differential, and the ascitic fluid total protein. If ascitic fluid infection is suspected, ascitic fluid should be cultured at the bedside. 1 Patients who drink alcohol should be strongly discouraged from further alcohol use. 5 Sodium restriction to 2,000 mg/day, together with spironolactone and furosemide, is the mainstay of therapy. Diuretic therapy should be initiated with single morning doses of spironolactone 100 mg and furosemide 40 mg administered orally. Titrate diuretic therapy every 3 to 5 days using the 100:40 mg dose ratio to attain adequate natriuresis and weight loss (reasonable daily weight loss goal is 0.5 kg).[5] Maximum daily doses are 400 mg spironolactone and 160 mg furosemide. This combination ratio is used because it usually maintains normokalemia. Fluid restriction, unless the serum sodium is less than 120 to 125 mEq/L (mmol/L), and bedrest are not recommended. Utilize the random spot urine test to confirm a sodium concentration that is greater than the potassium concentration as this correlates very well with a 24-hour urinary sodium excretion over the goal of 78 mmol/day. Monitor serum potassium and renal function frequently. Avoid rapid correction of asymptomatic hyponatremia in patients with cirrhosis. If tense ascites is present, paracentesis should be performed prior to institution of diuretic therapy and salt restriction. For patients who respond to diuretic therapy, this approach is preferred over the use of serial paracenteses. Discontinue diuretic therapy in patients who experience uncontrolled or recurrent encephalopathy, severe hyponatremia (serum sodium <120 mEq/L [mmol/L]) despite fluid restriction, or renal insufficiency (serum creatinine >2 mg/dL [177 μmol/L]). Serial paracenteses may be considered for patients with refractory ascites and albumin infusion of 6 to 8 g/L of fluid removed can be considered postparacentesis when paracentesis volumes exceed 5 L.

Patients with ascitic fluid PMN counts greater than or equal to 250 cells/mm³ (0.25 × 10⁹/L) should receive empiric antibiotic therapy with IV cefotaxime 2 g every 8 hours or a similar third-generation cephalosporin. Oral ofloxacin 400 mg twice daily may be an alternative option in patients without prior exposure to quinolones, vomiting, shock, severe encephalopathy, or serum creatinine over 3 mg/dL (265 μmol/L).[5] Patients with ascitic fluid PMN counts less than 250 cells/mm³ (0.25 × 10⁹/L) but with signs and symptoms of infection (symptoms such as abdominal pain, abdominal tenderness, and fever) should also receive empiric antibiotic treatment. Patients with ascitic fluid PMN counts greater than or equal to 250 cells/mm³ (0.250 × 10⁹/L) and suspicion of SBP should also receive 1.5 g of albumin per kilogram body weight within 6 hours of detection and 1 g of albumin per kilogram body weight on day 3 if they also have a serum creatinine over 1 mg/dL (88 μmol/L), blood urea nitrogen over 30 mg/dL (10.7 mmol/L), or total bilirubin over 4 mg/dL (68.4 μmol/L).

6 All patients who have survived an episode of SBP should receive long-term antibiotic prophylaxis with daily norfloxacin 400 mg or double strength trimethoprim–sulfamethoxazole.[5] Long-term prophylaxis should also be considered for the prevention of SBP in patients with low-protein ascites (<1.5 g/dL [15 g/L]) who also have one of the following: serum creatinine greater than or equal to 1.2 mg/dL (106 μmol/L), blood urea nitrogen greater than or equal to 25 mg/dL (8.9 mmol/L), serum sodium less than or equal to 130 mEq/L (mmol/L), or Child-Pugh score of greater than or equal to 9 with bilirubin greater than or equal to 3 mg/dL (51.3 μmol/L). Short-term prophylaxis (7 days) is indicated in patients with cirrhosis and GI hemorrhage. A summary of evidence-based treatment recommendations regarding ascites and SBP is found in Table 37-4.

Management of Hepatic Encephalopathy

Hepatic encephalopathy will occur in 30% to 40% of patients with cirrhosis at some point during the course of their disease.[31] The clinical manifestations of HE vary widely from subclinical alterations to coma. In addition to classification based upon underlying disease, HE is also classified based on severity, time course, and the presence of precipitating factors. To determine the severity of HE, a grading system that relates neurologic and neuromuscular signs can be used (Table 37-5). Time course of HE is classified as episodic, persistent, or recurrent. Recurrent HE refers to HE episodes which occur in time intervals less than 6 months apart. Persistent HE refers to behavioral symptoms which are always present and periodically interspersed with episodes of overt HE relapses. A precipitating factor or factors such as constipation, infection, diuretic overuse, GI bleeding, or electrolyte abnormalities can be identified in most episodic cases of HE related to cirrhosis, but spontaneous episodic HE can occur as well. The general approach to the management of HE is four pronged and includes the following: care for patients with altered consciousness, identify and treat any other causes besides HE for altered mental status, identify and treat any precipitating factors, and begin empirical HE treatment. Treatment for HE is primarily aimed at reducing ammonia blood concentrations through drug therapy aimed at inhibiting ammonia production or enhancing its removal. Additionally, treatment for HE should include avoidance and prevention of precipitating factors in an effort to avoid acute decompensation. In cases where a precipitant of episodic HE has been identified and adequately treated or removed, long-term prophylaxis against another acute HE episode may not be required. Otherwise, chronic therapy to prevent acute decompensation is often required.

Hyperammonemia

7 Treatment interventions to reduce ammonia blood concentrations are recommended in patients with HE. Decreasing ammonia blood concentrations by reducing the nitrogenous load from the gut remains a mainstay of therapy for patients with HE. Treatment options most commonly used to decrease ammonia load from the gut include nutritional management, nonabsorbable disaccharides, and antibiotics.

Guidelines for nutritional support of patients with liver disease have been published by the International Society for Hepatic Encephalopathy and Nitrogen Metabolism.[32] Protein withdrawal is a cornerstone of treatment for patients during acute episodes of HE.[31] However, prolonged restriction can lead to malnutrition and poorer prognosis among HE patients. Therefore, once successful reversal

TABLE 37-4 Evidence-Based Table of Selected Treatment Recommendations: Ascites and Spontaneous Bacterial Peritonitis

Recommendation	Grade
Ascites	
Paracentesis should be performed in patients with apparent new-onset ascites	IC
Sodium restriction of 2,000 mg/day should be instituted as well as oral diuretic therapy with spironolactone and furosemide	IIaA
Diuretic-sensitive patients should be treated with sodium restriction and diuretics rather than serial paracentesis	IIaC
Refractory ascites	
Serial therapeutic paracenteses may be performed	IC
Postparacentesis albumin infusion of 6-8 g/L of fluid removed can be considered if more than 5 L is removed during paracentesis	IIaA
Treatment of SBP	
If ascitic fluid PMN counts are >250 cells/mm³ (0.25 × 10⁹/L), empiric antibiotic therapy should be instituted (cefotaxime 2 g every 8 hours)	IA
If ascitic fluid PMN counts are <250 cells/mm³ (0.25 × 10⁹/L), but signs or symptoms of infection exist, empiric antibiotic therapy should be initiated while awaiting culture results	IB
Ofloxacin 400 mg twice daily may be substituted for cefotaxime in patients without vomiting, shock, grade II or higher encephalopathy, or serum creatinine >3 mg/dL (265 μmol/L) and if there is no prior exposure to quinolones	IIaB
If ascitic fluid polymorphonuclear leukocyte counts are >250 cells/mm³ (0.25 × 10⁹/L), clinical suspicion of SBP is present, and the patient has a serum creatinine >1 mg/dL (88 μmol/L), blood urea nitrogen >30 mg/dL (10.7 mmol/L), or total bilirubin over 4 mg/dL (68.4 μmol/L), 1.5 g/kg albumin should be infused within 6 hours of detection and 1 g/kg albumin infusion should also be given on day 3	IIaB
Prophylaxis against SBP	
Short-term antibiotic prophylaxis should be used for 7 days to prevent SBP in cirrhosis patients with GI hemorrhage	IA
Patients who survive an episode of SBP should receive long-term prophylaxis with either daily norfloxacin or trimethoprim–sulfamethoxazole	IA
Patients with low-protein ascites (<1.5 g/dL [15 g/L]) plus at least one of the following: serum creatinine ≥ 1.2 mg/dL (106 μmol/L), blood urea nitrogen ≥25 mg/dL (8.9 mmol/L), serum sodium ≤ 130 mEq/L (mmol/L), or Child–Pugh score of ≥ 9 with bilirubin ≥ 3 mg/dL (51.3 μmol/L) may also justifiably receive long-term norfloxacin or sulfamethoxazole/trimethoprim as prophylaxis	IA

Recommendation grading:
Class I—Conditions for which there is evidence and/or general agreement
Class II—Conditions for which there is conflicting evidence and/or a divergence of opinion
Class IIa—Weight of evidence/opinion is in favor of efficacy
Class IIb—Efficacy less well established
Class III—Conditions for which there is evidence and/or general agreement that treatment is not effective and/or potentially harmful
Level A—Data from multiple randomized trials or meta-analyses
Level B—Data derived from single randomized trial or nonrandomized studies
Level C—Only consensus opinion, case studies, or standard of care

Data from reference 5.

of HE symptoms is achieved, protein is added back to the diet in combination with other therapies until a target of 1.2 to 1.5 g/kg/day is reached. Vegetable-source and dairy-source protein may be preferable to meat-source protein because the latter contains a higher calorie-to-nitrogen ratio. Also, the higher fiber content of vegetable protein lowers colonic pH, increasing catharsis. Oral branched-chain amino acid formulations have been shown to improve symptoms in episodic HE and may be considered as alternative or add-on therapy in patients who do not respond to conventional measures.[33]

The use of lactulose, a nonabsorbable disaccharide, is standard therapy for both acute and chronic HE.[31] Lactulose, when administered orally through ingestion or a nasogastric tube, passes through the GI tract and reaches the colon unchanged. It can also be administered by retention enema. Lactulose is metabolized by gut flora into acetic acid and lactic acid, which lower colonic pH and create a cathartic effect. Lactulose administration lowers ammonia levels in the blood in several ways: (a) through creation of a laxative effect that reduces the time period available for ammonia absorption, (b) through leaching of ammonia from the circulation into the colon and increasing bacterial uptake of ammonia by colonic bacteria, and (c) through reducing ammonia production by the small intestine by interfering directly with the uptake of glutamine by the intestinal wall and its subsequent metabolism to ammonia.[34]

Inhibiting the activity of urease-producing bacteria with neomycin or metronidazole can decrease production of ammonia.[35] Additionally, neomycin inhibits glutaminase thereby further reducing ammonia production.[31] Neomycin at a dose of 1,000 mg every 6 hours for up to 6 days daily can be given during an acute episode

TABLE 37-5 Grading System for Hepatic Encephalopathy

Grade	Level of Consciousness	Personality/Intellect	Neurologic Abnormalities
Unimpaired	Normal	Normal	Normal
Minimal	No clinical evidence of change	No clinical evidence of change/alterations identified on psychometric or neuropsychological testing	No clinical evidence of change
I	Trivial lack of awareness; shortened attention span	Euphoria or anxiety; impairment of addition or subtraction	Altered sleep rhythm
II	Lethargic	Obvious personality changes; inappropriate behavior; apathy	Asterixis; dyspraxia; disoriented for time
III	Somnolent but arousable	Bizarre behavior	Responsive to stimuli; confused; gross disorientation to time and space
IV	Coma/unarousable	None	Does not respond to stimuli

Data from reference 31.

of HE.[35] For persistent HE, a dose of 1 to 2 g daily could be used with periodic renal and annual auditory monitoring since, despite poor absorption, chronic use of neomycin can lead to irreversible ototoxicity and nephrotoxicity. Metronidazole initiated at 250 mg twice daily may also produce a favorable clinical response in HE. However, neurotoxicity caused by impaired hepatic clearance of the drug may be problematic.

Rifaximin is a synthetic antibiotic structurally similar to rifamycin with a systemic absorption of only 0.4%.[34] It lowers blood ammonia levels and improves neuropsychiatric symptoms in HE. In a randomized, double-blind, placebo-controlled trial, patients in remission from recurrent HE were randomized to either rifaximin 550 mg twice daily or placebo for 6 months.[36] Rifaximin significantly reduced the risk of a recurrent episode of HE as well as hospitalization due to HE. Lactulose was used concomitantly in 90% of patients in this study. The incidence of adverse effects was similar between rifaximin and placebo with the most common serious adverse events reported being nausea and diarrhea.

Zinc can be deficient in cirrhotic patients, especially in cases of alcoholism.[35] Supplementation with elemental zinc at doses of 11 mg/day for men and 8 mg/day for women is recommended for patients with zinc deficiency.

Drugs Affecting Neurotransmission

The GABA-receptor complex is the primary inhibitory neural network within the CNS. An enhanced GABA-ergic tone and an increased amount of endogenous benzodiazepines may contribute to HE. Flumazenil 1 mg IV bolus may be considered for short-term therapy in refractory patients with suspected benzodiazepine intake, but cannot be recommended for routine clinical use.[13,31,35]

Alterations of dopaminergic neurotransmission have also been thought to play a role in the symptoms of HE, particularly the extrapyramidal signs. Improvements of extrapyramidal symptoms have been reported with bromocriptine therapy. Bromocriptine 30 mg twice daily is indicated for chronic HE treatment in patients who are unresponsive to other therapies. Prolactin levels may become elevated during bromocriptine treatment.[13,35]

Treatment Recommendations: Hepatic Encephalopathy

7 The mainstay of therapy of HE involves measures to lower blood ammonia concentrations and includes diet therapy, lactulose, and antibiotics alone or in combination with lactulose.[13,31,35] Other adjunctive therapies include zinc replacement in patients with zinc deficiency, flumazenil, and possibly bromocriptine.

In patients with episodic HE, protein is withheld or limited while maintaining the total caloric intake until the clinical situation improves. Then dietary protein is titrated back up based on tolerance, increasing gradually to a total of 1.2 to 1.5 g/kg/day.[31] Consider the substitution of meat-source protein with vegetable or dairy protein. Supplementation with elemental zinc at doses of 11 mg/day for men and 8 mg/day for women is recommended for long-term management in patients with cirrhosis who are zinc deficient.[35]

In episodic HE, lactulose is initiated at a dose of 45 mL orally every hour (or by retention enema: 300 mL lactulose syrup in 1 L water held for 60 minutes) until catharsis begins. The dose is then decreased to 15 to 45 mL orally every 8 to 12 hours and titrated to produce two to three soft stools per day for chronic therapy. The enema is retained for 1 hour with the patient in the Trendelenburg position. Monitor electrolytes periodically, follow patients for changes in mental status, and titrate to the number of stools as already described.

Rifaximin 550 mg twice daily plus lactulose has been proven superior to lactulose alone in patients with a history of recurrent HE.[36] Because of its more favorable adverse effect profile, rifaximin is now considered the next line of therapy for recurrent HE over either metronidazole or neomycin.[21] Rifaximin doses of 400 to 550 mg twice daily are utilized in chronic HE.[35] It is recommended that rifaximin be added on to lactulose therapy in recurrent HE following the second recurrence.[31]

Systemic Complications

In addition to the more common complications of chronic liver disease discussed earlier, other complications can occur, including hepatorenal syndrome, hepatopulmonary syndrome, coagulation disorders, and endocrine dysfunction.

Hepatorenal syndrome, which is a functional renal failure in the setting of cirrhosis, occurs in the absence of structural kidney damage.[37] It develops in patients with cirrhosis as a result of intense renal vasoconstriction, which results from extreme systemic vasodilation. The resultant reduction in blood supply to the kidneys causes avid sodium retention and oliguria. As liver disease progresses, systemic vasodilation worsens and, subsequently, increased renal vasoconstriction occurs and renal blood flow is further decreased. As this occurs, the heart's response becomes insufficient to maintain perfusion pressure, which the kidneys rely heavily on at this point to maintain adequate blood flow. Hepatorenal syndrome is common and develops in approximately 20% of hospitalized patients with cirrhosis.

Management of hepatorenal syndrome begins with a first step of discontinuing diuretics and any other medication that could potentially decrease effective blood volume and to expand the intravascular volume with IV albumin at a dose of 1 g/kg up to a maximum of 100 g.[21] Precipitating factors, such as infection, fluid loss, and blood loss, should be investigated and treated if found. Liver transplantation is the only definitive therapy for hepatorenal syndrome and the only therapy that will prolong survival. Therapies used to bridge patients until transplantation include arteriolar vasoconstrictor-based treatments with terlipressin or midodrine plus octreotide used in addition to IV albumin infusion as already discussed.

Hepatopulmonary syndrome affects somewhere between 5% and 32% of patients with cirrhosis.[38] This abnormality is characterized by a defect in arterial oxygenation, which is caused by the pulmonary vascular dilation that occurs in the presence of liver disease. Less commonly, pleural and pulmonary arteriovenous shunting can occur as well as portopulmonary venous anastomoses. These patients present with dyspnea on exertion, at rest, or both. Cirrhotic patients with these findings should be evaluated for hepatopulmonary syndrome, which is diagnosed based on the presence of arterial hypoxemia. Arterial hypoxemia is defined based on measurements of the partial pressure of oxygen that are performed with patients sitting and at rest. Testing for an increased alveolar–arterial oxygen gradient is also particularly important as this gradient can rise abnormally before the patient's partial pressure of oxygen measurement becomes abnormally low. Long-term management requires supportive therapy with supplemental oxygen. The prognosis for these patients is poor. Ultimately, liver transplantation offers the best chance for long-term recovery.

Correction of the coagulopathy is essential for patients actively bleeding. The pathophysiology of the coagulopathy is complex and involves impaired synthesis of clotting factors, excessive fibrinolysis, disseminated intravascular coagulation, thrombocytopenia, and platelet dysfunction. Acute therapy involves platelet transfusions for thrombocytopenia and fresh-frozen plasma for prolongation of the PT because of clotting factor deficiencies.[21]

The presence of cirrhosis can produce abnormal circulating levels of various hormones.[39] Hypogonadism, diabetes mellitus, osteoporosis, and thyroid disorders are among the endocrine disorders that may develop related to advanced liver disease. Erectile dysfunction related to hypogonadism can be treated with the administration of testosterone and the removal of causative factors such as alcohol.

Liver Transplantation

The complications seen in patients with chronic liver disease are essentially functional as a secondary effect of the circulatory and metabolic changes that accompany liver failure. Consequently, liver transplantation is the only treatment that can offer a cure for complications of end-stage cirrhosis.

PERSONALIZED PHARMACOTHERAPY

Cirrhosis modulates the behavior of drugs in the body by inducing kinetic alterations in drug absorption, distribution, and clearance.[40] Additionally, patients with cirrhosis may exhibit pharmacodynamic changes with increased sensitivity to the effects of certain drugs, namely, opiates, benzodiazepines, and nonsteroidal anti-inflammatory drugs. These pharmacodynamic changes are separate and distinct from the enhancement of drug effects seen in cirrhosis patients as a result of pharmacokinetic changes. Hepatic drug clearance is primarily dependent on protein binding, hepatic blood flow, and metabolic enzyme activity. The pathophysiologic changes that occur in patients with cirrhosis, including reduced liver blood flow, intrahepatic and extrahepatic portal-systemic shunting, diminished metabolic and synthetic function, and capillarization of the sinusoids, can have a significant impact on each of these factors. The consequence of these changes is a reduction in intrinsic metabolic activity, a reduction in the delivery of blood to the liver that decreases clearance and prolongs half-life, and a reduction in the degree of protein binding that increases the fraction of unbound drug in the serum. Finally, patients with cirrhosis frequently accumulate large amounts of interstitial fluid resulting in substantial changes in the volume of distribution, which also prolongs drug half-life. These changes occur most commonly in combination in patients with cirrhosis and are dynamic throughout the disease course. The effect that these changes will have depends on the drug and the type of biotransformation that the drug undergoes.

Drugs with a high extraction ratio (high-extraction drugs) are dependent on blood flow for metabolism, and the rate of metabolism will be sensitive to changes in blood flow. Drugs with a low extraction ratio (low-extraction drugs) are dependent on intrinsic metabolic activity for metabolism, and the rate of metabolism will reflect changes in intrinsic clearance and protein binding. Furthermore, hepatic biotransformation involves two types of metabolic processes: phase I reactions and phase II reactions. Phase I reactions involve the cytochrome P450 system and include hydrolysis, oxidation, dealkylation, and reduction reactions. Phase II reactions involve conjugation of the drug with an endogenous molecule, such as sulfate or amino acid, rendering it more water soluble and enhancing its elimination. Drugs metabolized by phase I reactions, especially oxidation, tend to be significantly impaired in patients with cirrhosis, whereas drugs eliminated by conjugation are relatively unaffected.

The variability and complexity of the interaction between the extent and severity of liver disease and individual characteristics of the drug make it difficult to predict the degree of pharmacokinetic perturbation in an individual patient. Unfortunately, there are no sensitive and specific clinical or biochemical markers that allow us to quantify the extent of liver insufficiency or the degree of metabolic activity. In addition, renal insufficiency and alterations that commonly accompany cirrhosis further complicate empiric dosing recommendations in these patients. Dosing recommendations are most commonly nonspecific, with recommendations labeled for patients with mild to moderate liver impairment. Dosing information for patients with more severe liver impairment is not available. As a result, when patients with cirrhosis require therapy with drugs that undergo hepatic metabolism (eg, benzodiazepines), monitoring response to therapy and anticipating drug accumulation and enhanced effects is essential. In the case of benzodiazepines, selection of an agent such as lorazepam, an intermediate-acting agent that is metabolized via conjugation and has no active metabolites, is easier to monitor than a drug such as diazepam, a long-acting benzodiazepine that is oxidized in the liver and has an active metabolite with a long half-life of its own.

EVALUATION OF THERAPEUTIC OUTCOMES

Table 37-6 summarizes the management approach for patients with cirrhosis and includes possible adverse drug effects. Cirrhosis is generally a chronic progressive disease that requires aggressive medical management to prevent or delay common complications. Table 37-6 also lists monitoring criteria that need to be carefully followed in order to achieve the maximum benefit from the medical therapies employed and prevent adverse effects. A therapeutic plan including therapeutic end points for each medical and diet therapy needs to be developed and discussed with the patient.

TABLE 37-6 Drug Monitoring Guidelines

Drug	Adverse Drug Reaction	Monitoring Parameter	Comments
Nonselective β-adrenergic blocker	Heart failure, bronchospasm, glucose intolerance	BP, HR Goal HR: 55-60 beats/min or maximal tolerated dose	Nadolol, propranolol, carvedilol
Octreotide	Bradycardia, hypertension, arrhythmia, abdominal pain	BP, HR, EKG, abdominal pain	
Vasopressin	Myocardial ischemia/infarction, arrhythmia, mesenteric ischemia, ischemia of the limbs, cerebrovascular accident	EKG, distal pulses, symptoms of myocardial, mesenteric, or cerebrovascular ischemia/infarction	
Spironolactone/furosemide	Electrolyte disturbances, dehydration, renal insufficiency, hypotension	Serum electrolytes (especially potassium), SCr, blood urea nitrogen, BP Goal sodium excretion: >78 mmol/day	Spot urine sodium concentration greater than potassium concentration correlates well with daily sodium excretion >78 mmol/day
Lactulose	Electrolyte disturbances	Serum electrolytes Goal number of soft stools per day: 2-3	
Neomycin	Ototoxicity, nephrotoxicity	SCr, annual auditory monitoring	
Metronidazole	Neurotoxicity	Sensory and motor neuropathy	
Rifaximin	Nausea, diarrhea		

BP, blood pressure; HR, heart rate; beats/min, beats per minute; EKG, electrocardiogram; SCr, serum creatinine; mmol, millimole.

ABBREVIATIONS

AASLD	American Association for the Study of Liver Diseases
ALT	alanine transaminase
AST	aspartate transaminase
EVL	endoscopic variceal ligation
GABA	γ-aminobutyric acid
GGT	γ-glutamyl transpeptidase
HE	hepatic encephalopathy
HVPG	hepatic venous pressure gradient
INR	international normalized ratio
MELD	Model for End-Stage Liver Disease
PMN	polymorphonuclear
PT	prothrombin time
SAAG	serum-ascites albumin gradient
SBP	spontaneous bacterial peritonitis
TIPS	transjugular intrahepatic portosystemic shunt

REFERENCES

1. Schuppan D, Afdhal NH. Liver cirrhosis. *Lancet* 2008;371(9615):838-851.
2. Guha IN, Iredale JP. Clinical and diagnostic aspects of cirrhosis. In: Rodés J, Benhamou J, Blei A, eds. *Textbook of Hepatology: From Basic Science to Clinical Practice.* 3rd ed. Malden, MA: Blackwell Publishing; 2007:604-619.
3. Chalasani NP, Hayashi PH, Bonkovsky HL, Navarro VJ, Lee WM, Fontana RJ on behalf of the Practice Parameters Committee of the American College of Gastroenterology. ACG clinical guideline: the diagnosis and management of idiosyncraticdrug-induced liver injury. Am J Gastroenterol advance online publication, 17 June 2014. Available at: http://gi.org/wp-content/uploads/2014/06/ACG_Guideline_Idiosyncratic_Drug-Induced_Liver_Injury_July_2014.pdf. (Accessed October 21, 2015)
4. Heron M. Deaths: Leading Causes for 2012. *Natl Vital Stat Rep* 2015;64(10):1-93.
5. Runyon BA. Management of adult patients with ascites due to cirrhosis: update 2012. Available at: http://www.aasld.org/sites/default/files/guideline_documents/adultascitesenhanced.pdf. (Accessed October 20, 2015)
6. Khalili M, Burman B. Liver disease. In: Hammer GD, McPhee SJ, eds. *Pathophysiology of Disease: An Introduction to Clinical Medicine.* 7th ed. New York: McGraw-Hill; 2010:385-426.
7. Friedman SL. Hepatic stellate cells: Protean, multifunctional, and enigmatic cells of the liver. *Physiol Rev* 2008;88:125-172.
8. Bosch J, Berzigotti A, Garcia-Pagan JC, et al. The management of portal hypertension: Rational basis, available treatments and future options. *J Hepatol* 2008;48:S68-S92.
9. Kashani A, Landaverde C, Medici V, et al. Fluid retention in cirrhosis: Pathophysiology and management. *Q J Med* 2008;101:71-85.
10. Bari K, Garcia-Tsao G. Treatment of portal hypertension. *World J Gastroenterol* 2012;18(11):1166-1175.
11. de Franchis R on behalf of the Baveno VI Faculty. Expanding consensus in portal hypertension report of the Baveno VI consensus workshop: Statifying risk and individualizing care for portal hypertension. *J Hepatol* 2015;63:743-752.
12. Cash WJ, McConville P, McDermott E, McCormick PA, Callender ME, McDougall NI. Current concepts in the assessment and treatment of hepatic encephalopathy. *Q J Med* 2010;103:9-16.
13. Blei AT, Cordoba J. Practice Parameters Committee of the American College of Gastroenterology. Hepatic encephalopathy. *Am J Gastroenterol* 2001;96:1968-1976.
14. Tropodi A, Mannucci PM. The coagulopathy of chronic liver disease. *N Engl J Med* 2011;365:147-156.
15. Heidelbaugh JJ, Bruderly M. Cirrhosis and chronic liver failure: Part I. Diagnosis and evaluation. *Am Fam Physician* 2006;74:756-762.
16. Giannini EG, Testa R, Savarino V. Liver enzyme alteration: A guide for clinicians. *Can Med Assoc J* 2005;172(3):367-379.
17. Cohen JA, Kaplan MM. The SGOT/SGPT ratio—An indicator of alcoholic disease. *Dig Dis Sci* 1979;24:835-838.
18. Pugh RNH, Murray-Lyon IM, Dawson JL, et al. Transection of the oesophagus for bleeding oesophagus varices. *Br J Surg* 1973;60:646-649.
19. About the MELD/PELD Calculator, http://optn.transplant.hrsa.gov/resources/allocation-calculators/meld-calculator/. (Accessed October 23, 2015)
20. MELD/PELD Calculator Documentation, https://www.unos.org/wp-content/uploads/unos/MELD_PELD_Calculator_Documentation.pdf. (Accessed October 23, 2015)
21. Garcia-Tsao G, Lim J, Members of the Veterans Affairs Hepatitis C Resource Center Program. Management and treatment of patients with cirrhosis and portal hypertension: Recommendations from the Department of Veterans Affairs Hepatitis C Resource Center Program and the National Hepatitis C Program. *Am J Gastroenterol* 2009;104:1802-1829.
22. Giannelli V, Lattanzi B, Thalheimer U, Merli M. Beta-blockers in liver cirrhosis. *Ann Gastroenterol* 2014;27(1):1-7.
23. Garcia-Tsao G, Sanyal AJ, Grace ND, et al. Prevention and management of gastroesophageal varices and variceal hemorrhage in cirrhosis. *Hepatology* 2007;46(3):922-938.
24. de Franchis R. Somatostatin, somatostatin analogues and other vasoactive drugs in the treatment of bleeding oesophageal varices. *Dig Liver Dis* 2005;36(Suppl 1):S93-S100.
25. Imperiale TF, Teran JC, McCullough AJ. A meta-analysis of somatostatin versus vasopressin in the management of acute esophageal variceal hemorrhage. *Gastroenterology* 1995;109(4):1289-1294.
26. Zheng M, Chen Y, Bai J, et al. Transjugular intrahepatic portosystemic shunt versus endoscopic therapy in the secondary prophylaxis of variceal rebleeding in cirrhotic patients meta-analysis update. *J Clin Gastroenterol* 2008;42(5):507-516.
27. Gluud LL, Langholz E, Drag A. Meta-analysis: Isosorbide-mononitrate alone or with either β-blockers or endoscopic therapy for the management of oesophageal varices. *Aliment Pharmacol Ther* 2010;32:859-871.
28. Garcia-Tsao G, Bosch J. Management of varices and variceal hemorrhage in cirrhosis. *N Engl J Med* 2010;362:823-832.
29. Gonzalez R, Zamora J, Gomez-Camarero J, Molinero LM, Bañares R, Albillos A. Meta-analysis: Combination endoscopic and drug therapy to prevent variceal rebleeding in cirrhosis. *Ann Intern Med* 2008;149:109-122.
30. Koulaouzidis A, Bhat S, Saeed AA. Spontaneous bacterial peritonitis. *World J Gastroenterol* 2009;15(9):1042-1049.
31. Vilstrup H, Amodio P, Bajaj J, et al. Hepatic encephalopathy in chronic liver disease: 2014 practice guideline by AASLD and EASL. Available at: https://www.aasld.org/sites/default/files/guideline_documents/hepaticencephenhanced.pdf. (Accessed October 23, 2015)
32. Amodio P, Bemeur C, Butterworth R, et al. The nutritional management of hepatic encephalopathy in patients with cirrhosis: ISHEN practice guidelines. *Hepatology* 2013;58:325-336.
33. Naylor CD, O'Rourke K, Detsky AS, Baker JP. Parenteral nutrition with branched chain amino acids in hepatic encephalopathy. A meta-analysis. *Gastroenterology* 1989;97:1033-1042.
34. Morgan MY, Blei A, Grüngreiff K, et al. The treatment of hepatic encephalopathy. *Metab Brain Dis* 2007;22:389-405.
35. Al Sibae MR, McGuire BM. Current trends in the treatment of hepatic encephalopathy. *Therapeutics and Clinical Risk Management* 2009;5:617-626.
36. Bass NM, Mullen KD, Sanyal A, et al. Rifaximin treatment in hepatic encephalopathy. *N Engl J Med* 2010;362:1071-1081.
37. Garcia-Tsao G, Parikh CR, Viola A. Acute kidney injury in cirrhosis. *Hepatology* 2008;48:2064-2077.
38. Rodriquez-Roisin R, Krowka MJ. Hepatopulmonary syndrome—A liver-induced lung vascular disorder. *N Engl J Med* 2008;358:2378-2387.
39. Minemura M, Tajri K, Shimizu Y. Systemic abnormalities in liver disease. *World J Gastroenterol* 2009;15(24):2960-2974.
40. Verbeeck RK. Pharmacokinetics and dosage adjustment in patients with hepatic dysfunction. *Eur J Clin Pharmacol* 2008;64:1147-1161.

Drug-Induced Liver Disease

e38

William R. Kirchain and Rondall E. Allen

KEY CONCEPTS

1. Through its normally functioning enzymes and processes the liver often causes a drug to become toxic through a process known as bioactivation.
2. Drug-induced liver disease (DILD) can have many different clinical presentations: idiosyncratic reactions, allergic hepatitis, toxic hepatitis, chronic active toxic hepatitis, toxic cirrhosis, and liver vascular disorders.
3. The mechanisms of DILD are diverse, representing many phases of biotransformation, and are susceptible to genetic polymorphism.
4. The assessment of a possible liver injury caused by drugs should include what is known in the literature, the timing involved, the clinical course, and, always, an exploration for preexisting conditions that may have encouraged the lesion's development.
5. Liver enzyme assays in serum can help to determine if a particular type of liver damage is present.
6. Monitoring for DILD must be tailored to the drug and the patient's potential risk factors.

INTRODUCTION

The number of drugs associated with adverse reactions involving the liver is extensive, but in clinical practice is dominated by alcohol, antibiotics, antiseizure medications and acetaminophen.[1] Complementary (herbal) medicines contribute disproportionately as well to this disease burden Drug-induced liver disease (DILD) is potentially fatal, often debilitating outcome of drug treatment. DILD is thought to be responsible for 11% to 13% of all cases of acute liver failure in the United States.[1,2]

Drug-induced liver disease accounts for as much as 20% of acute liver failure in pediatric populations and a similar percentage of adults with acute liver failure.[3] In approximately 75% of these cases, liver transplantation is ultimately required for patient survival.[4] Of patients who required liver transplantation according to the United Network for Organ Sharing, acetaminophen, isoniazid, antiepileptics, and antibiotics collectively account for just over 60% of cases.[5]

The liver's function affects every other organ system in the body; it in turn is exposed to every substance absorbed from the gut and every injected substance that enters the bloodstream. This chapter will first explore the underlying mechanisms in DILD. Then proceed to develop the key therapeutic skill required in recognizing and categorizing what is and what is not DILD.

MECHANSIMS OF DRUG-INDUCED DISEASES

Stimulation of Autoimmunity

Autoimmune injuries involve antibody-mediated cytotoxicity or direct cellular toxicity.[6,7] This type of injury occurs when enzyme–drug adducts migrate to the cell surface and form neoantigens. The liver plays host to all of the cells that make up the innate immune response system in the body along with Kupffer cells, which are a type of macrophage. These cells sit in anticipation around the hepatocytes, in the space of Disse and elsewhere waiting for antigens (or neoantigens) to present themselves. The neoantigens serve as targets for cytolytic attack by killer T-cells, and others.[8] Halothane, sulfamethoxazole, carbamazepine, nevirapine, fluoroquinolones, and antitumor necrosis factor (TNF) alpha inhibitors are associated with autoimmune injuries.[2,9] Stimulation of autoimmunity is often associated with fulminant presentations.

Dantrolene, isoniazid, phenytoin, nitrofurantoin, trazodone, and methyldopa are associated with a type of autoimmune-mediated disease in the liver called *chronic active hepatitis*.[10,11] Patients experience periods of symptomatic hepatitis followed by periods of convalescence, only to repeat the experience months later. It is a progressive disease with a high mortality rate and is more common in females than males. Antinuclear antibodies (ANA) appear in most patients. These drugs appear to form antiorganelle antibodies.[12] The exact identification of a causative agent is sometimes difficult as diagnosis requires multiple episodes occurring long after exposure to the offending drug.

Idiosyncratic Reactions

Idiosyncratic drug-related hepatotoxicity is rare and usually occurs in a small proportion of individuals. These adverse reactions are often categorized into allergic and nonallergic reactions. Allergic reactions represent 23% to 37% of all idiosyncratic drug-induce liver injuries and are characterized by fever, rash, eosinophilia, and granulomas.[11] They are usually dose-related and have a short latency period (less than 1 month). On re-exposure to the offending agent, there is a rapid recurrence of hepatotoxicity. Minocycline, nitrofurantoin, phenytoin, amoxicillin-clavulanate, sulfamethoxazole-trimethoprim, angiotensin-converting enzyme inhibitors, and allopurinol can cause allergic reactions.[2,11,13]

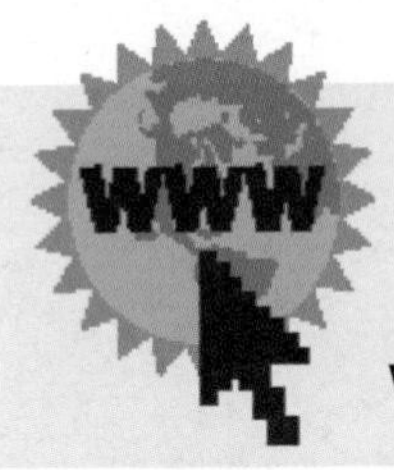

The complete chapter, learning objectives, and other resources can be found at **www.pharmacotherapyonline.com.**

39

Pancreatitis

Scott Bolesta and Patricia A. Montgomery

KEY CONCEPTS

ACUTE PANCREATITIS

1. Factors that can contribute to acute pancreatitis should be identified and corrected, including discontinuation of medications that could be potential causes.
2. Patients with acute pancreatitis should receive aggressive fluid replacement to reduce the risks of persistent systemic inflammatory response syndrome (SIRS) and organ failure.
3. Parenteral opioid analgesics are used to control abdominal pain associated with acute pancreatitis despite a lack of high quality evidence to support the practice.
4. Use of prophylactic antibiotics is not recommended in patients with acute pancreatitis without signs or symptoms of infection, including those with necrosis.

CHRONIC PANCREATITIS

5. Chronic pain, malabsorption with resultant steatorrhea, and diabetes mellitus are the hallmark symptoms and complications of chronic pancreatitis.
6. Pain from chronic pancreatitis may initially be treated with opioid analgesics, but adjuvant agents may be necessary as the disease progresses.
7. Reduction in dietary fat intake and pancreatic enzyme supplementation are the primary treatments for malabsorption due to chronic pancreatitis.
8. Enteric-coated pancreatic enzyme supplements are the preferred dosage form in the treatment of malabsorption and steatorrhea due to chronic pancreatitis.
9. The addition of a histamine$_2$-receptor antagonist or proton pump inhibitor to pancreatic enzyme supplementation may increase the effectiveness of enzyme therapy for malabsorption and steatorrhea due to chronic pancreatitis.

Pancreatitis is inflammation of the pancreas with variable involvement of regional tissues or remote organ systems.[1,2] Acute pancreatitis is characterized by severe pain in the upper abdomen and elevations of pancreatic enzymes in the blood.[2] In the majority of patients, acute pancreatitis is a self-limiting disease that resolves spontaneously without complications. Approximately 20% of adults with acute pancreatitis have a severe course.[1,2] Severe pancreatitis with either organ failure or infected necrosis is associated with a mortality of approximately 30% and it increases when both are present.[3] The risk for progression to chronic pancreatitis after an initial episode of acute pancreatitis is related to the etiology. Patients with acute pancreatitis due to gallstone disease have little risk for progression to chronic disease whereas patients with alcohol-related acute pancreatitis have a risk of 14% to 41% based on whether or not they continue to consume alcohol.[4]

Chronic pancreatitis is characterized by long-standing inflammation that eventually leads to a loss of pancreatic exocrine and endocrine functions.[5-7] It is a progressive disease that often goes unnoticed for many years. The usual initial presentation is complaints of chronic abdominal pain. Later in the disease process malabsorption with resultant steatorrhea occurs. This leads to malnutrition and weight loss. Finally, patients develop diabetes mellitus due to a loss of pancreatic endocrine function.[5,6]

EPIDEMIOLOGY

Acute pancreatitis is the most common gastrointestinal disorder causing hospitalization in the United States with admission rates of approximately 13 to 45 per 100,000 per year.[4,8] The risk for acute pancreatitis varies widely with geographic, etiologic (eg, alcohol consumption and smoking), environmental, and genetic factors. The incidence of acute pancreatitis has increased in the United States, which is likely related to an increase in obesity.[4] The annual incidence of chronic pancreatitis in the United States is 5 to 14 per 100,000, and the prevalence is 50 per 100,000.[7] The prevalence increases with age, with an average onset at 62 years, and it is 4.5 times more common in males than females.[7] Also, the prevalence of chronic pancreatitis varies widely based on geographic location.[5,6] There is also racial disparity with the disease, with African-Americans having 2 to 3 times the risk than Caucasians, and being more than twice as likely to be hospitalized.[7]

PANCREATIC EXOCRINE PHYSIOLOGY

The pancreas possesses both endocrine and exocrine functions. The islets of Langerhans, which contain the cells of the endocrine pancreas, secrete insulin, glucagon, somatostatin, and other polypeptide hormones. The exocrine pancreas is composed of acini and ductules that secrete about 2.5 L/day of isotonic fluid that contains water, electrolytes, and pancreatic enzymes necessary for digestion. Bicarbonate and other electrolytes are secreted primarily by the centroacinar (ductular) cells in order to neutralize gastric acid. Pancreatic juice is delivered to the duodenum via the pancreatic ducts (Fig. 39-1) where the alkaline secretion neutralizes gastric acid and provides an appropriate pH for maintaining the activity of pancreatic enzymes.[9]

The major pancreatic exocrine enzyme groups are as follows:

1. Amylolytic: amylase
2. Lipolytic: lipase, procolipase, prophospholipase A$_2$, and carboxylesterase
3. Proteolytic: trypsinogen, chymotrypsinogen, procarboxypeptidase, and proelastase
4. Nucleolytic: ribonuclease and deoxyribonuclease
5. Other: trypsin inhibitor

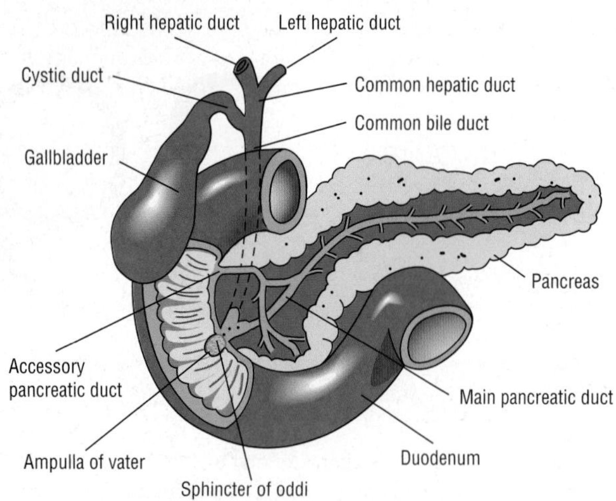

FIGURE 39-1 Anatomic structure of the pancreas and biliary tract.

Amylase is responsible for digestion of starches and glycogen through hydrolysis. The lipolytic enzymes break down triglycerides, cholesterol, and other fats in the digestive tract. Specifically, lipase hydrolyzes triglycerides into fatty acids and monoglycerides. Colipase and bile acids facilitate this process by allowing lipase to act on the hydrophobic surface of fat droplets in the mainly hydrophilic environment. Phospholipase A_2 and carboxylesterase continue to break down fatty acids, cholesterol, monoglycerides, and other products of fat digestion. Proteolytic enzymes digest proteins into oligopeptides and free amino acids, while nucleases break down nucleic acids.[9]

The production of proteolytic enzymes in the pancreas occurs in a manner that prevents self-digestion of the pancreas. These enzymes are synthesized within the acinar cells, stored in vacuoles, and secreted into the duodenum as zymogens (inactive enzymes). Enterokinase secreted by the duodenal mucosa converts trypsinogen to trypsin, which then activates all other proteolytic zymogens along with procolipase and prophospholipase A_2. Thus, two important mechanisms protect the pancreas from the potential degradative action of its own digestive enzymes. First, the synthesis of proteolytic enzymes as zymogens requires extrapancreatic activation by trypsin. Second, pancreatic juice contains a low concentration of trypsin inhibitor, which inactivates any autocatalytically formed trypsin within the pancreas. Proteolytic activity of trypsin in the intestinal lumen is not inhibited because the concentration of trypsin inhibitor is minimal. Lipase, amylase, ribonuclease, and deoxyribonuclease are secreted by the acinar cells in their active form.[9]

The regulation of exocrine pancreatic secretion is a complex interplay of neurohormonal feedback with three distinct phases. The first phase is the cephalic phase where the sight, smell, and taste of food produce pancreatic enzyme secretion through stimulus of the vagus nerve. Vasoactive intestinal peptide (VIP) and gastrin-releasing peptide (GRP) released from efferent vagus nerve terminals bind to receptors on the acinar cells stimulating enzyme release.[9] Water and bicarbonate are also released from ductal cells due to VIP stimulation. The gastric phase occurs due to gastric distension from food entering the stomach. This results primarily in secretion of digestive enzymes from the pancreas. Once chyme enters the duodenum, the intestinal phase begins. The chyme causes secretin to be released from the duodenal mucosa when its pH is less than 4.5. Secretin results in water and bicarbonate secretion from the pancreas to increase intestinal pH for stable lipolytic enzyme activity. Digestive enzymes are released from the pancreas due to the presence of fatty acids, peptides, amino acids, and glucose in the duodenum.[9]

The feedback mechanism for continued release of pancreatic enzymes involves the hormone cholecystokinin (CCK). When products of fat, protein, and starch digestion enter the upper small intestine, they stimulate release of CCK from I cells into the blood. Elevated levels of CCK in the serum activate a vasovagal reflex causing further release of VIP and GRP, leading to enhanced pancreatic enzyme secretion. Inhibition of this feedback loop is thought to be due to trypsin. After digestion is complete, unoccupied trypsin is thought to inhibit the release of CCK.[9] A more in-depth discussion of pancreatic physiology can be found elsewhere.[9]

ACUTE PANCREATITIS

Acute pancreatitis may be mild or may be associated with complications including organ failure and pancreatic necrosis. Prognosis and management vary according to the severity of the disease. There are several classification systems for acute pancreatitis that can be used to predict disease severity and outcomes. Some of these systems predict outcomes, but none have demonstrated superiority to the other.[10] In addition, it is not clear how management should change based on classification of severity.

Etiology

Table 39-1 lists the etiologic risk factors associated with acute pancreatitis. Obstruction caused by gallstones is the most common cause of acute pancreatitis in the United States, with alcohol abuse being the second most common. Abdominal obesity increases the risk for both gallstone- and non-gallstone-related acute pancreatitis. Moderate elevations in lipid levels are associated with non-alcohol related pancreatitis.[11] There is also an autoimmune form of pancreatitis.[12] Diabetes mellitus is also associated with an increase in acute pancreatitis as are autoimmune disorders such as inflammatory bowel disease.[4,13] Most remaining cases are classified as idiopathic.[2] Acute pancreatitis can occur as a result from undergoing an endoscopic retrograde cholangiopancreatography (ERCP) procedure and is more common following therapeutic ERCP than diagnostic, with overall rates up to 5.4%. Pregnancy is not considered a cause of acute pancreatitis; however, pregnant women develop pancreatitis as a result of a coincident process, most commonly cholelithiasis.[14] The reported incidence of acute pancreatitis in children has increased in recent years, and the common etiologies are biliary disease, medications, idiopathic, systemic disease, and trauma.[15]

TABLE 39-1 Etiologic Risk Factors Associated with Acute Pancreatitis

Structural	Gallstone disease, sphincter of Oddi dysfunction, pancreas divisum, pancreatic tumors
Toxins	Alcohol (ethanol) consumption, scorpion bite, organophosphate insecticides
Infectious	Bacterial, viral (including HIV and H1N1 influenza), parasitic
Metabolic	Hypertriglyceridemia, chronic hypercalcemia
Genetic	Cystic fibrosis, α_1-antitrypsin deficiency, hereditary (trypsinogen gene mutations)
Medications	See Table 39-2 for specific drugs
Iatrogenic	Abdominal surgery, ERCP
Kidney disease	Chronic kidney disease, dialysis-related
Trauma	Blunt abdominal trauma
Vascular	Vasculitis, atherosclerosis, cholesterol emboli, coronary artery bypass surgery
Other etiologies	Congenital, Crohn's disease, autoimmune, tropical, solid organ transplantation (eg, liver, kidney, heart), refeeding syndrome
Idiopathic	Undetermined cause

HIV, human immunodeficiency virus; ERCP, endoscopic retrograde cholangiopancreatography.

Data from references 15, 16, 31, and 33-35.

Medications

1 Factors that can contribute to acute pancreatitis should be identified and corrected, including discontinuation of medications that could be potential causes. Drug-induced acute pancreatitis should be considered when other causes have been excluded and there is a temporal relationship with the initiation of a medication that has been implicated as a cause. Most experts consider drug-induced pancreatitis to be rare. Published reports have reported 5.3% to 12.5% of hospital admissions for acute pancreatitis may be drug-induced.[17,18] However, it is possible that the difficulty in diagnosing drug-induced pancreatitis has led to an underestimation of the rate.[17,18] Most information on drug-induced acute pancreatitis is obtained from case reports, which do not provide reliable information on incidence. The most convincing case reports involve recurrence on rechallenge; however, rechallenge is rare, occurring only when alternative therapy is not available. Further complicating the evaluation of some reports is use of medications associated with pancreatitis in patient populations with an increased risk of pancreatitis.[19] Adverse events attributed to newly introduced medications may be reported more frequently.[20]

Many medications have been frequently reported to cause acute pancreatitis. There is a higher incidence of drug-induced acute pancreatitis in the United States in patients with human immunodeficiency virus (HIV) treated with antiretroviral therapy.[21] However, there was no increase in acute pancreatitis associated with antiretroviral use in a well-controlled trial including data from 33,742 person-years.[22] Pancreatitis due to azathioprine is reported more frequently in patients with Crohn's disease than patients taking the medication for other indications, suggesting an interaction between the disease and medication. Patients with Crohn's disease often take other medications that can cause pancreatitis, including 5-aminosalycilates, corticosteroids and sulfasalazine.[23] Patients with type 2 diabetes mellitus have an increased risk of acute pancreatitis. Case reports and some observational studies have linked antihyperglycemic agents, including metformin, sulfonylureas, and incretin mimetics, with pancreatitis. However, a meta-analysis did not find an increase in pancreatitis with incretin mimetics (such as exenatide and sitagliptin) compared to sulfonylureas, metformin or insulin.[24] Complicating comparisons between agents used to treat diabetes mellitus is that the medications are often used in obese patients and patients with different durations of disease, both of which may also influence disease-associated pancreatitis.[25,26]

There are numerous case reports of apparent drug-induced pancreatitis with statins. In contrast, a meta-analysis of lipid-lowering therapies found that statins were associated with a decreased number of acute pancreatitis cases.[27] However, pancreatitis was not a stated end point of any of the trials included and the issue remains controversial.

The onset of drug-induced pancreatitis after initiation of medications ranges from a few months to several years, with a median of 5 weeks; onset after rechallenge can occur within hours. The onset may differ according to the mechanism. Clinicians should be especially suspicious of a drug as a cause of acute pancreatitis in high-risk patients, such as those receiving immunomodulating drugs or who have HIV infection, the elderly, or those with diabetes mellitus.[28]

Mechanisms of drug-induced pancreatitis have been proposed for some medications but remain poorly defined. Possible mechanisms include direct toxic effects of the drug or its metabolites, hypersensitivity, drug-induced hypertriglyceridemia, and alterations of cellular function in the pancreas and pancreatic duct.[29] Ultimately, drug-induced pancreatitis causes damage to the pancreas, which produces a response similar to other causes of pancreatitis. It is prudent to withdraw a medication when an association is suspected.

Numerous drugs are believed to cause acute pancreatitis, but ethical and practical considerations prevent rechallenge with suspected agents. Table 39-2 lists specific agents associated with acute pancreatitis. Classification schemes consider factors such a case reports that include rechallenge, the number of case reports, consistency with respect to onset of symptoms following initiation of the suspect medication, and exclusion of other causes. Other classification systems have been developed that consider factors such as consistency in the temporal relationship.[30]

TABLE 39-2 Medications Associated with Acute Pancreatitis

Well-supported Association	Probable Association	Possible Association	
5-Aminosalicylic acid	Acetaminophen	Aldesleukin	Indinavir
Asparaginase	Atorvastatin	Amiodarone	Indomethacin
Azathioprine	Hydrochlorothiazide	Atorvastatin	Infliximab
Bortezomib	Ifosfamide	Asparaginase	Ketoprofen
Carbamazepine	Interferon α_{2b}	Calcium	Ketorolac
Cimetidine	Maprotiline	Ceftriaxone	Lipid emulsion
Corticosteroids	Methyldopa	Capecitabine	Liraglutide
Cisplatin	Oxaliplatin	Carboplatin	Lisinopril
Cytarabine	Simvastatin	Celecoxib	Mefenamic acid
Didanosine		Clozapine	Metformin
Enalapril		Cholestyramine	Metolazone
Erythromycin		Ciprofloxacin	Metronidazole
Estrogens		Clarithromycin	Nitrofurantoin
Furosemide		Clonidine	Omeprazole
Hydrochlorothiazide		Cyclosporine	Ondansetron
Mercaptopurine		Danazol	Paclitaxel
Mesalamine		Diazoxide	Pravastatin
Octreotide		Etanercept	Propofol
Olsalazine		Ethacrynic acid	Propoxyphene
Opiates		Exenatide	Rifampin
Pentamidine		Famciclovir	Sertraline
Pentavalent antimonials		Glyburide	Sitagliptin
Sulfasalazine		Gold therapy	Sorafenib
Sulfamethoxazole and trimethoprim		Granisetron	Sulindac
Sulindac		Ibuprofen	Zalcitabine
Tamoxifen		Imatinib	
Tetracyclines			
Valproic acid/salts			

Data from references 17-25 and 27-29.

Pathophysiology

The pathophysiology of acute pancreatitis is based on events that initiate injury and secondary events that establish and perpetuate the injury (Fig. 39-2). Gallstones, alcohol abuse, and other causes of pancreatitis produce different initial insults to the pancreas. However, the resulting pathophysiologic process may be similar and include a combination of autodigestion and inflammatory response. In acinar cells, the separation of zymogens and lysosomes can be disrupted, resulting in exposure of trypsinogen to lysosomal enzymes such as cathepsin B. The premature activation of trypsinogen to trypsin within the pancreas leads to activation of other digestive enzymes and autodigestion of the gland.[2]

In addition to activation of digestive enzymes within the pancrease, enzymes are also released into surrounding fat, vascular endothelium and other surrounding tissues and structures causing further damage and necrosis. Lipase damages fat cells, producing noxious substances that cause further pancreatic and peripancreatic injury. There may be an independent response from intra-acinar activation of inflammatory factors. The release of cytokines by acinar cells directly causes their injury and enhances the inflammatory response.[31] Injured acinar cells liberate chemoattractants that recruit neutrophils, macrophages, and other cells to the area of inflammation. These immune responses cause a systemic inflammatory response syndrome (SIRS). Vascular damage and ischemia causes the release of kinins, which makes capillary walls permeable and promotes tissue edema. The release of damaging oxygen-free radicals appears to correlate with the severity of pancreatic injury.[32] Finally, pancreatic infection may result from increased intestinal permeability and translocation of colonic bacteria.[33]

Clinical Presentation

Signs and Symptoms

The clinical presentation of acute pancreatitis varies depending on the severity of the inflammatory process and whether damage is confined to the pancreas or involves local and systemic complications (Table 39-3).[34]

Diagnosis

The diagnosis of acute pancreatitis requires two of the following three: upper abdominal pain, a serum lipase or amylase concentration at least three times greater than the upper limit of normal, or characteristic findings on imaging studies.[35,36] Lipase is more sensitive and specific than amylase and is the preferred laboratory test. Imaging studies are not necessary for diagnosis if the other two findings are positive. Contrast-enhanced computed tomography (CECT) of the abdomen may be used to confirm the diagnosis in patients with amylase or lipase that is not three times the upper limit of normal, or in sedated patients. The diagnosis of acute pancreatitis should also be considered when evaluating patients with SIRS (see Table 39-3).[36] For further information on laboratory tests and abdominal imaging, refer to Table 39-3. Pertinent history includes previous history of pancreatitis, gallstone disease, alcohol use, medication use, recent surgery or ERCP, hyperlipidemia, and family history. Magnetic resonance cholangiopancreatography (MRCP) is useful for detecting retained common bile duct stones. Laboratory tests should include liver enzymes, triglycerides and calcium. Transabdominal ultrasound of the right upper quadrant is recommended to assess for gallstones.[35,36]

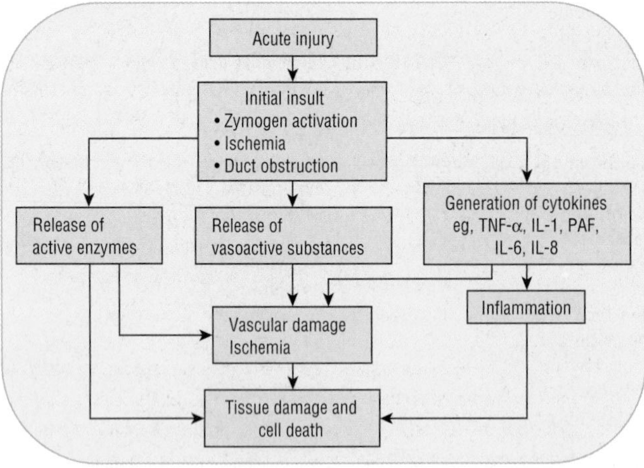

FIGURE 39-2 Pathophysiology of acute pancreatitis: initiating and secondary events. (IL-1β, interleukin-1β; IL-6, interleukin-6; IL-8, interleukin-8; PAF, platelet-activating factor; TNF-α, tumor necrosis factor-α.)

Prediction of severity of acute pancreatitis is useful for decisions involving the need for aggressive treatment, including admission to an intensive care unit. The risk for severe acute pancreatitis should be assessed on admission and on an ongoing basis.[37] Several scoring systems have been developed to assess the likelihood of severe disease.

Multiple scoring systems have been used to predict which patients with acute pancreatitis are at greatest risk for persistent organ failure.[38] This would be useful in determining aggressiveness of initial therapy as well as in developing clinical trials of interventions. However, development and validation of such systems remain an ongoing area of research. Scoring systems are developed based on retrospectively identified associations between clinical and laboratory findings and morbidity and mortality.[1,39] Many are too complicated for bedside use or rely on measurements that are not widely available. Some scoring systems have not been validated in prospective trials or have poor predictive ability.[38]

Ranson's criteria assesses 11 variables that must be monitored at the time of admission and during the initial 48 hours of hospitalization.[32] Severe acute pancreatitis is characterized by three or more criteria. Two separate groups have released recommendations for new classifications. The revised Atlanta Classification defines acute pancreatitis as mild disease (not associated with organ failure, local complications or systemic complications), moderately severe (transient organ failure, local complications or systemic complications) and severe (persistent organ failure).[40] In contrast, an international multidisciplinary group proposed using factors that have a causal association with severity (ie, distant organ failure or pancreatic necrosis) rather than events that may be associated with severity.[41] This determinant-based classification includes mild (no organ dysfunction or necrosis), moderate (sterile necrosis or transient organ dysfunction or both), severe (either infected necrosis or persistent organ dysfunction) and critical (infected necrosis and persistent organ dysfunction). The Acute Physiology and Chronic Health Evaluation II (APACHE II) system is a sensitive predictor of persistent organ failure in patients with acute pancreatitis; however, it is less specific than some scoring systems that were developed for acute pancreatitis.[42] Other tools for assessing the severity of acute pancreatitis include the Bedside Index of Severity in Acute Pancreatitis (BISAP), the Harmless Acute Pancreatitis Score (HAPS), and the Japanese Severity Score (JSS).

The accuracy of several scoring systems was assessed and none had consistent superiority to the others.[38] The IAP/APA guidelines recommend evaluation based on SIRS criteria.[36] Advantages of using SIRS criteria include ease of use and the widespread adoption of processes to ensure that it is routinely assessed.

Clinical Course and Prognosis

The clinical course of acute pancreatitis varies from a mild transitory disorder to a severe necrotizing disease. Mild acute pancreatitis is self-limiting and subsides spontaneously within 3 to 5 days. Mortality is influenced by etiology, as idiopathic and postoperative acute

TABLE 39-3 Presentation and Diagnosis of Acute Pancreatitis

General
• The patient may have acute mild symptoms or present with a severe acute attack with life-threatening complications.
Symptoms
• The patient may present initially with moderate abdominal discomfort to excruciating pain, nausea, shock, and respiratory distress. • Abdominal pain occurs in 95% of patients. The pain is usually epigastric and radiates to either of the upper quadrants or the back in two thirds of patients. In gallstone pancreatitis, the pain is typically sudden and quite severe and the intensity is often described as "knife-like" or "boring." The pain usually reaches its maximum intensity within 30 minutes and may persist for hours or days. Repositioning the patient relieves very little of the pain. In alcohol abuse and other cases, the onset of pain may be less abrupt and poorly localized. Pain may not be the dominant symptom if it is masked by multiorgan failure. • Nausea and vomiting occur in 85% of patients and usually follow the onset of abdominal pain. Vomiting does not provide relief of the abdominal pain.
Signs
• Marked epigastric or diffuse tenderness on palpation with rebound tenderness and guarding in severe cases. The abdomen is often distended and tympanic, with bowel sounds decreased or absent in severe disease. • Vital signs may be normal, but hypotension, tachycardia, and low-grade fever are often observed, especially with widespread pancreatic inflammation and necrosis. • Dyspnea and tachypnea are often signs of acute respiratory complications. Jaundice and altered mental status may be present and have multiple causes. Other signs of alcoholic liver disease may be present in patients with alcoholic pancreatitis.
Laboratory tests
• Leukocytosis is frequently present; hyperglycemia or hypoalbuminemia may be present. Liver transaminases, alkaline phosphatase, and bilirubin are usually elevated in gallstone pancreatitis and in patients with intrinsic liver disease. Elevated serum triglycerides may also be a possible etiology. • The hematocrit may be normal, but hemoconcentration results from multiple factors (eg, vomiting). In patients with third-space fluid loss, hemoconcentration is present and a reasonably accurate marker of severe disease. A hematocrit of greater than 47% (0.47) predicts severe acute pancreatitis and one of less than 44% (0.44) predicts mild disease. Further, failure to reverse hemoconcentration has been associated with pancreatic necrosis. • Blood urea nitrogen (BUN) that is elevated or rising over the first 24 hours has been associated with increased mortality. • The total serum calcium is usually normal initially, but hypocalcemia disproportionate to the hypoalbuminemia may develop. Marked hypocalcemia is an indication of severe necrosis and a poor prognostic sign. • The serum amylase concentration usually rises within 4-8 hours of the initial attack, peaks at 24 hours, and returns to normal over the next 8-14 days. Serum amylase concentrations greater than three times the upper limit of normal are highly suggestive of acute pancreatitis. Persistent elevations suggest extensive pancreatic necrosis and related complications. Normal concentrations may be observed if testing is delayed (ie, amylase may have returned to normal) or in patients with hyperlipidemic pancreatitis (ie, marked triglyceride elevations may interfere with amylase assay). In addition, many nonpancreatic diseases may be associated with hyperamylasemia, including salivary, kidney, hepatobiliary, metabolic, female reproductive tract, and neoplastic diseases. • Serum lipase is specific to the pancreas and concentrations are elevated and parallel the elevations in serum amylase. Levels remain elevated with pancreatic inflammation and return to normal when the inflammatory process resolves. Because of its longer half-life, elevations of serum lipase can be detected after the serum amylase has returned to normal. • Additional biomarkers: C-reactive protein (CRP) is a widely available test and levels greater than 150 mg/L at 48-72 hours predict severe acute pancreatitis with accuracy similar to that of APACHE II. Urinary trypsinogen activation peptide is specific for acute pancreatitis but not sensitive and not widely available. Procalcitonin has been studied for severity assessment as well as identification of patients with bacterial infection. • Thrombocytopenia and an increase in the international normalized ratio are seen in some patients with severe acute pancreatitis and associated liver disease.
Abdominal imaging
• Transabdominal ultrasound should be performed in all patients to detect dilated biliary ducts and stones in the gallbladder. • CECT is used if the diagnosis cannot be made from clinical and laboratory findings. It is less accurate for evaluating the gallbladder and biliary ducts. The test distinguishes interstitial from necrotizing pancreatitis, but does not distinguish between fat necrosis and acute fluid collection. Tests that are performed in the first few days may miss necrosis. Tests should be performed at least 72-96 after symptom onset; tests performed too early may result in unnecessary exposure to risk and increased cost. • Magnetic resonance imaging is used to grade the severity of acute pancreatitis, identify biliary duct problems that are not seen on CT, or if there are contraindications to CECT. Patients over the age of 40 with pancreatitis of an unknown etiology should be evaluated for pancreatic malignancy with CT or endoscopic ultrasonography.

APACHE, Acute Physiology and Chronic Health Evaluation; CECT, contrast-enhanced computed tomography; CT, computed tomography.

Data from reference 36.

pancreatitis have higher rates than gallstone- or alcohol-related disease. First and second occurrences also carry a higher mortality than subsequent episodes. Mortality increases with unfavorable early prognostic signs, local complications, and organ failure. Persistent organ failure is a greater risk than transient organ failure.[3] Severe pancreatitis with either organ failure or infected necrosis is associated with a mortality of approximately 30%, and increases when both are present.[3] Death during the first few days results from SIRS and multiorgan failure. When death occurs after this period, it is usually a result of infected necrosis, pancreatic abscess, and sepsis.[35,36,43]

Complications

Early complications are a result of SIRS and organ failure. The most common systemic complication of acute pancreatitis is respiratory failure.[40] In addition, patients may experience systemic complications due to exacerbation of pre-existing renal, lung or heart disease.[40] A second phase occurs in patients with moderately severe or severe disease. These patients have persistent organ failure and may have local complication including fluid collections that may become necrotic.[40] Long-term complications include glucose intolerance and recurrence of acute pancreatitis.[44,45]

There are also local complications that may occur, including interstitial pancreatitis (acute peripancreatic fluid collection and pancreatic pseudocysts) and collection of necrosis. These develop approximately 3 to 4 weeks after the initial attack. Pancreatic infections occur in 15% to 30% of those with pancreatic necrosis and are usually secondary infections of necrotic tissue.[34]

TREATMENT

Acute Pancreatitis

Desired Outcome

Treatment of acute pancreatitis is aimed at relieving abdominal pain and nausea, replacing fluids, correcting electrolyte, glucose, and lipid abnormalities, minimizing systemic complications, and managing pancreatic necrosis and infection. Management varies depending on the severity of the attack (Fig. 39-3). Patients with mild acute pancreatitis respond very well to the initiation of supportive care. Patients with severe acute pancreatitis should be treated aggressively and monitored closely.

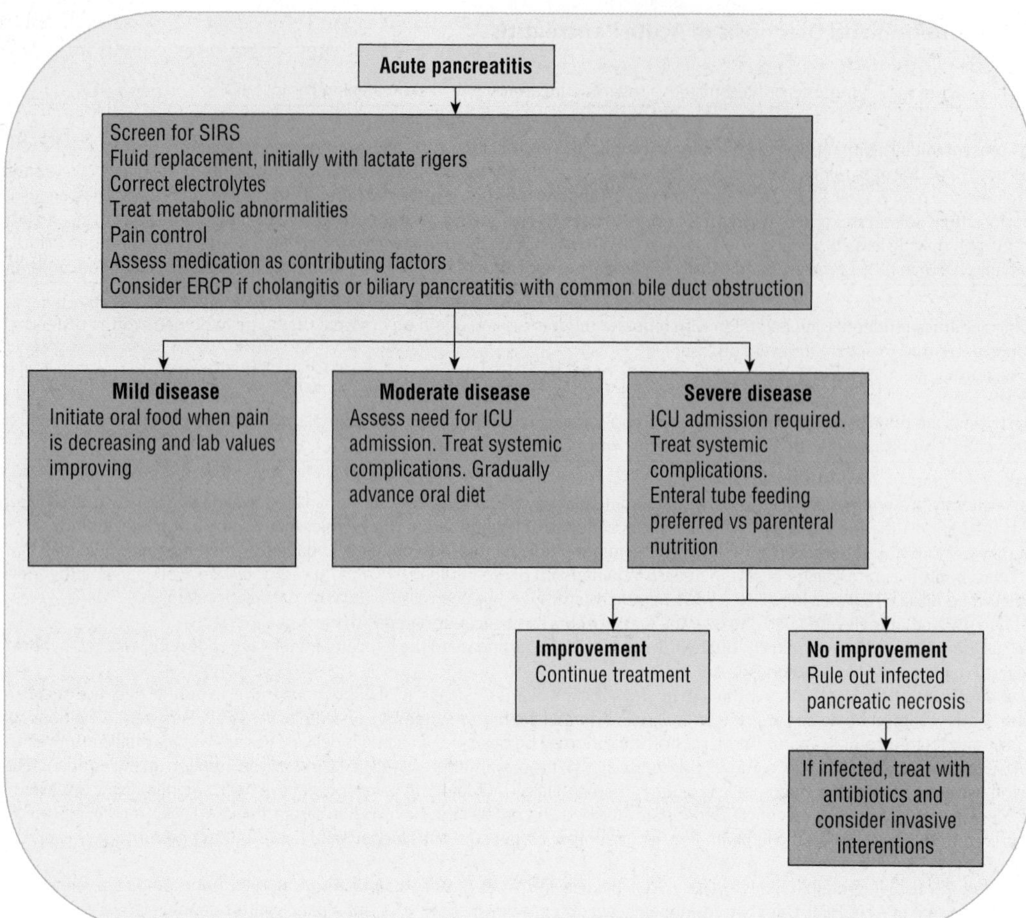

FIGURE 39-3 Algorithm of guidelines for evaluation and treatment of acute pancreatitis. (SIRS, systemic inflammatory response syndrome; ERCP, endoscopic retrograde cholangiopancreatography; ICU, intensive care unit.)

General Approach to Treatment

All patients with acute pancreatitis should receive supportive care, including IV fluid resuscitation, adequate nutrition, and effective relief of pain and nausea. Patients should be evaluated for admission to the intensive care unit. Patients predicted to follow a severe course may require treatment of systemic complications.[1] Fluid therapy is recommended and may help prevent organ failure.[36,46-52] Patients with pancreatitis and SIRS should be treated according to SIRS guidelines. IV potassium, calcium, and magnesium are used to correct electrolyte deficiency states. Insulin is used to treat hyperglycemia. Local complications resolve as the inflammatory process subsides. However, patients with necrotizing pancreatitis may require antibiotics and procedural intervention.[36,53] Medications listed in Table 39-2 should be discontinued if possible.

Nonpharmacologic Therapy

Nonpharmacologic therapy includes ERCP for removal of any underlying biliary tract stones, procedural interventions, and nutritional support. The need for admission to an intensive care unit should be addressed. Advances in minimally invasive surgical techniques are changing practice with respect to timing and approach to managing infected necrotizing pancreatitis, and may help lower the risk of mortality in the most critical patients.[37,53]

Nutrition and Probiotics

Nutritional support plays an important role in the management of patients with mild or severe disease as acute pancreatitis creates a catabolic state that promotes nutritional depletion. This can impair recovery, increase the risk of complications, and prolong hospitalization.[54] Patients with mild acute pancreatitis can begin oral feeding when pain is decreasing an inflammatory markers are improving. It is not necessary to withhold oral nutrition until lipase normalizes.[55] In severe or complicated disease, nutritional deficits develop rapidly and are complicated by tissue necrosis, organ failure, and surgery. Nutritional support should begin when it is anticipated that oral nutrition will be withheld for more than 1 week.[54] In the past, there was concern that enteral feeding stimulated pancreatic enzyme secretion and exacerbated the underlying disease. However, randomized controlled trials found that enteral nutrition results in a decrease in morality, multiple organ failure, and need for surgical intervention compared with parenteral nutrition.[54] Possible mechanisms for this include protection of the gut barrier and prevention of colonization with pathogenic bacteria, both of which may prevent translocation of bacteria and subsequent infection.[37] Therefore, enteral nutrition delivered via a nasogastric or nasojejunal tube is preferred over parenteral nutrition in patients with severe acute pancreatitis provided it can be tolerated. If enteral feeding is not possible or if the patient is unable to obtain sufficient nutrients, total parenteral nutrition should be implemented before protein and calorie depletion become advanced. ASPEN guidelines state that IV lipids are considered safe unless the serum triglyceride concentration is greater than 400 mg/dL (4.52 mmol/L) and the patient has a history of hyperlipidemia.[56]

Clinical trials do not support the use of probiotics in the treatment of acute pancreatitis, as they have not shown a benefit. One prospective randomized trial in patients with predicted severe acute pancreatitis showed an increase in mortality with probiotics compared with placebo.[57]

Pharmacologic Therapy

Patients with acute pancreatitis often require IV antiemetics for nausea. Those requiring ICU admission should be treated with antisecretory agents (such as famotidine or pantoprazole) if they are at risk of stress-related mucosal bleeding. Patients also require appropriate fluid resuscitation and pain management, but there is controversy surrounding both of these therapies. (see Fig. 39-3). Clinical trials have also failed to identify a group of patients that benefit from prophylactic antibiotics.

Fluid Resuscitation

Vasodilation from the inflammatory response, vomiting, and nasogastric suction contributes to hypovolemia and fluid and electrolyte abnormalities, thus necessitating replacement. 2 Patients with acute pancreatitis should receive aggressive fluid replacement to reduce the risks of persistent SIRS and organ failure. The IAP/APA guidelines recommend goal directed intravenous fluid with lactated Ringer's at an initial rate of 5 to 10 mL/kg/h while the ACG guidelines recommend 250 to 500 mL/h with crystalloids. Goals for fluid therapy are one or more of the following: heart rate less than 120/min, mean arterial pressure 65 to 85 mm Hg, urinary output greater than 0.5 to 1 mL/kg/h, invasive measures of stroke volume or intrathoracic blood volume, or hematocrit 35% to 44% (0.35-0.44) with transfusion of blood.[35,36]

Observational studies have identified both benefit (decreased mortality and organ failure) and harm (abdominal compartment syndrome) associated with early aggressive fluid administration. Most studies have compared standard therapy with aggressive fluid therapy over the first 24 hours retrospectively. One trial found that administration during the first 24 hours of at least one third the cumulative volume given over the first 72 hours was associated with a decrease in mortality.[47] A similar trial found a decrease in SIRS, organ failure at 72 hours, and length of stay in patients who received more fluid during the first 24-hour period than subsequent 24-hour periods.[51] In contrast, another study found that patients who received more than 3.1 L of fluid during the first 24 hours had higher rates of persistent organ failure, respiratory failure, and renal failure than those who received smaller volumes.[46] In a prospective, randomized trial, goal-directed fluid replacement therapy of 3 mL/kg/h for the first 20 hours did not result in a reduction in SIRS or C-reactive protein (CRP).[52] Replacement at rates of 10 to 15 mL/kg/h was associated with more abdominal compartment syndrome, mechanical ventilation, and sepsis in the first 2 weeks following presentation than standard therapy in another trial.[48]

Interpretation of these trials is complicated by the likelihood that sicker patients were given larger volumes of fluid. Studies of fluid resuscitation in acute pancreatitis suggest that some patients may not require aggressive fluid resuscitation, while others may require gradual fluid administration. For example, those with reduced cardiac reserve may do better if fluid is replaced over 72 hours rather than 24 to 48 hours.[50]

In addition to questions about the rate and volume of fluid that should be administered to patients with acute pancreatitis, there is also debate regarding which fluid is most appropriate. A small randomized trial found that goal-directed resuscitation with lactated Ringer's produced a reduction in SIRS and CRP at 24 hours compared with normal saline.[52] The study protocol used aggressive replacement with a bolus of 20 mL/kg of lactated Ringer's followed by 150 to 300 mL/h for the first 24 hours. If patients responded to this therapy as assessed by BUN, the rate could be reduced to 2 mL/kg/h. Patients with SIRS or sepsis should be resuscitated according to sepsis guidelines.[49]

Relief of Abdominal Pain

Parenteral opioid analgesics are used to control abdominal pain associated with acute pancreatitis despite a lack of high quality evidence to support the practice 3. A Cochrane review found a lack of studies to support any specific agent or class of agents for pain management in acute pancreatitis.[58]

Parenteral morphine is often recommended for pain control because it provides a longer duration of pain relief than other opioids. Although morphine increases biliary pressure, there is no evidence to indicate that it is contraindicated for use in acute pancreatitis. Patient-controlled analgesia should be considered in patients who require frequent opioid dosing (eg, every 2-3 hours).

Limitation of Systemic Complications and Prevention of Pancreatic Necrosis

There is currently no specific therapy to prevent the complications and necorosis associated with acute pancreatitis. The use of parenteral histamine^2-receptor antagonists or proton pump inhibitors does not improve the overall outcome of patients with acute pancreatitis.[34] Also, although somatostatin and its synthetic analog octreotide have been used to interrupt the inflammatory process of acute pancreatitis, there are insufficient data to support their routine use, and they are not recommended by guidelines.[35,36]

Antimicrobial use in Acute Pancreatitis

Antimicrobials have been widely studied in patients with acute pancreatitis, but there are still areas of uncertainty. Selective digestive tract decontamination uses oral minimally absorbed antibiotics, including polymyxin E, tobramycin, and amphotericin B, to eradicate intestinal flora, thereby reducing the likelihood of translocation.[59,60] This alternative to systemic antibiotics may be of benefit in reducing the risk of pancreatic infection, but randomized controlled trials in patients with acute pancreatitis are needed to confirm its effectiveness when compared with parenteral antibiotic prophylaxis.[59] The IAP/APA guidelines state that it may be effective but more studies are needed.[36]

Clinical **Controversy...**

The IAP/APA guidelines give a 2B recommendation (weak recommendation and moderate quality evidence) to the use of gut decontamination based on one randomized controlled trial. Due to many unanswered questions regarding efficacy and development of resistant organisms with this practice, the use of gut decontamination has not been widely implemented in clinical practice. Additional studies are needed before most clinicians begin utilizing it in the treatment of acute pancreatitis.

Several small, randomized clinical trials have compared antibiotic prophylaxis with no prophylaxis in patients with acute necrotizing pancreatitis with varying results. A meta-analysis found that prophylactic antibiotics do not reduce infected necrosis or mortality.[61] In addition, overuse of antibiotics increases microbial resistance. Use of prophylactic antibiotics is not recommended in patients with acute pancreatitis without signs or symptoms of infection, including those with necrosis 4.[35,36] However, empiric antimicrobial therapy may be considered in patients with necrosis who deteriorate or fail to improve with in 7 to 10 days.[35]

Because the source of bacterial contamination is most likely the colon, the antibiotic regimen for patients with known or suspected infected pancreatitis should be broad-spectrum, covering the range of enteric aerobic gram-negative bacilli and anaerobic microorganisms. Therapy should be initiated as soon as possible and not delayed in order to obtain cultures.[35,62] Imipenem–cilastatin (500 mg IV every 8 hours) has been widely used because of its good penetration into the pancreas and one positive prophylaxis study.[63] However, it has been replaced on many hospital formularies by one of the newer carbapenems (eg, meropenem). Fluoroquinolones, such as ciprofloxacin or levofloxacin, combined with metronidazole should be considered for penicillin-allergic patients.[64] Patients with infected necrotic pancreatitis are generally treated with a combination of invasive interventions and antibiotics. Antibiotics alone may be sufficient in some cases or at least delay the need for an invasive procedure long enough for the necrotic areas to be walled off.[62,65]

A high mortality associated with candidal infections in severe acute pancreatitis has led investigators to study strategies for identifying patients who might benefit from antifungal prophylaxis.[66] In a series of 479 patients with acute pancreatitis treated at one medical center, the strongest predictor of fungal infection was use of an antibiotic on admission (OR, 1.6; 95% CI, 1.4-1.8).[67] At this point, prophylactic antifungal therapy is not recommended for patients with acute pancreatitis.[35]

PostERCP Pancreatitis

The clinical characteristics of postERCP pancreatitis are similar to those of acute pancreatitis from other causes. In most cases, the disease course is mild and resolves in several days. The incidence of postERCP pancreatitis has decreased over the past 15 years, most likely due to better patient selection. Use of a pancreatic duct stent during the procedure is effective in reducing postERCP pancreatitis.[68] Several classes of medications have been studied for prevention of postERCP pancreatitis. The best data are with non-steroidal anti-inflammatory agents (NSAID).[69] Indomethacin suppositories decreased the incidence of postERCP pancreatitis by 46% in a population at increased risk.[70] This therapy was not associated with an increase in bleeding or renal failure. However, patients at increased risk for adverse effects from NSAIDs were excluded. A posthoc analysis of the data suggested that rectal indomethacin alone could be more cost-effective than use of a stent or stent plus indomethacin.[71]

CHRONIC PANCREATITIS

Chronic pancreatitis results from long-standing pancreatic inflammation resulting in irreversible destruction of pancreatic tissue with fibrin deposition, leading to a loss of exocrine and endocrine functions.[5-7] It has four different stages beginning with a preclinical inflammatory stage where patients remain asymptomatic or have indistinguishable symptoms.[5] In the second stage patients present with acute attacks that often resemble those of acute pancreatitis. The third stage consists of episodes of intermittent or constant abdominal pain. Finally, in the burnout stage patients present with diminished or absent pain, but develop malabsorption syndrome due to loss of pancreatic exocrine function and may develop diabetes mellitus from loss of endocrine function.

Etiology

Chronic alcohol consumption, especially heavy drinking, remains the leading cause of chronic pancreatitis in Western society, accounting for up to two-thirds of cases.[7,72,73] Generally, consumption of greater than or equal to 150 g/day of alcohol for greater than or equal to 15 years poses a significant risk of chronic pancreatitis.[7,73,74] Most of the remaining cases can be classified as idiopathic, while a small percentage of cases are due to rare causes, such as autoimmune, hereditary, and tropical pancreatitis.[6,7] Various genetic alterations have also been associated with the occurrence of chronic pancreatitis, including mutations of the following genes: protease serine 1 (trypsin 1) (*PRSS1*), serine peptidase inhibitor Kazal type 1 (*SPINK1*), and the cystic fibrosis transmembrane conductance regulator (*CFTR*).[6,7,73,74] There is also a demonstrated risk of chronic pancreatitis with

TABLE 39-4 Classification of Etiology and Risk Factors for Chronic Pancreatitis

M-ANNHEIM	
***M**ultiple*	Risk factors
Alcohol	Excessive consumption (>80 g/day), increased consumption (20-80 g/day), moderate consumption (<20 g/day)
Nicotine	Quantitated in pack years for current smokers
Nutritional factors	High-fat and protein diet, hyperlipidemia (especially hypertriglyceridemia)
Hereditary factors	Hereditary pancreatitis, familial pancreatitis, early and late-onset idiopathic pancreatitis, tropical pancreatitis, possible gene mutations (eg, *PRSS1*, *SPINK1*, and *CFTR*)
Efferent duct factors	Pancreas divisum, annular pancreas/congenital abnormalities, pancreatic duct obstruction (eg, tumors), posttraumatic pancreatic duct scars, sphincter of Oddi dysfunction
Immunologic factors	Autoimmune pancreatitis
Miscellaneous and rare factors	Hypercalcemia and hyperparathyroidism, chronic kidney disease, medications, toxins
TIGAR-O	
Toxic-metabolic	Alcohol, tobacco smoking, hypercalcemia, hyperlipidemia, chronic kidney disease, medications, toxins
Idiopathic	Early onset, late onset, tropical pancreatitis
Genetic mutations	*PRSS1*, *CFTR*, *SPINK1*, others
Autoimmune	Isolated, syndromic
Recurrent and severe associated acute pancreatitis	Postnecrotic (severe AP), vascular disease/ischemic, postirradiation
Obstructive	Pancreas divisum, sphincter of Oddi dysfunction, pancreatic duct obstruction (eg, tumor), posttraumatic pancreatic duct scars

PRSS1, cationic trypsinogen; *SPINK1*, serine protease inhibitor Kazal type 1; *CFTR*, cystic fibrosis transmembrane conductance regulator.

Used with permission from Conwell DL, Lee LS, Yadav D et al. American Pancreatic Association Practice Guidelines in Chronic Pancreatitis: Evidence-Based Report on Diagnostic Guidelines. Pancreas 2014;43(8).

cigarette smoking that appears to be dose-dependent and may contribute to mortality from chronic pancreatitis.[6,72,73,75,76] There are two classification systems for chronic pancreatitis that take into account the various risk factors associated with the disease (Table 39-4).[73]

Pathophysiology

Although the exact mechanism for the pathogenesis of chronic pancreatitis is unknown, several theories have been proposed. The oxidative stress theory proposes that the pancreas is exposed to by-products of mixed-function oxidases that lead to an inflammatory reaction.[74] Increased activity of hepatic and pancreatic oxidases may be due to increased exposure to substrates (eg, fat), inducers (eg, alcohol), or other substances. A toxic-metabolic theory focuses on alcohol as a primary causative agent where by-products of its metabolism in the pancreas lead to lipid accumulation in acinar cells and eventual fatty degeneration of the pancreas.[74] Ductal obstruction theories state that alcohol leads to obstruction of pancreatic ductals secondary to increased protein deposition and stone formation.[7,73] This leads to scarring of ductal epithelial cells, which potentiates further obstruction and eventually results in acinar atrophy and fibrin deposition. The final major theory suggests that periductular necrosis from repeated episodes of acute pancreatitis eventually leads to ductal obstruction and stone formation with subsequent acinar atrophy and fibrosis.[7,73]

Regardless of the pathophysiologic mechanism, several pieces of evidence now point to activation of pancreatic stellate cells as the cause of fibrin deposition in chronic pancreatitis. Various toxins, oxidative stress, and inflammatory mediators activate pancreatic stellate cells.[7,74,77] As an example, exposure of the pancreas to alcohol and its metabolites leads to the production of various mediators and proinflammatory cytokines, especially tumor necrosis factor-α and interleukin-1 and 6.[77] These then activate pancreatic stellate cells that initiate fibrinogenesis. Other mediators generated by the stellate cells themselves perpetuate continued stellate cell activation.

The pathogenesis of pain in chronic pancreatitis has long been thought to be the result of increased pancreatic parenchymal pressure from obstruction, inflammation, and necrosis.[7] However, evidence increasingly points to a neurogenic origin of pain. There is abnormal pain processing in the central nervous system of patients with chronic pancreatitis, with evidence of functional reorganization of the insular cortex.[7] Also, visceral nerves in these patients are sensitized. This may explain the hyperalgesia often experienced by these patients, and the need for various methods of pain management. Patients with chronic pancreatitis may also experience pain in areas distant to the pancreas due to impaired inhibition of somatic and visceral pain pathways.

Clinical Presentation

Chronic pain, malabsorption with resultant steatorrhea, and diabetes mellitus are the hallmark symptoms and complications of chronic pancreatitis (5). Although abdominal pain is the most common symptom at any stage, patients may present with various signs and symptoms depending on the stage of the disease. A more comprehensive list of the common signs and symptoms is presented in Table 39-5.

Diagnosis

The diagnosis of chronic pancreatitis is based primarily on presenting signs and symptoms in combination with either imaging or pancreatic function studies (see Table 39-5). Although histology would be the best diagnostic test, it is difficult and risky to perform and is generally not recommended.[74] Therefore, testing usually begins with noninvasive or invasive imaging studies. Abdominal ultrasonography and computed tomography (CT) may be used first, but are limited in their ability to produce detailed imaging of pancreatic ductal abnormalities.[73,78-80] Magnetic resonance imaging (MRI) with MRCP produces more detailed images of the pancreatic ducts.[73,78,79] While ERCP is the gold standard invasive study, it is rarely used due to inter- and intra-observer variability and the risk of postERCP pancreatitis, and endoscopic ultrasonography (EUS) is an equivalent alternative.[73,78,79] In addition to imagining studies, pancreatic function tests are used when imagining is inconclusive, as adjunctive diagnostic studies, or to quantify the degree of exocrine insufficiency.[78] The most sensitive studies are the secretin and CCK stimulation tests.[73,78,79] However, these are not widely available and are uncomfortable for patients. Indirect studies of pancreatic function are most sensitive during late chronic pancreatitis.[73]

TABLE 39-5 Signs, Symptoms, and Diagnosis of Chronic Pancreatitis

Signs
- Malnutrition (especially in chronic alcoholism)
- Abdominal mass (may indicate a pancreatic pseudocyst)
- Jaundice may be seen
- Splenomegaly (rare)

Symptoms
- Abdominal pain
  - Commonly in epigastric area
  - May radiate to the back
  - Described as deep and penetrating
  - May be relieved by bending/leaning forward or bringing knees to the chest
  - Often occurs with meals and at night
  - May be associated with nausea and vomiting
- Steatorrhea
  - Patients describe bulky or foul-smelling stools often with obvious oil droplets
  - Usually have an average of three to four stools per day
  - May be associated with deficiencies in fat-soluble vitamins
  - Watery diarrhea, excess gas, and abdominal cramps are uncommon
- Pancreatic diabetes mellitus
- Diarrhea (associated with steatorrhea)
- Weight loss
  - May be due to severe malabsorption or acute/chronic pain
  - Substantial loss may be due to associated or unrelated malignancy
- Osteoporosis (from vitamin D malabsorption and increased bone resorption)
- Dyspepsia

Laboratory studies
- CBC to rule out infection (ie, infected pseudocyst)
- Serum amylase and lipase
  - Low specificity for chronic pancreatitis
  - May be elevated in acute exacerbations
  - Usually are normal or only slightly elevated
- Total bilirubin, alkaline phosphatase, and hepatic transaminases may be elevated with ductal obstruction
- Fasting serum glucose
- Pancreatic function tests
  - Indirect
    - Serum trypsinogen (<20 ng/mL [or mcg/L] is abnormal)
    - Fecal elastase (<200 mcg/g of stool is abnormal)
    - Fecal chymotrypsin (<3 units/g of stool is abnormal)
    - Fecal fat estimation (>7 g/day is abnormal; need to collect 72 hours of stool)
    - ^{13}C-mixed triglyceride breath test (conducted over 6 hours; not available in United States)
  - Direct
    - Secretin stimulation (evaluates duodenal bicarbonate secretion)
    - Cholecystokinin stimulation (evaluates pancreatic lipase secretion)
- Serum albumin (may be low with malnutrition)
- Serum calcium (may be low with malnutrition)

Imaging studies
- Noninvasive
  - Abdominal ultrasound
  - Computed tomography (CT)
  - Magnetic resonance imaging (MRI) with Magnetic resonance cholangiopancreatography (MRCP)
- Invasive
  - Endoscopic ultrasonography (EUS)
  - Endoscopic retrograde cholangiopancreatography (ERCP)

CBC, complete blood count.

Data from references 5, 7, 73, 78, and 79.

Clinical Course and Prognosis

The clinical course of chronic pancreatitis depends on the etiology. Exocrine insufficiency occurs when lipase secretion is less than 10% of normal.[5,79] Patients with hereditary chronic pancreatitis typically have exocrine insufficiency occur at an early age, while those with alcohol related disease have exocrine insufficiency occur about 5 years after disease onset, with "burnout" of the pancreas in about 10 years.[79] Patients with early-onset idiopathic chronic pancreatitis have delayed progression to exocrine insufficiency compared to those with alcohol related or late-onset idiopathic disease.[79] Diabetes mellitus occurs later than exocrine insufficiency and has a reported prevalence of 70%.[81]

The life expectancy of patients with chronic pancreatitis is shorter than that of the general population.[4] However, death in patients with chronic pancreatitis most commonly results from other chronic diseases, infection, or malignancy.[4] One of the most significant complications of long-standing disease is pancreatic cancer. Patients with chronic pancreatitis are 13 times as likely as the general population to develop pancreatic cancer.[79] This risk increases depending on the etiology, with smokers having twice the risk.[79]

TREATMENT
Chronic Pancreatitis

Desired Outcome

The major goals in the treatment of uncomplicated chronic pancreatitis are relief of abdominal pain, treatment of any associated complications such as malabsorption and diabetes mellitus, and improvement in quality of life. Secondary goals include delaying development of complications and treating associated disorders such as depression and malnutrition.

General Approach to Treatment

Treatment of chronic pancreatitis and its complications involves various nonpharmacologic and pharmacologic interventions. Lifestyle modifications should include abstinence from alcohol and smoking cessation.[78-80,82] In addition, patients with steatorrhea may need to eat smaller, more frequent meals and reduce dietary fat intake.[5,79,83] The majority of patients require analgesics and pancreatic enzyme supplementation.[78-80,82] Pain can initially be controlled with medications, but may require more aggressive medical and surgical therapies as the disease progresses. Patients with malabsorption require pancreatic enzymes to reduce steatorrhea and maintain adequate nutrient absorption.[78-80] An antisecretory agent may be added to the regimen when enzymes alone provide an inadequate reduction in steatorrhea.[5,7,79,80]

Nonpharmacologic Therapy

In addition to medical management, the treatment of chronic pancreatitis includes both lifestyle and dietary modifications. Patients should be counseled to abstain from alcohol use, and smoking cessation should be advocated. Cessation of alcohol use may reduce pain in patients with alcoholic chronic pancreatitis, and hastens disease progression and reduces the risk of developing pancreatic cancer.[4,5,78-80,82] Smoking has been associated with more rapid progression of disease, so cessation should be advocated.[82] Patients with steatorrhea should be counseled to eat small and frequent meals.[79,83,84] A reduction in dietary fat is not needed routinely, but may be needed in those whose symptoms are uncontrolled with enzyme supplementation.[78] Consumption of a low-fat purified amino acid elemental diet may reduce pain in patients with chronic pancreatitis.[85] Supplementation with medium-chain triglycerides, which do not require lipolysis, should be considered for patients with steatorrhea who are unable to gain weight.[79,83] Enteral nutrition via a feeding tube is recommended for patients who cannot consume adequate calories, have continued weight loss, experience complications, or require surgery.[83] For patients with chronic pancreatitis requiring tube feeding, use of a jejunal feeding tube is the recommended.[83,84]

Invasive procedures and surgery are primarily used to treat uncontrolled pain and the associated complications of chronic pancreatitis. Stents placed via ERCP may be used to treat pancreatic duct strictures in order to relieve parenchymal pressure and reduce pain.[78,86] Extracorporeal shock wave lithotripsy can be used to break up pancreatic stones with ultrasonic vibration prior to removal by ERCP.[80,86] Blockade of pain signals through the celiac plexus may be achieved utilizing EUS.[78,80,86-88] The various complications of chronic pancreatitis that can be treated endoscopically include common bile duct strictures, duodenal obstructions, and pancreatic pseudocysts.[78,86] Various surgical techniques including total pancreatectomy may also be used to relieve pain associated with chronic pancreatitis.[78,80] Surgery is more effective at relieving pain than endoscopic procedures, but these trials have a number of limitations.[78,80,89] Finally, total pancreatectomy with transplantation of pancreatic islet cells to reduce the need for exogenous insulin is a possible option for the treatment of pain due to chronic pancreatitis.[78,80,90,91]

Pharmacologic Therapy
General Recommendations

Pharmacologic therapy of chronic pancreatitis is aimed at controlling pain, treating malabsorption and associated steatorrhea, and controlling diabetes mellitus. Once other causes have been excluded, weak opioid analgesics should be tried initially for pain management (Fig. 39-4).[5,78-80] Patients with inadequate relief from opioids should have adjuvant agents added to their regimen.[78-80,82] The addition of pancreatic enzyme supplements for pain control may also be considered in select patients.[5,78-80,82]

Most patients with malabsorption will require a modification in diet along with pancreatic enzyme supplementation in order to achieve adequate nutritional status and reduction in steatorrhea (Fig. 39-5). An antisecretory agent (such as ranitidine or omeprazole) should be added to the regimen when there is an inadequate response to enzyme therapy alone.[5,78-80] If these measures are ineffective, documentation of the diagnosis and exclusion of other diseases should be undertaken. Exogenous insulin is the primary pharmacologic agent used in the treatment of diabetes mellitus associated with chronic pancreatitis.[5,80,81] However, metformin may be initiated in early chronic pancreatitis, and has the added benefit of significantly reducing the risk pancreatic cancer.[81]

Relief of Chronic Abdominal Pain

Analgesics Pain from chronic pancreatitis may initially be treated with opioid analgesics, but adjuvant agent may be necessary as the

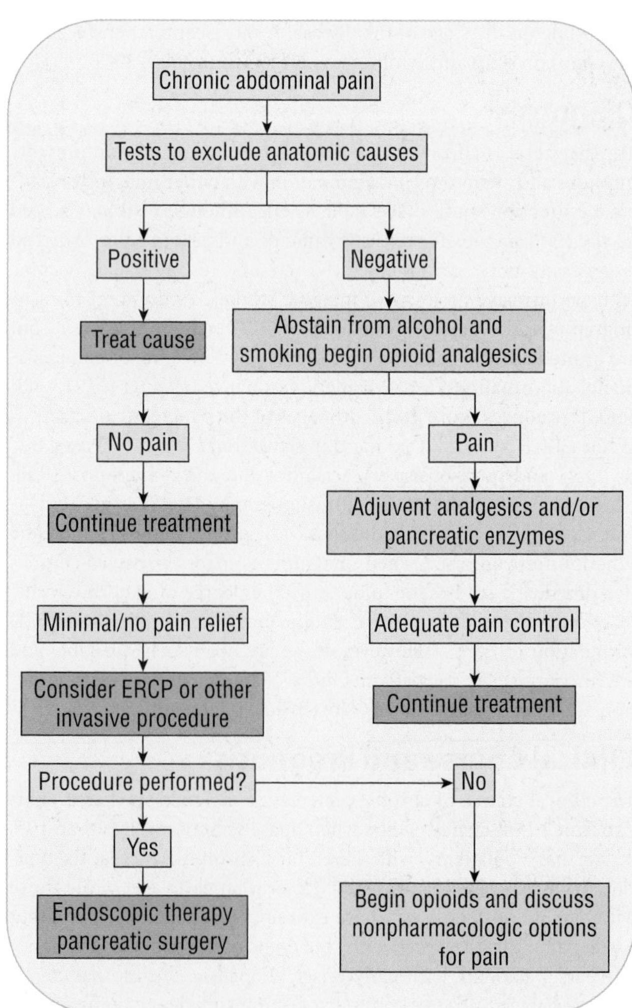

FIGURE 39-4 Algorithm for the treatment of abdominal pain in chronic pancreatitis. (ERCP, endoscopic retrograde cholangiopancreatography.)

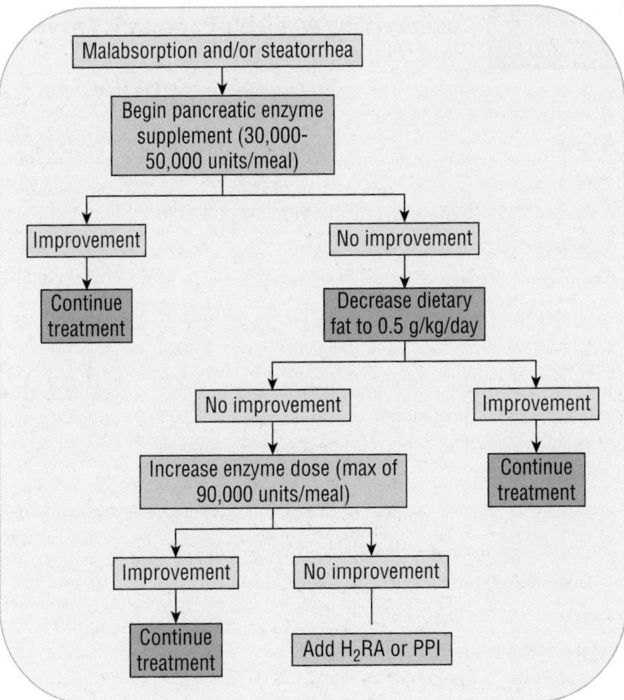

FIGURE 39-5 Algorithm for the treatment of malabsorption and steatorrhea in chronic pancreatitis. (H_2RA, histamine$_2$-receptor antagonist; PPI, proton pump inhibitor.)

disease progresses (6). Regimens should be individualized and should begin with the lowest effective dose. The dosage regimen should be maximized before adding or substituting agents. Analgesics should be scheduled around the clock rather than as needed in order to maximize efficacy. Scheduling short-acting analgesics prior to meals should help decrease postprandial pain. Less potent opioids should be used initially, and tramadol successfully treated pain in patients with chronic pancreatitis, but at a higher dose than that approved in the United States.[5,78-80] Severe pain will require the use of more potent opioids, such as oxycodone. Although opioids carry about a 10% to 30% risk of addiction in this population, their use should not be withheld.[5] Unless contraindicated, oral opioids should be used before parenteral, transdermal, or other dosage forms. The choice of agent should be based on cost, compliance, and avoidance of adverse drug events (eg, allergic reactions).

Pancreatic Enzymes Although pancreatic enzymes are primarily used to treat malabsorption associated with chronic pancreatitis, they are also used to treat pain from the disease. Relief of pain using pancreatic enzymes is thought to be due to their ability to break down CCK.[5,74,78,82] Normally, the release of CCK, which causes an increase in pancreatic secretion, is inhibited by trypsin. However, there is a decrease in the production of trypsin in patients with chronic pancreatitis. This leads to a loss of negative feedback on the release of CCK and thus an increase in pain due to unabated pancreatic secretion. The proteases in pancreatic enzyme supplements are thought to act as substitutes for endogenous trypsin, leading to a decrease in CCK release.

Despite this intuitive mechanism, mixed results have been found from trials investigating pancreatic enzyme supplements for the treatment of pain from chronic pancreatitis. This may be due to the differences between the various enzyme formulations used in the trials as well as the small number of subjects enrolled.[5,78,79,82] A Cochrane Collaborative review found no beneficial effect on pain relief.[92] However, trials that used non-enteric-coated enzyme formulations have demonstrated a benefit in the treatment of pain.[5,78,82] Enteric-coated formulations may not release enough proteases in the duodenum to inhibit CCK release. A trial of non-enteric-coated enzyme supplements may be used for patients with less advanced disease before more aggressive therapy is considered.[5,78,79,82] An alternative is to administer an enteric-coated product with an antisecretory agent in order to increase the amount of proteases available in the duodenum from these products (Table 39-6). However, no studies have been conducted using such a regimen for the treatment of pain from chronic pancreatitis.

Other Agents Various adjunctive agents are also used in patients experiencing pain from chronic pancreatitis. Selective serotonin reuptake inhibitors and tricyclic antidepressants are used both for treating the concomitant depression that often occurs in patients with chronic pancreatitis and for their potential effects on pain (see Table 39-6).[5] Gabapentin has been used as an adjunct to opioids.[5] Pregabalin significantly decreased maximum and average daily pain scores when studied in a prospective randomized trial in patients with chronic pancreatitis.[93] Evidence does not support use of octreotide for chronic pancreatitis pain.[5,78,82] There is evidence showing that patients with chronic pancreatitis have increased oxidative stress, and the use of antioxidants, such as selenium, vitamins C and E, and β-carotene, has demonstrated some benefit in relieving pain and improving quality of life in these patients.[94-96] However, evidence regarding their benefit remains variable and their widespread use in patients with chronic pancreatitis is not generally recommended.[78,79,82,97]

TABLE 39-6 Recommendations for the Pharmacologic Treatment of Chronic Pancreatitis

Treatment of chronic pain (oral drug regimens)

Opioids
- Tramadol: 50-100 mg every 4-6 hours, not to exceed 400 mg/day; has opioid-like effect; contraindicated in alcohol or hypnotic intoxication; be aware of drug interactions; expensive
- Codeine 30-60 mg every 6 hours; hydrocodone 5-10 mg every 4-6 hours; morphine sulfate (extended-release) 30-60 mg every 8-12 hours; oxycodone 5-10 mg every 6 hours; methadone 2.5-10 mg every 8-12 hours; hydromorphone 0.5-1 mg every 4-6 hours; fentanyl patch 25-100 mcg/h every 72 hours
- Risk of potentiation with alcohol; impaired respiration; constipation; hypotension; allergy
- Dosing is usually based on providing continuous pain relief; consider combining with acetaminophen; opioid dependence is common; abuse is a concern in alcoholics; tolerance may develop

Adjuvent agents
- Pregabalin: has the best evidence; begin with 75 mg twice daily; maximum dose of 300 mg twice daily
- Consider use selective serotonin reuptake inhibitors (eg, paroxetine), serotonin/norepinephrine reuptake inhibitors (eg, duloxetine) and tricyclic antidepressants in difficult-to-manage patients

Pancreatic enzymes
- Four to eight tablets/capsules of a preferred product (see Table 39-7) with each meal plus either a histamine$_2$-receptor antagonist or proton pump inhibitor; no clinical trials support such a regimen for pain management

Treatment of malabsorption and steatorrhea
- Start with pancreatic enzymes containing 30,000-50,000 USP units of lipase with each meal of a preferred product (see Table 39-7); administer dose during or just after meals
- Increase dose to a maximum of 90,000 USP units of lipase per meal
- Products containing enteric-coated microspheres or minimicrospheres may be more effective than other dose forms

Acid-suppression agents
- May improve efficacy of enzyme therapy for malabsorption and steatorrhea
- Use with either non-enteric-coated or enteric-coated formulations

USP, United States Pharmacopeia.

Data from references 5, 78, 79, 82, 93, and 99.

Treatment of Malabsorption

Reduction in dietary fat intake and pancreatic enzyme supplementation are the primary treatments for malabsorption due to chronic pancreatitis (7). Treatment should begin when steatorrhea is documented and persistent weight loss occurs despite initial dietary modifications. The combination of pancreatic enzymes and a reduction in dietary fat enhances the patient's nutritional status and reduces steatorrhea. Malabsorption is minimized if the concentration of lipase delivered to the duodenum with supplementation is about 10% of normal pancreatic output.[5] This requires that 30,000 to 50,000 units of lipase be administered with each meal to start (see Table 39-6).[78,80,98] In many cases the lipase dose will need to be increased due to insufficient lipolytic activity, but doses greater than 90,000 units per meal are not recommended.

There is little evidence regarding the optimal dosage form and administration of pancreatic enzyme supplements. Most studies have compared them with placebo rather than other enzyme products, and used quantitation of fat absorption or elimination as a primary measure of efficacy rather than weight gain.[99] Although they improve fat absorption, they may not completely eliminate steatorrhea.[99] However, they improve the quality of life of patients with chronic pancreatitis.[79] Since most exogenous lipase is rapidly and irreversibly destroyed at low intragastric pH, enteric-coated products are preferred for the treatment of malabsorption and steatorrhea (8). The enteric coating only dissolves at a pH greater than 5.5, which allows a sufficient quantity of enzymes to remain intact until dissolution of the coating in the duodenum.[79] However, enzymes must also be emptied from the stomach into the duodenum at the same rate and time as ingested food. The size of the enteric-coated enzyme preparation influences the rate of enzyme delivery to the duodenum.[5] Likewise, the administration time relevant to a meal influences the timing of enzyme delivery. Products that contain enzymes in small enteric-coated microspheres or minimicrospheres are often the best products because they are thought to mix effectively with chyme, thus leaving the stomach at a similar rate.[79,98] Also, the optimal administration time of enzymes containing minimicrospheres appears to be either with a meal or just after.[5,78,79,98]

Despite enzyme therapy, patients may continue to have steatorrhea and fail to gain sufficient weight. Compliance should be assessed in these patients as the number of capsules required with each meal can lead to noncompliance. Alternative products with higher lipase content can be tried in order to reduce the number of capsules needed. If this fails, the dose of lipase should be increased. Finally, addition of an antisecretory agent may be tried to increase the availability of active enzymes in the duodenum.[79,98]

Pancreatic Enzyme Supplements Six pancreatic enzyme products have been approved by the FDA since its 2004 mandate that any product marketed would need approval. Only two of these products are specifically approved for exocrine pancreatic insufficiency associated with chronic pancreatitis.[100,101] Dosage forms of approved products include regular-release tablets, enteric-coated beads, bicarbonate-buffered enteric-coated microspheres, enteric-coated minimicrospheres, and enteric-coated minitablets or microtablets encased in a cellulose or gelatin capsule (Table 39-7). Enzymes are easily administered to patients able to swallow the capsules or their contents. However, administration to patients with enteral feeding tubes presents a challenge. Products containing microspheres may be administered through feeding tubes in food or solutions with a pH of 4.5 or less.[98] Clinicians must be aware, however, that available products are not equivalent and should consider this before substituting products in patients who require administration through a nonoral route. Careful consideration should also be given to this issue in patient care facilities with limited formularies.

Adverse reactions from pancreatic enzyme supplements are generally benign. High doses can lead to nausea, diarrhea, and intestinal upset.[79] One of the more serious adverse effects of these products is fibrosing colonopathy. It occurs when the enzymes cause deposition of fibrin in the colon leading to colonic stricture. This reaction is uncommon and has been reported mostly in children with cystic fibrosis who received high doses of enzymes for prolonged periods.[79] Another concern with pancreatic enzymes is the risk of possible viral infection due to contamination of these porcine-derived products.[79,102] Finally, pancreatic enzymes and chronic pancreatitis have been associated with deficiencies in fat-soluble vitamins, and appropriate monitoring and supplementation, especially of vitamin D, should be instituted.[5,79]

TABLE 39-7 Commercially Available Pancreatic Enzyme (Pancrelipase) Preparations

	Enzyme Content Per Unit Dose (USP Units)		
Product	**Lipase**	**Amylase**	**Protease**
Tablets			
Viokace™ 10,440 lipase units	10,440	39,150	39,150
Viokace™ 20,880 lipase units	20,880	78,300	78,300
Enteric-coated beads			
Zenpep® 3,000 lipase units	3,000	16,000	10,000
Zenpep® 5,000 lipase units	5,000	27,000	17,000
Zenpep® 10,000 lipase units	10,000	55,000	34,000
Zenpep® 15,000 lipase units	15,000	82,000	51,000
Zenpep® 20,000 lipase units	20,000	109,000	68,000
Zenpep® 25,000 lipase units	25,000	136,000	85,000
Zenpep® 40,000 lipase units	40,000	218,000	136,000
Enteric-coated microspheres with bicarbonate buffer			
Pertzye™ 8,000 lipase units	8,000	30,250	28,750
Pertzye™ 16,000 lipase units	16,000	60,500	57,500
Enteric-coated minimicrospheres			
Creon® 3,000 lipase units	3,000	15,000	9,500
Creon® 6,000 lipase units	6,000	30,000	19,000
Creon® 12,000 lipase units	12,000	60,000	38,000
Creon® 24,000 lipase units	24,000	120,000	76,000
Creon® 36,000 lipase units	36,000	180,000	114,000
Enteric-coated minitablets/microtablets			
Pancreaze® 4,200 lipase units	4,200	17,500	10,000
Pancreaze® 10,500 lipase units	10,500	43,750	25,000
Pancreaze® 16,800 lipase units	16,800	70,000	40,000
Pancreaze® 21,000 lipase units	21,000	61,000	37,000
Ultresa™ 13,800 lipase units	13,800	27,600	27,600
Ultresa™ 20,700 lipase units	20,700	41,400	41,400
Ultresa™ 23,000 lipase units	23,000	46,000	46,000

USP, United States Pharmacopeia.

Clinical **Controversy...**

Adjuvant agents (such as pregabalin) for pain control in patients with chronic pancreatitis have not been widely studied, but are often utilized. Pregabalin has the best evidence of efficacy in this population, but it has only been studied in one prospective randomized trial. There is debate about the utilization of such agents for the treatment of pain associated with chronic pancreatitis because well-designed clinical trials demonstrating their efficacy are sparse.

Adjuncts to Enzyme Therapy The addition of a histamine$_2$-receptor antagonist or proton pump inhibitor to pancreatic enzyme supplementation may increase the effectiveness of enzyme therapy for malabsorption and steatorrhea (9). The beneficial effects of these agents result from an increase in gastric and duodenal pH.[79,80,98] This is thought to result in an increase in the amount of active enzymes available in the duodenum. Traditionally, their use has been advocated with non-enteric-coated enzyme products.[5,78] In fact, the only non-enteric-coated formulation currently approved by the FDA is indicated for administration with a proton pump inhibitor.[101] However, they are recommended to enhance the efficacy of both nonenteric-coated and enteric-coated formulations.[79,80]

PERSONALIZED PHARMACOTHERAPY

Some cases of drug-induced pancreatitis are associated with elevated concentrations of the causative medications, and it is possible that genetic differences in drug metabolism contribute to this. A pharmacogenetic analysis was performed in one case of drug-induced pancreatitis that was associated with high concentrations of clozapine.[103] However, the patient was not found to have any genetic variants that would affect the metabolism of clozapine. Diagnosis of acute pancreatitis in pregnant patients is complicated by normal increases in amylase and lipase of up to three times the normal limit in this population. Lipase is considered to be a more sensitive measure than amylase in this population. Contrast should be avoided in pregnant patients with acute pancreatitis.[14]

Although several genetic variations have been associated with the occurrence of chronic pancreatitis, variation in response to therapy related to these factors has not been studied. One cautionary note regarding pancreatic enzyme supplements is that they are all porcine-derived and thus contain purines. Therefore, they may increase uric acid levels and should be used cautiously in patients prone to the effects of hyperuricemia. This would include patients with a history of gout, impaired kidney function, and known hyperuricemia. One physiologic parameter affecting the efficacy of pancreatic enzyme supplements is GI transit. Non-enteric-coated formulations are preferred for patients with rapid gastrojejunal transit secondary to pancreatectomy associated with partial gastrectomy or vagotomy and gastroenteroscopy. These patients have hyposecretion of gastric acid and enteric-coated formulations would not be released early enough in the small intestine to confer a beneficial effect.[79]

EVALUATION OF THERAPEUTIC OUTCOMES

Acute Pancreatitis

Hydration status, serum electrolytes, pain control, and nutritional status should be assessed periodically in patients with mild acute pancreatitis, depending on the degree of abdominal pain and fluid loss. Patients with severe acute pancreatitis should receive intensive care and close monitoring of vital signs, fluid and electrolyte status, white blood cell count, blood glucose, lactate dehydrogenase, aspartate aminotransferase, serum albumin, hematocrit, BUN, serum creatinine, and international normalized ratio. Continuous hemodynamic and arterial blood gas monitoring is essential. Serum lipase, amylase, and bilirubin require less frequent monitoring. The patient should also be monitored for signs of infection, relief of abdominal pain, and adequate nutritional status. Severity of disease and patient response should be assessed using an evidence-based method.

Chronic Pancreatitis

The severity and frequency of abdominal pain should be assessed periodically in patients with chronic pancreatitis using a standardized scale in order to determine the efficacy of pain therapy. Patients receiving opioids should be prescribed laxatives on an as-needed or scheduled basis and be monitored for constipation. Patients receiving pancreatic enzymes for malabsorption should have their weight and stool frequency and consistency monitored periodically. More objective assessments of fecal fat content, such as the ^{13}C-mixed triglyceride breath test, can be utilized, but are usually unnecessary and impractical in general clinical practice.[5,79,93] Blood glucose must be closely monitored in patients with diabetes mellitus, and those with long-standing disease should receive appropriate monitoring for nephropathy, retinopathy, and neuropathy.[5]

ABBREVIATIONS

APACHE	Acute Physiology and Chronic Health Evaluation
BISAP	Bedside Index of Severity in Acute Pancreatitis
BUN	blood urea nitrogen
CCK	cholecystokinin
CECT	contrast-enhanced computed tomography
CFTR	cystic fibrosis transmembrane conductance regulator gene
CRP	C-reactive protein
CT	computed tomography
DPP-4	dipeptidyl peptidase-4
ERCP	endoscopic retrograde cholangiopancreatography
EUS	endoscopic ultrasonography
GLP-1	glucagon-like peptide-1
GRP	gastrin-releasing peptide
HAPS	Harmless Acute Pancreatitis Score
HIV	human immunodeficiency virus
ICU	intensive care unit
JSS	Japanese Severity Score
MRCP	magnetic resonance cholangiopancreatography
MRI	magnetic resonance imaging
NSAID	nonsteroidal antiinflammatory drug
PRSS1	protease serine 1 (trypsin 1) gene
SIRS	systemic inflammatory response syndrome
SPINK1	serine peptidase inhibitor Kazal type 1 gene
VIP	vasoactive intestinal peptide

REFERENCE

1. Anand N, Park JH, Wu BU. Modern management of acute pancreatitis. *Gastroenterol Clin North Am* 2012;41(1):1-8.
2. Lippi G, Valentino M, Cervellin G. Laboratory diagnosis of acute pancreatitis: In search of the Holy Grail. *Crit Rev Clin Lab Sci* 2012;49(1):18-31.
3. Petrov MS, Shanbhag S, Chakraborty M, Phillips AR, Windsor JA. Organ failure and infection of pancreatic necrosis as determinants of mortality in patients with acute pancreatitis. *Gastroenterology* 2010;139(3):813-820.
4. Yadav D, Lowenfels AB. The epidemiology of pancreatitis and pancreatic cancer. *Gastroenterology* 2013;144(6):1252-1261.
5. Forsmark CE. Chronic Pancreatitis. In: Feldman M, Friedman LS, Brandt LJ, eds. *Sleisenger and Fordtran's Gastrointestinal and Liver Disease: Pathophysiology, Diagnosis, Management*. 9th ed. Philadelphia: Saunders; 2010:985-1016.
6. Brock C, Nielsen LM, Lelic D, Drewes AM. Pathophysiology of chronic pancreatitis. *World J Gastroenterol* 2013;19(42):7231-7240.
7. Muniraj T, Aslanian HR, Farrell J, Jamidar PA. Chronic pancreatitis, a comprehensive review and update. Part I: Epidemiology, etiology, risk factors, genetics, pathophysiology, and clinical features. *Dis Mon* 2014;60(12):530-550.
8. Peery AF, Dellon ES, Lund J, et al. Burden of gastrointestinal disease in the United States: 2012 update. *Gastroenterology* 2012;143(5):1179-1187.
9. Pandol SJ. Pancreatic Secretion. In: Feldman M, Friedman LS, Brandt LJ, eds. *Sleisenger and Fordtran's Gastrointestinal and Liver Disease: Pathophysiology, Diagnosis, Management*. 9th ed. Philadelphia: Saunders; 2010:921-930.

10. Acevedo-Piedra NG, Moya-Hoyo N, Rey-Riveiro M, et al. Validation of the determinant-based classification and revision of the Atlanta classification systems for acute pancreatitis. *Clin Gastroenterol Hepatol* 2014;12(2):311-316.
11. Lindkvist B, Appelros S, Regner S, Manjer J. A prospective cohort study on risk of acute pancreatitis related to serum triglycerides, cholesterol and fasting glucose. *Pancreatology* 2012;12(4):317-324.
12. Sah RP, Pannala R, Chari ST, et al. Prevalence, diagnosis, and profile of autoimmune pancreatitis presenting with features of acute or chronic pancreatitis. *Clin Gastroenterol Hepatol* 2010;8(1):91-96.
13. Shen HN, Chang YH, Chen HF, Lu CL, Li CY. Increased risk of severe acute pancreatitis in patients with diabetes. *Diabet Med* 2012;29(11):1419-1424.
14. Ducarme G, Maire F, Chatel P, Luton D, Hammel P. Acute pancreatitis during pregnancy: A review. *J Perinatol* 2014;34(2):87-94.
15. Bai HX, Lowe ME, Husain SZ. What have we learned about acute pancreatitis in children? *J Pediatr Gastroenterol Nutr* 2011;52(3):262-270.
16. Baran B, Karaca C, Soyer OM, et al. Acute pancreatitis associated with H1N1 influenza during 2009 pandemic: A case report. *Clin Res Hepatol Gastroenterol* 2012;36(4):e69-e70.
17. Spanier BW, Tuynman HA, van der Hulst RW, Dijkgraaf MG, Bruno MJ. Acute pancreatitis and concomitant use of pancreatitis-associated drugs. *Am J Gastroenterol* 2011;106(12):2183-2188.
18. Vinklerova I, Prochazka M, Prochazka V, Urbanek K. Incidence, severity, and etiology of drug-induced acute pancreatitis. *Dig Dis Sci* 2010;55(10):2977-2981.
19. Nitsche CJ, Jamieson N, Lerch MM, Mayerle JV. Drug induced pancreatitis. *Best Pract Res Clin Gastroenterol* 2010;24(2):143-155.
20. Pezzilli R, Corinaldesi R, Morselli-Labate AM. Tyrosine kinase inhibitors and acute pancreatitis. *J Pancreas* 2010;11(3):291-293.
21. Fessel J, Hurley LB. Incidence of pancreatitis in HIV-infected patients: Comment on findings in EuroSIDA cohort. *AIDS* 2008;22(1):145-147.
22. Smith CJ, Olsen CH, Mocroft A, et al. The role of antiretroviral therapy in the incidence of pancreatitis in HIV-positive individuals in the EuroSIDA study. *AIDS* 2008;22(1):47-56.
23. Jasdanwala S, Babyatsky M. Crohn's disease and acute pancreatitis. A review of literature. *J Pancreas* 2015;16(2):136-142.
24. Li L, Shen J, Bala MM, et al. Incretin treatment and risk of pancreatitis in patients with type 2 diabetes mellitus: Systematic review and meta-analysis of randomised and non-randomised studies. *BMJ* 2014;348:g2366.
25. Yang L, He Z, Tang X, Liu J. Type 2 diabetes mellitus and the risk of acute pancreatitis: A meta-analysis. *Eur J Gastroenterol Hepatol* 2013;25(2):225-231.
26. Faillie JL, Azoulay L, Patenaude V, Hillaire-Buys D, Suissa S. Incretin based drugs and risk of acute pancreatitis in patients with type 2 diabetes: Cohort study. *BMJ* 2014;348:g2780.
27. Preiss D. Lipid-modifying therapies and risk of pancreatitis: A meta-analysis. *JAMA* 2012;308(8):804-811.
28. Nitsche C, Maertin S, Scheiber J, Ritter CA, Lerch MM, Mayerle J. Drug-induced pancreatitis. *Curr Gastroenterol Rep* 2012;14(2):131-138.
29. Jones MR, Hall OM, Kaye AM, Kaye AD. Drug-induced acute pancreatitis: A review. *Ochsner J* 2015;15(1):45-51.
30. Trivedi CD, Pitchumoni CS. Drug-induced pancreatitis: An update. *J Clin Gastroenterol* 2005;39(8):709-716.
31. Sah RP, Dawra RK, Saluja AK. New insights into the pathogenesis of pancreatitis. *Curr Opin Gastroenterol* 2013;29(5):523-530.
32. Forsmark CE, Baillie J. AGA Institute technical review on acute pancreatitis. *Gastroenterology* 2007;132(5):2022-2044.
33. Capurso G, Zerboni G, Signoretti M, et al. Role of the gut barrier in acute pancreatitis. *J Clin Gastroenterol* 2012;46 Suppl:S46-S51.
34. Lowenfels AB, Maisonneuve P, Sullivan T. The changing character of acute pancreatitis: Epidemiology, etiology, and prognosis. *Curr Gastroenterol Rep* 2009;11(2):97-103.
35. Tenner S, Baillie J, DeWitt J, Vege SS. American College of Gastroenterology guideline: Management of acute pancreatitis. *Am J Gastroenterol* 2013;108(9):1400-1415.
36. IAP/APA evidence-based guidelines for the management of acute pancreatitis. *Pancreatology* 2013;13(4 Suppl 2):e1-e15.
37. Talukdar R, Swaroop VS. Early management of severe acute pancreatitis. *Curr Gastroenterol Rep* 2011;13(2):123-130.
38. Mounzer R, Langmead CJ, Wu BU, et al. Comparison of existing clinical scoring systems to predict persistent organ failure in patients with acute pancreatitis. *Gastroenterology* 2012;142(7):1476-1482.
39. Wu BU. Prognosis in acute pancreatitis. *Can Med Assoc J* 2011;183(6):673-677.
40. Banks PA, Bollen TL, Dervenis C, et al. Classification of acute pancreatitis—2012: Revision of the Atlanta classification and definitions by international consensus. *Gut* 2013;62(1):102-111.
41. Dellinger EP, Forsmark CE, Layer P, et al. Determinant-based classification of acute pancreatitis severity: An international multidisciplinary consultation. *Ann Surg* 2012;256(6):875-880.
42. Yang CJ, Chen J, Phillips AR, Windsor JA, Petrov MS. Predictors of severe and critical acute pancreatitis: A systematic review. *Dig Liver Dis* 2014;46(5):446-451.
43. Wu BU, Banks PA. Clinical management of patients with acute pancreatitis. *Gastroenterology* 2013;144(6):1272-1281.
44. Das SL, Singh PP, Phillips AR, Murphy R, Windsor JA, Petrov MS. Newly diagnosed diabetes mellitus after acute pancreatitis: A systematic review and meta-analysis. *Gut* 2014;63(5):818-831.
45. Yadav D, O'Connell M, Papachristou GI. Natural history following the first attack of acute pancreatitis. *Am J Gastroenterol* 2012;107(7):1096-1103.
46. de-Madaria E, Soler-Sala G, Sanchez-Paya J, et al. Influence of fluid therapy on the prognosis of acute pancreatitis: A prospective cohort study. *Am J Gastroenterol* 2011;106(10):1843-1850.
47. Gardner TB, Vege SS, Chari ST, et al. Faster rate of initial fluid resuscitation in severe acute pancreatitis diminishes in-hospital mortality. *Pancreatology* 2009;9(6):770-776.
48. Mao EQ, Tang YQ, Fei J, et al. Fluid therapy for severe acute pancreatitis in acute response stage. *Chin Med J (Engl)* 2009;122(2):169-173.
49. Nasr JY, Papachristou GI. Early fluid resuscitation in acute pancreatitis: A lot more than just fluids. *Clin Gastroenterol Hepatol* 2011;9(8):633-634.
50. Trikudanathan G, Navaneethan U, Vege SS. Current controversies in fluid resuscitation in acute pancreatitis: A systematic review. *Pancreas* 2012;41(6):827-834.
51. Warndorf MG, Kurtzman JT, Bartel MJ, et al. Early fluid resuscitation reduces morbidity among patients with acute pancreatitis. *Clin Gastroenterol Hepatol* 2011;9(8):705-709.
52. Wu BU, Hwang JQ, Gardner TH, et al. Lactated Ringer's solution reduces systemic inflammation compared with saline in patients with acute pancreatitis. *Clin Gastroenterol Hepatol* 2011;9(8):710-717.
53. Rohan JD, Osman HG, Patel S. Advances in management of pancreatic necrosis. *Curr Probl Surg* 2014;51(9):374-408.
54. Al-Omran M, Albalawi ZH, Tashkandi MF, Al-Ansary LA. Enteral versus parenteral nutrition for acute pancreatitis. *Cochrane Database Syst Rev* 2010;(1):CD002837.
55. Teich N, Aghdassi A, Fischer J, et al. Optimal timing of oral refeeding in mild acute pancreatitis: Results of an open randomized multicenter trial. *Pancreas* 2010;39(7):1088-1092.
56. Mirtallo JM, Forbes A, McClave SA, Jensen GL, Waitzberg DL, Davies AR. International consensus guidelines for nutrition therapy in pancreatitis. *JPEN J Parenter Enteral Nutr* 2012;36(3):284-291.
57. Besselink MG, van Santvoort HC, Buskens E, et al. Probiotic prophylaxis in predicted severe acute pancreatitis: A randomised, double-blind, placebo-controlled trial. *Lancet* 2008;371(9613):651-659.
58. Basurto OX, Rigau CD, Urrutia G. Opioids for acute pancreatitis pain. *Cochrane Database Syst Rev* 2013;7:CD009179.
59. Lankisch PG, Lerch MM. The role of antibiotic prophylaxis in the treatment of acute pancreatitis. *J Clin Gastroenterol* 2006;40(2):149-155.
60. Luiten EJ, Bruining HA. Antimicrobial prophylaxis in acute pancreatitis: Selective decontamination versus antibiotics. *Baillieres Best Pract Res Clin Gastroenterol* 1999;13(2):317-330.
61. Villatoro E, Mulla M, Larvin M. Antibiotic therapy for prophylaxis against infection of pancreatic necrosis in acute pancreatitis. *Cochrane Database Syst Rev* 2010;(5):CD002941.
62. Freeman ML, Werner J, van Santvoort HC, et al. Interventions for necrotizing pancreatitis: Summary of a multidisciplinary consensus conference. *Pancreas* 2012;41(8):1176-1194.
63. Rokke O, Harbitz TB, Liljedal J, et al. Early treatment of severe pancreatitis with imipenem: A prospective randomized clinical trial. *Scand J Gastroenterol* 2007;42(6):771-776.
64. Schubert S, Dalhoff A. Activity of moxifloxacin, imipenem, and ertapenem against *Escherichia coli*, *Enterobacter cloacae*, *Enterococcus faecalis*, and *Bacteroides fragilis* in monocultures and mixed cultures in an in vitro pharmacokinetic/pharmacodynamic model simulating concentrations in the human pancreas. *Antimicrob Agents Chemother* 2012;56(12):6434-6436.

65. Mouli VP, Sreenivas V, Garg PK. Efficacy of conservative treatment, without necrosectomy, for infected pancreatic necrosis: A systematic review and meta-analysis. *Gastroenterology* 2013;144(2):333-340.
66. Hall AM, Poole LA, Renton B, et al. Prediction of invasive candidal infection in critically ill patients with severe acute pancreatitis. *Crit Care* 2013;17(2):R49.
67. Schwender BJ, Gordon SR, Gardner TB. Risk factors for the development of intra-abdominal fungal infections in acute pancreatitis. *Pancreas* 2015;44(5):805-807.
68. Choudhary A, Bechtold ML, Arif M, et al. Pancreatic stents for prophylaxis against post-ERCP pancreatitis: A meta-analysis and systematic review. *Gastrointest Endosc* 2011;73(2):275-282.
69. Badalov N, Tenner S, Baillie J. The Prevention, recognition and treatment of post-ERCP pancreatitis. *J Pancreas* 2009;10(2):88-97.
70. Elmunzer BJ, Scheiman JM, Lehman GA, et al. A randomized trial of rectal indomethacin to prevent post-ERCP pancreatitis. *N Engl J Med* 2012;366(15):1414-1422.
71. Elmunzer BJ, Higgins PD, Saini SD, et al. Does rectal indomethacin eliminate the need for prophylactic pancreatic stent placement in patients undergoing high-risk ERCP? Post hoc efficacy and cost-benefit analyses using prospective clinical trial data. *Am J Gastroenterol* 2013;108(3):410-415.
72. Yadav D, Hawes RH, Brand RE, et al. Alcohol consumption, cigarette smoking, and the risk of recurrent acute and chronic pancreatitis. *Arch Intern Med* 2009;169(11):1035-1045.
73. Conwell DL, Lee LS, Yadav D, et al. American Pancreatic Association Practice Guidelines in Chronic Pancreatitis: Evidence-based report on diagnostic guidelines. *Pancreas* 2014;43(8):1143-1162.
74. Braganza JM, Lee SH, McCloy RF, McMahon MJ. Chronic pancreatitis. *Lancet* 2011;377(9772):1184-1197.
75. Tolstrup JS, Kristiansen L, Becker U, Gronbaek M. Smoking and Risk of Acute and Chronic Pancreatitis Among Women and Men: A Population-Based Cohort Study. *Arch Intern Med* 2009;169(6):603-609.
76. Andriulli A, Botteri E, Almasio PL, Vantini I, Uomo G, Maisonneuve P. Smoking as a cofactor for causation of chronic pancreatitis: A meta-analysis. *Pancreas* 2010;39(8):1205-1210.
77. Talukdar R, Tandon RK. Pancreatic stellate cells: New target in the treatment of chronic pancreatitis. *J Gastroenterol Hepatol* 2008;23(1):34-41.
78. Muniraj T, Aslanian HR, Farrell J, Jamidar PA. Chronic pancreatitis, a comprehensive review and update. Part II: Diagnosis, complications, and management. *Dis Mon* 2015;61(1):5-37.
79. Afghani E, Sinha A, Singh VK. An overview of the diagnosis and management of nutrition in chronic pancreatitis. *Nutr Clin Pract* 2014;29(3):295-311.
80. Forsmark CE. Management of chronic pancreatitis. *Gastroenterology* 2013;144(6):1282-1291.
81. Ewald N, Hardt PD. Diagnosis and treatment of diabetes mellitus in chronic pancreatitis. *World J Gastroenterol* 2013;19(42):7276-7281.
82. Olesen SS, Juel J, Graversen C, Kolesnikov Y, Wilder-Smith OH, Drewes AM. Pharmacological pain management in chronic pancreatitis. *World J Gastroenterol* 2013;19(42):7292-7301.
83. Rasmussen HH, Irtun O, Olesen SS, Drewes AM, Holst M. Nutrition in chronic pancreatitis. *World J Gastroenterol* 2013;19(42):7267-7275.
84. Grant JP. Nutritional support in acute and chronic pancreatitis. *Surg Clin North Am* 2011;91(4):805-820.
85. Kataoka K, Sakagami J, Hirota M, Masamune A, Shimosegawa T. Effects of oral ingestion of the elemental diet in patients with painful chronic pancreatitis in the real-life setting in Japan. *Pancreas* 2014;43(3):451-457.
86. Kowalczyk LM, Draganov PV. Endoscopic therapy for chronic pancreatitis: Technical success, clinical outcomes, and complications. *Curr Gastroenterol Rep* 2009;11(2):111-118.
87. Puli SR, Reddy JB, Bechtold ML, Antillon MR, Brugge WR. EUS-guided celiac plexus neurolysis for pain due to chronic pancreatitis or pancreatic cancer pain: A meta-analysis and systematic review. *Dig Dis Sci* 2009;54(11):2330-2337.
88. Kaufman M, Singh G, Das S, et al. Efficacy of endoscopic ultrasound-guided celiac plexus block and celiac plexus neurolysis for managing abdominal pain associated with chronic pancreatitis and pancreatic cancer. *J Clin Gastroenterol* 2010;44(2):127-134.
89. Ahmed AU, Pahlplatz JM, Nealon WH, van GH, Gooszen HG, Boermeester MA. Endoscopic or surgical intervention for painful obstructive chronic pancreatitis. *Cochrane Database Syst Rev* 2012;1:CD007884.
90. Garcea G, Weaver J, Phillips J, et al. Total pancreatectomy with and without islet cell transplantation for chronic pancreatitis: A series of 85 consecutive patients. *Pancreas* 2009;38(1):1-7.
91. Bramis K, Gordon-Weeks AN, Friend PJ, et al. Systematic review of total pancreatectomy and islet autotransplantation for chronic pancreatitis. *Br J Surg* 2012;99(6):761-766.
92. Shafiq N, Rana S, Bhasin D, et al. Pancreatic enzymes for chronic pancreatitis. *Cochrane Database Syst Rev* 2009;(4):CD006302.
93. Olesen SS, Bouwense SA, Wilder-Smith OH, van GH, Drewes AM. Pregabalin reduces pain in patients with chronic pancreatitis in a randomized, controlled trial. *Gastroenterology* 2011;141(2):536-543.
94. Bhardwaj P, Garg PK, Maulik SK, Saraya A, Tandon RK, Acharya SK. A randomized controlled trial of antioxidant supplementation for pain relief in patients with chronic pancreatitis. *Gastroenterology* 2009;136(1):149-159.
95. Shah NS, Makin AJ, Sheen AJ, Siriwardena AK. Quality of life assessment in patients with chronic pancreatitis receiving antioxidant therapy. *World J Gastroenterol* 2010;16(32):4066-4071.
96. Grigsby B, Rodriguez-Rilo H, Khan K. Antioxidants and chronic pancreatitis: Theory of oxidative stress and trials of antioxidant therapy. *Dig Dis Sci* 2012;57(4):835-841.
97. Ahmed AU, Jens S, Busch OR, et al. Antioxidants for pain in chronic pancreatitis. *Cochrane Database Syst Rev* 2014;8:CD008945.
98. Trang T, Chan J, Graham DY. Pancreatic enzyme replacement therapy for pancreatic exocrine insufficiency in the 21(st) century. *World J Gastroenterol* 2014;20(33):11467-11485.
99. Waljee AK, Dimagno MJ, Wu BU, Schoenfeld PS, Conwell DL. Systematic review: Pancreatic enzyme treatment of malabsorption associated with chronic pancreatitis. *Aliment Pharmacol Ther* 2009;29(3):235-246.
100. *Creon (Pancrelipase)* [package insert]. North Chicago, IL: Abbott Laboratories; 2015.
101. *Viokace (Pancrelipase)* [package insert]. Birmingham, AL: Aptalis Pharma US Inc.; 2012.
102. Traynor K. First FDA-approved pancrelipase product may mark new era for providers, patients. *Am J Health Syst Pharm* 2009;66(12):1066, 1068.
103. Sani G, Kotzalidis GD, Simonetti A, et al. Development of asymptomatic pancreatitis with paradoxically high serum clozapine levels in a patient with schizophrenia and the CYP1A2*1F/1F genotype. *J Clin Psychopharmacol* 2010;30(6):737-739.

40

Viral Hepatitis

Paulina Deming

KEY CONCEPTS

1. Hepatitis A is transmitted via the fecal–oral route, most often from through travel to countries with high rates of hepatitis A, poor sanitation and hygiene, and overcrowded areas.
2. Hepatitis A causes an acute, self-limiting illness and does not lead to chronic infection. There are three stages of infection: incubation, acute hepatitis, and convalescence. Rarely, the infection progresses to liver failure.
3. Hepatitis A is vaccine preventable. In cases of acute infection, treatment consists of supportive care.
4. Hepatitis B causes both acute and chronic infection. Chronic infections are responsible for high rates of liver disease, liver cancer, and death.
5. Vaccination can prevent hepatitis B and is the most effective strategy in preventing complications of hepatitis B virus (HBV) infections. Prevention of hepatitis B infections focuses on immunization of all children and at-risk adults.
6. The purpose of anti-HBV drug therapy is for viral suppression and immune control and to prevent progression of liver disease and the complications associated with hepatitis B infections.
7. Initial therapy of chronic hepatitis B is with tenofovir or entecavir because these agents have a high barrier to resistance. Therapy is often long-term.
8. Patients undergoing immunosuppressive therapy should be screened for hepatitis B infections and may require hepatitis B therapy to reduce the risks of reactivating their hepatitis B infection.
9. Hepatitis C is an insidious, blood-borne infection. Increased screening of all patients born between 1945 and 1965 was implemented to help identify the many people unaware of their infection.
10. Hepatitis C infections can cause significant morbidity (including extrahepatic manifestations) and mortality. Patients with chronic hepatitis C are at risk for end-stage liver disease, cirrhosis, liver transplant, and death as a result of their infection.
11. The goal of anti-hepatitis C virus (HCV) drug treatment is cure. Drug therapy with direct acting antivirals optimized based on the infecting viral genotype, presence of cirrhosis and the patient's prior treatment experience.

The major hepatotrophic viruses responsible for viral hepatitis are hepatitis A, hepatitis B, hepatitis C, delta hepatitis, and hepatitis E. All share clinical, biochemical, immunoserologic, and histologic findings. Both hepatitides A and E are spread through fecal–oral contamination, whereas hepatitides B, C, and delta are transmitted parenterally. Infection with delta hepatitis requires coinfection with hepatitis B. Although the rates of acute infection have declined, viral hepatitis remains a major cause of morbidity and mortality with a significant impact on healthcare costs in the United States. Compared with human immunodeficiency virus (HIV), there are three to five times as many people infected with chronic viral hepatitis. In the United States, there is a general lack of knowledge among healthcare providers, social service providers, and the public regarding the risks of chronic hepatitis B and C infections.[1]

Unprecedented therapeutic advances have occurred with the treatment for hepatitis C with the approval of new agents, updated guidelines for care, and more novel therapies anticipated. For both hepatitides B and C, the challenge remains to increase awareness of the viral hepatic epidemic and to prevent the profound morbidity and mortality associated with chronic infection. This chapter focuses on hepatitides A, B, and C.

HEPATITIS A

Hepatitis A virus (HAV), or infectious hepatitis, is often a self-limiting and acute viral infection of the liver posing a health risk worldwide. The infection is rarely fatal. According to the Centers for Disease Control and Prevention (CDC), rates of reported cases of acute clinical hepatitis A infection in the United States continue to decline with 1,781 cases in 2013.[2] The significant declines in rates of acute HAV are associated with major vaccination campaigns that successfully reduced the incidence rate.

Epidemiology

Various patient groups are at increased risk for infection with HAV. Children pose a particular problem with the spread of the disease because they often remain asymptomatic and are infectious for longer periods of time than adults. The most likely patient group affected is household or close personal contacts of an infected person. (1) Infection primarily occurs through the fecal–oral route, by person-to-person, or by ingestion of contaminated food or water. Incidentally, HAV's prevalence is linked to regions with low socioeconomic status and specifically to those with poor sanitary conditions and overcrowding. International travel and immigration also mitigate potential exposure to the virus.

International travel, in particular travel to HAV endemic areas, continues to be a major risk factor for HAV infection. Other identified risk factors include sexual and household contact with an HAV-infected person, men who have sex with men (MSM), and persons who inject drugs (PWIDs).[2] Additional patient groups that are at risk include patients with chronic liver disease and persons working with nonhuman primates. In 2010, 75% of case reports of acute HAV reported no identifiable risk factor.[2] Among MSMs, specific sexual practices may be associated with an increased risk for infection.[3] Foodborne outbreaks also occur. In general, mortality rates are low but highest among persons 75 years or older.[2]

Despite low endemic rates and successful vaccination programs in the United States, travel to HAV endemic areas is a recognized risk for acquiring acute HAV infections. According to the CDC, the majority of travel-related cases correspond to travel to Central and South America and Mexico.[2] Most Americans traveling to Mexico do not consider that country to be a risk in part because of Mexico's proximity to the United States. Moreover, most tourists falsely believe that higher-end resorts imply safety and that short visits to foreign countries are not associated with a risk for infection. Travel related to international adoptions can also be of risk.

Etiology

Hepatitis A is an RNA virus of the *Picornaviridae* family. The virus is stable in the environment, including at low pH and in freezing to moderate temperatures.[4] Inactivation requires disinfecting with a 1:100 dilution of sodium hypochlorite (bleach) in tap water or heating foods to a minimum of 85°C (185°F) for 1 minute.[5] 1 Transmission occurs primarily through the fecal–oral route because HAV is shed in the feces of infected people.[6] Contaminated water or ice are common modes of transmission, as are any foods which may be prepared using contaminated water, including shellfish harvested from contaminated water.

Pathophysiology

HAV infection is usually acute, self-limiting, and confers lifelong immunity. HAV's life cycle in the human host classically begins with ingestion of the virus. Absorption in the stomach or small intestine allows entry into the circulation and uptake by the liver. Replication of the virus occurs within hepatocytes and gastrointestinal (GI) epithelial cells. New virus particles are released into the blood and secreted into bile by the liver. The virus is then either reabsorbed to continue its cycle or excreted in the stool. The enterohepatic cycle will continue until interrupted by antibody neutralization.[6]

Clinical Presentation

2 The incubation period of HAV is approximately 28 days, with a range of 15 to 50 days. Table 40-1 summarizes the clinical features of acute hepatitis A. Symptoms and severity of HAV vary according to age. Children younger than 6 years typically are asymptomatic and can shed the virus for long periods of time, serving as a reservoir for the spread of HAV. Peak fecal shedding of the virus precedes the onset of clinical symptoms and elevated liver enzymes. Acute hepatitis follows, beginning with the preicteric or prodromal period. The phase is marked by an abrupt onset of nonspecific symptoms; some very mild.[5] Other, more unusual symptoms include chills, myalgia, arthralgia, cough, constipation, diarrhea, pruritus, and urticaria. The phase generally lasts 2 months. There are no specific symptoms unique to HAV. Liver enzyme levels rise within the first weeks of infection, peaking approximately in the fourth week and normalizing by the eighth week. Conjugated bilirubinemia, clinically evident as dark urine, precedes the onset of the icteric period. GI symptoms may persist or subside during this time and some patients may have hepatomegaly. Duration of the icteric period varies and corresponds to disease duration, averaging between 7 and 30 days.[6]

TABLE 40-1 Clinical Presentation of Acute Hepatitis A

Signs and symptoms
- The preicteric phase brings nonspecific influenza-like symptoms consisting of anorexia, nausea, fatigue, and malaise.
- Abrupt onset of anorexia, nausea, vomiting, malaise, fever, headache, and right upper quadrant abdominal pain with acute illness.
- Icteric hepatitis is generally accompanied by dark urine, alcoholic (light-colored) stools, and worsening of systemic symptoms.
- Pruritus is often a major complaint of icteric patients.

Physical examination
- Icteric sclera, skin, and secretions
- Mild weight loss of 2-5 kg
- Hepatomegaly

Laboratory tests
- Positive-serum Ig M anti–HAV
- Mild elevations of serum bilirubin, γ-globulin, and hepatic transaminase (ALT and AST) values to about twice normal in acute anicteric disease
- Elevations of alkaline phosphatase, γ-glutamyl transferase, and total bilirubin in patients with cholestatic illness

ALT, alanine transaminase; AST, aspartate transaminase; HAV, hepatitis A virus; Ig, immunoglobulin.

The diagnosis of acute HAV is made through the immunoglobulin (Ig) M antibody to HAV (anti-HAV). IgM anti-HAV is detectable 5 to 10 days prior to symptomatic HAV infections in the majority of patients. The IgG anti-HAV replaces IgM and indicates host immunity following the acute phase of the infection.[5] Food and Drug Administration (FDA)-approved assays for serologic testing detect IgM anti-HAV only and total anti-HAV (IgM and IgG anti-HAV). Patients who have detectable total anti-HAV with a negative IgM have resolved their infection. Concentrations of antibody often fall to 10 to 100 times lower than what would be expected after a natural course of infection. Although a positive anti-HAV result confirms protection, undetectable concentration of anti-HAV may not necessarily imply that protective levels were not achieved.[5]

HAV does not lead to chronic infections. Some patients may experience symptoms for up to 9 months. Rarely, patients experience complications from HAV, including relapsing hepatitis, cholestatic hepatitis, and fulminant hepatitis. Fatalities from HAV are generally rare, although more likely in patients older than 50 years and in persons with preexisting liver disease.[5]

A diagnosis of HAV is based on clinical criteria of an acute onset of fatigue, abdominal pain, loss of appetite, intermittent nausea and vomiting, jaundice or elevated serum aminotransferase levels, and serologic testing for IgM anti-HAV. Serologic testing is necessary to differentiate the diagnosis from other types of hepatitis.

TREATMENT

Desired Outcomes

The majority of people infected with HAV can be expected to fully recover without clinical sequelae.[6] Nearly all individuals will have clinical resolution within 6 months of the infection, and a majority will have done so by 2 months. Rarely, symptoms persist for longer or patients relapse. The ultimate goal of therapy is complete clinical resolution. Other goals include reducing complications from the infection, normalization of liver function, and reducing infectivity and transmission. Prevention of HAV infection is important because significant costs are accrued during acute HAV infections, both from direct costs of hospitalizations and indirect costs from loss of work days.

General Approach to Treatment

3 Prevention and prophylaxis are keys to managing this vaccine preventable virus. No specific treatment options exist for HAV infections. Instead, patients should receive general supportive care. The importance of good hand hygiene cannot be overemphasized in preventing disease transmission. Passive immunity with Ig is used for preexposure and postexposure prophylaxis. Active immunity is achieved through vaccination. Vaccines were approved for use in 1995 and implemented in the routine vaccination of children, as well as at-risk adults, to reduce the overall incidence of HAV.[5]

Prevaccination serologic testing to determine susceptibility is generally not recommended. In some cases, testing may be cost-effective if the cost of the test is less than that of the vaccine and if the person is from a moderate to high endemic area and likely to have prior immunity. Similarly, because of high vaccine response, postvaccine serologic testing is not recommended.[5]

Prevention of Hepatitis A

HAV is easily preventable with vaccination. Because children often serve as reservoirs of the disease, vaccine programs have targeted children as the most effective means to control HAV. Two vaccines for HAV are available and are incorporated into the routine childhood vaccination schedule. In 2005, the FDA reduced the minimum age for the vaccines to 12 months. In response, the Advisory Committee on Immunization Practices (ACIP) recommended expanding vaccine coverage to all children, including catch-up programs for children living in areas without existing vaccination programs. The new recommendations were enacted in the attempt to further reduce HAV incidence rates and possibly to eradicate the virus.[5] Other updated ACIP guidelines included HAV vaccination for previously unvaccinated persons anticipating close personal contact with international adoptees from a country of high or intermediate endemicity. Complete HAV vaccination recommendations are available from the CDC (Table 40-2).

Routine prevention of HAV transmission includes regular hand washing with soap and water after using the bathroom, changing a diaper, and before food preparation. For travelers to countries with high endemic rates of HAV, even short-term stays in urban and upscale resorts are not risk-free.[5] In particular, contaminated water and ice, fresh produce, and any uncooked foods pose a risk.[6]

Vaccines to Prevent Hepatitis A

The inactivated virus vaccines licensed in the United States are the single-antigen HAVRIX® and VAQTA® and the combination of HAV and hepatitis B virus (HBV) antigen vaccine TWINRIX®. Both single-antigen vaccines are available for pediatric and adult use while the TWINRIX® is indicated for adults only (Table 40-3). The differences in the vaccines are in the use of a preservative and in expression of antigen content. VAQTA® is formulated without a preservative and uses units of HAV antigen to express potency. HAVRIX® and TWINRIX® use 2-phenoxyphenol as a preservative and antigen content is expressed as enzyme-linked immunosorbent assay (ELISA) units.[5] Although high seroconversion rates of more than or equal to 94% are achieved with the first dose, VAQTA® and HAVRIX® recommend a booster shot to achieve the highest possible antibody titers. Although seroconversion exceeds 90% for HAV after the first dose of TWINRIX®, the full three-dose series is required for maximal HBV seroconversion. An accelerated dosing schedule is available but requires four doses for optimal response. The combined vaccine offers the advantage of immunization against both types of hepatitis in a single vaccine.

TABLE 40-2 Recommendations for Hepatitis A Virus Vaccination

All children at 1 year of age.
Children and adolescents between 2 and 18 years who live in states or communities where routine hepatitis A vaccination has been implemented because of high disease incidence.
Persons traveling to or working in countries that have high or intermediate endemicity of infection.[a]
MSM.
Illegal drug users.
Persons with occupational risk for infection (eg, persons who work with HAV-infected primates or with HAV in a research laboratory).
Persons who have clotting factor disorders.
Persons with chronic liver disease.
All previously unvaccinated persons anticipating close personal contact (eg, household contact or regular babysitter) with an international adoptee from a country of high or intermediate endemicity within the first 60 days following the arrival of the adoptee.

HAV, hepatitis A virus; MSM, men who have sex with men,

[a]Travelers to Canada, Western Europe, Japan, Australia, or New Zealand are at no greater risk for infection than they are in the United States. All other travelers should be assessed for HAV risk.

From Centers for Disease Control and Prevention[7]

TABLE 40-3 Recommended Dosing of Hepatitis A Vaccines

Vaccine	Age (Years)	Dose of Hepatitis A Antigen	No. of Doses	Schedule
HAVRIX	1-18	720 ELISA units	2	0, 6-12 months
	≥19	1,440 ELISA units	2	0, 6-12 months
VAQTA	1-18	25 units	2	0, 6-18 months
	≥19	50 units	2	0, 6-18 months
TWINRIX[a]	≥18	720 ELISA units	3	0, 1, 6 months
	≥18 (accelerated schedule)	720 ELISA units	4	0, 7 days, 21-30 days, +12 months

ELISA, enzyme-linked immunosorbent assay.

[a]Combination hepatitis A and B vaccine, also contains 20 mcg of hepatitis B surface antigen and requires a three-dose schedule.

From Centers for Disease Control and Prevention[7]

In situations of postexposure prophylaxis, either the vaccine or Ig can be used. The use of the vaccine is advantageous as vaccination confers the benefit of long-term immunity against HAV; however, experience in patients older than 40 years or with underlying medical conditions is limited.[7] Both vaccines may be given concomitantly with Ig and the two brands are interchangeable for booster shots.[5]

Vaccine is recommended for international travel to areas of high or intermediate endemicity and can be given regardless of scheduled dates of departure. For older patients, immunocompromised, or any patients with chronic liver disease or any other chronic medical conditions traveling within 2 weeks, both Ig and vaccine are recommended.[7]

The most common side effects of the vaccines include soreness and warmth at the injection site, headache, malaise, and pain. More than 65 million doses of the vaccine have been administered and despite routine monitoring for adverse events, there are no data to suggest a greater incidence of serious adverse events among vaccinated people compared with nonvaccinated. The vaccine is considered safe.[5]

Immunoglobulin

Ig is used when preexposure or postexposure prophylaxis against HAV infection is needed in persons for whom vaccination is not an option. Vaccination is preferred for multiple reasons, including that it induces active immunity and therefore a longer time of protection against HAV than Ig.

A sterile preparation of concentrated antibodies against HAV, Ig provides protection by passive transfer of antibody. Ig is most effective if given in the incubation period of the infection. Receipt of Ig within the first 2 weeks of infection will reduce infectivity and moderate the infection in 85% of patients. Patients who receive at least one dose of the HAV vaccine at least 1 month prior to exposure do not need preexposure or postexposure prophylaxis with Ig.[5] Ig is available as both an intravenous (IV) and intramuscular (IM) injection, but for HAV exposure, only the IM is used.

Serious adverse events from Ig are rare. Anaphylaxis has been reported in patients with IgA deficiency. Patients who had an anaphylaxis reaction to Ig should not receive it. There is no contraindication for use in pregnancy or lactation.

Dosing of Ig is the same for adults and children. For postexposure prophylaxis and for short-term preexposure coverage of less than 3 months, a single dose of 0.02 mL/kg IM is given. For long-term preexposure prophylaxis of less than or equal to 5 months, a single dose of 0.06 mL/kg is used. Either the deltoid or gluteal muscle may be used. In children younger than 24 months, Ig can be given in the anterolateral thigh muscle.[5]

In most patients who were recently exposed to HAV and who had not been previously vaccinated, postexposure prophylaxis with vaccination is preferred. Ig prophylaxis is preferred in the following situations: patients are younger than 12 months or older than 40 years, are immunocompromised, have chronic liver disease or have underlying medical conditions, or for whom vaccine is contraindicated.[7]

Ig can be given concomitantly with the HAV vaccine. Although the antibody titer will be lower than if the vaccine were administered alone, the response is still protective and coadministration should be considered for the advantages of long-term HAV protection. However, Ig can interfere with the response of other live, attenuated vaccines and should be delayed.

Vaccine efficacy may be reduced in certain patient populations. In HIV-infected patients, greater immunogenic response may correlate with higher baseline CD4 cell counts. Patients with CD4 counts less than 200 cells/mm^3 ($<0.200 \times 10^9$/L) at vaccination have a reduced response rate. Moreover, patients with HIV/HCV coinfection may also have a lowered response.[8]

HEPATITIS B

4 Hepatitis B is highly infectious, approximately 50 to 100 times more so than HIV.[9] Although a vaccine was made available in 1981, HBV has acutely infected more than 2 billion people globally, leading to chronic infection in more than 240 million people.[9,10] Chronic infection with HBV is a major public health issue as it serves as a reservoir for continued HBV transmission and poses a significant risk of death resulting from liver disease including liver cirrhosis and hepatocellular carcinoma (HCC). According to the World Health Organization (WHO), an estimated 650,000 people per year die as a result of complications from HBV.[10] In the United States, estimates of prevalence and incidence of viral hepatitis are difficult because there is no national chronic hepatitis surveillance program.[1]

Epidemiology

According to the WHO, chronic HBV infections disproportionately affect low and middle-income countries.[9,10] Prevalence can vary regionally; however, areas commonly associated with high infectivity rates include sub-Saharan Africa, East Asia, followed by the Amazon and southern parts of Eastern and Central Europe.[10] Areas of high prevalence, approximately 45% of the global population, are of special concern because most infections are of infants and children and more than 90% of cases lead to a chronic carrier state. Myths and misinformation about HBV abound and can result in discrimination and social injustice.[1] There are approximately 1.4 million chronically infected HBV people in the United States. Rates of acute infection in the United States continue to decline and in 2013, an estimated 19,800 people developed new infections.[2] In 2013, the highest incidence rate was among persons aged 30 to 39 years and among non-Hispanic blacks. Data from a limited chronic surveillance program indicate Asian/Pacific Islanders account for the highest proportion of chronic HBV infections and HBV-related mortality.[2] Annually, 3,000 people die from chronic liver disease attributable to HBV.[1]

HBV is transmitted sexually, parenterally, and perinatally. In areas of high HBV prevalence, perinatal transmission from mother to infant at birth is most common, whereas in areas of intermediate prevalence, horizontal transmission from child to child is most common. Sexual contact, both homosexual and heterosexual, and injection-drug use are the predominant forms of transmission in low endemic countries such as the United States.[9] Concentration of HBV is high in blood, serum, and wound exudates of infected persons. Transmission occurs via blood-to-blood contact or semen or vaginal fluid of an infected person. The virus can be stable in the environment for at least 7 days and can cause infection during this time.[9] In the United States in 2013, no risk factor could be identified for the majority of acute infections with HBV. Among patients with identifiable risk factors, the most common risk is injection drug use, followed by sexual contact, specifically multiple sexual partners and MSM.[2] Other known risk factors include household contact of HBV-positive person.[2] Screening focuses on individuals at high risk for HBV (Table 40-4).[11]

TABLE 40-4 Persons at High Risk for HBV: Recommended Screening

Individuals From the Following Areas	Other Groups
Asia	US-born persons not vaccinated as infants whose parents were born in high HBV endemic regions
Africa	Household and sexual contacts of HBsAg-positive patients
South Pacific Islands	Persons who have ever injected drugs
Middle East (except Cyprus and Israel)	Persons with multiple sexual partners or history of STD
Malta	MSM
Spain	Inmates of correctional facilities
Arctic (indigenous populations of Alaska, Canada, Greenland)	Individuals with chronically elevated AST or ALT
South America: Ecuador, Guyana, Suriname, Venezuela, Amazon regions of Bolivia, Brazil, Colombia, Peru	Individuals with HIV or HCV
Eastern Europe (except Hungary)	Patients undergoing dialysis
Antigua and Barbuda, Dominica, Granada, Haiti, Jamaica, St. Kitts and Nevis, St. Lucia, Turks and Caicos	All pregnant women
	Persons requiring immunosuppressive therapy

ALT, alanine transaminases; AST, aspartate aminotransferase; HBsAg, hepatitis B surface antigen; HBV, hepatitis B virus; HCV, hepatitis C virus; HIV, human immunodeficiency virus; MSM, men who have sex with men; STD, sexually transmitted disease.

Data from references 11 and 14.

The mode of transmission has clinical implications because chronic infections are associated with infection acquired in younger patients, especially those infected perinatally and in early childhood.[9]

Clinical Controversy...

Between 2008 and 2014, at least 23 healthcare-associated HBV outbreaks were identified, resulting in 175 outbreak associated cases and more than 10,700 people notified for screening. Most outbreaks occurred in long-term care facilities and were linked to lapses in infection control. Inappropriate use of glucose meters without cleaning and disinfection was the suspected mode of transmission in most cases.

Etiology

The HBV is a DNA virus that preferentially replicates within the liver.[12] There are at least 10 HBV genotypes (GTs) (A-J) with distinct geographic and ethnic distribution. GT prevalence may depend on mode of transmission as types B and C are found in areas where vertical transmission is the primary mode of infection.[13] Additionally, various subtypes of GTs exist with varying clinical outcomes. Correlations between clinical outcomes and HBV GTs suggest infections with GT C are associated with more severe liver injury, including liver cirrhosis and progression to HCC. Resistance mutations may contribute to GT virulence and hence impact severity of liver disease in infection.[13-15] Testing for HBV GT is not currently recommended for clinical practice.[14]

Pathophysiology

On infection, replication of the virus begins by attachment of the virion to the hepatocyte cell surface receptors. The particles are transported to the nucleus where the DNA is converted into closed, circular DNA that serves as a template for pregenomic RNA. Viral RNA is then transcribed and transported back to the cytoplasm where it can alternatively serve as a reservoir for future viral templates or bud into the intracellular membrane with the viral envelope proteins and infect other cells.[13] The viral genome has four reading frames coding for various proteins and enzymes required for viral replication. Several of these proteins are used diagnostically (Table 40-5). The hepatitis B surface antigen (HBsAg) is the most abundant of the three surface antigens and is detectable at the onset of clinical symptoms. Its persistence past 6 months after initial detection corresponds to chronic infection and indicates an increased risk for cirrhosis, hepatic decompensation, and HCC. Development of antibody to HBsAg (anti-HBsAg) confers immunity to the virus and clearance of HBsAg is associated with favorable outcomes.[16] The precore polypeptide encodes for the secretory protein hepatitis B e antigen (HBeAg) and the hepatitis B core antigen (HBcAg) proteins. HBeAg is present in an acute infection and is replaced by antibodies (anti-HBeAg) once an infection is resolved. HBeAg was assumed to be a marker of viral replication and infectivity; however, it is now known that some viral mutants exist that are unable to have or have downregulated expression of HBeAg, although their ability to replicate is not affected.[14] HBeAg-negative mutants pose a particular clinical challenge because they are refractory to treatment. The HBcAg is a nucleocapsid protein that, when expressed on hepatocytes, promotes immune-mediated cell death. High levels of antibodies (IgM anti-HBcAg) are detectable during acute infections. Patients who respond to vaccine will have anti-HBsAg only.[7]

TABLE 40-5 Interpretation of Serologic Tests in Hepatitis B Virus

Tests	Result	Interpretation
HBsAg Anti-HBc Anti-HBs	(–) (–) (–)	Susceptible
HBsAg Anti-HBc Anti-HBs	(–) (+) (+)	Immune because of natural infection
HBsAg Anti-HBc Anti-HBs	(–) (c) (+)	Immune because of vaccination (valid only if test performed 1-2 months after third vaccine dose)
HBsAg Anti-HBc IgM anti-HBc Anti-HBs	(+) (+) (+) (–)	Acute infection
HBsAg Anti-HBc IgM anti-HBc Anti-HBs	(+) (+) (–) (–)	Chronic infection
HBsAg Anti-HBc Anti-HBs	(–) (+) (–)	Four interpretations possible: 1. Recovery from acute infection 2. Distant immunity and test not sensitive enough to detect low level of HBs in serum 3. Susceptible with false-positive anti-HBc 4. May have undetectable level of HBsAg in serum and be chronically infected

HBc, hepatitis B core; HBs, hepatitis B surface; HBsAg, hepatitis B surface antigen; IgM, immunoglobulin M.

From Centers for Disease Control and Prevention. Hepatitis B Serology. http://www.cdc.gov/ncidod/diseases/hepatitis/b/Bserology.htm.

HBV itself does not seem to be pathogenic to cells; rather, it is thought that the immune response to the virus is cytotoxic to hepatocytes.[13] The immune response is critical to viral clearance. If the response is weak, chronic infection is likely. Liver injury is likely caused by secondary, nonspecific inflammation activated by the initial cytotoxic lymphocyte response and as an attempt by the immune system to clear the virus by destroying HBV antigen—presenting hepatocytes. Destruction of hepatocytes results in release of circulating, and hence increased, alanine aminotransferase (ALT) levels.

Chronic Hepatitis B Virus

4 Patients who continue to have detectable HBsAg for more than 6 months have chronic HBV.[13] Chronic infections can be controlled in many cases, but cure is not possible because the HBV template is integrated into the host genome. The most predictive factor for developing a chronic infection is age. Perinatal infections almost always result in chronic infections because of immune tolerance to the virus. The risks of chronicity decline to a rate of 30% in infants and to less than 5% in adult-onset infections. Importantly, chronic HBV infections are differentiated into phases with varied serologic patterns and patients can progress from one phase to the next or experience an active infection after being in an inactive state.[14]

Clinical Presentation and Phases of Infection

The clinical symptoms and course of an HBV infection are indistinguishable from other types of viral hepatitis. Table 40-6 lists the clinical features of chronic HBV. Several phases of an HBV infection exist and are dynamic (Table 40-7).[15] During the initial or acute phase of an HBV infection in adults and older children, the HBV enters a 4- to 10-week incubation period, during which antibodies toward the HBV core are produced and the virus replicates profusely. Active viral replication results in high serum HBV DNA levels and HBeAg secretion. ALT levels may rise slightly, but most patients will remain asymptomatic. Symptoms, if they do occur, include fever, anorexia, nausea, vomiting, jaundice, dark urine, clay-colored or pale stools, and abdominal pain. Most neonates and children are anicteric and have no clinical symptoms; many adults are also asymptomatic.[9] HBsAg does not become detectable until after significant viremia. The initial phase is considered immunotolerant because no hepatic injury is sustained, as evidenced by generally normal ALT levels, and the virus replicates profusely. Patients are highly infectious during

TABLE 40-6 Clinical Presentation of Chronic Hepatitis B[a]

Signs and symptoms

- Easy fatigability, anxiety, anorexia, and malaise
- Ascites, jaundice, variceal bleeding, and hepatic encephalopathy can manifest with liver decompensation
- Hepatic encephalopathy is associated with hyperexcitability, impaired mentation, confusion, obtundation, and eventually coma
- Vomiting and seizures

Physical examination

- Icteric sclera, skin, and secretions
- Decreased bowel sounds, increased abdominal girth, and detectable fluid wave
- Asterixis
- Spider angiomata

Laboratory tests

- Presence of HBsAg >6 months
- Intermittent elevations of hepatic transaminase (ALT and AST) and HBV DNA >20,000 IU/mL ($>20 \times 10^6$ IU/L)
- Liver biopsies for pathologic classification as chronic persistent hepatitis, chronic active hepatitis, or cirrhosis

ALT, alanine transaminase; AST, aspartate transaminase; DNA, deoxyribonucleic acid; HBsAg, hepatitis B surface antigen; HBV, hepatitis B virus.

[a]Chronic hepatitis B can be present even without all the signs, symptoms, and physical examination findings listed being apparent.

TABLE 40-7 Patterns of Chronic Hepatitis B Virus Phases

State	HBeAg Status	ALT Level	HBV DNA IU/mL[a]	Other
Immune tolerant	+	WNL	>20,000	
Immune active	+	High	>2,000	
Immune control	–	WNL	<2,000	Anti-HBe +
Immune escape	–	High	>20,000	Anti-HBe +
Reactivation	±	High	>20,000	Associated with immunosuppressive states or therapies

ALT, alanine transaminase; DNA, deoxyribonucleic acid; HBeAg, hepatitis B e antigen; HBV, hepatitis B virus; WNL, within normal limits.

[a]Conversion factor for IU/mL to IU/L is 1,000.

this time.[15] In perinatally acquired infections, and in young children, the phase can last for decades—until adulthood.[15] Infected children pose a particular risk because they are often asymptomatic, undiagnosed, and highly infectious.

The immunoactive phase marks a decrease in HBV DNA levels with ongoing secretion of HBeAg. Patients are symptomatic with intermittent flares of hepatitis and marked increases in ALT levels. More frequent flares are associated with disease progression and reflect host immune response against HBV-infected hepatocytes, increased cell death in an attempt to clear the virus.[13] The phase can last a few weeks in acute disease, and for years in patients with chronic disease. As the host immune system attempts to gain control of the infection by stopping active viral replication, serum HBV DNA levels drop to undetectable, ALT levels normalize, and liver necroinflammation resolves.[13]

If the infection is self-limiting, HBV DNA quickly subsides, HBeAg disappears within weeks, and HBsAg usually resolves within 4 months. The final phase is seroconversion and is defined by the replacement of HBeAg with anti-HBeAg. Factors favoring seroconversion include female sex, older age, biochemical activity, and genotype (GT). Flares of hepatitis with ALT levels more than 5 times the upper limits of normal, compared with less than 5 times the upper limits of normal, correspond to increased immune system activity and precede seroconversion. Spontaneous HBeAg clearance is possible and is associated with older age, higher ALT, and infection with HBV GT B.[14] Patients who have achieved immune control over HBV will be HBeAg-negative, with detectable HBsAg and anti-HBeAg, normal ALT, and either low or undetectable levels of HBV DNA. This patient population usually experiences a more benign course of disease, with the possibility of long-term remission, even seroconversion, although reactivation is possible with the progression to cirrhosis and HCC. Up to 20% of patients in the inactive carrier state may revert to detectable HBeAg, emphasizing the need for lifelong follow-up to confirm quiescence.[14]

In a subset of patients, often in patients who are older, another phase of infection may occur which is described as the immune escape or HBeAg-negative chronic infection. This phase is linked to mutations of the virus resulting in a lack of production of HBeAg and is associated with worse outcomes.[10] Patients may have long periods of disease remission, but recurring flares of hepatitis with increased frequency and severity can progress to cirrhosis and HCC.

Reactivation of hepatitis B, defined as the recurrence or abrupt rise in HBV replication by an increase in serum HBV DNA of at least 1 $\log_{10}$ and a marked increase in transaminase levels, can occur and is well described in the literature in patients receiving cancer chemotherapy, steroids, and other immunosuppressive agents.[16,17] Reactivation can occur in anyone with a prior or current HBV exposure, but patients who are HBsAg positive are most likely to experience a reactivation.[17] The causes of reactivation include spontaneous mutations of the virus that allow it to escape immune control, development of resistance to HBV drug therapy or the cessation of HBV therapy, or changes in immunity, such as those that occur in patients undergoing immunosuppressive therapies or coinfection with HIV. Antiviral prophylactic therapy is often indicated to prevent reactivation.[10]

Cirrhosis

Cirrhosis results as the liver attempts to regenerate while in an environment of persistent inflammation. Most patients with compensated cirrhosis either are asymptomatic or have mild symptoms of epigastric pain. During cirrhosis, the liver enters a cycle of ongoing liver damage, fibrosis, and attempts at regeneration. The classical appearance of a small and knobby liver reflects the irreversible effect of nodules of regenerating cells integrated with infiltrates of inflammation-induced fibrous tissue. Both viral and clinical factors affect the outcome of cirrhosis (Table 40-8). Cirrhosis develops at an annual incidence rate of 2.1% to 3.5%.[13] The development of cirrhosis is mostly insidious and patients can remain stable for years before disease progression. An estimated 20% of all chronic hepatitis B patients develop complications of hepatic insufficiency and portal hypertension as their compensated cirrhosis progresses to decompensated cirrhosis within a 5-year period.[14]

Hepatocellular Carcinoma

HBV is a known risk factor for the development of HCC and in areas of high HBV endemicity, a major complication of the infection.[9] The development of HCC can be insidious, occurring in the absence of cirrhosis or in the presence of clinically silent, compensated cirrhosis. Many patients with HCC have no signs of cirrhosis.[14] The virus itself is not likely the causative agent of the cancer. In most cases, HCC develops after years of inflammatory processes provoked by ongoing HBV infection however HBV itself is an oncogenic virus.[10] Several factors influence the development of HCC, as well as predict survival (see Table 40-8). HCC is more prevalent in males; in older patients; in patients coinfected with HCV or delta hepatitis; in patients coinfected with HIV; in patients with diabetes; and in patients with serologic markings of past or present HBV infection, preexisting cirrhosis, or continued alcohol ingestion. Risks for death and decompensation increase with underlying liver disease. Serum ALT levels, on-going viral replication, and family history of HCC are also associated with progression.[10] Smoking is a risk factor among European and Asian patients.[18,19]

TABLE 40-8 Factors Associated with Hepatitis B Virus Cirrhosis and Disease Progression

Persistence of HBV serum DNA
Infection with genotype C
Coinfection with HCV, delta hepatitis, or HIV
Age at diagnosis
Severity of liver disease at diagnosis
Male sex
Frequency of severe hepatic flares
Alcohol use
Laboratory/physical findings of abnormal liver function
Obesity and metabolic disorders
Smoking

HBV, hepatitis B virus; HCV, hepatitis C virus; HIV, human immunodeficiency virus; DNA, deoxyribonucleic acid.

Data from references 13, 14, and 19.

Vaccine Prevention of Hepatitis B

5 The development of the HBV vaccine represented the first vaccine against a major human cancer.[10] Despite the availability of the HBV vaccine in 1982, rates of HBV did not decline in the early 1980s. Initial declines in incidence were likely attributable to behavioral changes among high-risk groups as a result of the acquired immune deficiency syndrome (AIDS) epidemic. A 94% decline in rates between 1990 and 2004 was seen in children and adolescents, which began with the initiation of screening of pregnant women and subsequent immunizations of infants and recommendations set forth in the 1990s to immunize adolescents. Regulations enacted by Occupational Safety and Health Administration (OSHA) further reduced overall U.S. rates by 75%.[12]

5 Prophylaxis against HBV can be achieved by vaccination or by passive immunity in postexposure cases with hepatitis B Ig. Vaccination is the most effective strategy to prevent infection and a comprehensive vaccination strategy has been implemented in the United States (Table 40-9). Vaccines use HBsAg for the antigen via recombinant DNA technology using yeast to prompt active immunity. More than 60 million adolescents and more than 40 million infants and children have received an HBV vaccine in the United States since 1982. The vaccine is considered safe. Since 2000, vaccines licensed in the United States contain either none or trace amounts of thimerosal as a preservative. Available vaccines include two single-antigen products and three combination products. The two single-antigen products are Recombivax® HB and Engerix-B®. TWINRIX® is a combination vaccine for HAV and HBV in adults. Comvax® and Pediarix® are used for children and are used for HBV along with other scheduled vaccines. Unlike the HAV vaccine, the HBV vaccine response is generally lower and often requires at least three doses for optimal protection.

TABLE 40-9 Recommendations for Hepatitis B Virus Vaccination

Infants
Adolescents including all previously unvaccinated children <19 years
All unvaccinated adults aged 19-59 with diabetes mellitus All unvaccinated adults at risk for infection
All unvaccinated adults seeking vaccination (specific risk factor not required)
Men and women with a history of other STDs and persons with a history of multiple sex partners (>1 partner/6 months)
MSM
Current or recent IDUs
Household contacts and sex partners of persons with chronic hepatitis B infection and healthcare and public safety workers with exposure to blood in the workplace
Clients and staff of institutions for the developmentally disabled
International travelers to regions with high or intermediate levels (HBsAg prevalence ≤2%) of endemic HBV infection
Recipients of clotting factor concentrates
STD clinic patients
HIV patient/HIV-testing patients
Drug abuse treatment and prevention clinic patients
Correctional facilities inmates
Chronic dialysis/ESRD patients including predialysis, peritoneal dialysis, and home dialysis patients
Persons with chronic liver disease

HBsAg, hepatitis B surface antigen; HBV, hepatitis B virus; HIV, human immunodeficiency virus; ESRD, end-stage renal disease; IDUs, injection drug users; MSM, Men who have sex with men; STDs, sexually transmitted diseases.

Data from reference 11.

Passive immunity in the form of anti-HBsAg offers temporary protection against HBV and is used in conjunction with the hepatitis B vaccine for postexposure prophylaxis.[12]

TREATMENT

Desired Outcomes

6 HBV infections are not curable; rather, the goals of therapy are to suppress HBV replication and prevent disease progression to cirrhosis and HCC. The loss of HBsAg is becoming an increasingly more important goal in therapy.

General Approach to Treatment

6 Response to therapy is monitored by biochemical, histologic, and virologic assessments (Table 40-10).[14] Maintenance of viral suppression is defined as durability of response. In HBeAg-positive patients, successful therapy includes loss of HBeAg status and seroconversion to anti-HBeAg. Other serologic markers are typically not evaluated in clinical trials. Recommendations for treatment consider the patient's age, serum HBV DNA and ALT levels, as well as histologic evidence and clinical progression of disease (Figs. 40-1 and 40-2). Not all chronic HBV patients are candidates for treatment. In general, treatment is indicated if the risk of liver-related morbidity and mortality is within the foreseeable future and the likelihood for achieving sustained viral suppression is high.[14] Some patients may be best managed with periodic monitoring for disease progression because the chances for therapeutic response are unlikely and do not outweigh the risks and costs associated with treatment. The major organizations providing guidelines on the management of HBV infections are the WHO, American Association for the Study

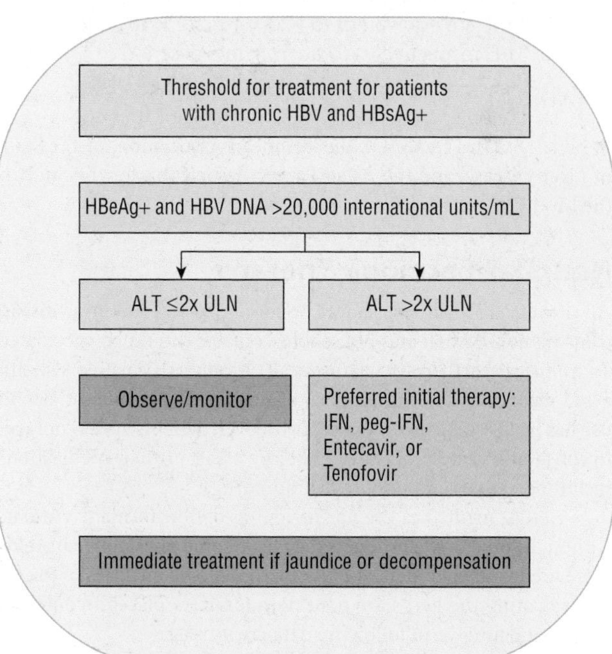

FIGURE 40-1 Suggested management algorithm for chronic hepatitis B virus infection based on the recommendations of the American Association for the Study of Liver Diseases. (ALT, alanine transaminases; HBeAg, hepatitis B e antigen; HBsAg, hepatitis B surface antigen; HBV, hepatitis B virus; DNA, deoxyribonucleic acid; IFN, interferon; peg-IFN, pegylated interferon; HBV DNA concentration of >20,000 IU/mL is equivalent to >20 × 10^6 IU/L.) *(Data from reference 14.)*

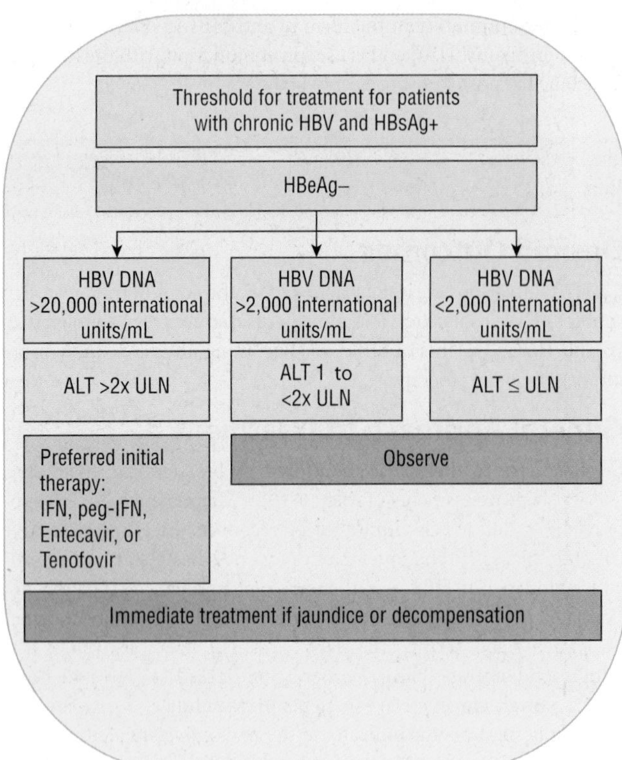

FIGURE 40-2 Suggested management algorithm based on the recommendations of the American Association for the Study of Liver Diseases for chronic hepatitis B virus–infected patients with cirrhosis. (ALT, alanine transaminases; HBeAg, hepatitis B e antigen; HBsAg, hepatitis B surface antigen; HBV, hepatitis B virus; DNA, deoxyribonucleic acid; IFN, interferon; peg-IFN, pegylated interferon; HBV DNA concentrations of >20,000, >2,000, and ≤2,000 IU/mL are equivalent to >20 × 10⁶, >2 × 10⁶, and ≤2 × 10⁶ IU/L, respectively.) *(Data from reference 14.)*

of Liver Diseases (AASLD), the European Association for the Study of Liver Disease, and the Asian Pacific Association for the Study of the Liver.[10,13-15]

Nonpharmacologic Therapy

All chronic HBV patients should be counseled on preventing disease transmission. Sexual and household contacts should be vaccinated. To minimize further liver damage, all chronic HBV patients should avoid alcohol and be immunized against HAV. No level of alcohol use has been established as safe.[14] Moreover, patients are encouraged to consult their medical provider before using any new medications, including herbals and nonprescription drugs.[14]

Herbal medicines are an intriguing option to many patients. Although some of the products may have some physiologic benefits, there are insufficient data and the methodologic qualities of the trials evaluating the herbs are poor. Randomized, placebo-controlled studies and long-term follow-up data are lacking.[20]

Pharmacologic Therapy

Because hepatic damage is sustained by ongoing viral replication, drug therapy aims to suppress viral replication by either immunomodulating agents or antivirals—the nucleos(t)ide agents (NAs). In the United States, the immune-mediating agents approved as first-line therapy are interferon (IFN)-alfa and pegylated (peg) IFN-alfa. The antiviral agents lamivudine, telbivudine, adefovir, entecavir, and tenofovir are all approved as first-line therapy options for chronic HBV.[14] A major difference in therapy is duration of use: IFN-based therapies are typically administered for a predefined duration, whereas NAs are used until a specific end point is achieved. For HBeAg-positive patients, treatment is recommended until HBeAg seroconversion and an undetectable HBV viral load are achieved and for 6 months of additional treatment. In HBeAg-negative patients, treatment should be continued until HBsAg clearance.[14]

Interferon

IFN-alfa therapy was the first approved therapy for treatment of HBV and improves long-term outcomes and survival. Acting as a host cytokine, it has antiviral, antiproliferative, and immunomodulatory effects in chronic HBV.[14] Several factors correlate with improved response to IFN therapy, including increased ALT and HBV DNA levels, high histologic activity score at biopsy, and being non-Asian. Asian patients tend to have more normal ALT levels in chronic infection; confounding the actual impact of ethnicity on infection.[14] The main mechanism of action of the IFNs is to enhance the host immune system to mount a defense against HBV.

Patients who respond to IFN therapy tend to have a more durable response than that seen with lamivudine, likely as a consequence of IFN's stimulation of the immune response for seroconversion. However, seroconversion with IFN therapy is most likely in patients with HBeAg positivity and who have persistent or intermittently elevated ALT. The duration of therapy is finite, although the optimal duration of treatment is unclear and some patients benefit from a prolonged course of therapy including up to 24 months.[14] Patients treated with IFN were historically treated with thrice-weekly IFN, which has largely been replaced by peg-IFN because of the benefits in ease of administration (once weekly injections) and improvements in efficacy. IFN-based therapies are still limited by multiple adverse effects. The high risk of infection precludes use of IFN in decompensated cirrhotic patients.[14] In patients with compensated cirrhosis, IFN appears to be safe and effective, although it can provoke hepatic flares and precipitate hepatic decompensation.[14] Because IFN is not directly acting on the virus and thus not susceptible to specific resistant mutations, it remains an option in treatment and ongoing clinical trials are investigating the use of either sequential or combination therapy with peg-IFN and NAs. The optimal role of IFN-based therapies in HBV treatment is not defined. IFN therapies remain an option in the United States.[14] However, due to the substantial side effects, need for monitoring, and toxicities of IFN-based therapies, IFN is not considered an option in resource-limited countries and not recommended as a first-line therapy by the WHO guidelines.[10]

Lamivudine

Lamivudine, an NA, has antiviral activity against both HIV and HBV but is not recommended as first-line therapy for chronic HBV infections. It is given at a dose of 100 mg by mouth daily and inhibits HBV DNA synthesis by being incorporated into growing DNA chains causing premature chain termination.[14] Normalization of ALT levels occurs gradually over 3 to 6 months in most patients. Additionally, fibrotic changes are reduced and may be reversed in some cases. Response to lamivudine is dependent on baseline ALT levels, with higher levels corresponding to greater likelihood of seroconversion.

TABLE 40-10 Definitions of Response in Hepatitis B Virus Therapy

Biochemical	Normalization of ALT
Histologic	Decrease in histology activity by at least 2 points as compared with baseline biopsy
Virologic	Undetectable HBV DNA and, in patients previously HBeAg positive, loss of HBeAg

ALT, alanine transaminase; DNA, deoxyribonucleic acid; HBV, hepatitis B virus; HBeAg, hepatitis B e antigen.

Seroconversion rates increase with duration of therapy and are at 50% by the fifth year of therapy.[14] Patients who can maintain long-term viral suppression have reduced and possibly reversed cirrhotic changes. However, lamivudine therapy is not without problems. There is no clear duration of treatment. Patients who are HBeAg-negative have a less than 20% viral suppression rate after 12 months of therapy.[14] Seroconversion rates are less than 20% after 1 year of therapy and will relapse in up to 58% of patients. Resistance is inevitable and can undermine the value of treatment. The emergence of resistant mutants increases with each subsequent year of therapy, with rates approaching 80% after 5 years of therapy, and is associated with returns of serum HBV DNA and elevated ALT levels.[21] Relapse is associated with reversion of histologic benefits.[14] In HBeAg-negative chronic hepatitis B, where therapy is long-term and the exact duration of therapy unknown, resistance is an especially daunting problem.[14] Patients on lamivudine therapy require monitoring for breakthrough infection. If patients have confirmed lamivudine-resistant mutations, therapy should be changed to include agents with activity against lamivudine-resistant HBV.[14]

Adefovir

Adefovir dipivoxil is an acyclic NA of adenosine monophosphate. The drug acts by inhibiting HBV reverse transcriptase and DNA polymerase and is effective in both wild-type and lamivudine-resistant HBV. It is dosed at 10 mg daily for 1 year in adults, although the optimal duration of therapy is unknown and some patients may benefit from a prolonged course of therapy.[14] Patients who are HBeAg-negative in particular are likely to benefit from prolonged treatment courses. Adefovir is well tolerated at the 10 mg daily dose. Previous reports of nephrotoxicity were associated with clinical trials where adefovir was dosed at 30 mg/day. In patients treated chronically at a dose of 10 mg daily, the incidence of nephrotoxicity was the same as placebo. Routine monitoring of serum creatinine is recommended every 3 months in patients at risk for renal insufficiency and in all patients treated for more than a year with adefovir.[14]

Resistance to adefovir has not been seen within the first year of therapy.[21] Resistant mutants have been identified and may be more likely in patients with prior lamivudine resistance.[14] In contrast, combination therapy with lamivudine and adefovir may decrease the risk of adefovir resistance.[22] Neither the optimal duration for combination therapy nor the optimal drug therapy in adefovir resistance is known.[14]

Adefovir's role in HBV therapy is unclear. It is no longer recommended as monotherapy by international guidelines.[10]

Entecavir

7 Entecavir is a guanosine NA that acts by inhibiting HBV replication at three different steps. An oral agent, it is more potent than lamivudine and adefovir in suppressing serum HBV DNA levels and is effective in lamivudine-resistant HBV.[14] Entecavir does have weak activity against HIV.[10] Rates of HBeAg seroconversion are higher in patients with elevated baseline ALT.[14] The drug is dosed at 0.5 mg daily for adults with treatment-naïve or non–lamivudine-resistant infections and at 1 mg daily in lamivudine-refractory patients. In treatment-naïve patients, entecavir resistance remains low, even after six years of therapy, demonstrating the high barrier to resistance of the drug.[21] However, treatment response in lamivudine-resistant patients is lower overall and more likely for the development of entecavir-resistant mutants especially if lamivudine is continued during entecavir therapy.[14] Patients on lamivudine who develop resistance and are switched to entecavir should stop lamivudine therapy.[14] Resistance to lamivudine is a risk factor for entecavir resistance.[21] In terms of safety, entecavir is comparable to lamivudine. Entecavir is considered to be a first-line agent for HBV therapy because of its efficacy and low rates of resistance.[10,14]

Telbivudine

Telbivudine is an HBV-specific NA that acts as a competitive inhibitor of viral reverse transcriptase and DNA polymerase to inhibit HBV DNA synthesis. Compared with lamivudine, telbivudine is a more potent suppressor of HBV DNA.[14] However, similar to lamivudine, telbivudine has a high rate of mutations that limits its efficacy. Moreover, telbivudine-resistant mutations are cross-resistant with lamivudine. Due to resistance concerns, telbivudine monotherapy has a limited role in the treatment of HBV and is not recommended as monotherapy by international guidelines.[10,14]

Tenofovir

7 Tenofovir is considered to be a first-line therapy in the treatment of HBV.[14] For HBV, it is available as a single-agent oral tablet. Tenofovir is similar to adefovir but without the nephrotoxicity seen with adefovir, permitting adult dosing to be 300 mg versus 10 mg of adefovir. The higher dosing strategy likely confers several advantages to tenofovir in comparison with adefovir. In lamivudine-resistant chronic hepatitis B, tenofovir showed an earlier and greater suppression of HBV DNA than adefovir. In studies of treatment-naïve patients on tenofovir for up to 3 years, no resistant mutations were detected.[27] Additional data suggest sustained viral suppression with regression of fibrosis and no resistance in patients treated with tenofovir for up to 7 years.[21,23] Viral suppression was seen in nearly all patients, regardless of HBeAg status.[23] No resistance was identified to tenofovir through the 7-year study period. Other studies have demonstrated good viral suppression with tenofovir in treatment-experienced patients. Tenofovir can overcome adefovir treatment failure, but adefovir mutants demonstrate some cross-resistance because viral suppression by tenofovir is reduced.[10,21]

Alternative Drug Treatments

Combination therapy has been proposed to increase drug effectiveness and to counter the issues of resistance. Potential disadvantages for combination therapy include costs, toxicity, and drug interactions. Currently no data exist that combination therapy of two antiviral agents improves effectiveness. IFN-based therapy, because it acts on the host immune system rather than the virus itself, poses an interesting option in overcoming viral resistance. Data for preventing resistance are mixed as complete suppression of resistance has not been achieved with combination therapy. Combination therapy with IFN and lamivudine creates less resistance than lamivudine monotherapy, but the combination did not change the posttherapy viral response in comparison to IFN monotherapy.[14] Given the toxicity profile of IFN, it is unlikely a combination therapy with IFN will be used.

Combination therapy with NA agents may offer a way to bypass IFN-induced toxicity and minimize resistance concerns; however, combination therapy is not frequently used as initial therapy. Many studies examined the role of sequential or add-on therapy, rather than comparing the effectiveness of monotherapy versus combination therapy in an otherwise treatment-naïve patient population. There may be a role for combination therapy, especially in patients with high initial viral loads or multiple underlying HBV resistance mutations.[24,25] Furthermore, in resource-limited areas where access to monotherapy may be cost-prohibitive, combination therapy may offer a strategy to reduce resistance and provide optimal HBV viral suppression.[21] There is also increasing interest in the use of combination therapy to prevent HBV recurrence in patients undergoing immunosuppressive therapies.

Combination therapy is not recommended as initial therapy. Current guidelines suggest combination therapy with two or more agents in patients who develop antiviral resistant HBV.[13-15] The AASLD recommends combination therapy with lamivudine or telbivudine plus adefovir, tenofovir, or entecavir for decompensated cirrhotic patients with chronic HBV regardless of HBV DNA levels or HBeAg status.[14]

Special Populations

Cirrhosis

The decision to treat cirrhotic patients depends on disease progression. Patients with decompensated cirrhosis require referral for liver transplant. The AASLD guidelines suggest lamivudine, telbivudine, adefovir, tenofovir, and entecavir are possible agents for use in cirrhotic patients (see Fig. 40-2).[14]

Clinical **Controversy...**

There is a variability in practice recommendations regarding the need and indications for HBV screening and prophylaxis across medical specialties. Even if patients are screened and antiviral prophylaxis is initiated, the optimal duration of antiviral therapy is unclear.

Coinfection with Hepatitis C Virus

In patients coinfected with HCV, the clinical practice is to treat the more dominant form of the hepatitis virus. There are no current recommendations on management of HBV/HCV coinfection. Previously published recommendations suggested treating HCV according to published guidelines and to consider the addition of entecavir or adefovir if HBV DNA levels remained stable or rose.[14]

Coinfection with Hepatitis D

Patients coinfected with hepatitis D, which requires infection with hepatitis B, may be treated with high-dose IFN-alfa or peg-IFN.[14] There is an overall paucity of data on HBV–HDV coinfection treatment. No NAs have demonstrated efficacy against HDV.[10]

Coinfection with Human Immunodeficiency Virus

In HIV-coinfected patients, therapy should be tailored specifically to the patient. Initiation of highly active antiretroviral therapy (HAART) in patients with cirrhosis is strongly recommended as it may improve overall survival. If the patient is being treated for HIV, certain regimens may be optimized to include drugs with efficacy against HBV, including tenofovir, emtricitabine, or lamivudine. [14]

Pediatric Patients

Although the majority of chronic HBV patients are adults, children may be treated. Lamivudine is indicated for children 2 years and older and IFN is approved for use in children 1 year and older. Entecavir is approved for children 2 years and older and adefovir for children 12 years and older. Tenofovir is approved for children 12 and older although for HIV, tenofovir may be used in children 3 years and older. Although peg-IFN-alfa does have indications for children 3 years and older, the approval is for the use in chronic hepatitis C infections.

Pregnant Females

Perinatal transmission of HBV is a major cause of chronic HBV. To prevent mother-to-child transmission, the use of lamivudine or telbivudine in the third trimester is recommended for women. Tenofovir is an alternative.[13]

Immunosuppressive or Cytotoxic Therapy

8 Patients who will undergo chemotherapy or immunosuppressive therapy should be assessed for risk of HBV. The American Gastroenterological Association publishes guidelines on antiviral prophylaxis.[26] According to their recommendations, patients who should receive antiviral prophylaxis because they are at high risk of HBV reaction are (1) HBsAg-positive or negative and anti-HBc-positive and undergoing B-cell depleting agents such as rituximab; (2) HBsAg-positive and anti-HBc-positive treated with anthracycline derivatives such as doxorubicin; (3) HBsAg-positive and anti-HBc-positive undergoing 10 to 20 mg prednisone daily or equivalent therapy or on high-dose (>20 mg prednisone daily or equivalent) corticosteroids for 4 weeks or more. Due to moderate risks of reactivation, other immunosuppressive therapies such as tumor necrosis factor alpha inhibitors, cytokine or integrin inhibitors, tyrosine kinase inhibitors, and corticosteroids are also identified as requiring antiviral prophylaxis in patients with specific HBV serological results.[26,27] The CDC recommends testing for hepatitis B for all patients who are to receive chemotherapy or other immunosuppressive agents.

8 Prophylactic therapy is recommended prior to initiation of cancer chemotherapy or immunosuppressive therapy. Patients who have undetectable HBV DNA and who are expected to be on treatment for 1 year or less should be treated for 6 months after completion of chemotherapy or immunosuppressive therapy.[27]

Resistance Concerns

Current guidelines favor the use of potent agents with low rates of resistance. Resistance potential in HBV is evaluated by an antiviral agent's genetic barrier to resistance, or the number of primary mutations needed for antiviral drug resistance to occur. Other factors include cross-resistance and drug potency. Viral suppression is important because the HBV virus requires ongoing viral replication in the setting of antiviral drug pressure to mutate. HBV therapy can be cost-prohibitive for many patients and can favor the use of lamivudine. Unfortunately lamivudine-based therapies are prone to resistance and may have long-term implications on viral activity, notably the concerns for development of vaccine-resistant mutants.[12,21]

Hepatitis B Virus Mutations

Although a DNA virus, HBV uses reverse transcriptase, similar to a retrovirus such as HIV. The similarities between HIV reverse transcriptase and HBV polymerase prompted the development of NAs for the treatment of HBV. IFN-based therapies, because they are immune-modulating and not directly antiviral, are not associated with resistance. However, long-term therapy with the NAs is problematic because of the high likelihood of developing HBV viral resistance given HBV's high replication rate and an estimated $10^{10\text{-}12}$ mutations generated daily.[10] In addition, HBV can archive drug-resistant mutations that allow the virus to quickly select the mutation if the antiviral agent is reintroduced. Cross-resistance amongst antiviral agents also occurs, further limiting therapeutic options. Lamivudine is most associated with resistance due to (1) its low barrier for developing resistance with a single mutation able to overcome the agent combined with (2) widespread use of lamivudine in some regions.[10]

Resistance to the NA agents occurs by alteration of the active site of the HBV DNA polymerase. Long-term use of lamivudine is associated with resistance mutations of this active site.[28] The incidence of lamivudine resistance increases with each subsequent year of therapy and may be associated with a more severe disease progression.[14] Cross-resistance occurs with HBV polymerase mutations to lamivudine also affecting telbivudine.[28] Other mutations include resistance to adefovir and entecavir. Based on clinical studies of NAs with up to 6 years of follow-up, patients on entecavir and tenofovir were the least likely to develop resistance.[21] As a result, both entecavir and tenofovir are the preferred first-line agents for HBV. The optimal management of patients with resistant HBV is not clear.

Another major factor in resistance is patient adherence to therapy. Studies on adherence suggest suboptimal adherence is common with approximately 40% of patients missing doses.[29] Moreover, in patients experiencing virologic breakthrough, studies have shown that 40% of cases were not related to antiviral drug resistance, emphasizing the impact of medication adherence on viral suppression.[30]

Personalized Pharmacotherapy

Vaccination for HBV is less effective than for HAV and requires multiple doses for improved response. Several host factors are implicated in a reduced response. Patients who are immunocompromised and patients on hemodialysis may require additional doses to induce antibody response. Some patients may require repeat vaccination.[31] Sleep deprivation may also contribute to decreased antibody response.[32]

HEPATITIS C

In the United States, approximately 3.2 million people are chronically infected with HCV.[1] HCV is approximately 5 times as common as HIV and is responsible for an estimated 10,000 chronic liver disease–associated deaths per year.[1] Most acute infections are asymptomatic and the course of the infection is insidious. As a result, many patients are not diagnosed until significant disease progression. Today's HCV disease burden is associated to the high numbers of patients infected in the 1980s. HCV was not easily identified and testing for the virus was not commonly implemented until the early 1990s. Historically, HCV treatment was plagued by significant side effects and profound laboratory abnormalities. Beginning in late 2013, HCV therapies evolved dramatically with all-oral regimens that are curative in the overwhelming majority of patients.

Epidemiology

HCV is the most common blood-borne pathogen. Since 2010, the number of acute HCV cases increased by over 151%, due to both improved surveillance and increase in incidence. There were 29,718 new HCV infections in 2013, primarily among young, white persons, living in nonurban areas, with a history of injection and opioid agonist use.[2] Since 2007, the number of deaths attributable to HCV exceeded the number of deaths due to HIV.[2,33] Considering that HCV infection is prevalent in high-risk populations such as prisoners, injection drug users (IDUs), and the homeless, and that this population is generally excluded from most surveys, the actual number of chronically infected people is significantly higher. Estimates vary, but approximately 45% to 85% of infected people may not be identified.[1,33,34] 9 10 The impact of undiagnosed and untreated HCV is expected to increase dramatically over the next 40 to 50 years with 1.76 million persons developing cirrhosis, 400,000 developing HCC, and 1 million persons dying from HCV-associated complications.[35] 10 Since 2013, the number of HCV-related deaths among adults between ages 55 and 64 years continues to increase. Targeted testing for HCV of persons born between 1945 and 1965, a recommendation by the CDC and the United States Prevention Services Task Force (USPSTF), attempts to address this rising epidemic.[36]

Transmission of HCV occurs through percutaneous exposure.[37] Injection-drug use is a major factor in the cycle of HCV transmission and the most common reason for new infections. In Indiana in 2015, an outbreak of 135 new cases of HIV among PWIDs identified coinfection with HCV in over 84% of patients.[38] Some experts also consider other illicit drug use, for example, intranasal cocaine, as a risk factor because of the possible contamination of drug paraphernalia not limited to syringes and needles. Unsafe injection practices are associated with HCV transmission and include tattoos received in a nonregulated setting and needle stick injuries. Less common routes of transmission include sexual transmission in particular among HIV-positive MSM and infants born to HCV-infected women. No specific sexual practices are associated with an increased risk of transmission.[39] Although sexual contact is considered an inefficient means of HCV transmission, multiple sexual partners and coinfection with sexually transmitted diseases, including HIV, increase the risk for HCV sexual transmission. Historically, blood transfusion posed a major risk for infection. Improved screening of blood in 1992 decreased the risk of transfusion-related HCV.[37] Healthcare-associated transmission is rare; however, unsafe injection practices as often identified as the cause of HCV transmission.

Although acute HCV infections are often not recognized and many progress to chronic infections, routine screening for infection is not recommended. The AASLD, in conjunction with the Infectious Diseases Society of America (IDSA) and the International Antiviral Society-USA (IAS-USA), publish on-line guidelines for testing, managing, and treating HCV (see www.hcvguidelines.org).[37] 9 In 2012, the CDC released recommendations to perform a one-time screening of all patients born between 1945 and 1965.[36] The recommendation was made due to the high rates of HCV in this birth cohort. The CDC estimates approximately 75% of adults with HCV were born in that age range.[36] Screening is also warranted in patients who are at high risk for infection, especially among PWIDs or who have a history of injection drug use (Table 40-11).[37] The risk of infection from other needle-borne exposures, such as tattooing and body piercing, is unclear and at this time not an indication for routine screening for HCV.[37]

The initial test for HCV infection is the anti-HCV or antibody test (Table 40-12). Patients who are antibody positive for HCV require confirmatory testing for HCV RNA to verify current HCV infection. Patients who are anti-HCV positive but who do not have a detectable HCV RNA do not have a current HCV infection and no further workup is required in the majority of cases.[40] Furthermore, it is important that the presence of antibody does not infer immunity and patients are at risk for HCV infection should they be reexposed.[41]

TABLE 40-11 Recommendations for Hepatitis C Virus Screening

Anyone born between 1945 and 1965
Current or past use of injection drug use
Coinfection with HIV
Received blood transfusions or organ transplantations before 1992
Received clotting factors before 1987
Patients who have ever been on hemodialysis
Patients with unexplained elevated ALT levels or evidence of liver disease
Healthcare and public safety workers after a needle-stick or mucosal exposure to HCV-positive blood
Children born to HCV-positive mothers
Sexual partners of HCV-positive patients

ALT, alanine transaminase; HCV, hepatitis C virus; HIV, human immunodeficiency virus.

Data from reference 62.

TABLE 40-12 Interpretation of Hepatitis C Virus Test Results

	Interpretation
HCV Antibody Nonreactive	No prior exposure to HCV If suspect recent HCV infection, test for HCV RNA
HCV Antibody Reactive	Prior or current exposure to HCV, requires further evaluation
HCV Antibody Reactive HCV RNA Negative	Prior HCV infection may indicate prior resolution or prior successful treatment
HCV Antibody Reactive HCV RNA Detectable	Indicates current, active infection

HCV, hepatitis C virus; RNA, ribonucleic acid.

Data from reference 40.

Etiology

HCV is a single-stranded RNA virus notable for lacking a proofreading polymerase and enabling frequent viral mutations.[41] The virus replicates within hepatocytes and, like hepatitis B, is not directly cytopathic. HCV replicates copiously posing an immense challenge for host immune control.[41] The implications of viral mutations on direct-acting antiviral (DAA) therapy for HCV is not well understood.

HCV is differentiated into six major GTs, numbered 1 to 6. GTs are further classified into subtypes (a, b, c, etc). The most widely distributed GTs are 1 and 2, with GT1 the most common. In the United States, most infections are caused by GT1a and GT1b, followed by GT2 and GT3. Although infection caused by any of the GTs can lead to cirrhosis, end-stage liver disease (ESLD), or HCC, the significance of the infecting GT is related to therapeutic response. Historically GT1 infections were least likely to respond to therapy, but with the release of DAAs, major advances in response are now possible. GT3 continues to pose a therapeutic challenge.

Pathophysiology

In most cases, an acute HCV infection leads to chronic infection. The immune response in an acute HCV infection is mostly insufficient to eradicate the virus. HCV poses a daunting challenge for immune control because of its rapid viral diversification. HCV genomic mutations are detectable within 1 year of infection. Resolved cases of HCV are defined by a vigorous T-cell response with highly active CD8 and persistent CD4 cell response. CD8 activity mediates protective immunity but requires the aid of CD4 cells to maintain the response during viral mutations.[41]

Clinical Presentation

In an acute HCV infection, most patients are asymptomatic and undiagnosed. HCV RNA is detectable within 1 to 2 weeks of exposure and levels rise quickly during the initial weeks. Approximately one-third of adults will experience some mild and nonspecific symptoms, including fatigue, anorexia, weakness, jaundice, abdominal pain, or dark urine.[42] Acute infections rarely progress to fulminant hepatitis, although the course can be severe and prolonged. If the infection is self-limiting, symptoms last several weeks as ALT and HCV RNA levels subside. Almost all patients, including immunosuppressed patients, will develop antibodies to HCV. Typically, antibodies are not detectable until either at the time of or shortly after the development of symptoms, limiting their usefulness in diagnosing an acute infection.[37]

Up to 85% of acutely infected patients will go on to develop a chronic HCV infection, defined as persistently detectable HCV RNA for 6 months or more. HCV RNA levels and ALT levels can fluctuate and even have periods of undetectable HCV RNA and normal ALTs. Most patients will have few, if any, symptoms. The most common symptom is persistent fatigue. Additional symptoms include right upper quadrant pain, nausea, or poor appetite. On physical examination, hepatomegaly is usually present. With advanced disease, stigmata of liver disease are evident, such as spider nevi, splenomegaly, palmar erythema, testicular atrophy, and caput medusae. However, almost all patients with chronic HCV will have some degree of necroinflammatory disease on liver biopsy. Chronic inflammation of the liver from chronic HCV infection may result in fibrosis. Fibrosis is defined by altered hepatic perfusion creating a distorted structure and affecting normal function. Fibrosis leads to cirrhosis, although the speed of fibrosis progression can vary.

10 The development of HCV cirrhosis poses a 30% risk over 10 years for the development of ESLD, as well as a 1% to 2% risk per year of developing HCC.[34] Progression to cirrhosis is the primary concern in patients infected with HCV for two decades or longer. Disease progression is not uniform or linear, making it difficult to identify which patients will have progressive liver damage and when. Other concomitant viral infections, comorbidities, and lifestyle factors can contribute to disease progression. On-going alcohol use, obesity, and metabolic syndrome can potentiate fibrosis.[37] Viral load is not a factor for disease progression and not associated with degree of fibrosis. Coinfection with HIV or HBV is associated with disease progression as is infection with HCV GT3.[37,43]

10 Although HCV is thought of as a liver disease, HCV is associated with extrahepatic manifestations, or HCV-associated systemic disease. The most common is cryoglobulinemia, a local deposition of immune complexes that cause vasculitis.[37] Typical manifestations involve the skin and internal organ damage, predominantly affecting the kidneys and associated with worsening renal function. Other systemic diseases associated with HCV include cardiovascular disease, diabetes, B-cell non-Hodgkin lymphoma, Sjögren syndrome, glomerulonephritis, arthritis, corneal ulcers, thyroid disease, neuropathies, and skin diseases such as vasculitis, porphyria cutanea tarda, and lichen planus.[44]

9 For many patients, a diagnosis of hepatitis C is incidental. Unfortunately, those patients who present with symptoms typically have advanced disease. Due to the profound morbidity and mortality associated with HCV, the overall lack of awareness of the HCV epidemic, and the advances in treatment, the CDC recommends testing for HCV for anyone born between 1945 and 1965.[36] Early diagnosis and treatment can prevent liver damage, cirrhosis, HCC, and death. The U.S. Preventative Task Force joined the CDC to recommend screening of HCV in the birth cohort and among high-risk individuals.[45]

TREATMENT

Desired Outcomes

11 The primary goal of therapy is to eradicate HCV infection. Virologic cure, or sustained virologic response (SVR), is defined as a nondetectable HCV RNA at least 12 weeks after completing HCV therapy. The definition of SVR changed as prior to the release of the DAAs, SVR was defined as nondetectable HCV RNA 24 weeks after completing treatment. Patients who achieve SVR will continue to have detectable HCV antibody, though this does not imply HCV immunity. Resolving the infection prevents the development of chronic HCV infection sequelae including ESLD, HCC, and death. Patients with extrahepatic manifestations of HCV are expected to benefit with reductions in symptoms and disease severity of their extrahepatic disease while experiencing improvements in quality of life measures.[37] As more patients are cured, the risk of transmission is expected to decline and reduce the long-term HCV disease prevalence.[37]

General Approach to Treatment

Although treatment for HCV is recommended for all HCV-infected persons, patients with advanced fibrosis, compensated cirrhosis, liver transplant recipients, and patients with severe extrahepatic HCV are recommended for urgent treatment.[37] Patients with fibrosis, HIV-HCV coinfection, HBV-HCV coinfection, other coexisting liver disease, debilitating fatigue, diabetes mellitus, and porphyria cutanea tarda are listed as high priority of treatment because of high risk for developing HCV complications. Importantly, there are no longer any clearly identified contraindications for HCV therapy. In some patients at high risk of transmitting HCV, HCV treatment may help reduce rates of HCV transmission.[37]

Before therapy is initiated, quantitative HCV testing and genotyping are performed. Quantitative amplification assays for HCV RNA are performed to confirm chronic HCV infection, can serve to identify candidates for a shortened duration of therapy, and are used to monitor virologic response once therapy is initiated. Genotyping is also necessary because duration of therapy varies depending on the infecting GT. An assessment of underlying liver disease is necessary to guide treatment options because the need for ribavirin and duration of therapy varies depending on the infecting GT. Although biopsy was previously recommended, less invasive tests can be used to stage liver disease. The less invasive tests include the use of routine tests and direct serum biomarkers and transient liver elastography. Moreover, the aspartate aminotransferase-to-platelet ratio index (also known as the APRI) or fibrosis-4 index can help identify patients with advanced fibrosis or cirrhosis.[37]

Nonpharmacologic Therapy

All chronic HCV patients should be vaccinated against hepatitis A and B. Lifestyle changes are an important factor in reducing health consequences in hepatitis C. Continued alcohol use is a known risk factor for disease progression and severity. There is no established lower limit of alcohol consumption at which disease progression is not seen. Obesity is also a factor and patients should be encouraged to eat a balanced diet and exercise regularly to maintain a normal weight. Progression of fibrotic changes is associated with obesity. Smoking may also contribute to disease progression. Marijuana smoking, especially daily use, is a risk factor for progression of liver disease in patients with HCV.[46,47] The use of herbal therapy is ineffective. Patients should be counseled on minimizing HCV transmission risks.

Pharmacologic Therapy

11 The treatment of chronic HCV was revolutionized with the approval of DAAs. Previously the treatment backbone included the injection of peg-IFN and was associated with a substantial side-effect profile. The current standard of care for all chronic HCV infections, regardless of GT, is an all-oral regimen. Table 40-13 lists current recommended therapeutic regimens for GT1 treatment-naïve patients. Current guidelines suggest a 12- or 24-week duration of therapy, depending on HCV GT and subtype (1a vs 1b). The need for concomitant ribavirin use varies. Patients who are treatment-experienced, in whom prior peg-IFN and ribavirin therapy failed, and who have cirrhosis may require either a longer treatment duration or the addition of ribavirin. There are few recommendations for patients who previously failed a protease inhibitor and the management of patients who failed DAAs is even less well understood. Table 40-14 provides a comparison of the DAAs.

Clinical **Controversy...**

Due in part to the high number of patients with HCV and the high cost of the medications, access to HCV therapies is often reserved for patients with more advanced liver disease. Patients with cirrhosis, however, often are more difficult to treat and may have lower SVR rates.

Ombitasvir/Paritaprevir/Ritonavir and/or Dasabuvir

The combination of ombitasvir/paritaprevir/ritonavir and dasabuvir is approved for HCV GT1 infections. Ritonavir does not have activity against HCV but is used to pharmacologically boost paritaprevir. The treatment duration and need for concomitant ribavirin use varies depends on the infecting HCV subtype. Patients with HCV GT1a require the use of ribavirin and for patients with HCV GT1a and cirrhosis, treatment includes ribavirin and is extended to 24 weeks. The need for ribavirin in HCV GT1a infections was demonstrated in the *PEARL-IV* study which found a lower SVR in patients who did not receive ribavirin at 90.2% versus 97% in patients who did receive ribavirin.[48] The *Turquoise-II* study demonstrated an improved SVR among patients treated for 24 weeks versus 12 weeks (94.2% vs 88.6%, respectively).[49] In contrast, patients without cirrhosis who had HCV GT1b infections were able to achieve high SVR with or without ribavirin, 99.5% versus 99%, in the *PEARL-III* study.[48] For HCV1b infections and underlying cirrhosis, the use of ribavirin is recommended, however, there does not seem to be any additional improvements in SVR by extending the duration of therapy from 12 to 24 weeks.[49,50]

The combination of ombitasvir/paritaprevir/ritonavir and ribavirin is approved for HCV GT4 infections. Unlike for HCV GT1, dasabuvir is not required for GT4 and thus the combination is packaged separately. The effectiveness of the regimen was studied in the PEARL-1 study, which showed SVR of 100% in patients treated with ribavirin, compared with 90.9% in patients without ribavirin.[51]

Overall, ombitasvir/paritaprevir/ritonavir with or without dasabuvir is well tolerated and has few laboratory abnormalities. Although ombitasvir/paritaprevir/ritonavir and dasabuvir can be used in cirrhosis, its use is limited to Child Turcotte Pugh Class A

TABLE 40-13 AASLD/IDSA Recommended Treatment Regimens for Treatment-Naïve Patients with Hepatitis C (in order of evidence, then alphabetically)

HCV Genotype	No Cirrhosis	Compensated Cirrhosis (CTP Class A)
1a	Elbasvir/Grazoprevir × 12 weeks* Ledipasvir/Sofosbuvir × 12 weeks Ombitasvir/Paritaprevir/ritonavir + Dasabuvir and ribavirin × 12 weeks Simeprevir + Sofosbuvir × 12 weeks Sofosbuvir/Velpatasvir × 12 weeks Daclatasvir + Sofosbuvir × 12 weeks	Elbasvir/Grazoprevir × 12 weeks* Ledipasvir/Sofosbuvir × 12 weeks Sofosbuvir/Velpatasvir × 12 weeks
1b	Elbasvir/Grazoprevir × 12 weeks Ledipasvir/Sofosbuvir × 12 weeks Ombitasvir/Paritaprevir/ritonavir + Dasabuvir and ribavirin × 12 weeks Simeprevir + Sofosbuvir × 12 weeks Sofosbuvir/Velpatasvir × 12 weeks Daclatasvir plus Sofosbuvir × 12 weeks	Elbasvir/Grazoprevir × 12 weeks Ledipasvir/Sofosbuvir × 12 weeks Ombitasvir/Paritaprevir/ritonavir + Dasabuvir and ribavirin × 12 weeks Sofosbuvir/Velpatasvir × 12 weeks
2	Sofosbuvir/Velpatasvir × 12 weeks	Sofosbuvir/Velpatasvir × 12 weeks
3	Daclatasvir + Sofosbuvir × 12 weeks Sofosbuvir/Velpatasvir × 12 weeks	Sofosbuvir/Velpatasvir × 12 weeks^ Daclatasvir + Sofosbuvir × 12 weeks^

CTP: Child Turcotte Pugh

*If no NS5A resistance detected; ^Pretreatment resistance testing recommended

Data from reference 37.

TABLE 40-14 Comparison of HCV Direct Acting Antivirals

Therapy	Component Drugs (Class)	Adult Dose	Use in Cirrhosis	Use in Renal Insufficiency	Adverse Effects	Comments
Harvoni®	90 mg ledipasvir (NS5A) with 400 mg sofosbuvir (NS5B)	1 tablet daily	Ok for use in all levels of liver disease	Not recommended	Headache, fatigue	Approved for HCV GT1, 4
Epclusa®	150 mg velpatasvir (NS5A) with 400 mg sofosbuvir (NS5B)	1 tablet daily	Ok for use in all levels of liver disease	Not recommended	Headache, fatigue	Approved for HCV GT1-6
Viekira Pak®	Pak contains: 2 tablets containing 12.5 mg ombitasvir (NS5A), 75 mg paritaprevir (NS3/4A) plus 50 mg ritonavir and 1 tablet with 250 mg dasabuvir (NS5B)	2 tablets once daily of combination and 1 dasabuvir tablet twice daily	Contraindicated in CTP Class B or C	Not recommended	Nausea, pruritus, insomnia	Approved for HCV GT1
Viekira XR®	Each tablet contains 200 mg dasabuvir (NS5B), 8.33 mg ombitasvir (NS5A), 50 mg paritaprevir (NS3/4A), and 33.3 mg ritonavir	3 tablets once daily	Contraindicated in CTP Class B or C	Not recommended	Nausea, pruritus, insomnia	Approved for HCV GT1
Zepatier®	50 mg elbasvir (NS5A) with 100 mg grazoprevir (NS3/4A)	1 tablet daily	Contraindicated in CTP Class B or C	Approved for use in all levels of renal insufficiency including hemodialysis	Fatigue, headache, nausea	Approved for HCV GT1 and 4; patients with HCV GT1a require baseline resistance testing
Daklinza®	60 mg daclatasvir (also available as 30 mg and 90 mg)	1 tablet daily	Ok for use in all levels of liver disease	Due to combined use with sofosbuvir, not recommended	Headache, fatigue	Approved for use with sofosbuvir; monotherapy not effective
Sovaldi®	400 mg sofosbuvir	1 tablet daily	Ok for use in all levels of liver disease	Not recommended	Headache, fatigue	As single agent, must be combined with another DAA; monotherapy not effective

CTP: Child Turcotte Pugh; DAA: direct acting antivirial; GT: genotype

cirrhosis as it is contraindicated in Class B and C cirrhosis. Patients must discontinue any ethinyl estradiol-containing medications prior to starting therapy with ombitasvir/paritaprevir/ritonavir because of expected elevations in ALT. The concomitant use of ribavirin adds side effects and is expected to exacerbate fatigue and skin reactions, as well as require more frequent laboratory monitoring. The use of ritonavir as a pharmacological booster adds additional drug-drug interaction concerns.

Sofosbuvir

Sofosbuvir was approved in 2013 for HCV GT1-4. Its use in GT1 and 4 was supplanted by the combination of ledipasvir/sofosbuvir which allowed for an IFN-free treatment. For HCV GT2, sofosbuvir in combination with ribavirin is highly effective and was the first all-oral, IFN-free HCV drug regimen available in the United States. Treatment duration is 12 weeks, however, a 16-week course of therapy is recommended in patients with cirrhosis.[37] The use of sofosbuvir for the treatment of HCV GT3 with ribavirin was effective although at substantially reduced SVR as compared to the treatment efficacy seen in other GTs. The preferred, most effective therapy for GT3 combines sofosbuvir and daclatasvir with or without ribavirin.[37] Sofosbuvir is well tolerated and has few drug-drug interactions. Symptomatic bradycardia was identified in patients treated with sofosbuvir and taking amiodarone in combination with other DAAs, thus this combination is not recommended.

Ledipasvir/Sofosbuvir

The fixed dose combination tablet of ledipasvir/sofosbuvir is approved for use in patients with HCV GT1. Ledipasvir is only available in combination with sofosbuvir. There are no differences in treatment whether patients have GT1a, 1b, or 4, however, there are differences in treatment duration depending on underlying cirrhosis.[52,53] Treatment-naïve patients with or without cirrhosis are recommended for a 12-week course of treatment; moreover, patients who are treatment-naïve and noncirrhotic who have a baseline viral load of less than 6 million IU/mL (6×10^9 IU/L)may be considered for an 8-week course of treatment with similar SVR as patients treated for 12 weeks (94% vs 95% SVR).[37,54] The use of ribavirin did not affect SVR rates and is not routinely recommended. In patients with underlying cirrhosis, ledipasvir/sofosbuvir is approved for 24 weeks of treatment, however, based on preliminary results of a multicenter study, the addition of ribavirin to ledipasvir/sofosbuvir allows for a 12-week course of therapy and is recommended by national guidelines.[37,55] National guidelines also recognize the use and efficacy of ledipasvir/sofosbuvir for treatment of HCV GT4 for a 12-week course of therapy.[37]

The combination of ledipasvir/sofosbuvir is well tolerated and can be used in patients with cirrhosis, including Child-Turcotte Pugh (CTP) Class A, B, and C cirrhosis. Its use in patients with renal insufficiency is limited to patients with an estimated glomerular filtration rate no less than 30 mL/min/1.73m^2. Headache and fatigue have been reported as side effects. Laboratory abnormalities are not frequently encountered. The drug-drug interaction potential is also limited although amiodarone use is not recommended because of the symptomatic bradycardia observed with the concomitant use of sofosbuvir, amiodarone, and other DAAs. Acid suppressive therapy poses a challenge to treatment because ledipasvir requires an acidic environment for absorption.

Daclatasvir

Daclatasvir is approved for use with sofosbuvir for HCV GT 1 and 3. It does have activity for other GTs. In both treatment-naïve and treatment-experienced patients with GT3, the combination was highly effective. In noncirrhotic patients the SVR was 96%.[56] The combination is recommended by national guidelines for a planned duration of therapy of 12 weeks.[37]

Daclatasvir is well tolerated. There are no dosing adjustments for renal or hepatic impairment. Daclatasvir is subject to various drug-drug interactions. Because it is used with sofosbuvir, it is also subject to warnings regarding serious bradycardia when co-administered with amiodarone. Daclatasvir is the first DAA available in varying dosage strengths: 30, 60, and 90 mg. The option to alter the strength allows for use with concomitant medications known or suspected affecting daclatasvir concentrations. The 30-mg strength allows for dosing in the presence of strong CYP3A inhibitors expected to increase the concentration of daclatasvir while the combined strength of 90 mg allows for use in the presence of moderate CYP3A inducers which would otherwise decrease daclatasvir concentrations.

Simeprevir

Simeprevir is a second-generation NS3/4A protease inhibitor. Simeprevir may be used in combination with sofosbuvir for treatment of HCV GT1. Increasingly, though, simeprevir's main role in therapy is in the retreatment of patients who failed DAA therapy. In these cases, HCV resistance testing is done prior to selecting the optimal retreatment strategy.

Sofosbuvir/Velpatasvir

Sofosbuvir/velpatasvir is the only HCV combination approved for use in HCV GT1-6. From the ASTRAL studies 99% SVR was achieved with sofobuvir/velpatasvir in patients with HCV GT1, 2, 4, 5, and 6, irrespective of prior treatment experience or whether patients had cirrhosis or not.[57] The combination was superior to sofosbuvir and ribavirin in achieving SVR for GT2 or 3.[58] In GT3 patients, pre-treatment resistance testing is recommended for any patients with cirrhosis or prior treatment experience and if a specific mutation is detected, ribavirin should be added.[37] Sofosbuvir/velpatasvir was well tolerated with few side effects or laboratory abnormalities. In a comparison of 12 weeks of sofosbuvir/velpatasvir with or without ribavirin in patients with HCV GT1, 2, 3, 4, or 6 and decompensated liver disease SVR was highest (94%) in patients treated with sofosbuvir/velpatasvir and ribavirin.[59] Most patients demonstrated an improvement in their liver disease as a result of treatment. Velpatasvir requires an acidic environment for absorption thus it is essential that patients are appropriately counseled to avoid the use of acid suppressive therapy while on sofosbuvir/velpatasvir.

Elbasvir/Grazoprevir

Elbasvir/grazoprevir is approved for use in patients with HCV GT1 and 4. In the C-EDGE study of treatment naïve patients with HCV GTs 1, 4, and 6, the overall SVR rate was 95%.[60] Among patients with HCV GT1a, SVR rates were lower than for GT1b and this difference was attributed to the presence of baseline resistance associated variants (RAVs). When comparing patients with GT1a vs 1b who did not have any RAVs, there was no difference in SVR (99 vs 100% SVR, respectively). However, for patients with baseline RAVs and GT1a, the SVR rated dropped to 58%. As a result, in patients with HCV GT1a pre-treatment resistance testing is required. If specific mutations are identified, patients can still be treated with elbasvir/grazoprevir but will require a 16-week course of therapy and the addition of ribavirin.[61] Elbasvir/grazoprevir is approved for use in patients with renal insufficiency including hemodialysis and demonstrated high SVR rates at 94%.[62]

Ribavirin

Ribavirin continues to be used in combination with DAAs, especially in difficult to treat patients such as those with prior treatment experience or with underlying cirrhosis. The mechanism of action of ribavirin is not well understood. Ribavirin is a synthetic guanosine analog and is ineffective as a monotherapy for HCV. The most common side effect of ribavirin is hemolytic anemia, necessitating close monitoring during HCV therapy. In addition, ribavirin is a teratogenic agent, Pregnancy Category X, and women of childbearing age as well as female partners of male patients who undergo HCV treatment with ribavirin need to practice two forms of contraception during HCV treatment and for 6 months after to avoid pregnancy.[37]

Special Populations

Clinical trials are conducted with a patient population that generally does not reflect the patient spectrum encountered in clinical practice. There are no contraindications to the treatment of PWIDs, prisoners, persons with substance abuse issues, or persons with psychiatric disorders. The sheer number of patients with HCV poses a challenge to access to treatment. Moreover, the costs of the medications are high, resulting in variable access to therapies.

Published recommendations for treatment in various populations are as follows.

Patients with Decompensated Cirrhosis

The presence of cirrhosis poses a substantial challenge in achieving SVR. Furthermore, the level of underlying cirrhosis limits the use of the DAAs. Patients with CTP Class B or C cirrhosis with decompensated cirrhosis are generally recommended to receive care from medical practitioners with expertise managing that level of liver disease. No dose adjustments for hepatic impairment are needed for ledipasvir/sofosbuvir, sofosbuvir, or daclatasvir. In contrast, ombitasvir/paritaprevir/ritonavir with or without dasabuvir or sofocbuvir/velpatasvir is contraindicated in CTP Class B or C.

Clinical **Controversy...**

Although HCV courses of therapy are predetermined, most patients receive medications in 4-week increments. Any delays in receipt of therapy risk the development of HCV resistance. Patients who develop resistance have very limited options for subsequent therapy. The impact of HCV DAA resistance will likely become increasingly important in HCV management. Although pretreatment-resistance testing is not currently recommended for most patients, resistance testing may be indicated for some treatment-experienced patients who failed therapy with DAAs.

Treatment-Experienced Patients

Patients do not have cirrhosis and who failed a previous course of peg-IFN and ribavirin can be retreated similarly to treatment-naïve patients. Patients who are treatment-experienced and have cirrhosis require either an extended duration of therapy or the addition of ribavirin, or both. There are limited data on the retreatment of patients who failed a prior course of therapy with the DAAs; however, the strategy of adding ribavirin and/or extending the treatment duration is recommended.[37] Additionally, most patients who failed DAA therapy require resistance testing.

Acute Exposures

Up to 50% of patients will spontaneously clear an HCV infection and the majority will do so within the first 6 months of exposure.[63] As a result, it is reasonable to defer HCV treatment for 6 months.[37] Once the decision is made to treat, the same regimens used for chronic HCV infections are recommended.[37]

Persons Who Inject Drugs

IDU is not a contraindication to therapy and treatment of PWIDs will be necessary to reduce HCV transmission.[64] Treatment of

PWIDs is recommended as part of a comprehensive harm-reduction effort, ideally in a multidisciplinary setting.[37,64] Studies in PWIDs suggest treatment outcomes are comparable to rates in non-IDU and reinfection rates among PWID are low.[65] However, access to HCV therapies is limited as many insurers refuse coverage of HCV therapies in the setting of active drug use.

Alcoholism

Because continued alcohol use affects disease progression and severity and thus response to therapy, the cessation of alcohol use during therapy is recommended. Moreover, a period of abstinence before initiation of therapy is also recommended.

End-Stage Renal Disease

Elbasvir/grazoprevir is currently the only HCV therapy approved for use in renal insufficiency, including hemodialysis.

HIV Coinfection

Current guidelines do not distinguish separate treatment recommendations for HIV–HCV coinfection; however, potential drug-drug interaction concerns between DAAs and HIV antivirals do merit careful scrutiny and may necessitate antiretroviral drug changes.[37] An important resource for screening of drug-drug interactions with DAAs is the University of Liverpool Web site—www.hep-druginteractions.org. Sofosbuvir has few clinically significant drug-drug interactions. Daclatasvir has potential for some drug-drug interactions; however, the option to adjust the dose of daclatasvir may mitigate the clinical significance of the interactions. Ledipasvir and velpatasvir increase tenofovir levels and may increase the risk of tenofovir-associated renal toxicity. The combination of ombitasvir/paritaprevir/ritonavir and dasabuvir includes ritonavir as a pharmacological booster; therefore HIV antiretrovirals which use ritonavir are not recommended or require dosing without ritonavir. Additional drug-drug interactions exist which may require changes in HIV antivirals. Treatment poses additional problems because of hepatotoxicity issues associated with HAART, hepatic complications from HIV-associated diseases, as well as flares in hepatitis as CD4 counts recover. The prognosis for an SVR is worse than in patients infected with HCV only. In general, treatment is recommended and both HIV and HCV therapies can be coadministered with the exception of didanosine and zidovudine. The combination of ribavirin and didanosine can result in fatal lactic acidosis. Ribavirin causes hemolytic anemia and when combined with zidovudine can result in severe anemia.

Children

Peg-IFN-alfa and ribavirin are approved in children however, due to concerns for use of peg-IFN and ribavirin in this population, and because children with chronic HCV often have mild liver disease, therapy is often deferred. The DAAs are approved in adults 18 and older.

Liver Transplant

Viral eradication prior to transplant is a goal for patients undergoing transplantation as it is associated with improved patient and graft survival. Viral suppression for at least 28 days prior to transplantation was associated with SVR. Among patients who are treated post-transplant, there are some drug-drug interaction concerns which may require increased monitoring and immunosuppressant dosing adjustments.

Prevention

No vaccine is available for HCV. It is unlikely that a vaccine will be developed in the near future because of the mutagenesis of the virus. Patients infected with HCV should be counseled on not being blood, organ, or semen donors. Although the likelihood of household transmission is small, patients should minimize risks by avoiding possible blood or mucus exposure, such as not sharing razors or toothbrushes and covering open wounds. Patients who continue to use illegal drugs should avoid sharing all drug paraphernalia, as risk of transmission is not limited to needles and syringes.

PERSONALIZED PHARMACOTHERAPY

It is currently not possible to definitively identify patients at risk for disease progression. Several factors may correlate with a decreased risk for chronicity and include host, virus, and environmental factors. Important host factors that minimize the risk of developing chronic infection include being younger than 40 years, female, non-black, not immunosuppressed, and with a symptomatic acute HCV infection. Being older than 20 years at infection triples the risk for chronic HCV. Blacks, especially black men, are more likely to develop chronic infection and have lower treatment responses.[63] Becoming symptomatic and having jaundice is associated with a lower likelihood of chronic infection, perhaps correlating to a stronger immune response to the acute infection. Finally, immunosuppressed patients, such as those with HIV, are more prone to chronic infection, although they are not inherently unable to clear the infection.[63] Similarly, disease progression is associated with increased age, male sex, continued alcohol intake, obesity, and HIV coinfection. Diabetes, as well as steatosis, may also potentiate fibrosis progression.[37]

Variation on a gene encoding for endogenous IFN, interleukin (IL) 28, has been described that is associated with a difference in response to treatment and may explain differences in response between patients of African American and European ancestry.[66] Patients who have the CC GT have higher rates of spontaneous clearance and higher rates of cure than patients who have IL GT CT or TT.[66] The DAA therapies have largely overcome the role of IL28 although this marker continues to be used in clinical studies.

Ribavirin-induced anemia can affect dosing strategies and is likely related to polymorphisms of the *ITPA* gene. The exact mechanism is not fully understood and the clinical relevance is not clear.

The use of IFN-based therapies targeting the host immune system's capacity to eradicate HCV minimized the role of HCV mutations and the potential for HCV resistance. With the approval of the DAAs, the role of resistance testing to guide treatment of HCV is expanding. Currently, baseline mutations affect patients with GT1a considering elbasvir/grazoprevir therapy. For GT3, all patients with cirrhosis or prior treatment experience require resistance testing. The impact of mutations is not well understood although combination therapies will likely be required to overcome various resistance mutations. Moreover, in order to minimize the development of resistance and optimize cure rates, it is imperative for patients to complete their HCV treatment regimens without interruptions.

ABBREVIATIONS

AASLD	American Association for the Study of Liver Diseases
ACIP	Advisory Committee on Immunization Practices
AIDS	acquired immune deficiency syndrome
ALT	alanine aminotransferase
Anti-HAV	antibody to hepatitis A virus
Anti-HBsAg	antibody to HBsAg
APRI	aminotransferase-to-platelet ratio index
CDC	Centers for Disease Control and Prevention
CTP	Child-Turcotte Pugh
CYP	cytochrome P450
DAA	direct-acting antiviral

ELISA	enzyme-linked immunosorbent assay
ESLD	end-stage liver disease
ETR	end-of-treatment response
GI	gastrointestinal
GT	genotype
HAART	highly active antiretroviral therapy
HAV	hepatitis A virus
HBcAg	hepatitis B core antigen
HBeAg	hepatitis B e antigen
HBsAg	hepatitis B surface antigen
HBV	hepatitis B virus
HCC	hepatocellular carcinoma
HCV	hepatitis C virus
HIV	human immunodeficiency virus
IAS-USA	International Antiviral Society-USA
IDSA	Infectious Diseases Society of America
IDU	injection drug users
IFN	interferon
Ig	immunoglobulin
IL	interleukin
IM	intramuscular
IV	intravenous
MSM	men who have sex with men
NAs	nucleos(t)ide analogs
OSHA	Occupational Safety and Health Administration
peg-IFN	pegylated interferon
PI	protease inhibitor
PWID	persons who inject drugs
SVR	sustained virologic response
USPSTF	United States Preventative Services Task Force
WHO	World Health Organization

REFERENCES

1. IOM (Institute of Medicine). *Hepatitis and Liver Cancer: A National Strategy for Prevention and Control of Hepatitis B and C.* Washington, DC; The National Academic Press: 2010.
2. Centers for Disease Control and Prevention. Viral Hepatitis Statistics and Surveillance—United States. 2013, Available at: http://www.cdc.gov/hepatitis/statistics/2013surveillance/index.htm. Accessed Sept. 1, 2015.
3. Workowski KA, Berman S; Centers for Disease Control and Prevention (CDC). Sexually transmitted diseases treatment guidelines, 2010. *MMWR Recomm Rep* 2010;59(RR-12):1-110.
4. Centers for Disease Control and Prevention. *CDC Health Information for International Travel 2014.* New York; Oxford University Press: 2014.
5. Centers for Disease Control and Prevention. Prevention of hepatitis A through active or passive immunizations: Recommendations of the Advisory Committee on Immunization Practices (ACIP). *MMWR Morb Mortal Wkly Rep* 2006;55(RR07):1-23.
6. Cuthbert JA. Hepatitis A. Old and new. *Clin Microbiol Rev* 2001;14:38-58.
7. Advisory Committee on Immunization Practices (ACIP) Centers for Disease Control and Prevention (CDC). Update: Prevention of hepatitis A after exposure to hepatitis A virus and in international travelers. Updated recommendations of the Advisory Committee on Immunization Practices (ACIP). *MMWR Morb Mortal Wkly Rep* 2007;56(41):1080-1084.
8. Jablonowska E, Kuydowicz J. Durability of response to vaccination against viral hepatitis A in HIV-infected patients: A 5-year observation. *Int J STD AIDS* 2014;25(10):745-750.
9. World Health Organization. Hepatitis B. Fact Sheet No. 204. 2015, Available at: http//www.who.int/mediacentre/factsheets/fs204/en/ Accessed Sept. 1, 2015.
10. World Health Organization. Guidelines for the prevention, care, and treatment of persons with chronic hepatitis B infection. 2015. Available at: http://apps.who.int/iris/bitstream/10665/154590/1/9789241549059_eng.pdf?ua=1&ua=1 Accessed Sept. 1, 2015.
11. Weinbaum CM, Williams I, Mast EE, et al. Centers for Disease Control and Prevention (CDC). Recommendations for identification and public health management of persons with chronic hepatitis B virus infection. *MMWR Morb Mortal Wkly Rep* 2008;57(RR-8):1-20.
12. Lapinski TW, Pogorzelska J, Flisiak R. HBV mutations and their clinical significance. *Adv Med Sci* 2012;57:18-22.
13. Liaw Y-F, Kao J-H, Piratvisuth T, et al. Asian-Pacific consensus statement on the management of chronic hepatitis B: A 2012 update. *Hepat Int* 2012;6:531-561.
14. Lok ASF, McMahon BJ. AASLD practice guidelines: Chronic hepatitis B: Update 2009. *Hepatology* 2009;50:661-662.
15. European Association for the Study of the Liver. EASL clinical practice guidelines: Management of chronic hepatitis B virus infection. *J Hepatol* 2012;57:167-185.
16. Manzano-Alonso ML, Castellano-Tortajada G. Reactivation of hepatitis B virus infection after cytotoxic chemotherapy or immunosuppressive therapy. *World J Gastroenterol* 2011;17:1531-1537.
17. Hwang JP, Vierling JM, Zelenetz AD, Lackey SC, Loomba R. Hepatitis B virus management to prevent reactivation after chemotherapy: A review. *Support Care Cancer* 2012;20:2999-3008.
18. Trichopoulos D, Bamia C, Lagiou P, et al. Hepatocellular carcinoma risk factors and disease burden in a European cohort: A nested case–control study. *J Natl Cancer Inst* 2011;103:1686-1695.
19. Koh WP, Robien K, Wang R, Govindarajan S, Yuan JM, Yu MC. Smoking as an independent risk factor for hepatocellular carcinoma: The Singapore Chinese Health Study. *Br J Cancer* 2011;105:1430-1435.
20. Zhang L, Wang G, Hou W, Li P, Dulin A, Bonkovsky HL. Contemporary clinical research of traditional Chinese medicines for chronic hepatitis B in China: An analytical review. *Hepatology* 2010;51:690-698.
21. Gish R, Jia J-D, Locarnini S, Zoulim F. Selection of chronic hepatitis B therapy with a high barrier to resistance. *Lancet Infect Dis* 2012; 12:341-354.
22. Vassiliadis TG, Giouleme O, Koumerkeridis G, et al. Adefovir plus lamivudine are more effective than adefovir alone in lamivudine-resistant HBeAg-chronic hepatitis B patients: A 4-year study. *J Gastroenterol Hepatol* 2010;25:54-60.
23. Buti M, Tsai N, Petersen J, et al. Seven-year efficacy and safety of treatment with tenofovir disoproxil fumarate for chronic hepatitis B virus infection. *Dig Dis Sci* 2015;60(5):1457-1464.
24. Lok AS, Trinh H, Carosi G, et al. Efficacy of entecavir with or without tenofovir disoproxil fumarate for nucleos(t)ide-naïve patients with chronic hepatitis B. *Gastroenterol* 2012;143:619-628.
25. Lim YS, Yoo BC, Byun KS, et al. Tenofovir monotherapy versus tenofovir and entecavir combination therapy in hepatitis B patients with multiple drug failure: results of a randomized trial. *Gut* 2015 Mar 23. doi: 10.1136/gutjnl-2014-308435. [Epub ahead of print]
26. Reddy RK, Beavers KL, Hammond SP, et al. American Gastroenterological Association Institute guideline on prevention and treatment of hepatitis B reactivation during immunosuppressive drug therapy. *Gastroenterol* 2015;148:215-219.
27. Perrillo RP, Gish R, Falck-Ytter YT. American Gastroenterological Association Institute technical review on prevention and treatment of hepatitis B virus reactivation during immunosuppressive drug therapy. *Gastroenterol* 2015;148:221-244.
28. Gupta N, Goyal M, Wu CH, Wu GY. The molecular and structural basis of HBV-resistance to nucleos(t)ide analogs. *J Clin Transl Hepatol* 2014;2:201-211.
29. Giang L, Selinger CP, Lee AU. Evaluation of adherence to oral antiviral hepatitis B treatment using structured questionnaires. *World J Hepatol* 2012;4:43-49.
30. Hongthanakorn C, Chotiyaputta W, Oberhelman K, et al. Current nucleos(t)ide analogue therapy for chronic hepatitis B. *Gut Liver* 2011;5:278-287.
31. Mast EE, Weinbaum CM, Fiore AE, et al. Advisory Committee on Immunization Practices (ACIP) Centers for Disease Control and Prevention (CDC). A comprehensive immunization strategy to eliminate transmission of hepatitis B virus infection in the United States. Recommendations of the Advisory Committee on Immunization Practices (ACIP) part II: Immunization of Adults. *MMWR Recomm Rep* 2006;55(RR-16):1-33.
32. Prather AA, Hall M, Fury JM, et al. Sleep and antibody response to hepatitis B vaccination. *Sleep* 2012;35:1063-1069.
33. Ly KN, Xing J, Klevens M, Jiles RB, Ward JW, Holmberg SD. The increasing burden of mortality from viral hepatitis in the United States between 1999 and 2007. *Ann Internal Med* 2012;156:271-278.
34. Ward J. Perspective: The hidden epidemic of hepatitis c virus in the United States: Occult transmission and burden of disease. *Top Antivir Med* 2013;21:15-19.
35. Rein DB, Wittenborn JS, Weinbaum CM, Sabin M, Smith BD, Lesesne SB. Forecasting the morbidity and mortality associated with prevalent cases of pre-cirrhotic chronic hepatitis C in the United States. *Dig Liver Dis* 2011;43:66-72.

36. Smith BD, Morgan RL, Beckett GA, et al. Centers for Disease Control and Prevention. Recommendations for the identification of chronic hepatitis C virus infection among persons born during 1945-1965. *MMWR Recomm Rep* 2012;61(RR-4):1-18.
37. AASLD/IDSA/IAS-USA. Recommendations for testing, managing, and treating hepatitis C. Available at: http://www.hcvguidelines.org. Accessed Sept. 15, 2015.
38. Conrad C, Bradley HM, Broz D, et al. Community outbreak of HIV infection linked to injection drug use of oxymorphone—Indiana, 2015. *MMWR* May 1, 2016;64(16):443-444.
39. Terrault NA, Dodge JL, Murphy EL, et al. Sexual transmission of HCV among monogamous heterosexual couples: The HCV partners study. *Hepatology* 2013;57:881-889.
40. Centers for Disease Control. Testing for HCV infection: An update of guidance for clinicians and laboratorians. *MMWR* 2013;62(18):362-365.
41. Kanto T, Hayashi N. Immunopathogenesis of hepatitis C virus infection: Multifaceted strategies subverting innate and adaptive immunity. *Intern Med* 2006;45:183-191.
42. Centers for Disease Control and Prevention. Hepatitis C FAQs for health professionals. Available at: http://www.cdc.gov/hepatitis/hcv/hcvfaq.htm Accessed Sept. 17, 2015.
43. Kanwal F, Kramer JR, Ilyas J, Duan Z, El-Serag HB. HCV genotype 3 is associated with an increased risk of cirrhosis and hepatocellular cancer in a national sample of U.S. Veterans with HCV. *Hepatology* 2014;60(1):98-105.
44. Sherman AC, Sherman KE. Extrahepatic manifestations of hepatitis C: Navigating CHASM. *Curr HIV/AIDS Rep* 2015;12(3):353-361.
45. U.S. Preventive Services Task Force. Final Update Summary: Hepatitis C: Screening. July 2015. Available at: http://www.uspreventiveservicestaskforce.org/Page/Document/UpdateSummaryFinal/hepatitis-c-screening Accessed Sept. 17, 2015.
46. Hezode C, Zafrani ES, Roudot-Thoraval F, et al. Daily cannabis use: A novel risk factor of steatosis severity in patients with chronic hepatitis C. *Gastroenterol* 2008;134:432-439.
47. Ishida JH, Peters MG, Jin C, et al. Influence of cannabis use on severity of hepatitis C disease. *Clin Gastroenterol Hepatol* 2008;6:69-75.
48. Ferenci P, Bernstein D, Lalezari J, et al. ABT-450/r-ombitasvir and dasabuvir with or without ribavirin for HCV. *N Engl J Med* 2014;370:1983-1992.
49. Poordad F, Hezode C, Trinh R, et al. ABT-450/r-ombitasvir and dasabuvir with ribavirin for hepatitis C with cirrhosis. *N Engl J Med* 2014;370:1973-1982.
50. Andreone P, Colombo MG, Enejosa JV, et al. ABT-450, ritonavir, ombitasvir and dasabuvir achieves 97% and 100% sustained virologic response with or without ribavirin in treatment-experienced patients with HCV genotype 1b infection. *Gastroenterol* 2014;147:359-365.
51. Hezode C, Asselah T, Reddy KR, et al. Ombitasvir plus paritaprevir plus ritonavir with or without ribavirin in treatment-naïve and treatment experienced patients with genotype 4 chronic hepatitis C virus infection (PEARL-1): A randomized, open-label trial. *Lancet* 2015;385:2502-2509.
52. Afdhal N, Zeuzem S, Kwo P, et al. for the ION-1 Investigators. Ledipasvir and sofosbuvir for untreated HCV genotype 1 infection. *N Engl J Med* 2014;370:1889-1898.
53. Afdhal N, Reddy KR, Nelson DR, et al. Ledipasvir and sofosbuvir for previously treated HCV genotype 1 infection. *N Engl J Med* 2014;370:1483-1493.
54. Kowdley KV, Gordon SC, Reddy KR, et al. Ledipasvir and sofosbuvir for 8 or 12 weeks for chronic HCV without cirrhosis. *N Engl J Med* 2014;370:1879-1888.
55. Flamm SL, Everson GT, Charlton M, et al. Ledipasvir/sofosbuvir with ribavirin for the treatment of HCV in patients with decompensated cirrhosis: Preliminary results of a prospective, multicenter study. 65th Annual Meeting of the American Association for the Study of Liver Diseases (AASLD). November 1-5, 2014; Boston, MA.
56. Nelson DR, Cooper JN, Lalezari JP, et al. All-oral 12-week treatment with daclatasvir plus sofosbuvir in patients with hepatitis C virus genotype 3 infection: ALLY-3 phase III study. *Hepatology* 2015;61(4):1127-1135.
57. Feld JJ, Jacobson IM, Hézode C, et al. Sofosbuvir and Velpatasvir for HCV Genotype 1, 2, 4, 5, and 6 Infection. *N Engl J Med.* 2015 Dec 31; 373(27):2599-2607.
58. Foster GR, Afdhal N, Roberts SK, et al. Sofosbuvir and Velpatasvir for HCV Genotype 2 and 3 Infection. *N Engl J Med.* 2015a Dec 31; 373(27):2608-2617.
59. Curry MP, O'Leary JG, Bzowej N, et al. Sofosbuvir and Velpatasvir for HCV in patients with Decompensated cirrhosis. NEJM 2015b: 373; 27: 2618-2628.
60. Zeuzem S, Ghalib R, Reddy KR et al. Grazoprevir-Elbasvir Combination Therapy for Treatment-Naive Cirrhotic and Noncirrhotic Patients With Chronic Hepatitis C Virus Genotype 1, 4, or 6 Infection: A Randomized Trial. *Ann Intern Med.* 2015;163(1):1-13.
61. Kwo P, Gane E, Peng C-Y, et al. P0886: Efficacy and safety of grazoprevir/elbasvir +/- RBV for 12 weeks in patients with HCV G1 or G4 infection who previously failed peginterferon/RBV: C-edge treatment-experienced trial. *J Hepatol.* 2015 Apr;62, Supplement 2: S674–S675.
62. Roth D, Nelson DR, Bruchfeld A et al. Grazoprevir plus elbasvir in treatment-naive and treatment-experienced patients with hepatitis C virus genotype 1 infection and stage 4-5 chronic kidney disease (the C-SURFER study): a combination phase 3 study. *Lancet.* 2015 Oct 17; 386(10003):1537-1545.
63. Kamal SM. Acute hepatitis C: a systematic review. *Am J Gastroenterol* 2008;103(5):1283-1297.
64. Doyle JS, Aspinall EJ, Hutchinson SJ, et al. Global policy and access to new hepatitis C therapies for people who inject drugs. *Int J Drug Policy* 2015 Jun 2. doi: 10.1016/j.drugpo.2015.05.008. [Epub ahead of print]
65. Aspinall EJ, Corson S, Doyle JS, et al. Treatment of hepatitis C virus infection among people who are actively injecting drugs: a systematic review and meta-analysis. *Clin Infect Dis* 2013;57(Suppl2):S80-S89.
66. Ge D, Fellay J, Thompson AJ, et al. Genetic variation in IL28B predicts hepatitis C treatment-induced viral clearance. *Nature* 2009;461:399-401.

Celiac Disease

41

Priti N. Patel and Robert A. Mangione

KEY CONCEPTS

1. Celiac disease is a chronic, small intestinal immune-mediated enteropathy caused by intolerance to gluten found in wheat, barley, rye, and other foods when a genetically predisposed person is exposed to the environmental trigger, gluten.
2. The prevalence of celiac disease is 0.7% in America and appears to be increasing in prevalence worldwide.
3. The integrity of the tissue junctions of the intestinal epithelium is compromised in patients with celiac disease; this enables gluten to reach the lamina propria. The presence of gluten in the lamina propria and an inherited combination of genes contribute to the heightened immune sensitivity to gluten that is found in patients with celiac disease.
4. The classic presenting symptom is diarrhea, which may be accompanied by abdominal pain or discomfort; however, it is noteworthy that during the past decade diarrhea has been reported as the main presenting symptom of celiac disease in less than 50% of cases.
5. Dermatitis herpetiformis is a skin manifestation of small intestinal immune-mediated enteropathy caused by exposure to dietary gluten.
6. The frequency of diagnosis of patients with celiac disease has increased; however, the majority of patients with this condition remain undiagnosed.
7. The confirmation of a diagnosis of celiac disease should be based on a combination of findings from the medical history, physical examination, serology, and duodenal biopsy. The recommended serologic marker that is used for screening patients is serum antitissue transglutaminase antibody.
8. Strict, lifelong adherence to a gluten-free diet is the only treatment for celiac disease that is currently available.
9. Clinicians must evaluate the patient with celiac disease for nutritional deficiencies (including folic acid, vitamin B_{12}, fat-soluble vitamins, iron, and calcium) due to malabsorption.

(1) Celiac disease is a small intestinal immune-mediated enteropathy caused by intolerance to ingested gluten, a storage protein found in wheat, barley, and rye. Genetic, environmental, and immune factors all play a role in the development of celiac disease. The mainstay of treatment of the disease is strict, lifelong adherence to a gluten-free diet.[1,2]

A disease resembling celiac disease was first described by a Greek physician in the second century AD.[3] In the mid-1900s, the connection between the ingestion of cereals and celiac disease was made. For many years, celiac disease was considered a disease of childhood with primarily GI symptoms. It is now recognized as a disease of all ages with varied presentation.

Celiac disease has also been known as celiac sprue, nontropical sprue, and gluten-sensitive enteropathy; however, these terms are currently not recommended. The non-specific use of celiac disease related terminology may lead to misunderstandings. It is therefore important that accepted terms associated with celiac disease be used, and understood when engaging in patient consultations or discussions with other healthcare providers. The publication of the Oslo Definitions has helped to address this concern.[1]

The disease is characterized by both GI and extraintestinal symptoms. Chronic inflammation caused by exposure to gluten leads to GI discomfort, nutrient malabsorption, and systemic complications. GI symptoms, including diarrhea, cramping, bloating, and flatulence, are the "classic" symptoms; however, a patient with celiac disease may initially present with a variety of extraintestinal symptoms. Patients with subclinical celiac disease have no or minimal symptoms but manifest mucosal damage on biopsy and have positive serologic testing. Patients with celiac disease classified as potential are asymptomatic patients who may show positive serology and have the human leukocyte antigen (HLA)-DQ2 and/or DQ8 haplotype, but have normal mucosa on biopsy.[1,4]

Adherence to a gluten-free diet is essential because it improves symptoms and prevents long-term complications of celiac disease, which include T-cell lymphomas, small bowel adenocarcinoma, and esophageal and oropharyngeal carcinomas.[5]

EPIDEMIOLOGY

(2) Originally thought to be a pediatric disease, celiac disease is now being diagnosed in increasing numbers of both adult and pediatric patients due to increased awareness and improved diagnostic techniques.[6] Celiac disease is common in Europe and North America. The prevalence of the disease is 0.71% to 0.79% in the United States, affecting up to 1% of non-Hispanic whites.[7,8] Similar to other autoimmune diseases, the prevalence of celiac disease is higher in females than in males at a rate of 1:2.8.[9] In Finland and the United States, the prevalence of celiac disease has increased fourfold during the past 50 years.[10] This finding has resulted from a true increase in the prevalence of the disease rather than simply an increase in the number of individuals who are diagnosed. While the reason for this increase is not known, it may be due to environmental factors such as the changing nature of gluten or other factors associated with diet.[11,12]

Celiac disease has been less well studied in other parts of the world. Previously believed to rarely occur in nonwhite populations, improved screening and diagnostic techniques now provide evidence that the prevalence of celiac disease in many non-Western nations is similar to that in Europe and North America.[13] In addition, in Asian countries where rice has traditionally been a staple, meals with rice are increasingly being replaced by a Western-style wheat-based diet. This transition in dietary preferences may lead to an increased prevalence of the disease in those populations.[12-14]

ETIOLOGY

Celiac disease is known to occur when a genetically predisposed person ingests gluten. Wheat gluten proteins exist in two fractions: gliadins and glutenins. Storage proteins similar to glutenins, called hordeins and secalins, are found in barley and rye, respectively. Table 41-1 refers to grains and other foods that do and do not contain gluten and related proteins. Ingestion of any of these proteins will lead to an autoimmune response in celiac disease patients. Wheat, barley, and rye are all derived from the Triticeae tribe of the grass (Gramineae) family. Oats, from the Aveneae tribe, are distantly related and therefore contain fewer disease-activating proteins.[16] One concern with oats is that they may be contaminated with gluten during the manufacturing process.[16]

Genetic factors, in combination with exposure to gluten, are necessary for the development of celiac disease. A concordance rate of 85% in monozygotic twins has been reported, indicating that genetics play a large role in the disease, but other factors also are likely to involved.[17,18]

Virtually all patients with celiac disease have variants of HLA-DQ2 or HLA-DQ8 molecules that are expressed on the surface of antigen-presenting cells.[4,5] Other non-HLA genes may also play a role in enhancing genetic susceptibility to celiac disease.[18]

Certain infectious agents and other compounds may contribute to the development of celiac disease. Both adenovirus and hepatitis C viruses are thought to act as triggers, whereas other agents, including *Campylobacter jejuni*, *Giardia lamblia*, rotavirus, and enterovirus infections, have been described in case reports as associated with celiac disease.[19] Various drugs, such as olmesartan, azathioprine, methotrexate, as well as others, have also been suggested to play a role in the development of sprue-like bowel disease.[3]

In Sweden, increased rates of diagnosis of celiac disease in the mid-1980s corresponded to a change in infant feeding practices where mothers reduced breast-feeding and introduced cereal into babies' diets earlier than had been previously in practice. Based on this finding, prolonged breast-feeding with introduction of gluten-containing grains during breast-feeding was recommended to help avoid the development of celiac disease.[20] However, multinational studies show that the timing of gluten introduction or duration of breastfeeding did not avoid the eventual diagnosis of celiac disease, even at children at higher risk due to the presence of one of the high risk HLA haplotypes.[21-24]

TABLE 41-1 Grains and Other Foods that Do and Do Not Contain Gluten

Contain Gluten	Do Not Contain Gluten
Wheat	Amaranth
Barley	Buckwheat
Rye	Corn
Bran	Flax
Graham flour	Millet
Spelt	Potato flour
Wheat germ	Quinoa
Triticale	Rice
Oats[a]	Sorghum
	Soybeans
	Tapioca
	Teff

[a]Oats are in a different plant family, but they have also been regarded as problematic, although the ingestion of certified pure gluten-free oats appears to be safe in most patients with celiac disease.[6] Due to the continued difference of opinion regarding the safety of oats, patients are generally advised to discuss the risks and benefits associated with consuming oats with their healthcare provider before they include oats in their diet.

PATHOPHYSIOLOGY

3 During normal digestion, peptides that remain from gastric or pancreatic digestion are broken down into amino acids, dipeptides, or tripeptides by the small intestinal brush-border membrane enzymes.[25] These GI proteases that are found in the intestinal lumen are one of the body's first defenses against potentially toxic dietary proteins.[15] The intestinal epithelium, with its intact intercellular tight junctions, functions as the primary barrier to the passage of macromolecules into the lamina propria. Gluten is unusually rich in the amino acids glutamine and proline, which enable part of the molecule to withstand the digestive processes. These peptides are kept within the GI tract and are primarily excreted before they can illicit an immune reaction. Small fractions of gluten do cross this important defense barrier in patients without celiac disease; however, the quantity of gluten that passes across the GI lining is generally insufficient to illicit a significant response from a normally functioning immune system.[25,26]

Events likely associated with the pathophysiology of celiac disease have been characterized as an interaction between gluten and immune, genetic, and environmental factors.[25] In celiac disease, the integrity of the tissue junctions of the intestinal epithelium is compromised, enabling gluten to reach the lamina propria through different routes. The presence of gluten in the lamina propria and an inherited combination of genes contribute to the heightened immune sensitivity to gluten found in patients with celiac disease (Table 41-2).[25] The notable immune response to gluten consists of both adaptive and innate immune responses that occur only in individuals who carry the HLA type DQ2 or in some populations DQ8.[25] The precise mechanism by which the immune system leads to damage of the intestinal lining of patients with celiac disease continues to be studied.

Clinical **Controversy...**

Non-celiac gluten sensitivity is a condition in which the ingestion of gluten results in morphological or symptomatic manifestations in the absence of celiac disease.[1] This disorder must therefore be considered in the differential diagnosis of celiac disease. It is noteworthy that symptoms

TABLE 41-2 Proposed Pathophysiology of Celiac Disease

- Enterocytes release the protein zonulin in response to the presence of indigestible fragments of gluten in the intestine
- Zonulin loosens the intercellular tight junctions
- Abundant quantities of gluten fragments cross the intestinal lining and accumulate under the enterocytes (epithelial cells)
- Gluten induces the enterocytes to secrete interleukin-15 (IL-15)
- IL-15 induces an immune response of intraepithelial lymphocytes against the enterocytes
- The damaged cells release the enzyme tissue transglutaminase (tTG), which modifies the gluten
- Antigen-presenting cells of the immune system join the modified gluten to human leukocyte antigen (HLA) molecules and display the resulting complexes to other immune cells (ie, helper T cells)
- Helper T cells that recognize the complexes secrete molecules that attract other immune cells, which may result in damage to the enterocytes
- Helper T cells spur killer T cells that directly attack the enterocytes
- B cells release antibody molecules that are targeted to gluten and tTG (the role that these antibodies play remains to be further clarified; however, they may cause further damage when they contact their targets on or near the enterocytes)
- Enterocytes are disabled or killed

Data from reference 25.

alone cannot reliably differentiate celiac disease from nonceliac gluten sensitivity. Therefore a diagnostic evaluation including celiac serology and small-intestinal biopsy (while the patient is including gluten in their diet) is needed. If these tests are negative, HLA-DQ typing is required to differentiate between the two disorders. Differentiating between these disorders is very important as it will impact upon the implications of the level of adherence to the gluten-free diet, approach to continued disease-state monitoring and evaluation, and the counseling of family members (as nonceliac disease sensitivity does not appear to have a strong hereditary basis).[5]

The primary toxic components of wheat gluten are a family of closely related proteins called gliadins.[25] The gliadin peptides induce changes in the epithelium through innate immunity and in the lamina propria through adaptive immunity.[25] Protected transport of gliadin peptides occurs in patients with celiac disease via a CD71-mediated transcytosis of immunoglobulin A (IgA)/gliadin peptides immune complexes from the lumen of the intestine to the lamina propria. In patients without celiac disease, the gliadin peptides are entirely degraded by lysosomal acid proteases during intestinal transcytosis. The abnormal expression of the IgA receptor CD71 at the apical side of the enterocytes that is found in celiac disease patients allows a protected retrotransport of serum immunoglobulin A (SIgA) gliadin immune complexes that could play an important role in triggering the immune activation that is characteristic of celiac disease. These researchers note that the normal function of SIgA (ie, the containment of harmful antigens in the intestinal lumen) is deficient in celiac disease. They further state that the fate of the immune complexes once absorbed is unknown; however, the complexes may bind to IgA receptors that are present on local antigen-presenting cells and trigger the activation of local memory CD4 T cells, which will perpetuate the inflammation.[27]

Tissue transglutaminase (tTG), a ubiquitous enzyme that catalyzes posttranslational modification of proteins and is released during inflammation, may play at least two crucial roles in celiac disease by serving as the main target autoantigen for antiendomysial enzymes and as a deaminating enzyme that raises the immunostimulatory effect of gluten. Expression and activity of tTG are raised in the mucosa of patients with celiac disease.[15] This enzyme, by deaminating glutamine to glutamic acid, makes the gliadin peptides become negatively charged and therefore more capable of fitting into pockets of the HLA-DQ2 (or HLA-DQ8) antigen-binding groove on the antigen-presenting cells.[15,28] Gliadin is presented to gliadin-reactive CD4 T cells through a T-cell receptor, which then results in the production of cytokines that cause tissue damage. This then leads to villous atrophy, crypt hyperplasia, and the expansion of antibody-producing B cells found in celiac disease.[28]

CLINICAL PRESENTATION

4 The recognition of celiac disease may be quite challenging due to the wide range of presenting symptoms, which includes patients who are asymptomatic.[15] Clinical manifestations of celiac disease also significantly vary according to age group (Table 41-3) in that pediatric patients are more likely to experience classic gastrointestinal symptoms while adults are more likely to have atypical symptoms.[29] Infants and young children generally experience diarrhea, abdominal distention, and failure to thrive. Vomiting, irritability, anorexia, and even constipation are also common in these young patients. Extraintestinal manifestations such as short stature, neurologic findings (eg, peripheral neuropathy, ataxia, seizure, migraine, and dementia), or anemia are often found in older children and adolescents.[29] The classic presenting symptom in adults is diarrhea, which may be accompanied by abdominal pain or discomfort; however, it is noteworthy that during the past decade diarrhea has been reported as the main presenting symptom of celiac disease in less than 50% of cases. Adults may exhibit iron-deficiency anemia or osteoporosis. Less common but important presentations of celiac disease in adults include abdominal pain, constipation, weight loss, neurologic symptoms, dermatitis herpetiformis, hypoproteinemia, hypocalcemia, and elevated liver enzymes. Some adults may be diagnosed as a result of having an endoscopy performed in response to their complaints of symptoms associated with gastroesophageal reflux.[28] Patients with celiac disease often experience symptoms for a long period of time and may experience multiple hospitalizations and undergo surgical procedures before celiac disease is diagnosed.[28]

5 Dermatitis herpetiformis is a skin manifestation of small intestinal immune-mediated enteropathy caused by the ingestion of gluten (Figs. 41-1 and 41-2).[1] It occurs more often in males and in patients 30 to 40 years old.[30] This extremely pruritic, bullous skin rash is generally found on the elbows, knees, buttocks, and scalp but

TABLE 41-3 Selected Signs and Symptoms of Celiac Disease

Children	Adults
Symptoms	Symptoms
• Fatigue	• Abdominal pain
• Bloating	• Chronic diarrhea
• Constipation	• Abdominal distension
• Abdominal pain	• Recurrent spontaneous abortion
• Chronic diarrhea	• Peripheral neuropathy
• Irritability	• Depression
• Vomiting	• Fatigue/malaise
Signs	• Ataxia
• Muscle wasting	Signs
• Failure to thrive/weight loss	• Weight loss
• Short stature	• Infertility
• Delayed puberty	• Dermatitis herpetiformis
• Osteopenia/osteoporosis	• Hepatitis
• Hepatitis	• Anemia
• Dental anomalies	• Aphthous ulcers
• Anemia	• Alopecia
	• Malignancy
	• Seizures
	• Osteopenia/osteoporosis
	• Arthritis

Data from reference 23.

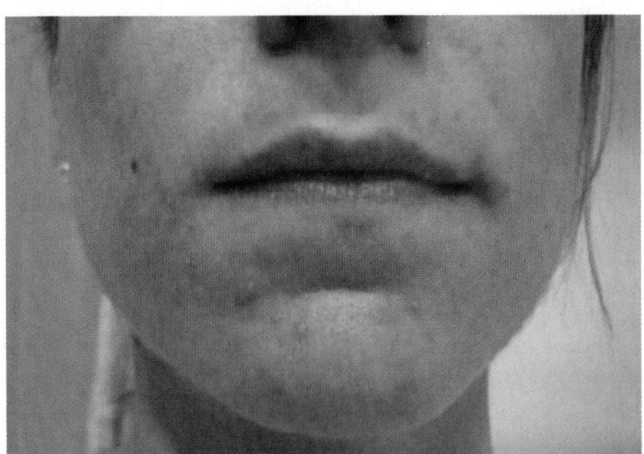

FIGURE 41-1 Photograph of dermatitis herpetiformis of the face. *(Copyright © American Pharmacists Association [APhA]. Reprinted by permission of APhA. Photographs provided by Peter H.R. Green, MD, Professor of Clinical Medicine, College of Physicians & Surgeons, Columbia University, New York.)*

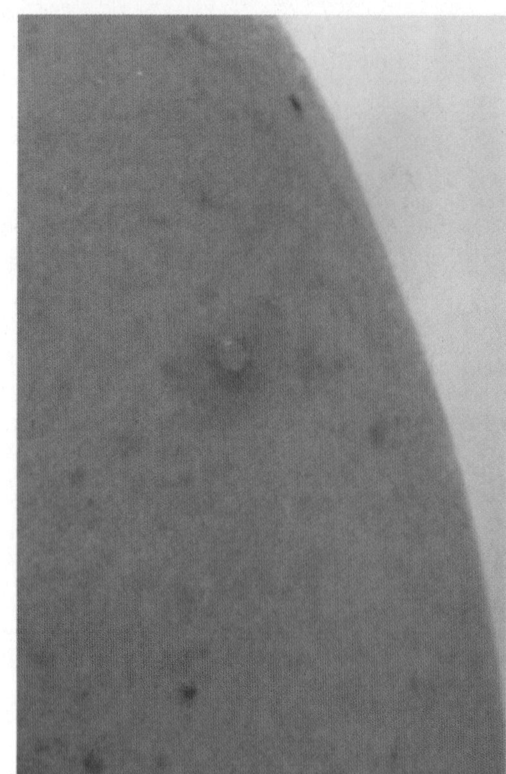

FIGURE 41-2 Photograph of bullous dermatitis herpetiformis. *(Copyright © American Pharmacists Association [APhA]. Reprinted by permission of APhA. Photographs provided by Peter H.R. Green, MD, Professor of Clinical Medicine, College of Physicians & Surgeons, Columbia University, New York.)*

can occur anywhere on the body.[30] Although dermatitis herpetiformis was once considered to be a skin disease that was often found in patients with celiac disease, researchers have also suggested that it is actually a cutaneous manifestation of gluten sensitivity.[30]

6 The diagnosis of celiac disease is based on clinical suspicion and confirmation with laboratory tests and duodenal biopsy.[5] Although the frequency of diagnosis of patients with celiac disease has increased, many patients with this condition remain undiagnosed.[5] This is particularly concerning as undiagnosed celiac disease has been associated with a nearly fourfold increased risk of death compared with subjects without serologic evidence of disease.[10]

Perhaps the most important initial step in making this diagnosis is for healthcare providers to recognize its many and diverse possible symptoms.[37] Only 11% of celiac disease cases are diagnosed in a timely manner, with an average reported period of 5.8 to 11.7 years from the onset of symptoms to the diagnosis.[32] Clinicians can help reduce the time from the onset of symptoms to the diagnosis of celiac disease by being aware of the common diseases that may also coexist with celiac disease (Table 41-4).[32]

Clinicians should also note that individuals with certain disorders are more likely to have celiac disease than the general population. Examples include other autoimmune diseases, such as thyroid disease, diabetes mellitus (type 1), multiple sclerosis, myasthenia gravis, Raynaud's disease, rheumatoid arthritis, Addison's disease, chronic active hepatitis, cystic fibrosis, scleroderma, and Sjögren's syndrome; Down's syndrome; neurologic conditions such as ataxia, epilepsy, and cerebral calcifications; and primary biliary cirrhosis. Although patients with these disorders are more frequently found to have celiac disease than the general population, these associated conditions are not believed to cause celiac disease.[15]

TABLE 41-4 Selected Common Misdiagnoses

Irritable bowel syndrome
Viral gastroenteritis
Lactose intolerance
Amoebic/parasitic infection
Inflammatory bowel disease
Psychological dysfunction
Gallbladder disease
Chronic fatigue syndrome
Gastroesophageal reflux disease
Allergies
Ulcers
Cystic fibrosis
Colitis

Data from reference 5.

Clinical **Controversy...**

The co-occurrence of celiac disease and type 1 diabetes mellitus is 5 to 7 times more prevalent than celiac disease alone.[33] The most common manifestations of celiac disease in patients with diabetes mellitus are gastrointestinal and diminished or impaired bone demineralization. Although these findings in diabetic patients may lead clinicians to test for celiac disease, testing for celiac disease in asymptomatic diabetes mellitus patients remains controversial.[5] A paucity of data exists clarifying the implications of celiac disease in adult patients with type 1 diabetes with respect to diabetes-related outcomes including glycemic control, lipids, microvascular complications, quality of life, and the effect of a gluten free diet. It is noteworthy however that researchers have reported that adults with undetected celiac disease and type 1 diabetes were found to have worse glycemic control and a higher prevalence of retinopathy and nephropathy.[34] The impact that effective treatment of celiac disease will have on the overall management of diabetes mellitus also needs to be studied further. Some researchers have suggested that an increase in absorption may lead to the need for increased insulin doses. (2) Careful patient monitoring is therefore always prudent.

7 Diagnostic testing for celiac disease must be performed while the patient continues to consume gluten.[5] A confirmed diagnosis of celiac disease requires both a positive finding on duodenal biopsy and a positive response to a gluten-free diet.[5] The identification of villous atrophy with small bowel endoscopy and biopsy is generally regarded as the diagnostic gold standard (although guidelines from the European Society of Paediatric Gastroenterology, Hepatology, and Nutrition suggest that a small intestinal biopsy may not be required in children with typical symptoms, titers of anti-tTG greater than 10 times the upper normal limit and predisposing HLA genotype).[35] Although villous atrophy is associated with celiac disease, clinicians must consider that this may also be found in other diseases, including giardiasis, autoimmune enteropathy, tuberculosis, Crohn's disease, intolerance to food other than gluten, intestinal lymphoma, and Zollinger-Ellison syndrome.[5]

The Marsh classification system is a standardized approach used by pathologists to describe the histologic changes seen in celiac disease. This classification includes ratings of Marsh I to IV with Marsh III being further subdivided into Marsh IIIa (partial villous atrophy), IIIb (subtotal villous atrophy), and IIIc (total villous atrophy). Most celiac disease patients (50%-60%) are placed in one of the Marsh III categories.[41] Histologic findings lead to a diagnosis that is followed by placing the patient on a gluten-free diet. Dermatitis herpetiformis is diagnosed by skin biopsy.[37]

Serologic test results provide clinicians with a useful noninvasive tool that helps to determine if symptomatic patients, or patients who are at risk for celiac disease, require a biopsy.[5] Available tests include those for antigliadin antibodies, connective tissue antibodies (antireticulum and antiendomysial antibodies), and antibodies against tTG. The most common serologic marker that is used for screening patients is IgA tTG antibodies.[5] Testing for gliadin antibodies is no longer utilized because of its low sensitivity and specificity for celiac disease.[5] Although serology is a good method to identify patients who will benefit from endoscopy and biopsy, negative serology should not preclude a biopsy examination in individuals for whom disease is suspected on clinical grounds.[5]

Genetic testing can be performed as a means of determining which family members of a diagnosed patient may develop the disease (the prevalence of celiac disease has been reported to be 10%-12% in first-degree relatives and is also higher than that found in the general population in second-degree relatives).[5] Patients and their family members can be tested for HLA-DQ2 and HLA-DQ8 as HLA-DQ2 is found in up to 95% of celiac disease patients, with most other patients being HLA-DQ8 positive.[5] Although nearly all celiac disease patients carry one of these alleles, they are also found in 30% to 40% of the general population. Therefore, when these alleles are absent, it is extremely unlikely that the individual has celiac disease (ie, the test has a high negative predictive value [NPV]).[5] A patient-administered saliva-based test for HLA-DQ2/DQ8 was released for direct sale to consumers but is not recommended for use in the diagnosis of celiac disease.[5]

TREATMENT

Desired Outcomes

Overall goals of treatment include relieving symptoms, healing the intestine, and reversing the consequences of malabsorption while enabling the patient to adhere to a healthy, interesting, and practical gluten-free diet.[27,45]

Nonpharmacologic

8 Table 41-5 presents a mnemonic that summarizes the major principles of the treatment of celiac disease. Strict lifelong adherence to a gluten-free diet is the only proven treatment for celiac disease.[15] Patients must recognize that adhering to a gluten-free diet includes not ingesting anything that contains gluten or has been contaminated with gluten. Wheat, barley, and rye must be avoided.[4] Although oats are in a different plant family, they have also been regarded to be problematic; however, the ingestion of certified pure gluten-free oats appears to be safe.[15] Due to the continued difference of opinion regarding the safety of oats, they should be added to the diet cautiously and with monitoring.[5] Patients must also commit to avoiding the ingestion of gluten found in nonfood items such as toothpaste, lip balm, lipstick, etc. A list of gluten-free grains can be found in Table 41-1.

TABLE 41-5 Mnemonic for Celiac Disease

C	Consultation with a skilled dietician
E	Education about the disease
L	Lifelong adherence to a gluten-free diet
I	Identifying and treating nutritional deficiencies
A	Access to an advocacy group
C	Continuous long-term followup by a multidisciplinary team

Data from reference 37.

Oral prescription drugs, nonprescription drugs, vitamin and mineral supplements, and health and beauty aids and cosmetics that have oral ingestion potential must not be overlooked as sources of gluten due to its presence in their formulation or due to contamination or contact.[38,39] Although clinicians have concluded that as little as 10 to 50 mg/day of gluten is the minimum dose required to produce measurable damage to the small intestinal mucosa, it is difficult to set a universal threshold given the individual variability among patients.[2,4,30]

The FDA determined the tolerable daily intake level for gluten in individuals with celiac disease to be 0.4 mg gluten/day for adverse morphologic effects and 0.015 mg gluten/day for adverse clinical effects and ruled in 2013 that foods labeled as gluten free must contain less than 20 ppm gluten.[40,41] Although the ruling pertains to food only, the concerns regarding low-level exposure emphasize why healthcare providers must check to determine whether prescription drugs contain gluten in their formulation or have been contaminated with gluten before these drugs are provided to the patient with celiac disease. Lack of reliable information can be confusing and although there are published lists of gluten-free drugs, it is often difficult to obtain information about the gluten content of medications.[42,43] In addition, it is important for clinicians to realize that conflicting data regarding drug absorption in patients with celiac disease requires careful selection and use of drugs in patients with celiac disease.

9 Newly diagnosed patients should be evaluated for nutritional deficiencies associated with vitamin and mineral malabsorption. This assessment should include assuring that the patient does not have deficiencies of folic acid, vitamin B_{12}, fat-soluble vitamins, iron, and calcium.[5] Monitoring for potential nutritional deficiencies should also continue during subsequent followup visits.

Most adults with celiac disease are found to have some degree of bone loss; therefore, all patients must be screened for osteoporosis or osteopenia.[30] Supplementing a calcium-rich gluten-free diet with calcium, magnesium, and vitamin D may arrest or reverse celiac decrease-related bone loss. Although their use has not been extensively studied in patients with celiac disease, bisphosphonates and other drugs have been prescribed for patients with bone disease.[44]

Implementing a gluten-free diet presents some challenges. Consultation with a registered dietician is recommended for dietary evaluation and education.[5] Patients are advised to initiate a complete gluten-free lifestyle immediately after diagnosis. Partial adherence to this diet is not adequate. In order to accomplish this objective, patients must be aware of what foods are gluten-free and when in doubt must know how to confirm whether a food contains gluten. Reading labels is extremely important; however, it may be difficult to identify hidden sources of gluten listed among the ingredients. Patients with celiac disease must also determine whether products were processed on equipment shared with wheat, barley, or rye. It may be necessary to call the manufacturers or check their website to obtain the needed information.[38]

Individuals with celiac disease must also be advised to maintain a gluten-free kitchen. A dedicated toaster, bread maker, waffle iron, and other appliances should be obtained for use in preparing gluten-free meals. Utensils and dishes must be carefully cleaned to avoid gluten contamination. Care must also be taken when dining in restaurants and homes of family and friends. The individuals who prepare and serve the food must be knowledgeable about gluten-free foods and food preparation.[30]

The economic burden associated with maintaining a gluten-free diet may present some challenges.[45,46] The relatively low availability and high cost of these foods contributes to the challenges associated with adhering to the required strict diet and may lead to varying degrees of noncompliance.[45,46] Patients also find that the extra cost associated with the special diet is not reimbursed by healthcare plans, and most policies do not pay for consultations with a dietician.[47] These challenges with compliance are particularly concerning as noncompliance with the gluten-free diet is associated with an increased mortality rate and compromised quality of life.[46] Patients are also encouraged to investigate their personal circumstances as to whether some of the costs of maintaining a gluten-free diet are eligible for approval as a tax deduction.[47]

Pharmacologic

Dietary avoidance of gluten remains the mainstay of treatment of celiac disease. Novel pharmacologic treatment modalities are under investigation. Most reports related to pharmacotherapy for celiac disease focus on the treatment of refractory disease.

In case reports, corticosteroids, azathioprine, cyclosporine, tacrolimus, infliximab, and alemtuzumab have been reported as effective treatments for refractory celiac disease. Patients characterized to have refractory celiac disease have persistent or recurrent malabsorptive symptoms and signs with villous atrophy despite maintaining a gluten-free diet for more than 12 months.[1] Less than 5% of adult patients are found to have refractory celiac disease.

Based on the pathophysiology of celiac disease, novel targets for the treatment of the disease have been identified: decreasing the antigenic load and modulation of the immune response. Methods of decreasing the antigenic load include blocking the activity of tTG, GI destruction of proline peptides via enzyme therapy, blocking the binding of deaminated proteins to HLA-DQ2 and HLA-DQ8, detoxification of gluten peptides, and decreasing intestinal permeability in patients with celiac disease, in particular through inhibition of zonulin.[3] Investigational tTG inhibitors have been developed; however, their safety is questioned due to the presence of the enzyme throughout the body and its role in many functions necessary for homeostasis.[49] In the area of gluten detoxification, gluten proteins were developed in which the proline residues were replaced by azidoprolines; these azidoproline residues bound to HLA-DQ2 but did not stimulate an autoimmune response.[50] A zonulin inhibitor, larazotide, was well tolerated and effective in a small study of patients with persistent symptoms despite a gluten free diet for 1 year.[51] A vaccine, Nexvax2, that modulates the immune response has passed phase 1b trials.[52]

Evaluation of Therapeutic Outcomes

Clinical improvement will often be observed within days or weeks of instituting the required diet.[28] Although dermatitis herpetiformis is also treated with the prescribed diet, these cutaneous lesions may not completely resolve for months to years after initiating dietary measures.[37]

Healthcare providers must also be mindful of conditions that are related to celiac disease and that are potential complications of the disease, including certain forms of cancer, neurologic manifestations, osteoporosis, depression, diabetes, infertility, as well as other autoimmune and related illnesses. Cancers that are of particular concern include thyroid cancer, adenocarcinoma of the small intestine, lymphoma (predominantly non-Hodgkin's lymphoma of any type), esophageal cancer, melanoma, and malignancies found in childhood.[4] Patients with celiac disease have also been found to have an increased risk of developing certain infectious diseases that include pneumococcal or staphylococcal sepsis and tuberculosis.[53] The immune system of celiac patients is not compromised as it is actually overactive. The risk of infections due to encapsulated organisms (pneumococcal pneumonia, meningococcal infections) arises from hyposplenism, which is common in active celiac disease. Therefore, patients over 50 years of age are advised to receive pneumococcal vaccine.[30] Annual influenza vaccine is advisable as this will reduce the incidence of secondary bacterial infections.[53] Increased hazard ratios (HRs) for death were found in individuals with biopsy-verified celiac disease, inflammation, and potential celiac disease (the absolute risks were small). Individuals undergoing small-intestinal biopsy in childhood had increased HRs for death. These researchers concluded that the main causes of death in patients they studied were cardiovascular disease and malignancy.[54]

ABBREVIATIONS

HLA	human leukocyte antigen
HR	hazard ratio
IgA	immunoglobulin A
NIH	National Institutes of Health
NPV	negative predictive value
SIgA	serum immunoglobulin A
tTG	tissue transglutaminase

REFERENCES

1. Ludvigsson JF, Leffler DA, Bai JC, et al. The Oslo definitions of celiac disease and related terms. *Gut* 2013;62:43-52.
2. Fasano A, Catassi C. Celiac disease. *N Engl J Med* 2012;367(25):2419-2426.
3. Freeman HJ. Celiac disease: A disorder emerging from antiquity, its evolving classification and risk, and potential new treatment paradigms. *Gut Liver* 2015;9(1):28-37.
4. Kelly CP, Bai JC, Liu E, et al. Advances in diagnosis and management of celiac disease. *Gastroenterology* 2015;148(6):1175-1186.
5. Rubio-Tapia A, Hill I, Kelly CP. ACG clinical guidelines: Diagnosis and management of celiac disease. *Am J Gastroenterol* 2013;108(5):656-676.
6. Gasbarrini G, Miele L, Malandrino N, et al. Celiac disease in the 21st century: Issues of under and overdiagnosis. *Int J Immunopathol Pharmacol* 2009;22(1):1-7.
7. Rubio-Tapia A, Ludvigsson JF, Brantner TL, et al. The prevalence of celiac disease in the United States. *Am J Gastroenterol* 2012;107: 1538-1544.
8. Mardini H, Westgate P. Racial differences in the prevalence of celiac disease in the US population: National Health and Nutrition Examination Survey (NHANES) 2009-2012. *Dig Dis Sci* 2015;60:1738-1742.
9. Ciccocioppo R, Kruzliak P, Cangemi GC, et al. The spectrum of differences between childhood and adulthood celiac disease. *Nutrients* 2015;7:8733-8751.
10. Rubio-Tapia A, Kyle RA, Kaplan EL, et al. Increased prevalence and mortality in undiagnosed celiac disease. *Gastroenterology* 2009;137:88-93.
11. Green PHR. Mortality in celiac disease, intestinal inflammation, and gluten sensitivity. *JAMA* 2009;302(11):1225-1226.
12. Kang JY, Kang AHY, Green A, et al. *Aliment Pharmacol Ther* 2013;38: 226-245.
13. Lionetti E, Gatti S, Puliverenti A, et al. Celiac disease from a global perspective. *Best Pract Res Clin Gastroenterol* 2015;29:365-379.
14. Cummins AG, Roberts-Thomson IC. Prevalence of celiac disease in the Asia-Pacific region. *J Gastroenterol Hepatol* 2009;24:1347-1351.
15. DiSabatino A, Corazza GR. Coeliac disease. *Lancet* 2009;373: 1480-1493.
16. Fric P, Gabrovska D, Nevoral J. Celiac disease, gluten-free diet, and oats. *Nutr Clin Care* 2011;69(2):107-115.
17. Nistico L, Fagnani C, Coto I, et al. Concordance, disease progression, and heritability of coeliac disease in Italian twins. *Gut* 2006;55:803-808.
18. Wolters VM, Wijmenga C. Genetic background of celiac disease and its clinical implications. *Am J Gastroenterol* 2008;103(1):190-195.
19. Plot L, Amital H. Infectious associations of celiac disease. *Autoimmun Rev* 2009;8:316-319.
20. Ivarsson A, Persson LA, Lystrom L, et al. Epidemic of coeliac disease in Swedish children. *Acta Paediatr* 2000;89(2):165-171.
21. Lionetti E, Castallenata S, Francavilla R, et al. *N Engl J Med* 2014;371: 1295-1303.
22. Vrienzing SL, Auricchio R, Bravi E, et al. Randomized feeding intervention in infants at high risk for celiac disease. *N Engl J Med* 2014;371(14):1304-1315.
23. Aronsson CA, Lee H, Liu E, et al. Age at gluten introduction and risk of celiac disease. *Pediatrics* 2015;135(2):239-245.
24. Jansen M, Tromp I, Kiefte-deJong JC, et al. Infant feeding and anti-tissue transglutaminase antibody concentrations in the generation R study. *Am J Clin Nutr* 2014;100:1095-1101.
25. Green PHR, Lebwohl B, Greywoode R. *J Allergy Clin Immunol* 2015;135(5):1099-1106.
26. Fasano A. Surprises from celiac disease. *Sci Am* 2009;301:54-61.

27. Heyman M, Menard S. Pathways of gliadin transport in celiac disease. *Ann N Y Acad Sci* 2009;1165:274-278.
28. Green PHR, Cellier C. Celiac disease. *N Engl J Med* 2007;357:1731-1743.
29. Vivas S, Vaquero L, Rodríguez-Martín L, et al. Age-related differences in celiac disease: Specific characteristics of adult presentation. *World J Gastrointest Pharmacol Ther* 2015;6(4):207-212.
30. Bolotin D, Petronic-Rosic V. Dermatitis herpetiformis part I: Epidemiology, pathogenesis, and clinical presentation. *J Am Acad Dermatol* 2011;64(6):1017-1024.
31. NIH consensus development conference on celiac disease. *NIH Consens State Sci Statements* 2004;21:1-23.
32. Thom S, Longo BM, Running A, Ashley J. Celiac disease: A guide to successful diagnosis and treatment. *J Nurse Pract* 2009;5:244-253.
33. Akirov A, Pinhas-Hamiel O. Co-occurrence of type 1 diabetes and celiac disease. *World J Diabetes* 2015;6(5):707-714.
34. Leeds JS, Hopper AD, Hadijivassiliou M, Tesfaye S, Sanders DS. High prevalence of microvascular complications in adults with type 1 diabetes and newly diagnosed celiac disease. *Diabetes Care* 2011;34(10):2158-2163.
35. Husby S, Koletzko S, Korponay-Szabo IR, et al. European Society for Pediatric Gastroenterology, Hepatology, and Nutrition guidelines for the diagnosis of coeliac disease. *J Pediatr Gastroenterol Nutr* 2012;54(1):136-160.
36. Kupfer SS. Making sense of Marsh. *Impact: A Publication of the University of Chicago Celiac Disease Center*. Chicago, IL: University of Chicago Celiac Disease Center, Fall; 2009:1-3.
37. Bolotin D, Petronic-Rosic V. Dermatitis herpetiformis part II: Diagnosis, management, and prognosis. *J Am Acad Dermatol* 2011;64(6):1027-1033.
38. Mangione RA, Patel PN. Caring for patients with celiac disease: The role of the pharmacist. *J Am Pharm Assoc* 2008;48(4):e125-e135.
39. Hlywiak KH. Hidden sources of gluten. *Pract Gastroenterol* 2008;32: 27-39.
40. Office of Food Safety Center of Food Safety and Applied Nutrition, Food and Drug Administration. Health Hazard Assessment for Gluten Exposure in Individuals with Celiac Disease: Determination of Tolerable Daily Intake Levels and Levels of Concern for Gluten. 2011. Available at: http://www.fda.gov/downloads/food/scienceresearch/researchaccess/riskassessmentsafetyassessment/ucm264152.pdf.
41. FDA. FDA defines "gluten free" for food labeling. Available at: http://www.fda.gov/NewsEvents/Newsroom/PressAnnouncements/ucm363474.htm. (Accessed November 10, 2015).
42. King AR. The impact of celiac sprue on patients' medication choices. *Hosp Pharm* 2009;44:105-106.
43. Mangione RA, Patel PN, Shin E, et al. Determining the gluten content of over the counter drugs: Information for patients with celiac disease. *J Am Pharm Assoc* 2011;51:734-737.
44. Tran T, Smith C, Mangione RA. Drug absorption in celiac disease. *Am J Health-Syst Pharm* 2013;70:2199-2206.
45. Krupa-Kozak U. Pathologic bone alterations in celiac disease: Etiology, epidemiology, and treatment. *Nutrition* 2014;30(1):16-24.
46. Lee A, Ng D, Zivin J, Green H. Economic burden of a gluten-free diet. *J Hum Nutr Diet* 2007;20:423-430.
47. Stevens L, Rashid M. Gluten-free and regular foods: A cost comparison. *Can J Diet Pract Res* 2008;69:147-150.
48. Alderman L. The expense of eating with celiac disease. *New York Times* August 15, 2009:B7.
49. Sanz Y. Novel perspectives in celiac disease therapy. *Mini Rev Med Chem* 2009;9:359-367.
50. Sanz Y, De Pama G, Laparra M. Unraveling the ties between celiac disease and intestinal microbiota. *Int Rev Immunol* 2011;30(4):207-218.
51. Leffler DA, Kelly CP, Green PH, et al. Larazotide acetate for persistent symptoms of celiac disease despite a gluten-free diet: A randomized controlled trial. *Gastroenterology* 2015;148(7):1311-1319.
52. ImmusanT. Celiac disease programs. Available at http://www.immusant.com/clinical-development/celiac-disease-programs.php. (Accessed November 10, 2015).
53. Ludvigsson JF, Montgomery SM, Ekbom A, et al. Small-intestinal histopathology and mortality risk in celiac disease. *JAMA* 2009;302: 1171-1178.
54. Picarelli A, Salvi I, Di Tola M, et al. Impact of gluten-free diet on quality of life in celiac disease patients. *Dig Liver Dis* 2009;41S:288.

Evaluation of Kidney Function

e42

Thomas C. Dowling

KEY CONCEPTS

1. The stage of chronic kidney disease (CKD) should be determined for all individuals based on the level of kidney function, independent of etiology, in accordance with the Kidney Disease: Improving Global Outcomes (KDIGO) classification system.
2. Persistent proteinuria indicates the presence of CKD and is associated with mortality and risk of end-stage renal disease (ESRD).
3. Quantitation of urine protein excretion, such as the measurement of a spot urine albumin-to-creatinine ratio, is critical for determining the severity of CKD and monitoring the rate of disease progression.
4. The glomerular filtration rate (GFR) is the single best indicator of kidney function.
5. Measurement of the GFR is most accurate when performed following the exogenous administration of iohexol, iothalamate, or radioisotopes such as technetium-99m diethylenetriamine pentaacetic acid (^{99m}Tc-DTPA).
6. Equations to estimate creatinine clearance (CL_{cr}) or GFR are commonly used in ambulatory and inpatient settings, and incorporate patient laboratory and demographic variables such as serum creatinine concentration (S_{cr}), cystatin C, age, sex, weight, and ethnicity.
7. Longitudinal assessment of GFR and albuminuria is important for monitoring the efficacy of therapeutic interventions, such as angiotensin-converting enzyme inhibitors and angiotensin receptor blockers, which are used to slow or halt the progression of kidney disease.
8. Assessments of kidney structure and function, such as radiography, computed tomography, magnetic resonance imaging, sonography, and biopsy, are predominantly used for determining the diagnosis of a given condition.

Chronic kidney disease (CKD) is an increasingly alarming worldwide health concern, with nearly 2 million people in the United States estimated to require hemodialysis or kidney transplantation by 2030.[1] In response to this widespread problem, standardized approaches are now used for the identification of individuals with CKD and their subsequent stratification into risk categories for the development of end-stage kidney disease (ESKD or ESRD) (see Chapter 44).[1,2] These efforts have heightened the awareness of the need for early identification of patients with CKD and the importance of monitoring the progression of kidney disease.

Assessment of kidney function using both qualitative and quantitative methods is an important part of the evaluation of patients and an essential characterization of individuals who participate in clinical research investigations. Estimation of creatinine clearance (CL_{cr}) has been considered the clinical standard for assessment of kidney function for nearly 50 years, and continues to be used as the primary method of stratifying kidney function in drug pharmacokinetic studies submitted to the United States Food and Drug Administration (FDA).[3,4] New equations to estimate glomerular filtration rate (GFR) are now used in many clinical settings to identify patients with CKD, and in large epidemiology studies to evaluate risks of mortality and progression to stage 5 CKD, that is, ESKD.[5,6] Other tests, such as urinalysis, radiographic procedures, and biopsy, are also valuable tools in the assessment of kidney disease, and these qualitative assessments are useful for determining the pathology and etiology of kidney disease. Urinalysis, for example, may give clues to the primary location, such as glomerular or tubular, of the renal disease. Follow-up studies, such as imaging procedures or kidney biopsy, may then further differentiate the specific cause, thereby guiding the selection of the optimal therapeutic intervention.

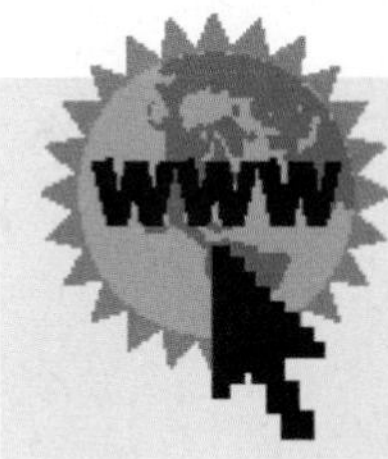

The complete chapter, learning objectives, and other resources can be found at **www.pharmacotherapyonline.com.**

43

Acute Kidney Injury

Jenana Halilovic and William Dager

KEY CONCEPTS

1. Three classification systems exist for staging severity of acute kidney injury (AKI): (a) Risk, Injury, Failure, Loss of Kidney Function, and End-Stage Kidney Disease (RIFLE), (b) Acute Kidney Injury Network (AKIN), and (c) Kidney Disease: Improving Global Outcomes (KDIGO) clinical practice guidelines. All three classification systems are based on separate criteria for serum creatinine (S_{cr}) and urine output.
2. AKI is a common complication in critically ill patients and is associated with high morbidity and mortality.
3. AKI has traditionally been categorized based on three types of injury: (a) prerenal—decreased renal blood flow, (b) intrinsic—structural damage within the kidney, and (c) postrenal—an obstruction within the urine collection system. However, recent advances in early detection of AKI with the availability of novel biomarkers has challenged this traditional classification and instead suggested distinguishing AKI in terms of functional change versus kidney damage.
4. Conventional formulas used to estimate glomerular filtration rate (eGFR) and creatinine clearance should not be used to estimate kidney function and adjust medication regimens in AKI patients.
5. The most effective prevention strategies for AKI include limiting exposure to nephrotoxic medications and maintaining adequate hydration with isotonic fluids.
6. Supportive management remains the primary approach to prevent or reduce complications associated with AKI or comorbid conditions. Supportive therapies include renal replacement therapy (RRT), nutritional support, avoidance of nephrotoxins, and blood pressure and fluid management.
7. For patients with prolonged or severe AKI, RRT is the cornerstone of support along with aggressive fluid and electrolyte management.
8. Drug dosing for AKI patients receiving continuous renal replacement therapy (CRRT) or sustained low-efficiency dialysis (SLED) is poorly characterized. Dosing requirements of agents primarily eliminated by the kidney may require individualization and require adjustment as renal function declines, and then subsequently increase as AKI resolves. Therapeutic drug monitoring should be utilized whenever possible for any agent with a narrow therapeutic index.
9. Diuretic resistance is a common phenomenon in the AKI patient and can be addressed with sodium restriction, combination diuretic therapy, or a continuous infusion of a loop diuretic.

INTRODUCTION

Acute kidney injury (AKI) is a clinical syndrome generally defined by an abrupt reduction in kidney function as evidenced by changes in, serum creatinine (S_{cr}), blood urea nitrogen (BUN), and urine output. The consequences of AKI can be serious, especially in hospitalized patients. Early recognition along with supportive therapy is the focus of management for those with established AKI, as there is no therapy that directly reverses the injury. Individuals at risk, such as those with history of chronic kidney disease (CKD), need to have their hemodynamic status carefully monitored and their exposure to nephrotoxins minimized. A thorough patient assessment including medical and surgical history, medication use, physical examination, and multiple laboratory tests is essential. Management goals include maintenance of blood pressure, fluid, and electrolyte homeostasis, all of which may be dramatically altered in the presence of AKI. Additional therapies designed to eliminate or minimize the insult that precipitated AKI include discontinuation of the offending drug (ie, the nephrotoxin), aggressive hydration, maintenance of renal perfusion, and renal replacement therapy (RRT).

In this chapter, the definition, classification, epidemiology, and common etiologies of AKI are presented. Methods to recognize and assess the extent of kidney function loss are also discussed. Finally, preventive strategies for patients at risk and management approaches for those with established AKI are reviewed.

DEFINITION AND CLASSIFICATION OF ACUTE KIDNEY INJURY

1 Three major classification systems have been developed to define and stage AKI in different patient populations. The *R*isk, *I*njury, *F*ailure, *L*oss of Kidney Function, and *E*nd-Stage Kidney Disease (RIFLE) was published in 2004 and the *A*cute *K*idney *I*njury *N*etwork (AKIN) criteria were developed in 2007.[1,2] Table 43-1 lists an overview of all classification systems. While generally similar, there are a few noteworthy differences: RIFLE defines AKI as an abrupt (1-7 days) but sustained (more than 24 hours) decrease in renal function from baseline while AKIN designates a 48-hour period for the decrease to occur. Also, AKIN removed RIFLE's last two classification components (Loss of Kidney Function and End-Stage Kidney Disease [ESKD]) from the staging system and instead places all patients receiving RRT automatically into AKIN stage 3. Finally, AKIN removed all estimated glomerular filtration rate (eGFR) criteria from its staging system and lowered the absolute increase in S_{cr} from 0.5 mg/dL (44 μmol/L) designated for the RIFLE-Risk class to 0.3 mg/dL (27 μmol/L) for AKIN stage 1.[1,2]

The Kidney Disease: Improving Global Outcomes (KDIGO) Clinical Practice Guidelines working group in 2012 proposed a staging system that shares many similarities with both RIFLE and

TABLE 43-1 RIFLE, AKIN, and KDIGO Classification Schemes for AKI[a]

RIFLE Category	S_{cr} and GFR[b] Criteria	Urine Output Criteria
Risk	S_{cr} increase to 1.5-fold or GFR decrease >25% from baseline	<0.5 mL/kg/h for ≥6 hours
Injury	S_{cr} increase to twofold or GFR decrease >50% from baseline	<0.5 mL/kg/h for ≥12 hours
Failure	S_{cr} increase to threefold or GFR decrease >75% from baseline, or S_{cr} ≥4 mg/dL (≥354 μmol/L) with an acute increase of at least 0.5 mg/dL (44 μmol/L)	Anuria for ≥12 hours
Loss	Complete loss of function (RRT) for >4 weeks	
ESKD	RRT >3 months	
AKIN Criteria	**S_{cr} Criteria**	**Urine Output Criteria**
Stage 1	S_{cr} increase ≥0.3 mg/dL (≥27 μmol/L) or 1.5- to 2-fold from baseline	<0.5 mL/kg/h for ≥6 hours
Stage 2	S_{cr} increase >2- to 3-fold from baseline	<0.5 mL/kg/h for ≥12 hours
Stage 3	S_{cr} increase >3-fold from baseline, or S_{cr} ≥4 mg/dL (≥354 μmol/L) with an acute increase of at least 0.5 mg/dL (≥44 μmol/L), or need for RRT	<0.3 mL/kg/h for ≥24 hours or anuria for ≥12 hours
KDIGO Criteria	**S_{cr} Criteria**	**Urine Output Criteria**
Stage 1	S_{cr} increase ≥0.3 mg/dL (≥27 μmol/L) or 1.5-1.9 times from baseline	<0.5 mL/kg/h for 6-12 hours
Stage 2	S_{cr} increase 2-2.9 times from baseline	<0.5 mL/kg/h for ≥12 hours
Stage 3	S_{cr} increase three times from baseline, or S_{cr} ≥4 mg/dL (≥354 μmol/L), or need for RRT, or eGFR[c] <35 mL/min/1.73 m² (<0.34 mL/s/m²) in patients <18 years	Anuria for ≥12 hours

AKI, acute kidney injury; AKIN, Acute Kidney Injury Network; ESKD, end-stage kidney disease; eGFR, estimated glomerular filtration rate; h, hours; KDIGO, Kidney Disease: Improving Global Outcomes; RIFLE, Risk, Injury, Failure, Loss of Kidney Function, and End-Stage Kidney Disease; RRT, renal replacement therapy; S_{cr}, serum creatinine.

[a]For all staging systems, the criterion that leads to worst possible diagnosis should be used.

[b]GFR calculated using the Modification of Diet in Renal Disease (MDRD) equation.

[c]GFR calculated using the Schwartz formula.

AKIN.[3] Their staging system, however, is extended in that it includes pediatric patients (younger than 18 years) in KDIGO Stage 3 for those with an eGFR of less than 35 mL/min/1.73 m² (0.34 mL/s/m²) as determined by the Schwartz formula.[3]

All three staging systems have been validated across different patient populations and their staging correlates closely with hospital mortality, cost, and length of stay. The KDIGO criteria seem to identify more patients with AKI and seem to be slightly more predictive of in-hospital mortality than either RIFLE or AKIN.[4-6] However, further studies are needed to definitely determine if one staging system is significantly better than the rest.

Since all three staging systems depend on S_{cr} and urine output as the main diagnostic criteria, they are associated with the same inherent weaknesses. An increase in S_{cr} is usually evident about 1 or 2 days after development of AKI. This lag time in S_{cr} rise may significantly delay diagnosis of AKI and adversely affect patient outcomes. Urine output reduction emerges earlier in AKI but is a very nonspecific marker. In fact, patients with AKI can be anuric (urine output less than 50 mL/day), oliguric (urine output less than 500 mL/day), or nonoliguric (urine output greater than 500 mL/day). Urine output will also vary with volume status, diuretic administration, and presence of obstruction.[7] Further, since all criteria are based on detecting an increase in S_{cr} from its baseline, a patient's renal function prior to the development of AKI needs to be known. If the baseline measure of S_{cr} is not available and the patient has no history of renal dysfunction, the Acute Dialysis Quality Initiative (ADQI), a workgroup composed of experts in nephrology and critical care, has suggested estimating the baseline S_{cr} value by using the four variable Modification of Diet in Renal Disease (MDRD) equation with an assumed normal eGFR of 75 mL/min/1.73 m².[1] However, this method needs to be interpreted with caution as it has been found to overestimate the incidence of AKI by as much as 40%.[8,9]

Use of small changes in S_{cr} to diagnose AKI has been associated with additional drawbacks. For example, AKI may be inappropriately diagnosed in patients with low baseline S_{cr} (less than 0.6 mg/dL [53 μmol/L]) when using definitions that incorporate percentage increases from baseline.[4] Also, diagnostic false-positive rates can be as high as because of inherent laboratory and biologic variabilities of creatinine.[10]

EPIDEMIOLOGY

The epidemiology of AKI varies widely depending on the patient population studied and the criteria used to evaluate the patient. While the disorder has a frequency of 2% in hospitalized noncritically ill patients, the prevalence among the critically ill is significantly higher, that is, 60%.[11,12] Common risk factors associated with AKI include the presence of CKD, diabetes, heart or liver disease, albuminuria, major surgery (especially cardiac surgery), acute decompensated heart failure, sepsis, hypotension, volume depletion (diarrhea, vomiting, or dehydration), medications (exposure to angiotensin-converting enzyme [ACE] inhibitors, angiotensin receptor blockers [ARBs], diuretics, aminoglycosides, etc.), advanced age, male gender, and African American race.[3,7,11,13-15]

(2) Increased mortality and morbidity are two well-recognized complications of AKI. Severity, duration, and frequency of AKI appear to be important predictors of poor patient outcomes. Any degree of AKI is associated with an increased risk of death, and the odds increase with the severity of the insult.[11,13,14] For survivors of AKI, the development of some degree of CKD and need for RRT are other important considerations.[16] In addition, AKI is associated with increased length of hospital stay, cost, readmission, ventilator days, and need for post-hospitalization care.[11,14,17]

ETIOLOGY

(3) The etiology of AKI can be divided into three broad categories based on the anatomic location of the injury associated with the precipitating factor(s). The management of patients presenting with this disorder is largely predicated on identification of the specific etiology responsible for the patient's AKI (Fig. 43-1). Traditionally, the causes of AKI have been categorized as (a) prerenal, which results from decreased renal perfusion in the setting of undamaged parenchymal tissue, (b) intrinsic, the result of structural damage to the kidney, most commonly the tubule from an ischemic or toxic insult, and (c) postrenal, caused by obstruction of urine flow downstream from the kidney (Fig. 43-2).

The risk of AKI increases substantially with decreasing glomerular filtration rate (GFR) and presence of albuminuria and

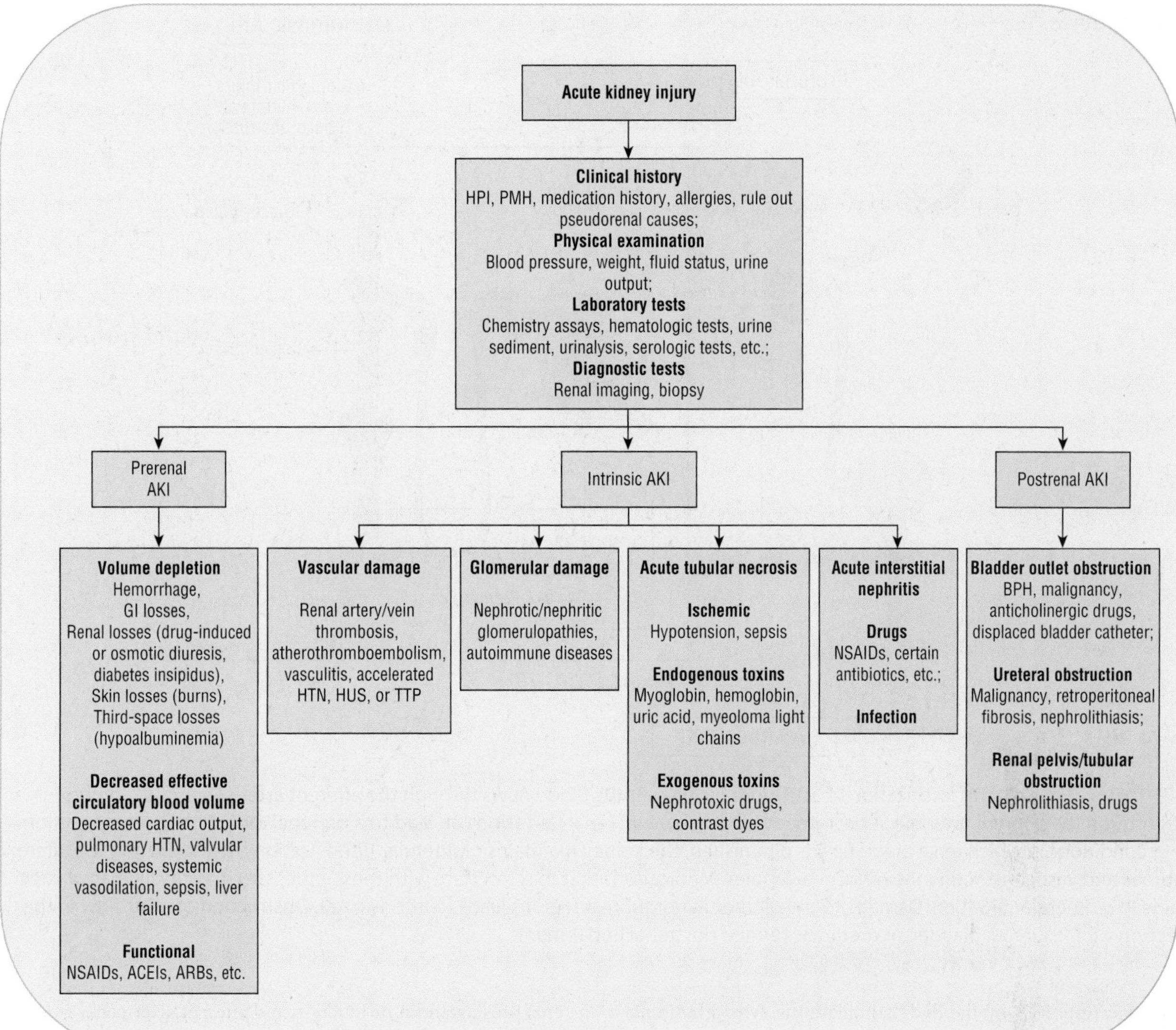

FIGURE 43-1 Classification of acute kidney injury (AKI) based on etiology. (ACEIs, angiotensin-converting enzyme inhibitors; ARBs, angiotensin receptor blockers; BPH, benign prostatic hyperplasia; HPI, history of present illness; HTN, hypertension; HUS, hemolytic uremic syndrome; NSAIDs, nonsteroidal anti-inflammatory drugs; PMH, past medical history; TTP, thrombotic thrombocytopenic purpura.)

underlying CKD.[15,18] A history of AKI has also been associated with high risk for developing additional episodes of AKI and subsequent complications such as advanced CKD.[19]

PATHOPHYSIOLOGY

The pathophysiologic processes involved in the development of the three traditional categories of AKI: prerenal AKI, intrinsic AKI, and postrenal AKI are described below. Pseudorenal kidney injury does not represent a true pathophysiologic process since it is associated with an alteration in laboratory measurement accuracy.

Pseudorenal Acute Kidney Injury

Pseudorenal AKI is characterized by a rise in either the BUN or the S_{cr}, which misleadingly may suggest the presence of renal dysfunction, when in fact GFR is not diminished. This could be the result of cross-reactivity of drugs or endogenous substances with the assay used to measure the BUN or S_{cr} or selective inhibition of the secretion of creatinine into the proximal tubular lumen by certain medications (see Chapter e42). A similar problem exists when urine output data are unreliable. Urine output may be either inaccurate (particularly in noncatheterized patients) or not reported at all. Since the urine output criteria for AKI staging are weight-based, some obese individuals may meet the definition of AKI without truly having any kidney impairment. Thus, clinical judgment should always be applied when interpreting laboratory results.

Prerenal Acute Kidney Injury

Prerenal AKI or prerenal azotemia results from hypoperfusion of the renal parenchyma, with or without systemic arterial hypotension. Renal hypoperfusion with systemic arterial hypotension may be caused by a decline in either the intravascular volume or the effective circulating blood volume. Intravascular volume depletion may result from several conditions, including hemorrhage, excessive gastrointestinal (GI) losses (severe vomiting or diarrhea), dehydration, extensive burns, and diuretic therapy. Effective circulating blood volume may be reduced in conditions associated with a decreased cardiac output and systemic vasodilation. Renal hypoperfusion without systemic hypotension is most commonly associated with bilateral renal artery occlusion or unilateral occlusion in a patient with a single functioning kidney.

Patients with a mild reduction in effective circulating blood volume or volume depletion are generally able to maintain a normal GFR by activating several compensatory mechanisms. Those initial

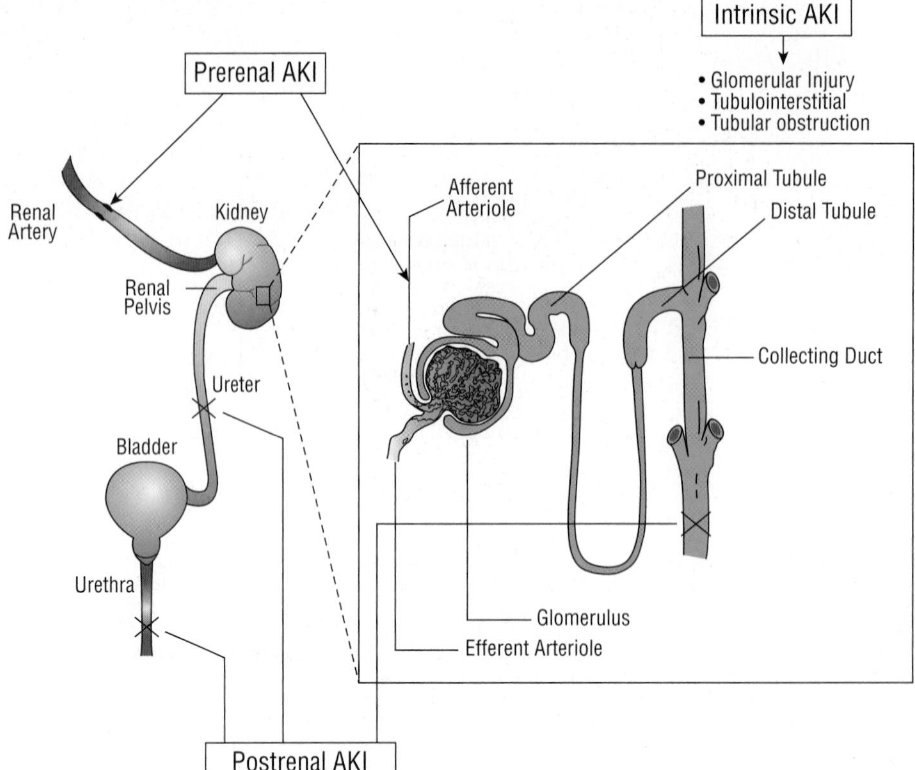

FIGURE 43-2 Physiologic classification of acute kidney injury (AKI). Blood flows through the afferent arteriole, to the glomerulus, and exits through the efferent arteriole. A decrease in blood flow and renal perfusion can lead to a prerenal reduction in renal function. Under conditions in which renal blood flow is diminished, the kidney maintains glomerular ultrafiltration by vasodilating the afferent arterioles and vasoconstricting the efferent arterioles. Medications that may interfere with these processes may result in an abrupt decline in glomerular filtration. Damage to the glomerular or tubular regions leads to intrinsic AKI. Obstruction of urine flow in the collecting tubule, ureter, bladder, or urethra is termed postrenal impairment.

physiologic responses by the body stimulate the sympathetic nervous and the renin–angiotensin–aldosterone system and release antidiuretic hormone if hypotension is present. These responses work together to directly maintain blood pressure via vasoconstriction and stimulation of thirst, which in conscious patients results in increased fluid intake, as well as sodium and water retention. Additionally, GFR may be maintained by afferent arteriole dilation (mediated by intrarenal production of vasodilatory prostaglandins, kallikrein, kinins, and nitric oxide) and efferent arteriole constriction (mainly mediated by angiotensin II). In concert, these homeostatic mechanisms are often able to maintain arterial pressure and renal perfusion, potentially averting the progression to AKI.[20] If, however, the decreased renal perfusion is severe or prolonged, these compensatory mechanisms may be overwhelmed, and prerenal AKI will be clinically evident.

Patients at risk for prerenal AKI are particularly susceptible to changes in the afferent and efferent arteriolar tone, as they may not be able to compensate as readily. Some drugs interfere with these renal adaptive responses, and the resulting reduction in the glomerular hydrostatic pressure precipitates an abrupt decline in GFR and is sometimes referred to as *functional AKI*. A common cause of this syndrome is a decrease in efferent arteriolar resistance as the result of initiation of an ACE inhibitor or ARB (see Chapter 46). For example, individuals with heart failure are often given an ACE inhibitor or ARB to help improve left ventricular function, but if the dose is titrated too rapidly, they may experience a decline in GFR. If the increase in the S_{cr} is less than 30% from baseline and potassium serum levels are within normal range, the medication can generally be continued. Nonsteroidal anti-inflammatory drugs (NSAIDs) may also initiate AKI in susceptible individuals due to their impact on renal prostaglandin production and afferent arteriolar vasodilation, which some patients rely on to maintain GFR.[21,22]

Sepsis is one of the leading clinical conditions associated with AKI. The traditional presumption that decreased renal hypoperfusion was responsible for reduced GFR has recently been questioned as new evidence indicates that there is little association between renal blood flow and GFR in patients with sepsis-induced AKI.[23] Instead, a complex interplay of different mechanisms may be involved in its pathogenesis; augmented vasoconstriction, capillary occlusion due to endothelial cell swelling, interaction of endothelial cells with leukocytes, and activation of coagulation. Simultaneously occurring renal inflammation and microcirculatory dysfunction further amplify these mechanisms. Recent studies have also found that apoptosis and tubular cell necrosis are rare during sepsis-induced AKI.[24-26] Instead, tubular epithelial cells develop adaptive responses, specifically downregulation of the cell function, in order to minimize energy demand and to ensure cell survival. This process also simultaneously results in reduced kidney function.

Intrinsic Acute Kidney Injury

Intrinsic AKI results from direct damage to the kidney and is categorized on the basis of the injured structures within the kidney: vasculature, glomeruli, tubules, and interstitium.

Renal Vasculature Damage

Occlusion of the larger renal vessels resulting in AKI is not common but can occur if large atheroemboli or thromboemboli occlude the bilateral renal arteries or one vessel of the patient with a single kidney. Atheroemboli most commonly develop during vascular procedures that cause atheroma dislodgement, such as angioplasty and aortic manipulations. Thromboemboli may arise from dislodgement of a mural thrombus in the left ventricle of a patient with severe heart failure or from the atria of a patient with atrial fibrillation. Renal artery thrombosis may occur in a similar fashion to coronary thrombosis, in which a thrombus forms in conjunction with an atherosclerotic plaque.

Although smaller vessels can also be obstructed by atheroemboli or thromboemboli, the damage is limited and the development of significant AKI is unlikely. However, these small vessels are susceptible to inflammatory processes that lead to microvascular damage and vessel dysfunction when the renal capillaries are affected. Neutrophils invade the vessel wall, causing damage that can include thrombus formation, tissue infarction, and collagen deposition within the vessel structure. Diffuse renal vasculitis can be severe and promote concomitant ischemic acute tubular necrosis (ATN). Untreated hypertension may also compromise renal microvascular blood flow, causing diffuse renal capillary damage.

Glomerular Damage

Only 5% of the cases of intrinsic AKI are of glomerular origin. The glomerulus is one of two capillary beds in the kidney. It serves to filter fluid and solute into the tubules while retaining proteins and other large blood components in the intravascular space. Because the glomerulus is a capillary system, similar damage in the renal vasculature as described above can occur by the same mechanisms. The pathophysiology and specific therapeutic approaches to glomerulonephritis are described in detail in Chapter 47.

Tubular Damage

Approximately 85% of all cases of intrinsic AKI are caused by ATN, of which 50% are a result of renal ischemia. The remaining 35% are the result of exposure to direct tubule toxins, which can be endogenous (myoglobin, hemoglobin, or uric acid) or exogenous (contrast agents, aminoglycosides, etc.) The tubules located within the medulla of the kidney are particularly at risk for ischemic injury, as this portion of the kidney is metabolically active and thus has high oxygen requirements, yet, as compared with the cortex, receives relatively low oxygen delivery. Thus, ischemic conditions caused by severe hypotension or exposure to vasoconstrictive drugs preferentially affect the tubules more than any other portion of the kidney.

The clinical evolution of ATN is characterized by four distinct phases: initiation, extension, maintenance, and recovery. Renal tubular epithelial cell injury is the hallmark of the initiation phase that results from vasoconstriction and ischemia, and leads to GFR reduction. Contrary to its name, ATN is not only characterized by necrosis and cell death but by a large spectrum of cellular injury that usually involves sublethal damage to the cells. The extent of injury depends not only on the severity and duration of ischemia but also on the sensitivity of renal cells to the insult which may vary based on the cells' metabolic demands, physical location within the kidney, degree of regional blood perfusion, oxygenation status, and membrane permeability. Further, alterations in cytoskeletal structure lead to a loss of epithelial polarity and barrier function. As a result, the glomerular filtrate starts leaking back into the interstitium and is reabsorbed into the systemic circulation. Additionally, urine flow is obstructed by accumulation of sloughed epithelial cells, cellular debris, and formation of casts.[27]

The extension phase is characterized by continued hypoxia following the initial ischemic event and an inflammatory response. Both events are more pronounced in the outer medullary region and the GFR continues to decrease. During the maintenance phase, GFR reaches a nadir during which cellular repair processes are initiated in an attempt to reestablish and maintain cellular and tubular integrity. The surviving cells undergo repair, migration, dedifferentiation, and proliferation. The maintenance phase is eventually followed by a recovery phase, during which new tubule cells are regenerated through redifferentiation and epithelial polarity is reestablished.[27]

Interstitial Damage

Acute interstitial nephritis (AIN) is an idiosyncratic delayed hypersensitivity immune reaction that is most commonly caused by drugs (see Chapter 46) and less commonly by infections, autoimmune diseases, or idiopathic causes. AIN is characterized by tubular and interstitial inflammation, and edema with lesions composed of mononuclear cells, with a predominance of lymphocytes (primarily CD4+ T lymphocytes) and monocytes or macrophages. The specific pathogenic process depends on the cause of AIN. Drug-induced disease is characterized by renal interstitial dendritic and renal tubular epithelial cells recognition of the offending agent as immunogenic and their activation of T lymphocytes which induce proinflammatory molecules. Once acute interstitial inflammation sets in, it can progress very rapidly to a more destructive fibrogenic process marked by increased interstitial matrix, ischemia, tubular atrophy, and interstitial fibrosis.[28] The prognosis of AIN varies widely as it is estimated that anywhere between 30% and 70% of patients may not recover their baseline renal function.[29] Patients who are at higher risk for permanent damage include elderly or those who develop more severe disease including azotemia, oliguria, or need for dialysis.[30] Delays in discontinuation of the offending drug and in initiating steroid treatment can also adversely affect recovery of kidney function.[31]

Postrenal Acute Kidney Injury

Postrenal AKI accounts for less than 5% of all cases of AKI and may develop as the result of obstruction at any level within the urinary collection system (see Fig. 43-1). However, if the obstructing process is above the bladder, it must involve both kidneys (one kidney in a patient with a single functioning kidney) to cause clinically significant AKI, as one functioning kidney can generally maintain a near-normal GFR. Bladder outlet obstruction, the most common cause of obstructive nephropathy, is often the result of a prostatic process (hypertrophy, cancer, or infection), producing a physical impingement on the urethra and thereby preventing the passage of urine. It may also be the result of an improperly placed urinary catheter. Blockage may also occur at the ureter level secondary to nephrolithiasis, blood clots, sloughed renal papillae, or physical compression by an abdominal process. Crystal deposition within the tubules from oxalate and some medications severe enough to cause AKI is uncommon, but it is possible in patients with severe volume contraction and in those receiving large doses of a drug with relatively low urine solubility (see Chapter 46). In these cases, patients have insufficient urine volume to prevent crystal precipitation in the urine. Extremely elevated uric acid concentrations from chemotherapy-induced tumor lysis syndrome can cause obstruction and direct tubular injury as well.[32] Where ever the location of the obstruction, urine will accumulate in the renal structures above the obstruction and cause increased pressure upstream. The ureters, renal pelvis, and calyces all expand, and the net result is a decline in GFR. If renal vasoconstriction ensues, a further decrement in GFR will be observed.

CLINICAL PRESENTATION

The initiating signs or symptoms of AKI are highly variable and largely dependent on the underlying etiology. It may be a change in urinary character (eg, decreased urine output or urine discoloration), sudden weight gain, or severe abdominal or flank pain. Early recognition and cause identification are critical, as they directly affect the outcome of AKI. One of the first steps in the diagnostic process is to determine if the change in renal function is acute, chronic, or the result of an acute change in a patient with known

CKD (also called acute-on-chronic renal failure). Patients should also be promptly evaluated for any changes in their fluid and electrolyte status. Patients presenting with AKI in the outpatient environment may have very nonspecific or seemingly unrelated symptoms so that the time of onset of the injury can be difficult to determine. On the other hand, AKI in hospitalized patients is often detected much earlier in its course due to frequent laboratory studies and daily patient assessment.

Patient Assessment

The assessment of a patient with AKI starts with a thorough review of his or her medical records, with a particular focus on chronic conditions, laboratory studies, procedures, and surgeries. An exhaustive review of prescription and nonprescription medicines, herbal products, and recreational drugs may help determine if AKI was potentially precipitated by drug ingestion.

During the initial patient evaluation, presumptive signs and symptoms of AKI need to be differentiated from a potential new diagnosis of CKD. A medical history for renal disease–related chronic conditions (eg, poorly controlled hypertension or diabetes mellitus), previous laboratory data documenting the presence of proteinuria or an elevated S_{cr}, and the finding of bilateral small kidneys on renal ultrasonography suggest the presence of CKD rather than AKI. However, it is important to note that patients with CKD may develop episodes of AKI as well. In that case, an abrupt rise in the patient's baseline S_{cr} is one of the most useful indicators of the presence of an acute insult to the kidneys. The staging of AKI should also be assessed including the initial insult and decline in renal function, stabilization of the decline in function, and recovery period.

An acute change in urinary habitus is another common and noticeable symptom associated with AKI. The presence of cola-colored urine is indicative of blood in the urine, a finding commonly associated with acute glomerulonephritis. In hospitalized patients, changes in urine output may be helpful in characterizing the cause of the patient's AKI. Acute anuria is typically caused by either complete urinary obstruction or a catastrophic event (eg, shock or acute cortical necrosis). Oliguria, which often develops over several days, suggests prerenal azotemia, whereas nonoliguric renal failure usually results from acute intrinsic renal failure or incomplete urinary obstruction.

Depending on the underlying cause of AKI, patients may present with a variety of symptoms affecting virtually any organ system of the body. Constitutional symptoms such as nausea, vomiting, fatigue, malaise, and weight gain are common but nonspecific. The onset of flank pain is suggestive of a urinary stone; however, if bilateral, it may suggest swelling of the kidneys secondary to acute glomerulonephritis or AIN. Complaints of severe headaches may suggest the presence of severe hypertension and vascular damage. The presence of fever, rash, and arthralgia may be indicative of drug-induced AIN or lupus nephritis.

A thorough physical examination is an important step in evaluating individuals with AKI, as clues regarding the etiology can be evident from the patient's head (eye examination) to toe (evidence of dependent edema) assessment. Evaluation of the patient's volume and hemodynamic status is critical as well, as it will guide management. For example, patients with prerenal AKI can present with either volume depletion or fluid overload. Volume depletion may be evidenced by the presence of postural hypotension, decreased jugular venous pressure (JVP), and dry mucous membranes. Fluid overload, on the other hand, is often reflected by elevated JVP, pitting edema, ascites, and pulmonary crackles.

Conventional Markers of Kidney Function

4 Commonly available laboratory tests used to evaluate the patient with renal insufficiency are described in Chapter e42. Over the past four decades, S_{cr} has been the most widely used laboratory test for estimating creatinine clearance (eCL_{cr}) and eGFR. However, there are several limitations associated with its use since it is affected by age, gender, muscle mass, diet, and hydration status. For example, patients with reduced creatinine production, such as those with low muscle mass, may have very low values (less than 0.6 mg/dL [53 μmol/L]); thus, the presence of a gradual rise to normal values (0.8-1.2 mg/dL [71-106 μmol/L]) may actually suggest the presence of AKI. However, in the presence of improved nutrition and a large muscle mass, a S_{cr} of 1.2 mg/dL (106 μmol/L) may be a true representation of a person's current renal status. Instead of using only the most current value to determine renal function, changes in the value from a patient's baseline need to be considered. S_{cr} is normally inversely proportional to GFR. However, rapid changes in GFR disrupt this equilibrium and make S_{cr} a very insensitive marker. In fact, changes in S_{cr} will lag behind the GFR's decline by 1 to 2 days due to slow accumulation, increased tubular secretion, and increased extrarenal clearance.[33,34] This can lead to a significant overestimation of the patient's GFR in the early stages of AKI and consequently a potential delay in the diagnosis of the syndrome.

An example of this phenomenon is illustrated by an acute renal artery thrombus that results in abrupt cessation of GFR in one kidney as a consequence of the complete obstruction of blood flow to that kidney. Although 5 minutes following the event GFR is decreased 50% (assuming the other kidney is functioning and unaffected), the S_{cr} remains unchanged. Assuming a standard daily creatinine production of about 20 mg/kg of lean body weight, one can expect about 1.4 g of creatinine production in a 24-hour period in a 70-kg individual. In pharmacokinetic terms, daily creatinine production is analogous to a continuous infusion, and GFR determines the elimination rate of creatinine. In a patient with normal renal function (GFR of 120 mL/min [2 mL/s]), the half-life of creatinine is 3.5 hours, with 95% of steady state achieved in about 14 hours. If GFR declines to 50%, 25%, or 10% of normal, the half-life of creatinine increases, resulting in prolongation of the time to reach 95% of steady state, specifically taking 1, 2, and 4 days, respectively.

Because S_{cr} steady-state values are assumed when one uses several GFR calculation methods, such as the Cockcroft-Gault, MDRD, and Chronic Kidney Disease Epidemiology Collaboration (CKD-EPI) equations, they should not be used to estimate GFR in AKI patients with unstable renal function. These equations will typically overestimate GFR when the AKI is worsening and underestimate it when the AKI is resolving. Instead, it may be useful to evaluate changes in S_{cr} values from the patient's baseline and also consider the S_{cr} sequence values to determine if renal function is potentially improving or worsening. The most recent S_{cr} reflects the time-averaged kidney function over the preceding time period. Several mathematical approaches to estimate GFR in patients with unstable S_{cr} that incorporate the principles of creatinine accumulation and elimination have been proposed and are discussed in detail in Chapter e42. However, these methods have not been extensively validated in the setting of AKI, and their value for adjusting medication dosing is questionable. Additionally, these equations are complex and are not commonly used in the clinical setting.

Two other widely available markers of renal function are BUN and urine output. The value of the BUN in AKI is very limited because urea production and renal clearance are heavily influenced by extrarenal factors such as critical illness, volume status, protein intake, and medications. Urine output measured over a specified period of time (eg, 4-24 hours) allows for short-term assessment of kidney function, but its utility is limited to cases in which it is significantly decreased. The presence of anuria suggests complete kidney failure, whereas oliguria indicates some degree of kidney damage. Urine output needs to be interpreted with caution, as it is dependent on several factors, such as hydration status and medications. As mentioned earlier in the chapter, a patient may have AKI and still maintain a normal urine output; this condition is referred to as *nonoliguric AKI*. Another approach to estimating renal function is to directly measure CL_{cr} over a short period of time, for example, 4 to 12 hours.[35] Although, potentially precise and fairly simple to do, its accuracy is questionable if the urine output is low or the urine collection is incomplete.

In addition to BUN and S_{cr}, selected blood and urine tests, and urinary sediment are routinely evaluated to differentiate the cause of AKI and guide patient management. For example, a complete blood cell count with differential can help rule out infectious causes of AKI. Serum electrolyte values may be abnormal because of the acute decline of the kidney's ability to regulate electrolyte excretion. Particular attention should be paid to serum potassium and phosphorus values, which can be markedly elevated and cause life-threatening complications. In individuals with normal renal function, the ratio between BUN and S_{cr} is usually less than 15:1 using conventional units (~60:1 using SI units). In the presence of prerenal AKI, reabsorption of BUN exceeds that of creatinine; thus, one often sees a ratio greater than 20:1 (greater than 100:1 for urea to creatinine ratio is commonly used when using parameters expressed in identical molar units).

Given the limited usefulness of solely using S_{cr} or BUN concentrations to differentiate the etiology of AKI, urinary electrolytes and osmolality should be determined, and both a microscopic and chemical analysis of the urine should be performed (Table 43-2). The finding of a high urinary specific gravity, in the absence of glucosuria or mannitol administration, suggests an intact urinary concentrating mechanism and that the cause of the patient's AKI is likely prerenal azotemia. The presence of urinary protein is often difficult to interpret, especially in the setting of acute or chronic renal failure. A patient with CKD may have a baseline proteinuria, thus clouding the clinical presentation, unless this is known at the time of AKI assessment. Classically, proteinuria is a hallmark of glomerular damage. However, tubular damage can also result in proteinuria, as the tubules are responsible for reabsorbing small proteins that are normally filtered by all glomeruli. The presence of blood also results in a positive urine protein test, so this confounder must always be assessed when a positive urine protein is obtained. Hematuria suggests acute intrinsic AKI secondary to glomerular injury, infection, or a kidney stone. On microscopic examination, the key findings are cells, casts, and crystals, and the presence of one or more of these may suggest specific etiologies of the AKI (Table 43-3). The finding of urinary crystals may indicate nephrolithiasis and a postrenal obstruction. If red blood cells or red blood cell casts are present, one should consider the presence of a physical injury to the glomerulus, renal parenchyma, or vascular beds. The finding of white blood cells or white blood cell casts suggests interstitial inflammation (ie, interstitial nephritis), which can be secondary to an allergic, granulomatous, or infectious process.

Simultaneous measurement of urine and serum electrolytes is also helpful in the setting of AKI (see Table 43-2). From these values, a fractional excretion of sodium (FE_{Na}) can be calculated. The equation for the calculation of the FE_{Na} is as follows:

$$FE_{Na} = \frac{\text{Excreted Na}}{\text{Filtered Na}} \times 100 = \frac{U_{vol} \times U_{Na}}{GFR \times S_{Na}} \times 100$$

where

$$GFR = \frac{U_{vol} \times U_{cr}}{S_{cr} \times t}$$

TABLE 43-2 Diagnostic Parameters for Differentiating Causes of AKI[a]

Laboratory Test	Prerenal AKI	Intrinsic AKI	Postrenal AKI
Urine sediment	Hyaline casts, may be normal	Granular casts, cellular debris	Cellular debris
Urinary RBC	None	2–4+	Variable
Urinary WBC	None	2–4+	1+
Urine Na (mEq/L or mmol/L)	<20	>40	>40
FE_{Na} (%)	<1	>2	Variable
Urine/serum osmolality	>1.5	<1.3	<1.5
Urine/S_{cr}	>40:1	<20:1	<20:1
BUN/S_{cr} (urea/S_{cr}, SI)	>20 (>100)	~15 (~60)	~15 (~60)
Urine specific gravity	>1.018	<1.012	Variable

AKI, acute kidney injury; BUN, blood urea nitrogen; FE_{Na}, fractional excretion of sodium; S_{cr}, serum creatinine; RBC, red blood cell; WBC, white blood cell.

[a]Common laboratory tests are used to classify the cause of AKI. Functional AKI, which is not included in this table, would have laboratory values similar to those seen in prerenal AKI. However, the urine osmolality-to-plasma osmolality ratios may not exceed 1.5, depending on the circulating levels of antidiuretic hormone. The laboratory results listed under intrinsic AKI are those seen in acute tubular necrosis, the most common cause of intrinsic AKI.

TABLE 43-3 Urinary Findings as a Guide to the Etiology of AKI

Type of Urinary Evaluation	Presence of	Suggestive of
Urinalysis	Leukocyte esterases	Pyelonephritis
	Nitrites	Pyelonephritis
	Protein	
	Mild (<0.5 g/day)	Tubular damage
	Moderate (0.5-3 g/day)	Glomerulonephritis, pyelonephritis, tubular damage
	Large (>3 g/day)	Glomerulonephritis, nephrotic syndrome
	Hemoglobin	Glomerulonephritis, pyelonephritis, renal infarction, renal tumors, kidney stones
	Myoglobin	Rhabdomyolysis-associated tubular necrosis
	Urobilinogen	Hemolysis-associated tubular necrosis
Urine sediment	Microorganisms	Pyelonephritis
Cells	Red blood cells	Glomerulonephritis, pyelonephritis, renal infarction, papillary necrosis, renal tumors, kidney stones
	White blood cells	Pyelonephritis, interstitial nephritis
	Eosinophils	Drug-induced interstitial nephritis, renal transplant rejection
	Epithelial cells	Tubular necrosis
Casts	Granular casts	Tubular necrosis
	Hyaline casts	Prerenal azotemia
	White blood cell casts	Pyelonephritis, interstitial nephritis
	Red blood cell casts	Glomerulonephritis, renal infarct, lupus nephritis, vasculitis
Crystals	Urate	Postrenal obstruction
	Calcium phosphate	Postrenal obstruction

AKI, acute kidney injury.

Thus:

$$FE_{Na} = \frac{U_{Na} \times S_{cr} \times 100}{U_{cr} \times S_{Na}}$$

where U_{vol} is urine volume; U_{cr} is urine creatinine concentration; U_{Na} is urine sodium; S_{cr} is serum creatinine concentration; S_{Na} is serum sodium concentration, which usually does not vary much; GFR is the glomerular filtration rate; and *t* is the time period over which the urine is collected.

The FE_{Na} is one of the better diagnostic parameters to differentiate the cause of AKI. A low urinary sodium concentration (less than 20 mEq/L [mmol/L]) and low FE_{Na} (less than 1%) in a patient with oliguria suggest that there is stimulation of the sodium-retentive mechanisms in the kidney and that tubular function is intact. These findings are most characteristic of prerenal azotemia. Unfortunately, diuretic use in the preceding days limits the usefulness of the FE_{Na} calculation by increasing natriuresis, even in hypovolemic patients. The fractional excretion of urea (FE_{Urea}), which can be calculated like FE_{Na}, is sometimes used as an alternative means to assess tubular function. The inability to concentrate urine results in a high FE_{Na} (greater than 2%), suggesting tubular damage as the primary cause of the intrinsic AKI. However, this is also not an absolute finding, as there are some intrinsic causes that can be associated with a low FE_{Na} (eg, contrast nephropathy, myoglobinuria, and interstitial nephritis). Highly concentrated urine (greater than 500 mOsm/kg [500 mmol/kg]) suggests stimulation of antidiuretic hormone and intact tubular function. These findings are consistent with prerenal azotemia.

Novel Biomarkers of Kidney Damage

A variety of biomarkers have been investigated to detect and predict the clinical outcomes of AKI. While they vary in their origin, function, distribution, and time of release following renal injury, the large majority are molecules that are released as a result of direct kidney cell damage. The performance of most biomarkers is variable and depends on the patient population, cause of AKI, presence of comorbidities, and timing of biomarker measurements. In general, their ability to detect AKI is significantly better within homogenous patient populations where the time of AKI is known than in heterogeneous populations with multiple comorbidities and unknown AKI time or cause such as critically ill patients. Even though some biomarker tests are now commercially available, these tests are not routinely available at most clinical practice sites. Lastly, there is still a barrier for clinical translation since there are little data available on the impact of the biomarker information on clinical decision making.[33,36]

Two of the most promising biomarkers studied in AKI are tissue inhibitor of metalloproteinases 2 (TIMP-2) and insulin-like growth factor binding protein 7 (IGFBP7). Both molecules inhibit specific proteins that result in G1 cell cycle arrest noted to occur during the very early phases of cellular stress or injury. The cell uses cell-cycle arrest as a protective mechanism to avoid cell division when potentially damaged. However, if the cells do not re-initiate the cell cycle and remain arrested, a fibrotic phenotype can develop instead. These findings are of importance as cell cycle arrest activation and deactivation may prove to be potential targets of therapeutic interventions in the future.[37] At this time, TIMP-2 and IGFBP7 have been validated in critically ill patients and noted to outperformed other biomarkers. In 2014, the combination of TIMP-2 and IGFBP7 was approved by the Food and Drug Administration (FDA) as the first point-of-care device to detect early AKI. The test called Nephrocheck® uses a fluorescent immunoassay and reveals test results expressed as an AKI risk score within 20 minutes. Scores over 0.3 $(ng/mL)^2/1,000$ indicate a patient is at greater risk for developing moderate to severe AKI within 12 hours of testing.[37] While TIMP-2 and IGFBP7 appear to be promising biomarkers, the cutoff value of 0.3 has a sensitivity of 92% but a specificity of only 46%.[38] In addition, the test's superior performance in critically ill patients was not reproducible in cardiac surgery patients raising the question of test's utility in various patient settings.[39]

One of the most studied biomarkers is neutrophil gelatinase–associated lipocalin (NGAL), a transporter protein found on cell surfaces of neutrophils and various epithelial cells. It is freely filtered by the glomeruli and reabsorbed by the proximal tubules. As a result, if proximal tubular injury occurs, urinary NGAL levels are expected to rise. Studies indicate that NGAL may be a valuable biomarker of AKI development across a range of clinical settings, including both children and adults, patients with contrast-induced nephropathy (CIN), critically ill, and cardiac surgery patients.[40] Also, the availability of commercial assays for both urine and serum NGAL may facilitate the use of this biomarker in multiple clinical settings. While NGAL has demonstrated promising results for the early recognition of AKI, it does have several limitations. Some comorbidities, especially CKD, may affect its results since CKD is associated with elevated serum and urinary NGAL levels. Also, NGAL synthesis increases in response to inflammatory triggers irrespective of the presence of AKI. Lastly, it was recently discovered that the total concentration of urinary NGAL represents a mixture of different molecular forms of NGAL with different cellular origins (renal tissue, neutrophils, and extrarenal tissue such as liver and lung), and the current assays are unable to distinguish the NGAL dimer that is specifically produced by the stressed renal tubular cells.[41]

The advances in our knowledge of AKI pathophysiology as well as the advent of biomarkers has prompted ADQI to propose the use of two new terms "functional change" and "kidney damage" instead of the traditional "prerenal, intrinsic, and postrenal" AKI definitions. Functional change refers to changes in glomerular and tubular function and includes markers such as S_{cr}, eGFR, and cystatin C. Kidney damage describes presence of tubular and/or glomerular injury and includes markers such as NGAL, TIMP-2, and IGFBP7. The rationale behind the proposed changes in terminology stems from a relatively new concept of subclinical kidney injury. According to this theory, kidney injury may be detected by changes in the plasma or urinary levels of specific biomarkers before overt changes in renal function (decreased eGFR or increased S_{cr}) have occurred. As a result, a patient may have kidney damage without a change in kidney function. These findings are significant because this patient group is at a greater risk of complications, a longer stay in intensive care unit, and has a higher risk of dying when compared with the group without kidney damage. Table 43-4 summarizes the relationship between functional change and kidney damage.[42,43]

Diagnostic Considerations

When the source of renal injury is unclear after a history, physical examination, and assessment of laboratory values, imaging techniques such as abdominal radiography, including the kidneys,

TABLE 43-4 Newly Proposed Classification of AKI Based on Functional and Kidney Damage Biomarkers

		Kidney Damage	
		No	**Yes**
Functional change	**No**	No functional change or damage; Biomarker negative RIFLE negative	Kidney damage without change in function Biomarker positive RIFLE negative
	Yes	Functional change but no kidney damage RIFLE positive Biomarker negative	Kidney damage with functional change RIFLE positive Biomarker positive

AKI, acute kidney injury; RIFLE, risk, injury failure, loss of function, and end stage renal disease.

ureters, and bladder (KUB), computed tomography (CT), and ultrasonography may be helpful. These may reveal small, shrunken kidneys indicative of CKD. Postrenal obstruction can often be identified with a renal ultrasonography and/or CT scan. Renal ultrasonography is also useful in detecting obstruction or hydronephrosis. Nephrolithiasis as small as 5 nm or a narrowing of the ureteral tract can be detected by ultrasonography or more sensitive tests, such as KUB and CT.

In cases in which the cause of AKI is not evident, renal biopsies are useful in determining the cause in most patients. Because of the associated risk of bleeding, a renal biopsy is rarely undertaken and should only be performed in those circumstances when a definitive diagnosis is needed to guide therapy, such as the precise etiology of glomerulonephritis (see Chapter 47).

PREVENTION OF ACUTE KIDNEY INJURY

Prevention of AKI is critical since there is no treatment to reverse the insult once it has developed. The risk of AKI can be reduced when the nonpharmacologic and pharmacologic therapies described below are used.

Desired Outcomes

The goals of AKI prevention are to (a) screen and identify patients at risk, (b) monitor high-risk patients until the risk has subsided, and (c) implement prevention strategies when appropriate.

General Approach to Prevention

5 The choice of preventive strategy depends on the cause of the renal insult. Clearly, avoidance of all potential causes of AKI is the most effective preventive method; however, it may not always be possible. Sometimes, the risk of renal injury is predictable, such as decreased perfusion secondary to coronary bypass surgery or secondary to the administration of a radiocontrast dye. In these situations, the potential insult to the kidneys cannot be avoided but may be preventable or minimized with aggressive hydration and avoidance or removal of any additional insults. In the outpatient setting, all healthcare professionals should educate the patient on preventive measures for AKI. Patients should receive counseling regarding their optimal daily fluid intake (~2 L/day) to avoid dehydration, especially if they are to receive a potentially nephrotoxic medication. In the inpatient setting, adequate hydration, standardized hemodynamic support in the critically ill, and avoidance of nephrotoxic medications are commonly recommended strategies for the prevention of AKI. Table 43-5 summarizes the recommendations published by KDIGO regarding recommended and not recommended therapies for the prevention of AKI.[3]

Nonpharmacologic Therapy

Hydration is one of the primary interventions that has consistently shown benefit and is routinely used in the prevention of AKI. Fluids have largely been studied in association with hemodynamic instability secondary to intravascular volume depletion as well as contrast administration before a radiologic procedure.

Hemodynamic instability increases the risk of AKI as it can lead to decreased renal perfusion and subsequent renal injury. Both isotonic crystalloids and colloid-containing solutions have been studied as means to replace intravascular volume. Among colloids, synthetic products such as hyperoncotic hydroxyethyl starch have been associated with renal dysfunction and should generally be avoided in patients at risk for AKI.[44] Albumin appears to be safe for the kidneys; however, it is more costly and does not provide better patient outcomes compared with isotonic saline.[45] As a result, KDIGO guidelines recommend isotonic crystalloids over colloids for intravascular volume expansion in patients at risk for AKI.[3]

Over the past several years, there has been a growing interest in the use of balanced solutions instead of isotonic saline. The main concerns associated with the use of large amounts of saline are hyperchloremic acidosis, interstitial edema, and fluid overload. The chloride content in isotonic saline is 1.5 times that of plasma (154 mEq/L [mmol/L]) which can lead to hyperchloremic metabolic acidosis. Hyperchloremia in turn can decrease renal artery blood flow and renal tissue perfusion. Further, saline infusions cause a greater increase in interstitial fluid volume than balanced solutions and this may result in a relatively greater increase in renal volume and thereby increased intracapsular pressure, decreased microvascular blood flow, and impaired renal function.[46] Balanced solutions (Plasmalyte and Sterofundin) have an electrolyte content that is closer to the plasma concentrations as chloride is partly replaced by bicarbonate precursors such as lactate, acetate, or gluconate. Some studies have demonstrated more favorable outcomes with balanced fluids, including a significantly lower risk of AKI and reduced need for RRT,

TABLE 43-5 KDIGO Recommendations for Prevention and Treatment of AKI

Drug	Indication	Recommended for Prevention	Recommended for Treatment	Comments
ANP	AKI	No (2C)	No (2B)	
Diuretics	AKI	No (1B)	No (2C)	Acceptable if managing concurrent fluid overload
Dopamine (1-3 mcg/kg/min)	AKI	No (1A)	No (1A)	
Fenoldopam	AKI CI-AKI	No (2C) No (1B)	No (2C)	
Isotonic saline IV	AKI CI-AKI	Yes (2B) Yes (1A)	Yes (2B)	For AKI: recommended in the absence of hemorrhagic shock
NAC	AKI CI-AKI	No (2D) Yes (2D)		For CI-AKI: give in combination with isotonic saline
RRT	AKI CI-AKI	 No (2C)	Yes (NG)	
Sodium bicarbonate IV	CI-AKI	Yes (1A)		
Theophylline	CI-AKI	No (2C)		
Vasopressors	AKI	Yes (1C)	Yes (1C)	Recommended in combination with fluids in vasomotor shock

AKI, acute kidney injury; ANP, atrial natriuretic peptide; CI-AKI, contrast-induced acute kidney injury; KDIGO, Kidney Disease: Improving Global Outcomes; NAC, *N*-acetylcysteine; RRT, renal replacement therapy.

Strength of recommendation levels: 1, recommended; 2, suggested; NG, not graded.

Quality of supporting evidence: A, high; B, moderate; C, low; D, very low.

while others have not.[47,48] Further randomized studies are needed to determine whether balanced solutions should replace isotonic saline as the mainstay of fluid resuscitation in critically ill patients.

CIN is a common cause of ATN in the inpatient setting (see Chapter 46 for a detailed discussion) and is typically characterized by an increase in S_{cr} starting at 12 hours up to 5 days after the radiologic procedure.[3] It is associated with increased mortality especially in individuals with CKD, diabetes, volume depletion, concurrent nephrotoxic drug therapy, or hemodynamic instability. Hydration is thought to counterbalance some of the deleterious effects of radiocontrast dyes by diluting the contrast media, preventing renal vasoconstriction that contributes to hypoxia and ischemia, and minimizing tubular obstruction. Sodium bicarbonate infusion has also been evaluated for the prevention of CIN. The hypothesized mechanism for protection is that sodium bicarbonate may reduce the formation of oxygen-free radicals by alkalinizing renal tubular fluid.[49] There is currently no agreement on which hydration regimen is more effective as some studies indicate lower incidences of CIN with sodium bicarbonate while others show lower CIN rates with isotonic saline.[50-52] The KDIGO guidelines currently recommend using either sodium bicarbonate or isotonic saline in high-risk individuals receiving radiocontrast media.[3]

Since there is no consensus on the optimal rate and duration of fluid infusions, CIN hydration protocols may vary. A common sodium bicarbonate regimen is 154 mEq/L (mmol/L) infused at 3 mL/kg/h for 1 hour before the procedure and at 1 mL/kg/h for 6 hours after the procedure.[50-52] The rate and duration of normal saline infusion also vary, but one frequently cited regimen is 1 mL/kg/h for 12 hours before and 12 hours after the procedure.[52] The rate of administration may need to be adjusted based on the patient's cardiopulmonary and volume status.

The role of oral hydration (defined as ingestion of a specific amount of water prior and after receiving radiocontrast media) is not as well established as intravenous hydration, however, it has been compared to the intravenous route and found to be as effective in reducing the risk of CIN.[53-55] However, this option is best reserved for outpatients, undergoing elective procedures, with either normal renal function or mild renal impairment. For inpatients or individuals who require emergent coronary angiography or radiological procedures with contrast exposures, IV hydration is still considered first-line treatment for prevention of CIN.[53]

Pharmacologic Therapy

Many pharmacologic therapies have been investigated for the prevention of AKI. Several therapies have shown either no benefit or an unacceptable safety profile.[3] For example, vasodilators such as dopamine and fenoldapam are not recommended due to lack of benefit and risk of hypotension.[57,58] Theophylline has also been studied because of its adenosine receptor antagonist properties, however, its modest benefit does not outweigh potential adverse effects such as tachycardia, tremor, and drug interactions.[3,59,60]

Per KDIGO guidelines, antioxidants (ascorbic acid and *N*-acetylcysteine [NAC]) and glycemic control with insulin may have a role in prevention of AKI for select patient populations and are described below.[3]

Ascorbic Acid

Ascorbic acid has mainly been studied for the prevention of CIN, as its antioxidant properties are thought to alleviate oxidative stress caused by CIN-associated ischemia reperfusion injury. While its excellent safety profile and low cost make it an attractive option, clinical studies have reported inconsistent results.[61-63] While the specific dosage regimens and route of administration vary between studies, one of the more frequently studied regimens consists of ascorbic acid 3 g orally before the procedure and 2 g orally twice daily for two doses after the procedure.[63] One meta-analysis demonstrated a small albeit significant reduction in the relative risk of CIN in patients undergoing coronary angiography.[64] While the KDIGO Work Group did not specifically provide recommendations on ascorbic acid, current literature indicates that ascorbic acid may be considered for the prevention of CIN since it is associated with minimal risks and a small protective effect.

N-Acetylcysteine

NAC is another antioxidant that has been widely studied in the prevention of CIN. However, its therapeutic benefit is thought to be quite modest and has not been consistently demonstrated.[51,65,66] A frequently quoted dosing regimen for prevention of CIN is 600 to 1,200 mg orally every 12 hours for 2 to 3 days, with the first two doses administered prior to contrast exposure. Due to its favorable safety profile and potential benefit, the KIDGO guidelines suggest using NAC in combination with IV isotonic saline in patients at risk for CIN.[3]

Glycemic Control

Glycemic control in critically ill patients is important as stress hyperglycemia and insulin resistance are common during critical illness and are associated with increased mortality. The causes of insulin resistance are multifactorial but include impaired glucose homeostasis due to loss of the kidney's metabolic function, and decreased hepatic and peripheral glucose uptake secondary to uremia. Several studies have found that hyperglycemia increases the risk of acute kidney injury, possibly by triggering oxidative stress within the kidneys via increased production of reactive oxygen species within the mitochondria.[67-69]

Critically ill patients with AKI are not only at increased risk for hyperglycemia but also hypoglycemia. Hypoglycemia can develop when insulin protocols are too aggressive and attempt to target normal blood glucose concentrations of 80 to 110 mg/dL (4.4-6.1 mmol/L). Patients with AKI or preexisting kidney disease are particularly susceptible to hypoglycemia as the kidneys are the primary metabolic site of insulin and also contribute significantly to gluconeogenesis.[67] Current KDIGO guidelines suggest using insulin therapy to target plasma glucose of 110 to 149 mg/dL (6.1-8.3 mmol/L).[3] Other guidelines such as the American Diabetes Association and the American Society of Parenteral and Enteral Nutrition have recommended a glycemic target range of 140 to 180 mg/dL (7.8-10.0 mmol/L) in critically ill patients.[70,71]

Clinical **Controversy...**

Automated, real-time electronic alert systems have the potential to improve recognition and management of AKI. While observational studies suggest that AKI alerts may increase frequency and timeliness of treatment, a recent single-center randomized controlled trial found no difference in clinical outcomes between patient groups who were assigned the electronic alert and those who were not. Further research is needed to determine whether AKI alerts and similar computerized decision-support initiatives are of value to the healthcare provider and if they can significantly improve care.

TREATMENT

6 Since there is no specific treatment that can reverse AKI or hasten its recovery, supportive measures that focus on hemodynamics, fluid balance, acid-base balance, and electrolyte homeostasis are the mainstays of therapy.

Desired Outcomes

Short-term goals of AKI management include minimizing the degree of insult to the kidney, reducing extrarenal complications, and expediting the patient's recovery of renal function. Therapy should focus on maintaining organ functions while sustaining mean arterial pressure. The ultimate goal is to have the patient's renal function restored to pre-AKI baseline. Table 43-5 summarizes the KDIGO clinical practice guidelines regarding recommended and not recommended therapies for the treatment of AKI.[3]

General Approach to Treatment

Identification and management of AKI should be prompt. Prerenal sources of AKI should be managed with hemodynamic support and volume replacement.[72] Postrenal therapy focuses on removing the cause of the obstruction. It is important to approach the treatment of established AKI with an understanding of the patient's comorbidities and baseline renal function. Loss of kidney function combined with other clinical conditions, such as cardiac and liver failure, is associated with higher mortality.[73] At times, the most efficacious remedy for AKI is management of the comorbid precipitating event. Presence of CKD indicates that the kidneys have less reserve, and there is a greater likelihood that full recovery may not occur. If AKI is severe, RRT may be necessary to maintain fluid, electrolyte, and acid-base balance while removing accumulating waste products or toxins.[72]

Pharmacologic and Nonpharmacologic Therapies

It should be emphasized again that the currently available pharmacologic and nonpharmacologic therapies are only supportive in nature and focus on managing complications such as fluid overload and acid-base/electrolyte imbalances. Maintaining an adequate fluid status is imperative and challenging at the same time. First-line therapies for volume resuscitation consist of crystalloids such as isotonic saline or balanced solutions. On the other hand, fluid overload is treated with loop diuretics or RRT. Patients with severe AKI are more likely to have concomitant acid-base and electrolyte derangements and thus are more likely to receive RRT. However, it is unclear whether RRT or conservative management should be preferred in patients with AKI. Randomized controlled-trials are currently underway to assess whether early initiation of RRT improves patient outcomes and reduces mortality.[74,75]

Hydration

The principal of fluid therapy is to maintain or restore effective intravascular volume to assure adequate tissue perfusion. Similarly to preventative hydration strategies, crystalloids such as isotonic saline or balanced solutions are preferred. At the same time, great care needs to be taken to avoid too liberal fluid administration which can result in interstitial edema, increased intra-abdominal pressure, renal venous congestion, and decreased GFR.[76] These processes have been associated with increased mortality and reduced recovery of renal function further exacerbate AKI and lead to additional fluid retention.[77] Thus, maintaining adequate fluid balance is a major challenge in AKI patients, particularly those who are critically ill. In addition, the patient should be monitored for body weight changes, fluid intake and urine output, pulmonary and peripheral edema, blood pressure (target mean arterial pressure ≥65 mm Hg), and serum electrolytes. Urine output more than or equal to 0.5 mL/kg/h is generally targeted during the initial fluid resuscitation phase.[78]

In patients with anuria or oliguria, slower rehydration, such as 250 mL boluses or 100 mL/h infusions of isotonic saline or a balanced crystalloid solution, should be considered to reduce the risk for pulmonary edema, especially if heart failure or pulmonary insufficiency exists. Isotonic saline has been associated with hyperchloremic metabolic acidosis, especially if the dehydration is accompanied by a severe electrolyte imbalance amenable to large and relatively rapid infusions. For example, if dehydration resulting from severe diarrhea is accompanied by metabolic acidosis as the result of bicarbonate losses, the optimal IV rehydration fluid would be 5% dextrose with 0.45% sodium chloride plus 50 mEq (mmol) of sodium bicarbonate per liter. This fluid will remain mostly in the intravascular space, providing the necessary perfusion pressure to the kidneys, as well as a substantial amount of bicarbonate to correct the acidosis.

If AKI is a result of blood loss or is complicated by symptomatic anemia, red blood cell transfusion to a hematocrit no higher than 30% (0.30) is the treatment of choice.[78] Although albumin is sometimes used as a resuscitative agent, its use should be limited to individuals with severe hypoalbuminemia (eg, liver disease and nephritic syndrome) who are resistant to crystalloid therapy. These patients have severe hypoalbuminemia-associated third spacing that complicates fluid management, and albumin may be useful in this setting.[79] In critically ill patients with vasomotor shock, vasopressors such as norepinephrine, vasopressin, or dopamine may be used in conjunction with fluids in order to maintain adequate hemodynamics and renal perfusion.[3]

Electrolyte Management

Hypernatremia and fluid retention are frequent complications of AKI. Total daily sodium intake should be monitored since excessive amounts may contribute to diuretic therapy failure. Since several commonly administered IV antibiotics such as metronidazole, ampicillin, piperacillin, and fluconazole contain significant amounts of sodium they can contribute to hypernatremia.

The most common electrolyte disorder encountered in AKI patients is hyperkalemia, as more than 90% of potassium is renally eliminated. Life-threatening cardiac arrhythmias may occur with serum potassium concentrations greater than 6 mEq/L (mmol/L), so frequent monitoring of potassium is essential. Some foods and medications such as oral phosphorous replacement powders (eg, Neutra-Phos and Neutra-Phos-K) and alkalinizers (Polycitra) contain substantial amounts of potassium (see Chapter 51). Some medications may promote potassium retention by the kidneys and should also be avoided or closely monitored (see Chapters 46 and 51).

Other electrolytes that require monitoring are phosphorus and magnesium. Both are eliminated by the kidneys and are not removed efficiently by dialysis. In the early stages of AKI, hyperphosphatemia may be more common than hypophosphatemia. Patients with significant tissue destruction (eg, trauma, rhabdomyolysis, and tumor lysis syndrome) may have substantial amounts of phosphorus released from the destroyed tissue. Calcium-containing antacids should be avoided to prevent precipitation of calcium phosphate in the soft tissues. Typically, the dietary intake of phosphorus and magnesium needs to be restricted. However, patients receiving prolonged RRT can develop deficiency states, particularly pediatric patients as a result of reduced body stores. In contrast to the patient with CKD, AKI patients do not usually develop calcium imbalance secondary to the limited duration of the illness. One exception to this is seen in patients who are receiving CRRT with citrate as the anticoagulant. Citrate binds to serum calcium and is typically infused before the dialyzer/hemofilter. Calcium chloride or calcium gluconate is administered prior to returning the blood to the patient, while the citrate that reaches the systemic circulation is subsequently metabolized by the liver. The goals of citrate anticoagulation are to maintain the circuit ionized calcium between 0.8 and 1.6 mg/dL (0.2 and 0.4 mmol/L), and the patient's systemic ionized calcium between 4.4 and 5.2 mg/dL (1.1-1.3 mmol/L).[3] Since severe hypocalcemia can result in arrhythmias or even death, frequent monitoring of unbound serum calcium concentrations is essential.

Nutritional Considerations in AKI

Nutritional management of critically ill patients with AKI can be extremely complex, as it needs to account for metabolic derangements resulting from both renal dysfunction and underlying disease processes, as well as the effects of RRT on nutrient balance. Stress, inflammation, and injury lead to hypermetabolic/hypercatabolic states and may alter the nutritional requirements. In addition, severe malnutrition found in up to 42% of patients with AKI is a risk factor for increased hospital mortality and length of stay.[78] Thus, patient outcomes can be significantly improved if the nutritional status is optimized.

Loss of the normal physiologic and metabolic functions of the kidney and the hypercatabolic response to stress and injury will have a significant impact on the metabolism of nutrients. Derangements in glucose, lipid, and protein metabolism result in hyperglycemia and insulin resistance, hypertriglyceridemia, protein catabolism, and negative nitrogen balance. The latter, in particular, is problematic to manage, as increased amino acid turnover and skeletal muscle breakdown lead to muscle wasting and malnutrition and do not respond well to increasing exogenous protein supplementation. The KDIGO guidelines currently recommend a caloric intake goal of 20 to 30 kcal/kg/day (84-126 kJ/kg/day); irrespective of the stage of renal impairment and preferentially through the enteral route. In the setting of noncatabolic AKI without need for dialysis, 0.8 to 1 g/kg/day of protein is suggested and 1 to 1.5 g/kg/day if patient is receiving RRT.[3] CRRT is associated with an increased removal of small water-soluble molecules such as amino acids and certain nutrients. As a result, hypercatabolic patients receiving CRRT will typically have higher protein requirements up to a maximum of 1.7 g/kg/day.[3]

Renal Replacement Therapy

7 RRT is often used to treat fluid overload, electrolyte and acid-base imbalances resulting from severe AKI. Multiple factors influence decisions to initiate dialysis including specific timing and type of modality.[80,81] The choice of continuous versus intermittent RRTs is a matter of considerable debate and usually depends on physician preference and the resources available at the hospital. The most common indications for initiation of RRT are summarized in Table 43-6.

Intermittent Hemodialysis Intermittent hemodialysis (IHD) is the most frequently used RRT. IHD machines are readily available in most acute care facilities, and healthcare workers are commonly familiar with their use. Hemodialysis treatments usually last 3 to 4 hours, with blood flow rates to the dialyzer typically ranging from 200 to 400 mL/min. Advantages of IHD include rapid removal of volume and solutes and thereby contribute to correction of most of the electrolyte abnormalities associated with AKI. The primary challenge is hypotension, typically caused by rapid removal of intravascular volume. Venous access for dialysis can be difficult in hypotensive patients and can limit the effectiveness of IHD, leading to ineffective solute clearance, lack of acidosis correction, continued volume overload, and delayed recovery because of further ischemic insults to the kidneys. If hemodialysis is carefully monitored and hypotension avoided, better patient outcomes can be achieved.[82] Patients with CKD stage 5 generally achieve adequate solute and volume control with three times weekly dialysis, but hypercatabolic, fluid-overloaded patients with AKI may require more frequent hemodialysis treatments. Chapter 45 provides a detailed explanation of the principles and processes of IHD.

TABLE 43-6 Common Indications for RRT

Indication for RRT	Clinical Setting
A: *acid-base abnormalities*	Metabolic acidosis (especially if pH <7.2)
E: *electrolyte imbalance*	Severe hyperkalemia and/or hypermagnesemia
I: *intoxications*	Salicylates, lithium, methanol, ethylene glycol, theophylline, phenobarbital
O: *fluid overload*	Fluid overload (especially pulmonary edema unresponsive to diuretics)
U: *uremia*	Uremia or associated complications (neuropathy, encephalopathy, pericarditis)

RRT, renal replacement therapy.

Continuous Renal Replacement Therapy CRRT is a viable approach to manage hemodynamically unstable patients with AKI. Several CRRT variants have been developed, including continuous venovenous hemofiltration (CVVH), continuous venovenous hemodialysis (CVVHD), and continuous venovenous hemodiafiltration (CVVHDF). They differ in the degree of solute and fluid clearance that can be clinically achieved as a result of the use of diffusion, convection, or a combination of both. A greater amount of solute removal and higher mean arterial pressures are observed during CCRT compared with IHD in critically ill patients with AKI.[83] In CVVH, solute and fluid clearance is primarily a result of convection, in which fluids containing solutes is removed, while replacement fluids absent of the solutes is replaced (Fig. 43-3). CVVHD provides extensive solute removal primarily by diffusion, in which solute molecules at a higher concentration (plasma) pass through the dialysis membrane to an area of lower concentration (dialysate). Also, some fluid is removed as a function of the ultrafiltration coefficient of the dialyzer and the patient's blood pressure. CVVHD potentially has a lower risk of clotting than CVVH because of reduced hemoconcentration, as there is less fluid removal during the process. CVVHDF combines both convection or hemofiltration and hemodialysis, achieving even higher solute and fluid removal rates (Fig. 43-3). The ultrafiltration rate is an important determinant of the effectiveness of all three forms of CRRT. In direct comparisons of ultrafiltration rates of 25 and 40 mL/kg/h or higher, no difference in mortality has been observed, and there was a tendency toward prolonged need for renal replacement in those who received the higher ultrafiltration rate.[84,85] Therefore, current KDIGO guidelines recommend an ultrafiltration rate of no more than 20 to 25 mL/kg/h during CRRT.[3]

Because of the reduced blood flow rates relative to IHD, CRRT-related thrombosis is a significant concern; thus, some form of anticoagulation is generally necessary for almost all patients. Typical anticoagulation is achieved by the administration of parenteral agents such as regional citrate (preferred if increased risk for bleeding is present), unfractionated heparin, low-molecular-weight heparin in some cases, or a direct thrombin inhibitor when other therapies are contraindicated.[3,86] Replacement fluids can be infused either just before or after the dialyzer/hemofilter. Infusing fluids after the hemofilter can result in hemoconcentration within the filter, a factor associated with an increased risk of thrombosis of the dialyzer. Replacing fluids before the filter reduces thrombosis risk, but it also reduces solute clearance.

Disadvantages of CRRT may include limited availability of the special equipment necessary to provide these treatments or the need for intensive nursing care, and the need to individualize the IV replacement, dialysate fluids, and drug therapy adjustments. There is also very little known about drug-dosing requirements for patients who are receiving CRRT.[87] CRRT use is most commonly considered for those patients with higher acuity because of their intolerance of IHD-associated hypotension. Current KDIGO guidelines suggest using CRRT over IHD in hemodynamically unstable patients.[3]

Hybrid Dialysis Therapies 8 An alternative to CRRT is extended-duration IHD or hybrid IHD therapies which have a

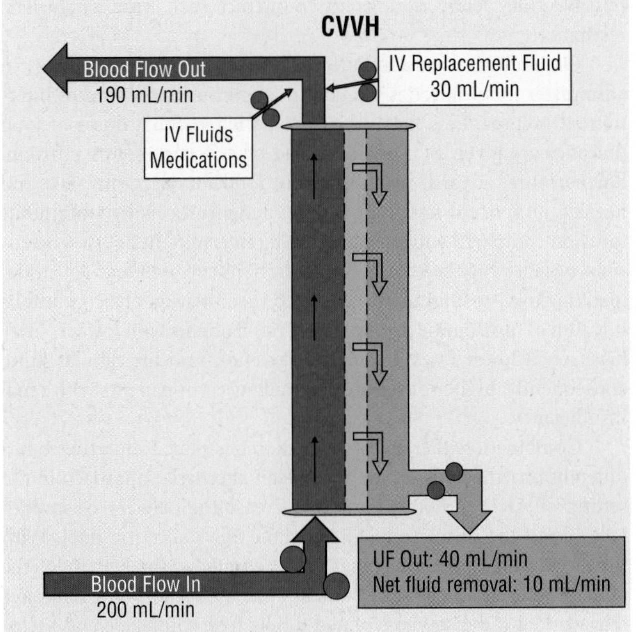

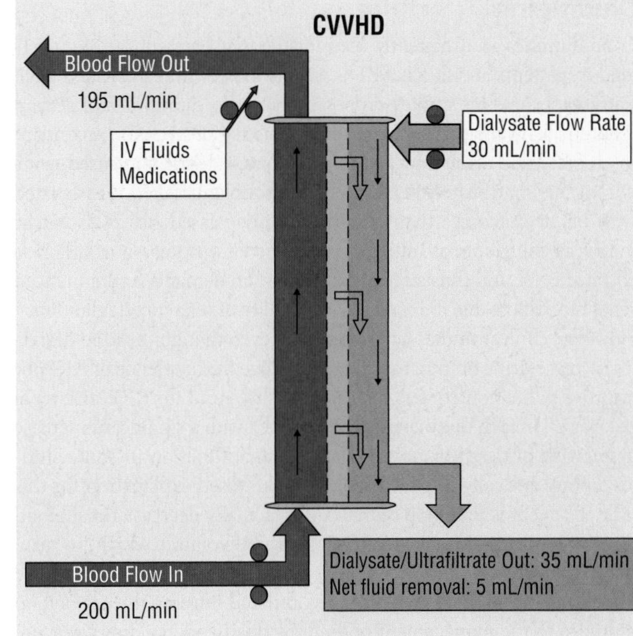

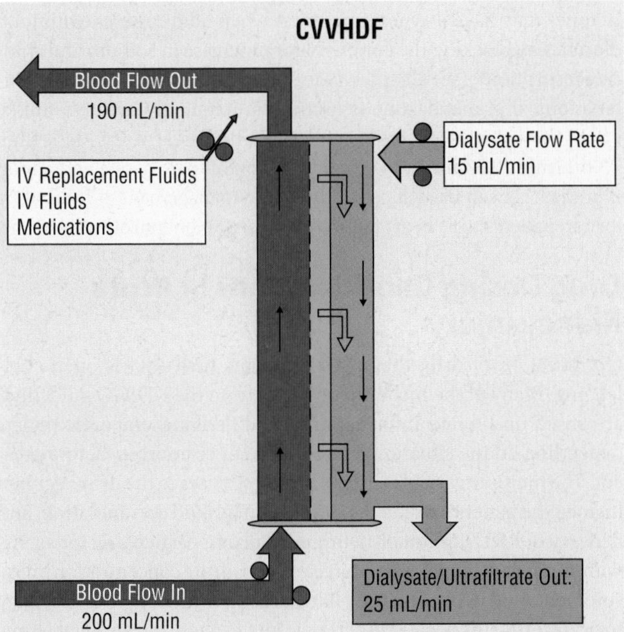

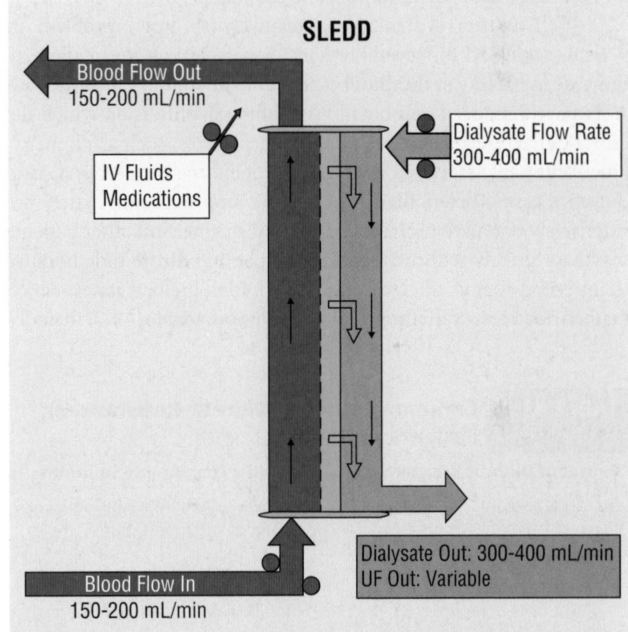

FIGURE 43-3 Several renal replacement therapies are commonly used in patients with acute kidney injury (AKI), including one of the three primary continuous renal replacement therapy (CRRT) variants: (a) continuous venovenous hemofiltration (CVVH), (b) continuous venovenous hemodialysis (CVVHD), (c) continuous venovenous hemodiafiltration (CVVHDF), and the hybrid intermittent hemodialysis therapy (d) sustained low-efficiency dialysis (SLED). The blood circuit in each diagram is represented in red, the hemofilter/dialyzer membrane is yellow, and the ultrafiltration/dialysate compartment is brown. Excess body water and accumulated endogenous waste products are removed solely by convection when CVVH is employed. With CVVHD, waste products are predominantly removed as the result of passive diffusion from the blood, where they are in high concentration to the dialysate. The degree of fluid removal that is accomplished by convection is usually minimal. CVVHDF uses convection to a degree similar to that employed during CVVH as well as diffusion, and thus is often associated with the highest clearance of drugs and waste products. Finally, SLED employs lower blood and dialysate flow rates than intermittent hemodialysis (IHD), but because of its extended duration, it is a gentler means of achieving adequate waste product and fluid removal.

variety of names, with the two most common being sustained low-efficiency dialysis (SLED) and slow, extended, daily dialysis (see Fig. 43-3).[88] These therapies use lower blood (150-200 mL/min) and dialysate (300-400 mL/min) flow rates with extended treatment periods of 6 to 12 hours. For critically ill patients with AKI, SLED appears comparable to CRRT for hemodynamic control.[82] Anticoagulation is still required, but the amount necessary compared with CRRT is lower. Although the use of hybrid hemodialysis therapies is increasing, our knowledge of their impact on drug removal is very limited.[89] Daily delivery of SLED presents challenges to clinicians prescribing drug and nutrition therapy, as most of the dosing guidelines are based on IHD given three times per week in CKD patients. Thus, application of these guidelines in patients with AKI may potentially yield suboptimal outcomes.

Diuretics

Loop diuretics are frequently used for the management of fluid overload in patients at risk for AKI as well as those with established AKI. Early experimental studies proposed that loop diuretics had several theoretical advantages: decreased risk of tubular obstruction secondary to an increased urine flow and flushing out of debris; increased urine output that may be beneficial in itself, as nonoliguric AKI is associated with better outcomes than oliguric AKI; decreased risk of ischemic injury as the result of inhibition of the sodium/potassium chloride cotransporter and thus a reduction in oxygen demand; and enhanced renal blood flow due to increased availability of renal prostaglandins.[90] However, clinical studies have found that even though the loop diuretics increase urine output, they neither reduce the incidence of AKI nor improve patient outcomes, such as mortality, need for RRT, and renal recovery.[90] In fact, they have been associated with a significant increase in the risk of death or nonrecovery of renal function in some studies among critically ill patients.[90,91] One proposed explanation for this lack of benefit is that loop diuretics may actually decrease renal blood flow by reducing effective circulating arterial volume, which, in turn, may stimulate the adrenergic and the renin–angiotensin systems.[92] Therefore, the KDIGO guidelines recommend limiting the use of loop diuretics to the management of fluid overload and avoiding their use for the sole purpose of prevention or treatment of AKI.[3]

9 Diuretic resistance is a relatively common problem in patients with AKI for several reasons. Excessive sodium intake may override the ability of the diuretics to eliminate sodium. Patients with ATN have a reduced number of functioning nephrons on which the diuretic may exert its action. Other clinical states, such as glomerulonephritis, are associated with heavy proteinuria. Intraluminal loop diuretics cannot exert their effect in the loop of Henle if they are extensively bound to proteins present in the urine. Still other patients may have greatly reduced bioavailability of oral furosemide because of intestinal edema, often associated with high preload states, which further reduces oral furosemide absorption. Table 43-7 includes possible therapeutic options to counteract each form of diuretic resistance.

TABLE 43-7 Common Causes of Diuretic Resistance in Patients with AKI

Causes of Diuretic Resistance	Potential Therapeutic Solutions
Excessive sodium intake (sources may be dietary, IV fluids, and drugs)	Remove sodium from nutritional sources and medications
Inadequate diuretic dose or inappropriate regimen	Increase dose, use continuous infusion or combination therapy
Reduced oral bioavailability (usually furosemide)	Use parenteral therapy, switch to oral torsemide or bumetanide
Nephrotic syndrome (loop diuretic protein binding in tubule lumen)	Increase dose, switch diuretics, use combination therapy
Reduced renal blood flow	
Drugs (NSAIDs, ACEIs, vasodilators)	Discontinue these drugs if possible
Hypotension	Intravascular volume expansion and/or vasopressors
Intravascular depletion	Intravascular volume expansion
Increased sodium resorption	
Nephron adaptation to chronic diuretic therapy	Combination diuretic therapy, sodium restriction
NSAID use	Discontinue NSAID
Heart failure	Treat heart failure, increase diuretic dose, switch to better-absorbed loop diuretic
Cirrhosis	Paracentesis
Acute tubular necrosis	Increase diuretic dose, diuretic combination therapy

ACEIs, angiotensin-converting enzyme inhibitors; NSAIDs, nonsteroidal anti-inflammatory drugs.

One effective technique to overcome diuretic resistance is to administer loop diuretics via continuous infusion instead of intermittent boluses. Less natriuresis occurs when equal doses of loop diuretics are given as a bolus instead of as a continuous infusion. Furthermore, adverse reactions from loop diuretics (myalgia and hearing loss) occur less frequently in patients receiving continuous infusion compared with those receiving intermittent boluses, ostensibly because higher serum concentrations are avoided. An initial loading dose is recommended prior to the initiation of a continuous infusion of furosemide or its equivalent.[91] Patients with low CL_{cr} may have much lower rates of diuretic secretion into the tubular fluid; consequently, higher doses are generally used in patients with renal insufficiency.

Combination therapy of loop diuretics plus a diuretic from a different pharmacologic class may be an alternative approach in the setting of AKI.[94,95] Loop diuretics increase the delivery of sodium chloride to the distal convoluted tubule and collecting duct. With time, these areas of the nephron compensate for the activity of the loop diuretic and increase sodium and chloride resorption. Diuretics that work at the distal convoluted tubule (chlorothiazide and metolazone) or the collecting duct (amiloride, triamterene, and spironolactone) may have a synergistic effect when administered with loop diuretics by blocking the compensatory increase in sodium and chloride resorption[95] (see Chapter 49 for more discussion). Of these combinations, oral metolazone is used most frequently because, unlike other thiazides, it produces effective diuresis at a Cr_{Cl} less than 20 mL/min (0.33 mL/s). The combination of metolazone and a loop diuretic has been used successfully in the management of fluid overload in patients with heart failure, cirrhosis, and nephrotic syndrome.

Drug Dosing Considerations in Acute Kidney Injury

Optimization of drug therapy for patients with AKI is often challenging. Many of the recommendations from the KDIGO guidelines are based on limited information and different therapeutic targets depending on the situation and concurrent co-morbid factors present. The multiple variables influencing responses to the drug regimen include the patient's residual drug clearance, fluid accumulation, and delivery of RRT. For renally eliminated drugs, particularly for agents with a narrow therapeutic range, serum drug concentration measurements and assessment of pharmacodynamic responses are likely to be necessary. If hepatic function is intact, choosing an agent eliminated primarily by the liver may be preferred. However, any renally eliminated active metabolites may accumulate to a point where they can elicit an undesired pharmacologic effect. Renal failure can also independently impair nonrenal drug elimination including metabolism.[96] Unfortunately, pharmacokinetic studies in patients with established AKI are fairly limited. Further, the use of dosing guidelines based on data derived from patients with stable CKD may not reflect the clearance and volume of distribution in critically ill AKI patients (see Chapter 48).[87] The inability to adequately dose drugs in critically ill patients with AKI requiring RRT may be one factor contributing to the lack of improving outcomes with newer RRT approaches.

Pharmacotherapy regimen decisions should further take into consideration four distinct phases of AKI described earlier, specifically initiation, extension, maintenance, and recovery phase. The initiation and extension phases occur right after the kidney insult. At this point, decisions on drug therapy should include the specific pharmacokinetics of the drug, the potential for increased risk for an adverse drug event, the goals of therapy, and therapeutic drug monitoring (if available). The severity and timing of the decline in renal function is relatively unpredictable so frequent monitoring and reevaluation of drug dosing is necessary. During the maintenance phase of AKI renal function has stabilized and drug therapy regimens may require less alterations. The third phase is recovery where AKI begins to resolve and there may be a need to increase the drug dose. Following the patient closely and recognizing trends for decreasing or increasing renal function along with adjustments in RRT in advance is important in achieving and maintaining drug therapy management goals.

Edema, which is common in AKI, can significantly increase the volume of distribution of many drugs, particularly water-soluble ones with relatively small volumes of distribution. Increased fluid distribution into the tissues (ie, sepsis and anasarca in heart failure) can also contribute to a larger volume of distribution for many drugs and thereby reduce the proportion of drug in the plasma that is available to be removed by RRT. Because AKI frequently occurs in critically ill patients, multisystem organ failure is often an accompanying problem. In addition to volume overload, reductions in cardiac output or liver function can significantly alter the pharmacokinetic profile of many drugs, such as vancomycin, aminoglycosides, and low-molecular-weight heparins.[87,97,98]

If rapid onset of activity is desired, a loading dose may be necessary to promptly achieve desired serum concentrations because the expanded volume of distribution and the prolonged elimination half-life extend the time (3.5 times the half-life) needed to reach steady-state concentrations. Maintenance dosing regimens should be reassessed frequently and be based on the patient's most current kidney function. A dose that provides the desired serum concentration on one day may be inappropriate a few days later if the patient's fluid status, RRT prescription, or renal function has changed dramatically.

Drug therapy individualization for the AKI patient who is receiving any form of RRT is complicated by the fact that patients with AKI may have a higher residual nonrenal clearance than patients with CKD who have a similar CL_{cr}.[87] Alterations in the activity of some, but not all, cytochrome P450 enzymes have been demonstrated in patients with CKD.[96] The nonrenal clearance of imipenem in patients with AKI (91 mL/min [1.52 mL/s]) is between the values observed in stage 5 CKD patients (50 mL/min [0.83 mL/s]) and those with normal renal function (130 mL/min [2.2 mL/s]).[96] This may be the result of less accumulation of uremic waste products that may alter hepatic function. If a patient with AKI has higher than anticipated nonrenal clearance, this would result in lower than expected, possibly subtherapeutic, serum concentrations. For example, to maintain comparable serum concentrations, the imipenem dose requirement in patients with AKI would be 2,000 mg daily as compared with the recommended dosage for patients with ESRD of 1,000 mg daily.[96] As AKI persists, the nonrenal clearance values appear to approach those observed in patients with CKD.[96] Another challenge is that much of the dosing-related data were acquired in patients with CKD, with initial pharmacokinetic assessments done after single-dose administration. The determination of pharmacokinetic parameters using a single-dose model may result in more rapid initial drug removal estimates secondary to distribution from the plasma to the tissue as well. Thus, application of dosing regimens derived from studies in patients with CKD and ESKD in addition to the use of more aggressive RRT approaches may result in under dosing of certain drugs and thereby contribute to less than optimal clinical outcomes.

Drug Dosing Considerations in Renal Replacement Therapy

There are marked differences between the different types of RRT and drug removal.[88,90,103] During CVVH, drug removal primarily occurs via convection/ultrafiltration (the passive transport of drug molecules at the concentration at which they exist in plasma water into the ultrafiltrate). Convective removal is most efficient for smaller agents, typically less than 15,000 Da (15 kDa) in size, and those that are primarily unbound in the plasma. The clearance of a drug by either of these methods is thus a function of the membrane permeability for the drug, which is called the sieving coefficient (SC), and the rate of ultrafiltrate formation (UFR). The pore size of the filter and surface charge relative to the molecule being removed may vary between different dialyzers. If diffusion of the drug is not dependent on the filter pore size, then the SC can be calculated as follows:

$$\text{SC} = \frac{2 \times C_{\text{UF}}}{C_a + C_v}$$

where C_a and C_v are the concentrations of the drug in the plasma going into and returning from the dialyzer/hemofilter, respectively, and C_{UF} is the concentration in the ultrafiltrate. The SC is often approximated by the fraction unbound (f_u) because this information may be more readily available. Thus, the clearance by CVVH can be calculated as

$$\text{Cl}_{\text{CVVH}} = \text{UFR} \times \text{SC}$$

or approximated as

$$\text{Cl}_{\text{CVVH}} = \text{UFR} \times f_u$$

In CVVHDF, clearance is a combination of both diffusion and convection. The $\text{Cl}_{\text{CVVHDF}}$ can be mathematically approximated, providing the blood flow rate is greater than 100 mL/min and the dialysate flow rate (DFR) is between 8 and 33 mL/min, as

$$\text{Cl}_{\text{CVVHDF}} = (\text{UFR} \times f_u) + \text{Cl}_{\text{diffusion}}$$

where $\text{Cl}_{\text{diffusion}}$ is the clearance via diffusion from plasma water to the dialysate. In the clinical setting, it is not possible to separate these two components (UFR and DFR) of $\text{Cl}_{\text{CVVHDF}}$. In essence, the $\text{Cl}_{\text{CVVHDF}}$ is calculated as the product of the combined ultrafiltrate and dialysate volume (V_{df}) and the concentration of the drug in this fluid (C_{df}) divided by the plasma concentration at the midpoint of the V_{df} collection period.

Individualization of therapy for a patient receiving CRRT is dependent on the patient's residual renal function and the clearance of the drug by the mode of CRRT. There are differences in the rate of drug removal, not only between the three primary modes of CRRT but also within each mode.[87,99] This is a result of differences in the filter membrane composition, variable degrees of drug binding to the membrane, and permeability characteristics of the membrane.[99,100] Primary factors that influence drug clearance during CRRT are thus the ultrafiltration rate, blood flow rate, and DFR. For example, clearance in CVVH is directly proportional to the ultrafiltration rate, whereas clearance during CVVHDF, which depends on both the ultrafiltration rate and the DFR, increases as either flow rate increases. An increase in the ultrafiltration flow rate (5-45 mL/min) and DFR (8.3-33.3 mL/min), however, can have dramatic effects on the clearance of agents such as ceftazidime during CVVH and CVVHD, respectively (Fig. 43-4).[100] Further, CRRT can rapidly remove excess fluid from edematous patients, thereby changing the volume of distribution (V_D) of drugs with limited distribution (low V_D suggesting a greater proportion in the plasma or extracellular fluid) fairly rapidly.[99] Drug clearances attained by IHD, CRRTs, and hybrid RRTs all differ from each other and must be added to any endogenous drug clearance that the patient generates.

Limitations of IHD-based dosing charts include variability in the patient's individual pharmacokinetic parameters, differences in the dialysis prescription, such as dialyzer blood flow or duration, and the use of new IHD dialyzers. The approach to hemodialysis may also change on a daily basis, especially in hemodynamically unstable individuals with AKI. This could include, for example, the

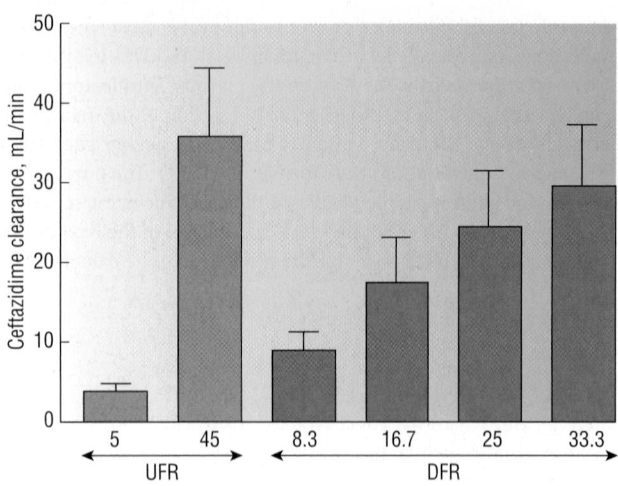

FIGURE 43-4 The effect of increasing ultrafiltration rate (UFR in milliliters per minute) and dialysate flow rate (DFR in milliliters per minute) on the clearance of ceftazidime. *(Data from reference 95.)*

type of dialyzer/filter used, the duration, the degree of hemofiltration compared with convection, and the blood flow rate. Individualization of a dosing regimen may require daily assessment of the clinical status of the patient and any planned or recently administered hemodialysis.

Overall, there are numerous potential pharmacokinetic and pharmacodynamic alterations to be aware of in the patient with AKI. Unfortunately, there is a dearth of data to quantify these changes, and even less evidence demonstrating that if one incorporates these considerations into patient care, the associated outcomes will be improved.

Clinical **Controversy...**

Dosing of antimicrobial agents in critically ill patients receiving CRRT or SLED is challenging. Although small pharmacokinetic studies are emerging to provide data to help address this problem, the variability in results from these studies is significant and makes it difficult for health care professionals to draw conclusions and apply these findings to the care of individual patients.

PERSONALIZED PHARMACOTHERAPY

In the presence of AKI, several processes may exist that can alter drug response such as impaired elimination, RRT-related drug removal, or physiologic alterations in pharmacodynamic response. Guidance from clinical trials on how to appropriately adjust drug regimens is limited. Thus, individualized pharmacotherapeutic regimens and frequent assessment is required to optimize patient outcomes. Changes in the patient's clinical condition including renal replacement regimens may require clinicians to make frequent dosage regimen adjustments. Information from yesterday's medical record review may not reflect what is happening today or will be needed for tomorrow. Patient frequently require more aggressive pharmacotherapy regimens initially because of altered pharmacokinetics that can be subsequently tapered if warranted. Clinicians should keep the overall clinical status of the patient in mind when developing management plans. Key to optimal patient outcomes includes maximizing prevention, early identification of AKI, timely implementation of supportive therapies, and frequent assessments and revisions of the care plan until the AKI has resolved.

EVALUATION OF THERAPEUTIC OUTCOMES

Vigilant monitoring of patients with AKI is essential, particularly in those who are critically ill. Table 43-8 summarizes the main monitoring parameters for patients with established AKI.

Once the laboratory-based tests (eg, urinalysis and FE_{Na} calculations) have been conducted to diagnose the cause of AKI, they usually do not have to be repeated. In established AKI, daily measurements of urine output, fluid intake, and weight should be performed. Vital signs should be monitored at least daily, more often if the acuity of illness warrants. Electrolytes, BUN, serum creatinine, and a complete blood cell count should be considered routine and measured at least daily for hospitalized patients.

Therapeutic drug concentration monitoring should be performed for drugs that have a narrow therapeutic index if results from these serum drug concentrations can be obtained in a timely fashion. The optimal time to measuring serum concentrations is patient-, drug-, and often clinician-specific; consensus is lacking. For patients receiving RRT measuring a serum drug concentration prior to hemodialysis has the advantage of allowing time for the result to be reported and the next dose calculated so that it can be administered shortly after dialysis. This is especially important if the desired pharmacologic effects are lost during or after hemodialysis is complete because the serum concentrations have become subtherapeutic. Knowledge based on previous observations of how a particular agent is removed for a given dialysis approach and a prehemodialysis serum concentration can assist in estimating the amount of the drug removed and predict the need for any postdialysis doses. Serum concentrations drawn after hemodialysis may reflect plasma concentrations that are transiently depressed until the drug can reequilibrate from the tissues (plasma rebound effect).

TABLE 43-8 Key Monitoring Parameters for Patients with Established AKI

Parameter	Frequency
Fluid intake & output	Every shift
Patient weight	Daily
Hemodynamics (blood pressure, heart rate, mean arterial pressure, etc.)	Every shift
Blood chemistries	
Sodium, potassium, chloride, bicarbonate, calcium, phosphate, magnesium	Daily
Blood urea nitrogen/serum creatinine	Daily
Drugs and their dosing regimens	Daily
Nutritional regimen	Daily
Blood glucose	Daily (minimum)
Serum concentration data for drugs	After regimen changes and after renal replacement therapy has been instituted
Times of administered doses	Daily
Doses relative to administration of renal replacement therapy	Daily
Urinalysis	
Calculate measured creatinine clearance	Every time measured urine collection performed
Calculate fractional excretion of sodium	Every time measured urine collection performed
Plans for renal replacement	Daily

The advantage of collecting a postdialysis sample is the greater accuracy in determining how much drug was removed during hemodialysis. The down side of this strategy is that it delays calculation and administration of the next dose and thus the reestablishment of the target concentration time profile.

CONCLUSION

The unique characteristics of AKI compared with CKD can lead to notable differences in how renal function is measured and how treatment regimens are developed. Most management approaches involve both prevention and support strategies, so as to minimize the potential for additional harm to the kidney. Understanding the constantly changing status inherent to AKI and how to adjust management regimens is a key component to optimizing therapy.

ABBREVIATIONS

ACE	angiotensin-converting enzyme
ADQI	Acute Dialysis Quality Initiative
AIN	acute interstitial nephritis
AKI	acute kidney injury
AKIN	Acute Kidney Injury Network
ARB	angiotensin receptor blocker
ATN	acute tubular necrosis
BUN	blood urea nitrogen
CIN	contrast-induced nephropathy
CKD	chronic kidney disease
CKD-EPI	Chronic Kidney Disease Epidemiology Collaboration
CL_{cr}	creatinine clearance
CRRT	continuous renal replacement therapy
CT	computed tomography
CVVH	continuous venovenous hemofiltration
CVVHD	continuous venovenous hemodialysis
CVVHDF	continuous venovenous hemodiafiltration
DFR	dialysate flow rate
GFR	glomerular filtration rate
GI	gastrointestinal
eCL_{cr}	estimating creatinine clearance
eGFR	estimated glomerular filtration rate
ESKD	end-stage kidney disease
FDA	Food and Drug Administration
FE_{Na}	fractional excretion of sodium
FE_{Urea}	fractional excretion of urea
GFR	glomerular filtration rate
IGFBP7	insulin growth like factor binding protein 7
IHD	intermittent hemodialysis
JVP	jugular venous pressure
KDIGO	Kidney Disease: Improving Global Outcomes
KUB	kidneys, ureters, and bladder
MDRD	Modification of Diet in Renal Disease
NAC	*N*-acetylcysteine
NGAL	neutrophil gelatinase–associated lipocalin
NSAID	nonsteroidal anti-inflammatory drug
RIFLE	Risk, Injury, Failure, Loss of Kidney Function, and End-Stage Kidney Disease
RRT	renal replacement therapy
SC	sieving coefficient
S_{cr}	serum creatinine
SLED	sustained low-efficiency dialysis
TIMP-2	tissue inhibitor of metalloproteinases 2
UFR	ultrafiltrate formation
HTN	hypertension

REFERENCES

1. Bellomo R, Ronco C, Kellum JA, et al. Acute renal failure—Definition, outcome measures, animal models, fluid therapy and information technology needs: The Second International Consensus Conference of the Acute Dialysis Quality Initiative (ADQI) Group. *Crit Care* 2004;8:R204-R212.
2. Mehta RL, Kellum JA, Shah SV, et al. Acute Kidney Injury Network: Report of an initiative to improve outcomes in acute kidney injury. *Crit Care* 2007;11:R31.
3. Kidney Disease: Improving Global Outcomes (KDIGO) Acute Kidney Injury Workgroup. KDIGO clinical practice guideline for acute kidney injury. *Kidney Int Suppl* 2012;2:1-138.
4. Zeng X, McMahon GM, Brunelli SM, et al. Incidence, outcomes, and comparisons across definitions of AKI in hospitalized individuals. *Clin J Am Soc Nephrol* 2014;9(1):12-20.
5. Fujii T, Uchino S, Takinami M, Bellomo R. Validation of the Kidney Disease Improving Global Outcomes criteria for AKI and comparison of three criteria in hospitalized patients. *Clin J Am Soc Nephrol* 2014(May);9(5):848-854.
6. Luo X, Jiang L, Du B, et al. A comparison of different diagnostic criteria of acute kidney injury in critically ill patients. *Crit Care* 2014(Jul);18(4):R144.
7. Bellomo R, Kellum JA, Ronco C. Acute kidney injury. *Lancet* 2012;380:756-766.
8. Siew ED, Matheny ME, Ikizler TA, et al. Commonly used surrogates for baseline renal function affect the classification and prognosis of acute kidney injury. *Kidney Int* 2010;77:536-542.
9. Zavada J, Hoste E, Cartin-Ceba R, et al. A comparison of three methods to estimate baseline creatinine for RIFLE classification. *Nephrol Dial Transplant* 2010;25:3911-3918.
10. Lin J, Fernandez H, Shashaty MG et al. False positive rate of AKI using consensus creatinine-based criteria. *Clin J Am Soc Nephrol* 2015(Oct);10(10):1723-1731.
11. Wonnecott A, Meran S, Amphlett B, et al. Epidemiology and outcomes in community-acquired versus hospital-acquired AKI. *Clin J Am Soc Nephrol* 2014(Jun);9(6):1007-1014.
12. Liangos O, Wald R, O'Bell JW, et al. Epidemiology and outcomes of acute renal failure in hospitalized patients: A national survey. *Clin J Am Soc Nephrol* 2006;1:43-51.
13. Piccinni P, Cruz DN, Gramaticopolo S et al. Prospective multicenter study on epidemiology of acute kidney injury in the ICU: A critical care nephrology Italian collaborative effort (NEFROINT). *Minerva Anestesiol* 2011(Nov);77(11):1072-1083.
14. Hoste EA, Bagshaw SM, Bellomo R, et al. Epidemiology of acute kidney injury in critically ill patients: the multinational AKI-EPI study. *Intensive Care Med* 2015(Aug);41(8):1411-1423.
15. Grams ME, Sang Y, Ballew SH, et al. A meta-analysis of the association of estimated GFR, albuminuria, age, race, and sex with acute kidney injury. *Am J Kidney Dis* 2015(Oct);66(4):591-601.
16. Coca SG, Singanamala S, Parikh CR. Chronic kidney disease after acute kidney injury: A systematic review and meta-analysis. *Kidney Int* 2012;81:442-448.
17. Horkan CM, Purtle SW, Mendu ML, et al. The association of acute kidney injury in the critically ill and postdischarge outcomes: a cohort study. *Crit Care Med* 2015(Feb);43(2):354-364.
18. Pannu N, James M, Hemmelgarn BR, et al. Modification of outcomes after acute kidney injury by the presence of CKD. *Am J Kidney Dis* 2011;58:206-213.
19. Thakar CV, Christianson A, Himmelfarb J, Leonard AC. Acute kidney injury episodes and chronic kidney disease risk in diabetes mellitus. *Clin J Am Soc Nephrol* 2011;6:2567-2572.
20. Badr KF, Ichikawa I. Prerenal failure: A deleterious shift from renal compensation to decompensation. *N Engl J Med* 1988;319:623-629.
21. Ungprasert P, Cheungpasitporn W, Crowson CS, Matteson EL. Individual non-steroidal anti-inflammatory drugs and risk of acute kidney injury: A systematic review and meta-analysis of observational studies. *Eur J Intern Med* 2015(May);26(4):285-291.
22. Zhang J, Ding EL, Song Y. Adverse effects of cyclooxygenase 2 inhibitors on renal and arrhythmia events: Meta-analysis of randomized trials. *JAMA* 2006(Oct);296(13):1619-1632.
23. Prowle JR, Ishikawa K, May CN, Bellomo R. Renal plasma flow and glomerular filtration rate during acute kidney injury in man. *Ren Fail* 2010(Jan);32(3):349-355.
24. Takasu O, Gaut JP, Watanabe E, et al. Mechanisms of cardiac and renal dysfunction in patients dying of sepsis. *Am J Respir Crit Care Med* 2013(Mar);187(5):509-517.

25. Gomez H, Ince C, De Backer D, et al. A unified theory of sepsis-induced acute kidney injury: Inflammation, microcirculatory dysfunction, bioenergetics, and the tubular cell adaptation to injury. *Shock* 2014(Jan);41(1):3-11.
26. Zarbock A, Gomez H, Kellum JA. Sepsis-induced acute kidney injury revisited: Pathophysiology, prevention, and future therapies. *Curr Opin Crit Care* 2014(Dec);20(6):588-595.
27. Basile DP, Anderson MD, Sutton TA. Pathophysiology of acute kidney injury. *Compr Physiol* 2012(Apr);2(2):1303-1353.
28. Krishnan N, Perazella MA. Drug-induced acute interstitial nephritis: Pathology, pathogenesis, and treatment. *Iran J Kidney Dis* 2015(Jan);9(1):3-13.
29. Praga M, Gonzalez E. Acute interstitial nephritis. *Kidney Int* 2010(Jun);77(11):956-961.
30. Raghavan R, Eknoyan G. Acute interstitial nephritis—A reappraisal and update. *Clin Nephrol* 2014(Sept);82(3):149-162.
31. Muriithi AK, Leung N, Valerie AM, et al. Biopsy-proven acute interstitial nephritis, 1993-2011: A case seris. *Am J Kidney Dis* 2014(Oct);64(4):558-566.
32. Frokiaer J, Zeidel ML. Urinary tract obstruction. In: Brenner BM, ed. *Brenner and Rector's The Kidney*, 9th ed. Philadelphia: WB Saunders, 2011:1382-1410.
33. Ostermann M. Diagnosis of acute kidney injury: Kidney Disease Improving Global Outcomes and beyond. *Curr Opin Crit Care* 2014(Dec);20(6):581-587.
34. Macedo E, Mehta RL. Measuring renal function in critically ill patients: Tools and strategies for assessing glomerular filtration rate. *Curr Opin Crit Care* 2013(Dec);19(6):560-566.
35. Baumann TJ, Staddon JE, Horst HM, Bivins BA. Minimum urine collection periods for accurate determination of creatinine clearance in critically ill patients. *Clin Pharm* 1987;6:393-398.
36. Wasung ME, Chawla LS, Madero M. Biomarkers of renal function, which and when? *Clin Chim Acta* 2015(Jan);438:350-357.
37. Kellum JA, Chawla LS. Cell-cycle arrest and acute kidney injury: The light and the dark sides. *Nephrol Dial Transplant* 2015;0:1-7.
38. Bihorac A, Chawla LS, Shaw AD, et al. Validation of cell-cycle arrest biomarkers for acute kidney injury using clinical adjudication. *Am J Respir Crit Care Med* 2014(Apr);189(8):932-939.
39. Wetz AJ, Richardt EM, Wand S, et al. Quantification of urinary TIMP-2 and IGFBP7: An adequate diagnostic test to predict acute kidney injury after cardiac surgery? *Crit Care* 2015(Jan);19:3.
40. Haase M, Bellomo R, Devarajan P, et al. Accuracy of neutrophil gelatinase-associated lipocalin (NGAL) in diagnosis and prognosis in acute kidney injury: A systematic review and meta-analysis. *Am J Kidney Dis* 2009;54:1012-1024.
41. Martensson J, Bellomo R. The rise and fall of NGAL in acute kidney injury. *Blood Purif* 2014;37(4):304-310.
42. McCullough PA, Shaw AD, Haase M, et al. Diagnosis of acute kidney injury using functional and injury biomarkers: workgroup statements from the tenth Acute Dialysis Quality Initiative Consensus Conference. *Contrib Nephrol* 2013;182:13-29.
43. Haase M, Kellum JA, Ronco C. Subclinical AKI – An emerging syndrome with important consequences. *Nat Rev Nephrol* 2012(Dec);8(12):735-739.
44. Zarychanski R, Abou-Setta AM, Turgeon AF, et al. Association of hydroxyethyl starch administration with mortality and acute kidney injury in critically ill patients requiring volume resuscitation: a systematic review and meta-analysis. *JAMA* 2013 (Feb);309(7):678-688.
45. Perel P, Roberts I. Colloids versus crystalloids for fluid resuscitation in critically ill patients. Cochrane Database Syst Rev 2012;6: CD000567.
46. Chowdhury AH, Cox EF, Francis ST, Lobo DN. A randomized, controlled, double-blind crossover study on the effects of 2-L infusions of 0.9% saline and Plasma-Lyte® 148 on renal blood flow velocity and renal cortical tissue perfusion in healthy volunteers. *Ann Surg* 2012(Jul);256(1):18-24.
47. Yunos NM, Bellomo R, Hegarly C, et al. Association between a chloride-liberal vs chloride-restrictive intravenous fluid administration strategy and kidney injury in critically ill adults. *JAMA* 2012(Oct);308(15):1566-1572.
48. Young P, Bailey M, Beasley R, et al. Effect of a Buffered Crystalloid Solution vs Saline on Acute Kidney Injury Among Patients in the Intensive Care Unit: The SPLIT Randomized Clinical Trial. *JAMA* 2015(Oct);314(16):1701-1710.
49. Andreucci M, Faga T, Pisani A, et al. Prevention of contrast-induced nephropathy through a knowledge of its pathogenesis and risk factors. *ScientificWorldJournal* 2014:823169.
50. Solomon R, Gordon P, Manoukian SV, et al. Randomized Trial of Bicarbonate or Saline Study for the Prevention of Contrast-Induced Nephropathy in Patients with CKD. *Clin J Am Soc Nephrol* 2015 (Sep);10(9):1519-24. Epub 2015 Jul 16.
51. Briguori C, Airoldi F, D'Andrea D, et al. Renal Insufficiency Following Contrast Media Administration Trial (REMEDIAL): A randomized comparison of 3 preventive strategies. *Circulation* 2007;115:1211-1217.
52. Klima T, Christ A, Marana I, et al. Sodium chloride vs. sodium bicarbonate for the prevention of contrast medium-induced nephropathy: A randomized controlled trial. *Eur Heart J* 2012;33:2071-2079.
53. Cheungpasitporn W, Thongprayoon C, Brabec BA, et al. Oral hydration for prevention of contrast-induced acute kidney injury in elective radiological procedures: A systematic review and meta-analysis of randomized controlled trials. *N Am J Med Sci* 2014(Dec);6(12):618-624.
54. Akyuz S, Karaca M, Kemaloglu Oz T, et al. Efficacy of oral hydration in the prevention of contrast-induced acute kidney injury in patients undergoing coronary angiography or intervention. *Nephron Clin Pract* 2014;128(1-2):95-100.
55. Hiremath S, Akbari A, Shabana W, et al. Prevention of contrast-induced acute kidney injury: is simple oral hydration similar to intravenous? A systematic review of the evidence. *PLoS One* 2013;8(3):e60009.
56. Cruz DN, Goh CY, Marenzi G, et al. Renal replacement therapies for prevention of radiocontrast-induced nephropathy: A systematic review. *Am J Med* 2012;125:66-78.e3.
57. Friedrich JO, Adhikari N, Herridge MS, Beyene J. Meta-analysis: Low-dose dopamine increases urine output but does not prevent renal dysfunction or death. *Ann Intern Med* 2005;142:280-224.
58. Bove T, Zangrillo A, Guarracino F, et al. Effect of fenoldopam on use of renal replacement therapy among patients with acute kidney injury after cardiac surgery: A randomized clinical trial. *JAMA* 2014(Dec);312(21):2244-2253.
59. Kelly AM, Dwamena B, Cronin P, et al. Meta-analysis: Effectiveness of drugs for preventing contrast-induced nephropathy. *Ann Intern Med* 2008;148:284-294.
60. Bagshaw SM, Ghali WA. Theophylline for prevention of contrast-induced nephropathy: A systematic review and meta-analysis. *Arch Intern Med* 2005;165:1087-1093.
61. Brueck M, Cengiz H, Hoeltgen R. Usefulness of N-acetylcysteine or ascorbic acid versus placebo to prevent contrast-induced acute kidney injury in patients undergoing elective cardiac catheterization: a single-center, prospective, randomized, double-blind, placebo-controlled trial. *J Invasive Cardiol* 2013(Jun);25(6):276-283.
62. Zhou L, Chen H. Prevention of contrast-induced nephropathy with ascorbic acid. *Intern Med* 2012;51(6):531-535.
63. Spargias K, Alexopoulos E, Kyrzopoulos S, et al. Ascorbic acid prevents contrast-mediated nephropathy in patients with renal dysfunction undergoing coronary angiography or intervention. *Circulation* 2004(Nov);110(18):2837-2842.
64. Sadat U, Usman A, Gillard JH, Boyle JR. Does ascorbic acid protect against contrast-induced acute kidney injury in patients undergoing coronary angiography: A systematic review with meta-analysis of randomized, controlled trials. *J Am Coll Cardiol* 2013(Dec);62(23):2167-2175.
65. Inda-Filho AJ, Caixeta A, Manggini M, Schor N. Do intravenous N-acetylcysteine and sodium bicarbonate prevent high osmolal contrast-induced acute kidney injury? A randomized controlled trial. *PLoS One* 2014(Sept);9(9):e107602.
66. Chousterman BG, Bouadma L, Moutereau S, et al. Prevention of contrast-induced nephropathy by N-acetylcysteine in critically ill patients: Different definitions, different results. *J Crit Care* 2013(Oct);28(5):701-719.
67. Fiaccadori E, Sabatino A, Morabito S, et al. Hyper/hypoglycemia and acute kidney injury in critically ill patients. *Clin Nutr* 2015(Apr); S0261-5614(15)00104-1.
68. Oezkur M, Wagner M, Weismann D, et al. Chronic hyperglycemia is associated with acute kidney injury in patients undergoing CABG surgery—A cohort study. *BMC Cardiovasc Disord* 2015(May)15:41.
69. Brownlee M. The pathobiology of diabetic complications: A unifying mechanism. *Diabetes* 2005(Jun);54(6):1615-1625.
70. McMahon MM, Nystrom E, Braunschweig C, et al. A.S.P.E.N clinical guidelines: Nutrition support of adult patients with hyperglycemia. *JPEN J Parenter Enteral Nutr* 2013(Jan);37(1):23-36.
71. American Diabetes Association. Standards of medical care in diabetes 2015. *Diabetes Care* 2015(Jan);38(Suppl 1):S80-S85.

72. Joslin J, Ostermann M. Care of the critically ill emergency department patient with acute kidney injury. *Emerg Med Int* 2012;2012:760623.
73. Kshatriya S, Kozman H, Siddiqui D, et al. The kidney in heart failure: Friend or foe? *Am J Med Sci* 2012(Sept);344(3):228-232.
74. Barbar SD, Binquet C, Monchi M, et al. Impact on mortality of the timing of renal replacement therapy in patients with severe acute kidney injury in septic shock: The IDEAL-ICU study (initiation of dialysis early versus delayed in the intensive care unit): Study protocol for a randomized controlled trial. *Trials* 2014(Jul);15:270.
75. Gaudry S, Hajage D, Schortgen F, et al. Comparison of two strategies for initiating renal replacement therapy in the intensive care unit: Study protocol for a randomized controlled trial (AKIKI). *Trials* 2015(Apr);16:170.
76. Godin M, Bouchard J, Mehta RL Fluid balance in patients with acute kidney injury: Emerging concepts. *Nephron Clin Pract* 2013;123(3-4):238-245.
77. Heung M, Wolfgram DF, Kommareddi M, et al. Fluid overload at initiation of renal replacement therapy is associated with lack of renal recovery in patients with acute kidney injury. *Nephrol Dial Transplant* 2012(Mar);27(3):956-961.
78. Dellinger RP, Levy MM, Carlet JM, et al. Surviving Sepsis Campaign: International guidelines for management of severe sepsis and septic shock: 2008. *Crit Care Med* 2008;36:296-327.
79. Vincent JL. Relevance of albumin in modern critical care medicine. *Best Pract Res Clin Anaesthesiol* 2009;23:183-191.
80. Macedo E, Mehta RL. Timing of dialysis initiation in acute kidney injury and acute-on-chronic renal failure. *Semin Dial* 2013(Nov-Dec); 26(6):675-681.
81. Hoste EA, Dhondt A. Clinical review: Use of renal replacement therapies in special groups of ICU patients. *Crit Care* 2012;16:201.
82. Fieghen HE, Friedrich JO, Burns KE, et al. The hemodynamic tolerability and feasibility of sustained low efficiency dialysis in the management of critically ill patients with acute kidney injury. *BMC Nephrol* 2010;11:32.
83. Cerda J, Ronco C. Modalities of continuous renal replacement therapies: Technical and clinical considerations. *Semin Dial* 2009 (Mar-Apr);22(2):114-122.
84. Bellomo R, Cass A, Cole L, et al. Intensity of continuous renal-replacement therapy in critically ill patients. *N Engl J Med* 2009;361:1627-1638.
85. Casey ET, Gupta BP, Erwin PJ, et al. The dose of continuous renal replacement therapy for acute renal failure: A systematic review and meta-analysis. *Ren Fail* 2010;32:555-561.
86. Tolwani AJ, Wille KM. Anticoagulation for continuous renal replacement therapy. *Semin Dial* 2009(Mar-Apr);22(2):141-145.
87. Heintz BH, Matzke GR, Dager WE. Antimicrobial dosing concepts and recommendations for critically ill adult patients receiving continuous renal replacement therapy or intermittent hemodialysis. *Pharmacotherapy* 2009;29:562-577.
88. Kielstein JT, Schiffer M, Hafer C. Back to the future: extended dialysis for treatment of acute kidney injury in the intensive care unit. *J Nephrol* 2010(Sep-Oct);23(5):494-501.
89. Dager WE. Filtering out important considerations for developing drug-dosing regimens in extended daily dialysis. *Crit Care Med* 2006;34:240-241.
90. Ho KM, Power BM. Benefits and risks of furosemide in acute kidney injury. *Anesthesia* 2010;65:283-293.
91. Nisula S, Kaukonen KM, Vaara ST, et al. Incidence, risk factors and 90-day mortality of patients with acute kidney injury in Finnish intensive care units: The FINNAKI study. *Intensive Care Med* 2013(Mar);39(3):420-428.
92. Ejaz AA, Mohandas R. Are diuretics harmful in the management of acute kidney injury? *Curr Opin Nephrol Hypertens* 2014(Mar);23(2):155-160.
93. Alqahtani F, Koulouridis J, Susantitaphong P, et al. A meta-analysis of continuous vs intermittent infusion of loop diuretics in hospitalized patients. *J Crit Care* 2014(Feb);29(1):10-17.
94. Karajala V, Mansour W, Kellum JA. Diuretics in acute kidney injury. *Minerva Anestesiol* 2009;75:251-257.
95. Jentzer JC, DeWald TA, Hernandez AF. Combination of loop diuretics with thiazide-type diuretics in heart failure. *J Am Coll Cardiol* 2010;56:1527-1534.
96. Vilay AM, Churchwell MD, Mueller BA. Clinical review: Drug metabolism and nonrenal clearance in acute kidney injury. *Crit Care* 2008;12:235.
97. Dager WE, King JH. Aminoglycosides in intermittent hemodialysis: Pharmacokinetics with individual dosing. *Ann Pharmacother* 2006;40:9-14.
98. Kane-Gill SL, Feng Y, Bobek MB, et al. Administration of enoxaparin by continuous infusion in a naturalistic setting: Analysis of renal function and safety. *J Clin Pharm Ther* 2005;30:207-213.
99. Churchwell MD, Mueller BA. Drug dosing during continuous renal replacement therapy. *Semin Dial* 2009;22:185-188.
100. Matzke GR, Frye RF, Joy MS, Palevsky PM. Determinants of ceftazidime clearance by continuous venovenous hemofiltration and continuous venovenous hemodialysis. *Antimicrob Agents Chemother* 2000;44: 1639-1644.

Chronic Kidney Disease

44

Joanna Q. Hudson and Lori D. Wazny

KEY CONCEPTS

1. Chronic kidney disease (CKD) is classified based on the cause of kidney disease, assessment of glomerular filtration rate, and extent of albuminuria.
2. The most common causes of category 5 CKD, often called end-stage renal disease (ESRD), are diabetes mellitus and hypertension.
3. Anemia of CKD is primarily the result of a deficiency in the production of endogenous erythropoietin by the kidney with iron deficiency as a contributing factor.
4. CKD-mineral and bone disorder (CKD-MBD) includes abnormalities in parathyroid hormone (PTH), fibroblast growth factor-23 (FGF-23), phosphorus, calcium, vitamin D, and bone turnover, and contributes to soft-tissue and extravascular calcifications.
5. Guidelines from the Kidney Disease: Improving Global Outcomes (KDIGO) provide information to assist healthcare providers in clinical decision making and the design of appropriate therapy to manage CKD progression and the associated complications.
6. Patient education plays a critical role in the appropriate management of patients with CKD and its associated complications. An interprofessional team structure is a rational approach to provide this education and effectively design and implement the recommended nonpharmacologic and pharmacologic interventions.
7. Angiotensin-converting enzyme inhibitors (ACEIs) and angiotensin receptor blockers (ARBs) are key pharmacologic treatments to delay progression of CKD associated with albuminuria because of their effects on renal hemodynamics to reduce intraglomerular pressure and proteinuria.
8. Management of anemia includes administration of erythropoiesis-stimulating agents (ESAs) (eg, epoetin alfa, darbepoetin alfa, methoxy polyethylene glycol-epoetin beta) and regular iron supplementation (oral or IV administration) to maintain hemoglobin concentration and prevent the need for blood transfusions. There is evidence indicating a higher risk of cardiovascular events when hemoglobin is targeted to a value of greater than 11 g/dL (110 g/L; 6.83 mmol/L).
9. Management of CKD-MBD includes dietary phosphorus restriction, phosphate-binding agents, vitamin D supplementation, and calcimimetic therapy.
10. Initiation of statins for primary prevention of hyperlipidemia in patients receiving dialysis is no longer recommended due to a lack of benefits from recent randomized controlled trials and meta-analyses.

INTRODUCTION

1 Chronic kidney disease (CKD) is defined as abnormalities in kidney structure or function, present for 3 months or longer, with implications for health.[1] For decades kidney disease was primarily considered to be present only when the patient's estimated or measured creatinine clearance (CLcr) was reduced to less than 50 mL/min (0.83 mL/s). In the 2000s a new classification system was proposed that incorporated glomerular filtration rate (GFR) and albuminuria. Documentation of the presence of structural changes in those with what previously would have been classified with normal kidney function (ie, CLcr or GFR >90 mL/min [>1.50 mL/s]) became the most sensitive indicator of CKD and was designated as category 1 CKD based on recommendations from the Kidney Disease: Improving Global Outcomes (KDIGO) guidelines for evaluation and management of CKD.[1] The KDIGO classification system is referred to as *CGA* staging (*C*ause, *G*FR, *A*lbuminuria). Table 44-1 outlines the KDIGO GFR categories. The KDIGO albuminuria categories are found in Chapter e42 and Table 44-6 in this chapter. A patient is classified with end-stage renal disease (ESRD) when their GFR is below 15 mL/min/1.73 m^2 (0.14 mL/s/m^2) and either chronic dialysis (Chapter 45) or kidney transplantation (Chapter 89) is needed to sustain life. Throughout this chapter CKD categories based on KDIGO classification will be used (eg, CKD 3a or CKD 5). The term CKD 5D indicates a patient with ESRD requiring dialysis as either hemodialysis (CKD 5HD) or peritoneal dialysis (CKD 5PD).

The prognosis of CKD is dependent on the following factors: (a) cause of kidney disease; (b) GFR at time of diagnosis; (c) degree of albuminuria; and (d) presence of other comorbid conditions. Patients with any of the following should be referred to a nephrologist for evaluation and collaborative management: persistent and significant albuminuria, progression of CKD (eg, a marked but nonacute decline in GFR), presence of unexplained urinary red cell casts, hypertension refractory to treatment (eg, ≥4 antihypertensive agents), persistent abnormalities of serum potassium, recurrent or extensive nephrolithiasis, GFR less than 30 mL/min/1.73 m^2 (0.29 mL/s/m^2), or hereditary kidney disease.[1]

Often complications of CKD are unrecognized or are inappropriately managed, and for many patients this contributes to significant morbidity, premature mortality, or a poorer prognosis if and when they develop CKD 5. Frequent complications of advanced CKD include altered sodium and water balance, hyperkalemia, metabolic acidosis, anemia, CKD-related mineral and bone disorder (CKD-MBD), and cardiovascular disease (CVD). This chapter primarily covers the pathophysiology and treatment of progressive CKD, anemia, CKD-MBD, and select cardiovascular (CV) complications. Table 44-2 lists other complications of advanced CKD not covered in detail in this chapter. The reader is referred to Chapters 49, 51, and 52 for a more detailed discussion of management and monitoring strategies for CKD patients with sodium and water balance abnormalities, hyperkalemia, and metabolic acidosis.

TABLE 44-1 Glomerular Filtration Rate Categories Based on KDIGO Classification

GFR Category[a]	GFR (mL/min/1.73 m^2 [mL/s/m^2])	Terms
1	>90 (>0.87)	Normal or high
2	60–89 (0.58–0.86)	Mildly decreased
3a	45–59 (0.43–0.57)	Mildly to moderately decreased
3b	30–44 (0.29–0.42)	Moderately to severely decreased
4	15–29 (0.14–0.28)	Severely decreased
5	<15 (<0.14)	Kidney failure

CKD, chronic kidney disease; GFR, glomerular filtration rate; KDIGO, Kidney Disease: Improving Global Outcomes.

[a]To meet criteria for CKD there must be a significant reduction in GFR (categories 3a-5) or there must also be evidence of kidney damage (categories 1 and 2) for 3 months or greater.

Data from reference 1.

TABLE 44-2 Other Complications of Chronic Kidney Disease[a]

Organ System or Complication	Clinical Manifestations
Amyloidosis	Accumulation of β_2-microglobulin Carpal tunnel syndrome
Blood and immune disorders	Bleeding diathesis Impaired cell-mediated immunity Lymphopenia Platelet dysfunction
Endocrine	Hypoglycemic episodes (result of decreased degradation of insulin by the kidney)
GI	Nausea, vomiting, anorexia (from uremia) Delayed gastric emptying Gastroesophageal reflux GI bleeding
Protein–energy wasting	Malnutrition
Neurologic	Peripheral neuropathies Restless leg syndrome Uremic encephalopathy
Uremic pruritus	Generalized itching predominantly of back, face, and extremity used for vascular access, but may affect any area May be more severe during or immediately after hemodialysis

[a]Not all inclusive.

EPIDEMIOLOGY

2 CKD is recognized as a significant global public health problem.[2] People with CKD experience high morbidity and mortality rates with a resulting economic burden to health-care systems due to hospitalizations and the high cost of chronic dialysis and kidney transplantation. From 1990 to 2013 the age-adjusted death rates attributable to CKD increased by 36.9% in 188 countries surveyed and CKD is now the 19th leading cause of life years lost.[3] Worldwide, an estimated 8% to 16% of the general population has CKD and 1.9 million patients are undergoing renal replacement therapy (hemodialysis, peritoneal dialysis, or kidney transplantation).[4,5] As a result, many countries have implemented public health initiatives to reduce the proportion of the population with CKD; increase the proportion of persons with CKD who know they have impaired kidney function; reduce the rate of new cases of ESRD and reduce mortality in persons with CKD.[6,7]

The prevalence of CKD increases with age to about 30% in people older than 70 years.[2] There is, however, some debate as to whether the GFR decline in older individuals as a consequence of the normal physiological aging process in the absence of proteinuria should truly be considered a *disease* necessitating the label of CKD.[8] Diabetes and hypertension are also important risk factors for CKD. A recent evaluation of type 1 diabetics in the Diabetes Control and Complications Trial (DCCT) and the Epidemiology of Diabetes Interventions and Complications (EDIC) studies reported that 17% to 25% of the participants developed diabetic chronic kidney disease (DCKD) after 30 years.[9] In patients with type 2 diabetes, a recent study from Spain noted a prevalence of 27%.[10] In the United States and other first-world countries, the leading cause of new ESRD cases is diabetes mellitus followed by hypertension (Fig. 44-1).[11]

Racial and socioeconomic disparities also exist. In the United States the rate of incident ESRD is 3.3 times greater for Blacks/African Americans and 1.5 times greater for Native Americans and Hispanics than for Whites.[11] The disparities are more striking among diabetics, with incidence rates of ESRD being approximately threefold higher in Blacks/African Americans and twofold higher in Hispanics. The rates of ESRD due to hypertension are also significantly higher among Blacks/African Americans than all other racial groups.[11] A survey in England found that high albuminuria was associated with low socioeconomic status even after adjustment for ethnicity, lifestyle, and clinical variables such as obesity, diabetes, hypertension, and smoking.[12] Greater prevalence of obesity, uncontrolled hypertension, and diabetes among nonwhite individuals are the most common reasons suggested for racial differences in albuminuria.[13] However, a study from Brazil found that the higher prevalence of CKD in individuals with lower educational status and

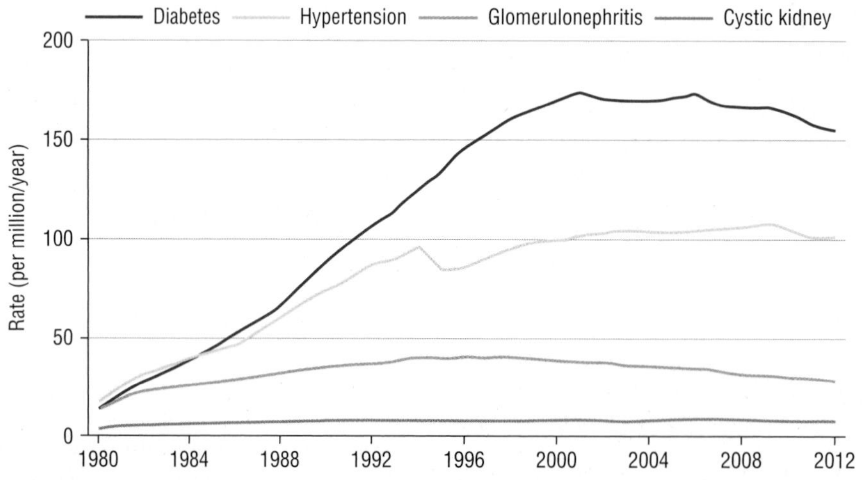

FIGURE 44-1 Incident rates of end-stage renal disease (ESRD) by primary diagnosis (1980-2012).[11]

in nonwhites could not be explained by differences in health-related factors.[14]

ETIOLOGY

Susceptibility and Initiation Risk Factors

Clinical and sociodemographic risk factors for susceptibility to and initiation of CKD are listed in Table 44-3 and are useful for identifying individuals at high risk of developing CKD.[15]

Progression Risk Factors

Progression risk factors are those associated with further decline in kidney function. Persistence of the underlying initiation factors (eg, diabetes mellitus, hypertension, glomerulonephritis) appears to be the most important predictor of progressive CKD. Other factors associated with progression include those that may be consequent to the underlying kidney disease (eg, hypertension, proteinuria) or independent of underlying kidney disease (eg, smoking, obesity).

Diabetes Mellitus

Achieving a hemoglobin A_{1C} (HbA1c) target of approximately 7% has been shown to prevent the surrogate endpoints of microalbuminuria and macroalbuminuria associated with diabetic chronic kidney disease (DCKD).[16,17] The original evidence to support this recommendation came from the type 1 diabetes DCCT trial and the long-term follow-up of these participants in the EDIC trial.[9] The evidence for individuals with type 2 diabetes comes from the United Kingdom Prospective Diabetes Study (UKPDS) and the Veterans Affairs Cooperative Study on Glycemic Control and Complications in Type 2 Diabetes Trial.[16] More recent trials in individuals with type 2 diabetes have also demonstrated reductions in new onset microalbuminuria or the development of macroalbuminuria with achievement of HbA1c less than 7% (0.07; 53 mmol/mol Hb).[18-20]

Hypertension

Data from the Prevention of Renal and Vascular End-stage Disease (PREVEND) study, a prospective, population-based cohort study in 6,894 people over a 4-year period, noted that the rate of eGFR decline was approximately 1.5 times higher in participants with hypertension.[21] The KDIGO guidelines for the management of blood pressure in CKD recommend the goal is to control blood pressure at all categories of CKD regardless of the underlying cause since early treatment of hypertension and achievement of target blood pressure have been demonstrated to slow the rate of progression of CKD.[22]

Proteinuria

Proteinuria, like hypertension, is an independent predictor of accelerated progression of CKD.[1] Proteinuria is also a risk factor for CV mortality and morbidity although there is some debate regarding the utility of proteinuria as a surrogate for more specific outcomes.[23-25]

Clinical Controversy...

Although proteinuria is associated with a faster rate of decline in kidney function, there is considerable controversy as to whether it is an appropriate surrogate endpoint for trials investigating therapies which slow progression of CKD. Critics of the use of proteinuria as a surrogate marker state that studies of ACEI or ARBs, which lower proteinuria, showed decreased risk of progression of CKD, but were not designed to test whether proteinuria itself was an appropriate target.[24] A recent meta-analysis of proteinuria as a surrogate marker suggested that data are limited and further assessment in prospective randomized controlled trials is needed.[25]

Smoking

Smoking is associated with an acute reduction in GFR and an increase in urinary albumin excretion, heart rate, and blood pressure, likely secondary to nicotine exposure.[26] Smoking is associated with kidney damage in the general population as well as in patients with diabetes and hypertension.[27] Smoking is also associated with an increase in CV events in people with CKD.[1]

Obesity

Population data from Kaiser Permanente revealed an increased risk of CKD 5 in overweight and obese subjects.[28] The risk of CKD 5 was directly related to the magnitude of obesity and remained even after adjustment for diabetes and hypertension. Another study showed that a body mass index (BMI) greater than or equal to 25 kg/m^2 at age 20 is associated with a threefold increase in risk of CKD compared with a BMI lower than 25 kg/m^2. Obesity (BMI ≥30 kg/m^2) among men and morbid obesity (BMI ≥35 kg/m^2) among women were associated with three- to fourfold increases in risk.[29] This finding has been supported by the results of a meta-analysis where the presence of kidney disease was associated with higher BMI and obesity led to more progressive loss of kidney function.[30]

Observational studies have shown obesity to be an independent risk factor for onset of CKD and a factor associated with the development of CKD secondary to focal and segmental glomerulosclerosis.[1,30-32] However, as evidenced by a meta-analysis, intentional weight loss in individuals with CKD was associated with decreases in proteinuria, systolic blood pressure, and stabilization in GFR during a mean follow-up of 7.4 months.[33] These data suggest that weight reduction be included as part of the treatment of CKD.

TABLE 44-3 Risk Factors for Susceptibility to and Initiation of Chronic Kidney Disease

Clinical Factors
Diabetes
Hypertension
Obesity
Autoimmune diseases
Systemic infections
Urinary tract infections
Urinary stones
Lower urinary tract obstruction
Neoplasia
Family history of CKD
Recovery from acute kidney injury
Reduction in kidney mass
Exposure to certain drugs
Low birth weight
Sociodemographic Factors
Older age
US ethnic minority status: African American, American Indian, Hispanic, Asian or Pacific Islander
Exposure to certain chemical and environmental conditions
Low income/education

Used with permission from Inker LA, Astor BC, Fox CH, et al. KDOQI US commentary on the 2012 KDIGO clinical practice guideline for the evaluation and management of CKD. *Am J Kidney Dis* 2014;63:713-735.

PATHOPHYSIOLOGY

Chronic Kidney Disease

Progression of CKD from category 1 to 5 occurs over decades in the majority of people, with the precise mechanism of kidney damage

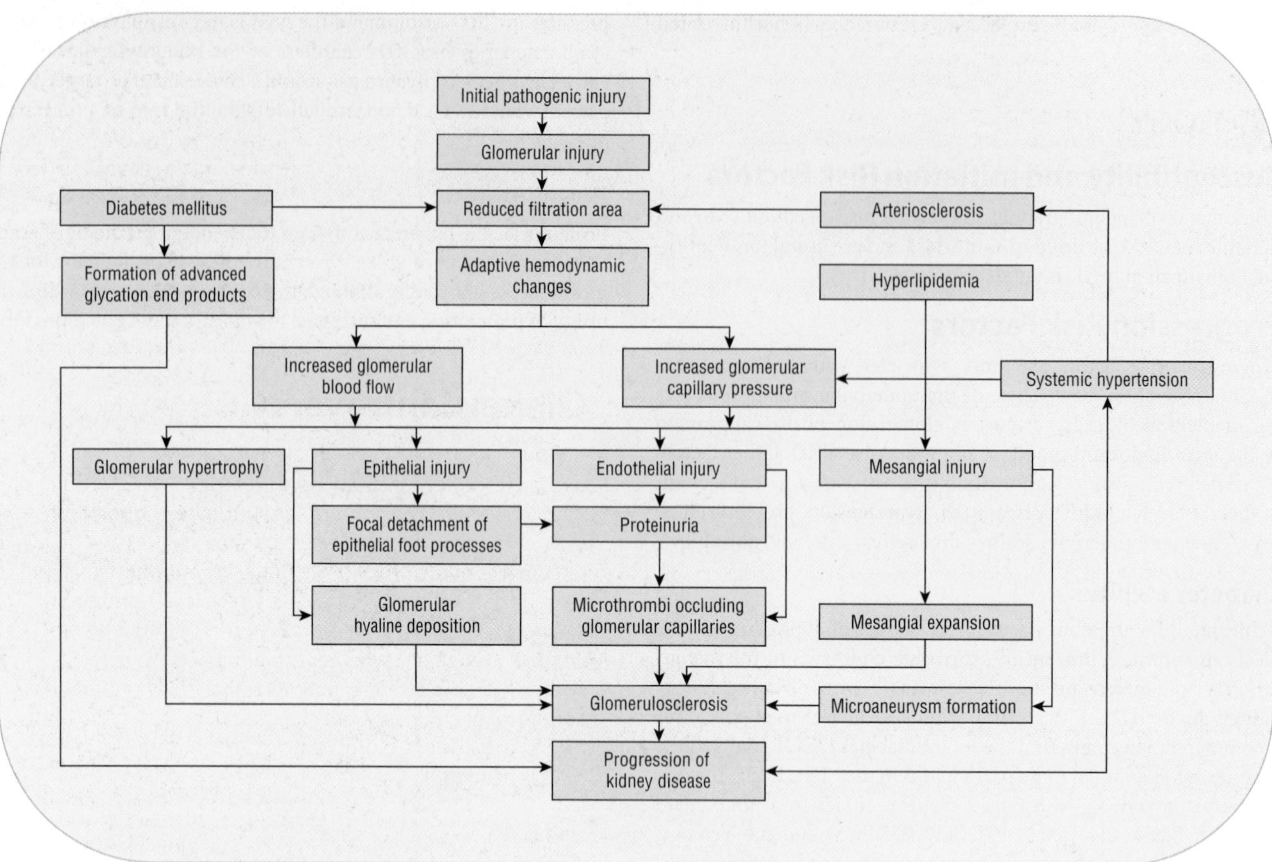

FIGURE 44-2 Proposed mechanisms of progression of kidney disease.

dependent on the etiology of the disease. As evidenced by the variety of initiation and progression factors, kidney damage can result from an array of heterogeneous causes. Diabetic CKD is characterized by glomerular mesangial expansion while with hypertensive nephrosclerosis, the kidney's arterioles have arteriolar hyalinosis. Polycystic kidney disease is characterized by the development and expansion of renal cysts.[34] While the initial structural damage depends on the primary disease affecting the kidney, the key elements of the pathway to ESRD are (a) loss of nephron mass, (b) glomerular capillary hypertension, and (c) proteinuria (Fig. 44-2).

Exposure to any of the initiation risk factors can result in loss of nephron mass. In response to the decrease in nephron function, the remaining nephrons compensate through the process of autoregulation. With nephron loss and the resulting reduction in perfusion pressure and GFR, renin release from the juxtaglomular apparatus increases and converts angiotensinogen to angiotensin I, which is then converted to angiotensin II (ATII). ATII is a potent vasoconstrictor of both afferent and efferent arterioles, but it preferentially affects the efferent arterioles, leading to increased pressure within the glomerular capillaries and consequent increased filtration fraction. Initially, this compensatory action may be adaptive and beneficial; however, over time it can lead to the development of intraglomerular hypertension and hypertrophy and a further decline in the number of functioning nephrons.[35] High intraglomerular capillary pressure impairs the size-selective function of the glomerular permeability barrier, resulting in increased urinary excretion of albumin and proteinuria. The development of intraglomerular hypertension usually parallels the development of systemic hypertension. ATII as well as aldosterone, may also mediate CKD progression through nonhemodynamic effects by increasing growth factors (eg, transforming growth factor beta [TGF-β]) and causing cellular proliferation and hypertrophy of the glomerular endothelial cells, epithelial cells, and fibroblasts ultimately resulting in further inflammation and fibrosis.[36]

Proteinuria alone may promote progressive loss of nephrons as a result of direct cellular damage. Filtered proteins such as albumin, transferrin, complement factors, immunoglobulins, cytokines, and ATII are toxic to kidney tubular cells. Numerous studies have demonstrated that the presence of these proteins in the renal tubule leads to increased production of inflammatory and vasoactive cytokines such as endothelin and monocyte chemoattractant protein-1 (MCP-1).[37] Proteinuria is also associated with the activation of complement components on the apical membrane of proximal tubules. Intratubular complement activation may be the key mechanism of damage in the progressive proteinuric nephropathies.[37] Furthermore, these events ultimately lead to scarring of the interstitium, progressive loss of structural nephron units, and a reduction in GFR.

Anemia of Chronic Kidney Disease

3 The primary cause of anemia of CKD is a decrease in production of erythropoietin, the glycoprotein hormone necessary for erythropoiesis (red blood cell production), by interstitial fibroblasts in the renal cortex of the kidney where approximately 90% of production occurs. In individuals with normal kidney function, plasma concentrations of erythropoietin increase exponentially in response to hypoxia; however, this response is lost as kidney disease progresses to CKD 3 and higher. The result is a normochromic (normal colored red cell), normocytic (normal size red cell) anemia (see Chapter 100).[38]

Iron deficiency is common in individuals with advanced kidney disease (ie, CKD 4 and 5) due to decreased gastrointestinal (GI) absorption of iron, inflammation, frequent blood testing, blood loss from hemodialysis (HD), and increased iron demands from erythropoiesis stimulating agent (ESA) therapy. It is the leading cause of resistance to ESAs and the reason frequent iron supplementation is necessary.[39] Hepcidin, a hormone produced by the liver directly inhibits the protein ferroportin that transports iron out of storage cells. When iron stores are high, hepcidin production is increased and results in a decrease in intestinal iron absorption, impairment of iron recycling from macrophages, and decreased mobilization of stored iron from hepatocytes. Hepcidin production is also induced by inflammation or infection. As a result, the increase in hepcidin in inflammatory conditions may lead to a sequestering of iron and ineffective red blood cell production. Conversely, hepcidin production is decreased when iron stores are low. The fact that hepcidin plays such a role in iron regulation has prompted the development of hepcidin antagonists to potentially alter iron transport.[40] At this time there are no commercially available agents.

Additional factors contributing to the development of anemia of CKD are the decreased red cell life span (from the normal of 120 days to approximately 60 days in individuals with CKD 5D), the effects of accumulation of uremic toxins and inflammatory cytokines, and vitamin B_{12} and folate deficiencies.[41]

Chronic Kidney Disease-Related Mineral and Bone Disorder

4 Disorders of mineral and bone metabolism are common in the CKD population and include abnormalities in PTH, calcium, phosphorus, vitamin D, fibroblast growth factor-23 (FGF-23), bone turnover, as well as soft-tissue calcifications. Historically these abnormalities have been described as characteristics of secondary hyperparathyroidism (sHPT) and renal osteodystrophy (ROD). The term CKD-MBD encompasses both of these abnormalities in mineral and bone metabolism as well as associated calcifications.[42]

The pathophysiology of CKD-MBD is complex (Fig. 44-3). Calcium and phosphorus homeostasis is mediated through the effects of PTH, 1,25-dihydroxyvitamin D_3 (calcitriol), and FGF-23 on bone, the GI tract, kidney, and the parathyroid gland. As kidney function declines, there is a decrease in phosphate elimination, which results in hyperphosphatemia and a decrease in serum calcium concentration. Hypocalcemia is the primary stimulus for secretion of PTH by the parathyroid glands. Hyperphosphatemia also increases PTH synthesis and release through its direct effects on the parathyroid gland and production of prepro-PTH messenger RNA.[43] In an attempt to normalize ionized calcium, PTH increases calcium reabsorption by the distal tubules and decreases phosphate reabsorption in the proximal tubules of the kidney (at least until the GFR falls to approximately 30 mL/min/1.73 m^2 [0.29 mL/s/m^2]) and also increases calcium mobilization from bone. FGF-23 production in bone also increases in response to high phosphate levels and promotes phosphate excretion by the kidney. The result is a relative normalization of calcium and phosphorus, at least in the early stages of CKD; however, this occurs at the expense of an elevated PTH and FGF-23 ("the trade-off hypothesis").[44] The increase in PTH is most notable when GFR is less than 60 mL/min/1.73 m^2 (0.58 mL/s/m^2) (CKD 3a and higher) and worsens as kidney function further declines.[43] With advanced kidney disease, the kidney fails to respond to PTH or to FGF-23 and abnormalities in calcium and phosphorus worsen. Over time the negative effects of sustained hyperparathyroidism on bone are realized as calcium resorption from bone persists.

1,25-dihydroxyvitamin D_3 or calcitriol promotes increased intestinal absorption of calcium and phosphorus, which helps normalize ionized calcium. Calcitriol also works directly on the parathyroid gland to suppress PTH production. The enzyme 1-α-hydroxylase is responsible for the final hydroxylation and conversion of the vitamin

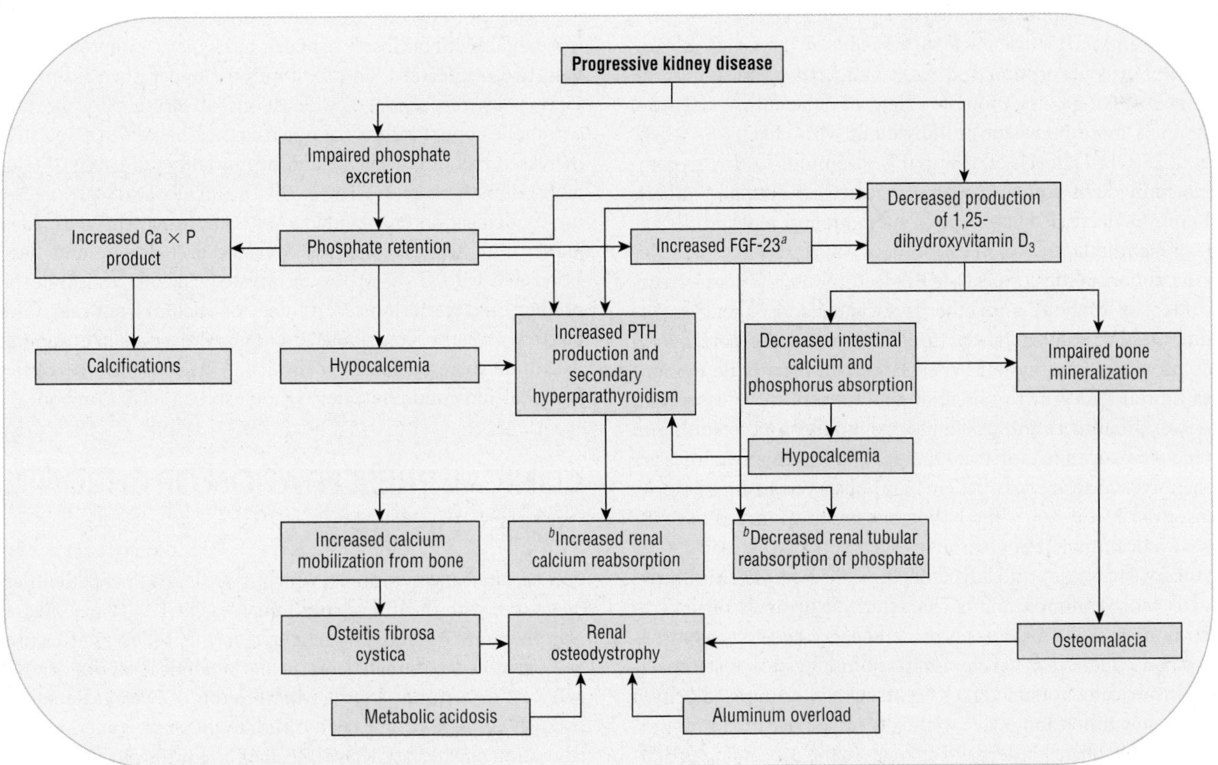

FIGURE 44-3 Pathophysiology of CKD-MBD. (Ca, calcium; FGF-23, fibroblast growth factor-23; PTH, parathyroid hormone.) [a]FGF-23 also increases in response to 1,25-dihydroxyvitamin D_3. [b]These adaptations are lost as kidney disease progresses.

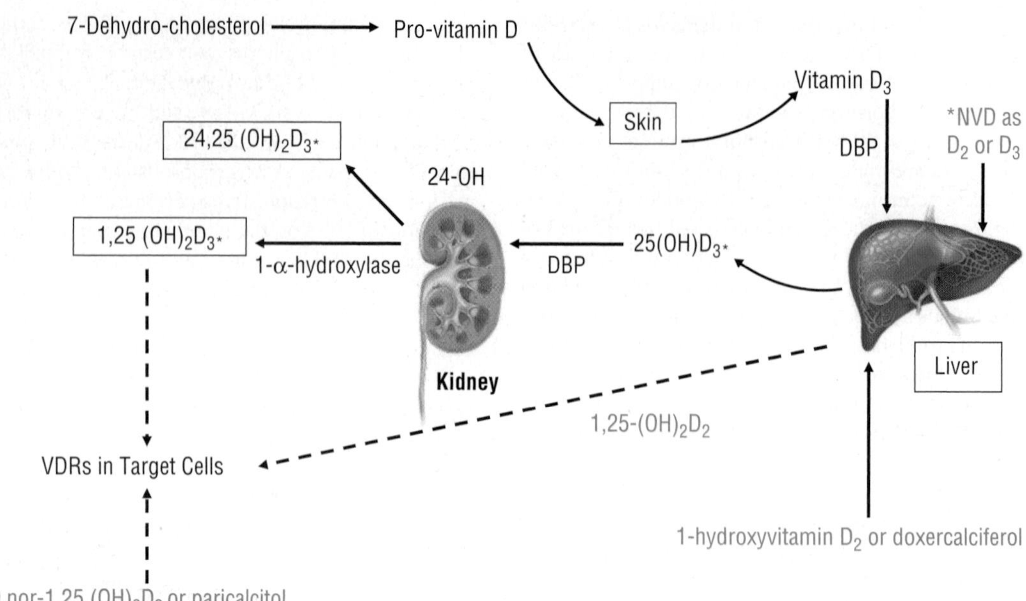

FIGURE 44-4 Vitamin D metabolism. (DBP, vitamin D binding protein; NVD, nutritional vitamin D; VDRs, vitamin D receptors.) Production of active vitamin D requires conversion of 7-dehydrocholesterol to cholecalciferol (vitamin D_3) by sunlight, followed by the first hydroxylation step in the liver to form 25-hydroxyvitamin D_3 or 25(OH)D_3, and the final conversion step in the kidney to form 1,25-dihydroxyvitamin D_3 or calcitriol. Within the kidney vitamin D may also be converted to an inactive form 24,25(OH)D_3. *If NVD is administered the resulting compound will be either a D_2 compound (as with ergocalciferol) or a D_3 compound (as with cholecalciferol). Paricalcitol and doxercalciferol are vitamin D analogs.

D precursor, 25-hydroxyvitamin D or 25(OH)D, to calcitriol in the kidney (Fig. 44-4). As kidney disease progresses, the concentrations of calcitriol decline due to loss of 1-α-hydroxylase activity. The resultant vitamin D deficiency leads to reduced intestinal calcium and phosphorus absorption and worsening hyperparathyroidism. Increases in FGF-23 also promote calcitriol deficiency.[45] Calcitriol deficiency is more prevalent in individuals with CKD 4-5.[46] Deficiency in 25(OH)D (levels of <30 ng/mL [<75 nmol/L]) is also common in individuals with CKD due to decreased dermal synthesis of vitamin D, decreased exposure to sunlight, and reduced dietary intake of vitamin D.[46]

The abnormalities of CKD-MBD lead to alterations in structural integrity of bone and other associated consequences. The continuous high rate of production of PTH by the parathyroid glands promotes parathyroid hyperplasia. Nodular tissue demonstrates more rapid growth potential and appears to be associated with fewer vitamin D and calcium-sensing receptors, resulting in resistance to exogenous calcitriol therapy.[43] Bone abnormalities are almost universal in dialysis patients and observed in the majority of those with CKD 3-5.[42] The bone abnormalities include osteitis fibrosa cystica (high bone turnover disease), osteomalacia (low bone turnover disease), and adynamic bone disease. Osteitis fibrosa cystica is most common and is characterized by areas of peritrabecular fibrosis. Bone marrow fibrosis and decreased erythropoiesis are also consequences of severe osteitis fibrosa cystica. Osteomalacia was historically noted in HD patients with aluminum toxicity, a finding less common today due to the decreased use of aluminum-containing phosphate binders and changes in the processing of dialysate solutions to decrease aluminum content. Adynamic lesions are characterized by low amounts of fibrosis or osteoid tissue and low bone formation rates. Multiple risk factors for the development of this bone disease include high concentrations of dialysate calcium along with high doses of calcium-containing phosphate binders, aggressive management with vitamin D therapy, diabetes, and aluminum toxicity.[42]

The morbidity and mortality of CKD patients is increased in individuals with both severe hypo- and hyperparathyroidism (ie, less than two or greater than nine times the upper normal limit for the PTH assay, respectively).[42] Elevations of serum phosphorus, even within the upper limits of the normal range, have been associated with increased risk of CV events and/or mortality (all-cause or CV mortality) in patients with CKD 3-5.[47] The incidence of calciphylaxis, or rapid calcification of subcutaneous tissue, in patients with advanced kidney disease has increased over the past decade and has been associated with CKD-MBD, an elevated calcium times phosphorus product, and warfarin use.[42,48] Intake of calcium from calcium-based binders may also contribute to coronary artery calcification. These data underscore the need to consider all the consequences of elevated PTH, calcium, and phosphorus, not just their effects on bone.

CLINICAL PRESENTATION OF CHRONIC KIDNEY DISEASE

CKD is often asymptomatic, which is a reason many patients are not diagnosed with the disease until they reach CKD 4 or 5 and are at or near the point of requiring renal replacement therapy. This problem has prompted automated reporting by clinical laboratories of the eGFR as determined by the Modification of Diet in Renal Disease (MDRD) equation or Chronic Kidney Disease Epidemiology Collaboration equation (CKD-EPI equation) for the purpose of identifying individuals with CKD earlier (see Chapter e42). Clinicians must understand how to interpret the eGFR and values for urine albumin excretion to appropriately stage individuals with CKD. Chapter e42 provides a detailed discussion of the methods available for detection of urinary albumin and protein.

CLINICAL PRESENTATION Stage 4 or 5 Chronic Kidney Disease

Symptoms

- Fatigue, weakness, shortness of breath, mental confusion, nausea and vomiting, bleeding, and loss of appetite, itching, cold intolerance, and peripheral neuropathies are common.

Signs

- Edema, weight gain (from accumulation of fluid), changes in urine output (volume and consistency), "foaming" of urine (indicative of proteinuria), and abdominal distension.

Laboratory Tests

- *Decreased*: eGFR, bicarbonate (metabolic acidosis), Hb/hematocrit (Hct) (anemia), transferrin saturation (TSat) and/or ferritin (iron deficiency; note: ferritin may be increased due to inflammatory conditions), vitamin D levels, albumin (malnutrition), glucose (may result from decreased degradation of insulin with impaired kidney function or poor oral intake), and calcium (in early stages of CKD).
- *Increased*: Serum creatinine, blood urea nitrogen, potassium, phosphorus, PTH, FGF-23, ACR, PCR blood pressure (hypertension is a common cause and result of CKD), glucose (uncontrolled diabetes is a cause of CKD), low-density lipoprotein (LDL) and triglycerides, and calcium (more likely in CKD 5).
- *Other*: May be hemoccult-positive if GI bleeding occurs secondary to uremia.

Other Diagnostic Tests

- Urine sediment abnormalities (hematuria, red blood cell and white blood cell casts, renal tubular epithelial cells)
- Pathologic abnormalities indicating glomerular, vascular, tubulointerstitial disease, or cystic and congenital diseases
- Structural abnormalities such as polycystic kidneys, renal masses, renal artery stenosis, cortical scarring due to infarcts and pyelonephritis, or small kidneys (common in more severe CKD) detected by imaging studies (eg, ultrasound, computed tomography, magnetic resonance imaging, angiography)

Diagnostic Considerations for Anemia of Chronic Kidney Disease

Signs and symptoms of anemia of CKD include fatigue, shortness of breath, cold intolerance, chest pain, tingling in the extremities, tachycardia, headaches, and general malaise. Since individuals with anemia of CKD may be asymptomatic, laboratory evaluation is commonly the initial approach to diagnosing anemia of CKD. According to the KDIGO guidelines Hb concentrations should be measured annually in CKD 3, biannually in CKD 4-5, and at least every 3 months in CKD 5D patients.[39] The diagnosis of anemia is made and further workup of anemia is required when the Hb is less than 13 g/dL (130 g/L; 8.07 mmol/L) for adult males and less than 12 g/dL (120 g/L; 7.45 mmol/L) for adult females.[39] As iron deficiency is the primary cause of resistance to treatment of anemia with ESAs, assessment of the iron status is necessary. The TSat provides information on iron immediately available for use in the bone marrow for red blood cell production and the serum ferritin is in indirect measure of storage iron. The TSat is calculated as follows: (serum iron/total iron-binding capacity [TIBC]) × 100. Transferrin is the carrier protein for iron and may be affected by nutritional status. Serum ferritin is an indirect measure of storage iron and an acute-phase reactant, meaning it may be elevated under certain inflammatory conditions and give a false indication of storage iron. Patients may be diagnosed with *absolute iron deficiency* when whole-body iron stores are low (low TSat and ferritin), or with *functional iron deficiency* when the TSat is low, but the serum ferritin is at or above goal. In this situation iron is not released rapidly enough to satisfy the demands for erythropoiesis and further evaluation is warranted. If the TSat and serum ferritin values are below the desired thresholds iron supplementation is warranted.

Additional workup should be done to evaluate other causes of anemia such as blood loss, deficiencies in vitamin B_{12} or folate, or other disease states that contribute to anemia, including human immunodeficiency virus infection and malignancies (see Chapter 100). Red blood cell indices (mean corpuscular volume, mean corpuscular Hb concentration), white blood cell count, differential and platelet count, and absolute reticulocyte count should also be assessed. A stool guaiac test should be performed to rule out GI bleeding. Measurement of serum erythropoietin concentrations is not generally useful since levels may fall into what is considered a "normal" range, but are insufficient relative to the degree of decline in Hb.

Diagnostic Considerations for Chronic Kidney Disease-Related Mineral and Bone Disorder

Symptoms of CKD-MBD are often not evident until significant skeletal damage has developed; consequently, prevention is the key to minimize the risk of long-term complications. When signs and symptoms such as bone pain and skeletal fractures are evident, the disease is not easily amenable to treatment. Thus the identification of biochemical or imaging abnormalities which typically precede clinical manifestations is an essential component of patient evaluation. The biochemical abnormalities of CKD-MBD that are commonly present in patients with CKD include alterations in serum phosphorus, calcium, PTH, and 25(OH)D. Because deficiency in the vitamin D precursor, 25(OH)D is common and has been associated with negative outcomes in the CKD population, measurement of 25(OH)D levels in patients with CKD 3-5D is suggested.[42] It should be noted, however, that the assay methods for 25(OH)D are not standardized, which creates a challenge regarding the clinical implications of abnormal values and limits its value as an indicator of therapeutic response.[49] The Vitamin D Standardization Program may help apply uniform laboratory measurement processes among manufacturers of assays and clinical and research laboratories. Current monitoring recommendations and goals of therapy are covered in the section on "Treatment of CKD-MBD."[50]

In addition to evaluating biochemical indices that define CKD-MBD, evaluation of bone architecture may be desirable. The gold standard test for diagnosing bone manifestations of CKD-MBD is a bone biopsy for histologic analysis; however, this is a very invasive test that is not easily performed. KDIGO guidelines recommend bone biopsy only in patients in whom the etiology is not clear or in those with a nontraditional biochemical presentation.[42] This includes patients experiencing unexplained fractures, persistent hypercalcemia, and possible aluminum toxicity. If aluminum concentrations are elevated (60-200 mcg/L [2.2-7.4 μmol/L]), a deferoxamine test should be done. KDIGO also suggests a bone biopsy be considered in CKD patients prior to beginning treatment with bisphosphonates since adynamic bone disease is a contraindication to the use of these agents. Bone biopsy findings are described on the basis of turnover rate, mineralization, and volume. Routine bone mineral density testing is not recommended in patients with CKD 3-5D since this test has not been shown to predict fracture risk and does not indicate the type of bone abnormality. CKD-MBD is also highly associated with vascular and soft-tissue calcifications, known risk factors for mortality; therefore, diagnostic testing for calcifications should be considered in the evaluation for CKD-MBD.[42]

TREATMENT
CKD

General Approach to Patient Care for Chronic Kidney Disease

Individuals with CKD should be evaluated frequently to assess the rate of progression of CKD, to identify the presence and causes of secondary complications and comorbid conditions, and to receive treatment for these complications prior to development of CKD 5D. Many nonpharmacologic and pharmacologic recommendations can be broadly applied as part of the general approach to care for all CKD patients Table 44-4.[1,22,51]

(5) Management of CKD should be based on the most current consensus guidelines and the best clinical practices such as those developed by KDIGO, which are based on evidence, when available, and expert recommendations. These recommendations should not replace clinical judgment, but rather provide a basis on which treatment decisions can be made in the context of both evidence and opinion. The secondary complications of CKD that are addressed in the currently available KDIGO clinical practice guidelines address evaluation and management of CKD, blood pressure, CKD-MBD, anemia, lipid management, hepatitis C in CKD, and glomerulonephritis. Table 44-5 provides a guide to the grading and strength of recommendations used in these guidelines. Where appropriate, comparisons with the Kidney Disease Outcome Quality Initiative (KDOQI) Guidelines will be made in this chapter.

(6) Appropriate management of CKD ideally involves an interprofessional approach to address the nonpharmacologic and pharmacologic interventions, dietary education, and social/financial concerns. Multiple chronic disease states, financial barriers, low health literacy, and psychosocial concerns are just a few of the unique challenges that necessitate comprehensive services. Furthermore, CKD 5D patients are prescribed an average of 10 to 12 medications, which increases the potential for medication-related problems (MRPs; eg, inappropriate dose or indication for a medication, adverse drug reactions).[52] The typical team in outpatient dialysis facilities includes physicians (nephrologists), nurses, dietitians, and social workers as mandated by the United States government. Although not mandated to be part of the care team, nephrology-trained pharmacists are active members of the care team in some CKD and especially dialysis settings in the United States and their inclusion has resulted in a reduction of MRPs.[52,53] In Canada, pharmacists' involvement is more standardized and pharmacists have a more clearly delineated role in the care of the CKD population.[54]

TABLE 44-4 Recommendations for Individuals with Chronic Kidney Disease

Nonpharmacologic
- Exercise 30 minutes five times per week [1D]
- Weight loss if BMI >25 kg/m^2 [1D]
- Smoking cessation [1D]
- Alcohol: Two standard drinks per day for men and one standard drink per day for women[a][2D]
- If hypertension: Low-sodium diet (<2 g/day, <90 mmol/day) [1C]

Pharmacologic
- Adjust medication doses for kidney function [1A]
- Seek pharmacist or medical advice before using over-the-counter medicines or nutritional protein supplements [1B]
- Herbal medicines are not recommended [1B]
- Temporarily discontinue potentially nephrotoxic/renally excreted drugs if eGFR <60 mL/min/1.73 m^2 in patients who are acutely unwell or hypovolemic (eg, metformin, RAAS blockers, diuretics, NSAIDs/COX II inhibitors, lithium, digoxin) [1C]
- Vaccines:
- Influenza yearly [1B]
- Pneumococcal vaccine if eGFR <30 mL/min/1.73 m^2, nephrotic syndrome, diabetes, or receiving immunosuppression. Single booster dose at year 5 [1B]
- Hepatitis B vaccine if eGFR <30 mL/min/1.73 m^2 and risk of progression of CKD [1B]
- ASA suggested for patients at risk for atherosclerotic events unless there is an increased bleeding risk [2B]
- Avoid oral phosphate-containing bowel preparations in people with a GFR <60 mL/min/1.73 m^2 (<0.58 mL/s/m^2) or in those known to be at risk of phosphate nephropathy [1A]

BMI, body mass index; CKD, chronic kidney disease; COX; cyclooxygenase; eGFR, estimated glomerular filtration rate; NSAIDs, nonsteroidal anti-inflammatory drugs; RAAS, renin–angiotensin–aldosterone system.

See Table 44-5 for definitions of evidence grading in brackets.

[a]Standard drink: 30 mL spirits, 100 mL wine, 285 mL full-strength beer, and 425 mL light beer.

Data from references 1, 22, and 51.

TABLE 44-5 KDIGO Guidelines: Grading and Strength of Recommendations

Grade	Description	Implications for Clinicians
Level 1	"We recommend"	Most patients should receive the recommended course of action.
Level 2	"We suggest"	Different choices will be appropriate for different patients. Each patient needs help arrive at a management decision consistent with her or his values and preferences.
Grade	**Quality of Evidence**	**Meaning**
A	High	We are confident that the true effect lies close to that of the estimate of the effect.
B	Moderate	The true effect is likely to be close to the estimate of the effect, but there is a possibility that it is substantially different.
C	Low	The true effect may be substantially different from the estimate of the effect.
D	Very low	The estimate of effect is very uncertain, and often will be far from the truth.

The strength of recommendation is indicated as Level 1, Level 2, or Not Graded. The quality of the supporting evidence is shown as A, B, C, or D.

Data from reference 1.

Pharmacists can provide comprehensive medication management (CMM) services and collaborate with community care coordinators and pharmacists. It is estimated that over 70% of MRPs could be prevented with integrated pharmacy services that include CMM.[55] Drug-dosing guidelines based on the degree of kidney function should be followed, and a complete medication history of prescription and nonprescription medications, as well as herbals and nutritional supplements, should be obtained and routinely updated. General recommendations for drug dosing in CKD patients were developed at a 2011 KDIGO conference and are presented in detail for CKD and dialysis patients in Chapter 48.[56] Appropriate measures should also be taken for patients with CKD to decrease the risk of nephrotoxicity from radiocontrast agents, antibiotics such as aminoglycosides, as well as from nonsteroidal anti-inflammatory drugs and ACEIs (Chapter 46).

Desired Outcome of CKD Treatment

The overall goal of therapy in CKD patients is to delay or prevent progression of the disease while minimizing the development or severity of associated complications. During CKD 4 planning for renal replacement therapy (HD or PD) should begin, including patient education about dialysis modalities and options for transplantation (Chapter 45). With CKD 5D the primary goal is to sustain and improve, if possible, the patient's quality of life and prevent adverse outcomes by aggressively managing complications of CKD.

Nonpharmacologic Therapy for CKD

Nonpharmacologic therapies for CKD include diet and lifestyle interventions targeted at reducing the risk factors for CKD progression.

Diet

There is no convincing or conclusive evidence that long-term protein restriction delays the progression of CKD.[1] Protein restriction to 0.8 g/kg/day is recommended only in patients with an eGFR less than 30 mL/min/1.73 m^2 (ie, CKD 4) with appropriate monitoring by a dietitian to avoid malnutrition.[1] High sodium intake can increase blood pressure and proteinuria, blunt the response to renin–angiotensin system blockade, and induce glomerular hyperfiltration; therefore, decreasing sodium intake to less than 2 g or 90 mEq (mmol) per day (corresponding to 5 g sodium chloride) is recommended, particularly in patients with preexisting hypertension or proteinuria (Table 44-4).[1]

Smoking Cessation, Exercise, and Weight Loss

Smoking cessation is encouraged to slow progression of CKD and to reduce the risk of CVD (Table 44-4). Clinicians should educate patients regarding the risks of smoking and institute appropriate therapeutic options, both nonpharmacologic and pharmacologic, for smoking cessation. These options are discussed in detail in Chapter 66. All individuals with CKD are encouraged to exercise at least 30 minutes five times per week and to achieve a BMI of 20 to 25 kg/m^2 if needed (see Chapter 144).[1]

Pharmacologic Therapy for CKD

Pharmacologic therapies used in slowing the progression of CKD include ACEIs and ARBs in patients with proteinuria as well as other antihypertensives used for achieving blood pressure targets. Glycemic control with oral hypoglycemic agents or insulin is also important for patients with diabetes mellitus.

Proteinuria

The antiproteinuric effect of ACEIs and ARBs is a class effect and not specific to any one agent.[22] For patients with hypertension, the primary goal is to achieve the target blood pressure while a secondary goal is to control proteinuria. For patients with DCKD, an ACEI or an ARB should be used as first-line therapy if the patient's urine albumin excretion is in category A2 or greater (ACR between 30-300 mg/g).

Specific dosing recommendations for ACEIs and ARBs for the treatment of proteinuria have not been established; consequently, the lowest recommended dose should be initiated. The dose is usually increased until albuminuria is reduced by 30% to 50% or side effects such as a greater than 30% decrease in eGFR or elevation in serum potassium occur (see Chapter 13). If patients exhibit a cough with an ACEI, a switch to an ARB is appropriate.

7 Evidence from clinical trials has confirmed the beneficial effects of ACEIs and ARBs on kidney function for DCKD. A meta-analysis has shown that the effects of ACEIs or ARBs on key CKD outcomes such as doubling of creatinine and prevention of progression of micro- to macroalbuminuria are equivalent and, thus, they can be used interchangeably.[57] A thorough discussion of dose, dose titration, monitoring, and adverse effects of ACEIs and ARBs is presented in Chapter 13.

The lack of response of some patients to ACEI or ARB therapy may be due to aldosterone escape from renin–angiotensin–aldosterone system (RAAS) blockade. Combination therapy with an ACEI plus an ARB produces a more complete blockade of the RAAS and results in a greater reduction in macroalbuminuria.[58] As a result, it was postulated that dual therapy would slow progression of CKD in the subset of patients who were already receiving the maximum dose of an ACEI or an ARB alone, but who still had macroalbuminuria.[59] The ONTARGET study first raised concerns with the use of an ACEI plus an ARB.[60] This study randomized 25,620 patients with established atherosclerotic vascular disease or diabetes with end-organ damage to telmisartan, ramipril, or a combination of the two drugs. The composite outcome of dialysis, renal transplantation, doubling of serum creatinine, or death occurred more frequently in patients receiving combination treatment than in either of the two other groups, despite a lower degree of albuminuria and less progression to microalbuminuria or macroalbuminuria. These findings led some to advise against the combination of these two agents; however, critics of the study argued that these findings cannot be extrapolated to individuals with proteinuric kidney disease as only 4% of patients in the study had overt proteinuria.[61] Combination therapy with an ACEI and an ARB in diabetic patients with CKD and macroalbuminuria in the VA NEPHRON D study revealed that ACEI plus ARB therapy increased the risk of acute kidney injury (12.2 vs 6.7 events per 100 person-years, $p < 0.001$) and hyperkalemia (6.3 vs 2.6 events per 100 person-years, $p < 0.001$) with no reduction in mortality.[62] Two other randomized controlled trials (ALTITUDE and a subgroup analysis of ORIENT) which employed various combinations of ACEI and ARB or aliskiren, a direct renin inhibitor, failed to show that dual blockade of the RAAS either slowed progression of CKD or decreased CV events.[63,64] Combination therapy in these trials was also associated with increased risks of hyperkalemia and acute kidney injury. Thus, the combination of an ACEI plus an ARB or aliskiren for the treatment of DCKD, even in patients with macroalbuminuria, is no longer recommended.

The concept of aldosterone escape has led to the search for other drug combinations to further suppress the RAAS in an effort to improve kidney outcomes. A Cochrane systematic review examined the addition of an aldosterone antagonist (spironolactone) to an ACEI or ARB (or both) in patients with CKD1-4.[65] Aldosterone antagonists significantly reduced proteinuria and blood pressure, but doubled the risk of hyperkalemia and significantly increased the risk of gynecomastia. However, it is unknown whether adding spironolactone to ACEI or ARB (or both) will reduce the risk of major CV events or ESRD. Another meta-analysis of spironolactone in DCKD reported similar results.[66] Dihydropyridine calcium channel blockers (CCBs) do not appear to have any beneficial effects beyond those attributable to reducing blood pressure. Nondihydropyridine agents (diltiazem and verapamil), however, have yielded beneficial effects on proteinuria, although not as profoundly as ACEIs.[67] The postulated mechanisms for this decrease in kidney injury include suppression of glomerular hypertrophy, inhibition of platelet aggregation, and a decrease in salt accumulation. These agents have been used to reduce proteinuria in combination with an ACEI or ARB despite the fact that there are limited data to support this strategy. In general, nondihydropyridine CCBs should be considered second-line antiproteinuric drugs when an ACEI or ARB is contraindicated or not tolerated (Figure 44-5).[68]

Endothelin-1 is present in the renal microvasculature, glomerular cells, and in the tubules, and exerts its actions via the endothelin A and B receptors. In type 2 diabetics a trial of the endothelin antagonist, avosentan was terminated early because of increased edema and heart failure.[69] The impact of atrasentan, another endothelin antagonist, on CKD progression when added to RAAS inhibitor therapy in patients with type 2 diabetes and CKD revealed that it significantly reduced albuminuria, blood pressure, LDL cholesterol, and triglycerides.[70] A longer trial examining the efficacy of atrasentan on preventing progression of DCKD is now underway, the Study of Diabetic Nephropathy with Atrasentan (SONAR), with results expected in 2018.[71]

Glomerulonephritis is the third leading cause of CKD and almost all of the many variants are associated with significant proteinuria. A thorough review of the epidemiology, pathophysiology, and treatment strategies is provided in Chapter 47.

Hypertension

Figure 44-5 provides an algorithm for the recommended blood pressure goals based on the degree of albuminuria present and the choice of antihypertensive agent. Previous guidelines suggested a target blood pressure of less than 130/80 mm Hg for all patients with CKD. A meta-analysis of 2,272 subjects with nondiabetic kidney disease concluded that no benefits in kidney, CV outcomes, or mortality were achieved in patients treated to a goal blood pressure of 125 to 130/75 to 80 mm Hg as compared with 140/90 mm Hg.[72] Subjects with proteinuria greater than 300 mg/day did benefit from the lower blood pressure target. The Systolic Blood Pressure Intervention Trial (SPRINT) assessed whether a lower systolic blood pressure goal of less than 120 mm Hg versus a target of less than 140 mm Hg was desirable.[73] Patients aged 50 years or older with a systolic blood

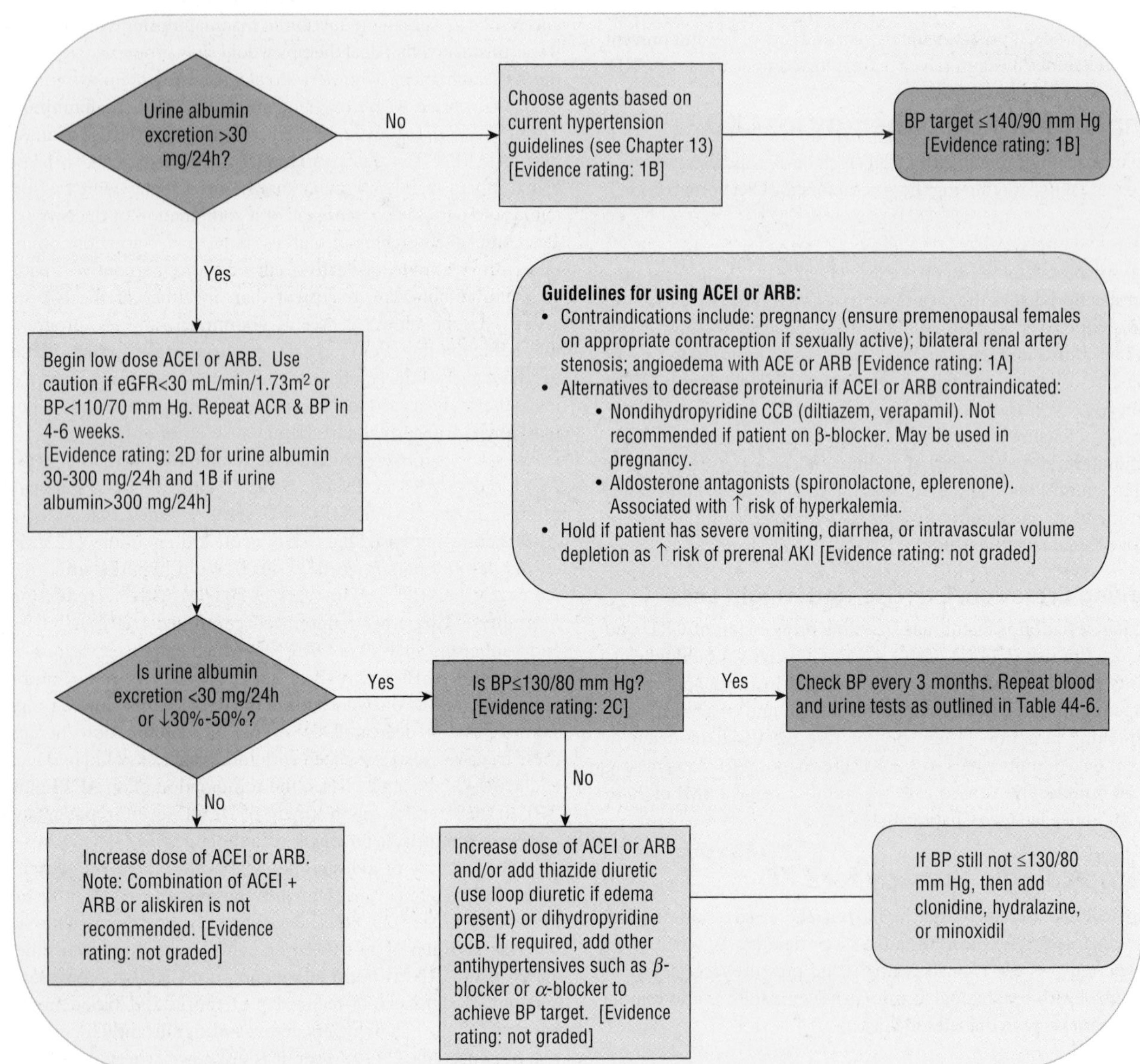

FIGURE 44-5 Treatment of hypertension in chronic kidney disease.[22] (ACEI, angiotensin-converting enzyme inhibitor; ACR, albumin-to-creatinine ratio; AKI, acute kidney injury; ARB, angiotensin receptor blocker; BP, blood pressure; CCB, calcium channel blocker; eGFR, estimated glomerular filtration rate.)

pressure of 130 to 180 mm Hg and an increased risk of CV events were included. CKD 3a to 4 patients (eGFR of 20-59 mL/min/1.73 m^2) were enrolled into this trial as they were considered to be at high CV risk (see chapter 13 for a discussion of non-CKD results). It is important to note that patients with a history of diabetes, category A3 proteinuria defined as greater than or equal to 1 g/24 hours of protein or albuminuria greater than or equal to 600 mg/24 hours, polycystic kidney disease, or a history of stroke were excluded. In the 2,646 participants with CKD, the composite renal outcome of a decrease in eGFR of 50% or more or the need for chronic dialysis or kidney transplantation was not significant over the 3.3 years duration of this trial. There were also potential harms to all participants (with and without CKD) in the intensive systolic blood pressure group that included significantly increased risks of syncope, hypotension, electrolyte abnormalities, AKI and CKD progression.[73] The current KDIGO Blood Pressure guidelines recommend a target blood pressure of less than or equal to 140/90 mm Hg for those with category A1 albuminuria.[22] In patients with category A2 and higher albuminuria, the target blood pressure is less than or equal to 130/80 mm Hg and first-line therapy with an ACEI or ARB is recommended.[22] If this regimen fails to achieve the target blood pressure, then the addition of a thiazide diuretic may be warranted.[74,75] KDIGO has started the process to review the SPRINT trial and other new data to determine if revisions to its blood pressure guideline are warranted.

Clinical **Controversy...**

It has been widely quoted that thiazide diuretics are not effective for blood pressure control for CKD 4 and 5, but there is limited evidence to support this statement. While salt and water excretion may initially account for their antihypertensive effect, long-term lowering of blood pressure appears to involve direct vasodilation that is not affected by kidney function. A number of small trials have demonstrated significant blood pressure lowering with systolic blood pressure reductions of 12 to 15 mm Hg in patients with CKD 4 and 5.[76] Various thiazide diuretics have been used including hydrochlorothiazide 25 mg daily, indapamide 1.5 to 5 mg daily, and chlorthalidone 25 mg daily. In addition, thiazides have also been combined with loop diuretics, such as furosemide 40 to 80 mg daily, with reductions in systolic blood pressure of 15 to 22 mm Hg so this combination may also have benefits.[76] A larger randomized controlled trial of the safety and efficacy of thiazides added to existing antihypertensives in individuals with CKD 4 and 5 is needed.

The choice of additional antihypertensive agents should be based on concomitant disease states and other compelling indications as discussed in Chapter 13. Patients and clinicians should be aware that targeting a blood pressure of less than 130/80 mm Hg will often require three or more drugs.

Diabetes

Patients with diabetes should be screened annually for CKD starting at the time of diagnosis of type 2 diabetes and 5 years after the diagnosis of type 1 diabetes by ordering a serum creatinine, eGFR, and a urine albumin-to-creatinine ratio (ACR).[51]

The management of diabetes in patients with CKD includes reduction of proteinuria and achievement of desired blood pressure and HbA1c (Chapter 74). The HbA1c target in this patient population should be 7% (0.07; 53 mmol/mol Hb); however, clinicians may consider a target greater than 7% (0.07; 53 mmol/mol Hb) if there is a risk of hypoglycemia or limited life expectancy (Evidence rating: 1A).[51] It should be noted that HbA1C measurements are based on an assumed red blood cell life span of 90 days. In CKD, the red blood cell life span is decreased, so HbA1c values may be falsely low.[51] Hence, in patients with CKD, the HbA1c should be interpreted along with the patient's home blood glucose readings before making a determination of diabetic control. It is also important to note that patients with CKD 3 and 4 are at higher risk of developing hypoglycemia because of the reduction in metabolism of insulin by the kidney as GFR declines. As a result, these patients may require reduced doses of oral or injectable hypoglycemic agents. Metformin can be continued in people with eGFR greater than or equal to 45 mL/min/1.73 m^2; reviewed in those with an eGFR 30 to 44 mL/min/1.73 m^2, and discontinued in individuals with an eGFR less than 30 mL/min/1.73 m^2 (Evidence level: not graded).[51] Dose adjustments or avoidance of other renally eliminated hypoglycemic agents may be necessary; the dosing, monitoring, and goals of therapies to treat diabetes mellitus is provided in Chapter 74 and an evidence-based approach to drug therapy individualization is presented in Chapter 48.

Personalized Pharmacotherapy

The clearance of all ACEIs (with the exception of fosinopril) is reduced in CKD; therefore, it is necessary to initiate therapy at lower initial doses and subsequently titrate the dose to achieve the optimal therapeutic effects such as decreased proteinuria and blood pressure. The antiproteinuric effects of ACEIs/ARBs are not necessarily attained at the same doses as the antihypertensive effects. Thus, individualization of therapy is required for patients who have reached their blood pressure goals yet require further reductions in urinary protein excretion.

Evaluation of Therapeutic Outcomes

Frequency of laboratory and urine testing based on CKD category and degree of albuminuria as defined by KDIGO is shown in Table 44-6. The monitoring necessary for patients with hypertension and diabetes is the same in the CKD population as it is in the non-CKD population, and readers should refer to the appropriate chapters in this textbook for further information.

Treatment
Secondary Complications

Anemia of CKD

Treatment of anemia often requires a combination of iron supplementation and ESA therapy to promote and maintain erythropoiesis and to achieve the individual patient goals.

Desired Outcome

The desired outcomes of anemia management are to increase oxygen-carrying capacity, decrease signs and symptoms of anemia, and decrease the need for blood transfusions. Hb is the preferred monitoring parameter for red blood cell production because, unlike Hct, its concentration is not affected by blood storage conditions and instrumentation used for analysis. Initiation of iron or ESA therapy is guided by the patient's Hb, TSat, and ferritin (Table 44-7).[39] The risk of mortality and CV events is higher in CKD patients treated to higher Hb target values with an ESA. There are discrepancies, however, in the FDA-approved labeling for ESAs and the KDIGO and KDOQI anemia guidelines in terms of when to initiate therapy and the target Hb.[39,77,78] Notably the KDOQI guidelines suggest a Hb range of 11 to 12 g/dL (110-120 g/L; 6.83-7.45 mmol/L) for all CKD patients, a target TSat of greater than 20% (>0.20), and a serum ferritin of greater than 100 ng/mL (mcg/L; >225 pmol/L) for CKD patients not requiring HD and greater than 200 ng/mL (mcg/L; >450 pmol/L) for CKD 5HD patients.

TABLE 44-6 Recommended Monitoring Intervals for Outcome Measure in Patients with Chronic Kidney Disease (Evidence Rating: Not Graded)

		Albuminuria Stage (based on ACR in mg/g)		
KDIGO GFR Category	eGFR (mL/min/1.73 m²)	A1: <30 mg/g (<3 mg/mmol)	A2: 30-300 mg/g (3-30 mg/mmol)	A3: >300 mg/g (>30 mg/mmol)
1	≥90	12 months	12 months	6 months
2	60-89	12 months	12 months	6 months
3a	45-59	12 months	6 months	4 months
3b	30-44	6 months	4 months	4 months
4	15-29	4 months	4 months	2-3 months
5	<15	1-3 months	1-3 months	1-3 months

Blood tests to monitor: CBC, Na, K, Cl, bicarbonate, urea, creatinine, and eGFR. If DKD, add HbA1C. Fasting lipid profile at least yearly. At CKD category 3b or later: also add albumin, calcium, phosphorus, parathyroid hormone, serum iron, TIBC, and ferritin.

Urine tests to monitor: ACR (or PCR if indicated), standard urinalysis, and urine culture and sensitivity only if symptoms suggestive of urinary tract infection.

Data from reference 1.

Despite associations of development of left ventricular hypertrophy (LVH) with worsening anemia, there are no prospective studies demonstrating that early and aggressive treatment improves CV end points or reduces LVH in CKD patients. Improvements in quality of life have been observed with increases in Hb in select populations, but such improvements must be weighed against reported risks associated with using ESAs to achieve near-normal Hb levels in the CKD population.[79]

Target Hemoglobin and Use of Erythropoiesis Stimulating Agents

The target range for Hb in the CKD population has been a topic of much debate. Although the benefits of achieving a normal or near normal Hb seemed rationale when ESAs became available in the late 1980s, the Normal Hematocrit Cardiac Trial (NHCT),[80,81] the Correction of Hb and Outcomes in Renal Insufficiency (CHOIR),[82] and the Cardiovascular Risk Reduction by Early Anemia Treatment with Epoetin Beta (CREATE)[83] trials later proved otherwise, and the suggested target Hb at the time of those trials of 11 to 12 g/dL (110-120 g/L; 6.83-7.45 mmol/L) was subsequently lowered. Several FDA advisories were released and changes were made to the precautions, black box warning, and dosing sections of ESA product labeling promoting more conservative use of ESAs.[84] The current labeling for all ESAs warns that dosing ESAs to target Hb levels greater than 11 g/dL (110 g/L; 6.83 mmol/L) for CKD patients increases the risk for death, serious CV reactions, and stroke. Practitioners are advised to consider ESAs in patients with CKD only when the Hb is below 10 g/dL (100 g/L; 6.21 mmol/L) and to individualize therapy to use the lowest ESA dose necessary to decrease the need for red blood cell transfusions.

Of concern is the fact that CHOIR demonstrated that targeting Hb levels above 11 g/dL (110 g/L; 6.83 mmol/L) with ESA therapy in individuals with CKD not requiring dialysis resulted in increased risk of mortality and CV events compared with patients maintained in a lower Hb range (trial was terminated early).[82] CREATE demonstrated no benefit of targeting a higher Hb target (13-15 g/dL [130-150 g/L; 8.07-9.31 mmol/L]) to reduce CV events in the non-dialysis CKD patients.[83] An increased risk of all-cause mortality with ESA treatment was also reported in a meta-analysis of nine randomized controlled trials that included over 5,100 CKD patients treated to Hb targets in the range of 12 to 16 g/dL (120-160 g/L; 7.45-9.93 mmol/L).[85] There was also a higher risk of dialysis access thrombosis and uncontrolled blood pressure in the higher Hb groups. Results from the Trial to Reduce Cardiovascular Events with Aranesp Therapy (TREAT) also failed to support a higher Hb.[86] In addition, there was also an almost twofold increase in the risk of stroke (5% in the

TABLE 44-7 KDIGO Recommendations for Initiation of Erythropoiesis Stimulating Agents and Iron in Anemia of Chronic Kidney Disease[a]

	ND-CKD	CKD 5HD and CKD 5PD	Pediatric CKD
ESA initiation	If Hb <10 g/dL (<100 g/L; <6.21 mmol/L). Consider rate of fall of Hb, prior response to iron, risk of needing a transfusion, risk of ESA therapy, and presence of anemia symptoms before initiating an ESA. [2C] Do not initiate if Hb ≥10 g/dL (≥100 g/L; ≥6.21 mmol/L). [2D]	Use ESAs to avoid drop in Hb to <9 g/dL (<90 g/L; <5.59 mmol/L) by starting an ESA when Hb is between 9 and 10 g/dL (90 and 100 g/L; 5.59 and 6.21 mmol/L). [2B]	Selection of Hb concentration at which to initiate ESA therapy should include consideration of potential benefits (eg, improvement in QOL, school attendance, avoidance of blood transfusions) and potential harms. [2D]
Hb level	Do not use ESAs to *intentionally* increase Hb above 13 g/dL (130 g/L, 8.07 mmol/L). [1A] Do not use ESAs to maintain Hb above 11.5 g/dL (115 g/L; 7.14 mmol/L). [2C]	Do not use ESAs to *intentionally* increase Hb above 13 g/dL (130 g/L, 8.07 mmol/L). [1A] Do not use ESAs to maintain Hb above 11.5 g/dL (115 g/L; 7.14 mmol/L). [2C]	Suggest Hb range of 11-12 g/dL (110-120 g/L, 6.83-7.45 mmol/L). [2D]
Iron initiation[b]	If TSat is ≤30% (≤0.30) and ferritin is ≤500 ng/mL (mcg/L; ≤1,120 pmol/L). [2C]	If TSat is ≤30% (≤0.30) and ferritin is ≤500 ng/mL (mcg/L; ≤1,120 pmol/L). [2C]	If TSat is ≤20% (≤0.20) and ferritin is ≤100 ng/mL (mcg/L; ≤225 pmol/L). [1D]

CKD, chronic kidney disease; ESA, erythropoiesis stimulating agent; Hb, hemoglobin; ND-CKD, nondialysis CKD patients; QOL, quality of life; TSat, transferrin saturation.

See Table 44-5 for definitions of evidence grading in brackets.

[a]The Kidney Disease Outcome Quality Initiative (KDOQI) Anemia Guidelines are discussed in the text.

[b]If TSat and serum ferritin are below suggested levels, consider iron supplementation if goal is to increase Hb and/or decrease ESA dose. *Note*: Serum ferritin is an acute-phase reactant-use clinical judgment when above 500 ng/mL (mcg/L; 1120 pmol/L).

Data from reference 39.

treatment group vs 2.6% in the placebo group), a finding that was not associated with baseline characteristics of the patients or other potential risk factors.[87] Those patients with a history of cancer in the higher Hb group also had a higher risk of death, a finding that requires additional investigation.

The overall negative CV outcomes observed with higher Hb targets in the randomized trials have prompted much discussion about the potential causes, including not only ESA dose and Hb target, but also the rate of rise in Hb and the variability in Hb over time (eg, degree of fluctuation in Hb).[88] Subsequent analysis of the CHOIR study showed that high-dose ESA use was associated with greater risk of death.[89] Those individuals able to achieve the target Hb in the CHOIR study did not have worse outcomes. Further analysis of the NHCT data also showed a reduction in mortality by 60% for those individuals who responded to epoetin therapy compared with nonresponders.[90] Such findings have led to discussion of whether hyporesponsiveness to ESAs due to other conditions such as inflammation may explain the higher event rates in this group of individuals.

Clinical **Controversy...**

Recommendations in the product labeling for ESAs differ from KDIGO and KDOQI guidelines with regard to the "target" Hb. The KDIGO expert panel considered the quality of the evidence regarding target Hb to be *low* or *very* low (2C or 2D grade recommendations). Clinicians should always take into account trends in Hb when adjusting ESA doses. Before making treatment decisions, the risks of ESA use and targeting Hb values greater than 11 g/dL (110 g/L; 6.83 mmol/L) must be weighed against the benefit of fewer blood transfusions.

Nonpharmacologic Therapy

Nonpharmacologic therapy for anemia of CKD includes maintaining adequate dietary intake of iron as well as folate and B_{12}. A relatively small amount of dietary iron, approximately 1 to 2 mg, is absorbed each day, primarily in the duodenum (see Chapter 101). Although there is some debate as to whether GI absorption of iron is significantly altered in patients with severe CKD, it is clear that oral intake from dietary sources alone is insufficient to meet the increased iron requirements from initiation of ESA therapy.

Pharmacologic Therapy

8 Pharmacologic therapy for anemia of CKD includes iron supplementation to prevent and correct iron deficiency and ESA therapy to correct erythropoietin deficiency. Iron supplementation is first-line therapy for anemia of CKD if iron deficiency is present, and for some patients the target Hb may be achieved without concomitant ESA therapy. For most individuals with advanced CKD, however, combined therapy with iron and an ESA will be necessary to achieve the target Hb.

Iron Supplementation

Iron supplements provide the elemental iron required for production of Hb and its subsequent incorporation in red blood cells, the net result of which is an increase in the transportation of oxygen to tissues. Iron supplementation is required for *absolute iron deficiency*, but may also be warranted in individuals with a TSat less than 30% (<0.30) and a ferritin less than 500 ng/mL (mcg/L; <1120 pmol/L) in whom an increase in Hb or a decrease in ESA dose is desired.[39]

Therapeutic Options Multiple oral and IV products are marketed in the United States as well as a newly approved dialysate iron formulation. Oral iron preparations include ferrous salts (ferrous sulfate, ferrous fumarate, and ferrous gluconate), polysaccharide iron complex, and carbonyl iron. These forms of iron differ in terms of the amount of elemental iron: ferrous sulfate (20%), ferrous gluconate (12%), ferrous fumarate (33%), iron polysaccharide (100%), and carbonyl iron (100%). A heme iron polypeptide formulation is also available and contains 12 mg of elemental iron. Numerous nonprescription as well as prescription products that contain these iron formulations are available (see Table 100-2). Approximately 10% of orally administered iron is absorbed in the duodenum and upper jejunum. Absorption of iron is decreased by food and achlorhydria. Some oral iron formulations also include ascorbic acid to enhance iron absorption.

Soluble ferric pyrophosphate citrate (Triferic) was approved in the United States in January 2015.[90] This iron compound is designed to be added to the dialysate used for HD and crosses from the dialysate to the blood side of the dialyzer by diffusion to allow for continuous iron administration during the procedure. Once in the systemic circulation ferric pyrophosphate binds directly to transferrin, bypassing the reticuloendothelial system, and is delivered to the bone marrow for use in red blood cell production. Studies performed to date have shown an increase in Hb concentration and a reduction in ESA dose and IV iron requirements, but no significant increase in ferritin or in nontransferrin bound iron.[91,92] These findings are important when considering the potential adverse effects associated with iron accumulation and free (unbound) iron. The role of this agent in treating anemia of CKD is yet to be determined as this agent is introduced in the clinical setting.

IV iron preparations are colloids that consist of an iron-containing core that is surrounded by a carbohydrate shell to stabilize the iron complex. Available agents differ in the size of the core and the composition of the surrounding carbohydrate. Such differences affect the rate of dissociation of iron from the complex, the rate of distribution, and the maximum tolerated dose and rate of infusion. Six IV iron products are currently available in the United States. (Table 44-8).

Either oral or IV administration of iron is recommended in non-HD patients (eg, CKD category 3 or higher and PD patients). Oral iron supplementation is more convenient since these patients do not have regular IV access; however, at some point they are likely to require IV iron supplementation to correct absolute iron deficiency, especially if they are receiving an ESA. The route of administration should be based on the severity of iron deficiency, availability of IV access, response to prior oral iron therapy, side effects, patient adherence to therapy, and cost. If oral therapy is initiated a 1- to 3-month trial is recommended to assess response. In patients with CKD 5HD GI absorption of iron is often inadequate to meet the increase in iron demand from ESA therapy and chronic blood loss. Thus the IV route is preferred for almost all HD patients.[39,78] IV administration is also recommended in the PD population, although the desire to preserve potential future venous access sites for HD (if needed) must be considered. Parenteral iron improves the responsiveness to ESA therapy and, thus, lower doses can be used to maintain the target Hb in HD patients.[39] Iron administration in patients with functional iron deficiency (ie, low TSat, high serum ferritin) is questionable. A trial of IV iron therapy may be warranted if the Hb is less than desired despite high dose ESA therapy.

Adverse Effects Adverse effects of oral iron are primarily GI in nature and include constipation, nausea, and abdominal cramping (see Chapter 100). These adverse effects are more likely as the dose is escalated and may be present in more than 50% of patients receiving 200 mg of elemental iron per day. These unfavorable effects often discourage patients from taking these medications on a chronic basis. Some of these GI side effects can be minimized if oral iron products are taken with food; however, food may decrease absorption of oral iron.

TABLE 44-8 IV Iron Preparations

Iron Compounds	Brand Names	Half-Life (Hours)	Molecular Weight (Daltons)	FDA-Approved Indications	FDA-Approved Dosing[a]	Dose Ranges (mg)[b]
Ferric carboxymaltose	Injectafer	7-12	150,000	Adult patients with intolerance to oral iron or who have had an unsatisfactory response to oral iron and in adult patients with CKD not on dialysis	Give 2 doses separated by at least 7 days of 750 mg per dose (if body weight is ≥50 kg) or 15 mg/kg per dose (if body weight is <50 kg) not to exceed 1,500 mg per course. Give either IV push (100 mg per min) or diluted in not more than 250 mL of 0.9 NaCl as an infusion over at least 15 minutes	750
Ferumoxytol	Feraheme	15	750,000	Adult patients with iron-deficiency anemia associated with chronic kidney disease	510 mg (17 mL) as a single dose, followed by a second 510 mg dose 3-8 days after the initial dose. Dilute in 50-200 mL of 0.9% NaCl or 5% dextrose and administer as an IV infusion over 15 minutes	510
Iron dextran	INFeD Dexferrum	40-60	96,000 265,000	Patients with iron deficiency in whom oral iron is unsatisfactory or impossible	100 mg over 2 minutes (25-mg test dose required) Note: Equation provided by manufacturer to calculate dose based on desired Hb	25-1,000
Iron sucrose	Venofer	6	43,000	Adult and pediatric CKD 5HD patients aged 2 years and older	Adult: 100 mg over 2-5 minutes or 100 mg in maximum of 100 mL of 0.9% NaCl over 15 minutes per consecutive HD session Pediatric: 0.5 mg/kg not to exceed 100 mg per dose over 5 minutes or diluted in 25 mL of 0.9% NaCl administered over 5-60 minutes (give dose every 2 weeks for 12 weeks)	25-1,000
				Adult and pediatric ND-CKD patients aged 2 years and older	Adult: 200 mg over 2–5 minutes on five different occasions within 14-day period. There is limited experience with administration of 500 mg diluted in a maximum of 250 mL of 0.9% NaCl over 3.5 to 4 hours on day 1 and day 14 Pediatric: see pediatric dosing for CKD 5HD (give dose every 4 weeks for 12 weeks)	
				Adult and pediatric CKD 5PD patients aged 2 years and older	Adult: Give 3 divided doses within 28 days as 2 infusions of 300 mg over 1.5 hours 14 days apart followed by one 400 mg infusion over 2.5 hours 14 days later. Dilute in a maximum of 250 mL of 0.9% NaCl Pediatric: see pediatric dosing for CKD 5HD (give dose every 4 weeks for 12 weeks)	
Sodium ferric gluconate	Ferrlecit	1	350,000	Adult and pediatric CKD 5HD patients aged 6 years and older receiving ESA therapy	Adult: 125 mg over 10 minutes or 125 mg in 100 mL of 0.9% NaCl over 60 minutes Pediatric: 1.5 mg/kg in 25 mL of 0.9% NaCl over 60 minutes; maximum dose 125 mg per dose	62.5-1,000

CKD, chronic kidney disease; ESA, erythropoiesis stimulating agent; ND-CKD, non-dialysis CKD patients.

[a]Monitor for 30 minutes following an infusion; KDIGO guidelines recommend monitoring for 60 minutes (1B recommendation for iron dextran, 2C recommendation for non-dextran products).

[b]With the exception of ferric carboxymaltose and ferumoxytol, small doses (eg, 25-150 mg/wk) are generally used for maintenance regimens. Larger doses (eg, 1 g) should be administered in divided doses.

Adverse effects of IV iron include allergic reactions, hypotension, dizziness, dyspnea, headaches, lower back pain, arthralgia, syncope, and arthritis. Some of these reactions, in particular hypotension, can be minimized by decreasing the dose or rate of infusion of iron. The most concerning potential consequence of IV iron administration is anaphylaxis. Serious reactions to iron dextran including respiratory complications and CV collapse have been reported in approximately 0.6% to 0.7% of patients.[39] Such reactions are believed to be partly a response to antibody formation to the dextran component. Adverse reactions have been reported more frequently in those receiving Dexferrum compared with INFeD and it should be noted that these iron dextrans products are not interchangeable.[39] Iron dextran products carry a black box warning of the risk of anaphylactic-type reactions, including fatalities, and a 25-mg test dose is required. A recent analysis of anaphylaxis risk in patients newly exposed to IV iron products (including dextran, gluconate, sucrose, or ferumoxytol) reported the highest risk for iron dextran with the lowest risk with iron sucrose.[93]

The non-dextran IV iron formulations have a better safety record than either of the iron dextran products. The labeling for these formulations also includes a warning of the risk of hypersensitivity reactions. Since the approval of ferumoxytol in 2009, there have been 79 cases of anaphylactic reactions, of which 18 were fatal.[94] Almost half of the cases occurred with the first dose and approximately 75% occurred during the infusion or within 5 minutes of completion. In July 2014, a warning was issued by Health Canada that ferumoxytol should not be used in patients allergic to other iron products given by injection or infusion, or in patents with multiple drug allergies. In November 2014, the Canadian product monograph for ferumoyxtol was also changed to indicate that this agent only be administered as an IV infusion over a minimum of 15 minutes and that administration by direct IV injection of the undiluted product is no longer recommended. In March 2015, the FDA required a black box warning for ferumoxytol stating that "fatal and serious hypersensitivity reactions including anaphylaxis have occurred" in patients receiving this agent.[95] It is also recommended that ferumoxytol not be administered IV push (as previously recommended), but should be diluted and administered as an IV infusion (see Table 44-8), and that the risks and benefits should be considered in patients with a history of multiple drug allergies. As a superparamagnetic oxide, ferumoxytol may alter the diagnostic ability of magnetic resonance imaging studies for up to 3 months after administration; therefore, they should be done prior to administration of ferumoxytol whenever possible.[95]

Long-term administration of IV iron also introduces a risk of iron overload. Deposition of excess iron may affect several organ systems, leading to hepatic, pancreatic, and cardiac dysfunction. Bone marrow biopsy provides the most definitive diagnosis of iron overload, but because it is an extremely invasive procedure, it is not widely employed in most clinical settings. Maintaining target serum ferritin and TSat values is the most reasonable approach to minimize the risk of iron toxicity. The challenge is in defining what should be the upper limit, particularly for serum ferritin, which may be elevated in inflammatory conditions and not reflective of true iron stores in such situations. If symptomatic overload does occur, iron chelating agents such as deferoxamine (Desferal), deferiprone (Ferriprox), deferasirox (Exjade), or phlebotomy may be necessary.[96]

Safety concerns and recent labeling changes for ESAs have led to increased use of IV iron in HD patients to maintain target Hb, TSat, and ferritin values while minimizing ESA use.[97] Furthermore, the bundled payment system adopted by the US Centers for Medicare and Medicaid Services (CMS) has contributed to higher IV iron use. This increase in iron utilization resulted in an upward shift in mean ferritin levels, from approximately 600 ng/mL (mcg/L; 1,350 pmol/L) in 2007 to 800 ng/mL (mcg/L; 1,800 pmol/L) in 2013.[97] The potential detrimental effect of increased iron exposure on patient outcomes is of concern even though there are no data confirming unequivocally that aggressive use of IV iron in CKD patients treated with ESA therapy increases patient morbidity or mortality.[98-102] Data from an observational study to assess the association between cumulative IV iron dose in a given time frame and mortality in 14,000 HD patients indicated that administration of cumulative IV iron doses below 1,050 mg or 2,100 mg within a relatively short time period (3-6 months) were not associated with a significant increase in all-cause, CV, or infection-related mortality.[98] Some studies found that IV iron contributed to infection,[99,100] whereas others refuted this assertion although they did indicate a link to increased oxidative stress.[101,102]

Clinical **Controversy...**

Although there are conflicting reports, some clinicians believe that exposure to iron may contribute to the risk of bacterial infection because iron is used by microorganisms for metabolic functions. KDIGO guidelines suggest that IV iron be avoided in patients with active systemic infections.[39] Healthcare providers should be aware of this controversy when deciding whether to initiate IV iron in patients with active infection.

Drug Interactions Drug interactions with oral iron are common. Iron absorption is decreased by other elements (eg, calcium in calcium-containing phosphate binders), medications that increase the pH of the GI tract such as proton pump inhibitors and H_2-antagonists, and antibiotics including doxycycline and tetracycline. Iron also decreases absorption of other drugs such as antibiotics (fluoroquinolones, doxycycline) (see Chapter 100).

Dosing and Administration If oral therapy is initiated, the recommended dose is 200 mg of elemental iron per day. With numerous oral agents to choose from, the best option is one that provides adequate elemental iron with the fewest number of dosage units required per day and the lowest incidence of adverse effects. KDIGO guidelines suggest a 1- to 3-month trial of oral therapy in the non-HD CKD population prior to initiating IV therapy.[39] For the HD population, IV therapy is preferred with administration of a 1-g course of IV iron (in divided doses) recommended to initially replete patients with an absolute iron deficiency. The amount per dose and rate at which to administer IV iron depends on the product (see Table 44-8). Typical repletion dosing regimens for IV iron are 100 mg as iron sucrose over 10 dialysis sessions or 125 mg of sodium ferric gluconate over 8 dialysis sessions. The 1-g course of IV iron may be repeated as needed with close monitoring of Hb and iron indices. Iron indices should not be measured within 1 week of receiving an IV iron dose. Without ongoing iron supplementation, many patients quickly become iron-deficient. To prevent iron deficiency, maintenance doses of IV iron can be administered in HD patients (eg, iron sucrose 25-100 mg/wk; sodium ferric gluconate 62.5-125 mg/wk).[39,78] As a general practice, if IV iron doses higher than those currently approved are needed, they should be infused over a longer period of time (eg, at least 2-4 hours) due to the risk of hypersensitivity reactions, hypotension, dizziness, and nausea. The newer agents, ferumoxytol and ferric carboxymaltose, differ in terms of how rapidly iron is released from the compound, which allows for higher single doses to be administered.

Administration of a 25-mg test dose is required for all iron dextran products. This test dose should be administered over at least 30 seconds for InFeD and 5 minutes for Dexferrum. It is recommended that patients be observed for at least 1 hour before administering the remainder of the dose. For this reason the non-dextran agents are more commonly used in the CKD population. Regardless of which IV iron agent is used all patients should be monitored for signs and symptoms of hypersensitivity for at least 30 minutes following completion of a dose. KDIGO clinical practice guidelines suggest monitoring patients for at least 60 minutes following administration of IV iron; a 1B recommendation for iron dextran products and a 2C recommendation for non-dextran forumulations.[39] These agents should only be administered when personnel and therapies are immediately available for the treatment of anaphylaxis and other hypersensitivity reactions.

Erythropoiesis-Stimulating Agent Therapy

Since FDA approval of epoetin alfa in 1989, ESA therapy has become an integral part of the care for patients with CKD. ESAs available

TABLE 44-9 Erythropoiesis-Stimulating Agents in Chronic Kidney Disease

Drug Name	Brand Name(s)	Starting Dose	Route of Administration	Half-Life (Hours)
Epoetin alfa	Epogen, Procrit	Adults: 50-100 units/kg three times per week Pediatrics: 50 units/kg three times per week	IV or SubQ	8.5 (IV) 24 (SubQ)
Darbepoetin alfa	Aranesp	Adults: ND-CKD: 0.45 mcg/kg once every 4 weeks CKD 5HD or CKD 5PD: 0.45 mcg/kg once per week or 0.75 mcg/kg every 2 weeks Pediatrics: 0.45 mcg/kg once weekly; may give 0.75 mcg/kg once every 2 weeks in ND-CKD patients	IV or SubQ	25 (IV) 48 (SubQ)
Methoxy PEG-epoetin beta	Mircera	All adult CKD patients: 0.6 mcg/kg every 2 weeks; Once Hb stabilizes, double the dose and administer monthly (eg, if administering 0.6 mcg/kg every 2 weeks, give 1.2 mcg/kg every month)	IV or SubQ	134 (IV) 139 (SubQ)

CKD, chronic kidney disease; ND-CKD, non-dialysis CKD patients; PEG, Polyethylene glycol; SubQ, subcutaneous.

in the United States are listed in Table 44-9. Methoxy polyethylene glycol (PEG)-epoetin beta was approved for treatment of anemia in CKD patients (including dialysis patients) in 2007. It was not marketed in the United States, however, until recently due to an injunction for patent infringement. It has been used in Europe since its approval in 2007.

Biosimilar ESAs are also expected in the US market in the near future. Biosimilars are nonbrand name products that are essentially replicas of the biologic drug. Biosimilar epoetin became available in Europe in 2007 after the expiration of patent protection for epoetin alfa in 2004.[103] The approval of biosimilars in the United States is expected since the patent for recombinant human erythropoietin expired in 2014.

Pharmacology and Mechanism of Action Epoetin alfa is a glycoprotein manufactured by recombinant DNA technology that has the same amino acid sequence as endogenous erythropoietin. Darbepoetin alfa has two additional *N*-linked carbohydrate chains that decrease the affinity for the erythropoietin receptor, but yield a longer duration of activity compared with erythropoietin. Methoxy PEG-epoetin beta was created by the addition of an amide bond between the N-terminal or ε-amino group of epoetin beta and methoxy polyethylene glycol butanoic acid. The compound, which is referred to as a continuous erythropoietin receptor activator (CERA), has a much longer half-life than the other ESAs. All ESAs have the same biologic activity as endogenous erythropoietin in that they bind to and activate the erythropoietin receptor to stimulate erythropoiesis.

Pharmacokinetics and Pharmacodynamics All available ESAs may be administered by either the IV or the subcutaneous (SubQ) route. Although bioavailability is less with SubQ than with IV administration, the prolonged absorption phase leads to an extended half-life (see Table 44-9). Thus the same target Hb can be achieved and maintained at SubQ epoetin doses 15% to 30% lower than IV doses.[39] The prolonged half-lives of darbepoetin alfa and methoxy PEG-epoetin beta offer the advantage of less-frequent dosing. This is of particular benefit for individuals with CKD who are not yet receiving dialysis and those receiving PD since these patients are not in a clinical setting as frequently as HD patients and do not have regular IV access.

The pharmacodynamic effect of ESAs is important to consider when evaluating response to therapy. With initiation of ESA therapy or a change in dose, the Hb may begin to rise as the result of demargination of reticulocytes; however, it takes approximately 10 days before erythrocyte progenitor cells mature and are released into the circulation. The Hb continues to increase until the life span of the cells stimulated by ESA therapy is reached (mean 2 months; range 1-4 months in patients with ESRD). At this point a new steady state is achieved (ie, the rate at which red blood cells are being produced equals the rate at which they are leaving the circulation). For this reason it is important to evaluate the Hb response over several weeks and not make dosing changes too soon.

Efficacy Patients will generally respond to ESA therapy in a dose-related fashion. The most common causes of resistance are iron deficiency, acute illness, inflammation, infection, chronic bleeding, aluminum toxicity, malnutrition, hyperparathyroidism, cancer, and chemotherapy.[39] Deficiencies in folate and vitamin B_{12} should also be considered as potential causes of resistance to ESA therapy, as both are essential for optimal erythropoiesis. Use of ACEIs and ARBs has also been associated with hyporesponsiveness to ESA therapy.[39]

Adverse Effects Hypertension is the most common adverse event reported with ESAs and may be associated with the rate of rise in Hb.[39] Hypertensive encephalopathy has also been observed. According to FDA-approved product labeling, ESAs should not be used in those with uncontrolled blood pressure. Protocols established in some clinical settings recommend withholding ESA therapy if blood pressure is above a defined threshold; however, others advocate more judicious use of antihypertensive agents and dialysis to control blood pressure. Seizures have occurred in patients treated with ESAs, particularly within the first 90 days of starting therapy. Thrombosis of the HD vascular access site and other thromboembolic events were reported when ESAs were used to target Hb greater than 13 g/dL (130 g/L; 8.07 mmol/L).[104-106] The potential for these adverse effects calls for close monitoring of the rate of rise in Hb, changes in blood pressure, and neurologic symptoms following initiation of therapy or a change in ESA dose.

Antibody-associated pure red cell aplasia (PRCA), caused by induction of antibodies directed against the ESA molecule, was reported in the late 1990s and early in 2000 and was primarily associated with subcutaneous administration of Eprex, an epoetin alfa formulation manufactured outside the United States.[107] This reaction was potentially a result of organic compounds being formed when the stabilizing agent polysorbate was used in combination with uncoated rubber stoppers in the prefilled syringes. There have been very few cases since changes in the packaging of this product were made; however, the cause of PRCA with this formulation has been disputed.[108] Of note, there have been reports of PRCA with methoxy PEG-epoetin beta.[104] This is important to consider since this agent has only recently been introduced to the US market. An evaluation for PRCA should be considered for patients receiving ESA therapy for more than 8 weeks who develop either a rapid decrease in Hb level (rate of 0.5-1 g/dL/wk [5-10 g/L/wk; 0.31-0.62 mmol/L/wk]) or require one to two blood transfusions per week, and have an absolute reticulocyte count of less than 10,000/μL (10×10^9/L) with a normal platelet and white blood cell count.[39] Discontinuation of ESA therapy is recommended if antibody-mediated PRCA develops because antibodies are cross-reactive and continued exposure may lead to anaphylactic reactions (a grade 1A recommendation).

ESAs have also been associated with a reduction in overall survival and increased risk of progression of certain tumor types among CKD patients (eg, head and neck). ESAs are not indicated in patients receiving myelosuppressive chemotherapy when the anticipated outcome is cure. These are important effects to consider when managing a CKD patients with an oncologic disorder.[109]

In 2010, the FDA required all ESAs to be prescribed and used under a risk management program, known as a risk evaluation and mitigation strategy (REMS). As part of the REMS, a Medication Guide explaining the risks and benefits of ESAs must be provided to all patients receiving ESAs.

Drug–Drug Interactions No significant drug interactions have been reported with the available ESAs.

Dosing and Administration Recommended starting doses of ESA are listed in Table 44-9. Less frequent dosing of epoetin alfa (eg, every 1-2 weeks) is effective and may be preferred for ND-CKD patients since these individuals are seen in the outpatient clinical setting on a relatively infrequent basis.[111] Subcutaneous dosing is also more convenient in this population and in PD patients who do not have regular IV access. Conversion tables for patients who are to be switched from epoetin alfa (units per week) to darbepoetin alfa (micrograms per week) are available in the labeling information for darbepoetin.[106] There is also a conversion chart for patients being converted from epoetin alfa or darbepoetin alfa to methoxy PEG-epoetin beta.[104]

When starting an ESA, Hb levels should be monitored at least monthly (weekly may be preferred) until stable and then monthly thereafter. Dose adjustments should be made based on Hb response with a goal of avoiding an excessively quick rise or the achievement of values above the recommend target values. An acceptable rate of increase in Hb is 1 to 2 g/dL (10-20 g/L; 0.62-1.24 mmol/L) per month. As a general rule, ESA doses should not be increased more frequently than every 4 weeks, although decreases in dose may occur more frequently in response to a rapid rate of rise in Hb. The dose should be reduced by at least 25% if the Hb increases by more than 1 g/dL (10 g/L; 0.62 mmol/L) in a 2-week period.[104-106] The dose should be reduced or temporarily discontinued if the Hb level approaches or exceeds 11 g/dL (110 g/L; 6.83 mmol/L) in dialysis patients or 10 g/dL (100 g/L; 6.21 mmol/L) in patients with CKD not requiring dialysis. KDIGO recommendations advocate a decrease in dose as opposed to withholding the ESA when a decrease in Hb concentration is desired (2C grade recommendatio)[39] A 25% increase in dose may be considered if the Hb has not increased by 1 g/dL (10 g/L; 0.62 mmol/L) after 4 weeks of ESA treatment and if no causes of hyporesponsiveness to the ESA have been identified. For patients who do not respond adequately over a 12-week escalation period, an increase in ESA dose is unlikely to improve response and may increase risks. Initial hyporesponsiveness to ESAs should be considered when there is no increase in Hb from baseline after the first month of appropriate weight-based dosing. In this situation escalations in ESA dose beyond double the initial weight-based dose should be avoided (a grade 2D recommendation). Acquired ESA hyporesponsiveness may be suspected when patients previously on a stable ESA dose require two increases in ESA doses up to 50% beyond the previously utilized stable dose.[39] In this situation repeat escalations in ESA dose beyond double the dose at which they had been stable should be avoided (a grade 2D recommendation). The lowest dose of ESA should be used to maintain an Hb level sufficient to reduce the need for red blood cell transfusions. Figure 44-6 provides an approach to management of anemia using ESAs and iron therapy in patients with CKD.

Transfusions and Adjunct Therapies

Red blood cell transfusions carry many risks and therefore should only be used in select situations, such as acute management of symptomatic anemia, following significant acute blood loss, and prior to surgical procedures that carry a high risk of blood loss, with the goal of preventing inadequate tissue oxygenation or cardiac failure. L-carnitine supplementation and vitamin C were previously suggested as adjunctive treatments of CKD anemia, but are not recommended because of the lack of evidence supporting improved anemia management with these therapies.[39]

Evaluation of Therapeutic Outcomes

Important therapeutic outcomes to monitor in patients with anemia of CKD include Hb, iron status, as well as the need for blood transfusions. Iron status should be assessed at least every 3 months in patients receiving a stable ESA regimen.[39] Iron status should be monitored more frequently (eg, every month) when initiating or increasing the ESA dose, following a course of IV iron, or when other factors put the patient at risk for iron loss (eg, bleeding). Hb levels should be monitored at least every 3 months in patients with CKD not on dialysis or CKD 5PD and at least monthly in CKD 5HD patients.[39] Hb should be monitored at least monthly in patients started on ESA therapy until the Hb is stable. Of note, FDA labelling for ESAs recommends weekly monitoring of Hb with initiation of therapy or a change in dose until the Hb is stable.[104-106]

Chronic Kidney Disease-Related Mineral and Bone Disorder

Management of PTH, phosphorus, and calcium is important in preventing CKD-MBD and CV and extravascular calcifications. Patients with CKD-MBD usually require a combination of dietary intervention, phosphate-binding medications, vitamin D, and calcimimetic therapy (for ESRD patients) to achieve these goals.

Desired Outcome

9 The desired outcomes for management of CKD-MBD are to "normalize" the biochemical parameters and prevent bone manifestations, CV and extravascular calcifications, and the associated morbidity and mortality with both nonpharmacologic and pharmacologic interventions. At present there are two guidance documents—KDOQI and KDIGO—that clinicians can use in their patient care decision-making process.[42,111] It should be noted that many of the recommendations in both documents are based on opinion or limited evidence given the lack of randomized controlled studies to evaluate treatment outcomes. The 2009 KDIGO clinical practice guidelines for CKD-MBD will be emphasized in this chapter with some comparisons made to KDOQI.

The KDIGO-recommended targets for calcium, phosphorus, and PTH and frequency of monitoring based on the CKD category are shown in Table 44-10. There are minor differences between KDIGO and KDOQI and with regard to recommendations for serum calcium (corrected for serum albumin): KDOQI recommends a more conservative calcium range (8.4-9.5 mg/dL, [2.10-2.38 mmol/L]) in ESRD patients based on an increased risk of soft-tissue and vascular calcifications.[111] The most appropriate strategy is to evaluate trends in corrected calcium to predict if hypercalcemia is a concern that warrants changes in therapy. The adoption

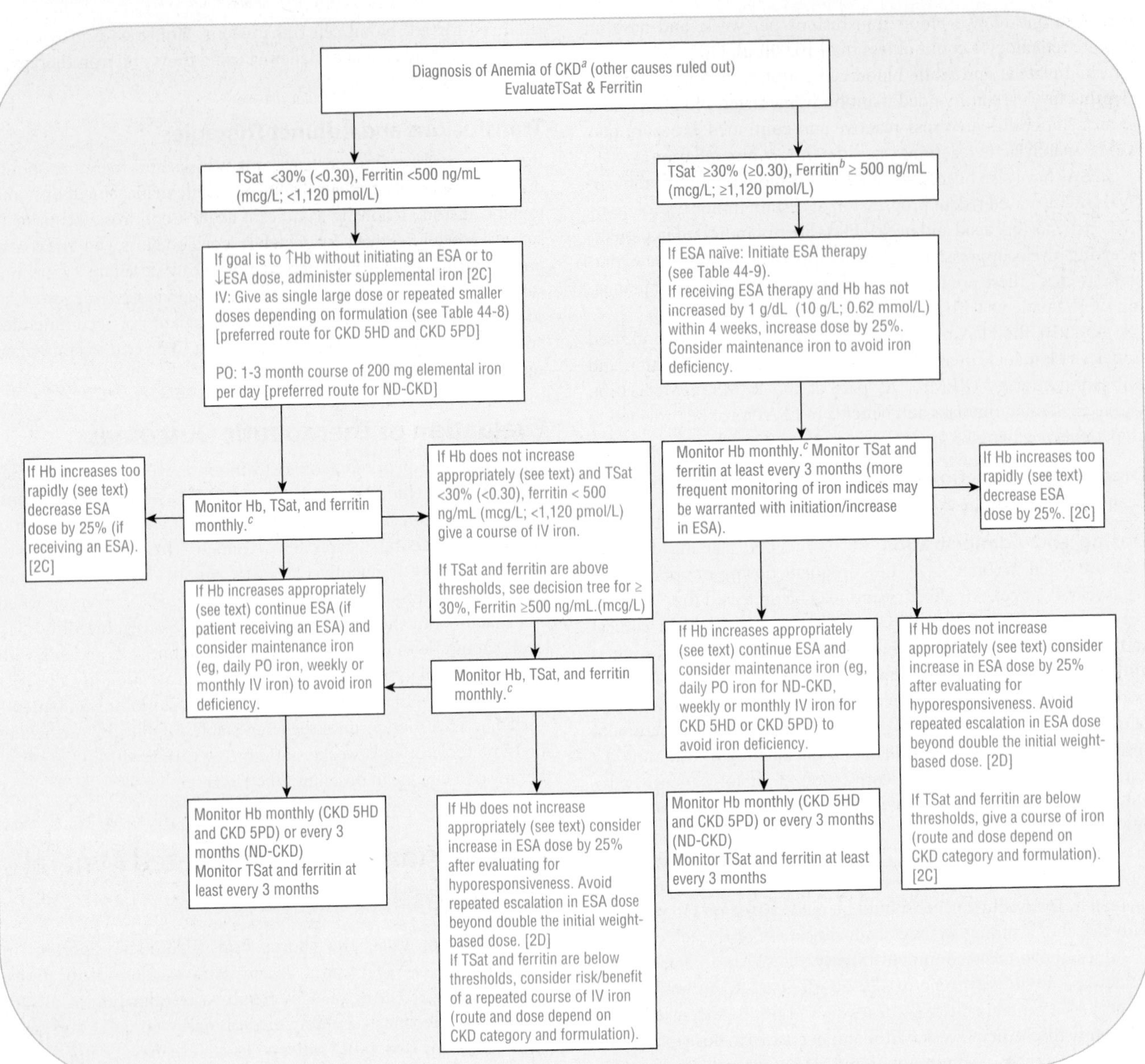

FIGURE 44-6 Algorithm for management of anemia of CKD in adults.[39,105] (CKD, chronic kidney disease; ESA, erythropoiesis-stimulating agent; Hb, hemoglobin; ND-CKD, non-dialysis CKD patients; TSat, transferrin saturation.) See Table 44-5 for definitions of evidence grading in brackets. [a]See Table 44-7 and text for discussion of Hb levels. [b]Clinical judgement should be used to determine if iron supplementation should be continued when ferritin >500 ng/mL (mcg/L; >1,120 pmol/L). [c]Weekly monitoring of Hb may be warranted. Wait at least 1 week after an IV dose of iron to measure TSat and ferritin.

by CMS of an *uncorrected* calcium value greater than 10.2 mg/dL (>2.55 mmol/L) as a quality measure starting in 2016 may influence patient care decisions and thereby reduce the prevalence of elevated calcium values.[112] Monitoring of alkaline phosphatase activity is also recommended in patients with CKD 4, 5, and ESRD as this test may serve as a gauge of a patient's response to therapy and/or bone turnover status. Avoiding the development of calciphylaxis is also important as treatment options for this complication once it develops are extremely limited.

Evaluation of Parathyroid Hormone

Clinicians involved in the care of patients with CKD should know which PTH assays are available in their facilities. PTH is secreted from the parathyroid gland as intact PTH, an 84-amino-acid peptide chain (1-84 PTH) that is biologically active, and as smaller carboxy-terminal PTH fragments.[113] Circulating levels of these fragments (eg, 7-84 PTH) may increase substantially in patients with CKD and actively antagonize the effects of 1 to 84 PTH. The available immunoradiometric assays measure not only the intact PTH molecule but also fragments, which may lead to overestimation of biologically active PTH. While correction factors have been proposed, they cannot be uniformly applied to all commercially available assays and thus inconsistent results are common. Because of the variability in PTH measurement and lack of evidence to support a specific target, it is not surprising that KDOQI and KDIGO both recommend monitoring trends in serum PTH to guide treatment decisions but have established different target ranges. KDIGO recommends that PTH values for ESRD patients be within two to nine times the upper limit of the normal range, which corresponds to a PTH of approximately 130 to 600 pg/mL [ng/L; 14-64 pmol/L]).[42] PTH values above 600 pg/mL (ng/L; 64 pmol/L) have been associated with higher CV mortality and hospitalizations.[114] In contrast, KDOQI recommends that PTH values should be between 150 and 300 pg/mL (ng/L; 16-32 pmol/L).[111]

TABLE 44-10 KDIGO Monitoring and Goals for Calcium, Phosphorus, and Parathyroid Hormone

	Chronic Kidney Disease Category[a]			
Parameter	**3**	**4**	**5**	**ESRD**
Corrected calcium[b]				
Monitoring frequency[c]	Every 6-12 months	Every 3-6 months	Every 1-3 months	Every 1-3 months
Goal	Maintain normal range [2D]	Maintain normal range [2D]	Maintain normal range [2D]	Maintain normal range [2D]
Phosphorus				
Monitoring frequency[c]	Every 6-12 months	Every 3-6 months	Every 1-3 months	Every 1-3 months
Goal	Maintain normal range [2C]	Maintain normal range [2C]	Maintain normal range [2C]	"Towards normal" [2C]
Intact PTH				
Monitoring frequency[c]	Based on baseline level and CKD progression	Every 6-12 months	Every 3-6 months	Every 3-6 months
Goal	Normal range[c]	Normal range[c]	Normal range[c]	2-9 times the upper normal limit [2C]

CMS, Centers for Medicare and Medicaid Services; QIP, Quality Incentive Program.

See Table 44-5 for definitions of evidence grading in brackets.

[a]Differences with Kidney Disease Outcome Quality Initiative (KDOQI) guidelines described in text.

[b]Corrected for albumin. Note: CMS finalized a rule that will use an uncorrected calcium level >10.2 mg/dL (>2.55 mmol/L) as a quality measure for the QIP starting in 2016.

[c]Not graded.

Data from reference 42.

Nonpharmacologic Therapy

Dietary Phosphorus Restriction

Dietary phosphorus restriction is a first-line intervention for management of hyperphosphatemia and should be initiated for most patients with CKD 3-5.[42,111,115] The KDOQI guidelines recommend phosphorus restriction to 800 to 1,000 mg/day when the upper levels of serum phosphorus are reached (opinion-based recommendation in CKD 3-5, evidence-based recommendation in ESRD).[111] This recommendation also applies to patients with PTH levels above the recommended range given the evidence that lowering phosphorus ingestion directly decreases PTH synthesis and secretion.[116] The challenge with dietary restriction of phosphorus is providing enough protein to prevent malnutrition, a common problem in the ESRD population because dialysis patients require a higher protein intake (1.2-1.3 g/kg/day) and foods high in phosphorus are generally high in protein. An additional consideration is the source of phosphorus, organic versus inorganic. Inorganic sources such as from frozen meals and processed foods include preservatives or additives used during food processing, whereas organic sources such as from meat and plant sources typically do not and may be a better option. One of the most common obstacles to dietary phosphorus restriction is patient nonadherence because of the poor palatability of the allowed foods. Regular counseling by a dietitian is necessary to design a realistic diet that works with the patient's lifestyle and considers nutritional goals.

Dialysis

HD and PD lower serum phosphorus and calcium, the extent of which is dependent on the concentration of each in the dialysate and the duration of dialysis. It is recommended that the dialysate calcium concentration be between 2.5 and 3 mEq/L (1.25 and 1.5 mmol/L) (a grade 2D recommendation).[42,110] Removal of phosphorus does occur with dialysis (approximately 2.5-3.5 g/wk, dependent on the dialysis prescription); however, dialysis alone does not usually control hyperphosphatemia.[117] Patients on daily HD or nocturnal HD who typically have longer and/or more frequent dialysis sessions may have better phosphorus control and require fewer phosphate-binding agents.

Parathyroidectomy

Parathyroidectomy is a therapeutic option for those patients with persistently elevated PTH associated with hypercalcemia and/or hyperphosphatemia who are refractory to medical therapy (a grade 2B recommendation).[42] KDOQI suggests considering a parathyroidectomy when the PTH level is persistently above (PTH >800 pg/mL [ng/L; >86 pmol/L], an opinion-based recommendation.[111] Surgical approaches include either subtotal parathyroidectomy or total parathyroidectomy with autotransplantation of parathyroid tissue to an accessible site, such as the forearm. Postoperative hypocalcemia, hypophosphatemia, and hypomagnesemia may occur because of a marked increase in bone production in relation to bone absorption ("hungry bone syndrome"). Following surgery frequent monitoring of calcium and phosphorus is necessary. Treatment with supplemental calcium and vitamin D may be required for weeks or months.

While a parathyroidectomy is indicated for refractory patients, these patients may experience significant morbidity following the procedure. In a study of over 4,400 ESRD patients who underwent a parathyroidectomy from 2007 to 2009, there was an increase in hospitalizations (particularly for acute myocardial infarction and dysrhythmia) and emergency room visits for treatment of hypocalcemia in the year following the procedure.[118] For some patients a parathyroidectomy may be ineffective and there is also the risk of oversuppression of PTH and prolonged hypocalcemia.[119]

Pharmacologic Therapy

Patients with CKD-MBD usually require a combination of dietary intervention, phosphate-binding medications, vitamin D, and calcimimetic therapy (for ESRD patients) to achieve goals.

Phosphate-Binding Agents

Patients with CKD, especially those with ESRD, typically require phosphate-binding agents in addition to dietary interventions to limit GI absorption and thereby control serum phosphorus. For many patients the pill burden with phosphate-binding agents affects nonadherence and efforts should be made to simplify their regimen when possible.

Pharmacology and Mechanism of Action Drugs that bind dietary phosphorous in the GI tract form insoluble phosphate compounds that are excreted in feces, thus reducing dietary phosphorus absorption. A variety of phosphate-binding agents are available including elemental calcium, iron, and lanthanum-containing compounds, and the nonelemental agent sevelamer (Table 44-11). Binding affinity varies depending on the binding agent (eg, calcium, iron, etc). Patients must be instructed to take these agents with meals to maximize the binding of phosphorus from dietary sources.

TABLE 44-11 Phosphate-Binding Agents for Treatment of Hyperphosphatemia in Chronic Kidney Disease Patients

Category	Drug	Brand Name	Compound Content	Starting Doses	Dose Titration[a]	Comments[b]
Calcium-based binders	Calcium acetate (25% elemental calcium)	PhosLo	25% elemental calcium (169 mg elemental calcium per 667 mg capsule)	1,334 mg three times a day with meals	Increase or decrease by 667 mg per meal (169 mg elemental calcium)	Comparable efficacy to calcium carbonate with lower dose of elemental calcium Approximately 45 mg phosphorus bound per 1 g calcium acetate Evaluate for drug interactions with calcium
		Phoslyra	667 mg calcium acetate per 5 mL			
	Calcium carbonate[c]	Tums, Os-Cal, Caltrate	40% elemental calcium	0.5-1 g (elemental calcium) three times a day with meals	Increase or decrease by 500 mg per meal (200 mg elemental calcium)	Dissolution characteristics and phosphate binding may vary from product to product Approximately 39 mg phosphorus bound per 1 g calcium carbonate Evaluate for drug interactions with calcium
Iron-based binders	Ferric citrate	Auryxia	210 mg tablets (= 1 g ferric citrate)	420 mg ferric iron three times daily with meals	Increase or decrease dose by 1 or 2 tablets per meal	May increase serum iron, ferritin, and TSat May cause discolored (dark) stools Evaluate for drug interactions with iron
	Sucroferric oxyhydroxide	Velphoro	500 mg chewable tablets	500 mg three times daily with meals	Increase or decrease by 500 mg per day	May cause discolored (dark) stools Evaluate for drug interactions with iron
Resin binders	Sevelamer carbonate	Renvela	800 mg tablet 0.8 and 2.4 g powder for oral suspension	800-1,600 mg three times a day with meals (once-daily dosing also effective)	Increase or decrease by 800 mg per meal	Also lowers low-density lipoprotein cholesterol Consider in patients at risk for extraskeletal calcification Risk of metabolic acidosis with sevelamer hydrochloride (less risk with carbonate formulation) May interact with cipro and mycophenolate mofetil
	Sevelamer hydrochloride	Renagel	400 & 800 mg caplets	800-1,600 mg three times a day with meals	Increase or decrease by 800 mg per meal	
Other elemental binders	Lanthanum carbonate	Fosrenol	500, 750, and 1,000 mg chewable tablets 750 and 1,000 mg oral powder	1,500 mg daily in divided doses with meals	Increase or decrease by 750 mg/day	Potential for accumulation of lanthanum due to GI absorption (long-term consequences unknown) Evaluate for drug interactions (eg, cationic antacids, quinolone antibiotics)
	Aluminum hydroxide	AlternaGel	Content varies (range 100-600 mg/unit)	300-600 mg three times a day with meals	Not for long-term use requiring titration	Not a first-line agent; risk of aluminum toxicity; do not use concurrently with citrate-containing products Reserve for short-term use (4 weeks) in patients with hyperphosphatemia not responding to other binders Evaluate for drug interactions

TSat, transferrin saturation.

[a]Based on phosphorus levels, titrate every 2 to 3 weeks until phosphorus goal reached.

[b]GI side effects are possible with all agents (eg, nausea, vomiting, abdominal pain, diarrhea, or constipation).

[c]Multiple preparations available that are not listed.

Efficacy Oral calcium compounds are well established as first-line agents for control of serum phosphorus. Calcium carbonate and calcium acetate are the primary preparations used. Calcium citrate is also available but is used less frequently since the citrate component increases aluminum absorption and may cause more GI side effects. Calcium carbonate is marketed in a variety of dosage forms and is relatively inexpensive. Unfortunately, many calcium carbonate products are considered food supplements and thus do not meet US Pharmacopeia (USP) disintegration and dissolution requirements. In general, nationally advertised brands do meet these requirements, but it is difficult to determine whether private labels or house brands conform to these standards. Variability in gastric pH may also affect disintegration or dissolution, and thus phosphate-binding efficacy. Calcium carbonate is more soluble in an acidic medium and should be administered prior to meals when stomach acidity is highest. In addition, acid-suppressing agents such as ranitidine and proton pump inhibitors may reduce the phosphate-binding activity of calcium carbonate by increasing gastric pH. Calcium acetate binds approximately twice as much phosphorus as calcium carbonate at comparable doses of elemental calcium.[111] Increased binding potency limits GI calcium absorption; however, calcium acetate is more soluble and therefore better absorbed than calcium carbonate in an alkaline pH. There is some evidence that calcium acetate may be less likely to cause hypercalcemia compared to carbonate.[111] For patients with hypocalcemia, calcium carbonate or calcium acetate may also be given as a calcium supplement taken between meals to promote calcium absorption. This is a common scenario for patients following a parathyroidectomy.

Hyperphosphatemia and vascular calcifications are associated with higher mortality.[42] There is evidence that chronic use of calcium-containing phosphate binders promotes progression of vascular calcification; however, not all studies support this finding and recent evidence suggests this effect may occur with non–calcium-containing binders as well. The effect of binder choice on mortality is also controversial. KDOQI guidelines suggest using a non–calcium-containing binder in dialysis patients with severe vascular or soft-tissue calcifications and that the total dose of elemental calcium provided by binders should not exceed 1,500 mg/day and the total daily intake of elemental calcium from all sources should not exceed 2,000 mg (opinion-based recommendations).[111] In general, KDIGO recommends that binder choice be made considering the CKD category and the risk of calcifications, and that calcium-based phosphate binders be restricted in patients with vascular calcifications and/or adynamic bone disease (a grade 2C recommendation).[42]

Sevelamer is a nonabsorbable, nonelemental hydrogel phosphate-binding agent approved for ESRD patients that effectively lowers phosphorus and has also been shown to lower LDL and increase HDL cholesterol. Sevelamer hydrochloride carries the risk of metabolic acidosis, a problem that has been overcome with development of the carbonate formulation. Sevelamer carbonate also comes in a powder formulation which is a good option for many patients unable to swallow tablets. Once-daily dosing of sevelamer carbonate powder has also been shown to significantly decrease phosphorus levels, although this regimen was not as effective as three times daily dosing.[120]

Lanthanum carbonate is a phosphate binder approved for patients with ESRD and has demonstrated efficacy in controlling phosphorus and maintaining PTH in the target range with less risk of hypercalcemia than calcium-containing binders.[42] The initial daily dose of 1,500 mg (administered in divided doses with meals) is often titrated to a range of 1,500 to 3,000 mg to maintain target phosphorus. The poor GI absorption, which limits systemic effects, and high binding capacity with phosphorus make this an attractive phosphate-binding agent, particularly when calcium-containing binders are not recommended due to hypercalcemia. Lanthanum is available as a chewable tablet, which may be appealing for some patients.

Ferric citrate and sucroferric oxyhydroxide are the newest iron-based phosphate-binding agents approved for ESRD patients. Sucroferric oxyhydroxide effectively lowers phosphorus over a long term (1-year) period and may have a lower pill burden compared to other agents.[121] It is also available as a chewable tablet. Ferric citrate effectively lowers phosphorus and also offers the potential advantage of increasing iron indices (TSat and ferritin) while lowering IV iron and ESA use.[122]

Aluminum salts were widely used in the 1980s as phosphate-binding agents because of their high binding potency. They should no longer be used as first-line agents, but rather reserved for acute treatment of severe hyperphosphatemia or used at low doses in combination with other binders in cases of hyperphosphatemia that is not responding to therapy with a single agent. According to KDOQI guidelines, the duration of aluminum therapy should be limited to 4 weeks if these agents are used at all.[111] Magnesium-containing antacids are also effective phosphate binders and may decrease the amount of calcium-containing binders necessary for control of phosphorus; however, their use is limited by the frequent occurrence of GI side effects (ie, diarrhea) and the potential for magnesium accumulation.

Adverse Effects Adverse effects of all available phosphate binders are generally limited to constipation, diarrhea, nausea, vomiting, and abdominal pain. The risk of hypercalcemia may necessitate restriction of calcium-containing binder use and/or a reduction in dietary intake. Aluminum binders have been associated with CNS toxicity and the worsening of anemia, whereas magnesium binder use may lead to hypermagnesemia and hyperkalemia (see Chapter 51); therefore, aluminum and magnesium are not recommended for regular use in patients with kidney disease. There has been a report of lanthanum tablets accumulating in the GI tract and causing severe complications in a patient who swallowed these tablets whole; therefore, it is important to counsel patients to chew these tablets.[123] The same counseling point applies for sucroferric oxyhydroxide.

Drug–Drug and Drug–Food Interactions Calcium-containing phosphate-binding agents interfere with the absorption of several oral medications that are commonly prescribed for CKD patients, including iron, zinc, and quinolone antibiotics. Coadministration of sevelamer with ciprofloxacin and mycophenolate did result in a reduction in bioavailability of these agents and they should be taken at least 2 hours before sevelamer. Coadministration of lanthanum with tetracyclines, fluoroquinolones, levothyroxine, or drugs known to bind with cationic antacids may result in decreased bioavailability of these agents. The iron containing products ferric citrate and sucroferric oxyhydroxide also have the potential for drug interactions due to the iron component. In general, it is rational to separate the administration time of oral medications for which a reduction in bioavailability has a clinically significant effect (eg, quinolones) from phosphate binders by at least 1 hour before or 3 hours after administration of the phosphate binder. Many phosphate binders are marketed as antacids or calcium supplements, and often CKD patients do not know why they have been prescribed these agents. Regular patient counseling is essential to improve adherence and minimize the potential for drug interactions.

Dosing and Administration Initial dosing regimens for phosphate-binding agents and suggested dose titration schemes are shown in Table 44-11. Doses should be titrated to achieve the recommended serum phosphorus concentrations in conjunction with dietary intervention and dialysis (for ESRD patients).

Vitamin D Therapy

Vitamin D compounds available in the United States include nutritional vitamin D [ergocalciferol (D_2) and cholecalciferol (D_3)], active vitamin D [calcitriol (D_3)], and vitamin D analogs [paricalcitol and doxercalciferol (both D_2)] (Table 44-12). Nutritional vitamin D

TABLE 44-12 Vitamin D Agents

Generic Name	Brand Name	Form of Vitamin D	Dosage Forms	Initial Dose[a]	Dosage Range	Frequency of Dosing
Nutritional Vitamin D						
Ergocalciferol	Drisdol	D_2	po	Varies based on 25(OH) D levels	400-50,000 international units	Daily (doses of 400-2,000 international units)
Cholecalciferol[b]	Generic	D_3	po			Weekly or monthly for higher doses (50,000 international units)
Vitamin D and Analogs						
Generic Name	**Brand Name**	**Form of Vitamin D**	**Dosage Forms**	**Initial Dose[a,c]**	**Dosage Range**	**Dose Titration[d]**
Calcitriol	Rocaltrol	D_3	po	0.25 mcg daily	0.25-5 mcg	Increase by 0.25 mcg/day at 4-8 week intervals
	Calcijex		IV	1-2 mcg three times per week	0.5-5 mcg	Increase by 0.5-1 mcg at 2 to 4 week intervals
Doxercalciferol[e]	Hectorol	D_2	po	ND-CKD: 1 mcg daily ESRD: 10 mcg three times per week	5-20 mcg	Increase by 0.5 mcg at 2-week intervals for daily dosing or by 2.5 mcg at 8-week intervals for three times per week dosing
			IV	ESRD: 4 mcg three times per week	2–8 mcg	Increase by 1-2 mcg at 8-week intervals
Paricalcitol	Zemplar	D_2	po	ND-CKD: 1 mcg daily or 2 mcg three times per week if PTH ≤500 pg/mL (ng/L; ≤54 pmol/L); 2 mcg daily or 4 mcg three times per week if PTH >500 pg/mL (ng/L; >54 pmol/L)	1-4 mcg	Increase by 1 mcg (for daily dosing) or 2 mcg (for three times per week dosing) at 2-4 week intervals
			IV	ESRD: 0.04-1 mcg three times per week	2.5-15 mcg	Increase by 2-4 mcg at 2-4 week intervals

ESRD, end-stage renal disease; ND-CKD, non-dialysis chronic kidney disease; PTH, parathyroid hormone.

[a]Dose ratios are as follows: 1:1 for IV paricalcitol to oral doxercalciferol, 1.5:1 for IV paricalcitol to IV doxercalciferol, and 1:1 for IV to oral calcitriol.

[b]Multiple preparations are available that are not listed.

[c]Daily orally dosing most common for non-hemodialysis CKD patients, IV dosing three times per week more often used in the hemodialysis population.

[d]Based on PTH, calcium and phosphorus levels. Decreases in dose are necessary if PTH is oversuppressed and/or if calcium and phosphorus are elevated.

[e]Prodrug that requires activation by the liver.

(NVD) is derived from dietary plant (D_2) and animal (D_3) sources, or from supplements. While this chapter focuses on the role of NVD and FDA-approved vitamin D formulations for the management of mineral homeostasis, there are several other therapeutic uses for vitamin D (eg, for CV and immune-related effects) and other analogs available outside the United States which are not discussed (eg, alfacalcidol).

Pharmacology and Mechanism of Action Vitamin D is a cholesterol derivative and is transported in the circulation by vitamin D binding protein. The process of vitamin D metabolism is shown in Fig. 44-4. Both endogenously synthesized D_3 and NVD compounds (as D_2 or D_3) are converted in the liver to 25(OH)D, by the 25-hydroxylase enzyme. The 25(OH)D form is subsequently converted to the biologically active form 1,25-dihydroxyvitamin D (either D_2 or D_3 depending on the parent compound) by the 1-α-hydroxylase enzyme. This conversion occurs primarily in the kidney, but this enzyme is also present in extrarenal tissues. It is not clear whether active vitamin D produced in extrarenal tissue exerts its effects only locally or contributes to the systemic endocrine functions. It is the concentration of 25(OH)D that is most commonly measured clinically to diagnose vitamin D deficiency.

Calcitriol and the vitamin D analogs bind to the vitamin D receptors (VDRs), which are located in many organ systems including the parathyroid glands, intestine, bone, kidney, heart, nervous, and immune systems. When vitamin D binds to the VDR there is a conformational change in the VDR that allows for interaction of the receptor with the retinoid X receptor (RXR), a transcriptional factor.[124] The VDR-RXR complex binds to DNA sequences in target genes to either promote or inhibit transcription depending on the organ system. Vitamin D inhibits or suppresses PTH synthesis and also stimulates absorption of serum calcium by intestinal cells. As a result, the serum calcium concentration is raised, which decreases PTH secretion by the parathyroid glands. The set point for calcium (ie, the calcium concentration at which PTH secretion is decreased by 50%), which is generally raised in those with CKD-MBD, is lowered when active vitamin D therapy is initiated. This results in a lower ionized calcium concentration becoming effective at suppressing secretion of PTH. Unfortunately, the enhanced GI absorption of calcium and phosphorus associated with calcitriol therapy may lead to hypercalcemia and hyperphosphatemia, which are associated with soft-tissue and vascular calcifications.

The unique interactions of vitamin D with the VDRs have led to the development of vitamin D analogs that vary in their affinity for the VDRs. Paricalcitol and doxercalciferol retain activity with vitamin D receptors on the parathyroid gland to effectively lower PTH, but have less risk of hypercalcemia and hyperphosphatemia due to their lower intestinal activity. Paricalcitol differs from calcitriol by the absence of the exocyclic carbon 19 and the fact that it is a vitamin D_2 derivative (19-nor-1,25-dihydroxyvitamin D_2). This compound is active as given. Doxercalciferol, however, is a prohormone that does require activation by CYP27 in the liver to form the major active D_2 metabolite 1,25-dihydroxyvitamin D_2 (see Fig. 44-4).

Pharmacokinetics Oral absorption of calcitriol occurs rapidly; therefore, both oral and IV therapies are reasonable options for treatment of CKD-MBD. The half-life of active calcitriol ranges from 15 to 38 hours in patients with ESRD.[125] The half-lives of paricalcitol and doxercalciferol are approximately 15 hours and 32 to 37 hours, respectively.[126,127] These agents are extensively bound to plasma proteins and not removed by dialysis.

Efficacy Calcitriol, paricalcitol, and doxercalciferol are all effective in lowering PTH in patients with CKD; however, the trade-off is the undesired effect of raising calcium and phosphorus concentrations due to increased intestinal absorption. Although these effects are less likely with paricalcitol and doxercalciferol, elevated calcium concentrations have been observed. An all-cause and CV survival benefit has also been reported with these agents in both CKD and ESRD patients.[128] It must be noted that these are observational studies and that prospective, randomized controlled trials are required to verify these survival benefits. When the effect of paricalcitol on left ventricular mass was evaluated in patients with CKD and mild to moderate LVH, no reduction in left ventricular mass was noted after 48 weeks of therapy.[129] A significant reduction in the urinary ACR was observed in CKD patients with type 2 diabetes receiving 2 mcg of oral paricalcitol daily compared with placebo.[130] These findings suggest potential new roles for vitamin D beyond suppression of PTH.

A review and meta-analysis in CKD patients (including ESRD patients) revealed that NVD supplementation was associated with an improvement in 25(OH)D levels and decreased PTH without significant hypercalcemia or hyperphosphatemia.[131] Suppression of secondary hyperparathyroidsim with NVD is most effective in patients with CKD 3. In ESRD patients, NVD has resulted in increased levels of 25(OH)D and a decrease in PTH, which suggests a potential role of extrarenal pathways of vitamin D activation; however, these patients typically also require active vitamin D or analog therapy. The survival benefit of correcting vitamin D deficiency with NVD in the CKD population is unknown.

Adverse Effects Although all agents are effective in suppressing PTH, they may cause hypercalcemia and hyperphosphatemia, an effect that is most likely with calcitriol. Oversuppression of PTH and inducement of adynamic bone disease are also distinct possibilities.

Drug–Drug and Drug–Food Interactions Cholestyramine may reduce the absorption of orally administered calcitriol and doxercalciferol. In vitro data suggest that paricalcitol is metabolized by the hepatic enzyme CYP3A4 and thus it has the potential to interact with other agents that are metabolized by this enzyme. Caution is also advised when CYP3A4 inhibitors are given to those receiving doxercalciferol since hydroxylation of this precursor agent may be inhibited.

Dosing and Administration Despite the lack of evidence, KDIGO guidelines support administering NVD to patients with CKD 3-5 and ESRD with vitamin D deficiency or insufficiency (a grade 2C recommendation).[42] KDOQI specifies that supplementation is warranted if the 25(OH)D level is less than 30 ng/mL (75 nmol/L).[111] The dose and duration of treatment are dependent on the severity of the deficiency: oral ergocalciferol 50,000 IU per week for 12 weeks, then monthly for 6 months for severe deficiency [25(OH)D levels <5 ng/mL, 12.5 nmol/L] and 50,000 IU monthly for 6 months for insufficiency [25(OH)D less than 30 ng/mL, 75 nmol/L]. Calcitriol, doxercalciferol, or paricalcitol should be administered when PTH remains elevated despite the achievement of adequate 25(OH)D levels.

Administration of calcitriol by either the oral or the IV route may utilize a daily (usually 0.25-1 mcg/day) or pulse dosing (0.5-2 mcg two to three times per week) approach. Logistically, IV dosing with doses administered three times per week is usually optimal in HD patients since this correlates with their in-center dialysis treatment schedule and IV therapy is covered in the bundled payment for dialysis (see the "Pharmacoeconomic Considerations" section). Oral therapy is more practical for non-dialysis CKD and PD patients. Recommended doses of calcitriol, doxercalciferol, and paricalcitol and suggested dose titration schemes are shown in Table 44-12. Prior to starting therapy, the serum calcium and phosphorus should be within the normal range. This does not mean that vitamin D therapy should be withheld or discontinued in all patients with elevated calcium and phosphorus values, but rather that use of agents with a lower risk of hypercalcemia and hyperphosphatemia and more prudent use of phosphate binders to lower calcium and phosphorus may be necessary in such patients. Dose adjustments of vitamin D should be made every 2 to 4 weeks based on PTH concentrations and trends in calcium and phosphorus.

Calcimimetics

Cinacalcet hydrochloride (Sensipar) is currently the only calcimimetic agent approved for treatment of secondary hyperparathyroidsim in CKD patients on dialysis.

Pharmacology and Mechanism of Action Cinacalcet acts by increasing the sensitivity of the calcium-sensing receptor located on the surface of the chief cells of the parathyroid gland to extracellular calcium, subsequently reducing PTH secretion. Cinacalcet does not increase intestinal calcium and phosphorus absorption. In fact, the reduction in PTH with cinacalcet is associated with a decrease in serum calcium.

Pharmacokinetics Cinacalcet peak concentrations are observed 2 to 6 hours following oral administration and its elimination half-life is approximately 30 to 40 hours. It has a large volume of distribution (approximately 1,000 L) and is 93% to 97% bound to plasma proteins, and thus removal by dialysis is likely negligible. It is metabolized by the liver, specifically by the cytochrome P450 isoenzymes CYP3A4, CYP2D6, and CYP1A2.[132]

Efficacy In clinical trials conducted predominantly in dialysis patients, cinacalcet significantly decreased PTH, calcium, and phosphorus, regardless of the severity of secondary hyperparathyroidsim.[42] In non-dialysis CKD patients it reduced PTH, but was associated with a high incidence of hypocalcemia and hyperphosphatemia; thus, this agent is not approved for use in non-dialysis CKD patients. Cinacalcet may be used as a single agent to control hyperparathyroidism in ESRD patients; however, combined therapy with vitamin D is often necessary to achieve target PTH, calcium, and phosphorus values. Cinacalcet plus low-dose active vitamin D increased coronary artery calcification scores but to a lesser degree than its comparator calcitriol alone.[133] A decrease in all-cause and CV mortality was also suggested by results of an observational study in HD patients prescribed cinacalcet in addition to vitamin D compared with those on vitamin D alone.[134] While these findings were promising, they were not supported by the EVOLVE trial (the Evaluation of Cinacalcet Therapy to Lower CV Events), a prospective study which revealed that cinacalcet did not significantly reduce the risk of all-cause mortality or major CV events in patients with CKD 5HD.[135]

Adverse Effects The most frequent adverse events associated with cinacalcet are nausea and vomiting. Since cinacalcet lowers serum calcium it should not be started if the serum calcium is less than the lower limit of normal, approximately 8.4 mg/dL (2.10 mmol/L). Serum calcium should be measured within 1 week after initiation or following a dose adjustment. Once the maintenance dose is established, serum calcium should be measured monthly. Potential manifestations of hypocalcemia include paresthesia, myalgia, cramping, tetany, and convulsions. Hypocalcemia may also lead to Q-T interval prolongation and ventricular arrhythmias, which further emphasizes the importance of regular calcium monitoring.[132]

Drug–Drug and Drug–Food Interactions Because cinacalcet is partially metabolized by cytochrome P450 CYP3A4, there is potential for drug interactions with agents that inhibit this pathway. Coadministration of cinacalcet and ketoconazole, a strong inhibitor of CYP3A4, resulted in a twofold increase in the area under the curve and maximum concentration. Cinacalcet is also a potent inhibitor of the enzyme CYP2D6. As a result, dose adjustments of concomitant medications that are predominantly metabolized by this enzyme and have a narrow therapeutic index, such as flecainide, thioridazine, vinblastine, and most tricyclic antidepressants (eg, amitriptyline), may be necessary.[132] Concurrent administration of cinacalcet with amitriptyline increased amitriptyline and nortriptyline (active metabolite) exposure by approximately 20% in CYP2D6-extensive metabolizers.

Food has been shown to increase absorption of cinacalcet by up to 82% compared with fasting; therefore, this medication should be taken with meals to achieve the maximal effect.[132]

Dosing and Administration The recommended starting dose of cinacalcet is 30 mg once daily. Calcium and phosphorus should be measured within 1 week and PTH should be measured within 1 to 4 weeks after starting cinacalcet or adjusting the dose. The dose should be titrated every 2 to 4 weeks to a maximum dose of 180 mg once daily until the desired PTH values are achieved and to maintain goal serum calcium concentrations. Patients with hepatic disease may require lower doses, since the cinacalcet half-life is approximately doubled in those with severe liver disease.[132] Cinacalcet is available as film-coated tablets containing 30, 60, or 90 mg.

Evaluation of Therapeutic Outcomes

The parameters listed in Table 44-10 should be evaluated to assess response to therapy. Of note, the shift in the treatment approach from the more conservative KDOQI guidelines to the KDIGO recommendations have led to changes in observed trends in these parameters. For example, PTH values have increased in most countries as a result of the higher range for PTH recommended by the more globally accepted KDIGO guidelines.[114] More definitive data on the effect of treatment approaches and achievement of target calcium, phosphorus, and PTH values on therapeutic outcomes are needed.

Pharmacoeconomic Considerations for Anemia and Chronic Kidney Disease-Related Mineral and Bone Disorder

The cost of medications to treat anemia and CKD-MBD is substantial.[11,136] In the United States insurance requirements for coverage of agents including ESAs, IV iron, and vitamin D analogs can be a major limitation to treatment of the CKD patient with anemia or MBD. The high cost of ESAs is a reason that legislation led to a *bundled* payment system for dialysis patients. The Medicare Modernization Act became effective in 2006 and provided for separately billable drugs such as ESAs, IV iron, IV vitamin D to be reimbursed based on the average sales price. The results of CHOIR and perceived overuse of ESAs later prompted Congress to reevaluate the reimbursement system, and in 2009 the bundled reimbursement system for dialysis was established (implemented in 2011), which included a composite rate for services and injectable drugs and oral equivalents. The primary goal of the bundled payment system was to decrease incentives for the overuse of previously separately reimbursable drugs, primarily ESAs because they were the most expensive and due to safety concerns with these agents.

Healthcare providers must consider the reimbursement structure with regard to ESA use and weigh the risks and benefits of ESA and IV iron treatment in individual patients when making decisions about anemia management. Since the introduction of erythropoietin in the late 1980s, the mean Hb rose from an average of 9.7 g/dL (97 g/dL, 6.02 mmol/L) in 1991 to a maximum of 12 g/dL (120 g/L, 7.45 mmol/L) in 2005 as weekly ESA doses increased from an average of approximately 7,300 units to over 19,000 units per week.[11,137] While doses have decreased since that time (to approximately 9,450 units per week in 2013) due to safety concerns, over 90% of US dialysis patients still receive an ESA.[11,138] On an international level (according to the Dialysis Outcomes and Practice Patterns Study Program) over 85% of CKD 5D patients use ESAs and 72% use IV iron.[138] Some observational studies also showed improved quality of life with Hb levels above 11 g/dL (110 g/L; 6.83 mmol/L).[79] It is clear now, however, that targeting Hb levels above 11 g/dL (110 g/L; 6.83 mmol/L) with ESA therapy increases risk of mortality and CV events and is associated with higher cost per quality-adjusted live-year (QALY) gained compared with patients maintained in a lower Hb range.[139] Patients may decide that risk of ESA therapy outweighs the benefits and is one reason a discussion with the patient (ie, as with the REMS program) is necessary. With the availability of biosimilars the cost of therapy is expected to decrease, although this will depend on the how these agents are accepted and adopted in clinical practice.[103]

The US payment system does affect treatment approaches for CKD-MBD. Oral ESRD drugs that do not have an IV equivalent, such as phosphate binders and cinacalcet, are outside the bundle and are reimbursable through Medicare part D, Medicaid or commercial prescription drug plans. These agents were to be included in the bundle in 2014, but their inclusion has been postponed until 2024. Since Medicare part D plans are administered through various insurance contractors with varying formularies and drug pricing tiers, the covered phosphate binder may be different depending upon the plan. From an international perspective approximately 80% of CKD 5D patients are prescribed phosphate binders, 70% vitamin D, and 17% cinacalcet.[138] The cost-effectiveness of phosphate binders, vitamin D, and cinacalcet on an international level have been evaluated; however, it is difficult to make conclusions about the value of such medications when data on hard outcomes such as mortality are limited.[140]

Cardiovascular Complications of Chronic Kidney Disease

Cardiovascular Disease

Patients with CKD are at increased risk of CVD, independent of the etiology of their kidney disease. This greater burden of CVD in patients with CKD is illustrated in Fig. 44-7. The prevalence of any form of CVD is double in CKD patients compared to patients without CKD (70% vs 35%).[141] Thirty percent of CKD patients had heart failure and 11% had a history of acute myocardial infarction. In contrast, the rates in non-CKD patients were 7% and 2%, respectively. This burden of CVD is associated with much higher mortality rates. For ESRD, adjusted rates of all-cause mortality are six to eight times greater than for individuals in the general population. In particular, cardiac death due to arrhythmia is the leading cause of death in this population.[141] Higher mortality and risk of CV events has also been observed in individuals with CKD 3 to 5.[142]

Traditional CVD risk factors present in patients with CKD include diabetes mellitus, dyslipidemia, hypertension, LVH, smoking, and obesity. Nontraditional risk factors include proteinuria, hyperhomocysteinemia, anemia, inflammation, and abnormal calcium and phosphate metabolism resulting in vascular calcification oxidative stress.[142] Unfortunately, the lack of randomized trials treating CVD in patients with CKD often leads to treatment decisions that are based on extrapolation from trials in non-CKD populations and from observational data in CKD.[143] However, the level of care

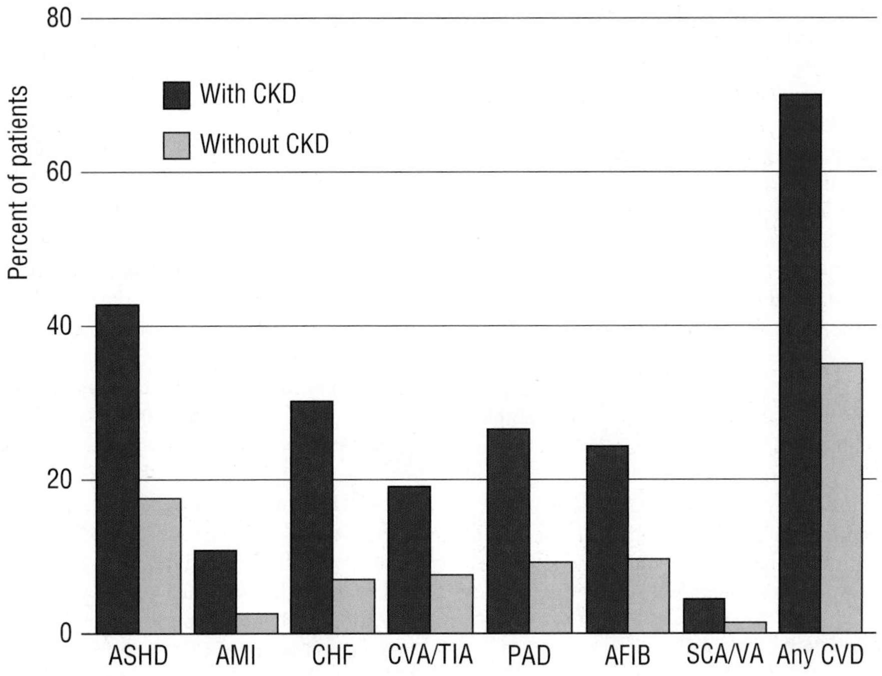

FIGURE 44-7 Cardiovascular disease in patients with or without CKD.[141] (AFIB, atrial fibrillation; AMI, acute myocardial infarction; ASHD, atherosclerotic heart disease; CHF, congestive heart failure; CKD, chronic kidney disease; CVA/TIA, cerebrovascular accident/transient ischemic attack; CVD, cardiovascular disease; PAD, peripheral arterial disease; SCA/VA, sudden cardiac arrest and ventricular arrhythmias.) Data Source: Medicare 5 percent sample. Patients aged 66 and older, alive, without end-stage renal disease, and residing in the U.S. on 12/31/2012 with fee-for-service coverage for the entire calendar year.

for ischemic heart disease offered to people with CKD should not differ from people without CKD (grade 1A recommendation) as there is evidence indicating that treatment of traditional risk factors in CKD patients is of benefit.[1] These patients should also receive the standard assessments and treatments such as statins for CKD 1-5 (nondialysis), beta-blockers, ACEIs/ARBs, and antiplatelet agents (see Chapter 16). Clinicians should note that in the diagnosis of acute coronary syndrome, elevated serum troponins should be interpreted with caution in individuals with a GFR less than 60 mL/min/1.73 m^2 (<0.58 mL/s/m^2) because these markers are often elevated as a result of reduced renal excretion (a grade 1B recommendation).[1]

Patients with CKD should receive standard heart failure therapies (Chapter 14); however, clinicians should be aware that RAAS blockade (eg, ACEI, ARB, spironolactone, eplerenone) and diuretic therapy (eg, furosemide, metolazone) may lead to significant changes in GFR and serum potassium concentrations. Such therapy should not be avoided, but closely monitored and put into the context of individual risks and benefits. With regard to the cardiac biomarkers of B-type natriuretic peptide (BNP) and N-terminal pro-BNP (NT-pro-BNP) in individuals with a GFR less than 60 mL/min/1.73 m^2 (<0.58 mL/s/m^2) (CKD 3a-5), it is recommended that serum concentrations be interpreted with caution with respect to diagnosis of heart failure and assessment of volume status (a grade 1B recommendation).[1]

Aspirin is recommended for secondary prevention in all patients with CKD based on decreased mortality in observational studies.[144,145] There is, however, controversy over the use of aspirin (ASA) for primary prevention in patients with CKD.[146-148]

Clinical **Controversy...**

The KDIGO guidelines state in one section that ASA is not recommended for primary prevention.[1] However, later in the guidelines it is stated that "adults with CKD at risk for atherosclerotic events be offered treatment with antiplatelet agents unless there is an increased bleeding risk that needs to be balanced against the possible CV benefits."[1] This position statement is derived from a post-hoc analysis of the Hypertension Optimal Treatment (HOT) trial which concluded that the increased risk of major bleeding appears to be outweighed by the substantial benefits of aspirin in individuals with CKD and hypertension.[146,147] As post-hoc analyses are hypothesis generating and should always be interpreted with caution, an editorial on the HOT trial CKD subgroup analysis made the following recommendations: (1) This study should not be taken as robust evidence in favor of aspirin therapy for primary prevention in CKD; (2)There is an urgent need for a prospective randomized controlled trial that includes patients with all categories of CKD and; (3) The risk of major bleeding as well as paradoxical thrombosis is a genuine concern when using aspirin for primary prevention in patients with CKD.[148]

Hyperlipidemia

CKD with or without nephrotic syndrome is frequently accompanied by abnormalities in lipoprotein metabolism (see Chapter 47).

A clear association between hypercholesterolemia, hypertriglyceridemia, and other lipoprotein changes in patients with CKD and CVD has not been demonstrated in large prospective studies because individuals with kidney disease are usually excluded from these trials. A low or declining serum cholesterol in patients with ESRD is associated with higher mortality, a paradoxical effect.[149] These findings beg the question of whether aggressive lipid lowering is warranted in this population.

Although the concentrations of LDL are not uniformly increased in patients with kidney disease, these patients appear to produce small, dense LDL particles that are more susceptible to oxidation and more atherogenic than larger LDL subfractions. Other lipid abnormalities include low HDL and increased triglycerides.[149] In patients with nephrotic syndrome, the major lipid abnormalities are elevation of plasma total and LDL cholesterol, with or without low HDL cholesterol, and elevated triglycerides. See Chapter 47 for a detailed discussion of the management of proteinuria in patients with glomerulonephritis.

The KDIGO Lipid Guidelines recommend that a complete fasting lipid profile be performed in all adults with newly identified CKD (a grade 1C recommendation).[150] Follow-up lipid levels are not recommended unless the information may alter management (eg, assessing adherence to therapy or assessing CV risk in a patient <50 years and not currently on a statin). Reduction in the risk of CV events in patients with CKD has only been demonstrated with statins or a statin plus ezetimibe combination.[150]

Statins in Chronic Kidney Disease

Statins have been shown to decrease mortality and CV events in CKD 1-5 patients, however, data are not as compelling in the ESRD population.[151] Although observational studies in HD patients receiving statins indicated a significant benefit, findings from prospective studies have not been encouraging. The 4D Trial, a 4-year study evaluating the effect of atorvastatin therapy on cardiac mortality in more than 1,200 HD patients with type 2 diabetes, showed no significant benefit in the composite end point compared with the placebo group.[152] In fact, there was a significantly greater relative risk (RR) of fatal stroke in the atorvastatin-treated patients. These findings do not support initiation of statin therapy in ESRD patients, especially those with type 2 diabetes. The findings with rosuvastatin were similar: despite a 43% reduction in cholesterol there was no significant change in the primary end points of death from CV causes, nonfatal MI, or nonfatal stroke.[153] The Study of Heart and Renal Protection (SHARP) trial was a primary prevention trial that evaluated the effects of combined simvastatin (20 mg) and ezetimibe (10 mg) compared with placebo on time to first major vascular event (nonfatal MI or cardiac death, any stroke, or revascularization) in patients with no history of MI or coronary revascularization and included patients with CKD (6,247) and ESRD (3,023).[154] In all patients receiving combined therapy during the 4.9-year follow up period, there was a significant 17% reduction in the RR of major vascular events and a 32% reduction in LDL in the patients who were assessed as compliant with therapy (two-thirds were compliant). While overall these results are positive, the study was not powered to evaluate whether the observed effect was significant in ESRD patients as a separate group. A subgroup analysis comparing dialysis versus non-dialysis and diabetic versus non-diabetic patients showed no differences in the RR of CV events even after adjustment for the reduction in LDL.

A recent meta-analysis of statins in dialysis patients indicated that they had no significant beneficial effect on major CV events, all-cause mortality, CV death, or myocardial infarction, and a trend toward increased strokes despite clinically relevant reductions in LDL cholesterol.[155] In contrast, a meta-analysis of statins in non-dialysis CKD showed significant reductions in major CV events, CV death, all-cause mortality; myocardial infarction but uncertain effects on stroke.[156]

The KDIGO Lipid guidelines[150] make the following recommendations:

1. In adults age 18-49 years with CKD but not treated with chronic dialysis or kidney transplantation, we suggest statin treatment in people with one or more of the following [Level 2A]: known coronary disease (myocardial infarction or coronary revascularization); diabetes mellitus; prior ischemic stroke; estimated 10-year incidence of coronary death or non-fatal myocardial infarction greater than 10%.
2. In adults age greater than 50 years with eGFR less than 60 ml/min/1.73 m^2 but not treated with chronic dialysis or kidney transplantation, we recommend treatment with a statin or statin/ezetimibe combination. [Level 1A]
3. In adults with dialysis-dependent CKD, we suggest that statins or statin/ezetimibe combination not be initiated. [Level 2A] However, in patients already receiving statins or statin/ezetimibe combination at the time of dialysis initiation, we suggest that these agents be continued. [Level 2C]

BOTTOM LINE

The incidence of CKD has recently declined but the prevalence continues to increase. Although efforts to delay progression of CKD including prudent use of ACEIs and ARBs are paramount, measures to diagnose and manage the associated secondary complications and comorbid conditions early in the course of the disease are also essential. Common complications of CKD 4 and 5 include anemia and CKD-MBD. CV complications are also prevalent in the population with CKD, and are the leading cause of mortality in patients with ESRD.

A multidisciplinary team structure is a rational approach to effectively design and implement individual patient care plans often required in the CKD population given the extensive nonpharmacologic and pharmacologic interventions. Thus pharmacists are well positioned to actively participate in the chronic disease and medication management of ambulatory CKD and dialysis patients as well as those who are hospitalized.

ABBREVIATIONS

ACEI	angiotensin-converting enzyme inhibitor
ACR	albumin-to-creatinine ratio
AKI	acute kidney injury
ARB	angiotensin receptor blocker
ATII	angiotensin II
BMI	body mass index
BNP	B-type natriuretic peptide
CCB	calcium channel blocker
CERA	continuous erythropoietin receptor activator
CHOIR	Correction of Hb and Outcomes in Renal Insufficiency
CKD	chronic kidney disease
CKD-EPI equation	Chronic Kidney Disease Epidemiology Collaboration equation
CLcr	Creatinine clearance
CMM	comprehensive medication management
CMS	Centers for Medicare and Medicaid Services
CREATE	Cardiovascular Risk Reduction by Early Anemia Treatment with Epoetin Beta
CV	cardiovascular
CVD	cardiovascular disease
DCCT	Diabetes Control and Complications Trial
DCKD	Diabetic Chronic Kidney Disease

EDIC	Epidemiology of Diabetes Interventions and Complications
eGFR	estimated glomerular filtration rate
ESA	erythropoiesis stimulating agent
ESRD	end-stage renal disease
FGF-23	fibroblast growth factor-23
GFR	glomerular filtration rate
GI	gastrointestinal
Hb	hemoglobin
Hct	hematocrit
HbA1c	glycated hemoglobin or hemoglobin A_{1c}
HD	hemodialysis
HOT	Hypertension Optimal Treatment
KDIGO	Kidney Disease: Improving Global Outcomes
KDOQI	Kidney Disease Outcomes Quality Initiative
LDL	low-density lipoprotein
LVH	left ventricular hypertrophy
MBD	mineral and bone disorder
MCP-1	monocyte chemoattractant protein-1
MDRD	Modification of Diet in Renal Disease
MRP	medication-related problem
ND-CKD	nondialysis CKD patients (CKD 1-5)
NHCT	Normal Hematocrit Cardiac Trial
NVD	nutritional vitamin D
25(OH)D	25-hydroxyvitamin D
PCR	protein-to-creatinine ratio
PRCA	pure red cell aplasia
PREVEND	Prevention of Renal and Vascular End-Stage Disease
PTH	parathyroid hormone
RAAS	renin–angiotensin–aldosterone system
REMS	risk evaluation and mitigation strategy
ROD	renal osteodystrophy
RR	relative risk
RXR	retinoid X receptor
sHPT	secondary hyperparathyroidism
SONAR	Study of Diabetic Nephropathy with Atrasentan
SPRINT	Systolic Blood Pressure Intervention Trial
TGF-β	transforming growth factor beta
TIBC	total iron-binding capacity
TREAT	Trial to Reduce Cardiovascular Events with Aranesp Therapy
TSat	transferrin saturation
UKPDS	United Kingdom Prospective Diabetes Study
USRDS	United States Renal Data System
VDRs	vitamin D receptors

REFERENCES

1. Kidney Disease: Improving Global Outcomes (KDIGO) CKD Work Group. KDIGO 2012 Clinical Practice Guideline for the Evaluation and Management of Chronic Kidney Disease. *Kidney Int Suppl* 2013;3:1-150.
2. Bruck K, Stel VS, Fraser S, et al. Translational research in nephrology: Chronic kidney disease prevention and public health. *Clinical Kidney Journal* 2015;8:647-655.
3. Murray CJ, Barber RM, Foreman KJ, et al. Global, regional, and national disability-adjusted life years (DALYs) for 306 diseases and injuries and healthy life expectancy (HALE) for 188 countries, 1990-2013: Quantifying the epidemiological transition. *Lancet* 2015;386:2145-2191.
4. Jha V, Garcia-Garcia G, Iseki K, et al. Chronic kidney disease: Global dimension and perspectives. *Lancet* 2013;382:260-272.
5. Anand S, Bitton A, Gaziano T. The gap between estimated incidence of end-stage renal disease and use of therapy. *PLoS ONE* 2013;8:e72860.
6. US Department of Health and Human Services. Healthy People 2020 Objectives for Chronic Kidney Disease. Available at: https://www.healthypeople.gov/2020/topics-objectives/topic/chronic-kidney-disease. Last Accessed, May 20, 2016.
7. Global Action Plan for the Prevention and Control of NCDs 2013-2020. WHO Press., 2013. Available at: http://www.who.int/nmh/events/ncd_action_plan/en/. Accessed January 2, 2016.
8. Winearls CG, Glassock RJ. Classification of chronic kidney disease in the elderly: Pitfalls and errors. *Nephron Clin Pract* 2011;119 Suppl 1:c2-4.
9. Nathan DM, Zinman B, Cleary PA, et al. Modern-day clinical course of type 1 diabetes mellitus after 30 years' duration: The diabetes control and complications trial/epidemiology of diabetes interventions and complications and Pittsburgh epidemiology of diabetes complications experience (1983-2005). *Arch Intern Med* 2009;169:1307-1316.
10. Rodriguez-Poncelas A, Garre-Olmo J, Franch-Nadal J, et al. Prevalence of chronic kidney disease in patients with type 2 diabetes in Spain: PERCEDIME2 study. *BMC Nephrol* 2013;14:46-2369-2314-2346.
11. U.S. Renal Data System, USRDS 2014 Annual Data Report: *Atlas of Chronic Kidney Disease and End-Stage Renal Disease in the United States*. Bethesda, MD: National Institutes of Health, National Institute of Diabetes and Digestive and Kidney Diseases; 2014.
12. Fraser SD, Roderick PJ, Aitken G, et al. Chronic kidney disease, albuminuria and socioeconomic status in the Health Surveys for England 2009 and 2010. *J Public Health (Oxf)* 2014;36:577-586.
13. Bryson CL, Ross HJ, Boyko EJ, Young BA. Racial and ethnic variations in albuminuria in the US Third National Health and Nutrition Examination Survey (NHANES III) population: Associations with diabetes and level of CKD. *Am J Kidney Dis* 2006;48:720-726.
14. Barreto SM, Ladeira RM, Duncan BB, et al. Chronic kidney disease among adult participants of the ELSA-Brasil cohort: Association with race and socioeconomic position. *J Epidemiol Community Health* 2015;10.1136/jech-2015-205834.
15. Inker LA, Astor BC, Fox CH, et al. KDOQI US commentary on the 2012 KDIGO clinical practice guideline for the evaluation and management of CKD. *Am J Kidney Dis* 2014;63:713-735.
16. National Kidney Foundation. KDOQI Clinical Practice Guideline for Diabetes and CKD: 2012 Update. *Am J Kidney Dis* 2012;60:850-886.
17. Williams ME, Garg R. Glycemic management in ESRD and earlier stages of CKD. *Am J Kidney Dis* 2014;63:S22-38.
18. Patel A, MacMahon S, Chalmers J, et al. Intensive blood glucose control and vascular outcomes in patients with type 2 diabetes. *N Engl J Med* 2008;358:2560-2572.
19. Ismail-Beigi F, Craven T, Banerji MA, et al. Effect of intensive treatment of hyperglycaemia on microvascular outcomes in type 2 diabetes: An analysis of the ACCORD randomised trial. *Lancet* 2010;376:419-430.
20. Duckworth W, Abraira C, Moritz T, et al. Glucose control and vascular complications in veterans with type 2 diabetes. *N Engl J Med* 2009;360:129-139.
21. Halbesma N, Jansen DF, Stolk RP, De Jong PE, Gansevoort RT, group PS. Changes in renal risk factors versus renal function outcome during follow-up in a population-based cohort study. *Nephrol Dial Transplant* 2010;25:1846-1853.
22. KDIGO Blood Pressure Work Group. KDIGO Clinical Practice Guideline for the Management of Blood Pressure in Chronic Kidney Disease. *Kidney Int Suppl* 2012;2:337-414.
23. Perkovic V, Verdon C, Ninomiya T, et al. The relationship between proteinuria and coronary risk: a systematic review and meta-analysis. *PLoS Med* 2008;5:e207.
24. Fried LF, Lewis J. Albuminuria is not an appropriate therapeutic target in patients with CKD: The con view. *Clin J Am Soc Nephrol* 2015;10:1089-1093.
25. Jun M, Turin TC, Woodward M, et al. Assessing the validity of surrogate outcomes for ESRD: A meta-analysis. *J Am Soc Nephrol* 2015;26:2289-2302.
26. Hogan SL, Vupputuri S, Guo X, et al. Association of cigarette smoking with albuminuria in the United States: the third National Health and Nutrition Examination Survey. *Ren Fail* 2007;29:133-142.
27. Orth SR, Hallan SI. Smoking: a risk factor for progression of chronic kidney disease and for cardiovascular morbidity and mortality in renal patients--absence of evidence or evidence of absence? *Clin J Am Soc Nephrol* 2008;3:226-236.
28. Hsu CY, McCulloch CE, Iribarren C, Darbinian J, Go AS. Body mass index and risk for end-stage renal disease. *Ann Intern Med* 2006;144:21-28.

29. Ejerblad E, Fored CM, Lindblad P, Fryzek J, McLaughlin JK, Nyren O. Obesity and risk for chronic renal failure. *J Am Soc Nephrol* 2006;17:1695-1702.
30. Wang Y, Chen X, Song Y, Caballero B, Cheskin LJ. Association between obesity and kidney disease: A systematic review and meta-analysis. *Kidney Int* 2008;73:19-33.
31. Eknoyan G. Obesity and chronic kidney disease. *Nefrologia* 2011;31(4):397-403.
32. Ritz E, Koleganova N, Piecha G. Is there an obesity-metabolic syndrome related glomerulopathy? *Curr Opin Nephrol Hypertens* 2011;20:44-49.
33. Navaneethan SD, Yehnert H, Moustarah F, Schreiber MJ, Schauer PR, Beddhu S. Weight loss interventions in chronic kidney disease: a systematic review and meta-analysis. *Clin J Am Soc Nephrol* 2009;4:1565-1574.
34. Skorecki K CG, Marsden P et al. *Brenner and Rector's The Kidney,* 10th ed. Philadelphia, PA: Elsevier; 2015.
35. Lopez-Novoa JM, Martinez-Salgado C, Rodriguez-Pena AB, Lopez-Hernandez FJ. Common pathophysiological mechanisms of chronic kidney disease: Therapeutic perspectives. *Pharmacol Ther* 2010;128:61-81.
36. Gajjala PR, Sanati M, Jankowski J. Cellular and molecular mechanisms of chronic kidney disease with diabetes mellitus and cardiovascular diseases as its comorbidities. *Front Immunol* 2015;6:340.
37. Abbate M, Zoja C, Remuzzi G. How does proteinuria cause progressive renal damage? *J Am Soc Nephrol* 2006;17:2974-2984.
38. Jelkmann W. Regulation of erythropoietin production. *J Physiol* 2011;589:1251-1258.
39. Kidney Disease: Improving Global Outcomes (KDIGO) Anemia Work Group. KDIGO Clinical Practice Guideline for Anemia in Chronic Kidney Disease. *Kidney Inter Suppl* 2012;2:279-335.
40. Coyne DW. Hepcidin: Clinical utility as a diagnostic tool and therapeutic target. *Kidney Int* 2011;80:240-244.
41. Kalantar-Zadeh K, Streja E, Miller JE, Nissenson AR. Intravenous iron versus erythropoiesis-stimulating agents: friends or foes in treating chronic kidney disease anemia? *Adv Chronic Kidney Dis* 2009;16:143-151.
42. KDIGO clinical practice guideline for the diagnosis, evaluation, prevention, and treatment of chronic kidney disease-mineral and bone disorder (CKD-MBD). *Kidney Int Suppl* 2009:S1-130.
43. Cunningham J, Locatelli F, Rodriguez M. Secondary hyperparathyroidism: Pathogenesis, disease progression, and therapeutic options. *Clin J Am Soc Nephrol* 2011;6:913-921.
44. Gutierrez OM. Fibroblast growth factor 23 and disordered vitamin D metabolism in chronic kidney disease: Updating the "trade-off" hypothesis. *Clin J Am Soc Nephrol* 2010;5:1710-1716.
45. Wolf M. Update on fibroblast growth factor 23 in chronic kidney disease. *Kidney Int* 2012;82:737-747.
46. Martin KJ, Gonzalez EA. Vitamin D supplementation in CKD. *Clin Nephrol* 2011;75:286-293.
47. Block GA. Therapeutic interventions for chronic kidney disease-mineral and bone disorders: focus on mortality. *Curr Opin Nephrol Hypertens* 2011;20:376-381.
48. Nigwekar SU, Kroshinsky D, Nazarian RM, et al. Calciphylaxis: risk factors, diagnosis, and treatment. *Am J Kidney Dis* 2015;66:133-146.
49. Jones G. Interpreting vitamin D assay results: Proceed with caution. *Clin J Am Soc Nephrol* 2015;10:331-334.
50. Binkley N, Sempos CT. Standardizing vitamin D assays: The way forward. *J Bone Miner Res* 2014;29:1709-1714.
51. KDOQI Clinical Practice Guideline for Diabetes and CKD: 2012 Update. *Am J Kidney Dis* 2012;60:850-886.
52. Mason NA. Polypharmacy and medication-related complications in the chronic kidney disease patient. *Curr Opin Nephrol Hypertens* 2011;20:492-497.
53. Pai AB, Cardone KE, Manley HJ, et al. Medication reconciliation and therapy management in dialysis-dependent patients: Need for a systematic approach. *Clin J Am Soc Nephrol* 2013;8:1988-1999.
54. Raymond CB, Wazny LD, Sood AR. Standards of clinical practice for renal pharmacists. *Can J Hosp Pharm* 2013;66:369-374.
55. Manley HJ, Barton-Pai A. Integrated pharmacy services: A necessary component for care of patients treated by long-term dialysis. *Am J Kidney Dis* 2013;62:445-447.
56. Matzke GR, Aronoff GR, Atkinson AJ, Jr., et al. Drug dosing consideration in patients with acute and chronic kidney disease-a clinical update from Kidney Disease: Improving Global Outcomes (KDIGO). *Kidney Int* 2011;80:1122-1137.
57. Strippoli GF, Bonifati C, Craig M, Navaneethan SD, Craig JC. Angiotensin converting enzyme inhibitors and angiotensin II receptor antagonists for preventing the progression of diabetic kidney disease. *Cochrane Database Syst Rev* 2006;(4):CD006257.
58. Tylicki L, Lizakowski S, Rutkowski B. Renin-angiotensin-aldosterone system blockade for nephroprotection: Current evidence and future directions. *J Nephrol* 2012;25:900-910.
59. Kunz R, Friedrich C, Wolbers M, Mann JF. Meta-analysis: Effect of monotherapy and combination therapy with inhibitors of the renin angiotensin system on proteinuria in renal disease. *Ann Intern Med* 2008;148:30-48.
60. Mann JF, Schmieder RE, McQueen M, et al. Renal outcomes with telmisartan, ramipril, or both, in people at high vascular risk (the ONTARGET study): A multicentre, randomised, double-blind, controlled trial. *Lancet* 2008;372:547-553.
61. Ruggenenti P, Remuzzi G. Proteinuria: Is the ONTARGET renal substudy actually off target? *Nat Rev Nephrol* 2009;5:436-437.
62. Fried LF, Emanuele N, Zhang JH, et al. Combined angiotensin inhibition for the treatment of diabetic nephropathy. *N Engl J Med* 2013;369:1892-1903.
63. Parving HH, Brenner BM, McMurray JJ, et al. Cardiorenal end points in a trial of aliskiren for type 2 diabetes. *N Engl J Med* 2012;367:2204-2213.
64. Imai E, Haneda M, Yamasaki T, et al. Effects of dual blockade of the renin-angiotensin system on renal and cardiovascular outcomes in type 2 diabetes with overt nephropathy and hypertension in the ORIENT: A post-hoc analysis (ORIENT-Hypertension). *Hypertens Res* 2013;36:1051-1059.
65. Bolignano D, Palmer SC, Navaneethan SD, Strippoli GF. Aldosterone antagonists for preventing the progression of chronic kidney disease. *Cochrane Database Syst Rev* 2014;4:Cd007004.
66. Hou J, Xiong W, Cao L, Wen X, Li A. Spironolactone add-on for preventing or slowing the progression of diabetic nephropathy: A meta-analysis. *Clin Ther* 2015;37:2086-2103.e2010.
67. Hart P, Bakris GL. Calcium antagonists: Do they equally protect against kidney injury? *Kidney Int* 2008;73:795-796.
68. Stanton RC. Clinical challenges in diagnosis and management of diabetic kidney disease. *Am J Kidney Dis* 2014;63:S3-21.
69. Mann JF, Green D, Jamerson K, et al. Avosentan for overt diabetic nephropathy. *J Am Soc Nephrol* 2010;21:527-535.
70. de Zeeuw D, Coll B, Andress D, et al. The endothelin antagonist atrasentan lowers residual albuminuria in patients with type 2 diabetic nephropathy. *J Am Soc Nephrol* 2014;25:1083-1093.
71. Study of Diabetic Nephropathy with Atrasentan (SONAR). Clinical Trials.gov. Available at: https://clinicaltrials.gov/ct2/show/NCT01858532?term=study+of+diabetic+nephropathy+with+atrasentan&rank=1. Accessed May 20, 2016.
72. Upadhyay A, Earley A, Haynes SM, Uhlig K. Systematic review: Blood pressure target in chronic kidney disease and proteinuria as an effect modifier. *Ann Intern Med* 2011;154:541-548.
73. Wright JT, Jr., Williamson JD, Whelton PK, et al. A randomized trial of intensive versus standard blood-pressure control. *N Engl J Med* 2015;373:2103-2116.
74. Dussol B, Moussi-Frances J, Morange S, Somma-Delpero C, Mundler O, Berland Y. A randomized trial of furosemide vs hydrochlorothiazide in patients with chronic renal failure and hypertension. *Nephrol Dial Transplant* 2005;20:349-353.
75. Turner JM, Bauer C, Abramowitz MK, Melamed ML, Hostetter TH. Treatment of chronic kidney disease. *Kidney Int* 2012;81:351-362.
76. Sinha AD, Agarwal R. Thiazides in advanced chronic kidney disease: Time for a randomized controlled trial. *Curr Opin Cardiol* 2015;30:366-372.
77. KDOQI Clinical Practice Guideline and Clinical Practice Recommendations for anemia in chronic kidney disease: 2007 update of hemoglobin target. *Am J Kidney Dis* 2007;50:471-530.
78. KDOQI Clinical Practice Guidelines and Clinical Practice Recommendations for Anemia in Chronic Kidney Disease. *Am J Kidney Dis* 2006;47:S11-145.
79. Kliger AS, Fishbane S, Finkelstein FO. Erythropoietic stimulating agents and quality of a patient's life: individualizing anemia treatment. *Clin J Am Soc Nephrol* 2012;7:354-357.
80. Besarab A, Bolton WK, Browne JK, et al. The effects of normal as compared with low hematocrit values in patients with cardiac disease who are receiving hemodialysis and epoetin. *N Engl J Med* 1998;339:584-590.
81. Besarab A, Goodkin DA, Nissenson AR. The normal hematocrit study—follow-up. *N Engl J Med* 2008;358:433-434.
82. Singh AK, Szczech L, Tang KL, et al. Correction of anemia with epoetin alfa in chronic kidney disease. *N Engl J Med* 2006;355:2085-2098.
83. Drueke TB, Locatelli F, Clyne N, et al. Normalization of hemoglobin level in patients with chronic kidney disease and anemia. *N Engl J Med* 2006;355:2071-2084.

84. FDA Drug Safety Communication: modified dosing recommendations to improve the safe use of erythropoiesis-stimulating agents (ESAs) in chronic kidney disease. Available at: http://www.fda.gov/Drugs/DrugSafety/ucm259639.htm. Last updated 6/24/2011.
85. Phrommintikul A, Haas SJ, Elsik M, Krum H. Mortality and target haemoglobin concentrations in anaemic patients with chronic kidney disease treated with erythropoietin: A meta-analysis. *Lancet* 2007;369:381-388.
86. Pfeffer MA, Burdmann EA, Chen CY, et al. A trial of darbepoetin alfa in type 2 diabetes and chronic kidney disease. *N Engl J Med* 2009;361:2019-2032.
87. Skali H, Parving HH, Parfrey PS, et al. Stroke in patients with type 2 diabetes mellitus, chronic kidney disease, and anemia treated with Darbepoetin Alfa: The trial to reduce cardiovascular events with Aranesp therapy (TREAT) experience. *Circulation* 2011;124:2903-2908.
88. Unger EF, Thompson AM, Blank MJ, Temple R. Erythropoiesis-stimulating agents--time for a reevaluation. *N Engl J Med* 2010;362:189-192.
89. Szczech LA, Barnhart HX, Inrig JK, et al. Secondary analysis of the CHOIR trial epoetin-alpha dose and achieved hemoglobin outcomes. *Kidney Int* 2008;74:791-798.
90. Triferic. Package Insert. Wixom, MI, Rockwell Medical, Inc.; 2015.
91. Gupta A, Amin NB, Besarab A, et al. Dialysate iron therapy: Infusion of soluble ferric pyrophosphate via the dialysate during hemodialysis. *Kidney Int* 1999;55:1891-1898.
92. Fishbane SN, Singh AK, Cournoyer SH, et al. Ferric pyrophosphate citrate (Triferic) administration via the dialysate maintains hemoglobin and iron balance in chronic hemodialysis patients. *Nephrol Dial Transplant* 2015;10.1093/ndt/gfv277.
93. Wang C, Graham DJ, Kane RC, et al. Comparative risk of anaphylactic reactions associated with intravenous iron products. *JAMA* 2015;314:2062-2068.
94. FDA drug safety communication: FDA strengthens warnings and changes prescribing instructions to decrease the risk of serious allergic reactions with anemia drug Feraheme (ferumoxytol). Available at: http://www.fda.gov/Drugs/DrugSafety/ucm440138.htm. Page last updated 4/2/2015. Last accessed Sept 23, 2015.
95. Feraheme. Package Insert. Waltham, MA, AMAG Pharmaceuticals, Inc.; 2015.
96. Flaten TP, Aaseth J, Andersen O, Kontoghiorghes GJ. Iron mobilization using chelation and phlebotomy. *J Trace Elem Med Biol* 2012;26:127-130.
97. U.S. Renal Data System, USRDS 2013 Annual Data Report: *Atlas of Chronic Kidney Disease and End-Stage Renal Disease in the United States,* Bethesda, MD: National Institutes of Health, National Institute of Diabetes and Digestive and Kidney Diseases; 2013.
98. Miskulin DC, Tangri N, Bandeen-Roche K, et al. Intravenous iron exposure and mortality in patients on hemodialysis. *Clin J Am Soc Nephrol* 2014;9:1930-1939.
99. Brookhart MA, Freburger JK, Ellis AR, Wang L, Winkelmayer WC, Kshirsagar AV. Infection risk with bolus versus maintenance iron supplementation in hemodialysis patients. *J Am Soc Nephrol* 2013;24:1151-1158.
100. Litton E, Xiao J, Ho KM. Safety and efficacy of intravenous iron therapy in reducing requirement for allogeneic blood transfusion: systematic review and meta-analysis of randomised clinical trials. *BMJ* 2013;347:f4822.
101. Susantitaphong P, Alqahtani F, Jaber BL. Efficacy and safety of intravenous iron therapy for functional iron deficiency anemia in hemodialysis patients: A meta-analysis. *Am J Nephrol* 2014;39: 130-141.
102. Ishida JH, Marafino BJ, McCulloch CE, et al. Receipt of intravenous iron and clinical outcomes among hemodialysis patients hospitalized for infection. *Clin J Am Soc Nephrol* 2015;10:1799-1805.
103. Fishbane S, Shah HH. The emerging role of biosimilar epoetins in nephrology in the United States. *Am J Kidney Dis* 2015;65:537-542.
104. Mircera. Package Insert. South San Francisco, CA: Hoffmann-La Roche, Inc.; October 2014.
105. Epogen. Package Insert. Thousand Oaks, CA: Amgen; December 2013.
106. Aranesp. Package Insert. Thousand Oaks, CA: Amgen; July 2015.
107. Macdougall IC, Roger SD, de Francisco A, et al. Antibody-mediated pure red cell aplasia in chronic kidney disease patients receiving erythropoiesis-stimulating agents: New insights. *Kidney Int* 2012;81:727-732.
108. Macdougall IC, Casadevall N, Locatelli F, et al. Incidence of erythropoietin antibody-mediated pure red cell aplasia: The Prospective Immunogenicity Surveillance Registry (PRIMS). *Nephrol Dial Transplant* 2015;30:451-460.
109. Hazzan AD, Shah HH, Hong S, Sakhiya V, Wanchoo R, Fishbane S. Treatment with erythropoiesis-stimulating agents in chronic kidney disease patients with cancer. *Kidney Int* 2014;86:34-39.
110. Pergola PE, Gartenberg G, Fu M, Sun S, Wolfson M, Bowers P. A randomized controlled study comparing once-weekly to every-2-week and every-4-week dosing of epoetin alfa in CKD patients with anemia. *Clin J Am Soc Nephrol* 2010;5:598-606.
111. Eknoyan G, Levin A, Levin NW. Bone metabolism and disease in chronic kidney disease. *Am J Kidney Dis* 2003;42:1-201.
112. Rivara MB, Ravel V, Kalantar-Zadeh K, et al. uncorrected and albumin-corrected calcium, phosphorus, and mortality in patients undergoing maintenance dialysis. *J Am Soc Nephrol* 2015;26:1671-1681.
113. Souberbielle JC, Roth H, Fouque DP. Parathyroid hormone measurement in CKD. *Kidney Int* 2010;77:93-100.
114. Tentori F, Wang M, Bieber BA, et al. Recent changes in therapeutic approaches and association with outcomes among patients with secondary hyperparathyroidism on chronic hemodialysis: The DOPPS study. *Clin J Am Soc Nephrol* 2015;10:98-109.
115. Dasgupta I, Shroff R, Bennett-Jones D, McVeigh G. Management of hyperphosphataemia in chronic kidney disease: Summary of National Institute for Health and Clinical Excellence (NICE) guideline. *Nephron Clin Pract* 2013;124:1-9.
116. Martin KJ, Gonzalez EA. Prevention and control of phosphate retention/hyperphosphatemia in CKD-MBD: What is normal, when to start, and how to treat? *Clin J Am Soc Nephrol* 2011;6:440-446.
117. Daugirdas JT. Removal of Phosphorus by Hemodialysis. *Semin Dial* 2015;28:620-623.
118. Ishani A, Liu J, Wetmore JB, et al. Clinical outcomes after parathyroidectomy in a nationwide cohort of patients on hemodialysis. *Clin J Am Soc Nephrol* 2015;10:90-97.
119. Wetmore JB, Liu J, Do TP, et al. Changes in secondary hyperparathyroidism-related biochemical parameters and medication use following parathyroidectomy. *Nephrol Dial Transplant* 2015 Aug 19 pii gfv291 [Epub ahead of print] 2015;10.1093/ndt/gfv291.
120. Fishbane S, Delmez J, Suki WN, et al. A randomized, parallel, open-label study to compare once-daily sevelamer carbonate powder dosing with thrice-daily sevelamer hydrochloride tablet dosing in CKD patients on hemodialysis. *Am J Kidney Dis* 2010;55:307-315.
121. Floege J, Covic AC, Ketteler M, et al. Long-term effects of the iron-based phosphate binder, sucroferric oxyhydroxide, in dialysis patients. *Nephrol Dial Transplant* 2015;30:1037-1046.
122. Lewis JB, Sika M, Koury MJ, et al. Ferric citrate controls phosphorus and delivers iron in patients on dialysis. *J Am Soc Nephrol* 2015;26: 493-503.
123. Moazzam AA, Boongird S. Ingestion of lanthanum carbonate tablets. *Am J Kidney Dis* 2013;62:844.
124. Wan LY, Zhang YQ, Chen MD, Liu CB, Wu JF. Relationship of structure and function of DNA-binding domain in vitamin D receptor. *Molecules* 2015;20:12389-12399.
125. Bailie GR, Johnson CA. Comparative review of the pharmacokinetics of vitamin D analogues. *Semin Dial* 2002;15:352-357.
126. Zemplar Injection Package Insert. North Chicago, IL: AbbVie, Inc.; 2013.
127. Hectorol Injection. Package Insert. Cambridge, MA: Genzyme Corporation; 2012.
128. Zheng Z, Shi H, Jia J, Li D, Lin S. Vitamin D supplementation and mortality risk in chronic kidney disease: A meta-analysis of 20 observational studies. *BMC Nephrol* 2013;14:199.
129. Thadhani R, Appelbaum E, Pritchett Y, Chang Y, et al. Vitamin D therapy and cardiac structure and function in patients with chronic kidney disease: The PRIMO randomized controlled trial. *JAMA* 2012;307:674-684.
130. de Zeeuw D, Agarwal R, Amdahl M, et al. Selective vitamin D receptor activation with paricalcitol for reduction of albuminuria in patients with type 2 diabetes (VITAL study): A randomised controlled trial. *Lancet* 2010;376:1543-1551.
131. Kandula P, Dobre M, Schold JD, Schreiber MJ, Jr., Mehrotra R, Navaneethan SD. Vitamin D supplementation in chronic kidney disease: A systematic review and meta-analysis of observational studies and randomized controlled trials. *Clin J Am Soc Nephrol* 2011;6:50-62.
132. Sensipar (cinacalcet HCl) Tablets Package Insert. Thousand Oaks, CA: Amgen Inc.; 2014.
133. Raggi P, Chertow GM, Torres PU, et al. The ADVANCE study: A randomized study to evaluate the effects of cinacalcet plus low-dose vitamin D on vascular calcification in patients on hemodialysis. *Nephrol Dial Transplant* 2011;26:1327-1339.
134. Block GA, Zaun D, Smits G, et al. Cinacalcet hydrochloride treatment significantly improves all-cause and cardiovascular survival in a large cohort of hemodialysis patients. *Kidney Int* 2010;78:578-589.

135. Chertow GM, Block GA, Correa-Rotter R, et al. Effect of cinacalcet on cardiovascular disease in patients undergoing dialysis. *N Engl J Med* 2012;367:2482-2494.
136. Yusuf AA, Howell BL, Powers CA, St Peter WL. Utilization and costs of medications associated with CKD mineral and bone disorder in dialysis patients enrolled in Medicare Part D. *Am J Kidney Dis* 2014;64:770-780.
137. U.S. Renal Data System, USRDS 2011 Annual Data Report: *Atlas of Chronic Kidney Disease and End-Stage Renal Disease in the United States*, Bethesda, MD: National Institutes of Health, National Institute of Diabetes and Digestive and Kidney Diseases; 2011.
138. 2012 Annual Report of the Dialysis Outcomes and Practice Patterns Study: Hemodialysis Data 1997-2011. Arbor Research Collaborative for Health AA, MI.
139. Clement FM, Klarenbach S, Tonelli M, Wiebe N, Hemmelgarn B, Manns BJ. An economic evaluation of erythropoiesis-stimulating agents in CKD. *Am J Kidney Dis* 2010;56:1050-1061.
140. Goto S, Komaba H, Fukagawa M, Nishi S. Optimizing the cost-effectiveness of treatment for chronic kidney disease-mineral and bone disorder. *Kidney Int Suppl* 2013;3:457-461.
141. Saran R, Li Y, Robinson B, et al. US Renal Data System 2014 Annual Data Report: Epidemiology of Kidney Disease in the United States. *Am J Kidney Dis* 2015;66:S1-305.
142. Ardhanari S, Alpert MA, Aggarwal K. Cardiovascular disease in chronic kidney disease: risk factors, pathogenesis, and prevention. *Adv Perit Dial* 2014;30:40-53.
143. Choi HY, Park HC, Ha SK. How do we manage coronary artery disease in patients with CKD and ESRD? *Electrolyte Blood Press* 2014;12:41-54.
144. Beattie JN, Soman SS, Sandberg KR, et al. Determinants of mortality after myocardial infarction in patients with advanced renal dysfunction. *Am J Kidney Dis* 2001;37:1191-1200.
145. McCullough PA, Sandberg KR, Borzak S, Hudson MP, Garg M, Manley HJ. Benefits of aspirin and beta-blockade after myocardial infarction in patients with chronic kidney disease. *Am Heart J* 2002;144:226-232.
146. Jardine MJ, Ninomiya T, Perkovic V, et al. Aspirin is beneficial in hypertensive patients with chronic kidney disease: A post-hoc subgroup analysis of a randomized controlled trial. *J Am Coll Cardiol* 2010;56:956-965.
147. Best PJ, Steinhubl SR, Berger PB, et al. The efficacy and safety of short- and long-term dual antiplatelet therapy in patients with mild or moderate chronic kidney disease: Results from the Clopidogrel for the Reduction of Events During Observation (CREDO) trial. *Am Heart J* 2008;155:687-693.
148. Wali RK. Aspirin and the prevention of cardiovascular disease in chronic kidney disease: Time to move forward? *J Am Coll Cardiol* 2010;56:966-968.
149. KDOQI Clinical Practice Guidelines for Cardiovascular Disease in Dialysis Patients. *Am J Kidney Dis* 2005;45:16-153.
150. KDIGO Clinical Practice Guideline for Lipid Management in Chronic Kidney Disease. *Kidney Int Suppl* 2013;3:259-305.
151. Palmer SC, Craig JC, Navaneethan SD, Tonelli M, Pellegrini F, Strippoli GF. Benefits and harms of statin therapy for persons with chronic kidney disease: A systematic review and meta-analysis. *Ann Intern Med* 2012;157:263-275.
152. Wanner C, Krane V, Marz W, et al. Atorvastatin in patients with type 2 diabetes mellitus undergoing hemodialysis. *N Engl J Med* 2005;353:238-248.
153. Fellstrom BC, Jardine AG, Schmieder RE, et al. Rosuvastatin and cardiovascular events in patients undergoing hemodialysis. *N Engl J Med* 2009;360:1395-1407.
154. Baigent C, Landray MJ, Reith C, et al. The effects of lowering LDL cholesterol with simvastatin plus ezetimibe in patients with chronic kidney disease (Study of Heart and Renal Protection): A randomised placebo-controlled trial. *Lancet* 2011;377:2181-2192.
155. Palmer SC, Navaneethan SD, Craig JC, et al. HMG CoA reductase inhibitors (statins) for dialysis patients. *Cochrane Database Syst Rev* 2013;9:CD004289.
156. Palmer SC, Navaneethan SD, Craig JC, et al. HMG CoA reductase inhibitors (statins) for people with chronic kidney disease not requiring dialysis. *Cochrane Database Syst Rev* 2014;5:CD007784.

Hemodialysis and Peritoneal Dialysis

45

Kevin M. Sowinski, Mariann D. Churchwell, and Brian S. Decker

KEY CONCEPTS

1. Hemodialysis (HD) involves the perfusion of blood and dialysate on opposite sides of a semipermeable membrane. Solutes are removed from the blood by diffusion and convection. Excess plasma water is removed by ultrafiltration.
2. Native arteriovenous (AV) fistulas are the preferred access for HD because of fewer complications and a longer survival rate. Venous catheters are plagued by complications such as infection and thrombosis and often deliver low blood flow rates.
3. Adequacy of HD can be assessed by the *Kt*/*V* and urea reduction ratio (URR). The National Kidney Foundation's Kidney Disease Outcomes Quality Initiative minimum goal *Kt*/*V* is greater than 1.2 per treatment and the URR is greater than 65%.
4. During HD, patients commonly experience hypotension and cramps. Other more serious complications include infection and thrombosis of the vascular access.
5. Peritoneal dialysis (PD) involves the instillation of dialysate into the peritoneal cavity via a permanent peritoneal catheter. The peritoneal membrane lines the highly vascularized abdominal viscera and acts as the semipermeable membrane. Solutes are removed from the blood across the peritoneum via diffusion and ultrafiltration. Excess plasma water is removed via ultrafiltration created by osmotic pressure generated by various dextrose or icodextrin concentrations.
6. Patients on PD are required to instill and drain, manually or via automated systems, several liters of fresh dialysate each day. The more exchanges completed each day results in greater solute removal.
7. Peritonitis is a common complication of PD. Initial empiric therapy for peritonitis should include intraperitoneal antibiotics that are effective against both gram-positive and gram-negative organisms.
8. Nasal carriage of *Staphylococcus aureus* is associated with an increased risk of catheter-related infections and peritonitis. Prophylaxis with intranasal mupirocin (twice a day for 5 days every month) or mupirocin (daily) at the exit site can effectively reduce *S. aureus* infections.

INTRODUCTION

The three primary treatment options for patients with end-stage renal disease (ESRD) are hemodialysis (HD), peritoneal dialysis (PD), and kidney transplantation. The United States Renal Data System (USRDS) is the national system that "collects, analyzes, and distributes" data relating to patients with ESRD or Stage 5 chronic kidney disease (CKD) in the United States and releases these data yearly.[1] According to the 2014 USRDS, at the end of 2012, there were 636,905 patients in the United States with ESRD. Of these, greater than 475,000 patients were being treated with HD or PD, and 186,303 had a functioning kidney transplant. In 2012, 114,813 new patients started therapy for ESRD (dialysis or transplantation) and more than 88,000 patients died. Greater than 90 percent of new dialysis patients are treated with HD. The number of patients treated with PD has decreased steadily since 2000.[1]

Since 1972, the cost of treating ESRD (both dialysis and kidney transplantation) has been covered by Medicare. The total cost of ESRD in 2012 was $42.5 million. This includes Medicare costs ($28.6 billion) and Medicare patient obligation costs, which together make up approximately 75% of all costs. Non-Medicare costs make up the remainder of the total disease costs. Total Medicare spending for ESRD rose by 3.5 percent in 2012. Medicare spending for ESRD does not include Part D expenditures, which were $2.16 billion in 2011. ESRD consumes a vastly disproportionate amount of resources. Approximately 1% of the patients in the Medicare program have ESRD, yet the ESRD program consumes nearly 6% of the Medicare budget. Although total spending for ESRD treatment continues to climb, per-patient spending (after adjusting for inflation) was nearly unchanged from 2011 to 2012.[1]

There are some positive signs as it relates to public health and ESRD. Although the total number of dialysis patients is increasing in the United States, the number of new dialysis patients per total population has stabilized or slightly decreased from the highest value observed in 1997. The prevalence of ESRD continues to climb, reflective of reduced mortality and enhanced patient care. The two primary diagnoses and underlying etiologies of kidney disease for new patients with ESRD are diabetes and hypertension.[1] Chapter 44 provides a thorough discussion on the epidemiology of chronic kidney disease.

This chapter serves as a primer on the principles and practice of dialysis and the complications associated with the delivery of dialysis treatments. The chapter focuses on HD and PD as the modalities most commonly employed for the management of ESRD (see Chapter 43 for a discussion of the role of renal replacement therapies in the management of acute kidney injury). The pertinent factors that should be considered before the initiation of dialysis are described. The morbidity and mortality associated with HD and PD are compared, as these considerations may influence the dialysis method chosen by patients and clinicians. The variants of HD and PD are detailed, and multiple types of vascular and peritoneal access used with each (ie, catheters and surgical techniques) are illustrated. The concept of dialysis adequacy for each modality is briefly reviewed. Finally, the clinical presentation of common complications of both dialytic therapies is presented, along with pertinent nonpharmacologic and pharmacologic therapeutic approaches. Information resources that describe the influence of CKD on patient's quality of life, as well as the patient perspective on dialysis and dialysis related therapies are presented to highlight the human consequences of chronic disease.

Morbidity and Mortality in Dialysis

Morbidity in patients receiving dialysis can be assessed in a number of different ways including tabulation of the number of hospitalizations per patient-year, the number of days hospitalized per patient per year, or the incidence of certain complications. The number of all-cause hospital admissions, 1.73 hospitalizations/patient year, has fallen in recent years. Trends in hospitalization demonstrate an increase in hospitalization as a consequence of infection and cardiovascular disease and a decrease in hospitalizations as a consequence of vascular access problems. Patients with a functioning kidney transplant have a lower rate of hospitalization and shorter length of stay. Hospitalizations are more frequent for whites than for blacks, and the frequency and duration increase with age in both dialysis modality groups.[1]

The life expectancy of U.S. dialysis patients is markedly lower than that of healthy subjects of the same age and sex. In those older than 65 years, the risk of dying is 2 to 3 fold higher in dialysis patients compared to those with diabetes, cancer, heart failure, or cardiovascular disease but not receiving dialysis.[1] Adjusted all-cause mortality is 6 to 8 fold greater for dialysis patients compared with age-matched individuals. Approximately 50% of deaths in dialysis patients are cardiovascular related. In fact, those with CKD are more likely to die from cardiovascular disease before they reach ESRD. Infections, usually related to the dialysis access, are the second most common cause of death in dialysis patients. Although mortality remains high in this patient population, the overall patient mortality rate has fallen among dialysis patients since 1991. Since that time, mortality has declined by 9% (1991-2002) and 26% (2003-2012). The reductions are dependent on treatment type, and are smallest for HD and greatest for transplantation. The changes in mortality rates are more impressive when the duration of a patient's time receiving dialysis is considered. For the first several months of dialysis therapy there is marked increase in mortality, followed by a reduction over the first 12 months. Mortality rates ultimately increase with time. In the United States, only 54% of HD patients and 65% of PD patients are alive 3 years after ESRD diagnosis and initiation of dialysis treatment.[1]

In addition to high morbidity and mortality, a dialysis patient's quality of life is generally poor. For example, restrictions caused by thrice weekly HD and/or associated treatments have been shown to impact many areas of a patient's life. These include but are not limited to, physical endurance, sex, employment, social life, and diet. Patients often complain of fatigue and fear of the unknown related to their disease and its progression. The PD patient or the home HD patient may have some freedom from these restrictions, but this freedom comes with its own constraints.

Indications for Dialysis

Since first published in 2002, The National Kidney Foundation's Kidney Disease Outcome Quality Initiative (KDOQI) has been the primary treatment guideline for CKD. Although the Kidney Diseases: Improving Global Outcomes (KDIGO) guidelines[2] published in 2013 now serve as a general update to the KDOQI guidelines, the 2006 version of the KDOQI guidelines established recommendations related to dialysis initiation. Planning for dialysis initiation when a patient's kidney function declines to CKD stage 4 (estimated glomerular filtration rate [eGFR] below 30 mL/min/1.73 m^2).[3] Beginning the preparation process at this point allows adequate time for proper education of the patient and family and for the creation of a suitable vascular or peritoneal access. For patients choosing HD, a permanent arteriovenous (AV) access (preferably a fistula) should be surgically created when eGFR falls below 25 mL/min/1.73 m^2, serum creatinine is greater than 4 mg/dL (354 μmol/L) or 1 year prior to the anticipated need for dialysis.[4] The KDIGO guidelines provide recommendations for referral to a specialist in kidney care services and for planning for RRT. The recommendation for timely referral is for patients with progressive CKD in whom the risk of kidney failure within 1 year is greater than 10% based upon validated risk prediction tools.[2]

> **Clinical Controversy...**
>
> There is debate over which dialysis treatment modality, HD or PD, is most desirable in terms of morbidity and mortality. There is further debate over which type of HD is more beneficial, standard in-center HD or intensive HD. Although most U.S. patients are treated with in-center HD, other therapies may provide more benefit.

The KDIGO guidelines and commentaries addressing them agree that the primary criterion for initiation of dialysis is the patient's clinical status, rather than a specific level of kidney function.[2,5] Namely, dialysis should be initiated when one or more of the following are present: signs or symptoms of kidney failure (eg, serositis, acid-base or electrolyte abnormalities, pruritis); inability to control volume status or blood pressure; a progressive deterioration in nutritional status or cognitive impairment. The guidelines suggest that these signs and symptoms tend to be evident once the patient's eGFR is in the range of 5 to 10 mL/min/1.73 m^2. The guidelines specifically indicate that RRT should be initiated to manage signs and symptoms and not to treat an arbitrary kidney function measurement.[2] The advantages and disadvantages of HD and PD are depicted in **Tables 45-1** and **45-2**, respectively. These factors, along with the patients' concomitant diseases, personal preferences, and support environments, are the principal determinants of the dialysis mode they will receive.[6] The timing of dialysis initiation is a compromise between maximizing patient quality of life by extending the dialysis-free period while avoiding complications that will decrease the length and quality of dialysis-assisted life.[3]

While the intent of this chapter is not to exhaustively compare and contrast HD and PD and the relative benefits of each, there is considerable debate in the literature regarding the mortality differences between HD and PD.[7] Most observational trials suggest that PD is associated with a survival advantage early in therapy, which wanes with increased treatment time. Prospective trials have reported conflicting results relative to efficacy of one modality over another.

TABLE 45-1 Advantages and Disadvantages of Hemodialysis

Advantages

1. Higher solute clearance allows intermittent treatment.
2. Parameters of adequacy of dialysis are better defined and therefore underdialysis can be detected early.
3. Technique failure rate is low.
4. Even though intermittent heparinization is required, hemostasis parameters are better corrected with hemodialysis than peritoneal dialysis.
5. In-center hemodialysis enables closer monitoring of the patient.

Disadvantages

1. Requires multiple visits each week to the hemodialysis center, which translates into loss of patient independence.
2. Disequilibrium, dialysis induced hypotension, and muscle cramps are common. May require months before the patient adjusts to hemodialysis.
3. Infections in hemodialysis patients may be related to the choice of membranes, the complement-activating membranes being more deleterious.
4. Vascular access is frequently associated with infection and thrombosis.
5. Decline of residual renal function is more rapid compared to peritoneal dialysis.

TABLE 45-2 Advantages and Disadvantages of Peritoneal Dialysis

Advantages

1. Hemodynamic stability due to slow ultrafiltration rate.
2. Higher clearance of larger solutes, which may explain good clinical status in spite of lower urea clearance.
3. Better preservation of residual renal function.
4. Convenient intraperitoneal route for administration of drugs such as antibiotics and insulin.
5. Suitable for elderly and very young patients who may not tolerate hemodialysis well.
6. Freedom from the "machine" gives the patient a sense of independence (for continuous ambulatory peritoneal dialysis).
7. Less blood loss and iron deficiency, resulting in easier management of anemia or reduced requirements for erythropoietin and parenteral iron.
8. No systemic heparinization required.
9. Subcutaneous vs intravenous erythropoietin or darbepoetin may reduce overall doses and be more physiologic.

Disadvantages

1. Protein and amino acid losses through peritoneum and reduced appetite from continuous glucose load and sense of abdominal fullness predispose patients to malnutrition.
2. Risk of peritonitis.
3. Catheter malfunction, exit site, and tunnel infection.
4. Inadequate ultrafiltration and solute clearance in patients with a large body size, unless large volumes and frequent exchanges are employed.
5. Patient burnout and high rate of technique failure.
6. Risk of obesity with excessive glucose absorption.
7. Mechanical problems such as hernias, dialysate leaks, hemorrhoids, or back pain are more common than HD.
8. Extensive abdominal surgery may preclude peritoneal dialysis.
9. No convenient access for intravenous iron administration.

If there is a survival advantage for PD, the consensus is that the advantage is early in therapy and not with continued therapy. Well-designed studies are extremely difficult to conduct in this population and thus the question of superiority of one modality over the other is controversial. Differences in outcomes may be related to a wide array of confounding factors, such as the dose of dialysis, baseline patient health status, physician bias in modality selection, patient compliance with dialysis and medication therapy, or other unknown factors. For example, healthier patients tend to be directed toward PD and factors such as age, duration of dialysis, and comorbidities play an important role in the complex relationship between patient outcomes and mortality.[8] Without clear distinction between modalities in terms of many important outcomes, the selection of the optimal therapy for a given patient is challenging. The selection of one modality over the other should be based upon patient motivation, desire, geographic distance from a HD unit, health care team preference, and patient education rather than survival advantages alone.

HEMODIALYSIS

Although HD was first successfully used in 1940, the procedure was not used widely until the Korean War in 1952. Permanent dialysis access was developed in the 1960s,[9] which allowed routine use of HD in patients with ESRD. Subsequent decades brought advances in dialysis technology, including the introduction of more efficient and biocompatible dialyzer membranes and safer techniques. HD is now the most common type of renal replacement therapy for patients with ESRD.

Principles of Hemodialysis

1 Hemodialysis consists of the perfusion of blood and a physiologic solution on opposite sides of a semipermeable membrane. Multiple substances, such as water, urea, creatinine, potassium, uremic toxins, and drugs, move from the blood into the dialysate, by either passive diffusion or convection as the result of ultrafiltration. Diffusion is the movement of substances down a concentration gradient. The rate of diffusion depends on the difference between the concentration of the solute in blood and dialysate, solute characteristics, ie, size, water solubility, and charge, the dialyzer membrane composition, and blood and dialysate flow rates. Diffusive transport is rapid for small solutes, but decreases with increasing molecular size. Other important diffusive solute transport factors include the membrane thickness, porosity and the steric hindrance between the membrane pores and solute. Ultrafiltration is the movement of water across the dialyzer membrane as a consequence of hydrostatic or osmotic pressure and is the primary means for removal of excess fluid. Convection occurs when dissolved solutes are "dragged" across a membrane with water transport. This occurs only if the pores in the dialyzer are large enough to allow them to pass along with water. Convection can be maximized by increasing the hydrostatic pressure gradient across the dialysis membrane, or by changing to a dialyzer that is more permeable to water transport. Diffusion and convection can be controlled independently, and thus a patient's HD prescription can be individualized to attain the desired degree of solute and fluid removal.

Hemodialysis Access

2 Obtaining and maintaining access to the circulation has been a challenge for long-term use and success of HD. Permanent access to the circulation may be accomplished by several techniques, including the creation of an AV fistula, an AV graft, or by the use of venous catheters (Fig. 45-1).[10] The native AV fistula is created by the anastomosis of a vein and artery (ie, the radial artery to the cephalic vein or the brachial artery to the cephalic vein). The native AV fistula has many advantages including providing the longest survival time of all blood-access devices and the lowest rate of complications such as infection and thrombosis. Patients with fistulas have increased survival and lower hospitalization rates compared to other HD patients. Finally, AV fistulas are the most cost-effective in terms of placement and long-term maintenance. Ideally, the most distal site (the wrist) is used to construct the first fistula; it is the easiest to create, and in the case of access failure, more proximal sites on the arm are preserved for later use. Unfortunately, fistulas require at least 1 to 2 months to mature before they can be routinely utilized for dialysis. Creation of an AV fistula however may be difficult in elderly patients and in patients with peripheral vascular disease, which is a particularly common comorbidity in patients with diabetes.

Synthetic AV grafts, usually made of polytetrafluoroethylene, are another permanent AV access option. These grafts require only 2 to 3 weeks before they can be routinely used. Their primary disadvantages are shorter survival of the graft, and higher rates of infection and thrombosis. The least-desirable and least permanent HD access option involves the placement of a central venous catheter. Venous catheters can be placed in the femoral, subclavian, or internal jugular veins. Their main advantage is that they can be used immediately and they are often used in small children, diabetic patients with severe vascular disease, the morbidly obese, and patients who have no viable sites for permanent AV access. Late referrals to a nephrology specialist and delayed placement of a more appropriate long-term access contribute to the use of venous catheters in chronic HD patients. The major problem with all venous catheters is they have a short life span and are more prone to infection and thrombosis than either AV grafts or fistulas. Furthermore, some catheters are not able to provide adequate blood flow rates, which can limit the deliverable dose of dialysis.[10-12] Regardless, tunneled dialysis catheters are used frequently because of the ease of insertion, pain-free dialysis needle placement and availability for immediate use. They are however associated with increased morbidity, mortality and cost.[13]

Hemodialysis Procedures

The HD system consists of an external vascular circuit through which the patient's blood is transferred in sterile polyethylene tubing

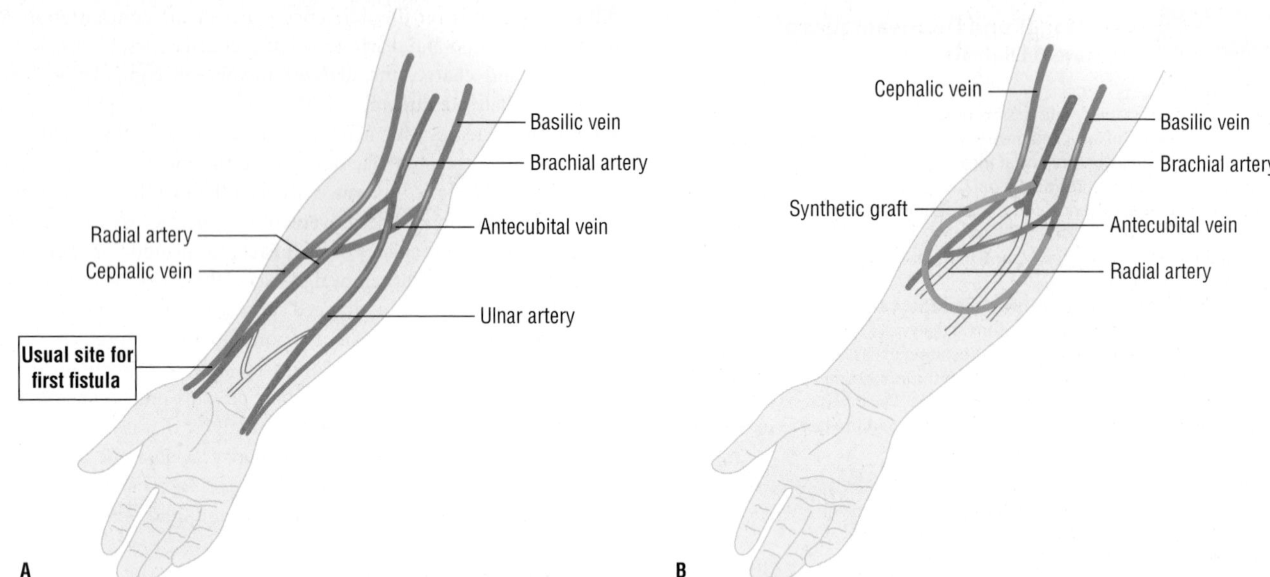

FIGURE 45-1 The predominant types of vascular access for chronic dialysis patients are (*A*) the arteriovenous fistula and (*B*) the synthetic arteriovenous forearm graft. The first primary arteriovenous fistula is usually created by the surgical anastomosis of the cephalic vein with the radial artery. The flow of blood from the higher-pressure arterial system results in hypertrophy of the vein. The most common AV graft (depicted in green) is between the brachial artery and the basilic or cephalic vein. The flow of blood may be diminished in the radial and ulnar arteries since it preferentially flows into the low pressure graft.

to the dialyzer via a mechanical pump (Fig. 45-2).[14] The patient's blood then passes through the dialyzer on one side of the semipermeable membrane and is returned to the patient. The dialysate solution, which consists of purified water and electrolytes, is pumped through the dialyzer countercurrent to the flow of blood on the opposite side of the semipermeable membrane. In most cases, systemic anticoagulation (with heparin) is used to prevent blood clotting in the HD circuit tubing. The process of dialysis results in the removal of metabolic waste products, medications, and water and replenishment of body buffers, such as acetate and bicarbonate.

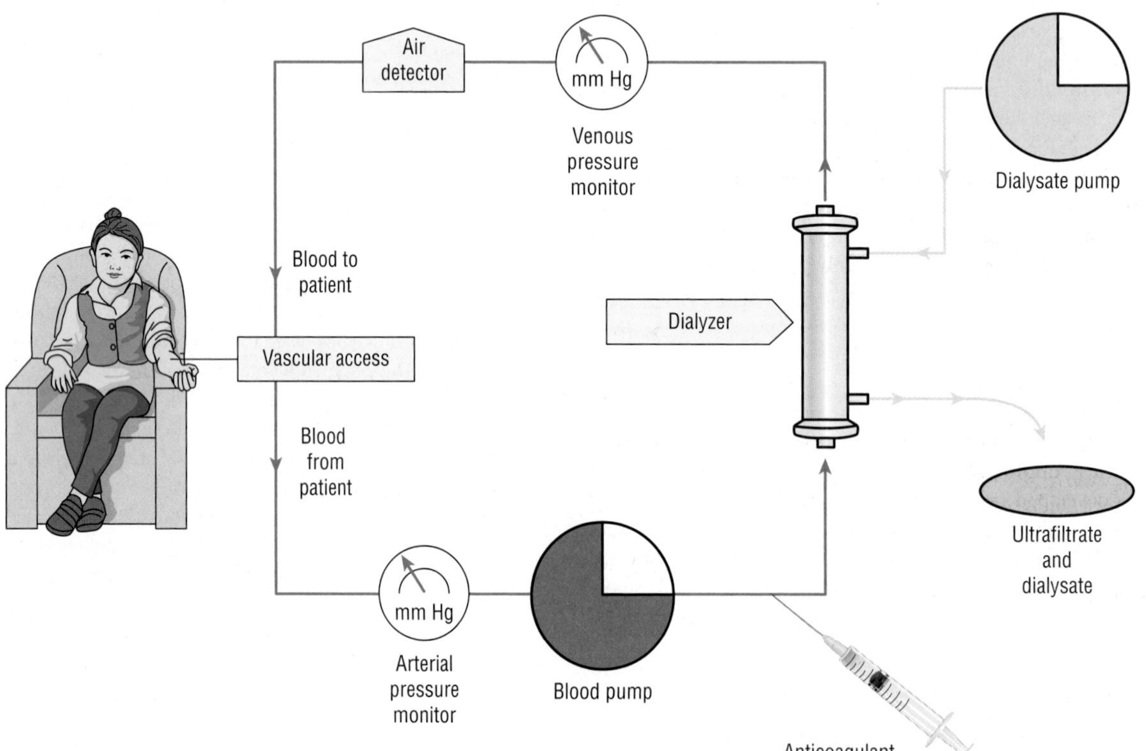

FIGURE 45-2 In hemodialysis, the patient's blood is pumped to the dialyzer at a rate of 300 to 600 mL/min. An anticoagulant (usually heparin) is administered to prevent clotting in the dialyzer. The dialysate is pumped at a rate of 500 to 1,000 mL/min through the dialyzer countercurrent to the flow of blood. The rate of fluid removal from the patient is controlled by adjusting the pressure in the dialysate compartment.

Hemodialfiltration (HDF) another variant of traditional HD enhances convective solute and water transport in addition to diffusive clearance to a much greater extent than high-flux HD.[15-17] When fluid losses exceed those desired for the patient, an IV infusion referred to as replacement fluid may be administered. HDF may improve outcomes due to its ability to remove middle molecular weight uremic solutes more efficiently than the other HD variants. Recent evidence suggests that HDF improves survival compared to conventional HD.[16,18] Preliminary information suggests that HDF enhances clearance of phosphate, beta-2 microglobulin and pro-inflammatory solutes. Currently, this procedure is not used extensively in the United States. Barriers to its use are the high cost and logistic issues associated with providing the fluid replacement needs.

Three categories of dialysis membranes have historically been utilized: low flux, high efficiency, and high flux. Low-flux and high-efficiency dialyzers, have small pores that limit clearance to relatively small molecules (size less than or equal to 500 daltons) such as urea and creatinine and are currently utilized for less than 20% of chronic HD procedures.[14] High-flux dialyzers are now used in the vast majority of patients because they are capable of removing high-molecular-weight endogenous substances, such as β_2-microglobulin, and medications such as vancomycin.[14,19] The primary reason to use high-flux membranes is that clearance of water as well as low- and high-molecular-weight substances is much greater allowing for shorter treatment times. To maximize the clearance capacity of high flux dialyzers the blood flow rates should be 400 to 600 mL/min, dialysate flow rates greater than 500 mL/min, which necessitates strict controls and active monitoring of the rate of fluid removal. Typically these dialyzers are composed of polysulfone, polymethylmethacrylate, polyamide, cellulose triacetate, and polyacrylonitrile.[14]

Hemodialysis is usually prescribed as three sessions weekly for 3 to 5 hours per session. These sessions are usually performed in "in-center" dialysis units. This is a large time commitment for any patient undergoing HD and results in substantial loss of control over their life. Several variants of HD have been explored in an effort to balance dialysis adequacy with patient outcomes and quality of life, including "intensive dialysis" procedures that increase dialysis frequency, enhance dialysis duration, or both.[20-22] Examples of these procedures include: 1) frequent HD (5-7 sessions/week), which can be frequent short (1.5-3 hours/session), frequent standard (3-5 hours/session), or frequent long sessions (longer than 5 hours/session); 2) long-session length regimens (more than 5 hours/session given 3 times/week or every other day; 3) short and standard frequent HD (also called daily HD); and 4) long frequent HD (or Nocturnal HD), typically performed at night. Many of these procedures that increase the frequency or duration of dialysis maybe associated with improved survival.[20-22] For example, in-center, thrice weekly HD was associated with a higher risk of the composite outcome of death, left-ventricular mass and change in health composite score than in-center six-times per week HD.[23] Intensive dialysis has been associated with reductions in left-ventricular mass and improved blood pressure control, both surrogates for improved cardiovascular outcomes, and improved phosphate removal. Lastly, and perhaps most importantly, these procedures are associated with a reduction in dialysis related symptoms and improved quality of life.[20-22] Despite the perceived advantages and more frequent use in other countries such as New Zealand and Canada, the use of home HD is uncommon in the United States, with less than 1% of dialysis patients receiving HD care at home.[1] Potential obstacles to home HD include patient factors (eg, lack of self-efficacy, fear of self-cannulation, fear of catastrophic event, and fear of lack of quality care), and a lack of awareness of the availability of this type of dialysis.[24,25] Finally, there are suggestions that patients receiving intensive dialysis may be at higher risk of access infections and need for vascular access procedures. Further clinical trials are needed to elucidate the role of these types of dialysis therapy.

Adequacy of Hemodialysis

The optimal dose of HD, the patient's dialysis prescription, is that amount of therapy above which there is no cost-effective increment in the patient's quality-adjusted life expectancy. The two primary goals of the dialysis prescription are to achieve the patient's dry weight and the adequate removal of endogenous waste products such as urea. Dry weight is the target postdialysis weight at which the patient is normotensive and free of edema. Measurement of urea removal, while imperfect, is the typical method used to quantify dialysis adequacy. Urea removal reflects the "delivered dose" of dialysis and is utilized as the surrogate for removal of other toxins.

The delivered or desired dose of dialysis in terms of solute removal can be expressed as the urea reduction ratio (URR) or the *Kt/V* (pronounced "K-T-over-V"). The URR is a simple concept and is easily calculated as:

$$\text{URR} = \frac{\text{Predialysis BUN} - \text{Postdialysis BUN}}{\text{Predialysis BUN}} \times 100$$

The URR is frequently used to measure the delivered dialysis dose, however, it does not account for the contribution of convective removal of urea. The *Kt/V* is a unitless index based on the dialyzer clearance of urea (*K*) in L/h multiplied by the duration of dialysis (*t*) in hours, divided by the urea distribution volume of the patient (*V*) in liters.[26] *Kt/V* is thus the fraction of the patient's total body water that is cleared of urea during a dialysis session. Urea kinetic modeling, using computer software, is the optimal means to calculate the *Kt/V*.[27] An in-depth discussion of the pros and cons of various methods of calculating and interpreting *Kt/V* is beyond the scope of this chapter. The reader is referred to other sources for more in-depth information.[26,27]

3 The KDOQI recommends that the minimally adequate delivered dose of dialysis is a *Kt/V* of 1.2 (equivalent to an average URR of 65%).[3] To achieve this goal, the recommended target prescribed *Kt/V* is 1.4 (equivalent to an average URR of 70%).[3] Lower doses of dialysis treatment are thought to be associated with increased morbidity and mortality. Many nephrologists believe that even greater doses of dialysis would have positive outcomes in dialysis patients, and so the average dose of dialysis has been increasing in the United States. In 2004, the mean delivered *Kt/V* as reported by the CPM was 1.55.[28] The results of HEMO study a prospective, randomized trial that assigned patients to either standard (*Kt/V* = 1.25) or high-dose (*Kt/V* = 1.65) dialysis with high-flux or low-flux membranes revealed that the risk of death was similar in both the standard and high-dose therapy and the low- and high-flux groups. Thus there does not appear to be any benefit in increasing the dose of dialysis above the current recommendations. The HEMO study only enrolled patients who were on traditional thrice-weekly dialysis, so the applicability of these findings to patients on more intensive regimens such as daily or nocturnal HD regimens remain to be determined.[29] However, intensive HD regimens may result in better blood pressure, anemia, and phosphate control.[29] In those relatively few patients who are below the adequacy goal, the deficiency may be related to patient compliance with the dialysis prescription (ie, ending dialysis early) or low blood flow rates caused by access stenosis or thrombosis, or due to the use of catheters. Adequate dialysis may not be achieved in some patients despite compliance and sufficient blood flow. For these patients there are two options to increase urea clearance: use a larger membrane or increase the treatment time.

Complications of Hemodialysis

4 Complications associated with HD therapy are significant and can limit therapy efficacy. These complications that occur during the actual therapy (intradialytic), as well as those associated with vascular access are discussed in this chapter.[30,31]

TABLE 45-3 Common Complications during Hemodialysis[37]

	Incidence (%)	Etiology/Predisposing Factors
Hypotension	20-30	Hypovolemia and excessive ultrafiltration
		Antihypertensive medications prior to dialysis
		Target dry weight too low
		Diastolic dysfunction
		Autonomic dysfunction
		Low calcium and sodium in dialysate
		High dialysate temperature
		Meal ingestion prior to or during dialysis
Hypertension	5-15	Plasma sodium concentration
		Intravascular volume
		Dialytic removal of antihypertensive medications
		Activation of the Renin Angiotensin Aldosterone system
Cramps	5-20	Muscle hypoperfusion due to ultrafiltration and hypovolemia
		Hypotension
		Electrolyte imbalance
		Acid-base imbalance
Nausea and vomiting	5-15	Hypotension
		Dialyzer reaction
Headache	5	Disequilibrium syndrome
		Caffeine withdrawal due to dialysis removal
Chest and back pain	2-5	Unknown
Pruritus	5	Inadequate dialysis
		Skin dryness
		Secondary hyperparathyroidism
		Abnormal skin concentrations of electrolytes
		Histamine release
		Mast cell proliferation
Fever and chills	<1	Endotoxin release; Infection of dialysis catheter

Hemodialysis Procedure Complications

The most common complications that occur during the HD procedure include hypotension, hypertension, cramps, nausea and vomiting, headache, chest pain, back pain, and fever or chills.[30,31] Table 45-3 lists these complications and their etiology and predisposing factors.

A decrease in blood pressure is often noted during HD, but a symptomatic decline in blood pressure that requires nursing or medical intervention can lead to a decrease in the effectiveness of this treatment.[31] Intradialytic hypotension (IDH) is primarily related to the rate and amount of fluid removed during[30,31] typical treatments, although other causes, as listed in Table 45-4, may also play a role.[30,31] Other symptoms such as nausea and cramping are often present during acute hypotensive episodes. The replacement of acetate with bicarbonate as the dialysate buffer, the use of volumetric ultrafiltration controllers, as well as individualized or modeled dialysate sodium concentrations have helped reduce the incidence of IDH. Sodium modeling uses a higher initial dialysate sodium concentration (145-155 mM) and tapers the sodium concentration down (135-140 mM) over the dialytic session. Dialytic treatment modifications such as sodium individualizing or modeling may decrease intradialytic weight gain and post-HD thirst decreasing hypotension related to aggressive dialytic fluid removal.[32-34]

TABLE 45-4 Management of Hypotension

Acute treatment	Place patient in Trendelenburg position
	Decrease ultrafiltration rate
	Give 100-200 mL bolus of normal saline intravenous
	Give 10-20 mL of hypertonic saline (23.4%) intravenous over 3-5 minutes
	Give 12.5 g mannitol
Prevention	
Nonpharmacologic	Accurately set "dry weight"
	Use steady constant ultrafiltration rate
	Keep dialysate sodium >serum sodium
	Lower dialysate temperatures
	Bicarbonate dialysate
	Avoid food before or during hemodialysis
Pharmacologic	Midodrine 2.5-10 mg orally 30 minutes before hemodialysis (start at 2.5 mg and titrate)
	Other options (limited evidence):
	Levocarnitine 20 mg/kg IV after hemodialysis
	Sertraline 50-100 mg daily
	Fludrocortisone 0.1 mg before hemodialysis
	DDAVP 1-2 intranasal sprays (150 mcg per spray)

Intradialytic or post-HD hypertension can occur in 5% to 15% of HD patients and may increase the risk of cardiovascular and all-cause mortality.[35] Underlying causes can include, not achieving postHD dry weight goal, over-estimation of dry weight, dialytic removal of antihypertensive medications or the activation of the renin-angiotensin system secondary to abrupt hypovolemia.[36]

Skeletal muscle cramps complicate 5% to 20% of HD treatments. Although the pathogenesis of cramps is multifactorial, plasma volume contraction and decreased muscle perfusion caused by excessive ultrafiltration are frequently the initiating events.[37] Pruritus, another complication that may appear to increase in severity during the HD treatment, is actually a complication of CKD and the management of this condition is discussed in Chapter 44.

Vascular Access Complications

The maintenance of vascular access patency is critical for HD patients. Aneurysm and stenosis are associated with AV fistulas and grafts, and these are resolved primarily by surgical intervention. Thrombosis and infection are the most common vascular access complications with the highest occurrence found in patients with a catheter compared with those with an AV graft or AV fistula.[31,38,39]

Vascular access dysfunction is usually identified by a decrease in blood flow through the access (blood flow less than 300 mL/min) over a period of days to weeks. Ultrasound, venography, or computed tomography scans can provide a definitive diagnosis.[39,40] Catheter thrombosis can form either inside (intrinsic) or outside (extrinsic) the catheter. The occlusion can form within the lumen at the tip or develop a fibrin sleeve around the catheter where this fibrin sleeve can serve as a nidus for infection and ultimately require catheter removal.[41,42]

Infection is a leading cause of mortality in HD patients.[1] The risk of sepsis-related death is 100 times greater in dialysis patients than the general population and those with an indwelling catheter have the highest risk.[42] Frequently, *Staphylococcus aureus* and coagulase-negative staphylococcus are the source of infection, but gram-negative bacterial and fungal causes must also be considered. Catheter-related infections develop at the insertion site, hub, or both. The infection source for long-term catheters such as a tunneled cuffed catheter is usually the hub where bacteria can enter the blood leading to a bloodstream infection.[39,42] Overall, HD access with a catheter is associated with higher rates of bacteremia, osteomyelitis, septic arthritis, endocarditis, thrombus and death, as well as increased treatment costs compared with an AV fistula or AV graft.[38,43]

Complications of CKD

HD patients are likely to have at least one additional co-morbid disease such as diabetes, hypertension, cardiovascular disease, or obesity (BMI greater than or equal to 30 kg/m^2 and older age, greater than or equal to 60). The pharmacotherapy management of most CKD complications and the multitude of co-morbid diseases that persist in HD patients are described in Chapter 44. The daily medication burden for HD patients is one of the highest for any chronic disease state, on average 11 medications (9 oral and 2 parenteral), which based on the oral medications alone results in a total burden of about 19 dosages per day. This burden is associated with a lower quality of life in HD patients.[44]

Management of Hemodialysis Complications

The management of HD complications are discussed in this section. The most common causes of HD complications and appropriate management are reviewed.

Hypotension

Acute management of (IDH) includes placing the patient in the Trendelenburg position, decreasing the ultrafiltration rate, lowering the dialysate temperature, modifying dialysate electrolyte concentrations, and/or administering normal or hypertonic saline.[30,33,34,37,45] IDH may not occur during each HD session and a patient's response to therapeutic modifications can be variable, which could necessitate modification of their HD prescription. Antihypertensive medications administered prior to HD therapy may contribute to IDH; therefore, a careful review of all medications including antihypertensive therapies is warranted. Patients with IDH should be counseled to take their blood pressure medications after HD.

Intradialytic hypotension is often due to an insufficient cardiac response to reduced circulating blood volume; therefore, most treatments are directed toward restoring or maintaining adequate blood vessel perfusion in these patients. For example, decreasing the dialysate temperature to 36.5°C (97.7°F) may help reduce core body temperature, which can decrease vasodilation.[40,45,46] If nonpharmacologic interventions are not adequate to prevent or reduce the incidence of symptomatic IDH, then pharmacologic interventions should be considered (see Table 45-4).

Oral midodrine (5 mg) given 2 to 3 times daily can increase blood pressure in HD patients with chronic hypotension on nondialysis days. It is important to note that the effects of midodrine are probably best in patients with hypotension related to autonomic dysfunction. Patients with peripheral vascular disease should be monitored for digital or lower limb ischemia.[47]

Other potential therapeutic agents for IDH include levocarnitine, sertraline and intra-nasal desmopressin acetate (DDAVP). Administration of levocarnitine (20 mg/kg IV at the end of each dialysis session) may reduce hypotensive episodes, particularly with carnitine deficiency.[48] High cost and limited efficacy precludes a strong recommendation for routine levocarnitine use. The administration of sertraline 50 mg daily titrated to 100 mg daily after 1 week improved systolic and diastolic blood pressure in a small trial.[49] An earlier study administered sertraline 50 mg daily and did not report an increase in post-HD blood pressure.[50] The mixed results do not support routine sertraline administration for hypotension. Overall, the use of DDAVP increased post-HD blood pressure and decreased the incidence of IDH.[51] In addition, fludrocortisone has been suggested as a potential agent for symptomatic hypotension. These medications have limited clinical evidence and should be used with caution in HD patients with IDH.

Hypertension

An increase in blood pressure either during or postHD may require a change in the delivery of a HD session, as well as changes in antihypertensive medications or adjustments to the timing of medication administration.[36] Carvedilol initiated at 6.25 mg twice daily and titrated up to 50 mg twice daily as tolerated significantly improved intradialytic hypertension in patients receiving HD. During HD sessions patients receiving carvedilol need to be monitored for bradycardia and hypotension. Although this small trial provides a possible treatment option for intradialytic hypertension initiation of carvedilol in HD patients requires careful titration and monitoring.

Muscle Cramps

Nonpharmacologic interventions related to dialytic therapy may help alleviate muscle cramps. These measures include adjusting the ultrafiltration rate to avoid hypotension, volume contraction or hypoosmolality. Other methods to reduce muscle cramps, including compression devices, moist heat, massage, exercise, stretching or muscle flexing should be considered first to minimize adverse consequences (Table 45-5).[30,31]

Both vitamin E and quinine can significantly reduce the incidence of muscle cramps.[52,53] Quinine is well tolerated, but rarely may cause temporary sight and hearing disturbances, thrombocytopenia, or gastrointestinal distress. Although, quinine sulfate is available as 324 mg capsule (Qualaquin, URL Pharma, Philadelphia, PA) it is only FDA approved for malaria. The FDA has warned against the off-label use of quinine for muscle cramps.[54] The dosage for HD-related muscle cramps is one capsule (324 mg) either at bedtime or 1 to 2 hours prior to HD.

Both vitamin E (400 mg) and vitamin C (250 mg) reduce the frequency of cramps in dialysis patients.[55] The combination of these two drugs had an additive effect. Although these data further strengthen the case for vitamin E, it is unclear what role oral vitamin C would play since many patients are on a renal multiple vitamin containing vitamin C. Furthermore, both vitamin C and vitamin E as long-term therapy must be used with caution since doses of vitamin E greater than 400 units per day have been reported to increase mortality and there is a risk of systemic oxalosis with the accumulation of a vitamin C metabolite, oxalate in HD patients. Pharmacologic interventions to diminish muscle cramps are limited and currently vitamin E has the strongest evidence-based efficacy and safety profile.

TABLE 45-5 Management of Cramps

Acute treatment	Give 100-200 mL bolus of intravenous normal saline
	Give 10-20 mL of intravenous hypertonic saline (23.4%) over 3-5 minutes
	Give 50 mL of 50% intravenous glucose (nondiabetic patients)
Prevention	
Nonpharmacologic	Accurately set "dry weight"
	Keep dialysate sodium >serum sodium
	Stretching exercises, massage, flexing or compression devices
Pharmacologic	Vitamin E 400 international units at bedtime.
	Quinine 324 mg daily (second-line therapy)

Vascular Access Thrombosis

Prevention of vascular access thrombus formation is a key to maintaining this lifeline for HD patients. Multiple oral and intravenous anticoagulant and antiplatelet agents and intravenous thrombolytic agents have been studied to ascertain their clinical value.

Clinical **Controversy...**

The use of oral anticoagulant or antiplatelet agents to maintain vascular access patency is controversial since the risk may be greater than the benefit. Studies have reported conflicting results and serious adverse reactions in HD patients that may increase morbidity and mortality.

Oral antiplatelet agents role in the prevention of vascular access thrombosis has been controversial since efficacy is not well-established and there is an increased risk of bleeding.[40,56,57] A trend toward maintaining primary AV graft patency has been shown with daily aspirin use.[56] Daily aspirin use also is associated with a lower rate of AV fistula failure and no increase in new GI bleeding.[58] The use of warfarin to maintain vascular access patency is controversial with some trials suggesting an increase in morbidity and mortality with the use of warfarin.[59-61] HD patients generally require a lower dose and are at a much higher risk of a major hemorrhagic event.[59,61]

The effect of fish oil supplementation, a combination of eicosapentaenoic acid (EPA) 400 mg and docosahexaenoic acid (DHA) 200 mg, on AV graft patency for 12 months after graft placement revealed that the loss of patency was lower in the fish oil (48%) than the placebo (62%). Fish oil thus may benefit some patients with an AV graft since time to thrombus was longer and thrombus rates were about half that of placebo.[62]

Catheter locking solutions with unfractionated heparin (UFH), recombinant tissue plasminogen activator (rt-PA), or sodium citrate instilled in each HD catheter lumen between HD sessions has been associated with a reduction in catheter thrombosis. Sodium citrate 4% is as effective as UFH but may offer a better safety profile at a reduced cost.[63] A systematic review and meta-analysis of randomized control trials of HD lock solutions containing UFH and citrate was associated with significantly fewer bleeding episodes.[64] UFH 5,000 units/mL twice weekly and recombinant tissue plasminogen activator (rt-PA) 1 mg per catheter lumen once weekly were instilled in patients receiving HD with a CVC. Alternating the catheter lock solution regimen with rt-PA significantly decreased catheter malfunction compared to the patients receiving UFH only for catheter patency. The cost of catheter replacement and hospitalization may offset the cost of once weekly administration of rt-PA.

The therapeutic alternatives for the management of venous catheter thrombosis are listed in Table 45-6. If a catheter-related thrombus is suspected, a forced saline flush should be used to clear the catheter, followed by installation of a thrombolytic. A number of studies have been published using alteplase and reteplase and initial reperfusion rates for both were approximately 90%, respectively.[65] The efficacy, safety, and cost of alteplase, reteplase, and tenecteplase were compared and venous catheter clearance rates, were similar with reteplase (88 ± 4%) and alteplase (81 ± 37%), but markedly lower with tenecteplase (41 ± 5%).[65] The cost analysis favored the use of reteplase; however, to attain these savings reteplase must be batch prepared and the fact that it is not currently FDA approved for this indication likely limits its use.[65]

Alteplase is available commercially and the only agent FDA approved, for venous catheter clearance and can be administered as a short dwell for 30 to 60 minutes, as a long dwell or left in the catheter between treatments. No difference in patency rates between the short or long dwells has been demonstrated. Alteplase has also been given as a short infusion 2 mg/h over 4 hours for a blocked catheter and 1 mg/h over 4 hours for sluggish blood flow. Infusions may theoretically be more efficacious than the dwell technique because the thrombus is only exposed to the thrombolytic at the very tip of the catheter. Another consideration is dwell versus push techniques for thrombolytic therapy, with recent data indicating a push protocol with alteplase is as effective and safe for managing HD catheter dysfunction and might be more practical than a dwell technique.[66]

TABLE 45-6 Management of Hemodialysis Catheter Thrombosis

Nonpharmacologic therapy
Forced saline flush
Referral to vascular surgeon
Pharmacologic therapy
Alteplase: instill 2 mg/2 mL per catheter lumen port; attempt to aspirate after 30 minutes; may repeat dose if catheter function is not restored in 120 minutes; longer durations of instillation have been used.
Reteplase: instill 0.4 units/0.4 mL in each lumen, attempt to aspirate after 20-30 minutes, may repeat if necessary.

Infection

HD patients who develop a fever during dialysis should immediately be evaluated for infection; blood cultures should be collected prior to the administration of any antibiotics. When an AV fistula infection is suspected, empiric broad-spectrum antibiotic therapy must be initiated usually with vancomycin plus an aminoglycoside. Antibiotic therapy, if the infection is confirmed, should continue for a total of 6 weeks and should be tailored to culture sensitivities. Unfortunately, a suspected infection in an AVG may require more than antibiotic therapy alone, and a surgical procedure to remove the infected graft material may be needed. A suspected infection in a temporary catheter may warrant catheter removal and a culture of the catheter tip should, if possible, be obtained.[41,67] Since catheter-related infections are more common than infections of an AV fistula or AVG, preventative care approaches are paramount. Preventative care includes minimizing the use and duration of catheters, proper disinfection and sterile technique, and the use of an antimicrobial ointment at the exit site (mupirocin 2%, povidone-iodine). Dialysis unit protocols that employ universal precautions, limit the manipulation of the catheter, utilize an antiseptic wash (tincture of iodine, chlorhexidine, etc.) for skin preparation, and the use of face masks by the patient and caregiver, can significantly reduce the incidence of catheter-related bacteremia.[41,67,68] Topical application of 2% mupirocin ointment to a tunneled HD catheter exit site after each HD session can increase infection-free days. However, there are concerns that the use of mupirocin prophylaxis may lead to the development of methicillin-resistant *S. aureus* (MRSA). A 6-year study that prospectively monitored HD patient catheter infection rates with a once-a-week application of a topical polysporin triple ointment (bacitracin/gramicidin/polymyxin B) to CVC exit sites did not reveal an increase in *S. aureus* resistance.[69] Alternative topical preparations to mupirocin to combat potential MRSA resistance are emerging and include octenidine dihydrochloride body wash, polyhexanide gel, and ethanol 70% combined with natural oil emollients.[70]

The Infectious Disease Society of America (IDSA) comprehensive guidelines regarding catheter care and the diagnosis and management of catheter-related infections[41,68] differ some from the KDOQI guidelines, which also provide an outline for patient care. Peripheral blood draws are often avoided in HD patients as an effort to protect potential or future HD vascular access sites. Thus blood cultures are generally obtained from the blood tubing connecting the catheter to the HD machine. A full-course of antimicrobial treatment is warranted if these blood cultures are found to be positive.[41,68]

Empiric therapy with coverage for both gram-positive and gram-negative bacteria should be initiated after the blood cultures are obtained. The incidence of MRSA bacteremia is high enough to warrant initial treatment with vancomycin for gram-positive coverage and either an aminoglycoside or third-generation cephalosporin for gram-negative coverage.[41,68] Therapy should be adjusted once blood cultures identify an organism. For example, if the isolated organism is methicillin-sensitive *S. aureus*, therapy IV cefazolin (20 mg/kg, rounded to the nearest 500 mg) after each dialysis session is recommended.[67,71] Antibiotic selection should be based on bacterial coverage and the ability to optimize pharmacokinetics by administering a dose after a HD treatment session without requiring additional dosages between HD sessions. Examples of antimicrobial agents that meet these objectives are vancomycin, cefazolin, ceftazidime, daptomycin, and aminoglycosides.[68,71]

The IDSA guidelines recommend that the infected catheter be removed if *S. aureus*, *Pseudomonas* species, or *Candida* species are identified as the infectious cause. Although removal of the catheter is warranted since up to 75% of patients have a recurrence of bacteremia after completing a course of antibiotics, this is not always possible and other options may need to be considered. Options such as replacing the catheter over a guidewire or using a catheter lock solution in conjunction with IV antibiotics have been suggested as an alternative.[41,68] Between 62% and 70% of catheters can be salvaged using catheter lock solutions in addition to systemic antibiotics.[41,68] The IDSA guidelines recommend the use of catheter lock solutions as adjunctive therapy after each dialysis session for 10 to 14 days in a patient whose catheter was not removed and bacteremia symptoms resolved in 2 to 3 days. The IDSA recommendations for antibiotic therapy are listed in Table 45-7.[41,68]

Microbial colonization of a catheter could affect patency and a patient's access to dialytic treatment. An examination of the catheter lock solutions, UFH 5,000 units/mL and tetra sodium EDTA, found an increased rate of microbial colonization with UFH but the tetra sodium EDTA solution had an increase rate of thrombosis.[72] An alternative to UFH and tetra sodium EDTA may be 4% sodium citrate to maintain catheter patency.[63,64,73]

TABLE 45-7 Management of Hemodialysis Access Infection[41,68]

I. Primary arteriovenous fistula
  A. Treat as subacute bacterial endocarditis for 6 weeks.
  B. Initial antibiotic choice should always cover gram-positive organisms, (eg, vancomycin 20 mg/kg IV with serum concentration monitoring or cefazolin 20 mg/kg IV 3 times per week or after each dialysis session).
  C. Gram-negative coverage is indicated for patients with diabetes, human immunodeficiency virus infection, prosthetic valves, or those receiving immunosuppressive agents, gentamicin 2 mg/kg IV with serum concentration monitoring.

II. Synthetic arteriovenous grafts
  A. Local infection—empiric antibiotic coverage for gram-positive, gram-negative, and *Enterococcus* (eg, gentamicin plus vancomycin then individualized after culture results available). Continue for 2 to 4 weeks.
  B. Extensive infection—antibiotics as above plus total resection.
  C. If access is less than 1 month old, antibiotics as above plus remove the graft.

III. Tunneled cuffed catheters (internal jugular, subclavian)
  A. Infection localized to catheter exit site.
    1. No drainage—topical antibiotics, (eg, mupirocin ointment).
    2. Drainage present—gram-positive antibiotic coverage, vancomycin 20 mg/kg IV with serum concentration monitoring or cefazolin 20 mg/kg IV three times per week.
  B. Bacteremia with or without systemic signs or symptoms.
    1. Gram-positive antibiotic coverage as in III.A.2.
    2. If symptomatic at 36 hours, remove the catheter.
    3. If stable and asymptomatic, change catheter and provide culture-specific antibiotic coverage for a minimum of 3 weeks.

Catheter locking has also been utilized to prevent infection and thrombosis in HD catheters.[73] A meta-analysis of randomized control trials of catheter-related bacteremia and antimicrobial lock solutions identified eight studies with 829 patients and more than 90,100 catheter days. Overall analysis found that the use of an antimicrobial lock solution significantly reduced the risk of a catheter-related infection (relative risk [RR] 0.32; 95% confidence interval [CI] 0.10-0.42).[73] A comparison of UFH 1,000 units/mL to the combination solution of 4% sodium citrate with gentamicin 320 mcg/mL (mg/L; 669 μmol/L) as a catheter lock solution significantly reduced the incidence of catheter related bloodstream infections.[74] The value of catheter lock solutions for treatment and prevention of catheter-related infections is increasingly becoming evident, but the possibility of antibiotic resistance with the wide use of antibiotics in catheter locks remains a concern. Currently, NKF-KDOQI does not recommend routine locking of catheters with antibiotics.

Clinical **Controversy...**

The use of a catheter lock solution containing an antimicrobial agent (ie, gentamicin) with citrate to prevent catheter related bloodstream infections is controversial since the risk of antimicrobial resistance may be greater than the benefit.

PERITONEAL DIALYSIS

Although the concept of peritoneal lavage has been described as far back as the 1700s, it wasn't until the 1920s that PD was first employed as an acute treatment for uremia. It was used infrequently during subsequent years until the concept of PD as a chronic therapy for ESRD was proposed in the 1960s. Over the ensuing years the number of patients receiving PD increased slowly until the early 1980s. At that time, several innovations in PD delivery systems were introduced, such as improved catheters and dialysate bags. These innovations led to improved outcomes, decreased morbidity, mortality and a corresponding increase in the use of PD as a viable alternative to HD for the treatment of ESRD. However, the worldwide use of PD has declined over the past decade.[6] Some patients, such as those with more hemodynamic instability (eg, hypotension) or significant residual renal function (RRF), and perhaps patients who desire to maintain a significant degree of self-care may be better suited to PD than to HD. Table 45-2 shows the advantages and disadvantages of PD.

Principles of Peritoneal Dialysis

5 The three basic components of HD—namely, a blood-filled compartment separated from a dialysate-filled compartment by a semipermeable membrane—are also present in PD.[75] In PD, the dialysate-filled compartment is the peritoneal cavity, into which dialysate is instilled via a peritoneal catheter that traverses the abdominal wall. The contiguous peritoneal membrane surrounds the peritoneal cavity. The cavity, which normally contains about 100 mL of lipid-rich lubricating fluid, can expand to a capacity of several liters. The peritoneal membrane that lines the cavity functions as the semipermeable membrane, across which diffusion and ultrafiltration occur. The peritoneal dialyzing membrane is comprised of a monocellular layer of peritoneal mesothelial cells, the basement membrane, and underlying connective and interstitial tissue. The peritoneal membrane has a total area that approximates body surface area (approximately 1-2 m^2). Blood vessels supplying and draining the abdominal viscera, musculature, and mesentery constitute the blood-filled compartment.

Unlike HD, the crucial components of PD cannot be manipulated to maximize solute and fluid removal. Because the blood is not in intimate contact with the dialysis membrane as it is in HD, metabolic waste products must travel a considerable distance to the dialysate-filled compartment. In addition, unlike HD, there is no easy method to regulate blood flow to the surface of the peritoneal membrane, nor is there a countercurrent flow of blood and dialysate to increase diffusion and ultrafiltration via changes in hydrostatic pressure. Similarly there is no easy means available to manipulate the peritoneal membrane. Thus, the available means to enhance PD clearance involve alterations in dialysate volume, dwell time, and the number of exchanges per day. For these reasons, PD is a much-less-efficient process per unit time as compared with HD, and must, therefore, be a virtually continuous procedure to achieve acceptable goals for clearance of metabolic waste products.

Peritoneal Dialysis Access

Access to the peritoneal cavity is via the placement of an indwelling catheter. Many types are available and Fig. 45-3 shows an example.[75] Most catheters are manufactured from silastic, which is soft, flexible, and biocompatible. A typical adult catheter is 40 to 45 cm long, 20 to 22 cm of which is inside the peritoneal cavity. Placement of the catheter is such that the distal end lies low in a pelvic gutter. The center section of the catheter has one or two cuffs made of a porous material that is tunneled inside the anterior abdominal wall so that the cuffs provide mechanical support and stability to the catheter, serves as a mechanical barrier to skin organisms, and prevents their migration along the catheter into the peritoneal cavity. The cuffs are placed at different sites surrounding the abdominal rectus muscle. The remainder of the central section of the catheter is tunneled subcutaneously before exiting the abdominal surface, usually a few centimeters below and to one side of the umbilicus.

The placement of the catheter exit site is one of the factors related to the development or prevention of exit-site infections and peritonitis. The external section of most peritoneal catheters ends with a Luer-Lok connector, which can be connected to a variety of administration sets. These catheters can be used immediately if necessary, provided small initial volumes are instilled; however, a maturation period of 2 to 6 weeks is preferred.

Peritoneal Dialysis Procedures

6 Several variants of PD are clinically utilized in the United States. All variants of PD require the placement of a dialysis solution to dwell in the peritoneal cavity for some period, removing the spent dialysate, and then repeating the process. The prescribed dose of PD may be altered by changing the number of exchanges per day, by altering the volume of each exchange, or by altering the strength of dextrose or other osmotic agent in the dialysate for some or all exchanges. Increasing any one of these variables increases the effective osmotic gradient across the peritoneum, leading to increased ultrafiltration and diffusion (solute removal). If the dwell time is extended, equilibrium may be reached, after which time there will be no further water or solute removal. In fact, after a critical period, reverse water movement may occur.[75] In a basic continuous ambulatory peritoneal dialysis (CAPD) system, the patient or caregiver is manually responsible for performing the prescribed number of dialysate exchanges. The patient is connected to a bag of prewarmed peritoneal dialysate via the PD catheter, by a length of tubing called a transfer set. The most common transfer set used is the Y transfer set which consists of a Y-shaped piece of tubing that is attached at its stem to the patient's catheter, leaving the remaining two limbs of the Y attached to dialysate bags, one filled with fresh dialysate and the other empty. The spent dialysate from the previous dwell is drained into the empty bag, and the peritoneum is subsequently refilled from the bag containing fresh dialysate. The Y set is then disconnected and the bag containing the spent fluid and the empty bag that had contained fresh dialysate are detached and discarded. Typically a patient instills 2 to 3 L of dialysate three times during the day with each exchange lasting 4 to 6 hours, and then a single dialysate exchange overnight lasting 8 to 12 hours. At the end of the prescribed dwell period a new Y set is attached and the process is repeated. The process of outflow, aseptic manipulation of the administration set and catheter, and inflow requires a total time of approximately 30 minutes.

Continuous ambulatory peritoneal dialysis involves performing the dialysate exchanges manually, whereas automated systems collectively termed automated peritoneal dialysis (APD) performs the exchanges with a device referred to as a cycler. APD systems are

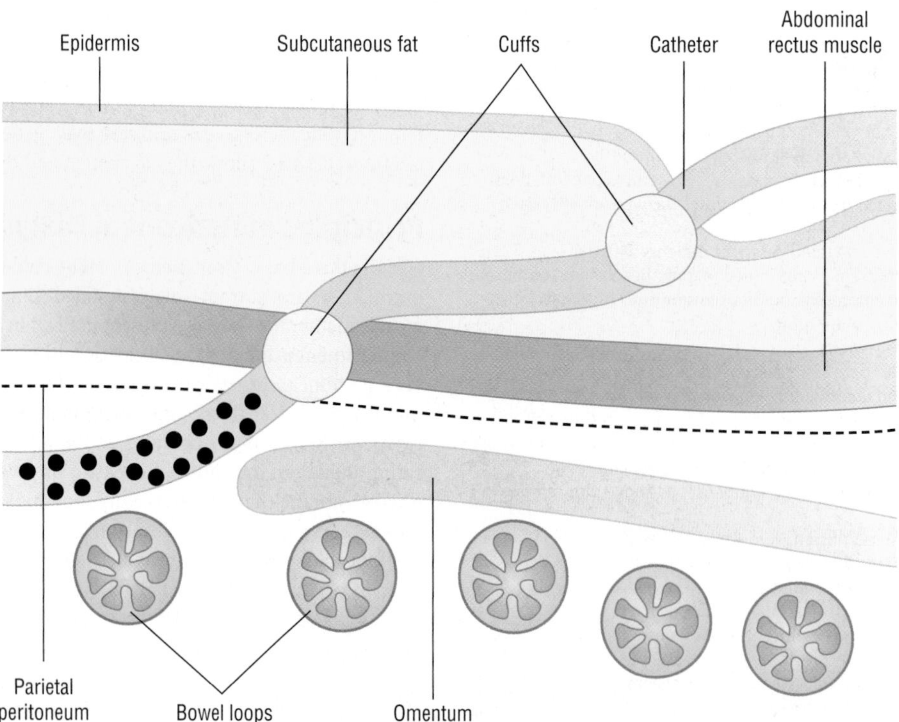

FIGURE 45-3 Diagram of the peritoneal dialysis catheter placement through the abdominal wall into the peritoneal cavity. *Data From Reference 37.*

designed for patients who are unable or unwilling to perform the necessary aseptic manipulations, and for those who require more dialysis. The device is set up in the evening, and the patient attaches the peritoneal catheter to it at bedtime. The machine performs several short-dwell exchanges (usually 1-2 hours) during the night. This permits a long cycle-free daytime dwell of up to 12 to 14 hours. Typical APD regimens involve total 24-hour exchanges of approximately 12 L, which include one or more daytime instillations and dwell periods.[76] This type of regimen is referred to as APD with a "wet" day. The APD variant, nightly intermittent PD, has a similar theme, except that the peritoneal cavity tends to be dialysate free during the day. This type of regimen is frequently referred to as APD with a "dry" day. A number of variants exist and depend largely on equipment availability, patient and prescriber preference, and whether the patient retains any RRF, which influences the quantity of dialysis prescribed.

The APD systems include continuous cycling PD, tidal PD, and nightly intermittent PD. The prototypic form of APD is usually a hybrid between CAPD and continuous cycling PD, in which some of the daily exchanges (usually the overnight exchanges) are completed using an automated device. Recent advances in PD procedures involve using continuous flow peritoneal dialysate.[77] This technique maintains a fixed intraperitoneal volume and rapid, continuous movement of dialysate into and out of the peritoneal cavity. To accomplish this, two PD catheters (an inlet and outlet catheter) and a means of generating a large volume of sterile dialysate are required. Dialysate is generated via conventional HD equipment or sorbent technology. In continuous flow peritoneal dialysate, clearance of small solutes is three to eight times greater than with APD, and approximates daily HD. Potential applications of continuous flow peritoneal dialysate include daily home dialysis, treatment of acute kidney injury in the intensive care unit, and ultrafiltration of ascites.

Peritoneal Dialysis Solutions

All forms of PD use dialysate solutions, which are commercially available in volumes of 1 to 3 L in flexible polyvinyl chloride plastic bags. It is beyond the scope of this chapter to exhaustively review all the options, but the most commonly used solutions which are commercially available contain glucose or icodextrin with varying concentrations of electrolytes, such as sodium (132 mEq/L [mmol/L]), chloride (96 mEq/L [mmol/L]), calcium (2.5-3.5 mEq/L [1.25-1.75 mmol/L]), magnesium (0.5 mEq/L [0.25 mmol/L]), and lactate (40 mEq/L [mmol/L]). These solutions may contain dextrose (1.5%, 2.5%, 3.86%, or 4.25%) or icodextrin (a glucose polymer) at a concentration of 7.5%. The dextrose solutions are hyperosmolar (osmolarity ranges from 345 to 484 mOsm/L) and induce ultrafiltration (removal of free water) by crystalline osmosis. Dextrose is not the ideal osmotic agent for peritoneal dialysate because these solutions are not biocompatible with peritoneal mesothelial cells or with peritoneal leukocytes. The cytotoxic effects on these cells are mediated by the osmolar load and the low pH of the solutions, as well as the presence of glucose degradation products formed during heat sterilization of these products. Icodextrin PD solution contains icodextrin, a starch-derived glucose polymer. It has an osmolality of 282 to 286 mOsm/L, which is isoosmolar with serum. Icodextrin produces prolonged ultrafiltration by a mechanism resembling colloid osmosis resulting in ultrafiltration volumes similar to those with 4.25% dextrose. Icodextrin may have fewer of the metabolic effects associated with dextrose, such as hyperglycemia and weight gain. It is indicated for use during the long (8-16 hours) dwell of a single daily exchange in CAPD and APD patients. Lower glucose degradation product dialysate solutions are also available with similar solute concentrations, but with pH of 7.3.[75,78] These newer, biocompatible dialysate solutions are described as less harmful to the peritoneal membrane and preserve RRF to a greater extent than currently available standard solutions.[79,80] Preservation of RRF in PD and HD patients is important as it has been shown to decrease mortality and increase the time to the first episode of peritonitis. However, the putative benefits of the biocompatible dialysate solutions have not been completely borne out: their use has not consistently slowed the rate of decline in glomerular filtration rate as compared to standard solutions, although the incidence of peritonitis has been lower.[81]

Adequacy of Peritoneal Dialysis

The adequacy of PD is determined by clinical assessment, solute clearance determination and fluid removal. As in HD, the clearance of urea can be quantified by calculating *Kt/V*. The calculations determine a daily *Kt/V*, which is then converted to a weekly value that is relevant to PD patients.

PD adequacy is a major issue that has received considerable attention. The most recent KDOQI guidelines recommend that patients on PD have a total *Kt/V* of at least 1.7 per week.[82] It is important to note that RRF may provide a significant component of the total *Kt/V*. Patients may commence PD with a residual CL_{cr} of approximately 9 to 12 mL/min (0.15-0.200 mL/s), which contributes a renal *Kt/V* of 0.2 to 0.4. Over a period of 1 to 2 years, if RRF progressively deteriorates the total *Kt/V* will progressively diminish unless PD *Kt/V* is increased (by increasing the prescribed dose of PD) to compensate for the reduced renal *Kt/V*.

For patients producing less than 100 mL urine per day, the weekly *Kt/V* dose of 1.7 must be provided entirely by peritoneal clearance. For patients producing greater than 100 mL urine per day, combined renal and peritoneal urea clearances must exceed the weekly *Kt/V* dose of 1.7.[82] The weekly *Kt/V* dose should be measured within the first month of PD initiation and at least once every 4 months thereafter. It is imperative to detect subtle decreases in RRF along with poor adherence to make necessary alterations to the prescribed PD dose to attain adequate clearance of waste products.

The KDOQI guidelines also stress the importance of preserving RRF in PD patients because it is associated with decreased mortality. Typical measures to preserve RRF include preferential use of angiotensin-converting enzyme inhibitors or angiotensin receptor blockers, regardless of blood pressure, and avoidance of medications or procedures that are associated with insults to the kidney (eg, nonsteroidal anti-inflammatory drugs, cyclooxygenase-2 inhibitors, aminoglycosides, intravenous iodinated radiocontrast dyes, withdrawal of immunosuppressant therapies from a transplanted kidney, hypovolemia, urinary tract obstruction, and hypercalcemia).[82]

Complications of Peritoneal Dialysis

Mechanical, medical, and infectious problems complicate PD therapy. Mechanical complications include kinking of the catheter and inflow and outflow obstruction; excessive catheter motion at the exit site, leading to induration and possible infection and aggravation of tissues; pain from impingement of the catheter tip on the viscera; or inflow pain resulting from a jet effect of too rapid dialysate inflow.

Table 45-8 lists the numerous medical complications of PD. An average PD patient absorbs up to 60% of the dextrose in each exchange. This continuous supply of calories leads to increased adipose tissue deposition, decreased appetite, malnutrition, and altered requirements for insulin in diabetic patients. Fibrin formation in dialysate is common and can lead to obstruction of catheter outflow. Infectious complications of PD are a major cause of morbidity and mortality and are the leading cause of technique failure and transfer from PD to HD. The two predominant infectious complications are peritonitis and catheter-related infections, which include both exit-site and tunnel infections.

Peritonitis

7 The incidence of peritonitis is influenced by connector technology, by the composition of patient populations, and by the use of APD versus CAPD. The incidence of peritonitis reported by most

TABLE 45-8 Medical Complications of Peritoneal Dialysis

Cause	Complication	Treatment
Glucose load	Exacerbation of diabetes mellitus	IP insulin
Fluid overload	Exacerbation of heart failure	Increase ultrafiltration
	Edema	Diuretics, if the patient has residual renal function
	Pulmonary congestion	
Electrolyte abnormalities	Hypercalcemia/Hypocalcemia	Alter dialysate calcium content
PD additives	Chemical peritonitis	Discontinue PD additives
Malnutrition	Albumin loss	Dietary changes
	Loss of amino acids	Parenteral nutrition
	Muscle wasting	Discontinue PD
	Increased adipose tissue	
Unknown	Fibrin formation in dialysate	IP heparin

IP, intraperitoneal; PD, peritoneal dialysis.

dialysis centers in the United States is about 1 episode every 24 patient-months, although it may be as low as 1 episode every 60 patient-months.[83] Within 1 year of starting CAPD, 40% to 60% of patients develop their first episode of peritonitis (although the incidence is significantly lower in APD patients).

Peritonitis is a major cause of catheter loss in PD patients. The clinical presentation and diagnosis is shown in Table 45-9. A statistically significant correlation between infectious complications and death rates has been reported: patients who had more than 1 peritonitis episode per year, 0.5 to 1 episode per year, or less than 0.5 episode per year, 50% died after 3, 4, and 5 years of therapy, respectively. It is important to note that these relationships are not necessarily cause and effect, as many of these patients succumb to cardiovascular events.[84]

Peritonitis has several imprecise definitions, but guidelines suggest that an elevated dialysate white blood cell count of greater than 100 per microliter (0.1×10^9/L) with at least 50% polymorphonuclear neutrophils indicates the presence of inflammation, of which peritonitis is the most likely cause.[85] A patient who presents with abdominal pain and a cloudy effluent is usually given a provisional diagnosis of peritonitis. Inherent in this definition is a number of false-positive and false-negative diagnoses, because a small percentage of patients with culture-proven peritonitis will have clear dialysate, and some patients, such as menstruating females, may have cloudy PD effluent

TABLE 45-9 Clinical Presentation and Diagnosis of Peritoneal Dialysis-Related Peritonitis

General
- Patients generally present with abdominal pain and cloudy effluent

Symptoms
- The patient may complain of abdominal tenderness, abdominal pain, fever, nausea and vomiting, and chills

Signs
- Cloudy dialysate effluent may be observed
- Temperature may or may not be elevated

Laboratory Tests
- Dialysate white blood cell count >100/mm^3 (>0.1×10^9/L), of which at least 50% are polymorphonuclear neutrophils
- Ram stain of a centrifuged dialysate specimen

Other Diagnostic Tests
- Culture and sensitivity of dialysate should be obtained

without clinical infection. Sterile culture peritonitis remains problematic; it is defined as an episode in which there is clinical suspicion of peritonitis, but for which the culture of the dialysate reveals no organism. There are several postulates for the high incidence (up to 20% of episodes) of culture-negative peritonitis. Many peritonitis-producing organisms are slime producers and may adhere to the peritoneal membrane or to the catheter surface and may be protected from exogenous antibiotics. Sufficient numbers of these bacteria may proliferate to cause peritoneal membrane inflammation and clinical peritonitis, but an inadequate number may seed into the peritoneal cavity to be recovered by conventional microbiologic techniques. In addition, free-floating planktonic bacteria may be rapidly phagocytosed by peritoneal white blood cells, thereby rendering them unavailable for culture.[86]

Contemporary methods have increased the recovery rate of organisms and decreased the culture-negative rate. Centrifugation is currently recommended as the optimum culture method. Centrifugation of a large volume of dialysate (50 mL), resuspension of the sediment in 3 to 5 mL of sterile saline, and subsequent inoculation in culture media produce a culture-negative rate less than 5%. If centrifuge equipment is not available, blood culture bottles can be directly injected with 5 to 10 mL of dialysate effluent. However, this method results in a culture-negative rate of up to 20%.[85]

The majority of infections are caused by gram-positive bacteria, of which *Staphylococcus epidermidis* is the predominant organism. There is no single predominant gram-negative organism. Together, gram-positive and gram-negative organisms account for 80% to 90% of all episodes of peritonitis, and constitute the spectrum against which initial empiric therapy is directed.[87]

Catheter-Related Infections

PD patients experience an exit-site infection approximately once every 24 to 48 months. Patients with previous infections tend to have a higher subsequent incidence. The majority of exit-site infections are caused by *S. aureus*. In contrast to peritonitis, *S. epidermidis* accounts for less than 20% of exit-site infections. Although gram-negative organisms, such as *Pseudomonas*, are less common, they can result in significant morbidity. The diagnostic characteristics of these infections are somewhat vague but generally include the presence of purulent drainage, with or without erythema at the catheter exit site. The risk of exit-site infections is increased several-fold in patients who are nasal carriers of *S. aureus*.[88]

Management

The management of PD related complications are discussed in this section.

Peritonitis

The International Society of Peritoneal Dialysis (ISPD) updated the Peritoneal Dialysis-Related Infections recommendations in 2010, which provide guidelines for treatments for peritonitis, tunneled and exit-site infections.[85] These PD related infections are associated with dialysis modality treatment failures and substantial morbidity and mortality; therefore appropriate pharmacotherapy treatment is essential (Fig. 45-4). The ISPD guidelines specifically address the importance of dialysis center antibiotic selection, the effect of RRF on antibiotic pharmacokinetics, and updated recommendations regarding the use of aminoglycosides and vancomycin in PD patients.[85] In 2011, ISPD published a position statement on reducing the risks of PD related infections that includes updates to the prevention of exit-site infections and routine care for PD patients.[89] There are also many institution specific guidelines, which may impact individual clinicians recommended treatment strategies.

Intraperitoneal (IP) administration of antibiotics remains the preferred delivery route over IV therapy. Antimicrobial dosing recommendations provided in the ISPD guidelines distinguish

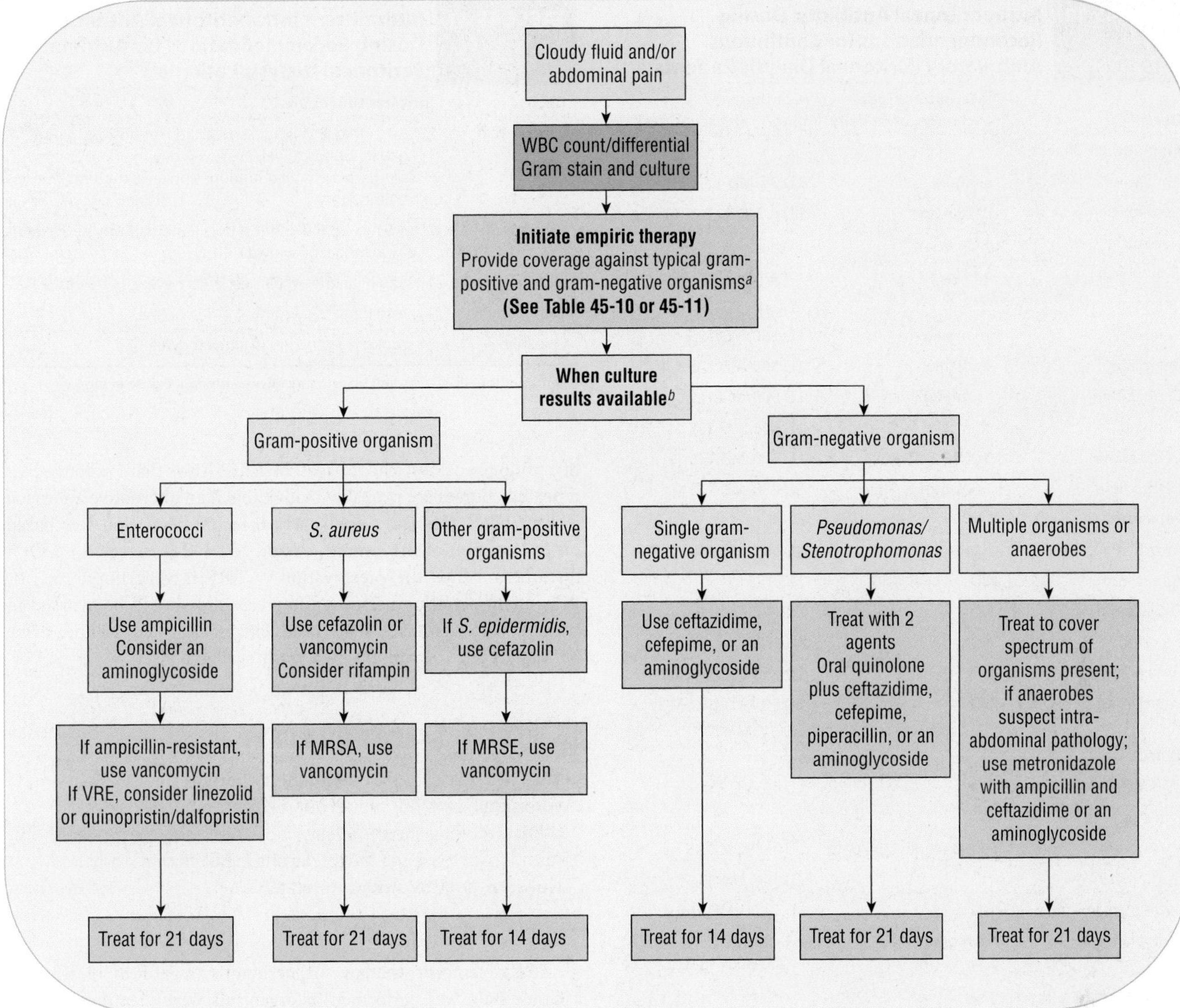

FIGURE 45-4 Pharmacotherapy recommendations for the treatment of bacterial peritonitis in peritoneal dialysis patients. [a]Choice of empiric treatment should be made based on the dialysis center's and the patient's history of infecting organisms and their sensitivities. [b]Final choice of therapy should always be guided by culture and sensitivity results. (MRSA, methicillin-resistant *Staphylococcus aureus;* MRSE, *methicillin-resistant Staphylococcus epidermidis; S. aureus, Staphylococcus aureus; S. epidermidis, Staphylococcus epidermidis;* VRE, vancomycin-resistant enterococci; WBC, white blood cell.)

between dosing for intermittent (one exchange per day) and continuous therapy (all exchanges). In addition, dosing recommendations are modified on the basis of the patient's PD modality (CAPD or APD) and whether the patient has RRF (urine output) greater than 100 mL/day.[85,89]

Following a single IP antibiotic dose the drug concentrations achieved in dialysate and serum differ between intermittent and continuous methods. Intermittent IP therapy necessitates that a sufficient amount of drug transfers from the peritoneal cavity to the systemic circulation, thus allowing drug to diffuse back into the peritoneum during drug-free dialysate dwell time(s). Therefore, once daily dosing requires drug(s) be added to the exchange with the longest dwell time to ensure maximum systemic exposure.

Continuous dosing recommendations may require a loading dose with the very first IP dose and a maintenance dose for each subsequent exchange. Vancomycin, aminoglycosides, and cephalosporins generally can be administered by either dosing method. It is recommended that a continuous dosing method be used for penicillins and fluoroquinolones. No matter which CAPD drug dosing method is used, the goal is to deliver and maintain adequate peritoneum drug concentrations. Intermittent or continuous dosing is effective for CAPD patients but IP dosing for APD patients may require a different dosing schedule. The rapid overnight dialysate exchanges with APD will increase solute clearance over a short time period. This appears to be particularly important for first generation cephalosporin agents. The ISPD guidelines recommend continuous dosing of a first-generation cephalosporin because of concerns over inadequate IP drug concentration during the shorter APD dialysate dwells. Another consideration would be to switch a patient to a CAPD regimen until treatment for peritonitis is completed. With regard to RRF, in patients with daily urine output greater than 100 mL, the dose of drugs that are renally eliminated should be empirically increased by 25%. The ISPD dosing recommendations for IP antibiotics in CAPD and APD patients are shown in Tables 45-10 and 45-11, respectively.[85]

The compatibility and stability of antibiotics added to peritoneal dialysate is another important consideration. In dextrose solutions, most antibiotic additives appear to be stable (usually defined as retaining at least 90% of initial activity) for about 1 week if refrigerated, or 1 to 2 days if left at room temperature. Recent data

TABLE 45-10 Intraperitoneal Antibiotic Dosing Recommendations for Continuous Ambulatory Peritoneal Dialysis Patients[85]

Drug	Intermittent (per exchange, once daily)	Continuous (mg/L, all exchanges)
Aminoglycosides		
Amikacin[a]	2 mg/kg	LD 25, MD 12
Gentamicin[a]	0.6 mg/kg	LD 8, MD 4
Netilmicin[a]	0.6 mg/kg	LD 8, MD 4
Tobramycin[a]	0.6 mg/kg	LD 8, MD 4
Cephalosporins		
Cefazolin[a]	15 mg/kg	LD 500, MD 125
Cefepime[a]	1,000 mg	LD 500, MD 125
Cephalothin[a]	15 mg/kg	LD 500, MD 125
Cephradine[a]	15 mg/kg	LD 500, MD 125
Ceftazidime[a]	1,000-1,500 mg	LD 500, MD 125
Ceftizoxime[a]	1,000 mg	LD 250, MD 125
Penicillins		
Azlocillin[a]	ND	LD 500, MD 250
Ampicillin[a]	ND	MD 125
Oxacillin[a]	ND	MD 125
Nafcillin[a]	ND	MD 125
Amoxicillin[a]	ND	LD 250-500, MD 50
Penicillin G[a]	ND	LD 50,000 units, MD 25,000 units
Quinolones		
Ciprofloxacin[a]	ND	LD 50, MD 25
Others		
Vancomycin[a]	15-30 mg/kg Q5-7d	LD 1,000, MD 25
Daptomycin	ND	LD 100, MD 20
Aztreonam[a]	ND	LD 1,000, MD 250
Teicoplanin Linezolid	15 mg/kg	LD 400, MD 20 Oral 200-300 mg q.d.
Antifungals		
Amphotericin B	NA	MD 1.5
Fluconazole	200 mg IP every 24-48 hours	
Combinations		
Ampicillin/sulbactam[a]	2 g q 12 h	LD 1,000, MD 100
Imipenem/cilastatin[a]	1 g twice daily	LD 500, MD 200
Quinupristin/dalfopristin[b]	25 mg/L in alternate bags	

LD, loading dose in mg; MD, maintenance dose in mg; NA, not applicable; ND, no data.

[a]Dosing of these drugs in patients with residual renal function (defined as more than 100 mL/day urine output) dose should be empirically increased by 25%.

[b]Given in conjunction with 500 mg IV twice daily.

suggests that cefazolin, ceftazidime, cefepime, vancomycin, gentamicin, tobramycin, netilmicin, and heparin are stable in icodextrin.[90] A concern with some compatibility and stability studies is that an assay of total drug concentration may include parent drug-degradation products in addition to active drug. Therefore, the solution may not retain sufficient pharmacologic activity. The systemic toxicities of IP regimens remain unclear, but are likely similar to those associated with IV and oral antibiotic administration. Intermittent (once-daily) IP dosing of drugs, such as aminoglycosides, may reduce the risk of systemic toxicity (ototoxicity and nephrotoxicity).[85] Due to controversial and conflicting clinical trial data the current ISPD guidelines state that there is no convincing evidence that short courses

TABLE 45-11 Intermittent Intraperitoneal Antibiotic Dosing Recommendations for Automated Peritoneal Dialysis Patients[85]

Drug	Intraperitoneal Dose
Vancomycin	LD: 30 mg/kg IP in longest dwell, repeat dosing 15 mg/kg IP in longest dwell every 3-5 days, (aim to keep serum trough concentrations above 15 mcg/mL [mg/L; 10 µmol/L])
Tobramycin	LD: 1.5 mg/kg IP in longest dwell, then 0.5 mg/kg IP each day in longest day dwell
Fluconazole	200 mg IP in one exchange per day every 24-48 hours
Cefepime	1 g IP in longest dwell
Cefazolin	20 mg/kg IP every day, in longest dwell

IP, Intraperitoneal; LD, loading dose in mg; MD, maintenance dose in mg.

of aminoglycosides lead to loss of RRF. Also, that prolonged or repeated courses are probably inadvisable if an alternative approach is available.[85] This latter controversial recommendation was based on the opinion of the committee and restated in a recent KDOQI document. Since the preservation of RRF is very important for PD patients, routine use of aminoglycosides should be avoided in patients with significant RRF (producing greater than 100 mL urine per day) if other antibiotic choices are available.[85]

Clinical **Controversy...**

The ISPD guidelines for peritonitis treatment state that patients with significant RRF should not receive aminoglycosides if other antibiotic choices are available. Aminoglycosides were found to increase the rate of decline in RRF in one study. However, another study refuted this claim.

Initial empiric therapy for peritonitis, regardless of whether a Gram stain was performed or organisms were identified, should include agents effective against both gram-positive and gram-negative organisms. Antibiotic selection should be based on a dialysis center's antibiogram or resistance patterns, a history of the patient's infections and the organism's antibiotic sensitivity profile. In many cases, a first-generation cephalosporin such as cefazolin in combination with a second drug that provides broader gram-negative coverage, such as ceftazidime, cefepime, or an aminoglycoside, will prove suitable. Patients with documented allergy to cephalosporin antibiotics can be treated with vancomycin and an aminoglycoside. High rates of methicillin resistance have been reported by many dialysis centers and vancomycin should be used as first-line therapy against gram-positive organisms for patients treated at these centers. Monotherapy with agents providing both gram-positive and gram-negative coverage is an alternative option. Both imipenem-cilastin and cefepime are effective in treating CAPD-related peritonitis.[91]

After culture and sensitivity results are obtained, antibiotic therapy should be adjusted appropriately (see Fig. 45-4). Tables 45-10 and 45-11 list doses for antibiotics. Treatment should be continued for 14 to 21 days. If the patient does not show signs of clinical improvement within 72 hours after antibiotic treatment is initiated, the culture should be repeated and the patient reevaluated. If the peritoneal dialysate white blood cell count remains high after 4 days of appropriate antibiotic therapy, clinicians should consider removing the peritoneal catheter, starting IV antibiotics and initiating HD for dialytic maintenance therapy.

Fungal peritonitis is associated with a poor prognosis and high morbidity and mortality. One problem with prospective assessment of antifungal regimens is the infrequency with which these infections occur. This makes it difficult to design and implement comparative studies. Most literature about antifungal treatment is therefore retrospective or limited to reports of local experience. As a result, the ISPD recommendations for treatment of fungal peritonitis are somewhat vague and treatment should be based on culture and sensitivity results. However, one area that has been clarified is the question as to whether the PD catheter should be removed. The ISPD recommendations are to remove the catheter immediately after identifying fungi. If the Gram stain indicates the presence of yeast, treatment may be initiated with amphotericin B and oral flucytosine. Once culture and sensitivity results are available, fluconazole, caspofungin, or voriconazole may replace amphotericin B. Treatment with these agents should be continued orally for an additional 10 days after catheter removal. It remains unclear whether there is any benefit from fungal prophylaxis. Recommendations are also provided for the treatment of mycobacterial, or tuberculous, peritonitis. Although this infection is a rare complication, it can be difficult to diagnose, and treatment requires multiple drugs.

Catheter-Site Infections

Topical antibiotics and disinfectants appear to be effective agents for the prevention of exit-site infections.[92] Gram-positive organisms should be treated with oral penicillinase-resistant penicillin or a first-generation cephalosporin such as cephalexin (**Fig. 45-5**). Rifampin may be added if necessary, in slowly resolving or particularly severe *S. aureus* infections. Vancomycin should be avoided in routine or empiric treatment of gram-positive catheter-related infections, but will be necessary for methicillin-resistant *S. aureus*. Gram-negative organisms should be treated with oral quinolones. The effectiveness of oral quinolones may be diminished owing to the chelation drug interactions with divalent and trivalent metal ions, which are commonly taken by dialysis patients. Administration of quinolones should occur at least 2 hours prior to these drugs. In cases where *Pseudomonas aeruginosa* is the pathogen, a quinolone should not be used as monotherapy. Options for a second antipseudomonal drug include the IP administration of aminoglycoside, ceftazidime, cefepime, piperacillin, imipenem-cilastatin or meropenem. In all cases antibiotics should be continued until the exit site appears normal; 2 to 3 weeks of therapy may be necessary. A patient with a catheter-related infection that progresses to peritonitis will usually require catheter removal.[85,89]

Prevention of Peritonitis and Catheter Exit-site Infections

8 Attempts to prevent peritonitis and catheter-related infections have included refinement of connector system technology (Luer-lok connectors), enhanced patient training techniques, and the use of prophylactic antibiotic regimens and vaccines. Several studies have examined the impact of antibacterial agents as prophylaxis against both peritonitis and tunnel-related infections. Intermittent rifampin 300 mg orally twice a day for 5 days, repeated every 3 months,

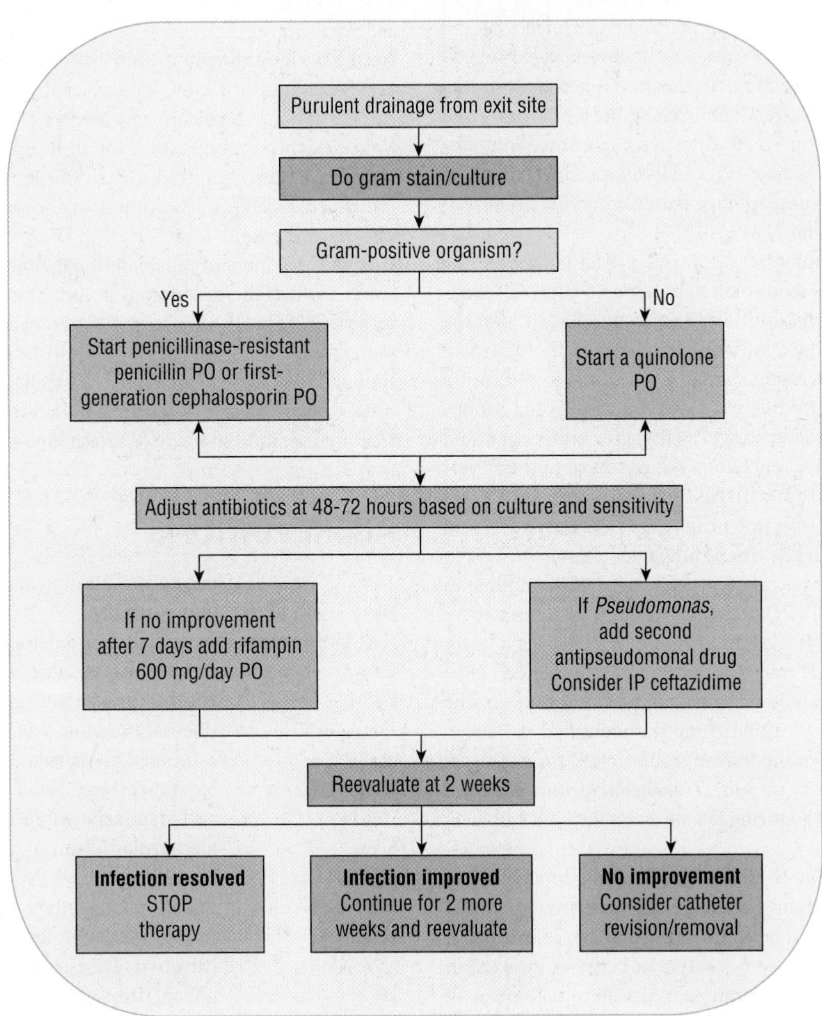

FIGURE 45-5 Management strategy of exit-site infections for peritoneal dialysis patients.[87] (IP, intraperitoneal; PO, orally.) *Data from reference 87.*

appears to decrease the number of catheter-related infections, but not the incidence of peritonitis. The efficacy of other antibiotic prophylaxis for peritonitis and catheter-related infections is limited. Long-term, extended-duration prophylaxis with penicillins or cephalosporins is not effective.[85,89]

Clinical **Controversy...**

Alternative topical agents have been studied to decrease PD exit-site infections but these topical agents have not been shown to be superior to mupirocin or gentamicin. Additionally, the clinician needs to assess the risk versus benefit based on the side effect profile of these agents.

Nasal carriage of *S. aureus* is associated with an increased risk of catheter-related infections and peritonitis.[85,89] In addition, diabetic patients and those on immunosuppressive therapy are at increased risk for *S. aureus* catheter infections. Prophylaxis with intranasal mupirocin (twice daily for 5-7 days every month), mupirocin (daily) at the exit site, or oral rifampin can effectively reduce *S. aureus* exit-site infections. Because of the minimal toxicity of mupirocin and the risk of rifampin resistance, mupirocin regimens are preferred.[85,89] However, it is important to note that *S. aureus* isolates with a high degree of resistance to mupirocin have been isolated from PD patients using prophylactic mupirocin at the peritoneal catheter exit site. A recent study did not observe resistance patterns with the use of mupirocin. Patients in this study applied mupirocin to the exit-site either once or thrice weekly. After 3 years exit-site infections and peritonitis rates were significantly lower in the thrice-weekly application group.[93] In addition, gentamicin cream applied daily to the exit site has been found to effectively reduce both *S. aureus* and *P. aeruginosa* exit-site infection.[85,89] However, a comparison of mupirocin 2% and gentamicin 0.1% creams for exit-site prophylaxis noted a decrease in gentamicin susceptibility patterns for *Enterobacteriaceace* (12%) and *Pseudomonas* (14%).[94]

A double-blinded, randomized controlled trial compared the use of the topical ointments mupirocin to polysporin triple (P^3; bacitracin, gramicidin and polymixin B) in PD patients ($n = 201$) for the prevention of PD-related infections. Patients applied the ointment to the exit-site with each dressing change and were followed for up to 18 months. No significant difference was found between groups for time to first PD-related infections ($P = 0.41$) for either agent but a significant increase in fungal infections was observed in the P^3 versus mupirocin group (7 vs 0; $P = 0.01$). The authors concluded that the use of P^3 for PD-related infection prophylaxis was not superior to mupirocin and may increase the risk of fungal infections.[95]

The use of polyhexanide was compared to povidone-iodine to prevent exit-site infections in PD patients in a single center prospective open label study ($n = 46$). After 12 months, there was a lower rate of overall infections ($P = 0.037$) and exit site infections ($P = 0.032$) with use of polyhexanide compared to povidine-iodine. The infection source in the polyhexanide group was identified as *P. aeruginosa* ($n = 3$) but in the povidine-iodine group ($n = 9$) three sources were identified as *S. aureus* ($n = 6$), *Corynebacterium jeikeium* ($n = 2$), *P. aeruginosa* ($n = 1$). During the study no infected catheters required removal.[96]

A multi-center open label trial to assess daily application at the exit site of antibacterial honey compared to standard care in **PD** patients ($n = 371$). Time to first peritonitis ($P = 0.97$) and time to first exit site infection ($P = 0.24$) were not different between groups but the honey group reported a higher rate of infection in patients with diabetes (*HR* 1.85 [1.05-3.24]; $P = 0.03$). Also, there was a higher rate of study withdrawal and skin rash in the honey group. The authors concluded that topical use of honey could not be recommended as routine therapy in PD patients.[97] These findings differ from previous smaller studies that examine the use of topical honey to prevent catheter related infections, which found medical-grade *Leptospermum* honey to be as effective as mupirocin in reducing catheter infections.[98]

TABLE 45-12 Patient Related Videos Relative to Dialysis Procedures and Therapies

Source	Web site (accessed 7/21/2015)
Baxter	http://www.youtube.com/renalinfo
Davita Inc.	http://www.davita.com/videos/
NxStage Medical, Inc.	http://www.nxstage.com/homehemodialysis/video-podcasts/patient-training
Fresenius Medical Care	http://www.ultracare-dialysis.com/Header1/LinksResources/VideoLibrary.aspx
National Kidney Foundation	http://www.youtube.com/watch?v=NHS0oyHR4vI&feature=plcp
NBC News	http://video.msnbc.msn.com/nightly-news/40856952#40856952

CONCLUSION

Because of the limitation of available kidneys for transplantation, HD and PD remain the most widely available and commonly used ESRD treatments. Despite continual advances in dialysis and transplantation, kidney disease is associated with significant morbidity and mortality. Given the lack of a true cure for kidney disease, emphasis has been placed on the prevention and early detection of kidney disease. Goals set by the KDOQI, the Healthy People 2020 initiative, and the Centers for Medicare and Medicaid Services' CPM Project provide guidance and direction for all healthcare practitioners. In fact, there have been significant reductions in the incidence rate of ESRD, enhanced timing and selection of the preferred access placement, and mortality and morbidity.[99,100] For patients with ESRD, a focus on quality of life and rehabilitation is now a valuable and viable goal toward which the nephrology community should direct its research resources. Several links to patient related videos that discuss CKD patient experiences are presented in Table 45-12. Although prevention of ESRD is the primary goal for clinicians and adequate access to renal transplantation is secondary, dialysis will likely be a part of the treatment paradigm for ESRD for many years to come.

ABBREVIATIONS

APD	automated peritoneal dialysis
AV	arteriovenous
CAPD	continuous ambulatory peritoneal dialysis
CL_{cr}	creatinine clearance
CPM	clinical performance measures
DHA	docosahexaenoic acid
eGFR	estimated glomerular filtration rate
EPA	eicosapentaenoic acid
ESRD	end-stage renal disease
GFR	glomerular filtration rate
HD	hemodialysis
HDF	hemodialfiltration
IDH	intradialytic hypotension
IDSA	Infectious Disease Society of America
IP	intraperitoneal
ISPD	The International Society of Peritoneal Dialysis
KDIGO	Kidney Diseases: Improving Global Outcomes
NKF-KDOQI	National Kidney Foundation's Kidney Disease/Dialysis Outcome Quality Initiative

PD	peritoneal dialysis
RRF	residual renal function
UFH	unfractionated heparin
URR	urea reduction ratio
USRDS	United States Renal Data System

REFERENCES

1. U.S. Renal Data System 2014 Annual Data Report: Atlas of End-Stage Renal Diseases in the United States. Bethesda, MD: National Institutes of Health, National Institutes of Diabetes and Digestive and Kidney Diseases; 2014.
2. KDIGO clinical practice guidelines for chronic kidney disease: Evaluation, classification, and stratification. *Kidney Int Suppl* 2013;3:1-150.
3. Clinical practice guidelines for hemodialysis adequacy, update 2006. *Am J Kidney Dis* 2006;48:S2-S90.
4. Yeun JY, Ornt DB, Depner TA. Hemodialysis. In: Taal MW, Chertow GM, Marsden PA, Skorecki K, Yu ASL and Brenner BM, eds. *Brenner & Rector's The Kidney*. 9th ed. Philadelphia: Elsevier Saunders; 2012: 2294-2346.
5. Andrassy KM. Comments on 'KDIGO 2012 Clinical Practice Guideline for the Evaluation and Management of Chronic Kidney Disease'. *Kidney Int* 2013;84:622-623.
6. Khawar O, Kalantar-Zadeh K, Lo WK, Johnson D, Mehrotra R. Is the declining use of long-term peritoneal dialysis justified by outcome data? *Clin J Am Soc Nephrol* 2007;2:1317-1328.
7. Sinnakirouchenan R, Holley JL. Peritoneal dialysis versus hemodialysis: Risks, benefits, and access issues. *Adv Chronic Kidney Dis* 2011;18:428-432.
8. Miskulin DC, Meyer KB, Athienites NV, et al. Comorbidity and other factors associated with modality selection in incident dialysis patients: The CHOICE Study. Choices for Healthy Outcomes in Caring for End-Stage Renal Disease. *Am J Kidney Dis* 2002;39:324-336.
9. Himmelfarb J, Ikizler TA. Hemodialysis. *N Engl J Med* 2010;363: 1833-1845.
10. Hayashi R, Huang E, Nissenson AR. Vascular access for hemodialysis. *Nat Clin Pract Nephrol* 2006;2:504-513.
11. Allon M, Asif A. Venous catheter access: The basics. In: Daugirdas JT, Blake PG and Ing TS, eds. *Handbook of Dialysis*. 5th ed. Philadelphia: Wolters Kluwer; 2014:121-136.
12. Vachharajani TJ, Wu S, Brouwer-Maier D, Asif A. Arteriovenous Fistulas and Grafts: The Basics. In: Daugirdas JT, Blake PG and Ing TS, eds. *Handbook of Dialysis*. 5th ed. Philadelphia: Wolters Kluwer; 2014:99-120.
13. Chan MR, Yevzlin AS. Tunneled dialysis catheters: Recent trends and future directions. *Adv Chronic Kidney Dis* 2009;16:386-395.
14. Ahmad S, Misra M, Hoenich N, Daugirdas JT. Hemodialysis apparatus. In: Daugirdas JT, Blake PG and Ing TS, eds. *Handbook of Dialysis*. 5th ed. Philadelphia: Wolters Kluwer; 2014:66-88.
15. Tattersall JE, Ward RA, Group E. Online haemodiafiltration: Definition, dose quantification and safety revisited. *Nephrol Dial Transplant* 2013;28:542-550.
16. den Hoedt CH, Mazairac AH, van den Dorpel MA, Grooteman MP, Blankestijn PJ. Effect of hemodiafiltration on mortality, inflammation and quality of life. *Contrib Nephrol* 2011;168:39-52.
17. Canaud B, Bowry S, Stuard S. Hemodiafiltration. In: Daugirdas JT, Blake PG and Ing TS, eds. *Handbook of Dialysis*. 5th ed. Philadelphia: Wolters Kluwer; 2014:321-332.
18. Mostovaya IM, Blankestijn PJ, Bots ML, et al. Clinical evidence on hemodiafiltration: A systematic review and a meta-analysis. *Semin Dial* 2014;27:119-127.
19. Schulman G. Clinical application of high-efficiency hemodialysis. In: Nissenson AR and Fine RN, eds. *Handbook of Dialysis Therapy*. 4th ed. Philadelphia: Saunders/Elsevier; 2008:481-497.
20. Nesrallah GE, Lindsay RM, Cuerden MS, et al. Intensive hemodialysis associates with improved survival compared with conventional hemodialysis. *J Am Soc Nephrol* 2012;23:696-705.
21. Schachter ME, Chan CT. Current state of intensive hemodialysis: A comparative review of benefits and barriers. *Nephrol Dial Transplant* 2012;27:4307-4313.
22. Hakim RM, Saha S. Dialysis frequency versus dialysis time, that is the question. *Kidney Int* 2014;85:1024-1029.
23. Group FHNT, Chertow GM, Levin NW, et al. In-center hemodialysis six times per week versus three times per week. *N Engl J Med* 2010;363:2287-2300.
24. Pipkin M, Eggers PW, Larive B, et al. Recruitment and training for home hemodialysis: Experience and lessons from the Nocturnal Dialysis Trial. *Clin J Am Soc Nephrol* 2010;5:1614-1620.
25. Cafazzo JA, Leonard K, Easty AC, Rossos PG, Chan CT. Patient-perceived barriers to the adoption of nocturnal home hemodialysis. *Clin J Am Soc Nephrol* 2009;4:784-789.
26. Daugirdas JT. Physiologic principles and urea kinetic modeling. In: Daugirdas JT, Blake PG and Ing TS, eds. *Handbook of Dialysis*. 5th ed. Philadelphia: Wolters Kluwer; 2014:25-58.
27. Daugirdas JT. Chronic Hemodialysis Prescription. In: Daugirdas JT, Blake PG and Ing TS, eds. *Handbook of Dialysis*. 5th ed. Philadelphia: Wolters Kluwer; 2014:192-214.
28. 2006 Annual Report, End Stage Renal Disease Clinical Performance Measures Project, in Department of Health and Human Services CMMS, Office of Clinical Standards of Quality (ed). National Institutes of Health, National Institutes of Diabetes and Digestive and Kidney Diseases, Baltimore, MD; 2006.
29. Pierratos A, Chan CT, McFarlane PA. Daily (quotidian) hemodialysis. In: Nissenson AR and Fine RN, eds. *Handbook of Dialysis Therapy*. 4th ed. Philadelphia: Saunders/Elsevier; 2008:352-363.
30. Davenport A. Intradialytic complications during hemodialysis. *Hemodial Int* 2006;10:162-167.
31. Sherman RA, Daugirdas JT, Ing TS. Complications during hemodialysis. In: Daugirdas JT, Blake PG and Ing TS, eds. *Handbook of Dialysis*. 5th ed. Philadelphia: Wolters Kluwer; 2014:215-236.
32. Thijssen S, Raimann JG, Usvyat LA, Levin NW, Kotanko P. The evils of intradialytic sodium loading. *Contrib Nephrol* 2011;171:84-91.
33. Gabutti L, Bianchi G, Soldini D, Marone C, Burnier M. Haemodynamic consequences of changing bicarbonate and calcium concentrations in haemodialysis fluids. *Nephrol Dial Transplant* 2009;24:973-981.
34. Zhou YL, Liu HL, Duan XF, Yao Y, Sun Y, Liu Q. Impact of sodium and ultrafiltration profiling on haemodialysis-related hypotension. *Nephrol Dial Transplant* 2006;21:3231-3237.
35. Park J, Rhee CM, Sim JJ, et al. A comparative effectiveness research study of the change in blood pressure during hemodialysis treatment and survival. *Kidney Int* 2013;84:795-802.
36. Denker MG, Cohen DL. Antihypertensive medications in end-stage renal disease. *Semin Dial* 2015;28:330-336.
37. Sherman R, Daugirdas J, Ing T. Complications during hemodialysis. In: Daugirdas J, Blake P and Ing T, eds. *Handbook of Dialysis*. 5th ed. Philadelphia: Wolters Kluwer; 2014:215-236.
38. Lok CE. Fistula first initiative: Advantages and pitfalls. *Clin J Am Soc Nephrol* 2007;2:1043-1053.
39. Hicks CW, Canner JK, Arhuidese I, et al. Mortality benefits of different hemodialysis access types are age dependent. *J Vasc Surg* 2015;61:449-456.
40. Clinical Practice Guidelines for Vascular Access: 2006. *Am J Kidney Dis* 2006;48:S176-S247.
41. O'Grady NP, Alexander M, Burns LA, et al. Guidelines for the prevention of intravascular catheter-related infections. *Am J Infect Control* 2011;39:S1-S34.
42. Bohlke M, Uliano G, Barcellos FC. Hemodialysis catheter-related infection: Prophylaxis, diagnosis and treatment. *J Vasc Access* 2015;16:347-355.
43. Xue H, Ix JH, Wang W, et al. Hemodialysis access usage patterns in the incident dialysis year and associated catheter-related complications. *Am J Kidney Dis* 2013;61:123-130.
44. Chiu YW, Teitelbaum I, Misra M, de Leon EM, Adzize T, Mehrotra R. Pill burden, adherence, hyperphosphatemia, and quality of life in maintenance dialysis patients. *Clin J Am Soc Nephrol* 2009;4: 1089-1096.
45. Chesterton LJ, Selby NM, Burton JO, McIntyre CW. Cool dialysate reduces asymptomatic intradialytic hypotension and increases baroreflex variability. *Hemodial Int* 2009;13:189-196.
46. Selby NM, McIntyre CW. A systematic review of the clinical effects of reducing dialysate fluid temperature. *Nephrol Dial Transplant* 2006;21:1883-1898.
47. Rubinstein S, Haimov M, Ross MJ. Midodrine-induced vascular ischemia in a hemodialysis patient: A case report and literature review. *Ren Fail* 2008;30:808-812.
48. Higuchi T, Abe M, Yamazaki T, et al. Levocarnitine improves cardiac function in hemodialysis patients with left ventricular hypertrophy: A randomized controlled trial. *Am J Kidney Dis* 2016;67(2):260-270. doi:10.1053/j.ajkd.2015.09.010.
49. Razeghi E, Dashti-Khavidaki S, Nassiri S, et al. A randomized crossover clinical trial of sertraline for intradialytic hypotension. *Iran J Kidney Dis* 2015;9:323-330.

50. Brewster UC, Ciampi MA, Abu-Alfa AK, Perazella MA. Addition of sertraline to other therapies to reduce dialysis-associated hypotension. *Nephrology (Carlton)* 2003;8:296-301.
51. Beladi-Mousavi SS, Beladi-Mousavi M, Hayati F, Talebzadeh M. Effect of intranasal DDAVP in prevention of hypotension during hemodialysis. *Nefrologia* 2012;32:89-93.
52. El-Hennawy AS, Zaib S. A selected controlled trial of supplementary vitamin E for treatment of muscle cramps in hemodialysis patients. *Am J Ther* 2010;17:455-459.
53. El-Tawil S, Al Musa T, Valli H, et al. Quinine for muscle cramps. *Cochrane Database Syst Rev* 2015;4:CD005044.
54. Houstoun M, Reichman ME, Graham DJ, et al. Use of an active surveillance system by the FDA to observe patterns of quinine sulfate use and adverse hematologic outcomes in CMS Medicare data. *Pharmacoepidemiol Drug Saf* 2014;23:911-917.
55. Khajehdehi P, Mojerlou M, Behzadi S, Rais-Jalali GA. A randomized, double-blind, placebo-controlled trial of supplementary vitamins E, C and their combination for treatment of haemodialysis cramps. *Nephrol Dial Transplant* 2001;16:1448-1451.
56. Dixon BS, Beck GJ, Dember LM, et al. Use of aspirin associates with longer primary patency of hemodialysis grafts. *J Am Soc Nephrol* 2011;22:773-781.
57. Dixon BS, Beck GJ, Vazquez MA, et al. Effect of dipyridamole plus aspirin on hemodialysis graft patency. *N Engl J Med* 2009;360: 2191-2201.
58. Hasegawa T, Elder SJ, Bragg-Gresham JL, et al. Consistent aspirin use associated with improved arteriovenous fistula survival among incident hemodialysis patients in the dialysis outcomes and practice patterns study. *Clin J Am Soc Nephrol* 2008;3:1373-1378.
59. Chan KE, Lazarus JM, Thadhani R, Hakim RM. Warfarin use associates with increased risk for stroke in hemodialysis patients with atrial fibrillation. *J Am Soc Nephrol* 2009;20:2223-2233.
60. Sood MM, Rigatto C, Bueti J, et al. Thrice weekly warfarin administration in haemodialysis patients. *Nephrol Dial Transplant* 2009;24:3162-3167.
61. Limdi NA, Beasley TM, Baird MF, et al. Kidney function influences warfarin responsiveness and hemorrhagic complications. *J Am Soc Nephrol* 2009;20:912-921.
62. Lok CE, Moist L, Hemmelgarn BR, et al. Effect of fish oil supplementation on graft patency and cardiovascular events among patients with new synthetic arteriovenous hemodialysis grafts: A randomized controlled trial. *JAMA* 2012;307:1809-1816.
63. Macrae JM, Dojcinovic I, Djurdjev O, et al. Citrate 4% versus heparin and the reduction of thrombosis study (CHARTS). *Clin J Am Soc Nephrol* 2008;3:369-374.
64. Zhao Y, Li Z, Zhang L, et al. Citrate versus heparin lock for hemodialysis catheters: A systematic review and meta-analysis of randomized controlled trials. *Am J Kidney Dis* 2014;63:479-490.
65. Hilleman D, Campbell J. Efficacy, safety, and cost of thrombolytic agents for the management of dysfunctional hemodialysis catheters: A systematic review. *Pharmacotherapy* 2011;31:1031-1040.
66. Vercaigne LM, Zacharias J, Bernstein KN. Alteplase for blood flow restoration in hemodialysis catheters: A multicenter, randomized, prospective study comparing "dwell" versus "push" administration. *Clin Nephrol* 2012;78:287-296.
67. Allon M. Treatment guidelines for dialysis catheter-related bacteremia: An update. *Am J Kidney Dis* 2009;54:13-17.
68. Mermel LA, Allon M, Bouza E, et al. Clinical practice guidelines for the diagnosis and management of intravascular catheter-related infection: 2009 Update by the Infectious Diseases Society of America. *Clin Infect Dis* 2009;49:1-45.
69. Battistella M, Bhola C, Lok CE. Long-term follow-up of the Hemodialysis Infection Prevention with Polysporin Ointment (HIPPO) Study: A quality improvement report. *Am J Kidney Dis* 2011;57:432-441.
70. Poovelikunnel T, Gethin G, Humphreys H. Mupirocin resistance: Clinical implications and potential alternatives for the eradication of MRSA. *J Antimicrob Chemother* 2015:2681-2692.
71. Fitzgibbons LN, Puls DL, Mackay K, Forrest GN. Management of gram-positive coccal bacteremia and hemodialysis. *Am J Kidney Dis* 2011;57:624-640.
72. Kanaa M, Wright MJ, Akbani H, Laboi P, Bhandari S, Sandoe JA. Cathasept Line Lock and Microbial Colonization of Tunneled Hemodialysis Catheters: A Multicenter Randomized Controlled Trial. *Am J Kidney Dis* 2015;66:1015-1023.
73. Labriola L, Crott R, Jadoul M. Preventing haemodialysis catheter-related bacteraemia with an antimicrobial lock solution: A meta-analysis of prospective randomized trials. *Nephrol Dial Transplant* 2008;23:1666-1672.
74. Moore CL, Besarab A, Ajluni M, et al. Comparative effectiveness of two catheter locking solutions to reduce catheter-related bloodstream infection in hemodialysis patients. *Clin J Am Soc Nephrol* 2014;9:1232-1239.
75. Correa-Rotter R, Cueto-Manzano A, Khanna R. Peritoneal dialysis. In: Skorecki K, Chertow GM, Marsden PA, Taal MW, Yu ASL and Brenner BM, eds. *Brenner and Rector's The Kidney*. 9th ed. Philadelphia: Elsevier Saunders; 2012:2347-2377.
76. Clinical Practice Recommendations For Peritoneal Dialysis Adequacy. *Am J Kidney Dis* 2006;48:S130-S158.
77. Diaz-Buxo JA. Continuous-flow peritoneal dialysis: Update. *Adv Perit Dial* 2004;20:18-22.
78. Yohanna S, Alkatheeri AM, Brimble SK, et al. Effect of neutral-pH, low-glucose degradation product peritoneal dialysis solutions on residual renal function, urine volume, and ultrafiltration: A systematic review and meta-analysis. *Clin J Am Soc Nephrol* 2015;10:1380-1388.
79. Thomas J, Teitelbaum I. Preservation of residual renal function in dialysis patients. *Adv Perit Dial* 2011;27:112-117.
80. Garcia-Lopez E, Lindholm B, Davies S. An update on peritoneal dialysis solutions. *Nat Rev Nephrol* 2012;8:224-233.
81. Johnson DW, Brown FG, Clarke M, et al. Effects of biocompatible versus standard fluid on peritoneal dialysis outcomes. *J Am Soc Nephrol* 2012;23:1097-1107.
82. Clinical Practice Guidelines for Peritoneal Dialysis Adequacy. *Am J Kidney Dis* 2006;48:S98-S129.
83. Troidle L, Finkelstein F. Treatment and outcome of CPD-associated peritonitis. *Ann Clin Microbiol Antimicrob* 2006;5:6.
84. Troidle L, Gorban-Brennan N, Finkelstein FO. Outcome of patients on chronic peritoneal dialysis undergoing peritoneal catheter removal because of peritonitis. *Adv Perit Dial* 2005;21:98-101.
85. Li PK, Szeto CC, Piraino B, et al. Peritoneal dialysis-related infections recommendations: 2010 update. *Perit Dial Int* 2010;30:393-423.
86. Piraino B, Bernardini J, Bender FH. An analysis of methods to prevent peritoneal dialysis catheter infections. *Perit Dial Int* 2008;28:437-443.
87. Piraino B, Bailie GR, Bernardini J, et al. Peritoneal dialysis-related infections recommendations: 2005 update. *Perit Dial Int* 2005;25:107-131.
88. Herwaldt LA, Boyken LD, Coffman S, Hochstetler L, Flanigan MJ. Sources of *Staphylococcus aureus* for patients on continuous ambulatory peritoneal dialysis. *Perit Dial Int* 2003;23:237-241.
89. Piraino B, Bernardini J, Brown E, et al. ISPD position statement on reducing the risks of peritoneal dialysis-related infections. *Perit Dial Int* 2011;31:614-630.
90. Ranganathan D, Naicker S, Wallis SC, Lipman J, Ratnajee SK, Roberts JA. Stability of antibiotics for intraperitoneal administration in extraneal 7.5% icodextrin peritoneal dialysis bags (Stab Study). *Perit Dial Int* 2015.
91. Wiggins KJ, Johnson DW, Craig JC, Strippoli GFM. Treatment of peritoneal dialysis-associated peritonitis: A systematic review of randomized controlled trials. *Am J Kidney Dis* 2007;50:967-988.
92. Mahaldar A, Weisz M, Kathuria P. Comparison of gentamicin and mupirocin in the prevention of exit-site infection and peritonitis in peritoneal dialysis. *Adv Perit Dial* 2009;25:56-59.
93. Cavdar C, Saglam F, Sifil A, et al. Effect of once-a-week vs thrice-a-week application of mupirocin on methicillin and mupirocin resistance in peritoneal dialysis patients: Three years of experience. *Ren Fail* 2008;30:417-422.
94. Pierce DA, Williamson JC, Mauck VS, Russell GB, Palavecino E, Burkart JM. The effect on peritoneal dialysis pathogens of changing topical antibiotic prophylaxis. *Perit Dial Int* 2012:525-530.
95. McQuillan RF, Chiu E, Nessim S, et al. A randomized controlled trial comparing mupirocin and polysporin triple ointments in peritoneal dialysis patients: The MP3 Study. *Clin J Am Soc Nephrol* 2012;7:297-303.
96. Nunez-Moral M, Sanchez-Alvarez E, Gonzalez-Diaz I, et al. Exit-site infection of peritoneal catheter is reduced by the use of polyhexanide. Results of a prospective randomized trial. *Perit Dial Int* 2014;34:271-277.
97. Johnson DW, Badve SV, Pascoe EM, et al. Antibacterial honey for the prevention of peritoneal-dialysis-related infections (HONEYPOT): A randomised trial. *Lancet Infect Dis* 2014;14:23-30.
98. Johnson DW, van Eps C, Mudge DW, et al. Randomized, controlled trial of topical exit-site application of honey (Medihoney) versus mupirocin for the prevention of catheter-associated infections in hemodialysis patients. *J Am Soc Nephrol* 2005;16:1456-1462.
99. Clinical Practice Guidelines for Vascular Access. *Am J Kidney Dis* 2006;48:S176-S247.
100. Mujais S, Story K. Peritoneal dialysis in the US: Evaluation of outcomes in contemporary cohorts. *Kidney Int Suppl* 2006:S21-S26.

Drug-Induced Kidney Disease

Thomas D. Nolin

46

KEY CONCEPTS

1 The initial diagnosis of drug-induced kidney disease (DIKD) typically involves detection of elevated serum creatinine (S_{cr}) and blood urea nitrogen, for which there is a temporal relationship between the toxicity and use of a potentially nephrotoxic drug.

2 Drug-induced kidney disease is best prevented by avoiding the use of potentially nephrotoxic agents for patients at increased risk for toxicity. However, when exposure to these drugs cannot be avoided, recognition of risk factors and specific techniques, such as hydration, may be used to reduce potential nephrotoxicity.

3 Acute tubular necrosis (ATN) is the most common presentation of DIKD in hospitalized patients. The primary agents implicated are aminoglycosides, radiocontrast media, cisplatin, amphotericin B, and osmotically active agents.

4 Angiotensin-converting enzyme inhibitors (ACEIs) and nonsteroidal antiinflammatory drugs (NSAIDs) are associated with hemodynamically mediated kidney injury, the pathogenesis of which is a decrease in glomerular capillary hydrostatic pressure.

5 Acute allergic interstitial nephritis (AIN) is observed in up to 27% of kidney biopsies performed for hospitalized patients with unexplained acute kidney injury (AKI). Clinical manifestations of AIN typically present approximately 14 days after initiation of therapy and include fever, maculopapular rash, eosinophilia, arthralgia, often with pyuria, hematuria, proteinuria, and oliguria.

INTRODUCTION

Numerous diagnostic and therapeutic agents have been associated with the development of drug-induced kidney disease (DIKD) or nephrotoxicity. It is a relatively common complication with variable presentations depending on the drug and clinical setting, inpatient or outpatient. Manifestations of DIKD may include acid–base abnormalities, electrolyte imbalances, urine sediment abnormalities, proteinuria, pyuria, and/or hematuria.[1] However, the most common manifestation of nephrotoxicity is a decline in the glomerular filtration rate (GFR) and a corresponding rise in serum creatinine (S_{cr}) concentrations. Initial diagnosis of nephrotoxicity is often delayed because it typically is based on the detection of elevated S_{cr}, for which there is a temporal relationship between the kidney injury (evidenced by the rise in S_{cr}) and exposure to the potentially nephrotoxic drug. This is consistent with contemporary definitions of acute kidney injury (AKI), which rely on either an abrupt increase in S_{cr} or an abrupt decline in urine output (see Chapters e42 and 43).[2]

Nephrotoxicity is often reversible if one discontinues the use of the offending agent, but in some cases it may evolve into AKI and may even progress to stage 5 chronic kidney disease (CKD). Currently, many different mechanisms are responsible for the pathogenesis of DIKD, and the introduction of new drugs with novel mechanisms of action provides the potential for the identification of new presentations of AKI and CKD. This chapter reviews the epidemiology, pathophysiology, risk factors, and basic principles of prevention of DIKD. Detailed discussions of these issues plus management strategies are presented for the most commonly used agents that have been associated with a moderate to high likelihood of DIKD.

EPIDEMIOLOGY

The incidence and characteristics of outpatient or community-acquired DIKD are not well understood since mild toxicity is often unrecognized in this setting. However, the acquisition of data regarding the pharmacoepidemiology of these effects has become more important as care increasingly shifts to the outpatient setting. The incidence of community-based AKI requiring dialysis is as high as 29.5 per 100,000 person years and 522.4 per 100,000 person years for patients not requiring dialysis.[3] Although the incidence of drug-induced AKI was not specifically reported, up to 20% of hospital admissions due to AKI have been attributed to nephrotoxicity acquired in the community setting.[4] The incidence of AKI is even higher in hospitalized patients and appears to be increasing over time.[3,5] As many as 22% of adults and 34% of children worldwide experience AKI during a hospital admission.[6] While up to 30% of critically ill patients experience AKI during their hospitalization, and 1 in 4 cases is associated with nephrotoxic medication exposure.[7] Indeed, drugs have been implicated in 26% of all cases of in-hospital AKI and as such are a recognized source of significant morbidity and mortality.[1]

1 Because the most common manifestation of DIKD is a decline in GFR leading to a rise in S_{cr} and BUN, the onset of toxicity in hospitalized, acutely ill patients is most often recognized by routine laboratory monitoring. Decreased urine output may also be an early sign of toxicity, particularly with radiographic contrast media, nonsteroidal antiinflammatory drugs (NSAIDs), and ACEIs. In the outpatient setting, nephrotoxicity is often recognized by the development of symptoms such as malaise, anorexia, vomiting, volume overload (shortness of breath or edema), and hypertension. S_{cr} or BUN concentrations and urine collection for creatinine clearance may subsequently be measured to quantify the degree of decline in GFR. Marked intrasubject between-day variability of S_{cr} values have been noted (±20% for values within the normal range; see Chapter e42). Furthermore, they may be altered as the result of dietary changes and initiation of drug therapy, which may interfere with the assay procedure. Nevertheless, changes in S_{cr} or urine output consistent with the diagnostic criteria for AKI (see Chapter 43), when correlated temporally with the initiation of drug therapy, are a common threshold for the identification of DIKD.[1]

CLINICAL PRESENTATION Drug-Induced Kidney Disease

General

- The most common manifestation is a decline in GFR leading to a rise in S_{cr} and BUN.
- Alterations in renal tubular function without loss of glomerular filtration may be evident.

Symptoms

- Patients may complain of malaise, anorexia, vomiting, shortness of breath, or edema, particularly in the outpatient setting.

Signs

- Decreased urine output may be an early sign of toxicity, particularly with radiographic contrast media, NSAIDs, and ACEIs, with progression to volume overload and hypertension.
- Proximal tubular injury: Metabolic acidosis with bicarbonaturia; glycosuria in the absence of hyperglycemia; and reductions in serum phosphate, uric acid, potassium, and magnesium due to increased urinary losses.
- Distal tubular injury: Polyuria from failure to maximally concentrate urine, metabolic acidosis from impaired urinary acidification, and hyperkalemia from impaired potassium excretion.

Laboratory Tests

- An abrupt (within 48 hours) reduction in kidney function defined as an absolute increase in S_{cr} of greater than or equal to 0.3 mg/dL (greater than or equal to 27 μmol/L), a percentage increase in S_{cr} of greater than or equal to 50% (1.5-fold from baseline) within 7 days, or a reduction in urine output (documented oliguria of less than 0.5 mL/kg/h for more than 6 hours), when correlated temporally with the initiation of drug therapy may indicate drug-induced AKI.[1]

Other Diagnostic Tests

- Urinary excretion of *N*-acetyl-*β*-D-glucosaminidase, *γ*-glutamyl transpeptidase, glutathione *S*-transferase, and interleukin (IL)-18 are markers of proximal tubular injury and have been used for the early detection of AKI in critically ill patients.
- Kidney injury molecule-1 (KIM-1) is expressed in the proximal tubule and is upregulated for patients with ischemic acute tubular necrosis (ATN), appearing in the urine within 12 hours after the ischemic insult.
- Neutrophil gelatinase-associated lipocalin (NGAL) protein may be detected in the urine within 3 hours of ischemic injury.

Nephrotoxicity may also be evidenced by primary alterations in renal tubular function without a corresponding loss of glomerular filtration. In this setting, urinary enzymes and low-molecular-weight proteins may be used as earlier and more specific biomarkers of nephrotoxicity compared with S_{cr} and BUN, which are relatively insensitive markers of kidney injury.[8,9] S_{cr} and BUN are used as surrogates of kidney function, not injury per se, and typically significant kidney injury must have occurred days before a rise in either is evident. The emergence of novel biomarkers of kidney injury represents an important opportunity for earlier detection of DIKD. Urinary excretion of KIM-1, *N*-acetyl-*β*-glucosaminidase, *γ*-glutamyl transpeptidase, glutathione *S*-transferase, NGAL, and interleukin-18 markers of proximal tubular injury have been used for the early detection of acute kidney damage in several patient populations.[8-10] For example, the transmembrane protein KIM-1 is upregulated for patients with ischemic ATN, appearing in the urine within 12 hours after the ischemic insult. Urinary *N*-acetylglucosamine (NAG) concentrations are a highly sensitive indicator of AKI and have been shown to detect AKI in critically ill patients up to 4 days prior to a rise in S_{cr} was observed. Similarly, urinary NGAL is an early marker of AKI, preceding a rise in S_{cr} by up to 3 days.[11]

Recently, the urinary cell-cycle arrest biomarkers insulin-like growth factor-binding protein 7 (IGFBP7) and tissue inhibitor of metalloproteinase 2 (TIMP-2) were shown to predict AKI in high-risk surgical patients,[12] and clinical outcomes (death and the need for dialysis) in critically ill adults.[13] To date, no clinical studies demonstrating the utility of IGFBP7 and TIMP-2 in detecting and/or minimizing DIKD have been reported, but several pre-clinical studies provide proof of principle for the potential clinical role and utility of monitoring TIMP or IGFBP for this purpose. For example, TIMP-1 is an effective biomarker of cisplatin-induced nephrotoxicity in human kidney cells,[14] and is useful in predicting aristolochic acid–induced kidney injury in rats.[15] In the future, urinary biomarkers may facilitate the earlier detection of kidney injury and diagnosis of nephrotoxicity and minimize the long-term consequences of this common drug-induced disorder.

PRINCIPLES FOR PREVENTION OF DRUG-INDUCED NEPHROPATHY

2 The primary principle for prevention of DIKD is to avoid the use of nephrotoxic agents for patients at increased risk for toxicity. Therefore, an awareness of potentially nephrotoxic drugs and knowledge of risk factors that increase renal vulnerability is essential.[16] Exposure to these drugs often cannot be avoided, so several interventions have been proposed to reduce the potential for the development of nephrotoxicity, for example, adjustment of medication dosage regimens based on accurate estimates of kidney function, and careful and adequate hydration to establish high urine flow rates.[17] Other preventative strategies are still theoretical and/or investigational and relate directly to the specific nephrotoxic mechanisms of a given drug.

The several specific drug-induced renal structural–functional alterations that are responsible for the vast majority of cases of DIKD are listed in Table 46-1. This chapter discusses the pathophysiologic mechanisms responsible for the development of DIKD with these agents in detail, along with clinical presentation, prevention strategies, therapeutic management approaches, and relevant monitoring plans.

TUBULAR EPITHELIAL CELL DAMAGE

3 Drugs that lead to renal tubular epithelial cell (RTEC) damage typically do so via direct cellular toxicity or ischemia. Damage is most often localized in the proximal and distal tubular epithelia

TABLE 46-1 Drug-Induced Kidney Structural–Functional Alterations

Tubular epithelial cell damage	
Acute tubular necrosis • Aminoglycoside antibiotics • Radiographic contrast media • Cisplatin, carboplatin • Amphotericin B • Cyclosporine, tacrolimus • Adefovir, cidofovir, tenofovir	• Pentamidine • Foscarnet • Zoledronate Osmotic nephrosis • Mannitol • Dextran • IV immunoglobulin
Hemodynamically mediated kidney injury	
• Angiotensin-converting enzyme inhibitors • Angiotensin II receptor blockers	• Nonsteroidal antiinflammatory drugs (NSAIDs) • Cyclosporine, tacrolimus • OKT3
Obstructive nephropathy	
Crystal nephropathy • Acyclovir • Sulfonamides • Indinavir • Foscarnet • Methotrexate	Nephrolithiasis • Sulfonamides • Triamterene • Indinavir Nephrocalcinosis • Oral sodium phosphate solution
Glomerular disease	
Minimal Change Disease • NSAIDs, COX-2 inhibitors • Lithium • Pamidronate • Interferon-α and -β Membranous Disease • NSAIDs • Penicillamine • Captopril	Focal Segmental Glomerulosclerosis • Pamidronate • Interferon-α and -β • Lithium • Sirolimus • Anabolic steroids
Tubulointerstitial disease	
Acute allergic interstitial nephritis • Penicillins • Ciprofloxacin • NSAIDs, cyclooxygenase-2 inhibitors • Proton pump inhibitors • Loop diuretics	Chronic interstitial nephritis • Cyclosporine • Lithium • Aristolochic acid Papillary necrosis • NSAIDs, combined phenacetin, aspirin, and caffeine analgesics
Renal vasculitis, thrombosis, and cholesterol emboli	
Vasculitis and thrombosis • Hydralazine • Propylthiouracil • Allopurinol • Penicillamine • Gemcitabine • Mitomycin C	Methamphetamines • Cyclosporine, tacrolimus • Adalimumab • Bevacizumab Cholesterol emboli • Warfarin • Thrombolytic agents

and is termed ATN when cellular degeneration and sloughing from proximal and distal tubular basement membranes are observed. This classically manifests as cellular debris-filled, RTECs and RTEC casts and/or muddy brown granular casts in the urinary sediment.[18] Specific indicators of proximal tubular injury include metabolic acidosis with bicarbonaturia; glycosuria in the absence of hyperglycemia; and reductions in serum phosphate, uric acid, potassium, and magnesium as a result of increased urinary losses.[19] Indicators of distal tubular injury include polyuria from failure to maximally concentrate urine (ie, nephrogenic diabetes insipidus), metabolic acidosis from impaired urinary acidification, and hyperkalemia from impaired potassium excretion.[20]

Acute Tubular Necrosis

Acute tubular necrosis is the most common presentation of DIKD in the inpatient setting. The primary agents associated with this type of injury are aminoglycosides, radiocontrast media, cisplatin, amphotericin B, foscarnet, and osmotically active agents such as immunoglobulins, dextrans, and mannitol.[21]

Aminoglycoside Nephrotoxicity

Incidence Aminoglycoside antibiotic-associated nephrotoxicity has been reported to occur in between 10% and 25% of patients receiving a therapeutic course.[22,23] Critically ill patients appear to have a higher risk for nephrotoxicity with reported rates as high as 58%.[24] The large variance is in part a result of the use of different definitions of toxicity, variability between agents in the class, and the risk factors present in the study population.

Clinical Presentation Clinical evidence of aminoglycoside-associated nephrotoxicity is typically seen within 5 to 7 days after initiation of therapy and manifests as a gradual progressive rise in S_{cr} and BUN and decrease in creatinine clearance.[23] Patients usually present with nonoliguria, that is, they maintain urine volumes greater than 500 mL/day and sometimes have microscopic hematuria and proteinuria.[21] Although renal magnesium wasting can occur (ie, daily excretion of more than 10-30 mg), the risk of symptomatic hypomagnesemia is generally low. Full recovery of kidney function is common if aminoglycoside therapy is discontinued immediately upon discovering signs of toxicity. However, severe AKI may develop occasionally, and for these individuals renal replacement therapy may be required (see Chapter 43). The diagnosis of aminoglycoside-associated nephrotoxicity is often difficult, particularly in critically ill patients with multiple comorbidities and is confounded by other factors that are independently associated with the development of AKI.[24] For instance, concurrent dehydration, sepsis, hypotension, ischemia, and use of other nephrotoxic drugs frequently contribute to AKI in patients who are receiving aminoglycosides.

Pathogenesis Aminoglycoside-associated ATN is primarily due to accumulation of high drug concentrations within proximal tubular epithelial cells, and subsequent generation of reactive oxygen species that produce mitochondrial injury, which leads to cellular apoptosis and necrosis.[22] This results in cell sloughing from proximal tubular basement membranes into the tubular lumen, which can result in tubular obstruction and back leakage of the glomerular filtrate across the damaged tubular epithelium. Toxicity is related to cationic charge of the drugs in this class, which facilitates their binding to negatively charged renal tubular epithelial membrane phospholipids in the proximal tubules, followed by intracellular transport and concentration in lysosomes. The number of cationic groups on the drug molecule appears to correlate with the degree of nephrotoxicity, which is consistent with the observation of higher rates of toxicity with neomycin versus gentamicin, followed by tobramycin, then amikacin.[23]

Risk Factors Multiple risk factors for aminoglycoside-associated nephrotoxicity have been identified: the aggressiveness of aminoglycoside dosing, synergistic toxicity as the result of combination drug therapy, and preexisting clinical conditions of the patient (Table 46-2).[22,24]

Prevention Aminoglycoside-associated ATN may be prevented by careful and cautious selection of patients and the use of alternative antibiotics whenever possible and as soon as microbial sensitivities are known. Commonly used alternatives include fluoroquinolones (eg, ciprofloxacin or levofloxacin) and third- or fourth-generation cephalosporins (eg, ceftazidime or cefepime). When aminoglycosides are necessary, gentamicin, tobramycin, and amikacin are most commonly used, but therapy should be selected to optimize antimicrobial efficacy. Furthermore, it is imperative to avoid volume depletion, limit the total aminoglycoside dose administered, and avoid concomitant therapy with other nephrotoxic drugs.[22] Future therapeutic alternatives may include new aminoglycoside congeners that retain the desired bactericidal activity and yet are devoid of nephrotoxicity, and may also include concurrent use of antioxidant compounds such as alpha-lipoic acid, vitamin E and *N*-acetylcysteine.[25,26]

TABLE 46-2 Potential Risk Factors for Aminoglycoside Nephrotoxicity

(A) Related to aminoglycoside dosing:
Large total cumulative dose
Prolonged therapy
Trough concentration exceeding 2 mg/L[a]
Recent previous aminoglycoside therapy
(B) Related to synergistic nephrotoxicity. Aminoglycosides in combination with
Cyclosporine
Amphotericin B
Vancomycin
Diuretics
Iodinated radiographic contrast agents
Cisplatin
NSAIDs
(C) Related to predisposing conditions in the patient
Preexisting kidney disease
Diabetes
Increased age
Poor nutrition
Shock
Gram-negative bacteremia
Liver disease
Hypoalbuminemia
Obstructive jaundice
Dehydration
Hypotension
Potassium or magnesium deficiencies

[a]The equivalent concentration in SI molar units are 4.3 μmol/L for tobramycin and 4.2 μmol/L for gentamicin.

Prospective, individualized pharmacokinetic monitoring has been associated with a decrease in the incidence of aminoglycoside-associated nephrotoxicity.[27] These studies, however, were often small and statistically underpowered. High-dose intermittent dosing of aminoglycosides, termed once daily dosing, used in combination with other antibiotics, has been intensively investigated as a practical cost-effective method to maintain antimicrobial efficacy while reducing the risk of AKI.[27,28] The reduction in incidence may be the result of limited proximal tubular aminoglycoside uptake during the transient, high-peak serum concentrations, and because of the presence of low aminoglycoside concentrations for a greater proportion of the dosing interval, which facilitates excretion of the aminoglycoside.[22] Although greater clinical efficacy and reduced nephrotoxicity may be realized with once daily compared with standard dosing, seriously ill, immunocompromised, and elderly patients, as well as those with preexisting kidney disease, are not ideal candidates for this approach.

Management Aminoglycoside use should be discontinued or the dosage regimen revised if AKI is evident (ie, there is an S_{cr} increase of 0.5 mg/dL [44 μmol/L] or more that is not attributable to another cause). Other nephrotoxic drugs should be discontinued if possible, and the patient should be maintained adequately hydrated and hemodynamically stable.[28] Short-term renal replacement therapy may be necessary, but ESRD is rarely the result of aminoglycoside toxicity alone.

Radiographic Contrast Media Nephrotoxicity

Incidence Radiographic contrast media-induced nephrotoxicity (CIN) is the third leading cause of hospital-acquired AKI, accounting for 10% to 13% of cases.[29] The incidence varies depending on the population studied and presence of risk factors; rising from less than 2% for patients with normal kidney function, to 17% in patients with impaired kidney function, and 23% to 50% of critically ill patients.[21,30,31] As the number of risk factors associated with CIN increases, there is a corresponding increase in the incidence of nephrotoxicity and mortality rates. A nearly 5-fold increased risk of death has been reported for patients who develop CIN compared with those who do not, with the highest mortality rates observed for patients who developed AKI and required renal replacement therapy. Specifically, in-hospital mortality for patients who developed CIN was 34% versus only 7% of patients who received contrast but did not develop AKI.[29] Moreover, a 2-year mortality rate of 81% has been observed for patients who developed CIN and required dialysis.[29]

Clinical Presentation Contrast media-induced nephrotoxicity is usually transient in nature, presenting most commonly as nonoliguria with kidney injury apparent within the first 24 to 48 hours after the administration of contrast. The S_{cr} concentration usually peaks between 3 and 4 days after exposure, with recovery after 7 to 10 days.[23] However, irreversible oliguric (urine volume less than 500 mL/day) AKI requiring dialysis has been reported in high-risk patients.[32] Urinalysis typically reveals tubular enzymuria with hyaline and granular casts but may also be completely void of casts. The urine sodium concentration and fractional excretion of sodium are frequently low, with the latter typically less than 1% (less than 0.01).

Pathogenesis The primary mechanisms by which contrast media induces nephrotoxicity are renal ischemia and direct cellular toxicity.[33] Renal ischemia likely results from systemic hypotension and simultaneous acute vasoconstriction caused by disruption of normal prostaglandin synthesis and the release of adenosine, endothelin, and other renal vasoconstrictors. Subsequently, a sustained reduction in renal blood flow of up to 25% that lasts for several hours immediately following contrast administration may be evident.[33] This reduced renal blood flow leads to a 50% reduction in oxygen partial pressure and renal ischemia, along with increased concentrations of contrast in the renal tubules, which exacerbates the direct cytotoxicity.[33,34] The extent of cellular toxicity is directly related to the duration of tubular cell exposure to contrast. Thus, preservation of high urinary flow rates with adequate hydration before, during, and after contrast administration is vital to keep renal blood flow as high as reasonably possible to minimize tubular cell exposure to the contrast agent.[34] In humans, plasma osmolality is normally between 275 and 290 mOsm/kg (mmol/kg). Since low- and high-osmolar contrast agents are hyperosmolar to plasma (ie, 600-800 mOsm/kg [mmol/kg] and ~2,000 mOsm/kg [mmol/kg], respectively), their use may result in osmotic diuresis, dehydration, renal ischemia, and increased blood viscosity caused by red blood cell aggregation.[35] Oxidative stress has also been implicated in the development of ATN after contrast administration, which may explain the possible benefit of the antioxidants *N*-acetylcysteine and ascorbic acid.[36]

Risk Factors Decreased renal blood flow exacerbates the ischemic and direct cytotoxic effects of contrast media on the renal tubules. Therefore, preexisting kidney disease, particularly in those with estimated GFR less than 60 mL/min/1.73 m^2 (less than 0.58 mL/s/m^2), is the most important risk factor, since lower GFR is associated with increasing levels of risk.[31] Other patient-specific risk factors include conditions associated with decreased renal blood flow (ie, congestive heart failure, dehydration/volume depletion, and hypotension), and patients with atherosclerosis and reduced effective circulating arterial blood volume appear to also have an elevated risk.[37,38] Diabetes is also a significant risk factor, likely due to coexisting kidney disease (diabetic nephropathy). The presence of multiple myeloma has traditionally been considered a relative contraindication for contrast use, but the risk appears to be associated with concomitant dehydration, kidney disease, or hypercalcemia rather than the diagnosis itself. Larger volumes or doses of contrast and the use of low- as well as high-osmolar contrast agents are also independent predictors of CIN.[37,38] Intraarterial administration of contrast confers greater risk than IV administration.[31] Lastly, concurrent use of nephrotoxins and drugs that alter renal hemodynamics such as NSAIDs and ACEIs also increases risk. Risk factors are additive, and there is a

TABLE 46-3 Recommended Interventions for Prevention of Contrast Nephrotoxicity[36-39]

Intervention	Recommendation	Recommendation Grade[a]
Contrast	• Minimize contrast volume/dose • Use noniodinated contrast studies • Use low- or iso-osmolar contrast agents	A-1 A-2 A-2
Medications	• Avoid concurrent use of potentially nephrotoxic drugs, eg, NSAIDs, aminoglycosides	A-2
Isotonic sodium chloride (0.9%)	• Initiate infusion 3-12 hours prior to contrast exposure and continue 6-24 hours postexposure • Infuse at 1-1.5 mL/kg/h adjusting postexposure as needed to maintain a urine flow rate of 150 mL/h • Alternatively, in urgent cases, initiate infusion at 3 mL/kg/h, beginning 1 hour prior to contrast exposure, then continue at 1 mL/kg/h for 6 hours postexposure	A-1
N-acetylcysteine	• Administer 600-1,200 mg by mouth (PO) every 12 hours, 4 doses beginning prior to contrast exposure (ie, 1 dose prior to exposure and 3 doses postexposure)	B-1

[a]*Strength of recommendations*: A, B, and C are good, moderate, and poor evidence to support recommendation, respectively. *Quality of evidence*: 1, evidence from more than 1 properly randomized, controlled trial; 2, evidence from more than 1 well-designed clinical trial with randomization, from cohort or case-controlled analytic studies or multiple time series, or dramatic results from uncontrolled experiments; 3, evidence from opinions of respected authorities, based on clinical experience, descriptive studies, or reports of expert communities.

proportional increase in the incidence of CIN and associated mortality as the number of risk factors increases.[38]

Prevention Contrast media-induced nephrotoxicity can be anticipated in the majority of patients who are at risk; so the use of preventative procedures is justified for virtually all patients. Table 46-3 lists the recommended interventions for prevention of contrast nephrotoxicity. All patients scheduled to receive contrast media should be assessed for risk factors, and the risk-to-benefit ratio should be considered.[29,37,38] High-risk patients can be identified by evaluating medical history and indication for the contrast study, along with their most recent S_{cr} concentrations. Nephrotoxicity is best prevented in high-risk patients by using alternative imaging procedures (eg, ultrasound, noncontrast magnetic resonance imaging, and nuclear medicine scans). However, if contrast media must be used, the smallest adequate volume should be administered.[29] If the ratio of the volume of contrast to be infused relative to the patient's creatinine clearance is greater than or equal to 3.7 (greater than or equal to 222 if creatinine clearance is expressed in units of milliliters per second), the likelihood of nephrotoxicity is markedly increased.[38] Therefore, in general, the volume of contrast administered should not be greater than twice the baseline estimated creatinine clearance.

Low-osmolar (600-800 mOsm/kg [mmol/kg]) nonionic (iohexol and iopamidol) and ionic (ioxaglate) contrast agents may be used to minimize the incidence of n ephrotoxicity. Standard hyperosmolar contrast media (eg, low- and high-osmolar agent) are not reabsorbed in the kidney and cause osmotic diuresis, which contributes to the renal toxicity observed with these agents. Low-osmolar contrast agents have less than half the osmolality of high-osmolar (~2,000 mOsm/kg [mmol/kg]) agents and are associated with less toxicity, especially when used for patients with preexisting kidney disease.[35] However, use of low-osmolar agents does not preclude the development of nephrotoxicity. Even low-osmolar agents are hyperosmolar relative to plasma, which is likely the reason they have been associated with greater nephrotoxicity than the iso-osmolar nonionic contrast agent iodixanol. Currently, the relative differences in nephrotoxicity between the class of low-osmolar agents and iodixanol are unclear.[38,39]

Clinical **Controversy...**

Some clinicians believe that low- or iso-osmolar contrast media should be used for virtually all patients at risk for toxicity. Others believe that the cost-to-benefit ratio of using low-osmolar contrast agents to prevent nephrotoxicity is questionable except for patients at high risk.

Volume expansion and correction of dehydration prior to contrast administration is a mainstay of preventive therapy.[34] Parenteral hydration with isotonic saline before and after contrast administration reduces the incidence of toxicity, particularly in high-risk patients, and is currently the most widely accepted preventative intervention.[38] Volume expansion may exert its beneficial effects through dilution of contrast media, prevention of renal vasoconstriction, preservation of high urine flow rates, decreased tubular cell exposure to contrast, and avoidance of tubular obstruction. Numerous clinical trials have compared the efficacy of hydration with isotonic saline to isotonic sodium bicarbonate for CIN prevention. Contradictory findings have been observed, and to date, there is no strong evidence of a benefit of sodium bicarbonate over saline. Thus, current guidelines recommend hydration with isotonic saline for CIN prevention.[38,39] The use of oral hydration is not currently recommended in lieu of parenteral hydration.[38,39]

N-acetylcysteine is a thiol-containing antioxidant that may effectively reduce the risk of developing CIN for patients with preexisting kidney disease. Despite the publication of dozens of clinical trials and meta-analyses, a therapeutic benefit of NAC has not been consistently demonstrated, and its therapeutic role remains controversial.[36] Although it is no longer recommended in CIN prevention guidelines,[38,39] it is still widely used, particularly in patients who are at high risk of toxicity.[23] The typical *N*-acetylcysteine dosing regimen for prevention of CIN is to give four doses of 600 mg to 1,200 mg orally every 12 hours, with the first dose administered prior to contrast exposure (see Table 46-3).[36] Finally, other nephrotoxic drugs should be discontinued if possible, and subsequent contrast studies appropriately timed to minimize cumulative toxicity.

Clinical **Controversy...**

Some clinicians believe that insufficient evidence exists to justify use of *N*-acetylcysteine for the prevention of contrast-induced nephrotoxicity, while others feel that its safety profile, ease of use, low cost, and potential for benefit are adequate justification for use for all patients.

Renal replacement therapy, including intermittent hemodialysis and continuous modalities, for example, continuous venovenous hemofiltration (CVVH), effectively removes iodinated contrast, and was considered by some to be a therapeutic option for the prevention of CIN. However, because of the logistical issues (eg, technical difficulty), potential infectious and noninfectious risks, high cost of renal replacement therapy, and lack of consistent clinical efficacy data, renal replacement therapy is not recommended.[31,39]

Management Currently there is no specific therapy available for managing established CIN. Care is supportive as described in Chapter 43. Kidney function (eg, S_{cr} and urine output), electrolytes (eg, sodium and potassium), and volume status should be closely monitored.

Cisplatin Nephrotoxicity

Incidence Cisplatin is one of the most important and widely used antineoplastic drugs for the treatment of solid tumors, often demonstrating exceptional efficacy (ie, cure rates over 90% in testicular cancers).[40] Unfortunately, the primary dose-limiting toxicity of platin-containing compounds is nephrotoxicity. Cisplatin nephrotoxicity occurs in up to one third of patients receiving the drug and is a significant cause of morbidity.[40,41] Carboplatin, a second-generation platinum analog, is associated with a lower incidence of nephrotoxicity than cisplatin and thus is the preferred agent in high-risk patients.[42]

Clinical Presentation Cisplatin administration results in impaired tubular reabsorption and decreased urinary concentration ability, leading to increased excretion of salt and water (ie, polyuria) within 24 hours of treatment. Polyuria persists, and a decrease in GFR evidenced by a rise in S_{cr} concentration may be seen within 72 to 96 hours after cisplatin administration.[43] S_{cr} peaks approximately 10 to 14 days after initiation of therapy, with recovery by 21 days.[44] As many as 25% of patients may have reversible elevations in S_{cr} and BUN for 2 weeks after cisplatin treatment. However, kidney damage is dose related and cumulative with subsequent cycles of therapy, so the S_{cr} concentration may continue to rise, and irreversible kidney injury may result.[42] Hypomagnesemia is a hallmark finding of cisplatin nephrotoxicity, due to impaired magnesium reabsorption and thus increased urinary losses.[45] Hypomagnesemia is often accompanied by hypocalcemia and hypokalemia and may be severe, leading to seizures, neuromuscular irritability, or personality changes. Urinalysis typically reveals leukocytes, RTECs, and granular casts.

Pathogenesis The pathogenesis of cisplatin nephrotoxicity is multifactorial in nature and likely begins with cellular uptake and accumulation of the drug in proximal tubular epithelial cells to concentrations that may reach five times the serum concentration.[46] Tubular cell exposure to cisplatin then activates a series of cell signaling pathways, including the mitogen-activated protein kinase (MAPK) pathway, p53, caspase, and the generation of reactive oxygen species, that collectively promote tubular cell injury and death via necrosis and/or apoptosis.[40,41] Simultaneous production of proinflammatory cytokines such as tumor necrosis factor-α (TNF-α) within tubular cells activates an inflammatory response, which may worsen the renal insult. Although tubular damage is evident in both the proximal and distal segments, the majority occurs in the proximal tubules and is followed by a progressive loss of glomerular filtration capacity and impaired distal tubular function. Renal biopsies generally reveal necrosis-apoptosis of proximal and distal tubules and collecting ducts, with no obvious morphological changes to the glomeruli.[44]

Risk Factors Risk factors include age more than 65 years, dehydration, preexisting kidney disease, renal irradiation, concurrent use of nephrotoxic drugs, large cumulative doses, and alcohol abuse.[47]

Prevention The best renoprotective strategy is a combination of interventions, including prospective dose reduction and decreased frequency of administration, which usually requires using the platin compounds in combination with other chemotherapeutic agents, avoiding concurrent use of other nephrotoxic drugs, and ensuring patients are euvolemic or somewhat hypervolemic prior to initiating treatment.[47,48] Vigorous hydration with isotonic saline should be used for all patients with a goal of maintaining at least 100 to 150 mL/h of urine output during and after cisplatin treatment. Hydration should be initiated 12 to 24 hours prior to and continued for 2 to 3 days after cisplatin administration at rates of 100 to 250 mL/h, as tolerated, to maintain a urine flow of 3 to 4 L/day.[43]

Amifostine, an organic thiophosphate that is converted to an active metabolite, chelates cisplatin in normal cells and reduces the nephrotoxicity, neurotoxicity, ototoxicity, and myelosuppression associated with cisplatin and carboplatin therapy. It is also thought to serve as a thiol donor, thereby reducing intracellular reactive oxygen species and corresponding oxidative stress that plays a critical role in the development of cellular injury.[41] Amifostine is FDA approved to reduce nephrotoxicity associated with repeated cisplatin treatment in patients with advanced ovarian cancer. Pretreatment with amifostine should be considered for patients who are at high risk for kidney injury, particularly patients who are elderly, volume depleted, have CKD, or are receiving other nephrotoxic drugs concurrently. The current recommended dose of amifostine is 910 mg/m^2 administered IV over 15 minutes, beginning 30 minutes prior to cisplatin administration. Common toxicities include acute hypotension, nausea, and fatigue.

Other renoprotective strategies include the use of hypertonic saline (eg, administration of each dose in 250 mL of 3% saline) to reduce tubular cisplatin uptake. Classic antioxidants such as ascorbic acid, thiol-based antioxidants such as α-lipoic acid and *N*-acetylcysteine, which reduce oxidative damage by acting as a sulfhydryl donor, and the disulfiram metabolite diethyldithiocarbamate to reduce cytochrome P450 2E1-mediated generation of hydroxyl radicals have also been evaluated.[46,49] Finally, reduced renal exposure can be achieved with the use of localized intraperitoneal administration in conjunction with systemic administration of sodium thiosulfate for those with peritoneal tumors.[43]

Management AKI caused by cisplatin therapy is usually partially reversible with time and supportive care, including dialysis. Kidney function indices should be closely followed, with S_{cr} and BUN concentrations checked daily. Serum magnesium, potassium, and calcium concentrations should be monitored daily and corrected as needed.[42] Hypocalcemia and hypokalemia may be difficult to reverse until hypomagnesemia is corrected. Progressive kidney disease caused by cumulative nephrotoxicity may be irreversible and in some cases may lead to ESRD and require chronic dialysis support.[42]

Amphotericin B Nephrotoxicity

Incidence Variable rates of amphotericin B nephrotoxicity have been reported that correspond in large part to the cumulative dose administered. Nephrotoxicity may be seen in nearly 30% of patients receiving median cumulative doses as low as 240 mg and reaches an incidence of greater than 80% when cumulative doses approach 5 g.[50-52] Although numerous studies demonstrate lower rates of nephrotoxicity with liposomal formulations compared with conventional amphotericin B, it is difficult to compare rates of toxicity between products and studies because of the variability in the study populations, doses administered, and inconsistent definitions of nephrotoxicity and methods of assessment.[50,51,53]

Clinical Presentation Dose-dependent nephrotoxicity is often evident after administration of cumulative doses of 2 to 3 g as nonoliguria, renal tubular potassium, sodium, and magnesium wasting, impaired urinary concentrating ability, and distal renal tubular acidosis.[23,53] Although the cumulative dose is a significant risk factor, the time to onset of kidney injury varies considerably, ranging from a few days to weeks. Tubular dysfunction usually manifests 1 to 2 weeks after treatment is begun, and potassium and magnesium replacement may be necessary.[50] This is typically followed by a decrease in GFR and a rise in S_{cr} and BUN concentrations. Consequently, kidney function indices should be closely followed, with

S_{cr} and BUN concentrations checked daily, and serum magnesium, potassium, and calcium concentrations monitored every other day and corrected as needed.

Pathogenesis Amphotericin B nephrotoxicity occurs predominantly via two mechanisms. The first is direct tubular epithelial cell toxicity resulting from interaction of amphotericin B with ergosterol in the cell membrane, leading to increased tubular cell membrane permeability, lipid peroxidation, and eventual necrosis of proximal tubular cells.[53] The second mechanism is afferent arteriolar vasoconstriction leading to a reduction in renal blood flow and GFR, and ischemic tubular injury.[23,53]

Risk Factors Risk factors that impact the likelihood of developing amphotericin B nephrotoxicity include preexisting kidney disease, large individual and cumulative doses, short infusion times, volume depletion, hypokalemia, increased age, and concomitant administration of diuretics and other nephrotoxins, including vancomycin and cyclosporine.[50,53]

Prevention Permanent decrements in GFR are best prevented by incorporating a low threshold (ie, if S_{cr} reaches 2 mg/dL [177 μmol/L] on 2 consecutive days) for stopping amphotericin B or switching to a liposomal formulation. Several lipid formulations of amphotericin B (eg, amphotericin B lipid complex, liposomal amphotericin B) are available and should be used in most high-risk patients as they reduce nephrotoxicity by enhancing drug delivery to sites of infection and reducing interaction with tubular epithelial cell membranes.[51,53] Nephrotoxicity can also be minimized by limiting the cumulative dose, increasing the infusion time, ensuring the patient is well hydrated, and avoiding concomitant administration of other nephrotoxins.[53] Administration of 1 L IV 0.9% sodium chloride daily during the course of therapy appears to reduce toxicity and a single infusion of saline 10 to 15 mL/kg prior to administration of each dose of amphotericin B are generally recommended.[53] A number of other antifungal agents such as itraconazole, voriconazole, and caspofungin are viable alternatives and are now routinely used in lieu of amphotericin B for patients at high risk of developing nephrotoxicity. Administration of the antioxidant *N*-acetylcysteine (600 mg orally twice daily in adults) during amphotericin treatment may be nephroprotective.[54]

Clinical **Controversy...**

Although liposomal formulations of amphotericin B are up to 200 times more expensive than conventional amphotericin B (ie, up to $1,000 per day vs $5 per day),[53] many clinicians recommend using liposomal formulations for all patients with CKD and those at risk for developing nephrotoxicity. Others maintain that the safety and efficacy of liposomal formulations are not yet established enough to warrant their use for all patients.

Management Amphotericin B nephrotoxicity is best treated by discontinuation of therapy and substitution of alternative antifungal therapy, if possible. Renal tubular dysfunction and glomerular filtration will improve gradually to some degree in most patients, but damage may be irreversible. Kidney function indices should be closely followed, with S_{cr} and BUN concentrations checked daily, and serum magnesium, potassium, and calcium concentrations should be monitored daily and corrected as needed.

Osmotic Nephrosis

Several drugs, including mannitol, low-molecular-weight dextran, hydroxyethyl starch, and radiographic contrast media, or drug vehicles, such as sucrose, maltose, and propylene glycol, are associated with osmotic nephrosis, which may rarely lead to ATN and AKI.[55] Since osmotic nephrosis does not necessarily negatively affect proximal tubular function, its presence may often go undetected in patients without overt signs of ATN. This likely contributes to the extremely low incidence of osmotic nephrosis reported for causative agents. IV immunoglobulin solutions containing hyperosmolar sucrose may cause osmotic nephrosis and AKI in 1% to 10% of cases, which is usually reversible shortly after discontinuing therapy.[56,57] Maltose-based IV immunoglobulin solutions have also been implicated in the development of osmotic nephrosis. Although IV immunoglobulin-induced AKI is the modern prototype for osmotic nephrosis, it is understood that the vehicle (ie, sucrose or maltose) is the culprit and not the immunoglobulins themselves.[57]

Clinical Presentation and Pathogenesis

The clinical presentation of osmotic nephrosis is often subtle. While tubular proteinuria or vacuolated tubular cells may be observed on urinalysis for patients with AKI, the definitive diagnosis of osmotic nephrosis is only made via a kidney biopsy.[56] IV immunoglobulin-induced AKI typically presents as oliguria after 2 to 4 days of treatment and may persist for up to 2 weeks. Kidney injury occurs via uptake of the offending agent through pinocytosis into proximal tubular epithelial cells, subsequent formation of vacuoles, and accumulation of lysosomes, which collectively results in an oncotic gradient and thus cellular swelling, tubular luminal occlusion, and compromised cellular integrity.[58] Renal replacement therapy may be necessary for up to 40% of patients developing osmotic nephrosis-associated AKI.[56] However, it is usually reversible, with nearly all patients recovering normal kidney function following withdrawal of the offending drug.

Risk Factors

Risk factors for osmotic nephrosis include excessive doses of offending agents, preexisting kidney disease, ischemia, older age (greater than 65 years), and concomitant use of other nephrotoxins. Nephrotoxicity may be prevented by limiting the dose, reducing the rate of infusion, and avoiding dehydration and concomitant nephrotoxins.[57,58]

HEMODYNAMICALLY MEDIATED KIDNEY INJURY

4 Hemodynamically mediated kidney injury generally refers to any cause of AKI resulting from an acute decrease in intraglomerular pressure, including "prerenal" states leading to reduced effective renal blood flow (eg, hypovolemia and congestive heart failure) and medications that affect the renin–angiotensin system.[23,59] The kidneys receive approximately 25% of resting cardiac output, which renders them particularly susceptible to alterations in renal blood flow and enhances their exposure to circulating drugs.[16,60] Within each nephron, blood flow and pressure are regulated by glomerular afferent and efferent arterioles to maintain intraglomerular capillary hydrostatic pressure, glomerular filtration, and urine output. Afferent and efferent arteriolar vasoconstrictions are primarily mediated by angiotensin II, whereas afferent vasodilation is primarily mediated by prostaglandins (Fig. 46-1). This specialized blood flow is precisely regulated by interrelations between arachidonic acid metabolites, natriuretic factors, nitric oxide, the sympathetic nervous system, the renin–angiotensin system, and the macula densa response to distal tubular solute delivery.[60] Drug-induced causes of hemodynamic kidney injury typically stem from constriction of glomerular afferent arterioles and/or dilation of glomerular efferent arterioles. ACEIs, angiotensin II receptor blockers (ARBs), and NSAIDs are the agents that have been most commonly implicated.[23,61]

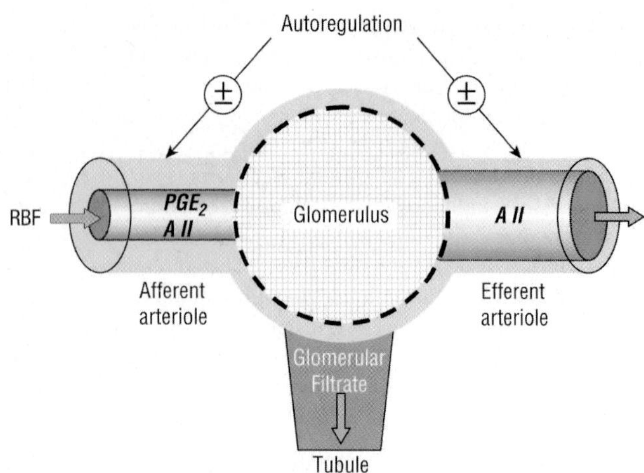

FIGURE 46-1 Normal glomerular autoregulation serves to maintain intraglomerular capillary hydrostatic pressure, glomerular filtration rate (GFR), and, ultimately, urine output. (A II, angiotensin II; PGE_2, prostaglandin E_2; RBF, renal blood flow.)

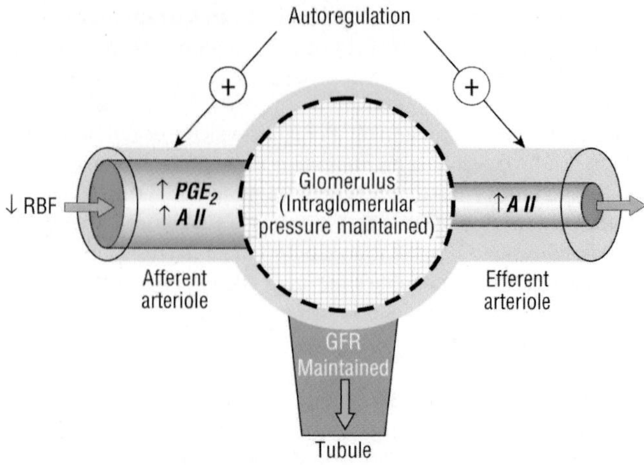

FIGURE 46-2 Glomerular autoregulation during "prerenal" states (ie, reduced blood flow). (A II, angiotensin II; GFR, glomerular filtration rate; PGE_2, prostaglandin E_2; RBF, renal blood flow.)

Angiotensin-Converting Enzyme Inhibitors and Angiotensin II Receptor Blockers

Angiotensin-converting enzyme inhibitors (ACEIs) and ARBs are extensively utilized for the management of hypertension and prevention of the progression of CKD even though they have been associated with the development of AKI.

Incidence

Patients with renal artery stenosis, volume depletion, and congestive heart failure and those with preexisting kidney disease, including diabetic nephropathy, are most likely to experience a significant decline in kidney function when therapy with one of these agents is initiated.[23] For example, up to 25% of hospitalized patients with congestive heart failure develop AKI within weeks after beginning treatment with ACEIs.[62] Moreover, ACEIs and ARBs are among the most commonly implicated medications in emergency hospitalizations, contributing to nearly 3% of emergency room visits for adverse drug events.[63]

Clinical Presentation

Therapy with ACEIs and ARBs will acutely reduce GFR; so a moderate rise in S_{cr} after initiation of therapy should be anticipated.[64] Importantly, a distinction must be made between a potentially detrimental reduction in GFR and a normal, predictable rise in S_{cr}. An increase in S_{cr} of up to 30% is commonly observed within 3 to 5 days of initiating therapy and is an indication that the drug has begun to exert its desired pharmacologic effect.[64] The increase in S_{cr} typically stabilizes within 1 to 2 weeks and is usually reversible upon stopping the drug. Furthermore, an association exists between acute increases in S_{cr} of less than or equal to 30% from baseline that stabilize within the first 2 months of initiating therapy and preservation of kidney function. The S_{cr} threshold for discontinuation of ACEI or ARB therapy is unclear. However, an increase in S_{cr} of more than 30% above baseline in the course of 1 to 2 weeks may necessitate discontinuation of the offending drug.[64]

Pathogenesis

Angiotensin-converting enzyme inhibitors—or ARB-mediated kidney injury is primarily the result of disruption of normal autoregulation of intraglomerular capillary hydrostatic pressure.[23] Normally, the kidney attempts to maintain GFR by dilating the afferent arteriole and constricting the efferent arteriole in response to a decrease in renal blood flow. During states of reduced blood flow, the juxtaglomerular apparatus increases renin secretion. Plasma renin converts angiotensinogen to angiotensin I, and ultimately angiotensin II by angiotensin-converting enzyme. Angiotensin II constricts the afferent and efferent arterioles, but has a greater effect on the efferent arterioles, resulting in a net increase in intraglomerular pressure.[60] Additionally, renal prostaglandins, prostaglandin E_2 in particular, are released and induce a net dilation of the afferent arteriole, thereby improving blood flow into the glomerulus. Together these processes maintain GFR and urine output (Fig. 46-2).

When ACEI therapy (eg, enalapril or ramipril) is initiated, the synthesis of angiotensin II is decreased, thereby preferentially dilating the efferent arteriole. This reduces outflow resistance from the glomerulus and decreases hydrostatic pressure in the glomerular capillaries, which alters Starling forces across the glomerular capillaries to decrease intraglomerular pressure and GFR. This in turn often leads to nephrotoxicity, particularly in the setting of reduced renal blood flow or effective arterial blood volume (Fig. 46-3), that is, prerenal settings (eg, congestive heart failure) in which glomerular afferent arteriolar blood flow is reduced and the efferent arteriole is vasoconstricted to maintain sufficient glomerular capillary hydrostatic pressure for ultrafiltration.[23]

Risk Factors

Patients at greatest risk are those dependent on angiotensin II and renal efferent arteriolar constriction to maintain blood pressure

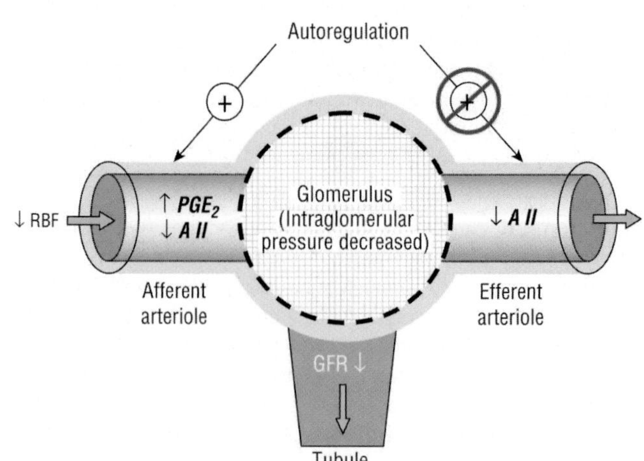

FIGURE 46-3 Pathogenesis of angiotensin-converting enzyme inhibitor (ACEI) nephropathy. (A II, angiotensin II; GFR, glomerular filtration rate; PGE_2, prostaglandin E_2; RBF, renal blood flow.)

and GFR. These include patients with bilateral renal artery stenosis or stenosis in a single kidney (ie, renal transplant); patients with decreased effective arterial blood volume (ie, prerenal states), especially those with decompensated congestive heart failure, volume depletion from excess diuresis or GI fluid loss, hepatic cirrhosis with ascites, and nephrotic syndrome; patients with preexisting kidney disease; and patients receiving concurrent nephrotoxic drugs, particularly other drugs that affect intraglomerular autoregulation such as NSAIDs.[23,61,65]

Prevention

Hemodynamically mediated AKI caused by ACEIs or ARBs is frequently preventable by recognizing the presence of preexisting kidney disease or decreased effective renal blood flow as a result of volume depletion, heart failure, or liver disease. A common strategy for at-risk patients is to initiate therapy with very low doses of a short-acting ACEI (eg, captopril 6.25 mg-12.5 mg), then gradually titrate the dose upward and convert to a longer-acting agent after patient tolerance has been demonstrated. Outpatients may be started on low doses of long-acting ACEIs (eg, enalapril 2.5 mg) with gradual dose titration every 2 to 4 weeks until the maximum dose or desired response is achieved.[64] Kidney function indices and serum potassium concentrations must be monitored carefully, daily for hospitalized patients and every 2 to 3 days for outpatients. Monitoring may need to be more frequent during outpatient initiation of ACEI or ARB therapy for patients with preexisting kidney disease, congestive heart failure, or suspected renovascular disease. Use of concurrent hypotensive agents and other drugs that affect renal hemodynamics (eg, NSAIDs, diuretics) should be discouraged and dehydration avoided.[64]

Management

Acute decreases in kidney function and the development of hyperkalemia usually resolve over several days after ACEI or ARB therapy is discontinued. Occasionally patients will require management of severe hyperkalemia, as described in detail in Chapter 51.

Angiotensin-converting enzyme inhibitors or ARB therapy may frequently be reinitiated, particularly for patients with congestive heart failure, after intravascular volume depletion has been corrected or diuretic doses reduced. Slight reductions in kidney function (maintenance of a S_{cr} concentration of 2-3 mg/dL [177-265 μmol/L]) may be an acceptable trade-off for hemodynamic improvement in certain patients with severe congestive heart failure or renovascular disease not amenable to revascularization.

Nonsteroidal Antiinflammatory Drugs and Selective Cyclooxygenase-2 Inhibitors

The overall safety of NSAIDs is evidenced by the nonprescription availability in the United States of several drugs in the class (eg, ibuprofen, naproxen, ketoprofen). Although potential adverse renal effects from nonprescription NSAIDs had been a concern, conventional nonselective NSAIDs and selective cyclooxygenase-2 (COX-2) inhibitors are unlikely to acutely affect kidney function in the absence of renal ischemia or excess renal vasoconstrictor activity. Nevertheless, given their general safety and widespread availability, NSAIDs are among the most commonly used drugs, with approximately 111 million prescriptions worldwide and 30 billion over-the-counter doses of NSAIDs administered annually in the United States.[66]

Incidence

The incidence of NSAID-induced kidney injury is unclear. Historical reports suggest that 500,000 to 2.5 million people develop some degree of NSAID nephrotoxicity in the United States annually.[67]

Clinical Presentation

Nonsteroidal antiinflammatory drug- and COX-2-induced AKI usually occurs within 2 to 7 days of initiating therapy,[59,66] particularly with a short-acting agent such as ibuprofen, or within days of some other precipitating event (eg, intravascular volume depletion). Patients typically present with complaints of diminished urine output, weight gain, and/or edema. Urine sodium concentrations (less than 20 mEq/L [mmol/L]) and fractional excretion of sodium (less than 1% [0.01]) are usually low, and BUN, S_{cr}, potassium, and blood pressure are typically elevated. The urine sediment is usually bland and unchanged from baseline but may show occasional RTECs and granular casts.[59,66]

Pathogenesis

The pathogenesis of NSAID- and COX-2-induced AKI lies in the disruption of normal intraglomerular autoregulation.[59] Specifically, NSAIDs inhibit cyclooxygenase (COX)-catalyzed synthesis of vasodilatory prostaglandins, including prostaglandins I_2 (prostacyclin) and E_2, from arachidonic acid.[66] These prostaglandins are synthesized in the renal cortex and medulla by vascular endothelial and glomerular mesangial cells, and their effects are primarily local and result in net afferent arteriolar vasodilation. Vasodilatory prostaglandins have limited activity in states of normal renal blood flow, but in states of decreased renal blood flow, their synthesis is increased and they serve a vital autoregulatory role in the protection against renal ischemia and hypoxia by antagonizing renal arteriolar vasoconstriction due to angiotensin II, norepinephrine, endothelin, and vasopressin. Thus, administration of NSAIDs in the setting of reduced renal blood flow will blunt the usual compensatory increase in prostaglandin activity, altering the normal autoregulatory balance in favor of renal vasoconstrictors, thereby promoting renal ischemia and a reduction in glomerular filtration.[66]

Risk Factors

Risk factors for NSAID- and COX-2-induced AKI include age more than 60 years, preexisting kidney disease, hepatic disease with ascites, congestive heart failure, intravascular volume depletion/dehydration, systemic lupus erythematosus, or concurrent treatment with diuretics, ACEIs, or ARBs.[61,65,66] The use of ACEIs, diuretics, and NSAIDs concurrently is associated with a greater than 30% increased risk for AKI, which increases to greater than 60% in patients over age 75 or with preexisting kidney disease.[61,65] The elderly are at higher risk because of multiple comorbidities, multiple-drug therapies, and reduced renal hemodynamics. Combined use of NSAIDs or COX-2 inhibitors and concurrent nephrotoxic drugs, particularly other drugs that affect intraglomerular autoregulation, should be avoided in high-risk patients.

Prevention

Nonsteroidal antiinflammatory drug- and COX-2 inhibitor-induced AKI can be prevented by recognizing high-risk patients, avoiding potent compounds such as indomethacin and using analgesics with less prostaglandin inhibition, such as acetaminophen, nonacetylated salicylates, aspirin, and possibly nabumetone. Nonnarcotic analgesics (eg, tramadol) may also be useful but do not provide antiinflammatory activity. When NSAID therapy is essential for high-risk patients, the minimal effective dose should be used for the shortest duration possible, and NSAIDs with short half-lives should be considered (eg, sulindac) along with optimal management of predisposing medical problems and frequent kidney function monitoring. Moreover, use of concurrent hypotensive agents and other drugs that affect renal hemodynamics (eg, ACEIs, ARBs, diuretics) should be discouraged in high-risk patients and dehydration avoided.[66]

Management

Nonsteroidal antiinflammatory drugs-induced AKI is treated by discontinuation of therapy and supportive care. Use of other nephrotoxic drugs should be avoided. Kidney injury is rarely severe, and kidney function generally recovers within 3 to 5 days.[59] Occasionally, the hemodynamic insult is sufficiently severe to cause ATN, which can prolong injury.

Cyclosporine and Tacrolimus

The calcineurin inhibitors cyclosporine and tacrolimus have dramatically enhanced the success of solid-organ transplantation. As many as 94% of kidney transplant patients are prescribed a calcineurin inhibitor-based immunosuppressive regimen.[68] Nephrotoxicity, however, remains a major dose-limiting adverse effect of both drugs. Although delayed chronic interstitial nephritis has also been reported,[69] acute hemodynamically mediated kidney injury is an important mechanism of calcineurin inhibitor-induced nephrotoxicity.

Incidence

Historically, reversible AKI occurred frequently in transplant recipients during the first 6 months of cyclosporine therapy. The 5-year risk of CKD after transplantation of a nonrenal organ ranges from 7% to 21%, depending on the type of organ transplanted, and the occurrence of CKD in these patients is associated with more than a fourfold increase in the risk of death.[70]

Clinical Presentation

The clinical presentation of acute nephrotoxicity associated with calcineurin inhibitors (ie, hemodynamically mediated AKI) is quite different from the presentation of chronic nephrotoxicity (see Chronic Interstitial Nephritis below).[71] AKI may occur within days of initiating therapy, manifesting as a rise in S_{cr} concentration and a corresponding decline in creatinine clearance. Hypertension, hyperkalemia, sodium retention, oliguria, renal tubular acidosis, and hypomagnesemia are frequently observed in the absence of urine sediment abnormalities or morphologic lesions.[68] On the other hand, renal biopsy may reveal thickening of arterioles, mild focal glomerular sclerosis, proximal tubular epithelial cell vacuolization and atrophy, and interstitial fibrosis. Biopsy is most useful to distinguish acute calcineurin inhibitor nephrotoxicity from acute cellular rejection of the transplanted kidney, the latter being evidenced by interstitial infiltrates composed of activated lymphocytes (see Chapter 90).[72]

Pathogenesis

The acute hemodynamic changes associated with calcineurin inhibitor nephrotoxicity result from an increase in potent vasoconstrictors including thromboxane A_2 and endothelin, activation of the renin–angiotensin and sympathetic nervous systems, as well as a reduction in the vasodilators nitric oxide, prostacyclin, and prostaglandin E_2.[68,70,71] The net effect is an imbalance in afferent and efferent tone, resulting in predominantly afferent vasoconstriction with reduced renal plasma flow and GFR. The mechanism of acute nephrotoxicity is generally thought to be dose related, since kidney function improves rapidly following dose reduction.[71]

Risk Factors

Risk factors include age over 65, higher dose, concomitant therapy with nephrotoxic drugs (particularly NSAIDs), and interacting drugs that inhibit calcineurin inhibitor metabolism and transport and thus increase systemic exposure, older kidney allograft age, salt depletion, diuretic use, and polymorphic expression of P-glycoprotein.[68,72]

Prevention

Because acute hemodynamically mediated kidney injury secondary to cyclosporine and tacrolimus appears to be concentration related, pharmacokinetic and pharmacodynamic monitoring is an important means of preventing toxicity.[68] However, the persistent presence of therapeutic or low cyclosporine concentrations does not totally preclude the development of nephrotoxicity. Calcium channel blockers may antagonize the vasoconstrictor effect of cyclosporine by dilating glomerular afferent arterioles and preventing acute decreases in renal blood flow and glomerular filtration.[68] Lastly, decreased doses of cyclosporine or tacrolimus, primarily when used in combination with other nonnephrotoxic immunosuppressants, may minimize the risk of toxicity, but this may increase the risk of chronic rejection.

Management

Acute kidney injury usually improves with dose reduction and treatment of contributing illness or the discontinuation of interacting drugs. CKD is usually irreversible, but progressive toxicity may be limited by discontinuation of cyclosporine (or tacrolimus) therapy or dose reduction, with the continuation of other immunosuppressants.[68,71] S_{cr} and BUN should be closely monitored (daily if possible), as should cyclosporine or tacrolimus concentrations, to ensure that serum concentrations are within the narrow therapeutic range.

OBSTRUCTIVE NEPHROPATHY

Numerous medications may cause obstructive nephropathy, or kidney injury from deposition or precipitation within the renal tubules and/or collecting system. For example, the precipitation of drug crystals in distal tubular lumens can lead to intratubular obstruction, interstitial nephritis, and occasionally superimposed ATN, collectively termed crystal nephropathy. Nephrolithiasis, the formation of stones within the kidney, results from abnormal crystal precipitation in the renal collecting system, potentially causing urinary tract obstruction with kidney injury. Several medications that have been associated with development of obstructive nephropathy are listed in Table 46-1.

Crystal Nephropathy

Incidence

The incidence of crystal nephropathy is unclear for most of the implicated agents because histologically confirmed cases are rare, and many drugs cause kidney injury via multiple mechanisms.[73] For example, AKI develops in approximately 2% of patients who receive high dose methotrexate, likely due to a combination of direct toxic effects and crystal nephropathy.[74,75] Similarly, crystalluria is observed in 20% of patients receiving indinavir, but the number of patients developing crystal nephropathy is unknown.[76]

Pathogenesis

Drugs may induce intratubular obstruction and AKI by direct (precipitation of the drug itself) and indirect means (ie, promoting release and precipitation of tissue-degradation products or cellular casts). For example, antineoplastic drugs may cause acute renal tubular obstruction indirectly by inducing tumor lysis syndrome, hyperuricemia, and intratubular precipitation of uric acid crystals.[47] The diagnosis is supported by a urine uric acid-to-creatinine ratio greater than 1. Uric acid precipitation can be prevented by vigorous hydration with normal saline, beginning at least 48 hours prior to chemotherapy, to maintain urine output 100 mL/h in adults. Administration of allopurinol 100 mg/m^2 thrice daily (maximum of 800 mg/day) started 2 to 3 days prior to chemotherapy, and urinary alkalinization to pH 7 may also be of value. In patients at high risk of developing tumor lysis syndrome (ie, large tumor burden, preexisiting kidney disease, and older age), a single fixed dose of 3 mg rasburicase may be beneficial.[77]

Drug-induced rhabdomyolysis is another form of indirect toxicity, which can lead to intratubular precipitation of myoglobin and, if severe, AKI.[78] The most common cause of drug-induced rhabdomyolysis is direct myotoxicity from 3-hydroxy-3-methylglutaryl-coenzyme A (HMG-CoA) reductase inhibitors or statins, including lovastatin and simvastatin.[79] The risk of rhabdomyolysis is increased when these drugs are administered concurrently with gemfibrozil, niacin, or inhibitors of the CYP3A4 metabolic pathway (eg, erythromycin and itraconazole).

Warfarin-related nephropathy (WRN) is characterized by glomerular hemorrhage with subsequent intratubular obstruction by red blood cell casts. Patients with underlying CKD appear to be at greatest risk. The incidence of WRN may be as high as 33% in CKD versus 16.5% in non-CKD patients. Other risk factors included age, diabetes mellitus, hypertension, and cardiovascular disease.[80]

Intratubular precipitation of drugs or their metabolites can also directly cause AKI. Precipitation of drug crystals is due primarily to supersaturation of a low urine volume with the offending drug or relative insolubility of the drug in either alkaline or acidic urine.[76] Volume depletion is an important risk factor for the development of AKI. Urine pH decreases to approximately 4.5 during maximal stimulation of renal tubular hydrogen ion secretion. Certain solutes can precipitate and obstruct the tubular lumen at this acid pH, particularly when urine is concentrated, such as for patients with volume depletion. For example, several antiviral drugs have been associated with intratubular precipitation and AKI.[81,82] Acyclovir is relatively insoluble at physiologic urine pH and is associated with intratubular precipitation in dehydrated oliguric patients.[76] Foscarnet complexation with ionized calcium may result in precipitation of calcium-foscarnet salt crystals in renal glomeruli, causing primarily a crystalline glomerulonephritis. The salt crystals may then secondarily precipitate in the renal tubules causing tubular necrosis.[23] The protease inhibitor indinavir has been associated with symptomatic crystalluria or nephrolithiasis in 20% to 33% of patients receiving chronic treatment.[76,82] Intratubular indinavir crystal precipitation can be prevented in most patients if the patient consumes adequate hydration to obtain a urinary output of at least 1,500 mL per day.[81] Sulfadiazine, when used at high doses, and methotrexate may also precipitate in acidic urine and can cause oligoanuric kidney injury.[76] Massive administration of ascorbic acid can also result in obstruction of renal tubules with calcium oxalate crystals, leading to "oxalate nephropathy".[76] Triamterene and the quinolone antibiotic ciprofloxacin may also precipitate in renal tubules and cause kidney injury.[23,73]

Kidney injury caused by intratubular precipitation of most tissue-degradation products or drugs and their metabolites can be largely prevented and possibly treated by administering the drug after vigorously prehydrating the patient, maintaining a high urine volume, and urinary alkalinization.[81,82]

NEPHROCALCINOSIS

Nephrocalcinosis is a clinical pathologic condition characterized by extensive tubulointerstitial precipitation and deposition of calcium phosphate crystals leading to marked tubular calcification.[83] It is most commonly seen in clinical conditions associated with hypercalcemia and hypercalciuria, such as hyperparathyroidism, malignancy, and less frequently increased intake of calcium or vitamin D. However, nephrocalcinosis can also result from hyperphosphatemia and hyperphosphaturia in the absence of hypercalcemia, as is known to occur for patients who have received oral sodium phosphate solution (OSPS) as a bowel preparation.[84]

Acute Phosphate Nephropathy

The term acute phosphate nephropathy was coined specifically to describe OSPS-induced nephrocalcinosis, as its pathogenesis is the result of increased phosphate intake rather than hypercalcemia.[84] Nephrocalcinosis is associated with use of OSPS for bowel preparation prior to GI procedures, and strong associations have recently been demonstrated between exposure to OSPS and a decline in kidney function, particularly in the elderly and those with preexisting kidney disease.[84,85]

Incidence

The incidence of acute phosphate nephropathy is between 1 in 1,000 and 1 in 5,000 exposures, translating to roughly 1,400 to 7,000 new cases annually.[86]

Clinical Presentation

Patients usually present with AKI several days to months after exposure to OSPS. Low-grade proteinuria (less than 1 g/day), normocalcemia, and bland urinary sediment are usually observed. Extensive deposition of calcium phosphate in the distal tubules and collecting ducts without glomerular or vascular injury is the hallmark of acute phosphate nephropathy.[76]

Risk Factors

Risk factors include advanced age, preexisting kidney disease, female sex, hypertension, diabetes, bowel conditions associated with prolonged intestinal transit, high sodium phosphate dosage, volume depletion, and medications that affect renal perfusion or function (eg, diuretics, lithium, NSAIDs, ACEIs, or ARBs).[84]

NEPHROLITHIASIS

Nephrolithiasis (formation of renal calculi or kidney stones) does not present as classic nephrotoxicity since GFR is usually not decreased. Drug-induced nephrolithiasis can be the result of abnormal crystal precipitation in the renal collecting system, potentially causing pain, hematuria, infection, or, occasionally, urinary tract obstruction with kidney injury. The overall prevalence of drug-induced nephrolithiasis is estimated to be 1% to 2% of all cases of nephrolithiasis.[82]

Kidney stone formation, possibly also accompanied by intratubular precipitation of crystalline material, has been a rare complication of drug therapy. Until the development of antiretroviral drugs, triamterene had been the drug most frequently associated with kidney stone formation, with a prevalence of 0.4%.[73] Sulfadiazine is a poorly soluble sulfonamide that may cause symptomatic acetylsulfadiazine crystalluria with stone formation and flank or back pain, hematuria, or kidney injury.[76] A high urine volume and urinary alkalinization to pH greater than 7.15 may be protective. Numerous other drugs have been implicated in the development of nephrolithiasis, including the antibacterial agents ciprofloxacin, amoxicillin, and nitrofurantoin, and various products containing ephedrine, norephedrine, pseudoephedrine, and melamine. Moreover, nephrolithiasis has become a well known complication of antiretroviral agents, including the protease inhibitors indinavir, atazanavir, nelfinavir, amprenavir, saquinavir, ritonavir and darunavir.[82]

GLOMERULAR DISEASE

Proteinuria, particularly nephrotic range proteinuria (defined as urine protein excretion greater than 3.5 g/day/1.73 m^2) with or without a decline in the GFR is a hallmark sign of glomerular injury (see Chapter 47). Glomerular injury associated with drug exposure is broadly classified into either direct cellular toxicity or immune mediated injury. Glomerular lesions associated with direct cellular toxicity include thrombotic microangiopathy (see Renal Vaculitis section), minimal change glomerular disease, and focal segmental glomerulosclerosis (FSGS). Lesions from immune-mediated injury include vasculitis (see Renal Vaculitis section) and membranous nephropathy.[87,88] Although drug-induced glomerular disease is uncommon, a variety of agents have been implicated.

Minimal Change Glomerular Disease

Drug-induced minimal change glomerular disease is frequently accompanied by interstitial nephritis and is most common during NSAID therapy. Lithium, pamidronate, interferon-α and interferon-β have also been implicated.[87] Patients present abruptly with nephrotic range proteinuria, hypoalbuminemia, and hyperlipidemia and rarely with hematuria and hypertension. The pathogenesis is unknown, but nephrotic range proteinuria as a consequence of NSAID therapy is frequently associated with a T-lymphocytic interstitial infiltrate, suggesting disordered cell-mediated immunity.[66] Proteinuria usually resolves rapidly after discontinuation of the offending drug, and a course of corticosteroids may help resolve the lesion. That said, the majority of adults with NSAID induced minimal change glomerular disease achieve complete remission over the course of several months, even in the absence of corticosteroid treatment.[87]

Focal Segmental Glomerulosclerosis

Focal segmental glomerulosclerosis is characterized by patchy areas (ie, only some glomeruli are partially affected by the disease) of glomerular sclerosis with interstitial inflammation and fibrosis (see Chapter 47). It represents a pattern of glomerular injury, not a disease per se, and is the final common pathway by which normal glomerular components are replaced by fibrous scar tissue. FSGS has been described in the setting of chronic heroin abuse (known as *heroin nephropathy*).[89] The pathogenesis is unknown but may include direct toxicity by heroin or adulterants and injury from bacterial or viral infections accompanying IV drug use. The bisphosphonates pamidronate and zoledronate, commonly used to treat osteoporosis, malignancy-associated hypercalcemia, and Paget's disease, are associated with the development of a particularly aggressive variant of FSGS called *collapsing glomerulopathy*.[87] It presents with massive proteinuria (greater than 8 g/day), and it is typically characterized by rising S_{cr} at diagnosis and rapid progression to ESRD. Patients receiving IV formulations, high doses, or prolonged therapy are at highest risk. Interferon-α, interferon-β, lithium, sirolimus, and anabolic steroids have also been associated with FSGS.

Membranous Nephropathy

Membranous nephropathy is the most common etiology of nephrotic syndrome in Caucasian adults.[88] It is characterized by subepithelial immune complex formation along glomerular capillary loops and, although rarely seen, has classically been associated with gold therapy, penicillamine, captopril, and NSAID use.[88] Patients present with nephrotic range proteinuria and microscopic hematuria, with hypertension and elevated S_{cr} apparent for patients with more advanced disease. The pathogenesis may involve damage to proximal tubule epithelium with antigen release, antibody formation, and glomerular immune complex deposition.[88] Proteinuria usually resolves slowly after discontinuing the offending drug. Patients who remain nephrotic after 6 months should be treated with a 6- to 12-month course of immunosuppressive therapy, which typically consists of prednisone with or without cyclophosphamide.

TUBULOINTERSTITIAL NEPHRITIS

Tubulointerstitial nephritis refers to diseases in which the predominant changes occur in the renal interstitium rather than the tubules. The presentation may be acute and reversible with interstitial edema, rapid loss of kidney function, and systemic symptoms or chronic and irreversible, associated with interstitial fibrosis and minimal to no systemic symptoms.[90]

Acute Allergic Interstitial Nephritis

Incidence

5 The incidence of drug-induced acute allergic interstitial nephritis (AIN) is unclear and likely varies with clinical setting. For example, pathology registries indicate AIN as the histologic lesion in only 2% to 5% of kidney biopsies, but from 10% to 27% of kidney biopsies performed in hospitalized patients with unexplained AKI demonstrate AIN.[59] Multiple drugs have been implicated in the development of AIN (Table 46-4). It usually manifests 2 weeks after exposure to a drug but may occur sooner if the patient was previously sensitized.[91]

TABLE 46-4 Drugs Associated with Allergic Interstitial Nephritis

Antimicrobials	
Acyclovir	Indinavir
Aminoglycosides	Rifampin
Amphotericin B	Sulfonamides
β-Lactams	Tetracyclines
Erythromycin	Trimethoprim–sulfamethoxazole
Ethambutol	Vancomycin
Diuretics	
Acetazolamide	Loop diuretics
Amiloride	Triamterene
Chlorthalidone	Thiazide diuretics
Neuropsychiatric	
Carbamazepine	Phenytoin
Lithium	Valproic acid
Phenobarbital	
Nonsteroidal antiinflammatory drugs	
Aspirin	Ketoprofen
Indomethacin	Phenylbutazone
Naproxen	Diclofenac
Ibuprofen	Zomepirac
Diflunisal	Cyclooxygenase-2 inhibitors
Piroxicam	
Miscellaneous	
Acetaminophen	Lansoprazole
Allopurinol	Methyldopa
Interferon-α	Omeprazole
Aspirin	*P*-aminosalicylic acid
Azathioprine	Phenylpropanolamine
Captopril	Propylthiouracil
Cimetidine	Radiographic contrast media
Clofibrate	Ranitidine
Cyclosporine	Sulfinpyrazone
Glyburide	Warfarin sodium
Gold	

Clinical Presentation

Although methicillin-induced AIN is the prototype for AIN, it is now recognized that AIN is associated with all β-lactam antibiotics (including cephalosporins) and numerous other antimicrobials. Clinical signs present approximately 14 days after initiation of therapy and include (with their approximate incidence) fever (27%-80%), maculopapular rash (15%-25%), eosinophilia (23%-80%), arthralgia (45%), and oliguria (50%).[91] Historically, systemic hypersensitivity findings of the classic triad of fever, rash, and arthralgia, often along with eosinophilia and eosinophiluria, were strongly suggestive of the diagnosis of AIN. However, it is now recognized that this constellation of findings is not consistently reliable as one or more are frequently absent. In fact, the triad is seen in only 5% to 10% of patients with AIN, so caution is warranted in basing diagnosis on hypersensitivity findings alone.[92] Eosinophilia alone is insensitive, and eosinophiluria is insensitive and nonspecific, so urinary eosinophils are not considered a useful sign of AIN and are no longer recommended as a diagnostic test.[92] Anemia, leukocytosis, and elevated immunoglobulin E levels may occur. Tubular dysfunction may be manifested by acidosis, hyperkalemia, salt wasting, and concentrating defects.[91]

Nonsteroidal antiinflammatory drugs-induced AIN has a different clinical presentation than that seen with most other drugs.[91] Patients are typically over 50 years of age (reflecting NSAID use for degenerative joint disease), the onset is delayed a mean of 6 months from initiation of therapy compared with 2 weeks with β-lactams, and fever, rash, and eosinophilia are typically not observed in patients with NSAID-induced AIN.[91] Concomitant nephrotic syndrome (proteinuria greater than 3.5 g/day) occurs in more than 70% of patients. Prompt diagnosis of AIN is important as discontinuation of the offending drug may prevent irreversible renal damage. Renal biopsy is the most definitive method for diagnosis.

Pathogenesis

The pathogenesis of the majority of cases of AIN is considered to be an allergic hypersensitivity response. This is supported by the fact that AIN is characterized as a diffuse or focal interstitial infiltrate of lymphocytes, eosinophils, and occasional polymorphonuclear neutrophils.[90] Granulomas and tubular epithelial cell necrosis are relatively common with drug-induced AIN. Occasionally a humoral antibody-mediated mechanism is implicated by the presence of circulating antibody to a drug hapten–tubular basement membrane complex, low serum complement levels, and deposition of immunoglobulin G and complement in the tubular basement membrane. More commonly, a cell-mediated immune mechanism is suggested by the absence of these findings and the presence of a predominantly T-lymphocyte.[90]

Risk Factors

No specific risk factors have been identified because these are idiosyncratic hypersensitivity reactions. Individuals with other drug allergies may have increased risk and warrant close monitoring.

Prevention

No specific preventive measures are known because of the idiosyncratic nature of these reactions. Patients must be monitored carefully to recognize the signs and symptoms because promptly discontinuing the offending drug often leads to full recovery.[91]

Management

Corticosteroid therapy is beneficial and should be initiated immediately or soon after diagnosis of AIN along with discontinuance of the offending drug to avoid the risk of incomplete recovery of kidney function. While various regimens have been used, high-dose oral prednisone 1 mg/kg/day for 4 to 6 weeks with a stepwise taper over the next 4 weeks may be considered. However, if there is no significant improvement in kidney function after 3 to 4 weeks of treatment, then steroids should be discontinued.[90] Typical kidney function indices (eg, S_{cr}, BUN) and signs and symptoms of AIN should be monitored closely for improvement.

Chronic Interstitial Nephritis

Lithium, analgesics, calcineurin inhibitors, aristolochic acid, and only a few other drugs have been reported to cause chronic interstitial nephritis, which is usually a progressive and irreversible lesion.

Lithium

Incidence The prevalence of non-dialysis-dependent CKD stemming from chronic lithium nephrotoxicity in the general population of patients treated with lithium is approximately 1%.[93,94] The prevalence of lithium-induced ESRD among all ESRD patients is between 0.2% and 0.8%.[93] Although several renal tubular lesions are associated with lithium therapy, an impaired ability to concentrate urine (nephrogenic diabetes insipidus) is seen in 20% of all patients receiving lithium therapy.[95]

Clinical Presentation Lithium-induced nephrotoxicity is typically asymptomatic and develops insidiously during years of therapy. Blood pressure is normal and urinary sediment is bland, making detection difficult until the disease progresses significantly.[96] It is usually recognized by rising BUN or S_{cr} concentrations or the onset of hypertension. Polydipsia (excessive thirst) and polyuria (excessive urination) are observed in 40% and 20%, respectively, of patients with nephrogenic diabetes insipidus (see Chapter 49). Although interstitial fibrosis may be observed as early as 5 years after beginning therapy, lithium-induced CKD usually occurs after 10 to 20 years of lithium treatment.[96]

Pathogenesis The precise mechanism of chronic lithium-induced nephrotoxicity is not well characterized. Impaired ability to concentrate urine is a result of a decrease in collecting duct response to antidiuretic hormone, which may be related to downregulation of aquaporin 2 water channel expression during lithium therapy.[96] Chronic tubulointerstitial nephritis attributed to lithium is evidenced most commonly by biopsy findings of interstitial fibrosis, tubular atrophy, and glomerular sclerosis. The pathogenesis may involve cumulative direct lithium toxicity since duration of therapy correlates with the decline in the GFR.[96]

Risk Factors Historically, the duration of lithium therapy and cumulative dose was considered the major determinants of chronic nephrotoxicity. However, this is now questionable, with some suggesting that long-term lithium therapy in the absence of episodes of acute intoxication is not nephrotoxic.[97] Increased age may also be a risk factor, but daily dose is not.[94,96]

Clinical **Controversy...**

Some clinicians believe that long-term lithium therapy is associated with nephrotoxicity even in the absence of acute episodes of intoxication. Others believe that duration of therapy is not an independent predictor of kidney injury.

Prevention Prevention of acute and chronic toxicity includes maintaining lithium concentrations as low as therapeutically possible, avoiding dehydration, and monitoring kidney function. It is unknown whether progression to CKD can be prevented by stopping lithium use when mild kidney injury is first recognized. This poses a dilemma as lithium is highly effective for affective disorders and the risks and potential benefits of discontinuing such a beneficial drug need to be carefully considered.[96] However, if lithium therapy is continued, kidney function must be monitored and therapy discontinued if it continues to decline. Amiloride has been used for prevention and treatment of lithium-induced nephrogenic diabetes insipidus, since it blocks epithelial sodium transport of lithium into the cortical collecting duct in the distal nephron.[96]

Management Symptomatic polyuria and polydipsia can be reversed by discontinuation of lithium therapy or ameliorated with amiloride 5 to 10 mg daily during continued lithium therapy (see Chapter 49). If polyuria does not resolve within 7 to 10 days of therapy, then the amiloride dose should be increased to 20 mg daily. Progressive chronic interstitial nephritis is treated by discontinuation of lithium therapy, adequate hydration, and avoidance of other nephrotoxic agents. Lithium serum concentrations, as well as kidney function indices, including urine output, BUN, and S_{cr}, should be monitored closely for resolution of signs and symptoms of toxicity.[96]

Cyclosporine and Tacrolimus

Delayed chronic tubulointerstitial nephritis, considered the Achilles' heel of calcineurin inhibitor-based immunosuppressive regimens, has been reported after several months of therapy and can result in irreversible kidney disease.[68,69] Toxicity is progressive and usually manifests as a slowly rising S_{cr} concentration and decreased creatinine clearance that may not reflect the severity of histopathologic changes. All three compartments of the kidney can be affected, evidenced by typical biopsy findings that include arteriolar hyalinosis, glomerular sclerosis, and a striped pattern of tubulointerstitial fibrosis.[69] The pathogenesis appears to involve sustained renal arteriolar endothelial cell injury and increased extracellular matrix synthesis, which ultimately result in chronic ischemia of the tubulointerstitial compartment because of increased release of endothelin-1, decreased production of nitric acid, and upregulation of transforming growth factor-β. Unlike acute nephrotoxicity, chronic toxicity is not dose dependent.[68,69]

Aristolochic Acid

Incidence Although the true incidence of aristolochic acid nephropathy is unknown, approximately 3% to 5% of patients who consume the natural product develop interstitial fibrosis with tubular atrophy.[98]

Clinical Presentation Patients with aristolochic acid nephropathy typically present with mild-to-moderate hypertension, mild proteinuria, glucosuria, and moderately elevated S_{cr} concentrations. Anemia and shrunken kidneys are also common on initial presentation.[99] The overwhelming majority of cases reported to date have been in women. The main pathologic lesions observed in the kidneys are interstitial fibrosis with atrophy and destruction of proximal tubules throughout the renal cortex; in general, the glomeruli are not affected. Perhaps the most remarkable feature of aristolochic acid nephropathy is the rate at which it progresses. In most individuals, ESRD requiring dialysis or transplantation develops within 6 to 24 months of exposure. An alarming high prevalence (approximately 40%-45%) of urothelial transitional cell carcinoma has been observed in Belgian patients who underwent renal transplantation.[98,99]

Pathogenesis Although the precise mechanism of aristolochic acid nephropathy and urothelial carcinoma has yet to be characterized. The major components of aristolochic acid are metabolized to mutagenic compounds called *aristolactam I* and *aristolactam II*, respectively, which have been demonstrated to form aristolochic acid–DNA adducts in humans. Recent data indicate that these adducts cause direct DNA damage and may lead to proximal tubular atrophy and apoptosis.[99]

Prevention The primary means of preventing aristolochic acid nephropathy appears to be the limitation of exposure to compounds containing aristolochic acids. Several countries, including the United States, United Kingdom, Canada, Australia, and Germany, have banned the use of *Aristolochia*-containing herbs.[99]

Papillary Necrosis

Papillary necrosis is a form of chronic tubulointerstitial nephritis characterized by necrosis of the renal papillae, the regions of the kidney where the collecting ducts enter the renal pelvis, which leads to progressive kidney disease. Papillary necrosis is associated with diabetes, sickle cell disease, obstruction and infection of the urinary tract, and most commonly analgesic use.[100]

Analgesic Nephropathy

Incidence Prototypical analgesic nephropathy is characterized by chronic tubulointerstitial nephritis with papillary necrosis.[100] Chronic excessive consumption of combination analgesics, particularly those containing phenacetin, was believed to be the major cause and led to the removal of phenacetin and phenacetin mixtures from most world markets. However, contemporary analgesics, particularly aspirin, acetaminophen, and NSAIDs, alone or in combination, are also associated with the development of analgesic nephropathy. The incidence of analgesic nephropathy has declined significantly since removal of phenacetin from many countries, with the prevalence estimated to now be less than 5% in the United States adult ESRD population.[100]

Clinical Presentation Analgesic nephropathy is a progressive disease that evolves slowly over several years.[100] It is difficult to recognize in the early stages of the disease because patients are often asymptomatic, and it may be underdiagnosed as a cause of ESRD. It is seen more commonly in women than men. Early manifestations are generally nonspecific and may include headache and upper GI symptoms; later manifestations include impaired urinary concentrating ability, dysuria, sterile pyuria, microscopic hematuria, mild proteinuria (less than 1.5 g/day), and lower back pain. As disease progresses, hypertension, atherosclerotic cardiovascular disease, renal calculi, and bladder stones are common, and pyelonephritis is a classic finding in advanced analgesic nephropathy. The most sensitive and specific diagnostic criteria include (a) a history of chronic daily habitual analgesic ingestion (daily use for at least 3-5 years); (b) IV pyelography, renal ultrasound, or renal computed tomography imaging, which reveals decreased renal mass and bumpy renal contours; (3) elevated S_{cr}, that is, up to 4 mg/dL (354 μmol/L); and (4) papillary calcifications.[100]

Pathogenesis Analgesic nephropathy originates in the papillary tip as a result of accumulated toxins, drugs and metabolites, decreased blood flow, and impaired cellular energy production. The metabolism of phenacetin to acetaminophen, which is then oxidized to toxic free radicals that are concentrated in the papilla, appears to be the initiating factor that causes toxicity by mechanisms analogous to acetaminophen hepatotoxicity via glutathione depletion.[101] Cortical interstitial nephritis develops secondary to papillary necrosis. Salicylates potentiate these effects by also depleting renal glutathione, and inhibiting prostaglandin-mediated vasodilation, thus further predisposing the renal medulla to ischemic injury.[101]

Risk Factors The epidemiology of analgesic use and analgesic nephropathy continues to evolve. The classic concept persists that risk for ESRD increases with cumulative consumption of combination analgesics, phenacetin, or acetaminophen and aspirin or NSAIDs. Caffeine contained in combination analgesics may increase risk, but the role is not clear.[100] Chronic use of therapeutic doses of NSAIDs or high-dose acetaminophen, but not aspirin or salicylates alone, can cause analgesic nephropathy.

Prevention Prevention has depended primarily on public health efforts to restrict the sale of phenacetin and combination analgesics. However, risk continues with ongoing availability of nonprescription combination analgesics containing aspirin, acetaminophen, and caffeine in the United States and throughout the world.

Individuals requiring chronic analgesic therapy may reduce risk by limiting the total dose, avoiding combined use of two or more analgesics, and maintaining good hydration to prevent renal ischemia and decrease the papillary concentration of toxic substances. Acetaminophen remains the preferred nonopiate analgesic for patients with preexisting kidney disease.

Management Treatment of established nephrotoxicity requires cessation of analgesic consumption.[101] This can prevent progression and may improve kidney function. Kidney function indices, including urine output, BUN, and S_{cr}, should be monitored every several months. Patients should also be monitored for the development of transitional cell carcinoma of the renal pelvis, calyces, ureters, and bladder, which may present years after analgesic nephropathy is diagnosed.

RENAL VASCULITIS, THROMBOSIS, AND CHOLESTEROL EMBOLI

Renal Vasculitis

Drug-induced renal vascular disease commonly presents as vasculitis, thrombotic microangiopathy, or cholesterol emboli.[88,102] Vasculitis implies inflammation of the vessel wall, capillaries, or glomeruli and is typically classified according to vessel size (ie, small, medium, or large vessel vasculitis). Small vessel vasculitides usually affect multiple organ systems, including the kidneys and lungs, and are associated with nonspecific inflammatory symptoms such as fever, malaise, myalgias, arthralgias, and weight loss. Numerous drugs are associated with the development of renal vasculitis, including hydralazine, propylthiouracil, allopurinol, phenytoin, sulfasalazine, penicillamine, and minocycline (see Table 46-1).[88,102] Most drug-induced cases of vasculitis, including hydralazine, propylthiouracil, allopurinol, penicillamine, and the anti-TNF-α drug adalimumab have been implicated in the development of antineutrophil cytoplasmic antibody (ANCA)-positive vasculitis.[88,102,103] Patients present with hematuria, proteinuria, oliguria, and red cell casts, frequently along with fever, malaise, myalgias, and arthralgias.[102] Treatment typically consists of withdrawing the offending drug and administration of corticosteroids or other immunosuppressive therapy, and usually leads to resolution of symptoms within weeks to months.

Thrombotic Microangiopathy

Thrombotic microangiopathy is characterized clinically by microangiopathic hemolytic anemia, fragmented red cells, and thrombocytopenia and pathologically by vascular endothelial proliferation, endothelial cell swelling, and intraluminal platelet thrombi in the small vessels, particularly affecting the renal and cerebral capillaries and arterioles.[87,104] The absence of inflammation in vessel walls distinguishes thrombotic microangiopathy from vasculitis. Numerous medications, including oral contraceptive agents, cyclosporine, tacrolimus, muromonab-CD3, many cancer chemotherapeutic agents including antiangiogenesis drugs (eg, bevacizumab, sunitinib, and sorafenib), mitomycin C, cisplatin, and gemcitabine, interferon-α, ticlopidine, clopidogrel, quinine, and several antimicrobial agents (eg, valacyclovir, penicillins, rifampin, and metronidazole) are associated with the development of thrombotic microangiopathy.[87,104] Patients may present with fever, neurological dysfunction, elevated S_{cr} and BUN, and hypertension, along with microangiopathic hemolytic anemia and thrombocytopenia. Kidney injury can be severe and irreversible, although corticosteroids, antiplatelet agents, plasma exchange, plasmapheresis, and high-dose IV immunoglobulin G have each induced clinical improvement.[104]

Cholesterol Emboli

Anticoagulants (particularly warfarin) and thrombolytics (eg, urokinase, streptokinase, and tissue-plasminogen activator) are associated with cholesterol embolization of the kidney.[105] These drugs act to remove or prevent thrombus formation over ulcerative plaques or may induce hemorrhage within clots, thereby causing showers of cholesterol crystals that lodge in small diameter arteries of the kidney (renal arterioles and glomerular capillaries). Cholesterol crystal emboli induce an endothelial inflammatory response, which leads to complete obstruction, ischemia, and necrosis of affected vessels within weeks to months after initiation of therapy.[105] Purple discoloration of the toes and mottled skin over the legs are important clinical clues. Treatment is supportive in nature, since kidney injury is generally irreversible.

PHARMACOECONOMICS

The pharmacoeconomic implications of DIKD are enormous. In general, an episode of AKI leads to higher hospital resource use, with increases in the median direct hospital cost of $2,600 and the hospital length of stay by 5 days.[106] An increase in S_{cr} of greater than or equal to 0.5 mg/dL (greater than or equal to 44 μmol/L) is independently associated with a 6.5-fold increase in the odds of death, a 3.5-day increase in length of hospital stay, and nearly $7,500 in excess hospital costs even after adjusting for age, sex, and measures of comorbidity.[107] Amphotericin B-induced AKI leads to a mean increased length of hospital stay of 8.2 days and adjusted additional costs of $29,823 per patient.[108] The major driver of the increased costs associated with contrast-induced AKI was the cost of the longer initial hospital stay. The increased availability of automated clinical decision support systems and computer-guided medication dosing for hospital inpatients may improve the safety of potentially harmful drugs and minimize the occurrence of nephrotoxicity in this setting, thereby potentially lowering the corresponding economic consequences.[108]

ABBREVIATIONS

ACEI	angiotensin-converting enzyme inhibitor
AIN	allergic interstitial nephritis
AKI	acute kidney injury
ARB	angiotensin II receptor blocker
ATN	acute tubular necrosis
BUN	blood urea nitrogen
CIN	contrast media-induced nephrotoxicity
CKD	chronic kidney disease
COX	cyclooxygenase
CVVH	continuous venovenous hemofiltration
DIKD	drug-induced kidney disease
ESRD	end-stage renal disease
FSGS	focal segmental glomerulosclerosis
GFR	glomerular filtration rate
IGFBP7	insulin-like growth factor-binding protein 7
KIM-1	kidney injury molecule-1
MAPK	mitogen-activated protein kinase
NGAL	neutrophil gelatinase-associated lipocalin
NSAID	nonsteroidal antiinflammatory drug
OSPS	oral sodium phosphate solution
RTEC	renal tubular epithelial cell
S_{cr}	serum creatinine
TIMP-2	inhibitor of metalloproteinase 2
WRN	warfarin-related nephropathy

REFERENCES

1. Mehta RL, Awdishu L, Davenport A, et al. Phenotype standardization for drug-induced kidney disease. *Kidney Int* 2015;88:226-234.
2. Thomas ME, Blaine C, Dawnay A, et al. The definition of acute kidney injury and its use in practice. *Kidney Int* 2015;87:62-73.
3. Siew ED, Davenport A. The growth of acute kidney injury: A rising tide or just closer attention to detail? *Kidney Int* 2015;87:46-61.
4. Elasy TA, Anderson RJ. Changing demography of acute renal failure. *Semin Dial* 1996;9:438-443.
5. Hsu RK, McCulloch CE, Dudley RA, Lo LJ, Hsu CY. Temporal changes in incidence of dialysis-requiring AKI. *J Am Soc Nephrol* 2013;24:37-42.

6. Susantitaphong P, Cruz DN, Cerda J, et al. World incidence of AKI: A meta-analysis. *Clin J Am Soc Nephrol* 2013;8:1482-1493.
7. Bentley ML, Corwin HL, Dasta J. Drug-induced acute kidney injury in the critically ill adult: Recognition and prevention strategies. *Crit Care Med* 2010;38:S169-S174.
8. van Meer L, Moerland M, Cohen AF, Burggraaf J. Urinary kidney biomarkers for early detection of nephrotoxicity in clinical drug development. *Br J Clin Pharmacol* 2014;77:947-957.
9. Gobe GC, Coombes JS, Fassett RG, Endre ZH. Biomarkers of drug-induced acute kidney injury in the adult. *Expert Opin Drug Metab Toxicol* 2015;11:1683-1694.
10. Chen LX, Koyner JL. Biomarkers in Acute Kidney Injury. *Crit Care Clin* 2015;31:633-648.
11. Vaidya VS, Ferguson MA, Bonventre JV. Biomarkers of acute kidney injury. *Annu Rev Pharmacol Toxicol* 2008;48:463-493.
12. Gocze I, Koch M, Renner P, et al. Urinary biomarkers TIMP-2 and IGFBP7 early predict acute kidney injury after major surgery. *PLoS One* 2015;10:e0120863.
13. Koyner JL, Shaw AD, Chawla LS, et al. Tissue Inhibitor Metalloproteinase-2 (TIMP-2)IGF-Binding Protein-7 (IGFBP7) levels are associated with adverse long-term outcomes in patients with AKI. *J Am Soc Nephrol* 2015;26:1747-1754.
14. Sohn SJ, Kim SY, Kim HS, et al. In vitro evaluation of biomarkers for cisplatin-induced nephrotoxicity using HK-2 human kidney epithelial cells. *Toxicol Lett* 2013;217:235-242.
15. Fuchs TC, Mally A, Wool A, Beiman M, Hewitt P. An exploratory evaluation of the utility of transcriptional and urinary kidney injury biomarkers for the prediction of aristolochic acid-induced renal injury in male rats. *Vet Pathol* 2014;51:680-694.
16. Perazella MA. Renal vulnerability to drug toxicity. *Clin J Am Soc Nephrol* 2009;4:1275-1283.
17. Ghane Shahrbaf F, Assadi F. Drug-induced renal disorders. *J Renal Inj Prev* 2015;4:57-60.
18. Perazella MA. The urine sediment as a biomarker of kidney disease. *Am J Kidney Dis* 2015;66:748-755.
19. Curthoys NP, Moe OW. Proximal tubule function and response to acidosis. *Clin J Am Soc Nephrol* 2014;9:1627-1638.
20. Subramanya AR, Ellison DH. Distal convoluted tubule. *Clin J Am Soc Nephrol* 2014;9:2147-2163.
21. Ettore B. Adverse effects of drugs on the kidney. *Eur J Intern Med* 2015;28:1-8.
22. Wargo KA, Edwards JD. Aminoglycoside-induced nephrotoxicity. *J Pharm Pract* 2014;27:573-577.
23. Pazhayattil GS, Shirali AC. Drug-induced impairment of renal function. *Int J Nephrol Renovasc Dis* 2014;7:457-468.
24. Oliveira JF, Silva CA, Barbieri CD, Oliveira GM, Zanetta DM, Burdmann EA. Prevalence and risk factors for aminoglycoside nephrotoxicity in intensive care units. *Antimicrob Agents Chemother* 2009;53:2887-2891.
25. Balakumar P, Rohilla A, Thangathirupathi A. Gentamicin-induced nephrotoxicity: Do we have a promising therapeutic approach to blunt it? *Pharmacol Res* 2010;62:179-186.
26. Asci H, Saygin M, Cankara FN, et al. The impact of alpha-lipoic acid on amikacin-induced nephrotoxicity. *Ren Fail* 2015;37:117-121.
27. Destache CJ. Aminoglycoside-induced nephrotoxicity—A focus on monitoring: A review of literature. *J Pharm Pract* 2014;27:562-566.
28. Pagkalis S, Mantadakis E, Mavros MN, Ammari C, Falagas ME. Pharmacological considerations for the proper clinical use of aminoglycosides. *Drugs* 2011;71:2277-2294.
29. Keaney JJ, Hannon CM, Murray PT. Contrast-induced acute kidney injury: How much contrast is safe? *Nephrol Dial Transplant* 2013;28:1376-1383.
30. Lefel N, Janssen L, le Noble J, Foudraine N. Sodium bicarbonate prophylactic therapy in the prevention of contrast-induced nephropathy in patients admitted to the intensive care unit of a teaching hospital: A retrospective cohort study. *J Intensive Care* 2016;4:5.
31. Weisbord SD, Palevsky PM. Contrast-associated Acute Kidney Injury. *Crit Care Clin* 2015;31:725-735.
32. McCullough PA. Contrast-Induced Nephropathy: Definitions, epidemiology, and implications. *Intervent Cardiol Clin* 2014;3:357-362.
33. Geenen RWF, Kingma HJ, van der Molen AJ. Pathophysiology of Contrast-Induced Acute Kidney Injury. *Intervent Cardiol Clin* 2014;3:363-367.
34. Rojkovskiy I, Solomon R. Intravenous and oral hydration: Approaches, principles, and differing regimens. *Intervent Cardiol Clin* 2014;3:393-404.
35. Aqeel I, Garcha AS, Rudnick MR. Relative nephrotoxicity of different contrast media. *Intervent Cardiol Clin* 2014;3:349-356.
36. Toso A, Leoncini M, Maioli M, Tropeano F, Bellandi F. Pharmacologic prophylaxis for Contrast-Induced Acute Kidney Injury. *Intervent Cardiol Clin* 2014;3:405-419.
37. Tao SM, Wichmann JL, Schoepf UJ, Fuller SR, Lu GM, Zhang LJ. Contrast-induced nephropathy in CT: Incidence, risk factors and strategies for prevention. *Eur Radiol* 2016;26(9):3310-3318.
38. Azzalini L, Spagnoli V, Ly HQ. Contrast-induced nephropathy: From pathophysiology to preventive strategies. *Can J Cardiol* 2016;32(2):247-255.
39. Guidelines on the use of iodinated contrast media in patients with kidney disease 2012: Digest version: JSN, JRS, and JCS Joint Working Group. *Circ J* 2013;77:1883-1914.
40. Yang Y, Liu H, Liu F, Dong Z. Mitochondrial dysregulation and protection in cisplatin nephrotoxicity. *Arch Toxicol* 2014;88:1249-1256.
41. Peres LA, da Cunha AD, Jr. Acute nephrotoxicity of cisplatin: Molecular mechanisms. *J Bras Nefrol* 2013;35:332-340.
42. Perazella MA. Onco-nephrology: Renal toxicities of chemotherapeutic agents. *Clin J Am Soc Nephrol* 2012;7:1713-1721.
43. Launay-Vacher V, Rey JB, Isnard-Bagnis C, Deray G, Daouphars M. Prevention of cisplatin nephrotoxicity: State of the art and recommendations from the European Society of Clinical Pharmacy Special Interest Group on Cancer Care. *Cancer Chemother Pharmacol* 2008;61:903-909.
44. Sanchez-Gonzalez PD, Lopez-Hernandez FJ, Lopez-Novoa JM, Morales AI. An integrative view of the pathophysiological events leading to cisplatin nephrotoxicity. *Crit Rev Toxicol* 2011;41:803-821.
45. Finkel M, Goldstein A, Steinberg Y, Granowetter L, Trachtman H. Cisplatinum nephrotoxicity in oncology therapeutics: Retrospective review of patients treated between 2005 and 2012. *Pediatr Nephrol* 2014;29:2421-2424.
46. dos Santos NA, Carvalho Rodrigues MA, Martins NM, dos Santos AC. Cisplatin-induced nephrotoxicity and targets of nephroprotection: An update. *Arch Toxicol* 2012;86:1233-1250.
47. Shirali AC, Perazella MA. Tubulointerstitial injury associated with chemotherapeutic agents. *Adv Chronic Kidney Dis* 2014;21:56-63.
48. Oh GS, Kim HJ, Shen A, et al. Cisplatin-induced kidney dysfunction and perspectives on improving treatment strategies. *Electrolyte Blood Press* 2014;12:55-65.
49. Santabarbara G, Maione P, Rossi A, Gridelli C. Pharmacotherapeutic options for treating adverse effects of Cisplatin chemotherapy. *Expert Opin Pharmacother* 2016;17(4):561-570.
50. Rocha PN, Kobayashi CD, de Carvalho Almeida L, de Oliveira Dos Reis C, Santos BM, Glesby MJ. Incidence, predictors, and impact on hospital mortality of Amphotericin B nephrotoxicity defined using newer acute kidney injury diagnostic criteria. *Antimicrob Agents Chemother* 2015;59:4759-4769.
51. Hamill RJ. Amphotericin B formulations: A comparative review of efficacy and toxicity. *Drugs* 2013;73:919-934.
52. Mistro S, Maciel Ide M, de Menezes RG, Maia ZP, Schooley RT, Badaro R. Does lipid emulsion reduce amphotericin B nephrotoxicity? A systematic review and meta-analysis. *Clin Infect Dis* 2012;54:1774-1777.
53. Bes DF, Rosanova MT, Sberna N, Arrizurieta E. Deoxycholate amphotericin B and nephrotoxicity in the pediatric setting. *Pediatr Infect Dis J* 2014;33:e198-e206.
54. Karimzadeh I, Khalili H, Sagheb MM, Farsaei S. A double-blinded, placebo-controlled, multicenter clinical trial of N-acetylcysteine for preventing amphotericin B-induced nephrotoxicity. *Expert Opin Drug Metab Toxicol* 2015;11:1345-1355.
55. Martensson J, Bellomo R. Are all fluids bad for the kidney? *Curr Opin Crit Care* 2015;21:292-301.
56. Dickenmann M, Oettl T, Mihatsch MJ. Osmotic nephrosis: Acute kidney injury with accumulation of proximal tubular lysosomes due to administration of exogenous solutes. *Am J Kidney Dis* 2008;51:491-503.
57. Dantal J. Intravenous immunoglobulins: In-depth review of excipients and acute kidney injury risk. *Am J Nephrol* 2013;38:275-284.
58. Nomani AZ, Nabi Z, Rashid H, et al. Osmotic nephrosis with mannitol: Review article. *Ren Fail* 2014;36:1169-1176.
59. Perazella MA, Luciano RL. Review of select causes of drug-induced AKI. *Expert Rev Clin Pharmacol* 2015;8:367-371.

60. Carlstrom M, Wilcox CS, Arendshorst WJ. Renal autoregulation in health and disease. *Physiol Rev* 2015;95:405-511.
61. Dreischulte T, Morales DR, Bell S, Guthrie B. Combined use of nonsteroidal anti-inflammatory drugs with diuretics and/or renin-angiotensin system inhibitors in the community increases the risk of acute kidney injury. *Kidney Int* 2015;88:396-403.
62. Cruz CS, Cruz LS, Silva GR, Marcilio de Souza CA. Incidence and predictors of development of acute renal failure related to treatment of congestive heart failure with ACE inhibitors. *Nephron Clin Pract* 2007;105:c77-c83.
63. Budnitz DS, Lovegrove MC, Shehab N, Richards CL. Emergency hospitalizations for adverse drug events in older Americans. *N Engl J Med* 2011;365:2002-2012.
64. St Peter WL, Odum LE, Whaley-Connell AT. To RAS or not to RAS? The evidence for and cautions with renin-angiotensin system inhibition in patients with diabetic kidney disease. *Pharmacotherapy* 2013;33:496-514.
65. Lapi F, Azoulay L, Yin H, Nessim SJ, Suissa S. Concurrent use of diuretics, angiotensin converting enzyme inhibitors, and angiotensin receptor blockers with non-steroidal anti-inflammatory drugs and risk of acute kidney injury: Nested case-control study. *BMJ* 2013;346:e8525.
66. Rahman S, Malcoun A. Nonsteroidal antiinflammatory drugs, cyclooxygenase-2, and the kidneys. *Prim Care* 2014;41:803-821.
67. Whelton A. Nephrotoxicity of nonsteroidal anti-inflammatory drugs: Physiologic foundations and clinical implications. *Am J Med* 1999;106:13S-24S.
68. Naesens M, Kuypers DR, Sarwal M. Calcineurin inhibitor nephrotoxicity. *Clin J Am Soc Nephrol* 2009;4:481-508.
69. Chapman JR. Chronic calcineurin inhibitor nephrotoxicity-lest we forget. *Am J Transplant* 2011;11:693-697.
70. Ojo AO, Held PJ, Port FK, et al. Chronic renal failure after transplantation of a nonrenal organ. *N Engl J Med* 2003;349:931-940.
71. Issa N, Kukla A, Ibrahim HN. Calcineurin inhibitor nephrotoxicity: A review and perspective of the evidence. *Am J Nephrol* 2013;37:602-612.
72. Pallet N, Djamali A, Legendre C. Challenges in diagnosing acute calcineurin-inhibitor induced nephrotoxicity: From toxicogenomics to emerging biomarkers. *Pharmacol Res* 2011;64:25-30.
73. Nasr SH, Milliner DS, Wooldridge TD, Sethi S. Triamterene crystalline nephropathy. *Am J Kidney Dis* 2014;63:148-152.
74. Garneau AP, Riopel J, Isenring P. Acute methotrexate-induced crystal nephropathy. *N Engl J Med* 2015;373:2691-2693.
75. Faught LN, Greff MJ, Rieder MJ, Koren G. Drug-induced acute kidney injury in children. *Br J Clin Pharmacol* 2015;80:901-909.
76. Herlitz LC, D'Agati VD, Markowitz GS. Crystalline nephropathies. *Arch Pathol Lab Med* 2012;136:713-720.
77. Jones GL, Will A, Jackson GH, Webb NJ, Rule S. British Committee for Standards in H. Guidelines for the management of tumour lysis syndrome in adults and children with haematological malignancies on behalf of the British Committee for Standards in Haematology. *Br J Haematol* 2015;169:661-671.
78. Petejova N, Martinek A. Acute kidney injury due to rhabdomyolysis and renal replacement therapy: A critical review. *Crit Care* 2014;18:224.
79. Zimmerman JL, Shen MC. Rhabdomyolysis. *Chest* 2013;144:1058-1065.
80. Brodsky SV, Nadasdy T, Rovin BH, et al. Warfarin-related nephropathy occurs in patients with and without chronic kidney disease and is associated with an increased mortality rate. *Kidney Int* 2011;80:181-189.
81. Kumar N, Perazella MA. Differentiating HIV-associated nephropathy from antiretroviral drug-induced nephropathy: A clinical challenge. *Curr HIV/AIDS Rep* 2014;11:202-211.
82. Izzedine H, Lescure FX, Bonnet F. HIV medication-based urolithiasis. *Clin Kidney J* 2014;7:121-126.
83. Shavit L, Jaeger P, Unwin RJ. What is nephrocalcinosis? *Kidney Int* 2015;88:35-43.
84. Markowitz GS, Perazella MA. Acute phosphate nephropathy. *Kidney Int* 2009;76:1027-1034.
85. Choi NK, Lee J, Chang Y, et al. Acute renal failure following oral sodium phosphate bowel preparation: A nationwide case-crossover study. *Endoscopy* 2014;46:465-470.
86. Markowitz GS, Radhakrishnan J, D'Agati VD. Towards the incidence of acute phosphate nephropathy. *J Am Soc Nephrol* 2007;18:3020-3022.
87. Markowitz GS, Bomback AS, Perazella MA. Drug-induced glomerular disease: Direct cellular injury. *Clin J Am Soc Nephrol* 2015;10:1291-1299.
88. Hogan JJ, Markowitz GS, Radhakrishnan J. Drug-induced glomerular disease: Immune-mediated injury. *Clin J Am Soc Nephrol* 2015;10:1300-1310.
89. Lan X, Rao TK, Chander PN, Skorecki K, Singhal PC. Apolipoprotein L1 (APOL1) Variants (Vs) a possible link between Heroin-associated Nephropathy (HAN) and HIV-associated Nephropathy (HIVAN). *Front Microbiol* 2015;6:571.
90. Krishnan N, Perazella MA. Drug-induced acute interstitial nephritis: Pathology, pathogenesis, and treatment. *Iran J Kidney Dis* 2015;9:3-13.
91. Perazella MA, Markowitz GS. Drug-induced acute interstitial nephritis. *Nat Rev Nephrol* 2010;6:461-470.
92. Perazella MA. Diagnosing drug-induced AIN in the hospitalized patient: A challenge for the clinician. *Clin Nephrol* 2014;81:381-388.
93. Bendz H, Schon S, Attman PO, Aurell M. Renal failure occurs in chronic lithium treatment but is uncommon. *Kidney Int* 2010;77:219-224.
94. Rej S, Herrmann N, Shulman K. The effects of lithium on renal function in older adults—A systematic review. *J Geriatr Psychiatry Neurol* 2012;25:51-61.
95. Alsady M, Baumgarten R, Deen PM, de Groot T. Lithium in the Kidney: Friend and Foe? *J Am Soc Nephrol* 2016;27(6):1587-1595.
96. Grunfeld JP, Rossier BC. Lithium nephrotoxicity revisited. *Nat Rev Nephrol* 2009;5:270-276.
97. Clos S, Rauchhaus P, Severn A, Cochrane L, Donnan PT. Long-term effect of lithium maintenance therapy on estimated glomerular filtration rate in patients with affective disorders: A population-based cohort study. *Lancet Psychiatry* 2015;2:1075-1083.
98. Debelle FD, Vanherweghem JL, Nortier JL. Aristolochic acid nephropathy: A worldwide problem. *Kidney Int* 2008;74:158-169.
99. Luciano RL, Perazella MA. Aristolochic acid nephropathy: Epidemiology, clinical presentation, and treatment. *Drug Saf* 2015;38:55-64.
100. De Broe ME, Elseviers MM. Over-the-counter analgesic use. *J Am Soc Nephrol* 2009;20:2098-2103.
101. Braden GL, O'Shea MH, Mulhern JG. Tubulointerstitial diseases. *Am J Kidney Dis* 2005;46:560-572.
102. Radic M, Martinovic Kaliterna D, Radic J. Drug-induced vasculitis: A clinical and pathological review. *Neth J Med* 2012;70:12-17.
103. Perez-Alvarez R, Perez-de-Lis M, Ramos-Casals M. Biologics-induced autoimmune diseases. *Curr Opin Rheumatol* 2013;25:56-64.
104. Izzedine H, Perazella MA. Thrombotic microangiopathy, cancer, and cancer drugs. *Am J Kidney Dis* 2015;66:857-868.
105. Scolari F, Ravani P. Atheroembolic renal disease. *Lancet* 2010;375:1650-1660.
106. Lameire NH, Bagga A, Cruz D, et al. Acute kidney injury: An increasing global concern. *Lancet* 2013;382:170-179.
107. Chertow GM, Burdick E, Honour M, Bonventre JV, Bates DW. Acute kidney injury, mortality, length of stay, and costs in hospitalized patients. *J Am Soc Nephrol* 2005;16:3365-3370.
108. Hug BL, Witkowski DJ, Sox CM, et al. Occurrence of adverse, often preventable, events in community hospitals involving nephrotoxic drugs or those excreted by the kidney. *Kidney Int* 2009;76:1192-1198.

Glomerulonephritis

Alan H. Lau

47

KEY CONCEPTS

1. Glomerulonephritis is a collection of glomerular diseases mediated by different immunologic pathogenic mechanisms, resulting in varied clinical presentation and therapeutic outcomes.
2. The signs and symptoms associated with glomerulonephritis are commonly nephrotic in nature and characterized by proteinuria. At times, there may be nephritic features, characterized by inflammatory injury.
3. Supportive treatments for edema, hypertension, hyperlipidemia, and intravascular thrombosis are important in reducing the complications associated with glomerulonephritis. These are especially important since specific and effective therapy for many types of glomerulonephritis are not available. Reduction of proteinuria can often improve long-term kidney and patient outcomes.
4. To maximize therapeutic benefits and minimize drug-induced complications, patients have to be monitored closely to assess their therapeutic responses as well as the development of any treatment-induced toxicities.
5. Among all the types of glomerulonephritis, minimal-change nephropathy is most responsive to treatment. Steroids can induce good responses in most patients during initial treatment as well as relapse.
6. Because of the lack of consistently effective treatment for primary focal segmental glomerular sclerosis, angiotensin-converting enzyme inhibitors or angiotensin receptor blockers are commonly used for patients with mild disease to control symptoms. Steroids and immunosuppressive agents are reserved for the management of patients with severe disease.
7. The optimal treatment for lupus nephritis depends on the underlying lesion and disease activity, as well as the severity and duration of the patient's condition.
8. The treatment of poststreptococcal glomerulonephritis is mainly supportive and symptomatic. Antibiotic therapy does not prevent subsequent disease development but may reduce the severity.

The precise pathogenetic mechanisms of many glomerular diseases remain unknown and the available therapeutic regimens are still far from optimal. This chapter provides an overview of the primary causes of glomerulonephritis with a focus on their etiology, the pathophysiologic mechanisms responsible for glomerular injury, and the clinical presentation of the eight predominant types of glomerulonephritis. Treatment options and monitoring approaches for each type of glomerulonephritis are also discussed.

Diabetes mellitus is an important secondary cause of glomerular injury and a thorough discussion of the pathophysiology and management of this condition can be found in Chapter 74.

NORMAL GLOMERULAR ANATOMY AND FUNCTION

The glomerulus, which is enclosed within the Bowman's capsule, consists of two important components: the capillary wall and the mesangium (Fig. 47-1). The capillary wall, which serves as the primary filtration barrier, consists of three well-defined layers: fenestrated endothelium, glomerular basement membrane (GBM), and epithelial cell layer. The epithelial cells, also known as podocytes, have specialized foot processes embedded in the outer layer of the GBM. It is across this barrier that plasma water flows and ultimately becomes the ultrafiltrate. Under normal conditions, the GBM functions as a compact hydrated gel of matrix proteins with a pore-like structure. The mesangium, which consists of mesangial cells embedded in an extracellular matrix, provides support for the glomerular capillaries and also modulates blood flow through the capillaries.

The unique capillary bed of the glomerulus allows small nonprotein plasma constituents up to the size of inulin, which has a molecular weight of 5.2 kDa, to pass freely while excluding macromolecules equal to or larger than albumin, which has a molecular weight of 69 kDa. The ease of solute passage through the glomerular membrane is impacted by both the size and charge of the solute. Fixed, negatively charged sites are found within all three layers of the glomerular capillary wall: the endothelium, the epithelium, and the GBM. The movement of negatively charged molecules is thus restricted more than that of neutral or positively charged molecules. Different glomerular diseases affect this size- and charge-selective barrier to different extents; consequently, glomerulopathies present with varied clinical features and solute-excretion patterns.

Some of the glomerular cells, such as the epithelial cells, have phagocytic function that can remove macromolecules trapped within the filtration barrier. They are also capable of synthesizing the GBM. In contrast, the mesangial cells regulate glomerular hemodynamics in response to angiotensin II and by producing prostaglandins. These cells also synthesize and respond to various cytokines and thus play a key role in immune-mediated glomerular diseases. Resident phagocytes in the mesangium are responsible for moving macromolecules trapped in the basement membrane into the urinary space. They are also involved in the development of both immune and nonimmune glomerular injury.

EPIDEMIOLOGY AND ETIOLOGY

In the United States in 2012, glomerulonephritis was the third most common cause of end-stage renal disease (ESRD), accounting for approximately 16% of all the living ESRD patients.

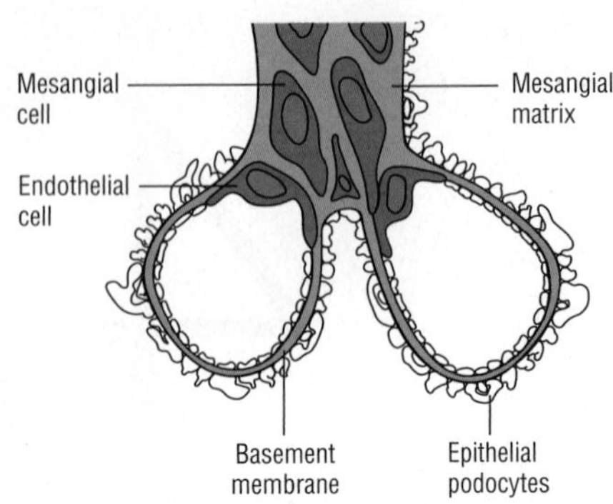

FIGURE 47-1 Microanatomy of the glomerulus.

About 9,100 patients (7.9% of all patients) develop stage 5 chronic kidney disease, which is also called ESRD, because of glomerulonephritis each year.[1] The life span of ESRD patients with glomerulonephritis is typically longer than those with other causes, such as diabetes and hypertension.

Humoral and cellular immunologic mechanisms participate in the pathogenesis of most glomerulonephritis. Abnormalities in coagulation and metabolism, as well as hereditary and vascular diseases, also contribute to glomerular damage. The histopathologic manifestations vary substantially among the different types of glomerulonephritis. An overview of the primary pathogenetic mechanisms is presented in this section, and specific abnormalities for each of the primary types of glomerulonephritis are presented in subsequent sections.

PATHOPHYSIOLOGY

1 The glomerular lesion may be diffuse (involving all glomeruli), focal (involving some but not all glomeruli), or segmental, also known as local (involving part of the individual glomerulus). The pathologic manifestations may also be described as proliferative (overgrowth of epithelium, endothelium, or mesangium), membranous (thickening of GBM), and/or sclerotic.

The glomerular capillary wall is particularly susceptible to immune-mediated injury. Antigens and antibodies tend to localize in the glomerulus, probably because of its high blood flow and capillary hydrostatic pressure. Parenchymal damage can be induced as a result of humoral- and cell-mediated immune reactions. Antibodies and sensitized T lymphocytes are the primary mediators of glomerular injury.[2,3] There is an increasing body of evidence to show that infections initiate most forms of glomerulonephritis through different simultaneous and/or sequential pathways that begin with the activation of innate immune response to result in autoimmunity.[4]

Production of antibodies to endogenous or exogenous antigens that are recognized as foreign is the first step in humoral immunologic damage to the glomerulus. Endogenous antigens may be intrinsic glomerular antigens, such as Heymann antigen on the epithelial cell or Goodpasture antigen on the GBM, or previously sequestered antigens, such as DNA or thyroglobulin. Exogenous antigens are most often viral, bacterial, parasitic, or fungal in origin. Antineutrophil cytoplasmic autoantibodies (ANCAs) (ie, autoantibodies that react to the cytoplasmic components of neutrophils and monocytes) are found in patients with idiopathic crescentic glomerulonephritis.

Complexes of antigens and antibodies may be formed in the circulation and then passively entrapped in the glomerular capillary or mesangium. Alternately, experimental antibodies may combine with endogenous glomerular antigens or exogenous antigens entrapped in the glomerulus to form complexes locally, or in situ.[3] The type and extent of glomerular damage depend on the location of the immune complex formation and the rate at which it is removed. Impaired removal facilitates the growth of the complex and thus increases the likelihood of glomerular damage.

Subsequent to antigen–antibody formation, a series of biologic events is triggered that ultimately leads to glomerular injury. Noninflammatory lesions can result from the binding of noncomplement-fixing antibody to the glomerular epithelial cell (mechanism 1) or from the activation of the complement system to form the C5b-9 membrane attack complex (mechanism 2).[3] Both mechanisms can damage the glomerular epithelial cell and result in capillary wall injury and proteinuria. Inflammatory lesions are induced by glomerular infiltration of circulating inflammatory cells such as neutrophils, monocytes/macrophages, and platelets (mechanism 3) or by proliferation of resident glomerular mesangial cells (mechanism 4), resulting in GBM damage.[3] The migration of neutrophils and monocytes to the glomerular tufts is promoted by chemoattractants such as complement fragments (C3a and C5a), platelet-activating factor, interleukin-8, and monocyte chemotactic protein-1.[5] Various cytokines, chemokines, and growth factors are then released to participate in the inflammatory process.[2]

T cells sensitized to glomerular antigen, macrophages, and resident mesangial cells are important participants in cell-mediated injury. Sensitized T cells can cause glomerular hypercellularity in the absence of antibody deposition.[2-5] Cytotoxic T cells may bind with the target cells and destroy them. Alternatively, a delayed-type hypersensitivity reaction may be initiated by activated T cells through the release of lymphokines to attract, activate, and transform monocytes into macrophages.[3] These humoral and cellular mediators, in conjunction with a host of toxic molecular entities including reactive oxygen species, proteinases, eicosanoids, and procoagulants, can alter the permeability, blood flow, and function of the glomeruli. Vascular constriction and occlusion follow and result in the eventual destruction of the glomeruli.

Acute forms of glomerular injury frequently lead to chronic kidney disease (CKD), even though the immune factors that induced the initial glomerular injury have been resolved. A variety of factors may participate in the progression of renal injury including, systemic and glomerular hypertension, high dietary protein intake, proteinuria, glomerular hypertrophy, hyperlipidemia, activation of the coagulation system, abnormalities of calcium and phosphorus homeostasis, and tubulointerstitial injury. The degree of proteinuria not only is an index of the severity of glomerular disease but also has been associated with an increased rate of progression of renal injury. Proteinuria is also accompanied by an increased flux of macromolecules across the mesangium. The mesangial overload may then lead to structural damage. The passage of serum components, such as complement, across the GBM may alter the integrity of the glomerular filtration barrier. The damaging effects of macromolecules other than albumin, such as immunoglobulins, lipoproteins, transferrin, and complement, have not yet been characterized.

CLINICAL PRESENTATION

2 Although patients with glomerular disease may present with an array of signs and symptoms, they are often categorized into one of two broad classifications: nephritic syndrome or nephrotic syndrome (Table 47-1). The unique clinical presentation characteristics of the predominant glomerulopathies are described in the individual disease sections, presented later in the chapter.

Nephritic syndrome reflects glomerular inflammation and frequently results in hematuria. White cells and cellular and granular casts are commonly found in the urine as well. In contrast, nephrotic syndrome results in few cells or cellular casts in the urine and initially, little or no reduction in glomerular filtration rate (GFR) may be noted.

Hematuria occurs when red blood cells leak through the openings of the GBM. The presence of red cell casts is highly indicative

CLINICAL PRESENTATION Nephritic and Nephrotic Syndromes

General

- The patients are generally not in acute distress

Symptoms

- The patients may not experience any major symptoms

Nephritic Signs

- Hematuria
- Hypertension and edema as renal function declines

Nephrotic Signs

- Edema
- Weight gain
- Fatigue

Laboratory Tests

- Proteinuria up to 3 g/day
- Pus, cellular and granular casts in urine is common
- Hypoproteinemia
- Hypercoagulable state for some patients
- Proteinuria, greater than 3.5 g/day/1.73 m^2
- Hyperlipidemia
- Lipiduria

of glomerulonephritis or vasculitis. The presence of dysmorphic red blood cells, those damaged as they pass through the openings in the GBM or as the result of osmotic injury, in the urine is suggestive of glomerular disease. The presence of proteinuria indicates a defect of the size- and/or charge-selective barriers within the GBM. Albuminuria, above the normal threshold of 30 to 300 mg/day, is associated with increased all-cause mortality, progression to ESRD as well as fatal and non-fatal cardiovascular events.[6] Normal urinary protein excretion is between 40 and 80 mg/day, with a maximum of 150 mg. Most of the albumin that enters the glomerular filtrate is either reabsorbed or catabolized by the tubular epithelium. The dipsticks that are commonly used to identify proteinuria detect only albumin; they become positive when protein excretion is more than 300 to 500 mg/day. They are therefore unable to detect the early stages of renal injury secondary to diabetes mellitus or hypertension, which often result in microalbuminuria with urinary albumin excretion ranges between 30 and 300 mg/day. Chemstrip Micral-Test II (Roche Diagnostics, Indianapolis, IN), a simple immunoassay on a dipstick, permits specific and semiquantitative determination of urinary albumin concentrations at five levels: 0, 10, 20, 50, and 100 mg/L. Another qualitative test, Micro-Bumintest (Bayer Diabetes Care, Mishawaka, IN), registers a positive reading when the urine albumin concentration is greater than 40 mg/L.

TABLE 47-1 Tendencies of Glomerular Diseases to Manifest Nephrotic and Nephritic Features

	Nephrotic Features	Nephritic Features
Minimal-change nephropathy	++++	–
Membranous nephropathy	++++	+
Diabetic glomerulosclerosis	++++	+
Amyloidosis	++++	+
Focal segmental glomerulosclerosis	+++	++
Mesangioproliferative glomerulonephritis	++	++
Membranoproliferative glomerulonephritis	++	+++
Proliferative glomerulonephritis	++	+++
Acute poststreptococcal glomerulonephritis	+	++++
Crescentic glomerulonephritis[a]	+	++++

[a]Can be immune complex-mediated, antiglomerular basement membrane antibody-mediated, or associated with antineutrophil cytoplasmic autoantibodies.

Hypertension is common among patients with glomerular diseases, as a result of renal salt retention and the resultant plasma volume expansion. In contrast, increased activity of vasoconstrictors such as angiotensin II is often the cause of chronic glomerular diseases. Scarring of the glomerulus resulting in regional ischemia is thought to be responsible for the hypertension. Activation of the sympathetic nervous system and the release of vasoconstrictor substances may also contribute.

Nephritic Syndrome

Glomerular bleeding resulting in hematuria is typical in nephritic syndrome. Dysmorphic red cells, especially acanthocytes, are a sensitive and specific marker of glomerular bleeding. The presence of pus and cellular and granular casts in the urine is common. The extent of proteinuria is variable. Patients with severe nephritic glomerular injury tend to have reduced GFR because of the reduced glomerular surface area available for filtration, as a result of constriction of the capillary lumen by proliferating mesangial or inflammatory cells.

Nephrotic Syndrome

Nephrotic syndrome is characterized by proteinuria greater than 3.5 g/day/1.73 m^2, hypoproteinemia, edema, and hyperlipidemia. A hypercoagulable state may also be present in some patients. The syndrome may be the result of primary diseases of the glomerulus, or be associated with systemic diseases such as diabetes mellitus, lupus, amyloidosis, and preeclampsia. Hypoproteinemia, especially hypoalbuminemia, results from increased urinary loss of albumin and an increased rate of catabolism of filtered albumin by proximal tubular cells. The compensatory increase in hepatic synthesis of albumin is insufficient to replenish the protein loss, probably because of malnutrition.

Edema formation in patients with nephrotic syndrome was traditionally thought to be driven by the reduced plasma oncotic pressure secondary to hypoalbuminemia. If the oncotic pressure was low, the movement of fluid from the vascular space to the interstitial compartment results in a reduction of the plasma volume, which can trigger compensatory renal sodium and water retention by activation of the renin–angiotensin–aldosterone axis, vasopressin, and the sympathetic nervous system (the "underfill" mechanism). However, since experimental data reveal that the plasma volume is actually normal or elevated, hypoalbuminemia may not cause edema until the serum albumin concentration is less than 2 g/dL (20 g/L).

In addition, the transcapillary oncotic pressure gradient is not as high as previously thought because increased lymphatic flow reduces the interstitial oncotic pressure by removing protein and fluid from the interstitium, thereby reducing the transcapillary oncotic pressure gradient. Instead, fluid retention is likely mediated by a primary increase in sodium reabsorption at the distal nephron, which is probably caused by tubular resistance to the action of atrial natriuretic peptide (the "overflow" mechanism).[7] Albuminuria greater than 3 g daily is associated with a significant increase in serum cholesterol concentrations for patients with primary glomerular disease.[8] Hyperlipidemia in nephrotic syndrome is characterized by elevated serum total cholesterol, triglyceride, very-low-density lipoprotein (VLDL), and low-density lipoprotein (LDL) cholesterol concentrations. The reduced plasma oncotic pressure as a result of hypoalbuminemia may lead to increased VLDL production and increased liver cholesterol synthesis, along with a decrease in LDL receptor activity, which can then lead to an increase in LDL cholesterol concentration. In addition, reduced serum albumin or the loss of a liporegulatory substance may result in reduced VLDL clearance.[9] Nephrotic patients with hyperlipidemia, especially those with concomitant hypertension, are presumed to have an increased risk for atherosclerotic vascular disease. Hyperlipidemia also promotes the progression of glomerular injury, as evidenced by glomerulosclerosis, mesangial expansion, and hyalinosis.[9,10]

Many patients with nephrotic syndrome have a hypercoagulable state as the result of defects in the function of several control proteins in the coagulation cascade. The concentration of the coagulation inhibitors antithrombin proteins C and S, along with increased concentrations of factors V, VIII, and fibrinogen as well as abnormal platelet function, may all contribute to the hypercoagulable state. The net result of these alterations in coagulation is an increased risk for arterial and venous thrombosis, especially in the deep and renal veins. As many as 25% of patients with membranous nephropathy may have renal vein thrombosis.

DIAGNOSTIC CONSIDERATIONS

Patients with suspected glomerular disease should undergo an extensive medical history to identify potential systemic causes (Table 47-2). Medication, environmental, and occupational histories may also help identify exposure to potentially nephrotoxic agents. A comprehensive physical examination and laboratory evaluation may reveal the presence of systemic diseases that may contribute to the development of glomerular disease (Fig. 47-2). In addition, the patient's age, gender, and ethnic background may be helpful in pinpointing the specific type of glomerular disease. For example, proliferative glomerulonephritis is more common in those less than 40 years of age, whereas the incidence of membranous glomerulonephritis is dramatically higher in those greater than 50 years of age.

Urinalysis can help differentiate the nephrotic or nephritic nature of the disease. The GFR may be used to determine the extent of glomerular damage. In the early stages of the disease, the GFR may remain normal. Initial injury to the glomerulus primarily lowers the permeability coefficient (K_f) of the GBM by reducing the surface area available for filtration. The reduced permeability is compensated by an elevation in the glomerular capillary hydrostatic pressure through afferent arteriolar dilation and efferent arteriolar constriction. Extensive glomerular damage may therefore be present before a substantial reduction of total GFR is evident.

Although the cause of glomerular disease may be established from clinical and laboratory evaluation, sometimes percutaneous renal biopsy is needed to provide a definitive diagnosis.

TABLE 47-2 Evaluation of Patients Suspected of Having Glomerular Disease

Medical history

To identify symptoms of medical conditions that may cause glomerular disease

- Diabetes mellitus
- Amyloidosis
- Systemic lupus erythematosus
- Other familial conditions associated with renal disease

To identify symptoms suggestive of nephrotic syndrome

- Reduced appetite
- Fatigue
- Weight gain
- Edema

Medication, environmental, and occupational histories

To identify possible exposure to potentially nephrotoxic drugs, toxins, or chemicals

Physical examination

To identify signs and symptoms associated with systemic diseases

- Hypertension
- Rash
- Arthritis
- Retinopathy
- Neuropathy
- Lymphadenopathy
- Hepatomegaly
- Malignancy

Laboratory evaluation

Urinalysis

- To determine nephrotic nature of glomerular disease
    - Proteinuria, >3.5 g/day/1.73 m^2
    - Lipiduria
- To determine nephritic nature of glomerular disease
    - Hematuria
    - Pyuria
    - Cellular, granular casts

Glomerular filtration rate

- To determine extent of glomerular damage

Other tests

- To identify type and etiology of glomerular disease
    - Serum complement concentration
    - Antinuclear and anti-DNA antibodies
    - Antistreptolysin antibodies
    - Circulating antiglomerular basement membrane antibodies
    - Cryoglobulins

Percutaneous renal biopsy

- To provide definitive diagnosis of glomerular disease

TREATMENT

General Approach to Treatment

In secondary glomerular diseases, such as poststreptococcal glomerulonephritis (PSGN), after the initiating factor is removed, the prognosis of the renal disease is often good. In contrast, the rates of renal function deterioration among the primary glomerulonephritides vary markedly. The majority of patients with minimal-change disease, IgA nephropathy, and membranous nephropathy have a good prognosis. However, those with focal segmental glomerulosclerosis (FSGS) who are resistant to therapy, as well as those with rapidly progressive glomerulonephritis (RPGN) who are untreated, are likely to experience rapid loss of renal function. In some instances, half of the renal function may be lost within a 3-month period. Some entities, such as minimal-change nephropathy, are very responsive to treatment while patients with membranous proliferative glomerulonephritis are rarely responsive to existing therapies.

Because of the variable clinical courses exhibited by the different glomerulonephritides, specific treatment approaches have been developed for each disease. The potential therapeutic benefits

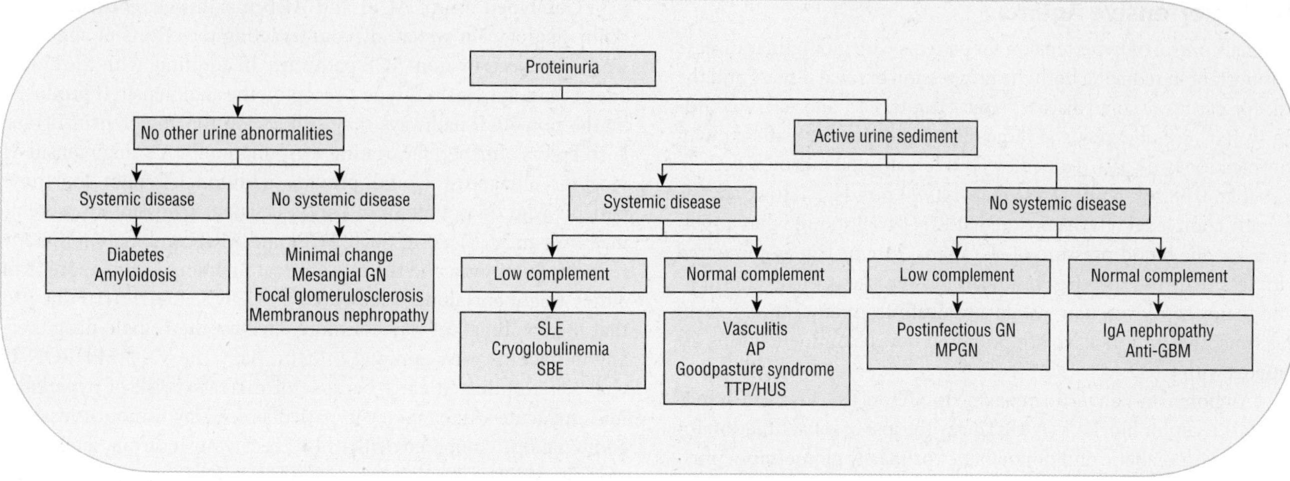

FIGURE 47-2 Clinical presentations of glomerulonephritis. (AP, anaphylactoid purpura; GBM, glomerular basement membrane; GN, glomerulonephritis; HUS, hemolytic uremic syndrome; IgA, immunoglobulin A; MPGN, membranoproliferative glomerulonephritis; SBE, subacute bacterial endocarditis; SLE, systemic lupus erythematosus; TTP, thrombotic thrombocytopenic purpura.)

of treatment regimens should always be weighed against the patient risks. When satisfactory regimens are not available to treat the primary disease, appropriate supportive measures should be employed: optimization of systemic and glomerular blood pressure, reducing proteinuria, and possibly controlling hyperlipidemia may all improve the long-term outcome as well as the quality of life of these patients.

Kidney Disease: Improving Global Outcomes (KDIGO) a global nonprofit foundation dedicated to improving the care and outcomes of kidney disease patients worldwide has promoted coordination, collaboration, and integration of initiatives to develop and implement clinical practice guidelines for many kidney diseases.[11] Many of these clinical practice guidelines are referenced in the ensuing sections which are focused on the treatment of individual primary glomerular diseases.

Nonpharmacologic Therapy

3 For patients with nephrotic syndrome, dietary measures involve restriction of sodium intake to 50 to 100 mEq/day (mmol/day),[12] protein intake of 0.8 to 1 g/day,[12,13] and a low-fat diet of less than 200 mg cholesterol per day. Total fat should account for less than 30% of daily total calories.[12] Sodium restriction is important not only in the control of edema, but also for the control of hypertension and proteinuria. Similarly, protein restriction not only helps to reduce proteinuria but also has a potential role in decreasing the progression of renal disease. Patients should also stop smoking because it is associated in a dose-dependent fashion with an increased risk for ESRD in men with primary inflammatory (immunoglobulin A glomerulonephritis) or noninflammatory (polycystic kidney disease) renal diseases.[14]

Because many immune factors are implicated in the pathogenesis of glomerulonephritis, plasmapheresis or plasma exchange, may be used to remove these mediators.[15] During the procedure, whole blood is removed from the body and centrifugation is used to separate the cellular elements from the plasma. The cells are then infused back to the patient after resuspension in saline or plasma substitute. The plasma proteins, presumably including the pathogenic immune factors, are thereby removed from the patient.

Pharmacologic Therapy

Immunosuppressive Agents

Immunosuppressive agents, alone or in combination, are commonly used to alter the immune processes that are responsible for several of the glomerulonephritides. Corticosteroids, in as a result of their immunosuppressive and antiinflammatory activities reduce the production and/or release of many substances that mediate the inflammatory process, such as prostaglandins, leukotrienes, platelet-activating factors, tumor necrosis factors, and interleukin-1 (IL-1). The immunosuppressive effects of corticosteroids are mediated through the inhibition of the release of IL-1 and tumor necrosis factor by activated macrophages, and interleukin-2 by activated T cells. In addition, the actions of migration-inhibiting factor and γ-interferon are inhibited. Cytotoxic agents, such as cyclophosphamide, chlorambucil, or azathioprine, are commonly used to treat glomerular diseases. Cyclosporine can reduce lymphokine production by activated T lymphocytes, and it may decrease proteinuria by improving the permselectivity of the GBM. Mycophenolate mofetil is useful in some glomerulonephritides because of its effects on T- and B-cell lymphocytes.

Several new agents, such as mTOR inhibitors (sirolimus and everolimus), monoclonal antibodies (rituximab, ocrelizumab, abatacept, and belimumab), imidazole nucleoside (mizoribine), and dihydroorotate dehydrogenase inhibitor (leflunomide), are now being evaluated for their usefulness to control the disease, preserve renal function, and improve patient outcome.[16]

Diuretics

Management of nephrotic edema involves salt restriction, bed rest, and use of support stockings and diuretics. However, severe salt restriction is difficult to achieve and prolonged bed rest can predispose nephrotic patients to thromboembolism. Hence the use of a loop diuretic such as furosemide is frequently required. Although the delivery of diuretic to the kidney tubules is normal, the presence of large amounts of protein in the urine promotes drug binding, and thereby reduces the availability of the diuretic to the luminal receptor sites. In addition, reduced sodium delivery to the distal tubule secondary to decreased glomerular perfusion may also alter diuretic effectiveness. Large doses of the loop diuretic, such as 160 to 480 mg of furosemide, may be needed for patients with moderate edema (see Chapter 49). In some instances, a thiazide diuretic or metolazone may be added to enhance natriuresis.[12,17] Alternatively, continuous IV infusion of a loop diuretic, such as furosemide 160 to 480 mg/day, may be employed.[18] For patients with morbid edema, albumin infusion may be used to expand plasma volume and increase diuretic delivery to the renal tubules, thus enhancing diuretic effect. However, it may precipitate congestive heart failure and may also reduce therapeutic response to steroids in patients with minimal-change nephropathy. For patients with significant edema, the goal of treatment should be a daily loss of 1 to 2 lb (0.45-0.9 kg) of fluid until the patient's desired weight has been obtained.

Antihypertensive Agents

Optimal control of hypertension for patients with glomerular disease is important in reducing both the progression of renal disease and the risk for cardiovascular disease[13] (see Chapters 13 and 44). According to JNC 8 guidelines, the target blood pressure for patients with chronic kidney disease defined by GFR less than 60 mL/min/1.73 m^2 (less than 0.58 mL/s/m^2) is less than 140/90 mm Hg.[19] However, the recently completed NIH-sponsored SPRINT trial showed that targeting a systolic blood pressure of less than 120 mm Hg, as compared with less than 140 mm Hg, resulted in lower rates of fatal and nonfatal major cardiovascular events and death from any cause.[20] As of this time, the authors have not proposed new recommendations for patients with CKD.

Angiotensin-converting enzyme inhibitors (ACEIs) and angiotensin II receptor blockers (ARBs) delay the loss of renal function for patients with diabetic and nondiabetic (primarily glomerulonephritis) renal diseases.[21] Nondihydropyridine calcium channel blockers (eg, diltiazem and verapamil) reduce proteinuria and preserve renal function and could be used as an additional agent. In contrast, the dihydropyridine calcium channel blockers (eg, nifedipine, amlodipine, or nisoldipine) are effective in lowering blood pressure, but without the benefit of proteinuria reduction.[22]

Antiproteinuria Agents

Dietary protein restriction reduces proteinuria and may minimize renal function deterioration. Secondary analysis of the Modification of Diet in Renal Disease Study for patients with moderate renal insufficiency (GFR of 25-55 mL/min/1.73 m^2 [0.24-0.53 mL/s/m^2]) revealed that reduced protein intake (0.66 g/kg/day) delayed the rate of GFR deterioration for patients with severe renal insufficiency (GFR of 13-24 mL/min/1.73 m^2 [0.13-0.23 mL/s/m^2]).[23] Consequently, modest protein restriction of 0.8 g/kg/day is reasonable for patients with moderate renal insufficiency. Decreasing dietary protein also reduces the intake of phosphorus and potassium. In many instances, the potential benefits of protein restriction have to be balanced against the nutritional deficiencies which may develop. For nondialyzed patients who have GFRs of less than 25 mL/min/1.73 m^2 (0.24 mL/s/m^2), dietary protein intake should be reduced to 0.6 g/kg/day.[14]

Angiotensin-Converting Enzyme Inhibitors and Receptor Blockers Since proteinuria is recognized to be an independent risk factor for renal function decline and cardiovascular disease, reducing proteinuria can retard renal function loss and delay the progression to ESRD.[21] Disruption of the renin-angiotensin system (RAS) by ACEI, ARB and direct renin inhibitors (DRIs) can all reduce angiotensin II.[24] The antiproteinuric effect of ACEIs is associated with a fall in filtration fraction, suggesting a reduction in intraglomerular pressure. ACEIs and ARBs may also have direct effects on podocytes, resulting in reduction of proteinuria and glomerular scarring.[21] In addition, angiotensin-converting enzyme (ACE) inhibition may also reduce the effect of angiotensin II on renal cell proliferation, thereby reducing sclerosis. These beneficial effects on proteinuria are beyond what can be attributed by the drug's antihypertensive effects (see Chapters 13 and 44).

Clinical **Controversy...**

Angiotensin-converting enzyme inhibitors and ARBs can reduce proteinuria through different mechanisms and combined use has been shown to be more effective than monotherapy. However, the risk of combination therapy has become a concern recently. Some clinicians therefore recommend the use of monotherapy while others consider the combination a powerful tool for renal preservation.

Combined use of ACEI and ARB maximizes blockade of the renin–angiotensin system by counteracting the effects of angiotensin II produced by non-ACE pathways. In addition, with the blockade of the angiotensin II type 1 receptor, the angiotensin II produced by the non-ACE pathways may still act on the angiotensin II type 2 receptors, further facilitating vasodilation.[21] An angiotensin II receptor antagonist would provide additional benefit for those patients who do not attain full and persistent remission of proteinuria with an ACEI alone. Such ACEI and ARB combination therapy reduces proteinuria and the rate of renal function decline more than either treatment alone.[25] However, the ONTARGET trial showed that the combination was not more effective than single-drug therapy in patients with minimal proteinuria.[26] The VA NEPHRON-D trial was terminated early because of increased risk of hyperkalemia and acute kidney injury in patients receiving lisinopril-losartan combination, compared with those receiving losartan monotherapy.[27] In addition, results of the ALTITUDE trial showed that adding the renin inhibitor aliskiren to ACEI or ARB monotherapy increased non-fatal strokes in type 2 diabetes patients with overt nephropathy.[26] In view of these findings, RAS blockage by dual therapy should be avoided because of potential increase in adverse effects, however, there are clinicians recommending the judious use of combination therapy to take advantage of the powerful proteinuria reduction.[24] It is anticipated that results from ongoing studies may help define the best use of these agents for renal protection.

A thorough review of the combined use of ACEs and ARBs for diabetic nephropathy and proteinuria reduction can be found in Chapter 44.

Nonsteroidal Antiinflammatory Agents Nonsteroidal antiinflammatory drugs (NSAIDs) probably reduce proteinuria through prostaglandin E_2 inhibition, resulting in a reduction of intraglomerular pressure, a decrease in GFR, and restoration of the barrier size selectivity of the GBM.[13] Indomethacin and meclofenamate, the two most evaluated NSAIDs have similar efficacy to ACEIs, and combined treatment with an ACEI results in additional proteinuria reduction.[28] However, adherence to a low-sodium diet or concurrent use of a diuretic is needed to maximize the antiproteinuric effect. Because of their potential for nephrotoxicity, especially for patients with preexisting CKD, long-term use of an NSAID for renoprotection is not commonly prescribed.[26]

Adrenocorticotropin A synthetic adrenocorticotropic hormone (ACTH) analog has been used in Europe for proteinuria reduction associated with nephrotic syndrome. It was reported to have effects similar to alternating months of steroids and cyclophosphamide.[29] Instead of the synthetic analog, a natural, purified ACTH gel is available in the United States and is approved by the FDA for inducing a remission of proteinuria of the idiopathic type or that due to lupus erythematosus. Favorable response was reported in an observation series of 21 patients in the United States.[30] However, the authors cautioned that the data were not derived from a controlled, randomized study and the patients had different glomerular diseases and the long-term effect was not reported.

Statins

It is important to treat patients with persistent nephrotic syndrome, especially those with high VLDL and LDL cholesterol levels (see Chapters 21 and 44). Therapy is especially needed for those with concurrent atherosclerotic cardiovascular disease, or with additional risk factors for atherosclerosis, such as smoking and hypertension.[8]

β-Hydroxy-β-methylglutaryl-coenzyme A (HMG-CoA) reductase inhibitors, also known as "statins" such as lovastatin, pravastatin, simvastatin, fluvastatin atorvastatin and rosuvastatin, are considered the treatment of choice.[31] They reduce total plasma cholesterol concentration, LDL cholesterol, and total plasma triglyceride concentrations.[8] Aside from the lipid-lowering effects, statins can reduce cardiovascular risk independent of serum lipid concentrations. Such 'pleiotropic' effects are mostly mediated through inhibition of protein prenylation, altering signaling pathways that regulate gene expression, membrane trafficking, cell proliferation, migration and apoptosis.[32] Renoprotection is conferred through the reduction of cell proliferation and mesangial matrix accumulation and their antiinflammatory and immunomodulatory effects.

Meta-analysis of published studies showed that statins appear to reduce renal function decline and slow the progression of proteinuria moderately. The beneficial effect may be dose-related and duration-dependent.[33] One analysis revealed that patients with cardiovascular disease were most likely to benefit, compared with those with diabetes or hypertensive nephropathy or glomerulonephritis.[34] In contrast, a large randomized, controlled trial (SHARP) with 9,438 participants showed that simvastatin 20 mg plus ezetimibe 10 mg did not affect the progression of ESRD, although the lipid reduction prevented major cardiovascular events in predialysis CKD patients.[35]

Based on the available data, statins should be used to treat the dyslipidemia; however, their effect on renal function preservation is not as clear. The PCSK9 inhibitors, alirocumab and evolocumab, may be especially useful in treating hypercholestermia in patients who have nephrotic syndrome and those on peritoneal dialysis, since they tend to have high PCSK9 concentrations.[36] However, the effect of these agents on renal function needs to be demonstrated in large clinical trials.

Anticoagulants

Renal vein thrombosis, pulmonary emboli, or other thromboembolic events are serious and common complications of nephrotic syndrome, and are frequently seen in those with membranous nephropathy. Although patients who have documented thromboembolic episodes should be anticoagulated with warfarin until remission of nephrotic syndrome, the use of prophylactic anticoagulation is controversial. A decision analysis study suggested that prophylactic anticoagulation is beneficial for patients with membranous nephropathy.[37] Prophylactic anticoagulation is not recommended for all patients; rather, a "selective" approach or individualized assessment should be conducted to identify those at high risk (ie, those with severe nephrotic syndrome and a serum albumin concentration less than 2-2.5 g/dL [less than 20-25 g/L]).[37] Also at risk are those who require prolonged bed rest, those receiving high-dose IV steroid therapy, and individuals who are dehydrated as well as postsurgical patients.[13]

Evaluation of Therapeutic Outcomes

The management of patients with glomerulonephritis involves specific pharmacologic therapy for the glomerular disease they have in addition to supportive measures to prevent and/or treat the pathophysiologic sequelae, namely, hypertension, edema, and progression of renal disease. Although the course of the disease, as well as the specific treatment regimens, varies the efficacy monitoring parameters are similar.

4 Patients should be monitored closely for therapeutic response as well as the development of treatment-related toxicities. Although the rate of renal function deterioration is an important indicator of the long-term success of treatment, resolution of nephrotic and nephritic signs and symptoms are also important short-term therapeutic targets (Table 47-3).

Serum creatinine concentration as well as creatinine clearance should be evaluated prior to and during treatment; 24-hour urine output should be collected to determine the extent of proteinuria. Alternatively, the daily urine protein excretion may be estimated from the urinary total protein-to-creatinine concentration ratio. After establishing the correlation between the 24-hour urinary protein excretion and the protein-to-creatinine ratio, single, random urine specimens may be used in place of a 24-hour urine collection. Blood pressure should be monitored at each visit to assess the need for and/or the adequacy of antihypertensive therapy. The clinical signs and symptoms of edema and fluid overload should be assessed at each clinic visit to gauge the need for diuretic intitation or dosage escalation. For patients with nephrotic syndrome, serum lipid concentrations should be monitored, at least quarterly. If the patient has hematuria, urinalysis and a complete blood count should be obtained. The clinician should also be aware of the patient's appetite and energy level, because these are indicators of the patient's overall well-being. Renal biopsy is occasionally needed to assess response to treatment and disease progression, to determine future treatment strategy, and to confirm the initial diagnosis.

TABLE 47-3 Monitoring Parameters to Assess Response to Glomerulonephritis Treatment

Renal function
Serum creatinine concentration
24-h urine collection for creatinine clearance determination
24-h urine collection for urinary protein excretion
Urine protein-to-creatinine ratio
Clinical signs and symptoms
Nephrotic syndrome
Proteinuria
Serum lipid concentrations
Edema
Nephritic presentations
Hematuria
Urinalysis
Complete blood count
Blood pressure
General well-being: appetite, energy level
Kidney biopsy to assess disease progression and response to therapy
Assessment of drug therapy adverse reactions and toxicities

The frequency of monitoring is dependent on the specific glomerulopathy and severity of the disease.

Patients receiving cytotoxic drug treatment should be evaluated to gauge their response and identify the presence of drug-related toxicities every week for a month and then monthly to quarterly there after. If a favorable response is obtained after a course of treatment, the patient may be evaluated every 3 to 4 months. The patient's renal function, proteinuria, urinalysis, blood pressure, lipid profile, and the overall state of health should be assessed during these regular follow-up visits.

Minimal-Change Nephropathy

Epidemiology and Etiology

Minimal-change nephropathy (also termed "nil disease") is most commonly observed in children, and accounts for 85% to 90% of all cases of nephrotic syndrome in children between 1 and 4 years of age. The percentage drops to less than 50% after age 10 and it accounts for less than 20% of all cases of idiopathic nephrotic syndrome in adults. Lipoid nephrosis is another term that has been used to describe this type of glomerular disease because lipids, as well as renal tubular cells, are found in the urine. Secondary causes of minimal-change nephropathy include drug exposure (eg, NSAIDs, lithium, and interferons), lupus, and various T-cell-related disorders, such as Hodgkin's disease and leukemias.

Pathophysiology

Minimal-change disease is characterized by the absence of definitive pathologic changes with light and immunofluorescence microscopy of a biopsy specimen. The characteristic lesion in patients with minimal-change disease, as visualized under electron microscopy, is the spreading and fusion of the foot processes of epithelial cells over an unchanged GBM. The pathogenesis of minimal-change disease is unknown, although some have proposed that altered cell-mediated immunologic response, specifically T-cell dysfunction or changes in the T-cell subpopulations, may be responsible. The activated lymphocytes are thought to secrete lymphokines that reduce the production of anions in the GBM and alter podocyte integrity. The permeability of the GBM to plasma albumin is increased as the result of the reduction of electrostatic repulsion. The loss of anionic charges also results in fusion of the epithelial cell foot processes.

Clinical Presentation

Most patients present initially with edema, frequently acute in onset, following a nonspecific upper respiratory tract infection, allergic reaction, or vaccinations, which might have activated T lymphocytes. Nephrotic syndrome with massive proteinuria (substantially more than 40 mg/m²/h for children and more than 3-3.5 g/day for adults), hypoalbuminemia, and hyperlipidemia is also common. The patient's weight may increase dramatically because of sodium and fluid retention. Nephritic features, such as gross hematuria, are uncommon. Hypertension and decreased renal function are uncommon in children but are frequently seen in older adults.

TREATMENT

Pharmacologic Therapy

Steroids

5 Minimal-change disease is most responsive to initial treatment with corticosteroids. In children, steroid therapy is expected to reduce proteinuria in approximately 90% of the patients and the 10-year renal survival rate exceeds 95%. Because of the excellent response to steroids and the prevalence of this glomerular disease in children, reduction of proteinuria secondary to steroid treatment is considered diagnostic for minimal-change disease without the need for biopsy. Prednisone is commonly administered at 60 mg/m²/day initially for 4 to 6 weeks. The dose is then reduced to 40 mg/m²/day every other day for 2 to 5 months, with dose tapering (Fig. 47-3).[38] Proteinuria will disappear in 50% of patients after 1 week and in 94% of patients after 4 weeks of treatment. Commonly, the initial episode is treated with an extended course (months) of therapy, followed by shorter treatment (weeks) for relapses.[39]

For adults, prednisone 1 mg/kg/day (maximum 80 mg) or alternate-day single dose therapy of 2 mg/kg (maximum of 120 mg) is given initially for a minimum of 4 weeks to maximum of 16 weeks and then tapered slowly with cessation by 6 months. 50% of the patients will respond after 4 weeks and an additional 10% to 25% will respond after 12 to 16 weeks of treatment.[40]

Relapse As many as 80% to 90% of the patients who respond to initial steroid therapy (steroid sensitive) will experience a relapse of proteinuria, within 6 to 12 months after disease onset. The risk of relapse is affected by the duration of initial steroid therapy.[12] Children who were asymptomatic with proteinuria diagnosed during routine urine screening tend to have less frequent relapses and a more favorable clinical course. In those who relapse, 50% to 65% may have steroid-responsive relapse episodes over the subsequent 3- to 5-years. The dose and duration of steroid treatment for relapse do not appear to influence the subsequent rate of relapse.[12] Commonly, 60 mg/m²/day of prednisone is given until the urine is free of protein for 3 days, followed by 4 weeks of alternate-day prednisone at 40 mg/m² per dose.[38]

Frequent Relapse Approximately 40% of children who are steroid responsive will experience frequent relapses or become steroid dependent, that is, requiring continuous low-dose alternate-day prednisone to maintain an extended relapse-free period.[38] A small number of patients eventually develop resistance to steroids, and a biopsy done at that time often reveals another pathology such as FSGS. It is controversial whether minimal-change disease progresses into FSGS or if FSGS was present at the time of initial clinical presentation.

Cytotoxic Agents

Cytotoxic agents are often considered for patients who are steroid resistant, as well as for those who require large doses of steroids to sustain remission (steroid dependent). These agents are also beneficial for pediatric patients who experience growth retardation secondary to chronic use of steroids. Cytotoxic agents are effective in inducing remission and the duration of remission tends to be longer than that induced by steroids. In those who relapse after cytotoxic therapy, they may regain or respond better to steroids than before.

Cyclophosphamide at 2 mg/kg/day for 8 to 12 weeks is very effective in inducing remission. Alternatively, chlorambucil at 0.1 to 0.2 mg/kg/day may be used. This agent, however, is associated with more adverse effects than cyclophosphamide. Azathioprine is no longer recommended since its effectiveness has not been substantiated in randomized trials.[38]

The immunosuppressive effect of cytotoxic agents can result in serious infections, which are the primary cause of death for patients with minimal-change nephropathy. Other toxicities associated with cyclophosphamide include gonadal fibrosis, which results in sterility, hemorrhagic cystitis, alopecia, and the potential development of malignancy in those on long-term treatment.

Calcineurin Inhibitors

Cyclosporine decreases lymphokine production by activated T lymphocytes and thereby reduces proteinuria by reversing the lymphokine-induced alterations in the anionic charge and permeability of the GBM to albumin. For patients with steroid-sensitive or steroid-dependent disease, cyclosporine induces remission in 80% to 85% of patients. However, the disease-free period is not often sustained, and relapse may occur as soon as the drug is tapered or discontinued. The steroid-sparing effect of cyclosporine is useful for steroid-dependent patients, especially those who have experienced significant adverse effects.

Tacrolimus has been used in children with frequent relapse and steroid dependence, to avoid the cosmetic side effects of cyclosporine. While randomized trials are not available to substantiate its use, it is believed that the efficacy is similar to cyclosporine based on one observational study.[41]

Dosage The usual starting dose of cyclosporine for remission induction is 4 to 5 mg/kg/day in 2 divided doses with the goal of achieving 12-hour trough serum concentrations of 80 to 150 ng/mL (mcg/L; 67-125 nmol/L). After achieving stable remission for 3 to 6 months, a lower serum concentration, perhaps at 60 to 80 ng/mL (mcg/L; 50-67 nmol/L), can be maintained to minimize cyclosporine-induced nephrotoxcity.[38] Therapy should be maintained for at least 12 months, since most patients experience relapse when treatment is stopped, especially those with a shorter duration of therapy. However, renal toxicity becomes a concern with longer term therapy. Tubulointerstitial lesions were found in 30% to 40% of patients after treatment of 12 months or more. Concuurent administration of ketoconazole can reduce the dose of cyclosporine, resulting in savings in drug cost with no compromise in efficacy.[42]

Adverse Events Adverse events such as hypertrichosis, and gingival hyperplasia are quite common. Long-term therapy may result in persistent hypertension and progressive renal failure.

Mycophenolate Mofetil

Mycophenolate mofetil is an immunosuppressant that can suppress T- and B-cell lymphocyte proliferation, B-lymphocyte antibody production, and expression of adhesion molecules. It is reported to have steroid-sparing effects and is useful in frequently relapsing, steroid-dependent and steroid-resistant patients, as well as in those who fail

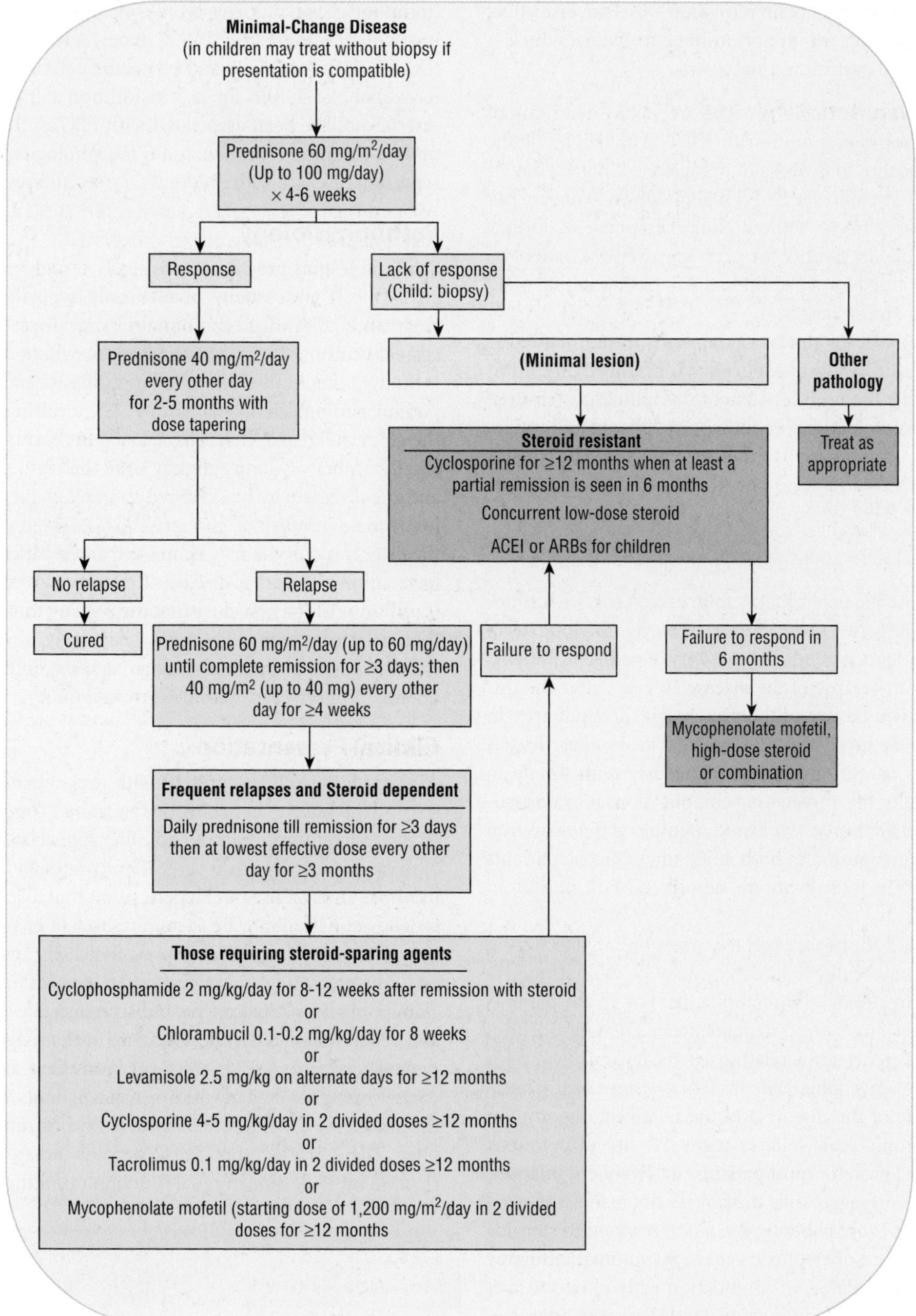

FIGURE 47-3 Treatment algorithm for minimal-change disease according to KDIGO guidelines. (*Data from references 38 and 40.*)

cytotoxic therapy.[43] KDIGO guidelines recommend a starting dose of 1,200 mg/m^2/day in 2 divided doses. Therapy should be maintained for at least 12 months since most will relapse when the treatment is stopped.[38] For those who experience relapse, treatment should be continued or another agent started to maintain the remission.

Rituximab

Rituximab has been found to reduce relapse rate and the need for prednisone and cyclosporine treatment in steroid dependent patients.[44] As an antiCD20 monoclonal antibody, it may act on the CD20+ B cells or CD17+ B or T cells, or exert a direct effect on the podocyte actin cytoskeleton.[45] At this time, due to the lack of randomized trial data and the potential for serious adverse effects, the KDIGO guidelines recommend rituximab be considered only for steroid-dependent children who have frequent relapses despite optimal combinations of prednisone and corticosteroid-sparing agents, and/or those who have serious adverse effects from such therapy.[38] Rituximab is not recommended for use in adult patients.

Levamisole

Levamisole, an immunostimulant, has been available for treatment for several decades. The drug is no longer available in the United States now; however, it is recommended by the KDIGO guidelines as a steroid-sparing agent.[38] Levamisole can promote the maturation of young T cells and restore their function as well as that of phagocytes. It may also inhibit the production of an immunosuppressive lymphokine. Levamisole was found to have a steroid-sparing effect and can enhance maintaining remission in children who had frequent relapse steroid-dependent nephrotic syndrome.[46] In addition, it is as effective as cyclophosphamide in reducing relapse rate and steroid dosages necessary to maintain remission.[47] The adverse effect of levamisole is uncommon and minor: mild neutropenia, which is generally reversible, and gastrointestinal upsets.

Steroid Resistant Nephrotic Syndrome While the definition of steroid resistance varies among studies, the KDIGO guidelines define it as a minimum exposure to 8 weeks of prednisone 2 mg/kg/day or 4 weeks of 60 mg/m^2/day, followed by 1.5 mg/kg/day or 40 mg/m^2 per dose alternate-day for 4 weeks without clinical response. A kidney biopsy would be needed to identify the pathology in these patients.[48] Steroids may be continued for an additional 4 weeks for a total of 12 weeks while awaiting biopsy results.

Calcineurin inhibitor for at least 12 months is recommended as initial therapy for steroid-resistant nephrotic syndrome. ACE inhibitors or ARBs should also be used concurrently to reduce proteinuria. If no response is observed after 6 months, mycophenolate mofetil, high-dose steroid or a combination of these agents should be considered. Available evidences do not support the use of cytotoxic agents and rituximab.[48]

Prognosis

Typically, minimal-change nephropathy follows a course with spontaneous remission (30%-40%) and relapse. However, the long-term prognosis of most patients is good. The majority of pediatric patients will not experience any relapse of the disease 10 years after the initial onset, and most will be free of the proteinuria after puberty. In adults, an 85% to 90% survival rate is seen 10 years after disease onset. Although this condition may spontaneously remit in up to 70% of untreated adults, life-threatening complications may be associated with untreated nephrotic syndrome. Significant deterioration in renal function is uncommon in both adult and pediatric patients and is observed only in those who are steroid resistant or steroid dependent.

Most children and adults are expected to respond well to steroid therapy. Resistance may be due to undetected FSGS lesion, underlying malignancy or treatment non-compliance. For those patients with frequent relapses and steroid-dependence, KDIGO guidelines do not indicate a preference for alkylating agents, levamisole, cyclosporine, tacrolimus or mycophenolate mofetil. Because of the overall favorable outcome of the disease and the relatively uncommon progression into chronic renal failure, aggressive use of cytotoxic agents is not indicated even for most patients with frequent relapses. Toxicities associated with aggressive therapy do not justify the need to induce remission in those patients who fail to respond to steroids and the nonaggressive use of cytotoxic agents. Symptomatic therapy with diuretics to control edema, in conjunction with a low-salt diet and albumin infusion as needed for acute development of anasarca, is often a more rewarding therapeutic approach. NSAIDs and ACEIs may also be used to reduce the proteinuria.

Focal Segmental Glomerulosclerosis

Etiology and Epidemiology

Focal segmental glomerular sclerosis is a clinicopathologic condition that can be idiopathic that is, primary or secondary to a variety of conditions such as sickle cell disease, cyanotic congenital heart disease, and morbid obesity which can induce hemodynamic stress on an initially normal nephron population and result in FSGS. FSGS accounts for less than 20% of the cases of idiopathic nephrotic syndrome in children and approximately 40% in adults;[49] however, it may account for 36% to 80% of the cases in African Americans, probably due to genetic predisposition. The incidence of FSGS has been rapidly increasing, so that it now is the most common glomerular disease that ultimately leads to ESRD. In the United States, FSGS is the most common etiology for proteinuria in African Americans and Hispanics. Severe glomerular injury can also be seen in patients with nephropathy associated with heroin abuse, human immunodeficiency virus (HIV) infection, and genetic mutations involving the podocin and WT1 genes. A recent case series identified the association of FSGS and proteinuria in bodybuilders after long-term anabolic steroid abuse.[50] In addition, heroin, pamidronate, and interferon have been associated with FSGS.[49] The primary and secondary sclerotic lesions may be morphologically similar, but they represent diseases with different courses and responses to therapy.

Pathophysiology

Sclerotic lesions are characteristically found in some of the glomeruli (focal) and usually involve only a portion of the glomeruli (segmental).[49] Similar to minimal-change disease, fusion of foot processes is commonly seen in those glomeruli that are not sclerotic. It is thought that both minimal-change disease and FSGS share similar pathogenetic mechanisms, with FSGS resulting in severe injury to the glomerular epithelial cells. During the early stage of FSGS, only a small number of glomeruli may have the segmental sclerotic lesion, and the disease may be confined to the juxtamedullary region. If an inadequate number of glomeruli are sampled during renal biopsy, the diagnosis of FSGS may be missed, or the patient may be thought to have minimal-change disease. Resistance to steroid therapy may thus be one of the first clues that the patient, indeed, has FSGS rather than minimal-change disease. Alternatively, a patient may have the steroid-sensitive minimal-change disease initially, which subsequently progresses to steroid-resistant FSGS.

Clinical Presentation

Almost all the patients present with proteinuria, and many of them have all the features of nephrotic syndrome. The proteinuria is nonselective, containing albumin and other higher-molecular-weight proteins, and is usually less severe when compared to patients who have minimal-change disease. Hypertension, microscopic hematuria, and renal dysfunction may be seen in up to half of the patients. Reduced renal function becomes more prevalent as the disease progresses.

The presenting clinical features in nephrotic adults with minimal-change nephropathy can be indistinguishable from that of FSGS, and renal biopsy is therefore critical in the diagnosis of adults with nephrotic syndrome. African Americans have a fourfold higher risk of developing FSGS than white or Asian patients. They tend to develop the disease earlier and present with nephrotic range proteinuria more often. They are less responsive to steroids and are more likely to experience a rapid decline in renal function, resulting in ESRD.

TREATMENT

Pharmacologic Therapy

The treatment of FSGS is controversial because of the lack of data from randomized, prospective, controlled trials.

Steroids

For patients with idiopathic FSGS and nephrotic syndrome, KDIGO guidelines recommend daily single dose of prednisone (1 mg/kg/day) or an alterntate-day dose regimen (2 mg/kg/day) for at least 4 weeks, up to a maximum of 16 weeks, or until complete remission, with subsequent tapering over 6 months after attaining complete remission.[51] Urinary protein excretion and serum albumin concentration should be monitored to assess efficacy. The median time to induce complete remission is 3 to 4 months, although 5 to 9 months may be needed in some patients. In general, 30% to 50% of all patients are expected to be resistant to steroids, after at least 4 months of therapy.

If the patient develops a relapse after an adequate response to the initial treatment, a second course of steroids is generally sufficient. In view of the lack of evidence specific for FSGS, the KDIGO recommendations for adults with minimal-change disease can be used to guide treatment of steroid-responsive primary FSGS. However, if relapse occurs frequently, cytotoxic agents or cyclosporine would be indicated.

Patients who are not nephrotic have a relatively favorable prognosis and thus their need for steroids or other immunosuppressive agents is unlikely. However, close follow-up and good blood pressure control with ACEIs/ARBs may be necessary to minimize disease progression.[49]

Most of the studies conducted predominantly included white patients. In a retrospective review of 72 patients that included 65 African American patients, steroid use was not associated with renal survival or the induction of proteinuria remission.[52] The initial creatinine level, blood pressure, and severity of renal lesions were significant predictors of renal survival. About one third of the patients who received steroids developed complications such as diabetes and significant weight gain.

Cytotoxic Agents

When used with steroids during initial therapy, cytotoxic agents were not found to offer any additional beneficial effect.[49,53] Randomized clinical trials are not available to support their use as first-line therapy.[51]

Calcineurin and Rapamycin Inhibitors

In patients with uncontrolled diabetes, psychiatric disorder, or severe osteoporosis, calcineurin inhibitors may be used as first-line therapy to avoid the potential steroid side effects on these conditions.[49,51] In steroid-resistant patients, KDIGO guidelines suggest using cyclosporine at 3 to 5 mg/kg/day in divided doses for at least 4 to 6 months. If there is a partial or complete remission, therapy may be continued for at least 12 months, followed by a slow taper.[51] Complete or partial remission was observed in 70% of patients, with a relapse rate of 47%.[54] Tacrolimus may also be used with similar effects.[55] The effect of sirolimus on proteinuria has been found to be conflicting; however, it may cause a rapid decline in GFR, and hence its use for FSGS is not recommended.[56]

Mycophenolate Mofetil

A randomized study in adult patients with FSGS and persistent nephrotic syndrome suggested that mycophenolate mofetil with low-dose prednisone might be beneficial for those who are unable to tolerate prolonged high-dose prednisone. Indeed comparable remission rates were found for both regimens.[57]

Mycophenolate mofetil has been reported to have favorable effects for patients who were steroid resistant. After inducing remission with high-dose IV methylprednisolone and oral cyclosporine, a combination of cyclosporine and mycophenolate, followed by mycophenolate alone, can sustain long-term remission, preserve renal function, and improve blood pressure control.[58] However, due to the varied experiences from different investigators, further studies are needed to define the role of this agent among the various treatment options.

Angiotensin-Converting Enzyme Inhibitors and Angiotensin II Receptor Blockers

6 Because of the lack of a consistently effective regimen for primary FSGS, many patients with mild disease are treated conservatively. ACEIs and ARBs are effective in reducing proteinuria and stabilizing renal function in many patients with primary or secondary FSGS. Control of blood pressure and hyperlipidemia are important as well.[49] For patients who have nephrotic range proteinuria, an elevated serum creatinine concentration, and interstitial scarring on biopsy, corticosteroids with or without immunosuppressive agents are often used as combination therapy.

Steroid-Resistant FSGS About 40% to 60% of patients with primary FSGS with nephrotic syndrome are resistant to steroid treatment. KDIGO guidelines suggest following the guidelines for relapsing minimal-change disease in this population of patients: Cyclosporine 3 to 5 mg/kg/day in divided doses be given for at least 4 to 6 months. Therapy should continue for at least 12 months, followed by slow taper, if there is a partial or complete remission. For those who are unable to tolerate cyclosporine, mycophenolate mofetil and high-dose dexamethasone should be considered, although data supporting efficacy is weak.[51] At present, there is insufficient evidence to support the use of alkylating agents, sirolimus, rituximab and ACTH. Randomized controlled trials are needed to clarify the role of these agents.

Prognosis

End-stage renal disease develops within 10 years in 10% or less of the adults and children who attained complete remission.[54] For those patients who are resistant to therapy, the rate of renal function deterioration to ESRD may be rapid, within 1 year, or slow, over as long as 10 to 20 years; approximately 50% develop ESRD within 10 years. Those patients with severe proteinuria (more than 10-15 g/day), high serum creatinine concentration at diagnosis, initial steroid resistance, or interstitial fibrosis on renal biopsy are likely to have a more rapid decline in renal function. Kidney transplantation is often indicated for those patients who develop ESRD; however, FSGS has recurred in 40% of the renal allografts soon after transplantation.[49] Children, nonblack race, and those with severe disease or rapid progression to ESRD prior to transplantation are more likely to experience a recurrence. The proteinuria may reappear within hours after transplantation, and graft failure may occur in one third to one half of the patients. High-dose IV methylprednisolone and cyclosporine may reduce recurrences. Rituximab may also be helpful in patients who fail to respond to plasmapheresis.[51] ACEIs and plasmapheresis are also used to prolong graft survival. The effectiveness of these therapies and the rapid recurrence of the disease in the transplanted kidney substantiate the possibility that a circulating humoral mediator is responsible for the nephropathy. Plasmapheresis to remove the mediator was found to be effective in inducing a remission.[49]

Membranous Nephropathy

Etiology and Epidemiology

Membranous nephropathy had been the most common disorder responsible for idiopathic nephrotic syndrome in adults. However, in a recent large survey of renal biopsy results, membranous nephropathy was the third most common type of GN (7.5%), after IgA nephropathy (22%) and FSGS (12.4%).[59] It is also a frequent cause of renal failure secondary to glomerulonephritis. The hallmark histologic features of membranous nephropathy are glomerular capillary wall thickening with subepithelial deposits under light and electron microscopy. Autoimmunity is responsible for most of the cases. Autoantibodies toward phospholipase A2 receptor (PLA2R) have been found in 80% of patients with idiopathic membranous nephropathy. In addition, antibodies against neutral endopeptidase (NEP) have been discovered in rare cases of neonatal membranous nephropathy.[60] The presence of bovine serum albumin (BSA) and anti-BSA antibodies in certain patients suggests that food antigens may be involved in the pathogenesis. Further, anti-PLA2R antibodies appear to predict disease activity and response to therapy.[60]

About 25% of adults and 80% of children have secondary causes. In the United States, the most common etiologies are autoimmune diseases (eg, lupus), infection (eg, hepatitis B and C), syphilis, neoplasm (eg, carcinoma of the lung, breast, GI tract, or kidney), and medications (eg, gold, penicillamine, or captopril). Malaria and schistosomiasis are common causes in other parts of the world. De novo membranous nephropathy can also occur in the allografts of renal transplant patients. Because the responses to therapy as well as the prognosis for idiopathic and secondary membranous nephropathy are different, it is important to identify any potential underlying causes for the nephropathy prior to treatment. Although this glomerular disease can occur at any age, the peak incidence is between ages 30 and 50 years and is especially likely in patients older than age 50 years who present with nephrotic syndrome.

Pathophysiology

Examination of kidney tissue under light microscopy reveals normal mesangium and normocellularity. The glomerular capillary wall may be thickened in well-developed lesions. In the advanced stage, the epithelial side of the capillary wall is markedly thickened, and intramembranous deposits are found. Progressive changes in capillary lumen patency parallel those in the GBM, resulting in glomerulosclerosis with capillary collapse and tubular atrophy in end-stage membranous nephropathy. Immunofluorescence microscopy shows strong capillary wall staining of IgG and C3 on the epithelial side of the basement membrane. Antibody-mediated immune injury appears to be the main pathogenetic mechanism. The immune complex can be formed in situ or deposited from circulating immune complexes.

Clinical Presentation

Most patients with membranous nephropathy present with heavy proteinuria (exceeding 3.5 g/day). Those patients excreting large amounts of IgG and α_1-microglobulin, indicating more significant tubulointerstitial damage, have a lower remission rate, and are more likely to progress toward renal failure.

The signs and symptoms are usually insidious in onset and may consist of anorexia, malaise, edema, anasarca, or ascites, and pericardial and pleural effusions may also be present. As a result of a hypercoagulable state, pulmonary embolism may develop but rarely results in death. The incidence of renal vein thrombosis varies from 5% to 62%, and membranous nephropathy should be suspected when there is a sudden onset of hematuria, loin pain, pulmonary embolus, fluctuating or worsening proteinuria or GFR, renal tubular acidosis, or an increase in leg edema. Hypertension is found in approximately 30% of patients and is more common in those with renal insufficiency.

In addition to heavy proteinuria, urinalysis often reveals lipiduria and oval fat bodies. Microhematuria is seen in fewer than 25% of patients, and gross hematuria and red cell casts are rare. In idiopathic membranous nephropathy, the serum complement concentrations are normal. Low levels of complement should alert one to search for secondary causes, such as lupus, hepatitis B infection, or an alternative diagnosis. Similarly, antinuclear antibodies, anti-DNA antibodies, rheumatoid factor, hepatitis B serologies, and serum cryoglobulins are generally negative in idiopathic membranous nephropathy. Occult malignancy has been found in as many as 10% of elderly patients with membranous nephropathy.

TREATMENT

The treatment of idiopathic membranous nephropathy is controversial and ranges from supportive therapy to immunosuppression. Conservative management of patients with mild disease includes edema control with salt restriction and diuretics[61] and reduction of proteinuria with protein restriction and ACEIs (Fig. 47-4).[11,62] Management of hypertension and hyperlipidemia is required for most patients, whereas prophylactic anticoagulation, despite having benefits shown to outweigh the risks, is usually given only for patients with renal vein thrombosis or documented pulmonary embolus.[37,62]

Pharmacologic Therapy

Due to the favorable long-term outcomes of patients presenting with mild disease, KDIGO guidelines recommend immunosuppressive therapy only for those with nephrotic syndrome, "severe, disabling or life-threatening symptoms" or with substantial elevation of serum creatinine within 6 to 12 months from time of diagnosis.[63] Since even partial remission of proteinuria improves long-term kidney and patient survival, inducing a lasting reduction of proteinuria is therefore the primary goal of treatment.

Steroids

Corticosteroids alone were ineffective in improving proteinuria remission rate in all controlled trials and in preventing progression.[64] The result of a meta-analysis also confirmed the lack of efficacy of steroids when used alone.[65]

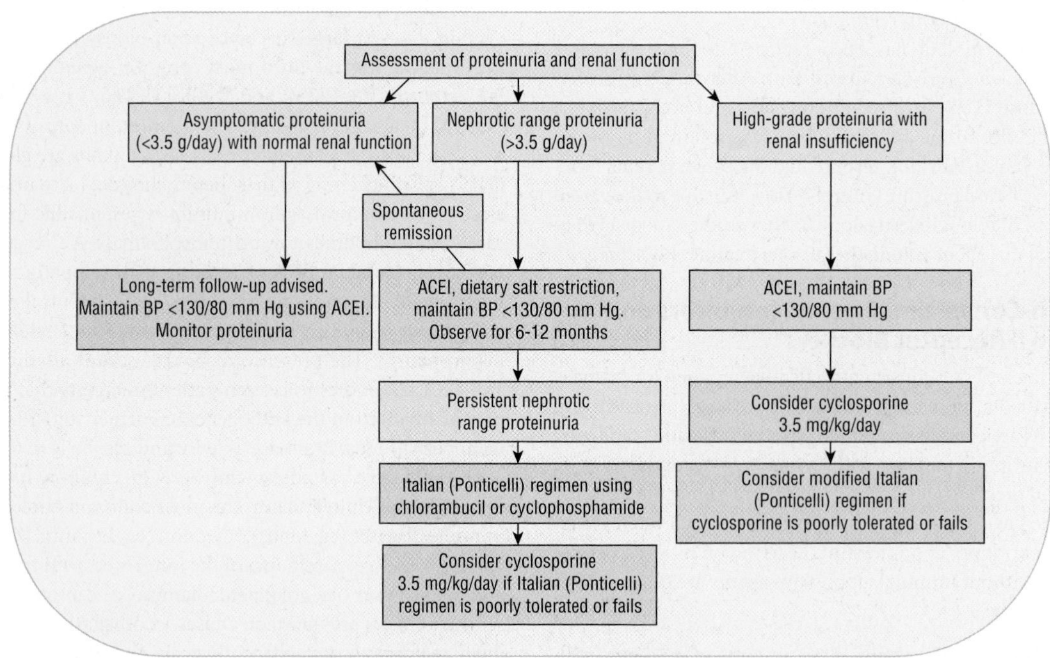

FIGURE 47-4 Treatment algorithm for idiopathic membranous nephropathy. *(Used with permission from Geddes CC, Cattran DC. The treatment of idiopathic membranous nephropathy. Semin Nephrol 2000;20:299-308. Copyright © 2000 Elsevier.)*

Cytotoxic Agents

Cytotoxic agents, when used in conjunction with corticosteroids, are effective in increasing the remission rate of proteinuria and preserving renal function.[11] KDIGO guidelines recommend therapy based on a regimen developed by Ponticelli and colleagues: IV methylprednisolone (1 g) for 3 days followed by oral methylprednisolone (0.5 mg/kg) for the subsequent 27 days of months 1, 3, and 5; oral chlorambucil (0.15-0.2 mg/kg) or cyclophosphamide (2.0 mg/kg/day) daily in months 2, 4, and 6.[63,66] The 10-year renal survival with this regimen was 92% compared with 60% in the control group receiving only symptomatic therapy. Cyclophosphamide is preferred over chlorambucil for initial therapy, since both agents resulted in similar rates of proteinuria remission and relapse, but with fewer serious side effects in those who received cyclophosphamide.[67]

Results from a meta-analysis of randomized, controlled trials affirmed that cytotoxic agents, but not steroids, are effective in reducing nephrotic-range proteinuria, with cyclophosphamide having fewer adverse effects than chlorambucil.[64]

Calcineurin Inhibitors

Cyclosporine is effective in reducing proteinuria and rate of renal function decline as well as inducing remission of nephrotic syndrome. KDIGO guidelines recommend using cyclosporine (3.5-5.0 mg/kg/day orally in two equally divided doses 12 hours apart, with prednisone 0.15 mg/kg/day) or tacrolimus (0.05-0075 mg/kg/day orally in two divided doses 12 hours apart, without prednisone) for at least 6 months for those patients who have contraindications to receiving the cyclical 'Ponticelli' steroid/alkylating agent combination.[63] After attaining a response, the dosage can be reduced at 4 to 8 week intervals to about 50% of the starting dose and this regimen should then be maintained for at least 12 months. Serum drug concentrations should be monitored during initial therapy and when there is an unexplained rise in serum creatinine. Cyclosporine trough concentrations of 125 to 175 ng/mL (mcg/L; 104-146 nmol/L) and 2-hour post-dose concentrations of 400-600 ng/mL (mcg/L; 333-499 nmol/L) are generally considered nontoxic. Long-term use of calcineurin inhibitors may increase blood pressure and result in nephrotoxicity, especially in patients with preexisting renal function impairment.

Alternative Therapeutic Options

Because spontaneous remission is common and only approximately 25% of patients with new-onset idiopathic membranous nephropathy ultimately develop ESRD in 20 to 30 years, it is prudent not to aggressively treat all patients at the onset of the disease. Patients who have a low risk for renal disease progression can be managed with observation and symptomatic therapy. Normalizing the blood pressure and reducing proteinuria with ACEIs and/or ARBs are important as both hypertension and proteinuria are independent risk factors for the progression of renal failure.[61] Patients with low risk for renal disease progression include children 2 to 16 years of age, adult males with proteinuria less than 2 g/day, or adult females with proteinuria less than 5 g/day and normal renal function.

In contrast, patients who have a high risk of developing renal failure, including those with proteinuria greater than 10 g/day with or without impaired renal function, and patients with symptomatic nephrotic syndrome with a plasma albumin of less than 2 g/dL (20 g/L) should be aggressively treated to induce remission. An alkylating agent such as cyclophosphamide or chlorambucil, combined with steroids, should be given to induce remission.

Recently, rituximab was shown to be effective in several small studies; however, randomized, controlled trials are not yet available to confirm its longer-term effects.[61,64] Treatment decisions should be made in light of the FDA black box warning for potentially fatal infusion reactions, mucocutaneous reactions as well as the risk for hepatitis B reactivation. Other monoclonal antibodies being evaluated include eculizumab, adalimumab, daclizumab, fresolimumab, belimumab and tocilizumab.[61]

Clinical **Controversy...**

Should mycophenolate mofetil be used in place of alkylating agent for initial treatment of idiopathic membranous nephropathy? Favorable results have been reported for mycophenolate mofetil by some investigators with conflicting efficacy by others.[64] It might be combined with steroid in place of an alkylating agent in the cyclical 'Ponticelli' regimen. However, the long-term efficacy of this combination has yet to be substantiated since relapse after mycophenolate mofetil treatment is frequent.

Tetracosactide, a synthetic analog of adrenocorticotropic hormone, as well as a natural highly purified ACTH gel, have been shown in small studies to offer favorable results.[68] Their mechanism of action in reducing proteinuria is not known. There might be a direct effect on podocytes since receptors for endogenous ACTH have been identified on the cells.

Relapse of Nephrotic Syndrome Occurs in 25% to 30% of patients within 5 years after treatment with alkylating agents and 40% to 50% within 1 year after CNIs. KDIGO guidelines suggest reinstitution of the same regimen used for inducing the initial remission.[63]

Clinical **Controversy...**

Should patients with membranous nephropathy be given prophylactic anticoagulation? Patients with idiopathic membranous nephropathy are prone to developing deep vein thrombosis and pulmonary artery embolism. The quality of evidence supporting prophylactic anticoagulation is low, mainly based on Markov modeling of anticipated benefits and risks derived from observational studies. KDIGO guidelines suggest prophylactic warfarin for patients with nephrotic syndrome, serum albumin less than 2.5 g/dL (less than 25 g/L) and additional risk factors, such as BMI more than 35 kg/m^2, history of thromboembolism, documented genetic predisposition, NYHA class III or IV congestive heart failure, recent abdominal or orthopedic surgery, prolonged immobilization.[63] However, the use of computerized algorithms in predicting morbidity and mortality has not been evaluated and there are many limitations that need to be considered.[69] Results from a randomized controlled trial are needed to elucidate the relative treatment benefits and risks.

Prognosis

The natural course of idiopathic membranous nephropathy is variable. Up to 30% of the patients experience spontaneous remission, commonly within 2 years of disease onset. Half of the remaining patients have persistent proteinuria with long-term preservation of renal function, while the other half has gradual loss of renal function. Heavy proteinuria (greater than 10 g/day), male gender, elevated serum creatinine concentration at the time of presentation; poorly controlled hypertension, advanced age at onset of disease, nonAsian race, certain human leukocyte antigen phenotypes, and tubulointerstitial fibrosis on initial renal biopsy are associated with progressive renal disease. A predictive algorithm, incorporating the level of proteinuria, initial creatinine clearance, as well as the slope of renal function decline over 6 months, has been developed to determine the risk for disease progression.[61]

In general, patients with idiopathic membranous nephropathy have a relatively benign course with mean 10-year survival of approximately 70%. Those who present with persistent nonnephrotic proteinuria seldom develop renal insufficiency and have a normal life expectancy. Fewer than 10% of patients develop a remitting and relapsing course. The prognosis for secondary membranous nephropathy depends on the underlying cause. Remission occurs when the infection resolves or when the causative medication is withdrawn. For patients with a transplanted kidney, both de novo and recurrent membranous nephropathy may occur. Patients with primary membranous nephropathy are more at risk. Recurrence is typically associated with nephrotic syndrome and a high risk of allograft failure from disease and/or rejection.

Membranoproliferative Glomerulonephritis

Etiology and Epidemiology

Membranoproliferative glomerulonephritis (MPGN) is one of the least-common renal morphologic entities that occur in older children and adults. Although it accounts for 7% to 10% of all case of biopsy-confirmed glomerulonephritis, MPGN is the third or fourth leading cause of ESRD among the primary glomerular diseases.[70] For some unclear reason, the incidence of MPGN has been decreasing over the past few decades in the United States and Europe. However, in Africa and Asia, idiopathic MPGN is still common, perhaps secondary to exposure to unrecognized infectious and parasitic agents.

Pathophysiology

Membranoproliferative glomerulonephritis is a "pattern of injury," rather than a specific disease, caused by many disorders.[11] The several types of MPGN are classified according to the pathologic features. Type I MPGN, also known as mesangiocapillary glomerulonephritis, is characterized by diffuse thickening of glomerular capillary walls and mesangial hypercellularity. Immune complexes are presumed to have a major role in the pathogenesis of type I MPGN, which is the most common type of primary, idiopathic MPGN.

Type II MPGN is also known as dense-deposit disease (DDD) because of the presence of dense deposits of C3 within the GBM, which gives rise to a ribbon-like appearance. Other variants of the disease include type III MPGN, which is seen rarely and consists of subendothelial and subepithelial deposits with lamination and disruption of the lamina densa of the GBM.

With the recent advances, MPGN is now classified according to the immunopathology, whether it is immune-complex-mediated or complement-mediated: Ig and C3 positive, C3 only or C3 dominant positive, and Ig and C3 negative.[70]

Clinical Presentation

Nephrotic syndrome is the most common presenting condition although some patients may also have a nephritic component (hematuria), hypertension, and progressive renal impairment. Hypocomplementemia is commonly seen.

TREATMENT

Pharmacological Treatment

Steroids and Cytotoxic Agents

Results from small uncontrolled studies suggest that certain patients may benefit from various immunosuppressive regimens. However, the lack of randomized, controlled studies makes it difficult to make strong treatment recommendations.[70] For patients with idiopathic MPGN, nephrotic syndrome, and progressive decline of kidney function, the KDIGO guidelines recommend using oral cyclophosphamide or mycophenolate plus low-dose alternate-day or daily steroids for initial therapy trial of no longer than 6 months.[11]

In those with normal kidney function, no active urinary sediment, and nonnephrotic range proteinuria, one may use ACEIs to control blood pressure and reduce proteinuria in light of the favorable long-term outcomes.[70] Patients with secondary MPGN should receive therapy directed against the primary etiology. Figure 47-5 presents an algorithm for a general approach for treatment and follow-up of MPGN.

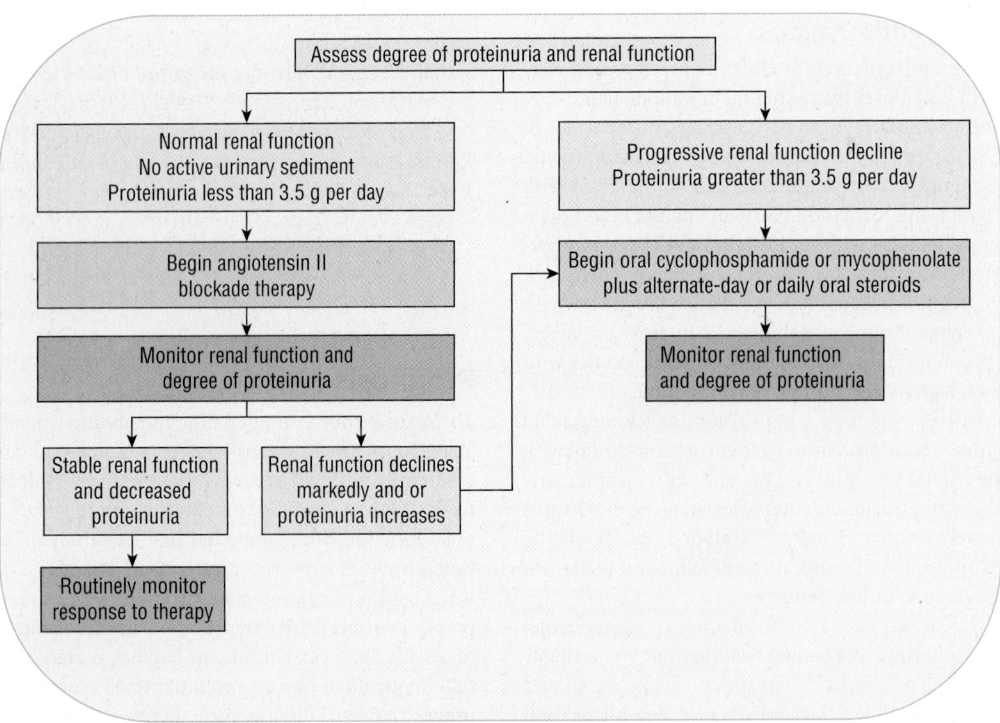

FIGURE 47-5 Treatment algorithm for membranoproliferative glomerulonephritis.

Antiplatelet Agents

Although several studies have shown dipyridamole and aspirin to reduce proteinuria, reduction of GFR decline was not generally observed.[71] Consequently, the efficacy of antiplatelet therapy for idiopathic MPGN remains in doubt.[11] Similarly, the ability of heparin and warfarin, in combination with steroids and cytotoxic agents, to reduce renal function decline was not confirmed to be sustained.

Alternative Therapeutic Agents

Since steroids are not known to be effective for type II disease other yet-to-be-proven strategies such as rituximab, eculizumab, sulodexide, and plasma infusion or exchange may be considered.[72] It is difficult to conduct large-scale controlled trials for MPGN because of the low incidence of the disease. Based on the available studies, many of the drugs evaluated do not have any consistent, beneficial effect on renal function and proteinuria. Renal transplantation is an alternative; however, the recurrence rate is close to 100% for type II MPGN and is approximately 20% to 30% for type I MPGN. Half of the allografts ultimately fail.

Prognosis

Type I MPGN is a slowly progressive disease that accounts for 80% of all MPGN, but only 5% to 15% of all cases of nephrotic syndrome seen in pediatric and adult patients. It occurs most frequently for patients between 5 and 30 years of age, and because remissions are rare, many patients eventually develop ESRD. The renal survival is 60% to 65% at 10 years, and the presence of nephrotic syndrome, interstitial disease, and hypertension are poor prognostic indicators.[72] Type II MPGN is a more aggressive disease that constitutes approximately 15% of all patients with MPGN. Only 20% of patients remain stable for more than a few years, and the median time before the development of ESRD is 7 years.

Immunoglobulin A Nephropathy

Etiology and Epidemiology

IgA nephropathy, also known as *Berger's disease*, was first described by Jean Berger in France in 1968. It now is the most common primary glomerulonephritis in the world and accounts for 10% of patients with ESRD in many countries. The prevalence among patients with glomerulonephritis or patients who had kidney biopsy varies from 30% to 35% to as high as 45% in Asia and 30% to 40% in Europe. In the United States, the overall prevalence is approximately 10% to 15% but is as high as 35% among Native Americans living in New Mexico.[73] These differences in prevalence may reflect variations in genetic predisposition, as well as the criteria used for urinary screening and kidney biopsy. The high biopsy rate tends to correlate with high frequency of the disease. Since the prevalence of clinically silent IgA nephropathy may be high, 16% in a study from Japan, the actual prevalence of the disease could be much higher than observed.[73]

IgA nephropathy is the most common primary glomerulapathy in young adult Caucasians[11] and is two to six times more common in males than in females. It is uncommon in blacks, both in the United States and in Africa.[73] IgA nephropathy was once thought to be a benign disease presenting with asymptomatic hematuria; however, its ability to present with any clinical syndrome associated with glomerular disease is now recognized. Some patients will develop ESRD over variable periods of time.

Pathophysiology

Primary IgA nephropathy is an immune-complex-mediated disease in which IgA deposits, either alone or with IgG, IgM or both as well as other pathologic lesions are found in kidney tissues. In contrast, Henoch–Schönlein purpura, a systemic disease that is believed to be closely linked to IgA nephropathy, shares similar immunohistologic findings in the kidneys. Both typically have vasculitis affecting the joints, skin, and GI tract, which may result from the same pathologic process of IgA nephropathy. The diagnosis of IgA nephropathy is established by the presence of mesangial IgA deposits upon immunofluorescence examination of the kidney biopsy. The IgA immune complex, composed of IgA antibody bound with an environmental antigen, such as a virus, bacteria, or food substances, is presumed deposited from the systemic circulation. Alternately, the complex may be formed in situ, with the IgA antibody bound with an endogenous antigen in the mesangium. In the mesangium, IgA can bind with receptors on the mesangial cells to induce proliferation and cytokine production. In addition, IgA can activate complement through the alternate pathway to induce glomerular damage. The extent of the injury depends on the characteristics of the IgA that favor mesangial deposition, the susceptibility of the mesangium toward deposition, the ability of the patient to mount an inflammatory response to the deposits, and the response of the kidney to the injury in a way that favors progressive renal damage. The key abnormalities and their implications on treatment was reviewed recently by Boyd et al.[74]

The Oxford histologic classification system has been developed to provide a uniform approach to biopsy evaluation and disease classification.[74,75] Further studies are needed to elucidate its ability to predict renal function loss and response to treatment.

Clinical Presentation

IgA nephropathy commonly presents in the second and third decades of life, but it can occur at any age. Many patients have microscopic hematuria and proteinuria for years, persistently or intermittently, during the early stages of the disease. In North America, about 75% of the patients present with gross hematuria concurrent with an infection, commonly in the upper respiratory or gastrointestinal tract.[73] The hematuria may occur 1 to 2 days after the onset of infection symptoms, which is different from the 10- to 14-day delay seen after the pharyngitis in PSGN. Proteinuria is common, and nephrotic range often indicates advanced disease. Hypertension and edema are infrequent but are common in PSGN.

Renal dysfunction is uncommon at the initial presentation; however, approximately 10% to 20% of the patients develop ESRD within 10 years, and 30% develop it after 20 years. The extent of proteinuria is one of the strongest predictors of poor long-term outcomes.[76] Uncontrolled hypertension, GFR reduction at disease presentation, and obesity are additional risk factors for developing renal failure.[11,76]

TREATMENT

General Approach to Treatment

Normotensive patients with normal renal function, isolated microhematuria, and minor proteinuria should be observed closely without specific treatment (Fig. 47-6).[76] Patients with minimal proteinuria of 0.5 to 1 g/day should receive optimized supportive therapy, using ACEIs or ARBs to attain BP of less than 130/80 mm Hg and urinary protein excretion of less than 500 mg/day.[27] However, the recently completed NIH-sponsored SPRINT trial showed that targeting a systolic blood pressure of less than 120 mm Hg, as compared with less than 140 mm Hg, resulted in lower rates of fatal and non-fatal major cardiovascular events and death from any cause.[20] As of this time, the authors do not have a separate recommendation for patients with CKD. Combined ACEI and ARB may be more effective than monotherapy; however, there is an increase in risk of adverse effects. For patients with persistent proteinuria greater than or equal to 1 g/day, the blood pressure goal would be less than 125/75 mm Hg, steroid therapy for 6 months should be used after 3 to 6 months of optimized supportive care and if the GFR is greater

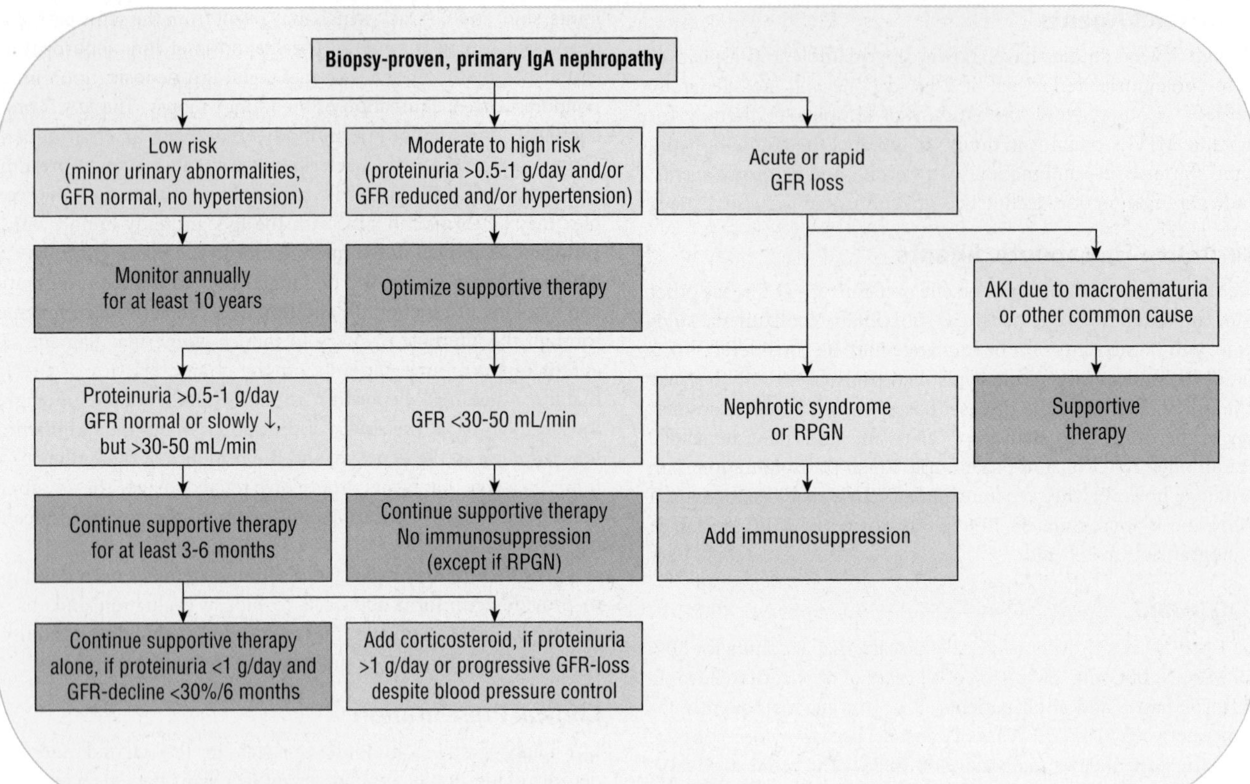

FIGURE 47-6 Treatment algorithm for biopsy-proven IgA nephropathy. Conversion form GFR units of mL/min to mL/s requires multiplication by 0.0167. *(Used with permission from Floege J, Eitner F. Current therapy for IgA nephropathy. J Am Soc Nephrol 2011;22:1785-1794.)*

than 50 mL/min/1.73 m^2 (greater than 0.48 mL/s/m^2).[77] Fish oil may be used if desired. Immunosuppression should not be used for patients with GFR less than 30 to 50 mL/min/1.73 m^2 (less than 0.29-0.48 mL/s/m^2) because of the lack of trials to demonstrate beneficial effects.[76] Comprehensive support must be continued in these patients in an attempt to stabilize the renal function.

Nonpharmacologic Therapy

Low-Gluten Diet and Tonsillectomy

Restriction of dietary gluten is effective for patients with celiac disease but not for patients with any identifiable nephritogenic antigens. Removal of the tonsils, which produce IgA$_1$ and may contribute to IgA nephropathy, may reduce proteinuria and hematuria, as shown in several small, nonrandomized trials in Japan.[74] However, such benefits were not seen in studies in Caucasians. Results from recent meta-analysis does not reveal efficacy when used alone.[78] The KDIGO guidelines therefore do not suggest using tonsillectomy for IgA nephropathy.[77] However, it may be helpful for patients who developed recurrent macroscopic hematuria as provoked by bacterial tonsillitis.

Pharmacological Therapy

Steroids

Corticosteroids with or without immunosuppressive agents have been used to treat IgA nephropathy for many years. A recent meta-analysis showed that steroid therapy is associated with reduction in proteinuria, risk for progression to ESRD, as well as the rate of renal function deterioration.[79] However, optimal antiproteinuric and antihypertensive therapy were not given in some of the studies.[77] Low-dose, short-term (less than 3 months) steroid therapy is not expected to yield favorable results. In contrast, larger doses of steroids (IV methylprednisolone 1 g/day for 3 days at months 1, 3, and 5 and oral prednisone 0.5 mg/kg every other day for 6 months) were able to reduce proteinuria and renal function deterioration.[80] However, the risk for toxicity with such high doses of steroid might be considered high by some, yet the side effects were reported as minor.[80] The KDIGO guidelines therefore suggest a 6-month course of steroid for patients with persistent proteinuria greater than or equal to 1 g/day, despite 3 to 6 months of optimized supportive care and GFR of greater than 50 mL/min/1.73 m^2 (greater than 0.48 mL/s/m^2).[77]

Cytotoxic Agents and Mycophenolate Mofetil

Several studies have evaluated the efficacy of azathioprine and cyclophosphamide. In some of the studies, cyclophosphamide was used in conjunction with dipyridamole, heparin, and warfarin. It is difficult to assess which of these agents contributed to the limited favorable effects observed. In addition, in many of these studies, blood pressure control and ACE inhibition were not always optimal. At present, there is no clear evidence to support the use of these cytotoxic agents for IgA nephropathy[76] except for those with crescentic IgA nephropathy with rapidly deteriorating kidney function.[77]

Clinical **Controversy...**

Fish oil has been recommended by some while others have advocated the first-line use of mycophenolate mofetil for the management of patients with IgA nephropathy.

Mycophenolate mofetil has been evaluated for treating IgA nephropathy on the premise that it may reduce IgA synthesis and mesangial uptake and/or suppress the effects of proinflammatory or profibrogenic mediators.[81] Favorable results were observed in two studies in China; however, no such beneficial effects were seen in studies from Belgium or the United States.[77] These heterogeneous results, possibly due to differences in ethnicity and achieved drug concentrations, and the potential for adverse effects preclude to the widespread use of mycophenolate for IgA nephropathy.[77]

Fish Oil

The third approach is to reduce glomerular inflammation and glomerulosclerosis induced by IgA deposits. Antiinflammatory agents, antiplatelet drugs, and anticoagulants have been tried without success to decrease the production or action of mediators responsible for IgA immune-complex-induced glomerular damage. However, the *n*-3 fatty acids in fish oil reduce the production or action of prostaglandins and leukotrienes, thus limiting the renal damage caused by inflammation, platelet aggregation, and vasoconstriction.[27] In a controlled trial on patients with heavy proteinuria and mildly impaired renal function, daily use of fish oil delayed the progression of renal failure with modest reduction in proteinuria.[82] A meta-analysis of five controlled studies indicated that a minor, but not statistically significant, beneficial effect on renal function may be observed.[83] Results from several recent studies failed to confirm the beneficial effects reported earlier, and further studies are needed to confirm the role as well as the optimal dose. In many of the studies, 4 to 12 g/day were given for two or more years. Some of the fish oil preparations are rich in cholesterol; thus, it is appropriate to monitor the LDL cholesterol levels for patients receiving therapy. In view of the conflicting study results and the very low-risk profile, the KDIGO guidelines suggest using fish oil for patients with persistent proteinuria of greater than or equal to 1 g/day, despite 3 to 6 months of optimized supportive care that includes ACEI or ARB and blood pressure control.[77]

Angiotensin-converting enzyme inhibitors and Angiotensin II receptor blockers

Because hypertension is a negative prognostic indicator of IgA nephropathy outcome and many of these patients already have left ventricular diastolic malfunction despite being normotensive, early antihypertensive intervention with ACEIs or ARBs is important.[73] Indeed, the KDIGO guidelines recommend using ACEI or ARBs for reducing proteinuria and blood pressure control.[76,77] Randomized controlled trials have shown that ACEIs and ARBs can reduce proteinuria and improve kidney function. However, the optimal duration of therapy for reducing the risk for ESRD is unknown. There are also no data to support if there is preference of ACEI over ARB, except perhaps a better side effect profile for ARB when compared with ACEI.[77] There are limited data to suggest that the combined use of ACEI with ARB may offer greater proteinuria reduction than monotherapy. However, further studies are needed to affirm such benefits for the combination therapy.

Alternative Therapeutic Approaches

Patients with IgA nephropathy have abnormal production of IgA and several different immunoglobulins. Immunoglobulins, administered IV initially and then intramuscularly, may have beneficial effects through immunomodulation, increased catabolism of autoantibodies, and blockade of receptors.[84] While favorable results were reported in one trial, large randomized controlled trials are needed to substantiate its efficacy.

Urokinase, danazol, dapsone, sodium cromoglycate, and plasma exchange have also been evaluated, but none is consistently effective nor shown to affect renal function. Cyclosporine, tacrolimus, sirolimus, and mizoribine have been evaluated in a limited number of studies; available results do not support its use for IgA nephropathy.

Antiplatelet agents are commonly used in Japan and rarely outside of Asia for IgA nephropathy.[85] A recent meta-analysis of seven trials (four in Japan and three in Hong Kong) revealed that these agents reduced proteinuria and stabilized renal function.[83] In view of the different agents and concurrent immunosuppressive regimens used among the trials, it would not be possible to derive a recommendation and the KDIGO guidelines do not recommend using these agents.[11]

Prognosis

The majority of the patients with IgA nephropathy have a clinically inconspicuous course and some may experience spontaneous remission. However, others may have an increase in proteinuria and decline in renal function. It is therefore important to follow the patients over a long period of time since progressive disease may appear in 30% of the patients.[76] Spontaneous remission is seen in only 10% to 25% of children and 5% to 7.5% of adults. Unfortunately, no therapy is known to be consistently effective for the treatment of IgA nephropathy. Because of the slow progression of the disease to ESRD, it is very difficult to conduct trials to evaluate the long-term effectiveness of specific treatments. Since the pathophysiological mechanisms of this disease are not well defined, it has been difficult to design and evaluate results of clinical trials.[74]

Urinary protein excretion and the mean arterial blood pressure at follow-up correlate well with the progression of disease. The risk of developing ESRD is proportional to the amount of proteinuria, under the influence of ACEI and ARB therapy, after 1 year of follow-up.[86] For those patients who develop end-stage renal failure, transplantation is appropriate, especially for young adults. Recurrence of IgA mesangial deposits in the renal allograft may occur in up to 50% of patients in 5 years and be universally present at 10 years or more posttransplant, but the recurrence of clinical disease is only approximately 10% to 15%.[73] There is also no correlation between the aggressiveness of the primary disease and the rate of recurrence. Use of ACEI may improve graft survival[87] while immunosuppression with corticosteroids, azathioprine, and/or cyclosporine is not expected to prevent the recurrent nephropathy.[76] The KDIGO guidelines do not address the treatment of recurrent IgA nephropathy in patients who have received a kidney transplant. Applying the guidelines for treating native-kidney IgA nephropathy seems to be reasonable.[73]

Lupus Nephritis

Etiology and Epidemiology

Glomerulonephritis is one of the most serious complications of systemic lupus erythematosus (SLE) and accounts for much of the morbidity and mortality of patients afflicted with the disease. SLE predominantly affects young women between 15 and 40 years of age, with an incidence of 1 in 2,000 women in the United States. African Americans are more susceptible; they develop the disease at a younger age, have nephritis earlier in the course, and are more likely to progress to end-stage kidney disease.

The renal manifestations of lupus nephritis (LN) are variable and encompass a wide spectrum of histopathologic lesions.[88] The underlying histopathology is associated with different prognoses and responses to therapy, which cannot be predicted solely based on clinical manifestations. Thus, a renal biopsy is required to assess the severity of the disease and to predict the short-term and long-term outcomes associated with therapy. Drugs, such as hydralazine and procainamide, are known to precipitate a lupus syndrome; however, they are unlikely to cause disease that affects the kidney.

Pathophysiology

Immune complex deposits, whether formed in the circulation or in situ, can be found in various regions of the glomerulus, as well as the peritubular interstitium and vasculature outside the glomerulus. Based on light, immunofluorescence, and electron microscopy findings, LN can be categorized into six ISN/RPS (International Society of Nephrology/Renal Pathology Society) classifications: I, minimal-mesangial LN; II, mesangial-proliferative LN; III, focal LN; IV, diffuse LN; V, membranous LN; and VI, advanced sclerosing LN.[89]

The hallmark feature in the pathogenesis of SLE is B-cell hyperactivity and the dysregulated production of autoantibodies against multiple antigens in the body, including DNA and various ribonucleoproteins.[88] The size and location of the immune complexes in the glomerulus correlate with the nature and severity of renal injury. Deposition of small numbers of stable immune complexes of intermediate size in the mesangium tends to produce less severe inflammation in the glomerulus. The sequestration of the immune complexes in the mesangium prevents them from activating inflammatory mediators. Hence, the lesion is noninflammatory in nature. In contrast, large numbers of intermediate-sized or large immune complexes result in infiltration of inflammatory cells and release of necrotizing enzymes. In addition, the kidney may also sustain damage through mechanisms related to thrombotic microangiopathy.

Clinical Presentation

Females have a higher risk for developing lupus, especially in the adult years. Nephritis is commonly seen within the first 4 years of diagnosis of SLE but may also be the first manifestation of the disease. The clinical presentation ranges from minimal hematuria and proteinuria to severe, rapidly progressive diffuse glomerulonephritis. Proteinuria is very common, and nephrotic syndrome is seen in most patients with membranous lesions. Microscopic hematuria is almost always present, whereas macroscopic hematuria, which commonly indicates severe renal involvement, is rare. Active urinary sediments (red cell casts, dysmorphic red cells, and hematuria) are suggestive of the diffuse proliferative lesion.[88] Hypertension is present in 25% to 45% of patients and is associated with a worse prognosis. Poor prognosis and higher risk for renal involvement were observed among African American, Hispanic, and Asian patients, compared with white and Puerto Rican–Hispanic patients.[11,90] Other conditions found to be associated with poor prognosis include elevated serum creatinine concentration, heavy proteinuria, anemia (hematocrit less than 26% [less than 0.26]), and disease onset during childhood or in those greater than 60 years of age. Most patients have hypocomplementemia and increased antibody titers for anti-double-stranded DNA, particularly those with focal or diffuse proliferative lesions. Serum creatinine concentration at the time of diagnosis is most predictive of short-term outcome.

TREATMENT

General Approach to Treatment

7 The choice of therapy depends on the underlying lesion and the activity, as well as the chronicity indices. Acute life-threatening disease involving multiple organs requires induction treatment that can suppress the disease promptly. In contrast, long-term management of chronic indolent disease requires therapy with more acceptable side-effect profiles. Corticosteroids are the cornerstone of therapy. However, for severe LN, primarily the diffuse proliferative type, alkylating agents may be needed to reduce or prevent the progression to ESRD. Newer alternatives with fewer side effects are now available.

Optimal blood pressure control is important. ACEIs or ARBs are commonly used to reduce proteinuria and blood pressure. It may also slow disease progression through reduction of inflammation and glomerular injury.[91] Patients with normal renal function and nonnephrotic range proteinuria (class I LN and II LN) typically do not require therapy, except for the management of extrarenal lupus manifestations.[92,91] The prognosis of these patients is generally good, and renal biopsy can be delayed. However, close follow-up of renal function and urinalysis is required.

Acute Induction Treatment

Steroids and Cytotoxic Agents

Patients with nephrotic range proteinuria, deteriorating renal function, and/or active urinary sediments require a renal biopsy to define the underlying lesion and determine the activity and chronicity of disease. Patients with class II LN with proteinuria greater than 3 g/day, class III LN and class IV LN should be treated with steroids: oral prednisone of up to 1 mg/kg, followed by tapering over 6 to 12 months or pulse IV methylprednisolone followed by low-dose oral steroids.[92]

Cyclophosphamide is used concurrently because it is a powerful B-cell inhibitor and can suppress the resynthesis of autoantibodies to normal levels. Combined use of IV cyclophosphamide and methylprednisolone is more effective than either agent alone in inducing remission.[92,93] Alternately, cyclophosphamide may be given orally, but it was found by some to have more adverse effects because of higher cumulative exposure.[91] Azathioprine has also been used instead; however, it was reported to result in higher relapse rate and renal function decline.[92] The risk for adverse events, such as infection, gonadal damage, amenorrhea, and cervical dysplasia, and malignancy is increased with the cytotoxic regimens.

Mycophenolate Mofetil

Several trials have found that mycophenolate mofetil with concurrent steroid therapy is an effective agent for induction therapy.[94] It was as effective as cyclophosphamide in inducing remission but with fewer side effects. A recent meta-analysis of the literature corroborates to the fact that it is an excellent agent for the induction of remission and that continued use may reduce risk for death or development of ESRD.[90] Several recent trials that included African Americans, who are known to have a poorer prognosis, also show that mycophenolate mofetil was more efficacious than IV cyclophosphamide and resulted in fewer adverse effects.[91,95] Based on these data, mycophenolate mofetil is now considered an alternative to cyclophosphamide as initial therapy for patients with class III LN and class IV LN. However, cyclophosphamide may be preferred for severe class III/IV LN since the long-term outcome is not as well established for mycophenolate[92] (Fig. 47-7).

Chronic Maintenance Treatment

Steroids and Cytotoxic Agents

Oral steroid is commonly used as a component of maintenance treatment (less than or equal to 10 mg/day prednisolone).[91,92] Alternate-day regimens are often used in children to minimize growth retardation. Monthly pulse IV steroids in conjunction with cyclophosphamide resulted in more sustained remission, fewer relapses, and no significant increase in side effects.[96] Meta-analysis shows this combination to be more beneficial than steroid or cyclophosphamide alone. Cyclophosphamide, because of its bladder and gonadal toxicity, has been given as monthly and then bimonthly IV injection, instead of daily administration, for 2 or more years. However, toxicity is still a concern.

The efficacy of mycophenolate or azathioprine as maintenance therapy was evaluated against cyclophosphamide. Patients receiving mycophenolate or azathioprine were found to have better outcome and fewer side effects than cyclophosphamide. They are recommended by the KDIGO guidelines for maintenance therapy.[92] Depending on the study, mycophenolate was found to be either equivalent or better than azathioprine.[97,98] However, the drug should not be used during pregnancy since many lupus patients are women of child-bearing age.

Calcineurin Inhibitors

Cyclosporine may reduce proteinuria, stabilize renal function, and improve kidney morphology. It has been shown to have comparable

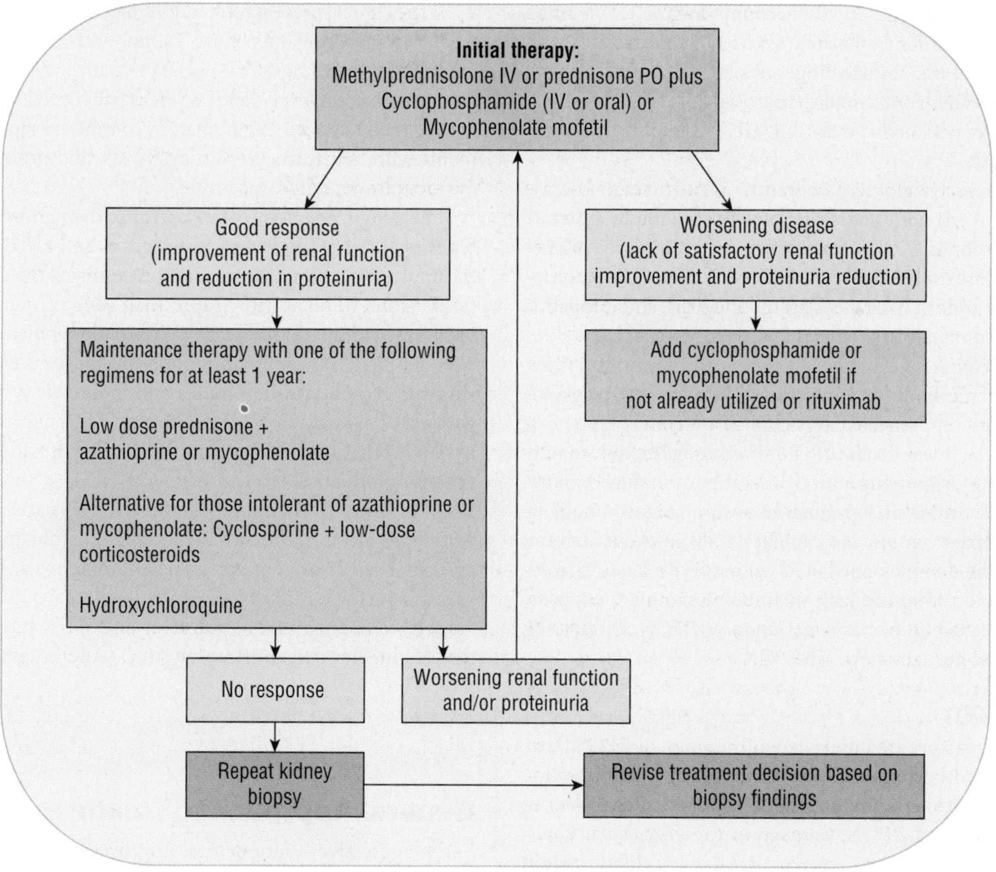

FIGURE 47-7 Treatment algorithm for class III (focal) and class IV (diffuse) lupus nephritis.

efficacy and safety with azathioprine in preventing relapse for patients with diffuse proliferative LN.[99] It is recommended by the KDIGO guidelines for those who cannot tolerate the side effects of azathioprine or mycophenolate. Once initiated therapy should be continued for at least 1 year after complete remission is attained.[92]

Hydroxychloroquine

The antimalarial agent hydroxychloroquine can inhibit the toll-like receptors that contribute to autoimmunity. It was reported to be protective against the onset of LN, relapse of the disease, development of ESRD, venous thrombosis, and also a beneficial effect on lipid profiles.[92] Hydroxychloroquine is recommended by KDIGO guidelines for all patients of any class for those receiving the drug should have annual eye examination for possible retinal toxicity, especially after 5 years of continuous use.

Alternative Therapeutic Agents

Many new agents have been developed to target the various pathways, costimulatory molecules, and immune mediators responsible for the pathologic autoantibody production.[90] Ocrelizumab is an antiCD20 monoclonal antibody being evaluated as an adjunctive induction agent.[91] Abatacept, a selective T-cell co-stimulation modulator, is being studied as add-on induction therapy to cyclophosphamide or mycophenolate regimens. Belimumab, a monoclonal antibody that inhibits B-lymphocyte stimulating protein, appears to offer some promising effects for LN.[100] Abatecept, which may selectively modulate the CD80/CD86:CD28 costimulatory signal,[100] acthar gel, an ACTH formulation,[29] laquinimod (TV-5600 or ABR-215062), a oral immunomodulator that is a quinoline-3-carboxamide derivative, mizoribine, an imidazole nucleoside that inhibits *de-novo* purine synthesis and leflunomide, a lymphocyte proliferation inhibitor, are also currently being evaluated to gauge their role in the management of LN.[16,91]

Prognosis

The prognosis of patients with class II disease is generally good, and often no specific treatment is needed. For patients with class V disease, KDIGO guidelines recommend using antiproteinuric and antihypertensive medications. Steroids and immunosuppressives are used for extrarenal manifestations of systemic lupus and also for those patients with persistent nephrotic range proteinuria.[92] The survival of patients with classes III and IV disease has improved during the last two to three decades to approximately 74% to 80% at 10 years.[88] With the recent use of mycophenolate mofetil, better understanding of the optimal cytotoxic regimens, the use of lower steroid dosages, and better management of complications such as hypertension, infections, hyperlipidemia, and other metabolic complications of the disease, the long-term outcome has become more favorable. Lupus patients with end-stage kidney disease on dialysis fare as well as those with nonlupus-related renal disease. In those patients who received a renal transplant, the allograft outcome of patients with LN is favorable and comparable to those without lupus. Recurrence of lupus in the renal allograft can occur but is usually of minor clinical importance.

Rapidly Progressive Glomerulonephritis

Etiology and Epidemiology

Rapidly progressive glomerulonephritis describes a clinicopathologic syndrome of rapid loss of renal function—usually a greater than 50% decrement of the GFR within 3 months. The predominant histologic finding of RPGN is extensive crescent formation, usually in more than 50% of the glomeruli. Hence, it is also known as *crescentic* glomerulonephritis. RPGN accounts for 2% to 7% of all renal biopsy findings and is responsible for up to 5% of patients with end-stage kidney disease. The age ranges of susceptible patients vary with the type of RPGN. For example, types I and II RPGN are more common in younger patients, whereas type III is seen more frequently in older individuals.

Rapidly progressive glomerulonephritis is not a single disease entity. A variety of glomerulonephritides with or without systemic diseases may present as RPGN, including anti-GBM glomerulonephritis, Goodpasture's syndrome, LN, PSGN, MPGN, IgA nephropathy, polyarteritis nodosa, Wegener's granulomatosis, and idiopathic crescentic glomerulonephritis.

Primary RPGN is categorized according to the immunofluorescence microscopic findings, indicating different immunopathogenesis, therapeutic approaches, and clinical outcomes. Type I is characterized by the linear localization of immunoglobulins, mainly IgG, along the GBM, signifying anti-GBM antibody-induced injury. Type II is defined by the coarse granular deposition of immunoglobulins and complement within the capillary walls and mesangium, indicating immune-complex–mediated injury. Type III is characterized by scanty or complete lack of immune complex deposits; consequently, it is also known as *pauci-immune RPGN.* Circulating ANCAs are often detected in type III RPGN.

Pathophysiology

Different etiologic factors are implicated as the cause of RPGN: toxins, drugs, viral and bacterial infections, neoplasms, autoimmune mechanisms, and various immunogenetic factors.[101] Regardless of the etiology and type of RPGN, damage in the glomerular capillary wall by both humoral and cellular pathways of inflammation is common. Activation of the terminal C5b-9 (membrane-attacking complex) of the complement system produces severe capillary wall injury. Proteinases and reactive oxygen species released by neutrophils and macrophages may result in severe glomerular injury. Platelets and the coagulation system are activated and result in capillary thrombosis. The ruptured capillaries release fibrinogen and procoagulants that may come into contact with thrombogenic tissue debris and lead to fibrinoid changes. In anti-GBM glomerulonephritis, the direct attack of the anti-GBM antibody on the GBM is responsible for the capillary wall injury.[101] For patients with ANCA-associated disease, the interaction of ANCAs with neutrophils and monocytes, which have been primed by concurrent infections or inflammatory processes, can lead to activation of these leukocytes and release of toxic oxygen species and lytic enzymes, resulting in vascular injury.

The disruption of the capillary wall allows movement of macrophages and other plasma constituents into Bowman's space and stimulates the formation of crescents, which are composed mainly of parietal epithelial cells, as well as macrophages and fibroblasts. Crescent formation indicates the severity of the glomerular capillary disease but not its pathogenesis.

Clinical Presentation

Among the crescentic glomerulonephritides, the pauci-immune RPGN (type III) is the most frequent, accounting for more than 50% of cases, whereas the anti-GBM antibody-mediated RPGN (type I) is the least frequent, occurring in roughly 10% to 20% of patients. 60% to 70% of patients with type 1 RPGN may have concurrent pulmonary hemorrhage and Goodpasture's syndrome, which is caused by antibodies directed against the pulmonary alveolar basement membrane. Most patients with immune-complex–mediated RPGN (type II) have collagen vascular disease, systemic infections, or a severe form of primary glomerular disease. Approximately 70% of patients with type III RPGN also present with evidence of systemic vasculitis, such as Wegener's granulomatosis and polyarteritis nodosa. Some patients have only renal manifestations and are said to have idiopathic crescentic glomerulonephritis or renal vasculitis.

The clinical presentation is dominated by progressive renal insufficiency with complaints of tea-colored urine, malaise, anorexia, low-grade fever, and migratory polyarthropathy. Type I RPGN is more common in younger patients, whereas patients with ANCA-mediated disease tend to be older.[102] Urinalysis commonly shows nephritic sediments with hematuria, erythrocyte casts, and proteinuria. However, overt nephrotic syndrome is rare.

Serologic analysis is very useful in distinguishing the different types of RPGN. The detection of serum anti-GBM antibodies with the appropriate clinical presentation confirms the diagnosis of anti-GBM glomerulonephritis. More than 80% of patients with pauci-immune or idiopathic crescentic glomerulonephritis have circulating ANCAs. ANCAs are autoantibodies specific for the cytoplasmic constituents of neutrophil granules and monocyte lysosomes. Patients with ANCA-associated disease limited to renal involvement often have P-ANCA (perinuclear staining), whereas patients with Wegener's granulomatosis tend to have C-ANCA (cytoplasmic staining). Both the anti-GBM antibody and the ANCAs are absent in patients with type II RPGN. Measurements of circulating immune complexes are not useful for making a specific diagnosis, but detection of specific serum antibodies known to mediate immune-complex-associated nephritis is helpful, using anti-DNA antibody as a marker for LN and elevated antistreptolysin O (ASO) titers for PSGN.

TREATMENT

General Approach to Treatment

Early aggressive therapy has improved the renal prognosis of patients with crescentic glomerulonephritis. The rapid deterioration of renal function and the paucity of a large number of patients make randomized controlled studies very difficult to conduct. Based on the available data, immunosuppressive therapy alone appears to be ineffective for type I RPGN, while types II and III RPGN respond well to high-dose steroid therapy.[101,103] Because of the differences in response, the therapeutic approaches for each type of RPGN are presented separately below.

Specific Approaches to Treatment

Antiglomerular Basement Membrane Glomerulonephritis (Type I)

Steroids and cyclophosphamide, in conjunction with plasma exchange, are recommended by the KDIGO guidelines in all patients with anti-GBM glomerulonephritis except those who are dialysis-dependent, have 100% crescent in biopsy sample, and do not have pulmonary hemorrhage.[11] Plasma exchanges remove the pathogenic anti-GBM antibodies in circulation and are conducted for 2 weeks or until the antibodies disappear. Steroids (prednisolone 1 mg/kg/day, tapered over 6 months) and cyclophosphamide (2-3 mg/kg/day for 3 months) are then given to prevent new antibody production.[102,103] Patients with mild disease generally respond well to plasma exchange alone or immunosuppression (steroid and/or cytotoxic agents). For patients with severe disease (poor renal function and extensive crescent formation), most are expected to respond to the combination of plasma exchange and steroid/cytotoxic drug therapy. Pulse IV administration of corticosteroids (methylprednisolone 30 mg/kg/day for 3 days) has been used successfully to alleviate pulmonary hemorrhage, but the results are not as convincing for glomerulonephritis.[91,94] Because of the rapid decline in renal function, diagnosis should be established early so that therapy can proceed without delay. When the serum creatinine concentration is 6 mg/dL (530 μmol/L) or above or the patient is oliguric or requires dialysis, the response to therapy is usually poor, and the patient should be treated conservatively.[93,94] Poor response should also be expected when crescents are found in more than 85% of the glomeruli.

Immune-Complex-Mediated Glomerulonephritis (Type II)

Patients with postinfectious RPGN generally have a favorable prognosis even without treatment. Complete spontaneous recovery occurs in 50% of cases, whereas chronic renal failure develops in 32%.[101] Pulse doses of methylprednisolone (30 mg/kg/day, every other day × 3), followed by oral prednisone (1 mg/kg/day, tapered over several months) and then tapering, are beneficial in type II RPGN, with a response rate of 85% for patients with acute disease and 70% in those with more chronic disease.[101,103] Plasmapheresis does not appear to provide any additional benefit.[103]

Antineutrophil Cytoplasmic Autoantibody-Associated Glomerulonephritis (Type III)

Combined use of high-dose corticosteroids and cyclophosphamide induces remission in more than 90% of patients.[104] IV cyclophosphamide, possibly because of the lower cumulative dose administered, is associated with fewer infectious complications while being as effective as the oral route in inducing remission; however, the risk of relapse may be higher.[105] Because approximately 30% of the patients may relapse, cyclophosphamide also has been used for maintenance therapy. Rituximab and corticosteroids are recommended by the KIDGO guidelines as an alternative initial treatment in patients without severe disease or in whom cyclophosphamide is contraindicated.[11]

Maintenance therapy, using azathioprine or mycophenolate mofetil, is recommended for at least 18 months in patients who remain in remission, except those who are dialysis-dependent and have no extrarenal manifestation of disease.[11] Trimethoprim-sulfamethoxazole is suggested to be used as an adjunct in patients with upper respiratory disease. However, etanercept is not recommended.

Mycophenolate mofetil and methotrexate are also being used, and they have been shown in limited studies to be effective.[103,105] Plasmapheresis is indicated for those with advanced kidney failure or diffuse pulmonary hemorrhage. However, its benefits for patients with better kidney function and mild to moderate disease is not clear.[11,105]

Renal Transplantation

Anti-GBM nephritis may recur in up to 55% of patients who received a renal transplant. However, only 25% of these patients showed clinical disease activity, with rare allograft failure. Because the frequency of recurrence and its severity are related to the presence of circulating anti-GBM antibody, it is recommended that transplantation should not be performed until the anti-GBM antibody is undetectable for at least 6 to 12 months. The recurrence rate of ANCA-associated nephritis is 17%, with the average time to relapse from transplantation of 31 months.[106]

Prognosis

Regardless of the type of RPGN, poor response to therapy and an ominous renal survival are expected if the patient presents with oliguria, has a serum creatinine concentration greater than 6 or 7 mg/dL (530 or 619 μmol/L), is dialysis dependent, or has a renal biopsy showing advanced chronic parenchymal disease.[104] For those patients who had received kidney transplant, recurrence of the disease is common.

Poststreptococcal Glomerulonephritis

Etiology and Epidemiology

PSGN and glomerulonephritis caused by other infectious agents, such as bacteria, viruses, and parasites, were once common. Improved sanitation, personal hygiene, medical care, and public health measures helped to decrease the incidence of group A streptococcal infection both in the United States and in other developed countries, resulting in a decline of PSGN. In contrast, glomerulonephritis secondary to other infectious agents, such as hepatitis C and HIV, is seen with increasing frequency.

PSGN is now the most common form of glomerulonephritis in children but is less common than the other types of glomerulonephritis in adults. PSGN is seen mostly in children aged between 5 and 15 years and is uncommon in children younger than 2 years of age and in adults older than 50 years of age. It normally follows pharyngeal or skin infection caused by the nephritogenic strains of group A streptococci; however, other strains of streptococci, such as groups C and G, have also been reported to cause PSGN. Streptococcal pharyngitis is more common in winter and early spring, whereas skin infection is frequently found in the summer. The risk for developing acute glomerulonephritis secondary to the nephritogenic strains of bacteria is approximately 10% to 15% for infected patients. However, three to four times more patients may experience a subclinical form of the disease.

Pathophysiology

Streptococcal antigens may induce changes in the glomerular components rendering them immunogenic or autologous IgG may be altered to become antigenic. Alternately, the streptococcal antigens may induce antibodies that react with glomerular antigens. In situ immune complexes are then formed and result in a complement-mediated inflammatory response. The kinin and coagulation cascades are activated, and chemotactic factors are released to recruit neutrophils and monocytes, resulting in acute glomerular lesions.

Examination of the acute PSGN kidneys reveals hypercellular glomeruli with proliferation of mesangial and endothelial cells. Infiltration of neutrophils, monocytes, and eosinophils is apparent within the capillary lumen and also in the mesangial areas. Crescent formation may be seen for patients with severe disease, and if found in more than 30% of the glomeruli, RPGN may be present concurrently.[107] The prognosis is generally poor for these patients, and complete recovery is unlikely. Immunofluorescence examination reveals diffuse granular deposits of IgG and C3 along the GBM and also in the mesangium.

Clinical Presentation

The nephritis is preceded by a latent period following a streptococcal infection. The latent period is commonly 7 to 14 days for pharyngitis and 14 to 28 days for skin infection. An acute nephritic syndrome then develops, commonly with hematuria and edema. Gross hematuria is seen in 70% of patients, and microscopic hematuria can be found in all patients. Hypertension is usually mild to moderate and results from sodium and water retention. Many patients have signs and symptoms associated with volume overload, which include dyspnea, orthopnea, and cough. Urinalysis of patients with PSGN reveals hematuria, dysmorphic red blood cells, and red cell casts. Proteinuria is common but often not in the nephrotic range. Renal function is frequently mildly impaired.

Throat or skin culture may be positive for group A streptococci, despite the latent period following the initial infection. However, antibiotic therapy may render the culture result negative. Serologic measurements of antibodies to different streptococcal antigens can confirm recent exposure to the infection. Titers that can be measured include ASO, antistreptokinase, antihyaluronidase (AHase), antideoxyribonuclease B (ADNase B), and antinicotyladenine dinucleotidase (NADase).[108] For most patients with streptococcal pharyngitis, the ASO titers begin to rise about 10 to 14 days later, peak at 3 to 4 weeks, and persist for several months before decreasing. The rise in ASO titers can be reduced by antibiotic treatment and may not be seen for patients with streptococcal skin infection in whom the streptolysin may be bound to skin lipids. ADNase B and AHase titers should be used instead because they are specific and are positive in the majority of patients. The streptozyme test is a combined assay for ASO, ADNase B, NADase, and AHase. Antibodies to other antigens such as zymogen, streptococcal cationic proteinase exotoxin B (SPEB), and plasmin receptor (Plr) were evaluated recently.[109]

Serum complement levels are often decreased for patients with PSGN. If the C3 level is depressed for more than 6 to 8 weeks, MPGN, LN, or glomerulonephritis related to endocarditis or occult visceral abscess should be suspected. Renal biopsy is not normally indicated unless the patient has prolonged hematuria, proteinuria, or depressed C3 level. Renal biopsy is needed to detect other types of glomerulonephritis such as lupus, RPGN, or MPGN.

TREATMENT

General Approach to Treatment

8 The treatment of PSGN is mainly supportive and symptomatic. Early antibiotic therapy does not prevent subsequent PSGN, but it may reduce the severity of the disease. It can, however, prevent the spread of the streptococcal infection to other family members. Antibiotic prophylaxis is not recommended because infected patients will develop long-lasting, often lifelong immunity against the strain of streptococci. Exposure to another nephritogenic strain of streptococci is possible, but unlikely.

Supportive measures should be used to control fluid volume and blood pressure. Because the hypertension is of the low-renin type, ACEIs and β-blockers are not expected to be useful. If the patient has crescentic disease, use of pulse steroids and/or immunosuppressive agents can be considered; however, the efficacy and safety of these agents have not been established for this condition.

Prognosis

The acute manifestations of PSGN are normally self-limited, and for more than 95% of patients renal function has returned to baseline within 3 to 6 weeks. Diuresis usually begins 7 to 10 days after onset of the acute episode, whereas hypertension and azotemia resolve in 1 to 2 acute. Gross hematuria lasts for 1 to 2 weeks, and proteinuria usually resolves within 6 months in more than 90% of children. However, microscopic hematuria may persist for up to 2 years. In general, children have more rapid recovery than adults. Prognosis is often better when PSGN occurs during an epidemic than in cases found sporadically. Most of the children will recover fully and be free from chronic complications of PSGN if they have no preexisting renal disorder, heavy proteinuria, or crescentic glomerular lesions or did not require hospitalization during the acute episode. In contrast, adult patients have a less favorable long-term outcome. As many as 50% of the patients may develop persistent proteinuria, hypertension, and renal insufficiency, with some resulting in end-stage renal failure.

CLINICAL BOTTOM LINE

A better understanding of the pathogenetic mechanisms leading to glomerular injury has led to marked improvements in the treatment of glomerulonephritis. However, the glomerulopathies are a heterogeneous group of immune disorders with different clinical courses, prognoses, and responses to current immunologic and nonimmunologic therapies. The optimal treatment strategy for individual patients should therefore be personalized based on the natural history and prognosis of each type of glomerulonephritis, the efficacy of different immunomodulation regimens in inducing disease remission and preserving renal function, as well as the characteristics of at-risk patients who warrant aggressive therapy. Judicious use of immunosuppressive agents with careful monitoring of their adverse effects cannot be overemphasized. In addition, treatment of the disease complications and control of factors that lead to progression of renal disease are important in reducing the morbidity and mortality of patients with glomerulonephritis. The KDIGO guidelines offer clinicians many evidence-based recommendations that are useful for making individual patient treatment decisions. Since few randomized controlled trials are available for many of the glomerulonephritis, specific recommendations and suggestions based on sound evidence are currently not available.

ABBREVIATIONS

ACE	angiotensin-converting enzyme
ACEI	angiotensin-converting enzyme inhibitors
ACTH	adrenocorticotropic hormone
ADNase B	antideoxyribonuclease B
AHase	antihyaluronidase
ANCA	antineutrophil cytoplasmic autoantibody
ARB	angiotensin II receptor blocker
ASO	antistreptolysin O
BSA	bovine serum albumin
DDD	dense-deposit disease
DRIs	direct renin inhibitors
ESRD	end-stage renal disease
GBM	glomerular basement membrane
GFR	glomerular filtration rate
FSGS	focal segmental glomerulosclerosis
HIV	human immunodeficiency virus
HMG-CoA	β-hydroxy-β-methylglutaryl-coenzyme A
LDL	low-density lipoprotein (cholesterol)
MPGN	membranoproliferative glomerulonephritis
NADase	antinicotyladenine dinucleotidase
NEP	neutral endopeptidase
NSAIDs	Nonsteroidal antiinflammatory drugs
PSGN	poststreptococcal glomerulonephritis
RAS	renin-angiotensin system
RPGN	rapidly progressive glomerulonephritis
SLE	systemic lupus erythematosus
VLDL	very-low-density lipoprotein (cholesterol)

REFERENCES

1. U.S. Renal Data System 2014 Annual Data Report. Minneapolis, MN: USRDS Coordinating Center. 2014. Available at: http://www.usrds.org.
2. Schena FP, Gesualdo L, Grandaliano G, and Montinaro V. Progression of renal damage in human glomerulonephritides: Is there sleight of hand in winning the game? *Kidney Int* 1997;52:1439-1457.
3. Couser WG. Mediation of immune glomerular injury. *J Am Soc Nephrol* 1990;1:13-29.
4. Couser WG, Johnson RJ. The etiology of glomerulonephritis: Roles of infection and autoimmunity. *Kidney Int* 2014;86:905-914.
5. Remuzzi G, Zoja C, Perico N. Proinflammatory mediators of glomerular injury and mechanisms of activation of autoreactive T cells. *Kidney Int Suppl* 1994;44:S8-S16.
6. Sjöblom P, Nystrom FH, Lanne T, et al. Microalbuminuria, but not reduced eGFR, is associated with cardiovascular subclinical organ damage in type 2 diabetes. *Diabetes Metab* 2014;40:49-55.
7. Schrier RW, Fassett RG. A critique of the overfill hypothesis of sodium and water retention in the nephrotic syndrome. *Kidney Int* 1998;53:1111-1117.
8. Warwick GL, Fox JG, Boulton-Jones JM. The relationship between urinary albumin excretion rate and serum cholesterol in primary glomerular disease. *Clin Nephrol* 1994;41:135-137.
9. Wheeler DC, Bernard DB. Lipid abnormalities in the nephrotic syndrome: Causes, consequences, and treatment. *Am J Kidney Dis* 1994;23:331-346.

10. Kaysen GA, De Sain-van der Verlden M. New insights into lipid metabolism in the nephrotic syndrome. *Kidney Int Suppl* 1999;71:S18-S21.
11. Cattran DC, Feehally J, et al. KDIGO clinical practice guidelines for glomerulonephritis. *Kidney Int Suppl* 2012;2:139-274.
12. Ponticelli C, Passerini P. Treatment of the nephrotic syndrome associated with primary glomerulonephritis. *Kidney Int* 1994;46:595-604.
13. Klahr S, Levey A, Beck G, et al. The effects of dietary protein restriction and blood pressure control on the progression of chronic renal disease. *N Engl J Med* 1994;330:877-884.
14. Orth SR, Stockmann A, Conradt C, et al. Smoking as a risk factor for end-stage renal failure in men with primary renal disease. *Kidney Int* 1998;54:926-931.
15. Clark WF. Plasma exchange for renal disease: Evidence and use 2011. *J Clin Apher* 2012;27:112-116.
16. Chan TM, Treatment of severe lupus nephritis: The new horizon. *Nat Rev Nephrol* 2015;11:46-61.
17. Fliser D, Schroter M, Neubeck M. Coadministration of thiazides increases the efficacy of loop diuretics even in patients with advanced renal failure. *Kidney Int* 1994;46:482-488.
18. Rudy DW, Voelker JR, Greene PK, et al. Loop diuretics for chronic renal insufficiency: A continuous infusion is more efficacious than bolus therapy. *Ann Intern Med* 1991;115:360-366.
19. James PA, Oparil S, Carter BL, et al. 2014 Evidence-based guideline for the management of high blood pressure in adults: Report from the panel members appointed to the Eighth Joint National Committee (JNC 8). *JAMA* 2014;311:507-520.
20. The SPRINT Research Group. A randomized trial of intensive versus standard blood-pressure control. *N Engl J Med* 2015;373:2103-2116.
21. Ruggenenti P1, Cravedi P, Remuzzi G. Mechanisms and treatment of CKD. *J Am Soc Nephrol* 2012;23:1917-1928.
22. Gashti CN, Bakris GL. The role of calcium antagonists in chronic kidney disease. *Curr Opin Nephrol Hypertens* 2004;18:155-161.
23. Levey AS, Adler S, Caggiula AW, et al. Effects of dietary protein restriction on the progression of advanced renal disease in the Modification of Diet in Renal Disease Study. *Am J Kidney Dis* 1996;27:652-663.
24. St Peter WL, Odum LE, Whaley-Connell AT. To RAS or not to RAS? The evidence for and cautions with renin-angiotensin system inhibition in patients with diabetic kidney disease. *Pharmacotherapy* 2013;33:496-514.
25. Ruggenenti P, Perticucci E, Cravedi P, et al. Role of remission clinics in the longitudinal treatment of CKD. *J Am Soc Nephrol* 2008;19:1213-1224.
26. Gentile G, Remuzzi G, Ruggenenti P. Dual renin-angiotensin system blockade for nephroprotection: Still under scrutiny. *Nephron* 2015;129:39-41.
27. Fried LF, Emanuele N, Zhang JH. Combined angiotensin inhibition for the treatment of diabetic nephropathy. *N Engl J Med* 2013;369:1892-1903.
28. Perico N, Remuzzi A, Sangalli F, et al. The antiproteinuric antagonism in human IgA nephropathy is potentiated by indomethacin. *J Am Soc Nephrol* 1998;9:2308-2317.
29. Ponticelli C, Passerini P, Salvadori M, et al. A randomized pilot trial comparing methylprednisolone plus a cytotoxic agent versus synthetic adrenocorticotropic hormone in idiopathic membranous nephropathy. *Am J Kidney Dis* 2006;47:233-240.
30. Bomback AS, Tumlin JA, Baranski J, et al. Treatment of nephrotic syndrome with adrenocorticotropic hormone (ACTH) gel. *Drug Des Dev Ther* 2011;5:147-153.
31. Stone NJ, Robinson JG, Lichtenstein AH, et al. 2013 ACC/AHA Guideline on the treatment of blood cholesterol to reduce atherosclerotic cardiovascular risk in adults. A Report of the American College of Cardiology/American Heart Association Task Force on Practice Guidelines. *Circulation* 2014;129(Suppl 2):S1-S45.
32. Kassimatis TI, Goldsmith DJ. Statins in chronic kidney disease and kidney transplantation. *Pharmacol Res* 2014;88:62-73.
33. Geng Q, Ren J, Song J. Meta-analysis of the effect of statins on renal function. *Am J Cardiol* 2014;114:562-570.
34. Turner JM, Bauer C, Abramowitz MK, et al. Treatment of chronic kidney disease. *Kidney Int* 2012;81:351-362.
35. Baigent C, Landray MJ, Reith C, et al. The effects of lowering LDL cholesterol with simvastatin plus ezetimibe in patients with chronic kidney disease (Study of Heart and Renal Protection): A randomized placebo-controlled trial. *Lancet* 2011;377:2181-2192.
36. Athyros VG, Katsiki N, Karagiannis A, et al. Statins can improve proteinuria and glomerular filtration rate loss in chronic kidney disease patients, further reducing cardiovascular risk. Fact or fiction? *Expert Opin Pharmacother* 2015;16:1449-1461.
37. Glassock RJ. Prophylactic anticoagulation in nephrotic syndrome: A clinical conundrum. *J Am Soc Nephrol* 2007;18:2221-2225.
38. Kidney Disease Improving Global Outcomes (KDIGO) Glomerulonephritis Work Group: KDIGO clinical practice guideline for glomerulonephritis. *Kidney Int* 2012;(Suppl 2):163-171.
39. Tune BM, Mendoza SA. Treatment of the idiopathic nephrotic syndrome: Regimens and outcomes in children and adults. *J Am Soc Nephrol* 1997;8:824-832.
40. Kidney Disease Improving Global Outcomes (KDIGO) Glomerulonephritis Work Group: KDIGO clinical practice guideline for glomerulonephritis. *Kidney Int* 2012;(Suppl 2):177-180.
41. Sinha MD, MacLeod R, Rigby E, et al. Treatment of severe steroid dependent nephrotic syndrome (SDNS) in children with tacrolimus. *Nephrol Dial Transplant* 2006;21:1848-1854.
42. El-Husseini A, El-Basuony F, Mahmoud I, et al. Impact of the cyclosporine-ketoconazole interaction in children with steroid-dependent idiopathic nephrotic syndrome. *Eur J Clin Pharmacol* 2006;62:3-8.
43. Hodson EM, Willis NS, Craig JC. Non-corticosteroid treatment for nephrotic syndrome in children. *Cochrane Database Syst Rev* 2008:CD002290.
44. Alsaran K, Grisaru S, Stephens D, et al. Levamisole vs. cyclophosphamide for frequently-relapsing steroid-dependent nephrotic syndrome. *Clin Nephrol* 2001;56:289-294.
45. Li Z, Duan C, He J, et al. Mycohenolate mofetil therapy for children with steroid-resistant nephrotic syndrome. *Pediatr Nephrol* 2010;25:883-888.
46. Ravani P, Magnasco A, Edefonti A, et al. Short-term effects of rituximab in children with steroid and calcineurin-dependent nephrotic syndrome: A randomized controlled trial. *Clin J Am Soc Nephrol* 2011;6:1308-1315.
47. Glassock RJ, Nachman PH, eds. *NephSAP Nephrology Self-Assessment Program* 2014;13:215-221.
48. Kidney Disease Improving Global Outcomes (KDIGO) Glomerulonephritis Work Group: KDIGO clinical practice guideline for glomerulonephritis. *Kidney Int* 2012;(Suppl 2):172-176.
49. D'Agati VD, Kaskel FJ, Falk RJ. Focal segmental glomerulosclerosis. *N Engl J Med* 2011;365:2398-2411.
50. Herlitz LC, Markowitz GS, Farris AB, et al. Development of focal segmental glomerulosclerosis after anabolic steroid abuse. *J Am Soc Nephrol* 2010;21:163-172.
51. Kidney Disease Improving Global Outcomes (KDIGO) Glomerulonephritis Work Group: KDIGO clinical practice guideline for glomerulonephritis. *Kidney Int* 2012;(Suppl 2):181-185.
52. Crook ED, Habeeb D, Gowdy O, et al. Effects of steroids in focal segmental glomerulosclerosis in a predominantly African-American population. *Am J Med Sci* 2005;330:19-24.
53. Goumenos DS, Tsagalis G, El Nahas AM, et al. Immunosuppressive treatment of idiopathic focal segmental glomerulosclerosis: A five-year follow-up study. *Nephron Clin Pract* 2006;104:c75-c82.
54. Frassinetti Castelo Branco Camurça Fernandes P, Bezerra Da Silva G Jr, De Sousa Barros FA, et al. Treatment of steroid-resistant nephrotic syndrome with cyclosporine: Study of 17 cases and a literature review. *J Nephrol* 2005;18:711-720.
55. Roberti I, Vyas S. Long-term outcome of children with steroid-resistant nephrotic syndrome treated with tacrolimus. *Pediatr Nephrol* 2010;25:1117-1124.
56. Cho ME, Hurley JK, Kopp JB. Sirolimus therapy of focal segmental glomerulosclerosis is associated with nephrotoxicity. *Am J Kidney Dis* 2007;49:310-317.
57. Gipson DS, Trachtman H, Kaskel FJ, et al. Clinical trial of focal segmental glomerulosclerosis in children and young adults. *Kidney Int* 2011;80:868-878.
58. Gellermann J, Ehrich JH, Querfeld U, et al. Sequential maintenance therapy with cyclosporin A and mycophenolate mofetil for sustained remission of childhood steroid-resistant nephrotic syndrome. *Nephrol Dial Transplant* 2012;27:1970-1978.
59. Zaza G, Bernich P, Lupo A. 'Triveneto' Register of Renal Biopsies (TVRRB): Renal biopsy in chronic kidney disease: Lessons from a large Italian registry. *Am J Nephrol* 2013;37:255-263.
60. Herrmann SMS, Sethi S, Fervenza FC. Membranous nephropathy: The start of a paradigm shift. *Curr Opin Nephrol Hypertens* 2012;21:203-210.
61. Waldman M, Austin HA III. Treatment of idiopathic membranous nephropathy. *J Am Soc Nephrol* 2012;23:1617-1630.
62. Geddes CC, Cattran DC. The treatment of idiopathic membranous nephropathy. *Semin Nephrol* 2000;20:299-308.

63. Kidney Disease Improving Global Outcomes (KDIGO) Glomerulonephritis Work Group: KDIGO clinical practice guideline for glomerulonephritis. *Kidney Int* 2012;(Suppl 2):186-197.
64. Waldman M, Austin III HA. Controversies in the treatment of idiopathic membranous nephropathy. *Nat Rev Nephrol* 2009;5:469-479.
65. Ponticelli C, Passerini P. Management of idiopathic membranous nephropathy. *Expert Opin Pharmacother* 2010;11:2163-2175.
66. Ponticelli C, Zucchelli P, Passerini P, et al. A 10-year follow-up of a randomized study with methylprednisolone and chlorambucil in membranous nephropathy. *Kidney Int* 1995;48:1600-1604.
67. Ponticelli C, Altieri P, Scolari F, et al. A randomized study comparing methylprednisolone plus chlorambucil versus methylprednisolone plus cyclophosphamide in idiopathic membranous nephropathy. *J Am Soc Nephrol* 1998;9:444-450.
68. Santoro D, Pellicano V, Visconti L, et al. Monoclonal antibodies for renal diseases: Current concepts and ongoing treatments. *Expert Opin Biol Ther* 2015;15:1119-1143.
69. Glassock RJ. Thrombo-prevention in membranous nephropathy: A new tool for decision making? *Kidney Int* 2014;85:1265-1266.
70. Sethi S, Fervenza FC. Membranoproliferative glomerulonephritis—A new look at an old entity. *New Engl J Med* 2012;366:1119-1131.
71. Levin A. Management of membranoproliferative glomerulonephritis: Evidence-based recommendations. *Kidney Int Suppl* 1999;70:S41-S46.
72. Smith RJ, Alexander J, Barlow PN, et al. New approaches to the treatment of dense deposit disease. *J Am Soc Nephrol* 2007;18:2447-2456.
73. Wyatt RJ, Julian BA. Immunoglobulin A nephropathy. *N Engl J Med* 2013;368:2402-2414.
74. Boyd JK, Cheung CK, Molyneux K, et al. An update on the pathogenesis and treatment of IgA nephropathy. *Kidney Int* 2012;81:831-843.
75. Barbour SJ, Reich HN. Risk stratification of patients with IgA nephropathy. *Am J Kidney Dis* 2012;59:865-873.
76. Floege J, Eitner F. Current therapy for IgA nephropathy. *J Am Soc Nephrol* 2011;22:1785-1794.
77. Kidney Disease Improving Global Outcomes (KDIGO) Glomerulonephritis Work Group: KDIGO clinical practice guideline for glomerulonephritis. *Kidney Int* 2012;(Suppl 2):209-217.
78. Wang Y, Chen J, Wang Y, et al. A meta-analysis of the clinical remission rate and long-term efficacy of tonsillectomy in patients with IgA nephropathy. *Nephrol Dial Transplant* 2011;26:1923-1931.
79. Strippoli GF, Maione A, Schena FP, et al. IgA nephropathy: A disease in search of a large-scale clinical trial to reliably inform practice. *Am J Kidney Dis* 2009;53:5-8.
80. Pozzi C, Andrulli S, Del Vecchio L, et al. Corticosteroids effectiveness in IgA nephropathy: Long-term results of a randomized, controlled trial. *J Am Soc Nephrol* 2004;15:157-163.
81. Lai KN. Future directions in the treatment of IgA nephropathy. *Nephron* 2002;92:263-270.
82. Donadio JV Jr, Grande JP, Bergstralh EJ, et al. The long-term outcome of patients with IgA nephropathy treated with fish oil in a controlled trial. Mayo Nephrology Collaborative Group. *J Am Soc Nephrol* 1999;10:1772-1777.
83. Dillon JJ. Fish oil therapy for IgA nephropathy: Efficacy and interstudy variability. *J Am Soc Nephrol* 1997;8:1739-1744.
84. Rasche FM, Keller E, Lepper PM, et al. High-dose intravenous immunoglobulin pulse therapy in patients with progressive immunoglobulin A nephropathy: A long-term follow-up. *Clin Exp Immunol* 2006;146:47-53.
85. Taji Y, Kuwahara T, Shikata S, et al. Meta-analysis of antiplatelet therapy for IgA nephropathy. *Clin Exp Nephrol* 2006;10:268-273.
86. Donadio JV, Bergstralh EJ, Grande JP, et al. Proteinuria patterns and their association with subsequent end-stage renal disease in IgA nephropathy. *Nephrol Dial Transplant* 2002;17:1197-1203.
87. Courtney AE, McNamee PT, Nelson WE, Maxwell AP. Does angiotensin blockade influence graft outcome in renal transplant recipients with IgA nephropathy? *Nephrol Dial Transplant* 2006;21:3550-3554.
88. Contreras G, Roth D, Pardo V, et al. Lupus nephritis: A clinical review for practicing nephrologists. *Clin Nephrol* 2002;57:95-107.
89. Weening JJ, D'Agati VD, Schwartz MM, et al. The classification of glomerulonephritis in systemic lupus erythematosus revisited. *Kidney Int* 2004;65:521-530.
90. Tsokos G. Systemic lupus erythematous. *New Engl J Med* 2011;365:2110-2121.
91. Bomback AS, Appel GB. Updates on the treatment of lupus nephritis. *J Am Soc Nephrol* 2010;21:2028-2035.
92. Kidney Disease Improving Global Outcomes (KDIGO) Glomerulonephritis Work Group: KDIGO clinical practice guideline for glomerulonephritis. *Kidney Int* 2012;(Suppl 2):221-232.
93. Gourley MF, Austin HA, Scott D, et al. Methylprednisolone and cyclophosphamide, alone or in combination, in patients with lupus nephritis. A randomized, controlled trial. *Ann Intern Med* 1996;125:549-557.
94. Walsh M, James M, Jayne D, Tonelli M, Manns BJ, Hemmelgarn BR. Mycophenolate mofetil for induction therapy of lupus nephritis: A systematic review and meta-analysis. *Clin J Am Soc Nephrol* 2007;2:968-975.
95. Appel GB, Contreras G, Dooley MA, et al. Mycophenolate mofetil versus cyclophosphamide for induction treatment of lupus nephritis. *J Am Soc Nephrol* 2009;20:1103-1112.
96. Illei GG, Austin HA, Crane M, et al. Combination therapy with pulse cyclophosphamide plus pulse methylprednisolone improves long-term renal outcome without adding toxicity in patients with lupus nephritis. *Ann Intern Med* 2001;135:248-257.
97. Houssiau FA, D'Cruz D, Sangle S. Azathioprine versus mycophenolate mofetil for long-term immunosuppression in lupus nephritis: Results from the MAINTAIN Nephritis Trial. *Ann Rheum Dis* 2010;69:2083-2089.
98. Dooley MA, Jayne D, Ginzler EM. Mycophenolate versus azathioprine as maintenance therapy for lupus nephritis. *N Engl J Med* 2011;365:1886-1895.
99. Griffiths B, Emery P, Ryan V. The BILAG multi-centre open randomized controlled trial comparing ciclosporin vs azathioprine in patients with severe SLE. *Rheumatology (Oxford)* 2010;49:723-732.
100. Glassock RJ, Nachman PH, eds. *NephSAP Nephrology Self-Assessment Program* 2014;13:258-272.
101. Couser WG. Rapidly progressive glomerulonephritis: Classification, pathogenetic mechanisms, and therapy. *Am J Kidney Dis* 1988;11:449-464.
102. Little MA, Pusey CD. Rapidly progressive glomerulonephritis: Current and evolving treatment strategies. *J Nephrol* 2004;17:10-19.
103. Bolton WK. Treatment of glomerular disease: ANCA-negative RPGN. *Semin Nephrol* 2000;20:244-255.
104. Jennette JC. Rapidly progressive crescentic glomerulonephritis. *Kidney Int* 2003;63:1164-1177.
105. de Groot K, Adu D, Savage CO. The value of pulse cyclophosphamide in ANCA-associated vasculitis: Meta-analysis and critical review. *Nephrol Dial Transplant* 2001;16:2018-2027.
106. Nachman PH, Segelmark M, Westman K, et al. Recurrent ANCA-associated small-vessel vasculitis after transplantation: A pooled analysis. *Kidney Int* 1999;56:1544-1550.
107. Couser WG, Johnson RJ. Postinfective glomerulonephritis. In: Neilson EG, Couser WG, eds. Immunologic Renal Diseases. 2nd ed. Philadelphia, PA: Lippincott-Raven; 2001:899-929.
108. Rodriguez-Iturbe B, Parra G. Glomerulonephritis associated with infection: Poststreptococcal glomerulonephritis. In: Massry SG, Glas-sock RJ, eds. Massry & Glassock's Textbook of Nephrology. 4th ed. Philadelphia, PA: Lippincott Williams & Wilkins; 2001:667-671.
109. Rodriguez-Iturbe B. Nephritis-associated streptococcal antigens: Where are we now? *J Am Soc Nephrol* 2004;15:1961-1962.

Drug Therapy Individualization for Patients with Chronic Kidney Disease

48

Marisa Battistella and Gary R. Matzke

KEY CONCEPTS

1. Chronic kidney disease (CKD) results in minimal alterations in the absorption or bioavailability of most drugs.
2. The volume of distribution (V_D) of many drugs is increased in the presence of acute and CKD as a consequence of volume expansion and/or reduced protein binding.
3. In addition to the expected decrement in renal clearance, nonrenal clearance (ie, gastrointestinal and hepatic drug metabolism) of several drugs is also reduced in CKD patients.
4. Individualization of a drug dosage regimen for a patient with reduced kidney function is based on the pharmacodynamic/pharmacokinetic characteristics of the drug, the patient's degree of residual renal function, and their overall clinical condition.
5. The drug dosing guidelines for CKD patients in many drug information resources are highly variable and many are not optimal for clinical use.
6. The effect of hemodialysis (HD) or peritoneal dialysis on drug elimination is dependent on the characteristics of the drug and the dialysis prescription.
7. HD clearance data can be used to guide the initial drug dosage regimen recommendation for HD patients; however, prospective monitoring of serum concentrations is often warranted especially for narrow therapeutic index drugs.

INTRODUCTION

Chronic kidney disease (CKD) is defined by the presence of abnormalities of kidney function or structure.[1] In its earliest stages it is characterized by either an estimated glomerular filtration rate (eGFR) less than 89 mL/min/1.73 m^2 or the persistence of one or more markers of kidney damage (eg, albuminuria) for more than 3 months in those with eGFR more than or equal to 90 mL/min/1.73 m^2. (see Chapters e42 and 44)[1] The Kidney Disease: Improving Global Outcomes (KDIGO) guidelines for evaluation and management of CKD eGFR and albuminuria categories are outlined in Tables 44-1 and 44-6. It is estimated that 10% to 15% of the global population has CKD and the number of deaths from CKD has risen by more than 80% in the past two decades.[2-4] The prevalence varies widely across the world in part because of true differences in the prevalence of CKD; heterogeneity of the laboratory methods used to detect CKD; environmental factors, public health policies, and genetics.[4] The incidence of CKD has more than doubled in the past 20 years in adults older than 65 years.[5] In part due to age-related reductions in kidney function, multiple medical comorbidities, and an increased use of medications that alter kidney function. Many drugs are predominantly eliminated by the kidney and even those that are highly metabolized may require dose adjustment in CKD patients to maximize therapeutic outcomes and to minimize adverse events. Medications which are predominantly renally eliminated unchanged (f_e) may accumulate in CKD patients, which can increase the risk of adverse effects. If 30% or more of a drug is eliminated unchanged in the urine, it will have a high likelihood of requiring dosage regimen adjustment in CKD patients, especially those with stage 3 to 5 disease.[6,7]

The pharmacokinetics of drugs with a fraction of drug eliminated unchanged in the urine less than 30% also may be affected and thus require a dose adjustment. In fact 32.2% of such drugs approved in the United States from 1998 to 2010 had a dosage-adjustment recommendation for CKD patients in the product labeling.[7] If there is no official dosage regimen recommendation in the product labeling, an adjustment may be calculated on the basis of the drug's f_e and the ratio of the patient's residual renal function relative to an age and gender normal value for estimated creatinine clearance (eCL$_{cr}$) or eGFR.[7,8] Despite increased conduction of renal studies by industry and improvements in approved product labeling language, challenges remain for dose adjustments in CKD patients especially for oncology and anti-retroviral agents.[7] Furthermore, physiologic and biochemical changes such as increased or decreased protein binding, altered cytochrome P450 enzyme activity, and transcellular transport systems that are associated with CKD may also independently impact serum and tissue drug concentrations and necessitate drug dosing adjustments.[6,9] Therefore in CKD patients, the dosage regimens of many drugs must be altered to prevent toxicity, without compromising the achievement of the desired therapeutic benefit.[6]

For medications that are extensively metabolized or for which dramatic changes in protein binding and/or distribution volume (V_D) have been noted, a complex adjustment strategy may need to be employed.[6,9] Despite extensive published evidence, dosing errors in CKD patients still occur at an alarming rate.[10-13] Studies have shown that the expanded use of electronic medical records has not resolved the need for clinician proactivity to optimize the use of medications in CKD patients; in these studies, up to 85% of the medications ordered had nephrotoxic potential and greater than 20% of the drugs ordered were not dose adjusted for the patient's kidney function.[14-16]

Clinicians thus will often need to design individualized therapeutic regimens to optimize achievement of the desired outcomes. In this chapter, the influence of CKD on absorption, distribution, metabolism and elimination of medications is characterized. A general approach to individualizing drug therapy for CKD patients is presented along with dosage recommendations for the most commonly used drugs in this patient population. Finally, the impact of chronic renal replacement therapy (ie, peritoneal dialysis and HD) on drug disposition is discussed and dosage recommendations for selected drugs are presented. Drug dosage regimen adjustment strategies for patients with acute kidney injury (AKI) including those who are receiving continuous renal replacement therapy are presented in Chapter 43.

PHARMACOKINETIC CHANGES IN CHRONIC KIDNEY DISEASE

The absorption, distribution, metabolism, and renal excretion of many drugs is altered by CKD. An understanding of why and how these processes are impacted by CKD provides a framework to project the influence of CKD on emerging drug therapies. In addition, when known, these effects can be factored into the clinician's dosage recommendations for individual CKD patients including those who are receiving chronic renal replacement therapy.

Drug Absorption

1 There is little quantitative information regarding the influence of CKD on drug absorption and bioavailability. The few studies evaluating the absorption of oral medications in CKD patients were not designed to provide an assessment of the drug's absolute bioavailability (eg, they did not include a comparison of the area under the concentration–time curve [AUC] after oral and intravenous [IV] administration of the drug). Rather, the principal outcomes that were documented were alterations in the peak concentration (C_{max}), time at which the peak concentration was attained (t_{max}), or the fractional amount of drug recovered in the urine in a finite time period.[17]

The absorption and bioavailability of some drugs is highly variable in CKD patients. The mechanisms responsible are multifactorial and include; drug interactions, delayed gastric emptying, and reduced gastric acidity. Decreased gastrointestinal (GI) motility secondary to gastroparesis in patients with diabetes may delay the t_{max} and may also reduce the C_{max}. For instance if a drug undergoes GI metabolism the slower transit time allows for more GI metabolism and thus lower C_{max} of the parent drug. Urea retention in CKD patients results in a high influx of urea into the gut, which in turn results in conversion of urea to ammonia by gastric urease. The subsequent increase in gastric pH may alter the dissolution or ionization properties of weakly basic drugs such as diazepam leading to changes in absorption.[18] A reduction in gastric acidity, that is, an increase in GI pH, associated with the concomitant administration of antacids, H_2-receptor antagonists, proton pump inhibitors, and phosphate binders has been associated with a reduction in bioavailability of several antibiotics and digoxin.[18] Finally antacids and vitamin supplements may decrease the bioavailability of some drugs as a result of the formation of insoluble salts or metal ion chelates.[19] Although this is not a disease-specific effect, since CKD patients are frequently taking these medications, the associated drug interactions will impact the absorption of other drugs. Edema of the GI tract, secondary to cirrhosis or congestive heart failure that may be present in CKD patients, can also decrease the absorption of some medications, such as oral furosemide for which a decrease from 50% to 10% has been reported.[19]

The bioavailablity of only a few drugs (eg, dextropropoxyphene, dihydrocodeine, felodipine, sertraline, and cyclosporine) has been documented to be increased in CKD patients.[20-22] For these drugs, the mechanism is a reduction in metabolism during the drug's first pass through the GI tract and liver. Drug interactions can also independently alter bioavailability. Bioflavonoids in grapefruit juice can inhibit cytochrome P450 3A4 and noncompetitively inhibit the metabolism of drugs metabolized by this enzyme; this interaction can increase the bioavailability of cyclosporine by as much as 20%.[23-25]

Distribution

2 A drug's volume of distribution reflects the extent of distribution throughout the body. The V_D of many drugs is increased in category G3a, G3b, G4, and G5 CKD patients as well as those with preexisting CKD who develop AKI (Table 48-1) and can lead to a reduction in serum drug concentrations.[6,9,26-28] This increase in V_D may be the result of pathophysiologic alterations in body composition, fluid overload secondary to excessive fluid administration or intake, decreased protein binding, or increased tissue binding. Decreased tissue binding of drugs in CKD patients may result in a reduction in V_D, which has been reported for only a few medications (eg, digoxin and pindolol).[26]

TABLE 48-1 Volume of Distribution of Selected Drugs in Patients with ESRD

Drug	Normal (L/kg)	ESRD (L/kg)	Change from Normal
Increased			
Amikacin	0.20	0.29	45%
Cefazolin	0.13	0.17	31%
Cefoxitin	0.16	0.26	63%
Ceftriaxone	0.28	0.48	71%
Cefuroxime	0.20	0.26	30%
Doripenem	0.25	0.47	88%
Dicloxacillin	0.08	0.18	125%
Erythromycin	0.57	1.09	91%
Furosemide	0.11	0.18	64%
Gentamicin	0.20	0.32	60%
Isoniazid	0.60	0.80	33%
Minoxidil	2.60	4.90	88%
Naproxen	0.12	0.17	42%
Phenytoin	0.64	1.40	119%
Trimethoprim	1.36	1.83	35%
Vancomycin	0.64	0.85	33%
Decreased			
Atenolol	1.20	0.90	25%
Chloraphenicol	0.87	0.60	31%
Ciprofloxacin	2.50	1.95	22%
Digoxin	7.30	4.00	45%
Ethambutol	3.70	1.60	57%
Methicillin	0.45	0.30	33%
Metoprolol	5.60	1.00	82%
Pindolol	2.10	1.10	48%
Propranolol	4.40	3.60	18%

ESRD, end-stage renal disease.
Data from references 26 and 28.

Variability in fluid status is a common issue in patients with severe CKD (category G4 and G5), especially those that are critically ill. Many critically ill patients receive large volumes of IV fluids for resuscitation from shock, and can subsequently develop edema, pleural effusions, or ascites. These therapeutic interventions, in addition to reduced water excretion due to AKI or CKD, often lead to an increase in a drug's V_D and a decrease in its serum concentrations. This is especially problematic with hydrophilic drugs, such as aminoglycosides and cephalosporins for which the V_D may be increased by up to 150%.[29,30]

Effect of Altered Plasma Protein Binding

Protein binding limits drug distribution as only unbound or "free" drug is able to cross cellular membranes and distribute outside the vascular space. Many drugs have been reported to exhibit altered protein binding in CKD patients.[31,32] Protein binding of many acidic drugs such as penicillins, cephalosporins, aminoglycosides, furosemide, and phenytoin is reduced secondary to hypoalbuminemia, qualitative changes in the conformation of the protein binding site, and/or competition for binding sites by other drugs, metabolites, and endogenous substances.[26,32] The result of a decrease in protein binding is an increase in the apparent V_D. A new equilibrium is ultimately established as a result of increased drug elimination/distribution, such that the unbound concentrations remain comparable to those observed in patients with normal renal function despite the fact that total concentrations are reduced. Thus, the net effect is an alteration in the relationship between total drug concentration and pharmacodynamic effect. For example, protein binding of phenytoin (90% protein-bound, primarily to albumin) is significantly reduced secondary to decreased plasma phenytoin binding affinity for albumin, as well as low serum albumin: these changes alter the relationship between total phenytoin concentration and desired and toxic effects.[31] The resulting increase in unbound fraction, from values of 10% in those with normal renal function to 20% or more in those with G5 CKD, results in increased hepatic clearance and decreased total concentrations. Thus, in patients with CKD, the therapeutic range based on total phenytoin concentration is shifted downward from normal values of 10 to 20 mg/L (mcg/mL; 40-79 μmol/L) to values as low as 4 to 8 mg/L (mcg/mL; 16-32 μmol/L). Since the unbound concentration therapeutic range is the same for all patients, 1 to 2 mg/L (mcg/mL; 4-8 μmol/L), this measurement provides the best target for individualizing phenytoin therapy in patients with CKD.

One can approximate the total phenytoin concentration that would be observed in category G5 CKD patients if they had normal plasma protein binding ($C_{\text{normal binding}}$). The estimated $C_{\text{normal binding}}$ total phenytoin concentration can then be interpreted in light of the usual total therapeutic range to assess the patient's response to therapy.[31]

For normal or low albumin (concentration expressed in g/dL) and category G5 CKD:

$$C_{\text{total normal binding}} = C_{\text{total reported}} / [(0.9)(0.48)\ (\text{albumin}/4.40)] + 0.1$$

where $C_{\text{normal binding}}$ = total phenytoin concentration that would be observed if patient had normal protein binding. C_{reported} = patient's total phenytoin concentration reported by laboratory (represents decreased plasma protein binding).

For albumin expressed in g/L the equation becomes:

$$C_{\text{total normal binding}} = C_{\text{total reported}} / [(0.9)(0.48)\ (\text{albumin}/44)] + 0.1$$

The principal binding protein for several basic drugs is α1-acid glycoprotein, an acute-phase reactant protein, whose plasma concentrations are increased in CKD patients.[6] As a result of this increase, the unbound fraction of some basic drugs (eg, bepridil, disopyramide) may be significantly decreased and the V_D increased in CKD patients, especially renal transplant and HD patients.[6]

Effect of Altered Tissue Binding

Distribution also may be affected by altered tissue binding of drugs in CKD patients; this is relatively rare and limited to few drugs, such as pindolol, ethambutol, and most notably digoxin.[26] The V_D of digoxin is decreased by up to 50% in patients with category G5 CKD, leading to elevated serum concentrations.[33] In this case, the absolute amount of digoxin bound to the receptor is reduced and the resultant serum digoxin concentration is higher than anticipated. Thus, in CKD patients, particularly in those with category G5, a "normal" total drug concentration may be associated with either an adverse reaction secondary to elevated unbound drug concentrations, or a subtherapeutic response because of an altered plasma-to-tissue drug concentration ratio. The monitoring of unbound drug concentrations in CKD patients is thus warranted for those drugs that have a narrow therapeutic range, are highly protein bound (unbound fraction of less than 20%), and for which marked variability in the unbound fraction has been reported (eg, phenytoin and disopyramide).

Effect of V_D Calculation Method

Finally, the method used to calculate the volume of distribution may be influenced by renal insufficiency. The three most commonly used volume of distribution terms are: volume of the central compartment (V_c), volume of the terminal phase (V_β and V_{area}), and volume of distribution at steady state (V_{ss}). The V_c for many drugs approximates extracellular fluid volume and thus may be increased or decreased by acute changes. Oliguric AKI is often accompanied by fluid overload and a resultant increased V_c for many drugs. The V_{area} or V_β represents the proportionality constant between plasma concentrations in the terminal elimination phase and the amount of drug remaining in the body. V_β is affected by both distribution characteristics, as well as by the terminal elimination rate constant. V_β and V_{ss} will often be similar in magnitude, with V_β being slightly larger. Because V_{ss} has the advantage of being independent of drug elimination, it is the most appropriate volume term to use when one desires to compare drug distribution volumes between patients with renal insufficiency and those with normal renal function.[34]

ELIMINATION

Elimination of a drug from the body is characterized in pharmacokinetic terms as total systemic clearance (CL_T), which is the sum of all organ clearances. Typically CL_T is defined simply as the sum of renal clearance (CL_R) and nonrenal clearance CL_{NR}.[6,9]

Renal Clearance

Kidney function is the most quantifiable determinant of drug clearance. It is important to note that the term "kidney function" includes the combined processes of glomerular filtration, tubular secretion, and reabsorption, as well as endocrine and metabolic functions. Alterations in any or all of these functions secondary to CKD may have a dramatic effect on drug disposition (see Chapter e42). Reduction in kidney mass, the number of functioning nephrons, renal blood flow, GFR, and/or the rate of tubular secretion and reabsorption all contribute to the decreased renal excretory capacity observed in those with CKD.

Renal clearance (CL_R) of a drug is the composite of GFR, tubular secretion, and reabsorption ($CL_R = [GFR \times f_u] + [CL_{secretion} - CL_{reabsorption}]$), where f_u is the fraction of the drug unbound to plasma proteins. Drug elimination by filtration occurs by diffusion; while tubular secretion and reabsorption are bidirectional processes that involve carrier-mediated renal transport systems.[35] Renal transport systems have been broadly classified on the basis of substrate selectivity into the anionic and cationic renal transport systems, which are responsible for the transport of a number of organic acidic and basic drugs, respectively (Table 48-3).[26,35] Several drugs are actively secreted by one or more of these transporter families, which include organic cationic (eg, famotidine, trimethoprim, and dopamine), organic anionic (eg, ampicillin, cefazolin, and furosemide), nucleoside (eg, zidovudine), and P-glycoprotein (Pgp) transporters (eg, digoxin, vinca alkaloids, and steroids).[35,36] Alterations in filtration, secretion, or reabsorption, secondary to CKD may have a dramatic effect on drug disposition: for drugs that are primarily filtered, a reduction in GFR will result in a proportional decrease in renal drug clearance.

Nonrenal Clearance

3 The effect of CKD on CL_{NR} is less clear than its impact on CL_R, but there has been an increased interest and plethora of new findings in this area in recent years.[26,36-38] CL_{NR} encompasses all routes of drug elimination, excluding renal excretion of unchanged drug, and includes hepatic and extrahepatic metabolism and altered transcellular transport pathways (see Tables 48-2 and 48-3). It is mediated largely by renal disease effects on many cytochrome P450 (CYP) metabolic

TABLE 48-2 Impact of ESRD on CL_{NR} of Selected Drugs

Drug Name	Decreased Change in CL_{NR}
Acyclovir	50%
Aztreonam	33%
Bupropion	↓
Captopril	50%
Carvedilol	↓
Cefotaxime	40%
Ceftriaxone	↓
Cimetidine	46%
Ciprofloxacin	33%
Doripenem	↓
Erythromycin	↓
Imipenem	58%
Isoniazid	↓
Ketorolac	↓
Losartan	↓
Lovastatin	↓
Metoclopramide	66%
Minoxidil	46%
Morphine	40%
Nicardipine	37%
Nimodipine	87%
Nortriptyline	↓
Procainamide	60%
Quinapril	↓
Raloxifene	↓
Repaglinide	↓
Rosuvastatin	↓
Simvastatin	↓
Valsartan	↓
Vancomycin	43%
Verapamil	54%
Warfarin	50%

CL_{NR}, nonrenal clearance; ESRD, end-stage renal disease.
↓ a decrease is documented but not quantified.
Data from references 9 and 26.

TABLE 48-3 Major Pathways of Nonrenal Drug CL

CL_{NR} Pathway	Selected Substrates
Oxidative Enzymes	
CYP	
1A2	Polycyclic aromatic hydrocarbons, caffeine, imipramine, theophylline
2A6	Coumarin
2B6	Nicotine, bupropion
2C8	Retinoids, paclitaxel, repaglinide
2C9	Celecoxib, diclofenac, flurbiprofen, indomethacin, ibuprofen, losartan, phenytoin, tolbutamide, *S*-warfarin
2C19	Diazepam, *S*-mephenytoin, omeprazole
2D6	Codeine, debrisoquine, desipramine, dextromethorphan, fluoxetine, paroxetine, duloxetine, nortriptyline, haloperidol, metoprolol, propranolol
2E1	Ethanol, acetaminophen, chlorzoxazone, nitrosamines
3A4/5	Alprazolam, midazolam, cyclosporine, tacrolimus, nifedipine, felodipine, diltiazem, verapamil, fluconazole, ketoconazole, itraconazole, erythromycin, lovastatin, simvastatin, cisapride, terfenadine
Conjugative Enzymes	
UGT	Acetaminophen, morphine, lorazepam, oxazepam, naproxen, ketoprofen, irinotecan, bilirubin
NAT	Dapsone, hydralazine, isoniazid, procainamide
Transporters	
OATP	
1A2	Bile salts, statins, fexofenadine, methotrexate, digoxin, levofloxacin
1B1	Bile salts, statins, fexofenadine, repaglinide, valsartan, olmesartan, irinotecan, bosentan
1B3	Bile salts, statins, fexofenadine, telmisartan, valsartan, olmesartan, digoxin
2B1	Statins, fexofenadine, glyburide
Pgp	Digoxin, fexofenadine, loperamide, irinotecan, doxorubicin, vinblastine, paclitaxel, erythromycin
MRP	
2	Methotrexate, etoposide, mitoxantrone, valsartan, olmesartan
3	Methotrexate, fexofenadine

CL_{NR}, nonrenal clearance; CYP, cytochrome P450; NAT, N-acetyltransferase; MRP, multidrug resistance protein; OATP, organic anion-transporting polypeptides; UGT, uridine diphophate-glucuronlytransferase.
Data from references 9, 26, 36, and 37.

enzymes, such as CYP3A, and transporters including Pgp, organic anion-transporting polypeptides (OATPs), and multidrug resistance-associated proteins in the GI tract and hepatobiliary system.[36,37]

Alterations of CYP 450 Enzyme Activity and Transporters

There is now good basic science and emerging clinical evidence which suggests that CKD may lead to alterations in nonrenal clearance of many medications as the result of alterations in the activities of uptake and efflux transporters as well as CYP enzymes in the liver and other organs[26,27,36,38] (see Tables 48-2 and 48-3). The effect(s) of renal insufficiency on nonrenal drug clearance appear to depend on whether the reduction in renal function is acute or chronic in nature. For example, higher residual nonrenal clearance for vancomycin, meropenem, and imipenem has been documented in patients with AKI compared to CKD patients, who have comparable CL_{cr}.[39-42] In humans with renal insufficiency, the activities of CYPs appear to be relatively unaffected. It was reported that CYP3A4 activity was reduced,[26,37,38,43] but recent data indicate that OATP uptake activity is reduced and thus the perceived changes in CYP3A4 activity were likely due to altered transporter activity, not an alteration in CYP activity. The reduction of nonrenal clearance of several drugs that are metabolized by a CYP pathway as well as transported in CKD category G4 or G5 patients supports this premise (see Table 48-3). These studies must be interpreted with caution, however, because concurrent drug intake, age, smoking status, and alcohol intake were often not taken into consideration. Furthermore, pharmacogenetic variations in drug-metabolizing enzymes that may have been present in the individual before the onset of AKI or CKD must also be considered.[26,37,38] This differential effect on individual enzymes may help explain some of the conflicting reports of whether drug metabolism is altered in the presence of CKD. CYP3A activity as measured by the erythromycin breath test (EBT) is 28% lower in category G5 patients as compared with healthy controls.[44] Although baseline CYP3A activity was lower in these patients, the increase in CYP3A activity observed following enzyme induction with rifampin was similar.[44] Nolin and colleagues subsequently reported that EBT results are reduced more in those end-stage renal disease (ESRD) patients with higher blood urea nitrogen concentrations and that HD is associated with an acute improvement in the patient's metabolic activity.[43] These data suggest that CKD has a detrimental effect on this important pathway of hepatic drug metabolism in humans.

Prediction of the effect of renal insufficiency on the metabolism of a particular drug is difficult and there is no quantitative strategy to predict changes for one drug based on data from another even if they are in the same pharmacologic class. However, some qualitative insight can be gained if one knows what enzyme is involved in the metabolism of the drug of interest and how the enzyme or transporter is affected by the presence of CKD.

Accumulation of Metabolites

Category G4 and G5 CKD patients who are receiving chronic drug therapy may experience significant accumulation of metabolite(s) as well as the parent compound if their ultimate route of elimination is via glomerular filtration. Metabolites of several drugs have been reported to have significant pharmacologic and/or toxicologic activity.[45,46] However, the pharmacokinetics and pharmacodynamics of metabolites are not often fully elucidated during the drug development process. In a sense, the patient with severe CKD is being exposed to a new pharmacologic entity since the sum of the serum concentrations of the metabolite and the parent compound maybe markedly different than those reported in patients with normal renal function.

The metabolite may have pharmacologic activity similar to that of the parent drug and thus contribute significantly to clinical response; that is true, for example, of oxypurinol, the active metabolite of allopurinol. Another example is morphine; the liver rapidly metabolizes morphine, into active metabolites, morphine-3-glucuronide (M3G) and morphine-6-glucuronide (M6G) which readily cross the blood-brain barrier and bind to opiate receptors, exerting strong analgesic effects. In CKD patients, morphine is metabolized more slowly, and these active metabolites increase, making prolonged narcosis and respiratory depression more likely.[47] Alternatively, the metabolite may have qualitatively dissimilar pharmacologic action; for example, normeperidine has CNS stimulatory activity that reportedly produces seizures, whereas meperidine has CNS depressant actions.[48] Because of the multiplicity of potential interactions of compounds that are primarily metabolized, the practical consequences of metabolite accumulation are difficult to predict and are most often identified in those patients at risk serendipitously.

PHARMACOGENOMICS

Over the past two decades, genome-wide analyses have identified genetic variants that are associated with the risk of several diseases,[49,50] although most confer a very low discriminatory and predictive values.[51,52] Thus how CKD patients respond to medications is a consequence of alterations in pharmacokinetics and pharmacodynamics as well as pharmacogenomics.[50,53-58] Genotyping information is becoming more widely available than phenotyping data and this is generating demands for a more individualized approach to pharmacotherapy. Genotypic characterization now serves as the basis for dosing recommendations for some drugs,[59-61] and more than 120 US Food and Drug Administration (FDA)-approved drugs have pharmacogenomic information in their labeling, including fluoropyrimidines, codeine, Selective serotonin reuptake inhibitors (SSRIs), tricyclic antidepressants, β-blockers, opiates, neuroleptics, antiarrhythmic agents, and statins.[61] However, the promise of pharmacogenomics has not always translated into improvements in patient care.[62,63]

One example of the real-life challenges associated with application of pharmacogenomics data is the anticoagulant, warfarin. Pharmacogenetic-based dosing of warfarin was associated with a significantly higher percentage of time in therapeutic range (TTR) compared to that achieved with standard dosing during initiation of warfarin therapy (67.4% vs 60.3%).[64] However, this improvement was not considered clinically significant. Moreover, the results of the study by Kimmel et al,[65] suggested that genotype-guided dosing of warfarin did not improve anticoagulation control during the initiation of warfarin therapy as compared with initiating warfarin using a clinically predicted maintenance dose.[65] Among 1,015 patients assigned to usual care or usual care plus genotype, international normalized ratio (INR) results showed that the mean percentage of time in the therapeutic range at 4 weeks was 45.2% in the genotype-guided group and 45.4% in the usual care group.[65] Moreover, rates of the combined outcome of any INR of 4 or more, major bleeding, or thromboembolism did not differ significantly according to dosing strategy.[65] Thus, at present, there is insufficient data to warrant genomic testing in persons with CKD to guide drug therapy. Future work will focus on the use of both pharmacokinetic and pharmacogenomic testing to improve drug dosing for CKD patients.

PHARMACODYNAMICS

CKD can affect multiple organ systems and consequently the response to a given drug many change beyond that predicted upon pharmacokinetic changes alone. For example, several studies have shown that enoxaparin dosage reduction is required in category G4 and G5 CKD patients.[66,67] This appears to be due to the accumulation of uremic toxins which results in complex disturbances of the coagulation system leading to an increase in bleeding. Therefore it seems that dosage adjustment based on kidney function such as eGFR may not always lead to optimal anticoagulation outcomes in CKD patients.

Successful antibiotic or antiviral treatment of CKD patients requires not only consideration of pharmacokinetic profiles, but also the drugs' pharmacodynamics, which links measures of drug exposure (such as peak and trough serum concentrations, and AUC) to bacteriologic activity.[68] Most antibiotics demonstrate concentration-dependent or time-dependent bacterial killing. In general, for concentration-dependent antibiotics such as fluroquinolones or aminoglycosides, a high ratio of the peak serum concentration to the minimum inhibitory concentration (MIC, the minimum concentration required to inhibit bacterial growth) has been associated with increased likelihood of clinical success; whereas for time-dependent antibiotics such as cephalosporins, the percentage of the dosing interval spent above the MIC is the most important pharmacodynamic parameter to maximize clinical success. This has led to the utilization of prolonged infusions or even in some cases to continuous infusions. Thus it is necessary to administer anti-infective drugs with a time-dependent action more frequently whereas anti-infective drugs with a concentration-dependent action should be administered with a higher maintenance dose and potentially a prolonged dosage interval to increase efficacy while minimizing toxicity. Therefore both the pharmacodynamics and pharmacokinetics of drugs may need to be considered when initiating antimicrobial therapy in CKD patients. Pharmacodynamic modeling, however, doesn't accurately predict clinical success in some patient settings.[69] Thus large prospective clinical studies are needed to assure that this approach truly enhances patient outcomes.

Estimation of Kidney Function for Drug Dosage Regimen Individualization

Accurate assessment of kidney function is an essential component of determining appropriate drug dosing regimens. Because of the invasive nature and technical difficulties of directly measuring GFR in clinical settings, many equations for estimating GFR have been proposed. A detailed discussion of the pros and cons of estimating equations for GFR (Table e42-6) and creatinine clearance (Table e42-7) are presented in Chapter e42. The Cockcroft Gault (CG) equation has been the most commonly used method to estimate kidney function for drug dosing purposes for over 40 years.[70,71] The modification of diet in renal disease (MDRD) and the chronic kidney disease epidemiology collaboration equation (CKD-EPI) have been developed primarily for the identification and classification of CKD patients.[72,73]

The automated reporting of eGFR in the clinical setting has led some practitioners to consider substituting eGFR in place of eCL_{cr} for renal dose adjustments. Others argue that use of the MDRD and CKD-EPI equations for drug dosing are not appropriate given that the pharmacokinetic studies were performed using estimated creatinine clearance via the CG equation.[74,75] Furthermore, many studies have highlighted discordance between drug dosing recommendations based on these equations.[76-81] These studies have compared dosing recommendations based on the three different equations for commonly used drugs in CKD patients. Average discordance rates for the MDRD Study and CG equations were between 20% and 30%.[76-80] Another study which evaluated eight antimicrobial dosing regimens based on CKD-EPI, MDRD, and CG demonstrated overall discordance rates were 15% to 25% between CG and CKD-EPI and 7% to 12% between MDRD and CKD-EPI.[81] Major limitations with these studies include, equations were not compared to gold standard such as measured GFR and the studies did not assess drug levels or clinical outcomes. Although Stevens et al described average concordance rates for the MDRD study and CG equations to measured GFR to be 88% and 85%, respectively; this was a simulation study and they did not evaluate drug levels or patient outcomes.[82]

Serum cystatin C has also been proposed as an alternative marker to estimate GFR, either alone or in combination with serum creatinine. Multiple equations have been proposed to estimate GFR from age, gender, race, and muscle mass based on cystatin C measurements (Table 42-6)[82-86], however, their use in drug dosing is limited to a few studies with carboplatin, topotecan, and cefuroxime.[87-90]

Therefore, none of these equations for estimating GFR should be used as the sole determinant for drug dosing decision making. Potential discrepancies in kidney function estimates and corresponding drug dosing regimens necessitate careful consideration of the risk: benefit ratio of each approach within the context of the complete clinical picture of the patient. Since most drug dosage regimen recommendations are based on broad categorical ranges of kidney function, the impact of an eGFR of 40 mL/min/1.73 m^2 versus 50 mL/min/1.73 m^2 is likely of no clinical significance. Furthermore these estimating equations for GFR are based on a standard 1.73 m^2 body surface area (BSA); thus for an individual patient, the BSA must be determined separately so that the eGFR can be expressed in milliliters per minute (mL/min).[74] Nevertheless, regardless of the kidney function estimating equation that was used and published dosing recommendation guidelines that were consulted, clinical judgment will ultimately prevail in the determination of which regimen is best for the patient and feasible to administer given the available dosage forms.

Drug Dosing Information Resources

Prior to 1998, there were no official guidelines regarding when and how to conduct pharmacokinetic and pharmacodynamic studies of a new drug in patients with impaired kidney function. The 1998 FDA guidance on pharmacokinetic studies in patients with impaired kidney function recommended use of renal dosage adjustment categories derived from creatinine clearance (CL_{cr}).[91] This was based on the rationale that CL_{cr} was widely used in patient care settings as a measure of renal function, and thus more practical than most other alternatives as a criterion for adjusting drug dosage. Since then both the FDA and the European Medicine Agency (EMA) have issued updated guidance documents on the conduct of pharmacokinetic studies in patients with impaired kidney function.[92,93] The adoption of the 1998 FDA guidance has resulted in improved availability of pharmacokinetic and drug dosing recommendations for drugs which have high (greater than 30%) fraction of the drug eliminated renally unchanged.[7] It appears that there have been significant improvements over the past 15 years in the frequency and rigor with which pharmacokinetic studies have been conducted in the setting of kidney dysfunction.

The 2010 proposed revision to the 1998 FDA guidance recommended: (a) conducting studies for nonrenally as well as renally eliminated drugs, (b) conducting studies in patients receiving HD, (c) conducting studies to evaluate pharmacokinetics of therapeutic proteins in patients with renal insufficiency, (d) categorizing renal function based on eGFR (using the MDRD equation) or CL_{cr} (using the CG equation), and (e) modifications to how the results of renal impairment studies are presented in the official drug label.[93] Furthermore, several recent publications have offered suggestions to pharmaceutical industry and regulatory agencies regarding assessment of kidney function and which populations of patients should be included in the pharmacokinetic studies of new chemical entities during the drug development process.[94,95] These papers present population pharmacokinetics and physiologically based pharmacokinetic models that will assist in providing optimal dosing recommendations for new chemical entities in development in subjects with kidney dysfunction. Finally, the Kidney Disease: Improving Global Outcomes (KDIGO) held a conference to investigate these issues and propose recommendations for practitioners, researchers, and those involved in drug development and regulatory affairs. The conference generated 37 recommendations for clinical practice, 32 recommendations for future research, and 24 recommendations for regulatory agencies to enhance the quality of pharmacokinetic and pharmacodynamic information available to clinicians.[96]

Drug Dosing Regimens for CKD Patients

4 The initial or "loading" dose for CKD patients should be the same as the dose recommended for those with normal renal function unless the drug's V_D is known to be altered in the presence of CKD or a concomitant disease then the dose should be increased proportionally (see Table 48-1). Rapid achievement of therapeutic drug concentrations is important in many patient care situations and thus it is better to start therapy aggressively rather than conservatively. Maintenance dosage regimen guidelines for CKD patients in FDA- or EMA-approved product labeling should be the foundation for ongoing therapy.[96] However, if such information is not available or if there is marked variance between these two agencies' recommendations, the approach depicted in Table 48-4 for designing a dosage regimen for a patient with CKD can be used. In either case, the design of the optimal dosage regimen is dependent on the availability of an accurate characterization of the relationship between the pharmacokinetic parameters of the drug and renal function and an accurate assessment of the patient's renal function.

Most dosage adjustment guidelines have proposed the use of a fixed dose or interval for patients with broad ranges of renal function that are different from those that are the foundation of the CKD staging scheme (see Chapter 44).[9,17,28,74,97-103] Indeed, normal renal function has often been ascribed to anyone who has a CL_{cr} greater than 80 to 90 mL/min/1.73 m^2 (greater than 0.77-0.87 mL/s/m^2), even though the population normal CL_{cr} values range from 115 to 125 mL/min per 1.73 m^2 (greater than 1.11-1.20 mL/s/m^2) (see Chapter e42). The approved product labeling dosage adjustment recommendations and secondary references often use different ranges to represent mild, moderate, and severe renal insufficiency.[74] The predominant ranges for mild, moderate, and severe renal insufficiency can be defined as a CL_{cr} of 60 to 89 mL/min (1-1.48 mL/s), CL_{cr} of 30 to 59 mL/min (0.5-0.99 mL/s), and CL_{cr} of 10 to 29 mL/min (0.17-0.49 mL/s), respectively (Table 48-5). ESRD is usually

TABLE 48-4 Stepwise Approach to Adjust Drug Dosage Regimens for Patients with Renal Insufficiency

Step 1	Obtain history and relevant demographic/clinical information	Ask/obtain patient medical history including: Prescription medication Over-the-counter medication Recreational drugs Tobacco and alcohol use History of renal disease Height Weight
Step 2	Determine the degree of renal insufficiency	Measure serum creatinine and/or cystatin C Determine eGFR or CL_{cr} for drug dosing based best available methodology Order 24-hour urine collection for measured CL_{cr} if necessary
Step 3	Review the medication list	Ensure medications are all indicated Evaluate for potential drug interactions Identify drugs which need to dosage regimen adjusted
Step 4	Individualize treatment regimen for identified medications	Ascertain best initial dosage regimen from FDA- or EMA-approved product labelling For narrow therapeutic range drugs—calculate dosage regimen based on pharmacokinetic characteristics of the drug and the patient's renal function Titrate the dose of drugs to patient effect, if applicable
Step 5	Avoid nephrotoxic drugs	Discontinue or avoid prescription of nephrotoxic medications if possible
Step 6	Monitor	Monitor drug serum concentrations (if available) to guide further therapy Monitor parameters of drug response and toxicity Monitor renal function every 3-5 days for acute therapies and monthly or quarterly for chronic medications
Step 7	Reassess	Reassess the patient to evaluate drug efficacy and safety Revise regimen based on drug response or change in patient condition (including renal function)

CL_{cr}, creatinine clearance; eGFR, estimated glomerular filtration rate; EMA, European Medicine Agency; FDA, Food and Drug Administration.

defined as a CL_{cr} of less than 10 mL/min (0.17 mL/s). Each of these categories encompasses a broad range in renal function, and thus the recommended drug regimen may not be optimal for all patients whose renal function lies within the given category of renal function.

5 FDA-approved drug labels, and commonly used drug information sources such as American Hospital Formulary Service Drug Information,[97] Goodman and Gilman's the Pharmacological Basis of Therapeutics,[17,103] the British National Formulary,[98] and Drug Prescribing in Renal Failure,[99] are excellent sources of information about a drugs' pharmacokinetic characteristics. In some cases, however, they yield marked variation in recommendations and the paucity of details of the methods used to generate the dosing advice have

TABLE 48-5 GFR Categories Based on KDIGO Classification

GFR Category[a]	GFR (mL/min/1.73 m²) [mL/s/m²])	Terms
1	>90 (>0.87)	Normal or high
2	60-89 (0.58-0.86)	Mildly decreased
3a	45-59 (0.43-0.57)	Mildly to moderately decreased
3b	30-44 (0.29-0.42)	Moderately to severely decreased
4	15-29 (0.14-0.28)	Severely decreased
5	<15 (<0.14)	Kidney failure

GFR, glomerular filtration rate; KDIGO, Kidney Disease: Improving Global Outcomes.
[a]To meet criteria for CKD there must be a significant reduction in GFR (categories 3a-5) or there must also be evidence of kidney damage (categories 1 & 2) for 3 months or greater. Adapted from reference 96.

resulted in some clinicians cautioning against their routine clinical use[104,105] (Table 48-6). In addition, none of these sources consistently provide the explicit relationships of the kinetic parameters of interest (total body clearance [CL], elimination rate constant [k], and V_D) with a continuous index of renal function, such as eCL_{cr} or eGFR. To find this information, one may need to identify the original research study that assessed the drug's disposition or a comprehensive review article on the class of drugs of interest. This is a time-consuming process that may be difficult to carry out for each drug and patient combination in real time.

Dr. Luzius Dettli is often credited for being the first to systematically approach the issue of drug dosing for those with impaired kidney function.[106] The "Dettli Method" is a graphic means to generate drug dosing recommendations based on the linear relationship between the elimination rate constant of a given renally cleared drug and a patient's creatinine clearance:

$$k = k_{NR} + (\alpha \times CL_{cr})$$

where k is the elimination rate constant of the drug based on a first-order one compartment model, k_{NR} is the nonrenal elimination rate constant, and α is a constant relating the renal drug elimination rate constant to the patient's creatinine clearance (CL_{cr}). This approach assumes that the overall elimination rate constant (or clearance) declines linearly with CL_{cr}, and that the nonrenal elimination rate constant (or CL_{NR}) remains constant as kidney function declines. While the first assumption generally holds true for drugs that are mainly renally cleared, the second assumption is flawed, as the functional expression of many drug metabolizing enzymes and drug transporters is reduced in patients with kidney disease.[36,37]

Ideally, one should be able to identify a relationship between CL or k with an estimated GFR or CL_{cr}, such as those depicted in Table 48-7. This information, along with the patient's estimated CL_{cr} or GFR, is the foundation upon which one can formulate a therapeutic regimen to attain the desired drug concentration time profile and ultimately the therapeutic outcome when approved product labeling information is not available.

If specific literature recommendations and/or the relationship of kinetic parameters to estimated GFR or CL_{cr} are not available, then one can estimate the CL or k of the CKD patient with the method of Rowland and Tozer,[8] provided the fraction of the drug that is eliminated renally unchanged (f_e) in subjects with normal renal function is known.[107] This approach assumes that the change in CL and k are proportional to ${}_{e}CL_{cr}$, that the renal disease does not alter the drug's metabolism, that the metabolites, if formed, are inactive and nontoxic, that the drug obeys first-order (linear) kinetic principles, and that it is adequately described by a one-compartment model.

TABLE 48-6 Comparison of Secondary References Used for Drug Dosing in CKD

Resource	Pros	Cons
Aronoff's Drug Prescribing in Renal Failure[99]	- Exclusive focus on drug dosing in renal dysfunction - Information provided for IHD, PD, CRRT - Tables include drug PK and dosage adjustment based on CrCl (>50, 10-50, <10 mL/min [>0.83, 0.17-0.83, <0.17 mL/s]) - Tables for both adult and pediatric dosing provided - Concise, easy to use - References to primary literature provided	- Hard copy only - Updated every few years; information may not be most current, newer drugs may not be included - Some dosage recommendations are not feasible for dialysis patients (ie, q 36 hours dosing interval)
The Renal Drug Handbook[100]	- Contains information on clinical use of drugs, drug PK, dose in normal renal function, dose adjustment in CKD, drug interactions and administration - Specific to CKD patients	- Updated every few years information may not be most current, newer drugs may not be included - References not provided
Lexicomp[101]	- Easy to access with a subscription - Accessible via mobile device - Easy to navigate - Concise information - Dose adjustment in CKD provided (HD and PD)	- Difficult to navigate at first - No specific focus on CKD patients - References to primary literature for dosing not provided
Micromedex[102]	- Easy to access with a subscription - Accessible via mobile device - Comprehensive, detailed information (both "in-depth" and "quick") - Dose adjustment in CKD provided (both HD and PD)	- Difficult to navigate - Can be slow - No specific focus on CKD patients - References to primary literature for dosing not provided
American Hospital Formulary Service (AHFS)[97]	- Detailed drug monographs - "Dosage in Renal and Hepatic Impairment/Special Populations" section for each drug listed - Available online with a subscription - Online version updated regularly, print version updated yearly	- Hard copy version can be difficult to navigate, cumbersome - Information on dose adjustment in CKD is minimal - No specific focus on CKD patients - References to primary literature for dosing not provided

CKD, chronic kidney disease; CrCl, creatinine clearance; CRRT, continuous renal replacement therapy; HD, hemodialysis; IHD, intermittent hemodialysis; PD, peritoneal dialysis; PK, pharmacokinetics.

Data from references 97, 99, 100 to 105.

If these assumptions are true, which is rarely the case, then the kinetic parameter/dosage-adjustment factor (Q) can be calculated as:

$$Q = 1 - [f_e\,(1 - \text{KF})]$$

where KF is the ratio of the patient's eCL_{cr} or eGFR to the assumed normal value of 120 mL/min (equivalent to 2 mL/s). Thus for a drug that is 85% eliminated renally unchanged in a patient who has an eCL_{cr} of 10 mL/min (0.17 mL/s), the Q factor would be:

$$\begin{aligned} Q &= 1 - [0.85[1 - (10/120)]] \\ &= 1 - [0.85(0.85(0.92)] \\ &= 1 - 0.78 \\ &= 0.22 \end{aligned}$$

TABLE 48-7 Relationship Between CL_{cr} and CL of Selected Drugs

Drug	Total Body Clearance[a]
Acyclovir	CL = 3.37 (CL_{cr}) + 0.41
Amikacin	CL = 0.6 (CL_{cr}) + 9.6
Aztreonam	CL = 0.8 (CL_{cr}) + 26.6
Cefazolin	CL = 0.34 (CL_{cr}) + 6.6
Ceftazidime	CL = 1.15 (CL_{cr}) + 10.6
Ciprofloxacin	CL = 2.83 (CL_{cr}) + 363
Digoxin	CL = 0.88 (CL_{cr}) + 23
Ganciclovir	CL = 1.24 (CL_{cr}) + 8.57
Gentamicin	CL = 0.983 (CL_{cr})
Imipenem	CL = 1.42 (CL_{cr}) + 54
Lithium	CL = 0.20 (CL_{cr})
Ofloxacin	CL = 1.04 (CL_{cr}) + 38.7
Piperacillin	CL = 1.36 (CL_{cr}) + 1.50
Tobramycin	CL = 0.801 (CL_{cr})
Vancomycin	CL = 0.69 (CL_{cr}) + 3.7

CL, total body clearance; CL_{cr}, creatinine clearance.

[a]Clearance in mL/min can be converted to mL/s through multiplication by 0.0167.

The best method for dosage regimen adjustment must then be selected. Specifically, one must determine whether the desired goal is the maintenance of a similar peak, trough, or average steady-state drug concentration or if there is a clearly defined pharmacodynamic endpoint such as the time above the MIC (eg, cephalosporins) or the ratio of the AUC relative to the MIC (eg, fluoroquinolones).[108] If there is a significant relationship between peak concentration and clinical response (eg, aminoglycosides)[109] or toxicity[107] (eg, phenobarbital and phenytoin), then attainment of the specific target values is critical. If, however, no specific target values for peak or trough concentrations have been reported (eg, antihypertensive agents and benzodiazepines), then a regimen goal of attaining the same average steady-state concentration is likely to be appropriate.

The principal choices to attain the desired average steady-state concentration profile are to decrease the dose or prolong the dosing interval. If the size of the dose is reduced while the dosing interval remains unchanged, the desired average steady-state concentration will be similar; however, the peak will be lower and the trough higher (Fig. 48-1). Alternatively, if the dosing interval is increased and the dose size remains unchanged, the peak and trough concentrations in the patient with reduced renal function will be similar to those in the patient with normal renal function. This dosage adjustment method is often recommended because it is likely to yield cost savings as a result of a reduction in nursing and pharmacy time, as well as a reduction in the supplies associated with frequent drug administration. Finally, the dose and dosing interval may both need to be changed to allow the administration of a clinically feasible dose (500 mg vs a calculated value of 487 mg) or a practical dosing interval, for example, 12 hours instead of 17 hours.

If the relationship between the pharmacokinetic parameters of the drug and renal function are known, the first step in the process is to estimate the drug disposition parameters in the patient with renal insufficiency. The dosage-adjustment factor (Q) calculated as the ratio of the estimated k or CL of the patient relative to subjects with normal renal function is then used to determine the dose or dosing interval alterations necessary for the patient.

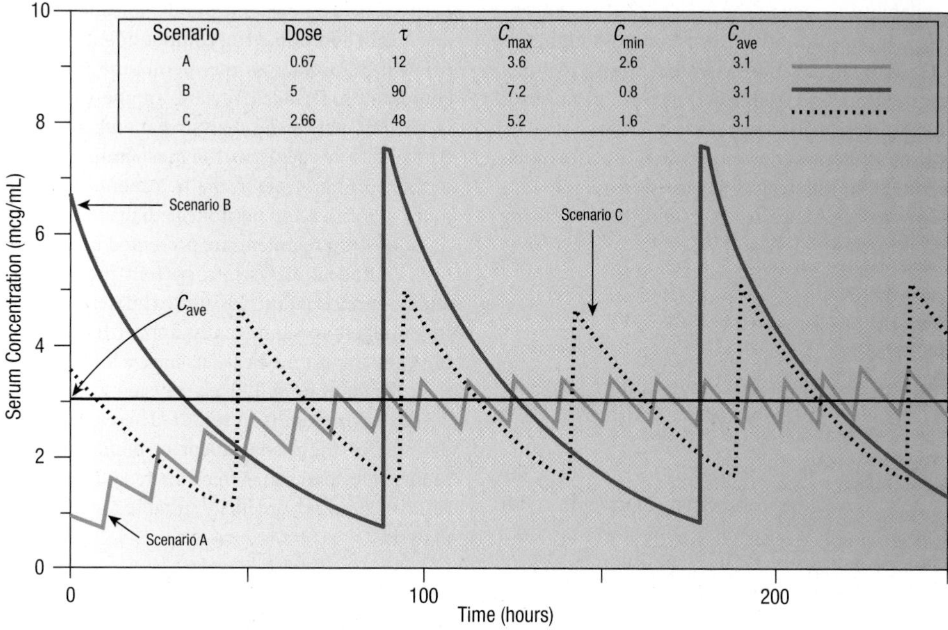

FIGURE 48-1 Although the average steady-state concentrations (C_{ave}) are identical regardless of which dosage-adjustment strategy one decides to implement, the concentration–time profile will be markedly different if one changes the dose and maintains the dosing interval (τ) constant (*Scenario A*), versus changing the dosing interval and maintaining the dose constant (*Scenario B*) or changing both (*Scenario C*).

First, the relationship between drug clearance and CL_{cr} (expressed in conventional units of mL/min) is required; these relationship equations have been reported for several drugs (Table 48-7). How one can apply the relationship between a patient's renal function and pharmacokinetic characteristics of ciprofloxacin, a commonly used antibiotic for the treatment of infections in CKD and dialysis patients to develop and individualized dosage recommendation are illustrated in Table 48-8 and briefly highlighted here. The first step is to calculate the CL of ciprofloxacin for a subject with normal renal function (CL_{norm}) and CL for the patient with CKD (CL_{CKD}) to obtain the ratio of the predicted clearance values (Q) which can be used to calculate the new dosing regimen.

It is also important to consider other characteristics of antibiotics, such as the most relevant MICs and concentrations associated with toxicities and adverse events, before modifying a dosage regimen.[110] Ciprofloxacin, a concentration-dependent antibiotic has an associated concentration-dependent post antibiotic effect, in which bactericidal action continues for a period of time after the antibiotic concentration falls below the MIC. The peak concentration and AUC determine efficacy of these antibiotics. Therefore extending the interval but keeping the same dose allows for this pharmacodynamic action. Furthermore, extending the interval without increasing the dose will achieve high concentrations of ciprofloxacin without an accumulation of drug that could cause dose-dependent toxicities such as seizures.[110]

If the V_D of a drug is significantly altered in CKD patients or if one desires to attain a specific maximum or minimum concentration, the estimation of a dosage regimen becomes more complex. If the relationship between V_D and CL_{cr} has been characterized, then V_D may be estimated. If one assumes that a one-compartment linear model can describe the drug, the predicted V_D may then be used with the predicted k of the drug to yield an adjusted-dosing interval and IV dose.

For orally administered drugs, the τ_f can be calculated and the dose can be approximated from the following equations as:

$$\tau_f = [(-1/k_f)[\ln(C_{min}/C_{max})]] + t_{peak}$$

$$\text{Dose } p_o = [F\, C_p^{\tau}\, V_D\, (ka - k)] \,/\, [ka\, (e^{-kt}/1 - e^{-k\tau})(e^{-kat}/1 - e^{-ka\tau})]$$

TABLE 48-8 Stepwise Approach to Calculating a Dosage Regimen Based on Drug's Pharmacokinetic Characteristics and Patient's Renal Function

	Steps	Calculation Examples with Ciprofloxacin
Step 1	Calculate total body clearance of drug in a subject with normal renal function (CL_{norm}); CL_{cr} = 120 mL/min	CL_{norm} = [2.83 (CL_{cr})] + 363 CL_{norm} = [2.83(120)] + 363 CL_{norm} = 702.6 mL/min per 1.73 m²
Step 2	Calculate total body clearance of drug in a subject with renal insufficiency (CL_{fail})	In patient with CL_{cr} = 15 mL/min CL_{fail} = [2.83(CL_{cr})] + 363 CL_{fail} = [2.83(15)] + 363 CL_{fail} = 405.5 mL/min per 1.73 m²
Step 3	Calculate the quotient (Q) for a subject with renal insufficiency	$Q = CL_{fail}/CL_{norm}$ Q = 702.6/405.5 Q = 0.58
Step 4	Calculate the maintenance dose (D_f) or adjusted dosing interval (τ_f) in a subject with renal insufficiency; D_n = normal dose; τ_n = normal dosing interval	D_n = 500 mg; τ_n = 12 h $D_f = D_n \times Q$ D_f = 500 mg × 0.58 D_f = 290 mg $\tau_f = \tau_n/Q$ τ_f = 12/0.58 τ_f = 20.7 h
Step 5	Choose dosing adjustment: 1. Maintain D_n and use τ_f 2. Maintain τ_n and use D_f	Dosing adjustments: 1. 500 mg every 21 h 2. 290 mg every 12 h
Step 6	Calculate D_f based on practical dosing interval (τ_p), which is selected	D_n = 500 mg; τ_f = 21 h; τ = 24 h (selected to limit missed doses) $D_f = (D_n \times Q \times \tau_p)/\tau_n$ D_f = (500 mg × 0.58 × 24)/12 D_f = 580 mg
Step 7	Recommend dosing regimen (dependent on product availability and limited risk of missed doses)	500 mg every 24 h

CL_{cr}, creatinine clearance.

Creatinine clearance in mL/min can be converted to mL/s through multiplication by 0.0167. Clearance in mL/min per 1.73 m² can be converted to mL/s/m² through multiplication by 0.00963.

where F equals bioavailability, C'_p equals the desired plasma concentration at time t, and k_a is the absorption rate constant. Although, this approach allows for the individualization of an oral dosage regimen for attainment of specific peak and trough serum concentrations it is rarely used in clinical practice. This is in part due to the paucity of data on the absorption rate constant of individual drug formulations. Thus many assume that the drug is absorbed extremely rapidly, in which case one can approximate the τ_f and the dose using equations originally proposed for IV dosing as:

$$\tau_f = (-1/k_f)[\ln (C_{min}/C_{max})]$$

$$\text{Dose } p_o = V_D \times (C_{max} - C_{min})$$

These principles have been used by several investigators to derive dosage recommendations for many commonly used drugs for CKD patients (Tables 48-9 and 48-10).[99-102,111-114]

It should be noted, however, that in most dosing guidelines, the "usual" dose or dose for "normal renal function" represents eGFR greater than 50 mL/min/1.73 m^2. This assumption, however, could lead to dosing errors for patients with eGFRs of 60 mL/min/1.73 m^2 versus 90 mL/min/1.73 m^2 versus 130 mL/min/1.73 m^2. In fact, augmented renal clearance (ARC) defined as CL_{cr} greater than 130 mL/min/1.73 m^2 has been associated with subtherapeutic antibiotic concentrations and patient outcomes when standard doses of antibiotics were administered.[115-117] Although more research has been performed in the past 10 years in the critically ill, clinicians need to be aware of the potential to under dose these patients because of their augmented renal function and thus need to consider the use of higher doses especially for antibiotics and antivirals.

DRUG DOSAGE REGIMEN DESIGN FOR PATIENTS RECEIVING RENAL REPLACEMENT THERAPY

Continuous renal replacement therapies are used for the management of fluid overload and the removal of uremic toxins in patients with AKI and other conditions. Several forms of continuous renal replacement therapy in clinical use today are extensively described in Chapter 43 and several dosage regimen individualization approaches are also presented in that chapter. Which of these therapies will be optimal for a given patient is dependent on several factors, including bleeding risk, degree of hypercatabolism, acid–base balance, and experience of the healthcare provider team. The rationale and approaches for delivery of renal replacement therapy for those with ESRD are described in Chapter 45.

This next section will describe drug dosing regimens for patients on peritoneal dialysis and HD, including short-daily hemodialysis (SDHD) and nocturnal hemodialysis (NHD).

Peritoneal Dialysis

Peritoneal dialysis, like other dialysis modalities, has the potential to affect drug disposition; however, drug therapy individualization is often less complicated in these patients as a result of the limited drug clearances achieved with the variants of this procedure (see Chapter 45). In general, HD is more effective in removing drugs than peritoneal dialysis such that if a drug is not removed by HD, it is unlikely to be significantly removed by peritoneal dialysis. Many of the factors that are important in determining drug dialyzability for other treatment modalities pertain to peritoneal dialysis as well.[118,119] Factors that influence drug dialyzability by peritoneal dialysis include drug-specific characteristics such as molecular weight, solubility, degree of ionization, protein binding, and V_D. The intrinsic properties of the peritoneal membrane that affect drug removal include blood flow and peritoneal membrane surface area, which is approximately equal to the body surface area. There is an inverse relationship between peritoneal drug clearance and molecular weight, protein binding, and V_D. In addition, drug compounds that are ionized at physiologic pH will diffuse across the membrane more slowly than unionized compounds. Detailed reviews of the disposition of several drugs in chronic peritoneal dialysis patients are reported elsewhere.[120,121] Anti-infective agents are the most commonly studied drugs because of their primary role in the treatment of peritonitis.[120,122] The treatment priorities for peritoneal dialysis peritonitis and the recommended drug regimens are presented in detail in Chapter 45.

Peritoneal dialysis, in current practice, is often prescribed to attain a urea clearance of approximately 10 mL/min (0.17 mL/s), so it is unlikely to significantly impact the CL of any drug.[96] In addition, since most medications have a larger molecular size than urea, their resultant CL will likely be even lower: probably between 5 and 7.5 mL/min (0.08-0.13 mL/s). Therefore, drug dosing recommendations for the management of conditions other than peritonitis, reported for patients with estimated CL_{cr} or GFR of 10 to 15 mL/min (0.17-0.25 mL/s), are likely suitable for patients receiving peritoneal dialysis.[99]

Hemodialysis

Although many hemodialyzers have been introduced in the past 20 years and more than 100 different ones were available in North America in 2015, the effect of HD on drug disposition is rarely reevaluated after it is initially reported. Thus, most of the literature, especially for older medications, probably represents an underestimation of the impact of HD on a drug's disposition.[123]

6 The impact of HD on a patient's drug therapy is dependent on several factors, including the physicochemical characteristics of the drug, the dialysis conditions, and the clinical situation for which dialysis is performed. Drug-related factors that affect dialyzability include the molecular weight or size, degree of protein binding, and V_D.[6] The vast majority of dialysis filters in use in North America up until the mid-1990s were composed of cellulose, cellulose acetate, or regenerated cellulose (cuprophane), and they were generally impermeable to drugs with a molecular weight greater than 1,000 Da.[123] Dialysis membranes in the 21st century are predominantly composed of semisynthetic or synthetic materials (eg, polysulfone, polymethylmethacrylate, or polyacrylonitrile). These high-flux dialysis membranes have larger pore sizes and more closely mimic the filtration characteristics of the human kidney. This allows the passage of most solutes, including drugs (eg, vancomycin) that have a molecular weight of 20,000 Da or less.[123,124] Therefore drugs such as vancomycin (1,450 Da) will be more easily removed with high flux dialyzers. An increase in removal has also been reported with several other drugs that have lower molecular weights such as ceftzadine.[123] Some drugs that are cleared in high-flux dialysis but not through conventional dialysis include: carbamazepine, cisplatin, enoxaparin, ranitidine, valproic acid, sorafenib, and tramadol.[96] Therefore, it is likely that many dosing recommendations for HD patients made prior to this change underestimate the impact of HD on drug removal. If this is the case some have suggested that the dosage of many of these older drugs may need to be increased by as much as 25% to 50% due to enhanced dialytic clearance.[96] Therefore therapeutic drug monitoring for drugs such as aminoglycosides and vancomycin should be performed to ensure adequate dosing for patients on HD.

Drugs that are small but highly protein bound (ie, greater than 90%) are not well dialyzed because both of the principal binding proteins, α_1-acid glycoprotein and albumin, have a very high molecular weight. For example, the molecular weight of albumin is 60,000 Da; thus a drug such as apixaban which is 90% bound to plasma proteins would not be removed by HD. Finally, those drugs that are widely distributed, with V_D greater than 2 L/kg such as ciprofloxacin, are poorly removed by HD.

TABLE 48-9 Drug Dosing Guidelines for Nonantibiotics Commonly Used by CKD Patients

Drug	Regimen for Normal Renal Function	Glomerular Filtration Rate (mL/min)[a] 30-50	10-30	<10	IHD Dosing
Amlodipine	5 mg daily	No Adjustment Necessary			
Apixaban	Indication dependent; 2.5-10 mg BID	50-25 mL/min: 100%	<25 mL/min: Not Recommended	Not Recommended	5 mg BID 2.5 mg BID if age > 79 years or body weight <61 kg[3]
Aripiprazole	2-5 mg daily	No Adjustment Necessary			
Atenolol	50-100 mg daily	100%	50 mg q 24 h	25 mg q 24 h	25-50 mg three times weekly
Atorvastatin	10 mg daily	No Adjustment Necessary			
Bumetanide	0.5-2 mg q 8-12 h	No Adjustment Necessary			
Canagliflozin	100-300 mg daily	Not Recommended	Avoid[1]	Avoid[1]	Avoid[1]
Dabigatran	Indication dependent; Starting Dose: 75-110 mg MD: 150-220 mg daily	50-15 mL/min: 75 mg BID	Not Recommended	Not Recommended	Not Recommended
Digoxin	Indication: dependent; LD: 1-1.5 mg MD: 0.125-0.5 mg q 24 h	LD: 100%, MD: 25%-50% q 24 h	LD: 100%, MD: 25%-75% q 24 h	LD: 50%, MD: 10%-25% q 48 h	LD: 50%, MD: 10%-25% q 48 h
Diltiazem	30 mg q 6-8 h (oral regular)	No Adjustment Necessary			
Duloxetine	30-60 mg daily	100%	Avoid	Avoid	Avoid
Esomeprazole	20-40 mg daily	No Adjustment Necessary			
Exenatide (immediate release)	5-10 mcg q 12 h	100%[b]	Avoid	Avoid	Avoid
Famotidine	20-40 mg daily	50% daily	50% daily	25%-50% daily	25%-50% daily or 20-40 mg q 48-72 h
Furosemide	Individualize	No Adjustment Necessary			
Gabapentin	300-600 mg q 8 h	200-700 mg q 12 h	200-700 mg q 24	100-300 mg q 24	LD: 300 mg, MD: 100-300 mg q 24 Post-HD: 100-300 mg
Glipizide	5-10 mg daily	50%	50%	50%	50%
Glyburide	2.5-5 mg daily	Use with caution	Use with caution	Use with caution	Not recommended
Hydralazine (oral)	25-50 mg q 6 h	q 8 h	q 8 h	q 8-12 h	q 8-12 h
Hydrochlorothiazide	25-50 mg daily	100%	100%	Avoid[c]	Avoid[c]
Insulin	Variable	75%	75%	50%	50%
Lansoprazole	15-60 mg daily	No Adjustment Necessary			
Linagliptin	5 mg daily	No Adjustment Necessary			
Lisinopril	10 mg daily	50%-75%	50%	25%	25%
Metformin	0.5-1 g q 12 h	25%-50%	25%	Avoid	Avoid
Metoprolol	25-200 mg q 12 h	No Adjustment Necessary			
Olmesartan	20-40 mg daily	No Adjustment Necessary			
Pantoprazole (oral)	40 mg q 12 h	No Adjustment Necessary			
Pravastatin	10-40 mg daily	100%	10 mg q 24 h	10 mg q 24	10 mg q 24
Pregabalin	300 mg/day	50%	25%	10%-25%	10%-25% Post-HD: 50-75 mg
Ramipril	2.5-10 mg daily	50%	50%	25%	25%
Ranitidine	150-300 mg daily (oral)	150 mg q 24 h	150 mg q 24 h	75 mg q 24 h	75 mg q 24 h
Rivaroxaban	Treatment dependent; 10-20 mg daily	15-50 mL/min: 15 mg daily	<15 mL/min: Avoid	Avoid	Avoid
Rosuvastatin	5-40 mg daily	100%	5–10 mg daily[d]	5-10 mg daily[d]	5-10 mg daily[d]
Simvastatin	10-40 mg daily	100%	100%	5 mg q 24 h	5 mg q 24
Sitagliptin	100 mg daily	50%	25%	25%	25%
Spironolactone	50-100 mg/daily	Usual dose, q 12-24 h	Usual dose, q 12-24 h	Not Recommended	Not Recommended
Venlafaxine	75 mg daily	25%-50%	25%-50%	25%-50%	50%
Zopiclone	5-7.5 mg daily	3.75-5 mg daily	3.75-5 mg daily	3.75-5 mg daily	3.75-5 mg daily

IHD, intermittent hemodialysis; LD, loading dose; MD, maintenance dosing.

% = percentage of usual dose.

[a]The range following glomerular filtration rate (GFR) indicates the use of the dose that corresponds to that range of GFR in patients not on dialysis. GFR in mL/min can be converted to mL/s through multiplication by 0.0167.

[b]Caution should be used when initiating or escalating dose.

[c]Should not be used with CL_{cr} <30 mL/min (<0.5 mL/s), but are effective with loop diuretics.

[d]Initial dose should be 5 mg daily and titrate as needed to a maximum dose of 10 mg daily.

Data from references 9, 26, 97, 99, 100 to 102.

TABLE 48-10 Antibiotic and Antifungal Drug Dosing Recommendations

Drug	Regimen for Normal Renal Function	Glomerular Filtration Rate (mL/min)[a] 30-50	10-30	<10	IHD Dosing
Amoxicillin	0.5-1.0 g q 8	q 8-12 h	q 12 h	q 24 h	0.25-0.5 g q 24 h
Amoxicillin/clavulanate	500/125 mg q 8 h	q 8-12 h	q 12 h[b]	q 12 h[b]	q 12-24 h[b]
Ampicillin	1-2 g q 6 h	q 6-12	q 6-12	q 12-24	1 g q 12 h
Ampicillin/sulbactam	1.5-3 g q 6-8 h	q 8 h	q 12 h	q 12-24 h	q 12-24 h
Azithromycin	250-500 mg q 24 h	100%	100%	100%	100%
Caspofungin	50-70 mg IV q 24 h	100%	100%	100%	100%
Cefazolin	1-2 g q 8 h	q 8-12 h	0.5-1 g q 12 h	0.5-1 g q 24 h	15-20 mg/kg q 48-72
Cefepime	2 g q 8-12 h	q 12-24 h	1-2 g q 24 h	0.5-1 g q 24 h	1-2 g q 48-72 h
Ceftriaxone	1 g q 24 h	100%	100%	100%	100%
Ceftazidime	1-2 g q 8-12h	q 12-24 h	q 12-24 h	q 24-48 h	1 g after dialysis
Cefuroxime	750 mg-1.5 g q 6-8 h	q 8 h	q 8-12 h	q 12-24 h	Dose after dialysis
Cephalexin	250-1,000 mg q 6 h	500 mg q 8–12 h	500 mg q 8–12 h	250-500 mg q 12-24 h	250 mg q 12-24 h
Ciprofloxacin	400 mg q 8-12 h (IV)	q 8-12 h	q 24 h	q 24 h	200-400 q 24
	500-750 mg q 12 h (oral)	50%-75%	50%-75%	50%	50%
Clarithromycin	250-500 mg q 12 h	100%	100%	100%	No data on supplemental dosing. Dose after dialysis.
Clindamycin	150-450 mg q 6 h	100%	100%	100%	No supplement for dialysis
Doripenem	500 mg q 8 h	250 mg q 8 h	250 mg q 12 h	250 mg q 12 h	250 mg q 24 h[c]
Ertapenem	1 g q 24 h	100%	50%	50%	50%
Fidaxomicin	200 mg po bid	100%	100%	100%	No dose adjustment in IHD
Imipenem	0.5 g q 6 h	0.5 g q 8 h	0.5 g q 12 h	0.25 g q 12 h	0.25-0.5 g q 12 h
Itraconazole	100-400 mg q 24 h	Limited data. Consider dose adjustment.	Limited data. Consider dose adjustment.	Limited data. Consider dose adjustment.	Limited data; not removed by dialysis
Levofloxacin	500-750 mg q 24 h	50%	50%	25%-50%	25%-50%
		q 24 h	q 24-48 h	q 48 h	q 48-72 h
Linezolid	600 mg q 12 h	100%	100%	100%	No adjustment in IHD
Meropenem	1 g q 8 h	1 g q 12 h	0.5-1 g q 12 h	0.5 g q 24 h	1 g q 48-72 h
Metronidazole	250-500 mg q 8-12 h	100%	100%	100%	Dose after dialysis
Moxifloxacin	400 mg q 24 h	100%	100%	100%	100%
Penicillin G	1-4 million U q 4-6 h	75%	75%	25%-50%	LD: usual dose MD: 25%-50% q 4-6 h or 50%-100% q 8-12 h
Piperacillin/tazobactam[d]	3.375-4.5 g q 6 h	2.25-3.375 g q 6 h	2.25-3.375 g q 8-12 h	2.25 g q 8-12	125 g q 8-12 h
Tobramycin[e]	5-7 mg/kg q 24 h	5-7 mg/kg q 36-48 h	IND	IND	1.5-2 mg/kg q 48-72 h and then IND
Trimethoprim/ sulfamethoxazole[f]	2.5-5 mg/kg q 6-12 h	q 6-12 h	q 12-24 h	q 24 h	2.5-10 mg/kg/day or 5-20 mg/kg three times weekly
Vancomycin[e,g]	15-20 mg/kg q 8-12 h	q 24 h	IND	IND	LD: 15-25 mg/kg MD: 5-10 mg/kg (after IHD)
Voriconazole[h]	Weight <40 kg: 100 mg PO q 12 h Weight >40 kg: 200 mg PO q 12 h	100%	100%	100%	100%

IND, individualize based on concentration monitoring; IHD, intermittent hemodialysis; LD, loading dose; MD, maintenance dosing; MU, million units; NC, no change.

[a]The range following glomerular filtration rate (GFR) indicates the use of the dose that corresponds to that range of GFR in patients not on dialysis. GFR in mL/min can be converted to mL/s through multiplication by 0.0167.

[b]Extended release and 875 mg tablets are not recommended.

[c]For infection caused by *Pseudomonas aeruginosa*, should be dosed 500 mg IV q 12 h on day 1, then 500 mg IV q 24 h.

[d]First dosage modification should be made at a GFR of ≤40 mL/min (≤0.67 mL/s). Second dosage modification should be made at a GFR of <20 mL/min (<0.33 mL/s).

[e]Dosing in critically ill patients should be individualized based on pharmacokinetic monitoring.

[f]Dosed based on trimethoprim component.

[g]A vancomycin loading dose of 25-30 mg/kg (based on actual body weight) should be considered for all patients. In patients with a GFR ≤ 30 mL/min (≤0.5 mL/s), subsequent doses of 15 to 20 mg/kg should be given when the serum concentration falls below 10 mg/L or 20 mg/L (6.9 or 14 μmol/L) (depending on the site of infection and MIC of organism).

[h]Intravenous formulation of voriconazole not recommended, as the vehicle it is prepared in can be nephrotoxic.

Data from references 9,97,99,100 to 102,107,108,114,120 to 123.

The HD procedure, be it acute for the management of AKI, intermittent three times a week or daily for an extended period or some combination thereof for the management of category G5 CKD patients can dramatically affect the total body clearance of a medication.[123] The primary factors that vary between patients are the composition of the dialysis filter, the filter surface area, the blood, dialysate and ultrafiltration flow rates, and whether or not the dialysis unit reuses the dialysis filter.

Overall, the impact of HD on drug therapy is highly variable and thus one cannot assume that a certain percentage of a drug is removed with each dialysis session; neither should a "yes" or "no" answer regarding the dialyzability of a drug be considered sufficient information to make therapeutic decisions, since this provides no quantification of the impact of HD. Characteristics of the dialysis procedure that was utilized in the drug study, such as membrane composition and surface area and blood and dialysis flow rates, are thus critical data that should be known before one uses the published HD clearance data to prospectively design a drug dosing regimen for a HD patient.

If drug concentrations can be measured in the clinical setting the quantitative impact of HD on drug disposition can be calculated in one of several ways.[6] The most commonly utilized means for assessing the effect of HD is to calculate the dialyzer clearance (CL_D) of the drug. The CL^p_D from blood can be calculated as $CL^p_D = Q_p [(A_p - V_p)/A_p]$, where Q_b is the blood flow through the dialyzer and Q_p is the plasma flow, which equals Q_b (1 − hematocrit) and, A_p is the plasma concentration of drug entering the dialyzer, and V_p is the plasma concentration of the drug leaving the dialyzer. This clearance calculation most accurately reflects dialysis drug clearance as most drugs do not significantly penetrate red blood cells or bind to formed blood elements. However, for drugs that readily partition into and out of erythrocytes, this equation would likely underestimate HD clearance. Furthermore, one must keep in mind that venous plasma concentrations may be artificially high and CL^p_D will be low if plasma water is removed from the blood at a faster rate than the drug. This tends to occur when extensive ultrafiltration is performed simultaneously with diffusion during dialysis.[96]

The following principles may be used to generate a drug dosage regimen recommendation for HD patients, if none is available in FDA or EMA product labeling, by using a value of CL_D that is reported in the literature.[6,17,123] Because clearance terms are additive, the total clearance during dialysis can be calculated as the sum of the patient's residual renal and nonrenal clearance during the interdialytic period (CL_{RES}) and dialyzer clearance (CL_D):

$$CL_T = CL_{RES} + CL_D$$

The half-life during the period between dialysis treatments and during dialysis can then be calculated from the following relationships using an estimate of the drug's V_D, which can be obtained from the literature:[6,107]

$$t_{1/2,\text{off HD}} = 0.693(V_D/CL_{RES})$$

$$t_{1/2,\text{on HD}} = 0.693(V_D/CL_{RES} + CL_D)$$

Once the key pharmacokinetic parameters have been estimated/calculated, they may be used to simulate the plasma concentration–time profile of the drug for the individual patient and then one can ascertain how much drug to administer and when. This approach to drug therapy individualization can be accomplished in a stepwise fashion assuming first-order elimination of the drug and a one-compartment model.

CLINICAL CASE EXAMPLE Dosage Regimen Calculation for a Hemodialysis patient

A 54-year-old critically ill woman with ESRD was transferred to a medical intensive care unit from the general medical unit, where she was febrile with a temperature of 39°C (102.2°F). Her weight was 64 kg (141 lb) and her height was 65 in (165 cm). She had a residual CL_{cr} of 5 mL/min (0.083 mL/s), and was receiving high-flux dialysis (F80 polysulfone dialyzer) for 4 hours on Mondays, Wednesdays, and Fridays. She was started on vancomycin for a methicillin-resistant *Staphylococcus aureus* (MRSA) catheter-associated bacteremia and her first dose of 1,000 mg was administered at the end of her HD treatment. The first step is to estimate this patient's pharmacokinetic parameters of vancomycin on the basis of published population data.[125] The V_D in this patient can be estimated to be 54.4 L (0.85 L/kg × 64 kg), and her residual total body clearance (CL_{RES}) estimated from the relationship between CL and CL_{cr} [$CL_{RES} = (0.69 \times CL_{cr}) + 3.7$] is 7.15 mL/min (0.12 mL/s) or 0.43 L/h. The k can be approximated as:

$$\begin{aligned} k &= CL_{RES}/V_D \\ &= 0.43\ \text{L/h}/54.4\ \text{L} \\ &= 0.0079\ \text{h}^{-1} \end{aligned}$$

The HD clearance of vancomycin (CL_D) is dependent on the dialyzer and a value of 120 mL/min (2 mL/s; 7.2 L/h) is a reasonable estimate for this dialyzer.[125,126]

One now can predict what the plasma concentrations of vancomycin will be over the next 24 to 48 hours, assuming the infusion time for the drug (t') was 1 hour. The concentration at the end of the 1-hour infusion (C_{max}) would be:

$$\begin{aligned} C_{max} &= \frac{(\text{Dose}/t')(1-e^{-kt'})}{CL_{RES}} \\ &= \frac{(1{,}000\ \text{mg/h})(1-e^{-(0.0079)1})}{0.43\ \text{L/h}} \\ &= (2{,}325.58\ \text{mg/L})(0.0078) \\ &= 18.1\ \text{mg/L} \end{aligned}$$

The plasma concentration prior to the next dialysis session (C_{bD}), which is 44 hours away can be calculated as:

$$\begin{aligned} C_{bD} &= C_{max} \times e{-}(CL_{RES}/V_D) \times t \\ &= 18.1 \times e{-}0.0079 \times 44 \\ &= 12.8\ \text{mg/L} \end{aligned}$$

and the concentration 4 hours later after dialysis (C_{aD}) can be calculated as:

$$\begin{aligned} C_{aD} &= C_{bD} \times e^{-[(CL_{RES} + CL_D)/V_D] \times t} \\ &= 12.8 \times e^{-[(0.43 + 7.2)/54.4] \times 4} \\ &= 12.8 \times e^{-0.14 \times 4} \\ &= 7.3\ \text{mg/L} \end{aligned}$$

On the basis of these data, the second dose which should be administered after the second dialysis session should be increased as one generally desires to maintain

(Continued)

CLINICAL CASE EXAMPLE Dosage Regimen Calculation for a Hemodialysis patient (*Continued*)

vancomycin trough concentrations between 15 and 20 mg/L (10-14 μmol/L) for a MRSA catheter-associated bacteremia.[111,127] The patient received a vancomycin dose of 1,500 mg 4 hours after the end of the second dialysis session. The increase in serum concentration at the end of this 1-hour infusion (C_{change}) can thus be estimated:

$$C_{change} = \frac{(\text{Dose}/t')(1-e^{-kt'})}{CL_{RES}}$$

$$= \frac{(1{,}500\text{ mg/h})\left(1-e^{-(0.0079)1}\right)}{0.43\text{ L/h}}$$

$$= (3{,}488.4\text{ mg/L})(0.0078) = 27.2\text{ mg/L}$$

Thus the C_{max} would be approximately 34 mg/L (24 μmol/L), the sum of the residual concentration from the first dose of approximately 7 mg/L (5 μmol/L) and the C_{change}. The plasma concentration prior to the third dialysis session (C_{bD}), which is 40 hours away can be estimated as:

$$C_{bD} = C_{max} \times e^{-(CL_{RES}/V_D) \times t}$$

$$= 34\text{ mg/L} \times e^{-0.0079 \times 40}$$

$$= 24.8\text{ mg/L}$$

and the concentration 4 hours later after the third dialysis (C_{aD}) can be estimated as:

$$C_{aD} = C_{bD} \times e^{-[(CL_{RES} + CL_D)/V_D] \times t}$$

$$= 24.8 \times e^{-[(0.43 + 7.2)/54.4] \times 4}$$

$$= 24.8 \times e^{-0.14 \times 4}$$

$$= 14.2\text{ mg/L}$$

This higher dose would be considered by many to have achieved too high of concentrations since the lowest value during the majority of the dosing interval exceeded 24.8 mg/L (17.1 μmol/L).

For medications with a narrow therapeutic index (eg, vancomycin, phenytoin, and gentamicin), therapeutic drug monitoring (eg, plasma concentration measurements and dialyzer clearance estimation) should be utilized to guide drug dosing.[6] The ultimate reason for measuring the plasma concentrations of antibacterial agents is to individualize the patient's dosage regimen to achieve a bacteriologic cure while preventing adverse effects and preserving residual renal function. Thus there remains one important step in the case above: the calculation of the dose the patient should receive after the second dialysis session. Vancomycin dosing is primarily based on attaining desired trough concentrations, usually between 15 and 20 mg/L (10-14 μmol/L). Peak concentrations are rarely used and not recommended to derive dosing recommendations and adjustments; however, for this patient example, a desired peak concentration of 30 mg/L (21 μmol/L), the midpoint of the recommended range of 20 to 40 mg/L (14-28 μmol/L) could be utilized to calculate a dose.[111]

Assuming the desired peak concentration of 30 mg/L (21 μmol/L) and trough concentration was 15 mg/L (10 μmol/L), the postdialysis dose this patient would need can then be calculated using the simplified approach below, because the $t_{1/2}$ is extremely prolonged relative to the infusion time, and thus minimal drug is eliminated during the post HD infusion period:

$$\text{Dose} = V_D \times (C_{max} - C_{min})$$

$$= 40\text{ L} \times (30 - 15)$$

$$= 600\text{ mg}$$

7 It is common practice in most HD units to administer drugs after the patient has received dialysis on the premise that it is desirable to minimize the loss of drug that would result from the additional clearance during HD. Certainly, administration of antihypertensive agents and vasoactive drugs should be avoided in the hours prior to a HD session to minimize the likelihood of hypotension. In some cases, medications for pain are given on a precise schedule and thus the medication would be given to the patient irrespective of the time on dialysis. The administration of traditional doses of tobramycin (1.5 mg/kg) or vancomycin (1,000 mg) during dialysis has been associated with markedly lower AUCs than those observed when the same dose was administered postdialysis; consequently, higher dosage regimens are usually necessary to compensate for the additional loss of drug during the dialysis procedure. Furthermore, emerging pharmacokinetic and pharmacodynamic considerations suggest that it may be optimal approach to administer some drugs, such as aminoglycosides[128,129] and vancomycin during or immediately prior to the start of a dialysis treatment.[130,131] Two evaluations of predialysis and one of intradialytic dosing of aminoglycosides indicate that similar peak concentrations, a prime indicator of efficacy, can be obtained in these scenarios relative to those observed with postdialysis dosing.[128] The AUC during the dosing interval and the subsequent predialysis concentrations were noted to be significantly reduced and thus the risk of ototoxicity and further renal injury may be minimized. The best dosing schedule, a dose roughly twice that traditionally employed for postdialysis administration, in the 26 patients evaluated by Teigen et al, resulted in the achievement of the desired peak and AUC in approximately 90% of patients.[128]

Performing HD immediately after dosing might also be a good option for several anticancer drugs. The predialysis administration of a normal dose makes sense when the patient undergoes HD 2 to 12 hours later. This strategy delivers the desired maximum plasma concentration effect while minimizing patient exposure to the toxic drug or metabolite effects.[132-135]

Alternative Hemodialysis Modalities

Short-daily and nocturnal HD are two alternative HD techniques. Both modalities are administered 6 to 7 days a week but differ primarily in the duration of the treatment and blood-flow rate. SDHD is typically for 2 hours per session; nocturnal HD occurs overnight for 6 to 8 hours but at lower blood and dialysate flow rates.[136]

Nocturnal Hemodialysis

NHD use is increasing since there is increased evidence of benefits over conventional thrice-weekly HD[137-139] (Chapter 45). NHD has demonstrated improvements in hypertension, left ventricular hypertrophy, quality of life related to burden and effects of kidney disease, and malnutrition compared to conventional HD.[137,138] In addition,

North American studies suggest that survival is significantly better in NHD than conventional HD and possibly similar to survival after kidney transplantation.[140,141]

NHD is performed over 5 to 8 hours on 3 to 7 nights per week thus receive between 24 and 45 hours of dialysis per week, versus 12 hours with conventional HD.[136] The longer dialysis duration removes a higher quantity of solute and fluid, more closely mimicking the human physiological state when compared with conventional HD.[136] There is a paucity of data when it comes to drug dosing with this modality; however, the principles of drug dosing discussed above with intermittent HD can also be applied here. Although there is an increase in dialysis hours, which would suggest an increase in drug removal, the blood and dialysate flow rates are slower and thus drug clearance per unit of time will be less. This has been shown in a study with cefazolin where the cefazolin clearance during NHD was slightly lower (CL = 1.65 L/h) than during high-flux intermittent HD (CL = 1.85 L/h);[141] however, a greater percentage of cefazolin was removed in 8 hours of NHD (80%) than conventional 4-hour high-flux HD (60%). The investigators concluded that a dosing regimen of a 2-g loading dose followed by 1g IV after each NHD was sufficient to achieve concentrations 6 × MIC for *Staphylococcus* species for at least 70% of the dosing interval.[141]

Short-Daily Hemodialysis

SDHD involves 2 hours of dialysis, 6 days of the week, and has been associated with improved control of blood pressure and phosphorus, decreased medication requirements, decrease in left ventricular mass, and improved quality of life.[142,143] It has also shown a trend toward prolonged survival because of these improvements in clinical outcomes. As in the case with NHD, there is also limited data on drug dosing with this modality; however, the general principles of drug dosing for HD also apply here. In SDHD, the number of dialysis sessions per week and blood and dialysate flow rates are similar to intermittent HD, which may suggest similar drug removal. However, for certain medications (smaller size and decreased V_D, and protein binding) drug removal may be increased.

This has been shown in a study with cefazolin where the cefazolin clearance rate in SDHD was slightly higher than the value observed during high-flux intermittent HD; in fact the amount of cefazolin removed in 2 hours of SDHD was similar to that after 4 hours of high-flux HD.[144] The investigators concluded that a dosing regimen of 1 g after each SDHD was sufficient to achieve concentrations 8 × MIC for *Staphylococcus* species for at least 90% of the dosing interval.[144] Therefore, it appears that the same amount of medication given over the entire week for patients on intermittent HD could also be given to patients on SDHD but in smaller amounts administered more frequently. For instance, in intermittent HD, the cefazolin dose is typically 2 g IV after each HD for a total of 6 g per week; whereas in SDHD, the dose would be 1 g IV daily (ie, for 6 days) after each HD.

Overall small solute removal is more efficient if the frequency of HD is increased. Therefore, SDHD and NHD therapies yield different clearance values compared to intermittent three times per week HD. Furthermore, prolonged HD such as in the case of NHD, results in less rebound of drug concentrations after the termination of dialysis. This likely occurs because the rate of transfer from the peripheral to central compartment relative to the rate of diffusive removal is lower. Therefore, careful monitoring of drug therapy is necessary when these newer modalities are used to avoid potential errors in designing drug dosing regimens.

CONCLUSION

Subtherapeutic responses to drugs in patients with renal insufficiency are often misinterpreted and not recognized. The adverse outcomes associated with inappropriate drug dosing have rarely been quantified but warrant future investigations. The utilization of FDA or EMA drug dosage recommendations in official prescribing information should be used for the initiation of therapy in most clinical situations. However, critically ill individuals especially those with preexisting CKD likely have marked pharmacokinetic variability and may require the use of pharmacokinetic principles in conjunction with reliable population pharmacokinetic estimates to determine the optimal drug dosage regimen design. Individualization of all drugs with a narrow therapeutic index for AKI and CKD patients should be undertaken whenever clinical therapeutic monitoring tools are available. The key action step is to use the knowledge we have to improve patient outcomes. The lack of dosage adjustment for CKD patients in ambulatory and hospital environments is an unfortunate reminder of how far we still have to go to optimize the therapy of CKD patients.[10-14,145]

Clinicians should therefore be aware of all the possible alternations in pharmacokinetics of drug, what processes are likely to be altered in renal failure and tailor pharmacotherapy accordingly to ensure that CKD patients receive maximal benefits from their drug therapy while minimizing potential adverse outcomes.

ABBREVIATIONS

A_b	concentration of drug in blood going into the dialyzer (arterial side)
AKI	acute kidney injury
A_p	concentration of drug in plasma going into the dialyzer (arterial side)
AUC_{0-t}	the area under the predialyzer plasma concentration–time curve during hemodialysis
ARC	augmented renal clearance
BSA	body surface area
C_{aD}	plasma concentration after dialysis
C_{bD}	plasma concentration prior to the next dialysis session
CG	Cockcroft–Gault
CKD	chronic kidney disease
CKD-EPI	Chronic Kidney Disease Epidemiology Collaboration Equation
CL	total body clearance
CL^b_D	dialyzer clearance from blood
CL_{cr}	creatinine clearance
CL_D	dialyzer clearance
CL_{fail}	clearance of a drug in patients with impaired renal function
CL_{norm}	clearance of a drug in patients with normal renal function
CL_{NR}	clearance nonrenal
CL^p_D	dialyzer clearance from plasma
CL_R	net renal excretion
CL^r_D	recovery clearance of dialyzer
$CL_{reabsorption}$	tubular reabsorption
CL_{RES}	residual drug clearance in a dialysis patient
$CL_{secretion}$	tubular secretion
CL_T	total clearance during dialysis
C_{max}	peak drug concentration
C_{min}	trough drug concentration
C_{ss}	average steady-state plasma concentration
CYP	cytochrome P450

D_f	maintenance dose for a patient with renal insufficiency
D_n	dose for a patient with normal renal function
EBT	erythromycin breath test
eCLcr	estimated creatinine clearance
eGFR	estimated glomerular filtration rate
EMA	European Medicine Agency
ESRD	end-stage renal disease
f_e	fraction of drug eliminated unchanged in the urine
f_u	fraction of drug unbound to plasma proteins
GFR	glomerular filtration rate
HD	hemodialysis
INR	international normalized ratio
k	elimination rate constant
k_{DD}	elimination rate constant during dialysis
KDIGO	Kidney Disease: Improving Global Outcomes
KF	ratio of the patient's CL_{cr} to the assumed normal value of 120 mL/min (2 mL/s)
k_{ID}	elimination rate constant between dialysis sessions (interdialytic)
MDRD	modification of diet in renal disease equation
MIC	minimum inhibitory concentration
MRSA	methicillin-resistant *Staphylococcus aureus*
NHD	nocturnal hemodialysis
Q	kinetic parameter/dosage-adjustment factor
Q_b	blood flow through the dialyzer
Q_p	plasma flow through the dialyzer = Q_b (1 – hematocrit)
R	the total amount of drug recovered unchanged in the dialysate
SSRIs	selective serotonin reuptake inhibitors
t'	infusion time of drug
Δt	time in hours between two measured concentrations
$t_{1/2}$	half-life
$t_{1/2,\text{on HD}}$	half-life during dialysis
$t_{1/2,\text{off HD}}$	half-life off dialysis
τ_f	dosing interval in a patient with renal failure
τ_p	practical dosing interval for a patient with renal failure
τ_n	dosing interval in a patient with normal renal function
t_{max}	time-to-peak drug concentration
TTR	time in therapeutic range
V_{area}	volume of distribution area
V_b	blood concentration of drug leaving the dialyzer
V_β	volume of terminal phase (serum protein)
V_c	volume of the central compartment
V_D	volume of distribution
V_{ss}	volume of distribution at steady state

REFERENCES

1. Stevens PE, Levin A. Kidney Disease: Improving Global Outcomes Chronic Kidney Disease Guideline Development Work Group M. Evaluation and Management of Chronic Kidney Disease: Synopsis of the Kidney Disease: Improving Global Outcomes. *Ann Intern Med* 2012:825-830.
2. Mills KT, Xu Y, Zhang W, et al. A systematic analysis of worldwide population-based data on the global burden of chronic kidney disease in 2010. *Kidney Int* 2015;88:950-957.
3. Radhakrishnan J, Remuzzi G, Saran R, et al. Taming the chronic kidney disease epidemic: A global view of surveillance efforts. *Kidney Int* 2014;86:246-250.
4. Brück K, Stel VS, Gambaro G, et al. CKD Prevalence Varies across the European General Population. *J Am Soc Nephrol* 2015. doi:ASN.2015050542.
5. National Kidney and Urologic Diseases Information Clearinghouse (NKUDIC). Kidney Disease Statistics for the United States. U.S. Department of Health and Human Services Available at: http://kidney.niddk.nih.gov/kudiseases/pubs/kustats/November 2012. Accessed February 1, 2016.
6. Matzke GR, Comstock TJ. Influence of renal disease and dialysis on pharmacokinetics. In: Evans WE, Schentag JJ, Burton ME, eds. *Applied Pharmacokinetics: Principles of Therapeutic Drug Monitoring*, 4th ed. Baltimore, MD: Lippincott Williams & Wilkins, 2005:187-212.
7. Matzke GR, Dowling TC, Marks SA, et al. Influence of kidney disease on drug disposition: An assessment of industry studies submitted to the FDA for new chemical entities 1999–2010. *J Clin Pharmacol* 2015. doi:10.1002/jcph.604.
8. Rowland M, Tozer TN. *Clinical Pharmacokinetics: Concepts and Applications*, 3rd ed. Philadelphia, PA: Lea & Febiger, 1995:156-183.
9. Matzke GR, Dowling TD. Dosing concepts in renal dysfunction. In: Murphy JE, ed. *Clinical Pharmacokinetics Pocket Reference*, 5th ed. Bethesda, MD: American Society of Health-System Pharmacists, 2011:427-443.
10. Farag A, Garg AX, Li L, et al. Dosing errors in prescribed antibiotics for older persons with CKD: a retrospective time series analysis. *Am J Kidney Dis* 2014;63:422-428.
11. Chang F, O'Hare AM, Miao Y, et al. Use of renally inappropriate medications in older veterans: A National Study. *J Am Geriatr Soc* 2015;63:2290-2297.
12. Muller C, Mimitrov Y, Imhoff O, et al. Oral antidiabetics use among diabetic type 2 patients with chronic kidney disease. Do nephrologists take account of recommendations? *J Diabetes Complications* 2016. doi: 10.1038/clpt.2008.59.
13. Via-Sosa MA, Lopes N, March M. Effectiveness of a drug dosing service provided by community pharmacists in polymedicated elderly patients with renal impairment—a comparative study. *BMC Fam Pract* 2013;14:96.
14. Chertow GM, Lee J, Kuperman GJ, et al. Guided medication dosing for inpatients with renal insufficiency. *JAMA* 2001;286:2839-2844.
15. Salomon L, Deray G, Jaudon MC, et al. Medication misuse in hospitalized patients with renal impairment. *Int J Qual Health Care* 2003;15:331-335.
16. Aronoff GR, Aronoff JR. Drug prescribing in kidney disease: can't we do better? *Am J Kidney Dis* 2014;3:382-383.
17. Thummel KE, Shen DD, Isoherranen N. Appendix II. Design and optimization of dosage regimens: Pharmacokinetic data. In: Brunton LL, Chabner BA, Knollmann BC, eds. *Goodman & Gilman's The Pharmacological Basis of Therapeutics*, 12th ed. New York, NY: McGraw-Hill 2011.
18. Ramezani A, Raj DS. The gut microbiome, kidney disease, and targeted interventions. *J Am Soc Nephrol* 2014;25:657-670.
19. Etemad B. Gastrointestinal complications of renal failure. *Gastroenterol Clin North Am* 1998;27:875-892.
20. Matzke GR, Frye RF. Drug administration in patients with renal insufficiency. *Drug Saf* 1997;16:205-231.
21. Gibson TP, Giacomini KM, Briggs WA, et al. Propoxyphene and norpropoxyphene plasma concentrations in the anephric patient. *Clin Pharmacol Ther* 1980;27:665-670.
22. Barnes JN, Williams AJ, et al. Dihydrocodeine in renal failure: Further evidence for an important role of the kidney in the handling of opioid drugs. *BMJ* 1985;290:740-742.
23. Min DI, Ku YM, Perry PJ, et al. Effect of grapefruit juice on cyclosporine pharmacokinetics in renal transplant patients. *Transplantation* 1996;62:123-125.
24. Ueda N, Yoshimura R, Umene-Nakano W, et al. Grapefruit juice alters plasma sertraline levels after single ingestion of sertraline in healthy volunteers. *World J Biol Psychiatry* 2009;10:832-835.
25. Bailey DG, Arnold JM, Bend JR, et al. Grapefruit juice-felodipine interaction: reproducibility and characterization with the extended release drug formulation. *Br J Clin Pharmacol* 1995;40:135.
26. Verbeeck RK, Musuamba FT. Pharmacokinetics and dosage adjustment in patients with renal dysfunction. *Eur J Clin Pharmacol* 2009;65:757-773.

27. Olyaei AJ, Steffl JL. A quantitative approach to drug dosing in chronic kidney disease. *Blood Purif* 2011;31:138-145.
28. Olyaei AJ, Bennett WM. Drug dosing in the elderly patients with chronic kidney disease. *Clin Geriatr Med* 2009;25:459-527.
29. Brunner M, Pernerstorfer T, Mayer BX, et al. Surgery and intensive care procedures affect the target site distribution of piperacillin. *Crit Care Med* 2000;28:1754-1759.
30. Álvarez-Lerma F, Grau S. Management of antimicrobial use in the intensive care unit. *Drugs* 2012;72:447-470.
31. Winter ME. Phenytoin and fosphenytoin. In *Clinical Pharmacokinetics*. 5th ed. Murphy J, editor. Bethesda MD: American Society of Health System Pharmacists; 2012.
32. Meijers BKI, Bemmers B, Verbeke B, et al. A review of albumin binding in CKD. *Am J Kidney Dis* 2008;51:839-850.
33. Job ML. Digoxin. In: Murphy JE, ed. *Clinical Pharmacokinetics Pocket Reference,* 5th ed. Bethesda, MD: American Society of Health-System Pharmacists, 2012:139-147.
34. Koup JR. Disease states and drug pharmacokinetics. *J Clin Pharmacol* 1989;29:674-679.
35. Masereeuw R, Russel FGM. Therapeutic implications of renal anionic drug transporters. *Pharmacol ther* 2010;126:200-216.
36. Yeung CK, Shen DD, Thummel KE, et al. Effects of chronic kidney disease and uremia on hepatic drug metabolism and transport. *Kidney Int* 2014;85:522-528.
37. Naud J, Nolin TD, Leblond FA, et al. Current understanding of drug disposition in kidney disease. *J Clin Pharmacol* 2012;52:10S-22S.
38. Nolin TD, Unruh ML. Clinical relevance of impaired nonrenal drug clearance in ESRD. *Sem Dialysis* 2010;23:482-485.
39. Macias WL, Mueller BA, Scarim SK. Vancomycin pharmacokinetics in acute renal failure: preservation of nonrenal clearance. *Clin Pharmacol Ther* 1991;50:688-694.
40. Heinemeyer G, Link J, Weber W, et al. Clearance of ceftriaxone in critical care patients with acute renal failure. *Intensive Care Med* 1990;16:448-453.
41. Mueller BA, Scarim SK, Macias WL. Comparison of imipenem pharmacokinetics in patients with acute or chronic renal failure treated with continuous hemofiltration. *Am J Kidney Dis* 1993;21:172-179.
42. Vilay AM, Churchwell MD, Mueller BA. Drug metabolism and clearance in acute kidney injury. *Crit Care* 2008;12:235.
43. Nolin TD, Appiah K, Kendrick SA, et al. Hemodialysis acutely improves hepatic CYP3A4 metabolic activity. *J Am Soc Nephrol* 2006;17:2363-2367.
44. Dowling TC, Briglia AE, Fink JC, et al. Characterization of hepatic cytochrome P4503A activity in patients with end-stage renal disease. *Clin Pharmacol Ther* 2003;73:427-434.
45. Yuan R, Venitz J. Effect of chronic renal failure on the disposition of highly hepatically metabolized drugs. *Int J Clin Pharmacol Ther* 2000;38:245-253.
46. Murphy EJ. Acute pain management for the patient with concurrent renal or hepatic disease. *Anaesth Intensive Care* 2005;33:311-322.
47. Osborne R, Joel S, Grebenik K, et al. The pharmacokinetics of morphine and morphine glucuronides in kidney failure. *Clin Pharmacol Ther* 1993;54:158-167.
48. Szeto HH, Inturrisi CE, Houde R, et al. Accumulation of normeperidine, an active metabolite of meperidine, in patients with renal failure of cancer. *Ann Intern Med* 1977;86:738-741.
49. Hardy J, Singleton A. Genomewide association studies and human Disease. *N Engl J Med* 2009;360:1759-1768.
50. Godman B, Finlayson AE, Cheema PK, et al. Personalizing health care: Feasibility and future implications. *BMC Med* 2013;11:179-202.
51. Kraft P, Hunter DJ. Genetic risk prediction-are we there yet? *N Engl J Med* 2009;360:1701-1703.
52. Janssens AC, van Duijn CM. Genome-based prediction of common diseases: Advances and prospects. *Hum Mol Genet* 2008;17:R166-R173.
53. Drozda K, Müller DJ, Bishop JR. Pharmacogenomic testing for neuropsychiatric drugs: Current status of drug labelling, guidelines for using genetic information, and test options. *Pharmacotherapy* 2014;34:166-184.
54. Patel JN. Application of genotype-guided cancer therapy in solid tumors. *Pharmacogenomics* 2014;15:79-93.
55. Becker ML, Pearson ER, Tkáč I. Pharmacogenetics of oral antidiabetic drugs. *Int J Endocrinol* 2013:686315, 2013.
56. Needham M, Mastaglia FL: Statin myotoxicity: A review of genetic susceptibility factors. *Neuromuscul Disord* 2014;24:4-15.
57. Kawaguchi-Suzuki M, Frye RF. The role of pharmacogenetics in the treatment of chronic hepatitis C infection. *Pharmacotherapy* 2014;34:185-201.
58. Weeke P, Roden DM. Applied pharmacogenomics in cardiovascular medicine. *Annu Rev Med* 2014;65:81-94.
59. Carr DF, O'Meara H, Jorgensen AL, et al. SLCO1B1 genetic variant associated with statin-induced myopathy: a proof-ofconcept study using the clinical practice research datalink. *Clin Pharmacol Ther* 2013;94:695-701.
60. Crews KR, Gaedigk A, Dunnenberger HM, et al. Clinical Pharmacogenetics Implementation Consortium (CPIC) guidelines for codeine therapy in the context of cytochrome P450 2DG (CYP2D6) genotype. *Clin Pharmacol Ther* 2012;91:321-326.
61. U.S. Food and Drug Administration: Table of pharmacogenomic biomarkers in drug labeling. Available at: www.fda.gov/drugs/scienceresearch/researchareas/pharmacogenetics/ucm083378.htm. Accessed February 1, 2016.
62. Kazi DS, Garber AM, Shah RU, et al. Cost-effectiveness of genotype-guided and dual antiplatelet therapies in acute coronary syndrome. *Ann Intern Med* 2014;160:221-232.
63. Patel HN, Ursan ID, Zueger PM, et al. Stakeholder views on pharmacogenomic testing. *Pharmacotherapy* 2014;34:151-165.
64. Pirmohamed Munir, Burnside Girvan, et al. A randomized trial of genotype-guided dosing of warfarin. *N Engl J Med* 2013;369:2294-2303.
65. Kimmel SE, French B, Kasner SE, et al. A pharmacogenetic versus a clinical algorithm for warfarin dosing. *N Engl J Med* 2013;369:2283-2293.
66. Bazinet A, Almanric K, Brunet C, et al. Dosage of enoxaparin among obese and renal impairment patients. *Thromb Res* 2005;116:41-50.
67. Hulot JS, Vantelon C, Urien S, et al. Effect of renal function on the pharmacokinetics of enoxaparin and consequences on dose adjustment. *Ther Drug Monit* 2004;26:305-310.
68. Ambrose PG, Bhavnani SM, Rubino CM, et al. Pharmacokinetics-pharmacodynamics of antimicrobial therapy: it's not just for mice anymore. *Clin Infect Dis* 2007;44:79-86.
69. Fish DN, Kiser TH. Correlation of pharmacokinetic/pharmacodynamic-derived predictions of antibiotic efficacy with clinical outcomes in severely ill patients with Pseudomonas aeruginosa pneumonia. *Pharmacother* 2013;33:1022-1034.
70. Nyman HA, Dowling TC, Hudson JQ, et al. Comparative Evaluation of the Cockcroft-Gault Equation and the Modification of Diet in Renal Disease (MDRD) Study Equation for Drug Dosing: An Opinion of the Nephrology Practice and Research Network of the American College of Clinical Pharmacy. *Pharmacother* 2011;31:1130-1144.
71. Cockcroft DW, Gault MH. Prediction of creatinine clearance from serum creatinine. *Nephron* 1976;16:31-41.
72. Levey AS, Bosch JP, Lewis JB, et al. A more accurate method to estimate glomerular filtration rate from serum creatinine: a new prediction equation. *Ann Intern Med* 1999;130:461-470.
73. Levey AS, Stevens LA, Schmid CH, et al. A new equation to estimate glomerular filtration rate. *Ann Intern Med* 2009;150:604-612.
74. Dowling TC, Matzke GR, Murphy JE, Burckart GJ. Evaluation of renal drug dosing: Prescribing information and clinical pharmacist approaches. *Pharmacotherapy* 2010;30:776-786.
75. Steffl JL, Bennett W, Olyaei AJ. The old and new methods of assessing kidney function. *J Clin Pharmacol* 2012;52:63S-71S.
76. Wargo KA, Eiland EH, Hamm W, et al. Comparison of the modification of diet in renal disease and Cockcroft-Gault equations for antimicrobial dosage adjustments. *Ann Pharmacother* 2006;40:1248-1253.
77. Gill J, Malyuk R, Djurdjev O, et al. Use of GFR equations to adjust drug doses in an elderly multi-ethnic group—A cautionary tale. *Nephrol Dial Transpl* 2007;22:2894-2899.
78. Golik MV, Lawrence KR. Comparison of dosing recommendations for antimicrobial drugs based on two methods for assessing kidney function: Cockcroft–Gault and modification of diet in renal disease. *Pharmacotherapy* 2008;28:1125-1132.
79. Melloni C, Peterson ED, Chen AY, et al. Cockcroft-Gault versus modification of diet in renal disease: importance of glomerular filtration rate formula for classification of chronic kidney disease in patients with non–ST-segment elevation acute coronary syndromes. *J Am Coll Cardiol* 2008;51:991-996.
80. Hermsen ED, Maiefski M, Florescu MC, et al. Comparison of the modification of diet in renal disease and Cockcroft–Gault equations for dosing antimicrobials. *Pharmacotherapy* 2009;29:649-655.
81. Wargo KA, English TM. Evaluation of the chronic kidney disease epidemiology collaboration equation for dosing antimicrobials. *Ann Pharmacother* 2010;44:439-446.

82. Stevens LA, Nolin TD, Richardson MM, et al. Comparison of drug dosing recommendations based on measured GFR and kidney function estimating equations. *Am J Kidney Dis* 2009;54:33-42.
83. Rule AD, Bailey KR, Lieske JC, et al. Estimating the glomerular filtration rate from serum creatinine is better than from cystatin C for evaluating risk factors associated with chronic kidney disease. *Kidney Int* 2013;83:1169-1176.
84. Matsushita K, Mahmoodi BK, Woodward M, et al. Comparison of risk prediction using the CKD-EPI equation and the MDRD study equation for estimated glomerular filtration rate. *JAMA* 2012;307:1941-1951.
85. Shlipak MG, Matsushita K, Ärnlöv J, et al. Cystatin C versus creatinine in determining risk based on kidney function. *N Engl J Med* 2013;369:932-943.
86. Inker LA, Schmid CH, Tighiouart H, et al. Estimating glomerular filtration rate from serum creatinine and cystatin C. *N Engl J Med* 2012;367:20-29.
87. Schmitt A, Gladieff L, Lansiaux A, et al. A universal formula based on cystatin C to perform individual dosing of carboplatin in normal weight, underweight, and obese patients. *Clin Cancer Res* 2009;15:3633-3639.
88. Viberg A, Lannergård A, Larsson A, et al. A population pharmacokinetic model for cefuroxime using cystatin C as a marker of renal function. *Br J Clin Pharmacol* 2006;62:297-303.
89. Hoppe A, Séronie-Vivien S, Thomas F, et al. Serum cystatin C is a better marker of topotecan clearance than serum creatinine. *Clin Cancer Res* 2005;11:3038-3044.
90. Thomas F, Séronie-Vivien S, Gladieff L, et al. Cystatin C as a new covariate to predict renal elimination of drugs. *Clin Pharmacokinet* 2005;44:1305-1316.
91. US Food Drug Administration. Guidance for industry: pharmacokinetics in patients with imparied renal function-study design, data analysis and impact on dosing and labelling199. Available at: http://www.fda.gov/downloads/Drugs/GuidanceComplianceRegulatoryInformation/Guidances/ucm072127.pdf. Accessed February 1, 2016.
92. European Medicines Agency. 2014 Guideline on the evaluation of the pharmacokinetics of medicinal products in patients with decreased renal function. Available at: http://www.ema.europa.eu/docs/en_GB/document_library/Scientific_guideline/2009/09/WC500003123.pdf. Accessed February 1, 2016.
93. US Food Drug Administration. Guidance for industry: pharmacokinetics in patients with imparied renal function-study design, data analysis and impact on dosing and labelling 2010. Available at: http://www.fda.gov/downloads/Drugs/GuidanceComplianceRegulatoryInformation/Guidances/ucm072127.pdf. Accessed February 1, 2016.
94. Tortorici MA, Cutler D, Zhang L, et al. Design, conduct, analysis, and interpretation of clinical studies in patients with impaired kidney function. *J Clin Pharmacol* 2012;52:109S-1018S.
95. Tortorici MA, Cutler DL, Hazra A, et al. Emerging areas of research in the assessment of pharmacokinetics in patients with chronic kidney disease. *J Clin Pharmacol* 2015;55:241-250.
96. Matzke GR, Aronoff GR, Atkinson AJ Jr, et al. Drug dosing consideration in patients with acute and chronic kidney disease—A clinical update from Kidney Disease: Improving Global Outcomes (KDIGO). *Kidney Int* 2011;80:1122-1137.
97. McEvoy GK, Snow EK, Miller J, et al. American Hospital Formulary Service, Drug Information. Bethesda, MD: American Society of Health-System Pharmacists, 2016.
98. Joint Formulary Committee. *British National Formulary,* 64th ed. London: British Medical Association and Royal Pharmaceutical Society of Great Britain, 2004.
99. Aronoff GR, Bennett WM, Berns JS, et al. *Drug Prescribing in Renal Failure: Dosing Guidelines for Adults and Children,* 5th ed. Philadelphia, PA: American College of Physicians-American Society of Internal Medicine, 2007.
100. The Renal Drug Handbook. The UK Pharmacy Group [Internet]. 2014. Available at: http://www.ayurvedavignan.in/freeEbooks/Renal-Drug-Handbook.pdf. Accessed Febbruary 21, 2016.
101. Takamoto CK. Pediatric and Neonatal Lexi-Drugs. Lexi-Comp, Inc. 2015.
102. Micromedex 2.0 Truven Health Analytics Inc [Internet]. 2015.
103. Hilal-Dandan R, Brunton L. *Goodman and Gilman Manual of Pharmacology and Therapeutics,* 2nd ed. New York, NY: McGraw Hill Medical, 2014.
104. Mountford CM, Lee T, de Lemos J, et al. Quality and usability of common drug information databases. *Can J Hosp Pharm* 2010;63:130.
105. Vidal L, Shavit M, Fraser A, et al. Systematic comparison of four sources of drug information regarding adjustment of dose for renal function. *BMJ* 2005;331:263-266.
106. Dettli LC. Drug dosage in patients with renal disease. *Clin Pharmacol Ther* 1974;16:274-280.
107. Matzke GR, Clermont G. Clinical pharmacology and therapeutics. In: Murray PT, Brady HR, Hall JB, eds. *Intensive Care in Nephrology.* Boca Raton, FL: Taylor & Francis, 2006:245-265.
108. Eyler RF, Mueller BA. Antibiotic pharmacokinetic and pharmacodynamic considerations in patients with kidney disease. *Adv Chronic Kidney Dis* 2010;17:392-403.
109. Craig WA. Pharmacokinetic/pharmacodynamic parameters: rationale for antibacterial dosing of mice and men. *Clin Infect Dis* 1998:1-10.
110. Kushner JM, Peckman HJ, Snyder CR. Seizures associated with fluoroquinolones. *Ann Pharmacother* 2001;35:1194-1198.
111. Rybak MJ, Lomaestro BM, Rotschafer JC, et al. Vancomycin therapeutic guidelines: A summary of consensus recommendations from the Infectious Diseases Society of America, the American Society of Health-System Pharmacists, and the Society of Infectious Diseases Pharmacists. *Clin Infect Dis* 2009;49:325-327.
112. Drusano GL. Pharmacokinetic optimisation of β-lactams for the treatment of ventilator-associated pneumonia. *Eur Respir Rev* 2007;16:45-49.
113. Gilbert B, Robbins P, Livornese LL Jr. Use of antibacterial agents in renal failure. *Infect Dis Clin North Am* 2009;23:899-924.
114. Heintz BH, Matzke GR, Dager WE. Antimicrobial dosing concepts and recommendations for critically ill adult patients receiving continuous renal replacement therapy or intermittent hemodialysis. *Pharmacotherapy* 2009;29:562-577.
115. Udy AA, Varghese JM, Altukroni M, et al. Subtherapeutic initial β-lactam concentrations in select critically ill patients: association between augmented renal clearance and low trough drug concentrations. *CHEST Journal* 2012;142:30-39.
116. Claus BOM, Hoste EA, Colpaert K, et al. Augmented renal clearance is a common finding with worse clinical outcome in critically ill patients receiving antimicrobial therapy. *J Crit Care* 2013;28:695-700.
117. Hobbs AL, Shea KM, Roberts KM, et al. Implications of augmented renal clearance on drug dosing in critically ill patients: A focus on antibiotics. *Pharmacother* 2015;35:1063-1075.
118. Janknegt R, Nube MJ. A simple method for predicting drug clearances during CAPD. Available at: http://www.pdiconnect.com/content/5/4/254.2.full.pdf+html. Accessed February 1, 2016.
119. Maher JF: Influence of continuous ambulatory peritoneal dialysis on elimination of drugs. Available at: http://www.pdiconnect.com/content/7/3/159.full.pdf. Accessed February 1, 2016.
120. Manley HJ, Bailie GR. Automated Peritoneal Dialysis Symposium: Treatment of Peritonitis in APD: Pharmacokinetic Principles. *Sem Dialysis* 2002;15:418-421.
121. Taylor CA III, Abdel-Rahman E, Zimmerman SW, et al. Clinical pharmacokinetics during continuous ambulatory peritoneal dialysis. *Clin Pharmacokinet* 1996;31:293-308.
122. Li PK, Szeto CC, Piraino B, et al. Peritoneal dialysis-related infections recommendations: 2010 update. *Perit Dial Int* 2010;30:393-423.
123. Matzke GR. Status of Hemodialysis of Drugs in 2002. *J Pharm Pract* 2002;15:405-418.
124. Cheung AK. Hemodialysis and hemofiltration. In: Greenberg A, Cheung AK, Coffman TM, Falk RJ, Jennette JC, eds. *Primer on Kidney Disease,* 5th ed. Philadelphia, PA: WB Saunders; 2008.
125. Matzke GR. Buby J. Vancomycin. In: Murphy JE, ed. *Clinical Pharmacokinetics Pocket Reference,* 5th ed. Bethesda, MD: American Society of Hospital Pharmacists; 2011.
126. Launay-Vacher V, Izzedine H, Mercadal L, et al. Clinical review: Use of vancomycin in haemodialysis patients. *Critical Care* 2002;6:313.
127. Liu C, Bayer A, Cosgrove SE, et al. Clinical practice guidelines by the Infectious Diseases Society of America for the treatment of methicillin-resistant *Staphylococcus aureus* infections in adults and children. *Clin Infect Dis* 2011;52:1-38.
128. Teigen MM, Duffull S, Dang L, et al. Dosing of gentamicin in patients with end-stage renal disease receiving hemodialysis. *J Clin Pharmacol* 2006;46:1259-1267.
129. Mohamed OHK, Wahba IM, Watnick S, et al. Administration of tobramycin in the beginning of the hemodialysis session: a novel intradialytic dosing regimen. *Clin J Am Soc Nephrol* 2007;2:694-699.
130. Zelenitsky SA, Ariano RE, McCrae ML, et al. Initial vancomycin dosing protocol to achieve therapeutic serum concentrations in patients undergoing hemodialysis. *Clin Infect Dis* 2012;55:527-533.
131. Ariano RE, Fine A, Sitar DS, et al. Adequacy of a vancomycin dosing regimen in patients receiving high-flux hemodialysis. *Am J Kidney Dis* 2005;46:681-687.

132. Kamata H, Asano K, Soejima K, et al. Appropriate hemodialysis scheduling based on therapeutic drug monitoring of carboplatin in a patient with lung cancer and chronic renal failure. *Gan to Kagaku Ryoho* 2009;36:1529-1532.
133. Oguri T, Shimokata T, Inada M, et al. Pharmacokinetic analysis of carboplatin in patients with cancer who are undergoing hemodialysis. *Cancer Chemother Pharmacol* 2010;66:813-817.
134. Haubitz M, Bohnenstengel F, Brunkhorst R, et al. Cyclophosphamide pharmacokinetics and dose requirements in patients with renal insufficiency. *Kidney Int* 2002;61:1495-1501.
135. Koolen SL, Huitema AD, Jansen RS, et al. Pharmacokinetics of gemcitabine and metabolites in a patient with double-sided nephrectomy: A case report and review of the literature. *Oncologist* 2009;14:944-998.
136. Kooistra MP. Frequent prolonged home haemodialysis: three old concepts, one modern solution. *Nephrol Dial Transpl* 2003;18:16-18.
137. Culleton BF, Walsh M, Klarenbach SW, et al. Effect of frequent nocturnal hemodialysis vs conventional hemodialysis on left ventricular mass and quality of life: A randomized controlled trial. *JAMA* 2007;298:1291-1299.
138. Jefferies HJ, Virk B, Schiller B, et al. Frequent hemodialysis schedules are associated with reduced levels of dialysis-induced cardiac injury (myocardial stunning). *Clin J Am Soc Nephrol* 2011;6:1326-1332.
139. Johansen KL, Zhang R, Huang Y, et al. Survival and hospitalization among patients using nocturnal and short daily compared to conventional hemodialysis: A USRDS study. *Kidney Int* 2009;76:984-990.
140. Pauly RP, Gill JS, Rose CL, et al. Survival among nocturnal home haemodialysis patients compared to kidney transplant recipients. *Nephrol Dial Transpl* 2009;24:2915-2919.
141. Law V, Walker S, Dresser L, et al. Optimized dosing of cefazolin in patients treated with nocturnal home hemodialysis. *Am J Kidney Dis* 2014;64:479-480.
142. FHN. Trial Group. In-center hemodialysis six times per week versus three times per week. *N Engl J Med* 2010;363:2287-2300.
143. Culleton BF, Asola MR. The impact of short daily and nocturnal hemodialysis on quality of life, cardiovascular risk and survival. *J Nephrol* 2011;24:405.
144. Palmer K, Walker S, Jassal V, et al. Pharmacokinetics study of cefazolin in short daily hemodialysis. *Am J Kidney Dis* 2015;65:A64.
145. van Dijk EA, Drabbe NRG, Kruijtbosch M, et al. Drug dosage adjustments according to renal function at hospital discharge. *Ann Pharmacother* 2006;40:1254-1260.

Disorders of Sodium and Water Homeostasis

49

Katherine H. Chessman and Jason Haney

KEY CONCEPTS

1. Blood volume and serum osmolality which are essential for normal cellular function are tightly regulated in the human body. Water balance determines the serum sodium concentration, and sodium balance determines water status.
2. Hypovolemic hypotonic hyponatremia is relatively common in patients taking thiazide diuretics; however, thiazide-induced hyponatremia is usually mild and relatively asymptomatic.
3. Euvolemic (isovolemic) hyponatremia is most often caused by the syndrome of inappropriate secretion of antidiuretic hormone (SIADH). Common causes of SIADH include certain cancers, central nervous system (CNS) and pulmonary disorders, and some drugs.
4. Symptoms of hypo- or hypernatremia are usually neurologic and range from weakness, lethargy, restlessness, irritability, twitching, and confusion to seizures, coma, and death. Symptom severity depends on both the magnitude of the change in the serum sodium concentration and the rate at which it changes.
5. Treatment goals in patients with either hypo- or hypernatremia should include cautious correction of the serum sodium concentration and, when appropriate, restoration of a normal extracellular fluid (ECF) volume. Too rapid correction of the serum sodium can result in cerebral edema, seizures, neurologic damage, osmotic demyelination syndrome, and possibly death. To minimize the risk of these complications, the serum sodium concentration should be corrected at a rate not to exceed 6 to 12 mEq/L (mmol/L) in 24 hours, depending on the rate of change in the serum sodium concentration.
6. Asymptomatic or mildly symptomatic hyponatremia should be managed conservatively with treatment directed at the underlying cause. Intravenous (IV) infusion of 0.9% sodium chloride (NaCl) is most often used to correct the serum sodium concentration in patients with hypovolemic hypotonic hyponatremia and moderate to severe symptoms. A 3% NaCl infusion may be used cautiously in patients with moderate to severe symptoms and euvolemic or hypervolemic hypotonic hyponatremia (along with a loop diuretic).
7. Hypernatremia is always hypertonic and most commonly occurs when increased water or hypotonic fluid losses are not offset by increased water intake.
8. Hypovolemic hypernatremia is relatively common in patients taking loop diuretics. After symptoms of hypovolemia are corrected with 0.9% NaCl, the free water deficit should be replaced.
9. Patients with central diabetes insipidus (DI) can be treated with desmopressin acetate, with a goal to decrease urine volume to less than 2 L per day while maintaining a normal or near normal serum sodium concentration. Patients with nephrogenic DI should be treated by correcting the underlying cause, when possible, and sodium restriction in conjunction with a thiazide diuretic to decrease the ECF volume by approximately 1 to 1.5 L.
10. Edema develops as a primary defect in the kidney's ability to adjust sodium reabsorption or as a response to a decreased effective circulating volume. It is usually first detected in the feet or pretibial areas of ambulatory patients. Pulmonary edema, evidenced by auscultatory crackles, can be life-threatening.
11. Diuretics are the primary pharmacologic means for minimizing edema. Diuretic resistance often can be overcome by using an increased dose or by using a combination of a loop diuretic and a thiazide or thiazide-like diuretic.

1 Blood volume and serum osmolality which are essential for normal cellular function are tightly regulated. Blood volume is a determinant of effective tissue perfusion which is required to deliver oxygen and nutrients to and remove metabolic waste products from tissues. Serum osmolality, the primary determinant of which is sodium concentration, is an important determinant of intracellular fluid (ICF) volume. Maintenance of normal ICF volume is particularly critical in the brain, which is 80% water, and where alterations, especially rapid changes, can result in significant dysfunction and potentially death.

Simply put, water balance determines the serum sodium concentration, and sodium balance determines the volume status. Thus, the homeostatic mechanisms for controlling blood volume are focused on controlling sodium balance, and, in contrast, the homeostatic mechanisms for controlling serum osmolality are focused on controlling water balance. Disorders of sodium and water homeostasis are common, caused by a variety of diseases, conditions, and drugs, and potentially serious. This chapter reviews the etiology, classification, clinical presentation, and therapy for disorders of sodium and water homeostasis.

SODIUM AND WATER HOMEOSTASIS

The average daily sodium intake of those consuming western diets far exceeds the usual requirement of 1.5 g per day.[1] Appropriately functioning kidneys excrete the excess to maintain the serum sodium concentration and osmolality within a very tight range. The kidney can also conserve sodium during periods of low sodium intake or in the presence of excessive losses. Both hypo- and hypernatremia are syndromes of altered serum tonicity and cell volume that reflect a change in the ratio of total exchangeable body sodium to total body water (TBW). TBW comprises 45% to

60% of body weight and is distributed primarily into two compartments: the intracellular compartment or intracellular fluid (ICF; two-thirds [67%] of TBW) and the extracellular compartment or extracellular fluid (ECF; one-third [33%] of TBW). Serum (plasma) volume is approximately 17% of the ECF volume. Sodium and its accompanying anions (chloride and bicarbonate) comprise more than 90% of the ECF osmolality; whereas ICF osmolality is primarily determined by the concentration of potassium and its accompanying anions (mostly organic and inorganic phosphates). The intra- and extracellular sodium and potassium concentrations are maintained by the sodium–potassium–adenosine triphosphatase (Na^+-K^+-ATPase) pump. Most cell membranes are freely permeable to water, allowing the free flow of water between compartments, keeping the ICF and ECF osmolalities equal.

Effective osmoles are solutes that cannot freely cross cell membranes, such as sodium and potassium. The ECF concentration of effective osmoles determines its tonicity, which directly affects water distribution between the ECF and ICF. Addition of an isotonic solution (eg, 0.9% NaCl) to the ECF will result in no change in intracellular volume because there will be no change in the effective ECF osmolality. However, addition of a hypertonic solution (eg, 3% NaCl) to the ECF will result in a decrease in ICF (cell) volume. Conversely, addition of a hypotonic solution (eg, 0.45% NaCl) to the ECF will result in an increase in ICF (cell) volume. Table 49-1 summarizes the composition of commonly used IV solutions and their respective distribution into the ICF and ECF compartments following administration.

Edelman's equation (simplified) defines serum sodium (Na_S) as a function of the total exchangeable sodium and potassium in the body and the TBW: $Na_S = Na_{total\ body} + K_{total\ body}/TBW$, where $Na_{total\ body}$ is the total body sodium content; $K_{total\ body}$ is the total body potassium content; and TBW is the total body water in liters.[2,3] The serum sodium concentration is tightly regulated and thus usually varies by no more than 3%. Regulation of serum sodium occurs via mechanisms that control its determinants: serum osmolality and blood volume. The kidney regulates water excretion through a hypothalamic feedback mechanism, such that the serum osmolality remains relatively constant (275-290 mOsm/kg [mmol/kg]) despite day-to-day variations in water intake. While serum osmolality is primarily determined by the sodium concentration, glucose and blood urea nitrogen (BUN) may contribute significantly at times. Serum osmolality can be estimated as:

$$Osm_S = (2 \times Na_S) + (glucose_S/18) + (BUN/2.8)$$

where Osm_S is the serum osmolality in mOsm/kg; Na_S is the serum sodium concentration in mEq/L; $glucose_S$ is the serum glucose concentration in mg/dL; BUN is the blood urea nitrogen concentration in mg/dL; and 18 and 2.8 are the factors needed to convert from a weight measurement (mg/dL) to a concentration (mmol/L) for glucose and BUN, respectively. Thus, when using SI units the equation becomes:

$$Osm_S = (2 \times Na_S) + glucose_S + BUN$$

where Osm_S is the serum osmolality in mmol/kg; and Na_S, $glucose_S$, and BUN are their respective concentrations in mmol/L.

Arginine vasopressin (AVP), commonly known as antidiuretic hormone (ADH), is synthesized in the hypothalamus and secreted by the posterior pituitary in response to both osmotic and nonosmotic regulators. When the serum osmolality increases by as little as 1% to 2%, AVP is released and binds to vasopressin 2 (V2) receptors on the basolateral surface of renal tubular epithelial cells, resulting in the insertion of water channels (aquaporin 2) into the apical tubular lumen surface of the cell.[4] Water can then pass through the cell into the peritubular capillary space where it is reabsorbed into the systemic circulation. The increase in AVP release also stimulates thirst as an additional means to return serum osmolality toward normal. The combined effect of increased water intake and decreased water excretion (kidney's response to AVP) results in a decrease in the serum osmolality and inhibition of further AVP secretion, once the serum osmolality is restored to normal.

Nonosmotic AVP release occurs when osmoreceptors in the brain detect a 6% to 10% reduction in the effective circulating blood volume or arterial blood pressure. The effective circulating volume is that part of the ECF responsible for organ perfusion. A decrease in the effective circulating volume (more accurately, the blood pressure associated with that volume) activates arterial baroreceptors in the carotid sinus and glomerular afferent arterioles, resulting in stimulation of the renin–angiotensin system and increased angiotensin II synthesis. Angiotensin II stimulates both nonosmotic AVP release and thirst. This volume stimulus can override osmotic inhibition of AVP release. Water conservation then restores the effective circulating volume and blood pressure at the expense of producing a decreased serum osmolality and hyponatremia.[4] While hyponatremia and hypernatremia can be associated with conditions of high, low, or normal ECF sodium and volume, both conditions most commonly result from abnormalities of water homeostasis. To understand treatment options, it is important to note the distinction between *dehydration* (hypertonicity) and *hypovolemia*. Dehydration refers to a loss of TBW producing hypertonicity while hypovolemia (volume depletion) is a deficit in ECF volume.[5,6] Although these terms are often used interchangeably, they are reflective of different processes.

TABLE 49-1 Composition of Common IV Solutions

						Distribution		
Solution	**Dextrose**	**[Na⁺] (mEq/L or mmol/L)**	**[Cl⁻] (mEq/L or mmol/L)**	**Osmolality (mOsm/kg or mmol/kg)**	**Tonicity**	**% ECF**	**% ICF**	**Free water (mL/1,000 mL)**
Dextrose 5% in water	5 g/dL (50 g/L)	0	0	253	Hypotonic	33	67	1,000 mL
0.45% NaCl[a]	0	77	77	154	Hypotonic	67	33	500 mL
Lactated Ringer's	0	130	105	273	Isotonic	97	3	0 mL
0.9% NaCl[b]	0	154	154	308	Isotonic	100	0	0 mL
3% NaCl[c]	0	513	513	1,026	Hypertonic	100	0	–2,331 mL

Cl^-, chloride; ECF, extracellular fluid; ICF, intracellular fluid; IV, intravenous; Na^+, sodium; NaCl, sodium chloride.

[a]Also referred to as "half normal saline."

[b]Also referred to as "normal saline."

[c]This hypertonic solution will result in osmotic removal of water from the intracellular space.

HYPONATREMIA

Epidemiology and Etiology

Hyponatremia, generally defined as a serum sodium concentration less than 135 mEq/L (mmol/L), is the most common electrolyte abnormality encountered in clinical practice in both adults and children.[2,6-9] Although the prevalence is not well established and varies with the patient population studied, it has been estimated to be as high as 28% at the time of admission to an acute care hospital. The prevalence of mild hyponatremia (serum sodium concentration less than 136 mEq/L [mmol/L]) was 42% (28% on admission, 14% during admission); 6.2% of patients evaluated (2.5% on admission, 3.7% during admission) had values less than 126 mEq/L (mmol/L); and only 1.2% (0.5% on admission, 0.7% during admission) had values less than 116 mEq/L (mmol/L). The incidence of hyponatremia (serum sodium concentration less than 136 mEq/L [mmol/L]) was reported to be 21% in patients seen in ambulatory hospital clinics and 7% in community clinics.[10] Drug-induced hyponatremia, especially that associated with thiazide diuretics[11,12] and psychotropic medications,[13,14] is common. Advancing age (older than 30 years) also appears to be a risk factor for hyponatremia, independent of sex.[10]

Residents in nursing homes have a twofold higher incidence of hyponatremia than that observed in age-matched, community-dwelling individuals.[6] More than 75% of these hyponatremic episodes were precipitated by increased intake of hypotonic oral or IV fluids. Similarly, ingestion of excessive volumes of hypotonic fluids (water, sports drinks) has been identified as a key risk factor in the development of exercise-associated hyponatremia in athletes.[15] In one study, women runners had a threefold higher rate of hyponatremia; however, smaller body size and longer racing time, not sex, were the principal factors accounting for the increased incidence.[16]

Recognition of the high prevalence of hyponatremia is essential because this condition is associated with significant morbidity and mortality.[4,17-20] Transient or permanent brain dysfunction in patients with hyponatremia can result from either the acute effects of hypoosmolality or too rapid correction of hypoosmolality. Hyponatremia is predominantly the result of an excess of extracellular water relative to sodium because of impaired water excretion. The kidney normally has the capacity to excrete large volumes of dilute urine after ingestion of a water load. Nonosmotic AVP release, however, can lead to water retention and a decrease in the serum sodium concentration, despite a decrease in both serum and intracellular osmolality. Causes of nonosmotic AVP release include hypovolemia and decreased effective circulating volume as seen in patients with chronic heart failure (HF), nephrosis, and cirrhosis. The syndrome of inappropriate secretion of antidiuretic hormone (SIADH), a common cause of hyponatremia, is associated with some cancers, especially small cell lung cancer, and central nervous system (CNS) damage (eg, traumatic brain injury, meningitis). The pathophysiology, clinical features, and management of hyponatremia are discussed further.

Pathophysiology

Hyponatremia can be associated with normal, increased, or decreased serum osmolality, depending on its cause. Figure 49-1 provides an algorithm for evaluating patients with hyponatremia.[2,21] Hyponatremia in a patient with a normal measured serum osmolality can be seen in those with markedly elevated serum lipids or proteins (hyperproteinemia, multiple myeloma) when flame photometry is the method used to measure the sodium concentration. This *pseudohyponatremia* is an artifact because the elevated lipids or proteins account for a larger than usual proportion of the total sample volume, reducing the percentage of water in the serum (Fig. 49-2). Because sodium is distributed in the water component only, the measured serum sodium concentration will be falsely decreased. The measurement of serum osmolality is not affected, leading to a discrepancy between the calculated and measured serum osmolality. When sodium concentration is measured via ion-selective electrodes, pseudohyponatremia has not been noted because all serum samples are diluted and a constant distribution between water and the solid phase of serum is assumed when the serum sodium concentration is calculated. If the measurement of serum osmolality is

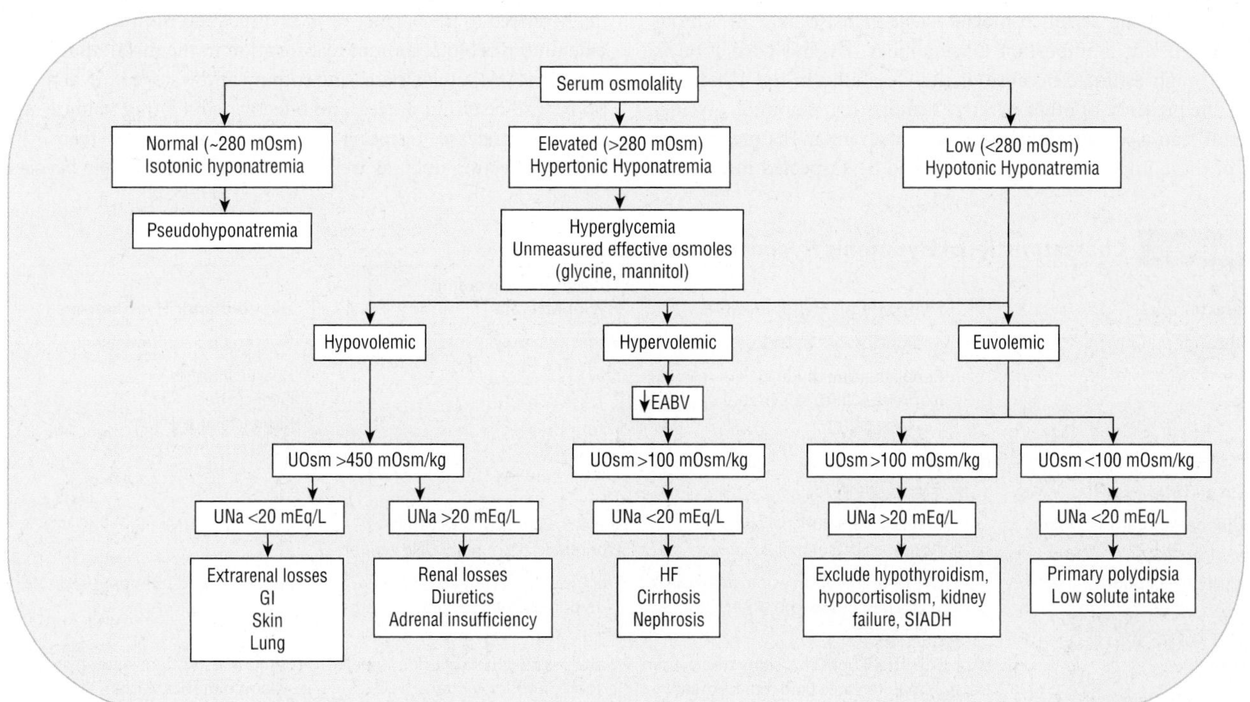

FIGURE 49-1 Diagnostic algorithm for the evaluation of hyponatremia. (HF, heart failure; EABV, effective arterial blood volume; GI, gastrointestinal; SIADH, syndrome of inappropriate secretion of antidiuretic hormone; UNa, urine sodium concentration [values in mEq/L are numerically equivalent to mmol/L]; UOsm, urine osmolality [values in mOsm/kg are numerically equivalent to mmol/kg].)

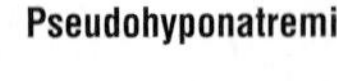

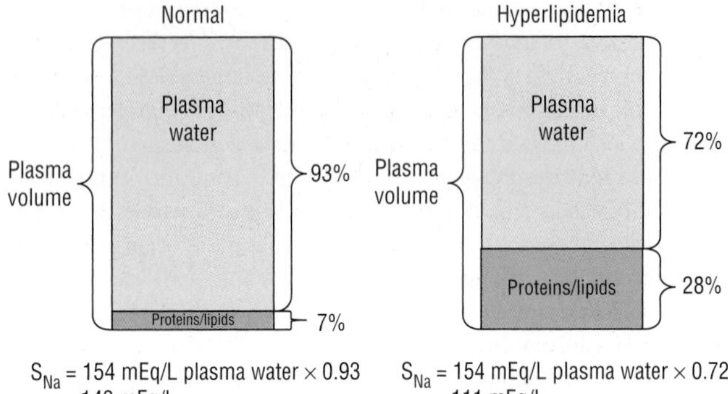

FIGURE 49-2 Elevated lipids or proteins result in a larger discrepancy between the volume of the sample and serum water, leading to a falsely low measurement of the serum sodium concentration when using the method of flame photometry. (S_{Na}, serum sodium concentration [values in mEq/L are numerically equivalent to mmol/L].)

not available, direct potentiometery using a blood gas analyzer will yield the true sodium concentration.[21]

Hyponatremia associated with an increased serum osmolality, hypertonic hyponatremia, is due to the presence of excess, effective osmoles (other than sodium) in the ECF. This type of hyponatremia is most frequently encountered in patients with hyperglycemia. The elevated serum glucose concentration causes diffusion of water from the cells (ICF) into the ECF, thereby decreasing the ICF volume, expanding the ECF volume, and diluting the existing sodium resulting in a decreased serum sodium concentration. The volume of distribution (V_d) of glucose is a complex function of insulin activity, glucose distribution time, ECF volume, and glucose concentration. Using a clinically relevant glucose V_d of 0.3 to 0.5 L/kg, one would predict a 1.5 to 1.9 mEq/L (mmol/L; mean, 1.7 mEq/L [mmol/L]) decrease in the serum sodium concentration for every 100 mg/dL (5.6 mmol/L) increase in the serum glucose concentration above 100 mg/dL (5.6 mmol/L) or 0.29 mmol/L for every 1 mmol/L decrease, and the serum osmolality will increase by 2 mOsm/kg (mmol/kg).[5,22] It is important to remember that this correction is only a rough estimate because of the variability in the V_d of glucose. The presence of other effective osmoles (eg, mannitol, glycine, sorbitol) can also cause hypertonic hyponatremia. The presence of one of these unmeasured osmoles should be suspected in patients with hypertonic hyponatremia when there is a significant osmolal gap, defined as the difference between the measured and calculated serum osmolality.

Hyponatremia associated with decreased serum osmolality, hypotonic hyponatremia, is the most common form of hyponatremia and has many potential causes (Table 49-2). Clinical assessment of ECF volume is an important step in the diagnostic evaluation of a patient with hypotonic hyponatremia. Categorization of these patients into one of three groups (decreased, increased, or clinically normal ECF volume) is the essential first step in identifying the pathophysiologic mechanisms responsible for the hyponatremia and developing an appropriate treatment plan.

Hypovolemic Hypotonic Hyponatremia

Most patients with ECF volume contraction lose fluids that are hypotonic relative to serum and thus can become "transiently" hypernatremic. This scenario includes patients with fluid losses caused by diarrhea, excessive sweating, and diuretics. This transient hypernatremic hyperosmolality results in osmotic AVP release and thirst. If sodium and water losses continue, the resultant hypovolemia results in more AVP release. Patients who then drink water (a hypotonic fluid) or who are given hypotonic IV fluids retain water, and hyponatremia develops. These patients will typically have a urine osmolality greater than 450 mOsm/kg (mmol/kg), reflecting AVP action leading to formation of concentrated urine. The urine sodium concentration will be less than 20 mEq/L (mmol/L) when sodium losses are extrarenal (eg, diarrhea), and greater than 20 mEq/L (mmol/L) in patients with renal sodium losses (eg, thiazide diuretic use or adrenal insufficiency).[23]

2 Hypotonic hyponatremia is relatively common in patients taking thiazide diuretics.[12,21,24] Thiazide diuretic-induced hyponatremia is usually mild and relatively asymptomatic, but occasionally it can be severe and symptomatic.[24] Hyponatremia typically develops within 2 weeks of diuretic initiation, but can occur at any time during therapy, particularly after dosage increases or if other causes of hyponatremia are present.[20,24] Elderly women are at the greatest risk for thiazide diuretic-induced hyponatremia.[21,24]

The mechanism of thiazide diuretic-induced hyponatremia is likely related to the balance of their direct and indirect effects. Thiazide diuretics block sodium reabsorption in the distal tubules of the renal cortex, thereby increasing sodium and water removal from the body. The resulting decrease in effective circulating volume stimulates AVP release, resulting in increased free water reabsorption in the collecting duct, as well as increased water intake because of

TABLE 49-2 Characteristics of Hypotonic Hyponatremic States

Characteristics	Hypovolemic Hyponatremia	Euvolemic (Isovolemic) Hyponatremia	Hypervolemic Hyponatremia
Water and sodium	Sodium loss >> water loss	Water gain only	Water gain >sodium gain
Causes	Renal: thiazide diuretics Nonrenal: diarrhea, cerebral salt-wasting	SIADH	Heart Failure Liver cirrhosis Kidney failure
Effect on TBW	↓↓	↑	↑↑
Effect on TBNa	↓	↔	↑↑
Additional laboratory findings	Renal: UOsm high, UNa high Nonrenal: UOsm high, UNa low	Renal: UOsm low, UNa variable Nonrenal: UOsm high, UNa variable	UOsm high, UNa high
Clinical presentation	Orthostasis, hypotension, tachycardia, dry mucous membranes, CNS changes	Depends on severity of hyponatremia: seizures, lethargy	Peripheral and pulmonary edema, variable blood pressure
Treatment	0.9% NaCl until vital signs stable; then maintenance fluid replacement (D5/0.45% NaCl); sodium replacement if cerebral salt wasting; vaptan contraindicated	Water restriction; demeclocycline; loop diuretics; vaptan	Sodium restriction; water restriction; loop diuretics; vaptan

CNS, central nervous system; a SIADH, syndrome of inappropriate antidiuretic hormone; TBW, total body weight.

stimulation of thirst. Hyponatremia develops when the net result of these effects is the loss of more sodium than water.

Conversely, hyponatremia occurs infrequently with loop diuretics due to their different site of action. Loop diuretics block sodium reabsorption in the ascending limb of the loop of Henle. This action decreases medullary osmolality; thus, when loop diuretic use decreases effective circulating volume and stimulates AVP release, less water reabsorption occurs in the collecting ducts than would occur if the osmolality of the renal medulla were normal. Thiazide diuretics do not alter medullary osmolality because they act in the renal cortex. In addition, most loop diuretics have a shorter half-life than thiazides, and patients can usually replete the urinary sodium and water losses prior to taking the next dose, thereby minimizing AVP stimulation.[25]

Cerebral/renal salt wasting syndrome is a rare condition observed in patients with intracranial disorders such as subarachnoid bleeding and traumatic brain injury, but it can occur in patients without CNS pathology. It results in decreased ECF volume due to profound natriureis. A very high urine sodium concentration, high serum urea, orthostatic hypotension, low central venous pressure, and high urine output suggests cerebral salt wasting rather than SIADH.[21,26]

Euvolemic Hypotonic Hyponatremia

3 Euvolemic (isovolemic) hypotonic hyponatremia is associated with a normal or slightly decreased ECF sodium content and increased TBW and ECF volume. The ECF volume increase is usually not sufficient to cause peripheral or pulmonary edema or other signs of volume overload, and thus patients appear euvolemic upon physical examination. Euvolemic hyponatremia is most often caused by SIADH.

In SIADH, water intake exceeds the kidney's capacity to excrete water, either because of increased AVP release via nonosmotic and/or nonphysiologic processes or enhanced sensitivity of the kidney to AVP. In most patients with SIADH, the urine osmolality will be greater than 100 mOsm/kg (mmol/kg), and the urine sodium concentration will be greater than 20 mEq/L (mmol/L) due to ECF volume expansion (see Table 49-2).

The most common causes of SIADH include tumors such as small cell lung or pancreatic cancer, CNS disorders (eg, head trauma, stroke, meningitis, pituitary surgery), and pulmonary disease (eg, tuberculosis, pneumonia, acute respiratory distress syndrome). Patients with kidney and adrenal insufficiency or hypothyroidism can also present with euvolemic hyponatremia, and the evaluation of patients with suspected SIADH should always include consideration of these disorders. A number of drugs can cause SIADH by enhancing AVP release or its effect on the kidney, or by other mechanisms[13,17,27] (Table 49-3). The differential diagnosis of euvolemic hypotonic hyponatremia also includes primary or psychogenic polydipsia. Patients with this disorder drink more water (usually more than 20 L/day) than the kidneys can excrete as solute-free water. However, unlike in SIADH, AVP secretion is suppressed, resulting in a urine osmolality that is less than 100 mOsm/kg (mmol/kg). The urine sodium is typically low (less than 15 mEq/L [mmol/L]) as a result of dilution.[4,14] Hyponatremia can develop even with more modest water intakes in patients who ingest very low-solute diets.

Hypervolemic Hypotonic Hyponatremia

Hyponatremia associated with ECF volume expansion occurs in conditions in which both the kidney's sodium and water excretion are impaired. Patients with cirrhosis, HF, or nephrotic syndrome have an expanded ECF volume and edema, but a decreased effective arterial blood volume. This decreased volume results in renal sodium retention, and eventually ECF volume expansion and edema. At the same time, there is nonosmotic stimulation of AVP release and water retention in excess of sodium retention, which perpetuates the hyponatremic state.

TABLE 49-3 Potential Causes of SIADH

Drug-Induced		Nondrug-Induced
Barbiturates Bromocriptine Carboplatin Cisplatin Clofibrate Haloperidol Monoamine oxidase inhibitors	Nicotine Opioids Phenothiazines Thioridazine Thiothixene Tricyclic antidepressants	Malignancy (lung, pancreatic, duodenal) CNS (trauma, tumor, meningitis, hemorrhage, stroke) Pulmonary (pneumonia, ARDS, TB) Postoperative state Nausea Anxiety
Increased sensitivity to ADH		
Acetaminophen AVP analogs (desmopressin) Lamotrigine	NSAIDs Oxytocin Tolbutamide	
Mixed or uncertain mechanism		
ACE inhibitors Carbamazepine Chlorpropamide Cyclophosphamide Ecstasy	Moxifloxacin Omeprazole SSRIs Vinca alkaloids	

ACE, angiotensin-converting enzyme; ARDS, acute respiratory distress syndrome; AVP, arginine vasopressin; CNS, central nervous system; NSAIDs, nonsteroidal anti-inflammatory drugs; SIADH, syndrome of inappropriate antidiuretic hormone; SSRIs, selective serotonin receptor inhibitors; TB, tuberculosis.

Clinical **Controversy...**

Traditional maintenance fluids for children provide dextrose and potassium in a hypotonic solution such as 0.45% NaCl or 0.2% NaCl. Concern for the development of hyponatremia has led some clinicians to advocate for the use of isotonic solutions such as 0.9% NaCl for "maintenance" fluids to reduce the incidence of hyponatremia. Isotonic fluids may, in fact, be appropriate for some hospitalized children, but it is important to remember that 'maintenance' fluids are appropriate when used as intended for children who are euvolemic, with no excess ongoing fluid losses and normal kidney function. Excess administration of isotonic fluids can result in sodium overload and metabolic acidosis.

Clinical Presentation

4 Patients with chronic (lasting longer than 48 hours) mild hyponatremia (serum sodium concentration 125-134 mEq/L [mmol/L]) are usually asymptomatic, with hyponatremia often being discovered incidentally when serum electrolytes are measured for other purposes.[28] Mild symptoms of hyponatremia frequently go unnoticed by both clinicians and patients.[18,29] Chronic, mild hyponatremia however has been associated with impairment of attention, posture, and gait, all of which contribute to a substantially increased fall risk. Even "asymptomatic" patients, when formally tested, have impaired attention and gait to a degree that is comparable to symptoms seen with a blood alcohol level of 0.06% (13 mmol/L).[18,30,31]

Patients with moderate (serum sodium concentration 115-124 mEq/L [mmol/L]), severe (serum sodium concentration 110-114 mEq/L [mmol/L]), or rapidly developing hypotonic hyponatremia often present with a range of neurologic symptoms resulting from hypoosmolality-induced brain cell swelling. Classic neurologic symptoms include nausea, malaise, headache, lethargy, restlessness,

CLINICAL PRESENTATION Hyponatremia

General

- Patients are usually asymptomatic.
- Symptoms are primarily neurologic.
- Presence and severity of symptoms depend on the magnitude and rapidity of onset of hyponatremia.
- Other symptoms may be present depending on the etiology of the hyponatremia (eg, dry mucous membranes, tachycardia, and hypotension with hypovolemia).

Symptoms

- Mild: Nausea and malaise
- Moderate: Headache, lethargy, restlessness, disorientation
- Severe: Seizures, coma, respiratory arrest, brainstem herniation, death

Laboratory Tests

- Serum sodium concentration less than 135 mEq/L (mmol/L)
- Plasma osmolality and urine sodium concentration can be helpful
- Other tests: Serum glucose and lipids and kidney and thyroid function tests

and disorientation. In severe cases, seizures, coma, respiratory arrest, brainstem herniation, and death can occur.

The presence and severity of these symptoms depend on both the degree of the hyponatremia and the rate at which it develops. The magnitude of the hyponatremia is important because serum osmolality decreases in direct proportion to the serum sodium concentration, and water movement into brain cells increases as serum osmolality decreases. The rate of change of the serum osmolality is important because brain cells are not able to rapidly adjust intracellular osmolality to minimize cellular volume changes.[3,32] When a decline in serum osmolality causes water movement into brain cells, inorganic Cl^- and K^+, and organic osmolytes, such as taurine, glutamate, and myoinositol, move out of the cells to decrease intracellular osmolality and minimize intracellular water shifts.[31] The components of this adaptive mechanism occur over different time frames, with sodium and potassium efflux occurring within minutes to hours and organic osmolyte efflux occurring within hours to days.[32,33] Maximal compensation for decreased serum osmolality typically requires up to 48 hours. Thus, acute changes in serum osmolality are more likely to be associated with symptoms. Concurrent respiratory failure and hypoxemia increase the risk of adverse neurologic outcomes because hypoxemia diminishes the brain's capacity to actively transport solute out of cells, leading to a higher incidence of cerebral edema.[32,33] Children and women have poorer clinical outcomes than adults and men, respectively. For example, post menopausal women with acute hypervolemic hypotonic hyponatremia have a 25-fold higher risk of death or permanent neurological damage than men.[34] Hyponatremia is a severe risk factor for morbidity and mortality in patients with HF and cirrhosis.[4]

In addition to neurologic symptoms, patients with hypovolemic hyponatremia present with signs and symptoms of hypovolemia, including dry mucous membranes, decreased skin turgor, tachycardia, decreased jugular venous pressure, hypotension, and orthostatic hypotension. These findings are often helpful in identifying the type of hyponatremia present.

5 The brain's adaptation to a chronic change in the serum osmolality leads to development of neurologic symptoms if hyponatremia (hypoosmolality) is corrected too rapidly. The combination of the adaptive decrease in intracellular osmolality and rapid increase in serum osmolality results in rapid and excessive water movement out of the brain cells and ICF volume depletion. Thus, too rapid correction of the serum sodium concentration can lead to an acute decrease in brain cell volume, which contributes to the pathogenesis of *osmotic demyelination syndrome* (ODS), or central pontine myelinolysis.[4,35] Demyelinated lesions seen on magnetic resonance imaging most often occur in the central pons, but ODS can extend to extrapontine structures.[23] Patients with ODS may develop hyperreflexia, para- or quadriparesis, parkinsonism, pseudobulbar palsy, *locked-in syndrome* (a condition in which a patient is aware and awake but cannot move or communicate verbally due to complete paralysis of nearly all voluntary muscles in the body except for the eyes), or death in approximately 1 to 7 days.[2,16,36] Patients with a significant degree of cerebral adaptation (eg, chronic serum sodium concentration less than 110 mEq/L [mmol/L]) to hypotonic hyponatremia are at highest risk of developing ODS because as these patients have lower intracellular osmolalities at the initiation of therapy, there is a greater decrease in intracellular volume in brain cells when the serum osmolality is raised too rapidly.[35] Other concomitant conditions that increase the risk of ODS include alcoholism, liver failure, orthotopic liver transplantation, potassium depletion, and malnutrition. Thus, if duration of hyponatremia is unknown, then it is generally safer to treat as if it is chronic when developing an initial treatment plan.

TREATMENT

6 General guidelines for the treatment of patients with hyponatremia are shown in Table 49-4.[2,22,24,27,37] Application of these principles to the treatment of various forms of hypotonic hyponatremia is discussed in the following sections.

Desired Outcome

Regardless of the type or cause of hyponatremia, treatment goals for all patients are to resolve the underlying cause of the sodium and ECF volume imbalance, if possible, and to safely correct the sodium and water derangements. The treatment plan for a patient with hyponatremia depends on the underlying cause and the severity of symptoms. Patients with an acute onset of hyponatremia or severe symptoms require more aggressive therapy to correct the hypotonicity. The initial goal for these patients is to increase serum tonicity just enough to control severe symptoms; this typically requires only a small increase (5%) in serum sodium concentration. Once

TABLE 49-4 General Guidelines for Treatment of Hyponatremia

- For both short- and long-term management, treat the underlying cause of hyponatremia.
- Appropriate treatment of hypotonic hyponatremia requires balancing the risks of hyponatremia vs the risk of ODS.
- Patients who acutely develop moderate to severe hyponatremia and/or patients who have severe symptoms are at greatest risk and potentially benefit most from more rapid correction of hyponatremia.
- Correction of hypovolemic hypotonic hyponatremia is usually best accomplished with 0.9% NaCl, as these patients have both sodium and water deficits.
- Active correction of euvolemic and hypervolemic hypotonic hyponatremia in patients who do not require rapid correction is usually best accomplished by water restriction. Demeclocycline, AVP vasopressin 2-receptor antagonists (*vaptans*), or 0.9% NaCl plus a loop diuretic (furosemide, bumetanide) can be used if the initial response to water restriction is not adequate.
- In patients with severe symptoms, 3% NaCl (possibly combined with a loop diuretic) should initially be used to more rapidly correct the hyponatremia. A loop diuretic can be administered concurrently with 3% NaCl to enhance the serum sodium correction by increasing free water excretion.
- Long-term management will be required for patients in whom the underlying cause of hyponatremia cannot be corrected. Depending on the cause, water restriction, increasing sodium intake, and/or an AVP antagonist (vaptan) may be used.

AVP, arginine vasopressin; ODS, osmotic demyelination syndrome.

severe symptoms have abated, then continued serum sodium correction should be achieved at a controlled rate. Patients who are asymptomatic or who have only mild to moderate symptoms do not require rapid correction of the serum sodium concentration. Treatment is dictated by the underlying etiology. In all cases, the goal is to avoid an increase in the serum sodium concentration of more than 12 mEq/L (mmol/L) in 24 hours or 0.5 mEq/L (mmol/L) per hour.[2,4,21,28,37] However, when duration of hyponatremia is unknown, a correction rate of no more than 6 to 8 mEq/L (mmol/L) or 0.33 mEq/L/h (mmol/L/h) is prudent to avoid ODS.[2]

ACUTE OR SEVERELY SYMPTOMATIC HYPOTONIC HYPONATREMIA

A patient who has or is at high risk of experiencing severe symptoms caused by hyponatremia should receive either 3% NaCl (513 mEq/L [mmol/L]) or 0.9% NaCl (154 mEq/L [mmol/L]) until severe symptoms resolve.[2,6,24,29,38] Resolution of severe symptoms frequently requires only a small (approximately 5%) increase in serum sodium concentration; although, some clinicians suggest that the initial safe target should be a serum sodium concentration of approximately 120 mEq/L (mmol/L).[6,39] The relative concentrations of urine sodium and potassium (osmotically effective urine cations) must be compared with those of the infusate in planning a treatment regimen for patients with hypotonic hyponatremia. For the serum sodium concentration to increase after a NaCl infusion, the sodium concentration of the infusate must exceed the sum of the urinary sodium and potassium concentrations to produce an effective net free-water excretion.

Patients with SIADH often have urinary concentrations of osmotically effective cations that exceed the sodium concentration of 0.9% NaCl. In this case, use of isotonic NaCl can actually worsen hyponatremia.[40] These patients should be preferentially treated with 3% NaCl. The relatively high urinary sodium concentration in patients with SIADH is due to ECF expansion, which minimizes sodium reabsorption along the nephron. When the urine osmolality exceeds 300 mOsm/kg (mmol/kg), it is generally advisable to administer an IV loop diuretic, not only to increase solute-free water excretion but also to prevent volume overload, which can result from hypertonic sodium chloride. Intravenous furosemide 20 to 40 mg every 6 hours or bumetanide 0.5 to 1 mg every 2 to 3 hours for several doses is generally sufficient to prevent volume overload and to decrease the urinary concentration of osmotically active cations to less than 150 mEq/L (mmol/L). If intermittent loop diuretic doses are not sufficient to manage edema, then continuous infusions have been used. Either furosemide 20 to 40 mg given intravenously followed by a 10 to 40 mg/h infusion or bumetanide 1 mg given intravenously followed by a 0.5 to 2 mg/h infusion can be used.

Patients with hypovolemic hypotonic hyponatremia can be treated with 0.9% NaCl. In contrast to patients with SIADH, patients with this condition avidly reabsorb sodium throughout the nephron because the effective circulating blood volume is decreased. Thus, the urine sodium concentration is often less than 20 mEq/L (mmol/L), substantially less than the sodium content of 0.9% NaCl. While the use of 3% NaCl will correct hyponatremia in these patients, it will not correct the hypovolemia; thus, its use should be reserved for patients with severe symptoms requiring very rapid correction of the serum sodium concentration.

Acute hypervolemic hypotonic hyponatremia is particularly problematic to manage because the sodium and volume needed to minimize the risk of cerebral edema or seizures can worsen already compromised liver, heart, or kidney function. These patients generally should be treated with 3% NaCl and initiation of fluid (water) restriction. Loop diuretic therapy will also likely be required to facilitate urinary free water excretion.

Determination of a Sodium Chloride Infusion Regimen

Multiple methods for determining the correct NaCl infusion regimen for a patient with hyponatremia can be used.[2,4,21,24,36,38,39] These empiric approaches provide an initial estimate of the correct infusion regimen. Several complex equations have been derived, but improved outcomes using these equations have not been demonstrated.[24,36]

One common approach is to estimate the change in serum sodium concentration resulting from the infusion of 1 L of 3% or 0.9% NaCl. An example of this approach is shown in Table 49-5. Another method involves calculating the sodium deficit, then replacing one-third of the deficit in the first 6 hours and the remaining two-thirds over the following 24 to 48 hours or longer depending on the acuity of the decrease in the serum sodium concentration. Sodium deficit can be calculated using the following equation: Na deficit (mEq or mmol) = $[(Na_D - Na_S) \times TBW]$

where Na_D is the goal or desired serum sodium (usually 120-125 mEq/L [mmol/L] to avoid too rapid or over correction); Na_S is the patient's current serum sodium concentration; and, TBW is the patient's current TBW calculated as shown in Table 49-5.

Using these methods, the appropriate infusion volume for a given patient can be estimated using the desired proportion of the estimated change that would result from a 1-L infusion or the amount of fluid needed to provide the calculated sodium deficit, respectively. The final step is to calculate an appropriate infusion rate for the calculated volume that will increase the serum sodium concentration by 6 to 12 mEq/L (mmol/L) in 24 hours (see table 49-5). Using desmopressin in combination with 3% NaCl to minimize the risk of treating hyponatremia has been suggested but is generally not recommended.[2]

TABLE 49-5 Assessment and Treatment of Euvolemic Hyponatremia

Change in serum sodium concentration after an IV fluid bolus

$$\Delta Na_S = (Na_{IV} - Na_S) / (TBW + volume_{IV})$$

ΔNa_S, change in serum sodium concentration; Na_{IV}, sodium concentration of infusate (eg, 154 mEq/L [mmol/L] for 0.9% NaCl; 513 mEq/L [mmol/L] for 3% NaCl); Na_S, initial serum sodium concentration; TBW, total body water (L); and $volume_{IV}$, volume of infused fluid (L)

TBW can be estimated as:

- Children and men younger than 70 years: 0.6 L/kg × wt (kg)
- Men older than 70 years and women younger than 70 years: 0.5 L/kg × wt (kg)
- Women older than 70 years: 0.45 L/kg × wt (kg)
- Dehydrated, older patients: 0.4 L/kg × wt (kg)

where wt is the current body weight

Clinical Example

A 66-year-old man (weight, 70 kg [154 lb]; height, 178 cm [5 ft 10 in]) presents with nausea, headache, and confusion which developed over the past 3 days. Ten days ago, he began taking carbamazepine for trigeminal neuralgia. His serum sodium concentration on admission to the emergency department was 109 mEq/L (mmol/L). He is diagnosed with SIADH.

Plan of Care

1. Discontinue carbamazepine (the likely etiology of his SIADH).
2. Admit to the hospital for correction of hyponatremia.
3. Increase the serum sodium concentration by no more than 6 to 12 mEq/L (mmol/L) during first 24 hours and no higher than 120 mEq/L (mmol/L); thus, the goal is to increase the sodium concentration by 11 mEq/L (mmol/L).
4. Due to degree of hyponatremia (less than 110 mEq/L [mmol/L]) and the presence of moderate to severe symptoms, give 3% NaCl.

Calculate the change in serum sodium after 1 L infusion of 3% NaCl:

$$\Delta Na_S = (513\ mEq/L - 109\ mEq/L)/[(0.5\ L/kg \times 70\ kg) + 1\ L] = 11.2\ mEq/L \text{ or } 1.12\ mEq/100\ mL$$

(Note: In SI units, the calculation is the same using mmol/L rather than mEq/L.) Infusion of 1 L of 3% NaCl will result in a 11.2 mEq/L (mmol/L) rise in the serum sodium concentration. An 11 mEq/L (mmol/L) increase is desired; thus, the appropriate infusion volume is 982 mL [(11 mEq/L/11.2 mEq/L) × 1,000 mL] or [(11 mmol/L/11.2 mmol/L) × 1,000 mL].

(Note: The approach to this calculation would be similar if 0.9% NaCl was used, except that for each 1 L infusion, the expected increase in serum sodium concentration would be only 1.25 mEq/L (mmol/L), and an infusion volume of approximately 8.8 L would be required to achieve the targeted serum sodium concentration.)

5. Moderate to severe symptoms: serum sodium concentration should be increased by approximately 1.5 mEq/L/h (mmol/L/h) over the first 2 to 4 hours of treatment for a total of 3 to 6 mEq/L [mmol/L] or until the symptoms have resolved. An initial infusion rate of 114 mL/h for the first 2 to 4 hours is needed.
6. Check serum sodium concentration every 1 to 3 hours.
7. Once symptoms subside, continue infusion rate at approximately 23 to 31 mL/h for the next 20 to 22 hours, to slowly correct hyponatremia. Monitor serum sodium concentration every 4 hours or more often if serum sodium is rapidly changing.

Clinical **Controversy...**

Clinicians often disagree whether or not to administer 3% NaCl to patients with symptomatic hypotonicity. An Advantage of 3% NaCl is more rapid correction of serum sodium concentration with a smaller infusion volume. The disadvantage of 3% NaCl is a higher risk of too rapid correction of serum sodium concentration causing ODS. The clinician must carefully consider the cause and the rapidity of development of the patient's hyponatremia as well as the relative risk of slower correction of the hyponatremia versus the development of ODS.

Evaluation of Therapeutic Outcomes

Patients with severely symptomatic hypotonic hyponatremia should be admitted to the intensive care unit (ICU) or other setting where frequent monitoring of neurologic symptoms and volume status is feasible. Examination of the heart, lungs, and neurologic status should be performed frequently during the initial 12 hours of therapy. The serum sodium concentration should be measured at least every 2 to 4 hours, and the urine osmolality, sodium, and potassium should be measured every 4 to 6 hours over the first day of therapy so that the infusion rate can be adjusted to avoid increasing the serum sodium too rapidly.[2]

NONEMERGENT HYPOVOLEMIC HYPOTONIC HYPONATREMIA

Most patients with hypovolemic hypotonic hyponatremia are either asymptomatic or have only mild-to-moderate symptoms so they do not require rapid correction of their hyponatremia. Many of these patients are at higher risk of developing ODS if serum sodium correction occurs too rapidly because they have chronic hyponatremia that has been maximally compensated for by the brain's osmotic adaptation. Treatment of these patients should include correction of the underlying condition, if possible, and administration of 0.9% NaCl to correct the hypovolemia. This solution will replace the existing sodium and water deficits, and its use carries a lower risk of too rapid correction than using 3% NaCl.

The ECF deficit can be estimated based on sex, change in body weight, and age. One method to estimate the ECF deficit and an example of its use is shown in Table 49-6. If the patient's previous weight is not known, the ECF deficit can be roughly estimated based on clinical signs and symptoms. The presence of hyponatremia suggests an ECF deficit of 5% or more, whereas the presence of orthostatic hypotension suggests an ECF deficit of at least 10% to 15%. An isotonic solution (0.9% NaCl or Lactated Ringer's) would be optimal to correct the patient's volume deficit because essentially 100% of it will remain in the ECF space (see Table 49-1). The overriding initial treatment goal is to restore effective circulating volume; thus, it might be necessary to infuse 0.9% NaCl at 200 to 400 mL/h until symptoms of hypovolemia improve. The infusion rate can then be decreased to 100 to 150 mL/h so that the serum sodium concentration increases by no more than 6 to 12 mEq/L (mmol/L) or 0.5 to 1 mEq/L/h (mmol/L/h) over the initial 24 hours. Fluids should be given rapidly enough and in sufficient quantity to restore and maintain adequate tissue perfusion without overloading the cardiovascular system. The patient's underlying heart and kidney function will determine how well fluid replacement is tolerated. For example, infusion of 0.9% NaCl at a rate greater than 250 mL/h should be used cautiously in patients with left ventricular dysfunction or severe kidney dysfunction.

It is important to recognize that the rate of increase in the serum sodium concentration can substantially increase once hypovolemia has been corrected if infusion rates are not adjusted appropriately.[2] When the ECF volume is restored, AVP secretion will stop,

TABLE 49-6 Assessment and Treatment of Hypotonic Hypovolemic Hyponatremia

Calculating ECF Deficit

$$\text{ECF deficit (mL)} = \text{ECF}_{normal} - \text{ECF}_{current}$$

where ECF volume = 0.33 × TBW

Clinical Example

A 75-year-old woman (height, 168 cm [5 ft 6 in]; usual weight, 50 kg [110 lb]) was started on hydrochlorothiazide 25 mg once daily 10 days ago for hypertension. She presents with complaints of mild nausea and dizziness when she stands up. Her current weight is 45 kg (99 lb). Upon physical examination she has dry mucous membranes and orthostatic hypotension. Her serum sodium concentration is 126 mEq/L (mmol/L).

Calculate the ECF deficit

ECF deficit = (50 kg × 0.4 L/kg × 0.33) − (45 kg × 0.4 L/kg × 0.33) = 660 mL

(Note: TBW = 0.4 L/kg used because she is a dehydrated older patient; see Box 49-1)

Calculate the expected increase in the serum sodium after infusion of 1 L of 0.9% NaCl (see Box 49-1):

ΔNa_S with 1 L of infusate = [154 mEq/L − 126 mEq/L]/ [(0.4 L/kg × 45 kg) + 1 L] = 1.47 mEq/L (mmol/L)

The patient's serum sodium concentration will be 127.5 mEq/L (mmol/L) following the infusion of 1 L 0.9% NaCl

Treatment goals: Restore effective circulating volume and correct serum sodium concentration

Treatment plan:

1. Infuse 0.9% NaCl at 200 to 250 mL/h until symptoms of hypovolemia improve; then decrease infusion to 150 to 200 mL/h so that the serum sodium concentration increases by no more than 6 to 12 mEq/L (mmol/L) or 0.5 to 1 mEq/L/h (mmol/L/h) over the initial 24 hours. Rate depends on patient status.
2. Hold thiazide diuretic until volume status is restored.
3. Consider restarting diuretic at lower dose, for example, 12.5 mg once daily, if needed.

and a rapid water diuresis can ensue, which can potentially result in an increase in the serum sodium concentration at a rate greater than desired. Estimation of the patient's ECF deficit at the start of therapy can be helpful. If the serum sodium concentration is observed to be increasing at a rate greater than 0.5 mEq/L/h (mmol/L/h), the infusate can be changed to 0.45% NaCl, and the infusion rate set to one that slows the rate of increase in the serum sodium concentration. In general, 0.45% NaCl should not be infused alone as this solution is hypo-osmolar (osmolality is 154 mOsm/L), and its infusion may result in red blood cell hemolysis. Most often, Dextrose 5%/0.45% NaCl is infused to provide an isotonic solution. Potassium depletion or repletion can also affect hyponatremia and its correction. One mEq (mmol) of retained potassium equals 1 mEq (mmol) retained sodium; thus, if concomitant hypokalemia is corrected at the same time as the hyponatremia, too rapid correction of hyponatremia can occur.[2]

Evaluation of Therapeutic Outcomes

Patients presenting with evidence of volume depletion should be reexamined frequently during the initial few hours of therapy. The serum sodium concentration should be measured every 2 to 4 hours to allow timely adjustment of the rate and composition of IV fluids to avoid too rapid increase in the serum sodium concentration. In patients with a history of HF or kidney insufficiency, 0.9% NaCl should be administered judiciously with frequent cardiopulmonary assessments so that the infusion rate can be appropriately decreased at the earliest sign of pulmonary congestion.

NONEMERGENT EUVOLEMIC HYPOTONIC HYPONATREMIA

The fact that an individual's neurological performance is restored to normal with correction of hyponatremia provides a rationale for therapeutic management of all patients to maintain their serum sodium concentration at or above 130 mEq/L (mmol/L), if possible. Long-term management is thus required for patients in whom the underlying cause of hyponatremia is not readily correctable.

The treatment of SIADH always involves restricting water and correcting the underlying cause (see Table 49-2). Drugs that could be contributing should be identified and discontinued. The goal of treatment is to induce negative water balance by restricting water intake to less than 1,000 to 1,200 mL/day, such that water losses from insensible sources (skin and lung) and from obligate urine and stool losses exceed intake. Daily insensible water losses via skin and lungs are approximately 900 mL/day; whereas approximately 200 mL and a minimum of 500 mL/day is lost in stool and urine, respectively. Because approximately 850 mL of water per day is ingested in food, and an additional 350 mL are generated from oxidative processes, this degree of water restriction should result in a negative water balance of several hundred milliliters per day. Other therapy goals include keeping the serum sodium concentration between 125 and 130 mEq/L (mmol/L) to prevent symptoms of hypotonicity and avoiding iatrogenic hypo- or hypervolemia.

Patients with chronic SIADH who are unable to restrict water sufficiently to maintain the serum sodium between 120 and 125 mEq/L (mmol/L) can be treated by increasing solute intake with NaCl and/or administration of a loop diuretic. NaCl tablets increase the obligatory daily solute excretion, which augments the kidney's capacity for water excretion. The goal is to increase the daily solute intake and excretion to approximately 900 mOsm (mmol) per day. Because an average diet contains approximately 600 mOsm (mmol), 9 g of NaCl would be required to increase the osmolar excretion to 900 mOsm/day (mmol/day) (each 1 g NaCl tablet contains 17 mmol of sodium and 17 mmol of chloride). Because ECF volume expansion is an expected adverse effect, a loop diuretic should be administered concurrently to avoid pulmonary and peripheral edema. Loop diuretics will also enhance water excretion by limiting the formation of the medullary concentration gradient.

Demeclocycline is a treatment option in patients with SIADH whose serum sodium concentration is not adequately controlled by water restriction alone or as an alternative to water restriction. Demeclocycline, a semisynthetic tetracycline antibiotic, essentially causes nephrogenic diabetes insipidus by inhibiting tubular AVP activity, resulting in increased free water excretion. The use of demeclocycline in SIADH is largely based on clinical experience rather than data from clinical trials.[41] The usual demeclocycline dosage is 300 mg given orally two to four times daily. Because of its delayed onset of action (3-6 days), this agent has no role in the acute management of severe hyponatremia, and dosage adjustments should be made no more frequently than every 3 to 4 days.[42] Demeclocycline should not be used in patients with liver disease or compromised fluid intake, who are at high risk for demeclocycline-induced renal tubular toxicity and acute kidney failure,[42,43] in children younger than 8 years because it can interfere with tooth and bone development, and in pregnant women.

The usual therapeutic options of water restriction, loop diuretic, and increased sodium intake have recently been augmented with the introduction of the vaptans. These agents can be used to treat SIADH, as well as other causes of euvolemic and hypervolemic hypotonic hyponatremia.[42,44-49]

Blockade of AVP binding can occur at one or more of its three distinct receptors: V1, predominantly found in the liver, CNS, and cardiomyocytes; V2, located in the distal nephron; and V3, located in the anterior pituitary and pancreas. Selective V2-receptor antagonism prevents aquaporin-2 water channel transport to the apical surface, thereby decreasing AVP-dependent water reabsorption in the collecting duct. The inhibition of AVP activity leads to excretion of large volumes of water, decreased urine osmolality, and thus an increase in the serum sodium concentration.[4] These positive outcomes are achieved without significantly increasing electrolyte excretion; thus, these agents also have been called "aquaretics." Vaptans are not effective in patients with stage 4 or 5 chronic kidney disease.[49] New compounds are being investigated, but only two vaptans are currently marketed in the United States.

Conivaptan (Vaprisol®, Astellas Pharma US, Inc., North Brook, IL), a mixed vasopressin V1- and V2-receptor antagonist, is FDA-labeled for use in the treatment of acute euvolemic and hypervolemic hyponatremia in hospitalized patients. Its utility in the treatment of chronic hyponatremia is limited because it is only available as an IV formulation, is a moderate CYP3A4 inhibitor, and is not FDA-labeled for use in patients with HF.

Tolvaptan (Samsca®, Otsuka Pharmaceutical Co, Ltd, Tokyo, Japan) is an oral, nonpeptide selective AVP V2-receptor blocker with a greater affinity for the V2 receptor than endogenous AVP. It is FDA-labeled for use in the treatment of clinically significant (serum sodium concentration less than 125 mEq/L [mmol/L]) euvolemic or hypervolemic hyponatremia or less marked symptomatic hyponatremia that is unresponsive to other therapeutic interventions in patients with HF, cirrhosis, and SIADH. It appears to be safe and effective when given alone at promoting aquaresis and raising serum sodium concentration by 3.6 mEq/L (mmol/L) at 4 days and 4.4 mEq/L (mmol/L) at 30 days in both short- and intermediate-term studies (SALT-1 and SALT-2), respectively.[46,50] However, the average fluid intake was approximately 2 L per day for patients in these studies which may have limited tolvaptan's efficacy. The percent of patients with normal serum sodium concentrations (greater than 135 mEq/L [mmol/L]) at one month was 53% (SALT-1) and 58% (SALT-2) for tolvaptan versus 25% (both studies) for placebo. When used alone, tolvaptan appears to be superior to furosemide or water restriction, and when given in combination with furosemide, synergistic effects have been noted.[51] Approximately 15% of patients do not significantly respond to vaptan therapy.[52] Therapeutic resistance or failure with vaptan therapy could be due to high circulating AVP concentrations, AVP-independent impaired urinary dilution, excessive water intake, or an activating V2-receptor mutation causing nephrogenic SIADH.[49] There are currently no pharmacogenomic data for the G protein-coupled receptor family of AVP receptors or any of the available vaptans that can be used to individualize therapy.[53]

Tolvaptan is primarily metabolized to inactive metabolites by CYP3A4 and less than 1% is eliminated unchanged in the urine; thus clinicians should avoid its use in those receiving potent CYP3A4 inhibitors (eg, ketaconazole, clarithromycin, itraconazole, ritonivir). Concomitant therapy with P-glycoprotein inhibitors and grapefruit juice has also been noted to result in increased serum tolvaptan concentrations. For example, digoxin steady-state concentrations increased 20%, peak concentrations increased approximately 30%, and renal clearance decreased 59% when given concomitantly with tolvaptan (60 mg/day).[54] Conversely, the optimal benefits of tolvaptan therapy may not be realized and the dosage may need to be increased in patients who are receiving potent CYP3A4 inducers (eg, phenytoin, phenobarbital, St. John's Wort). Dose linearity has been observed within the therapeutic range, and based on its terminal half-life (5-12 hours after 7 days or more of therapy), minimal accumulation occurs.[55,56] The usual starting tolvaptan dosage is 15 mg given orally once daily. Tolvaptan has an oral bioavailabilty of about 56%, and its activity peaks at 2 to 4 hours after the dose. For patients who can not take tolvaptan tablets orally, the tablets can be crushed, suspended in water and administered via a nasogastric tube, but a 25% mean decrease in the tolvaptan area under the concentration-time curve has been demonstrated in healthy adults with this administration method.[57] If, after 24 hours, a greater increase in serum sodium concentration is needed, the dosage may be increased to 30 mg once daily, and after another 24 hours, to a maximum of 60 mg once daily. Tolvaptan therapy is contraindicated in those patients needing rapid correction of their serum sodium concentration, those unable to sense or respond appropriately to thirst, patients with hypovolemic hyponatremia, patients taking strong CYP3A4 inhibitors, and patients who are anuric. Vaptan use should be avoided with hypertonic saline (eg, 3% NaCl) due to the risk of too rapid and/or overcorrection of the serum sodium concentration. Among clinical trial participants who had a serum sodium concentration less than 125 mEq/L (mmol/L) at the start of tolvaptan therapy, the most common adverse events were thirst, dry mouth, weakness, constipation, hyperglycemia, and urinary frequency; although, these adverse events have rarely necessitated therapy discontinuation. Reversible hepatic transaminase elevations have also been reported. However, irreversible liver damage was reported in three patients in a large clinical trial evaluating the use of tolvaptan in patients with autosomal dominant polycystic kidney disease.[58] The dosages in this trial were two to four times higher than those used for hyponatremia and the length of therapy was longer than 30 days. As a result, the FDA issued a warning that tolvaptan should not be used for more than 30 days; should not be used by anyone with liver disease, including cirrhosis; and if any sign of liver injury occurs during therapy, it should be stopped. To reduce the ODS risk, the FDA-approved labeling includes a boxed warning stating that tolvaptan therapy should begin or resume only in a hospital where the patient's serum sodium concentration can be closely monitored. A medication guide is included in the package insert given to all patients with each prescription.

The vaptans have dramatic effects on water excretion, and the marketing of tolvaptan represented the first significant breakthrough in the therapy of hyponatremia and disorders of fluid homeostasis since the introduction of loop diuretics. However, the role of vaptans in the clinical management of patients with SIADH and HF is still unclear, especially given their high cost.[49] It is still unknown if vaptans decrease length of hospitalization, rehospitalization rates, morbidity, or increase quality of life. The association between copeptin peptide concentrations and tolvaptan response was recently investigated in patients with HF and may help determine the most appropriate patients for vaptan use.[59,60]

Evaluation of Therapeutic Outcomes

The serum sodium concentration should be measured every 24 to 48 hours after water restriction is initiated until it stabilizes at a concentration at or above 125 mEq/L (mmol/L). A continued decline in the serum sodium concentration would indicate either nonadherence to the prescribed water restriction or the need for stricter restriction. Serum sodium concentration should be monitored every 4 hours after tolvaptan administration. When the serum sodium has increased by 6 to 8 mEq/L (mmol/L), oral water or IV Dextrose 5% in water (D_5W) should be given to replace urine output to minimize the risk of overcorrecting the serum sodium concentration and development of ODS. In the SALT trials, only 1.8% of patients exceeded the daily limit for changes in serum sodium; however, most of the patients had serum sodium concentrations greater than 130 mEq/L (mmol/L) and were protected from overcorrection by thirst, so the risk of sodium overcorrection in clinical practice may be greater.[46] Once the serum sodium concentration is stable at 125 mEq/L (mmol/L) or higher, the patient should be evaluated every 2 to 4 weeks to assess neurologic status and to obtain serum and urine sodium, potassium, and osmolality. Volume status assessments (eg, blood pressure, mucous membranes, skin turgor, and heart and lung examination) should also be done, particularly in patients who are being treated with NaCl tablets and/or loop diuretics.

NONEMERGENT HYPERVOLEMIC HYPOTONIC HYPONATREMIA

The initial treatment goals for patients with asymptomatic or minimally symptomatic hypotonic hyponatremia and an expanded ECF volume include achieving a negative water balance while minimizing rapid changes in cell volume until the serum sodium concentration is at or above 125 mEq/L (mmol/L). Management involves correction of the underlying cause, when possible, as well as water restriction to an intake of less than 1,000 to 1,200 mL/day. Additionally, dietary sodium intake should be restricted to 1,000 to 2,000 mg/day, depending on the degree of ECF volume expansion and edema.

The severity of hypervolemic hypotonic hyponatremia is directly related to the severity of HF and is associated with poorer short- and long-term prognoses once serum sodium concentrations fall below 137 mEq/L (mmol/L).[61,62] Patients with hypervolemic hypotonic hyponatremia caused by HF should be treated with measures that can potentially improve cardiac contractility and effective circulating volume, thereby limiting nonosmotic AVP release. Therapeutic options include digitalis or afterload reduction with angiotensin-converting enzyme inhibitors (ACEIs) or angiotensin II receptor blockers (ARBs). Of these, only ACEIs have been shown in clinical trials to be of benefit in partially correcting hyponatremia in patients with HF[63]; however, correction of sodium with ACEIs has not been shown to lead to better outcomes.[64] No specific ACEI offers any particular advantage for this indication, and the dosage should be titrated to keep the systolic blood pressure between 100 and 130 mm Hg. Dose-limiting adverse effects of ACEIs include hyperkalemia (serum potassium concentration greater than 5.5 mEq/L [mmol/L]) and impaired kidney function. The benefits and risks of continuing ACEI use must be weighed carefully in each case, but a decrease in glomerular filtration rate (GFR) of less than 30% that stabilizes within 2 months of beginning ACEI therapy generally does not require ACEI dosage reduction or discontinuation.[61]

Other potentially treatable causes of asymptomatic hyponatremia associated with an expanded ECF volume include nephrotic syndrome and cirrhosis. ACEIs can be used to decrease proteinuria in patients with nephrotic syndrome, leading to partial correction of hypoalbuminemia and to a decrease in nonosmotic AVP release. Patients with advanced cirrhosis can benefit from placement of a transjugular intrahepatic portosystemic shunt, which can increase the effective circulating volume and thus reduce nonosmotic AVP release. This procedure can potentially exacerbate or precipitate hepatic encephalopathy and should be avoided in patients with a history of encephalopathy.

Vaptans have also been used for the treatment of hypervolemic hypotonic hyponatremia in patients with HF or cirrhosis.[44,46,65,68] As previously mentioned, an FDA warning was issued regarding the use of tolvaptan in patients with liver dysfunction due to the potential for further liver injury.[58] Conivaptan would not be an ideal choice for patients with cirrhosis due to its mixed antagonism of the V1 and V2 receptors. Blockade of the V1 receptor in such patients may worsen hypotension, increase bleeding risk, and compromise kidney function.[68] The effectiveness of tolvaptan in the short-term management of HF patients with hypervolemic hyponatremia has been evidenced by decreased body weight, increased urine output, decreased pulmonary capillary wedge pressure, and decreased urine osmolality.[69-74] Long-standing beneficial effects, reduction in hospitalization or death, or slowed progression of HF have not been observed in several pivotal trials, and the recommended duration of tolvaptan use is only 30 days.[71,73-75] Prolonged tolvaptan use leads to increased endogenous AVP concentration, and this overstimulation of V1A receptors could lead to increased afterload and HF progression.[76] However, no worsening of left ventricular dilatation has been observed after 52 weeks of tolvaptan therapy (30 mg daily).[75] The 2013 American College of Cardiology Foundation/American Heart Association (ACCF/AHA) guidelines recommend short-term use of vaptans in hospitalized patients who have volume overload and persistent severe hyponatremia and who are at risk for or having cognitive symptoms despite fluid restriction and optimization of guideline-directed medical therapy.[77]

Clinical **Controversy...**

Despite FDA labeling, tolvaptan may be considered in patients with end stage liver disease who are awaiting liver transplantation in order to normalize serum sodium concentrations. The benefit of avoiding rapid perioperative correction of hyponatremia outweighs the likely negligible effect of tolvaptan-related hepatotoxicity in such patients. Additonally, it is reasonable to continue treatment until liver transplantation even if beyond 30 days.

Evaluation of Therapeutic Outcomes

Patients being treated for hypervolemic hypotonic hyponatremia should initially be evaluated on a daily basis for lung congestion, ascites, peripheral edema, and signs or symptoms of hyponatremia. The serum sodium concentration should be measured daily until it stabilizes at or above 125 mEq/L (mmol/L) following initiation of water restriction. If vaptan therapy is initiated, serum sodium concentrations should be monitored every 4 hours to minimize sodium overcorrection and the development of ODS. Patients should be assessed 1 week following discharge, and then every 2 to 4 weeks to assess compliance with water restriction and other treatment measures, volume status, and hyponatremia-related symptoms.

HYPERNATREMIA

Epidemiology and Etiology

7 Hypernatremia, defined as a serum sodium concentration greater than 145 mEq/L (mmol/L), is always associated with hypertonicity and cellular dehydration, resulting from a deficit of water relative to ECF sodium content. This hypertonic state is a potent stimulus for AVP secretion and activation of the thirst mechanism. Therefore, hypernatremia is most commonly observed in patients with an impaired thirst response or in those who can not access water. Young infants and children, intubated mechanically ventilated patients or comatose patients, the elderly, and disabled patients with an impaired sensorium or functional status are therefore at highest risk for this disorder.[78] Hypernatremia generally occurs in sicker patients and has a higher mortality.[79] The incidence of hypernatremia in general medical–surgical hospitalized patients and patients in ICUs has been estimated to be at least 1% and as high as 26%, respectively.[10,80-83] In 92% of 130 ICU cases in a matched case–control study,

TABLE 49-7 Characteristics of Hypernatremic States

Characteristics	Hypovolemic Hypernatremia	Euvolemic (Isovolemic) Hypernatremia	Hypervolemic Hypernatremia
Water and sodium	Water loss >> sodium loss	Water loss only	Sodium gain > water gain
Causes	Renal: osmotic diuresis, diuretic use, postoperative diuresis, high-output acute tubular necrosis	Congenital or acquired DI Nephrogenic DI Primary polydipsia	Sodium overload (eg, 3% NaCl, sodium bicarbonate, salt tablets, concentrated tube feedings, hypertonic dialysate, sodium-containing medications)
Effect on TBW	↓↓	↓	↑
Effect on TBNa	↓	↔	↑↑
Laboratory findings in addition to hypernatremia	Renal: UOsm high, UNa high Non-renal: UOsm high, UNa low	Renal: UOsm low, UNa variable Non-renal: UOsm high, UNa variable	UOsm high, UNa high
Clinical presentation	Orthostasis, hypotension, tachycardia, dry mucous membranes	Depends on severity of hypernatremia; seizures, lethargy	Peripheral and pulmonary edema, variable blood pressure
Treatment	0.9% NaCl until vital signs stable, then free water replacement	Free water replacement, AVP, AVP analogue	Free water replacement with loop diuretic; may require hemodialysis to remove volume

DI, diabetes insipidus; TBW, total body weight;

hypernatremia was iatrogenic: the result of too little free water and too much hypertonic solution along with increased renal water loss.[84]

Clinical outcomes in patients with hypernatremia, as in hyponatremia, depend on the severity of the increase and the rapidity with which it developed. In children, mortality from acute hypernatremia developing in less than 72 hours ranges from 10% to 70%. In contrast, chronic hypernatremia, defined as that which develops over 3 or more days, has a mortality rate of only 10%.[85] In adults, an acute increase in serum sodium concentration to greater than 160 mEq/L (mmol/L) is associated with a 75% mortality rate. In contrast to children, adults in whom hypernatremia develops at a slower rate still have a high mortality rate of approximately 60%.[38] Hypernatremia in adults is often associated with a serious underlying illness, which likely contributes to the higher mortality rate.

Pathophysiology

Hypernatremia most often results from water loss by either renal or extrarenal mechanisms. Hypernatremia can also result from administration of hypertonic or isotonic fluids or excess sodium ingestion. Patients develop hypovolemic, hypervolemic, or isovolemic hypernatremia depending on the relative magnitude of sodium and water loss or gain caused by the underlying condition (Table 49-7).

Water loss commonly occurs as a result of insensible losses (evaporative water loss through the skin and lungs) in patients deprived of water. Hospitalized patients who are febrile or receiving mechanical ventilation are often treated with IV fluids containing insufficient free water to replace insensible losses. Hypernatremia can be observed in patients with hypotonic GI losses (diarrhea, vomiting, gastric suctioning) or in patients who have been exposed to high temperatures who suffer large water losses from both sweat and insensible losses.

A water diuresis can also be caused by diabetes insipidus (DI), which can be classified as either central DI (decreased AVP secretion) or nephrogenic DI (decreased kidney response to AVP). Patients with untreated DI excrete large volumes (3-20 L/day) of dilute urine, resulting in hypernatremia. Possible causes of DI are listed in Table 49-8.

Hypertonic NaCl administration can result in hypernatremia and an expanded ECF volume. This type of hypernatremia is typically iatrogenic and can follow excess sodium bicarbonate administration, use of hypertonic NaCl enemas, or intrauterine injection of hypertonic sodium chloride. Normal ECF osmolality is 275 to 290 mOsm/kg (mmol/kg); whereas these *isotonic* solutions, Lactated Ringer's and 0.9% NaCl, are 273 mOsm/kg (mmol/kg) and 308 mOsm/kg (mmol/kg), respectively (see Table 49-1). Excessive 0.9% NaCl infusions may lead to sodium accumulation, particularly if a dilute urine is excreted.[86] Patients with hyperaldosteronism rarely present with an expanded ECF and mild hypernatremia. A common cause of hypernatremia in the ICU patient is sodium intake from IV and enteral fluids and medications.[79,87] Sodium balance should be carefully monitored in critically ill patients to avoid iatrogenic hypernatremia.

Clinical Presentation

Hypernatremia results in movement of water from the ICF to the ECF. Patients with central DI often present with sudden onset of polyuria, whereas patients with nephrogenic DI develop polyuria more gradually. Symptoms seen in patients with hypernatremia are similar to those seen with hyponatremia and primarily due to decreased neuronal (brain) cell volume. Symptoms of mild to moderate hypernatremia (hypertonicity) include weakness, lethargy, restlessness, irritability, twitching, and confusion. More severe or

TABLE 49-8 Causes of DI

Central	Nephrogenic
Familial[a]	Familial
Unreplaced insensible losses	• Inherited aquaporin-2 defect
• Skin	• Inherited vasopressin V2-receptor defect
• Lung	Hypercalcemia (chronic)
Hypodipsia	Hypokalemia
Neurogenic	Kidney disease
• Neurosurgery	Drug-induced
• Tuberculosis	• Cidofovir
• Head trauma	• Lithium toxicity
• CNS malignancy/cyst	• Amphotericin B
• Hypoxic encephalopathy	• Demeclocycline
• Ethanol ingestion (transient)	• Foscarnet
• Sarcoidosis	• Ifosfamide
• Sheehan syndrome[b]	• Vaptans
	• Methoxyflurane

AVP, arginine vasopressin; CNS, central nervous system; DI, diabetes insipidus.

[a]60 mutations in the AVP gene cause neurohypophyseal DI from U.S. National Library of Medicine. Genetics Home Reference. AVP. *http://ghr.nlm.nih.gov/gene/AVP*.

[b]Postpartum hypopituitarism caused by severe bleeding during childbirth.

CLINICAL PRESENTATION Hypernatremia

General

- Increase in serum sodium concentration and osmolality causes acute water movement from the ICF to the ECF.
- Decreased volume in the brain can cause cerebral vein rupture, leading to focal intracerebral and subarachnoid hemorrhages and possible irreversible neurologic damage.

Symptoms

- Mild: Lethargy, weakness, confusion, restlessness, irritability
- Moderate: Twitching
- Severe: Seizures, coma, death; usually requires an acute elevation in the plasma sodium concentration to 160 mEq/L (mmol/L) or higher
- Serum sodium concentrations greater than 180 mEq/L (mmol/L) are associated with a high mortality rate
- Other symptoms depend on etiology of hypernatremia: postural hypotension, tachycardia, dry mucous membranes, diminished skin turgor, reduced or increased urine output
- Signs and symptoms may be difficult to detect because many patients with this condition have underlying neurologic disease

Laboratory tests

- Serum sodium concentration greater than 145 mEq/L (mmol/L)
- Urine osmolality may be helpful in diagnosing the cause

rapidly developing hypernatremia can lead to seizures, coma, and/or death. As discussed in the hyponatremia section, neurons adapt to ECF tonicity changes by decreasing or increasing the concentration of inorganic (potassium, chloride) and organic (glutamate, taurine, and myoinositol).[3,33] ECF hypertonicity results in generation of intracellular organic osmolytes within 24 hours of onset leading to an increase in ICF tonicity that then draws water into brain cells, limiting the decrease in cell volume. Patients with chronic hypernatremia are therefore less likely to present with symptoms compared to patients with acute hypernatremia.

Hypernatremia is often associated with serious underlying illness, and signs and symptoms related to the illness are often present. Patients with a history of severe diarrhea or vomiting can present with ECF volume depletion. Elderly patients deprived of water after sustaining a stroke or hip fracture often present with mental status changes and other signs of ECF volume depletion. Clinically detectable ECF volume depletion, however, might not be evident until the serum sodium concentration exceeds 160 mEq/L (mmol/L) because these patients primarily have water loss, two-thirds of which is derived from the ICF. The urine is concentrated, osmolality often exceeds 450 mOsm/kg (mmol/kg), as a result of both osmotic and nonosmotic AVP release. The first step in evaluating patients with hypernatremia is the clinical assessment of the ECF and urine volume and the serum and urine osmolality (Fig. 49-3). Assessment of the ECF volume status is commonly imprecise. It is important to note that volume status is not defined by just one value or number, such as blood pressure.

Patients with a contracted ECF volume and a low urine output include those who have sustained insensible water losses that exceed intake, as well as those with extrarenal losses of hypotonic fluids. On physical examination, the patient will have postural hypotension, diminished skin turgor, and delayed capillary refill. Lactic acidosis

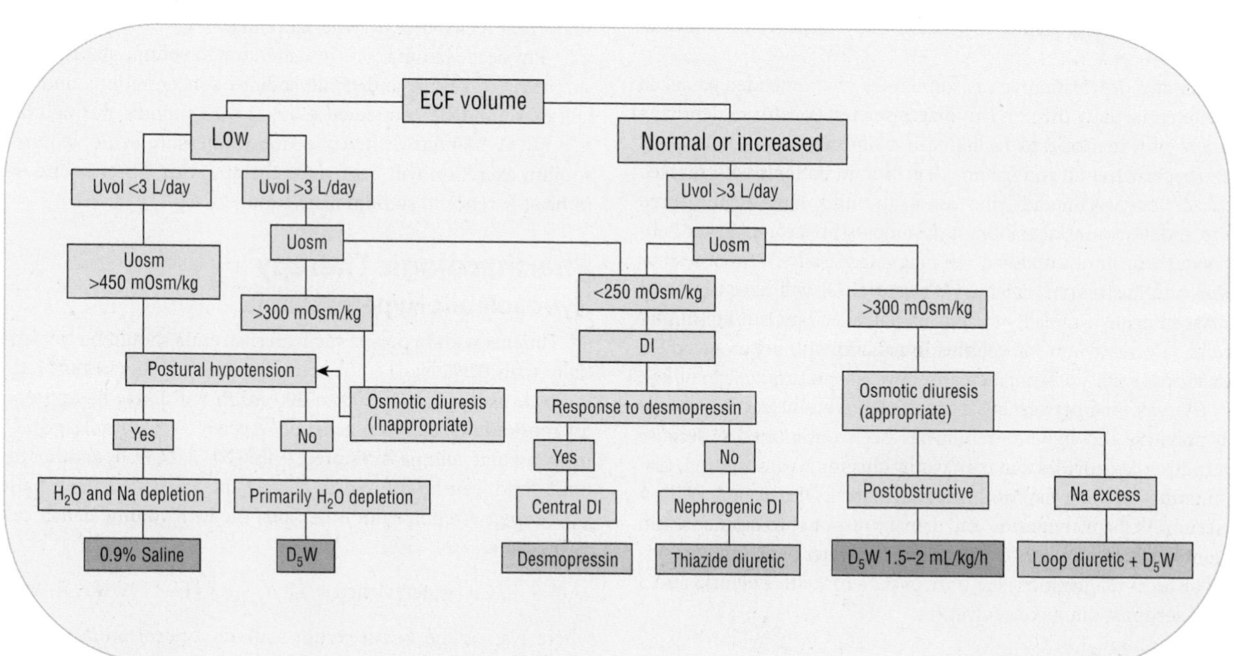

FIGURE 49-3 Diagnostic and treatment algorithm for hypernatremia. (D_5W, Dextrose 5% in water; DI, diabetes insipidus; ECF, extracellular fluid; H_2O, water; Na, sodium; Uosm, urine osmolality [values in mOsm/kg are numerically equivalent to mmol/kg]; Uvol, daily urine volume.) See the text for guidelines regarding calculations of infusion rates for IV solutions.

and low mixed venous oxygen saturation, indicating decreased tissue perfusion, may be present. The daily urine output is typically less than 1 L.

A multicenter, case–control study examined the clinical presentation of hypernatremia in 150 elderly patients in geriatric care facilities.[88] Low blood pressure, tachycardia, dry oral mucosa, decreased skin turgor, and recent changes in consciousness were all more common in patients with hypernatremia than in controls. In this patient population, the presence of signs of dehydration was variable, with orthostatic hypotension and decreased subclavicular and forearm skin turgor present in at least 60% of patients. Abnormal subclavicular and thigh skin turgor, dry oral mucosa, and recent change in consciousness were significantly and independently associated with hypernatremia.

Osmotic Diuresis

In the presence of an ongoing osmotic diuresis, patients will have a urine volume greater than 3 L/day. Excessive urinary excretion of glucose, sodium, urea, or an exogenously administered solute (eg, mannitol) can be identified either by history or by direct measurement of serum and urinary concentrations of the suspected solute. Patients with postobstructive diuresis, such as those with bladder outlet obstruction caused by prostatic hypertrophy, are usually volume expanded as a result of retained excess solute because of a decline in the GFR. The osmotic diuresis that follows obstruction resolution is appropriate in that it promotes excretion of the excess retained solute.

Patients with severe hyperglycemia may have a measured low sodium concentration (hyponatremia) but a high corrected sodium concentration (hypernatremia). Patients with severe hyperglycemia present with signs of volume depletion, and the diuresis is inappropriate as it further exacerbates the degree of ECF volume contraction associated with hyperglycemia. The estimated (or corrected) serum sodium concentration can be calculated by adding 1.7 mEq/L (mmol/L) for every 100 mg/dL (5.6 mmol/L) increase in the serum glucose concentration before estimating the water deficit (see Box 49-1).[6]

Diabetes Insipidus

Patients with DI tend to maintain a normal ECF volume as long as they are conscious and have free access to water. Patients typically have only a slight increase in the serum sodium concentration (usually 141-145 mEq/L [mmol/L]), and a daily urine volume greater than 3 L.

A water deprivation test is sometimes recommended to aid in the differential diagnosis.[38,83] This diagnostic test consists of depriving a patient of water for 8 to 12 hours in a supervised setting to avoid severe hypernatremia and volume depletion in patients with marked polyuria. Body weight and urine osmolality and volume are measured before and after administration of desmopressin acetate (4 mcg subcutaneously or intravenously or 10 mcg intranasally).[86] After desmopressin administration, patients with central DI will have a prompt increase in urine osmolality to approximately 600 mOsm/kg (mmol/kg) and a decrease in urine volume. In patients with nephrogenic DI, the urine osmolality will not increase above 300 mOsm/kg (mmol/kg).

The value of performing a water deprivation test in patients with polyuria and hypernatremia has been questioned.[87] Because hypernatremia provides a maximal stimulus for AVP secretion, discriminating between nephrogenic and central DI can be based on the serum AVP concentration and urinary response to desmopressin without the need for water deprivation. The water deprivation test is likely to be of diagnostic value only in patients with polyuria and a normal serum sodium concentration.

Sodium Overload

Patients who have ingested large amounts of sodium (more than 4 tablespoons table salt [1,400 mEq or mmol sodium]) or who have received more than 5 L of hypertonic fluids are volume expanded; although, this volume may not always be clinically evident as edema. Volume expansion results in an osmotic diuresis, polyuria, and a urine osmolality greater than 300 mOsm/kg (mmol/kg). The excess sodium will be excreted in the urine in patients with normal perfusion and kidney function; with organ dysfunction, volume expansion will occur.

Clinical Controversy...

The relative merits of the various drug treatment options, including thiazides and nonsteroidal anti-inflammatory drugs (NSAID), for nephrogenic DI have not been well studied. The choice of agent is therefore subject to clinician preference. It is unclear if there is a significant difference among these agents in the risk of clinically important decreases in GFR when they are used to produce a mild ECF volume deficit.

TREATMENT

Desired Outcomes

Treatment goals for patients with hypernatremia include correcting the serum sodium concentration to 145 to 150 mEq/L (mmol/L) at a rate that restores and maintains brain cell volume as close to normal as possible and normalizing the ECF volume, if indicated. Adequate treatment should result in the resolution of symptoms associated with hypovolemia, but hypernatremia is often undertreated in adults. Although inadvertent overcorrection is more common with hyponatremia, careful titration of fluids and medications should minimize the adverse effects from too rapid correction of the serum sodium concentration. Rapid correction can result in movement of excessive water into brain cells, resulting in cerebral edema, seizures, neurologic damage, and potentially death. However, these complications have almost exclusively been reported in young children with chronic hypernatremia of at least 48 hours duration and serum sodium concentrations greater than 150 mEq/L (mmol/L).[3] Water replacement and dietary sodium restriction can be necessary to prevent recurrence of hypernatremia.

Physical examination with attention to volume status and measurement of serum and urine sodium concentrations and osmolalities should be completed every 2 to 3 months during chronic therapy. A 24-hour urine collection to measure urine volume and sodium excretion will help guide therapy with diuretics and determine adherence to sodium restriction.

Pharmacologic Therapy

Hypovolemic Hypernatremia

8 Patients with hypovolemic hypernatremia should be treated initially with 0.9% NaCl until hemodynamic stability is restored. An initial infusion rate of 200 to 300 mL/h will likely be appropriate for most adults; children generally receive 10 to 20 mL/kg/h. Once intravascular volume is restored, 0.45% NaCl, D_5W, or another hypotonic fluid, can be infused to correct the water deficit. In patients with hypernatremia from water loss, the ECF volume deficit can be estimated as:

$$\text{ECF (water) deficit} = \text{TBW}_{\text{current}} \times [1 - (140/\text{Na}_{\text{S1}})]$$

where Na_{S1} is the initial serum sodium concentration (in mEq/L [mmol/L]); and 140 is the normal or goal serum sodium concentration in mEq/L (mmol/L). Although this formula provides an estimate of the water deficit caused by pure free water loss, it underestimates the deficit in patients with hypotonic fluid loss.[2]

The appropriate correction rate depends on the rapidity with which the hypernatremia developed. Hypernatremia developing in only a few hours can be initially corrected at a rate of approximately 1 mEq/L (mmol/L) per hour, whereas a rate of 0.5 mEq/L (mmol/L) per hour or less should be used when hypernatremia has developed more slowly.[2,3,28] The correction should generally be limited to no more than 10 to 12 mEq/L (mmol/L) per day.[2,3,37] Renal replacement therapy may be initiated for severe cases in patients with kidney failure. NaCl should be added to the replacement fluid/dialysate to achieve the same sodium content as the goal serum sodium concentration in order to avoid rapid overcorrection and cerebral edema.[79]

The serum sodium concentration and fluid status should be monitored every 2 to 3 hours during the first 24 hours of treatment in patients with symptomatic hypernatremia to permit appropriate adjustment of the hypotonic fluid infusion rate. After symptoms resolve and the serum sodium concentration is less than 148 mEq/L (mmol/L), assessing serum sodium concentrations every 6 to 12 hours and fluid status every 8 to 24 hours is generally adequate.

Recurrent iatrogenic hypernatremia can be prevented by avoiding infusing too much hypertonic solution, providing adequate amounts of maintenance fluids, and replacing ongoing abnormal losses. The standard maintenance fluid for adults and children weighing 40 kg or more is Dextrose 5%/0.45% NaCl with 20 mEq (mmol) KCl/L. Children weighing less than 40 kg typically receive Dextrose 5%/0.2% NaCl with 20 mEq (mmol) KCl/L, except infants younger than 3 months who may receive Dextrose 10%/0.2% NaCl with 20 mEq (mmol) KCl/L. Estimating daily fluid requirements and calculation of an appropriate maintenance fluid rate is discussed in Chapter 141.

Treatment of hyperglycemia-induced osmotic diuresis consists of correcting the hyperglycemia with insulin, as well as administering 0.9% NaCl until signs of ECF volume depletion resolve. Once hemodynamic stability is restored, the free water deficit should be corrected as described above.

Hypernatremia in patients undergoing a postobstructive diuresis should be treated with infusion of hypotonic fluids (eg, 0.45% NaCl) at a rate of approximately 1.5 mL/kg per hour. Because this solution is hypotonic, care should be taken to avoid infusing it alone to prevent hemolysis. The common practice of administering IV or oral fluids to replace urine output on a 1:1 volume basis tends to perpetuate the diuresis and generally should be avoided. Some clinicians use a 0.5:1 volume replacement for this reason.

Central Diabetes Insipidus

9 Patients with central DI should generally receive AVP replacement therapy with desmopressin, an AVP analog.[2,28] Because of variable absorption of orally administered desmopressin, central DI is best treated with the intranasal formulation, 1-desamino-8-D-arginine vasopressin (DDAVP); however, oral tablets are available and are useful in some patients. The initial intranasal DDAVP dosage should be 10 mcg once daily, titrated to 20 mcg twice daily based on serum sodium concentration. Each insufflation of intranasal DDAVP (100 mcg/mL) delivers 10 mcg of desmopressin acetate.[89] A rhinal tube delivery system is preferred in patients requiring doses that are not in increments of 10 mcg. Patients commonly prefer oral tablets due to the ease of administration, but not all patients adequately respond to the oral formulation. The bioavailability of DDAVP is approximately 5%. A 0.1 mg tablet is equivalent to 2.5 to 5 mcg of nasal spray but retitration is often required when transitioning between dosage forms due to the unpredictable response. Subcutaenous or IV desmopressin may be administered in cases when the intranasal and oral routes are not feasible.

The desmopressin dose should be adjusted to achieve adequate urinary concentration during sleep to prevent nocturia, a daily urine volume of approximately 1.5 to 2 L, and a normal or near normal serum sodium concentration. The mean duration of action of intranasal DDAVP is 7 to 9 hours. The serum sodium concentration should be measured at 24 hours and every 3 to 4 days during the initial dose titration period, and then every 2 to 4 months. Desmopressin administration results in nonsuppressible AVP activity and presents a risk of water intoxication with excess water retention. Patients using desmopressin should be aware of signs and symptoms of both hyponatremia and hypervolemia. Patients who experience water intoxication may minimize the risk of a second episode by delaying one desmopressin dose each week until polyuria and thirst develop, thus demonstrating the continued need for desmopressin therapy.[28]

TABLE 49-9 Drugs Used to Manage Central and Nephrogenic DI

Drug	Indication	Dose
Desmopressin acetate	Central and nephrogenic	5-20 mcg intranasally q 12-24 h
Chlorpropamide	Central	125-250 mg orally daily
Carbamazepine	Central	100-300 mg orally twice daily
Clofibrate	Central	500 mg orally four times daily
Hydrochlorothiazide	Central and nephrogenic	25 mg orally q 12-24 h
Amiloride	Lithium-related nephrogenic	5-10 mg orally daily
Indomethacin	Central and nephrogenic	50 mg orally q 8-12 h

DI, diabetes insipidus.

Additionally, several medications with antidiuretic properties have been used successfully in the management of central and nephrogenic DI (Table 49-9). They can be used as adjunctive therapy or as an alternative to DDAVP.

Nephrogenic Diabetes Insipidus

In patients with nephrogenic DI, concomitant hypercalcemia and hypokalemia, if present, should be corrected, and any medications that potentially contribute to the pathogenesis should be discontinued, if possible.[91,92] Because the ongoing urinary losses are essentially free water, patients with nephrogenic DI should receive hypotonic fluids to avoid excess NaCl intake and worsening hypernatremia. Water or milk should be given enterally or, if necessary, intravenous D_5W can be given intravenously at a rate that slightly exceeds the urine output with a goal to normalize the serum sodium concentration at a rate of less than 0.5 mEq/L/h (mmol/L/h).[93] One key goal in treating nephrogenic DI is to induce a mild ECF deficit (1-1.5 L) with a thiazide diuretic and dietary sodium restriction (85 mEq [mmol] Na^+ or 2,000 mg NaCl per day), which can decrease urine volume by as much as 50% (see Table 49-9). This ECF deficit will increase proximal tubule water reabsorption, decrease the filtrate volume delivered to the distal nephron, and decrease urine volume. In a patient with a maximally dilute urine osmolality (100 mOsm/kg [mmol/kg]), each gram of salt that is avoided will reduce the obligatory urine output by 360 mL because 1 g of table salt provides an osmolar load of approximately 36 mOsm.[93] Indomethacin, 50 mg given orally three times daily, potentiates AVP activity and can be used as adjunctive therapy in patients able to tolerate the GI side effects.

Sodium Overload

Treatment of sodium overload consists of administration of D_5W and a loop diuretic to facilitate excretion of the excess sodium. The infusate volume needed to correct the water deficit and hypernatremia at an appropriate rate can be estimated as described previously. Furosemide, 20 to 40 mg given intravenously every 6 hours, should also be administered.

The serum sodium concentration should initially be measured at least every 2 to 4 hours, and the diuretic continued until signs of ECF volume overload (pulmonary congestion and edema) resolve. The serum sodium concentration can be determined every 6 to 12 hours once the serum sodium concentration is less than 148 mEq/L (mmol/L) and symptoms of hypertonicity have resolved.

EDEMA

10 The development of edema is usually due to heart, kidney, or liver failure, or a combination of these conditions; although, it can develop secondary to a rapid decrease in serum albumin concentration along with excess fluid intake such as seen in the setting of burns or trauma.[94,95] Blood volume is constantly monitored to ensure adequate tissue perfusion. A decline in the effective circulating volume (actually the blood pressure resulting from that volume) results in decreased kidney sodium and water excretion. Under these conditions, the kidneys retain all the water and sodium ingested until the effective circulating volume is restored to near normal. An increase in dietary sodium is accompanied by an increase in water intake caused by the initial increase in serum osmolality and stimulation of thirst. The resultant increase in ECF volume augments kidney perfusion, resulting in a transient increase in GFR which leads to enhanced sodium filtration and excretion. These homeostatic mechanisms are crucial for maintaining sodium balance, as retention of just a few milliequivalents (millimoles) of sodium per day can eventually lead to an expanded ECF volume and edema formation.

Pathophysiology

Edema can be defined as a clinically detectable increase in interstitial fluid volume. In adults, edema formation is indicative of an interstitial volume increase of at least 2.5 to 3 L. Edema develops when excess sodium is retained either as a primary defect in renal sodium excretion or as a response to a decrease in the effective circulating volume despite a normal or expanded ECF volume. An increase in the capillary hydrostatic pressure because of ECF volume expansion or an increase in central venous pressure can lead to edema formation. Edema may also occur when there is an alteration in Starling forces within the capillary.[94] The Starling equation denotes the relationship between factors affecting fluid movement between the capillary and interstitium and is discussed in detail in Chapters 23 and 24.

Edema may develop rapidly in those with an acute decompensation in myocardial contractility, which leads to an elevation in pulmonary venous pressure that is transmitted back to the pulmonary capillaries and ultimately results in acute pulmonary edema. Edema may also develop insidiously as in the case of renal sodium and water retention due to diminished effective circulating volume, which leads to increased ECF volume and edema formation in both peripheral and pulmonary interstitial tissues.

Edema is the classical presentation in patients with nephrotic syndrome. There are two theories posited to explain edema in nephrotic syndrome: the *underfill* and the *overfill* hypothesis.[94] The underfill hypothesis states that decreased oncotic pressure from hypoalbuminemia (most pronounced with a serum albumin concentration <2 g/dL [20 g/L]) leads to excess filtration of fluid from the intravascular space to the interstitial space (*third spacing*) causing hypovolemia, kidney hypoperfusion, activation of the renin–angiotensin–aldosterone system, and secondary renal sodium retention. The overfill hypothesis is simply that primary renal sodium retention leads to edema. Both of these mechanisms contribute to edema formation. Distinguishing the predominant mechanism in individual patients with nephrotic syndrome is clinically important, as patients that are primarily underfilled will likely have worsening hypovolemia and an elevated serum creatinine after initially tolerating diuresis.

Patients with cirrhosis initially develop ascites as a result of splanchnic vasodilation resulting in an increase in the pressure in the portal circulation (portal hypertension). The combination of portal hypertension and splanchnic vasodilation increases capillary pressure and permeability and facilitates the accumulation of ascites (fluid in the abdominal cavity; third spacing). Ascites can cause a decrease in effective circulating ECF volume and activation of the sympathetic nervous system and the renin–angiotensin–aldosterone system, leading to secondary hyperaldosteronism. The subsequent renal sodium retention leads to worsened ascites and edema.[94]

Clinical Presentation

Edema is usually first detected in the feet or pretibial area of ambulatory patients and in the presacral area of bed-bound individuals. Edema is described as "pitting" when a depression created by exerting pressure for several seconds over a bony prominence, such as the tibia, does not rapidly refill. Edema severity should be rated on a semi-quantitative scale of 1+ to 4+ depending on the depth of the pit: 1+ = 2 mm; 2+ = 4 mm; 3+ = 6 mm; and 4+ = 8 mm.

The extent of the edema should also be quantified according to the areas involved. Pretibial edema, for example, should be quantified according to how far it extends up the lower leg (eg, one-third up the lower leg). Pulmonary edema, an increase in lung interstitial and alveolar water, is often evidenced by crackles (rales) upon auscultation. Rales should be quantified according to how far the crackles extend from the dependent portion of the lung(s). So, for example, edema limited to the ankles and feet would indicate less severe edema than edema that extends halfway up the lower legs, and crackles limited to the base of both lungs in an upright person would indicate less severe pulmonary edema than crackles throughout both lung fields. *Anasarca* is a term used to refer to a massive amount of edema that is generalized throughout the body.

TREATMENT

General Approach

Treatment goals for hypervolemic hypernatremia are to minimize edema and to improve organ function, as well as to relieve accompanying symptoms (eg, dyspnea, abdominal distention). Importantly, the presence of edema does not always dictate the need for pharmacologic (diuretic) therapy. Severe pulmonary edema however requires immediate pharmacologic treatment because it is life-threatening. Other forms of edema may be treated gradually, with a comprehensive approach that includes not only diuretics but also sodium and water restriction and treatment of the underlying disease. Sodium intake should generally be restricted to 1,000 to 2,000 mg/day. A slow, more judicious approach in non-life-threatening situations will help minimize complications of diuretic therapy and excessive diuresis, including impaired perfusion, azotemia, and impaired cardiac output due to a fall in the left ventricular end-diastolic filling pressure. Fluid should be removed cautiously in patients with cirrhosis and ascites but no peripheral edema. A maximum of 300 to 500 mL/day can be safely mobilized in patients with isolated ascites before the resultant decreased serum volume leads to elevated BUN and possibly hepatorenal syndrome.[96]

Pharmacologic Therapy

11 Diuretics are the primary pharmacologic therapy for edema when treatment of the underlying disease and sodium and water restriction are insufficient. Diuretics can be categorized according to the site in the nephron where sodium reabsorption is inhibited.

TABLE 49-10 Characteristics of Thiazide Diuretics

Diuretic	Duration of Action	Initial Daily Dose(s)	Sequential Nephron Blockade	Maximum Total Daily Dose
Chlorothiazide	6-12 h	250-500 mg once or twice	500-1,000 mg once plus loop diuretic	1,000 mg
Chlorthalidone	24-72 h	12.5-25 mg once		100 mg
Hydrochlorothiazide	6-12 h	25 mg once or twice	25-100 mg once or twice plus loop diuretic	200 mg
Indapamide	36 h	2.5 mg once		5 mg
Metolazone	12-24 h	2.5 mg once	2.5-10 mg plus loop diuretic	20 mg

Loop diuretics (furosemide, bumetanide, torsemide and ethacrynic acid) inhibit the sodium–potassium–chloride (Na^+–K^+–$2Cl^-$) carrier in the loop of Henle, while thiazide diuretics (hydrochlorothiazide, chlorothiazide, chlorthalidone, and metolazone) inhibit the Na^+–Cl^- carrier in the distal tubule. Potassium-sparing diuretics inhibit the sodium channel in the cortical collecting duct either directly (triamterene and amiloride) or by interfering with aldosterone activity (spironolactone and eplerenone). A diuretic's efficacy in edema therapy depends on: the amount of filtered sodium normally reabsorbed at its site of action; the amount of sodium reabsorbed distal to its site of action; adequate drug delivery to the site of action; and the amount of sodium reaching the site of action.

All diuretics act by inhibiting sodium reabsorption in the renal tubules; thus they increase fractional excretion of sodium (FeNa). Loop diuretics are the most potent diuretics, as evidenced by the fact that they increase peak FeNa from normal (1% [0.01] or less) to 20% to 25% (0.20-0.25). Thiazide- and potassium-sparing diuretics are less potent and increase peak FeNa only to 3% to 5% (0.03-0.05) and 1% to 2% (0.01-0.02), respectively.[25] Although a large portion of the filtered sodium is reabsorbed in the proximal nephron, the efficacy of proximal-acting diuretics (eg, acetazolamide) is limited by excess fluid and sodium reabsorption in the loop of Henle. Furthermore, sodium reabsorption by the distal tubule can compensate for reduced reabsorption in the loop of Henle when sodium intake is high.

The pharmacogenomics of diuretic therapy, particularly the thiazides, have been studied extensively in the area of hypertension therapy.[97,98] Multiple variants involving the different diuretic sites of action have been identified, but no clinically significant differences in outcomes have been demonstrated in large randomized studies.[99] Perhaps a more complex predictive model utilizing pharmacodynamic as well as pharmacokinetic and pharmacogenomic information will be necessary to predict significantly different responses and outcomes due to the potential for compensatory mechanisms in other parts of the nephron.[94] Genetic testing is currently not a practical option to guide diuretic treatment because there are no commercially available tests that identify these gene variants.

The effectiveness of thiazide and loop diuretics is dependent on drug concentrations in the tubular lumen. These diuretics are delivered to the tubular lumen via active transport by the proximal tubular cells. Osmotic diuretics are freely filtered into the tubular lumen in the proximal tubule; whereas, spironolactone gains access to mineralocorticoid receptors in the cortical collecting duct through diffusion from the systemic circulation.

A threshold concentration of loop or thiazide diuretic must be delivered to the respective site of action to achieve a natriuresis.[25] Once this threshold concentration is achieved, a further diuretic dose increase will not elicit an increase in diuretic response. Thus, a "ceiling dose" for these diuretics is recognized. Administration of 40 mg of furosemide intravenously to a normal subject will result in excretion of 200 to 250 mEq (mmol) of sodium in 3 to 4 L of urine over a 3- to 4-hour period.[25]

Loop diuretics, except torsemide, have a rapid action but short half-life requiring administration every 2 to 3 hours while thiazide diuretics have a longer half-life allowing for less frequent (once daily) dosing (Table 49-10). Table 49-11 lists the maximal effective doses and dosing intervals for loop diuretics in patients with cirrhosis, HF, nephrotic syndrome, and those with reduced kidney function.

Patients with kidney insufficiency often require larger diuretic doses to achieve adequate drug concentrations at the site of action. The natriuretic response is decreased in patients with kidney insufficiency because the filtered sodium load falls proportionately as GFR declines. This decrease in the GFR can be partially overcome by administering diuretics more frequently or by using a continuous infusion, a method commonly used in critically ill patients. The latter will limit the effect of postdiuretic sodium retention in the distal nephron. Table 49-12 lists initial continuous infusion rates based on creatinine clearance and maximum infusion rates.

TABLE 49-11 Characteristics of Loop Diuretics

Diuretic	Dosing Interval	Normal	Cirrhosis	HF	Nephrotic Syndrome	GFR 10-50 mL/min [0.17-0.83 mL/s]	GFR <10 mL/min (<0.17 mL/s)	Maximum Total Daily Dose
Furosemide								
IV	6-8 h	10-40 mg	40 mg	40-80 mg	120 mg	80 mg	200 mg	200 mg or 160 mg/h
Oral	6-8 h	20-80 mg	80 mg	80-160 mg	240 mg	160 mg	320-400 mg	600 mg
Bumetanide								
IV/oral	6-8 h	1 mg	1 mg	2-3 mg	3 mg	2-3 mg	8-10 mg	10 mg
Torsemide								
IV/oral	24 h	15-20 mg	10-20 mg	20-50 mg	50 mg	20-50 mg	50-100 mg	200 mg

HF, heart failure; GFR, glomerular filtration rate.

[a]Although these doses are considered maximal doses, higher doses may be required due to insufficient quantities in the renal tubular fluid.[73]

TABLE 49-12 Continuous Infusion Rates for Loop Diuretics

Drug	Initial Infusion Rate based on Creatinine Clearance			Maximum Infusion Rate	
	<25 mL/min (<0.42 mL/s)	25-75 mL/min (0.42-1.25 mL/s)	>75 mL/min (>1.25 mL/s)	Undiluted Bolus	Continuous Infusion
Bumetanide	1-2 mg/h	0.5-1 mg/h	0.5 mg/h	5 mg/min	0.17 mg/min[a] (up to 5 mg)
Furosemide	20-40 mg/h	10-20 mg/h	10 mg/h	40 mg/min	4 mg/min
Torsemide	10-20 mg/h	5-10 mg/h	5 mg/h	100 mg/min	3.1 mg/h[b]

[a]Doses of 2 to 5 mg may be given over 30 to 60 minutes in 500 mL of a suitable infusion fluid.

[b]Studies used a 100-mg total daily dose as a 25-mg injection over 2 minutes (25% of total daily dose) followed by an infusion of 3.1 mg/h over 24 hours (75% of total daily dose).

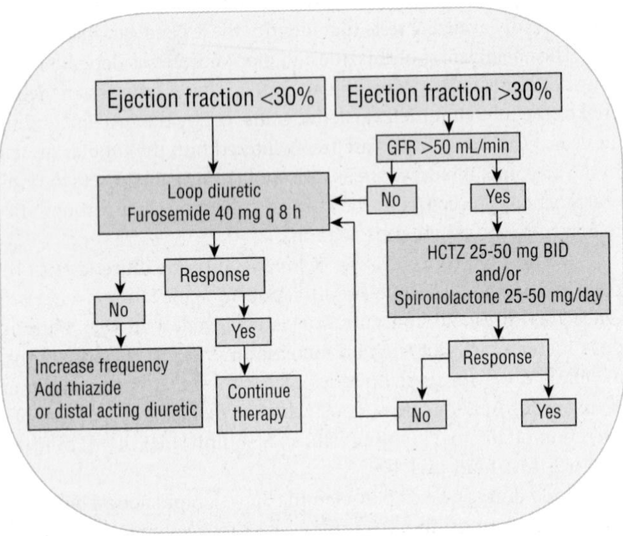

FIGURE 49-4 Therapeutic algorithm for diuretic use in patients with heart failure. (GFR, glomerular filtration rate [50 mL/min is equivalent to 0.83 mL/s]; HCTZ, hydrochlorothiazide.)

Loop diuretic resistance can be caused by pronounced sodium reabsorption in the distal nephron when sodium absorption in the loop of Henle is blocked. If sodium intake is not restricted, this distal sodium reabsorption can compensate entirely for loop-diuretic induced sodium loss. Patients with diuretic-resistant edema can be treated with both a loop diuretic and metolazone, a thiazide-type diuretic. Metolazone should be given first and allowed sufficient time to start blocking distal sodium reabsorption in order to maximize the loop diuretic's efficacy. Another mechanism of diuretic resistance is impaired diuretic delivery to the site of action. Patients with HF and a normal GFR may have impaired oral furosemide absorption. An adequate diuresis is most readily sustained by increasing the frequency of diuretic administration, but a higher dose may also be effective (Fig. 49-4). Absorption of orally administered loop diuretics can be compromised by GI edema and delayed gastric emptying, conditions often seen in critically ill patients. Inadequate drug concentrations at the site of action can also be caused by decreased perfusion as might be seen in patients with decompensated HF or those with decreased kidney perfusion. Due to extensive albumin binding (more than 95%), very little of these agents reach the tubule lumen by filtration, and they are almost exclusively transported into the proximal tubule lumen by active secretion via the organic acid secretory pathway.[25] Human studies, however, have demonstrated that when albumin binding is inhibited by concurrent sulfasoxazole administration, diuretic resistance persists, suggesting a decrease in intrinsic tubular sensitivity to loop diuretics.[100] This impaired natriuretic response can be overcome by using higher diuretic doses to increase unbound drug delivery to the secretory site in the nephron.[101] Decreased intrinsic diuretic activity with repeated dosing may also play a role in the development of diuretic resistance. Whether this is mediated by the first two mechanisms or as a mechanism to prevent hypovolemia is not well understood. Combinations of loop diuretics with distally acting diuretics are generally necessary to promote a natriuresis that exceeds distal tubular sodium reabsorption for those with nephrotic syndrome (Fig. 49-5).

Secondary hyperaldosteronism from activation of the renin–angiotensin–aldosterone system plays a major role in the pathogenesis of edema in patients with cirrhosis. Therefore, these patients

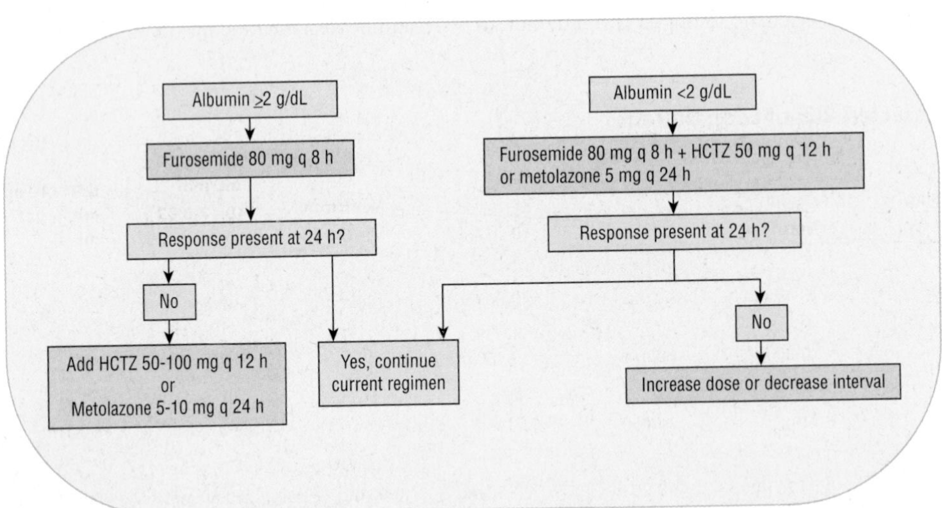

FIGURE 49-5 Therapeutic algorithm for diuretic therapy in patients with nephrotic syndrome. Albumin concentration of 2 g/dL is equivalent to 20 g/L. (HCTZ, hydrochlorothiazide.)

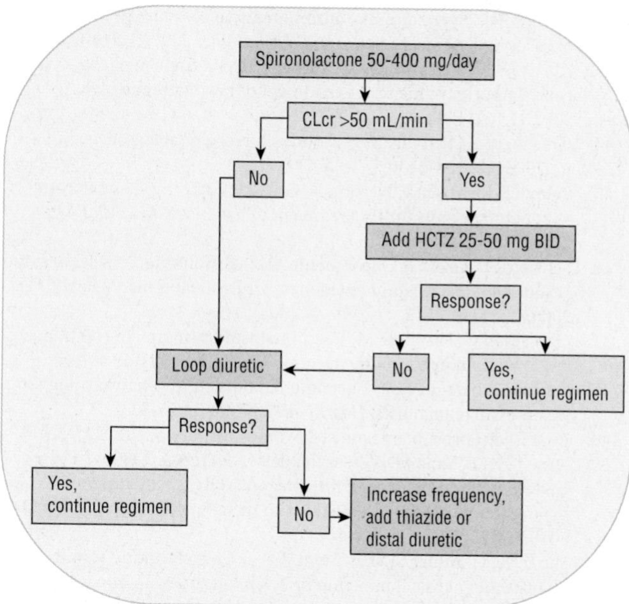

FIGURE 49-6 Therapeutic algorithm for diuretic use in patients with cirrhosis. (CLcr, creatinine clearance [50 mL/min is equivalent to 0.83 mL/s]; HCTZ, hydrochlorothiazide.)

should initially be treated with an aldosterone antagonist (eg, spironolactone) in the absence of impaired GFR and hyperkalemia (Fig. 49-6). Thiazides can then be added for patients with a creatinine clearance greater than 50 mL/min (0.83 mL/s). For those whose edema remains diuretic resistant, a loop diuretic can be used instead of the thiazide. Patients with impaired GFR (creatinine clearance less than 40 mL/min [0.67 mL/s]) can require a loop diuretic, with addition of a thiazide in those who do not achieve adequate diuresis.[95,100]

Complications of loop and thiazide diuretic therapy include hypokalemia, excess ECF volume loss (hypovolemia), calcium imbalance (hypocalcemia with loop, hypercalcemia with thiazide), hypo- or hypernatremia (hyponatremia with thiazides, hypernatremia with loop), hypomagnesemia, metabolic alkalosis, and hyperuricemia. Patients with refractory edema treated with high-dose synergistic combinations are at highest risk for developing hypokalemia.[11] Thiazide-induced hypercalcemia can occur, particularly in patients with mild subclinical hyperparathyroidism. Loop diuretics cause hypercalciuria and can lead to bone disorders when used chronically. Chronic therapy with potassium-sparing diuretics can cause a mild metabolic acidosis and hyperkalemia. Patients with moderate to severe kidney dysfunction or those receiving NSAIDs, ACEIs, or angiotensin receptor blockers are at highest risk for hyperkalemia. In addition, spironolactone can cause reversible gynecomastia in about 10% of men receiving it, and in about 50% of men receiving 150 mg/day or more. This side effect, however, has not been associated with eplerenone, another aldosterone antagonist.[102]

Evaluation of Therapeutic Outcomes

Patients should be monitored by careful history and intermittent physical examinations to detect signs and symptoms of edema as well as adverse effects. Physical examination should include measurement of blood pressure and pulse in either supine or seated positions and after standing for 2 to 3 minutes. ECF volume can be estimated based on the height of the jugular venous pressure, extent of edema, heart and lung auscultation, and skin turgor. Follow-up monitoring (10-14 days after therapy initiation) should include determinations of serum sodium, potassium, chloride, bicarbonate, magnesium, calcium, BUN, serum creatinine, and uric acid. A new steady state will have developed over that time period and further fluctuations in ECF volume and electrolyte balance generally do not occur in the absence of a change in clinical status, diuretic dosage, or dietary intake. Repeated blood tests are not necessary at every visit unless there is a change in the patient's clinical status.

ABBREVIATIONS

ACEI	angiotensin-converting enzyme inhibitor
AVP	arginine vasopressin, also known as vasopressin, antidiuretic hormone, or ADH
ATPase	adenosine triphosphatase
BUN	blood urea nitrogen
D_5W	Dextrose 5% in water
DDAVP	1-desamino-8-D-arginine vasopressin
DI	diabetes insipidus
ECF	extracellular fluid
FeNa	fractional excretion of sodium
GFR	glomerular filtration rate
HF	heart failure
ICU	intensive care unit
IV	intravenous
NSAID	nonsteroidal anti-inflammatory drug
ODS	osmotic demyelination syndrome
SIADH	syndrome of inappropriate secretion of antidiuretic hormone
TBW	total body water
Vaptan	vasopression 2 receptor antagonist
V_d	volume of distribution

REFERENCES

1. Panel on Dietary Reference Intakes for Electrolytes and Water, Standing Committee on the Scientific Evaluation of Dietary Reference Intakes, Food and Nutrition Board. Dietary Reference Intakes for water, potassium, sodium, chloride, and sulfate, 2005. Available at: http://www.nap.edu/read/10925/chapter/1. Last accessed October 30 2015.
2. Androgué HJ, Madias NE. The challenge of hyponatremia. *J Am Soc Nephrol* 2012;23:1140-1148.
3. Sterns RH. Disorders of plasma sodium causes, consequences, and correction. *N Engl J Med* 2015;372:55-65.
4. Schrier RW. The science behind hyponatremia and its clinical manifestations. *Pharmacotherapy* 2011;31(5 Pt 2):9S-17S.
5. Bhave G, Neilson EG. Volume depletion versus dehydration: how understanding the difference can guide therapy. *Am J Kidney Dis* 2011;58:302-309.
6. Upadhyay A, Jaber BL, Madias NE. Incidence and prevalence of hyponatremia. *Am J Med* 2006;119(7A):S30-S35.
7. Upadhyay A, Jaber BL, Madias NE. Epidemiology of hyponatremia. *Semin Nephrol* 2009;29(3):227-238.
8. Patterson JH. The impact of hyponatremia. *Pharmacother* 2011;31(5 Pt 2):5S-8S.
9. Hoorn EJ, Geary D, Robb M, Halperin ML, Bohn D. Acute hyponatremia related to intravenous fluid administration in hospitalized children: an observational study. *Pediatr* 2004;113:1279-1284.
10. Hawkins RC. Age and gender as risk factors for hyponatremia and hypernatremia. *Clin Chim Acta* 2003;337:169-172.
11. Sarafidis PA, Georgianos PI, Lasaridis AN. Diuretics in clinical practice. Part II: Electrolyte and acid-base disorders complicating diuretic therapy. *Expert Opin Drug Saf* 2010;9:259-273.
12. Chow KM, Szeto CC, Wong, TY-H, et al. Risk factors for thiazide-induced hyponatremia. *Q J Med* 2003;96:911-917.

13. Jacob S, Spinler SA. Hyponatremia associated with selective serotonin reuptake inhibitors in older adults. *Ann Pharmacother* 2006;40:1618-1622.
14. Meulendijks D, Mannesse CK, Jansen PA, et al. Antipsychotic-induced hyponatremia: A systematic review of the published evidence. *Drug Saf* 2010;33:101-114.
15. Hew-Butler T, Rosner MH, Fowkes-Godek S, et al. Statement of the Third International Exercise-associated Hyponatremia Consensus Development Conference, Carlsbad, California, 2015. *Clin J Sport Med* 2015;25:303-320.
16. Almond CSD, Shin AY, Fortescue EB, et al. Hyponatremia among runners in the Boston Marathon. *N Engl J Med* 2005;352:1550-1556.
17. Koczmara C, Wade AW, Skippen P, et al. Hospital-acquired acute hyponatremia and reports of pediatric deaths. *Dynamics* 2010;21:21-26.
18. Rondon-Berrios H, Bert T. Mild chronic hyponatremia in the ambulatory setting: significance and management. *Clin J Am Soc Nephrol* 2015;10:2268-78.
19. Asadollahi K, Beeching N, Gill G. Hyponatremia as a risk factor for hospital mortality. *Q J Med* 2006;99:877-880.
20. Friedman B, Cirulli J. Hyponatremia in critical care patients: frequency, outcome, characteristics, and treatment with vasopressin V2-receptor antagonist tolvaptan. *J Crit Care* 2013;28:219.e1-219.e12.
21. Spasovski G, Vanholder R, Allolio B, et al. Clinical practice guideline on diagnosis and treatment of hyponatraemia. *Eur J Endo* 2014;170:G1-G47.
22. Palmer BF, Clegg DJ. Electrolyte and acid-base disturbances in patients with diabetes mellitus. *N Engl J Med* 2015;373:548-559.
23. Kurtz I, Nguyen MK. Evolving concepts in the quantitative analysis of the determinants of the plasma water sodium concentration and the pathophysiology and treatment of dysnatremias. *Kidney Int* 2005;68:1982-1993.
24. Reynolds RM, Seckl JR. Hyponatremia for the clinical endocrinologist. *Clin Endocrinol* 2005;63:366-374.
25. Sarafidis PA, Georgianos PI, Lasaridis AN. Diuretics in clinical practice. Part I: Mechanisms of action, pharmacological effects and clinical indications of diuretic compounds. *Expert Opin Drug Saf* 2010;9:243-257.
26. Oh JY, Shin JI. Syndrome of inappropriate antidiuretic hormone secretion and cerebral/renal salt wasting syndrome: similarities and differences. *Front Pediatr* 2015;2:146. doi: 10.3389/fped.2014.00146.
27. Liamis G, Milionis H, Elisaf M. A review of drug-induced hyponatremia. *Am J Kidney Dis* 2008;52:144-153.
28. Reynolds RM, Padfield PL, Seckl JR. Disorders of sodium balance. *BMJ* 2006;332:702-705.
29. Decaux G. Is asymptomatic hyponatremia really asymptomatic? *Am J Med* 2006;119(7A):S79-S82.
30. Kinsella S, Moran S, Sullivan MO, et al. Hyponatremia independent of osteoporosis is associated with fracture occurrence. *Clin J Am Soc Nephrol* 2010;5:275-280.
31. Ayus JC, Morits ML. Bone disease as a new complication of hyponatremia: Moving beyond brain injury. *Clin J Am Soc Nephrol* 2010;5:167-168.
32. Sterns RH, Silver SM. Brain volume regulation in response to hypoosmolality and its correction. *Am J Med* 2006;119(7A):S12-S16.
33. Fisher SK, Heacock AM, Keep RF, Foster DJ. Receptor regulation of osmolyte homeostasis in neural cells. *J Physiol* 2010;18:3355-3364.
34. Ayus JC, Arrief AI. Chronic hyponatremic encephalopathy in post-menopausal women—association of therapies with morbidity and mortality. *JAMA* 1999;281:2299-2304.
35. Murase TM, Sugimura Y, Takefuji S, et al. Mechanisms and therapy of osmotic demyelination. *Am J Med* 2006;119(7A):S69-S73.
36. Nguyen MK, Kurtz I. A new quantitative approach to the treatment of the dysnatremias. *Clin Exp Nephrol* 2003;7:125-137.
37. Ellison DH. Core curriculum in nephrology: Disorders of sodium and water. *Am J Kidney Dis* 2005;46:356-361.
38. Kraft MD, Btaiche IF, Sacks GS, Kudsk KA. Treatment of electrolyte disorders in adult patients in the intensive care unit. *Am J Health Syst Pharm* 2005;62:1663-1682.
39. Liamis G, Kalogirou M, Saugos V, Moses E. Therapeutic approach in patients with dysnatremias. *Nephrol Dial Transplant* 2006;21:1564-1569.
40. Decaux G, Soupart A. Treatment of symptomatic hyponatremia. *Am J Med Sci* 2003;326:25-30.
41. Miell J, Dhanjal P, Jamookeeah C. Evidence for the use of demeclocycline in the treatment of hyponatremia secondary to SIADH: a systematic review. *Int J Clin Pract* 2015; doi: 10.1111/ijcp.12713. Last accessed October 2015.
42. Cawley MJ. Hyponatremia: current treatment strategies and the role of vasopressin antagonists. *Ann Pharmacother* 2007;41:840-850.
43. Curtis NJ, van Heyningen C, Turner JJ. Irreversible nephrotoxicity from demeclocycline in the treatment of hyponatremia. *Age Ageing* 2002;31:151-152.
44. Greenberg A, Verbalis JG. Vasopressin receptor antagonists. *Kidney Int* 2006;69:2124-2130.
45. Palm CP, Pistrosch F, Herbrig K, Gross P. Vasopressin antagonists as aquaretic agents for the treatment of hyponatremia. *Am J Med* 2006;119(7A):S87-S92.
46. Schrier RW, Gross P, Gheorghiade M, et al. Tolvaptan, a selective oral vasopressin V2-receptor antagonist, for hyponatremia. *N Engl J Med* 2006;355:2099-2112.
47. Oghlakian G, Klapholz M. Vaospressin and vasopressin receptor antagonists in heart failure. Cardiol Rev 2009;17:10-15.
48. Costello-Boerrigter LC, Boerrigter G, Burnett JC. Pharmacology of vasopressin antagonists. *Heart Fail Rev* 2009;14:75-82.
49. Berl T. Vasopressin antagonists. *N Engl J Med* 2015;372:2207-2216.
50. Rozen-Zvi B, Yahav D, Gheorghiade M, Korzets A, Leibovici L, Gafter U. Vasopressin receptor antagonists for the treatment of hyponatremia: systematic review and meta-analysis. *Am J Kidney Dis* 2010;56:325-337.
51. Shoaf SE, Graumer SL, Briemont P, et al. Pharmacokinetic and pharmacodynamic interaction between tolvaptan, an ono-peptide AV antagonist and furosemide or hydrochlorthiazide. *J Cardiovasc Pharmacol* 2007;50:213-222.
52. Decaux G. V2-antagonists for the treatment of hyponatraemia. *Nephrol Dial Transplant* 2007;22:1853-1855.
53. Rosskopf D, Michel MC. Pharmacogenomics of G protein-coupled receptor ligands in cardiovascular medicine. *Pharmacol Rev* 2008;60:513-535.
54. Shoaf SE, Ohzone Y, Ninomiya S, et al. In vitro P-glycoprotein interactions and steady-state pharmacokinetic interactions between tolvaptan and digoxin in healthy subjects. *J Clin Pharmacol* 2011:51:761-769.
55. Hauptman PJ, Zimmer C, Udelson J, et al. Comparison of two doses and dosing regimens of tolvaptan in congestive heart failure. *J Cardiolvasc Pharmacol* 2005;46:609-614.
56. Ambrosy A, Goldsmith SR, Gheorghiade M. Tolvaptan for the treatment of heart failure: A review of the literature. *Exp Opin Pharmacother* 2011;12:961-976.
57. McNeely EB, Talameh JA, Adams Jr KF, et al. Relative bioavailability of tolvaptan administered via nasogastric tube and tolvaptan tablets swallowed intact. *Am J Health-Syst Pharm* 2013;70:1230-1237.
58. Torres VE, Chapman AB, Devuyst O, et al. Tolvaptan in patients with autosomal dominant polycystic kidney disease. *NEJM* 2012;367:2407-2418.
59. Adams KF, Glotzer J, Lee AK, Schwartz T et al. Pilot study of the relationship of ambient copeptin to the aquaretic effects of tolvaptan in patients with heart failure [ACC.15 abstract 1183-193]. *J Am Coll Cardiol.* 2015;65:(10S):A917.
60. Adams KF. Tolvaptan treatment to reverse worsening outpatient heart failure: possible role of copeptin in identifying responders (TROUPER). In: ClinicalTrials.gov [Internet]. Bethesda (MD): National Library of Medicine (US). 2000- [cited 2016 Aug 29]. Available from: https://clinicaltrials.gov/ct2/show/NCT02476409 NLM Identifier: NCT02476409.
61. Lee WH, Packer M. Prognostic importance of serum sodium concentration and its modification by converting-enzyme inhibition in patients with severe chronic heart failure. *Circulation* 1986;73:257-267.
62. Klein L, O'Connor CM, Leimberger JD, et al; OPTIME-CHF Investigators. Lower serum sodium is associated with increased short-term mortality in hospitalized patients with worsening heart failure: results from the Outcomes of a Prospective Trial of Intravenous Milrinone for Exacerbations of Chronic Heart Failure (OPTIME-CHF) study. *Circulation* 2005;111:2454-2460.
63. Bakris GL, Weir MR. Angiotensin-converting enzyme inhibitor-associated elevation of creatinine: Is this a cause for concern? *Arch Intern Med* 2000;160:685-693.
64. Baldasseroni S, Urso R, Orso F, et al. Relation between serum sodium levels and prognosis in outpatients with chronic heart failure: neutral effect of treatment with beta-blockers and angiotensin-converting enzyme inhibitors: data from the Italian network on congestive heart failure (IN-CHF database). *J Cardiovasc Med* 2011;12:723-731.
65. Gerbes AL, Gulberg V, Gines P, et al. Therapy of hyponatremia in cirrhosis with a vasopressin receptor antagonist: A randomized double-blind multicenter trial. *Gastroenterology* 2003;124:933-939.

66. Berl T, Quittnet-Pelletier F, Verbalis JG, et al. Oral tolvaptan is safe and effective in chronic hyponatremia. *J Am Soc Nephrol* 2010;21:705-712.
67. Human T. Current therapeutic options for hyponatremia: indications, limitations, and confounding variables. *Pharmacotherapy* 2011;31(5 Pt 2):18S-24S.
68. Urso C, Brucculeri S, Caimi G. Employment of vasopressin receptor antagonists in management of hyponatraemia and volume overload in some clinical conditions. *J Clin Pharm Ther* 2015;40:376-385.
69. Dixon MB, Lien YH. Tolvaptan and its potential in the treatment of hyponatremia. *Therapeut Clin Risk Management* 2008;4:1149-1155.
70. Gheorghaide M, Niazi I, Quyang J, et al. Vasopressin V2-receptor blockage with tolvaptan in patients with chronic heart failure: Results from a double-blind randomized trial. *Circulation* 2003;107:2690-2696.
71. Gheorghaide M, Gattis WA, O'Connor CM, et al. Effects of tolvaptan, a vasopressin antagonist, in patients hospitalized with worsening heart failure: A randomized controlled trial. *JAMA* 2004;291:1963-1971.
72. Gheorghiade M, Konstam MA, Burnett JC Jr, et al. Short-term clinical effects of tolvaptan, an oral vasopressin antagonist, in patients hospitalized for heart failure: The EVEREST Clinical Status Trials. *JAMA* 2007;297:1332-1343.
73. Konstam MA, Gheorghiade M, Burnett JC Jr, et al. Effects of oral tolvaptan in patients hospitalized for worsening heart failure: The EVEREST Outcome Trial. *JAMA* 2007;297:1319-1331.
74. Udelson JE, Orlandi C, Quyang J, et al. Acute hemodynamic effects of tolvaptan, a vasopressin V2 receptor blocker, in patients with symptomatic heart failure and systolic dysfunction: an international, multicenter, randomized, placebo-controlled trial. *J Am Coll Cardiol* 2008;52:1540-1545.
75. Udelson JE, McGrew FA, Flores E, et al. Multicenter, randomized, double-blind, placebo-controlled study on the effect of oral tolvaptan on left ventricular dilation and function in patients with heart failure and systolic dysfunction. *J Am Coll Cardiol* 2005;49:2151-2159.
76. Costello-Boerrigter LC, Smith WB, Boerrigter G, et al. Vasopressin-2-receptor antagonism augments water excretion without changes in renal hemodynamics or sodium and potassium excretion in human heart failure. *Am J Physiol Renal Physiol* 2005;290:F273-F278.
77. Yancy CW, Jessup M, Bozkurt B, et al. American College of Cardiology Foundation/American Heart Association Task Force on Practice Guidelines. 2013 ACCF/AHA guideline for the management of heart failure: a report of the American College of Cardiology Foundation/American Heart Association Task Force on practice guidelines. *Circulation* 2013;128:e240-e327.
78. Al-Absi A, Gosmanova EO, Wall BM. A clinical approach to the treatment of chronic hypernatremia. *Am J Kidney Dis* 2012;60:1032-1038.
79. Overgaard-Steensen C, Ring T. Clinical review: Practical approach to hyponatraemia and hypernatraemia in critically ill patients. *Crit Care* 2013;17:206. Available at: http://ccforum.com/content/17/1/206. Last accessed October 2015.
80. Waite MD, Fuhrman SA, Badawi O, Zuckerman IH, Franey CS. Intensive care unit-acquired hypernatremia is an independent predictor of increased mortality and length of stay. *J Crit Care* 2013;28:405-412.
81. Palevsky PM, Bhagrath R, Greenberg A. Hypernatremia in hospitalized patients. *Ann Intern Med* 1996;124:197-203.
82. Aiyagari V, Deibert E, Diringer MN. Hypernatremia in the neurologic intensive care: How high is too high? *J Crit Care* 2006;21:163-172.
83. Stelfox HT, Ahmed SB, Khandwala F, et al. The epidemiology of intensive care unit-acquired hyponatraemia and hypernatraemia in medical-surgical intensive care units. *Crit Care* 2008;12:R162. Available at: http://ccforum.com/content/12/6/R162. Last accessed October 2015.
84. Hoom EJ, Betjes MG, Weigel J, Zietse R. Hypernatremia in critically ill patients: Too little water and too much salt. *Nephrol Dial Transplant* 2008;23:1562-1568.
85. Moritz ML, Ayus JC. The changing pattern of hypernatremia in hospitalized children. *Pediatrics* 1999;104:435-439.
86. Lindner G, Funk GC. Hypernatremia in critically ill patients. *J Crit Care* 2013;28:216.e11-216.e20. Available at: http://dx.doi.org/10.1016/j.jcrc.2012.05.001. Last accessed October 2015.
87. Buckley MS, Leblanc JM, Cawley MJ. Electrolyte disturbances associated with commonly prescribed medications in the intensive care unit. *Crit Care Med* 2010;38:S253-S264.
88. Chassagne P, Druesne L, Capet C, Menard JF, Bercoff E. Clinical presentation of hypernatremia in elderly patients: A case control study. *J Am Geriatr Soc* 2006;54:1225-1230.
89. Saifan C, Nasr R, Mehta S, et al. Diabetes insipidus: a challenging diagnosis with new drug therapies. ISRN Nephrol 2013:797620. Available at: http://dx.doi.org/10.5402/2013/797620. Last accessed October 12, 2015.
90. Moritz ML. A water deprivation test is not indicated in the evaluation of hypernatremia [letter]. *Am J Kidney Dis* 2005;46:1150-1151.
91. Sands JM, Bichet DG. Nephrogenic diabetes insipidus. *Ann Intern Med* 2006;144:186-194.
92. Garofeanu CG, Weir M, Rosas-Arellano P, et al. Causes of reversible nephrogenic diabetes insipidus: A systematic review. *Am J Kidney Dis* 2005;45:626-637.
93. Bockenhauer D, Bichet DG. Pathophysiology, diagnosis and management of nephrogenic diabetes insipidus. *Nat Rev Nephrol* 2015;11:576-588.
94. Siddall EC, Radhakrishnan J. The pathophysiology of edema formation in the nephrotic syndrome. *Kidney Int* 2012;82:635-642.
95. Somberg JC, Molnar J. Therapeutic approaches to the treatment of edema and ascites: The use of diuretics. *Am J Ther* 2009:16:98-101.
96. Pockros PJ, Reynolds TB. Rapid diuresis in patients with ascites from chronic liver disease: the importance of peripheral edema. *Gastroenterology* 1986;90:1827-1833.
97. Thorn CF, Ellison DH, Turner ST, Altman RB, Klein TE. PharmGKB summary: diuretics pathway, pharmacodynamics. *Pharmacogenet Genomics* 2013;23:449-453.
98. Peters BJ, Klungel OH, de Boer A, Ch Stricker BH, Maitland-van der Zee AH. Pharmacogenetics of cardiovascular drug therapy. *Clin Cases Miner Bone Metab* 2009;6:55-65.
99. Voora D, Ginsburg GS. Clinical application of cardiovascular pharmacogenetics. *J Am Coll Cardiol* 2012;60:9-20.
100. Agarwal R, Gorski JC, Sundblad K, Brater DC. Urinary protein binding does not affect response to furosemide in patients with nephrotic syndrome. *J Am Soc Nephrol* 2000;11:1100-1105.
101. Ellison DH. Edema and the clinical use of diuretics. In: Greenberg A, ed. *Primer on Kidney Diseases*, 5th ed. Philadelphia, PA: WB Saunders, 2009:135-147.
102. Nappi JM, Sieg A. Aldosterone receptor antagonists in patients with chronic heart failure. *Vasc Heal Risk Manag* 2011;7:353-363.

Disorders of Calcium and Phosphorus Homeostasis

50

Amy Barton Pai

KEY CONCEPTS

1. Severe acute hypercalcemia can result in cardiac arrhythmias, whereas chronic hypercalcemia can lead to calcium deposition in soft tissues including blood vessels and the kidney.
2. The correction of hypercalcemia can include multiple pharmacotherapeutic modalities such as hydration, diuretics, bisphosphonates, and steroids, depending on the etiology and acuity of the hypercalcemia.
3. Hypocalcemia is typically associated with an insidious onset; however, some drugs such as cinacalcet are associated with rapid decreases in serum calcium.
4. Acute treatment of hypocalcemia requires calcium supplementation whereas chronic management may require other therapies such as vitamin D to maintain serum calcium values.
5. Hyperphosphatemia occurs most frequently in patients with chronic kidney disease (CKD).
6. Treatment of nonemergent hyperphosphatemia includes the use of phosphate binders to decrease absorption of phosphorus from the gastrointestinal (GI) tract.
7. Hypophosphatemia is a relatively common complication among critically ill patients.
8. Treatment of acute hypophosphatemia usually requires IV supplementation of phosphorous salts.

INTRODUCTION

Disorders of calcium and phosphorus are common complications of multiple acute and chronic diseases. These disorders are frequently seen in the acute care setting; however, they are also often present in ambulatory patients, usually in a less severe state. The consequences of electrolyte disorders can range from asymptomatic to life-threatening, requiring hospitalization and emergent treatment. The maintenance of fluid and electrolyte homeostasis requires adequate functioning and modulation by multiple hormones on tissues of multiple organ systems.

There are many common drug therapies that can disturb the normal homeostatic mechanisms that maintain calcium and phosphorous balance. In addition, with some drug therapies, toxicity is enhanced when underlying electrolyte disorders are present. Drug-induced disorders typically respond well to discontinuation of the offending agent(s); however, additional therapies are sometimes required to correct the disorder. This chapter reviews the etiology, classification, clinical presentation, and therapy for the most common disorders of calcium and phosphorus homeostasis.

DISORDERS OF CALCIUM HOMEOSTASIS

The maintenance of physiologic calcium concentrations in the intracellular and extracellular spaces is vital for the preservation and function of cell membranes; propagation of neuromuscular activity; regulation of endocrine and exocrine secretory functions; blood coagulation cascade; platelet adhesion process; bone metabolism; muscle cell excitation/contraction coupling; and mediation of the electrophysiologic slow-channel response in cardiac and smooth-muscle tissue.

The disorders of calcium homeostasis are related to the calcium content of the extracellular fluid (ECF), which is tightly regulated and comprises less than 0.5% of the total body stores of calcium. Skeletal bone contains more than 99% of total body stores of calcium.[1] ECF calcium is moderately bound to plasma proteins (40%), primarily albumin.[2] Ionized or free calcium is the physiologically active form and is the fraction that is homeostatically regulated.[3] Extracellular calcium, however, is most commonly measured as the total serum calcium level, which includes both bound and unbound calcium.[2] The normal total calcium serum concentration range is 8.5 to 10.5 mg/dL (2.13-2.63 mmol/L).[3]

Proper assessment of total serum calcium concentrations includes measurement of the patient's serum albumin concentration. Hypoalbuminemia, which can be associated with many chronic disease states, is probably the most common cause of "laboratory hypocalcemia." Patients remain asymptomatic because the unbound or ionized fraction of serum calcium remains normal (normal range, 4.4-5.4 mg/dL [1.10-1.35 mmol/L]). A corrected total serum calcium (S_{ca}) concentration can be calculated based on the measured total serum calcium and the difference between a patient's measured albumin concentration and the normative value of 4 g/dL (40 g/L) by the following equations:

$$\text{Corrected } S_{ca}\ (\text{mg/dL}) = \text{Measured } S_{ca}\ (\text{mg/dL}) + (0.8 \times [4\ \text{g/dL} - \text{measured albumin (g/dL)}])$$

or

$$\text{Corrected } S_{ca}\ (\text{mmol/L}) = \text{Measured } S_{ca}\ (\text{mmol/L}) + (0.02 \times [40\ \text{g/L} - \text{measured albumin (g/L)}])$$

The concentration of ionized calcium is closely regulated by the interactions of parathyroid hormone (PTH), phosphorus, vitamin D, and calcitonin (Fig. 50-1). PTH increases serum calcium concentrations by stimulating calcium release from bone, increasing renal tubular reabsorption, and enhancing absorption in the gastrointestinal (GI) tract secondary to increased renal production of 1,25-dihydroxy vitamin D_3. Vitamin D directly increases serum calcium, as well as phosphorus concentrations, by increasing GI absorption. Indirectly, it can also lead to calcium release from bone and reduced renal excretion. Calcitonin inhibits osteoclastic bone resorption. Its plasma concentrations are increased when ionized calcium concentrations are

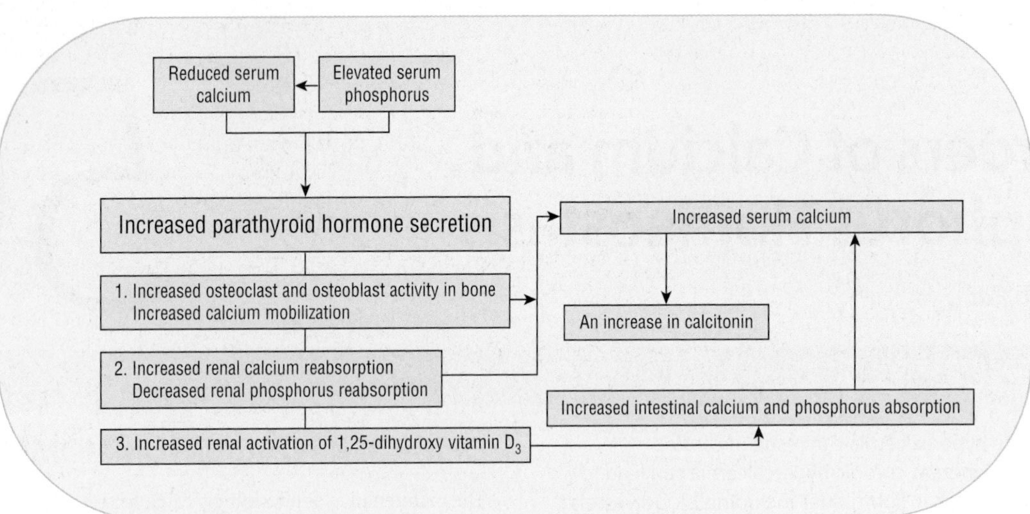

FIGURE 50-1 Homeostatic mechanisms to maintain serum calcium concentrations.

high as the body attempts to return the calcium level to the normal range. Disruption of these homeostatic mechanisms results in the clinical manifestations of hypercalcemia or hypocalcemia.

Alteration of the concentration of albumin or its binding of calcium can be expected to change the unbound fraction of total serum calcium. The most significant cause of changes in calcium binding to albumin is a change in ECF pH. In the presence of acute metabolic alkalosis the fraction of calcium bound to albumin is increased, thus reducing the plasma concentration of ionized calcium. This can result in symptomatic hypocalcemia; that is, paresthesia, muscle cramping and spasms, memory loss, and seizures.[1] Conversely, metabolic acidosis decreases calcium binding to albumin and results in increased ionized calcium. Hypoalbuminemic states are probably the most common cause of "laboratory hypocalcemia." When the albumin level is decreased, the ionized calcium concentration can be normal, although total serum calcium concentration is low. Each 1 g/dL (10 g/L) drop in the serum albumin concentration below 4 g/dL (40 g/L) will result in a decrease of total serum calcium concentration by 0.8 mg/dL (0.20 mmol/L).[2] This approach of calculating an albumin-adjusted calcium concentration has been found to overestimate the degree of hypercalcemia and usually fails to identify hypocalcemia in critically ill patients; therefore, ionized calcium values should be used to assess calcium status in these patients.[3,4,5]

HYPERCALCEMIA

There are multiple and diverse causes of hypercalcemia (total serum calcium more than 10.5 mg/dL [more than 2.63 mmol/L]) (Table 50-1). The most common causes of hypercalcemia are cancer and primary hyperparathyroidism.

Epidemiology and Etiology

The reported incidence of primary hyperparathyroidism in the United States ranges from 10 to 30 cases per 100,000 people.[6] Hypercalcemia of cancer occurs in approximately 15% to 70% of cancer patients at some time during the course of their disease and is dependent on tumor type.[7] Cancer-associated hypercalcemia is predominantly encountered in hospitalized patients, whereas primary hyperparathyroidism accounts for the vast majority of cases in the outpatient setting.[8,9]

Pathophysiology

Hypercalcemia is the result of one or a combination of three primary mechanisms: increased bone resorption, increased GI absorption, or increased tubular reabsorption by the kidneys (see Fig. 50-1).

Many tumors secrete PTH-related protein (PTHrP), which binds to the PTH receptors in bone and renal tissues, leading to increased bone resorption and renal tubular reabsorption.[10] Tumors can also secrete substances such as vitamin D, transforming growth factor, interleukins, prostaglandins, interferon, tumor necrosis factor, and granulocyte-macrophage colony-stimulating factor, which are associated with the development of hypercalcemia.[7] Hypercalcemia of malignancy is a common complication of squamous cell carcinomas of the lung, head, and neck, hematologic malignancies such as multiple myeloma and T-cell lymphomas, and carcinomas of ovary, kidney, bladder, and breast. The most frequent types of malignancy associated with hypercalcemia are carcinomas of the lung and breast.[7] Breast and squamous cell lung carcinomas secrete PTHrP which binds to the type I PTH receptor (PTHR1) and enhances bone resorption.[10,11] In contrast, up to 40% of patients with multiple myeloma develop hypercalcemia principally as the result of osteoclast-mediated bone destruction.[7]

Primary hyperparathyroidism is the most common cause of chronic hypercalcemia in the general population. Benign parathyroid adenomas account for 80% to 85% of these cases of

TABLE 50-1 Etiologies of Hypercalcemia

Neoplasms	**Medications**
Bone metastasis	Thiazides
Breast	Lithium
Multiple myeloma	Vitamin D
Lymphoma	Vitamin A
Leukemia	Calcium
Humoral induced	Aluminum/magnesium antacids
Ovary	Theophylline
Kidney	Tamoxifen
Pheochromocytoma	Ganciclovir
Multiple endocrine neoplasia	**Granulomatous disease**
Lung	Sarcoidosis
Head and neck	Tuberculosis
Esophagus	Cryptococcus
Cervix	Berylliosis
Lymphoproliferative disease	Histoplasmosis
Hyperparathyroidism	Coccidioidomycosis
Primary	Leprosy
Tertiary	**Endocrine disease**
Miscellaneous	Adrenal insufficiency
Immobilization	Hyperthyroidism
Paget's disease	Acromegaly
Familial hypocalciuric hypercalcemia	
Adolescence	
Rhabdomyolysis	

hyperparathyroidism, parathyroid hyperplasia accounts for 15%, and parathyroid carcinoma is the cause in less than 1% of cases.[8]

Other causes of chronic hypercalcemia include medications, endocrine and granulomatous disorders, physical immobilization, high bone-turnover states (adolescence and Paget disease), and rhabdomyolysis. Increased GI absorption can be the result of excessive ingestion of vitamin D analogs, calcium supplements, and lithium. Lithium and vitamin A therapy can increase bone resorption, whereas increased renal tubular reabsorption of calcium can occur with thiazide and lithium therapy. The exact mechanism of lithium-induced hypercalcemia is not known but may include competitive inhibition of calcium influx into cells, increasing the threshold sensitivity of the calcium-sensing receptor (CaSr) and subsequent inhibition of PTH gene transcription.[11] Addison disease, acromegaly, and thyrotoxicosis are endocrine disorders that can lead to hypercalcemia because of increased renal tubular reabsorption and increased bone resorption. Milk-alkali syndrome is the term applied to those situations where an individual develops hypercalcemia following the ingestion of calcium and absorbable alkali (eg, calcium carbonate) and is a frequent cause of hypercalcemia in patients who are not on dialysis.[12,13] Finally, the granulomatous disorders (sarcoidosis, tuberculosis, histoplasmosis, and leprosy) are associated with hypercalcemia secondary to an increase in GI and renal tubular absorption as the result of granuloma production of 1,25-dihydroxy vitamin D_2.[14]

Clinical **Controversy...**

Prevalent use of calcium and vitamin D supplementation has increased the frequency of hypercalcemia. This risk ultimately needs to be balanced with evidence of improved outcomes associated with supplementation of calcium and vitamin D.

Clinical Presentation

Patients with mild-to-moderate hypercalcemia, that is, total serum calcium concentrations above the upper threshold of normal but less than 13 mg/dL (3.25 mmol/L) or ionized calcium concentrations less than 6 mg/dL (1.50 mmol/L) can often be asymptomatic. This is typically the case for the vast majority of patients who have drug-induced hypercalcemia or primary hyperparathyroidism.[14,15] In fact, one study noted normocalcemia in approximately 20% of patients with a diagnosis of primary hyperparathyroidism, suggesting target tissue resistance to PTH.[15]

1 The presenting signs and symptoms of severe hypercalcemia that occur if the total serum calcium concentration is more than 13 mg/dL (more than 3.25 mmol/L) may differ depending on the acuity of onset.[2] Hypercalcemia of malignancy usually develops quickly and is accompanied by a classic symptom complex of anorexia, nausea and vomiting, constipation, polyuria, polydipsia, and nocturia.[7] Polyuria and nocturia secondary to a urinary-concentrating defect constitute some of the most frequent renal effects of hypercalcemia.[14] Hypercalcemic crisis is characterized by an acute elevation of total serum calcium to a value more than 15 mg/dL (more than 3.75 mmol/L), acute renal insufficiency, and obtundation (inability to arouse).[15,16] If untreated, hypercalcemic crisis can progress to oliguric renal failure, coma, and life-threatening ventricular arrhythmias.[14] The primary complications associated with chronic hypercalcemia (hyperparathyroidism) include metastatic calcification, hypercalciuria, and chronic renal insufficiency secondary to interstitial nephrocalcinosis.[14]

Calcium and/or calcium–phosphorus complex deposition in blood vessels and multiple organs is a complication of chronic hypercalcemia and/or concomitant hyperphosphatemia and hyperparathyroidism. Calcium deposits in atherosclerotic lesions contribute to cardiac disease.[17] Intracardiac and arterial calcifications have been found in patients with Paget disease who have normal renal function. It is hypothesized that similar calcification processes occur in both bone and vascular tissue, leading to cardiovascular diseases including heart failure, systolic hypertension, and ischemic heart disease.[18]

The electrocardiographic changes associated with hypercalcemia include shortening of the QT interval and coving of the ST-T wave.[14] Very high serum calcium concentrations can cause T-wave widening, indicating a repolarization defect that may be associated with spontaneous ventricular tachyarrhythmias.[14] Hypertension and arrhythmias have occurred in the setting of hypercalcemia. The effects of digoxin on cardiac conduction including lowering of the excitation threshold, shortening of the effective refractory period, and increased atrioventricular refractoriness can be potentiated by hypercalcemia.[19]

CLINICAL PRESENTATION Hypercalcemia

General

- The signs and symptoms of hypercalcemia depend on the severity and on the rapidity of onset.

Symptoms

- Symptoms include fatigue, weakness, anorexia, depression, anxiety, cognitive dysfunction, vague abdominal pain, and constipation. Renal symptoms can include polyuria, polydipsia, and nocturia. Rarely, severe hypercalcemia leads to acute pancreatitis.

Signs

- Renal: Nephrolithiasis; renal tubular dysfunction, particularly decreased concentrating ability; and acute and chronic renal insufficiency
- Cardiovascular: Hypercalcemia also directly shortens the myocardial action potential, which is reflected in a shortened QT interval and coving of the ST-T wave. Spontaneous ventricular tachyarrhythmias and elevations in blood pressure have also been reported. Chronic hypercalcemia can lead to cardiac calcification
- Musculoskeletal: Rheumatologic complaints related to hyperparathyroidism include gout, pseudogout, and chondrocalcinosis

Laboratory Tests

- Serum calcium concentrations of more than 10.5 mg/dL (more than 2.63 mmol/L) are considered to represent hypercalcemia. Patients with values up to 13 mg/dL (3.25 mmol/L) are generally considered to have mild or moderate hypercalcemia, whereas those with values greater than this indicate the presence of severe hypercalcemia.

Nephrolithiasis

Nephrolithiasis (kidney stones) and nephrocalcinosis (calcium deposits in the kidney) are the primary renal complications arising from long-standing hypercalcemia, as the result of primary hyperparathyroidism. Stone formation is dependent on a favorable milieu within the kidney or urinary tract, such as oversaturation of the urine and/or reduced concentrations of endogenous inhibitors of crystal formation (eg, citrate or pyrophosphate). It is estimated that hyperparathyroidism accounts for 2% to 8% of all patients with calcium stones.[20,21] Of note, in those patients with low glomerular filtration rates (GFRs), the 24-hour urinary calcium will actually diminish secondary to decreased production of 1,25-dihydroxy vitamin D_2. However, the fractional excretion of calcium might increase.[21] Sarcoidosis is the other hypercalcemic condition frequently associated with calcium stones.[14] Other causes of nephrolithiasis with calcium-containing stones include hypocitraturia, renal tubular acidosis, hyperoxaluria, and hyperuricosuria, which are conditions that are prevalent among bariatric surgery patients.[22,23] Stone formers who have primary hyperparathyroidism are more likely to be women, older than 50 years, and have a family history of multiple endocrine disorders.[20] High dietary sodium intake can also raise urinary calcium concentrations, perhaps due to a reduction in calcium reabsorption in the kidney, thus predisposing patients to calcium stones. Although chronic renal failure can be the ultimate result of persistent stones, it is the primary cause of renal disease in less than 2% of the end-stage renal disease population.

TREATMENT

Desired Outcome

The indications for the treatment of acute hypercalcemia are dependent on the severity of hypercalcemia, acuity of its development, and presence or absence of symptoms requiring emergent treatment (eg, necrotizing pancreatitis). The therapeutic intervention plan should be crafted to reverse signs and symptoms, restore normocalcemia within hours to days depending on acuity, and correct or manage the underlying cause of hypercalcemia.

General Approach

Chronic hypercalcemia is usually caused by an underlying medical condition or prescribed pharmacotherapies that can be resolved by successful treatment of the condition or withdrawal of the offending agent resulting in a decrease in serum calcium within days or weeks. Acute hypercalcemic episodes induced by malignancies may be mitigated by chemotherapy and/or radiation treatment. Effective surgical or drug treatment of primary hyperparathyroidism should reduce serum calcium concentrations as well as reduce the development of long-term complications such as vascular complications, chronic kidney disease (CKD), and kidney stones. For treatment of nephrolithiasis the goal in management of serum calcium is prevention of stone formation and diameter. The reduction of serum calcium should be targeted at the underlying disease state causing hypercalcemia (eg, using cinacalcet for primary hyperparathyroidism). Hypercalcemic crisis and acute symptomatic severe hypercalcemia should be considered medical emergencies and treated immediately (Fig. 50-2).

These patients may require immediate-acting interventions to promptly reduce the serum calcium concentration if electrocardiographic (ECG) changes, neurologic manifestations, or pancreatitis are present. Pharmacologic therapy consisting of volume expansion and enhancement of urinary calcium excretion with loop diuretics is usually the initial management strategy. Hemodialysis against a zero- or low-calcium dialysate solution should be considered for patients with severely impaired renal function (CKD stage 4 or 5) who cannot tolerate large fluid loads and in whom diuretics have limited efficacy.[14]

Effective treatment of moderate to severe hypercalcemia in the absence of life-threatening symptoms begins with attention to the underlying disorder and correction of associated fluid and electrolyte abnormalities. Patients with primary hyperparathyroidism may require surgery, particularly if they have systemic manifestations.

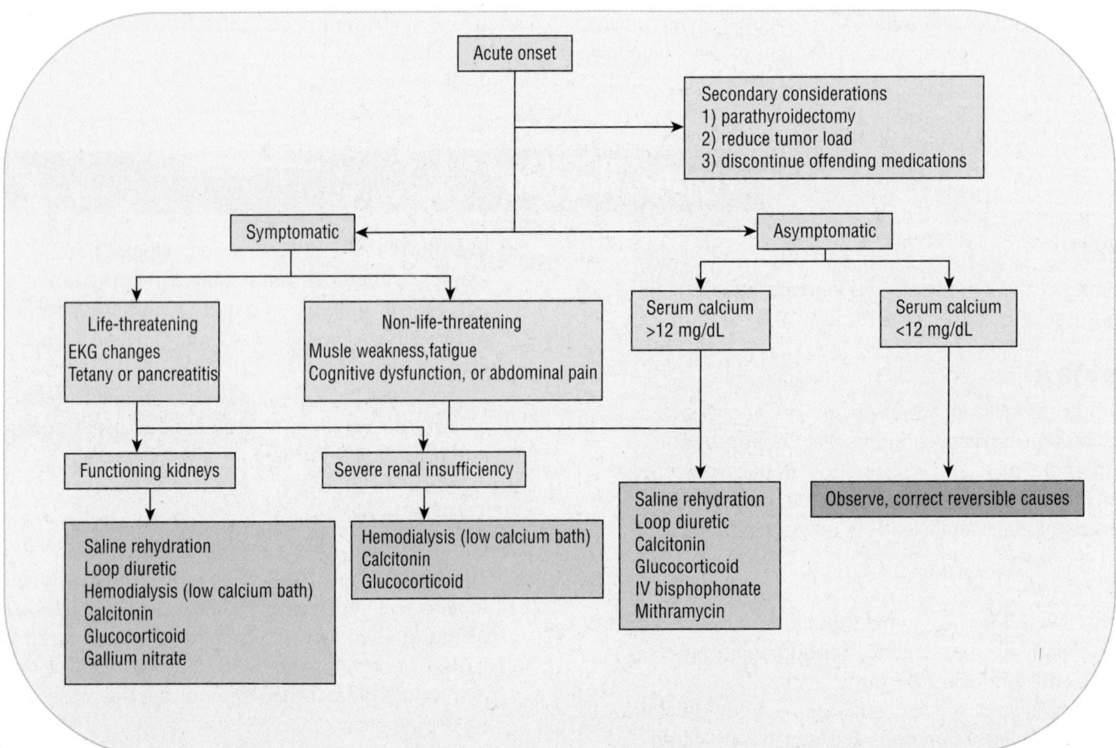

FIGURE 50-2 Pharmacotherapeutic options for the acutely hypercalcemic patient. Serum calcium of 12 mg/dL is equivalent to 3 mmol/L.

Patients with malignancy often require surgical or chemotherapeutic reduction of tumor load to control the exogenous supply of cytokines and hormones (eg, PTHrP) that cause hypercalcemia. In contrast, patients with drug-induced hypercalcemia generally respond to discontinuation of the offending agent.

Pharmacologic Therapy

Sympotomatic Patient Management

2 For those patients with normal to moderately impaired renal function (CKD stages 3a, 3b, and 4), the cornerstone of initial first-line treatment of severe, acute hypercalcemia or hypercalcemic crisis is volume expansion with normal saline to increase natriuresis and ultimately urinary calcium excretion (Table 50-2). Patients with symptomatic hypercalcemia are often extracellular volume depleted secondary to vomiting and polyuria; thus rehydration with saline-containing fluids is necessary to interrupt the stimulus for sodium and calcium reabsorption in the renal tubule.[24] Rehydration can be accomplished by the rapid infusion of 1 to 2 L of normal saline followed by a maintenance infusion at 250 to 300 mL/h, until the patient is fluid resuscitated and serum calcium approaches the upper limit of the normal range.[24] The precise rate depends on concomitant conditions (primarily cardiovascular and renal) and magnitude of hypercalcemia. The saline infusion rate can be decreased to a rate that approximates the patient's intake of oral or IV fluids. See Chapter 49 for a thorough discussion of how to calculate water deficit and monitor patient's response to saline infusion. Loop diuretics such as furosemide (40-80 mg IV every 1-4 hours) can also be instituted to increase urinary calcium excretion.[24] Loop diuretics block calcium (and sodium) reabsorption in the thick ascending limb of the loop of Henle and augment the calciuric effect of saline alone. Rehydration prior to loop diuretic use is critical because if dehydration persists or becomes worse, the serum calcium can actually increase because of enhanced proximal tubule calcium reabsorption.[25] The primary role for loop diuretics is to minimize the development of volume overload from the administration of saline. (Fig. 50-2 and Table 50-2). Despite its common use there is little evidence that supports the efficacy of furosemide in tratement of hypercalcemia.[25] Potassium chloride, 10 to 20 mEq/L (10-20 mmol/L), should be considered for addition to the saline infusion after rehydration is accomplished to prevent the development of hypokalemia that is a common adverse effect of aggressive diuretic therapy. Serum magnesium levels should also be monitored, and magnesium replacement instituted if magnesium concentrations fall below 1.8 mg/dL (0.74 mmol/L). Rehydration with saline and administration of furosemide may result in normalization total serum calcium within 24 to 48 hours, however, rebound hypercalcemia can occur.[25] Hemodialysis with low or zero calcium dialysate is a treatment option in the case of failure or when calcium concentrations are life threatening. It should be noted that preparing a patient for hemodialysis takes time to achieve vascular access, thus, this approach is best suited for patients already receiving hemodialysis chronically.

Asymptomatic Patient Managment

Calcitonin In those patients in whom saline hydration therapy is contraindicated (eg, those with severe chronic heart failure [CHF] or moderate-to-severe renal dysfunction), short-term therapy with calcitonin is a viable alternative agent to initiate reduction of serum calcium levels within 24 to 48 hours. Calcitonin has a rapid onset of action (within 1-2 hours); however, the degree and extent of serum calcium level reduction are often unpredictable.[2]

Subcutaneous administration of salmon calcitonin, 50 to 100 international units daily or three times weekly, has been used to manage mild hypercalcemia in patients with Paget disease.[26] The intranasal formulation of calcitonin has been used in doses of 200 to 400 international units daily; unfortunately, this has resulted in only mild decreases in serum calcium. The lack of significant efficacy of the synthetic intranasal formulation is the result of the lower potency and shorter duration of action as compared to salmon calcitonin.

Pharmacology Calcitonin decreases serum calcium concentrations, primarily by inhibiting bone resorption. It can also reduce renal tubular reabsorption of calcium, thus promoting calciuresis.[26] Calcitonin from salmon sources is most commonly administered subcutaneously or intramuscularly (for larger volumes) in a starting dose of 4 units/kg every 12 hours.

Adverse Effects The side effects from IV administered calcitonin (facial flushing, nausea, and vomiting) limit patient acceptability. Allergic reactions, although rare, do occur; therefore, a test dose (intradermal injection of 0.1 mL of a 10 units/mL solution) is recommended prior to starting therapy. If marked erythema and/or wheal formation does not occur within 15 minutes after administration, therapy can begin. Salmon calcitonin therapy is associated with tachyphylaxis caused by antibody formation to foreign proteins or molecules resembling the calcitonin polypeptide.[27] Tachyphylaxis has been primarily documented in patients receiving therapy for more than 4 months and thus might not be clinically significant in the acute care setting. The addition of corticosteroid therapy or conversion to human calcitonin increases effectiveness.[2]

TABLE 50-2 Drug Dosing Table for Hypercalcemia

Drug/Brand Name	Starting Dosage	Time Frame to Initial Response	Monitoring and Special Population Considerations
0.9% saline ± electrolytes	200-300 mL/h	24-48 hours	Electrolyte abnormalities; fluid overload CI in renal insufficiency; congestive heart failure
Loop diuretics Furosemide/Lasix® Bumetandide/Bumex® Torsemide/Demadex®	40-80 mg IV q 1-4 h of furosemide or equivalent	N/A	Electrolyte abnormalities (potassium and magnesium) CI in patients with allergy to sulfas (use ethacrynic acid)
Calcitonin/Miacalcin®	4 units/kg q 12 h SC/IM 10-12 units/h IV	1-2 hours	Facial flushing, nausea/vomiting, allergic reaction, CI in patients with allergy to calcitonin
Pamidronate/Aredia®	30-90 mg IV over 2-24 hours	2 days	Fever, fatigue, skeletal pain, CI in renal insufficiency
Zoledronate/Zometa®	4-8 mg IV over 15 minutes	1-2 days	Fever, fatigue, skeletal pain, CI in renal insufficiency
Glucocorticoids	40-60 mg oral prednisone equivalents daily	3-5 days	Diabetes; osteoporosis; infection, CI in patients with serious infections; hypersensitivity

CI, contraindicated; SC, subcutaneous.

Bisphosphonates Bisphosphonates block bone resorption very efficiently, render the hydroxyapatite crystal of bone mineral resistant to hydrolysis by phosphatases, and also inhibit osteoclast precursors from attaching to the mineralized matrix, thus blocking their transformation into mature functioning osteoclasts.[14,28] The antiresorptive properties of this class of agents can provide long-term control of serum calcium and are the first-line therapy for cancer-associated hypercalcemia.

Pharmacology The first line bisphosphonates to treat hypercalcemia are pamidronate and zoledronic acid.[29] The usual dose of pamidronate is 30 to 90 mg as an IV infusion given over 2 to 24 hours. Pamidronate also has the advantage of single-day therapy.[29] Zoledronic acid is a high-potency bisphosphonate with demonstrated effectiveness in the treatment of hypercalcemia of malignancy. Complete response has been reported in 88.4% to 86.7% of zoledronate- versus 69.7% of pamidronate-treated patients.[30,31] Zoledronic acid IV doses of 4 to 8 mg given over 15 minutes have resulted in normalization of serum calcium concentrations.[30] IV infusions of 0.02 or 0.04 mg/kg diluted in 5% dextrose (given over 20-50 minutes) have also been effective.[32] The onset of serum calcium concentration decline is slower with bisphosphonate therapy (concentrations begin to decline in 2 days and reach a nadir in 7 days); thus calcitonin therapy or other interventions may be necessary if rapid serum level reduction is required.[29] Duration of normocalcemia varies, but usually does not exceed 2 to 3 weeks. It appears to be dependent on the severity and treatment response of the underlying malignancy.[7] The duration of response has been suggested to be longer with zoledronate (4-5 weeks), although the data are sparse.[32]

Adverse Effects Fever is a common side effect of IV bisphosphonate therapy. Although oral bisphosphonates are useful for the treatment of bone turnover in Paget disease, there are insufficient data to suggest their use for the initial treatment of hypercalcemia. The use of oral bisphosphonates for maintenance therapy in patients predisposed to hypercalcemia (malignancy) has been successful in some cases.[33] The safety of continuous bisphosphonate therapy in patients with moderate-to-severe renal insufficiency is currently unknown. Renal function monitoring (serum creatinine) is advised with the use of bisphosphonates, as cases of renal function decline and acute tubular necrosis have been reported.[34,35] Although there are no published guidelines for frequency of serum creatinine monitoring, it is advisable to evaluate serum creatinine within a week after the infusion and just prior to the next scheduled dose. Osteonecrosis of the jaw is evidenced by an area of exposed bone in the maxillofacial or mandibular region that does not heal within 8 weeks after diagnosis.[29] Higher potency bisphosphonates and longer durations of therapy are associated with increased risk.[36]

Denosumab

Pharmacology Denosumab is a monoclonal antibody that inhibits the receptor activator of nuclear factor kappa-light-chain-enhancer of activated B cells (NF-κB) ligand (RANKL), a principal mediator of osteoclast survival. Denosumab is FDA-approved for the treatment hypercalcemia of malignancy.[37] An open-label, trial evaluated the value of denosumab in patients with hypercalcemia of malignancy (with or without bone metastases) who were refractory to intravenous bisphosphonate therapy, that is, their corrected serum calcium remained above 12.5 mg/dL (3.13 mmol/L) after more than 7 days of therapy.[37] Sixty-four percent of patients who received 120 mg of denosumab subcutaneously on days 1, 8, achieved a corrected serum calcium less than or equal to 11.5 mg/dL (less than or equal to 2.88 mmol/L) within 10 days which is considered an appropriate duration for time to clinical response. Denosumab has also been reported to successfully treat hypercalcemia after successful stem cell transplantation and restitution of osteoclast function in patients with osteopetrosis, a heritable disorder associated with defective osteoclast function.[38]

Adverse Effects Denosumab has been associated with osteonecrosis of the jaw.[39] Athough the renal impairment has not been shown to affect the pharmacodynamics and pharmacokinetics of denosumab, severe, symptomatic hypocalcemia has been reported in CKD patients receiving the drug.[40] This may be due to induction of a hungry bone-like syndrome and warrants careful monitoring.[41]

Corticosteroids Prednisone or an equivalent agent is usually effective in the treatment of hypercalcemia resulting from multiple myeloma, leukemia, lymphoma, sarcoidosis, and hypervitaminoses A and D.[14,28,42] Steriods are effective because they reduce GI calcium absorption.[42] Corticosteroids may also prevent tachyphylaxis to salmon calcitonin.[26] Daily doses of 40 to 60 mg of prednisone or the equivalent have effectively normalized serum calcium values within 3 to 5 days followed by a reduction in urinary calcium excretion within 7 to 10 days. The disadvantages of corticosteroid therapy are its relatively slow onset of action and the potential for diabetes mellitus, osteoporosis, and increased susceptibility to infection.[43]

Cinacalcet The calcimimetic agent cinacalcet is approved for management of parathyroid carcinoma and primary hyperparathyroidism.[44,45] It binds to the CaSr, and increases the sensitivity for receptor activation by extracellular calcium. This results in reduced PTH and serum calcium concentrations.[44,45] Cinacalcet administered at a starting dose of 30 mg orally twice daily has been used for the treatment of hypercalcemia secondary to parathyroid carcinoma. The dosage is titrated every 2 to 4 weeks in 30-mg increments until the desired serum calcium level is achieved. The maximum approved dosage is 90 mg three to four times daily. Patients should have serum calcium measured within 1 week after starting or increasing the dose of this agent.[46] The role of cinacalcet in the management of nephrolithiasis is still controversial. Patients were randomly assigned to receive potassium citrate alone, allopurinol or allopurinol with cinacalet. Stone number and diameter was reduced compared to baseline in patients who received the combination regimen with cinacalcet in both hypercalcemic and normocalcemic patients.[47]

Pharmacoeconomic Considerations

For treatment of asymptomatic hypercalcemia from a pharmacoeconomic standpoint corticosteroids are very inexpensive, however, the low cost of the drug may be offset by the multitude of long-term side effects and potential need for additional treatment. Calcitonin is only suitable for very short-term therapy and thus long-term pharmacoeconimic analyses have not been done. The introduction of denosomab and it's demonstrated efficacy in preventing and delaying skeletal related adverse events while reducing hypocalcemia has stimulated cost-effectiveness analyses.[48] Denosumab and zoledronic acid in hormone refractory prostate cancer with bone metastatses showed that the incremental total costs per skeletal-related adverse event avoided for denosomab were $71,027 over a 1-year period and $51,319 over a 3-year period.[48] This suggests that denosomab may be a costly alternative to zoledronic acid and formulary restrictions with specific patient criteria may be judicious. Additional considerations for choice of therapy evaluated in a survey of more than 200 physicians included co-pay costs and patient assistance program availablity for these agents.[49]

Nephrolithiasis Chronic Hypercalcuria and Hypercalemia

Patients who develop nephrolithiasis from hypercalciuria are most often treated with sodium citrate to prevent stone formation, thiazide diuretics to decrease urinary calcium excretion, or shock wave lithotripsy (Table 50-3). There are multiple approaches to treating

TABLE 50-3 Treatment of Nephrolithiasis Associated with Chronic Hypercalcemia and Hypercalciuria

Intervention	Indications	Comments
Extracorporeal Shock Wave Lithotripsy		
Uses sound waves to break up stones, which then can pass spontaneously	Obstruction of the urinary tract, especially with stones >5 mm	Consider adjunctive use of potassium citrate to inhibit aggregation of residual fragments
Prevention of Stone Formation		
Alkalinizing agents	Treatment for nonemergent active stones. Can also be used for prevention	Potassium citrate preferred over sodium citrate as it decreases urinary calcium, inhibits calcium oxalate precipitation, and increases urinary citrate more
Potassium citrate PO 20 mEq twice daily		
Sodium citrate PO 20-30 mEq twice daily		
Decrease Urinary Calcium Excretion		
Thiazide diuretics	Prevention	Drug of choice in patients with low bone density
Hydrochlorothiazide (Hydrodiuril®) PO 50 mg every day		
Indapamide (Lozol®) PO 25 mg every day		
Chlorthalidone (Hygroton®) PO 25 mg every day		
Binding Intestinal Calcium		
Cellulose sodium phosphate (Calcibind)	Prevention for those with absorptive hypercalciuria	Alternative to thiazides if intolerant or ineffective, monitor bone density
Calcium binding ion-exchange resin that decreases GI absorption of calcium: PO 5 g twice daily with oxalate restriction		
Inhibition of Crystal Formation		
Phyllanthus niruri plant extract	Prevention, after shock wave lithotripsy	Commercial preparations with *P. niruri* as the sole ingredient can be difficult to obtain
Inhibits calcium oxalate stone formation by incorporating glycosaminoglycans into the calculi: PO 2 g daily		
Low-Calcium Diet		
Less than 400 mg/day	Prevention	Monitor bone density prior to and periodically during treatment, limit oxalate restriction, can increase hyperoxaluria, data suggest that high calcium intake may actually be more beneficial

and preventing future nephrolithiasis issues which include stone removal or disintegration, using medications to dissolve or prevent stone formation as well as dietary interventions to prevent stone formation.[23] Procedures such as shockwave lithotripsy are effective in disintegrating stones and subsequently allowing for their urinary removal, however, the procedure is painful and expensive. Urinary alkalinizing agents such as potassium or sodium citrate prevent growth of stone diameter, increasing the likelihood of spontaneous passage. These agents can also be used for prevention but are available in liquid form and must be taken consistently multiple times per day to maintain an alkaline urine.[20] Thiazide diuretics decrease urinary calcium excretion and reduce the potential for crystal formation and are commonly used for prevention.[23] Other agents such as calcium binding resins, natural plant extracts (*Phyllanthus niruri*) and reduction of dietary calcium have limited evidence that they offer a successful prevention strategy.

HYPOCALCEMIA

3 Hypocalcemia occurs infrequently in the outpatient setting and is most common in elderly, malnourished patients and those who have received sodium phosphate as a bowel preparation agent.

Epidemiology

The incidence of hypocalcemia in intensive care unit patients ranges from 70% to 90% based on total serum calcium values less than 8.5 mg/dL (2.13 mmol/L) to 15% to 50% based on the observation of ionized calcium concentrations less than 4.4 mg/dL (1.10 mmol/L).[4] Emergent treatment of hypocalcemia is rarely warranted unless life-threatening symptoms are present (eg, frank tetany or seizures).

Pathophysiology

Hypocalcemia is the result of alterations in the effect of PTH and vitamin D on the bone, gut, and kidney (see Fig. 50-1). The primary causes of hypocalcemia are postoperative hypoparathyroidism and vitamin D deficiency. Other causes include magnesium deficiency, thyroid surgery, medications, hypoalbuminemia, blood transfusions, peripheral blood progenitor cell harvesting, tumor lysis syndrome, and mutations in the CaSr.[50-55] PTH concentrations are elevated in conditions of hypocalcemia, with the exception of hypoparathyroidism and hypomagnesemia.[56]

Vitamin D Deficiency

Vitamin D and its metabolites play an important role in the maintenance of extracellular calcium concentrations and in normal skeletal structure and mineralization. Vitamin D is necessary for the optimal absorption of calcium and phosphorus. On a worldwide basis, the most common cause of chronic hypocalcemia is nutritional vitamin D deficiency. In malnourished populations, manifestations include rickets and osteomalacia. Nutritional vitamin D deficiency is uncommon in Western societies because of the fortification of milk with ergocalciferol. The most common cause of vitamin D deficiency in Western societies is GI disease.[14] Gastric surgery, chronic pancreatitis, small-bowel disease, intestinal resection, and bypass surgery are associated with decreased concentrations of vitamin D and its metabolites.[14] Vitamin D replacement therapy might need to be administered by the IV route if poor oral bioavailability is noted. Decreased production of 1,25-dihydroxyvitamin D_3 can occur as a result of a hereditary defect resulting in vitamin D-dependent rickets.[56] Recently, polymorphisms of the vitamin D receptor have been identified, and these genetic variations can contribute to increased risk of rickets associated with vitamin D and calcium deficient diets, especially in certain African and East Asian populations.[57] It also can occur secondary to CKD if there is insufficient production of the 1-α-hydroxylase enzyme for the production of the 1,25-dihydroxy vitamin D_3. Treatment of hypocalcemia associated with CKD is reviewed in Chapter 44.

Hypomagnesemia

Hypomagnesemia of any cause can be associated with severe symptomatic hypocalcemia that is unresponsive to calcium replacement therapy (see Chapter 51). Reduced serum magnesium concentrations can impair PTH secretion and induce resistance of target organs to the actions of PTH.[14] Normalization of serum calcium concentrations in these patients is thus dependent on appropriate replacement of magnesium.

Hungry Bone Syndrome

An acute, symptomatic rapid fall in total serum calcium concentration (to values less than 7 mg/dL [less than 1.75 mmol/L]) is common in patients who have recently had a parathyroidectomy or thyroidectomy. Hypocalcemia in these postsurgical patients is generally transient in nature.[56] The "hungry bone syndrome" is a condition of profound hypocalcemia whereby the bone avidly incorporates calcium and phosphorus from the blood in an attempt to recalcify bone.[58] Serum calcium concentrations should be monitored every 6 hours during the 24 to 48 hours following such surgeries, and pharmacologic doses of calcium can be necessary to prevent or minimize the drop in serum calcium. Additionally, mild-to-moderate hypocalcemia can be a long-term consequence of parathyroidectomy in hemodialysis patients.[56]

Drug-Induced Hypocalcemia

Drug-induced hypocalcemia has been reported in patients receiving furosemide, calcitonin, bisphosphonates, denosomab, oral sodium phosphate solutions, polyethylene glycol bowel preparation solutions, cinacalcet, fluoride, ketoconazole, and pentamidine.[40,46,59,60]

Oral phosphorus therapy, commonly used to treat patients with malabsorption syndromes caused by GI diseases, can also result in hypocalcemia. The anticonvulsants phenobarbital and phenytoin cause hypocalcemia by increasing catabolism of vitamin D and thereby impairing calcium release from bone and reducing intestinal calcium absorption.[50] Drugs that cause hypomagnesemia (aminoglycosides, amphotericin B, cyclosporine, diuretics, foscarnet, and cisplatin) are also associated with an increased risk of hypocalcemia.[61] Chelating agents in blood (citrate) and in radiographic contrast media (ethylenediaminetetraacetate) can also cause transient hypocalcemia.[50,51,62] Concentrated citrate is increasingly being used in hemodialysis catheter locks and to anticoagulate the dialysis circuit during continuous renal replacement therapy.[63] Symptomatic hypocalcemia (ionized calcium less than 2.4 mg/dL [less than 0.60 mmol/L]) has been reported in patients exposed to citrate solutions, which appears to be related to the concentration of the citrate solution.[64] Injection of citrate solutions greater than the volume of the dead space of the catheter lumen or accidental injection of citrate catheter lock solutions that are not intended for systemic

CLINICAL PRESENTATION Hypocalcemia

General

- Acute hypocalcemia may result in rapid decreases in serum ionized calcium. Parathyroidectomy and thyroidectomy are also associated with a rapid reduction in serum calcium. In chronic hypocalcemia vitamin D deficiency should be considered.

Symptoms

- The symptoms of hypocalcemia include tetany, paresthesia, muscle cramps, and laryngeal spasms. Chronic hypocalcemia is usually associated with depression, anxiety, memory loss, and confusion.

Signs

- Neurologic: The hallmark of acute hypocalcemia is tetany, which is characterized by neuromuscular irritability including seizure potential. Extrapyramidal disorders, mainly parkinsonism but also dystonia, hemiballismus, choreoathetosis, and oculogyric crises occur in 5% to 10% of patients with idiopathic hypoparathyroidism. Chvostek and/or Trousseau signs can be elicited during physical examination.
- Dermatologic: The skin can be dry, puffy, and coarse. Other dermatologic manifestations can include hyperpigmentation, dermatitis, eczema, and psoriasis. Hair and skin signs including coarse, brittle, and sparse hair with patchy alopecia and brittle nails can also appear.
- Ophthalmologic: Cataract development has been reported to occur with hypocalcemia.
- Dental manifestations: These are usually associated with the presence of chronic hypocalcemia in early development. Signs include dental hypoplasia, failure of tooth eruption, defective enamel and root formation, and abraded carious teeth.
- Cardiovascular: Hypotension, decreased myocardial performance, and CHF have been reported. A prolonged QT interval, arrhythmias, and bradycardia can also occur but are more common with acute or very severe hypocalcemia.
- GI: Steatorrhea can be associated with chronic hypocalcemia.
- Musculoskeletal: Myopathy has been reported.
- Endocrine: Hypocalcemia alone can impair insulin release. In addition, idiopathic hypoparathyroidism can be associated with polyglandular autoimmune syndromes.

Laboratory Tests

- Serum calcium levels of less than 8.5 mg/dL (2.13 mmol/L) are considered to represent hypocalcemia if ionized calcium values are also less than 4.4 mg/dL (1.1 mmol/L).

administration have been associated with serious cardiovascular problems such as hypotension or cardiac arrest.[65]

Hypoparathyroidism

Hypoparathyroidism can be caused by autoimmune disease, congenital defects, or iatrogenically by inadvertent removal of some or all of the parathyroid glands during thyroidectomy or from damage with radiation therapy. Chronic hypoparathyroidism produces an insidious development of hypocalcemia and thus most patients remain asympotomatic. The chronic hypocalcemia may ultimately present as visual impairment secondary to cataracts.[66]

Clinical Presentation

The clinical manifestations of hypocalcemia are quite variable. The more acute the drop in ionized calcium concentration, the more likely the patient will develop symptoms.[3] Increases in plasma pH enhance the binding of calcium to albumin and thus alkalosis can result in rapid decreases in ionized calcium. Concomitant hypomagnesemia, hypokalemia, hyponatremia, and additive side effects from prescribed medications also increase the likelihood of symptomatic presentation.

Hypocalcemia can manifest as neuromuscular, central nervous system (CNS), dermatologic, and cardiac sequelae.[14] Acute hypocalcemia is more likely to manifest as neuromuscular (paresthesia, muscle cramps, tetany, and laryngeal spasm) and cardiovascular symptoms, whereas chronic hypocalcemia often presents as CNS (eg, depression, anxiety, memory loss, confusion, hallucinations, and tonic–clonic seizures) and dermatologic symptoms (hair loss, grooved and brittle nails, and eczema).[50] The hallmark sign of acute hypocalcemia is tetany caused by enhanced peripheral neuromuscular irritability.[14] Tetany manifests as paresthesia around the mouth and in the extremities, muscle spasms and cramps, carpopedal (hands and feet) spasms, and rarely as laryngospasm and bronchospasm.[14] Chvostek and/or Trousseau signs can be elicited during physical examination.[50] Chvostek sign is elicited by tapping the facial nerve anterior to the ear and eliciting twitching of facial muscles. Trousseau sign is elicited by inflating a blood pressure cuff above systolic blood pressure for 3 minutes and observing whether a carpal spasm is induced.

The cardiovascular manifestations of hypocalcemia result in ECG changes characterized by a prolonged QT interval and symptoms of decreased myocardial contractility often associated with congestive heart failure (CHF).[50] Both acute and chronic hypocalcemia can result in a reversible syndrome characterized by acute myocardial failure or refractory CHF. Other cardiovascular manifestations include arrhythmias, bradycardia, and hypotension that are unresponsive to fluid and pressor administration.[50]

Clinical **Controversy...**

Bariatric surgery is associated with malabsorption of calcium. There are limited data regarding the differential impact the various bariatric procedures have on calcium absorption and what if any adverse consequences develop.[23]

TREATMENT

Desired Outcome

4 The goals of therapy for patients with normal renal function are the resolution of signs and symptoms of hypocalcemia, restoration of normocalcemia, management of associated electrolyte abnormalities, and treatment of the underlying cause of hypocalcemia. The goals for patients with CKD are different and are discussed in detail in Chapter 44. Asymptomatic hypocalcemia associated with hypoalbuminemia requires no treatment because ionized (physiologically active) plasma calcium concentrations are normal. Treatment of hypocalcemia is dependent on identification of the pathogenesis of the underlying disorder, acuteness of onset, and presence and severity of symptoms.

Pharmacologic Therapy

Treatment of hypocalcemia is driven by acuity of onset and how significant the ionized calcium is below the normal range. The first approach to treatment is to evaluate causes that will dictate corrective action. Acute symptomatic hypocalcemia will nearly always require parenteral administration of soluble calcium salts (Fig. 50-3).

Acute Treatment

The initial therapeutic intervention for patients with acute symptomatic hypocalcemia is to administer 100 to 300 mg of elemental calcium IV slowly over 10 to 30 minutes.[66] This can be accomplished by the administration of 1 g of calcium chloride (27% elemental calcium) or 2 to 3 g of calcium gluconate (9% elemental calcium). Calcium gluconate is generally preferred over calcium chloride for peripheral venous administration because calcium gluconate is less irritating to veins. Calcium should not be infused at a rate greater than 60 mg of elemental calcium per minute because severe cardiac dysfunction, including ventricular fibrillation, can result, thus electrocardiogram monitoring is recommended.[61] IV calcium administration should be used with caution in patients receiving digitalis glycosides because of the possibility of bradycardia or atrioventricular (A–V) block.[66] The bolus dose of calcium is only effective for 1 to 2 hours and should be followed by a continuous infusion of elemental calcium at a rate of 0.5 to 2 mg/kg per hour.[61] Serum calcium should rise by approximately 1.2 to 2 mg/dL (0.30-0.50 mmol/L).[66] The calcium concentrations should be monitored every 4 to 6 hours during IV infusions. The ionized calcium concentration usually normalizes within 4 hours, and the maintenance infusion rate of elemental calcium can then be decreased to 0.3 to 0.5 mg/kg per hour to maintain the desired calcium concentration.[66] Calcium should not be added to bicarbonate- or phosphate-containing solutions because of the possibility of precipitation.[61] Treatment of chronic hypoparathyroidism with parathyroid hormone formulations such as teriparatide has been shown to better maintain serum calcium concentrations and normalize urinary calcium.[67]

Chronic Treatment

Once acute hypocalcemia is corrected by parenteral administration, further treatment modalities should be individualized according to the cause of hypocalcemia. If hypomagnesemia is present, magnesium supplementation is indicated until concentrations normalize which will promote successful calcium supplementation regardless of route. (see Chapter 51). Hypocalcemia secondary to hungry bone syndrome following parathyroidectomy has been attenuated by pretreatment with bisphosphonates.[68] Asymptomatic and chronic hypocalcemia associated with hypoparathyroidism and vitamin D-deficient states can be managed by oral calcium and vitamin D supplementation (see Chapter 44). Therapy is begun with 1 to 3 g/day of elemental calcium.[61] Average maintenance doses range from 2 to 8 g of elemental calcium per day in divided doses. If serum calcium does not normalize, a vitamin D preparation may need to be added. In patients with achlorhydria a solution of 10% (1-30 mL) calcium chloride orally every 8 hours can raise serum calcium.[61]

Treatment of chronic asymptomatic hypocalcemia associated with vitamin D-deficient states should be individualized. In patients with malabsorption, vitamin D requirements vary markedly, and large doses can be required. In contrast, vitamin D deficiency associated with anticonvulsant medication can be corrected with smaller

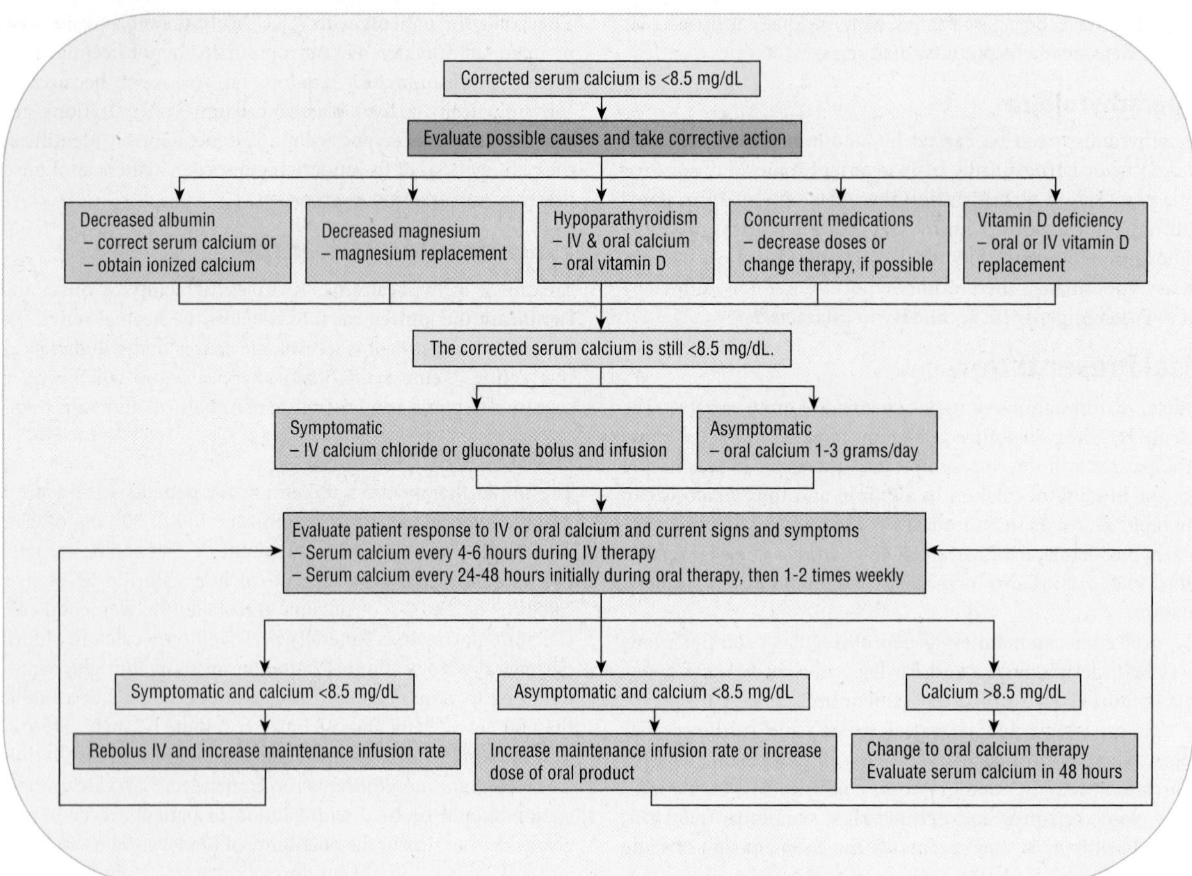

FIGURE 50-3 Hypocalcemia diagnostic and treatment algorithm. Serum calcium of 8.5 mg/dL is equivalent to 2.13 mmol/L.

doses of vitamin D. Oral doses of 1,25-dihydroxy vitamin D_3 usually range from 0.5 to 3 mcg daily.[61] The usual initial oral dose of ergocalciferol is 50,000 international units daily.[61] Vitamin D doses are usually adjusted approximately every 4 weeks. Vitamin D deficiency is highly prevalent especially in areas of low sun exposure and limited dietary sources of vitamin D.[69] New data suggest that current dietary recommendations are not sufficient to maintain 25-hydroxy vitamin D_3 concentrations at or above 32 mcg/L (80 nmol/L).[69] The treatment of vitamin D deficiency associated with CKD generally requires the administration of 1,25-dihydroxy vitamin D_3 or another synthetic vitamin D_2 analog such as paricalcitol or doxercalciferol. Patients who have reduced 25-hydroxylase activity (eg, hepatic disease) can also require treatment with calcitriol (1,25-dihydroxy vitamin D_3). In selected cases, increasing calcium ingestion can be required if vitamin D replacement alone is ineffective in returning calcium concentrations to normal.

Clinical **Controversy...**

Some data have shown that animal source vitamin D_3 (cholecalciferol) is more efficacious at raising serum 25(OH) D concentrations compared with plant source vitamin D_2 (ergocalciferol). However, higher loading and maintenance doses of cholecalciferol are required to maintain serum 25, OH vitamin D concentrations.

Adverse Effects

Adverse effects of oral calcium and vitamin D supplementation include hypercalcemia and hypercalciuria, especially in the hypoparathyroid patient, in whom the renal calcium-sparing effect of PTH is absent. Hypercalciuria can increase the risk of calcium stone formation and nephrolithiasis in susceptible patients. One maneuver to help prevent calcium stones is to maintain the urine calcium excretion below 300 mg per day. Intermittently monitoring of 24-hour urine collections for total calcium excretion can help minimize the occurrence of hypercalciuria. The addition of thiazide diuretics for patients at risk for stone formation can result in an increase in tubular calcium reabsorption and reduction of vitamin D requirements.[61] (see Table 50-3)

DISORDERS OF PHOSPHORUS HOMEOSTASIS

Inorganic phosphorus in the form of phosphate is an essential element in phospholipid cell membranes, nucleic acids, and phosphoproteins, which are required for mitochondrial function.[1] Phosphorus regulates the intermediary metabolism of carbohydrates, fats, and proteins. Phosphorus also regulates enzymatic reactions including glycolysis, ammoniagenesis, and the 1-hydroxylation of 25-hydroxyvitamin D_3.[1,70] In addition, phosphorus is required for the generation of 2,3-diphosphoglycerate (2,3-DPG) in red blood cells, which is required for normal oxygen–hemoglobin dissociation and delivery of oxygen to the tissues.[1] Phosphorus is the source of the high-energy bonds of adenosine triphosphate (ATP), thus fueling a wide variety of physiologic processes, including muscle contractility, electrolyte transport, neurologic function, and other important biochemical reactions.[1] Considering its diverse biologic importance, it is not difficult to appreciate the clinical implications of disorders of phosphorus homeostasis.

Phosphate, the major intracellular anion, is present in living organisms mainly as organic phosphate esters such as 2,3-DPG, adenosine, guanosine triphosphate, and fructose 1,6-diphosphate.[1] Only a small fraction of intracellular phosphorus exists as inorganic phosphate; however, this fraction is critical because it is the source from which ATP is resynthesized.[1] The majority of inorganic phosphate is located in the extracellular space where it is the prime determinant of intracellular phosphate; thus, small increments in the organic phosphate levels can profoundly alter both the extracellular and intracellular phosphate levels. Metabolic disturbances (acidosis, alkalosis, and ketoacidosis), hydrogen ion shifts, and hormones (PTH, calcitonin, cortisol, and vitamin D) all can cause transcellular shifts in phosphorus concentrations. Because of these phenomena, the serum phosphorus level does not accurately reflect total body stores.[71]

The typical Western diet provides a daily intake of 800 to 1,600 mg of phosphorus. Approximately 60% to 80% of this is absorbed in the GI tract by passive and active transport (vitamin D-mediated). PTH, 1,25-dihydroxy vitamin D_3, and low-phosphate diets mediate increased absorption. Decreased absorption occurs under conditions of increased dietary intake of phosphorus and magnesium, glucocorticoid therapy, and hypothyroidism. The normal serum phosphorus concentration in adults is 2.5 to 4.5 mg/dL (0.81-1.45 mmol/L) and for children younger than 12 years it is 4 to 5.6 mg/dL (1.29-1.81 mmol/L). Influx via the GI tract and bone and tubular reabsorption by the kidney are the most important regulators of steady-state serum phosphorus concentrations. Renal excretion of phosphorus is a two-step process: glomerular filtration and proximal tubular reabsorption by passive transport coupled to sodium. Under normal conditions, 85% to 90% of filtered phosphate is reabsorbed, the majority in the early proximal tubule. Renal tubular reabsorption of phosphate is inhibited by PTH and 1,25-dihydroxy vitamin D_3.[71] There are increasing data in the literature that indicate fibroblast growth factor 23 (FGF23) is a key regulator of phosphate homeostasis.[72] FGF23 acts principally to decrease tubular reabsorption of phosphate and inhibit 1-α-hydroxylase, thereby reducing the concentration of active vitamin D. FGF23-mediated receptor activation requires klotho, a transmembrane protein. The tissue specificity for FGF23 effects appears to be defined by klotho–FGF23 coexpression. Conversely, phosphate reabsorption in the renal tubule is increased by growth hormone, insulin, and insulin-like growth factor 1.[1] Internal phosphorus balance (transcellular phosphate distribution) is also of importance in the maintenance of normal serum phosphate. The serum phosphate concentration can vary by as much as 2 mg/dL (0.65 mmol/L) throughout the day, primarily as the result of changes in carbohydrate intake, insulin secretion, and diurnal variation.[1]

Hyperphosphatemia

Hyperphosphatemia typically results from either CKD, acute kidney injury (AKI), or endogenous intracellular phosphate release. Hyperphosphatemia occurs frequently in patients with AKI and is a nearly universal finding in those with advanced CKD (eg, stages 4 and 5). Tumor lysis syndrome, a complication of chemotherapy associated with massive lysis of cells and release of intracellular contents is also associated with hyperphoshatemia. The incidence of tumor lysis syndrome is highest among patients treated for acute lymphoblastic leukemia, acute myeloid leukemia and Burkitt's lymphoma[53] (see Chapter 134). Other causes of hyperphosphatemia include hemolysis and rhabdomyolysis.

Pathophysiology

5 The most common cause of hyperphosphatemia is a reduction in renal tubular reabsorption of phosphate when GFR is markedly inpaired (eg, GFR less than 25 mL/min/1.73 m^2 [less than 0.24 mL/s/m^2]).[70,71] Retention of phosphate decreases vitamin D synthesis and induces hypocalcemia, which leads to an increase in PTH, a finding that can be seen in those with stage 2 to 3 CKD. This physiologic response inhibits further tubular reabsorption of phosphorus as the kidney attempts to correct hyperphosphatemia and normalize serum calcium concentrations. Patients with excessive exogenous phosphate administration or who experience massive tissue breakdown or cell lysis in the setting of acute renal failure can rapidly develop moderate-to-severe hyperphosphatemia (serum phosphate more than 6.5 mg/dL [more than 2.10 mmol/L]).[71] Severe hyperphosphatemia (serum phosphate more than 7 mg/dL [more than 2.26 mmol/L]) is commonly encountered in patients with CKD, especially those with GFRs less than 15 mL/min per 1.73 m^2 (0.14 mL/s/m^2) (see Chapter 44).

Hyperphosphatemia caused by an increase in renal tubular reabsorption associated with hypoparathyroidism and associated decreases in PTH, is usually less severe than that observed in patients with severe renal failure or excessive exogenous or endogenous introduction of phosphate into the ECF. Acromegaly (mediated by growth hormone) and thyrotoxicosis (mediated by catecholamines) can also cause hyperphosphatemia by increasing tubular phosphate reabsorption.

Exogenous Phosphate Loads Iatrogenic causes of hyperphosphatemia have been widely reported, and clinicians should be aware of the phosphorus content of IV, oral, and rectally administered products.[73] Although less-well recognized, oral and rectal administration of phosphate-containing solutions such as sodium phosphate (Fleet Phospho-Soda) can also result in severe and life-threatening hyperphosphatemia, especially in patients with moderate and severe CKD.[60,73] The risk of mortality is dependent on the amount of phosphorus absorbed from the administered product; however, fatalities have occurred at low phosphate concentrations.[73] Acute phosphate nephropathy and renal failure have also been reported with the use of oral sodium phosphate bowel preparations. In 2008, the FDA issued a safety warning regarding the use of these products in patients at risk (the elderly, those with CKD) or on medications known to effect renal hemodynamics (eg, diuretics, nonsteroidal anti-inflammatory drugs [NSAIDs], or renin–angiotensin–aldosterone system inhibitors).[74] Acute phosphorus poisoning as a result of ingestion of laundry detergents is a rare and often unrecognized cause of elevated phosphate concentrations.

Rapid Tissue Catabolism Any disorder that results in necrosis of skeletal muscle (ie, rhabdomyolysis) can generate the release of large amounts of intracellular phosphate into the systemic circulation. This condition is frequently associated with AKI (see Chapter 43) and thus severe hyperphosphatemia can develop because of increased endogenous phosphate release coupled with the impaired proximal tubule reabsorption such that phosphaturic hormones (eg, PTH, FGF23) become ineffective. Bowel infarction, malignant hyperthermia, and severe hemolysis are also conditions that can increase endogenous release of phosphate.

Moderate hyperphosphatemia is also commonly observed in patients undergoing treatment for acute leukemia and lymphomas.[53] Chemotherapeutic treatment of acute lymphoblastic leukemia can result in the release of large amounts of phosphate into the systemic circulation secondary to lysis of lymphoblasts. Initiation of chemotherapy for Burkitt lymphoma results in tumor lysis syndrome, a rapid lysis of malignant cells that results in hyperphosphatemia, hyperuricemia, hyperkalemia, and hypocalcemia.[53]

Acid–Base Disorders Lactic acidosis and diabetic ketoacidosis can trigger the transcellular shift of endogenous intracellular phosphate into the extracellular space and thereby dramatically increases serum phosphorous concentrations.[75] After the institution of treatment, serum phosphate levels should be checked hourly as they can decrease rapidly, and patients can ultimately develop hypophosphatemia.

Clinical Presentation

The severe acute onset of hyperphosphatemia can result in calcium and phosphate complexation and lead to the precipitation of calcium phosphate crystals in soft tissues, and within the kidney tht can result in nephrolithiasis or obstructive uropathy. Extravascular calcification can result in band keratopathy, "red eye," pruritus, and periarticular calcification, especially in CKD patients. In addition, soft-tissue calcifications in the conjunctiva, skin, heart, cornea, lung, gastric mucosa, and kidney have been observed, primarily in CKD patients with chronic disordered mineral metabolism.[71] Extracellular phosphate can form insoluble nanoparticles with both calcium and fetuin-A which are referred to as calciprotein particles.[1] Calcium-phosphate crystals are likely to form in vivo when the product of the serum calcium and phosphate concentrations exceeds 50 to 60 mg^2/dL^2 (4-4.8 $mmol^2/L^2$). Serum phosphate concentrations greater than 6.5 mg/dL (2.10 mmol/L) have been independently associated with increased morbidity and mortality in patients on maintenance hemodialysis.[76] Other symptoms associated with moderate-to-severe hyperphosphatemia include nausea, vomiting, diarrhea, lethargy, and seizures. The major effects of long-term hyperphosphatemia are related to the development of hypocalcemia (caused by phosphate inhibition of renal 1-α-hydroxylase) and its related consequences, as well as vascular and organ damage resulting from the deposition of calcium-phosphate crystals. Hyperphosphatemia associated with CKD can result in renal osteodystrophy because of overproduction of PTH. This condition is discussed in detail in Chapter 44.

TREATMENT

Desired Outcome

Management of patients with acutely elevated serum phosphate concentrations should be directed at avoiding GI and neurologic symptoms and preventing deposition in the urinary tract to avoid the development of AKI. The treatment of hyperphosphatemia is focused on returning serum phosphate concentrations to the normal or near normal (for those with CKD) range, with the hope that one can minimize the long-term cardiovascular consequences of calcium-phosphate deposition in the vasculature. The Kidney Disease Improving Global Outcomes (KDIGO) clinical practice guidelines suggest that for patients with CKD stages 3 to 5, serum phosphorus should be maintained in the normal range. In dialysis-dependent patients with stage 5 CKD, KDIGO suggests lowering elevated phosphorus levels toward the normal range.[77] (See Table 44-10.)

Pharmacologic Therapy

Severe symptomatic hyperphosphatemia manifesting as hypocalcemia and tetany may be treated by the IV administration of calcium. Although this can seem counterintuitive and many consider it controversial for a patient with a phosphate of 16 mg/dL (5.17 mmol/L) and a calcium of 7 mg/dL (1.75 mmol/L) (the calcium–phosphorus product is 112 mg^2/dL^2 [9 $mmol^2/L^2$]), correction of severe hypocalcemia is of primary importance because of the critical nature of this disorder. If calcium concentrations are not critically low, the initial management strategy should include limitation of all exogenous sources of phosphate and efforts to block further absorption should be initiated. Hemodialysis can be initiated if the patient remains symptomatic despite these interventions.[61]

6 In general, the most effective way to treat nonemergent hyperphosphatemia is to decrease phosphate absorption from the GI tract by implementing phosphate-binding therapy and altering the dietary content of phosphorous.[71] Antacids containing divalent and trivalent cations (calcium, lanthanum, magnesium, iron, and aluminum), or sevelamer are the agents most frequently used in the prevention and treatment of hyperphosphatemia (see Table 44-11).[78] Long-term treatment with aluminum hydroxide and aluminum carbonate should be discouraged because the use of these agents has been associated with anemia, CNS disorders, and bone disease.[78] Short-term therapy with these agents is effective and safe. Aluminum, calcium, and magnesium agents are available in oral suspension formulations, which can aid administration in acutely ill patients who are receiving enteral nutrituion. The most frequent adverse effect from phosphate-binding agents (especially calcium) is constipation. Calcium salts are the preferred phosphate-binding agents except when there is concomitant hypercalcemia. Therapy with the polymer agent (sevelamer) or lanthanum carbonate might avoid the detrimental effects associated with the other agents. The iron-based binder offers the potential advantage of enhancing iron absorption (ferric citrate coordination complex) and reduced pilled burden (sucroferric oxyhydroxide).[79]

Hypophosphatemia

Mild-to-moderate hypophosphatemia is usually asymptomatic and associated with serum phosphate concentrations of 1 to 2 mg/dL (0.32-0.65 mmol/L), whereas severe hypophosphatemia that is frequently symptomatic is correlated with serum phosphorus concentrations of less than 1 mg/dL (0.32 mmol/L).[80]

Incidence

Hypophosphatemia has been observed in approximately 1% to 3% of the laboratory screening panels of patients who have been admitted to a hospital.[80] The incidence in hospitalized critically

CLINICAL PRESENTATION Hyperphosphatemia

General

- Serum phosphate concentration is primarily determined by the ability of the kidneys to reabsorb phosphate; therefore, hyperphosphatemia is uncommon in patients with normal kidney function.

Symptoms

- Acute symptoms include GI disturbances, lethargy, obstruction of the urinary tract, and rarely seizures. Symptoms associated with chronic hyperphosphatemia include "red eye" and pruritus.

Signs

- The elevated calcium-phosphate product results in precipitation in arteries, joints, soft tissues, and the viscera. This can result in tissue necrosis, termed calciphylaxis or calcemic uremic arteriopathy.

Laboratory Tests

- Serum phosphate levels more than 4.5 mg/dL (more than 1.45 mmol/L) represent hyperphosphatemia.

ill patients is 18% to 28%.[80] Unlike its severe form, mild or moderate hypophosphatemia seldom causes recognizable signs and symptoms.[78]

Pathophysiology 7 Hypophosphatemia can be the result of decreased GI absorption, reduced tubular reabsorption, or extracellular to intracellular redistribution.[1] Although mild-to-moderate hypophosphatemia is common and can occur in inpatients and outpatients, severe hypophosphatemia is predominantly encountered in the acute care setting and can be associated with life-threatening symptoms, including seizures, coma, and rhabdomyolysis (Table 50-4).

TABLE 50-4 Conditions Associated with the Development of Hypophosphatemia

Decreased GI absorption
Phosphate-binding drugs
Sucralfate
Calcium carbonate
Aluminum/magnesium antacids
Sevelamer
Lanthanum carbonate
Decreased dietary phosphorus intake
Glucocorticoids
Vitamin D deficiency/resistance
Hypoparathyroidism
Chronic diarrhea
Steatorrhea
Reduced tubular reabsorption
Hyperparathyroidism (primary and secondary)
Elevated FGF23
Recovery from burns
Rickets
Malignant neoplasms
Fanconi syndrome
Acute volume expansion
Metabolic acidosis
Renal transplantation
Vitamin D deficiency and/or resistance
Diuretics
Acetazolamide
Osmotic agents
Glucocorticoids
Sodium bicarbonate
Internal redistribution
Refeeding syndrome
Parenteral nutrition
Parathyroidectomy (hungry bone syndrome)
Alcoholism
Respiratory alkalosis
Diabetic ketoacidosis (correction)
Dextrose solutions
Insulin
Catecholamines
Anabolic steroids
Glucagon
Calcitonin
Erythropoietin

Decreased GI Absorption Phosphate-binding substances such as sucralfate, calcium carbonate, sevelamer, lanthanum carbonate, sucroferric oxyhydroxide, ferric citrate coordination complex, and aluminum- or magnesium-containing antacids have the potential to bind large amounts of phosphorus in the gut, thereby preventing absorption. If phosphate-binding agents are ingested on a chronic basis in conjunction with a dietary phosphorus deficiency, hypophosphatemia can result.[81] Patients who are receiving long-term phosphate-binding agents, those with peptic ulcer disease or CKD, and those who may be predisposed to moderate hypophosphatemia (alcoholics) are at highest risk for the development of severe hypophosphatemia. Hyperparathyroidism can cause hypophosphatemia as a result of decreased GI absorption of dietary phosphorus.

Decreased Tubular Reabsorption Reduced tubular reabsorption of phosphate can occur in hyperparathyroid (primary and secondary) patients with normal renal function and those with vitamin D deficiency or elevated FGF23 concentrations. Elevated PTH levels lead to an increase in serum calcium concentrations and decreased serum phosphate concentrations. Serum phosphorus is decreased as the result of a reduction in renal tubular reabsorption.[75] Recovery from extensive third-degree burns is associated with development of an anabolic state as stress levels decrease and nutritional therapies take effect as well as a marked diuretic phase associated with an impressive renal loss of phosphate.[82] Because phosphate is rapidly incorporated into the new cells, this can contribute to the severity of the hypophosphatemia. Drugs that cause increased renal elimination of phosphate include diuretics (acetazolamide and osmotic diuretics), glucocorticoids, and sodium bicarbonate.[81] In a recent analysis, the IV iron formulation ferric carboxymaltose was associated with the development of hypophosphatemia (in 51% of patients treated, and 13% of cases were severe (serum phosphorus less than 1 mg/dL [less than 0.32 mmol/L]) and prolonged.[83] The mechanism is unclear, however, iron deficiency itself is associated with elevated FGF-23.[84]

Cellular Redistribution Rapid refeeding of malnourished patients with high-carbohydrate, high-calorie diets with inadequate amounts of supplemental phosphate can result in severe symptomatic hypophosphatemia. This phenomenon is especially prevalent in patients with other underlying risk factors for the development of hypophosphatemia, such as alcoholism.[82] The etiology of severe hypophosphatemia associated with hyperalimentation and nutritional recovery can be separated into two phases: acute, rapid hypophosphatemia secondary to intracellular shifts of phosphate resulting from glucose-induced insulin secretion; and the gradual decrease in serum phosphate concentration over 5 to 10 days secondary to tissue repair in the presence of phosphate deprivation.[85] The development of severe hypophosphatemia secondary to hyperalimentation can be prevented by the administration of 12 to 15 mmol of phosphate per liter of hyperalimentation solution or 15 mmol per 1,000 calories (4.2 kJ) of dextrose.[85] Transcellular shifts in phosphate also occur after parathyroidectomy, causing severe hypocalcemia and hypophosphatemia because of hungry bone syndrome (deposition of phosphate and calcium in the bone).

Severe and prolonged respiratory alkalosis (a result of hyperventilation, pain, anxiety, and sepsis) can cause hypophosphatemia.[80] Respiratory alkalosis is thought to contribute significantly to the hypophosphatemia observed during alcohol withdrawal.[71] Although patients with diabetic ketoacidosis may present with hyperphosphatemia, the institution of therapy to correct it can cause serum phosphate concentrations to decrease rapidly as phosphate shifts back into the intracellular compartment. In addition, the acidosis associated with the diabetic ketoacidotic state can cause a decomposition of organic compounds inside the cell and a release of inorganic phosphate into the plasma and subsequently into the urine.[86] The combination of intracellular phosphate breakdown and the shift of phosphate into cells on initiation of treatment can lead to severe hypophosphatemia. Drugs associated with transcellular shifts in phosphate include dextrose solutions, glucagon, insulin, catecholamines, calcitonin, erythropoietic agents, and anabolic steroids.

Chronic ethanol abusers are prone to a variety of serum electrolyte disorders including hypocalcemia, hypomagnesemia, hypokalemia, and hypophosphatemia. The etiology of hypophosphatemia in the alcoholic patient is multifactorial. Malnutrition, poor dietary intake, diarrhea, vomiting, and the use of phosphate-binding antacids can all contribute to the hypophosphatemia of alcoholism.[87] In addition, serum phosphate concentrations may decrease after hospitalization in the alcoholic patient with the institution of dextrose-containing IV fluids as a result of an intracellular shift of phosphate.[85,87] Hyperventilation associated with the alcohol withdrawal syndrome can also contribute to the development of hypophosphatemia.[85] Alcoholic patients are particularly susceptible to the complications of hypophosphatemia such as rhabdomyolysis, which is often seen during withdrawal or refeeding.[85] Thus, serum phosphate concentrations should be routinely monitored in alcoholic patients.

Clinical Presentation

The clinical manifestations of severe hypophosphatemia are diverse and many organ systems can be affected. It is likely that two primary biochemical abnormalities are responsible for most of the clinical manifestations of severe hypophosphatemia.[80] First, intracellular energy stores may be decreased secondary to depletion of intracellular ATP. This can result in disruptions in cellular function. Second, reduced red blood cell 2,3-DPG concentrations are associated with a shift to the left of the oxyhemoglobin saturation curve. This shift is associated with a decrease in the release of oxygen to peripheral tissues (secondary to increased oxygen affinity for hemoglobin) and may result in tissue hypoxia.[80] These metabolic disorders can be seen in a wide variety of organ systems.

Neurologic manifestations of severe hypophosphatemia can result in a metabolic encephalopathy syndromecharacterized by irritability, apprehension, weakness, numbness, paresthesia, dysarthria, confusion, obtundation, seizures, and coma has been described in patients with severe hypophosphatemia.[82,85] Neuropsychiatric disturbances include apathy, delirium, hallucinations, and paranoia. Peripheral neuropathy and symptoms resembling Guillain–Barré syndrome have also been reported.[85]

Severe hypophosphatemia can result in significant dysfunction of skeletal muscle ranging from myalgia, bone pain, and weakness, with chronic hypophosphatemia, to potentially fatal rhabdomyolysis with severe acute hypophosphatemia.[82] Laboratory evaluations can help distinguish between chronic and acute on chronic hypophosphatemia. Elevated alkaline phosphatase, normal creatine phosphokinase, and normal to low phosphate and calcium are present in cases of chronic hypophosphatemia. In contrast, hyperkalemia, hyperuricemia, elevated blood urea nitrogen and creatinine, hypercalcemia, and myoglobinuria are often present in cases in which rhabdomyolysis complicates the acute or chronic hypophosphatemia.[76] Hypophosphatemia can result in acute respiratory failure secondary to respiratory muscle weakness and diaphragmatic contractile dysfunction. Thus, frequent assessment of serum phosphate concentration is indicated in patients at risk for respiratory failure.[80] Likewise, adequate treatment of hypophosphatemia in respiratory failure can aid in successful weaning from the ventilator.[80] Dysphagia and ileus have also been attributed to hypophosphatemia.[80]

Myocardial dysfunction has been reported to be impaired in the setting of hypophosphatemia and has resulted in congestive cardiomyopathy. This has been reported in alcoholics, and postoperative and intensive care patients. Depletion of cardiac ATP stores has been hypothesized as the cause of this syndrome[88] Arrhythmias have also been reported in patients with hypophosphatemia. Because hypophosphatemia is a potentially reversible cause of heart failure, it should be considered in patients who experience an acute deterioration in ventricular function.

Hematologic manifestations of hypophosphatemia include decreased levels of 2,3-DPG, decreased red blood cell ATP, and

CLINICAL PRESENTATION Hypophosphatemia

General

- Major conditions associated with symptomatic hypophosphatemia are chronic alcoholism, IV hyperalimentation without adequate phosphate supplementation, and the chronic ingestion of antacids. Severe hypophosphatemia can also be seen during treatment of diabetic ketoacidosis and with prolonged hyperventilation.

Symptoms

- Except for the effects on mineral metabolism, the symptoms of hypophosphatemia are caused by two consequences (reduction of red cell 2,3-DPG and reduction of intracellular ATP levels), and can impact virtually all organ systems. The symptoms are predominantly neurological and can include irritability, apprehension, weakness, numbness, paresthesia, and confusion. Severe acute development of hypophosphatemia can result in seizures or coma.

Signs

- The initial response of bone to hypophosphatemia contributes to hypercalcemia and hypercalciuria. Prolonged hypophosphatemia can also result in rickets and osteomalacia.
- Neurologic: Severe hypophosphatemia can lead to a metabolic encephalopathy.
- Cardiopulmonary: Impaired myocardial contractility, respiratory failure secondary to ATP depletion, CHF, new onset or worsening of an existing condition.
- Musculoskeletal: Proximal myopathy, dysphagia, and ileus have been reported. Acute hypophosphatemia superimposed on preexisting severe phosphate depletion can lead to rhabdomyolysis.
- Hematologic: Alterations in the hematopoietic system can also occur, resulting in hemolysis, reduction in phagocytotic and granulocyte chemotactic ability, as well as defective clot retraction and thrombocytopenia.

Laboratory Tests

- Serum phosphate levels less than 2.4 mg/dL (less than 0.78 mmol/L) are indicative of hypophosphatemia; however, symptomatic hypophosphatemia typically is not evident until serum phosphate less than 1 mg/dL (less than 0.32 mmol/L).

membrane rigidity.[88] When red blood cell ATP decreases cells become spherocytic and rigid, and are trapped and destroyed in the spleen.[88] Therefore, hemolysis can be a manifestation of severe hypophosphatemia. Reduction in ATP content of white blood cells can result in mobility, chemotaxis, phagocytosis, and bactericidal dysfunction.[88,85] These changes can contribute to an increased risk of infection in hypophosphatemic patients.

Finally, prolonged hypophosphatemia may result in osteopenia and osteomalacia because of enhanced osteoclastic resorption of bone and limited crystallization constituents (phosphate), respectively.[87]

TREATMENT

Desired Outcomes

The goals of therapy are the reversal of signs and symptoms of hypophosphatemia, normalization of serum phosphate concentrations, and management of underlying conditions. Awareness of the clinical situations in which hypophosphatemia is anticipated (alcoholism, diabetic ketoacidosis, and parenteral nutrition) is of vital importance in preventing iatrogenic hyperphosphatemia due to overly aggressive therapy. The routine addition of phosphate (12-15 mmol/L) to IV parenteral nutrition solutions is important for the prevention of severe hypophosphatemia in hospitalized patients.

Pharmacologic Therapy

Pharmacologic treatment for hypophosphatemia will typically involve phosphorus salt supplementation. The acuity and other electrolyte conditions dictate the salt, formulation, and route of administration (Table 50-5).

Severe Hypophosphatemia

8 Patients with severe (less than 1 mg/dL [less than 0.32 mmol/L]) or symptomatic hypophosphatemia should be treated with parenteral phosphate replacement. Thus, dosage and infusion recommendations, as well as response to parenteral phosphate replacement, are highly variable.[89] The infusion of 15 mmol of phosphate in 250 mL of 5% dextrose or 0.9% sodium chloride over 3 hours is a safe and effective treatment for severe hypophosphatemia.[87] Mean increases in serum phosphate of 0.5 to 0.8 mg/dL (0.16-0.26 mmol/L) have been reported. Doses of 0.2 to 0.6 mmol/kg of phosphate can be given over 1 to 3 hours in patients without hypercalcemia (serum calcium more than 10.5 mg/dL [more than 2.63 mmol/L]).[89] Other authors recommend a wider dosage range of 0.08 to 0.64 mmol/kg body weight (5-45 mmol in a 70-kg [154 lb] patient) given over 4 to 12 hours.[90] IV phosphate therapy produces the desired increase in serum phosphate at 24 hours in 20% to 80% of patients. Response is dependent on the degree of phosphate depletion and replacement dose administered.[87] The initial success is often followed in 48 to 72 hours by recurrent hypophosphatemia, necessitating close monitoring of serum phosphate and repeated administration of phosphate products as warranted.

Adverse Effects of Parenteral Phosphate Parenteral phosphate supplementation is associated with risks of hyperphosphatemia, metastatic soft tissue deposition of calcium-phosphate product, hypomagnesemia, hypocalcemia, and hyperkalemia or hypernatremia (dependent on which IV phosphate formulation is administered). Inappropriate administration of large doses of parenteral phosphate over relatively short time periods has resulted in symptomatic hypocalcemia and soft-tissue calcification.[1] The rate of infusion and choice of initial dosage should therefore be based on severity of hypophosphatemia, presence of symptoms, and coexistent medical conditions. Patients should be closely monitored with frequent (every 6 hours) serum phosphate determinations for 48 to 72 hours after starting IV therapy. It can be necessary to continue administration of IV phosphate for several days in some patients, although other patients may be able to tolerate an oral maintenance regimen. Monitoring should also include assessment of serum potassium, calcium, and magnesium concentrations. Hypomagnesemia secondary to intracellular shifts occurs frequently (27%-80%) in severely hypophosphatemic patients.[78] Therapy with parenteral phosphate should be undertaken with great caution and at reduced dosage for patients with hypercalcemia or renal dysfunction.[85]

TABLE 50-5 Phosphorus Replacement Therapy

Product (Salt)	Phosphate Content	Initial Dosing Based on Serum K
Oral Therapy (Potassium Phosphate + Sodium Phosphate)		
Neutra-Phos® (7 mEq/packet each of Na and K)	250 mg (8 mmol)/packet	Serum K >5.5 mEq/L (mmol/L) one packet three times daily
Neutra-Phos-K® (14.25 mEq/packet of K)	250 mg (8 mmol)/packet	Serum K >5.5 mEq/L (mmol/L); not recommended
K-Phos Neutral® (13 mEq/tablet Na and 1.1 mEq/tablet K)	250 mg (8 mmol)/tablet	Serum K >5.5 mEq/L (mmol/L) one tablet three times daily
Uro-KP-Neutral® (10.9 mEq/tablet Na and 1.27 mEq/tablet K)	250 mg (8 mmol)/tablet	Serum K >5.5 mEq/L (mmol/L) one tablet three times daily
Fleets Phospho-soda® (sodium phosphate solution)	4 mmol/mL	Serum K >5.5 mEq/L (mmol/L) 2 mL three times daily
IV Therapy		
Sodium PO_4 (4 mEq/mL Na)	3 mmol/mL	Serum K >3.5 mEq/L (mmol/L) 15-30 mmol IVPB
Potassium PO_4 (4.4 mEq/mL K)	3 mmol/mL	Serum K <3.5 mEq/L (mmol/L) 15-30 mmol IVPB

IVPB, IV piggy back; K, potassium; Na, sodium; PO_4, phosphate.

Mild-to-Moderate Hypophosphatemia

Mild-to-moderate or asymptomatic hypophosphatemia can be treated by the administration of oral phosphate salts in doses of 1.5 to 2 g (50-60 mmol) daily in divided doses (see Table 50-5). Phosphate concentrations should be monitored daily, with the goal of correcting the reduced phosphate concentration in approximately 7 to 10 days. The primary dose-limiting adverse effect associated with oral phosphate replacement is the development of osmotic diarrhea. Patients with mild-to-moderate hypophosphatemia and moderate-to-severe renal insufficiency should receive reduced daily oral doses (ie, 1 g or approximately 30 mmol of phosphate) with careful monitoring of serum phosphate concentration because they are predisposed to phosphate retention. In addition to phosphate supplementation for hypophosphatemia, dipyridamole can decrease renal phosphate leaking and increase serum phosphate. Doses of 75 mg four times daily have resulted in increases in serum 1,25-dihydroxy vitamin D_3 and decreases in serum calcium and urolithiasis events.[81]

CLINICAL BOTTOM LINE

Initial treatment strategy should be based on acuity of onset and severity of symptoms. Because the etiologies of calcium and phosphate disorders are diverse, it is important to integrate the known or anticipated consequences of concomitant diseases into the treatment strategy. The patient's medication history should be comprehensively assessed to determine whether the electrolyte abnormality may be drug induced. After resolution or treatment of the acute calcium or phosphate disorder, the medication regimen should be evaluated periodically. This proactive interventional approach will facilitate the management of mild disorders in the community and can reduce the need for hospitalization.

ABBREVIATIONS

ATP	adenosine triphosphate
CHF	congestive heart failure
CKD	chronic kidney disease
FGF23	fibroblast growth factor 23
2,3-DPG	2,3-diphosphoglycerate
NSAID	nonsteroidal anti-inflammatory drug
PTH	parathyroid hormone
PTHrP	PTH-related protein
S_{ca}	serum calcium

REFERENCES

1. Brown RB, Razzaque MS. Dysregulation of phosphate metabolism and conditions associated with phosphate toxicity. *Bonekey Rep* 2015 Jun 3; 4:705.
2. French S, Subauste J, Geraci S. Calcium abnormalities in hospitalized patients. *South Med J* 2012 Apr;105(4):231-237.
3. Baird GS. Ionized calcium. *Clin Chim Acta* 2011 Apr 11;412(9-10): 696-701.
4. Steele T, Kolamunnage-Dona R, Downey C, Toh CH, Welters I. Assessment and clinical course of hypocalcemia in critical illness. *Crit Care* 2013 Jun 4;17(3):R106.
5. Byrnes MC, Huynh K, Helmer SD, et al. A comparison of corrected serum calcium levels to ionized calcium levels among critically ill surgical patients. *Am J Surg* 2005;189:310-314.
6. Marcocci C, Cetani F. Clinical practice. Primary hyperparathyroidism. *N Engl J Med* 2011;365(25):2389-2397.
7. Rizzoli R, Body JJ, Brandi ML, et al; International Osteoporosis Foundation Committee of Scientific Advisors Working Group on Cancer-Induced Bone Disease. Cancer-associated bone disease. *Osteoporos Int* 2013 Dec;24(12):2929-2953.
8. Fraser WD. Hyperparathyroidism. *Lancet* 2009;374:145-158.
9. McMahan J. A case of resistant hypercalcemia of malignancy with a proposed treatment algorithm. *Ann Pharmacother* 2009;43:1532-1538.
10. McCauley LK, Martin TJ. Twenty-five years of PTHrP progress: From cancer hormone to multifunctional cytokine. *J Bone Miner Res* 2012;27(6):1231-1239.
11. Rifai MA, Moles JK, Harrington DP. Lithium-induced hypercalcemia and parathyroid dysfunction. *Psychosomatics* 2001;42:359-361.
12. Picolis MK, Lavis VR, Orlander PR. Milk-alkali is a major cause of hypercalcemia. *Clin Endocrinol (Oxf)* 2005;63:566-576.
13. Machado MC, Bruce-Mensah A, Whitmire M, Rizvi AA. Hypercalcemia Associated with Calcium Supplement Use: Prevalence and Characteristics in Hospitalized Patients. *J Clin Med* 2015 Mar 9; 4(3):414-424.
14. Moe SM. Disorders involving calcium, phosphorus and magnesium. *Prim Care* 2008;35:215-237, v-vi.
15. Shlapack MA, Rizvi AA. Normocalcemic primary hyperparathyroidism: Characteristics and clinical significance of an emerging entity. *Am J Med Sci* 2012;343(2):163-166.
16. Ahmad S, Kuraganti G, Steenkamp D. Hypercalcemic crisis: a clinical review. *Am J Med* 2015 Mar;128(3):239-245.
17. Karwowski W, Naumnik B, Szczepaski M, Myliwiec M. The mechanism of vascular calcification—A systematic review. *Med Sci Monit* 2012;18(1): RA1-RA11.
18. Towler DA, Demer LL. Thematic series on the pathobiology of vascular calcification: An introduction. *Circ Res* 2011;108(11):1378-1380.
19. Vella A, Gerber TC, Hayes DL, et al. Digoxin, hypercalcemia and cardiac conduction. *Postgrad Med* 1999;75:554-556.
20. Rejnmark L, Vestergaard P, Mosekilde L. Nephrolithiasis and renal calcifications in primary hyperparathyroidism. *J Clin Endocrinol Metab* 2011;96(8):2377-2385.
21. Silverberg SJ, Clarke BL, Peacock M, et al. Current issues in the presentation of asymptomatic primary hyperparathyroidism: Proceedings of the Fourth International Workshop. *J Clin Endocrinol Metab* 2014 Oct;99(10):3580-9435.
22. Ramaswamy K, Killilea DW, Kapahi P, Kahn AJ, Chi T, Stoller ML. The elementome of calcium-based urinary stones and its role in urolithiasis. *Nat Rev Urol* 2015 Sep 1.
23. Tarplin S, Ganesan V, Monga M. Stone formation and management after bariatric surgery. *Nat Rev Urol* 2015 May;12(5):263-270.
24. Minisola S, Pepe J, Piemonte S, Cipriani C. The diagnosis and management of hypercalcaemia. *BMJ* 2015 Jun 2;350:h2723.
25. LeGrand SB, Leskuski D, Zama I. Narrative review: Furosemide for hypercalcemia: An unproven yet common practice. *Ann Intern Med* 2008 Aug 19;149(4):259-263.
26. Inzerillo AM, Zaidi M, Huang CL. Calcitonin: Physiological actions and clinical applications. *J Pediatr Endocrinol Metab* 2004;17:931-940.
27. Grauer A, Ziegler R, Raue F. Clinical significance of antibodies against calcitonin. *Exp Clin Endocrinol Diabetes* 1995;103:345-351.
28. Stewart AF. Hypercalcemia associated with cancer. *N Engl J Med* 2005;352:373-379.
29. Van Poznak CH, Temin S, Yee GC, et al. American Society of Clinical Oncology. American Society of Clinical Oncology executive summary of the clinical practice guideline update on the role of bone-modifying agents in metastatic breast cancer. *J Clin Oncol* 2011 Mar 20; 29(9):1221-1227.
30. Wellington K, Goa KL. Zoledronic acid: A review of its use in the management of bone metastases and hypercalcemia of malignancy. *Drugs* 2003;63:417-437.
31. Major P, Lortholary A, Hon J, et al. Zoledronic acid is superior to pamidronate in the treatment of hypercalcemia of malignancy: A pooled analysis of two randomized, controlled clinical trials. *J Clin Oncol* 2001;19:558-567.
32. Body JJ, Lortholary A, Romieu G, et al. A dose-finding study of zoledronate in hypercalcemic cancer patients. *J Bone Miner Res* 1999;14:1557-1561.
33. Costa L, Lipton A, Coleman RE. Role of bisphosphonates for the management of skeletal complications and bone pain from skeletal metastases. *Support Cancer Ther* 2006;3:143-153.
34. Banerjee D, Asif A, Striker L, et al. Short-term, high-dose pamidronate-induced acute tubular necrosis: The postulated mechanisms of bisphosphonate nephrotoxicity. *Am J Kidney Dis* 2003;41:E18.
35. Markowitz GS, Fine PL, Stack JI, et al. Toxic acute tubular necrosis following treatment with zoledronate (Zometa). *Kidney Int* 2003;64: 281-289.
36. Allen MR. Medication-Related Osteonecrosis of the Jaw: Basic and Translational Science Updates. *Oral Maxillofac Surg Clin North Am* 2015 Nov;27(4):497-508.
37. Hu MI, Glezerman IG, Leboulleux S, et al. Denosumab for treatment of hypercalcemia of malignancy. *J Clin Endocrinol Metab* 2014 Sep;99(9): 3144-3152.
38. Shroff R, Beringer O, Rao K, Hofbauer LC, Schulz A. Denosumab for post-transplantation hypercalcemia in osteopetrosis. *N Engl J Med* 2012;367(18):1766-1767.
39. You TM, Lee KH, Lee SH, Park W. Denosumab-related osteonecrosis of the jaw: A case report and management based on pharmacokinetics. *Oral Surg Oral Med Oral Pathol Oral Radiol* 2015 Nov;120(5):548-553.
40. Lambe G, Malvathu R, Thomas HM, Graves A. Hypocalcaemic tetany occurring post a single denosumab dose in a patient with stage 4 chronic kidney disease, followed by calcium- and calcitriol-induced hypercalcaemia. *Nephrology (Carlton)* 2015 Aug;20(8):583-584.
41. Martín-Baez IM, Blanco-García R, Alonso-Suárez M, et al. Severe hypocalcaemia post-denosumab. *Nefrologia* 2013;33(4):614-615.
42. Ziegler R. Hypercalcemic crisis. *J Am Soc Nephrol* 2001;12(Suppl 17): S3-S9.
43. Silverman SL, Lane NE. Glucocorticoid-induced osteoporosis. *Curr Osteoporos Rep* 2009;7:23-26.
44. Silverberg SJ, Rubin MR, Faiman C, et al. Cinacalcet hydrochloride reduces the serum calcium concentration in inoperable parathyroid carcinoma. *J Clin Endocrinol Metab* 2007;92:3803-3808.
45. Messa P, Alfieri C, Brezzi B. Clinical utilization of cinacalcet in hypercalcemic conditions. *Expert Opin Drug Metab Toxicol* 2011;7(4):517-528.
46. Sensipar® (cinacalcet HCl) [package insert]. Thousand Oaks, CA: Amgen, Inc., 2014.
47. Brardi S, Cevenini G, Verdacchi T, Romano G, Ponchietti R. Use of cinacalcet in nephrolithiasis associated with normocalcemic or hypercalcemic primary hyperparathyroidism: Results of a prospective randomized pilot study. *Arch Ital Urol Androl* 2015 Mar 31;87(1):66-71.
48. Xie J, Namjoshi M, Wu EQ, Parikh K, Diener M, Yu AP, Guo A, Culver KW. Economic evaluation of denosumab compared with zoledronic acid in hormone-refractory prostate cancer patients with bone metastases. *J Manag Care Pharm* 2011 Oct;17(8):621-643.

49. Arellano J, Hauber AB, Mohamed AF, et al. Physicians' preferences for bone metastases drug therapy in the United States. *Value Health.* 2015 Jan;18(1):78-83.
50. Khan A, Fong J. Hypocalcemia: Updates in diagnosis and management for primary care. *Can Fam Physician* 2012;58(2):158-162.
51. Chung HS, Cho SJ, Park CS. Effects of liver function on ionized hypocalcaemia following rapid blood transfusion. *J Int Med Res.* 2012;40(2):572-582.
52. Kishimoto M, Ohto H, Shikama Y, et al. Treatment for the decline of ionized calcium levels during peripheral blood progenitor cell harvesting. *Transfusion* 2002;42:1340-1347.
53. Wilson FP, Berns JS. Tumor lysis syndrome: new challenges and recent advances. *Adv Chronic Kidney Dis* 2014 Jan;21(1):18-26.
54. Filopanti M, Corbetta S, Barbieri AM, Spada A. Pharmacology of the calcium sensing receptor. *Clin Cases Miner Bone Metab* 2013 Sep; 10(3):162-165.
55. Choi KH, Shin CH, Yang SW, Cheong HI. Autosomal dominant hypocalcemia with Bartter syndrome due to a novel activating mutation of calcium sensingreceptor, Y829C. *Korean J Pediatr* 2015 Apr;58(4):148-153.
56. Peacock M. Calcium metabolism in health and disease. *Clin J Am Soc Nephrol* 2010;5:S23-S30.
57. Kitanaka S, Isojima T, Takaki M, et al. Association of vitamin D-related gene polymorphisms with manifestation of vitamin D deficiency in children. *Endocr J* 2012;59(11):1007-1014.
58. Tachibana S, Sato S, Yokoi T, et al. Severe hypocalcemia complicated by postsurgical hypoparathyroidism and hungry bone syndrome in a patient with primary hyperparathyroidism, Graves' disease, and acromegaly. *Intern Med* 2012;51(14):1869-1873.
59. Maalouf NM, Heller HJ, Odvina CV, et al. Bisphosphonate-induced hypocalcemia: Report of 3 cases and review of the literature. *Endocr Pract* 2006;12:48-53.a
60. Kan WC, Wang HY, Chien CC, Tan CK, Lin CY, Su SB. Intermediate bioelectrolyte changes after phospho-soda or polyethylene glycol precolonoscopic laxatives in a population undergoing health examinations. *Nephrol Dial Transplant* 2012 Feb;27(2):752-757.
61. Kelly A, Levine MA. Hypocalcemia in the critically ill patient. *J Intensive Care Med* 2013 May-Jun;28(3):166-177.
62. Choyke PL, Knopp MV. Pseudohypocalcemia with MR imaging contrast agents: A cautionary tale. Radiology 2003;227:639-646.
63. Yon CK, Low CL. Sodium citrate 4% versus heparin as a lock solution in hemodialysis patients with central venous catheters. *Am J Health Syst Pharm* 2013 Jan 15;70(2):131-136.
64. Morgan DJ, Ho KM. Profound hypocalcaemia in a patient being anticoagulated with citrate for continuous renal replacement therapy. *Anaesthesia* 2009 Dec;64(12):1363-1366.
65. Polaschegg HD, Sodemann K. Risks related to catheter locking solutions containing concentrated citrate. *Nephrol Dial Transplant* 2003;18:2688-2689.
66. De Sanctis V, Soliman A, Fiscina B. Hypoparathyroidism: from diagnosis to treatment. *Curr Opin Endocrinol Diabetes Obes* 2012 Dec; 19(6):435-442.
67. Cusano NE, Rubin MR, Irani D, Sliney J Jr, Bilezikian JP. Use of parathyroid hormone in hypoparathyroidism. *J Endocrinol Invest* 2013 Dec;36(11):1121-1127.
68. Lee I, Sheu WH, Tu ST, et al. Bisphosphonate pretreatment attenuates hungry bone syndrome postoperatively in subjects with primary hyperparathyroidism. *J Bone Miner Metab* 2006;24:255-258.
69. Hollis BW. Circulating 25-hydroxy vitamin D levels indicative of vitamin D sufficiency: Implications for establishing a new effective dietary intake recommendation for vitamin D. *J Nutr* 2005;135:317-322.
70. Blaine J, Chonchol M, Levi M. Renal control of calcium, phosphate, and magnesium homeostasis. *Clin J Am Soc Nephrol* 2015 Jul 7; 10(7):1257-72.
71. Felsenfeld AJ, Levine BS, Rodriguez M. Pathophysiology of Calcium, Phosphorus, and Magnesium Dysregulation in Chronic Kidney Disease. *Semin Dial* 2015 Aug 25.
72. Kocełak P, Olszanecka-Glinianowicz M, Chudek J. Fibroblast growth factor 23--structure, function and role in kidney diseases. *Adv Clin Exp Med* 2012 May-Jun;21(3):391-401.
73. Adamcewicz M, Bearelly D, Porat G, Friedenberg FK. Mechanism of action and toxicities of purgatives used for colonoscopy preparation. *Expert Opin Drug Metab Toxicol* 2011;7(1):89-101.
74. FDA requires new safety measures for oral sodium phosphate products to reduce risk of acute kidney injury risk associated with both prescription and over-the-counter (OTC) products. Available at: http://www.fda.gov/NewsEvents/Newsroom/PressAnnouncements/2008/ucm116988.htm Accessed: 24 October 2015.
75. Kamel KS, Halperin ML. Acid-base problems in diabetic ketoacidosis. *N Engl J Med.* 2015 May 14;372(20):1969-1970.
76. Block GA, Klassen PS, Lazarus JM, et al. Mineral metabolism, mortality and morbidity in maintenance hemodialysis. *J Am Soc Nephrol* 2004;15:2208-2218. Accessed: 24 October 2015.
77. KDIGO Clinical Practice Guidelines for the Diagnosis, Evaluation, Prevention, And Treatment Of Chronic Kidney Disease-Mineral And Bone Disorder (CKD-MBD). Chapter 4.1: Treatment of CKD-MBD targeted at lowering high serum phosphorus and maintaining serum calcium. *Kidney Int* 2009;76(Suppl 113):S50-S99.
78. Hutchison AJ, Smith CP, Brenchley PE. Pharmacology, efficacy and safety of oral phosphate binders. *Nat Rev Nephrol* 2011;7(10):578-589.
79. Pai AB, Jang S, Wegryzn N. Iron-based phosphate binders-a new element for treatment of hyperphosphatemia in kidney disease. *Expert Opin Metab Toxicol* 2015 Nov 16:1-13.
80. Chang WT, Radin B, McCurdy MT. Calcium, magnesium, and phosphate abnormalities in the emergency department. *Emerg Med Clin North Am* 2014 May;32(2):349-366.
81. Liamis G, Milionis HJ, Elisaf M. Medication-induced hypophosphatemia: A review. *QJM* 2010;103(7):449-459.
82. Subramanian R, Khardori R. Severe hypophosphatemia. Pathophysiologic implications, clinical presentation, and treatment. *Medicine (Baltimore)* 2000;79:1-78.
83. Hardy S, Vandemergel X. Intravenous iron administration and hypophosphatemia in clinical practice. *Int J Rheumatol* 2015;2015:468675.
84. Wolf M, White KE. Coupling fibroblast growth factor 23 production and cleavage: iron deficiency, rickets, and kidney disease. *Curr Opin Nephrol Hypertens* 2014 Jul;23(4):411-419.
85. Amanzadeh J, Reilly RF. Hypophosphatemia: An evidence-based approach to its clinical consequences and management. *Nat Clin Pract Nephrol* 2006;2:136-148.
86. Konstantinov NK, Rohrscheib M, Agaba EI, Dorin RI, Murata GH, Tzamaloukas AH. Respiratory failure in diabetic ketoacidosis. *World J Diabetes* 2015 Jul 25;6(8):1009-1023.
87. Felsenfeld AJ, Levine BS. Approach to treatment of hypophosphatemia. *Am J Kidney Dis* 2012 Oct;60(4):655-661.
88. Gaasbeek A, Meinders AE. Hypophosphatemia: an update on its etiology and treatment. *Am J Med* 2005 Oct;118(10):1094-1101.
89. Agarwal B, Walecka A, Shaw S, Davenport A. Is parenteral phosphate replacement in the intensive care unit safe? *Ther Apher Dial* 2014 Feb;18(1):31-36.
90. Clark CL, Sacks GS, Dickerson RN, et al. Treatment of hypophosphatemia in patients receiving specialized nutrition support using a graduated dosing scheme: Results from a prospective clinical trial. *Crit Care Med* 1995;23:1504-1511.

Disorders of Potassium and Magnesium Homeostasis

51

Rachel W. Flurie and Donald F. Brophy

KEY CONCEPTS

1. Potassium regulates many biochemical processes in the body and is a key cation for electrical action potentials across cellular membranes.
2. In patients with concomitant hypokalemia and hypomagnesemia, it is imperative to correct the hypomagnesemia before the hypokalemia.
3. Potassium chloride is the preferred potassium supplement for the most common causes of hypokalemia.
4. Hyperkalemia is a common occurrence in patients with acute kidney injury or chronic kidney disease.
5. Hypomagnesemia is commonly caused by excessive gastrointestinal (GI) or renal magnesium wasting.
6. Hypermagnesemia is predominantly observed in patients with acute or chronic kidney disease.
7. Severe hypermagnesemia may affect the neuromuscular and cardiovascular systems.

Potassium and magnesium are electrolytes that are responsible for numerous metabolic activities. Disorders of these electrolytes are frequently seen in both the acute care and community ambulatory care settings. Therefore, clinicians need a firm understanding of the etiology, pathophysiology, symptoms, pharmacotherapy, and monitoring of these disorders. This chapter describes the homeostatic mechanisms that are responsible for the maintenance of normal potassium and magnesium serum concentrations. The clinical disorders responsible for the development of hyperkalemia, hypermagnesemia, hypokalemia, and hypomagnesemia are also reviewed.

POTASSIUM

Potassium is the most abundant cation in the body, with estimated total-body stores of 3,000 to 4,000 mEq (mmol).[1] Ninety-eight percent of this amount is contained within the intracellular compartment, and the remaining 2% is distributed within the extracellular compartment. The sodium-potassium adenosine triphosphatase (Na^+-K^+-ATPase) pump located in the cell membrane is responsible for the compartmentalization of potassium. This pump is an active transport system that maintains increased intracellular stores of potassium by transporting sodium out of the cell and potassium into the cell at a ratio of 3:2. Consequently, the pump maintains a higher concentration of potassium inside the cell.

The normal serum concentration range for potassium is 3.5 to 5 mEq/L (mmol/L), whereas the intracellular potassium concentration is approximately 150 mEq/L (mmol/L).[2] Approximately 75% of the intracellular potassium is located in skeletal muscle; the remaining 25% is located in the liver and red blood cells. Extracellular potassium is distributed throughout the serum and interstitial space. Potassium is dynamic in that it is constantly moving between the intracellular and extracellular compartments according to the body's needs. Thus, the serum potassium concentration alone does not accurately reflect the total-body potassium content.

1 Potassium has many physiologic functions within cells, including protein and glycogen synthesis and cellular metabolism and growth. It is also a determinant of the electrical action potential across the cell membrane.[1] The ratio of the intracellular-to-extracellular potassium concentration is the major determinant of the resting membrane potential across the cell membrane. Thus, the resting membrane potential is greatly affected by variations in extracellular potassium concentration. Serum potassium concentrations outside the normal range can have disastrous effects on neuromuscular activity, in particular cardiac conduction. Hypo- and hyperkalemia are both associated with potentially fatal cardiac arrhythmias, along with other neuromuscular disturbances. Finally, potassium is integral to maintaining blood pressure, prevention of stroke, and potentially other cardiovascular diseases.[3] Both the National High Blood Pressure Education Program and the Institute of Medicine recommend potassium supplementation as a strategy for preventing and treating hypertension.[4-5]

Control of Potassium Homeostasis

Potassium homeostasis, the maintenance of serum potassium within the normal range, is affected by dietary intake, GI and urinary excretion, hepatic and muscular sequestration, hormones, acid–base balance, body fluid tonicity, central and peripheral circadian clocks, and a highly integrated feedback mechanism.[6,7] Together, these mechansisms usually maintain total-body potassium content within a narrow window without appreciable changes in the serum potassium concentration.[6] Deviations in serum potassium concentrations outside of the normal range are a result of nonhomeostatic processes that are not sensitive to changes in potassium balance.[6] The recommended adequate intake of dietary potassium in the United States is approximately 120 mEq/day (mmol/day); yet the typical American adult only consumes 56% of this recommended amount.[8] Potassium is considered to be a nutrient of concern, because of its beneficial effects on blood pressure, reduction in the risk of kidney stones, and decrease of bone loss.[9] Potassium is abundant in fruits, vegetables, meats, whole grains, and milk products. Most dietary potassium is absorbed, with only 10 to 20 mEq/day (mmol/day) eliminated in feces. The amount eliminated in the feces increases, however, in patients with diarrhea and in those with chronic kidney disease (CKD).[7]

The kidney is the primary route of potassium elimination. Potassium is freely filtered, but almost all of it is reabsorbed passively in the proximal tubule and the thick ascending limb of the loop of Henle.[9] Therefore, urinary potassium excretion is primarily determined by potassium secretion from the luminal cells of the distal tubule and collecting duct. Although the amount of potassium filtered by the glomerulus approaches 700 mEq (mmol) per day, only approximately 10% to 20% is actually excreted in the urine.[9]

However, this amount can vary based on dietary intake, serum potassium concentration, and aldosterone activity. For example, more potassium is renally excreted in conditions that result in high aldosterone activity (eg, dehydration) when the body is attempting to conserve sodium or when there is an increase in dietary potassium intake.

Hormones such as insulin, catecholamines, and aldosterone dramatically affect potassium homeostasis. Insulin is the most important hormonal mediator of potassium balance because it stimulates the cellular Na^+-K^+-ATPase pump to increase transport of potassium into liver, muscle, and adipose tissue.[6] There is a complex negative feedback loop in which insulin secretion tightly regulates serum potassium concentrations: an increase of only a few tenths of a milliequivalent (mmol) of potassium stimulates pancreatic insulin secretion in an attempt to prevent hyperkalemia from developing.[1] If hyperkalemia does occur, glucagon is released from the liver to protect against insulin-induced hypoglycemia. Conversely, hypokalemia inhibits insulin secretion, a finding that explains why some patients receiving diuretics develop hyperglycemia.

An elevation in circulating catecholamines such as epinephrine usually results in the intracellular movement of potassium by two mechanisms.[9] Stimulation of the β-receptor, which directly activates the Na^+-K^+-ATPase pump and glycogenolysis, which raises blood glucose concentrations, thereby increasing insulin secretion. This dual mechanism is often used therapeutically in patients with hyperkalemia to normalize serum potassium concentrations.

Aldosterone, a mineralocorticoid that is secreted from the adrenal glands in response to high serum potassium concentrations, promotes urinary potassium excretion. Aldosterone acts on the distal tubule and collecting duct to promote the reabsorption of sodium and water in exchange for potassium. It also increases potassium permeability and transport across the luminal membrane of the nephron by stimulating cellular Na^+-K^+-ATPase pump activity.[7]

Changes in acid–base status significantly affect the serum potassium concentration. For example, the infusion of metabolic inorganic acids, such as hydrochloric acid, results in an increase in serum potassium. The body compensates for excessive hydrogen ions by moving them from the serum into the cell in exchange for intracellular potassium, to maintain electroneutrality. The processes by which this occurs are highly complex and involve cellular H^+-K^+-ATPase pumps and both Na^+-HCO_3^- and K^+-HCO_3^- cotransporters.[10] The efflux of potassium into the serum can result in hyperkalemia. A commonly quoted approximation of the pH effect is that for every 0.1 unit decrease in pH, serum potassium concentration increases by 0.6 to 0.8 mEq/L (mmol/L) (with a wide range of 0.2 to 1.7).[11] This is often referred to as *false hyperkalemia* because there is not a true excess of total-body potassium. Metabolic acidosis associated with lactic acidosis and ketoacidosis does not result in hyperkalemia, because both cations and anions enter the cell, thus maintaining electroneutrality.[1] Respiratory acidosis also does not significantly affect the serum potassium concentration.

Conversely, metabolic alkalosis has been associated with hypokalemia. As a result of a net loss of hydrogen ion from the serum, intracellular hydrogen ions enter the serum to increase the acidity of the blood. To maintain electroneutrality, extracellular potassium ions are shifted intracellularly. This creates a relative deficiency of potassium in the serum. Serum potassium decreases approximately 0.6 mEq/L (mmol/L) for each 0.1 unit increase in blood pH. This is frequently termed *false hypokalemia* because there is not a true deficiency in total-body potassium.

Finally, hyperosmolality can result in enhanced movement of potassium from the cell into the extracellular fluid. This occurs most likely because of the associated cell shrinkage and water loss, which increases the intracellular-to-extracellular potassium gradient.[4] This is seen in conditions such as diabetic ketoacidosis. Conversely, hypoosmolality does not seem to affect potassium distribution.

HYPOKALEMIA

Epidemiology

Hypokalemia (defined as a serum potassium concentration less than 3.5 mEq/L [mmol/L]) is a commonly encountered electrolyte abnormality in clinical practice. Hypokalemia is often categorized as mild (serum potassium 3.1-3.5 mEq/L [mmol/L]), moderate (serum potassium 2.5-3 mEq/L [mmol/L]), or severe (less than 2.5 mEq/L [mmol/L]).[2] When hypokalemia is detected, the diagnostic workup should evaluate the patient's comorbid disease states and concomitant medications. Hypokalemia is virtually nonexistent in healthy adults. This is due in part to the relatively high potassium content in the typical Western diet as well as the body's effective potassium-sparing mechanisms, which tightly regulate the serum potassium concentration. However, as many as 20% of hospitalized patients and up to 40% of patients taking thiazide diuretics will develop hypokalemia.[2]

While transient hypokalemia may be thought of as merely a laboratory abnormality, there are serious potential consequences associated with persistent hypokalemia. Recent data suggest that hypokalemia increases mortality in patients with chronic heart failure or CKD, populations typically thought to be more sensitive to the effects of hyperkalemia.[12] In fact, even mild hypokalemia in patients with CKD appears to confer a greater risk of death compared with those with mild to moderate hyperkalemia.[13]

Etiology and Pathophysiology

Hypokalemia results when there is a total-body potassium deficit, or when serum potassium is shifted into the intracellular compartment. Total-body deficits occur in the setting of poor dietary intake of potassium, or when there are excessive renal and GI losses of potassium. Maintaining a consistent dietary intake of potassium is important because the body has no effective method for storing potassium. At steady state, potassium excretion matches potassium intake; approximately 90% of ingested potassium is renally excreted, whereas 10% is excreted in feces.[9] This underscores the importance of eating a well-balanced diet. Elderly patients with chronic diseases and those undergoing surgery are at increased risk for developing hypokalemia because of insufficient intake or losses resulting from surgery.

Many drugs can cause hypokalemia by a variety of mechanisms including intracellular potassium shifting and increased renal or stool losses (Table 51-1). The most common cause of drug-induced hypokalemia is loop and thiazide diuretic administration as these agents inhibit renal sodium reabsorption, which results in increased sodium delivery to the distal tubule. Consequently, hypokalemia

TABLE 51-1 Mechanism of Drug-Induced Hypokalemia

Transcellular Shift	Enhanced Renal Excretion	Enhanced Fecal Elimination
β_2-Receptor agonists	Diuretics	Laxatives
Epinephrine	Acetazolamide	Sodium polystyrene sulfonate
Albuterol	Thiazides	Phenolphthalein
Terbutaline	Indapamide	Sorbitol
Fomoterol	Metolazone	Patiromer
Salmeterol	Furosemide	
Isoproterenol	Torsemide	
Ephedrine	Bumetanide	
Pseudoephedrine	Ethacrynic acid	
Tocolytic agents	High-dose penicillins	
Ritodrine	Nafcillin	
Nylidrin	Ampicillin	
Theophylline	Penicillin	
Levothyroxine	Mineralocorticoids	
Decongestants	Miscellaneous	
Caffeine	Aminoglycosides	
Insulin overdose	Amphotericin B	
Verapamil overdose	Cisplatin	
Barium overdose		

develops because the distal tubule selectively reabsorbs sodium, and excretes potassium. Second, because diuretics result in vascular volume contraction, aldosterone is secreted that further promotes the renal excretion of potassium. If concomitant potassium supplements are not provided to patients receiving loop and thiazide diuretics, mild to moderate hypokalemia is inevitable.

The second most common etiology of hypokalemia is excessive loss of potassium-rich GI fluid as a result of diarrhea and/or vomiting. The typical potassium loss in feces is approximately 10 mEq (mmol) per day.[7] In diarrheal states, this amount increases proportionally with the volume of stool output. A case report of a patient with secretory diarrhea reported fecal potassium losses of 130 to 170 mEq/L (mmol/L).[14] Vomiting also accounts for substantial potassium losses, which have been estimated to be as high as 30 to 50 mEq (mmol) per liter of vomitus.[15] Metabolic alkalosis which often develops in those with severe diarrhea and vomiting as a result of loss of these bicarbonate-rich fluids causes an intracellular shift of potassium, which lowers the serum concentration of potassium even further. Prolonged diarrhea and vomiting tend to affect children and elderly patients profoundly because their kidneys are unable to effectively maintain adequate fluid status.

2 Hypomagnesemia, which is present in more than 50% of cases of clinically significant hypokalemia, contributes to the development of hypokalemia because it reduces the intracellular potassium concentration and promotes renal potassium wasting.[16] While the precise mechanism of the accelerated renal loss is unknown, many believe that the intracellular potassium concentration may decrease because hypomagnesemia impairs the function of the Na^+-K^+-ATPase pump thereby promoting potassium wasting. Alternatively, the combination of increased sodium delivery to the distal tubule, elevated aldosterone concentrations, and hypomagnesemia may cause the renal outer medullary potassium channels to excrete more potassium.[16] What is clear is that hypokalemia and hypomagnesemia often coexist as a result of drugs (diuretic administration) or disease states (diarrhea). When concomitant hypokalemia and hypomagnesemia occur, the magnesium deficiency should be corrected first, otherwise full repletion of the potassium deficit is difficult.

TREATMENT

Desired Outcomes

The goals of hypokalemia management are to prevent and/or treat serious life-threatening complications, normalize the serum potassium concentration, identify and correct the underlying cause of hypokalemia, and finally prevent overcorrection of the serum potassium concentration.

General Approach to Therapy

The general approach to therapy depends on the degree and rapidity with which hypokalemia developed and the presence of signs and symptoms. Serum potassium concentrations between 3.5 and 4 mEq/L (mmol/L) are a sign of early potassium depletion. No pharmacologic therapy is recommended; however, patients should be encouraged to increase their dietary intake of potassium-rich foods. When the serum potassium concentration is between 3 and 3.5 mEq/L (mmol/L), the patient's concomitant conditions and therapies will largely determine whether pharmacologic therapy should be initiated. Most patients will not have signs or symptoms if serum potassium concentrations remain greater than 3 mEq/L (mmol/L). The presence of signs or symptoms with mild hypokalemia warrants the intiation of potassium supplementation. Oral potassium supplementation should be initiated in patients with underlying cardiac conditions that predispose them to cardiac arrhythmias. Patients with serum potassium concentrations less than 3 mEq/L (mmol/L) should always be treated to achieve values between 4 and 4.5 mEq/L (mmol/L). In asymptomatic patients, oral therapy is the preferred route of administration. Intravenous (IV) potassium may be necessary in symptomatic patients with severe depletion, or in patients who are intolerant to oral supplementation. In patients with concomitant moderate to severe hypomagnesemia, the magnesium deficit should be corrected before potassium supplementation is started.[2,9]

CLINICAL PRESENTATION Hypokalemia

General

- The signs and symptoms of hypokalemia are usually nonspecific and highly variable between patients.

Symptoms

- Symptoms are dependent on the degree of hypokalemia and its rapidity of onset.
- Mild hypokalemia is often asymptomatic.
- Moderate hypokalemia is associated with cramping, weakness, malaise, and myalgias.

Signs

- Cardiovascular: In severe hypokalemia, electrocardiogram (ECG) changes often include ST-segment depression or flattening, T-wave inversion, and U-wave elevation. Clinical arrhythmias include heart block, atrial flutter, paroxysmal atrial tachycardia, ventricular fibrillation, and digitalis-induced arrhythmias.
- Musculoskeletal: Cramping and impaired muscle contraction.

Laboratory Tests

- Serum potassium concentration below 3.5 mEq/L (mmol/L) is diagnostic. Hypomagnesemia (serum magnesium concentration below 1.7 mg/dL [1.4 mEq/L; 0.70 mmol/L]) can also be present.

Nonpharmacologic Therapy

The best and most abundant sources of dietary potassium supplementation are fresh fruits and vegetables, fruit juices, and meats (Table 51-2). Increased dietary intake of foods with high potassium content, however, is not recommended long term because it can add unwanted calories to the patient's diet. Moreover, dietary potassium is almost entirely coupled with phosphate, rather than chloride, so it is not as effective in correcting potassium loss associated with hypochloremic conditions such as vomiting, nasogastric suctioning, and diuretic therapy. Salt substitutes that contain potassium chloride are another effective, inexpensive source of potassium and because they provide chloride as well they are frequently recommended.

TABLE 51-2 Foods that Are High in Potassium

High content (>250 mg)	Very high content (>500 mg)
Kidney beans, cooked	Potato, baked, flesh and skin
Lentils, cooked	Sweet potato, baked in skin
Soybeans, green, cooked	Juice, canned
Lima beans, cooked	Prunes
Soybeans, mature, cooked	Carrot
Pinto beans, cooked	Tomato
Lentils, cooked	Tomato paste
Halibut, cooked	Tomato puree
Rockfish, Pacific, cooked	Beet greens, cooked
Cod, Pacific, cooked	White beans, canned
Tuna, yellowfin, cooked	Plain yogurt, nonfat or low-fat
Rainbow trout, cooked	Clams, canned
Evaporated milk, nonfat	
Low-fat (1%) or reduced fat (2%) chocolate milk	
Skim milk (nonfat)	
Low-fat milk or buttermilk (1%)	
Orange juice, fresh	
Bananas	
Peaches, dried, uncooked	
Prunes, stewed	
Apricots, dried, uncooked	
Plantains, cooked	
Tomato sauce	
Pork loin, center rib, lean, roasted	
Spinach, cooked	

TABLE 51-3 General Consensus Guidelines for Potassium Replacement

Guideline	Comment
Potassium replacement therapy should accompany dietary consumption of potassium-rich foods.	Potassium-rich foods often cannot completely replace potassium associated with chloride losses (vomiting, diuretics, or nasogastric suction) because it is almost entirely coupled to phosphate. Furthermore, increasing dietary intake of these foods can lead to unwanted weight gain.
Potassium replacement is recommended for sodium-sensitive and hypertensive patients.	A high-sodium diet often results in excessive urinary potassium excretion.
Potassium replacement is recommended in patients who are subject to vomiting, diarrhea, or diuretic/laxative abuse.	These conditions promote excessive renal and GI potassium loss.
Potassium supplementation is best administered orally in divided doses over several days to achieve full repletion.	
Laboratory measurement of serum potassium is convenient, but not always accurate.	Clinicians should be aware of the factors that result in transcellular potassium shifts. Monitoring 24-hour urinary potassium excretion can be necessary in high-risk patients.
Patient adherence to potassium replacement can be increased with compliance-enhancing regimens.	Microencapsulated products have no bitter smell or aftertaste and have much better GI tolerance. Regimens should be made as simple as possible to follow.
A potassium dosage of 20 mEq/day (mmol/day) is usually sufficient to prevent hypokalemia from occurring. Doses of 40-100 mEq (mmol) are usually sufficient to treat hypokalemia.	

Pharmacologic Therapy

Formal guidelines for potassium supplementation were last published by the National Council on Potassium in Clinical Practice in 2000 (Table 51-3).[17] These guidelines provide a comprehensive framework for potassium administration as a prophylactic and therapeutic replacement for many patient populations. When deciding how to design the optimal regimen, one must consider: (a) the patient's normal, that is, baseline potassium concentration; (b) underlying medical conditions that can affect potassium balance; (c) concomitant medications that can affect potassium balance; (d) the patient's dietary salt intake; and (e) the patient's ability to comply with the therapeutic regimen.[17]

A general rule for potassium replacement is that for every 1 mEq/L (mmol/L) decrease of serum potassium below 3.5 mEq/L (mmol/L), there is a corresponding total-body potassium deficit of 100 to 400 mEq (mmol). Because of the wide variance in projected deficits, each patient's therapy must be individualized and adjustments made on the basis of the patient's signs, symptoms, and frequent measurements of serum potassium. In the acute care setting, the administration of 10 mEq (mmol) of IV or oral potassium should increase the serum potassium concentration by 0.1 mEq/L (mmol/L). This approximation is used as a basis for dose calculations, with frequent measurements of serum potassium to avoid overestimation. In patients receiving chronic loop or thiazide diuretic therapy, 40 to 100 mEq (mmol) of oral potassium supplementation can correct mild to moderate potassium deficits. Doses up to 120 mEq (mmol) can be required in more severe deficiencies. When providing oral potassium supplementation, the total daily dose should be divided into three to four doses to minimize the development of GI side effects. Patients receiving diuretics can become chronically hypokalemic and can benefit from combination potassium-sparing diuretic therapy.

3 Whenever possible, potassium supplementation should be administered by mouth. Three salts are available for oral potassium supplementation: chloride, phosphate, and bicarbonate. Potassium phosphate should be used when the patient is both hypokalemic and hypophosphatemic; potassium bicarbonate is most commonly used when potassium depletion occurs in the setting of metabolic acidosis. Potassium chloride, however, is the primary salt form used because it is the most effective treatment for the most common causes of potassium depletion (ie, diuretic and diarrhea-induced) as these conditions are associated with potassium and chloride losses.

Potassium chloride can be administered in either tablet or liquid formulations (Table 51-4). The liquid forms are generally less expensive; however, patient compliance can be low because of their strong, unpleasant taste. Liquid forms should be used when a rapid reponse to supplementation is desired. Two sustained-release solid dosage forms are currently available in the United States: a wax-matrix formulation, and a microencapsulated formulation. The microencapsulated tablet is generally preferred because it is associated with less GI irritation. IV potassium use should be limited to: (a) severe cases of hypokalemia (serum concentration less than 2.5 mEq/L [mmol/L]); (b) patients exhibiting signs and symptoms such as ECG changes or muscle spasms; or (c) patients unable to tolerate oral therapy. IV supplementation is more dangerous than oral therapy because it is more likely to result in hyperkalemia, phlebitis, and pain at the site of infusion.

The vehicle in which IV potassium is administered is important. Whenever possible, potassium should be prepared in saline-containing

TABLE 51-4 Differences Among Oral Potassium Supplements

Supplement	Comment
Controlled-release microencapsulated tablet	Disintegrates better in GI tract; fewer GI erosions as compared to wax-matrix tablets
Encapsulated controlled-release microencapsulated particles	Fewer erosions as compared to wax-matrix tablets
Potassium chloride elixir	Inexpensive, poor taste, poor compliance, immediate effect
Potassium chloride effervescent tablets for solution	More expensive than elixir, convenient
Wax-matrix extended-release tablets	Easier to swallow; more GI erosions as compared to other therapies

solutions (eg, 0.9%-0.45% sodium chloride [NaCl]). Dextrose-containing solutions stimulate insulin secretion, which can cause intracellular shifting of potassium, worsening the patient's hypokalemia, and should be avoided whenever possible. Generally, 10 to 20 mEq (mmol) of potassium is diluted in 100 mL 0.9% NaCl for IV administration. These concentrations are safe when administered through a peripheral vein over an hour. When infusion rates exceed 10 mEq/h (mmol/h) ECG monitoring should be performed to detect cardiac changes. The serum potassium concentration should be evaluated following the infusion of each 30 to 40 mEq (mmol) to guide further potassium replacement administration. Multiple doses of potassium can be repeated as needed until the serum potassium concentration normalizes. To allow adequate time for the potassium to equilibrate between the intra- and extracellular spaces, one should wait at least 30 minutes from the end of each infusion and care should be taken to avoid sampling from the same line in which the potassium was infused, as this can result in a spuriously high potassium concentration.

In cases of severe potassium depletion, patients can require as much as 300 to 400 mEq/day (mmol/day). In this instance, it is common practice to dilute 40 to 60 mEq (mmol) in 1,000 mL 0.45% NaCl and infuse at a rate not exceeding 40 mEq/h (mmol/h). The total 24-hour dose should not exceed 400 mEq (mmol). This should be performed in an intensive care unit under continuous ECG monitoring. Because of the high potassium concentration, and the risk for burning pain and peripheral venous sclerosis, the infusion should be through a central venous catheter into a large vein (eg, superior vena cava) but care must be taken not to place the tip of the catheter into the right atrium.[18] Directly delivering high potassium concentrations into the heart can result in cardiac arrhythmias. Given the volume required to infuse this dose of potassium, this infusion strategy might be impractical in certain clinical situations (eg, patients requiring fluid restriction). A reasonable approach is to split the potassium dose between the oral and IV routes. For example, if a symptomatic patient requires 120 mEq (mmol) of potassium, the clinician can give 60 mEq (mmol) as the immediate-release potassium liquid, and the other 60 mEq (mmol) can be given through the IV route (20 mEq/100 mL/h [mmol/100 mL/h] in three doses). When giving large potassium doses, serum monitoring should be performed following the administration of half the dose to guide the need for additional potassium. This can also help avoid the development of hyperkalemia.

In the rare circumstances when cardiac arrest from hypokalemia is imminent, IV bolus dosing of potassium 10 mEq (mmol) over 5 minutes can be initiated and repeated once, if necessary.[18]

Alternative Therapies

Potassium-sparing diuretics are a viable alternative to chronic exogenous potassium supplementation, especially when patients are concomitantly receiving drugs that are known to deplete potassium (eg, diuretics). Spironolactone inhibits the effect of aldosterone in the renal distal convoluted tubule, thereby decreasing potassium elimination in the urine. Spironolactone is especially effective as a potassium-sparing agent in patients with primary or secondary hyperaldosteronism. Amiloride and triamterene are reasonable second-line agents that act by an aldosterone-independent but unknown mechanism.

Spironolactone is available as 25-, 50-, and 100-mg tablets. The usual starting dose is 25 to 50 mg daily, and can be titrated to a maximum dose of 400 mg/day. The potassium-retaining effects generally take 48 hours to be evident. Principle adverse effects include hyperkalemia, gynecomastia, breast tenderness, and impotence in men. Triamterene is available as 50- and 100-mg capsules. The usual starting dose is 50 mg twice daily, which can be titrated to 100 mg twice daily. Triamterene is also available as a combination product with hydrochlorothiazide (37.5/25 mg, 50/25 mg, or 75/50 mg) and is commonly used for the treatment of hypertension. Common side effects include hyperkalemia, sodium depletion, and metabolic acidosis. The usual starting dose of amiloride is 5 mg daily; however, 10 mg can be given in those with severe hypokalemia. This is also available as a combination product with hydrochlorothiazide 50 mg. The most common side effects are hyperkalemia and metabolic acidosis.

Concomitant use of potassium supplementation with potassium-sparing diuretics is generally not necessary and when used there is a significant risk of hyperkalemia, especially in patients with CKD or diabetes mellitus.

Evaluation of Therapeutic Outcomes

Serum potassium concentrations should be monitored regularly while the patient is receiving potassium supplementation. For ambulatory patients receiving prophylactic potassium supplementation during diuretic therapy, the serum potassium and magnesium concentrations, as well as renal function should be monitored every 1 to 2 months. In hospitalized patients receiving oral therapy for mild hypokalemia, the potassium concentration should be monitored every 2 to 3 days. If it does not increase by at least 1 mEq/L (mmol/L) within 96 hours, the clinician should suspect concomitant magnesium depletion. Patients receiving IV potassium supplementation require close ECG monitoring if the infusion rate is greater than 20 mEq/h (mmol/h): doses greater than this should be administered only in the presence of continuous ECG monitoring. Additionally, the patient should have potassium concentrations obtained halfway through, and 30 minutes following completion of the total potassium dose to guide further potassium administration. Finally, the patient should be assessed for adverse effects such as pain at the infusion site or phlebitis.

Clinical Bottom Line

Hypokalemia is a frequent medical condition caused by both biological processes as well as drug therapy. While mild hypokalemia is frequently asymptomatic, severe hypokalemia can cause fatal cardiac dysrhythmias, particularly in patients with underlying cardiac disease. Patients receiving drugs that cause potassium wasting (eg, thiazide or loop diuretics), should be closely followed for the development of hypokalemia and appropriate potassium supplementation should be started when necessary. Generally oral potassium is sufficient for the management of mild hypokalemia; IV potassium shoud be reserved for severe deficiency, and its use should be monitored closely.

HYPERKALEMIA

Hyperkalemia, defined as a serum potassium concentration greater than 5 mEq/L (mmol/L), can be further classified according to its severity: mild hyperkalemia (5.1-5.9 mEq/L [mmol/L]), moderate hyperkalemia (6-7 mEq/L [mmol/L]), and severe hyperkalemia (above 7 mEq/L [mmol/L]).[17]

Epidemiology

4 Hyperkalemia is much less common than hypokalemia. In fact, if all patients with AKI and CKD were excluded, the prevalence of hyperkalemia would be less than 1% in the rest of the population. The incidence of hyperkalemia in hospitalized patients is highly variable, and reports have ranged from 1% to 10%.[19] Most cases of hyperkalemia are the result of overcorrection of hypokalemia with IV potassium supplements. Severe hyperkalemia occurs more commonly in elderly patients with renal insufficiency who have been receiving chronic oral potassium supplementation.

Etiology and Pathophysiology

Hyperkalemia develops when potassium intake exceeds excretion (true hyperkalemia) (ie, elevated total-body stores), or when the transcellular distribution of potassium is disturbed (ie, normal total-body stores). The four primary causes of hyperkalemia—(a) increased potassium intake, (b) decreased potassium excretion, (c) tubular unresponsiveness to aldosterone, and (d) redistribution of potassium into the extracellular space—are discussed further.

Hyperkalemia Associated with Increased Potassium Intake

Hyperkalemia in this setting is almost always associated with renal insufficiency. Patients with stage 4 or 5 CKD and dialysis patients who are noncompliant with dietary potassium restrictions often present with life-threatening hyperkalemia. Many of these patients do not realize that fresh fruits and vegetables contain large amounts of potassium. Anecdotally, in many dialysis centers the incidence of hyperkalemia peaks during the summer months, when fresh garden produce is available. Another common dietary source associated with the development of hyperkalemia is potassium chloride salt substitutes. Many dialysis patients are instructed to use salt substitutes to avoid excessive sodium intake in an attempt to control volume overload. These patients unwittingly become hyperkalemic because these products contain approximately 10 to 15 mEq (mmol) potassium per gram, or 200 mEq (mmol) per tablespoon. Finally, some over-the-counter herbal and alternative medicine products may contain significant amounts of potassium. It is thus essential for patients with CKD to receive education regarding dietary sources of potassium as well as information on the potassium content of herbal products when available.

Hyperkalemia Associated with Decreased Renal Potassium Excretion

Normally functioning kidneys excrete 90% of the daily potassium intake. Therefore, when the kidney is unable to excrete potassium appropriately, as in AKI and stage 4 to 5 CKD, potassium is retained and often results in hyperkalemia. Finally, because aldosterone is responsible for potassium excretion via the renal cortical collecting duct, medications and disesaes that inhibit this process contribute to hyperkalemia.[20]

Severe hyperkalemia is more common in AKI than in CKD because patients are often hypercatabolic and have underlying disorders, such as rhabdomyolysis or tumor lysis syndrome, which result in release of potassium from injured or lysed cells.[21] Severe hyperkalemia is rare in stable stage 1 to 4 CKD patients, perhaps because of enhanced GI and renal potassium excretion.[22] Data suggest that hyperkalemia directly stimulates renal potassium excretion through an effect that is independent of, and additive to, that of aldosterone.[22] Although the overall incidence of hyperkalemia is higher in patients with CKD when compared with patients without CKD, due to these adaptive mechanisms and patients' decreased susceptibility to cardiac effects of chronic hyperkalemia, they have a lower mortality rate than other patient populations.[23] Renal excretion of potassium is also inhibited by various endocrinologic disorders, including adrenal insufficiency, Addison disease, and selective hypoaldosteronism. All of these disorders involve a decreased production of aldosterone, which results in the retention of potassium.

Several drugs have profound effects on the kidney's ability to regulate potassium. Five drug classes in particular: angiotensin-converting enzyme inhibitors (ACEIs), angiotensin-II receptor blockers (ARBs), direct renin inhibitors, potassium-sparing diuretics, and prostaglandin inhibitors such as nonsteroidal anti-inflammatory drugs (NSAIDs). Although hyperkalemia is typically dose-dependent, the rates of hyperkalemia have been reported to range from 2% to 10% in most clinical trials.[24-26] Other commonly used drugs that can cause hyperkalemia are digoxin, cyclosporine, tacrolimus, trimethoprim–sulfamethoxazole, heparin, and pentamidine.

Tubular Unresponsiveness to Aldosterone

Sickle cell anemia, systemic lupus erythematosus, and amyloidosis, can produce a defect in renal tubular potassium secretion, possibly as the result of an alteration in the aldosterone-binding site.

Redistribution of Potassium into the Extracellular Space

The efflux of potassium from within the cell into the extracellular space, which is associated with no change in total-body potassium stores, is often observed in the presence of metabolic acidosis, diabetes mellitus, CKD, or lactic acidosis. β-Blockers can also result in a transcellular potassium shift.

The serum potassium concentration can also be falsely elevated in some conditions and not reflect the actual in vivo potassium concentration, that is, pseudohyperkalemia. Pseudohyperkalemia occurs most commonly in the setting of extravascular hemolysis of red blood cells. When a blood specimen is not processed promptly and cellular destruction occurs, intracellular potassium is released into the serum. It can also occur in conditions of thrombocytosis or leukocytosis. If severe hyperkalemia is found in a patient who is asymptomatic with an otherwise normal laboratory report, the hyperkalemia is most likely pseudohyperkalemia, and a repeat blood sample should be collected. Truly elevated potassium concentrations are normally associated with other laboratory abnormalities, such as low carbon dioxide (acidosis) or elevated blood urea nitrogen and creatinine concentrations (indicating renal insufficiency).

CLINICAL PRESENTATION Hyperkalemia

General

- Related to the effects of excessive potassium on neuromuscular, cardiac, and smooth muscle cell function.

Symptoms

- Frequently asymptomatic.
- The patient might complain of heart palpitations or skipped heartbeats.

Signs

- ECG changes (Fig. 51-1)

Laboratory Tests

- Serum potassium concentration above 5.0 mEq/L (mmol/L) is diagnostic.

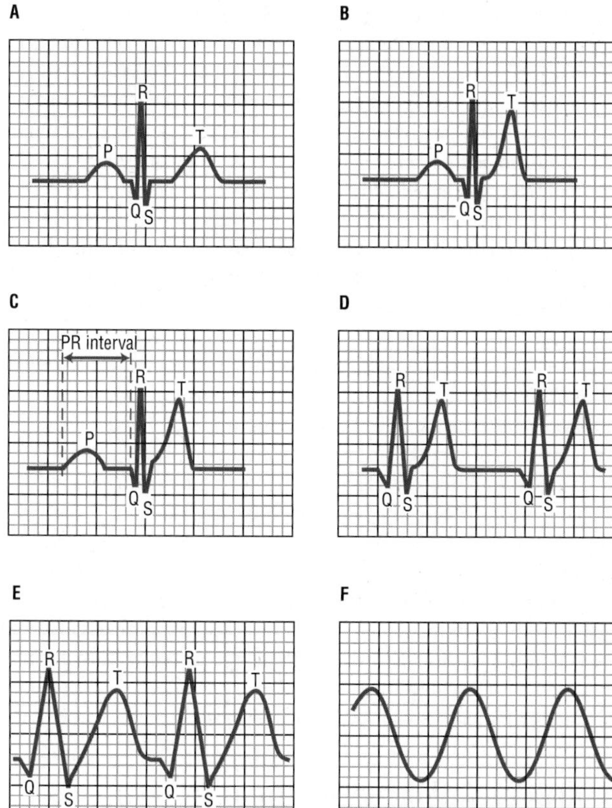

FIGURE 51-1 The earliest electrocardiographic manifestation of hyperkalemia is an increase in the rate of ventricular repolarization, which results in a peaking of the T wave at serum potassium concentrations of ~5.5 to 6 mEq/L (mmol/L) (*B*), relative to the normal ECG presentation (*A*). Further increases in the serum potassium concentration above 6 mEq/L (mmol/L) result in conduction delays through the His-Purkinje system, the atrial myocardium, and the ventricular myocardium. The ECG manifestations of these conduction delays and the sequence in which they occur are a widening of the PR interval (*C*), delay through the His-Purkinje system, a loss of the P wave (*D*), delay through the atrial myocardium, a widening of the QRS complex (*E*), and delay through the ventricular myocardium. Finally, there is a merging of the QRS complex with the T wave (*F*), which results in a sine-wave appearance.

TREATMENT

Desired Outcomes

The goals of therapy for the treatment of hyperkalemia are to antagonize adverse cardiac effects, reverse signs and symptoms that are present, and return the serum and total-body stores of potassium to normal. The optimal treatment approach is dependent on the severity of hyperkalemia, the rapidity of its development, and the patient's clinical condition. Although ECG changes are directly proportional to the plasma potassium concentration and its rate of increase, they may not be present in all patients. In contrast, ventricular fibrillation may be the first cardiac manifestation of hyperkalemia in some patients.[27] Asymptomatic patients with mild hyperkalemia usually require no specific therapy other than dietary education to control intake, and monitoring of serum potassium daily if an inpatient or weekly if an outpatient to assure resolution.

Severe hyperkalemia (above 7 mEq/L [mmol/L]) or moderate hyperkalemia (6-6.9 mEq/L [mmol/L]), when associated with clinical symptoms or ECG changes, requires immediate treatment. Initial treatment should be focused on antagonism of the cardiac membrane actions of hyperkalemia (eg, administration of calcium). Secondarily, one should attempt to decrease extracellular potassium concentration by promoting its intracellular movement (eg, with insulin, β_2-receptor agonists, or sodium bicarbonate) or enhance its removal from the body by hemodialysis: the oral administration of cation-exchange resins, and/or the use of loop diuretics may aslo be considered in some patients. In any case, the underlying cause of hyperkalemia should be identified and reversed, and exogenous potassium must be withheld.

General Approach to Treatment

A treatment approach for patients with hyperkalemia is outlined in Fig. 51-2. In patients who have acute ECG changes, IV calcium should be administered to prevent or treat any cardiac manifestations of hyperkalemia. At the same time, the serum potassium concentration should be rapidly decreased to below 5 mEq/L (mmol/L) within minutes by administering drugs that cause an intracellular shift of potassium, followed by the initation of those that increase the elimination of potassium from the body.[27] If the patient is asymptomatic, rapid correction may not be necessary and will likely depend on the clinical context associated with the rise in serum potassium concentration. If one anticipates the need to reduce total-body potassium stores, an ion exchange resin (eg, sodium polystyrene sulfonate [SPS]) that results in removal of potassium from the body over several hours to days may be initiated shortly after the

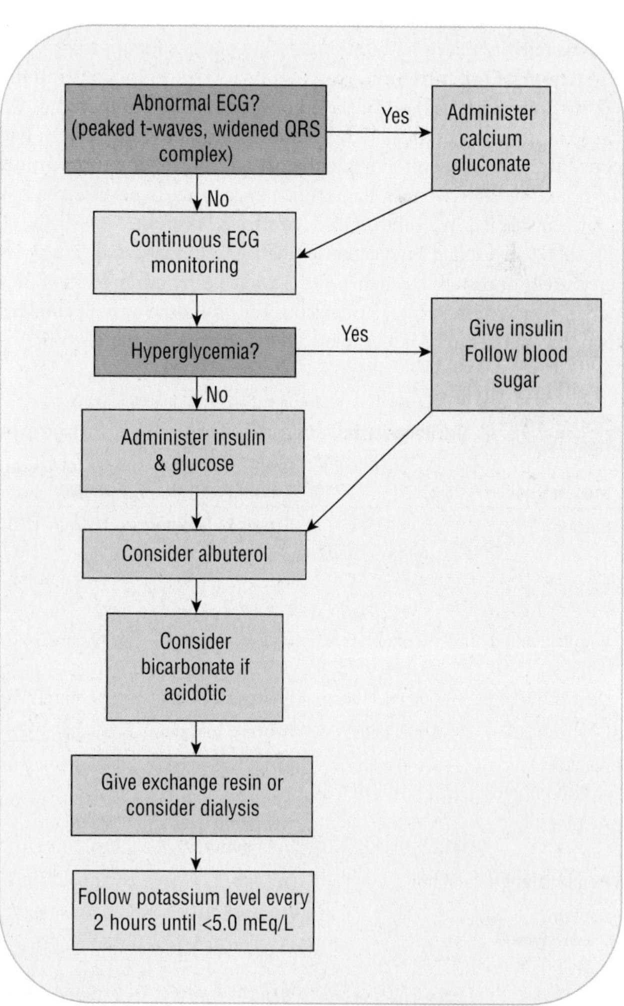

FIGURE 51-2 Treatment approach for hyperkalemia. (Serum potassium of 5.0 mEq/L is equivalent to 5.0 mmol/L.)

emergent care has been instituted. Recently, two cation exchange agents with a similar effect have emerged. Patiromer (Veltassa™) is a potassium binder approved for the treatment of hyperkalemia and sodium zirconium cyclosilicate (ZS-9) is pending approval for a similar indication.

Nonpharmacologic Therapy

A recent study suggested that hemodialysis patients who ingested foods supplemented with glycyrrhetinic acid, the active ingredient in licorice, were better able to maintain plasma potassium concentrations within the normal range compared with hemodialysis patients given placebo.[28,29] Glycyrrhetinic acid inhibits the enzyme 11β-hydroxy-steroid dehydrogenase II, thereby increasing cortisol availability in the colon. The net result is enhanced potassium elimination in the feces. Other nonpharmacologic therapies, specifically available for dialysis-dependent patients are the tailoring of their intermittent dialysis or hemofiltration therapy to include a low potassium dialysate to enhance the removal of potassium (see Chapter 45).

Pharmacologic Therapy

There are several drug therapy options to lower the serum potassium concentration. The optimal regimen for a given patient is dependent on the rapidity and degree of lowering that is necessary. Table 51-5 provides an overview of the available therapies and their respective onset and duration of action.

While specific treatment recommendations vary, it is generally accepted that asymptomatic patients with potassium concentrations below 6 mEq/L (mmol/L) can be treated conservatively. In patients with normal renal function, or those with stage 3 or 4 CKD, this typically involves the administration of furosemide to promote urinary potassium excretion. When given IV at a dosage of 40 to 80 mg, urine flow usually increases within minutes and persists for approximately 4 to 6 hours. Oral furosemide can also be used, keeping in mind the IV:PO dose ratio (1:2) and delayed onset of action compared to IV. Close monitoring of the patient's volume status and other electrolyte concentrations is required while the patient is receiving furosemide. Of note, the effectiveness of diuretics in treating hyperkalemia has not been studied in a randomized, controlled fashion.

SPS (Kayexalate®) is a cation-exchange resin that can be administered orally or rectally by enema. SPS is available in powder form or prepackaged as a 33% sorbitol suspension. The oral route is more effective than the enema and is better tolerated by patients. As the resin passes through the intestines, each gram of SPS exchanges 1 mEq (mmol) of sodium for 1 mEq (mmol) of potassium, which is in a relatively higher concentration in the large intestine. The onset of action of SPS is within 1 hour, and it can be repeated every 4 hours as needed. The sorbitol component of the suspension promotes the excretion of the cationically modified potassium exchange resin by inducing diarrhea. The usual oral SPS dose is 15 to 60 g in the 33% sorbitol suspension.

There have been several reports of colonic necrosis with the use of SPS.[30,31] In 2009, the U.S. Food and Drug Administration (FDA) mandated a boxed warning for SPS due to reports of colonic necrosis and other serious GI toxicities.[32] The GI toxicities were believed to be associated with the 70% sorbitol; however, there are also reports of GI toxicity when the 33% sorbitol solution was administered. A common finding in these reports was that toxicity occurred most commonly in patients who had recently undergone GI surgery or had a current or history of bowel dysfunction. This FDA warning was updated in 2011. A recent commentary provided some needed perspective on the role of SPS in treating hyperkalemia.[33] While the authors echoed the FDA warning, they found little risk to using the SPS 33% sorbitol suspension or SPS powder mixed in water for oral administration. These authors recommended that the retention enema route of administration be abandoned given the risk of side effects and the fact that the enema route appears to be less effective compared with oral administration. Additionally, SPS use is contraindicated in patients with bowel dysfunction.

Clinical **Controversy...**

In 2015, the FDA issued a safety communication requiring the drug manufacturer to conduct studies to investigate the potential of SPS to bind to other orally administered medications. This comes after *in vitro* binding studies of another potassium binding agent, patiromer, demonstrated that the drug bound about half of the oral medications tested, which could affect their absorption and efficacy. The FDA recommends prescribers and patients consider separating the dose of SPS from other oral medications by 6 hours and that they monitor the patient's clinical response closely. Based on the manufacturer's studies, there may be mandated updates to the drug label to include information about these interactions.[34]

TABLE 51-5 Therapeutic Alternatives for the Management of Hyperkalemia

Medication	Dose	Route of Administration	Onset/Duration of Action	Acuity	Mechanism of Action	Expected Result
Calcium	1 g	IV over 5-10 minutes	1-2 min/10-30 min	Acute	Raises cardiac threshold potential	Reverses electrocardiographic effects
Furosemide	20-40 mg	IV	5-15 min/4-6 h	Acute	Inhibits renal Na^+ reabsorption	Increased urinary K^+ loss
Regular insulin	5-10 units	IV or SC	30 min/2-6 h	Acute	Stimulates intracellular K^+ uptake	Intracellular K^+ redistribution
Dextrose 10%	1,000 mL (100 g)	IV over 1-2 hours	30 min/2-6 h	Acute	Stimulates insulin release	Intracellular K^+ redistribution
Dextrose 50%	50 mL (25 g)	IV over 5 minutes	30 min/2-6 h	Acute	Stimulates insulin release	Intracellular K^+ redistribution
Sodium bicarbonate	50-100 mEq (50-100 mmol)	IV over 2-5 minutes	30 min/2-6 h	Acute	Raises serum pH	Intracellular K^+ redistribution
Albuterol	10-20 mg	Nebulized over 10 minutes	30 min/1-2 h	Acute	Stimulates intracellular K^+ uptake	Intracellular K^+ redistribution
Hemodialysis	4 hours	N/A	Immediate/variable	Acute	Removal from serum	Increased K^+ elimination
Sodium polystyrene sulfonate	15-60 g	Oral or rectal	1 h/variable	Nonacute	Resin exchanges Na^+ for K^+	Increased K^+ elimination
Patiromer	8.4-25.2 g	Oral	Hours/variable	Nonacute	Resin exchanges Ca^{++} for K^+	Increased K^+ elimination

In symptomatic patients, or in those with severe hyperkalemia, emergency care is indicated. Initial therapy in this setting is the administration of IV calcium chloride or gluconate 1 g to protect the heart from life-threatening arrhythmias.[27] Calcium antagonizes the cardiac membrane effect of hyperkalemia by reducing the electrical threshold potential for cardiac myocytes and reverses ECG changes within minutes. IV calcium should not be given to patients receiving digoxin as it can lead to digoxin toxicity. Its duration of action is 30 to 60 minutes, and it can be repeated as needed based on ECG findings. IV calcium can be given as either the chloride or gluconate salt; each is available as a 10% solution by weight. Calcium chloride provides approximately three times more calcium than equal volumes of the gluconate salt; however, it can cause tissue necrosis if extravasation occurs. For this reason, calcium gluconate is more commonly administered, with the standard dose being 10-mL IV bolus over 5 to 10 minutes.

Rapid correction of hyperkalemia may necessitate the administration of drugs that result in an intracellular shift of potassium, such as insulin and dextrose, sodium bicarbonate, and a β_2-adrenergic receptor agonist (eg, albuterol). The treatment of choice depends on the underlying medical disorders accompanying hyperkalemia. For example, in patients with concomitant metabolic acidosis, a sodium bicarbonate bolus or infusion of 50 to 100 mEq (mmol) is the preferred therapy. Sodium bicarbonate helps correct the metabolic acidosis by raising the extracellular pH, in addition to causing a rapid intracellular potassium shift. It should be noted that sodium bicarbonate is much less effective when hyperkalemia is not related to metabolic acidosis.[1] Sodium bicarbonate is also less effective in patients with end-stage renal disease (ESRD), in whom a decrease in serum potassium may not be seen for as long as 4 hours. Sodium bicarbonate can also lead to sodium and volume overload in patients with stage 4 or 5 CKD. Administration of a rapid-acting (eg, Insulin lispro 10 units IV) or regular insulin (10 units IV) and dextrose (10% or 50%) is an effective method of reducing potassium. Insulin increases the activity of the Na^+-K^+-ATPase pump, thereby intracellularly shifting potassium. Glucose should be given with insulin unless the serum glucose is above 250 mg/dL (13.9 mmol/L) because hypoglycemia can develop as a result of the effects of the insulin therapy. An IV bolus of 10 units of regular insulin and 25 g of dextrose usually lowers the serum potassium concentration by 0.6 mEq/L (mmol/L) in dialysis-dependent patients.[32] β_2-adrenergic agonists have a dual mechanism for lowering serum potassium. First, they stimulate the Na^+-K^+-ATPase pump to promote intracellular potassium uptake. Second, they stimulate pancreatic β-receptors to increase insulin secretion. Albuterol can be administered via IV (0.5 mg given over 15 minutes) or via nebulizer (10-20 mg nebulized over 10 minutes).

However, it should be noted that injectable albuterol is not available in the United States. In ESRD patients, decreases in plasma potassium concentration of 0.6 mEq/L (mmol/L) and 1 mEq/L (mmol/L) can be anticipated after inhalation of 10 and 20 mg of albuterol, respectively. Of note, the doses of inhaled albuterol used for hyperkalemia are at least four times higher than those typically used for bronchospasm. There are important limitations with albuterol therapy, most notably variable bioavailability via the inhaled route (leading to potential over- or underdosing and unpredictability of response) and second, cardiac side effects such as tachycardia, which are undesirable in patients who already have an abnormal ECG. Furthermore, as many as 40% of patients may be resistant to the hypokalemic effects of albuterol and patients already receiving a nonselective β_2-receptor antagonist may not respond. Therefore, albuterol should not be used alone for the urgent treatment of hyperkalemia in CKD patients.[27]

A Cochrane Review evaluated the emergency treatment of hyperkalemia.[35] Many of the reviewed studies were small, and not all intervention groups had sufficient data for meta-analysis to be performed. Most of the data were from nonrandomized, noncontrolled observational studies and case reports. However, given these limitations, inhaled and nebulized β-agonists, and IV insulin and glucose were all deemed effective. The combination of nebulized β-agonists with IV insulin and glucose appeared to be more effective than either agent alone. The meta-analysis results were equivocal for IV bicarbonate, and notably, SPS was not effective by 4 hours. Given the limitations of this Cochrane Review, clinicians should exercise caution when extrapolating these findings to clinical practice. Nonetheless, the Cochrane database review corroborates the approach detailed in Fig. 51-2.

Frequently, management of hyperkalemia will be based on the clinician's personal judgment or institutional protocols. A recent prospective chart review examined how hyperkalemia was treated in an academic teaching hospital.[36] Overall, 95% of the patients received SPS, 21% received insulin, 21% received IV calcium, and less than 10% of patients received bicarbonate, albuterol, or hemodialysis. Combination therapy was given to 21% of patients, with SPS and insulin being the most common.

In nonhospitalized patients who have experienced chronic increases in serum potassium concentration, long-term management of hyperkalemia is focused on dietary restriction of potassium-rich foods and supplements, reducing and avoiding medications that impair renal potassium excretion, and using diuretics or other medications to counteract the effects of medications that increase serum potassium concentrations. Medications used for chronic conditions that are known to cause hyperkalemia include NSAIDs, ACEIs, ARBs, direct renin inhibitors, and aldosterone antagonists. These typically result in asymptomatic hyperkalemia without the need for emergent therapies. To prevent hyperkalemia, clinicians may attempt to lower the dose or switch to another medication without hyperkalemia as a side effect (eg, calcium channel blocker). However, medications that inhibit the renin–angiotensin–aldosterone system (RAAS) have significant beneficial effects on morbidity and mortality in patients with chronic diseases such as diabetes mellitus, congestive heart failure, and CKD. Therefore reducing or avoiding the use of these medications to prevent hyperkalemia is not often appropriate. The use of a combination of ACEI and ARB is generally avoided due to the increased risk of hyperkalemia.[37] Aldosterone antagonists have a different mechanism of action and their use in combination with an ACEI or ARB is considered acceptable. A recent study found that the extent of hyperkalemia was greater with a combination ACEI and aldosterone antagonist than a combination ACEI and ARB in patients with diabetic nephropathy, suggesting an extrarenal mechanism of this adverse effect in aldosterone antagonists.[38]

Using existing polymeric exchange resins (eg, SPS) in outpatient settings is not ideal given the risk of adverse effects and unknown efficacy.[31] Recently, two new cation exchange agents have emerged as potential therapies for acute and short-term treatment of outpatients with mild hyperkalemia. Veltassa™ (patiromer) is a nonabsorbable polymer that exhanges calcium for potassium in the intestine to increase fecal elimination of potassium. Two major studies examined its efficacy in lowering serum potassium concentrations. A phase 3 clinical trial consisting of a 4-week initial treatment phase and an 8-week randomized, placebo-controlled withdrawal phase assessed the response in adults with stage 3 or 4 CKD on stable doses of RAAS inhibitors.[39] A majority of patients in the initial phase achieved normokalemia. During the withdrawal phase, patiromer continued to decrease serum potassium concentrations (estimated mean reduction of 0.72 mEq/L (mmol/L)) whereas placebo had no effect on serum potassium concentration. In a phase 2 dose-finding study that included a similar patient population, normokalemia was maintained with patiromer in 77% to 95% of patients, depending on the degree of hyperkalemia at baseline.[40] Patiromer comes as 8.4, 16.8, and 25.2 g packets for oral suspension. The package insert cautions that it should not be used to treat life-threatening hyperkalemia due to its delayed onset of action.[41] Additionally, patiromer has been shown in *in vitro* studies to bind to many oral medications, which could lead to decreased absorption of other mediations and loss of efficacy. Therefore, it is recommended to administer other oral medications at least 6 hours before or after patiromer.[41] If this is not possible, alternative regimens should be considered.

Sodium zirconium cyclosilicate (ZS-9) is a nonabsorable inorganic compound that selectively enhances potassium excretion by the intestinal route. Two phase 3, randomized, placebo-controlled trials have assessed the efficacy of ZS-9 in lowering serum potassium concentrations in adult outpatients with asymptomatic mild to moderate hyperkalemia. Both trials found that ZS-9 significantly decreased serum potassium concentrations 48 hours after administration compared to placebo, with an average decrease of approximately 1 mEq/L (mmol/L) for the 10 g dose.[42,43] A majority of the patients maintained normokalemia during maintenances phases of 15 and 28 days, despite a high incidence of patients with CKD, congestive heart failure, diabetes mellitus, and use of RAAS inhibitors. The most common adverse effect in the ZS-9 group was edema, likely from the exchange of sodium for potassium.

Clinical **Controversy...**

For both ZS-9 and patiromer, efficacy in producing normokalemia in the short-term has been shown in outpatients on RAAS inhibitors who have asymptomatic mild to moderate hyperkalemia. It remains to be seen whether the effects are sustainable in the long-term or whether either agent can be used in the acute treatment of hospitalized patients. These agents should presently not be used in acute treatment of hyperkalemia, but may be appropriate for outpatient treatment in combination with nonpharmacological strategies.

Evaluation of Therapeutic Outcomes

The frequency and rigor with which one evaluates patients to ascertain if they have achieved the desired therapeutic outcomes depends on the severity and acuity of hyperkalemia. For example, cautious waiting is more common for those with mild or moderate asymptomatic hyperkalemia compared to those with acute symptomatic, severe hyperkalemia. Many drugs such as ACEIs, ARBs, direct renin inhibitors, and spironolactone result in asymptomatic hyperkalemia and changes in dosage or to a different agent may be all that is warranted. In patients with normal renal function, once these drugs are initiated and the dose titrated, clinicians should check the potassium concentration at least monthly. For those patients with renal dysfunction, monitoring should be biweekly until the dose is stabilized.

In patients who have acute symptomatic hyperkalemia (eg, ECG changes), frequent potassium concentration and ECG monitoring is warranted. The patient should receive continuous ECG telemetry monitoring until the serum potassium concentration decreases below 5 mEq/L (mmol/L), and the ECG abnormalities resolve. Similarly, while the patient is receiving emergent therapy, serial serum potassium concentrations should be obtained hourly until the potassium concentration decreases below 5 mEq/L (mmol/L). For patients who receive insulin and dextrose therapy for hyperkalemia, blood glucose monitoring should be performed hourly or more frequently if patients demonstrate signs and symptoms of hypoglycemia. For patients who receive large doses of sodium bicarbonate therapy for hyperkalemia, an arterial blood gas or serum chemistry profile should be obtained to assess their acid–base status. Furthermore, the patient should be evaluated for signs of fluid overload secondary to the high sodium load. Patients receiving albuterol therapy should be questioned regularly regarding the development of palpitations and tachycardia. The patient's medication records should be reviewed to assure the patient is not receiving drug therapy that increases the serum potassium concentration. Furthermore, the patient should be questioned regarding the occurrence of diarrheal stool output.

Clinical Bottom Line

Hyperkalemia commonly occurs in patients with reduced kidney function or other metabolic disturbances. It can rapidly evolve into a medical emergency; therefore, prompt identification and appropriate pharmacotherapy is needed. In patients with mild hyperkalemia, potassium binding resins or loop diuretics may be useful, and should be used as first-line therapy. In severe hyperkalemia with ECG changes, IV calcium should be given to protect against cardiac dysrhythmias. Additionally rapid-acting therapies such as IV insulin and β_2-adrenergic agonists are indicated to move potassium intracellularly.

DISORDERS OF MAGNESIUM HOMEOSTASIS

Magnesium plays a central role in cellular function and is an important cofactor in more than 300 biochemical reactions in the body, especially those systems that are dependent on adenosine triphosphate. Mitochondrial function, protein synthesis, cell membrane function, parathyroid hormone secretion, and glucose metabolism are just a few important functions affected by magnesium.[44] It is the fourth most abundant extracellular cation and the second most abundant intracellular cation, after potassium. Disorders of magnesium homeostasis are commonly encountered in clinical situations and most frequently are manifested as alterations in cardiovascular and neuromuscular function. Life-threatening conditions such as paralysis and cardiac arrhythmias can occur, making the proper recognition and treatment of these problems of paramount importance. Altered magnesium balance also plays a key role in chronic disease states such as diabetes mellitus, CKD, osteoporosis, development of kidney stones, as well as heart and vascular disease.[45]

Magnesium is principally distributed in bone (67%) and muscle (20%). Because of its predominantly intracellular distribution, measurement of magnesium in the extracellular compartment may not accurately reflect the total-body magnesium content. The majority of magnesium in the extracellular fluid is in the ionized form as only 30% is bound to serum proteins. The normal range for serum magnesium is 1.4 to 1.8 mEq/L (1.7-2.3 mg/dL or 0.70-0.95 mmol/L).

The recommended daily dietary magnesium intake for adults is approximately 420 mg/day and 320 mg/day for men and women, respectively. The maintenance of magnesium homeostasis depends on the balance between intake and output. Ingested magnesium (30%-40%) is absorbed in the small bowel. The absorption of magnesium decreases as the dietary intake increases. Reductions in absorption have also been noted in the elderly and those with CKD. A small amount is present in intestinal secretions and reabsorbed in the sigmoid colon. The kidneys play a major role in maintaining magnesium balance. Approximately 95% of the filtered magnesium is reabsorbed, thus in most patients less than 5% is excreted in the urine.[38] Renal magnesium handling is unique in that approximately 20% of the filtered magnesium is reabsorbed in the proximal tubule; the majority (up to 70%) of reabsorption occurs in the thick ascending limb of the loop of Henle. This explains why loop diuretics often cause profound urinary magnesium wasting. The remaining 10% is reabsorbed in the distal convoluted tubule.[46] Unlike most other important electrolytes, there is no hormonal regulation of the distribution of magnesium between bone and circulating or intracellular magnesium pools. Because of this, both hypomagnesemia and hypermagnesemia commonly occur.

CLINICAL PRESENTATION Hypomagnesemia

General

- The dominant organ systems affected by hypomagnesemia are the neuromuscular and cardiovascular systems.

Symptoms

- Neuromuscular symptoms such as tetany, twitching, and generalized convulsions are common.
- Cardiac symptoms include heart palpitations.

Signs

- Neuromuscular: Presence of Chvostek sign, Trousseau sign, tremor, and tetany.
- Cardiovascular: Cardiac arrhythmias (ventricular fibrillation, torsade de pointes, or digoxin-induced arrhythmias), sudden cardiac death, and hypertension can be present. ECG abnormalities include widened QRS complex and peaked T waves with mild hypomagnesemia; and prolonged PR interval, progressive widening of QRS complex, and flattened T waves with moderate to severe hypomagnesemia.

Laboratory Tests

- Serum magnesium concentration less than 1.4 mEq/L (1.7 mg/dL [0.70 mmol/L]). Serum potassium and calcium concentrations can also be low.

HYPOMAGNESEMIA

Epidemiology

Hypomagnesemia is a common problem in both ambulatory and hospitalized patients. Although the exact prevalence is difficult to estimate, it has been reported that up to 65% of intensive care unit patients are magnesium-deficient. Although serum magnesium concentrations are not a reliable index of total-body magnesium content, they remain the primary diagnostic tool to evaluate body stores.

Hypomagnesemia is associated with an increase in mortality in critically ill patients. There are limited data regarding the incidence and associated risks of hypomagnesemia in hospitalized general medicine patients, even though they are at an increased risk of hypomagensemia given the presence of comorbidities such as congestive heart failure, CKD, and diabetes mellitus. A recent study reported a 20% incidence of hypomagensemia in hospitalized general medicine patients, which was associated with increased mortality compared to normomagnesemic patients (17.2% vs 7.2%, respectively).[47]

Etiology and Pathophysiology

5 Hypomagnesemia is usually associated with disorders of the intestinal tract or kidney.[48] Drugs or conditions that interfere with intestinal absorption or increase renal excretion of magnesium can result in hypomagnesemia (Table 51-6). Decreased intestinal absorption as a result of small bowel disease is the most common cause of hypomagnesemia worldwide. These disorders include regional enteritis, radiation enteritis, ulcerative colitis, acute and chronic diarrhea, pancreatic insufficiency and other malabsorptive syndromes, small-bowel bypass surgery, and chronic laxative abuse. Proton pump inhibitors, especially when used chronically, can cause hypomagnesemia through impaired intestinal absorption. Hypomagnesemia is commonly associated with alcoholism, where the etiology is multifactorial, including reduced intake, pancreatic insufficiency, chronic vomiting and diarrhea, and urinary magnesium wasting.

Primary renal magnesium wasting can be caused by a defect in renal tubular magnesium reabsorption, or inhibition of sodium reabsorption in those segments in which magnesium transport follows passively. The former condition is associated with hypercalciuria, nephrolithiasis, and progressive renal disease, while the latter is associated with Gitelman and Bartter syndromes.[48] Much more common than these is renal magnesium wasting secondary to thiazide and loop diuretics. Other commonly used drugs that can cause renal magnesium wasting include aminoglycosides, amphotericin B, cyclosporine, digoxin, tacrolimus, cisplatin, pentamidine, and foscarnet.[49]

TREATMENT

Desired Outcomes

The treatment goals in the management of hypomagnesemia are (a) resolution of the signs and symptoms, (b) restoration of normal magnesium concentrations, (c) correction of concomitant electrolyte abnormalities, and (d) identification and correction of the underlying cause of magnesium depletion.

General Approach to Treatment

Nearly all of the data regarding magnesium replacement therapy have been derived from relatively old data in acutely ill, hospitalized patients. Magnesium supplementation can be given by the oral, intramuscular (IM), or IV route. The severity of the magnesium depletion and the presence of severe signs and symptoms should dictate the route of administration. Because IM administration is painful, it should be reserved for those patients with severe hypomagnesemia and limited venous access. IV bolus administration is associated with flushing, sweating, and a sensation of warmth; thus bolus administration should be avoided if possible. Additionally, because calcium forms a complex with the sulfate moiety, which is then excreted, large amounts of IV magnesium sulfate should be administered with caution to hypocalcemic patients, as it can further exacerbate calcium deficiency.[45] There have been no clinical trials assessing the optimal regimen for magnesium replacement; however, it is widely accepted that 8 to 12 g of magnesium sulfate be administered, in divided doses, in the first 24 hours followed by 4 to 6 g/day for 3 to 5 days to adequately replete body stores in those with severe hypomagnesemia.[50] Even if severe magnesium depletion is present, approximately 50% of the administered dose is excreted in the urine. Consequently, magnesium replacement should be performed over 3 to 5 days, and continued supplementation should be provided for patients unable to eat. Table 51-7 lists the commonly used magnesium oral supplements and their respective elemental magnesium content.

Nonpharmacologic Therapy

There are currently no nonpharmacologic options for the management of hypomagnesaemia.

TABLE 51-6 Causes of Hypomagnesemia

GI
Reduced intake
Protein-calorie malnutrition
Prolonged parenteral fluid administration without magnesium
Alcoholism
Reduced absorption
Primary hypomagnesemia
Malabsorption syndromes (eg, tropical sprue, celiac disease, radiation enteritis, or intestinal lymphectasia)
Short-bowel syndrome (eg, small-bowel resection or ileal bypass)
Pancreatic insufficiency
Proton pump inhibitors (long-term use)
Increased loss
Excessive vomiting
Prolonged nasogastric suction
Excessive laxative use
Intestinal and biliary fistulas
Prolonged diarrhea (ulcerative colitis, Crohn disease, or cancer of the colon)
Renal
Primary tubular disorders
Primary renal magnesium wasting
Bartter syndrome
Renal tubular acidosis
Diuretic phase of acute tubular necrosis
Postobstructive diuresis
Postrenal transplant diuresis
Glomerulonephritis
Pyelonephritis
Drug-induced renal losses
Aminoglycosides
Amphotericin B
Cyclosporine
Tacrolimus
Diuretics
Digitalis
Cisplatin
Pentamidine
Foscarnet
Hormone-induced renal losses
Primary hyperparathyroidism
Hyperthyroidism
Aldosteronism
"Hungry bone syndrome" after parathyroidectomy
Internal redistribution
Diabetic ketoacidosis
Glucose, amino acid, or insulin administration
Massive blood transfusion (citrate)
Pancreatitis with lipedema (magnesium soap)
Other
Excessive sweating and lactation
Hypercalcemia and hypercalciuria
Phosphate depletion
Chronic alcoholism
Extracellular fluid volume expansion

Pharmacologic Therapy

It is currently controversial whether all asymptomatic patients require magnesium supplementation when serum magnesium concentration falls below the normal range. In particular, it has been suggested that for patients with type 2 diabetes mellitus, hypomagnesemia contributes to diabetic complications by affecting glucose transport and insulin secretion and utilization. Indeed, it has been shown that oral magnesium supplementation in type 2 diabetic patients with hypomagnesemia improves insulin sensitivity and metabolic control.[51] Others suggest that hypomagnesemia is more likely a consequence of diabetes mellitus. Possible mechanisms of hypomagensemia in these patients include reduced GI absorption, enhanced renal excretion secondary to an increased filtered magnesium load and tubular flow, and reduced tubular reabsorption.

TABLE 51-7 Common Magnesium Products and Their Elemental Magnesium Content

Product	Elemental Magnesium Content
Magnesium oxide	242 mg in a 400-mg tablet
Magnesium hydroxide	167 mg in a 400-mg tablet or 5-mL oral suspension
Magnesium chloride	64 mg in each 535-mg tablet
Magnesium citrate	48 mg in each 5 mL of the oral solution
Magnesium gluconate	27 mg in a 500-mg tablet
Magnesium lactate	84 mg in an 84 mg-tablet

Metabolic abnormalities such as hypokalemia, hypophosphatemia, and metabolic acidosis may also contribute to its development.[52] While it seems reasonable to provide a supplement for diabetic patients with low serum magnesium concentrations, clinical trials have yet to prove that supplementation leads to improved clinical outcomes.

Should treatment be warranted, those patients with serum magnesium concentrations greater than 1 mEq/L (1.2 mg/dL [0.5 mmol/L]) can be treated with oral supplements. Oral supplementation is preferred because magnesium uptake is a slow process that may require prolonged administration. Several magnesium products are available, including magnesium-containing antacids or laxatives, comprising a variety of magnesium salts in tablet or capsule formulations. Many of the oral products contain very little magnesium, which necessitates three or four doses per day. As expected, diarrhea is the most common dose-limiting side effect of oral therapy, which can greatly reduce patient compliance. Therefore, sustained-release magnesium products are preferred as they not only improve patient compliance, but also reduce the occurrence of GI side effects.

In cases of severe magnesium depletion (serum concentrations less than 1 mEq/L [less than 1.2 mg/dL; less than 0.5 mmol/L]), or if signs and symptoms are present regardless of the serum concentration, IV magnesium should be administered. A dose of 4 to 6 g in 50 to 100 mL (maximum concentration 1 g/10 mL) should be administered in divided doses over 12 to 24 hours and repeated as necessary in order to maintain magnesium concentrations above 1 mEq/L (1.2 mg/dL [0.5 mmol/L]). Doses of 2 to 4 g in 50 mL infused over 1 hour are frequently used clinically; however, these result in transient benefit because of the extensive renal excretion, and usually have to be repeated daily over 3 to 5 days for adequeate repletion. Therapy should be continued until the signs and symptoms have completely resolved. In patients with renal insufficiency, some have reduced the does by 25% to 50%.

Clinical **Controversy...**

Hypomagnesemia in patients with type 2 diabetes may be associated with impaired insulin and glucose utilization. Other data suggest that hypomagnesemia is a consequence of diabetes itself. Supplementation in hypomagnesemic diabetes patients increases insulin sensitivity and metabolic control, but its effect on clinical outcomes has yet to be elucidated.

Evaluation of Therapeutic Outcomes

In patients with acute, asymptomatic mild to moderate hypomagnesemia, serum magnesium concentrations should be obtained at least daily during their hospitalization. Patients receiving oral magnesium therapy should be questioned regarding GI tolerance and the occurrence of diarrhea. Patients being treated for symptomatic severe hypomagnesemia should have their serum magnesium concentration monitored hourly until the serum concentration reaches 1.5 mEq/L (1.8 mg/dL [0.75 mmol/L]) and the symptoms resolve. At that point, the serum magnesium concentration can be monitored every 6 to 12 hours for the next 24 hours while receiving magnesium supplementation. Once the magnesium concentration is stable in the normal range, a concentration can be obtained daily. It should be reiterated that it typically takes 3 to 5 days to fully replete total-body magnesium stores. Patients receiving oral magnesium-containing antacids or supplements should be asked regularly about the occurrence of diarrhea.

Clinical Bottom Line

Hypomagnesemia is generally associated with kidney or GI tract disorders. In cases of mild, chronic magnesium loss, oral magnesium preparations can be used; however, the dose-limiting side effect is diarrhea. For more severe cases of hypomagnesemia, IV magnesium sulfate can be safely administered. Repeated doses may be needed as IV magnesium is rapidly eliminated in urine. In such cases, close monitoring of serum magnesium concentrations is needed.

HYPERMAGNESEMIA

Epidemiology

6 Hypermagnesemia (serum magnesium greater than 2 mEq/L [greater than 2.4 mg/dL; greater than 1 mmol/L]) is a rare occurrence that is generally seen in patients with stage 4 or 5 CKD when magnesium intake exceeds the excretory capacity of the kidneys. Elderly patients are prone to hypermagnesemia because of their reduced glomerular filtration rate (GFR) and because of their tendency to consume magnesium-containing antacids and vitamins.

Etiology and Pathophysiology

Because magnesium excretion decreases as GFR declines, serum magnesium concentrations tend to increase in patients with moderate to severe CKD. Indeed, magnesium concentrations steadily increase as the GFR decreases below 30 mL/min/1.73 m^2. As long as the patient maintains a normal diet, the serum magnesium concentration typically stabilizes at approximately 2.5 mEq/L (3 mg/dL [1.25 mmol/L]). If patients with stage 4 or 5 CKD are taking concomitant magnesium-containing antacids, the serum concentration can approach 6 mEq/L (7.3 mg/dL [3 mmol/L]), a value associated with signs and symptoms of toxicity. Critically ill patients with multiorgan system failure receiving enteral or parenteral nutrition are also prone to develop hypermagnesemia. Finally, the parenteral treatment of eclampsia with magnesium sulfate can lead to hypermagnesemia. Table 51-8 lists other causes of hypermagnesemia.

TABLE 51-8 Causes of Hypermagnesemia

Decreased renal excretion
Acute renal failure
CKD with exogenous intake
Excessive intake
Treatment of toxemia of pregnancy
Ureteral irrigants (hemiacidrin)
Cathartics
Other
Lithium therapy
Hypothyroidism
Milk-alkali syndrome
Addison disease
Viral hepatitis
Acute diabetic ketoacidosis

CKD, chronic kidney disease.

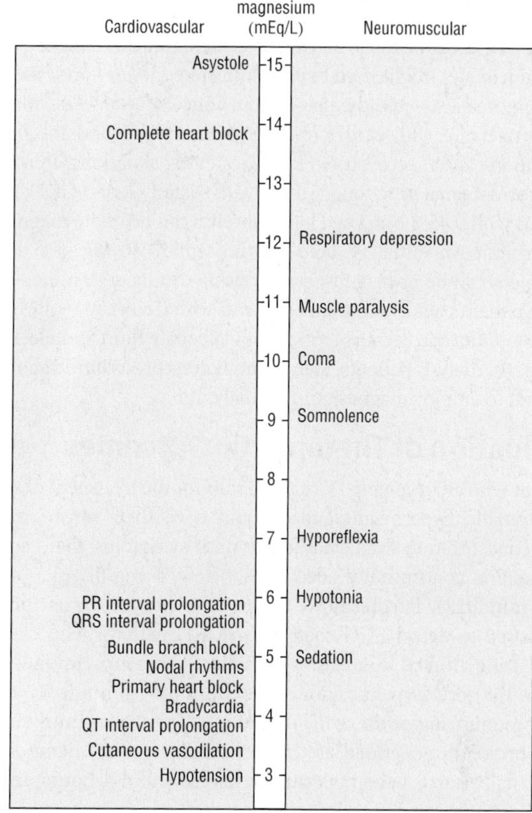

FIGURE 51-3 Clinical findings associated with hypermagnesemia. (Serum magnesium levels in mmol/L can be determined by multiplying the serum magnesium value expressed in mEq/L by 0.5.)

Clinical Presentation

7 The signs and symptoms of hypermagnesemia reflect magnesium's action on the neuromuscular and cardiovascular systems.[50,53] The main symptoms include lethargy, confusion, dysrhythmias, and muscle weakness. Symptoms are rare when the serum concentration is below 4 mEq/L (4.9 mg/dL [2 mmol/L]) (Fig. 51-3).

TREATMENT

Desired Outcome

The goals of therapy are to (a) reverse the neuromuscular and cardiovascular manifestations of hypermagnesemia, (b) decrease the magnesium concentration toward normal values, and (c) identify and treat the underlying cause of hypermagnesemia.

Nonpharmacologic Therapy

There are currently no nonpharmacologic options for the management of hypermagnesemia.

Pharmacologic Therapy

There are three primary means of treating hypermagnesemia: (a) reduce magnesium intake, (b) enhance elimination of magnesium, and (c) antagonize the physiologic effects of magnesium. The optimal treatment regimen for the management of hypermagnesemia depends on the severity of the patient's signs and symptoms and the degree of serum concentration elevation. IV elemental calcium doses of 100 to 200 mg directly antagonize the neuromuscular and cardiovascular effects of hypermagnesemia. Oral calcium is not effective because of its relatively poor bioavailability and slow onset of action. The clinical effect of calcium is immediate, but the effect is transient; hence, repeated IV doses of 100 to 200 mg of elemental calcium (eg, 2 g of calcium gluconate) might need to be administered hourly until the signs or symptoms abate and the magnesium concentration is normalized. Supportive care with cardiac pacing, vasopressors, and mechanical ventilation can be necessary in life-threatening situations. In patients with normal renal function, or those with stage 1, 2, or 3 CKD, forced diuresis with 0.45% NaCl and loop diuretics can promote magnesium elimination. An initial IV bolus of furosemide 40 mg or a similar equivalent can be used. Subsequent dosing can be determined based on the patient's clinical response. Patients with CKD can require long-term loop diuretic therapy to maintain adequate fluid and electrolyte balance. In dialysis patients, their hemodialysis prescription should be changed to employ magnesium-free dialysate.

Evaluation of Therapeutic Outcomes

Patients who are receiving IV calcium salts for the treatment of severe, symptomatic hypermagnesemia should have their serum magnesium concentration evaluated hourly until symptoms abate and the magnesium concentration decreases below 4 mg/dL (3.3 mEq/L [1.64 mmol/L]). Furthermore, the patient should be continuously monitored to detect ECG changes. In CKD patients who can produce urine, forced diuresis with saline and furosemide should reduce the serum magnesium concentration within 6 to 12 hours. Close monitoring of the urine output and physical examination for signs of volume overload are important. Emergency hemodialysis will usually correct the hypermagnesemia within 4 hours and is a reasonable option for those who are currently receiving hemodialysis. To prevent further episodes of hypermagnesemia, the patient should receive dietary education regarding foods and beverages that contain large quantities of magnesium (Table 51-9).

TABLE 51-9 Magnesium Content of Selected Foods

Food	Elemental Magnesium Content per Serving (mg)
Halibut, cooked, 3 oz (85g)	90
Almonds, dry roasted, 1 oz (28g)	80
Spinach, boiled, one-half cup (~125mL)	78
Cashews, dry roasted, 1 oz (28g)	74
Peanuts, oil roasted, one-fourth cup (~60 mL)	63
Shredded wheat cereal, two large biscuits	61
Soymilk, plain or vanilla, 1 cup (~250mL)	61
Black beans, cooked, one-half cup (~125mL)	60
Edamame, shelled, cooked, one-half cup (~125mL)	50
Peanuts, dry roasted, 1 oz (28g)	50
Peanut butter, smooth, 2 tablespoons (~30 mL)	49
Bread, whole wheat, 2 slices	46
Avocado, cubed, 1 cup (~250mL)	44
Potato, baked with skin, 3.5 oz (~100g)	43
Yogurt, plain, low fat, 8 oz (~225g)	42
Rice, brown, cooked, one-half cup (~125 mL)	42
Breakfast cereals, fortified with 10% of the daily value for magnesium	40
Instant oatmeal, 1 cup (~250 mL)	36
Kidney beans, canned, one-half cup (~125 mL)	35
Banana, 1 medium	32

Clinical Bottom Line

Hypermagnesemia is generally associated with advanced CKD. Severe cases of hypermagnesemia can result in neurologic symptoms or cardiac dysrhythmias. Should these symptoms occur, IV calcium can counteract these effects. Forced diuresis with saline and loop diuretics is useful in lowering magnesium in patients with mild to moderate renal dysfunction; hemodialysis should be reserved for ESRD patients.

PERSONALIZED PHARMACOTHERAPY

As discussed throughout the chapter, there are numerous patient considerations that must be taken into account when designing appropriate pharmacotherapy for potassium and magnesium disorders. At this time, there are no genetic, genomic, or pharmacokinetic factors that are used to personalize pharmacotherapy for the treatment of these electrolyte disorders.

ABBREVIATIONS

ACEI	angiotensin-converting enzyme inhibitor
AKI	acute kidney injury
ARB	angiotensin-II receptor blocker
CKD	chronic kidney disease
ECG	electrocardiogram
ESRD	end-stage renal disease
FDA	Food and Drug Administration
GFR	glomerular filtration rate
GI	gastrointestinal
IM	intramuscular
IV	intravenous
NSAID	nonsteroidal anti-inflammatory drug
RAAS	renin–angiotensin–aldosterone system
SPS	sodium polystyrene sulfonate

REFERENCES

1. Palmer BF, Dubose TD. Disorders of potassium metabolism. In: Schrier RW, ed. *Renal and Electrolyte Disorders*, 7th ed. Philadelphia, PA: Lippincott Williams & Wilkins, 2010;137-165.
2. Pepin J, Shields C. Advances in diagnosis and management of hypokalemic and hyperkalemic emergencies. *Emerg Med Pract* 2012;14(2):1-20.
3. D'Elia L, Barba G, Cappuccio FP, Strazzullo P. Potassium intake, stroke, and cardiovascular disease: A meta-analysis of prospective studies. *J Am Coll Cardiol* 2011;57:1210-1219.
4. Whelton PK, He J, Appel LJ, et al. Primary prevention of hypertension: Clinical and public health advisory from the National High Blood Pressure Education Program. *JAMA* 2002;288:1882-1888.
5. Food and Nutrition Board, Institute of Medicine. *Panel on Dietary Reference Intakes for Electrolytes and Water. Dietary Reference Intakes for Water, Potassium, Sodium, Chloride, and Sulfate*. Washington, DC: National Academies Press; 2005.
6. Gumz ML, Rabinowitz L, Wingo CS. An integrated view of potassium homeostasis. *N Engl J Med* 2015;373:60-72.
7. Palmer BF. Regulation of potassium homeostasis. *Clin J Am Soc Nephrol* 2015;10:1050-1060.
8. U.S. Department of Agriculture and U.S. Department of Health and Human Services. *Dietary guidelines for Americans, 2010*. 7th ed. Washington, DC: U.S. Government Printing Office; December 2010.
9. Malnic G, Giebisch G, Muto S, Wang W, Bailey MA, Satlin LM. Regulation of K^+ excretion. In: Alpern RJ, Moe OW, eds. *Seldin and Giebisch's the Kidney*, 5th ed. Amsterdam: Elsevier; 2013;1659-1715.
10. Aronson PS, Giebisch G. Effects of pH on potassium: new explanations for old observations. *J Am Soc Nephrol* 2011;22:1981-1989.
11. Adrogue HJ, Madias NE. Sodium and potassium in the pathogenesis of hypertension. *N Engl J Med* 2007;356:1966-1978.

12. Bowling CB, Pitt B, Ahmed MI, et al. Hypokalemia and outcomes in patients with chronic heart failure and chronic kidney disease. *Circ Heart Fail* 2010;3:253-260.
13. Korgaonkar S, Tilea A, Gillespie BW, et al. Serum potassium and outcomes in CKD: Insights from the RRI CKD cohort study. *J Am Soc Nephrol* 2010;5:762-769.
14. Van Dinter TG, Fuerst FC, Richardson CT, et al. Stimulated active potassium secretion in a patient with colonic pseudo-obstruction: A new mechanism of secretory diarrhea. *Gastroenterol* 2005;129:1268-1273.
15. Gennari FJ. Hypokalemia. *N Engl J Med* 1998;339:451-458.
16. Huang CL, Kuo E. Mechanism of hypokalemia in magnesium deficiency. *J Am Soc Nephrol* 2007;18:2649-2652.
17. Cohn JN, Kowey PR, Whelton PK, Prisant LM. New guidelines for potassium replacement in clinical practice: A contemporary review by the National Council on Potassium in Clinical Practice. *Arch Intern Med* 2000;160:2429-2436.
18. 2005 American Heart Association Guidelines for Cardiopulmonary Resuscitation and Emergency Cardiovascular Care. Part 10.1. Life threatening emergencies. *Circulation* 2005;112:IV-121-IV-125.
19. Nyirenda MJ, Tang JI, Padfield PL, Seckl JR. Hyperkalemia. *Br Med J* 2009;339:b4114.
20. Schaefer TJ, Wolford RW. Disorders of Potassium. *Emerg Med Clin N Am* 2005;23:723-747.
21. Chmielewski CM. Hyperkalemic emergencies: Mechanisms, manifestations and management. *Crit Care Nurs Clin North Am* 1998;10:449-458.
22. Gennari FJ, Segal AS. Hyperkalemia: An adaptive response in chronic renal insufficiency. *Kidney Int* 2002;62:1-9.
23. Einhorn LA, Zhan M, Hsu VD, et al. The frequency of hyperkalemia and its significance in chronic kidney disease. *Arch Int Med* 2009;169:1156-1162.
24. Packer M, Poole-Wilson PA, Armstrong PE, et al. Comparative effects of low and high doses of the angiotensin-converting enzyme inhibitor, lisinopril, on morbidity and mortality in chronic heart failure. *Circulation* 1999;100:2312-2318.
25. Pfeffer MA, Swedberg K, Granger CB, et al. Effects of candesartan on mortality and morbidigy in patients with chronic heart failure: the CHARM-Overall programme. *Lancet* 2003;759-766.
26. Zannad F, McMurray JJV, Krum H, et al. Eplerenone in patients with systolic heart failure and mild symptoms. *N Engl J Med* 2011;364:11-21.
27. Weisberg LS. Management of severe hyperkalemia. *Crit Care Med* 2008;36:3246-3251.
28. Farese S, Jruse A, Pasch A, et al. Glycyrrhetinic acid food supplementation lowers serum potassium concentration in chronic hemodialysis patients. *Kidney Int* 2009;76:877-884.
29. Ferrari P. Licorice: A sweet alternative to prevent hyperkalemia in dialysis patients? *Kidney Int* 2009;76:811-812.
30. McGowan CE, Saha S, Chu G, et al. Intestinal necrosis due to sodium polystyrene sulfonate (Kayexalate) in sorbitol. *South Med J* 2009;102:493-497.
31. Sterns RH, Rojas M, Bernstein P, Chennupati S. Ion-exchange resin for the treatment of hyperkalemia: Are they safe and effective? *J Am Soc Nephrol* 2010;21:733-735.
32. Kayexalate (Sodium Polystyrene Sulfonate) Powder Boxed Warning. 2012, http://www.fda.gov/Safety/MedWatch/SafetyInformation/ucm186845.htm.
33. Watson M, Abbott KC, Yuan CM. Damned if you do, damned if you don't: Potassium binding resins in hyperkalemia. *Clin J Am Soc Nephrol* 2010;5:1723-1726.
34. Kayexalate (Sodium Polystyrene Sulfonate): Drug Safety Communication. 2015. http://www.fda.gov/Safety/MedWatch/SafetyInformation/SafetyAlertsforHumanMedicalProducts/ucm468720.htm.
35. Mahoney BA, Smith WAD, Lo DS, et al. Emergency interventions for hyperkalemia. Cochrane Database Syst Rev 2005;18:CD003235.
36. Fordjour KN, Walton T, Doran JJ. Management of hyperkalemia in hospitalized patients. *Am J Med Sci* 2014;347:93-100.
37. Phillips CO, Kashani A, Ko DK, Francis G, Krumholz HM. Adverse effects of combination angiotensin II receptor blockers plus angiotensin-converting enzyme inhibitors for left ventricular dysfunction. *Arch Intern Med* 2007;167:1930-1936.
38. Van Buren PN, Adams-Huet B, Nguyen M, Molina C, Toto RD. Potassium handling with dual renin-angiotensin system inhibition in diabetic nephropathy. *Clin J Am Soc Nephorl* 2014;9:295-301.
39. Weir MR, Bakris GL, Bushinsky DA, et al. Patiromer in patients with kidney disease and hyperkalemia receiving RAAS inhibitors. *N Engl J Med* 2015;372:211-221.
40. Bakris GL, Pitt B, Weir MR, et al. Effect of patiromer on serum potassium level in patients with hyperkalemia and diabetic kidney disease; The AMETHYST-DN randomized clinical trial. *J Am Med Assoc* 2015;314:151-161.
41. Veltassa™ [package insert]. Redwood City, CA: Relypsa, Inc; 2015.
42. Packham DK, Rasmussen HS, Lavin PT, et al. Sodium zirconium cyclosilicate in hyperkalemia. *N Engl J Med* 2015;372:222-231.
43. Kosiborod M, Rasmussen HS, Lavin P, et al. Effect of sodium zirconium cyclosilicate on potassium lowering for 28 days among outpatients with hyperkalemia; The HARMONIZE randomized clinical trial. *J Am Med Assoc* 2014;12:2223-2233.
44. Spiegel DM. Normal and abnormal magnesium metabolism. In: Schrier RW, ed. *Renal and Electrolyte Disorders*, 7th ed. Philadelphia, PA: Lippincott Williams & Wilkins; 2010;229-250.
45. Musso CG. Magnesium metabolism in health and disease. *Int Urol Nephrol* 2009;41:357-362.
46. Blaine J, Chonchol M, Levi M. Renal control of calcium, phosphate, and magnesium homeostasis. *Clin J Am Soc Nephrol* 2015;10:1257-1272.
47. Wolf F, Hilewitz A. Hypomagnesaemia in patients hospitalised in internal medicine is associated with increased mortality. *Int J Clin Pract* 2014;68:111-116.
48. Martin KJ, Gonzalez EA, Slatopolsky E. Clinical consequences and management of hypomagnesemia. *J Am Soc Nephrol* 2009;20:2291-2295.
49. Atsmon J, Dolev E. Drug-induced hypomagnesaemia. *Drug Saf* 2005;28:763-788.
50. Ayuk J, Gittoes NJL. Treatment of hypomagnesemia. *Am J Kidney Dis* 2014;63(4):691-695.
51. Rodriguez-Moran M Guerrero-Romero F. Oral magnesium supplementation improves insulin sensitivity and metabolic control in type 2 diabetes subjects. *Diabetes Care* 2003;26:1147-1152.
52. Pham PCT, Pham PMT, Pham SV, Miller JM, Pham PTT. Hypomagnesemia in patients with type 2 diabetes. *Clin J As Soc Nephrol* 2007;2:366-373.
53. Jahnen-Dechent W, Ketteler M. Magnesium basics. *Clin Kidney J* 2012;5[Suppl 1]:i3-i14.

Acid–Base Disorders

John W. Devlin and Gary R. Matzke

52

KEY CONCEPTS

1 The kidney plays a central role in the regulation of acid–base homeostasis through the excretion or reabsorption of filtered bicarbonate (HCO_3^-), the excretion of metabolic fixed acids, and the generation of new HCO_3^-.

2 Arterial blood gases (ABGs), along with serum electrolytes, physical findings, medical and medication history, and the clinical condition of the patient, are the primary tools to determine the cause of an acid–base disorder and to design and monitor a course of therapy.

3 Each acid-base disturbance has a compensatory response that attempts to correct the HCO_3^--to-$PaCO_2$ ratio toward normal and mitigate the change in pH. The respiratory compensatory response to metabolic disturbances is initiated rapidly whereas the metabolic compensatory response to respiratory disturbances occurs more slowly.

4 Metabolic acidosis and metabolic alkalosis are generated by a primary change in the serum bicarbonate concentration. In metabolic acidosis, bicarbonate is lost or a nonvolatile acid is gained, whereas metabolic alkalosis is characterized by a gain in bicarbonate or a loss of nonvolatile acid.

5 Renal tubular acidosis (RTA) refers to a group of disorders characterized by impaired tubular renal acid handling despite normal or near-normal glomerular filtration rates. These patients often present with hyperchloremic metabolic acidosis.

6 Although respiratory compensation for a primary metabolic acidosis begins rapidly (within 15-30 minutes) it does not reach a steady state for 12 to 24 hours after the onset of metabolic acidosis.

7 Primary therapy of most acid–base disorders must include treatment or removal of the underlying cause, not just correction of the pH and electrolyte disturbances.

8 Potassium supplementation is always necessary for patients with chronic metabolic acidosis, as the bicarbonaturia resulting from alkali therapy increases renal potassium wasting.

9 Effective treatment of the underlying cause of some organic acidoses (eg, ketoacidosis) can result in bicarbonate regeneration within hours thus mitigating the need for alkali therapy.

10 Loss of gastric acid from vomiting or nasogastric suctioning may lead to hypochloremia and hyperbicarbonatemia and may often lead to a metabolic alkalosis.

11 Aggressive diuretic therapy can produce a metabolic alkalosis, and the accompanying hypokalemia can be serious.

12 A patient's response to volume replacement can be predicted by the urine chloride concentration and permits the differential diagnosis of metabolic alkalosis.

13 Management of these disorders usually consists of treatment of the underlying cause of mineralocorticoid excess. In patients in whom the mineralocorticoid excess cannot be corrected, chronic pharmacologic therapy can be required.

14 In most cases of acute metabolic acidosis, such as following cardiopulmonary arrest, sodium bicarbonate therapy is not indicated and can be detrimental. Blood gas analysis should guide therapy.

INTRODUCTION

Acid–base disorders are common and often serious disturbances that can result in significant morbidity and mortality. This chapter reviews the mechanisms responsible for the maintenance of acid–base balance and the laboratory analyses that aid clinicians in their assessment of acid–base disorders. The pathophysiology of the four primary acid–base disturbances is presented, evidence-based therapeutic options are reviewed, and management guidelines to optimize the outcome of patients with one of these disorders are presented. Given that medications are a frequent cause of acid–base abnormalities and that acid–base abnormalities are often preventable, clinicians must anticipate drug-related problems to avoid or minimize the clinical consequences of acid–base disorders, and when necessary, design appropriate treatment regimens.

ACID–BASE CHEMISTRY

An acid (in this equation, hydrochloric acid) is a substance that can *donate* protons (hydrogen ion [H^+]):

$$\text{(Acid) HCl} \rightarrow H^+ + \text{Chloride ion (Cl)}$$

A base (in this equation, ammonia [NH_3]) is a substance that can *accept* protons (hydrogen ion [H^+]):

$$\text{Ammonia } (NH_3) + H^+ \rightarrow NH^+_4 \text{ (base)}$$

The acid–base pairs commonly encountered in clinical practice are listed in Table 52-1.

The acidity of body fluids is quantified in terms of the hydrogen ion concentration. By convention, the degree of acidity is expressed as pH, or the negative logarithm (base 10) of the hydrogen ion concentration. Thus, hydrogen ion concentration and pH are inversely related. Normally, the pH of blood is maintained at 7.40 ([H^+] of 4×10^{-8} M) with a range of 7.35 to 7.45. A pH of less than 6.7 ([H^+] of 2×10^{-7} M), representing a fivefold increase in hydrogen ion concentration, or greater than 7.7 ([H^+] of 2×10^{-8} M), representing a 50% decrease in hydrogen ion concentration, is considered incompatible with life.

The hydrogen ion concentration in blood may not be indicative of that in other body compartments. For example, the pH within cells, within the cerebrospinal fluid, or on the surface of bone can all be altered without causing an alteration in blood pH.[1] Recognizing this caveat, the acid–base status of the body is usually analyzed based

TABLE 52-1 Acid–Base Pairs

Carbonic acid/bicarbonate	H_2CO_3/HCO_3^-
Monobasic/dibasic phosphate	H_2PO_4/HPO_4^-
Ammonium/ammonia	NH_4^+/NH_3
Lactic acid/lactate	$H_6C_3O_2/H_5C_3O_2^-$

on measurement of blood pH. Alterations in blood pH serve as the basis for the diagnosis of acid–base disorders.

Because the dissociation of acid–base pairs is an equilibrium reaction, the relationship between hydrogen ion concentration or pH and the relative concentrations of the acid and base can be described mathematically in terms of the dissociation constant for the acid–base buffer pair. When expressed as a logarithmic relationship, where p*K* is the negative logarithm of the dissociation constant *K*, this is known as the Henderson–Hasselbalch equation:

$$pH = pK + \log([base]/[acid])$$

BUFFERS

The ability of a weak acid and its corresponding anion (base) to resist change in the pH of a solution with the addition of a strong acid or base is referred to as *buffering*. An acid–base pair is most efficient in functioning as a buffer at a pH close to its p*K*. The principal extracellular buffer is the carbonic acid/bicarbonate (H_2CO_3/HCO_3^-) system. Other physiologic buffers include plasma proteins, hemoglobin, and phosphates. Because the isohydric principle requires that all buffer systems remain in chemical equilibrium, the complex buffering of biologic fluids can be analyzed based on a single buffer pair.

The carbonic acid/bicarbonate buffer system plays a unique role in acid–base homeostasis. In addition to being the most abundant extracellular buffer, the components of this buffer pair exist under dynamic regulation by the body. In the presence of carbonic anhydrase, carbonic acid, [H_2CO_3], is in equilibrium with carbon dioxide (CO_2) gas. Changes in ventilation that alter the partial pressure of CO_2 (PCO_2) in the blood regulate the carbonic acid level in the blood. The bicarbonate concentration is independently regulated by the kidney. Because the p*K* for the carbonic acid/bicarbonate system is 6.1, the relationship between pH, carbonic acid, and bicarbonate concentrations can be described by the Henderson–Hasselbalch equation. The concentration of carbonic acid is directly proportional to the amount of CO_2 dissolved in blood, which is equal to the product of PCO_2 and its solubility in physiologic fluids ($PCO_2 \times 0.03$ for PCO_2 expressed in mm Hg or $PCO_2 \times 0.226$ for PCO_2 expressed in kPa). This term can, therefore, be substituted into the equation below in place of [H_2CO_3].

$$pH = 6.1 + ([HCO_3^-]/[H_2CO_3])$$

$$pH = 6.1 + \log([HCO_3^-]/[PCO_2 \times 0.03]) \text{ for } PCO_2 \text{ in mm Hg}$$

or

$$pH = 6.1 + \log([HCO_3^-]/[PCO_2 \times 0.226]) \text{ for } PCO_2 \text{ in kPa}$$

Thus, hydrogen ion concentration and pH are determined not by the absolute amounts of bicarbonate and PCO_2 present but by their ratio.[1] Under normal physiologic conditions, the kidneys maintain the serum bicarbonate at approximately 24 mEq/L (mmol/L), whereas the lungs maintain the PCO_2 at approximately 40 mm Hg (5.3 kPa). The normal physiologic pH is thus 7.4:

$$pH = 6.1 + \log[24/(0.03 \times 40)] \text{ (or } pH = 6.1 + \log[24/(0.226 \times 5.3)])$$

$$pH = 6.1 + 1.3 = 7.4$$

If, in response to an acid load, the serum bicarbonate concentration were to decrease to 12 mEq/L (mmol/L), the predicted pH would be:

$$[HCO_3^-] = 12 \text{ mEq/L (mmol/L)}$$

$$PCO_2 = 40 \text{ mm Hg (5.3 kPa)}$$

$$pH = 6.1 + \log[12/0.03 \times 40] \text{ or}$$

$$pH = 6.1 + \log[12/(0.226 \times 5.3)]$$

$$pH = 6.1 + 1.0 = 7.1$$

However, the normal respiratory response to an acid load is hyperventilation. As a result, if the PCO_2 decreased to approximately 26 mm Hg (3.5 kPa), the change in pH would be less:

$$[HCO_3^-] = 12 \text{ mEq/L (mmol/L)}$$

$$PCO_2 = 26 \text{ mm Hg (3.5 kPa)}$$

$$pH = 6.1 + \log[12/0.03 \times 26]$$

$$\text{(or } pH = 6.1 + \log[12/(0.226 \times 3.5)])$$

$$pH = 6.1 + 1.19 = 7.29$$

Thus, the physiologic regulation of both PCO_2 and [HCO_3^-] permits the carbonic acid/bicarbonate system to provide more effective buffering of the extracellular fluids (ECFs) than could be achieved on the basis of chemical buffering alone.

REGULATION OF ACID–BASE HOMEOSTASIS

Cellular metabolism results in the production of large quantities of hydrogen that need to be excreted to maintain acid–base balance. In addition, small amounts of acid and alkali are also presented to the body through the diet. The bulk of acid production is in the form of CO_2, with the average adult producing approximately 15,000 mmol of CO_2 each day from the catabolism of carbohydrate, protein, and fat.[2] When respiratory function is normal, the amount of CO_2 produced metabolically is equal to the amount lost by respiration, and the blood CO_2 concentration remains constant.

Digestion of dietary substances and tissue metabolism also result in the production of nonvolatile acids. These acids are derived primarily from the sulfur-containing amino acids cysteine and methionine, as well as from ingested sulfur. In addition, phosphates are generated from the metabolism of proteins and phospholipids. Neutral substances such as glucose can also be incompletely metabolized to intermediates, such as lactic and pyruvic acid, and fatty acids can be incompletely metabolized to acetoacetic acid and β-hydroxybutyric acid. These dietary and metabolic fixed acids are excreted primarily by the kidney to maintain acid–base homeostasis. On average, daily fixed acid excretion is approximately 0.8 mEq/kg per day (mmol/kg per day).[3]

Three processes, each of which varies in its onset, collectively maintain acid–base balance: extracellular buffering, ventilatory regulation of carbon dioxide elimination, and renal regulation of hydrogen ion and bicarbonate excretion. Extracellular buffering occurs rapidly and is the body's first defense against a sudden increase in hydrogen ion concentration. Hyperventilation then results in a decrease in PCO_2, returning blood pH toward normal. Finally, over a period of day(s), the kidney will excrete the excess hydrogen ion and acid–base balance will return to normal.

Extracellular Buffering

The body's buffering system can be divided into three components: bicarbonate/carbonic acid, proteins, and phosphates. The bicarbonate buffer is the most important of the body's buffers, because: (a) there is more bicarbonate present in the ECF than any other buffer component; (b) the supply of CO_2 is unlimited; and (c) the acidity of ECF can be regulated by controlling either the bicarbonate concentration or the PCO_2.

Carbonic acid represents the respiratory component of the buffer pair because its blood concentration is directly proportional to the PCO_2, which is determined by ventilation. Bicarbonate represents the metabolic component because the kidney may alter its concentration by reabsorption, generating new bicarbonate, or altering elimination.[1] The bicarbonate buffer system easily adapts to changes in acid–base status by alterations in ventilatory elimination of acid (PCO_2) and/or renal elimination of base (HCO_3^-).

The phosphate buffer system consists of serum inorganic phosphate (3.5-5 mg/dL [1.13-1.62 mmol/L]), intracellular organic phosphate, and calcium phosphate in bone. Extracellular phosphate is present only in low concentrations, so its usefulness as a buffer is limited; however, as an intracellular buffer, phosphate is more useful. Calcium phosphate in bone is relatively inaccessible as a buffer, but prolonged metabolic acidosis will result in the release of phosphate from bone.

Intracellular and extracellular proteins also act as buffering systems. The charged side chains of amino acids provide the buffering action. Because the concentration of protein is much greater intracellularly than extracellularly, protein is much more important as an intracellular buffer.

Respiratory Regulation

The second process involved in maintenance of acid–base homeostasis is ventilatory regulation of CO_2 elimination. Both the rate and depth of ventilation can be varied to allow for excretion of CO_2 generated by diet and tissue metabolism. Medullary chemoreceptors in the brainstem sense changes in PCO_2 and pH and modulate the control of breathing. Increasing minute ventilation (the total amount of air exhaled over a 1-minute period), by increasing respiratory rate and/or tidal volume (the amount of air exhaled in one breath), will increase CO_2 excretion and decrease the blood PCO_2. Conversely, decreasing minute ventilation decreases CO_2 excretion and increases blood PCO_2. This system rapidly adjusts within minutes to changes in acid–base balance.[1]

Renal Regulation

1 Bicarbonate is freely filtered at the glomerulus because it is a small ion. The bicarbonate load delivered to the nephron is approximately 4,500 mEq/day (mmol/day). To maintain acid–base balance, this entire filtered bicarbonate load must be reabsorbed. Bicarbonate reabsorption occurs primarily in the proximal tubule (Fig. 52-1). In the tubular lumen, filtered bicarbonate combines with hydrogen ion, secreted by the apical sodium ion (Na^+)–H^+-exchanger, to form carbonic acid. The carbonic acid is rapidly broken down to CO_2 and water by carbonic anhydrase, an enzyme located on the luminal surface of the brush border membrane. The CO_2 then diffuses into the proximal tubular cell, where it reforms carbonic acid in the presence of intracellular carbonic anhydrase. The carbonic acid dissociates to form hydrogen ions that can again be secreted into the tubular lumen, and bicarbonate that exits the cell across the basolateral membrane and enters the peritubular capillary.

Excretion of metabolic fixed acids and generation of new HCO_3^- is achieved in nearly equal parts by renal ammoniagenesis and distal tubular hydrogen ion secretion. Ammoniagenesis plays a critical role in acid-base homeostasis, with ammonium (NH_4^+) excretion comprising approximately 50% of renal net acid excretion. Ammonium is generated from the deamination of glutamine in the proximal tubule. For each ammonium ion excreted in the urine, one bicarbonate ion is regenerated and returned to the circulation.[3]

Distal tubular hydrogen ion secretion accounts for the remaining 50% of net acid excretion (Fig. 52-2). In the distal tubular cell, CO_2 combines with water in the presence of intracellular carbonic anhydrase to form carbonic acid, which dissociates to H^+ and HCO_3^-. The H^+ is actively transported into the tubular lumen by a H^+–adenosine triphosphatase (ATPase). The bicarbonate exits the cell across the basolateral membrane and enters the circulation.[1]

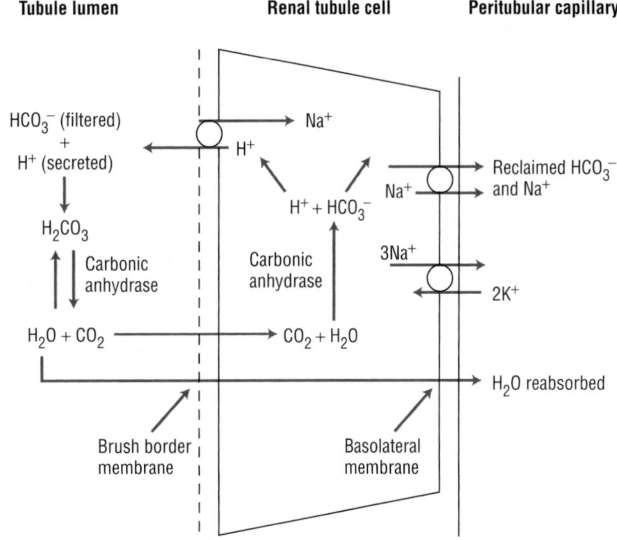

FIGURE 52-1 Proximal tubular bicarbonate reabsorption. In the tubular lumen, filtered bicarbonate (HCO_3^-) combines with hydrogen ion (H^+) secreted by an apical sodium ion (Na^+)–H^+ exchanger to form carbonic acid (H_2CO_3). The carbonic acid is rapidly broken down to carbon dioxide (CO_2) and water by carbonic anhydrase located on the luminal surface of the brush border membrane. The CO_2 then diffuses into the proximal tubular cell, where it reforms carbonic acid in the presence of intracellular carbonic anhydrase. The carbonic acid dissociates the former hydrogen ion that can again be secreted into the tubular lumen, and bicarbonate that exits the cell across the basolateral membrane and enters the peritubular capillary.

ACID–BASE DISTURBANCES

2 Alterations in blood pH are designated by the suffix "-emia"; *acidemia* is an arterial blood pH less than 7.35 and *alkalemia* is an arterial blood pH more than 7.45. The pathophysiologic processes

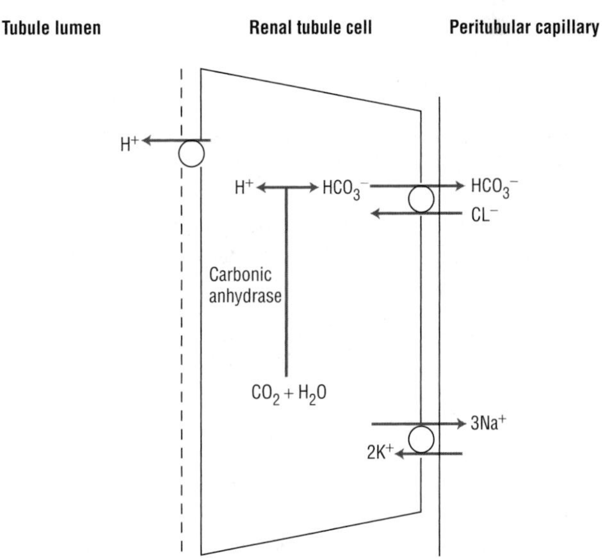

FIGURE 52-2 Collecting duct acid excretion. Hydrogen ion (H^+) and bicarbonate (HCO_3^-) are generated intracellularly from carbon dioxide (CO_2) and water, in the presence of intracellular carbonic anhydrase. The hydrogen ion is actively secreted into the tubular lumen by H^+–ATPase located in the apical (luminal) membrane. Bicarbonate exits the cell across the basolateral membrane and enters the peritubular capillary. (Cl^-, chloride ion; Na^+, sodium ion.)

TABLE 52-2 Interpretation of Simple Acid–Base Disorders

Acid–Base Disorder	pH	Primary Disturbances	Compensation
Acidosis			
Respiratory	Decrease	Increase $PaCO_2$	Increase HCO_3^-
Metabolic	Decrease	Decrease HCO_3^-	Decrease $PaCO_2$
Alkalosis			
Respiratory	Increase	Decrease $PaCO_2$	Decrease HCO_3^-
Metabolic	Increase	Increase HCO_3^-	Increase $PaCO_2$

HCO_3^-, bicarbonate; $PaCO_2$, partial pressure of carbon dioxide from arterial blood.

TABLE 52-3 Normal Blood Gas Values

	Arterial Blood	Mixed Venous Blood
pH	7.40 (7.35-7.45)	7.38 (7.33-7.43)
PO_2	80-100 mm Hg (10.6-13.3 kPa)	35-40 mm Hg (4.7-5.3 kPa)
SaO_2	95% (0.95)	70-75% (0.70-0.75)
PCO_2	35-45 mm Hg (4.7-6.0 kPa)	45-51 mm Hg (6.0-6.8 kPa)
HCO_3^-	22-26 mEq/L (mmol/L)	24-28 mEq/L (mmol/L)

HCO_3^-, bicarbonate; PCO_2, partial pressure of carbon dioxide; PO_2, partial pressure of oxygen; SaO_2, saturation of arterial oxygen.

that result in alterations in blood pH are designated by the suffix "-osis." These disturbances are classified as either metabolic or respiratory in origin. In metabolic acid–base disorders, the primary disturbance is in the plasma bicarbonate concentration. Metabolic acidosis is characterized by a decrease in the plasma bicarbonate concentration whereas in metabolic alkalosis the plasma bicarbonate concentration is increased. Respiratory acid–base disorders are caused by alterations in alveolar ventilation that produce corresponding changes in the partial pressure of carbon dioxide from arterial blood ($PaCO_2$). In respiratory acidosis, the $PaCO_2$ is elevated; in respiratory alkalosis, it is decreased. 3 Each disturbance has a compensatory (secondary) response that attempts to correct the HCO_3^--to-$PaCO_2$ ratio toward normal and mitigate the change in pH (Table 52-2). Although the time course of the respiratory compensatory response to metabolic disturbances is rapid, the metabolic compensation for respiratory disturbances is slow. As a result, respiratory disturbances are characterized as acute (minutes to hours in duration), indicating that there has not been sufficient time for metabolic compensation, or chronic (days), indicating that sufficient time for metabolic compensation has elapsed.

CLINICAL ASSESSMENT OF ACID–BASE STATUS

4 A blood gas is measured to determine not only a patient's acid–base status but also their oxygenation. Under normal circumstances, the pH difference between arterial and mixed venous blood is not clinically significant. However, the oxygenation difference between arterial and mixed venous blood is always substantial. Arterial samples are designated with the letter "a" (eg, partial pressure of oxygen from arterial blood [PaO_2] and $PaCO_2$), whereas mixed venous samples are labeled with the letter "v" or not labeled (eg, partial pressure of oxygen from venous blood [PvO_2] and partial pressure of carbon dioxide from venous blood [$PvCO_2$]). The normal values for arterial and venous blood gases are shown in Table 52-3. Arterial blood reflects how well the blood is being oxygenated by the lungs (an accurate measurement of PaO_2), whereas venous blood reflects how much oxygen tissues are using. Arterial blood rather than venous blood should be used whenever possible because venous blood obtained from an extremity can provide misleading information. If metabolism in the extremity is altered by hypoperfusion, exercise, infection, or some other cause, the difference in the amount of dissolved oxygen between arterial and venous blood can be dramatic. The venous pH and PCO_2 during cardiopulmonary resuscitation might be significantly lower and higher, respectively, than the arterial pH and arterial PCO_2. This indicates a severe tissue acidosis from CO_2 accumulation caused by hypoperfusion.

Analysis of Arterial Blood Gas Data

ABGs provide an assessment of the patient's acid–base status.[2,3] Low pH values (less than 7.35) indicate an acidemia, whereas high pH values (more than 7.45) indicate an alkalemia (Fig. 52-3). In a metabolic acidosis, the pH is decreased in association with a decreased serum bicarbonate concentration and a compensatory decrease in $PaCO_2$. In a respiratory acidosis while the pH is decreased, the $PaCO_2$ is elevated. The serum bicarbonate concentration is variable, depending on whether it is an acute disturbance (minimal increase in serum bicarbonate) or a chronic respiratory acidosis (substantial increase in serum bicarbonate). In a metabolic alkalosis, the pH is elevated in association with an increased bicarbonate concentration and a compensatory increase in $PaCO_2$. In a respiratory alkalosis, while the pH is also elevated, the $PaCO_2$ is decreased. As with respiratory acidosis, the metabolic compensation is variable: a minimal decrease in serum bicarbonate is often noted in acute respiratory alkalosis while a larger decrease in [HCO_3^-] is common with chronic respiratory alkalosis. Although each measurement has a normal range (see Table 52-3), it is often easiest to consider the midpoint of each range as the normal value. This would correlate to a pH of 7.4,

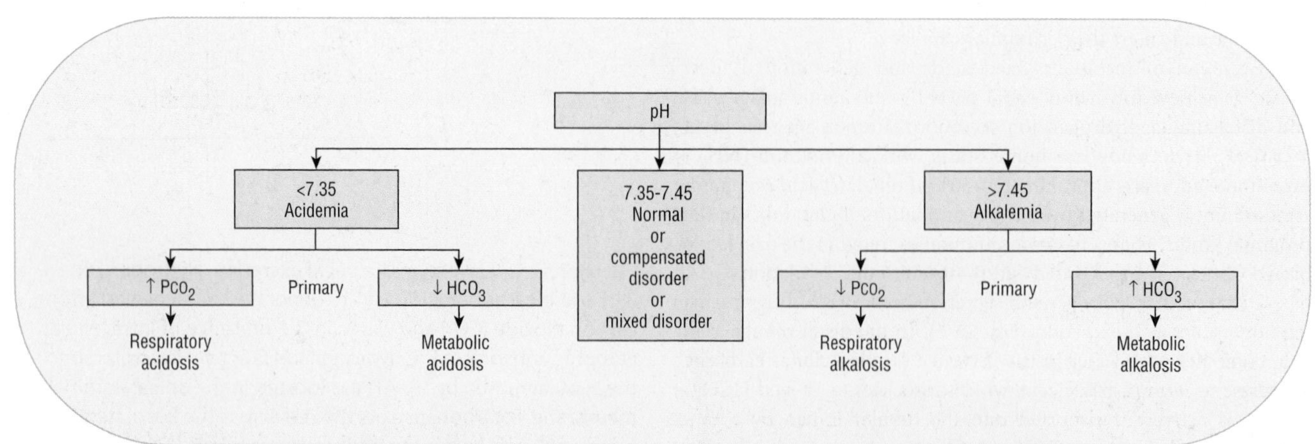

FIGURE 52-3 Analysis of arterial blood gases. (HCO_3^-, bicarbonate; PCO_2, partial pressure of carbon dioxide.)

TABLE 52-4 Steps in Acid–Base Diagnosis

1. Obtain ABGs and electrolytes simultaneously
2. Compare [HCO_3^-] on ABG and electrolytes to verify accuracy
3. Calculate SAG
4. Is acidemia (pH <7.35) or alkalemia (pH >7.45) present?
5. Is the primary abnormality respiratory (alteration in $PaCO_2$) or metabolic (alteration in HCO_3)?
6. Estimate compensatory response (Table 52-7)
7. Compare change in [Cl^-] with change in [Na^+]

[Cl^-], chloride ion; [HCO_3^-], bicarbonate; [Na^+], sodium ion; $PaCO_2$, partial pressure of carbon dioxide from arterial blood; SAG, serum anion gap.

$PaCO_2$ of 40 mm Hg (5.3 kPa), and HCO_3^- of 24 mEq/L (mmol/L). Steps in acid–base interpretation are described in Table 52-4.

When ABGs differ significantly from those expected on the basis of the patient's clinical condition and previous laboratory determinations, additional venous blood samples should be drawn to assess plasma electrolyte concentrations. The bicarbonate calculated from the patient's $PaCO_2$ and pH of the blood gas should be compared with the measured total CO_2 content (the amount of CO_2 gas extractable from plasma, consisting of HCO_3^-, H_2CO_3, and PCO_2). Ordinarily, the blood gas bicarbonate value is approximately 1 to 2 mEq/L (mmol/L) less than total CO_2 content.[3] If these values do not correspond, the results should be interpreted with caution because the difference can reflect an error in the blood collection or storage of the sample, or in the calibration of the blood gas analyzer.

METABOLIC ACID–BASE DISORDERS

Metabolic Acidosis

Metabolic acidosis is characterized by a decrease in pH as the result of a primary decrease in serum bicarbonate concentration.

Pathophysiology

Metabolic acidosis can result from the buffering (consumption of HCO_3^-) of an exogenous acid, an organic acid accumulating because of a metabolic disturbance (eg, lactic acid or ketoacids), or the progressive accumulation of endogenous acids secondary to impaired kidney function (eg, phosphates and sulfates).[4,5] The serum HCO_3^- can also be decreased as the result of a loss of bicarbonate-rich body fluids (eg, diarrhea, biliary drainage, or pancreatic fistula) or occur secondary to the rapid administration of non-alkali–containing IV fluids (dilutional acidosis).[4]

The serum anion gap (SAG), as defined below, can be used to infer whether an organic or mineral acidosis is present.

$$SAG = [Na^+] - [Cl^-] - [HCO_3^-]$$

To maintain electroneutrality, the total concentration of cations in the serum must equal the total concentration of anions.

$$[Na^+] + [UCs] = ([Cl^-] + [HCO_3^-]) + [UAs]$$

The cation concentration is equal to the sodium concentration plus that of "unmeasured" cations (UCs), predominantly magnesium, calcium, and potassium. The anion concentration is equal to the concentrations of chloride, bicarbonate, and "unmeasured" anions (UAs), including proteins, sulfates, phosphates, and organic anions. Therefore, as the result of the combination of the two equations above, the SAG can be expressed as:

$$SAG = [UAs] - [UCs]$$

The normal SAG is approximately 9 mEq/L (mmol/L), with a range of 3 to 11 mEq/L (mmol/L). This value is lower than the value of 12 mEq/L (mmol/L) cited in the literature in the past because of changes in the instrumentation for measurement of serum electrolytes.[3] Increases in the anion gap (AG) to values in excess of 17 to 20 mEq/L (mmol/L) are indicative of the accumulation of unmeasured anions in ECF.[5]

These unmeasured anions are generated as the result of the consumption of HCO_3^- by endogenous organic acids such as lactic acid, acetoacetic acid, or β-hydroxybutyric acid or from the ingestion of toxins such as methanol or ethylene glycol. The degree of elevation in the SAG is dependent on the clearance of the anion, as well as the multiple factors that influence HCO_3^- concentrations. Thus, the SAG is a relative rather than an absolute indication of the cause of metabolic acidosis. The SAG can also be elevated in the metabolic acidosis because of kidney disease, as the result of the accumulation of various organic anions, phosphates, and sulfates.

In hyperchloremic metabolic acidosis, bicarbonate losses from the ECF are replaced by chloride, and the SAG remains normal. This decrease in bicarbonate may be due to gastrointestinal (GI) tract losses, dilution of bicarbonate in the ECF as the result of the addition of sodium chloride solutions or chloride-containing acids. Common causes of metabolic acidosis with an increased or a normal SAG are listed in Table 52-5.

Hyperchloremic Metabolic Acidosis

Hyperchloremic metabolic acidosis can result from increased GI bicarbonate loss, renal bicarbonate wasting, impaired renal acid excretion, or exogenous acid gain.[4] GI disorders such as diarrhea, biliary, or pancreatic drainage through either a surgical drain or fistula can result in the loss of large volumes of bicarbonate-containing fluids.

TABLE 52-5 Common Causes of Metabolic Acidosis

Increased Serum Anion Gap	Normal Serum Anion Gap/ Hyperchloremic States
Lactic acidosis	**GI bicarbonate loss**
Lactic acidosis (see Table 52-6)	Diarrhea
Renal failure (acute or chronic)	External pancreatic or small bowel drainage (fistula)
Methanol ingestion	Ureterosigmoidostomy, ileostomy
Ethylene glycol ingestion	**Drugs**
Salicylate overdose	Cholestyramine (bile acid diarrhea)
Starvation	Magnesium sulfate (diarrhea)
	Calcium chloride (acidifying agent)
	RTA
	Hypokalemia
	Proximal renal tubular acidosis (type II)
	Distal renal tubular acidosis (type I)
	Carbonic anhydrase inhibitors (eg, acetazolamide)
	Drug-induced hypokalemia
	Amphotericin B
	Furosemide
	Ifosfamide
	Lithium
	Hyperkalemia
	Generalized distal nephron dysfunction (type IV)
	Mineralocorticoid deficiency or resistance
	Tubulointerstitial disease
	Drug-induced hyperkalemia
	Potassium-sparing diuretics (amiloride, spironolactone, triamterene)
	Trimethoprim
	Pentamidine
	Heparin
	ACE inhibitors and receptor blockers
	NSAIDs
	Cyclosporin A
	Other
	Acid ingestion (ammonium chloride, hydrochloric acid, hyperalimentation)
	Expansion acidosis (rapid saline administration)

ACE, angiotensin converting enzyme; GI, gastrointestinal; NSAIDs, nonsteroidal anti-inflammatory drugs; RTA, renal tubular acidosis.

Severe diarrhea, the most common cause of hyperchloremic metabolic acidosis, can lead to a daily loss of 5 to 10 L of fluid containing 100 to 140 mEq/L (mmol/L) of sodium, 20 to 40 mEq/L (mmol/L) of potassium, 80 to 100 mEq/L (mmol/L) of chloride, and 30 to 50 mEq/L (mmol/L) of bicarbonate.[4] Patients who have undergone ureteral diversion into the sigmoid colon or isolated ileal loop can also develop a hyperchloremic metabolic acidosis. This is the result of a net loss of bicarbonate, given that chloride is reabsorbed and bicarbonate is secreted by GI epithelial cells in the presence of the urine that is retained in the colon or bowel loop.

Hyperchloremic metabolic acidosis caused by renal bicarbonate wasting is the defining disturbance in proximal renal tubular acidosis (RTA) and is a complication of therapy with carbonic anhydrase inhibitors, particularly when they are administered for more than 24 to 48 hours.[4,6] During the treatment of diabetic ketoacidosis, renal loss of β-hydroxybutyrate and acetoacetate, which would otherwise be metabolized to yield bicarbonate, can contribute to the development of hyperchloremic metabolic acidosis.[7,8] Impaired renal acid excretion that occurs as a result of distal tubular dysfunction in patients with distal RTAs can also occur in patients with moderate to severe kidney disease from other causes. The metabolic acidosis observed in patients with kidney disease is initially hyperchloremic but can progress to an anion-gap acidosis as kidney disease progresses and sulfates, phosphates, and other anions accumulate.[4] Hyperchloremic metabolic acidosis can also result from the exogenous administration of acid (hydrochloric acid, ammonium chloride) or the unbuffered administration of acid salts from the amino acids in total parenteral nutrition fluids.[9]

Renal Tubular Acidosis

5 Renal tubular disorders can involve the proximal tubule, with a resultant failure to reabsorb filtered bicarbonate, or affect acid excretion in the distal tubule. The distal RTAs are the most common, and are all characterized by impaired net acid excretion. The distal RTAs are subdivided into those that are associated with hypokalemia (type I) and those associated with hyperkalemia (type IV). Type II represents proximal RTA (see further). Type III is extremely rare and will not be discussed.

Patients with classic distal (type I) RTA have impaired hydrogen ion secretion and are unable to excrete the daily acid load necessary to maintain acid–base balance.[4,5] These patients are unable to maximally acidify their urine (ie, attain urine pH less than 5.5), even in the face of an acid challenge. Type I RTA may be the result of a primary tubular defect or develop secondary to a wide variety of disorders including hypercalcemia, multiple myeloma, systemic lupus erythematosus, Sjögren syndrome, sickle-cell disease, and kidney transplant rejection, or following the administration of amphotericin B, ifosfamide or lithium.[10,11] The primary form of this disorder usually occurs in children and can result in severe acidosis, slowed growth, nephrocalcinosis, and kidney stones.[7,9] In adults, clinical complications include osteomalacia, nephrocalcinosis, and recurrent kidney stones. The hypokalemia associated with classic distal (type I) RTA results from secondary hypoaldosteronism associated with volume depletion. The renal potassium wasting decreases considerably if bicarbonate therapy is administered.

The hyperkalemic distal (type IV) RTAs are a heterogeneous group of disorders characterized by hypoaldosteronism or generalized distal tubule defects. The most common form of type IV RTA is hyporeninemic hypoaldosteronism. This syndrome is most commonly associated with diabetic nephropathy, but can also be seen in a variety of other disorders, including chronic interstitial nephritis, sickle-cell disease, human immunodeficiency virus (HIV) nephropathy, and obstructive uropathy. The clinical presentation of this syndrome is often exacerbated by drugs that can interfere with the renin–angiotensin–aldosterone axis, such as β-adrenergic blockers, angiotensin-converting enzyme (ACE) inhibitors, angiotensin receptor blockers, and nonsteroidal anti-inflammatory drugs (NSAIDs). Heparin can induce the syndrome by inhibiting adrenal aldosterone biosynthesis. Patients with this form of RTA are able to maximally acidify their urine (urine pH less than 5.5).[10] The primary defect in acid excretion is impaired ammoniagenesis caused by decreased kidney function. Hyperaldosteronism predisposes to the development of hyperkalemia, which results in further impairment of ammoniagenesis. Treatment to control the hyperkalemia is usually sufficient to reverse the metabolic acidosis, and mineralocorticoid replacement is frequently unnecessary.

Hyperkalemic distal (type IV) RTA resulting from generalized distal tubule defects is less common than hyporeninemic hypoaldosteronism but is more common than classic distal (type I) RTA. Patients with this defect have impaired tubular potassium secretion in addition to impaired urinary acidification (urine pH more than 5.5, despite acidemia or acid loading). Urinary obstruction is the most frequent cause of this disorder, which can also be associated with sickle-cell nephropathy, systemic lupus erythematosus, HIV nephropathy, analgesic abuse nephropathy, amyloidosis, kidney transplant rejection, and chronic cyclosporine nephrotoxicity.

Proximal (type II) RTA is characterized by defects in proximal tubular reabsorption of bicarbonate. Normally, more than 85% of filtered bicarbonate is reabsorbed in the proximal tubule. Defects in proximal tubular bicarbonate reabsorption result in increased delivery of bicarbonate to the distal nephron, which has a limited capacity for bicarbonate reabsorption. As a result, at a normal serum bicarbonate concentration, the filtered bicarbonate load is incompletely reabsorbed, and is lost in the urine. As the serum bicarbonate concentration decreases, the filtered load of bicarbonate is proportionately decreased. A new equilibrium is established in which the kidney is able to reabsorb the filtered bicarbonate load, albeit at a reduced serum bicarbonate concentration. Thus, patients with proximal RTA present with a chronic, nonprogressive hyperchloremic metabolic acidosis. These patients are able to acidify their urine in response to an acid load, but develop bicarbonaturia at a reduced serum bicarbonate concentration following bicarbonate loading. The impaired bicarbonate reabsorption results in salt wasting and secondary hyperaldosteronism. Hypokalemia, which can be severe, usually develops as a result of the hyperaldosteronism and bicarbonaturia.[4,11] Unlike patients with classic distal (type I) RTA, the hyperkalemia if present in proximal RTA is exacerbated by alkali replacement. Proximal RTA can develop as an isolated defect, or it can be associated with generalized proximal tubular dysfunction (Fanconi syndrome), with impaired proximal tubular glucose, phosphate, and amino acid reabsorption. Proximal RTA usually presents as an acquired disorder, secondary to a variety of diseases (amyloidosis, multiple myeloma, or nephrotic syndrome) or exposure to toxins (lead, cadmium, mercury, or outdated tetracyclines). Pharmacologic therapy with carbonic anhydrase inhibitors produces an iatrogenic form of proximal RTA.

Elevated Anion Gap Metabolic Acidosis

Metabolic acidosis with an increased SAG commonly results from increased endogenous organic acid production.[12] In lactic acidosis, lactic acid accumulates as a by-product of anaerobic metabolism.[13] Accumulation of the ketoacids β-hydroxybutyric acid and acetoacetic acid defines the ketoacidosis of uncontrolled diabetes mellitus, alcohol intoxication, and starvation (Table 52-5).[8] In advanced kidney disease, accumulation of phosphate, sulfate, and organic anions is responsible for the increased SAG, which is usually less than 24 mEq/L (mmol/L).[2] The severe metabolic acidosis seen in myoglobinuric acute kidney injury caused by rhabdomyolysis may be caused by the metabolism of large amounts of sulfur-containing amino acids released from myoglobin.

The presence of mild elevations in the SAG cannot be automatically attributed to the presence of a high SAG metabolic acidosis.

Elevations in the SAG are commonly seen in hospitalized patients, especially those who are critically ill.[14] A variety of factors can contribute to this nonspecific elevation in the SAG, including the presence of alkalemia, which increases the anionic charge of albumin and other plasma proteins. The usefulness of the SAG as a marker of acid–base status is dependent on proper interpretation of a patient's clinical status.[5,11] Despite these limitations, when the SAG exceeds 20 to 25 mEq/L (mmol/L) a significant organic acidosis is likely to be present.[12-14]

High anion gap metabolic acidosis can develop in many clinical settings, including uncontrolled diabetes mellitus (see Chapter 74), alcohol intoxication (see Chapters 37 and 66), and starvation (see Chapter 64).[8,10,15] Toxic ingestions of methanol and ethylene glycol are also associated with high anion gap metabolic acidosis and can be differentiated from other causes of SAG because of the presence of an elevated osmolar gap.[15] The mechanisms responsible for the development of acidosis in these settings are diverse.[14]

Lactic Acidosis Lactic acidosis is one of the most common causes of high SAG metabolic acidosis and can impact approximately 1% of hospitalized patients. Lactic acid is the end product of anaerobic metabolism of glucose (glycolysis).[13] In normal individuals, lactic acid derived from pyruvate enters the circulation in small amounts and is promptly removed by the liver. In the liver, and to a lesser extent in the kidney, lactic acid is reoxidized to pyruvic acid, which is then metabolized to CO_2 and H_2O. The normal plasma lactate concentration in healthy subjects is approximately 1 mEq/L (mmol/L).[1,2,13] The diagnosis of lactic acidosis should be considered in all patients with metabolic acidosis associated with an increased SAG. Lactic acidosis is considered to be present when lactate concentrations exceed 4 to 5 mEq/L (mmol/L) in an acidemic patient.

Classically, lactic acidosis has been differentiated into disorders associated with tissue hypoxia (type A lactic acidosis) and disorders associated with deranged oxidative metabolism (type B lactic acidosis), although the distinction between them is blurred (Table 52-6).[13] The etiologies of lactic acidosis can also be categorized on the basis of changes in lactate production and/or utilization.[7,12] Metabolic disturbances can result in increased tissue pyruvate production or impaired utilization, with proportional increases in lactate concentrations. Increased lactate production is more commonly associated with alterations in tissue redox state, resulting in preferential conversion of pyruvate to lactate. During anaerobic metabolism, reduced nicotinamide adenine dinucleotide accumulates, driving the conversion of pyruvate to lactate and increasing the lactate-to-pyruvate ratio. States of enhanced metabolic activity (eg, grand mal seizures, strenuous exercise, or hyperthermia), decreased tissue oxygen delivery (eg, severe anemia, hypoxia, circulatory shock, or carbon monoxide poisoning), or impaired oxygen utilization (eg, cyanide toxicity) all are associated with lactic acidosis. Impaired hepatic clearance of lactate, as seen in hypoperfusion states, liver failure, and alcohol intoxication, can also result in lactic acidosis.

Cardiovascular and septic shock, with resultant tissue hypoperfusion, are the most common causes of lactic acidosis.[13] Poor tissue perfusion and hypoxia influence enzymatic pyruvate and lactate metabolism to stimulate anaerobic glycolysis and to decrease lactate utilization. This leads to hyperlactatemia and lactic acidosis. The mortality rate of this type of lactic acidosis can be as high as 80% and correlates with the degree of hyperlactatemia.

Lactic acidosis associated with liver disease, toxins, and congenital enzyme deficiency can be caused by deranged oxidative metabolism or impaired lactate clearance.[2-4,13,15] The exact role of diabetes mellitus in the induction of lactic acidosis is not clear.[7,8] It may involve a decrease in pyruvate dehydrogenase activity, the enzyme responsible for pyruvate metabolism. Lactic acidosis in neoplastic disease is uncommon and reported mostly in patients with myeloproliferative disorders. Leukocytes and neoplastic cells in general have high rates of glycolysis. In the case of a large tumor or tightly packed bone marrow, oxygenation can be decreased, favoring the accumulation of lactate. Lactic acidosis has been reported in patients with massive liver tumors, and it has been postulated that the liver uptake of lactate is decreased in these patients. Lactic acidosis associated with seizures is usually transient and occurs because of excessive muscle activity.[13]

A number of medications can cause lactic acidosis.[9,10,13,16-23] Two of the most common medications associated with the development of lactic acidosis are nucleoside-analog reverse transcriptase inhibitors (NRTIs) (3.9 cases per 1,000 person-years) and metformin (0.03 cases per 1,000 person-years).[16,17] The proposed mechanism of NRTI-induced lactic acidosis is the inhibition of the enzyme DNA polymerase gamma that is responsible for mitochondrial DNA synthesis.[16] Disruption of this enzyme can inhibit the transport of lactate into the mitochondria, leading to an accumulation in the cytoplasm. Stavudine is the NRTI most frequently associated with lactic acidosis; however, the combination of stavudine and didanosine confers the highest risk. Lactic acidosis has been rarely reported with tenofovir, lamiduvine and abacavir.

The primary suspected mechanism for metformin-induced lactic acidosis is inhibition of liver gluconeogenesis as the result of its inhibitory effects on pyruvate carboxylase, which is necessary for the conversion of pyruvate to glucose.[7,17,18] Other possible pathways for metformin-associated lactic acidosis include a decrease in both hepatic intracellular pH and cardiac output, an increase in lactate production in the gut, and increased renal loss of bicarbonate.[7,17,18] Risk factors for metformin-induced lactic acidosis include impaired kidney function, liver disease, dehydration, advanced age, alcohol consumption, and supratherapeutic dosing. Metformin should be discontinued during periods of tissue hypoxia (eg, myocardial infarction, sepsis), for 3 days after contrast media has been administered or 2 days before general anesthesia administration. In the latter two cases, metformin should only be reinstituted when the patient's kidney function is stable.

Linezolid inpairs mitcochondrial function and has been rarely reported to cause lactic acidosis, usually after prolonged (more than or equal to 4 weeks) therapy.[19] The weight loss combination medication phentermine-topiramate (Qysmia®) has been reported to cause lactic acidosis.[20]

Propylene glycol is commonly used as a solubilizing agent in IV drug preparations (eg, lorazepam, pentobarbital) and is predominantly metabolized to lactic acid via the hepatic enzyme alcohol

TABLE 52-6 Causes of Lactic Acidosis

Primary decrease in tissue oxygenation
Shock
Severe anemia
Congestive heart failure
Asphyxia
Carbon monoxide poisoning
Deranged oxidative metabolism
Medications
Catecholamines
Linezolid
Metformin
Nalidixic acid
NRTIs (abacavir, lamivudine, tenofovir)
Overdose (iron, isoniazid, salicylates, theophylline)
Propofol infusion syndrome
Propylene glycol toxicity (IV lorazepam, IV pentobarbital)
Sodium nitroprusside (secondary to cyanide toxicity)
Streptozocin
Diabetes mellitus
Malignancy
Seizures
Methanol, ethanol, or ethylene glycol
Disorders associated with inborn errors of metabolism

dehydrogenase.[21,22] The administration of large doses of propylene glycol, particularly to patients with impaired kidney or liver function, can lead to a lactic acidosis with an osmolar gap. Thus, serial measurement of the osmolar gap can be used to detect propylene glycol accumulation.[21,22]

Reports of the association between propofol and lactic acidosis were initially described in children.[23] This association is now recognized in adults and has come to be known as the propofol-related infusion syndrome. In addition to lactic acidosis, cardiac failure, rhabdomyolysis, and acute kidney injury have been observed primarily because of uncoupling of oxidative phosphorylation and impaired oxidation of free fatty acids. This syndrome is most frequently seen in patients receiving propofol at high doses (more than 5 mg/kg/h) for more than 2 days.

Clinical Presentation

Chronic metabolic acidosis is usually not associated with severe acidemia and is relatively asymptomatic. The major manifestations are bone demineralization with the development of rickets in children and osteomalacia and osteopenia in adults.[4,24] In infants and children, chronic metabolic acidosis is associated with growth failure and short stature and can be associated with nonspecific symptoms including anorexia, nausea, weight loss, and muscle weakness.

Severe metabolic acidosis is usually associated with acute processes. The manifestations of severe acidemia (pH less than 7.20) involve the cardiovascular, respiratory, and central nervous system (CNS). Hyperventilation is often the first sign of metabolic acidosis. At a pH of 7.2, pulmonary ventilation increases approximately fourfold, and an eightfold increase has been noted at a pH of 7.[3,25] Respiratory compensation can occur as Kussmaul respirations— the deep, rapid respirations seen commonly in patients with diabetic ketoacidosis. In extremely severe acidosis (pH less than 6.8), CNS function is disrupted to such a degree that the respiratory center is depressed.

CNS depression correlates more closely with spinal fluid pH than with blood pH. For this reason, neurologic symptoms tend to occur more frequently and to a greater degree in patients with respiratory acidosis because the CO_2 accumulated in the respiratory form readily crosses the blood–brain barrier to cause acidosis in the CNS.[4] Because of the slow penetration of administered bicarbonate into the CNS, the CNS pH fails to normalize as rapidly as blood pH. Therefore patients continue to hyperventilate because of sustained CNS acidity, and severe respiratory alkalosis can occur. Sustained lowering of the $PaCO_2$ within 12 to 36 hours is to be anticipated during the correction of any metabolic acidosis.[4]

Systemic acidosis can cause peripheral arteriolar dilatation, characterized by flushing, a rapid heart rate, and wide pulse pressure. Initially, cardiac output can be increased, but as acidosis becomes more severe, myocardial contractility becomes impaired, and cardiac output decreases. The effects of vagal stimulation are also enhanced at pH levels lower than 7.1, probably as a consequence of inhibition of acetylcholinesterase. This increases the danger of vagally mediated bradycardia and heart block during acidosis.

GI symptoms of metabolic acidosis include loss of appetite, nausea, and vomiting. Severe acidosis (pH less than 7.1) interferes with carbohydrate metabolism and insulin utilization, and results in hyperglycemia. Metabolic acidosis alters potassium homeostasis and contributes to the development of hyperkalemia. The magnitude of the effect on serum potassium depends on the type of acidosis: Acidosis caused by mineral acids (eg, hydrochloric acid) is associated with a greater change in potassium levels than acidosis caused by organic acids (eg, lactic acidosis), in which the increase in potassium attributable to the acidosis per se is minimal.

Compensation

6 The patient's primary means to compensate for metabolic acidosis is to increase carbon dioxide excretion by increasing the respiratory rate. This results in a decrease in $PaCO_2$. This ventilatory compensation results from stimulation of the respiratory center by changes in cerebral bicarbonate concentration and pH.[1,25] For every 1-mEq/L (mmol/L) decrease in bicarbonate concentration below the average of 24, the $PaCO_2$ decreases by approximately 1 to 1.5 mm Hg (0.13-0.20 kPa) from the normal value of 40 (5.3 kPa) (Table 52-7).

The anticipated $PaCO_2$ associated with a given bicarbonate concentration for patients with uncomplicated metabolic acidosis can be calculated as:[25]

$$PaCO_2 = (1.5 \times [HCO_3^-] + 8) \pm 2 \text{ for } PaCO_2 \text{ in mm Hg}$$

$$(PaCO_2 = (0.2 \times [HCO_3^-] + 1.1) \pm 0.3 \text{ for } PaCO_2 \text{ in kPa})$$

For example, 95% of patients with a plasma bicarbonate of 16 mEq/L (mmol/L) should have an arterial PCO_2 of 30 to 34 mm Hg (4.0-4.5 kPa). An observed arterial PCO_2 within this range is consistent with physiologic respiratory compensation for a metabolic acidosis and suggests that there is no respiratory disturbance.

CLINICAL PRESENTATION Metabolic Acidosis

General

- The patient usually is relatively asymptomatic if the acidosis is acute and mild. In those with severe acidemia (pH less than 7.15-7.20), the cardiovascular, respiratory, and CNS systems can be affected.

Symptoms

- The patient may complain of loss of appetite, nausea, and vomiting.

Signs

- Cardiac: Flushing, a rapid heart rate, wide pulse pressure, and an increase in cardiac output can be seen initially. This can be followed by a reduction in cardiac output, blood pressure, and liver and kidney blood flow.
- Cerebral: Obtundation or coma.
- Metabolic: Insulin resistance; increased protein degradation; increased metabolic demands.
- GI: Nausea, vomiting, loss of appetite.
- Respiratory: Dyspnea, hyperventilation with deep, rapid respirations is seen in those with severe acidosis.
- Chronic acidemia causes bone demineralization with the development of rickets in children and osteomalacia and osteopenia in adults.

Laboratory Tests

- Serum CO_2 is low. Hyperglycemia and hyperkalemia are common. Patients with a pH of less than 7.2 are deemed to have a severe acidosis.

TABLE 52-7 Guidelines for Initial Interpretation of Acid–Base Disorders

Acidosis	
Metabolic	$PaCO_2$ (in mm Hg) should decrease by 1.3 times the fall in plasma [HCO_3^-] (in mEq/L or mmol/L)
Acute respiratory	The plasma [HCO_3^-] should increase by 0.1 times the increase in $PaCO_2$ ± 3 (in mm Hg)
Chronic respiratory	The plasma [HCO_3^-] should increase by 0.35 times the increase in $PaCO_2$ ± 4 (in mm Hg)
Alkalosis	
Metabolic	$PaCO_2$ (in mm Hg) should increase by 0.4-0.6 times the rise in plasma [HCO_3^-] (in mEq/L or mmol/L)
Acute respiratory	The plasma [HCO_3^-] should decrease by 0.2 times the decrease in $PaCO_2$ (in mm Hg), but usually not to < 18 mEq/L (mmol/L)
Chronic respiratory	The plasma [HCO_3^-] should fall by 0.35 times the decrease in $PaCO_2$ (in mm Hg), but usually not to < 14 mEq/L (mmol/L)

HCO_3^-, bicarbonate; $PaCO_2$, partial pressure of carbon dioxide from arterial blood.

In contrast, if the PCO_2 is less than 30 mm Hg (4.0 kPa), a superimposed respiratory alkalosis can be present, whereas if the PCO_2 is greater than 34 mm Hg (4.5 kPa), a superimposed respiratory acidosis is likely present.

TREATMENT

7 Asymptomatic patients with mild to moderate degrees of acidemia (plasma bicarbonate of 12-20 mEq/L [mmol/L]; pH 7.2-7.4) do not require emergent therapy. They can usually be managed with gradual correction of the acidemia, over a period of days to weeks, using oral sodium bicarbonate or other alkali preparations (Table 52-8). In all forms of chronic metabolic acidosis, primary therapy should be directed at treating the underlying disease state. GI pathology should be treated to reduce ongoing bicarbonate losses, and factors that exacerbate RTA should be treated. If acidemia persists, alkali therapy should be instituted with the goal of normalization of blood pH. The loading dose (LD) of alkali to initially correct the acidemia can be calculated as follows:

$$\text{LD (mEq or mmol/L)} = (V_D\ HCO_3^- \times \text{body weight [BW]}) \times (\text{desired } [HCO_3^-] - \text{current } [HCO_3^-])$$

where V_D is the volume of distribution of bicarbonate.[4]

For a 60-kg patient with a serum bicarbonate of 15 mEq/L (mmol/L), the LD is calculated thus:

$$\text{LD (mEq)} = (0.5 \text{ L/kg} \times 60 \text{ kg}) \times (24 \text{ mEq/L} - 15 \text{ mEq/L})$$
$$= 30 \text{ L} \times 9 \text{ mEq/L}$$
$$= 270 \text{ mEq/L (mmol/L)}$$

The calculated LD of alkali should be administered over several days to avoid volume overload from the accompanying sodium load. For this scenario, a regimen of 60 to 70 mEq (mmol) three times a day for 3 to 5 days should result in an increase in HCO_3^- levels toward normal. In addition to the calculated LD, supplemental alkali must also be provided to replace ongoing losses, which can be approximated to be 2 mEq/kg (mmol/kg) per day or 40 mEq (mmol) three times a day. In patients with associated volume depletion, bicarbonate replacement can be provided simultaneous with volume resuscitation by substituting bicarbonate for chloride in IV crystalloid solutions.

In patients with chronic metabolic acidosis because of GI bicarbonate losses, maintenance therapy should provide sufficient alkali to replace ongoing bicarbonate losses. The magnitude of this replacement is variable and can be substantial (more than 10 mEq/kg [mmol/kg] per day). In addition, associated losses of other electrolytes, such as potassium and magnesium, may need to be replaced (see Chapter 51).

Proximal (type II) RTA is a bicarbonate-wasting disorder that requires the administration of large maintenance doses of alkali (10-15 mEq/kg [mmol/kg] per day). As alkali replacement raises

TABLE 52-8 Therapeutic Alternatives for Oral Alkali Replacement

Generic Name	Trade Name(s)	Milliequivalents of Alkali	Dosage Form(s)	Comment
Shohl's solution (sodium citrate/citric acid)	Bicitra (Willen)	1 mEq Na/mL; equivalent to 1 mEq bicarbonate	Solution (500 mg Na citrate, 334 mg citric acid/5 mL)	Citrate preparations increase absorption of aluminum
Sodium bicarbonate	Various (eg, Sodamint)	3.9 mEq bicarbonate/tablet (325 mg)	325 mg tablet	Bicarbonate preparations can cause bloating because of CO_2 production
		7.8 mEq bicarbonate/tablet (650 mg)	650 mg tablet	
	Baking soda (various)	60 mEq bicarbonate/tsp (5 g/tsp)	Powder	
Potassium citrate	Urocit-K (Mission)	5 mEq citrate/tablet	5 mEq tablet	See above
Potassium bicarbonate/potassium citrate	K-Lyte (Bristol)	25 mEq bicarbonate/tablet	25 mEq tablet (effervescent)	
	K-Lyte DS (Bristol)	50 mEq bicarbonate/tablet (double strength)	50 mEq tablet (effervescent)	See above
Potassium citrate/citric acid	Polycitra-K (Willen)	2 mEq K/mL; equivalent to 2 mEq bicarbonate	Solution (1,100 mg K citrate, 334 mg citric acid/5 mL)	See above
		30 mEq bicarbonate/unit dose packet	Crystals for reconstitution (3,300 mg K citrate, 1,002 mg citric acid/unit dose packet)	
Sodium citrate/potassium citrate/citric acid	Polycitra (Willen) Polycitra-LC (Willen)	1 mEq K, 1 mEq Na/mL; equivalent to 2 mEq bicarbonate	Syrup (Polycitra) solution (Polycitra-LC) (Both contain 550 mg K citrate, 500 mg Na citrate, 334 mg citric acid/5 mL)	See above

the serum bicarbonate concentration toward normal, the proximal tubule's capacity to reabsorb bicarbonate is overwhelmed, and renal bicarbonate wasting increases. In children, aggressive therapy of proximal RTA is necessary to avoid growth retardation and osteopenia. Because this is generally a mild, nonprogressive acidosis in adults, the benefit of alkali therapy is frequently outweighed by the risks of increased potassium wasting. In patients with classic distal (type I) RTA, maintenance therapy usually requires only enough alkali to buffer the amount of acid generated from dietary intake and metabolism. This usually approximates 1 to 3 mEq/kg per day (mmol/kg per day).

8 After initial potassium deficits are replaced, ongoing potassium supplementation may not be required, as renal potassium losses decrease following initiation of appropriate alkali therapy. The use of potassium alkali salts can, however, be desirable in patients with associated nephrolithiasis, because sodium salts can increase urinary calcium excretion.

The metabolic acidosis associated with hyperkalemic distal (type IV) RTA with hyporeninemic-hypoaldosteronemia that is often seen in patients with diabetes mellitus can be corrected by the treatment of hyperkalemia alone (see Chapter 51). The use of supplemental alkali (1-2 mEq/kg [mmol/kg] per day) to increase sodium intake and stimulate distal tubular potassium secretion can be beneficial. A minority of patients require the administration of pharmacologic amounts of fludrocortisone.[4] Type IV RTA resulting from a generalized distal tubular disorder often responds to low doses of alkali (1.5-2.0 mEq/kg [mmol/kg] per day).[4,11] Corrections of the acidosis along with modest dietary potassium restriction (to 1 mEq/kg [mmol/kg] per day) will often result in the maintenance of serum potassium concentrations of 5 mEq/L (mmol/L) or less.

Acute Severe Metabolic Acidosis

9 The management of life-threatening acute metabolic acidosis (plasma bicarbonate of 8 mEq/L [mmol/L] and pH less than 7.20) is dependent on the underlying cause and the patient's cardiovascular status. In some cases, patients will require emergent hemodialysis therapy (see Chapter 45). Patients with hyperchloremic acidosis (eg, diarrhea-induced) are unable to regenerate bicarbonate, and the generation of new bicarbonate by the kidneys can require several days before one can observe a meaningful change in their status.[4] Thus IV alkali therapy is often required for these patients.

Although conventional wisdom recommends the use of alkali replacement in patients with severe acidemia because of the deleterious effects of acidemia on circulatory function,[2,4,7,8] studies have not demonstrated that its administration improves patient outcomes.[26,27] Alkali therapies may either improve or worsen clinically relevant endpoints such as [H^+], $PaCO_2$, lactate concentrations, and cardiac output. The specific patient populations most likely to benefit or be harmed from alkalinizing therapy are presented in Table 52-9.

There are several therapeutic alternatives available for the acute correction of severe metabolic acidosis. Sodium acetate, sodium citrate, and sodium lactate are unreliable sources of alkali because their alkalinizing effect is dependent on their oxidative conversion to bicarbonate by the liver. This process is often impaired in critically ill patients, especially those with hepatic disease or circulatory failure. Although sodium bicarbonate is the most widely used IV alkalotic agent,[4] several studies suggest that it is frequently ineffective and can actually be deleterious, especially in patients with lactic acidosis.[27-28] Among the two remaining alternatives, (Dichloroacetate [DCA]) is investigational and not available in most clinical settings. Tromethamine, or THAM, is a carbon dioxide—consuming, commercially available solution that buffers respiratory as well as metabolic acids.

TABLE 52-9 Patient Populations Likely to Benefit or Suffer from Alkalinizing Therapy

Patients with Potential for Benefit	Patients with Potential for Harm
Distal (type 1) renal tubular acidosis	Hypernatremia
Severe hypochloremic metabolic acidosis secondary to diarrhea or surgical diversion	Hypervolemia
	Acute renal failure
	Congestive heart failure
Specific poisonings and intoxications (eg, salicylate overdose with metabolic acidosis)	Pulmonary disease resulting in decreased ventilation
	Acute lung injury where lung-protective ventilation strategy is used
	Diabetic ketoacidosis

Clinical **Controversy...**

The role of alkali therapy in patients with severe lactic acidosis is controversial. Treatment should be directed at the underlying causes as serial bicarbonate administration is often not effective and in some settings can be deleterious.

Sodium Bicarbonate

While sodium bicarbonate administration provides fluid and electrolyte replacement and increases arterial pH, neither animal nor clinical studies demonstrate an improvement in cardiac function, organ perfusion, or intracellular pH.[8,26-30] In addition, sodium bicarbonate administration can actually have paradoxical adverse effects on intracellular pH. When bicarbonate is given by IV infusion, the carbon dioxide generated diffuses more readily than bicarbonate across cell membranes and into cerebrospinal fluid. Therefore, the intracellular pH can actually be decreased by administration of bicarbonate.[4,28,31,32]

Excessive sodium bicarbonate administration can result in (a) a shift of the oxyhemoglobin saturation curve to the left, thereby impairing oxygen release from hemoglobin to tissues; (b) sodium and water overload, with subsequent pulmonary congestion and hypernatremia; (c) paradoxical tissue acidosis as a result of the production of CO_2 that freely diffuses into myocardial and cerebral cells[32]; and (d) decreased ionized calcium with a resultant decrease in myocardial contractility. If there is an endogenous source of bicarbonate, such as can occur in the case of ketoacidosis or lactic acidosis, a bicarbonate "overshoot" can develop because the ketoacids (acetoacetic acid and β-hydroxybutyric acid) or lactic acid are converted in the liver to bicarbonate once the underlying cause of acidosis is corrected.[7,8,13] Alkalosis can also result if too much sodium bicarbonate is administered too quickly.

If IV sodium bicarbonate is used, one must be mindful that the goals are to increase, not normalize, pH (to approximately 7.20) and plasma bicarbonate (to 8-10 mEq/L [mmol/L]). There is no calculative method that will assure attainment of these goals with a given dose of sodium bicarbonate because of the multiplicity of competing processes that can affect acid–base status (eg, vomiting, potential increases in endogenous acid production, and kidney disease) and the marked variability in the volume of distribution of bicarbonate (50% of body weight in patients with mild acidosis to approximately 100% in those with severe acidosis).[4,30,31] The dose of sodium bicarbonate may be calculated using a distribution volume of 50% of body weight for all patients to avoid overtreatment.[31] The total dose calculated as described previously in the RTA section should be administered as an infusion over one-half to several hours.

Follow-up monitoring of ABGs, beginning no sooner than 30 minutes after the end of the infusion, should be used to guide further therapeutic decisions.

Clinical **Controversy...**

Although it has been recommended that sodium bicarbonate be administered to raise the arterial pH to approximately 7.20, in an effort to prevent complications such as ventricular tachyarrhythmia, there are no controlled clinical trials demonstrating that sodium bicarbonate administration is significantly better than general supportive care in reducing morbidity and mortality in these patients.[5, 8, 27, 28]

Bicarbonate therapy is generally not necessary for patients with cardiac arrest, even if the initial arrest was unmonitored. The American Heart Association's Advanced Cardiac Life Support (ACLS) provider manual states that sodium bicarbonate is not useful or effective during resuscitation in hypoxic patients with lactic acidosis.[30] Additionally, sodium bicarbonate is considered to be not useful or effective in those who are undergoing prolonged resuscitation with effective ventilation.[4,29] Furthermore, if sodium bicarbonate is used, it should be used only after defibrillation, cardiac compression, support of ventilation including intubation, and drug therapies such as epinephrine and antiarrhythmic agents have been employed.[30] The initial dose of sodium bicarbonate in this situation is (1 mEq/kg [mmol/kg]) administered by rapid, direct IV injection.[30] Subsequent doses of sodium bicarbonate should be based on measurements of arterial blood pH and $PaCO_2$ given the propensity for it to cause alkalemia.[28,29]

Tromethamine

THAM, available as a 0.3 N solution, is a highly alkaline, sodium-free organic amine that acts as a proton acceptor to prevent or correct acidosis.[4,33] THAM combines with hydrogen ions from carbonic acid to form bicarbonate and a cationic buffer. THAM also acts as an osmotic diuretic to increase urine flow, urine pH, and the excretion of fixed acids, CO_2, and electrolytes. At pH 7.4, 30% of THAM is not ionized and therefore can penetrate into cells and neutralize acidic anions of the intracellular fluid. Intracellular pH increases have been noted within 1 hour after the infusion of THAM. There is, however, no clinical or physiologic evidence that this action is beneficial, or that THAM is more efficacious than sodium bicarbonate.[31,33]

When THAM is used, it must be administered slowly, with careful monitoring to avoid alkalosis. The usual empiric dosage range for THAM is 1 to 5 mmol/kg administered IV over 1 hour, but doses up to 1.25 mmol/kg can be given over 5 to 15 minutes in acute situations. The dose of THAM can be individualized using the following equation[31]:

$$\text{Dose of THAM (in mL)} = 1.1 \times \text{BW (in kg)} \times \text{base deficit}$$

where base deficit = normal $[HCO_3^-]$ − current $[HCO_3^-]$.

The need for additional THAM is determined by serial measurements of the serum bicarbonate concentration and calculation of the base deficit. Large doses can cause respiratory depression as a result of an increase in blood pH and a decrease in $PaCO_2$ concentration.[31] THAM solution is highly alkaline and can cause severe inflammation, vascular spasm, or tissue damage (necrosis, sloughing, pain, chemical phlebitis, or thrombosis) if infiltration occurs. Hyperkalemia, hypoglycemia, hypocalcemia, and impaired coagulation have also been reported.[31] This agent should only be used with extreme caution in patients with severe liver or kidney failure.

Dichloroacetate

DCA, another investigational agent, facilitates aerobic lactate metabolism by stimulating the activity of lactate dehydrogenase, thus reversing hyperlactatemia and elevating blood pH.[34-37] DCA, when compared to conventional management in controlled studies, however, has not been shown to improve hemodynamic parameters or clinical outcomes.[34-37] DCA can cause mild drowsiness and peripheral neuropathy that can be ameliorated or prevented with thiamine supplementation.[31] The future role of DCA in the management of metabolic acidosis, particularly lactic acidosis, remains to be clarified.[13]

Metabolic Alkalosis

Pathophysiology

Metabolic alkalosis is a simple acid–base disorder that presents as alkalemia (increased arterial pH) with an increase in plasma bicarbonate.[1,2] It is an extremely common entity in hospitalized patients with acid–base disturbances. Under normal circumstances, the kidney is readily able to excrete an alkali load. Thus evaluation of patients with metabolic alkalosis must consider two separate issues: (a) the initial process that generates the metabolic alkalosis; and (b) alterations in kidney function that maintain the alkalemic state.[38,39]

10 The generation of metabolic alkalosis can also result from excessive losses of hydrogen ions from the kidneys or stomach or from a gain secondary to the ingestion or administration of bicarbonate-rich fluids. Gastric juice, rich in chloride and hydrogen ions, is secreted at a rate of less than 50 mL/h in the basal state, but can increase up to fivefold with stimulation.[3] In the gastric parietal cells, the hydrogen ion and bicarbonate are generated from CO_2 and water.[3,39] The hydrogen ion is secreted into gastric fluid, and the bicarbonate is retained in the ECF. Normally, an amount of bicarbonate equal to the bicarbonate generated in the stomach is eliminated in the alkaline pancreatic and small-bowel secretions, maintaining hydrogen ion balance. With vomiting and nasogastric suctioning, the hydrogen ion is lost externally and metabolic alkalosis results. Diarrhea, as seen with secretory villous adenomas and other secretory diarrheas, often results in excessive GI losses of chloride-rich, bicarbonate-poor fluid, and thus leads to the generation of metabolic alkalosis.

11 Diuretic agents acting on the thick ascending limb of the loop of Henle (eg, furosemide, bumetanide, and torsemide) and distal convoluted tubule (eg, thiazides) have most commonly been associated with the generation of metabolic alkalosis.[3,40] These agents promote the excretion of sodium and potassium almost exclusively in association with chloride, without a proportionate increase in bicarbonate excretion. Collecting duct hydrogen ion secretion is stimulated directly by the increased luminal flow rate and sodium delivery, and indirectly by intravascular volume contraction, which results in secondary hyperaldosteronism. Renal ammoniagenesis can also be stimulated by concomitant hypokalemia, further augmenting net acid excretion.

Increased renal acid excretion can also be the result of excess mineralocorticoid activity. Elevated mineralocorticoid levels directly stimulate collecting duct hydrogen ion secretion and indirectly increase ammoniagenesis by causing hypokalemia.[1,3,38,41] Increased mineralocorticoid activity can result from Cushing syndrome, primary hyperaldosteronism, or hyperaldosteronism secondary to increased renin activity (eg, malignant hypertension). In Bartter and Gitelman syndromes, defects in sodium transport in the loop of Henle (Bartter) or distal convoluted tubule (Gitelman) lead to hypokalemia, secondary hyperaldosteronism, and metabolic alkalosis.[41] In Liddle syndrome, enhanced sodium reabsorption by the cortical collecting duct epithelial sodium channel results in a syndrome of pseudohyperaldosteronism.[38,39] Administration of high doses of penicillins (eg, ticarcillin) can produce metabolic alkalosis because they act as nonreabsorbable anions.[10] High concentrations of poorly reabsorbable anions in the distal renal tubule increase luminal flow rate and luminal electronegativity, which enhances the secretion of potassium and hydrogen ions and results in hypokalemia and metabolic alkalosis.

Metabolic alkalosis can also be generated by the gain of exogenous alkali. This can be seen as a result of bicarbonate administration or from the infusion of organic anions that are metabolized to bicarbonate, such as acetate, lactate, and citrate. The milk-alkali syndrome was historically a common cause of metabolic alkalosis in patients with peptic ulcer disease secondary to the ingestion of large quantities of milk products and antacids. With the advent of alternative therapies for dyspeptic syndromes that are far more effective than milk, this syndrome is now rarely seen.

Metabolic alkalosis is predominantly maintained because of an abnormality in kidney function. Normally, the kidneys are capable of excreting all of the excess bicarbonate presented to them, even during periods of increased bicarbonate loads.[2] As the serum bicarbonate concentration increases, the filtered bicarbonate load exceeds the maximal rate for bicarbonate reabsorption, and the excess bicarbonate is excreted in the urine. Under normal circumstances, the excess bicarbonate is rapidly excreted, and metabolic alkalosis does not occur or is corrected in a matter of hours.[38]

12 Bicarbonate excretion becomes impaired via several mechanisms, which collectively contribute to the maintenance phase of metabolic alkalosis.[38] In general, these mechanisms can be divided into volume-mediated processes (sodium chloride-responsive) and volume-independent processes (sodium chloride-resistant) that are predominantly associated with excess mineralocorticoid activity and hypokalemia (Table 52-10).[1,3] Intravascular volume depletion perpetuates metabolic alkalosis a number of different ways. A decrease in the glomerular filtration rate reduces the filtered load of bicarbonate at any given serum concentration, thereby decreasing the kidney's ability to excrete a bicarbonate load. Although this can play a role in patients with chronic kidney disease, it is also an important factor in patients in whom intravascular volume contraction accompanies metabolic alkalosis. Decreased effective arterial blood volume also enhances proximal and distal tubular sodium reabsorption. Sodium reabsorption must be coupled with reabsorption of an anion, such as chloride or bicarbonate, or exchange with a cation, such as potassium or hydrogen, to maintain charge neutrality. In the proximal tubule, increased sodium reabsorption stimulates bicarbonate reabsorption. In the distal nephron, enhanced sodium reabsorption, particularly in the setting of hypokalemia, stimulates hydrogen ion secretion.

Mineralocorticoid excess also plays a significant role in the maintenance of metabolic alkalosis. In patients with volume-responsive metabolic alkalosis, intravascular volume depletion stimulates aldosterone secretion. As discussed earlier, excess mineralocorticoid activity can also underlie the generation of metabolic alkalosis. In either situation, the increased mineralocorticoid effect stimulates collecting duct hydrogen ion secretion. Metabolic alkalosis can also be maintained by persistent hypokalemia, enhancing proximal tubular bicarbonate reabsorption, stimulating ammoniagenesis, and increasing distal tubular hydrogen ion secretion.[38]

TABLE 52-10 Causes of Metabolic Alkalosis Differentiated on the Basis of Their Responsiveness to Sodium Chloride

Sodium chloride-responsive (urinary chloride concentration <10 mEq/L [mmol/L])
GI disorders
Vomiting
Gastric drainage
Villous adenoma of the colon
Chloride diarrhea
Diuretic therapy
Correction of chronic hypercapnia
Cystic fibrosis
Excessive bicarbonate therapy of an organic acidosis
Mild/moderate potassium deficiency
Sodium chloride-resistant (urinary chloride concentration >20 mEq/L [mmol/L])
Excess mineralocorticoid activity
Hyperaldosteronism
Cushing syndrome
Bartter syndrome
Gitelman syndrome
Excessive black licorice intake
Profound potassium depletion
Magnesium deficiency
Liddle syndrome
Estrogen therapy
Unclassified
Alkali administration
Milk-alkali syndrome
Massive blood or plasma protein fraction transfusion
Nonparathyroid hypercalcemia
Carbohydrate refeeding after starvation
Large doses of penicillin

Clinical Presentation

There are no unique signs or symptoms associated with mild-to-moderate metabolic alkalosis, but patients may complain of symptoms related to the underlying cause of the disorder (eg, muscle weakness with hypokalemia or postural dizziness with volume depletion).[38,39] They may have a history of vomiting, gastric drainage, or diuretic use, all of which contribute to the development of metabolic alkalosis. Severe alkalemia (blood pH more than 7.60) has been associated with cardiac arrhythmias, particularly in patients with heart disease, hyperventilation, and hypoxemia.[38] Neuromuscular irritability can be present, with signs of tetany or hyperactive reflexes, possibly caused by the decreased ionized calcium concentration that occurs secondary to the increase in pH. This decrease in ionized calcium may be caused by a conformational change in the albumin molecules to which the calcium is bound, resulting in increased binding, or by decreased competition from hydrogen ions for binding sites on the albumin molecule. Mental confusion, muscle cramping, and paresthesia can also occur. Lastly, patients will be more difficult to liberate from mechanical ventilation.

Compensation

The respiratory response to metabolic alkalosis is hypoventilation, which results in an increased $PaCO_2$. Respiratory compensation is initiated within hours when the central and peripheral chemoreceptors sense an increase in pH. The $PaCO_2$ increases 6 to 7 mm Hg (0.8-0.9 kPa) for each 10 mEq/L (mmol/L) increase in bicarbonate, up to a $PaCO_2$ of approximately 50 to 60 mm Hg (6.7-8.0 kPa) (see Table 52-7) before hypoxia sensors react to prevent further hypoventilation.[1,25] If the $PaCO_2$ is normal or less than normal, one should consider the presence of a superimposed respiratory alkalosis, which can be secondary to fever, gram-negative sepsis, or pain.

TREATMENT

Because the body tolerates alkalemia far less well than acidemia, treatment of metabolic alkalosis is nearly always required and should be aimed at correcting the factor(s) responsible for the maintenance of the alkalosis.[38] For example, vomiting should be treated with antiemetics, gastric losses of hydrogen ions during nasogastric suction can be modulated by giving histamine blockers such as ranitidine or proton pump inhibitors such as omeprazole, and reducing or discontinuing diuretic therapy.[38,42] Metabolic alkalosis will persist until the renal mechanism responsible for maintaining the disorder is corrected, despite the fact that the original cause of the elevated plasma bicarbonate may have resolved. For example, hypovolemia should be treated with sodium chloride to allow excretion of bicarbonate by the kidney. However, patients with severely

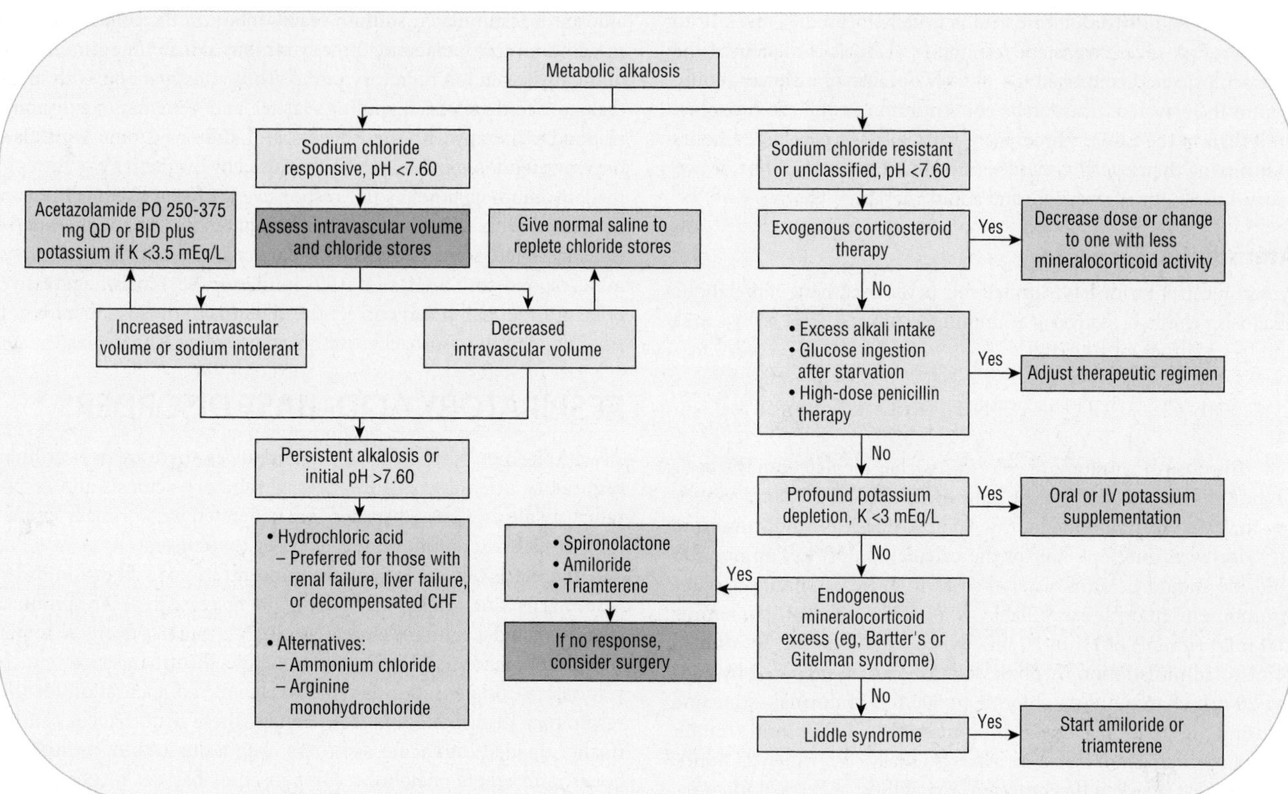

FIGURE 52-4 Treatment algorithm for patients with primary metabolic alkalosis. (BID, twice daily; CHF, chronic heart failure; K, potassium [serum potassium in mEq/L is numerically equivalent to mmol/L]; PO, orally; QD, every day.)

compromised cardiovascular function may not be able to tolerate this therapeutic approach. In situations such as this and/or the presence of life-threatening alkalosis, some have advocated reduction in pH by control of ventilation.[38] Although controlled hypoventilation, sometimes using inspired CO_2 with supplemental oxygen to prevent hypoxia can be lifesaving,[2] this approach is not universally accepted.[38] Therapy for metabolic alkalosis can be conceptualized on the basis of the sodium chloride responsiveness of the disorders as shown in Fig. 52-4.

Sodium Chloride-Responsive Metabolic Alkalosis

Sodium chloride-responsive disorders usually result from volume depletion and chloride loss, which can accompany severe vomiting, prolonged nasogastric suction, and diuretic therapy. Initially, therapy is directed at expanding intravascular volume and replenishing chloride stores. Sodium and potassium chloride-containing solutions should be administered to patients who can tolerate the volume load.[2,38] Patients with metabolic alkalosis who are volume overloaded or intolerant to volume administration because of congestive heart failure can benefit from the carbonic anhydrase inhibitor acetazolamide. This agent inhibits the action of carbonic anhydrase, thereby inhibiting renal bicarbonate reabsorption. Unfortunately, it also increases the renal losses of potassium and phosphate. Administration of acetazolamide (250-375 mg once or twice daily) can promote a sufficient bicarbonate diuresis and return the pH toward normal.[43] However, because the clinical effectiveness of the drug declines as the HCO_3^- concentration decreases, only rarely will this approach fully correct the alkalosis.[38]

Acidifying agents including hydrochloric acid, ammonium chloride, and arginine monohydrochloride can be used to treat severe (pH more than 7.6) symptomatic metabolic alkalosis.[44,45] In general, this management is reserved for patients who are unresponsive to conventional fluid and electrolyte management or who are unable to tolerate the requisite volume load because of decompensated congestive heart failure or advanced kidney disease.[44] Alternatively, hemodialysis using a low-bicarbonate dialysate can be used for the rapid correction of metabolic alkalosis.

Hydrochloric Acid

Hydrochloric acid is usually infused IV via a large central vein as a 0.1 to 0.25 N HCl solution in either 5% dextrose or normal saline, although sterile water has also been used. Extemporaneously prepared solutions can be made by adding 100 to 250 mEq (mmol) of HCl through a 0.22-mm filter into a glass container of saline or dextrose. Hydrochloric acid can also be added to parenteral nutrient solutions and administered via a central line without serious degradation of proteins.[31] The rate of infusion should be 100 to 125 mL/h (10-25 mEq/h [mmol/h]), with frequent monitoring of ABGs. To prevent overcorrection, the infusion should be stopped when the arterial pH decreases to 7.50.[38]

The dose of hydrochloric acid can be based on an estimate of the total body chloride deficit:[31]

$$\text{Dose HCl (in mEq or mmol)} = [0.2 \text{ L/kg} \times \text{BW (in kg)}] \times [103 - \text{observed serum chloride}]$$

where the estimated chloride space is 0.2 times the body weight, and the average serum chloride is 103 mEq/L (mmol/L). Alternatively, the dose can be calculated based on the estimated base deficit:[31]

$$\text{Dose HCl (in mEq or mmol)} = [0.5 \text{ L/kg} \times \text{BW (in kg)}] \times (\text{desired } [HCO_3^-] - \text{observed } [HCO_3^-])$$

Clinical **Controversy...**

At present, there are no comparative data that address the relative accuracy of these two formulas for determining the dose of hydrochloric acid.

The dose of hydrochloric acid is usually infused IV over 12 to 24 hours.[31] A severe transient respiratory acidosis can occur if the hydrochloric acid is infused too quickly because of a slower reduction of the elevated bicarbonate concentration in the cerebrospinal fluid than in the ECF. Improvement is usually seen within 24 hours of initiating therapy. ABGs and serum electrolytes should be drawn every 4 to 8 hours to evaluate and adjust therapy.

Ammonium Chloride

Ammonium chloride has a limited role in the treatment of metabolic alkalosis. The liver converts ammonium chloride (NH_4Cl) to urea and free hydrochloric acid[31]:

$$2NH_4Cl + 2HCO_3^- \rightarrow CO(NH_2)_2 + CO_2 + 3H_2O + 2Cl^-$$

The dose of ammonium chloride can be calculated on the basis of the chloride deficit using the same method as for HCl and assuming that 20 g ammonium chloride will provide 374 mEq (mmol) of H^+. However, only one half of the calculated dose of ammonium chloride should be administered so as to avoid ammonia toxicity. Ammonium chloride is available as a 26.75% solution containing 100 mEq (mmol) of H^+ in 20 mL, which should be further diluted prior to administration. A dilute solution can be prepared by adding 20 mL of ammonium chloride to 500 mL of normal saline and infusing the solution at a rate of no more than 1 mEq/min (mmol/min). Improvement in metabolic status is usually seen within 24 hours. CNS toxicity, marked by confusion, irritability, seizures, and coma, has been associated with more rapid rates of administration. Ammonium chloride must be administered cautiously to patients with impaired kidney or hepatic function. In patients with impaired hepatic function, decreased conversion of ammonia to urea can result in increased ammonia levels and worsened encephalopathy. In patients with kidney disease, the increased urea synthesis can exacerbate uremic symptoms.[31,38]

Arginine Monohydrochloride

Arginine monohydrochloride at a dose of 10 g/h given IV has been used to treat metabolic alkalosis, although it was never FDA-approved for this purpose.[31] Like ammonium chloride, arginine must undergo metabolism by the liver to produce hydrogen ions, with a conversion of 100 g to 475 mEq (mmol) of H^+. Unlike ammonium chloride, arginine combines with ammonia in the body to synthesize urea; thus it can be used in patients with relative hepatic insufficiency. Patients with kidney disease should not receive arginine monohydrochloride because it can significantly elevate blood urea nitrogen and is associated with severe hyperkalemia.[31,38] The increase in potassium is caused by arginine-induced shifts of potassium from the intracellular to the extracellular space. One recent study of critically ill children with metabolic alkalosis resistant to standard treatment practices found that acetazolamide was more efficacious in resolving the alkalosis than arginine.[45]

Sodium Chloride-Resistant Metabolic Alkalosis

13 Management of these disorders usually consists of treatment of the underlying cause of the mineralocorticoid excess. For patients taking a corticosteroid, a dosage reduction or a switch to a corticosteroid with less mineralocorticoid activity (eg, methylprednisolone) should be considered. Patients with an endogenous source of excess mineralocorticoid activity can require surgery or the administration of spironolactone, amiloride, or triamterene.[2,14,38]

Spironolactone is a competitive antagonist of the mineralocorticoid receptor. Amiloride and triamterene are potassium-sparing diuretics that inhibit the epithelial sodium channel in the distal convoluted tubule and collecting duct. All three agents inhibit aldosterone-stimulated sodium reabsorption in the collecting duct. In addition, spironolactone directly inhibits aldosterone stimulation of the hydrogen ion secretory pump. Thus, most patients with mineralocorticoid excess, including Bartter and Gitelman syndromes, respond to therapy with these agents.[38,41] Liddle syndrome, which is a form of pseudohypoaldosteronism caused by overactivity of the epithelial sodium channel, is not responsive to spironolactone but can be treated with either amiloride or triamterene. Although experience is limited, some patients with Bartter and Gitelman syndromes may respond to NSAIDs or ACE inhibitors.[46,47] Finally, aggressive potassium repletion can correct the alkalosis in those who have not responded to the approaches outlined above (see Chapter 51).

RESPIRATORY ACID–BASE DISORDERS

As with the metabolic acid–base disturbances, there are two cardinal respiratory acid–base disturbances: respiratory acidosis and respiratory alkalosis. These disorders are generated by a primary alteration in CO_2 excretion, which changes the concentration of CO_2, and therefore the carbonic acid concentration in body fluids.[1,48] A primary reduction in $PaCO_2$ causes an increase in pH (respiratory alkalosis), and a primary increase in $PaCO_2$ causes a decrease in pH (respiratory acidosis). Unlike the metabolic disturbances, for which respiratory compensation is rapid, metabolic compensation for the respiratory disturbances is slow. Hence, these disturbances can be further divided into acute disorders, with a duration of minutes to hours, and where metabolic compensation has yet to occur, and chronic disorders that have been present long enough for metabolic compensation to be complete.

Respiratory Alkalosis

Respiratory alkalosis is characterized by a primary decrease in $PaCO_2$ that leads to an elevation in pH. The $PaCO_2$ decreases when the excretion of CO_2 by the lungs exceeds the metabolic production of CO_2. It is the most frequently encountered acid–base disorder, occurring physiologically in normal pregnancy and in persons living at high altitudes.[1] Respiratory alkalosis also occurs frequently among hospitalized patients (Table 52-11).

Pathophysiology

A decrease in $PaCO_2$ occurs when ventilatory excretion exceeds metabolic production. Because endogenous production of CO_2 is relatively constant, negative CO_2 balance is primarily caused by an increase in ventilatory excretion of CO_2 (hyperventilation). The metabolic production of CO_2, however, can be increased during periods

TABLE 52-11 Causes of Respiratory Alkalosis

Central stimulation of respiration
Anxiety
Pain
Fever
Brain tumors, vascular accidents
Head trauma
Pregnancy
Progesterone
Catecholamines, theophylline, nicotine
Salicylates
Hypoxemia or tissue hypoxemia
High altitude
Decreased $PaCO_2$
Pneumonia
Pulmonary edema
Severe anemia
Peripheral stimulation of respiration
Pulmonary emboli
Asthma

$PaCO_2$, partial pressure of carbon dioxide from arterial blood.

of stress or with excess carbohydrate administration (eg, parenteral nutrition). Hyperventilation can develop from an increase in neurochemical stimulation via either central or peripheral mechanisms, or be the result of voluntary or mechanical (iatrogenic) hyperventilation.

A decrease in $PaCO_2$ can occur in patients with cardiogenic, hypovolemic, or septic shock because oxygen delivery to the carotid and aortic chemoreceptors is reduced. This relative deficit in PaO_2 stimulates an increase in ventilation. The hyperventilation in sepsis is also mediated via a central mechanism. Hyperventilation-induced respiratory alkalosis with an elevation in cardiac index and hypotension without peripheral vasoconstriction can therefore be an early sign of sepsis.

Clinical Presentation

Although most patients are asymptomatic, respiratory alkalosis can cause adverse neuromuscular, cardiovascular, and GI effects.[2,3,48] During periods of decreased $PaCO_2$, there is a decrease in cerebral blood flow, which can be responsible for symptoms of light-headedness, confusion, decreased intellectual functioning, syncope, and seizures. Nausea and vomiting can occur, probably as a result of cerebral hypoxia. In severe respiratory alkalosis, cardiac arrhythmias can occur because of sensitization of the myocardium to the arrhythmogenic effects of circulating catecholamines.[2,29] Acute respiratory alkalosis has no effect on blood pressure or cardiac output in awake individuals. Anesthetized patients, however, can experience a decrease in both cardiac output and blood pressure, possibly owing to the lack of a tachycardic response.[29]

The concentration of serum electrolytes can also be altered secondary to the development of respiratory alkalosis. The serum chloride concentration is usually slightly increased, and serum potassium concentration can be slightly decreased. Clinically significant hypokalemia can be a consequence of extreme respiratory alkalosis, although the effect is usually very small or negligible.[2,29] Serum phosphorus concentration can decrease by as much as 1.5 to 2.0 mg/dL (0.48-0.65 mmol/L) because of the shift of inorganic phosphate into cells. Reductions in the blood ionized calcium concentration can be partially responsible for symptoms such as muscle cramps and tetany. Approximately 50% of calcium is bound to albumin, and an increase in pH results in an increase in binding.[29]

Compensation

The initial response of the body to acute respiratory alkalosis is chemical buffering: hydrogen ions are released from the body's buffers—intracellular proteins, phosphates, and hemoglobin—and titrate down the serum bicarbonate concentration. This process occurs within minutes. Acutely, the bicarbonate concentration can be decreased by a maximum of 3 mEq/L (mmol/L) for each 10-mm Hg (1.3 kPa) decrease in $PaCO_2$ (see Table 52-7).[24] When only physicochemical buffering has occurred, the disturbance is referred to as acute respiratory alkalosis.

Metabolic compensation occurs when respiratory alkalosis persists for more than 6 to 12 hours. In response to the alkalemia, proximal tubular bicarbonate reabsorption is inhibited, and the serum bicarbonate concentration decreases. Renal compensation is usually complete within 1 to 2 days. The renal bicarbonaturia, as well as decreased NH_4^+ and titratable acid excretion, are direct effects of the reduced $PaCO_2$ and pH on renal reabsorption of chloride and bicarbonate.[2,29] The acuity of the respiratory alkalosis can be assessed on the basis of the degree of renal compensation (see Table 52-7). In fully compensated respiratory alkalosis, the bicarbonate concentration decreases by 4 mEq/L (mmol/L) below 24 for each 10-mm Hg (1.3 kPa) drop in $PaCO_2$. For example, a sustained decrease in $PaCO_2$ of 20 mm Hg (2.7 kPa) will lower serum bicarbonate from 24 to 16 mEq/L (mmol/L) with a resultant pH of 7.46. Bicarbonate concentrations differing from those anticipated using the preceding guidelines suggest a mixed acid–base disorder.

TREATMENT

Because most patients with respiratory alkalosis, especially chronic cases, have few or no symptoms and pH alterations are usually mild (pH not exceeding 7.50), treatment is often not required.[29,50] The first consideration in the treatment of acute respiratory alkalosis with pH more than 7.50 is the identification and correction of the underlying cause. Relief of pain, correction of hypovolemia with IV fluids, treatment of fever or infection, treatment of salicylate overdose, and other direct measures can prove effective. A rebreathing device, such as a paper bag, can be useful in controlling hyperventilation in patients with the anxiety/hyperventilation syndrome.[57] Oxygen therapy should be initiated in patients with severe hypoxemia. Patients with life-threatening alkalosis (pH more than 7.60), particularly if it is a mixed respiratory and metabolic condition, tend to have complications, such as arrhythmias or seizures, which can require mechanical ventilation with sedation and/or paralysis to control hyperventilation.

Respiratory alkalosis in patients receiving mechanical ventilation is usually iatrogenic. It can often be corrected by decreasing either the set respiratory rate or tidal volume, although other measures can also be employed. The use of a capnograph and spirometer in the breathing circuit enables a more precise adjustment of the ventilator settings. Another method of treating respiratory alkalosis is to increase the amount of dead space in the ventilator circuit by placing a known length of tubing between the artificial airway and the "T" piece of the ventilator. This results in "rebreathing" of

CLINICAL PRESENTATION Respiratory Alkalosis

General

- The patient is usually asymptomatic if the condition is chronic and mild.

Symptoms

- The patient may complain of light-headedness, confusion, muscle cramps and tetany, and decreased intellectual functioning.
- Nausea and vomiting can occur, probably as a result of cerebral hypoxia.

Signs

- In severe respiratory alkalosis pH more than 7.60
  - Syncope and seizures
  - Cardiac arrhythmias
  - Hyperventilation

Laboratory Tests

- Serum chloride concentration is usually slightly increased. Serum ionized calcium, potassium, and phosphorus concentration can be decreased.

TABLE 52-12 Causes of Acute Respiratory Acidosis

Central
Drugs (anesthetics, opioids, sedatives)
Stroke
Head injury
Infection
Status epilepticus
Perfusion abnormalities
Massive pulmonary embolism
Cardiac arrest
Airway and pulmonary abnormalities
Airway obstruction: Foreign body, laryngeal edema
Aspiration of vomitus
Asthma
COPD
Severe pulmonary edema
Severe pneumonia
ARDS
Smoke inhalation
Pneumothorax
Neuromuscular abnormalities
Brainstem or cervical cord injury
Guillan–Barré syndrome
Myasthenia gravis
Mechanical ventilator
Ventilator malfunction
Inadequate frequency or tidal volume settings
Large dead space
Total parenteral nutrition (increased CO_2 production)

ARDS, adult respiratory distress syndrome; COPD, chronic pulmonary obstructive disease.

expired gas, and therefore an increase in the inspired carbon dioxide concentration, which should increase the carbon dioxide tension of the patient, correcting the respiratory alkalosis. In patients breathing more rapidly than the ventilator settings, sedation with or without paralysis can be employed.

Respiratory Acidosis

Pathophysiology

Respiratory acidosis occurs when the lungs fail to excrete CO_2 resulting in a lower pH. This can be the result of conditions that centrally inhibit the respiratory center, diseases that interfere with pulmonary perfusion or neuromuscular function, and intrinsic airway or parenchymal pulmonary disease (Table 52-12). Acute respiratory acidosis with hypoxemia, hypercarbia, and acidosis is life-threatening. Those disorders that produce an increase in $PaCO_2$ and hypoxemia to a degree compatible with life (eg, chronic obstructive pulmonary disease), with or without oxygen therapy, can result in chronic respiratory acidosis (Table 52-13).

TABLE 52-13 Causes of Chronic Respiratory Acidosis

Neuromuscular abnormalities
Brainstem infarct
Obesity-hypoventilation (Pickwickian) syndrome
Tumors
Poliomyelitis
Multiple sclerosis
Diaphragmatic paralysis
Pulmonary abnormalities
Chronic obstructive pulmonary disease
Kyphoscoliosis
Interstitial pulmonary disease
Overzealous parenteral feeding

These patients can function normally without noticeable neurologic defects with $PaCO_2$ concentrations in the range of 90 to 100 mm Hg (12-13.3 kPa) (normal, 40 mm Hg [5.3 kPa]), provided that adequate oxygenation is maintained.[48]

Clinical Presentation

Respiratory acidosis can produce neurologic symptoms, including altered mental status, abnormal behavior, seizures, stupor, and coma. Hypercapnia can mimic stroke or CNS tumors by producing headache, papilledema, focal paresis, and abnormal reflexes. These CNS symptoms are attributable to the vasodilator effects of CO_2 in the brain that result in an increase in cerebral blood flow.[2] The CNS response to hypercapnia is extremely variable between patients and is most influenced by the acuity of presentation. Given that chronic hypercapnia blunts the usual respiratory stimulus of an elevated $PaCO_2$, hypoxemia rather than hypercapnia provides the primary ventilatory stimulus in patients with severe chronic respiratory acidosis.[48]

The degree to which cardiac contractility and heart rate are altered depends on the severity of the acidosis and the rapidity with which it develops. Modest acute hypercapnia ($PaCO_2$ of 50-55 mm Hg [6.7-7.3 kPa]) stimulates a stress-like response, with elevated catecholamines and corticosteroid hormone levels, and can result in increased cardiac output and pulmonary artery pressure.[29] As the severity increases, cardiac output declines and vascular resistance decreases leading to refractory hypotension in some patients.[2]

In respiratory acidosis, the serum potassium concentration increases modestly secondary to cellular shifts. The increases are less than those seen with inorganic metabolic acidosis and are difficult to predict for individual patients.

Compensation

The body responds to acute respiratory acidosis with chemical buffering. The increase in $PaCO_2$ results in increased carbonic acid levels.

CLINICAL PRESENTATION Respiratory Acidosis

General

- The patient is usually symptomatic.

Symptoms

- The patient may complain of confusion or difficulty thinking and headache.

Signs

- In severe respiratory acidosis.
- Cardiac: Increased cardiac output if moderate that decreases if severe. Refractory hypotension can be present in some patients.
- CNS: Abnormal behavior, seizures, stupor, and coma. Papilledema, focal paresis, and abnormal reflexes can also be present.

Laboratory Tests

- Serum potassium concentration can be modestly increased. Hypercapnia can be moderate ($PaCO_2$ of 50-55 mm Hg [6.7-7.3 kPa]) to severe ($PaCO_2$ of more than 80 mm Hg [more than 10.6 kPa]). Hypoxia (PaO_2 is less than 70 mm Hg [less than 9.3 kPa]) is often present.

The carbonic acid dissociates, releasing hydrogen ions, which are buffered by nonbicarbonate buffers (ie, proteins, phosphate, and hemoglobin) and bicarbonate. Thus, on the basis of physicochemical factors, increases in $PaCO_2$ raise the serum bicarbonate concentration. In general, in acute respiratory acidosis, the bicarbonate concentration increases by 1 mEq/L (mmol/L) above 24 for each 10 mm Hg (1.3 kPa) increase in $PaCO_2$ above 40 (5.3 kPa) (see Table 52-7).

Metabolic compensation occurs when respiratory acidosis is prolonged beyond 12 to 24 hours. In response to hypercapnia and acidemia, proximal tubular bicarbonate reabsorption, ammoniagenesis, and distal tubular hydrogen secretion are enhanced, resulting in an increase in the serum bicarbonate concentration that raises the pH toward normal. Renal compensation for chronic hypercapnia generally results in the plasma bicarbonate concentration increasing by 4 mEq/L (mmol/L) above 24 for each 10 mm Hg (1.3 kPa) increase in $PaCO_2$ above 40 (5.3 kPa) (see Table 52-7). The new steady state in acid–base values is generally achieved within 5 days of the onset of hypercapnia in dogs; the time interval necessary for compensation in humans has not been established.

TREATMENT

The treatment of respiratory acidosis is dependent on the chronicity of the patient's condition. Respiratory decompensation in patients with chronic elevations in $PaCO_2$ is frequently seen in those with acute infections and those recently started on narcotic analgesics or oxygen therapy.[29] Aggressive treatment of these conditions can offer considerable benefit and should be initiated. Furthermore, tranquilizers and sedatives should be avoided and supplemental oxygen, if used, should be minimized.

Acute Respiratory Acidosis

14 When carbon dioxide excretion is severely impaired ($PaCO_2$ more than 80 mm Hg [more than 10.6 kPa]) and/or life-threatening, hypoxia is present (PaO_2 less than 40 mm Hg [less than 5.3 kPa]); the immediate therapeutic goal is to provide adequate oxygenation. Under these circumstances, hypoxia, not acidemia, is the principal threat to life. A patent airway needs to be established, which can necessitate intubation. Excessive secretions must be cleared from the airway and oxygen administered to restore adequate oxygenation. Mechanical ventilation is usually required.

The underlying cause of the acidosis should be treated aggressively (ie, bronchodilators for treatment of severe bronchospasm; narcotic or benzodiazepine antagonists to reverse the deleterious effects of these agents on the respiratory center). Bicarbonate administration is rarely necessary in the treatment of respiratory acidosis. Furthermore, rapid correction of acidosis with bicarbonate can eliminate the patient's respiratory drive or precipitate metabolic alkalosis. Cautious use of alkali (bicarbonate or THAM) can restore the responsiveness of bronchial muscles to β-adrenergic agonists and thus can be beneficial for those patients with severe bronchospasm.[29] ABGs should be monitored closely to ensure that the respiratory acidosis is resolving without creating a metabolic alkalosis as the result of compensatory elevation in HCO_3^- and decrease in $PaCO_2$. ABGs should be obtained every 2 to 4 hours during the acute phase and less frequently (every 12-24 hours) as the acidosis improves.

Acute Respiratory Acidosis in a Compensated Chronic Respiratory Acidotic Patient

Patients with a history of chronic respiratory acidosis (ie, those with chronic obstructive pulmonary disease) can experience an acute worsening of their respiratory acidosis. This can result in severe life-threatening hypoxemia. As with acute respiratory acidosis, the goals of therapy are maintenance of a patent airway and adequate oxygenation. Individuals with chronic respiratory acidosis are routinely able to tolerate a low PaO_2 and an elevated $PaCO_2$ because of compensation (increased number of red blood cells, hemoglobin content, and 2,3-diphosphoglycerate). The drive to breathe in these patients is dependent on hypoxemia rather than hypercarbia. Administration of oxygen to a patient with chronic respiratory acidosis can eliminate this drive to breathe and result in the syndrome of carbon dioxide narcosis. In this case, if the PaO_2 is 50 mm Hg (6.7 kPa), no oxygen treatment is necessary. If the PaO_2 is less than 50 mm Hg (less than 6.7 kPa), oxygen therapy should be initiated carefully using a controlled flow of oxygen.[2]

ABGs should be checked periodically to ensure adequate oxygenation. If the $PaCO_2$ increases during oxygen therapy, it can be a sign of impending carbon dioxide narcosis and oxygen therapy may need to be discontinued. The underlying cause of the acute exacerbation should be aggressively managed. Pulmonary infections should be treated with the appropriate antibiotics and bronchodilators administered as necessary. Excess secretions should be cleared from the airway to allow proper gas exchange. This can involve increasing oral fluid intake to decrease the viscosity of secretions, deep breathing, and postural drainage, suction, or bronchoscopy.

MIXED ACID–BASE DISORDERS

Diagnosis

The diagnosis of a mixed disorder depends on an understanding of the appropriate quantitative response of the compensatory mechanisms for each of the simple acid–base disturbances.[2,3,25] To diagnose mixed disorders, one must know how each of the four simple disorders alters pH, $PaCO_2$, and (HCO_3^-) (see Table 52-7). If a given set of blood gases does not decrease within the range of expected responses for a simple acid–base disturbance, a mixed disorder should be suspected. In addition to laboratory information, a thorough history and physical examination of the patient will often lead to the diagnosis, even before the laboratory data are available. Examples of common mixed disturbances follow.

Mixed Respiratory Acidosis and Metabolic Acidosis

A mixed respiratory and metabolic acidosis disturbance is characterized by a failure of compensation. The respiratory disorder prevents the compensatory decrease in $PaCO_2$ expected in the defense against metabolic acidosis. The metabolic disorder prevents the buffering and renal mechanisms from raising the bicarbonate concentration as expected in the defense against respiratory acidosis. In the absence of these compensatory mechanisms, the pH decreases markedly.

Mixed respiratory and metabolic acidosis may develop in patients with cardiorespiratory arrest, in those with chronic lung disease who are in shock, and in metabolic acidosis patients who develop respiratory failure. When treating this mixed disorder, clinicians need to respond to both the respiratory and metabolic acidosis. Improved oxygen delivery must be initiated to improve hypercarbia and hypoxia. Mechanical ventilation may be needed to reduce $PaCO_2$. During the initial stage of therapy, appropriate amounts of alkali should be given to reverse the metabolic acidosis (see "Treatment," "Metabolic Acidosis" above).

Mixed Respiratory Alkalosis and Metabolic Alkalosis

The combination of respiratory and metabolic alkalosis is the most common mixed acid–base disorder. This mixed disorder occurs frequently in critically ill surgical patients with respiratory alkalosis caused by mechanical ventilation, hypoxia, sepsis, hypotension, neurologic damage, pain, or drugs, and with metabolic alkalosis caused by vomiting or nasogastric suctioning and massive blood transfusions. It can also occur in patients with hepatic cirrhosis who hyperventilate, receive diuretics, or vomit, as well as in patients with chronic respiratory acidosis and an elevated plasma bicarbonate concentration who are placed on mechanical ventilation and undergo a rapid decrease in $PaCO_2$.

The renal excretion of bicarbonate that usually occurs as compensation for the respiratory alkalosis is prevented by the complicating metabolic alkalosis. Likewise, the retention of $PaCO_2$ expected to compensate for metabolic alkalosis is prevented by the primary respiratory alkalosis. The failure of compensation that occurs with mixed respiratory and metabolic alkalosis can result in a severe alkalemia.

Administration of sodium chloride and potassium chloride solutions will help correct the metabolic component of a mixed respiratory and metabolic alkalosis, and adjustment of the ventilator and/or treatment of an underlying process that is causing hyperventilation can correct or ameliorate the respiratory component of this mixed disorder.

Mixed Metabolic Acidosis and Respiratory Alkalosis

This mixed disorder is often seen in patients with advanced liver disease, salicylate intoxication, and pulmonary-renal syndromes. The respiratory alkalosis will decrease the $PaCO_2$ beyond the appropriate range for the respiratory compensation usually seen with metabolic acidosis. The plasma bicarbonate concentration also decreases below the level expected in compensation for a simple respiratory alkalosis. In a sense, the defense of pH for either disorder alone is enhanced; thus the pH can be normal or close to normal, with a low $PaCO_2$ and a low (HCO_3^-). Treatment of this disorder should be directed at the underlying cause. Because of the enhanced compensation, the pH is usually closer to normal than in either of the two simple disorders.

Mixed Metabolic Alkalosis and Respiratory Acidosis

This mixed disorder often occurs in patients with chronic obstructive pulmonary disease and chronic respiratory acidosis who are treated with salt restriction, diuretics, and possibly glucocorticoids. When diuretics are initiated, the plasma bicarbonate may increase because of increased renal bicarbonate generation and reabsorption, providing mechanisms for both generating and maintaining metabolic alkalosis. The elevated pH diminishes respiratory drive and may therefore worsen the respiratory acidosis.

Although the pH may not deviate significantly from normal, treatment may need to be initiated to maintain PaO_2 and $PaCO_2$ at acceptable levels. Because it is often difficult to correctly identify this mixed disorder, it is helpful to observe the patient's response to discontinuation of diuretics and administration of sodium and potassium chloride.[2,25] The $PaCO_2$ will normalize if the patient has a simple metabolic alkalosis, but it will be minimally affected in the setting of a mixed disorder. Treatment should be aimed at decreasing the plasma bicarbonate with sodium and potassium chloride therapy, thereby allowing the renal excretion of retained bicarbonate from the diuretic-induced metabolic alkalosis. This therapy should be used cautiously to avoid exacerbating any underlying congestive heart failure.

CLINICAL BOTTOM LINE

Acid–base disorders are a common and widespread problem, and clinicians can play a key role in identifying, preventing, and properly treating them. Acid–base disorders do not occur only in the intensive care unit setting. Patients in ambulatory and extended care settings have many chronic conditions and drug therapies that commonly affect acid–base balance. Thus clinicians in all practice settings should strive to identify patients at high risk for developing drug-related problems that affect acid–base balance and to undertake appropriate prevention and treatment measures to improve the quality of life of their patients.

ABBREVIATIONS

BW	body weight
DCA	dichloroacetate
ECF	extracellular fluid
H^+	hydrogen ion
HCO_3^-	bicarbonate
H_2CO_3	carbonic acid
HIV	human immunodeficiency virus
NH_4^+	ammonium
$PaCO_2$	partial pressure of carbon dioxide from arterial blood
PaO_2	partial pressure of oxygen from arterial blood
pH	the negative logarithm (base 10) of the hydrogen ion concentration
pK	the negative logarithm of the dissociation constant
$PvCO_2$	partial pressure of carbon dioxide from venous blood
PvO_2	partial pressure of oxygen from venous blood
RTA	renal tubular acidosis
SAG	serum anion gap
THAM	tromethamine (Tris[hydroxymethyl]-aminomethane)
UCs	unmeasured cations
UAs	unmeasured anions

REFERENCES

1. Berend K, de Vries AP, Gans RO. Physiological approach to assessment of acid-base disturbances. *N Engl J Med* 2014;37:1434-1445.
2. Palmer BF, Perazella MA, Choi MJ. American Society of Nephrology Quiz and Questionnaire 2013: electrolyte and acid-base. *Clin J Am Soc Nephrol* 2014;9:1132-1137.
3. Seifter JL. Integration of acid-base and electrolyte disorders. *N Engl J Med* 2014;371:1821-31.
4. Kraut JA, Madias NE. Metabolic acidosis: Pathophysiology, diagnosis and management. *Nat Rev Nephrol* 2010;6:274-285.
5. Albert MS, Dell RB, Winters RW. Quantitative displacement of acid–base equilibrium in metabolic acidosis. *Ann Intern Med* 1964;66:312-322.
6. Chadra V, Alon US. Hereditary renal tubular disorders. *Semin Nephrol* 2009;29:399-411.
7. Palmer BF, Clegg DJ. Electrolyte and acid-base disturbances in patients with diabetes mellitus. *N Eng J Med* 2015;373:548-559.
8. Kamel KS, Halperin ML. Acid-base problems in diabetic ketoacidosis. *N Engl J Med* 2015;372:546-554.
9. Dounousi E, Zikou X, Koulouras V, et al. Metabolic acidosis during parenteral nutrition: pathophysiological mechanisms. *Indian J Crit Care Med* 2015;19:270-274.
10. Kitterer D, Schwab M, Alscher MD, et al. Drug-induced acid-base disorders. *Pediatr Nephrol* 2015;30:1407-1423.
11. Reddy P. Clinical approach to renal tubular acidosis in adult patients. *Int J Clin Pract* 2011;65:350-360.
12. Kraut JA, Nagami GT. The serum anion gap in the evaluation of acid-base disorders: What are its limitations and can its effectiveness be improved? *Clin J Am Soc Nephrol* 2013;8:2018-2024.
13. Kraut JA, Madias NE. Lactic acidosis. *N Engl J Med* 2014;371:2309-2319.
14. Al Jaghbeer M, Kellum JA. Acid-base disturbances in intensive care unit patients: etiology, pathophysiology and treatment. *Nephrol Dial Transplant* 2015;30:1104-1111.
15. Wiener SW. Toxicologic acid-base disorders. *Emerg Med Clin North Am* 2014;32:149-165.
16. Margolis AM, Heverling H, Pham PA, et al. A review of the toxicity of HIV medications. *J Med Toxicol* 2014;10:26-39.
17. Kajbaf F, Lalau JD. Mortality rate in so-called 'metformin-associated lactic acidosis": A review of the data since the 1960s. *Pharmacoepidemiol Drug Saf* 2014;23:1123-1127.
18. Lalau JD. Lactic acidosis induced by metformin: Incidence, management and prevention. *Drug Saf* 2010;33:727-740.
19. Kishor K, Dhasmana N, Kamble SS, et al. Linezolid induced adverse drug reactions–an update. *Curr Drug Metab* 2015;16:553-559.
20. Woloshin S, Schwartz LM. The new weight-loss drugs, lorcaserin and phentermine-topiramate: slim pickings? *JAMA Intern Med* 2014;174:615-619.
21. Horinek EL, Kiser TH, Fish DN, et al. Propylene glycol accumulation in critically ill patients receiving intravenous lorazepam infusions. *Ann Pharmacother* 2009;43:1964-1971.

22. Pillai U, Hothi JC, Bhat ZY. Severe propylene glycol toxicity secondary to use of anti-epileptics. *Am J Ther* 2014;21:106-109.
23. Mirrakhimov AE, Voore P, Halytskyy O, et al. Propofol infusion syndrome: A clinical update. *Crit Care Res Pract* 2015;260:385-393.
24. Chauhan V, Kelepouris E, Chauban N, et al. Current concepts and management strategies in chronic kidney disease-Mineral and bone disorders. *South Med J* 2012;1045:479-485.
25. Adrogues HJ. Mixed acid–base disturbances. *J Nephrol* 2006; 19(Suppl 9):S97-S103.
26. Kim HJ, Son YK, An WS. Effect of sodium bicarbonate administration on mortality in patients with lactic acidosis: A retrospective analysis. *PLoS One* 2013;8:e65283.
27. Velissaris D, Karamouzos V, Ktenopoulos N, et al. The use of sodium bicarbonate in the treatment of acidosis in sepsis: A literature update on a long-term debate. *Crit Care Res Pract* 2015 (Epub 2015 July 20).
28. Adrogue HJ, Rashad MN, Gorin AB, et al. Assessing acid–base status in circulatory failure: Differences between arterial and central venous blood. *N Engl J Med* 1989;320:1312-1316.
29. Gomez H, Kellum JA. Understanding acid-base disorders. *Crit Care Clin* 2015;31:849-860.
30. Callaway CW, Soar J, Aibiki M, et al. Part 4: Advanced Life Support: 2015 International Consensus on Cardiopulmonary Resuscitation and Emergency Cardiovascular Care Science With Treatment Recommendations. *Circulation* 2015;132(16 Suppl 1):S84-145.
31. McEvoy GK, Litvak K, Welsh OH, et al. American Hospital Formulary Service, Drug Information. Bethesda, MD: American Society of Health-System Pharmacists, 2015.
32. Geraci MJ, Klipa D, Heckman MG, et al. Prevalence of sodium bicarbonate-induced alkalemia in cardiopulmonary arrest patients. *Ann Pharmacother* 2009;43:1245-1250.
33. Hoste EA, Colpaert K, Vanholder RC, et al. Sodium bicarbonate versus THAM in ICU patients with mild metabolic acidosis. *J Nephrol* 2005;18:303-307.
34. Stacpoole PW, Wright EC, Baumgartner TG, et al. A controlled clinical trial of dichloroacetate for treatment of lactic acidosis. *N Engl J Med* 1992;327:1564-1569.
35. Stacpoole PW, Nagaraja NV, Hutson AD. Efficacy of dichloroacetate as a lactate-lowering drug. *J Clin Pharmacol* 2003;43:683-691.
36. Vary TC, Siegel JH, Zechnich A, et al. Pharmacologic reversal of abnormal glucose regulation, BCAA utilization, and muscle catabolism in sepsis by dichloroacetate. *J Trauma* 1988;28:1301-1311.
37. Shangraw RE, Lohan-Mannion D, Hayes A, et al. Dichloroacetate stabilizes the intraoperative acid–base balance during liver transplantation. *Liver Transpl* 2008;14:989-998.
38. Soifer JT, Kim HT. Approach to metabolic alkalosis. *Emerg Med Clin North Am* 2014;32:453-463.
39. Gennari FJ. Pathophysiology of metabolic alkalosis: A new classification based on the centrality of stimulated collecting duct ion transport. *Am J Kidney Dis* 2011;58:626-636.
40. Mikhalidis G, Mikhailidis DP, Elisaf M. Acid–base and electrolyte abnormalities observed in patients receiving cardiovascular drugs. *J Cardiovasc Pharmacol Ther* 2003;8:267-279.
41. Graziani G, Fedeli C, Moroni L, et al. Gitelman syndrome: Pathophysiological and clinical aspects. *QJM* 2010;103:741-748.
42. Barton CH, Vaziri ND, Ness RL, et al. Cimetidine in the management of metabolic alkalosis induced by nasogastric drainage. *Arch Surg* 1979;1:70-74.
43. Mazur JE, Devlin JW, Peters MJ, et al. Single versus multiple doses of acetazolamide for metabolic alkalosis in critically ill medical patients: A randomized, double-blind trial. *Crit Care Med* 1999;27:1257-1261.
44. Rowlands BJ, Tindall SF, Elliot DJ. The use of dilute hydrochloric acid and cimetidine to reverse severe metabolic alkalosis. *Postgrad Med J* 1978;54:118-123.
45. Heble DE, Oschman A, Sandritter TL. Comparison of arginine hydrochloride and acetazolamide for the correction of metabolic alkalosis in pediatric patients. *Am J Ther* 2014 (Epub 2014 Nov 6). DOI: 10.1097/MJT.0000000000000147.
46. Hene RJ, Koomans HA, Dorhout Mees EJ, et al. Correction of hypokalemia in Bartter's syndrome by enalapril. *Am J Kidney Dis* 1987;9:200-205.
47. Vinci JM, Gill JR Jr, Bowden RE, et al. The Kallikrein-Kinin system in Bartter's syndrome and its response to prostaglandin synthetase inhibition. *J Clin Invest* 1987;61:1671-1682.
48. Guerin C, Nesme P, Leray V, et al. Quantitative analysis of acid-base disorders in patients with chronic respiratory failure in stable or unstable respiratory condition. *Respir Care* 2010;55:1453-1463.

Evaluation of Neurologic Illness

e53

Melody Ryan, Stephen J. Ryan, and Susan C. Fagan

KEY CONCEPTS

1. Accurate diagnosis of neurological disorders leads to effective pharmacotherapy.
2. The clinical neurologic history and examination are the cornerstones of neurologic diagnosis and management.
3. The neurologic history and examination are directed at localization of the disease process so that evaluation and management may be planned appropriately.
4. Appropriate history taking and examination techniques are useful for monitoring and evaluating the pharmacotherapeutic plan.
5. After forming the differential diagnosis, appropriate testing helps pinpoint the correct diagnosis.

(1) Accurate diagnosis of neurological disorders leads to effective pharmacotherapy. This diagnosis is built upon history, a detailed neurological examination, and appropriate testing. To contribute most effectively to the care of patients with neurologic illness, one must understand the tools used in the diagnosis and management of these patients. In addition, clinicians must be able to gather their own data through history taking and a targeted neurologic examination to ensure optimal pharmacotherapy in neurologic patients. (2) Despite technologic advances that have led to the development of sensitive diagnostic tests in neuroscience, the clinical neurologic history and examination are still the cornerstones of neurologic diagnosis and management.[1]

SIGNS AND SYMPTOMS OF NEUROLOGIC DISORDERS

(2) As in all of medicine, obtaining an accurate and complete history is of utmost importance in the evaluation of neurologic diseases. In many instances, the diagnosis can be made on the basis of the history, and the neurologic examination can be tailored to optimally evaluate the patient and confirm the diagnosis.[1] Open-ended questions allow the patient to provide the salient history without leading the patient toward preconceived diagnoses. Obtaining an accurate history may be difficult because a number of neurologic diseases may affect patients' communication and memory. Details obtained from the family or other observers support and further expand the data obtained from the patient during history taking; additionally family history can be helpful in diagnosis.[1] Through the patient's history, one can determine the main symptoms, location, onset (acute, subacute, or chronic), progression over time (maximal at onset or steadily gaining intensity), and associated illnesses or risk factors for neurologic disease.[2] The history should also identify factors that might precipitate or ameliorate the symptoms.[2] Each complaint of the patient should be thoroughly investigated while taking the history. See Table e53-1 for questions to assist the clinician in obtaining the neurologic history.

As part of the history, special attention should be given to the medication history. It is important to determine current medications, doses, dosing schedule (times, relationship to other medications, and relationship to meals), duration, and adherence. Additionally, adverse effects should be recorded in detail. Past and recently discontinued medications as well as any medications used previously, including reasons for discontinuation, to treat the main complaints may also be important. Clinicians should also consider if the patient's symptoms may be drug-induced.

Additional history is necessary for pediatric patients. History may be obtained from the patients, guardians, or caretakers rather than the child in most cases.[3] The child should be allowed to provide as much history as he/she is developmentally able to do so. Because of the differing developmental stages of children, the amount of information the child is able to provide will vary with age. Family history is particularly important because some pediatric illnesses have an inherited genetic cause.[3] History of the pregnancy, including maternal illnesses, medication or toxin exposures, and complications, should be noted.[3] Details of labor and delivery including duration, method of delivery, and complications may also be important.[3] Developmental history requires comparison of the child's developmental stage to standard age-related developmental milestones.[3]

THE NEUROLOGIC EXAMINATION

A general physical examination is important because it can reveal evidence of systemic disease that may secondarily affect the nervous system.[2] The neurologic examination is one component of a complete general physical examination. (3) A detailed neurologic examination is an extremely important tool for localizing a lesion within the nervous system.

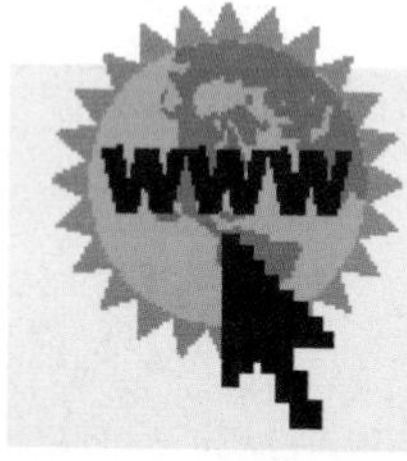

The complete chapter, learning objectives, and other resources can be found at **www.pharmacotherapyonline.com.**

54

Alzheimer Disease

Emily P. Peron, Patricia W. Slattum, Kacie E. Powers, and Sarah E. Hobgood

KEY CONCEPTS

1. Alzheimer disease (AD) is the most common form of dementing illness, and the prevalence of AD increases with each decade of life.
2. The etiology of AD is unknown, and current pharmacotherapy neither cures nor arrests the pathophysiology.
3. Neuritic plaques and neurofibrillary tangles (NFTs) are the pathologic hallmarks of AD; however, the definitive cause of this disease is yet to be determined.
4. Alzheimer disease affects multiple areas of cognition and is characterized by a gradual onset with a slow, progressive decline.
5. A thorough physical examination (including neurologic examination), as well as laboratory and imaging studies, is required to rule out other disorders and diagnose AD before considering drug therapy.
6. Pharmacotherapy for AD focuses on impacting three domains: cognition, behavioral and psychiatric symptoms, and functional ability.
7. Nondrug therapy and social support for the patient and family are the primary treatment interventions for AD.
8. Cholinesterase inhibitors and memantine are used to treat cognitive symptoms of AD; other medications have been suggested to be beneficial because of their potential preventive or cognitive effects.
9. Appropriate management of vascular disease risk factors may reduce the risk for developing AD and may prevent the worsening of dementia in patients with AD.
10. A thorough behavioral assessment and plan with careful examination of environmental factors should be conducted before initiating drug therapy for behavioral symptoms.

"I now begin the journey that will lead me into the sunset of my life."
Ronald Reagan

Alzheimer disease (AD), first characterized by Alois Alzheimer in 1907, is a gradually progressive dementia affecting cognition, behavior, and functional status. The exact pathophysiologic mechanisms underlying AD are not entirely known, and no cure exists.[1] Although drugs may reduce AD symptoms for a time, the disease is eventually fatal.

Alzheimer disease profoundly affects the family as well as the patient. The need for supervision and assistance increases until the late stages of the disease, when AD patients become totally dependent on a caregiver for all of their basic needs. These are the all-too-common experiences of the millions of people in the United States who care for someone with AD. To address the growing AD crisis facing the United States, the first national strategic plan, the National Alzheimer's Plan, was released in 2012 with the goals of coordinating efforts across the federal government to prevent and treat AD, increase public awareness, and improve the quality of care and support for patients and their caregivers.[2] The U.S. Department of Health and Human Services released an update to this strategic plan in 2015 that includes a timeline for achieving its goal of preventing and effectively treating AD by 2025.[2]

EPIDEMIOLOGY

1 Alzheimer disease is the most common cause of dementia, accounting for approximately 60% of cases in persons over age 65 years.[3] Its prevalence among dementia patients increases to 80% if AD lesions in conjunction with other pathologic brain lesions are considered.[3-5] Table 54-1 lists the most common types of dementia. Dementia can result from multiple etiologies. This chapter focuses exclusively on dementia of the Alzheimer type; however, the reader is encouraged to use the nonpharmacologic approaches and management of behavioral problems outlined in this chapter as a general treatment approach for other types of dementia that may share similar features with AD.

Approximately 5.3 million Americans have AD.[3,6] By the year 2050, one in five people will be older than age 65 years, and the number of AD patients is projected to be 13.8 million (Fig. 54-1).[6] Most cases present in persons older than age 65 years, but approximately 4% of cases occur in persons younger than age 65 years. Onset can be as early as age 30 years, resulting in the arbitrary age classifications of early-onset (age less than 65 years) and late-onset (age 65 years and older).[5]

Increasing age is the greatest risk factor for AD, but AD is not a normal part of aging. The prevalence of AD increases exponentially with age, affecting approximately 11% of people age 65 years and older and 32% of people age 85 years and older.[3] Factors determining age of onset and rate of progression remain largely undefined.

Survival following AD diagnosis is typically 4 to 8 years but may be as long as 20 years. It is the fifth leading cause of death for those age 65 years and older in the United States. AD may not cause death directly. The most common cause of death in patients with AD is pneumonia, possibly resulting from swallowing difficulties and immobility in the terminal stage of the disease.[3] Those diagnosed with AD spend, on average, more years in the most severe stage of the disease than any other stage, and much of this time is spent in a nursing home.[3]

TABLE 54-1 Common Types of Dementia in Late Life

Alzheimer disease
Vascular dementia
Dementia with Lewy bodies
Mixed dementia
Other (eg, Parkinson disease dementia, Frontotemporal dementia, Huntington disease, Creutzfeldt–Jakob disease)
Potentially reversible causes of cognitive dysfunction (eg, normal pressure hydrocephalus, thyroid dysfunction, vitamin B_{12} deficiency, delirium, depression, Wernicke–Korsakoff syndrome)

Data from References 2 and 123.

ETIOLOGY

Etiology and Genetics

2 The exact etiology of AD is unknown; however, several genetic and environmental factors have been explored as potential causes. Genetic factors have been linked to both early- and late-onset AD.

Dominantly inherited forms of AD account for less than 1% of cases.[7,8] More than half of early-onset, dominantly inherited cases of AD can be attributed to alterations on chromosomes 1, 14, or 21. The majority and most aggressive early-onset cases are attributed to mutations of a gene located on chromosome 14, which produces a protein called presenilin 1.[9] A structurally similar protein, presenilin 2, is produced by a gene on chromosome 1. Both presenilin 1 and presenilin 2 encode for membrane proteins that may be involved in amyloid precursor protein (APP) processing. Scientists have identified more than 160 mutations in presenilin genes, and these mutations appear to result in reduced activity of γ-secretase, an enzyme important in β-amyloid peptide (Aβ) formation.[9] APP is encoded on chromosome 21. Only a small number of early-onset familial AD cases have been associated with mutations in the APP gene, resulting in overproduction of Aβ or an increase in the proportion of Aβ ending at residue 42.[9]

Genetic susceptibility to late-onset AD is primarily linked to the apolipoprotein E (*APOE*) genotype. There are three major subtypes or alleles of *APOE* (eg, **2*, **3*, and **4*). Inheritance of the *APOE*4* allele is believed to account for much of the genetic risk in late-onset AD. The mechanism through which *APOE*4* confers an increased risk is unknown, although *APOE*4* is associated with factors that may contribute to AD pathology, such as abnormalities in mitochondria, cytoskeletal dysfunction, and low glucose usage.[5]

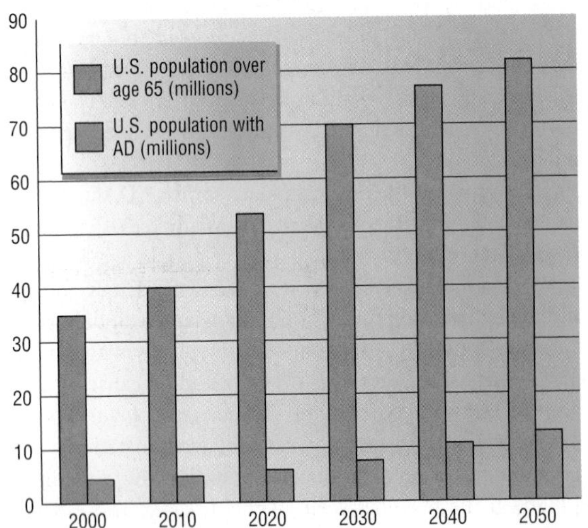

FIGURE 54-1 Our aging population. The percentage of the U.S. population older than age 65 years and the percentage with AD projected from years 2000 to 2050.[1,6] *(Estimates based on data from references 1 and 6.)*

The risk for AD is twofold to threefold higher in individuals with one *APOE*4* allele and 12-fold higher in individuals with two *APOE*4* alleles compared to those with no *APOE*4* alleles.[10] Moreover, onset of symptoms occurs at a relatively younger age as compared with patients having zero or only one copy of *APOE*4* in their genotype[10] Of note, the *APOE*4* allele is not diagnostic of AD or even essential for disease presence. Moreover, as of 2015, more than 25 different genetic loci have been discovered that are known to be associated with late-onset AD.[11,12] Genetic explanatory factors continue to be investigated.[12]

Environmental and Other Factors

A number of environmental factors are associated with an increased risk of AD, including age, decreased reserve capacity of the brain (reduced brain size, low educational level, and reduced mental and physical activity in late life), head injury, Down syndrome, depression, mild cognitive impairment (MCI), and risk factors for vascular disease (hypercholesterolemia, hypertension, atherosclerosis, coronary heart disease, smoking, elevated homocysteine, obesity, metabolic syndrome, and diabetes).[3,5] Whether these vascular risk factors are true causal risk factors for AD contributing to AD pathology, or whether they result in cerebrovascular pathology that, in turn, contributes to the symptoms of AD, remains to be established.

The incidence of AD rises with increasing age, and AD may develop in individuals over the course of decades,[3] suggesting that AD is a disease most people are in the process of developing throughout adulthood. The debate about whether dementia is a distinct disease or part of aging remains unresolved. An in-depth discussion of the aging—AD controversy is not possible in this chapter; it is reviewed elsewhere.[13,14]

PATHOPHYSIOLOGY

3 The signature lesions in AD are amyloid plaques and neurofibrillary tangles (NFTs) located in the cortical areas and medial temporal lobe structures of the brain.[4] Along with these lesions, degeneration of neurons and synapses, as well as cortical atrophy occurs. Plaques and NFTs may also be present in other diseases, even in normal aging, but at least in younger demographics there tends to be a higher burden of plaques and NFTs in AD-affected subjects than there is in age-matched controls. Several mechanisms have been proposed to explain changes in the brain that result in symptoms of AD, including misfolding of proteins (Aβ aggregation and deposition leading to the formation of plaques and hyperphosphorylation of tau protein leading to NFT development); synaptic failure and depletion of neurotrophin and neurotransmitters; and mitochondrial dysfunction (oxidative stress, impaired insulin signaling in the brain, vascular injury, inflammatory processes, loss of calcium regulation, and defects in cholesterol metabolism).[4]

Amyloid Cascade Hypothesis

Amyloid plaques are extracellular lesions found in the brain and cerebral vasculature. Plaques largely consist of Aβ. Aβ peptides consisting of 36 to 43 amino acids are produced via processing of a larger protein, APP. Aβ_{42} is less common than other Aβ peptides, but is prone to aggregation and plaque formation.[4] The amyloid cascade hypothesis states that there is an imbalance between the production and clearance of Aβ peptides resulting in aggregation that causes accumulation of Aβ ultimately leading to AD.[4] Studies on early-onset AD and patients with Down syndrome led to the formulation of the amyloid cascade hypothesis. Recent versions of the amyloid cascade hypothesis assume Aβ that is not sequestered in plaques actually drives the disease.[4] Even so, the amyloid cascade hypothesis seems most applicable in cases of early-onset, autosomal dominant AD. It is not clear whether it is reasonable to etiologically extrapolate to the late-onset form (which afflicts the vast majority of those affected). Whether individuals with late-onset AD also carry genetic variations that promote a primary Aβ amyloidosis remains to be shown. If this turns out not to be the case, the possibility that amyloidosis in late-onset AD is secondary to a more upstream event will require consideration. Before this conceptual conundrum is laid to rest, however, the amyloid cascade hypothesis will likely undergo a therapy-based practical test. If treatments that efficiently reduce Aβ production or remove brain Aβ fail to arrest disease progression, it would argue amyloidosis is not the primary pathology in most of those with AD.

Neurofibrillary Tangles

At the same time as Aβ was being identified in plaques, other researchers showed that NFTs are commonly found in the cells of the hippocampus and cerebral cortex in persons with AD and are composed of abnormally hyperphosphorylated tau protein. Tau protein provides structural support to microtubules, the cell's transportation and skeletal support system.[4] When tau filaments undergo abnormal phosphorylation at a specific site, they cannot bind effectively to microtubules, and the microtubules collapse. Without an intact system of microtubules, the cell cannot function properly and eventually dies. The density of the NFTs correlates with the severity of the dementia.[4] NFTs are found in other dementing illnesses besides AD, and may represent a common method by which various inciting factors culminate in cell death.[4]

Inflammatory Mediators

Inflammatory or immunologic paradigms are often viewed as a corollary of the amyloid cascade hypothesis. Certainly, brain amyloid deposition associates with local inflammatory and immunologic alterations. This led some to propose that inflammation is relevant to AD neurodegeneration.[4] Inflammatory/immunologic hypotheses argue that although Aβ may have direct neurotoxicity, at least some of its toxicity might actually be an indirect consequence of an Aβ protofibril-induced microglia activation and astrocyte recruitment. This inflammatory response may represent an attempt to clear amyloid deposition; however, it is also associated with release of cytokines, nitric oxide, and other radical species, and complement factors that can both injure neurons and promote ongoing inflammation.[4] Indeed, levels of multiple cytokines and chemokines are elevated in AD brains, and certain proinflammatory gene polymorphisms are reported to be associated with AD.[4]

Consistent with these molecular observations are epidemiologic data suggesting that exposure to nonsteroidal antiinflammatory drugs (NSAIDs) may reduce AD risk.[15] However, multiple prospective short duration trials of NSAIDs in AD prevention and of NSAIDs as AD treatment have been disappointing.[4,16]

The Cholinergic Hypothesis

Multiple neuronal pathways are destroyed in AD. Neuronal damage can be seen in conjunction with plaque structures.[4] Widespread cell dysfunction or degeneration results in a variety of neurotransmitter deficits, with cholinergic abnormalities being the most prominent.[4] Loss of cholinergic activity correlates with AD severity. In the late stage of AD, the number of cholinergic neurons is reduced, and there is loss of nicotinic receptors in the hippocampus and cortex. Presynaptic nicotinic receptors control the release of acetylcholine, as well as other neurotransmitters important for memory and mood, including glutamate, serotonin, and norepinephrine.[4]

The discovery of vast cholinergic cell loss led to the development of a cholinergic hypothesis of the pathophysiology of AD. The cholinergic hypothesis targeted cholinergic cell loss as the source of memory and cognitive impairment in AD. Consequently, it was presumed that increasing cholinergic function would improve symptoms of memory loss. This approach is flawed because cholinergic cell loss appears to be a secondary consequence of AD pathology, not the disease-producing event, and cholinergic neurons are only one of many neuronal pathways destroyed in AD. Simple addition of acetylcholine cannot compensate for the loss of neurons, receptors, and other neurotransmitters lost during the course of the illness. Thus the goal is to minimize or improve symptoms through augmentation of neurotransmission at remaining synapses.

Other Neurotransmitter Abnormalities

Although the cholinergic system has received particular attention in AD pharmaceutical research, deficits also exist in other neuronal pathways. For example, serotonergic neurons of the raphe nuclei and noradrenergic cells of the locus ceruleus are lost, while monoamine oxidase type B activity is increased. Monoamine oxidase type B is found predominantly in the brain and in platelets, and is responsible for metabolizing dopamine. In addition, abnormalities appear in glutamate pathways of the cortex and limbic structures, where a loss of neurons leads to a focus on excitotoxicity models as possible contributing factors to AD pathology.

Glutamate is the major excitatory neurotransmitter in the cortex and hippocampus. Many neuronal pathways essential to learning and memory use glutamate as a neurotransmitter, including the pyramidal neurons (a layer of neurons with long axons carrying information out of the cortex), hippocampus, and entorhinal cortex. Glutamate and other excitatory amino acid neurotransmitters have been implicated as potential neurotoxins in AD.[17] Dysregulated glutamate activity is thought to be one of the primary mediators of neuronal injury after stroke or acute brain injury. Although intimately involved in cell injury, the role of excitatory amino acids in AD is as yet unclear; however, blockade of *N*-methyl-D-aspartate (NMDA) receptors decreases activity of glutamate in the synapse and may hypothetically lessen the degree of cellular injury in AD.

Brain Vascular Disease and High Cholesterol

There is growing evidence of a causal association between cardiovascular disease and its risk factors and the incidence of AD. Cardiovascular risk factors that are also risk factors for dementia include hypertension, hypercholesterolemia, and diabetes.[18] Brain vascular disease may augment the cognitive impairment observed for a given amount of AD pathology in the brain. Dysfunctional blood vessels may impair nutrient delivery to neurons and reduce clearance of Aβ from the brain.[4] Vascular disease may accelerate amyloid deposition and increase amyloid toxicity to neurons.[4] Midlife hypertension is adversely associated with AD, while late-life hypertension may show an inverse association with AD.[19] Mechanistically, the increased risk of AD seen among patients with prediabetes and diabetes may be a result of microvascular damage or direct neurotoxicity related to increased glucose and insulin levels.[19] Disturbances in insulin-signaling pathways, both in the periphery and the brain, have been linked to AD. Insulin may also regulate the metabolism of Aβ and tau protein.[20]

Research has found multiple links between cholesterol and AD. *APOE* is synthesized in the liver, central nervous system, and cerebrospinal fluid (CSF) and is responsible for transporting cholesterol in the blood through the brain. It is carried by low-density lipoprotein into neurons and binds to NFTs. *APOE*4* is associated with increasing deposition of Aβ and is thought to act as an accelerating modulator in vascular dementia. Elevated cholesterol levels in brain neurons may alter membrane functioning and result in the cascade leading to plaque formation and AD.

Other Mechanisms

Other hypotheses proposed to explain AD pathogenesis include oxidative stress, mitochondrial dysfunction, and loss of estrogen. Each of these mechanisms may contribute to AD pathogenesis, but the extent of the contribution is uncertain. There is a growing body of evidence of a role for oxidative stress and the accumulation of free radicals in the brain of AD patients.[4] Some epidemiologic studies suggest vitamin E, and possibly the combination of vitamin E and vitamin C, may reduce AD risk while others do not.[4] Mitochondrial dysfunction may result in disruption of energy metabolism in the neuron.[4,21-23] The role of estrogen in cognitive aging and dementia continues to be an active area of investigation. Despite convincing evidence that estrogens affect the brain in ways that would be expected to improve cognitive aging and reduce the risk of AD, the results of clinical studies have been largely disappointing.[21] A single common mechanism for producing AD does not exist. Regardless of the source, however, the features remain the same: degeneration of neurons in higher brain areas; accumulation of NFTs and amyloid plaques; profound destruction of cholinergic pathways; and an insidious dementia, slowly progressive until death.

TABLE 54-2 Stages of Alzheimer Disease

Stage	Description
Mild (MMSE score 26–21)	Patient has difficulty remembering recent events. Ability to manage finances, prepare food, and carry out other household activities declines. May get lost while driving. Begins to withdraw from difficult tasks and to give up hobbies. May deny memory problems
Moderate (MMSE score 20–10)	Patient requires assistance with activities of daily living. Frequently disoriented with regard to time (date, year, and season). Recall for recent events is severely impaired. May forget some details of past life and names of family and friends. Functioning may fluctuate from day to day. Patient generally denies problems. May become suspicious or tearful. Loses ability to drive safely. Agitation, paranoia, and delusions are common
Severe (MMSE score 9–0)	Patient loses ability to speak, walk, and feed self. Incontinent of urine and feces. Requires care 24 hours a day, 7 days a week

MMSE, Mini-Mental State Examination.

Data from References 38 *and* 124.

CLINICAL PRESENTATION AND DIAGNOSIS

4 The onset of AD is almost imperceptible, without abrupt changes in cognition or function. Deficits occur progressively over time, affecting multiple areas of cognition.[3,23] For treatment and assessment purposes, it is helpful to divide AD symptoms into two basic categories: cognitive symptoms and noncognitive (behavioral) symptoms. Cognitive symptoms are present throughout the illness, whereas behavioral symptoms are less predictable. Table 54-2 summarizes the stages of AD.

Diagnosis

A family member often first brings memory complaints to the attention of a primary care clinician. Up to 75% of patients who meet criteria for dementia are not given a diagnosis in the primary care setting, leading some to believe that an appropriate screening tool may be helpful in aiding diagnosis and leading to earlier treatment.[24] Despite the phenomenon of underdiagnosis, the U.S. Preventative Services Task Force concluded that there are insufficient data to recommend for or against cognitive screening for AD because it could not be determined if the benefits outweigh the risks.[24] Screening is being promoted as part of the Medicare Annual Wellness Visit by the Alzheimer's Association (AA).[25] The Mini-Mental State Examination (MMSE) is a widely used 30-point assessment tool for AD; because of its copyrighted status, however, the MMSE must either be administered from memory or paid for by the user. Alternatives to the MMSE include the Mini-Cog, the St. Louis University Mental Status Exam (SLUMS), and the Montreal Cognitive Assessment (MoCA).[26]

Until recently the only way to confirm a clinical diagnosis of AD was through direct examination of brain tissue at autopsy or biopsy. Several criteria have been used in clinical practice and research for the detection and diagnosis of dementia, including the *Diagnostic and Statistical Manual of Mental Disorders*, Fifth Edition (DSM-5) criteria,[27] the Agency for Healthcare Research and

CLINICAL PRESENTATION Alzheimer Disease

General

- The patient may have vague memory complaints initially, or the patient's significant other may report that the patient is "forgetful." Cognitive decline is gradual over the course of illness. Behavioral disturbances may be present in moderate stages. Loss of daily function is common in advanced stages.

Symptoms

Cognitive

- Memory loss (poor recall and losing items)
- Aphasia (circumlocution and anomia)
- Apraxia
- Agnosia
- Disorientation (impaired perception of time and unable to recognize familiar people)
- Impaired executive function

Noncognitive

- Depression, psychotic symptoms (hallucinations and delusions)
- Behavioral disturbances (physical and verbal aggression, motor hyperactivity, uncooperativeness, wandering, repetitive mannerisms and activities, and combativeness)

Functional

- Inability to care for self (dressing, bathing, toileting, and eating)

Laboratory Tests

- Rule out vitamin B_{12} and folate deficiency
- Rule out hypothyroidism with thyroid function tests
- Blood cell counts, serum electrolytes, liver function tests

Other Diagnostic Tests

- Computed tomography (CT) or magnetic resonance imaging (MRI) scans may aid diagnosis

Quality (AHRQ) Guidelines,[28] the American Academy of Neurology Guidelines,[29] the National Institute of Neurological Disorders and Stroke (NINDS) criteria,[30] and the National Institute of Neurological and Communicative Disorders and Stroke (NINCDS) and the Alzheimer's Disease and Related Disorders Association (ADRDA) Criteria.[31] In 2011, revisions to the NINCDS-ADRDA Criteria for the clinical diagnosis of AD were recommended by the National Institute on Aging (NIA) and the AA.[32] DSM-5 provides criteria for diagnosis of minor and major neurocognitive disorders, with specific criteria for neurocognitive disorders due to AD.[27] The new NIA-AA criteria view AD as a spectrum beginning with a preclinical phase progressing to increasingly severe clinical stages of AD. Three workgroups formulated diagnostic criteria for the dementia phase,[33] the symptomatic, predementia phase (MCI),[34] and the asymptomatic, preclinical phase of AD.[35] The preclinical phase has been further broken down into three stages—Stage 1 (asymptomatic cerebral amyloidosis), Stage 2 (asymptomatic amyloidosis plus neurodegeration), and Stage 3 (amyloidosis plus neurodegeneration plus subtle cognitive/behavioral decline).[35] As U.S. guidelines are being updated, groups from Europe and the U.K. have published guidance documents in the meantime.[36,37]

Clinical **Controversy...**

Publication of the DSM-5 has changed the diagnostic criteria for AD, including the elimination of MCI and amendments to other terminology. Patients diagnosed and educated using the NIA-AA dementia staging recommendations may require assimilation to the new DSM-5 approach, which describes a spectrum of minor to major neurocognitive disorder rather than a diagnosis of dementia of the Alzheimer type. Controversy surrounds the potential implications for patients to process their diagnosis and its implications and the added burden placed on healthcare professionals to interpret the new criteria themselves. Despite the DSM update, many clinicians continue to educate patients and their loved ones using previous diagnostic criteria to enhance understanding. Clearly, translation of the new criteria and its terminology into widely used medical jargon will require time, money, and a commitment on the part of healthcare professionals and health systems.

At this time, AD is primarily a clinical diagnosis, but this will likely change in coming years as brain imaging, CSF, and other AD biomarkers become increasingly available for routine clinical use. The patient's examination should suggest that cognitive decline from a previously higher baseline has occurred. The history should corroborate this, and further indicate that cognitive decline has reached the point where changes in social or occupational functioning are present. It is possible to administer a sophisticated exam that defines cognitive domain strengths and weaknesses and enables a neuroanatomic localization of the observed deficits. When approached in this way, the exam can indicate a pattern of cognitive decline that is consistent with AD, and assist with rendering a diagnosis that is as much a diagnosis of inclusion as it is of exclusion.

Discussing the diagnosis of dementia is potentially distressing for patients and their loved ones, especially at first. Most people, however, prefer to be told about a dementia diagnosis, as it allows them to appropriately plan for the future and access necessary support and treatment services in the meantime.[38]

Objectively defining social or occupational dysfunction can prove tricky in the older patient who may be retired, and who may also lead a socially restricted lifestyle for reasons of frailty. For such patients, the minimal requirement is to establish a change in activities of daily living. Early on, this usually involves a change in instrumental activities of daily living (handling finances and organizing medications) rather than basic activities of daily living (hygiene and dressing). Some AD subspecialists use a detailed, standardized, semistructured interview of a nonpatient informant as the most critical piece of the diagnostic evaluation.[39]

5 For patients who meet criteria for dementia (whether the underlying cause is ultimately felt to be AD or not), current recommendations from the American Academy of Neurology include a neuroimaging study (CT or MRI), as well as a serologic evaluation that includes blood cell counts, serum electrolytes, liver function tests, a test of thyroid function, and a vitamin B_{12} level.[29] When circumstances suggest AD is not the leading entity on the differential diagnosis, other neurologic tests such as CSF analysis or electroencephalogram can occasionally be justified. Neuropsychological testing is also optional, but can prove quite useful for the diagnosis of AD by helping to establish a neuroanatomical localization for the patient's cognitive deficits.

Almost any medication can contribute to cognitive impairment in vulnerable individuals, but certain classes of medication are more commonly implicated. Benzodiazepines and other sedative hypnotics, anticholinergics, opioid analgesics, antipsychotics, and anticonvulsants have been associated with cognitive impairment.[40,41] NSAIDs, histamine H_2-receptor antagonists, digoxin, amiodarone, antihypertensives, and corticosteroids have been implicated in cases of delirium.[32] Because medications are a reversible cause of cognitive symptoms, medication review and management are essential.

Guidelines from the U.S., U.K., and Europe currently recommend that structural imaging (noncontrast enhanced CT or, ideally, MRI) be performed in the evaluation of patients with suspected dementia.[42] Efforts to define the role of other AD diagnostic tests are ongoing. Positron emission tomography scanning may reveal a pattern of hypometabolism typical of AD, but by itself the diagnostic accuracy of positron emission tomography scanning still lags behind that of the clinical examination and history.[35] *APOE* genotyping by itself is also insufficient to make or break a diagnosis of AD, but demonstrating an *APOE*4* allele in a suspected patient increases the specificity of the diagnosis and can help predict which patients with MCI are most likely to progress to a diagnosis of AD over the next several years.[43] Unless the patient developed dementia prior to age 60 years and also had a parent that developed AD before age 60 years, presenilin 1, presenilin 2, or APP genotyping is usually not indicated.

Mild Cognitive Impairment

It has long been recognized that aging individuals experience changes in cognitive function. MCI constitutes a syndromic designation that categorizes patients with cognitive complaints insufficient to warrant a diagnosis of dementia. The NIA-AA diagnostic criteria specifically address the diagnosis of MCI.[34] Persons diagnosed with MCI carry a 10% to 15% chance per year of progressing to an AD diagnosis.[44] What clinicians are likely seeing in most people with MCI is the initial manifestation of a progressive degenerative dementia that will eventually meet AD diagnostic criteria.[34,44] However, it is important to note that not everyone meeting MCI criteria will develop AD; the rate of progression of MCI to dementia remains uncertain.[45] As the MCI designation is increasingly applied, MCI criteria continue to evolve.[34,44]

TREATMENT

Desired Outcomes

6 The primary goal of treatment in AD is to symptomatically treat cognitive difficulties and preserve patient function as long as possible. Secondary goals include managing psychiatric and behavioral sequelae. Current AD treatments have not been shown to prolong

life, cure AD, or halt or reverse the pathophysiologic processes of the disorder.[39]

General Treatment Approach

Clinical trials have consistently demonstrated modest benefits of early and continuous treatment with cholinesterase inhibitors.[46] Memantine added in moderate to severe disease may also provide benefit. Following this approach allows for maximal maintenance of cognition and activities of daily living. A symptomatic approach is used to treat behavioral symptoms as they arise.

Provision of education to the patient and family at the time of diagnosis, including discussion of the course of illness, realistic expectations of treatment, and the importance of legal and financial planning, are essential to appropriate treatment.

Nonpharmacologic Therapy

7 Alzheimer disease has a profound effect on both the patient and family, so appropriate treatment is needed. Nonpharmacologic interventions are the current primary interventions for management of AD, and medications should be used in the context of multimodal interventions. Behavioral and psychiatric symptoms are among the most challenging and distressing symptoms of the disease and may be the determining factor in a family's decision to seek institutional care. Symptoms, such as sleep disturbances, wandering, urinary incontinence, agitation, and aggression in patients with dementia are best managed using behavioral interventions rather than medications whenever possible.[46,47]

Upon initial diagnosis, the patient and caregiver should be educated on the course of illness, prognosis, available treatments, legal decisions, and quality-of-life issues. Caregiving strategies, including stress-management techniques and support group options, should also be discussed. Caregiver education and support programs have been shown to improve caregiver skill, knowledge, confidence, and quality-of-life, and even delay time to nursing home placement for their loved one.[48] Table 54-3 lists basic principles of care for the AD patient. The general approach to nonpharmacologic strategies for behavioral symptoms is to identify the symptom, identify causative factors, and adapt the caregiving environment to remedy the situation.[3] Environmental triggers may include noise, glare, and too much background distraction, including television. Personal discomfort may also trigger behaviors, so it is important to monitor for pain, hunger, thirst, constipation, full bladder, fatigue, infections, skin irritation, comfortable temperature, fears, and frustrations.[49] Medical comorbidity is a major source of functional and cognitive impairment in patients with AD, so general health maintenance is warranted.[3] Interventions should redirect the patient's attention rather than be confrontational and should specifically address known triggers. Creating a calm environment and removing stressors and triggers is key. Other nonpharmacologic approaches include exercise, light therapy, music therapy, reminiscence therapy, aroma therapy, relaxation techniques, validation therapy, massage and touch therapy, and multisensory stimulation.[50] Caregivers should be referred to support services, such as the AA, for assistance in developing nonpharmacologic strategies for managing difficult behaviors.

The caregiver must be prepared to face the changes in life that will occur, and acceptance rarely comes easily. Denial on the part of the patient and rationalization on the part of the family are common. The clinician should encourage the family to address legal and financial matters and designate a durable power of attorney for execution of financial and medical decisions once the patient is incompetent. The caregiver will need to address issues such as respite services to provide time for rest, relaxation, and conduct of personal business. Eventually, the caregiver will need to face critical and difficult questions with respect to institutionalization. Local resources, such as the AA, can provide detailed information regarding support services. Table 54-4 lists this and other referral sources for caregivers.

Education, communication, and planning are key nonpharmacologic components of caring for a patient with AD. Preparation in the early stages of illness may lessen some of the caregiver stress as the illness progresses.

TABLE 54-3 Basic Principles of Care for the Patient with Alzheimer Disease

- Consider vision, hearing, or other sensory impairments
- Find optimal level of autonomy and adjust expectations for patient performance over time
- Avoid confrontation. Remain calm, firm, and supportive if the patient becomes upset
- Maintain a consistent, structured environment with stimulation level appropriate to the individual patient
- Provide frequent reminders, explanations, and orientation cues. Employ guiding, demonstration, and reinforcement
- Reduce choices, keep requests and demands of the patient simple, and avoid complex tasks that lead to frustration
- Bring sudden declines in function and the emergence of new symptoms to professional attention

Data from References 2 and 77.

TABLE 54-4 Resources for Caregivers of Persons with Alzheimer Disease

The following organizations provide educational literature and information on diagnosis, treatment, social support, and ongoing research in Alzheimer disease:
U.S. Administration on Aging, National Family Caregiver Support Program *http://www.aoa.gov*
National Institute on Aging Alzheimer's Disease Education & Referral Center (ADEAR) *http://www.nia.nih.gov/alzheimers*
The Alzheimer's Association *http://www.alz.org*
The Alzheimer's Research Forum *http://www.alzforum.org*
AARP *http://www.aarp.org*
National Family Caregivers Association *http://www.thefamilycaregiver.org*
Family Caregiver Alliance *http://www.caregiver.org*
ElderCare Online *http://www.ec-online.net*

Pharmacologic Therapy

Pharmacotherapy for Cognitive Symptoms

8 Table 54-5 presents pharmacologic treatment recommendations for managing cognitive symptoms in AD. Cholinesterase inhibitors and NMDA-receptor antagonists are indicated for treatment of AD. Current guidelines recommend initiation of cholinesterase inhibitors for AD with no preference for a specific agent.[46] Donepezil, rivastigmine, and galantamine are indicated in mild to moderate AD; donepezil is also indicated in severe disease. Despite inconclusive evidence for early intervention, cholinesterase inhibitors are commonly prescribed off-label prior to formal diagnosis of AD.[51] Memantine is indicated for moderate to severe AD; current evidence does not support its use in earlier stages of the disease.[52] Additional benefit may be achieved when memantine is added to cholinesterase

TABLE 54-5 Pharmacologic Treatment Options for Cognitive Symptoms in Alzheimer Disease

- In mild to moderate disease, consider therapy with a cholinesterase inhibitor:
  - Donepezil or
  - Rivastigmine or
  - Galantamine
- Titrate to recommended maintenance dose as tolerated
- In moderate to severe disease, consider adding antiglutamatergic therapy:
  - Memantine
- Titrate to recommended maintenance dose as tolerated
- Alternatively, consider memantine or cholinesterase inhibitor therapy alone
- Behavioral symptoms may require additional pharmacologic approaches

Data from References 1 and 52.

inhibitor therapy in moderate to severe AD.[52] There is no evidence supporting combination therapy of more than one cholinesterase inhibitor. No head-to-head trials comparing memantine monotherapy to cholinesterase inhibitor therapy have been conducted to date.

Disagreement exists about how best to determine effectiveness of treatments for AD. Selection of qualitative versus quantitative assessment may bias a clinician's impression of response. Subtle changes are often detected only by psychometric testing. Because no standard has been suggested to define the effectiveness of medications for AD, great variation exists between clinicians, and the duration of treatment ranges from months to years. Realistic expectations for treatment success may include slowed decline in behavioral, functional, and cognitive abilities and delayed long-term care placement.[53] An initial dramatic improvement in symptoms is unlikely but may be reported by a minority of patients or their caregivers.[54]

Unfortunately, clinical trials have failed to provide answers to key questions in treating AD patients. Information from clinical trials is insufficient to know if a cholinesterase inhibitor dose–response relationship exists, or if additional cognitive improvement may be gained by increasing to the maximum tolerated dose, rather than continuing with the usual recommended daily dosage. Guidance in extrapolating data related to changes in cognition is needed, so that a reasonable duration of clinical treatment with cholinesterase inhibitors and NMDA-antagonists can be determined. One concern is that those who respond to treatment may lose the benefits of that treatment once the medication is stopped.[55] Gaps in treatment have been linked with worse cognitive outcomes in clinical trial extension studies;[56] in a more recent observational study there was no increased risk of institutionalization or death associated with gaps in cholinesterase inhibitor therapy.[57] Regardless, dosing regimens should be simplified and patient/caregiver preferences considered in an effort to improve adherence and persistence.

In natural disease progression studies, scores on the Alzheimer's Disease Assessment Scale—Cognition (ADAS-cog) have been shown to worsen (increase) by an average of less than or equal to five points over 1 year in mild dementia and 7 to 11 points annually in moderate dementia. Based on these findings, the general consensus is that a four-point change in the ADAS-cog represents a clinically significant change.[46] Therefore, if a pharmacotherapeutic agent decreases the ADAS-cog score by four points, one could think of this as having delayed progression of disease symptoms by 6 months. The usefulness of the ADAS-cog in clinical practice is limited because of the time required for administration; it is much more practical to assess changes in disease severity using the MMSE. An untreated patient has an average decline of two to four points in MMSE score per year. Successful treatment would reflect a decline of less than two points a year. It is reasonable to change to a different cholinesterase inhibitor if the decline in MMSE score is greater than two to four points after 1 year with the initial agent.[58]

8 **Cholinesterase Inhibitors** In the early 1980s, researchers began to examine means to enhance cholinergic activity in patients with AD by inhibiting the hydrolysis of acetylcholine through reversible inhibition of cholinesterase. Tacrine was the first such drug to be examined in a systematic fashion. However, tacrine was fraught with significant side effects, including hepatotoxicity, which severely limited its usefulness. Tacrine is no longer available in the United States market, having been replaced by safer, more tolerable cholinesterase inhibitors. The newer cholinesterase inhibitors donepezil, rivastigmine, and galantamine show similar modest symptomatic improvements in cognitive, global, and functional outcomes in patients with mild to moderate AD, and duration of benefit varies from 3 to 24 months.[59,60] One open-label extension study of galantamine showed benefit beyond the 24-month mark.[61]

The mechanism of action differs slightly between drugs in this class.[58] Donepezil specifically and reversibly inhibits acetylcholinesterase. Rivastigmine inhibits both butyrylcholinesterase and acetylcholinesterase. Galantamine is a selective, competitive, reversible acetylcholinesterase inhibitor and also enhances the action of acetylcholine on nicotinic receptors. The clinical relevance of these differences is unknown.

Choice of cholinesterase inhibitor therapy for an individual patient is based primarily on ease of use, patient preference, cost, and safety issues, such as potential for drug interactions. Pharmacokinetic properties should also be considered, as rivastigmine and galantamine have short half-lives (1.5 and 7 hours, respectively) compared to donepezil (70 hours). As such, if rivastigmine or galantamine treatment is interrupted for several days or longer, the patient should be restarted at the lowest dose and titrated to the current dose. This is true for all formulations of these drugs, including the rivastigmine transdermal patch.[62-64] Dosing strategies for cholinesterase inhibitors and memantine are summarized in Table 54-6.

Adverse drug reactions and corresponding monitoring parameters are described in Table 54-7. Cholinesterase inhibitors have similar adverse event profiles, and this class of drugs is generally well-tolerated. The most frequent adverse events associated with these agents are mild to moderate GI symptoms (eg, nausea, vomiting, and diarrhea).[45] Gradual dose titration over several months can improve tolerability.[26] Alternatives to the immediate-release tablet/capsule dosage form are available for patients who have complex dosing regimens, tolerability issues, or difficulty swallowing, though cost may be prohibitive until they are generically available. Patients and caregivers should be cautioned against abrupt discontinuation of cholinesterase inhibitor therapy, as this can lead to worsening cognition and behavior in some patients.[65] Concurrent use of anticholinergic medications with cholinesterase inhibitors should be avoided and nonpharmacologic interventions employed to manage urinary incontinence, if possible.[66]

Depending on individual patient response, tolerability, and preference, switching to an alternate dosage form of cholinesterase inhibitor agent may be necessary during the course of AD treatment. Manufacturer recommendations for switching between dosage forms of the same drug are specified in the prescribing information, but the optimal procedure for switching between agents remains uncertain. When switching from one cholinesterase inhibitor to another due to side effect intolerance, a washout period is recommended.[54] Length of the washout period may vary based on drug pharmacokinetics and time to side effect resolution.[54,58] Some patients who fail to respond to donepezil, rivastigmine, or galantamine, may respond when switched to a different drug; in the case of lack of initial benefit, an overnight switch is preferred to minimize potential for clinical deterioration.[54,58] To clarify, loss of benefit over time may not be an appropriate reason to switch cholinesterase inhibitors, as the progressive nature of AD is likely to become more noticeable over time.[58] Indeed, initiation of memantine may be a more appropriate next step as patients progress in their disease course.[58]

8 **Antiglutamatergic Therapy** Memantine is the only NMDA-antagonist currently available. At concentrations achieved at least under in vitro conditions, memantine blocks glutamatergic neurotransmission by antagonizing NMDA receptors. Glutamate is an excitatory neurotransmitter in the brain implicated in long-term potentiation, a neuronal mechanism important for learning and memory.[67] Blocking NMDA receptors can mitigate excitotoxic neurotoxicity and potentially provide neuroprotection (as has been suggested in animal models); however, there is currently no clinical evidence to indicate memantine confers neuroprotection in AD.[68]

Memantine is currently indicated for use in moderate to severe AD. Its use has been studied in patients with moderate and severe AD as monotherapy and in combination with donepezil with favorable results on cognition and function.[52] Studies of memantine alone and in combination with cholinesterase inhibitors in mild AD performed to date have provided insufficient evidence to support an indication for mild AD.[52]

TABLE 54-6 Dosing of Drugs Used for Cognitive Symptoms

Drug	Brand Name	Initial Dose	Usual Range	Special Population Dose	Other
Cholinesterase Inhibitors					
Donepezil	Aricept, Aricept ODT	5 mg daily in the evening	5-10 mg daily in mild to moderate AD 10-23 mg daily in moderate to severe AD	No dosage adjustments recommended	Available as: tablet, ODT Can be taken with or without food Weight loss associated with 23 mg daily dose
Rivastigmine	Exelon, Exelon Patch	1.5 mg twice daily (capsule, oral solution) 4.6 mg/day (transdermal patch)	3-6 mg twice a day (capsule, oral solution) 9.5-13.3 mg/day (transdermal patch)	Capsule/oral solution: Renal impairment, hepatic impairment, or low body weight (≤50 kg [<110 lb]): Patients may be able to only tolerate lower doses Transdermal patch: Mild to moderate hepatic impairment or low body weight: consider maximum daily dose of 4.6 mg every 24 hours	Available as: capsule, oral solution, transdermal patch Take with meals Also indicated for Parkinson disease dementia Application of multiple transdermal patches at same time associated with hospitalization and death
Galantamine	Razadyne, Razdyne ER	4 mg twice daily (tablet, oral solution) 8 mg daily in the morning (extended-release capsule)	8-12 mg twice a day (tablet, oral solution) 16-24 mg (extended-release capsule)	Moderate renal or hepatic impairment: maximum daily dose of 16 mg Severe renal or hepatic impairment: not recommended	Available as: tablet, oral solution, extended-release capsule Take with meals
***N*-methyl-D-aspartate (NMDA) Receptor Antagonist**					
Memantine	Namenda, Namenda XR	5 mg daily 7 mg daily (extended-release capsule)	10 mg twice daily 28 mg daily (extended-release capsule)	Severe renal impairment: recommended maintenance dose of 5 mg twice daily (tablet, oral solution) or 14 mg daily (extended-release capsule) Severe hepatic impairment: administer with caution	Available as: tablet, oral solution, extended-release capsule Can be taken with or without food Can open extended-release capsule and sprinkle contents on applesauce for ease of administration
Cholinesterase Inhibitor + NMDA Receptor Antagonist					
Memantine + Donepezil	Namzaric	28 mg/10 mg	14-28 mg/10 mg daily	Severe renal impairment: 14 mg/10 mg daily	Available as: memantine extended-release and donepezil capsule Can be taken with or without food Can open capsule and sprinkle contents on applesauce for ease of administration

ODT, orally disintegrating tablet.

Data from References 62-64, 69, 70, 125, and 126.

In its tablet or oral solution form, memantine should be initiated at 5 mg once a day and titrated weekly in 5 mg intervals to the target maintenance dose of 10 mg twice daily. The extended-release capsule form of memantine is to be initiated at 7 mg daily and titrated up to a maximum of 28 mg daily. Dose titration is achieved in 7 mg intervals with at least 1 week between dose adjustments. Dosing of 5 mg twice daily (tablet and oral solution) or 14 mg daily (extended-release capsule) is recommended in patients with severe renal impairment (creatinine clearance of 5-29 mL/min [0.08-0.49 mL/s]).

Overall, memantine has been well-tolerated in clinical trials. The most common adverse events include headache, constipation, confusion, and dizziness. Memantine has 100% bioavailability regardless of administration with or without food. Protein binding is relatively low (45%). Memantine is not metabolized by the liver and does not inhibit cytochrome P450 activity. It is primarily excreted unchanged in the urine, and the half-life of memantine ranges from 60 to 80 hours.[69,70]

Role of Combination Therapy Combination therapy with memantine added to cholinesterase inhibitor therapy is generally prescribed for patients with moderate to severe AD. The rationale for this add-on therapy is that the drug classes have different mechanisms of action.

Combination therapy has been supported in several randomized controlled trials (RCTs) and reviews.[71] Combination therapy has been shown to slow cognitive and functional decline to a statistically significant degree compared to cholinesterase inhibitor monotherapy or no treatment.[71] One trial randomized patients with moderate to severe AD already receiving stable donepezil treatment to either memantine or placebo. At the end of this 6-month trial, patients randomized to receive memantine (combination therapy) had significantly better outcomes in measures of cognition, function, behavior, and global status than those continued on donepezil monotherapy. The group randomized to receive memantine also had a lower rate of discontinuation due to adverse events versus placebo.[72] Based on data from this study and others, memantine may have a role in mitigating GI adverse events associated with cholinesterase inhibitors.[46]

In 2014, a combination product containing memantine extended-release and donepezil was approved by the U.S. Food and Drug Administration (FDA) for moderate to severe dementia in patients already stabilized on memantine and donepezil. As drug effectiveness was based on bioequivalence with the two active ingredients, the package insert separately lists the most common side effects of memantine extended-release (headache, diarrhea, and dizziness) and donepezil (diarrhea, anorexia, vomiting, nausea,

TABLE 54-7 Monitoring Drug Therapy for Cognitive Symptoms

Drug	Adverse Drug Reaction	Monitoring Parameter	Comments
Galantamine	Serious skin reactions (Stevens-Johnson syndrome and acute generalized exanthematous pustulosis)	Appearance of skin rash	Discontinue galantamine at first sign of skin rash, unless clearly not drug-related If signs/symptoms are suggestive of a serious reaction, consider alternative treatment and do not rechallenge
Rivastigmine	Allergic dermatitis	Application site reaction spread beyond patch size, evidence of a more intense local reaction (increasing erythema, edema, papules, vesicles), and if symptoms do not improve within 48 hours of patch removal	Discontinue rivastigmine if evidence of disseminated allergic dermatitis appears Patients sensitized by exposure to the transdermal patch may not be able to take rivastigmine by mouth either; allergy testing and close medical supervision recommended
Cholinesterase inhibitors	Dizziness, syncope, bradycardia, atrial arrhythmias, myocardial infarction, angina, seizures, sinoatrial and atrioventricular block	Report of dizziness or falls, pulse, blood pressure, and postural blood pressure change	Dizziness is usually mild, transient, and not related to cardiovascular problems Routine pulse checks at baseline, monthly during titration, and every 6 months thereafter
Cholinesterase inhibitors	Nausea, vomiting, diarrhea, anorexia, and weight loss	Weight and GI complaints	Take with food to decrease GI upset Usually transient, dose-related GI adverse effects seen with drug initiation, dosage titration, or drug switch Debilitated patients or those weighing <55 kg (<121 lb) may be more likely to experience GI adverse effects and significant weight loss, particularly when rivastigmine is prescribed or when titrating to donepezil 23 mg GI adverse effects less prominent with transdermal versus oral rivastigmine
Cholinesterase inhibitors	Peptic ulcer disease, GI bleeding	Signs or symptoms of active or occult GI bleeding	Of particular concern for patients at increased risk of developing ulcers, such as those with a history of ulcer disease or concurrently taking NSAIDs
Cholinesterase inhibitors	Insomnia, vivid/abnormal dreams, nightmares	Complaints of sleep disturbances, daytime drowsiness	Donepezil can be taken in the morning to decrease risk of sleep disturbances
Memantine	Headache, confusion, dizziness, hallucinations	Report of dizziness or falls, hallucinations	Confusion may be observed during dose titration and is usually transient Memantine may mitigate GI adverse effects associated with cholinesterase inhibitor therapy
Memantine	Constipation	GI complaints	

NSAIDs, nonsteroidal antiinflammatory drugs.

Data from References 3, 46, 62-64, 69, 70, 125, and 126.

and ecchymosis). The fixed-dose combination product comes in two strengths, and dosage reduction is recommended in the case of severe renal impairment. No dosage adjustments are needed in patients with mild or moderate renal or hepatic impairment. The drug has not been studied in patients with severe hepatic impairment.

Clinical **Controversy...**

In light of the irreversible nature of AD and prolonged benefits seen with long-term use of cholinesterase inhibitors alone and in combination with memantine,[71] the question of when, if ever, to stop drug therapy for AD remains controversial. In the case of AD, treatment benefits are not always evident, and the combined perception of slowed progression and fear of deterioration can lead patients to be prescribed drug therapy from diagnosis to death. One could choose to withdraw medications until the time of nursing home placement; then, however, it is possible that drug therapy could help manage behavioral disturbances of AD. Some clinicians will recommend withdrawing AD drug therapy if the patient significantly deteriorates in cognition or function, while others wait until the patient has lost all cognitive and functional abilities. As such, side effects, cost, and family request factor heavily into drug therapy discontinuation decisions. If cholinesterase inhibitors are discontinued and cognition worsens or behavioral issues emerge, the drugs can be restarted.

Effect of Current Treatments on Neurodegenerative Processes AD is a progressive disorder. Affected individuals typically experience some degree of cognitive decline and histologic change years (if not decades) before a diagnosis is made. Therefore, the ideal treatment will be one that not only reverses symptoms by enhancing cognitive function (a symptomatic treatment), but also arrests the neurodegeneration-relevant molecular processes that underlie cognitive decline (a disease-modifying treatment).

Clinical trials for AD prompt consideration of whether positive outcomes suggest either a symptomatic or disease-modifying effect. Any rapid performance improvement in cognitive ability, activities of daily living, or behavioral end points is indicative of a symptomatic effect. All cholinesterase inhibitor agents and memantine demonstrate this pattern. On the other hand, arrest of decline or a sustained reduction in the slope of decline would argue the presence of a disease-modifying effect. It has not been possible to unequivocally demonstrate this in trials of the currently approved treatments. Long-duration, double-blind, placebo-controlled trials to evaluate whether cholinesterase inhibitors, with or without memantine, have disease-modifying effects are difficult to perform, because doing so would require continuing a placebo arm over an extended period, well beyond demonstration of symptomatic benefit. Also, subject attrition over an extended study would complicate both intent-to-treat and observed case analyses.

With the currently approved AD drug treatments, pivotal placebo-controlled trials were followed by open-label extension studies. Published studies have lasted as long as 5 years, and as part of these studies, decline in the treatment group was compared with "projected" placebo groups based on the placebo groups followed during the 6-month randomized phase of the efficacy study, as well as natural history cohorts from the precholinesterase inhibitor therapy era. Although analyses of this sort conclude that, for up to at least 5 years, persons receiving treatment exceed their projected nontreatment cognitive performance, no convincing evidence of a disease-modifying effect emerges.[61,73-76]

Management of Brain Vascular Health 9 Guidelines for the care of patients with AD support the management of vascular brain disease and its associated risk factors as part of the treatment of AD.[77] There is a growing body of evidence that brain vascular disease plays a role in the progression of dementia. For a given level of AD pathology, vascular disease in the brain may add to the degree of cognitive impairment.[78] Management of brain vascular disease includes monitoring blood pressure, glucose, cholesterol, and homocysteine and initiation of appropriate interventions.[78] Elevated homocysteine levels are associated with vascular disease. Some studies also suggest an association with brain atrophy, NFTs, and AD, but there remains insufficient evidence of a benefit of B vitamin supplementation on cognitive function in patients with AD at this time.[1,19,79]

The World Health Organization and Alzheimer's Disease International encourage primary prevention through public health campaigns targeting smoking, underactivity, midlife obesity, midlife hypertension, and diabetes.[80] Adherence to the Mediterranean Diet (MeDi) or Dietary Approaches to Stop Hypertension (DASH) diet may reduce the risk of cognitive impairment or decline.[19,79] Physical activity is an important component of vascular brain health and has been shown in some short-term studies to be associated with a reduced risk of cognitive impairment as well.[19] Of note though is that most positive trial findings have been from cognitively healthy older adults.[19,79]

While appropriate management of vascular disease risk factors may reduce the risk for developing AD,[81] insufficient evidence exists to draw definitive conclusions on the association between risk factor modification and risk of AD.[19,78]

Other Potential Treatment Approaches Estrogen replacement has been studied extensively for the treatment and prevention for AD. Most, but not all, retrospective epidemiologic studies show a lower incidence of AD in women who took estrogen replacement therapy postmenopausally. Prospective clinical trials have not supported the use of estrogen as a treatment for cognitive decline, and longer trials tend to suggest harm. Overall, the evidence does not support the use of estrogen to treat or prevent dementia.[82] Although phytoestrogens, found in soy-containing foods and soy-derived dietary supplements, have been suggested for the treatment or prevention of dementia, there are no clinical trials supporting the use of these treatments for dementia.[82]

Antiinflammatory Agents Retrospective epidemiologic studies suggest a protective effect against AD in patients who have taken NSAIDs. The benefits of antiinflammatory agents have been less compelling in prospective clinical studies. NSAIDs have had no cognitive benefit in AD patients or else benefits so minimal the risk of harm exceeds the potential benefit.[83] Because there is a lack of compelling data and also a significant incidence of adverse effects, particularly gastritis and the possibility of GI bleeds, NSAIDs and prednisone are not recommended for general use in the treatment or prevention of AD.[83]

Lipid-Lowering Agents An AD protective effect has been postulated for lipid-lowering agents, particularly the 3-hydroxy-3-methylglutaryl-coenzyme A-reductase inhibitors. Longitudinal epidemiologic studies suggest an association between elevated midlife total cholesterol levels and AD.[18] Increased risk of dementia does not appear to be associated with hypercholesterolemia in late life however.[18] Other studies note that the incidence of AD is lower in patients who have taken either a statin or another lipid-lowering agent, but not in patients who were taking other cardiovascular medications.[18] It is important to note that not all epidemiologic studies suggest an association between cholesterol and AD.[18]

Randomized controlled trials of statin therapy given in late life to patients at risk for vascular disease indicate that statins do not prevent AD.[84] Four randomized placebo-controlled trials of statin therapy indicated no significant benefit of statin therapy in patients with probable or possible AD.[84] Interestingly, cognitive impairment has been recognized as a rare adverse event associated with statin therapy. More research is needed to understand the complex relationship between cholesterol, statin therapy, and cognitive functioning. For now these agents should be reserved for patients who have other indications for their use.

Dietary Supplements Dietary supplements are widely used for the prevention and treatment of AD, and available evidence has been reviewed.[85-88] A detailed discussion of the many nutraceuticals, herbal products, and medical foods that have been promoted for the prevention and treatment of AD is beyond the scope of this chapter. The more commonly used dietary supplements are described here.

Vitamin E Based on pathophysiologic theories involving oxidative stress and the accumulation of free radicals in AD, significant interest has evolved regarding the use of antioxidants in the treatment of AD. Two RCTs have evaluated the effects of vitamin E supplementation (1,000 IU twice daily) in patients with AD.[89] The first studied patients with moderate AD for 2 years and demonstrated a significant delay in the time to institutionalization in the treatment group compared to placebo. The second trial studied the efficacy of α-tocopherol, memantine or their combination in delaying clinical progression of AD in patients taking an acetylcholinesterase inhibitor with mild to moderate AD (mean follow-up time of 2.3 years) and showed a reduced annual rate of decline in ADLs in those treated with vitamin E but no cognitive benefits. No significant side effects were reported between treatment groups in either study; however, a meta-analysis found that high-dose vitamin E increases mortality in supplemented subjects.[90] In addition, vitamin E had no benefit in patients with MCI in the progression to AD.[91] In light of these findings, there is insufficient evidence to recommend vitamin E supplementation for the treatment of AD. Vitamin E remains under investigation for the prevention of AD.

Ginkgo biloba *Ginkgo biloba* for the prevention and treatment of AD has been extensively studied. Proposed mechanisms for Ginkgo's use in AD include its potential to increase blood flow, decrease blood viscosity, antagonize platelet-activating factor receptors, increase anoxia tolerance, inhibit monoamine oxidase, and serve as an antioxidant. Active ingredients in *Ginkgo biloba* include flavonoids, the Ginkgo flavone glycosides, and bioflavonoids. Most studies reporting benefit in patients with cognitive impairment or dementia have studied a standardized extract, EGb 761, in doses of 240 mg/day for 22 to 26 weeks.[92] The clinical significance of the modest benefits detected is unclear, and direct comparisons to cholinesterase inhibitors or memantine are lacking. A large trial of *Ginkgo biloba* in which the 120 mg twice a day dose was studied did not reduce either the overall incidence rate of dementia or AD incidence in elderly individuals with normal cognition or MCI.[93] Another large trial found that the long-term use of *Ginkgo biloba* extract did not reduce the risk of progression to AD among older adults suffering from memory complaints compared with placebo.[94] Side effects reported from EGb 761 studies were typically mild, including nausea, vomiting, diarrhea, headaches, dizziness, palpitations, restlessness, and weakness. Because EGb also has a potent antiplatelet effect, it should be avoided by individuals taking anticoagulant or antiplatelet therapies, and should be used cautiously in patients taking NSAIDs.[94,95]

Huperzine A It is an alkaloid isolated from the Chinese club moss, *Huperzia serrata*. It reversibly inhibits acetylcholinesterase and is administered orally in doses of 50 to 200 mcg two to four times daily. Short-term clinical studies suggest huperzine A shows efficacy in the symptomatic treatment of AD compared to placebo, but more studies are needed to determine its place in therapy. The current consensus is that huperzine A has not been adequately studied for use in AD, its consistent potency and purity in commercially available products remains a concern, and potential side effects could be significant, especially in those taking cholinesterase inhibitors.[96]

Polyphenols Several epidemiological studies have demonstrated that moderate ingestion of wine, but not distilled spirits, is associated with a lower incidence of AD.[86] One of the components of red wine, resveratrol, has been the focus of research related to dementia. Resveratrol, a phenolic compound with antioxidant properties, is found commonly in foods such as grapes, peanuts, chocolate, blueberries, and red wine. Resveratrol's proposed benefits in AD are to prevent reactive oxygen species-induced Aβ production and apoptosis-mediated neurodegeneration.[86] A Phase II randomized, double-blind, placebo-controlled study of resveratrol 500 mg daily for 13 weeks followed by 1,000 mg daily for 39 weeks in patients with mild to moderate AD found alterations in plasma and CSF biomarkers, but further studies are needed to establish the clinical significance of these changes.[97]

The polyphenol curcumin (turmeric) is a spice used in Indian curry that has antioxidant and antiinflammatory properties and has been proposed as one explanation for the lower incidence of AD in India compared to the United States.[98] Curcumin may prevent or treat AD by decreasing amyloid plaque formation, clearing existing plaques, and chelating metal ions.[98] Early studies with curcumin in AD did not provide evidence supporting its benefit in AD, but this may have been due to the poor oral availability of curcumin, insufficient dosing, and short duration of the trials. Synthetic formulations of curcumin as well as pharmaceutical modifications of the naturally occurring curcumin are being developed to improve the bioavailability of curcumin.[98] Studies are ongoing to evaluate the efficacy, safety, and dosing of curcumin for the treatment of AD.

Medical Foods Several medical foods have been studied for the treatment of MCI or AD. Medical foods constitute a unique category that consists of ingestible entities specifically intended for the treatment of diseases that have "specific nutritional requirements" and in which the medical food may manipulate disease-relevant pathophysiology. Although medical foods regulatory approval standards are not as rigorous as those required for approvals of new medications, medical foods are obtained only by prescription. The only medical food studied in mild to moderate AD is AC1202 (Axona), a mixture of medium-chain fatty acids, consisting primarily of the C8 fatty acid caprylic acid.[99] AC1202 is converted by the liver to a ketone body, β-hydroxybutyrate, which is released into the blood stream. β-hydroxybutyrate crosses the blood–brain barrier and can be used as an oxidative phosphorylation substrate by neuronal mitochondria. Support for AC1202 efficacy in the treatment of AD comes mostly from a phase IIb trial in which subjects randomized to 40 mg/day of AC1202 for 45 days performed relatively better on the ADAS-cog than did subjects randomized to a placebo.[100] A subanalysis of these data revealed that this benefit was entirely driven by subjects who did not have an *APOE*4* allele. For *APOE*4* carriers, ADAS-cog performance between subjects receiving AC1202 and placebo were comparable at all time points studied. GI-related side effects were common, but in general side effects were felt to be mild. Coconut oil is a source of caprylic acid, but does not contain sufficient quantities to meet the needs of a person with AD.[85] Coconut oil continues to be used by some patients as a less expensive alternative to AC1202 however.

Tramiprosate Tramiprosate (homotaurine), or Alzhemed, showed promise as a treatment for AD in early development. In animal studies, homotaurine demonstrated the ability to interfere with amyloid plaque formation and subsequent degeneration of neuronal cells. Phase III trials were disappointing, and the FDA declined to approve marketing of homotaurine as a prescription drug. Homotaurine is naturally occurring in seaweed, and is now available as the dietary supplement Vivimind for age-associated memory impairment.[67]

Omega-3 Fatty Acids Arguments that omega-3 fatty acids found in fish oil, such as docosahexaenoic acid and eicosapentaenoic acid, could benefit AD subjects have existed for some years. A large prospective, placebo-controlled trial of docosahexaenoic acid in AD subjects was recently reported. For the most part, results were disappointing, and although it could not be ruled out that population subsets did benefit, the primary study end points were negative.[101] There is insufficient evidence at this time to recommend docosahexaenoic acid for the treatment of AD.

Drugs and Treatment Strategies in Development New drug development is focused on disease-modifying and prevention strategies and falls broadly into several categories: treatments designed to reduce levels of brain Aβ or manipulate its configuration, treatments targeting tau protein, antiinflammatory approaches, and therapies to address insulin resistance in the brain. Although many potential new drugs have advanced to early clinical studies, there have been no new agents entering the market since 2004. Progress has been made in developing novel biomarkers and improving clinical trial designs, but results of clinical trials remain disappointing.[102]

Reducing Aβ Formation To reduce brain amyloid levels, approaches to both reducing Aβ production and enhancing its removal have been and still are undergoing evaluation. Aβ is produced through enzymatic processing of APP by two enzyme complexes, the β- and γ-secretases. β-Secretase inhibitors have entered phase II and III human trials and promising agents remain in the pipeline.[103] Agents that specifically inhibit γ-secretase have proved to be problematic both from a side-effect perspective, as γ-secretase is also critical for processing Notch3, a protein of developmental importance and perhaps brain maintenance, and also from an efficacy perspective. Stimulation of α-secretase blocks the formation of Aβ and generates neuroprotective peptide that is another strategy to reduce Aβ. Therapies aimed at activating α-secretase are currently under investigation.[104]

Increasing Aβ Clearance Immunotherapy approaches have been studied as a way to enhance Aβ removal. Active and passive immunization have been most widely studied immunotherapy approaches for AD over the past decade. Active immunization involves administering a vaccine containing antigens designed to cause antibody generation in the patient. In passive immunization, exogenous antibodies are administered. In both cases the goal is for the antibodies to clear amyloid plaques from the brain of patients with AD. An advantage of active immunization is that a small number of vaccine administrations results in a long-term antibody response. Research on active immunization strategies has been hampered by variability in response among patients, serious and persistent adverse events, and potentially reduced immune response by a senescent immune system; however, this remains an active area of research.[105] Passive immunization approaches with polyclonal and monoclonal antibodies allow for reproducible administration and rapid clearance of the antibodies, but have the disadvantage of requiring repeated administration. Although some agents for passive immunization have failed in Phase III clinical trials (bapineuzumab and solanezumab) due to lack of efficacy, others remain under active investigation.[105]

Preventing Aβ Aggregation Proponents of the amyloid cascade hypothesis claim the species of Aβ that is most likely to prove relevant to AD neurodegeneration are Aβ oligomers formed through limited aggregation of Aβ monomers. Tramiprosate was designed to prevent Aβ oligomer formation and tested clinically in a large phase III trial. No evidence of efficacy was seen.[106] Other agents targeted at this mechanism, including inositol, remain under clinical investigation. Metals such as zinc, copper, and iron play a role in Aβ aggregation. Metal chelators are also being developed for potential treatment of AD.[106]

Targeting Tau Targeting tau has been challenging, and thus far there are few therapeutic options in clinical trials. One approach is to administer small molecular weight compounds such as the dye methylene blue that inhibit formation of tau oligomers and fibrils and thus prevent tau aggregation.[103] Another approach is inhibition of kinase-mediated phosphorylation since tau hyperphosphorylation leads to tau dysfunction and aggregation. Agents studied included lithium and valproate, but trials results were disappointing.[103] Immunotherapy is also under investigation, with the first clinical investigation of vaccines targeting misfolded, truncated tau underway.[103]

Reducing Oxidative Stress and Inflammation in the Brain Inflammation, oxidative stress, and mitochondrial dysfunction in chronic neurodegenerative disorders contribute to the neuronal dysfunction and loss that occurs in these conditions. Production of Aβ and hyperphosphorylated tau may simply be downstream cell responses to the cycle of inflammation and oxidative stress that eventually overwhelms the neuron's ability to compensate. Targeting the upstream oxidative stress and inflammation is an active area of investigation. Nutriceuticals and vitamins, as well as antiinflammatory medications (etanercept, prednisone, ibuprofen, indomethacin, naproxen, celecoxib, rofecoxib, atorvastatin, simvastatin, rosuvastatin, pravastatin, rosiglitazone, and the mitochondrial stabilizer latrepirdine) have shown promising results in preclinical studies and early clinical investigations, but subsequent clinical trials have often been conflicting or negative.[107] One possible explanation is that the benefit from these agents may be in primary prevention before damage is severe enough that symptoms of cognitive decline are evident.[107]

Targeting Insulin Resistance in the Brain Low levels of insulin and insulin resistance in the brain are associated with cognitive impairment and AD. Individuals with type 2 diabetes have a twofold higher risk of developing AD.[108] One of the actions of insulin in the brain is to modulate the levels of Aβ, leading researchers to explore this area for potential treatment opportunities. One promising approach is a new class of diabetes medications, glucagon-like peptide-1 receptor agonists. Liraglutide has been shown to reduce amyloid production and protect neurons from resulting damage in animal models, and early clinical trials are ongoing.[106] Early clinical studies with intranasal insulin showed improvement in memory and daily functioning in patients with MCI and mild or moderate AD.[109] A large multicenter trial of this treatment strategy is underway.[108]

Suggestions of efficacy in phase II trials in no way ensure efficacy will be seen in phase III trials. This caveat seems especially pertinent in AD drug development, as phase II trials of flurbiprofen, tramiprosate, rosiglitazone, latrepirdine, bapineuzumab, and solanezumab all reported some evidence of efficacy that did not bear out in phase III studies. Obviously, successful development of new AD treatments depends on elucidating AD's true underlying pathophysiology. One reason for the failure of so many AD therapies may be that current strategies do not target the pathways that ultimately result in AD. Another reason may be that medications are being initiated when the disease has already progressed too far to be reversed.[103] New approaches include studying amyloid-blocking agents in patients with genetic predisposition to early-onset AD before symptoms are present and studying patients with biomarkers of disease risk or presymptomatic signs of disease to determine the potential value of new treatments. Prevention trials are currently underway in both genetically determined AD and sporadic AD.[103]

Pharmacotherapy of Noncognitive Symptoms

Most patients with AD manifest noncognitive symptoms at some point in the illness.[110] These symptoms can be roughly divided into three categories: (1) psychotic symptoms, (2) inappropriate or disruptive behavior, and (3) depression. Effective management of these problems is important because behavioral symptoms are distressing to both the patient and the caregiver, necessitate increased caregiver supervision and patience, and are a leading reason for nursing home placement.

(10) Strategies for treatment of psychotic or behavioral symptoms should include nonpharmacologic interventions first, then pharmacologic interventions only when necessary. Behaviors, such as agitation, aggression, delusions, hallucinations, repetitive vocalizations, and wandering, may be caused by medications, medical illness (eg, pain, constipation, dehydration, and infection), environmental precipitants, poor caregiving, physical/verbal abuse, and unmet physical or psychological needs. These possible underlying causes should be explored and corrected when possible before initiating drug therapies.[110] The need for medications may exist when neuropsychiatric symptoms are of sufficient severity to cause significant distress to the patient or caregiver, interfere with function or cause disability, impede delivery of necessary care, or pose a danger to self or others and have not responded to nonpharmacologic interventions.[46,110,111] The balance between risks of the medication and expected benefits must be acceptable to the patient or surrogate decision maker. Medications should be used cautiously, with adequate monitoring for efficacy and adverse events.

Despite the high prevalence of noncognitive symptoms in AD, relatively little research has been conducted in these patients. To date, no drug has been approved by the FDA for the treatment of behavioral disturbances in patients with dementia. Because of limited clinical data, treatment is primarily empiric, with side-effect profiles used as a guide in selecting the appropriate treatment. Psychotropic medications with anticholinergic effects should be avoided because they may actually worsen cognition and interfere with cholinesterase inhibitor therapy.

General guidelines governing pharmacologic therapy can be summarized as follows: reserve for situations where nonpharmacologic therapies have failed, use reduced doses, monitor closely, titrate dosage slowly, minimize the duration of therapy, and document carefully. Treatment should be considered as temporary.[110,111] Caregivers may have unrealistic expectations regarding the effects of psychotropic medications, and the anticipated benefits and risks of therapy should be clearly explained. Disruptive behaviors and delusions wax and wane with disease progression, and some behaviors (eg, wandering, hoarding, screaming, and repetitive behaviors) lack evidence of response to medication.[112] Attempts to slowly taper and discontinue medication should be undertaken regularly in minimally symptomatic patients, as behaviors often fluctuate, changing in character and intensity over time, and the medication may no longer be providing a benefit.[110]

Cholinesterase Inhibitors and Memantine Clinical trials with cholinesterase inhibitors have reported modest benefit in managing neuropsychiatric symptoms, although these are generally not the primary outcomes studied in the trials, and the clinical significance is controversial.[110] Cholinesterase inhibitors may not significantly reduce agitation when administered to patients experiencing acute agitation.[113] Memantine shows modest behavioral benefits as well in trials of patients with moderate to severe dementia, either alone or in combination with cholinesterase inhibitors;[110] however, a recent trial of memantine specifically evaluating the effect of memantine to treat agitation in patients with AD found no difference compared to placebo.[114] These benefits should be considered along with cognitive benefits in treatment decisions and weighed against the side effects associated with these medications. Long-term effects on behavior have not been demonstrated to date, and further research is needed.

Antipsychotics Antipsychotics are often used in the management of neuropsychiatric symptoms in AD despite efforts by CMS and other groups to reduce their use in nursing homes.[115] There is modestly convincing evidence that most of the atypical antipsychotics provide some benefit for particular neuropsychiatric symptoms, but these data have been insufficient to gain FDA approval as an indication for the management of behavioral symptoms in AD. More than 15 RCTs have evaluated atypical antipsychotics for behavioral symptoms of dementia, with more than 5,000 patients participating and treatment durations of 8 to 12 weeks for most trials. Based on one systematic review and meta-analysis, aripiprazole (three trials), risperidone (five trials) but not olanzapine (five trials) showed benefit for managing behavioral symptoms of dementia. Studies of quetiapine (three trials) could not be statistically combined due to methodological differences in inclusion criteria and outcomes assessed, so the evidence for quetiapine was insufficient for evaluation. The analysis showed that lower efficacy was associated with having less severe cognitive impairment and having psychosis.[110] Similar results were noted in a second meta-analysis, except that olanzapine showed efficacy for treating the symptoms of aggression and agitation, but not psychosis.[110] In a double-blind, placebo-controlled trial of 421 outpatients with AD and psychosis, aggression, or agitation randomized to receive olanzapine, quetiapine, risperidone, or placebo for up to 36 weeks, there were no significant differences among the treatments in time to discontinuation of treatment or improvement based on the Clinical Global Impression–Change (CGI-C) response. The investigators concluded that adverse effects offset advantages in the efficacy of atypical antipsychotic drugs for treatment of psychosis, aggression, or agitation in patients with AD.[116] Adverse events are common with atypical and typical antipsychotics in patients with AD. Adverse events associated with atypical antipsychotics include somnolence, extrapyramidal symptoms, abnormal gait, worsening cognition, cerebrovascular events, and increased risk of death.[110] In 2005, the FDA mandated the addition of a "black box warning" to all atypical antipsychotics due to increased risk of mortality in older adults with dementia-related psychosis. Compared to atypical agents, typical antipsychotics are more commonly associated with more severe extrapyramidal effects and hypotension. In 2008, the FDA "black box warning" for increased mortality in older adults treated for dementia-related psychosis was expanded to include typical antipsychotics.[117] Chapter 67 includes a more detailed discussion of antipsychotic adverse events. Overall, there is a modest expectation of treatment benefit and potential for significant harm associated with antipsychotic use in patients with AD. Individual risk and benefit must be considered when initiating therapy. Prescribing of antipsychotics in AD should be restricted to patients with severe symptoms that have not responded to other measures, and treatment should be tapered as early as possible.[111] Diligent monitoring during treatment is essential, as is frequent reassessment of continued need. A meta-analysis of RCTs of antipsychotic discontinuation showed no significant difference in change in severity of behavioral and psychological symptoms of dementia upon discontinuation compared to the continuation group.[118]

Antidepressants Depressive symptoms are common in patients with AD. Apathy is seen in 48% to 92% of individuals with dementia, and clinically significant depression occurs in approximately 32% with mild dementia, 23% with moderate disease, and 18% in the severe stage of the dementia.[119] Some trials have studied the efficacy of antidepressants in treating depression in patients with AD, but the results are conflicting.[110] Small sample size, short duration of treatment, and differing measures of therapy outcomes limit comparison across studies and may account in part for conflicting study results.[119] Improvement in patients receiving placebo is also common. In practice, treatment with selective serotonin reuptake inhibitors (SSRIs) is initiated most commonly in patients with AD, based on side-effect profile and evidence of efficacy;[110] however, a study comparing sertraline, mirtazapine, and placebo found no benefit for these agents in treating depression in patients with dementia.[120] Among the SSRIs, the best evidence exists for sertraline and citalopram.[110] Serotonergic function may also play a role in some of the other behavioral symptoms of AD, such as agitation, and some studies support the use of SSRIs in the management of these behaviors, even in the absence of depression.[110] Clinical trials are needed to compare the efficacy of SSRIs to atypical antipsychotics. Tricyclic antidepressants have efficacy similar to the SSRIs but should generally be avoided because of their anticholinergic activity.[110] Chapter 68 has a more complete discussion of treatment of depression.

Clinical **Controversy...**

The appropriate use of medications—and antipsychotics in particular—for the management of behavioral disturbances in patients with dementia continues to be controversial. Nonpharmacologic approaches are considered first-line therapy, but evidence for individual nonpharmacologic strategies is often lacking. Additionally, commonly cited institutional barriers to implementing nonpharmacologic approaches include education and training, staffing resources and time, and availability of necessary supplies or equipment. Overcoming these barriers may be challenging and costly initially, but doing so is an important first step in minimizing reliance on and potentially inappropriate use of medications for behavioral disturbances in AD.

Miscellaneous Therapies Because antipsychotic and antidepressant therapy have shown only modest efficacy and pose the potential for undesirable side effects, medications traditionally used to treat disruptive behaviors and aggression in other psychiatric and neurologic disorders have been suggested as potential alternatives. These alternatives include benzodiazepines and anticonvulsants.[110]

Benzodiazepines have been used to treat anxiety, agitation, and aggression, but the benefit is unclear. There are no RCTs that have investigated the use of benzodiazepines for the management of behavioral disturbances in AD.[110]

Because benzodiazepine use is associated with impaired cognition, respiratory depression, oversedation, and increased risk of falls in patients with AD, their routine use is not advised, except on an "as needed basis" for infrequent acute episodes of agitation.[110] "Mood stabilizer" anticonvulsants, such as carbamazepine, valproic acid, and gabapentin, may be appropriate alternatives, but evidence is conflicting.[110] More rigorous placebo-controlled studies are needed to determine the relative efficacy and place in therapy for these medication alternatives.

Noncognitive symptoms are often the most difficult aspect of AD for the caregiver. When nonpharmacologic approaches fail, selected antipsychotics and antidepressants have been useful for effective management of behavioral, psychotic, and depressive symptoms, thereby easing caregiver burden and allowing the patient to spend additional time at home. All too often, however, nonpharmacologic measures are not implemented appropriately and medication overuse is an ongoing problem. Adverse events remain an important concern in this population as well.

PERSONALIZED THERAPY

At this time there are no specific recommendations regarding the choice of agent or dosing regimen for current cognitive enhancing therapies based on genotype or other biomarkers. There is a great deal of attention among AD researchers to identify biomarkers for AD, and recommendations are likely to evolve over time as we better understand the underlying pathophysiology of AD and the predictors of patient response.

Given the exponentially increasing number of individuals and families facing the diagnosis of AD, the National Institutes of Health, FDA, pharmaceutical companies, and nonprofit organizations have joined together in an "Accelerating Medicines Partnership." Contributing almost 130 million dollars over the next 5 years, these groups will combine forces to create networks, share data, and manage clinical trials (http://www.nih.gov/science/amp/alzheimers.htm).

Recommendations for patients with renal or hepatic dysfunction or low body weight are detailed in Table 54-6. It is important to consider that most patients with AD are older adults and therefore may be taking multiple medications for other acute and chronic health conditions. The potential for adverse events due to drug interactions increases as the number of medications increases.

EVALUATION OF THERAPEUTIC OUTCOMES

An evaluation of therapeutic outcomes in the patient with AD begins with a thorough assessment at baseline and a clear definition of therapeutic goals. Cognitive status, physical status, functional performance, mood, and behavior all need to be evaluated before initiation of drug therapy. The clinician should interview both the patient and the caregiver to assess response to drug therapy. In evaluating response to cognitive agents, the clinician should ask questions about the patient's ability to perform daily functional tasks and about mood and behavior, as well as questions about memory and orientation. Objective assessments (eg, MMSE for cognition, Bristol Activities of Daily Living Scale for function, Neuropsychiatric Inventory for behavioral disturbances) can be used to quantify changes in symptoms and function.[121]

Because target symptoms of psychiatric disorders may respond differently in dementia patients, a detailed list of symptoms to be treated should be documented in the pharmacotherapy plan to aid in monitoring. These could include, for example, "striking at spouse because patient believes spouse is an impostor," "verbal threats and refusal to allow clothes to be changed," and so on, as opposed to documenting vague symptoms such as "aggression" or "delusions." To make an accurate assessment of depression, multiple symptoms (eg, sleep, appetite, and activity and interest levels) need to be assessed in addition to the patient's stated mood.

The patient should be observed carefully for potential side effects of drug therapy. The specific side effects to be monitored and the method and frequency of monitoring should be documented. Patients should be monitored for therapeutic effect 8 weeks after initiation of therapy and at least every 6 months thereafter.[122] However, patients must be treated for an adequate duration to see a therapeutic effect from a given intervention. The effects of cognition-enhancing medications will not necessarily be obvious, and a treatment period of several months to a year may be necessary before it can be determined whether therapy is beneficial. Cognitive effects of the drug are often noticed only as a plateauing during treatment or as deterioration following drug discontinuation. In general, cognitive agents should be continued if the patient is demonstrating no change in clinical status. However, if there is doubt, the medication can be slowly tapered and discontinued, and the patient monitored off the drug for 4 to 6 weeks to determine the need for continued therapy.

ABBREVIATIONS

AA	Alzheimer's Association
Aβ	β-Amyloid peptide
AD	Alzheimer disease
ADAS-cog	Alzheimer's Disease Assessment Scale—Cognition
ADRDA	Alzheimer's Disease and Related Disorders Association
AHRQ	Agency for Healthcare Research and Quality
APOE	apolipoprotein E
APP	amyloid precursor protein
CGI-C	Clinical Global Impression–Change
CSF	cerebrospinal fluid
CT	computed tomography
DASH	Dietary Approaches to Stop Hypertension
DSM-5	Diagnostic and Statistical Manual of Mental Disorders, Fifth Edition
FDA	Food and Drug Administration
MCI	mild cognitive impairment
MeDi	Mediterranean Diet
MMSE	Mini-Mental State Examination
MoCA	Montreal Cognitive Assessment
MRI	magnetic resonance imaging
NFT	neurofibrillary tangle
NIA	National Institute on Aging
NINCDS	National Institute of Neurological and Communicative Disorders and Stroke
NINDS	National Institute of Neurological Disorders and Stroke
NMDA	*N*-methyl-D-aspartate
NSAID	nonsteroidal antiinflammatory drug
RCT	randomized controlled trial
SLUMS	St. Louis University Mental Status Exam
SSRI	selective serotonin reuptake inhibitor

REFERENCES

1. Ballard C, Gauthier S, Corbett A, et al. Alzheimer's disease. *Lancet* 2011;377:101-131.
2. U.S. Department of Health and Human Services. National Plan to Address Alzheimer's Disease: 2015 update. Available at: *https://aspe.hhs.gov/sites/default/files/pdf/107031/NatlPlan2015.pdf.* (Last accessed, January 12, 2016)
3. Alzheimer's Association. 2016 Alzheimer's Disease Facts and Figures. Available at: http://www.alz.org/documents_custom/2016-facts-and-figures.pdf (Last accessed, July 22, 2016)
4. Querfurth HW, LaFerla FM. Alzheimer's disease. *N Engl J Med* 2010;362:329-344.
5. Reitz C, Brayne C, Mayeux R. Epidemiology of Alzheimer disease. *Nat Rev Neurol* 2011;7:137-152.
6. Hebert LE, Weuve J, Scherr PA, Evans DA. Alzheimer disease in the United States (2010-2050) estimated using the 2010 census. *Neurology* 2013;80:1778-1783.
7. Bekris LM, Yu C-E, Bird TD, Tsuang DW. Genetics of Alzheimer disease. *J Geriatr Psychiatry Neurol* 2010;23:213-227.
8. Bertram L, Tanzi RE. The genetics of Alzheimer's disease. *Prog Mol Biol Transl Sci* 2012;107:79-100.
9. Williamson J, Goldman J, Marder KS. Genetic aspects of Alzheimer disease. *Neurologist* 2009;15:80-86.
10. Kim J, Basak JM, Holtzman DM. The role of apolipoprotein E in Alzheimer's disease. *Neuron* 2009;63:287-303.
11. Lambert JC, Ibrahim-Verbaas CA, Harold D, et al. Meta-analysis of 74,046 individuals identifies 11 new susceptibility loci for Alzheimer's disease. *Nat Genet* 2013;45:1452-1458.
12. Sims R, Williams J. Defining the genetic architecture of Alzheimer's disease: Where next? *Neurodegener Dis* 2016;16:6-11.
13. Kern A, Behl C. The unsolved relationship of brain aging and late-onset Alzheimer disease. *Biochim Biophys Acta* 2009;1790:1124-1132.
14. Duncan GW. The aging brain and neurodegenerative diseases. *Clin Geriatr Med* 2011;27(4):629-644.
15. Trepanier CH, Milgram NW. Neuroinflammation in Alzheimer's disease: Are NSAIDs and selective COX-2 inhibitors the next line of therapy? *J Alzheimers Dis* 2010;21:1089-1099.
16. Wang J, Tan L, Wang H-F, et al. Anti-inflammatory drugs and risk of Alzheimer's disease: An updated systematic review and meta-analysis. *J Alzheimers Dis* 2015;44:385-396.
17. Danysz W, Parsons CG. Alzheimer's disease, β-amyloid, glutamate, NMDA receptors and memantine—searching for the connections. *Br J Pharmacol* 2012;167:324-352.

18. Dickstein DL, Walsh J, Brautigam H, et al. Role of vascular risk factors and vascular dysfunction in Alzheimer's disease. *Mt Sinai J Med* 2010;77:82-102.
19. de Bruijn RFAG, Ikram MA. Cardiovascular risk factors and future risk of Alzheimer's disease. *BMC Med* 2014;12:130.
20. Dineley KT, Jahrling JB, Denner L. Insulin resistance in Alzheimer's disease. *Neurobiol Dis* 2014;72 Pt A:92-103.
21. Henderson VW. Action of estrogens in the aging brain: Dementia and cognitive aging. *Biochim Biophys Acta* 2010;1800:1077-1083.
22. Swerdlow RH. Brain aging, Alzheimer's disease, and mitochondria. *Biochim Biophys Acta* 2011;1812:1630-1639.
23. Galvin JE, Sadowsky CH. Practical guidelines for the recognition and diagnosis of dementia. *J Am Board Fam Med* 2012;25:367-382.
24. Moyer VA. Screening for cognitive impairment in older adults: U.S. Preventive Services Task Force recommendation statement. *Ann Intern Med* 2014;160:791-797.
25. Cordell CB, Borson S, Boustani M, et al. Alzheimer's Association recommendations for operationalizing the detection of cognitive impairment during the Medicare Annual Wellness Visit in a primary care setting. *Alzheimers Dement* 2013;9:141-150.
26. Rabins PV, Blass DM. Dementia. *Ann Intern Med* 2014;161:ITC1. Doi: 10.7326/0003-4819-161-3-201408050-01002.
27. American Psychiatric Association. *Diagnostic and Statistical Manual of Mental Disorders: DSM-5*. 5th ed. Washington, DC: American Psychiatric Association; 2013.
28. Costa PT Jr, Williams TF, Somerfield M, et al. Early identification of Alzheimer's disease and related dementias. Clinical Practice Guideline, Quick Reference Guide for Clinicians, No. 19. AHCPR Publication No. 97–0703. Rockville, MD: U.S. Department of Health and Human Services, Public Health Service, Agency for Health Care Policy and Research; 1996.
29. Knopman DS, DeKosky ST, Cummings JL, et al. Practice parameter: Diagnosis of dementia (an evidence-based review). Report of the Quality Standards Subcommittee of the American Academy of Neurology. *Neurology* 2001;56:1143-1153.
30. Román GC, Tatemichi TK, Erkinjuntti T, et al. Vascular dementia: Diagnostic criteria for research studies. Report of the NINDS-AIREN International Workshop. *Neurology* 1993;43:250-260.
31. McKhann G, Drachman D, Folstein M, et al. Clinical diagnosis of Alzheimer's disease: Report of the NINCDS-ADRDA Work Group under the auspices of Department of Health and Human Services Task Force on Alzheimer's disease. *Neurology* 1984;34: 939-944.
32. Jack CR, Albert MS, Knopman DS, et al. Introduction to the recommendations from the National Institute on Aging-Alzheimer's Association workgroups on diagnostic guidelines for Alzheimer's disease. *Alzheimers Dement* 2011;7:257-262.
33. McKhann GM, Knopman DS, Chertkow H, et al. The diagnosis of dementia due to Alzheimer's disease: Recommendations from the National Institute on Aging-Alzheimer's Association workgroups on diagnostic guidelines for Alzheimer's disease. *Alzheimers Dement* 2011;7:263-269.
34. Albert MS, DeKosky ST, Dickson D, et al. The diagnosis of mild cognitive impairment due to Alzheimer's disease: Recommendations from the National Institute on Aging-Alzheimer's Association workgroups on diagnostic guidelines for Alzheimer's disease. *Alzheimers Dement* 2011;7:270-279.
35. Sperling RA, Aisen PS, Beckett LA, et al. Toward defining the preclinical stages of Alzheimer's disease: Recommendations from the National Institute on Aging-Alzheimer's Association workgroups on diagnostic guidelines for Alzheimer's disease. *Alzheimers Dement* 2011;7:280-292.
36. Schmidt R, Hofer E, Bouwman FH, et al. EFNS-ENS/EAN Guideline on concomitant use of cholinesterase inhibitors and memantine in moderate to severe Alzheimer's disease. *Eur J Neurol* 2015;22:889-898.
37. National Institute for Health and Care Excellence. *Donepezil, Galantamine, Rivastigmine and Memantine for the Treatment of Alzheimer's Disease*. London, UK: NICE; 2011. NICE technology appraisal guidance TA217.
38. Robinson L, Tang E, Taylor JP. Dementia: Timely diagnosis and early intervention. *BMJ* 2015;350:h3029.
39. Fillenbaum GG, Peterson B, Morris JC. Estimating the validity of the clinical Dementia Rating Scale: The CERAD experience. Consortium to Establish a Registry for Alzheimer's disease. *Aging (Milano)* 1996;8:379-385.
40. Moore AR, O'Keeffe ST. Drug-induced cognitive impairment in the elderly. *Drugs Aging* 1999;15:15-28.
41. Gray SL, Anderson ML, Dublin S, et al. Cumulative use of strong anticholinergics and incident dementia: A prospective cohort study. *JAMA Intern Med* 2015;175:401-407.
42. Harper L, Barkhof F, Scheltens P, et al. An algorithmic approach to structural imaging in dementia. *J Neurol Neurosurg Psychiatry* 2014;85:692-698.
43. Schipper HM. Apolipoprotein E: Implications for AD neurobiology, epidemiology and risk assessment. *Neurobiol Aging* 2011;32: 778-790.
44. Geda YE. Mild cognitive impairment in older adults. *Curr Psychiatry Rep* 2012;14:320-327.
45. Lin JS, O'Connor E, Rossom RC, et al. Screening for cognitive impairment in older adults: An evidence update for the U.S. Preventive Services Task Force. Evidence Report No. 107. AHRQ Publication No. 14-05198-EF-1. Rockville, MD: Agency for Healthcare Research and Quality; 2013.
46. Sadowsky CH, Galvin JE. Guidelines for the management of cognitive and behavioral problems in dementia. *J Am Board Fam Med* 2012;25(3):350-366.
47. Gitlin LN, Kales HC, Lyketsos CG. Nonpharmacologic management of behavioral symptoms in dementia. *JAMA* 2012;308: 2020-2029.
48. Mittelman MS, Bartels SJ. Translating research into practice: Case study of a community-based dementia caregiver intervention. *Health Aff (Millwood)* 2014;33:587-595.
49. Alzheimer's Association. Challenging Behaviors. Available at: *http://www.alz.org/documents_custom/statements/challenging_behaviors.pdf*. (Last accessed, January 12, 2016)
50. O'Neil M, Freeman M, Christensen V, et al. Non-pharmacological interventions for behavioral symptoms of dementia: A systematic review of the evidence. VA-ESP Project #05-225;2011.
51. Roberts JS, Karlawish JH, Uhlmann WR, et al. Mild cognitive impairment in clinical care: A survey of American Academy of Neurology members. *Neurology* 2010;75:425-431.
52. Rabins PV, Rovner BW, Rummans T, et al. Guideline watch (October 2014): Practice guideline for the treatment of patients with Alzheimer's disease and other dementias. Available at: *http://psychiatryonline.org/pb/assets/raw/sitewide/practice_guidelines/guidelines/alzheimerwatch.pdf*. (Last accessed, January 12, 2016)
53. Howard R, McShane R, Lindesay J, et al. Nursing home placement in the Donepezil and Memantine in Moderate to Severe Alzheimer's Disease (DOMINO-AD) trial: Secondary and post-hoc analyses. *Lancet Neurol* 2015;14:1171-1181.
54. Stahl SM. *Prescriber's Guide: Stahl's Essential Psychopharmacology*. 5th ed. New York, NY: Cambridge University Press; 2014.
55. Rainer M, Mucke HA, Krüger-Rainer C, et al. Cognitive relapse after discontinuation of drug therapy in Alzheimer's disease: Cholinesterase inhibitors versus nootropics. *J Neural Transm* 2001;108:1327-1333.
56. Gaudig M, Richarz U, Han J, et al. Effects of galantamine in Alzheimer's disease: Double-blind withdrawal studies evaluating sustained versus interrupted treatment. *Curr Alzheimer Res* 2011;8:771-780.
57. Pariente A, Fourrier-Réglat A, Bazin F, et al. Effect of treatment gaps in elderly patients with dementia treated with cholinesterase inhibitors. *Neurology* 2012;78:957-963.
58. Massoud F, Desmarais JE, Gauthier S. Switching cholinesterase inhibitors in older adults with dementia. *Int Psychogeriatr* 2011;23:372-378.
59. Birks JS, Chong LY, Grimley Evans J. Rivastigmine for Alzheimer's disease. *Cochrane Database of Syst Rev* 2015;9:CD001191.
60. Buckley JS, Salpeter SR. A Risk-Benefit Assessment of Dementia Medications: Systematic Review of the Evidence. *Drugs Aging* 2015;32:453-467.
61. Raskind MA, Peskind ER, Truyen L, et al. The cognitive benefits of galantamine are sustained for at least 36 months: A long-term extension trial. *Arch Neurol* 2004;61:252-256.
62. *Razadyne (Galantamine Hydrobromide)*. Titusville, NJ: Janssen Pharmaceuticals, Inc.; 2013. Package insert.
63. *Exelon (Rivastigmine Tartrate)*. East Hanover, NJ: Novastis Pharmaceuticals Corp.; 2015. Package insert.
64. *Exelon Patch (Rivastigmine Transdermal System)*. East Hanover, NJ: Novastis Pharmaceuticals Corp.; 2015. Package insert.
65. Bidzan L, Bidzan M. Withdrawal syndrome after donepezil cessation in a patient with dementia. *Neurol Sci* 2012;33:1459-1461.
66. Sink KM, Thomas J, Xu H, et al. Dual use of bladder anticholinergics and cholinesterase inhibitors: Long-term functional and cognitive outcomes. *J Am Geriatr Soc* 2008;56:847-853.

67. Herrmann N, Chau SA, Kircanski I, Lanctôt KL. Current and emerging drug treatment options for Alzheimer's disease: A systematic review. *Drugs* 2011;71:2031-2065.
68. Fonseca-Santos B, Gremião MPD, Chorilli M. Nanotechnology-based drug delivery systems for the treatment of Alzheimer's disease. *Int J Nanomedicine* 2015;10:4981-5003.
69. *Namenda (Memantine Hydrochloride)*. St. Louis, MO: Forest Pharmaceuticals, Inc.; 2013.
70. *Namenda Extended-release Capsules (Memantine Hydrochloride)*. St. Louis, MO: Forest Pharmaceuticals, Inc.; 2014.
71. Deardorff WJ, Feen E, Grossberg GT. The use of cholinesterase inhibitors across all stages of Alzheimer's disease. *Drugs Aging* 2015;32:537-547.
72. Tariot PN, Farlow MR, Grossberg GT, et al. Memantine treatment in patients with moderate to severe Alzheimer disease already receiving donepezil: A randomized controlled trial. *JAMA* 2004;291:317-324.
73. Rogers SL, Doody RS, Pratt RD, Ieni JR. Long-term efficacy and safety of donepezil in the treatment of Alzheimer's disease: Final analysis of a US multicentre open-label study. *Eur Neuropsychopharmacol* 2000;10:195-203.
74. Farlow MR, Lilly ML; ENA713 B352 Study Group. Rivastigmine: An open-label, observational study of safety and effectiveness in treating patients with Alzheimer's disease for up to 5 years. *BMC Geriatr* 2005;5:3.
75. Reisberg B, Doody R, Stöffler A, et al. A 24-week open-label extension study of memantine in moderate to severe Alzheimer disease. *Arch Neurol* 2006;63:49-54.
76. Doody RS, Geldmacher DS, Gordon B, et al, Donepezil Study Group. Open-label, multicenter, phase 3 extension study of the safety and efficacy of donepezil in patients with Alzheimer disease. *Arch Neurol* 2001;58:427-433.
77. Lyketsos CG, Colenda CC, Beck C, et al. Position statement of the American Association for Geriatric Psychiatry regarding principles of care for patients with dementia resulting from Alzheimer disease. *Am J Geriatr Psychiatry* 2006;14:561-572.
78. Gorelick PB, Scuteri A, Black SE, et al. Vascular contributions to cognitive impairment and dementia: A statement for healthcare professionals from the American Heart Association/American Stroke Association. *Stroke* 2011;42:2672-2713.
79. Anstey KJ, Eramudugolla R, Hosking DE, et al. Bridging the translation gap: From dementia risk assessment to advice on risk reduction. *J Prev Alzheimer's Di* 2015;2:189-198.
80. World Health Organization and Alzheimer's Disease International. Dementia: A Public Health Priority. Available at: *http://apps.who.int/iris/bitstream/10665/75263/1/9789241564458_eng.pdf*. (Last accessed, January 12, 2016)
81. Middleton LE, Yaffe K. Promising strategies for the prevention of dementia. *Arch Neurol* 2009;66:1210-1215.
82. Henderson VW. Alzheimer's disease: Review of hormone therapy trials and implications for treatment and prevention after menopause. *J Steroid Biochem Mol Biol* 2014;142:99-106.
83. Jaturapatporn D, Isaac MG, McCleery J, Tabet N. Aspirin, steroidal and non-steroidal anti-inflammatory drugs for the treatment of Alzheimer's disease. *Cochrane Database Syst Rev* 2012;2:CD006378.
84. McGuinness B, Craig D, Bullock R, et al. Statins for the treatment of dementia. *Cochrane Database Syst Rev* 2014;7:CD007514.
85. Wollen KA. Alzheimer's disease: The pros and cons of pharmaceutical, nutritional, botanical, and stimulatory therapies, with a discussion of treatment strategies from the perspective of patients and practitioners. *Altern Med Rev* 2010;15:223-244.
86. Shah RC. Medical foods for Alzheimer's disease. *Drugs Aging* 2011;28:421-428.
87. Howes MJ, Perry E. The role of phytochemicals in the treatment and prevention of dementia. *Drugs Aging* 2011;28:439-468.
88. Kim HG, Oh MS. Herbal medicines for the prevention and treatment of Alzheimer's disease. *Curr Pharm Des* 2012;18:57-75.
89. La Fata G, Weber P, Mohajeri MH. Effects of vitamin E on cognitive performance during ageing and in Alzheimer's disease. *Nutrients* 2014;6:5453-5472.
90. Miller ER, Pastor-Barriuso R, Dalal D, et al. Meta-analysis: High-dosage vitamin E supplementation may increase all-cause mortality. *Ann Intern Med* 2005;142:37-46.
91. Petersen RC, Thomas RG, Grundman M, et al. Vitamin E and donepezil for the treatment of mild cognitive impairment. *N Engl J Med* 2005;352:2379-2388.
92. Tan MS, Yu JT, Tan CC, et al. Efficacy and adverse effects of ginkgo biloba for cognitive impairment and dementia: A systematic review and meta-analysis. *J Alzheimers Dis* 2015;43:589-603.
93. DeKosky ST, Williamson JD, Fitzpatrick AL, et al. Ginkgo biloba for prevention of dementia: A randomized controlled trial. *JAMA* 2008;300:2253-2262.
94. Vellas B, Coley N, Ousset PJ, et al. Long-term use of standardised Ginkgo biloba extract for the prevention of Alzheimer's disease (GuidAge): A randomised placebo-controlled trial. *Lancet Neurol* 2012;11:851-859.
95. Weinmann S, Roll S, Schwarzbach C, et al. Effects of Ginkgo biloba in dementia: Systematic review and meta-analysis. *BMC Geriatr* 2010;10:14.
96. Yang G, Wang Y, Tian J, Liu JP. Huperzine A for Alzheimer's disease: A systematic review and meta-analysis of randomized clinical trials. *PLoS One* 2013;8:e74916.
97. Pasinetti GM, Wang J, Ho L, et al. Roles of resveratrol and other grape-derived polyphenols in Alzheimer's disease prevention and treatment. *Biochim Biophys Acta* 2015;1852:1202-1208.
98. Brondino N, Re S, Boldrini A, et al. Curcumin as a therapeutic agent in dementia: A mini systematic review of human studies. *Sci World J* 2014;2014:1-6.
99. Cummings JL, Isaacson RS, Schmitt FA, Velting DM. A practical algorithm for managing Alzheimer's disease: What, when, and why? *Ann Clin Transl Neurol* 2015;2:307-323.
100. Henderson ST, Vogel JL, Barr LJ, et al. Study of the ketogenic agent AC-1202 in mild to moderate Alzheimer's disease: A randomized, double-blind, placebo-controlled, multicenter trial. *Nutr Metab (Lond)* 2009;6:31.
101. Cederholm T, Salem N, Palmblad J. ω-3 fatty acids in the prevention of cognitive decline in humans. *Adv Nutr* 2013;4:672-676.
102. Cummings JL, Morstorf T, Zhong K. Alzheimer's disease drug-development pipeline: Few candidates, frequent failures. *Alzheimers Res Ther* 2014;6:37.
103. Hampel H, Schneider LS, Giacobini E, et al. Advances in the therapy of Alzheimer's disease: Targeting amyloid beta and tau and perspectives for the future. *Expert Rev Neurother* 2015;15:83-105.
104. Macleod R, Hillert E-K, Cameron RT, Baillie GS. The role and therapeutic targeting of α-, β- and γ-secretase in Alzheimer's disease. *Futur Sci OA* 2015;1:1-16.
105. Lannfelt L, Relkin NR, Siemers ER. Amyloid-β-directed immunotherapy for Alzheimer's disease. *J Intern Med* 2014;275:284-295.
106. Jia Q, Deng Y, Qing H. Potential therapeutic strategies for Alzheimer's disease targeting or beyond β-amyloid: Insights from clinical trials. *Biomed Res Int* 2014;2014:837157.
107. Haas C. Strategies, development, and pitfalls of therapeutic options for Alzheimer's disease. *J Alzheimers Dis* 2012;28:241-281.
108. Friedrich MJ. New research on Alzheimer treatments ventures beyond plaques and tangles. *JAMA* 2012;308:2553-2555.
109. Craft S, Baker LD, Montine TJ, et al. Intranasal insulin therapy for Alzheimer disease and amnestic mild cognitive impairment: A pilot clinical trial. *Arch Neurol* 2012;69:29-38.
110. Kales HC, Gitlin LN, Lyketsos CG. Assessment and management of behavioral and psychological symptoms of dementia. *BMJ* 2015;350:h369.
111. Ngo J, Holroyd-Leduc JM. Systematic review of recent dementia practice guidelines. *Age Ageing* 2015;44:25-33.
112. Cohen-Mansfield J, Jensen B, Resnick B, Norris M. Knowledge of and attitudes toward nonpharmacological interventions for treatment of behavior symptoms associated with dementia: A comparison of physicians, psychologists, and nurse practitioners. *Gerontologist* 2012;52:34-45.
113. Howard RJ, Juszczak E, Ballard CG, et al. Donepezil for the treatment of agitation in Alzheimer's disease. *N Engl J Med* 2007;357:1382-1392.
114. Fox C, Crugel M, Maidment I, et al. Efficacy of memantine for agitation in Alzheimer's dementia: A randomised double-blind placebo controlled trial. *PLoS One* 2012;7:e35185.
115. Chiu Y, Bero L, Hessol NA, et al. A literature review of clinical outcomes associated with antipsychotic medication use in North American nursing home residents. *Health Policy* 2015;119:802-813.
116. Schneider LS, Dagerman K, Insel PS. Efficacy and adverse effects of atypical antipsychotics for dementia: Meta-analysis of randomized, placebo-controlled trials. *Am J Geriatr Psychiatr*. 2006;14:191-210.
117. Food and Drug Administration. Information for Healthcare Professionals: Conventional Antipsychotics. Available at: *http://www.fda.gov/Drugs/DrugSafety/PostmarketDrugSafetyInformationforPatientsandProviders/ucm124830.htm*. (Last accessed, January 12, 2016)
118. Pan YJ, Wu CS, Gau SSF, et al. Antipsychotic discontinuation in patients with dementia: A systematic review and meta-analysis of

published randomized controlled studies. *Dement Geriatr Cogn Disord* 2014;37:125-140.
119. Desai AK, Schwartz L, Grossberg GT. Behavioral disturbance in dementia. *Curr Psychiatry Rep* 2012;14:298-309.
120. Banerjee S, Hellier J, Dewey M, et al. Sertraline or mirtazapine for depression in dementia (HTA-SADD): A randomised, multicentre, double-blind, placebo-controlled trial. *Lancet* 2011;378:403-411.
121. Sheehan B. Assessment scales in dementia. *Ther Adv Neurol Disord* 2012;5:349-358.
122. Raetz J, v d Luft E. FPIN's clinical inquiries. Monitoring therapy for patients with Alzheimer's disease. *Am Fam Physician* 2007;75:1703-1704.
123. Simmons BB, Hartmann B, Dejoseph D. Evaluation of suspected dementia. *Am Fam Physician* 2011;84:895-902.
124. Folstein MF, Folstein SE, McHugh PR. Mini-mental state. A practical method for grading the cognitive state of patients for the clinician. *J Psychiatr Res* 1975;12:189-198.
125. *Aricept (Donepezil Hydrochloride)*. Woodcliff Lake, NJ: Eisai Inc.; 2015. Package insert.
126. *Namzaric Capsules (Memantine Hydrochloride Extended Release and Donepezil Hydrochloride)*. Cincinnati, OH: Forest Pharmaceuticals, Inc.; 2015. Package insert.

55

Multiple Sclerosis

Jacquelyn L. Bainbridge, Augusto Miravalle, and Pei Shieen Wong

KEY CONCEPTS

1. The etiology of multiple sclerosis (MS) is unknown, but it appears to be autoimmune in nature. Currently there is no cure.
2. Multiple sclerosis is characterized by central nervous system (CNS) demyelination and axonal damage.
3. Multiple sclerosis is classified by the nature of progression over time into several categories, which have different clinical presentations and responses to therapy.
4. Although studies do not support the general use of any of the FDA-approved disease-modifying therapies (DMTs), except mitoxantrone, in patients with progressive forms of the illness, information derived from multiple studies suggests younger patients with progressive illness and those with either superimposed acute relapses or enhancing lesions on magnetic resonance imaging (MRI) scans may benefit from some of the presently used DMTs.
5. Diagnosis of MS requires evidence of dissemination of lesions over time and in multiple parts of the CNS and/or optic nerve, and is made primarily on the basis of clinical symptoms and examination. Diagnostic criteria also allow for the use of MRI, spinal fluid evaluation, optical coherence tomography, and evoked potentials to aid in the diagnosis.
6. Exacerbations or relapses of MS can be disabling. When this is the case, exacerbations and relapses are treated with high-dose glucocorticoids, such as methylprednisolone intravenous (IV), with onset of clinical response typically within 3 to 5 days.
7. Treatment of relapsing-remitting multiple sclerosis (RRMS) with the DMTs interferon-β (IFN-β) (Avonex, Betaseron, Rebif, Extavia), glatiramer acetate (Copaxone), natalizumab (Tysabri), mitoxantrone (Novantrone), fingolimod (Gilenya), teriflunomide (Aubagio), dimethyl fumarate (Tecfidera), and alemtuzumab (Lemtrada) can reduce annual relapse rate, lessen severity of relapses, slow progression of changes on MRI scans, slow progression of disability, and slow cognitive decline. In addition, they have been shown to reduce the likelihood of developing a second attack after a first clinically isolated syndrome (CIS) consistent with MS.
8. In most cases, treatment with DMTs should begin promptly after the diagnosis of RRMS, or after a CIS if the brain MRI is suggestive of high risk of further attacks. Natalizumab and other choices that have been associated with problematic adverse events should be reserved for those patients who have failed one or more standard therapies and those with poor prognostic signs.
9. The definition of treatment inadequacy for RRMS remains unclear, and therapy changes after "treatment failure" should be individualized.
10. Patients suffering with MS frequently have symptoms such as spasticity, bladder dysfunction, fatigue, neuropathic pain, cognitive dysfunction, and depression that can require treatment. Patients must be counseled that DMTs will not relieve these symptoms. Depression is common in MS and can pose the risk of suicide.

Multiple sclerosis (MS) is an inflammatory disease of the central nervous system (CNS) that affects approximately 1 in 200 women and fewer men in the United States.[1] The term "multiple sclerosis" refers to two characteristics of the disease: numerous affected areas of the brain and spinal cord producing multiple neurologic symptoms that accrue over time, and the characteristic plaques or sclerosed areas that are the hallmark of the disease.

(1) Although MS was first described almost 140 years ago, the cause remains a mystery, and a cure is still unavailable. Nevertheless, many advances have been made in treating and managing the disease complications and improving the quality-of-life of affected individuals.

EPIDEMIOLOGY

Epidemiologic aspects of MS have been reviewed in many publications.[1-5] MS affects approximately 2.3 million people worldwide.[6] MS is usually diagnosed between the ages of 15 and 45 years; peak incidence occurs in the fourth decade. Women are afflicted more than men by a ratio of 2:1. Men usually develop the first signs of MS at a later age than women, and are more likely to develop a progressive form of the disease. The most important factors in determination of risk for developing the disease are geography, age, environmental influences, and genetics. In general, disease prevalence is higher the greater the distance from the equator; within the United States the prevalence of MS is higher in states above the 37th parallel. Recent studies, however, suggest a waning latitude gradient as demonstrated by a substantial increase in MS incidence in Mediterranean regions. Rising incidence of MS in females appears to be associated with urbanization.[7]

Multiple sclerosis occurs more frequently in whites of Scandinavian ancestry than in other ethnic groups. In addition, an inverse relationship between MS risk and 25-hydroxyvitamin D levels has been proposed.[1,8]

ETIOLOGY

The exact cause of MS is still unknown, but the disease is thought to develop in genetically susceptible individuals, that are exposed to random events and environmental factors that could trigger immune mediated CNS damage. Genetic variation accounts for approximately 30% of the overall disease risk, and with the advent of genome-wide association studies (GWASs), more than 100 distinct genetic regions have been identified as being associated with MS, collectively explaining approximately one-third of the genetic component of the condition. However, nongenetic factors have a proportionately larger contribution than genetic factors to immunological heterogeneity. Environmental determinants of risk in MS are still under investigation, but there are interesting advances in our understanding of the epidemiology of MS. To date, the reported environmental factors implicated in MS variably, but not exclusively, include vitamin D deficiency, human cytomegalovirus infection, Epstein–Barr virus (EBV), Human Herpesvirus (HHV)-6, smoking, high levels of dietary sodium, and circadian disruption.

It is thought that genetically susceptible individuals below 15 years of age who have lived in a high-risk area for at least 2 years and were exposed to a crucial environmental agent are at risk for developing MS. Interestingly, an individual who migrates from a low- to high-risk area prior to the age of 15 years acquires the same chance of developing MS as those who live in a high-risk area all their lives.[2] If the move is made from a high- to a low-risk area, the individual retains the high risk if the move is made after the age of 15 years, but acquires the lower risk if the move is made prior to this age.[2] Smoking cigarettes has been associated with both an increased risk of developing MS and with more severe progression of disability.[5,9]

Although no clear association has been identified, certain viral or bacterial infections might participate in the pathogenesis of MS by initiating or activating autoreactive immune cells in genetically susceptible individuals, leading to subsequent demyelination. Evidence to support a viral etiology includes increased immunoglobulin G (IgG) synthesis in the CNS, increased antibody titers to certain viruses, and epidemiologic studies that indicate a childhood exposure factor, suggesting that "viral" infections may precipitate exacerbations. In addition, viruses have been shown to cause diseases with prolonged incubation periods, myelin destruction, and a relapsing-remitting course in both humans and experimental animal models.[1,10]

Although numerous viruses have a hypothetical proposed association with MS, the greatest evidence supports EBV. Autoreactive T-cells could be activated by EBV through molecular mimicry, whereby sequence similarities between EBV and self-peptides are sufficient to result in the cross-activation of autoreactive T- or B-cells. Other potential mechanisms of demyelination include enhanced breakdown and presentation of self-antigens, expression of viral superantigens, or bystander activation.[11] Antibody titers to Epstein–Barr nuclear antigen (EBNA) complex are higher in MS patients versus controls, especially if blood is collected 5 years or more before onset. These titers increase over time in MS patients (controls are unchanged), and a fourfold increase in EBNA titers over time results in a threefold increased risk of developing MS (almost an 18-fold increase in those with first samples before age 20).[12] Interestingly, one paper notes individuals positive for human leukocyte antigen *(HLA) DRB1*1501* have a 24-fold increased risk of developing MS when they also have antibodies to certain epitopes within EBNA-1 compared with others.[13] This is consistent with a genetic-environmental interaction. In addition, anti-EBNA titers have been associated with RRMS, conversion of CIS to clinically definite multiple sclerosis (CDMS, confirmed diagnosis of MS), and with magnetic resonance imaging (MRI) measures such as gadolinium-enhancing lesions, change in T2 lesion volume (r = 0.27; P = 0.044), and Expanded Disability Status Scale (EDSS) score (r = 0.3; P = 0.035). Zivadinov et al. also found anti-EBNA and anti-vascular cell adhesion (VCA) titers associated with gray matter atrophy in MS.[14] While Serafini et al. have claimed to identify evidence of abortive infection in a significant number of MS patients,[15] others have not been able to replicate these findings.[16] The majority of data would lead to a conclusion that exposure to EBV is somehow associated with developing MS, but does not support the concept of an active or aborting EBV infection directly causing MS.

The familial recurrence rate of MS is approximately 5%, with siblings being the most commonly reported relationship,[4] and a concordance rate among monozygotic twins of approximately 25%. This is consistent with the idea that an environmental agent is important in the etiology of MS, but also suggests a role for one or more genes. Genes that lie within the major histocompatibility complex (MHC), which is located on the sixth chromosome in humans, have been linked to MS.[1,4] Recent data show a significant association of risk with mutations in the interleukin-2α (IL-2α) and interleukin-7α (IL-7α) receptor genes.[17-19] African Americans are significantly less likely to be diagnosed with MS compared with whites, although there is emerging evidence that they are more likely to have a severe disease course[20] and respond less to interferon (IFN) therapy.[21] A locus on chromosome 1 may be associated with increased susceptibility in African Americans.[22]

PATHOPHYSIOLOGY

An important feature to consider when understanding pathophysiology of MS and its potential clinical applications is the concept that immune cell infiltration from the periphery is a prominent feature of early-stage MS. Peripheral immune cells can enter the CNS parenchyma by direct crossing of the blood–brain barrier, the subarachnoid space, or from the choroid plexus across the blood-cerebrospinal fluid (CSF) barrier.

2 Once in the CNS, immune cells promote neurodegeneration by stripping of the myelin sheath surrounding CNS axons. This activity is associated with an inflammatory, perivenular infiltrate consisting of T and B lymphocytes, macrophages, antibodies, and complement.[10] Demyelination renders axons susceptible to damage, which becomes irreversible when they are severed. Irreversible axonal damage correlates with disability and can be visualized as hypointense lesions, or "black holes," on T1-weighted MRI.[23,24]

Peripheral immune cells, along with activated CNS-resident microglia and astrocytes, promote demyelination as well as oligodendrocyte and neuroaxonal injury. This is mediated through direct cell contact-dependent mechanisms and the action of soluble inflammatory and neurotoxic mediators. The exact trigger for activation of T-cells in the periphery remains unclear, but the T-cells in MS patients recognize myelin basic protein (MBP), proteolipid protein, myelin oligodendrocyte glycoprotein, and myelin-associated glycoprotein. T-helper subtypes can be either pathogenic or protective in MS. Furthermore, theory holds that certain T-cell subsets are not terminally differentiated, but instead engender a level of plasticity that allows for their conversion from pathogenic to protective and vice versa under certain conditions (Fig. 55-1).[25]

A new concept of T-cell entry into the CNS suggests that the initial lymphocyte invasion in MS may proceed through the ventricles, toward the choroid plexus along a CCL 20 gradient that attracts activated Th17 (T-helper) cells.[26] The actual mediator of myelin and axonal destruction has not been established, but may reflect a combination of macrophages, antibodies, destructive cytokines, and reactive oxygen intermediates. In patients with stable or mild disease, increased numbers of cells are found that express messenger RNA (mRNA) for transforming growth factor-β (TGF-β) and interleukin-10 (IL-10) compared with patients with severe disease. Conversely, a reduction in the number of T-regulatory (Treg) cells, which exhibit suppressor activity, is associated with active MS and can be found in patients with progressive disease. It should be noted,

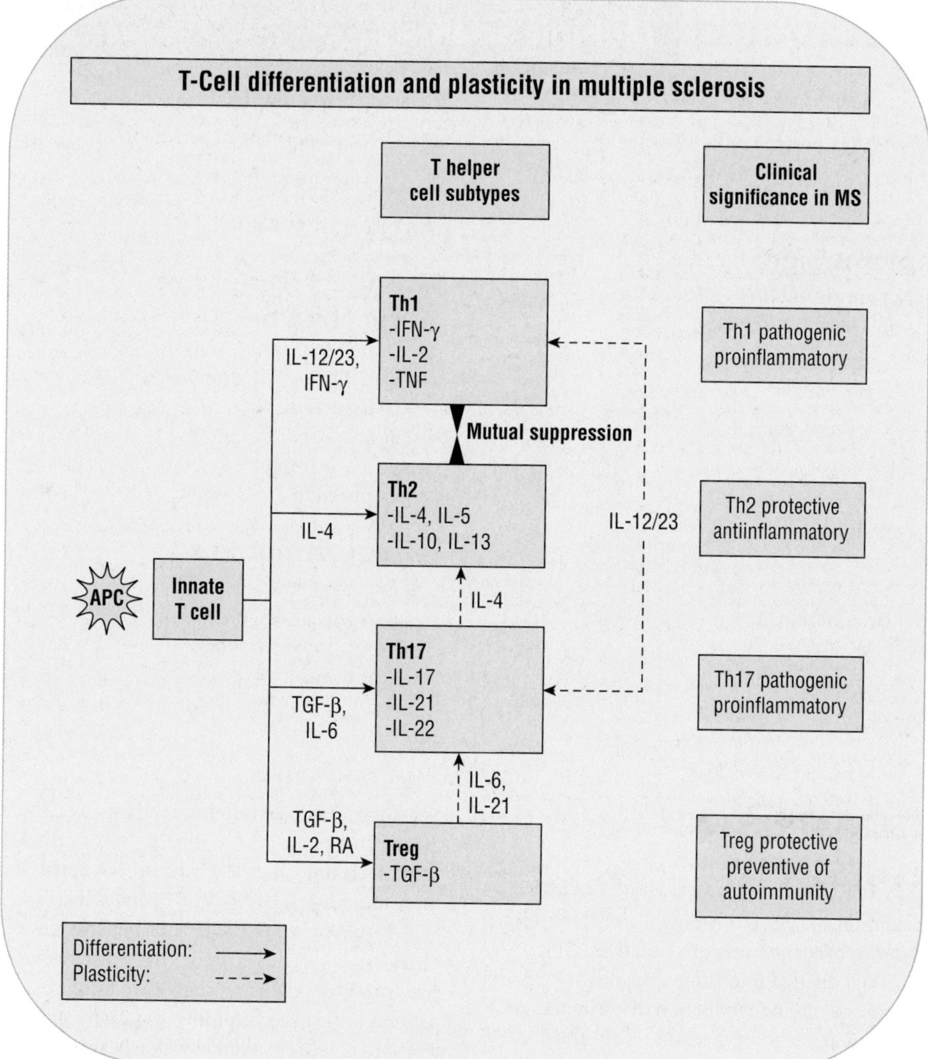

FIGURE 55-1 Upon interaction with an antigen-laden APC and specific cytokines, the innate T-cells undergo differentiation into a few lineages (subtypes). Four subtypes significant for MS pathophysiology are illustrated here (Th1, Th2, Th17, and Treg). Th1 and Th17 are proinflammatory, Th2 is antiinflammatory, and Treg is regulatory. Th1 and Th2 are mutually suppressive and are relatively stable differentiated subtypes. In contrast, Th17 and Treg subtypes are recently found to exhibit "plasticity." In other words, they can undergo phenotypic conversion to another T-cell subtype (Th1 or Th2) in the presence of specific cytokine conditions. This plasticity of Th17 and Treg is the immunologic basis for development of therapeutic agents to favor the production of suitable Th subtypes for combating microbial invasion and also concurrently achieving neurocellular recovery after an infection.[25] (APC, antigen presenting cell.)

however, that Treg ratios do not always correlate with disease activity. Of note, experimental evidence associates high 25-hydroxyvitamin D levels with improved Treg function, favoring the Th2 phenotype in the Th1/Th2 balance.[27] Finally, the significance of one of the immunological hallmarks of MS, the intrathecal synthesis of multiple clones of immunoglobulins, remains unclear. The antigen(s) against which these immunoglobulins are directed remain unknown, but do not appear to include common CNS myelin antigens.[28] The complex interplay of a variety of cells, antibodies, and cytokines remains to be elucidated.

It is well accepted that MS lesions are heterogeneous, which may be due in part to differences in the stage of evolution of the lesions over time, differences in underlying immunopathogenesis, or a combination. Acute lesions show demyelination and axonal destruction with lymphocytic activity consistent with an inflammatory state. In contrast chronic lesions display less inflammatory lymphocytes with active remyelination.[10] As the disease progresses, immune cell infiltration wanes, perhaps due to adaptive immune cell exhaustion from chronic antigen exposure. Chronic CNS-intrinsic inflammation and neurodegeneration continues independent of peripheral immune activation. As a consequence, meningeal tertiary lymphoid-like structures, which have specifically been documented in secondary progressive disease, may contribute to late-stage inflammation in patients with this form of MS.

Although traditional descriptions have focused on white matter as the sole location of MS lesions, more recent studies have clearly identified cortical and subcortical gray matter lesions both pathologically[29] and radiographically.[30] In addition, a subset of patients with progressive MS are noted to have abnormalities consistent with B-cell follicles in the meninges.[31]

Just as the full dimensions of the neuropathology are uncertain, so is the pathogenesis of the MS lesion. Substantial evidence suggests it is an autoimmune process directed against myelin and oligodendrocytes, the cells that make myelin[10] (Fig. 55-2).

CLINICAL PRESENTATION Multiple Sclerosis

General

- Most patients with MS present with nonspecific complaints. Many have problems with their vision or paresthesias

Primary Symptoms/Signs

- Visual complaints/optic neuritis
- Gait problems and falls
- Paresthesias
- Pain
- Spasticity
- Weakness
- Ataxia
- Speech difficulty
- Psychological changes
- Cognitive changes
- Fatigue
- Bowel/bladder dysfunction
- Sexual dysfunction
- Tremor

Laboratory Tests

- MS is a diagnosis of exclusion
- MRI
- CSF studies
- Evoked potentials

Secondary Symptoms

- Recurrent UTIs
- Urinary calculi
- Decubiti and osteomyelitis
- Osteoporosis
- Respiratory infections
- Poor nutrition
- Depression

Tertiary Symptoms

- Financial problems
- Personal/social problems
- Vocational problems
- Emotional problems

CLINICAL PRESENTATION AND COURSE OF ILLNESS

3 The clinical presentation of MS is extremely variable among patients and typically varies over time in a given patient. The signs and symptoms of MS can be divided into three categories. Primary symptoms are a direct consequence of conduction disturbances produced by demyelination and axonal damage, and reflect the area of the CNS that is damaged. Secondary symptoms are complications resulting from primary symptoms. For example, urinary retention, a primary symptom, can lead to frequent urinary tract infections (UTIs), a secondary symptom. Tertiary symptoms relate to the effect of the disease on the patient's everyday life.[32]

The clinical course of CDMS is classified into four categories.[33] At the onset of symptoms, about 85% of patients have exacerbations—new symptoms lasting at least 24 hours and separated from other new symptoms by at least 30 days—followed by remissions (complete or incomplete). Exacerbations are frequently referred to as relapses or attacks. This course is called RRMS; the first clinical presentation is typically CIS. During the RRMS phase, there is a correlation between new brain MRI lesions and clinical attacks, but typically there are many more new MRI lesions than new clinical symptoms. In RRMS patients, attack frequency tends to decrease over time and becomes independent of the development of progressive disabilities.[34] Neurologic recovery following an exacerbation is often quite good early in the disease course, but following repeated relapses, recovery tends to be less complete. In addition, there is a new concept of a radiologically isolated syndrome (RIS), referring to individuals who have clinical scenarios not typical of MS, yet obtain MRI scans for other reasons (eg, headache) and have radiological signs suggestive of MS. Some percentage of these patients convert to RRMS over time,[35] although when to start DMT remains unclear and varies by practice.

Approximately 10% to 20% of RRMS patients have a benign course, characterized by few relapses, often sensory, with minimal disability accruing over time. Most RRMS patients eventually enter a progressive phase in which attacks and remissions are difficult to identify. This is referred to as secondary-progressive multiple sclerosis (SPMS). Disability tends to accumulate more significantly during this phase of the illness. New brain MRI lesions, especially those seen only after the injection of contrast media, are less common, and brain atrophy and T1 holes increase.[36]

4 Approximately 15% of patients never have discrete phases of attacks and remissions but have progressive disease from the outset, known as primary-progressive multiple sclerosis (PPMS). These patients will have symptoms, especially spastic paraparesis that may worsen rapidly or relatively slowly over time, and accrue progressively more disability. Patients with PPMS are diagnosed at a later age, with the number of males roughly equal to that of females. In general, PPMS patients tend to have a worse prognosis than those who present initially with RRMS, although data suggest progression is variable.[37] Many clinical trials have suggested that a significant portion of patients with PPMS do not receive benefit from studied therapies. However, a study using rituximab suggests a subgroup of PPMS patients who are less than 51 years of age and have at least one gadolinium-enhancing lesion may benefit from this therapy.[38] Finally, a small percentage of patients may have a mixture of both progression and relapses, referred to as progressive-relapsing multiple sclerosis (PRMS). These patients are generally treated as relapsing patients.

Progression of the illness throughout the lifetime can be measured in many ways. The most widely used clinical rating scale is the EDSS, which uses a numerical value ranging from 0 (no disability) to 10 (death) to evaluate neurologic functions.[39] The limitations of this scale are the relative insensitivity to clinical changes not involving impairment of ambulation, such as changes in cognition, fatigue, and affect. Other tools, such as the multiple sclerosis functional composite (MSFC), are being evaluated for increased sensitivity and utility in describing changes in MS-related disability over time.[40] Increasingly, MRI is being used as an index of both disease activity and progression.[10] Specifically, the appearance of new lesions or changes in lesion number, size, and volume are being used as outcome measures in research studies. Optical coherence tomography measures the retinal neural fiber layer thickness, and may also be a measurable sign of pathological progression over time.[41]

The unpredictable nature of MS makes it impossible to anticipate when an exacerbation will occur. However, certain factors,

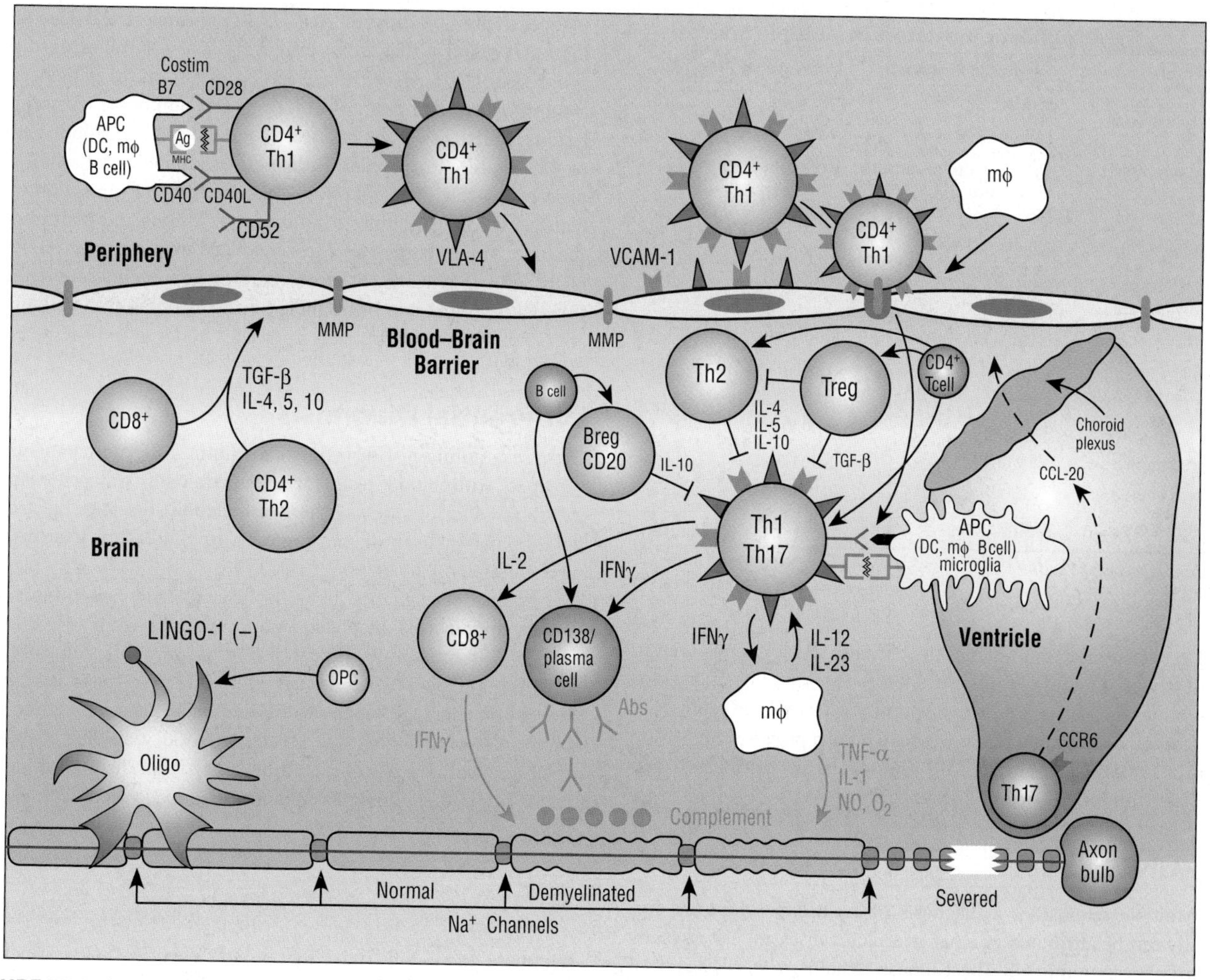

FIGURE 55-2 Autoimmune theory of the pathogenesis of multiple sclerosis (MS). In MS, the immunogenic cells tend to be more myelin-reactive, and these T-cells produce cytokines mimicking a Th1-mediated proinflammatory reaction. T-helper cells (CD4$^+$) appear to be key initiators of myelin destruction in MS. These autoreactive CD4$^+$ cells, especially of the T-helper cell type 1 (Th1) subtype, are activated in the periphery, perhaps following a viral infection. The activation of T- and B-cells requires two signals. The first signal is the interaction between MHC and APC (macrophage, dendritic cell, and B-cell). The second signal consists of the binding between B7 on the APC and CD28 on the T-cell for T-cell activation. Similarly, CD40 expressed on APCs and CD40L expressed on T-cells interact to signal the proliferation of B-cells within the blood–brain barrier following the entry to T-cells. The T-cells in the periphery express adhesion molecules on their surfaces that allow them to attach and roll along the endothelial cells that constitute the blood–brain barrier. The activated T-cells also produce MMP that help to create openings in the blood–brain barrier, allowing entry of the activated T-cells past the blood–brain barrier and into the CNS. Once inside the CNS, the T-cells produce proinflammatory cytokines, especially interleukins (ILs) 1, 2, 12, 17, and 23, tumor necrosis factor-α (TNF-α), and interferon-γ (INF-γ), which further create openings in the blood–brain barrier, allowing entry of B-cells, complement, macrophages, and antibodies. The T-cells also interact within the CNS with the resident microglia, astrocytes, and macrophages, further enhancing production of proinflammatory cytokines and other potential mediators of CNS damage, including reactive oxygen intermediates and nitric oxide. The role of modulating, or downregulating, cytokines such as IL-4, IL-5, IL-10, and transforming growth factor-β (TGF-β) also has been described. These cytokines are the products of CD4$^+$, CD8$^+$, and Th1-cells.[10] New pathogenic mechanisms involve, but are not limited to, receptor-ligand mediated T-cell entry via choroid plexus (CCR6-CCL20 axis),[26] coupling of key receptor-ligands for inhibition of myelination/demyelination (LINGO-1/NOGO66/p75 or TROY complex, Jagged-Notch signaling). (Ag, antigens; APC, antigen presenting cell; DC, dendrite cell; IgG, immunoglobulin G; MΦ, macrophage; Na$^+$, sodium ion; MMP, matrix metalloproteinases; MHC, major histocompatibility complex; OPC, oligodendrocyte precursor cell; VLA, very late antigen; VCAM, vascular cell adhesion molecule.)

including infections, heat (including fever), sleep deprivation, stress, malnutrition, anemia, concurrent organ dysfunction, exertion, and childbirth, may aggravate symptoms or lead to an attack. Interestingly, many patients experience a significant reduction in relapses during the third trimester of pregnancy, followed by a relative increase postpartum.[42]

Between 60% and 80% of individuals diagnosed with the MS have been reported to be sensitive to environmental heat. Clinically, increased body temperature might result in worsening of previous neurological deficits, including fatigue and decreased muscular endurance. Blurred vision, known as Uthoff's phenomenon, is caused by increased body temperature due to physical exercise or physical restraint. Body temperature influences nerve impulses, which are blocked or slowed down in a damaged nerve. After normalization of the temperature, signs and symptoms improve or disappear.

Multiple sclerosis usually does not directly diminish life expectancy, although the development of secondary complications such as pneumonia or septicemia (secondary to aspiration in those with swallowing difficulties, decubitus ulcers, or UTIs) or rapid progression of primary lesions affecting respiratory function can lead to a shorter

TABLE 55-1 Prognostic Indicators in Multiple Sclerosis

Indicator	Favorable Prognosis	Unfavorable Prognosis
Age at onset	<40 years	>40 years
Gender	Female	Male
Initial symptoms	Optic neuritis or sensory symptoms	Motor or cerebellar symptoms; polysymptomatic
Disability	Late	Early
Attack frequency in early disease	Low	High
Course of disease	Relapsing/remitting	Progressive
Recovery after first event	Good	Poor
T2 lesions	Low load	High load
T1 black hole lesions	Low rate	High rate
Growth of lesions	Slow	Rapid
Locations of lesions	Single	Multiple

Data from references 48 and 49.

than expected life span. Most of the decrease in life span is seen in patients with rapidly progressive disease. Suicide rates as high as seven times that seen in the general population have been reported.[43] Clinical and demographic factors used to predict prognosis of MS are listed in Table 55-1.[5,44] Several MRI features also have been shown to correlate with progression of disease (see below).[45-47]

DIAGNOSIS

5 Multiple sclerosis is a diagnosis of exclusion; symptoms frequently can be attributed to other neurologic diseases, just as many syndromes can mimic MS. The diagnosis remains primarily a clinical one that requires demonstration of "lesions separated in space and time," referring to the occurrence of at least two episodes of neurologic disturbance reflecting distinct sites of CNS damage that cannot be explained by another mechanism.[50] An international panel of MS experts established the McDonald criteria,[50] which allows brain MRI lesions, CSF abnormalities, and visual-evoked potential (VEP) studies to substitute for clinical lesions in defining "separated in space and time" A reevaluation of the McDonald criteria has simplified the use of these laboratory studies.[45] In the new scheme, diagnostic categories are MS, possible MS (for those individuals at high risk of developing MS), and not MS; these new criteria allow for earlier diagnosis.[45] Newer, simpler MRI criteria defining dissemination in space and time may be somewhat more sensitive and equally specific.[51-53] A consensus panel of the American Association of Neurology endorses the utility of MRI for diagnostic purpose,[47] and the US FDA has approved several of the immunotherapies to be used after a single attack (CIS) of demyelination in the context of an appropriately abnormal brain MRI. A proposed set of criteria now being considered will allow for earlier diagnosis in patients with CIS to establish "dissemination in space and time" with a single MRI. Therefore, patients will need to have lesions in different areas of their CNS with at least one enhancing lesion that correlates with clinical symptomatology. By fulfilling these criteria, a patient can be diagnosed with CDMS.

Laboratory Studies

To date, there are no tests specific for MS. Evidence provided by MRI of the brain and spine,[46,47] CSF evaluation (presence of increased oligoclonal bands and increased IgG), evoked potentials,[45,50] and optic coherence tomography,[54] used in conjunction with the physical examination and history, aids in establishing the diagnosis of MS. MRI, the most valuable diagnostic tool, produces images of the brain and spine that reflect damage that is characteristic of MS plaques in multiple areas of the CNS. MRI is the preferred technique for establishing a diagnosis, prognosis, and for following disease progression. Optic neuritis, a lesion or lesions on the optic nerve, is a common first symptom of MS. A greater number of T2-weighted lesions (called *T2 burden of disease*) on MRI following optic neuritis or CIS appears to correlate with the development of disability and progression to CDMS.[46] Lesions that enhance after injection of the contrast media gadolinium indicate new lesions and disruption of the blood–brain barrier and are associated with early conversion to CDMS in CIS patients.[46,55] However, they do not correlate well over time with progression of disability. Brain atrophy, even early in the course of the illness, probably correlates better with progression of disability.[47]

Differential Diagnosis

Because a number of disorders can mimic MS, most patients are screened with blood tests for rheumatologic, collagen-vascular, infectious, and sometimes inherited metabolic diseases. Electromyography may help in diagnosing amyotrophic lateral sclerosis and neuropathies.

Magnetic resonance imaging, used to rule out tumors and cervical spondylosis, may also lead to evaluations for MS in many patients with little or no clinical history of MS. While some of these patients may have MRI scans suggestive of MS (so-called RIS), most have nonspecific MRI scans with identifiable causes for their scan abnormalities, including age greater than 50 years, hypertension, and migraine.[56] The use of established criteria for distinguishing MS lesions from other etiologies enhances diagnostic accuracy.

TREATMENT

Treatment of MS falls into three broad categories: (1) treatment of exacerbations, (2) DMTs, and (3) symptomatic therapies. Treatment of exacerbations will shorten the duration and possibly decrease the severity of the attack. DMTs alter the course of the illness, and diminish progressive disability over time. Symptomatic management of the disease is of utmost importance to maintain the patient's quality-of-life. Although different treatment modalities have been studied in the last 30 years, many older trials had flawed designs. As there are no universally accepted treatment algorithms, treatments vary among clinicians and centers. Perhaps more importantly, treatment decisions are frequently based on the wishes and goals of individual patients rather than evidence-based algorithms. One potential algorithm for the immunotherapy of CDMS is shown in Fig. 55-3.

Desired Outcomes

The main goals of treatment are to improve patients overall quality-of-life and minimize long-term disability. Treatment goals are attained by altering MS exacerbations or relapses, decreasing the number of white matter lesions and black holes on MRI, averting brain atrophy, and ultimately halting disease progression. This can be achieved by early recognition of the disease and immediate utilization of FDA-approved DMTs.

General Approach to Treatment

The severity of symptoms at initial presentation will determine whether an induction or escalation algorithm will be assigned to an individual patient. When FDA-approved drugs do not alter the naturally progressive disease, investigational agents or non–FDA-approved medications, such as rituximab, may be used. As a general rule, MS affects patients in their most productive years of life. Practitioners must work with their patients to set realistic expectations over their lifetime and develop a long-term treatment and management plan. With disease progression, patients are likely

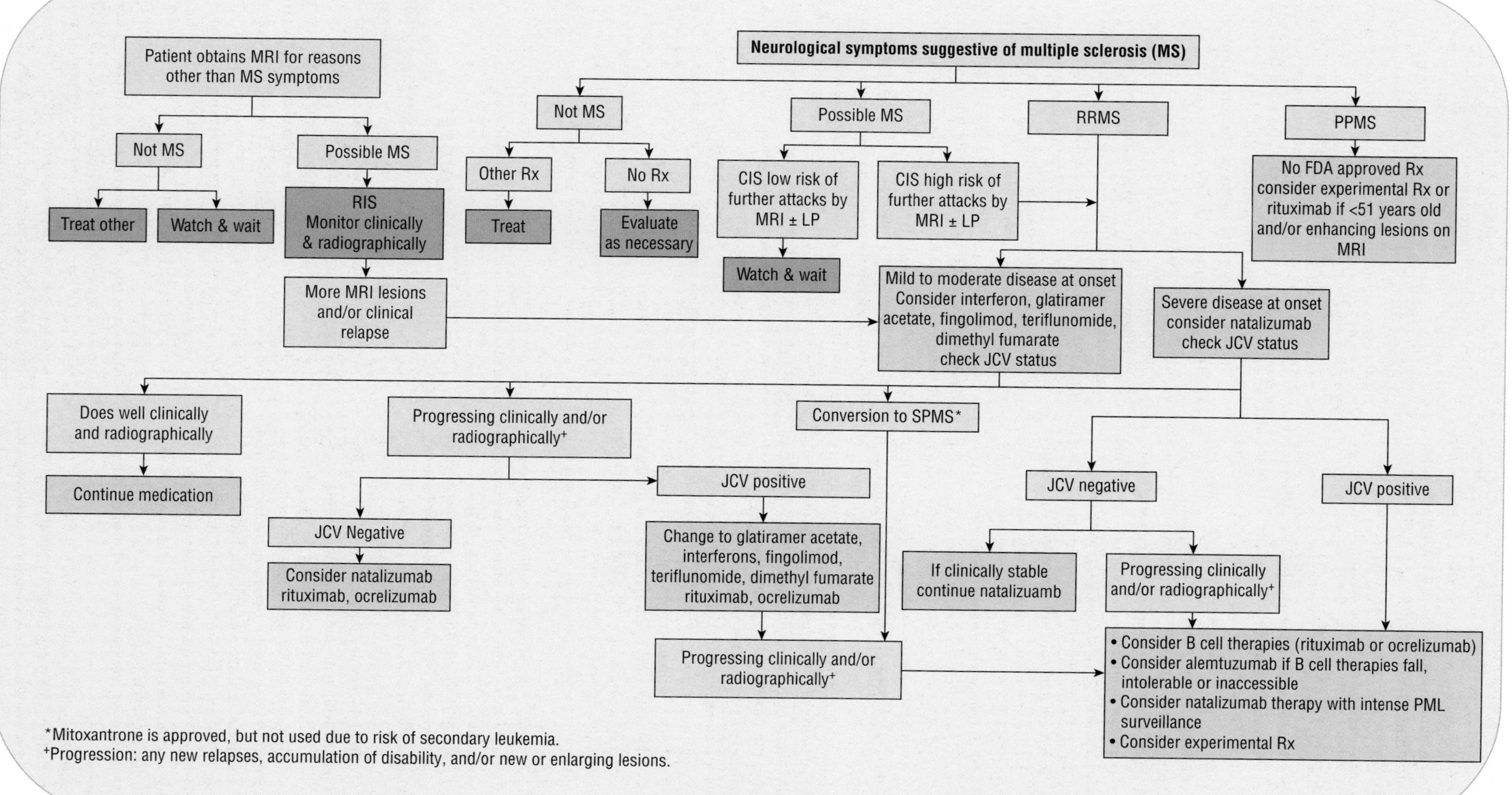

FIGURE 55-3 Algorithm for management of clinically definite multiple sclerosis.

to acquire secondary and tertiary symptoms of MS. In clinical trials, high nonadherence rates are reported as an important issue for potential treatment failure. Potential reasons identified for nonadherence are lack of perceived benefit, cost, adverse effects, depression, and undesirable routes of administration (eg, subcutaneous, intramuscular injection, intravenous [IV]). With the advance of FDA-approved medications to treat MS, patients are experiencing fewer relapses, slower disease progression, and improved quality-of-life.

Treatment of Exacerbations

6 Exacerbations are the hallmark of early RRMS. Although recovery after relapses is in general complete, over time a substantial accumulation of disability occurs. Controversy exists about the relationship between relapses and subsequent accumulation of disability. Frequent relapses (more than three relapses per year in the first 2 years after diagnosis) have shown consistent positive correlation with later development of neurological disability. Generally, mild exacerbations that do not produce functional decline may not require treatment. Decisions to treat relapses are usually substantiated by patient expectations, prior experience with corticosteroids, and predicted course of recovery. Generally accepted indications are based on mono- or polysymptomatic presentations; relapses that localize to the optic nerve, spinal cord, or brainstem; functional limitations that affect activities of daily living; and symptoms that continue to worsen over a period of 2 weeks. When functional ability is affected, the standard intervention is IV injection of high-dose corticosteroids. The American Academy of Neurology (AAN) recommends that if treatment with steroids is warranted, it is best to use IV methylprednisolone.[57] The mechanism of action for corticosteroids in MS is unknown, but it is speculated that steroids improve recovery by decreasing edema in the area of demyelination. IV methylprednisolone has been shown to shorten the duration of exacerbations; it may also delay repeat attacks for up to 2 years after optic neuritis,[57] although it has not been shown to definitively affect disease progression.[58] In some circumstances, equipotent doses of oral prednisone can be substituted for IV methylprednisolone. Interestingly, adrenocorticotropic hormone (ACTH) is the only agent that is FDA approved for treatment of MS exacerbation treatment, although it is rarely used due to cost and availability.

Methylprednisolone doses range from 500 to 1,000 mg/day, given IV. Duration of therapy is variable and can range from 3 to (rarely) 10 days, depending on clinical response. Functional recovery after an exacerbation is more rapid if corticosteroids are initiated within 2 weeks of symptom onset. If improvement occurs, it usually begins after 3 to 5 days. Short-term use is often accompanied by sleep disturbance, a metallic taste in the mouth, and rarely, gastrointestinal (GI) upset. Patients with diabetes mellitus or a predilection to diabetes mellitus may have significant elevations of blood sugar, requiring the use of insulin. Longer durations of IV methylprednisolone therapy are associated with acne and fungal infections, mood alteration, and, rarely, GI hemorrhage (especially in hospitalized patients or in those taking aspirin). If methylprednisolone is not available, equipotent doses of dexamethasone have been used as a substitute, although this is not well supported in the literature.

A small number of patients have more severe attacks, manifested by hemiplegia, paraplegia, or quadriplegia. If these patients fail to improve with aggressive steroid therapy, plasma exchange (PLEX) every other day for seven treatments can be beneficial for approximately 40% of patients, or intravenous immunoglobulin (IVIG) can be given.

A "pseudoexacerbation" is an episode with symptoms consistent with an exacerbation, but precipitated by something other than the natural course of the disease. A pseudoexacerbation can be precipitated by heat, infections (eg, UTIs), or stress (emotional or physical); these must be ruled out before exacerbation treatment is initiated or DMTs are altered.

Disease-Modifying Therapy

7 Indications and dosing of DMTs are shown in Table 55-2. MS is a complex, heterogeneous disease with clear variability in pathogenesis between patients and within patients over time. As a result, treatment decisions are usually based on clinical predictors of disease severity, our incomplete understanding of the mechanism of action of currently available therapies, and the safety and tolerability profile of the medications. There is some degree of agreement that use of escalation approaches early in the course of the disease, with safer yet partially effective medications, is useful. Currently, FDA-approved first-generation therapies (self-injected medications that decrease annualized relapse rate by about 30% and decrease the formation of new white matter lesion) include four IFN formulations (five brand names), and glatiramer acetate (a non-IFN). The first-generation DMTs are not immediately efficacious for patient symptoms. However, their efficacy is noted approximately 1 to 2 years after starting therapy. In addition to first-generation DMTs, the FDA has approved natalizumab, mitoxantrone, fingolimod, teriflunomide, dimethyl fumarate, and alemtuzumab for the treatment of relapsing forms of MS. Mitoxantrone also has an FDA indication for progressive or worsening MS.

8 In some patients with poor prognostic factors and poor clinical presentation, natalizumab, fingolimod, teriflunomide, and dimethyl fumarate may be prescribed as initial therapy, as opposed to starting first generation DMTs that are associated with less serious side-effect risk. This type of algorithm would be considered an induction therapy, where you concentrate all therapeutic efforts in the early phases of disease. Drugs used to treat MS can be considered either immunomodulatory (able to alter the immune signals without cytotoxic effect or bone marrow suppression) or immunosuppressive (able to alter the immune system through a direct cytotoxic activity or bone marrow suppression). However, these agents have a higher risk-to-benefit ratio based on their safety profile.[59] Adverse drug reactions and monitoring parameters of DMTs are shown in Table 55-3.

It is important to note that the efficacy of the DMTs may vary considerably between individual patients and for any given patient at different points in time. Moreover, patients with MS may have different tolerance for side effects and risks, as well as preference for different routes of administration. Therefore, access to the full range of options is critical in order for patients with MS and their clinicians to make optimal treatment decisions.

Clinical **Controversy...**

Current MS therapies target inflammatory activity, defined by clinical relapses and MRI lesions, as a way to impact disability development. So, the absence of clinical and MRI activity are accepted paradigms of disease-free status in treated patients. The development of highly effective therapies is allowing neurologists to consider their use early on the course of the disease in order to prevent permanent disability. However, certain therapies (natalizumab, fingolimod, dimethyl fumarate) have an inherent increased risk of serious complications (eg, PML). For that reason, it is imperative to consider risk benefit assessments regularly in the care of MS patients. The rationale behind escalating therapy is that treatment starts with safer drugs and moves on to more effective therapies if the ongoing treatment fails. In the escalating approach, glatiramer acetate and interferon betas are regarded as first-line drugs, whereas immunosuppressants (natalizumab, fingolimod, dimethyl fumarate, alemtuzumab) are considered second-line drugs. The concept of induction treatment with highly effective therapies early on in the course of the disease followed by long-term maintenance treatment has attracted considerable attention. Given that all the immunosuppressants that are currently available present potentially serious side effects, the induction strategy has generally been reserved for patients with very active and aggressive disease from onset. In general, there is acceptance on defining treatment success, and that is by the absence of any clinical evidence of progression (eg, relapses, progression of disability, and new MRI findings). However, controversy arises because there is a lack of biomarkers to reveal the extent of tissue damage in MS. In the coming years, new MRI techniques should help us to identify those RRMS patients, especially individuals without any real disability, who are most at risk of developing destructive CNS lesions with or without first-line therapy and who are therefore more eligible for an early and more aggressive treatment strategy.

TABLE 55-2 Disease Modifying Therapy

Drug	Brand Name	Indication	Initial Dose	Usual Dose	Comment
First generation agents					
Self-injectables					
Interferon-β_{1a}	Avonex	Relapsing forms of MS	30 mcg (6 million international units) IM once weekly	30 mcg IM once weekly	Avonex is considered as a low potency interferon Cost per year[a]: $78,530
Interferon-β_{1a}	Rebif	Relapsing forms of MS	22 mcg SQ three times a week	22 or 44 mcg SQ three times a week	Rebif is considered as a high potency interferon Cost per year[a]: $84,766
Interferon-β_{1b}	Betaseron, Extavia	Relapsing forms of MS	250 mcg (8 million international units) SQ every other day	250 mcg SQ every other day	Betaseron/Extavia is considered as a high potency interferon Pregnancy category C Cost per year[a]: $83,276/$73,504 (Betaseron/Extavia)
Pegylated Interferon-β_{1a}	Plegridy	RRMS	6.3 mcg SQ day 1, then 94 mcg SQ on day 15, then 125 mcg SQ on day 29, then 125 mcg SQ every 14 days	125 mg SQ every 14 days	Pregnancy category C Can premedicate or concurrently use an antipyretic/analgesic for flu-like symptoms Cost per year[a]: 157,040
Glatiramer acetate	Copaxone Glatopa	CIS, RRMS	20 mg SQ once daily or 40 mg SQ three times a week	20 mg SQ once daily or 40 mg SQ three times a week	Pregnancy category B Cost per year[a]: $89,213 (Copaxone 20 mg/day), $78,125 (Copaxone 40 mg three times a week), $78,991 (Glatopa 20 mg/day)
IV infusion					
Mitoxantrone	Novantrone	SPMS, PRMS, and worsening RRMS	12 mg/m^2 IV every 3 months	12 mg/m^2 IV every 3 months	Lifetime dose should not exceed 140 mg/m^2 Pregnancy category D
Second generation agents					
Oral agents					
Fingolimod	Gilenya	Relapsing forms of MS	0.5 mg orally once daily	0.5 mg orally once daily	REMS Pregnancy category C Cost per year[a]: $85,136
Teriflunomide	Aubagio	Relapsing forms of MS	7 mg orally once daily	7 or 14 mg orally once daily	Pregnancy category X Cost per year[a]: $79,438 Cholestyramine and charcoal accelerate teriflunomide elimination
Dimethyl fumarate	Tecfidera	Relapsing forms of MS	120 mg delayed release twice daily for 7 days	240 mg delayed release twice daily	Pregnancy category C Cost per year: $79,716
IV infusion					
Natalizumab	Tysabri	Relapsing forms of MS	300 mg IV every 4 weeks	300 mg IV every 4 weeks	REMS Pregnancy category C Cost per year[a]: $5,468
Alemtuzumab	Lemtrada	RRMS	1st treatment course: 12 mg/day IV for 5 consecutive days (60 mg total dose) 2nd treatment course: 12 mg/day IV for 3 consecutive days (36 mg total dose) administered 12 months after 1st treatment course		May premedicate with high dose corticosteroid (1,000 mg methylprednisolone or equivalent) immediately prior to infusion for first 3 days Also administer herpes viral prophylaxis starting on first day of treatment and continued for at least 2 months after completion of treatment or until CD4$^+$ count is at least 200 cells/μL (0.2×10^9/L), whichever occurs last Pregnancy category C REMS Total treatment cost[a]: $158,000
Self-injectable					
Daclizumab	Zinbryta	Relapsing forms of MS	150 mg SQ once monthly	150 mg SQ once monthly	REMS Cost per year: $98,400

CIS, clinically isolated syndrome; IM, intramuscular; PRMS, primary relapsing multiple sclerosis; REMS, Risk Evaluation and Mitigation Strategy; RRMS, relapsing remitting multiple sclerosis; SPMS, secondary progressive multiple sclerosis; SQ, subcutaneous.

[a]Cost: Cost as reported in Red Book, Not all drug companies publish average wholesale price (AWP), and those are calculated in accordance with Truven Health Analytics AWP Policy. Does not include nursing, pharmacy, and technical fees.

TABLE 55-3 Adverse Drug Reactions and Monitoring Parameters

Drug	Adverse Drug Reaction	Monitoring Parameter	Comments
Interferon-β_{1a}	Depression, flu-like symptoms, leukopenia, injection site reactions	Electrolytes, CBC, LFTs, thyroid function, LVEF, depression LFTs at baseline, 1 month, and every 3 months for a year, and every 6 months thereafter	Avoid use in untreated severe depression
Interferon-β_{1b}	Depression, injection site reactions, leukopenia, flu-like symptoms	Electrolytes, CBC, LFTs, thyroid function, depression	Avoid use in untreated severe depression More frequent injection site reactions reported
Glatiramer acetate	Injection site reactions, infection, hypersensitivity, chest tightness, urticaria	MRI, tissue necrosis, postinjection reaction	Chest tightness, urticaria can occur at any dose
Mitoxantrone	Bone marrow suppression, neutropenia, cardiotoxicity, AML, nausea, vomiting, diarrhea, alopecia	CBC, ECG, LVEF, LFTs	Secondary leukemia Lifetime maximum dose due to cardiac toxicity
Natalizumab	PML, depression, fatigue, respiratory infection, arthralgia, hepatotoxicity	JCV antibody, infection, MRI, LFTs	Risk of PML Risk of IRIS when discontinued due to PML
Fingolimod	Lymphocytopenia, macular retinal edema, AV block, infection, headache	CBC, ECG, varicella zoster antibody, blood pressure, ophthalmic examination, LFTs	Requires first dose observation Contraindicated in patients receiving Class I and III antiarrhythmic drugs and those with recent cardiac disease,[a] second and third degree AV block Ketoconazole increases fingolimod serum concentration (3A4 inhibition) Vaccine efficacy may be decreased
Teriflunomide	Steven–Johnson syndrome, liver failure, neutropenia, respiratory infection, activation of TB, alopecia, neuropathy	CBC, LFTs, blood pressure, pregnancy, TB test	Contraindicated in severe hepatic impairment Possibility of TB reactivation Active metabolite of leflunomide
Dimethyl fumarate	Flushing, rash, pruritus, GI discomfort, lymphocytopenia, increased LFTs, albuminuria	CBC, LFTs	Taking with food decreases incidence of flushing
Alemtuzumab	Infusion reactions, infections (nasophyaryngitis, UTI, URI, herpes viral infections), autoimmune disorders, thyroid disorders, immune-mediated thrombocytopenic purpura, Goodpasture syndrome	CBC, thyroid function, antibodies to varicella zoster virus, HPV screening, serum creatinine, TB prior to treatment, infusion reactions, skin exams, urinalysis	May premedicate with high dose corticosteroid (1,000 mg methylprednisolone or equivalent) immediately prior to infusion for first 3 days. Also administer herpes viral prophylaxis starting on first day of treatment and continued for at least 2 months after completion of treatment or until CD4+ count is at least 200 cells/μL (0.2×10^9/L), whichever occurs last Contraindicated with HIV infection Birth control should be used during treatment and for 4 months after each treatment course Breastfeeding not recommended during treatment and for 4 months following each treatment course
Daclizumab	Upper respiratory tract infection, depression, rash, pharyngitis, increased ALT	LFTs & bilirubin (prior to treatment then monthly during treatment & for 6 months after the last dose) Contraindicated in hepatic disease or hepatic impairment	Live vaccines are not recommended during treatment and up to 4 months after discontinuation Evaluate for tuberculosis prior to treatment

AML, acute myeloid leukemia; CBC, complete blood count; ECG, electrocardiogram; LVEF, left ventricular ejection fraction; IRIS, immune reconstitution inflammatory syndrome; PML, progressive multifocal leukoencephalopathy; LFT, liver function test.

[a]Cardiac disease including myocardial infarction, unstable angina, stroke, transient ischemic attack, and heart failure NYHA Class III/IV.

Interferon-β_{1b} and Interferon-β_{1a}

IFN-β_{1b} (Betaseron, Extavia) was the first agent proven to favorably alter the natural course of the illness (Table 55-4).[60] Although the exact mechanism of action is unknown, effect of IFN-β_{1b} in MS may be caused by its immunomodulating properties, including the ability to augment suppressor cell function and reduce IFN-γ secretion by activated lymphocytes, its macrophage-activating effect, and its ability to downregulate the expression of IFN-γ–induced class II MHC gene products on antigen-presenting glial cells. IFN suppresses T-cell proliferation and may decrease blood–brain barrier permeability by decreasing matrix metalloproteinases.[60] IFN-β also increases the production of regulatory CD56 (bright) natural killer cells and Treg cells.[61] In general, all IFNs exert these actions in the periphery and at the blood–brain barrier level.

IFN-β_{1b} is a nonglycosylated synthetic analog of recombinant IFN-β that is produced in *Escherichia coli*. IFN-β_{1b} is administered subcutaneously every other day at a dose of 250 mcg (8 million international units). Clinical trials have demonstrated that at these doses, IFN-β_{1b} significantly reduces annual relapse rate and MRI burden of disease compared with placebo. No significant differences were noted between the IFN and placebo-treated groups with respect to clinical disability.[60] Betaseron is packaged in partially premixed syringes with a new formulation that does not require refrigeration and can be used with an autoinjector. In 2009, an additional IFN product was introduced with the trade name Extavia; Extavia is the same medicinal product as Betaseron.

IFN-β_{1a} (Avonex, Rebif) is a natural-sequence glycosylated IFN produced in Chinese hamster ovary cells. Avonex is administered as a 30-mcg dose (6 million international units) intramuscularly once weekly. Rebif is made in a very similar fashion to Avonex but given as either 22 or 44 mcg subcutaneously three times weekly. Both are supplied in a 0.5-mL prefilled syringe and should be refrigerated, but remain stable at room temperature for 30 days. Rebif may have lower immunogenicity and a slightly better side-effect profile.[62]

TABLE 55-4 Evidenced-Based Recommendations for Disease Modifying Treatment of Multiple Sclerosis

Recommendations	Recommendation Grades[a]
Interferon-β	
• Interferon-β has been shown to reduce attack rates in patients with MS or those with CIS who are at high risk of developing MS	A-I
• It is appropriate to consider IFN-β for any patient with clinically definite MS or who already has RRMS or SPMS and is still experiencing relapses	A-I
• The effectiveness of IFN-β in patients with SPMS but without relapses is uncertain	U-I
• Route of administration of IFN-β products is probably not clinically important with regards to efficacy; however, the side-effect profile does differ	B-II
• Rate of production of neutralizing antibodies is probably less with IFN-β_{1a} than with IFN-β_{1b}	B-I
• Presence of neutralizing antibodies may be associated with a reduction in the clinical effectiveness of IFN-β treatment	C-I
Glatiramer acetate	
• Glatiramer acetate has been shown to reduce the attack rate in patients with RRMS	A-I
• Treatment with glatiramer acetate may slow sustained disability progression in RRMS	C-I
Mitoxantrone	
• Mitoxantrone probably reduces the attack rate in patients with relapsing forms of MS	B-II, III
• Mitoxantrone may have a beneficial effect on disease progression in MS	C-II, III
Natalizumab	
• Natalizumab decreases clinical relapse rate, Gd-enhancing lesions, and new T2 lesions	A-I
• Natalizumab in RRMS positively changes measures of disease severity such as EDSS progression rate and changes lesions on MRI in RRMS	A-I

CIS, Clinically isolated syndrome; RCT, randomized controlled trial; RRMS, relapsing-remitting multiple sclerosis; SPMS, secondary-progressive multiple sclerosis.

[a]Strength of recommendations: A: established. B: probable. C: possible. U: inadequate data to support recommendation.

Quality of evidence: Class I, evidence from one or more prospective, randomized, controlled clinical trial; Class II, evidence from cohort or RCT not meeting criteria for class I; Class III, evidence from other controlled trials; Class IV, evidence from uncontrolled studies, case reports, case series, or expert opinion.

Data from references 60 and 124.

When given 30 mcg intramuscularly once weekly for 2 years, patients receiving IFN-β_{1a} (Avonex) demonstrated, compared with placebo, statistically significant reductions (approximately one-third) in annual relapse rate as well as disease progression, defined as a confirmed decrease of one point on the EDSS.[63] When disease progression was assessed by MRI studies, patients receiving active drug had significantly fewer new enhancing lesions compared with placebo-treated patients. Similar results were seen with higher dose (44 mcg), more frequent administration (three times weekly), and subcutaneous injection of IFN-β_{1a} (Rebif).[60] Other studies reveal significant effects on slowing brain atrophy[64] and the progression of cognitive decline[63] in patients treated with Avonex. These observations show that IFN-β possesses significant disease-modifying activity.

Pegylated IFN-β_{1a} (Plegridy) was approved by FDA for treatment of relapsing forms of MS in August 2014. The attachment of polyethylene glycol (PEG) polymer chains to the interferon molecules results in a longer half-life and allows for less frequent dosing. Peg-IFN-β_{1a} is given by subcutaneous injections once every 2 weeks. Results from the pivotal study ADVANCE demonstrated significant reduction in annualized relapse rates (35.6%), reduction of new lesions on MRI scans and reduction of risk of disability progression (as measured by EDSS scale) when compared to placebo.[65]

Side effects are similar with all the IFNs. Baseline CBCs, platelet determinations, and LFTs should be documented before starting therapy, at 1 month, every 3 months for 1 year, and every 6 months thereafter. Small percentages of patients develop depressed cell counts and liver enzyme elevations that are usually transient and respond to discontinuation of therapy. Rarely patients have developed true liver failure requiring liver transplant, and package inserts for IFN-β products have been altered to reflect this risk. The most common adverse effects include injection-site redness and swelling, menstrual irregularities, flu-like symptoms (eg, fever, chills, and myalgias), and rarely injection-site necrosis. The flu-like side effects are seen in most patients and typically occur for up to 24 hours after injection and typically abate within 1 to 3 months after starting the injections, but can persist in some patients. Injection-site reactions are probably worse with IFN-β_{1b}, can occur at any time, and can be lessened by using appropriate injection technique, including site rotation, topical lidocaine, application of ice before and after the injection, or use of an autoinjector. Injecting the medications at body temperature (place under armpits to warm) will decrease injection-site pain. By taking the injection at night prior to bed time the patient may sleep through most of the flu-like symptoms; nonsteroidal antiinflammatory agents or acetaminophen taken before and at regular intervals for 24 hours after administration can alleviate the flu-like symptoms. Initiation of one-quarter or one-half the standard dose, with increase to full dosage over 1 to 2 months, is also beneficial in reducing flu-like side effects.[66] Some authors suggest that because of the transient immune activation that can occur following the introduction of IFN-β, a short burst of oral prednisone can alleviate some adverse effects.[66]

Less commonly reported side effects include transient shortness of breath or tachycardia, thyroid dysfunction, and neutralizing antibodies. Although depression is a common finding in MS patients, all the IFNs, especially IFN-β_{1b}, can produce depressive symptoms. Clinicians must monitor patients carefully for signs of depression. Patients who develop depression should be monitored closely for suicide risk. Most patients will not feel better or have improvement in MS symptoms when taking IFNs, and many will experience side effects; thus, adherence can become a major issue. Finally, safety data on IFN-β in pregnancy and lactation are lacking. Abortifacient activity in primates has been noted, and until adequate safety data are available, women should be counseled as to appropriate contraception while using these products.

Glatiramer Acetate (Copaxone)

Glatiramer acetate (formerly known as copolymer-1) is a synthetic polypeptide consisting of L-alanine, L-glutamic acid, L-lysine, and L-tyrosine. Although the precise mechanism of action of this compound is unknown, glatiramer acetate appears to mimic the antigenic properties of MBP.[67] This agent also may act by directly binding to MHC class II receptors and inhibiting binding of MBP peptides to T-cell receptor complexes.[67] Glatiramer acetate has demonstrated that it induces Th2 (antiinflammatory) lymphocytes in experimental allergic encephalomyelitis.[67] This is thought to contribute to "bystander" suppression at the site of the MS lesion and thereby reduction of inflammation, demyelination, and axonal damage.[60] Glatiramer acetate may also suppress T-cell activation; recent studies suggest that it may be associated with a neuroprotective effect by inducing brain-derived neurotrophic factor.[68]

Given as a daily 20 mg or three times weekly 40-mg subcutaneous dose, glatiramer acetate appears to have a relatively mild adverse effect profile. Mild pain and pruritus at the injection site are the most frequent patient complaints. Approximately 10% of patients experience a one-time transient reaction consisting of chest tightness, flushing, and dyspnea beginning several minutes after injection and lasting usually no longer than 20 minutes. The postinjection reaction can occur with any dose, and is not limited to the first injection. If patients have no history or evidence of coronary artery disease, they may be assured these reactions are almost always self-limited and benign. Multicenter trials with glatiramer acetate have demonstrated significant reductions in mean annual relapse rate (approximately 29%), comparable with the IFNs.[60] An extension trial, completed after the original, pivotal 2-year study, suggests that glatiramer acetate may slow the progression of disability in patients with RRMS.[60] Glatiramer acetate also delays development of T1 holes on brain MRIs;[69] long-term uncontrolled data show that it remains safe and effective for individuals who continue to take it over 10 years.[70] Glatiramer acetate needs to be stored in the refrigerator but can be kept at room temperature for up to 1 week.

On Jan 28, 2014, the FDA approved glatiramer acetate (Copaxone) 40 mg/mL administered three times weekly by subcutaneous injection for the treatment of RRMS based largely on the results of the Glatiramer Acetate Low-frequency Admnistration (GALA) study.[71] This placebo-controlled trial in treatment-naïve patients demonstrated significant reduction in mean annual relapse rate (approximately 34%), reduction of new T2 lesions as well as T1 lesions, and comparable safety profile. Another open-label study Glatiramer Acetate low frequency safety and patient experience (GLACIER), further demonstrated comparable efficacy with favorable injection-related adverse events and convenience profile when patients were switched from glatiramer acetate 20 mg daily to 40 mg three times weekly.[72]

Clinical **Controversy...**

The US Food and Drug Administration approved a generic equivalent of daily glatiramer acetate 20 mg in April 2015. It has been launched in the United States as a disease-modifying therapy for people with relapsing forms of MS and CIS.

The mechanism of action of glatiramer acetate is unique. It does not appear to depend on general or selective immunosuppression in any form, but rather mediates its effects in MS through immunoregulatory pathways. It acts as an antigen, yet the precise mechanism of action remains to be fully elucidated, and no validated pharmacokinetic or pharmacodynamic biomarkers exist. In order to better characterize glatiramer acetate's biological impact, genome-wide expression studies were conducted with a human monocyte (THP-1) cell line. Consistent with previous literature, branded glatiramer acetate upregulated antiinflammatory markers (eg, IL10), and modulated multiple immune-related pathways. Despite some similarities, significant differences were observed between expression profiles induced by branded glatiramer acetate and a differently manufactured glatiramoid purported to be a generic. These observations suggest differential biological impact by the two glatiramoids and warrant further investigation.

Natalizumab (Tysabri)

Natalizumab is a partially humanized monoclonal antibody directed at the cell surface adhesion molecule $\alpha_4\beta$-integrin (also known as very-late antigen 1, VLA-1). Natalizumab works by attaching to VLA-1 and blocking its interaction with its ligand on CNS endothelium vascular cell adhesion molecule 1 (VCAM-1). Thus, activated lymphocytes are denied entry past the blood–brain barrier. In a phase II study, compared with placebo, natalizumab significantly reduced the number of new gadolinium-enhancing lesions by more than 90%, and diminished relapses.[73] In a 2-year phase III trial (A Randomized, Placebo-Controlled Trial of Natalizumab for Relapsing Multiple Sclerosis [AFFIRM]), compared with placebo, annual relapse rate was reduced by more than 60%, gadolinium-enhancing lesions were lessened by more than 90%, and progression of disability was significantly delayed.[74] In a separate 2-year, phase III trial (The Safety and Efficacy of Natalizumab in Combination with Interferon Beta-1a in Patients with Relapsing Remitting Multiple Sclerosis [SENTINEL]) in patients already taking IFN-β_{1a} (Avonex), those who had natalizumab added had a relapse rate reduction of more than 50% and gadolinium-enhancing lesion reduction of 84% compared with patients who continued with IFN-β_{1a} alone.[75] In these trials, natalizumab was infused IV every 4 weeks and was relatively well tolerated, although approximately 1% of patients developed infusion reactions, and 6% developed neutralizing antibodies that diminished the efficacy of the drug.

On November 23, 2004, the FDA approved natalizumab for use in relapsing MS in patients with inadequate response or intolerance to other MS therapies with the stipulation that the studies would continue. In February 2005, Biogen and Elan voluntarily removed natalizumab from the market after receiving reports of two patients (one patient from the SENTINEL trial, and one patient in a Crohn's disease study), who died after developing progressive multifocal leukoencephalopathy (PML), a rare brain infection most commonly seen in patients with human immunodeficiency virus.[76-78] One other patient who developed PML in the SENTINEL trial survived.[76-78] Further safety analysis did not identify other cases, so on March 9, 2006, an FDA advisory panel reviewing the data suggested reapproval of natalizumab for use in relapsing patients with a mandatory Risk Evaluation and Mitigation Strategy (REMS) program called TOUCH. On June 5, 2006, the FDA reapproved use of natalizumab in the United States with a black-box warning about PML. The estimated risk for developing PML is low. Three factors appear to impact the overall risk of developing PML while receiving natalizumab therapy: duration of treatment (24 months or longer), history of John Cunningham virus (JCV) infection, and prior use of immunosuppressive therapies (mycophenolate mofetil, alemtuzumab, efalizumab, and rituximab).[79,80] A two-step enzyme-linked immunosorbent assay (ELISA, STRATIFY TEST) is available for qualitative detection of serum antibodies to the JCV, offering a false-negative rate of 2.5%.[79,80]

Plasma exchange has been utilized to help clear the drug more rapidly from the blood of patients who develop PML.[81] An acute syndrome, referred to as immune reconstitution inflammatory syndrome (IRIS), has been associated with acute neurological deterioration after PLEX, requiring the use of steroids.[82]

Natalizumab is indicated for relapsing forms of MS to delay the accumulation of physical disability and decrease the number of relapses in patients who have a documented inadequate response or intolerance to traditional MS therapies. Patients receiving natalizumab must be enrolled in the TOUCH program. The overall predicted seroconversion rate for JCV is 2% to 3% per year. For that reason, the current recommendation is to screen patients at baseline and every 6 months with a JCV test while receiving natalizumab therapy.[83]

Fingolimod (Gilenya)

Approved September 21, 2010, fingolimod is the first oral DMT for MS. It has a unique mechanism of action as a sphingosine 1-phosphate receptor agonist. Fingolimod exhibits its immunosuppressant properties by sequestering circulating lymphocytes into secondary lymphoid organs and reduces the infiltration of T lymphocytes and macrophages into the CNS. It may have neuroprotective effects. In clinical trials it decreased annualized relapse rates by approximately 52% compared to IFN-β_{1a}. After 7 years of continuous fingolimod therapy, approximately 92% of patients were free of gadolinium-enhancing lesions, although this data used the 1.25 mg dose and the recommended dose approved by the FDA is 0.5 mg once daily.

Major side effects include pronounced first dose bradycardia and, rarely, bradyarrhythmia or atrioventricular block, infections, macular edema, a decrease in forced expiratory volume over

1 second in patients with previously compromised lung function, elevation of liver enzymes, and a sustained increase of approximately 1 to 2 mm Hg in systolic and diastolic blood pressure. Rare cases of lymphoma have also been identified. The reversal of lymphopenia can take 2 to 4 weeks after discontinuation of the drug. It is recommended that all patients starting fingolimod treatment be monitored for signs of bradycardia for at least 6 hours after the first dose. The FDA also recommends hourly pulse and blood pressure monitoring for all patients starting treatment, with electrocardiogram monitoring prior to dosing and at the end of the observation period or continued until all symptoms resolve. The period should extend past 6 hours in patients at higher risk, in some cases overnight. Additionally, the package insert requires a new 6-hour observation period in patients who have discontinued and wish to restart therapy. The recommendation varies depending on the time of discontinuation and days of therapy missed. To reduce risks related to bradycardia or atrioventricular block, extended monitoring is now recommended in patients with certain preexisting conditions such as QT prolongation. This is also a concern in patients receiving concomitant drugs that slow the heart rate or atrioventricular conduction, drugs that cause QT interval prolongation, and those who have a known risk for torsades. The following class Ia and class III antiarrhythmic agents are contraindicated with concurrent use of fingolimod: quinidine, procainamide, disopyramide, amiodarone, bretylium, sotalol, ibutilide, azimilide, dofetilide, and dronedarone.[84] PML has been reported with fingolimod use in three patients after 3 years of exposure as of September 2015.

Additional monitoring recommendations include baseline CBCs, LFTs, ophthalmologic examinations, and ECG in patients with known heart problems. To date, one important drug interaction has been reported with concomitant use of ketoconazole and fingolimod. Ketoconazole has been shown to increase the area under the curve by 70%. If a live vaccine is to be administered to a patient (Zostavax, Flumist, YF-VAX, etc.), consider doing so prior to starting fingolimod or wait until 2 months after discontinuation.

Teriflunomide (Aubagio)

Teriflunomide is an oral immunomodulatory agent, which was FDA approved on September 12, 2012 for the treatment of relapsing forms of MS. The medication works by inhibiting dihydroorotate dehydrogenase to prevent the proliferation of peripheral lymphocytes (T and B cells). The reduction of activated lymphocytes in the CNS reduces the inflammation and demyelination, which occurs in patients with MS. Teriflunomide is the active metabolite of leflunomide, an agent approved for the treatment of rheumatoid arthritis; however, teriflunomide is dosed as 7 or 14 mg orally once daily.

O'Connor et al. studied 1,088 patients with CDMS. Patients receiving 7 or 14 mg daily of teriflunomide had a statistically significant reduction in annualized relapse rate compared with placebo (relative risk reductions: 31.2% and 31.5%; $P = 0.0002$ and 0.0005, respectively). The risk of disability progression was statistically significantly reduced for those receiving 14 mg of teriflunomide daily (hazard ratio reduction: 29.8%; $P = 0.0279$).[85]

In a 36-week randomized, double-blinded, placebo-controlled study in 179 MS subjects with relapse, the primary outcome was the average number of unique active lesions per MRI scan during treatment. A statistically significant reduction in the primary endpoint was reported for both 7 and 14 mg of teriflunomide compared with placebo (0.98 and 1.06; $P = 0.0052$ and 0.0234, respectively).[86]

Although teriflunomide is not metabolized by CYP 450 enzymes, it inhibits CYP2C8 and induces CYP1A2. This medication is also a substrate for the breast cancer resistant protein (BCRP). Thus, inhibitors of BCRP (cyclosporine) may increase serum concentrations of teriflunomide. Additionally, teriflunomide inhibits OATP1B1 and OAT3, however, the significance of these drug interactions is unknown at this time. Studies found that concomitant use of warfarin and teriflunomide resulted in a 25% decrease in international normalized ratio (INR), rendering the need for close monitoring. When teriflunomide is coadministered with estradiol and levonorgestrel, the mean maximum serum concentration and area under the curve are increased.

The most common adverse effects seen with teriflunomide are increases in LFTs, alopecia, nausea, diarrhea, influenza, headache, and paresthesias.

Teriflunomide carries a black-box warning because of the risk of hepatotoxicity and teratogenicity (based on animal data). Monitoring for teriflunomide includes LFTs, within 6 months prior to initiating teriflunomide and monthly for the first 6 months. Animal studies have found that oral teriflunomide resulted in fetal malformations and embryolethality in female rats as well as reduced sperm count in male rats. Therefore, teriflunomide is contraindicated in pregnancy and in women of childbearing potential not using reliable contraception. Patients who become pregnant during therapy or within 2 years after discontinuation of therapy should enroll in the Aubagio Pregnancy Registry and consider a cholestyramine washout. Additionally, men taking this medication with partners who wish to become pregnant may consider a cholestyramine washout to reduce serum drug levels, as this drug may remain in the blood for up to 2 years after discontinuation. Teriflunomide may activate tuberculosis so a negative skin test or treatment of the disease must be documented prior to starting therapy.

Dimethyl Fumarate (Tecfidera)

Dimethyl fumarate has an unknown mechanism of action; however, it is an in vitro nicotinic acid receptor agonist and an in vivo activator of the nuclear factor (erythroid-derived 2)-like 2 (Nrf2) pathway that is involved in cellular response to oxidative stress. It is approved by the FDA for relapsing forms of MS. Dimethyl fumarate is metabolized by esterases in the GI tract, blood, and tissues. There are no known drug interactions. It is classified as pregnancy category C. Dimethyl fumarate is dosed initially at 120 mg (delayed release) orally twice daily. After 7 days, the dose should be increased to 240 mg (delayed release) orally twice daily. Laboratory monitoring includes a CBC prior to starting therapy and within 6 months of initiating treatment and annually. Side effects include lymphocytopenia (2%-6%), increased LFTs, and flushing (40%), which should improve over 1 month and is decreased by taking it with food. Two cases of PML have been reported in patients treated with dimethyl fumarate as of September 2015. Rash, abdominal pain, diarrhea, nausea, and vomiting have also been reported. GI side effects decrease over 1 month and respond to symptomatic treatment. It is unclear if slowing the dose escalation may decrease the risk of GI side effects.

In the "Efficacy and Safety Study of Oral Dimethyl Fumarate (BG-12) with Active Reference in Relapsing Remitting Multiple Sclerosis (CONFIRM)" dimethyl fumarate decreased the annualized relapse rate by 44% and 51% with twice daily or three times daily dosing, respectively.[87] In "The Determination of the Efficacy and Safety of Oral BG-12 in Relapsing-Remitting MS" the annualized relapse rate decreased by 47% and 52% with 240 mg twice daily or three times daily dosing, respectively.[88]

Clinical **Controversy...**

Progressive multifocal leukoencephalopathy is caused by the reactivation of the JCV, a common virus to which many people have been exposed. PML has emerged in MS patients as a consequence of certain treatments including natalizumab, fingolimod, and dimethyl fumarate. At this time, there have been two cases of PML in MS patients receiving dimethyl fumarate and three cases in patients receiving fingolimod.

Even though it is premature to determine the exact risk stratification of PML with new oral agents, it is very likely that the presence of positive JCV serology, duration of therapy, and prolonged lymphopenia are factors to consider in making therapeutic decisions.

Alemtuzumab (Lemtrada)

Alemtuzumab is a humanized monoclonal antibody against CD52 approved for the therapy of RRMS. Alemtuzumab has proven high efficacy in clinical phase II and III trials, where INF-β_{1a} was used as active comparator. CD52 is a glycosylphosphatidylinositol (GPI)-anchored protein consisting of 12 amino acids expressed at high levels on T and B lymphocytes, and to a lesser extent on monocytes, macrophages, and eosinophil granulocytes. Within a few minutes after infusion alemtuzumab leads to depletion of CD52 positive cells through antibody-dependent cell-mediated cytolysis (ADCC) and complement-dependent cytolysis (CDC).

The two Phase III trials, CARE-MS I[89] and II,[90] were randomized, rater-blinded studies with subcutaneous IFN-β_{1a} as active comparator designed to test clinical application of alemtuzumab. CARE-MS I included 581 treatment-naïve RRMS patients, whereas CARE-MS II enrolled 637 RRMS patients with breakthrough disease under previous DMTs. Alemtuzumab demonstrated a significant reduction in relapses compared to IFN-β_{1a} therapy (0.18 vs 0.39 = 54.9% ARR reduction in CARE-MS I; 0.26 vs 0.52 = 49.4% ARR reduction in CARE-MS II; each with $p < 0.0001$). However, a significant reduction in 6-month accumulation of disability was observed in CARE-MS II (42% reduction; 21% with IFN-β_{1a} vs 13% with alemtuzumab; $p < 0.01$), but not in CARE-MS I (11% with IFN-β_{1a} vs 8% with alemtuzumab; $p = 0.22$). The latter might be attributed to the unexpectedly low rate of disability progression in the IFN-β_{1a} group, indicating a relatively underpowered trial. MRI measures also proved superiority of alemtuzumab with significantly less gadolinium-enhancing lesions, new or enlarging T2 lesions and brain atrophy. Significantly more alemtuzumab than IFN-β_{1a} treated patients were free of any clinical disease (CARE-MS I: 74% vs 56%, $p < 0.0001$; CARE-MS II: 60% vs 41%; $p < 0.0001$) and free of any clinical and MRI disease activity (CARE-MS I: 39% vs 27%, $p < 0.01$; CARE-MS II: 32% vs 14%; $p < 0.0001$).

The high efficacy of alemtuzumab contrasts with its considerable high risks. Infusion Associated Reactions (IARs) affect over 90% of patients. Most are mild to moderate and consisted of headache, rash, pyrexia, and nausea. Respiratory tract and urinary tract infections are common. The accumulation of herpes infections during the CARE-MS studies led to the implementation of prophylactic acyclovir treatment (0-4 weeks after alemtuzumab infusion) significantly reducing infection rates. Moreover, there are single case reports of spirochetal gingivitis, pyogenic granuloma, esophageal candidiasis, tuberculosis, and listeria meningitis; the latter leading to dietary advice to avoid, for example, unpasteurized cheese.[91] No cases of PML have been reported to date.

Secondary autoimmune disease affects approximately 30% to 40% of patients, predominantly impairing thyroid function. Thyroid autoimmune disease mainly comprised hyperthyroidism, hypothyroidism, goiter, and thyroiditis. There is also a small but serious risk of immune thrombocytopenia (ITP). This complication can occur at any time ranging from 1 to 34 months post-alemtuzumab administration. Additionally, glomerulonephritis and single cases of autoimmune neutropenia, hemolytic anemia, and type 1 diabetes have been reported.[91] Extensive monitoring and early intervention allow for an appropriate risk management.

According to the labeling information, 12 mg of alemtuzumab are infused for five consecutive days in the first course and for 3 days in the second course 1 year later. Currently, alemtuzumab therapy is approved for the initial two courses. Concomitant corticosteroids, antihistamine, and antipyretic drugs are utilized with the infusion in order to avoid IARs.

Mitoxantrone (Novantrone)

Mitoxantrone, a member of the anthracenedione family, is approved by the FDA for reducing neurologic disability and the frequency of clinical relapses in patients with SPMS (chronic), PRMS, or worsening RRMS.[92] The MRI outcomes, however, were not as robust as those typically seen in the trials of relapsing patients alone.[93] Mitoxantrone is administered as a brief (5- to 15-minute) IV infusion dosed at 12 mg/m^2 every 3 months. An evaluation of left ventricular ejection fraction and ECG are required prior to administration of each dose, and if signs or symptoms of congestive heart failure develop. The maximum allowable lifetime cumulative dose of mitoxantrone is 140 mg/m^2. Other potential side effects noted are nausea, alopecia, menstrual disorder, amenorrhea, upper respiratory tract infection, UTIs, and leukemia. The role that mitoxantrone will ultimately play in the treatment of MS remains unclear, because potential cardiac toxicity limits its long-term use. More recent estimates also suggest the risk of leukemia may be as high as 1 in 145 patients, which has significantly decreased interest in its use for MS patients.[94] In addition, although patients with SPMS were included in the mitoxantrone in multiple sclerosis (MIMS—effect of mitoxantrone on MRI in progressive MS) trial, resulting in FDA approval for use in SPMS, there was no substudy documenting slowing of progression specifically in this subgroup of patients.[92,93] Thus, support for use of mitoxantrone in this context is lacking.[94]

Remaining Questions for Disease-Modifying Therapy

9 Despite encouraging results from well-conducted clinical trials, several relevant issues remain. Important questions in the use of the DMTs include when to begin therapy, which agent to initiate, and when to switch and stop therapies. The MS Coalition has developed an evidence-based paper, which is endorsed by the Americas Committee for Treatment and Research in Multiple Sclerosis (ACTRIMS), to provide guidance on the use of DMT in MS. Key recommendations regarding treatment and access considerations are summarized in Table 55-5.[95]

TABLE 55-5 Key Recommendations on Treatment and Access Considerations

- Initiation of therapy with an FDA-approved disease-modifying treatment is recommended as soon as possible following a definite diagnosis of relapsing MS, and can also be considered for selected patients with a first clinical attack consistent with MS where other potential causes have been excluded as well as patients with progressive MS with clinical relapses and/or inflammatory activity
- Choice of initial or alternative disease modifying therapy is complex and should be collaboratively done by the treating clinician and the patient
- Therapy is to be continued indefinitely, unless there is clear lack of benefit, intolerable side effects, inadequate patient compliance, new data that reveal other reasons for cessation, or better therapy becomes available
- Absence of relapses while on treatment should not justify discontinuation of treatment
- When switching disease modifying therapy due to suboptimal response, an agent with an alternative mechanism of action should be chosen
- Patient and clinician access to all available therapies is necessary due to significant variability in the MS population such as response to therapies, contraindications, risk tolerance, and compliance that may be influenced by route of administration and/or side effects
- Patient access to medication should not be limited by the frequency of relapses, age or other personal characteristics, or level of disability and should not be withheld to allow for determination of coverage by payers, as this puts the patient at increased risk for recurrent disease activity

Data from reference 95.

Decisions about the use of any medication rest on determination of the severity of the illness, the efficacy of the medication, side effects, and costs related to the therapy. Clearly, these drugs slow the course of the illness but do not suppress it completely, and in some individuals, there is no apparent benefit. There is now, however, overwhelming evidence that the vast majority of untreated patients will have progressive disease over time. Pathologic data clearly show that even in acute lesions there is significant axonal damage that is essentially irreversible. MRI data show that 80% to 90% of all new enhancing lesions are asymptomatic, suggesting that a "quiet" clinical course does not necessarily mean there is not ongoing disease activity that ultimately will lead to cognitive deficits and progressive spastic paraparesis.

It is clear that very early therapy is effective. In patients with CIS and two or more T2 lesions on brain MRI (ie, at high risk for developing CDMS), placebo-controlled studies with all three of the IFN agents and glatiramer acetate have shown significant delay in a second attack and positive outcomes on a variety of MRI measures (BENEFIT, Betaseron in Newly Emerging Multiple Sclerosis for Initial Treatment; CHAMPS, Controlled High Risk Subjects Avonex Multiple Sclerosis Prevention Study; and ETOMS, Early Treatment of Multiple Sclerosis).[60,96] Thus, very early therapy is potentially warranted, and IFN-β_{1b}, IFN-β_{1a} (Avonex), and glatiramer acetate are approved by the FDA for use after CIS in those patients with abnormal MRIs consistent with demyelination. The MS Coalition recommends that patients with relapsing disease should be initiated on an FDA-approved DMT as soon as possible following diagnosis.[95]

A second major issue is which drug to use in which patient. There has not been a single, randomized study comparing DMTs with one another in a similar patient population at the same time.[97] In the case of the first generation self-injectables, the pivotal, placebo-controlled trials produced results that were more similar than different when comparing across trials, including a nearly identical one-third reduction in relapse rate for all four drugs over 2 years. A small number of studies suggested higher dose, more frequent administration of IFN may be more efficacious than lower dose, less frequent administration.[98,99] Other studies argue against this,[100,101] and recent studies note no significant difference in outcomes between standard and double dose IFN-β_{1b} and glatiramer acetate,[102] and no difference between IFN-β_{1a} (Rebif) and glatiramer acetate.[103]

A concern with all three IFN products that further muddies our understanding of the clinical differences between IFN products is the development of neutralizing antibodies. In clinical trials, 30% to 40% of patients receiving IFN-β_{1b} developed antibodies directed against the drug.[104] In these patients, the exacerbation rate was similar to that in placebo-treated patients. In patients on IFN-β_{1b}, neutralizing antibodies can occur as early as 3 to 6 months and as late as 18 months. This product tends to be the most antigenic.[105] With IFN-β_{1a}, neutralizing antibodies were found in 22% of early trials of Avonex, but later studies reported that only 2% to 5% of treated patients developed antibodies; this decrease was caused by a formulation change of the drug making it the least antigenic.[101,105] Percentages of antibody formation for Rebif (approximately 12%) are intermediate, therefore moderately antigenic occuring in the first 9 to 15 months of treatment similar to Avonex.[60,104,105] Neutralizing antibodies are seen in approximately 6% of patients treated with natalizumab, and the antibodies seem to diminish efficacy.[75] The long-term clinical significance of these findings is still not completely clear, although three recent studies have further confirmed the effect of neutralizing antibodies on relapses, MRI lesions, and progression of disability.[105-108] Whether these antibodies are truly cross-reactive between products is unknown, as is the duration during which antibodies can be detected. There are no general consensus guidelines regarding when to test for neutralizing antibodies, which assay to use, or what titer cutoff to apply to patients in clinical settings.[109] An important question is whether production of antibodies might be diminished with treatments such as corticosteroids.

8 We now have experience for more than two decades with MS patients taking DMTs, yet they continue to have more relapses, more lesions on MRI, more disability, and ongoing slippage into SPMS.[110] There is no accepted definition of treatment inadequacy, although the Canadian Multiple Sclerosis Research Council has suggested a relatively simple approach that incorporates the elements of relapse rate, new MRI lesions, and change on the EDSS.[111] If a patient develops significant and persistent IFN antibodies, movement to a non-IFN (glatiramer acetate, natalizumab, fingolimod, teriflunomide, dimethyl fumarate, mitoxantrone, or possibly rituximab[112]) is reasonable. A second option is addition of an immunosuppressant agent, such as monthly methylprednisolone,[113] azathioprine, methotrexate, or mycophenolate. As noted above, the addition of natalizumab to IFN-β_{1a} was effective, but produced rare cases of PML, and thus, this combination should not be used. The addition of a statin agent may worsen MS[114] although these results are not definitive.

Symptomatic Management

10 Many of the symptoms of MS do not require pharmacologic management or do not respond to it. This section addresses the primary symptoms in which pharmacologic management may be of benefit (Table 55-6).[32,111,115,116,118,121] See the preceding section on the treatment of exacerbations for a discussion of optic neuritis.

Gait Difficulties and Spasticity

Problems with gait can be caused by spasticity, weakness, ataxia, defective proprioception, or a combination of these factors. Spasticity often presents late in disease and is amenable to pharmacologic intervention, whereas physical therapy may be required in treating gait disturbances caused by other factors. Spasticity is encountered commonly and tends to affect the legs more markedly than the arms. Spasticity can result in falls; however, in the later stages of the disease, the increased muscle tone of a spastic limb often lends pseudo strength to patients with underlying weakness. Therefore, when using muscle relaxants, one must be careful not to decrease the tone to an extent that ambulation is actually hindered.[32,115] Baclofen (Lioresal), a short acting γ-aminobutyric acid (GABA) analog, is the preferred agent and usually is started in dosages of 10 mg three times daily and titrated upward to achieve the desired response. Most patients achieve a satisfactory response with dosages between 40 and 80 mg/day; however, dosages higher than the recommended daily maximum of 80 mg are required by some patients.[32,115] A wearing-off is common, due to the relatively short duration of action. Continuous intrathecal administration of baclofen (Gablofen) may be an option for patients unable to tolerate or unresponsive to oral therapy. Baclofen should not be discontinued abruptly to avoid the possibility of seizures.[115]

Another effective agent with a different mechanism of action is tizanidine (Zanaflex). This short-acting, α-adrenergic agonist acts in the CNS to reduce spasticity by increasing presynaptic inhibition of motor neurons. It appears to have efficacy comparable with that of baclofen.[115] Dosage must be titrated slowly over 2 to 4 weeks, starting with 4 mg at bedtime, with adjustments based on clinical response. Effective tolerated dosages have ranged from 2 to 36 mg/day. Sedation, dizziness, and dry mouth are the most commonly reported adverse effects, but hypotension also can occur, as well as a rare but severe hepatotoxicity. Tizanidine can be added in small dosages to baclofen, sometimes creating better results and making possible smaller doses of each drug.

In patients who are unable to tolerate baclofen or tizanidine, diazepam (Valium; 2-10 mg/day), clonazepam (Klonopin; 1-3 mg/day), or dantrolene sodium (Dantrium; 100-400 mg/day) may be considered as alternatives, but they generally are less effective than either baclofen or tizanidine. Mild spasticity also may respond to moderately high doses of gabapentin (Neurontin; 1,800-3,600 mg/day). Tiagabine (Gabitril 8-56 mg/day) may be useful in some patients

TABLE 55-6 Treatment of Selected Primary MS Symptoms

Spasticity	Bladder Symptoms	Sensory Symptoms	Fatigue
Baclofen	Propantheline	Carbamazepine	Amantadine
Dantrolene	Oxybutynin	Phenytoin	Antidepressants
Diazepam	Dicyclomine	Amitriptyline or other TCAs	Modafinil
Tizanidine	DDAVP	Gabapentin	Methylphenidate
Tiagabine	Self-catheterization	Lamotrigine	Dextroamphetamine
Gabapentin	Imipramine or amitriptyline	Pregabalin	Armodafinil
Pregabalin	Prazosin	Duloxetine	
Botulinum toxin type A	Botulinum toxin type A		
Dalfampridine	Solifenacin		
	Darifenacin		
	Trospium		
	Hyoscyamine		

DDAVP, desmopressin acetate; TCA, tricyclic antidepressant.

Data from references 32, 111, 115, 116, 118, and 121.

with spasticity, but side effects can prohibit its use. Pregabalin (Lyrica; 75-300 mg/day) has similar features and mechanism of actions as gabapentin, although pregabalin is approximately three times more potent and does not saturate the L-transporter system in the GI tract, so it may prove useful in the treatment of spasticity in MS patients.

Botulinum toxin type A (Botox; dose depending on the muscles injected) has been shown to be effective in alleviating spasticity.[32] The amount of toxin required to exert an effect on spasticity is often too excessive to use safely in the larger muscles; therefore, its use is best limited to smaller areas of focal muscle spasm.

An alternative approach to gait disruption employs K^+ channel blockers such as 4-aminopyridine (4-AP), which can potentiate synaptic transmission and increase muscle twitch tension. In 2010, the FDA approved the use of a long-acting proprietary version of 4-AP, dalfampridine (Ampyra; 20 mg/day) to improve walking speed in patients with MS. Studies have shown that dalfampridine may improve walking speed by approximately 25% in responders.[116,117] In other countries, dalfampridine is referred to as fampridine.[117] A REMS program is in place to manage risks associated with dalfampridine use.

Safety concerns with the use of dalfampridine include the risk of seizures, particularly when patients exceed the maximum dose of 10 mg twice daily, and is contraindicated in patients with a history of seizures. It is important to educate patients on not taking compounded 4-AP with dalfampridine, which is the comparable extended release product. Additionally, the drug should not be chewed, crushed, or cut. If the patient misses a dose, they should take it immediately upon recognition and never double up on the dose, due to the risk of seizures. Commonly reported side effects of dalfampridine include UTIs, insomnia, dizziness, headaches, and balance disorders.

Tremor

Cerebellar symptoms such as tremor can be troubling and difficult to control. Medications that can be helpful include propranolol, primidone, and isoniazid.

Bowel and Bladder Symptoms

Patients commonly complain of incontinence, urgency, frequency, and nocturia, which are indications of a hyperreflexic bladder (ie, inability to store urine). A number of anticholinergic agents are used to treat this problem if symptoms are mild. In addition, tricyclic antidepressants have been used for their anticholinergic properties to treat this condition. With all anticholinergic agents, great care must be used to avoid falls, decreased cognition, and constipation, which is worsened by the patient's natural instinct to limit fluid intake. Antimuscarinic agents are also used to treat incontinence. Patients with significant sphincter detrusor dyssynergia may benefit from the oral use of α-adrenergic blockers or intramuscular use of botulinum toxin type A (Botox; dose depends on the muscles injected) to relax the internal sphincter (see Chapter e86).

Intermittent self-catheterization and the crede maneuver with or without a concomitant anticholinergic agent are recommended in patients with large postvoid residual volumes (more than 100 mL) or when the urinary problem is hyporeflexic in nature (failure to empty). Cholinergic agents (bethanechol) may be useful in patients with a hyporeflexive bladder. Patients with large post-void residual volumes are at risk for developing UTIs and often are prescribed urinary acidifiers such as vitamin C or antiseptics such as methenamine mandelate to prevent infections. Antibiotics used for UTI prophylaxis include sulfamethoxazole/trimethoprim, cephalexin, cinoxacin, and nitrofurantoin.

Constipation is the most common bowel complaint. Many medications (eg, narcotics, anticholinergics) in common use may worsen this problem, as may voluntary water restriction in those patients with urinary urgency and incontinence. Increases in dietary fiber and hydration may alleviate this problem, but in some instances laxatives or enemas may be necessary (see Chapter 36).

Major Depression

Major depression is common in patients with MS, and the risk of suicide may be increased markedly compared with healthy subjects.[118] Patients should be monitored closely for the development of major depressive symptomatology and treated accordingly (see Chapter 68). IFN products and natalizumab should be used cautiously in patients with significant depression.

Sensory Symptoms

Numbness and paresthesia are frequent sensory complaints but usually do not require treatment. Some MS patients may develop acute or chronic pain syndromes[115] such as trigeminal neuralgia and painful dysesthesias, for which treatment is necessary (see Chapter 60).

Sexual Dysfunction

Sexual dysfunction in both men and women are common in MS, and counseling should be offered to both partners. Phosphodiesterase inhibitors or Alprostadil, a prostaglandin E1, can be very effective in men with MS who have erectile dysfunction (see Chapter 84). Viagra is currently being studied in females with MS and sexual dysfunction. In patients needing antidepressant therapy for whom sexual dysfunction is a concern, bupropion is preferable to selective serotonin reuptake inhibitors as it has a much lower incidence of sexual side effects.

Fatigue

Fatigue, one of the most common complaints in MS patients, can be severely disabling, but treatment is often overlooked. Typically present in the mid to late afternoon, it can increase with heat exposure, exertion, intercurrent infection, spasticity, weakness, and depression. Amantadine hydrochloride (100 mg twice daily) is used often and may offer significant relief.[32,111] Methylphenidate (Ritalin) and related products, and dextroamphetamine (Dexedrine) are used commonly for fatigue in MS. Modafinil (Provigil), 200 mg daily, up to 400 mg daily may be helpful for MS-related fatigue. The *R*-enantiomer of modafinil is armodafinil (Nuvigil) dosed at 150 or 250 mg daily, which reaches peak concentrations more quickly with potentially fewer side effects than modafinil. In patients suffering from both depression and fatigue, a more activating antidepressant such as fluoxetine may be employed.

Cognition

Cognitive dysfunction is common in MS, affecting up to 50% or more of patients. It generally manifests itself as word-finding difficulties and problems with concentration and short-term memory. Cognitive dysfunction can be treated with stimulants or cholinesterase inhibitors.

Pseudobulbar Palsy

Pseudobulbar palsy is a condition caused by progressive degeneration of the corticobulbar tract in patients with MS. Symptoms include dysarthria, dysphonia, dysphagia, and sudden, inappropriate, uncontrollable, emotional outbursts such as crying or laughing. Dextromethorphan/quinidine 20 mg/10 mg is used for the treatment of this pseudobulbar affect. The recommended dosing for this combination medication is one capsule daily for 1 week, followed by one capsule twice daily. The mechanism of action is unknown. The rationale for utilization of this combination is that dextromethorphan is rapidly metabolized by CYP2D6, and quinidine inhibits the CYP2D6 enzyme to increase the serum concentration of dextromethorphan.

Complementary and Alternative Therapies for MS

Approximately 33% to 80% of patients with MS use complementary and alternative medicine (CAM) instead of, or in addition to, disease-modifying and symptomatic therapies.[119] Common CAM therapies include diet and dietary supplements such as vitamins, minerals, and herbs. Antioxidant supplements vitamin A, C, E, α-lipoic acid, coenzyme Q10, grape seed, pine bark extracts, mangosteen, and acai have suggestive evidence of benefiting MS patients. However, for patients with MS, there is a theoretical risk associated with taking antioxidant supplements owing to their ability to stimulate the immune system (T-cells and macrophages). Stimulating the immune system in patients with MS could be counterproductive, possibly worsening or exacerbating their disease, and may counteract the effects of immunomodulators. Other immune-stimulating supplements that should be used with caution are garlic, ginseng (Asian and Siberian), Echinacea, cat's claw, astragalus, alfalfa, and stinging nettle.[120]

The American Academy of Neurology recently updated evidence-based recommendations for the use of CAM in MS[119] (Table 55-7). Oral cannabis extract is established as effective treatment for spasticity and pain (Level A). Tetrahydrocannabinol (THC) and Sativex oromucosal spray may also reduce symptoms of spasticity and pain. (Level B). Of note, the safety and interactions with

TABLE 55-7 AAN Evidence-based Recommendations on CAM Therapies in MS

CAM Therapy	Type of MS	Symptoms and Reported Use	Effective	Ineffective	Recommendation Level
Oral cannabis extract	RRMS, SPMS, PPMS, MSU	Symptoms of spasticity and pain	x		A
	RRMS,SPMS, PPMS	Signs of Spasticity (short-term), tremor (short-term)		x	B
	MSU	Signs and symptoms of spasticity (long-term)	x		C
	RRMS, SPMS, PPMS, MSU	Bladder symptoms, urge incontinence			U
Synthetic THC	RRMS, SPMS, PPMS	Symptoms of spasticity, pain	x		B
	RRMS, SPMS, PPMS	Signs of spasticity (short-term), tremor (short-term)		x	B
	MSU	Signs and symptoms of spasticity (long-term)	x		C
	RRMS, SPMS, PPMS, MSU	Bladder symptoms, urge incontinence, central neuropathic pain			U
Sativex oromucosal spray	MSU	Symptoms of spasticity, pain, urinary frequency	x		B
		Signs of spasticity, incontinence episodes		x	B
		Tremor		x	C
		Anxiety/sleep, cognition, QOL, fatigue			U
Smoked cannabis	RRMS, SPMS, MSU	Spasticity, pain, balance and posture, cognition			U
Ginkgo biloba	RRMS, SPMS, PPMS	Fatigue	x		C
		Cognitive function		x	A
Lofepramine plus phenylalanine with B_{12} (Cari Loder regimen)	RRMS, SPMS, PPMS	Disability, symptoms, depression, fatigue		x	C
Reflexology	MSU	Paresthesia	x		C
		Pain, HRGOL, disability, spasticity, fatigue, cognition, bowel/bladder function, depression, anxiety, insomnia			U
Bee venom	RRMS, SPMS	MRI lesion number and volume, relapses, disability, fatigue, HRQOL		x	C
Magnetic therapy	RRMS, SPMS, PPMS	Fatigue	x		B
		Depression		x	B
Low-fat diet with omega-3 supplementation	RRMS	Relapses, disability, MRI lesions, fatigue, QOL		x	B

CAM, complementary and alternative medicine; HRQOL, health-related QOL; MS, multiple sclerosis; MSU, MS type unspecified; PCE, oral cannabis extract; PPMS, primary progressive MS; QOL, quality-of-life; RRMS, relapsing remitting MS; SPMS, secondary progressive MS; THC, tetrahydrocannabinol. A, established as effective or ineffective; B, probably effective or ineffective; C, possibly effective or ineffective; U, insufficient evidence to determine effectiveness or ineffectiveness.

Data from reference 119.

concurrent MS disease-modifying therapies (DMTs) has not been studied. There are limited data to support the effectiveness and safety of most of the CAM therapies for MS. However, for patients with MS who are willing to try new approaches with limited evidence, CAM may be a consideration in some cases. Healthcare providers can be a source of objective information regarding the use of CAM for MS and can assist their patients in making the best decision.[120]

Vaccine Recommendations

A yearly flu shot is recommended for all patients with MS, including patients on any of the DMTs. The intranasal influenza vaccine, FluMist, which is a live, attenuated vaccine, is not recommended for patients with MS, however. As DMTs suppress the immune system, a patient taking one of these medications is at increased risk for developing an infection of the strain of virus given in the vaccine. Live virus vaccines are also more likely to cause an increase in MS disease activity than inactivated virus vaccines. Finally, it is unknown whether there are any direct interactions between DMTs and the intranasal influenza vaccine.[121] This information can likely be extrapolated to other vaccines, so if a patient is in need of a vaccination of any kind, "killed" virus vaccines are recommended.

Patients opting to take fingolimod who are varicella zoster virus antibody negative should receive the varicella zoster virus immunization (even though it is a live attenuated vaccine) at least 2 months prior to beginning fingolimod. This should allow time to mount an antibody response prior to immunosuppression with fingolimod.

Personalized Pharmacotherapy

The initial presentation of MS differs between individuals. When a patient is newly diagnosed modifiable risk factors may be considered prior to selecting therapy. Some of these modifiable risk factors include vitamin D deficiency, excess body weight, and smoking. Vitamin D deficiency has been associated with the risk of developing MS, and higher vitamin D levels may reduce MRI brain activity and thus reduce relapse rates.[8] Excess body weight is also associated with a higher risk of developing MS.[122] Smoking is associated with the development of MS, disability, MRI abnormalities, and conversion to CDMS (51%-75% in 3 years).[9,123]

Treatments available for MS need to be individualized based on the initial symptomatology, MRI presentation, and the risk associated with the chosen therapy. Essentially when patients present, they can be given a modestly effective therapy with a low side-effect profile (eg, IFNs and glatiramer acetate) or a more aggressive therapy with a higher risk profile (natalizumab, fingolimod, or dimethyl fumarate). The weighing of the risks and benefits is ultimately dependent on a patient's presentation or progression of disease, along with comorbid conditions such as depression.

The importance of adherence cannot be underestimated in patients taking DMTs. Nonadherence has been reported anywhere between 17% and 50%. The reason many patients stop taking their DMTs is multifactorial, and includes perceived lack of efficacy, side effects, undesirable route of administration, and depression. Patients who remain adherent to their DMTs generally remain employed full-time compared with those who are nonadherent. It is crucial that we establish realistic expectations for our patients on DMTs. Overall, untreated MS patients generally relapse about every 6 months, whereas treated patients relapse about every 2 to 5 years. Adherence is the key to successful treatment of MS.

EVALUATION OF THERAPEUTIC OUTCOMES

Response to treatment of acute exacerbations of MS is commonly seen within days. With respect to DMTs, it is important for the clinician to recognize that over the short term (days to weeks), little or no apparent benefit may be noted by either patient or clinician. Evaluation of therapeutic outcomes, such as decreased MS exacerbations and hospitalizations or perhaps slowed disease progression and disability (as measured using scales such as EDSS), must be conducted over a period of months to years. Patients should be provided with realistic goals and expectations of these treatment options and encouraged to participate in the evaluation of therapeutic response. Initially, it may be important to reevaluate patients at relatively short time intervals to monitor for adverse effects.

Safety monitoring of patients on IFN includes regular laboratory monitoring, patient observation, and questioning for adverse effects or changing disability, and regular neurologic examinations. Laboratory monitoring for individuals on IFN therapy should include a CBC, platelet count, and LFTs. These should be completed at baseline, every 3 months for 1 year, and every 6 months thereafter. Glatiramer acetate requires no laboratory monitoring. Teriflunomide requires a transaminase, bilirubin, CBC, tuberculin skin test, and blood pressure prior to initiating therapy and alanine aminotransferase monthly for 6 months after starting. Teriflunomide is associated with renal failure and increased serum potassium; therefore, patients should be monitored as needed. Dimethyl fumarate requires a CBC prior to starting therapy and within 6 months of treatment initiation and annually and LFTs. Natalizumab, fingolimod, and alemtuzumab have REMS programs to monitor safety.

In addition to counseling patients regarding the adverse effects associated with these drugs, clinicians should actively encourage patients to adhere with their prescribed regimens.

ACKNOWLEDGMENT

The authors acknowledge Felecia Hart, PharmD, Rebecca Barnhart, PharmD, and Joan Kaufman, illustrator, for their contributions to this chapter.

ABBREVIATIONS

AAN	American Academy of Neurology
ACTH	adrenocorticotropic hormone
ADCC	antibody-dependent cell-mediated cytolysis
4-AP	4-aminopyridine
BCRP	breast cancer resistant protein
CAM	complementary and alternative medicine
CBC	complete blood count
CD	cluster of differentiation
CDC	complement-dependent cytolysis
CDMS	clinically definite multiple sclerosis
CIS	clinically isolated syndrome
CNS	central nervous system
CSF	cerebrospinal fluid
DMT	disease-modifying therapy
EBNA	Epstein–Barr nuclear antigen
EBV	Epstein–Barr virus
ECG	electrocardiogram
EDSS	expanded disability status scale
GI	gastrointestinal
GPI	glycosylphosphatidylinositol
GWAS	genome-wide association study
HHV	Human Herpesvirus
HLA	human leukocyte antigen
IAR	infusion associated reaction
IFN	interferon
IgG	immunoglobulin G
IL	interleukin
INR	international normalized ratio
IRIS	immune reconstitution inflammatory syndrome
ITP	immune thrombocytopenia

IV	intravenous
IVIG	intravenous immunoglobulin
JCV	John Cunningham virus
LFT	liver function test
MBP	myelin basic protein
MHC	major histocompatibility complex
MIMS	mitoxantrone in multiple sclerosis
MRI	magnetic resonance imaging
MS	multiple sclerosis
MSFC	multiple sclerosis functional composite
PEG	polyethylene glycol
PLEX	plasma exchange
PML	progressive multifocal leukoencephalopathy
PPMS	primary-progressive multiple sclerosis
PRMS	progressive-relapsing multiple sclerosis
REMS	Risk Evaluation and Mitigation Strategy
RIS	radiologically isolated syndrome
RRMS	relapsing-remitting multiple sclerosis
SPMS	secondary-progressive multiple sclerosis
TGF	transforming growth factor
Th	T-helper cells
THC	tetrahydrocannabinol
Treg	T-regulatory cells
UTI	urinary tract infection
VCA	vascular cell adhesion
VCAM	vascular cell adhesion molecule
VEP	visual-evoked potential
VLA-1	very-late antigen 1

REFERENCES

1. Ascherio A, Munger K. Epidemiology of multiple sclerosis: From risk factors to prevention. *Semin Neurol* 2008;28:17-28.
2. Goodin DS. The causal cascade to multiple sclerosis: A model for MS pathogenesis. *PLoS One* 2009;4:e4565.
3. Oksenberg JR, Baranzini SE, Sawcer S, Hauser SL. The genetics of multiple sclerosis: SNPs to pathways to pathogenesis. *Nat Rev Genet* 2008;9:516-526.
4. Ebers GC. Environmental factors and multiple sclerosis. *Lancet Neurol* 2008;7:268-277.
5. Healy BC, Ali EN, Guttmann CRG, et al. Smoking and disease progression in multiple sclerosis. *Arch Neurol* 2009;66:858-864.
6. National MS Society. *Fact sheet multiple sclerosis*; 2015. Available at: http://www.nationalmssociety.org/NationalMSSociety/media/MSNationalFiles/Brochures/Brochure-Just-the-Facts.pdf. (Accessed Dec. 17, 2015)
7. Kotzamani D, Panou T, Mastorodemos V, et al. Rising incidence of multiple sclerosis in females associated with urbanization. *Neurology* 2012;78(22):1728-1735.
8. Munger KL, Levin LI, Hollis BW. Serum 25-hydroxyvitamin D levels and risk of multiple sclerosis. *JAMA* 2006;296:2832-2838.
9. Zivadinov R, Weinstock-Guttman B, Hashmi K, et al. Smoking is associated with increased lesion volumes and brain atrophy in multiple sclerosis. *Neurology* 2009;73(7):504-510.
10. Frohman EM, Racke MK, Raine CS. Multiple sclerosis—The plaque and its pathogenesis. *N Engl J Med* 2006;354:942-955.
11. Owens GP, Bennett JL. Trigger, pathogen, or bystander: The complex nexus linking Epstein–Barr virus and multiple sclerosis. *Mult Scler* 2012;18(9):1204-1248.
12. Levin LI, Munger KL, Rubertone MV, et al. Temporal relationship between elevation of Epstein–Barr virus antibody titers and initial onset of neurological symptoms in multiple sclerosis. *JAMA* 2005;293:2496-2500.
13. Sundstrom P, Nystrom M, Ruuth K, et al. Antibodies to specific EBNA-1 domains and HLA DRB1*1501 interact as risk factors for multiple sclerosis. *J Neuroimmunol* 2009;215(1-2):102-107.
14. Zivadinov R, Zorzon M, Weinstock-Guttman B, et al. Epstein–Barr virus is associated with grey matter atrophy in multiple sclerosis. *J Neurol Neurosurg Psychiatry* 2009;80(6):620-625.
15. Serafini B, Rosicarelli B, Franciotta D, et al. Dysregulated Epstein–Barr virus infection in the multiple sclerosis brain. *J Exp Med* 2007;204:2899-2912.
16. Willis SN, Stadelmann C, Rodig SJ, et al. Epstein–Barr virus infection is not a characteristic feature of multiple sclerosis brain. *Brain* 2009;132:3318-3328.
17. Hafler DA, Compston A, Sawcer S, et al. Risk alleles for multiple sclerosis identified by a genomewide study. *N Engl J Med* 2007;357:851-862.
18. D'Netto MJ, Ward H, Morrison KM, et al. Risk alleles for multiple sclerosis in multiplex families. *Neurology* 2009;72:1984-1988.
19. Maier LM, Lowe CE, Cooper J, et al. IL2RA genetic heterogeneity in multiple sclerosis and type 1 diabetes susceptibility and soluble interleukin-2 receptor production. *PLoS Genet* 2009;5:e1000322.
20. Cree BA, Khan O, Bourdette D, et al. Clinical characteristics of African Americans versus Caucasian Americans with multiple sclerosis. *Neurology* 2004;63:2039-2045.
21. Cree BA, Al-Sabbagh A, Bennett R, et al. Response to interferon beta-1a treatment in African American multiple sclerosis patients. *Arch Neurol* 2005;62:1681-1683.
22. Reich D, Patterson N, DeJager PL, et al. A whole-genome admixture scan finds a candidate locus for multiple sclerosis susceptibility. *Nat Genet* 2005;37:1113-1118.
23. Trapp BD, Peterson J, Ransohoff RM, et al. Axonal transection in the lesions of multiple sclerosis. *N Engl J Med* 1998;338:278-285.
24. Truyen L, van Wuesberghe JHTM, Barkof F, et al. Accumulation of hypointense lesions ("black holes") on T_1 spin echo MRI correlates with disease progression in multiple sclerosis. *Neurology* 1996;47:1469-1476.
25. Pirko I, Lucchinetti CF, Sriram S, Bakshi R. Gray matter involvement in multiple sclerosis. *Neurology* 2007;68:634-642.
26. Zivadinov R, Minagar A. Evidence for gray matter pathology in multiple sclerosis: A neuroimaging approach. *J Neurol Sci* 2009;282:1-4.
27. Magliozzi R, Howell O, Vora A, et al. Meningeal B-cell follicles in secondary progressive multiple sclerosis associate with early onset of disease and severe cortical pathology. *Brain* 2007;130:1089-1104.
28. Reboldi A, Coisne C, Baumjohann D, et al. C-C chemokine receptor 6-regulated entry of T_H-17 cells into the CNS through the choroid plexus is required for the initiation of EAE. *Nat Immunol* 2009;10:514-523.
29. Zhou L, Chong MMW, Littman DR. Plasticity of CD4+ T-cell lineage differentiation. *Immunity* 2009;30:646-655.
30. Smolders J, Thewissen M, Peelen E, et al. Vitamin D status is positively correlated with regulatory T cell function in patients with multiple sclerosis. *PLoS One* 2009;4:e6635.
31. Owens GP, Bennett JL, Lassmann H, et al. Antibodies produced by clonally expanded plasma cells in multiple sclerosis cerebrospinal fluid. *Ann Neurol* 2009;65:639-649.
32. Schapiro RT. Managing symptoms of multiple sclerosis. *Neurol Clin* 2005;23:177-187.
33. Lublin FD, Reingold SC, Cohen JA, et al. Defining the clinical course of multiple sclerosis. *Neurology* 2014;83:278-286.
34. Confavreux C, Vukusic S. Natural history of multiple sclerosis: A unifying concept. *Brain* 2006;129(3):606-616.
35. Lebrun C, Bensa C, Debouverie M, et al. Association between clinical conversion to multiple sclerosis in radiologically isolated syndrome and magnetic resonance imaging, cerebrospinal fluid, and visual evoked potential: Follow-up of 70 patients. *Arch Neurol* 2009;66:841-846.
36. Zivadinov R, Zorzon M. Is gadolinium enhancement predictive of the development of brain atrophy in multiple sclerosis? A review of the literature. *J Neuroimaging* 2002;12:302-309.
37. Tremlett H, Paty D, Devonshire V. The natural history of primary progressive MS in British Columbia, Canada. *Neurology* 2005;65:1919-1923.
38. Hawker K, O'Connor P, Freedman MS, et al. Rituximab in patients with primary progressive multiple sclerosis: Results of a randomized double-blind placebo-controlled multicenter trial. *Ann Neurol* 2009;66:460-471.
39. Kurtzke JF. Rating neurologic impairment in multiple sclerosis: An expanded disability status scale (EDSS). *Neurology* 1983;33:1444-1452.
40. Rudick RA, Cutter G, Reingold S. The multiple sclerosis functional composite: A new clinical outcome measure for multiple sclerosis trials. *Mult Scler* 2002;8:359-365.
41. Gordon-Lipkin E, Chodkowski B, Reich DS, et al. Retinal nerve fiber layer is associated with brain atrophy in multiple sclerosis. *Neurology* 2007;69:1603-1609.
42. Lee M, O'Brien P. Pregnancy and multiple sclerosis. *J Neurol Neurosurg Psychiatry* 2008;79:1308-1311.

43. Sadovnick AD, Eisen K, Ebers GC, Paty DW. Cause of death in patients attending multiple sclerosis clinics. *Neurology* 1991;41:1193-1196.
44. Swanson JW. Multiple sclerosis: Update in diagnosis and review of prognostic factors. *Mayo Clin Proc* 1989;64:577-586.
45. Polman CH, Reingold SC, Edan G, et al. Diagnostic criteria for multiple sclerosis: 2005 revisions to the "McDonald Criteria." *Ann Neurol* 2005;58:840-846.
46. Frohman EM, Goodin DS, Calabresi PA, et al. The utility of MRI in suspected MS. Report of the Therapeutics and Technology Assessment Subcommittee of the American Academy of Neurology. *Neurology* 2003;61:1332-1338.
47. Fisher E, Rudick R, Simon J, et al. Eight-year follow-up study of brain atrophy in patients with MS. *Neurology* 2002;59:1412-1420.
48. Fisniku LK, Brex PA, Altmann DR, et al. Disability and T2 MRI lesions: A 20-year follow-up of patients with relapse onset of multiple sclerosis. *Brain* 2008;131(Pt3):808-817.
49. Confavreux C, Vukusic S. Accumulation of irreversible disability in multiple sclerosis from epidemiology to treatment. *Clin Neurol Neurosurg* 2006;108(3):327-332.
50. McDonald W, Compston A, Edan G, et al. Recommended diagnostic criteria for multiple sclerosis: Guidelines from the international panel on diagnosis of multiple sclerosis. *Ann Neurol* 2001;50:121-127.
51. Dalton C, Brex P, Miszkiel K, et al. New T_2 lesions enable an earlier diagnosis of multiple sclerosis in clinically isolated syndromes. *Ann Neurol* 2003;53:673-676.
52. Swanton JK, Rovira A, Tintore M, et al. MRI criteria for multiple sclerosis in patients presenting with clinically isolated syndromes: A multicentre retrospective study. *Lancet Neurol* 2007;6:677-686.
53. Lo CP, Kao HW, Chen SY, et al. Prediction of conversion from clinically isolated syndrome to clinically definite multiple sclerosis according to baseline MRI findings: A comparison of revised McDonald criteria and Swanton modified criteria. *J Neurol Neurosurg Psychiatry* 2009;80:1107-2209.
54. Galetta KM, Calabresi PA, Frohman EM, Balcer LJ. Optical coherence tomograph (OCT): Imaging the visual pathway as a model for neurodegeneration. *Neurotherapeutics* 2011;8(1):117-132.
55. Berger T, Rubner P, Schautzer F, et al. Antimyelin antibodies as a predictor of clinically definite multiple sclerosis after a first demyelinating event. *N Engl J Med* 2003;349:139-145.
56. Carmosino MJ, Brousseau KM, Arciniegas DB, et al. Initial evaluations for multiple sclerosis in a university multiple sclerosis center: Outcomes and role of magnetic resonance imaging in referral. *Arch Neurol* 2005;62:585-590.
57. Kaufman DI, Trobe JD, Eggenberger ER, Whitaker JN. Practice parameter: The role of corticosteroids in the management of acute monosymptomatic optic neuritis. Report of the Quality Standards Subcommittee of the American Academy of Neurology. *Neurology* 2000;54:2039-2044.
58. Zivadinov R, Rudick RA, De Masi R, et al. Effects of IV methylprednisolone on brain atrophy in relapsing-remitting MS. *Neurology* 2001;57:1239-1247.
59. Kinkel PR, Miravalle A. Current guidelines and standard treatments of RR-MS. 2011. Addressing Unmet Medical Needs in Relapsing-Remitting Multiple Sclerosis. Available at: *http://www.futuremedicine.com*. doi:10.2217/ebo.11.111:6-25. Accessed date, July 27, 2016.
60. Goodin DS, Frohman EM, Garmany GP, et al. Disease-modifying therapies in multiple sclerosis: Report of the Therapeutics and Technology Assessment Subcommittee of the American Academy of Neurology and the Multiple Sclerosis Council for Clinical Practice Guidelines. *Neurology* 2002;58:169-178.
61. Vandebark AA, Huan J, Agotsch M, et al. Interferon-beta-1a increases CD56 (bright) natural killer cells and CD4+CD25+ Foxp3 expression in subjects with multiple sclerosis. *J Neuroimmunol* 2009;215:125-128.
62. Giovannoni G, Barbarash O, Casset-Semanaz F, et al. Safety and immunogenicity of a new formulation of interferon beta-1a (Rebif New Formulation) in a Phase IIIb study in patients with relapsing multiple sclerosis: 96-week results. *Mult Scler* 2009;15:219-228.
63. Fischer JS, Priore RL, Jacobs LD, et al. Neuropsychological effects of interferon-β-la in relapsing multiple sclerosis. *Ann Neurol* 2000;48:885-892.
64. Simon JH, Jacobs L, Campion M, et al. A longitudinal study of brain atrophy in relapsing MS. *Neurology* 1999;58:139-145.
65. Calabresi PA, Kieseier BC, Arnold DL, et al. Pegylated interferon beta-1a for relapsing-remitting multiple sclerosis (ADVANCE): A randomized, phase 3 double-blind study. *Lancet Neurol* 2014;13:657-665.
66. Frohman E, Phillips T, Kokel K, et al. Disease-modifying therapy in multiple sclerosis: Strategies for optimizing management. *Neurology* 2002;8:227-236.
67. Racke MK, Lovett-Racke AE, Karandikar NJ. The mechanism of action of glatiramer acetate treatment in multiple sclerosis. *Neurology* 2010;74(Suppl 1):S25-S30.
68. Azoulay D, Vachapova V, Shihman B, et al. Lower brain-derived neurotrophic factor in serum of relapsing remitting MS. Reversal by glatiramer acetate. *J Neuroimmunol* 2005;167:215-218.
69. Fillippi M, Rovaris M, Rocca MA, et al. Glatiramer acetate reduces the proportion of new MS lesions evolving into "black holes." *Neurology* 2001;57:731-733.
70. Ford CC, Johnson KP, Lisak RP, et al. A prospective open-label study of glatiramer acetate: Over a decade of continuous use in multiple sclerosis patients. *Mult Scler* 2006;12:309-320.
71. Khan O, Rieckmann P, Boyko A, et al. Three times weekly glatiramer actate in relapsing-remitting multiple sclerosis. *Ann Neurol* 2013;73:705-13.
72. Wolinsky JS, Borresen TE, Dietrich DW, et al. GLACIER: An open-label, randomized, multicenter study to assess the safety and tolerability of glatiramer acetate 40 mg three times weekly verus 20 mg daily in patients with relapsing-remitting multiple sclerosis. *Mult Scler Relat Disord* 2015;4:370-376.
73. Miller DH, Khan OA, Sheremata WA, et al. A controlled trial of natalizumab for relapsing multiple sclerosis. *N Engl J Med* 2003;348:15-23.
74. Polman CH, O'Conor PW, Havrdova E, et al. A randomized, placebo-controlled trial of natalizumab for relapsing multiple sclerosis (AFFIRM). *N Engl J Med* 2006;354:899-910.
75. Rudick RA, Stuart WH, Calabresi PA, et al. Natalizumab plus interferon beta-1a for relapsing multiple sclerosis (SENTINEL). *N Engl J Med* 2006;354:911-923.
76. Kleinschmidt-DeMasters BK, Tyler KL. Progressive multifocal leukoencephalopathy complicating treatment with natalizumab and interferon beta-1a for multiple-sclerosis. *N Engl J Med* 2005;353:369-374.
77. Langer-Gould A, Atlas SW, Green AJ, et al. Progressive multifocal leukoencephalopathy in a patient treated with natalizumab. *N Engl J Med* 2005;353:375-381.
78. Van Assche G, Van Ranst M, Sclot R, et al. Progressive multifocal leukoencephalopathy after natalizumab therapy for Crohn's disease. *N Engl J Med* 2005;353:362-368.
79. Gorelik L, Lerner M, Bixler S, et al. Anti-JC virus antibodies: Implications for PML risk stratification. *Ann Neurol* 2010;68:295-303.
80. Bozic C, Richman S, Plavina T, et al. Anti-John Cunningham virus antibody prevalence in multiple sclerosis patients: Baseline results of STRATIFY-1. *Ann Neurol* 2011;70(5):742-750.
81. Khatri BO, Man S, Giovannoni G, et al. Effect of plasma exchange in accelerating natalizumab clearance and restoring leukocyte function. *Neurology* 2009;72:402-409.
82. Lindå H, von Heijne A, Major EO, et al. Progressive multifocal leukoencephalopathy after natalizumab monotherapy. *N Engl J Med* 2009;361:1081-1087.
83. Sadiq SA, Puccio LM, Brydon EW. JCV detection in multiple sclerosis patients treated with natalizumab. *J Neurol* 2010;257:954-958.
84. U.S. Food and Drug Administration. FDA Drug Safety Communication: Revised recommendations for cardiovascular monitoring and use of multiple sclerosis drug Gilenya fingolimod. FDA 2013. Available at: http://www.fda.gov/Drugs/DrugSafety/ucm303192.htm. (Accessed Dec. 17, 2015)
85. O'Connor P, Wolinsky JS, Confavreux C, et al. Randomized trial of oral teriflunomide for relapsing multiple sclerosis. *N Engl J Med* 2011;365(14):1293-1303.
86. O'Connor PW, Li D, Freedman MS, et al. A Phase II study of the safety and efficacy of teriflunomide in multiple sclerosis with relapses. *Neurology* 2006;66(6):894-900.
87. Kita M, Fox RJ, Phillips JT, et al. Effects of BG-12 (dimethyl fumarate) on health-related quality of life in patients with relapsing-remitting multiple sclerosis: Findings from the CONFIRM study. *Mult Scler* 2014;20(2):253-257.
88. Gold R, Kappos L, Arnold DL, et al. Placebo-controlled phase 3 study of oral BG-12 for relapsing multiple sclerosis. *N Engl J Med* 2012;367(12):1098-1107.
89. Cohen JA, Coles AJ, Arnold DL, et al. Alemtuzumab versus interferon β 1a as first-line treatment for patients with relapsing-remitting multiple sclerosis: A randomised controlled phase 3 trial. *Lancet* 2012;380:1819-1828. doi:10.1016/S0140-6736(12)61769-3.

90. Coles AJ, Twyman CL, Arnold DL, et al. Alemtuzumab for patients with relapsing multiple sclerosis after disease-modifying therapy: A randomised controlled phase 3 trial. *Lancet* 2012;380:1829-1839. doi: 10.1016/S0140-6736(12)61768-1.
91. Havrdova E, Horakova D, Kovarova I. Alemtuzumab in the treatment of multiple sclerosis: Key clinical trial results and considerations for use. *Ther Adv Neurol Disord* 2015;8:31-45. doi: 10.1177/1756285614563522.
92. Hartung HP, Gonsette R, Konig N, et al. Mitoxantrone in progressive multiple sclerosis, a placebo-controlled, double-blind, randomized, multicentre trial. *Lancet* 2002;360:2018-2025.
93. Krapf H, Morrissey SP, Zenker O, et al. Effect of mitoxantrone on MRI in progressive MS. Results of the MIMS trial. *Neurology* 2005;65:690-695.
94. Martinelli V, Bellantonio P, Bergamaschi R, et al. Incidence of acute leukaemia in multiple sclerosis patients treated with mitoxandrone: A multicentre retrospective Italian study. *Neurology* 2009;73:330-333.
95. Costello K, Halper J, Kalb R, et al. The use of disease-modifying therapies in multiple sclerosis. A consensus Paper by the Multiple Sclerosis Coalition. Available at: http://www.nationalmssociety.org/getmedia/5ca284d3-fc7c-4ba5-b005-ab537d495c3c/DMT_Consensus_MS_Coalition_color. (Accessed Dec. 17, 2015)
96. Freedman MS, Kappos L, Polman CH, et al. Betaseron in newly emerging multiple sclerosis for initial treatment (BENEFIT): Clinical outcomes. *Neurology* 2006;(Suppl 2):A61.
97. Vartanian T. An examination of the results of the EVIDENCE, INCOMIN, and phase III studies of interferon beta products in the treatment of multiple sclerosis. *Clin Ther* 2003;1:105-118.
98. Durelli L, Verdun E, Bergui M, et al. Every-other-day interferon-β-1b versus once-weekly interferon-β-1a for multiple sclerosis: Results of a 2-year prospective randomized multicentre study (INCOMIN). *Lancet* 2002;359:1453-1460.
99. Panitch H, Goodin D, Francis G, et al. Randomized, comparative study of interferon-β-1a treatment regimens in MS. The EVIDENCE Trial. *Neurology* 2002;59:1496-1506.
100. Koch-Henriksen N, Sorensen PS, Christensen T, et al. A randomized study of two interferon-beta treatments in relapsing-remitting multiple sclerosis. *Neurology* 2006;66:1056-1060.
101. Clanet M, Radue E, Kappos L, et al. A randomized, double-blind, dose-comparison study of weekly interferon-β-1a in relapsing MS. *Neurology* 2002;59:1507-1517.
102. O'Connor P, Filippi M, Arnason B, et al. 250 mcg or 500 mcg interferon beta-1b versus 20 mg glatiramer acetate in relapsing-remitting multiple sclerosis: A prospective, randomised, multicentre study. *Lancet Neurol* 2009;8:889-897.
103. Mikol DD, Barkhof F, Chang P, et al. Comparison of subcutaneous interferon beta-1a with glatiramer acetate in patients with relapsing multiple sclerosis (the Rebif vs. Glatiramer Acetate in Relapsing MS Disease [REGARD] study): A multicentre, randomised, parallel, open-label trial. *Lancet Neurol* 2008;7:903-914.
104. Namaka M, Pollitt-Smith M, Gupta A, et al. The clinical importance of neutralizing antibodies in relapsing-remitting multiple sclerosis. *Curr Med Res Opin* 2006;22:223-239.
105. Bertolotto A. Neutralizing antibodies to interferon beta: Implications for the management of multiple sclerosis. *Curr Opin Neurol* 2004;17:241-246.
106. Francis GS, Rice GP, Alsop JC, et al. Interferon beta 1a in MS: Results following development of neutralizing antibodies in PRISMS. *Neurology* 2005;65:48-55.
107. Kappos L, Clanet M, Sandberg-Wollheim M, et al. Neutralizing antibodies and efficacy of interferon beta-1a: A 4-year controlled study. *Neurology* 2005;65:40-47.
108. Giovannoni G, Goodman A. Neutralizing anti-IFN-beta antibodies: How much more evidence do we need to use them in practice? *Neurology* 2005;65:6-8.
109. Goodin DS, Frohman EM, Hurwitz B, et al. Neutralizing antibodies to interferon beta: Assessment of their clinical and radiographic impact: An evidence report. *Neurology* 2007;67:977-984.
110. Kappos L, Polman C, Pozzilli C, et al. Final analysis of the European multicenter trial on IFNβ-1b in secondary-progressive MS. *Neurology* 2001;57:1969-1975.
111. Freedman MS, Patry DG, Grand'Maison F, et al. Treatment optimization in multiple sclerosis. *Can J Neurol Sci* 2004;31: 157-168.
112. Hauser SL, Waubant E, Arnold DL, et al. B-cell depletion with rituximab in relapsing-remitting multiple sclerosis. *N Engl J Med* 2008;358:676-688.
113. Sorensen PS, Mellgren SI, Svenningsson A, et al. NORdic trial of oral methylprednisolone as add-on therapy to interferon beta-1a for treatment of relapsing-remitting multiple sclerosis (NORMIMS study): A randomised, placebo-controlled trial. *Lancet Neurol* 2009;8:519-529.
114. Birnbaum G, Cree B, Altafullah I, et al. Combining beta interferon and atorvastatin may increase disease activity in multiple sclerosis. *Neurology* 2008;71:1390-1395.
115. Mitchell G. Update on multiple sclerosis therapy. *Med Clin North Am* 1993;77:231-249.
116. Goodman AD, Brown TR, Krupp LB, et al. Sustained-release oral fampridine in multiple sclerosis: A randomised, double-blind, controlled trial. *Lancet* 2009;373:732-738.
117. Egeberg M, Oh CY, Bainbridge JL. Clinical overview of dalfampridine: The agent with a novel mechanism of action to help with gait disturbances. *Clinical Therapeutics* 2012;34:2185-2194.
118. Stenager EN, Stenager E, Koch Henriksen N, et al. Suicide and multiple sclerosis: An epidemiological investigation. *J Neurol Neurosurg Psychiatry* 1992;55:542-545.
119. Yadav V, Bever C Jr, Bowen J, et al. Summary of evidence-based guideline: complementary and alternative medicine in multiple sclerosis: report of the guideline development subcommittee of the American Academy of Neurology. *Neurology* 2014;82: 1083-1092.
120. Bowling AC. *Optimal Health with Multiple Sclerosis: A Guide to Integrating Lifestyle, Alternative, and Conventional Medicine.* New York, NY: Demos; 2014.
121. National MS Society. News Detail, 2009. Available at: http://nationalmssociety.org/news/news-detail/index.aspx?nid=2115. (Accessed Dec. 17, 2015)
122. Munger KL, Chitnis T, Ascherio A. Body size and risk of MS in two cohorts of US women. *Neurology* 2009;73(19):1543-1550.
123. Hedstrom AK, Baarnhielm M, Olsson T, Alfredsson L. Tobacco smoking, not Swedish snuff use, increases the risk of multiple sclerosis. *Neurology* 2009;73(9):696-701.
124. Goodin et al. Assessment: the use of natalizumab (Tysabri) for the treatment of multiple sclerosis (an evidence-based review): report of the Therapeutics and Technology Assessment Subcommittee of the American Academy of Neurology. *Neurology* 2008;71:766-773.

56

Epilepsy

Viet-Huong V. Nguyen, Christine B. Baca, Jack J. Chen, and Susan J. Rogers

KEY CONCEPTS

1. Accurate classification and diagnosis of seizure type/epilepsy syndrome, including mode of seizure onset, is critical to selection of appropriate pharmacotherapy.
2. The goal of pharmacotherapy is seizure freedom with minimal side effects, and two-thirds to 80% percent of patients can achieve this.
3. Patients who do not respond to drug therapy should be referred to a comprehensive epilepsy center to determine if nonpharmacologic treatments such as surgery are potential options.
4. Patient specific treatment goals should be identified as early as possible, and patient characteristics such as age, comorbid conditions, ability to adhere with the prescribed regimen, presence or absence of insurance coverage, gender, child-bearing ability, and ethnicity should be considered.
5. If the therapeutic goal is not achieved with monotherapy, a second antiseizure drug (ASD), preferably with a different mechanism of action, can be added, or a switch to an alternative single ASD can be made.
6. Pharmacotherapy of epilepsy is highly individualized and requires titration of the dose to optimize ASD therapy (maximal seizure control with minimal or no side effects).
7. Newer ASDs appear to have comparable efficacy to older ASDs and are perhaps better tolerated.
8. Despite numerous drug trials, 20% to 35% of patients will have unsatisfactory control with ASDs.

Epilepsy is a common neurologic condition in which a person is prone to recurrent epileptic seizures. There are many types of epilepsies characterized by different seizure types, ranging in severity and etiologies. While the specific pathophysiologic mechanisms behind different epilepsies are complex, the underlying general pathophysiologic process at the heart of all epilepsies is disturbed regulation of electrical activity in the brain resulting in synchronized and excessive neuronal discharge.

Beyond seizures, people with epilepsy face many challenges. It is important to recognize the coexisting health conditions and psychosocial effects of epilepsy. Patients with epilepsy may display neurodevelopmental delay, cognitive impairment, and often suffer from comorbid depression and anxiety.[1] Furthermore, patients with epilepsy may face educational and vocational challenges, have difficulties with independent living, and be victims of stigma and common public misunderstanding.[2] Such comorbid and psychosocial issues must be taken into account when treating and caring for patients with epilepsy. Indeed, the International League Against Epilepsy (ILAE) defines epilepsy not only as "a chronic condition of the brain characterized by an enduring propensity to generate epileptic seizures" but also by "the neurobiological, cognitive, psychological, and social consequences of this condition."[3] Clinicians treating epilepsy must try to address these common issues and comorbidities. Drug therapy should be selected to not only reduce the frequency of seizures as much as possible, but also with the goal of minimizing side effects, addressing coexisting health and social conditions, and enhancing quality of life (QOL).

EPIDEMIOLOGY

Epilepsy is the fourth most common neurologic disorder globally and in the United States following stroke, migraine, and Alzheimer's disease.[4] According to the World Health Organization (WHO), more than 65 million people worldwide suffer from epilepsy with 2.4 million people being diagnosed with epilepsy each year.[2] In the United States, approximately 2.2 million people suffer from epilepsy with 150,000 new cases being diagnosed each year.[4] Worldwide, the prevalence of epilepsy is believed to range from 1% to 3% and in the United States the prevalence is estimated at 1%.[4]

Epilepsy is a chronic disease and can present at all ages. One in 26 people in the United States will be diagnosed with epilepsy at some point in their lives across the age spectrum.[5] However, the highest number of new cases (incidence) will occur in childhood and in the geriatric population. The number of cases in childhood has been reported to be as high as 82.8 per 100,000 children compared to 40 to 70 cases per 100,000 in the general population.[6,7] Among children, epilepsy is most highly prevalent in children under 5 years of age with the highest number of new cases occurring under 2 years of age.[7] The high frequency of epilepsy in the elderly is now also being recognized with 1.5% of people older than 65 being affected by epilepsy in the United States.[2]

The majority of patients with epilepsy have a good prognosis and will be able to attain seizure freedom and enjoy normal life expectancy.[2] However overall, the mortality rate of patients with epilepsy is 2 to 3 times that of the general population and life expectancy in some of these patients is reduced.[2] This increase in mortality has been attributed to a wide variety of reasons including sudden unexplained death in epilepsy (SUDEP).[2]

Although all individuals with epilepsy experience seizures, not all individuals who experience seizures will be diagnosed with epilepsy. Some seizures are provoked and occur as a result of systemic, toxic, or metabolic insults such as drug overdose; alcohol, barbiturate or benzodiazepine withdrawal; or acute neurologic (eg, brain hemorrhage) or systemic illnesses (eg, hypocalcemia, hypoglycemia, uremia, and eclampsia). Some patients will have seizures only associated with fever (eg, febrile seizures). These seizures do not constitute epilepsy, as they are a symptom of the provoking insult and do not constitute "an enduring predisposition to generate epileptic seizures," once the provoking insult is removed or treated. For example, seizures provoked by transient high-temperature fevers will not recur when the patient is afebrile. Therefore, it is possible to have a seizure and to not have epilepsy.

Each year, 120 per 100,000 people in the United States will be evaluated for a newly recognized seizure whether it be provoked or unprovoked, but only 40 to 70 cases per 100,000 will be diagnosed with epilepsy. At least 10% of the general population will have at least one seizure from *any* cause in their lifetime. Furthermore, 8% of the general population will have at least one unprovoked seizure.[2]

Clinical **Controversy...**

SUDEP is the sudden, unexpected death of someone with epilepsy, who was otherwise healthy. Each year, more than 1 out of 1,000 people with epilepsy die from SUDEP. If seizures are uncontrolled, the risk of SUDEP increases to more than 1 out of 150. Seizure severity appears to be the strongest risk factor for SUDEP. Other potential risk factors include gender, seizure etiology, and younger age at onset. Sudden deaths are rare in children, but are the leading cause of death in young adults with uncontrolled seizures. The exact mechanisms underlying SUDEP are unclear, but recent research suggests there may be a cardiac mechanism involved.[2]

ETIOLOGY

Thousands of medical conditions can cause epilepsy, from genetic mutations to acquired injury (eg, stroke or traumatic brain injury). The most common causes vary depending on population. For instance, childhood-onset epilepsy is predominantly caused by genetic issues, while epilepsy with onset in older age is most often caused by acquired structural injury (eg, stroke or traumatic brain injury). In 2014, the ILAE issued a new report on etiologically based diagnoses. In this report they identified epilepsy etiologies that could be generally classified into six categories reviewed here: (1) genetic; (2) structural; (3) infectious; (4) metabolic; (5) immune; and (6) unknown.[8] These categories are not mutually exclusive as many epilepsies having etiologies that can belong to two or more categories.

Epilepsies with genetic etiology usually present in infancy or childhood. Examples of genetic epilepsies are Juvenile Myoclonic Epilepsy (JME) associated with many different mutations including mutations in EF-hand containing protein-1 (EFHC1), Dravet Syndrome associated with mutations in sodium channel, voltage gated, type I alpha subunit (SCN1A), and Childhood Absence Epilepsy (CAE) associated with many different mutations in T-type Ca^{2+} channels and GABA receptor subunits.[9-12] Prior to 2010, genetic epilepsies have historically been labeled primary generalized epilepsy or idiopathic generalized epilepsy (IGE), as there were no clear structural brain abnormalities that could be found to be responsible for the epilepsy.[13,14] However, it is now recognized that most of these disorders have abnormalities at the molecular level and are genetic in origin and have thus been reclassified as genetic epilepsies.[14,15] Genetic etiologies cannot be acquired.

Structural etiologies can be of acquired or genetic origin and refer to abnormalities visible on structural neuroimaging.[8,15] Common epilepsies caused by structural abnormalities include mesial temporal lobe epilepsy and post-traumatic epilepsy. Mesial temporal lobe epilepsy is a common type of adult-onset epilepsy and is responsible for many of the drug resistant epilepsies seen in tertiary care epilepsy clinics. In mesial temporal lobe epilepsy, sclerosis occurs in the hippocampus, the main structure of the mesial temporal lobe and is characterized by glial scarring, reduced hippocampal volume seen on magnetic resonance imaging (MRI), and decreased cellular density seen on biopsy.[16] Traumatic brain injury from blunt force injury or stroke may cause structural lesions in the brain that may also cause epilepsy.[17] Prior to 2010, epilepsies with structural etiologies were referred to as symptomatic epilepsies.[14]

The most common epilepsy etiology worldwide is infectious and is generally acquired.[17] An infectious etiology refers to a patient who develops epilepsy as the sequelae of an infection, and not to a patient who is experiencing seizures in the setting of acute infection such as meningitis or encephalitis. In developing countries, the most common epilepsy is acquired from neurocysticercosis, a tapeworm in pork that infects the brain when ingested, causing subsequent structural injury that promotes the development of epilepsy.[17]

Metabolic and immune etiologies are less common, although they are increasingly being recognized and understood. Metabolic etiologies refer to a range of metabolic disorders that are associated with epilepsy such as Lafora disease, which is associated with abnormal glycogen metabolism and subsequent development of insoluble glycogen inclusion bodies resulting in epilepsy.[18] A range of immune epilepsies are also being recognized, such as anti-*N*-methyl-D-aspartate (anti-NMDA) receptor encephalitis which causes autoimmune-mediated central nervous system (CNS) inflammation and resulting epilepsy.[19] Both etiologies carry specific treatment implications that are currently evolving.

Lastly, patients can also present with unprovoked seizures that do not have an identifiable cause, and thus by definition have epilepsy of unknown cause.[8] Prior to 2010, these epilepsies were known as cryptogenic epilepsies.[14] These epilepsies may be due to an as yet unidentified gene or may be the consequence of an as yet unrecognized structural or metabolic disorder.

Risk Factors and Seizure Triggers

Separate from etiology are epilepsy risk factors and seizure triggers. While certain risk factors may suggest a predisposition to epilepsy, they are not necessarily the causative agent. Epilepsy risk factors include premature birth with small gestational weight, perinatal injury (eg, anoxia), history of alcohol withdrawal seizures, history of febrile seizures, and family history of seizures.[20] The presence of such risk factors aid in establishing the diagnosis of epilepsy and may help in identifying the underlying epilepsy etiology.

Many factors have been shown to trigger seizures in susceptible individuals. Two of the best known seizure triggers are hyperventilation and photostimulation (eg, flashing lights or rapidly changing or alternating images) in certain genetic epilepsies including JME and CAE.[21] Physical and emotional stress, sleep deprivation, sensory stimuli, and hormonal changes occurring around the time of menses, puberty, or pregnancy have been associated with the onset of or an increased frequency of seizures.[21] Drugs including theophylline, alcohol, high-dose phenothiazines, antidepressants (especially bupropion), and street drug use have been associated with lowering seizure threshold and provoking seizures.[21]

PATHOPHYSIOLOGY

The underlying general pathophysiologic process at the heart of all epilepsies is neuronal hyperexcitability and hypersynchronization. Initially during a seizure, a small number of hyperexcitable neurons fire abnormally in synchrony. Normal membrane conductances and inhibitory synaptic currents break down, and excess excitability spreads, either locally to produce a localized focal seizure or more widely to produce a generalized seizure. This onset is propagated by physiologic pathways and networks to involve adjacent or remote areas. The clinical manifestations depend on the site of the focus, the degree of irritability of the surrounding area of the brain, and the intensity of the impulse.[22]

Hyperexcitability occurs because there is an enhanced predisposition of a neuron to depolarize and discharge when stimulated. Hyperexcitability may result from a number of mechanisms. Among these mechanisms, alterations in the number, type, and biophysical properties of voltage- or ligand-gated K^+, Na^+, Ca^{2+}, and Cl^- ion channels in neuronal membranes may play a significant role.[23] While mutations in these ion channels have been found to be associated with multiple different epilepsies, the exact nature of these alterations likely differ between epilepsies and are not fully elucidated. A large number of antiseizure drugs (ASDs) have mechanisms of actions that act on these specific ion channels, highlighting the importance of these channels in promoting hyperexcitability. For instance, carbamazepine and phenytoin reduce excitability by slowing Na^+ channel recovery from inactivation, thereby preventing hyperexcitable neurons from rapidly and repetitively firing and blocking firing in a use-dependent fashion.[24] Ezogabine acts on K^+ channels and enhances transmembrane potassium currents, thereby stabilizing the resting membrane potential and reducing excitability.[25] Benzodiazepines bind to the gamma subunit of the $GABA_A$ receptor leading to an increase in chloride ion conductance and inhibition of action potentials.[24]

Other mechanisms of epileptogenesis, which may play roles in hyperexcitability, are related to alterations in vesicle trafficking and neurotransmitter release. For instance, synaptic vesicle protein 2-A, a protein responsible for fusion of vesicles to the membrane, has been found to be upregulated in certain models of epilepsy, and is the target of the ASD levetiracetam.[25] Alterations in neurotransmitter uptake and metabolism may also play a role. Vigabatrin, an irreversible inhibitor of γ-aminobutyric acid transaminase (GABA-T), the enzyme responsible for the metabolism of the inhibitory neurotransmitter GABA, works on this possible mechanism, increasing GABA and promoting inhibition.[24]

There are many other possible mechanisms which promote hyperexcitability including: (a) biochemical modifications of receptors; (b) modulation of second messaging systems and gene expression; and (c) changes in extracellular ion concentrations.[23,26] However, hyperexcitability that results simply in increased firing of random individual neurons by itself does not result in epileptic seizures. Epileptic seizures result only when there is also synchronization of excessive neuronal firing.[27] The intrinsic organization of local circuits of certain cerebral structures including the hippocampus, the neocortex and the thalamus contribute to synchronization and promote generation of epileptiform activity.[27,28] Modifications in the ratio and function of inhibitory circuits in these structures play an important role in promoting epileptogenesis, as a large number of these neurons are interconnected and can become simultaneously inhibited, and then synchronously excited. Although under normal circumstances, these neurons are asynchronous, it is believed that under abnormal circumstances, they become synchronous and act as pacemakers promoting epileptiform activity. Furthermore, sprouting and reorganization of neuronal projections in abnormal tissue may also lead to a chronic susceptibility to seizures.[27] Therefore, both excitation and inhibitory connections lie at the heart of the pathophysiologic mechanisms behind epileptogenicity.

CLASSIFICATION OF SEIZURES, EPILEPSIES, AND EPILEPSY SYNDROMES

An epileptic seizure is defined as a transient occurrence of signs and/or symptoms due to abnormal excessive or synchronous neuronal activity in the brain.[3] Because a seizure is a symptom that occurs within the disease or the syndrome, it is important to understand that the classification of seizures is separate from the classification of epilepsies and epilepsy syndromes. In some cases the classification of seizures will be very similar to the epilepsy classification. In other cases there will be many seizure types occurring within an epilepsy syndrome. 1 Regardless, these classifications are important to distinguish because medication choices, treatment strategies (eg, epilepsy surgery) and prognosis may differ depending on these classifications. Classification strategies and seizure/epilepsy terminology has changed over the years.[13-15] Revised terminology as well as older terminology for classification of seizures and epilepsy will be reviewed in these sections. It is still important to be familiar with older terminology, as many practitioners continue to use this terminology and because much of the prior literature in epilepsy references this terminology. Throughout this chapter, we will try to use revised terminology where appropriate and refer to older terminology only when the referenced literature requires we do so.

Classification of Seizures—Mode of Onset

Epileptic seizures can manifest physically in a variety of ways and can range from intense involuntary repetitive muscular contractions (eg, convulsions) to subtle alterations in sensation or consciousness. Due to the wide range of seizure types that may present it is often difficult to describe and classify seizures. However, in general, most seizures can be classified by their mode of onset and can be divided broadly into two categories: (1) generalized and (2) focal.[15] In the broadest terms, generalized *onset* seizures begin in *both* hemispheres of the brain, while focal *onset* seizures begin in only *one* hemisphere of the brain. Understanding seizure onset is important, as it is the fundamental characteristic by which to classify seizures. Recognizing mode of seizure onset has significant treatment and prognostic implications. For instance, patients with generalized onset seizures may have seizure exacerbation when treated with certain ASDs (eg, treating a patient who has CAE with carbamazepine).[29] Likewise, patients with focal onset seizures who are drug resistant may be good candidates for surgical resection, while patients with generalized onset seizures are not.

Focal Onset Seizures

Focal seizures may be further characterized by whether impairment or alteration of consciousness occurs. Impairment of consciousness is usually defined by loss of awareness of external stimuli or by the inability to respond to external stimuli in a purposeful and appropriate manner. When consciousness is not impaired and when awareness and responsiveness are retained, such seizures are termed focal seizures without dyscognitive features under the newest classification system released by the ILAE in 2010.[15] These seizures correspond to what has historically been termed simple partial seizures, as by definition consciousness is not impaired.[13] When impairment of consciousness occurs during a focal onset seizure, such seizures are termed focal seizures *with* dyscognitive features.[15] These seizures correspond to what have historically been termed *complex partial seizures* (CPS).[13] Focal dyscognitive seizures may have similar clinical signs and symptoms as those described for focal nondyscognitive seizures (see Clinical Presentation section), but the essential feature that distinguishes them is the presence of impaired consciousness.

Focal seizures may spread beyond the one hemisphere of the brain to the contralateral hemisphere to involve both hemispheres. When both hemispheres of the brain become involved, the seizure is said to have generalized. During generalization, the person usually becomes unconscious and may display bilateral convulsive features such as tonic-clonic motor features (see Clinical Presentation section for further details). Under the 2010 ILAE classification system, focal seizures that generalize into GTC seizures are now referred to as focal seizures evolving to a bilateral convulsive seizure which is considered to be a more precise and descriptive term. Such seizures have historically been referred to as CPS with *secondary* generalization.[15,30]

Generalized Onset Seizures

Generalized *onset* seizures begin in *both* hemispheres of the brain and have previously been referred to as primary generalized seizures. The ILAE now recognizes six types of generalized onset seizures including (1) absence seizures, (2) myoclonic seizures, (3) tonic-clonic seizures, (4) clonic seizures, (5) tonic seizures, and (6) atonic seizures.[15,31] Like secondarily generalized seizures, generalized onset seizures typically have clinical manifestations that indicate involvement of both hemispheres (eg, motor manifestations are bilateral and symmetric). Recognizing the difference between generalized onset seizures and secondarily generalized seizures may be difficult, but certain distinguishing features such as presence of aura and characteristic findings on electroencephalogram (EEG) aid in distinguishing between the two (see Clinical Presentation section for more details).

Classification of Epilepsies and Epileptic Syndromes

In 1989, the ILAE defined an epileptic syndrome as an epileptic disorder characterized by a cluster of signs and symptoms customarily occurring together.[14] These include such characteristics as type of seizure, etiology, anatomy, precipitating factors, age of onset, severity, chronicity, diurnal and circadian cycling, and sometimes prognosis. These syndromes have historically been classified along two main axes with the first axis separating epilepsies with generalized seizures from epilepsies with partial or focal seizures. Partial or focal seizures were then further subcategorized based on etiology. Many practitioners continue to categorize epilepsies along these axes. This distinction is important, as many practitioners also base initial ASD selection according to these axes. ASDs that can be used in both axes are often considered broad-spectrum ASDs. Narrow spectrum ASDs can only be used in one axis or in particular seizure types or epilepsy syndromes.

In 2010, the ILAE defined four categories by which to organize the epilepsies and epilepsy syndromes according to specificity of the diagnosis.[15] These categories are: (1) the electroclinical syndromes which have the most specific diagnoses and are distinct clinical entities that are reliably identified by a cluster of characteristics such as symptoms, signs, age of onset, EEG characteristics, and seizure types; (2) epilepsies with distinctive constellations/surgical syndromes which do not meet the criteria of an electroclinical syndrome yet can and should be recognized based on clinical features; (3) epilepsies attributed to and organized by structural-metabolic causes which are nonsyndromic epilepsies that do not fit into a specific electroclinical syndrome and which would have previously been termed "symptomatic focal epilepsies"; and (4) epilepsies of unknown cause which would have previously been termed "cryptogenic" epilepsies. Epilepsy classification and seizure classification are still evolving. This classification schema for seizures and epilepsy syndromes and epilepsies is depicted in Fig. 56-1 and Table 56-1. It is important to be familiar with older as well as revised terminology for classification of epilepsies and epilepsy syndromes.

TABLE 56-1 2010 ILAE Electroclinical Syndromes and Other Epilepsies

I. **Electroclinical Syndromes** (and common examples arrange by age at onset)
Infancy:
West Syndrome
Dravet Syndrome
Childhood:
Febrile Seizure Plus (FS+)
Lennox-Gastaut Syndrome
Childhood Absence Epilepsy
Adolescent-Adult:
Juvenile Myoclonic Epilepsy (JME)
Progressive Myoclonic Epilepsy (PME—including Lafora)
Epilepsy with Generalized Tonic-Clonic Seizures Alone

II. **Distinctive Constellations** (and common examples):
Mesial Temporal Lobe Epilepsy with Hippocampal Sclerosis

III. **Epilepsies Attributed to and Organized by Structural-Metabolic Causes** (and common examples):
Malformations of Cortical Development
Tuberous Sclerosis
Tumor
Trauma
Strokes

IV. **Epilepsies of Unknown Cause**

Data from reference 15.

CLINICAL PRESENTATION

Characteristics of Focal Seizures

Focal seizures without dyscognitive features may manifest clinically in a variety of ways and may be further characterized by one or more features including motor or autonomic symptoms.[15] Such symptoms will vary depending on where the abnormal firing occurs. For example, seizures may manifest as alterations in motor functions such as clonic movements (eg, twitching or jerking) of the arm, shoulder, face, or leg indicating seizure activity in motor pathways. Sensory or somatosensory symptoms may also occur, such as feelings of numbness or tingling or a feeling of déjà vu, indicating parietal or temporal lobe seizure activity. Visual disturbances or hallucinations may also indicate seizure activity involving the occipital lobe, while ringing or buzzing sounds in the ears may indicate seizure activity in auditory areas of the brain. Autonomic symptoms such as sweating, salivation, or pallor may also occur, indicating seizure activity in autonomic areas of the brain. In all the above examples of focal nondyscognitive seizures, only a portion of the brain is affected during the seizure, and the person retains consciousness, awareness, and responsiveness.[15,31]

The hallmark of focal dyscognitive seizures is amnesia to the event. Depending on the area of the brain involved, focal dyscognitive seizures may have similar clinical signs and symptoms as that described except with impairment of consciousness. The patient

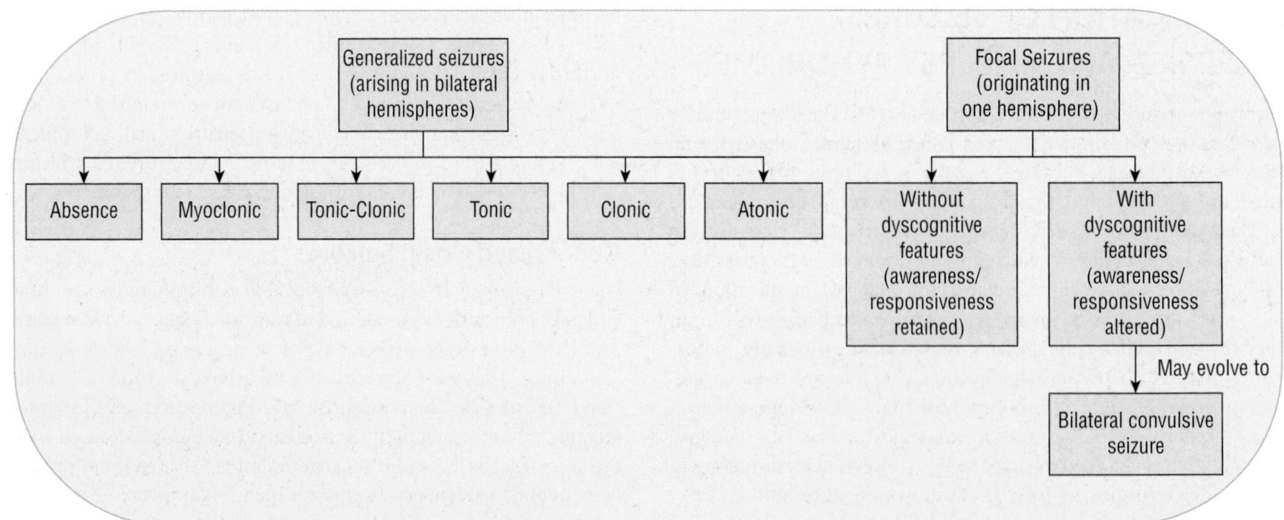

FIGURE 56-1 2010 ILAE Revised Terminology for Classification of Seizures.

may still be able to perform routine tasks such as walking, although such movements are not purposeful or planned and after the event is over the patient may not recall their actions. The patient may also be able to respond to questions during the seizure, although they may not respond appropriately. The degree of alteration in awareness and responsiveness may be so subtle that witnesses may sometimes not be able to recognize that anything is overtly wrong. For example, during these seizures the patient may simply display behavioral arrest and stare off into space for a minute. They may also display subtle automatisms such as lip smacking, chewing, or picking at their clothing unpurposefully. On the other hand, some patients may display extreme aberrations of behavior, and some are even mistakenly diagnosed as having psychotic episodes. After the seizure (postictal period), the patient may display altered consciousness, drowsiness, confusion, or even paranoia for a variable period of time and frequently go into a deep sleep.[15,30]

Focal seizures are sometimes followed by convulsive seizures. During convulsive or generalized tonic-clonic (GTC) seizures, the patient experiences loss of consciousness, followed by a sudden sharp tonic contraction of muscles with a subsequent period of rigidity and clonic movements oftentimes described as jerking of the arms and legs. During the seizure, the patient may cry or moan, due to muscles in the larynx being activated. The patient may also lose sphincter control with bladder and/or bowel incontinence or bite the tongue. Postictally, after the patient regains consciousness, the patient may experience confusion, drowsiness, lack of coordination, soreness throughout the body, and amnesia for the event.

Focal seizures evolving to a bilateral convulsive seizure have clinical features that differentiate it from generalized onset convulsive seizures (eg, seizures with onset in bilateral brain hemispheres). For instance, in some cases of secondarily generalized seizures, patients will describe somatosensory symptoms as a "warning" prior to the convulsive seizure. These warnings are frequently termed auras, which are by definition restricted focal epileptic discharges. Auras are subjective and may be sensory or experiential. Sensory auras may include feelings of tingling, numbness, flashing lights, odors, tastes, and epigastric distress. Experiential auras include feelings of fear, depression, joy, anger, or memory phenomena such as feelings of familiarity (déjà vu) or unfamiliarity (jamais vu). Auras are focal nondyscognitive seizures which may progress to focal dyscognitive seizures and then to seizures with bilateral convulsions.[15,31] Other features that aid in distinguishing generalized-onset seizures from secondarily generalized seizures are age of onset, family history of seizures, the presence of genetic mutations, and findings on EEG, computed tomography (CT), and MRI that are beyond the scope of this chapter.

Characteristics of Generalized Seizures

Clinical descriptions of the six types of generalized onset seizures recognized by the ILAE including (1) absence seizures, (2) myoclonic seizures, (3) clonic seizures, (4) tonic seizures, (5) tonic-clonic seizures, and (6) atonic seizures are described hereunder:

1. Generalized absence seizures are manifested by a sudden onset interruption of ongoing activities, a blank stare, and possibly a brief upward rotation of the eyes indicating the abrupt onset and offset of impaired consciousness. The staring and behavioral arrest lasts 2 to 30 seconds during which time the patient is unaware of the environment and unresponsive. The patient has neither a warning that the seizure is going to occur, nor does the patient have postictal confusion or lethargy after the seizures. After cessation of the seizure, the patient will often return to the previous activity as if nothing had happened. These absence seizures generally occur in young children through adolescence. It is important to differentiate these seizures from focal dyscognitive seizures. In general, absence type seizures are much more brief then the staring spells associated with focal dyscognitive seizures and have minimal post-ictal manifestations.[15,31]
2. Myoclonic seizures are characterized by brief, shock-like muscle contractions commonly referred to as jerks. These jerks can occur as a single jerk or as a series of jerks with each jerk typically lasting only milliseconds. These jerks are synchronous and display bilateral features usually involving the whole body simultaneously, although they can be asymmetric and confined to body parts. They are not associated with an alteration in consciousness and are typically worse in the late evening or early morning either prior to going to sleep or soon after awakening.[15,31]
3. Generalized clonic seizures are seizures involving bilaterally rhythmic jerking that are more sustained and rhythmic than that seen in a myoclonic seizure.[15,31]
4. Generalized tonic seizures involve bilaterally increased tone or "stiffening" of the limbs typically lasting seconds to a minute.[15,31]
5. Generalized onset tonic-clonic seizure is a seizure consisting of an initial tonic phase followed by a clonic phase. It is important to remember that GTC seizures can also be secondarily generalized and that these seizures must be differentiated from generalized onset tonic-clonic seizures.[15,31]
6. In contrast to tonic seizures in which there is a sudden onset of increased tone, a sudden loss of muscle tone occurs in *atonic seizures*. Atonic seizures are not preceded by myoclonic or tonic features and can be very brief. They often occur in patients with intellectual impairment. They may present as a head drop, the dropping of a limb, or a slumping to the ground (due to loss of postural tone). These patients often wear protective headware to prevent trauma. Atonic seizures are the hallmark of Lennox-Gastaut Syndrome.[15,10,31]

Diagnosis

Epilepsy is a clinical diagnosis, meaning that it is a diagnosis made on the basis of medical signs and patient-reported symptoms, rather than any one diagnostic test. As previously noted, the ILAE has defined epilepsy as a "disease characterized by an enduring predisposition to generate epileptic seizures and by the neurobiological, cognitive, psychological, and social consequences of this condition."[3] However, this definition is theoretical and not sufficiently detailed for the purposes of diagnoses. Therefore, in 2014 the ILAE developed a practical (operational) definition of epilepsy, designed for use by doctors and patients.[32] According to the ILAE, a person is considered to have epilepsy if they meet any of the following conditions: (1) at least two unprovoked (or reflex) seizures occurring greater than 24 hours apart; (2) one unprovoked (or reflex) seizure and a probability of further seizures similar to the general recurrence risk (at least 60%) after two unprovoked seizures, occurring over the next 10 years; or (3) diagnosis of an epilepsy syndrome.[32]

When a person presents with possible epilepsy, the most important initial step in clinical evaluation is to get a detailed description of the event. In most cases, the healthcare provider will not be in a position to witness a seizure. Many patients (particularly those with focal dyscognitive seizures or focal seizures evolving to bilateral convulsions) are amnestic to the actual seizure event, and obtaining an adequate description from a witness is critically important. Firstly, the presence of an aura should be determined. If the presence of an aura can be confirmed, it becomes very likely that the seizure is focal. The presence of ictal motor, sensory, or autonomic features should all be noted. The degree of mental status impairment during the event should be determined. Tongue biting, cheek biting, and bladder or bowel incontinence during the seizures should be asked about

CLINICAL PRESENTATION Epilepsy

Recall That:

- Focal (eg, partial) seizures may present with just motor symptoms (twitching or shaking, usually one-sided) or just sensory symptoms (numbness, tingling, usually one-sided)
- Focal dyscognitive (eg, complex partial) seizures are associated with altered consciousness or impairment in awareness
- Absence seizures can be almost nondetectable with only very brief (seconds) periods of altered consciousness
- Convulsive (eg, GTC) seizures are major convulsive episodes and are always associated with a loss of consciousness

Some Pertinent Questions to Ask

- Was there any warning that something was going to happen? What were the warning signs?
- Were there any abnormal movements or shaking?
- Was there loss of bowel or bladder function?
- Did you bite your tongue?
- Was there any post-event confusion?
- How much of the event do you remember?
- How long did the event last?
- How often do you have these events?

Signs

- Interictally (between seizure episodes), there are typically no objective or pathognomonic signs

Laboratory Tests

- There are currently no diagnostic laboratory tests for epilepsy
- In some cases, particularly following generalized convulsive seizures, serum prolactin levels obtained within 10 to 20 minutes can be transiently elevated[33]
- Laboratory tests can be done to rule out treatable causes of seizures (eg, hypoglycemia, altered electrolyte concentrations, infections, etc.) that do not represent epilepsy

Other Diagnostic Tests

- An abnormal epileptiform EEG is found in only approximately 50% of the patients who have epilepsy. Sometimes several EEGs must be obtained before convincing epileptiform activity is detected. Video EEG is the gold standard for diagnosing epilepsy and involves admission to the hospital and recording video and EEG until the patient has a typical event. However, this is not the standard for most patients and is generally reserved for cases unresponsive to medication or difficult to characterize.[34,35]
- Brain MRI is indicated in patients with epilepsy. MRI is the preferred imaging technique to identify structural abnormalities (eg, sclerosis in the mesial temporal lobes and traumatic brain injury).[35]
- A computed tomography (CT) scan typically is not helpful except in the initial evaluation for a brain tumor, cerebral bleeding, or gross anatomical injury.[35]

Epilepsy-Related Health Screening

- Screening for comorbid medical, psychiatric, and neurodevelopmental conditions commonly coexisting with epilepsy is useful.[35]
- Common conditions that are typically screened for in patients with epilepsy include depression (and suicidal ideation), learning and development in children, and bone health.[35]

and the seizure time course noted. Finally, postictal phenomena (eg, fatigue, headaches, confusion, and psychosis) should be assessed.

Beyond the actual ictal event, age of onset of seizures, frequency of, and evolution of the seizures over time must be assessed. Although seizures tend to be stereotyped within an individual, the clinical presentation of the seizure may change over time or with treatment. Furthermore, triggers should be identified because avoiding them may have a significant impact on seizure control. Seizures that result in injuries should also be noted and mental health problems should be identified.

Accurate diagnosis also depends on the neurologic examination and diagnostic techniques such as electroencephalography (EEG) and brain imaging. The EEG can identify abnormal brain wave patterns that are associated with certain seizure types and epilepsy syndromes and is one of the most important diagnostic tests that can be performed for patient with epilepsy. Brain imaging with either CT or MRI can detect structural lesions that can aid in the diagnosis of seizures and epilepsy types. Though CT is commonly initially performed in a patient who presents with a first seizure, an MRI is preferred for validation of an epilepsy diagnosis.

TREATMENT

Desired Outcomes

Antiseizure drug therapy is the mainstay of epilepsy treatment. However, ASDs are symptomatic treatment only. None have been proven to have any disease modifying properties, and no ASDs are curative. Surgery is the only possibly curative therapy, and only a select number of patients qualify for surgery. Therefore, the majority of patients will be on life-long ASD therapy. 2 The goal of ASD therapy is to eliminate symptoms (eg, seizures) with minimal side effects. In most patients the goal is complete seizure freedom. However, in 20% to 35% of patients this may not be possible, and seizure control must be balanced with QOL goals.

Treatment goals can change over time.[36] For those who cannot obtain seizure freedom despite these therapies, more obtainable goals should be established (eg, decrease in the number of seizures and minimized drug adverse effects).

Clinical **Controversy...**

Currently available drugs used in the treatment of epilepsy are commonly called antiepileptic drugs (AEDs). However, all currently available drugs act to prevent seizures only. None of the currently available AEDs have been proven to have any disease modifying or antiepileptogenic properties. Therefore, there is controversy as to whether such drugs should be labeled AEDs or antiseizure drugs (ASDs). In this chapter, we refer to drugs used in epilepsy treatments as ASDs. However, it is important to recognize that AED is a commonly used term that is often used interchangeably with ASD.

General Approach to Treatment

The general approach to treatment involves assessment of seizure type and frequency, identification of treatment goals, development of a care plan, and a plan for follow-up evaluation. During the assessment phase, it is critical to establish an accurate diagnosis of the seizure type and epilepsy classification. Once the assessment is complete and the most accurate epilepsy diagnosis is made for patients with new onset seizures, the choice is whether to use drug therapy and, if so, which one.

Once the decision to initiate therapy has been determined, patient-specific treatment goals must be identified. The drug treatments of first choice depend on the type of epilepsy as well as patient characteristics such as age, gender, comorbid medical conditions, susceptibility to adverse effects, ability to comply with a prescribed regimen, and insurance coverage.

When starting ASD therapy, monotherapy is preferred.[37] Polytherapy should be considered for those patients who cannot achieve seizure freedom on ASD monotherapy. Those who have unsatisfactory control despite multiple drug treatment may be candidates for vagal nerve stimulators, surgery, or ketogenic diet.

Once the care plan is established and an ASD is selected, patient education and assurance of patient understanding of the plan is essential. Detailed directions regarding titration, what to do in the event of a treatment-emergent side effect, and what to do if a seizure occurs must be provided to patients. Providing the patient with a seizure and side-effect diary will assist in the follow-up and evaluation phase.

At the follow-up stage of treatment (which can be done in the hospital, clinic, pharmacy, or by phone), the treatment goals must be reviewed. If the goal has been achieved, new goals should be identified. For example, if convulsive seizures are now controlled, the goal may be to control focal seizures. If a patient fails to respond to the first ASD, trials with other ASDs should be attempted as appropriate. Patient adherence, drug efficacy, and safety of treatment should be taken into account. For a patient with long-standing epilepsy, adequacy of the current medication regimen should be routinely evaluated.

When seizures are not controlled, medication nonadherence must always be considered as it is the single most common reason for treatment failure. It is estimated that up to 60% of patients with epilepsy are nonadherent.[38] The rate of nonadherence is increased by the complexity of the drug regimen and by doses taken three and four times a day.[38] Frequent uncontrolled seizures can also predispose a patient to nonadherence secondary to confusion over whether the drug was taken. Nonadherence is not influenced by age, sex, psychomotor development, or seizure type.[12]

When to Start Antiseizure Drugs

If a patient presents after a single isolated seizure, one of three treatment decisions can be made: (1) treat, (2) possibly treat, or (3) do not treat. These decisions are based on the probability of the patient having a second seizure. For patients with no risk factors, normal MRI, and normal EEG, the probability of a second seizure is less than 10% in the first year and approximately 21% by the end of 2 years. If risk factors are present, the probability of seizure recurrence is 26% in the first year and 41% by the end of the second year.[39]

Some clinicians start ASD treatment after the first seizure, whereas others start ASD treatment after one unprovoked seizure with a definite abnormal epileptiform EEG. Others do not initiate treatment until a second, unprovoked seizure has occurred. The decision on whether to start ASD therapy depends on the provider and on patient-specific factors such as patient's lifestyle and preferences. However, patients who have had two or more unprovoked seizures should be started on ASDs.[32]

When to Stop Antiseizure Drugs

The ASDs used to control seizures may not need to be given for a lifetime. Polypharmacy can be reduced, and some patients can discontinue ASDs altogether. The drug considered least effective or the agent deemed most responsible for adverse effects should be discontinued first. In some cases, decreasing the number of ASDs can decrease side effects and increase cognitive abilities.[40] This improvement in cognition may be small, especially if the patient is on a drug that primarily affects psychomotor speed with less effect on higher-order cognitive functioning.

Factors favoring successful withdrawal of ASDs include a seizure-free period of 2 to 4 years, complete seizure control within 1 year of onset, an onset of seizures after age 2 but before age 35, and a normal neurologic examination and EEG.[41,42] Factors associated with a poor prognosis in discontinuing ASDs, despite a seizure-free interval, include a history of a high frequency of seizures, repeated episodes of status epilepticus (SE), a combination of seizure types, and development of abnormal mental functioning.[41,42] The American Academy of Neurology (AAN) has issued guidelines for discontinuing ASDs in seizure-free patients.[43] After assessing the risks and benefits to both the patient and society, ASD withdrawal can be considered in a patient meeting the following profile: seizure free for 2 to 5 years, a history of a single type of focal seizure or primary generalized seizures, a normal neurologic exam and normal IQ, and an EEG that has normalized with treatment. When these factors are present, the relapse rate at 1 year is expected to be 35% and 29% at 2 years.[44] ASDs can be restarted in patients who relapse after ASD withdrawal. Seizure freedom can be regained for most patients who restart ASDs although not for all.[42]

Antiseizure drug withdrawal should be done gradually. Some patients will have a recurrence of seizures as the ASDs are withdrawn. Sudden withdrawal can be associated with the precipitation of SE. Withdrawal seizures are of particular concern for agents such as benzodiazepines and barbiturates, and these ASDs should be withdrawn more slowly over a period of many months.

Nonpharmacologic Therapy

Nonpharmacologic therapy for epilepsy includes diet, surgery, and vagus nerve stimulation (VNS) among other modalities. A vagal nerve stimulator is an implanted medical device that is Food and Drug Administration (FDA) approved for use as adjunctive therapy in reducing the frequency of seizures in adults and adolescents older than 12 years of age with partial-onset seizures that are refractory to ASDs. It is also used off-label in the treatment of refractory primary generalized epilepsy. The mechanisms of antiseizure actions of VNS are unknown. Human clinical studies have shown that VNS changes the cerebrospinal fluid (CSF) concentration of inhibitory and stimulatory neurotransmitters and activates specific areas of the brain that generate or regulate cortical seizure activity through increased blood flow. There is experimental evidence to suggest that the anticonvulsant effect of VNS is mediated by the locus coeruleus.[45]

The VNS device is relatively safe. It may also have a positive effect on mood and behavior, often independent of seizure reduction.[46] The most common side effect associated with stimulation is hoarseness, voice alteration, increased cough, pharyngitis, dyspnea, dyspepsia, and nausea. Serious adverse effects reported include infection, nerve paralysis, hypoesthesia, facial paresis, left vocal cord paralysis, left facial paralysis, left recurrent laryngeal nerve injury, urinary retention, and low-grade fever. In the VNS studies, the percentage of patients who achieved a 50% or greater reduction in their seizure frequency (responders) ranged from 23% to 50% at 3 months.[47,48] VNS effects are not noted immediately and are more long term. VNS is also unlikely to lead to seizure freedom but may allow for reduced seizure frequency and reduced medication burden.[49]

3 Surgery is the treatment of choice in selected patients with refractory focal epilepsy, especially those patients with seizures originating from the temporal lobe. A 2001 randomized controlled trial focusing on temporal lobe epilepsy, found that 58% of patients who underwent surgery were seizure free at 1 year compared to 8% of patients who did not undergo surgery.[50] A second randomized controlled study, initiated to evaluate the efficacy of early surgery versus continued medical management in patients who had failed two ASD trials, showed that 11 of 15 patients who had undergone surgery were seizure free at 2 year follow-up, compared to none in the medical therapy group.[51] Certain factors have been found to predict good outcomes in surgical patients including presence of a focal brain lesion on MRI, presence of unilateral mesial temporal sclerosis, presence of a localized temporal lobe positron emission tomography (PET) abnormality (even if brain MRI is normal), concordant EEG data showing location of ictal onset and shorter preoperative seizure duration.[52-54] The last finding is important to emphasize, as it is imperative to identify possibly drug-resistant patients with epilepsy quickly and to refer them to an epilepsy center as soon as possible. Epilepsy surgery is not without risk. Learning and memory can be impaired postoperatively, and general intellectual abilities are also affected in a small number of patients.[54] Patients may need to continue ASD therapy for a period of time following successful epilepsy surgery, but dosage reduction may be achievable.[55]

The ketogenic diet, devised in the 1920s, is high in fat and low in carbohydrates and protein, and it leads to acidosis and ketosis. Protein and calorie intake are set at levels that will meet requirements for growth. Most of the calories are provided in the form of heavy cream and butter. No sugar is allowed. Vitamins and minerals are supplemented. Medium-chain triglycerides can be substituted for the dietary fats. Fluids are also controlled. It requires strict control and parent compliance. Although some centers find the diet useful for medically refractory epilepsy patients, particularly those with certain etiologies such as GLUT1 deficiency, others have found that it is poorly tolerated by patients. Long-term effects include kidney stones, increased bone fractures, and adverse effects on growth.[56] An international consensus statement has been published, which offers recommendations employing various forms of the ketogenic diet which may be more tolerable, including the use of the modified Atkins diet and the Low Glycemic Index Treatment.[57] Subsequent data support the use of these variations in the ketogenic diet, as well as the medium chain triglyceride ketogenic diet in select patients.[58]

Pharmacologic Therapy

4 Selection and optimization of ASD therapy first requires consideration of the seizure type, epilepsy classification, and epilepsy etiology, as an ASD must be effective for the specific seizure type and epilepsy or epilepsy syndrome being treated. Patient characteristics such as age, gender, medical conditions must also be considered, as different patient groups may be better suited to receive one ASD over another, not only because of seizure type but also because of susceptibility or relative risk for certain adverse effects (eg, children may be more susceptible to neuropsychiatric adverse effects, women of child-bearing potential should not be on teratogenic drugs, and the elderly may be more susceptible to adverse effects on cognition). Furthermore, patients with comorbid conditions, such as migraine headache, tremor, or neuropathy, may benefit from the use of particular ASDs that can also treat that condition. Also of extreme importance to consider is a patient's ability to adhere to a prescribed regimen and insurance coverage, as these factors can influence nonadherence to the regimen or cause financial hardship if the medicine is expensive and not covered. Ultimately, ASD effectiveness is the result of the interaction of each of these factors.

ASD Selection

When selecting an ASD, the following should be considered:

1. ASD effectiveness for the specific seizure type, epilepsy, or epilepsy syndrome
2. Selection of an ASD with the most tolerable adverse effect profile, considering patient specific factors including age and gender
3. Selection of an ASD that can also treat the patient's other comorbid conditions
4. Ability to comply with a regimen (eg, three or four times daily dosing) and insurance coverage, as this can affect ASD adherence and effectiveness
5. Interactions with other medications
6. Need for therapeutic levels to be reached quickly (eg, avoid ASDs which require slow titration such as lamotrigine or topiramate)

5 Once an ASD has been selected, start with a low dose, and gradually titrate to a moderate dose goal, taking into account the patient's response to treatment. If the patient is seizure free with no adverse effects at a moderate therapeutic dose, then no further increase in dose is necessary. If the patient continues to have seizures at this moderate dose, titrating the patient to a maximum dose is recommend. If the first ASD monotherapy is ineffective, or if the patient experiences intolerable adverse effects, adding a second AED and then tapering and discontinuing the ineffective or intolerable first ASD is appropriate. Selecting an ASD with a different mechanism of action than the first intolerable or ineffective ASD may increase the likelihood of success.[59] If the second ASD is ineffective, polytherapy may be indicated, and an adjunctive ASD should be gradually titrated on. Selection of an adjunctive ASD with a different or complementary mechanism of action is the basis behind rational polytherapy and is recommended, although there is no clear evidence in humans to support this. A suggested algorithm for a general approach to the treatment of epilepsy is shown in Fig. 56-2.

6 Some patients, such as elderly patients who are sensitive to falls, sedation, and other neurocognitive side effects, need to have ASDs titrated much more slowly and start at much lower initial doses. In such cases, a slow titration can last over many weeks or months and may have a lower goal dose. In other patients, such as patients with multiple recent seizures, a therapeutic dose needs to be reached much more quickly, and a more rapid titration over days instead of weeks is appropriate. For such patients, loading doses, either administered orally or intravenously, may be indicated. When loading, it is important to select ASDs that can be administered safely as loading doses (eg, lamotrigine requires titration and should not be used in patients who require loading to reach therapeutic levels quickly).

Efficacy and Effectiveness

7 There are more than 20 ASDs available in the United States and worldwide for the treatment of epilepsy. Efficacy of ASDs as monotherapy or as add-on treatment in epilepsy is generally established through clinical trials. However, monotherapy efficacy has not been studied for all agents. Although many newer ASDs have been tested only as add-on treatment, many providers will use most ASDs off-label as monotherapy in clinical practice.

Due to the paucity of well-designed, properly conducted, randomized, controlled trials for comparing ASDs, there is a lack of quality evidence to describe comparative efficacy and effectiveness of ASDs. Evidence for comparable effectiveness is primarily available for older agents and some newer agents.[29] Generally speaking, however, the newer ASDs appear to have comparable efficacy to the older agents and are perhaps better tolerated, but we do not have quality evidence to decisively conclude that. What has become obvious is that individuals respond differently to each AED, and that an understanding of each of these agents is needed to optimize therapy for individual patients.

The evidence we do have for long-term effectiveness was summarized in 2013 by the ILAE who reviewed evidence for initial ASD monotherapy in six age-related seizure types and two epilepsy syndromes. Some ASDs including carbamazepine, ethosuximide, gabapentin, levetiracetam, oxcarbazepine, phenytoin, valproic acid, and zonisamide, have strong enough evidence to be labeled as efficacious or effective, or as probably efficacious or effective as initial monotherapy in certain seizure types, while others have weaker evidence and can only be labeled as possibly or potentially efficacious or effective.[59] Furthermore, there is limited evidence that some ASDs may possibly or potentially precipitate or aggravate certain seizure types, and therefore it is suggested that they should be used with caution in those patients (eg, carbamazepine and phenytoin in generalized onset tonic-clonic seizure types or carbamazepine, gabapentin, oxcarbazepine, phenytoin, tiagabine, and vigabatrin among others in children with absence or in JME).[29] The ILAE findings are summarized in Table 56-2. Also included in Table 56-2 are evidenced-based treatment recommendations from the American Academy of Neurology (AAN)-American Epilepsy Society (AES) and recommendations

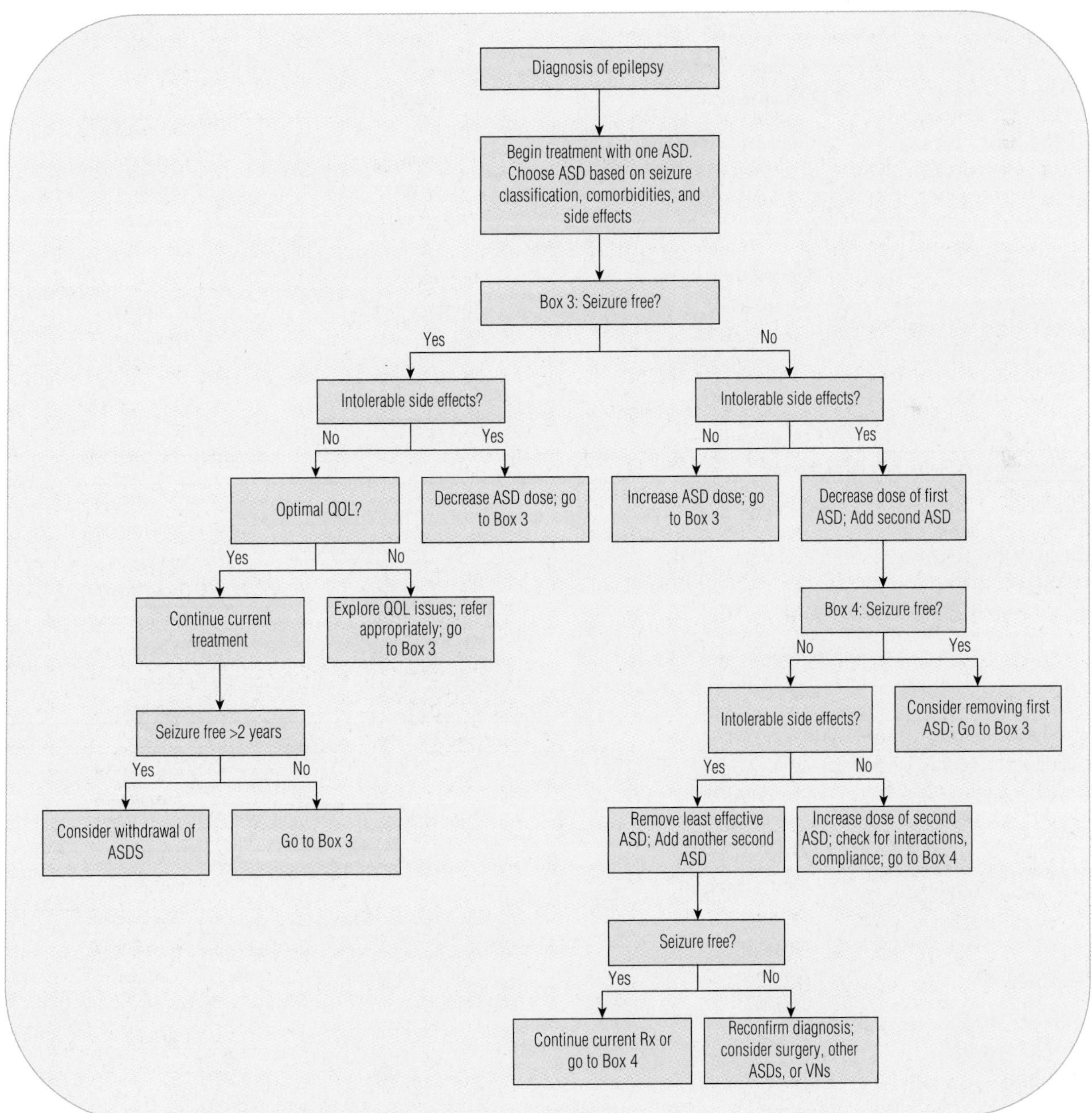

FIGURE 56-2 Algorithm for the treatment of epilepsy (ASD, antiseizure drug; QOL, quality of life).

TABLE 56-2 Drugs of Choice for Specific Seizure Disorders

Seizure Type	Effective Drugs[a]	Alternative Drugs[b]	Comments
Focal Onset Seizures (Newly Diagnosed)			
US Guidelines[60,61]	*Adults and adolescents:* Carbamazepine Gabapentin Oxcarbazepine Phenobarbital Phenytoin Topiramate Valproic acid		*FDA approved:* Carbamazepine Lacosamide Phenobarbital Phenytoin Topiramate Valproic acid
ILAE Guidelines[29]	*Adults:* Carbamazepine Phenytoin* Valproic acid* Levetiracetam Zonisamide	*Adults:* Gabapentin Lamotrigine Oxcarbazepine Phenobarbital Topiramate Vigabatrin	*Potentially efficacious* Carbamazepine Primidone **side effects* make these ASDs unpopular first choices
	Children: Oxcarbazepine	*Children:* Phenobarbital Phenytoin Topiramate Valproic acid Carbamazepine	*Potentially efficacious* Clonazepam Clobazam Lamotrigine Vigabatrin Zonisamide
	Elderly: Gabapentin Lamotrigine	*Elderly:* Carbamazepine	*Potentially efficacious:* Topiramate Valproic acid
U.S. Expert Panel 2005[62]	Carbamazepine Lamotrigine Oxcarbazepine	Levetiracetam	
Focal Onset Seizures (Refractory Monotherapy)			
US Guidelines[60,61]	Lamotrigine Oxcarbazepine Topiramate		*FDA approved:* Carbamazepine Lamotrigine Oxcarbazepine Phenobarbital Phenytoin Topiramate Valproic acid
Focal Onset Seizures (Refractory Adjunct)			
US Guidelines[60,61]	*Adults:* Gabapentin Lamotrigine Levetiracetam Oxcarbazepine Tiagabine Topiramate Zonisamide *Children:* Gabapentin Lamotrigine Oxcarbazepine Topiramate		*FDA approved:* Carbamazepine Gabapentin Lamotrigine Levetiracetam Oxcarbazepine Phenobarbital Phenytoin Pregabalin Tiagabine Valproic acid Vigabatrin Zonisamide

(continued)

TABLE 56-2 Drugs of Choice for Specific Seizure Disorders (*Continued*)

Seizure Type	Effective Drugs[a]	Alternative Drugs[b]	Comments
Generalized Seizures Absence (Newly Diagnosed)			
US Guidelines[60,61]	Lamotrigine		*FDA approved:* Ethosuximide Valproic acid
ILAE Guidelines[29]	Ethosuximide Valproic Acid	Lamotrigine	Gabapentin is ineffective
US Expert Panel 2005[62]	Ethosuximide Valproic acid	Lamotrigine	
Generalized Onset (Tonic-Clonic)			
US Guidelines[60,61]	Topiramate		*FDA approved:* Lamotrigine Levetiracetam Topiramate Perampanel
ILAE Guidelines[29]	*Adults* None	*Adults:* Carbamazepine* Lamotrigine Oxcarbazepine Phenobarbital Phenytoin* Topiramate Valproic acid *Children:* Carbamazepine* Phenobarbital Phenytoin* Topiramate Valproic acid	*may precipitate other generalized seizures—use w/caution *Potential Efficacy:* Oxcarbazepine *may precipitate other generalized seizures—use w/caution
US Expert Panel 2005[62]		Lamotrigine Topiramate	
Juvenile Myoclonic Epilepsy			
ILAE Guidelines[29]	None	Clonazepam Lamotrigine Levetiracetam Valproic acid Zonisamide	
US Expert Panel 2005[62]	Valproic acid	Levetiracetam Topiramate Zonisamide	

ILAE, International League Against Epilepsy.

[a]Includes probably effective drugs based on Level A or B evidence.

[b]Includes possibly effective drugs based on less than Level A or B evidence.

Data from references 29, 60, 62 and 63.

from a US panel of experts, which included more recent drug treatment data compared to the AAN-AES recommendations.[29,60-62.]

Drug Resistance

8 Approximately 65% of patients can be expected to be maintained on one ASD and be considered well controlled, although not necessarily seizure free.[36] The percentage of patients who are seizure free on one drug varies by seizure type. After 12 months of treatment, the percentage who are seizure free is highest for those who have only GTC seizures (48%-55%), lowest for those who have only focal seizures (23%-26%), and intermediate for those with mixed seizure types (25%-32%).[63] Polytherapy with two or more ASDs is appropriate for those patients who cannot achieve seizure freedom on ASD monotherapy. Of the 35% of patients with unsatisfactory control on monotherapy, 10% will be well controlled with a two-drug treatment. Of the remaining 25%, 20% will continue to have unsatisfactory control despite greater than two drug treatment and are deemed to be drug resistant.[36] In 2009, the ILAE issued a consensus definition for drug resistant epilepsy which defined drug resistance as "failure of adequate trials of two tolerated and appropriately chosen and used AED schedules (whether as monotherapies or in combination) to achieve sustained seizure freedom."[64]

Pharmacokinetic and Drug-Drug Interactions

An appreciation of pharmacokinetic variability (Table 56-3) is necessary when selecting drug treatment. Knowledge of ASD metabolic pathways as well as inducer or inhibitory effects on liver enzymes (Table 56-4) can aid in the optimization of ASD therapy. Pharmacokinetic interactions are a common complicating factor in ASD selection. Interactions can occur in any of the pharmacokinetic processes: absorption, distribution, metabolism, or elimination. Caution should be used when ASDs are added to or withdrawn from a drug regimen.

Adverse Effects

Individual ASDs have their own unique adverse effect profile. However, there are some common adverse effects shared by ASDs as a class. Since all ASDs act on the CNS to exert their antiseizure effects, CNS side effects are among the most common adverse effects of ASDs and include sedation, dizziness, blurred or double vision, difficulty with concentration, and ataxia. ASD effects on cognition are of particular concern. Barbiturates in particular appear to cause more cognitive impairment than other commonly used ASDs (although in children it paradoxically causes hyperactivity).[65] In general, newer agents have less effects on cognition, although topiramate is known to cause substantial cognitive impairment.[66] In many cases, these effects can be avoided by titrating the dose upward very slowly or can be alleviated by decreasing the dose. Patients changed from polytherapy to monotherapy may also demonstrate improvement in cognition.

Concentration-dependent effects are common and troublesome but not usually life-threatening. It is important to note that patients dosed and maintained within "therapeutic ranges" are also capable of experiencing toxicities to ASDs.[67] More uncommon are idiosyncratic side effects which are generally not concentration-dependent. Most idiosyncratic reactions are mild, but they can be serious and even life threatening if the hypersensitivity involves one or more organ systems. Perhaps the most widely recognized idiosyncratic reactions are ASD-induced drug rashes. As discussed earlier, some rashes can progress to Steven Johnsons Syndrome (SJS)/Toxic Epidermal Necrolysis (TEN). Other serious but rare idiosyncratic side effects include hepatitis or blood dyscrasias. Acute organ failure due to an idiosyncratic reaction, when it occurs, generally occurs within the first 6 months of ASD therapy.[68] In any patient, laboratory assessment, including white blood cell (WBC) counts and liver function tests, may be reasonable if the patient reports an unexplained illness (eg, lethargy, vomiting, fever, or rash). ASD treatment itself may sometimes worsen seizures and can represent a paradoxical toxic effect of the drug.[65]

Antiseizure drugs are often used life-long and as such, adverse effects associated with long-term use have been recognized. One such adverse effect of chronic ASD treatment is osteomalacia and osteoporosis.[69,70] The effects on bone can range from asymptomatic high-turnover disease with findings of normal bone mineral density, to markedly decreased bone mineral density sufficient to warrant the diagnosis of osteoporosis. It has been hypothesized that certain drugs, including phenytoin, phenobarbital, carbamazepine,

TABLE 56-3 Antiseizure Drug Pharmacokinetic Data

ASD	$t_{1/2}$ (Hours)	Time to Steady State (Days)	Unchanged (%)	V_D (L/kg)	Clinically Important Metabolite	Protein Binding (%)
Carbamazepine	12 M; 5-14 Co	21-28 for completion of autoinduction	<1	1-2	10,11-epoxide	40-90
Clobazam	36-42	7-14	3	1.4	*N*-desmethylclobazam	80-90
Eslicarbazepine	13-20	4-5	67%	0.87	oxcarbazepine	<40
Ethosuximide	A 60; C 30	6-12	10-20	0.67	No	0
Ezogabine	7-11	3-4	36%	2-3	*n*-Acetyl metabolite	80
Felbamate	16-22	5-7	50	0.73-0.82	No	~25
Gabapentin[a]	5-40[b]	1-2	100	0.65-1.04	No	0
Lacosamide	13	3	40	0.6	No	<15
Lamotrigine	25.4 M	3-15	10	1.28	No	40-50
Levetiracetam	7-10	2		0.7	No	<10
Oxcarbazepine	3-13	2		0.7	10-Hydroxycarbazepine	40
Perampanel	105	14-21	74-80	77 L	No	95%-96%
Phenobarbital	A 46-136; C 37-73	14-21	20-40	0.6	No	50
Phenytoin	A 10-34; C 5-14	7-28	<5	0.6-8.0	No	90
Pregabalin	A 6-7[b]	1-2	90	0.5	No	0
Primidone	A 3.3-19; C 4.5-11	1-4	40	0.43-1.1	PB	20
Rufinamide	6-10	2	4	0.8-1.2	No	26-35
Tiagabine	5-13		Negligible		No	95
Topiramate	18-21	4-5	50-70	0.55-0.8 (male); 0.23-0.4 (female)	No	15
Valproic acid	A 8-20; C 7-14	1-3	<5	0.1-0.5	May contribute to toxicity	90-95 binding saturates
Vigabatrin	5-8	N/A	80	0.8	No	0
Zonisamide	24-60	5-15	35	0.8-1.6	No	40-60

A, adult; ASD, antiseizure drug; C, child; Co, combination therapy; M, monotherapy; N/A, not applicable since effect depends on inhibiting enzyme; PB, phenobarbital; V_D, volume of distribution.

[a]The bioavailability of gabapentin is dose-dependent.

[b]Half-life depends on renal function.

Data from references 24, 90, and package inserts 88, 92, 94, 101, 105, 110, 113, 117, 119.

TABLE 56-4 Antiseizure Drug Elimination Pathways and Major Effects on Hepatic Enzymes

Antiepileptic Drugs	Major Hepatic Enzymes	Renal Elimination (%)	Induced	Inhibited
Carbamazepine	CYP3A4; CYP1A2; CYP2C8	<1	CYP1A2; CYP2C; CYP3A; GT	None
Clobazam	CYP3A4; CYP2C19; CYP2B6	0	CYP3A4 (weak)	CYP2D6
Eslicarbazepine	Undergoes hydrolysis	<90% parent drug >60% active metabolite	GT (mild)	CYP2C19
Ethosuximide	CYP3A4	12-20	None	None
Ezogabine	GT; acetylation	85	None	None
Felbamate	CYP3A4; CYP2E1; other	50	CYP3A4	CYP2C19; β-oxidation
Gabapentin	None	Almost completely	None	None
Lacosamide	CYP2C19	70	None	None
Lamotrigine	GT	10	GT	None
Levetiracetam	None (undergoes nonhepatic hydrolysis)	66	None	None
Oxcarbazepine (MHD is active oxcarbazepine metabolite)	Cytosolic system	1 (27 as MHD)	CYP3A4; CYP3A5; GT	CYP2C19
Perampanel	CYP3A4/5; CYP1A2; CYP2B6	Undefined	CYP3A4/5;GT	CYPA3A4/5
Phenobarbital	CYP2C9; other	25	CYP3A; CYP2C; GT	None
Phenytoin	CYP2C9; CYP2C19	5	CYP3A; CYP2C; GT	
Pregabalin	None	100	None	None
Rufinamide	Hydrolysis	2	CYP3A4 (weak)	CYP2E1 (weak)
Tiagabine	CYP3A4	2	None	None
Topiramate	Not known	70	CYP3A (dose dependent)	CYP2C19
Valproate	GT; β-oxidation	2	None	CYP2C9; GT epoxide hydrolase
Vigabatrin	None	Almost completely	CYP2C9	None
Zonisamide	CYP3A4	35	None	None

CYP, cytochrome P450 isoenzyme system; GT, glucuronyltransferase.

Data from references 24, 90, and package inserts 88, 92, 94, 101, 105, 110, 113, 117, 119.

oxcarbazepine, felbamate, and valproic acid, may interfere with vitamin D metabolism.[71] It is currently unknown whether other ASDs also cause these effects. Patients receiving these drugs should receive supplemental vitamin D and calcium, as well as bone mineral density testing if other risk factors for osteoporosis are present.

Role of Serum Concentration Monitoring

Serum concentrations of the older ASDs should be viewed as a tool with which to optimize therapy for an individual patient, not as a therapeutic end point in itself. The serum concentration is a target that should be correlated with clinical response. The desired outcome is the cessation of seizures without side effects. Seizure control can occur before the "minimum" of the published therapeutic range is achieved, and side effects can appear before the "maximum" of the range is achieved. Some patients may need and tolerate concentrations beyond the maximum. The therapeutic range for ASDs can be different for different seizure types. Serum concentrations may need to be higher to control focal dyscognitive seizures than to control tonic–clonic seizures. Clinicians should define a therapeutic range for an individual patient above which there are side effects and below which the patient experiences seizures. Then serum levels can be useful to document lack of efficacy, loss of efficacy, noncompliance, and to determine how much room there is to increase a dose based on expected toxicity. Depending on the ASD, serum levels can also be useful in patients with significant renal and/or hepatic disease, patients taking multiple drugs, and women who are pregnant or taking OCs. Therapeutic concentration ranges have not been clearly defined for some of the second-generation ASDs.[67]

PERSONALIZED PHARMACOTHERAPY

The most important aspect of ASD therapy is tailoring the choice of drug to the individual patient. Besides seizure type(s) and concomitant medical problems (including hepatic function, renal function, and concurrent medications), patient specific characteristics that must be considered include age, gender, child-bearing ability, and ethnicity. Therapeutic considerations in these groups are discussed hereunder.

Therapeutic Considerations in the Elderly and Young

Use of ASDs in the elderly and young can pose special challenges. The elderly are often on many different medications which may contribute to increased sensitivity to neurocognitive effects as well as increased possibility of drug-drug interactions with ASDs that affect the cytochrome P450 (CYP450) system (eg, carbamazepine, phenytoin, and valproic acid). Hypoalbuminemia is also common in the elderly, and highly albumin-bound ASDs (eg phenytoin and valproic acid) can be problematic.[67] The elderly also experience body mass changes, such as an increase in fat to lean body mass or decrease in body water, which can affect the drug volume of distribution and elimination half-life.[67] In addition, the elderly may have compromised renal or hepatic function that require ASD dosage adjustment.[67] Lamotrigine is often considered the medication of choice in elderly patients with focal-onset seizures, as results from a VA cooperative trial found that it had equal efficacy to carbamazepine and gabapentin and was better tolerated than carbamazepine.[73]

For neonates and infants, an increase in the total body water to fat ratio and a decrease in serum albumin and α-acid glycoprotein can result in volume of distribution changes that affect ASD elimination half-life. Additionally, infants up to the age of 3 years have decreased renal elimination of ASDs, with neonates being the most affected. Hepatic activity is also reduced in neonates and infants, but by age 2 to 3 years, hepatic activity then becomes more robust than that seen in adults. Therefore, whereas neonates and infants require lower doses of ASDs, children require higher doses than that seen in adults. Therapeutic drug monitoring becomes especially important in the young, even though the definitions of therapeutic blood levels are less certain in these patients than in adults.[67]

Therapeutic Considerations in Women (and Men)

Estrogen and progesterone are among the many hormones that can influence brain electrical excitability. Estrogen has a slight proconvulsant effect, whereas progesterone exerts a mild anticonvulsant effect.[21] In some women, vulnerability to seizures is highest just before and during the menstrual flow (catamenial seizures) and at the time of ovulation, and is believed to be due to a slight increase of estrogen relative to progesterone, or due to progesterone withdrawal and changes in the estrogen-to-progesterone ratio.[21] The risk of catamenial seizures is estimated be anywhere from 10% to 70% in women with epilepsy.[21] In such women, conventional ASDs should be used as primary agents, but intermittent supplementation with higher dose of ASD or benzodiazepines should be considered. Acetazolamide has also been used during catamenial periods, but with variable and limited success. Hormonal therapy with progestational agents, particularly cyclic natural progesterone therapy, may be effective in certain subsets of patients.[72]

At menopause, seizures often improve in frequency, particularly in women with a catamenial seizure pattern. However, for those women who need hormone replacement therapy, it has been reported that conjugated equine estrogens plus 2.5 mg of medroxyprogesterone acetate may increase the frequency of epileptic seizures. Therefore a hormone replacement therapy that consists of just a single estrogenic compound, such as 17-β-estradiol, along with a natural progesterone, may be recommended for women with disruptive menopausal symptoms.[74]

Antiseizure drugs may also have an effect on endogenous and exogenous hormones. Enzyme-inducing ASDs increase the metabolism of estrogen, progesterone, and testosterone and increase production of sex hormone-binding globulin, leading to decreases in the free fraction of these hormones endogenously. These alterations lead to disturbances in the regulation of the hypothalamic–pituitary–adrenal axis and contribute to reproductive endocrine disorders including menstrual irregularity, infertility, sexual dysfunction, and in some patients polycystic ovary syndrome (PCOS).[75] Valproic acid, in particular, may affect sex hormone concentrations causing hyperandrogenism and polycystic changes, especially in women who have gained weight or those who start valproic acid at age less than 20 years.[75]

Exogenously, enzyme-inducing ASDs (eg, carbamazepine and topiramate and oxcarbazepine at higher doses, and possibly clobazam, felbamate, lamotrigine, and rufinamide) can cause treatment failures in women taking oral contraceptives (OCs) due to increased metabolism of ethinyl estradiol and progestin. Medroxyprogesterone depot injections and hormone-releasing intrauterine systems on the other hand, are not similarly affected by ASDs, and it is unclear if there is an effect of ASDs on the transdermal contraceptive patch or the emergency contraceptive pill. A supplemental or alternative form of birth control (eg, IUD) is advised if breakthrough bleeding occurs in woman taking certain types of ASDs (eg, enzyme-inducing ASDs) and OCs, and it has been suggested that women use twice the normal dose of emergency contraception.[76]

Antiseizure drugs may also have reproductive endocrine effects in men. Data suggests that men with epilepsy have reduced fertility, and that carbamazepine, oxcarbazepine, and valproic acid are associated with sperm abnormalities in these men. In addition, valproic acid seems to cause testicular atrophy resulting in reduced testosterone volume. Levetiracetam on the other hand, appears to slightly increase serum testosterone. Various ASDs have also been anecdotally reported to affect libido and sexual function in both men and women.[76]

Therapeutic Considerations for Pregnancy and Breastfeeding

Pregnancy and epilepsy is a particularly complex topic. The goal of treatment in pregnant women with epilepsy is to achieve the best possible control of seizure with the minimal adverse effects for both the mother and the child. Epilepsy-related complications during pregnancy include possible changes in seizure frequency, fluctuating ASD plasma levels, and possible teratogenic effects of ASDs.[77-79]

Despite multiple reports of both increased and decreased seizure frequency during pregnancy, a recent practice parameter update issued by the AAN found that there was inconclusive evidence to conclude that changes in seizure frequency occurred during pregnancy.[77] What was concluded however, was that women with epilepsy who were seizure free for at least 9 months to 1 year prior to pregnancy, had a very high probability (84%-92%) of remaining seizure free during pregnancy.[77] It should be noted, however, that if seizures are increasing during pregnancy, a commonly over-looked reason for this increase is nonadherence in a normally adherent patient, due to concerns about the potential adverse drug effects on the developing fetus.[80]

Fluctuations in ASD concentration may be caused by physiologic changes that occur during pregnancy including reduced gastric motility, nausea and vomiting, increased drug distribution, increased renal elimination, altered hepatic enzyme activity as well as changes in protein binding during pregnancy.[76] Physiologic changes, such as changes in protein binding, can begin as early as the first 10 weeks of pregnancy, and may require up to 4 weeks postpartum to normalize (eg, protein binding in carbamazepine, phenobarbital, and phenytoin). Fluctuations in ASD plasma concentrations due to increased ASD clearance has been found to be true for lamotrigine, carbamazepine, phenytoin, oxcarbazepine, levetiracetam.[78] Clinical consequences of ASD fluctuations are variable and some women will not experience increased seizure frequency despite fluctuating levels. Women on lamotrigine however have been found to undergo a 40% decrease in the ratio of plasma lamotrigine concentration to dose, resulting in deterioration of seizure control in approximately 75% of pregnant patients.[76] It is therefore recommended that ASD levels, particularly lamotrigine levels, be monitored closely during pregnancy, and to increase doses if needed over the course of the pregnancy with rapid decrease in the postpartum period. Of note, fluctuations have also been reported for phenobarbital, valproic acid, primidone, and ethosuximide, although strong evidence for this is lacking.[78]

Adverse pregnancy outcomes associated with ASD use include an increased risk of major congenital malformations (MCMs) compared to nonepileptic women.[79] This risk is believed to be due to ASD exposure and not maternal seizures, as infants born to women with epilepsy who do not take ASDs have the same risk of birth defects as infants born to seizure-free women (2%-3%).[80] The most concerning effects are found with the use of valproic acid which is associated with a risk of MCMs that is 3.5 to 4 times that of offspring from nonepileptic women, especially if taken during the first trimester of pregnancy.[79] Furthermore there is an increased risk of neurodevelopmental deficits, including effects on cognition in children exposed to valproic acid *in utero*.[79] These effects are dose-dependent, and the risk of major congenital malformation significantly increases at 600 mg/day, with the greatest risk observed at doses that exceed 1,000 mg/day.[66] However, individual susceptibility is genetically determined, and teratogenicity can occur at much lower doses in some persons. Due to these findings, it is recommended that valproate should preferably not be used in epilepsy and that withdrawal of valproate or switch to an alternative treatment should be considered in these patients. When valproate is used, doses should not exceed 500 to 600 mg/day.[66]

Data on teratogenic risk with the newer agents are limited, although topiramate was recently reclassified from pregnancy category C to D due to an increased association with cleft palate (it may also have a negative effect on birth weight and cause increases in hypospadias).[66,81] In general, higher ASD doses, higher ASD serum concentrations, polytherapy (especially polytherapy with valproate), and a family history of birth defects appear to increase the teratogenic risk of ASDs.[79] As such, the risk of birth defects is believed to have gone down with decreasing doses and decreasing use of polytherapy. Deciding on the most effective single-drug treatment prior to conception is vitally important. Teratogenic effects of ASD must always be considered when choosing ASDs for women of reproductive age, even when they do not plan on becoming pregnant, as many unplanned pregnancies occur and MCMs generally occur early in pregnancy before women know that they are pregnant. With proper counseling and management, more than 90% of these pregnancies will still have satisfactory outcomes. Updated practice parameters are available to aid in the counseling and management of pregnant women with epilepsy.[77-79,81]

Teratogenic effects may possibly be prevented by adequate folate intake, although strong data are lacking.[81] However, as the risk of MCM is possibly decreased by folic acid supplementation, prenatal vitamins with folic acid (0.4-5 mg/day) are recommended for women of child-bearing potential who are taking ASDs.[81] Higher folate doses should be used in women with a history of a previous pregnancy with a neural tube defect or taking valproic acid. Additionally, some ASDs may possibly cause neonatal hemorrhagic disorder. There is a lack of strong evidence to determine if prenatal vitamin K supplementation can reduce this complication. However, vitamin K 10 mg/day is often administered orally to the mother during the last month of pregnancy and/or administered parenterally to the newborn at delivery.[81]

Some ASDs pass into the breast milk. ASDs with less protein binding will accumulate more in breast milk. Treatment with ASDs is not necessarily a reason to discourage breastfeeding, although ASD concentrations are measureable in breastfeeding infants. In fact, an argument could be made that since ASDs should rarely be discontinued abruptly, breastfeeding allows for a downward titration of a medication that the baby was exposed to for the past 9 months. Infants born to women taking any ASD (particularly barbiturates or benzodiazepines) should be closely observed for signs of excess sedation, irritability, or poor feeding.[81,82]

Therapeutic Considerations in Asians and South Asians

A common idiosyncratic side effect of ASDs is rash. However, in some cases, the rash can quickly progress to SJS, TEN, or Drug Reactions with Eosinophilia and Systemic Symptoms (DRESS) which are severe and life threatening conditions. Studies have found that there is a strong association between the presence of an inherited variant of the *HLA-B* gene, *HLA-B*1502*, in these populations, and the risk of developing SJS/TEN with carbamazepine (and possibly phenytoin, lamotrigine, and oxcarbazepine as well).[83,84] This *HLA-B* variant is found in up to 15% of individuals from many Asian, Southeast Asian and South Asian populations including Hong Kong, Thailand, Malaysia, Philippines, Taiwan, North China, India, and to a much lesser extent Japan and Korea. The variant is largely absent in individuals not of Asian origin. Testing for *HLA-B*1502* may be recommended for patients in these populations who may need to be initiated on carbamazepine, phenytoin, lamotrigine, or oxcarbazepine therapy. If positive, these ASDs should generally be avoided in these patients. In addition, the *HLA* genotype *HLA-A*3101* has also been found to be associated with multiple carbamazepine-induced cutaneous reactions in Chinese, Japanese, and European populations.[83] It should be noted that many *HLA-B*1502*-positive and *HLA-A*3101*-positive patients treated with ASDs will not develop SJS/TEN or other hypersensitivity reactions, and these reactions can still occur infrequently in *HLA-B*1502*-negative and *HLA-A*3101*-negative patients of any ethnicity. Of those who do experience SJS/TEN with carbamazepine, 90% will have this reaction within the first few months of treatment.[83]

Clinical Considerations with Specific Drugs

Tables 56-5 and 56-6 list specific data (including adverse effects and dosing) for each of the commonly used ASDs. Here we summarize the pharmacology, advantages and disadvantages, and perspectives on the place in therapy of some specific ASD.

Clinical **Controversy...**

A warning on suicidal behavior and ideation accompanies all ASDs. This is based on pooled analyses of almost 200 placebo-controlled trials of 11 different ASDs showing that patients randomized to an ASD had approximately twice the risk of suicidal thinking or behavior compared to patients randomized to placebo. The estimated incidence of suicidal ideation was low, less than 0.5% of patients on ASDs compared to 0.24% of patients on placebo. While some believed that this risk is nonsignificant, responsible providers must carefully assess this risk when evaluating their patients for ASD therapy, especially as depression and anxiety are common comorbid conditions in epilepsy. Patients and caregivers should be informed that ASDs increase the risk of suicidal thoughts and should be advised to be on the alert for any unusual changes in mood or behavior.

Carbamazepine

Mechanism of Action Carbamazepine acts primarily by enhancing fast inactivation of voltage-gated Na^+ channels. Interaction with voltage-gated Ca^{2+} and K^+ channels may also contribute.[85]

Pharmacokinetics Absorption of carbamazepine immediate-release (IR) tablets is slow and erratic with large variability in the peak-to-trough concentrations of up to 40% due to its low water solubility. Suspension is absorbed faster than the tablets.[86] There is no first-pass metabolism. Food, especially fat, may enhance the bioavailability of carbamazepine. Controlled-release (Tegretol-XR) and sustained-release (Carbatrol) preparations are also available, and if dosed every 12 hours, they are bioequivalent to the immediate-release tablets dosed every 6 hours. Compared with carbamazepine IR tablets, both these formulations have lower peaks and higher troughs, which may decrease side effects and improve QOL and seizure control. Patients should be told to take Tegretol-XR with food and that the casing will be excreted in the feces. It cannot be broken or crushed. Tegretol-XR and Carbatrol appear to be bioequivalent; however, there is less variability in the absorption of Carbatrol.[87]

Carbamazepine is a neutral and highly lipophilic drug that is highly protein bound to α_1-acid glycoprotein and albumin. The major metabolite of carbamazepine is carbamazepine-10,11-epoxide, which has anticonvulsant activity, and is affected by concurrent use of other enzyme-inducing or enzyme-inhibiting drugs (eg, valproate and felbamate).

TABLE 56-5 Antiseizure Drug Side Effects and Monitoring

Drug	Adverse Drug Reaction Acute Side Effects: Concentration Dependent	Adverse Drug Reaction Acute Side Effects: Idiosyncratic	Chronic Side Effects
Carbamazepine	Diplopia Dizziness Drowsiness Nausea Unsteadiness Lethargy	Blood dyscrasias Rash (HLA antigen testing may be relevant to avoid Stevens-Johnson or toxic epidermal necrolysis)	Hyponatremia Metabolic bone disease (monitor Vit D and serum calcium)
Clobazam	Somnolence Sedation Pyrexia Ataxia	Drooling Aggression Irritability Constipation	
Eslicarbazepine	Dizziness Ataxia Somnolence/fatigue Cognitive changes Visual changes	Rash	Hyponatremia
Ethosuximide	Ataxia Drowsiness GI distress (avoid by multiple daily dosing) Unsteadiness Hiccoughs	Blood dyscrasias Rash	Behavior changes Headache
Ezogabine	Dizziness Somnolence Fatigue Confusion Vertigo Tremors Blurred vision	Urinary retention QT prolongation (get baseline ECG and during treatment) Euphoria	Blue gray skin discoloration Retinal abnormalities
Felbamate	Anorexia Nausea Vomiting Insomnia Headache	Aplastic anemia (follow CBC) Acute hepatic failure (follow liver enzymes)	Not established
Gabapentin	Dizziness Fatigue Somnolence Ataxia	Pedal edema	Weight gain
Lacosamide	Dizziness Vertigo Headache Nausea Vomiting PR interval increase (get baseline ECG and during treatment)	Liver enzyme elevation	Not established
Lamotrigine	Diplopia Dizziness Unsteadiness Headache	Rash (slower titration of dose may decrease chance of occurrence)	Not established
Levetiracetam	Sedation Behavioral disturbance	Psychosis (rare but more common in elderly or persons with mental illness)	Not established
Oxcarbazepine	Sedation Dizziness Ataxia Nausea	Rash	Hyponatremia

(Continued)

TABLE 56-5 Antiseizure Drug Side Effects and Monitoring (*Continued*)

	Adverse Drug Reaction Acute Side Effects		
Drug	**Concentration Dependent**	**Idiosyncratic**	**Chronic Side Effects**
Perampanel	Severe behavior changes Dizziness Ataxia/falls Somnolence/fatigues	Rash	Weight gain
Phenobarbital	Ataxia Hyperactivity Headache Unsteadiness Sedation Nausea	Blood dyscrasias Rash	Behavior changes Connective tissue disorders Intellectual blunting Metabolic bone disease Mood change Sedation
Phenytoin	Ataxia Nystagmus Behavior changes Dizziness Headache Incoordination Sedation Lethargy Cognitive impairment Fatigue Visual blurring	Blood dyscrasias Rash (HLA antigen testing may be relevant to avoid Stevens-Johnson or toxic epidermal necrolysis) Immunologic reaction	Behavior changes Cerebellar syndrome (occurs high serum levels) Connective tissue changes Skin thickening Folate deficiency Gingival hyperplasia Hirsutism Coarsening of facial features Acne Cognitive impairment Metabolic bone disease (monitor Vit D and serum calcium) Sedation
Pregabalin	Dizziness Somnolence Incoordination Dry mouth Blurred vision	Pedal edema Creatine kinase elevation Decrease platelets	Weight gain
Primidone	Behavior changes Headache Nausea Sedation Unsteadiness	Blood dyscrasias Rash	Behavior change Connective tissue disorders Cognitive impairment Sedation
Rufinamide	Dizziness Nausea Vomiting Somnolence	Multiorgan hypersensitivity Status epilepticus Leukopenia QT shortening	Not established
Tiagabine	Dizziness Fatigue Difficulties concentrating Nervousness Tremor Blurred vision Depression Weakness	Spike-wave stupor	Not established
Topiramate	Difficulties concentrating Psychomotor slowing Speech or language problems Somnolence, fatigue Dizziness Headache	Metabolic acidosis Acute angle glaucoma Oligohydrosis	Kidney stones Weight loss
Valproic acid	GI upset Sedation Unsteadiness	Acute hepatic failure Acute pancreatitis Alopecia	Polycystic ovary-like syndrome (increase incidence in females <20 years or overweight) Weight gain

(*Continued*)

TABLE 56-5 Antiseizure Drug Side Effects and Monitoring (*Continued*)

Drug	Adverse Drug Reaction Acute Side Effects: Concentration Dependent	Adverse Drug Reaction Acute Side Effects: Idiosyncratic	Chronic Side Effects
	Tremor		Hyperammonemia
	Thrombocytopenia		Menstrual cycle irregularities
Vigabatrin	Permanent vision loss Fatigue Somnolence Weight gain Tremor Blurred vision	Abnormal MRI brain signal changes (infants with infantile spasms) Peripheral neuropathy Anemia	Permanent vision loss (greater frequency, adults vs. children vs. infants)
Zonisamide	Sedation	Rash (is a sulfa drug)	Kidney stones
	Dizziness	Metabolic acidosis	Weight loss
	Cognitive impairment	Oligohydrosis	
	Nausea		

Data from references 24, 90, and package inserts 88, 92, 94, 101, 105, 110, 113, 117, 119.

Carbamazepine induces its own metabolism (autoinduction). Its half-life starts decreasing 3 to 5 days after initiation of therapy, and induction is complete within 21 to 28 days (although reversal of autoinduction is rapid upon discontinuation). Therefore, initial therapeutic concentrations may fall out of range despite good adherence. Carbamazepine also displays diurnal variation in its serum level with evening levels lower than morning levels. Carbamazepine is cleared significantly faster in females than males and in Caucasians compared to African Americans, and therefore variable dosing may be needed.[86]

Adverse Effects Neurosensory side effects are the most common (35%-50% of patients) especially during initiation of therapy and can dissipate with continued treatment, dose adjustment or use of the controlled-release or sustained-release formulation. Food may help with nausea caused by a local effect of the drug on the gastrointestinal (GI) tract, but discontinuation may be required if nausea comes from any brainstem effect. Importantly, carbamazepine can cause hyponatremia (although less so than with oxcarbazepine), especially in the elderly, and monitoring of serum sodium is recommended.[85]

The incidence of leukopenia can be as high as 10% but is usually transient, even when the drug is continued, and can be caused by a redistribution of WBCs rather than a decrease in their production.[85] In about 2% of patients, leukopenia is persistent, but therapy is generally continued unless the WBC count drops to less than 2,500/mm^3 (2.5×10^9/L) and the absolute neutrophil count drops to less than 1,000/mm^3 (1×10^9/L).

Drug Interactions Carbamazepine has significant drug interactions and can induce the metabolism of other drugs. Additionally, CYP3A4 inhibitors may potentially increase carbamazepine serum concentrations.

Dosing and Administration During initiation, it must be remembered that carbamazepine clearance increases with time. The initial adult dose is 400 mg/day and may be increased by 200 mg at weekly intervals. For those patients who need to reach therapeutic levels more quickly, the dose may be increased by 200 mg every few days. However, faster titrations may increase the risk for rash, and this should be monitored. Extended-release preparations can be dosed twice a day while immediate-release preparations require doses to be given four times a day.

Advantages Carbamazepine has been well studied and is also available in liquid dosage forms and extended release and controlled release preparations. Compared with other first-generation ASDs, carbamazepine causes minimal cognitive impairment.

Disadvantages It induces its own metabolism, which complicates dosage titration. It also has many drug interactions including interactions which may increase its active metabolite causing toxicity. Carbamazepine also has known teratogenicity and chronic use has been associated with decreases in bone mineral density and 25-hydroxy (OH) vitamin D.

Place in Therapy Carbamazepine is a commonly used ASD and is considered first-line in many seizure types as it is well studied. It is FDA approved for use in patients with focal onset seizures, GTC seizures, and mixed seizure types. It may worsen absence seizures and possibly precipitate or aggravate tonic-clonic seizures in patients with other generalized seizure types.

Clobazam

Mechanism of Action Clobazam is a 1, 5-chlorinated benzodiazepine derivative that potentiates GABA's effect at the subunit of the $GABA_A$ receptor, increasing the chloride current by increasing chloride channel opening.[24]

Pharmacokinetics The drug is metabolized in the liver to the primary active metabolite *N*-desmethylclobazam which achieves plasma concentrations three to five times higher than clobazam with 1/5 the activity and elimination half-lives of 36 to 42 hours and 71 to 82 hours, respectively.[24]

Adverse Effects CNS effects are the most common side effects. Abrupt discontinuation may cause a withdrawal syndrome which consists of convulsions, psychosis, hallucinations, behavioral disorder, tremor, and anxiety; milder symptoms can present as dysphoria, anxiety, and insomnia.[24]

Drug Interactions Clobazam inhibits CYP2D6 and may affect metabolism of other drugs in this pathway. It is also a weak inducer of CYP3A4 and may lower the serum levels of some OCs.[24]

Dosing and Administration Patients weighing less than or equal to 30 kg are started at 5 mg/day and increased slowly to 20 mg/day, while those weighing more than 30 kg are started at 10 mg/day and increased slowly to 40 mg/day; doses greater than 5 mg should be given in two divided doses. Dosing in geriatric patients is initiated as in patients weighing less than or equal to 30 kg, but increased up to 40 mg depending on the weight of the patient. Poor metabolizers of CYP2C19 are dosed like geriatric patients.[24]

TABLE 56-6 Antiseizure Drug Dosing and Target Serum Concentration Ranges

Drug	Brand Name	Initial or Starting Dose	Usual Range or Maximum Dose	Comments Target Serum Concentration Range
Barbiturates				
Phenobarbital	Various	1-3 mg/kg/day (10-20 mg/kg LD)	180-300 mg	10-40 mcg/mL[a] (43-172 μmol/L)
Primidone	Mysoline	100-125 mg/day	750-2,000 mg	5-10 mcg/mL (23-46 μmol/L)
Benzodiazepines				
Clobazam	Onfi	≤30 kg 5 mg/day; >30 kg 10 mg/day	≤30 kg up to 20 mg; >30 kg up to 40 mg	0.03-0.3 ng/mL (0.1-1.0 nmol/L)
Clonazepam	Klonopin	1.5 mg/day	20 mg	20-70 ng/mL (67-233 pmol/L)
Diazepam	Valium	PO: 4-40 mg IV: 5-10 mg	PO: 4-40 mg IV: 5-30 mg	100-1,000 ng/mL (0.4-3.5 μmol/L)
Lorazepam	Ativan	PO: 2-6 mg IV: 0.05 mg/kg IM: 0.05 mg/kg	PO: 10 mg IV: 0.05 mg/kg	10-30 ng/mL (31-93 nmol/L)
Hydantoin				
Phenytoin	Dilantin	PO: 3-5 mg/kg (200-400 mg) (15-20 mg/kg LD)	PO: 300-600 mg	Total: 10-20 mcg/mL (40-79 μmol/L) Unbound: 0.5-3 mcg/mL (2-12 μmol/L)
Succinimide				
Ethosuximide	Zarontin	500 mg/day	500-2,000 mg	40-100 mcg/mL (282-708 μmol/L)
Other				
Carbamazepine	Tegretol Tegretol XR	400 mg/day	400-2,400 mg	4-12 mcg/mL (17-51 μmol/L)
Eslicarbazepine	Aptiom	400 mg/day	800-1,600 mg	Not defined
Ezogabine	Potiga	300 mg/day	1,200 mg	Not defined
Felbamate	Felbatol	1,200 mg/day	3,600 mg	30-60 mcg/mL (126-252 μmol/L)
Gabapentin	Neurontin	300-900 mg/day	4,800 mg	2-20 mcg/mL (12-117 μmol/L)
Lacosamide	Vimpat	100 mg/day	400 mg	Not defined
Lamotrigine	Lamictal Lamictal XR	25 mg every other day if on VPA; 25-50 mg/day if not on VPA	100-150 mg if on VPA; 300-500 mg if not on VPA	4-20 mcg/dL (16-78 μmol/L)
Levetiracetam	Keppra Keppra XR	500-1,000 mg/day	3,000-4,000 mg	12-46 mcg/mL (70-270 μmol/L)
Oxcarbazepine	Trileptal Oxtellar XR	300-600 mg/day	1,200-2,400 mg	3-35 mcg/mL (MHD) (12-139 μmol/L)
Perampanel	Fycompa	2 mg/day	8-12 mg	Not defined
Pregabalin	Lyrica	150 mg/day	600 mg	Not defined
Rufinamide	Banzel	400-800 mg/day	3,200 mg	Not defined
Tiagabine	Gabitril	4-8 mg/day	80 mg	0.02-0.2 mcg/mL (0.05-0.5 μmol/L)
Topiramate	Topamax Trokendi XR	25-50 mg/day	200-1,000 mg	5-20 mcg/mL (15-59 μmol/L)
Valproic acid	Depakene Depakote DR/ER Depacon	15 mg/kg (500-1,000 mg)	60 mg/kg (3,000-5,000 mg)	50-100 mcg/mL (347-693 μmol/L)
Vigabatrin	Sabril	1,000 mg/day	3,000 mg	0.8-36 mcg/mL (6-279 μmol/L)
Zonisamide	Zonegran	100-200 mg/day	600 mg	10-40 mcg/mL (47-188 μmol/L)

IM, intramuscular; LD, loading does; MHD, 10-monohydroxy-derivative; PO, orally; VPA, valproic acid.

[a]Units mcg/mL and mg/L are numerically equivalent, and units of ng/mL and mcg/L are numerically equivalent.

Data from references 24, 90, and package inserts 88, 92, 94, 101, 105, 110, 113, 117, 119.

Advantages Clobazam is more efficacious than clonazepam in the treatment of LGS. Though tolerance can develop to benzodiazepines, 30% of patients do not develop tolerance to clobazam, so the drug can often be used for years.

Disadvantages It is a class IV controlled substance. Patients must be carefully weaned off the drug to avoid significant withdrawal symptoms. The drug is much less effective than clonazepam in treatment of myoclonic jerks and absence seizures.

Place in Therapy It is FDA approved for adjunctive treatment of seizures associated with LGS. However, it may also have a role in focal onset epilepsies and other generalized onset epilepsies after failure of other agents.

Eslicarbazepine

Mechanism of Action Eslicarbazepine prolongs the inactivation phase of voltage-gated Na^+ channels. It is structurally similar to carbamazepine and oxcarbazepine but is different at the 10, 11 position and does not form the carbamazepine-10, 11-epoxide.[24,89]

Pharmacokinetics Eslicarbazepine is a prodrug that undergoes hydrolysis to S-licarbazepine and is subsequently glucuronidated and renally excreted. Unlike oxcarbazepine, which is metabolized to both S- and R-licarbazepine, eslicarbazepine is extensively converted to S-licarbazepine (eslicarbazepine). The half-life is about 24 hours. Eslicarbazepine is highly bioavailable, and food has no effect. It is not highly protein bound and is extensively metabolized by hydrolytic first pass metabolism with no clinically relevant effects on most CYP enzymes and only a moderately inhibitory effect on CYP2C19. It moderately induces UGT1A1 mediated glucuronidation. Dosage adjustment is needed in patients with creatinine clearance of less than 50 mL/min (0.83 mL/s).[89]

Adverse Effects The most common adverse effects include dizziness and somnolence. Nausea, headache, diplopia, vomiting, fatigue, vertigo, ataxia, blurred vision, and tremor were also commonly reported. Like carbamazepine or oxcarbazepine, hyponatremia can occur but is less common. Eslicarbazepine may increase the PR interval on the ECG.[89]

Drug Interactions Carbamazepine, phenobarbital, phenytoin, and primidone can induce enzymes that metabolize eslicarbazepine. Eslicarbazepine can inhibit CYP2C19 and affect plasma concentration of drugs metabolized by this isoenzyme.[89]

Dosing and Administration Eslicarbazepine is initiated with a starting dose of 400 mg as a single daily dose. It may be increased by 400 mg/day on a weekly basis to a maximum dose of 1,200 mg/day.[89]

Advantages Eslicarbazepine has once daily dosing and may cause less hyponatremia than oxcarbazepine. Eslicarbazepine has potentially less CNS adverse effects than oxcarbazepine.

Disadvantages It is a new drug, and further data on its effectiveness is needed.

Place in Therapy Eslicarbazepine is FDA approved as monotherapy or adjunctive treatment for focal onset seizures. It is the newest ASD and should be reserved for failure of other ASD agents.

Ethosuximide

Mechanism of Action Inhibition of T-type Ca^{2+} channels[24,90]

Pharmacokinetics Absorption is unaffected by food, and metabolism occurs in the liver by hydroxylation to inactive metabolites with some evidence of nonlinear pharmacokinetics at higher concentrations.[24,90]

Adverse Effects Nausea and vomiting are reported in up to 40% of patients, which may be minimized by administration of smaller and more frequent doses.[24]

Drug Interactions Valproic acid may inhibit ethosuximide's metabolism, but only if the metabolism of ethosuximide is near saturation.[24]

Dosing and Administration Titration over 1 to 2 weeks to maintenance doses of 20 mg/kg/day usually results in therapeutic concentrations. Once-a-day therapy is efficacious; however, GI distress appears to be dose related, and the total daily dose is usually divided into two equal doses.[24]

Advantages This drug is very effective in the treatment of CAE and is well tolerated.

Disadvantages Ethosuximide has a very narrow spectrum of activity.

Place in Therapy Ethosuximide is a first-line treatment for absence seizures.

Ezogabine

Mechanism of Action The primary mechanism of action of ezogabine is as a selective positive allosteric opener of KCNQ2-5 channels, which stabilizes the resting membrane potential and reduces brain excitability.[24,91]

Pharmacokinetics Ezogabine's oral bioavailability is 60%; high fat food increases its maximal blood drug concentration (C_{max}) 38%. Ezogabine has a 30% lower trough serum level in the evening than in the morning. The drug undergoes glucuronidation and acetylation with the major metabolite, *n*-acetyl metabolite (NAMR) being less active than the parent compound in animal models. Elderly subjects show a 40% to 50% higher area under the drug concentration time curve (AUC) and a 30% higher half-life compared to younger subjects, and therefore dosage reduction is recommended.[92]

Adverse Effects Ezogabine can cause abnormalities of the retina usually after long term use (eg, 4 years) with features similar to those seen in retinal pigment dystrophies known to cause vision loss. Because of this potential vision loss, ezogabine is recommended only after several alternatives have been tried. Urinary retention can also occur, usually within the first 6 months, and caution is advised in persons with benign prostatic hypertrophy, those on anticholinergics, or those persons unable to communicate clinical symptoms. Ezogabine can also cause QT prolongation, usually within 3 hours of administration, and caution is advised when using with other QT prolonging drugs and in persons with congestive heart failure, ventricular hypertrophy, hypokalemia, or hypomagnesemia. Lastly, ezogabine can cause blue or gray-blue skin discoloration predominantly around the lips or in the nailbeds of fingers and toes and sometimes also face, legs, palate, sclera, and conjunctiva usually occurring 2 or more years after treatment at doses of 900 mg or greater. Consequences and reversibility of this adverse effect are unknown, but discontinuation should be considered if this occurs. Otherwise, CNS effects are the most common side effects.[92]

Drug Interactions Ezogabine can increase lamotrigine clearance by 22% and decrease AUC by 18% while NAMR may inhibit renal clearance of digoxin. Ezogabine serum levels may be reduced 35% by phenytoin and 31% by carbamazepine. Lastly, alcohol may increase systemic exposure, C_{max} and AUC, of ezogabine, resulting in an increase in adverse drug effects.[92]

Dosing and Administration Ezogabine is initiated at 300 mg/day dosed three times a day, with dosage increases of 150 mg every week until a goal dose of 600 to 1,200 mg/day is reached.[92]

Advantages Ezogabine works by an entirely different mechanism than other ASDs and therefore may be valuable when added to another ASD as adjunctive therapy.

Disadvantages Ezogabine is a class V controlled substance. The drug may interfere with both urine and serum bilirubin clinical lab assays causing falsely elevated readings. It is dosed three times per day. Most importantly, it's potential for vision loss, and other unique adverse effects including urinary retention, skin discoloration, and QT prolongation are disadvantages for use.

Place in Therapy Ezogabine is approved as adjunctive treatment for focal onset seizures. Due to the potential for vision loss, ezogabine is recommended only after several alternatives have been tried.

Felbamate

Mechanism of Action Felbamate inhibits *N*-methyl-D-aspartate (NMDA) glutamate receptors and modulates $GABA_A$ receptors. At higher doses it may modulate voltage-gated Na^+ channels and inhibit high-voltage gated Ca^{2+} channels.[93,94]

Pharmacokinetics

Felbamate is unaffected by food or antacids. Approximately 40% to 50% of a felbamate dose is metabolized by hydroxylation and conjugation pathways in the liver, and the remainder is excreted unchanged in the urine. It displays linear pharmacokinetics.[93,94]

Adverse Effects Felbamate is associated with potentially fatal idiosyncratic reactions including aplastic anemia (1 in 3,000 patients) and acute liver failure (1 in 10,000 patients) with reported onset between 68 and 354 days of therapy. The risk for aplastic anemia may be increased in women, those with a history of cytopenia, ASD allergy or significant toxicity, viral infection, and/or immunologic problems.[93] Use of felbamate now requires signed written consent. Otherwise, the most common side effects are insomnia, nausea, and headache (sometimes severe). Anorexia and weight loss are also common and may be especially problematic in children and in patients with diminished caloric intake.[93,94]

Drug Interactions Felbamate can induce or inhibit the metabolism of the older AEDs. Interactions between warfarin and felbamate have also been reported.[93,94]

Dosing and Administration Felbamate is initiated at doses of 1,200 mg/day in 3 to 4 divided doses and can be increased at 1- to 2-week intervals to 2,400 mg/day and then to 3,600 mg/day.[93]

Advantages Felbamate has a unique mechanism of action and a broad spectrum of activity (eg, useful in atonic seizures of LGS and focal seizures).

Disadvantages Use is limited by the risk of possibly fatal aplastic anemia and hepatotoxicity.

Place in Therapy Felbamate is approved as either monotherapy or adjunctive therapy in patients with focal onset seizures with or without generalization, and for the treatment of seizures associated with LGS in children. Its use is reserved for patients not responding to other ASDs.

Gabapentin

Mechanism of Action Gabapentin elevates human brain GABA levels, possibly via alterations in GABA synthesis or reversal of the neuronal GABA transporter, resulting in nonvesicular release of GABA. Gabapentin appears to bind to an amino acid carrier protein and to act at a unique receptor. It binds to the $\alpha 2\delta$ subunit of Ca^{2+} channels which is believed to underlie its antinociceptive effects.[24]

Pharmacokinetics Gabapentin is a substrate of the L-amino acid carrier protein in the gut and in the CNS which actively transports the drug across membranes.[95] Binding is saturable causing dose-dependent bioavailability that varies considerably between patients.[96] Food does not affect absorption.[97] Concentrations in human CSF are 5% to 35% of plasma levels, and tissue concentrations are approximately 80% of plasma levels. Gabapentin is renally eliminated, and dosage adjustments may be necessary in patients with significantly impaired renal function.[24]

Adverse Effects CNS effects, as well as weight gain, are the most common side effects seen with gabapentin. Aggressive behavior has been reported in children.[98] A withdrawal reaction characterized by anxiety, insomnia, nausea, sweating, and increased pain has also been reported with abrupt discontinuation in patients taking it for pain.

Drug Interactions There is a 10% reduction in the clearance of gabapentin in patients taking cimetidine and a 20% reduction in the bioavailability if aluminum antacids are taken simultaneously with gabapentin, although this may not be clinically significant.[24]

Dosing and Administration Typical starting doses of gabapentin are 300 mg at bedtime on the first day, increasing to 900 mg/day over 3 days. Faster titration rates (eg, starting at 300-900 mg three times daily) have been well tolerated.[99] Data suggest gabapentin should be given at least four times a day when the total daily dose is 3,600 mg or greater.[100] It does not appear to be absorbed rectally. Patients on hemodialysis should receive an initial 300- to 400-mg dose with 200 to 300 mg given after every 4 hours of hemodialysis.

Advantages It has a broad therapeutic index with minimal CNS adverse effects and few drug interactions. Doses can be escalated rapidly. It is available in a liquid dosage form.

Disadvantages It is oftentimes considered a poorly efficacious ASD. However, it is well tolerated, and studies in elderly patients suggest it may be as efficacious as lamotrigine in this population.

Place in Therapy Gabapentin is FDA approved for patients with focal onset seizures with or without secondary generalization in patients 3 years and older. It is usually considered a second-line agent for patients with focal seizures who have failed initial treatment, although it may have a role in new-onset focal epilepsy in the elderly. It may be most useful in treating epilepsies with comorbid conditions such as neuropathic pain.

Lacosamide

Mechanism of Action Lacosamide is a functionalized amino acid that enhances slow inactivation of voltage-gated Na^+ channels, stabilizing hyperexcitable neuronal membranes and inhibiting repetitive neuronal firing. It may also bind to collapsin response mediator protein (CRMP-2 involved in neuronal differentiation and axonal outgrowth), although the clinical significance of this is unclear.[24,101]

Pharmacokinetics Lacosamide is almost completely absorbed after oral administration, and bioavailability is not affected by food. There is a linear relationship between daily doses and serum concentrations up to 800 mg/day. Moderate hepatic and renal impairment have both been shown to increase systemic drug exposure up to approximately 40%.[24,101]

Adverse Effects CNS and GI effects, such as dizziness, nausea, diplopia, and ataxia, are the most common side effects seen with lacosamide. These effects are dose related and may occur more commonly in patients receiving concomitant treatment with other Na^+ channel inhibitors. The drug can also cause a small increase in median PR interval on the electrocardiogram (ECG).[24,101]

Drug Interactions Lacosamide blood levels are decreased by approximately 15% to 20% by enzyme-inducing ASDs.[33] It is a substrate of CYP2C19; however, there are no known drug interactions between lacosamide and drugs metabolized by CYP2C19 including OCs.[24,101]

Dosing and Administration The starting dose is 100 mg/day given in two divided doses. The dose is increased by 100 mg/day every week until a daily dose of 200 to 400 mg has been reached. Studies have shown that a dose of 600 mg daily may be efficacious for some patients, but at the expense of more CNS side effects.[24,101]

Advantages An IV form of lacosamide is available for short-term replacement that appears to be safe, well tolerated, and easy to administer as well as a liquid dosage form. It also has a novel mechanism of action.[24,101]

Disadvantages Lacosamide is a class V controlled substance.[101]

Place in Therapy Lacosamide is approved as monotherapy or adjunctive treatment for focal onset seizures. Due to ease of use, including availability of intravenous loading and lack of drug interactions, it has become a first-line agent among many providers, although there is no strong evidence to support this. Although many providers use it first-line, it is only available as brand and due to cost should be reserved as second-line or third-line therapy after failure of other equally efficacious, less expensive ASDs.[24,101]

Lamotrigine

Mechanism of Action Lamotrigine inhibits voltage-gated Na^+ channels; it also modulates high voltage-gated Ca^{2+} channels, modulates hyperpolarization-activated cation (HCN) channels, and attenuates release of glutamate and to a lesser extent, GABA and dopamine.[24,102]

Pharmacokinetics Lamotrigine is completely and rapidly absorbed, and absorption is unaffected by food. Rectal bioavailability is approximately 50% of that of the oral dosage forms. Lamotrigine clearance is higher in children and lower in the elderly compared with young adults. Severe hepatic disease can influence lamotrigine pharmacokinetics. Its half-life is also prolonged in renal failure. If a patient is on hemodialysis, approximately 17% of the dose can be removed by hemodialysis, with the half-life being reduced to approximately 13 hours.[24,102]

Adverse Effects Lamotrigine can cause rash, which usually appears in the first 3 to 4 weeks of therapy and is more likely to occur if the patient has had a prior rash to another ASD.[103] The rash typically is generalized, erythematous, and morbilliform, although SJS can occur. Some rashes can necessitate the withdrawal of lamotrigine. Risk factors for the emergence of more serious rashes appear to be concomitant use of valproic acid and situations where high initial doses or rapid dosage escalation is used. When dosed appropriately, the incidence of rash is similar to that of carbamazepine and phenytoin. The incidence is higher in children than in adults.[104] Otherwise, the most common side effects are CNS related.

Drug Interactions Valproic acid substantially inhibits the metabolism of lamotrigine, with maximal inhibition occurring at valproic acid doses and serum concentrations of 500 mg/day and 40 to 50 mcg/mL (mg/L; 277-347 μmol/L) respectively.[105] A pharmacodynamic interaction can occur with concurrent carbamazepine therapy, causing an increase in CNS side effects.[105] Lamotrigine does not inhibit liver enzymes and has a low potential for pharmacokinetic interactions with other drugs although such interactions are still possible. It has been found to decrease the bioavailability of the progesterone component (levonorgestrel) of a combination OC by 19%, although the clinical relevance of this interaction is unclear.[106] Concomitant treatment with OCs can lead to a reduction in the serum concentrations of lamotrigine because of an induction of lamotrigine glucuronidation by ethinyl estradiol.[107] In addition, lamotrigine serum levels can significantly increase during the week off OC treatment in some patients.[107]

Dosing and Administration In patients who are taking enzyme-inducing drugs, lamotrigine can be started more rapidly than in patients receiving valproic acid. The maintenance doses are also different. For patients on monotherapy, lamotrigine should be started at 25 mg daily for 2 weeks, increased to 25 mg twice daily for 2 weeks, and then increased by 50 mg/day every 2 weeks until the goal dose of 200 to 400 mg/day is reached. For patients on concomitant valproic acid, lamotrigine should be started at doses of 25 mg every other day for 2 weeks, then 25 mg daily for 2 weeks, and then increased by 25 mg/day every 2 weeks until goal doses of 100 and 200 mg/day are reached. For patients on concomitant enzyme inducing ASDs such as carbamazepine or phenytoin, lamotrigine should be started at 50 mg daily for 2 weeks, then increased to 50 mg twice daily for 2 weeks, then increased by 100 mg/day every 2 weeks until goal doses of 300 to 500 mg/day are reached. Removal of inducers from a lamotrigine regimen may necessitate decreases in lamotrigine dose, whereas removal of valproic acid can necessitate an increase in the lamotrigine dose.[105]

Advantages Lamotrigine is potentially a broad-spectrum ASD, having efficacy in focal onset seizures and several types of generalized seizures. Pediatric dosage forms are available as a chewable dispersible tablet and an oral disintegrating tablet, and it is also available as an extended release product for once daily dosing. Besides rash, it is generally well tolerated in children, adults, and elderly patients.

Disadvantages Lamotrigine is associated with rash, and the initial doses must be low (especially if the patient is on valproic acid) and escalated slowly to maximize safety. Because of the need for slow titration, it is not a good agent for patients who need to reach therapeutic ASD levels quickly.

Place in Therapy Lamotrigine is broad spectrum and is approved as both monotherapy and adjunctive treatment in patients with focal onset seizures and can be considered first- or second-line therapy. It is also approved for primary GTC seizures and for primary generalized seizures of LGS.[105] The elderly may experience less cognitive effects than with other ASDs.[66] Its use is mainly limited by its slow titration and risk of rash.

Levetiracetam

Mechanism of Action Levetiracetam binds to synaptic vesicle protein SV2A, in presynaptic terminals and prevents neurotransmitter release.[108]

Pharmacokinetics Absorption of levetiracetam is rapid and complete and not significantly affected by food.[109] Renal elimination of unchanged parent drug accounts for the majority of clearance (66%), with the remainder being metabolized via nonhepatic enzymatic hydrolysis to inactive metabolites. Levetiracetam clearance appears to be approximately 40% higher in children than in adults. Patients with severe liver cirrhosis should initially receive one-half the recommended starting dose because of a 57% decrease in clearance. Levetiracetam is excreted into breast milk in potentially clinically important amounts.[24,104]

Adverse Effects Levetiracetam is extremely well tolerated. CNS effects are the most common side effects seen with levetiracetam, and they are usually mild. In children and young adults, agitation, irritability, or somnolence/lethargy are the most frequently reported CNS side effects.[24,110]

Drug Interactions It does not significantly interact with other AEDs, warfarin, digoxin, or OCs.[24,110]

Dosing and Administration Typically the initial dose is 500 mg given twice daily. The dose may be increased by 500 to 1,000 mg every 1 to 2 weeks. Doses above the maximum FDA approved 3,000 mg/day are often used. To minimize CNS side effects, dosing may be initiated at 250 mg twice daily, especially in the elderly. Levetiracetam can be loaded orally or intravenously. Doses can be converted on a 1:1 basis.[24,110]

Advantages Levetiracetam has a novel mechanism of action, is well tolerated, has no significant drug interactions and can be loaded when therapeutic levels need to be reached quickly.

Disadvantages Behavioral problems can limit therapy in some patients.

Place in Therapy Levetiracetam is FDA approved as adjunctive therapy in the treatment of focal onset seizures in patients 12 years of age or older although it is routinely used as first-line monotherapy. It is also approved for adjunctive treatment of myoclonic seizures in patients with JME and as adjunctive treatment of primarily generalized seizures in patients with IGE (eg, genetic generalized epilepsies).[24,110]

Oxcarbazepine

Mechanism of Action Oxcarbazepine is structurally related to carbamazepine and is a prodrug that is rapidly converted to the active 10-monohydroxy derivative (MHD). Like carbamazepine, oxcarbazepine and MHD block voltage-gated Na^+ channels, and also modulate Ca^{2+} and K^+ currents, although it displays differing affinities for these ion channels compared to carbamazepine. Whereas carbamazepine may modulate L-type Ca^{2+} channels, oxcarbazepine appears to modulate N- and P-type Ca^{2+} channels,[103] although the clinical significance of these difference is unclear.[111,112]

Pharmacokinetics Oxcarbazepine is completely absorbed, and MHD is inactivated by glucuronide conjugation and eliminated by the kidneys. Oxcarbazepine and MHD do not undergo autoinduction, and the relationship between dose and serum concentration is linear. Children 2 to 6 years of age need larger doses to achieve the same serum concentration, suggesting a more rapid clearance, whereas elderly patients may have decreased renal elimination. Patients with significant renal impairment may require a dosage reduction.[13,24]

Adverse Effects CNS effects are the most frequent side effects seen with oxcarbazepine especially at doses greater than 1,200 mg/day and in the elderly, although in comparative trials oxcarbazepine generally caused fewer side effects than phenytoin, valproic acid, or carbamazepine. Hyponatremia has been reported in up to 25% of patients and occurs more often in elderly patients and in patients receiving concomitant sodium-depleting drugs such as diuretics. Hyponatremia occurs less frequently in children. Monitoring serum Na^+ levels and for symptoms of hyponatremia are recommended. Approximately 25% to 30% of patients who develop a rash with carbamazepine will experience a similar reaction with oxcarbazepine.[24,113]

Drug Interactions Oxcarbazepine decreases the bioavailability of ethinyl estradiol and levonorgestrel and may cause contraceptive failure. Unlike carbamazepine, there are no interactions between cimetidine, erythromycin, or warfarin, and oxcarbazepine. Oxcarbazepine dosed greater than 1,200 mg can cause a 40% increase in the concentration of phenytoin, consistent with inhibition of CYP 2C19. Oxcarbazepine treatment may also modestly reduce lamotrigine serum concentrations, suggesting induction of UGT isozymes. The replacement of carbamazepine with oxcarbazepine may result in a drug interaction because an enzyme-inducing drug is being removed.[24,113,114]

Dosing and Administration Dosing in adults can be initiated at 300 to 600 mg/day in two divided doses and increased by 300 mg/day every 3 days or weekly to a recommended dose of 1,200 mg/day (although doses of up to 2,400 mg/day are recommended in conversion to monotherapy). In children 4 years of age and older, the dose can be initiated at 8 to 10 mg/kg/day and increased by 5 mg/kg every 3 days up to 60 mg/kg/day. Doses up to 60 mg/kg/day have also been used in infants and children younger than 4 years of age.[106] In patients being converted from carbamazepine, the typical maintenance dose of oxcarbazepine is 1.5 times the carbamazepine dose (or less if the carbamazepine is dosed high due to autoinduction).[24,113,115]

Advantages There is strong evidence for its effectiveness in seizure disorders. It is also effective in patients not demonstrating a response to carbamazepine, and its efficacy is comparable with that of carbamazepine, phenytoin, and valproic acid. It may also be better tolerated than phenytoin as monotherapy.[116]

Disadvantages There are more reports of hyponatremia with oxcarbazepine. About 30% of patients who had carbamazepine-induced rash will also have rash with oxcarbazepine. Enzyme-inducing drugs can increase the clearance of MHD.

Place in Therapy Oxcarbazepine is FDA approved for use as monotherapy or adjunctive therapy in the treatment of focal seizures in adults and children as young as 4 years of age and can be considered first-line.

Perampanel

Mechanism of Action Perampanel is a highly selective noncompetitive AMPA-type glutamate receptor antagonist.[117]

Pharmacokinetics Perampanel is rapidly and almost completely absorbed. It is highly protein bound (95%) and eliminated primarily via CYP3A4 metabolism to an inactive metabolite with an elimination half-life of about 100 hours. Its clearance is increased twofold to threefold when given with enzyme-inducing ASDs.[117]

Adverse Effects The most common adverse effects include dizziness, somnolence, headache, and ataxia. Perampanel has an FDA boxed warning pertaining to monitoring of psychiatric, behavioral, mood, or personality changes which may be life-threatening.[117]

Drug Interactions Serum levels of perampanel are decreased by enzyme inducing ASDs. It displays modest enzyme inducing properties of its own at the high end of its dose range (12 mg/day).[117]

Dosing and Administration Perampanel is initiated with starting doses of 2 mg/day and titrated by 2 mg/day on a weekly basis to a maximum dose of 12 mg/day. If the patient is taking enzyme inducing ASDs, the dose should be initiated at 4 mg/day. In hepatic failure, the dose should be increased every 2 weeks, and the target dose is decreased to 4 to 6 mg/day.[117]

Advantages Perampanel has a novel mechanism of action and can be dosed once per day.

Disadvantages There is limited experience with perampanel.

Place in Therapy Perampanel is approved for focal onset seizure with or without secondary generalization in patients with epilepsy 12 years of age or older. It is also approved for primary GTC seizures in patients 12 years of age or older.[117] It is a new drug and should be reserved for use after failure of other ASDs.

Phenobarbital

Mechanism of Action Phenobarbital potentiates the action of GABA on $GABA_A$ receptors by prolonging the opening of the GABA receptor-chloride ionophore complex. It also depresses normal excitatory synaptic transmission by inhibiting glutamate release through an effect on P/Q type high-voltage activated Ca^{2+} channels and blocking AMPA/Kainate receptors.[24,118]

Pharmacokinetics Phenobarbital is hepatically metabolized by CYP2C9 (major), CYP2C19, and CYP2E1 to two inactive metabolites although approximately 25% is renally cleared with a half-life of 70 to 130 hours. It is an inducer of many CYP proteins, including CYP1A2, CYP2B6, CYP2A6, CYP2C8, CYP2C9, and CYP3A4 and induces metabolism. It also induces lamotrigine metabolism by inducing UGT1A4 enzyme. Usual adult therapeutic levels are between 10 and 40 mcg/mL (mg/L; 43-172 μmol/L). Side effects including sedation occur commonly at higher dosage levels.[24,118]

Adverse Effects The most common side effects are somnolence, dizziness, decreased coordination, impaired cognition, mental confusion, depressed affect, and behavior problems seen in children. Long-term use is associated osteomalacia, megaloblastic anemia, and folate deficiency. Serious side effects include hepatotoxicity, and serious dermatologic effects such as SJS and TEN.[24,118]

Drug Interactions Phenobarbital increases the metabolism of clobazam, midazolam, and lamotrigine and decreases their serum levels but may increase *or* decrease phenytoin serum levels. Felbamate, oxcarbazepine, phenytoin, and valproate may inhibit the metabolism of phenobarbital, thereby increasing phenobarbital serum levels. Common drugs that interact with phenobarbital include amitriptyline, citalopram, cyclosporine, haloperidol, felodipine, nifedipine, propranolol, verapamil, and warfarin.[24,118]

Dosing and Administration The initial starting dose of phenobarbital in adults is 60 mg/day and can be titrated up to a target dose of 100 to 300 mg/day over several weeks.[24,118]

Advantages Phenobarbital is an effective ASD and has been in use for the longest period of time and is readily available worldwide.

Disadvantages Phenobarbital causes much sedation.

Place in Therapy Due to the availability of better tolerated ASDs with fewer drug interactions, phenobarbital should be reserved for second line use in focal onset and generalized seizures.

Phenytoin

Mechanism of Action Phenytoin inhibits voltage-gated Na^+ channels.[24]

Pharmacokinetics The pharmacokinetics of phenytoin are complex, and the reader is referred to a more extensive review for a more in-depth understanding.[119] The oral absorption of phenytoin may be saturable at higher doses above 400 mg. Absorption following IM administration is erratic and delayed, and IM injections are painful; however, IM fosphenytoin absorption is rapid and well tolerated. Phenytoin is highly protein bound, and it is essential to know the patient's serum albumin level when interpreting serum phenytoin concentrations.[120] Significant renal dysfunction will also alter phenytoin protein binding, whereas obesity increases the volume of distribution. Phenytoin is metabolized in the liver by parahydroxylation mainly by CYP2C9 and CYP2C19.[24] Phenytoin displays Michaelis–Menten pharmacokinetics, and the metabolism of phenytoin saturates at doses used clinically, so that a small change in dose can result in a disproportionally large increase in serum concentrations, potentially leading to toxicity.[119] This can also occur at low serum concentrations in some patients. Phenytoin metabolism may also decrease in the elderly although this been challenged.[121]

Adverse Effects CNS effects are the most frequent side effects seen with phenytoin. Most of these effects usually are transient and can be minimized by slow dosage titration. At very high concentrations of greater than 50 mcg/mL (mg/L; 200 μmol/L), phenytoin can exacerbate seizures. Phenytoin has multiple side effects associated with chronic use including gingival hyperplasia (minimized by good oral hygiene), vitamin D deficiency, osteomalacia, carbohydrate intolerance, immunologic disturbances, hypothyroidism, and peripheral neuropathy. Phenytoin is associated with rare hypersensitivity and idiosyncratic reactions resulting in rashes, SJS, pseudolymphoma, bone marrow suppression, lupus-like reactions, and hepatitis.[24,122]

Drug Interactions Phenytoin has numerous drug interactions. It is an inducer of both CYP450 and UGT isozymes. The absorption of phenytoin can be increased or decreased with the administration of food depending on the composition of the meal. The bioavailability of phenytoin suspension can be decreased in patients receiving continuous enteral nutrient tube feedings.[24] Phenytoin decreases folic acid absorption. Replacement of folic acid can reduce phenytoin concentration and result in loss of efficacy.[24]

Dosing and Administration Immediate-release capsules and liquid dosage forms are available, although the extended-release capsule is most often used. Only the extended-release capsules should be dosed once daily. An oral loading dose (eg, 20 mg/kg), should be divided into 3 to 4 doses and given at 4 to 6-hour intervals to therapeutic levels of between 10 and 20 mcg/mL (mg/L; 40-79 μmol/L).[124] When adjusting dosages based on levels one can increase the daily dose by 100 mg if the serum levels are less than 7 mcg/mL (mg/L; 28 μmol/L), by 50 mg if the serum levels are between 7 and 12 mcg/mL (mg/L; 28-48 μmol/L), and by 30 mg if serum levels are greater than 12 mcg/mL (mg/L; 48 μmol/L).[123] A common maintenance dose is 300 mg/day. One should also remember that 100 mg of phenytoin acid is equal to 92 mg of phenytoin sodium. Intravenous and IM administration of phenytoin is available although IM is not recommended. Fosphenytoin is a prodrug for phenytoin, has less side effects, and is available intravenously (see chapter on status epilepticus for more information on phenytoin and fosphenytoin IV).

Advantages After more than 66 years, phenytoin's risk-to-benefit ratio is well established. It is available intravenously for emergent situations.

Disadvantages Phenytoin has numerous side effects associated with chronic use. It has a relatively narrow therapeutic window, and dose titration is complicated by Michaelis–Menten kinetics. There are also many drug interactions associated with its metabolism and protein binding. It can also be present in breast milk and it crosses the placenta.

Place in Therapy Phenytoin is FDA approved for focal onset seizures and GTC seizures. It may exacerbate seizures in generalized epilepsies and should be avoided in those epilepsies. It has known efficacy and has long been used as a first line ASD for many seizure types. However, known side effects with chronic use may limit its use, and its place in therapy is being reevaluated as newer ASDs with fewer side effects become more common.

Pregabalin

Mechanism of Action Pregabalin is structurally related to gabapentin and binds to the $\alpha^2\delta$ subunit of voltage-gated Ca^{2+} channels which possibly results in decreased release of the excitatory neurotransmitters glutamate, noradrenaline, substance P, and calcitonin gene-related peptide.[24]

Pharmacokinetics Pregabalin is a substrate of the L-amino acid carrier protein in the CNS. It does not display dose-dependent bioavailability, and bioavailability is unaffected by food.[125] Pregabalin is eliminated renally as unchanged drug, and dosage adjustment is required in patients with significantly impaired renal function. In anuric patients, 50% of the dose is removed by 4 hours of hemodialysis.

Adverse Effects CNS effects, as well as weight gain, are the most frequently reported side effects seen with pregabalin. It is unknown if pregabalin causes aggressive behavior in children. A withdrawal reaction characterized by anxiety, nervousness, and irritability has been noted in patients being treated for generalized anxiety upon abrupt discontinuation of the drug.[125]

Drug Interactions Drug interactions are unlikely.

Dosing and Administration Pregabalin is started at doses of 150 mg/day divided into twice or thrice daily intervals. Doses can be increased by 50 to 100 mg/day every 1 to 2 weeks. Doses greater than 600 mg/day are uncommon. The manufacturer recommends that patients with end-stage renal disease maintained on hemodialysis receive a 25 to 75 mg daily dose with 25 to 75 mg given after every 4 hours of hemodialysis.[24]

Advantages Pregabalin is somewhat more potent than gabapentin without the dose-limiting GI absorption properties. It has minimal CNS side effects and no drug interactions.

Disadvantages Pregabalin is a class V controlled substance. Like gabapentin it can cause weight gain and peripheral edema, especially as the dose is increased.

Place in Therapy Pregabalin is FDA approved for focal onset seizures in adults. It has been used as monotherapy, although generally it is reserved for patients who have failed initial treatment with other ASDs or for patients who also have chronic neuropathic pain or generalized anxiety disorder.[24]

Rufinamide

Mechanism of Action Rufinamide is a triazole derivative that suppresses neuronal hyperexcitability through prolongation of the inactivation phase of voltage-gated Na^+ channels.[126]

Pharmacokinetics Rufinamide is slowly absorbed (T_{max} of 4-6 hours) with decreasing absorption at higher doses (85% at 600 mg). Absorption is improved when taken with food. It is extensively metabolized by primary biotransformation via carboxylesterases with no active metabolites. The drug may have a higher clearance in children.[126]

Adverse Effects CNS effects are the most common side effects and are dose-dependent. Rufinamide may increase the incidence of convulsions in some patients, and may precipitate SE. Multiorgan hypersensitivity has occurred within 4 weeks of starting treatment in patients younger than 12 years of age.

Drug Interactions Rufinamide is a weak inhibitor of CYP2E1 and a weak inducer of CYP3A4. It is responsible for a modest increase in the clearance of carbamazepine, lamotrigine, phenobarbital, and phenytoin. This effect may be greater in children than adults. Similarly, carbamazepine, phenytoin, primidone, and phenobarbital significantly increase the clearance of rufinamide. Valproic acid significantly decreases the clearance of rufinamide and elevates serum levels by 70%.[24]

Dosing and Administration The initial dose of rufinamide is 400 to 800 mg/day given in divided doses with an increase in dose every other day until a maximum dose of 45 mg/kg/day or 3,200 mg/day (whichever is less) is obtained.

Advantages The drug is effective for seizures associated with LGS without causing cognitive and psychiatric adverse effects. The dose can be rapidly escalated.

Disadvantages Drug interactions are common with rufinamide, and patients with LGS are usually on multiple medications. The drug has caused convulsions and SE in some patients.

Place in Therapy Rufinamide is FDA approved as an adjunctive agent for seizures in LGS and is efficacious in the treatment of tonic-atonic seizures. It should be reserved for use after patients have failed other ASDs.

Tiagabine

Mechanism of Action Tiagabine is a potent specific inhibitor of GABA transporter type 1 (GAT1), and enhances GABA by decreasing its removal from the synaptic space and prolonging inhibitory postsynaptic potentials.[127]

Pharmacokinetics Tiagabine is well absorbed, and there is a linear relationship between dose and serum concentrations. Children eliminate tiagabine slightly faster than adults. Hepatic impairment causes higher and more prolonged plasma concentrations of the drug, although renal dysfunction does not change its pharmacokinetics.[127] Tiagabine evening levels are lower than morning levels.

Adverse Effects Tiagabine has increased the incidence of nonconvulsive SE in patients with chronic refractory partial epilepsy, and there are reports of SE or new-onset seizures occurring in patients without a history of epilepsy.[128,129] Otherwise, mild and transient CNS and GI effects are the most frequent side effects, mostly occurring during dose titration and can be alleviated with food which slows absorption.[128]

Drug Interactions Tiagabine is displaced from protein by naproxen, salicylates, and valproate but does not itself displace phenytoin, valproic acid, amitriptyline, tolbutamide, or warfarin.[127]

Dosing and Administration The initial dose of 7.5 to 15 mg/day is given in divided doses and is increased by 5 to 10 mg/day weekly to a minimum effective dose of 30 mg/day, although individuals on enzyme-inducing drugs may require doses up to 50 to 60 mg/day.

Advantages It has a unique mechanism of action with few drug interactions.

Disadvantages Tiagabine has been associated with an increase in seizure frequency and SE.

Place in Therapy Tiagabine is FDA approved as adjunct therapy for patient with focal seizures with or without generalization. It should be reserved for those who have failed other therapies due to the potential to cause seizures and SE in some patients.

Topiramate

Mechanism of Action Topiramate has multiple modes of action involving voltage-dependent Na^+ channels, $GABA_A$-receptor subunits, high-voltage Ca^{2+} channels, and kainate/α-amino-3-hydroxy-5-methylisoxazole-4-propionic acid (AMPA) subunits. It also inhibits carbonic anhydrase, which may have some antiseizure effects but is likely not a major mechanism of action.[130]

Pharmacokinetics Although generally considered to have linear absorption and elimination pharmacokinetics, there is saturable binding to erythrocytes that may affect C_{max} and AUC.[131] Approximately 50% of the dose is excreted renally unchanged and should be dose adjusted in renally impaired patients. Renal tubular reabsorption may affect elimination. Metabolism is increased 50% when given with enzyme-inducing ASDs.

Adverse Effects CNS effects are frequently reported including word-finding difficulties and problems with cognition, occurring more often during rapid titration and at higher doses.[132,133] Kidney stones occur in 1.5% of patients (2-4 times that of the general population), and patients should be encouraged to maintain adequate fluid intake. Topiramate can also cause metabolic acidosis at doses as low as 50 mg/day, especially in patients with renal disease, severe respiratory disorders, diarrhea, surgery, and in patients on the ketogenic diet.[132]

Drug Interactions Topiramate can increase phenytoin serum concentrations in some patients due to decreasing CYP2C19 metabolism, although the extent of its effect depends on whether the patient is a "poor metabolizer" phenotype. Topiramate can modestly increase the clearance of valproic acid and increase formation of toxic metabolites. It also increases the clearance of ethinyl estradiol in a dose-dependent manner, although doses of less than 200 mg/day are unlikely to alter OC pharmacokinetics. Topiramate also slightly increases the clearance of digoxin.[134]

Dosing and Administration Topiramate should be titrated slowly to avoid adverse events. Doses can be initiated at 25 mg/day and increased by 25 to 50 mg/day every 1 to 2 weeks. For patients on other ASDs, doses greater than 400 mg/day do not appear to lead to improved efficacy and can cause increased adverse effects.[24,135]

Advantages Topiramate has multiple mechanisms of action and is a broad-spectrum ASD. Elimination is primarily renal, although hepatic metabolism occurs at higher doses.

Disadvantages With rapid dosage escalation, topiramate can compromise cognitive functioning, including impaired word finding and impaired short-term memory. Therefore, initial doses should be low, and titration must be slow. Renal stones and weight loss have been associated with topiramate use.

Place in Therapy Topiramate is FDA approved as monotherapy or adjunctive therapy for focal onset seizures is patients 2 years or older. It is also approved for the treatment of tonic–clonic seizures in primary generalized epilepsy and generalized seizures in patients with LGS. It can be considered first- or second-line therapy but use is limited by CNS effects and slow titration. It has benefit in patients with comorbid migraines or obesity.

Valproic Acid/Divalproex Sodium

Mechanism of Action Valproic acid may potentiate postsynaptic GABA responses, may have a direct membrane-stabilizing effect, and may affect Na^+ and K^+ channels.[136]

Pharmacokinetics Valproic acid is completely absorbed orally,[136] although the rate of absorption differs among preparations. Peak concentrations occur in 0.5 to 1 hour with the syrup, 1 to 3 hours with the capsule, and 2 to 6 hours with the enteric-coated tablet.[136] Divalproex is composed of sodium valproate and valproic acid in a 1:1 molar relationship and dissociates to the valproate ion in the GI tract.

Valproic acid is extensively bound to albumin, and the valproic acid free fraction will increase as the total serum concentration increases. Because binding is saturable, monitoring of free fractions, although uncommon, may be better than total concentrations, especially at higher concentrations or in patients with hypoalbuminemia.

The primary pathway of valproic acid metabolism is β-oxidation, although up to 40% of a dose may be excreted as the glucuronide. At least 10 metabolites of valproic acid have been identified, some with weak anticonvulsant activity, and at least one metabolite (4-ene-VPA), which may be increased with concomitant enzyme-inducing drugs, may be responsible for the reported hepatotoxicity.[136] Valproic acid has lower evening serum levels than morning levels. It crosses into the placenta and concentrations may be up to five times higher in cord serum blood than in the mother due to higher binding in the fetal compartment.[137]

Adverse Effects GI side effects including nausea, vomiting, anorexia, as well as weight gain are most commonly reported (20%). Pancreatitis is rare. GI complaints may be minimized by food or by giving the enteric-coated or ER formulation. Alopecia and hair changes are temporary, and hair growth returns even with continued dosing. Weight gain can be significant for many patients and is associated with an increase in fasting insulin and leptin serum levels,[138] possibly due to the inhibition of insulin metabolism by the liver[139] and leading to the development of insulin resistance in obese patients.[136]

Serious hepatotoxicity has occurred with most deaths in patients younger than 2 years of age, occurring early in the course of therapy, in children with mental retardation and receiving multiple ASDs (as ASDs can alter valproic acid metabolism and lead to development of possible toxic metabolites). Hyperammonemia is common (50%) but does not necessarily imply liver damage. Valproic acid has also been shown to alter carnitine metabolism, and it is possible that carnitine deficiency may cause both liver toxicity and hyperammonemia[140] but routine carnitine supplementation is not generally supported.[141] Thrombocytopenia is also common especially at concentrations greater than 100 mcg/mL (mg/L; 693 μmol/L) and may occur more frequently in children than adults.[142]

Drug Interactions Highly protein-bound drugs (eg, free fatty acids and aspirin) can displace valproic acid. Valproic acid can inhibit specific CYP450 isozymes, epoxide hydrolase, and UGT isozymes. Valproic acid decreases clearance of phenobarbital and lamotrigine by 30% to 50% and can lead to phenobarbital and lamotrigine toxicity. OCs may also increase the clearance of valproic acid and lower serum levels by 20%.[65] In addition, carbapenems, especially meropenem, can lower valproic acid levels.[143]

Dosing and Administration Once-daily dosing is possible with extended-release divalproex, but more frequent dosing is the norm due to reports of breakthrough seizures on once daily dosing. The concentration-dose ratio decreases with increasing dose probably because of increasing free concentrations and a resulting increase in clearance. Valproic acid is available as a soft gelatin capsule, an enteric-coated tablet, a syrup, a "sprinkle capsule," an extended-release formulation designed for once-daily dosing, and an IV formulation.[136] This parenteral formulation must not be given IM because it can cause tissue necrosis. The sprinkle capsule, designed to be opened and mixed with food, has a slower rate of absorption, which results in fewer fluctuations in the peak-to-trough ratio. The syrup is absorbed more rapidly than any solid dosage form. The enteric-coated divalproex tablet is not sustained-release but reduces GI distress and delays absorption. Dosing may be initiated at 10 to 15 mg/kg/day and increased by 5 to 10 mg/kg weekly. Valproate may be intravenously loaded at a dose of 15 to 20 mg/kg. Depakote-ER is approximately 15% less bioavailable than the enteric-coated divalproex sodium delayed-release.

Advantages Valproic acid is available in multiple dosage formulations, has a wide therapeutic index, and is considered a broad-spectrum ASD. It is also used in other neurologic or psychiatric disorders (eg, migraine headache and bipolar disorder).

Disadvantages Valproic acid causes significant weight gain and has other side effects, such as alopecia, tremor, pancreatitis, PCOS, and thrombocytopenia, and it is teratogenic. It also has multiple drug–drug interactions as an enzyme inhibitor.

Place in Therapy Valproic acid is first-line therapy for generalized seizures, including myoclonic, atonic, and absence seizures. It can be used as both monotherapy and adjunctive therapy for focal-onset seizures, and it is very useful in patients with mixed seizure disorders. Its use is limited by potential long-term side effects such as weight gain and teratogenicity.

Vigabatrin

Mechanism of Action Vigabatrin is an amino acid that is a structural analog of GABA and is a selective, irreversible inhibitor of GABA-transaminase, the enzyme that degrades GABA, thereby increasing GABA levels in the CNS.[144]

Pharmacokinetics Vigabatrin undergoes virtually no metabolism and is excreted unchanged in the urine dosage. No dose adjustment is required for renally impaired patients. Food has no effect on its absorption. Duration of effect is not related to serum levels and is directly related to regeneration of the GABA-transaminase enzyme. Children have a higher vigabatrin clearance than adults and require higher mg/kg doses.[65]

Adverse Effects Vigabatrin may aggravate seizures, particularly absence and myoclonic seizures in patients with generalized epilepsies. Patients with history of depression, psychosis, or behavioral disturbances may be at greater risk to develop psychiatric effects.[144] Vigabatrin causes progressive, irreversible, bilateral concentric visual field constriction in a high percentage of patients. It may also reduce visual acuity in a dose-related and life exposure-related manner. Vigabatrin is associated with weight gain and edema, peripheral neuropathy, somnolence, and fatigue. In up to 11% of patients (up to age 3 years) treated with high doses of the drug for infantile spasms, MRI findings have been strongly suggestive of intramyelinic edema in select brain areas. These findings appear to be reversible, and their significance is unclear.[145]

Drug Interactions Vigabatrin induces CYP2C9 and therefore decreases phenytoin plasma levels by approximately 20% and possibly increases serum carbamazepine by 10%.

Dosing and Administration The initial dose is 1,000 mg/day given in two divided doses. Doses are increased by 500 mg/day weekly until 3,000 mg/day is reached. The dose in infants and children for infantile spasms is 50 mg/kg/day given in two divided doses with an increase by 25 to 50 mg/kg/day every 3 days to a maximum dose of 150 mg/kg/day.

Advantages Vigabatrin is first-line for infantile spasm and has been widely studied.

Disadvantages Adverse effects are significant, and it is available only through a restricted distribution program (SHARE program), which requires providers and patients to register. Vision should be checked at baseline and every 3 months for up to 6 months after drug discontinuation.

Place in Therapy It is a first-line agent for infantile spasms, particularly those with tuberous sclerosis as the etiology. It is a third-line adjunctive agent for refractory focal onset epilepsy.

Zonisamide

Mechanism of Action Zonisamide, a sulfonamide, exerts its antiepileptic effect by inhibition of slow Na^+ channels and T-type Ca^{2+} channels, and possibly by inhibition of glutamate release. Like topiramate, it also has a weak carbonic anhydrase inhibitory effect.[146]

Pharmacokinetics Zonisamide is well absorbed and reaches a maximum concentration in 2 to 5 hours. It is metabolized by CYP450 system, although it has minimal drug interactions, and 30% is excreted unchanged in the urine. It crosses the placenta, and the concentration in breast milk is similar to that in the plasma.[146]

Adverse Effects Common CNS effects include sedation and effects on cognition especially with rapid dose escalation. Paresthesias, modest weight loss, oligohidrosis with effects on body temperature control are also reported. Hypersensitivity reactions can occur (0.02% of patients), and it should be used with caution (if at all) in patients with sulfonamide allergies. A 2.6% incidence of symptomatic kidney stones has been reported.[147]

Drug Interactions Zonisamide does not inhibit or induce the CYP450 system.

Dosing and Administration Zonisamide is given once or twice daily. Once-daily dosing of zonisamide causes greater fluctuations in serum concentrations and perhaps more side effects, and therefore it should be dosed twice daily at doses of greater than 400 mg/day. It can be initiated at 100 mg once daily and the dose should be increased by 100 mg/day every 1 to 2 weeks to response. Doses greater than the FDA approved maximum of 600 mg/day are uncommon.

Advantages Zonisamide has multiple mechanisms of action and may be a broad-spectrum ASD with minimal drug interactions and can be dosed once daily. There is broad international experience with this drug especially in Asian populations, and patients may experience modest weight loss.

Disadvantages Cognitive impairment can limit its use, especially with rapid dose escalation. It should be avoided in patients allergic to "sulfa drugs." Renal stones may limit its use.

Place in Therapy Zonisamide is approved for the adjunctive treatment of focal onset seizures and may be considered first-line. However, it may be potentially effective in a variety of focal onset and generalized onset seizure types.

EVALUATION OF THERAPEUTIC OUTCOMES

Clinical response is more important than the serum drug concentrations and involves identifying the number and type of seizures and adverse effects. Patients should record the severity and the frequency of seizures in a seizure diary, and there should be a decrease with treatment. Patients and family should be questioned regularly to determine whether patients are truly seizure free. Patients should also be monitored long term for comorbid conditions, social adjustment (including QOL assessments), drug interactions, and adherence. Periodic screening for comorbid neuropsychiatric disorders, such as depression and anxiety, is also important.

Outcomes are focusing increasingly more on optimal QOL. The AAN has developed quality performance measures for the clinician that define a high quality of care of these patients. Among those performance measures, it is important to remember to counsel patients about ASD side effects, initiate discussion about depression, and assess their knowledge about referral of the intractable epilepsy patient for surgery. Besides seizure control and ASD side effects, factors that can impact QOL in epilepsy patients and which should be addressed include issues about driving, economic security, forming relationships, epilepsy safety such as precautions when swimming, social isolation, and social stigma.

ABBREVIATIONS

AAN	American Academy of Neurology
AES	American Epilepsy Society
AMPA	α-amino-3-hydroxy-5-methylisoxazole-4-propionic acid
ASD	antiseizure drug
AUC	area under the drug concentration time curve
CAE	Childhood Absence Epilepsy
C_{max}	maximal blood drug concentration
CNS	central nervous system
CPS	complex partial seizure
CRMP	collapsin response mediator protein
CSF	cerebrospinal fluid
CT	computed tomography
DRESS	Drug Reactions with Eosinophilia and Systemic Symptoms
ECG	electrocardiogram
EEG	electroencephalogram
EFHC1	EF-hand containing protein-1
GABA	γ-aminobutyric acid
GI	gastrointestinal
GTC	generalized tonic-clonic
IGE	idiopathic generalized epilepsy
ILAE	International League Against Epilepsy
IM	intramuscular
IQ	intelligence quotient
LGS	Lennox-Gastaut Syndrome
JME	Juvenile Myoclonic Epilepsy
MCMs	major congenital malformations
MHD	monohydroxy derivative
MRI	magnetic resonance imaging
NMDA	*N*-methyl-D-aspartate
OC	oral contraceptive
PCOS	polycystic ovary syndrome
PET	positron emission tomography
PME	Progressive Myoclonic Epilepsy
QOL	quality of life
SE	status epilepticus
SJS	Steven Johnsons Syndrome

SP	simple partial
SUDEP	sudden unexplained death in epilepsy
TEN	Toxic Epidermal Necrolysis
T_{max}	time to maximal blood drug concentration
VNS	vagus nerve stimulation
WBC	white blood cell

REFERENCES

1. Kerr MP, Mensah S, Besag F, et al. International consensus clinical practice statements for the treatment of neuropsychiatric conditions associated with epilepsy. *Epilepsia* 2011;52:2133-2138.
2. England MJ, Liverman CT, Schultz AM, et al. A summary of the Institute of Medicine report: Epilepsy across the spectrum: Promoting health and understanding. *Epilepsy Behav* 2012;25(2):266-276.
3. Fisher RS, van Emde Boas W, Blume W, et al. Epileptic seizures and epilepsy: Definitions proposed by the international league against Epilepsy (ILAE) and the International Bureau for Epilepsy (IBE). *Epilepsia* 2005;46(4):470-2.
4. Avanzini G, Beghi E, de Boer H, et al. Neurological disorders: A public health approach (dementia, epilepsy, headache disorders, multiple sclerosis). *Neurological Disorders: Public Health Challenges.* 2012:41-110.
5. Hesdorfer DC, Logroscino G, Benn EK, et al. Estimating risk for developing epilepsy: A population based study in Rochester, Minnesota. *Neurology* 2011:76(1):23-27.
6. Hauser WA. Seizure disorders: The changes with age. *Epilepsia* 1992:33(S4):6-14.
7. Salpekar J, Byrne M, Ferrone G. Epidemiology and common comorbidities of epilepsy in childhood. In: Wheless JW, ed. *Epilepsy in Children and Adolescents.* Chichester, UK: John Wiley & Sons, Ltd.; 2012:5-15.
8. Scheffer IE, Berkovic SF, Capovilla G, et al. The Organization of the Epilepsies: Report of the ILAE Commission on Classification and Terminology. Available at: http://www.ilae.org/Visitors/Centre/Organization.cfm. (Accessed Oct 31, 2015)
9. Suzuki T, Delgado-Escueta AV, Aguan K, et al. Mutations in EFHC1 cause juvenile myoclonic epilepsy. *Nat Genet* 2004;36(8):842-849.
10. Nieh SE, Sherr EH. Epileptic encephalopathies: New genes and new pathways. *Neurotherapeutics* 2014;11:796-806.
11. Macdonald RL, Kang JQ, Gallagher MJ. Mutations in $GABA_A$ receptor subunits associated with genetic epilepsies. *J Physiol* 2010;588(11):1861-1869.
12. Tanaka M, Olsen RW, Medina MT, et al. Hyperglycosylation and reduced GABA currents of mutated GABRB3 polypeptide in remitting childhood absence epilepsy. *Am J Hum Genet* 2008;82(6):1249-1261.
13. Commission on Classification and Terminology of the International League Against Epilepsy. Proposal for revised clinical and electroencephalographic classification of epileptic seizures. *Epilepsia* 1981;22:489-501.
14. Commission on Classification and Terminology of the International League Against Epilepsy. Proposal for revised classification of epilepsies and epileptic syndromes. *Epilepsia* 1989;30:389-399.
15. Berg AT, Scheffer IE. New concepts in classification of the epilepsies: Entering the 21st century. *Epilepsia* 2011:52(6):1058-1062.
16. Malmgren K, Thom M. Hippocampal sclerosis—origins and imaging. *Epilepsia* 2012;53(S4):19-33.
17. Shorvon SD. The causes of epilepsy: Changing concepts of etiology of epilepsy over the past 150 years. *Epilepsia* 2011;52(6):1033-1044.
18. Minassian BA, Lee JR, Herbrick J-A, et al. Mutations in a gene encoding a novel protein tyrosine phosphatase cause progressive myoclonus epilepsy. *Nature Genet* 1998;20:171-174.
19. Nabbout R. Autoimmune and inflammatory epilepsies. *Epilepsia* 2012:53(S4):19-33.
20. Hesdorffer DC. Risk factors. In: Engel J, Pedley TA, eds. *Epilepsy: A Comprehensive Text Book.* 2nd ed. Philadelphia, PA: Lippincott Williams & Wilkins; 2008:57-63.
21. Jallon P, Zifkin BF. Seizure precipitants. In: Engel J, Pedley TA, eds. *Epilepsy: A Comprehensive Text Book.* 2nd ed. Philadelphia, PA: Lippincott Williams & Wilkins; 2008:77-80.
22. Najm IM, Moddel G, Janigro D. Mechanisms of epileptogenesis and experimental models of seizures. In: Wyllie E, ed. *The Treatment of Epilepsy.* 4th ed. Philadelphia, PA: Lippincott Williams & Wilkins; 2006:91-102.
23. Engel J. Mechanisms of neuronal excitation and synchronization: The neuron. *Seizures and Epilepsy.* 2nd ed. New York, NY: Oxford University Press; 2013:56-72.
24. Engel J. Antiseizure drugs. *Seizures and Epilepsy.* 2nd ed. New York, NY: Oxford University Press; 2013:541-602.
25. Rogawski MA, Bazil CW. New molecular targets for antiepileptic drugs: 2, SV2A, and Kv7/KCNQ/M potassium channels. *Curr Neurol Neurosci Rep* 2008;8(4):345-352.
26. Engel J. Mechanisms of neuronal excitation and synchronization: Glial influences. *Seizures and Epilepsy.* 2nd ed. New York, NY: Oxford University Press; 2013:73.
27. Engel J, Mechanisms of neuronal excitation and synchronization: Neuronal networks. *Seizures and Epilepsy.* 2nd ed. New York, NY: Oxford University Press; 2013:73-81.
28. Huguenard JR, McCormick DA. Thalamic synchrony and dynamic regulation of global forebrain oscillations. *Trends Neurosc* 2007;30:350-356.
29. Glauser T, Ben-Menachem E, Bourgeois B, et al. Updated ILAE evidence review of antiepileptic drug efficacy and effectiveness as initial monotherapy for epileptic seizures and syndromes. *Epilepsia* 2013;54(3):551-563.
30. Noachtar S, Peters AS. Semiology of epileptic seizures: A critical review. *Epilepsy Behav* 2009;15(1):2-9.
31. Foldvary-Schaefer N, Unnwongse K. Localizing and lateralizing features of auras and seizures. *Epilepsy Behav* 2011;20(2): 160-166.
32. Fisher RS, Acevedo C, Arzimanoglou A, et al. A practical clinical definition of epilepsy. *Epilepsia* 2014;55(4):475-482.
33. Chen DK, So YT, Fisher RS. Use of serum prolactin in diagnosing epileptic seizures. Report of the therapeutic and technology assessment subcommittee of the American Academy of Neurology. *Neurology* 2005;65:668-675.
34. Bouma HK, Labos C, Gore GC, Wolfson C, Keezer MR. The diagnostic accuracy of routine electroencephalography after a first unprovoked seizure. *Eur J Neurol* 2016;23(3):455-463.
35. Fountain NB, Van Ness PC, Swain-Eng R, et al. Quality improvement in neurology: AAN epilepsy quality measures: Report of the Quality Measurement and Reporting Subcommittee of the American Academy of Neurology. *Neurology* 2011;76(1):94-99.
36. Kwan P, Brodie MJ. Early identification of refractory epilepsy. *N Engl J Med* 2000;342:314-319.
37. Louis EK, Rosenfeld WE, Bramley T. Antiepileptic drug monotherapy: The initial approach in epilepsy management. *Current Neuropharm* 2009;7:77-82.
38. Garnet WR. Antiepileptic drug treatment: Outcomes and adherence. *Pharmacotherapy* 2000;20:191s-199s.
39. Krumholz A, Wiebe S, Gronseth GS, et al. Evidence-based guideline: Management of an unprovoked first seizure in adults. *Neurology* 2015;84:1705-1712.
40. Duncan JS, Shorvon SD, Trimble MR. Effects of removal of phenytoin, carbamazepine, and valproate on cognitive function. *Epilepsia* 1990;31:584-591.
41. Anderson T, Brathen G, Person A, et al. A comparison between one and three years of treatment in uncomplicated childhood epilepsy: A prospective study. The EEG as a predictor of outcome after withdrawal of treatment. *Epilepsia* 1997;38:228-232.
42. Chadwick D, Taylor J, Johnson T. Outcomes after seizure recurrence in people with well-controlled epilepsy and the factors that influence it. The MRC antiepileptic drug withdrawal group. *Epilepsia* 1996;37:1043-1050.
43. Practice parameter: A guideline for discontinuing antiepileptic drugs in seizure-free patients—summary statement. Report of the Quality Standards Subcommittee of the American Academy of Neurology. *Neurology* 1996;47(2):600-602.
44. Berg AT, Shinnar S. Relapse following discontinuation of antiepileptic drugs: A meta-analysis. *Neurology* 1994;44:601-608.
45. Krahl SE, Clark KB, Smith DC, et al. Locus coeruleus lesions suppress the seizure-attenuating effects of vagus nerve stimulation. *Epilepsia* 1998;39:709-714.
46. Shuchman M. Approving the vagus-nerve stimulator for depression. *N Engl J Med* 2007;356:1604-1607.
47. Salinsky MC, Uthman BM, Ristanovic RK, et al. Vagus nerve stimulation for the treatment of medically intractable seizures: Results of a 1 year open extension trial. *Arch Neurol* 1996;53:1176-1180.

48. Handforth A, Degiorgio CM, Schachter SC, et al. Vagus nerve stimulation therapy for partial-onset seizures: A randomized active controlled trial. *Neurology* 1998;51(1):48-55.
49. Rolston JD, Englot DJ, Wang DD, Shih T, Chang EF. Comparison of seizure control outcomes and the safety of vagus nerve, thalamic deep brain, and responsive neurostimulation: Evidence from randomized controlled trials. *Neurosurgical Focus* 2012;32(3):E14.
50. Wiebe S, Blume WT, Girvin JP, Eliasziw M; Effectiveness and Efficiency of Surgery for Temporal Lobe Epilepsy Study Group. A randomized, controlled trial of surgery for temporal-lobe epilepsy. *N Engl J Med* 2001;345(5):311-318.
51. Engel J, McDermott MP, Wiebe S, et al. Early surgical therapy for drug-resistant temporal lobe epilepsy. *JAMA* 2012;307:922-930.
52. TI Jeong SW, Lee SK, Hong KS, Kim KK, Chung CK, Kim H. Prognostic factors for the surgery for mesial temporal lobe epilepsy: Longitudinal analysis. *Epilepsia* 2005;46(8):1273-1279.
53. Janszky J, Janszky I, Schulz R, et al. Temporal lobe epilepsy with hippocampal sclerosis: Predictors for long-term surgical outcome. *Brain* 2005;128(Pt 2):395-404.
54. Jeha LE, Najm IM, Bingaman WE, et al. Predictors of outcome after temporal lobectomy for the treatment of intractable epilepsy. *Neurology* 2006;66(12):1938-1940.
55. Berg AT, Vickrey GB, Langfitt JT, et al. Reduction of AEDs in postsurgical patients who attain remission. *Epilepsia* 2006;47:64-71.
56. Groesbeck DK, Blum RM, Kossoff EH. Long-term use of the ketogenic diet: Outcomes of 28 children with over 6 years diet duration. *Neurology* 2006;66(Suppl 2):A41.
57. Dossoff EH, Zupec-Kania BA, Amark PE, et al. Optimal clinical management of children receiving the ketogenic diet: Recommendations of the International Ketogenic Diet Study Group. *Epilepsia* 2009;50:304-317.
58. Miranda MJ, Turner Z, Magrath G. Alternative diets to the classical ketogenic diet—Can we be more liberal? *Epilepsy Res* 2012;100:278-285.
59. Brigo F, Ausserer H, Tezzon F, Nardone R. When one plus one makes three: The quest for rational antiepileptic polytherapy with supraadditive anticonvulsant efficacy. *Epilepsy Behav* 2013;27(3):439-442.
60. French JA, Kanner AM, Bautista J, et al. Efficacy and tolerability of the new antiepileptic drugs: I. Treatment of new onset epilepsy. *Neurology* 2004;62:1252-1260.
61. French JA, Kanner AM, Bautista J, et al. Efficacy and tolerability of the new antiepileptic drugs: II. Treatment of refractory epilepsy. *Neurology* 2004;62:1261-1273.
62. Karceski S, Morrell MJ, Carpenter D. Treatment of epilepsy in adults: Expert opinion. *Epilepsy Behav* 2005;7:S1-S64.
63. Mattson RH, Cramer JA, Collins JF. Prognosis for total control of complex partial and secondarily generalized tonic-clonic seizures. Department of Veterans Affairs Epilepsy Cooperative Studies No. 118 and No. 264. *Neurology* 1996;46:68-76.
64. Kwan P, Arzimanoglou A, Berg AT, et al. Definition of drug resistant epilepsy: Consensus proposal by the ad hoc Task Force of the ILAE Commission on Therapeutic Strategies. *Epilepsia* 2010;51(6):1069-1077.
65. Perucca P, Gilliam FG. Adverse effects of antiepileptic drugs. *Lancet* 2012;11:792-802.
66. Wlodarczyk BJ, Palacios AM, George TM, Finnell RH. Antiepileptic drugs and pregnancy outcomes. *Am J Med Genet* 2012;158A:2071-2090.
67. Patsalos PN, Berry DJ, Bourgeois BFD, et al. Antiepileptic drugs-best practice guidelines for therapeutic drug monitoring: A position paper by the subcommission on therapeutic drug monitoring, ILAE Commission on Therapeutic Strategies. *Epilepsia* 2008;49:1239-1276.
68. Dreifuss FE, Langer DH, Moline KA, Maxwell JE. Valproic acid hepatic fatalities-experience since 1984. *Neurology* 1989;39:201-207.
69. Pack AM, Morrell MJ, McMahon DJ, et al. Bone health in young women with epilepsy after one year of antiepileptic drug monotherapy. *Neurology* 2008;70:1586-1593.
70. Lado F, Spiegel R, Masur JH, et al. Value of routine screening for bone demineralization in an urban population of patients with epilepsy. *Epilepsy Res* 2008;78:155-160.
71. Wang Z, Lin YS, Zheng XE, et al. An inducible cytochrome P4503A4-dependent vit D catabolic pathway. *Mol Pharmacol* 2012;81:498-509.
72. Herzog AG. Progesterone therapy in women with epilepsy: A 3-year follow-up. *Neurology* 1999;52(9):1917-1918.
73. Rowan AJ, Ramsay ER, Collins JF, et al. New onset geriatric epilepsy: A randomized study of gabapentin, lamotrigine, and carbamazepine. *Neurology* 2005;64:1868-1873.
74. Harden CL, Pulver MC, Ravdin L, et al. The effect of menopause and perimenopause on the course of epilepsy. *Epilepsia* 1999;40(10):1403-1407.
75. Verrotti A, D'Egidio C, Mohn A, et al. Antiepileptic drug, sex hormones, and PCOS. *Epilepsia* 2011;52:199-211.
76. Savers A, Harden CL. Gender issues for drug treatment. In: Engel J and Pedley TA, eds. *Epilepsy: A Comprehensive Text Book*. 2nd ed. Philadelphia, PA: Lippincott Williams & Wilkins; 2008:1263-1269.
77. Harden CL, Hopp J, Ting TY, et al. Practice parameter update: Management issues for women with epilepsy—focus on pregnancy (an evidence-based review): Obstetrical complications and change in seizure frequency. *Neurology* 2009;73:126-132.
78. Harden CL, Hopp J, Ting TY, et al. Practice parameter update: Management issues for women with epilepsy—focus on pregnancy (an evidence-based review): Obstetrical complications and change in seizure frequency. *Neurology* 2009;73:126-132.
79. Harden CL, Meador KJ, Pennell PB, et al. Management issues for women with epilepsy—Focus on pregnancy (an evidence-based review): II. Teratogenesis and perinatal outcomes. *Neurology* 2009;50:1237-1246.
80. Williams J, Myson V, Steward S, et al. Self discontinuation of AEDs in pregnancy: Detection by hair analysis. *Epilepsia* 2002;43(8):824-831.
81. Tomson T, Marson A, Boon P, et al. Valproate in the treatment of epilepsy in women and girls. Pre-Publication Summary of Recommendations from a joint Task Force of ILAE-Commission on European Affairs* and European Academy of Neurology (EAN)** Available at: http://www.ilae.org/visitors/news/documents/ValproateCommentILAE-0315.pdf. (Accessed Oct 31, 2015)
82. Harden CL, Pennell PB, Koppel BS, et al. Management issues for women with epilepsy—Focus on pregnancy (an evidence-based review): III. Vitamin K, folic acid, blood levels, and breast-feeding: Report of the Quality Standards Subcommittee and Therapeutics and Technology Assessment Subcommittee of the American Academy of Neurology and the American Epilepsy Society. *Epilepsia* 2009;50:1247-1255.
83. Meador KJ, Baker GA, Browning N, et al. Effects of breastfeeding in children of women taking antiepileptic drugs. *Neurology* 2010;75:1954-1960.
84. Tegretol [package insert]. East Hanover, NJ: Novartis Pharmaceuticals Corp.; September 2015.
85. Garnett WR, Bainbridge JL, Johnson SL. Carbamazepine. In: Murphy J, ed. *Clinical Pharmacokinetics*. 4th ed. Bethesda, MD: American Society of Health-Systems Pharmacists; 2008:121-138.
86. Marino SE, Birbaum AK, Leppik IE, et al. Steady-state carbamazepine pharmacokinetics following oral and stable-labeled intravenous administration in epilepsy patients: Effects of race and sex. *Clin Pharmacol Ther* 2012;91:483-488.
87. Ficker DM, Privitera M, Krauss G, et al. Improved tolerability and efficacy in epilepsy patients with extended-release carbamazepine. *Neurology* 2005;65:593-595.
88. Onfi [package insert]. Deerfield, IL: Lundbeck Inc.; October 2011.
89. Aptiom [package insert]. Marlborough, MA: Sunovion Pharmaceuticals; August 2015.
90. Garnett WR, Bainbridge JL, Johnson SL. Ethosuximide. In: Murphy J, ed. *Clinical Pharmacokinetics*. Bethesda, MD: American Society of Health-Systems Pharmacists; 2008:153-159.
91. Gunthorpe MJ, Large CH, Sankar R. The mechanism of action of retigabine (ezogabine), a first-in-class K channel opener for the treatment of epilepsy. *Epilepsia* 2012;53:412-424.
92. Potiga [package insert]. Research Triangle Park, NC: GlaxoSmithKline and Valeant Pharmaceuticals North America; June 2011.
93. Pellock JM, Perhach JL, Sofia RD. Felbamate. In: Levy RH, Mattson RH, Meldrum BS, et al., eds. *Antiepileptic Drugs*. 5th ed. Philadelphia, PA: Lippincott Williams & Wilkins; 2002:301-318.
94. Felbatol [package insert]. Somerset, NJ: Meda Pharmaceuticals; July 2011.
95. Luer MS, Hamani C, Dujovny M, et al. Saturable transport of gabapentin at the blood-brain barrier. *Neurol Res* 1999;21:559-562.
96. Gidal BE, Radulovic LL, Kruger S, Rutecki P, Pitterle M, Bockbrader HN. Inter- and intrasubject variability in gabapentin (GBP) absorption and absolute bioavailability. *Epilepsy Res* 2000;40:123-127.
97. Gidal BE, Maly MM, Kowalski JW, Rutecki PA, Pitterle ME, Cook DE. Gabapentin absorption: Effect of mixing with foods of varying macronutrient content. *Ann Pharmacother* 1998;32:405-408.
98. Lee DO, Steingard RJ, Cesena M, et al. Behavioral side effects of gabapentin in children. *Epilepsia* 1996;37:87-90.

99. McLean MJ, Gidal BE. Gabapentin in the treatment of epilepsy: A dosing review. *Clin Ther* 2003;25:1382-1406.
100. Gidal BE, DeCerce J, Bockbrader HR, et al. Gabapentin bioavailability: Effect of dose and frequency of administration in adult patients with epilepsy. *Epilepsy Res* 1998;31:91-99.
101. Vimpat [package insert]. Smyrna, GA: UCB, Inc.; August 2014.
102. Gilman JT. Lamotrigine: An antiepileptic agent for the treatment of partial seizures. *Ann Pharmacother* 1995;29:144-151.
103. Hirsch LJ, Weintraub DB, Buchsbaum R, et al. Predictors of lamotrigine-associated rash. *Epilepsia* 2006;47:318-322.
104. Messenheimer JA. Rash in adult and pediatric patients treated with lamotrigine. *Can J Neurol Sci* 1998;25:S14-S18.
105. Lamictal [package insert]. Research Triangle Park, NC: GlaxoSmithKline; May 2015.
106. Sidhu J, Bulsara S, Job S, Philipson R. A bi-directional pharmacokinetic interaction study of lamotrigine and the combined oral contraceptive pill in healthy subjects [abstract]. *Epilepsia* 2004;45(S7):330.
107. Christensen J, Petrenaite V, Atterman J, et al. Oral contraceptives induce lamotrigine metabolism: Evidence from a double-blind, placebo-controlled trial. *Epilepsia* 2007;48:484-489.
108. Lynch BA, Lambeng N, Nocka K, et al. The synaptic vesicle protein SV2A in the binding site for the antiepileptic drug levetiracetam. *Proc Natl Acad Sci USA* 2004;101:9861-9866.
109. Fay MA, Sheth RD, Gidal BE. Oral absorption kinetics of levetiracetam: The effect of mixing with food or enteral nutrition. *Clin Ther* 2005:27:594-598.
110. Keppra [package insert]. Smyrna, GA: UCB, Inc.; September 2013.
111. Ambrosio AF, Soares-Da-Silva P, Carvalho CM, Carvalho AP. Mechanisms of action of carbamazepine and its derivatives, oxcarbazepine, BIA 2-093 and BIA 2-024. *Neurochem Res* 2002;27:121-130.
112. Kalis MM, Huff NA. Oxcarbazepine, an antiepileptic agent. *Clin Ther* 2001;23:680-700.
113. Trileptal [package insert]. East Hanover, NJ. Novartis Pharmaceuticals; July 2014.
114. May TW, Ramback B, Jurgens U. Influence of oxcarbazepine and methsuximide on lamotrigine concentrations in epileptic patients with and without valproic acid comedication: Results of a retrospective study. *Ther Drug Monit* 1999;21:175-181.
115. Pina-Garza JE, Espinoza R, Nordli D, et al. Oxcarbazepine adjunctive therapy in infants and young children with partial seizures. *Neurology* 2005;65:1370-1375.
116. Muller M, Marson AG, Williamson PR. Oxcarbazepine versus phenytoin monotherapy for epilepsy. *Cochrane Database Syst Rev* 2006;2:CD003615.
117. Fycompa [package insert]. Woodcliff Lake, NJ: Eisai Inc.; June 2015.
118. Tozer TN, Winter ME. Phenytoin. In: Evans WE, Schentag JJ, Jusko WJ, eds. *Applied Pharmacokinetics*. 3rd ed. Spokane, WA: Applied Therapeutics; 1992:1-44.
119. Dilantin [package insert]. New York, NY: Pfizer; April 2009.
120. Anderson GD, Pak C, Doane KW, et al. Revised Winter-Tozer equation for normalized phenytoin concentrations in trauma and elderly patients with hypoalbuminemia. *Ann Pharmacother* 1997;31:279-284.
121. Ahn JE, Cloyd JC, Brundage RC, et al. Phenytoin half-life and clearance during maintenance therapy in adults and elderly patients with epilepsy. *Neurology* 2008;71:38-43.
122. Bruni J. Phenytoin and other hydantoins: Adverse effects. In: Levy RH, Mattson RH, Meldrum BS, et al., eds. *Antiepileptic Drugs*. 5th ed. Philadelphia, PA: Lippincott Williams & Wilkins; 2002:605-610.
123. Privitera MD. Clinical rules for phenytoin dosing. *Ann Pharmacother* 1993;27:1169-1173.
124. Ben-Menachem E. Pregabalin pharmacology and its relevance to clinical practice. *Epilepsia* 2004;45(Suppl 6):13-18.
125. Shneker BF, McAuley JW. Pregabalin: A new neuromodulator with broad therapeutic indications. *Ann Pharmacother* 2005;39:2029-2037.
126. Perucca E, Cloyd J, Critchley D, Fuseau E. Rufinamide: Clinical pharmacokinetics and concentration response relationships in patients with epilepsy. *Epilepsia* 2008;49:1123-1141.
127. Schachter SC. Tiagabine: Current status and potential clinical applications. *Expert Opin Investig Drugs* 1996;5:1377-1387.
128. Leppik IE. Tiagabine: The safety landscape. *Epilepsia* 1995;36:S10-S13.
129. Koepp MJ, Edwards M, Collins J, et al. Status epilepticus and tiagabine therapy revisited. *Epilepsia* 2005;46:1625-1632.
130. Ferraro TN, Buono RJ. The relationship between the pharmacology of antiepileptic drugs and human gene variation. *Epilepsy Behav* 2005;7:18-36.
131. Gidal BE, Lensmeyer GL. Therapeutic drug monitoring of topiramate: Evaluation of the saturable distribution between erythrocytes and plasma in whole blood using an optimized HPLC method. *Ther Drug Monit* 1999;21:567-576.
132. Shorvon SD. Safety of topiramate: Adverse events and relationship to dosing. *Epilepsia* 1996;37(S2):S18-S22.
133. Mula M, Trimble M, Thompson P, et al. Topiramate and word-finding difficulties in patients with epilepsy. *Neurology* 2003;60:1104-1107.
134. Gidal BE. Topiramate: Drug interactions. In: Levy RH, Mattson RH, Meldrum BS, et al., eds. *Antiepileptic Drugs*. 5th ed. Philadelphia, PA: Lippincott Williams & Wilkins; 2002:735-739.
135. Privitera M, Fincham R, Penry J, et al. Topiramate placebo-controlled dose-ranging trial in refractory partial epilepsy using 600-, 800-, and 1,000-mg daily dosages. *Neurology* 1996;46(6):1678-1683.
136. Davis R, Peters DH, McTavish D. Valproic acid: A reappraisal of its pharmacological properties and clinical efficacy in epilepsy. *Drugs* 1994;47:332-372.
137. Ornoy A. Valproic acid in pregnancy: How much are we endangering the embryo and fetus? *Reprod Toxicol* 2009;28:1-10.
138. Greco R, Latini G, Chiarelli F, et al. Leptin, ghrelin, and adiponectin in antiepileptic patients treated with valproic acid. *Neurology* 2005;65;1808-1809.
139. Pylvanen V, Pakarinen A, Knip M, Isojaervi J. Characterization of insulin secretion in valproate-treated patients with epilepsy. *Epilepsia* 2006;47:1460-1464.
140. Genton P, Gelissse P. Valproic acid: Adverse effects. In: Levy RH, Mattson RH, Meldrum BS, et al., eds. *Antiepileptic Drugs*. 5th ed. Philadelphia, PA: Lippincott Williams & Wilkins; 2002:837-851.
141. Gidal BE, Inglese CM, Meyer JM, Pitterle ME, Antonopolous J, Rust RS. Diet and valproate mediated transient hyperammonemia: Effect of L-carnitine supplementation in children with epilepsy. *Pediatr Neurol* 1997;16:301-305.
142. Gerstner T, Teich M, Bell N, et al. Valproate-associated coagulopathies are frequent and variable in children. *Epilepsia* 2006;47:1136-1143.
143. Anonymous. Comparison of carbapenem antibiotics. *Pharmacist's Lett/Prescriber's Lett* 2007;23(12):231205.
144. Ben-Menachem E, Dulac O, Chiron C. Vigabatrin. In: Engel J, Pedley TA, eds. *Epilepsy: A Comprehensive Textbook*. 2nd ed. Philadelphia, PA: Lippincott Williams & Wilkins; 2008:1683-1693.
145. Shorvon SD. Drug treatment of epilepsy in the century of the ILAE: The second 50 years, 1959-2009. *Epilepsia* 2009;50(Suppl 3):93-130.
146. Welty TE. Zonisamide. In: Wyllie E, ed. *The Treatment of Epilepsy*. 4th ed. Philadelphia, PA: Lippincott Williams & Wilkins; 2006:891-899.
147. Lee BI. Zonisamide: Adverse effects. In: Levy RH, Mattson RH, Meldrum BS, et al., eds. *Antiepileptic Drugs*. Philadelphia, PA: Lippincott Williams & Wilkins; 2002: 892-898.

57

Status Epilepticus

Stephanie J. Phelps and James W. Wheless

KEY CONCEPTS

1. Status epilepticus (SE) is a neurologic emergency that may be associated with significant morbidity and mortality.
2. Generalized convulsive status epilepticus (GCSE) is defined as any recurrent or continuous seizure activity lasting longer than 30 minutes in which the patient does not regain baseline mental status. Any seizure that does not stop within 5 minutes should be aggressively treated as impending SE.
3. There are two types of SE, GCSE and nonconvulsive status epilepticus (NCSE). GCSE is the most common type and can be divided into four stages: (1) impending, (2) established, (3) refractory, and (4) super-refractory.
4. Although the pathophysiology of GCSE is unknown, experimental models have shown that there is a dramatic decrease in γ-aminobutyric acid–mediated inhibitory synaptic transmission and that glutamatergic excitatory synaptic transmission sustains the seizures.
5. During prolonged GCSE, $GABA_A$ receptors move from the synaptic membrane into the cytoplasm where they become functionally inactive. A loss of these receptors on the synaptic surface may result in time-dependent pharmacoresistance to benzodiazepines.
6. The main purpose of treatment is to prevent or decrease morbidity and mortality of prolonged seizures. Pharmacologic treatment needs to be rapid and aimed at terminating both electrical and clinical seizures. The probability of poorer outcomes increases with increased length of electrographic seizure activity.
7. Lorazepam is the preferred benzodiazepine in treatment of GCSE because of its efficacy and long duration of action in the central nervous system (CNS). Midazolam is the preferred benzodiazepine for intramuscular (IM) and intranasal (IN) administration.
8. Although practice is slowly moving to other anticonvulsants, the hydantoins (phenytoin and fosphenytoin) continue to be the long-acting anticonvulsants used most frequently. Either phenytoin or fosphenytoin should be given concurrently with benzodiazepines.
9. If GCSE is not controlled by two anticonvulsants, the GCSE is considered to be refractory. In these cases, anesthetic doses of midazolam, pentobarbital, ketamine, or propofol may be used.

(1) Status epilepticus (SE) is a common neurologic emergency that is associated with brain damage and death. The Commission on Classification and Terminology and the Commission on Epidemiology of the International League Against Epilepsy (ILAE) have recently proposed a new definition: Conceptually, SE results from the failure of the mechanisms responsible for seizure termination or from the initiation of mechanisms, which lead to abnormally, prolonged seizures. There are two operational dimensions to this new definition. First, the length of the seizure and the time point (5 minutes) beyond which the seizure should be regarded as "continuous seizure activity." Second, is the time of ongoing seizure activity after which there is a risk of long-term consequences (30 minutes). Both time points are based on animal experiments and clinical research; hence, these time points should be considered the best estimates currently available.[1] (2) The traditional definition defines SE as (a) any seizure lasting longer than 30 minutes whether or not consciousness is impaired or (b) recurrent seizures without an intervening period of consciousness between seizures.[2] Clinically, this definition has limited use, as the average seizure is less than 2 minutes; and only 40% of seizures lasting 10 to 29 minutes cease without treatment.[3] Pharmacoresistance and mortality significantly increase with prolonged seizure duration.[2] (2) Therefore, aggressive treatment of seizures lasting 5 minutes or more is strongly recommended. (3) SE can present in several forms (Table 57-1), including generalized convulsive status epilepticus (GCSE) and nonconvulsive status epilepticus (NCSE).

Nonconvulsive status epilepticus occurs in 25% of those with SE and is characterized by a fluctuating or continuous "epileptic twilight" state that produces altered consciousness and/or behavior (eg, lethargy and decreased mental function).[4] An electroencephalogram (EEG) is the most important diagnostic and management tool.[4] In most instances, a benzodiazepine and/or valproate remain drugs of choice.[4] Although intravenous (IV) hydantoin, levetiracetam, or phenobarbital can be tried in nonresponders, general anesthesia is usually not appropriate.[4]

(3) This chapter will focus on GCSE, which is the most common and severe form of SE. GCSE can be divided into four stages: (1) impending, (2) established, (3) refractory, and (4) super-refractory (Table 57-2).[5] It is characterized by repeated primary or secondary generalized seizures that involve both hemispheres of the brain, results in a loss of consciousness, and are associated with a persistent postictal state.

EPIDEMIOLOGY

The worldwide and United States incidence ranges between 1.2 to 5 million and 100,000 to 152,000 cases each year, respectively.[2] GCSE has no predilection for gender or socioeconomic status but does occur more frequently in nonwhites across all ages.[6] Most GCSE occurs in individuals with no history of epilepsy; however, approximately 5% of adults and 10% to 25% of children with epilepsy will develop GCSE.[7] The incidence is highest in those younger than 1 year of age and in those older than 60 years of age.

TABLE 57-1 International Classification of Status Epilepticus

Convulsive		Nonconvulsive	
International	**Traditional Terminology**	**International**	**Traditional Terminology**
Generalized SE • Tonic–Clonic[a,b] • Tonic[c] • Clonic[c] • Myoclonic[b] • *Erratic*[d]	Grand mal, epilepticus convulsivus	Absence[c]	Petit mal, spike-and-wave stupor, spike and-slow-wave or 3/s spike-and-wave, epileptic fugue, epilepsia minora continua, epileptic twilight, minor SE
Secondary generalized SE[a,b] • Tonic • Partial seizures with secondary generalization		Partial SE[a,b] Simple partial Somatomotor Dysphasic Other types Complex partial	Focal motor, focal sensory, epilepsia partialis continua, adversive SE Elementary Temporal lobe, psychomotor, epileptic fugue state, prolonged epileptic stupor, prolonged epileptic confusional state, continuous epileptic twilight state

SE, status epilepticus.

[a]Most common in older children.

[b]Most common in adolescents and adults.

[c]Most common in infants and young children.

[d]Most common in neonates.

ETIOLOGY

Precipitating events for GCSE vary and generally reflect different populations and referral patterns. Most episodes in individuals with epilepsy occur because of acute anticonvulsant withdrawal, a metabolic disorder or concurrent illness, or progression of a preexisting neurologic disease. Common etiologies and mortality rates are shown in Table 57-3.[6,8] Precipitating events are divided into those with or without neurologic structural lesions or those with a precipitating injury or insult. Cases with structural lesions or those with a specific neurologic insult are associated with a poor prognosis.

There are major differences in etiologies for pediatric and adult patients (see Table 57-3). During their first few weeks of life, infants who are born to addicted mothers can develop drug withdrawal seizures. Other neonates can develop GCSE because of pyridoxine deficiency, which should resolve within hours following IV pyridoxine (100 mg). Acute encephalopathy and metabolic disorders are the major causes of GCSE in those younger than 1 year of age. In young children, the cause is often a nonspecific illness such as fever and/or a viral illness. The most frequent precipitating events in adults are cerebrovascular disease, rapid anticonvulsant withdrawal, and low anticonvulsant serum concentrations. Cerebrovascular disease is the leading cause in those who have their first seizures after age 60. Prescription, over-the-counter, herbal, and recreational drugs should be considered in anyone with new-onset GCSE.

MORBIDITY AND MORTALITY

Generalized convulsive status epilepticus is harmful to the brain. While most contend that the GCSE is responsible for the damage, it is unknown if the morbidity results from the underlying etiology or the GCSE. Regardless of the inducing stimulus, neuronal damage in animal models is evident following 30 to 60 minutes of GCSE, and most progress to develop epilepsy following a prolonged seizure.

TABLE 57-2 Stages of Generalized Convulsive Status Epilepticus

	Stage	Definition
Stage 1 (0-30 minutes)	Impending GCSE	an acute condition characterized by continuous seizures for at least 5 minutes, or by two seizures without full recovery of consciousness between them
Stage 2 (30-60 minutes)	Established GCSE	an acute condition characterized by continuous seizures for at least 30 minutes, or by 30 minutes of intermittent seizures without full recovery of consciousness between events
Stage 3 (>120 minutes)	Refractory GCSE	an acute condition characterized by continuous seizures despite initial treatment with 2-3 AEDs
Stage 4 (>24 hours)	Super-refractory GCSE	an acute condition characterized by seizures that continue 24 hours or longer after the administration of anesthesia, including cases in which SE recurs on reduction or withdrawal of anesthesia

AED, antiepileptic drug; GCSE, generalized convulsive status epilepticus; SE, status epilepticus.

TABLE 57-3 Etiology and Mortality for Pediatric and Adult Cases of Status Epilepticus

Etiology	Mortality Number of Cases (%) $n = 200$ Cases of Pediatric SE	Mortality Number of Cases (%) $n = 512$ Cases of Adult SE
Type I (no Structural Lesion)		
Infection	55 (5)	6 (35)
CNS infection	11 (0)	2 (20)
Metabolic	20 (5)	12 (36)
Low AED levels	16 (0)	24 (7)
Alcohol	0 (0)	13 (8)
Idiopathic	6 (0)	13 (18)
Type II (Structural Lesion)		
Anoxia/hypoxia	27 (13)	14 (65)
CNS tumor	3 (50)	5 (22)
CVA	5 (0)	26 (27)
Drug overdose	5 (0)	3 (23)
Hemorrhage	5 (11)	4 (35)
Trauma	13 (0)	3 (23)
Remote causes[a]	33 (5)	7 (13)

AED, antiepileptic drug; CVA, cerebrovascular accident; SE, status epilepticus. Percentages do not add up to 100% because some patients had multiple etiologies.

[a]More than half of remote causes were congenital malformations and CVA in pediatric and adult patients, respectively.

Data from references 6 and 8.

Interestingly, inhibiting the seizure-induced neuronal damage does not prevent the development of epilepsy, suggesting that the seizures themselves may be harmful. It is hard to establish a relationship between GCSE and long-term outcomes because it is difficult to weigh the effects of seizure type, etiology, duration, concurrent physiologic events, and therapy or lack thereof. It has been shown that patients with a history of prolonged febrile seizures who later developed epilepsy share similar histopathologic changes (ie, hippocampal sclerosis) to those found in animal models of GCSE.[9,10] In these cases, the period between the initial GCSE and the first epileptic seizure may be months to decades, suggesting a possible link between GCSE and the development of epilepsy. Importantly, studies of GCSE show that the currently available anticonvulsants do not reproducibly prevent the development of epilepsy following prolonged seizures.[9,11]

Patients who develop epilepsy following prolonged GCSE are less likely to experience remission of their seizures and may have decreased cognitive and memory function, mental retardation, or neurologic deficits when compared to those who develop epilepsy and subsequently have GCSE.[2] Most studies have found that younger children, the elderly, and those with preexisting epilepsy have a higher propensity for sequelae. Unless accompanied by an underlying neurologic abnormality, febrile SE is less likely to be associated with sequelae.

Estimated mortality in the United States following GCSE ranges between 22,000 and 42,000 individuals per year,[8] with rates up to 16% in children,[12] 20% in adults,[2] and 38% in the elderly.[6] When compared with other populations, neonates have a higher mortality and more neurologic sequelae.

Table 57-3 summarizes the etiology and corresponding mortality rates for GCSE.[6,8] Interestingly, the mortality associated with many etiologies is significantly greater in adults than in children. Unresponsive patients may die from GCSE, but more frequently they die from the acute illness that precipitated the GCSE. For example, patients with serious central nervous system (CNS) structural changes (eg, hemorrhage and stroke) have a poor prognosis, compared to those with no structural lesion.

Outcome is affected by the time between onset of GCSE and the initiation of treatment and the duration of the seizure. Mortality significantly increases with increased seizure duration (eg, 2.6% for seizures 10-29 minutes, 19% for seizures lasting greater than 30 minutes, and 32% for seizures lasting greater than 60 minutes).[3,8] Mortality has decreased over the past decade and probably reflects a recognition of the need to initiate sequenced therapy using large doses as soon as possible.

PATHOGENESIS

Seizures occur when the excitatory neurotransmission overcomes inhibitory impulses in one or more brain regions. After a single, brief, generalized tonic–clonic seizure (less than 5 minutes), the seizure threshold is significantly elevated. The brain's inhibitory mechanisms restore the balance of normal neurotransmission and prevent runaway excitation. Although it is unknown why the mechanisms that control normal brain homeostasis fail, when seizures occur in close succession or the magnitude of the proconvulsant stimulus is severe, compensatory mechanisms can be overwhelmed, and seizures become self-sustaining.

4 While the exact cellular mechanisms are unknown, it appears that seizure initiation is caused by an imbalance between excitatory (eg, glutamate, calcium, sodium, substance P, and neurokinin B) and inhibitory neurotransmission (eg, γ-aminobutyric acid [GABA], adenosine, potassium, neuropeptide Y, opioid peptides, and galanin).[13] $GABA_A$-mediated inhibition becomes less effective while glutamate excitatory actions are enhanced. These alterations have implications to understanding how GCSE progresses to refractory disease and impacts decisions related to sequencing antiepileptic medications.

Most of what is known has focused on gated ion channels. GCSE is largely caused by glutamate acting on postsynaptic *N*-methyl-D-aspartate (NMDA) and α-amino-3-hydroxy-5-methylisoxazole-4-propionate (AMPA)/kainate receptors.[13] During GCSE, NMDA subunits are recruited to the synaptic membrane where they form additional receptors that are proconvulsant. Glutamate activation of the NMDA and AMPA receptors causes opening of the gated calcium and sodium channels, which lead to neuronal depolarization.[13] Sustained depolarization may maintain GCSE and eventually cause neuronal death through calcium-, free radical-, and kinase-mediated events.[14] Although drugs acting as NMDA and AMPA receptor antagonists seem attractive, it is likely that glutamate is not the sole mechanism for sustaining GCSE and that other mechanisms become increasingly important as the duration of seizures increases.

Within minutes of repetitive seizures receptor trafficking (eg, metabotropic GABA and glutamate receptors) occurs. $GABA_A$ postsynaptic receptors control chloride channels to produce hyperpolarization (inhibition) of the postsynaptic cell membrane.[14] These receptors have binding sites for GABA and select anticonvulsants (eg, phenobarbital and benzodiazepines) and enhance $GABA_A$-mediated chloride inhibitory currents. It was previously thought that a decrease in presynaptic GABA led to prolonged seizures; however, it is currently held that GABA concentrations increase during the early phases of GCSE and continue to be elevated during late GCSE. During prolonged seizures postsynaptic $GABA_A$ receptors experience endocytosis. This results in a decrease in the number of γ_2 and $\beta_{2\text{-}3}$ subunits as the receptors move from the synaptic membrane into the cytoplasm where they are functional inactive. These modifications of $GABA_A$ receptors may decrease response to both endogenous GABA and GABA agonists.[13] 5 The γ_2 subunit is associated with benzodiazepine effectiveness; hence, a loss of these on the synaptic surface would result in time-dependent pharmacoresistance to benzodiazepine. Clinically, the relative potencies of benzodiazepines can be reduced up to 20-fold if seizures persist for more than 30 minutes.[14] For this reason, a benzodiazepine should always be combined with another drug that acts at a different site. A similar phenomenon occurs with sodium channel antagonists (phenytoin); however, the magnitude of resistance is less.

PATHOPHYSIOLOGY

As GCSE persists, complex pathophysiologic and biochemical changes lead to systemic alterations, progression of motor phenomena, and development of specific EEG findings.[15] Two distinct and predictable phases have been identified. Phase I occurs during the first 30 minutes of seizure activity, and phase II immediately follows.[15] Although these systemic complications affect the prognosis of GCSE, a prolonged seizure can destroy neurons independent of these events.[14] In fact, the systemic effects of induced seizures in animals can be blocked, but the damage to the neocortex, cerebellum, and hippocampus persists.

During phase I, each seizure markedly increases plasma epinephrine, norepinephrine, and steroid concentrations, which can cause hypertension, tachycardia, and cardiac arrhythmias Within minutes, arterial systolic pressures can rise to above 200 mm Hg, and heart rate can increase by 83 beats per minute.[15] Mean arterial pressure does not fall below 60 mm Hg (8.0 kPa); hence, cerebral perfusion pressure is not compromised. In animals, cerebral blood flow is also increased, thereby protecting neurons from hypoxic injury.

In the presence of a hypoxic myocardium, seizure-induced increases in sympathetic and parasympathetic stimulation of the heart can result in ventricular arrhythmias.[15] Autonomic neuron stimulation can cause a release of insulin and glucagon. Concurrently, circulating catecholamines cause an elevation of hepatic cyclic adenosine monophosphate, producing glycogenolysis. Although the patient can be hyperglycemic initially, serum glucose begins to fall.[15]

Seizure-induced muscular contractions and hypoxia cause lactic acid release, which can produce severe acidosis that may be accompanied by hypotension and shock. Muscle contractions can be so severe that rhabdomyolysis with secondary hyperkalemia and acute tubular necrosis can occur. The airway can be obstructed, causing the patient to become cyanotic or hypoxic. Additionally, an increase in salivation and tracheal and pulmonary secretions can cause aspiration pneumonia. Although transient pleocytosis can develop, it should not be attributed to SE until infectious causes have been eliminated. Between seizures, the EEG slows, and blood pressure normalizes. Although metabolic demands are increased, the brain is able to adequately compensate.

When seizures exceed 30 minutes (phase II), the EEG ictal discharge and clonic motor activity become continuous, and the patient begins to decompensate.[15] Despite elevated levels of catecholamines, the patient can become hypotensive. During this time, autoregulation of cerebral blood flow becomes dependent on mean arterial pressure and begins to fail. There continues to be an excessive consumption of oxygen and glucose; however, compensatory mechanisms are no longer able to meet demands.

During Phase II, the serum glucose concentration may be normal or decreased. Profound hypoglycemia, secondary to hyperinsulinemia, can occur in those with hepatic dysfunction or reduced glycogen stores.[15] Hyperthermia and respiratory deterioration with hypoxia and ventilatory failure can develop. Metabolic and biochemical complications, including respiratory and metabolic acidosis, hyperkalemia, hyponatremia, and azotemia, may develop. There is increased sweating and salivation.

CLINICAL PRESENTATION AND DIAGNOSIS

Accurate diagnosis requires observation, physical examination, laboratory assessment, EEG, and neurologic imaging. The nature and duration of the seizure should be obtained, but a diagnosis of GCSE should not be made until a clinician has observed a seizure. Most patients have an altered consciousness that ranges from obtunded to marked lethargy and somnolence with pronounced eyes-open unresponsiveness and waxy rigidity. Motor features can include muscle contractions, extensor or flexor posturing, and spasms. Over time, the clinical manifestations become less apparent. This has important ramifications, in that seizures appear to have terminated without treatment or when an ineffective therapy is given.

In addition to an assessment of language and cognitive abilities, the physical and neurological examinations should assess motor, sensory, and reflex abnormalities, pupillary response, asymmetry, and posturing. The patient should also be examined for secondary injuries (eg, tongue lacerations, shoulder dislocations, and head and facial trauma).

Laboratory tests are essential to the diagnosis of various etiologies. Hypoglycemia, hyponatremia, hypernatremia, hypomagnesemia, hypocalcemia, and renal failure all can cause seizures. A urine drug screen can help eliminate illicit drug use or drug overdose. Serum drug concentration(s) should be obtained in those on chronic anticonvulsants, as low concentrations can reflect partial adherence or rapid drug withdrawal. A baseline serum concentration is necessary to determine whether a loading dose of a specific anticonvulsant is required. Assessment of other laboratory parameters (eg, hematology and chemistries to include albumin, renal function, and hepatic function) that affect anticonvulsant dosing also can be useful. An EEG is a valuable diagnostic tool, particularly in those with prolonged GCSE in whom clinically apparent seizures are not always evident, but therapy should not be delayed while awaiting testing or results.

CLINICAL PRESENTATION GCSE

Symptoms

- Impaired consciousness (eg, lethargy to coma)
- Disorientation once GCSE is controlled
- Pain associated with injuries (eg, tongue lacerations, shoulder dislocations, back pain, myalgias, headache, and head trauma)

Early Signs

- Generalized convulsions
- Acute injuries or CNS insults that cause extensor or flexor posturing
- Hypothermia or fever suggestive of intercurrent illnesses (eg, sepsis or meningitis)
- Incontinence
- Normal blood pressure or hypotension and respiratory compromise

Late Signs

- Clinical seizures may or may not be apparent
- Pulmonary edema with respiratory failure
- Cardiac failure (dysrhythmias, arrest, and cardiogenic shock)
- Hypotension or hypertension
- Disseminated intravascular coagulation, multisystem organ failure
- Rhabdomyolysis
- Hyperpyrexia

Initial Laboratory Tests

- Complete blood count (CBC) with differential
- Serum chemistry profile (eg, electrolytes, calcium, magnesium, glucose, serum creatinine, alanine aminotransferase [ALT], and aspartate aminotransferase [AST])
- Urine drug/alcohol screen
- Blood cultures
- Arterial blood gas to assess for metabolic and respiratory acidosis, oxygenation
- Serum drug concentration if previous anticonvulsant suspected or known

Other Diagnostic Tests

- Spinal tap if CNS infection suspected
- EEG should be obtained on presentation and once clinical seizures are controlled
- CT with and without contrast
- MRI
- Radiograph if indicated to diagnose fractures

Clinical Presentation GCSE

Once seizures have stopped, it is important to determine if the patient is febrile or has a systemic or CNS infection. Many physiologic consequences of GCSE (eg, leukocytosis, pleocytosis, and hyperthermia) produce symptoms that can be confused with other conditions. If a CNS infection is suspected, a spinal tap should be performed, and empiric antibiotics should be started. If vascular, neoplastic, or infectious etiologies are suspected, computed tomography (CT) or magnetic resonance imaging (MRI) should be obtained once the seizures are controlled.

TREATMENT

Various treatments are available for the management of GCSE. These range from abortion of impending SE with rescue medications to the use of pharmacologic and nonpharmacologic therapies for GCSE and refractory/resistant SE.

Desired Outcomes

6 Short-term desired outcomes include (a) immediate termination of all clinical and electrical seizure activity, (b) no clinically significant adverse effects, and (c) lack of recurrent seizure activity. The long-term outcomes involve minimizing or avoiding pharmacoresistant epilepsy and/or the development of neurologic sequelae that significantly impact quality of life.

Nonpharmacologic Therapy

The time of seizure onset should be noted. Vital signs should be assessed, an adequate and protected airway should be established, ventilation should be maintained, and oxygen should be administered (Fig. 57-1).

Hyperthermia, if present, should be aggressively treated (eg, rectal acetaminophen and cooling blanket). Febrile GCSE is common in the pediatric patient, and normalization of body temperature helps minimize neurologic morbidity.

Intravenous access should be established. Laboratory studies including serum glucose and electrolyte levels (including calcium and magnesium), complete blood count, and renal and hepatic function tests should be performed. Anticonvulsant serum concentration should be obtained as needed, and a urine drug screen should be performed if there is suspicion of ingestion.

Although hypoglycemia rarely causes GCSE, adults and children with a blood glucose less than 60 mg/dL (3.3 mmol/L) should receive 50 mL of a 50% dextrose solution, and 1 mL/kg of a 25% dextrose solution, respectively.[2,6] Because Wernicke's encephalopathy can develop in alcoholics, adults should receive IV thiamine (100 mg) prior to glucose.[2] Serum glucose concentration should be determined to assess the need for further supplementation. For children younger than 12 to 18 months of age, a trial of pyridoxine (Vitamin B6) should be initiated until metabolic causes have been ruled out.

If infection is suspected, blood cultures, lumbar puncture, and urinalysis may be needed. Antibiotic administration does not need to wait until after the lumbar puncture if the patient is medically unstable. Patients with persistent GCSE should also have frequent arterial blood gas determinations to assess for metabolic acidosis, which should be treated with sodium bicarbonate if the pH is less than 7.2. Assisted ventilation should be used to correct respiratory acidosis.

Because electrical seizures may persist in the absence of overt clinical motor manifestations, an EEG should be performed in patients who continue to have altered consciousness after clinical control of their seizures. Patients with persistent GCSE should also have continuous EEG monitoring.

Pharmacologic Therapy: Impending and Established GCSE

When a seizure does not stop within 5 minutes, or when doubt exists regarding the diagnosis, patients should be treated as if they have GCSE (see Fig. 57-1). There are four immediate goals: (a) patient stabilization, including adequate oxygenation, preservation of cardiorespiratory function, and management of systemic complications; (b) accurate diagnosis of the subtype of GCSE and identification of precipitating factors; (c) termination of clinical and electrical seizures as early as possible; and (d) prevention of seizure recurrence. The benzodiazepines, hydantoins, and barbiturates are the most commonly used classes of anticonvulsants for the initial treatment of GCSE; however, there are no class I data to support recommendations for most anticonvulsants in established, refractory, and super-refractory GCSE.[16]

Benzodiazepines

The benzodiazepines are effective initial therapy in most patients and should be administered as soon as possible. Generally, one or two IV doses will terminate seizures within 2 to 3 minutes.[2,5] All benzodiazepines are effective; therefore, preference is determined by differences in pharmacokinetics, route of administration, pharmacoeconomics, adverse-effect profile, and current availability.

Diazepam is extremely lipophilic with a large volume of distribution (1-2 L/kg). Although it initially distributes into the brain within seconds, it rapidly redistributes into fat, causing its CNS half-life to be less than 1 hour and its duration of effect to be less than 30 minutes. The rapid decrease in brain concentration and pharmacoresistance can cause seizure recurrence; hence, a longer-acting anticonvulsant (eg, phenytoin or phenobarbital) should also be given immediately after diazepam. Dosing can be found in Table 57-4.

7 Most practitioners consider IV-administered lorazepam the benzodiazepine of choice for impending or established GCSE (see Table 57-4).[2,5] A Cochrane Database Review concluded that lorazepam is as effective, but safer than diazepam in children.[17] Another Cochrane Database Review that included pediatric and adults data noted no difference in death, requirements for ventilator support, or adverse effects between the two agents; however, when compared to diazepam, there was a significantly lower risk of persistent seizures with lorazepam.[18]

Lorazepam is less lipid soluble than diazepam and takes longer to achieve peak concentrations in the brain; however, its minimal redistribution into fat results in a longer duration of action in the CNS, which can provide seizure protection for up to 24 hours.[1,5] It also has a higher-affinity binding to the benzodiazepine receptor than diazepam.

Patients chronically on a benzodiazepine (eg, clobazam and clonazepam) might have developed tolerance and could require large doses. Diazepam and lorazepam contain propylene glycol, which can cause dysrhythmia and hypotension if administered too rapidly (Table 57-5). They also cause vein irritation; therefore, the parenteral product should be diluted with an equal volume of compatible diluent before administration. Because of slow and erratic absorption, standard parenteral formulations should not be given IM.

Unfortunately, there are insufficient data comparing IV lorazepam to IV midazolam in GCSE. Midazolam has an extremely short half-life, and maintenance doses must be given by continuous infusion (see Table 57-4). Because of its increased solubility, midazolam has a more reliable IM absorption than either diazepam or lorazepam. A recent study showed that when emergency personnel give IM midazolam as first-line treatment in the prehospital setting, it was superior to IV lorazepam for cessation of seizures, requirement for intensive care unit (ICU) admission, and subsequent hospitalization.[19] There was not a difference in recurrent seizures or adverse effects.

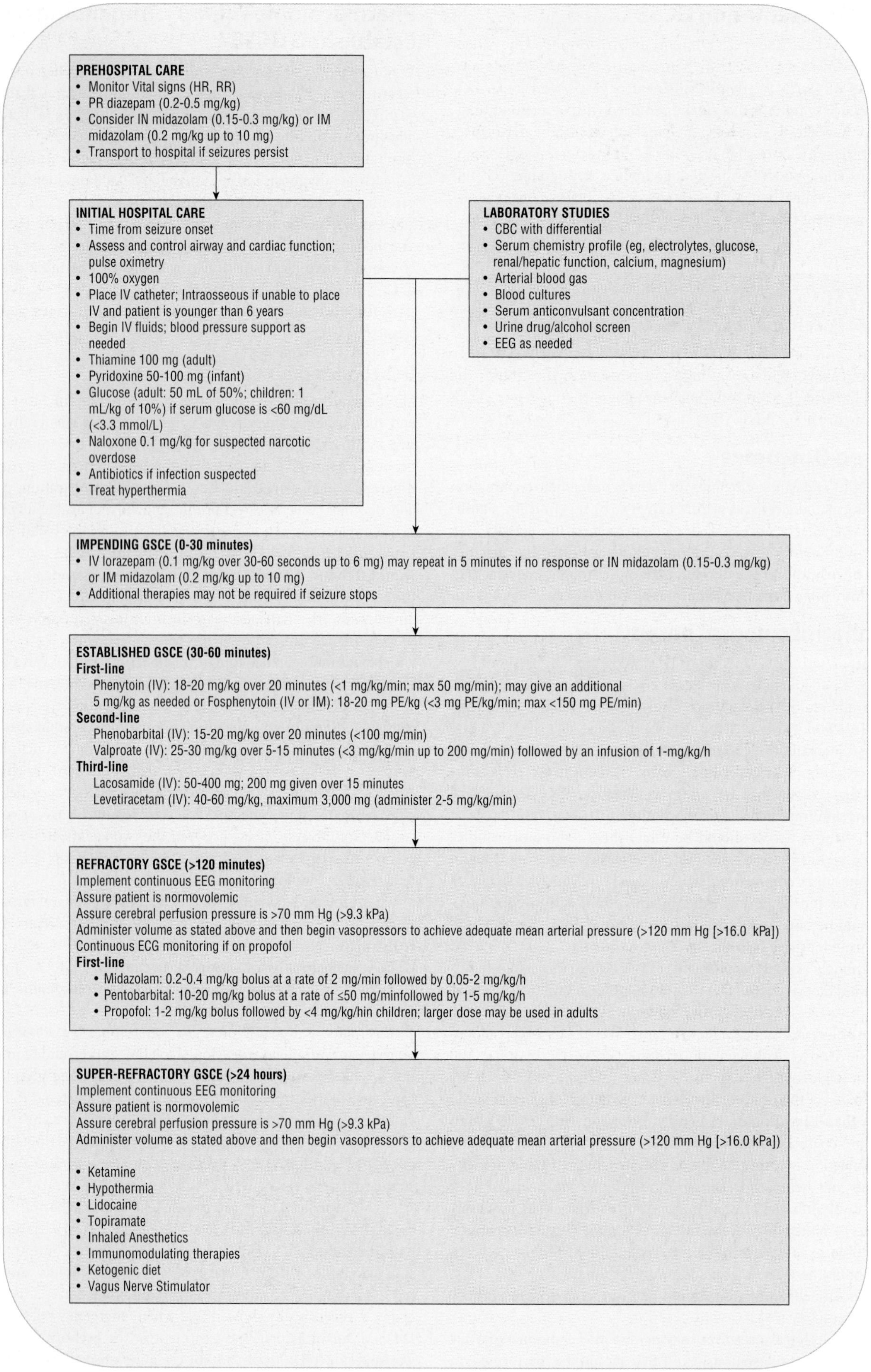

PREHOSPITAL CARE
- Monitor Vital signs (HR, RR)
- PR diazepam (0.2-0.5 mg/kg)
- Consider IN midazolam (0.15-0.3 mg/kg) or IM midazolam (0.2 mg/kg up to 10 mg)
- Transport to hospital if seizures persist

INITIAL HOSPITAL CARE
- Time from seizure onset
- Assess and control airway and cardiac function; pulse oximetry
- 100% oxygen
- Place IV catheter; Intraosseous if unable to place IV and patient is younger than 6 years
- Begin IV fluids; blood pressure support as needed
- Thiamine 100 mg (adult)
- Pyridoxine 50-100 mg (infant)
- Glucose (adult: 50 mL of 50%; children: 1 mL/kg of 10%) if serum glucose is <60 mg/dL (<3.3 mmol/L)
- Naloxone 0.1 mg/kg for suspected narcotic overdose
- Antibiotics if infection suspected
- Treat hyperthermia

LABORATORY STUDIES
- CBC with differential
- Serum chemistry profile (eg, electrolytes, glucose, renal/hepatic function, calcium, magnesium)
- Arterial blood gas
- Blood cultures
- Serum anticonvulsant concentration
- Urine drug/alcohol screen
- EEG as needed

IMPENDING GSCE (0-30 minutes)
- IV lorazepam (0.1 mg/kg over 30-60 seconds up to 6 mg) may repeat in 5 minutes if no response or IN midazolam (0.15-0.3 mg/kg) or IM midazolam (0.2 mg/kg up to 10 mg)
- Additional therapies may not be required if seizure stops

ESTABLISHED GSCE (30-60 minutes)

First-line

Phenytoin (IV): 18-20 mg/kg over 20 minutes (<1 mg/kg/min; max 50 mg/min); may give an additional 5 mg/kg as needed or Fosphenytoin (IV or IM): 18-20 mg PE/kg (<3 mg PE/kg/min; max <150 mg PE/min)

Second-line

Phenobarbital (IV): 15-20 mg/kg over 20 minutes (<100 mg/min)

Valproate (IV): 25-30 mg/kg over 5-15 minutes (<3 mg/kg/min up to 200 mg/min) followed by an infusion of 1-mg/kg/h

Third-line

Lacosamide (IV): 50-400 mg; 200 mg given over 15 minutes

Levetiracetam (IV): 40-60 mg/kg, maximum 3,000 mg (administer 2-5 mg/kg/min)

REFRACTORY GSCE (>120 minutes)

Implement continuous EEG monitoring

Assure patient is normovolemic

Assure cerebral perfusion pressure is >70 mm Hg (>9.3 kPa)

Administer volume as stated above and then begin vasopressors to achieve adequate mean arterial pressure (>120 mm Hg [>16.0 kPa])

Continuous ECG monitoring if on propofol

First-line
- Midazolam: 0.2-0.4 mg/kg bolus at a rate of 2 mg/min followed by 0.05-2 mg/kg/h
- Pentobarbital: 10-20 mg/kg bolus at a rate of ≤50 mg/minfollowed by 1-5 mg/kg/h
- Propofol: 1-2 mg/kg bolus followed by <4 mg/kg/hin children; larger dose may be used in adults

SUPER-REFRACTORY GSCE (>24 hours)

Implement continuous EEG monitoring

Assure patient is normovolemic

Assure cerebral perfusion pressure is >70 mm Hg (>9.3 kPa)

Administer volume as stated above and then begin vasopressors to achieve adequate mean arterial pressure (>120 mm Hg [>16.0 kPa])

- Ketamine
- Hypothermia
- Lidocaine
- Topiramate
- Inhaled Anesthetics
- Immunomodulating therapies
- Ketogenic diet
- Vagus Nerve Stimulator

FIGURE 57-1 **Algorithm for the treatment of GCSE.** BP, blood pressure; CBC, complete blood count; EEG, electroencephalogram; GCSE, generalized convulsive status epilepticus; HR, heart rate; PR, per rectum; RR, respiratory rate. [a]Because variability exists in dosing, monitor serum concentration. [b]If seizure is controlled, begin maintenance doses and optimize using serum concentration monitoring.

TABLE 57-4 Dosing of Medications Used in the Initial Treatment of GCSE

Drug (Route)	Brand name	Initial Dose (Maximum Dose)	Maintenance Dose	Comments
Diazepam (IV)	Valium plus generic			
Adult		0.25 mg/kg[a,b,c] (20 mg)	Not used	Given IV at a rate not to exceed 5 mg/min
Pediatric		0.25-0.5 mg/kg[a,c] (20 mg)	Not used	
Fosphenytoin (IV)	Cerebyx plus generic			
Adult		20-25 mg PE/kg	4-5 mg PE/kg/day	Given IV at a rate not to exceed 150 mg PE/min in adults and 3 mg PE/kg/min in pediatric patients
Pediatric		20-25 mg PE/kg	5-10 mg PE/kg/day	
Lorazepam (IV)	Ativan plus generic			
Adult		4 mg[b,c] (6 mg)	Not used	Given IV at a rate not to exceed 2 mg/min in adult and pediatric patients
Pediatric		0.1 mg/kg[a,c] (6 mg)	Not used	
Midazolam (IV, IM)	Versed plus generic			
Adult		200 mcg/kg[a,d] (10mg)	50-500 mcg/kg/h[e]	Given IV at a rate 0.5-1 mg/min in adults and over 2-3 minutes in pediatric patients
Pediatric		150 mcg/kg[a,d] (10 mg)	60-120 mcg/kg/h[e]	
Phenobarbital (IV)	Generic			
Adult		10-20 mg/kg[e]	1-4 mg/kg/day[e]	Given IV at a rate not to exceed 100 mg/min in adults and 30 mg/min in pediatric patients
Pediatric		15-20 mg/kg[e]	3-5 mg/kg/day[e]	
Phenytoin (IV)	Dilantin plus generic			
Adult		20-25 mg/kg[f]	4-5 mg/kg/day[e]	Given IV at a rate not to exceed 50 mg/min[g] in adults and 3 mg/kg/min (max 50 mg/min) in pediatric patients
Pediatric		20-25 mg/kg[f]	5-10 mg/kg/day[e]	

GCSE, generalized convulsive status epilepticus; PE, phenytoin equivalents.

[a]Doses can be repeated every 10 to 15 minutes until the maximum dosage is given.

[b]Initial doses in the elderly are 2 to 5 mg.

[c]Larger doses can be required if patients chronically on a benzodiazepine (eg, clonazepam).

[d]Can be given by the intramuscular, rectal, or buccal routes.

[e]Titrate dose as needed.

[f]Administer additional loading dose based on serum concentration.

[g]The rate should not exceed 25 mg/min in elderly patients and those with known atherosclerotic cardiovascular disease.

Recent studies have focused on aborting impending SE via transmucosally delivered benzodiazepine when IV and/or IM administration may be difficult or impossible (eg, home setting, extended care, and paramedic).[5,20] Benzodiazepines have been given via the rectal, intranasal, and buccal routes. Rectal absorption of diazepam is rapid but varies significantly (50%-100%) due to first-pass metabolism and is difficult to administer in the home environment. Buccal and sublingual routes also bypass gastric and hepatic first pass metabolism, but bioavailability can be incomplete as the drug is often swallowed. Buccal administration is easily accomplished, and the volume of fluid is small enough (eg, 2-5 mL) that aspiration is unlikely. While successful administration is unlikely due to muscular contractions of the jaw and clenching of teeth, a Cochrane Database Review concluded that buccal midazolam is more effective than rectal diazepam in children.[17]

Intranasally administrated benzodiazepines readily cross the nasal mucosa and the blood-brain barrier to produce a rapid rise in both serum and cerebrospinal fluid concentrations.[5,20] In fact, serum concentrations are comparable to those noted following IV injection. When compared to rectally administered diazepam, all studies have concluded that intranasal midazolam results in higher serum concentrations, faster onset of action, more effective seizure control and fewer adverse effects.[5]

Although most reports have used a variety of delivery systems (eg, drops, sprays, and atomization devices), the lack of standardization in delivery and availability of a commercial kit has not impacted efficacy. Because the dose must be administered in a 100 to 200 μL spray or solution, this route can only be used for products that are highly concentrated and have good aqueous solubility. It is imperative to account for medication that will remain in the dead space within the syringe and atomizer tip by overfilling the syringe with 0.1 mL of medication.

Medication should be drawn up at the time it is needed and not stored in a plastic syringe, as this may negatively impact efficacy as medication leaches into the plastic.

Effective delivery is best achieved by briskly compressing the syringe plunger to distribute the drug as a mist rather than as larger droplets that may aggregate and run out of the nose or down the back of the throat, rendering it ineffective.[20] By delivering *half* of the dose into each nostril the surface area available for absorption is doubled. Upper airway infections, the extent of nasal mucosa irritation, and differences in the amount of spray that is swallowed may all impact absorption. However, the variability in the amount absorbed after nasal administration should be comparable to that after oral administration.

Clinical **Controversy...**

The positioning of midazolam among the medications used to treat GCSE is changing. It is now recommended that midazolam be a first-line anticonvulsant for intramuscular (IM) or intranasal (IN) administration for out-of-hospital treatment, when IV access cannot be established. Its intranasal use in the hospital setting for the management of acute seizures is also increasing, and it may eventually replace IV administration in the emergency department.

Although rare, brief cardiorespiratory depression can necessitate assisted ventilation or require intubation (see Table 57-5).

TABLE 57-5 Adverse Drug Reactions and Monitoring of Patients Receiving Drugs for GCSE

Drug	Adverse Drug Reaction	Monitoring Parameters	Comments
Diazepam	Hypotension and cardiac arrhythmias	Vital signs and ECG during administration	Propylene glycol causes hypotension and cardiac arrhythmias when administered too rapidly; hypotension may occur with large doses
Fosphenytoin	Hypotension and cardiac arrhythmias; paresthesia, pruritus	Vital signs and ECG during administration	Hypotension is less than that noted with phenytoin, as this product does not contain propylene glycol; pruritus generally involves the face and groin areas, is dose and rate related, and subsides 5-10 minutes after infusion
Lidocaine	Fasciculations, visual disturbances, tinnitus, seizures		Occur at serum concentrations between 6 and 8 mg/L (25.6-34.1 μmol/L); seizures >8 mg/L (>34.1 μmol/L)
Lorazepam	Apnea, hypotension, bradycardia, cardiac arrest, respiratory depression, metabolic acidosis, and renal toxicity	Vital signs and ECG during administration; HCO_3 and serum creatinine; cumulative dose of propylene glycol	Accumulation of propylene glycol during prolong continuous infusions may cause acidosis
Pentobarbital	Hypotension	Vital signs and ECG during administration	Rate of infusion should be slower or dopamine should be added if hypotension occurs
Phenytoin	Hypotension and cardiac arrhythmia; nystagmus	Vital signs and ECG during administration	Propylene glycol causes hypotension and cardiac arrhythmias when administered too rapidly. Large loading doses are generally not given to elderly individuals with preexisting cardiac disease or in critically ill patients with marginal blood pressure. The infusion rate should be slowed if the QT interval widens or if hypotension or arrhythmias develop; horizontal nystagmus suggests serum concentration above the reference range and toxicity; if a serum phenytoin concentration validates this, the dose should be decreased
Phenobarbital	Hypotension, respiratory, and CNS depression	Vital signs and mental status; EEG if used in anesthesia doses	Contains propylene glycol; if hypotension occurs, slow the rate of administration or begin dopamine; apnea and hypopnea can be more profound in patients treated initially with benzodiazepines
Propofol	Progressive metabolic acidosis, hemodynamic instability, and bradyarrhythmias	Vital signs, ECG, osmolar gap; EEG if used in anesthesia doses	Referred to as propofol-related infusion syndrome, which can be fatal
Topiramate	Metabolic acidosis	Acid base status (serum bicarbonate)	Extremely rare

CNS, central nervous system; ECG, electrocardiogram; EEG, electroencephalogram.

This is especially true if a benzodiazepine is used concomitantly with a barbiturate; however, cardiorespiratory depression is more likely due to ongoing seizures than benzodiazepines. Hypotension secondary to a reduction in vasomotor tone can occur following large doses.[5]

Clinical **Controversy...**

The choice of which long-acting anticonvulsant to give following the initial benzodiazepine is controversial. For decades phenytoin has been used to prevent and treat seizures that recur after treatment with a benzodiazepine; however, no studies have documented the superiority of a hydantoin over other anticonvulsants. One meta-analysis concluded that evidence does not support the use of phenytoin as a first-line agent. Thus, it is questionable if a hydantoin should be administered alone, in larger doses, or at all when seizures recur following benzodiazepine administration.

Phenytoin

8 A hydantoin is the second-line agent in GCSE that is unresponsive to the benzodiazepines or in seizures that recur after successful treatment with a benzodiazepine.[2,21] It is effective in terminating seizures when first-line agents fail and continue to be recommended for this purpose in recent guidelines[21]; however, it has been noted to be inferior to lorazepam, phenobarbital, or diazepam plus phenytoin at stopping GCSE within 20 minutes of infusion.[22,23] Despite a meta-analysis that concluded evidence does not support the use of phenytoin as a first or second-line agent,[24] it continues to be used.

Phenytoin has a long half-life (20-36 hours) and causes less respiratory depression and sedation than the benzodiazepines or phenobarbital; however, it cannot be delivered rapidly enough to be considered a first-line single agent.[2,5] Injectable phenytoin should be diluted to less than or equal to 5 mg/mL in normal saline. Microcrystals will precipitate if it is mixed in a glucose-containing solution. The vehicle (40% propylene glycol) can cause administration-related hypotension and cardiac arrhythmias (see Table 57-5). For this reason, the maximum rate of infusion is limited (see Table 57-4).

Suggested IV loading doses are provided in Table 57-4. A reduction in the loading dose is recommended for elderly patients, and a larger loading dose is required in obese individuals.[25] If the patient has been on phenytoin prior to admission and the serum concentration is known, this should be considered in determining a loading dose. Although some advocate the administration of an additional 5 mg/kg dose in those with unresponsive GCSE, there is no evidence that this will be beneficial. This practice can cause concentrations to exceed the reference range and produce toxicity. Because phenytoin has poor lipid solubility and enters the brain slowly, it can take up to 60 minutes before the pharmacodynamic effect is apparent. This delay is important when considering administration of a second loading dose. Therapeutic serum concentrations, 10 to 20 mg/L (40-79 μmol/L), generally do not persist more than 24 hours; hence, maintenance doses (see Table 57-4) should be started within 12 to 24 hours of the loading dose.

Phenytoin has an alkaline pH, which may cause pain and burning during infusion; phlebitis can occur with chronic infusion, and tissue necrosis is likely on infiltration. IM administration is not recommended because absorption is delayed and erratic, and phenytoin can crystallize in tissue. Although oral loading doses have been used in patients not actively seizing, it may take 4 to 12 hours before adequate serum concentrations are obtained; thus, this practice is not recommended.

Fosphenytoin

Fosphenytoin, a water-soluble phosphate ester, has no known pharmacologic activity. It is converted rapidly (7-15 minutes) and completely (100%) to phenytoin by blood and tissue phosphatases after IV and IM dosing.[26] The conversion delay was a concern initially; however, this time is offset by high protein binding, saturable binding at high concentrations, and the rapid rate of infusion.[26] It does not contain propylene glycol and is compatible with most common IV fluids.

Fosphenytoin should be dosed using phenytoin equivalents (PE), thereby obviating the need for interconversion between phenytoin and fosphenytoin. The loading dose and rates of administration of fosphenytoin can be found in Table 57-4. Because of delays in achieving adequate phenytoin serum concentrations, a loading dose should not be given IM unless IV access is impossible.

Fosphenytoin serum concentrations have no value. Serum phenytoin concentrations should be used for therapeutic drug monitoring, and the desired serum concentration range is the same as that for phenytoin. Fosphenytoin cross reacts with some phenytoin immunoassays causing an overestimation of phenytoin concentration; hence, blood should not be obtained for at least 2 hours after IV and 4 hours after IM administration.[26]

Phenobarbital

Phenobarbital has biphasic distribution into body organs. During phase I, the drug distributes into highly vascular organs, but does not distribute into the brain. With the exception of fat, phenobarbital distributes throughout the body during phase II; hence, lean body mass should be used in calculating doses in obese patients.[27] Although the highest brain concentrations occur 12 to 60 minutes after an IV dose,[27] seizures are controlled within minutes of the loading dose.[23] Despite two studies that found phenobarbital to be as effective as phenytoin, lorazepam, or diazepam plus phenytoin in patients with GCSE,[22,23] and a meta-analysis noting that no evidence to support the use of phenytoin as a first-line agent[24] phenobarbital continues to be given after a benzodiazepine plus phenytoin has failed.

The loading and maintenance dose are given in Table 57-4. When necessary, larger loading doses (30 mg/kg) have been used in neonates without adverse effects. If the initial loading dose does not stop the seizures within 20 to 30 minutes, an additional 10 to 20 mg/kg can be given. If seizures continue, a third 10 mg/kg load can be given.[28] Phenobarbital exhibits first-order linear pharmacokinetics, and there is no maximum dose beyond which further doses are likely to be ineffective. Once GCSE is controlled, the maintenance dose should be started within 12 to 24 hours. Although injectable phenobarbital contains propylene glycol, it can be given more rapidly than phenytoin (see Table 57-4). While it can be given IM, its rate of absorption is too slow to be effective. Adverse drug reactions and monitoring can be found in Table 57-5.[2,5]

Pharmacologic Therapy: Refractory GCSE

9 When adequate doses of a benzodiazepine, hydantoin, or barbiturate have failed, the condition is termed *refractory*.[5] Approximately 10% to 15% of patients will develop refractory GCSE, and approximately 30% whose seizures are "clinically" controlled will have persistent electrical manifestations after administration of these anticonvulsants. When a patient develops refractory GCSE, an intense search should be performed for an acute or progressive cause.

While the goal is to stop electrical epileptiform activity, there is no consensus regarding the anticonvulsant of choice, sequencing of therapy, or treatment of refractory GCSE. Most recommend the administration of anesthetic doses of midazolam, pentobarbital, or propofol, while other approaches include the use of valproate, levetiracetam, lacosamide, or topiramate. Doses for these agents can be found in Table 57-6.

Benzodiazepines

Although time-dependent pharmacoresistance to benzodiazepines may occur in refractory GCSE, some advocate that anesthetic doses of midazolam should be the first-line agent in refractory GCSE. Table 57-6 shows the loading and maintenance doses of midazolam.[29] Most patients respond to these doses within an hour. Most studies used termination of seizures on EEG as the endpoint for success; however, EEG burst suppression is rarely achieved with the recommended doses of midazolam. Tachyphylaxis rapidly develops within 24 to 48 hours; hence, the dose is often increased to prevent seizure relapse.[5]

Clinical **Controversy...**

During prolonged seizures the number of γ_2 and $\beta_{2\text{-}3}$ subunits on the $GABA_A$ receptors decrease as the receptors move from the synaptic membrane into the cytoplasm where they are functionally inactive. These modifications may decrease effectiveness of both endogenous GABA and GABA agonists and result in time-dependent pharmacoresistance to benzodiazepines. Following SE that persist more than 30 minutes, the relative potencies of benzodiazepines can be reduced up to 20-fold. For this reason, some believe that that anesthetic doses of midazolam should be the first-line agent in refractory GCSE. If a benzodiazepine is used, it should always be combined with another drug that acts at a different site.

After initial control, seizures have been observed to recur in 6% to 19% of patients. There is no specific protocol for tapering of midazolam, but some suggest a seizure-free period of 24 to 48 hours followed by decreasing by 1 to 2 mcg/kg/min every 15 minutes.[5] Maintaining the patient's phenytoin and phenobarbital serum concentration(s) above 20 mg/L (79 μmol/L) and 40 mg/L (172 μmol/L), respectively enhances successful discontinuation.

Because of midazolam's short half-life, patients can return to consciousness more rapidly than those receiving larger doses of more sedating anticonvulsants (eg, phenytoin and phenobarbital). Generally, continuous-infusion midazolam has been well tolerated, with few cases of hypotension and respiratory depression. Hypotension and poikilothermia can occur and can require supportive therapies. When adverse effects do occur, patients recover quickly. The availability of a pharmacological antidote for benzodiazepines, flumazenil, lends to the safe use of midazolam.

Valproate

The IV dosage form approved by the FDA is not labeled for GCSE. IV valproate and continuous infusion diazepam are comparable in GCSE.[29,30] One meta-analysis noted that valproate controlled refractory SE sooner than diazepam; however, there was no difference within 30 minutes of administration.[31] There was also no difference in control of GCSE between valproate and phenytoin.[32] A second meta-analysis noted that there is sufficient evidence to use valproate as first-line therapy in those with SE refractory to benzodiazepines.

TABLE 57-6 Dosing of Medications Used to Treat Refractory or Supr-Refractory GCSE

Drug (Brand Name)	Initial Dose (Maximum Dose)	Maintenance Dose	Comments
Ketamine (generics)			
Adult	1-4 mg	1-5 mg/kg/h	
Pediatric	0.5-2 mg/kg	1-10 mg/kg/h	
Lacosamide (Vimpat)			
Adult	200-400 mg	200 mg bid	Administer IV over 15 minutes, monitor serum concentrations
Pediatric	4-6 mg/kg	6-8 mg/kg/day, given twice a day	
Levetiracetam (Keppra plus generics)			
Adult	2,000-3,000 mg	1,000 mg thrice a day	Administer IV over 5-15 minutes
Pediatric	40-60 mg/kg	40-60 mg/kg/day, given twice or thrice a day	
Lidocaine (generics)			
Adult	50-100 mg	1.5-3.5 mg/kg/h	Administer IV in ≤2 minutes
Pediatric	1 mg/kg (maximum 3-5 mg/kg in the first hour)	1.2-3 mg/kg/h	
Midazolam (Versed plus generic)			
Adult	200 mcg/kg[a]	50-500 mcg/kg/h[b]	Initial dose may be given IM; administer IV over 0.5-1 mg/min; continuous-infusion rate should be increased every 15 minutes in those who do not respond and should be guided by EEG response; development of tachyphylaxis can require frequent increases in dose; decrease dose by 1 mcg/kg/min every 2 hours once GCSE is controlled
pediatric	150 mcg/kg[a]	60-120 mcg/kg/h[b]	
Pentobarbital (generics)			
Adult	10-20 mg/kg	1-5 mg/kg/h[b]	Over 1-2 hours, rate of infusion should be slowed or dopamine should be added if hypotension occurs; gradually titrate dose upward until there is evidence of burst suppression on EEG (ie, isoelectric EEG) or prohibitive adverse effects occur. Twelve hours after a burst suppression is obtained, the rate should be titrated downward every 2-4 hours
Pediatric	15-20 mg/kg	1-5 mg/kg/h[b]	
Propofol (Diprivan plus generic)			
Adult	2 mg/kg	5-10 mg/kg/h[b]	Over 10 seconds in adults and 20-30 seconds in pediatric patients
Pediatric	3 mg/kg	2-4 mg/kg/h[c]	
Topiramate (Topamax plus generic)			
Adult	300-500 mg	400-1,600 mg/day	Given orally in divided dose every 12 hours. Doses as large as 25 mg/kg/day for 2-5 days have been used in children. Monitor serum bicarbonate levels and serum concentrations
Pediatric	5-10 mg/kg	5-10 mg/kg/day, given thrice a day	
Valproate (Depacon plus generic)			
Adult	15-30 mg/kg	1-4 mg/kg/h[b]	Administer at 3 mg/kg/min; and follow by a continuous or intermittent infusion; larger doses may be required in those on hepatic enzyme inducers, monitor serum concentrations
Pediatric	20-25 mg/kg	1-4 mg/kg/h[b], or give every 4-6 hour	

EEG, electroencephalogram; GCSE, generalized convulsive status epilepticus; IM, intramuscular; IV, intravenous.

[a]Doses can be repeated twice at 10 to 15 minute intervals until the maximum dosage is given.

[b]Titrate dose as needed.

[c]Generally recommended not to exceed a dose of 4 mg/kg/h and a duration of 48 hours.

A number of loading and continuous-infusion doses (see Table 57-5) have been used in both adult and pediatric patients. Although the manufacturer originally recommended IV valproate be given no faster than 20 mg/min, much faster rates have been studied (40 mg/min; 2-10 mg/kg/min) and are used for administration of the loading dose. One study suggested the need to consider the effects of enzyme-inducing anticonvulsants when dosing and recommended that the continuous-infusion rate be determined by the presence of concurrent anticonvulsants (no inducers present, 1 mg/kg/h; one or more inducers [eg, phenytoin and phenobarbital], 2 mg/kg/h; and inducers and pentobarbital coma, 4 mg/kg/h).[33] In general, IV valproate has been well tolerated, with no cases of respiratory depression. Hemodynamic instability is extremely rare, but patients' vital signs should be monitored closely during the loading dose for hypotension.

Clinical **Controversy...**

The role and position of the newer anticonvulsants as first-line agents in SE remains controversial. At this time, evidence supports the use of valproate and levetiracetam in refractory SE. Insufficient evidence exists to support using lacosamide and topiramate. That said, selection of an agent is complicated by the shortages in the availability of some first-line medications. There is a clear consensus that if the traditional antiepileptic drug does not work, an anesthetic agent may be indicated.

Levetiracetam and Lacosamide

Historically, levetiracetam was used in cases of super-refractory SE, but it is being used earlier due to medication shortages that have made traditional drugs unavailable. IV levetiracetam has been used for GCSE and has been noted to be as effective as IV lorazepam in aborting seizures and preventing recurrence.[34-36] When compared to phenytoin, levetiracetam was equally effective at terminating seizures and preventing recurrence at 24 hours.[36] One meta-analysis noted that sufficient evidence exist to support the use of levetiracetam as first-line therapy in those refractory to benzodiazepines.[24] Levetiracetam is not hepatically metabolized and is minimally protein bound, which makes drug–drug interactions unlikely. Doses for IV levetiracetam are noted in Table 57-5. Doses larger than 3,000 mg/day do not increase efficacy.

Although effective in refractory GCSE, literature supporting the use of lacosamide comes from case reports or case series. Two meta-analyses noted there is insufficient evidence to support the routine use of lacosamide in benzodiazepine-resistant GCSE.[24,37,38]

Pentobarbital

If the patient has refractory disease, anesthetizing the patient to suppress the cerebral ictal discharge is recommended.[5,21] Although it is likely that the patient is already being mechanically ventilated, intubation and respiratory support are mandatory during barbiturate coma, along with continuous EEG monitoring (see Table 57-5). A short-acting barbiturate (ie, pentobarbital or thiopental) is preferred because it allows a more rapid reversal of coma.

Although barbiturates are frequently used, there are no controlled trials to support this practice. A meta-analysis comparing studies involving midazolam, propofol, and pentobarbital in refractory GCSE found overall response rates were significantly greater in those treated with pentobarbital compared to midazolam or propofol.[39] The recurrence of seizures was also less frequent with pentobarbital and propofol. Mortality rates were similar for the three drugs, but significant hypotension was more common with pentobarbital.

Several sources note that the initial loading dose of pentobarbital is 5 mg/kg; however, this dose is inadequate to achieve the serum concentrations (40 mg/L; 172 μmol/L) necessary to induce an isoelectric EEG (see Table 57-6).[37] Although the duration of barbiturate coma in most studies has been 2 to 3 days, it has been used safely for 53 days in an 18-year-old patient.[40] To avoid complications (eg, pneumonia and pulmonary edema), pentobarbital should be discontinued as soon as possible. The risk of seizure recurrence is minimized if other anticonvulsants are at therapeutic concentrations before pentobarbital is withdrawn. Because pentobarbital is a potent hepatic enzyme inducer, doses of most concurrent anticonvulsants will need to be larger than usual maintenance doses, and the patient will need to be monitored for side effects as deinduction occurs and anticonvulsant concentrations increase. This can take up to 1 month after pentobarbital's discontinuation.

Propofol

Propofol is extremely lipid soluble, has a large volume of distribution, and has a very rapid onset of action. Its extremely short half-life promotes easy titration and rapid awakening on drug discontinuation. Although several studies have compared propofol and barbiturates, most studies were underpowered. Its efficacy appears to be comparable to midazolam for refractory GCSE.[39,41] Propofol is given as a loading dose that is followed by a continuous infusion. The loading dose can be repeated every 3 to 5 minutes until the desired clinical response is obtained. Once EEG burst suppression is achieved, the dose should be reduced.

Adverse drug reactions can be found in Table 57-6. Prolonged infusions greater than 4 mg/kg/h have been associated with propofol-related infusion syndrome (PRIS).[42,43] Signs and symptoms of PRIS include progressive metabolic acidosis, hemodynamic instability, and bradyarrhythmias that are refractory to aggressive pharmacological treatments. It may occur with or without the presence of hepatomegaly, rhabdomyolysis, or lipemia. A retrospective case series of 41 patients with refractory GCSE noted that 10% had sudden unexplained cardiorespiratory arrests, and 35% had non-life-threatening features of PRIS.[43] Propofol may be proconvulsant in some patients and involuntary myoclonic movements have been reported.

Vital signs, should be carefully monitored, and continuous electrocardiogram (ECG) should assess for dysrhythmias. While no guidelines have been proposed for laboratory monitoring, it would seem advisable to assess serum lactic acid, serum triglycerides, serum creatinine, creatine kinase, and hepatic enzymes in patients receiving doses larger than 4 mg/kg/h and/or those receiving therapy for more than 48 hours.

Pharmacologic Therapy: Super-Refractory GCSE

Ketamine

Because medications targeting GABA may be less effective in prolonged GCSE, NMDA-targeted agents such as ketamine have been investigated. Ketamine may increase the number of NMDA receptor to increase glutamate's effect and may also possesses an antagonistic effect on NMDA receptors. A summary of the findings appears in recently published review papers.[5,44] Ketamine appears to be a reasonable agent to consider in refractory GCSE that has failed general anesthesia, especially in those with cardiac instability. Doses can be found in Table 57-6. An advantage of ketamine is its ability to maintain arterial blood pressure, pulse rate, and cardiac output. It may cause hallucinations upon awakening, increased salivation, and increased intraocular and intracranial pressures.

Topiramate

Topiramate has been given orally in adults and in children with GCSE and should be implemented at full therapeutic doses and divided three times a day (see Table 57-6).[5,45] To administer nasogastrically, the tablets should be crushed, mixed with water, and administered via syringe into the nasogastric tube. Response tends to be delayed hours to days. Once seizures are controlled, the dose should be tapered to a normal age/weight-appropriate maintenance dosage.

Aggressive implementation of large doses may cause hyperchloremic, non-anion gap, metabolic acidosis due to inhibition of type II and IV carbonic anhydrase enzymes. Dose does not appear to be the sole determinate, as it has been noted following small doses and after overdoses. If metabolic acidosis occurs, it can be treated with citrates, with a goal of maintaining a serum bicarbonate of at least 20 mEq/L (mmol//L).[5]

Lidocaine

Currently, weak evidence supports the use of lidocaine in refractory or supra-refractory SE. Lidocaine has been used in refractory GCSE, but is not recommended unless other agents have failed.[46] It is administered IV (see Table 57-5) and has a rapid onset of action. Although the reference serum concentration range for the antiarrhythmic effects of lidocaine is 2 to 6 mg/L (8.5-25.6 μmol/L), the reference range for GCSE has not been established. Serum lidocaine concentrations should be monitored to avoid drug accumulation and toxicity (see Table 57-6).

Inhaled Anesthetics

Today inhaled anesthetics are not used until other approaches fail, and only a few studies have used inhaled anesthetics (particularly isoflurane) for the treatment of refractory SE.[47,48] Halothane, isoflurane, and other inhaled anesthetics can produce EEG suppression; however, these gases are difficult to deliver outside the operating room and require an anesthesiologist. No proven advantages have been shown over traditional anticonvulsants (eg, barbiturate coma or continuous-infusion benzodiazepine), and these gases can increase intracranial pressure. If used, dosing is titrated to obtain EEG burst suppression.

Although concentrations required to maintain burst suppression are variable, isoflurane generally stops seizure at concentrations of 0.5% to 3%, which are not ordinarily associated with hemodynamic effects. Isoflurane can induce hypotension, so close hemodynamic monitoring is necessary, with administration of isotonic fluids and vasopressors as needed.

Immunomodulating therapies

The use of corticosteroids and IV immune globulin is based upon animal data that suggest the development of super-refractory GCSE may be due to antibodies directed against the voltage-gated potassium channels and the NMDA receptor.[48] There is also mounting evidence that inflammation plays a role in epileptogenesis, specifically the activation of select inflammatory signaling pathways (eg, interleukin-1 receptor/toll-like receptor [IL-1R/TLR]). Steroids may also decrease blood-brain barrier opening and reverse GABAergic inhibition.

Little evidence supports the use of steroids; however, in the absence of contraindications, a trial of large doses of steroids (eg, 1 g/day of IV prednisolone for 3 days followed by 1 mg/kg/day in four divided doses) should be used in patients with an unidentified etiology for the super-refractory GCSE. Patients who respond should continue long-term steroids, IV immunoglobulins, and other immunomodulatory agents such as cyclophosphamide or rituximab.

Hypothermia

Controlled hypothermia reduces excitatory transmission and epileptic discharges and reduces brain edema, cerebral metabolic rate, oxygen utilization, and ATP consumption. Few studies have assessed the efficacy or safety of hypothermia in refractory GCSE.[47,49-51] Despite a resurgence in use, a recent meta-analysis suggested that only level D evidence supports the use of hypothermia in refractory SE.[52]

When used, a core body temperature of about 32°C to 35°C is targeted for at least 24 to 48 hours. It may or may not be given in combination with barbiturate anesthetics.[47] Cardiovascular and coagulation parameters, biochemistry and acid-base balance, and serum lactate should be monitored. Hypothermia may significantly reduce the clearance of several drugs, including anesthetics and antiepileptics, resulting in a need for monitoring of serum concentrations.[5]

Ketogenic Diet

A small number of reports have shown that an orally or intravenously administered ketogenic diet in a 4:1 ratio of fat to combined protein and carbohydrate should be tried in severe cases of super-refractory SE.[47,52] Before initiating the diet, metabolic disorders as a possible etiology should be eliminated. Close monitoring of total daily fluid, ketosis, and potential complications is essential. If a metabolic acidosis develops, treatment is suggested to maintain serum bicarbonate levels greater than 18 to 20 mEq/L (mmol/L).[47]

Vagus Nerve Stimulator

Acute placement of a vagus nerve stimulator has been used in both pediatric and adult patients with refractory SE.[48] Currently its use for refractory SE is not recommended, as only grade D evidence suggest improvement in generalized refractory SE.[53]

PERSONALIZED PHARMACOTHERAPY

If the patient has been on phenytoin, phenobarbital, valproate, or levetiracetam prior to admission, a stat serum concentration should be obtained and the results considered in determining a loading dose or redosing. A serum concentration should be obtained in any patient who is unresponsive to therapy or who exhibits concentration-associated adverse drug reactions. Pharmacogenetics produces differences in metabolic pathways and rate of drug metabolism, which can influence efficacy or toxicity. Obviously, a patient who is a poor metabolizer would theoretically have changes in drug metabolism based on expression of specific isoenzymes. For example, many Asians have decreased CYP2C19 activity; therefore, they may respond to lower doses of diazepam. If one were concerned about benzodiazepine-associated adverse effects in this population, lorazepam would be preferred.

Although a patient may have an alteration in gene expression that could be important in development of refractory SE or in response to various anticonvulsants, there are no data to support that this is important in GCSE and no evidence to support a change in treatment protocol based on underlying genetics.

While HLA-B*1502 has been associated with severe skin reactions in patients receiving phenytoin, this is applicable to chronic and not acute, single dose therapy. Recently, CYP2C variants that included CYP2C9*3, which is known to reduce drug clearance, were identified as important genetic factors associated with phenytoin-related severe cutaneous adverse reactions.[54]

Drug resistance factors have also been identified in human epileptogenic tissue that has been removed surgically. Multidrug resistance proteins (P-glycoprotein) are localized to endothelial cells in brain capillaries and associated astroglia. Since multidrug resistance factors are localized to abnormal tissues, they appear to have little or no effect on systemic pharmacokinetic parameters of a drug, but may affect the local distribution of the drug within the target epileptogenic areas. If a role in refractory human epilepsy is confirmed, drugs that inhibit P-glycoprotein (eg, verapamil) may prove useful. That said, no reports have suggested that such an association exists.

EVALUATION OF THERAPEUTIC OUTCOMES

Initial success is defined as termination of all clinical and electrical seizure activity, but ultimate success is measured by the patient's subsequent quality of life. The morbidity and mortality associated with GCSE are affected by the underlying etiology; however, morbidity and mortality can be minimized by the rapid implementation of a rational therapeutic plan. An EEG is an extremely important tool that not only allows practitioners to determine when abnormal electrical activity has been aborted, but also can assist in determining which anticonvulsant was effective. Because many of the anticonvulsants affect the cardiorespiratory system, it is imperative that vital signs (eg, heart rate, respiratory rate, and blood pressure) be monitored during drug loading and infusion. Finally, it is imperative that the infusion site be assessed for any evidence of infiltration before and during administration of phenytoin. Information regarding the patient's past medical and drug history and imaging studies (eg, MRI) also can help to determine if there is a defined etiology for the original episode of GCSE. This information then can be used to guide future medication therapy, as well as help in determining if the patient is at risk for a poor outcome.

ABBREVIATIONS

AMPA	α-amino-3-hydroxy-5-methyl-isoxazole-4-propionate
CNS	central nervous system
CT	computed tomography
ECG	electrocardiogram
EEG	electroencephalogram, electroencephalography
GABA	γ-aminobutyric acid
GCSE	generalized convulsive status epilepticus
ICU	intensive care unit
IL-1R/TLR	interleukin-1 receptor/toll-like receptor
ILAE	International League Against Epilepsy

IM	intramuscular
IN	intranasal
IV	intravenous
MRI	magnetic resonance imaging
NCSE	nonconvulsive status epilepticus
NMDA	N-methyl-D-aspartate
PE	phenytoin equivalents
PRIS	propofol-related infusion syndrome
SE	status epilepticus

REFERENCES

1. Trinka E, Cock H, Hesdorffer D, et al. A definition and classification of status epilepticus—Report of the ILAE Task Force on Classification of Status Epilepticus. *Epilepsia* 2015;56(10):1515-1523. doi: 10.1111/epi.13121.
2. Lowenstein DH, Alldredge BK. Status epilepticus. *N Engl J Med* 1998;338:970-976.
3. DeLorenzo RJ, Garnett LK, Towne AR, et al. Comparison of status epilepticus with prolonged seizure episodes lasting from 10 to 29 minutes. *Epilepsia* 1999;40:164-169.
4. Maganti R, Gerber P, Drees C, Chung S. Nonconvulsive status epilepticus. *Epilepsy Behav* 2008;12:572-586.
5. Alford EL, Wheless JW, Phelps SJ. Treatment of generalized convulsive status epilepticus in pediatric patients. *J Pediatr Pharmacol Ther* 2015;20:260-289.
6. DeLorenzo RJ, Pellock JM, Towne AR, Boggs J. Epidemiology of status epilepticus. *J Clin Neurophysiol* 1995;12:316-325.
7. Shorvon S. The management of status epilepticus. *J Neurol Neurosurg Psychiatry* 2001;70(Suppl 2):II22-II27.
8. DeLorenzo RJ, Towne AR, Pellock JM, Ko D. Status epilepticus in children, adults, and the elderly. *Epilepsia* 1992;33:S15-S25.
9. Pitkanen A. Efficacy of current antiepileptics to prevent neurodegeneration in epilepsy models. *Epilepsy Res* 2002;50:141-160.
10. Wasterlain CG, Mazarati AM, Naylor D, et al. Short-term plasticity of hippocampal neuropeptides and neuronal circuitry in experimental status epilepticus. *Epilepsia* 2002;45(Suppl 5):20-29.
11. Temkin NR. Antiepileptogenesis and seizure prevention trials with anti-epileptic drugs: Meta-analysis of controlled trials. *Epilepsia* 2001;42:515-524.
12. Singh RK, Gaillard WD. Status epilepticus in children. *Curr Neurol Neurosci Rep* 2009;9:137-144.
13. Wasterlain CG, Chen JWY. Mechanistic and pharmacologic aspects of status epilepticus and its treatment with new antiepileptic drugs. *Epilepsia* 2008;49:63-73.
14. Pitkänen A, Nehlig A, Brooks-Kayal AR, et al. Issues related to development of antiepileptogenic therapies. *Epilepsia* 201;54(Suppl 4): 35-43.
15. Lothman E. The biochemical basis and pathophysiology of status epilepticus. *Neurology* 1990;40:13-23.
16. Trinka E, Höfler J, Leitinger M, Brigo F. Pharmacotherapy for status epilepticus. *Drugs* 2015;75:1499-1521.
17. Appleton R, Macleod S, Martland T. Drug management for acute tonic–clonic convulsions including convulsive status epilepticus in children. *Cochrane Database Syst Rev* 2008;3:CD001905.
18. Prasad M, Krishnan PR, Sequeira R, Al-Roomi K. Anticonvulsant therapy for status epilepticus. *Cochrane Database Syst Rev* 2014;9:1-88.
19. Shlbergleit R, Durkalski V, Lowenstein D, et al. Intramuscular versus intravenous therapy for prehospital status epilepticus. *N Engl J Med* 2012;366:591-600.
20. Humphries LK, Eiland LS. Treatment of acute seizures: Is intranasal midazolam a viable option? *J Pediatr Pharmacol Ther* 2013;18:79-87.
21. Capovilla G, Beccaria F, Beghi E, et al. Treatment of convulsive status epilepticus in childhood: Recommendations of the Italian League Against Epilepsy. *Epilepsia* 2013;54(Suppl 7):23-34.
22. Shaner DM, McCurdy SA, Herring MO, Gabor AJ. Treatment of status epilepticus: A prospective comparison of diazepam and phenytoin versus phenobarbital and optional phenytoin. *Neurology* 1988;38:202-207.
23. Treiman DM, Meyers PD, Walton NY, et al. A comparison of four treatments for generalized convulsive status epilepticus. Veterans Affairs Status Epilepticus Cooperative Study Group. *N Engl J Med* 1998;339:792-798.
24. Yasiry Z, Shorvon SD. The relative effectiveness of five antiepileptic drugs in treatment of benzodiazepine-resistant convulsive status epilepticus: A meta-analysis of published studies. *Seizure* 2014;2:167-174.
25. Abernethy DR, Greenblatt DJ. Phenytoin disposition in obesity: Determination of loading dose. *Arch Neurol* 1985;42:468-471.
26. Fischer JH, Patel TV, Fischer PA. Fosphenytoin: Clinical pharmacokinetics and comparative advantages in the acute treatment of seizures. *Clin Pharmacokinet* 2003;42:33-58.
27. Dodson WE, Rust RS. Phenobarbital: Absorption, distribution, and excretion. In: Levy R, Mattson R, Meldrum B, eds. *Antiepileptic Drugs*. 4th ed. New York: Raven Press; 1995:379-387.
28. Crawford TO, Mitchell WG, Fishman LS, Snodgrass SR. Very-high-dose phenobarbital for refractory status epilepticus in children. *Neurology* 1988;38:1035-1040.
29. Abend NS, Diugos DJ. Treatment of refractory status epilepticus: Literature review and a proposed protocol. *Pediatr Neurol* 2008;38:377-390.
30. Chen WB, Gao R, Su Y, et al. Valproate versus diazepam for generalized status epilepticus: A pilot study. *Eur J Neurol* 2011;18:1391-1396.
31. Mehta V, Singhi P, Singhi S. Intravenous sodium valproate versus diazepam infusion for the control of refractory status epilepticus in children: A randomized controlled trial. *J Child Neurol* 2007;22:1191-1197.
32. Liu X, Wu Y, Chen Z, et al. A systematic review of randomized controlled trials on the therapeutic effect of intravenous sodium valproate in status epilepticus. *Int J Neurosci* 2012;12:277-283.
33. Hovinga CA, Chicella MF, Rose DF, et al. Use of IV valproate in three pediatric patients with nonconvulsive or convulsive status epilepticus. *Ann Pharmacother* 1999;33:579-584.
34. Rossetti AO, Bromfield EB. Determinants of success in the use of oral levetiracetam in status epilepticus. *Epilepsy Behav* 2006;8:651-654.
35. Misra UK, Kalita J, Maurya PK. Levetiracetam versus lorazepam in status epilepticus: A randomized, open labeled pilot study. *J Neurol* 2012;25:645-648.
36. Chakravarthi S, Goyal MK, Modi M, et al. Levetiracetam versus phenytoin in management of status epilepticus. *J Clin Neurosci* 2015;22:959-963.
37. Trinka E. What is the evidence to use new intravenous AEDs in status epilepticus? *Epilepsia* 2011;52(Suppl 8):35-38.
38. Paquette V, Culley C, Greanya ED, Ensom MH. Lacosamide as adjunctive therapy in refractory epilepsy in adults: A systematic review. *Seizure* 2015;25:1-17.
39. Claassen J, Hirsch LJ, Emerson RG, Mayer SA. Treatment of refractory status epilepticus with pentobarbital, propofol, or midazolam: A systematic review. *Epilepsia* 2002;43:146-153.
40. Mirski MA, Williams MA, Hanlet DF. Prolonged pentobarbital and phenobarbital coma for refractory generalized status epilepticus. *Crit Care Med* 1995;23:400-404.
41. Brown LA, Levin GM. Role of propofol in refractory status epilepticus. *Ann Pharmacother* 1998;32:1053-1059.
42. Timpe EM, Eichner SF, Phelps SJ. Propofol-related infusion syndrome in critically ill pediatric patients: Coincidence, association, or causation? *J Pediatr Pharmacol Ther* 2006;11:17-42.
43. Iyer VN, Hoel R, Rabinstein AA. Propofol infusion syndrome in patients with refractory status epilepticus: An 11-year clinical experience. *Crit Care Med* 2009;37:3024-3030.
44. Dorandeu F, Dhote F, Barbier L, et al. Treatment of status epilepticus with ketamine, are we there yet? *CNS Neurosci Ther* 2013;19:411-427.
45. Shelton CM, Alford EL, Storgion S, et al. Enteral topiramate in a pediatric patient with refractory status epilepticus: A case report and review of the literature. *J Pediatr Pharmacol Ther* 2014;19:317-324.
46. Zeiler FA, Zeiler KJ, Kazina CJ, et al. Lidocaine for status epilepticus in adults. *Seizure* 2015;31:41-48.
47. Wheless JW. Treatment of refractory convulsive status epilepticus in children: Other therapies. *Semin Pediatr Neurol* 2010;17:190-194.
48. Zeiler FA, Zeiler KJ, Teitelbaum J, et al. Modern inhalational anesthetics for refractory status epilepticus. *Can J Neurol Sci* 2015;42:106-115.
49. Rossetti AO. What is the value of hypothermia in acute neurologic diseases and status epilepticus? *Epilepsia* 2011;52(Suppl 8):64-66.
50. Zeiler FA, Zeiler KJ, Teitelbaum J, et al. Therapeutic hypothermia for refractory status epilepticus. *Can J Neurol Sci* 2015;42:221-229.
51. Bennett AE, Hoesch RE, DeWitt LD, et al. Therapeutic hypothermia for status epilepticus: A report, historical perspective, and review. *Clin Neurol Neurosurg* 2014;126:103-109.
52. O'Connor SE, Ream MA, Richardson C, et al. The ketogenic diet for the treatment of pediatric status epilepticus. *Pediatr Neurol* 2014;50:101-103.
53. Zeiler FA, Zeiler KJ, Teitelbaum J, et al. VNS for refractory status epilepticus. *Epilepsy Res* 2015;112:100-113.
54. Chung WH, Chang WC, Lee YS, et al; Taiwan Severe Cutaneous Adverse Reaction Consortium; Japan Pharmacogenomics Data Science Consortium. Genetic variants associated with phenytoin-related severe cutaneous adverse reactions. *JAMA* 2014;312:525-534.

Acute Management of the Brain Injury Patient

58

Bradley A. Boucher and G. Christopher Wood

KEY CONCEPTS

1. Cerebral ischemia is the key pathophysiologic event triggering secondary neuronal injury following severe traumatic brain injury (TBI). Intracellular accumulation of calcium is postulated to be a central pathophysiologic process in amplifying and perpetuating secondary neuronal injury via inhibition of cellular respiration and enzyme activation.
2. *Guidelines for the Management of Severe Brain Injury*, published by the Brain Trauma Foundation (BTF)/American Association of Neurological Surgeons (AANS), serve as the foundation on which clinical decisions in managing adult neurotrauma patients are based; comparable guidelines for infants, children, and adolescents have also been published.
3. Correcting and preventing early hypotension (systolic blood pressure [SBP] less than 90 mm Hg) and hypoxemia (PaO_2 less than 60 mm Hg [8.0 kPa]) are primary goals during the initial resuscitative and intensive care of severe TBI patients.
4. Nonpharmacologic treatment in the management of intracranial hypertension includes raising the head of the bed 30°, short-term mild hyperventilation ($PaCO_2$ 30-35 mm Hg [4.0-4.7 kPa]), ventricular drainage if a ventriculostomy is present, and decompressive surgery.
5. The principal monitoring parameter for severe TBI patients within the intensive care environment is intracranial pressure (ICP). Cerebral perfusion pressure (CPP) is also a critical monitoring parameter and should be maintained between 50 and 70 mm Hg (6.7 and 9.3 kPa) (greater than 40 mm Hg [5.3 kPa] in pediatric patients) through the use of fluids, vasopressors, and/or ICP normalization therapy.
6. Nonspecific pharmacologic treatment in the management of intracranial hypertension should include analgesics, sedatives, antipyretics, and paralytics under selected circumstances.
7. Specific pharmacologic treatment in the management of intracranial hypertension includes mannitol, hypertonic saline, furosemide, and high-dose pentobarbital. Neither routine use of corticosteroids nor aggressive hyperventilation (ie, $PaCO_2$ less than 25 mm Hg [3.3 kPa]) should be used in the management of intracranial hypertension.
8. Use of phenytoin for the prophylaxis of posttraumatic seizures usually should be discontinued after 7 days if no seizures are observed.
9. Numerous investigational strategies targeted at limiting injury and/or stimulating axonal repair following severe TBI have been employed, but no proven therapeutic benefits have been identified.

Traumatic brain injury (TBI) is currently the leading cause of death and disability among children and young adults in the industrialized world.[1] A focus on TBI prevention, improved acute care, and rehabilitation must remain national priorities. This chapter summarizes TBI epidemiology and pathophysiology, and highlights the major guidelines and systematic reviews of the literature pertaining to the management of severe TBI patients.

EPIDEMIOLOGY

It is estimated that approximately 1.7 million persons sustain a TBI each year in the United States equating to a TBI every 15 seconds.[1] Among these individuals, 275,000 require hospital admission, and 53,000 die annually.[1] Importantly, an estimated 5.3 million Americans currently live with disabilities as a result of their TBI, highlighting the enormous physical and emotional toll of this health care problem.[2] The economic effects of acute neurotrauma are also enormous, with estimates of direct and indirect spending on TBI patients requiring hospitalization of $76.5 billion in the United States in 2010.[2] Economic costs to society from lost productivity are also massive, especially considering the young age of many TBI patients.[2] Falls are the leading cause of TBI (35.2%), while firearm-related and motor vehicle accidents result in the greatest number of TBI-related hospitalizations and deaths overall.[1,2] Death rates from TBI are highest in patients aged 75 years or older.[1]

PRIMARY AND SECONDARY BRAIN INJURY PATHOPHYSIOLOGY

The neurologic sequelae of brain trauma can occur instantaneously as a consequence of the primary injury or can result from secondary injuries that follow within minutes, hours, or days.[3] Primary injury involves the external transfer of kinetic energy to various structural components of the brain (eg, neurons, nerve synapses, glial cells, axons, and cerebral blood vessels). The biomechanical forces responsible for primary brain injury can be classified broadly as contact (eg, blunt-object blow, penetrating-missile injuries) and acceleration/deceleration (eg, instantaneous brain movements following motor vehicle accidents).[4] Contact forces commonly result in skull fractures, brain contusions, and/or hemorrhages. Primary injuries are categorized further as focal (eg, contusions, hematomas) or diffuse.[4] The latter usually are associated with shearing or stretch forces, which primarily affect axons within the brain (ie, diffuse axonal injury).[4] The type of primary injury (ie, focal vs diffuse) is a major factor as to which of the secondary injury mechanisms discussed below will predominate following a TBI; however, many patients, especially those involved in high-speed accidents, sustain both types of injury.[4]

1 A complex sequence of pathophysiologic events precipitated by primary brain injury may seriously disrupt the normal central

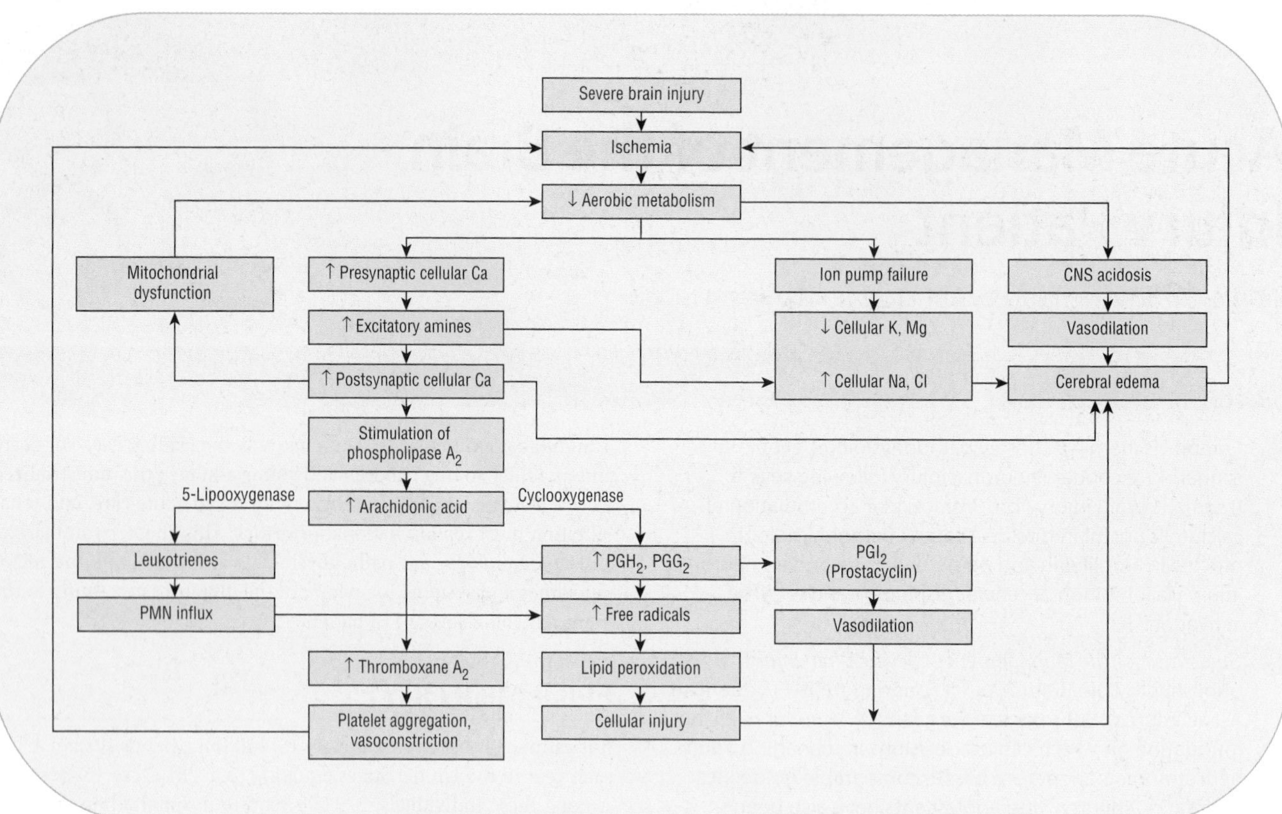

FIGURE 58-1 Schematic illustration of the cascade of biochemical events proposed to occur following severe neurotrauma (secondary brain injury). (Ca, calcium; Cl, chloride; CNS, central nervous system; K, potassium; Mg, magnesium; Na, sodium; PMN, polymorphonucleocyte; PGH_2, prostaglandin H_2; PGG_2, prostaglandin PGG_2; PGI_2, prostaglandin PGI_2).

nervous system (CNS) balance between oxygen supply and demand resulting in a metabolic crisis.[5,6] Hypotension in particular during the early posttraumatic period is a major contributor to this imbalance and a primary determinant of outcome. The end result of this imbalance may be cerebral ischemia, the key pathophysiologic event triggering secondary injury.[5] Figure 58-1 is a simplified schematic of the processes that constitute secondary brain injury and their various interrelationships. The brain is particularly susceptible to ischemia because of its normally high resting energy requirement and its limited capacity to store oxygen, glucose, and adenosine triphosphate (ATP).[3] These phenomena can result in imbalances in cerebral oxygen delivery (CDO_2) and consumption ($CMRO_2$), processes that are closely autoregulated under normal circumstances.[5] Factors that can diminish cerebral oxygen supply following brain injury include cerebral edema, expanding mass lesions (eg, epidural, subdural, and intracerebral hematomas), cerebral vasospasm, and loss of vasoregulatory control. Vasogenic cerebral edema can develop as a consequence of cerebral capillary endothelial damage and disruption of the blood–brain barrier.[6] Cytotoxic cerebral edema is a consequence of loss of cell wall integrity that accompanies ischemia or hypoxia with accumulation of lactic acid secondary to anaerobic metabolism.[6] With cytotoxic and vasogenic edema comes expansion of the intracellular and extracellular fluid spaces, respectively. Elevated intracranial pressure (ICP) is the most detrimental consequence of cerebral edema formation and occurs as the brain tissue volume increases within the nondistensible skull. A significant increase in ICP may further compromise cerebral blood flow (CBF) and extend cytotoxic edema. Hence an increase in ICP can be self-perpetuating unless this cycle is reversed. Hypoxemia can further exacerbate local decreases in cerebral oxygen supply following acute respiratory failure and systemic hypotension. Metabolic demand also can increase following neurotrauma secondary to seizures, agitation, and temperature elevation.[7,8]

The two distinctive end points along the spectrum of secondary neuronal injury are: (a) energy-independent cellular necrosis characterized by membrane cell lysis, edema, and inflammation, and (b) energy-independent apoptosis that leads to cell shrinkage and cell membrane dissolution.[4] Apoptosis, which is also known as programmed cell death, requires a cascade of intracellular events for completion of cell death.[4] The loss of ionic homeostasis is postulated to be a key event in fostering secondary brain injury following cerebral ischemia. Cellular influx of sodium, chloride, magnesium, and water with a corresponding efflux of potassium secondary to cytotoxic edema and Na^+-K^+-ATPase pump dysfunction.[3] An influx of calcium into the presynaptic terminal ends of damaged neurons is mediated by N-type voltage-sensitive calcium channels. This influx is postulated to stimulate excessive release of the excitatory amines glutamate and aspartate from the affected neurons. These amines then accumulate in the neuronal synaptic cleft in the presence of cellular energy failure.[3] The result is ongoing stimulation of postsynaptic cells, which can result in an extension of neurotoxicity and cell death. Influx of calcium and additional sodium is stimulated by activation of ionophore receptors including the *N*-methyl-D-aspartate (NMDA) receptor.[4] Calcium influx and its intracellular accumulation initiate a number of events that amplify and perpetuate secondary neuronal injury. High intracellular concentrations of calcium result in mitochondrial dysfunction, which further inhibits cellular respiration, a process already affected by ischemic and/or hypoxic insults.[3-5]

A second major deleterious effect of calcium is to stimulate activation of autodestructive enzymes, including phospholipases, endonucleases, and proteases, such as the caspase family of enzymes.[4]

CLINICAL PRESENTATION Acute Brain Injury

General

- Level of consciousness on admission ranges from awake and alert to completely unresponsive (ie, Glasgow Coma Scale [GCS] 15-3, respectively).

Symptoms

- Posttraumatic amnesia (eg, greater than 1 hour), increasing dizziness, a moderate-to-severe headache, nausea/vomiting, limb weakness, or paresthesia may indicate more severe injury.

Signs

- Cerebrospinal fluid (CSF) otorrhea or rhinorrhea, seizures, or unequal or unreactive pupils may indicate more severe injury.
- A rapid deterioration in mental status strongly suggests the presence of an expanding lesion within the skull.
- Severe TBI may be accompanied by significant alterations or instability in vital signs, including abnormal breathing patterns (eg, apnea, Cheyne–Stokes respiration, tachypnea), hypertension, or bradycardia.

Laboratory Tests

- Arterial blood gases (ABGs) indicating hypoxia (ie, decreased PaO_2) or hypercapnia (ie, increased $PaCO_2$) may indicate compromised ventilation.
- A positive blood ethanol concentration and/or positive urine drug screen indicates that drug intoxication may be affecting the patient's mental status in addition to the TBI.
- Electrolyte disturbances can cause alterations in mental status, and their effects may interfere with assessment of neurological status relative to brain lesion.

Other Diagnostic Tests

- Computed tomography (CT) of the head is an important diagnostic tool for detecting the presence of mass lesions and structural signs of edema (eg, midline shift, compressed ventricles).

The effect of phospholipase A_2 stimulation includes formation of several arachidonic acid metabolites derived from membrane lipids: thromboxane A_2, prostaglandins, and leukotrienes. The subsequent effects of these metabolites are lipid peroxidation and the formation of reactive oxygen species.[3-5] Data suggest that this event occurs very early after injury (eg, before hospitalization), which may limit the effectiveness of exogenously administered antioxidants.

Cell-mediated injury involving inflammatory mediators (eg, proinflammatory cytokines) and nitric oxide activation is yet another possible mechanism involved in secondary neuronal injury.[5,6] Among the cell lines implicated are polymorphonuclear neutrophils, platelets, endothelial cells, and macrophages. Noteworthy is that limited data suggest that activation of some inflammatory mediators may actually be beneficial such that the relative balance of the mediators rather than absolute concentrations may be the most significant pathophysiologic factor following TBI. Stimulation of platelet aggregation, vasodilation, and vasoconstriction also may occur.[5]

CLINICAL PRESENTATION

The GCS was designed over 40 years ago and is still the most widely used system to grade the arousal and functional capacity of the cerebral cortex.[7] The GCS defines the level of consciousness according to eye opening, motor response, and verbal response (Table 58-1). A GCS score of 15 corresponds to a normal neurologic examination based on eye, motor, and verbal responses. A GCS score of 3 to 8, 9 to 12, and 13 to 15 is consistent with severe, moderate, and mild or minor brain injury, respectively.[7] The possibility of ethanol or drug intoxication, hypotension, hypoxia, postictal state, hypoglycemia, electrolyte imbalances, or hypothermia altering the neurologic examination always should be considered. Because opiates, sedatives, and neuromuscular blockers affect the neurologic examination, they should not be administered until the initial examination is complete if at all possible. Simple, rapidly attainable clinical variables that are predictive of poor outcomes include patient age, presence of hypotension, increased ICP, decreased GCS score (especially the motor score), pupillary reactivity, and findings on a CT scan of the head that include the presence and size of a hematoma, subarachnoid hemorrhage, midline shift, and compression of the ventricular cisterns.[9]

GENERAL TRAUMATIC BRAIN INJURY TREATMENT PRINCIPLES

2 In July 1995, the Brain Trauma Foundation (BTF) published an extensive document entitled *Guidelines for the Management of Severe Brain Injury* as a joint initiative with the Guidelines Committee of the American Association of Neurological Surgeons (AANS) and the Joint Section on Neurotrauma and Critical Care of the AANS and the Congress of Neurological Surgeons, with subsequent revision in 2000. A third revision was released in 2007.[10] This landmark publication constitutes the most widely accepted series of evidence-based

TABLE 58-1 Glasgow Coma Scale

Response	Score
Eyes	
Open spontaneously	4
To verbal command	3
To pain	2
No response	1
Best motor response	
To verbal command	
Obeys	6
To painful stimulus (pressure to nailbeds)	
Localizes pain	5
Flexion, withdrawal	4
Flexion, abnormal (decorticate rigidity)	3
Extension (decerebrate rigidity)	2
No response	1
Best verbal response	
(Arouse patient with painful stimulus if necessary)	
Oriented and converses	5
Disoriented and converses	4
Inappropriate words	3
Incomprehensible sounds	2
No response	1
Total	3-15

standards, guidelines, and options for the care of severe TBI patients in the United States.[11] Recommendations are reported as Level I (standards), Level II (guidelines), or Level III (options) based on the corresponding classes of evidence. As important are the data documenting that compliance with the BTF/AANS guidelines can result in improved outcomes relative to mortality rate, functional outcome scores, length of hospitalization, and cost. Since then, guidelines addressing prehospital TBI management[12] and surgical management[13] have been published. Furthermore, TBI management guidelines for infants, children, and adolescents were developed in 2003 with a second edition published in 2012.[14] The recommendations emanating from these published guidelines on TBI management and various published systematic reviews will be highlighted throughout the remaining portion of this chapter. Until further clinical studies become available, recommendations from the published guidelines should serve as the foundation on which all clinical decisions in managing severe TBI are based. Nonetheless, it should be noted that the majority of the guidelines are based on Class II evidence (primarily prospective clinical trials) and Class III evidence (primarily retrospective clinical trials). Few Class I evidence studies (ie, prospective, randomized, controlled trials) are available for treatment of TBI. The pharmacologic management of TBI is summarized in Table 58-2. Recommendations provided in this chapter pertain to adults and children unless specifically noted to the contrary.

Desired Outcomes

The overall goal in TBI management is not only reduction in morbidity and mortality, but also optimization of long-term functional outcome for these patients. This requires careful attention to the following short-term therapeutic goals: (a) establishment of an adequate airway and maintenance of ventilation and circulation during the initial period of resuscitation and evaluation, (b) maintenance of balance between CDO_2 and $CMRO_2$, (c) prevention or attenuation of secondary neuronal injury, and (d) prevention and/or treatment of associated medical complications.

Initial Resuscitation

The first priority in the unconscious patient is the establishment of an airway, which ensures adequate oxygenation and prevents aspiration.[7] Thereafter, restoration and maintenance of systolic blood pressure (SBP) between 120 and 140 mm Hg is desired since admission SBP outside this range is associated with increased mortality.[15] 3 In particular, correcting and preventing early hypotension (SBP less than 90 mm Hg in adults) and hypoxia (PaO_2 less than 60 mm Hg [8.0 kPa]) are essential, because these two factors are among the most powerful predictors of outcome.[8-10] Isotonic saline (0.9% normal saline) and lactated Ringer's solution have been traditionally used as initial resuscitation fluids of choice in TBI patients. However, some clinicians believe that hypertonic saline (eg, 3% or 7.5% saline) is beneficial in the resuscitation of TBI patients. Clinical studies have yielded equivocal results relative to superiority over isotonic solutions.[8,16] Regardless, no clear consensus exists as to the optimal initial resuscitation fluid. While albumin therapy may be considered an alternative to crystalloid fluid resuscitation, a retrospective analysis of 460 TBI patients revealed an increase in mortality (33.2%) compared with those patients receiving 0.9% normal saline.[17] Vasopressors and inotropic agents may be needed to maintain an adequate mean arterial pressure (MAP) if hypotension persists after adequate restoration of intravascular volume. Figure 58-2 is an algorithm summarizing treatment priorities in the initial management of acute TBI.

Postresuscitative Care

Following successful resuscitation, priorities shift toward diagnostic evaluation of intracranial and extracranial injuries and emergent surgical intervention as needed. In many patients, evacuation of intracranial hematomas (ie, epidural, subdural, and intracerebral hematomas) is essential to control ICP and improve outcome. Elevation of depressed skull fractures and debridement of penetrating wound tracts are other important emergent surgical procedures in TBI patients. 4 Decompressive craniectomies (ie, removal of variable amount of skull bone) with or without temporal or frontal lobectomy may be considered in patients with increases in ICP refractory to more conservative measures.[5] The beneficial effects of routine decompressive surgery in adult TBI patients to date are controversial.[18] However, a recent pivotal randomized trial, while demonstrating acute effectiveness in ICP control using decompressive craniectomy, also found worse long-term outcomes compared with controls. This latter study calls into question the routine use of decompressive craniectomy in patients with refractory ICP.[19] Continuous ICP monitoring (eg, intraventricular catheter, intraparenchymal fiberoptic catheter) is indicated in salvageable patients with a GCS score of 3 to 8 after resuscitation with an abnormal admission CT scan. In addition, continuous ICP monitoring is indicated in high-risk severe TBI patients with a normal CT scan and two of the following criteria: age older than 40 years, motor posturing, or SBP less than 90 mm Hg.[10] Intraventricular catheters have a

TABLE 58-2 Pharmacologic Management of TBI

Hyperosmolar therapy
Mannitol is effective for control of raised ICP at doses of 0.25-1 g/kg body weight (Level II).
Hypertonic saline is effective in small studies, but no guideline recommendation is given in adults. In pediatric patients, hypertonic saline should be considered in severe TBI associated with intracranial hypertension (Level II).
Infection prophylaxis
Periprocedural antibiotics for intubation should be administered to reduce the incidence of pneumonia (based largely on a single study) (Level II).
Routine prophylactic antibiotic use for ventricular catheter placement is not recommended to reduce infection (Level III).
Deep venous thrombosis prophylaxis
LMWH or low-dose unfractionated heparin should be used in combination with mechanical prophylaxis. However, there is an increased risk of expansion of intracranial hemorrhage (Level III).
Anesthetics, analgesics, and sedatives
Prophylactic administration of barbiturates to reduce burst suppression ECG is not recommended (Level II).
High-dose barbiturate administration is recommended to control elevated ICP refractory to maximum standard medical and surgical treatment in adults. Hemodynamic stability is essential before and after barbiturate therapy (Level II). In pediatric patients, high-dose barbiturate therapy can be used to treat refractory intracranial hypertension in hemodynamically stable patients (Level III).
Propofol is recommended for the control of ICP, but not for improvement in mortality or 6-month outcomes. High-dose propofol can produce significant morbidity (Level II).
Antiseizure prophylaxis
Prophylactic use of phenytoin or valproate is not recommended for preventing late PTS (>7 days) (Level II).
Anticonvulsants are indicated to decrease the incidence of early PTS (within 7 days of injury) (Level II).
Corticosteroids
The use of steroids is not recommended for improving outcome or reducing ICP in adults or pediatric TBI patients. In patients with moderate or severe TBI, high-dose methylprednisolone is associated with increased mortality and is contraindicated (Level II).

ECG, electrocardiogram; ICP, intracranial pressure; LMWH, low-molecular weight heparin; PTS, posttraumatic seizures; TBI, traumatic brain injury.

Level I: Recommendation based on a high level of clinical certainty from Class I evidence (eg, good quality randomized controlled trial [RCT]).

Level II: Recommendation based on a moderate level of clinical certainty from Class II evidence (eg, moderate quality RCT; good quality cohort; good quality case–control).

Level III: Clinical certainty has not been established based on Class III evidence (eg, poor quality RCT; moderate or poor quality cohort; moderate or poor quality case–control; case series, databases, or registries).

Data from reference 10, 14.

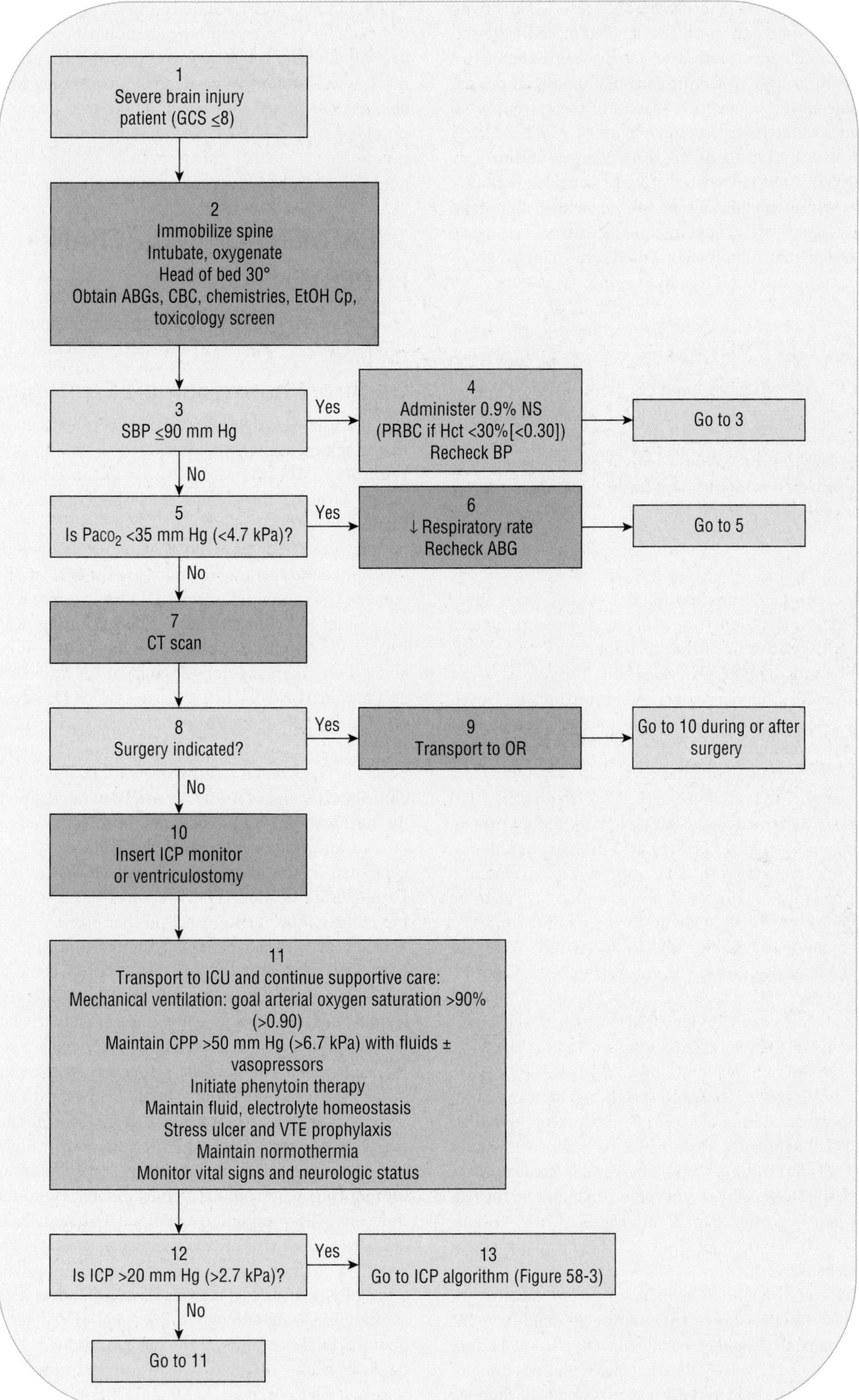

FIGURE 58-2 Algorithm for the acute management of the TBI patient. (ABG, arterial blood gas; BP, blood pressure; CBC, complete blood count; CPP, cerebral perfusion pressure; CT, computed tomography; EtOH Cp, ethanol plasma concentration; GCS, Glasgow coma scale; Hct, hematocrit; ICP, intracranial pressure; ICU, intensive care unit; NS, normal saline; OR, operating room; $PaCO_2$, partial pressure of arterial blood carbon dioxide; PRBC, packed red blood cells; SBP, systolic blood pressure.) *(Reprinted with permission from Wood CG, Boucher BA. Acute Management of the Traumatic Brain Injury Patient. In: Richardson M, Chant C, Chessman KH, et al., eds.* Pharmacotherapy Self-Assessment Program, *7th ed. Neurology and Psychiatry. Lenexa, KS: American College of Clinical Pharmacy, 2012:143-4.)*

therapeutic advantage over the alternatives but are associated with a higher complication rate and can be difficult to place in the setting of the swollen brain. Specifically, CSF can be drained using this device as a means to lower ICP. Continuous ICP monitoring is the only means to objectively evaluate the success of therapies used to decrease ICP.[7] Once the ICP exceeds 20 to 25 mm Hg (2.7-3.3 kPa), therapy should be initiated to decrease ICP below 20 mm Hg (2.7 kPa).[10,14,20,21] While used extensively in TBI patients and advocated within consensus guidelines, a randomized controlled trial did not demonstrate a superior outcome in patients with ICP managed with an intraparenchymal monitor compared with patients treatment based on imaging and clinical examination.[22]

Clinical **Controversy...**

Continuous ICP monitoring has been the mainstay of managing selected severe TBI patients for decades. This management practice is now being questioned based on data suggesting no improvement in outcome with ICP monitoring compared with treatment based on imaging and clinical examination.

Jugular venous oxygen saturation ($SjvO_2$) monitoring is advocated by some practitioners for detection of global cerebral hypoxia (ie, adequacy of CBF relative to $CMRO_2$), although it is technically difficult to achieve consistent results.[7] Hence its use remains confined predominantly to academic centers and for research purposes. The use of brain tissue oxygen monitoring is another alternative to $SjvO_2$ to measure oxygen diffusion in TBI patients.[7] Cerebral microdialysis is yet another technique that has been used successfully as a research tool to measure the cerebral extracellular chemistry of TBI patients.[7] Biochemical markers (eg, S-100 calcium-binding protein B, neuron-specific enolase, glial fibrillary acid protein, serum substance P[23]) have been suggested to have utility in diagnosing and monitoring TBI patients.[24,25] However, no clear role has yet to be defined for such markers with each having assorted limitations.[24,25]

5 Another important monitoring parameter for severe TBI patients within the intensive care environment is the CPP. The CPP is the difference between MAP and ICP (ie, CPP = MAP − ICP). Maintenance of an acceptable CPP has been postulated to be critical in reducing cerebral ischemia and secondary injury. The BTF/AANS guidelines recommend maintaining a range of CPP between 50 and 70 mm Hg (6.7 and 9.3 kPa) and specifically indicate avoiding CPP values less than 50 mm Hg (6.7 kPa).[10] Current guidelines also recommend that aggressive attempts to maintain CPP greater than 70 mm Hg (9.3 kPa) in adults should be avoided because of the risk of the acute respiratory distress syndrome.[10] In children, the recommended CPP goal is greater than 40 mm Hg (5.3 kPa).[14] Despite being commonly used, the optimal approach to CPP management continues to be debated.

The goal CPP can be achieved by increasing MAP through the use of fluids and/or vasopressors or by lowering elevated ICP. The goal of volume expansion should be euvolemia as well as avoidance of a hypoosmolar state and negative fluid balance.[7,14] If the hemoglobin is below 7 g/dL (70 g/L; 4.34 mmol/L), transfusion of packed red blood cells (PRBCs) is indicated. Nevertheless, liberal transfusions should be avoided since using a hemoglobin target goal of 10 g/dL (100 g/L; 6.21 mmol/L) has been associated with higher incidence of thromboembolic events without an improvement in neurologic outcome based on a recent randomized trial.[26] However, more data are needed before these findings can be applied to all TBI patients.[8] Furthermore, use of erythropoietin was not associated with an improved neurologic outcome in the same trial.[26] Volume status should be targeted to a central venous pressure of 7 to 12 cm H_2O (0.7-1.2 kPa) if invasive monitoring is employed. After achievement of euvolemia, the patient's head should be elevated at 30 degrees to promote venous drainage and decrease ICP. If restoration of the intravascular volume is inadequate in elevating MAP to an acceptable level, hypertension should be induced using vasopressors (eg, norepinephrine, phenylephrine, dopamine).[7] Patients should be monitored for renal dysfunction, lactic acidosis, and signs of peripheral ischemia when vasopressors are used, especially in large doses.

TREATMENT OF INTRACRANIAL HYPERTENSION

Several general and specific pharmacologic and nonpharmacologic strategies are used in the treatment of intracranial hypertension.

General Pharmacologic Strategies

6 The use of analgesics and sedatives has an important primary role in the management of intracranial hypertension (Fig. 58-3 and Table 58-3). This is related directly to the association of pain, agitation, excessive muscle movement, and resisting mechanical ventilation with transient increases in ICP. Paralytics are a secondary option in refractory patients.[27] Nonetheless, there is no strong evidence that one agent is superior to another relative to affecting outcome in patients with severe TBI based on a recent systematic review of randomized clinical trials.[28] Effects on ICP, CPP, and MAP are variable.[29] Morphine sulfate is the most commonly used analgesic and sedative in this setting.[10,28] Noteworthy is that bolus doses of opiates may increase ICP by increasing CBF.[28] However, while continuous infusions of fentanyl and sufentanil are gaining in popularity, their use also may be associated with mild elevations in ICP.[10,28] Propofol has become the sedative of choice in TBI patients among many clinicians because of its ease of titration, rapidly reversible effects on discontinuation, and possible neuroprotective effects.[10] Although it is used for sedation in infants and children who are mechanically ventilated in the intensive care unit (ICU) setting, the Food and Drug Administration (FDA) requires that the manufacturer labeling contains specific information that propofol is not approved for sedation of pediatric patients admitted to an ICU. One of the biggest safety concerns with the use of propofol is the propofol infusion syndrome (PRIS) characterized by hyperkalemia, hepatomegaly, lipemia, metabolic acidosis, myocardial failure, rhabdomyolysis, renal failure, and death in some cases.[10] While initially reported in children, PRIS can also occur in adults. Doses greater than 5 mg/kg/hour and infusion exceeding 48 hours should be used with extreme caution.[10] Triglyceride concentrations also should be monitored in patients receiving prolonged propofol infusions and/or high dosages of propofol considering its lipid emulsion formulation and the potential for inducing hypertriglyceridemia under these conditions. Increased mortality with propofol in an animal TBI study has also raised concerns regarding use of this sedative in TBI patients.[30] Alternative sedatives include short-acting benzodiazepines (eg, midazolam), especially if there is a reasonable suspicion of alcohol withdrawal as the underlying etiology of the agitation,[31] intermittent low-dose pentobarbital, ketamine,[32] dexmedetomidine,[33] or etomidate (particularly useful in rapid-induction anesthesia). The potential for these agents to decrease MAP and CPP must be monitored closely. Additionally, the cumulative sedative effects of longer-acting drugs, especially benzodiazepines, must be taken into account. The use of any sedative agent also must be weighed against its potential to obscure the neurologic examination of the patient. Interference with the neurologic examination is also a problem with paralytic agents.

Hyperventilation

4 The practice of prolonged aggressive hyperventilation ($PaCO_2$ less than 25 mm Hg [3.3 kPa]) to decrease ICP is no longer recommended.[10]

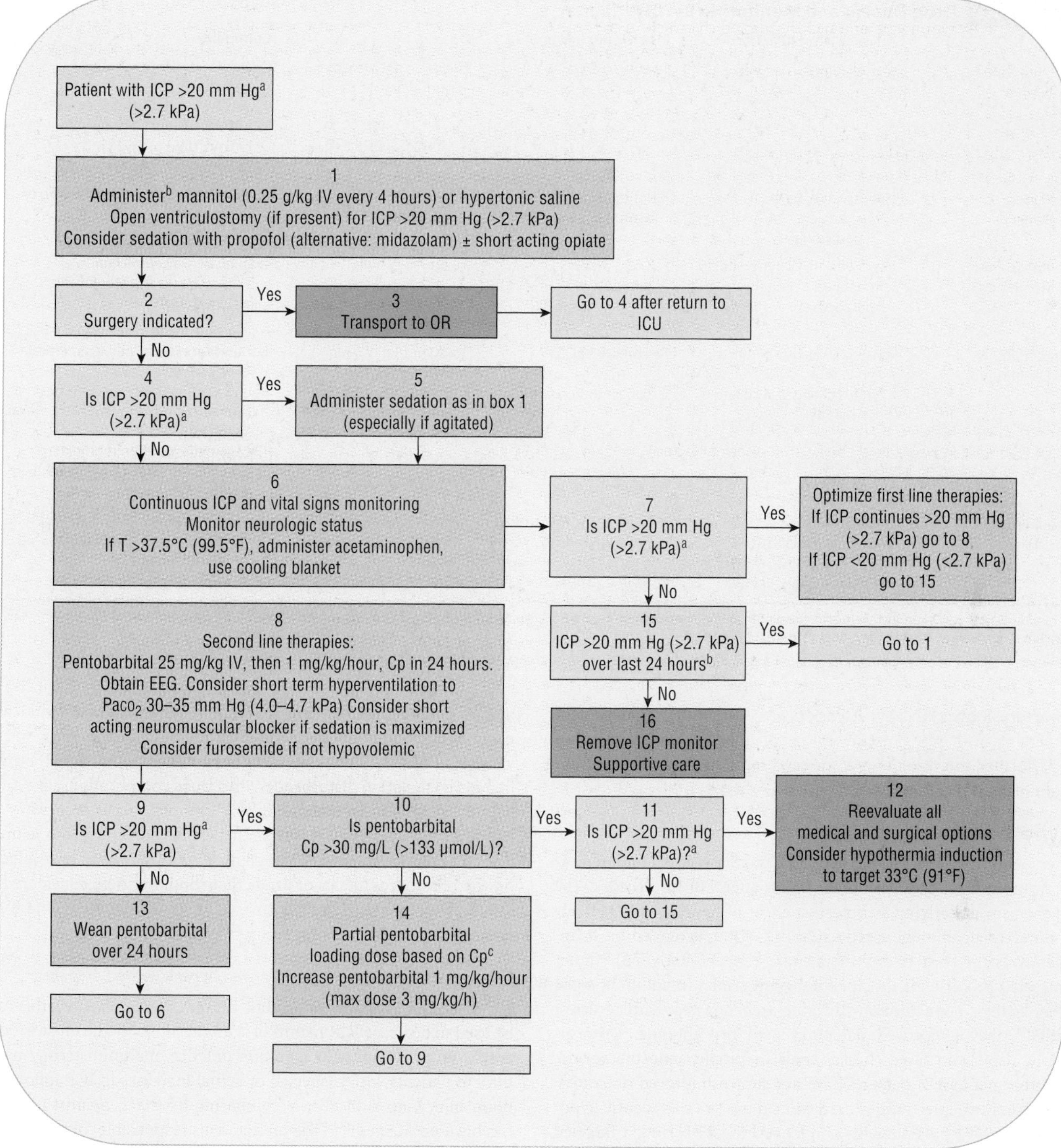

FIGURE 58-3 Algorithm for the management of increased ICP. [a]Treatment thresholds: ICP 20 to 29 mm Hg (2.7-3.9 kPa) for >15 minutes; ICP 30 to 39 mm Hg (4.0-5.2 kPa) for >2 minutes; ICP more than or equal to 40 mm Hg (≥5.3 kPa) for more than 1 minute. Note: Transient increases may occur following respiratory procedures (eg, suctioning, chest physiotherapy, bronchoscopy, and intubation). [b]Hold if serum osmolality is more than 320 mOsm/kg (320 mmol/kg). [c]Partial pentobarbital loading dose (mg) = (30 mg/L – measured Cp) (1 L/kg × wt[kg]) (pentobarbital concentration in μmol/L must first be divided by 4.439 to convert to mg/L). (Cp, plasma concentration; EEG, electroencephalogram; ICP, intracranial pressure; ICU, intensive care unit; OR, operating room; PaCO2, partial pressure of arterial blood carbon dioxide.) *(Reprinted with permission from Wood CG, Boucher BA. Acute Management of the Traumatic Brain Injury Patient. In: Richardson M, Chant C, Chessman KH, et al., eds.* Pharmacotherapy Self-Assessment Program, *7th ed. Neurology and Psychiatry. Lenexa, KS: American College of Clinical Pharmacy, 2012:143-4.)*

Hyperventilation acutely decreases systemic and cerebral $PaCO_2$. The resulting hypocapnia, in turn, induces cerebral vasoconstriction, thereby decreasing CBF and cerebral blood volume (CBV). For decades, it was a widely held belief that a reduction in CBV and any accompanying decrease in ICP were beneficial. Nonetheless, a comprehensive literature review concluded that there are no data demonstrating improved outcomes using this therapeutic intervention.[34] Hyperventilation should be avoided during the first 24 hours following acute TBI when CBF is often critically reduced according to the most current BTF/AANS guidelines.[10] 7 Hyperventilation for brief periods with a goal of 30 to 35 mm Hg (4.0-4.7 kPa) nonetheless may be considered a temporary maneuver in the setting of

TABLE 58-3 Drug Dosing and Monitoring in TBI Patients

Drug	Adverse Drug Reactions	Monitoring Parameter	Dosing	Comments
Levetiracetam (Keppra)	CNS changes	Seizures, SCr	500 mg IV Q12 h (dose during first 14 days)	Caution in patients with renal dysfunction If used for active seizures: increase to 1,000 mg every 12 hours after 14 days, then to 1,500 mg every 12 hours after 28 days
Mannitol (Generic)	Hypotension, renal dysfunction, hyperosmolality	ICP, CPP, BP, serum osmolality, Na, UO, SCr	0.25 to 1 g/kg IV every 2-4 hours	Avoid in patients with renal failure or CHF
Pentobarbital (Nembutal)	Hypotension, GI hypomotility, induction of hepatic drug metabolism	ICP, CPP, BP, EEG, GI function	10 mg/kg IV over 30 minutes, then 5 mg/kg over 3 hours, then 1 mg/kg/h	Administer via central line. General dose range for infusion is 1-3 mg/kg/h
Phenytoin (Dilantin)	Hypotension, dysrhythmias, nystagmus, ataxia, mental status changes, exfoliative dermatitis	Seizures, BP, ECG, phenytoin concentrations, skin	15-20 mg/kg IV over 60 minutes, then 5 mg/kg/day divided every 8 hours or every 12 hours	Administer <50 mg/min; use central line if available Round loading doses up to nearest 250 mg, round maintenance doses up to nearest 25 mg Trauma patients often require higher doses (ie, >6 mg/kg/day) to achieve therapeutic concentrations
Propofol (Diprivan)	Hypotension, hyperkalemia, metabolic, acidosis, rhabdomyolysis, renal failure, hepatomegaly, lipemia	ICP, CPP, BP, SCr, K, arterial pH, triglycerides, lactate	General range: 0.5-3 mg/kg/h titrated to desired effect	Avoid doses greater than 5 mg/kg/h or prolonged infusions; not approved for use in children

BP, blood pressure; CHF, congestive heart failure; CPP, cerebral perfusion pressure; ECG, electrocardiogram; EEG, electroencephalogram; GI, gastrointestinal; ICP, intracranial pressure; K, potassium; Na, sodium; SCr, serum creatinine; UO, urine output.

The reader is referred to other appropriate chapters regarding other drugs not listed in this table.

refractory intracranial hypertension or in the initial management of patients with signs of cerebral herniation.[10] If hyperventilation is performed, the use of $SjvO_2$ or cerebral tissue oxygen perfusion monitoring is recommended.[10]

Hypothermia

Therapeutic hypothermia has been an attractive strategy for attempting to minimize secondary brain injury after TBI for decades. The mechanism underlying a protective effect of hypothermia is likely multifactorial, although a reduction in $CMRO_2$ is offered most frequently as the basis of any therapeutic benefits. Early TBI studies suggested promise for therapeutic hypothermia. In addition, some other patient populations with brain ischemia (eg, cardiac arrest patients) have improved outcomes with hypothermia. Unfortunately, data from large clinical trials of prophylactic therapeutic hypothermia in TBI patients have not shown improved outcomes. The first of two large randomized clinical trials of therapeutic hypothermia in 392 patients with nonpenetrating TBI using a targeted temperature of 33°C (91°F) revealed no improvement in outcome compared with the normothermic group.[10] In addition, more hypotension was observed in the therapeutic hypothermia group. The second major multicenter study focused on early cooling (ie, ≤2.5 hours) to 35°C (95°F), then 48 hours at 33°C (91°F) followed by gradual rewarming.[35] The control group was treated under normothermic conditions. This study was discontinued after enrollment of 108 patients because of futility with poorer outcomes including death observed in the hypothermic group. Based on the clinical evidence to date, prophylactic therapeutic hypothermia is not recommended as a routine neuroprotective strategy in patients with TBI.[7] Nevertheless, a report emanating from five critical care societies would not recommend for or against therapeutic hypothermia (ie, "targeted temperature management") based on available data.[36] Furthermore, a recent systematic review of therapeutic hypothermia in TBI found some evidence supporting its use.[37] In pediatric patients, moderate hypothermia within 8 hours of TBI should be considered in patients with intracranial hypertension.[14] Noteworthy is that a large, multicenter study of hypothermia for ICP reduction in TBI patients (Eurotherm3235Trial) is currently underway that may provide additional insights on the use of this therapeutic intervention in adults.[38] Potential side effects of therapeutic hypothermia include coagulation disturbances, infectious complications, and cardiac arrhythmias. An increase in ICP also may occur secondary to hypothermia-associated shivering that can be prevented with neuromuscular blocking agents. Therapeutic hypothermia can have effects on the pharmacokinetics of drugs that should also be considered.[39] Specifically, cardiac output decreases by 7% for every 1°C (1.8°F) decrease in core body temperature.[40]

Osmotic Agents

7 Although a number of osmotic diuretics (eg, urea, glycerol) can be used to decrease ICP, mannitol is unquestionably the most widely employed.[10,41] Despite the common practice of administering mannitol to patients with suspected or actual increases in ICP following brain injury, no clinical trial comparing its effects against placebo has been performed.[29,42] The mechanisms responsible for mannitol's beneficial effects likely relate to (a) an immediate plasma-expanding effect that reduces blood viscosity and increases CBF and (b) establishment of an osmotic concentration gradient across an intact blood–brain barrier that decreases ICP as water diffuses from the brain into the intravascular compartment.[10] Recommended doses of mannitol typically range from 0.25 to 1 g/kg IV every 2 to 4 hours.[10,41] Increased ICP is reduced within minutes following mannitol administration, and the duration of action ranges from 90 minutes to 6 hours depending on the dose and the clinical conditions that are present.[10] In order to maximize benefit and minimize adverse events, it has been suggested that mannitol be administered as a bolus and not as a continuous infusion in this setting. However, more recent analyses conclude that there is no demonstrable benefit using one administration approach over the other.[10]

Several adverse effects are associated with mannitol.[41] In addition to hypotension resulting from its diuretic effect, a reversible acute renal dysfunction may occur in patients with previously normal renal function after long-term, large-dose administration, especially in patients with advanced age and preexisting renal dysfunction based on data in patients with intracranial hemorrhage.[43] As such, mannitol should be avoided in patients with acute kidney injury or chronic kidney diseases. Acute exacerbation of underlying congestive heart failure and pulmonary edema also may occur following rapid intravascular volume expansion. Furosemide is recommended as an alternative diuretic for lowering ICP in these latter patient groups.

While hypertonic saline solutions have been advocated by some as a resuscitative fluid following TBI as previously mentioned, solutions ranging from concentrations of 2% to 23.4% have also been used to acutely lower increased ICP.[44] Not only do hypertonic saline solutions create an osmotic gradient in favor of reducing cerebral edema, but evidence suggests that they may also have beneficial vasoregulatory, immunologic, and neurochemical effects as well.[44] Plasma expansion may also lead to an increase in CBF. It is noteworthy, however, that the 2007 BTF guidelines do not recommend hypertonic saline due to a lack of supporting evidence.[10] Nevertheless, two recent meta-analyses also suggested that hypertonic saline may be modestly more effective than mannitol.[44,45] In contrast, two clinical trials of equimolar doses of mannitol versus 7.45% and 15% hypertonic saline, respectively, revealed similar effects between the regimens in TBI patients.[46,47] In most studies, the goal of therapy was to treat an elevated ICP. However, in some studies the goal of therapy was to increase the serum sodium regardless of ICP. If used in this way, hypertonic saline should target serum sodium concentration less than 160 mEq/L (160 mmol/L) since additional benefit is unlikely at higher concentrations.[41]

Barbiturates

7 High-dose barbiturate therapy (ie, barbiturate coma) has been used for decades in the management of increased ICP despite a lack of evidence documenting beneficial effects on patient morbidity and mortality.[48] Nonetheless, based largely on beneficial outcomes observed in a randomized clinical trial published in 1988, BTF/AANS and pediatric guidelines recommend that high-dose barbiturate therapy be considered in hemodynamically stable severe TBI patients refractory to maximal medical ICP-lowering therapy and decompressive surgery.[10,14] A recent study indicated survival at a discharge of 40% (22 of 55) and good functional outcomes in 68% of survivors (13 of 19 evaluable patients) at 1 year in this TBI patient subset receiving high-dose barbiturate therapy.[49] Prophylactic use of barbiturates is not advocated in light of insufficient evidence supporting this practice and the potential for adverse events (eg, hypotension).[10,14,48] The mechanism responsible for the cerebral protective effects of barbiturates is generally attributed to suppression of cerebral metabolism thereby cerebral metabolic demands and CBV.[48] Prior to inducing a barbiturate coma, the severe TBI patient must be mechanically ventilated with continuous monitoring of arterial blood pressure, electrocardiogram (ECG), and ICP. Pentobarbital is the most commonly used barbiturate for this indication, although thiopental also has been used. Pentobarbital should be administered as an IV loading infusion totaling 25 mg/kg (ie, 10 mg/kg over 30 minutes and then 5 mg/kg per hour for 3 hours), followed by a maintenance infusion of 1 to 2 mg/kg per hour.[10] If the SBP falls during the loading or maintenance infusions, the rate should be slowed temporarily and blood pressure support initiated. The goal of a barbiturate coma is to maintain ICP and CPP at the previously discussed target thresholds in addition to achieving a pentobarbital steady-state concentration of between 30 and 40 mg/L (133 and 178 mmol/L) (despite poor correlation between serum concentrations and outcome) and electroencephalography (EEG) burst suppression.[10] Initiation of barbiturate therapy withdrawal can occur when ICP has been controlled satisfactorily for 24 to 48 hours. Barbiturates should be tapered over 24 to 72 hours to prevent ICP spikes.

Side effects associated with high-dose barbiturate therapy involve primarily the cardiovascular system. Hypotension caused by peripheral vasodilation may occur, necessitating decreasing the barbiturate dose or the administration of fluids and vasopressors to maintain blood pressure. A systematic review of the literature suggested that one of every four patients receiving barbiturate therapy will develop hypotension.[48] Gastrointestinal (GI) effects of barbiturates include decreased GI muscular tone and decreased amplitude of contraction. On emergence from coma, there may be a period of GI hypermotility. Care should be taken to avoid extravasation of pentobarbital and thiopental solutions because severe tissue damage may occur. Barbiturates should be administered by continuous infusion through a central line dedicated for this purpose. The potential for barbiturates to induce the hepatic drug metabolism of concurrent medications should be also considered. Lastly, the potential for prolonged interference with the neurologic examination of TBI patients must be considered prior to the initiation of high-dose barbiturate therapy.

Corticosteroids

7 Although corticosteroids are effective in preventing or reducing cerebral edema in patients with nontraumatic conditions producing vasogenic edema, studies in TBI patients have not demonstrated the ability of corticosteroids to lower ICP or improve outcome.[10,14] Specifically, use of corticosteroids following TBI has been associated with increased mortality and complications, including GI bleeding, glucose intolerance, electrolyte abnormalities, and infection. The largest investigation to date was known as the corticosteroid randomization after significant head injury (CRASH) study.[50] In this study, 10,008 patients with a GCS score less than or equal to 14 were randomized to receive a 48-hour continuous infusion of methylprednisolone or placebo. Results of this study indicated a higher risk of death within 2 weeks of enrollment (relative risk 1.18) in those patients receiving corticosteroids compared with patients receiving placebo (*P* less than 0.001).[50] Based on this and several other major randomized trials, the BTF/AANS adult and pediatric guidelines recommend that high-dose corticosteroids not be used in patients with moderate to severe TBI.[10,14]

TREATMENT AND PROPHYLAXIS OF COMPLICATIONS

In addition to specific management of TBI problems such as intracranial hypertension, the potential for secondary complications must also considered in addition to rendering general supportive care. Development and implementation of clinical pathways for consistency of care, and clinical investigation of neuroprotective agents are important in advancing TBI treatment in the future.

Posttraumatic Seizures

It is generally agreed that adult patients who have experienced one or more seizures following a moderate-to-severe TBI should receive anticonvulsant therapy to avoid increases in $CMRO_2$ that occur with the onset of subsequent seizures and to prevent the development of (sometimes subclinical) status epilepticus with associated increase in mortality.[10] Initial therapy in these persons should consist of incremental IV doses of diazepam (5-40 mg adults, 0.1-0.5 mg/kg infants and children) or lorazepam (2-8 mg adults, 0.03-0.1 mg/kg infants and children) to terminate any active seizure activity, followed by IV phenytoin to prevent seizure recurrence. Phenytoin dosing regimens for adults and pediatric patients include an IV loading dose of 15 to 20 and 10 to 15 mg/kg, respectively, followed by a maintenance dose of 5 mg/kg per day. Alternatively, fosphenytoin, a water-soluble phosphate ester of phenytoin, can be administered IV or intramuscularly using the same doses, specified as phenytoin equivalents (PE). The merits of preventive anticonvulsant therapy in patients who have not had a seizure postinjury historically have been more controversial. Risk factors for early posttraumatic seizures (less than 7 days after injury) include a GCS score of less than 10, a cortical contusion, a depressed skull fracture, a subdural hematoma, an epidural hematoma, an intracerebral hematoma, a penetrating head wound, or a seizure within the first 24 hours of injury.[10] In a landmark randomized, placebo-controlled study, the incidence of early posttraumatic seizures in patients receiving placebo was 14.2% compared with 3.6% in patients receiving phenytoin (*P* less than 0.05) without a significant increase in drug-related side effects.[51] (8) Thus, it is recommended that phenytoin (or alternatively carbamazepine) should be used to prevent seizures in TBI patients at high risk for the first 7 days after injury.[10,51] Recommendations in pediatric TBI patients state that phenytoin may be used in the first 7 days postinjury to prevent early seizures.[14] Interestingly, recent data suggest that phenytoin may not decrease early posttraumatic seizures and may diminish functional outcome after blunt TBI, challenging this longstanding practice.[52]

Clinical **Controversy...**

Prophylactic phenytoin therapy for TBI patients deemed at risk of posttraumatic seizures has been a traditional management strategy for decades. Recent data challenge this practice based on failure of phenytoin to decrease posttraumatic seizures and possibly diminish functional outcomes in TBI patients.

Valproate therapy is not recommended based on a trend for higher mortality in a study comparing valproate-treated patients with those receiving phenytoin short-term therapy.[51] Levetiracetam is a potentially attractive option;[53,54] however, the drug should be used cautiously because it is not approved as monotherapy for seizures, and effectiveness in patients with TBI has not been studied in a large randomized clinical trial. Furthermore, the cost-effectiveness of levetiracetam versus phenytoin favors phenytoin.[55,56] A high-quality, randomized, clinical trial demonstrating superiority is needed before levetiracetam displaces phenytoin as the drug of choice following TBI. Nonetheless, if used in TBI patients, the potential for increased levetiracetam systemic clearance should be considered in dosing this agent.[57] The benefits of prophylactic anticonvulsants beyond 7 days have not been demonstrated, and thus their use for this indication is not recommended.[10,14] Unfortunately, despite reducing the incidence of early seizures following brain injury, no beneficial effects have been documented for anticonvulsants on patient mortality or long-term disability.[10,51] This is particularly disconcerting considering that the long-term risk of epilepsy after TBI has been documented up to 10 years or longer based on the results of a recent population-based cohort study.[58]

Supportive Care

While normalizing ICP and maintaining an adequate CPP are the highest priorities in preventing secondary injury following severe TBI, attention also must be given to preventing and/or treating systemic and extracranial complications.[10] One such complication is systemic hypertension. Antihypertensives that can be used include IV labetalol, nicardipine, and enaliprilat.[7] Fluid and electrolyte management is another important area of focus in the critically ill TBI patient. Common electrolyte disturbances in TBI patients that should be monitored and treated aggressively include hyponatremia, hypomagnesemia, hypokalemia, and hypophosphatemia. Aggressive nutritional support of the TBI patient is another important therapeutic consideration. Evidence suggests that early feeding of TBI patients (ie, by 7 days) may be associated with a trend toward better outcomes in terms of survival and disability.[7,10,59] Early enteral nutrition, in particular, within 48 hours is associated with better survival and better outcome at 1 month postinjury based on a recent retrospective study of severe TBI patients compared with matched controls who did not receive early enteral nutrition.[60] Hyperglycemia (glucose ≥160 mg/dL [8.9 mmol/L]) is also common in patients with TBI and is associated with worse outcomes.[61] Nevertheless, intensive insulin therapy versus conventional glucose control should not be used since it is associated with adverse effects on brain glucose metabolism[62] and poor outcomes.[63] Infectious complications commonly encountered in severe TBI patients include nosocomial pneumonia, sepsis, urinary tract infections, and meningitis. Treatment of these potentially devastating infections should be aggressive, with careful attention being paid to antibiotic blood–brain barrier penetration for intracranial infections. Hyperthermia also should be avoided in TBI patients because patients with elevated temperatures have poorer outcomes than normothermic patients.[64,65] Hence aggressive maintenance of a core temperature of less than 37.5°C (99.5°F) using acetaminophen, nonsteroidal anti-inflammatory drugs (NSAIDs), and cooling blankets is indicated for patients following severe TBI. Other important therapeutic interventions include acute gastritis prophylaxis, and prevention of decubiti and contractures. Prevention of thromboembolic events is also extremely important supportive care in TBI patients since the incidence of a deep venous thrombosis is higher in TBI patients compared with patients without brain injury.[66] This can be accomplished with the use of intermittent pneumatic compression devices (preferred) or graduated compression stockings initially. Thereafter, the decision to start systemic therapy (eg, low-molecular weight heparin) depends on multiple factors. Generally, patients who had relatively minor bleeding on the initial CT scan and good ICP control can have pharmacological prophylaxis started within 24 to 48 hours postinjury.[67,68] Data suggest that TBI patients with an intracranial hemorrhage can have systemic anticoagulation prophylaxis safely and effectively (ie, reduced deep venous thromboses) initiated 24 hours after a follow-up CT scan shows no worsening of bleeding in patients with an intracranial hemorrhage.[69] However, a recent evidence-based review recommends waiting 72 hours for patients at moderate to high-risk of intracranial hemorrhage postinjury.[67] Regardless of initiation time, prophylaxis is continued until they are ambulatory.[10,70,71] Nevertheless, systemic anticoagulation must be used with caution in patients with more severe intracerebral hemorrhage, or in patients who may need to undergo craniotomy early in their course. Monitoring for a coagulopathy is important in any severe TBI patient, since the incidence is high (greater than 30%), and coagulopathy is associated with a significantly longer ICU length of stay and an almost 10-fold increase in mortality based on data from a recent study.[72] Low platelet count was the strongest predictor of intracranial bleeding progression compared with other coagulation tests in isolated TBI patients based on a recent retrospective study.[73] Reversal of coagulopathy with recombinant factor VIIa in critically ill trauma patients with TBI is popular among some practitioners despite lacking an approved indication or large clinical trials demonstrating its safety and efficacy in TBI patients.[74-76] Tranexamic acid is a less expensive hemostatic alternative to recombinant factor VIIa. However, more data are needed to determine the role of this agent in isolated TBI patients before it is used routinely despite being generally advocated in bleeding trauma patients.[77-79] A study known as CRASH-3 is currently underway investigating the role of early administration tranexamic acid in TBI patients with intracranial bleeding.[80]

Clinical **Controversy...**

Tranexamic acid is an antifibrinolytic agent that has been demonstrated to improve mortality in bleeding trauma patients. It is unclear if tranexamic acid should be administered to TBI patients with isolated intracranial bleeding.

Clinical Pathways/Guideline Implementation

Use of clinical pathways and formal TBI management guidelines have been demonstrated to improve TBI patient outcomes and reduce institutional resource utilization.[81,82] A cost–benefit analysis revealed that adoption of the BTF guidelines resulted in an increase of more than 3,600 adult severe TBI patients surviving at least 1 day from the more than 23,000 patients with severe TBI admitted annually to U.S. hospitals. Furthermore, patients having a good outcome based on their Glasgow Outcome Scale (GOS) increased from 35% to 66% with an overall estimated annual cost savings exceeding $4 billion.[83] Few practitioners would dispute the overall importance of integrating current evidence-based management guidelines into clinical practice as a means to optimize care and improve the functional outcome of TBI patients.

Investigational Therapy

9 The steady decrease in morbidity and mortality following severe neurotrauma over the past 30 years can be attributed largely to expeditious and aggressive management of events resulting in secondary injury (ie, ischemia, hypoxia, increased ICP) using conventional treatment strategies. Numerous neuroprotective agents targeting specific pathophysiologic processes that are theorized to occur following severe TBI have been investigated over the past decade in an attempt to further enhance the prospects for a meaningful recovery. Prominent among these strategies have been attempts to modulate calcium influx through the administration of calcium antagonists[84] and glutamate antagonists including magnesium, and the use of antioxidants/free radical scavengers.[85] Inhibitors of inflammatory mediators also are under consideration as neuroprotective agents.[86] Unfortunately, none of these agents to date has demonstrated a significant reduction in morbidity or mortality following severe TBI in phase III clinical trials. More recently there was immense enthusiasm for progesterone as a neuroprotective agent based on two moderately sized clinical studies that demonstrated improved outcome following acute TBI.[87] However, results of two subsequent large prospective trials of progesterone in patients with acute TBI were halted early due to lack of improving functional outcomes dashing hopes for this promising therapy.[88,89] In contrast, interest continues to exist for erythropoietin-stimulating agents as neuroprotective agents.[85] One prospective clinical trial comparing the erythropoiesis-stimulating agent (ESA), darbepoetin alfa, in severe TBI patients also demonstrated significantly improved survival in those receiving the darbepoetin compared with matched patients not receiving an ESA.[90] Other agents that have may have beneficial effects in TBI based on limited clinical or epidemiologic data include 3-hydroxy-3-methylglutaryl (HMG) coenzyme A reductase inhibitors[91] and β-blockers.[92] However, confirmation of the benefits from either drug class will require additional prospective, randomized, clinical trials in TBI patients. Miscellaneous agents being considered as viable neuroprotective agents based on experimental TBI studies including calpain inhibitors, the immunosuppressant, cyclosporine,[85] as well as inhibitors of caspases (enzymes involved in apoptosis). Others have proposed that stimulation of axonal repair processes versus limiting injury may be the most fruitful neuroprotective pathway for future investigations.[85,93] Acknowledging the complexities surrounding acute TBI, a broad-based, multidisciplinary approach is undoubtedly needed before breakthrough therapies are identified for this multifaceted, catastrophic condition.[94,95] The BRAIN Initiative—Brain Research Through Advancing Neurotechnologies, a Presidential and National Institutes of Health focused program aimed at revolutionizing understanding of the human brain launched in 2014 exemplifies the commitment to this extremely important yet daunting task.[96]

Other Treatment Strategies

The concept of administering commercially available CNS-active agents for nonapproved indications in TBI patients should presently be considered investigative therapy. One example is the use of CNS stimulants in the management and rehabilitation of TBI patients. Data supporting this approach are equivocal.[85] Another example is the use of Parkinson disease medications (eg, amantadine, bromocriptine, carbidopa/levodopa) in severe TBI patients in an attempt to enhance dopamine release and inhibit reuptake within the injured region of the brain. The results of a multicenter, prospective, double-blind, randomized, placebo controlled trial of amantadine, which was conducted in nonpenetrating TBI patients, were recently published.[97] Patients were enrolled 4 to 16 weeks after their TBI. The amantadine-treated patients had a significantly faster recovery and favorable rehabilitation outcomes compared with placebo. Unfortunately, the two groups became indistinguishable relative to neurologic improvement following taper of amantadine. Regardless, this agent holds excellent promise in TBI patients during the postinjury rehabilitation period. Cholinergic agents such as donepezil have also undergone limited investigation in TBI patients.[98] Antidepressants represent yet another class of agents that has been studied in TBI patients.[98] While intuitively appealing, use of psychostimulants to improve cognitive outcomes in TBI patients should be done cautiously with perhaps the lone exception of amantadine until large, well-controlled studies demonstrating beneficial effects are available. Additionally, the timing of administration of these drugs is controversial; the potential for cardiovascular side effects in the face of uncertain benefit would suggest that these drugs should be reserved for the postacute phase of treatment (ie, weeks to months postinjury).

PERSONALIZED PHARMACOTHERAPY

There are several opportunities for personalized pharmacotherapy in severe TBI patients. The most common general pharmacokinetic challenge is that TBI patients have a larger volume of distribution and more rapid hepatic clearance of drugs than most other patient populations. These pharmacokinetic changes often make the optimizing of phenytoin and, less commonly, pentobarbital concentrations very difficult. As such, recommendations for phenytoin and pentobarbital dosing are weight based, and in the case of phenytoin, usually higher than the 300 mg/day dose that is commonly seen in ambulatory patients. Pharmacodynamically, there can be wide interpatient variability in the efficacy of pharmacologic and nonpharmacologic interventions for ICP control. For some patients, there is a high degree of trial and error to find the best combination of interventions that are effective and not contraindicated by other factors. Lastly, the decision to start pharmacologic deep venous thrombosis prophylaxis may also be highly personalized depending on CT findings, neurologic progress, ICP control, and the possible need for surgery.

EVALUATION OF THERAPEUTIC OUTCOMES

The process for evaluation of therapeutic outcomes is summarized in Table 58-4. Patients with severe TBI require ICU monitoring initially with the goals of maintaining or reestablishing neurologic and systemic homeostasis as well as readily detecting any neurologic deterioration. This requires frequent evaluation of the patient's neurologic status (eg, GCS) and measurement of vital signs, urine

TABLE 58-4 Evaluation of Therapeutic Outcomes

General	GCS: Record hourly initially, decrease frequency as neurologic status stabilizes Vital signs (BP, HR, RR, temperature): Record hourly initially, decrease frequency as neurologic status stabilizes UO: Record hourly initially, decrease frequency as neurologic status stabilizes Arterial oxygen saturation: Continuously while in ICU
Risk of increased ICP	ICP: Record hourly, decrease frequency as ICP stabilizes <20 mm Hg (2.7 kPa) (usually not until 48-72 hours postinjury at a minimum) CPP: Record hourly, decrease frequency as CPP stabilizes in the desired range[a]
Laboratory tests	Ethanol concentration and urine drug screen: On admission ABGs: Daily at a minimum while intubated, repeated as needed based on pulmonary instability requiring ventilator setting changes CBC: Daily while in ICU Serum electrolytes (Na, K, Cl): Daily while in ICU. Serum sodium and osmolality may be monitored as frequently as every 6 hours if osmotherapy (mannitol, furosemide, hypertonic saline) is being used Minerals (Mg, Ca, P): Daily initially until concentrations stable
Radiologic procedures	CT scan: Postresuscitation initially with repeat scan(s) as needed based on degree of neurologic instability (eg, decrease in GCS) or initial CT appearance

ABG, arterial blood gas; BP, blood pressure; Ca, calcium; CBC, complete blood count; Cl, chloride; CPP, cerebral perfusion pressure; CT, computed tomography; GCS, Glasgow Coma Scale; HR, heart rate; ICP, intracranial pressure; K, potassium; Mg, magnesium; Na, sodium; P, phosphorus; RR, respiratory rate; UO, urine output.

[a]Continuous monitoring mandated initially if technologically feasible.

output, and arterial oxygen saturation (as well as ICP in patients with an ICP monitor in place). Furthermore, careful attention must be paid to the potential for development of a variety of electrolyte, mineral, and acid–base disturbances; coagulopathies; and infections by obtaining various laboratory tests on a daily basis initially. The intensity of monitoring will be a function of the relative degree of neurologic and hemodynamic stability of the patient in the hours and days following the neurologic insult. Lastly, radiologic tests (eg, CT scans) are essential not only for the initial diagnostic evaluation of TBI patients but also as means to evaluate the etiology for any subsequent neurologic deterioration.

ABBREVIATIONS

AANS	American Association of Neurological Surgeons
ABG	arterial blood gas
ATP	adenosine triphosphate
BTF	Brain Trauma Foundation
CBF	cerebral blood flow
CBV	cerebral blood volume
CDO_2	cerebral oxygen delivery
$CMRO_2$	cerebral oxygen consumption
CPP	cerebral perfusion pressure
CSF	cerebrospinal fluid
CT	computed tomography
ECG	electrocardiogram
EEG	electroencephalography
ESA	erythropoiesis-stimulating agent
FDA	Food and Drug Administration
GCS	Glasgow Coma Scale
GI	gastrointestinal
GOS	Glasgow Outcome Scale
HMG	3-hydroxy-3-methylglutaryl
ICP	intracranial pressure
ICU	intensive care unit
MAP	mean arterial pressure
NMDA	*N*-methyl-D-aspartate
NSAID	nonsteroidal antiinflammatory drug
PIS	propofol infusion syndrome
PRBCs	packed red blood cells
SBP	systolic blood pressure
$SjvO_2$	jugular venous oxygen saturation
TBI	traumatic brain injury

REFERENCES

1. Coronado VG, Xu L, Basavaraju SV, et al. Surveillance for traumatic brain injury-related deaths-United States, 1997-2007. *MMWR Surveill Summ* 2011;60(5):1-32.
2. Prevention CfDCa. CDC grand rounds: Reducing severe traumatic brain injury in the United States. *MMWR Morb Mortal Wkly Rep* 2013;62(27):549-552.
3. Prins M, Greco T, Alexander D, Giza CC. The pathophysiology of traumatic brain injury at a glance. *Dis Model Mech* 2013;6(6):1307-1315.
4. Andriessen TM, Jacobs B, Vos PE. Clinical characteristics and pathophysiological mechanisms of focal and diffuse traumatic brain injury. *J Cell Mol Med* 2010;14(10):2381-2392.
5. Algattas H, Huang JH. Traumatic Brain Injury pathophysiology and treatments: Early, intermediate, and late phases post-injury. *Int J Mol Sci* 2014;15(1):309-341.
6. Hinson HE, Rowell S, Schreiber M. Clinical evidence of inflammation driving secondary brain injury: A systematic review. *J Trauma Acute Care Surg* 2015;78(1):184-191.
7. Frattalone AR, Ling GS. Moderate and severe traumatic brain injury: Pathophysiology and management. *Neurosurg Clin N Am* 2013;24(3):309-319.
8. Stocchetti N, Taccone FS, Citerio G, et al. Neuroprotection in acute brain injury: An up-to-date review. *Crit Care* 2015;19:186.
9. Tasaki O, Shiozaki T, Hamasaki T, et al. Prognostic indicators and outcome prediction model for severe traumatic brain injury. *J Trauma* 2009;66(2):304-308.
10. Bratton SL, Chestnut RM, Ghajar J, et al. Guidelines for the managment of severe head injury. The Brain Trauma Foundation. The American Association of Neurological Surgeons. The Joint Section on Neurotrauma and Critical Care. *J Neurotrauma* 2007;24 Suppl 1: S1-S106.
11. Alarcon JD, Rubiano AM, Chirinos MS, et al. Clinical practice guidelines for the care of patients with severe traumatic brain injury: A systematic evaluation of their quality. *J Trauma Acute Care Surg* 2013;75(2):311-319.
12. Gabriel EJ, Ghajar J, Jagoda A, et al. Guidelines for prehospital management of traumatic brain injury. *J Neurotrauma* 2002;19(1):111-174.
13. Bullock MR, Chesnut R, Ghajar J, et al. Guidelines for the surgical management of traumatic brain injury. *Neurosurgery* 2006;58(3):S2 1-62.
14. Kochanek PM, Carney N, Adelson PD, et al. Guidelines for the acute medical management of severe traumatic brain injury in infants, children, and adolescents-second edition. *Pediatr Crit Care Med* 2012;13 Suppl 1:S1-82.
15. Fuller G, Hasler RM, Mealing N, et al. The association between admission systolic blood pressure and mortality in significant traumatic brain injury: A multi-centre cohort study. *Injury* 2014;45(3):612-617.
16. Gantner D, Moore EM, Cooper DJ. Intravenous fluids in traumatic brain injury: What's the solution? *Curr Opin Crit Care* 2014;20(4):385-389.

17. Cooper DJ, Myburgh J, Heritier S, et al. Albumin resuscitation for traumatic brain injury: is intracranial hypertension the cause of increased mortality? *J Neurotrauma* 2013;30(7):512-518.
18. Sahuquillo J, Martinez-Ricarte F, Poca MA. Decompressive craniectomy in traumatic brain injury after the DECRA trial. Where do we stand? *Curr Opin Crit Care* 2013;19(2):101-106.
19. Cooper DJ, Rosenfeld JV, Murray L, et al. Decompressive craniectomy in diffuse traumatic brain injury. *N Engl J Med* 2011;364(16):1493-1502.
20. Alali AS, Fowler RA, Mainprize TG, et al. Intracranial pressure monitoring in severe traumatic brain injury: results from the American College of Surgeons Trauma Quality Improvement Program. *J Neurotrauma* 2013;30(20):1737-1746.
21. Dawes AJ, Sacks GD, Cryer HG, et al. Intracranial pressure monitoring and inpatient mortality in severe traumatic brain injury: A propensity score-matched analysis. *J Trauma Acute Care Surg* 2015;78(3):492-501; discussion 501-492.
22. Chesnut RM, Temkin N, Carney N, et al. A trial of intracranial-pressure monitoring in traumatic brain injury. *N Engl J Med* 2012;367(26):2471-2481.
23. Lorente L, Martin MM, Almeida T, et al. Serum substance P levels are associated with severity and mortality in patients with severe traumatic brain injury. *Crit Care* 2015;19:192.
24. Neher MD, Keene CN, Rich MC, et al. Serum biomarkers for traumatic brain injury. *South Med J* 2014;107(4):248-255.
25. Stein DM, Kufera JA, Lindell A, et al. Association of CSF biomarkers and secondary insults following severe traumatic brain injury. *Neurocrit Care* 2011;14(2):200-207.
26. Robertson CS, Hannay HJ, Yamal JM, et al. Effect of erythropoietin and transfusion threshold on neurological recovery after traumatic brain injury: A randomized clinical trial. *JAMA* 2014;312(1):36-47.
27. Sanfilippo F, Santonocito C, Veenith T, et al. The role of neuromuscular blockade in patients with traumatic brain injury: A systematic review. *Neurocrit Care* 2015;22(2):325-334.
28. Roberts DJ, Hall RI, Kramer AH, et al. Sedation for critically ill adults with severe traumatic brain injury: A systematic review of randomized controlled trials. *Crit Care Med* 2011;39(12):2743-2751.
29. Meyer MJ, Megyesi J, Meythaler J, et al. Acute management of acquired brain injury part II: an evidence-based review of pharmacological interventions. *Brain Inj* 2010;24(5):706-721.
30. Thal SC, Timaru-Kast R, Wilde F, et al. Propofol impairs neurogenesis and neurologic recovery and increases mortality rate in adult rats after traumatic brain injury. *Crit Care Med* 2014;42(1):129-141.
31. Gu JW, Yang T, Kuang YQ, et al. Comparison of the safety and efficacy of propofol with midazolam for sedation of patients with severe traumatic brain injury: A meta-analysis. *J Crit Care* 2014;29(2):287-290.
32. Zeiler FA, Teitelbaum J, West M, Gillman LM. The ketamine effect on ICP in traumatic brain injury. *Neurocrit Care* 2014;21(1):163-173.
33. Wang X, Ji J, Fen L, Wang A. Effects of dexmedetomidine on cerebral blood flow in critically ill patients with or without traumatic brain injury: A prospective controlled trial. *Brain Inj* 2013;27(13-14):1617-1622.
34. Meyer MJ, Megyesi J, Meythaler J, et al. Acute management of acquired brain injury part I: An evidence-based review of non-pharmacological interventions. *Brain Inj* 2010;24(5):694-705.
35. Clifton GL, Valadka A, Zygun D, et al. Very early hypothermia induction in patients with severe brain injury (the National Acute Brain Injury Study: Hypothermia II): A randomised trial. *Lancet Neurol* 2011;10(2):131-139.
36. Nunnally ME, Jaeschke R, Bellingan GJ, et al. Targeted temperature management in critical care: A report and recommendations from five professional societies. *Crit Care Med* 2011;39(5):1113-1125.
37. Crossley S, Reid J, McLatchie R, et al. A systematic review of therapeutic hypothermia for adult patients following traumatic brain injury. *Crit Care* 2014;18(2):R75.
38. Andrews PJ, Sinclair LH, Harris B, et al. Study of therapeutic hypothermia (32 to 35 degrees C) for intracranial pressure reduction after traumatic brain injury (the Eurotherm3235Trial): Outcome of the pilot phase of the trial. *Trials* 2013;14:277.
39. Empey PE, de Mendizabal NV, Bell MJ, et al. Therapeutic hypothermia decreases phenytoin elimination in children with traumatic brain injury. *Crit Care Med* 2013;41(10):2379-2387.
40. Varon J. Therapeutic hypothermia: Implications for acute care practitioners. *Postgrad Med* 2010;122(1):19-27.
41. Ropper AH. Hyperosmolar therapy for raised intracranial pressure. *N Engl J Med* 2012;367(8):746-752.
42. Wakai A, McCabe A, Roberts I, Schierhout G. Mannitol for acute traumatic brain injury. *Cochrane Database Syst Rev* 2013;8:CD001049.
43. Kim MY, Park JH, Kang NR, et al. Increased risk of acute kidney injury associated with higher infusion rate of mannitol in patients with intracranial hemorrhage. *J Neurosurg* 2014;120(6):1340-1348.
44. Mortazavi MM, Romeo AK, Deep A, et al. Hypertonic saline for treating raised intracranial pressure: Literature review with meta-analysis. *J Neurosurg* 2012;116(1):210-221.
45. Kamel H, Navi BB, Nakagawa K, et al. Hypertonic saline versus mannitol for the treatment of elevated intracranial pressure: A meta-analysis of randomized clinical trials. *Crit Care Med* 2011;39(3):554-559.
46. Francony G, Fauvage B, Falcon D, et al. Equimolar doses of mannitol and hypertonic saline in the treatment of increased intracranial pressure. *Crit Care Med* 2008;36(3):795-800.
47. Sakellaridis N, Pavlou E, Karatzas S, et al. Comparison of mannitol and hypertonic saline in the treatment of severe brain injuries. *J Neurosurg* 2011;114(2):545-548.
48. Roberts I, Sydenham E. Barbiturates for acute traumatic brain injury. *Cochrane Database Syst Rev* 2012;12:CD000033.
49. Marshall GT, James RF, Landman MP, et al. Pentobarbital coma for refractory intra-cranial hypertension after severe traumatic brain injury: Mortality predictions and one-year outcomes in 55 patients. *J Trauma* 2010;69(2):275-283.
50. Roberts I, Yates D, Sandercock P, et al. Effect of intravenous corticosteroids on death within 14 days in 10008 adults with clinically significant head injury (MRC CRASH trial): Randomised placebo-controlled trial. *Lancet* 2004;364(9442):1321-1328.
51. Temkin NR. Preventing and treating posttraumatic seizures: The human experience. *Epilepsia* 2009;50 Suppl 2:10-13.
52. Bhullar IS, Johnson D, Paul JP, et al. More harm than good: Antiseizure prophylaxis after traumatic brain injury does not decrease seizure rates but may inhibit functional recovery. *J Trauma Acute Care Surg* 2014;76(1):54-60; discussion 60-51.
53. Kruer RM, Harris LH, Goodwin H, et al. Changing trends in the use of seizure prophylaxis after traumatic brain injury: a shift from phenytoin to levetiracetam. *J Crit Care* 2013;28(5):883 e889-813.
54. Zafar SN, Khan AA, Ghauri AA, Shamim MS. Phenytoin versus Leviteracetam for seizure prophylaxis after brain injury - A meta analysis. *BMC Neurol* 2012;12:30.
55. Cotton BA, Kao LS, Kozar R, Holcomb JB. Cost-utility analysis of levetiracetam and phenytoin for posttraumatic seizure prophylaxis. *J Trauma* 2011;71(2):375-379.
56. Pieracci FM, Moore EE, Beauchamp K, et al. A cost-minimization analysis of phenytoin versus levetiracetam for early seizure pharmacoprophylaxis after traumatic brain injury. *J Trauma Acute Care Surg* 2012;72(1):276-281.
57. Spencer DD, Jacobi J, Juenke JM, et al. Steady-state pharmacokinetics of intravenous levetiracetam in neurocritical care patients. *Pharmacotherapy* 2011;31(10):934-941.
58. Christensen J, Pedersen MG, Pedersen CB, et al. Long-term risk of epilepsy after traumatic brain injury in children and young adults: A population-based cohort study. *Lancet* 2009;373(9669):1105-1110.
59. Wang X, Dong Y, Han X, et al. Nutritional support for patients sustaining traumatic brain injury: A systematic review and meta-analysis of prospective studies. *PLoS One* 2013;8(3):e58838.
60. Chiang YH, Chao DP, Chu SF, et al. Early enteral nutrition and clinical outcomes of severe traumatic brain injury patients in acute stage: A multi-center cohort study. *J Neurotrauma* 2012;29(1):75-80.
61. Liu-DeRyke X, Collingridge DS, Orme J, et al. Clinical impact of early hyperglycemia during acute phase of traumatic brain injury. *Neurocrit Care* 2009;11(2):151-157.
62. Vespa P, McArthur DL, Stein N, et al. Tight glycemic control increases metabolic distress in traumatic brain injury: A randomized controlled within-subjects trial. *Crit Care Med* 2012;40(6):1923-1929.
63. Graffagnino C, Gurram AR, Kolls B, Olson DM. Intensive insulin therapy in the neurocritical care setting is associated with poor clinical outcomes. *Neurocrit Care* 2010;13(3):307-312.
64. Badjatia N. Hyperthermia and fever control in brain injury. *Crit Care Med* 2009;37(7 Suppl):S250-257.
65. Bohman LE, Levine JM. Fever and therapeutic normothermia in severe brain injury: An update. *Curr Opin Crit Care* 2014;20(2):182-188.
66. Reiff DA, Haricharan RN, Bullington NM, et al. Traumatic brain injury is associated with the development of deep vein thrombosis independent of pharmacological prophylaxis. *J Trauma* 2009;66(5):1436-1440.
67. Abdel-Aziz H, Dunham CM, Malik RJ, Hileman BM. Timing for deep vein thrombosis chemoprophylaxis in traumatic brain injury: An evidence-based review. *Crit Care* 2015;19:96.

68. Phelan HA, Wolf SE, Norwood SH, et al. A randomized, double-blinded, placebo-controlled pilot trial of anticoagulation in low-risk traumatic brain injury: The Delayed Versus Early Enoxaparin Prophylaxis I (DEEP I) study. *J Trauma Acute Care Surg* 2012;73(6):1434-1441.
69. Farooqui A, Hiser B, Barnes SL, Litofsky NS. Safety and efficacy of early thromboembolism chemoprophylaxis after intracranial hemorrhage from traumatic brain injury. *J Neurosurg* 2013;119(6):1576-1582.
70. Koehler DM, Shipman J, Davidson MA, Guillamondegui O. Is early venous thromboembolism prophylaxis safe in trauma patients with intracranial hemorrhage. *J Trauma* 2011;70(2):324-329.
71. Scudday T, Brasel K, Webb T, et al. Safety and efficacy of prophylactic anticoagulation in patients with traumatic brain injury. *J Am Coll Surg* 2011;213(1):148-153; discussion 153-144.
72. Talving P, Benfield R, Hadjizacharia P, et al. Coagulopathy in severe traumatic brain injury: A prospective study. *J Trauma* 2009;66(1):55-61; discussion 61-52.
73. Joseph B, Aziz H, Zangbar B, et al. Acquired coagulopathy of traumatic brain injury defined by routine laboratory tests: which laboratory values matter? *J Trauma Acute Care Surg* 2014;76(1):121-125.
74. DeLoughery EP, Lenfesty B, DeLoughery TG. A retrospective case control study of recombinant factor VIIa in patients with intracranial haemorrhage caused by trauma. *Br J Haematol* 2011;152(5):667-669.
75. Perel P, Roberts I, Shakur H, et al. Haemostatic drugs for traumatic brain injury. *Cochrane Database Syst Rev* 2010(1):CD007877.
76. Yuan Q, Wu X, Du ZY, et al. Low-dose recombinant factor VIIa for reversing coagulopathy in patients with isolated traumatic brain injury. *J Crit Care* 2015;30(1):116-120.
77. Roberts I, Shakur H, Ker K, et al. Antifibrinolytic drugs for acute traumatic injury. *Cochrane Database Syst Rev* 2012;12:CD004896.
78. Yutthakasemsunt S, Kittiwatanagul W, Piyavechvirat P, et al. Tranexamic acid for patients with traumatic brain injury: A randomized, double-blinded, placebo-controlled trial. *BMC Emerg Med* 2013;13:20.
79. Zehtabchi S, Abdel Baki SG, Falzon L, Nishijima DK. Tranexamic acid for traumatic brain injury: A systematic review and meta-analysis. *Am J Emerg Med* 2014;32(12):1503-1509.
80. Dewan Y, Komolafe EO, Mejia-Mantilla JH, et al. CRASH-3 - tranexamic acid for the treatment of significant traumatic brain injury: Study protocol for an international randomized, double-blind, placebo-controlled trial. *Trials* 2012;13:87.
81. Hesdorffer DC, Ghajar J. Marked improvement in adherence to traumatic brain injury guidelines in United States trauma centers. *J Trauma* 2007;63(4):841-847; discussion 847-848.
82. Marion DW. Evidenced-based guidelines for traumatic brain injuries. *Prog Neurol Surg* 2006;19:171-196.
83. Faul M, Wald MM, Rutland-Brown W, et al. Using a cost-benefit analysis to estimate outcomes of a clinical treatment guideline: Testing theBrain Trauma Foundation guidelines for the treatment of severe traumatic brain injury. *J Trauma* 2007;63(6):1271-1278.
84. Xu GZ, Wang MD, Liu KG, et al. A meta-analysis of treating acute traumatic brain injury with calcium channel blockers. *Brain Res Bull* 2013;99:41-47.
85. Diaz-Arrastia R, Kochanek PM, Bergold P, et al. Pharmacotherapy of traumatic brain injury: state of the science and the road forward: Report of the Department of Defense Neurotrauma Pharmacology Workgroup. *J Neurotrauma* 2014;31(2):135-158.
86. Shakur H, Andrews P, Asser T, et al. The BRAIN TRIAL: A randomised, placebo controlled trial of a Bradykinin B2 receptor antagonist (Anatibant) in patients with traumatic brain injury. *Trials* 2009;10:109.
87. Ma J, Huang S, Qin S, You C. Progesterone for acute traumatic brain injury. *Cochrane Database Syst Rev* 2012;10:CD008409.
88. Skolnick BE, Maas AI, Narayan RK, et al. A clinical trial of progesterone for severe traumatic brain injury. *N Engl J Med* 2014;371(26):2467-2476.
89. Wright DW, Yeatts SD, Silbergleit R, et al. Very early administration of progesterone for acute traumatic brain injury. *N Engl J Med* 2014;371(26):2457-2466.
90. Talving P, Lustenberger T, Inaba K, et al. Erythropoiesis-stimulating agent administration and survival after severe traumatic brain injury: A prospective study. *Arch Surg* 2012;147(3):251-255.
91. Wible EF, Laskowitz DT. Statins in traumatic brain injury. *Neurotherapeutics* 2010;7(1):62-73.
92. Alali AS, McCredie VA, Golan E, et al. Beta blockers for acute traumatic brain injury: A systematic review and meta-analysis. *Neurocrit Care* 2014;20(3):514-523.
93. Krieger DW. Therapeutic drug approach to stimulate clinical recovery after brain injury. *Front Neurol Neurosci* 2013;32:76-87.
94. Manley GT, Maas AI. Traumatic brain injury: An international knowledge-based approach. *JAMA* 2013;310(5):473-474.
95. Becker-Barroso, E. A rally for traumatic brain injury research. *Lancet Neurol* 2013;12(12):1127.
96. BRAIN Initative. http://www.braininitiative.nih.gov/index.htm: National Institutes of Health; 2014 [cited 2015 June 23, 2015].
97. Giacino JT, Whyte J, Bagiella E, et al. Placebo-controlled trial of amantadine for severe traumatic brain injury. *N Engl J Med* 2012;366(9):819-826.
98. Meyer MJ, Megyesi J, Meythaler J, et al. Acute management of acquired brain injury Part III: An evidence-based review of interventions used to promote arousal from coma. *Brain Inj* 2010;24(5):722-729.

59

Parkinson Disease

Jack J. Chen and Khashayar Dashtipour

KEY CONCEPTS

1. Awareness and continuous surveillance of motor and nonmotor symptoms in combination with thoughtful consideration of initial and adjunctive therapies with adjustment of drug dosing throughout the course of idiopathic Parkinson disease (PD) is required to optimize long-term therapeutic outcomes, minimize adverse effects, and improve quality of life.
2. The optimal time to start drug therapy varies. In general, treatment should be initiated when the disease begins to interfere with activities of daily living, employment, or quality of life.
3. Surgery is reserved for patients who require additional symptomatic relief or control of motor complications despite receiving medically optimized therapy.
4. Anticholinergic medication can be useful for mild symptoms of PD but, due to anticholinergic side effects, should be used with caution in the elderly and in those with preexisting cognitive difficulties.
5. As monotherapy, amantadine and monoamine oxidase type B (MAO-B) inhibitors provide symptomatic benefit, but less than that of dopamine agonists or carbidopa/levodopa (L-dopa).
6. Carbidopa/L-dopa is the most effective medication for symptomatic treatment and eventually all patients with PD will require it.
7. Most carbidopa/L-dopa–treated patients will develop motor complications (eg, fluctuations and dyskinesias).
8. MAO-B inhibitors and catechol-*O*-methyl-transferase inhibitors are useful add-on therapies to attenuate motor fluctuations in carbidopa/L-dopa–treated patients.
9. Amantadine is a useful add-on agent to attenuate dyskinesias.
10. Dopamine agonists are effective and, compared to L-dopa, associated with less risk of developing motor complications but more risk of causing psychiatric symptoms, such as hallucinations and impulse control disorders.

The presence of tremor at rest, rigidity, bradykinesia, and postural instability (instability of balance) are considered the hallmark motor features of idiopathic Parkinson disease (PD), a disorder of the extrapyramidal system. These clinical features of PD were adeptly described in 1817 by James Parkinson.[1]

EPIDEMIOLOGY

Up to 1 million individuals in the United States have PD. The approximate annual incidence of PD (ie, number of persons diagnosed with PD per year) is age-dependent and ranges from 10 per 100,000 persons in the sixth decade of life (ie, 50-59 years) to 120 per 100,000 persons in the ninth decade of life (ie, 80-89 years).[2] Likewise, the prevalence of PD also increases with age, affecting less than 0.5% of people in their 60s and 2.5% of those older than 80 years.[3] The usual age at time of diagnosis ranges between 55 and 65 years. Overall, a higher preponderance of PD is reported among males.[3]

ETIOLOGY

PD occurs sporadically and the true etiology is unknown. At the cellular level, degeneration of dopaminergic neurons (axons and soma) projecting from the substantia nigra pars compacta (SNc) to the striatum (caudate nucleus and putamen) are a hallmark of PD.[4] Additionally, neurons in autonomic ganglia, enteric nervous system, limbic system, olfactory bulb, spinal cord, and neocortex are affected. The underlying mechanisms are interconnected and multifaceted with involvement of toxic biochemical reactions (excitotoxicity, nitric oxide toxicity, oxidative stress), abnormal cellular and cell death signaling pathways (apoptosis, inflammation), dysfunctional organelles (lysosomes, mitochondria), and dysfunctional protein degradation systems (autophagy, ubiquitin proteasomal system) resulting in cytoplasmic protein (α-synuclein) accumulation.[5] Several of these mechanisms result in excessive production of free radicals which exert stress on cells by damaging membranes and organelles. The SNc and the striatum are regions characterized by high levels of oxidative stress due to dopamine degradation and the Fenton reaction (Fig. 59-1). Normally, intrinsic antioxidants (eg, glutathione) buffer against oxidant stress, but in PD, this buffer might be impaired or overwhelmed. Pathologic findings reveal a correlation between the extent of nigrostriatal dopamine loss and the severity of certain PD motor features (eg, bradykinesia). At the time of PD onset, the estimate losses of SNc neurons and striatal dopamine content are 30% and 50%, respectively.[6] The loss of striatal dopamine exceeds the loss of SNc cell bodies because cellular degeneration begins in the distal presynaptic axon terminals and proceeds over time toward the cell body/soma (ie, "dying back" axonopathy).[6]

Aging, genetic constitution, and environmental factors likely increase an individual's risk for PD.[7,8] Epidemiologic research links environmental factors (eg, chronic exposure to pesticides), with an elevated risk. Interestingly, cigarette smoking and caffeine consumption are consistently associated with a lower risk.[9,10] Genetic polymorphisms and epigenetics also modify an individual's risk for PD. It is known that pesticide exposure and genetic forms of parkinsonism (eg, *leucine-rich repeat kinase 2 [LRRK2]*, *parkin*, *PTEN-induced putative kinase 1 [PINK1]*) are associated with mitochondrial dysfunction and oxidative stress.

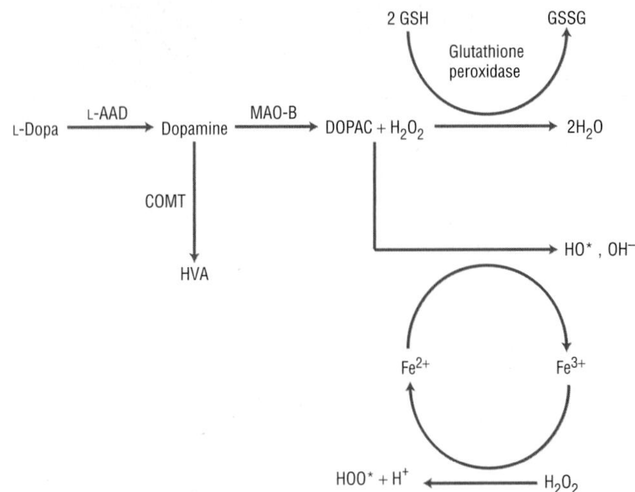

FIGURE 59-1 Dopamine metabolism results in hydrogen peroxide (H_2O_2) formation. In the Fenton reaction, H_2O_2 accepts an electron from ferrous iron (Fe^{2+}) to produce ferric iron (Fe^{3+}) and the hydroxyl radical (HO*). Fe^{3+} is reduced back to Fe^{2+} by another molecule of H_2O_2, forming a hydroperoxyl radical (HOO*). The radicals damage cell membranes and organelles (eg, mitochondria) and also induce apoptotic signaling. (COMT, catechol-*O*-methyl transferase; DOPAC, 3,4-dihydroxyphenylacetic acid; GSH, glutathione; GSSG, glutathione disulfide; H^+, proton; H_2O, water; HVA, homovanillic acid; L-AAD, L-aromatic amino acid decarboxylase; OH^-, the hydroxide ion; MAO-B, monoamine oxidase B.)

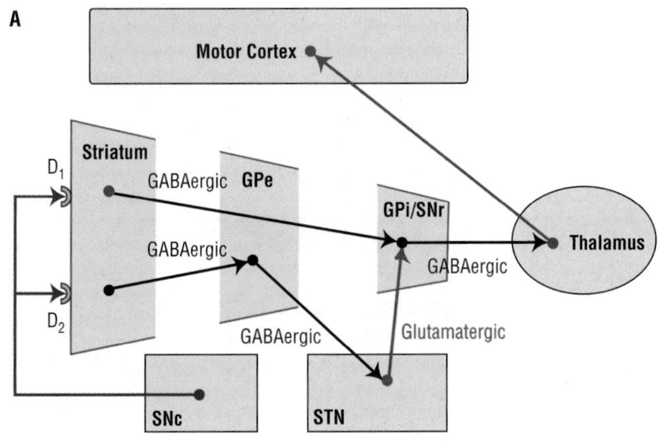

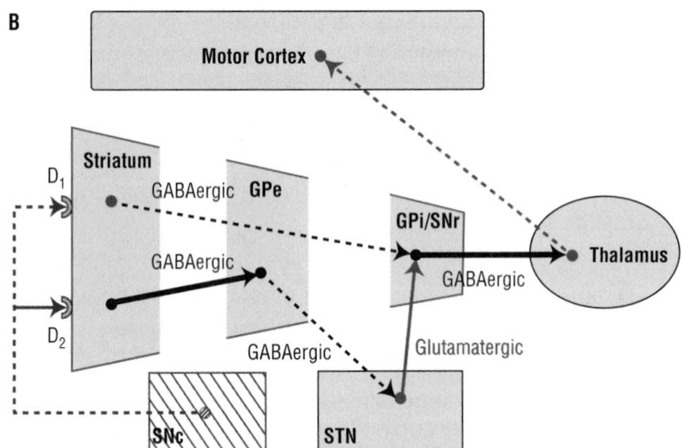

FIGURE 59-2 *A.* Dopaminergic pathways of the basal ganglia–thalamocortical circuit. Activation of D_1 and D_2 receptors results in depolarization and hyperpolarization, respectively, of postsynaptic neurons. (Red dots and lines represent excitatory input; black dots and lines represent inhibitory input) *B.* In Parkinson disease, degeneration of presynaptic nigrostriatal neurons results in inhibition of the thalamocortical circuit and reduced signaling to the motor cortex. (*Dashed lines* represent reduction of neurotransmitter activity; GPe, globus pallidus externa; GPi, globus pallidus interna; SNc, substantia nigra pars compacta; SNr, substantia nigra pars reticulata; STN, subthalamic nucleus.)

PATHOPHYSIOLOGY

A function of the basal ganglia (composed of subcortical structures including the substantia nigra, striatum, globus pallidus, and subthalamic nucleus) is to regulate voluntary movement. These subcortical structures exist in duplicate, with one structure on each side of the midline. The substantia nigra consists of two parts: the SNc and pars reticulata (SNr). Neuronal projections from the SNc to the striatum are referred to as the *nigrostriatal pathway.* The striatum conveys signals to the SNr, via the dopamine$_1$ (D_1) direct and the dopamine$_2$ (D_2) indirect pathways (Fig. 59-2a). The SNr (which is closely linked to the globus pallidus interna [GPi]) receives signals from the striatum and conveys final processed signals to the thalamus, which serves as the "gateway" to the motor cortex. When examining the basal ganglia circuitry, it is important to note that striatal D_1 receptors are coupled to adenylate cyclase and mediate postsynaptic depolarization, thus D_1 receptor activation results in stimulation of the striatal GABAergic neurons.[11] In contrast, striatal D_2 receptors are coupled to a guanosine triphosphate-binding protein and mediate postsynaptic hyperpolarization, thus D_2 receptor activation results in inhibition of striatal GABAergic neurons.[11] In PD, reduced dopaminergic activation of D_1 and D_2 receptors and the sequential downstream effect on signaling pathways results in a net inhibitory tone on the thalamus (Fig. 59-2b). Dopaminergic therapies help restore functional activity within the D_1 and D_2 pathways with the latter primarily responsible for mediating clinical improvements.

Within the SNc, histopathologic features of PD are (1) depigmentation of dopamine-producing neurons (ie, loss of SNc neurons) and (2) presence of Lewy bodies (cytoplasmic filamentous aggregates composed of the protein α-synuclein) in the remaining neurons.[4] Lewy bodies appear in association with adjacent gliosis (ie, a response of glial cells to injury) and the formation and spread of Lewy pathology is proposed to occur in stages. In the premotor stage of PD, Lewy bodies are found in the medulla oblongata, locus coeruleus, raphe nuclei, enteric nervous system, and olfactory bulb. This provides anatomic correlates to observations that mood (eg, anxiety, depression) and peripheral symptoms (eg, constipation, impaired olfaction) are present in premotor stages of PD. Evidence suggests that Lewy pathology develops peripherally in the enteric nervous system and olfactory system and may spread anterogradely or retrogradely to the brain.[12] With the development of Lewy pathology in the midbrain (particularly the SNc), motor features begin to emerge. In advanced stages, Lewy pathology spreads to the cortex, and this may correlate with cognitive and additional behavior changes. Lewy pathology has also been shown to spread into adjacent healthy neurons in a prion-like manner.

CLINICAL PRESENTATION Idiopathic Parkinson Disease

General Features

- The patient exhibits bradykinesia and at least one of the following: resting tremor, rigidity, or postural instability. Asymmetry of motor features is supportive.

Motor Symptoms

- The patient experiences hypokinetic movements, decreased manual dexterity, difficulty arising from a seated position, diminished arm swing during ambulation, dysarthria (slurred speech), dysphagia (difficulty with swallowing), festinating gait (tendency to pass from a walking to a running pace), flexed posture, "freezing" at initiation of movement, hypomimia (reduced facial animation), hypophonia (reduced voice volume), and micrographia (Fig. 59-3).

Autonomic and Sensory Symptoms

- The patient experiences bladder dysfunction, constipation, diaphoresis, fatigue, olfactory impairment, orthostatic intolerance, pain, paresthesia, paroxysmal vascular flushing, seborrhea, sexual dysfunction, and sialorrhea (drooling).

Mental Status Changes

- The patient experiences anxiety, apathy, bradyphrenia (slowness of thought processes), cognitive impairment, depression, and hallucinosis/psychosis (typically drug-induced).

Sleep Disturbances

- The patient experiences excessive daytime sleepiness, insomnia, obstructive sleep apnea, and rapid eye movement (REM) sleep behavior disorder.

Laboratory Tests

- No laboratory tests are available to diagnose PD.

Other Diagnostic Tests

- Genetic testing is not routinely helpful.
- Neuroimaging may be useful for excluding other diagnoses.
- Medication history should be obtained to rule out drug-induced parkinsonism.

The synaptic organization of the basal ganglia also involves a variety of other neurotransmitters and neuromodulators, including acetylcholine, adenosine, enkephalins, γ-aminobutyric acid (GABA), glutamate, serotonin, and substance P. The potential role for drug modulation of these other neurotransmitters and receptor types is an active area of research and novel drug discovery.[13]

Atypical parkinsonian disorders such as multiple system atrophy and progressive supranuclear palsy are characterized by damage to postsynaptic striatal neurons and dopamine receptors. Therefore, dopaminergic therapies are less efficacious in atypical parkinsonism.

CLINICAL PRESENTATION

The clinical diagnosis of PD is based on the presence of bradykinesia and at least one of three other features: muscular rigidity, resting tremor, and postural instability (Table 59-1).[14] Asymmetry of motor features is a supportive finding. It is important to note that tremor is not always present at the time of diagnosis, and postural instability typically occurs in later stages of PD. Overall, a diagnosis of PD can be made with a high level of confidence in a patient who has bradykinesia (along with rest tremor and/or rigidity), prominent asymmetry, and a good response to dopaminergic therapy. For the diagnosis of PD, other conditions must be reasonably excluded (see Table 59-1). Medication-induced parkinsonism can mimic PD and is the second most common form of parkinsonism. It is important to assess for recent use of medications, especially drugs that block D_2 receptors, such as antipsychotics (eg, haloperidol), metoclopramide, or phenothiazine antiemetics (eg, prochlorperazine).[15] Neurologic conditions that can be mistaken for PD include atypical parkinsonisms and tremor disorders (eg, dystonic tremor, essential tremor). Because the management and prognosis of PD differs from these other conditions, obtaining an accurate diagnosis is important. When the diagnosis is in doubt, referral to a movement disorders specialist is recommended. Currently, efforts are underway to develop and validate diagnostic tools based on personalized clinical, laboratory, imaging, and genomics data.

PD develops insidiously and progressively worsens over many years. Tremor of an upper extremity occurring at rest (and occasionally an action or postural tremor) is often the sole presenting complaint; however, only two-thirds of patients with PD have tremor on diagnosis, and some never develop this sign. Tremor in PD is present most commonly in the hands, sometimes with a characteristic pill-rolling motion. Less commonly, tremor may involve the jaw or legs. Like other motor features of PD, resting tremor often begins unilaterally and becomes bilateral with disease progression. Stressful or emotional (either negative or positive) situations often increase the tremor amplitude and severity. Usually, tremor is absent during sleep. Although resting tremor is visibly noticeable in PD and may cause social embarrassment for the patient, it often is the least physically disabling of the motor features.

Rigidity is the increased muscular resistance to passive range of motion and most commonly affects the upper and lower extremities, and occasionally the neck. If tremor is present in the affected extremity, the rigidity is associated with a cogwheel or ratchet-like quality upon examination. Facial muscles also are affected, resulting in hypomimia that may be erroneously interpreted as apathy, depression, or unfriendliness.

Hypokinesia is decreased movement and often described as either bradykinesia (slowness of movement) or akinesia (absence of movement). Movement in PD is often slow throughout an intended action, and difficulty with the initiation of movement also occurs. A progressive slowing and decline in dexterity may impair tasks such as hand clapping, finger tapping, and handwriting (Fig. 59-3). Intermittent immobility or akinesia (freezing) is another common characteristic. Freezing is especially likely to occur in situations such as when walking through a narrow doorway or initiating a turn.

Currently, the clinical diagnosis of PD relies on motor findings; however, researchers have identified markers associated with

TABLE 59-1 Diagnostic Criteria and Differential Diagnosis for Parkinson Disease

Parkinson Disease
Step 1: Presence of bradykinesia and at least one of the following: resting tremor, rigidity, or postural instability
Step 2: Exclude other types of parkinsonism or tremor disorders (see Differential Diagnosis)
Step 3: Presence of at least three supportive positive criteria:
• Asymmetry of motor signs/symptoms
• Unilateral onset
• Progressive disorder
• Resting tremor
• Excellent response to carbidopa/L-dopa
• L-dopa response for 5 years or longer
• Presence of L-dopa dyskinesias
Differential Diagnosis
Essential tremor
Pharmacotoxicity (drug-induced)
Antiemetics (eg, metoclopramide, prochlorperazine)
Antipsychotics (eg, chlorpromazine, fluphenazine, haloperidol, olanzapine, risperidone, thioridazine)
Other drugs (α-methyldopa, cinnarizine, flunarizine, tetrabenazine)
Environmental toxicity (eg, manganese, organophosphates)
Infections (eg, human immunodeficiency virus, subacute sclerosing panencephalitis)
Metabolic disorder (eg, hypothyroidism, parathyroid abnormalities)
Neoplasms, strokes, traumatic lesions involving the nigrostriatal pathways
Normal-pressure hydrocephalus
Parkinsonism with other neuronal system degenerations
Corticobasal ganglionic degeneration
Dementia with Lewy bodies
Multiple-system atrophies
Progressive supranuclear palsy
Familial (hereditary) parkinsonism
Autosomal dominant
α-Synuclein gene mutation (*PARK1* and *PARK4*)
L-responsive dystonia
Leucine-rich repeat kinase 2 (LRRK2) mutation
Rapid-onset dystonia parkinsonism (DYT12)
Spinocerebellar ataxias (SCA2, SCA3)
Autosomal recessive
Wilson disease
Young-onset parkinsonism (DJ-1, parkin, PINK1)
X-linked recessive
Fragile X tremor/ataxia syndrome (FXTAS)
Lubag (DYT3 or Filipino dystonia parkinsonism)

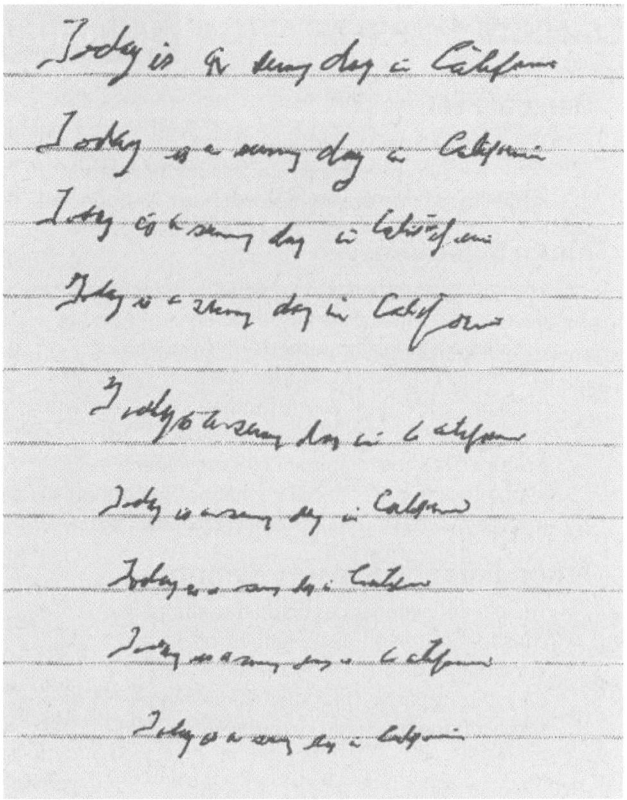

FIGURE 59-3 Example of micrographia in a patient with Parkinson disease. As the sentence, "Today is a sunny day in California" is repeatedly handwritten, progressive diminution of letter size occurs (micrographia). The height of each lined row is approximately 5/16 inches (8 mm). *(Used with permission from Jack J. Chen, PharmD.)*

the premotor stage of PD, such as REM sleep behavior disorder, and olfactory impairment.[16] Such markers may someday aid in very early detection of PD (before onset of motor impairment).

Postural instability, most common in advanced stages of PD, is one of the most disabling problems of PD because it increases the fall risk and is least amenable to pharmacotherapy. Testing for impaired postural responses by means of the pull test (in which a patient is unable to recover balance after sudden backward displacement at the shoulders) can help identify the risk for falling. Many patients with impaired postural responses also have tendencies for propulsive gait with difficulty halting their steps while in motion (festination) and freezing, which also increases the risk of falling.

Nonmotor symptoms are common in PD and must be identified, assessed, managed, and monitored (Table 59-2). These include anxiety, cognitive impairment, constipation, daytime sleepiness, depression, drooling, dysphagia, falling, fatigue, impulsivity, insomnia, orthostatic hypotension, overactive bladder, pain, hallucinations/psychosis, REM sleep behavior disorder, and restless legs syndrome.[17] As a component of managing these nonmotor symptoms, it is important to maintain continuous surveillance of prescription and nonprescription medications for potential side effects that can exacerbate, mimic, or precipitate nonmotor symptoms. If feasible, any identified offending medication should be removed.

TREATMENT

Desired Outcomes

The goal in the management of PD is to improve motor and nonmotor symptoms so that patients are able to maintain the best possible quality of life.[18] Specific objectives to consider when selecting an intervention include preservation of the ability to perform activities of daily living; employment; improvement of mobility; minimization of adverse effects and treatment complications, putative disease modification; and improvement of nonmotor features. To accomplish some of these objectives, consultation with a specialist is helpful (eg, movement disorders, pharmacotherapy, physical therapy, psychiatry, and sleep medicine).

General Approach to Treatment

① ② Awareness and surveillance of motor and nonmotor symptoms in combination with thoughtful selection of initial and adjunctive therapies with adjustment of drug dosing throughout the course of PD is required to optimize long-term therapeutic outcomes, minimize adverse effects, and improve quality of life. The optimal time to start drug therapy in PD varies, but in general, treatment should be initiated when the disease begins to interfere with activities of daily living, employment, or quality of life. Figure 59-4 illustrates a general

TABLE 59-2 Nonmotor Symptoms and Possible Treatments

Symptom	Possible Treatments
Anxiety	Cognitive behavioral therapy, selective serotonin reuptake inhibitors, venlafaxine, minimize "off" times.
Cognitive impairment	Eliminate anticholinergic agents. Add cholinesterase inhibitor.
Constipation	Fiber, hydration, exercise, laxatives, stool softeners.
Daytime sleepiness	Proper night time sleep hygiene, reduce dose of dopamine agonist, referral to sleep specialist to rule out apnea and sleep disorders.
Depression	Selective serotonin reuptake inhibitor, newer-generation serotonin norepinephrine reuptake inhibitor, cognitive behavioral therapy.
Drooling	Local injection of botulinum toxin, atropine sublingual drop, glycopyrrolate, ipratropium sublingual spray.
Dysphagia	Referral to speech therapist, dysphagia diet, avoid anticholinergic medications, manage dry mouth.
Fatigue	Caffeine, armodafinil, modafinil, proper night time sleep hygiene, referral to sleep specialist to rule out sleep disorder.
Falling	Referral to physical therapy; assistance with ambulation, minimize risk for bone fractures, treat osteoporosis.
Hallucinations/psychosis	Eliminate adjunctive medications, especially anticholinergic agents and dopamine agonists. Add clozapine, quetiapine, pimavanserin.
Impulse control disorder	Discontinue dopamine agonist or add clozapine, quetiapine, or naltrexone
Insomnia	Nonbenzodiazepine $GABA_A$ agonists, trazodone.
Orthostatic hypotension	Reduce dose of alpha-blockers, dopamine agonist, diuretics, vasodilators. Abdominal compression, add salt and water to diet, water boluses, fludrocortisone, midodrine, droxidopa, pyridostigmine.
Overactive bladder	Behavioral therapies (eg, bladder training, fluid management, pelvic floor muscle exercises), antimuscarinic agents, mirabegron, intradetrusor injections of botulinum toxin.
Pain	Treatment as per type of pain (eg, dystonic, musculoskeletal, neuropathic), minimize "off" times, appropriate referral to orthopedics, physical therapy, pain specialist, rheumatology.
REM sleep behavior disorder	Clonazepam, melatonin.
Restless legs syndrome	Dopamine agonist at bedtime; gabapentin.

GABA, γ-aminobutyric acid; REM, rapid eye movement.

treatment approach for early and advanced PD. Table 59-3 summarizes antiparkinsonian medications and dosing, and Table 59-4 summarizes monitoring parameters for potential adverse reactions. Treatment guidelines and monographs are updated frequently to keep up with new information and changes in treatment paradigms.[17,19-21] Additionally, general guidelines and recommendations for geriatric health maintenance and disease prevention (eg, bone health, routine vaccinations, vitamin and mineral supplementations) should also be observed.

Clinical **Controversy...**

For younger patients with mild PD, the question of when to initiate L-dopa therapy is a matter of debate. Proponents for the L-dopa sparing strategy cite evidence indicating that (1) this approach is associated with a reduced risk of developing motor complications, such as fluctuations and dyskinesias and (2) initial monotherapy with a dopamine agonist or MAO-B inhibitor provides benefits that are sufficient for symptomatic management of mild PD. Opponents of this strategy recommend that L-dopa should be the drug of choice for initial therapy in mild PD because (1) L-dopa is inexpensive, more effective, and potent; (2) dopamine agonists are associated with more side effects; and (3) once L-dopa is added, dopamine agonists no longer provide a preventive effect on development of motor complications. For older patients (ie, older than 65 years), most clinicians would agree that initial therapy should begin with L-dopa. Overall, clinical necessity and not age should be the major deciding factor for selection of initial drug therapy. Ultimately, the best approach for guiding therapeutic interventions is to take into consideration the patient's disability, comorbidities, and potential side effects and to align decisions with the patient's goals and expectations.

Nonpharmacologic Therapy

Surgical Therapy

3 Currently, surgery should be considered an adjunct to pharmacotherapy when patients are experiencing frequent motor fluctuations or disabling dyskinesia or tremor despite an optimized medical regimen. There are several patient-selection criteria for surgery, including a diagnosis of L-dopa–responsive PD and absence of cognitive impairment. Anatomic targets include the thalamus, GPi, and the subthalamic nucleus (STN). Bilateral, chronic, high-frequency electrical stimulation, also known as deep-brain stimulation (DBS), is the preferred surgical modality.[22]

In DBS surgery, a battery-powered neurostimulator is implanted subcutaneously below the clavicle and provides constant electrical stimulation, via electrode wires, to the targeted brain structure. Thalamic DBS is very effective for suppressing tremor (specifically arm tremor), but it does not significantly improve the other parkinsonian features (bradykinesia, rigidity, motor fluctuations, or dyskinesias). Both STN and GPi DBS are associated with improvements in tremor, rigidity, bradykinesia, motor fluctuations, dyskinesia, and activities of daily living, however, STN DBS allows for greater reduction in medications.[23] As with pharmacotherapy, DBS uncommonly improves gait or postural instability.

DBS procedures require routine adjustment of the electrical stimulation parameters (eg, voltage, frequency, and pulse width) to achieve optimal control while minimizing side effects. The electrical stimulation parameters (or "electrical dosage") are adjusted via a programmable handheld device to meet each patient's needs and are performed by physicians as well as other trained individuals, including nurse practitioners and clinical pharmacists.

Cell-based restorative procedures such as implantation of dopamine-producing cells (ie, human fetal mesencephalon tissue or retinal pigmented epithelial cells) into the striatum have yielded disappointing clinical results.[24] However, other biotherapies, such as

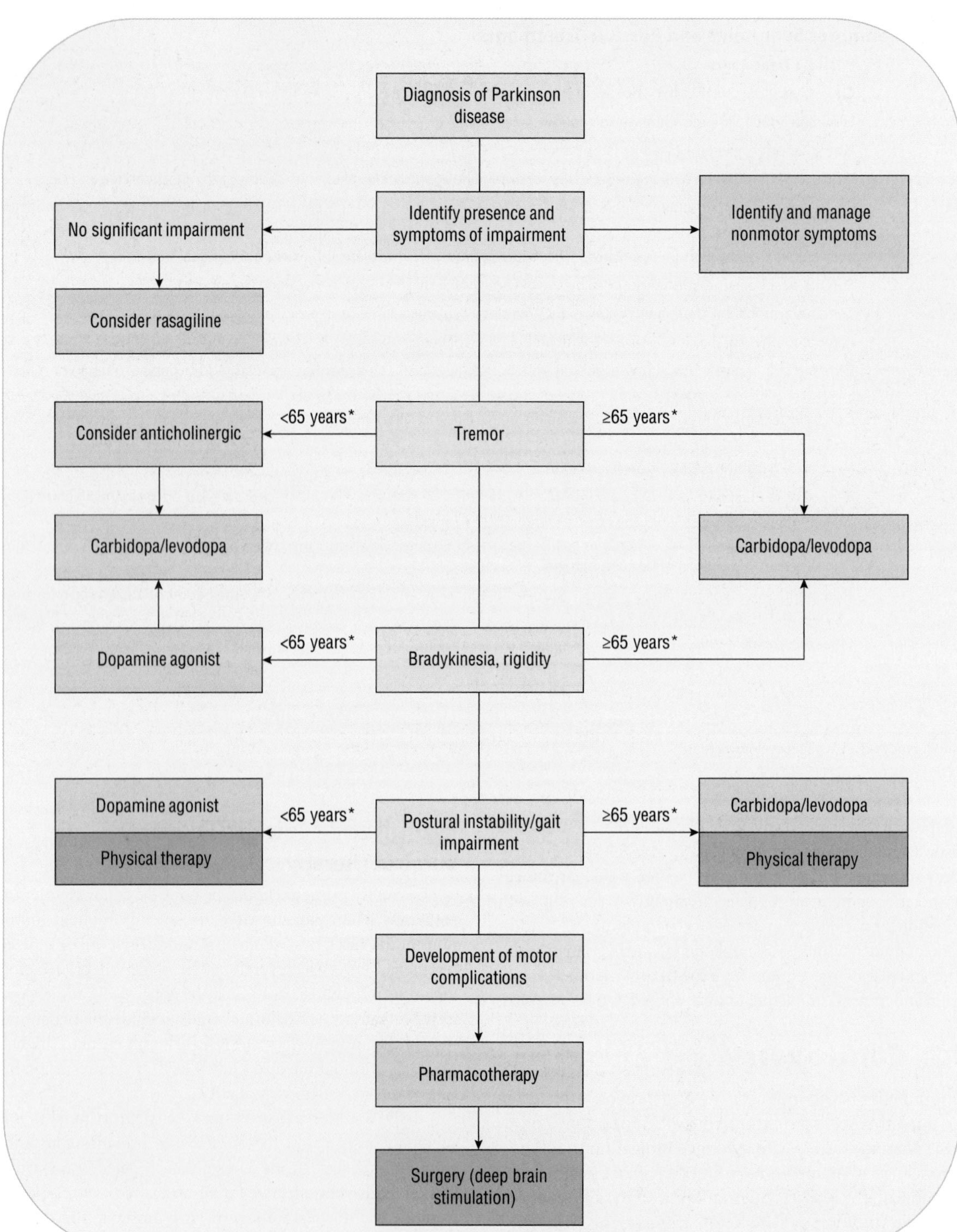

FIGURE 59-4 General approach to the management of early to advanced Parkinson disease. *Age is not the sole determinant for drug choice. Other factors such as cognitive function and overall tolerability of drug (especially in the elderly) should be considered.

stem cell and gene-based approaches, are currently under investigation and remain highly experimental. Of note, gene delivery of neurotrophic factor directly into the putamen and substantia nigra in patients with advanced PD has not demonstrated benefit.[25]

Pharmacologic Therapy

Anticholinergic Medications

4 Because dopamine provides negative feedback to acetylcholine neurons in the striatum, the degeneration of nigrostriatal dopamine neurons also results in a relative increase of striatal cholinergic interneuron activity. This increased cholinergic activity is believed to contribute to the tremor of PD. The anticholinergic drugs (eg, benztropine and trihexyphenidyl) are considered effective against tremor, but no more so than dopaminergic agents.[18] Sometimes dystonic symptoms associated with PD are also improved by anticholinergic agents. Use of anticholinergic agents is limited due to the development of intolerable side effects (eg, anticholinergic effects), necessitating drug discontinuation. Common adverse effects include blurred vision, confusion, constipation, dry mouth, memory difficulty, sleepiness, and urinary retention (see Table 59-4). Younger patients are better able to tolerate anticholinergic side effects,

TABLE 59-3 Dosing of Drugs Used in Parkinson Disease[a]

Generic Name	Trade Name	Starting Dose[b] (mg/day)	Maintenance Dose[b] (mg/day)	Dosage Forms (mg)
Anticholinergic Drugs				
Benztropine	Cogentin	0.5-1	1-6	0.5, 1, 2
Trihexyphenidyl	Artane	1-2	6-15	2, 5, 2/5 mL
Carbidopa/Levodopa Products				
Carbidopa/L-dopa	Sinemet	300[c]	300-2,000[c]	10/100, 25/100, 25/250
Carbidopa/L-dopa ODT	Parcopa	300[c]	300-2,000[c]	10/100, 25/100, 25/250
Carbidopa/L-dopa CR	Sinemet CR	400[c]	400-2,000[c]	25/100, 50/200
Carbidopa/L-dopa IR/ER	Rytary	435[c]	435-2,450[c]	23.75/95, 36.25/145, 48.75/195, 61.25/245[d]
Carbidopa/L-dopa enteral suspension	Duopa	1,000[c]	1,000-2,000[c]	4.63/20 per mL
Carbidopa/L-dopa/entacapone	Stalevo	600[e]	600-1,600[e]	12.5/50/200, 18.75/75/200, 25/100/200, 31.25/125/200, 37.5/150/200, 50/200/200
Carbidopa	Lodosyn	25	25-75	25
Dopamine Agonists				
Apomorphine	Apokyn	1-3	3-12	30/3 mL[f]
Bromocriptine	Parlodel	2.5-5	15-40	2.5, 5
Pramipexole	Mirapex	0.125	1.5-4.5	0.125, 0.25, 0.5, 1, 1.5
Pramipexole ER	Mirapex ER	0.375	1.5-4.5	0.375, 0.75, 1.5, 3, 4.5
Ropinirole	Requip	0.75	9-24	0.25, 0.5, 1, 2, 3, 4, 5
Ropinirole XL	Requip XL	2	8-24	2, 4, 6, 8, 12
Rotigotine	Neupro	2	2-8	1, 2, 3, 4, 6, 8
COMT Inhibitors				
Entacapone	Comtan	200-600	200-1,600	200
Tolcapone	Tasmar	300	300-600	100, 200
MAO-B Inhibitors				
Rasagiline	Azilect	0.5-1	0.5-1	0.5, 1
Selegiline	Eldepryl	5-10	5-10	5
Selegiline ODT	Zelapar	1.25	1.25-2.5	1.25, 2.5
Miscellaneous				
Amantadine	Symmetrel	100	200-300	100, 50/5 mL

COMT, catechol-*O*-methyltransferase; CR, controlled release; IR/ER, immediate-release/extended-release; MAO, monoamine oxidase; ODT, orally disintegrating tablet.

[a]Marketed in the United States for Parkinson disease.

[b]Dosages may vary.

[c]Dosages expressed as L-dopa component.

[d]Dosages of Rytary were developed to avoid confusion with other oral carbidopa/L-dopa products that contain L-dopa in multiples of 50 mg.

[e]Dosages expressed as entacapone component.

[f]Sterile solution of subcutaneous injection with supplied pen injector.

whereas, this drug class is avoided in patients with advanced age, preexisting cognitive deficits, and dysphagia.

Amantadine

5 Although amantadine can be used for managing tremor, rigidity, and bradykinesia, it is most often used for management of L-dopa–induced dyskinesia.[21] Amantadine is typically administered 300 mg/day in divided doses. An amantadine controlled-release formulation (ADS-5102) is in Phase III testing for treatment of L-dopa–induced dyskinesias. The precise mechanism of action of amantadine for management of PD is unknown, but enhancement of dopamine release from presynaptic terminals and inhibition of glutamatergic *N*-methyl-D-aspartate (NMDA) receptors are implicated. The anti-dyskinetic properties of amantadine are presumed to be mediated by antiglutamate properties which, in the setting of dyskinesias, appears to dominate over dopaminergic properties. Amantadine is eliminated renally, and a reduced dose should be administered when renal dysfunction is present (100 mg/day with creatinine clearances of 30-50 mL/min [0.50-0.84 mL/s], 100 mg every other day for creatinine clearances of 15-29 mL/min [0.25-0.49 mL/s], and 200 mg every 7 days for creatinine clearances of less than 15 mL/min [0.25 mL/s], and patients on hemodialysis).

Side effects of amantadine include confusion, dizziness, dry mouth, and hallucinations. The elderly are particularly prone to develop confusion. Not uncommonly, amantadine may cause livedo reticularis, a reversible condition characterized by diffuse mottling of the skin affecting the upper or lower extremities and often accompanied by lower-extremity edema (see Table 59-4).

Carbidopa/L-Dopa

6 L-Dopa is the immediate precursor of dopamine and, in combination with a peripherally acting L-amino acid decarboxylase inhibitor (carbidopa or benserazide), remains the most effective drug for the symptomatic treatment of PD.[21] In the United States, L-Dopa is combined with carbidopa. L-Dopa crosses the blood–brain barrier, whereas carbidopa does not. Carbidopa reduces the unwanted peripheral conversion of L-dopa to dopamine. As a result, increased amounts of L-dopa are transported into the brain, and peripheral

TABLE 59-4 Monitoring of Potential Adverse Reactions to Drug Therapy for Parkinson Disease

Generic Name	Adverse Drug Reaction	Monitoring Parameter	Comments
Amantadine	Confusion	Mental status; renal function	Reduce dosage; adjust dose for renal impairment
	Livedo reticularis	Lower extremity examination; ankle edema	Reversible upon drug discontinuation
Benztropine	Anticholinergic effects, confusion, drowsiness	Dry mouth, mental status, constipation, urinary retention, vision	Reduce dosage; avoid in elderly and in those with a history of constipation, memory impairment, urinary retention
Trihexyphenidyl	See benztropine	See benztropine	See benztropine
Carbidopa/L-dopa	Drowsiness	Mental status	Reduce dose
	Dyskinesias	Abnormal involuntary movements	Reduce dose; add amantadine
	Nausea	Nausea	Take with food
COMT Inhibitors			
Entacapone	Augmentation of L-dopa side effects; also diarrhea	See carbidopa/L-dopa; also bowel movements	Reduce dose of L-dopa; antidiarrheal agents
Tolcapone	See entacapone; also liver toxicity	See carbidopa/L-dopa; also ALT/AST	See carbidopa/L-dopa; also at start of therapy and for every dose increase, ALT and AST levels at baseline and every 2-4 weeks for the first 6 months of therapy; afterward monitor based on clinical judgment.
Dopamine Agonists			
Apomorphine	Drowsiness	Mental status	Reduce dose
	Nausea	Nausea	Premedicate with trimethobenzamide
	Orthostatic hypotension	Blood pressure, dizziness upon standing	Reduce dose
Bromocriptine	See pramipexole; also pulmonary fibrosis	Mental status; also chest radiograph	Reduce dose; chest radiograph at baseline and once yearly
Pramipexole	Confusion	Mental status	Reduce dose
	Drowsiness	Mental status	Reduce dose
	Edema	Lower extremity swelling	Reduce dose or discontinue medication
	Hallucinations/delusions	Behavior, mental status	Reduce dose or discontinue medication
	Impulsivity	Behavior	Discontinue medication
	Nausea	Nausea	Titrate dose upward slowly; take with food
	Orthostatic hypotension	Blood pressure, dizziness upon standing	Reduce dose
Ropinirole	See pramipexole	See pramipexole	See pramipexole
Rotigotine	See pramipexole; also skin irritation at site of patch application	See pramipexole; also skin examination	See pramipexole; rotate patch application site
MAO-B Inhibitors			
Rasagiline	Nausea	Nausea	Take with food
Selegiline	Agitation/confusion	Mental status	Reduce dose
	Insomnia	Sleep	Administer dose earlier in day
	Hallucinations	Behavior, mental status	Reduce dose
	Orthostatic hypotension	Blood pressure, dizziness upon standing	Reduce dose

ALT, alanine aminotransferase; AST, aspartate aminotransferase; COMT, catechol-*O*-methyltransferase; MAO, monoamine oxidase.

adverse effects of dopamine, such as nausea, are reduced. In the SNc, L-dopa is converted to dopamine by the enzyme L-amino acid decarboxylase and inactivated by the enzymes MAO and catechol-*O*-methyltransferase (COMT) (**Figs. 59-1** and 59-5).

6 Regardless of what the initial therapeutic agent is, ultimately all patients with PD will require L-dopa. With regard to carbidopa, about 75 mg/day is required to sufficiently inhibit the peripheral activity of L-amino acid decarboxylase, but some patients require more. Therefore, the usual initial maintenance carbidopa/L-dopa regimen is 25/100 mg three times daily. As the motor features of PD become progressively more severe, use of higher dosages is required. There is no maximum allowable total daily L-dopa dose; however, in patients with severe PD, the usual maximal dose tolerated is approximately 1,000 to 1,500 mg/day. Slow buildup of dose (eg, increments of 100 mg L-dopa per week) can help minimize treatment-emergent side effects, such as drowsiness and nausea (see Table 59-4).

For patients with difficulty swallowing intact tablets, an orally disintegrating tablet (ODT) preparation of carbidopa/L-dopa is available. Although the ODT formulation rapidly dissolves on contact with saliva, the carbidopa/L-dopa does not undergo transmucosal absorption and the dissolved drug in saliva must be swallowed for absorption in the proximal duodenum. Additionally, carbidopa/L-dopa is available in a capsule formulation containing immediate-release (IR) and extended-release (ER) beads (ie, Rytary) which can be sprinkled on food (eg, apple sauce).

Pharmacokinetics There is marked intra- and intersubject variability in the time to peak plasma concentrations after oral carbidopa/L-dopa, and this may in part be attributed to differences in gastric emptying. L-Dopa is absorbed in the proximal duodenum by a saturable large neutral amino acid transport system. Competition for this transporter by dietary (or pharmaceutical) large neutral amino acids (eg, leucine, phenylalanine) may result in reduced

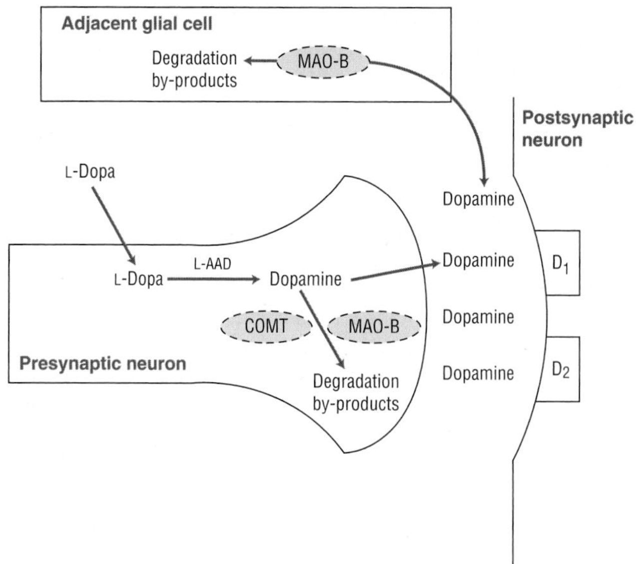

FIGURE 59-5 Dopamine synthesis and metabolism within the striatal neurons. See also Fig. 59-1 for additional details. (COMT, catechol-O-methyl transferase; D_1–D_2, dopamine receptors; L-AAD, L-aromatic amino acid decarboxylase; L-Dopa, levodopa; MAO-B, monoamine oxidase B.)

L-dopa bioavailability. However, for patients with early PD, this interaction is generally not significant.

L-Dopa is not bound to plasma proteins. Active transport across the blood–brain barrier also occurs by the large neutral amino acid transporter system. In advanced PD, special diets involving protein restriction may improve L-dopa responsiveness and are sometimes implemented. A metabolite of L-dopa, 3-O-methyldopa, also competes for transport, but it is not clear how this affects L-dopa clinical response.

When peripheral decarboxylation of L-dopa is inhibited by carbidopa, 3-O-methylation (via COMT) becomes the predominant catabolic pathway. The elimination half-life of L-dopa is about 1 hour, and this is extended to about 1.5 hours with the addition of carbidopa. With the addition of a COMT inhibitor such as entacapone to carbidopa/L-dopa, the elimination half-life is extended to about 2 to 2.5 hours.

It is important to note that the controlled release (ie, Sinemet CR) and IR/ER carbidopa/L-dopa formulations (ie, Rytary) are 70% and 75% bioavailable, respectively, compared to standard IR carbidopa/L-dopa. Manufacturer-provided dosage conversion recommendations are available to guide dosing conversions between carbidopa/L-dopa formulations.

7 Motor Complications of L-Dopa Long-term L-dopa therapy is associated with a variety of motor complications, of which end-of-dose "wearing off" (motor fluctuations) and L-dopa peak-dose dyskinesias are the two most commonly encountered.[26] These motor complications can become disabling and a challenge to manage. The approximate risk of developing either motor fluctuations or dyskinesia is 10% per year of L-dopa therapy.[27,28] However, motor complications can occur as early as 6 months after starting L-dopa therapy, especially if excessive doses are used initially.[29] Table 59-5 lists the common motor complications associated with long-term treatment with L-dopa and suggested initial management strategies. Initiating therapy with the CR form of carbidopa/L-dopa (ie, Sinemet CR) does not reduce the development of motor complications compared with IR carbidopa/L-dopa.[19]

7 End-of-Dose Wearing Off The terms "off" and "on" refer to periods of poor movement (ie, return of tremor, rigidity, or slowness) and good movement, respectively. End-of-dose wearing off prior to a dose of medication is a common type of response fluctuation. This phenomenon is related to the increasing loss of neuronal storage capability for dopamine as well as the short half-life of L-dopa. Initially, exogenous L-dopa is taken up by the remaining SNc neurons, converted to dopamine, and stored in synaptic vesicles. With progressive loss of SNc neurons and storage capacity, patients become more dependent on exogenous carbidopa/L-dopa. Hence the peripheral pharmacokinetic properties of L-dopa increasingly become the determinant of central dopamine synthesis. With advancing PD, the duration of action of a single carbidopa/L-dopa dose progressively shortens, and in some cases may produce benefits for as little as 1 hour. As a result, carbidopa/L-dopa needs to be given more frequently. In addition to administering L-dopa doses more frequently, other options are available (see Table 59-5). In particular, the addition of the COMT inhibitor entacapone or the MAO-B inhibitor rasagiline extends the action of L-dopa, and either should be considered.[19] A dopamine agonist (eg, pramipexole, ropinirole, or rotigotine) also can be added to a carbidopa/L-dopa regimen for management of wearing off. The older CR L-dopa product (ie, Sinemet CR) has been investigated for management of motor fluctuations, but the evidence is not compelling.[19] A newer IR/ER carbidopa/L-dopa formulation (ie, Rytary) contains beads that dissolve at different rates. Following administration, therapeutic L-dopa levels are rapidly achieved and are maintained for 4 to 5 hours providing efficacy for management of motor fluctuations.[30] Also in development, is a novel controlled-release, biodegradable, gastroretentive dosage form consisting of a carbidopa/L-dopa-polymer matrix strip folded like an accordion within a capsule. After administration, the "accordion" strip unfolds and is retained in the stomach due to its larger unfolded dimension which prevents passage through the pyloric sphincter.

Carbidopa/L-dopa enteral suspension is effective and safe for patients with advanced PD experiencing persistent, on/off fluctuations.[31] This carbidopa/L-dopa enteral suspension is contained within a medication cassette reservoir and infusion into the small intestine is achieved by a portable pump device. This treatment is semi-invasive as it requires placement, through the abdominal wall, of a percutaneous endoscopic gastrostomy tube along with a jejunal extension. The drug infusion typically runs for 16 continuous hours per day and is turned off at night.

For acute off episodes, a subcutaneously administered short-acting dopamine agonist, apomorphine, provides a rapid onset of effect (within 20 minutes), and it is administered as needed.[32] An investigational L-dopa inhaled powder formulation (CVT-301) is in clinical testing and administered "as needed" for acute off episodes.

TABLE 59-5 Common Motor Complications and Possible Initial Treatments

Effect	Possible Treatments
End-of-dose "wearing off" (motor fluctuation)	Increase frequency of carbidopa/L-dopa doses; add either COMT inhibitor or MAO-B inhibitor or dopamine agonist; add or switch to extended release carbidopa/L-dopa (ie, Rytary)
"Delayed on" or "no on" response	Give carbidopa/L-dopa on empty stomach; use carbidopa/L-dopa ODT; avoid carbidopa/L-dopa SR; use apomorphine subcutaneous
Start hesitation ("freezing")	Increase carbidopa/L-dopa dose; add a dopamine agonist or MAO-B inhibitor; utilize physical therapy along with assistive walking devices or sensory cues (eg, rhythmic commands, stepping over objects)
Peak-dose dyskinesia	Provide smaller doses of carbidopa/L-dopa; reduce dose of adjunctive dopamine agonist; add amantadine

COMT, catechol-O-methyltransferase; MAO, monoamine oxidase; ODT, orally disintegrating tablet; SR, sustained release.

Although not commonly performed, sipping small amounts of carbidopa/L-dopa solution very frequently throughout the day is also a method for managing on/off fluctuations. A solution that is stable for 72 hours at room temperature can be prepared by adding 10 crushed tablets of carbidopa/L-dopa 10/100 (or 25/100) mg and 2 g crystalline ascorbic acid to 1 L of water.[33]

Often, off episodes occur during the night, and patients will awaken in an off state (as a consequence of an overnight decline of drug levels). Bedtime administration of a dopamine agonist or a drug formulation that provides sustained drug levels overnight (eg, carbidopa/L-dopa CR or IR/ER, ropinirole XL, pramipexole ER, rotigotine transdermal patch) can help reduce nocturnal off episodes and improve functioning upon awakening.

Nonadherence to medications also contributes to the frequency of off episodes. Therefore, engaging and supporting patients and caregivers in overcoming barriers to medication adherence is important.

"Delayed-On" and "No-On" Response "Delayed-on" or "no-on" (a delayed or absent onset of drug effect, respectively) responses to individual doses of carbidopa/L-dopa can be a result of delayed gastric emptying or decreased absorption in the duodenum. Chewing a tablet or crushing it and then drinking a full glass of water or using the ODT formulation on an empty stomach can help mitigate effects of delayed gastric emptying. Additionally, subcutaneously administered apomorphine may be used as rescue therapy for delayed-on or no-on periods. A drug-free period ("drug holiday") may be initiated in an attempt to modify postsynaptic dopamine receptors and thus decrease unpredictable off states. Although not commonly performed because of discomfort (to the patient) and medical risks, when drug holidays are performed, it should be under close medical supervision.

Freezing "Freezing," or a sudden, episodic akinesia of the lower extremities, may occur and will interfere with ambulation and increase the risk of falls. Patients may report that their "feet suddenly feel stuck to the floor" during ambulation or that they have difficulty initiating steps (start hesitation) or turns (turn hesitation). Freezing often is exacerbated by anxiety or when perceived obstacles (eg, doorways, turnstiles) are encountered. Management consists of physical therapy along with use of assistive walking devices and sensory cues.

9 ***Dyskinesias*** Another complication of L-dopa therapy is "on" period dyskinesias (involuntary choreiform movements involving usually the neck, trunk, and lower/upper extremities). Among all the antiparkinson medications, dyskinesias are specific to L-dopa therapy. If patients report "shakiness," it is important to clarify if they are referring to tremor or dyskinesias. Dyskinesias usually are associated with peak striatal dopamine levels (peak-dose dyskinesia) and, simplistically, can be thought of as too much movement secondary to extension of the L-dopa pharmacologic effect. Lowering the dose of carbidopa/L-dopa to counteract dyskinesias should be attempted. However, the use of a lower dose may result in suboptimal control of parkinsonian features, thus, necessitating addition of another antiparkinson agent (eg, dopamine agonist). Glutamate overactivity may also be involved, as suggested by the dyskinesia improvement observed with amantadine (NMDA receptor antagonist) and other antiglutamate ligands.[34] Less commonly, dyskinesias also can develop during the rise and fall of L-dopa effects (the dyskinesia–improvement–dyskinesia or diphasic pattern of response). For severe dyskinesias (despite pharmacologically optimized therapy), surgery should be considered.

"Off-Period" Dystonia In PD, dystonias (sustained muscle contractions) can occur and more commonly affect a distal lower extremity (eg, clenching of toes or involuntary turning of a foot). Dystonias often occur in the early morning hours (as a result of waning drug levels) and improve with the first carbidopa/L-dopa dose of the day. Remedies for early morning dystonia include bedtime administration of a long-acting dopamine agonist, long-acting carbidopa/L-dopa, or baclofen. Additionally, focal injections of botulinum toxin type A or B are effective for persistent focal dystonias. Focal dystonias can also occur as L-dopa peak dose effect and management is similar to that of dyskinesias.

Monoamine Oxidase B Inhibitors

5 Two selective MAO-B inhibitors, rasagiline and selegiline, are available for management of PD. The selective inhibition of MAO-B in the brain interferes with the degradation of dopamine and results in prolonged dopaminergic activity. Both drugs contain a propargylamine moiety, which is essential for conferring irreversible ("suicide") inhibition of MAO-B. At therapeutic doses, these agents preferentially inhibit MAO-B over MAO-A.

A common concern with use of these agents is the potential for interactions with drugs that possess serotonergic activity. Concomitant use of MAO-B inhibitors with meperidine and other selected opioid analgesics is contraindicated because of a small risk of serotonin syndrome. However, concomitant use of serotonergic antidepressants is not contraindicated, and these drugs can be used concomitantly when clinically warranted.[35]

5 8 Selegiline, also known as L-deprenyl, is marketed for extending L-dopa effects and is typically administered 5 mg twice daily. Selegiline is also available as an ODT formulation administered 1.25 to 2.5 mg once daily. A transdermal formulation of selegiline is also available but is not indicated for PD. As monotherapy in early PD, selegiline provides modest improvements in motor function.[2] In advanced PD, adjunctive use of selegiline can provide up to 1 hour of extra on time for patients with wearing off, although the data are inconsistent.[19] This inconsistent effect may be explained, in part, by poor and erratic bioavailability of selegiline.

As an amphetamine pharmacophore, selegiline undergoes first-pass hepatic metabolism (predominantly via cytochrome P450 [CYP450] 2B6 and 2C19) to end products of L-methamphetamine and L-amphetamine. Adverse effects of selegiline are minimal but can include agitation, insomnia (especially if administered at bedtime), hallucinations, and orthostatic hypotension (see Table 59-4). Selegiline also increases the peak effects of L-dopa and can worsen preexisting dyskinesias or psychiatric symptoms such as delusions. With the selegiline ODT formulation, first-pass hepatic metabolism is bypassed as a consequence of transmucosal absorption of the drug. Hence, bioavailability is improved and formation of amphetamine metabolites is reduced.

5 8 Rasagiline is a second-generation, irreversible, selective MAO-B inhibitor administered at 0.5 or 1 mg once daily.[36] Rasagiline is effective as monotherapy in early PD and also as add-on therapy for managing motor fluctuations in advanced PD. For the management of motor fluctuations, the efficacy of rasagiline appears similar to that of entacapone, offering approximately 1 hour of extra on time during the day. Consequently, when an adjunctive agent is required for managing motor fluctuations, rasagiline is considered a first-line agent (as is entacapone).[19] Rasagiline is well tolerated with minimal gastrointestinal (GI) or neuropsychiatric side effects. Rasagiline is metabolized by hepatic CYP1A2 to aminoindan, which is inactive and devoid of amphetamine-like properties.[36]

MAO-B inhibitors with a propargylamine molecular scaffolding have been investigated for neuroprotective properties (clinically referred to as *disease modification*). MAO-B inhibitors possess antiapoptotic properties, and MAO-B inhibition diverts dopamine degradation to an alternate route (ie, COMT) that does not generate free radicals (see Figs. 59-1 and 59-5). To date, clinical studies to demonstrate disease modification with MAO-B inhibitors have yielded inconclusive results.

Clinical **Controversy...**

The optimal timing to initiate drug therapy in patients newly diagnosed with PD is a subject of debate. The traditional approach is to initiate symptomatic therapy when there is evidence of functional impairment. However, others believe that early treatment with a dopaminergic agent, in the absence of functional impairment, acts to alleviate stress on intrinsic compensatory mechanisms, and greater long-term benefit is derived. Randomized controlled studies designed to specifically address this approach have not been conducted, and there is insufficient information on whether treatment in the absence of functional impairment has an acceptable risk-benefit profile or whether this is cost-effective.

Catechol-*O*-Methyltransferase Inhibitors

8 Two COMT inhibitors, entacapone and tolcapone, have been developed to extend the effects of L-dopa and are indicated for managing wearing off. Both reduce the peripheral conversion of L-dopa to dopamine, thus enhancing central L-dopa bioavailability. Consequently, in the absence of L-dopa, they have no effect on PD symptoms. COMT inhibitors increase L-dopa area under the curve by approximately 35% and, for patients with wearing off, can increase on time by about 1 to 2 hours.[19]

Tolcapone inhibits both peripheral and central COMT. Its use is limited by reports of fatal hepatotoxicity, such that strict monitoring of hepatic function, especially during the first 6 months of therapy, is required (see Table 59-4). Because of the hepatotoxicity risk, tolcapone is reserved for patients with fluctuations that are not responding to other therapies.

Entacapone has a shorter half-life than tolcapone, and 200 mg needs to be given with each dose of carbidopa/L-dopa up to a maximum of eight times per day. A triple-combination product of carbidopa/L-dopa/entacapone offers convenience for some patients (ie, fewer tablets to administer). Unlike tolcapone, entacapone is not associated with hepatotoxicity. Entacapone is considered one of the first-line choices for adjunctive therapy to manage motor fluctuations.[19]

With both agents, augmentation of dopaminergic adverse effects may occur and generally are manageable by reduction of the carbidopa/L-dopa dosage. Patients should be advised that other adverse effects include brownish-orange urinary discoloration and delayed onset of diarrhea (weeks to months later).

Dopamine Agonists

Dopamine agonists fall into two pharmacologic subtypes: ergot-derived agonists (bromocriptine) and the nonergot agonists (apomorphine, pramipexole, ropinirole, and rotigotine).[37] Nonergot dopamine agonists have a better safety profile and are more commonly used. Dopamine agonists stimulate dopamine receptors (eg, D_1, D_2, D_3) and are useful as monotherapy in mild-moderate PD, and also as adjuncts to carbidopa/L-dopa therapy to reduce off time in patients with motor fluctuations.[19]

10 Compared with long-term carbidopa/L-dopa therapy, dopamine agonist significantly reduce the risk of developing motor complications.[38,39] For younger patients, who are more likely to develop motor complications, dopamine agonists are preferred over carbidopa/L-dopa. For older patients, dopamine agonists should be used conservatively due to greater likelihood for development of intolerable side effects. For patients with cognitive problems or dementia, dopamine agonists should be avoided.

Common adverse effects of dopamine agonists include nausea, confusion, drowsiness, hallucinations, lower-extremity edema, and orthostatic hypotension (see Table 59-4). When initiating therapy, a slow dose titration is required to minimize development of adverse effects, particularly nausea. The addition of a dopamine agonist to carbidopa/L-dopa therapy also can induce dyskinesias, especially in patients with preexisting dyskinesias. Less common but serious adverse effects include impulsive and compulsive behaviors (eg, pathologic gambling or shopping; paraphilia), delusions/psychosis, and sleep attacks (sudden, unexpected episodes of sleep). Hallucinations and delusion should be managed using a systematic approach that starts with dose reduction or discontinuation of the dopamine agonist, and if needed, addition of an atypical antipsychotic medication such as clozapine, pimavanserin, or quetiapine.[17,20] Involvement of caregivers in surveillance for potential adverse effects of dopamine agonists, particularly development of delusions, hallucinations, and impulsive behaviors, facilitates earlier detection and management.

Pramipexole is initiated at a dose of 0.125 mg three times a day and increased every 5 to 7 days, as tolerated, to a maximum of 1.5 mg three times a day. An extended-release pramipexole formulation is also available. Immediate-release ropinirole is initiated at 0.25 mg three times a day and increased by 0.25 mg three times a day on a weekly basis to a maximum of 24 mg/day. An extended-release ropinirole formulation also is available.

Pramipexole is renally excreted with an 8- to 12-hour half-life. The initial dosage must be adjusted in renal insufficiency (0.125 mg twice daily for creatinine clearances of 35-59 mL/min [0.58-0.99 mL/s], 0.125 mg once daily for creatinine clearances of 15-34 mL/min [0.25-0.57 mL/s]). Ropinirole has a 6-hour half-life and is metabolized by CYP1A2. Potent inhibitors (eg, fluoroquinolone antibiotics) and inducers (eg, cigarette smoking) of this enzyme likely will lead to alterations in ropinirole clearance. Rotigotine transdermal patch is initiated at 2 mg once daily and increased weekly by 2 mg increments to achieve desired therapeutic effect. The rotigotine transdermal patch provides continuous release of drug over a 24-hour period.[40] Patch application sites should be rotated to minimize skin irritation and rash. Rotigotine disposition is not affected by hepatic or renal impairment, and CYP-mediated drug interactions are not significant.

Apomorphine is an aporphine alkaloid originally derived from morphine, but lacks narcotic properties.[32] Because of poor oral bioavailability due to extensive hepatic first-pass metabolism, apomorphine is administered subcutaneously. Apomorphine is indicated for patients with advanced PD who are experiencing intermittent off episodes despite optimized therapy. Upon subcutaneous administration, apomorphine produces an "on" response within 20 minutes. The effective dose ranges from 2 to 6 mg per injection. Sites of injection (abdomen, upper arm, and upper thigh) should be rotated to avoid development of subcutaneous nodules. Apomorphine elimination half-life is approximately 40 minutes, and the duration of benefit can be up to 100 minutes. Nausea and vomiting are common side effects, and prior to the initiation of apomorphine, patients should be premedicated with the antiemetic trimethobenzamide.

PERSONALIZED PHARMACOTHERAPY

Currently, there are no pharmacogenomic parameters used to guide PD pharmacotherapy. Personalized therapy should take into account patient-specific factors including age; comorbidities; severity of functional impairment; nonmotor symptoms; patient preferences, therapeutic goals and outcomes; employment status; drug tolerability; presence of cognitive impairment or motor complications; need for skilled assistance; and health-related economics. The lowest dose of antiparkinson medication that provides satisfactory symptomatic results should be used, and for patients already on carbidopa/L-dopa, optimization of the regimen should be attempted before adding adjunctive agents. With the increasing motor disability, emergence of medication side effects, and changes in severity of nonmotor symptoms, therapy adjustments (eg, dose reductions, medication addition or discontinuation) are expected, and desired therapeutic endpoints should be routinely reassessed.

For mild functional impairment, initial monotherapy may be initiated with an MAO-B inhibitor, such as rasagiline, with the addition of other therapeutic agents as PD motor symptoms progressively worsen. Dopamine agonist monotherapy provides greater symptomatic benefit for patients with mild to moderate impairment. However, dopamine agonists are less well tolerated, especially in older patients. For patients who are older, cognitively impaired, intolerant of dopamine agonists, or experiencing moderate or severe functional impairment, carbidopa/L-dopa is preferred. Ultimately, all patients will require the use of carbidopa/L-dopa (either as monotherapy or in combination with other agents). With the development of motor fluctuations, patients should administer carbiopa/L-dopa more frequently. Alternatively, addition of a COMT inhibitor, MAO-B inhibitor, or dopamine agonist to the carbidopa/L-dopa regimen should be considered. For management of carbodopa/L-dopa–induced peak-dose dyskinesias, a reduction in L-dopa dose and/or addition of amantadine should be considered. Surgery is considered only in patients who need more symptomatic control or who are experiencing severe motor complications despite pharmacologically optimized therapy.

The treatment plan evolves as the disease progresses and must include consideration of short-term symptomatic relief as well as long-term effects. Patient education should be communicated with realistic optimism. For example, it should be explained that although there is no cure for PD, modern medicine has many medications that can provide relief of symptoms. Nonpharmacologic interventions such as exercise should be encouraged, and problematic nonmotor features of PD should always be addressed.

EVALUATION OF THERAPEUTIC OUTCOMES

1 Comprehensive medication management with optimization of medications related to PD improves patient outcomes.[41] Routine evaluation and monitoring of motor and nonmotor symptoms should occur every 3 to 6 months for patients on a stable treatment regimen. With the changes in pharmacotherapy (eg, drug addition, discontinuation, dose change), follow-up monitoring for efficacy and side effects should occur within 1 or 2 weeks and may occur via telephone. Table 59-6 lists the monitoring parameters for PD therapy. Patient and caregiver satisfaction is an important component of evaluating therapeutic outcomes. Toward this end, establishing appropriate treatment expectations is important. Patients and caregivers should be educated that symptoms of PD often progresses with time, and adjustments to the medication regimen will be required to manage motor and nonmotor features. Additionally, some symptoms do not respond to pharmacotherapy (eg, freezing, gait, and postural instability). Assessment of the patient's general level of functioning, including activities of daily living and mobility, is important to determine when medication adjustments or physical therapy interventions are needed. It is also important to be aware of and adhere to the general guidelines and recommendations for geriatric health maintenance and disease prevention (eg, bone health, routine vaccinations, and vitamin and mineral supplementations).

Patients and caregivers can participate in treatment by recording medication administration times as well as the duration of on and off times that can be reviewed at each visit. Periodic review of all prescription and nonprescription medications that the patient is taking should be performed to identify use of medications with side effects that can exacerbate PD motor and nonmotor features. For example, D_2 blockers (such as metoclopramide and typical antipsychotics) can worsen motor features and should be avoided. If the patient reports memory problems, medications with anticholinergic properties should be avoided.

Nonmotor symptoms must be identified, assessed, managed, and monitored. These include anxiety, cognitive impairment, constipation, daytime sleepiness, depression, drooling, dysphagia, fatigue, falls, hallucinations/psychosis, impulsivity, insomnia, orthostatic hypotension, overactive bladder, pain, REM sleep behavior disorder, and restless legs syndrome. Screening for anxiety or depressive disorders will help determine if antidepressant or antianxiety therapy is needed. If falling is a problem, it is important to investigate whether falls are secondary to insufficient motor control, orthostatic hypotension, or drug side effects, such as dizziness. The former may necessitate an increase in dose of antiparkinson agents, and the latter two conditions, a reduction in drug dosage. Physical therapy is also helpful for strengthening ambulation and balance skills to minimize falls. The patient should be questioned about any difficulties with their antiparkinson medications, including presence of adverse effects. Recommendations always should be made in view of the patient's perception of the severity of symptoms and effect on quality of life.

TABLE 59-6 Monitoring Parkinson Disease Therapy

1. Monitor medication administration times. Educate the patient that immediate-release carbidopa/L-dopa is absorbed best on an empty stomach but is commonly taken with food to minimize nausea. Avoid administration of conventional selegiline in the late afternoon or evening to minimize insomnia.
2. Monitor to ensure that the patient and/or caregivers understand the prescribed medication regimen. For example, they should understand that catechol-O-methyltransferase inhibitors work by enhancing the effect of L-dopa and that the patient should not discontinue medication without notifying the clinician.
3. Monitor and inquire specifically about dose-by-dose effects of medication, including response to doses of medication and the presence of dyskinesias, wearing-off effects, dizziness, nausea, orthostasis, or visual hallucinations. Offer suggestions to help alleviate these, or encourage the patient to discuss them with the clinician.
4. Monitor caregiver involvement and facilitation for early detection of abnormal behaviors, dyskinesias, falls, hallucinations, impulsivity, memory problems, mood changes, and sleep disorders.
5. Monitor for nonadherence and, if present, inquire for possible reasons (eg, dosing convenience, financial issues, and adverse effects) and offer suggestions.
6. Monitor for presence of drugs that can exacerbate idiopathic Parkinson disease motor features (eg, D_2 receptor blockers).
7. Monitor for presence of drugs that can exacerbate nonmotor symptoms. Evaluate whether the presence of an anticholinergic agent is causing confusion or cognitive impairment.

ABBREVIATIONS

COMT	catechol-*O*-methyltransferase
CR	controlled release
CYP450	cytochrome P450
D_1	dopamine receptor subtype 1
D_2	dopamine receptor subtype 2
DBS	deep-brain stimulation
ER	extended release
GABA	γ-aminobutyric acid
GI	gastrointestinal
GPi	globus pallidus interna
IR	immediate release
L-dopa	levodopa
MAO	monoamine oxidase
NMDA	*N*-methyl-D-aspartate
ODT	orally disintegrating tablet
PD	Parkinson disease
REM	rapid eye movement
SNc	substantia nigra pars compacta
SNr	substantia nigra pars reticulate
STN	subthalamic nucleus

REFERENCES

1. Parkinson J. *An Essay on the Shaking Palsy.* London: Sherwood, Neely, and Jones; 1817:1-66.
2. Kasten M, Chade A, Tanner CM. Epidemiology of Parkinson's disease. *Handb Clin Neurol* 2007;83:129-151.
3. Pringsheim T, Jette N, Frolkis A, et al. The prevalence of Parkinson's disease: A systematic review and meta-analysis. *Mov Disord* 2014;29:1583-1590.
4. Jellinger KA. The pathomechanisms underlying Parkinson's disease. *Expert Rev Neurother* 2014;14:199-215.
5. Dias V, Junn E, Mouradian MM. The role of oxidative stress in Parkinson's disease. *J Parkinsons Dis* 2013;3:461-491.
6. Burke RE, O'Malley K. Axon degeneration in Parkinson's disease. *Exp Neurol* 2013;246:72-83.
7. Coppedè F. Genetics and epigenetics of Parkinson's disease. *Scientific World J* 2012;2012:489830.
8. Dick FD, De Palma G, Ahmadi A, et al. Geoparkinson study group. Environmental risk factors for Parkinson's disease and parkinsonism: The Geoparkinson study. *Occup Environ Med* 2007;64:666-672.
9. Costa J, Lunet N, Santos C, et al. Caffeine exposure and the risk of Parkinson's disease: A systematic review and meta-analysis of observational studies. *J Alzheimers Dis* 2010;20(Suppl 1):S221-S238.
10. Chen H, Huang X, Guo X, et al. Smoking duration, intensity, and risk of Parkinson disease. *Neurology* 2010;74:878-884.
11. Smith Y, Bevan MD, Shink E, Bolam JP. Microcircuitry of the direct and indirect pathways of the basal ganglia. *Neuroscience* 1998;86:353-387.
12. Hansen C, Li JY. Beyond α-synuclein transfer: pathology propagation in Parkinson's disease. *Trends Mol Med* 2012;18:248-255.
13. Stayte S, Vissel B. Advances in non-dopaminergic treatments for Parkinson's disease. *Front Neurosci* 2014;8:113.
14. Jankovic J. Parkinson's disease: Clinical features and diagnosis. *J Neurol Neurosurg Psychiatry* 2008;79:368-376.
15. López-Sendón JL, Mena MA, de Yébenes JG. Drug-induced parkinsonism in the elderly: Incidence, management and prevention. *Drugs Aging* 2012;29:105-118.
16. Postuma RB, Gagnon JF, Bertrand JA, et al. Parkinson risk in idiopathic REM sleep behavior disorder: Preparing for neuroprotective trials. *Neurology* 2015;84:1104-1113.
17. Seppi K, Weintraub D, Coelho M, et al. The Movement Disorder Society Evidence-Based Medicine Review Update: Treatments for the non-motor symptoms of Parkinson's disease. *Mov Disord* 2011;26(Suppl 3):S42-S80.
18. Chen JJ, Swope DM. Pharmacotherapy for Parkinson's disease. *Pharmacotherapy* 2007;27(12 Pt 2):161S-173S.
19. Pahwa R, Factor SA, Lyons KE, et al. Quality Standards Subcommittee of the American Academy of Neurology. Practice parameter: Treatment of Parkinson's disease with motor fluctuations and dyskinesia (an evidence-based review): Report of the Quality Standards Subcommittee of the American Academy of Neurology. *Neurology* 2006;66:983-995.
20. Miyasaki JM, Shannon K, Voon V, et al. Quality Standards Subcommittee of the American Academy of Neurology. Practice Parameter: Evaluation and treatment of depression, psychosis, and dementia in Parkinson's disease (an evidence-based review): Report of the Quality Standards Subcommittee of the American Academy of Neurology. *Neurology* 2006;66:996-1002.
21. Fox SH, Katzenschlager R, Lim SY, et al. The Movement Disorder Society Evidence-Based Medicine Review Update: Treatments for the motor symptoms of Parkinson's disease. *Mov Disord* 2011;26(Suppl 3):S2-S41.
22. Larson PS. Deep brain stimulation for movement disorders. *Neurotherapeutics* 2014;11:465-474.
23. Liu Y, Li W, Tan C, et al. Meta-analysis comparing deep brain stimulation of the globus pallidus and subthalamic nucleus to treat advanced Parkinson disease. *J Neurosurg* 2014;121:709-718.
24. Drouin-Ouellet J, Barker RA. The challenges of administering cell-based therapies to patients with Parkinson's disease. *Neuroreport* 2013;24:1000-1004.
25. Bartus RT, Kordower JH, Johnson EM Jr, et al. Post-mortem assessment of the short and long-term effects of the trophic factor neurturin in patients with α-synucleinopathies. *Neurobiol Dis* 2015;78:162-71.
26. Khan TS. Off spells and dyskinesias: Pharmacologic management of motor complications. *Cleve Clin J Med* 2012;79(Suppl 2):S8-S13.
27. Stocchi F. Prevention and treatment of motor complications. *Parkinsonism Relat Disord* 2003;9(Suppl 2):S73-S81.
28. Pahwa R, Lyons KE. Options in the treatment of motor fluctuations and dyskinesias in Parkinson's disease: A brief review. *Neurol Clin* 2004;22(Suppl 3):S35-S52.
29. Parkinson Study Group. Levodopa and the progression of Parkinson's disease. *N Engl J Med* 2004;351:2498-2508.
30. Hauser RA, Hsu A, Kell S, et al. IPX066 ADVANCE-PD investigators. Extended-release carbidopa-levodopa (IPX066) compared with immediate-release carbidopa-levodopa in patients with Parkinson's disease and motor fluctuations: A phase 3 randomised, double-blind trial. *Lancet Neurol* 2013;12:346-356.
31. Olanow CW, Kieburtz K, Odin P, et al. The LCIG Horizon Study Group. Continuous intrajejunal infusion of levodopa-carbidopa intestinal gel for patients with advanced Parkinson's disease: a randomised, controlled, double-blind, double-dummy study. *Lancet Neurol* 2014;13:141-149.
32. Chen JJ, Obering C. Apomorphine in the management of motor fluctuations associated with Parkinson's disease. *Clin Ther* 2005;27:1710-1724.
33. Pappert EJ, Buhrfiend C, Lipton JW, et al. Levodopa stability in solution: Time course, environmental effects, and practical recommendations for clinical use. *Mov Disord* 1996;11:24-26.
34. Johnson KA, Conn PJ, Niswender CM. Glutamate receptors as therapeutic targets for Parkinson's disease. *CNS Neurol Disord Drug Targets* 2009;8:475-491.
35. Panissett M, Chen JJ, Rhyee SH, et al. Serotonin toxicity association with concomitant antidepressants and rasagiline treatment: retrospective study (STACCATO). *Pharmacotherapy* 2014;34:1250-1258.
36. Chen JJ, Swope DM, Dashtipour K. Comprehensive review of rasagiline, a second-generation monoamine oxidase inhibitor, for the treatment of Parkinson's disease. *Clin Ther* 2007;29:1825-1849.
37. Blandini F, Armentero MT. Dopamine receptor agonists for Parkinson's disease. *Expert Opin Investig Drugs* 2014;23:387-410.
38. Rascol O, Brooks DJ, Korczyn AD, et al. A five-year study of the incidence of dyskinesia in patients with early Parkinson's disease who were treated with ropinirole or levodopa. 056 Study Group. *N Engl J Med* 2000;342:1484-1491.
39. Parkinson Study Group. Pramipexole vs levodopa as initial treatment for Parkinson's disease: A 4-year randomized controlled trial. *Arch Neurol* 2004;61:1044-1053.
40. Chen JJ, Swope DM, Dashtipour K, Lyons KE. Transdermal rotigotine: A clinically innovative dopamine receptor agonist for the management of Parkinson's disease. *Pharmacotherapy* 2009;29:1452-1467.
41. Schröder S, Martus P, Odin P, Schaefer M. Impact of community pharmaceutical care on patient health and quality of drug treatment in Parkinson's disease. *Int J Clin Pharm* 2012;34:746-756.

60

Pain Management

Chris M. Herndon, Jennifer M. Strickland, and James B. Ray

KEY CONCEPTS

1. It is important, whenever possible, to ask patients if they have pain, to identify the source of pain, and to assess the characteristics of the pain.
2. Patients taking analgesics should be monitored for response and side effects, particularly respiratory depression, sedation and constipation associated with opioids.
3. Oral analgesics are preferred over other dosage forms whenever feasible, but it is important to adjust the route of administration to the needs of the patient.
4. Equianalgesic doses are useful as a guide when converting from one agent to another, but further dose titration usually is required to achieve treatment goals.
5. Doses must be individualized for each patient and administered for an adequate duration of time. Around-the-clock regimens should be considered for acute and chronic pain. As needed regimens should be used for breakthrough pain or when acute pain displays wide variability and/or has subsided greatly.
6. For chronic pain that has a maladaptive inflammatory and/or neuropathic component, anticonvulsants, topical analgesics, tricyclic antidepressants, serotonin-norepinephrine reuptake inhibitors, and opioids should be considered based on evidence based recommendations when available.
7. Whenever possible, a multidisciplinary approach and nonpharmacologic strategies should be used.
8. Placebo therapy should not be used as an attempt to diagnose psychogenic pain.
9. Etiology of pain may not always be identifiable.

INTRODUCTION

If we know that pain and suffering can be alleviated, and do nothing about it, then we ourselves, become the tormentors.

– Primo Levi[1]

Humans have always known and sought relief from pain.[2] Today, pain's impact on society still is great, and pain complaints remain a primary reason patients seek medical advice.[3]

Regrettably, many healthcare providers do not receive adequate training in the treatment of pain. Understanding the pathophysiology of pain and maintaining a thorough understanding of both pharmacologic and nonpharmacologic treatment modalities are important factors in addressing pain control.

DEFINITION

Pain is defined as: "an unpleasant sensory and emotional experience associated with actual or potential tissue damage or described in terms of such damage."[4] Pain is subjective, however, and many clinicians define pain as "whatever the patient says it is."

EPIDEMIOLOGY

Data presented in the recently released Institute of Medicine report, "Relieving Pain in America" suggests that greater than 100 million persons in the United States live with chronic pain.[5] Given that greater than 50% of persons reporting low back pain in the previous 3 months also reported interference with basic and complex activities, it is not surprising that the estimated economic burden of chronic pain alone exceeds 500 billion dollars (US) annually.[5] In 1 year, an estimated 25 million Americans will experience acute pain due to injury or surgery, and one third will experience severe chronic pain at some point in their lives.[3] Unfortunately, despite much public attention, pain often remains inadequately or inappropriately treated.[6,7]

PHYSIOLOGY AND PATHOPHYSIOLOGY

The pathophysiology of pain involves complex interactions between neural and immune networks within the peripheral and central nervous system (CNS) in response to afferent sensory stimuli that produces the conscious experience we know as pain. It can be physiologic and protective (adaptive) or pathophysiologic and harmful (maladaptive).[8]

Adaptive Pain

The pain experienced from touching something too cold, hot, or sharp is called nociceptive pain, a primitive evolutionary mechanism to protect our body from actual or potential tissue damage from external noxious stimuli. Pain that occurs as a result of unavoidable tissue damage (trauma or surgery) creates sensitization at and adjacent to the site of tissue injury. This process also engages the immune system, and is called inflammatory pain. Nociceptive and inflammatory pain are both adaptive and protective. The physiological processing of pain occurs within a neurotransmission circuit via a number of steps known as transduction, conduction, transmission, perception, and modulation.[8]

Transduction

The first step leading to the sensation of pain is stimulation of nerve fiber receptors known as *nociceptors*. These receptors are found in both somatic and visceral structures and help to discriminate between noxious and innocuous stimuli. Nociceptors are activated and subsequently sensitized by mechanical, thermal, and chemical stimuli.[8] The underlying mechanism of these noxious stimuli (which in and of themselves may sensitize/stimulate the receptor) may be the release/activation of numerous cytokines and chemokines that sensitize and/or activate the nociceptors[8,9] (Fig. 60-1).

Conduction

Receptor activation, involving voltage-gated sodium channels, leads to the generation of action potentials that are conducted along

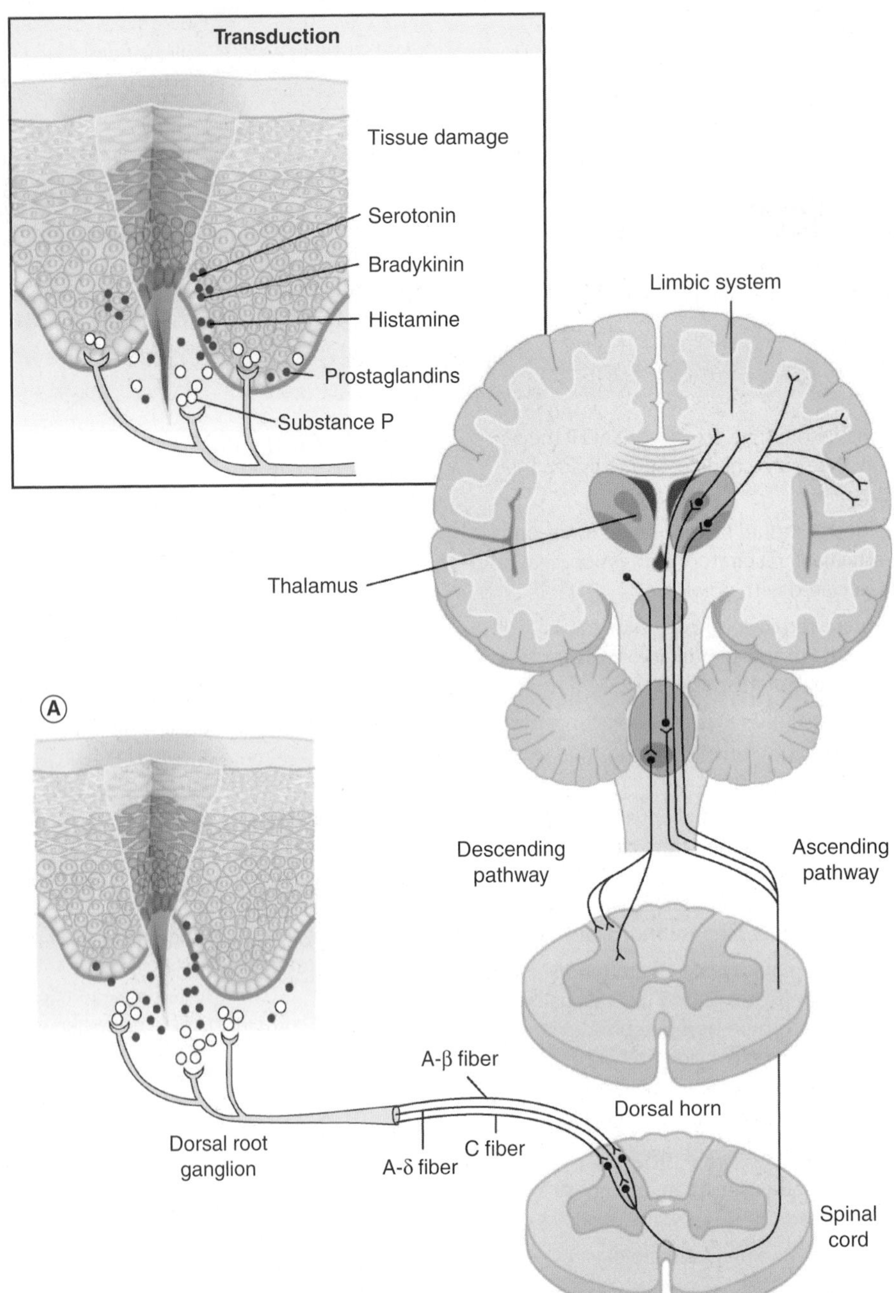

FIGURE 60-1 Schematic representation of nociceptive pain. *(Used with permission from Pasero C, Portenoy R. Neurophysiology of pain and analgesia and the pathophysiology of neuropathic pain. In: McCaffery M, Pasero C, eds. Pain Assessment and Pharmacologic Management. St. Louis: Mosby, 2011:4-5. Copyright © 2011 with permission from Elsevier.)*

afferent A-δ and C-nerve fibers to the spinal cord.[11,12] Stimulation of large-diameter, sparsely myelinated A-δ fibers evokes sharp, well-localized pain, whereas stimulation of unmyelinated, small-diameter C fibers produces aching, poorly localized pain.[10]

Transmission

These afferent, nociceptive pain fibers synapse in various layers (laminae) of the spinal cord's dorsal horn, releasing excitatory neurotransmitters, such as glutamate and substance P. N-type voltage-gated calcium channels regulate the release of these excitatory neurotransmitters. The complex array of events that influence pain can be explained in part by the interactions between neuroreceptors and neurotransmitters that take place in this synapse. Pain signals reach the brain through a host of ascending spinal cord pathways, which include the spinothalamic tract.[10] Other sensory information is also carried along these pathways. Thus, pain is influenced by many factors supplemental to nociception, which prevents simple schematic representation. The thalamus acts as a relay station within the brain. As these pathways ascend and pass the impulses to higher cortical structures, pain can be processed further.[10]

Perception

At this point in transmission, pain is thought to become a conscious experience that takes place in higher cortical structures. The physiology surrounding perception is complex and not well understood, but we know cognitive and behavioral functions can modify pain. Thus relaxation, distraction, meditation, and guided mental imagery may strongly influence pain perception and decrease pain.[11,12] In contrast conditions such as depression or anxiety often worsens pain.[13]

Modulation

The brain and spinal cord modulate pain through a number of intricate processes. Pain transmission may be facilitated by neurotransmitters such as glutamate or substance P to make the signals stronger and pain more intense. The signal can also be attenuated/inhibited by descending pathways that consist of endogenous opioids (eg, enkephalins, and β-endorphins) γ-aminobutyric acid (GABA), norepinephrine, or serotonin.[14,15] Like exogenous opioids, endogenous peptides bind to opioid receptor sites and modulate the transmission of pain impulses.[14] Blockade of *N*-methyl-D-aspartate (NMDA) receptors may increase the μ-receptors' responsiveness to opiates.[16]

Immune System Impact on Pain Signaling

Over the past two decades research has demonstrated that a two-way communication exists between neurons and immune cells within the CNS, especially astrocytes and microglia. Microglia are the equivalent of a macrophage within the CNS.[16,17] Activation of microglia within the CNS in response to nerve injury (both in the periphery and CNS) leads to a complex cascade of events that appears to be responsible for the ongoing pain seen in neuropathic pain conditions. Activated microglia may also play a partial role in the development of opioid tolerance and opioid-induced hyperalgesia. Evidence is emerging that the interface between immune cells and neurons in the CNS plays a significant role in the maintenance of chronic pain and offers a new frontier of potential therapeutic targets in active research.[18]

Maladaptive (Pathophysiologic) Pain

Pathophysiologic pain is distinctly different from nociceptive pain in that it becomes disengaged from noxious stimuli or healing and often is described in terms of chronic pain. This type of pain is a result of damage or abnormal functioning of the peripheral nervous system (PNS) and/or CNS.[11] Maladaptive pain can be neuropathic, in which there is ongoing peripheral nerve injury (eg, postherpetic neuralgia, diabetic neuropathy or chemotherapy-induced neuropathy) or in the CNS (eg, following an ischemic stroke or with multiple sclerosis). Maladaptive pain may also be centralized, where no nerve injury or inflammation exists, but a centrally mediated disturbance in pain processing within the CNS leads to pain hypersensitivity and subsequently spontaneous pain. Classic examples are fibromyalgia, irritable bowel syndrome, temporomandibular joint disorder and chronic tension headaches. Chronic pain states are often mixed with all three mechanisms (nociceptive, neuropathic, and centralized) present within the same patient.[19] These pain syndromes are frequently under-recognized and difficult to treat. Additionally, reported pain is often not commensurate with physical examination findings or imaging results, which may result in undertreatment and ultimately inadequate pain relief.

The mechanism responsible for pain of this nature may be the nervous system's endogenous dynamic nature. Nerve damage or certain disease states may cause both peripheral (eg, alteration in nociceptive nerve fiber sensitivity, alteration of sodium channels, collateral sprouting of nerve fibers) and central (eg, hyperexcitability of central neurons or central sensitization, NMDA-glutamate receptor activation, central disinhibition) changes in neurotransmission leading to increased pain.[14,16] Pain circuits rewire themselves both anatomically and biochemically (often referred to as neural plasticity), and this produces a mismatch between pain stimulation and inhibition, potentially resulting in a progressive increase in the discharge of dorsal horn neurons.[20] The end result is chronic pain, where patients may present with episodic or continuous pain transmission (often described as burning, tingling, shock like, or shooting), exaggerated painful response to normally noxious stimuli (hyperalgesia), and/or painful response to normally non-noxious stimuli (allodynia).[9,10,21] This change over time may help to explain why this type of pain often manifests long after the actual nerve-related injury or when no actual injury is identified.

CLASSIFICATION OF PAIN

1 It is helpful in guiding assessment and treatment of pain to classify or subdivide the presenting symptoms into types of pain. There are numerous ways of classifying pain, such as by type of pain (eg, nociceptive, neuropathic, inflammatory), by pain intensity (eg, mild, moderate, or severe), or most commonly by duration of pain (eg, acute, subacute, or chronic pain).

Acute Pain

Acute pain can be a useful physiologic process, serving its adaptive purpose by warning individuals of disease states and potentially harmful situations. Unfortunately, severe, unremitting, undertreated acute pain may outlive its biologic usefulness, and produce many deleterious effects. Aside from unnecessary suffering, untreated and undertreated acute pain has also been associated with numerous metabolic, hemodynamic and hemostatic changes and has been shown to increase one's risk for the development of chronic pain syndromes.[22] Acute pain is typically short in duration, lasting less than 3 to 6 months. It is often due to an identifiable cause and is usually nociceptive in nature with common causes including surgery, acute illness, trauma, labor, medical procedures, and cancer or cancer treatment.[23]

Chronic Pain

Under normal conditions, acute pain subsides quickly as the healing process decreases the pain-producing stimuli; however, in some instances, pain persists for months to years, leading to a chronic pathophysiologic pain state with features quite different from those of acute pain (Table 60-1).[23] In many cases, the exact etiology of pain may not always be identifiable. Chronic pain can be classified as either being associated with cancer (cancer pain) or from noncancer etiologies (chronic noncancer pain). Chronic noncancer pain is often a result of changes to nerve function and transmission thus making treatment more challenging.[24]

Cancer Pain

Pain associated with potentially life-threatening conditions is often called malignant pain or in the case of cancer, cancer pain.[25] This type of pain includes both chronic and acute (eg, breakthrough pain) components and often has multiple etiologies. It is pain caused by the disease itself (eg, tumor invasion and organ obstruction), treatment (eg, chemotherapy, radiation, and surgical incisions), or diagnostic

TABLE 60-1 Characteristics of Acute and Chronic Pain

Characteristic	Acute Pain	Chronic Pain
Relief of pain	Highly desirable	Highly desirable
Dependence and tolerance to medication	Unusual	Common
Psychological component	Usually not present	Often a major problem
Organic cause	Common	May not be present
Environmental/family issues	Small	Significant
Insomnia	Unusual	Common component
Treatment goal	Cure	Functionality
Depression	Uncommon	Common

Data from references 23 and 27.

procedures (eg, biopsy).[25] Regardless of pain duration, or suspected underlying etiology, a standardized approach to evaluation of a pain complaint is imperative.

CLINICAL PRESENTATION

A patient-oriented approach is essential, and pain evaluation methods should not differ from those used in other medical conditions.[26] 1 Therefore, a comprehensive history and physical examination are imperative to evaluate underlying diseases and other possible contributing factors.[23] This includes asking if the patient has pain and identifying the source when possible; however, the absence of a discreet etiology should not preclude appropriate treatment.[23] A baseline characterization of pain can be obtained by assessing the attributes outlined in Table 60-2.[27]

TREATMENT

Desired pain management outcomes include both nonpharmacologic and pharmacologic strategies.

TABLE 60-2 Assessment of Pain

Onset and duration	When did pain begin and how long has it been since the pain began?
Palliative factors	What makes the pain better?
Provocative factors	What makes the pain worse?
Quality	Describe the pain.
Location	Where is the pain?
Severity/intensity	How does this pain compare with other pain you have experienced?
Temporal factors	Does the intensity of the pain change with time?

Data from reference 23.

Desired Outcomes

The primary goal of pain treatment depends on the type of pain present and should be tailored to individual patients and circumstances. 2 3 For example, a desired outcome in the acute postoperative setting may be to achieve a level of pain relief that allows the patient to attain certain functional goals, such as deep breathing

CLINICAL PRESENTATION Pain

Acute Pain

General

- Look for obvious distress (eg, trauma). In infants, presentation may include changes in feeding habits and/or increased fussiness. Those with dementia may exhibit changes in eating habits, increased agitation, calling out, and/or facial grimacing. Attention also must be given to mental/emotional factors that alter the pain threshold. Anxiety, depression, fatigue, anger, and fear, in particular, are noted to lower this threshold, whereas rest, mood elevation, sympathy, diversion, and understanding raise the pain threshold

Symptoms

- Can be described as sharp, dull, shock like, tingling, shooting, radiating, fluctuating in intensity, and varying in location (these occur in a timely relationship with an obvious noxious stimuli)

Signs

- Hypertension, tachycardia, diaphoresis, mydriasis, and pallor, but these signs are *not diagnostic*
- In some cases there are no obvious physical signs
- Comorbid conditions usually not present
- Outcome of treatment generally predictable

Laboratory Tests

- Pain is always subjective
- There are no specific laboratory tests for pain
- Pain is best diagnosed based on patient description and history

Chronic Pain

General

- Can appear to have no noticeable suffering. Attention also must be given to mental/emotional factors that alter the pain threshold. Anxiety, depression, fatigue, anger, and fear, in particular, are noted to lower this threshold; whereas rest, mood elevation, sympathy, diversion, and understanding raise the pain threshold

Symptoms

- Can be described as sharp, dull, shock-like, tingling, shooting, radiating, fluctuating in intensity, and varying in location (these often occur without a temporal relationship with an obvious noxious stimuli)
- Over time, the pain stimulus may cause symptoms that completely change (eg, sharp to dull and obvious to vague)

Signs

- Hypertension, tachycardia, diaphoresis, mydriasis, and pallor are seldom present
- In most cases there are no obvious signs
- Comorbid conditions often present (eg, insomnia, depression, and anxiety)
- Outcome of treatment often unpredictable

Laboratory Tests

- Pain is always subjective
- Pain is best diagnosed based on patient description and history
- There are *no* specific laboratory tests for pain; however, history and/or diagnostic proof of past trauma (eg, computed tomography) may be helpful in diagnosing etiology. General labs that may be considered include vitamin D, thyroid stimulating hormone (generalized or widespread pain), and B12 (neuropathic pain)

Data from reference 23.

or participation in physical therapy. In comparison, the goals in chronic noncancer pain are to improve or maintain the patient's level of functioning, decrease pain perception, reduce the use of medications when possible, and improve the patient's quality of life. And finally, in cancer pain or other forms of malignant pain, the goal is to provide patients with adequate pain relief such that they can tolerate diagnostic and therapeutic manipulation and permit the patient to function at a level that will allow freedom of movement and choice while minimizing adverse effects of chosen analgesics.[25]

Nonpharmacologic Therapy

The use of nonpharmacologic therapies in the management of pain should always be considered first line therapy, either alone or in combination with appropriate analgesics. Physical manipulation, application of heat or cold, massage, biofeedback, cognitive behavioral therapy, relaxation, acupuncture, and exercise are all modalities with variable efficacy for both acute and chronic pain.[28] Implanted spinal cord stimulators have also been found to be somewhat beneficial in some chronic neuropathic pain conditions.[29] The evidence basis for many of the nonpharmacologic approaches is evolving and the results of these approaches can have varied efficacy based on the skill of the individual applying the modality, as well as the type of pain being treated.

Transcutaneous electrical nerve stimulation (TENS), a commonly used nonpharmacologic therapy, may reduce pain by enhancing natural descending inhibitory pathways within the CNS. Evidence to date suggests that the frequency of the electrical stimulation delivered, presence or absence of systemic analgesics and the type of underlying pain may affect the overall efficacy of this treatment.[30]

Simple interventions (eg, education or introductory information about expected discomfort or pain after certain procedures) reduce patient distress and help to reduce postprocedure pain.[31] Psychological techniques (eg, cognitive-behavioral therapy, relaxation training, and mindfulness-based stress reduction) have proven effective in reducing pain-related disability and improving global functioning in patients with numerous types of chronic pain.[32] 7 Partnering with other clinicians who are familiar with the use of effective nonpharmacologic modalities should always be considered whenever possible to help reduce the overall reliance on pharmacologic approaches, especially opioids.

Pharmacologic Treatment—Appropriate Patient Selection

Pharmacologic treatment is often considered the cornerstone of pain management. Proper agent selection using a benefit-to-risk assessment is crucial when determining the optimal therapeutic plan for an individual patient. The potential for benefit with each pharmacologic option as well as the risk of adverse effects must be assessed.

Patient Selection Considerations in Acute Pain

2 4 5 6 8 The World Health Organization (WHO) recommends a three-step ladder approach using nonopioids as initial treatment and escalating to either "weak" or "strong" opioids based on mild, moderate, or severe pain intensity ratings, respectively. However, patient specific factors (e.g., renal or liver dysfunction which may limit nonopioid alternatives), may lead clinicians to initiate therapy with an opioid to optimize pain relief while minimizing adverse effects.

Patient Selection Considerations in Chronic Noncancer Pain

7 8 9 In all cases of chronic noncancer pain, an integrated systematic approach (such as that often provided by specialty pain providers), with a strong emphasis on patient–clinician relationships, is essential. Patients and clinicians must realize that optimal treatment may take months or even years to achieve. Although opioids continue to be commonly utilized in the management of chronic noncancer pain and can be effective for individual patients, limited data is available supporting the long-term safety and efficacy of these agents.[33] Thus, there is significant debate regarding the benefit of chronic opioid therapy for chronic pain. Chronic opioid therapy in this setting requires careful patient selection to evaluate whether the benefit of therapy outweighs the potential risks in the individual patient. Steps should be taken to identify and manage risks (eg, misuse and abuse) prior to initiating opioid therapy and risk mitigation strategies (eg, treatment agreements that outline patient and provider responsibilities and expectations, urine drug testing) should commonly be employed.[34] "Universal precautions" for pain have been suggested as a method to standardize the assessment and ongoing management of chronic pain with opioids and incorporate many of these principles.[7] 9 Placebo should never be considered as a reasonable option for the management of pain regardless of risk factors.

Pharmacologic Treatment

Nonopioid Agents

Analgesia should be initiated with the most effective analgesic agent having the fewest side effects. Acetaminophen and nonsteroidal anti-inflammatory drugs (NSAIDs) are often preferred first-line therapies in the treatment of mild-to-moderate pain, although the efficacy of acetaminophen has recently been called into question (Table 60-3).[35,36] The exact mechanism of acetaminophen is not completely understood but likely involves central prostaglandin modulation.[37] NSAIDs inhibit formation of varying prostaglandins produced in response to noxious stimuli, thereby decreasing the pain impulses received by the CNS.[29] Acetaminophen is generally indicated as a first-line therapy in some pain-related disease states, such as osteoarthritis, although prompt reassessment should occur to evaluate effectiveness. NSAIDs may be particularly useful in the management of cancer-related bone pain and for short-term relief in the management of chronic low back pain.[38]

Studies comparing the efficacy of individual NSAIDs have failed to identify greater efficacy of any NSAID compared to another. Therefore, the choice of a particular agent often depends on availability, cost, pharmacokinetics, pharmacologic characteristics, and the side-effect profile. Because of the large interpatient variability in response to individual NSAIDs, it is considered rational therapy to switch to another member of this class if there is inadequate response after a sufficient therapeutic trial of any single agent.[39] The duration of a sufficient trial has not been well defined; however, typically, an NSAID should be continued for a minimum of 1 month prior to evaluating the need to switch agents. Chronic use of NSAIDs may result in gastrointestinal (GI), renal, and cardiac toxicity. Topical NSAIDs may offer similar efficacy as oral NSAIDs with improved safety and tolerability in the treatment of small or superficial joint arthritis.[40] Appropriate patient selection for NSAID therapy is critical to ensure optimal benefit while minimizing potential adverse effects.

Opioid Agents

Opioids are often the next step in the management of acute pain and cancer-related chronic pain (Figure 60-3). This medication class may also be an effective treatment option in the management of chronic noncancer pain; however, this continues to be increasingly controversial. When a trial of opioids is warranted, each trial should not be done without a complete assessment of the pain complaint, including an assessment of the patient's functionality and risk factors for opioid misuse and abuse.[34,41]

Opioid choice should be based on patient acceptance; analgesic effectiveness; as well as pharmacokinetic, pharmacodynamic, and side-effect profiles with these attributes provided in Tables 60-4 and 60-5.[42]

TABLE 60-3 Adult FDA-Approved Nonopioid Analgesics (Includes Only FDA-Approved Agents for Pain)

Class and Generic Name (Brand Name)	Approximate Half-Life (h)	Usual Dosage Range (mg)	Maximal Dose (mg/day)
Salicylates			
Acetylsalicylic acid[a]—aspirin (various)	0.25	325-1,000 every 4-6 h	4,000
Choline and magnesium trisalicylate (various)	9-17	1,000-1,500 every 12 h 750 every 8 h (elderly)	3,000
Diflunisal (Dolobid, various)	8-12	500-1,000 initial 250-500 every 8-12 h	1,500
Salsalate (various)	1	1,000 every 12 h or 500 every 6 h	3,000
Para-aminophenol			
Acetaminophen[a] (Oral—Tylenol, various; Parenteral—Ofirmev)	2-3	325-1,000 every 4-6 h	4,000[b] Dosing for peds lower based on weight
Fenamates			
Meclofenamate (various)	0.8-3.3	50-100 every 4-6 h	400
Mefenamic acid (Ponstel)	2	Initial 500, 250 every 6 h (max. 7 days)	1,000[c]
Pyranocarboxylic acid			
Etodolac (various) (immediate release)	7.3	200-400 every 6-8 h	1,000 1,200 with extended-release product
Acetic acid			
Diclofenac potassium (Cataflam, various, Flector [patch] Voltaren Gel, Pennsaid [solution])	1.9	In some patients, initial 100, 50 three times per day Patch available—to be applied twice daily to painful area (intact skin only), Gel and solution dosing joint specific	150[d]
Propionic acids			
Ibuprofen[a] (Motrin, Caldolor, various)	2-2.5	200-400 every 4-6 h Injectable, 400-800 every 6 h (infused over 30 min)	3,200[e] 2,400[e] 1,200[f]
Fenoprofen (Nalfon, various)	3	200 every 4-6 h	3,200
Ketoprofen (various)	2	25-50 every 6-8 h	300 200 with extended-release product
Naproxen (Naprosyn, Anaprox, various)	12-17	500 initial 500 every 12 h or 250 every 6-8 h	1,000[c]
Naproxen sodium[a] (Aleve, various, combined with esomeprazole [Vimovo])	12-17	In some patients, 440 initial[f] 220 every 8-12 h[f]	660[f]
Pyrrolizine carboxylic acid			
Ketorolac—parenteral (Toradol, various)	5-6	30[g]-60 (single IM dose only) 15[g]-30 (single IV dose only) 15[g]-30 every 6 h (IV dose) (max. 5 days)	30[g]-60 15[g]-30 60[g]-120
Ketorolac—oral, indicated for continuation with parenteral only (various)	5-6	10 every 4-6 h (max. 5 days, which includes parenteral doses) In non-elderly patients, initial oral dose of 20	40
Ketorolac—nasal spray, indicated for acute, moderate to moderately severe pain		1 spray (15.75 mg) in each nostril every 6-8 h in adults < 65 yr and weight ≥ 50 kg	126
Pyrazoles			
Celecoxib (Celebrex)	11	Initial 400 followed by another 200 on first day, then 200 twice daily (note some recommend maintenance doses of 200 mg/day due to cardiovascular concerns)	400

FDA (Food and Drug Administration); h (hours); IM (intramuscular); IV (intravenous).

[a]Available both as an over-the-counter preparation and as a prescription drug.

[b]Some experts believe 4,000 mg may be too high. OTC max dose 3,000 mg daily, lower with weight based dosing in pediatric patients.

[c]Up to 1,250 mg on the first day.

[d]Up to 200 mg on the first day.

[e]Some individuals may respond better to 3,200 mg as opposed to 2,400 mg, although well-controlled trials show no better response; consider risk versus benefits when using 3,200 mg/day.

[f]Over-the-counter dose.

[g]Dose for elderly and those under 50 kg (110 lb).

Data from references 39 and 42.

TABLE 60-4 Opioid Analgesics, Central Analgesics, Opioid Antagonist

Class and Generic Name (Brand Name)	Chemical Source	Relative Histamine Release	Route*	Equianalgesic Dose in Adults (mg)	Approximate Onset (min)/Half-Life (h)
Phenanthrenes (morphine-like agonists)					
Morphine (Embeda[i] various)	Naturally occurring	+++	IM/IV	10	10-20/2
			PO	30	
Hydromorphone (Dilaudid, Exalgo, various)	Semisynthetic	+	IM	1.5	10-20/2-3
			PO	7.5	
Oxymorphone (Numorphan, Opana)	Semisynthetic	+	IM	1	10-20/2-3
			PO	10	
Levorphanol (various)	Semisynthetic	+	IM	Variable	10-20/12-16
			PO	Variable	
Codeine (various)	Naturally occurring	+++	IM	15-30[a]	
			PO	15-30[a]	10-30/3
Hydrocodone (available as combination, single entity extended release—Hysingla ER, Zohydro ER)	Semisynthetic	N/A	PO	5-10[a]	30-60/4
Oxycodone (OxyContin[i], Oxecta[i], Xtampza, Xartemis XR [oxycodone & acetaminophen])	Semisynthetic	+	PO	15-30[b]	30-60/2-3
Phenylpiperidines (meperidine-like agonists)					
Meperidine (Demerol, various)	Synthetic	+++	IM/IV	75	10-20/3-5
			PO	300[b]; not recommended	
Fentanyl (Sublimaze, Duragesic, Lazanda, Abstral, Fentora, Subsys, OTFC, Ionsys, various)	Synthetic	+	IM	0.125[c]	7-15/3-4
			Transdermal	Variable[d]	
			Buccal, transmucosal, sublingual, nasal inhaled	Variable[d]	
Diphenylheptanes (methadone-like agonists)					
Methadone	Synthetic	+	IM/IV	Variable[e] (acute)	
(Dolophine, various)			PO	Variable[e] (acute)	30-60/12-190
			IM	Variable[e] (chronic)	
			PO	Variable[e] (chronic)	
Agonist–antagonist derivatives					
Pentazocine (Talwin, various)	Synthetic	N/A	IM	Not recommended	
			PO	50[a]	15-30/2-3
Butorphanol (Stadol, various)	Synthetic	N/A	IM	2	10-20/3-4
			Intranasal	1[a] (one spray)	
Nalbuphine (Nubain, various)	Synthetic	N/A	IM/IV	10	<15/5
Buprenorphine (Buprenex, Butrans, Suboxone, Belbuca, Subutex, various)	Synthetic	N/A	IM Transdermal Sublingual	0.3 Variable Variable	10-20/2-3
Antagonist					
Naloxone (Narcan, various)	Synthetic	N/A	IV	0.4-2[f]	1-2 (IV), 2-5 (IM)/0.5-1.3
Methylnaltrexone (Relistor)	Synthetic	N/A	SC	Variable	
Naltrexone (Revia)	Synthetic	N/A	PO		
Alvimopan (Entereg)	Synthetic	N/A	PO	12 mg QD-Q12	15 doses
Naloxegol (Movantik)	Synthetic	N/A	PO	12.5-25 mg QD	120/6-11

(continued)

TABLE 60-4 Opioid Analgesics, Central Analgesics, Opioid Antagonist (*Continued*)

Class and Generic Name (Brand Name)	Chemical Source	Relative Histamine Release	Route*	Equianalgesic Dose in Adults (mg)	Approximate Onset (min)/Half-Life (h)
Central analgesics					
Tramadol (Ultram, Rybix, Ryzolt, ConZip, various)	Synthetic	N/A	PO	50-100[a,g,h]	<60/5-7
Tapentadol (Nucynta)	Synthetic	N/A	PO	50-100[a,g,h]	Within 60/4

IM, intramuscular; IV, intravenous; N/A, not available; PO, oral.

*The IM route should be avoided whenever possible—produces significant pain with administration and rate and extent of absorption is highly variable. If IV route is unavailable then administer subcutaneously (SC).

[a]Starting dose only (equianalgesia not shown).

[b]Starting doses lower (oxycodone 5-10 mg, meperidine 50-150 mg).

[c]Equivalent PO morphine dose = variable.

[d]For breakthrough pain only. Equianalgesic dose conversion should be avoided for Transmucosal Immediate Release Fentanyl (TIRF) products.

[e]The equianalgesic dose of methadone when compared with other opioids will decrease progressively the higher the previous opioid dose. Caution should be exercised when initiating in opioid naïve patients.

[f]Starting doses to be used in cases of opioid overdose.

[g]First day of dosing may administer second dose 1 hour after first dose.

[h]Onset of action may differ for long-acting formulations. Ceiling dose recommendations exist and may differ from immediate release dosing recommendations.

[i]FDA approved as abuse-deterrent formulation.

Data from reference 42.

The pharmacologic activity of opioids depends on their affinity for and action at central and peripheral opiate receptors.[43] Therapeutic activities and side effects for this medication class range from those exhibited by the opiate agonists (eg, morphine) to those seen with the opiate antagonists (eg, naloxone). Partial agonists and antagonists (eg, nalbuphine) compete with agonists for opiate receptor sites and, depending on the inherent agonist and antagonist properties, exhibit mixed agonist–antagonist activity.[43] This may result in analgesia with fewer undesirable side effects. Efficacy and side effects also may further differ among opioid agents because of receptor subtype variability.[44] This μ-receptor (MOR) subtype variability may explain why some patients respond differently to certain opioids, specifically MOR agonists.[44]

The effects of the opioid analgesics are relatively selective, and at normal therapeutic concentrations, do not affect other sensory modalities.[43] While sensations of touch and proprioception are preserved; undesirable side effects may increase as the dose is escalated (Table 60-6).[43] Patients in severe pain may receive high doses of opioids with relatively no unwanted side effects, but as the pain subsides, even very low doses may not be tolerated.[45] Frequently, when opioids are administered, pain is not eliminated, but its unpleasantness is decreased.[43] Patients report that although their pain is still present, it no longer bothers them.

Opioids share related pharmacologic attributes and exert a profound effect on the CNS and GI tract.[43] Mood changes, sedation, nausea, vomiting, decreased GI motility, constipation, respiratory depression, dependence, and tolerance are evident in varying degrees with all agents.[39,45] Tolerance to side effects (except to constipation) often develops over time.[43,45] Some differences exist between the opioids in regards to incidence of side effects, which may assist in selection of the most appropriate agent. 3 4 5 The route of administration depends on individual patient needs, with the oral route being preferred. However, the onset of analgesic effect for oral medications is approximately 45 minutes, and the peak effect usually occurs 1 to 2 hours after administration.[39] This delay must be considered when immediate relief is needed in the management of acute pain. Therefore, in some scenarios, such as acute severe pain (eg, pain crisis) or when the patient is unable to take oral medications, alternative routes of therapy, such as intravenous (IV) administration, may be preferred. The relative potency, defined by the equianalgesic dose, of opioids differs greatly (see Table 60-4). 4 5 Equianalgesic dose tables are often based on single-dose studies without regard for patient variability and should be used only as a guide, with further dose titration frequently required.[46]

Although true opioid allergies are rare, Table 60-4 can also be used when treating a patient who has a documented hypersensitivity to opioids. Most reactions, such as itching or rash, are due to the associated histamine release from cutaneous mast cells and not a true allergic or immunoglobulin-E (IgE) or T-cell response.[47] Although caution is always advised, a decrease in potential cross-sensitivity is thought to exist when moving from one opioid structural class to another.[48] The classes are phenanthrenes (morphine-like agonists), phenylpiperidines (meperidine-like agonists), and diphenylheptanes (methadone-like agonists). When considering cross-sensitivity, the mixed agonist–antagonist and partial agonist class acts much like the morphine-like agonists.[49]

2 5 In the initial stages of acute pain, analgesics should be given around the clock. This should commence after administering a typical starting dose and titrating up or down, depending on the patient's degree of pain and demonstrated side effects (eg, sedation). As needed schedules may produce wide swings in analgesic plasma concentrations resulting in alternating states of uncontrolled pain and sedation. This may initiate a vicious cycle where increasing amounts of pain medications are needed for relief. 5 As the painful state subsides and the need for medication decreases, as needed schedules may be appropriate, which may also be useful in patients who present with pain that is intermittent or sporadic in nature (Fig. 60-2). As the painful state subsides and the need for medication decreases, as-needed schedules may be appropriate, which may also be useful in patients who present with pain that is intermittent or sporadic in nature (Fig. 60-2). When opioids are used in the management of persistent chronic pain, such as in oncology, around-the-clock administration schedules should be utilized (Fig 60-3). As needed opioids should be used in conjunction with around-the-clock regimens for times when patients experience breakthrough pain, which is a brief, transitory, exacerbation of moderate to severe pain typically occurring in patients with underlying persistent pain that may otherwise be controlled.[25,39,46]

Continuous IV infusion of opioids should be reserved for opioid-tolerant patients.[50] An alternative method is patient-controlled analgesia (PCA), which is a technique in which patients can self-administer a preset dose of an IV opioid via a pump electronically interfaced with a timing device. Compared with traditional as needed opioid dosing, PCA yields better pain control, improved patient satisfaction, and relatively few differences in side effects.[50,51]

Administration of opioids directly into the CNS (eg, epidural and intrathecal/subarachnoid routes) may also be used by

TABLE 60-5 Dosing Guidelines

Agent(s)	Doses (Use Lowest Effective Dose, Titrate Up or Down Based on Patient Response, Opioid Tolerant Patients May Need Dose Modification)	Notes
NSAIDs/acetaminophen/aspirin	Use lowest effective dose for the shortest duration possible (see Table 69-3)	Used in mild-to-moderate pain
		May use in conjunction with opioid agents to decrease doses of each
		Regular alcohol use and acetaminophen may result in liver toxicity
		Care must be exercised to avoid overdose when combination products containing these agents are used
		Underlying renal impairment, hypovolemia, and heart failure may predispose to nephrotoxicity
Morphine	PO 5-30 mg every 4 h[a]	Drug of choice in severe pain
	IM 5-20 mg every 4 h[a]	Use immediate-release product with SR product to control breakthrough pain in cancer patients
	IV 5-15 mg every 4 h[a]	Typical patient controlled analgesia IV dose is 1 mg with a 10-minute lock out interval
	SR 15-30 mg every 12 h (may need to be every 8 h in some patients)	Every 24-hour products available use caution in renally-compromised patients
	Rectal 10-20 mg every 4 h[a]	
Hydromorphone	PO 2-4 mg every 4-6 h[a]	Use in severe pain
	XR 8 mg to 64 mg every 24 h IM 1-2 mg every 4-6 h[a]	More potent than morphine; otherwise, no advantages
	IV 0.5-2 mg every 4 h[a]	Typical patient controlled analgesia IV dose is 0.2 mg with a 10-minute lock out interval
	Rectal 3 mg every 6-8 h[a]	Every 24-hour product (Exalgo) available
Oxymorphone	IM 1-1.5 mg every 4-6 h[a]	Use in severe pain
	IV 0.5 mg every 4-6 h[a]	No advantages over morphine
	PO immediate-release 5-10 mg every 4-6 h[a]	Use immediate-release product with controlled-release product to control breakthrough pain in cancer or chronic pain patients
	PO extended-release 5-10 mg every 12 h[a]	Manufacturer recommends 5 mg every 12 h in opioid-naïve patients Take ER on empty stomach
Levorphanol	PO 2-3 mg every 6-8 h[a] (Levo-Dromoran)	Use in severe pain
	PO 2 mg every 3-6 h[a] (Levorphanol Tartrate)	Extended half-life useful in cancer patients
	IM 1-2 mg every 6-8 h[a]	In chronic pain, wait 3 days between dosage adjustments
	IV 1 mg every 3-6 h[a]	
Codeine	PO 15-60 mg every 4-6 h[a]	Use in mild to moderate pain
	IM 15-60 mg every 4-6 h[a]	Weak analgesic; analgesic prodrug
Hydrocodone	PO 5-10 mg every 4-6 h[a]	Use in moderate/severe pain
Oxycodone	PO 5-15 mg every 4-6 h[a]	Use in moderate/severe pain
	Controlled release 10-20 mg every 12 h	
		Use immediate-release product with controlled-release product to control breakthrough pain in cancer or chronic pain patients CR reformulated to deter abuse
Meperidine	IM 50-150 mg every 3-4 h[a]	Use in severe pain
	IV 5-10 mg every 5 min prn[a]	Oral not recommended
		Do not use in renal failure
		May precipitate tremors, myoclonus, and seizures
		Monoamine oxidase inhibitors can induce hyperpyrexia and/or seizures or opioid overdose symptoms
Fentanyl	IV 25-50 mcg/h	Used in severe pain
	IM 50-100 mcg every 1-2 h[a]	**Do not use transdermal in acute pain**
	Transdermal 25 mcg/h every 72 h	Transmucosal for breakthrough cancer pain in patients already receiving or tolerant to opioids
	Transmucosal (Actiq/OTFC Lozenge and Onsolis buccal film) 200 mcg may repeat × 1, 30 min after first dose is started, then titrate	**Always start with lowest dose despite daily opioid intake. Product specific titration recommendations exist**
	Transmucosal (Fentora Buccal Tablet) 100 mcg, may repeat × 1, 30 min after first dose is started, then titrate	

(continued)

TABLE 60-5 Dosing Guidelines (*Continued*)

Agent(s)	Doses (Use Lowest Effective Dose, Titrate Up or Down Based on Patient Response, Opioid Tolerant Patients May Need Dose Modification)	Notes
	Intranasal (Lazanda Spray) 100 mcg (one spray) in one nostril. Wait 2 h prior to redosing	
	Sublingual (Subsys Spray) 100 mcg (1 spray). Wait 4 h prior to redosing	
	Sublingual (Abstral Tablet) 100 mcg tablets placed sublingually. Must wait 2 h prior to redosing	
Methadone	PO 2.5-10 mg every 8-12 h[a]	Effective in severe chronic pain
	IM 2.5-10 mg every 8-12 h[a]	
		Some chronic pain patients can be dosed every 12 h
		Equianalgesic dose of methadone when compared with other opioids will decrease progressively the higher the previous opioid dose. Avoid dose titrations more frequently than weekly in chronic pain maintenance
Pentazocine	PO 50-100 mg every 3-4 h[b] (max. 600 mg daily, for those 50 mg tablet containing 0.5 mg of naloxone)	Second-line agent for moderate-to-severe pain May precipitate withdrawal in opiate-dependent patients Parenteral doses not recommended
	PO 25 mg every 4 h[b] (max. 150 mg daily, for those 25 mg tablet containing 325 mg of acetaminophen)	
Butorphanol	IM 1-4 mg every 3-4 h[b]	Second-line agent for moderate-to-severe pain
	IV 0.5-2 mg every 3-4 h[b]	May precipitate withdrawal in opiate-dependent patients
	Intranasal 1 mg (1 spray) every 3-4 h[b]	
	If inadequate relief after initial spray, may repeat in other nostril × 1 in 60-90 min	
	Max. 2 sprays (one per nostril) every 3-4 h[b]	
Nalbuphine	IM/IV 10 mg every 3-6 h[b] (max. 20 mg dose, 160 mg daily)	Second-line agent for moderate-to-severe pain May precipitate withdrawal in opiate-dependent patients Used frequently in low doses to treat/prevent opioid-induced pruritus
Buprenorphine	IM 0.3 mg every 6 h[b]	Second-line agent for moderate-to-severe pain
	Slow IV 0.3 mg every 6 h[b]	May precipitate withdrawal in opiate-dependent patients
		Transdermal delivery systems (5, 7.5, 10, 15, 20 mcg/h) available for every 7 day administration. Detailed manufacturer dosing conversion recommendations exist
	May repeat × 1, 30-60 min after initial dose	Naloxone may not be effective in reversing respiratory depression
Naloxone	IV IM 0.4-2 mg	When reversing opiate side effects in patients needing analgesia, dilute and titrate (0.1-0.2 mg every 2-3 min) so as not to reverse analgesia
Tramadol	PO 50-100 mg every 4-6 h[a]	Maximum dose for nonextended-release, 400 mg/24 h; maximum for extended release, 300 mg/24 h
	If rapid onset not required, start 25 mg/day and titrate over several days	Decrease dose in patient with renal impairment and in the elderly
	Extended release PO 100 mg every 24 h	
Tapentadol	PO 50-100 mg every 4-6 h[a]	First day of therapy may administer second dose after the first within 1 h Maximum dose first day 700 mg, max. dose thereafter 600 mg (max. dose for CR 500 mg)

CR, controlled release; ER, extended release; IM, intramuscular; IV, intravenous; NSAID, nonsteroidal antiinflammatory drug; PO, oral; prn, as needed; SR, sustained release; HCL, hydrochloride.

[a]May start with an around-the-clock regimen and switch to prn if/when the painful signal subsides or is episodic.

[b]May reach a ceiling analgesic effect.

Data from references 39, 42, and 46.

anesthesiology pain consult services in the control of acute, chronic noncancer, and cancer pain (Table 60-7); and is useful in more difficult to control pain states.[52] Due to reports of respiratory depression, pruritus, nausea, vomiting, urinary retention, and hypotension, these methods of analgesia require careful monitoring and are best used by experienced practitioners. Respiratory depression is of concern and can occur within minutes with intrathecal fentanyl or manifest as late as 19 hours after a single dose of intrathecal morphine. Guidelines mandate respiratory monitoring for at least 24 hours after a single dose of intrathecal or epidural morphine with standing orders for naloxone (opioid antagonist) for full or partial reversal.[53] Analgesia and side effects are evident at even lower doses when opioids are administered intrathecally instead of epidurally. This form of analgesia is often administered as a continuous-infusion and/or on a patient-controlled basis. When given simultaneously with intrathecal or epidural local anesthetics such as bupivacaine, opioid analgesics have been proven relatively safe and effective. All agents administered directly into the CNS should be preservative free.

Opioids

Morphine and Congeners Despite the availability of several newer agents, morphine remains the prototype opiate analgesic.

TABLE 60-6 Major Adverse Effects of the Opioid Analgesics

Effect	Manifestation
Mood changes	Dysphoria, euphoria
Somnolence	Sedation, inability to concentrate
Stimulation of chemoreceptor trigger zone	Nausea, vomiting
Respiratory depression	Decreased respiratory rate
Decreased gastrointestinal motility	Constipation
Increase in sphincter tone	Biliary spasm, urinary retention (varies among agents)
Histamine release	Urticaria, pruritus, rarely exacerbation of asthma due to bronchospasm (varies among agents)
Tolerance	Larger doses for same effect
Dependence	Withdrawal symptoms upon abrupt discontinuation
Addiction	Genetic predisposition leads to loss of control of drug use, continued use despite harm, compulsion to use, cravings
Hypogonadism	Fatigue, depression, loss of analgesia, sexual dysfunction, amenorrhea (women)
Sleep	Disrupts sleep-wake cycle, causes dose-dependent rapid eye movement (REM) suppression

Data from references 39 and 42.

As new opioid and nonopioid compounds are developed, their efficacy and side-effect profiles are typically compared against morphine as the standard. Using the equianalgesic tables, clinicians often refer to "oral morphine equivalents" when describing efficacy of other opioids. Many clinicians consider morphine the first-line agent when treating moderate-to-severe pain due to its relative low cost, broad clinical experience, and abundant dosage forms/strengths.

2 Side effects can be numerous, particularly when morphine is first initiated or when doses are significantly increased. Morphine causes nausea and vomiting through direct stimulation of the chemoreceptor trigger zone, decreased peristalsis, and a vestibular mechanism.[43] Opioid-induced nausea typically subsides over time with continued dosing, although this side-effect may be incredibly troublesome to patients, especially following surgery.[54] Although euphoria and dysphoria have been reported, morphine's unpleasant effects are more prominent when administered to patients not experiencing pain.[43,45] As doses of morphine are increased, the respiratory center becomes less responsive to carbon dioxide, causing progressive respiratory depression.[45] This effect is less pronounced in patients being treated for severe or chronic pain, although concurrent administration with other respiratory depressants, such as benzodiazepines, may greatly enhance this adverse effect.[41] Respiratory depression often manifests as a decrease in respiratory rate (although minute volume and tidal exchange also are affected) and is further compounded because the cough reflex is also depressed.[43] More recently, end-tidal capnography has become commonplace as a means to monitor opioid-induced respiratory depression, especially in those at increased risk.[55] Morphine-induced respiratory depression can be reversed by the opioid antagonist, naloxone. In patients with underlying pulmonary dysfunction or sleep disordered breathing, caution must be exercised when opioids are used, as these patients are already using compensatory breathing mechanisms and are at risk for further respiratory compromise. Caution is also urged when combining opiate analgesics with alcohol or other CNS depressants (ie, benzodiazepines), because this combination is potentially harmful and possibly lethal.[43]

Therapeutic doses of morphine have minimal effects on blood pressure, cardiac rate, or cardiac rhythm when patients are supine; however, morphine does produce venous and arteriolar vessel dilation, potentially resulting in orthostatic hypotension, and hypovolemic patients may be more susceptible to morphine-induced cardiovascular changes (eg, decreases in blood pressure).[45] Because morphine prompts a decrease in myocardial oxygen demand in ischemic cardiac patients, it is often used to treat pain associated with myocardial infarction, although this practice has been called into question due to the potential for increased mortality.[56]

Morphine decreases the propulsive contractions of the GI tract resulting in constipation.[57] Morphine-induced spasms of the sphincter of Oddi have also been observed; however, the clinical significance of this is unclear. Urinary retention is another significant side effect of morphine and should be routinely assessed. Morphine-induced histamine release often manifests as pruritus, and may even exacerbate bronchospasm in patients with a history of asthma.[39] Therapeutic doses of morphine are not contraindicated in head injury, but drug-induced respiratory depression can increase intracranial pressure. Thus, caution is advised in head trauma patients who are not mechanically ventilated because morphine may increase intracranial pressures and cloud the neurologic examination results.[43]

Morphine is metabolized to two major metabolites, morphine-3-glucuronide (M3G) and morphine-6-glucuronide (M6G). M6G contributes to analgesia, whereas M3G may contribute to unwanted side effects. The metabolites are renally cleared and can accumulate in patients with renal impairment, contributing to greater side effects.[43] Most clinicians recommend avoiding morphine in renally compromised patients (ie, creatinine clearance less than or equal to 30 mL/min [less than or equal to 0.5 mL/s]). Morphine also inhibits the release of gonadotropin-releasing hormone from the hypothalamus, thus decreasing plasma testosterone and cortisol (opioid-induced hypogonadism), whereas male patients may present with symptoms of erectile dysfunction, decreased libido, and decreased analgesic efficacy.[58] Women may experience alopecia, amenorrhea, and depressed mood, as well as decreased analgesic efficacy. Recommendations for clinical replacement of these hormones in patients using chronic opioid therapy are not well defined.[58] While the clinical meaning has not clearly been elucidated, morphine and other opioids, depending on the situation being used, may either enhance or inhibit the immune system.[39,43]

4 Hydromorphone is more potent than morphine, but its overall pharmacologic profile parallels that of morphine. Some clinicians believe hydromorphone is associated with fewer side effects, especially pruritus, compared with other opioids. However, the research is limited and does not conclusively demonstrate this difference. Oxymorphone can be administered orally and by injection. Although extended-release and immediate-release oral products are available, it offers no pharmacologic advantage over morphine. Patients must be counseled to take the extended-release oxymorphone without food as high fat meals may greatly increase absorption, resulting in an increased risk of toxicity. Levorphanol has an extended half-life, but its overall therapeutic effects are similar to the other agents in this class.

Codeine is a commonly used opiate for the treatment of mild-to-moderate pain. It often is combined with other analgesic products (eg, acetaminophen). Unfortunately, it has the same propensity to produce side effects as morphine. Hydrocodone is perhaps the most commonly prescribed opiate and is available orally as immediate-release combined with nonopioid analgesics, as well

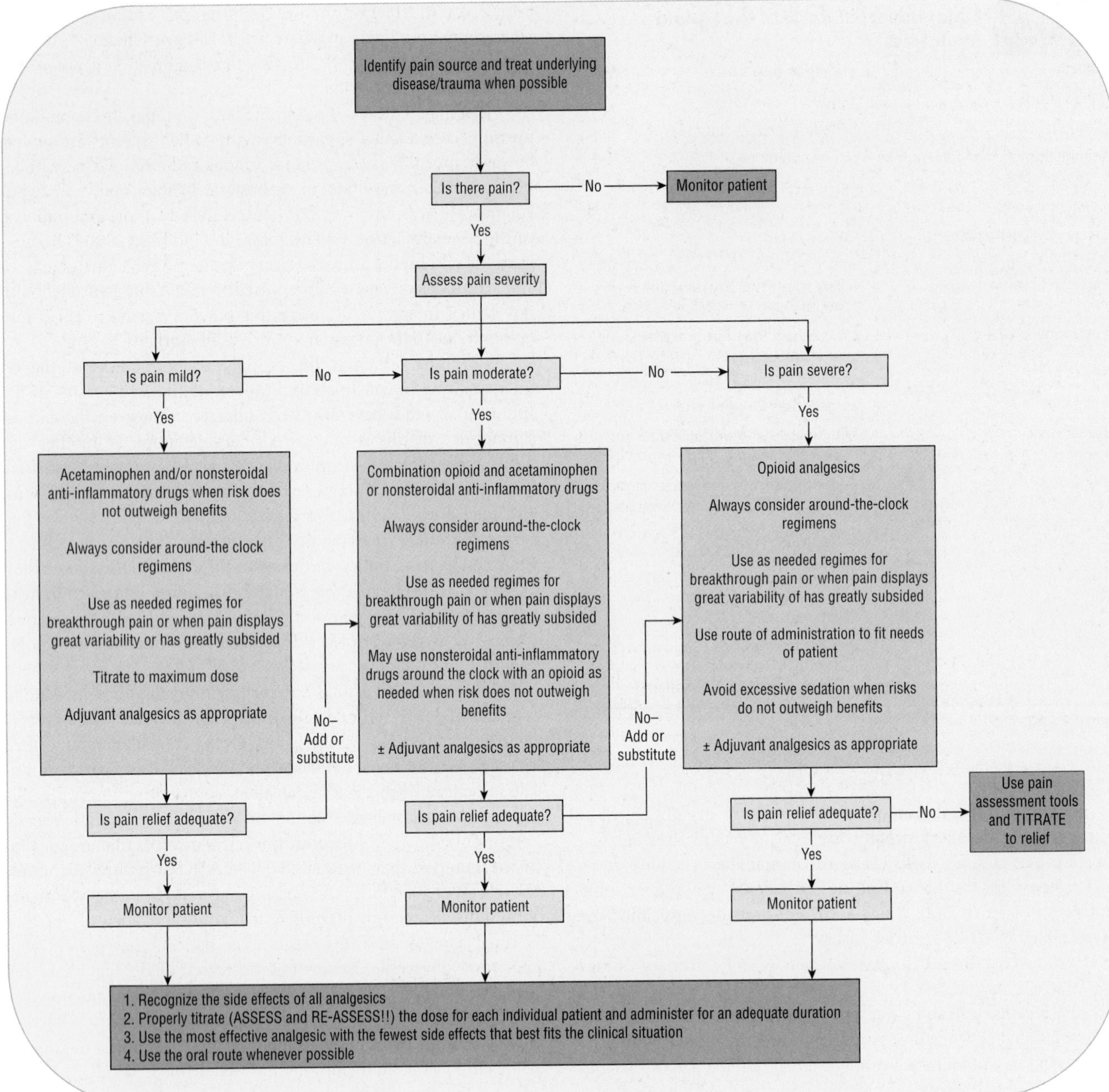

FIGURE 60-2 Algorithm for acute pain. *(Data from Omnicare, Inc., Acute Pain Pathway.)*

as extended-release formulations. Its pharmacologic properties are similar to those of morphine. Oxycodone is a useful oral analgesic for moderate-to-severe pain. This is especially true when the product is used in combination with nonopioids. Although oxycodone shares basic morphine characteristics, the availability of an immediate-release and controlled-release oral dosage form also makes it very useful in chronic pain as well as acute pain.

Meperidine and Congeners (Phenylpiperidines) The prototype phenylpiperidine, meperidine, has a pharmacologic profile comparable with that of morphine; however, it is not as potent and has a shorter analgesic duration. Meperidine offers no analgesic advantage over morphine, has greater toxicity (CNS hyperirritability caused by its renally eliminated metabolite normeperidine), and should be limited in use, especially in elderly patients, those with renal dysfunction, or for prolonged treatment durations.[39] In particular, avoid long-term usage and use in patients at greatest risk for toxicity (eg, elderly patients and those with renal dysfunction).[59]

Fentanyl is a synthetic opioid structurally related to meperidine that is used often in anesthesiology as an adjunct to general anesthesia. This agent is significantly more potent and faster acting than meperidine (see Table 60-4). It can be administered parenterally, transmucosally, sublingually, intranasally, and transdermally.[46]

Methadone and Congeners Methadone has gained considerable popularity as an analgesic due to its oral efficacy, extended duration of action, and low cost. Properties unique to methadone, compared with other opioids, include the S-isomer's ability to antagonize NMDA receptors, agonist effects at the kappa opioid receptor (KOR) and delta opioid receptor (DOR), as well as the blockade of serotonin and norepinephrine reuptake.[60] These properties may prove useful in

TABLE 60-7 Intraspinal Opioids

Agent	Single Dose (mg)	Onset of Pain Relief (min)	Duration of Pain Relief (h)	Continual Infusion Dose (mg/h)
Epidural route				
Morphine	1-6	30	6-24	0.1-1
Hydromorphone	0.8-1.5	5-8	4-8	0.1-0.3
Fentanyl	0.025-0.1	5	2-8	0.025-0.1
Sufentanil	0.01-0.06	5	2-4	0.01-0.05
Subarachnoid route				
Morphine	0.1-0.3	15	8-34	–
Fentanyl	0.005-0.025	5	3-6	–

Note: Doses above should not be interpreted as equianalgesic doses for conversion to or from the specific opioid or route of administration.

Data from reference 39.

the treatment of neuropathic and chronic pain. However, few trials have thoroughly evaluated methadone's risks versus benefits.[41,60] Epidemiologic studies suggest a growing number of methadone-related deaths, and cardiac arrhythmias have been associated with this medication, particularly at higher doses or when used concurrently with other agents that prolong QTc intervals. Recommendations exist for specific echocardiogram monitoring for methadone; however, concerns exist regarding their applicability.[60] The equianalgesic dose of methadone may decrease with higher doses of the comparator opioid, complicating conversions from other opioids to methadone. Methadone should not be titrated more frequently than every 5 to 7 days due to its unpredictable potency and variable half-live.[46,60]

Clinical **Controversy...**

Some clinicians believe that methadone should be tried before other opioids in many chronic pain conditions where an opioid is warranted because they believe that neuropathic pain is often a component. Other clinicians believe that sustained-released morphine or oxycodone is better first choice.

Opioid Agonist–Antagonist Derivatives This analgesic class produces analgesia and has the potential for less respiratory depression than opioid agonists as they exert their analgesic activity via the KOR and either block or act as partial agonists at the MOR.[43] Agents in this class are considered to have a lower abuse potential than morphine, but psychotomimetic responses (eg, hallucinations and dysphoria), limited analgesic effect, and a propensity to initiate withdrawal in opioid-dependent populations have precluded their widespread clinical use. Both butorphanol and nalbuphine are available parenterally, with butorphanol also available as an intranasal spray. Nalbuphine is gaining popularity as a treatment for MOR agonist associated pruritus.[61]

Buprenorphine is a pharmacologically rich opioid, which exhibits KOR antagonism, and several MOR related actions, including partial agonism. Buprenorphine also displays agonist properties at the opioid receptor-like 1 receptor (ORL-1) which may have clinical ramifications in prevention of tolerance, euphoria/reward, and hyperalgesia.[62] Buprenorphine is available as a sublingual tablet, a once-weekly transdermal patch, or in combination with naloxone as a sublingual film. When buprenorphine/naloxone sublingual film is prescribed for opioid use disorder, a special DEA license is required by the prescriber.[63]

Central-Acting Opioids Tramadol and tapentadol are the only centrally acting analgesics currently available in the United States. Tramadol binds to MOR receptors and inhibits serotonin, and, to a lesser extent, norepinephrine reuptake.[64] Tapentadol also binds the MOR receptor, but inhibits largely norepinephrine reuptake. Tramadol is indicated for the relief of moderate to moderately severe pain, while tapentadol is indicated for moderate-to-severe acute pain and diabetic peripheral neuropathy.[14,43]

Both tramadol and tapentadol have side-effect profiles similar to that of the previously mentioned opioid analgesics (eg, dizziness, nausea, somnolence, and constipation). Tapentadol has not been systematically evaluated in patients with seizures, and it should be used with caution in these patients. Seizure risk may be elevated in patients taking tramadol.[65] In general, tramadol may have a place in treating patients with chronic pain, especially neuropathic pain, while tapentadol may be useful in the management of acute pain and the controlled release product may have a role in chronic pain treatment (eg, diabetes-related nerve pain).[66,67] It is important to note that tapentadol is significantly more potent than tramadol and these agents should not be used interchangeably.

Opioid Antagonists The opioid antagonist naloxone binds competitively to opioid receptors but does not produce an analgesic or opioid side-effect response. Therefore, it is used most often to reverse the toxic effects of agonist- and agonist–antagonist-derived opioids. Other opioid antagonists exist, including naltrexone, naloxegol, and methylnaltrexone. Naltrexone's use is primarily limited to addiction medicine, while naloxegol and methylnaltrexone are peripherally acting only and used for opioid-induced constipation.[68]

With the growing prevalence of heroin and prescription opioid abuse related overdoses, pharmacists are increasingly being called upon to assist in the prevention of these deaths. Several States have legislation pending allowing for pharmacists to both prescribe and administer naloxone to those suspected of experiencing an opioid overdose. Naloxone may be administered intranasally or intramuscularly in these situations, and an intramuscular autoinjector, similar to that of the epinephrine devices, has recently become available.[69]

Tolerance, Hyperalgesia, Physical Dependence, Addiction, and Pseudoaddiction A barrier that consistently causes clinicians to misjudge and mistreat pain is the misunderstanding of opioid tolerance, hyperalgesia, physical dependence, addiction, and pseudoaddiction. Tolerance is the reduction of drug effect over time as a result of exposure to the drug.[45] It develops at different rates and with great patient variability. However, with stable disease, opioid dose may stabilize over time. Hyperalgesia is an increased sensitivity to pain secondary to increased opioid doses that can be seen with rapid opioid escalation or high dose administration.[70] The mechanism or true clinical impact of this phenomenon is not currently understood. Opioid physical dependence is characterized by an abstinence syndrome following administration of an antagonist drug or abrupt dose reduction/discontinuation of an opioid.[45] Clinicians must understand that physical dependence and tolerance are not equivalent to addiction; and with chronic opioid use, physical dependence is expected.[45] Many definitions and classifications exist to describe the biopsychosocial phenomenon of addiction. The American Society of Addiction Medicine (ASAM) defines addiction as a "primary, chronic disease of brain reward, motivation, memory, and related circuitry" leading to biological, psychological, social and spiritual manifestations.[71] Addiction is characterized by cravings, resulting in an inability to abstain from continued drug use despite harm and impairment in behavioral control. Individually, these behaviors are often described as aberrant, although patients may display aberrant behaviors (eg, medication-related behaviors that are inconsistent with strict adherence to the prescribed treatment) that are not a result of an underlying addiction.[7] A baseline assessment and ongoing evaluation of these behaviors and an individual's risk of misuse, abuse, and addiction is critical to mitigate risks of chronic opioid therapy and ensure patient safety.[72] Higher risk for opioid misuse or abuse is associated with a personal substance abuse, misuse, addiction, or diversion history, a significant family history of substance abuse, and presence of underlying psychiatric diagnosis.[41] Modifications to the treatment plan should be stratified based on patient risk, including baseline and random drug screens, patient–provider treatment agreements, pill counts, a smaller prescription supply, and regular assessment of aberrant behaviors. Combining these approaches with regular and ongoing assessments of pain and functionality may result in improved outcomes.[41]

Coanalgesics

Coanalgesics represent a diverse group of pharmacologic agents with individual characteristics that make them useful in the management of pain, but typically are not classified as analgesics. Examples of coanalgesics include antidepressants and anticonvulsants. 6 Chronic pain that has a neuropathic component (eg, diabetic neuropathy) often requires coanalgesic therapy (Table 60-8). Anticonvulsants (eg, gabapentin, pregabalin, which may decrease neuronal excitability), tricyclic antidepressants and serotonin and norepinephrine reuptake inhibitor antidepressants (eg, nortriptyline, duloxetine, venlafaxine—which block the reuptake of serotonin and norepinephrine, thus enhancing pain inhibition), and topically applied local anesthetics (which decrease nerve stimulation) all have demonstrated efficacy in managing various chronic pain conditions.[73]

Clinical Controversy...

Many clinicians believe that some chronic painful conditions (eg, osteoarthritis) should never be treated with opioids; whereas others believe that when other modalities are not effective or seem to pose more of a risk to that particular patient than does conventional therapy (eg, NSAIDs), then opioids are necessary.

In the management of cancer pain, radiopharmaceuticals (eg, strontium-89 or samarium), corticosteroids, and bisphosphonates are useful coanalgesics in treating bone pain (Fig. 60-3).[74] Although antihistamines and amphetamines have been used as coanalgesics, they have demonstrated only limited success.

Multimodal Therapy

Commonly, multimodal therapy may be employed to optimize either acute or chronic pain management. Multimodal therapy is the concomitant use of different therapeutic interventions with the intent of obtaining additive therapeutic effects. Multimodal analgesia, one type of multimodal therapy, includes combining medications from different analgesic classes (eg, combination therapy with opioids and nonopioids or coanalgesics).[14,45] This often results in analgesia superior to that produced by either agent alone. Multimodal analgesia may also permit the use of lower doses and provide a more favorable side-effect profile, for example when NSAIDs are prescribed with opioids yielding an "opioid sparing" effect.

Regional Analgesia

Regional analgesia with properly administered local anesthetics can provide relief of both acute and chronic pain (Table 60-9).[75]

TABLE 60-8 Opioids to Avoid/Exercise Caution

Drug	Caution	Notes
Codeine	Do not use—especially in children and breastfeeding	Codeine is a prod rug, must be converted by CYP 2D6 to morphine to produce analgesia. High degree of polymorphism of 2D6, ultra-rapid metabolism = toxicity, poor metabolism = no analgesia
Meperidine	Do not use	Short duration of analgesia requiring frequent dosing Produces non-analgesic, toxic metabolite normeperidine, accumulation results in seizures, risk of accumulation increased in renal insufficiency
Agonist/Antagonist agents	Caution	Can produce opioid withdrawal in patients chronically taking opioid. Higher rate of psychomimetic reactions compared to other opioids
Tramadol	Caution—especially in elderly or in renal dysfunction	Tramadol is a pro-drug, must be converted by CYP 2D6 to desmethyl-tramadol (M1) to produce analgesia. High degree of polymorphism of 2D6, ultra-rapid metabolism = toxicity, poor metabolism = no analgesia Risk of seizure, risk of serotonin syndrome, risk of hypoglycemia

Data from references 59, 64, 65 and 80.

TABLE 60-9 Local Anesthetics[a]

Agent (Brand Name)	Onset (min)	Duration (h)
Esters		
Procaine (Novocain, various)	2-5	0.25-1
Chloroprocaine (Nesacaine, various)	6-12	0.5
Tetracaine (Pontocaine)	≤15	2-3
Amides		
Mepivacaine (Polocaine, various)	3-5	0.75-1.5
Bupivacaine (Marcaine, various)	5	2-4
Bupivacaine liposomal (Exparel—wound infiltration only)	variable	24 local 96 systemic
Lidocaine (Xylocaine, various)	<2	0.5-1
Prilocaine (Citanest)	<2	1-2
Ropivacaine[b] (Naropin)	10-30	0.5-6

[a]Unless otherwise indicated, values are for infiltrative anesthesia.

[b]Epidural administration.

Data from reference 42.

These agents can be positioned by injection (eg, in joints, in the epidural or intrathecal space, along nerve roots, or in a nerve plexus) or topically. Lidocaine in the form of a patch has proven effective in treating focal neuropathic pain.[76] Regional nerve blocks with local anesthetics may effectively relieve pain. Although rare, elevated plasma concentrations of local anesthetics can cause CNS excitation and depression, including dizziness, tinnitus, drowsiness, disorientation, muscle twitching, seizures, and respiratory arrest.[75] Cardiovascular adverse effects include myocardial depression, hypotension, decreased cardiac output, heart block, bradycardia, arrhythmias, and cardiac arrest. Disadvantages of such methods include the need for skillful technical application, need for frequent administration, and highly specialized follow-up procedures.

Clinical **Controversy...**

Some clinicians believe that daily opioid doses in chronic noncancer patients should be limited because the risk of potential abuse and that the adverse effects may outweigh the benefits. In fact, some guidelines have even incorporated recommendations to limit doses to less than 90 mg of morphine or its daily equivalent (Centers for Disease Control). Other clinicians believe that by carefully screening patients for risks of abuse, frequent monitoring, identifying targeted pain symptoms, utilizing pain treatment "agreements," and distinctly outlining the treatment plans with patients, opioids can be titrated to effect, based on symptoms with no defined maximum dose.

SPECIAL POPULATIONS

The elderly and the young are at a higher risk for undertreatment because of inability to communicate or rate their pain. It is in these cases that parent or caregiver input becomes paramount to identify changes in behavior, which might suggest pain (eg, fussy, inconsolable, changes in eating patterns, crying out, or agitation). When patients cannot verbalize their pain (eg, coma), monitoring behaviors (eg, agitation) and physiologic signs and symptoms (eg, heart rate) is appropriate.

7 In addition, those living with chronic, debilitating, and life-threatening illnesses need specialized pain control and care that is palliative in nature.[77] Although care must be taken in these populations to ensure that proper individualized treatment plans follow accepted guidelines, the key concepts in pain management as outlined in this chapter are the guiding tenets in maximizing pain control.[78,79]

PERSONALIZED PHARMACOTHERAPY

Recent research has illustrated genetic differences in pain transmission and response inter-individually as well as between genders, ages, and ethnicity. More interesting is the pharmacogenomic variability of analgesic response to both opioid and nonopioid analgesics. Genotyping (eg, CYP 2D6, CYP 2B6) may be useful when considering the addition of an opioid metabolized via one of these enzymes.

Codeine, oxycodone, hydrocodone, and methadone, as well as several of the SSRIs and SNRIs, are all either converted to active or inactive metabolites via one of these enzyme pathways.[80] Individuals who possess a variant allele for one or more of these enzymes may have unexpected outcomes, including greater than expected toxicity or side effects and lower than expected efficacy, depending on the individual genotype and phenotype. Frequency of genetic variation differs by ethnicity and gene. For example, up to 10% to 15% of the general population may be phenotypically poor metabolizers of CYP2D6, while 20% of Africans may be poor metabolizers and 30% of Arabs are ultra-rapid metabolizers.[81] This may be especially relevant for opioids in which much of the analgesic activity relies on conversion to an active metabolite from a relatively inactive parent (ie, codeine and tramadol). Recent data suggests high rates of variant metabolism in patients evaluated for genetic variation in CYP2C9, CYP2C19, and CYP2D6, with over 50% of patients expressing a variant in two or more genes.[82]

In some cases, genotype results may further help to explain cases where patients require higher doses to achieve adequate analgesia. For example, early published data suggests that variants in opioid-receptor subtypes, specifically MOR-1 (OPRM1 gene), may predict efficacy and dosing requirements for some opioids such as morphine or hydromorphone.[83,84]

EVALUATION OF THERAPEUTIC OUTCOMES

2 5 Consistent monitoring for effectiveness (eg, pain relief and adequate functionality) and adverse effects (eg, sedation) is critical in optimizing therapeutic outcomes. Numerous validated scoring tools exist (eg, numeric rating scale, visual analog scale, etc.); however, the tools need to be appropriate for the type of pain being evaluated, used consistently, and with good clinical judgment.[23,26] Pain management efficacy, any change in pain, and medication side effects (eg, opioid-induced sedation or constipation) must be assessed and reassessed on a regular basis. Frequency of reassessment should be dictated by the medication's route of administration, duration of action, various pharmacokinetic factors, or other concomitant therapies. Postoperative pain and acute exacerbation of cancer pain may need to be assessed hourly, whereas chronic noncancer pain may require only daily or less frequent assessment. Pain intensity assessment is vital in acute pain, whereas functionality becomes more of an issue in chronic pain. Quality of life must be assessed on a regular basis in all patients. Many advocate using the four "A"s (analgesia, activity, aberrant drug behavior, and adverse effects) as key assessment measures for any patient with chronic pain.

It is important to note that often objective signs are lacking for pain evaluation. Acute pain may result in increased sympathetic tone (eg, hypertension, tachycardia, and tachypnea); however, this response is usually diminished as acute pain progresses to chronic pain. The clinician must rely on the patient's description of their pain.

2 All opioids can cause constipation. The best management of constipation is prevention. Patients should be counseled on the proper intake of fluids and fiber. A stimulating laxative should be added with chronic opioid use. 7 CNS depressants (eg, alcohol and benzodiazepines) amplify CNS depression when used with opioid analgesics, and use of these combinations should be discouraged when possible. When the combinations are used, patients should be monitored closely.

Clinical **Controversy...**

Some clinicians believe that opioid risk evaluation and mitigation strategies, which consist of mandatory care-giver enrollment, prescriber training, patient medication guides, and patient prescriber agreements, as outlined by the Federal Food and Drug Administration will decrease opioid misuse and lead to better patient care. Others feel this leads to increased costs and becomes a barrier to effective pain therapy.

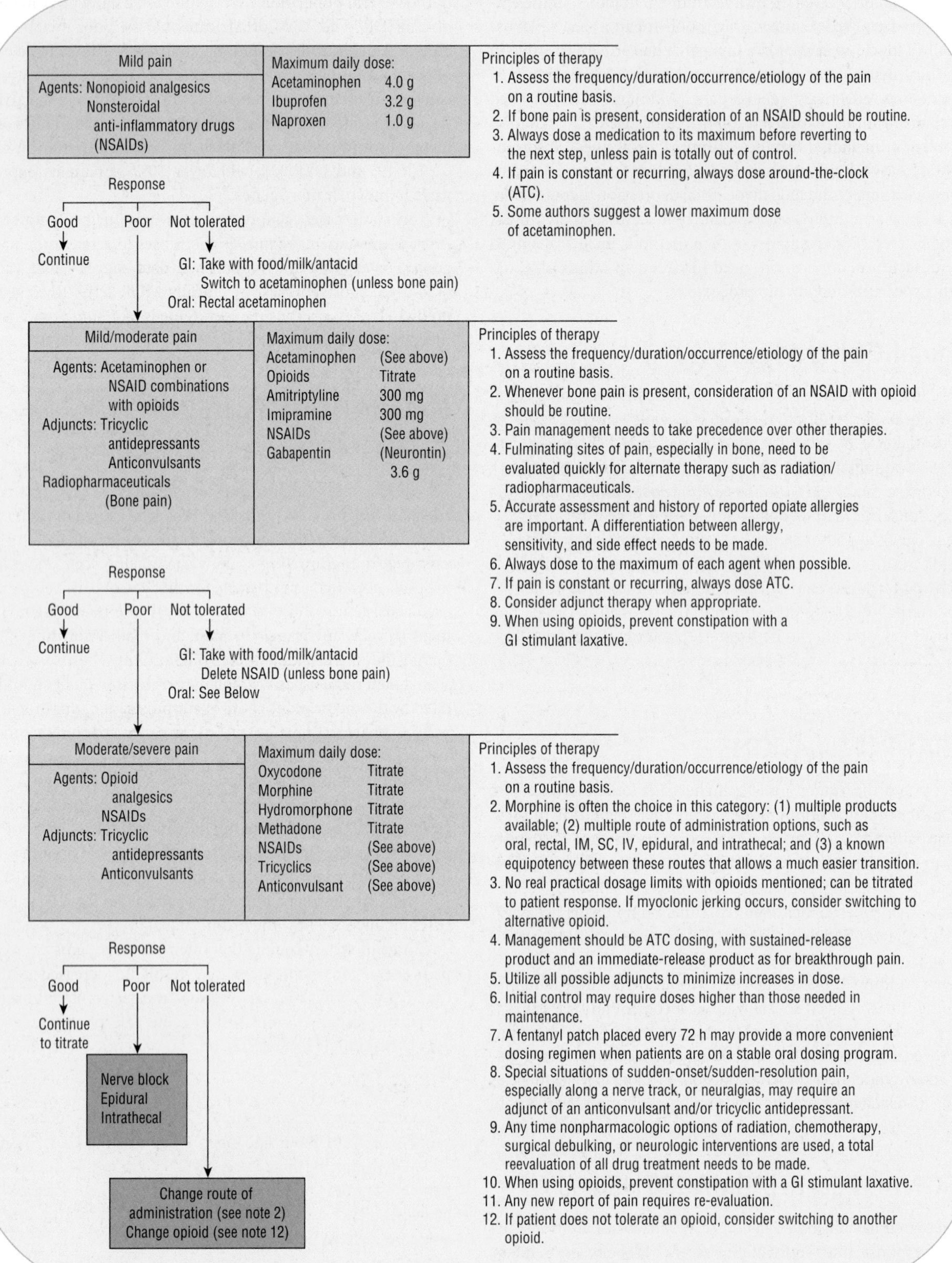

FIGURE 60-3 Algorithm for pain management in oncology patients. *(Data from the Kaiser Permanente Algorithm for Pain Management in Patients with Advanced Malignant Disease.)*

ABBREVIATIONS

ASAM	American Society of Addiction Medicine
CNS	central nervous system
COX-2	cyclooxygenase-2
CYP	cytochrome P450
DOR	delta opioid receptor
GABA	γ-aminobutyric acid
GI	gastrointestinal
IgE	immunoglobulin-E
IM	intramuscular
IV	intravenous
KOR	kappa opioid receptor
M3G	morphine-3-glucuronide
M6G	morphine-6-glucuronide
MOR	μ-opioid receptor

NMDA	*N*-methyl-D-aspartate
NSAIDs	nonsteroidal antiinflammatory drugs
OPRM1	opioid receptor, μ-1 gene subtype
ORL-1	opioid receptor-like receptor (nociceptin receptor)
PCA	patient-controlled analgesia
PNS	peripheral nervous system
TENS	transcutaneous electrical nerve stimulation
WHO	World Health Organization

REFERENCES

1. Primo Levi Quote. Available at: http://www.medscape.org/viewarticle/461612. (Accessed July, 2012)
2. Stimmel B. *Pain, Analgesia, and Addiction: The Pharmacology of Pain* New York, NY: Raven Press; 1983.
3. Blackwell DL, Lucas JW, Clarke TC. Summary health statistics for U.S. adults: National health interview survey, 2012. *Vital Health Stat 10* 2014;(260):1-161.
4. IASP (International Association for the Study of Pain). Classification of Chronic Pain, Second Edition (Revised): 2012. Available at: http://www.iasp-pain.org/PublicationsNews/Content.aspx?ItemNumber=1673&navItemNumber=677. (Accessed July 9, 2015)
5. IOM (Intitute of Medicine). *Relieving Pain in America: A Blueprint for Transforming Prevention, Care, Education, and Research* Washington, D.C.: National Academies Press; 2011.
6. Humble SR, Dalton AJ, Li L. A systematic review of therapeutic interventions to reduce acute and chronic post-surgical pain after amputation, thoracotomy or mastectomy. *Eur J Pain* 2015;19(4):451-465.
7. Webster LR, Fine PG. Approaches to improve pain relief while minimizing opioid abuse liability. *J Pain.* 2010;11(7):602-611.
8. Woolf CJ. What is this thing called pain? *J Clin Invest* 2010;120(11):3742-3744.
9. Gold MS, Gebhart GF. Peripheral pain mechanisms and nociceptor sensitization. In: Fishman SM, Ballantyne JC, Rathmell JP, eds. *Bonica's Pain Management* Baltimore, MD: Wolters Kluwer Health; 2010:24-34.
10. Fong A, Schug SA. Pathophysiology of pain: A practical primer. *Plast Reconstr Surg* 2014;134(4 Suppl 2):8S-14S.
11. Uman LS, Birnie KA, Noel M, et al. Psychological interventions for needle-related procedural pain and distress in children and adolescents. *Cochrane Database Syst Rev* 2013;10:CD005179.
12. Wetherell JL, Afari N, Rutledge T, et al. A randomized, controlled trial of acceptance and commitment therapy and cognitive-behavioral therapy for chronic pain. *Pain* 2011;152(9):2098-2107.
13. Tsatali M, Papaliagkas V, Damigos D, Mavreas V, Gouva M, Tsolaki M. Depression and anxiety levels increase chronic musculoskeletal pain in patients with Alzheimer's disease. *Curr Alzheimer Res* 2014;11(6):574-579.
14. Pasero C, Portenoy R. Neurophysiology of pain and analgesia and the pathophysiology of neuropathic pain. In: McCaffery M, Pasero C, eds. *Pain Assessment and Pharmacologic Management* St. Louis, MO: Mosby; 2011:1-12.
15. Randich A, Ness T. Modulation of spinal nociceptive processing. In: Fishman SM, Ballantyne JC, Rathmell JP, eds. *Bonica's Pain Management* Baltimore, MD: Wolters Kluwer Health; 2010.
16. Woolf CJ. Central sensitization: Implications for the diagnosis and treatment of pain. *Pain* 2011;152(3 Suppl):S2-15.
17. Scholz J, Woolf CJ. The neuropathic pain triad: Neurons, immune cells and glia. *Nat Neurosci* 2007;10(11):1361-1368.
18. Grace PM, Hutchinson MR, Maier SF, Watkins LR. Pathological pain and the neuroimmune interface. *Nat Rev Immunol* 2014;14(4):217-231.
19. Clauw DJ. Fibromyalgia: A clinical review. *Jama* 2014;311(15):1547-1555.
20. Apkarian AV, Baliki MN, Farmer MA. Predicting transition to chronic pain. *Curr Opin Neurol* 2013;26(4):360-367.
21. Apkarian AV. Pain and brain changes. In: Benzon HT, Rathmell JP, Wu CL, eds. *Raj's Practical Management of Pain* Philadelphia, PA: Mosby; 2008:151-173.
22. Hanley MA, Jensen MP, Smith DG, Ehde DM, Edwards WT, Robinson LR. Preamputation pain and acute pain predict chronic pain after lower extremity amputation. *J Pain* 2007;8(2):102-109.
23. McCaffery M, Herr K, Pasero C. Assessment. In: Pasero C, McCaffery M, eds. *Pain Assessment and Pharmacologic Management* St. Louis, MO: Mosby Elsevier; 2011.
24. Latremoliere A, Woolf CJ. Central sensitization: A generator of pain hypersensitivity by central neural plasticity. *J Pain* 2009;10(9):895-926.
25. Swarm RA, Abernethy AP, Anghelescu DL, et al. Adult cancer pain. *J Natl Compr Canc Netw* 2013;11(8):992-1022.
26. Breivik H, Borchgrevink PC, Allen SM, et al. Assessment of pain. *Br J Anaesth* 2008;101(1):17-24.
27. Twycross RG. Pain and analgesics. *Curr Med Res Opin* 1978;5(7):497-505.
28. Chou R, Huffman LH, American Pain Society, American College of Physicians. Nonpharmacologic therapies for acute and chronic low back pain: A review of the evidence for an American Pain Society/American College of Physicians clinical practice guideline. *Ann Intern Med* 2007;147(7):492-504.
29. Boldt I, Eriks-Hoogland I, Brinkhof MW, de Bie R, Joggi D, von Elm E. Non-pharmacological interventions for chronic pain in people with spinal cord injury. *Cochrane Database Syst Rev* 2014;11:CD009177.
30. Vance CG, Dailey DL, Rakel BA, Sluka KA. Using TENS for pain control: The state of the evidence. *Pain Manag* 2014;4(3):197-209.
31. O'Donnell KF. Preoperative pain management education: A quality improvement project. *J Perianesth Nurs* 2015;30(3):221-227.
32. Darnall BD. Minimize opioids by optimizing pain psychology. *Pain Manag* 2014;4(4):251-253.
33. Chou R, Deyo R, Devine B, et al. *The effectiveness and risks of long-term opioid treatment of chronic pain* Agency for Healthcare Research Quality; September 2014. Publication No. 14-E005-EF.
34. Nuckols TK, Anderson L, Popescu I, et al. Opioid prescribing: A systematic review and critical appraisal of guidelines for chronic pain. *Ann Intern Med* 2014;160(1):38-47.
35. Moore RA, Derry S, Wiffen PJ, Straube S, Aldington DJ. Overview review: Comparative efficacy of oral ibuprofen and paracetamol (acetaminophen) across acute and chronic pain conditions. *Eur J Pain* 2015;19(9):1213-1223.
36. Machado GC, Maher CG, Ferreira PH, et al. Efficacy and safety of paracetamol for spinal pain and osteoarthritis: Systematic review and meta-analysis of randomised placebo controlled trials. *BMJ* 2015;350:h1225.
37. Aronoff DM, Oates JA, Boutaud O. New insights into the mechanism of action of acetaminophen: Its clinical pharmacologic characteristics reflect its inhibition of the two prostaglandin H2 synthases. *Clin Pharmacol Ther* 2006;79(1):9-19.
38. Roelofs PD, Deyo RA, Koes BW, Scholten RJ, van Tulder MW. Nonsteroidal anti-inflammatory drugs for low back pain: An updated Cochrane review. *Spine (Phila Pa 1976).* 2008;33(16):1766-1774.
39. APS (American Pain Society). *Principles of Analgesic Use in the Treatment of Acute Pain and Cancer Pain* 6th ed. Glenview, IL: American Pain Society; 2008.
40. Roth SH, Fuller P. Diclofenac topical solution compared with oral diclofenac: A pooled safety analysis. *J Pain Res* 2011;4:159-167.
41. Chou R, Fanciullo GJ, Fine PG, et al. Clinical guidelines for the use of chronic opioid therapy in chronic noncancer pain. *J Pain.* 2009;10(2):113-130.
42. Wolters Kluwer Health. online.lexi.com. Accessed December 4, 2015.
43. Yaksh TL, Wallace MS. Opioids, analgesia, and pain management. In: Brunton LL, Chabner BA, Knollman BC, eds. *The Pharmacological Basis of Therapeutics* 12th ed. New York, NY: McGraw-Hill; 2011:481-525.
44. Pasternak GW. Molecular insights into mu opioid pharmacology: From the clinic to the bench. *Clin J Pain* 2010;26(Suppl 10):S3-9.
45. Pasero C, Quinn TE, Portenoy RD. Physiology and pharmacology of opioids analgesics. In: McCaffery M, Pasero C, eds. *Pain Assessment and Pharmacologic Management* St. Louis, MO: Mosby; 2011:283-300.
46. McPherson ML. *Demystifying Opioid Conversion Calculations* Bethesda, MD: American Society of Health-System Pharmacists; 2010.
47. Topaz M, Seger DL, Lai K, et al. High Override Rate for Opioid Drug-allergy Interaction Alerts: Current Trends and Recommendations for Future. *Stud Health Technol Inform* 2015;216:242-246.
48. DeDea L. Prescribing opioids safely in patients with an opiate allergy. *JAAPA* 2012;25(1):17.
49. Woodall HE, Chiu A, Weissman DE. Opioid allergic reactions. *J Palliat Med* 2008;11(5):776-777.
50. American Society of Anesthesiologists Task Force on Acute Pain M. Practice guidelines for acute pain management in the perioperative setting: An updated report by the American Society of Anesthesiologists Task Force on Acute Pain Management. *Anesthesiology* 2012;116(2):248-273.

51. McNicol ED, Ferguson MC, Hudcova J. Patient controlled opioid analgesia versus non-patient controlled opioid analgesia for postoperative pain. *Cochrane Database Syst Rev* 2015;6:CD003348.
52. Bujedo BM, Santos SG, Azpiazu AU. A review of epidural and intrathecal opioids used in the management of postoperative pain. *J Opioid Manag* 2012;8(3):177-192.
53. American Society of Anesthesiologists Task Force on Neuraxial O, Horlocker TT, Burton AW, et al. Practice guidelines for the prevention, detection, and management of respiratory depression associated with neuraxial opioid administration. *Anesthesiology* 2009;110(2):218-230.
54. Jokinen J, Smith AF, Roewer N, Eberhart LH, Kranke P. Management of postoperative nausea and vomiting: How to deal with refractory PONV. *Anesthesiol Clin* 2012;30(3):481-493.
55. Conway A, Douglas C, Sutherland J. Capnography monitoring during procedural sedation and analgesia: A systematic review protocol. *Syst Rev* 2015;4:92.
56. Meine TJ, Roe MT, Chen AY, et al. Association of intravenous morphine use and outcomes in acute coronary syndromes: Results from the CRUSADE Quality Improvement Initiative. *Am Heart J* 2005;149(6):1043-1049.
57. Herndon CM, Jackson KC 2nd, Hallin PA. Management of opioid-induced gastrointestinal effects in patients receiving palliative care. *Pharmacotherapy* 2002;22(2):240-250.
58. Birthi P, Nagar VR, Nickerson R, Sloan PA. Hypogonadism associated with long-term opioid therapy: A systematic review. *J Opioid Manag* 2015;11(3):255-278.
59. Latta KS, Ginsberg B, Barkin RL. Meperidine: a critical review. *Am J Ther* 2002;9(1):53-68.
60. Chou R, Cruciani RA, Fiellin DA, et al. Methadone safety: A clinical practice guideline from the American Pain Society and College on Problems of Drug Dependence, in collaboration with the Heart Rhythm Society. *J Pain.* 2014;15(4):321-337.
61. Somrat C, Oranuch K, Ketchada U, Siriprapa S, Thipawan R. Optimal dose of nalbuphine for treatment of intrathecal-morphine induced pruritus after caesarean section. *J Obstet Gynaecol Res* 1999;25(3):209-213.
62. Davis ML. Twelve reasons for considering buprenorphine as a frontline analgesic in the management of pain. *J Support Oncol* 2012;10(6):209-219.
63. Weeks WB, O'Connell MJ. Buprenorphine Waivers For Physicians. *Health Aff (Millwood)* 2015;34(8):1428.
64. Young JW, Juurlink DN. Tramadol. *CMAJ.* 2013;185(8):E352.
65. Nelson LS, Juurlink DN. Tramadol and hypoglycemia: One more thing to worry about. *JAMA Intern Med* 2015;175(2):194-195.
66. Elling C, Galic M, Steigerwald I. Tapentadol prolonged release in the treatment of neuropathic pain related to diabetic polyneuropathy. *Lancet Neurol* 2015;14(7):684-685.
67. Russell IJ, Kamin M, Bennett RM, Schnitzer TJ, Green JA, Katz WA. Efficacy of tramadol in treatment of pain in fibromyalgia. *J Clin Rheumatol* 2000;6(5):250-257.
68. Chey WD, Webster L, Sostek M, Lappalainen J, Barker PN, Tack J. Naloxegol for opioid-induced constipation in patients with noncancer pain. *N Engl J Med* 2014;370(25):2387-2396.
69. Coe MA, Walsh SL. Distribution of naloxone for overdose prevention to chronic pain patients. *Prev Med* 2015;80:41-43.
70. Chen L, Sein M, Vo T, et al. Clinical interpretation of opioid tolerance versus opioid-induced hyperalgesia. *J Opioid Manag* 2014;10(6):383-393.
71. ASAM. Public policy statement: Definition of addiction. 2011. (Accessed September 24, 2015)
72. Cheatle MD. Prescription Opioid Misuse, Abuse, Morbidity, and Mortality: Balancing Effective Pain Management and Safety. *Pain Med* 2015;16(Suppl 1):S3-8.
73. Attal N, Cruccu G, Baron R, et al. EFNS guidelines on the pharmacological treatment of neuropathic pain: 2010 revision. *Eur J Neurol* 2010;17(9):1113-e1188.
74. Mitra R, Jones S. Adjuvant analgesics in cancer pain: A review. *Am J Hosp Palliat Care* 2012;29(1):70-79.
75. Melton S, Spencer S. Regional anesthesia techniques for acute pain management. In: Fishman SM, Ballantyne JC, Rathmell JP, eds. *Bonica's Pain Management* Baltimore, MD: Wolters Kluwer Health; 2010:723-754.
76. Finnerup NB, Attal N, Haroutounian S, et al. Pharmacotherapy for neuropathic pain in adults: A systematic review and meta-analysis. *Lancet Neurol* 2015;14(2):162-173.
77. Levy MH, Back A, Benedetti C, et al. NCCN clinical practice guidelines in oncology: Palliative care. *J Natl Compr Canc Netw* 2009;7(4):436-473.
78. American Geriatrics Society Panel on Pharmacological Management of Persistent Pain in Older P. Pharmacological management of persistent pain in older persons. *J Am Geriatr Soc* 2009;57(8): 1331-1346.
79. Tobias JD. Acute pain management in infants and children-Part 1: Pain pathways, pain assessment, and outpatient pain management. *Pediatr Ann* 2014;43(7):e163-168.
80. Crews KR, Gaedigk A, Dunnenberger HM, et al. Clinical Pharmacogenetics Implementation Consortium guidelines for cytochrome P450 2D6 genotype and codeine therapy: 2014 update. *Clin Pharmacol Ther* 2014;95(4):376-382.
81. Sistonen J, Sajantila A, Lao O, Corander J, Barbujani G, Fuselli S. CYP2D6 worldwide genetic variation shows high frequency of altered activity variants and no continental structure. *Pharmacogenet Genomics* 2007;17(2):93-101.
82. Verbeurgt P, Mamiya T, Oesterheld J. How common are drug and gene interactions? Prevalence in a sample of 1143 patients with CYP2C9, CYP2C19 and CYP2D6 genotyping. *Pharmacogenomics* 2014;15(5):655-665.
83. Boswell MV, Stauble ME, Loyd GE, et al. The role of hydromorphone and OPRM1 in postoperative pain relief with hydrocodone. *Pain Physician* 2013;16(3):E227-235.
84. Walter C, Lotsch J. Meta-analysis of the relevance of the OPRM1 118A>G genetic variant for pain treatment. *Pain* 2009;146(3): 270-275.

Headache Disorders

61

Deborah S. Minor and T. Kristopher Harrell

KEY CONCEPTS

1. Acute migraine therapies should provide consistent, rapid relief and enable the patient to resume normal activities at home, school, or work.
2. A stratified care approach, in which the selection of initial treatment is based on headache-related disability and symptom severity, is the preferred treatment strategy for the migraineur.
3. Strict adherence to maximum daily and weekly doses of anti-migraine medications is essential.
4. Preventive therapy should be considered in the setting of recurring migraines that produce significant disability; frequent attacks requiring symptomatic medication more than twice per week; symptomatic therapies that are ineffective, contraindicated, or produce serious side effects; and uncommon migraine variants that cause profound disruption and/or risk of neurologic injury.
5. The selection of an agent for headache prophylaxis should be based on individual patient response, tolerability, convenience of the drug formulation, and coexisting conditions.
6. Each prophylactic medication should be given an adequate therapeutic trial (usually 6 months) to judge its maximal efficacy.
7. A general wellness program and consideration of headache triggers should be included in the management plan.
8. After an effective abortive agent and dose have been identified, subsequent treatments should begin with that same regimen.

Headache is one of the most common complaints encountered by healthcare practitioners and among the top five principal reasons given by adults 18 to 44 years of age for visiting US emergency departments.[1] It can be symptomatic of a distinct pathologic process or can occur without an underlying cause. In 2013, the International Headache Society (IHS) updated its classification system and diagnostic criteria for headache disorders, cranial neuralgias, and facial pain[2] (Table 61-1). Designed to facilitate headache diagnosis in clinical practice and research, the IHS classification provides more precise definitions and standardized nomenclature for both the primary (tension-type, migraine, and cluster headache) and secondary (symptomatic of organic disease) headache disorders. This chapter focuses on the management of the primary headache disorders.

Most recurrent headaches are the result of a benign chronic primary headache disorder.[3] Less often, headaches are symptomatic of a serious underlying medical condition, such as infection, cerebral hemorrhage, or brain mass lesion. The peak prevalence of tension-type and migraine headache, the most common of the primary headache disorders, occurs during the most productive years of life (18-54 years of age).[3,4] Despite the prevalence of these disorders and their associated disability, studies indicate that most headache sufferers do not obtain appropriate medical care for their headaches.[4,6] An improved understanding of the diagnosis and pathophysiologic mechanisms of the primary headache disorders, particularly migraine, has led to the development of medications capable of providing rapid relief from moderate to severe attacks. However, a thorough evaluation of the headache history is essential to establish an accurate headache diagnosis and identify patients who can benefit from these specific therapeutic options.

MIGRAINE HEADACHE

Epidemiology

Results of the American Migraine Prevalence and Prevention Study indicate that 17.1% of women and 5.6% of men in the United States experience one or more migraine headaches per year. The prevalence of migraine varies considerably by age and gender, but the epidemiologic profile has remained stable over the past 8 years. Gender differences in migraine prevalence have been linked to menstruation, but these differences persist beyond menopause. Prevalence is highest in both men and women between the ages of 18 and 44 years and is inversely related to income and educational attainment. In the American Migraine Prevalence and Prevention Study, 93% of those with migraine reported some headache-related disability, and 54% were severely disabled or needed bedrest during an attack.[4,5] A number of neurologic and psychiatric disorders as well as cardiovascular diseases, including stroke, epilepsy, major depression, sleep apnea, obesity, and anxiety disorder, show increased comorbidity with migraine.[6,7] Whether this relationship is causal or representative of a common pathophysiologic mechanism is unknown. The economic burden of migraine is substantial; however, the indirect costs from work-related disability far exceed the direct costs associated with treatment.[8,9]

Etiology And Pathophysiology

The etiologic and pathophysiologic mechanisms of migraine are not completely understood. According to earlier theories, the migraine aura was caused by intracerebral arterial vasoconstriction followed by reactive extracranial vasodilation and associated headache. Studies of regional blood flow in the brain do not support this hypothesis, and previous vascular and neural theories of migraine development have merged into a combined theory of neurovascular mechanisms. Most clinicians now believe that the pathogenesis of migraine may be related to complex dysfunctions in neuronal and broad sensory processing.[2,6,10]

The pain and symptoms of migraine may be understood as a combination of altered perceptions resulting from neural

TABLE 61-1 International Headache Society Classification System: Focus on Migraine Headache

Migraine
Migraine without aura
Migraine with aura
Migraine with typical aura (lasting less than 1 hour) with or without headache
Migraine with brainstem aura
Hemiplegic migraine (familial, sporadic)
Retinal migraine (repeated attacks of monocular visual disturbance)
Chronic migraine (occurring on 15 or more days/mo for more than 3 months)
Complications of migraine
Status migrainous (debilitating attack lasting for more than 72 hours)
Persistent aura without infarction (symptoms persisting for more than 1 week)
Migrainous infarction (aura symptoms associated with an ischemic brain lesion)
Migraine aura-triggered seizure
Probable migraine with or without aura
Episodic syndromes that may be associated with migraine
Recurrent gastrointestinal disturbance (cyclical vomiting syndrome or abdominal migraine)
Benign paroxysmal vertigo
Benign paroxysmal torticollis
Tension-type headache
Cluster headache and other trigeminal autonomic cephalalgias
Other primary headaches
Headache attributed to head and/or neck trauma
Headache attributed to cranial or cervical vascular disorder
Headache attributed to nonvascular intracranial disorder
Headache attributed to a substance or its withdrawal
Headache attributed to infection
Headache attributed to disorder of homeostasis
Headache or facial pain attributed to disorder of cranium, neck, eyes, ears, nose, sinuses, teeth, mouth, or other facial or cervical structure
Headache attributed to psychiatric disorder
Cranial neuropathies and facial pains
Other headache disorders, not elsewhere classified or unspecified

Adapted from Headache Classification Committee of the International Headache Society. The international classification of headache disorders, 3rd ed. Cephalalgia 2013;33(9):629-808.

suppression and activation of subcortical structures and trigeminal systems. Migraine pain is believed to result from activity within the trigeminovascular system, a network of visceral afferent fibers that arises from the trigeminal ganglia and projects peripherally to innervate the pain-sensitive intracranial extracerebral blood vessels, dura mater, and large venous sinuses[11] (Fig. 61-1). These fibers also project centrally, terminating in the trigeminal nucleus caudalis in the brain stem and upper cervical spinal cord, and thus provide a pathway for nociceptive transmission from meningeal blood vessels into higher centers of the central nervous system (CNS). Activation of trigeminal sensory nerves triggers the release of vasoactive neuropeptides, including calcitonin gene-related peptide (CGRP), neurokinin A, and substance P, from perivascular axons. The released neuropeptides interact with dural blood vessels to promote vasodilation and dural plasma extravasation, resulting in neurogenic inflammation. Orthodromic conduction along trigeminovascular fibers transmits pain impulses to the trigeminal nucleus caudalis, where information is relayed further to higher cortical pain centers. Continued afferent input can result in sensitization of these central sensory neurons, producing a hyperalgesic state that responds to previously innocuous stimuli and maintains the headache.[6,10-12]

Aura occurs in a subgroup of migraineurs and also with the other primary headache disorders. The neurologic changes of the aura parallel those that occur during cortical spreading depression, a neuronal event characterized by a wave of depressed electrical activity that advances across the brain cortex at a rate consistent with the spread of aura symptoms.[6,10] Cortical spreading depression can cause inflammation and activation of the trigeminal nucleus caudalis. It is not clear whether this cortical spreading depression and the aura are the substrate of pain or actually trigger the presentation of migraine.[6,12]

Genetic factors seem to play an important role in susceptibility to migraine attacks. Studies in monozygotic twins suggest approximately 50% heritability of migraine with a multifactorial polygenic basis.[13] Although it is possible for any individual to experience a migraine attack, it is recurrence in the migraineur that is abnormal. Attack occurrence and frequency are governed by CNS sensitivity to migraine-specific triggers or environmental factors. Migraineurs appear to have a lowered threshold of response to specific environmental circumstances as a result of genetic factors that govern the balance of CNS excitation and inhibition at various levels. Thus, trigger factors can be viewed as modulators of the genetic set point that predisposes to migraine headache.[13,14] The hyperresponsiveness of the migrainous brain may be the result of an inherited abnormality in calcium and/or sodium channels and sodium/potassium pumps that regulate cortical excitability through the release of serotonin (5-hydroxytryptamine [5-HT]) and other neurotransmitters. Increased levels of excitatory amino acids such as glutamate and alterations in levels of extracellular potassium also can affect the migraine threshold and initiate and propagate the phenomenon of cortical spreading depression.[6,13-16]

5-HT has long been implicated as an important mediator of migraine headache. Specific populations of 5-HT receptor subfamilies appear to be involved in the pathophysiology and treatment of migraine headache. Acute antimigraine drugs such as the ergot alkaloids and triptan derivatives are agonists of vascular and neuronal 5-HT_1 receptor subtypes, resulting in vasoconstriction of meningeal blood vessels and inhibition of vasoactive neuropeptide release and pain signal transmission.[6,15] Drugs used for migraine prophylaxis also modulate neurotransmitter systems.[10] These actions and benefits in migraine management are consistent with the current understanding of migraine pathophysiology and neurovascular disorders.

Clinical Presentation

The migraine attack has been divided into several phases. *Premonitory symptoms* are experienced by 12% to 79% of migraineurs in the hours or days before the onset of headache.[2,6] The previously popular terms *prodrome* and *warning symptoms* should be avoided because these are often used mistakenly to include aura.[2] Premonitory symptoms vary widely among migraineurs but usually are consistent within an individual. Neurologic symptoms (eg, allodynia, phonophobia, photophobia, hyperosmia, and difficulty concentrating) are common, but psychological (eg, anxiety, depression, euphoria, irritability, drowsiness, fatigue, hyperactivity, and restlessness), autonomic (eg, polyuria, diarrhea, and constipation), and constitutional (eg, stiff neck, yawning, thirst, food cravings, and anorexia) symptoms also are reported.[2,6,16]

The migraine *aura*, a complex of positive and negative focal neurologic symptoms that precedes or accompanies an attack, is experienced by approximately 25% of migraineurs on some occasions.[2,16] The aura typically evolves over 5 minutes or longer and lasts less than 60 minutes. Headache usually occurs within 60 minutes of the end of the aura. Occasionally, aura symptoms begin at the onset

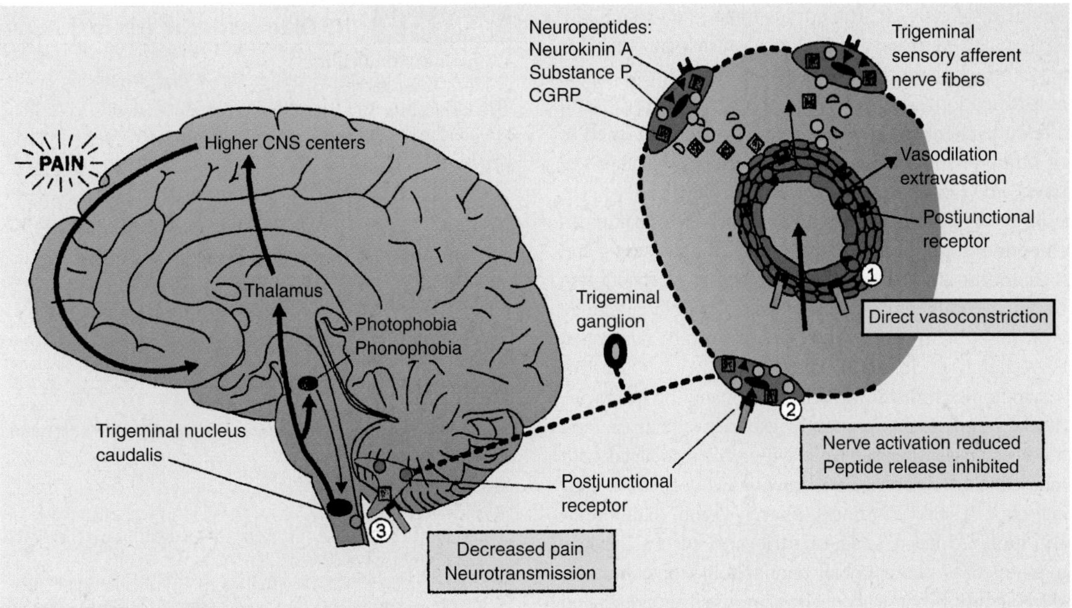

FIGURE 61-1 The pathophysiology of migraine headache. Vasodilation of intracranial extracerebral blood vessels (possibly the result of an imbalance in the brainstem) results in the activation of the perivascular trigeminal nerves that release vasoactive neuropeptides to promote neurogenic inflammation. Central pain transmission may activate other brainstem nuclei, resulting in associated symptoms (nausea, vomiting, photophobia, and phonophobia). The antimigraine effects of the 5-HT$_{1B/ID}$ receptor agonists are highlighted at areas 1, 2, and 3. (CGRP, calcitonin gene-related peptide.) *(Reprinted from the Lancet, Vol. 351, Ferrari MD, Migraine, 1043-1051, Copyright © 1998, with permission from Elsevier.)*

CLINICAL PRESENTATION Migraine Headache

General

- Migraine is a common, recurrent, severe headache that interferes with normal functioning. It is a primary headache disorder divided into two major subtypes, migraine without aura and migraine with aura.

Symptoms

- Migraine is characterized by recurring episodes of throbbing head pain, frequently unilateral, that when untreated can last from 4 to 72 hours. Migraine headaches can be severe and associated with nausea, vomiting, and sensitivity to light, sound, and/or movement. Not all symptoms are present in every attack.
- In the headache evaluation, diagnostic alarms should be identified. These include: acute onset of the "first" or "worst" headache ever, accelerating pattern of headache following subacute onset, onset of headache after age 50 years, headache associated with systemic illness (eg, fever, nausea, vomiting, stiff neck, and rash), headache with focal neurologic symptoms or papilledema, and new-onset headache in a patient with cancer or human immunodeficiency virus (HIV) infection.

Signs

- A stable pattern, absence of daily headache, positive family history for migraine, normal neurologic examination, presence of food triggers, menstrual association, long-standing history, improvement with sleep, and subacute evolution are all signs of migraine headache. Aura can signal the migraine headache but is not required for diagnosis.

Laboratory Tests

- In selected circumstances and secondary headache presentation, serum chemistries, urine toxicology profiles, thyroid function tests, Lyme disease studies, and other blood tests such as a complete blood count, antinuclear antibody titer, erythrocyte sedimentation rate, and antiphospholipid antibody titer can be considered.

Diagnostic Tests

- Perform a general medical and neurologic physical examination. Check for abnormalities: vital signs (fever, hypertension), funduscopy (papilledema, hemorrhage, and exudates), palpation and auscultation of the head and neck (sinus tenderness, hardened or tender temporal arteries, trigger points, temporomandibular joint tenderness, bruits, nuchal rigidity, and cervical spine tenderness), and neurologic examination (identify abnormalities or deficits in mental status, cranial nerves, deep tendon reflexes, motor strength, coordination, gait, and cerebellar function). Consider neuroimaging studies in patients with abnormal neurologic examination findings of unknown etiology and in those with additional risk factors warranting imaging.

of headache or during the attack. The aura is most often visual and frequently affects half the visual field.[2] Visual auras vary in their complexity and can include both positive (scintillations, photopsia, teichopsia, or fortification spectrum) and negative (scotoma and hemianopsia) features. Sensory and motor aura symptoms, such as paresthesias or numbness involving the arms and face, dysphasia or aphasia, weakness, and hemiparesis, also are reported.[2,16]

Migraine *headache* pain is usually gradual in onset, peaking in intensity over a period of minutes to hours and lasting between 4 and 72 hours. Pain can occur anywhere in the face or head but most often involves the frontotemporal region. The headache is typically unilateral and throbbing or pulsating in nature; however, pain can be bilateral at onset or become generalized during the course of an attack.[2,16] Gastrointestinal (GI) symptoms almost invariably accompany the headache. During an attack, migraineurs frequently experience nausea, and emesis sometimes occurs. Other systemic symptoms associated with the headache phase include anorexia, food cravings, constipation, diarrhea, abdominal cramps, nasal stuffiness, blurred vision, diaphoresis, facial pallor, and localized facial, scalp, or periorbital edema. Sensory hyperacuity, manifested as photophobia, phonophobia, or osmophobia, is reported frequently. Because headache pain usually is aggravated by physical activity, most migraineurs seek a dark, quiet room for rest and relief. Impaired concentration, depression, irritability, fatigue, or anxiety often accompanies the headache. Once headache pain wanes, patients may experience a *resolution phase* characterized by feeling tired, exhausted, irritable, or listless. Impaired concentration may continue, as well as scalp tenderness or mood changes. Some patients experience depression and malaise, whereas others can feel unusually refreshed or euphoric.[2,16] The reader is referred to the IHS classification and recent reviews for descriptions of the classic migraine variants and other migraine subtypes[2,16] (see Table 61-1).

Although headaches have many potential causes, most are considered to be primary headache disorders. A comprehensive headache history is the most important element in establishing the clinical diagnosis of migraine.[2,6,17] A thorough headache history always should be obtained, and information collected should include age at onset, attack frequency and timing, duration of attacks, precipitating or aggravating factors, ameliorating factors, description of neurologic symptoms, characteristics of the headache pain (quality, intensity, location, and radiation), associated signs and symptoms, treatment history, family and social history, and the impact of headaches on daily life.

Secondary headache can be identified or excluded based on the headache history, as well as the results of general medical and neurologic examinations. Diagnostic and laboratory testing also can be warranted in the setting of suspicious headache features or an abnormal examination. The routine use of neuroimaging (computed tomography or magnetic resonance imaging) generally is not indicated in patients with migraine and a normal neurologic examination, but should be considered in patients with an unexplained abnormal neurologic examination or an atypical headache history. Because migraine headaches usually begin by the second or third decade of life, headaches beginning after age 50 years suggest an organic etiology such as a mass lesion, cerebrovascular disease, or temporal arteritis.[2,3,16] Table 61-2 lists the IHS diagnostic criteria for migraine with and without aura.[2]

TABLE 61-2 IHS Diagnostic Criteria for Migraine

Migraine without aura

At least five attacks

Headache attack lasts 4-72 hours (untreated or unsuccessfully treated)

Headache has at least two of the following characteristics:

- Unilateral location
- Pulsating quality
- Moderate or severe intensity
- Aggravation by or avoidance of routine physical activity (ie, walking or climbing stairs)

During headache at least one of the following:

- Nausea, vomiting, or both
- Photophobia and phonophobia
- Not attributed to another disorder

Migraine with aura (classic migraine)

At least two attacks

Migraine aura fulfills criteria for typical aura, hemiplegic migraine, retinal migraine or brainstem aura

Not attributed to another disorder

Typical aura

Fully reversible visual, sensory, or speech symptoms (or any combination) but no motor weakness

Homonymous or bilateral visual symptoms including positive features (eg, flickering lights, spot, lines) or negative features (eg, loss of vision) or unilateral sensory symptoms including positive features (eg, pins and needles) or negative features (ie, numbness), or any combination

At least two of the following:

- At least one symptom that develops gradually over a minimum of 5 minutes or different symptoms that occur in succession or both
- Each symptom lasts for at least 5 minutes and for no longer than 60 minutes
- Headache that meets criteria for migraine without aura begins during the aura or follows aura within 60 minutes

IHS, International Headache Society.

Adapted from Headache Classification Committee of the International Headache Society. The international classification of headache disorders, 3rd ed. Cephalalgia 2013;33(9):629-808.

TREATMENT
Migraines

Desired Outcome

Clinicians who care for migraineurs must appreciate the impact of this painful and debilitating disorder on the life of the patient, the patient's family, and the patient's employer. Treatment strategies must address both immediate and long-term goals. (1) Acute migraine therapies should provide consistent, rapid relief and enable the patient to resume normal activities at home, school, or work. Recurrence of symptoms and treatment-related adverse effects should be minimal. Ideally, patients should be able to manage their own headaches effectively without a medical visit. In addition, migraineurs should take an active role in the creation of a long-term formal management plan. An individualized approach to treatment can result in a reduction in attack frequency and severity, thus minimizing headache-related disability and emotional distress and improving the patient's quality of life. Goals of long-term and acute treatment of migraine are listed in Table 61-3.[15,17,18]

General Approach To Treatment

Nonpharmacologic and pharmacologic interventions are available for the management of migraine headache; however, drug therapy remains the mainstay of treatment for most patients. Pharmacotherapeutic management of migraine can be acute (ie, symptomatic or abortive) or preventive (ie, prophylactic). When choosing acute or preventive therapies, the clinician should consider the patient's response to specific medications and their tolerability, as well as coexisting illnesses that can limit treatment choices. Abortive or acute therapies can be migraine-specific (eg, ergots and triptans) or nonspecific (eg, analgesics, antiemetics, nonsteroidal antiinflammatory drugs [NSAIDs], and corticosteroids) and are most effective at relieving pain and associated symptoms when administered at the onset of migraine[15,17,18] (Table 61-4). (2) A stratified care approach in which the selection of initial treatment is based on headache-related disability and symptom severity is the preferred treatment strategy for the migraineur.[15,17] Because attack severity varies in individuals,

TABLE 61-3 Goals of Therapy in Migraine Management

Goals of long-term migraine treatment
Reduce migraine frequency, severity, and disability
Reduce reliance on poorly tolerated, ineffective, or unwanted acute pharmacotherapies
Improve quality of life
Prevent headache
Avoid escalation of headache medication use
Educate and enable patients to manage their disease
Reduce headache-related distress and psychological symptoms
Goals for acute migraine treatment
Treat migraine attacks rapidly and consistently without recurrence
Restore the patient's ability to function
Minimize the use of backup and rescue medications[a]
Optimize self-care for overall management
Be cost-effective in overall management
Cause minimal or no adverse effects

[a]Rescue medications are defined as medications used at home when other treatments fail that permit the patient to get relief without a visit to the physician's office or emergency department.

Data from references 15, 17, and 18.

patients may be advised to use nonspecific agents for mild to moderate headache not causing disability while reserving migraine-specific medications for more severe attacks. The absorption and efficacy of orally administered drugs can be compromised by gastric stasis or nausea and vomiting that accompany migraine. Pretreatment with antiemetic agents or the use of nonoral treatment (eg, suppositories, nasal sprays, or injections) is advisable when nausea and vomiting are severe.[15,19]

The frequent or excessive use of acute migraine medications can result in a pattern of increasing headache frequency and drug consumption known as *medication-overuse headache* (or *rebound headache*).[2,6] The syndrome appears to evolve as a self-sustaining headache-medication cycle in which the headache returns as the medication wears off, leading to the consumption of more drug for relief. The headache history often reflects the gradual onset of an atypical daily or near-daily headache with superimposed episodic migraine attacks. Medication overuse is one of the most common causes of chronic daily headache.[20,21] Agents most commonly implicated in this syndrome include simple and combination analgesics and opiates. Triptans are also implicated.[2,6,22] Discontinuation of the offending agent leads to a gradual decrease in headache frequency and severity and a return of the original headache characteristics. Although detoxification usually can be accomplished on an outpatient basis, hospitalization can be necessary for the control of refractory rebound headache and other withdrawal symptoms (eg, nausea, vomiting, asthenia, restlessness, and agitation).[20,21] 3 Regulation of nociceptive systems and renewed responsiveness to therapy usually occur within 2 months following medication withdrawal.[2] Most experts recommend limiting use of acute migraine therapies to *fewer than 10 days per month* to avoid the development of medication-overuse headache.[2,22,23]

Preventive migraine therapies are administered on a daily basis to reduce the frequency, severity, and duration of attacks and improve responsiveness to symptomatic migraine therapies[8,24,25] (Table 61-5). 4 Preventive therapy should be considered in the setting of recurring migraines that produce significant disability despite acute therapy; frequent attacks occurring more than twice per week with the risk of developing medication-overuse headache; symptomatic therapies that are ineffective or contraindicated, or produce serious side effects; uncommon migraine variants that cause profound disruption and/or risk of permanent neurologic injury (eg, hemiplegic migraine, basilar migraine, and migraine with prolonged aura); and patient preference to limit the number of attacks.[22,26] Preventive therapy also may be administered preemptively or intermittently when headaches recur in a predictable pattern (eg, exercise-induced migraine or menstrual migraine).[26] The evidence to support the various agents used for migraine prophylaxis has recently been reviewed. Only propranolol, timolol, divalproex sodium, and topiramate are currently approved by the FDA for the indication, although other agents have established or probable efficacy. 5 Guidelines identify which agents might be effective, but there is insufficient evidence as to how to choose one therapy over another. Thus, the selection of an agent typically is based on its side effect profile and the patient's coexisting/comorbid conditions.[17,24,25] 6 A therapeutic trial of 2 to 3 months is necessary to achieve clinical benefit, but some reduction in attack frequency can be evident by the first month of therapy. Maximal benefits are typically observed by 6 months of treatment.[14,24,26] Drug therapy should be initiated with low doses and gradually increased until a therapeutic effect is achieved or side effects become intolerable. Drug doses for migraine prophylaxis are often lower than those necessary for other indications.[25,26] Overuse of acute headache medications will interfere with the effects of preventive treatment.[2,17] Prophylactic treatment usually is continued for at least 6 to 12 months after the frequency and severity of headaches have diminished. After that time, based on discussions with the patient, gradual tapering or discontinuation may be reasonable.[22,24] Many migraineurs experience fewer and less severe attacks for lengthy periods following discontinuation of prophylactic medications or taper to a lower dose. Figures 61-2 and 61-3 identify treatment and management algorithms for migraine headache.

Nonpharmacologic Therapy

Nonpharmacologic therapy of acute migraine headache is limited but can include application of ice to the head and periods of rest or sleep, usually in a dark, quiet environment. Recommendations for the preventive management of migraine typically suggest that patients identify and avoid individual factors or triggers that consistently provoke migraine attacks[2,3,17,27] (Table 61-6). Changes in estrogen levels associated with menarche, menstruation, pregnancy, menopause, oral contraceptive use, and other hormone therapies can trigger, intensify, or alleviate migraine.[3] A headache diary that records the frequency, severity, and duration of attacks can facilitate identification of migraine triggers. 7 In appropriate situations, some patients may learn to cope with triggers after a process of controlled exposure and approach/confront strategies.[27,28] Patients also can benefit from adherence to a wellness program that includes regular sleep, exercise, and eating habits, smoking cessation, and limited caffeine intake. Behavioral interventions, such as relaxation therapy, biofeedback (often used in combination with relaxation therapy), and cognitive therapy, are preventive treatment options for patients who prefer nondrug therapy or when symptomatic therapies are poorly tolerated, contraindicated, or ineffective.[17]

Clinical **Controversy ...**

Most migraineurs have triggers for the acute attack, at least occasionally, and are generally advised to avoid these as part of management to reduce the frequency of attacks. However, research evaluating the efficacy and usefulness of trigger avoidance is almost nonexistent. Triggers may change over time in the life of the migraineur and be modified by preventive medication. Trigger avoidance can also impose severe lifestyle restrictions and more stress. Avoidance may ultimately not allow for desensitization from the trigger and the subsequent development of relative immunity.[27,28]

TABLE 61-4 Dosing of Acute Migraine Therapies[a]

Drug	Dose	Usual Range/Comments
Analgesics		
Acetaminophen (Tylenol)	1,000 mg at onset; repeat every 4-6 hours as needed	Max. daily dose is 4 g
Acetaminophen 250 mg/aspirin 250 mg/ caffeine 65 mg (Excedrin Migraine)	2 tablets at onset and every 6 hours	Available over-the-counter as Excedrin Migraine
Nonsteroidal antiinflammatory drugs		
Aspirin	500-1,000 mg every 4-6 hours	Max. daily dose is 4 g
Ibuprofen (Motrin)	200-800 mg every 6 hours	Avoid doses >2.4 g/day
Naproxen sodium (Aleve, Anaprox)	550-825 mg at onset; can repeat 220 mg in 3-4 hours	Avoid doses >1.375 g/day
Diclofenac (Cataflam, Voltaren)	50-100 mg at onset; can repeat 50 mg in 8 hours	Avoid doses >150 mg/day
Ergotamine tartrate		
Oral tablet (1 mg) with caffeine 100 mg (Cafergot)	2 mg at onset; then 1-2 mg every 30 minutes as needed	Max. dose is 6 mg/day or 10 mg/wk; consider pretreatment with an antiemetic
Sublingual tablet (2 mg) (Ergomar)		
Rectal suppository (2 mg) with caffeine 100 mg (Cafergot, Migergot)	Insert 1/2 to 1 suppository at onset; repeat after 1 hour as needed	Max. dose is 4 mg/day or 10 mg/wk; consider pretreatment with an antiemetic
Dihydroergotamine		
Injection 1 mg/mL (D.H.E. 45)	0.25-1 mg at onset IM, IV or subcutaneous; repeat every hour as needed	Max. dose is 3 mg/day or 6 mg/wk
Nasal spray 4 mg/mL (Migranal)	One spray (0.5 mg) in each nostril at onset; repeat sequence 15 minutes later (total dose is 2 mg or 4 sprays)	Max. dose is 3 mg/day; prime sprayer 4 times before using; do not tilt head back or inhale through nose while spraying; discard open ampules after 8 hours
Serotonin agonists (triptans)		
Sumatriptan (Imitrex)		
Injection	6 mg subcutaneous at onset; can repeat after 1 hour if needed	Max. daily dose is 12 mg
Oral tablets	25, 50, 85 or 100 mg at onset; can repeat after 2 hours if needed	Optimal dose is 50-100 mg; max. daily dose is 200 mg; combination product with naproxen, 85 mg/500 mg
Nasal spray	5, 10, or 20 mg at onset; can repeat after 2 hours if needed	Optimal dose is 20 mg; max. daily dose is 40 mg; single-dose device delivering 5 or 20 mg; administer one spray in one nostril
Zolmitriptan (Zomig, Zomig-ZMT)		
Oral tablets	2.5 or 5 mg at onset as regular or orally disintegrating tablet; can repeat after 2 hours if needed	Optimal dose is 2.5 mg; max. dose is 10 mg/day Do not divide ODT dosage form
Nasal spray	5 mg (one spray) at onset; can repeat after 2 hours if needed	Max. daily dose is 10 mg/day
Naratriptan (Amerge)	1 or 2.5 mg at onset; can repeat after 4 hours if needed	Optimal dose is 2.5 mg; max. daily dose is 5 mg
Rizatriptan (Maxalt, Maxalt-MLT)	5 or 10 mg at onset as regular or orally disintegrating tablet; can repeat after 2 hours if needed	Optimal dose is 10 mg; max. daily dose is 30 mg; onset of effect is similar with standard and orally disintegrating tablets; use 5-mg dose (15 mg/day max.) in patients receiving propranolol
Almotriptan (Axert)	6.25 or 12.5 mg at onset; can repeat after 2 hours if needed	Optimal dose is 12.5 mg; max. daily dose is 25 mg
Frovatriptan (Frova)	2.5 or 5 mg at onset; can repeat in 2 hours if needed	Optimal dose 2.5-5 mg; max. daily dose is 7.5 mg (3 tablets)
Eletriptan (Relpax)	20 or 40 mg at onset; can repeat after 2 hours if needed	Max. single dose is 40 mg; max. daily dose is 80 mg
Miscellaneous		
Metoclopramide (Reglan)	10 mg IV at onset	Useful for acute relief in the office or emergency department setting
Prochlorperazine (Compazine)	10 mg IV or IM at onset	Useful for acute relief in the office or emergency department setting

ODT, orally disintegrating tablet.

[a]Limit use of symptomatic medications to fewer than 10 days/mo when possible to avoid medication-overuse headache.

Data from references 15, 19, and 31.

TABLE 61-5 Dosing of Prophylactic Migraine Therapies

Drug	Initial Dose	Usual Range	Comments
β-Adrenergic antagonists			
Atenolol[a] (Tenormin)	50 mg/day	50-200 mg/day	
Metoprolol[b] (Toprol, Toprol XL)	100 mg/day in divided doses	100-200 mg/day in divided doses	Dose short-acting 4 times a day and long-acting 2 times a day; available as extended release
Nadolol[a] (Corgard)	40-80 mg/day	80-240 mg/day	
Propranolol[b] (Inderal, Inderal LA)	40 mg/day in divided doses	40-160 mg/day in divided doses	Dose short-acting 2-3 times a day and long-acting 1-2 times a day; available as extended release
Timolol[b] (Blocadren)	20 mg/day in divided doses	20-60 mg/day in divided doses	
Antidepressants			
Amitriptyline[a] (Elavil)	10 mg at bedtime	20-50 mg at bedtime	
Venlafaxine[a] (Effexor, Effexor-XR)	37.5 mg/day	75-150 mg/day	Available as extended release; increase dose after 1 week
Anticonvulsants			
Topiramate[b] (Topamax)	25 mg/day	50-200 mg/day in divided doses	As effective as amitriptyline, propranolol or valproate; increase by 25 mg/wk
Valproic acid/divalproex sodium[b] (Depakene, Depakote, Depakote ER)	250-500 mg/day in divided doses, or daily for extended release	500-1,500 mg/day in divided doses, or daily for extended release	Monitor levels if compliance is an issue
Nonsteroidal antiinflammatory drugs			
Ibuprofen[a] (Motrin)	400-1,200 mg/day in divided doses	Same as initial dose	Use intermittently, such as for menstrual migraine prevention; daily or prolonged use may lead to medication-overuse headache and is limited by potential toxicity
Ketoprofen[a] (Orudis)	150 mg/day in divided doses	Same as initial dose	
Naproxen sodium[a] (Aleve, Anaprox)	550-1,100 mg/day in divided doses	Same as initial dose	
Serotonin agonists (triptans)			
Frovatriptan[b] (Frova)	2.5 mg/day or 5 mg/day in divided doses	Same as initial dose	Taken in the perimenstrual period to prevent menstrual migraine
Naratriptan[a] (Amerge)	2 mg/day in divided doses	Same as initial dose	
Zolmitriptan[a] (Zomig)	5-7.5 mg/day in divided doses	Same as initial dose	
Miscellaneous			
Histamine[a] (Histatrol)	1-10 ng two times/wk	Same as initial dose	May cause transient itching and burning at injection site
Magnesium[a]	400 mg/day	800 mg/day in divided doses	May be more helpful in migraine with aura and menstrual migraine
MIG-99[a] (feverfew)	10-100 mg/day in divided doses	Same as initial dose	Withdrawal may be associated with increased headaches
Petasites[b]	100-150 mg/day in divided doses	150 mg/day in divided doses	Use only commercial preparations, plant is carcinogenic
Riboflavin[a]	400 mg/day in divided doses	400 mg/day in divided doses	Benefit only after 3 months

[a]Level B—probably effective (1 Class I or 2 Class II studies).

[b]Level A—established efficacy (≥2 Class I studies).

As per Ameican Academy of Neurology therapeutic classification of evidence, Silberstein and Holland, et al. and Holland and Silberstein, et al. Neurology 2012;78:1337-1345 and 78:1346-1353.

Data from references 24 and 35.

PHARMACOLOGIC MANAGEMENT OF ACUTE MIGRAINE

Analgesics and NSAIDs

Simple analgesics and NSAIDs are effective medications for the management of many migraine attacks (see Table 61-4). They offer a reasonable first-line choice for treatment of mild to moderate migraine attacks or severe attacks that have been responsive in the past to similar NSAIDs or nonopiate analgesics. Of the NSAIDs, aspirin, diclofenac, ibuprofen, ketorolac, naproxen sodium, tolfenamic acid, and the combination of acetaminophen plus aspirin and caffeine have demonstrated the most consistent evidence of efficacy.[15,19] Evidence for other NSAIDs is either limited or inconsistent. Although some

Clinical **Controversy ...**

A stratified care approach, in which the selection of initial treatment is based on headache-related disability and symptom severity, is the most recommended treatment strategy for the migraineur. This approach assumes that greater severity is a risk factor for failure of symptomatic treatments and reflects the need for more specific treatment, such as a triptan. However, recent reviews support the efficacy of aspirin and other NSAIDs in acute migraine, regardless of pre-treatment headache intensity, and with efficacy comparable to oral triptans.[29,30]

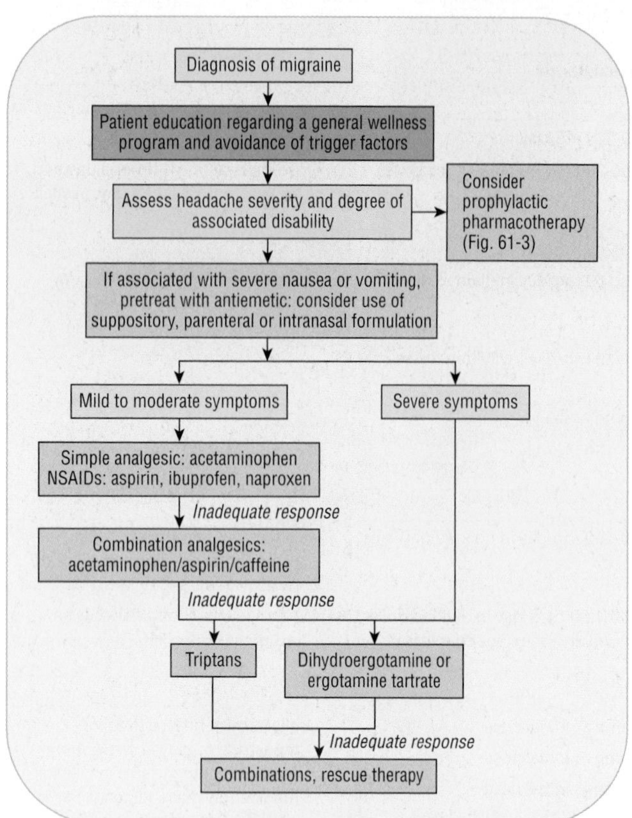

FIGURE 61-2 Treatment algorithm for migraine headaches.

TABLE 61-6 Commonly Reported Triggers of Migraine

Food triggers
Alcohol
Caffeine/caffeine withdrawal
Chocolate
Fermented and pickled foods
Monosodium glutamate (eg, in Chinese food, seasoned salt, and instant foods)
Nitrate-containing foods (eg, processed meats)
Saccharin/aspartame (eg, diet foods or diet sodas)
Tyramine-containing foods
Environmental triggers
Glare or flickering lights
High altitude
Loud noises
Strong smells and fumes
Tobacco smoke
Weather changes
Behavioral–physiologic triggers
Excess or insufficient sleep
Fatigue
Menstruation, menopause
Sexual activity
Skipped meals
Strenuous physical activity (eg, prolonged overexertion)
Stress or post-stress

Data from references 3, 17, 27, and 28.

patients may observe benefits, acetaminophen alone is not generally recommended for migraine because the scientific support is not optimal.[18] Comparisons with other pharmacotherapeutic classes are limited; however, studies support the comparable efficacy of NSAIDs and triptans in acute migraine. Baseline headache intensity does not predict the success or failure of aspirin or other NSAIDs.[29,30] There are no studies comparing the relative efficacy of different NSAIDs.[19]

Nonsteroidal antiinflammatory drugs appear to prevent neurogenically mediated inflammation in the trigeminovascular system through the inhibition of prostaglandin synthesis. Metoclopramide can speed the absorption of analgesics and alleviate migraine-related nausea and vomiting.[15] Suppository analgesic preparations are an option when nausea and vomiting are severe.[19] Acute NSAID therapy is associated with gastrointestinal (GI) (eg, dyspepsia, nausea, vomiting, and diarrhea) and CNS (eg, somnolence, dizziness) side effects. NSAIDs should be avoided or used cautiously in patients with previous ulcer disease, renal disease, or hypersensitivity to aspirin.[18,19]

The nonprescription combination of acetaminophen, aspirin, and caffeine was approved for the treatment of migraine in the United States because of its proven efficacy in relieving migraine pain and associated symptoms.[15,18] Aspirin and acetaminophen are also available in prescription combination products containing a short-acting barbiturate (butalbital) or narcotic (codeine). No randomized, placebo-controlled studies support the efficacy of butalbital-containing

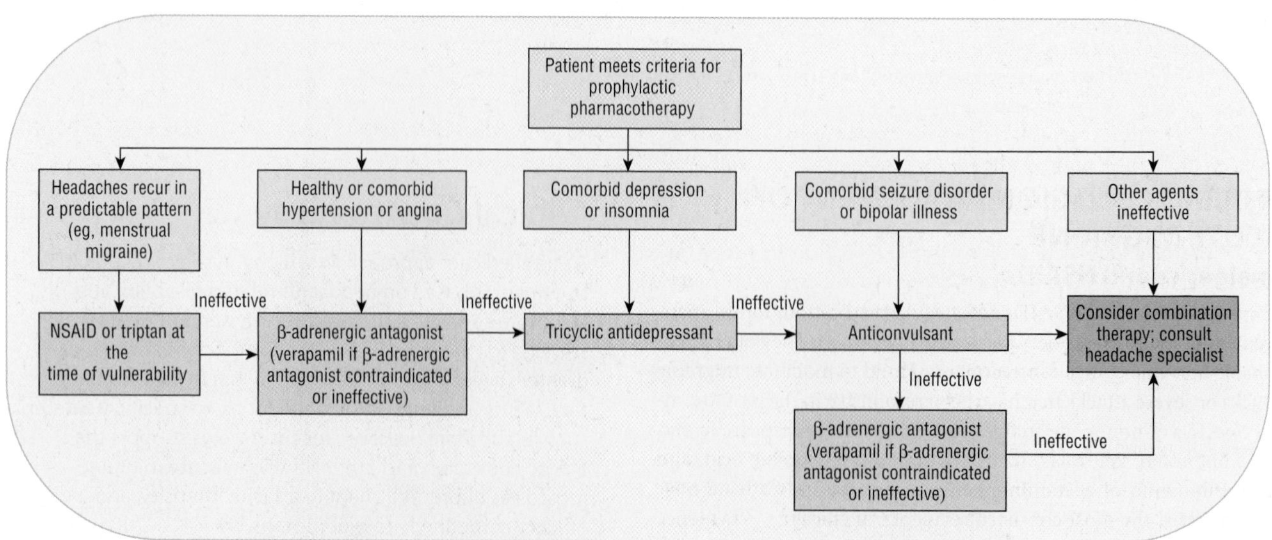

FIGURE 61-3 Treatment algorithm for prophylactic management of migraine headaches. (NSAID, nonsteroidal antiinflammatory drug.)

products in the treatment of migraine. The use of butalbital-containing analgesics or narcotics should be limited because of concerns about overuse, medication-overuse headache, and withdrawal.[18,19,23] Although frequent consumption of aspirin or acetaminophen alone can result in medication-overuse headache, combination analgesics appear to pose a greater risk.[19,23]

Opiate Analgesics

The use of narcotic analgesic drugs (eg, meperidine, butorphanol, oxycodone, and hydromorphone) in migraine treatment is controversial, and evidence for use is generally negative. Opiates have no vasopressor or antiinflammatory effects and can cause central sensitization, increasing the risk of medication-overuse headache and interfering with the efficacy of other treatments even with intermittent use.[15,23] Use should generally be reserved for patients with moderate to severe infrequent headaches in whom conventional therapies are contraindicated or as "rescue medication" after patients have failed to respond to conventional therapies.[18] Opioid therapy should be supervised closely because of the risk of sedation and the potential for abuse.[15,23]

Antiemetics

Adjunctive antiemetic therapy is useful for combating the nausea and vomiting that accompany migraine headaches and the medications used to treat attacks (eg, ergotamine tartrate). A single dose of an antiemetic, such as metoclopramide, chlorpromazine, or prochlorperazine, administered 15 to 30 minutes before ingestion of oral abortive migraine medications is often sufficient. Suppository preparations are available when nausea and vomiting are particularly prominent. Metoclopramide is also useful to reverse gastroparesis and improve absorption from the GI tract during severe attacks.[15,18]

In addition to antiemetic effects, dopamine antagonist drugs also have been used successfully as monotherapy for the treatment of intractable headache (see Table 61-4). Prochlorperazine administered by the IV and intramuscular routes and IV metoclopramide provided more effective pain relief than placebo. Chlorpromazine and droperidol also have provided relief of migraine headache when administered parenterally at doses of 12.5 to 37.5 and 2.5 to 5 mg, respectively. The precise mechanism of action for these agents is unknown. The dopamine antagonists offer an alternative to the narcotic analgesics for the treatment of refractory migraine. Drowsiness and dizziness were reported occasionally, and extrapyramidal side effects were reported infrequently in migraine trials. Droperidol has a risk for QT prolongation.[18,19,23]

Miscellaneous Nonspecific Medications

Corticosteroids can be considered as rescue therapy for status migrainous (a severe, continuous migraine that can last up to 1 week).[18] IV or intramuscular dexamethasone at a dose of 10 to 25 mg has also been used as an adjunct to abortive therapy.[19]

Limited studies suggest a role for intranasal lidocaine in the treatment of acute migraine headache. Intranasal lidocaine, one to four drops of a 4% solution, provides rapid pain relief within 15 minutes of administration, but headache recurrence is common. Adverse effects generally are limited to local irritation, an unpleasant taste, and numbness of the throat.[18]

IV valproate 500 to 1,000 mg and magnesium sulfate 1,000 mg are nonsedating options for use in acute migraine treatment.[23] Future studies might establish a more defined role for these agents in migraine management.

Ergot Alkaloids and Derivatives

Ergotamine tartrate and dihydroergotamine can be considered for the treatment of moderate to severe migraine attacks (see Table 61-4). These drugs are nonselective 5-HT_1 receptor agonists that constrict intracranial blood vessels and inhibit the development of neurogenic inflammation in the trigeminovascular system.[15] Central inhibition of the trigeminovascular pathway is also reported as well as agonist activity at dopaminergic receptors. Venous and arterial constriction occur with therapeutic doses, but ergotamine tartrate exerts more potent arterial effects than dihydroergotamine.[15,19,23]

Ergotamine tartrate is available for oral, sublingual, and rectal administration. Oral and rectal preparations contain caffeine to enhance absorption and potentiate analgesia. Ergotamine use is limited because of issues of efficacy and side effects. Dosage requirements should be titrated strictly to establish an effective but subnauseating dose for future attacks. Despite clinical use since 1926, evidence supporting the efficacy of ergotamine in migraine is inconsistent.[19]

Dihydroergotamine is available for intranasal and parenteral administration by the intramuscular, subcutaneous, and IV routes.[23] Parenteral dihydroergotamine was viewed previously as inpatient or emergency department treatment for moderate to severe migraine or intractable headache, but patients can be trained to self-administer dihydroergotamine intramuscularly or subcutaneously. Mixing with 1% or 2% lidocaine can reduce burning at the injection site. Clinical opinion suggests its use is relatively safe and effective when compared with other migraine therapies.[15,18]

Nausea and vomiting (resulting from stimulation of the chemoreceptor trigger zone) are among the most common adverse effects of the ergotamine derivatives. Pretreatment with an antiemetic agent should be considered with ergotamine and IV dihydroergotamine therapy. Other common side effects include abdominal pain, weakness, fatigue, paresthesias, muscle pain, diarrhea, and chest tightness. Rarely, symptoms of severe peripheral ischemia (ergotism), including cold, numb, painful extremities, continuous paresthesias, diminished peripheral pulses, and claudication, can result from the vasoconstrictor effects of the ergot alkaloids. Gangrenous extremities, myocardial infarction, hepatic necrosis, and bowel and brain ischemia have also been reported. Dihydroergotamine is rarely associated with such side effects. Triptans and ergot derivatives should not be used within 24 hours of each other.[15,19] Ergotamine derivatives are contraindicated in patients with renal or hepatic failure; coronary, cerebral, or peripheral vascular disease; uncontrolled hypertension; and sepsis; and in women who are pregnant or nursing. Dihydroergotamine does not appear to cause rebound headache, but dosage restrictions for ergotamine tartrate should be observed strictly to prevent this complication.[19,23]

Serotonin Receptor Agonists (Triptans)

Introduction of the 5-HT receptor agonists, or triptans, represented a significant advance in migraine pharmacotherapy. The first member of this class, sumatriptan, and the second-generation agents zolmitriptan, naratriptan, rizatriptan, almotriptan, frovatriptan, and eletriptan are selective agonists of the 5-HT_{1B} and 5-HT_{1D} receptors. Relief of migraine headache is the result of three key actions: normalization of dilated intracranial arteries through enhanced vasoconstriction, inhibition of vasoactive peptide release from perivascular trigeminal neurons, and inhibition of transmission through second-order neurons ascending to the thalamus.[15,31] These agents also display varying affinity for 5-HT_{1A}, 5-HT_{1E}, and 5-HT_{1F} receptors. The triptans are appropriate first-line therapy for patients with mild to severe migraine and are used for rescue therapy when nonspecific medications are ineffective.[31]

Sumatriptan, the most extensively studied acute therapy, is available for subcutaneous, oral, and intranasal administration. Subcutaneous sumatriptan is consistently superior to placebo in alleviating migraine headache and associated symptoms, with relief reported in 70% of patients at 2 hours in a meta-analysis of placebo-controlled studies.[31] In addition to enhanced efficacy, subcutaneous sumatriptan has a more rapid onset of action when compared with the oral formulation. The subcutaneous injection is packaged as an autoinjector device for self-administration by patients. Intranasal

TABLE 61-7 Pharmacokinetic Characteristics of Triptans

Drug	Half-Life (hours)	Time to Maximal Concentration (t_{max})	Bioavailability (%)	Elimination
Almotriptan	3-4	1.4-3.8 hours	80	MAO-A, CYP3A4, CYP2D6
Eletriptan	4-5	1-2 hours	50	CYP3A4
Frovatriptan	25	2-4 hours	24-30	Mostly unchanged, CYP1A2
Naratriptan	5-6	2-3 hours	63-74	Largely unchanged, CYP450 (various isoenzymes)
Rizatriptan	2-3		45	MAO-A
Oral tablets		1-1.2 hours		
Disintegrating		1.6-2.5 hours		
Sumatriptan	2			MAO-A
SC injection		12-15 minutes	97	
Oral tablets		2.5 hours	14	
Nasal spray		1-2.5 hours	17	
Zolmitriptan	3		40-48	CYP1A2, MAO-A
Oral		2 hours		
Disintegrating		3.3 hours		
Nasal		4 hours		

CYP, cytochrome P450; MAO-A, monoamine oxidase type A.
Data from references 15, 23, and 31.

sumatriptan provides a faster onset of effect than the oral formulation and produces similar rates of response in placebo-controlled studies.[19,31]

Selection of a triptan is based on characteristics of the headache, convenience of dosing, and the patient's preference. At all marketed doses, the oral triptans are effective and well tolerated. The triptans differ in their pharmacokinetic and pharmacodynamic profiles (Table 61-7). In general, triptans can be divided into those with a faster onset and higher efficacy and those with a slower onset and lower efficacy. A recent meta-analysis summarizes the efficacy and tolerability of the oral triptans across published and unpublished studies. Using 100 mg of sumatriptan as the reference dose and based on 2-hour response rates, at doses recommended by the manufacturer, most of the triptans evaluated had similar therapeutic gains; frovatriptan and naratriptan were the exceptions with lower efficacy. Compared with other triptans, frovatriptan and naratriptan have the longest half-lives, the slowest onset of action, and less headache recurrence. This may make them more suitable for patients who have migraine attacks of a slow onset and longer duration. Faster-acting triptans are more efficacious when a rapid onset is necessary. Subcutaneous, intranasal, or orally dissolving tablets may be useful in patients with prominent early nausea or vomiting or those who have difficulty in swallowing tablets. Despite the fact that oral absorption can be delayed during migraine attacks, most patients prefer oral formulations.[15,23,29,31]

Clinical response to the triptans can vary considerably among individual patients. Individual responses cannot be predicted, and if one triptan fails, a patient can be switched successfully to another triptan.[15] 8 After an effective agent and dose have been identified, subsequent treatments should begin with that same regimen. Combination therapy may also improve response rates and diminish migraine recurrence. A proprietary formulation of sumatriptan 85 mg plus naproxen 500 mg in a single tablet was more effective in clinical trials for headache relief and sustained pain-free response than either agent as monotherapy.[15,19]

Side effects to the triptans are common but usually mild to moderate in nature and of short duration. Adverse effects are consistent among the class and include paresthesias, fatigue, dizziness, flushing, warm sensations, and somnolence. Local side effects are reported with the subcutaneous (minor injection site reactions) and intranasal (taste perversion, nasal discomfort) routes. Up to 25% of patients receiving a triptan consistently report "triptan sensations," including tightness, pressure, heaviness, or pain in the chest, neck, or throat. The mechanism of these symptoms is unknown, but a cardiac source of pain seems unlikely in most patients.[31] However, all triptans are partial agonists of human 5-HT coronary artery receptors in vitro, resulting in a small but significant vasoconstrictor response. Adverse cardiac events are rare with only isolated cases of myocardial infarction and coronary vasospasm with ischemia reported. The triptans are contraindicated in patients with a history of ischemic heart disease (eg, angina pectoris, Prinzmetal's angina, or previous myocardial infarction), uncontrolled hypertension, and cerebrovascular disease. Patients at risk for unrecognized coronary artery disease should use triptans with caution. Postmenopausal women, men older than 40 years of age, and patients with uncontrolled risk factors should receive a cardiovascular assessment prior to triptan use and have initial doses administered under medical supervision. Triptans are also contraindicated in patients with hemiplegic and basilar migraine and should not be used routinely in pregnancy.[19,31] The triptans should not be given within 24 hours of the ergotamine derivatives. Administration of sumatriptan, rizatriptan, and zolmitriptan within 2 weeks of therapy with monoamine oxidase inhibitors (MAOIs) is not recommended. Eletriptan should not be administered with cytochrome P450 3A4 inhibitors such as macrolide antibiotics, antifungals, and some antiviral therapies. Concomitant therapy with the selective serotonin reuptake inhibitors (SSRIs) or serotonin-norepinephrine reuptake inhibitors (SNRIs) (eg, duloxetine, venlafaxine, and mirtazapine) can potentially cause 5-HT syndrome. Regulatory agencies caution against concurrent administration, although it appears the likelihood of CNS adverse events is extremely low. The potential risk of these combinations should be carefully considered and discussed with the patient.[15,19,32] Frequent use of the triptans has been associated with the development of medication-overuse headache.[18,31]

Prophylactic Pharmacolgic Therapy

β-Adrenergic Antagonists

β-Adrenergic antagonists are among the most widely used drugs for migraine prophylaxis. Metoprolol, propranolol, and timolol have established efficacy in controlled clinical trials, reducing the frequency of attacks by 50% in greater than 50% of patients.[24,26] Atenolol and nadolol are also probably effective, while nebivolol and pindolol are possibly effective (see Table 61-5).[24] Because the relative efficacy of the individual agents has not been established, selection of a β-blocker can be based on β-selectivity, convenience of the formulation, and tolerability. Although their precise mechanism of antimigraine action is unknown, β-blockers may raise the migraine threshold by modulating adrenergic or serotonergic neurotransmission in cortical or subcortical pathways. Although not first-line treatment for hypertension, β-blockers may be useful along with other therapy in patients with comorbid hypertension or angina. Side effects can include drowsiness, fatigue, sleep disturbances, vivid dreams, memory disturbance, depression, impotence, bradycardia, and hypotension. β-Blockers should be used with caution in patients with congestive heart failure, peripheral vascular disease, atrioventricular conduction disturbances, asthma, depression, and diabetes.[24,26]

Clinical **Controversy …**

To determine maximal clinical benefits, a therapeutic trial of 6 months is recommended when initiating treatment for episodic migraine prevention. Despite this recommendation, most migraine prevention studies have relatively brief treatment durations of only 12 to 16 weeks. Long-term scientifically sound assessments and evaluations of migraine preventive treatments are needed to further define their role in clinical care.[24]

Antidepressants

The beneficial effects of antidepressants in migraine are independent of their antidepressant activity and may be related to downregulation of central 5-HT_2 receptors, increased levels of synaptic norepinephrine, and enhanced endogenous opioid receptor actions.[33] The tricyclic antidepressant (TCA) amitriptyline and SNRI venlafaxine have demonstrated efficacy in placebo-controlled and comparative studies and are classified as probably effective for migraine prophylaxis (see Table 61-5).[24,26] Use of other antidepressants is based primarily on clinical and anecdotal experience. There are insufficient or conflicting data to support or refute the efficacy of other antidepressants, such as protriptyline, fluoxetine, or fluvoxamine, for migraine prophylaxis.[24]

Anticholinergic side effects are common with TCAs and limit use of these agents in patients with benign prostatic hyperplasia and glaucoma. Evening doses are preferred because of associated sedation. Increased appetite and weight gain can occur. Orthostatic hypotension and cardiac toxicity (slowed atrioventricular conduction) also are reported occasionally.[24,26] The most common side effects reported with venlafaxine are nausea, vomiting, and drowsiness. Again, the potential risk of 5-HT syndrome should be considered in patients using SSRIs or SNRIs along with a triptan.[24,32]

Anticonvulsants

Anticonvulsant medications have emerged as important therapeutic options for migraine prophylaxis with valproate, divalproex, and topiramate all having established efficacy.[24] The beneficial effects of these agents are likely caused by multiple mechanisms of action, including enhancement of γ-aminobutyric acid (GABA)-mediated inhibition, modulation of the excitatory neurotransmitter glutamate, and inhibition of sodium and calcium ion channel activity.[33] Anticonvulsants are particularly useful in migraineurs with comorbid seizures, anxiety disorder, or bipolar illness.[24,26] The efficacy of sodium valproate and divalproex sodium (a 1:1 molar combination of valproate sodium and valproic acid) has been demonstrated in multiple placebo-controlled studies. In most trials for headache prophylaxis, there were no significant differences in treatment-emergent side effects between these agents and placebo. Nausea and vomiting, the most common early side effects, are self-limited and appear to be less common with divalproex sodium and gradual titration of doses. Alopecia, tremor, asthenia, somnolence, and weight gain are also complaints.[24,26] The extended-release formulation of divalproex sodium is administered once daily and is better tolerated than the enteric-coated formulation. Hepatotoxicity is the most serious side effect of valproate therapy, but the risk appears to be low in migraineurs (eg, patients older than 10 years of age who are receiving monotherapy and have no underlying metabolic or neurologic disorder). Baseline liver function tests should be obtained, but routine followup studies are not necessary in asymptomatic adults on monotherapy. Regular followup is necessary, however, for dosage adjustments and monitoring of effects. Valproate is contraindicated in pregnant women (owing to potential teratogenicity) and patients with a history of pancreatitis or chronic liver disease.[24,26]

Topiramate is the most extensively studied medication to date for migraine prophylaxis. Efficacy and improvements in health-related quality of life including daily work, home, and social activities have been demonstrated in several placebo-controlled studies.[17] To minimize adverse effects, topiramate should be initiated at a low dose and slowly titrated upward. The benefits of topiramate are observed as early as 2 weeks after initiation of therapy, with significant reductions in migraine frequency within the first month. Approximately 50% of patients treated to target doses are responders (50% or greater reduction in mean headache frequency). Treatment-emergent adverse events associated with topiramate include paresthesia, fatigue, anorexia, diarrhea, weight loss, hypesthesia, difficulty with memory, language problems, taste perversion, and nausea. Paresthesia is the most common adverse event, occurring in about half of patients at target doses. Weight loss, occurring in 9% to 12% of patients, is a unique adverse effect, as weight gain is a common reason to discontinue other preventive medications. Topiramate should be used with caution or avoided in patients with a history of kidney stones or cognitive impairment.[24,26]

Preliminary studies suggest a role for other anticonvulsants for migraine prevention. Carbamazepine is possibly effective, and a recent study evaluated gabapentin, but data are insufficient to determine efficacy. Lamotrigine is classified as possibly or probably ineffective.[24]

Nonsteroidal antiinflammatory drugs

Nonsteroidal antiinflammatory drugs are modestly effective for reducing the frequency, severity, and duration of migraine attacks, but potential GI and renal toxicity limit the daily or prolonged use of these agents. Consequently, NSAIDs have been used intermittently to prevent headaches that recur in a predictable pattern, such as menstrual migraine. Administration of NSAIDs in the perimenstrual period can be beneficial in women with true menstrual migraine. NSAIDs should be initiated up to 1 week prior to the expected onset of headache and continued for no more than 10 days.[26,34] If long-term NSAID therapy is initiated, monitoring of renal function and occult blood loss is necessary. For migraine prevention, the evidence for efficacy is strongest for naproxen and weakest for aspirin.[24,26]

Triptans

Triptans are also useful for the prevention of menstrual migraine. Frovatriptan has established efficacy, while naratriptan and zolmitriptan are probably effective. The triptan is usually started 1 or

2 days before the expected onset of headache and continued during the period of vulnerability.[24,26] A separate indication for pure menstrual migraine is currently being deliberated by regulatory authorities.[24]

Miscellaneous Prophylatic Agents

At least two placebo-controlled studies show that petasites, an extract from the butterbur plant *Petasites hybridus*, is an effective preventive treatment for migraine.[26,35] A double-blind, placebo-controlled study demonstrated the probable efficacy of riboflavin (vitamin B_2) 400 mg daily in migraine prophylaxis. Riboflavin was well tolerated and associated with 50% or greater improvement in attack frequency in 54% of patients. However, the benefits of therapy became significant only after 3 months.[26,35] The relatively stable extract of feverfew (*Tanacetum parthenium*), MIG-99, is the most studied herbal preparation for migraine prevention. MIG-99 is classified as probably effective, reducing migraine frequency by 1.9 attacks per month.[35] Clinical trials evaluating various formulations of magnesium for migraine prevention have yielded mixed results, but there is probable efficacy.[26,35] CNS levels of magnesium are known to be significantly low during migraine attacks. Magnesium supplementation may be particularly effective for prevention of menstrual migraine.[34] Subcutaneous histamine has been compared with placebo, sodium valproate, and topiramate, with favorable results indicating probable efficacy in improving headache frequency, duration, and intensity. Transient burning and itching at the injection site were the only reported side effects with histamine administration.[35]

Other agents are possibly effective and may be considered for migraine prevention.[24,35] The angiotensin-converting enzyme inhibitor lisinopril and the angiotensin II receptor blocker candesartan provided effective migraine prophylaxis in recent double-blind, placebo-controlled, crossover studies of these agents.[24,26] Although use is limited by side effects, clonidine and guanfacine have also demonstrated possible efficacy.[24] Coenzyme Q10 was effective for migraine prevention and well tolerated in a small, randomized, double-blind, controlled study.[26,35] In one study, cyproheptadine (4 mg/day) was as effective as propranolol (80 mg/day) in reducing migraine frequency, duration, and severity, while the combination was more effective in attack frequency reduction.[24,35]

The calcium channel blockers, primarily verapamil, have been widely used for preventive treatment, although evidence supporting their use is inadequate or conflicting.[24,26] Extensive clinical experience and the ease of use of verapamil suggest a possible role in migraine prevention. Side effects of verapamil can include constipation, hypotension, bradycardia, atrioventricular block, and exacerbation of congestive heart failure.[24]

Localized injections of botulinum toxin type A have been used for various conditions and pain syndromes, including migraine headache. However, no consistent, statistically significant benefits have been found with migraine. The American Academy of Neurology concludes that botulinum toxin is probably ineffective.[26] Further study is needed to confirm the clinical utility and comparative efficacy for many of these miscellaneous agents in the prevention of migraine.

Personalized Pharmacotherapy

Although migraine is widely recognized as a disease that exacts an enormous toll on the sufferer, healthcare providers often do not recognize the degree and scope of functional impairment imposed by migraine on the individual.[17] Approximately 1 out of every 6 healthcare visits for migraine occurs in the emergency department, though management in this setting is often suboptimal. The use of opioids for the acute treatment of migraine in the emergency department is increasing, and the likelihood of unnecessary radiation exposure is greater.[5] Although most episodic migraine sufferers take medications for their headaches, only 2 in 3 patients who have been diagnosed and consulted with a healthcare provider use migraine-specific treatments. Just 11% of those eligible for use of medications to prevent migraine currently use them, although approximately 38% would benefit from prophylaxis.[14] Because many migraineurs who receive inadequate care experience substantial levels of pain and disability, improvement in migraine diagnosis, care, and treatment potentially could result in lower direct and indirect costs of the disease.

Effective communication and education of headache patients regarding required behavior changes and appropriate use of acute and prophylactic pharmacotherapy is essential. Healthcare professionals should inquire about and address coexisting conditions that may contribute to headache presentation or successful acute and preventive management. Decisions for treatment should be individualized, with consideration of frequency and severity of headache episodes, level of disability, trigger factors, coexisting conditions, tolerability of the available agents, and the patient's lifestyle and preferences.[17,24]

Medications with the highest level of efficacy should be used for treatment. Migraine management should be individualized on the basis of the patient's clinical presentation and medical history. Therapy should usually be initiated with the lowest effective dose and then titrated upward until clinical benefits are achieved, in the absence of adverse events. Medications that increase headache frequency or severity should be avoided. Many patients try nonpharmacologic or nonprescription treatments for headache management either before or concurrently with other drug therapy. Patients may not know how to take these products optimally and often need instructions and dosing limits.

Analgesics and NSAIDs can be considered the drugs of choice if effective for infrequent mild to moderately severe attacks. The triptans or dihydroergotamine can be used if initial therapies prove ineffective or as first-line therapy in moderate to severe migraine headache. Abortive therapy should be instituted early in the course of the attack to optimize efficacy and minimize migraine-related pain and disability. Preventive therapy should be considered in the setting of recurring migraines that produce significant disability; frequent attacks requiring symptomatic medication more than twice per week; symptomatic therapies that are ineffective or contraindicated, or produce serious side effects; and uncommon migraine variants that cause risk of neurologic injury. Efficacy of any prescribed prophylactic regimen should be reassessed periodically. Therapeutic interventions require an adequate trial to achieve clinical benefit and often as long as 6 months for assessment of maximal benefit. A prolonged headache-free interval could allow for gradual dosage reduction and discontinuation of therapy.

A formal management plan and maintaining a headache diary are necessary for the patient and provider to evaluate therapy, headache impact, and medication consumption. Oversights can lead to decreased efficacy of medications resulting in repeat dosing and polypharmacy, decreased compliance, increased emergency visits, increased "doctor shopping," and, perhaps, increased use of expensive diagnostic procedures and inpatient services. Patients with stratified care targeted to their needs have higher headache response rates, shorter disability times, less health service utilization, and less loss of productivity.[19,26,35]

TENSION-TYPE HEADACHE

Epidemiology

Tension-type headache is the most common type of primary headache, with an estimated 1-year prevalence ranging from 38% to 86%.[3,36] Prevalence peaks in the fourth decade and is higher among women. The incidence decreases with age.[36] Although most tension-type headache sufferers experience some degree of functional impairment during their attacks, few sufferers seek medical attention, likely because they have infrequent attacks. Infrequent episodic tension-type headache (defined as fewer than one episode per month) is experienced by 64% of sufferers, while 22% have frequent episodic tension-type headache (episodes on 1-14 days/mo). The prevalence of chronic tension-type headache (15 or more days/mo, perhaps without recognizable episodes) is estimated at 0.9% to 2.2%.[2,36] Risk factors associated with a poor outcome in tension-type headache include coexisting migraine, sleep problems, anxiety, poor stress management, and the presence of chronic tension-type headache.[36]

Pathophysiology

Although tension-type headache is the most common type of headache, it is the least studied of the primary headache disorders, and there is limited understanding of key pathophysiologic concepts.[2,36] Some evidence supports that migraine and tension-type headaches represent a continuum of headache severity with similarities in mechanisms and pathophysiology. However, more recently, tension-type headache has been recognized as a distinct disorder.[2] The mechanism of pain in chronic tension-type headache is thought to originate from myofascial factors and peripheral sensitization of nociceptors. Central mechanisms also are involved, with heightened sensitivity of pain pathways in the CNS.[36] Mental stress, nonphysiologic motor stress, a local myofascial release of irritants, or a combination of these may be the initiating stimulus. Following activation of supraspinal pain perception structures, a self-limiting headache results in most individuals owing to central modulation of the incoming peripheral stimuli. Chronic tension-type headache can evolve from episodic tension-type headache in predisposed individuals due to a change in central circuits and nociceptive processing along the brain stem reflex pathway and subsequent sensitization of the CNS.[36] It is likely that other pathophysiologic mechanisms also contribute to the development of tension-type headache.

Clinical Presentation

Premonitory symptoms and aura are absent with tension-type headache. The pain usually is mild to moderate in intensity and often is described as a dull, nonpulsatile tightness or pressure.[2,36] Bilateral pain is most common, classically described as having a "hatband" pattern. Associated symptoms generally are absent, but mild photophobia or phonophobia may be reported. The disability associated with tension-type headache typically is minor in comparison with migraine headache, and routine physical activity does not affect headache severity.[2,36] Palpation of the pericranial or cervical muscles can reveal tender spots or localized nodules in some patients.[2] Tension-type headache is classified as either episodic (infrequent or frequent) or chronic based on the frequency and duration of the attacks.[2]

TREATMENT
Tension-Type Headaches

General Approach To Treatment

The vast majority of episodic tension-type headache sufferers self-medicate with nonprescription medications and do not consult a healthcare professional. Although pharmacologic and nonpharmacologic treatments are available, simple analgesics and NSAIDs are the mainstay of acute therapy. Most agents used for tension-type headache have not been studied in controlled clinical trials.[37,38]

Nonpharmacologic Therapy

Psychophysiologic therapy and physical therapy have been used in the management of tension-type headache. Behavioral treatments can consist of cognitive-behavioral therapy (ie, stress management), relaxation training, and biofeedback.[37] These therapies (alone or in combination with pharmacotherapy) can result in a 33% to 64% reduction in headache activity. Relaxation training combined with biofeedback is more effective than other behavioral therapy options.[39] Evidence supporting physical therapeutic options, such as heat or cold packs, ultrasound, electrical nerve stimulation, stretching, exercise, massage, acupuncture, manipulations, ergonomic instruction, and trigger point injections or occipital nerve blocks, is somewhat inconsistent. However, individual patients may benefit from selected modalities in reducing the frequency of tension-type headache or during an acute episode.[38,39]

Pharmacologic Therapy

Simple analgesics (alone or in combination with caffeine) and NSAIDs are effective for the acute treatment of most mild to moderate tension-type headaches. Acetaminophen, aspirin, diclofenac, ibuprofen, naproxen, ketoprofen, and ketorolac have demonstrated efficacy in placebo-controlled and comparative studies.[38] Failure of nonprescription agents can warrant therapy with prescription drugs. The combination of aspirin or acetaminophen with butalbital or, rarely, codeine can be effective options in selected patients; however, use of butalbital and codeine combinations should be avoided when possible owing to the high potential for overuse and dependency. Acute medications should be taken for episodic tension-type headache not more than 3 days (butalbital-containing), 9 days (combination analgesics), or 15 days (NSAIDs) per month to prevent the development of medication-overuse or chronic tension-type headache.[38] There is no evidence to support the efficacy of muscle relaxants in the management of episodic tension-type headache.[38] Preventive treatment is appropriate for most patients with chronic tension-type headache and should be considered in those with frequent episodic tension-type headache if frequency (more than 2 per week), duration (greater than 3-4 hours), or severity results in medication overuse or substantial disability.[39] The principles of preventive treatment for tension-type headache are similar to those for migraine headache. TCAs are prescribed most often for prophylaxis, but other drugs also can be selected after consideration of comorbid medical conditions and respective side effect profiles. SSRIs are not effective in patients with tension-type headache who do not have depression. Limited studies support the use of the SNRIs mirtazapine and venlafaxine in patients with chronic tension-type headache and without depression.[37,39] Topiramate, gabapentin, and tizanidine may have benefits in chronic tension-type headache; however, confirmation is needed from randomized clinical trials. Data from small randomized studies suggest that trigger point injections of lidocaine may reduce headache frequency with frequent episodic or chronic tension-type headache. Injection of botulinum toxin into pericranial muscles has demonstrated inconsistent efficacy in the prophylaxis of tension-type headache and because of this, it is of uncertain benefit.[39]

CLUSTER HEADACHE

Epidemiology

Cluster headache, the most severe of the primary headache disorders, is characterized by attacks of excruciating, unilateral head pain that occur in series lasting for weeks or months (ie, cluster periods) separated by remission periods usually lasting months or years.[2,40] Cluster headaches can be episodic or chronic.[2] Cluster headache is relatively uncommon among the primary headache disorders, but the exact prevalence is uncertain. Estimates from pooled population studies show a lifetime prevalence of 124 per 100,000 or 0.12%.[40,41] The male-to-female ratio for cluster headache is approximately 4:1 with age of onset typically in the third to fifth decade. Greater than 65% of patients with cluster headache are tobacco smokers or have a history of smoking. Tobacco cessation does not, however, seem to improve the course of cluster headaches. Recent genetic epidemiologic surveys support a predisposition for cluster headache can exist in certain families.[40,41]

Pathophysiology

The etiologic and pathophysiologic mechanisms of cluster headache are not completely understood. Neuroimaging studies performed during acute attacks have demonstrated activation of the ipsilateral hypothalamic gray area, implicating the hypothalamus as a modulator of cluster headaches. The hypothalamus secondarily activates trigeminal-autonomic reflexes, leading to the ipsilateral pain and cranial autonomic features characteristic of cluster headache.[40,41] The cyclic and circadian rhythmicity of attacks also implicates a pathogenesis of hypothalamic dysfunction.[41] There is some evidence that cluster headache may result from inflammation of the nerves traversing the cavernous sinus resulting in injury to sympathetic fibers of the internal carotid artery.[41]

Clinical Presentation

One hallmark of cluster headaches is the circadian rhythm of painful attacks. Episodic cluster headaches are the most common cluster headache subtype in both men and women, occurring in up to 90% of patients.[41] In episodic cluster headaches, attacks occur daily for a week to several months, followed by long pain-free intervals.[40,41] Periods of remission average 2 years in length but have been reported to be from 2 months to 20 years in duration. Approximately 10% of patients have chronic symptoms with attacks recurring for over 1 year without remission or with remission periods of less than 1 month.[40,41]

Cluster headache attacks occur commonly at night and more commonly in the spring and fall. Attacks occur suddenly, with pain peaking quickly after onset and generally lasting 15 to 180 minutes.[40] The pain is excruciating, penetrating, and of a boring intensity in orbital, supraorbital, and temporal unilateral locations.[40,41] The headache is accompanied by cranial autonomic symptoms such as conjunctival injection, lacrimation, nasal stuffiness, rhinorrhea, eyelid edema, facial sweating, and miosis/ptosis, which resolve with resolution of the headache. Most sufferers of cluster headaches also describe restlessness or agitation. Whereas migraine patients retreat to a quiet, dark room, cluster headache patients generally sit and rock or pace about the room clutching their head.[40,41] Auras are not present with cluster headaches. During the cluster period, attacks occur from once every other day to eight times per day.[40,41] Specific diagnostic criteria for cluster headaches are provided within the IHS classification system.[2]

TREATMENT
Cluster Headaches

As in migraine, therapy for cluster headaches involves both abortive and prophylactic therapy. Abortive therapy is directed at managing the acute attack. Prophylactic therapies are started early in the cluster period in an attempt to induce remission. Patients with chronic cluster headache can require prophylactic medications indefinitely.

Abortive Therapy

Oxygen

The standard acute treatment of cluster headache is inhalation of 100% oxygen by nonbreather facial mask at a rate of at least 12 L/min for 15 minutes.[42-44] Repeat or frequent administration over a short period of time should be avoided, as overuse may increase the frequency or merely delay rather than abort the attack in some patients.[42,43] No side effects have been reported with the use of oxygen, but caution should be used for those who smoke or have chronic obstructive pulmonary disease.

Triptans

The quick onset of subcutaneous and intranasal triptans makes them safe and effective abortive agents for cluster headaches. Subcutaneous sumatriptan (6 mg) is the most effective agent. Nasal sprays are less effective but may be better tolerated in some patients. Adverse events reported in cluster headache patients are similar to those seen in migraineurs. Orally administered triptans have limited use in cluster attacks because of their relatively slow onset of action; oral zolmitriptan (10 mg), however, was beneficial in patients with episodic cluster headache, with 60% experiencing mild or no pain at 30 minutes.[42,44]

Ergotamine Derivatives

All forms of ergotamine have been used in cluster headaches, although no controlled clinical trials support their use.[42,44] In clinical use, IV dihydroergotamine may be given as a bolus followed by repeated administration over several days to break the cycle of frequent attacks.[42] Ergotamine tartrate also has provided effective relief of cluster headache attacks when administered sublingually or rectally.[42] Dosing guidelines are similar to those for migraine headache therapy.

Prophylactic Therapy

Verapamil

The preferred first-line treatment for prevention of cluster headaches is verapamil, a calcium channel blocker with antianginal and antiarrhythmic properties.[43,44] The beneficial effects of verapamil often appear within 2 to 3 weeks of therapy. A typical suggested dosage range is from 360 to 960 mg/day, starting with a dose of 240 mg/day. Rarely, patients with refractory cluster headaches are treated with doses as high as 1,200 mg/day. In such patients, an electrocardiogram should be obtained as the dose is increased, due to concerns for bradycardia or heart block.[42,44]

Lithium

Lithium carbonate is effective for episodic and chronic cluster headache attacks and can be used as an alternative to or in combination with verapamil.[44] A positive response is seen in up to 78% of patients with chronic cluster headache, and in up to 63% of patients with episodic cluster headache.[42] The usual dose is 600 to 1,200 mg/day, with a suggested starting dose of 300 mg twice daily.[44] Optimal plasma lithium levels for prevention of cluster headache have not been established, but levels should be monitored and maintained between 0.6 and 1.2 mEq/L (0.6 and 1.2 mmol/L).[42]

Initial side effects are mild and include tremor, lethargy, nausea, diarrhea, and abdominal discomfort. Thyroid and renal function must be monitored during lithium therapy. Lithium should be administered with caution to patients with significant renal or cardiovascular disease, dehydration, pregnancy, or concomitant diuretic or NSAID use.[42,44]

Corticosteroids

Although there are few clinical trials evaluating the use of corticosteroids in cluster headache management, they have been used effectively for inducing remission.[42] Therapy is initiated with at least 5 days of 60 to 100 mg/day prednisone and then tapered by a dose reduction of approximately 10 mg/day. To avoid steroid-induced complications, long-term use is generally not recommended. Headaches can recur when therapy is tapered or discontinued.[42,44]

Miscellaneous Agents

Other therapies that have been used in the acute management of cluster headache include intranasal lidocaine and subcutaneous octreotide. Limited studies or case reports also support the use of divalproex sodium, topiramate, indomethacin, and intranasal capsaicin.[42-44]

Neurosurgical interventions to relieve chronic cluster headaches in patients refractory to pharmacologic therapy should be considered for some with debilitating headaches.[40,44] Neurostimulation has gained attention in the last several years.[42,45] Deep brain stimulation of the posterior hypothalamus and occipital nerve stimulation studies have shown positive results in small clinical trials.[42,45]

EVALUATION OF THERAPEUTIC OUTCOMES

Patients should be monitored for frequency, intensity, and duration of headaches, as well as any change in the headache pattern. To this end, patients should be encouraged to keep a headache diary to document the frequency, severity, and duration of attacks, as well as response to medication and potential trigger factors. Careful monitoring is essential to initiate the most appropriate pharmacotherapy, document therapeutic successes and failures, identify medication contraindications, and prevent or minimize adverse events. Patients using acute therapies should be monitored for frequency of use of prescription and nonprescription medications to identify potential medication-overuse headache. Patient counseling is necessary to allow for proper medication use (eg, self-injection with sumatriptan), to encourage early use of medications in the headache cycle, and to enhance patient compliance. Strict adherence to dosing guidelines should be stressed to minimize potential toxicity. Patterns of abortive medication use can be documented to establish the need for prophylactic therapy. Prophylactic therapies also should be monitored closely (every 3-6 months until stable) for adverse reactions, abortive therapy needs, adequate dosing, and compliance. Consultation with other healthcare practitioners should be encouraged when changes in headache patterns or medication use occur.

ABBREVIATIONS

CGRP	calcitonin gene-related peptide
CNS	central nervous system
FDA	Food and Drug Administration
GABA	γ-aminobutyric acid
GI	gastrointestinal
5-HT	serotonin, 5-hydroxytryptamine
IHS	International Headache Society
MAOI	monoamine oxidase inhibitor
NSAIDs	nonsteroidal antiinflammatory drugs
SNRI	serotonin-norepinephrine reuptake inhibitor
SSRI	selective serotonin reuptake inhibitor
TCA	tricyclic antidepressant

REFERENCES

1. Weiss AJ, Wier LM, Stocks C, Blanchard J. Overview of emergency department visits in the United States, 2011. Statistical Brief #174. June 2014. Agency for Health Care Policy and Research, Rockville, MD. Available at: http://www.hcup-us.ahrq.gov/reports/statbriefs/sb174-Emergency-Department-Visits-Overview.pdf. (Accessed August 9, 2015)
2. Headache Classification Committee of the International Headache Society. The international classification of headache disorders, 3rd ed. *Cephalalgia* 2013;33(9):629-808.
3. Bajwa ZH, Wootton RJ. Evaluation of headache in adults. *UpToDate* 2015;3:1-21, Available at: www.uptodate.com. Accessed August 9, 2015.
4. Smitherman TA, Burch RC, Sheikh H, Loder E. The prevalence, impact, and treatment of migraine and severe headaches in the United States: A review of statistics from national surveillance studies. *Headache* 2013;53:427-436.
5. Burch RC, Loder S, Loder E, Smitherman TA. The prevalence and burden of migraine and severe headache in the United States: Updated statistics from government health surveillance studies. *Headache* 2015;55:21-34.
6. Bigal ME, Ferrari M, Silberstein SD, et al. Migraine in the triptan era: Lessons from epidemiology, pathophysiology, and clinical science. *Headache* 2009;49:S21-S33.
7. Bigal ME, Kurth T, Hu H, et al. Migraine and cardiovascular disease. *Neurology* 2009;72:1864-1871.
8. Stokes M, Becker WJ, Lipton RB, et al. Cost of health care among patients with chronic and episodic migraine in Canada and the USA: Results from the International Burden of Migraine Study (IBMS). *Headache* 2011;51:1058-1077.
9. Steiner TJ, Birbeck GL, Jensen RH, et al. Headache disorders are third cause of disability worldwide. *J Headache Pain* 2015;16:58.
10. Sprenger T, Goadsby PJ. Migraine pathogenesis and state of pharmacological treatment options. *BMC Med* 2009;7(71):1-5.
11. Ferrari MD. Migraine. *Lancet* 1998;351:1043-1051.
12. Akerman S, Holland PR, Goadsby PJ. Diencephalic and brainstem mechanisms in migraine. *Nature* 2011;12:570-584.
13. Silberstein SD, Dodick DW. Migraine genetics: Part II. *Headache* 2013;53:1218-1229.
14. Lipton RB, Silberstein SD. Episodic and chronic migraine headache: Breaking down barriers to optimal treatment and prevention. *Headache* 2015;S2:103-122.
15. Da Silva AN, Tepper SJ. Acute treatment of migraines. *CNS Drugs* 2012;10:823-839.
16. Cutrer FM, Bajwa ZH. Pathophysiology, clinical manifestations, and diagnosis of migraine in adults. *UpToDate* 2015;20:1-18. Available at: www.uptodate.com. Accessed August 9, 2015.
17. Buse DC, Rupnow FT, Lipton RB. Assessing and managing all aspects of migraine: Migraine attacks, migraine-related functional impairment, common comorbidities, and quality of life. *Mayo Clin Proc* 2009;84(5):422-435.
18. Matchar DB, Young WB, Rosenberg JA, et al. Evidence-based guidelines for migraine headache in the primary care setting: Pharmacological management of acute attacks. The U.S. Headache Consortium. 2000. Available at: www.aan.com/professionals/practice/guidelines. (Accessed August 9, 2015)
19. Bajwa ZH, Sabahat A. Acute treatment of migraine in adults. *UpToDate* 2015;37:1-19. Available at: www.uptodate.com. Accessed August 9, 2015.
20. Garza I, Schwedt TJ. Medication overuse headache: Etiology, clinical features, and diagnosis. *UpToDate* 2015;9:1-8. Available at: www.uptodate.com. Accessed August 9, 2015.
21. Garza I, Schwedt TJ. Medication overuse headache: Treatment and prognosis. *UpToDate* 2015;11:1-14. Available at: www.uptodate.com. Accessed August 9, 2015.
22. MacGregor EA. Migraine. *Ann Intern Med* 2013;159:ITC5-1.
23. Tepper SJ, Spears RC. Acute treatment of migraine. *Neurol Clin* 2009;27:417-427.
24. Silberstein SD, Holland S, Freitag F, et al. Evidence-based guideline update: Pharmacological treatment for episodic migraine prevention in adults: Report of the Quality Standards Subcommittee of the American Academy of Neurology and the American Headache Society. *Neurology* 2012;78:1337-1345.
25. Rizzoli P. Preventive pharmacotherapy in migraine. *Headache* 2014;54:364-369.
26. Bajwa ZH, Smith JH. Preventive treatment of migraine in adults. *UpToDate* 2015;25:1-16. Available at: www.uptodate.com. Accessed August 9, 2015.
27. Martin PR. Behavioral management of migraine headache triggers: Learning to cope with triggers. *Curr Pain Headache Rep* 2010;14:221-227.
28. Martin PR. Behavioral management of the triggers of recurrent headache: A randomized controlled trial. *Behav Res Ther* 2014;64:1-11.
29. Magis D, Schoenen J. Treatment of migraine: Update on new therapies. *Curr Opin Neurol* 2011;24:203-210.
30. Lampl C, Voelker M, Steiner TJ. Aspirin is first-line treatment for migraine and episodic tension-type headache regardless of headache intensity. *Headache* 2012;52:48-56.
31. Loder E. Triptan therapy in migraine. *N Engl J Med* 2010;363:63-70.
32. Center for Drug Evaluation and Research. FDA Public Health Advisory: Combined Use of 5-Hydroxytryptamine Receptor Agonists (Triptans), Selective Serotonin Reuptake Inhibitors (SSRIs) or Selective

Serotonin/Norepinephrine Reuptake Inhibitors (SNRIs) May Result in Life-Threatening Serotonin Syndrome. 2011. Available at: www.fda.gov/cder/drug/advisory. Accessed August 9, 2015.
33. Matthew NT. Dynamic optimization of chronic migraine treatment. *Neurology* 2009;72(Suppl 1):S14-S20.
34. Calhoun AH. Estrogen-associated migraine. *UpToDate* 2015;16:1-14. Available at: www.uptodate.com. Accessed August 9, 2015.
35. Holland S, Silberstein SD, Freitag F, et al. Evidence-based guideline update: NSAIDs and other complementary treatments for episodic migraine prevention in adults: Report of the Quality Standards Subcommittee of the American Academy of Neurology and the American Headache Society. *Neurology* 2012;78:1346-1353.
36. Taylor FR. Tension-type headache in adults: Pathophysiology, clinical features, and diagnosis. *UpToDate* 2015;3:1-15. Available at: www.uptodate.com. Accessed August 9, 2015.
37. Bendtsen L, Jensen R. Treating tension-type headache: An expert opinion. *Expert Opin Pharmacother* 2011;12(7):1099-1109.
38. Taylor FR. Tension-type headache in adults: Acute treatment. *UpToDate* 2015;9:1-9. Available at: www.uptodate.com. Accessed August 9, 2015.
39. Taylor FR. Tension-type headache in adults: Preventive treatment. *UpToDate* 2015;10:1-12. Available at: www.uptodate.com. Accessed August 9, 2015.
40. Nesbitt AD, Goadsy PJ. Cluster headache. *BMJ* 2012;344:e2407.
41. May A. Cluster headache: Epidemiology, clinical features, and diagnosis. *UpToDate* 2015;12:1-16. Available at: www.uptodate.com. Accessed August 9, 2015.
42. May A. Cluster headache: Treatment and prognosis. *UpToDate* 2015;20:1-14. Available at: www.uptodate.com. Accessed August 9, 2015.
43. Martelletti P. Cluster headache management and beyond. *Expert Opin Pharmacother* 2015;16(10)1411-1415.
44. Tfelt-Hansen PC, Jensen RH. Management of cluster headache. *CNS Drugs* 2012;26(7):571-580.
45. Wolter T, Kaube H. Neurostimulation for chronic cluster headache. *Ther Adv Neurol Disord* 2012;5(3):175-180.

Assessment of Psychiatric Disorders

e62

Mark E. Schneiderhan, Leigh Anne Nelson, and Steven Bauer

KEY CONCEPTS

1. Patients with psychiatric conditions are treated in all healthcare settings. All clinicians can apply the basic skills of the psychiatric assessment to provide the best care for their patients.
2. The *Diagnostic and Statistical Manual of Mental Disorders, Fifth Edition (DSM-5)* and the *Pocket Guide to the DSM-5 Diagnostic Exam* provides clinicians with a standardized approach for the initial assessment and follow up of patients with mental health conditions.
3. The World Health Organization's *International Classification of Diseases and Related Health Problems (ICD)* classification is currently used in both mental health and nonmental health settings for billing purposes.
4. Clinicians should be prepared to gather both the mental and physical health history from their patients. Obtaining a release of information (ROI) from patients to communicate with other healthcare providers or significant others is necessary when there are multiple providers.
5. Patient interviews should be conducted in an atmosphere that ensures the comfort, privacy, and safety of both the patient and the clinician. Effective listening skills and the application of open-ended questions are essential in the interview process and therapeutic relationship. Motivational interviewing (MI) can empower patients to participate and design achievable treatment goals.
6. If a patient is in crisis, the clinician may feel some apprehension about asking certain assessment questions. Knowing what specific questions to ask can help facilitate inquiry about sensitive areas, such as delusional thinking and suicidality.
7. A thorough current and past medication history, including allergies and side effects, is a cornerstone of effective medication management. The medication history should be assessed for safety (eg, contraindications and drug interactions), tolerability (eg, side effects), efficacy (eg, response of target symptoms and adequate dosage and duration), and adherence (eg, affordability).
8. Baseline mental status examination (MSE), psychiatric rating scales, and psychological/neuropsychological tests are useful tools in diagnosing and monitoring the severity of symptoms and response to treatments of psychiatric disorders.
9. Although there are no diagnostic tests for psychiatric disorders, physical and laboratory assessments can help the rule out drug-induced or medical causes that may produce similar or overlapping symptoms.
10. Psychiatric rating scales, cognitive testing (neuropsychiatric rating scales), and psychological testing provide objective measures of psychiatric symptoms, adverse side effects, memory, and intellectual capacity and are often used in research and clinical settings.

INTRODUCTION

1 Patients with mental health conditions often have comorbid physical illnesses, therefore, communication between multiple providers is necessary to prevent serious medical and/or medication-related consequences. Often care coordination between mental health and primary care services is required.[1] A good psychiatric assessment can identify the need for coordinated care and should be included as part of the full patient assessment in all healthcare settings. A psychiatric assessment should not be limited to the clinical setting. In many communities, basic mental health assessment education programs are being offered in efforts to reduce stigma and to help the public understand and even respond to signs of psychiatric illness and substance use disorders.[2] Along with traditional assessments used across all medical specialties (eg, laboratory tests, medical history, physical examination), mental health clinicians rely on communication skills and use validated assessments that are perhaps less objective in nature and less familiar to nonmental health practitioners. This chapter provides a basic overview of appropriate assessment techniques used by clinicians to develop individualized treatment plans for patients with psychiatric conditions. Readers needing greater depth than the materials provided in this chapter are referred to other sources.[3-10]

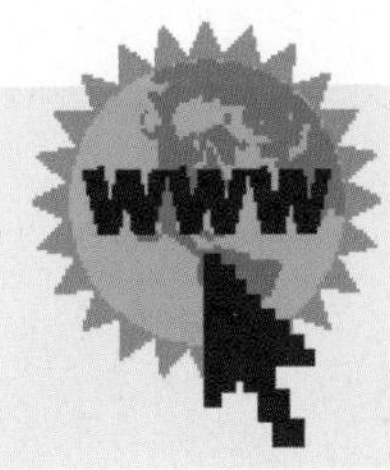

The complete chapter, learning objectives, and other resources can be found at **www.pharmacotherapyonline.com.**

Attention Deficit/Hyperactivity Disorder

63

Julie A. Dopheide and Steven R. Pliszka

KEY CONCEPTS

1. Untreated or ineffectively treated childhood attention deficit/hyperactivity disorder (ADHD) can lead to poor school performance, poor socialization, and increased risk for traffic accidents, psychiatric comorbidities, unemployment, and incarceration during adolescence and adulthood.
2. ADHD is 40% to 90% genetic in origin, and it is associated with decreased brain volume, a delay in cortical thickening, and dysregulation of the "default mode network," a brain system that regulates attention, prioritization of information, memory, and impulse control.
3. Symptoms of inattention or hyperactivity and impulsivity or all three must be present during childhood and cause functional impairment in two different settings for 6 months to meet diagnostic criteria for ADHD.
4. Prior to initiating pharmacotherapy, overall physical and mental health and psychiatric comorbidities must be assessed, and goals of treatment must be set.
5. Preschoolers, school-age children, adolescents, and adults with ADHD all can benefit from nonpharmacologic interventions that include a healthy diet, education on ADHD, and potentially effective cognitive and behavioral treatments.
6. The psychostimulants, methylphenidate, dexmethylphenidate, lisdexamfetamine or amphetamine salts, are the most effective pharmacologic treatment options for all ages with a rapid therapeutic effect, typically within 1 or 2 hours of an effective dose.
7. α_2-Adrenergic agonists such as extended-release preparations of guanfacine and clonidine are less effective than stimulants as monotherapy and are used as stimulants in youth to improve symptom control, particularly oppositional behaviors and insomnia.
8. When ADHD coexists with other neuropsychiatric conditions, such as anxiety disorders, major depression, autism spectrum disorder (ASD) or Tourette's disorder, it is optimal to treat the most functionally impairing disorder first (whether it is ADHD or the co-occurring condition) and then treat the second disorder.
9. When ADHD coexists with bipolar disorder, it is necessary to first stabilize the mood with lithium, an anticonvulsant, or an atypical antipsychotic before adding an ADHD-specific medication such as a psychostimulant.
10. Atomoxetine is a good option to manage ADHD symptoms in adolescents and adults with substance use disorders. It has a delayed onset of effect (2-4 weeks), but it has no abuse potential.

INTRODUCTION

Once considered primarily a childhood disorder, attention deficit/hyperactivity disorder (ADHD) is now known to persist into adolescence for 75% and into adulthood for approximately 50% of individuals.[1-3] The American Academy of Pediatrics (AAP) considers ADHD a chronic condition that requires ongoing management.[1,2] Functionally impairing inattention, impulsivity, and hyperactivity in the ADHD brain have been correlated with neuroanatomical and functional brain changes.[4,5] It is unusual for an individual to display signs of the disorder in all settings or even in the same setting at all times; however, there is a persistent pattern of symptoms that persists for 6 months or more.[4,6] Co-occurring anxiety, mood disorders, learning disabilities, medical conditions, and substance abuse must be considered in assessment and treatment. Behavioral interventions and medications are effective for all ages, but there are special considerations for treatment plan development and monitoring in each age group.[1-4,7]

The psychiatric assessment of a child requires obtaining information from the child, parents, caregivers, and teachers.[1,4,8] Treating children with psychotropic drugs requires a very different approach than treating adults. Children undergo neurologic, physiologic, and psychosocial changes throughout development. Age-related pharmacodynamic and pharmacokinetic differences can alter drug disposition and response. Psychotropic drug treatment of children is intended to control symptoms or behaviors that impair learning and development.[1,2,4,5] Children may not be able to articulate symptom response or adverse effects of a medication. (1) Adolescents and adults with ADHD may not have been diagnosed and treated during childhood, putting them at greater risk for the psychosocial consequences of ADHD including unemployment, unstable relationships, substance abuse, and incarceration.[1-4,9-11]

EPIDEMIOLOGY

ADHD is the most well-known and researched neurodevelopmental disorder of childhood. It is present in approximately 5% to 6% of children and approximately 2% to 3% of adults.[6,12] A 30-year epidemiological study showed that the actual prevalence of ADHD has not increased during the past 10 years, despite U.S. Centers for Disease Control (CDC) reports of increasing diagnosis.[12,13] When consistent diagnostic criteria from the *Diagnostic and Statistical Manual of Mental Disorders* (DSM-5) are applied, the prevalence of ADHD for children and adolescents is similar among countries globally, at approximately 5.5%.[12,13] ADHD is more prevalent in males than females with a ratio of 2:1 in children and 1.6:1 in adults.[6] In 2012, 5 million children in the United States or 10% of those aged 3 to 17 years were diagnosed with ADHD; almost twice the actual rate according to worldwide prevalence studies. Non-Hispanic Caucasian and black children were more likely diagnosed with ADHD compared with children of Hispanic or Asian descent.[13]

Increasing rates of ADHD diagnosis in the United States is likely a factor associated with the observed increased prescribing of ADHD medications. A Food and Drug Administration (FDA) study analyzed pediatric prescribing records from 59,000 retail pharmacies to compare prescribing rates in 2010 with those in 2002 in children aged 0 to 17 years for several therapeutic areas including antibiotics, proton-pump inhibitors, antidepressants, and ADHD medications. Overall pediatric prescribing decreased 7% over the 8 years studied, but prescriptions for ADHD medications increased by 46%. Methylphenidate was the most commonly prescribed drug in the ADHD category, but usage remained constant from 2002 to 2010, whereas usage of amphetamine products dropped by 15%.[14] Usage of dexmethylphenidate, lisdexamfetamine, and guanfacine increased from 2002 to 2010, while usage of atomoxetine in youth decreased.[14] The 2011 National survey of children's health queried parents and found that 11% of youth aged 4 to 17 years had ever been given the diagnosis of ADHD, and two-thirds were currently taking ADHD medication.[15]

A large U.S. pharmacy benefits management company, Express Script's, analysis of pharmacy claims representing 400,000 privately insured individuals younger than 65 years showed that ADHD medication use increased by 35.5% for all age groups between 2008 and 2012. The number of adults using ADHD medications was up 53.4% from 2008 to 2012. Children still received a higher percentage of ADHD prescriptions compared to adults; 80% of these were stimulants. Geography significantly impacted ADHD medication prescribing. In 2012, the number of U.S. citizens on ADHD medications was highest in the South at 3.6% and lowest in the West at 2.2%. South Carolina had the highest utilization with 5% of residents taking ADHD medications.[16] Health care professionals and teachers should recommend thorough assessment of ADHD by an experienced clinician using standardized criteria and investigating all possible causes of inattention, impulsivity, and hyperactivity in order to avoid overdiagnosis and potentially inappropriate treatment.

ETIOLOGY AND PATHOPHYSIOLOGY

(2) Both genetic and environmental factors are implicated in the pathogenesis of ADHD. Children with fetal alcohol syndrome, lead poisoning, and meningitis have a higher incidence of ADHD compared to nonaffected children.[4,17] Obstetric adversity, maternal smoking, and adverse parent–child relationships are factors known to increase the risk of ADHD.[4,17]

Genetic studies show ADHD runs in families, with heritability estimated to be between 40% and 90%.[18,19] ADHD is considered a polygenic disorder meaning risk is not transferred on just a few key genes but rather hundreds or even thousands of genetic variants are thought to be involved modulating risk for symptom expression. Patients may have copies or deletions in the genome that cover multiple genes called copy number variants (CNV). These CNV studies have implicated a number of systems in ADHD: cholinergic receptors, and genes for central nervous system (CNS) development,[19] on an area of chromosome 15q13,[20,21] as well as glutamate metabotropic receptors.[18,22] Thus, the pathophysiology of ADHD may go well beyond the catecholamine systems that have been the focus of most studies to date. There is a continuum of genetic risk for ADHD, as some individuals inherit just a few symptoms and are considered clinically "subthreshold" while others present with more severe symptomatology meeting full DSM-5 criteria for ADHD.[19]

Some of the same genes that code for ADHD are involved in the heritability of autism spectrum disorder (ASD) and Tourette's disorder supported by the clinical observation that 30% to 80% of youth with ASD meet criteria for ADHD and 50% to 60% of patients with Tourette's disorder have impairing ADHD symptoms.[23,24]

Structural and functional brain changes are part of the pathophysiology of ADHD. Smaller brain volumes and a delay in cortical thickening have been documented in children with ADHD and in those who still meet criteria for the symptoms of ADHD in adulthood.[25,26] This delay in cortical thickening is thought to contribute to the difficulty with prioritizing attention and tasks; while a lack of connectivity between the prefrontal cortex and precuneus (located in the midline of the parietal lobe) is associated with the failure of suppression of the default mode network, causing lapses in attention and poor impulse control.[18,25]

(2) Alterations in the "default mode" attention network have been found in adults with ADHD.[18] The default mode network consists of the medial prefrontal cortex, medial parietal lobe or precuneus, as well as the posterior cingulate. These areas are active during the "resting state" when attention is not engaged; this system is actively suppressed during active attention. A lack of connectivity between the prefrontal cortex and precuneus is associated with failure of suppression of the default mode network, causing lapses in attention and inhibitory control.[18] Therapeutic doses of stimulants that are recommended for the treatment of ADHD have been shown to normalize these structural and functional brain deficits, while improving symptoms of inattention and impulsivity.[5,25] By explaining the biological basis of ADHD as a brain disorder with genetic causes and some modifiable risk factors, clinicians can help families to better understand ADHD and minimize its negative impact on outcomes.

CLINICAL PRESENTATION ADHD

General

- Onset of symptoms must be before 12 years of age.

Symptoms

- Six or more of the symptoms must be present for 6 months; significant impairment must be seen in two or more settings (eg, home and school); symptoms must be documented by parent, teacher, and clinician. Only five symptoms are required in older adolescents and adults (age 17 and older).
- *Inattention:*
  - Often fails to give close attention to details or makes careless mistakes in schoolwork, at work, or during other activities (eg, overlooks or misses details, or work is inaccurate)
  - Often has difficulty sustaining attention in play activities or tasks (eg, has difficulty remaining focused during lectures, conversations, or lengthy reading)

(Continued)

CLINICAL PRESENTATION ADHD (*Continued*)

- Often has difficulty organizing tasks and activities (eg, poor time management, disorganized work, fails to meet deadlines)
- Avoids tasks that require sustained mental effort (eg, schoolwork, reviewing lengthy papers or preparing reports)
- Often does not seem to listen when spoken to directly (eg, mind seems to wander)
- Often does not follow through on instructions and fails to finish schoolwork, chores, or duties in the workplace
- Is easily distracted by extraneous stimuli (may include unrelated thoughts)
- Is often forgetful in daily activities (eg, doing chores, returning calls, paying bills)
- Loses things necessary for activities (eg, school materials, keys, wallet)

- *Hyperactivity and impulsivity:*
    - Often fidgets with hands or feet or squirms in seat
    - Often leaves seat when remaining seated is expected
    - Often runs about or climbs excessively at inappropriate times (in adolescents or adults may be limited to feeling restless)
    - Often has difficulty playing quietly
    - Often blurts out answers before a question is completed (also finishes the sentences of others; cannot wait for turn in conversation)
    - Often interrupts or intrudes on others; may take over what others are doing

Data from American Psychiatric Association. Disorders usually first evident in infancy, childhood or adolescence. In: Diagnostic and Statistical Manual of Mental Disorders, Fifth Edition. Arlington, VA, American Psychiatric Association, 2013:59-66.

CLINICAL PRESENTATION

The AAP guideline for the diagnosis, evaluation, and treatment of ADHD in children and adolescents recommends an evaluation for any child between ages 4 and 18 years who presents with academic or behavioral problems and symptoms of inattention, hyperactivity, or impulsivity.[AAP11] 3 At least six symptoms of inattention or hyperactivity and impulsivity causing impairment in more than one major setting (eg, home, school) for 6 months and an onset of symptoms before age 12 are currently required by the DSM-5 for a diagnosis of ADHD in children 4 to 12 years only. Only five symptoms are required for older adolescents and adults (age 17 and over).[6] Validated rating scales, such as the Connors Rating Scales—revised (CRS-revised), and the Vanderbilt ADHD diagnostic scale are recommended for objective symptom ratings from parents and teachers in different age groups.[1,2,4,5,27] To make a diagnosis of ADHD, the clinician should rule out alternative causes of symptoms (learning disability, situational stressor) and assess for other conditions that may coexist with ADHD including oppositional defiant and conduct disorders, tics, ASD, sleep and mood disorders.[4,6,28]

Preschoolers (3 to 5 Years)

The DSM-5 diagnostic criteria for ADHD can be applied to preschool-age children, although it may be difficult to document symptoms in multiple settings with different caregivers if the child does not attend preschool.[1,6,9] Enrollment in a qualified preschool and a parent training program is often recommended. Both can help parents develop reasonable expectations for their child's development and foster the development of management skills for problem behaviors. Although methylphenidate has been found safe and effective for ADHD in 4- and 5-year-olds, behavioral interventions are recommended first. Medications can be considered when the child has moderate to severe symptoms unresponsive to behavioral interventions. The clinician needs to weigh the risks of starting medication at an early age against the harm of delaying diagnosis and treatment.[1,2,29]

School Age (6 to 11 Years)

Most cases of ADHD are first realized during ages 6 to 9 years, with the child having difficulty academically and/or socially in school and at home. Most children have combined inattentive and hyperactive or impulsive symptoms that cause functional impairment. This period is crucial to the child's success in school, socialization, and the development of his or her sense of self; therefore, accurate diagnosis and treatment is critical. Comorbid oppositional defiant disorder (ODD), conduct disorder, and aggression are indicators that the child is at greater risk for delinquency and substance abuse in adolescence.[9,30] This is the most well-studied age group, with strong data showing benefits of recognition and treatment with behavioral interventions and medications.[2,4]

Adolescents (12 to 18 Years)

Hyperactivity decreases in adolescents, and inattention and impulsivity are the more prominent functionally impairing symptoms. There may be fewer numbers of symptoms of ADHD in adolescence, but the symptoms present cause significant functional impairment.[6,7,94] Higher rates of delinquency, drug and alcohol use, and psychiatric comorbidity have been documented in adolescents with ADHD compared with those without ADHD.[1,2,9,11] Assessment for substance abuse and risk of diversion must be considered before starting stimulant medications. Speeding and increased motor vehicle accidents occur at higher rates in teens with ADHD compared with those without the disorder.[1-3,7,9]

Adults

The presence of multiple comorbid conditions, particularly conduct or mood disorder, can increase the likelihood of ADHD chronicity into adulthood. DSM-5 criteria for ADHD in childhood also apply to adults. Inattentive symptoms are the most common and functionally impairing in adults, but hyperactive/restless and impulsive symptoms are experienced by many and are associated with higher rates of bipolar disorder and psychosis.[3] Cognitive deficits (eg, executive functioning, working memory, task prioritization, lower IQ) have been documented in adults with ADHD in addition to a greater risk for unstable relationships, unemployment, psychiatric hospitalization, and incarceration compared with those without ADHD.[3,10,11] The Adult ADHD Self-Report Scale (ASRS.v1.1) can be a useful screening tool as a first step to a more thorough diagnosis with an experienced clinician. Gathering collateral information from family and friends is recommended to either support or refute the diagnosis.[31,32]

TREATMENT

ADHD-specific cognitive and behavioral interventions are increasingly recognized as necessary components of an overall treatment plan aimed at symptom relief and optimal functioning. Several studies show combining medications with behavioral interventions produces the greatest symptom relief and the best outcomes.[2,33-36]

Desired Outcomes

4 Specific goals of treatment or desired outcomes must be identified (eg, able to sit in chair for 20 minutes; completes homework assignments, or no longer blurts out comments in class without being called upon). For adults, the desired outcome may be to read an entire newspaper before starting another project, improving safety while driving, or successfully completing tasks on time at work.[36-37]

Nonpharmacologic Therapy

Educational, Cognitive, and Behavioral Interventions

5 Education on ADHD as a biologic disorder with brain-derived causes is essential for destigmatizing ADHD and improving treatment acceptance. Parent training and behavioral interventions such as positive rewards for good behavior and structured limit setting are recommended as first-line interventions before medication trials in preschoolers (3- to 5-year-olds) with ADHD. Behavioral interventions for ADHD are described in Table 63-1. It is crucial to get parents, teachers, and clinicians involved to coordinate care and provide consistent behavioral management for the child at home and at school. School-age children (6-11 years) also benefit from these behavioral interventions in addition to strategies, such as breaking up homework assignments into shorter, manageable segments. Although it varies by state, children and adolescents with ADHD may qualify for an individualized educational program (IEP) that allows for more time to take an exam, preferred seating, and modified work assignments.[1,2,31] It is noteworthy that most studies comparing behavioral intervention with stimulant therapy in youth found a much stronger effect on ADHD core symptoms from stimulants.[1,2,5,31] Combined behavioral and stimulant therapy resulted in greater improvements on academic and conduct measures in some studies with greater parent and teacher satisfaction ratings. Lower doses of stimulant were effective when behavioral interventions were administered according to several studies.[2,35]

5 Recommended behavioral interventions for adolescents and adults include keeping an external organizer (eg, smart phone, notebook with "to-do" lists) and breaking up activities into short, manageable tasks. Recognizing triggers for distraction and making a point of thinking before acting are useful interventions and are recommended during cognitive behavioral therapy (CBT) sessions designed to manage adult ADHD.[34,38] Controlled studies have shown that ADHD-specific CBT was more effective than psychoeducation and relaxation in adults with ADHD whose symptoms were only partially responsive to medication.[34] Similarly, adults with ADHD who partially responded to medications benefited more from a group-administered metacognition program (2 h/wk over 12 weeks) compared with supportive therapy sessions administered for the same amount of time.[38] Yoga, meditation, and some dietary supplements have been recommended for ADHD as well, but they should not take the place of more established effective treatments, such as medications and cognitive interventions.[39]

TABLE 63-1 Behavioral Interventions for ADHD

Age	Description of Intervention	Typical Outcomes
Preschool and school age	Parent and family education on ADHD Training on behavioral modification Classroom management instruction for teachers	Improved parental understanding and satisfaction Improved compliance with parental commands Improved teacher satisfaction
Adolescent	Break up homework assignments into manageable segments. Structured schedule; organizer	Completion of assignments improves; improved self-esteem and sense of self
Adolescent and adult	ADHD-specific cognitive behavioral therapy Metacognitive therapy	Improved productivity and vocational success Improved relationships

ADHD, attention deficit/hyperactivity disorder.

Data from references 2, 4, 7, 29 and 33.

Dietary Interventions

Extensive research has evaluated dietary interventions for ADHD, primarily in children with some adolescent data. When iron and zinc are supplemented in youth with known deficiencies, the therapeutic benefit of stimulant therapy can be enhanced, frequently allowing lower effective doses.[40,41] Omega-3 supplements can benefit some individuals with few side effects, but results are not consistently better than placebo. Although scientific evidence is lacking, there is a universal belief among families that the avoidance of sugar and artificial sweeteners improves ADHD symptoms. The attention paid to sugar avoidance and healthy diet is the more likely reason for improved behavior. An overall healthy diet with the proper balance of protein, fresh produce, and fiber is recommended.[41]

Clinical Controversy...

Studies are mixed regarding the long-term outcome of ADHD-specific pharmacotherapy. Do the long-term benefits in academic performance, health, occupational, psychosocial, and quality of life outcomes outweigh the risks? The longest U.S. naturalistic study over 8 years, the multimodal treatment study of children with ADHD (MTA) study, found that there was no long-term benefit in those who continued pharmacotherapy compared to those who did not [42,43] yet a German study showed 34% decrease in accidental severe brain injury in those treated with stimulant or atomoxetine for an average of 3.5 years compared to youth with ADHD who were untreated.[44] A 9-year Danish study showed lower rates of hospital contacts in youth who began treatment for ADHD before age 10 and slightly lower criminality.[45]

Pharmacologic Therapy

Figure 63-1 is an algorithm for drug selection in the treatment of ADHD.

Stimulants

Stimulants are considered first-line therapy in most cases of ADHD; however, comorbid conditions impact the drug selection process. Pharmacotherapy should be considered whenever a thorough

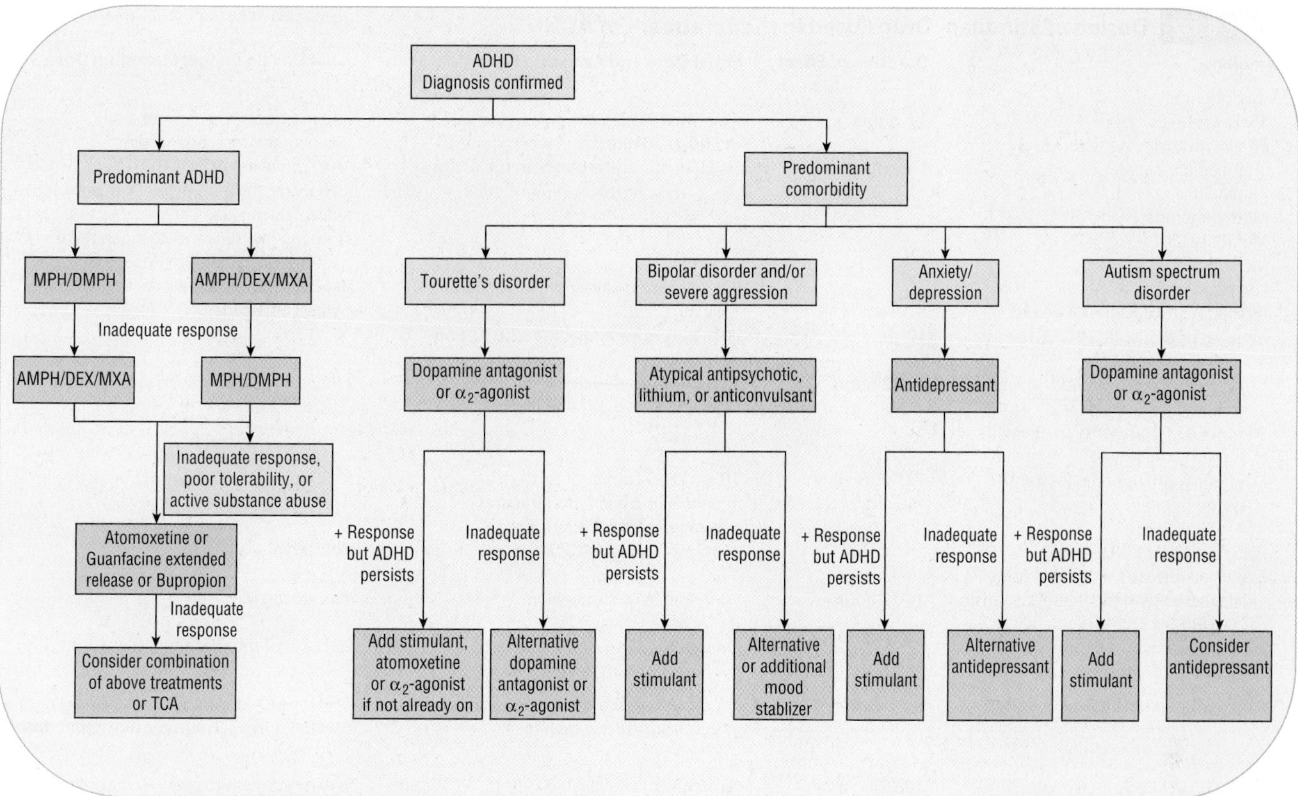

FIGURE 63-1 Algorithm for drug selection in the management of attention deficit/hyperactivity disorder (ADHD). Treat predominant disorder first, reassess, and consider alternative or adjunct medications for optimal symptom control. (DEX, dextroamphetamine; DMPH, dexmethylphenidate; MPH, methylphenidate; MXA, mixed amphetamine salts; AMPH, amphetamine; TCA, tricyclic antidepressant.) (*Data from References 2, 4, 5, 47, and 79.*)

diagnostic assessment results in a diagnosis of ADHD. Several studies demonstrate the superiority of stimulants over behavioral interventions in alleviating core symptoms of ADHD.[4,37]

Treatment for ADHD may decrease the rate of some serious injuries in youth. Investigators evaluated a large German healthcare database (reflecting 20% of the population) and found no difference in overall injury rates in children between ages 3 and 17 years with ADHD treated with stimulant or atomoxetine compared with those not treated; however, there was a 34% decrease in severe brain injury in the treated group.[44]

Improvement in academic performance has been associated with stimulant treatment of ADHD. A National Institutes of Health (NIH) study of 594 fifth graders with ADHD showed those medicated (greater than 90% took stimulants) had 2.9 points higher math scores and 5.4 points higher reading scores compared with unmedicated children.[46] Another study involving 363 children between ages 10 and 18 years with ADHD showed medication improved but did not normalize cognition.[47]

6 Stimulants (eg, methylphenidate, dexmethylphenidate, mixed amphetamine salts, and dextroamphetamine) are the most effective drug treatment options, with an effect size of 0.9 compared with nonstimulant drug treatment options whose effect sizes range from 0.5 to 0.7 signifying lower efficacy.[2,4,48] Methylphenidate and amphetamines block dopamine and norepinephrine reuptake; amphetamines also increase catecholamine release.[49] Both drugs inhibit monoamine oxidase (MAO), amphetamines more potently than methylphenidate.[49] Because different stimulants work through slightly different mechanisms, the lack of response to one chemical class of stimulant (eg, methylphenidate or dexmethylphenidate) does not preclude response to another class (eg, dextroamphetamine including lisdexamfetamine or mixed amphetamine salts).[5,37]

Stimulant dosing should be titrated for maximum individual efficacy and minimum side effects (Table 63-2).[2,4,5,50]

Clinical **Controversy...**

Stimulants are regularly prescribed for ADHD beyond the FDA's recommended daily maximum dose. This practice has not been studied, and therefore the clinical impact of such a practice is unknown. Short-term studies evaluating therapeutic benefits of doses at the high end of the FDA-approved therapeutic range show greater efficacy in managing aggression for example.[66] Conversely, a 9-year study shows 1.8x greater risk of adverse cardiac events in patients taking stimulants at the high end of the dosing range.[65]

With immediate-release stimulants, most patients require a two or three times daily dosing schedule because of the short half-lives and duration of action of these drugs (2-4 hours for methylphenidate and dexmethylphenidate and ~4 to 6 hours for dextroamphetamine or mixed amphetamine salts).[2,4,5] Drug response is maximal during the absorption phase, is evident in 15 to 30 minutes, and lasts 2 to 6 hours.[4,5]

Drug delivery systems of once-daily products (amphetamine aspartate, amphetamine sulfate, dextroamphetamine sulfate, and dextroamphetamine saccharate [Adderall XR]; methylphenidate [Concerta]; methylphenidate [Daytrana]; dexmethylphenidate [Focalin XR]; methylphenidate [Metadate CD]; and methylphenidate long-acting [Ritalin LA]) provide 8 to 12 hours of symptom control.[2,4,5,48,51] Concerta uses an oral osmotic (OROS) controlled-release delivery

TABLE 63-2 Dosing of Stimulant Drugs Used in the Treatment of ADHD

Stimulant	Duration of Effect	Initial Dose and Available Strengths	Usual Dosing Range; Maximum Dose
Methylphenidate C-II[a]			
Short-acting IR Ritalin, methylin, generics[b]	3-5 hours	5 mg two or three times daily; increase by 5-10 or 20 mg/day at weekly intervals	5-20 mg two or three times a day; maximum dose: 60 mg/day
Intermediate-acting Ritalin SR[b] Methylphenidate SR[b] Metadate ER[b] Methylin ER[b]	3-8 hours	SR, ER doses; corresponds to the IR dose	20-40 mg every AM or 40 mg every AM and 20 mg in the early afternoon; maximum dose: 60 mg/day 20-40 mg every AM and 20 mg in the early afternoon; maximum dose: 60 mg/day
Long-acting Ritalin LA 50% IR, 50% ER beads[b]	8-10 hours	20 mg every AM; available as 10, 20, and 30 mg	20-60 mg/day, given every AM; maximum dose: 60 mg/day
Metadate CD 30% IR, 70% ER beads[b]	10-12 hours	20 mg every AM; available as 20, 30, and 40 mg	
Concerta (OROS controlled-release delivery)[b] ER inner compartments coated with IR methylphenidate	10-12 hours	18 mg every AM; available as 18, 27, 36, and 54 mg; 90% bioavailability of IR	27-72 mg/day, given every AM; maximum dose: 72 mg/day
Daytrana methylphenidate transdermal system[b]	12 hours when worn for 9 hours	10 mg (12.5 cm²) applied to clean, dry area on hip each morning and removed after 9 hours	10-30 mg (12.5-37.5 cm²). Drug active for 3 hours after patch removal
Aptensio XR 40% IR, 60% ER Extended release methylphenidate[b]	10-12 hours	10 mg; available as 10, 20, 30, 40, 50, and 60 mg capsules	Max: 60 mg daily
Quillavant extended release suspension 20% IR/80% ER[b]	10-12 hours	10-20 mg in AM suspension	Max: 60 mg daily
Must be reconstituted by pharmacist to 25 mg/5 mL concentration		Only studied in 6- to 12-year-olds	Stable for 4 months after reconstituted
Dexmethylphenidate (Focalin) C-II[b]	3-5 hours	2.5 mg every AM or twice daily; available as 2.5, 5, and 10 mg tablets	5-10 mg/day given twice a day; maximum initial dose: 7.5 mg/day; maximum dose: 20 mg/day
Focalin XR 50% IR, 50% ER beads[b]	10-12 hours	5 mg every AM; available as 5, 10, 15, 25, 30, 35, and 40 mg capsules	5-40 mg/day, given every AM maximum dose: 30 mg/day for children and adolescents; maximum 40 mg/day for adults
Mixed amphetamine salts C-II (dextroamphetamine and levoamphetamine 3:1 ratio)			
Short-acting IR (Adderall, mixed amphetamine generics)[c]	4-6 hours	2.5 – 5mg every am to twice daily; Available in 5, 10, 7.5, 12.5, 15, 20, 30mg tablet	5-40mg; Max: 40mg/day
Amphetamine C-II (dextroamphetamine and levoamphetamine ratio 1:1)[c] Evekeo,	6-10 hours	2.5 -5mg every am to twice daily; Available in 5 and 10mg tablets	5-20mg; Max: 40mg/day
Long-acting XR (Adzenys XR-ODT) dextroamphetamine and levoamphetamine ratio 3:1[d]	10-12 hours	3.1, 6.3, 9.4, 12.5, 15.7, 18.8, extended release oral disintegrating tablets 3.1mg Adzenys ODT ~ 5mg of Adderall XR	3.1 – 18.8mg/day; Max: 18.8mg/day
Dyanavel XR 2.5mg/ml Dextroamphetamine and levoamphetamine ratio 3.2:1[d]	10-12 hours	2.5mg/1ml oral suspension 2.5mg of suspension ~ 4mg of mixed amphetamine salts	5 – 20mg/day; Max: 20mg/day
Mixed amphetamine salts C-II Extended release capsule (Adderall XR) dextroamphetamine and levoamphetamine ratio 3:1[d]	10-12 hours	5 – 10mg every am; available as 5, 10, 20, 30mg extended release capsule	5 - 30mg; Max: 30mg/day
Dextroamphetamine C-II	4-6 hours	2.5 mg every AM once- or twice-daily dosing	10-40 mg/day (divided in two doses)
Short-acting Dextroamphetamine generics[c] Dexedrine, Zenzedi[c]	3-5 hours	2.5 mg every AM to two or three times daily dosing	10-40 mg/day given twice daily
Intermediate-acting Dexedrine Spansule[d] *Long-acting*	5-8 hours	Available as 5, 10, and 15 mg 5 mg every AM; available as 5 and 10 mg	5-30 mg every day or 5-15 mg twice daily; maximum: 40 mg/day
Lisdexamfetamine (Vyvanse)[d] (prodrug converted to dextroamphetamine)	10-12 hours	Available as 20, 30, 40, 50, 60, and 70 mg capsules	Start at low end; titrate weekly to response; give in AM Slower onset compared with other dextroamphetamine products

ER, extended release; IR, immediate release; OROS, osmotically released oral delivery system; SR, sustained release; XR, extended release.

[a]The Drug Enforcement Administration label C-II, schedule II refers to significant abuse potential.

[b]Methylphenidate and dexmethylphenidate products are FDA approved in ≥6 years old.

[c]Immediate release amphetamine and dextroamphetamine products are FDA approved in ≥3 years old.

[d]Extended release amphetamine and dextroamphetamine products are FDA approved in ≥6 years old.

Data from references 2, 4, 5, 27, 52 and stimulant product package inserts or Daily Med.

system, whereas other oral preparations use combinations of immediate-release and extended-release beads.[2,4,5] Concerta is a nondeformable tablet, and it should not be given to children with gastrointestinal (GI) narrowing because of the risk of obstruction. Methylphenidate transdermal system provides 12 hours of symptom control when worn for 9 hours.[2,48,51] Methylphenidate extended release suspension was only studied in 6- to 12-year-olds, and it can be an advantage for children with trouble swallowing pills.[52] Older wax-matrix sustained-release (SR) products (eg, Ritalin SR) are less effective and infrequently used.[4,5] Once-daily stimulant formulations are the preferred treatment for ADHD in most individuals due to convenience and better medication adherence.[4,5,53] Immediate-release formulations have the advantage of lower cost, less insomnia, and potentially fewer growth effects versus extended-release products.[4,30] Adolescents and adults with ADHD are also responsive to stimulants.[2,4,37] Methylphenidate is effective in adolescents and adults in doses up to 1.5 mg/kg daily.[3,5,37] Lisdexamfetamine is a prodrug conjugated to an amino acid that requires cleavage during metabolism to the active dextroamphetamine. It has a longer time to onset of effect but may provide a smoother blood level compared with extended-release formulations. It is intended to pose less abuse potential.[48]

Administration of stimulant medications with food can delay the absorption and subsequently delay the onset of therapeutic effect by 30 minutes to 1 hour for immediate-release preparations, and 1 to 2 hours for extended-release preparations.[50] Total bioavailability of stimulant can be decreased by 10% to 30% with coadministration of food, more so for beaded formulations of extended-release stimulant compared with OROS methylphenidate or lisdexamfetamine.[50]

Adverse Effects The most common adverse effects of stimulants and their management strategies are listed in Table 63-3.[54] At least 15 cases of priapism, (painful prolonged erection) associated with stimulant use have been reported to the FDA in boys with a mean age of 12.5 years. A few cases of priapism have been reported with atomoxetine, and all cases require immediate medical attention.[55a] FDA has received at least 51 reports of skin discoloration, also known as chemical leukoderma that may not be reversible.[55b]

Psychiatric, cardiac, and growth effects of stimulants have been extensively studied and are compared to other treatment options in the sections below.

Psychiatric Although considered rare, the FDA has added warnings to the labeling of all ADHD medications (ie, stimulants, atomoxetine, α_2-adrenergic agonists) regarding three broad categories of psychiatric adverse effects: psychosis, mood disturbance (ie, irritability, lability, or depression), and severe anxiety or panic attacks. Treatment-emergent psychosis is estimated to occur in approximately 1.5% of youth treated with stimulant medications based on placebo-controlled trials.[30,56] Hallucinations involving visual or tactile sensations of insects, snakes, or worms were typical in children, with adolescents and adults experiencing hallucinations and delusions.[57] Sadness from stimulants may in part be genetically mediated, as an association was found between two (CES1) (SNP) markers and the occurrence of sadness in 77 youth taking immediate-release methylphenidate for ADHD.[58] There is also evidence to suggest that preschool-aged youth are more susceptible to sadness, irritability, and mood lability with stimulant treatment compared with adolescents and adults.[30,54]

Case reports of atomoxetine-associated mania and psychosis exist, but the risk is less well-characterized versus stimulants. Both stimulant and atomoxetine have the potential to cause or exacerbate mania, anxiety, panic attacks, or depression. Stimulants and atomoxetine should not be given to manage attention in individuals with primary psychotic illnesses such as schizophrenia or schizoaffective disorder due to the high risk of worsening psychosis.[30,57]

Clonidine and guanfacine are much less likely than stimulants or atomoxetine to cause psychosis, mania, or anxiety, but treatment-emergent irritability, depression, and nightmares have been reported.[59,60,61] When psychiatric adverse effects occur, dose reduction or cessation of therapy and supportive treatment is recommended.[30]

Cardiac Stimulants, atomoxetine, and α_2-adrenergic agonists have well-described cardiac and cardiovascular side effects that are not significant for most youth but can be intolerable in some, particularly in those with existing cardiac/cardiovascular disease. Clinical trial data show that children who take stimulants for ADHD can have an increased heart rate by 3 to 10 beats/min and/or increased systolic blood pressure by 3 to 8 mm Hg, and increased diastolic blood pressure by 2 to 14 mm Hg.[30] Atomoxetine treatment has been associated with increased heart rate at an average of approximately 4 beats/min and increased systolic or diastolic blood pressure of 2 to 4 mm Hg.[62] Clonidine and guanfacine may cause dose-related

TABLE 63-3 Stimulant Adverse Effects and Their Management

Adverse Effect	Recommendation/Management Strategy
Common	
Reduced appetite, weight loss	Give high-calorie meal when stimulant effects are low (at breakfast or at bedtime), or consider cyproheptadine at bedtime
Stomachache	Administer stimulant on a full stomach; lower dose if possible
Insomnia	Give dose earlier in the day; lower the last dose of the day or give it earlier; consider a sedating medication at bedtime (guanfacine, clonidine, melatonin, or cyproheptadine)
Headache	Divide dose, give with food, or give an analgesic (eg, acetaminophen or ibuprofen)
Rebound symptoms	Consider longer-acting stimulant trial, atomoxetine, or antidepressant
Irritability/jitteriness	Assess for comorbid condition (eg, bipolar disorder); reduce dosage; consider mood stabilizer or atypical antipsychotic
Uncommon to Rare	
Dysphoria	Reduce dosage; reassess diagnosis; consider alternative therapy
Skin discoloration (chemical leukoderma)	Counsel regarding risk before using methylphenidate patch
Zombie-like state	Reduce dosage or change stimulant medication
Tics or abnormal movements	Reduce dosage; consider alternative medication
Priapism (painful erection)	Obtain medical assistance immediately; consider alternative treatment
Hypertension, pulse fluctuations	Reduce dosage; change medication
Hallucinations	Discontinue stimulant; reassess diagnosis; mood stabilizer and/or antipsychotic may be needed

Data from references 3, 4, 27, 30, 55, 84.

bradycardia and lowered blood pressure in youth that may prevent upward titration in addition to modest widening of the QTc interval (5-7 msec) that warrants monitoring, particularly if the child takes another agent known to prolong QTc such as an antidepressant or antipsychotic.[30,60]

Reports of sudden unexplained death associated with stimulant treatment for ADHD prompted the U.S. Agency for Healthcare Research and Quality to conduct two studies of large healthcare databases in order to compare rates of sudden cardiac death, heart attack, and stroke in those taking stimulants with those not taking stimulants. The first study of 1.2 million 2- to 24-year-olds (mean age at baseline 11.1 years) taking stimulants for an average of 2.1 years showed that 3.1 per 100,000 experienced a serious cardiac event. This was no greater than rates in the general population.[63] The second study included 150,000 users of stimulants aged 25 to 64 years each matched to two nonusers of stimulants (443,000). This study in adults found no greater risk of sudden death, heart attack, or stroke in stimulant users versus nonstimulant users.[64] The relatively short duration of use and overall good health of those studied may have biased the results. These studies add to earlier findings showing no increased risk of serious cardiac events with stimulant use, and, therefore, no restriction in stimulant use has been recommended.[63,64]

Stimulant products should be used with caution in pediatrics and in adults with known structural cardiac abnormalities. The American Heart Association recommends careful screening of all children and adolescents prior to initiating pharmacologic therapy for ADHD, including a medical and family history and physical examination.[30] The physician should consider a baseline electrocardiogram (ECG) if history suggests cardiovascular disease.[30]

A 9.5-year prospective cohort study of children with ADHD found that although rare, adverse cardiovascular events were twice as likely to occur in stimulant users as in nonusers.[65] There were 111 cardiovascular events in the 8,300 children with ADHD. Hypertension, heart disease not otherwise specified, and cardiovascular disease not otherwise specified comprised 62% of adverse cardiac events, arrhythmias comprised 23%, while cardiac arrest accounted for less than 1% of events.[30] The same investigators looked at national rates of stimulant use (n = 714,258) and found 1.8 times greater risk of a cardiovascular events in those taking stimulant with greater risk of adverse cardiac events on higher doses of stimulant compared with lower doses.[65]

Growth Two reviews that analyzed approximately 32 studies indicated that stimulant treatment of ADHD can affect growth, but the effects are minimal or insignificant for most children. A study of 579 children showed a decrease of approximately 1 cm/y (~0.5 in) in height over 1 to 3 years of continuous treatment with methylphenidate and a weight deficit of 3 kg (6.6 lb) in the first year of treatment and 1.2 kg (2.6 lb) in the second year of treatment.[4,5] Amphetamine products may be associated with more growth effects than methylphenidate according to separate studies.[4,5] Proposed mechanisms of stimulant effects on growth include alterations in growth hormone or growth factor, decreased thyroxine secretion, and suppression of appetite leading to reduced caloric intake.[4,30] Two case–control studies, with approximately 140 boys and 110 girls, assessed growth effects after taking stimulant medication over a 10-year period and found no significant effect on growth in boys or girls taking stimulants compared with matched controls not taking stimulant. The average duration of stimulant use was 7.5 years.[30]

In most cases, children should be given a drug-free trial every year.[4,30] Time off stimulant appears to lessen stimulant growth suppressant effects, but evidence is lacking to firmly determine the impact of drug holidays on growth.[4,37] Consideration must be given to the risks of negative effects on learning, socialization, and self-image while off stimulant therapy when determining the frequency and duration of the drug-free trial.[4,30] Drug dosage often varies from year to year, largely because of age-related pharmacokinetic changes. As a child develops, hepatic metabolism slows, and volume of distribution increases.[50]

Nonstimulants

Extended-release guanfacine and extended-release clonidine are less effective alternatives to the stimulants for treatment of ADHD in children and adolescents. Clonidine and guanfacine are approved by the FDA as monotherapy and as adjuncts to stimulants for improving overall response and for managing behavioral symptoms and insomnia associated with ADHD. Unlike guanfacine and clonidine, atomoxetine is also approved in adults. Atomoxetine is generally considered less effective than stimulants, but there is evidence to show that some patients preferentially respond to atomoxetine over stimulants.[37] Potential advantages of atomoxetine and α_2-adrenergic agonists relative to stimulants include no abuse potential, less potential for growth effects, and less sleep disturbance.[4,30] See Table 63-4 for dosing.

Atomoxetine Atomoxetine is a selective norepinephrine reuptake inhibitor that should be taken in divided doses in the morning or late afternoon by children for improved tolerability.[67] Adults can take it once daily, usually in the morning.[3,67] Placebo-controlled, short-term trials (6-12 weeks) have shown that atomoxetine is effective in reducing ADHD symptoms in children, teens, and adults, and long-term studies show ongoing benefit and safety for children and adolescent responders out to 4 years.[68] A controlled trial comparing atomoxetine, OROS methylphenidate, and placebo over 6 weeks in 6 to 16-year-old patients showed that both drugs were significantly better than placebo at improving ADHD symptoms, but OROS methylphenidate was superior to atomoxetine.[4,37] There was evidence for a preferential response to atomoxetine in some individuals.[37]

Atomoxetine has a significantly slower onset of therapeutic effect than stimulants (2-4 weeks vs 1-2 hours with an effective stimulant dose), and full benefit may not be seen for 6 to 12 weeks.[4,37] Atomoxetine is sometimes combined with a stimulant in partially responsive patients based on limited data from open trials and case series describing fewer late-day rebound effects and better sleep when atomoxetine is given in the evening; however, adverse effects are additive.[4,37,67] A new norepinephrine reuptake inhibitor, edivoxetine has shown some benefit for managing ADHD in children; more studies are needed.[69]

Atomoxetine Adverse Effects Possible adverse effects of atomoxetine and their management are similar to those of stimulants, including upset stomach and psychiatric and cardiac adverse effects (see Table 63-4). Atomoxetine has less growth suppression risk compared with stimulants, but it has a greater risk of fatigue, sedation, and dizziness compared with stimulants or bupropion. Studies show that adults experience overall similar adverse effects as youth but they are less likely to report decreased appetite and are more likely to report urinary hesitation/retention and sexual side effects (decreased libido and erectile disturbances) compared to youth.[37,67] Unlike stimulants, atomoxetine labeling includes a bolded warning of potential for severe liver injury following reports in two patients. Continuation studies have not shown evidence for liver toxicity with long-term use; however, a case of idiosyncratic liver toxicity requiring liver transplantation in a 10-year-old boy was reported.[68,70]

Atomoxetine is the only FDA-approved ADHD medication with a labeled warning for new-onset suicidality, 0.4% in atomoxetine-treated patients versus 0% in patients receiving placebo.[30] Despite this statistic, atomoxetine treatment is not thought to increase the risk of suicidality beyond the increased risk associated with having ADHD.[30]

α_2-Adrenergic Agonists Guanfacine and clonidine are central α_2-adrenergic agonists, acting both presynaptically to inhibit norepinephrine release and postsynaptically to increase blood flow in the prefrontal cortex. Increased blood flow in the prefrontal cortex has been shown to enhance working memory and executive functioning.

TABLE 63-4 Dosing and Adverse Effect Monitoring of Nonstimulant Drugs for ADHD

Drug	Dosing Range and Titration Schedule	Adverse Effect Monitoring
Atomoxetine (Strattera)	≤70 kg (≤154 lb): start at 0.3-0.5 mg/kg every AM or twice daily, maximum: 1.4 mg/kg/day; ≥70 kg (≥154 lb): start at 40 mg every AM or divided twice daily, maximum: 100 mg/day	Nausea, anorexia, ↑ blood pressure, ↑ pulse, insomnia, fatigue, sedation, severe liver injury (rare), suicidality
Bupropion (Wellbutrin SR, XL)	50-300 mg/day; 3 mg/kg/day by end of week 1; can increase to 6 mg/kg/day or maximum of 300 mg/day as tolerated	Nausea, insomnia, rash, tics; dose-related risk of seizures
Antipsychotics (for comorbid aggression, mood disorders, tics, or irritability associated with ASD)		
Aripiprazole[a] (Abilify)	2-5 mg daily; can titrate weekly as tolerated to response (usual range: 5-20 mg/day)	Nausea, restlessness, insomnia extrapyramidal symptoms, dizziness, sedation
Haloperidol[a] (Haldol)	0.5-1 mg twice daily; can titrate every 3-4 days as tolerated to response (usual range: 0.5-5 mg/day)	Extrapyramidal symptoms, dizziness, ↑ serum prolactin, sedation
Olanzapine[a] (Zyprexa)	2.5-5 mg every day; can titrate every 3-4 days as tolerated to response (usual range: 7.5-15 mg/day)	Sedation, severe weight gain, restlessness, extrapyramidal symptoms Diabetes, marked hyperlipidemia (never a first-line treatment)
Quetiapine[a] (Seroquel)	25-50 mg twice daily; can titrate every 3-4 days as tolerated to response (usual range: 200-600 mg/day)	Sedation, dizziness, weight gain, diabetes, hyperlipidemia
Risperidone[a] (Risperdal)	0.25-0.5 mg twice daily; can titrate every 3-4 days as tolerated to response (1-4 mg/day)	Extrapyramidal symptoms, dizziness, ↑ serum prolactin, decreased skeletal bone mass, hepatotoxicity, weight gain Diabetes, hyperlipidemia
Ziprasidone[a] (Geodon)	10-20 mg twice daily; can titrate every 3-4 days as tolerated to response (usual range: 40-160 mg/day)	Nausea, restlessness, insomnia extrapyramidal symptoms, sedation, QTc prolongation
Other		
Clonidine (Catapres) or clonidine extended release XR (Kapvay)	0.05 mg two or four times daily; can increase as tolerated to 0.1-0.4 mg/day. For XR, give 0.1 mg at bedtime; may increase by 0.1 mg weekly; maximum: 0.4 mg/day given twice a day if dose >0.2 mg/day	Sedation, dizziness, heart block (check ECG), constipation, headache, upper abdominal pain
Guanfacine (Tenex) or guanfacine extended release XR (Intuniv)	0.5 once or twice daily; can increase as tolerated to 1-4 mg/day. Max: 4 mg/day in children/adolescents For XR, give 1 mg in the AM; titrate weekly to response Max: 4 mg/day in children; 7 mg/day in adolescents	Same as above with potentially lower risk of sedation. Effective dose higher in heavier children

ADHD, attention deficit/hyperactivity disorder; ASD, autism spectrum disorder; ECG, electrocardiogram; SR, sustained release; XL, extended length.

[a]Short-term use (1–4 months) only for severe aggression associated with ADHD; may be longer if comorbidity such as bipolar disorder, Tourette's disorder, or autism spectrum disorder.

Data from references 4,30,60,61,75,76,78.

Both interact with a multitude of neurotransmitter systems, including catecholamine, indolamine, and α_2-receptors on parasympathetic neurons, opioids, imidazole, and amino acid systems.[49]

Guanfacine has a longer elimination half-life and duration of action (18 hours) compared with clonidine (12 hours), and its greater selectivity for the α_{2a}-receptor, compared with clonidine, imparts less sedation and dizziness.[60] 7 Clonidine and guanfacine are not as effective as stimulants for monotherapy treatment (effect size 0.22-0.58 vs 0.8-1.2 for stimulants).[60] In addition to being approved as monotherapy, extended-release clonidine and guanfacine are FDA approved as adjuncts to stimulants. Both are prescribed frequently as adjuncts to reduce disruptive behavior, control aggression, or improve sleep in youth.[4,60] Neither have been studied sufficiently for ADHD in adults.

Guanfacine XR can be given once daily during monotherapy while clonidine XR should be given twice daily for optimal symptom coverage. Both are considered acceptable second-line agents for children and adolescents unresponsive to or unable to tolerate stomach upset or insomnia with stimulant medications. Extended-release guanfacine and clonidine are more sedating than stimulants or atomoxetine; therefore, sleepiness during the school day requires careful monitoring.[60]

α_2-Adrenergic Agonist Adverse Effects The most common side effects of clonidine and guanfacine are dose-dependent sedation, hypotension, and constipation.[2,4,60] Sedation usually subsides after 2 to 3 weeks of therapy.[4,60] Clinical trials show a mean decrease of 3 to 5 mm Hg in blood pressure with mean heart rate decrease of 3 to 5 beats/min. Heart block and sudden death have been reported rarely with α_2-adrenergic agonists. Further analysis revealed that these events occurred in the context of polypharmacy and/or congenital heart malformation. Prescreening for existing cardiac problems and increased monitoring when combining medications is warranted.[30,60]

Bupropion Bupropion, a monocyclic antidepressant, is a weak dopamine and norepinephrine reuptake inhibitor with no significant direct effect on serotonin or MAO. Its active metabolites augment noradrenergic and dopaminergic function. Investigations with bupropion in children demonstrated efficacy greater than placebo in two controlled trials and efficacy comparable with methylphenidate (n = 15 children) in another controlled trial.[4,5] Bupropion has been found beneficial for adolescents with depression and ADHD. For adults with ADHD, the number needed to treat (NNT) is between 4 and 5 compared with "2" with stimulant therapy.[51] Bupropion causes less appetite suppression and weight loss compared with stimulants but has a greater risk of seizures.[4,51]

Bupropion Adverse Effects Bupropion's adverse effects include nausea, which can resolve over time or with slower dosage titration, and rash, which can require discontinuation of therapy if severe (see Table 63-4). Bupropion should not be used in children with a seizure or eating disorder because of unacceptable risk of seizures in these patients. It can cause or exacerbate tics.[4,37,71]

Lithium and Anticonvulsants Lithium and anticonvulsants are used increasingly to control aggression and explosive behavior in patients with a diagnosis of ADHD who are not responsive or are only partially responsive to treatment with a stimulant. Some patients actually can have childhood-onset bipolar disorder or combined ADHD–bipolar disorder.[4,72,73] Valproate is the most well-studied anticonvulsant for aggression associated with ADHD. Dosing starts in low divided doses with titration over 1 to 2 weeks to therapeutic response.[72,74]

Antipsychotics Conventional antipsychotics such as chlorpromazine and haloperidol can improve symptoms of hyperactivity and impulsivity, but their negative effects on learning, cognitive functioning, and the significant risk of extrapyramidal side effects (eg, dystonia and tardive dyskinesia) limit their usefulness.[75]

Second-generation antipsychotics such as risperidone, olanzapine, quetiapine, ziprasidone, and aripiprazole have been used to control severe aggression in refractory cases of ADHD, particularly if conduct disorder (CD) or bipolar disorder coexists.[72,73] They pose a lower risk of extrapyramidal side effects compared with conventional agents, but they can cause metabolic side effects such as hyperlipidemia, hyperglycemia, and weight gain in addition to hyperprolactinemia.[75-77] Ziprasidone has the lowest risk of metabolic side effects among these second-generation antipsychotics. Risperidone is the most well studied for aggression associated with ADHD,[77] but because it has the most potent dopamine antagonism, it poses the highest risk of hyperprolactinemia and associated early puberty, gynecomastia, galactorrhea, amenorrhea, and decreased bone density.[75,78] Aripiprazole is least likely to elevate prolactin due to its dopamine agonist effects.[75]

Comorbidity

8 Individuals with ADHD often present with comorbid conditions (Fig. 63-1). If multiple drugs are started simultaneously, it is impossible to determine the impact of each drug. The predominance and urgency of symptoms guide the drug selection process. For example, if a child presents as severely anxious or depressed with associated attentional problems, then an antidepressant should be initiated first with monitoring to determine if attentional symptoms improve.[2,4,71] When a child presents with severe ADHD and associated anxiety or depression, a stimulant should be initiated to treat the more severe ADHD. If ADHD symptoms improve significantly, but anxiety or depression persists, then an antidepressant can be added.[2,4,37,71] Studies show that stimulants do not routinely make anxiety disorders worse, but they might not improve symptoms either.[5,37] 9 Bipolar disorder may be difficult to distinguish from ADHD because inattention, hyperactivity, and impulsivity are common with both conditions. When ADHD is diagnosed in an individual with bipolar disorder, the mood must be stabilized first with lithium, an anticonvulsant, or an atypical antipsychotic before considering an ADHD-specific treatment.[72,73]

ADHD and ASD ASD is estimated to occur in 20% to 50% of youth with ADHD and 30% to 80% of youth with ASD exhibit symptoms of inattention.[79] Impairments can range from mild to severe with poor language development, poor social skills, sensory over-responsivity, emotional dysregulation, inattention, impulsivity, irritability, oppositional behavior, and aggression.[79] There are few studies to guide treatment of ADHD in individuals with ASD. Only one double-blind, 4-week crossover trial showed methylphenidate improved ADHD symptoms in 34 of 66 children with ASD (51%); however, 18% of these children discontinued during the 8-week open-continuation phase because of irritability. Sleep changes, poor appetite, diarrhea, anxiety, depression, and headache were also reported.[79]

Available evidence shows that stimulants are less effective and less well-tolerated for managing ADHD in youth with more severe forms of ASD.[79] If a stimulant trial is initiated, the child with ASD should be monitored carefully for worsening stereotypies, obsessional symptoms, sleep difficulties, poor appetite, irritability, or the emergence of seizures. Atomoxetine was only slightly better than placebo in managing ADHD symptoms in children with ASD according to a controlled trial in 97 children, ages between 6 and 17 years, during 8 weeks.[79] Clonidine and guanfacine have small, uncontrolled studies only showing benefit for improving attention and decreasing aggressive/impulsive behavior in children with ASD.[79]

ADHD and Epilepsy Patients with ADHD are two to three times more likely to experience seizures than age-matched peers, and ADHD is the most common comorbidity in youth with epilepsy.[30] Fortunately, while there are a few reports of worsening seizure frequency, most studies show methylphenidate is safe and effective for managing ADHD in youth with epilepsy. The child should be stabilized and seizure-free on an anticonvulsant prior to initiation of the stimulant as stimulants are known to lower the seizure threshold. The impact of atomoxetine, clonidine, and guanfacine on seizure frequency requires further study.[30]

ADHD and Substance Abuse Genetics, age (14- to 25-year-olds), psychosocial factors, and comorbidities all influence one's risk for drug and alcohol abuse.[9,80] ADHD itself is a known risk factor for the development of a substance use disorder. A review of 27 longitudinal studies that followed children with and without ADHD into adolescence or adulthood found that compared with control subjects without ADHD, children with ADHD were (1) nearly three times more likely to report nicotine dependence in adolescence/adulthood, (2) almost two times more likely to meet diagnostic criteria for alcohol abuse or dependence, (3) approximately 1.5 times more likely to meet criteria for marijuana use disorder, (4) twice as likely to develop cocaine abuse or dependence, and (5) more than 2.5 times more likely to develop a substance use disorder overall.

Parents frequently express concern that treating their child with a stimulant, particularly early treatment, may increase the risk of substance abuse. Follow-up studies show that stimulant therapy for ADHD neither increases nor decreases the risk of subsequent drug or alcohol abuse.[9,80] There is evidence that individuals initiating treatment early (before age 8), are less likely to use substances than those who have delayed onset of treatment. Behavioral therapy may also confer some protection against substance use and delinquency.[9,80] 10 Atomoxetine, an α_2-agonist, or bupropion are preferred agents for individuals with ADHD and active substance use disorders.

Comorbid conditions including depression, anxiety, low self-esteem, conduct disorder, and antisocial personality disorder all increase the risk for developing a substance use disorder in an individual with ADHD.[9,80] These comorbidities also increase the risk for delinquency and incarceration that can prevent treatment and lead to ongoing substance abuse. As youth with ADHD transition to adolescence, parents and clinicians should pay attention to whether the teen could be at risk for substance abuse or inappropriate use of their prescribed medication.[5,81,82]

Several studies have evaluated protective factors against substance abuse and delinquency for youth both with and without ADHD. These studies found that a quality parent-youth relationship, involving good communication, regular time together, consistent rules, and sharing of information (eg, how the child or adolescent spends free time and who his or her friends are) can be effective in deterring alcohol and substance abuse in youth with or without ADHD.[9,80,83] Youth support groups at high schools, such as the Gay/Straight Alliance (GSA), are credited with assisting schools with achieving lower rates of illicit drug use and the misuse of prescription ADHD medications compared with schools without GSAs.[83]

ADHD and ODD/CD Causes of ODD, CD, and associated severe aggression in youth are multifactorial with psychosocial adversity factors contributing along with comorbidities that could include a learning disability, ADHD, disruptive mood dysregulation disorder (DMDD), or bipolar disorder.[73,76,77,80] Experts consider psychosocial interventions that include parent training and support for the child's family an essential part of the treatment plan for youth with ADHD, co-occurring with ODD or CD.[27]

Effectively managing ADHD with stimulant or atomoxetine has the most evidence for improving associated ODD symptoms in youth, although clonidine or guanfacine may also be effective.[7,27,60] Once treated, ODD may be less likely to develop into the more severe CD. A study in aggressive 6- to 13-year-olds with ADHD found that systematic weekly methylphenidate titration to an average dose of 52 mg/day along with behavioral therapy resulted in optimal symptom control without the need for antiaggressive medications such as risperidone or quetiapine.[66] This prevents exposure to the risk of atypical antipsychotic side effects such as weight gain, diabetes, hyperprolactinemia, and extrapyramidal side effects. Studies in adolescents taking OROS methylphenidate found most of them needed between 54 and 72 mg/day for optimal therapeutic benefit.[66]

Studies in adolescents and adults with ADHD show that doses of stimulant above the recommended daily maximum are frequently needed for optimal symptom control prompting the American Academy of Child and Adolescent Psychiatry to publish an "off-label maximum dosage of 100 mg/day for methylphenidate and 60 mg/day for dextroamphetamine and mixed amphetamine salts." These dosage ranges appear in the academy's practice parameter on the treatment of ADHD.[3,27]

Unfortunately optimizing ADHD-specific medication such as stimulant or atomoxetine is not universally effective for aggression and over half of youth with ADHD and ODD/CD need more than one medication for optimal symptom control.[77] The treatment of severe childhood aggression (TOSCA) study showed that adding risperidone 1 to 3 mg daily to parent training, behavioral therapy, and optimized stimulant in 168 youth (mean age 9) with ADHD and either ODD or CD resulted in moderate improvement in aggression. Adverse effects documented over the 9-week study included nausea, elevation in prolactin, and weight gain.[77]

ADHD and Tourette's Disorder ADHD occurs in 50% to 60% of youth with chronic tics or Tourette's disorder, and 20% of children with ADHD go on to develop chronic tics or Tourette's disorder.[24,84] Until recently, experts cautioned that stimulants should not be first-line treatments for ADHD in youth with tic disorders due to the stimulant's ability to increase central dopaminergic and noradrenergic activity, potentially exacerbating tics. There is less need for concern according to investigators who conducted a meta-analysis of 22 placebo-controlled trials involving 2,385 children with ADHD and Tourette's disorder. The analysis showed that stimulants were not more likely to worsen tics than placebo, and the association between stimulants and new-onset tics was more coincidental than a cause and effect relationship.[84] The timing of tic development in the context of ADHD may have led clinicians to inappropriately attribute new onset tics to stimulant treatment. Epidemiologic studies show that when ADHD and Tourette's co-occur, symptoms of ADHD present 2 to 3 years before tics emerge. Tourette's disorder is known for fluctuating symptom severity with tics worsening and remitting in an unpredictable pattern, further diminishing the ability to accurately attribute tic causality.[24,84]

A double-blind, placebo-controlled trial compared methylphenidate or clonidine monotherapy with combination methylphenidate and clonidine in patients with ADHD and Tourette's disorder. Combination therapy demonstrated the greatest benefit in reducing symptoms of ADHD and tics (P less than 0.0001).[4] Clonidine appeared most helpful for impulsivity and hyperactivity, whereas methylphenidate was most helpful for inattention. All treatments were well tolerated, but sedation was common (28%) in those receiving clonidine.[4]

Clonidine or guanfacine alone is a less effective alternative to stimulants in the treatment of children with Tourette's disorder and ADHD. Guanfacine was administered to 34 children (mean age 10.4 years), with ADHD and tic disorder during an 8-week, placebo-controlled trial at a dose of 1.5 to 3 mg/day. Tic severity decreased by 31% in the guanfacine group compared with 0% in the placebo group.[4] There was a mean improvement of 37% on the teacher-rated ADHD scale compared with 8% improvement with placebo.

Atomoxetine, when studied for 16 to 18 weeks, appears to be an effective treatment for ADHD and tics in pediatric patients with comorbid Tourette syndrome or chronic motor tic disorder. For instance, in 148 children and adolescents, randomized to up to 18 weeks of atomoxetine (0.5-1.5 mg/kg/day) or placebo, improvements were observed both in the severity of ADHD (effect size = 0.6) and tics (effect size = 0.3).[68]

Individuals with Tourette's disorder and ADHD are more prone to disruptive behaviors including poor frustration tolerance, aggression, and impulsivity, often requiring behavioral interventions and medications that may include second-generation antipsychotics.[24] Second-generation antipsychotics such as risperidone, aripiprazole, and ziprasidone have evidence from controlled trials to support their use in managing motor and vocal tics associated with Tourette disorder, however, aripiprazole is the only agent currently FDA-approved for managing Tourette's disorder.[24]

Personalized Pharmacotherapy

Factors that should be taken into account to personalize pharmacotherapy for ADHD include age, co-occurring conditions including substance abuse, effectiveness of treatment, side-effect sensitivities, and patient or family preference. An individual's ability to metabolize a drug and the drug's pharmacokinetic profile and drug-interaction potential should also be considered. To date, genomic studies have not provided information to guide clinical practice.

Pharmacokinetic and Drug Interactions

Methylphenidate is de-esterified prior to elimination and is less likely to have metabolic drug interactions compared with mixed amphetamine salts. Gender has been shown to influence the absorption of methylphenidate, with males having increased bioavailability compared with females.[50] Variability in dosage requirements for amphetamine salts, atomoxetine, and bupropion, can be due to interpatient variability in plasma concentration achieved at a given dose. All are metabolized via cytochrome P450 (CYP) 2D6, and bioavailability and half-life can be four to eight times greater in those taking a CYP2D6 inhibitor (eg, bupropion, fluoxetine, or paroxetine) or in poor metabolizers. For example, atomoxetine's half-life is 5 hours in extensive metabolizers and 19 hours in poor metabolizers.[4] Over time, dosage adjustments may be necessary for any medication in order to compensate for age-related changes in distribution and metabolism.

EVALUATION OF THERAPEUTIC OUTCOMES

Careful documentation of baseline symptoms and complaints over a 1-month predrug period is essential to the evaluation of therapeutic and adverse outcomes. Investigation regarding family history of psychiatric disorders and cardiac disease is essential to determine risk for related adverse drug reactions and to implement appropriate monitoring.[2,30] Baseline symptoms can be measured using videotapes, clinician rating scales (eg, ADHD Rating Scale IV, Vanderbilt ADHD Diagnostic Scale), or both. In addition, height, weight, and eating and sleeping patterns should be recorded at baseline and every 3 months.[4,27,30]

After the initiation and titration of any drug treatment, it is necessary that parents, teachers, and clinicians assess the overall functioning of the child or adult using standardized rating scales to determine if significant therapeutic benefit justifies continuing medication.[2,4,27] Therapeutic effects of the stimulants include decreased motor activity and impulsivity and increased attention span.[2,4,5,27] This suggests that stimulants are indicated for ADHD symptoms and not for primary learning disorders. The benefits of drug therapy must outweigh the potential for adverse effects to justify continued treatment.[2,4,27]

There is a lack of standardized assessment tools for adults; however, the adult ADHD screening tool can be useful.[32] Short-term studies (1 year or less) in adults with ADHD show that treatment with stimulants improves subjective quality of life. Long-term studies are needed to better assess the risk versus benefit of stimulant therapy on psychosocial and health outcomes.[85]

Atomoxetine, α_2-adrenergic agonists, and bupropion also require monitoring to detect changes in appetite, weight, and sleep patterns, as well as pulse and blood pressure. A therapeutic trial of atomoxetine or bupropion consists of 6 weeks at maximum tolerated doses unless response occurs at a lower dose.[2,4,27] Atomoxetine's full therapeutic benefit may continue to build over weeks to months, but if there is no significant benefit in the initial 6 weeks, it is unlikely that atomoxetine will be effective; therefore it can be tapered off.[68]

When guanfacine or clonidine is given, careful clinical monitoring for fatigue, dizziness, and autonomic changes (eg, blood pressure and pulse) is recommended.[30,60] The American Heart Association has stated that ECG monitoring is not required for α_2-adrenergic agonists treatment in children, although many clinicians continue to assess for ECG changes, particularly if there is a family history of cardiac disease, if the patient is taking other agents that impact cardiac function, or if clinical symptoms warrant.[30,45] When discontinuing treatment, clonidine and guanfacine should be withdrawn slowly (0.05 mg clonidine/0.5 mg guanfacine reductions every 3-7 days) to prevent rebound hypertension or behavioral dyscontrol.[59,60] A therapeutic trial requires 1 to 2 months to assess therapeutic response, although increased sleep usually occurs immediately.[59,60]

Evaluation of therapeutic outcomes is particularly important when antipsychotics are used in youth as the U.S. Office of Inspector general's peer review psychiatrists found quality of care concerns in 67% of 475 medical records of youth receiving antipsychotics through Medicaid.[86] Among the biggest problems were lack of appropriate indications and lack of appropriate monitoring to ensure safety. Baseline weight, lipids, and fasting glucose should be monitored every 6 months in addition to the need to monitor for extrapyramidal symptoms and hyperprolactinemia.[8,75,86]

ABBREVIATIONS

AAP	American Academy of Pediatrics
ADHD	attention deficit/hyperactivity disorder
ASD	autism spectrum disorder
CBT	cognitive behavioral therapy
CD	conduct disorder
CNS	central nervous system
CNV	copy number variants
CRS-revised	Connor's Rating Scales—revised
CYP	cytochrome P450
DMDD	disruptive mood dysregulation with dysphoria
DSM-5	*Diagnostic and Statistical Manual of Mental Disorders* (fifth edition)
ECG	electrocardiogram
FDA	Food and Drug Administration
GI	gastrointestinal
IEP	individualized educational program
MAO	monoamine oxidase
MTA	multimodal treatment study of children with ADHD
NIH	National Institutes of Health
NNT	number needed to treat
ODD	oppositional defiant disorder
OROS	osmotically released oral delivery system
SR	sustained release
TOSCA	Treatment of Severe Aggression Study
TCA	tricyclic antidepressant

REFERENCES

1. American Academy of Pediatrics, Subcommittee on Attention-Deficit/Hyperactivity Disorder, Steering Committee on Quality Improvement and Management. ADHD: Clinical practice guideline for the diagnosis, evaluation, and treatment of attention-deficit/hyperactivity disorder in children and adolescents. *Pediatrics* 2011;128:1007-1022.
2. American Academy of Pediatrics (AAP) Algorithm Pediatrics. Supplemental information: implementing the key action statements: An algorithm and explanation for process of care for the evaluation, diagnosis, treatment, and monitoring ADHD in children and adolescents. *Pediatrics* 2011;(suppl):S11-S21.
3. Wilens TE, Morrison NR, Prince J. An update on the pharmacotherapy of attention deficit/hyperactivity disorder in adults. *Expert Rev Neurother* 2011;11(10):1443-1465.
4. Dopheide JA, Pliszka SR. Attention deficit hyperactivity disorder: An update. *Pharmacotherapy* 2009;29(6):656-679.
5. Pliszka SR. Psychostimulants. In: Rosenberg DR, West GS, eds. *Pharmacotherapy of Child and Adolescent Psychiatric Disorders*. Sussex, UK: Wiley-Blackwell; 2012:65-104.
6. American Psychiatric Association. *Diagnostic and Statistical Manual of Mental Disorders*. Fifth Edition (DSM-5). Arlington, VA: American Psychiatric Publishing; 2013.
7. Childress AC, Barry SA. Pharmacotherapy of ADHD in Adolescents. *Drugs* 2012;72(3):309-325.
8. Texas Department of Family and Protective Services Web site. 2013. Psychotropic Medications. A Guide to Medical Services at CPS. (Utilization parameters for children and youth in foster care.) Available at: http://www.dfps.state.tx.us/Child_Protection/Medical_Services/guide-psychotropic.asp. Accessed May 7, 2015.
9. Molina BS, Pelham WE Jr. Attention-deficit/hyperactivity disorder and risk of substance use disorder: developmental considerations, potential pathways, and opportunities for research. *Annu Rev Clin Psychol* 2014;10:607-639.
10. Young S, Moss D, Sedgwick O, et al. A meta-analysis of the prevalence of attention deficit hyperactivity disorder in incarcerated populations. *Psychol Med* 2014;45:247-258.
11. Biederman J, Petty CR, Monuteaux MC, et al. Adult psychiatric outcomes of girls with ADHD: 11 year follow-up in a longitudinal case-control study. *Am J Psychiatry* 2010;167:409-417.
12. Polanczyk G, Willcutt EG, Salum GA, et al. ADHD prevalence estimates across three decades: an updated systematic review and meta-regression analysis. *Int J Epidemiol* 2014;43(2):434-442.
13. Bloom B, Jones LI, Freeman G. Summary health statistics for U.S. children: National Health Interview Survey, 2012. National Center for Health Statistics. *Vital Health Stat 10* (258). 2013.
14. Chai G, Governale L, McMahon AW, et al. Trends of outpatient prescribing in US children, 2002-2010. *Pediatrics* 2012;130(1):23-31.
15. Visser SN, Danielson MLL, Bitsko RH, et al. Trends in the parent-report of health care provider-diagnosed and medicated ADHD: United States, 2003-2011. *J Am Acad Child Adolesc Psychiatry* 2014;53(1):34-46.
16. Austerman J, Muzina DJ. US Medication Trends for ADHD: An Express Scripts Report. Available at: http://lab.express-scripts.com/publications/turning-attention-to-adhd-report. March 2014, Accessed on August 28, 2015.
17. Thapar A, Cooper M, Jefferies R, et al. What causes attention deficit hyperactivity disorder? *Arch Dis Child* 2012;97:260-265.
18. Friedman LA, Rapoport JL. Brain development in ADHD. *Curr Opin Neurobiol* 2015;30:106-111.
19. Stergiakouli E, Martin J, Hamshere ML, et al. Shared genetic influences between ADHD traits in children and clinical ADHD. *J Am Acad Child Adolesc Psych* 2015;54(4):322-327.
20. Williams NM, Franke B, Mick E, et al. Genome-wide analysis of copy number variants in attention deficit hyperactivity disorder: The role of rare variants and duplications at 15q13.3. *Am J Psychiatry* 2012;169:195-204.
21. Scerif G, Baker K. Annual research review: Rare genotypes and childhood psychopathology uncovering diverse developmental mechanisms of ADHD risk. *J Child Psychology and Psychiatry* 2015;56(3):251-273.
22. Elia J, Glessner JT, Wang K, et al. Genome-wide copy number variation study associates metabotropic glutamate receptor gene networks with attention deficit hyperactivity disorder. *Nat Genet* 2012;44:78-84.

23. van der Meer JM, Oerlemens AM, van Steijn DJ, et al. Are autism spectrum disorder and attention-deficit/hyperactivity disorder different manifestations of one overarching disorder? Cognitive and symptom evidence from a clinical and population-based sample. *J Am Acad Child Adolesc Psychiatry* 2012;51(11):1160-1172.
24. Murphy TK, Lewin AB, Storch EA, et al. Practice parameter for the assessment and treatment of children and adolescents with tic disorders. *J Am Acad Child Adolesc Psychiatry* 2013;52(12):1341-1359.
25. Cubillo A, Halari R, Smith A, et al. A review of fronto-striatal and fronto-cortical brain abnormalities in children and adults with attention deficit hyperactivity disorder (ADHD) and new evidence for dysfunction in adults with ADHD during motivation and attention. *Cortex* 2012;48:194-215.
26. Proal E, Riesse PT, Klein RT, et al. Brain gray matter deficits at 33-year follow-up in adults with ADHD established in childhood. *Arch Gen Psychiatry* 2011;68(11):1122-1134.
27. Pliszka SR, Bernet W, Bukstein O, et al. American Academy of Child and Adolescent Psychiatry Work Group on Quality Issues. Practice parameter for the assessment and treatment of children and adolescents with ADHD. *J Am Acad Child Adolesc Psychiatry* 2007;46:894-921.
28. Dopheide JA. Autism Spectrum Disorder. In: Eiland LS, Todd TJ eds. *Advanced Pediatric Therapeutics*. Pediatric Pharmacy Advocacy Group, Memphis, TN: Allen press copyright; 2015:1-8.
29. Kaplan A, Adesman A. Clinical diagnosis and management of ADHD in preschool children. *Curr Opin Pediatr* 2011;23:684-692.
30. Schneider BN, Enenbach M. Managing the risks of ADHD treatment. *Curr Psychiatry Reports* 2014;479:1-8.
31. Brownlie EB, Lazare K, Beitchman J. Validating a self-report screen for ADHD in early adulthood using child and teacher ratings. *J Atten Disord* 2012;16(6):467-477.
32. New York University Medical School, Harvard Medical School, World Health Organization. *Adult ADHD Self-Report Scale (ASRS-v1.1) Symptom Checklist Instructions*. Available at: http://webdoc.nyumc.org/nyumc/files/psych/attachments/psych_adhd_checklist.pdf. Accessed August 29, 2015.
33. Watson SM, Richels C, Michalek AP, Raymer A. Psychosocial treatments for ADHD: A systemic appraisal of the evidence. *J Atten Disord* 2015;19(1):3-10.
34. Safren SA, Sprich S, Mimiaga MJ, et al. Cognitive behavioral therapy vs. relaxation with educational support for medication-treated adults with ADHD and persistent symptoms. *JAMA* 2010;304(8):875-880.
35. Pelham WE, Burrows-MacLean, Gnagy EM, et al. A dose-ranging study of behavioral and pharmacological treatment in social settings for children with ADHD. *J Abnorm Child Psychol* 2014;42:1009-1031.
36. Hirvikovski T, Waaler E, Alfredsson J, et al. Reduced ADHD symptoms in adults with ADHD after structured skills training group: Results from a randomized controlled trial. *Behav Res Ther* 2011;49:175-185.
37. Kaplan G, Newcorn JH. Pharmacotherapy for child and adolescent attention-deficit hyperactivity disorder. *Pediatr Clin North Am* 2011;58:99-120.
38. Solanto MV, Marks DJ, Wasserstein J, et al. Efficacy of meta-cognitive therapy for ADHD. *Am J Psychiatry* 2010;167:958-968.
39. Bader A, Adesman A. Complementary and alternative therapies for children and adolescents with ADHD. *Current Opinion in Pediatrics* 2012;24(6):760-769.
40. Turner CA, Xie D, Zimmerman BM, Carlarge CA. Iron status in toddlerhood predicts sensitivity to psychostimulants in children. *J Atten Disord* 2012;16(4) 295-303.
41. Millichap JG, Yee MM. The diet factor in attention deficit hyperactivity disorder. *Pediatrics* 2012;129:330-337.
42. Swanson JM, Arnold LE, Kraemer H, et al. Evidence, interpretation, and qualification from multiple reports of long-term outcomes in the Multimodal Treatment study of Children With ADHD (MTA): Part I: Executive summary. *J Atten Disord* 2008;12:4-14.
43. Molina BSG, Hinshaw SP, Swanson JM, et al. The MTA at 8-years: Prospective follow-up of children treated for combined-type ADHD in a multisite study. *J Am Acad Child Adolesc Psychiatry* 2009;48(5):484-500.
44. Mikolajczyk R, Horn J, Biomath D, et al. Injury prevention by medication among children with ADHD: A case-only study. *JAMA Pediatrics* 2015;169(4):391-395.
45. Dalsgaard S, Nielsen HS, Simonsen M. Consequences of ADHD medication use for children's outcomes. *J of Health Economics* 2014;37:137-151.
46. Scheffler RM, Brown TT, Fulton BD, et al. Positive association between attention-deficit/hyperactivity disorder medication use and academic achievement during elementary school. *Pediatrics* 2009;123:1273-1279.
47. Gualitieri CT, Johnson L. Medications do not necessarily normalize cognition in ADHD patients. *J Atten Disord* 2008;11:459-469.
48. Brams M, Moon E, Pucci M, et al. Duration of effect of long-acting stimulant preparations throughout the day. *Curr Med Res Opin* 2010;26(8):1809-1825.
49. Wilens TE. Mechanism of agents used for ADHD. *J Clin Psychiatry* 2006;67(Suppl 8):32-37.
50. Ermer JC, Adeyi BA, Pucci ML. Pharmacokinetic variability of long-acting stimulants in the treatment of children and adults with attention-deficit hyperactivity disorder. *CNS Drugs* 2010;24:1009-1025.
51. Faraone SV, Glatt SJ. A comparison of the efficacy of medications for adult ADHD using meta-analyses of effect sizes. *J Clin Psychiatry* 2010;71(6):754-763.
52. Quillivant XR—an extended release oral suspension of methylphenidate. *Med Lett Drugs Ther* 2013;55(1409):10-11.
53. Palli SR, Kamble PS, Chen H, Aparasu RR. Persistence of stimulants in children and adolescents with attention-deficit/hyperactivity disorder. *J Child Adolesc Psychopharmacol* 2012;22(2):139-148.
54. Clavenna A, Bonati M. Safety of medicines used for ADHD in children. *Arch Dis Child* 2014;99:866-872.
55. U.S. Food and Drug Administration Drug Safety Communication—Methylphenidate. Available at: http://www.fda.gov/Drugs/DrugSafety/InformationbyDrugClass/ucm283449.htm reports of priapism and leukoderma. Accessed November 1, 2015.
56. Mosholder AD, Gelperin K, Hammad TA, et al. Hallucinations and other psychotic symptoms associated with the use of ADHD drugs in children. *Pediatrics* 2009;123(2):611-616.
57. Kraemer M, Uekerman J, Wiltfang J, et al. Methylphenidate-induced psychosis in adult ADHD: Report of 3 new cases and review of the literature. *Clin Neuropharmacol* 2010;33(4):204-206.
58. Johnson KA, Barry E, Lambert D, et al. Methylphenidate side effect profile is influenced by genetic variation in the ADHD-Associated CES1 Gene. *J Child and Adolescent Psychopharmacology* 2013;23(10):655-664.
59. Faraone SV, McBurnett K, Sallee FR, et al. Guanfacine extended release: A novel treatment for ADHD in children and adolescents. *Clin Therapeutics* 2013;35(11):1778-1793.
60. Hirota T, Schwartz S, Correll CU. Alpha-2 agonists for attention-deficit/hyperactivity disorder in youth: a systematic review and meta-analysis of monotherapy and add-on trials to stimulant therapy. *J Am Acad Child Adolesc Psychiatry* 2014;53(2):153-173.
61. Guanfacine extended release package insert. Available at: www.Intuniv.com, Intuniv-Shire, Wayne PA, U.S. Inc. Accessed November 1, 2015.
62. Fredriksen M, Halmoy A, Faraone SV, et al. Long-term efficacy and safety of treatment with stimulants and atomoxetine in adult ADHD: A review of controlled and naturalistic studies. *European Neuropsychopharmacol* 2013;23:508-527.
63. Cooper WO, Habel LA, Sox CM, et al. ADHD drugs and serious cardiovascular events in children and young adults. *N Engl J Med* 2011;365:1896-1904.
64. Habel LA, Cooper WO, Sox CM, et al. ADHD medications and risk of serious cardiovascular events in young and middle-aged adults. *JAMA* 2011;306(24):2673-2683.
65. Dalsgaard S, Kvist AP, Leckman JF, et al. Cardiovascular safety of stimulants in children with ADHD: A nationwide prospective cohort study. *J Child Adolescent Psychopharmacology* 2014;24(6):302-310.
66. Blader JC, Pliszka SR, Jensen PS, et al. Stimulant response and stimulant refractory aggressive behavior. *Pediatrics* 2010;126:e796-e806.
67. Wietecha LA, Ruff DD, Allen AJ, et al. Atomoxetine tolerability in pediatric and adult patients receiving different dosing schedules. *J Clin Psychiatry* 2013;74(12):1217-1223.
68. Savill NC, Buitelaar JK, Anand E, et al. The efficacy of atomoxetine for the treatment of children and adolescents with attention-deficit/hyperactivity disorder: A comprehensive review of over a decade of clinical research. *CNS Drugs* 2015;29(2):131-151.
69. Lin DY, Kratochvil CJ, Xu W, et al. A randomized trial of edivoxetine in pediatric patients with attention-deficit/hyperactivity disorder. *J Child Adolesc Psychopharmacol* 2014;24(4):190-200.
70. Erdogen A, Ozcay F, Piskin E. Idiosyncratic liver failure probably associated with atomoxetine. *J Child Adolesc Psychopharmacol* 2011;21(2):295-297.
71. Dopheide JA. Recognizing and treating depression in children and adolescents. *Am J Health Syst Pharm* 2006;63:233-243.
72. Geller B, Tillman R, Bolhofner K, et al. Pharmacologic and non-drug treatment of child bipolar 1 disorder during prospective 8-year follow-up. *Bipolar Disord* 2010;12:164-171.

73. Carlson GA, Klein DN. How to understand divergent views on bipolar disorder in youth. *Annu Rev Clin Psychology* 2014;10:529-551.
74. Blader JC, Schooler NR, Jensen PS, et al. Adjunctive divalproex versus placebo for children with ADHD and aggression refractory to stimulant monotherapy. *Am J Psychiatry* 2009;166:1392-1401.
75. Seida JC, Schouten JR, Boylan K, et al. Antipsychotics for children and young adults: A comparative effectiveness review. *Pediatrics* 2012;129:e771-e784.
76. Linton D, Barr AM, Honer WG, Procyshyn RM. Antipsychotic and psychostimulant drug combination therapy in attention deficit/hyperactivity and disruptive behavior disorders: A systematic review of efficacy and tolerability. *Curr Psychiatry Rep* 2013;15(5):355.
77. Aman MG, Bukstein OG, Gadow KD, et al. What does risperidone add to parent training and stimulant for severe aggression in child ADHD? *J Am Acad Child Adolesc Psychiatry* 2014;53(1):47-60.
78. Calarge CA, Burns TL, Schlechte JA, et al. Longitudinal examination of the skeletal effects of selective serotonin reuptake inhibitors and risperidone. *J Clin Psychiatry* 2015;76(5):607-613.
79. Dopheide J. Autism Spectrum Disorder. In: Eiland L & Todd T, eds. *Advanced Pediatric Therapeutics*. Published by Pediatric Pharmacy Advocacy Group (PPAG) copyright; 2015: Chapter 36.
80. Harstad E, Levy S. Committee on Substance Abuse. Attention-deficit/hyperactivity disorder and substance abuse. *Pediatrics* 2014;134(1):e293-e301.
81. Wilens TE, Morrison NR. The intersection of ADHD and substance abuse. *Curr Opin Psychiatry* 2011;24:280-285.
82. Rabiner DL. Stimulant prescription cautions: Addressing misuse, diversion and malingering. *Curr Psychiatry Rep* 2013;15(7):375.
83. Heck NC, Livingston NA, Flentje A, et al. Reducing risk for illicit drug use and prescription drug misuse: High school gay-straight alliances and lesbian, gay, bisexual, and transgender youth. *Addict Behav* 2014;39(4):824-828.
84. Cohen SC, Mulqueen JM, Ferracioli-Oda, et al. Meta-analysis: Risk of tics associated with psychostimulant use in randomized placebo-controlled trials. *J Am Acad Child Adolesc Psychiatry* 2015;54(9):728-736.
85. Surman CBH, Hammerness PG, Pion K, et al. Do stimulants improve functioning in adults with ADHD: a review of the literature. *European Neuropsychopharmacology* 2013;23:528-533.
86. Department of Health and Human Services (HHS), Office of Inspector General. *Second-Generation Antipsychotic Drug Use among Medicaid-Enrolled Children: Quality of Care Concerns*. HHS Web site. Available at: https://oig.hhs.gov/oei/reports/oei-07-12-00320.pdf. Accessed March 15, 2015.

Eating Disorders

64

Steven C. Stoner and Valerie L. Ruehter

KEY CONCEPTS

1. Eating disorders, while no longer considered a controversial psychiatric illness, remain difficult to treat, as comparative effectiveness trials are limited, study methods and outcome measures vary, and patients are often resistant to accepting treatment.
2. The fifth edition of the *Diagnostic and Statistical Manual of Mental Disorders* (DSM-5) separates binge-eating disorder (BED) as an individual eating disorder diagnosis and replaces the category of Eating Disorders Not Otherwise Specified with Specified and Unspecified Feeding and Eating Disorders.
3. Despite strong genetic associations for the development of eating disorders as established in monozygotic and dizygotic twin studies, a clear association with a specific genetic linkage or mutation has not been identified.
4. Shifting between eating disorder diagnostic categories is possible, especially when symptom remission is not achieved with treatment.
5. Psychiatric comorbidities are common with all forms of eating disorders, and the differential diagnosis should generally include evaluation for depression, schizophrenia, generalized anxiety, obsessive–compulsive disorder (OCD), and personality disorders.
6. During the process of caloric restoration, calories must be gradually introduced to prevent the potentially fatal complication known as refeeding syndrome. Failure to restore calories quickly enough may result in an unfeeding syndrome.
7. Mortality resulting from suicide in individuals with eating disorders is not uncommon, and clinicians must monitor closely for suicidality and educate appropriately as they would during the treatment of patients with major depressive disorder taking antidepressants.
8. The current preferred treatment approach for anorexia nervosa (AN) includes a minimum of 6 months of psychotherapy, preferably cognitive behavioral therapy (CBT) in adults and family-based therapy in children.
9. Despite limited data, antidepressants are the preferred pharmacologic intervention for the acute and maintenance phases of bullemia nervosa (BN) in combination with nonpharmacologic treatments.
10. There is growing sentiment that severe and enduring AN exists and that the focus should be on the impact of the disorder and improving quality of life instead of on treating medical symptoms.

Eating disorders are widely accepted as serious mental illnesses. The spectrum of eating disorders encompasses several complex diseases, with most sharing the pathologic feature of over-evaluation of body shape and weight. Eating disorders arise from the complex interaction between environmental, societal, developmental, psychosocial, genetic, and biologic factors. It is estimated that 5 to 10 million women and 1 million men in the United States alone have an eating disorder. The urbanization of society, social pressure, and obsession with perfection and being thin have led to an increasing prevalence of eating disorders, with a median age of onset between 18 and 21 years, though estimates in adolescent studies suggest median ages of onset between 12 and 13 years.[1,2] Anorexia nervosa (AN), bulimia nervosa (BN), and binge-eating disorder (BED) are the most prevalent forms of eating disorders.[3]

1 Despite an improved understanding of these cognitively and emotionally disabling and potentially fatal disorders, treatment remains difficult. Pharmacologic intervention is a small part of a comprehensive treatment plan that emphasizes psychotherapy, notably cognitive behavioral therapy (CBT) in adults and family therapy in younger patients.

EPIDEMIOLOGY

Anorexia Nervosa

Anorexia nervosa impacts an estimated 0.9% to 2% of women in the United States, occurring predominantly in girls and young women (90%), and usually presenting during adolescent years (median onset 12.3 years of age).[1,2] The estimated 12-month prevalence of the disorder in the general population is 0.4% of females with a smaller percentage in males.[2,3] Longitudinal management of AN is difficult, as patients are often resistant to weight restoration plans, and psychiatric comorbidities exist in over 50% of those with AN.[2] Rates of relapse requiring hospitalization within 1 year exceed 30%, and crude mortality rates are estimated at 5%.[3-5]

The promotion of the virtues of being thin is also a potentially negative environmental factor. Many internet and online communities inappropriately promote healthy lifestyle aspects of anorexia and being thin as a means of being in control and successful, while also serving as a means of support.[6]

Bulimia Nervosa

Bulimia Nervosa also occurs predominantly in girls and young women (90%) and usually presents in later adolescence or early adult life.[2] Between 1% and 4.6% of adolescent and young adult females meet the diagnostic criteria for BN, with lifetime prevalence estimates of 1.5% of females and 0.5% of men.[1-3,7,8]

Binge-Eating Disorder

Binge-Eating Disorder often presents in adolescence but can also present later in life.[3] BED is more common in females with a lifetime prevalence of 2.8% in adults and 1.6% in adolescents.[1,9] The 12-month prevalence rate is an estimated 1.6% in females and 0.8% in males.[3,10] CBT and interpersonal psychotherapy are the preferred treatments, although antidepressants and lisdexamfetamine have demonstrated benefits.[11]

Other Specified and Unspecified Feeding and Eating Disorders

2 According to the DSM-5, the new categories of Specified and Unspecified Feeding and Eating Disorders apply to cases where symptoms result in distress, but do not meet full diagnostic criteria for any feeding or eating disorders.[3] Examples listed within these categories include atypical AN, BN (lower frequency), BED (lower frequency), purging disorder, and night eating syndrome (NES).[3]

Night eating syndrome is common in obesity clinic populations, often accompanied by depressive symptoms. The syndrome is defined by repetitive night eating that includes eating after having been asleep or excessive food consumption following evening meals.[3,12] NES affects an estimated 1.5% of the general population with a high prevalence of obesity and psychiatric comorbidities.[13] Patients with NES are reported to benefit from antidepressant therapy, most notably sertraline 50 to 200 mg daily or escitalopram 5 to 20 mg daily.[12,14]

Additionally, DSM-5 includes Pica, Avoidant/Restrictive Food Intake Disorder, and Rumination Disorder as stand-alone diagnoses' within Feeding and Eating Disorders.[3]

ETIOLOGY AND PATHOPHYSIOLOGY

The exact etiology of eating disorders remains unknown; however it is most likely a combination of genetic, biologic, developmental, and environmental factors. The biologic basis for eating disorders is difficult to delineate because it is unclear if the biologic changes are caused by or are a result of the aberrant eating behavior.

Structural and functional brain imaging studies utilizing computerized tomography (CT) and magnetic resonance imaging (MRI) have yielded a number of inconclusive findings. AN has been linked with the development of enlarged cortical sulci, ventricles, inter-hemispheric fissure and reductions in grey matter (amygdala, hippocampus, cingulate cortex, and putamen). Findings examining white matter volume changes have not produced consistent results.[15] Dystrophic abnormalities in the cerebrum have also been noted with weight loss, though normalization occurs with weight gain.[15] Abnormalities of the hypothalamic–pituitary–gonadal, hypothalamic–pituitary–adrenal, and hypothalamic–pituitary–thyroid axes are described as potential causes of AN. Amenorrhea is found in the majority of females with anorexia, providing support for the association with gonadotropin; however amenorrhea as a required symptom was removed with the release of DSM-5.[3,8]

Serotonin, norepinephrine, and dopamine have been studied extensively with well-described roles in controlling eating behaviors. Special emphasis has been placed on the role of serotonin (5-HT), specifically noting reduced cerebrospinal fluid (CSF) basal concentrations of 5-hydroxyindoleacetic acid (5-HIAA), the principle metabolite of 5-HT, as well as increased binding of 5-HT_{1A} receptors and reduced binding of 5-HT_{2A} receptors in different regions within the central nervous system (CNS). Reduced dietary intake of certain foods leads to reduced levels of tryptophan, which is required for the development of 5-HT.[16-18] There is evidence suggesting that 5-HT and dopamine function remain abnormal after weight restoration, with 5-HT activity being abnormally high in patients recovered from AN, while 5-HT_{2A} receptors are reduced and dopamine receptors are increased following recovery.[16-18]

Complicating the study of these abnormalities is that their dysfunction is thought to be secondary to weight loss. Another molecular genetic target of study is brain-derived neurotrophic factor (BDNF), which is also being studied in other diseases such as depression.[18]

3 There are strong genetic influences in AN and likely associations in both BN and BED. In addition, there is a high degree of premorbid anxiety and obsessive tendencies, which are also symptoms of disorders with suspected genetic associations. Twin studies have shown concordance of ~55% and 35% in monozygotic twins and 5% and 30% in dizygotic twins for AN and BN, respectively.

Genetic-based linkage studies have examined multiple single nucleotide peptides to identify predictors for developing AN, which may subsequently help identify appropriate pharmacologic treatments. Studies to date have identified possible associations with chromosomes #1, #2, #3, #4, and #13; however, there are no consistent findings to date, and studies are limited by low sample size.[16,19,20] Genetic mutation studies have focused on polymorphisms of the 5-HT_{2A} receptor.[21] One acquired hereditary abnormality being studied is the presence of low-function alleles associated with the 5-HT transporter (*5-HTTLPR*) and 5-HT_{2A} receptor gene (*–1438G/A*), with findings suggesting an association with poor treatment response.[22] Recent work has also associated estrogen receptor I gene (ESRI) with the restrictive form of AN.[23]

Emphasis is also placed on environmental factors such as social stress and psychological and developmental issues related to dysfunctional family relationships that may trigger abnormal eating behaviors. Athletes are at risk for eating disorders, especially female gymnasts, ballet dancers, figure skaters, distance runners, swimmers, male wrestlers, and body builders.[24]

DIAGNOSTIC CRITERIA AND CLINICAL PRESENTATION

Anorexia nervosa and BN occur together in ~30% to 64% of patients with eating disorders, thus appearing as a continuum of symptoms making careful medical and psychiatric assessment at baseline essential.[25] 4 Patients who initially present with either AN or BN may alternate from one to the other, especially in cases where remission is not achieved. Figure 64-1 demonstrates similar and unique features of both disorders.

The use of purging methods is not limited to BN. Self-induced vomiting is the most common form of purging behavior.[26] Laxative abuse is another form of purging common in both AN and BN, used by an estimated 3% to 70% of patients.[26-28] Although ineffective as a weight-loss strategy, laxative abuse is often used in combination with other behaviors, including exercise, diuretics, enemas, and saunas. Within the diagnostic framework of AN, laxative abuse is most common in those identified with the purging subtype.[26] Psychiatric symptoms of depression, anxiety, and borderline personality disorder are also reported in those who abuse laxatives.[26-28]

Depression, schizophrenia, obsessive–compulsive disorder (OCD), and conversion disorders should be included in the differential diagnosis of AN, BN, and BED as eating abnormalities can be a component or share similar symptoms of these illnesses. The salient differences are the overriding drive for thinness, disturbed body image, increased energy directed at losing weight, and binge eating episodes that are relatively specific for eating disorders. Most patients with eating disorders experience relief of psychiatric symptoms on refeeding.[10]

Anorexia Nervosa

The presentation of AN includes a recent period of weight loss as well as associated behaviors to promote this such as vomiting, limiting food intake, and excessive exercise. Current diagnostic criteria for AN include the restriction of energy intake relative to requirements that leads to low body weight contextually as it relates to age, sex, developmental trajectory, and physical health.[3] The *DSM-5*

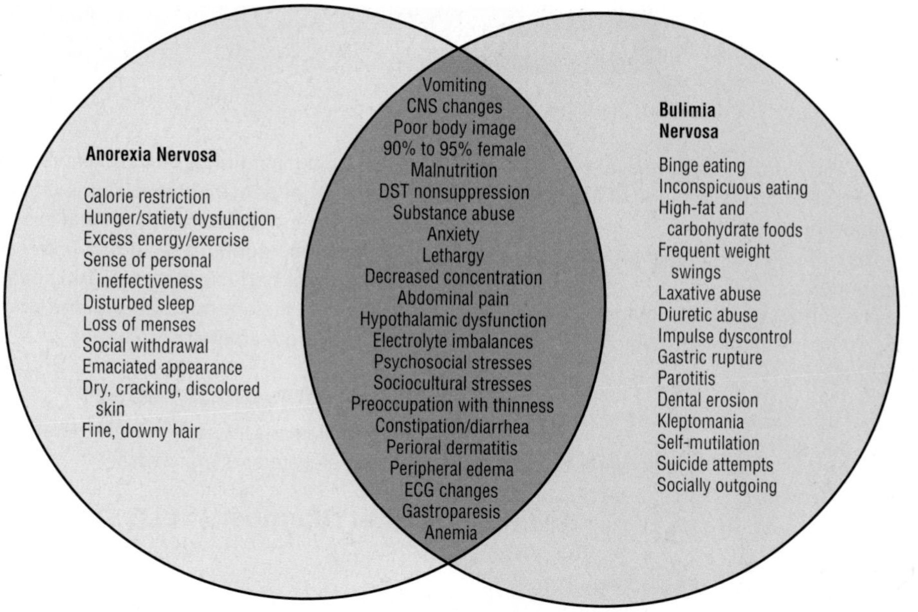

Anorexia Nervosa

Calorie restriction
Hunger/satiety dysfunction
Excess energy/exercise
Sense of personal ineffectiveness
Disturbed sleep
Loss of menses
Social withdrawal
Emaciated appearance
Dry, cracking, discolored skin
Fine, downy hair

Vomiting
CNS changes
Poor body image
90% to 95% female
Malnutrition
DST nonsuppression
Substance abuse
Anxiety
Lethargy
Decreased concentration
Abdominal pain
Hypothalamic dysfunction
Electrolyte imbalances
Psychosocial stresses
Sociocultural stresses
Preoccupation with thinness
Constipation/diarrhea
Perioral dermatitis
Peripheral edema
ECG changes
Gastroparesis
Anemia

Bulimia Nervosa

Binge eating
Inconspicuous eating
High-fat and carbohydrate foods
Frequent weight swings
Laxative abuse
Diuretic abuse
Impulse dyscontrol
Gastric rupture
Parotitis
Dental erosion
Kleptomania
Self-mutilation
Suicide attempts
Socially outgoing

FIGURE 64-1 Signs and symptoms of anorexia nervosa and bulimia nervosa. (DST, dexamethasone suppression test; ECG, electrocardiogram.)

further classifies AN as restricting type (restricting food intake with no binge eating or purging behavior over the past 3 months) or binge eating/purging type, in which patients regularly participate in bingeing or purging over the prior 3 months.[3] The severity of AN is based upon body mass index (BMI) in adults and BMI percentiles in children and adolescents. Comorbid psychiatric conditions, such as major depression, are frequent but should initially be considered secondary to starvation and not a true mood disorder. Specific risk factors for AN include being female, having a sibling with AN, the presence of mood disorders in family members, and co-morbid anxiety, personality, or substance use disorders.[29]

5 Psychiatric comorbidity is common, as up to 75% of patients have a primary mood disorder, and there is also an association with personality disorders (eg, oppositional defiant disorder) and anxiety disorders, such as social phobia and OCD.[2,30] The lifetime prevalence of OCD in patients with AN is reported to be as high as 40% compared to 2.5% in the general population.[30-32] The impact that psychiatric comorbidity has on treatment outcomes of AN is unknown, but it is important to understand that deprivation of food may contribute to both mood and cognitive fluctuations.

Bulimia Nervosa

The core feature of BN is recurrent episodes of binge eating (an excessive intake of calorie-laden food over a short period of time). Most have normal weight, although they might fluctuate between being underweight and overweight. Patients lack control over their eating and participate in recurrent compensatory behavior to prevent weight gain. These behaviors may include self-induced vomiting;

CLINICAL PRESENTATION Anorexia Nervosa

General

- Restriction of energy intake that leads to low body weight and self-evaluation that is influenced by perceptions of weight and body shape.

Symptoms

- Patients have obsessions and fears about eating and gaining weight.
- They complain about feeling full even when they have eaten very little food.
- Denial of symptoms, failure to recognize low body weight, and low self-esteem.
- Patients often feel ineffective and have a lack of self-control.

Signs

- Weakness, lethargy, cachexia, amenorrhea, vomiting, restricted food intake, inappropriate exercise, delayed sexual development, edema, delayed gastric emptying, constipation, abdominal pain, bradycardia, hypotension, osteoporosis, dry cracking skin, lanugo, callus on dorsum of hand, cold intolerance, perioral dermatitis, and erosion of dental enamel.

Laboratory Abnormalities

- Hypokalemia, hypochloremia, hypothyroidism, hypophosphatemia, hypokalemic alkalosis, hypomagnesemia, metabolic acidosis, blood urea nitrogen, hepatic enzymes, leukopenia, thrombocytopenia, anemia, QT interval prolongation, bradycardia, hypercholesterolemia, and bone mineral density.

Other Diagnostic Tests

- Nonspecific electroencephalogram (EEG) changes.

CLINICAL PRESENTATION Bulimia Nervosa

General

- Patients binge eat and stop when they have abdominal pain or self-induced vomiting or are interrupted by another person.
- They have a pattern of severe dieting followed by binge eating episodes.
- They are concerned about their body image but do not have the drive to thinness, which is a characteristic of AN.

Symptoms

- Patients do not eat regular meals and do not feel satiety at the end of a meal.
- They may use purging methods such as laxatives for weight control.
- They have guilt, depression, and self-disparagement after binges.
- Social isolation can result from frequent bingeing.
- Chaotic and troubled personal relationships and substance abuse are common.

Signs

- Bingeing, vomiting, salivary gland inflammation, erosion of dental enamel, callus on dorsum of hand, perioral dermatitis, dental caries, parotid gland enlargement, abdominal pain, upper end of normal body weight or slightly overweight, frequent weight fluctuations, and diminished masticatory ability.

Laboratory Abnormalities

- Hypokalemia, hypochloremic metabolic acidosis, and elevated serum amylase.

Other Diagnostic Tests

- None

misuse of laxatives, diuretics, enemas, or other medications; strict dieting or fasting; or excessive exercise. To meet *DSM-5* criteria, the binges and compensatory behaviors must occur on average at least once weekly for 3 months.[3] BN can further be differentiated by purging type (regularly engages in self-induced vomiting or the misuse of laxatives, diuretics, or enemas) or non-purging type (uses other inappropriate compensatory behaviors, such as fasting or excessive exercise, but does not engage in purging activities).[3]

Patients typically binge and vomit at least once daily. Caloric intake varies, but patients can consume between 5,000 and 20,000 cal (20,920 and 83,680 J) during a single binge. Patients tend to consume foods that are easy to ingest, do not require much chewing or preparation, and are high in carbohydrates or fat. Binge eating is typically secretive and precipitated by a stressful event, followed by post-binge remorse. Binges often last less than 2 hours but can extend to more than 8 hours. To compensate for the excessive caloric intake, many patients fast for prolonged periods, exercise compulsively, purge, or abuse laxatives.

Psychiatric comorbidity includes depression (up to 80%), poor impulse control, and substance abuse. Approximately 30% to 37% of bulimic patients have a personal history of substance abuse.[33] Kleptomania and borderline and avoidant personality disorders are also frequently observed.[30,34] Patients also commonly steal laxatives and comfort items, such as candies and clothes.[8]

Binge-Eating Disorder

Patients with BED present with recurrent episodes of bingeing without the compensatory behaviors associated with AN or BN. It is estimated that 5% to 10% of patients seeking treatment for obesity have BED. Comorbid psychotic disorders are common and reported in greater than 70% of BED patients. Depression and low self-esteem are common, but self-deprecating focus on body image is less severe than in AN or BN.[32,35] Diagnostic criteria for BED requires recurrent episodes of binge eating (eating an amount of food in a specific period of time that is larger than what most people would eat in a similar situation and a sense of lack of control over eating during the episode).[3] The binge-eating episodes are required to be associated with at least three of the following: eating more rapidly than normal; eating until feeling uncomfortably full; eating large amounts of food when not physically hungry; eating alone because of embarrassment of how much is being eaten; and feeling disgusted with oneself, depressed, or guilty after the episode. The severity of BED is determined by the number of binge-eating episodes per week (1-3 = mild; 4-7 = moderate; 8-13 = severe; 14 or more = extreme).[3]

MEDICAL COMPLICATIONS OF EATING DISORDERS

The potential medical complications of eating disorders involve multiple organ systems. The type of medical complication encountered is dependent on the type and frequency of the eating disorder behavior. Cardiac complications may occur and can include arrhythmias such as sinus bradycardia, cardiac muscle atrophy, orthostatic hypotension, decreased cardiac output, arrhythmia, and QTc interval prolongation.[36,37] 6 During caloric restoration, there is a potential risk for developing refeeding syndrome, which can progress to fatal cardiovascular collapse. This risk is reduced by the gradual versus rapid reintroduction of calories.

Metabolic (metabolic acidosis and metabolic alkalosis) and electrolyte disturbances (eg, hypokalemia, hypomagnesemia, and hypocalcemia) and dehydration are often seen. Elevations in bicarbonate levels during periods of hypokalemia can be an indication that the patient is inducing vomiting or using dietary weight-loss medications. Non-anion-gap acidosis has also been reported with the abuse of laxative agents. Additionally, both acute and chronic renal failures have been reported.

Gastrointestinal (GI), oropharyngeal, and dental complications are frequent, as are general complaints of lethargy and fatigue. Evidence of Russell's sign may be present signified by skin lesions on the fingers used to induce vomiting.

Hormonal changes related to the hypothalamic–pituitary–gonadal axis resulting from starvation are seen. These abnormalities include effects on estradiol, the gonadotropins (eg, luteinizing hormone, follicle-stimulating hormone, and gonadotropin-releasing hormone), thyroid function, adrenal function, and growth

CLINICAL PRESENTATION Binge-Eating Disorder

General

- Repeated episodes of binge-eating that includes a lack of self-control and eating an amount of food that is beyond what most people would eat.
- Episodes of binge-eating may include rapid eating, a sense of fullness to the point of being uncomfortable, eating when not hungry, eating alone secondary to feeling embarrassed, and a sense of self-disgust, depression, or guilt.

Symptoms

- Episodes of binge-eating
- Lack of self-control
- Rapid consumption of food
- Feeling full and eating when not hungry
- Isolation and guilt/depression

Signs

- Obesity
- History of weight loss followed by weight gain
- Binge-eating without compensatory purging
- Psychiatric (eg, depression, anxiety) and medical complications (eg, GERD, hypertension) are not uncommon.

Laboratory Abnormalities

- Elevated lipids, glucose, and hemoglobin A1C, abnormal electrolytes, increased weight.

Other Diagnostic Tests

- None

hormone.[8,36] Specific to female athletes is the female athlete triad, defined by the development of irregular menses, osteoporosis, and disordered eating.[36,38] An athlete may experience only one or two components of the triad, or all three.[39] Osteopenia and osteoporosis are potential long-term complications of suppressed estrogen. The restoration of weight, specifically in AN, reverses the bone loss, although estrogen supplementation does not appear to be effective.[40] In all cases, the preferred method to address these issues is the normalization of nutrition. The impact on female fertility is not well studied, although the ability to carry a pregnancy to term or to give birth to a child of average birth weight appears reduced.

Chronic starvation can contribute to brain atrophy. Decreases in white matter and CSF volumes return to normal after a healthy weight is achieved, but gray matter loss can persist.[10,41,42]

Obesity is common in patients with binge eating disorder and may also be present in patients with BN, placing these patients at an increased risk of medical co-morbidities including Type II diabetes mellitus and hypertension.[25] Assessment should include measurement of weight, height, pulse rate, blood pressure, and calculation of BMI. Random glucose and ECG should be done as medically indicated.[25]

A thorough physical and laboratory evaluation, as described in Table 64-1, is essential to determine the severity of medical complications.[3,10,25,54]

TABLE 64-1 Physical and Laboratory Assessment of Eating Disorders

Evaluation	Target Symptoms
Pulse	Bradycardia, Tachycardia
Blood pressure	Hypotension, orthostasis
Height/weight	Underweight for size and age/body mass index
Respiratory rate	Rapid if heart failure occurs during refeeding
Temperature	Hypothermia, cold intolerance
Electrocardiogram	ST depression, flat T waves, U waves, increased QT interval, atrioventricular block
GI	Hypoactive bowel sounds, gastritis, abdominal distention
Skin	Dryness, scaling, lanugo, hair loss, calluses on fingers and hands
Menses	Amenorrhea
Complete blood count	Leukopenia, anemias, thrombocytopenia
Electrolytes	Hypokalemia, hypomagnesemia, hyponatremia, hypophosphatemia, or hyperphosphatemia
pH	Metabolic alkalosis (acidosis if laxative abuse)
Amylase	Elevated; pancreatitis rare
Liver	Hypoalbuminemia, elevated γ-glutamyl transferase if alcohol abuse, elevated AST
Thyroid	Low to low normal, but not true thyroid disease
Cortisol	Elevated with lack of suppression on dexamethasone suppression test
Bone density	Osteoporosis, Osteopenia
Renal	Reduced eGFR (< 60 mL/min [1 mL/s])
Endocrine	Hypoglycemia

Data from references 3, 10, 25, and 54.

TREATMENT

Desired Outcomes

The goals for patients with eating disorders are to reduce distorted body image; restore and maintain healthy body weight; establish normal eating patterns; improve psychological, psychosocial, and physical problems; resolve contributory family problems; enhance compliance; and prevent relapse.[10] Specific to BED is the additional goal of weight loss.

Prognosis

Anorexia Nervosa

The long-term prognosis of patients with AN is not clear, as the majority of studies focus only on patients receiving treatment. The course of the disorder most commonly consists of a single episode with subsequent return to normal weight, although patients can still experience issues with disturbed body image, disordered eating, and other psychiatric problems.[10] Some patients experience an unremitting course leading to death, whereas others suffer episodically.

Remission rates appear to be a function of time in treatment, as the lowest rates of remission are reported in shorter-duration follow-up trials, while remission rates near 80% have been reported in longer-term follow-up studies at 8 and 16 years.[43] Despite this, it is estimated that up to 20% remain chronically ill despite weight normalization, return of menses, and improved eating behaviors.[44] The prognosis is more favorable with longer follow-up care and younger age of onset, whereas a poorer prognosis is associated with chronic illness, lower initial weight, poor family relationships, obsessive–compulsive personality symptoms, and the presence of bulimia or purging behavior.[21,44-46]

7 Crude mortality rates appear to be lower than historically projected; the estimated mortality rate is 2.8% to 4%. When death occurs, it is most often the result of cardiac arrest or suicide.[3,43,44]

Bulimia Nervosa

The prognosis of BN, although not well studied, appears to be better than that of AN. Patients with milder presenting symptoms who are treated as outpatients tend to do better, whereas those with electrolyte imbalances, esophagitis, dental caries, and salivary gland enlargement have a more complicated course.[8] The presence of psychiatric comorbidity and greater general psychiatric symptom severity has been determined to be poor prognostic indicators. Longer rates of follow-up tend to have higher rates of remission, reaching 70% or higher with 5 to 20 years of follow-up. However, it is important to note that even in cases in which patients respond, they continue to exhibit symptoms that wax and wane, sometimes meeting full criteria for diagnosis of BN or sub-threshold forms of BN on the basis of insufficient frequency and/or duration of disordered eating behavior. Total absence of symptoms is an uncommon outcome, and residual symptoms predispose the patient to relapse.[43] The actual definition of recovery varies, as once-a-month binge–purge episodes are considered by some to be recovery if their episodes were previously more frequent, whereas other clinicians consider a patient recovered only when there is complete absence of these behaviors.[46]

Binge Eating Disorder

Of all of the eating disorders, BED has the least amount of long-term follow-up data associated with it. Studies to date suggest higher remission rates (25%-80%) in 1- and 4-year follow-up studies compared with findings in AN and BN longitudinal studies. These numbers are irrespective of treatment selected and treatment during the follow-up time frame studied. Estimated crude mortality rates range from 0% to 3% with a cumulative mortality rate reported at 0.5%.[43]

General Approach to Treatment

Treatment plans are individualized based on the severity of specific core features of the eating disorder and comorbid medical and psychiatric conditions. Psychiatrists, physician assistants, nurses, nutrition specialists, psychologists, and pharmacists play a role in the care of these complex patients. The absence of an adequate support system of family and friends can contribute to failed treatment. A critical first step is to determine the severity of illness, as that drives both the intensity and the setting for delivery of care. Hospitalization is generally reserved for the most severely ill patients. Some criteria for hospitalization are outlined in Table 64-2.[3,10,21,24,53] Medications are part of the comprehensive treatment strategy for eating disorders, but are rarely recommended as the sole treatment.[47-49] Comparative, double-blind, placebo-controlled trials are sparse, and most are limited by small sample sizes, ambivalent patient attitudes toward treatment, medical complications, and high dropout rates.[50]

TABLE 64-2 Considerations for Hospitalization of Patients with Eating Disorders

- Rapid weight loss or BMI <12
- Reduced oral intake of food (sudden and persistent)
- Medical complications (eg, edema) and metabolic abnormalities (eg, hypoproteinemia) from bingeing, purging, and starvation (eg, heart rate <40 beats/min, heart rate >120 beats/min, blood pressure <90/60 mm Hg, glucose <60 mg/dL [<3.3 mmol/L], potassium <3 mEq/L [<3 mmol/L], or inability to maintain core temperature)
- Co-occurring psychiatric symptoms, notably suicidal ideation, self-harm, psychotic depression, or substance abuse and dependence
- Nonresponsive to outpatient treatment (after 3-4 months) and poor motivation to recover
- Demoralization or nonfunctional family
- Denial of severity of abnormal eating behaviors
- Continuous supervision required to prevent purging (vomiting or laxative abuse)

Data from references 3, 10, 21, 24, and 54.

Anorexia Nervosa

Nonpharmacologic Treatments

8 Evidence supports that psychotherapy based treatments have the greatest likelihood of eliciting a response in AN patients.[10,25,51,52] However, the specific type of psychotherapy that is preferred varies and may include CBT, dialectical behavioral therapy, focal psychodynamic therapy, behavioral management, specialist supportive clinical management, interpersonal psychotherapy, nutritional counseling, and family therapy.[10,25,30,51-55] In younger patients, family therapy is the preferred first-line therapy.[56] Patients of lower age, those with shorter duration of illness, with restrictive type AN, who are employed, who are not taking psychotropic medications, and with better social adjustment may have improved outcomes.[55] Current guidelines suggest at least 6 months of psychotherapy is preferred, though studies of at least 1 year in duration have demonstrated favorable outcomes by reducing relapse rates.[25,52,53] CBT helps the patient overcome distorted thinking, including self-worth as measured by body image, feelings of being fat despite evidence to the contrary, and denial. CBT also teaches patients how to use strategies besides eating to cope.

Interpersonal psychotherapy focuses on interpersonal relationships and functioning, whereas CBT provides positive reinforcement for weight gain.[31] A combined approach of interpersonal psychotherapy and CBT is also a reasonable treatment approach.[51] Many psychiatric symptoms in an acutely ill patient, such as depression and anxiety, diminish or disappear with weight restoration. Initial treatment is directed toward restoring a healthy weight, especially in inpatient settings where target weights are often more rapidly achieved.[30] After medical stability and appropriate weight are reached, therapy can be redirected toward addressing ongoing interpersonal problems, weight maintenance, cognitive restructuring, and skill development for relapse prevention.[25] Oral refeeding, initially with liquid formulas if necessary, is the most common approach to weight restoration.

In severe cases when a patient refuses to eat, nasogastric refeeding is preferred over IV bolus dosing in part because it can allow for higher initial caloric intake and has been associated with reductions in length of inpatient hospitalizations and increased rate of weight gain without an increase in complications.[57] Total parenteral nutrition is reserved only for the management of severely malnourished patients and if other refeeding methods fail. The decision to administer total parenteral nutrition must be made carefully, because of the potentially devastating psychological effect on patients who do not wish to gain weight.

Current clinical evidence suggests a controlled weight gain of 0.9 to 1.4 kg (2-3 lb) per week in inpatient settings and 0.2 to 0.5 kg (0.5-1 lb) per week in outpatient settings.[3,49,58] Refeeding recommendations vary between younger patients and adults and are considered controversial. An acceptable approach for younger patients is to begin refeeding at 800 to 1,000 cal/day (3347-4184 J/day), while others suggests a more aggressive approach.[59] Adults may be considered for refeeding initiation in the range of 1,000 to 1,600 cal/day (4184-6694 J/day)

(30-40 cal/kg/day [126-167 J/kg/day]) with slow titration (every other day) upwards (100-200 cal/day [419-837 J/day]) until they begin to demonstrate sustained weight gain or achieve target weights.[10,53,60] This can require the intake of an additional 3,500 to 7,000 cal (14,644-29,288 J) per week.[53] Slow refeeding has long been considered important to prevent psychological and medical consequences, including the severe electrolyte disturbance that results from insulin surges known as refeeding syndrome, which can result in death. A criticism is that too conservative of an approach results in further weight loss early in treatment (unfeeding syndrome), contributing to a failure to achieve nutritional recovery goals.[61]

Pharmacologic Therapy

Antidepressants Although many studies examined the role of antidepressants in the treatment of AN, they often have small sample sizes and large confidence intervals.[63] Antidepressants currently have no role in the acute treatment of AN, unless there is another clinical indication present.[10,21,47]

Data suggest that medication is ineffective, especially in cases where the patient is below their expected weight. Thus, antidepressants should be initiated only if depression, anxiety, obsessions, or compulsions persist after the target weight is achieved.[21,58] The duration of treatment when antidepressants are used in this manner is unclear, but one study showed benefit in treated patients for 1 year, and current guidelines suggest 9 to 12 months of therapy.[10,25,51-53] Antidepressants, along with psychotherapy, have been used to help maintain weight and prevent relapse, but data supporting this are limited.[63] Most clinicians prefer the selective serotonin reuptake inhibitor (SSRI) antidepressants because they are better tolerated and have greater cardiovascular safety than tricyclic antidepressants (TCAs) and monoamine oxidase inhibitors (MAOIs).[10,25,51,52] Because these patients are sensitive to anticholinergic and cardiovascular effects, if TCAs or MAOIs are used, low starting doses and slow titration toward an effective dose are appropriate. The risk of cardiotoxicity in a malnourished population must not be underestimated, and a baseline electrocardiogram (ECG) should be obtained before initiation of these agents.

Fluoxetine continues to be the most widely studied SSRI in AN. Most clinicians initiate at low doses, for example, 20 mg/day, and increase to a maximum of 60 mg/day based on response and tolerability.[60,62,63] Some controversy exists regarding when antidepressant therapy should be initiated. During the starvation phases of anorexia, the majority of clinical trials suggest that antidepressants are ineffective, partly due to reduced tryptophan levels, though debate remains as to their effectiveness once weight restoration has occurred. Evidence from a 52-week, randomized, placebo-controlled clinical trial of 93 patients with the treatment arm receiving doses from 20 to 80 mg/day after weight restoration showed no difference between fluoxetine and placebo for time to relapse.[64]

Antipsychotics First- and second-generation antipsychotics have been utilized as a treatment for AN, specifically targeting anxiety and obsessive and paranoid thoughts related to weight gain. First-generation antipsychotics contributed to BMI gains, but provided little benefit overall at reducing other core symptoms, and the associated adverse events were considered to outweigh the benefits. Second-generation antipsychotics have provided an additional alternative for treating AN, with reports of improvement in weight gain and reductions in symptoms such as depression, anxiety, and obsessive–compulsiveness. Most of the data are from case reports or small trials in both adolescents and adults using risperidone 0.5 to 2.5 mg daily, olanzapine 2.5 to 10 mg daily, and quetiapine 50 to 800 mg daily.[65-69] Olanzapine in combination with day hospital treatment has been shown to be more effective than day hospital treatment alone in achieving greater weight gain and reducing obsessive symptoms.[68] In addition, an outpatient study examining olanzapine versus placebo, independent of concurrent psychotherapy, demonstrated significant improvement in BMI.[70] While some benefits have been reported, not all positive findings have been replicated, and caution is urged, as there is likely an increased susceptibility to some of the physiologic effects of antipsychotic medications. Optimal treatment duration is unknown, as most of the larger studies are less than or equal to 3 months in duration.

Miscellaneous Agents Metoclopramide can be helpful in reducing bloating, early satiety, and abdominal pain commonly found in AN, but it does not affect weight gain.[10] Low-dose, short-acting benzodiazepines (0.25 mg alprazolam or 0.5 mg lorazepam) given before meals are useful when severe anxiety limits eating.[10] Estrogen replacement has been used, but restoring menses through refeeding is a preferred approach to minimize bone density loss. Supplementation with zinc is also being studied to assist with weight restoration.[51]

Clinical **Controversy...**

There is widespread disagreement about the most appropriate rate of refeeding. An approach that is too aggressive may increase the risk of developing "refeeding syndrome" while utilizing a conservative approach may result in delays in patients achieving proper weight restoration.

Bulimia Nervosa

Nonpharmacologic Therapy

Outpatient-based treatment is most often recommended except in extreme cases (see Table 64-2). The nondrug strategies used in BN are similar to those used with AN, and they are equally critical to success. CBT has the strongest evidence supporting its benefit in managing BN.[25,51,53] Current treatment guidelines suggest that CBT should consist of 16 to 20 sessions over a 4- to 5-month period.[25,53] Data suggests that 30% to 50% of individuals who receive CBT for BN are abstinent from binge eating and purging behaviors by conclusion of the treatment.[71] Interpersonal psychotherapy also plays a role and has a moderate degree of evidence to support its use, but it is considered less effective than CBT.[10,22] A 2014 study demonstrated that CBT was more effective in relieving binging and purging than psychoanalytic psychotherapy and was generally faster in alleviating eating disorder features and general psychopathology.[72] Nutritional counseling, planned meals, and self-monitoring can help interrupt the binge–purge cycle. Family therapy in bulimic patients is less critical than with AN, as these patients tend to be older. A recent study suggested that CBT-guided self-care was a more effective treatment approach in adolescents than family therapy. Programs using motivational teaching and self-help guides based on CBT have shown promise.[31,75-77] When such programs have been combined with medication, for example, fluoxetine, enhanced response has been reported.[78] Online delivery of CBT may provide an acceptable treatment alternative for patients who have limited access.[73,74] Data support the use of 12-step programs, but they should not be used as monotherapy.[10,21] Adjunctive interventions, such as acupuncture and yoga, targeting symptoms of anxiety and depression need further study.[79,80]

Pharmacologic Therapy

Antidepressants 9 Antidepressants are used in the acute and maintenance phases of BN adjunctively with nonpharmacologic approaches. A wide array of antidepressants, including TCAs, MAOIs, trazodone, serotonin–norepinephrine reuptake inhibitors (SNRIs), bupropion, and SSRIs, have been studied. Additionally, several reviews analyzing this body of literature have been published, although there continues to be limited placebo-controlled, randomized, double-blind clinical studies.[21,47,81] Antidepressants are reported to reduce depression, anxiety, obsessions, and impulsive behaviors, such as binge eating and purging, and improve eating habits, although their impact on body dissatisfaction remains unclear. The presence of comorbid mood disorders is not necessary for a response in patients with BN.

The benefit appears to be more robust in the acute phase of the illness, as relapse despite continued antidepressant use is common in patients who are in or near remission.[21,49] Antidepressant response usually occurs in 6 to 8 weeks, and reduction in frequency of binge–purge behavior has been as high as 73% and as low as zero.[47] Abstinence rates (elimination of bingeing and purging behaviors) with short-term use range from 0% to 68%. More data are needed to determine the long-term benefits of antidepressants for preventing relapse of bulimia symptoms. One trial evaluating the impact of fluoxetine versus placebo in the maintenance phase showed a better outcome in patients receiving fluoxetine 60 mg/day, although high dropout rates in both groups blurred the overall benefit.[82]

Selective serotonin reuptake inhibitors are the preferred agents because of their tolerability and because they have been studied in the largest number of patients. Fluoxetine remains the only medication with FDA approval for BN. Efficacy of other SSRI agents is still lacking, but an alternative SSRI may be considered in clinical practice for patients who do not respond to fluoxetine.[81] Tolerability is the primary criterion for selecting an antidepressant in the treatment of BN because of patients' heightened sensitivity to adverse effects and the lack of a clear difference in efficacy between the classes. Even though there is a suggestion that MAOIs produce the most robust effect, the risk of using these medications in impulsive patients limits their use.[49] SNRIs have shown promising results; however, the data supporting their use are limited to case reports. Bupropion, a norepinephrine–dopamine reuptake inhibitor, is contraindicated in bulimic patients because of the increased risk of seizures.

Before initiating pharmacologic therapy, a careful baseline physical examination, ECG, and laboratory workup are essential. Underlying ECG changes secondary to hypokalemia or bradycardia and atrioventricular block from starvation can be present. There is potential for fatal outcomes secondary to cardiac arrest or suicide. All antidepressants can cause seizures; thus, a careful risk–benefit assessment is warranted if the patient has predisposing factors such as a personal or family history of seizures, cerebrovascular disease, or alcohol or sedative–hypnotic withdrawal.

Doses in the treatment of BN are similar to those in patients treated for depression, although at the higher end of the range. Readers are referred to Chapter 68 for antidepressant dosing ranges. For fluoxetine, the higher end of the dosing range, 60 mg/day, can be necessary for response.[83] With all agents, most clinicians initially target the bottom to the middle of the dosing range and increase the dose if there is an inadequate response. Slow titration is needed to allow time to develop tolerance to adverse effects. If TCAs are used, serum concentration monitoring is recommended to ensure that absorption is not compromised by purging.

The time for antidepressant onset of effect in BN is unclear. In the absence of data, the definition of a therapeutic trial from the depression literature (4-8 weeks at a therapeutic dose) should be used. A 2010 report by Sysko et al. identified that response (defined as greater than 60% reduction in binge eating or vomiting frequency) by week 3 is a positive predictor of eventual treatment response.[84] Because the majority of subjects will not experience a complete remission, and there are few data on predictors of response or whether switching to another class will improve response, a clear and specific target should be stated initially.[17]

Optimal duration of treatment after response is poorly defined, although most clinicians treat for 9 months to 1 year and then reevaluate. The evidence is mixed as to whether any early benefit is sustained; hence, the decision to continue treatment should be made based on both initial response and the maintenance of that benefit. If the symptoms return within a few months after antidepressant discontinuation, then the treatment may need to be reinitiated. Figure 64-2 describes criteria for medication use in BN.

Miscellaneous Agents Because of the lack of evidence demonstrating their benefit, lithium and traditional anticonvulsants are reserved for bulimic patients with comorbid bipolar disorder.[10,85] Randomized, placebo-controlled trials with topiramate have demonstrated reduced binge/purge frequency and weight loss versus placebo, although side effects including cognitive impairment and paresthesia may hinder medication adherence.[86,87] Low-dose benzodiazepines before meals can help reduce anxiety associated with refeeding, although long-term use is not warranted because of the risk of abuse and dependence. One double-blind trial with ondansetron has shown benefit, but there are insufficient data to recommend a specific role for this agent.[88] One small, open-label, pilot study of zonisamide showed it to be effective in BN, but due to study limitations, the results should be considered preliminary, and further data are needed to confirm its role in treatment.[89] Data are conflicting on the opiate antagonist naltrexone with only modest improvement seen at high doses, but naltrexone is not recommended due to risk of elevated hepatic transaminases.[65] Antipsychotics and appetite suppressants do not play a role in managing core symptoms of BN.[21]

Nonpharmacologic versus Pharmacologic Approaches

The combination of pharmacologic and nonpharmacologic measures appears to produce the best chance for a positive outcome for patients with BN.[53] Antidepressants, specifically SSRIs, are the drug class of choice in bulimic patients, whereas other medications are reserved for patients with comorbid psychiatric conditions. Only in unusual circumstances should patients be treated with antidepressants alone. Evidence suggests the greatest benefit is during the acute phase of treatment, whereas data are mixed regarding their role in the prevention of relapse.

Binge Eating Disorder

Nonpharmacologic Therapy

Individual and group CBT are universally accepted as the nonpharmacologic treatment interventions of choice, specifically aimed at reducing the number binge eating episodes though not likely to significantly improve weight loss.[52,90] Interpersonal therapy (IPT) has recently demonstrated comparable efficacy to CBT at 1-, 2-, and 5-year follow-up reviews.[91,92] Dialectical behavior therapy (DBT) is also an appropriate psychotherapy treatment intervention, though not considered first-line.[91,92] Weight loss focused treatment programs are generally considered to be the most effective nonpharmacologic intervention to reduce weight, specifically in those who are obese.[93]

Pharmacologic Therapy

The stimulant lisdexamfetamine, antidepressants, and anticonvulsants are the pharmacologic agents that are most extensively studied in BED. Antidepressants have demonstrated efficacy as monotherapy at reducing binge eating, decreasing BMI, and improving depressed mood during the acute phases of the illness compared with placebo, but they can also be used in combination with CBT to augment response.[25,65,94-96] The SSRIs citalopram (20 mg-60 mg in clinical trials, however doses above 40 mg are not recommended), escitalopram (10 mg-30 mg), fluvoxamine (up to 200 mg), fluoxetine (40 mg-80 mg), sertraline (100 mg-200 mg), are associated with some level of improvement in BED related symptoms.[94-97] This includes a reduction in binge frequency, a reduction in BMI, improved mood symptoms, and reduced obsessive compulsive symptoms, though not all studies have included each of these outcome measures in their methodology.[97] The results from two different meta-analyses

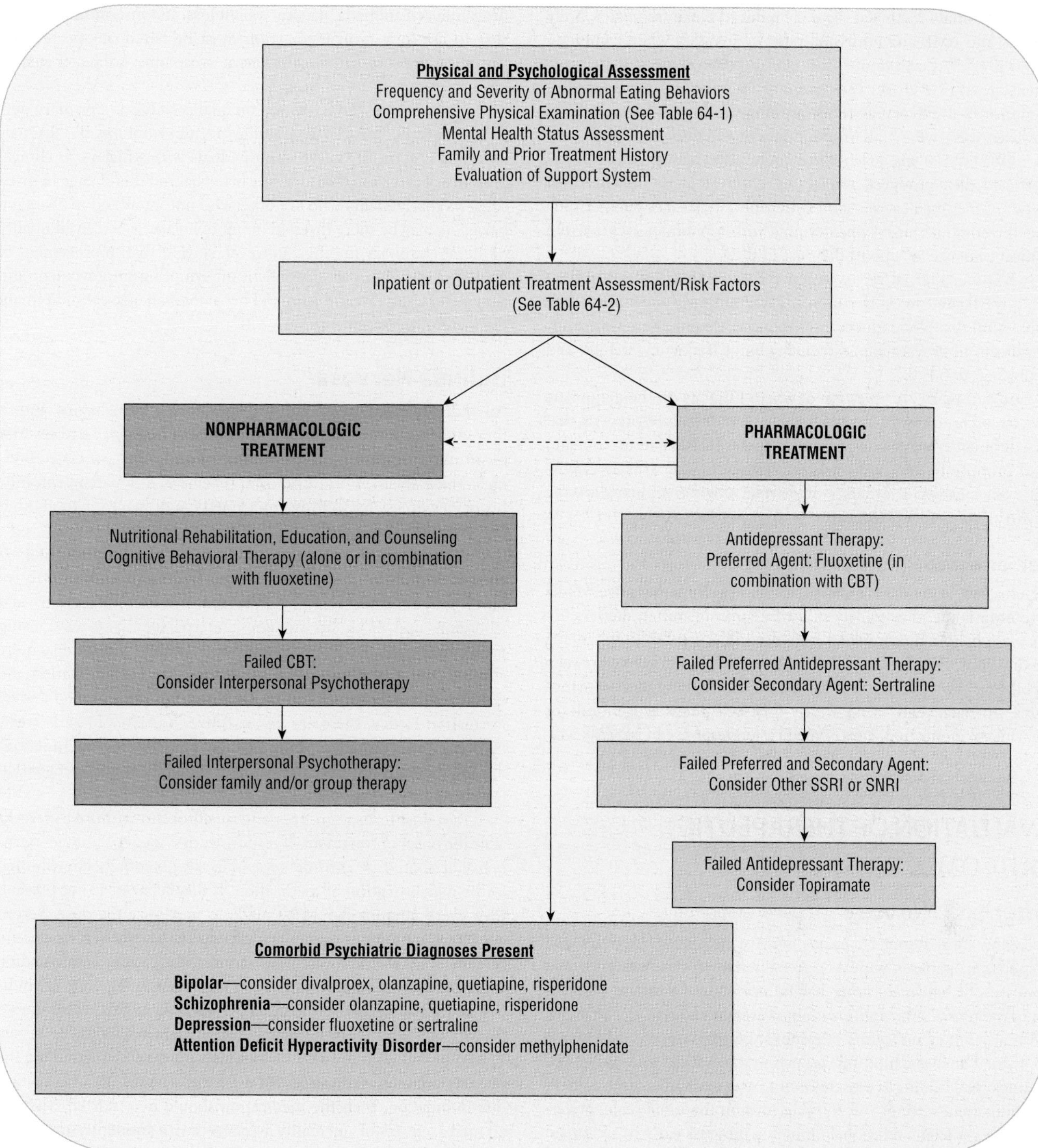

FIGURE 64-2 Bulimia nervosa treatment algorithm. (CBT, cognitive behavioral therapy; SNRI, serotonin–norepinephrine reuptake inhibitor; SSRI, selective serotonin reuptake inhibitor.)

suggest that antidepressants have higher remission rates when compared with placebo.[81] The majority of the data are with SSRIs given at antidepressant doses.[97]

Atomoxetine (40 mg-120 mg) and venlafaxine (75 mg-300 mg) have evidence to support improvement in BED symptoms. Specific benefit was reduction in binge frequency, reduced BMI, weight loss, and improved mood symptoms.[97]

Lisdexamfetamine is a prodrug of dextroamphetamine and is FDA approved for the treatment of moderate to severe BED (30 mg initially and titrated to 50 mg-70 mg daily). Clinical trials demonstrated reductions in numbers of binge days per week, a greater percentage of patients with global clinical improvement, a higher percentage achieving a 4-week cessation of binge episodes, and improvement in obsessive compulsive psychometric measures.[98]

Clinical **Controversy...**

Lisdexamfetamine has recently gained FDA approval for the treatment of BED; however, in many cases it is not utilized as a first-line therapy. The limitations to its use as a first-line agent for BED relate to safety concerns (eg, possible abuse, cardiac arrhythmia).

Topiramate 25 to 300 mg daily reduced binge frequency, body weight, and BMI, and remission rates were higher when combined with CBT.[99,100] Zonisamide (100-600 mg/day) alone and in combination with CBT over the course of 16-week and 1-year studies demonstrated efficacy at reducing binge eating and weight loss; however, there were high dropout rates due to intolerability.[81]

Orlistat 120 mg given three times daily, along with calorie-restricted diet, produced weight reduction in obese patients with BED.[101] Other medications used to treat obesity, such as phentermine and the combination of phentermine with topiramate lack current clinical evidence to support their use in BED.

Another alternative, chromium picolinate (600-1,000 mcg/day) was investigated in BED patients. Results from a small, 6-month trial found that blood glucose was reduced, though there were non-significant improvements in reducing binge frequency, weight, and depressed mood.[102]

In summary, the question of where BED fits on the diagnostic spectrum continues to be explored. Current literature suggests that two different types of pharmacologic agents (SSRIs and topiramate) hold promise in the short term, but long-term data are lacking. As with other eating disorders, nonpharmacologic treatments are the key to a successful outcome.

Personalized Pharmacotherapy

Results from genetic variation studies are largely inconclusive. While serotonin is the most widely studied neurotransmitter, there is not an overwhelmingly consistent response to the serotonin-enhancing medications. Often response is simply a reduction in behaviors such as bingeing and purging, but not a complete amelioration of symptoms. To date, there is no widely accepted pharmacogenomic or pharmacokinetic predictors of medication response in patients with eating disorders.

EVALUATION OF THERAPEUTIC OUTCOMES

Anorexia Nervosa

A combination of subjective and objective measures is used to assess response in patients with AN. A reduction in the frequency and severity of abnormal eating habits, normalized exercise patterns and laboratory tests, and a sustained weight close to age-matched normals are key indicators of response. A diary recording exercise frequency, menses, food intake, patterns of eating, and associated feelings while eating is a useful tool to track progress, especially in the outpatient setting. Weekly weigh-ins on the same scale, preferably at a clinician's office, help monitor progress early in treatment and reduce the focus on weight and anxiety caused by the variability found among different scales. Follow-up laboratory tests and ECGs are not part of routine monitoring unless the patient is restricting food intake, is purging, or continues to lose weight despite treatment. Inpatients require daily assessment of weight and caloric intake, vital signs, and urine output because of the severity of their illness. They also can need monitoring of bathroom privileges early in their care. A healthy weight gain of not more than 0.2 to 0.5 kg (0.4-1.1 lb) per week toward a goal of 90% to 95% of normal weight or a BMI greater than 18.5 kg/m^2 is a critical sign of treatment success. A patient's use of coping skills and contingencies for dealing with stress, other than manipulating food consumption, also should be assessed. Antidepressants can assist in alleviation of persistent depression, anxiety, and obsessions, after weight restoration. Improvement in mood is expected to occur within 8 weeks. Patients receiving TCAs should be evaluated for dry mouth, constipation, hypotension, and sedation. Patients receiving SSRIs should be monitored for agitation, drug-induced anorexia, nausea, weight loss, and insomnia. The decision to use long-term medication must be based on specific and sustained improvement in the target symptoms, balanced against adverse effects.

10 Recent research focused on quality of life as a primary outcome measure compared to targeting specific symptoms of AN. Quality of life is generally lower in individuals with a history or clinical presence of an eating disorder. The belief behind this change in focus suggests that patients who are otherwise not interested in changing behaviors may be more invested in improving their perceived quality of life. Preliminary findings, however, suggest that improvement in quality of life is in part dependent on symptom improvement and weight gain, thus weight gain and behavioral change should remain the focus of treatment.[103]

Bulimia Nervosa

An individualized treatment and monitoring plan begins with a thorough assessment describing the baseline frequency and severity of treatment-responsive target symptoms and other associated findings. The assessment must be comprehensive, as a patient can hide his or her illness by shifting from one type of behavior to another (eg, exercise to purging).

A comprehensive assessment includes a description of psychiatric symptoms, physical findings, frequency and severity of binge–purge episodes, laxative and ipecac use, exercise patterns, and laboratory and ECG abnormalities. Interpersonal and relationship problems should also be evaluated. Some findings indicating a more chronic course of illness, such as salivary gland inflammation and erosion of dental enamel, can take months to reverse or might never normalize. Hence, these are not sensitive indicators of early treatment response. Data describing a patient's baseline level of functioning and previous response to treatment should be used to set goals in the current treatment plan.

Response to an antidepressant usually occurs within 4 to 8 weeks after the onset of treatment. If response does not occur, binge–purge behavior should be considered as a factor potentially contributing to the malabsorption of medication. If this behavior is not present, then every attempt should be made to maximize the dose. Serum concentration monitoring, when appropriate as with TCAs, should be done periodically (every 3-6 months if a patient is responding and tolerating the medication, or more frequently if clinically indicated). Evaluation of previously described adverse effects also should be part of the monitoring plan. If the patient responds, he or she should be followed for 6 to 12 months, and then reassessed for the need for ongoing medication. If the patient relapses after medication discontinuation, then the medication should be restarted. There is an increased risk of suicidality associated with antidepressant use in major depression, thus suicidality assessments should be included following their initiation, especially early in therapy. Please refer to Chapter 68 for further details and more comprehensive information related to antidepressant use.

Eating disorder patients who are outpatients present a particular challenge to clinicians. Impulsivity associated with BN can increase the risk for suicide. Prescriptions should be limited to small supplies. In addition, pharmacists should be alert to persons who make large or frequent purchases of laxatives or ipecac syrup, as this is an indicator of possible bulimic behaviors.

ABBREVIATIONS

5-HIAA	5-hydroxyindoleacetic acid
5-HT	serotonin
5-HTTLPR	serotonin transporter

AN	anorexia nervosa
BDNF	brain-derived neurotrophic factor
BED	binge-eating disorder
BMI	body mass index
BN	bulimia nervosa
CBT	cognitive behavioral therapy
CNS	central nervous system
CSF	cerebrospinal fluid
CT	computerized tomography
DBT	dialectical behavior therapy
DSM-5	*Diagnostic and Statistical Manual of Mental Disorders* (fifth edition)
ECG	electrocardiogram
EEG	electroencephalogram
ESRI	estrogen receptor I gene
GI	gastrointestinal
IPT	interpersonal therapy
MAOI	monoamine oxidase inhibitor
MRI	magnetic resonance imaging
NES	night eating syndrome
OCD	obsessive–compulsive disorder
SNRI	serotonin–norepinephrine reuptake inhibitor
SSRI	selective serotonin reuptake inhibitor
TCA	tricyclic antidepressant

REFERENCES

1. Hudson JI, Hiripi E, Pope HG Jr, Kessler RC. The prevalence and correlates of eating disorders in the national comorbidity survey replication. *Biol Psychiatry* 2007;61:348-358.
2. Swanson AA, Crow SJ, Le Grange D, et al. Prevalence and correlates of eating disorders in adolescents. *Arch Gen Psychiatry* 2011;68(7):714-723.
3. American Psychiatric Association. *Diagnostic and Statistical Manual of Mental Disorders, 5th ed.* Arlington, VA: American Psychiatric Press; 2013:329-360.
4. Pike KM. Long-term course of anorexia nervosa: Response, relapse, remission, and recovery. *Clin Psychol Rev* 1998;18:447-475.
5. Crow SJ, Peterson CV, Swanson SA, et al. Increased mortality in bulimia nervosa and other eating disorders. *Am J Psychiatry* 2009;166:1342-1346.
6. Rodgers RF, Skowron S, Chabrol H. Disordered eating and group membership among members of a pro-anorexic online community. *Eur Eat Disorders Rev* 2012;20:9-12.
7. Hoek H, van Hoeken D. Review of the prevalence and incidence of eating disorders. *Int J Eat Disord* 2003;34:383-386.
8. Sadock BJ, Sadock VA, eds. *Kaplan and Sadock's Synopsis of Psychiatry: Behavioral Sciences/Clinical Psychiatry*, 9th ed. Philadelphia: Lippincott Williams & Wilkins; 2003:739-750.
9. McElroy SL, Guerdjikova AI, Mori N, O'Melia AM. Current pharmacotherapy options for bulimia nervosa and binge eating disorder. *Expert Opin Pharmacother* 2012;13(14):2015-2026.
10. American Psychiatric Association. Treatment of patients with eating disorders, 3rd ed. *Am J Psychiatry* 2006;163(7 Suppl):4-54.
11. Reas DL, Grilo CM. Current and emerging drug treatments for binge eating disorder. *Expert Opin Pharmacother* 2014;19(1):99-142.
12. O'Reardon JP, Allison KC, Martino NS, et al. A randomized, placebo-controlled trial of sertraline in the treatment of night eating syndrome. *Am J Psychiatry* 2006;163:893-898.
13. Fischer S, Meyer AH, Herman E, et al. Night eating syndrome in young adults: Delineation from other eating disorders and clinical significance. *Psychiatry Res* 2012;200:494-501.
14. Allison KC, Studt SK, Berkowitz RI, et al. An open-label efficacy trial of escitalopram for night eating syndrome. *Eat Behav* 2013;14:199-203.
15. Phillipou A, Rossell SL, Castle DJ. The neurobiology of anorexia nervosa: A systematic review. *Aust N Z J Psychiatry* 2014;48(2): 128-152.
16. Kaye WH. Neurobiology of anorexia and bulimia nervosa. *Physiol Behav* 2008;94:121-135.
17. Frank GK, Bailer UF, Henry SE, et al. Increased dopamine D2/D3 receptor binding after recovery from anorexia nervosa measured by positron emission tomography and [11c]raclopride. *Biol Psychiatry* 2005;58:908-912.
18. Ribases M, Gratacos M, Fernandez-Aranda F, et al. Association of BDNF with anorexia, bulimia, age of onset of weight loss in six European populations. *Hum Mol Genet* 2004;13(12):1205-1212.
19. Pinheiro AP, Bulik CM, Thornton LM, et al. Association study of 182 candidate genes in anorexia nervosa. *Am J Med Genet B Neuropsychiatr Genet* 2010;153B:1070-1080.
20. Grave RD. Eating disorders: Progress and challenges. *Eur J Intern Med* 2011;22:153-160.
21. Fairburn CG, Harrison PJ. Eating disorders. *Lancet* 2003;361:407-416.
22. Steiger H, Joober R, Gauvin L, et al. Serotonin-system polymorphisms (5-HTTLPR and -1438G/A) and responses of patients with bulimic syndromes to multimodal treatments. *J Clin Psychiatry* 2008;69:1565-1571.
23. Versini A, Ramoz N, Le Strat Y, et al. Estrogen receptor I gene is associated with restrictive anorexia nervosa. *Neuropsychopharmacology* 2010;35:1818-1825.
24. Powers PS. Initial assessment and early treatment options for anorexia nervosa and bulimia nervosa. *Psychiatr Clin North Am* 1996;19:639-655.
25. Hay P, Chinn D, Forbes D, et al. Royal Australian and New Zealand College of Psychiatrists clinical practice guidelines for the treatment of eating disorders. *Aust N Z J Psychiatry* 2014;48(11):977-1008.
26. Tozzi F, Thornton LM, Mitchell J, et al. Features associated with laxative abuse in individuals with eating disorders. *Psychosom Med* 2006;68:470-477.
27. Garner DM, Garner MV, Rosen LW. Anorexia nervosa "restrictors" who purge: Implications for subtyping anorexia nervosa. *Int J Eat Disord* 1993;13:171-185.
28. Shroff H, Reba L, Thornton LM, et al. Features associated with excessive exercise in women with eating disorders. *Int J Eat Disord* 2006;39:454-461.
29. Steinhausen HC, Jakobsen, Helenius D, et al. A nation-wide study of the family aggregation and risk factors in anorexia nervosa over three generations. *Int J Eat Disord* 2015;48:1-8.
30. Jordan J, Joyce PR, Carter FA, et al. Specific and nonspecific comorbidity in anorexia nervosa. *Int J Eat Disord* 2008;41:47-56.
31. Halmi KA. Eating disorders: Anorexia nervosa, bulimia nervosa, and obesity. In: Hales RE, Yudofsky SC, eds. *Essentials of Clinical Psychiatry*, 3rd ed. Washington, DC: American Psychiatric Press; 1999:667-685.
32. Braun DL, Sunday SR, Halmi KA. Psychiatric comorbidity in patients with eating disorders. *Psychol Med* 1994;24:859-867.
33. Herzog DB, Keller MB, Sacks NR, et al. Psychiatric comorbidity in treatment seeking anorexics and bulimics. *J Am Acad Child Adolesc Psychiatry* 1992;31:810-818.
34. O'Brien KM, Vincent NK. Psychiatric comorbidity in anorexia and bulimia nervosa: Nature, prevalence, and causal relationships. *Clin Psychol Rev* 2003;23:53-74.
35. Grilo CM, White MA, Masheb RM. DSM-IV psychiatric disorder comorbidity and its correlates in binge eating disorder. *Int J Eat Disord* 2009;42(3):228-234.
36. Rome ES, Ammerman, S. Medical complications of eating disorders: An update. *J Adolesc Health* 2003;33:418-426.
37. Meczekalski B, Podfigurna-Stopa A, Katulski K. Long-term consequences of anorexia nervosa. *Maturitas* 2013;75:215-220.
38. Birch K. Female athlete triad. *Br Med J* 2005;330(7485):244-246.
39. Mendelsohn FA, Warren MP. Anorexia, bulimia, and the female athlete triad: Evaluation and management. *Endocrinol Metab Clin North Am* 2010;39:155-167.
40. Mehler PS, MacKenzie TD. Treatment outcomes of osteopenia and osteoporosis in anorexia nervosa: A systematic review of the literature. *Int J Eat Disord* 2009;42(3):195-201.
41. Kingston K, Szmukler G, Andrews D, et al. Neuropsychological and structural brain changes in anorexia nervosa before and after refeeding. *Psychol Med* 1996;26:15-28.
42. Lambe EK, Katzman DK, Mikulis DJ, et al. Cerebral gray matter volume deficits after weight recovery from anorexia nervosa. *Arch Gen Psychiatry* 1997;54:537-542.
43. Keel PK, Brown TA. Update on course and outcome in eating disorders. *Int J Eat Disord* 2010;43:195-204.
44. Steinhausen HC. The outcome of anorexia nervosa in the 20th century. *Am J Psychiatry* 2002;159(8):1284-1293.
45. Fichter MM, Quadflieg N. Six year course of bulimia nervosa. *Int J Eat Disord* 1997;22:361-384.

46. Yu J, Agras WS, Bryson S. Defining recovery in adult bulimia nervosa. *Eat Disord* 2013;21:379-394.
47. Mitchell JE, de Zwaan M, Roerig JL. Drug therapy for patients with eating disorders. *Curr Drug Targets CNS Neurol Disord* 2003;2:17-29.
48. Bacaltchuk J, Hay P. Antidepressants versus placebo for people with bulimia nervosa. *Cochrane Database Syst Rev* 2003;(4):CD003391 [updated November 2005].
49. Nakash-Eisikovits O, Dierberger A, Westen D. A multidimensional meta-analysis of pharmacotherapy for bulimia nervosa: Summarizing the range of outcomes in controlled clinical trials. *Harv Rev Psychiatry* 2002;10:190-211.
50. Halmi KA, Agras WS, Crow S, et al. Predictors of treatment acceptance and completion in anorexia nervosa: Implications for future study designs. *Arch Gen Psychiatry* 2005;62:776-781.
51. Yager J, Devlin MJ, Halmi KA, et al. *Guideline Watch (August 2012): Practice Guideline for the Treatment of Patients with Eating Disorders.* 3rd ed. Available at: http://psychiatryonline.org/pb/assets/raw/sitewide/practice_guidelines/guidelines/eatingdisorders-watch.pdf. (Accessed October 8, 2015)
52. Watson HJ, Bulik CM. Update on the treatment of anorexia nervosa: Review of clinical trials, practice guidelines, and emerging interventions. *Psychol Med* 2013;43:2477-2500.
53. National Collaborating Centre for Mental Health. *Eating Disorders: Core Interventions in the Treatment and Management of Anorexia Nervosa, Bulimia Nervosa and Related Eating Disorders.* London: British Psychological Society and Royal College of Psychiatrists; 2004:1-36.
54. Le Grange, D, Fitzsimmons-Craft EE, Crosby RD, et al. *Predictors and moderators of outcome for severe and enduring anorexia nervosa. Behav Res Ther* 2014;56:91-98.
55. Zipfel S, Wild B, Grob G, et al. Focal psychodynamic therapy, cognitive behavior therapy, and optimised treatment as usual in outpatients with anorexia nervosa (ANTOP study): Randomized controlled trial. *Lancet* 2014;383:127-137.
56. Lock J, La Via MC. Practice parameter for the assessment and treatment of children and adolescents with eating disorders. *J Am Acad Child Adolesc Psychiatry* 2015;54(5):412-425.
57. Agostino H, Erdstein J, De Meglio G. Shifting paradigms: Continuous nasogastric feeding with high caloric intakes in anorexia nervosa. *J Adolesc Health* 2013;53:590-594.
58. Zerbe KJ. Multimodal treatment of severe eating disorders. *Essent Psychopharmacol* 2000;3:1-17.
59. Rocks T, Pelly F, Wilkinson P. Nutrition therapy during initiation of refeeding in underweight children and adolescent inpatients with anorexia nervosa: A systematic review of the evidence. *J Acad Nutr Diet* 2014;114:897-907.
60. Yager J, Anderson AE. Anorexia nervosa. *N Engl J Med* 2005;353(14):1481-1488.
61. Garber AK, Mauldin K, Michihata N, et al. Higher calorie diets increase rate of weight gain and shorten hospital stay in hospitalized adolescents with anorexia nervosa. *J Adolesc Health* 2013;53:579-584.
62. Bulik CM, Berkman ND, Brownley KA, et al. Anorexia nervosa treatment: A systematic review of randomized controlled trials. *Int J Eat Disord* 2007;40:310-320.
63. Kaye WH, Nagata T, Weltzin TE, et al. Double-blind placebo-controlled administration of fluoxetine in restricting- and restricting-purging-type anorexia nervosa. *Biol Psychiatry* 2001;4:644-652.
64. Walsh BT, Kaplan AS, Attia E, et al. Fluoxetine after weight restoration in anorexia nervosa: A randomized controlled trial. *JAMA* 2006;295(22):2605-2612.
65. Flament MF, Bissada H, Spettigue W. Evidence-based pharmacotherapy of eating disorders. *Int J Neuropsychopharmacol* 2012;15:189-207.
66. Dunican KC, DelDotto D. The role of olanzapine in the treatment of anorexia nervosa. *Ann Pharmacother* 2007;41:111-115.
67. Mehler-Wex C, Romanos M, Kirchheiner J, Schulze UME. Atypical antipsychotics in severe anorexia nervosa in children and adolescents—Review and case reports. *Eur Eat Disord Rev* 2008;16:100-108.
68. Bissada H, Tasca GA, Barber AM, Bradwejn J. Olanzapine in the treatment of low body weight and obsessive thinking in women with anorexia nervosa: A randomized, double-blind, placebo-controlled trial. *Am J Psychiatry* 2008;165:1281-1288.
69. Powers PS, Klabunde M, Kaye W. Double-blind placebo-controlled trial of quetiapine in anorexia nervosa. *Eur Eat Disord Rev* 2012;20:331-334.
70. Attia E, Kaplan AS, Walsh BT, et al. Olanzapine versus placebo for outpatients with anorexia nervosa. *Psychol Med* 2011;41:2177-2182.
71. Glasofer DR, Devlin MJ. Cognitive behavioral therapy for bulimia nervosa. *Psychotherapy* 2013;50(4):537-542.
72. Poulsen S, Lunn S, Daniel SIF, et al. A randomized controlled trial of psychoanalytic psychotherapy or cognitive-behavioral therapy for bulimia nervosa. *Am J Psychiatry* 2014;171(1):109-116.
73. Ruwaard J, Lange A, Broeksteeg J, et al. Online cognitive-behavioural treatment of bulimic symptoms: A randomized controlled trial. *Clin Psychol Psychother* 2013;20(4):308-318.
74. Bulik CM, Marcus MD, Zerwas S, et al. CBT4BN versus CBTF2F: Comparison of online versus fact-to-face treatment for bulimia nervosa. *Contemp Clin Trials* 2012;33(5):1056-1064.
75. Schmidt U, Lee S, Beecham J, et al. A randomized controlled trial of family therapy and cognitive behavior therapy guided self-care for adolescents with bulimia nervosa and related disorders. *Am J Psychiatry* 2007;164:591-598.
76. Mitchell JE, Agras S, Crow S, et al. Stepped care and cognitive-behavioural therapy for bulimia nervosa: Randomized trial. *Br J Psychiatry* 2011;198:391-397.
77. Wilson GT, Zandberg LJ. Cognitive-behavioral guided self-help for eating disorders: Effectiveness and scalability. *Clin Psychol Rev* 2012;32:343-357.
78. Walsh BT, Fairburn CG, Mickley D, et al. Treatment of bulimia nervosa in a primary care setting. *Am J Psychiatry* 2004;161:556-561.
79. Fogarty S, Harris D, Zaslawski C, et al. Acupuncture as an adjunct therapy in the treatment of eating disorders: A randomized cross-over pilot study. *Complement Ther Med* 2010;18:233-240.
80. Carei TR, Fyfe-Johnson AL, Breuner CC, Brown MA. Randomized controlled clinical trial of yoga in the treatment of eating disorders. *J Adolesc Health* 2010;46:346-351.
81. Hay PJ, Claudino AM. Clinical psychopharmacology of eating disorders: A research update. *Int J Neuropsychopharmacol* 2012;15:209-222.
82. Romano SJ, Halmi KA, Sarkar NP, et al. A placebo-controlled study of fluoxetine in continued treatment of bulimia nervosa after successful fluoxetine treatment. *Am J Psychiatry* 2002;159:96-102.
83. Fluoxetine Bulimia Nervosa Collaborative Study Group. Fluoxetine in the treatment of bulimia nervosa: A multicenter, placebo-controlled, double-blind trial. *Arch Gen Psychiatry* 1992;49:139-147.
84. Sysko R, Sha N, Wang Y, et al. Early response to antidepressant treatment in bulimia nervosa. *Psychol Med* 2010;40:999-1005.
85. McElroy SL, Kotwal R, Hudson JI, et al. Zonisamide in the treatment of binge eating disorder: An open-label, prospective trial. *J Clin Psychiatry* 2004;65(1):50-56.
86. Hoopes SP, Reimherr FW, Hedges DW, et al. Treatment of bulimia nervosa with topiramate in a randomized, double-blind, placebo-controlled trail, part 1: Improvement in binge and purge measures. *J Clin Psychiatry* 2003;64(11):1335-1341.
87. Nickel C, Tritt K, Muehlbacher M, et al. Topiramate treatment in bulimia nervosa patients: A randomized, double-blind, placebo-controlled trial. *Int J Eat Disord* 2005;38(4):295-300.
88. Faris PL, Kim SW, Meller WH, et al. Effect of decreasing afferent vagal activity with ondansetron on the symptoms of bulimia nervosa: A randomized double-blind trial. *Lancet* 2000;355:792-797.
89. Guerdjikova AI, Blom TJ, Martens BE, et al. Zonisamide in the treatment of bulimia nervosa: An open-label, pilot, prospective study. *Int J Eat Disord* 2013;46(7):747-750.
90. Vocks S, Tuschen-Caffier B, Pietrowsky R, et al. Meta-analysis of the effectiveness of psychological and pharmacological treatments for binge eating disorder. *Int J Eat Disord* 2010;43(3):205-217.
91. Hilbert A, Bishop ME, Stein RI, et al. Long-term efficacy of psychological treatments for binge eating disorder. *Br J Psychiatry* 2012;200(3):232-237.
92. Kass AE, Kolko RP, Wilfley DE, et al. Psychological treatments for eating disorders. *Curr Opin Psychiatry* 2013;26(6):549-555.
93. Grilo CM, Masheb RM, Wilson GT. Cognitive-behavioral therapy, behavioral weight loss, and sequential treatment for obese patients with binge eating disorder: A randomized controlled trial. *J Consult Clin Psychol* 2001;79(5):675-685.
94. Devlin MJ, Goldfein JA, Petkova E, et al. Cognitive behavioral therapy and fluoxetine as adjuncts to group behavioral therapy for binge eating disorder. *Obes Res* 2005;13(6):1077-1088.
95. Kaplan AS. Academy for Eating Disorders international conference on eating disorders. *Expert Opin Investig Drugs* 2003;12:1441-1443.
96. McElroy SL, Casuto LS, Nelson EB, et al. Placebo-controlled trial of sertraline in the treatment of binge eating disorder. *Am J Psychiatry* 2000;157:1004-1006.
97. Aigner M, Treasure J, Kaye W, et al. World Federation of Societies of Biological Psychiatry (WFSBP) guidelines for the pharmacologic treatment of eating disorders. *World J Biol Psychiatry* 2011;12:400-443.

98. McElroy SL, Hudson JI, Mitchell, JE, et al. Efficacy and safety of lisdexamfetamine for treatment of adults with moderate to severe binge-eating disorder. A randomized clinical trial. *JAMA Psychiatry* 2015;72(3):235-246.
99. McElroy SL, Hudson JI, Capece JA, et al. Topiramate for the treatment of binge-eating disorder associated with obesity: A placebo-controlled study. *Biol Psychiatry* 2007;61:1039-1048.
100. Claudino AM, de Oliveira IR, Appolinario JUC, et al. Double-blind, randomized, placebo-controlled trial of topiramate plus cognitive-behavior therapy in binge-eating disorder. *J Clin Psychiatry* 2007;8:1324-1332.
101. Golay A, Laurent-Jaccard A, Habicht F, et al. Effect of orlistat in obese patients with binge eating disorder. *Obes Res* 2005;13(10):1701-1708.
102. Brownley KA, Von Holle A, Hamer RM, et al. A double-blind, randomized pilot trial of chromium picolinate for binge-eating disorder: Results of the binge eating and chromium (BEACh) study. *J Psychosom Res* 2013;75:36-42.
103. Bamford B, Barras C, Sly R, et al. Eating disorder symptoms and quality of life: Where should clinicians place their focus in severe and enduring anorexia nervosa. *Int J Eat Disord* 2015;48:133-138.

Substance-Related Disorders I: Overview and Depressants, Stimulants, and Hallucinogens

65

Paul L. Doering and Robin Moorman Li

KEY CONCEPTS

1. Problems related to abuse of chemical substances can occur acutely (eg, respiratory arrest from using heroin) or after some length of time (eg, dependence or withdrawal from continued use of an opiate). The treatment approach is distinctly different depending on the type of problem.
2. Certain drugs of abuse are marketed via the Internet and other unregulated outlets using names that would not immediately identify the substance as a dangerous drug. Health professionals must stay abreast of the latest marketing ruse to conceal the true nature of the substance.
3. Synthetic chemists are constantly developing new drugs of abuse with pharmacology that mimics that of established controlled substances. Often, the dangers of these substances are greater than that of the parent compound.
4. For a few drugs, there is a specific antidote that can be used in cases of overdoses. For others, treatment is symptomatic and supportive. Early recognition and treatment of acute drug intoxications can make a huge difference in the ultimate outcome for the patient.
5. Withdrawal from certain classes of drugs (eg, benzodiazepines or barbiturates) can be life-threatening, and steps must be taken to ensure that discontinuation or dose reduction is gradual and that it takes place in closely supervised settings.
6. While there is much research focusing on drugs to treat the underlying addictive processes, to date the successes have been few. Whereas methadone, levo-α-acetylmethadol (LAAM), and buprenorphine are used for narcotic maintenance, the logical approach at present should center on prevention and using pharmacotherapies like buprenorphine to wean patients off of opioids altogether.
7. While the goal of therapy for substance dependence is to wean patients from a drug or drug category altogether, this is often difficult to do. For some, the treatment strategy is to manage the chemical dependency to allow the patient to lead as normal a life as is possible. This may require the substitution of one drug for the primary drug of dependency.
8. Pharmacotherapy of substance-related disorders is most often adjunctive to other modes of therapy such as counseling and intense psychotherapy.

The book of *Ecclesiastes* wisely reminds us that "[W]hat has been will be again, what has been done will be done again; there is nothing new under the sun."[1] It is doubtful that the author of these sage words was referring to the repeating cycle of substance abuse, but when it comes to this subject there rarely *is* anything new under the sun, and this metaphor aptly applies.

Psychoactive drug use dates back to prehistoric times and the Neolithic era (8,500-4,000 BC) where the earliest human use of psychoactive substances consisted almost exclusively of plants and fruits whose mood-altering qualities were accidentally discovered but subsequently deliberately grown.[2]

Ancient civilizations (4,000 BC-400 AD) such as the Sumerians, Egyptians, Indians, Chinese, and South Americans used opium, alcohol, cannabis, peyote, psychedelic mushrooms, and coca leaves. The Middle Ages (400-1,400) saw the use of psychoactive plants, such as belladonna and psilocybin mushroom, used by witches and shamans for healing and spiritual purposes, and distilled alcohol, coffee, tea, and opium spread along the trade routes.[2]

Almost 5,000 years ago at the Temple of Imhotep, a center for treating mental illness, opium was used in an attempt to cure the mentally ill by inducing vision, performing rituals, and praying to the gods.[2] Hippocrates, the father of medicine, recommended opium as a painkiller and as a treatment of female hysteria.[2] Evidence of the inhalation of cannabis smoke can be found in the 3rd millennium BC, as indicated by charred cannabis seeds found in a ritual fire at an ancient burial site in present-day Romania.[3] In 2003, a leather basket filled with cannabis leaf fragments and seeds was found next to a 2,500- to 2,800-year-old mummified shaman in the northwestern Xinjiang Uygur Autonomous Region of China.[4] Thousands of years later, nearly every one of these drugs is still used today in one form or another for their mind-altering effects.

For any textbook to remain relevant, it must give emphasis to *current* information in any given content area. This means that space previously budgeted to one subject must give way to more recent trends. For example, if this chapter was written in the late 1960s, great attention would be given to the use and abuse of lysergic acid diethylamide (LSD) or methamphetamine.[5,6] If it was written in the late 1970s, the epidemic abuse of hydromorphone (Dilaudid) would be featured.[7] Sadly, hydromorphone has regained a prominent position in the sprawling landscape of drug abuse and addiction.

In the mid-to late-1970s great attention would be given to the abuse of methaqualone (Quaalude).[8] Somewhere along the way, the abuse of pentazocine would take center stage.[9] Amphetamine abuse has come, gone, and come back again.[10] γ-Hydroxybutyric acid (GHB) made a sudden and dramatic appearance on the scene, but its use has lessened in the past years.[11] The current epidemic of prescription drug abuse has skyrocketed its way into prominence. Hallucinogens such as dimethyltryptamine (DMT) and phenylethylamine derivatives are making a strong comeback.

By no means does this suggest that these above-mentioned drugs have disappeared, but instead many have taken a back seat to other, more commonly encountered drugs. For this reason, this rewrite of the present chapter and the one to follow will leave out some of the information from previous editions. The interested reader should consult prior editions of this textbook for information about these substances.

TERMINOLOGY USED IN SUBSTANCE ABUSE

The lack of a common vocabulary in substance abuse treatment and prevention leads to several problems. Wide arrays of terms are in common use, many without precise meaning. This lack of universal agreement on language hampers effective communication among professionals and leads to difficulties in formulating public policy and administering third-party reimbursement programs.

In 2003, the Liaison Committee on Pain and Addiction, a collaborative effort of the American Academy of Pain Medicine, the American Pain Society, and the American Society of Addiction Medicine (ASAM), developed definitions related to the use of medications for the treatment of pain consistent with current understanding of relevant neurobiology, pharmacology, and appropriate clinical practice. While other classification systems are currently in use, the following definitions have been approved by each of the three collaborating organizations. The following definitions resulted from this consensus development committee[12]:

1. *Addiction* is a primary, chronic, neurobiologic disease, with genetic, psychosocial, and environmental factors influencing its development and manifestations. It is characterized by behaviors that include one or more of the following five Cs: *c*hronicity, impaired *c*ontrol over drug use, *c*ompulsive use, *c*ontinued use despite harm, and *c*raving.
2. *Drug abuse* is a maladaptive pattern of substance use characterized by repeated adverse consequences related to the repeated use of the substance. Examples include failure to fulfill important obligations at work, school, or home; repeated use creating physical danger, such as driving under the influence; legal problems; and social or interpersonal problems such as arguments and fights.
3. *Physical dependence* is a state of adaptation that is manifested by a drug class–specific withdrawal syndrome that can be produced by abrupt cessation, rapid dose reduction, decreasing blood level of the drug, and/or administration of an antagonist.
4. *Tolerance* is a state of adaptation in which exposure to a drug induces changes that result in a diminution of one or more of the drug's effects over time.

EPIDEMIOLOGY

Illicit drug use, including the misuse of prescription medications, affects the health and well-being of millions of Americans. Cardiovascular disease, stroke, cancer, infection with the human immunodeficiency virus (HIV), hepatitis, and lung disease can all be affected by drug use. Some of these effects occur when drugs are used at high doses or after prolonged use. However, other adverse effects can occur after only one or a few occasions of use. Addressing the impact of substance use alone is estimated to cost Americans more than $600 billion each year.

National Survey On Drug Use and Health

The National Survey on Drug Use and Health (NSDUH)[13] is the primary source of statistical information on the use of illegal drugs by the U.S. population. Conducted by the federal government since 1971, the survey collects data from a representative sample of the population at their place of residence.

The National Survey on Drug Use and Health obtains information on nine categories of illicit drugs: marijuana (including hashish), cocaine (including crack), heroin, hallucinogens, and inhalants, as well as the nonmedical use of prescription-type pain relievers, tranquilizers, stimulants, and sedatives.

In 2014, an estimated 27.0 million Americans aged 12 or older were current (past month) illicit drug users, meaning that they had used an illicit drug during the month prior to the survey interview. This corresponds to about 1 in 10 Americans (10.2%). The most commonly used illicit drug in the past month was marijuana, which was used by 22.2 million people aged 12 or older. An estimated 6.5 million people reported nonmedical use of psychotherapeutic drugs in the past month, including 4.3 million nonmedical users of prescription pain relievers.

Although nonmedical pain reliever use continued to be the second most common type of illicit drug use in 2014, the percentage of people aged 12 or older in 2014 who were current nonmedical users of pain relievers (1.6%) was lower than the percentages in most years from 2002 to 2012, but it was similar to the percentage in 2013.

The use of many types of other illicit drugs has not increased in recent years. However, the percentage of people aged 12 or older in 2014 who were current heroin users was higher than the percentages in most years from 2002 to 2013.

Approximately 21.5 million people aged 12 or older in 2014 had a substance use disorder (SUD) in the past year, including 17.0 million people with an alcohol use disorder, 7.1 million with an illicit drug use disorder, and 2.6 million who had both an alcohol use and an illicit drug use disorder.

Monitoring The Future Study

Every year the Institute for Social Research at the University of Michigan conducts its Monitoring the Future Study (MTFS), supported under a series of research grants from the National Institute on Drug Abuse.[14]

A main purpose of this research is to study changes in the beliefs, attitudes, and behavior of young people in the United States which requires frequent reassessment to identify the rapidly changing patterns.[14]

The 2014 MTF survey encompassed about 41,600 8th-, 10th-, and 12th-grade students in 377 secondary schools nationwide.[14] Annual marijuana prevalence peaked among 12th graders in 1979 at 51%, following a rise that began during the 1960s. In the ensuing years rates have gone up and down in 8th, 10th, and 12th graders. Daily use increased in all three grades after 2007, reaching peaks in 2011 (at 1.3% in 8th), 2013 (at 4.0% in 10th), and 2011 (at 6.6% in 12th), before declining modestly since. Daily prevalence rates in 2014 were 1.0%, 3.4%, and 5.8%, respectively. Researchers postulate that the increase of smoking marijuana is partly attributable to the national debate over medical use of cannabis which may make the drugs seem safer to teenagers.[14]

Synthetic marijuana (see below) which contains designer chemicals included in the cannabinoid family (common names are K-2, Spice, and Blaze) has been of increasing concern both because of its adverse effects and its high rates of use, first documented by this study in 2011. Annual prevalence at that time was found to be 11.4%, making synthetic marijuana the second most widely used class of illicit drug after marijuana among 12th graders. Despite the Drug Enforcement Administration's (DEA) intervention, use among 12th graders remained unchanged in 2012 at 11.3%, which suggests either that compliance with the new scheduling had been limited or that producers of these products succeeded in continuing to change their chemical formulas to avoid using the ingredients that had been scheduled. In 2012, for the first time, 8th and 10th graders were asked about their use of synthetic marijuana; annual prevalence rates were 4.4% and 8.8%, respectively. Use in all 3 grades dropped in 2013, and the decline was sharp and significant among 12th graders. The declines continued into 2014 and were significant for both 10th and 12th graders.

ECONOMIC IMPACT OF SUBSTANCE ABUSE

Substance abuse and addiction have an enormous impact on the economy. Annual costs of illicit drug use are estimated at more than $11 billion for health care and $182 billion for crime and lost productivity.[15]

ACUTE VERSUS CHRONIC PROBLEMS

1 Misuse of chemical substances causes problems of two types: those that occur acutely and those that arise after continued use of a drug. Acute problems are usually predictable, given the pharmacology of the drug. Chronic abuse of chemical substances can cause a wide array of physical, psychological, and psychiatric morbities. The substance-induced disorders discussed here mainly include intoxication and withdrawal.

1 The essential feature of substance dependence is the continued use of the substance despite adverse substance-related problems. The criteria for substance dependence are the same for each of the drugs or drug classes, varying only to fit the unique pharmacologic properties of each drug. Patients who take prescribed drugs for appropriate medical indications and in correct doses may still show tolerance, physical dependence, and withdrawal symptoms if the drug is stopped abruptly rather than being tapered. Tolerance and physical dependence are inevitable consequences of chronic treatment with opioids and certain other drugs, but by themselves, tolerance and physical dependence do not imply "addiction." According to the *Diagnostic and Statistical Manual of Mental Disorders, Fifth Edition*, (*DSM-5*)[16] the overall category of substance-induced disorders includes intoxication, withdrawal, and other substance/medication-induced mental disorders (eg, substance-induced psychotic disorder, substance-induced depressive disorder). To meet *DSM-5* criteria for the diagnosis of SUD, at least two of the following must occur within a 12-month period:

1. The specific substance is often taken in larger amounts or over a longer period than was intended.
2. There is a persistent desire or unsuccessful efforts to cut down or control use of the substance.
3. A great deal of time is spent in activities necessary to obtain, use, or recover from the effects of the substance.
4. Craving, or a strong desire or urge to use the substance.
5. Recurrent use of the substance resulting in a failure to fulfill major role obligations at work, school, or home.
6. Continued substance use despite having persistent or recurrent social or interpersonal problems caused or exacerbated by the effects of substance.
7. Important social, occupational, or recreational activities are given up or reduced because of the use of the substance.
8. Recurrent substance use in situations in which it is physically hazardous.
9. Use of the substance is continued despite knowledge of having a persistent or recurrent physical or psychological problem that is likely to have been caused or exacerbated by the substance.
10. Tolerance, as defined by either of the following:
    a. A need for markedly increased amounts of the substance to achieve intoxication or desired effect.
    b. Markedly diminished effect with continued use of the same amount of the substance.
11. Withdrawal, as manifested by either of the following:
    a. The characteristic withdrawal syndrome for the substance of the criteria set for a given substance.
    b. The substance (or a closely related one) is taken to relieve or avoid withdrawal symptoms.

The DSM-5 does not use the word *addiction* in its classification scheme, although it is in common usage in many countries to describe severe problems related to compulsive and habitual use of substances. The more neutral term *SUD* is used to describe the wide range of the disorder, from a mild form to a severe state of chronically relapsing, compulsive drug taking. Some clinicians will choose to use the word addiction to describe more extreme presentations, but the word is omitted from the official DSM-5 SUD diagnostic terminology because of its uncertain definition and its potentially negative connotation.

Intoxication refers to the development of a substance-specific syndrome after recent ingestion and presence in the body of a substance, and it is associated with maladaptive behavior during the waking state caused by the effect of the substance on the central nervous system (CNS). Examples include belligerence, mood lability, impaired judgment, and impaired social or occupational functioning. Evidence for recent intake of the substance can be obtained from the history, physical examination, or laboratory examination. The most common changes involve disturbances in perception, wakefulness, attention, thinking, judgment, motor behavior, and interpersonal behavior.

As with most illnesses, the course and prognosis of the disorders of substance use and dependence are variable. Getting patients who are drug dependent to stop using drugs is very difficult, and many patients return to drug use even after treatment. It has been reported that as many as 75% of treated, substance-dependent patients will relapse at least once. Many patients, however, are able to obtain recovery with treatment and continued care in 12-step programs such as Alcoholics Anonymous or Narcotics Anonymous. Substance dependence or addiction can be viewed as a chronic illness that can be controlled successfully with treatment but cannot be cured and is associated with a high relapse rate. Without treatment, the course can progress to life-threatening severity, resulting from the effects of the drug, drug contaminants, or medical complications of use.[18] Although an in-depth discussion of the mechanism of drug addiction is beyond the scope of this chapter, the interested reader is directed to a review article that presents the current understanding of the biology of drug addiction.[17]

CNS DEPRESSANTS

Opiates and Opioids

Deaths from prescription opioids have reached epidemic levels in the past decade. The number of overdose deaths is now greater than the number of deaths from heroin and cocaine combined. In 2014, an estimated 6.5 million Americans aged 12 or older were current nonmedical users of psychotherapeutic drugs, representing 2.5% of the population aged 12 or older. Estimates of current nonmedical use of prescription psychotherapeutic drugs among the population aged 12 or older has largely been driven by the nonmedical use of prescription pain relievers. In 2014, about two thirds of the current nonmedical users of psychotherapeutic drugs who were aged 12 or older reported current nonmedical use of pain relievers. This represents 1.6% of the population aged 12 or older. Nonmedical users of pain relievers in 2014 were lower than the percentages in most years from 2002 to 2012, but it was similar to the percentage in 2013. A few years back, The Centers for Disease Control and Prevention (CDC) noted that, between 1997 and 2007, drug company distribution of prescription opioid analgesics increased 627%. The quantity of prescription painkillers sold to pharmacies, hospitals, and doctors' offices was 4 times larger in 2010 than in 1999. According to the CDC, enough of these drugs are currently distributed for every American to take 5 mg Vicodin every 4 hours for 3 weeks.[19,20]

Stated differently, enough prescription opioids were prescribed in 2010 to medicate every American adult around-the-clock for a month.[21] Distribution by drug companies rose from 96 mg/person in 1997 to 698 mg/person in 2007. Although most of these drugs were prescribed for a medical purpose, many ended up in the hands of people who misused or abused them. Each day, almost 7,000 people are treated in emergency departments (ED's) for using these drugs in a manner other than as directed. Deaths from prescription painkillers have also quadrupled since 1999, killing more than 16,000 people in the United States in 2013.[21]

Many states report problems with "pill mills," where doctors prescribe large quantities of opioids to people without medical justification. Some people also obtain prescriptions from multiple prescribers by "doctor shopping."

Clinical **Controversy...**

There is considerable debate about the appropriate use of prescribed opiates and how this might contribute to the overuse or abuse of these same drugs for nonmedicinal purposes. Not all decisions that physicians and other prescribers make are going to be correct. Likewise, pharmacists are going to occasionally make the wrong decision by either declining to fill a prescription that is proper and appropriate or by filling one that is bogus. In the final analysis, mistakes in judgment are going to be made in both directions. Given this fact, in which direction should the health professional err? Should health practitioners give the patient the benefit of the doubt, writing or filling the prescription, even if their decision ultimately turns out to be wrong? Or should the mandate be in the other direction: refuse to prescribe pain medicines or refuse to fill the prescriptions, even when, in truth, the prescription is appropriate and valid? Most healthcare professional assume that complaints of pain are real and prescribe accordingly.

Nearly every state has authorized prescription drug monitoring programs (PDMPs), and most are operational at this time. PDMPs are electronic systems for the monitoring of controlled substances and drugs of concern dispensed in the state or dispensed to an address in the state. PDMPs aim to detect and prevent the diversion and abuse of prescription drugs at the retail level, where no other automated information collection system exists, and to allow for the collection and analysis of prescription data more efficiently than states without such a program can accomplish.

In 2011 NSDUH indicated that illicit drug use is 16.2% among pregnant teens and 7.4% among pregnant women aged 18 to 25 years.[13] From 2009 to 2012, incidence of Neonatal Abstinence Syndrome (NAS), defined as a withdrawal syndrome that occurs in opioid-exposed infants shortly after birth, increased nationally from 3.4 (95% confidence interval [CI]: 3.2-3.6) to 5.8 (95% CI 5.5-6.1) per 1,000 hospital births, reaching a total of 21,732 infants with the diagnosis. Aggregate hospital charges for NAS increased from $732 million to $1.5 billion (*P*<0.001), with 81% attributed to state Medicaid programs in 2012.[23] NAS incidence varied by geographic census division, with the highest incidence rate (per 1,000 hospital births) of 16.2 (95% CI 12.4-18.9) in the East South Central Division (Kentucky, Tennessee, Mississippi and Alabama) and the lowest in West South Central Division Oklahoma, Texas, Arkansas and Louisiana 2.6 (95% CI 2.3-2.9).[24]

Methadone

More than 30% of prescription opioid deaths involve methadone, even though only 2% of painkiller prescriptions are for this drug. Six times as many people died of methadone overdoses in 2009 than a decade before.[25]

Studies using medical examiner data suggested that more than three-quarters of methadone overdoses involved persons who were not enrolled in programs treating opioid addiction with methadone and that most persons who overdosed were using it without a prescription.[26]

Still, more than 4 million methadone prescriptions were written for pain in 2009, despite US Food and Drug Administration (FDA) warnings about the risks associated with this drug.

Methadone has pharmacologic properties unique among opioids, and as a result, a lack of knowledge about methadone among practitioners and patients has been identified as a factor contributing to the increased number of deaths observed in recent years.[28] Methadone's elimination half-life (8-59 hours) is longer than its duration of analgesic action (4-8 hours). In an FDA advisory issued in November 2006,[29] healthcare professionals were reminded that methadone's peak respiratory depressant effects typically occur later, and persist longer than its peak analgesic effects. The advisory notes that during treatment initiation, methadone's full analgesic effect is usually not attained until 3 to 5 days of dosing.

Deaths have been reported during conversion from chronic, high-dose treatment with other opioid agonists to methadone. It is critical to understand the pharmacokinetics of methadone when converting patients from other opioids to methadone. Particular vigilance is necessary during treatment initiation, during conversion from one opioid to another, and during dose adjustments. Also, there are pharmacokinetic and pharmacodynamic drug interactions between methadone and many other drugs. Thus drugs administered concomitantly with methadone should be evaluated for interaction potential.[29]

Heroin

The threat posed by heroin in the United States is serious and has increased since 2007. Heroin is available in larger quantities, used by a larger number of people, and is causing an increasing number of overdose deaths. In 2013, 8,620 Americans died from heroin-related overdoses, nearly triple the number in 2010. Increased demand for, and use of, heroin is being driven by both increasing availability of heroin in the U.S. market and by some controlled prescription drug (CPD) abusers using heroin. CPD abusers who begin using heroin do so chiefly because of price differences, but also because of availability, and the reformulation of OxyContin®, a commonly abused prescription opioid.

Also, high purity batches of heroin sold in certain markets are causing users to accidentally overdose. There is an increase in new heroin initiates, many of whom are young and inexperienced. Abusers of prescription opioids (drugs with known compositions and concentrations) initiating use of heroin may encounter, an illicitly-manufactured drug with varying purities, dosage amounts, and adulterants; and the use of highly toxic heroin adulterants such as fentanyl in certain markets (see below). Further, heroin addicts who have stopped using heroin for a period of time (due to rehabilitation programs, incarceration, etc.) and subsequently return to using heroin are particularly susceptible to overdose, because their tolerance for the drug has decreased.

Heroin availability is increasing in areas throughout the United States. Availability levels are highest in the Northeast and in areas of the Midwest, according to law enforcement reporting. According to National Seizure System (NSS) data, heroin seizures in the United States increased 81% over 5 years, from 2,763 kg in 2010 to 5,014 kg in 2014. Traffickers are also transporting heroin in larger amounts. The average size of a heroin seizure in 2010 was 0.86 kg; in 2014, the average heroin seizure was 1.74 kg.[30]

Between 1980s and 1990s, the purity of the heroin brought into the United States increased significantly. In 1981, the average retail-level purity of heroin was 10%. By 1999, that had increased to an average of 40%. During the same time, the price per gram decreased greatly. In 1981, the average price per gram of pure heroin was $3,260 in 2012 U.S. dollars (USD) at the retail-level; by 1999, that price had decreased to $622 (2012 USD). Since that time, heroin prices have remained low, and heroin purity levels, while fluctuating, have remained elevated.[30]

When heroin is higher in purity, it can be snorted or smoked, which broadens its appeal. Many people who would never consider injecting a drug were introduced to heroin by inhalation. In the 1990s, the drug largely lost the stigma associated with injecting, and a new population of heroin users emerged. High-purity heroin is still commonly inhaled and, according to treatment officials, remains a common method of administration by new heroin initiates.

Current cocaine users outnumbered heroin users by approximately 5 times in 2013, but heroin-involved overdose deaths were almost twice those of cocaine. Deaths involving heroin are also increasing at a much faster rate than for other illicit drugs, more than tripling between 2007 (2,402) and 2013 (8,260).

Fentanyl

Fentanyl, a synthetic and short-acting opioid analgesic, is 50-100 times more potent than morphine and approved for managing acute or chronic pain associated with advanced cancer. Although pharmaceutical fentanyl can be diverted for misuse, most cases of fentanyl-related morbidity and mortality have been linked to illicitly manufactured fentanyl and fentanyl analogs, collectively referred to as non-pharmaceutical fentanyl (NPF). NPF is sold via illicit drug markets for its heroin-like effect and often mixed with heroin and/or cocaine as a combination product—with or without the user's knowledge—to increase its euphoric effects.

In March 2015, the DEA issued a nationwide alert identifying fentanyl as a threat to public health and safety. The National Heroin Threat Assessment Summary, noted that beginning in late 2013 and throughout 2014, several states have reported spikes in overdose deaths due to fentanyl and its analog acetyl-fentanyl.

Similar to previous fentanyl overdose outbreaks, most of the more than 700 fentanyl-related overdose deaths reported to DEA during this timeframe were attributable to illicitly-manufactured fentanyl—not diverted pharmaceutical fentanyl—and either mixed with heroin or other diluents and sold as a highly potent form (sometimes under the street name "China White"). The DEA report noted that the true number of fentanyl deaths is most likely higher because many coroners' offices and state crime laboratories do not test for fentanyl or its analogs unless given a specific reason to do so.[32]

Fentanyl poses a significant danger to public health workers, first responders, and law enforcement personnel that may unwittingly come into contact with it either by absorbing through the skin or accidental inhalation of airborne powder. In August 2015, New Jersey law enforcement officers conducting a narcotics field test on an illicit substance experienced shortness of breath, dizziness, and respiratory distress after coming into contact with an unknown substance, which forensic laboratory testing determined to be a mix of cocaine, heroin, and fentanyl.[32]

Benzodiazepines And Other Sedative-Hypnotics

Emergency department visits involving benzodiazepines clearly outnumber those involving any of the other types of psychotherapeutic agents. The Drug Abuse Warning Network (DAWN)[33] estimates that 408,021 ED visits associated with nonmedical use of pharmaceuticals involved benzodiazepines in 2010 (the last year such data is available).[15] This is a dramatic increase from 2004 in which there were 170,471 ED visits attributed to benzodiazepines.

Because all benzodiazepines have abuse and dependence liability, patients cannot be switched from one benzodiazepine to another in hopes of decreasing a pattern of drug abuse or dependence behavior. Zolpidem, a nonbenzodiazepine, nonbarbiturate sedative, has been suggested to have little liability for physical dependence, but tolerance and withdrawal have been reported in association with its use as well.[33] Recent reports in the lay press have linked use of zolpidem to sleep walking, erratic driving, binge eating, and other similarly bizarre activities.

Benzodiazepines generally do not cause life-threatening respiratory depression (unless taken with other sedatives), as do the barbiturate-like drugs.[34] Long-term use of even therapeutic doses of benzodiazepines can cause physical dependence and withdrawal symptoms after abrupt discontinuation.[34] Occurrence of hallucinations or seizures would indicate severe physical withdrawal.

Gradual tapering of dosage is also associated with less withdrawal and rebound anxiety than abrupt discontinuation. Treatment of sedative-hypnotic and benzodiazepine intoxication is summarized in Table 65-1. For additional information on benzodiazepine withdrawal, refer to Chapter 70.

CLINICAL PRESENTATION Benzodiazepine Intoxication and Withdrawal

General

- The intoxicated patient may be in acute distress in overdoses or when benzodiazapines are combined with alcohol.
- Patients in withdrawal may also be in acute distress and should be treated with a benzodiazepine taper to prevent seizures.

Symptoms

- The patient may experience memory impairment, drowsiness, visual disturbances, confusion, and gastrointestinal disturbances. Patients may appear intoxicated, with slurred speech, poor coordination, swaying, and bloodshot eyes, with or without the odor of alcohol.
- Withdrawal symptoms include agitation and restlessness, dizziness, flu-like symptoms, impaired memory and concentration, nausea and vomiting, nightmares, visual disturbances, convulsions, and hallucinations.

Signs

- Hypotension or nystagmus may be observed, and urinary retention may occur.

Laboratory Tests

- Qualitative testing to confirm presence of benzodiazepines is useful for diagnostic purposes, but quantitative plasma concentrations are usually not clinically useful.

TABLE 65-1 Pharmacologic Treatment of Substance Intoxication

Drug Class	Nonpharmacologic Therapy	Pharmacologic Therapy	Level of Evidence[a,b]
Benzodiazepines	Support vital functions	Flumazenil 0.2 mg/min IV initially, repeat up to 3 mg max.	AI
Alcohol, barbiturates, and sedative-hypnotics (nonbenzodiazepines)	Support vital functions	None	B3
Opiates	Support vital functions	Naloxone 0.4-2 mg IV every 3 minutes	A1
Cocaine and other CNS stimulants	Monitor cardiac function	Lorazepam 2-4 mg IM every 30 minutes to 6 hours as needed for agitation	B2
		Haloperidol 2-5 mg (or other antipsychotic agent) every 30 minutes to 6 hours as needed for psychotic behavior	B3
Hallucinogens, marijuana, and inhalants	Reassurance; "talk-down therapy"; support vital functions	Lorazepam and/or haloperidol as above	B3
Phencyclidine	Minimize sensory input	Lorazepam and/or haloperidol as above	B3

[a]Strength of recommendations, evidence to support recommendation, A, good; B, moderate; C, poor.

[b]Quality of evidence: 1, evidence from more than 1 properly randomized, controlled trial; 2, evidence from more than one well-designed clinical trial with randomization, from cohort or case-controlled analytic studies or multiple time series; or dramatic results from uncontrolled experiments; 3, evidence from opinions of respected authorities, based on clinical experience, descriptive studies, or reports of expert communities.

Data from references 91 and 111.

Carisoprodol

Carisoprodol is a prescription drug marketed since 1959 and used in primary care settings for the treatment of musculoskeletal conditions associated with muscle spasms and back pain. Its effectiveness for this use has been questioned.[35]

It is marketed in the United States as Soma as well as many generic versions. It is both structurally and pharmacologically related to meprobamate, a schedule IV substance. In fact, a substantial percentage of the drug is metabolized to meprobamate,[35] a drug with barbiturate-like properties.

In legitimate medical practice carisoprodol is used as an adjunct to rest, physical therapy, and other measures for relief of acute, painful musculoskeletal conditions.[35] Adverse effects are mostly related to the CNS: drowsiness, dizziness, vertigo, ataxia, tremor, agitation, irritability, headache, depressive reactions, syncope, and insomnia. Carisoprodol may also adversely affect cardiovascular (tachycardia, postural hypotension, and facial flushing), gastrointestinal (nausea, vomiting, hiccup, and epigastric distress), and hematologic systems. Carisoprodol overdose has resulted in stupor, coma, shock, respiratory depression, and death.[35]

The number of carisoprodol-related ED visits involving misuse or abuse by patients aged 50 or older tripled between 2004 and 2009 (from 2,070 to 7,115 visits). The majority of ED visits involving carisoprodol also involved other pharmaceuticals (77%); the most common combinations involved narcotic pain relievers (55%) and benzodiazepines (47%).[33]

Recognizing that prolonged abuse of carisoprodol at high dosage can lead to tolerance, dependence, and withdrawal,[35] DEA issued a final rule to classify carisoprodol as a Schedule IV controlled substance effective from January 11, 2012.[36]

Dextromethorphan

Dextromethorphan abuse is one of the most common (and most dangerous) examples of over-the-counter (OTC) drug abuse.[37] Intoxication from consuming large doses of cough syrup is known on the street as "robodosing" or "robotripping." Handfuls of cough and cold remedies are sometimes called "skittles" because they look similar to the popular fruit candy. Dextromethorphan creates a depressant and sometimes profound hallucinogenic effect when taken in large doses. Since the drug is available OTC, it is easily procured by adolescents. Those who use the cough syrup to get high are sometimes called "syrup heads."

High doses induce effects that include hyperexcitability, lethargy, ataxia, slurred speech, diaphoresis, hypertension, nystagmus, and mydriasis. When taken at much higher doses, it acts as a dissociative anesthetic, similar to phencyclidine (PCP, "angel dust") and ketamine ("Special K"). These are the effects sought by those who use the drug to get high. At these high doses, dextromethorphan also is a CNS depressant.[38]

The recommended treatment for acute overdoses of dextromethorphan is naloxone. Although reports of its efficacy are mixed, it may be helpful in reversing the CNS depressant and neurologic effects.[38]

CNS STIMULANTS

Cocaine

Cocaine is perhaps the most behaviorally reinforcing of all drugs of abuse. Clinicians estimate that approximately 10% of people who begin to use the drug recreationally will go on to serious, heavy use. Once having tried cocaine, an individual cannot predict or control the extent to which he or she will continue to use the drug.

The most characteristic pharmacologic effect of cocaine is stimulation of the CNS. In the CNS, cocaine appears to mediate its effects primarily by blocking reuptake of catecholamine neurotransmitters such as norepinephrine and dopamine.

Cocaine is absorbed rapidly from virtually all sites of application. For many years, cocaine has been administered as the hydrochloride salt form, usually by inhalation, but also by injection. In the last 18 to 20 years, as the purity of cocaine hydrochloride obtained on the street declined, many users converted the cocaine hydrochloride to cocaine base, also known as "crack" or "rock." Smoking the drug leads to almost instant absorption and intense euphoria. Peak plasma concentrations of more than 900 ng/mL (mcg/L; 3.0 μmol/L) have been achieved following inhalation of cocaine base vapors, compared with concentrations of only 150 to 200 ng/mL (mcg/L; 0.49-0.66 μmol/L) achieved after inhalation of similar amounts of pure cocaine hydrochloride powder.[39]

The high from snorting can last 15 to 30 minutes, whereas that from smoking can last 5 to 10 minutes. Increased use can reduce the period of stimulation. An appreciable tolerance to the high can develop, and many addicts report that they seek but fail to achieve as much pleasure as they did from their first exposure. Scientific evidence suggests that the powerful neuropsychologic reinforcing property of cocaine is responsible for an individual's continued use despite harmful physical and social consequences.

Research has helped clarify certain patterns of cocaine use, such as combining cocaine and alcohol. Such drug use would seem counterintuitive because cocaine is a CNS stimulant, and alcohol a CNS depressant. In the presence of alcohol, cocaine is metabolized to cocaethylene, a longer-acting but potent psychoactive compound compared to the parent drug.[40,41] The risk of death from cocaethylene is greater than from cocaine. The cocaine-alcohol combination is one of the most commonly identified among individuals who come to hospital EDs with acute substance abuse problems.

Cocaine is metabolized and eliminated rapidly. The elimination half-life of cocaine is approximately 1 hour, and the duration of effect is very short.[39] The short duration of effect provides a powerful incentive for repeated use of the drug. Many users experience intense drug use cycling, sometimes lasting days, characterized by rapidly repeating doses of cocaine until their supply is exhausted. Laboratory monkeys, given a choice between food and cocaine around the clock for 8 days, consistently choose cocaine.

Complications of cocaine use frequently involve cardiovascular events.[42,43] Cocaine is a psychotomimetic drug, sometimes even at nontoxic doses. A kindling phenomenon has been described with cocaine in which neuronal function becomes altered with each dose of the drug. The psychosis is qualitatively very similar to a paranoid schizophrenic psychosis.[44] Although there is some controversy as to whether cocaine is associated with physical withdrawal on abrupt discontinuation, most clinicians feel that there is a characteristic syndrome of withdrawal effects, although they are not life-threatening.

Amphetamine, Methamphetamine, and Other Stimulants

The physiologic and psychologic effects of amphetamines and other stimulants are qualitatively similar to those of cocaine—they diminish fatigue, increase alertness, and suppress appetite. Pharmacologically, amphetamines increase the activity of catecholamine neurotransmitters (eg, norepinephrine and dopamine) by increasing release and by inhibiting the degradative enzyme monoamine oxidase.

Methamphetamine is used orally, intranasally, rectally, by intravenous injection, and by smoking. Immediately after inhalation or intravenous injection, the methamphetamine user experiences an intense sensation, called a "rush" or "flash," that lasts only a few minutes and is described as extremely pleasurable.[45]

Because methamphetamine elevates mood, people who experiment with it tend to use it with increasing frequency and in increasing doses, although this was not their original intent. The timing and intensity of the "rush" that accompanies the use of methamphetamine, which is a result of the release of high levels of dopamine in the brain, depend in part on the method of administration.[45] Specifically, the effect is almost instantaneous when smoked or injected, whereas it takes approximately 5 minutes after snorting or 20 minutes after oral ingestion.[39,45] Prolonged use of methamphetamine can result in a tolerance for the drug and increased use at higher dosage levels, creating dependence. Such continual use of the drug with little or no sleep may lead to an extremely irritable and paranoid state. Discontinuing use of methamphetamine often results in a state of depression, as well as fatigue, anergia, and some types of cognitive impairment that can last from 2 days to several months.[45]

Negative consequences of methamphetamine abuse range from anxiety and insomnia to convulsions, paranoia, and brain damage. Methamphetamine-induced caries, or "meth mouth" is a characteristic pattern of dental decay commonly observed in patients that smoke methamphetamine.[46]

In addition to the many direct effects on methamphetamine users are the indirect impacts on individuals and society. Flammable ingredients that include acetone, red phosphorous, ethyl alcohol, and lithium metal are used in methamphetamine cookers, often with disastrous results. Fires and explosions often ensue, resulting in severe burns and uncovering laboratories to local law enforcement. Children of methamphetamine abusers are at high risk of neglect and abuse, and pregnant women's use of methamphetamine can cause growth retardation, premature birth, and developmental disorders in neonates. Treatment for methamphetamine dependence is very difficult, and has a low success rate.[45]

According to the 2014 National Drug Threat Survey,[46] 31.8% of responding agencies indicated methamphetamine was the greatest drug threat in their areas. Also, 40.6% of responding agencies indicated that methamphetamine is highly available, meaning the drug is easily obtained at any time. The majority of methamphetamine available in the United States is Mexico-produced.[46]

The vast majority of methamphetamine laboratories seized in the United States are the small capacity production laboratories, also

CLINICAL PRESENTATION Amphetamine Intoxication and Withdrawal

General

- Amphetamine intoxication is an acute condition that may result in death. Pharmacotherapy may be indicated for symptomatic control of seizures.
- Patients may experience withdrawal symptoms for several days, but are usually not in acute distress. Treatment of withdrawal is supportive in nature. Pharmacotherapy is not effective to treat the symptoms of amphetamine withdrawal.

Symptoms

- Depression, altered mental status, drug craving, dyssomnia, and fatigue are all symptoms of withdrawal.
- Amphetamine intoxication may present as increased wakefulness, increased physical activity, decreased appetite, increased respiration, hyperthermia, and euphoria. Other CNS effects include irritability, insomnia, confusion, tremors, convulsions, anxiety, paranoia, chest pain, and aggressiveness. Hyperthermia and convulsions can result in death.

Signs

- Patients with amphetamine intoxication may present with tachycardia, hypertension, or stroke.

Laboratory Tests

- A qualitative urine screening for drugs of abuse is used for diagnostic purposes. Confirmatory blood tests with gas chromatography and mass spectrophotometry or liquid chromatography coupled tandem mass spectrometry may be used for verification.

known as "one-pot" or "shake-and-bake" or "mom-and-pop" laboratories. These laboratories produce small amounts of methamphetamine—generally one to three grams per laboratory—generally for personal use or use among a small group of people.[46]

In this process, ephedrine or pseudoephedrine is extracted from OTC cold and allergy tablets. Producers mix pseudoephedrine and other household items in a plastic soda-type bottle. The chemical reaction that produces methamphetamine reduces the ephedrine. Indeed, a synonym for methamphetamine is desoxy-ephedrine.[46]

Pharmacists should be wary of persons wishing to purchase large quantities of products containing nonprescription sympathomimetic products. As a precaution, federal legislation now mandates that pseudoephedrine-containing products be kept behind a counter, and suitable identification must be shown before they can be purchased.

Because the reaction is exothermic, this method of production is highly volatile and dangerous, and is susceptible to error resulting in fires or explosions. It also exposes bystanders to dangerous, sometimes lethal, chemicals. Although these laboratories produce very small amounts of methamphetamine, they produce large amounts of toxic waste. The DEA estimates that one pound of methamphetamine produced by a small capacity lab can produce five to six pounds of toxic waste.

Ecstasy and Other Methamphetamine Analogs

Several dozen analogs of amphetamine and methamphetamine are mildly hallucinogenic. Two methamphetamine analogs of most concern are 3,4-methylenedioxyamphetamine and especially 3,4-methylenedioxymethamphetamine (MDMA or Ecstasy). The annual prevalence of Ecstasy declined significantly in 2014 from the previous year in all three grades, dropping from 4.1% to 3.5%. Over the past dozen years, the use of Ecstasy has changed quite a bit, with peak incidence in 2001 at 6.7% and decreasing each year until 2014.[14]

The effects of MDMA usually last approximately 4 to 6 hours. Users of the drug say that it produces profoundly positive feelings, empathy for others, elimination of anxiety, and extreme relaxation. MDMA is also said to suppress the need to eat, drink, or sleep, enabling users to endure 2- to 3-day parties. Consequently, MDMA use sometimes results in severe dehydration or exhaustion. MDMA generally reduces inhibitions and creates a sense of euphoria, but it also can evoke anxiety and paranoia. Heavier doses generate depression, irrationality, and psychosis. Users claim they experience feelings of closeness with others and a desire to touch them.

MDMA use can result in a variety of acute psychiatric disturbances, including panic, anxiety, depression, and paranoid thinking. Physical symptoms include muscle tension, nausea, blurred vision, faintness, chills, and sweating. MDMA also increases the heart rate and blood pressure. Other effects include hyperthermia, dehydration, vomiting, tremors, loss of control over body movements, insomnia, convulsions, rapid eye movements, and teeth and jaw clenching.[47]

MDMA is perceived to be a harmless drug by many of its users, based in part on the fact that the risk of death is low compared with other drugs such as heroin and cocaine. However, mounting evidence points to neurotoxic effects of MDMA, involving a complex and incompletely understood mechanism. MDMA has been shown to destroy serotonin-producing neurons in animals, but further research is needed to understand the mechanism behind this loss of serotonin following MDMA exposure.[47]

Researchers have found that heavy MDMA users have memory problems that persist for at least 2 weeks after they have stopped using the drug.[48,49] McCann and colleagues[50,51] conducted several studies to determine the effects of MDMA use on cognitive performance. MDMA users and controls were found to perform similarly on several cognitive tasks. However, MDMA subjects had significant performance deficits on a sustained-attention task requiring arithmetic calculations, a task requiring complex attention and incidental learning, a task requiring short-term memory, and a task of semantic recognition and verbal reasoning. The authors believe that their data provide further evidence that MDMA is neurotoxic to brain serotonin neurons in humans, and the behavioral data suggest that brain serotonin injury is associated with subtle but significant cognitive deficits.

Manufacturers of illicit drugs sometimes substitute other, potentially more dangerous substances for the one the buyer is expecting. Other suppliers produce products adulterated with chemical byproducts of the incomplete processing of active ingredients. One such chemical, *para*-methoxyamphetamine, is a drastically more potent hyperthermic agent than MDMA, and deaths have been attributed to this agent.[52]

"Molly" (for "molecular") is a purified form of MDMA that is typically ingested orally, or may be added to marijuana and smoked.[53] This form of MDMA is popular due to a faster time to peak, a reported cleaner feeling of euphoria, and a reported more subtle "come down" period. "Molly" is also rumored as a safer form of MDMA, since it supposedly contains no adulterants commonly found in the tablet form of MDMA.[53]

A very engaging and insightful article on the possible medical uses of MDMA was published recently[54] and the interested reader is encouraged to read it.

Synthetic Cathinones (A.K.A., Bath Salts)

2 Bath salts are a family of structurally related sympathomimetic, synthetic, designer drugs, known collectively as cathinones. Despite being marketed as "bath salts" or "plant food" and labeled "not for human consumption," people use these substances for their amphetamine or cocaine like effects. The name "bath salts" appears to have been selected to disguise the true nature of these substances. They are available in small quantities (milligram or one-half gram packages) and obviously are not the same as legitimate commercial bath products that are used for taking a soothing bath. Since the time of their appearance in the recreational drug market, there have been numerous confirmed cases of abuse, dependence, severe intoxication, and deaths related to the consumption of synthetic cathinones.[55]

Catha edulis (Khat) is an evergreen slow-growing shrub or tree native to Ethiopia and cultivated in East Africa and the South West Arabian Peninsula that in recent years has been grown widespread in Europe as well.[56]

In areas where it is grown people use the fresh vegetable material (leaves, stems, and flower buds) of this plant for its stimulant effects. The fresh khat leaves contain 62 alkaloids, and two of these, cathine and cathinone, have been demonstrated to have amphetamine-like effects. Like amphetamines, cathine and cathinone are CNS stimulants, but their potency is less. Several studies have shown that the chronic use of this plant may produce various harmful effects, such as increased incidence of acute coronary vasospasm and myocardial infarction, esophagitis, gastritis, oral keratotic lesions, and liver toxicity.[56]

Most of the synthetic cathinones, first appearing as recreational drugs in the mid-2000s, are a ring-substituted cathinone closely related to the phenethylamine family. The synthetic cathinones are the beta-keto analogues of natural cathinone and differ from amphetamines by the presence of a ketone oxygen group at the beta-position.[56]

3 The pharmacology of these substances has not been extensively studied, but available information shows that these molecules may also inhibit monoamine oxidase. Within the class of synthetic cathinones there are considerable differences in pharmacology. The synthetic cathinones, pyrovalerone and methylenedioxypyrovalerone (MDPV), are highly potent and selective catecholamine transporter inhibitors but not substrate releasers. Mephedrone, methylone,

ethylone, butylone, and naphyrone act as nonselective monoamine uptake inhibitors, similar to cocaine and, with the exception of naphyrone, also release serotonin, similar to MDMA. Cathinone and methcathinone are selective catecholamine uptake inhibitors and releasers, similar to their non-β-keto analogs amphetamine and methamphetamine.[56]

Case reports have revealed a variety of adverse effects associated with the use of bath salts, including tachycardia, hypertension, diabetic ketoacidosis, delusions, paranoid psychosis, hyperthermia, dizziness, agitation, headaches, hyponatremia, acute liver failure, and suicide. Fatal intoxication has been associated with members of this class of drugs.[56] One report[57] by the Substance Abuse and Mental Health Services Administration (SAMHSA) reveals that bath salts were linked to an estimated 22,904 visits to hospital EDs in 2011.

The report shows that about two-thirds (67%) of ED visits involving bath salts also involved the use of another drug. Only 33% of the bath salts-related visits to EDs involved just the use of bath salts; 15% of the visits involved combined use with marijuana or synthetic forms of marijuana, and 52% involved the use of other drugs.[57]

A particularly potent synthetic cathinone burst upon the scene in late 2014 and early 2015.[58,59] Known by its street name, "flakka" a single dose is about a tenth of a gram and costs just $4 to $5. People who take more than this small amount—either accidentally or purposefully—risk powerful side effects that include accelerated heart rate, anxiety, paranoia, agitation, and psychosis.[58]

The drug is particularly prevalent in some counties in Florida, Submissions for testing to the Florida Department of Law Enforcement's crime labs have grown from 38 in 2013 to 228 in 2014.[59] At the Broward County Florida Sheriff's Office laboratory, flakka submissions grew from fewer than 200 in 2014 to 275 in just the first three months of 2015. By August, 2015 there had been at least 33 deaths linked to the substance in the preceding 10 months.[59]

On July 9, 2012, President Barack Obama signed a law that classified certain synthetic cathinones and classes of related chemicals as Schedule I Controlled Substances.[57] Flakka and 9 similar drugs were placed into Schedule I on March 7, 2014, pursuant to the temporary scheduling provisions of the Controlled Substances Act.

HALLUCINOGENS

Lysergic acid diethylamide

The drugs commonly classified as hallucinogens are LSD, psilocybin, DMT, mescaline, and other related compounds. LSD is one of the most potent mood-changing chemicals. It is manufactured from lysergic acid, which is found in ergot, a fungus that grows on rye and other grains.

Pharmacologically, LSD and related drugs stimulate both presynaptic (5-hydroxytryptamine $[5\text{-HT}]_{1A}$ and 5-HT_{1B}) and postsynaptic (5-HT_2) serotonin receptors in the brain, which functionally can cause either agonist or antagonist effects on serotonin activity. Precisely how the hallucinogens exert their effects remains unclear. LSD is an extraordinarily potent compound, producing observable CNS effects at doses as low as 25 mcg. For an in-depth review of LSD, the reader is directed to a review by Passie and colleagues.[61] An interesting article on the history, current status, and future uses of LSD has been recently published.[62]

Designer Drugs

2 The past few years have witnessed the (re)-emergence of a number of very potent substances from three categories of drugs: the phenethylamine, the piperazines, and the tryptamines.[63] These drugs are marketed largely through Internet sales, and are abused by people of all ages. They are illegally manufactured or synthesized in clandestine laboratories; many designer drugs are offered as a "research chemical," "not for human consumption."

Phenethylamines are ingested for their stimulant and hallucinogenic effects on the CNS. One group of the phenethylamine category that has received attention in recent years contains 2,5-dimethyoxy or 2C derivatives, such as 4-bromo-2,5-dimethyoxyphenethylamine (2C-B) or 2,5-dimethyoxy-4-iodophenethylamine (2C-I).

Due to their stimulant and hallucinogenic effects, piperazines have entered the club or party scene. Piperazines of concern include N-benzylpiperazine (BZP), 1-(3-trifluoromethylphenyl)-piperazine (TFMPP), and 1-(3-chlorophenyl)-piperazine (meta-chlorophenylpiperazine, mCPP). While mCPP is found in the illicit market, it is also a metabolite and starting material for the synthesis of several prescription drugs (eg, trazodone and nefazadone).[63]

Many of these emerging drugs have been added to DEA's drugs and chemicals of concern list, and two drugs—BZP and TFMPP—appeared on the list of top 25 drugs reported to National Forensic Laboratory Information System (NFLIS) in 2008 (BZP only), 2009, and 2010.[64] For example, N,N-dimethyltryptamine (DMT), occurs naturally. South American snuffs and brews like Ayahuasca, prepared from a jungle vine (*Banisteriopsis caapi*), have been used in ancient medicinal and ritualistic practices that continue today. Like piperazines, tryptamines are hallucinogenic substances that are taken orally, or more rarely by smoking, snorting, or injection. Commonly abused tryptamines include DMT and 5-methoxy-N, N-diisopropyltryptamine (5-MeO-DIPT). Several of the drugs presented in this NFLIS Special Report have been named and federally scheduled under the Controlled Substances Act.

MARIJUANA

Marijuana continues to be the most commonly used illicit drug in the United States. An estimated 22.2 million Americans aged 12 or older in 2014 were current users of marijuana.[13] This number of past month marijuana users corresponds to 8.4% of the population aged 12 or older. The percentage of people aged 12 or older who were current marijuana users in 2014 was higher than the percentages from 2002 to 2013. According to the most recent MTFS[14] current daily marijuana use, defined as use on 20 or more occasions in the last 30 days, has fluctuated widely since the MTFS began. Among 12th-grade respondents, it rose from 6.0% in 1975 to 10.7% in 1978, declined to 1.9% by 1992, and then began to increase again. Current daily use reached 6.6% in 2011, the highest prevalence seen in three decades (ie, since 1981). In 2014 daily use of marijuana was at 5.8%. It is estimated that 3.8% of the world's population used cannabis in the last year.[65]

Most users smoke marijuana in hand-rolled cigarettes (joints), while some use pipes or water pipes (bongs). Marijuana cigars called blunts have also become popular.[14] To make blunts, users slice open cigars and replace the tobacco with marijuana.

Marijuana's effects begin immediately after the drug enters the brain and last from 1 to 3 hours. If marijuana is consumed in food or drink, the short-term effects begin more slowly, usually within 30 minutes to 1 hour, and last longer, for as long as 4 hours. Smoking marijuana delivers several times more of its major active ingredient, Δ-9-tetrahydrocannabinol (THC) into the blood than does eating or drinking the drug.

Marijuana Potency

The principal psychoactive component of marijuana is THC. Hashish, the dried resin of the top of the plant, is much more potent than the plant itself. Increasingly sophisticated growing techniques have resulted in plants of greater potency.

The Potency Monitoring Project, funded by the National Institute on Drug Abuse, studies samples of drugs that have been confiscated by law enforcement personnel. The Project issues a Quarterly Report that publishes average concentrations of THC for various types of cannabis specimens. The specimens of domestically

CLINICAL PRESENTATION Marijuana Intoxication

General Symptoms

- Patients intoxicated with marijuana may experience euphoria, sensory intensification, increased appetite, apathy, hallucinations, and dry mouth. Occasionally, marijuana use produces anxiety, fear, distrust, or panic.

Signs

- Tachycardia and conjunctival congestion may be observed in patients intoxicated with marijuana.

Laboratory Tests

- Although the duration of effect of marijuana may be only several hours, THC is detectable on toxicologic screening for up to 4 to 5 weeks, especially in chronic users.

eradicated cannabis are sent to the project from state and local drug labs. In addition, specimens of seized cannabis are sent from DEA's field forensic labs.

In 1995, the average THC potency of leaf marijuana was 3.96%; in 2013, the average THC potency was 12.55%. In the 1990s, the average THC content of hash oil, a type of marijuana concentrate, ranged from 13% to 16%; today the average THC content of hash oil is 52%; one recent sample tested at 82%.[46]

The abuse of marijuana concentrates ("wax," "butane honey oil," etc.) is increasing throughout the United States. These concentrates can be abused using e-cigarettes or consumed in edibles, and have significantly higher THC levels than leaf marijuana. Highly flammable butane gas is used to extract the THC from the marijuana leaf, and has resulted in explosions, injuries, and deaths.[46,66]

Harmful Effects of Marijuana

Marijuana has been used widely and is believed by many to be a relatively harmless, nonaddictive intoxicant. The DSM-5 has a classification called Cannabis Use Disorder.[16] New to DSM-5 is the recognition that abrupt cessation of daily or near-daily cannabis use often results in the onset of a cannabis withdrawal syndrome. Common symptoms of withdrawal include irritability, anger or aggression, anxiety, depressed mood, restlessness, sleep difficulty, and decreased appetite or weight loss. Although typically not as severe as alcohol or opiate withdrawal, the cannabis withdrawal syndrome can cause significant distress and contribute to difficulty quitting or relapse among those trying to abstain.

Scientific research has found that 1 in 10 marijuana users will become addicted to the drug. And if one begins in adolescence, that number rises to 1 in 6.[67] Acutely, marijuana has many of the effects of alcohol—sedation, a decrease in reactivity and ability to perform complex tasks, and disinhibition. Endocrine effects including amenorrhea, decreased testosterone production, and inhibition of spermatogenesis have been demonstrated. Marijuana is associated with an amotivational syndrome characterized by a behavioral pattern of apathy, dullness, impaired judgment, decreased concentration and memory, loss of interest in personal hygiene, and a general reduction of goal-directed behavior.[68]

Science confirms that the adolescent brain, particularly the part of the brain that regulates the planning of complex cognitive behavior, personality expression, decision making, and social behavior, is not fully developed until the early to mid-20s. Developing brains are especially susceptible to all of the negative effects of marijuana and other drug use.[69]

One of the most well designed studies[70] on marijuana and intelligence, released in 2012, found that marijuana use reduces IQ by as much as eight points by age 38 among people who started using marijuana regularly before age 18 but then stopped. The purpose of the study was to test the association between persistent cannabis use and neuropsychological decline and determine whether decline is concentrated among adolescent-onset cannabis users. Participants were members of the Dunedin Study, a prospective study of a birth cohort of 1,037 individuals followed from birth (1972/1973) to age 38 years. Cannabis use was ascertained in interviews at ages 18, 21, 26, 32, and 38 years. Neuropsychological testing was conducted at age 13 years, before initiation of cannabis use, and again at age 38 years, after a pattern of persistent cannabis use had developed. Persistent cannabis use was associated with neuropsychological decline broadly across domains of functioning, even after controlling for years of education. Informants also reported noticing more cognitive problems for persistent cannabis users. Impairment was concentrated among adolescent-onset cannabis users, with more persistent use associated with greater decline. Further, cessation of cannabis use did not fully restore neuropsychological functioning among adolescent-onset cannabis users. Findings are suggestive of a neurotoxic effect of cannabis on the adolescent brain and highlight the importance of prevention and policy efforts targeting adolescents.[70]

A recent study found that the prevalence of marijuana use among U.S. adults doubled over the past decade.[71] Face-to-face interviews conducted in surveys of 2 nationally representative samples of U.S. adults: the National Epidemiologic Survey on Alcohol and Related Conditions (data collected April 2001-April 2002; $N = 43{,}093$) and the National Epidemiologic Survey on Alcohol and Related Conditions-III (data collected April 2012-June 2013; $N = 36{,}309$). In total, 79,000 people were interviewed on alcohol use, drug use and related psychiatric conditions during the 2001-2002 and 2012-2013 surveys.[71]

The percentage of Americans who reported using marijuana in the past year more than doubled between 2001-2002 and 2012-2013, and the increase in marijuana use disorder during that time was nearly as large. Past year marijuana use rose from 4.1% to 9.5% of the U.S. adult population, while the prevalence of marijuana use disorder rose from 1.5% to 2.9%.[71]

In this study, approximately 30% of people who used marijuana in the past year met criteria for marijuana use disorder during 2012 to 2013, as defined by the DSM-5. About 3 in 10 people who use marijuana met the criteria for addiction.[71]

When examined by age, young adults (ages 18-29) were found to be at highest risk for marijuana use and marijuana use disorder, with use increasing from 10.5% to 21.2% and disorder increasing from 4.4% to 7.5% over the past decade.[71]

Marijuana and Driving

Studies have shown that marijuana impairs driving performance, increasing lane weaving, and that since the legalization of medical marijuana in Colorado, drivers involved in fatal motor vehicle crashes are significantly more likely to test positive for marijuana use.[72,73]

As marijuana and alcohol are frequently used together, more research is needed to understand the effects of combined use.

Studies suggest that using marijuana and alcohol together impairs driving more than either substance alone, and that alcohol use may increase the absorption of THC, the psychoactive chemical found in marijuana.[72]

Along with the increased prevalence of marijuana smoking, rates of driving under the influence of cannabis have also risen in recent years. Studies show that approximately 6% to 11% of fatal accident victims test positive for THC. In many of these cases alcohol is detected as well.[74] A systematic review and meta-analysis was conducted to determine whether the acute consumption of cannabis by drivers increases the risk of motor vehicle collisions.[75] The report included nine studies. The authors conclude that acute cannabis consumption is associated with an increased risk of a motor vehicle crash, especially for fatal collisions. Another meta-analysis showed an estimated odds ratios relating marijuana use to crash risk reported in included studies ranged from 0.85 to 7.16.[76]

Medical Marijuana

Since 1996, 23 states now have medical marijuana laws, and four states, as well as the District of Columbia, have legalized marijuana for recreational use. Some believe that the widespread use of medical marijuana is a thinly veiled strategy for the future legalization of recreational as well as medicinal use. Vague state laws governing medical marijuana have allowed recreational users of the drug to take advantage of marijuana dispensaries. Obtaining a license to use marijuana is not difficult. For example, on the boardwalk of Venice Beach, California, pitchmen dressed in marijuana green clothing approach passers-by with offers of a $35, 10-minute evaluation for a medical marijuana recommendation for everything from cancer to appetite loss.[77]

Clinical **Controversy...**

The mere mention of the words "medical marijuana" is bound to evoke strong emotions among laypersons and healthcare professionals alike. While the federal government continues to enforce laws that make possession and use of marijuana illegal, regardless of the intended purpose, at last count twenty-three states now have medical marijuana laws and four states, as well as the District of Columbia, have legalized marijuana for recreational use. While the safety and efficacy of marijuana to treat certain identifiable medical conditions has been confirmed, many other uses are supported by anecdote or limited clinical experience. However, the debate involves much more than whether cannabis works or not to treat illness. Instead, there are political, social, economic, and religious considerations that cloud the controversy over whether marijuana should be legalized for medical purposes. This debate is bound to continue for years to come.

Designing and conducting adequate research studies of the beneficial effects of marijuana present some methodological challenges.[78] Smoked marijuana varies by dose, due to individual differences in absorption and metabolism in the liver, as well as puff frequency, depth of inhalation, and retention of inhaled smoke. Two comprehensive and dispassionate reviews[79,80] of medical marijuana have been published, and the reader is encouraged to consult these for further information.

Synthetic Cannabinoids

3 Over the past several years, recreational use of synthetic cannabinoid compounds has been increasing in the United States. Known colloquially as "K2," "Spice," "Aroma," "Mr. Smiley," "Zohai," "Eclipse," "Black Mamba," "Red X Dawn," "Blaze," and "Dream," these products were not listed as controlled substances until somewhat recently. As a result, they were available at gas stations, convenience stores, and on the Internet.

Following identification of THC in 1964 and the CB l and CB 2 cannabinoid receptors in the 1980s, there was a pharmaceutical effort to synthesize cannabinoid receptor agonists for potential therapeutic indications like nausea and pain. The largest structural group of synthetic cannabinoid receptor agonists is the JWH compounds named after John W. Huffman, an organic chemist at Clemson University, who synthesized many of these compounds.[81] The vast majority of these efforts never reached commercial fruition. However, independent chemists now use this publicly available research to produce synthetic cannabinoids.

Synthetic cannabinoids produce a combination of adverse effects that resemble intoxication from Δ-9-THC, the psychoactive component of marijuana. However, synthetic cannabinoids appear to be more potent and may stay active in the body longer than Δ-9-THC. The adverse effects of synthetic cannabinoids include severe agitation, anxiety, nausea, vomiting, tachycardia, elevated blood pressure, tremors, seizures, hallucinations, paranoid behavior, and nonresponsiveness. After regular consumption, withdrawal signs and symptoms have been observed. Death after use of synthetic cannabinoids has also been reported.[76]

3 Currently there are over 100 compounds referred to as "synthetic marijuana."[82] The finished salable products consist of psychoactively inert dry plant material sprayed or otherwise mixed with these synthetic cannabinoid receptor agonists.[83,84]

Symptoms of synthetic cannabinoid toxicity are similar to the euphoric and psychoactive effects of marijuana with additional sympathomimetic symptoms, including severe agitation and anxiety, extreme tachycardia, hypertension, nausea and vomiting, muscle spasms, seizures, tremors, diaphoresis, and restlessness. Intense hallucinations and psychotic episodes, and suicidal and other harmful thoughts and/or actions have also been reported.[85,86] Cohen et al. published one of the first articles in the medical literature describing the effects of synthetic cannabinoid intoxication.[87]

Gunderson et al. have published a systematic review of the effects of synthetic cannabinoids and their psychosocial implications.[88] Additional information on synthetics can be found at the web site of the U.S. Office of National Drug Control Policy.[89]

INHALANTS

Inhalants are a diverse group of substances that include volatile solvents, gases, and nitrites that are sniffed, snorted, huffed, or bagged to produce intoxicating effects similar to those of alcohol. These substances are found in common household products such as glues, lighter fluid, cleaning fluids, paint products, nail polish remover, gasoline, rubber glue, waxes, and varnishes. Chemicals found in these products include toluene, benzene, methanol, methylene chloride, acetone, methylethyl ketone, methylbutyl ketone, trichloroethylene, and trichloroethane. The gas used as a propellant in canned whipped cream and in small metallic containers called "whippets" (used to make whipped cream) is nitrous oxide or "laughing gas."

Space limitation prevents an in-depth discussion of inhalants, and the interested reader is referred to past editions of this text or at the NIDA website.[90]

TREATMENT

Acute Drug Intoxications

4 Treatment of drug intoxication, summarized in Table 65-1, is primarily supportive. Vital functions are maintained while waiting for the drug to be eliminated. Whenever possible, drug therapy should

CLINICAL PRESENTATION Opioid Intoxication and Withdrawal

General

- Onset of the acute phase of withdrawal ranges from a few hours after stopping heroin to 3 to 5 days after stopping methadone. The duration of withdrawal ranges from 3 to 14 days.
- Opioid withdrawal is not fatal unless there is a concurrent medical problem of major concern.
- The presence of delirium should raise the question of concurrent withdrawal from another drug, such as alcohol, or another cause of delirium possibly secondary to drug use.

Symptoms

- During withdrawal, patients can experience piloerection, insomnia, muscle aches, and yawning. While intoxicated, patients can experience euphoria, dysphoria, apathy, sedation, or attention impairment.

Signs

- Fever, lacrimation, diaphoresis, or diarrhea may be observed during withdrawal. Motor retardation, slurred speech, and miosis may be observed during intoxication.

Laboratory Tests

- Treatment is based more on clinical presentation because plasma opioid levels may not be clinically useful.

Other Diagnostic Tests

- Arterial blood gases, pulse oximetry, and pulmonary function tests are useful to assess respiratory depression.

be avoided because psychotropic drug therapy has the potential for worsening a toxic reaction to another psychoactive agent; however, when patients are agitated, combative, assaultive, hallucinating, or delusional, drug therapy may be required. Toxicology screens are useful in the evaluation and treatment process, but knowledge of the metabolism of the suspected drug and its excretion patterns is important for proper interpretation of test results.

Flumazenil can be used to reverse toxic effects of benzodiazepines. Naloxone can be used to reverse the effects of opiates. The usual dosage for naloxone in acute opiate toxicity is 0.4 to 2 mg intravenously, given approximately every 3 minutes as necessary. In some instances a naloxone infusion could be administered since the half-life of the opiate is likely to be longer than that of naloxone (Table 65-2). Although naloxone is effective in reversing opiate overdose, it also can precipitate physical withdrawal in physically dependent patients. An excellent comprehensive review of the management of opioid analgesic overdose was published in 2012.[91]

Intoxication with stimulants, including cocaine, is treated pharmacologically only if the patient is overtly psychotic and agitated.[92,93] Injectable benzodiazepines, usually lorazepam 2 to 4 mg intramuscularly every 30 minutes to 6 hours as necessary, can be used for agitation. Antipsychotic drugs can be used on a short-term basis, primarily in patients with psychotic symptoms, and usually at relatively low doses, such as haloperidol 2 to 5 mg intramuscularly every 30 minutes to 6 hours as necessary, followed by 5 to 15 mg orally per day in single or divided doses if the patient is still psychotic after initial treatment.[92]

An evidence-based guideline gives precise recommendations for treating the cardiovascular complications of cocaine abuse and provides insight into the epidemiology, pathophysiology, treatment, and prognosis of the cardiac effects of cocaine.[94] Seizures generally are treated supportively. Intravenous lorazepam or diazepam can be used if seizures progress to status epilepticus.[92]

Hallucinogen intoxication is treated in a manner similar to stimulant intoxication. Drug therapy often can be avoided because patients can respond to careful reassurance, or so-called talk-down therapy. When necessary, short-term antianxiety and/or antipsychotic drug therapy can be used, as described previously.

Withdrawal

5 Treatment of drug withdrawal is the primary indication for drug therapy in substance-related disorders. Goals of drug therapy include prevention of progression of withdrawal to life-threatening severity and enabling the patient to be sufficiently comfortable

TABLE 65-2 How to Use a Naloxone Infusion

1. If a naloxone bolus (start with 0.04 mg IV and titrate) is successful, administer two thirds of the effective bolus dose per hour by IV infusion; frequently reassess the patient's respiratory status
2. If respiratory depression is not reversed after the bolus dose:
   Intubate the patient, as clinically indicated
   Administer up to 10 mg of naloxone as an IV bolus. If the patient does not respond, do not initiate an infusion
3. If the patient develops withdrawal after the bolus dose:
   Allow the effects of the bolus to abate
   If respiratory depression recurs, administer half of this new bolus dose and begin an IV infusion at two thirds of the initial bolus dose per hour.
   Frequently reassess the patient's respiratory status
4. If the patient develops withdrawal signs or symptoms during the infusion:
   Stop the infusion until the withdrawal symptoms abate
   Restart the infusion at half the initial rate; frequently reassess the patient's respiratory status
   Exclude withdrawal from other xenobiotics
5. If the patient develops respiratory depression during the infusion:
   Readminister half of the initial bolus and repeat until reversal occurs
   Increase the infusion by half of the initial rate; frequently reassess the patient's respiratory status
   Exclude continued absorption, readministration of opioid, and other etiologies as the cause of the respiratory depression

Data from reference 112.

CLINICAL PRESENTATION Cocaine Intoxication and Withdrawal

General

- In overdoses, cocaine is a CNS and cardiac stimulant. Cocaine-related deaths are often a result of cardiac arrest or seizures followed by respiratory arrest.

Symptoms

- Symptoms of intoxication include motor agitation, elation, euphoria, grandiosity, loquacity, hypervigilance, sweating or chills, nausea, and vomiting.
- Symptoms of withdrawal include fatigue, sleep disturbances, nightmares, depression, and changes in appetite.
- High doses of cocaine and/or prolonged use can trigger paranoia.

Signs

- Tachycardia, mydriasis, and either elevated or lowered blood pressure may be observed with overdose. Cardiac abnormalities (eg, arrhythmias) and respiratory depression may be observed with overdose. Bradyarrhythmias, myocardial infarction, and tremors may be observed in acute withdrawal. Prolonged cocaine snorting can result in ulceration of the mucous membranes of the nose and can damage the nasal septum enough to cause it to collapse.

Laboratory Tests

- Qualitative urine screening tests for drugs of abuse are useful, followed by confirmatory testing if necessary. Levels of the primary metabolite, benzoylecgonine, may help diagnose acute cocaine toxicity.

Other Diagnostic Tests

- Abnormal electroencephalograms may be observed with patients in acute withdrawal.

and functional to participate in a behavioral treatment program and supportive drug therapy. The clinician should remember that withdrawal is usually part of a substance dependence disorder. In drug therapy for withdrawal, it is important to avoid reinforcing the patient's drug-seeking and drug-use behavior to the extent possible. Patients must be educated to deal with the stress of withdrawal without seeking drugs. Treatment of drug withdrawal is summarized in Table 65-3.

CNS Depressant Withdrawal

Benzodiazepines

5 Treatment of benzodiazepine withdrawal is very similar to the treatment of alcohol withdrawal. The major difference in management is the length of treatment.[95] The onset of withdrawal symptoms in patients physically dependent on the long-acting benzodiazepines can be delayed up to 7 days after discontinuation of the drug. A common approach in detoxification of such patients is to initiate treatment at usual dosages (chlordiazepoxide orally 50 mg 3 times a day; lorazepam orally 2 mg 3 times a day) and to maintain the initial dosage for 5 days, with gradual tapering over an additional 5 days. Detoxification in patients physically dependent on shorter-acting benzodiazepines is similar to treatment of alcohol withdrawal.[95]

Among the benzodiazepines, alprazolam has been suggested to be more difficult to taper and discontinue than the other benzodiazepines.[95] A longer, more gradual taper of the benzodiazepine used for detoxification can be needed. With all benzodiazepines, protracted minor abstinence symptoms—such as anxiety, insomnia, irritability, sensitivity to light and sound, and muscle spasms—can remain for several weeks in patients with a history of long term exposure, even after the acute phase of benzodiazepine withdrawal is complete.[95]

Opiates

Opiate withdrawal syndrome is similar to a severe case of influenza. It is not life-threatening unless there is a concurrent life-threatening medical condition. Observable signs of withdrawal should be noted before initiation of drug therapy. Characteristic signs and symptoms of opiate withdrawal include pupillary dilatation, lacrimation,

TABLE 65-3 Treatment of Withdrawal from Some Common Drugs of Abuse

Drug or Drug Class	Pharmacologic Therapy	Level of Evidence[a,b]
Benzodiazepines		
Short to intermediate acting	Lorazepam 2 mg three to four times a day; taper over 5-7 days	A1
Long-acting	Lorazepam 2 mg three to four times a day; taper over additional 5-7 days	A1
Barbiturates	Pentobarbital tolerance test; initial detoxification at upper limit of tolerance test; decrease dosage by 100 mg every 2-3 days	B3
Opiates	Methadone 20-80 mg orally daily; taper by 5-10 mg daily or buprenorphine 4-32 mg orally daily, or clonidine 2 mcg/kg three times a day × 7 days; taper over additional 3 days	A1 (methadone and buprenorphine) B1 (clonidine)
Mixed-substance withdrawal		
Drugs are cross-tolerant	Detoxify according to treatment for longer-acting drug used	B3
Drugs are not cross-tolerant	Detoxify from one drug while maintaining second drug (cross-tolerant drugs), then detoxify from second drug	B3
CNS stimulants	Supportive treatment only; pharmacotherapy often not used; bromocriptine 2.5 mg three times a day or higher may be used for severe craving associated with cocaine withdrawal	B2

[a]Strength of recommendations, evidence to support recommendation, A, good; B, moderate; C, poor.

[b]Quality of evidence: 1, evidence from more than 1 properly randomized, controlled trial; 2, evidence from more than one well-designed clinical trial with randomization, from cohort or case-controlled analytic studies or multiple time series; or dramatic results from uncontrolled experiments; 3, evidence from opinions of respected authorities, based on clinical experience, descriptive studies, or reports of expert communities.

Data from reference 45, 91 and 111.

rhinorrhea, piloerection ("gooseflesh"), yawning, sneezing, anorexia, nausea, vomiting, and diarrhea. Seizures do not occur. Onset and duration of withdrawal symptoms and the time of peak occurrence depends on the half-life of the drug involved. Typically heroin withdrawal reaches a peak within 36 to 72 hours of discontinuation and can last for 7 to 10 days. For methadone, symptoms peak at 72 hours but can last for 2 weeks or more.

In the past, drug therapy for opioid withdrawal had typically been methadone, a synthetic opiate. Methadone is administered in decreasing doses over a period not exceeding 30 days (short-term detoxification) or 180 days (long-term detoxification). With methadone there were limited provisions for take-at-home dosing of methadone because of concern about the diversion of these drugs to illicit use.[96,97]

The American Society of Addiction Medicine recently published a practice guideline for the use of medication in the treatment of addiction involving opioid use.[98]

Use Of Buprenorphine In Opiate Withdrawal and Maintenance

6 In 2002, buprenorphine was approved for opioid withdrawal. Prior to the passage of the federal Drug Addiction Treatment Act (DATA) of 2000,[99] office-based management of opioid dependence was illegal because existing federal laws prohibited physicians from prescribing narcotics for the sole purpose of maintaining a patient in a narcotic-addicted state.

Sublingual buprenorphine is available in the United States in three formulations. When buprenorphine with naloxone is administered sublingually, the naloxone component produces no clinically significant effect; however, after parenteral administration, naloxone-induced opioid antagonism occurs resulting in symptoms of withdrawal.[100,101]

The single ingredient and naloxone combination tablet formulations were introduced in the United States in January 2003, and a mucoadhesive combination film formulation was introduced in September 2010. In the combination tablets and film, naloxone is incorporated in a fixed ratio (1 mg naloxone per 4 mg buprenorphine) to deter abuse by parenteral routes, such as nasal insufflation ("snorting") or injection.

To qualify to prescribe buprenorphine, physicians must be board certified in addiction medicine/psychiatry or hold other special credentials, and physicians are required to obtain 8 hours of authorized training before they can prescribe medications for office-based treatment of opioid dependence.[99] DATA 2000, as amended in December 2006, specifies that an individual physician may have a maximum of 30 patients on opioid therapy at any one time for the first year. One year after the date on which a physician submitted the initial notification, the physician may submit a second notification of the need and intent to treat up to 100 patients.[99]

Medically supervised withdrawal with buprenorphine consists of an induction phase and a dose-reduction phase. Best practice guidelines collectively called Treatment Improvement Protocols (TIPs) are periodically issued for treatment of SUDs. TIP 40 (the guideline for the Use of Buprenorphine in the Treatment of Opioid Addiction),[102] provides consensus- and evidence-based guidance on the use of buprenorphine.

The statement recommends that patients dependent on short-acting opioids (eg, hydromorphone, oxycodone, and heroin) be inducted directly onto buprenorphine/naloxone tablets. The use of buprenorphine (either as buprenorphine monotherapy or buprenorphine/naloxone combination treatment) to taper off long-acting opioids should be considered only for those patients who have evidence of sustained medical and psychosocial stability, and should be undertaken in conjunction and in coordination with patients' overall opioid treatment programs (OTPs).[93]

6 7 Maintenance treatment with buprenorphine for opioid addiction consists of three phases: (1) induction, (2) stabilization, and (3) maintenance.[101] Induction is the first stage of buprenorphine treatment and involves helping patients begin the process of switching from the opioid of abuse to buprenorphine. The goal of the induction phase is to find the minimum dose of buprenorphine at which the patient discontinues or markedly diminishes use of other opioids and experiences no withdrawal symptoms, minimal or no side effects, and no craving for the drug of abuse. The consensus panel recommends that the buprenorphine/naloxone combination be used for induction treatment (and for stabilization and maintenance) for most patients. The consensus panel further recommends that initial induction doses be administered as observed treatment; further doses may be thereafter provided via prescription. To minimize the chances of precipitating withdrawal, patients who are transferring from long-acting opioids (eg, methadone, sustained-release morphine, and sustained-release oxycodone) to buprenorphine should be inducted using buprenorphine monotherapy, but switched to buprenorphine/naloxone soon thereafter. Induction protocols are shown in Figure 65-1.

The stabilization phase begins when a patient is experiencing no withdrawal symptoms, is experiencing minimal or no side effects, and no longer has uncontrollable cravings for opioid agonists. Dosage adjustments may be necessary during early stabilization, and frequent contact with the patient increases the likelihood of compliance. The longest period that a patient is on buprenorphine is the maintenance phase. This period may be indefinite. During the maintenance phase, attention must be focused on the psychosocial and family issues that have been identified during the course of treatment as contributing to a patient's addiction.[102]

Some other issues related to opioid abuse that need to be addressed during maintenance treatment include, but are not limited to, the following:[102]

- Psychiatric comorbidity
- Somatic consequences of drug use
- Family and support issues
- Structuring of time in prosocial activities
- Employment and financial issues
- Legal consequences of drug use
- Other drug and alcohol abuse

A systematic review was published in 2009[94] evaluating the withdrawal component of buprenorphine treatment, including 21 studies involving 1,736 participants. The major comparisons for buprenorphine were with methadone (5 studies) and clonidine or lofexidine (12 studies). Five studies compared different rates of buprenorphine dose reduction.

The authors concluded that severity of withdrawal is similar for withdrawal managed with buprenorphine and withdrawal managed with methadone, but withdrawal symptoms may resolve more quickly with buprenorphine. It appears that completion of withdrawal treatment may be more likely with buprenorphine relative to methadone (RR 1.18; 95% CI, 0.93-1.49; $P = 0.18$) but more studies are required to confirm this.[103]

A more recent study[104] was published examining outcomes over 42 months in the Prescription Opioid Addiction Treatment Study (POATS). POATS was a multi-site clinical trial lasting up to 9 months, examining different durations of buprenorphine-naloxone treatment plus standard medical management for prescription opioid dependence, with participants randomized to receive or not receive additional opioid drug counseling. Telephone interviews were administered approximately 18, 30, and 42 months after main-trial enrollment.

At Month 42, 31.7% were abstinent from opioids and not on agonist therapy; 29.4% were receiving opioid agonist therapy, but met no symptom criteria for current opioid dependence; 7.5%

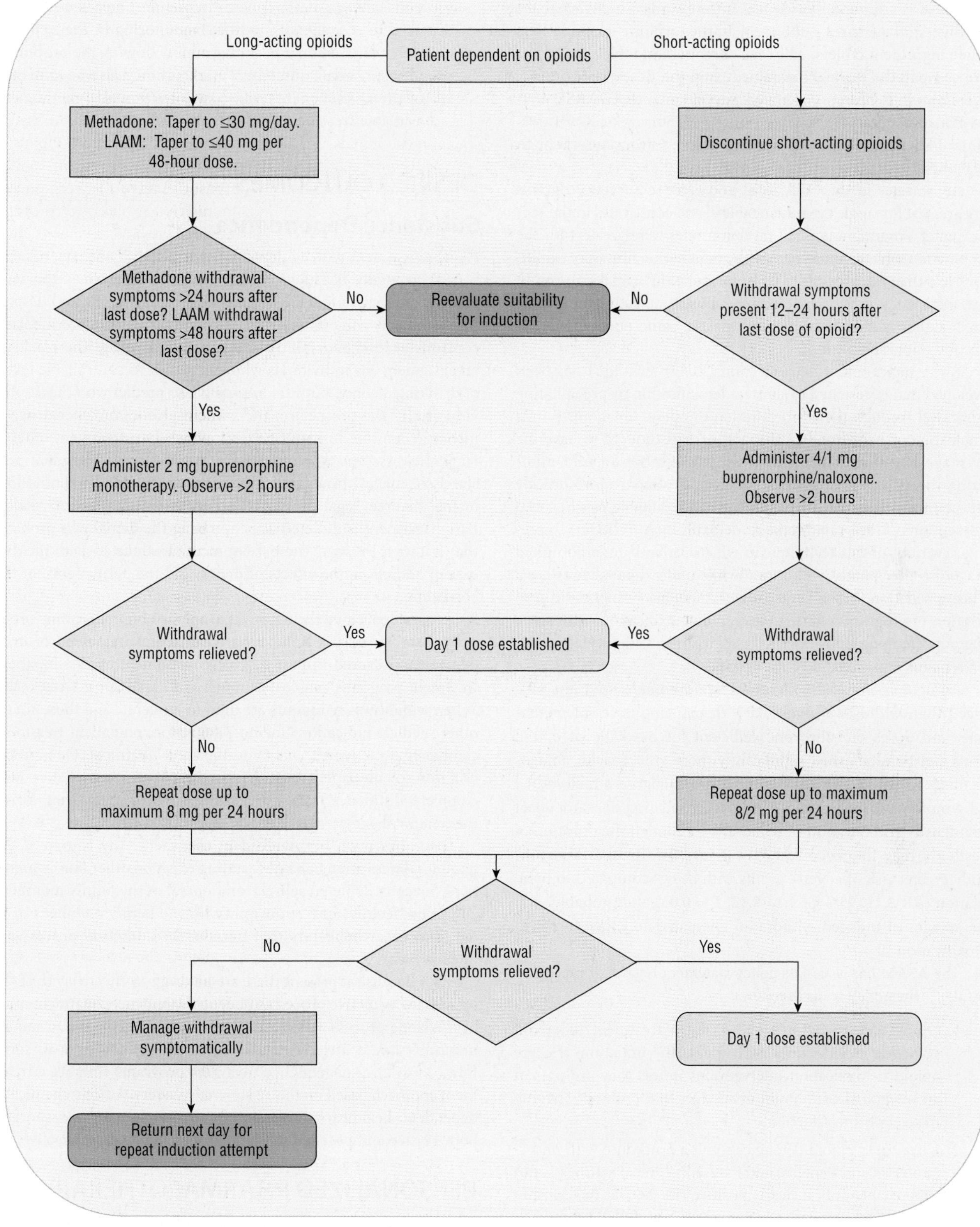

FIGURE 65-1 Determining the induction dose for days 1 to 2 of buprenorphine therapy.

were using illicit opioids while on agonist therapy; and the remaining 31.4% were using opioids without agonist therapy. Participants reporting a lifetime history of heroin use at baseline were more likely to meet DSM-IV criteria for opioid dependence at month 42 (OR = 4.56, 95% CI = 1.29-16.04, $p < .05$). Engagement in agonist therapy was associated with a greater likelihood of illicit-opioid abstinence. Eight percent ($n = 27/338$) used heroin for the first time during follow-up; 10.1% reported first-time injection heroin use.

The authors concluded that long-term outcomes for those dependent on prescription opioids demonstrated clear improvement from baseline. However, a subset exhibited a worsening course, by initiating heroin use and/or injection opioid use.

Unfortunately, buprenorphine itself can be abused, and in fact, abuse is common worldwide. In one study[105] rates of abuse and diversion of three sublingual buprenorphine formulations (single ingredient tablets; naloxone combination tablets and film) were compared. Data were obtained from the Researched Abuse, Diversion, and Addiction-Related Surveillance (RADARS®) System Poison Center, Drug Diversion, OTP, Survey of Key Informants' Patients (SKIP), and College Survey Programs through December 2012.

Abuse rates in the OTP, SKIP, and College Survey Programs were greatest for single ingredient tablets, and abuse rates in the Poison Center Program and illicit diversion rates were greatest for the combination tablets. Abuse rates with combination film were significantly less than rates for either tablet formulation in all programs. In some instances, the film version can be abuse by injecting the soluble film.[105] Other studies have reported on the same phenomenon of injection of the soluble film.[97]

5 A rapid opioid detoxification (ROD) technique has been developed that is designed to shorten detoxification by precipitating withdrawal through the administration of opioid antagonists such as naloxone or naltrexone.[107] This approach is thought to have the advantage of getting patients through detoxification rapidly, minimizing the risk of relapse, and initiating treatment more quickly with naltrexone maintenance combined with suitable psychosocial interventions. Ultra-rapid opioid detoxification (UROD) represents a variant of this technique in which patients undergo opioid antagonist–precipitated withdrawal while under general anesthesia or heavy sedation. In the United States, there has been a rapid proliferation of programs offering ultrarapid detoxification, with some programs charging up to $15,000 per treatment. Rapid detoxification remains unproven and controversial.

Antagonist-induced withdrawal is more intense but less prolonged than withdrawal managed with reducing doses of methadone, and doses of naltrexone sufficient for blockade of opioid effects can be established significantly more quickly with antagonist-induced withdrawal than withdrawal managed with clonidine and symptomatic medications. The level of sedation does not affect the intensity and duration of withdrawal, although the duration of anesthesia may influence withdrawal severity. There is a significantly greater risk of adverse events with heavy, compared to light, sedation (RR 3.21, 95% CI 1.13-9.12, $P = 0.03$) and probably with this antagonist-induced withdrawal compared to other forms of detoxification.[107]

The ASAM has issued its policy statement regarding rapid and UROD.[108] The policy reads as follows:

1. Opioid detoxification alone is not a treatment of opioid addiction. ASAM does not support the initiation of acute opioid detoxification interventions unless they are part of an integrated continuum of services that promote ongoing recovery from addiction.
2. Ultra-rapid opioid detoxification is a procedure with uncertain risks and benefits, and its use in clinical settings is not supportable until a clearly positive risk-benefit relationship can be demonstrated. Further research on UROD should be conducted.
3. Although there is medical literature describing various techniques of ROD, further research into the physiology and consequences of ROD should be supported so that patients may be directed to the most effective treatment methods and practices.
4. Prior to participation in any particular modality of opioid detoxification, a patient should be provided with sufficient information to allow him/her to provide informed consent. This should include information about the risks of termination of a treatment of prescribed agonist medications such as methadone or buprenorphine, as well as the need to comply with medical monitoring of their clinical status for a defined period of time following the procedure to ensure a safe outcome. Patients should also be informed of the risks, benefits and costs of alternative methods of available treatment.

DESIRED OUTCOMES

Substance Dependence

8 The treatment of drug dependence is primarily behavioral. The patient generally is taught that complete abstinence is the only realistic alternative to a life of uncontrollable drug use and despair that ultimately will end in death, and that there is no intermediate, controllable level of drinking or use of another drug. There may be an extremely few individuals who can return to controllable levels of drinking alcohol, but it is impossible to predict who these individuals are. The prospect of life without alcohol or other drugs is incomprehensible to many patients. Entry into treatment often is facilitated by some type of leverage that the drug-dependent person associates with negative consequences, such as potential loss of job, divorce, legal problems, or deteriorating physical health. Early treatment is directed at penetrating the denial of a problem that is always present. The patient must be educated as to the disease of addiction, the effects of drugs, and the permanence of the condition.

As evidenced by the approval of the two buprenorphine products, there has been a trend toward outpatient treatment for drug dependence, caused in part by cost-containment efforts. Inpatient treatment programs can cost as much as $20,000 for a 4-week stay. When withdrawal symptoms are mild to moderate and there are no other medical indications for hospitalization, outpatient treatment can be an attractive alternative to inpatient treatment. One critical criterion for outpatient treatment is the patient's compliance with complete abstinence from the dependence-producing drug during the treatment experience.

Families must be involved in treatment. The course of the patient's illness often has a devastating effect on other family members. Severely depleted self-esteem, denial of the family member's addiction, feelings of responsibility for the family member's drug use, and other behaviors that parallel the addiction process are often present.

8 Because at present there are no drugs to effectively treat the underlying addictive processes of drug dependence, treatment must be a lifelong process. Aftercare, or what is now being called *continued care,* should include regular and frequent treatment in some form. Most drug-dependence treatment programs embrace a treatment approach based on the 12 steps to recovery. Among chemically dependent healthcare professionals, treatment that incorporates both 12-step and peer-led self-help groups can be most effective.

PERSONALIZED PHARMACOTHERAPY

The notion of using pharmacogenetic testing to individualize the treatment of substance abuse disorders is relatively new, but studies of several genes have yielded significant findings.[100] Several gene variants have been shown to influence individual response to pharmacotherapy for drug addiction, notably in the μ opioid receptor gene OPRM1 A118G (rs561720), polymorphisms of CYP2A6, and ANKK1 Taq1A. It remains to be seen how this genetic information will be incorporated into clinical practice. Prospective studies evaluating the use of genetic testing in a clinical setting and the effect on treatment outcome are warranted to further evaluate the benefits and risks of this approach.[109,110]

ABBREVIATIONS

5-HT	5-hydroxytryptamine
ASAM	The American Society of Addiction Medicine
BZP	N-benzylpiperazine
CDC	Centers for Disease Control and Prevention
CNS	central nervous system
CPD	controlled prescription drug
DATA	Drug Addiction Treatment Act
DAWN	Drug Abuse Warning Network
DEA	Drug Enforcement Administration
DMT	dimethyltryptamine
DSM-5	*Diagnostic and Statistical Manual of Mental Disorders, Fifth Edition*
ED	emergency department
FDA	US Food and Drug Administration
GHB	γ-hydroxybutyrate
HIV	human immunodeficiency virus
LAAM	levo-α-acetylmethadol
LSD	lysergic acid diethylamide
mCPP	1-(3-chlorophenyl)-piperazine (meta-chlorophenylpiperazine)
MDA	3,4-methylenedioxyamphetamine
MDMA	3,4-methylenedioxymethamphetamine
MDPV	methylenedioxypyrovalerone
MTFS	Monitoring the Future Study
NA	Narcotics Anonymous
NAS	Neonatal Abstinence Syndrome
NFLIS	National Forensic Laboratory Information System
NPF	non-pharmaceutical fentanyl
NSDUH	National Survey on Drug Use and Health
NSS	National Seizure System
OTC	over-the-counter
OTP	opioid treatment programs
PCP	phencyclidine
PDMP	prescription drug monitoring program
POATS	Prescription Opioid Addiction Treatment Study
REM	rapid eye movement
ROD	rapid opioid detoxification
SAMHSA	Substance Abuse and Mental Health Services Administration
SKIP	Survey of Key Informants' Patients
SUD	substance use disorder
TFMPP	1-(3-trifluoromethylphenyl)-piperazine
THC	Δ9-tetrahydrocannabinol
TIPS	Treatment Improvement Protocols
UROD	ultra-rapid opioid detoxification
USD	US dollars

REFERENCES

1. Ecclesiastes 1:9 New International Version. Available at: http://www.biblegateway.com/passage/?search=Ecclesiastes%201:9&version=NIV. (Accessed September 3, 2012)
2. Inaba DS, Cohen WE. *Uppers, Downers, All Arounders: Physical and Mental Effects of Psychoactive Drugs*, 8th ed. CNS Productions, Inc.; 2014.
3. Rudgley Richard. *The Lost Civilizations of the Stone Age*. New York: Free Press; 2000:138.
4. Jiang HE, Xiao Li X, Zhaod YX, et al. A new insight into Cannabis sativa (Cannabaceae) utilization from 2500-year-old Yanghai Tombs, Xinjiang, China. *J Ethnopharmacol* 2006;108:414-422.
5. Frosch WA, Robbins ES, Stern M. Untoward reactions to lysergic acid diethylamide (LSD) resulting in hospitalization. *N Engl J Med* 1965;273(23):1235-1239.
6. James IP. A methylamphetamine epidemic? *Lancet* 1968;1(7548):916.
7. Lindberg DK. A word of warning: Marked increase in hydromorphone (Dilaudid) addiction. *J Fla Med Assoc* 1978;65:822.
8. Bridge TP, Ellinwood EH Jr. Quaalude alley: A one-way street. *Am J Psychiatry* 1973;130:217-219.
9. Finkelstein IS. Pentazocine abuse. *JAMA* 1973;224:249.
10. Derlet RW, Rice P, Horowitz BZ, Lord RV. Amphetamine toxicity: Experience with 127 cases. *J Emerg Med* 1989;7(2):157-161.
11. Bechtel LK, Holstege CP. Criminal poisoning: Drug-facilitated sexual assault. *Emerg Med Clin North Am* 2007;25:499-525.
12. Savage SR, Joranson DE, Covington EC, et al. Definitions related to the medical use of opioids: Evolution towards universal agreement. *J Pain Symptom Manage* 2003;26:655-667.
13. Center for Behavioral Health Statistics and Quality. Behavioral health trends in the United States: Results from the 2014 National Survey on Drug Use and Health (HHS Publication No. SMA 15-4927, NSDUH Series H-50). 2015. Available at: http://www.samhsa.gov/data/. (Accessed September 13, 2015)
14. JohnstonL D, O'Malley PM, Miech RA, et al. *Monitoring the Future national Survey Results on Drug Use: 1975-2014: Overview, Key Findings on Adolescent Drug Use*. Ann Arbor: Institute for Social Research, The University of Michigan; 2015.
15. US Department of Justice, National Drug Intelligence Center. *The Economic Impact of Illicit Drug Use on American Society*. Report 2011-Q0317-002. Washington, DC: US Dept of Justice; 2011:1-50. Available at: www.justice.gov/archive/ndic/pubs44/44731/44731p.pdf. (Accessed May 8, 2015)
16. American Psychiatric Association: *Statistical Manual of Mental Disorders*, 5th ed. Arlington, VA: American Psychiatric Association. Available at: http://dx.doi.org/10.1176/appi.books.9780890425596.dsm16. (Accessed October 20, 2015)
17. Koob GF, Volkow ND. Neurocircuitry of addiction. *Neuropsychopharmacology* 2010;35:217-238. Erratum in *Neuropsychopharmacology* 2010;35:1051.
18. Center for Behavioral Health Statistics and Quality. *Behavioral Health Trends in the United States: Results from the 2014 National Survey on Drug Use and Health* (HHS Publication No. SMA 15-4927, NSDUH Series H-50). 2015. Available at: http://www.samhsa.gov/data/. (Accessed October 29, 2015)
19. Centers for Disease Control and Prevention. Prescription Painkiller Overdoses in the US. Available at: http://www.cdc.gov/VitalSigns/pdf/2011-11-vitalsigns.pdf. (Accessed October 3, 2015)
20. Public Health Grand Rounds. Centers for Disease Control and Prevention. February 17, 2011. Available at: http://www.cdc.gov/about/grand-rounds/archives/2011/pdfs/PHGRRx17feb2011.pdf. (Accessed October 5, 2015)
21. Centers for Disease Control and Prevention. National Vital Statistics System mortality data. 2015. Available at: http://www.cdc.gov/nchs/deaths.htm. (Accessed October 29, 2015)
22. Substance Abuse and Mental Health Services Administration. *Results from the 2012 National Survey on Drug Use and Health: Summary of National Findings*. NSDUH Series H-46, HHS Publication No. (SMA) 13-4795. Rockville, MD: Substance Abuse and Mental Health Services Administration; 2013.
23. Patrick SW, Schumacher RE, Benneyworth BD, et al. Neonatal abstinence syndrome and associated health care expenditures: United States, 2000-2009. *JAMA* 2012;307:1934-1940. Epub 2012 Apr 30.
24. Patrick SW, Davis MM, Lehman CU, et al. Increasing incidence and geographic distribution of neonatal abstinence syndrome: United States 2009 to 2012. *J Perinatol* 2015;35:650-655. doi:10.1038/jp.2015.36; published online 30 April 2015.
25. Vital Signs: Risk for Overdose from Methadone Used for Pain Relief—United States, 1999–2010. Centers for Disease Control and Prevention. Available at: http://www.cdc.gov/mmwr/preview/mmwrhtml/mm6126a5.htm. (Accessed October 29, 2015)
26. Substance Abuse and Mental Health Services Administration. Data summary: Methadone mortality, a 2010 reassessment. Rockville, MD: US Department of Health and Human Services, Substance Abuse and Mental Health Services Administration; 2010. Available at: http://www.dpt.samhsa.gov/pdf/methadone_mortality_data_2010.pdf. (Accessed October 29, 2015)
27. Vital signs: Risk for overdose from methadone used for pain relief—United States, 1999-2010. *MMWR Morb Mortal Wkly Rep* 2012;61:493-497.
28. Methadone-Associated Overdose Deaths; Factors Contributing to Increased Deaths and Efforts to Prevent Them. United States Government Accounting Office Report to Congressional Requesters. GAO-09-341. March 26, 2009. Available at: http://www.gao.gov/new.items/d09341.pdf. (Accessed October 29, 2015)
29. U.S. Food and Drug Administration. Information for Healthcare Professionals: Methadone. Issued November 27,

2006. Available at: http://www.fda.gov/Drugs/DrugSafety/PostmarketDrugSafetyInformationforPatientsandProviders/ucm142841.htm. (Accessed October 29, 2015)

30. National Heroin Threat Assessment Summary. DEA Intelligence Report. April 2015. Available at: http://www.dea.gov/divisions/hq/2015/hq052215_National_Heroin_Threat_Assessment_Summary.pdf. (Accessed October 29, 2015)
31. Increases in Fentanyl Drug Confiscations and Fentanyl-related Overdose Fatalities, CDC HEALTH ADVISORY CDCHAN-00384 October 26, 2015. Available at: http://emergency.cdc.gov/han/han00384.asp#_edn5 (Accessed October 29, 2015)
32. DEA Issues Nationwide Alert on Fentanyl as Threat to Health and Public Safety. March 8, 2015. Available at: http://www.dea.gov/divisions/hq/2015/hq031815.shtml. (Accessed October 29, 2015)
33. Substance Abuse and Mental Health Services Administration, Center for Behavioral Health Statistics and Quality. The DAWN Report: Highlights of the 2010 Drug Abuse Warning Network (DAWN) Findings on Drug-Related Emergency Department Visits. Rockville, MD: Substance Abuse and Mental Health Services Administration, July 2; 2012.
34. National Center for Health Statistics. National Hospital Ambulatory Medical Care Survey: 2009 Emergency Department Summary Tables. Available at: http://www.cdc.gov/nchs/data/ahcd/nhamcs_emergency/2009_ed_web_tables.pdf and http://www.cdc.gov/nchs/fastats/ervisits.htm. (Accessed October 2, 2015)
35. Reeves RR, Burke RS, Kose S. Carisoprodol: Update on abuse potential and legal status. *South Med J* 2012;105(11):619-623. doi: 10.1097/SMJ.0b013e31826f5310.
36. Department of Justice, Drug Enforcement Administration. 21 CFR Part 1308. Schedules of Controlled Substances: Placement of Carisoprodol Into Schedule IV 21. Available at: http://www.deadiversion.usdoj.gov/fed_regs/rules/2011/fr1212_10.htm. (Accessed October 2, 2015)
37. Reissig CJ, Carter LP, Johnson MW, et al. High doses of dextromethorphan, an NMDA antagonist, produce effects similar to classic hallucinogens. *Psychopharmacology (Berl)*. 2012;223(1):1-15. Epub 2012 Apr 13.
38. Chyka PA, Erdman AR, Manoguerra AS, et al. American Association of Poison Control Centers. Dextromethorphan poisoning: An evidence-based consensus guideline for out-of-hospital management. *Clin Toxicol (Phila)* 2007;45:662-677.
39. Allain F, Minogianis EA, Roberts DCS, Samaha AN. How fast and how often: The pharmacokinetics of drug use are decisive in addiction. *Neurosci Biobehav Rev* 2015;56:166-179. doi: 10.1016/j.neubiorev.2015.06.012. Epub 2015 Jun 24.
40. Laizure SC, Parker RB. Pharmacodynamic evaluation of the cardiovascular effects after the coadministration of cocaine and ethanol. *Drug Metab Dispos* 2009;37:310-314.
41. Graziani M, Nencini P, Nisticò R. Genders and the concurrent use of cocaine and alcohol: Pharmacological aspects. *Pharmacol Res* 2014 Sep;87:60-70. doi: 10.1016/j.phrs.2014.06.009. Epub 2014 Jun 24.
42. Phillips K, Luk A, Soor GS, et al. Cocaine cardiotoxicity: A review of the pathophysiology, pathology, and treatment options. *Am J Cardiovasc Drugs* 2009;9:177-196.
43. McCord J, Jneid H, Hollander JE, et al. American Heart Association Acute Cardiac Care Committee of the Council on Clinical Cardiology. Management of cocaine-associated chest pain and myocardial infarction: A scientific statement from the American Heart Association Acute Cardiac Care Committee of the Council on Clinical Cardiology. *Circulation* 2008;117:1897-1907. Epub 2008 Mar 17.
44. Mahoney III JJ, Kalechstein AD, De La Garza II R, et al. Presence and persistence of psychotic symptoms in cocaine-versus methamphetamine-dependent participants. *Am J Addict* 2008;17:83-98.
45. Radfar SR, Rawson RA. Current research on methamphetamine: Epidemiology, medical and psychiatric effects, treatment, and harm reduction efforts. *Addict Health* 2014 Summer-Aut umn;6(3-4):146-154.
46. Hamamoto DT, Rhodus NL. Methamphetamine abuse and dentistry. *Oral Dis* 2009;15:27-37.
45. Shoptaw SJ, Kao U, Heinzerling K. Treatment for amphetamine withdrawal. *Cochrane Database Syst Rev* 2009:CD003021.
46. U.S. Department Of Justice National Drug Threat Assessment 2014. DEA-DCT-DIR-002-15. Available at: http://www.dea.gov/resource-center/dir-ndta-unclass.pdf. (Accessed October 29, 2015)
47. Parrott AC. MDMA, serotonergic neurotoxicity, and the diverse functional deficits of recreational 'Ecstasy' users. *Neurosci Biobehav Rev* 2013;37(8):1466-1484. doi: 10.1016/j.neubiorev.2013.04.016. Epub 2013 May 6.
48. Skelton MR, Williams MT, Vorhees CV. Developmental effects of 3,4-methylenedioxymethamphetamine: A review. *Behav Pharmacol* 2008;19: 91-111.
49. Indlekofer F, Piechatzek M, Daamen M. Reduced memory and attention performance in a population-based sample of young adults with a moderate lifetime use of cannabis, ecstasy and alcohol. *J Psychopharmacol* 2009;23(5):495-509.
50. McCann UD, Kuwabara H, Kumar A, et al. Persistent cognitive and dopamine transporter deficits in abstinent methamphetamine users. *Synapse* 2008;62:91-100.
51. McCann UD, Szabo Z, Vranesic M, et al. Positron emission tomographic studies of brain dopamine and serotonin transporters in abstinent (+/-)3,4-methylenedioxymethamphetamine ("ecstasy") users: Relationship to cognitive performance. *Psychopharmacology (Berl)* 2008;200:439-450.
52. Nicol JJ, Yarema MC, Jones GR, et al. Deaths from exposure to paramethoxymethamphetamine in Alberta and British Columbia, Canada: A case series. *CMAJ Open* 2015;3(1):E83-E90. doi: 10.9778/cmajo.20140070.
53. Kahn DE, Ferraro N, Benveniste RJ. Three cases of primary intracranial hemorrhage associated with "Molly", a purified form of 3,4-methylenedioxymethamphetamine (MDMA). *J Neurol Sci* 2012;323(1-2):257-260. doi: 10.1016/j.jns.2012.08.031. Epub 2012 Sep 19.
54. McMillan, K. Is Ecstasy the Key to Treating Women with PTSD? Some say yes—and that the prescription could come as early as 2021. Marie Claire Magazine September 2015. Available at: http://www.marieclaire.com/health-fitness/news/a15553/mdma-ecstasy-drug-ptsd-treatment/. (Accessed October 29, 2015)
55. Banks ML, Worst TJ, Rusyniak DE, et al. Synthetic cathinones ("bath salts"). *J Emerg Med* 2014;46(5):632-642. doi: 10.1016/j.jemermed.2013.11.104. Epub 2014 Feb 22.
56. Katz DP, Bhattacharya D, Bhattacharya S, et al. Synthetic cathinones: "a khat and mouse game". *Toxicol Lett* 2014;229(2):349-356. doi: 10.1016/j.toxlet.2014.06.020. Epub 2014 Jun 25.
57. "Bath Salts" Were Involved in over 20,000 Drug-Related Emergency Department Visits in 2011. The DAWN Report, September 17, 2013. Available at: http://www.samhsa.gov/newsroom/press-announcements/201309170400). (Accessed October 15, 2015).
58. Kaizaki A, Tanaka S, Numazawa S. New recreational drug 1-phenyl-2-(1-pyrrolidinyl)-1-pentanone (alpha-PVP) activates central nervous system via dopaminergic neuron. *J Toxicol Sci* 2014;39(1):1-6.
59. Casale JF and Hays PA. The Characterization of α-Pyrrolidinopentiophenone. U.S. Department of Justice, Drug Enforcement Administration, Special Testing and Research Laboratory. *Microgram J* 2015;9(1):33-38.
60. One Hundred Twelfth Congress of the United States of America. Synthetic Drug Abuse Prevention Act of 2012. Senate Bill 3187, the Food and Drug Administration Section 1152. Addition Of Synthetic Drugs To Schedule I of the Controlled Substances Act. January 3, 2012.
61. Passie T, Halpern JH, Stichtenoth DO, et al. The pharmacology of lysergic acid diethylamide: A review. *CNS Neurosci Ther* 2008 Winter;14(4):295-314.
62. Smith DE, Raswyck GE, Davidson LD. From Hofmann to the Haight Ashbury, and into the future: The past and potential of lysergic acid diethlyamide. *J Psychoactive Drugs* 2014;46(1):3-10.
63. Emerging 2C-Phenethylamines, Piperazines, and Tryptamines in NFLIS, 2006-201 U.S. Drug Enforcement Administration, Office of Diversion Control. National Forensic Laboratory Information System Special Report: Emerging 2C-Phenethylamines, Piperazines, and Tryptamines in NFLIS, 2006-2011. Springfield, VA: U.S. Drug Enforcement Administration. 2012. Available at: http://www.deadiversion.usdoj.gov/nflis/spec_rpt_emerging_2012.pdf. (Accessed October 29, 2015)
64. U.S. Drug Enforcement Administration, Office of Diversion Control. (2015). National Forensic Laboratory Information System: Year 2014 Annual Report. Springfield, VA: U.S. Drug Enforcement Administration.
65. United Nations Office on Drugs and Crime, World Drug Report 2015 (United Nations publication, Sales No. E.15.XI.6). Available at: https://www.unodc.org/documents/wdr2015/World_Drug_Report_2015.pdf. (Accessed October 29, 2015)
66. University of Mississippi, National Center for Natural Products Research, Research Institute of Pharmaceutical Sciences. Quarterly Report #124, 2014.
67. Storr CL, Wagner FA, Chen CY, et al. Childhood predictors of first chance to use and use of cannabis by young adulthood. *Drug Alcohol*

Depend 2011;117(1):7-15. doi: 10.1016/j.drugalcdep.2010.12.023. Epub 2011 Feb 1.

68. Cherek DR, Lane SD, Dougherty DM. Possible amotivational effects following marijuana smoking under laboratory conditions. *Exp Clin Psychopharmacol* 2002;10:26-38.
69. Mills KL, Lalonde F, Clasen L, et al. Developmental changes in the structure of the social brain in late childhood and adolescence. *Soc Cogn Affect Neurosci* 2014;9(1):123-31. doi: 10.1093/scan/nss113.
70. Meier MH, Caspi A, Ambler A, et al. Persistent cannabis users show neuropsychological decline from childhood to midlife. *Proc Natl Acad Sci U S A* 2012;109(40):E2657-E2664. doi: 10.1073/pnas.1206820109. Epub 2012 Aug 27.
71. Hasin DS, Saha TD, Kerridge BT, et al. Prevalence of marijuana use disorders in the United States between 2001-2002 and 2012-2013. *JAMA Psychiatry* 2015;21:1-9. doi: 10.1001/jamapsychiatry.2015.1858. [Epub ahead of print].
72. Hartman RL, Brown TL, Milavetz G, et al. Cannabis effects on driving lateral control with and without alcohol. *Drug Alcohol Depend* 2015;154:25-37. doi: 10.1016/j.drugalcdep.2015.06.015. Epub 2015 Jun 23.
73. Sewell RA, Poling J, Sofuoglu M. The effect of cannabis compared with alcohol on driving. *Am J Addict* 2009;18:185-193.
74. Asbridge M, Hayden JA, Cartwright JL. Acute cannabis consumption and motor vehicle collision risk: Systematic review of observational studies and meta-analysis. *BMJ* 2012;344:e536. doi: 10.1136/bmj.e536.
75. Li MC, Brady JE, DiMaggio CJ, et al. Marijuana use and motor vehicle crashes. *Epidemiol Rev* 2012;34(1):65-72. [Epub October 4, 2011].
76. Bosker WM, Kuypers KP, Theunissen EL, et al. Medicinal Δ(9) -tetrahydrocannabinol (dronabinol) impairs on-the-road driving performance of occasional and heavy cannabis users but is not detected in Standard Field Sobriety Tests. *Addiction* 2012;107(10):1837-1844. doi: 10.1111/j.1360-0443.2012.03928.x. Epub 2012 Jul 12.
77. Marijuana Only for the Sick? A Farce, Some Angelenos Say. New York Times, Oct7, 2012). NORIMITSU ONISHI. Available at: http://www.nytimes.com/2012/10/08/us/california-fight-to-ensure-marijuana-goes-only-to-sick.html?_r=0. (Accessed October 28, 2015)
78. Farley SB, Reissig CJ. Methodological challenges with marijuana research in the U.S. *Drug Alcohol Depend* 2015;146:e274.
79. Hill KP. Medical marijuana for treatment of chronic pain and other medical and psychiatric problems: A clinical review. *JAMA* 2015;313(24):2474-2483. doi: 10.1001/jama.2015.6199.
80. Whiting PF, Wolff RF, Deshpande S, et al. Cannabinoids for medical use: A systematic review and meta-analysis. *JAMA* 2015;313(24): 2456-2473. doi: 10.1001/jama.2015.6358.
81. Federation of American Scientists. Synthetic Drugs: Overview and Issues for Congress. Available at: http://www.fas.org/sgp/crs/misc/R42066.pdf. (Accessed April 3, 2012)
82. Substance Abuse and Mental Health Services Administration, Center for Behavioral Health Statistics and Quality. (October 16, 2014). *Update: Drug-Related Emergency Department Visits Involving Synthetic Cannabinoids*. Rockville, MD.
83. European Monitoring Centre for Drugs and Drug Addiction. Action on new drugs briefing paper: Understanding the 'spice' phenomenon. 2009. Available at: http://www.emcdda.europa.eu/drugsituation/new-drugs. (Accessed May 16, 2011)
84. Brents LK, Prather PL. The K2/Spice phenomenon: Emergence, identification, legislation and metabolic characterization of synthetic cannabinoids in herbal incense products. *Drug Metab Rev* 2014;46(1):72-85. doi: 10.3109/03602532.2013.839700. Epub 2013 Sep 24.
85. Mills B, Yepes A, Nugent K. Synthetic Cannabinoids. *Am J Med Sci* 2015;350(1):59-62. doi: 10.1097/MAJ.0000000000000466.
86. U.S. Drug Enforcement Administration, Office of Diversion Control. *National Forensic Laboratory Information System: Year 2014 Annual Report*. Springfield, VA: U.S. Drug Enforcement Administration; 2015.
87. Cohen J, Morrison S, Greenberg J, Saidinejad M. Clinical presentation of intoxication due to synthetic cannabinoids. *Pediatrics* 2012;129:e1064-e1067. doi: 10.1542/peds.2011-1797. Epub 2012 Mar 19.
88. Gunderson EW, Haughey HM, Ait-Daoud N, et al. "Spice" and "K2" herbal highs: A case series and systematic review of the clinical effects and biopsychosocial implications of synthetic cannabinoid use in humans. *Am J Addict* 2012;21:320-326. doi: 10.1111/j.1521-0391.2012.00240.x. Epub 2012 Apr 23.
89. Office of National Drug Control Policy, The White House. (n.d.). Synthetic drugs (a.k.a. K2, Spice, bath salts, etc.). Available at: https://www.whitehouse.gov/ondcp/ondcp-fact-sheets/synthetic-drugs-k2-spice-bath-salts. (Accessed October 29, 2015)
90. Inhalant Abuse. National Institute on Drug Abuse Research Report Series. NIH Publication Number 10-3818 Printed May 1999, Revised July 2010. Available at: http://casaa.unm.edu/ctn/ctn%20mod%20tool%20kit/General%20Information/Inhalants/NIDA%20Research%20Report%20-%20Inhalants.pdf. (Accessed October 29, 2015)
91. Boyer EW. Management of opioid analgesic overdose. *N Engl J Med* 2012;367:146-155.
92. Mathias S, Lubman DI, Hides L. Substance-induced psychosis: A diagnostic conundrum. *J Clin Psychiatry* 2008;69:358-367.
93. Phillips K, Luk A, Soor GS, et al. Cocaine cardiotoxicity: A review of the pathophysiology, pathology, and treatment options. *Am J Cardiovasc Drugs* 2009;9(3):177-196. doi: 10.2165/00129784-200909030-00005.
94. McCord J, Jneid H, Hollander JE, et al. Management of cocaine-associated chest pain and myocardial infarction: A scientific statement from the American Heart Association Acute Cardiac Care Committee of the Council on Clinical Cardiology. *Circulation* 2008;117:1897-1907.
95. Lader M, Tylee A, Donoghue J. Withdrawing benzodiazepines in primary care. *CNS Drugs* 2009;23:19-34. doi: 10.2165/0023210-200923010-00002.
96. Soyka M, Kranzler HR, van den Brink W, et al. The World Federation of Societies of Biological Psychiatry (WFSBP) guidelines for the biological treatment of substance use and related disorders. Part 2: Opioid dependence. WFSBP Task Force on Treatment, Guidelines for Substance Use Disorders. *World J Biol Psychiatry* 2011;12:160-187.
97. Amato L, Minozzi S, Davoli M, Vecchi S. Psychosocial and pharmacological treatments versus pharmacological treatments for opioid detoxification. *Cochrane Database Syst Rev* 2011(Sep);(9):CD005031.
98. Kampman K1, Jarvis M. American Society of Addiction Medicine (ASAM) National Practice Guideline for the Use of Medications in the Treatment of Addiction Involving Opioid Use. *J Addict Med* 2015;9(5):358-367. doi: 0.1097/ADM.0000000000000166.1
99. Drug Addiction Treatment Act of 2000 (DATA), Title XXXV of the Children's Health Act of 2000 (Pub L No. 106–310, 116 Stat 1222). Available at: http://buprenorphine.samhsa.gov/fulllaw.html. (Accessed October 29, 2015)
100. CSAT Buprenorphine information center. The Center for Substance Abuse Treatment (CSAT), Substance Abuse and Mental Health Services Administration (SAMHSA). Available at: http://buprenorphine.samhsa.gov/. (Accessed October 29, 2015)
101. Mattick RP, Breen C, Kimber J, Davoli M. Buprenorphine maintenance versus placebo or methadone maintenance for opioid dependence. *Cochrane Database Syst Rev* 2014;2:CD002207. doi: 10.1002/14651858.CD002207.pub4.
102. TIP 40 Center for Substance Abuse Treatment. *Clinical Guidelines for the Use of Buprenorphine in the Treatment of Opioid Addiction. Treatment Improvement Protocol (TIP) Series 40*. DHHS Publication No. (SMA) 04-3939. Rockville, MD: Substance Abuse and Mental Health Services Administration; 2004. Available at: http://www.ncbi.nlm.nih.gov/bookshelf/br.fcgi?book=hssamhsatip&part=A72248. (Accessed November 8, 2012)
103. Gowing L, Ali R, White JM. Buprenorphine for the management of opioid withdrawal. *Cochrane Database Syst Rev* 2009 Jul 8;(3):CD002025. doi: 10.1002/14651858.CD002025.pub4.
104. Weiss RD, Potter JS, Griffin ML, et al. Long-term outcomes from the National Drug Abuse Treatment Clinical Trials Network Prescription Opioid Addiction Treatment Study. *Drug Alcohol Depend* 2015;150:112-119. doi: 10.1016/j.drugalcdep.2015.02.030. Epub 2015 Mar 6.
105. Lavonas EJ, Severtson SG, Martinez EM, et al. Abuse and diversion of buprenorphine sublingual tablets and film. *J Subst Abuse Treat* 2014;47(1):27-34. doi: 10.1016/j.jsat.2014.02.003. Epub 2014 Mar 3.
106. White N, Flaherty I, Higgs P, Larance B, et al. Injecting buprenorphine-naloxone film: Findings from an explorative qualitative study. *Drug Alcohol Rev* 2015;34(6):623-629. doi: 10.1111/dar.12308. Epub 2015 Jul 14.
107. Gowing L, Ali R, White JM. Opioid antagonists under heavy sedation or anaesthesia for opioid withdrawal. *Cochrane Database Syst Rev* 201020;(1):CD002022. doi: 10.1002/14651858.CD002022.pub3.
108. American Society of Addiction Medicine. Public Policy Statement on Rapid and Ultra Rapid Opioid Detoxification. Adopted by the American Society of Addiction Medicine Board of Directors April 2000 as Public Policy Statement on Opioid Antagonist Agent Detoxification under Sedation or Anesthesia (OADUSA); rev. April; 2005. Available at: http://www.asam.org/docs/publicy-policy-statements/1rod-urod—rev-of-oadusa-4-051.

pdf?sfvrsn=0#search="rapid detoxification". (Accessed October 29, 2015)

109. Sturgess JE, George TP, Kennedy JL, et al. Pharmacogenetics of alcohol, nicotine and drug addiction treatments. *Addict Biol* 2011;16(3):357-376. doi: 10.1111/j.1369-1600.2010.00287.x. Epub 2011 Mar 1.
110. Crist RC, Berrettini WH. Pharmacogenetics of OPRM1. *Pharmacol Biochem Behav* 2014;123:25-33. doi: 10.1016/j.pbb.2013.10.018. Epub 2013 Nov 5.
111. Ruiz P, Strain EC. *Lowinson and Ruiz's Substance Abuse: A Comprehensive Textbook*. 5th ed. Riverwoods, IL: Lippincott Williams & Wilkins; 2011:1074.
112. Nelson LS, Olsen D. Opioids. In: Nelson LS, Olsen D, eds. *Goldfrank's Toxicologic Emergencies, Tenth Edition*, McGraw-Hill Education. Available at: http://accesspharmacy.mhmedical.com/content.aspx?bookid=1163§ionid=64552562. (Accessed December 11, 2015)

Substance-Related Disorders II: Alcohol, Nicotine, and Caffeine

66

Paul L. Doering and Robin Moorman Li

KEY CONCEPTS

1. Tobacco is the number one preventable cause of death in the United States.
2. In the United States from 2010 to 2012, alcohol poisoning was attributed to an estimated 6 deaths per day in men between the ages of 35 to 64.
3. Pharmacogenomic studies have identified genotypic and functional phenotypic variants that either serve to protect patients or predispose them toward alcohol dependence.
4. Except at very high and very low blood concentrations, the metabolism of alcohol is considered to follow zero-order pharmacokinetics, and this has important implications for the time course in which alcohol can exert its effects.
5. Disulfiram, naltrexone, and acamprosate are FDA-approved drug therapies for the treatment of alcohol dependence. The clinical utility of these agents to improve sustained abstinence remains controversial. Relapse is common.
6. More than three quarters of smokers are nicotine dependent. Tobacco dependence is a chronic condition that requires repeated interventions.
7. A systematic Cochrane review completed in 2012 showed all forms of nicotine replacement therapy were effective in reducing the amount smoked and achieving abstinence.
8. It has been suggested a quit date should be set 1 week following initiating varenicline therapy. Studies now show a flexible quit date is efficacious and safe.
9. Caffeinism is the term coined to describe the clinical syndrome produced by acute or chronic overuse of caffeine. As many as one in five adults consume doses of caffeine generally considered large enough to cause clinical symptoms.
10. Energy drinks are now popular particularly among adolescents and emerging adults. There are now safety concerns surrounding the use of these drinks due to the doubling of emergency room visits from 2000 to 2011 secondary to adverse reactions.

(1) Alcohol, nicotine, and caffeine are considered by most to be socially acceptable drugs, yet they impose an enormous social and economic cost on our society. Approximately 480,000 deaths in the United States each year are attributable to tobacco use, making tobacco the number one preventable cause of death and disease the United States.[1] The three leading causes of death attributable to smoking include lung cancer, chronic obstructive pulmonary disease, and ischemic heart disease.[1]

(2) In 2013, heavy drinking was reported by 6.3% of the population aged 12 or older, or 16.5 million people.[2] Approximately one quarter (22.9%) of persons aged 12 or older participated in binge drinking at least once in the 30 days prior to the National Survey on Drug Use and Health (NSDUH) in 2013 which is very similar to the 23% reported in 2012.[2] The World Health Organization estimates that in 2012, there were approximately 3.3 million people worldwide who died from alcohol consumption.[3] Long-term alcohol abuse often leads to chronic disease. A causal relationship between alcohol abuse and at least 200 types of chronic disease or injury has been established (eg, esophageal cancer, liver cancer, and cirrhosis of the liver, epileptic seizures, homicide, and motor vehicle accidents) worldwide.[3] Nationally, between the years of 2010 to 2012, there were approximately 2,200 deaths caused by alcohol poisoning in patients greater than 15 years old. It has been calculated that during this time period, there were an average of 6 deaths per day predominately in men between the ages of 35 to 64 caused by alcohol poisoning.[4]

Caffeine is currently the most widely used psychoactive substance in the world. In the United States, 80% to 90% of adults regularly consume behaviorally active doses of caffeine.

ALCOHOL

Epidemiology of Alcohol Use

Approximately half of Americans aged 12 or older reported being current drinkers of alcohol according to the NSDUH in 2013 (52.2%) which translates to an estimated 136.9 million people.[2] In 2013, heavy drinking was reported by 6.3% of the population aged 12 or older, meaning that they drank five or more drinks on the same occasion on at least 5 different days in the past month.[2]

The Disease Model of Addiction as Applied to Alcoholism

The disease concept of addiction, using alcoholism as a model, states that addiction is a disease, and that individuals who suffer from the disease do not choose to contract the disease any more than someone who suffers from heart disease or diabetes mellitus chooses to contract that illness. A *disease* is defined as "any deviation from or interruption of the normal structure or function of any part, organ, or system (or combination thereof) of the body that is manifested by a characteristic set of symptoms and signs and whose etiology, pathology, and prognosis may be known or unknown."[5] Diagnostic criteria for alcoholism have changed in the recent release of the *Diagnostic and Statistical Manual of Mental Disorders*, fifth edition (DSM-5). The DSM-5 now refers to alcohol use disorder (AUD) rather than having 2 separate disorders, alcohol abuse and alcohol dependence, which were listed in the DSM-4.[6] Based on DSM-5, AUD requires meeting 2 of the 11 criteria during a 12-month period. Severity is determined based on the number of criteria met and subsequently classified as mild (2-3 symptoms), moderate (4-5 symptoms), or severe (6 or more symptoms). Comparison of the criteria between DSM-4 and DSM-5 shows most criteria are very similar with the exception of elimination of legal problems and addition of craving in the criteria for DSM-5.[7,8]

TABLE 66-1 Genotypic, Phenotypic, and Environmental Factors That Increase Alcohol-Dependence Risk

Susceptibility Genes	Phenotype	Environment
Regions on chromosomes 1 and 4 that code for the following receptors: $GABA_A$ Serotonin 1b DRD4 Tryptophan hydroxylase Neuropeptide Y Gene that codes for: ALDH2 5HTTLPR	Personality traits that include: Novelty seeking Impulsivity Aggression Depression Maximum number of alcoholic drinks consumed per day	Religious background Urban residence (vs rural) History of sexual abuse Being single Having deceased parents

ALDH2, aldehyde dehydrogenase 2; DRD4, type 4 dopamine receptor gene; GABA, γ-aminobutyric acid; 5HTTLPR, 5 hydroxytryptamine transporter.

Data from references 9 and 12.

3 It has long been recognized that alcohol dependence is heritable, as 50% of first-degree relatives of alcoholics become alcohol-dependent themselves.[9,10] A recent quantitative meta-analysis evaluated heritability of AUD's on twin and adoption studies and determined similar results: 0.49 (95% confidence interval [CI] 0.47-0.54).[11] Pharmacogenomic research continues to work to identify genetic variations leading to not only variations in responses to alcohol, but also the responses to the effects of the pharmacological treatment of AUDs.[10] Large-scale pharmacoepidemiologic studies have further elucidated the environmental risk factors that are associated with either protective effects or predisposition toward alcoholism (Table 66-1).[12]

Pharmacology and Pharmacokinetics of Alcohol

Alcohol as a Drug

Alcohol is a CNS depressant that affects the CNS in a dose-dependent fashion, producing sedation that progresses to sleep, unconsciousness, coma, surgical anesthesia, and finally fatal respiratory depression and cardiovascular collapse. Alcohol affects endogenous opiates and several neurotransmitter systems in the brain, including γ-aminobutyric acid (GABA), glutamine, and dopamine. Alcohol is available in a variety of concentrations in various alcoholic beverages. There is approximately 14 g of alcohol in a 12-oz (355 mL) can of beer (approximately 5%), 5 oz (148 mL) of nonfortified wine (approximately 12%), or one shot (1.5 oz [44 mL]) of 80-proof whiskey (40%).[13] Full consumption of this amount will cause an increase in blood alcohol level of approximately 20 to 25 mg/dL (4.3 to 5.4 mmol/L) in a healthy 70-kg (154 lb) male, although this varies with the time frame over which the alcohol is consumed, the type of alcoholic beverage, whether food is consumed along with it, and many patient variables. The lethal dose of alcohol in humans is variable, but deaths generally occur when blood alcohol levels are greater than 400 to 500 mg/dL (87-109 mmol/L).[14]

Pharmacokinetics

Absorption of alcohol begins in the stomach within 5 to 10 minutes of oral ingestion. The onset of clinical effects follows fairly rapidly. Peak serum concentrations of alcohol usually are achieved 30 to 90 minutes after finishing the last drink, although it is variable depending on the type of alcoholic beverage consumed, what and when the person last ate, and other factors.[15]

More than 90% of alcohol in the plasma is metabolized in the liver by 3 enzyme systems that operate within the hepatocyte. The remainder is excreted by the lungs and in urine and sweat. Alcohol is metabolized to acetaldehyde by alcohol dehydrogenase in the cell. In turn, acetaldehyde is metabolized to carbon dioxide and water by the enzyme aldehyde dehydrogenase. A second pathway for oxidation of alcohol uses catalase, an enzyme located in the peroxisomes and microsomes. The third enzyme system, the microsomal alcohol oxidase system, has a role in the oxidation of alcohol to acetaldehyde. These last two mechanisms are of lesser importance than the alcohol dehydrogenase–aldehyde dehydrogenase system.[15,16]

4 The metabolism of alcohol generally is said to follow zero-order pharmacokinetics.[17] This can, in fact, be an oversimplification because at very high or very low concentrations of alcohol, the metabolism can follow first-order pharmacokinetics.[17] On average, the blood alcohol concentration (BAC) is lowered from 15 to 22.2 mg/dL (3.3-4.8 mmol/L) per hour in the nontolerant individual, assuming that the individual is in the postabsorptive state (Table 66-2). Alcohol has a volume of distribution of 0.6 to 0.8 L/kg, representing the total body water.[17]

Clinical Indicators of Chronic Alcohol Abuse

The CAGE questionnaire is a commonly used tool for detecting individuals more likely to be abusing alcohol and therefore at greater risk for alcohol withdrawal. CAGE is a mnemonic for four questions: (a) Do you ever feel the need to *c*ut down on your alcohol use? (b) Have you ever been *a*nnoyed by others telling you that you drink too much? (c) Have you ever felt *g*uilty about your drinking or something you did while drinking? (d) Do you ever have an "*e*ye opener"? A positive response to two or more of these four questions suggests an increased likelihood of alcohol abuse with an average sensitivity of 0.71 (71%) and an average specificity of 0.90 (90%).[18]

TABLE 66-2 Specific Effects of Alcohol Related to BAC

BAC (%)[a] (mmol/L)	Effect
0.02-0.03 (4-8)	No loss of coordination, slight euphoria, and loss of shyness
0.04-0.06 (9-14)	Feeling of well-being, relaxation, lower inhibitions, sensation of warmth. Euphoria. Some minor impairment of reasoning and memory, lowering of caution
0.07-0.09 (15-21)	Slight impairment of balance, speech, vision, reaction time, and hearing. Euphoria. Judgment and self-control are reduced, and caution, reason, and memory are impaired. It is illegal to operate a motor vehicle in some states at this level
0.10-0.125 (22-27)	Significant impairment of motor coordination and loss of good judgment. Speech can be slurred; balance, vision, reaction time, and hearing impaired. Euphoria. It is illegal to operate a motor vehicle at this level of intoxication
0.13-0.15 (28-34)	Gross motor impairment and lack of physical control. Blurred vision and major loss of balance. Euphoria is reduced, and dysphoria is beginning to appear
0.16-0.20 (35-43)	Dysphoria (anxiety, restlessness) predominates; nausea can appear. The drinker has the appearance of a "sloppy drunk"
0.25 (54)	Needs assistance in walking; total mental confusion. Dysphoria with nausea and some vomiting
0.30 (65)	Loss of consciousness
≥0.40 (>87)	Onset of coma, possible death caused by respiratory arrest

BAC, blood alcohol concentration.

[a]Grams of ethyl alcohol per 100 mL of whole blood.

Data from references 20 and 21.

The Alcohol Use Disorders Identification Test (AUDIT) is a validated 10-question screening tool originally developed to screen for alcohol dependence, problems associated with alcohol use, and the amount and frequency of alcohol consumption in adults in the primary care setting.[19] This screening tool can be completed by the patient or can be completed via an interview with a health care provider. AUDIT scores greater than 8 out of a possible 40 indicate moderate issues with alcohol, and anything greater than 16 indicates greater problems with alcohol requiring subsequent counseling and monitoring. If scores are higher than 20, then further evaluation for alcohol dependence is indicated. The AUDIT tool, as well as a short version of AUDIT (AUDIT-C), has been used within a broad range of patient population samples and is an appropriate first step in identifying patients struggling with alcohol issues.[19]

Acute Effects of Alcohol

At lower serum concentrations, euphoria and disinhibition may be noted. Slurred speech, altered perception of the environment, impaired judgment, ataxia, incoordination, nystagmus, and hyperreflexia may occur. As plasma levels increase, combative and destructive behavior may occur. With higher levels still, somnolence and respiratory depression may ensue.[20] The typical effects of various BACs are shown in Table 66-2, although effects vary from individual to individual.

Alcohol Poisoning

Acute alcohol poisoning usually occurs with rapid consumption of large quantities of alcoholic beverages. With sustained drinking of moderate amounts of alcohol, the user passes out before a toxic dose of alcohol can be ingested, and/or the person vomits to rid the stomach of its toxic reservoir. With rapid drinking, the person may fall asleep or pass out without vomiting, allowing continued alcohol absorption from the gastrointestinal (GI) tract until fatal BACs are achieved.[21]

Laboratory Studies

In the emergency room, a BAC should be ordered in any patient in whom alcohol ingestion is suspected, regardless of the presenting complaint. For clinical purposes, most laboratories report BAC in units of mg/dL or mmol/L. In legal cases, results are reported in percentage (grams of ethyl alcohol per 100 mL of whole blood). Along with a BAC, a complete blood count to assess for anemia, complete metabolic panel, serum magnesium to assess electrolytes, serum glucose, and renal and liver function should be ordered. If the diagnosis is unclear, if the intoxication seems atypical, or when there is suspicion of multiple drug ingestions, a complete toxicologic screen to rule out the presence of other substances may be useful.[22]

Treatment

Alcohol-Related Disorders

Desired Outcomes Goals for alcohol-dependent persons trying to decrease or discontinue alcohol intake include: (a) the prevention and treatment of withdrawal symptoms (including seizures and delirium tremens) and medical or psychiatric complications, (b) long-term abstinence after detoxification, and (c) entry into ongoing medical and alcohol-dependence treatment.

Alcohol Withdrawal

Pharmacologic Therapy Following the completion of a baseline assessment by using a validated tool, such as the Clinical Institute Withdrawal Assessment for Alcohol, revised (CIWA-Ar),[23] symptom-triggered treatment with a benzodiazepine is the current standard of care in alcohol detoxification to manage and minimize symptoms and avoid progression to the more severe stages of withdrawal. Trials comparing different benzodiazepines demonstrated that all appear similarly efficacious in reducing signs and symptoms of withdrawal.[24,25]

Although benzodiazepines are the standard of care, other agents have been evaluated for efficacy in the treatment of alcohol withdrawal. A Cochrane review of the efficacy and safety of

CLINICAL PRESENTATION Alcohol Intoxication and Withdrawal

General

- Acute alcohol detoxification and withdrawal after chronic alcohol abuse is a serious condition that can require hospitalization and adjunctive pharmacotherapy. At very high BAC, death is possible.

Symptoms

- The intoxicated patient can present with slurred speech and ataxia. The patient can be sedated or unconscious. As BACs decrease rapidly, nausea, vomiting, and hallucinations can ensue. Delirium and seizures are the most severe symptoms.
- An evaluation should be completed using the Clinical Institute Withdrawal Assessment for Alcohol, revised (CIWA-Ar) to document the patients baseline symptoms.

Signs

- The intoxicated patient can present with nystagmus.
- In withdrawal, the patient can present with tachycardia, diaphoresis, or hyperthermia.

Laboratory Tests

- In the emergency department, a BAC should be ordered when alcohol ingestion is suspected. Clinical laboratories typically report BAC in units of milligrams per deciliter or millimoles per liter. A whole blood alcohol level of 150 mg/dL (33 mmol/L) reported in the hospital corresponds to 0.15% BAC obtained by law enforcement.
- A complete blood count to assess for anemia, complete metabolic panel along with magnesium to assess electrolytes, glucose, renal, and liver function.
- A complete toxicologic screen to rule out the presence of other substances can be useful.

Other Diagnostic Tests

- Differentiate acute alcohol intoxication from other medical illnesses (eg, head trauma).
- Order computed tomography (CT) on any patient with focal neurologic findings, failure to improve, new-onset seizures, or mental status out of proportion to degree of intoxication.

pharmacological options in treating alcohol withdrawal syndrome was published in 2011. A total of 7,333 patients were included in this review, and the medications evaluated included benzodiazepines, baclofen, anticonvulsants, psychotropic analgesic nitrous oxide (PAN), and gamma hydroxybutyrate. Efficacy was determined based on the impact on alcohol withdrawal seizures. Benzodiazepines were more efficacious when compared to both placebo (RR 0.16; 95% CI 0.04-0.69) and antipsychotics (RR 0.24; 95% CI 0.07-0.88). Within the benzodiazepine class comparison, no benzodiazepine was statistically shown to have better efficacy, although there was a trend for better efficacy with chloridazepoxide.[26]

Treatment Regimens

Front-Loading Therapy One approach to managing alcohol withdrawal includes initially using a high dose of a long-acting benzodiazepine, such as diazepam 10 to 20 mg or chlordiazepoxide 100 mg, and administering repeat doses approximately every 1 to 2 hours until the patient is sedated.[22] It is reported that an average of three doses of these long-acting benzodiazepines is commonly utilized to achieve adequate sedation. It is important for providers to monitor the patients carefully for benzodiazepine toxicity such as over sedation, respiratory depression, and delirium. Additionally, this approach should be used with extreme caution in elderly patients or patients who have liver disease since the elimination rate will be extended leading to increased risk of toxicity.[22]

Symptom-Triggered Therapy With symptom-triggered therapy, medication is given only when the patient has symptoms and CIWA-Ar score is 8 or above.[22] This approach results in treatment that is shorter, potentially avoiding oversedation and allowing the clinician to focus on specific therapy for alcohol dependence.[24,25] Various benzodiazepines have been used in this therapy including diazepam, chlordiazepoxide, and lorazepam depending on factors including the patient's age and liver function. The patient is then reassessed hourly utilizing the CIWA-Ar score. If the score remains above 8, the patient can continue to receive the dose of selected benzodiazepine. If the score is lower than 8 and the patient appears stable, the time frame for assessment and repeat treatment can extend to 4 to 8 hours (Table 66-3).[27]

Fixed-Schedule Therapy Over the years, benzodiazepines given regularly at a fixed dosing interval have been used for alcohol withdrawal. The major problem with this approach is under dosing of the benzodiazepine because of cross-tolerance (see Table 66-3). Current guidelines take exception with this rigid approach, urging clinicians to allow for some degree of individualization within fixed-schedule therapy.[24,25]

Treatment of Alcohol Withdrawal Seizures Alcohol withdrawal seizures do not require treatment with an anticonvulsant drug unless they progress to status epilepticus, because seizures usually end before diazepam or another drug can be administered.[25] Phenytoin, which is not cross-tolerant to alcohol, does not prevent or treat withdrawal seizures, and without an IV loading dose, therapeutic blood levels of phenytoin are not reached until acute withdrawal is complete. Patients experiencing seizures should be treated supportively. An increase in the dosage and slowing of the tapering schedule of the benzodiazepine used in detoxification or a single injection of a benzodiazepine may be necessary to prevent further seizure activity. Patients with a history of withdrawal seizures can be predicted to experience an especially severe withdrawal syndrome. In such patients, a higher initial dosage of a benzodiazepine and a slower tapering period of 7 to 10 days are advisable.

Treatment of Nutritional Deficits and Electrolyte Abnormalities Fluid status should be carefully assessed, and fluid, electrolyte, and vitamin abnormalities should be corrected. Hydration can be necessary in patients with vomiting, diarrhea, increased body temperature, or severe agitation. Alcoholics often have electrolyte imbalances because of inadequate nutrition and fluid volume related to antidiuretic hormone inhibition. Hypokalemia can be corrected with oral potassium supplementation as long as renal function is adequate. Thiamine (vitamin B_1) is often depleted in alcoholics, and supplementation is standard because it can prevent the development of the Wernicke-Korsakoff syndrome (eg, mental confusion, eye movement disorders, and ataxia [poor motor coordination]). An initial dose of 100 mg IV or IM is commonly used. In practice, thiamine is usually given 100 mg once daily orally, IV, or intramuscularly for 3 to 5 days (see Table 66-3).[25]

Alcohol hypoglycemia usually occurs in the absence of overt liver disease, and it is more likely if the patient is fasting or exercising or is sensitive to alcohol; it is less likely if the patient is obese. The alcohol directly interferes with hepatic gluconeogenesis, but not glycogenolysis. The energy required for metabolism of alcohol is diverted away from the energy needed to take up lactate and pyruvate—substrates for gluconeogenesis. So, patients who drink alcohol can become hypoglycemic once glycogen stores are depleted. Neurologic symptoms of hypoglycemia can be confused with alcohol intoxication, and in the inpatient setting, blood glucose should be monitored regularly.[25]

Treatment Settings Alcohol withdrawal treatment can take place in hospitals, inpatient detoxification units, or outpatient settings. Only patients with mild to moderate symptoms should be considered for outpatient treatment, and it is a good idea to have a responsible, sober person available to help the patient monitor symptoms and administer medications. Patients with a strong craving for alcohol, those concurrently using other drugs, and those with a history of seizures or delirium tremens are not good candidates for outpatient treatment. Pharmacologic agents used in the treatment of alcohol withdrawal are summarized in Table 66-3.[24,25]

Pharmacologic Management of Alcohol Dependence

5 In the United States, disulfiram, naltrexone, once-monthly injectable extended-release naltrexone, and acamprosate are the only four drugs that are FDA-approved for the treatment of alcohol dependence. Disulfiram acts as a deterrent to the resumption of drinking, and naltrexone is a competitive opioid antagonist that has been shown to reduce cravings for alcohol. Acamprosate is a GABA ergic agonist that modulates alcohol cravings (Table 66-4).[7] Other drugs, including nalmefene, baclofen, bupropion, various serotonergic agents (including selective serotonin reuptake inhibitors and vascular serotonin-3 [5-HT_3] receptor antagonists), topiramate, gabapentin, and lithium, also have been used either abroad or in the United States off-label for alcohol dependence. A Cochrane review of 25 studies with 2,641 patients was completed to evaluate a variety of anticonvulsants, including gabapentin, topiramate, oxcarbazepine, valproate, levetiracetam, pregabalin, and carbamazepine, to determine efficacy in the treatment of alcohol dependence. These agents did perform better than placebo when comparing the number of drinks per day and average heavy drinking days but there was insufficient evidence that these agents led to an increased number of patients abstaining from alcohol. The conclusion was there is insufficient evidence of efficacy to support the use of anticonvulsant treatment of alcohol dependence.[30]

Disulfiram

Disulfiram deters a patient from drinking by producing an aversive reaction if the patient drinks. In the absence of alcohol, disulfiram has minimal effects. It inhibits aldehyde dehydrogenase in the biochemical pathway for alcohol metabolism, allowing acetaldehyde to accumulate. The resulting increase in acetaldehyde causes severe facial flushing, throbbing headache, nausea and vomiting, chest pain, palpitations, tachycardia, weakness, dizziness, blurred vision,

TABLE 66-3 Dosing and Monitoring of Pharmacologic Agents Used in the Treatment of Alcohol Withdrawal

Drug	Dose Per Day (Unless Otherwise Stated)	Indication	Monitoring	Duration of Dosing	Level of Evidence for Efficacy[a]
Multivitamin	1 tablet	Malnutrition	Diet	At least until eating a balanced diet at caloric goal	B3
Thiamine	50-100 mg	Deficiency	CBC, WBC, nystagmus	Empiric × 5 days. More if evidence of deficiency	B2
Crystalloid fluids (typically D5–0.45 NS with 20 mEq (20 mmol) of KCl per liter)	50-100 mL/hour	Dehydration	Weight, electrolytes urine output, nystagmus if dextrose	Until intake and outputs stabilize and oral intake is adequate	A3
Clonidine oral (Catapres)	0.05-0.3 mg Consider dose reduction in the elderly	Autonomic tone rebound and hyperactivity	Shaking, tremor, sweating, blood pressure	3 days or less	B2
Clonidine transdermal (Catapres-TTS)	TTS-1 to TTS-3 Consider dose reduction in the elderly	Autonomic tone rebound and hyperactivity	Shaking, tremor, sweating, blood pressure	1 week or less. One patch only	B3
Labetalol	20 mg IV every 2 hours as needed; dosage reduction (eg, by about 50% for oral dosage) is advised in patients with hepatic impairment	Hypertensive urgencies and above	Blood pressure target	Individual doses as needed	B3
Antipsychotics, haloperidol (Haldol)	2.5 to 5 mg every 4 hours	Agitation unresponsive to benzodiazepines, hallucinations (tactile, visual, auditory, or otherwise), or delusions	Subjective response plus rating scale (CIWA-AR or equivalent)	Individual doses as needed	B1
Antipsychotics, atypical		Agitation unresponsive to benzodiazepines, hallucinations, or delusions in patients intolerant of conventional antipsychotics	Subjective response plus rating scale (CIWA-AR or equivalent)	Individual doses as needed in addition to scheduled antipsychotic	C3
Quetiapine (Seroquel)	25-200 mg; dosage adjustment is necessary in hepatic impairment				
Aripiprazole (Abilify)	5-15 mg				
Benzodiazepines		Tremor, anxiety, diaphoresis, tachypnea, dysphoria, seizures	Subjective response plus rating scale (CIWA-AR or equivalent)	Individual doses as needed. Underdosing is more common than overdosing	A2
Lorazepam (Ativan)	0.5-2 mg				
Chlordiazepoxide (Librium)	5-100 mg				
Clonazepam (Klonopin)	0.5-2 mg				
Diazepam (Valium)	2.5-10 mg				
Alcohol oral		Prevent withdrawal	Subjective signs of withdrawal	Wide variation	C3
Alcohol IV		Prevent withdrawal	Subjective signs of withdrawal	Wide variation	C3

CBC, complete blood count; CIWA-AR, Clinical Institute Withdrawal Assessment for Alcohol, Revised; D5, dextrose 5%; KCl, potassium chloride; NS, normal saline; WBC, white blood cell count.

[a]Strength of recommendations, evidence to support recommendation: A, good; B, moderate; C, poor.

Quality of evidence: 1, evidence from more than one properly randomized controlled trial; 2, evidence from more than one well-designed clinical trial with randomization, from cohort or case–control analytic studies or multiple time series, or dramatic results from uncontrolled experiments; 3, evidence from opinions of respected authorities, based on clinical experience, descriptive studies, or reports of expert communities.

Data from references 22, 28, and 29.

confusion, and hypotension. Severe reactions including myocardial infarction, congestive heart failure, cardiac arrhythmia, respiratory depression, convulsions, and death can occur, particularly in vulnerable individuals.[7]

Naltrexone

Naltrexone, an opiate antagonist available in the United States since 1984 for the treatment of opioid dependence, blocks the effects of exogenous opioids. In 1994, the FDA approved its use in the treatment of alcohol dependence. Naltrexone is thought to attenuate the reinforcing effects of alcohol, and those who consume alcohol while taking naltrexone report feeling less intoxicated and having less craving for alcohol.[7] Evidence suggests that genetics plays a role in the clinical response to naltrexone, as the efficacy of naltrexone treatment varies greatly among individuals. In previous preliminary studies, Asp40 polymorphism in the μ-opioid receptor gene demonstrated increased response to naltrexone with lower rates of relapse to heavy drinking. In a recent double blind, randomized, controlled clinical trial evaluating naltrexone in comparison to placebo, 221 patients were stratified by genotype. It was found that Asp40 allele does not have a significant effect on the response rate for naltrexone treatment,[31] but further studies are needed.

Naltrexone should not be given to patients currently dependent on opiates because it can precipitate a severe withdrawal syndrome.

TABLE 66-4 Dosing and Monitoring of Pharmacologic Agents Used in the Treatment of Alcohol Dependence

Drug	Dosage Range Per Day	Indication	Monitoring	Duration of Dosing	Level of Evidence for Efficacy[a]
Disulfiram (Antabuse)	250-500 mg; used with extreme caution in patients with hepatic cirrhosis or insufficiency	Deterrence	Facial flushing, liver enzymes	Indefinite	B2
Acamprosate (Campral)	999-1,998 mg and higher (333 mg tablets) Dosage adjustment necessary in renal impairment	Craving	Patient-reported craving, renal function	Indefinite	A1
Naltrexone (ReVia)	50-100 mg; dosage adjustment may be needed in renal and liver impairment	Craving	Patient-reported craving	Indefinite	A1
Naltrexone (Vivitrol)	380 mg intramuscularly once every 4 weeks Risk of hepatotoxicity lower compared to oral formulation due to lack of first pass effect	Craving	Patient-reported craving	Indefinite	B2
Mood stabilizers (eg, lamotrigine [Lamictal], topiramate [Topamax], carbamazepine [Tegretol], valproic acid [Depakote])	Seizure disorder doses	Craving	Patient-reported craving, plasma drug levels	Indefinite	B2
Antidepressants (eg, clomipramine [Anafranil], bupropion [Wellbutrin], doxepin [Sinequan], fluoxetine [Prozac])	Depression doses	Craving, depression, anxiety	Patient-reported craving	Indefinite	B2

[a]Strength of recommendations: A, B, and C, good, moderate, and poor evidence to support recommendation, respectively.

Quality of evidence: 1, evidence from more than one properly randomized controlled trial; 2, evidence from more than one well-designed clinical trial with randomization, from cohort or case–control analytic studies or multiple time series, or dramatic results from uncontrolled experiments; 3, evidence from opinions of respected authorities, based on clinical experience, descriptive studies, or reports of expert communities.

Data from references 28 and 29.

Naltrexone should be used with caution in patients with moderate to severe renal impairment. Although naltrexone is associated with dose-related hepatotoxicity, this generally occurs at doses higher than those recommended for treatment of alcohol dependence, and elevated liver enzyme levels generally normalize upon discontinuation of naltrexone. It is recommended that baseline and periodic liver function tests should be completed one to three months after initiation of therapy and then continued annually.[32] Nevertheless, it is considered contraindicated in patients with hepatitis, liver failure, or serum aminotransferase levels greater than 5 times normal.[7]

A review of 50 randomized controlled studies, which included approximately 7,800 patients, showed the most common side effects were nausea and daytime sedation. Efficacy was measured by the decrease in drinking days and also the amount of heavy drinking. Results showed there was approximately a 4% decrease in drinking days, and the risk of heavy drinking decreased to 83% compared to placebo (NNT = 9). The usual starting dose of oral naltrexone is 50 mg/day, but doses of 100 mg/day have been used and studied.[33]

In April 2006, the FDA approved Vivitrol, a once-monthly intramuscular naltrexone formulation. The usual effective dose is 380 mg IM each month.[34] Extended-release formulations reduce the likelihood of forgetting or choosing not to take medication, assuring that once the patient receives an injection, he or she will be "adherent" for the next month.[34]

Criticism has been leveled at the extended-release dosage form, suggesting that naltrexone's benefit may be limited to less severe alcohol dependence, and exclusively to reduction in heavy drinking rather than abstinence. Pettinati et al[34] report the results of a study in alcohol-dependent patients who had higher baseline severity, as measured by: (a) the Alcohol Dependence Scale or (b) having been medically detoxified in the week before randomization. Higher severity alcohol-dependent patients, when receiving 380 mg (n = 50) of the extended-release compound compared with placebo (n = 47), had significantly fewer heavy-drinking days during the study (hazard ratio = 0.583; P = 0.0049) and showed an average reduction of 37.3% in heavy-drinking days compared with 27.4% for placebo-treated patients (P = 0.039). The authors contend that their data support the efficacy of extended-release naltrexone 380 mg in relatively higher severity alcohol dependence for both reduction in heavy drinking and maintenance of abstinence.[34]

Acamprosate

Acamprosate is a glutamate modulator at the *N*-methyl-D-aspartate receptor that reduces alcohol craving. Acamprosate, approved in the United States in 2004, had been available in Europe for many years. Patients treated with acamprosate are more successful in maintaining abstinence from alcohol versus placebo. Acamprosate is well tolerated, with GI adverse effects most common.

A Cochrane review of 24 randomized controlled trials (RCTs) with 6,915 participants[35] found that, compared with placebo, acamprosate significantly reduced the risk of any drinking (RR 0.86; 95% CI 0.81-0.91; NNT 9.09; 95% CI 6.66-14.28) and significantly increased the cumulative abstinence duration (mean difference 10.94 days [95% CI 5.08-16.81]), while secondary outcomes did not reach statistical significance. Diarrhea was the only side effect that was more frequently reported with acamprosate than placebo (risk difference 0.11 [95% CI 0.09-0.13]; NNTB 9.09 [95% CI 7.69-11.11]). Table 66-4 shows dosing information for this and the other options used in treating alcohol dependence.

NICOTINE

Since 1964 when the first Surgeon General's report on smoking was released, the number of adults who smoke has decreased from 42.4% in 1965[36] to 17.1% in March 2014,[37] and now there are more former smokers than current smokers.[1] This trend has been aided by the clinical guidelines for tobacco use and dependence which were released in 2000 and last updated in 2008.[38] Telephone quitlines are also available in every state, and more patients are increasingly referred to smoking cessations counseling services. There is also a growing number of Internet and mobile phone text messaging programs to reach the teenage and young adult population to promote smoking cessation.[39,40]

Despite proven effectiveness of pharmacological and counseling services to aid in sustained smoking cessation, cigarette smoking continues to be the leading cause of preventable morbidity and mortality in the United States. Data from the 2013 National Health Interview Survey[41] found that the overall percent of current smokers from the years 2005 to 2013 in adults (18 years old and older) decreased from 20.9 to 17.8. It was determined this represents 3 million fewer smokers in 2013 compared with 2005, but this decline has not been uniform across all subsets of the population.[42] The Healthy People 2020 target is currently set for the prevalence of smoking to be less than or equal to 12%, and based on the current rate of decline, this target will not be met. Healthy People 2020 also calls for greater utilization of tobacco use counseling within ambulatory settings to improve smoking cessation rates with the goal of increasing the cessation attempts from 48% in 2008 to 80% by 2020.[43]

Epidemiology of Tobacco Use

The NSDUH reported in 2013 that an estimated 25.5% (66.9 million) of the US population's 12 years of age and older people used a tobacco product at least once in the month prior to being interviewed. In addition, 55.8 million Americans were current cigarette smokers, 12.4 million smoked cigars, 8.8 million used smokeless tobacco, and 2.3 million smoked pipes.[44] Comparing age groups, adults between the ages of 18 and 25 years have the highest rate of cigarette use (37%), but it is encouraging to see the rates continue to decrease each year since 2002 when 45.3% of young adults were using cigarettes. Within youth aged 12 to 17, use of cigarettes also continued to decline from 15.2% in 2002 to 7.8% in 2013.[44]

Data trends from the 2013 NSDUH continue to show smoking prevalence varies based on the level of education. The highest percentage of adults who admitted to smoking was adults who had not completed high school (33.6%). The lowest rate of smoking was seen in adults who graduated from college (11.2%). Results from the NSDUH also showed cigarette smoking was higher in unemployed adults (40.1%) in comparison to adults who were employed full time (22.8%).[44]

Economic Impact of Smoking

The direct healthcare expenditures associated with smoking range between $289 and $333 billion a year for both direct medical care of adults and indirect costs such as lost productivity.[1] Medicaid patients' smoking rates are substantially higher in comparison to the general population. Smoking-attributable medical expenditures are estimated at 11% of Medicaid program expenditures.[45]

Health Risks of Smoking

Cigarette smoking substantially increases the risk of (a) cardiovascular diseases, such as stroke, sudden death, and heart attack; (b) nonmalignant respiratory diseases including emphysema, asthma, chronic bronchitis, and chronic obstructive pulmonary disease; (c) lung cancer; and (d) other cancers.[1] Exposure to environmental tobacco smoke (*passive exposure*) has been cited as the cause of lung cancer, stroke, and coronary heart disease in adults.[46,47] Children who are exposed to environmental smoke have a higher risk of respiratory infection, asthma, and ear infections than those who are not exposed. Sudden infant death syndrome occurs more often in infants whose mothers smoked during pregnancy than in offspring of nonsmoking mothers. The harmful effects of smoking on reproduction and pregnancy include reduced fertility and fetal growth, as well as increased risk of ectopic pregnancy and spontaneous abortion.[46]

Pharmacology of Nicotine

Nicotine is a ganglionic cholinergic agonist with pharmacologic effects that are highly dependent on dose. These effects include central and peripheral nervous system stimulation and depression, respiratory stimulation, skeletal muscle relaxation, catecholamine release by the adrenal medulla, peripheral vasoconstriction, and increased blood pressure, heart rate, cardiac output, and oxygen consumption. Cigarette smoking or low doses of nicotine produce an increased alertness and increased cognitive functioning by stimulating the cerebral cortex. At higher doses, nicotine stimulates the "reward" center in the limbic system of the brain.[48]

When nicotine is ingested, a feeling of pleasure and relaxation can occur. Repetitive exposure to nicotine leads to neuroadaptation, which builds tolerance to the initial effects. An accumulation of nicotine in the body leads to a more substantial withdrawal reaction if cessation is attempted. Common symptoms experienced during withdrawal can include anxiety, difficulties concentrating, irritability, and strong cravings for tobacco.[49] Onset of these withdrawal symptoms usually occurs within 24 hours and can last for days, weeks, or longer. This powerful force of nicotine addiction is one reason smokers who attempt to achieve smoking cessation have a high rate of relapse, and only 3% remain abstinent 6 months following the quit date.[51]

Treatment

Desired Outcomes

Ideally, we would hope that all smokers quit, and that young people never take up the habit. Unfortunately, this is unlikely to happen. The Healthy People 2020 target setting the prevalence of smoking at less than or equal to 12% is a realistic and achievable goal.[43]

Nicotine Dependence

Agency for Healthcare Research and Quality Clinical Practice Guideline: Treating Tobacco Use and Dependence The Agency for Healthcare Research and Quality (AHRQ) periodically convenes expert panels to develop clinical guidelines for healthcare practitioners. Because of the widespread prevalence of smoking-related illnesses, its related morbidity and mortality, and the economic burden imposed, the agency convened a panel of experts in 1994 to develop guidelines on the treatment of tobacco addiction. The resultant guideline for smoking cessation was updated in 2008,[38] and no further updates have been released at the time of this writing.

The guideline suggests strategies for appropriate treatments for every patient. Because effective treatments for tobacco dependence

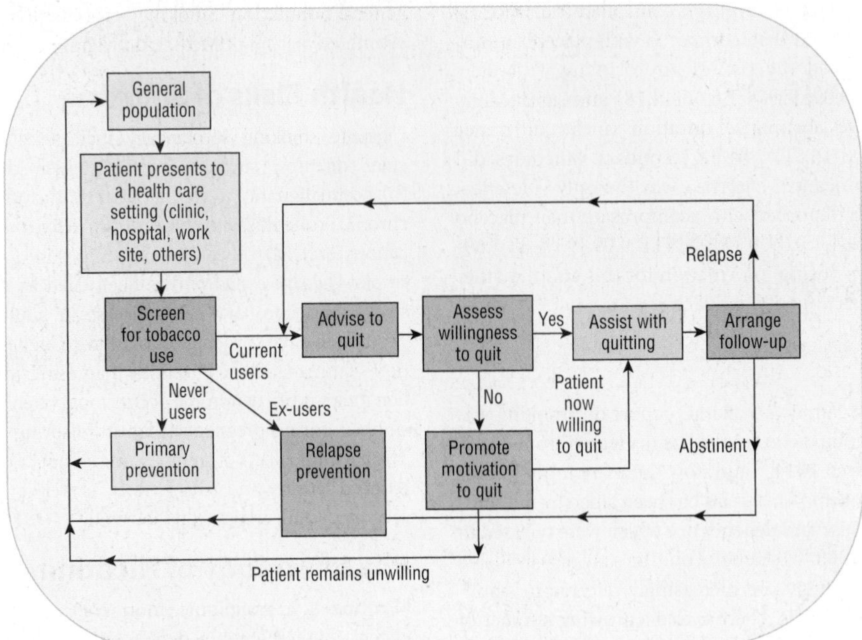

FIGURE 66-1 Model for treatment of tobacco use and dependence.

now exist, every patient should receive at least minimal treatment every time he or she visits a clinician (Figs. 66-1 and 66-2).

The guideline identified a number of key findings that clinicians should use:

1. 6 Tobacco dependence is a chronic condition that often requires repeated intervention. However, effective treatments exist that can produce long-term or permanent abstinence.
2. Because effective tobacco-dependence treatments are available, every patient who uses tobacco should be offered at least one of these treatments.
3. It is essential that clinicians and healthcare delivery systems (including administrators, insurers, and purchasers) institutionalize the consistent identification, documentation, and treatment of every tobacco user who is seen in a healthcare setting.
4. Brief tobacco-dependence treatment is effective, and every patient who uses tobacco should be offered at least brief treatment.
5. There is a strong dose–response relationship between the intensity of tobacco-dependence counseling and its effectiveness. Treatments involving person-to-person contact (via individual, group, or proactive telephone counseling) are consistently effective, and their effectiveness increases with treatment intensity (eg, minutes of contact).
6. Three types of counseling and behavioral therapies were found to be especially effective and should be used with all patients who are attempting tobacco cessation:

- Provision of practical counseling (problem-solving/skills training)
- Provision of social support as part of treatment (intratreatment social support)
- Help in securing social support outside treatment (extra-treatment social support)

Numerous effective pharmacotherapy options for smoking cessation now exist (Table 66-5). Seven first-line pharmacotherapy options reliably increase long-term smoking abstinence rates: sustained-release (SR) bupropion, nicotine gum, nicotine inhaler,

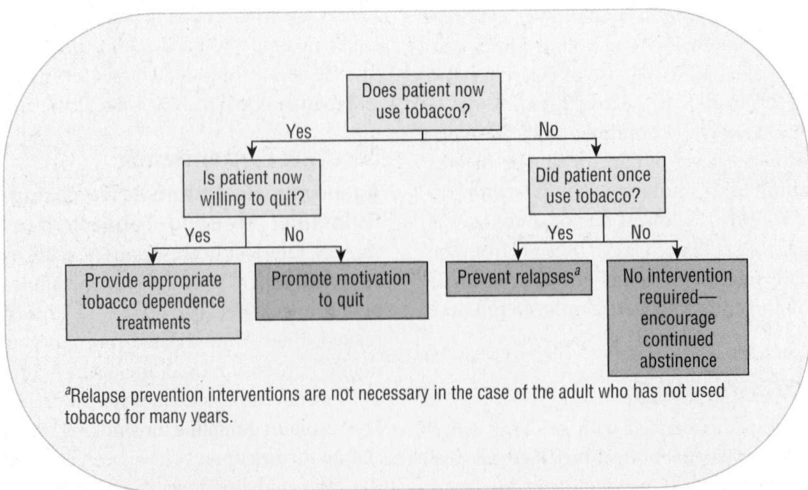

FIGURE 66-2 Algorithm for treating tobacco use.

CLINICAL PRESENTATION Nicotine Withdrawal

General

- The patient may experience anxiety, but may not be in acute distress. Symptoms can wax and wane over time.

Symptoms

- The patient may complain of cravings, difficulty concentrating, frustration, irritability, and impatience. Hostility, insomnia, and restlessness can also occur.

Signs

- Increased skin temperature can be present.

nicotine lozenge, nicotine nasal spray, nicotine patch, and varenicline. Combinations of these should be considered if a single agent has failed.

Two second-line pharmacotherapy options are considered efficacious and can be considered by clinicians if first-line options are not effective: clonidine and nortriptyline.[38] Tobacco-dependence treatments are both clinically effective and cost-effective relative to other medical and disease prevention interventions. As such, insurers and purchasers should ensure all insurance plans include as a reimbursed benefit the counseling and pharmacotherapeutic treatments that are identified as effective in this guideline, as well as clinician reimbursement for providing tobacco-dependence treatment just as they are reimbursed for treating other chronic conditions.

Other Factors Important to the Success of a Smoking-Cessation Strategy

The AHRQ expert panel emphasized the importance of the type and intensity of the contact with the counselor to the success

TABLE 66-5 Dosing and Monitoring of Pharmacologic Agents Used for Smoking Cessation

Drug	Place in Therapy	Dosage Range	Duration	Comments/Monitoring Parameters	LOEE[a]
Bupropion SR[b,c] (Zyban)	First-line	Titrate up to 150 mg orally twice daily. May require reduced initial dose in elderly	3-6 months	Patients receiving both bupropion and a nicotine patch should be monitored for hypertension	A1
Clonidine[c,d] (Catapres)	Second-line	Titrate to response; 0.2-0.75 mg/day. Consider dose reduction in the elderly	6-12 months	Monitor baseline electrolyte and lipid profiles, renal function, uric acid, complete blood count, and blood pressure	B2
Nicotine polacrilex (gum)[b] (Nicorette)	First-line	Initial dose depends on smoking history: 2-4 mg every 1-8 hours	12 weeks (taper down over time)	Heart rate and blood pressure should be monitored periodically during nicotine replacement therapy	A1
Nicotine inhaler[b] (Nicotrol)	First-line	24-64 mg/day (total daily dose)	3-6 months (taper down over time)	Heart rate and blood pressure should be monitored periodically during nicotine replacement therapy	A1
Nicotine nasal spray[b] (Nicotrol NS)	First-line	8-40 mg/day (total daily dose)	14 weeks (taper down over time)	Heart rate and blood pressure should be monitored periodically during nicotine replacement therapy	A1
Nicotine patch[b] (NicoDerm, Nicotrol)	First-line	Initial dose depends on smoking history: 7-21 mg topically once daily	6 weeks (taper down over time)	Heart rate and blood pressure should be monitored periodically during nicotine replacement therapy	A1
Nortriptyline[c,d] (Aventyl)	Second-line	Titrate up to 75-100 mg orally daily	6-12 months	Dry mouth, blurred vision, and constipation are dose-dependent adverse effects	B2
Varenicline[c] (Chantix)	First-line	Titrate up to 1 mg orally twice daily. If CrCl <30 mL/min (0.5 mL/s), 0.5 mg once per day	3-6 months	Monitor renal function, especially in elderly patients. Nausea, headache, insomnia are dose-dependent adverse effects	A1

LOEE, level of evidence for efficacy.

[a]Strength of recommendations, evidence to support recommendation: A, good; B, moderate; C, poor.

Quality of evidence: 1, evidence from more than one properly randomized controlled trial; 2, evidence from more than one well-designed clinical trial with randomization, from cohort or case–control analytic studies or multiple time series, or dramatic results from uncontrolled experiments; 3, evidence from opinions of respected authorities, based on clinical experience, descriptive studies, or reports of expert communities.

[b]Nicotine replacement therapies can be combined with each other and/or bupropion to increase long-term abstinence rates.

[c]Do not abruptly discontinue. Taper up initially, and taper off once therapy is complete.

[d]Clonidine and nortriptyline are not FDA-approved for smoking cessation.

Data from reference 38.

of the intervention. When interventions last for more than 10 minutes, the increase in cessation rates is much better than when interventions do not involve contact with a professional. Group and individual counseling are more effective than no intervention in increasing abstinence rates. Self-help materials (e.g., handouts, pamphlets, and brochures) without any direct physical contact are not effective.[52] Interventions are more successful when they include social support and training in general problem-solving skills, stress management, and relapse prevention. The number of treatment sessions offered is also important. Providing at least four or more sessions, longer than 10 minutes in length, and if possible providing treatments from multiple types of clinicians have proven higher success rates compared with less intensive interventions.[38] A Cochrane analysis reviewed 38 trials, which included approximately 15,000 patients who received a combination of pharmacotherapy treatment and behavioral support either in person or through telephone support. It was determined based on the results of these trials the addition of behavioral support could improve the chances of cessation from 10% to 25%.[53] Although comprehensive behavioral interventions have been shown to be more effective in helping people quit smoking and remain abstinent, less intensive treatments are beneficial as well. Even minimal contacts lasting less than 3 minutes including the steps known as the 5 A's: Ask, Advise, Assess, Assist, and Arrange are more successful in increasing cessation rates than intervention involving no contact.[38]

Motivational interviewing is a form of counseling to help patients identify barriers for making a behavior change. A meta-analysis[54] of 28 studies published between 1997 and 2014, including over 16,000 smokers who underwent motivational interviewing as part of the smoking cessation program, found that motivational interviewing with standard care or brief cessation advice did improve quit rates modestly. Subgroup analysis found that motivational interviewing was most effective when completed in shorter sessions by general practitioners.

Other forms of interventions have been identified as effective to improve smoking cessation rates. Telephone-based quitlines which are operated by the National Cancer Institute and offered in all 50 states, the District of Columbia, Puerto Rico, and Guam via 1-800-QUIT-NOW provide various options such as recorded messages, counseling services, mailed materials, counselor follow up services, and access to pharmacotherapy options for smoking cessation.[55] Physicians are also offered a referral process to the quitlines to improve time efficiency by suggesting the patients call the quitline, or by faxing or emailing a referral. Studies evaluating this process have identified combining the physician visit with a referral to a quit line has been effective in improving quit rates.[56] Quitlines are also now included with the graphic warning labels on the cigarette packages to help improve utilization of the counseling services. The use of technology to further enhance counseling opportunities has also increased over the years including websites, text messaging, social networking, and smart phone applications although further studies are needed to determine what format is the most effective.[57]

Counseling alone can be effective, but counseling efficacy is further augmented by the addition of pharmacotherapy. In a meta-analysis that included 150 trials with more than 50,000 participants using one or more of the five forms of nicotine replacement therapy (NRT) including nicotine gum, nasal spray, transdermal patches, sublingual tablets/lozenges, or inhaler, it was found that the use of NRT significantly increased the rate of cessation by 50% to 70% compared with placebo. Although counseling is suggested by guidelines, it was shown that NRT is effective independent of counseling services.[58]

Pharmacologic Therapy for Smoking Cessation

All patients attempting to quit should be encouraged to use effective pharmacotherapy agents for smoking cessation except in the presence of special circumstances. First line agents include NRT, sustained release bupropion hydrochloride, and varenicline tartrate.[38] As with other chronic diseases, the most effective treatment of tobacco dependence encompasses multiple modalities. Pharmacotherapy is a vital element of a multicomponent smoking cessation program that should always include nonpharmacologic components. The role of pharmacotherapy in smoking cessation is summarized in Table 66-5.

Nicotine Replacement Therapy

7 In 2012, a systematic review[58] was performed to determine the effectiveness of the different forms of NRT (eg, chewing gum, transdermal patches, nasal spray, inhalers, and tablets) in achieving abstinence or a sustained reduction in the amount smoked. The review showed that all of the commercially available forms of NRT were effective for smoking cessation and increased quit rates by 50% to 70%.

Nicotine Gum Clinicians should offer 4-mg rather than 2-mg nicotine gum to highly dependent smokers.[38] The 2-mg gum is recommended for patients smoking fewer than 25 cigarettes per day, whereas the 4-mg gum is recommended for patients smoking 25 or more cigarettes per day. Generally, the gum should be used for up to 12 weeks, no more than 24 pieces chewed per day. Gum should be chewed slowly until a peppery or minty taste emerges and then "parked" between cheek and gums to facilitate nicotine absorption through the oral mucosa. Acidic beverages (eg, coffee, juices, or soft drinks) interfere with the buccal absorption of nicotine, so eating and drinking anything except water should be avoided for 15 minutes before and during chewing. Instructions to chew the gum on a fixed schedule (at least one piece every 1-2 hours) for at least 1 to 3 months can be more beneficial than ad libitum use.[38]

Nicotine Patch The nicotine patch is available both as a nonprescription medication and as a prescription drug, and it approximately doubles long-term abstinence rates over those produced by placebo interventions.[58] Treatment of 8 weeks or less has been shown to be as efficacious as longer treatment periods. It has also been shown combining the nicotine patch with an oral formulation such as the nicotine gum which allows ad libitum nicotine delivery can improve the overall cessation without significant increased risk for harm.[59] Clinicians should consider starting treatment on a lower patch dose in patients smoking 10 or fewer cigarettes per day.[38] The 16- and 24-hour patches have shown a possible benefit in comparison to the standard dose patches which could be considered for heavier smokers.[58] A patch should be applied as soon as the patient wakes on the quit day and at the start of each day thereafter. The patient should place a new patch on a relatively hairless location, typically between the neck and waist. There are no restrictions on activity while using the patch. Patients who experience sleep disruption should remove the 24-hour patch prior to bedtime or use the 16-hour patch.[38]

Nicotine Nasal Spray Nicotine nasal spray more than doubles long-term abstinence rates when compared with a placebo spray. It is available exclusively as a prescription medication. A dose of nicotine nasal spray consists of one 0.5-mg delivery to each nostril (1 mg total). Initial dosing should be one to two doses per hour, increasing as needed for symptom relief. The minimum recommended treatment is 8 doses per day, with a maximum limit of 40 doses per day (5 doses per hour). Recommended duration of therapy is 3 to 6 months. Patients should not sniff, swallow, or inhale through the nose while administering doses because this increases irritating effects.[38]

Nicotine Lozenge The nicotine lozenge is available as a 2-mg and a 4-mg dose. The 2-mg lozenge is recommended for patients who normally smoke their first cigarette later than 30 minutes after awakening, and the 4-mg lozenge is recommended for smokers who smoke within 30 minutes of waking. The duration of treatment is 12 weeks. It is recommended no more than 20 lozenges should be used in 1 day.[38] The most common side effect of the lozenge is nausea. As with the nicotine gum, acidic beverages (eg, coffee, juices, or soft drinks) interfere with the buccal absorption of nicotine, so eating and drinking anything except water should be avoided for 15 minutes before and during use of the lozenge.[38]

Instructing Patients in the Use of NRT Compliance with NRT improves when the patient is presented a clear rationale for its use and a realistic expectation about the response. It should be explained to the patient that nicotine is responsible for addiction and discontinuation of the nicotine causes craving for cigarettes, tension, irritability, sadness, problems with sleep, and difficulty concentrating. The patient should be told using the patch results in less desire to smoke and provides an opportunity for a new nonsmoker to practice all the new nonsmoking skills without being burdened by craving. The patient should understand that with smoking, there are naturally peaks and valleys in the amount of nicotine in the bloodstream. With the patch, there is a steady gradual rise in the blood nicotine concentration that levels off and remains constant for much of the day, and then gradually decreases while the person is asleep.[38]

Side Effects Nicotine-replacement products have relatively few side effects. Nausea and light-headedness are possible symptoms of nicotine overdose that warrant a reduction of the nicotine dose. The most frequent side effect with the nicotine patch is skin irritation related to the adhesive or the medium containing nicotine and not to the nicotine itself. Approximately 50% of patients report skin irritation during the course of treatment with the patch. The patch site can be rotated to diminish this problem. Switching to a different brand of patch can alleviate the problem because different products use different adhesives or media. The gum can be used instead of the patch when the skin irritation is severe. Less than 5% of patients were forced to discontinue therapy because of skin reactions.[38]

Duration Those who commit to quitting smoking using NRT should be told that treatment for up to 3 months is common.[60] However, some patients will experience severe withdrawal even beyond this time period; thus, long-term use of NRT might be indicated. Long-term use of NRT has not been linked to any safety concerns and is supported by the 2008 updated US Public Health Service Guidelines.[38]

Non-Nicotine Options

Bupropion Bupropion inhibits neuronal reuptake and potentiates the effects of norepinephrine and dopamine. Although its precise mechanism in smoking cessation is not well understood, dopamine has been associated with the rewarding effects of addictive substances. The AHRQ panel concluded that SR bupropion is an efficacious smoking cessation treatment that patients should be encouraged to use.[38]

Contraindications for bupropion use include current or past seizure disorders, a history of monoamine oxidase inhibitor use over the last 14 days, and a history of anorexia nervosa or bulimia. Along with multiple other precautions listed in the product labeling, current alcohol use, use of medications that lower seizure threshold (eg, antidepressants and antipsychotics), and depression are possible concerns when using this medication.[38] In 2009, the FDA required manufacturers of Zyban (bupropion) and generic manufacturers to add new boxed warnings and to develop a medication guide highlighting the risk of serious neuropsychiatric symptoms in patients using this product. Possible symptoms include depressed mood, agitation, anxiety, hostility, changes in behavior, suicidal thoughts and behavior, and attempted suicide.[38] A meta-analysis[61] involving 65 trials utilizing bupropion for smoking cessation showed that bupropion significantly increased the incidence of long-term cessation when used as a sole agent in 44 separate trials. Other trials that used bupropion as an add-on agent with NRT did not show additional benefit in improving cessation rates.[61]

For smoking cessation, the manufacturer recommends a dosage of 150 mg once daily for 3 days and then twice daily for 7 to 12 weeks or longer, with or without NRT. Patients are instructed to stop smoking during the second week of treatment and are encouraged to use counseling and support services along with the medication. For maintenance therapy, consider SR bupropion 150 mg twice daily for up to 6 months.[38]

Varenicline (Chantix) Varenicline acts at sites in the nicotine-affected brain in two ways: by providing nicotine effects to ease withdrawal symptoms and by blocking the effects of nicotine from cigarettes if they resume smoking. Specifically, varenicline is a partial agonist that binds selectively to α_4-β_2-nicotinic acetylcholine receptors with a greater affinity than nicotine. When bound to the receptor, the drug blocks nicotine from binding and also evokes a response but to a lesser degree than nicotine. The stimulation of the receptor results in release of dopamine and thus provides a type of "reward" that can decrease craving and withdrawal symptoms.[62]

8 The recommended dosage for varenicline is 0.5 mg daily for 3 days, increase to 0.5 mg twice daily for 3 days, and then increase to 1 mg twice daily for a standard 12-week treatment. It is suggested the quit date should be set for 1 week after initiating varenicline, but recent studies have shown allowing a flexible quit date is also efficacious and safe. If abstinence has not been achieved after the 12-week treatment, then a second 12-week treatment may be prescribed.[63]

Varenicline is listed as a first-line agent in the 2008 clinical guidelines on treating tobacco use and dependence. Fourteen trials comparing varenicline with placebo, three of which also had a comparison with bupropion, were reviewed in a meta-analysis.[64] Varenicline resulted in an over two fold increased likelihood of long-term smoking cessation compared with counseling alone. The most common side effect seen in these studies was mild to moderate nausea over a short period of time following treatment initiation.

Since 2006, when varenicline was approved by the FDA, alarming numbers of adverse effects, including suicidal thoughts, erratic behavior, and aggressive behavior, have been reported. The large number of reports led to the release of a Public Health Advisory by the FDA in February 2008.[65] The advisory stressed the importance of screening for any type of psychiatric illness or any behavior changes after starting varenicline. A boxed warning along with an update of the medication guide from the manufacturer was required by the FDA.[66] The FDA sponsored two epidemiologic studies that evaluated the neuropsychiatric adverse events linked to the use of varenicline. These studies had multiple limitations, and although the studies did not show an increased risk of hospitalization secondary to neuropsychiatric events, it is important for both healthcare professionals and patients to be aware of the possible risks associated with the use of varenicline.[67] Specific warnings stress patients should report any history of psychiatric illness and any changes in behavior or mood immediately to their prescribing practitioner.[68] Since the addition of the boxed warning, there have been additional reports of adverse reactions when mixing varenicline with alcohol, including decreased tolerance to the effects of alcohol and unusual behavior. There have also been some rare reports of seizures predominately in the first month of treatment with varenicline in patients with well-controlled seizure disorder or no history of seizures.[68]

Additionally, in 2011, the FDA issued a safety communication reporting cardiovascular adverse events, including myocardial infarctions, which were seen in a higher number of patients receiving varenicline compared with placebo.[69] A meta-analysis[70] was completed which included over 7,000 patients enrolled in randomized, controlled, double-blind, placebo controlled trials greater than or equal to 12 weeks in duration. The goal of this meta-analysis was to study the cardiovascular safety by evaluating the number of occurrences of major adverse cardiac events and the timing of these events. Although a trend for increased risk of cardiac events was observed in this analysis, the increased risk was not found to be statistically significant.[70] The current recommendation from the FDA is to evaluate the risk versus benefit of using varenicline[71] since there is a greater than twofold increased likelihood of long-term smoking cessation compared with nonpharmacologic treatment when using varenicline.[64] It has been shown varenicline was more effective in helping patients to achieve smoking cessation and maintain abstinence for up to 1 year than placebo.[72]

Clinical **Controversy...**

It has been well established that smoking during pregnancy can lead to adverse outcomes during the pregnancy including miscarriage, placental abruption, preterm delivery, and low birth rate leading to a higher risk of infant morbidity and mortality.[38] In 2012, a Cochrane review of 6 trials utilizing NRT in 1,745 pregnant women concluded there was insufficient evidence to support efficacy or safety in using NRT in pregnancy. (RR 1.3; 95% CI 0.93-1.9).[73] In 2014, the SNIPP trial, a randomized, double blind, placebo controlled, parallel group, multicenter trial included 402 pregnant women who were randomized into NRT with nicotine patches or placebo treatment from quit day until delivery. Nicotine patches did not improve cessation rates compared to placebo, although the incidences of serious adverse effects were not higher for the NRT treatment group.[74] The SNAPP trial evaluated 1,050 pregnant smokers who were randomized to NRT or placebo and followed at multiple endpoints including 1 month after starting therapy, at delivery, and at 6, 12, and 24 months following delivery.[75] NRT was effective during the first month, but subsequently efficacy was equal to placebo with regards to smoking cessation. Children involved in the study showed no difference in birth weight or respiratory issues, but the children randomized into the NRT group did have fewer developmental problems compared to the placebo group. In a 2015 retrospective population-based study, over 2,500 children with maternal exposure to NRT during pregnancy were shown not to have experienced adverse effects linked to NRT.[76] Although it is clear more research is needed, the current recommendations are similar to the 2008 guidelines. Behavioral therapy should be attempted, but if this fails then the risks and benefits of NRT should be discussed, and initiation of the NRT and proper monitoring should be considered if appropriate based on the individual patient.[38]

Comparison of NRT and Non-Nicotine Options

A systematic review and multiple treatment meta-analysis was performed using a Bayesian model to evaluate the effect of high-dose and standard-dose NRT, combination NRT, bupropion, and varenicline.[77] The primary outcome included smoking abstinence at 4, 12, 26, and 52 weeks following the set quit date. The standard- and high-dose NRT patch, bupropion, and varenicline were shown to be superior to placebo and controls on a consistent basis. Varenicline was shown to be statistically more effective in achieving smoking abstinence compared with the other agents except at 6 months when compared with high-dose NRT patches and combination therapy. It is difficult to identify which agent is more effective over another at this time, since other considerations, such as cost and specific patient factors must also be taken into account.[77] Furthermore, a meta-analysis was performed which included 12 Cochrane reviews between 2008 and 2012, 267 trials, and 101,000 smokers to evaluate benefits and risks associated with the first line pharmacotherapy agents including: NRT, varenicline, and bupropion. Additionally, other agents including nortriptyline and clonidine were also evaluated in this review. All first line smoking cessation agents were found to be superior to placebo, and varenicline was found to be superior to both single forms of NRT (OR 2.88; 95% CI 2.40-3.37) and to bupropion (OR 1.59; 95% CI 1.29-1.96) and is equally effective in comparison to combination NRT (OR 1.06; 95% CI 0.75-1.48). Bupropion and NRT were equal in efficacy. In regards to safety, there were no excessive neuropsychiatric events or cardiovascular events with bupropion (neuropsychiatric events data: RR 0.88; 95% CI 0.31-2.50; cardiovascular data: RR 0.77; 95% CI 0.37-1.59) and no excessive neuropsychiatric events with varenicline (RR 0.53; 95% CI 0.17-1.67) and no statistically significant cardiovascular events. (RR 1.26; 95% CI 0.62-2.56).[78]

Second-Line Medications

Second-line medications are pharmacotherapy options for which there is evidence of efficacy for treating tobacco dependence, but which have a more limited role than first-line medications because (a) the FDA has not approved them for treatment of tobacco dependence and (b) there are more concerns about potential side effects than with first-line medications.[38] Second-line treatments should be considered for use on a case-by-case basis after first-line treatments have been used or considered.

Clonidine It has been found that clonidine is efficacious as a smoking cessation treatment. It can be used off-label as a second-line agent to treat tobacco dependence. A meta-analysis of six trials showed that clonidine increased smoking cessation rates by 9% (RR 1.63, CI 1.22-2.18).[78] There are reports of dose-dependent side effects, particularly sedation and hypotension. It should be noted that abrupt discontinuation of clonidine can result in symptoms, such as nervousness, agitation, headache, and tremor, accompanied or followed by a rapid rise in blood pressure and elevated catecholamine levels.[38] Doses have varied significantly, from 0.15 to 0.75 mg/day orally and from 0.1 to 0.2 mg/day transdermally, without a clear dose–response relationship to cessation. Most commonly reported side effects include dry mouth, drowsiness, dizziness, sedation, and constipation. Clonidine will lower blood pressure in most patients; thus, blood pressure should be monitored.[38]

Nortriptyline It is also considered to be efficacious as a second-line agent for tobacco dependence. Therapy is initiated 10 to 28 days before the quit date to allow it to reach steady state at the target dose. Trials have initiated treatment at a dose of 25 mg/day, increasing gradually to a target dose of 75 to 100 mg/day. Duration of treatment used in smoking cessation trials has been approximately 12 weeks. A recent meta-analysis of 6 trials with 975 patients showed that nortriptyline as a sole agent does show similar efficacy to NRT and has also been effective in increasing long-term cessation rates.[61] Most commonly reported side effects include sedation, dry mouth, blurred vision, urinary retention, light-headedness, and tremor.[38]

Future Treatments Work continues on the development of vaccines to treat nicotine addiction. Vaccines are designed to produce antibodies that bind to nicotine and prevent it from entering the brain. As a result, the positive stimulus in the brain that is normally caused by nicotine is no longer present, thereby taking away the physical motivation for smoking.[79] Multiple vaccines have been in development including NicVAX, NicQb, and Niccine, but clinical trial results utilizing the first generation of nicotine vaccines have been disappointing. It is postulated the vaccines have not been able to produce the antibody levels needed to achieve clinical efficacy, and the challenges presented by patient individual variability have also been detrimental.[79] Research is needed to further develop next-generation vaccines in hopes that this will become a treatment option for smoking cessation in the future.

Personalized Pharmacotherapy The genetics associated with nicotine addiction is very complex and continues to be studied with great interest. Many phenotypes and corresponding genes have been identified which affect smoking behavior, including nicotine dependence, daily cigarette consumption, onset of smoking, smoking cessation success, and withdrawal symptoms.[80] Studies continue to evaluate the effects of polymorphisms in various genes and the effect this has on the efficacy of pharmacotherapy treatment options. Additionally, genetic variability in nicotine metabolism continues to be evaluated since variations in Cytochrome P450 2A6 leads to different addiction rates to nicotine and responses to NRT.[80] Further understanding of these variations will prove helpful in creating a personalized pharmacotherapy plan to improve smoking cessation rates.

Electronic Nicotine Delivery Systems The electronic nicotine delivery systems (ENDS; also known as e-cigarettes or electronic cigarettes) are designed to deliver a propylene glycol or glycerol product with a combination of nicotine, flavorings, and/or other chemicals through an aerosol. Using this device is commonly referred to as "vaping." It has been suggested that using the products instead of smoking traditional cigarettes can eliminate the exposure to most of the toxins commonly seen in traditional cigarettes.[81] The range of nicotine delivered to the user can vary according to the product type and brand, but can also be affected by the temperature and the specific delivery system.[82] At the time of this writing, no ENDS has been approved by the FDA as a cessation aid, although these products have gained popularity as a cessation aid. A review of 2 studies which included 600 people indicated the use of e-cigarettes with nicotine improved the chances of long term smoking cessation compared with e-cigarettes without nicotine. To date, there are not enough studies comparing e-cigarettes with nicotine to traditional NRT options for smoking cessation. The evidence for efficacy of e-cigarettes with nicotine for smoking cessation is low, and further studies are needed. Additionally, the safety of e-cigarettes has not been studied to determine the risks associated with the chemicals used in these devices, the amount of nicotine exposure delivered, nor the risk of second-hand exposure to the chemicals emitted while vaping. The popularity of these agents is also concerning since younger individuals might feel this is a safer alternative to smoking and become addicted to nicotine through this method.

Clinical **Controversy...**

A huge debate continues regarding e-cigarettes. The e-cigarettes are viewed as a better choice over traditional cigarettes by some since the user will not be exposed to the carcinogens associated with smoking traditional cigarettes. However, there are other concerns associated with e-cigarette including possible dangers associated with propylene glycol or glycerol and added flavorings that are included in these products. Additionally, e-cigarettes can appeal to adolescents due to the belief that e-cigarettes are safer and varieties of flavors offered in these products can be very appealing as well. Exposure of the developing brain to nicotine could increase the risk of developing a nicotine addiction. A recent study has shown that exposure to e-cigarettes did increase the likelihood of using other tobacco products including traditional cigarettes and other forms of tobacco within the following year of e-cigarette exposure. Further studies are needed to clarify the benefits of e-cigarettes compared to the risks.[83]

CAFFEINE

9 Caffeine is the most widely consumed behaviorally active substance in the world, generating an increased sense of well-being, happiness, energy, alertness, and sociability.[84] Caffeinism is the term coined to describe the clinical syndrome produced by acute or chronic overuse of caffeine. The syndrome usually is characterized by CNS and peripheral manifestations, most notably anxiety, psychomotor alterations, sleep disturbances, mood changes, and psychophysiologic complaints. As many as one in five adults consumes doses of caffeine generally considered large enough to cause clinical symptoms.[84]

Pharmacologically, the risk of developing meaningful clinical manifestations becomes high when intake exceeds 500 mg/day. Drinking traditional coffee, it could be assumed this level of caffeine might not be reached. This helps explain why, up until recently, deaths from acute ingestions of caffeine were virtually nonexistent. However, pure caffeine powder has become available via the Internet,[85] and some individuals have been using it by the teaspoonful. One teaspoonful of the bulk powder is estimated to be equivalent to 25 to 30 cups of coffee. The "recommended dose" is 1/64th to 1/16th of a teaspoonful, which is equivalent to 2 cups of coffee, and exceeding this dose has led to toxicity including life threatening cardiac arrhythmias and death. Due to this risk, efforts are being made to regulate powdered caffeine, which currently is available for purchase without regulation.[85]

Caffeine has been proposed as a "model of drug abuse" despite the facts that its sale is largely unrestricted and that heavy consumption of caffeine-containing beverages is not considered to be drug abuse. The following information represents a broad overview of dependence, withdrawal, and tolerance. The reader interested in more information is urged to consult the exhaustive review by Juliano et al.[84]

Epidemiology of Caffeine Use and Abuse

Recently, data from the What We Eat in America/National Health and Nutrition Examination Survey (NHANES) was evaluated on caffeine consumption in the United States through caffeinated beverages, foods, and energy drinks. This data showed that 89% of men and women in the United States consume caffeine daily, predominantly through caffeinated beverages (98%). The most common caffeinated beverage was coffee (64%), tea, and soft drinks were less popular (16% and 18%, respectively). The intake of caffeine averaged 186 mg/day, and over half of the consumers ingested this amount in one consumption.[86] Caffeine intake among children, adolescents, and young adults is prevalent from foods and beverages based on the 1999 to 2010 NHANES data analyzing ages of participants from 2 years old to 22 years old. It was found that 73% consumed caffeine, although the caffeine consumption overall remained similar through the years, the choice of beverages has changed from predominately soda in 1999 to 2000 to a combination of soda, sweetened coffee, and energy drinks in 2009 to 2010.[87]

Energy Drinks

A number of energy drinks containing caffeine, taurine, vitamins, and sugar which are sold under brand names such as Red Bull, Monster Energy, Rockstar, NOS, and Amp, continue to gain popularity among adolescents and emerging adults. It is now estimated that 30% to 50% of this population are now using these products.[88] The amount of caffeine in 1 can of Red Bull (8.4 oz [250 mL]) includes 77 mg of caffeine, although other products can contain higher amounts of caffeine depending on the size of the container. The energy shot, a 2 ounce (60 mL) product, claims to contain the "same amount of caffeine as a cup of coffee" and also includes a variety of B vitamins and other products claimed to improve energy.[89] Since these products commonly include natural ingredients such as ginkgo, they are regulated by the 1994 Dietary Supplement and Education Act and are not required to disclose how much caffeine is in the product.

10 Many questions on the safety of the use of these products have been raised due to the increase in emergency department visits which doubled from 2007 to 2011.[90] Reports submitted to the FDAs Center for Food Safety and Applied Nutrition from 2004 to 2012 included over 20 reports on adverse reactions to Red Bull, including cardiac symptoms, anxiety, aggression, and convulsions.[91] Additionally, there are multiple case reports of cardiovascular events including atrial fibrillation, ST-elevation myocardial infarctions, and fatal ventricular arrhythmias in adolescents following energy drink consumption.

Several manufacturers were marketing alcoholic beverages containing caffeine. In 2010, the FDA requested that the manufacturers remove the caffeine from their products. Unfortunately, mixing the energy drinks with alcohol remains popular and has been proven dangerous because the high levels of caffeine can reduce awareness and mask the typical depressant effects of alcohol, giving the consumer a false sense of competence leading to poor decision making such as drunk driving or other increased risky behavior.[92]

Differential Diagnosis

The DSM-5 has 4 caffeine-related diagnoses including: caffeine intoxication, caffeine withdrawal, other caffeine-induced disorders which include both caffeine induced sleep and anxiety disorders, and unspecified caffeine-related disorder which includes symptoms, which might be attributed to caffeine use, but does not fit in any of the other categories. DSM-5 does not currently list a diagnosis of caffeine use disorder (CUD), but it has been identified as an area which needs further research to determine if CUD should become an official diagnosis.[8]

The diagnostic criteria for caffeine intoxication include recent consumption of caffeine normally exceeding 250 mg and 5 or more symptoms during or shortly after consumption of caffeine. The symptoms of caffeine intoxication will usually decrease over 24 hours as the caffeine is eliminated from the body. Consumption of very high doses of caffeine could be dangerous and require immediate medical attention.[8]

Caffeine withdrawal is a new diagnosis in the DSM-5. It occurs after the abrupt cessation of chronic caffeine use and can occur even with low doses of caffeine in some patients. The diagnosis of caffeine withdrawal requires 3 of the 5 listed symptoms, including headache (most common), marked fatigue or drowsiness, altered mood (depressed, irritable, and dysphoric), difficulty in concentrating, or flu-like symptoms including nausea, vomiting, muscle pain/stiffness (Table 66-6). The extent and severity of withdrawal can vary individually but normally will be more severe with higher chronic doses of caffeine.[8]

TABLE 66-6 DSM-5 Diagnostic Criteria for Caffeine Withdrawal

Criteria
Prolonged daily use of caffeine

Abrupt cessation or decreased use in caffeine leading to at least three of the following symptoms after 24 hours of cessation
• Concentration problems
• Mood changes: dysphoric mood, depressed mood, irritability
• Dramatic fatigue or drowsiness
• Headache
• Flu-like symptoms
  • Nausea
  • Vomiting
  • Muscle pain/stiffness

Symptoms negatively impact areas of functioning such as social or occupational functioning.
Symptoms experienced cannot be explained by other concurrent medical conditions.

Data from reference 8.

Pharmacology of Caffeine

Caffeine is rapidly and completely absorbed from the GI tract, reaching a peak blood level within 30 to 60 minutes after oral ingestion. It easily crosses the blood–brain barrier, and levels achieved in the brain are proportional to the dose administered.[93] The half-life of caffeine in humans is approximately 4 to 6 hours in healthy nonsmoking adults. Smoking will result in a shorter half-life, and liver dysfunction and pregnancy will extend the half-life.[93] Overdoses of caffeine are now more common due to the wide availability of energy drinks. Caffeine increases the heart rate and force of cardiac contraction and also has a strong diuretic effect. Due to the stimulating properties of caffeine, nervousness, agitation, and insomnia may occur. More serious reactions could include cardiac arrhythmias, hypotension, and convulsions.[94] The key factor promoting caffeine use and dosage increases can be the drug's reinforcing effect on pleasure and reward centers of the brain. Caffeine's pharmacologic actions appear comparable (although less potent) with those of other stimulants, such as amphetamines and cocaine.[93]

Caffeine Dependence

Research has shown that abstinence from caffeine induces a distinct withdrawal syndrome.[95] In a structured psychiatric interview, subjects who self-identified as having problems with caffeine use were evaluated for features of a *DSM-IV-TR* diagnosis of drug dependence. Those judged to be caffeine dependent manifested at least three of four criteria (eg, tolerance, withdrawal, persistent desire, or an unsuccessful attempt to reduce consumption and persistent use despite adverse psychological or physical consequences). Of 99 people screened, 27 were evaluated by means of a structured psychiatric

CLINICAL PRESENTATION Caffeine Intoxication

General

- The patient may not be in acute distress.

Symptoms

- The patient may complain of nausea, vomiting, diarrhea, and psychomotor agitation, and can appear restless, nervous, and excited.

Signs

- The patient can present with facial flushing, diuresis, and muscle twitching.
- Tachycardia or cardiac arrhythmias can also occur.

Laboratory Tests

- Caffeine serum concentrations are rarely used clinically.

interview modified for the diagnosis of caffeine dependence; 16 of those subjects (59%) met the criteria. In a second phase of the study, 11 of the 16 caffeine-dependent individuals participated in a 2-day, double-blind, crossover study of caffeine deprivation. Nine showed evidence of caffeine withdrawal during the placebo phase.

Caffeine Withdrawal

The frequency of the caffeine withdrawal syndrome is not well known, but it may be common. Withdrawal can occur when individuals who previously consumed caffeine on a regular basis suddenly discontinue its intake or reduce the dose.[84] The syndrome is characterized by the occurrence of headache, drowsiness, fatigue, and sometimes impaired psychomotor performance, difficulty concentrating, nausea, excessive yawning, and craving. These symptoms usually appear within 18 to 24 hours after discontinuation, corresponding to the time required for the drug to be cleared from the body.

The caffeine withdrawal headache is somewhat unique, starting with a sense of fullness in the head and progressing to throbbing and diffuse pain that is made worse by movement. The maximum intensity of the pain occurs 3 to 6 hours after beginning.

When caffeine is reintroduced, relief of withdrawal symptoms tends to occur within 30 to 60 minutes. Reintroduction of caffeine appears to be the most effective "treatment" for the caffeine withdrawal syndrome.[84]

Effect on Sleep

Caffeine interferes with sleep in most nontolerant individuals.[84] Tolerant people are much less likely to self-report sleep abnormalities, or they may sense that the insomnia has disappeared altogether. To illustrate, 53% of those consuming less than 250 mg/day agreed that caffeine before bedtime would prevent sleep, compared with 43% of those consuming 250 to 749 mg/day and only 22% of those taking 750 mg/day or more. Even though the higher-level consumers denied that caffeine interferes with their sleep, studies done in the sleep laboratory confirm that caffeine consumers do have greater sleep latency, more frequent awakenings, and altered sleep architecture, and that these effects are dose related.

Caffeine during Pregnancy

Over the years, there has been much discussion on whether or not caffeine intake during pregnancy is harmful to the developing fetus. Results of research have been mixed, but in general, caffeine has not been shown to be a potent and consistent teratogen. Kuczkowski[96] published an evidence-based review highlighting the implications of caffeine intake in pregnancy and offering recommendations for practitioners providing peripartum care to expectant mothers who consume caffeine. The author concluded that, for the healthy pregnant adult, moderate daily caffeine intake at a dose level up to 400 mg/day is not associated with adverse effects, such as general toxicity, cardiovascular effects, effects on bone status and calcium balance, changes in adult behavior, increased incidence of cancer, or effects on fertility. The study did not identify any significant positive associations between maternal caffeine consumption and cardiovascular malformations. The March of Dimes advises women to limit their caffeine intake to less than 200 mg/day. This recommendation was prompted by the results of a population-based prospective cohort study published in March 2008,[97] showing that pregnant women consuming 200 mg or more of caffeine a day had double the risk of miscarriage compared with those who had no caffeine. Criticism of this study was swift to follow, and its conclusions have been called into question. A Cochrane systematic review[98] points out that authors of some observational studies have concluded that caffeine intake is harmful to the fetus. The review concludes that there is insufficient evidence from RCTs to support any reason to avoid caffeine during pregnancy. Unfortunately, this review is based on only two published controlled trials.

Caffeine and Headaches

A Norwegian study[99] investigated the association between caffeine consumption and headache in the general adult population. Results were based on cross-sectional data from 50,483 (55%) out of 92,566 invited participants aged greater than or equal to 20 years. A weak but significant association (OR 1.16; 95% CI 1.09-1.23) was found between high caffeine consumption and infrequent headaches. In contrast, headache for greater than 14 days/mo was less likely among individuals with high caffeine consumption compared with those with low caffeine consumption. The authors speculate that their results may indicate that high caffeine consumption changes chronic headache into infrequent headache due to the analgesic properties of caffeine. Alternatively, chronic headache sufferers tend to avoid intake of caffeine to not aggravate their headaches, whereas individuals with infrequent headache are less aware that high caffeine use can be a cause.

Treatment

Desired Outcomes

Many people drink coffee, tea, and other caffeinated beverages without problems. When adverse health effects occur (eg, insomnia, headaches, anxiety, AND palpitations), it may be necessary to cut down on the amount of caffeine ingested or to eliminate it altogether to achieve the goal of elimination of these symptoms.

Caffeinism

Caffeinism is treated by reducing or discontinuing the drug. It may be necessary to wean the patient off the drug gradually because going "cold turkey" can produce such serious symptoms that the drug must be restarted. Decaffeinated beverages can be substituted slowly for the caffeinated type. However, relapses are less likely to occur when the drug is discontinued all at once, probably because of the considerable self-discipline required to continue weaning the drug when one knows that an increase in dose will cause the symptoms to abate.

CLINICAL PRESENTATION Caffeine Withdrawal

General

- The patient may not be in acute distress.

Symptoms

- The patient may complain of headache, nausea, vomiting, drowsiness, poor concentration, depressed mood.
- The patient reports the symptoms are adversely affecting overall social/occupational functioning and/or leading to distress.

Laboratory Tests

- Caffeine serum concentrations are rarely used clinically.

ABBREVIATIONS

AHRQ	Agency for Healthcare Research and Quality
AUD	Alcohol Use Disorder
AUDIT	Alcohol Use Disorders Identification Test
AUDIT-C	Alcohol Use Disorders Identification Test consumption questions
BAC	blood alcohol concentration
CIWA-AR	Clinical Institute Withdrawal Assessment for Alcohol, Revised
CT	computed tomography
CUD	Caffeine Use Disorder
DSM-IV-TR	*Diagnostic and Statistical Manual of Mental Disorders, Fourth Edition, Text Revision*
DSM-5	*Diagnostic and Statistical Manual of Mental Disorders, Fifth Edition*
ENDS	Electronic Nicotine Delivery Systems
GABA	γ-aminobutyric acid
GI	gastrointestinal
5-HT_3	serotonin-3 receptor
NHANES	National Health and Nutrition Examination Survey
NRT	nicotine replacement therapy
NSDUH	National Survey on Drug Use and Health
PAN	psychotropic analgesic nitrous oxide
RCT	randomized controlled trial
SNIPP	Study of Nicotine Patch in Pregnancy
SNAPP	Smoking Nicotine and Pregnancy
SR	sustained release

REFERENCES

1. U.S. Department of Health and Human Services. The Health Consequences of Smoking—50 Years of Progress: A Report of the Surgeon General. (http://www.cdc.gov/tobacco/data_statistics/sgr/50th-anniversary/index.htm), Atlanta: U.S. Department of Health and Human Services, Centers for Disease Control and Prevention, National Center for Chronic Disease Prevention and Health Promotion, Office on Smoking and Health, 2014.
2. Substance Abuse and Mental Health Services Administration, Results from the 2013 National Survey on Drug Use and Health: Summary of National Findings, NSDUH Series H-48, HHS Publication No. (SMA) 14-4863. Rockville, MD: Substance Abuse and Mental Health Services Administration, 2014.
3. World Health Organization, Department of Mental Health and Substance Abuse. Global Status Report on Alcohol and Health. Geneva: World Health Organization. *http://www.who.int/substance_abuse/publications/global_alcohol_report/msbgsruprofiles.pdf.* Last accessed, July 24, 2015.
4. Kanny D, Brewer R, Mesnick J, et al. Vital signs: alcohol poisoning deaths—United States 2010-2012. *MMWR* 2015;63(53):1238-1242. http://www.cdc.gov/mmwr/preview/mmwrhtml/mm6353a2.htm?s_cid=mm6353a2_w. Last accessed, July 10, 2015.
5. Genung V. Understanding the neurobiology, assessment, and treatment of substances of abuse and dependence: a guide for the critical care nurse. *Crit Care Nurs Clin North Am* 2012;24:117-130.
6. Dawson D, Goldstein R, Grant B. Differences in the profiles of DSM IV and DSM-5 alcohol use disorders: implications for clinicians. *Alcohol Clin Esp Res* 2013;37(S1):E305-E313.
7. Substance Abuse and Mental Health Services Administration and National Institute on Alcohol Abuse and Alcoholism, Medication for the treatment of alcohol use disorder: a brief guide. HHS Publication No. (SMA) 15-4907. Rockville, MD: Substance Abuse and Mental Health Services Administration, 2015.
8. American Psychiatric Association. Diagnostic and statistical manual of mental disorders, Fifth Edition, DSM-5. Arlington: American Psychiatric Association. 2013.
9. Enoch M. Genetic influences on the development of alcoholism. *Curr Psychiatry Resp* 2013;15(11):412. doi:10.1007/s11920-013-0412-1.
10. Jones J, Comer S, Kranz H. The pharmacogenetics of alcohol use disorder. *Alcoholism Clin Exp Res* 2015;39(3):391-402.
11. Verhulst B, Neale M, Kendler K. The heritability of alcohol use disorders: a meta-analysis of twin and adoption studies. *Psychologic Med* 2015;54:1061-1072.
12. Agrawal A, Verweij KJ, Gillespie NA, et al. The genetics of addiction—a translational perspective. *Transl Psychiatry* 2012;2:e140. doi:10.1038/tp.2012.54.
13. Chan L, Anderson G. Pharmacokinetic and pharmacodynamics drug interactions with ethanol (alcohol). *Clin Pharmacokinet* 2014;53:1115-1136.
14. Kugelberg FC, Jones AW. Interpreting results of ethanol analysis in postmortem specimens: a review of the literature. *Forensic Sci Int* 2007;165:10-29.
15. Zakhari S. Overview: how is alcohol metabolized by the body? *Alcohol Res Health* 2006;29:245-254.
16. Nassir F, Ibdah J. Role of mitochondria in alcoholic liver disease. *Would J Gastroenterol* 2014;20(9):2136-2142.
17. Jones AW. Evidence-based survey of the elimination rates of ethanol from blood with applications in forensic casework. *Forensic Sci Int* 2010;200:1-20 [Epub March 20, 2010].
18. Dhalla S, Kopec JA. The CAGE questionnaire for alcohol misuse: a review of reliability and validity studies. *Clin Invest Med* 2007;30:33-41.
19. Lundin A, Hallgren M, Balliu N, Forsell Y. The use of alcohol use disorders identification test (AUDIT) in detecting alcohol use disorder and risk drinking in the general population: validation of AUDIT using schedules for clinical assessment in Neuropsychiatry. *Alcohol Clin Exp Res* 2015;39(1):158-165.
20. Dubowski K. Stages of acute alcohol influence/intoxication. http://www.drugdetection.net/PDF%20documents/Dubowski%20-%20stages%20of%20alcohol%20effects.pdf. Last accessed, July 27, 2015.
21. National Institute on Alcohol Abuse and Alcoholism. Alcohol overdose: the dangers of drinking too much. http://pubs.niaaa.nih.gov/publications/AlcoholOverdoseFactsheet/Overdosefact.htm. Last accessed, July 27, 2015.
22. Perry E. Inpatient management of acute alcohol withdrawal syndrome. *CNS Drugs* 2014;28:401-410.
23. Sulivan JT, Sykora K, Schneiderman J, et al. Assessment of alcohol withdrawal: the revised clinical institute withdrawal assessment for alcohol scale (CIWA-Ar). *Br J Addict* 1989;84:1353-1357.
24. Mayo-Smith MF. Pharmacological management of alcohol withdrawal. A meta-analysis and evidence-based practice guideline. American Society of Addiction Medicine Working Group on Pharmacological Management of Alcohol Withdrawal. *JAMA* 1997;278:144-151.
25. Mayo-Smith MF, Beecher LH, Fischer TL, et al. Working Group on the Management of Alcohol Withdrawal Delirium, Practice Guidelines Committee, American Society of Addiction Medicine. Management of alcohol withdrawal delirium. An evidence-based practice guideline. *Arch Intern Med* 2004;164:1405-1412 [Erratum. Arch Intern Med 2004;164:2068].
26. Amato L, Minozzi S, Davoli M. Efficacy and safety of pharmacological interventions for the treatment of the Alcohol Withdrawal Syndrome. *Cochrane Database Syst Rev* 2011, Issue 6. Art. No.: CD008537. doi:10.1002/14651858.CD008537.pub2.
27. McMicken D, Liss JL. Alcohol-related seizures. *Emerg Med Clin North Am* 2011;29:117-124.
28. Garbutt JC. The state of pharmacotherapy for the treatment of alcohol dependence. *J Subst Abuse Treat* 2009;36:S15-S23 [quiz S24--S25].
29. Frank J, Jayaram-Lindstrom N. Pharmacotherapy for alcohol dependence: status of current treatments. *Current Opinion in Neurobiology* 2013;23:692-699.
30. Pani PP, Trogu E, Pacini M, Maremmani I. Anticonvulsants for alcohol dependence. *Cochrane Database Syst Rev* 2014, Issue 2. Art. No.: CD008544. doi:10.1002/14651858.CD008544.pub2.
31. Oslin D, Leong S, Lynch K, et al. Naltrexone vs. Placebo for the treatment of alcohol dependence. *JAMA Psychiatry* 2015;72(5):430-437.
32. Robinson S, Meeks T, Geniza C. Medication for alcohol use disorder: which agents work best? *Current Psychiatry* 2014;13(1):22-29.

33. Rosner S, Hackl-Herrwerth A, Leucht S, et al. Opioid antagonists for alcohol dependence. *Cochrane Reviews* 2010, Issue 12. Article No. CD001867. doi:10.1002/14651858.
34. Pettinati HM, Silverman BL, Battisti JJ, et al. Efficacy of extended-release naltrexone in patients with relatively higher severity of alcohol dependence. *Alcohol Clin Exp Res* 2011;35(10):1804-1811. doi:10.1111/j.1530-0277.2011.01524.x [Epub May 16, 2011].
35. Rösner S, Hackl-Herrwerth A, Leucht S, et al. Acamprosate for alcohol dependence. *Cochrane Database Syst Rev* 2010;(9):CD004332.
36. Cigarette Smoking United States 1965-2008 Jan 14, 2011 60(01); 109-113. http://www.cdc.gov/mmwr/preview/mmwrhtml/su6001a24.htm#fig. Last accessed, July 29, 2015.
37. Early release of selected estimates based on data from the National Health Interview Survey, January-March 2014. http://www.cdc.gov/nchs/data/nhis/earlyrelease/earlyrelease201409_08.pdf. Last accessed, August 18, 2015.
38. Fiore MC, Baily WC. Treating Tobacco Use and Dependence. Clinical Practice Guidelines. Rockville, MD: U.S. Department of Health and Human Services, Public Health Service, June 2000 [updated May 2008].
39. Pierce J, Cummins S. Quitlines and nicotine replacement for smoking cessation: do we need to change policy? *Annu Rev Public Health* 2012;33:341-356.
40. Jamal A, Dube SR, Malarcher AM, et al. Centers for Disease Control and Prevention. Tobacco use screening and counseling during physician office visits among adults—National Ambulatory Medical Care Survey and National Health Interview Survey, United States, 2005-2009. *MMWR Morb Mortal Wkly Rep* 2012;61(Suppl):38-45.
41. King B, Dube S, Kaufmann R, et al. Centers for Disease Control and Prevention. Vital signs: Current cigarette smoking among adults aged 18 years—United States, 2005-2010. *MMWR Morb Mortal Wkly Rep* 2011;60(35):1207-1212.
42. Jamal A, Agaku I, O'Connor E, et al. Centers for Disease Control and Prevention. Vital signs: current cigarette smoking among adults—United States. 2005-2013. *MMWR Morb Mortal Wkly Rep* 2014;63(47):1108-1112. http://www.cdc.gov/mmwr/pdf/wk/mm6404.pdf. Last accessed, July 29, 2015.
43. HealthyPeople2020. Reduce cigarette smoking by adults. http://www.healthypeople.gov/2020/topics-objectives/topic/tobacco-use/objectives. Last accessed, July 29, 2015.
44. National Survey on Drug Use and Health: Summary of National Findings 2013: http://www.samhsa.gov/data/sites/default/files/NSDUHresultsPDFWHTML2013/Web/NSDUHresults2013.pdf. Last accessed, August 13, 2015.
45. Armour BS, Finkelstein EA. State-level Medicaid expenditures attributable to smoking. *Prev Chronic Dis* 2009;6:A84.
46. U.S. Department of Health and Human Services. The Health Consequences of Involuntary Exposure to Tobacco Smoke: A Report of the Surgeon General. Atlanta, GA: U.S. Department of Health and Human Services, Centers for Disease Control and Prevention, Coordinating Center for Health Promotion, National Center for Chronic Disease Prevention and Health Promotion, Office on Smoking and Health, 2006, *http://www.surgeongeneral.gov/library/secondhandsmoke/report/citation.pdf*. Last accessed, August 13, 2015.
47. Centers for Disease Control and Prevention. Vital signs: Disparities in Nonsmokers' Exposure to Secondhand Smoke-United States, 1999-2012. *MMWR Morb Mortal Wkly Rep* 2015;64(4):103-108. http://www.cdc.gov/mmwr/pdf/wk/mm6404.pdf. Last accessed, July 29, 2015.
48. Balfour DJ. Neuroplasticity within the mesoaccumbens dopamine system and its role in tobacco dependence. *Curr Drug Targets CNS Neurol Disord* 2002;1:413-421.
49. Benowitz N. *Nicotine Addiction NEJM* 2010;362:2295-2303.
50. Benowitz NL. Clinical pharmacology of nicotine implications for understanding, preventing, and treating tobacco addiction. *Clin Pharmacol Ther* 2008;83:531-541.
51. Benowitz N. Pharmacology of nicotine: addiction, smoking-induced disease, and therapeutics. *Annu Rev Pharmacol Toxicol* 2009;49:57-71.
52. Ranney L, Melvin C. Systematic review: smoking cessation intervention strategies for adults and adults in special populations. *Ann Intern Med* 2006;145:845-856.
53. Stead LF, Lancaster T. Behavioral interventions as adjuncts to pharmacotherapy for smoking cessation. *Cochrane Database Syst Rev* 2012;12:CD009670. doi:10.1002/14651858. CD009670.pub2.
54. Lindson-Hawley N, Thompson TP, Begh R. Motivational interviewing for smoking cessation. *Cochrane Database Syst Rev* 2015, Issue 3. Art. No.: CD006936. doi:10.1002/14651858. CD006936.pub3.
55. Lichtenstein E, Zhu S, Tedeschi G. Smoking cessation quitlines. *Am Psychol* 2010 May-June;65(4):252-261.
56. Rothemich SF, Woolf SH, Johnson R, et al. Promoting primary care smoking cessation support with quitlines: the QuitLink Randomized Controlled Trial. *Am J Prev Med* 2010;38:367-374.
57. Chen Y, Madan J, Welton N, et al. Effectiveness and cost-effectiveness of computer and other electronic aids for smoking cessation: a systematic review and network meta-analysis. *Health Technol Assess* 2012;16(38). doi:10.3310/hta16380.
58. Stead LF, Perera R, Bullen C, et al. Nicotine replacement therapy for smoking cessation. *Cochrane Database Syst Rev* 2012, Issue 11. Art. No.: CD000146. doi:10.1002/14651858.CD000146.pub4.
59. Carpenter M, Jardin B, Burris J, et al. Clinical strategies to enhance the efficacy of nicotine replacement therapy for smoking cessation: a review of the literature. *Drugs* 2013;73:407-426.
60. McRobbie H, Thornley S. The importance of treating tobacco dependence. *Rev Esp Cardiol* 2008;6:620-628.
61. Hughes JR, Stead LF. Antidepressants for smoking cessation. *Cochrane Database Syst Rev* 2014;(1):CD000031.
62. Williams J. Review of varenicline for tobacco dependence: panacea or plight? *Expert Opin Pharmacother* 2011;12:1799-1812.
63. Rennard S, Hughes J, Cinciripini P, et al. A randomized placebo-controlled trial of varenicline for smoking cessation allowing flexible quite dates. *Nicotine Tob Res* 2012;14(3):343-350.
64. Cahill K, Stead LF, Lancaster T. Nicotine receptor partial agonists for smoking cessation. *Cochrane Database Syst Rev* 2012;4:CD006103.
65. FDA Public Health Advisory. Important Information on Chantix (Varenicline). 2008, http://www.fda.gov/Drugs/DrugSafety/PostmarketDrugSafetyInformationforPatientsandProviders/DrugSafetyInformationforHeathcareProfessionals/PublicHealthAdvisories/ucm051136.htm. Last accessed, August 13, 2015.
66. FDA Public Health Advisory. FDA Requires New Boxed Warnings for the Smoking Cessation Drugs Chantix and Zyban. 2009, http://www.fda.gov/Drugs/DrugSafety/PostmarketDrugSafetyInformationforPatientsandProviders/DrugSafetyInformationforHeathcareProfessionals/PublicHealthAdvisories/ucm169988.htm. Last accessed, August 13, 2015.
67. FDA Drug Safety Communication: Safety Review Update of Chantix (Varenicline) and Risk of Neuropsychiatric Adverse Events. October 24, 2011, http://www.fda.gov/Drugs/DrugSafety/ucm276737.htm. Last accessed, August 13, 2015.
68. FDA Drug Safety Communication: FDA updates label for stop smoking drug Chantix (varenicline) to include potential alcohol interaction, rare risk of seizures, and studies of side effects on mood, behavior, or thinking http://www.fda.gov/Drugs/DrugSafety/ucm436494.htm. Last accessed, July 15, 2015.
69. Food and Drug Administration. FDA Drug Safety Communication: Chantix (Varenicline) may Increase the Risk of Certain Cardiovascular Adverse Events in Patients with Cardiovascular Disease. July 2011, http://www.fda.gov/Drugs/Drugsafety/ucm259161.htm. Last accessed, July 15, 2015.
70. Ware J, Vetrovec GW, Miller A, et al. Cardiovascular safety of varenicline: patient-level meta-analysis of randomized, blinded, placebo-controlled trials. *Am J Ther* 2013;20(3):235-246.
71. FDA Drug Safety Communication: safety review update of Chantix (varenicline) and risk of cardiovascular adverse events. http://www.fda.gov/Drugs/DrugSafety/ucm330367.htm. Last accessed, July 21, 2015.
72. Food and Drug Administration. FDA Drug Safety Communication: Chantix (Varenicline) may increase the risk of certain cardiovascular adverse events in patients with cardiovascular disease. July 2011, http://www.fda.gov/Drugs/Drugsafety/ucm259161.htm. Last accessed, July 21, 2015.
73. Coleman T, Chamberlain C, Davey M, et al. Pharmacological interventions for promoting smoking cessation during pregnancy. *Cochrane Database Syst Rev* 2012;(9):Art. No: CD010078.
74. Berlin I, Grange G, Jacob N, Tanguy M. Nicotine patches in pregnant smokers: randomized, placebo, controlled, multicenter trial of efficacy. *BMJ* 2014 Mar 11;348:g1622. http://www.bmj.com/content/bmj/348/bmj.g1622.full.pdf.
75. Cooper S, Taggar J, Lewis S, et al. Effect of nicotine patches in pregnancy on infant and maternal outcomes at 2 years: follow up from the randomized double-blind placebo-controlled SNAP trial. *Lancet Respir Med* 2014;2:728-737.
76. Dhalwani N, Szatkowski L, Coleman T, et al. Nicotine replacement therapy in pregnancy and major congenital anomalies in offspring. *Pediatrics* 2015;135(5):859-867.

77. Mills E, Wu P, Lockhart I, et al. Comparisons of high dose and combination nicotine replacement therapy, varenicline, and bupropion for smoking cessation: a systematic review and multiple treatment meta-analysis. *Ann Med* 2012;44:588-597.
78. Cahill K, Stevens S, Perera R, Lancaster T. Pharmacological interventions for smoking cessation: an overview and network analysis (review). *Cochrane Database Syst Rev* 2013;5:CD009329.
79. Pentel P, LeSage M. New directions in nicotine vaccine design and use. *Adv Pharmacol* 2014;69:553-580.
80. Tiili E, Hirvonen A. Can Genetics help in treatment of smoking addiction? *Curr Pharmacogen Person Med* 2013;11:216-223.
81. McRobbie H, Bullen C, Hartmann-Boyce J, Hajek P. Electronic cigarettes for smoking cessation and reduction. *Cochrane Database Syst Rev* 2014;12:1-58.
82. Trehy ML, Ye W, Hadwiger M, et al. Analysis of electronic cigarette cartridges refill solutions, and smoke for nicotine and nicotine related impurities. *J Liquid Chromatogr Relat Techol* 2011;34:1442-1458.
83. Leventhal A, Strong D, Kirkpatrick M, et al. Association of electronic cigarette use with initiation of combustible tobacco product smoking in early adolescence. *JAMA* 2015;314(7):700-707.
84. Juliano LM, Evatt DP, Richards BD, Griffiths RR. Characterization of individuals seeking treatment for caffeine dependence. *Psychol Addict Behav* 2012;26:948-954. doi:10.1037/a0027246.
85. Laskowski L, Henesch J, Nelson L, et al. Start me up! Recurrent ventricular tachydysrhythmias following intentional concentrated caffeine ingestion. *Clinical Toxicology* 2015;53(8):830-833.
86. Fulgoni V, Keast D, Lieberman H. Trends in intake and sources of caffeine in the diets of US adults: 2001-2010. *Am J Clin Nutr* 2015. doi:10.3945/ajcn.113.080077.
87. Branum A, Rossen L, Schoendorf K. Trends in caffeine intake among US children and adolescents. *Pediatrics* 2014;133(3):386-393.
88. Seifert S, Schaechter J, Hershorin E, Lipshultz S. Health effects of energy drinks on children, adolescents, and young adults. *Pediatrics* 2011;127(3):511-528.
89. 5 hour energy website: http://5hourenergy.com/facts/ingredients/. Last accessed, August 10, 2015.
90. Substance Abuse and Mental Health Services Administration, Center for Behavioral Health Statistics and Quality. January 10, 2013. The DAWN Report: Update on Emergency Department Visits Involving Energy Drinks: A Continuing Public Health Concern. Rockville, MD. http://archive.samhsa.gov/data/2k13/DAWN126/sr126-energy-drinks-use.htm. Last accessed, August 10, 2015.
91. CFSAN Adverse Event Reporting System: Voluntary Reports on Red Bull Energy Drink January 1, 2004 through October 23, 2012. http://www.fda.gov/downloads/AboutFDA/CentersOffices/OfficeofFoods/CFSAN/CFSANFOIAElectronicReadingRoom/UCM328525.pdf. Last accessed, August 10, 2015.
92. Weldy R. Risks of alcoholic energy drinks for youth. *JABFM* 2010;23:555-558.
93. Benowitz N. Clinical pharmacology of caffeine. *Ann Rev Med* 1990;41:277-288.
94. Wolk B, Ganetsky M, Babu K. Toxicity of energy drinks. *Curr Opin Pediatr* 2012;24:243-251.
95. Strain EC, Mumford GK, Silverman K, Griffiths RR. Caffeine dependence syndrome. Evidence from case histories and experimental evaluations. *JAMA* 1994;272:1043-1048.
96. Kuczkowski KM. Caffeine in pregnancy. *Arch Gynecol Obstet* 2009;280:695-698.
97. Weng X, Odouli R, Li DK. Maternal caffeine consumption during pregnancy and the risk of miscarriage: a prospective cohort study. *Am J Obstet Gynecol* 2008;198:279.e1-279.e8.
98. Jahanfar S, Jaafar SH. Effects of restricted caffeine intake by mother on fetal, neonatal and pregnancy outcome. *Cochrane Database Syst Rev* 2013, Issue 2. Art. No.: CD006965. doi:10.1002/14651858.CD006965.pub3.
99. Hagen K, Thoresen K, Stovner LJ, Zwart JA. High dietary caffeine consumption is associated with a modest increase in headache prevalence: results from the Head-HUNT Study. *J Headache Pain* 2009;10:153-159.

Schizophrenia

M. Lynn Crismon, Rania S. Kattura, and Peter F. Buckley

67

KEY CONCEPTS

1. Although multiple neurotransmitter dysfunctions are involved in schizophrenia, the etiology is more likely mediated by multiple subcellular processes that are influenced by different genetic polymorphisms.
2. The clinical presentation of schizophrenia is characterized by positive symptoms, negative symptoms, and impairment in cognitive functioning.
3. Comprehensive care for individuals with schizophrenia must occur in the context of a multidisciplinary mental healthcare environment that offers comprehensive psychosocial services in addition to psychotropic medication management.
4. A thorough patient evaluation (eg, history, mental status examination, physical examination, psychiatric diagnostic interview, and laboratory analysis) should occur to establish a diagnosis of schizophrenia and to identify potential co-occurring disorders, including substance abuse and general medical disorders.
5. Given that it is challenging to differentiate among antipsychotics based on efficacy, side effect profiles become important in choosing an antipsychotic for an individual patient.
6. Pharmacotherapy guidelines should emphasize antipsychotics monotherapies that optimize efficacy-to-side effect ratios before progressing to medications with greater side effect risks. Combination regimens should only be used in the most treatment-resistant patients.
7. Adequate time on a given medication at a therapeutic dose is the most important variable in predicting medication response.
8. Long-term maintenance antipsychotic treatment is necessary for the vast majority of patients with schizophrenia in order to prevent relapse.
9. Thorough patient and family psychoeducation should be implemented, utilizing motivational interviewing methods that focus on patient-driven outcomes in an effort to allow patients to achieve life goals.
10. Pharmacotherapy decisions should be guided by systematic monitoring of patient symptoms, preferably with the use of brief symptom rating scales and systematic assessment of potential adverse effects.

Schizophrenia is one of the most complex and challenging of psychiatric disorders. It represents a heterogeneous syndrome of disorganized and bizarre thoughts, delusions, hallucinations, inappropriate affect, and impaired psychosocial functioning. From the time that Kraepelin first described dementia praecox in 1896 until publication of the *Diagnostic and Statistical Manual of Mental Disorders, Fifth Edition* (*DSM-5*) in 2013, the description of this illness has continuously evolved.[1] Scientific advances that increase our knowledge of central nervous system (CNS) physiology, pathophysiology, and genetics will likely improve our understanding of schizophrenia in the future.

EPIDEMIOLOGY

The lifetime prevalence of schizophrenia ranges from 0.3% to 0.7%.[1] The worldwide prevalence of schizophrenia is fairly similar among most cultures. Schizophrenia most commonly has its onset in late adolescence or early adulthood and rarely occurs before adolescence or after the age of 40 years. Although the prevalence of schizophrenia is equal in males and females, the onset of illness tends to be earlier in males. Males most frequently have their first episode during their early 20s, whereas with females it is usually during their late 20s.[1]

ETIOLOGY

Although the etiology of schizophrenia is unknown, research has demonstrated various abnormalities in brain structure and function.[2] However, these changes are not consistent among all individuals with schizophrenia. The cause of schizophrenia is likely multifactorial, that is, multiple pathophysiologic abnormalities can play a role in producing the similar but varying clinical phenotypes we refer to as schizophrenia.

A neurodevelopmental model has been evoked as one possible explanation for the etiology of schizophrenia.[2] This model proposes that schizophrenia has its origins in some as yet unknown in utero disturbance, possibly occurring during the second trimester of pregnancy. Evidence for this is provided by the abnormal neuronal migration demonstrated in studies of brains from people with a diagnosis of schizophrenia. This "schizophrenic lesion" can result in abnormalities in cell shape, position, symmetry, connectivity, and functionality to the development of abnormal brain circuits.[2] Changes are consistent with a cell migration abnormality during the second trimester of pregnancy, and some studies associate upper respiratory infections during the second trimester of pregnancy with a higher incidence of schizophrenia.[3] Other studies associate low birth weight (LBW; less than 2.5 kg [5.5 lb]), obstetric complications, or neonatal hypoxia with schizophrenia.[2] Maternal stress, perhaps related to the effects of circulating glucocorticoids in utero, may be a risk factor for schizophrenia. Maternal "stress" could derive from a variety of external and internal noxious events (malnutrition, infection, etc.). The resulting secondary "synaptic disorganization" associated with such insults is thought not to produce overt clinical manifestations of psychosis until adolescence or early adulthood because this is the corresponding time period of neuronal maturation. Recent attempts to link neurotramsitter abnormalities with a neurodevelopmental model are discussed under pathophysiology.[4]

Although studies show decreased cortical thickness and increased ventricular size in the brains of many patients with schizophrenia, this occurs in the absence of widespread gliosis.[2] One hypothesis is that obstetric complications and hypoxia, in combination with a genetic predisposition, could activate a glutamatergic cascade that results in increased neuronal pruning. It is hypothesized that this genetic predisposition may be related to genes controlling *N*-methyl-D-aspartate (NMDA) receptor activity. As a part of the normal neurodevelopmental process, pruning of dendrites occurs. In normal individuals, approximately 35% of the peak number of dendrites at 2 years of age has been pruned by the time the person reaches mid adolescence. Studies have shown a higher percentage of pruning in individuals with schizophrenia. Furthermore, synaptic pruning predominantly involves glutamatergic dendrites. Hypoxia or other prenatal insult can result in a decreased number of basal neurons from which to start, and glutamatergic activation can exaggerate the pruning process.[2,3] Studies have shown an increased susceptibility to immune/autoimmune disorders in schizophrenia, as well as abnormalities of autoantibodies and cytokine functioning.[5] The immune hypothesis of schizophrenia emphasizes integration of mental and physical well-being.

Numerous studies have shown neuropsychological abnormalities and impairment in reaching normal motor milestones and abnormal movements in young children who later develop schizophrenia.[2] Abnormalities in brain function occur long before the onset of psychotic symptomatology and provide empirical evidence for schizophrenia being a neurodevelopmental disorder.[2] However, the progressive clinical deterioration in many patients suggests that this illness can also have a neurodegenerative component. This is consistent with recent brain imaging studies that show deteriorative brain changes in patients with frequent relapses.[2,6] These changes may be most pronounced among adolescents with early onset schizophrenia.[7] Schizophrenia may be an illness exhibiting neurodegenerative propensity based on a vulnerable neurodevelopmental predisposition.[2,7] Although a specific abnormality has not been discovered, evidence suggests a genetic basis for schizophrenia, and at least part of this may be epigenetic. Although the risk of developing schizophrenia is 0.6% to 1.9% in the US population, the risk is approximately 10% if a first-degree relative has the illness and 3% if a second-degree relative has the illness.[2] If both parents have schizophrenia, the risk of producing an offspring with schizophrenia increases to approximately 40%. Twin studies in dizygotic twins report that the risk of the second twin developing schizophrenia, if one twin has the illness, is between 12% and 14%. However, in monozygotic twins the risk increases to 48%.[2] Adoption studies indicate that the risk for schizophrenia lies with the biologic parents, and environmental changes during the child's developmental stages do not alter this. If schizophrenia occurs in siblings, the onset of illness tends to occur at the same age in each, thus lessening the possibility of an environmental precipitant.

Numerous approaches have been utilized to study the genetics of schizophrenia, including genome-wide association studies (GWAS), copy number variant (CNV) studies, and gene candidate studies.[8] Genetic etiologies in schizophrenia are likely heterogeneous, but present with similar clinical phenotypes, and involve epigenetic interactions.[8] GWAS have identified nearly 20 genetic loci that reach genome-wide significance ($P = 5 \times 10^{-8}$), but only some of these have been replicated in multiple studies.[8] GWAS indicate susceptible genes for schizophrenia on chromosome 6, and common genes underlying psychosis on zinc finger protein 804A (*ZNF804A*), voltage-dependent Ca channel (*CACN1A2*), neurogranin (*NRGN*), and polybromo 1 (*PBRM1*).[6,8] Of major interest is the finding that polymorphisms of the complement component 4 (*C4*) genes on chromosome 6 may be implicated in the abnormal dendritic pruning seen in individuals with schizophrenia.[9] Risk for schizophrenia has been demonstrated in CNV studies for deletions on chromosomes 1, 15, and 22. Polymorphism in the 158 valine/methionine (158*Val/Met*) alleles of the catecholamine-*O*-methyl transferase (*COMT*) gene may explain some of the frontal lobe functional deficits in a subset of individuals with schizophrenia.[6] Other recent studies have shown abnormalities in several genes that code for neurodevelopment and for trophic factors.[10,11] For example, dysbindin is a neurodevelopmental protein gene that is found on chromosome 6, and it has been termed a *NMDA-related schizophrenia susceptibility gene*.[12] Alleles associated with decreased dysbindin ribonucleic acid (RNA) in the dorsolateral prefrontal cortex have been reported in patients with schizophrenia and their families.[12] Another recent GWAS of a large pedigree showed an increased signal at chromosome 8p, close to the gene that encodes for neuregulin—another neurodevelopmental gene. Interest is burgeoning regarding how genetic vulnerability might interact with environmental stressors.[6] It is also important to appreciate that there is an overlap—both clinically and biologically—between schizophrenia and mood disorders. Indeed, one "mega genome with association study" found broad overlap in single nucleotide polymorphisms (SNPs) from chromosomes 3, 10, and 12, across schizophrenia, bipolar disorder, and major depression. Two of these SNPs were at loci related to the pathophysiology calcium-channels.[10] Another study showed '108' potential risk loci associated with schizophrenia. Those related to calcium-channel genes as well as glutamatergic genes are immune-related genes.[11] Thus, the epigenetic risk in schizophrenia may be for a spectrum of mental disorders with other factors assisting in determining the clinical phenotype.

PATHOPHYSIOLOGY

Most recent studies have found decreases in gray matter and increases in ventricular size in individuals with schizophrenia. Although some of these changes may be associated with chronic antipsychotic use, particularly with first generation antipsychotics, studies in first break, treatment-naïve individuals also show decreased grey matter. A meta-analysis of systematic reviews conducted since the year 2000 found consistent decreases in gray matter in multiple brain areas, including the frontal lobes, cingulate gyri, and medial temporal regions among others. A corresponding increase in ventricular size was also observed as well as decreased white matter in the corpus callosum.[13] A recent longitudinal study of high-risk youth showed a substantially greater decrease in grey matter in high-risk youth who progressed to psychosis than in high-risk youth who did not progress to psychosis and in normal controls.[14] Changes in hippocampal volume may correspond with impairment in neuropsychological testing.[2,6] Rather than a decrease in the number of neurons in affected brain areas, a decrease in axonal and dendritic communications between cells can result in a loss of connectivity that can be important with respect to neuronal adaptivity and CNS homeostasis.[2,6] These changes are likely consistent with the evidence for abnormal neuronal pruning.[2]

Although a DA-receptor defect likely exists in schizophrenia, this is an over simplification. Presynaptic changes in dopaminergic neurons occur as well, and this is consistent with the neurodevelopmental model that has been proposed.[4,6] Numerous positron emission tomography (PET) studies have shown regional brain abnormalities, including increased glucose metabolism in the caudate nucleus and decreased blood flow and glucose metabolism in the frontal lobe and left temporal lobe.[2] This may indicate dopaminergic hyperactivity in the head of the caudate nucleus and dopaminergic hypofunction in the frontotemporal regions. PET studies using dopamine-2 (D_2)-specific ligands suggest increased densities of D_2 receptors in the head of the caudate nucleus with decreased densities in the prefrontal cortex.[2,6] However, a meta-analysis showed an increase in presynaptic DA synthesis and release in the striatum with only a small increase in $D_{2/3}$ receptor availability.[15] PET studies assessing dopamine-1 (D_1)

function suggest that subpopulations of patients with schizophrenia may have decreased densities of D_1 receptors in the caudate nucleus and the prefrontal cortex. Hypofrontality can be associated with lack of volition and cognitive dysfunction, core features of schizophrenia. It is unknown whether these changes represent a primary event or secondary processes related to other pathophysiologic abnormalities in schizophrenia. Because of the heterogeneity in the clinical presentation of schizophrenia, it has been suggested that the DA hypothesis may be more applicable to "neuroleptic-responsive psychosis," with multiple different etiologies possibly being responsible for causing schizophrenia.[2,4,6] Attempts have been made to develop relationships between these abnormal findings and behavioral symptoms present in patients with schizophrenia. The positive symptoms are possibly more closely associated with DA-receptor hyperactivity in the mesocaudate, whereas negative symptoms and cognitive impairment are most closely related to DA-receptor hypofunction in the prefrontal cortex. Presynaptic D_1 receptors in the prefrontal cortex are thought to be involved in modulating glutamatergic activity, and this can be important with regard to working memory in individuals with schizophrenia.[2,4,6]

A recent commentary attempts to link different neurotransmitter alterations with different phases of schizophrenia.[4] Krystal hypothesizes that a Predrome Phase is associated with glutamategic synaptic dysfunction resulting in a glutamate signaling defect. This deficit is partially compensated for by a down regulation of gamma-amino-butyric acid (GABA) and synaptic proliferation, producing the Prodromal Phase of Schizophrenia. The GABA deficit results in less inhibition of excitatory circuits to dopaminergic projections, producing dopaminergic dysfunction, the onset of psychosis and the Syndrome Phase. The degree of dopamine dysfunction may well be associated with more severe disease.[6] Associated loss of grey matter compounds the synaptic deficits, leading to the Chronic Phase.[4] Clinical support for this hypothesis is based on a recent exploratory analysis indicating that the glutamatergic receptor (mGluR2/3) agonist methionil improves symptoms of schizophrenia in early disease but not in later disease.[16]

The glutamatergic system is one of the most widespread excitatory neurotransmitter systems in the brain. Alterations in its function, either hypoactivity or hyperactivity, can result in toxic neuronal reactions.[4] Dopaminergic innervation from the ventral striatum decreases the limbic system's inhibitory activity (perhaps through GABA interneurons); thus, dopaminergic stimulation increases arousal. The corticostriatal glutamate pathways have the opposite effect, inhibiting dopaminergic function from the ventral striatum, therefore allowing the limbic system to have increased inhibitory activity. Descending glutamatergic tracts interact with dopaminergic tracts directly as well as through GABA interneurons. Glutamatergic deficiency produces symptoms similar to those of dopaminergic hyperactivity and possibly those seen in schizophrenia. It is proposed that schizophrenia may involve some in utero assault that leads to a developmental defect in NMDA receptor function—so-called NMDA hypofunction. This defect is proposed to have latent clinical expression with the psychotic manifestations from NMDA hypofunction not being seen until late adolescence or early adulthood. MicroRNAs, small noncoding RNAs, are critical to neurodevelopment as well as to regulation of adult neuronal processes. NMDA-regulated microRNA miR-132 is significantly downregulated in individuals with schizophrenia as compared with controls. Several genes are regulated by miR-132, and this altered expression may be related to NMDA hypofunction and the abnormal synaptic pruning seen in the brains of individuals with schizophrenia.[17]

1 Schizophrenia is a complex disorder, and multiple etiologies likely exist. Based on current knowledge, it is naive to think that any currently proposed etiology can adequately explain the genesis of this complex disease. Molecular research involving genetically determined subtle changes in microRNA, G proteins, protein metabolism, and other subcellular processes can eventually identify the biologic disturbances associated with schizophrenia.[2,17] Moreover, the development of distinct biomarkers will help tease out specific phenocopies of schizophrenia as well as the boundaries between psychosis and mood disorders.[18] The advent of regenerative medicine and the application of stem cell research to schizophrenia also holds promise to disentangle the pathobiology of this enigmatic disorder.[19]

CLINICAL PRESENTATION

Schizophrenia is the most common functional psychosis, and great variability occurs in clinical presentation. Despite numerous attempts to portray a stereotype in movies and on television, the stereotypic person with schizophrenia essentially does not exist. Moreover, schizophrenia is not a "split personality." It is a chronic disorder of thought and affect with the individual having a significant disturbance in interpersonal relationships and ability to function in society.

The first psychotic episode can be sudden in onset with few premorbid symptoms, or commonly can be preceded by withdrawn, suspicious, peculiar behavior (schizoid). During acute psychotic episodes, the patient loses touch with reality, and in a sense, the brain creates a false reality to replace it. Acute psychotic symptoms can include hallucinations (especially hearing voices), delusions (fixed false beliefs), and ideas of influence (beliefs that one's actions are controlled by external influences). Thought processes are disconnected (loose associations), the patient may not be able to carry on logical conversation (alogia), and can have simultaneous contradictory thoughts (ambivalence). The patient's affect can be flat (no emotional expression), or it can be inappropriate and labile. The patient is often withdrawn and inwardly directed (autism). Uncooperativeness, hostility, and verbal or physical aggression can be seen because of the patient's misperception of reality. Self-care skills are impaired, and the patient is frequently dirty and unkempt, and in general has poor hygiene. Sleep and appetite are often disturbed. When the acute psychotic episode remits, the patient typically has residual features. This is an important point in differentiating schizophrenia from other psychotic disorders. Although residual symptoms and their severity vary, patients can have difficulty with anxiety management, suspiciousness, and lack of volition, motivation, insight, and judgment. Therefore, they often have difficulty living independently in the community. Because of poor anxiety management and suspiciousness, they are frequently withdrawn socially, and have difficulty forming close relationships with others. In addition, impaired volition and motivation contribute to poor self-care skills and make it difficult for the patient with schizophrenia to maintain employment.

Patients with schizophrenia frequently experience a lack of historicity, or difficulty in learning from their experiences. They can repeatedly make the same mistakes in social conduct and situations requiring judgment. They have difficulty understanding the importance of treatment, including medications, in maintaining their ability to function in society. Therefore, they tend to discontinue medications and other treatments, and this increases the risk of relapse and rehospitalization. The co-occurrence of substance abuse (predominantly alcohol or polysubstance—alcohol, cannabis, and cocaine) in patients with schizophrenia is very common and is another frequent reason for relapse and hospitalization.[1] This effect can be caused by direct toxic effects of these drugs on the brain,[20] but is also caused by the medication nonadherence that is associated with substance abuse. Some drugs of abuse—most notably cannabis—have been associated with a higher prevalence of schizophrenia.[20,21]

Although the course of schizophrenia is variable, the long-term prognosis for many patients is poor. It is marked by intermittent acute

TABLE 67-1 Schizophrenia Symptom Clusters

Positive	Negative	Cognitive
Suspiciousness	Affective flattening	Impaired attention
Unusual thought content (delusions)	Alogia	Impaired working memory
Hallucinations	Anhedonia	Impaired executive function
Conceptual disorganization	Avolition	

Data from references 1, 20, 23, 25.

psychotic episodes and impaired psychosocial functioning between acute episodes, with most of the deterioration in psychosocial functioning occurring within 5 years after the first psychotic episode.[20] By late life, the patient can appear "burned out," that is, the patient ceases to have acute psychotic episodes, but residual symptoms persist. In a subpopulation of patients, probably 5% to 15%, psychotic symptoms are nearly continuous, and response to antipsychotics is poor.[20]

Schizophrenia is a chronic disorder, and the patient's history must be carefully assessed for dysfunction that has persisted for longer than 6 months. After their first episode, patients with schizophrenia rarely have a level of adaptive functioning as high as before the onset of the disorder. The *DSM-5* should be consulted for the complete criteria for a diagnosis of schizophrenia.[1] The DSM-5 also asks the clinician to specify the episode severity for schizophrenia after having the diagnosis for at least 1 year and whether the patient is presenting with catatonia.[1]

2 The *DSM-5* classifies the symptoms of schizophrenia into two categories: positive and negative. Greater emphasis is being placed on a third symptom category, cognitive dysfunction (Table 67-1).[20] The areas of cognition found to be abnormal in schizophrenia include attention, working memory, and executive function. Positive symptoms have traditionally attracted the most attention and are the ones most improved by antipsychotics. However, negative symptoms and impairment in cognition are more closely associated with poor psychosocial function. Along with these characteristic features of schizophrenia, many patients also have comorbid psychiatric and general medical disorders.[20] These include depression, anxiety disorders, substance abuse, and general medical disorders such as respiratory disorders, cardiovascular disorders, and metabolic disturbances. These comorbidities substantially complicate the clinical presentation and course of schizophrenia.

It has been suggested that symptom complexes can correlate with prognosis, cognitive functioning, structural abnormalities in the brain, and response to antipsychotic drugs. Negative symptoms and cognitive impairment can be more closely associated with prefrontal lobe dysfunction and positive symptoms with temporolimbic abnormalities. Many patients demonstrate both positive and negative symptoms. Patients with negative symptoms frequently have more antecedent cognitive dysfunction, poor premorbid adjustment, low level of educational achievement, and a poorer overall prognosis.[20]

TREATMENT

Desired Outcome

Pharmacotherapy is a mainstay of treatment in schizophrenia, and it is impossible to effectively implement psychosocial rehabilitation programs without antipsychotic treatment in the majority of patients.[20] 3 A pharmacotherapeutic treatment plan should be developed that delineates drug-related aspects of therapy. Most deterioration in psychosocial functioning occurs during the first 5 years after the initial psychotic episode, and treatment should be particularly assertive during this period.[20] The individualized treatment plan created for each patient should have explicit end points defined, including realistic goals for the target symptoms most likely to respond, and the relative time course for response.[23] Other desired outcomes include avoiding unwanted side effects (SEs), integrating the patient back into the community, increasing adaptive functioning to the extent possible, and preventing relapse.

Nonpharmacologic Therapy

Psychosocial rehabilitation programs oriented toward improving patients' adaptive functioning are the mainstay of nondrug treatment for schizophrenia. These programs can include case management, psychoeducation, targeted cognitive therapy, basic living skills, social skills training, basic education, work programs, supported housing, and financial support. In particular, programs aimed at employment and housing have been the more effective interventions and are considered "best practices." Programs that involve families in the care and life of the patient have been shown to decrease rehospitalization and improve functioning in the community. For particularly low-functioning patients, assertive intervention programs, referred to as *active community treatment* (ACT), are effective in improving patients' functional outcomes. ACT teams are available on a 24-hour basis and work in the patient's home and place of employment to provide comprehensive treatment, including medication, crisis intervention, daily living skills, and supported employment and housing.[20] Medication treatment cannot be successful without proper attention to these other aspects of care. People with schizophrenia need comprehensive care, with coordination of services across psychiatric, addiction, medical, social, and rehabilitative services. The level of coordination in the United States is often insufficient, and patients become at risk to "fall through the cracks." National policy documents have called for greater coordination of care.[22] Other countries have highlighted more robust primary and secondary preventative approaches, highlighting early identification, ease of access to care, and staging of disease management.[23] The National Institute of Mental Health (NIMH) Recovery After Initial Schizophrenia Episode (RAISE) study found that four core interventions ("personalized medication management, family psychoeducation, resilience-focused individual therapy, and supported employment and education") significantly improved the quality of life over a 24 month period for individuals with early schizophrenia as compared to usual community care.[24]

Emphasis is growing on the role that the patient plays in a recovery-based system of care, where the person's lifetime aspirations and goals become the center of care, rather than symptom reduction being the primary focus. This recovery-based approach recognizes the strengths and resilience of people with schizophrenia.[24] It also acknowledges how people with schizophrenia can be a support to others who are coping with the illness.[24] It is important to frame clinical decision making in the context of a mutual process involving patient and clinician—rather than a unilateral "here's a prescription ... please take these tablets" approach. It is increasingly recognized that cognitive behavioral therapy can help some patients. Computer-based therapies and social media related approaches are emerging to help people with schizophrenia. Cognitive remediation—which uses computer-based cognitive retraining techniques—has been shown to be of benefit (not FDA approved at time of writing).[25] It is probable that social media and mobile technology strategies may be harnessed to improve communications, medication adherence, and potentially detect early warning signs of impending relapse in patients with schizophrenia. A list of psychotherapeutic approaches to the treatment of schizophrenia is given in Table 67-2.

Pharmacologic Therapy

4 The importance of initial accurate diagnostic assessment cannot be overemphasized. A thorough mental status examination (MSE), psychiatric diagnostic interview, physical, and neurologic

TABLE 67-2 Psychotherapeutic Approaches to the Treatment of Schizophrenia

Individual	Group	Cognitive Behavioral
Supportive/counseling Personal therapy Social skills therapies Vocational sheltered employment rehabilitation therapies	Interactive/social	Cognitive behavioral therapy Compliance therapy

Data from references 20, 24, 25, 31.

examination, complete family and social history, and laboratory workup must be performed to confirm the diagnosis and exclude general medical or substance-induced causes of psychosis. Laboratory tests, biologic markers, and commonly available brain imaging techniques do not assist in the diagnosis of schizophrenia or selection of medication. A pretreatment patient workup not only is important in excluding other pathology, but also serves as a baseline for monitoring potential medication-related side effects, and should include vital signs, complete blood count, electrolytes, hepatic function, renal function, electrocardiogram (ECG), fasting serum glucose, hemoglobin A1c, serum lipids, thyroid function, and urine drug screen.

Both first-generation antipsychotics (FGAs) and second-generation antipsychotics (SGAs) are used in the treatment of schizophrenia.[26-28] Since no absolute criterion distinguishes atypical (second-generation) from typical (traditional or FGA) antipsychotics, and no universally accepted definition exists for an atypical antipsychotic. *Second-generation antipsychotic* is a more appropriate term. Common to all definitions is the ability of the drug to produce antipsychotic response with few or no acutely occurring extrapyramidal side effects (EPS). Other attributes that have been ascribed to some SGAs include enhanced efficacy (particularly for negative symptoms and cognition), absence or near absence of propensity to cause tardive dyskinesia, and lack of effect on serum prolactin.[29] To date, the only approved SGA that fulfills all of these criteria is clozapine.[29] The major factor in distinguishing among antipsychotics is adverse effects.[26-29] The major advantage of SGAs is their lower risk of neurologic side effects, particularly effects on movement. However, this is offset by increased risk of metabolic side effects with some SGAs, including weight gain, hyperlipidemias, and diabetes mellitus. (5) Side effect profiles differ among antipsychotics, and this information in combination with individual patient characteristics should be used in deciding which drug to use in an individual patient.

Results from the Clinical Antipsychotic Trials of Intervention Effectiveness (CATIE) study, primarily in patients with chronic schizophrenia, indicate that olanzapine, compared with quetiapine, risperidone, ziprasidone, and the FGA perphenazine, had modest, but not statistically significant, superiority in maintenance therapy with treatment persistence as the primary clinical outcome.[30] However, increased metabolic adverse effects occurred with olanzapine. Another major study of patients early on in their illness also highlights the high rate of cardiometabolic disturbances and the need to tailor treatment early in the course of the illness.[31,32]

No known differences exist in efficacy between low- and high-potency FGAs. Previous patient or family history of response to an antipsychotic is helpful in the selection of an agent. Table 67-3 lists antipsychotics and their usual dosage ranges.

Published Guidelines and an Algorithm Example

(6) Figure 67-1 outlines a suggested pharmacotherapeutic algorithm for schizophrenia. This algorithm is based on information from four evidence-based guidelines, the Psychopharmacology Algorithm Project at the Harvard Medical School Department of Psychiatry, South Shore Program,[27,28] the 2009 update of the practice guideline from the American Psychiatric Association (APA),[33] the 2009 update of the Patient Outcomes Research Team (PORT) guidelines,[26] and the 2012 update of the guidelines from the World Federation of Biological Psychiatry.[29] These sources were augmented with results from recent published clinical trials.

Stage 1A of the treatment algorithm applies to those patients experiencing their first acute episode of schizophrenia. Studies suggest that SGAs result in greater treatment retention and are more effective in preventing a second episode in first episode patients than FGAs. In addition, SGAs carry a reduced risk of EPS.[29] Among the SGAs, only aripiprazole, olanzapine, quetiapine, risperidone, and ziprasidone have evidence of efficacy in first episode patients. Olanzapine is not recommended in first episode because of weight gain and metabolic side effects.[26-29]

Quetiapine is associated with less time to rehospitalization than other compared SGAs and also causes greater weight gain so it is not recommended in Stage 1A. This leaves aripiprazole, risperidone, and ziprasidone as the evidence based options in first episode patients (Stage 1A).[27,28] Of these, aripiprazole and ziprasidone produce the least weight gain. Because of the sensitivity to antipsychotic-induced EPS in first-episode patients, antipsychotic dosing should be initiated at the lower end of the dose range.[39]

A recent study in first episode patients showed that long-acting risperidone injectable was more effective than oral risperidone in preventing relapse over a 1 year period.[34] In fact, the relapse rate was six times higher in the oral risperidone group than with the long-acting injectable. Based upon this study, long-acting risperidone can also be considered a treatment option for first episode patients. If long acting risperidone is going to be used, patients should first be stabilized on oral risperidone. As indicated in the nonpharmacological treatment section, it is critical that enriched psychosocial programs be implemented along with appropriate pharmacotherapy.

Clinical **Controversy...**

Although studies do not demonstrate a difference in acute response rates between SGAs and FGAs in first episode schizophrenia, better patient retention rates and a longer time to second episode are associated with the use of SGAs. While the World Federation of Psychiatry Guidelines and the Harvard guidelines favor the SGAs as first-line antipsychotics, the PORT guidelines offer no preference. All four sets of guidelines recommend not using olanzapine in patients with their first episode of schizophrenia.

Stage 1B addresses pharmacotherapy of a patient who was previously treated with an antipsychotic, and treatment is being restarted because the patient stopped taking the medication. If the patient experienced a robust improvement in symptoms, good tolerability, and the patient is positive about taking the previous antipsychotic, then that medication can be restarted. Otherwise, a medication from Stage 2 should be used. Stage 2 addresses pharmacotherapy in a patient who had inadequate clinical improvement with the antipsychotic used in stage 1A or 1B, or the patient responded but subsequently had a relapse while taking medication. Stage 2 recommends antipsychotic monotherapy with a FGA or SGA not used in Stage 1.[26-29] Because of safety concerns and the need for white blood cell (WBC) monitoring, clozapine is not generally recommended at Stage 2.[26-29] However, clozapine has superior efficacy in decreasing suicidal behavior, and it should be considered at stage 2 for the suicidal patient.[26] Clozapine can also be considered at stage 2 in patients with a history of violence or comorbid substance

TABLE 67-3 Available Antipsychotics and Dosage Ranges

Generic Name	Trade Name	Starting Dose (mg/day)	Usual Dosage Range (mg/day)	Comments
First-Generation Antipsychotics				
Chlorpromazine	Thorazine	50-150	300-1,000	Most weight gain among FGAs
Fluphenazine	Prolixin	5	5-20	
Haloperidol	Haldol	2-5	2-20	Higher dropout rate in first episode
Loxapine	Loxitane	20	50-150	
Loxapine inhaled	Adasuve	10	10	Maximum 10 mg per 24 hours Approved REMS program only
Perphenazine	Trilafon	4-24	16-64	
Thioridazine	Mellaril	50-150	100-800	Significant QTc prolongation
Thiothixene	Navane	4-10	4-50	
Trifluoperazine	Stelazine	2-5	5-40	
Second-Generation Antipsychotics				
Aripiprazole	Abilify	5-15	15-30	
Asenapine	Saphris	5	10-20	Sublingual only, no food or drink for 10 minutes after administration of the dose
Brexpiprazole	Rexulti	1	2-4	
Cariprazine	Vraylar	1.5	1.5-6	Due to long half-life, steady-state is not reached for several weeks
Clozapine	Clozaril	25	100-800	Check plasma level before exceeding 600 mg
Iloperidone	Fanapt	1-2	6-24	Care with dosing in CYP2D6 slow metabolizers
Lurasidone	Latuda	20-40	40-120	Take with food; ≥350 calories (≥1,460 J)
Olanzapine	Zyprexa	5-10	10-20	Avoid in first episode because of weight gain
Paliperidone	Invega	3-6	3-12	Bioavailability increased when administered with food
Quetiapine	Seroquel	50	300-800	
Quetiapine XR	Seroquel XR	300 mg	400-800	
Risperidone	Risperdal	1-2	2-8	
Ziprasidone	Geodon	40	80-160	Take with food, ≥500 calories (≥2,100 J)

Note: In first-episode patients, starting dose and target dose should generally be 50% of the usual dose range. See Long-Acting Injectable Antipsychotics in text for dosing of these agents.

Data from reference 29, 40, 58-60, 63, 69, 116.

abuse.[26] If a patient has unacceptable side effects with the antipsychotic used during Stage 1A, Stage 1B, or Stage 2, then an alternate antipsychotic for that stage should be chosen.

Long acting injectable (LAIs) antipsychotics may be considered at Stage 2. LAIs have been traditionally used in patients with a pattern of poor medication adherence, but it has been suggested that their use may be more successful if used earlier in the course of schizophrenia before patients develop a pattern of nonadherence.[26,29,35]

In stage 3 the recommended treatment is clozapine.[26-29]

In stage 4, only minimal evidence exists for any treatment option for those patients who do not have adequate symptom improvement with clozapine. However, a recent placebo controlled trial showed that ziprasidone 80 mg/day added to clozapine significantly improved negative symptoms and general psychopathology as compared with placebo, and a recent small trial demonstrated efficacy for electroconvulsive therapy (ECT) augmentation of clozapine.[36,37] Additional treatment options that are tried, again with minimal evidence, include mood stabilizer augmentation, and another antipsychotic combined with clozapine.[26,29,38] The use of antipsychotic combinations is controversial, as limited evidence supports increased efficacy for combination antipsychotic treatment.[26,29,38]

Predictors of Response

Obtaining a thorough medication history is important, and previous antipsychotic treatment should help guide the selection of drug therapy, in that either a good prior response favors the use of the same agent or a negative prior response suggests the selection of a dissimilar drug. Nonprescription and illicit drug use can influence psychiatric presentation and thus diagnosis or antipsychotic response. Amphetamines and other CNS stimulants, cocaine, corticosteroids, digitalis glycosides, indomethacin, marijuana, pentazocine, phencyclidine, and other drugs can induce psychosis in susceptible individuals or exacerbate psychosis in patients with preexisting psychiatric illness.[1,20,21,29] Patients with schizophrenia who continue to abuse alcohol or drugs usually have a poor response to medications and a poor prognosis. Alcohol, caffeine, and nicotine use may potentially result in drug interactions with antipsychotics.

Individual differences in patient response have been either proposed or identified, which can be clinically useful predictors of response.[20] Acute onset and short duration of illness, presence of acute stressors or precipitating factors, later age of onset, family history of affective illness, and good premorbid adjustment as reflected in stable interpersonal relationships or employment are all predictors of good response.[20]

Although controversial, affective symptoms can correlate with an overall good response. Negative symptoms and neuropsychological deficits related to cognition and neurologic soft signs can correlate with poor antipsychotic response.[20] A patient's subjective response within the first 48 hours after being administered an FGA can be associated with drug responsiveness.[38] An initial dysphoric response, demonstrated by stating a dislike of the medication, or feeling worse or zombie-like, combined with anxiety or akathisia-like symptoms, is associated with poor drug response, adverse effects, and nonadherence.

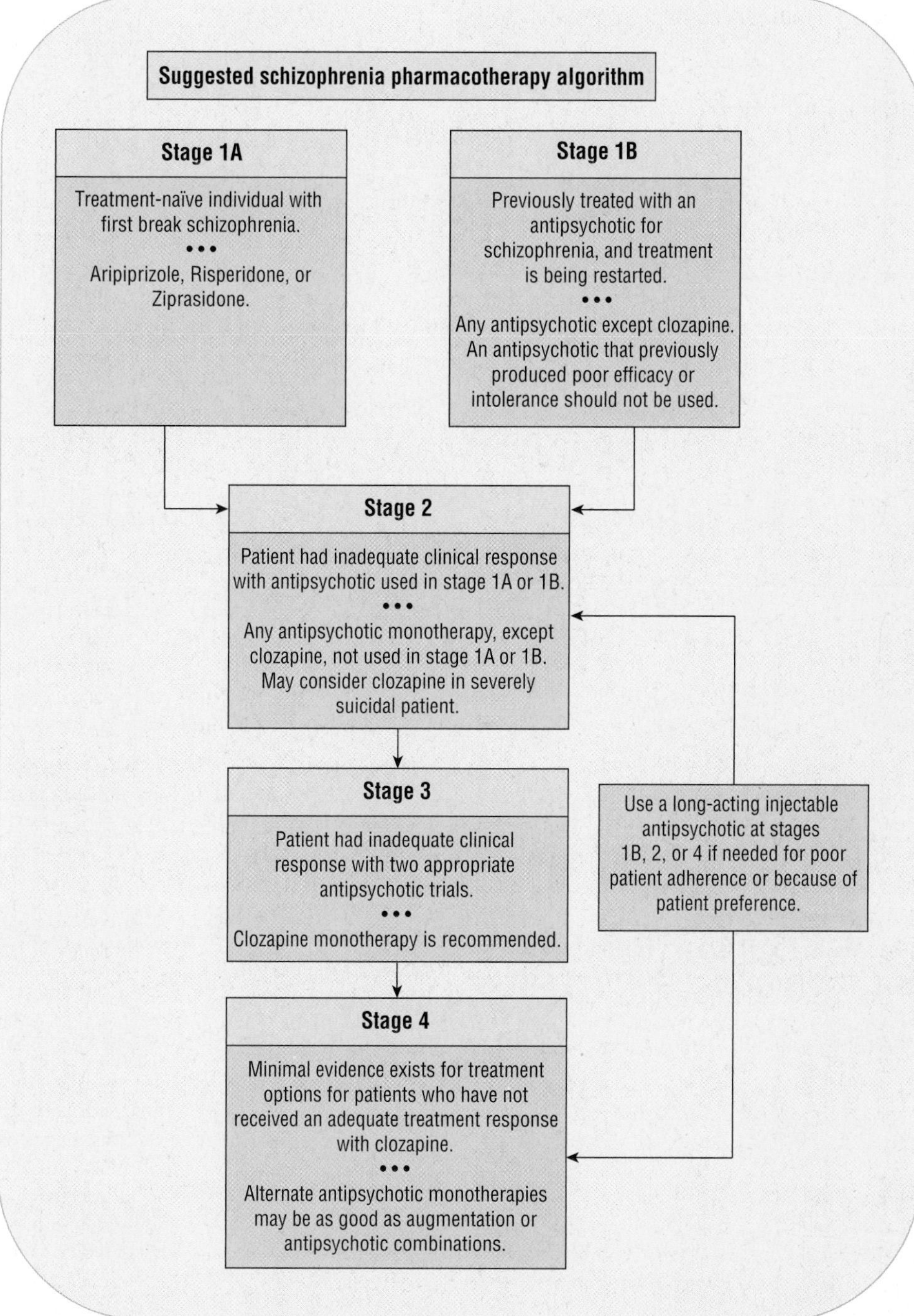

FIGURE 67-1 Suggested pharmacotherapy algorithm for treatment of schizophrenia. Schizophrenia should be treated in the context of an interprofessional model that addresses the psychosocial needs of the patient, necessary psychiatric pharmacotherapy, psychiatric co-occurring mental disorders, treatment adherence, and any medical problems the patient may have. See the text for a description of the algorithm stages. *(Data from references 26-30.)*

The importance of developing a therapeutic alliance between the patient and the clinician cannot be underestimated. Patients who form positive therapeutic alliances are more likely to be adherent with all aspects of therapy, experience a better outcome at 2 years, and require smaller antipsychotic doses.[20]

A certain minority of patients fails to benefit from antipsychotic therapy, and their psychosocial functioning can actually worsen.

Initial Treatment in an Acute Psychotic Episode

The goals during the first 7 days of treatment should be decreased agitation, hostility, combativeness, anxiety, tension, and aggression, and normalization of sleep and eating patterns. The usual recommendation is to initiate therapy and to titrate dose over the first few days to an average effective dose, unless the patient's physiologic status or history indicates that this dose can result in unacceptable adverse effects. Because of its strong alpha one (α_1) receptor antagonism and resulting risk of hypotension, iloperidone and clozapine should be titrated more slowly than other antipsychotics. Table 67-4 lists the usual dosage range, and an average dose is typically midrange. Because of increased sensitivity to side effects, particularly EPS, in first-episode psychotic patients, typical dosing ranges are approximately 50% of the doses used in chronically ill individuals.[26,29] If "cheeking" of medication is suspected, liquid formulations and orally disintegrating tablets of different antipsychotics are available. If a patient has shown absolutely no improvement after 2 weeks at a therapeutic dose then later clinical response is

TABLE 67-4 Summary of Available Long Acting Injectable (LAI) Antipsychotics

Medication Name Parameter	Fluphenazine Decanoate	Haloperidol Decanoate	Risperidone LAI Risperdal Consta	Paliperidone Palmitate		Olanzapine Pamoate Zyprexa Relprevv	Aripiprazole Monohydrate Abilify Maintena	Aripiprazole Lauroxil Aristada
				Invega Sustenna	Invega Trinza			
FDA Approved Indication	Schizophrenia	Schizophrenia	Schizophrenia Bipolar I Disorder maintenance	Schizophrenia Schizoaffective Disorder	Schizophrenia	Schizophrenia	Schizophrenia	Schizophrenia
Dose Range (mg)	12.5-100	20-450	12.5-50	39-234	273-819	150-405	160-400	441-882
PO Overlap	None	4 weeks (none if loading); use PO dose patient was taking prior to injection	3 weeks after first injection Use PO dose patient was taking prior to injection	None	None	None	2 weeks PO dose ranges from 10 to 20 mg/day	21 days PO over lap after first injection
Recommended maximum dose	100 mg every 2-3 weeks	450 mg every 4 weeks	50 mg every 2 weeks	234 mg every 4 weeks	819 mg every 3 months	300 mg every 2 weeks or 405 mg every 4 weeks	400 mg monthly	882 mg monthly
Initiation or Loading	Can Load	Can Load	None	Initiation required	None required, dose used depends on last Invega Sustenna dose as follows: If 78 mg give 273 mg If 117 mg give 410 mg If 156 mg give 546 mg If 234 mg give 819 mg	Initiation required	None	None required, dose depends on PO dose as follows: If 10 mg/day PO give 441 mg per month IM If 15 mg/day PO give 662 mg per month IM If 20 mg PO give 882 mg per month
Time to peak	8-24 hours	4-11 days	4-5 weeks	13 days	30-33 days	<1 week	5-7 days	5-6 days
T_{ss}	2-3 months	2-3 months	6-8 weeks	36 days		3 months	3-4 months	4 mos.
Injection Site Gluteal	Yes	Yes	Yes	Yes after 2nd dose	Yes	Yes	Yes	Yes for all dose strengths
Deltoid	Yes	Yes	Yes	Yes	Yes	No	No	Yes, but only 441 mg dose
Injection Method/Technique		Z-Track				Standard		
Notes			A starting dose of 12.5 mg is recommended in patients with hepatic or renal impairment	Avoid use in patients with moderate to severe renal impairment (CrCl <50 mL/min [<0.83 mL/s])	Requires at least a 4 month trial with Invega Sustenna Not recommended in patients with moderate or severe renal impairment (CrCl <50 mL/min[<0.83 mL/s])	Monitor for PDSS Subject to REMS	Maintenance dose reduced to 300 mg if patient experiences adverse events. Dose adjustment needed in CYP2D6 slow metabolizers. Avoid use in patients taking CYP 3A4 inhibitors >14 days	May require up to 2 weeks of PO trial to establish tolerability to aripiprazole before initiating LAI Avoid use of strong CYP2D6 and 3A4 inhibitors on 662 mg and 882 mg dose, no adjustment needed for 441mg dose

PO, Oral; T_{ss}, Time to steady-state; CrCl, Creatine Clearance; IM, intramuscular; LAI, Long Acting Injectable.

Data from references 29, 34, 41, 42, 45-47.

unlikely, and moving to the next treatment stage in the algorithm is recommended.[20,39]

Clinical **Controversy...**

Minimal research evidence supports the use of antipsychotic doses beyond the dose range in the FDA-approved product labeling. However, clinicians frequently titrate doses above the approved range, and frequently attest to symptom improvement when this is done. It is unclear whether the observed symptom improvement is due to the increased dose, time on the antipsychotic, or just pure chance. If higher than recommended doses are used, treatment should be time limited (eg, 6-12 weeks), and a brief clinical rating scale should be used to monitor for potential change in symptoms.

Although some clinicians believe that larger daily doses are necessary in more severely symptomatic patients, data are not available to support this practice. Some symptoms, such as agitation, tension, aggression, and increased motor activity, may respond more quickly, but side effects can be more common with higher doses. However, interindividual differences in dosage and patient response do occur. In partial but inadequate responders who are tolerating the chosen antipsychotic, it may be reasonable to titrate above usual dose ranges. However, this tactic should be time-limited (ie, 2-4 weeks), and if the patient does not achieve further improvement, either the dose should be decreased or an alternative treatment strategy should be tried. In general, rapid titration of antipsychotic dosage is not indicated.[20,26] However, intramuscular (IM) antipsychotic administration (eg, aripiprazole 5.25-9.75 mg IM, haloperidol 2-5 mg IM, olanzapine 2.5-10 mg IM, or ziprasidone 10-20 mg IM) can be used to assist in calming a severely agitated patient. Agitation can be manifested as loud, physically or verbally threatening behavior, motor hyperactivity, or physical aggression. Although this technique can assist in calming an acutely agitated psychotic patient, it does not improve the extent of remission, or time to remission, or the length of hospitalization. Haloperidol IM for treatment of acute aggression is associated with a higher incidence of EPS than using an injectable SGA. If the patient is receiving an antipsychotic within the usual therapeutic range, the use of lorazepam 2 mg IM as needed in combination with the maintenance antipsychotic is a rational alternative to an injectable antipsychotic. Hypotension, respiratory depression, CNS depression, and death have been reported with injectable lorazepam in combination with either olanzapine or clozapine; thus, parenteral lorazepam is not recommended in combination with either of these antipsychotics.[29,33]

The initial Risk Evaluation and Mitigation Strategy (REMS) for inhaled loxapine powder was approved by the Food and Drug Administration (FDA) with an indication of treatment of acute agitation associated with schizophrenia or bipolar disorder. Because of the risk of bronchospasm, pulmonary distress, and pulmonary arrest, the medication can only be administered in a healthcare facility and through the FDA-approved REMS. Before administration, patients must be screened for a history of asthma, chronic obstructive pulmonary disease, or other lung disease associated with bronchospasm, and use is limited to one 10 mg inhaled dose per 24-hour period.[40] It is not known whether inhaled loxapine offers any therapeutic advantages in acute agitation compared with currently available IM or oral products.

Stabilization Therapy

Improvement is usually a slow but steady process over 6 to 12 weeks or longer. During the first 2 to 3 weeks, goals should include increased socialization and improvement in self-care habits and mood. Improvement in formal thought disorder should follow and can take an additional 6 to 8 weeks to respond. Patients who are early in the course of their illness can experience a more rapid resolution of symptoms than individuals who are more chronically ill. In general, if a patient has shown no improvement after 2 weeks of treatment at therapeutic doses, or has achieved only a partial decrease in positive symptoms within 12 weeks at adequate doses, then the next algorithm stage should be considered. In more chronically ill patients, symptoms may continue to improve over 3 to 6 months. During acute stabilization, usual FDA-labeled doses of SGAs are recommended (see Table 67-4).[26-29] An optimum dose of the chosen drug should be estimated in the initial treatment plan. If the patient begins to show adequate response at a particular dose, then the patient should remain at this dosage as long as symptoms continue to improve. (7) In general, adequate time on a therapeutic antipsychotic dose is the most important factor in predicting medication response. However, if necessary, dose titration can continue within the therapeutic range every 1 or 2 weeks as long as the patient has no side effects.

Before changing medications in a poorly responding patient, the following should be considered: Were the initial target symptoms indicative of schizophrenia or did they represent manifestations of a different diagnosis, a long-standing behavioral problem, a substance abuse disorder, or a general medical condition? Is the patient adherent with pharmacotherapy? Are the persistent symptoms poorly responsive to antipsychotics (eg, impaired insight or judgment, or fixed delusions)? How does the patient's current status compare with response during previous exacerbations? Would this patient potentially benefit from a change to a different treatment stage (Fig. 67-1)? Does this patient have a treatment-resistant schizophrenia?

The conclusion that a partially responding patient has achieved as much symptomatic improvement as possible is one that must be made with great care. Treatment goals must be realistic. Medications are effective at decreasing many of the symptoms of schizophrenia (and are thus referred to as palliative), but they are not curative, and all symptoms may not abate. Although one should aim to achieve none to minimal residual positive symptoms with effective treatment, it is still unclear what a realistic goal is with regard to maximum improvement in negative symptoms.

It is important to screen patients for co-occurring mental disorders, and their presence can become more apparent during the stabilization or maintenance phases of schizophrenia treatment. Examples include substance abuse disorders, depression, obsessive-compulsive disorder, and panic disorder. As co-occurring disorders will limit symptom and functional improvement and increase the risk of relapse, it is critical that treatment for the co-occurring disorder be implemented in combination with evidence-based treatment for schizophrenia.

Maintenance Treatment

Maintenance drug therapy prevents relapse, as shown in numerous double-blind studies. The average relapse rate after 1 year is 18% to 32% with active drug (including some nonadherent patients) versus 60% to 80% for placebo.[26-29] Thus avoiding relapses is a major goal of treatment.[26-29]

After treatment of the first psychotic episode in a patient with schizophrenia, medication should be continued for at least 12 months after remission.[26-29] (8) Many schizophrenia experts recommend that patients with robust medication response be treated for at least 5 years. In chronically ill individuals, continuous or lifetime pharmacotherapy is necessary in the majority of patients to prevent relapse. This should be approached with the lowest effective dose of the antipsychotic that is likely to be tolerated by the patient.[26-29]

Antipsychotics should be tapered slowly before discontinuation. Abrupt discontinuation of antipsychotics, especially clozapine, can result in withdrawal symptoms, felt to be a manifestation of rebound cholinergic outflow. Insomnia, nightmares, headaches, GI symptoms (eg, abdominal cramps, stomach pain, nausea, vomiting, and diarrhea), restlessness, increased salivation, and sweating are reported. Although available evidence does not indicate a best way to switch from one antipsychotic to another, it is often recommended to taper and discontinue the first antipsychotic over at least 1 to 2 weeks while the second antipsychotic is initiated and the dose titrated.[29] Tapering needs to occur more slowly with clozapine.[29]

Long-Acting Injectable Antipsychotics

Traditionally, long-acting antipsychotics have been primarily used for patients who are unreliable in taking oral medication on a daily basis. More recently, it has been suggested to offer LAIs to patients as a treatment option earlier in treatment before they develop a pattern of nonadherence.[35] As indicated earlier, one study showed LAI risperidone to be more effective in preventing relapse in patients with their first episode of schizophrenia.[34]

Before declaring a patient nonadherent, it should be determined whether the patient's medication nonadherence is because of side effects. If so, an alternative medication with a more favorable side effect profile should be considered before a long-acting injectable antipsychotic. The patient's motivation for treatment is a major factor influencing outcome. Conversion from oral therapy to a long-acting injectable is most successful in patients who have been stabilized on oral therapy.

Paliperidone palmitate is a long-acting injectable (LAI) that has the advantage of once-monthly injections and easy conversion from oral to IM treatment.[41] Similarly, aripiprazole monohydrate and aripiprazole lauroxil LAI are once monthly injections that require 2 and 3 weeks of oral antipsychotic overlap respectively.

Olanzapine pamoate monohydrate is a LAI administered every 2 or 4 weeks. It is associated with a postinjection delirium/sedation syndrome (PDSS) occurring in approximately 2% of patients.[42] The symptoms of PDSS are similar to those of an oral olanzapine overdose and include delirium like symptoms, sedation, as well as changes in level of consciousness. Delirium is the most commonly reported symptom in PDSS cases. The risk of occurrence does not appear related to dose or duration of treatment. One hypothesis is that its occurrence may be associated with accidental entry of the drug into the bloodstream.[42] In 2013, the FDA issued a warning regarding sudden death of two patients who received olanzapine LAI.[43] A follow up to this report indicated that the cause of the sudden deaths was inconclusive.[44] The product labeling contains an FDA boxed warning regarding PDSS. Olanzapine pamoate is subject to REMS, and the FDA labeling limits the availability of olanzapine LAI to a restricted distribution program. The injection must be administered in a registered healthcare facility, and the patient must be observed by a health professional for at least 3 hours after administration and must not drive or operate machinery for that day.[42]

Conversion from an oral antipsychotic to a LAI medication should start with stabilization on an oral dosage form of the same agent, for a short trial (3-7 days), to determine whether the patient tolerates the medication without significant side effects. With long-acting risperidone, measurable serum concentrations are not seen until approximately 3 weeks after single-dose administration. Thus, it is important that the oral antipsychotic be administered for at least 3 weeks after beginning the injections. Dose adjustments are recommended to be made no more often than once every 4 weeks.[45] The recommended starting dose with risperidone LAI is 25 mg, and clinical experience suggests that titration to doses greater than or equal to 37.5 mg per injection may be necessary for maintenance treatment. Long-acting risperidone has demonstrated efficacy, with an optimal dose range between 25 and 50 mg given IM every 2 weeks. Doses above 50 mg every 2 weeks are not recommended, as research indicates no greater clinical efficacy but more EPS.[45]

Paliperidone palmitate (Invega Sustenna) can be injected into either the deltoid or the gluteal muscle, and treatment is initiated with 234 mg on day 1 and 156 mg a week later. No overlap with oral drug is necessary. Monthly IM doses are then titrated according to response within a range of 39 to 234 mg.[41] A 3 month formulation of paliperidone palmitate (Invega Trinza) is approved for the management of schizophrenia and significantly delays time to relapse compared with placebo. This 3 month formulation provides the longest dosing interval currently available but requires patients to be treated for at least 4 months with Invega Sustenna prior to its initiation. The first Invega Trinza dose is based on the previous 1 month injection dose as shown in Table 67-5.[45] Olanzapine pamoate monohydrate is recommended for deep gluteal injection, and the initial injectable dose varies from 210 to 405 mg depending on the oral olanzapine daily maintenance dose and the frequency of injectable administration. The official product information should be consulted regarding preparation and administration information.[41,42]

Aripiprazole monohydrate LAI is administered as a single intramuscular injection in the gluteal or deltoid muscle once a month at a starting and maintenance dose of 400 mg. If the patient does not tolerate the 400 mg dose, the next injection can be reduced to 300 mg. After the first injection of aripiprazole monohydrate LAI, a 14 day overlap with oral aripiprazole (10-20 mg/day) or any other antipsychotic is recommended.[41] Aripiprazole lauroxil LAI is administered as a single intramuscular injection in the deltoid (441 mg dose only) or gluteal (441 mg, 662 mg, or 882 mg, once a month). The 882 mg dose can be administered every 6 weeks however. As mentioned earlier, oral overlap is needed for 3 weeks with this LAI formulation.[46]

For fluphenazine decanoate, the simplest dosing conversion method recommends 1.2 times the oral fluphenazine daily dose for stabilized patients, rounding up to the nearest 12.5-mg interval, administered in weekly doses for the first 4 to 6 weeks; or 1.6 times the oral daily dose for more acutely ill patients.[47] Subsequently, fluphenazine decanoate can be administered once every 2 to 3 weeks. Oral fluphenazine can be overlapped for 1 week. Fluphenazine decanoate can be administered subcutaneously, though it is usually administered by intramuscular injection in the deltoid or gluteal muscle.[41] For haloperidol decanoate, the first dose should be 10 to 20 times the oral haloperidol daily dose, and the maintenance dose is typically 10 to 15 times the oral dose once monthly. The initial injection is limited to 100 mg followed by the remaining balance of the first monthly dose given 3 to 7 days later.[41] An oral haloperidol overlap is recommended for the first month. Table 67-4 provides a summary of LAIs discussed in this chapter.

Methods to Enhance Patient Adherence

It is often challenging for individuals with chronic illnesses to maintain appropriate medication adherence, and partial adherence is a reality in the treatment of all chronic illnesses.[29] Individuals with serious mental disorders have somewhat higher nonadherence rates than those with general medical disorders, with the following explanations provided: denial of illness, lack of insight, grandiosity or paranoia, no perceived need for medication, perceived lack of input into choice of medication or dosage, side effects, misperceived "allergies," too many medications prescribed, or too many doses prescribed daily. It is estimated that half of patients with schizophrenia or schizoaffective disorder take their medication less than 70% of the time.[29] Clinicians should expect partial medication adherence to be the norm. This should be approached in a positive, nonjudgmental manner, with the clinician actively engaging the patient in care and using motivational interviewing techniques as mechanisms to enhance therapeutic alliance and patient adherence.

Numerous different methods have been used in an attempt to improve treatment adherence of patients with schizophrenia. Interventions that provide continuous focus on adherence and that are of long duration have shown benefit. These should incorporate problem solving techniques and be accompanied by technical learning aids. It has been suggested that programs need to include a focus on patient-driven outcomes, and not just medication adherence.

TABLE 67-5 Pharmacokinetic Parameters of Selected Antipsychotics

Drug	Bioavailability (%)	Half-Life	Major Metabolic Pathways	Active Metabolites
Selected First-Generation Antipsychotics (FGAs)				
Chlorpromazine	10-30	8-35 hours	FMO3, CYP3A4	7-Hydroxy, others
Fluphenazine	20-50	14-24 hours	CYP2D6	?
Fluphenazine decanoate		14.2 ± 2.2[a] days	CYP2D6	
Haloperidol	40-70	12-36 hours	CYP1A2, CYP2D6, CYP3A4	Reduced haloperidol
Haloperidol decanoate		21 days	CYP1A2, CYP2D6, CYP3A4	Reduced haloperidol
Perphenazine	20-25	8.1-12.3 hours	CYP2D6	7-OH-perphenazine
Second-Generation Antipsychotics (SGAs)				
Aripiprazole	87	48-68 hours	CYP2D6, CYP3A4	Dehydroaripiprazole
Aripiprazole Lauroxil		29.2-34.9 days	CYP2D6. CYP3A4	Dehydroaripiprazole
Aripiprazole Monohydrate		29.9-46.5 days	CYP2D6, CYP3A4	Dehydro-aripiprazole
Asenapine	<2 orally 35 SL Nonlinear	13-39 hours	UGT1A4, CYP1A2	None known
Brexpiprazole	95	91 hours	CYP2D6, CYP3A4	DM-3411
Cariprazine		2-4 days, DDCAR 1-3 weeks	CYP2D6, CYP3A4	Desmethyl cariprazine [DCAR], Didesmethyl cariprazine [DDCAR]
Clozapine	12-81	11-105 hours	CYP1A2, CYP3A4, CYP2C19	Desmethylclozapine
Iloperidone	96	18-33 hours	CYP2D6, CYP3A4	P88
Lurasidone	10-20	18 hours	CYP3A4	ID-14233 and ID-14326
Olanzapine	80	20-70 hours	CYP1A2, CYP3A4, FMO3	*N*-Glucuronide; 2-OH-methyl; 4-*N*-oxide
Olanzapine LAI		30 days	CYP1A2, CYP3A4, FMO3	*N*-Glucuronide; 2-OH-methyl; 4-*N*-oxide
Paliperidone ER	28	23 hours	Renal unchanged (59%) CYP3A4 and multiple pathways	None known
Paliperidone palmitate		25-49 days	Renal unchanged (59%) CYP3A4 and multiple pathways	None known
Paliperidone Palmitate ER		84-89 days (deltoid) 118-139 days (gluteal)	Renal unchanged (59%) CYP3A4 and multiple pathways	None known
Quetiapine	9 ± 4	6.88 hours	CYP3A4	N-desalkylquetiapine
Quetiapine XR		7 hours	CYP3A4	N-desalkylquetiapine
Risperidone	68	3-24 hours	CYP2D6	9-OH-risperidone
Risperidone Consta		3-6 days	CYP2D6	9-OH-risperidone
Ziprasidone	59	4-10 hours	Aldehyde oxidase, CYP3A4	None

UGT, UDP glucuronosyltransferases genes; FMO3, flavin containing monooxygenase 3 gene; SL, sublingual.

[a]Based on multiple-dose data. Single-dose data indicate a β-half-life of 6-10 days.

Data from references 40-42, 45-47, 58-61, 63-64, 69, 116, 130.

For example, interventions should include efforts to allow patients to achieve life goals and function. This requires that programs be tailored to the needs of individual patients.[48] Psychoeducation strategies should include motivational interviewing techniques in individual counseling as well as group activities. 9

Some studies suggest that compliance therapy, targeted cognitive behavioral therapy focusing on medication adherence, can improve patient adherence, but the success seen in early studies has not been consistently replicated.[48]

Groups facilitated by trained individuals who have the illness are alleged to be more effective in enhancing awareness and acceptance of schizophrenia and necessary treatment than groups led only by professionals. Active involvement of family members further increases the likelihood of patient adherence with treatment. In addition to programs provided by community mental health centers, support groups operated by consumer groups such as the National Alliance on Mental Illness (NAMI) are available in most urban areas. In the hospital, self-medication administration can reinforce the patient's perception of his or her active role in treatment. When patients miss outpatient appointments, active outreach interventions must be implemented to enhance patient engagement in treatment.[48]

Management of Treatment-Resistant Schizophrenia

In general, "treatment resistant" describes a patient who has had inadequate symptom response from multiple antipsychotic trials.[26-29] Traditionally, treatment resistance has been defined as lack of improvement in positive symptoms, but it can be defined by poor improvement in negative symptoms, or even by medication intolerance. Between 10% and 30% of patients receive minimal symptomatic improvement after multiple FGA monotherapy trials.[26-29] An additional 30% to 60% of patients have partial but inadequate improvement in symptoms or unacceptable side effects associated with antipsychotic use.[26-29] In those patients failing two or more pharmacotherapy trials, a treatment-refractory evaluation should be performed to reexamine diagnosis, substance abuse, medication adherence, and psychosocial stressors. Targeted cognitive behavioral therapy or other psychosocial augmentation strategies should be considered.[29]

Clozapine Only clozapine has shown superiority over other antipsychotics in randomized clinical trials for the management of treatment-resistant schizophrenia. Most other SGAs have either not been studied in treatment-refractory patients or have been evaluated in small open trials. In a seminal study, clozapine was effective in approximately 30% of patients with treatment-resistant schizophrenia, compared with only 4% treated with a combination of chlorpromazine and benztropine.[49] The definition of treatment resistance requires two treatment failures with either FGAs or SGAs. Other treatment candidates for clozapine include those patients with severe suicidality, aggressive behavior, or those who cannot tolerate neurologic side effects of even conservative doses of other antipsychotics.

Clinical **Controversy...**

Although clozapine is the only treatment that has evidence of proven benefit in patients with treatment-resistant schizophrenia, and its use in treatment-resistant schizophrenia is recommended in all treatment guidelines, it is underutilized by clinicians in practice. Although the reasons for its underutilization are not totally understood, factors may include clinician fear of clozapine's potential adverse effects, the Absolute Neutrophil Count (ANC) monitoring required by the FDA, and mental health treatment systems that do not support use of the drug and the required ANC monitoring.

Symptomatic improvement with clozapine in the treatment-resistant patient often occurs slowly, and as many as 60% of patients may improve if clozapine is used for up to 6 months. This, in combination with clozapine's adverse effect profile, provides sufficient information to conclude that clozapine is not a panacea for schizophrenia. Polydipsia and hyponatremia (psychogenic water drinking) is a frequent problem among treatment-resistant patients, and clozapine reportedly decreases water drinking and increases serum sodium in such patients.[27,29]

Because of the risk of orthostatic hypotension, clozapine is usually titrated more slowly than other antipsychotics, particularly on an outpatient basis. If a 12.5-mg test dose does not produce hypotension, then clozapine 25 mg at bedtime is recommended, increased to 25 mg twice a day after 3 days, and then increased in 25 to 50 mg/day increments every 3 days until a dose of at least 300 mg/day is reached. Because high doses are associated with significantly increased side effects, including seizures, a clozapine serum concentration is recommended before exceeding 600 mg/day. If the clozapine serum concentration is less than 350 ng/mL (mcg/L; 1.07 μmol/L), then the dose should be increased as side effects allow, to achieve this serum concentration.[29]

Augmentation and Combination Strategies Little empirical evidence exists to guide treatment decisions for patients who do not respond to clozapine.[26,29] Augmentation therapy involves the addition of a nonantipsychotic drug to an antipsychotic drug in a poorly or partially responsive patient, whereas combination treatment involves using two antipsychotics simultaneously.

In a small, single blind, randomized trial, 50% of patients demonstrated clinically significant improvement in symptoms with ECT augmentation of clozapine, compared with no responders in the clozapine monotherapy group. When the patients in the clozapine monotherapy group received ECT, 47% demonstrated clinically significant improvement.[37]

Mood stabilizers are frequently used as an augmentation strategy. Lithium does not enhance antipsychotic effect but may improve labile affect and agitated behavior in selected patients.[27-28] Valproic acid and carbamazepine have also been used. A large placebo-controlled trial supports faster symptom improvement, but no difference in maintenance treatment, when divalproex was used in combination with either olanzapine or risperidone.[50] Enzyme induction with carbamazepine can cause a decrease in antipsychotic serum concentrations and potentially worsen psychotic symptoms in some patients.[29] The 2009 PORT recommendations do not endorse the use of mood stabilizer augmentation in treatment-resistant patients.[26]

Only limited data are available to support antidepressant augmentation of antipsychotics.[29] Consistently positive results have been reported when using selective serotonin reuptake inhibitors (SSRIs) to treat obsessive-compulsive symptoms that worsen or arise during clozapine treatment.

Combining an FGA with an SGA and combining different SGAs have been suggested as intervention strategies for treatment-resistant patients. Pharmacodynamically, there is limited rationale to explain how combinations of antipsychotics would produce enhanced efficacy, but increased side effects, particularly increased EPS, metabolic effects, and hyperprolactinemia, are possible results.[51] Clinically, scant evidence exists to prove that antipsychotic combinations are superior to monotherapy, and the 2009 PORT recommendations do not support their use.[26] However, a recent placebo controlled trial indicated that ziprasidone added to clozapine improved negative symptoms and general psychopathology.[36] This topic remains highly contentious, and clinicians' practice is not aligned with available evidence. In general, a series of antipsychotic monotherapies, including clozapine, are preferred over antipsychotic combinations,[26] and it is observed that clozapine is itself associated with lower rates of polypharmacy over time.[52] However, when clozapine fails to produce desired outcomes, a time-limited combination trial is sometimes considered.[27,29] Such antipsychotic combination treatment trials should be time-limited (eg, maximum 12 weeks) and the patient carefully evaluated with rating scales for changes in symptomatology. If no apparent improvement is observed, then one of the medications should be tapered and discontinued. However, if the patient has a partial response (greater than or equal to 20% improvement in positive symptoms) after 12 weeks with combination treatment, medications should be titrated to doses at the upper end of the therapeutic range, and treatment should continue for an additional 12 weeks before a change in treatment is considered.

Clinical **Controversy...**

Insufficient evidence exists to support the routine use of antipsychotic combination treatment, and guidelines such as PORT do not recommend this practice, even in patients with treatment-resistant schizophrenia. However, a recent small placebo controlled trial showed improvement in negative and general psychopathology when ziprasidone was added to clozapine. A small recent, single blinded study found improvement when ECT was added to clozapine. Although we have insufficient evidence regarding the treatment of patients who are clozapine nonresponders, a few positive studies are beginning to emerge. Clinical guidelines may lag behind the current research, and busy clinicians are often unable to keep up with the current biomedical literature. In difficult to treat patients, clinicians must weigh the evidence from available guidelines versus the need to treat seriously ill patients with treatment resistant illnesses.

Violence in Schizophrenia

Most patients with schizophrenia do not exhibit violent behavior—perhaps this is even surprising given the severity and stress of hearing voices, being paranoid, etc. That said, patients with schizophrenia are more likely to be violent than the general population. Risk factors for violence include those associated with violence in the general population (eg, childhood trauma and exposure to violence, alcohol and substance abuse, psychopathy, and access to firearms) and (to some lesser extent) psychotic symptoms.[53] Results from a meta-analysis indicate that most of the risk of violence is associated with co-occurring substance abuse.[54] Patients are at risk to become violent when they relapse and so keeping patients with schizophrenia clinically stable is a major consideration. Some states even have outpatient commitment laws where patients at risk of violence are "forced" to get ongoing care, and if they default, they are sent back to the hospital. Patients who are really dangerous are invariably contained either in the legal system itself or legally as "forensic" patients where they are held by court order in a psychiatric facility.

Antipsychotic Mechanism of Action

The exact mechanism of action of antipsychotics is unknown. It has been suggested that antipsychotics be classified into three different categories: (a) typical or traditional (high D_2 antagonism and low serotonin-2 receptor [5-HT_{2A}] antagonism); (b) atypical (moderate to high D_2 antagonism and high 5-HT_{2A} antagonism); and (c) atypical clozapine-like (low D_2 antagonism and high 5-HT_{2A} antagonism).[55] With the exception of aripiprazole and brexipiprazole, all current SGAs have a greater affinity for 5-HT_{2A} receptors than D_2 receptors, and brexipiprazole shows stronger antagonism of the 5-HT_{2A} receptor than aripiprazole.[55,56] Brexipiprazole also demonstrates higher affinity for the serotonin-1A (5-HT_{1A}) receptor compared to aripiprazole but with less intrinsic D_2 activity than aripiprazole.[56]

Prospective studies of antipsychotic receptor binding in humans have used PET scans to examine neurotransmitter receptor binding at steady state, 12 hours postdose in small numbers of individuals. It has been proposed that at least 60% to 65% D_2 receptor occupation is necessary to decrease positive psychotic symptoms, whereas blockade of approximately 77% or more of D_2 receptors is associated with EPS.[55] FGAs are DA receptor antagonists with high affinity for D_2 receptors. During chronic treatment with these agents, between 70% and 90% of D_2 receptors in the striatum are usually occupied. In contrast, during clozapine treatment only 38% to 47% of D_2 receptors are occupied, even with high doses. Newer SGAs have variable D_2 binding. With low-dose risperidone (2-5 mg/day), D_2 binding ranges from 60% to 79%, but with doses greater than 6 mg daily, binding commonly exceeds the 77% threshold associated with the development of EPS. Risperidone 2 mg/day produces 5-HT_{2A} binding greater than 70%, and with 4 mg/day it is nearly 100%.[55,57] Olanzapine 10 to 20 mg/day produces D_2 binding ranging from 71% to 80%, whereas at 30 to 40 mg/day, it ranges from 83% to 88%. At 5 mg/day, 5-HT_{2A} receptors are near saturation of binding.[55,57] Ziprasidone has the highest 5-HT_{2A}-to-D_2 affinity ratio of any of the currently available antipsychotics. It is also a potent serotonin-1A (5-HT_{1A}) agonist.[55]

Quetiapine has the lowest D_2 binding. At doses of 300 to 600 mg/day, 12-hour post dose D_2 binding ranges from 0% to 27%. Even at quetiapine 800 mg/day, only 30% of D_2 receptors are occupied. At these same daily doses, 45% to 90% of 5-HT_{2A} receptors are occupied. However, when quetiapine D_2 binding is examined 2 to 3 hours postdose, 58% and 64% of receptors were occupied with 400 and 450 mg, respectively. Transient blockade of DA receptors may be adequate to produce antipsychotic effect, but long-term D_2 blockade is required for production of EPS and sustained hyperprolactinemia. Low D_2 binding, and thus atypicality, can be directly associated with how rapidly the antipsychotic disassociates from the D_2 receptor.[55,57] Aripiprazole and brexpiprazole, partial agonists at D_2 receptors, represent a further elaboration of the DA hypothesis of antipsychotic action.[55,56]

Iloperidone has high affinity for D_2, dopamine-3 (D_3), and 5-HT_{2A} receptors, and moderate affinity for dopamine-4 (D_4), serotonin-6 (5-HT_6), serotonin-7 (5-HT_7), and α_1-receptors.[58] Asenapine has high affinity for 5-HT_{2A} and D_2 receptors as well as for α_1- and histamine-1 receptors. D_2 occupancy of approximately 80% is predicted to occur with a sublingual dose of 5 to 10 mg twice daily.[59] Cariprazine has high affinity for D_2 and D_3 receptors as a partial agonist, with the D_3 potency being significantly greater than D_2. It is also a partial agonist at 5-HT_{1A} receptors and an antagonist at serotonin-1B (5-HT_{1B}) receptors.[60] It is clear that the SGAs differ in their mechanisms of action and most likely in the manner in which they produce an atypical clinical profile.

The primary therapeutic effects of antipsychotics are thought to occur in the limbic system, including the ventral striatum, whereas EPS are thought to be related to DA blockade in the dorsal striatum. 5-HT_{2A} antagonism in combination with modest D_2 blockade leads to release of DA in the prefrontal cortex, and this is one explanation for the decrease in negative symptoms and improvement in cognition reported with atypical antipsychotics.[55]

Antipsychotics vary in their effects on other neurotransmitter receptor systems.[55] Although the significance of these different mechanisms on efficacy is unclear, they do potentially explain differences in side effect profiles. These differences in pharmacodynamic profiles point out that the SGAs are not all alike, and patients obtaining an inadequate clinical response (either efficacy or side effects) with one antipsychotic may have a superior response on an alternate drug. Thus, serial SGA monotherapy trials should be tried in patients receiving a suboptimal clinical response (see Fig. 67-1).

Pharmacokinetics

As a class, antipsychotics are highly lipophilic and highly bound to membranes and plasma proteins. They distribute readily into most tissues with a high blood supply and can accumulate in tissues; therefore, they have large volumes of distribution.[61] Most antipsychotics are largely metabolized, primarily through the cytochrome P450 (CYP) pathways in the liver, except for ziprasidone, which is largely metabolized by aldehyde oxidase. Fluphenazine, perphenazine, and risperidone are metabolized through CYP2D6, and thus are susceptible to polymorphic metabolism.[62] This is also one of the major pathways for the metabolism of aripiprazole, brexpiprazole and iloperidone.[58,63] Thirty to 35% of Africans and Asians are slow to intermediate metabolizers. Approximately 0% to 5% of African Americans, 1% of Asians, and 5% to 10% of whites are poor metabolizers.[62,64] In addition, some people of Swedish descent and up to 30% of those from Northern Africa may be ultrarapid metabolizers.[64] Polymorphisms in CYP1A2 can potentially result in a decrease in the metabolic rate of clozapine, and increased clozapine metabolic rate in smokers has been linked to a specific genotype.[62] The possibility of genetic polymorphism should be considered when dosing and monitoring the clinical effects of antipsychotics.[62,65] Table 67-5 outlines the prominent metabolic pathways of selected antipsychotics.

Asenapine is unique in that it has less than 2% bioavailability after oral administration, but has a bioavailability of approximately 35% sublingually—the FDA-approved route of administration. Eating and drinking within 10 minutes after sublingual administration will reduce bioavailability, and bioavailability decreases with single doses above 10 mg.[59,64]

Most antipsychotics have fairly long elimination half-lives, generally 24 hours or more, with the exception of quetiapine and ziprasidone, which have short half-lives.[61,64] Among the SGAs, only clozapine has an established therapeutic serum concentration, with efficacy being associated with a clozapine plasma concentration greater than 350 ng/mL (mcg/L; 1.07 μmol/L).[61] Whether a potential maximum therapeutic clozapine serum concentration exists is unknown. Clozapine serum concentration should be obtained before exceeding 600 mg daily, in patients who develop unusual or severe adverse side effects, in patients who are taking concomitant medications that can cause drug interactions, in patients who have age or pathophysiologic changes suggesting a change in pharmacokinetics, or for assessment of patient adherence.[61,64]

Adverse Effects

Table 67-6 presents the relative incidence of common categories of antipsychotic side effects. Side effects are discussed below with respect to organ system affected. A general approach to monitoring and assessing side effects requires prospective monitoring by

TABLE 67-6 Relative Side Effect Incidence of Commonly Used Antipsychotics[a,b]

	Sedation	EPS	Anticholinergic	Orthostasis	Weight Gain	Prolactin
Aripiprazole	+	+	+	+	+	+
Asenapine	+	++	±	++	+	+
Brexpiprazole	+	+	+	+	+	+
Chlorpromazine	++++	+++	+++	++++	++	+++
Clozapine	++++	+	++++	++++	++++	+
Fluphenazine	+	++++	+	+	+	++++
Haloperidol	+	++++	+	+	+	++++
Iloperidone	+	±	++	+++	++	+
Lurasidone	+	+	+	+	±	±
Olanzapine	++	++	++	++	++++	+
Paliperidone	+	++	+	++	++	++++
Perphenazine	++	++++	++	+	+	++++
Quetiapine	++	+	+	++	++	+
Risperidone	+	++	+	++	++	++++
Thioridazine	++++	+++	++++	++++	+	+++
Thiothixene	+	++++	+	+	+	++++
Ziprasidone	++	++	+	+	+	+

EPS, extrapyramidal side effects. Relative side effect risk: ±, negligible; +, low; ++, moderate; +++, moderately high; ++++, high.

[a]Side effects shown are relative risk based on doses within the recommended therapeutic range.

[b]Individual patient risk varies depending on patient-specific factors.

clinicians, preferably using a thorough review of systems approach. Patient-oriented self-rated side effect scales can be helpful, as many patients with schizophrenia do not readily complain of side effects.

With the variety of antipsychotics available, using an alternative antipsychotic should be considered in patients who complain of poorly tolerated side effects. Because medication side effects are one of the primary predictors of patient nonadherence, the clinician should take advantage of the treatment options currently available in an attempt to improve patient outcomes. As we learn more about relative side effect risks (eg, weight gain, glucose intolerance, QTc prolongation, acute EPS, and tardive dyskinesia), it will be necessary to regularly reconsider which antipsychotics should be considered first-line treatment alternatives.

Endocrine System DA blockade in the tuberoinfundibular tract results in increased prolactin levels as DA is the major prolactin-inhibiting factor. Hyperprolactinemia may occur in up to 71% of patients diagnosed with schizophrenia and treated with FGAs or SGA. US based studies show no gender difference in incidence of antipsychotic induced hyperprolactinemia, however UK based studies suggest women are twice as likely to experience antipsychotic induced hyperprolactinemia than men (52% vs 26% respectively).[66,67] The major side effects associated with hyperprolactinemia are gynecomastia, galactorrhea, menstrual irregularities, decreased libido, and sexual dysfunction. Although the clinical significance is unclear, chronic hyperprolactinemia has been associated with decreased bone mineral density.[68] Tolerance does not appear to develop to antipsychotic-induced hyperprolactinemia. Newer antipsychotics including asenapine, iloperidone, and lurasidone have not been shown to induce clinically meaningful changes in prolactin levels.[58,59,69] Switching to an SGA that has minimal sustained effect on prolactin is a reasonable treatment option. A recent meta-analysis suggests that augmentation with aripiprazole 5 to 30 mg daily may help reduce risperidone induced hyperprolactinemia.[70]

Weight gain is frequently reported in both adults and children receiving antipsychotics.[71] Although the exact mechanism is uncertain, weight gain has been associated with antihistaminic effects, antimuscarinic effects, and blockade of 5-HT_{2C} receptors including 5-HT_{2C} receptor polymorphism. However, dietary factors and activity levels can play a significant role in this population, as well as re-nourishment after a period of poor self-care. In particular, significant weight gain, defined by the FDA as greater than or equal to 7% of the baseline body weight, after 1 year of treatment has been seen in as many as 80% of patients treated with olanzapine, 58% treated with risperidone, 50% treated with quetiapine, and 21% treated with iloperidone.[58,72] The risk of weight gain may be greater in patients with their first psychotic episode. A recent meta-analysis evaluating antipsychotic induced weight changes in first episode psychosis showed an overall clinically significant increase in weight and body mass index (BMI) in short and long term use of antipsychotics compared with placebo. In the same meta-analysis, olanzapine, and clozapine were associated with the greatest weight changes over time, while ziprasidone showed no clinically significant weight changes. Ziprasidone and aripiprazole, as well as newer agents asenapine and lurasidone, are associated with minimal weight gain.[59,69]

The risk of cardiovascular-related mortality is higher in individuals with schizophrenia,[72,74] and this is further aggravated by drug-related weight gain and the high prevalence of smoking. Additionally, obesity is a risk factor for diabetes mellitus.[71] Weight gain during treatment is concerning for patients and a major reason for poor medication adherence.[75]

Several different genetic variations have been correlated with predisposition for antipsychotic-associated weight gain. A meta-analysis of all genetic studies looking at the −759 C/T promoter region polymorphism of the *5-HT_{2C}* receptor gene confirmed an association of 5-HT_{2C} in antipsychotic-induced weight gain.[76] Polymorphisms in leptin and leptin receptor genes have also been linked with clozapine- and olanzapine-associated weight gain.[77] Alpha-2a-adrenergic receptor gene, G protein β_3 subunit gene, melanocortin-4-receptor (*MC4R*), methylenetetrahydrofolate reductase (*MTHFR*) and brain-derived neurotrophic factor (*BDNF*) gene have been genetic targets; however, results are inconsistent as to whether a relationship exists with these polymorphisms and antipsychotic-associated weight gain.[77,78]

Several approaches have been recommended to address weight gain. Stroup et al. have shown that switching the antipsychotic to another agent with less weight gain liability is one choice.[79] Metformin has been shown to be effective in treating antipsychotic induced weight gain with a meta-analysis indicating an average of a 3.17 kg weight loss compared with placebo.[80] Dietary restriction, exercise, and behavior modification programs are reported to be successful. Both the Reducing Weight and Diabetes Risk in an Underserved Population (STRIDE) and the Randomized Trial of Achieving Healthy Lifestyles in Psychiatric Rehabilitation (ACHIEVE) clinical trials showed behavioral weight loss interventions resulted in significant weight loss in patients with mental illness receiving antipsychotics. The STRIDE study also showed reductions in fasting glucose over 6 and 12 month periods using such interventions.[78,81,82] An American Diabetes Association consensus task force recommends consideration of a change in antipsychotic if a patient gains more than 5% of baseline body weight after starting the drug.[83]

Clinical **Controversy...**

Although weight gain with antipsychotics is a major challenge in psychiatry, no clear consensus currently exists regarding how to address weight gain in these patients. Medications such as metformin have been shown to decrease weight in patients taking SGAs, and studies have shown that multipronged behavioral interventions result in weight loss in such patients. Although it is tempting to use medication in attempt to achieve weight loss, multipronged behavioral interventions including diet and exercise offer health benefits beyond just losing weight.

Patients with schizophrenia have a higher prevalence of type 2 diabetes compared to patients without schizophrenia. Beyond this, antipsychotics may adversely affect glucose levels in diabetic patients. The extent to which these effects are related to drug-induced weight gain is unclear.[71] Data collected from the FDA MedWatch Drug Surveillance System for clozapine, olanzapine, quetiapine, and risperidone indicate that nearly 60% of new-onset diabetes occurred within the first 6 months of treatment initiation.[72] Clozapine and olanzapine have the highest risk of new-onset diabetes followed by risperidone and then quetiapine. Although less likely than with the other SGAs, inadequate data are available to accurately estimate the risk with ziprasidone and aripiprazole.[72] In a study comparing first episode patients compared with healthy controls, the greatest increases in glucose impairment occurred during the first 14 weeks of treatment, with olanzapine being the greatest contributor.[81] The 2009 PORT guidelines do not recommend olanzapine as a first-line antipsychotic option due to its side effect profile.[26] The FDA approved product labeling for all SGAs reflects the increased risk of diabetes mellitus in patients taking these medications. Designing care models and standards for managing diabetes in patients with schizophrenia is important in addressing this major health problem.

Cardiovascular System

Orthostatic Hypotension Orthostatic hypotension is thought to be caused by α-adrenergic blockade, and may occur in up to 75% of treated patients.[84] Clozapine and quetiapine had the highest incidence of orthostatic hypotension in the CATIE study, and iloperidone appears to have the highest risk among newer SGAs.[84] Orthostatic hypotension can occur in any patient, but diabetic patients with preexisting cardiovascular disease and the elderly seem particularly predisposed. Other risk factors may include older age, dehydration and presence of alcoholic neuropathy.[84,85] Antipsychotic combination treatment has been reported to result in a greater risk of orthostasis.[84,85] Patients should be advised to avoid sudden positional changes to allow for adaptation. Tolerance to this effect may occur within 2 to 3 months. If not, lower doses or a change to an antipsychotic with less α-blockade can be attempted. Fluid resuscitation or increasing salt intake may also help minimize orthostatic blood pressure changes.[84]

Electrocardiographic Changes Among the antipsychotics, thioridazine is most likely to cause electrocardiographic (ECG) changes. ECG changes include increased heart rate (through sinus tachycardia from anticholinergic effects, or reflex tachycardia from α-adrenergic blockade), flattened T waves, ST segment depression, and prolongation of QT and PR intervals. The most clinically important of these potential changes is prolongation of the QTc interval, which has been associated with ventricular arrhythmias, including torsade de pointes syndrome. This is thought to occur as a result of blockade of the cardiac delayed potassium rectifier channel as well as impairment in autonomic function.[85,86] Thioridazine has been shown to prolong the QTc on average approximately 20 milliseconds longer than haloperidol, risperidone, olanzapine, or quetiapine.[86] Thioridazine's effect on QTc prolongation is dose related, and has led to a boxed warning in the FDA-approved product labeling. In the same study, ziprasidone prolonged the QTc by approximately 10 milliseconds or about one half of the effect of thioridazine.[87] A recent comprehensive review was not able to stratify the degree of QTc prolongation of nine different SGAs.[88] Iloperidone however, is subject to polymorphic metabolism and there may be an increased risk of QTc prolongation in CYP2D6 slow metabolizers.[58] High IV doses of haloperidol elevate the risk for QTc prolongation, and it has a boxed warning in the FDA approved labeling.[89] Although the precise point at which QTc prolongation becomes clinically dangerous is unclear, the risk for arrhythmia escalates when the QTc interval exceeds 500 milliseconds, or is 60 milliseconds above the baseline QTc.[85,90] Accordingly, it has been recommended to discontinue a medication associated with QTc prolongation if the interval consistently exceeds 500 milliseconds. A recent comprehensive review suggests that QTc intervals greater than or equal to 450 milliseconds and/or a 30 milliseconds increase in QTc interval from baseline are predictors of a drug's risk to cause torsades.[88]

While QTc prolongation may predict torsade de pointes, it rarely happens in the absence of other risks factors, including patients greater than 60 years, female gender, those with preexisting cardiac or cerebrovascular disease (including bradycardia, second- or third-degree AV block, and congenital long QTc syndrome), hepatic impairment, hypokalemia, hypomagnesemia, concomitant medications that prolong the QTc interval, metabolic inhibition by another medication, and preexisting QTc prolongation.[87-89] For patients over the age of 50 years of age, a pretreatment ECG is recommended, as are baseline serum potassium and magnesium levels.

Sudden Cardiac Death A large retrospective analysis found that the risk of sudden cardiac death (SCD) with use of FGAs and SGAs was twice that of nonusers, with risk increasing with escalated dose.[87,91] It has been estimated that 15 cases of SCD occur per 10,000 years of antipsychotic exposure.[86] Meta-analysis has conferred a lack of evidence for differential effects on cardiovascular mortality favoring one class of antipsychotics over the other.[87,91] A recent case cross over study involving over 17,000 patients showed that use of antipsychotics was associated with a 1.53 fold increase in ventricular arrhythmia or SCD. The magnitude of effect was greatest among patients who received antipsychotics for a short term (less than 28 days).[92] Nonetheless, prospectively designed studies are needed to confirm a dose-dependent increase in cardiovascular sudden death with antipsychotic use, and to determine whether certain antipsychotics are associated with a greater risk than others.

Lipid Changes Treatment with at least some SGAs and phenothiazines appears to be associated with elevations in serum triglycerides and cholesterol. Oxidation of apolipoprotein B lipoproteins and elevations in sterol regulatory element binding protein-controlled gene expression are among the purported mechanisms by which these lipid changes occur during antipsychotic treatment.[93] Among the SGAs, less risk for change in serum lipid or cholesterol levels has been associated with risperidone, ziprasidone, aripiprazole, asenapine, iloperidone, and lurasidone.[59,69,72,74] In the CATIE trial, olanzapine was associated with greater and significant adverse effects on metabolic parameters, including lipids, blood glucose, and body weight versus the other study treatments, but these differences in tolerability did not affect discontinuation rates.[30]

The occurrence of weight gain, diabetes, and lipid abnormalities during antipsychotic therapy is consistent with the development of metabolic syndrome (ie, syndrome X). Cohorts of patients with schizophrenia have shown elevated prevalence of metabolic syndrome as compared with general population cohorts. Prevalence rates of metabolic syndrome in US populations treated with antipsychotics range from 28% to 60%, with 40.9% reported in the prospectively designed CATIE trial.[94]

Metabolic syndrome consists of raised triglycerides (greater than or equal to 150 mg/dL [1.70 mmol/L]), low HDL cholesterol (less than or equal to 40 mg/dL [1.03 mmol/L] for males, less than or equal to 50 mg/dL [1.29 mmol/L] for females), elevated fasting glucose (greater than or equal to 100 mg/dL [5.6 mmol/L]), blood pressure elevation (greater than or equal to 130/85 mm Hg), and weight gain (abdominal circumference greater than 102 cm [40 in] for males, greater than 89 cm [35 in] in females).[72,74] These abnormalities dictate an important role for general health screening and monitoring in patients with schizophrenia, and prompt intervention when such abnormalities occur. The propensity of individual antipsychotics to produce metabolic disturbances should be considered in the context of individual patient risk factors at the time of drug selection.

Anticholinergic Effects Patients receiving antipsychotics or antipsychotics in combination with anticholinergics can experience anticholinergic side effects (eg, dry mouth, constipation, tachycardia, blurred vision, inhibition or impairment of ejaculation, urinary retention, or impaired memory). These side effects are particularly seen when low-potency FGAs are used, and in elderly patients who are especially sensitive to these effects. Of the SGAs, clozapine, and olanzapine have moderately high rates of causing anticholinergic effects. Constipation, caused by slowed peristaltic movement and decreased intestinal fluid content, should be closely monitored and treated, especially in the elderly. Paralytic ileus and necrotizing enterocolitis can also occur.

CNS

Extrapyramidal System Extrapyramidal symptoms is an umbrella term used to describe antipsychotic induced movement side effects due to excess dopamine blockade in the nigrostriatal pathway. These symptoms include: dystonia, akathisia, pseudoparkinsonism, and tardive dyskinesia, which are explained in detail below.

Dystonia—a state of abnormal tonicity, sometimes described simplistically as a severe, "muscle spasm.[95] More accurately, dystonias are prolonged tonic contractions, with a rapid onset, usually within 24 to 96 hours of initiating or increasing the dose of an antipsychotic. They can be life-threatening, as in the case of pharyngeal–laryngeal dystonias, and can contribute to patient nonadherence with their medications. Types of dystonic reactions include trismus, glossospasm, tongue protrusion, pharyngeal–laryngeal dystonia, blepharospasm, oculogyric crisis, torticollis, and retrocollis. Dystonic reactions occur primarily with FGAs. Risk factors include younger patients (especially males), the use of high-potency agents, and high dosage. The overall incidence from the 1960s to the mid-1970s ranged from 2.3% to 10%, but as higher-potency traditional antipsychotics became more widely used, the rate increased to as high as 64%.

Intramuscular or IV anticholinergics (Table 67-7) or benzodiazepines are the treatments of choice for dystonia. Benztropine 2 mg or diphenhydramine 50 mg can be given intramuscularly or IV. Diazepam 5 to 10 mg by slow IV push or lorazepam 1 to 2 mg intramuscularly is a treatment alternative. Relief is typically seen within 15 to 20 minutes of an intramuscular injection and within 5 minutes of IV administration. The antipsychotic can be continued, with concomitant short-term use of oral anticholinergic agents. In general, prophylactic anticholinergic medications are not recommended routinely with all FGAs. However, prophylaxis is reasonable when using high-potency FGAs (eg, haloperidol or fluphenazine) in young men, and in patients with a history of dystonia.[95] Dystonias can also be minimized by the use of lower initial FGA doses. Anticholinergics are good choices for prophylaxis, whereas amantadine has not been proven effective for this purpose. The risk of dystonia is greatly reduced with SGAs.

TABLE 67-7 Agents Used to Treat Extrapyramidal Side Effects

Generic Name	Equivalent Dose (mg)	Daily Dosage Range (mg)
Antimuscarinics		
Benztropine[a]	1	1-8[b]
Biperiden[a]	2	2-8
Trihexyphenidyl	2	2-15
Antihistaminic		
Diphenhydramine[a]	50	50-400
Dopamine Agonist		
Amantadine	NA	100-400
Benzodiazepines		
Lorazepam[a]	NA	1-8
Diazepam	NA	2-20
Clonazepam	NA	2-8
β-Blockers		
Propranolol	NA	20-160

NA, Not applicable.

[a]Injectable dosage form can be given intramuscularly for relief of acute dystonia.

[b]In treatment-refractory cases, dosage can be titrated to 12 mg/day with careful monitoring; nonlinear pharmacokinetics have been reported.

Akathisia—defined as the inability to sit still and having functional motor restlessness. The most accurate diagnosis is made by combining subjective complaints with objective symptoms (pacing, shifting, shuffling, or tapping feet). Subjectively, patients may describe a feeling of inner restlessness or disquiet or a compulsion to move or remain in constant motion. Akathisia occurs in 20% to 40% of patients treated with high-potency FGAs.[95,96] It is frequently accompanied by dysphoria. In severe cases, akathisia may be mistaken for aggression and if left untreated, akathisia has been linked to causing insomnia, increased suicidality and development of tardive dyskinesia.[97]

Akathisia responds poorly to anticholinergics.[96] Traditionally, reduction in antipsychotic dosage has been considered the best intervention; however, this might not be a realistic goal in an acutely psychotic patient. A logical alternative is to switch to an antipsychotic with a lower risk of akathisia, or an antipsychotic previously used in the patient without adverse effect. Akathisia can occasionally occur with SGAs, particularly aripiprazole and risperidone. Quetiapine and clozapine appear to have the lowest risk of producing akathisia.[96,97]

Benzodiazepines have been used for treatment of akathisia, but the high prevalence of co-occurring substance abuse in schizophrenia discourages their prescribing.[96] The β-blockers (eg, propranolol in doses up to 160 mg daily, nadolol in doses up to 80 mg daily, and metoprolol in β_2-selective doses of 100 mg daily or less) are reported as effective.[95,96] Emerging literature suggests that agents with antagonist activity at the 5-HT_2 receptor may be protective against akathisia and may be used for its management. Examples of such agents include cyproheptadine, mirtazapine, and trazodone.[95,97]

Pseudoparkinsonism—is produced by D_2 blockade in the nigrostriatum, resembling idiopathic Parkinson's disease. A patient with pseudoparkinsonism can present with any of four cardinal symptoms: (a) akinesia, bradykinesia, or decreased motor activity including difficulty initiating movement, as well as extreme slowness, mask-like facial expression, micrographia, slowed speech, and decreased arm swing; (b) tremor, known as pill-rolling type, that is predominant at rest and decreases with movement, usually involving the fingers and hands, although tremors can also be seen in the arms, legs, neck, head, and chin; (c) cogwheel rigidity, seen as the patient's limbs yielding in jerky, ratchet-like fashion when passively moved by the examiner; and (d) postural abnormalities and instability manifested as stooped posture, difficulty in maintaining stability when changing body position, and a gait that ranges from slow and shuffling to festinating. Fatigue and weakness can be noted, as well as oral abnormalities including dysphagia, dysarthria, and abnormal palmomental and glabellar reflexes. The overall incidence of pseudoparkinsonism from FGAs ranges from 15.4% to 36%, depending on the drug and dose. Akinesia alone can be seen in 59% of patients on high-potency FGAs. Other risk factors include increasing age and possibly female gender. The onset of symptoms is typically 1 to 2 weeks after initiation of antipsychotic therapy or a dose increase.[95,96]

The efficacy of anticholinergic medications in treating symptoms of pseudoparkinsonism is well established.[95,96] Recent meta-analyses and trial data, such as a secondary analysis of data from the Cost Utility of the Latest Antipsychotic drugs in Schizophrenia Study (CUtLASS-1) and CATIE studies, did not report marked differences in rates of EPS between FGAs and SGAs when FGA treatments were accompanied by appropriate use of anticholinergic medications.[98]

Anticholinergic dosing for pseudoparkinsonism is outlined in Table 67-7. Diphenhydramine produces more sedation than the other agents. Symptoms typically begin to resolve within 3 to 4 days after initiation of treatment, but a minimum of at least 2 weeks of treatment is normally required for full response. All of the anticholinergics have been abused for their euphoriant effects.[99] Amantadine may be as efficacious for pseudoparkinsonism as anticholinergics, but with significantly less effect on memory function.[96] Rotigotine, a dopamine agonist, is effective at doses ranging from 2 to 8 mg per day, and without worsening positive or negative symptoms of schizophrenia.[100] Prophylactic use of these agents against pseudoparkinsonism is less convincing compared with dystonias, and is unnecessary when using SGAs.[96] The long-term treatment of pseudoparkinsonism with antiparkinsonism medication is somewhat controversial. An attempt should be made to taper and discontinue these agents 6 weeks to 3 months after symptom resolution. If symptoms reappear, then switching to a SGA should be considered. The risk of pseudoparkinsonism with SGAs is low. When risperidone is used in doses greater than 6 mg/day, the risk of pseudoparkinsonism symptoms approaches that with FGAs. Quetiapine, aripiprazole, and clozapine are reasonable alternatives in a patient experiencing EPS with other SGAs.[96,98]

Tardive Dyskinesia (TD)—is a syndrome characterized by abnormal involuntary movements occurring late in onset in relation to initiation of antipsychotic therapy. It is sometimes irreversible and continues to be a controversial issue.

The classic description of tardive dyskinesia is the buccal–lingual–masticatory (BLM) syndrome, or orofacial movements. The onset of BLM movements is usually insidious. Typically, they are the first detectable signs of tardive dyskinesia which begin with mild forward, backward, or lateral movements of the tongue. If the disorder progresses, more obvious or frank BLM movements appear, including tongue thrusting, rolling, or fly-catching movements, and chewing or lateral jaw movements. Tardive dyskinesia symptoms can interfere with the patient's ability to chew, speak, or swallow. Further complications include oral ulcerations, inability to wear dentures, and inflammation and loosening of mandibular joints. Eating difficulties and malnutrition can be severe complications. Weight loss can be seen in patients with esophageal or respiratory manifestations. Facial movements include frequent blinking, brow arching, grimacing, upward deviation of the eyes, and lip smacking. Involvement of the extremities sometimes occurs, with the appearance of restless choreiform and distal athetosis of limbs including twisting, spreading, flexion and extension of fingers, toe tapping, and toe dorsiflexion. Unusual posture, hyperextension, pelvic thrusting, axial hyperkinesia ballismus, exaggerated lordosis, rocking, and swaying are occasionally observed. Among the differential diagnoses are withdrawal dyskinesias occurring after short-term use of antipsychotics, spontaneous orofacial dyskinesias in the elderly, orofacial dyskinesias in the edentulous, Huntington's disease, congenital torsion dystonia, and stereotypic movements associated with schizophrenia. Orofacial movements are more common in older patients, whereas the truncal axial movements are classically reported in young adults. Movements can worsen with stress, decrease with sedation, and disappear during sleep. Concentration on motor tasks or attempts to suppress the movements can actually increase them.[101]

Early signs of tardive dyskinesia can be reversible but if allowed to persist, they can become irreversible, even with drug discontinuation. When the antipsychotic dose is decreased or tapered and discontinued, worsening of abnormal movements may occur, followed by possible slow improvement after months or years if the patient remains on lower doses or discontinues treatment. No standardized diagnostic criteria for tardive dyskinesia are available. Abnormal involuntary movements can be detected early through physical assessment and the use of rating scales. Available rating scales include the Abnormal Involuntary Movement Scale (AIMS) and the Dyskinesia Identification System: Condensed User Scale (DISCUS).[102] Neither scale is diagnostic in itself.

Risk factors include increasing age, the occurrence of acute EPS, poor antipsychotic drug response, diagnosis of organic mental disorder, diabetes mellitus, mood disorders, and possibly female gender.[101] Duration of antipsychotic therapy, daily dosage, and possibly total cumulative dosage are probably the most significant risk factors. Polymorphisms of the D_2, D_3, 5-HT_{2C} receptor, and the superoxide dismutase-2 genes have all been implicated in varying the risk of TD with antipsychotic use.[101] Overall morbidity and mortality are greater in tardive dyskinesia patients.

With FGAs, the reported prevalence of TD ranges from 20% to 50%.[101] In first episode schizophrenia, the incidence is estimated at about 5% per year, with the overall prevalence ranging from 20% to 25% with long-term treatment. Among the elderly, the overall risk of TD is higher.[96] Tardive dyskinesia is not always permanent, with remission of symptoms observed in 25% of patients after 5 years of continued treatment.[29,96]

With SGAs, a systematic review of 12 studies lasting 1 year or more found the overall risk of tardive dyskinesia to be approximately 2.98% per year in nonelderly adults as compared with 7.7% for FGAs.[103] Although lower than the FGAs, the PORT guidelines report no difference in the risk of TD among SGAs.[26,29]

Prevention of tardive dyskinesia is important, as treatment of the movements once they occur is difficult. One of the more compelling arguments for the first-line use of SGAs is their lower risk of TD.[27-29] Regular neurologic examinations (AIMS or other scales) should be performed at baseline and at least quarterly to assess for possible early signs of tardive dyskinesia. At the first signs of tardive dyskinesia, the need for continuing antipsychotic treatment should be assessed. In such situations, if the patient is taking an FGA and continuing treatment is indicated, the medication should be switched to a SGA.

Numerous drugs have been used in an attempt to treat tardive dyskinesia. In two controlled trials lasting 22 to 52 weeks, clozapine decreased abnormal involuntary movements.[26,29] Although some treatment guidelines recommend switching antipsychotic therapy to clozapine as a favored first-line pharmacotherapeutic strategy in patients with moderate to severe dyskinesias, others do not support this.[31,96,104] A guideline developed by the American Academy of Neurology recommends short-term treatment of TD with either clonazepam or ginkgo biloba based upon randomized clinical trial data. However, long-term treatment data are lacking.[104]

Sedation and Cognition Chlorpromazine, thioridazine, clozapine, olanzapine, and quetiapine are the most sedating antipsychotics. Administration of most or all of the daily dosage at bedtime can decrease daytime sedation and in some patients eliminate the need for hypnotic agents. Sedation occurs early in treatment and can decrease over time. Over-sedation can play a large role in cognitive, perceptual, and motor dysfunction. However, positive effects of medication on cognition are seen with chronic administration, evidenced by improvements in tasks involving visual motor skills, attention to task, and working memory. Compared with FGAs, several studies have shown cognitive benefits of SGAs. However, results from the CATIE trial showed no differences in cognitive improvement between SGAs and the FGA perphenazine.[105] Comparative effects of different SGAs on cognition are as yet unclear, but available studies suggest that different SGAs can have effects on varying cognitive domains.[27,29,]

As discussed in Long-Acting Injectable Antipsychotics section, olanzapine pamoate monohydrate injectable is associated with a postinjection sedation/delirium syndrome.[42-44]

Seizures An increased risk of drug-induced seizures occurs in patients receiving antipsychotics as these agents decrease the seizure threshold. However, this risk is greater if the following predisposing factors are present: preexisting seizure disorder, history of drug-induced seizure, abnormal electroencephalogram (EEG), and preexisting CNS pathology or head trauma. Seizures are more closely associated with higher doses of antipsychotics, rapid dosage titrations, and when treatment is initiated. When an isolated seizure occurs, a dosage reduction in the antipsychotic is first recommended; routine prophylactic use of anticonvulsant therapy is not recommended. Although spontaneously occurring seizures have been reported with most antipsychotics, the highest potential risk for an antipsychotic-related seizure is with clozapine or chlorpromazine. If a change in antipsychotic therapy is required because of a drug-induced seizure, risperidone, thioridazine, haloperidol, pimozide, trifluoperazine, and fluphenazine are associated with the lowest potential.[96]

Thermoregulation Poikilothermia, the body temperature adjusting to the ambient temperature, can be a serious side effect of antipsychotic therapy in temperature extremes.[106] Hyperpyrexia can be a danger in hot weather or during exercise. Inhibition of sweating, a result of anticholinergic properties impairing the peripheral mechanisms of heat dissipation, can contribute to this problem, which in its severest form can lead to heat stroke. Hypothermia is a risk in cold temperatures, particularly in the elderly. All patients receiving antipsychotics should be educated about these potential problems. Thermoregulatory problems are reportedly more common with the use of low-potency FGAs and can occur with the more anticholinergic SGAs.

Neuroleptic Malignant Syndrome Neuroleptic malignant syndrome (NMS) occurs in 0.5% to 1% of patients receiving FGAs. NMS can occur more frequently in patients receiving high-potency FGAs, injectable or depot FGAs, and in patients who are dehydrated, with physical exhaustion, or organic mental disorders. Additionally, young to middle aged men as well as postpartum women are at elevated risk for NMS.[107] Although less common, NMS has been reported with SGAs, including clozapine. The onset of symptoms varies from early in treatment to months later. It develops rapidly, over the course of 24 to 72 hours. NMS can occur after antipsychotic discontinuation, especially when depot agents are used. Possible mechanisms of NMS include disruption of the central thermoregulatory process or excess production of heat secondary to skeletal muscle contractions. The differential diagnosis includes heat stroke, lethal catatonia, anesthetic-associated malignant hyperthermia, anticholinergic toxicity, and monoamine oxidase inhibitor drug interactions. Cardinal signs and symptoms of NMS are body temperature exceeding 38°C (100.4°F), altered level of consciousness, autonomic dysfunction (tachycardia, labile blood pressure, diaphoresis, tachypnea, or urinary or fecal incontinence), and rigidity. Laboratory evaluation, although nonspecific, frequently shows leukocytosis with or without a left shift, increases in creatine kinase (CK), aspartate aminotransferase, alanine aminotransferase, lactate dehydrogenase, and myoglobinuria.[96,106]

Treatment should begin with antipsychotic discontinuation and supportive care. In many cases that alone is effective. The role of adjunctive agents is unclear, yet they are often used. The DA agonist bromocriptine reduces rigidity, fever, or CK in up to 94% of patients, whereas the use of amantadine has been successful in up to 63% of patients. Dantrolene has been used as a skeletal muscle relaxant, with positive effects on temperature, heart rate, respiratory rate, and CK in up to 81% of patients.[96,106] Wide recognition and rapid antipsychotic discontinuation has drastically reduced mortality from 20% 25 years ago to 4% in the mid-1990s.

Many patients with schizophrenia, despite having had NMS, will require future antipsychotic pharmacotherapy. A review of antipsychotic rechallenges suggests that the risk of rechallenge is acceptable in most patients, provided that the patient is observed for an extended period of time (2 weeks or more is suggested) without antipsychotics, that there is careful monitoring and slow dose titration, and that the patient is maintained on the lowest possible dose.[96] A different antipsychotic, a SGA or a low-potency FGA, should be used for rechallenge following an episode of NMS.

Psychiatric Side Effects Antipsychotic-induced akathisia, akinesia, and dysphoria can have unfortunate sequelae, resulting in what has been termed *behavioral toxicity*.[38] Akinesia, characterized by "diminished spontaneity," results in symptoms of apathy and withdrawal, often mistaken for the negative symptoms of schizophrenia; these patients can actually appear depressed. Delirium and psychosis are reported with larger doses of FGAs or combinations of anticholinergics with FGAs. Chronic confusion and disorientation can occur in the elderly as a result of antipsychotic treatment.[108] Unfortunately, the link is not always made with antipsychotic therapy, and the patient is misdiagnosed with delirium from a different etiology. This clinical presentation, called a *pseudodementia*, may be reversible upon discontinuation of the antipsychotic.

Ophthalmologic Effects Anticholinergic effects of antipsychotics or concomitant antiparkinson medications can exacerbate narrow-angle (angle-closure) glaucoma. Antipsychotics with low anticholinergic effects should be used in such individuals, and they should be appropriately monitored.[109]

Opaque deposits in the cornea and lens occur with chronic phenothiazine treatment, most frequently with chlorpromazine. Although visual acuity is not usually affected, periodic ophthalmologic examinations are frequently recommended in patients receiving long-term treatment with phenothiazines, as fully formed cataracts are possible.[109]

Because of cataract development and lenticular changes in animals, baseline and periodic eye examinations are recommended in the product labeling for quetiapine. However, quetiapine's effects on lens opacity was found to be no different than risperidone in a 2 year comparative trial.[110] Retinitis pigmentosa can result from use of thioridazine doses greater than 800 mg daily. It is caused by melanin deposits and can result in permanent visual impairment or blindness.

Genitourinary System Urinary hesitancy and retention, secondary to anticholinergic effects, are reported with low-potency FGAs and with clozapine. Men with benign prostatic hypertrophy are especially prone to this effect.[111] Reducing the antipsychotic dose or switching to an antipsychotic with less anticholinergic activity may help manage this side effects. Alternatively, bethanecol can be used to treat antipsychotic induced urinary hesitancy and retention.

Urinary incontinence is thought to be caused by α-blockade, and among the SGAs, it appears to be particularly problematic with clozapine. The incidence has been reported to be as high as 44%, and it can be persistent in 25% of patients. Female gender, and previous urinary incontinence can be risk factors for developing this side effect.[112]

Although inadequately studied, multiple mechanisms are likely responsible for sexual dysfunction, including dopaminergic blockade, hyperprolactinemia, histaminergic blockade anticholinergic effects, and α-adrenergic blockade. Unmedicated individuals with schizophrenia report decreased libido. Most but not all studies show a relationship between hyperprolactinemia and sexual dysfunction, including decreased libido, erectile dysfunction, difficulty achieving orgasm, and ejaculatory abnormalities. Risperidone produces at least as much sexual dysfunction as FGAs; while other SGAs, with weak effects on prolactin, produce less sexual dysfunction. Patients experiencing sexual dysfunction with FGAs or risperidone should be switched to an SGA with less effect on prolactin.[113]

Priapism, a sustained and painful erection which is unprovoked and persists for longer than an hour, is increasingly reported with antipsychotic medication use. This is believed to occur as a result of α_1-adrenergic receptor blockade, leading to intracavernosal blood stasis.[114] This can evolve into a urologic emergency, due to the ischemic nature of the priapism. If left untreated, priapism may lead to permanent impotence.

Hematologic System Transient leukopenia can occur during initial treatment with antipsychotics; however, it typically does not progress to be clinically significant.[115] Agranulocytosis reportedly occurs in 0.01% of patients receiving FGAs, and more frequently with chlorpromazine and thioridazine. The three antipsychotics with the highest relative risk for neutropenia in rank order are clozapine, chlorpromazine, and olanzapine.[115] The onset is usually within the first 8 weeks of therapy. If the absolute neutrophil count (ANC) is less than 500/μL (0.5×10^9/L) the antipsychotic should be discontinued and the ANC monitored closely until it returns to normal. Agranulocytosis can initially manifest as a local infection, with sore throat, leukoplakia, erythema, and ulcerations of the pharynx. These symptoms in any patient receiving antipsychotics should signal the immediate need for an ANC. If the ANC is less than 500/μL (0.5×10^9/L) the drug should be discontinued immediately and the patient monitored closely for the development of secondary infections. Isolated rare cases of thrombocytopenia and eosinophilia have also been reported.

Agranulocytosis with clozapine significantly limits the usefulness of this agent, and it is only available through the Clozapine REMS Program.[116] The risk of developing neutropenia or agranulocytosis with clozapine is approximately 3% and 0.8%, respectively.[115] Increasing age and female gender are associated with greater risk. The baseline ANC must be at least 1,500/μL (1.5×10^9/L) in order to start clozapine. Weekly ANC monitoring for the first 6 months of therapy is mandated in the FDA-approved product labeling. After this time, if the patient's ANC remains greater than 1,500/μL (1.5×10^9/L) the labeling allows ANC monitoring to be decreased to every 2 weeks for the next 6 months. After this, monitoring can be decreased to monthly if all ANCs remains greater than 1,500/μL (1.5×10^9/L). If at any time the ANC drops to less than 500/μL (0.5×10^9/L) clozapine must be discontinued and the ANC monitored daily until it is greater than 1,500/μL (1.5×10^9/L). The FDA approved product labeling should be consulted for more detailed information regarding ANC monitoring, including monitoring for mild and moderate leukopenia and recommendations for patients with benign ethnic neutropenia.[116]

Dermatologic System Allergic reactions are rare and usually occur within 8 weeks of initiating therapy, manifesting as maculopapular, erythematous, pruritic rashes that are evident on the face, neck, trunk, or extremities. Contact dermatitis, including the oral mucosa, has been reported in patients and medical personnel exposed to FGA liquid formulations. The risk of oral mucosal reactions can be decreased by mixing the FGA concentrate in a sufficient quantity of a nonacidic liquid and swallowing it quickly. Care should be taken in the handling and preparation of liquid FGAs. Recently, the FDA added a warning for ziprasidone to its labelling regarding the risk for a rare but fatal skin reaction called *Drug Reaction with Eosinophilia and Systemic Symptoms* (DRESS).[117]

Phenothiazines can absorb ultraviolet light, resulting in the formation of free radicals, which can have damaging effects on the skin. All antipsychotics can cause photosensitivity resulting in erythema and sunburn. Exposure to sunlight should be limited, and patients should be educated about the use of a maximally blocking sunscreen, hats, protective clothing, and sunglasses.[115]

Blue-gray or purplish skin coloration in areas exposed to sunlight occurs in patients receiving higher doses of low-potency phenothiazines during long-term administration, especially with chlorpromazine. It commonly occurs with concurrent corneal or lens pigmentation.

Miscellaneous Adverse Effects A sometimes troubling side effect with clozapine is sialorrhea (drooling), which is typically prominent at night.[118] This side effect can affect up to 54% of patients receiving clozapine. The mechanism of clozapine-induced drooling is unclear, however two theories exist. The first involves muscarinic receptor activity and clozapine's imbalanced binding affinity to this receptor. The other involves clozapine's alpha antagonist activity at the salivary glands leaving unopposed beta-receptor stimulation and hence hyper-salivation.[118] Anticholinergics such as benztropine and atropine, and α-agonists such as clonidine have been used to treat clozapine-related sialorrhea.[118]

Toxicity with Overdose

Acute overdose with antipsychotics rarely results in serious symptomatology. Mild intoxication manifests as sedation, hypotension, and miosis, whereas with severe intoxication, agitation and delirium can typically progress to motor retardation, seizures, cardiac arrhythmias, respiratory arrest, and coma. Dystonias and pseudoparkinsonism symptoms also occur. Supportive measures, gastric lavage, and activated charcoal are recommended. Induction of emesis can be difficult because of effects on the chemoreceptor trigger zone. Dialysis is ineffective due to antipsychotics' high degree of drug–protein binding. Phenytoin or sodium bicarbonate is useful in the treatment of quinidine-like cardiac conduction effects on the QRS or QTc interval. Physostigmine is not generally recommended to reverse anticholinergic toxicity because of deleterious effects on arrhythmias and seizure threshold.[119]

Use in Pregnancy and Lactation

Minimal data exist regarding the effects of pregnancy on schizophrenia and its treatment. However, disorganized thought processes, impaired cognition, and negative symptoms can have a detrimental effect on the functioning and self-care of the mother, and therefore adversely affect the fetus.[120] Currently available data assessing the risk of teratogenesis with antipsychotic agents are insufficient. Epidemiologic studies show a slightly increased risk of birth defects with low-potency FGAs. Haloperidol is the best studied of all antipsychotics, and no relationship between its use and teratogenicity has been found. One study indicates a greater than twofold elevated risk of preterm birth in women with schizophrenia taking FGAs as compared with unaffected mothers not taking antipsychotics.[120]

Although increasing information regarding the safety of SGAs in pregnancy is becoming available, very few large studies and very few prospective studies have been performed to evaluate possible teratogenicity of SGAs. One large registry data study performed in Sweden found a significantly increased risk of cardiovascular defects with antipsychotic exposure; however, when stratifying by antipsychotic class, it was found that all defects were found in those exposed to FGAs, while no cardiovascular defects were reported with SGAs.[121] A meta-analysis of 12 studies found a greater risk of first trimester birth defects with SGAs, but no specific abnormality. An increased risk of preterm birth was also present in the SGA treated group. However, healthy women composed the control group in these studies, and the underlying disease state being treated with a SGA is an important confounder.[122] Thus, large, well-controlled studies are needed to determine the safety of SGAs during pregnancy.

Other potential interest in studying early and late exposure to antipsychotics include postnatal and gestational complications. Weight gain associated with olanzapine and clozapine and the potential risk of gestational diabetes should be considered in drug selection.[123] A recent retrospective cohort study reported nearly twofold odds of gestational diabetes in women who used antipsychotics during pregnancy, and this was confirmed by a population cohort study.[123,124] In addition, an increased risk of hypertension in women taking antipsychotics during pregnancy as well as venous thromboembolism have been reported.

Risk of neonatal EPS is increased with in utero exposure to FGAs, with effects in the infant lasting for 3 to 12 months after birth.[125] In February 2011, the FDA issued a safety announcement informing healthcare professionals that the pregnancy section of drug labels had been updated for the entire antipsychotic class, highlighting the potential risk for EPS and withdrawal symptoms in newborns whose mothers were treated with antipsychotics during their third trimester.[125] Symptoms of neonatal withdrawal reported to the FDA included agitation, hypertonia, hypotonia, tremor, somnolence, respiratory distress, and feeding disorder.

The risk of antipsychotic use must be weighed against the benefits of pharmacotherapy in pregnant women experiencing disorganized thoughts, delusions about change in body image or pregnancy, or who are unable to provide adequate prenatal care.[120,125] A national pregnancy exposure registry monitors pregnancy outcomes in women exposed to atypical antipsychotics during pregnancy. This registry can be accessed at http://womensmentalhealth.org/clinical-and-research-programs/pregnancyregistry/atypicalantipsychotic.

Antipsychotics appear in breast milk with milk-to-plasma ratios of 0.5:1. However, 1 week after delivery, clozapine milk concentrations were found to be as much as 279% of serum concentrations. Its use during breast-feeding is not recommended due to the risk of bone marrow suppression.[126] Aripiprazole and quetiapine have the most data regarding their use in breastfeeding and are generally considered safe.[126] Information regarding olanzapine use in breastfeeding is inconclusive. First generation antipsychotics are detected in breast milk, however haloperidol, perphenazine, and trifluoperazine have not been reported to cause clinically evident adverse effects. Infants exposed to chlorpromazine through breast milk have been reported to be drowsy and lethargic. The co-administration of chlorpromazine and haloperidol is reported to result in developmental delays at 12 to 18 months of age.[127] Although not contraindicated, the lowest dosage for antipsychotics should be used in the mother, and the infant carefully monitored for antipsychotic adverse events such as EPS, sedation, seizures and developmental delays.[126]

Drug Interactions

Most drug interactions occur because of pharmacodynamic or pharmacokinetic interactions. Common examples of pharmacodynamic interactions resulting in enhanced effect include the excess sedation that can occur when antipsychotics are used concomitantly with other medications that have sedative side effects. Additive antimuscarinic effects can be seen when antipsychotics are used with other medications possessing antimuscarinic effects, potentially resulting in urinary retention, constipation, blurred vision, or other anticholinergic side effects.[38,128] Both combined sedative and anticholinergic effects from multiple medications can result in impaired cognition, particularly in the elderly and other patients predisposed to such problems.[128] Patients are more likely to experience symptomatic orthostatic hypotension when an antipsychotic is used with other medications that cause orthostasis. Metoclopramide is prescribed for treating esophageal reflux; it is a DA antagonist, and patients are more likely to experience akathisia and other EPS if it is used concomitantly with antipsychotics.[129] Although some SSRIs can interact with antipsychotics through enzyme inhibition, they can also interact through pharmacodynamic mechanisms. 5-HT_2 receptors are present on the presynaptic dopaminergic neuron, and their activation leads to decreased DA release from the presynaptic terminal. Increased availability of 5-HT through SSRI effect can activate these receptors, decrease DA release, and add to the dopaminolytic effects of antipsychotics.[130] In the absence of enzyme inhibition, SSRIs can still precipitate akathisia or EPS when added to a patient stabilized on an antipsychotic. A potentially more dangerous interaction can occur when medications that slow myocardial conduction, and thus prolong the QTc interval, are used in combination with antipsychotics having the same effect.[130] Careful monitoring should occur with medications that prolong the QTc interval, as well as when antipsychotics with this effect are combined with diuretics.[130]

Asenapine inhibits CYP2D6, and is the only SGA that has been shown to significantly affect the pharmacokinetics of other medications.[59] Table 67-6 lists the known major pathways involved in the metabolism of SGAs. Risperidone is metabolized primarily by CYP2D6 to its active metabolite, 9-OH-risperidone (paliperidone), which is thought to have a similar pharmacodynamic profile.[130] Although paliperidone is primarily eliminated renally unchanged, potent inducers of CYP3A4 can cause a potential need for dosage adjustment.[64,130] CYP1A2 is the primary isoenzyme for metabolism of asenapine with CYP3A4 also being a significant pathway.[64,130]

Based on current information, inhibitors of CYP1A2 have the greatest potential for causing interactions with clozapine and olanzapine, and some concern with asenapine.[130] Examples include cimetidine, fluvoxamine, and fluoroquinolone antibiotics (ie, ciprofloxacin) to varying degrees. To date, however, no serious inhibition interactions have been reported with olanzapine, which may be a result of olanzapine's wide therapeutic index. Carbamazepine has been reported to increase olanzapine elimination by as much as 50%.[130] Cigarette smoking is a potent inducer of CYP1A2, and one would expect lower mean olanzapine serum concentrations in smokers compared with those in nonsmokers.

Because of the risk of seizures with higher clozapine tissue concentrations, interactions that inhibit clozapine's metabolism are potentially significant. In particular, fluvoxamine increases clozapine serum concentrations by an average of two to threefold and up to fivefold.[130] Ciprofloxacin, other fluroquinolones, fluoxetine and erythromycin can also increase clozapine serum concentrations.[130] Smoking has been associated with a 33% to 55% increase in clozapine clearance.[130] If a patient taking clozapine stops smoking, the resulting increase in clozapine serum concentration could be associated with seizures.[64] Carbamazepine can also induce clozapine metabolism and lead to lower serum concentrations.[130]

A study with the potent CYP3A4 inhibitor ketoconazole showed minimal effects on ziprasidone single-dose pharmacokinetics, with only a 33% mean increase in the ziprasidone area under the time-versus-concentration curve.[130] These results are consistent with data suggesting that aldehyde oxidase is the major metabolic pathway for ziprasidone, with only 30% to 35% being metabolized by CYP3A4.[130]

Modest elevations of aripiprazole serum concentration occur in the presence of ketoconazole or quinidine, which inhibit CYP3A4 and 2D6, respectively. Ketoconazole has a profound effect on decreasing lurasidone metabolism, and it is recommended that they not be used concomitantly.[69,130] Carbamazepine has been reported to decrease aripiprazole serum concentrations.[130]

Since iloperidone is metabolized through CYP2D6 and 3A4, its clearance can be impaired by inhibitors of these pathways. Since iloperidone prolongs the QTc interval, these types of interactions have the potential to be clinically significant. For example, it is recommended that the iloperidone dose be decreased by 50% when used with CYP2D6 inhibitors such as fluoxetine or paroxetine.[58,130]

Table 67-8 summarizes potential antipsychotic drug interactions.

Personalized Pharmacotherapy

Pharmacotherapy must be individualized for each person with schizophrenia. With the possible exception of iloperidone, no laboratory tests are generally available that will predict a patient's response to treatment. Past response to treatment, potential adverse effects, patient personal preference, and medication price are the primary variables that should be used in selecting an antipsychotic that is included in stages 1A, 1B, or 2 of the treatment algorithm. In the CATIE study, the number one reason for drug discontinuation was the patient not wanting to take that medication any more, and the second most common reason was adverse effects.[30] These two factors should be carefully considered in antipsychotic selection. Medication dosage must also be individualized within the usual dose ranges. Careful consideration must also be given to concomitant medications that may interact with the antipsychotic and necessitate a change in dosage.

Preliminary data suggest a relationship between different genetic markers and clinical improvement as well as QTc prolongation in patients treated with iloperidone. [131] Substantial interest exists regarding the potential utility of pharmacogenetic monitoring in the pharmacotherapy of schizophrenia. Increasing relationships are being identified between specific genetic polymorphisms and both the pharmacodynamics and pharmacokinetics of different antipsychotics. However, no convincing data have demonstrated that clinical outcomes are superior when using routine pharmacogenetic monitoring in the pharmacotherapy of schizophrenia, nor have cost-effectiveness studies of its use been performed.[132] Although promising for the future, routine pharmacogenetics monitoring in schizophrenia is not currently recommended. It will be important to learn to what extent schizophrenia treatment will realize the aspirations of personalized medicine as other areas of medicine are moving toward.[133]

TABLE 67-8 Common Potential Drug Interactions with Antipsychotic Medications

Mechanism of Interaction	Examples of Interacting Drugs or Other Substances		Clinical Effect
Pharmacodynamic Drug Interactions with Antipsychotics			
Muscarinic receptor blockade	*Anticholinergics* Benztropine Diphenhydramine Trihexyphenidyl		↑ Anticholinergic SE [Blurred vision, Constipation, Impaired Cognition, and Urinary retention]
Additive or synergistic sedation	*Sedatives* Benzodiazepines Concomitant AP Diphenhydramine Melatonin and melatonin agonists Mirtazapine Trazodone TCAs Hypnotics Opiates *Anticholinergics* Benztropine Diphenhydramine Trihexyphenidyl Mirtazapine		↑ sedation Lethargy Impaired cognition Impaired psychomotor activity ↑ Risk of accidents
DA antagonist use for different indication	Metoclopramide		↑ EPS
Cardiovascular interactions			
QTc prolongation	Amitriptyline Clomipramine Imipramine Citalopram Fluorquinolone antibiotics	Procainamide Quinidine	↑ Risk of ECG changes and dysrhythmias
Electrolyte changes	Diuretics		↑ Risk of ECG changes and dysrhythmias
Stimulation of presynaptic 5-HT receptors on DA neuron	SSRIs		↑ EPS
Sympatholytics: α-blockade-↓ NE release	Clonidine Methyldopa Prazosin, Nitric oxide containing products		↑ Hypotension
↑ DA receptor binding	Antipsychotics		↑ SEs, particularly EPS

(continued)

TABLE 67-8 Common Potential Drug Interactions with Antipsychotic Medications (*Continued*)

Mechanism of Interaction	Examples of Interacting Drugs or Other Substances			Clinical Effect
Pharmacokinetic Drug Interactions with Antipsychotics				
Substrate Antipsychotic and Mechanism of Action		**Inhibitor or Inducer**		**Clinical Effect**
Aripiprazole, brexipiprazole, Cariprazine, and iloperidone				
Inhibition of AP metabolism (CYP2D6, CYP3A4)	*Antidepressants* Bupropion Clomipramine Doxepin Duloxetine Fluoxetine Fluvoxamine Paroxetine Sertraline *HIV protease inhibitors* Indinavir Nelfinavir Ritonavir	*Anti-infectives* Ciprofloxacin Clarithromycin Erythromycin Fluconazole Ketoconazole Itraconazole *Antipsychotics* Asenapine Chlorpromazine Haloperidol Perphenazine Thioridazine	*Miscellaneous* Ciprofloxacin Chlorpheniramine Cimetidine Cocaine Diltiazem Diphenhydramine Cimetidine Grapefruit juice Haloperidol Hydroxyzine Methadone Quinidine Ticlopidine Verapamil	↑ AP effect ↑ SE
Induction of AP metabolism	*Antiepileptics* Carbamazepine Oxcarbazepine Phenobarbital Phenytoin	*Anti-infectives* Rifampin *Miscellaneous* Glucocorticoids Modafinil	*Herbals* St. John's wort	↓ AP effect
Asenapine Eating food or drinking liquids within 10 minutes of asenapine sublingual administration will decrease bioavailability				
Inhibition of AP metabolism (CYP1A2)	*Antidepressants* Fluvoxamine	*Anti-infectives* Ciprofloxacin Fluroquinolones	*Miscellaneous* Amidarone Cimetidine	↑ AP effect ↑ SE
Induction of AP metabolism	*Anti-infectives* Nafcillin	*Miscellaneous* Broccoli Brussels sprouts Chargrilled meat Smoking tobacco	*Miscellaneous* Insulin Modafinil Omeprazole	↓ AP effect
Pharmacokinetic Drug Interactions with Antipsychotics				
Substrate Antipsychotic and Mechanism of Action		**Inhibitor or Inducer**		***Clinical Effect***
Brexpiprazole (see Aripiprazole above) *Clozapine*				
Inhibition of AP metabolism (CYP3A4, CYP1A2, CYP2C19)	*Antidepressants* Fluoxetine Fluvoxamine *HIV protease inhibitors* Indinavir Nelfinavir Ritonavir *Anticonvulsants* Felbamate Oxcarbazepine	*Anti-infectives* Ciprofloxacin Clarithromycin Erythromycin Fluconazole Fluroquinolones Ketoconazole Itraconazole Nafcillin	*Miscellaneous* Amidarone Diltiazem Cimetidine Grapefruit juice Haloperidol Modafinil Omeprazole Ticlopidine Topiramate Verapamil Cimetidine	↑ AP effect ↑ SE
Induction of AP metabolism	*Antiepileptics* Carbamazepine Phenobarbital Phenytoin	*Anti-infectives* Rifampin *Miscellaneous* Glucocorticoids Insulin Modafinil Omeprazole Smoking tobacco	*Herbals* St. John's wort	↓ AP effect

(*Continued*)

TABLE 67-8 Common Potential Drug Interactions with Antipsychotic Medications (*Continued*)

Mechanism of Interaction	Examples of Interacting Drugs or Other Substances			Clinical Effect
Haloperidol				
Inhibition of AP metabolism (CYP2D6, CYP3A4, CYP1A2)	*Antidepressants* Bupropion Doxepin Duloxetine Fluoxetine Fluvoxamine Paroxetine Sertraline *HIV protease inhibitors* Indinavir Nelfinavir Ritonavir Sequinavir	*Anti-infectives* Ciprofloxacin Clarithromycin Erythromycin Fluconazole Fluoroquinolones Ketoconazole Itraconazole *Antipsychotics* Chlorpromazine Perphenazine	*Miscellaneous* Amiodarone Chlorpheniramine Cimetidine Diltiazem Diphenhydramine Quinidine Diphenhydramine Cimetidine Grapefruit juice Hydroxyzine Methadone Quinidine Verapamil	↑ AP effect ↑ SE
Induction of AP metabolism	*Anticonvulsants* Carbamazepine Oxcarbazepine Phenobarbital Phenytoin	*Anti-infectives* Nafcillin Rifampin *Miscellaneous* Broccoli Brussels sprouts Chargrilled meat Glucocorticoids Insulin Modafinil Omeprazole Modafinil	*Herbals* St. John's wort Tobacco smoking	↓ AP effect
Iloperidone (see Aripiprazole above)				
Olanzapine				
Inhibition of AP metabolism (CYP3A4 and CYP1A2)	*Antidepressants* Fluoxetine (norfluoxetine) Fluvoxamine *HIV protease inhibitors* Indinavir Nelfinavir Ritonavir	*Anti-infectives* Ciprofloxacin Clarithromycin Erythromycin Fluconazole Fluoroquinolones Ketoconazole Itraconazole	*Miscellaneous* Amiodarone Cimetidine Diltiazem Cimetidine Grapefruit juice Verapamil	↑ AP effect ↑ SE
Induction of AP metabolism	*Antiepileptics* Carbamazepine Oxcarbazepine Phenobarbital Phenytoin *HIV protease inhibitors* Efavirenz Nevirapine	*Anti-infectives* Nafcillin Rifampin Miscellaneous Broccoli Brussels sprouts Chargrilled meat Glucocorticoids Insulin Modafinil Omeprazole	*Herbals* St. John's wort Smoking tobacco	↓ AP effect
Paliperidone				
The bioavailability of paliperidone is significantly increased when it is taken with food. Although this could increase paliperidone effect, including adverse effects, the clinical significance is undetermined. Only potent CYP3A4 (eg, carbamazepine, rifampin, St. John's wort) inducers appear to increase paliperidone metabolism and affect dose requirements				
Pharmacokinetic Drug Interactions with Antipsychotics				
Substrate Antipsychotic and Mechanism of Action		**Inhibitor or Inducer**		**Clinical Effect**
Lurasidone and quetiapine Inhibition of AP metabolism (CYP3A4)	*Antidepressants* Fluoxetine (norfluoxetine) Fluvoxamine Nefazodone *HIV protease inhibitors* Indinavir Nelfinavir Ritonavir Sequinavir	*Anti-infectives* Ciprofloxacin Clarithromycin Erythromycin Fluconazole Ketoconazole Itraconazole	*Miscellaneous* Amiodarone Cimetidine Diltiazem Grapefruit juice Verapamil	↑ AP effect ↑ SE

(continued)

TABLE 67-8 Common Potential Drug Interactions with Antipsychotic Medications (*Continued*)

Mechanism of Interaction	Examples of Interacting Drugs or Other Substances			Clinical Effect
Induction of AP metabolism	*Antiepileptics* Carbamazepine Oxcarbazepine Phenobarbital Phenytoin *HIV protease inhibitors* Efavirenz Nevirapine	*Anti-infectives* Rifampin *Miscellaneous* Glucocorticoids Modafinil	*Herbals* St. John's wort	↓ AP effect
Lurasidone AUC and C_{max} increase by two and threefolds when given with at least 350 calories, (1460 J) of food regardless of fat content.				
Perphenazine and risperidone Note: Because risperidone's metabolite formed through CYP2D6 metabolism is active (paliperidone), the clinical significance of metabolic drug interactions with risperidone is unclear				
Inhibition of AP metabolism (CYP2D6)	*Antidepressants* Bupropion Clomipramine Doxepin Duloxetine Fluoxetine Paroxetine Sertraline *Antipsychotics* Chlorpromazine Haloperidol (reduced haloperidol) Perphenazine	*Miscellaneous* Amiodarone Cimetidine Chlorpheniramine Cocaine Diphenhydramine Cimetidine Haloperidol Hydroxyzine Methadone Quinidine		↑ AP effect ↑ SE
Induction of AP metabolism (via CYP3A34, a minor pathway for risperidone)	Dexamethasone Rifampin			↓ AP effect
Ziprasidone The bioavailability of ziprasidone is increased twofold when it is taken with food. Consistent administration with food is recommended				

AP, antipsychotic; DA, dopamine; EPS, extrapyramidal symptoms; 5-HT, serotonin; SE, side effect; SSRI, serotonin selective reuptake inhibitor; TCAs, tricyclic antidepressants, AUC, Area Under the Curve; C_{max}, maximum plasma concentration; NE, norepinephrine.

Data from references 29, 41, 42, 45-47, 58-60, 63-64, 69, 115, 128-130.

Given that no antipsychotic has proven superiority with regard to efficacy in the treatment of schizophrenia (with the exception of clozapine in treatment resistance), cost should be a factor in antipsychotic selection. Aripiprazole, clozapine, olanzapine, quetiapine, risperidone, ziprasidone, and all FGAs have generic equivalents available, and this should be a factor in selecting an antipsychotic.

Clinical **Controversy...**

Approximately 32% of people presenting with prodromal symptoms will go on to have a florid psychosis within 3 years.[136] Early identification of people who exhibit the prodrome of schizophrenia, raises the possibility that intervening early might either avert psychosis altogether or at best, alter its course. This is a major international focus of research, and while intuitive, it is currently not clear that prodrome identification is easily done, offers effective treatment options that are ethically justified, or alters the course of schizophrenia.

Evaluation of Therapeutic Outcomes

Assessment of response has traditionally been done subjectively or empirically (a relative sense of how the clinician feels the patient is doing). A formal MSE is used to structure the patient interview and focus on items related to appearance, mood, sensorium, intellectual functioning, and thought processes. However, the MSE is neither specific nor quantitative for the measurement of drug response. 10 Clinicians should be trained to use simple, standardized psychiatric rating scales to assist in objectively rating patient drug responses.[134] The Brief Psychiatric Rating Scale (BPRS) and the Positive and Negative Symptom Scale (PANSS) were developed for use in clinical trials as research tools to quantify symptom improvement seen with antipsychotic treatment. Objectively, the use of a numeric indicator (eg, 20%, 30%, or 40% reduction in BPRS score) has been used to quantify overall symptom reduction and classify patients according to different degrees of response. However, these types of rating scales are too long and unwieldy to be routinely used within the time constraints of most clinical practices. Symptom scales used in clinical practice must be sufficiently brief to be used during an ordinary clinic visit (eg, 15-30 minutes) while measuring both positive and negative symptoms, and being sufficiently representative of overall symptomatology. The four-item Positive Symptom Rating Scale (PSRS) and the Brief Negative Symptom Assessment are brief scales that meet such criteria (Table 67-9).[134] A brief rating scale of positive symptoms, such as the PSRS, should be used at baseline before starting pharmacotherapy, and at each time response to pharmacotherapy is assessed.

Clinical **Controversy...**

Psychiatry is one of the few specialties in medicine in which measurement is not a routine component of patient care. Although biologic measures do not currently exist in psychiatry, symptoms associated with a patient's illness can be measured and quantified. Although increasing evidence attests to the benefits of quantifying symptom severity, the use of symptom rating scales remains uncommon in clinical practice.

TABLE 67-9 Brief Clinical Assessments for Monitoring Antipsychotic Response in Schizophrenia

4-Item Positive Symptom Rating Scale (PSRS)								
Use each item's anchor points to rate the patient								
1. Suspiciousness	NA[a]	1	2	3	4	5	6	7
2. Unusual thought content	NA	1	2	3	4	5	6	7
3. Hallucinations	NA	1	2	3	4	5	6	7
4. Conceptual disorganization	NA	1	2	3	4	5	6	7
Each item is scored from 1 (not present) to 7 (extremely severe)							SCORE:	
Brief Negative Symptom Assessment (BNSA)								
Use each item's anchor points to rate the patient								
1. Prolonged time to respond	1	2	3	4	5	6		
2. Emotion: Unchanging facial expression, blank, expressionless face	1	2	3	4	5	6		
3. Reduced social drive	1	2	3	4	5	6		
4. Poor grooming and hygiene	1	2	3	4	5	6		
Each item is scored from 1 (normal) to 6 (severe)					SCORE:			

[a]NA, not able to be assessed.
Data from reference 134.

TABLE 67-10 Antipsychotic Adverse Effects and Monitoring Parameters

Adverse Reaction	Monitoring Parameter	Frequency	Comments
Adverse Effect Monitoring Parameters for all Antipsychotic Medications			
Akathisia	Ask about restless or anxiety. Observe patient for restlessness. Barnes Akathisia Scale can also be used	Every visit	
Anticholinergic side effects	Ask patient about constipation, blurry vision, urinary retention, or unusual dry mouth	Every visit	
Glucose intolerance	FBS or HbA1c	At baseline, after 3 months, and if normal, then annually	
Hyperlipidemia	Lipid profile	At baseline, after 3 months, and if normal, then annually	
Orthostatic hypotension	Ask patient about dizziness on standing. If present, check BP and HR in sitting and standing positions	Every visit	The degree of orthostatic change in BP to produce symptoms varies. In general, a BP change of 20 mm Hg or more is significant
Hyperprolactinemia	In women, ask about expression of milk from the breast and menstrual irregularities. In men, ask about breast enlargement or expression of milk from nipples. If symptoms present, check serum prolactin level	Every visit	In the absence of symptoms, there is no need to monitor serum prolactin
Sedation	Ask patient about unusual sedation or sleepiness	Every visit	
Sexual dysfunction	Ask patient about decreased sexual desire, difficulty being aroused, or problems with orgasm	Every visit	Patients with schizophrenia have more sexual dysfunction than the normal population. Compare symptoms with medication-free state
Tardive dyskinesia	Standardized rating scale such as the AIMS or the DISCUS	At baseline, and then every 3 months for FGAs and every 6 months for SGAs	
Weight gain	Measure body weight, BMI, and waist circumference	At baseline, monthly for the first 3 months, and then quarterly	Waist circumference is the single best predictor of cardiac morbidity
Adverse Effect Monitoring Parameters for Specific Antipsychotics			
Agranulocytosis	White blood cell (WBC) and absolute neutrophil counts (ANC)	At baseline, weekly for 6 months, then every 2 weeks for 6 months, and then monthly	Clozapine only

(*continued*)

TABLE 67-10 Antipsychotic Adverse Effects and Monitoring Parameters (*Continued*)

Adverse Reaction	Monitoring Parameter	Frequency	Comments
Sialorrhea or excess drooling	Ask patient about problems with excess drooling, waking in the morning with a wet ring on his or her pillow. Visual observation of the patient for drooling	Every visit	Clozapine only
Bronchospasm, respiratory distress, respiratory depression, respiratory arrest	Before administration, patients must be screened for a history of asthma, chronic obstructive pulmonary disease, or other lung disease associated with bronchospasm. Monitor patient every 15 minutes for a minimum of 1 hour after drug administration for signs and symptoms of bronchospasm (ie, vital signs and chest auscultation). Only one 10 mg dose can be given every 24 hours	Every dose administration	Inhaled loxapine only. Can only be administered in approved healthcare facilities registered in REMS program
Postinjection sedation/delirium syndrome	Observation of the patient for at least 3 hours after drug administration. Monitor for possible sedation, altered level of consciousness, coma, delirium, confusion, disorientation, agitation, anxiety, or other cognitive impairment	Every dose administration	Long-acting olanzapine pamoate monohydrate only. Can only be administered in approved healthcare facilities registered in REMS program

Similarly, the pharmacotherapeutic plan should include specific monitoring parameters for side effects (Table 67-10). The plan should include how the potential side effect will be evaluated, and the frequency of assessment. Given the risk of weight gain, diabetes, and lipid abnormalities associated with many of the SGAs, a consensus task force led by the American Diabetes Association recommends the following baseline parameters before beginning antipsychotics: family history, weight, height, BMI, waist circumference, blood pressure, fasting plasma glucose, and fasting lipid profile.[83] They also recommend follow-up monitoring of these parameters after beginning or changing SGAs. Weight should be monitored monthly for the first 3 months, and quarterly thereafter. The other parameters should be assessed at the end of 3 months and then annually. Self-assessments can be a useful adjunct in treating the patient. Although the patient with schizophrenia may not always be accurate in evaluating symptom severity, the use of patient self-assessments increases patient engagement in care, enhances therapeutic alliance, and gives the clinician an opportunity to identify misconceptions the patient may have regarding symptoms associated with the illness, medication side effects, and the like.[135] Traditionally, clinicians have often accepted partial symptom response in schizophrenia as success, and have not been aggressive in attempting to achieve greater symptomatic remission. The advent of multiple different SGAs with varying side effect profiles should encourage clinicians to be more assertive in attempting to achieve symptom remission. This is consistent with an increasing focus on remission as a goal of treatment and evolving recovery movements with an emphasis on consumerism in the care of the severely mentally ill.[22]

ABBREVIATIONS

α_1	alpha one adrenergic receptor
ACHIEVE	Randomized Trial of Achieving Healthy Lifestyles in Psychiatric Rehabilitation
ACT	active community treatment
AIMS	Abnormal Involuntary Movement Scale
ANC	absolute neutrophil count
AP	antipsychotic
APA	American Psychiatric Association
AUC	area under the curve
β_2	beta-2 adrenergic receptor
BDNF	brain-derived neurotrophic factor
BLM	buccal–lingual–masticatory
BMI	body mass index
BP	blood pressure
BPRS	Brief Psychiatric Rating Scale
C4	complement component 4 genes
CACN1A2	voltage-dependent Ca channel 1A2
CATIE	Clinical Antipsychotic Trials of Intervention Effectiveness
CK	creatine kinase
CNS	central nervous system
CNV	copy number variant
COMT	catecholamine-*O*-methyl transferase
C_{max}	maximum plasma concentration
CUtLASS-1	Cost Utility of the Latest Antipsychotic drugs in Schizophrenia Study
CYP	cytochrome P450
D_1	dopamine-1 receptor
D_2	dopamine-2 receptor
D_3	dopamine-3 receptor
D_4	dopamine-4 receptor
DA	dopamine
DISCUS	Dyskinesia Identification System: Condensed User Scale
DRESS	Drug Reaction with Eosinophilia and Systemic Symptoms
DSM-5	*Diagnostic and Statistical Manual of Mental Disorders, Fifth Edition*
ECG	electrocardiogram or electrocardiographic
ECT	electroconvulsive therapy
EEG	electroencephalogram
EPS	extrapyramidal side effect
FBS	fasting blood sugar
FDA	Food and Drug Administration
FGA	first-generation antipsychotic
FMO3	flavin containing monooxygenase 3 gene
GABA	γ-aminobutyric acid
GWAS	genome-wide association studies

5-HT	serotonin or 5-hydroxytryptamine
5-HT_{1A}	serotonin-1A receptor
5-HT_{2}	serotonin-2 receptor
5-HT_{2A}	serotonin-2A receptor
5-HT_{2C}	serotonin-2C receptor
5-HT_{6}	Serotonin-6 receptor
5-HT_{7}	Serotonin-7 receptor
HR	heart rate
IM	intramuscular
LAI	Long acting injectable
LBW	low birth weight
MC4R	Melanocortin-4-Receptor
MTHFR	methylenetetrahydrofolate reductase
MSE	mental status examination
NAMI	National Alliance on Mental Illness
NE	norepinephrine
NIMH	National Institute of Mental Health
NMDA	*N*-methyl-D-aspartate
NMS	neuroleptic malignant syndrome
NRGN	neurogranin
PANSS	Positive and Negative Symptom Scale
PDSS	Post-injection delirium/sedation syndrome
PET	positron emission tomography
PORT	Patient Outcomes Research Team
PBRM1	polybromo 1
PSRS	Positive Symptom Rating Scale
RAISE	Recovery After Initial Schizophrenia Episode
REMS	Risk Evaluation and Mitigation Strategy
RNA	ribonucleic acid
SCD	sudden cardiac death
SEs	side effects
SGA	second-generation antipsychotic
SNP	single nucleotide polymorphism
SSRI	selective serotonin reuptake inhibitor
STRIDE	Reducing Weight and Diabetes Risk in an Underserved Population
TCA	tricyclic antidepressant
UGT	UDP glucuronosyltransferases genes
158*Val/Met*	158 valine/methionine
WBC	white blood cell
ZNF804A	zinc finger protein 804A

REFERENCES

1. American Psychiatric Association. Schizophrenia spectrum and other psychotic disorders. In: *Diagnostic and Statistical Manual of Mental Disorders*. 5th ed. Arlington, VA: American Psychiatric Association; 2013:87-122.
2. Weinberger D, Levitt P. Schizophrenia as a neurodevelopmental disorder. In: Weinberger DR, Harrison P, eds. *Schizophrenia*, 3rd ed. Oxford, UK: Wiley-Blackwell; 2011:326-348.
3. Miller BJ, Culpepper N, Rapaport MH, Buckley P. Prenatal inflammation and neurodevelopment in schizophrenia: A review of human studies. *Prog Neuropsychopharmacol Biol Psychiatry* 2013;42:92-100.
4. Krystal JH, Anticevic. Toward illness phase-specific pharmacotherapy for schizophrenia. *Biol Psychiatry* 2015;78:738-740.
5. Benros ME, Nielsen PR, Nordentoft M, et al. Autoimmune diseases and severe infections as risk factors for schizophrenia: A 30-year population-based register study. *Am J Psychiatry* 2011;168:1303-1310.
6. Howes OD, Murray RM. Schizophrenia: An integrated sociodevelopmental cognitive model. *Lancet* 2014;383:1677-1687.
7. Arango C, Rapado-Castro M, Reig S, et al. Progressive brain changes in children and adolescents with first-episode psychosis. *Arch Gen Psychiatry* 2012;69(1):16-26.
8. Lee KW, Woon PS, Teo YY, Sim K. Genome wide studies (GWAS) and copy number variation (CNV) studies of the major psychoses: What have we learnt? *Neurosci Biobehav Rev* 2012;36:556-571.
9. Sekar A, Bialas AR, de Rivera H, et al. Schizophrenia risk from complex variation of complement component 4. *Nature* 2016;530:177-183. doi: 10.1038/nature16549.
10. Cross-Disorder Group of the Psychiatric Genomics Consortium. Identification of risk loci with shared effects on five major psychiatry disorders: A genome-wide analysis. *Lancet* 2013;381(9875):1371-1379.
11. Schizophrenia Working Group of the Psychiatric Genomics Consortium. Biological insights from 108 schizophrenia-associated genetic lock. *Nature* 2014;511(7510):421-427.
12. Kantrowitz J, Javitt DC. Glutamatergic transmission in schizophrenia: From basic research to clinical practice. *Curr Opin Psychiatry* 2012;25:96-102.
13. Shepherd AM, Laurens KR, Matheson SL, et al. Systematic meta-review and quality assessment of the structural brain alterations in schizophrenia. *Neurosci Biobehav Rev* 2012;36:1342-1356.
14. Cannon TD, Chung Y, He G, et al. North American Prodrome Longitudinal Study Consortium. Progressive reduction in cortical thickness as psychosis develops: A multisite longitudinal neuroimaging study of youth at elevated clinical risk. *Biol Psychiatry* 2015;77(2):147-157.
15. Howes OD, Kambeitz J, Kim E, et al. The nature of dopamine dysfunction in schizophrenia and what this means for treatment. *Arch Gen Psychiatry* 2012;69:776-786.
16. Kinon BJ, Millen BA, Zhang L, McKinzie DL. Exploratory analysis for a targeted patient population responsive to the metabotropic glutamate 2/3 receptor agonist pomaglumetad methionil in schizophrenia. *Biol Psychiaty* 2015;78:754-762.
17. Miller BH, Zeier Z, Lanz TA, et al. MicroRNA-132 dysregulation in schizophrenia has implications for both neurodevelopment and adult brain function. *PNAS* 2012;109:3125-3130.
18. Clementz BA, Sweeney J, Keshavan MS, Pearlson G, Tamminga CA. Using biomarker batteries. *Biol Psychiatry* 2015;77(2):90-92.
19. Wright R, Rethelyi JM, Gage FG. Enhancing induced pluripotent stem cell models of schizophrenia. *JAMA Psychiatry* 2014;71(3):334-335.
20. Castle DJ, Buckley PF. *Schizophrenia*. Oxford, UK: Oxford University Press; 2008.
21. Kerner B. Comorbid substance use disorders in schizophrenia: A latent class approach. *Psychiatry Res* 2015;225:395-401.
22. Committee on Crossing the Quality Chasm: Adaptation to Mental Health and Addictive Disorders. *Improving the Quality of Health Care for Mental and Substance-Use Conditions: Quality Chasm Series*. Rockville, MD: Institute of Medicine, National Academies Press; 2005.
23. McGorry PD. The next stage for diagnosis: Validity through utility. *World Psychiatry* 2013;12(3):213-214.
24. Kane JM, Robinson DG, Schooler NR, et al. Comprehensive versus usual community care for first-episode psychosis: 2-Year outcomes from the NIMH RAISE early treatment program. *Am J Psychiatry* 2015;173:362-372. Oct 20:appiajp201515050632.
25. Saperstein AM, Kurtz MM. Current trends in the empirical study of cognitive remediation for schizophrenia. *Can J Psychiatry* 2013;58(6):311-318.
26. Buchanan RW, Kreyenbuhl J, Kelly DL, et al. The 2009 schizophrenia PORT psychopharmacological treatment recommendations and summary statements. *Schizophr Bull* 2010;36:71-93.
27. Osser DN, Roudsari MJ, Manschreck T. The psychopharmacology algorithm project at the Harvard South Shore Program: An update on schizophrenia. *Harvard Review of Psychiatry* 2013;21:18-40.
28. Osser DN (ed.). Psychopharmacology Algorithm Project at the Harvard Medical School Department of Psychiatry, South Shore Program. Available at: *http://www.psychopharm.mobi*. (Accessed November 23, 2015).
29. Hasan A, Falkai P, Wobrock T, et al. World Federation of Societies of Biological Psychiatry (WFSBP) guidelines for the biological treatment of schizophrenia, part 1: Update 2012 on the acute treatment of schizophrenia and the management of treatment resistance. *World J Biol Psychiatry* 2012;13:318-378.
30. Lieberman JA, Stroup S. The NIMH-CATIE schizophrenia study: What did we learn? *Am J Psychiatry* 2011;168:770-775.
31. Kane JM, Schooler NR, Marcy P, Correll CU, Brunette MF, Mueser KT, et al. The RAISE early treatment program for first-episode psychosis: Background, rationale, and study design. *J Clin Psychiatry* 2015;76(3):240-246.
32. Correll CU, Robinson DG, Schooler NR, et al. Cardiometabolic risk in patients with first-episode schizophrenia spectrum disorders: Baseline results from the RAISE-ETP Study. *JAMA Psychiatry* 2014;71(12):1350-1363.

33. Dixon LB, Perkins B, Calmas C. Guideline watch (September 2009): Practice guideline for the treatment of patients with schizophrenia. Psychiatry Online. *http://psychiatryonline.org/content.aspx?bookid=28§ionid=1682213.*
34. Subotnik KL, Casaus LR, Ventura J, et al. Long-acting injectable risperidone for relapse prevention and control of breakthrough symptoms after a recent first episode of schizophrenia. *JAMA Psychiatry* 2015;72:822-829.
35. Carpenter WT, Buchanan RW. Expanding therapy with long-acting antipsychotic medication in patients with schizophrenia. *JAMA Psychiatry* 2015;72:745-746.
36. Muscatello MR, Pandolfo G, Mico U, Lamberti Castronuovo E, Abenavoli E, Spina E, et al. Augmentation of clozapine with ziprasidone in refractory schizophrenia: A double-blind, placebo-controlled study. *J Clin Psychopharmacol* 2014;34(1):129-133.
37. Petrides G, Matur C, Braga RJ, et al. Electroconvulsive therapy augmentation in clozapine-resistant schizophrenia: A prospective, randomized study. *Am J Psychiatry* 2015;172:52-58.
38. Miyamoto S, Jarskog LF, Fleischhacker WW. Schizophrenia: When clozapine fails. *Curr Opin Psychiatry* 2015;28:243-248.
38a. Van Putten T, Marder SR. Behavioral toxicity of antipsychotic drugs. *J Clin Psychiatry* 1987;48(Suppl 9):13-19.
39. Samara MT, Leucht C, Leeflang MM, et al. Early improvement as a predictor of later response to antipsychotics in schizophrenia: A diagnostic test review. *Am J Psychiatry* 2015;172:617-629.
40. Initial REMS Approval. NDA 022549, ADASUVE (Loxapine) Inhalation Powder. Approved Risk and Mitigation Strategies (REMS). U.S. Food and Drug Administration. *http://www.fda.gov/downloads/AdvisoryCommittees/CommitteesMeetingMaterials/Drugs/PsychopharmacologicDrugsAdvisoryCommittee/UCM282900.pdf.*
41. Citrome L. New second-generation long-acting injectable antipsychotics for the treatment of schizophrenia. *Expert Rev Neurother* 2013;13:767-783.
42. Prescribing information. Zyprexa Relprevv. Indianapolis, IN: Lilly USA, December 14, 2014.
43. FDA Drug Safety Communication: FDA is investigating two deaths following injection of long-acting antipsychotic Zyprexa Relprevv (olanzapine pamoate). Available at: *http://www.fda.gov/Drugs/DrugSafety/ucm356971.htm.* Published 6/18/2013; (Accessed July 04, 2015).
44. FDA Drug Safety Communication: FDA review of study sheds light on two deaths associated with the injectable schizophrenia drug Zyprexa Relprevv (olanzapine pamoate). Available at: *http://www.fda.gov/downloads/Drugs/DrugSafety/UCM439343.*pdf. Published 3/23/2015; (Accessed July 04, 2015).
45. Prescribing information. *Invega Trinza.* Titusville, NJ: Janssen Pharmaceuticals Inc., May, 2015.
46. Prescribing information. *Aristada.* Waltham, MA: Alkermes Inc., October 2015.
47. Ereshefsky L, Saklad SR, Jann MW, et al. Future of depot neuroleptic therapy: Pharmacokinetics and pharmacodynamic approaches. *J Clin Psychiatry* 1984;45(5 pt. 2):50-59.
48. Barkhof E, Meijer CJ, de Sonneville LMJ, et al. Interventions to improve adherence to antipsychotic medications in patients with schizophrenia—A review of the past decade. *Eur Psychiatry* 2012;27:9-18.
49. Kane J, Honigfeld G, Singer J, et al. Clozapine for the treatment-resistant schizophrenic: A double-blind comparison with chlorpromazine. *Arch Gen Psychiatry* 1988;45:789-796.
50. Casey DE, Daniel DG, Wassef AA, et al. Effect of divalproex combined with olanzapine or risperidone in patients with an acute exacerbation of schizophrenia. *Neuropsychopharmacology* 2003;28:182-192.
51. Kapur S, Roy P, Daskalakis J, Remington G. Increased dopamine D_2 receptor occupancy and elevated prolactin level associated with addition of haloperidol to clozapine. *Am J Psychiatry* 2001;158:311-314.
52. Velligan DI, Carroll C, Lage MJ, Fairman K. Outcomes of Medicaid beneficiaries with schizophrenia receiving clozapine only or antipsychotic combinations. *Psychiatr Serv* 2015;66(2):127-133.
53. Buckley P, Citrome L, Nichita C, Vitacco M. Psychopharmacology of aggression in schizophrenia. *Schizophr Bull* 2011;37:930-936.
54. Fazel S, Gulati G, Linsell L, Geddes J, Grann M. Schizophrenia and violence: Systematic review and meta-analysis. *PLoS Med* 2009;6(8):e1000120.
55. Miyamoto S, Miyake N, Jarskog LF, Fleischhacker WW, Lieberman JA. Pharmacological treatment of schizophrenia: A critical review of the pharmacology and clinical effects of current and future therapeutic agents. *Mol Psychiatry* 2012;17:1206-1227.
56. Maeda K, Sugino H, Akazawa H, et al. Brexpiprazole I: In vitro and in vivo characterization of a novel serotonin-dopamine activity modulator. *J Pharmacol Exp Ther* 2014;350:589-604.
57. Kapur S, Zipursky RB, Remington G. Clinical and theoretical implications of 5-HT_2 and D_2 receptor occupancy of clozapine, risperidone, and olanzapine in schizophrenia. *Am J Psychiatry* 1999;156:286-293.
58. Citrome L. Iloperidone for schizophrenia: A review of the efficacy and safety profile for this newly commercialized second-generation antipsychotic. *Int J Clin Pract* 2009;63:1237-1248.
59. Citrome L. Asenapine for schizophrenia and bipolar disorder: A review of the efficacy and safety profile for this newly approved sublingually absorbed second-generation antipsychotic. *Int J Clin Pract* 2009;63:1762-1784.
60. McCormack PL. Cariprazine: First global approval. *Drugs* 2015;75:2035-2043.
61. Mauri MC, Volonteri LS, Colasanti A, et al. Clinical pharmacokinetics of atypical antipsychotics: A critical review of the relationship between plasma concentrations and clinical response. *Clin Pharmacokinet* 2007;46:359-388.
62. Pouget JG, Shams TA, Tiwari, Muller DJ. Pharmacogenetics and outcome with antipsychotic drugs. *Dialogues Clin Neurosci* 2014;16:555-566.
63. Prescribing information. *Rexulti.* Tokyo, Japan: Otsuka pharmaceutical Co, Ltd July, 2015.
64. Preskorn SH. Clinically important differences in the pharmacokinetics of the ten newer atypical antipsychotics: Part 2. Metabolism and elimination. *J Psychiatr Pract* 2012;18:361-368.
65. Brennan MD. Pharmacogenetics of second-generation antipsychotics. *Pharmacogenomics.* 2014;15:869-84.
66. Milano W, D'Acunto CW, De Rosa M, et al. Recent clinical aspects of hyperprolactinemia induced by antipsychotics. *Rev Recent Clin Trials* 2011;6(1):52-63.
67. Wong-Anuchit C. Clinical management of antipsychotic-induced hyperprolactinemia. *Perspect Psychiatr Care* 2015;52:145-152. doi: 10.1111/ppc.12111. [Epub ahead of print]
68. Kinon BJ, Liu-Seifert H, Stauffer VL, Jacob J. Bone loss associated with hyperprolactinemia in schizophrenia. *Clin Schizophr Relat Psychoses* 2013;7:114-123.
69. Citrome L. Lurasidone for schizophrenia: A review of the efficacy and safety profile for this newly approved second-generation antipsychotic. *Int J Clin Pract* 2011;65:189-210.
70. Meng M, Li W, Zhang S, et al. Using aripiprazole to reduce antipsychotic-induced hyperprolactinemia: Meta-analysis of currently available randomized controlled trials. *Shanghai Arch Psychiatry* 2015;27(1):4-17.
71. Correll CU, Manu P, Olshanskiy V, et al. Cardiometabolic risk of second-generation antipsychotic medications during first-time use in children and adolescents. *JAMA* 2009;302:1765-1773.
72. Monteleone P, Martiadis V, Maj M. Management of schizophrenia with obesity, metabolic and endocrinological disorders. *Psychiatr Clin North Am* 2009;32:775-794.
73. Tek C, Kucukgoncu S, Guloksuz S, Woods SW, Srihari VH, Annamalai A. Antipsychotic induced weight Gain in First Episode Psychosis patients: A Meta-Analysis of Differential effects of antipsychotic medications. *Early Interv Psychiatry* 2015;10:193-202. doi: 10.1111/eip.12251. [Epub ahead of print]
74. Ganguli R, Strassing M. Prevention of metabolic syndrome in serious mental illness. *Psychiatr Clin North Am* 2011;34(1):109-125.
75. Velligan DI, Weiden PJ, Sajatovic M, et al. The expert consensus guideline series: Adherence problems in patients with serious and persistent mental illness. *J Clin Psychiatry* 2009;70:1-48.
76. De Luca V, Mueller DJ, de Bartolomeis A, et al. Association of the HTR2C gene and antipsychotic induced weight gain: A meta-analysis. *Int J Neuropsychopharmacol* 2007;10(5):697-704.
77. Kao AC, Muller DJ. Genetics of antipsychotic-induced weight gain: Update and current perspectives. *Pharmacogenomics* 2013;14:2067-2083.
78. Shams TA, Müller DJ. Antipsychotic-induced weight gain: Genetics, epigenetics and biomarkers reviewed. *Curr Psychiatry Rep* 2014;16(10):473. doi:10.1007/s11920-014-0473-9.
79. Stroup TS, McEvoy JP, King KD, et al. Schizophrenia trials network. A randomized trial comparing the effectiveness of switching from olanzapine, quetiapine, or risperidone to aripiprazole to reduce metabolic risk: Comparison of antipsychotics for metabolic problems (CAMP). *Am J Psychiatry* 2011;168:947-956.
80. Mizuno Y, Suzuki T, Nakagawa A, et al. Pharmacological strategies to counteract antipsychotic-induced weight gain and metabolic adverse

effects in schizophrenia: A systematic review and meta-analysis. *Schizophr Bull* 2014;1385-13403.

81. Wani RA, Dar MA, Margoob MA, Rather YH, Haq I, Shah MS. Diabetes mellitus and impaired glucose tolerance in patients with schizophrenia, before and after antipsychotic treatment. *J Neurosci Rural Pract* 2015;6(1):17-22.
82. Green CA, Yarborough BJ, Leo MC, Yarborough MT, Stumbo SP, Janoff SL, et al. The STRIDE weight loss and lifestyle intervention for individuals taking antipsychotic medications: A randomized trial. *Am J Psychiatry* 2015;172(1):71-81.
83. American Diabetes Association. Consensus development conference on antipsychotic drugs and obesity and diabetes. *Diabetes Care* 2004;27:596-601.
84. Gugger J. Antipsychotic pharmacotherapy and orthostatic hypotension: Identification and management. *CNS Drugs* 2011;25:659-671.
85. Leung JY, Barr AM, Procyshyn RM, Honer WG, Pang CC. Cardiovascular side-effects of antipsychotic drugs: The role of the autonomic nervous system. *Pharmacol Ther* 2012 Aug;135(2):113-22.
86. Nielsen J, Graff C, Kanters J, et al. Assessing QT interval prolongation and its associated risks with antipsychotics. *CNS Drugs* 2011;25:473-490.
87. Mackin P. Cardiac side effects of psychiatric drugs. *Hum Psychopharmacol* 2008;23:3-14.
88. Hasnain M, Vieweg WVR. QTc interval prolongation and torsades de pointes associated with second generation antipsychotics and antidepressants: A comprehensive review. *CNS Drugs* 2014;28:887-920.
89. Wenzel-Seifert K, Wittmann M, Haen E. QTc prolongation by psychotropic drugs and the risk of torsade de pointes. *Dtsch Arztebl Int* 2011;108:687-693.
90. Shah AA, Aftab A, Coverdale J. QTc prolongation with antipsychotics: Is routine ECG monitoring recommended? *J Psychiatr Pract* 2014;20(3):196-206.
91. Weinmann S, Read J, Aderhold V. Influence of antipsychotics on mortality in schizophrenia: Systematic review. *Schizophr Res* 2009;113(1):1-11.
92. Wu CS, Tsai YT, Tsai HJ. Antipsychotic drugs and the risk of ventricular arrhythmia and/or sudden cardiac death: A nationwide case-crossover study. *J Am Heart Assoc* 2015;4(2). pii: e001568. doi: 10.1161/JAHA.114.001568.
93. Ferno J, Skrede S, Vik-Mo AO, et al. Lipogenic effects of psychotropic drugs: Focus on the SREBP system. *Front Biosci* 2011;16:49-60.
94. McEvoy JP, Meyer JM, Goff DC, et al. Prevalence of the metabolic syndrome in patients with schizophrenia: Baseline results from the Clinical Antipsychotic Trials of Intervention Effectiveness (CATIE) schizophrenia trial and comparison with national estimates from NHANES III. *Schizophr Res* 2005;80(1):19-32.
95. Burkhard PR. Acute and subacute drug-induced movement disorders. *Parkinsonism Relat Disord* 2014;20S1:S108-S112.
96. Haddad PM, Dursun SM. Neurological complications of psychiatric drugs: Clinical features and management. *Hum Psychopharmacol* 2008;23:15-26.
97. Agarkar S, Anthony D, Ferrando S. Risk of Akathisia associated with Atypical Antipsychotics. *J Neuropsychiatry Clin Neurosci* 2013;25(1):E46-E47.
98. Peluso M, Lewis S, Barnes T, et al. Extrapyramidal motor side-effects of first and second-generation antipsychotic drugs. *Br J Psychiatry* 2012;200:387-392.
99. Caplan JP, Epstein LA, Quinn DK, et al. Neuropsychiatric effects of prescription drug abuse. *Neuropsychol Rev* 2007;17:363-380.
100. Di Fabio R, De Filippis S, Cafariello C, Penna L, Marianetti M, Serrao M, et al. Low doses of rotigotine in patients with antipsychotic-induced parkinsonism. *Clin Neuropharmacol* 2013;36(5):162-165.
101. Aquino CCH, Lang AE. Tardive dyskinesia syndromes: Current concepts. *Parkinsonism Relat Disord* 2014;20S1:S113-S117.
102. Sprague RL, Kalachnik JE. Reliability, validity, and a total score cutoff for the Dyskinesia Identification System Condensed User Scale (DISCUS) with mentally ill and mentally retarded populations. *Psychopharmacol Bull* 1991;27:51-58.
103. Correll CU, Schenk EM. Tardive dyskinesia and new antipsychotics. *Curr Opin Psychiatry* 2008;21:151-156.
104. Bhidayasiri R, Fahn S, Gronseth GS, et al. Evidence-based guideline: Treatment of tardive syndromes: report of the guideline development subcommittee of the American Academy of Neurology. *Neurology* 2013;81:463-469.
105. Keefe RS, Bilder RM, Davis SM, et al. Neurocognitive effects of antipsychotic medications in patients with chronic schizophrenia in the CATIE trial. *Arch Gen Psychiatry* 2007;64:633-647.
106. Paden MS, Franjic L, Halcomb SE. Hyperthermia caused by drug interactions and adverse reactions. *Am J Health Syst Pharm* 2013;70:34-42.
107. Robottom B, Shulam LM, Weiner WJ. Drug induced movement disorders: Emergencies and management. *Neurol Clin* 2012;30:309-320.
108. Jackson N, Doherty J, Coulter S. Neuropsychiatric complications of commonly used palliative care drugs. *Postgrad Med J* 2008;84:121-126.
109. Li J, Tripathi RC, Tripathi BJ. Drug-induced ocular disorders. *Drug Saf* 2008;31:127-141.
110. Laties AM, Flach AJ, Baldycheva I, et al. Cataractogenic potential of quetiapine versus risperidone in long-term treatment of patients with schizophrenia or schizoaffective disorder: A randomized open-label, ophthalmologist-masked, flexible-dose, non-inferiority trial. *J Psychopharmacol* 2015;29:69-79.
111. Verhamme KM, Sturkenboom MC, Stricker BH, Bosch R. Drug-induced urinary retention: Incidence, management, and prevention. *Drug Saf* 2008;31:373-388.
112. Saddichha S, Kumar M. Antipsychotic-induced urinary dysfunction: Anticholinergic effect or otherwise? *BMJ Case Rep* 2009; doi: 10.1136/bcr.02.2009.1547. Epub 2009 May 21.
113. Rettenbacher MA, Hofer A, Ebenbichler C, et al. Prolactin levels and sexual adverse effects in patients with schizophrenia during antipsychotic treatment. *J Clin Psychopharmacol* 2010;30:711-715.
114. Andersohn F, Schmedt N, Weinmann S, et al. Priapism associated with antipsychotics: Role of alpha1 adrenoceptor affinity. *J Clin Psychopharmacol* 2010;30:68-71.
115. Hasan A, Falkai P, Wobrock T, et al. World Federation of Societies of Biological Psychiatry (WFSBP) guidelines for biological treatment of schizophrenia, part 2: Update 2012 on the long-term treatment of schizophrenia and management of antipsychotic induced side effects. *World J Biol Psychiatry* 2013;14:2-44.
116. Clozapine FDA prescribing information. Teva Pharmaceuticals, revised 11/2015.
117. FDA Drug Safety Communication: FDA reporting mental health drug ziprasidone (Geodon) associated with rare but potentially fatal skin reactions: 2014, Available at: *http://www.fda.gov/Drugs/DrugSafety/ucm426391.htm*. (Accessed June 1, 2015).
118. Bird AM, Smith TL, Walton AE, Current treatment strategies for clozapine-induced sialorrhea. *Ann Pharmacother* 2011;45:667-75.
119. Levine M, Ruha AM. Overdose of atypical antipsychotics: Clinical presentation, mechanisms of toxicity and management. *CNS Drugs* 2012;26:601-611.
120. Lin HC, Chen IJ, Chen YH, et al. Maternal schizophrenia and pregnancy outcome: Does the use of antipsychotics make a difference? *Schizophr Res* 2010;116(1):55-60.
121. Einarson A, Boskovic R. Use and safety of antipsychotic drugs during pregnancy. *J Psychiatr Pract* 2009;15(3):183-192.
122. Terrana N, Koren G, Pivovarov J, Etwel F, Nulman I. Pregnancy outcomes following in utero exposure to second-generation antipsychotics: A systematic review and meta-analysis. *J Clin Psychopharmacol* 2015;35:559-565.
123. Bodén R, Lundgren M, Brandt L, et al. Antipsychotics during pregnancy: Relation to fetal and maternal metabolic effects. *Arch Gen Psychiatry* 2012;69:715-721.
124. Vigod SN, Gomes T, Wilton AS, Taylor VH, Ray JG. Antipsychotic drug use in pregnancy: High dimensional, propensity matched, population based cohort study. *BMJ* 2015;359. h2298 doi 10.1136/bmj.h2298.
125. Antipsychotics and Pregnancy, Safety Announcement. U.S. Food and Drug Administration, 2011. Available at: *http://www.fda.gov/Drugs/DrugSafety/ucm243903.htm*.
126. Parikh T, Goyal D, Scarff JR, Lippmann S. Antipsychotic drugs and safety concerns for breast-feeding infants. *South Med J* 2014;107(11):686-688.
127. Yoshida K, Smith B, Craggs M, et al. Neuroleptic drugs in breast milk: A study of pharmacokinetics and of possible adverse effects in breast fed infants. *Psychol Med* 1998;28:81-91.
128. Ereshefsky L. Drug–drug interactions with the use of psychotropic medications. *CNS Spectr* 2009;14(Suppl 8):1-8.
129. Gaertner J, Ruberg K, Schlesiger G, Frechan S, Voltz R. Drug interactions in palliative care—it's more than cytochrome P450. *Palliat Med* 2012;26:813-825.
130. Kennedy WK, Jann MW, Kutscher EC. Clinically significant drug interactions with atypical antipsychotics. *CNS Drugs* 2013;27:1021-1048.

131. Fijal BA, Stauffer VL, Kinon BJ, et al. Analysis of gene variants previously associated with iloperidone response in patients with schizophrenia who are treated with risperidone. *J Clin Psychiatry* 2012;73:367-371.
132. Pouget JG, Shams TA, Tiwari AK, Muller DJ. Pharmacogenetics and outcome with antipsychotic drugs. *Dialogues Clin Neurosci* 2014;16:555-566.
133. Rubin R. Precision medicine: The future or simply politics? *JAMA* 2015;313(11):1089-1091.
134. Velligan DI, Lopez L, Castillo DA, et al. Interrater reliability of using brief standardized outcome measures in a community mental health setting. *Psychiatr Serv* 2011;62:558-560.
135. Velligan DI, Weiden PJ, Sajatovic M, et al. Strategies for addressing adherence problems for patients with serious and persistent mental illness: Recommendations from the expert guideline series. *J Psychiatr Pract* 2010;16:306-324.
136. van Os J. The many continua of psychosis. *JAMA Psychiatry* 2014;71(9):985-986.

68

Major Depressive Disorder

Christian J. Teter, Judith C. Kando, and Barbara G. Wells

KEY CONCEPTS

1. Extensive treatment guidelines are available to assist in the treatment of major depressive disorder, including medication management. Clinicians treating individuals with major depressive disorder should be familiar with these guidelines.
2. When evaluating a patient for the presence of depression, it is essential to rule out medical causes of depression and drug-induced depression.
3. The goals of treatment for depression are the resolution of current symptoms (ie, remission) and the prevention of further episodes of depression (ie, relapse or recurrence).
4. When counseling patients with depression who are receiving antidepressant medications, the patient should be informed that adverse effects might occur immediately, while resolution of symptoms may take 2 to 4 weeks or longer. Adherence to the treatment plan is essential for a successful outcome, and tools to help increase medication adherence should be discussed with each patient.
5. Antidepressants are generally considered equally efficacious in groups of patients with major depressive disorder. Therefore, other factors, such as age, side effect profile, and past history of response, are used to guide the selection of antidepressants.
6. When determining if a patient has been nonresponsive to a particular pharmacotherapeutic intervention, it must be determined whether the patient has received an adequate dose for an adequate duration and whether the patient has been medication adherent.
7. Pharmacogenetic tests (eg, the FDA-approved AmpliChip to evaluate CYP2D6 and CYP2C19 polymorphisms) are now commercially available. However, there are no standard or well-accepted recommendations for the use of pharmacogenetic testing as it relates to antidepressant treatment of major depressive disorder.
8. When evaluating response to an antidepressant, in addition to target signs and symptoms, the clinician must consider quality-of-life issues, such as role, social, and occupational functioning. In addition, the tolerability of the agent should be assessed because the occurrence of side effects may lead to medication nonadherence, especially given the chronicity of the disease and need for long-term medication management.

A diagnosis of major depressive disorder (MDD) is given when an individual experiences one or more major depressive episodes without a history of a manic or hypomanic episode. A major depressive episode is defined by the criteria listed in the *Diagnostic and Statistical Manual of Mental Disorders, Fifth Edition* (*DSM-5*).[1] Depression is associated with significant functional disability, morbidity, and mortality. Newer generations of antidepressants, such as the selective serotonin reuptake inhibitors (SSRIs), are effective and better tolerated than older agents, such as the tricyclic antidepressants (TCAs) and the monoamine oxidase inhibitors (MAOIs). In addition, substantial efforts have been undertaken to improve the ability of clinicians to recognize and appropriately treat the signs and symptoms of depression. This chapter focuses exclusively on the diagnosis and treatment of MDD.

(1) In the absence of well-accepted evidence-based medicine for the medication management of MDD, the reader is referred to the *Practice Guideline for the Treatment of Patients with Major Depressive Disorder*, which is available at *www.psych.org*. This extensive document (now available in its third iteration) is a practical guide to the management of depression based on the best available data as well as clinical consensus.[2] Alternatively, the reader should refer to the British Association of Psychopharmacology (BAP) guidelines, which provide a complementary data-driven viewpoint on antidepressant treatment for MDD.[3]

EPIDEMIOLOGY

The true prevalence of depressive disorders in the United States is unknown. The National Comorbidity Survey Replication found that 16.2% of the population studied had a history of MDD in their lifetime, and more than 6.6% had an episode within the past 12 months.[4] Women have a higher risk of depression than men from early adolescence until their mid-50s, with a lifetime rate that is 1.7 to 2.7 times greater.[5] Although depression can occur at any age, adults 18 to 29 years of age experience the highest rates of major depression during any given year.[4] The estimated lifetime prevalence of major depression in individuals aged 65 to 80 recently was reported to be 20.4% in women and 9.6% in men.[6] Depressive disorders are common during adolescence, with comorbid substance abuse, suicide attempts, and deaths occurring frequently in these young patients.[7,8] Depressive disorders and suicide tend to occur within families. For example, approximately 8% to 18% of patients with major depression have at least one first-degree relative (father, mother, brother, or sister) with a history of depression, compared with 5.6% of those without depression.[9] Furthermore, first-degree relatives of patients with depression are 1.5 to 3 times more likely to develop depression than normal controls.[1,9] A recent meta-analysis found that the heritability of liability for major depression was 37%, whereas the remaining 63% of the variance in liability was due to individual-specific environment.[10] Therefore, MDD is relatively common, occurs more frequently in women than in men, and prevalence is influenced by both genetic and environmental factors.

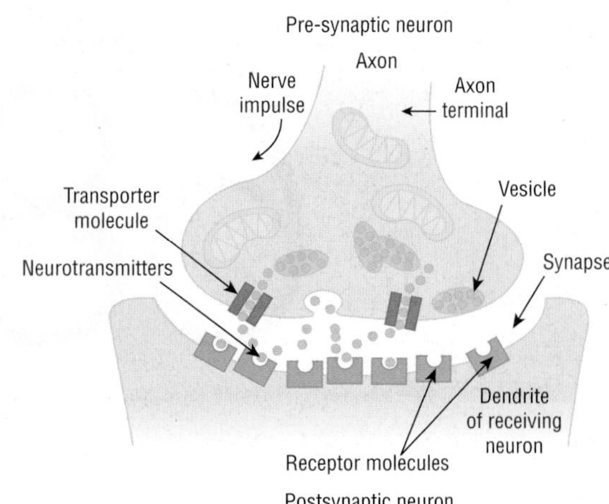

FIGURE 68-1 Monoamine neurotransmitter (NT) regulation at the neuronal level. NTs carry messages between cells. Each NT generally binds to a specific receptor, and this coupling initiates a cascade of events. NTs are reabsorbed back into nerve cells by reuptake pumps (ie, transporter molecules) at which point they may be recycled for later use or broken down by enzymes. For their primary mechanism of action, most antidepressants are thought to inhibit the transporter molecules and allow more NT to remain in the synapse. *(Reproduced from Mind Over Matter. NIH Publication No. 09-7423. The National Institute on Drug Abuse, National Institutes of Health, U.S. Department of Health and Human Services. Printed 2009.)*

ETIOLOGY

The etiology of depressive disorders is too complex to be totally explained by a single social, developmental, or biologic theory. Several factors appear to work together to cause or precipitate depressive disorders. The symptoms reported by patients with MDD consistently reflect changes in brain monoamine neurotransmitters (NTs), specifically norepinephrine (NE), serotonin (5-HT), and dopamine (DA).[11,12] See Figure 68-1 for a visual explanation of how these monoamine NTs are regulated at the level of the neuron and within the synapse.

PATHOPHYSIOLOGY

Several years before the introduction of antidepressants, the cause of depression was linked to decreased brain levels of the NTs NE, 5-HT, and DA, although the actual cause remains unknown. This biogenic amine hypothesis evolved as a result of several observations made in the early 1950s. It was noted that the antihypertensive drug reserpine depleted neuronal storage granules of NE, 5-HT, and DA and produced clinically significant depression in 15% or more of patients.[13]

Although the reuptake blockade of monoamines (eg, NE, DA, and 5-HT) occurs immediately on administration of an antidepressant, the clinical antidepressant effects (ie, measurable improvement) are generally delayed by weeks.[11,14] This delay may be the result of a cascade of events from receptor occupancy to gene transcription.[15] This delay in onset of action has caused researchers to focus on the adaptive changes induced by antidepressants. Accordingly, theories that focus on adaptive (or chronic) changes in amine receptor systems have emerged. In the mid-1970s, it was recognized that chronic, but not acute, administration of antidepressants to animals caused desensitization of NE-stimulated cyclic adenosine monophosphate synthesis. In fact, for most antidepressants, downregulation of β-adrenergic receptors accompanies this desensitization.[16] Studies of many antidepressants have demonstrated that either desensitization or downregulation of NE receptors corresponds to a clinically relevant time course for antidepressant effects.[11] Other studies have revealed desensitization of presynaptic 5-HT_{1A} autoreceptors following chronic administration of antidepressants.[17] Thus, a theory based on changes in receptor sensitivity provides a cogent explanation of the delayed onset of therapeutic response of antidepressant drugs. The dysregulation hypothesis incorporates the diversity of antidepressant activity with the adaptive changes occurring in receptor sensitization over several weeks. In this theory, emphasis is placed on a failure of homeostatic regulation of NT systems rather than on absolute increases or decreases in their activities. According to this hypothesis, effective antidepressant agents restore efficient regulation to the dysregulated NT system.[18]

The 5-HT/NE link hypothesis maintains that both the serotonergic and noradrenergic systems are involved in an antidepressant response.[16] This hypothesis is consistent with the rationale of the postsynaptic alteration theory of depression, which emphasizes the importance of β-adrenergic receptor downregulation for achieving an antidepressant effect.[16] Furthermore, both serotonergic and noradrenergic medications downregulate β-adrenergic receptors, and there is a link between 5-HT and NE.[16] This implies that medications that are effective in the treatment of depression act at both of these NT systems.

Traditional explanations of the biologic basis of depressive disorders have focused largely on NE and 5-HT; however, most of the evidence that coalesced into the biogenic amine hypothesis of depression does not clearly distinguish between NE and DA. There is an abundance of evidence suggesting that DA transmission is decreased in depression and that agents that increase dopaminergic transmission have been found to be effective antidepressants.[19] Specifically, studies suggest that increased DA transmission in the mesolimbic pathway accounts for at least part of the mechanism of action of antidepressant medications.[19] The mechanisms by which antidepressant drugs alter DA transmission remain unclear, but may be mediated either directly by dopaminergic changes or indirectly by primary actions at NE or 5-HT terminals. The complexity of the interaction between 5-HT, NE, and DA is gaining greater appreciation, but a more in-depth understanding of the precise mechanism is needed. Furthermore, the availability of dopaminergic-based first-line and augmentation antidepressant strategies has been slowly growing (eg, bupropion, high-dose venlafaxine, aripiprazole, and most recently brexpiprazole).

More recent insight into the many possible mechanisms underlying depressive disorders comes from studies on brain-derived neurotrophic factor (BDNF). BDNF is a growth factor protein that regulates the differentiation and survival of neurons. A growing body of evidence suggests this process might be disrupted in depressive disorders. More specifically, chronic stress and an associated increase in glucocorticoids such as cortisol may cause a disruption of BDNF expression in the hippocampus. This process may be prevented, or possibly even reversed, by antidepressant medications.[20] This relatively recent theory has not been firmly established; however, if validated, it will demonstrate that antidepressants may help prevent deleterious effects of chronic stress and depressive symptoms. It also highlights the fact that antidepressants may work by a mechanism that is not yet evident at this time, as we continue to learn more about the complexities of major depression and its treatment.

Biologic Markers

Investigators continue to search for biologic or pharmacodynamic (PD) markers to assist in the diagnosis and treatment of depressed patients. Although no biologic marker has been discovered, several biologic abnormalities are present in many depressed patients. Approximately 45% to 60% of patients with major depression have a neuroendocrine abnormality, including hypersecretion of cortisol or a lack of cortisol suppression after dexamethasone administration (ie, a positive dexamethasone suppression test). In fact, it has been suggested that the inability of the brain to suppress the hypothalamic–pituitary–adrenal (HPA) axis and the associated stress response could lead to the pathophysiology and symptoms of depression.[21] According to this theory, there is a disruption somewhere in the normal negative feedback system that controls cortisol levels (see Fig. 76-3 for a representation of this negative feedback system). There are many potential negative consequences of excess circulating cortisol, including disruption in BDNF expression as discussed above.

Unfortunately, the high rate of false-positive and false-negative results associated with neuroendocrine abnormalities in depressed patients limits the usefulness of testing for these markers, and has led to their relative lack of use in clinical practice. However, they still provide a clue to the potential pathophysiology of depressive disorders, which may lead us to more effective treatment options.

CLINICAL PRESENTATION

2 When a patient presents with depressive symptoms, it is necessary to investigate the possibility of a contributing medical or drug-induced etiology. All depressed patients should have a complete physical examination, mental status examination, and basic laboratory workup, including a complete blood count with differential, thyroid function tests, and electrolyte determinations, to identify any potential medical problems. A listing of all possible medical conditions associated with depression is beyond the scope of this chapter. The *DSM-5* describes a diagnostic category for both "Depressive Disorder Due to Another Medical Condition" and "Substance/Medication-Induced Depressive Disorder,"[1] which are common causative factors for depressive symptoms. For example, multiple medical conditions (eg, stroke, Parkinson disease, traumatic brain injury, and hypothyroidism) have strong associations with the development of depressive symptoms.[1] Furthermore, individuals experiencing withdrawal from substances of abuse (eg, cocaine) commonly present with depressive symptoms.[1]

Table 68-1 lists medications commonly associated with causing or exacerbating depressive symptoms.[2,22,23] A complete medication review should be performed because several medications (in addition to those listed in Table 68-1) may contribute to depressive symptoms. Once a medical condition or concomitant medication has been ruled out as the cause of the depressive symptoms, the patient should be evaluated for MDD. According to the *DSM-5*, a single major depressive episode is characterized by five (or more) of the symptoms described in Table 68-2. At least one of the symptoms is depressed mood (often an irritable mood in children or adolescents) or loss of interest or pleasure in nearly all activities.[1] These symptoms must have been present nearly every day for at least 2 weeks and must represent a change from the patient's previous level of functioning. The DSM-5 *omits* the bereavement exclusion that appeared in earlier DSM editions. Some feel that this omission opens the door to misdiagnosis of normal grief as MDD. The diagnostic code for MDD is determined by whether this is a single or recurrent depressive episode, current severity, presence of psychotic features, and remission status. The diagnosis can be followed by specifiers that apply to the current episode. The possible specifiers include anxious distress, mixed features (ie, presence of some manic/hypomanic features), melancholic features, atypical features, mood-congruent or incongruent psychotic features, catatonia, peripartum onset, and seasonal pattern. The clinician must consider presenting symptoms, their duration, and the patient's current level of social, occupational, or other important areas of functioning. Significant stressors or life events may trigger depression in some individuals but not others, and there may be an important precipitant at the beginning of the disorder.[1]

TABLE 68-1 Selected Medications Associated with Drug-Induced Depressive Symptoms

Acne treatment
Isotretinoin
Anticonvulsants
Levetiracetam
Topiramate
Vigabatrin
Antimigraine agents
Triptans
Cardiovascular medications
β-Blocker
Clonidine
Methyldopa
Reserpine
Hormonal therapy
Gonadotropin-releasing hormone
Oral contraceptives
Steroids (eg, prednisone)
Tamoxifen
Immunologic agents
Interferons
Smoking cessation medications
Varenicline

Data from references 2, 22, 23.

Depression Rating Scales

Instruments to assess the severity of depressive symptoms can be used for both clinical and research purposes. For example, the Montgomery-Åsberg Depression Rating Scale (MADRS) is a clinician-administered scale that is commonly used in drug trials given its sensitivity to change.[24] Some depression rating scales are self-administered. For example, the Beck Depression Inventory (BDI) takes only 5 to 10 minutes to complete by the respondent.[25] For a more detailed explanation for both of these instruments, as well as other rating scales and evaluation approaches, refer to Chapter e62.

Emotional Symptoms

A major depressive episode is characterized by a persistent, diminished ability to experience pleasure. A loss of interest and pleasure in usual activities, hobbies, or work is common. Patients appear sad or depressed, and they are often pessimistic and believe that nothing will help them feel better. Anxiety symptoms are present in almost 90% of depressed outpatients. The presence of feelings of worthlessness or inappropriate guilt may identify patients at risk for suicide.[26] Patients often have guilt feelings that are unrealistic, and these may reach delusional proportions. Patients may feel that they deserve punishment and may view their present illness as a punishment. A patient suffering from major depression with psychotic features may hear voices (auditory hallucinations) saying that he or she is a bad person and that he or she should commit suicide. Depression with psychotic features may require hospitalization, especially if the patient becomes a danger to self or others.

Physical Symptoms

Physical symptoms often motivate patients, especially the elderly, to seek medical attention. Chronic fatigue is a common complaint, with a decreased ability to perform normal daily tasks. Fatigue often appears worse in the morning and does not improve with rest. Complaints of pain, especially headache, often accompany fatigue.

Sleep disturbances generally present as frequent early morning awakening with difficulty returning to sleep. This may coexist

TABLE 68-2 DSM-5 Diagnostic Criteria for Major Depressive Disorder

A. Five (or more) of the following symptoms have been present during the same 2-week period and represent a change from previous functioning; at least one of the symptoms is either (1) depressed mood or (2) loss of interest or pleasure.
Note: Do not include symptoms that are clearly attributable to another medical condition.
1. Depressed mood most of the day, nearly every day, as indicated by either subjective report (eg, feels sad, empty, and hopeless) or observation made by others (eg, appears tearful). (**Note:** In children and adolescents, can be irritable mood.)
2. Markedly diminished interest or pleasure in all, or almost all, activities most of the day, nearly every day. (as indicated by either subjective account or observation.)
3. Significant weight loss when not dieting or weight gain (eg, a change of more than 5% of body weight in a month), or decrease or increase in appetite nearly every day. (**Note:** In children, consider failure to make expected weight gain.)
4. Insomnia or hypersomnia nearly every day.
5. Psychomotor agitation or retardation nearly every day. (observable by others, not merely subjective feelings of restlessness or being slowed down.)
6. Fatigue or loss of energy nearly every day.
7. Feelings of worthlessness or excessive or inappropriate guilt (which may be delusional) nearly every day. (not merely self-reproach or guilt about being sick.)
8. Diminished ability to think or concentrate, or indecisiveness, nearly every day (either by subjective account or as observed by others.)
9. Recurrent thoughts of death (not just fear of dying), recurrent suicidal ideation without a specific plan, or a suicide attempt or a specific plan for committing suicide.

B. The symptoms cause clinically significant distress or impairment in social, occupational, or other important areas of functioning.

C. The episode is not attributable to the physiological effects of a substance or to another medical condition.
Note: Criteria A–C represent a major depressive episode.
Note: Responses to a significant loss (eg, bereavement, financial ruin, losses from a natural disaster, a serious medical illness or disability) may include the feelings of intense sadness, rumination about the loss, insomnia, poor appetite, and weight loss noted in Criterion A, which may resemble a depressive episode. Although such symptoms may be understandable or considered appropriate to the loss, the presence of a major depressive episode in addition to the normal response to a significant loss should also be carefully considered. This decision inevitably requires the exercise of clinical judgment based on the individual's history and the cultural norms for the expression of distress in the context of loss.
In distinguishing grief from a major depressive episode (MDE), it is useful to consider that in grief the predominant affect is feelings of emptiness and loss, while in MDE it is persistent depressed mood and the inability to anticipate happiness or pleasure. The dysphoria in grief is likely to decrease in intensity over days to weeks and occurs in waves, the so-called pangs of grief. These waves tend to be associated with thoughts or reminders of the deceased. The depressed mood of MDE is more persistent and not tied to specific thoughts or preoccupations. The pain of grief may be accompanied by positive emotions and humor that are uncharacteristic of the pervasive unhappiness and misery characteristic of MDE. The thought content associated with grief generally features a preoccupation with thoughts and memories of the deceased, rather than the self-critical or pessimistic ruminations seen in MDE. In grief, self-esteem is generally preserved, whereas in MDE feelings of worthlessness and self-loathing are common. If self-derogatory ideation is present in grief, it typically involves perceived failings vis-à-vis the deceased (eg, not visiting frequently enough, not telling the deceased how much he or she was loved). If a bereaved individual thinks about death and dying, such thoughts are generally focused on the deceased and possibly about "joining" the deceased, whereas in MDE such thoughts are focused on ending one's own life because of feeling worthless, undeserving of life, or unable to cope with the pain of depression.

D. The occurrence of the major depressive episode is not better explained by schizoaffective disorder, schizophrenia, schizophreniform disorder, delusional disorder, or other specified and unspecified schizophrenia spectrum and other psychotic disorders.

E. There has never been a manic episode or a hypomanic episode.
Note: This exclusion does not apply if all of the manic-like or hypomanic-like episodes are substance-induced or are attributable to the physiological effects of another medical condition.

with difficulty falling asleep and frequent nighttime awakening. Less frequently, depressed patients complain of increased sleep (hypersomnia), although they experience daytime exhaustion or fatigue. Recognition and management of sleep disturbances among depressed patients is crucial, as it has been estimated that approximately 60% to 90% of patients experiencing MDD report sleep disturbances.[27]

Appetite disturbances, including complaints of decreased appetite, often result in substantial weight loss, especially in the elderly.[28] Some patients lose 2 lb (0.9 kg) or more per week without dieting. Other patients, especially in the ambulatory setting, may overeat and gain weight, although they actually may not enjoy eating.

Patients may present with a variety of other symptoms such as GI issues, cardiovascular complaints (eg, palpitations), or muscle fatigue. Patients frequently present with a loss of sexual interest or libido.[29]

Intellectual or Cognitive Symptoms

Intellectual or cognitive symptoms include a decreased ability to concentrate, slowed thinking, and a poor memory for recent events. Patients may appear confused and indecisive. Depression should be considered when cognitive symptoms are present in the elderly.[28]

Psychomotor Disturbances

Patients may appear noticeably slowed or retarded in physical movements, thought processes, and speech (psychomotor retardation). Conversely, depression may be accompanied by psychomotor agitation, manifesting as purposeless, restless motion (eg, pacing, wringing of hands, or outbursts of shouting).

SUICIDE RISK EVALUATION AND MANAGEMENT

As of 2013, the Centers for Disease Control and Prevention listed suicide as the 10th leading cause of death among Americans and the 2nd leading cause of death among 25- to 34-year-olds.[30] All patients diagnosed with MDD should be assessed for suicidal thoughts. Factors associated with an increased risk for suicide include psychiatric and substance use disorders, adolescence and younger age adults, physical illness, recent stressful life event, childhood trauma, hopelessness, and male gender.[31] Those with a higher level of risk have high degrees of suicidal intent and describe more specific plans, in particular, plans that are violent and irreversible.[31] It is important to remember that the risk of suicide in those recovering from major depression may increase as they develop the energy and capacity to act on a plan made earlier in a course of illness. Additionally, despite factors to help identify those at greatest risk, it remains very difficult to predict suicidality in any given individual. Therefore, when suicidal intent is suspected, it is important to ask, "Are you thinking about harming or killing yourself?" If the risk is significant, the patient must be referred immediately to an appropriate healthcare professional. Additionally, certain depression rating scales, such as the MADRS discussed above, include questions that target suicidality, which may help identify those patients at risk.

In September 2004, the FDA required manufacturers of antidepressants to add a boxed warning stating that antidepressants increase the risk of suicidal thinking and behavior in short-term studies in children and adolescents with depressive disorders. These risks have become a new source of concern among those treating their patients with antidepressants. In order to help deal with the confusion these risks have caused, experts have recommended the following:[32]

1. It is especially important to closely monitor patients for suicidal ideation and behavior at the beginning of treatment and among younger patients.
2. Discuss the possibility that adverse events may occur, including behavioral agitation or anger, and encourage patients to seek help should this occur.
3. Deal with the subject of suicide directly.

It is important to note that there is little evidence to suggest that withholding antidepressant treatment decreases the risk of eventual suicide and may actually increase the risk. Furthermore, it may be that longer-term medication is needed for any protective effects against suicidality.[32]

In May 2007, the FDA released additional requests to the makers of antidepressants that the black box warning regarding suicidality be expanded to include warnings about the increased risk of suicidality (thinking and behavior) in young adults 18 to 24 years of age, during the initial stages of treatment.

In contrast to some of the concerns discussed above, recent evidence suggests that fluoxetine and venlafaxine may be associated with a "protective" effect from suicidality among adults and older patients; however, among youth, the medications lacked this apparent protective effect. It should be noted that this recent research did not find that fluoxetine and venlafaxine increased the risk of suicidality among youth.[33] The complex relationships between antidepressant use and suicidality will continue to be explored with the hopes of more unequivocal recommendations.

TREATMENT

Desired Outcomes

3 The goals of treatment for depression are the resolution of current symptoms (ie, remission) and the prevention of further episodes of depression (ie, relapse or recurrence). Whether or not to hospitalize the patient is often the first decision that is made in consideration of the patient's risk of suicide, physical state of health, social support system, and presence of a psychotic depression.

General Approach to Treatment

There are three phases of treatment for patients with MDD: (a) the *acute* phase lasting approximately 6 to 12 weeks in which the goal is remission (ie, absence of symptoms); (b) the *continuation* phase lasting 4 to 9 months after remission is achieved, in which the goal is to eliminate residual symptoms or prevent relapse (ie, return of symptoms within 6 months of remission); and (c) the *maintenance* phase lasting at least 12 to 36 months in which the goal is to prevent recurrence (ie, a separate episode of depression).[2,34] The duration of antidepressant therapy depends on the risk of recurrence. The risk of recurrence increases as the number of past episodes increases. Some investigators recommend lifelong maintenance therapy for persons at greatest risk for recurrence (persons younger than 40 years of age with two or more prior episodes and persons of any age with three or more prior episodes).[2] An alternative approach is to treat for at least 2 years in patients considered to be at high risk for relapse.[3] The decision as to "when" and "how" to taper/discontinue an antidepressant regimen is always going to depend on patient- and medication-specific variables, and is briefly discussed below.

Clinical **Controversy...**

There are no universally agreed upon approaches (eg, dose over time-course) for tapering antidepressants to discontinuation. However, research suggests there may be no advantage to shorter versus longer duration tapers. For example, a small study ($n = 28$) demonstrated that 3-day and 14-day antidepressant tapers resulted in similar rates of discontinuation symptoms according to the Discontinuation Emergent Signs and Symptoms checklist.[113] The precise rate of the antidepressant taper is typically influenced by many variables (eg, medication half-life, patient sensitivity to withdrawal symptoms). Therefore, the clinician (and patient) must carefully monitor for discontinuation signs and symptoms and for a return of depressive symptoms. Regardless of the taper approach employed in a given situation, monitoring the patient's status is essential throughout (and for days to weeks following) the taper period.

4 Educating the patient and their support system (eg, family and friends) regarding the delay in antidepressant effects and the importance of adherence should occur before and during the entire course of treatment. The treatment of MDD generally includes nonpharmacologic and pharmacologic strategies, which are discussed in further detail below.

Nonpharmacologic Therapy

In addition to pharmacologic interventions, psychotherapy should be employed whenever the patient is able and willing to participate. Psychotherapy alone is not recommended for the acute treatment of patients with severe and/or psychotic MDD. However, if the depressive episode is mild to moderate in severity, psychotherapy may be the first-line therapy.[35] The effects of psychotherapy and antidepressant medications are considered to be additive. Combined treatment may be advantageous for patients with partial responses to either treatment alone and for those with a chronic course of illness. However, for uncomplicated, nonchronic MDD, combined treatment may provide no unique advantage.[35] Cognitive therapy, behavioral therapy, and interpersonal psychotherapy appear equally effective.[35] Maintenance psychotherapy as the sole treatment to prevent recurrence generally is not recommended. Often, medication alone may prevent a depressive recurrence during the maintenance phase.[35]

Electroconvulsive therapy (ECT) is a safe and effective treatment for certain severe mental illnesses, including MDD. Patients with depression are candidates for ECT when a rapid response is needed, risks of other treatments outweigh potential benefits, there is a history of poor response to antidepressants and a history of good response to ECT, and the patient expresses a preference for ECT. Guidelines developed by the American Psychiatric Association (APA) include indications and contraindications for the appropriate use of ECT, procedures for obtaining informed consent, and issues in administering ECT. A more recent nonpharmacologic approach is repetitive transcranial magnetic stimulation (rTMS), which has demonstrated efficacy in treating MDD and does not require anesthesia as does ECT.[36]

Physical activity has long been recommended for individuals with many ailments, and recent data suggest benefits in depressed patients.

For example, positive preliminary findings led to the Treatment with Exercise Augmentation for Depression (TREAD) study, which is a study designed to confirm the promising initial findings. Recently published findings from this study showed that 16 kcal (67 kJ) per kilogram per week (KKW) exercise was associated with greater remission rates compared with 4 KKW, when both were used as augmentation to an SSRI.[86] The task force concluded that integrating exercise into the MDD treatment plan is medically appropriate and confers many well-accepted health benefits.

Pharmacologic Therapy

Antidepressants are considered first-line treatment for a moderate to severe depressive episode,[3] and they can be classified in several ways, including by chemical structure and the presumed mechanism of antidepressant activity. Although the link between the presumed mechanism of drug action and antidepressant response is tenuous, this classification has the advantage of being based on established pharmacology and clearly explains some of the common, but expected, adverse effects. The knowledgeable clinician can use these facts to tailor treatment to individual patient needs and thereby optimize treatment outcome. Currently available antidepressants, including dosing guidance, are provided in Table 68-3.[2,14,34,37-40]

5 Studies have found that antidepressants are of *equivalent efficacy* in groups of patients when administered in comparable doses. Because one cannot predict which antidepressant will be the most effective in an individual patient, the initial choice is made empirically. Factors that often influence the choice of an antidepressant include the patient's history of response, history of familial antidepressant response, patient's concurrent medical illnesses and medications, presenting symptoms (eg, fatigue as compared with insomnia), potential for drug–drug interactions, adverse events profile, patient preference, and drug cost. Although the pathophysiology of major depression remains elusive, the clinician can now select from multiple approved drug therapies with presumed different mechanisms of action as highlighted in Table 68-4.[2,14,34,39-42] Failure to respond to one antidepressant class or one antidepressant drug within a class does not predict a failed response to another drug class or another drug within the same class. Approximately 50% to 60% of patients with varying types of depression improve with acute drug therapy, compared with about 30% to 40% who improve with placebo.[3,43]

Selective Serotonin Reuptake Inhibitors

The efficacy of SSRIs is superior to placebo and comparable to other classes of antidepressants in treating patients with major depression.[2,34] SSRIs are generally chosen as *first-line antidepressants* due to their safety in overdose and improved tolerability. Furthermore, the decision as to which SSRI to use *within* the class is typically based on the nuances of each medication, such as differences in drug interaction profile and pharmacokinetic (PK) parameters (eg, half-life), or due to cost considerations. These concepts will be discussed in greater detail later in this chapter. Evidence suggests that two of the SSRIs, escitalopram and sertraline, demonstrate the 'best' efficacy/side effect profile compared to other newer-generation antidepressants.[44]

Serotonin–Norepinephrine Reuptake Inhibitors (SNRIs)

Tricyclic Antidepressants Although TCAs are effective in treating all depressive subtypes, their use has diminished greatly due to the availability of equally effective therapies that are much safer in overdose and better tolerated. All TCAs potentiate the activity of NE and 5-HT by blocking their reuptake. However, the potency and selectivity of TCAs for the inhibition of reuptake of NE and 5-HT vary greatly among these agents (see Table 68-4). Because TCAs affect other receptor systems (eg, cholinergic, histaminergic, and α-adrenergic systems, adverse events are reported frequently during TCA therapy.[14]

Newer-Generation SNRIs Venlafaxine inhibits 5-HT reuptake at low doses, and NE reuptake at higher doses; thus, it is referred to as an SNRI. Desvenlafaxine, the primary active metabolite of venlafaxine, is also an SNRI approved to treat depressive disorders. Duloxetine is an SNRI with both 5-HT and NE reuptake inhibition across all doses. Some studies suggest that the SNRIs may be associated with higher rates of response and remission than other antidepressants; however, most of these studies involved venlafaxine, and not all studies support this conclusion.[41] A report from the Agency for Healthcare Research and Quality (AHRQ) found that discontinuation rates secondary to lack of efficacy are 34% lower (odds ratio = 0.66, 95% CI = 0.47-0.93) for venlafaxine compared with those for SSRIs.[45] This is consistent with the BAP guidelines, which discuss the possibility of a slight (ie, large numbers needed to treat; NNT) efficacy advantage for venlafaxine (in addition to escitalopram/sertraline as discussed above) compared to other antidepressants.[3]

The most recent SNRI to be FDA-approved is levomilnacipran. It is too soon to determine its place in the pharmacotherapy for MDD; however, a pharmacological mechanism that makes it relatively unique among the SNRIs is greater potency at inhibiting NE reuptake as compared to 5-HT reuptake.[46]

Mixed Serotonergic Medications (Mixed 5-HT)

Trazodone and nefazodone have dual actions on serotonergic neurons, acting as both 5-HT_2 antagonists and 5-HT reuptake inhibitors. They may also enhance 5-HT_{1A}-mediated neurotransmission.[14] Trazodone blocks α_1-adrenergic and histaminergic receptors leading to increased side effects (eg, dizziness and sedation) that limit its use as an antidepressant. Recently, a longer-acting extended-release preparation of trazodone was approved by the FDA. This extended-release trazodone preparation has the potential to demonstrate a more tolerable side effect profile compared to its immediate-release predecessor. Nefazodone's use as an antidepressant has declined after reports of hepatic toxicity began to emerge. The FDA-approved nefazodone labeling includes a black box warning describing rare cases of liver failure. Trazodone and nefazodone are effective agents in treating major depression; however, both of them carry risks that limit their usefulness. Generic, immediate-release trazodone is often used adjunctively (in low doses) to induce sleep among depressed patients who are taking other antidepressant medications.

Recently, vilazodone became the first combination SSRI and 5-HT_{1A} receptor partial agonist to be approved for the treatment of MDD based on two 8-week, placebo-controlled MDD trials.[47] More recently, the *multi-modal* serotonergic medication, vortioxetine, was FDA approved for the treatment of MDD. The place for these two serotonin-based medications in the management of depression has yet to be determined. However, based upon their *multi-modal* mechanisms of action and the possibility of other neurotransmitter involvement (especially with vortioxetine), it has been proposed that vilazodone may be particularly efficacious for depressed patients experiencing anxiety while vortioxetine may help patients suffering from depression accompanied by cognitive difficulties.[48,49]

Norepinephrine and Dopamine Reuptake Inhibitor (NDRI)

Bupropion has no appreciable effect on the reuptake of 5-HT, but it inhibits both the NE and DA reuptake pumps.[17,42] These pharmacologic properties make bupropion unique among all currently available antidepressants.

Serotonin and α_2-Adrenergic Receptor Antagonists

Mirtazapine enhances central noradrenergic and serotonergic activity through the antagonism of central presynaptic α_2-adrenergic autoreceptors and heteroreceptors.[50] Furthermore, it antagonizes 5-HT_2 and 5-HT_3 receptors as well as histamine receptors. The antagonism of 5-HT_2 and 5-HT_3 receptors has been linked to lower

TABLE 68-3 Adult Dosing Guidance for Currently Available Antidepressant Medications

Drug (Brand Name)	Initial Dose (mg/day)	Usual Dosage Range (mg/day)	Comments (eg, Maximum Daily Dosage, Suggested Therapeutic Plasma Concentration)[a]
Selective Serotonin Reuptake Inhibitors (SSRIs)			
Citalopram (Celexa)	20	20-40	Doses >40 mg/day not recommended due to QT prolongation risk; maximum 20 mg/day for CYP2C19 poor metabolizers or coadministration with CYP2C19 inhibitors; 20 mg/day recommended for patients older than 60 years of age
Escitalopram (Lexapro)	10	10-20	Maximum 20 mg/day; dose may be increased to maximum daily dose after at least 1 week if needed; 5 mg tablet available for unique circumstances
Fluoxetine (Prozac)	20	20-60	Maximum 80 mg/day; dose may be increased in 20 mg increments; doses of 5 or 10 mg/day have been used as initial therapy; doses >20 mg/day may be given in a single daily dose or divided twice daily
Fluvoxamine (Luvox)	50	50-300	Maximum 300 mg/day; daily doses >100 mg total dose should be divided twice daily, with the larger dose given at night Maximum 300 mg/day (ER formulation)
Paroxetine (Paxil)	20	20-50	Maximum 50 mg/day (IR formulation); titrate 10 mg/day increments weekly Maximum 62.5 mg/day (CR formulation); titrate 12.5 mg/day increments weekly
Sertraline (Zoloft)	50	50-200	Maximum 200 mg/day; titrate 25 mg/day increments weekly
Serotonin–Norepinephrine Reuptake Inhibitors (SNRIs)			
Newer-generation SNRIs			
Desvenlafaxine (Pristiq)	50	50	Doses up to 400 mg/day have been studied; however, AEs are increased and no additional benefit has been shown at doses exceeding 50 mg/day. Dose reductions or discontinuation may be required if sustained hypertension occurs
Duloxetine (Cymbalta)	30	30-90	Maximum 120 mg/day (given once or twice daily); doses exceeding 60 mg/day not shown to provide increased efficacy for the treatment of MDD
Venlafaxine (Effexor)	37.5-75	75-225	Maximum 375 mg/day (IR); maximum 225 mg/day (ER); may increase in increments up to 75 mg/day at a minimum of every 4 days. Dose reductions or discontinuation may be required if sustained hypertension occurs
Levomilnacipran (Fetzima)	20	40-120	Initial dose (20 mg) for 2 days before dose increases are recommended at intervals of two or more days. Dose adjustment or discontinuation may be required if sustained elevated heart rate or hypertension occurs
Tricyclic antidepressants (TCAs)			
Amitriptyline (Elavil)	25	100-200	Maximum 300 mg/day for MDD; depending on the total dose, it may be given as a single daily dose at bedtime or in divided doses throughout the day; Therapeutic serum level 100-250 ng/mL (mcg/L; 370-925 nmol/L); parent drug plus metabolite (ie, nortriptyline)
Desipramine (Norpramin)	25	100-200	Maximum 300 mg/day; Suggested therapeutic concentration range for combined imipramine + desipramine: 150-300 ng/mL (mcg/L; 550-1,100 nmol/L)
Doxepin (Sinequan)	25	100-200	Maximum 300 mg/day; may be given in a single daily dose at bedtime (if tolerated) or in divided doses throughout the day; a single dose should not exceed 150 mg
Imipramine (Tofranil)	25	100-200	Maximum 300 mg/day; may be given in a single daily dose at bedtime (if tolerated) or in divided doses throughout the day; Suggested therapeutic concentration range for combined imipramine + desipramine: 150-300 ng/mL (mcg/L; 550-1,100 nmol/L)
Nortriptyline (Pamelor)	25	50-150	Maximum 150 mg/day; total daily may be given as a single daily dose (if tolerated) or 25 mg doses given three to four times daily; Therapeutic serum level 50-150 ng/mL (mcg/L; 190-570 nmol/L)
Norepinephrine and Dopamine Reuptake Inhibitor (NDRI)			
Bupropion (Wellbutrin)	150 (75 mg given twice daily)	150-300	Please see text for proper dosing, which can help decrease seizure risk; Maximum 450 mg/day (IR, ER), 400 mg/day (SR); ER dosed once daily; SR dosed once or twice daily; IR may be dosed up to three times daily
Mixed Serotonergic Effects (Mixed 5-HT)			
Nefazodone (Serzone)	100	200-400	Maximum 600 mg/day; daily doses should be divided twice daily
Trazodone (Desyrel; Oleptro)	50	150-300	Maximum 600 mg/day; IR daily dose should be divided three times daily and may increase by 50 mg/day increments every 3-7 days; ER dose titration initiated at 150 mg at bedtime and can be increased 75 mg/day every 3 days
Vilazodone (Viibryd)	10	20-40	Target dose 20-40 mg/day unless coadministered with CYP3A4 inhibitor (dose not to exceed 20 mg/day). Dose titration: 10 mg/day for 7 days, 20 mg/day for 7 days, and then may increase to 40 mg/day. Dose must be taken with food to ensure adequate drug absorption and bioavailability.
Vortioxetine (Brintellix)	10	20	Maximum 20 mg/day; US studies demonstrated better treatment effects at the higher dose
Serotonin and α_2-Adrenergic Antagonist			
Mirtazapine (Remeron)	15	15-45	Maximum 45 mg/day; may increase dose no more frequently than every 1-2 weeks; dose adjustment may be required for renal impairment
Monoamine Oxidase Inhibitors (MAOIs)			
Phenelzine (Nardil)	15	30-90	Early phase recommended dosing: 15 mg three times daily; dosing may be increased to 90 mg/day based on tolerance and response; Maintenance phase: dose should be reduced over several weeks to a daily dose as low as 15 mg/day or 15 mg every other day
Selegiline (transdermal) (Emsam)	6	6-12	Not to exceed 12 mg/24 hours; dose may be increased by 3 mg/day increments every 2 weeks; transdermal delivery system designed to deliver dose continuously over a 24-hour period
Tranylcypromine (Parnate)	10	20-40	Maximum 60 mg/day; divided dosing; if no response after 2 weeks, increase by 10 mg increments at 1- to 3-week intervals; Medication cross-taper: allow at least 1 medication-free week, an then initiate tranylcypromine at 50% of usual starting dose for at least 1 week

AE, adverse effects; CR, continuous release; ER, extended release; IR, immediate release; MDD, major depressive disorder; SR, sustained release.

[a]SI conversion for cases where reference ranges are for a mixture of parent drug and active metabolite is calculated based on a 1:1 ratio.

Data from references 2, 14, 34, 37-40, 46, 57, 65.

TABLE 68-4 Relative Potencies of Norepinephrine and Serotonin Reuptake Blockade and Selected Side Effect Profile of Antidepressants

	Reuptake Antagonism						
	NE	**5-HT**	**ACh Effects**	**Sedation**	**OH**	**Seizures**[a]	**Conduction Changes**[a]
Selective Serotonin Reuptake Inhibitors (SSRIs)							
Citalopram	0	++++	0	+	0	++	++
Escitalopram	0	++++	0	0	0	0	0
Fluoxetine	+	++++	0	0	0	++	0
Fluvoxamine	0	++++	0	+	0	++	0
Paroxetine	++	++++	+	+	0	++	0
Sertraline	0	++++	0	0	0	++	0
Serotonin–Norepinephrine Reuptake Inhibitors (SNRIs)							
Duloxetine[b]	+++	++++	+	0	+	0	0
Levomilnacipran[c]	++++	+++	+	0	0	0	0
Venlafaxine[d] and desvenlafaxine	+++	++++	+	+	0	++	+
Tricyclic Antidepressants (TCAs)							
Amitriptyline	++	++++	++++	++++	+++	+++	+++
Desipramine	++++	++	++	++	++	++	++++
Doxepin	++	++	+++	++++	++	+++	++
Imipramine	++	++++	+++	+++	++++	+++	+++
Nortriptyline	++++	++	++	++	+	++	++
Mixed Serotonergic (Mixed 5-HT)							
Nefazodone	0	++	0	+++	+++	++	+
Trazodone	0	++	0	++++	+++	++	+
Vilazodone	0	++++	0	+	0	++	0
Norepinephrine and Dopamine Reuptake Inhibitor (NDRI)							
Bupropion[e]	+	0	+	0	0	++++	+
Serotonin and α_2-Receptor Antagonist							
Mirtazapine	0	0	+	++	++	0	+

++++, high; +++, moderate; ++, low; +, very low; 0, absent or not adequately studied.

Ach, anticholinergic; OH, orthostatic hypotension.

[a]These are uncommon side effects of antidepressant drugs, particularly when used at normal therapeutic doses; they may be dose-dependent, resulting in corresponding dose restrictions. (eg, citalopram 40 mg/day maximum due to QTc prolongation concerns.)

[b]Duloxetine: balanced 5-HT and NE reuptake inhibition.

[c]Levomilnacipran: greater potency at NE reuptake inhibition compared to 5-HT.

[d]Venlafaxine: primarily 5-HT at lower doses, NE at higher doses, and DA at very high doses.

[e]Bupropion: also blocks dopamine reuptake.

Data from references 2,14,34,37-40,46,65.

anxiety and GI side effects, respectively. Blockade of histamine receptors is associated with the sedative properties of mirtazapine.[17]

Monoamine Oxidase Inhibitors

MAOIs increase the concentrations of NE, 5-HT, and DA within the neuronal synapse through inhibition of the MAO enzyme. Similar to TCAs, chronic therapy causes changes in receptor sensitivity (ie, downregulation of β-adrenergic, α-adrenergic, and serotonergic receptors).[51] The MAOIs phenelzine and tranylcypromine are nonselective inhibitors of MAO-A and MAO-B. A selegiline transdermal patch was approved by the FDA for treatment of MDD that allows inhibition of MAO-A and MAO-B in the brain, yet has reduced effects on MAO-A in the gut[37] (see tyramine interactions with MAOIs below).

Adverse Effects

Selective Serotonin Reuptake Inhibitors The SSRIs have a low affinity for histaminic, α_1-adrenergic, and muscarinic receptors, and therefore they produce fewer anticholinergic and cardiovascular adverse effects than the TCAs, and are not usually associated with significant weight gain.[52-54] The most common adverse effects, which generally are mild and short-lived, are gastrointestinal (GI) symptoms (eg, nausea, vomiting, and diarrhea), sexual dysfunction in both males and females, headache, and insomnia.[53] It should be noted that medications which augment serotonergic function, such as the SSRIs, may cause clinically relevant impairment in all three stages of the human sexual response.[55] A discontinuation or withdrawal syndrome may occur if SSRIs are abruptly discontinued. However, the longer the half-life of the drug and its active metabolite, the less likely a withdrawal syndrome will occur.[54,56] Although SSRIs are known to improve the anxiety symptoms associated with depression, a few patients experience an increase in anxiety symptoms or agitation early in treatment. Lastly, despite their excellent safety profile, there have been growing concerns with the SSRIs. For example, citalopram has been linked to a dose-dependent increase in QT interval that requires careful attention to maximum dosages.[57] This dose-dependent increase in QT interval may also be associated with escitalopram.[58]

Serotonin–Norepinephrine Reuptake Inhibitors The TCAs affect several NTs and produce a wide range of pharmacologic actions, including several unwanted, but expected, adverse effects. The most commonly occurring side effects are dose-related and are associated with blockade of cholinergic receptors (anticholinergic effects) and include dry mouth, constipation, blurred vision, urinary retention, dizziness, tachycardia, memory impairment, and, at higher doses, delirium.[59] Although some tolerance does develop to these adverse effects, they have the potential to impact patient adherence, particularly in the elderly and those receiving long-term maintenance therapy. Additional adverse effects that may lead to TCA nonadherence include weight gain and sexual dysfunction.[60]

Orthostatic hypotension is a common, dose-related, and potentially problematic adverse effect that has been attributed to the affinity of the TCAs for adrenergic receptors.[61] TCAs also cause cardiac conduction delays and may induce heart block in patients with a preexisting conduction disorder. TCA overdose can produce severe arrhythmias.[61] Furthermore, the FDA released a warning in December 2009 that the desipramine prescribing information will be changed to reflect an increased risk of death in patients receiving desipramine who have a *family history* of sudden cardiac death, cardiac dysrhythmias, and cardiac conduction disturbances. More on this reaction can be found at the FDA's MedWatch website. Therefore, caution should be exercised when prescribing these agents, especially in higher doses, to patients with clinically significant cardiac disease, and to patients with a family history of a cardiac event.

The most commonly reported adverse effects with venlafaxine are similar to those of SSRIs and may be dose-related; they include nausea, sexual dysfunction, and activation.[2] However, recent evidence strongly suggests that venlafaxine is associated with a higher incidence of nausea and vomiting compared with the SSRIs.[45] Venlafaxine may also cause a dose-related increase in diastolic blood pressure, and baseline blood pressure is not a useful predictor of the occurrence of this phenomenon. Blood pressure should be monitored regularly during venlafaxine therapy, and dosage reduction or discontinuation may be necessary if sustained hypertension occurs.[62] This is also true of levomilnacipran, given the increases in blood pressure (and heart rate) that have been documented in levomilnacipran clinical trials.[46]

Duloxetine was relatively well tolerated in short-term clinical trials; however, experience in long-term studies and in a larger population of patients will more clearly define its risks and benefits. The most commonly reported adverse events were nausea, dry mouth, constipation, decreased appetite, insomnia, and increased sweating.[41] According to the AHRQ report cited above, there were higher discontinuation rates secondary to side effects associated with both duloxetine and venlafaxine compared with the SSRI class of antidepressants.[45]

Mixed Serotonergic Medications Trazodone and nefazodone have minimal anticholinergic effects and comparatively less 5-HT agonist side effects (eg, sexual dysfunction), but they can cause orthostatic hypotension. Sedation, cognitive slowing, and dizziness are the most frequent dose-limiting side effects associated with trazodone.[51] Common adverse effects associated with nefazodone include light-headedness, dizziness, orthostatic hypotension, and somnolence. Due to the previously discussed potential for hepatic injury associated with nefazodone use, treatment should not be initiated in individuals with active liver disease or with elevated baseline serum transaminases. A rare but potentially serious adverse effect of trazodone is priapism, which is reported to occur in approximately 1 in 6,000 male patients. Some cases have required surgical intervention (1 in 23,000), and permanent impotence may result.[63] There have been no reports of priapism associated with nefazodone use in men, but there is a published case report of nefazodone-induced clitoral priapism.[63] Vilazodone is associated with GI side effects (eg, diarrhea and nausea), dizziness, insomnia, and decreased libido (particularly among men).[64] The most pronounced side effects associated with vortioxetine are GI related (eg, nausea and constipation). There also appeared to be a greater incidence of "treatment emergent sexual dysfunction" among men at the highest vortioxetine dose (20 mg/day) compared to placebo.[65]

Norepinephrine and Dopamine Reuptake Inhibitor Adverse effects associated with bupropion include nausea, vomiting, tremor, insomnia, dry mouth, and skin reactions. The occurrence of seizures in patients taking bupropion appears to be strongly dose-related, and may be increased by predisposing factors such as history of prior seizure activity, severe alcohol withdrawal, head trauma, and CNS tumor. Additionally, bupropion use is contraindicated in patients with eating disorders such as bulimia and anorexia, as these patients are prone to electrolyte abnormalities and are therefore at higher risk for seizure activity. At daily doses of 450 mg (the FDA-approved maximum dose) or less, the incidence of seizures is 0.4%.[66] Due to its pharmacologic profile (ie, proadrenergic), bupropion may cause activation or agitation in some patients.[17] Bupropion is associated with less sexual dysfunction compared with the SSRIs.[45]

Serotonin and α_2-Adrenergic Receptor Antagonists The most common adverse effects of mirtazapine are somnolence, weight gain, dry mouth, and constipation. Certain side effects associated with mirtazapine (eg, somnolence and weight gain in particular) are likely due to mirtazapine's relatively strong antihistaminergic properties.[27] Furthermore, side effects such as weight gain may be less with larger mirtazapine doses due to different mechanisms of action at different doses,[54] such as increased noradrenergic transmission as the dose is increased. Weight gain associated with mirtazapine after 6 to 8 weeks is in the range of 0.8 to 3 kg.[45] Mirtazapine should be considered as an option for those patients who experience sexual dysfunction following antidepressant treatment, which may be due to mirtazapine's ability to antagonize postsynaptic serotonergic receptors and/or its pro-noradrenergic effects.

Monoamine Oxidase Inhibitors The most common adverse effect of MAOIs is postural hypotension; this is more likely to occur with phenelzine than with tranylcypromine and may be minimized through divided dosage scheduling. Other common adverse effects include weight gain and sexual side effects (eg, decreased libido and anorgasmia).[2] Phenelzine has mild to moderate sedating effects, while tranylcypromine may exert a stimulating effect, and therefore insomnia can occur. In addition, fever, myoclonic jerking, and brisk deep tendon reflexes may occur.[67]

Hypertensive crisis, a potentially serious and life-threatening but rare adverse reaction, may occur when MAOIs are taken concurrently with certain foods, especially those high in tyramine, or some medications. Examples of potentially high tyramine foods and medications that should be avoided or used with caution are provided in Table 68-5.[39,40] Ten milligrams of tyramine can cause a marked pressor effect, and 25 mg can result in a serious hypertensive crisis. These incidents may culminate in cerebrovascular accident and death. Symptoms of hypertensive crisis include occipital headache, stiff neck, nausea, vomiting, sweating, and sharply elevated blood pressure. Hypertensive crises can be treated with antihypertensive agents such as captopril.[68] Education of patients taking MAOIs regarding dietary and medication restrictions is extremely important.

Serotonin Syndrome (SS) Any antidepressant that increases serotonergic neurotransmission can be associated with SS. The typical triad of symptoms seen in SS includes mental status changes, autonomic instability, and neuromuscular abnormalities. However, SS has been identified in cases without all three of these symptoms being present. Therefore, alternative approaches to the well-accepted SS triad have been suggested. For example, it has been proposed that the presence of any of the following symptom clusters is highly diagnostic of SS: (a) tremor + hyperreflexia, (b) spontaneous clonus,

TABLE 68-5 Dietary and Medication Restrictions for Patients Taking Monoamine Oxidase Inhibitors[a]

Foods	
Aged cheese[b]	Liver (chicken or beef, more than 2 days old)
Sour cream[c]	Raisins
Yogurt[c]	Pods of broad beans (fava beans)
Cottage cheese[c]	Yeast extract and other yeast products
American cheese[c]	Soy sauce
Mild Swiss cheese[c]	Chocolate[e]
Wine[d] (especially Chianti and sherry)	Coffee[e]
Beer	Ripe avocado
Sardines	Sauerkraut
Canned, aged, or processed meats	Licorice
Monosodium glutamate	
Medications	
Amphetamines	Levodopa
Appetite suppressants	Local anesthetics containing sympathomimetic vasoconstrictors
Asthma inhalants	Meperidine
Buspirone	Methyldopa
Carbamazepine	Methylphenidate
Cocaine	Other antidepressants[f]
Cyclobenzaprine	Other MAOIs
Decongestants (topical and systemic)	Reserpine
Dextromethorphan	Rizatriptan
Dopamine	Stimulants
Ephedrine	Sumatriptan
Epinephrine	Sympathomimetics
Guanethidine	Tryptophan

[a]According to the FDA-approved prescribing information for the transdermal selegiline patch, patients receiving the 6-mg/24-hour dose are not required to modify their diet. However, patients receiving the 9- or 12-mg/24-hour dose are still required to follow the dietary restrictions similar to the other MAOIs.

[b]Clearly warrants absolute prohibition (eg, English Stilton, blue, Camembert, and cheddar).

[c]Up to 2 oz (~60 g) daily is acceptable.

[d]Three ounce white wine or a single cocktail is acceptable.

[e]Up to 2 oz (~ 60 mL) daily is acceptable: larger amounts of decaffeinated coffee are acceptable.

[f]Tricyclic antidepressants may be used with caution by experienced clinicians in treatment-resistant populations.

Data from references 39,40.

(c) muscle rigidity + temperature greater than 38°C (100.4°F) + ocular clonus or inducible clonus, (d) ocular clonus + agitation or diaphoresis, and (e) inducible clonus + agitation or diaphoresis.[69,67]

Pharmacokinetics and Pharmacodynamics

The PK of the antidepressants is summarized in Table 68-6.[39-41,70-72] The diversity of SSRIs is evident not only in their chemical structures but also in their PK profiles.[70,73] The unique PK attributes of each SSRI can be used to guide treatment. For example, the long half-life of fluoxetine and its active metabolite norfluoxetine may be beneficial in instances of partial nonadherence (eg, missed doses). Conversely, caution must be taken to monitor for drug–drug interactions prior to combining another medication with fluoxetine. SSRIs are extensively distributed to the tissues, and all, with the possible exception of citalopram and sertraline, may have a nonlinear pattern of drug accumulation with long-term administration.[52,73] Therefore, the relationship between the dose and observed effect (eg, side effect) may change over time for the nonlinear SSRIs, and this needs to be considered during treatment.

Bioavailability is low (30%-70%) for most TCAs as a result of the first-pass hepatic effect, which shows great interindividual variation.[74] The TCAs have a large volume of distribution and concentrate in brain and cardiac tissue in laboratory animals. They are bound extensively and strongly to plasma albumin, erythrocytes, α_1-acid glycoprotein, and lipoprotein.[74] The major metabolic pathways are demethylation, aromatic and aliphatic hydroxylation, and glucuronide conjugation. Enterohepatic cycling has been described.[74,75] Metabolism of TCAs is linear within the usual dosage range. The elimination half-lives of the TCAs can vary greatly among individual patients.[74]

Venlafaxine is metabolized to an active metabolite, *O*-desmethylvenlafaxine, which contributes to the overall pharmacologic effect,[76] and has received FDA approval as an antidepressant. As might be expected, different formulations of venlafaxine with different PK profiles have led to different adverse effect profiles. For example, venlafaxine extended-release formulation, with its sustained plasma concentrations, has been associated with higher rates of sexual dysfunction among men (37%) compared with the immediate-release formulation (6%).[76]

Bupropion is metabolized to multiple active metabolites (see Table 68-6). There are currently three formulations of bupropion (immediate release, sustained release, and extended release), which are considered bioequivalent.[77] The bupropion peak plasma concentrations are lower for the sustained-release formulation of bupropion, and it is believed this may contribute to a lower seizure risk with that formulation.[78]

Mirtazapine undergoes extensive biotransformation to several metabolites[79] and is primarily eliminated in the urine (renal elimination). However, these metabolites are present at such low plasma concentrations as to minimally contribute to the overall pharmacologic profile of mirtazapine. Levomilnacipran is another newer-generation antidepressant with renal excretion playing a major role in its elimination.

Altered Pharmacokinetics In patients with cirrhosis, the half-lives of fluoxetine and norfluoxetine increased to 7.6 and 12 days, respectively.[73] Patients with hepatic impairment had a twofold increase in plasma concentrations of paroxetine.[80] Similarly, in patients with mild stable cirrhosis, the half-life of sertraline was 2.5 times greater than in patients without liver disease.[81] Patients with renal impairment had a twofold to fourfold increase in paroxetine plasma concentrations compared with normal volunteers.[80] Plasma concentrations of SSRIs in the elderly are reported to be greater than in younger patients.[73]

Factors that influence TCA plasma concentrations include disease states, genetics, age, cigarette smoking, and concurrent drug administration. Hepatic disease may result in increased TCA plasma concentrations.[38] Renal failure does not alter nortriptyline metabolism, but the 10-hydroxy metabolite may accumulate, and protein binding may be diminished, with resulting enhanced sensitivity to the drug.[74] Clinicians should be alert to the possibility of higher-than-expected plasma concentrations of some TCAs in the elderly.

The clearance of venlafaxine, mirtazapine, and their metabolites may be reduced among patients with hepatic or renal disease,[71] and doses should be adjusted accordingly. Elderly patients may require a dose reduction with mirtazapine.[71]

Plasma Concentration and Clinical Response

For the newer antidepressants, a strong correlation has not been established between plasma concentration and clinical response or adverse effects. Studies in acutely depressed patients have demonstrated a correlation between antidepressant effect and plasma concentrations for some TCAs. There are four TCAs (amitriptyline, nortriptyline, desipramine, and imipramine) with evidence to support an association between plasma concentrations and clinical response. However, the best established therapeutic range is for nortriptyline (50-150 ng/mL [190-570 nmol/L]),[38] which appears to

TABLE 68-6 Pharmacokinetic Properties of Antidepressants

Generic Name	Elimination Half-Life[a]	Time of Peak Plasma Concentration (Hours)	Plasma Protein Binding (%)	Percentage Bioavailable	Clinically Important Metabolites
Selective Serotonin Reuptake Inhibitors (SSRIs)					
Citalopram	33 hours	2-4	80	≥80	None
Escitalopram	27-32 hours	5	56	80	None
Fluoxetine	4-6 days[b]	4-8	94	95	Norfluoxetine[e]
Fluvoxamine	15-26 hours	2-8	77	53	None
Paroxetine	24-31 hours	5-7	95		None
Sertraline	27 hours	6-8	99	36[c]	None
Serotonin–Norepinephrine Reuptake Inhibitors (SNRIs)					
Desvenlafaxine	11 hours	7.5	30	80	None
Duloxetine	12 hours	6	90	50	None
Levomilnacipran	12 hours	6-8	22	92	None
Venlafaxine	5 hours	2	27-30	45	*O*-Desmethyl-venlafaxine
TCAs					
Amitriptyline	9-46 hours	1-5	90-97	30-60	Nortriptyline
Desipramine	11-46 hours	3-6	73-92	33-51	2-Hydroxy-desipramine
Doxepin	8-36 hours	1-4	68-82	13-45	Desmethyl-doxepin
Imipramine	6-34 hours	1.5-3	63-96	22-77	Desipramine
Nortriptyline	16-88 hours	3-12	87-95	46-70	10-Hydroxy-nortriptyline
Mixed Serotonergic (Mixed 5-HT)					
Nefazodone	2-4 hours	1	99	20	*meta*-Chlorophenyl-piperazine
Trazodone	6-11 hours	1-2	92	[d]	*meta*-Chlorophenyl-piperazine
Vilazodone	25 hours	4-5	>95	72[e]	
Vortioxetine	66 hours	7-11	98	75	
Norepinephrine/Dopamine Reuptake Inhibitor (NDRI)					
Bupropion	10-21 hours	3	82-88	[d]	Hydroxy-bupropion Threohydro-bupropion Erythrohydro-bupropion
Serotonin and α_2-Adrenergic Antagonists					
Mirtazapine	20-40 hours	2	85	50	None

[a]Biologic half-life in slowest phase of elimination.

[b]Four to 6 days with chronic dosing; norfluoxetine, 4-16 days.

[c]Increases 30%-40% when taken with food.

[d]No data available.

[e]Take with food to increase area under the curve concentrations by greater than 60%.

Data from references 39-41, 46, 65, 70-72.

demonstrate a curvilinear plasma concentration–response relationship. See Table 68-3 for a listing of suggested therapeutic plasma concentration ranges.

It must be noted that the patient's clinical response, not plasma concentration, dictates dosage adjustments. Some patients with plasma concentrations outside the suggested therapeutic plasma concentration range respond, whereas others are nonresponsive regardless of their plasma concentration.

Plasma Concentration Monitoring

Because of interindividual variations in plasma concentrations achieved by a given dose, interpretation of plasma concentrations can be very difficult for the TCAs.[38] Although plasma level monitoring is not performed routinely, some indications include inadequate response, relapse, serious or persistent adverse effects, use of higher-than-standard doses, suspected toxicity, elderly patients, pregnant patients, cardiac disease, suspected nonadherence, suspected PK drug interactions, and change in the manufacturer of the product. If plasma concentration monitoring is used to detect nonadherence, a cutoff as low as 30 ng/mL (mcg/L; ~110 nmol/L) for the TCAs has been suggested to avoid confusion with low bioavailability or unusually rapid metabolism. Blood samples for plasma concentration determinations should be obtained at steady state, usually after a minimum of 1 week at constant dosage. Sampling should be performed during the drug elimination phase, usually in the morning, 12 hours after the last dose. Samples collected in this manner are comparable for patients on once-, twice-, or thrice-daily regimens.[74]

Drug Interactions

Drug–drug interactions fall into two broad categories: PK or PD drug interactions. In contrast to the SSRIs, which have potential for both PK and PD interactions, other newer-generation antidepressants such as venlafaxine, duloxetine, mirtazapine, and bupropion have drug interactions that are primarily PD. This may be

TABLE 68-7 Second- and Third-Generation Antidepressants and Cytochrome (CYP) P450 Enzyme Inhibitory Potential

	CYP Enzyme			
Drug	**1A2**	**2C**	**2D6**	**3A4**
Bupropion	0	0	+	0
Citalopram	0	0	+	NA
Duloxetine	0	0	+++	0
Escitalopram	0	0	+	0
Fluoxetine	0	++	++++	++
Fluvoxamine	++++	++	0	+++
Mirtazapine	0	0	0	0
Nefazodone	0	0	0	++++
Paroxetine	0	0	++++	0
Sertraline	0	++	+	+
(des)-Venlafaxine	0	0	0/+	0

++++, high; +++, moderate; ++, low; +, very low; 0, absent.

Data from references 39, 40, 52, 70-72.

partly explained by the relative lack of cytochrome P450 inhibition among these newer agents compared with that among SSRIs (see Table 68-7).[39,40,52,70-72]

Pharmacokinetic Drug Interactions Drug–drug interactions may occur when an SSRI is coadministered with another drug metabolized through the cytochrome P450 system. Two of the isoenzymes of the cytochrome P450 system, 2D6 and 3A4, are responsible for the metabolism of more than 80% of currently marketed drugs.[72] The ability of an SSRI, or any antidepressant, to inhibit or induce the activity of these enzymes will be a significant contributory factor in determining its capability to cause a PK drug interaction when administered concomitantly. Table 68-7 shows the cytochrome P450 enzyme inhibitory potential of the second- and third-generation antidepressant agents. In patients receiving a stable dose of any medication known to interact with SSRIs, if an SSRI is to be initiated, the starting dose should be low and titrated carefully to evaluate the potential importance of the interaction.

Because the TCAs are metabolized in the liver through the cytochrome P450 system, they may interact with other drugs that modify hepatic enzyme activity or hepatic blood flow. TCAs are also extensively protein bound, which can cause drug interactions through displacement from protein-binding sites. Many commonly used medications can interact when given concurrently with TCAs. Due to their frequent coadministration, a common drug interaction occurs between the TCAs and certain SSRIs, such as paroxetine and fluoxetine. These drugs are known to inhibit cytochrome P450 (eg, CYP2D6) with the resultant increase in TCA plasma concentrations.

As nefazodone use has been severely limited due to its potential to induce liver toxicity, and trazodone is primarily used as a non-FDA-approved hypnotic at low doses, neither of these agents are likely to be involved in clinically significant drug interactions. However, it should be noted that nefazodone is a potent inhibitor of cytochrome P450 3A4.[72]

Pharmacodynamic Drug Interactions Certain PD drug interactions that may occur with SSRIs are concerning and require close monitoring. For example, the combination of an SSRI with another drug that augments serotonergic function (eg, linezolid) can lead to SS, which is characterized by symptoms such as clonus, hyperthermia, and mental status changes,[69] although these symptoms are not unanimously agreed upon; therefore, a washout period of 2 to 5 weeks (depending on the half-life of the SSRI) may be necessary before the initiation of another serotonergic medication. Lastly, the TCAs, SNRIs, and SSRIs can also potentially be involved in SS as described within Adverse Effects above and in Table 68-8.[39,40]

There are two types of pharmacodynamic drug interactions that may occur between antidepressant medications and NSAIDs. First, increased risk for abnormal bleeding (eg, upper GI and intracranial hemorrhage) associated with the combined use of antidepressants and NSAIDs is a potentially very serious pharmacodynamic interaction that has been reported in the literature.[82,83] This first PD interaction is likely mediated by serotonergic mechanisms that occur at the platelet level. Second, recent research, in both mice and humans, suggests the possibility that NSAIDs may lessen the efficacy of SSRIs. A recent editorial in the *American Journal of Psychiatry* provided a thoughtful discussion on the topic.[84] At this time evidence is insufficient to draw firm conclusions. However, given the volume of prescriptions for both NSAIDs and SSRIs, this is an area of pharmacotherapy that certainly deserves further research and thoughtful prescribing practices.

Lastly, refer to Monoamine Oxidase Inhibitors under Adverse Effects above and Table 68-5 to read more about the hypertensive crisis that may result following the coadministration of MAOIs and other medications that increase vasopressor response (eg, amphetamines). Notably, MAOIs and TCAs may be coadministered safely in refractory patients with apparent increased efficacy compared with monotherapy; however, severe reactions (eg, hypertensive crisis) and fatalities have occurred.[2,74] Therefore, this combination should be used sparingly by experienced clinicians and monitored extremely carefully.

Alternative Pharmacotherapy

The APA Task Force on Complementary and Alternative Medicine (CAM) recently provided consensus-based recommendations on the use of CAM for the treatment of MDD.[85] While these recommendations are not the focus of this chapter, clinicians treating patients with MDD should be cognizant of them.

Omega-3 Fatty Acids It appears from the literature reviewed by the task force that eicosapentaenoic acid (EPA) and docosahexaenoic acid (DHA) omega-3 fatty acids can be used as augmentation in the treatment of MDD. Furthermore, EPA alone or the combination of EPA/DHA is likely more effective than DHA alone.

St. John Wort There is a lack of consensus regarding St. John's wort for the treatment of MDD. Furthermore, St. John's wort induces hepatic metabolic enzymes and is associated with significant drug interactions. Therefore, the APA Task Force conservatively states that St. John's wort may be reasonable for some individuals with mild to moderate MDD. It should be noted, that the BAP guidelines state a "standardized" preparation of St. John's wort "could be considered"

TABLE 68-8 Selected Drug Interactions of Newer-Generation Antidepressants

Antidepressant	Interacting Drug/Drug Class	Effect
Selective Serotonin Reuptake Inhibitors		
Citalopram and escitalopram	MAOIs	Potential for hypertensive crisis, serotonin syndrome, delirium
	Linezolid (*MAOI effects*)	Serotonin syndrome
	Sibutramine	Serotonin syndrome
	Triptans	Serotonin syndrome
Fluoxetine	Alprazolam	Increased plasma concentrations and half-life of alprazolam; increased psychomotor impairment
	Antipsychotics (eg, haloperidol and risperidone)	Increased antipsychotic concentrations; increased extrapyramidal side effects
	β-Adrenergic blockers	Increased metoprolol serum concentrations; increased bradycardia; possible heart block
	Carbamazepine	Increased plasma concentrations of carbamazepine; symptoms of carbamazepine toxicity
	Linezolid (*MAOI effects*)	Serotonin syndrome
	MAOIs	Potential for hypertensive crisis, serotonin syndrome, delirium
	Phenytoin	Increased plasma concentrations of phenytoin; symptoms of phenytoin toxicity
	TCAs	Markedly increased TCA plasma concentrations; symptoms of TCA toxicity
	Sibutramine	Serotonin syndrome
	Triptans	Serotonin syndrome
	Thioridazine	Thioridazine C_{max} increased; prolonged QTc interval
Fluvoxamine	Alosetron	Increased alosetron AUC (sixfold) and half-life (threefold)
	Alprazolam	Increased AUC of alprazolam by 96%, increased alprazolam half-life by 71%; increased psychomotor impairment
	β-Adrenergic blockers	Fivefold increase in propranolol serum concentration; bradycardia and hypotension
	Carbamazepine	Increased plasma concentrations of carbamazepine; symptoms of carbamazepine toxicity
	Clozapine	Increased clozapine serum concentrations; increased risk for seizures and orthostatic hypotension
	Diltiazem	Bradycardia
	MAOIs	Potential for hypertensive crisis, serotonin syndrome, delirium
	Methadone	Increased methadone plasma concentrations; symptoms of methadone toxicity
	Ramelteon	Increased AUC (190-fold) and C_{max} (70-fold)
	Sibutramine	Serotonin syndrome
	TCAs	Increased TCA plasma concentration; symptoms of TCA toxicity
	Theophylline and caffeine	Increased serum concentrations of theophylline or caffeine; symptoms of theophylline or caffeine toxicity
	Thioridazine	Thioridazine C_{max} increased; prolonged QTc interval
	Warfarin	Increased hypoprothrombinemic response to warfarin
Paroxetine	Antipsychotics (eg, haloperidol, risperidone)	Increased antipsychotic concentrations; increased CNS and extrapyramidal side effects
	β-Adrenergic blockers	Increased metoprolol serum concentrations; increased bradycardia; possible heart block
	Linezolid (*MAOI effects*)	Serotonin syndrome
	MAOIs	Potential for hypertensive crisis, serotonin syndrome, delirium
	TCAs	Markedly increased TCA plasma concentrations; symptoms of TCA toxicity
	Sibutramine	Serotonin syndrome
	Triptans	Serotonin syndrome
	Thioridazine	Thioridazine C_{max} increased; prolonged QTc interval
Sertraline	Linezolid (*MAOI effects*)	Serotonin syndrome
	MAOIs	Potential for hypertensive crisis, serotonin syndrome, delirium
	Sibutramine	Serotonin syndrome
	Triptans	Serotonin syndrome
Serotonin–Norepinephrine Reuptake Inhibitors		
Venlafaxine and desvenlafaxine	MAOIs	Potential for hypertensive crisis, serotonin syndrome, delirium
	Sibutramine	Serotonin syndrome
	Triptans	Serotonin syndrome
Duloxetine	MAOIs	Potential for hypertensive crisis, serotonin syndrome, delirium
	Sibutramine	Serotonin syndrome
	Thioridazine	Thioridazine C_{max} increased; prolonged QTc interval
	Triptans	Serotonin syndrome
Levomilnacipran	CYP3A4 inhibitors	Clinically relevant increases in levomilnacipran plasma concentrations may occur
	MAOIs	Potential for hypertensive crisis, serotonin syndrome
Mixed Serotonergic (mixed 5-HT)		
Vilazodone	CYP3A4 inhibitors	Maximum vilazodone dose 20 mg with coadministration of potent CYP3A4 inhibitor
Vortioxetine	CYP2D6 inhibitors	May need to reduce vortioxetine dose by half with coadministration of potent CYP2D6 inhibitor
Serotonin and α-2-Adrenergic Antagonist		
Mirtazapine	Carbamazepine	Mirtazapine concentration decreased (60%)
	MAOIs	Theoretically, central serotonin syndrome could occur
Norepinephrine and Dopamine Reuptake Inhibitor		
Bupropion	MAOIs	Potential for hypertensive crisis
	Medications that lower seizure threshold	Increased incidence of seizures

NOTE: any medication that augments serotonergic function may impact bleeding risk and should be used with caution in patients receiving NSAIDs or other medications with hematologic effects.

AUC, area under the time concentration curve; C_{max}, maximum concentration; MAOI, monoamine oxidase inhibitor.

Data from references 2, 39, 40, 46, 65.

in patients with mild to moderate MDD, if other first-line medications are not an option.[3]

S-Adenosyl-L-Methionine (SAMe) The use of SAMe received a favorable review by the APA Task Force. However, the final consensus was that more rigorous studies need to confirm the efficacy of SAMe for treating MDD. In agreement, the BAP guidelines state that evidence is developing for use of SAMe as an augmentation strategy in the treatment of MDD.[3]

Folate The three compounds in this category are (a) folic acid, (b) folinic acid, and (c) 5-methyltetrahydrofolate (5-MTHF). These folate compounds are involved in the synthesis of key NTs, such as 5-HT. The task force states that augmentation with these compounds is reasonable, but more work is needed to clarify which subgroup of patients may achieve the greatest response. For example, in one study, only women responded to folic acid augmentation of fluoxetine treatment.

Special Populations

Elderly Patients Depression in the elderly is a major public health problem. Many elderly depressed patients are inadequately treated, or depression is missed or mistaken for another disorder, such as dementia. In the elderly, depressed mood, the typical signature symptom of depression, may be less prominent than other depressive symptoms such as loss of appetite, cognitive impairment, sleeplessness, anergia, and loss of interest in and enjoyment of the normal pursuits of life. Older adults may not recognize common symptoms associated with depression such as anhedonia (inability to experience pleasure), fatigue, and concentration difficulties. Somatic (physical) complaints are quite frequently the presenting symptoms in elderly depressed patients. Appropriate recognition and treatment of depression in the elderly is extremely important. In fact, individuals 65 years of age and older have a very high rate of suicidality. Increased suicide attempts in the depressed elderly may be due to access to firearms, diminished cognitive functioning, sleep disruptions, poor social interactions, and inattention among primary caregivers.[87]

Before initiating antidepressant treatment, a complete physical examination should be performed. In prescribing antidepressants, elderly patients may be either overtreated or undertreated. Overtreatment occurs when age-related PK and PD factors are overlooked. Undertreatment results from an overly conservative approach as a result of the patient's advanced age or concurrent medical problems. SSRIs are usually selected as first-choice antidepressants in the elderly, and this may enable the clinician to avoid some of the problematic adverse effects commonly associated with TCAs (eg, sedative, anticholinergic, and cardiovascular side effects). Furthermore, there is evidence to suggest that the long-term use of antidepressants such as SSRIs in the elderly, administered with either psychotherapy or clinical management, may prevent a depressive relapse.[88] Bupropion and venlafaxine are often selected because of milder anticholinergic and less frequent cardiovascular side effects.[89] Mirtazapine has been shown to be an effective antidepressant in the elderly (at least 65 years of age) and better tolerated than the SSRI paroxetine; furthermore, secondary measures of anxiety and sleep were improved following mirtazapine administration.[90] Regardless of the specific antidepressant chosen, the effect sizes for antidepressants as a pharmacological class (as compared to placebo) may be smaller in older patients than in younger adult populations.[3]

Pediatric Patients Accumulating evidence indicates that childhood depression occurs quite commonly. Symptoms of depression in the young may vary from accepted diagnostic criteria and include several nonspecific symptoms such as boredom, anxiety, failing adjustment, and sleep disturbance.[91]

Data collected under controlled conditions that support the efficacy of antidepressants in children and adolescents are sparse, and no antidepressant, except fluoxetine and escitalopram, is FDA-approved for the treatment of depression in patients younger than 18 years of age, although other antidepressants (eg, sertraline) have been studied in this population.[92]

The use of antidepressants in children and adolescents was complicated when, in March 2004, the FDA issued a black box warning in the product labeling for antidepressant medications warning clinicians and patients of the increased risk for suicidal ideation and behavior when antidepressants are used in this population. However, several retrospective longitudinal reviews of the use of antidepressants in children found no significant increase in the risk of suicide attempts or deaths.[93-95] Furthermore, adolescents suffering from depression who remain untreated may successfully commit suicide.[96,97] Further study is needed to resolve this important clinical dilemma.

Several cases of sudden death have been reported in children and adolescents taking antidepressants, such as desipramine. A baseline electrocardiogram (ECG) is recommended before initiating treatment with a TCA in children and adolescents, and many clinicians recommend an additional ECG when steady-state plasma concentrations are achieved.[98]

The treatment of depression in children remains challenging, as depression can be difficult to diagnose and treat once identified. Furthermore, differences in efficacy between medication and placebo may be small and nonsignificant in children below the age of 13 years.[3] However, antidepressants (in particular, the SSRIs) remain viable treatment options when prescribed and monitored appropriately.

Pregnant and Lactating Patients The crucial decision as to whether to use antidepressants during pregnancy continues to be debated and must always include a risk-benefit analysis based upon the available evidence at the time of treatment.[99] There are findings that both support and refute the decision to use antidepressants during pregnancy.[100-102] For example, approximately 14% of pregnant women develop a serious depression during pregnancy.[100] Furthermore, it has been documented that women who discontinued antidepressant therapy were five times more likely to have a relapse during their pregnancy than were women who continued treatment.[102] In contrast, another study found that prenatal exposure to SSRIs was associated with an increased risk of low birth weight and respiratory distress, and that this relationship remained after accounting for maternal illness severity.[100] A study by Chambers et al. reported a sixfold greater likelihood of the occurrence of persistent pulmonary hypertension of newborn infants exposed to an SSRI after the 20th week of gestation.[101] These are selected examples of studies on either the pro or con "side" of the argument and a full exploration of the conflicting literature on this topic is beyond the scope of this chapter.

A recent editorial on the use of antidepressants in pregnancy lists four therapeutic principles to guide the clinician in treating women during pregnancy: (a) Pregnancy does not protect against the occurrence of depression, and the likelihood of relapse is very high in untreated women with recurrent illness. (b) Maternal depression adversely affects child development, and prenatal depression may adversely affect the offspring. (c) When attempting to balance benefit and risk, transient postnatal behavioral abnormalities in the offspring of treated mothers must not be assumed to portend long-term compromise. (d) SSRIs, the most commonly used and best-tolerated treatment for depression, carry a small but significant risk for a serious medical consequence.[103]

In September 2009, the APA and the American College of Obstetricians and Gynecologists released a report discussing the treatment of depression during pregnancy. One of the prominent conclusions of this report was that *both* antidepressant treatment and untreated depression have been associated with potential problems during pregnancy. However, studies to date have not been able to adequately control for all the necessary variables involved in birth outcomes (eg, maternal depressive disorder) and more work needs to be done.[104]

In summary, the risks and benefits of drug therapy during pregnancy must always be weighed, and concerns about the risks of untreated depression during pregnancy should be considered. These include the possibility of low birth weight secondary to poor maternal weight gain, suicidality, potential for hospitalization, potential for marital discord, inability to engage in appropriate obstetric care, and difficulty caring for other children.[105] Several different approaches exist for dealing with pregnancy and antidepressant use. First, discontinuation of an antidepressant before conception is an option for women who are stable and appear likely to remain well while not taking antidepressant medication. Second, continuation of the antidepressant until conception may be reasonable. For those who have a history of depressive relapse after medication discontinuation, the antidepressant should be continued throughout pregnancy.

Further evaluations of the newer antidepressants are needed to fully understand the risks associated with their use at various stages of the gestational period. There is some recent evidence to suggest there may be less risk associated with particular antidepressants (eg, sertraline) compared to others (eg, paroxetine and fluoxetine) during early pregnancy.[106]

There is a great deal of uncertainty regarding long-term antidepressant exposure during breastfeeding due to the lack of data. However, both sertraline and paroxetine appear in relatively low concentrations in breast milk and in samples taken from infants.[107] Again, the risks of not treating depression in a pregnant or breastfeeding woman should not be underestimated or minimized.

Relative Resistance and Treatment-Resistant Depression

The majority of "treatment-resistant" depressed patients are likely the result of inadequate therapy (relative resistance). This theory is supported by data from the National Institute of Mental Health (NIMH) Sequenced Treatment Alternatives to Relieve Depression (STAR*D) study, which is generally considered to be one of the premier antidepressant trials among patients with depressive disorders.[108] This study showed that one in three depressed patients who previously did not achieve remission using an antidepressant became symptom free with the help of an additional medication (eg, bupropion SR) and one in four achieved remission after switching to a different antidepressant (eg, venlafaxine XR). Furthermore, patients can be switched to another medication within the same class. For example, patients in the STAR*D study not responding to an initial SSRI were shown to be as likely to respond to another SSRI as they were to a medication from a different class.[109] Consistent with the STAR*D findings, the BAP guidelines place a higher level of confidence in both augmentation and switching strategies, compared to dose increase approaches.[3]

Although several different definitions for treatment-resistant depression have been proposed, the most widely accepted is depression that has not achieved remission even after two optimal antidepressant trails.[110] More than 40% of patients with MDD being treated with antidepressants meet these criteria.[110] Three pharmacologic approaches that have been used with success for treatment-resistant depression include the following:

1. The current antidepressant may be stopped and a trial with another agent initiated (ie, switching). For example, the STAR*D trial compared switching to mirtazapine (up to 60 mg/day) versus nortriptyline (up to 200 mg/day) after two consecutive failed medication treatments.[111] In the mirtazapine group, 12.3% of patients met the remission criterion of a score of 7 or less on the Hamilton Rating Scale for Depression (HAM-D), while 19.8% of nortriptyline patients met this criterion at the end of 14 weeks.
2. The current antidepressant can be augmented by the addition of another agent such as lithium, or another antidepressant can be added (ie, combination antidepressant treatment). For example, the STAR*D trial evaluated the addition of lithium or triiodothyronine (T_3) to current antidepressant treatment. After approximately 10 weeks, T_3 augmentation resulted in higher remission rates (24.7%) compared with lithium (15.9%). However, the differences between these two augmentation strategies were modest and not statistically significant.[110] Although T3 and lithium demonstrated similar remission rates in this seminal trial, the BAP guidelines provide a stronger recommendation rating for lithium (ie, "A") compared to T3-based approaches (ie, "B").[3]
3. The use of atypical antipsychotic agents to augment the antidepressant response. Aripiprazole was the first atypical antipsychotic to receive FDA approval for adjunctive use in adults with MDD. Aripiprazole and quetiapine have been recommended as first-line agents to augment an antidepressant medication.[3] More recently, brexpiprazole was FDA-approved for this indication.

The APA practice guideline for the treatment of patients with MDD offers guidance for managing patients who fail to respond. These guidelines advise that if patients fail to respond to medication after 6 to 8 weeks, a reappraisal of the treatment regimen should be considered.[2] Partial responders should consider changing the dose, augmenting the antidepressant, or adding psychotherapy or ECT. For those with no response, options include changing to a second antidepressant or the addition of psychotherapy or ECT. Again, the BAP guidelines suggest that stronger evidence exists for switching or augmentation strategies compared to dose increases in patients with inadequate antidepressant response.[3] Comorbid medical or psychiatric conditions should be identified and treated because they may complicate treatment.

6 Before changing a patient's treatment, the clinician is advised to evaluate the adequacy of the medication dosage and adherence with the prescribed regimen. Issues to be addressed in assessing the patient who has not responded to treatment include the following:

1. Is the diagnosis correct?
2. Does the patient have a psychotic depression?
3. Has the patient received an adequate dose and adequate duration of treatment?
4. Do adverse effects preclude adequate dosing?
5. Has the patient adhered to the prescribed regimen?
6. Was a stepwise approach to treatment used?
7. Was treatment outcome adequately measured?
8. Is there a coexisting or preexisting medical or psychiatric disorder?
9. Are there other factors that interfere with treatment?

Clinical **Controversy...**

Low dose buprenorphine has been assessed for treatment resistant depression (TRD) among adults age 50 years and older.[114] The average buprenorphine dose used in this study was very low (0.4 mg/day) compared to buprenorphine for other conditions, such as opioid dependence. This low dose was provided by the authors as one explanation for the lack of "clinically significant physiologic or psychological withdrawal" when buprenorphine was tapered. Obviously, pharmacological approaches such as buprenorphine for TRD would need to be carefully monitored for misuse or diversion behaviors. However, it is possible that such approaches could provide relief for patients suffering from TRD. Clearly, more study is needed.

Clinical Application

A suggested algorithm for the management of uncomplicated MDD is shown in Figure 68-2. Recommended initial doses and dosage ranges are shown in Table 68-3. Antidepressant doses are generally titrated upwards depending on symptom response and adverse effects. Table 68-3 provides some medication-specific guidelines for dose titration. It is important to remember that 3 to 4 weeks is usually required before a mood-elevating response is seen. A 6-week trial at a maximum dosage is considered an adequate trial.[2] It is crucial to counsel the patient about the expected lag time before the onset of clinical response. Patients uneducated in this regard often fail to adhere to their prescribed regimens.

Some of the newer-generation antidepressant dosing regimens are particularly important from a safety standpoint. For example, bupropion must be carefully dosed in order to reduce seizure risk. Bupropion IR formulation is usually initiated at 75 mg twice daily, and this dose may be increased to 100 mg three times daily after a few days. Most patients will respond at 300 mg/day; however, an increase to 450 mg/day, given as 150 mg three times daily, may be considered in patients with no or partial response after several weeks of treatment at 300 mg/day. Additionally, both a 12-hour and a 24-hour sustained-release formulation are available, allowing for less frequent dosing. More recently, a maximum citalopram dose of 40 mg has been recommended, given increased QT prolongation at higher doses. Again, it should be noted that caution must be used with any dose regimen of TCAs or MAOIs. According to the FDA-approved prescribing information for the transdermal selegiline patch, patients receiving the 6-mg/24-hour dose are not required to modify their diet. However, patients receiving the 9- or 12-mg/24-hour dose are required to follow the dietary restrictions similar to the other MAOIs.

Caution is urged when dosing antidepressants in special populations. For example, in elderly patients, as a general rule, dosing

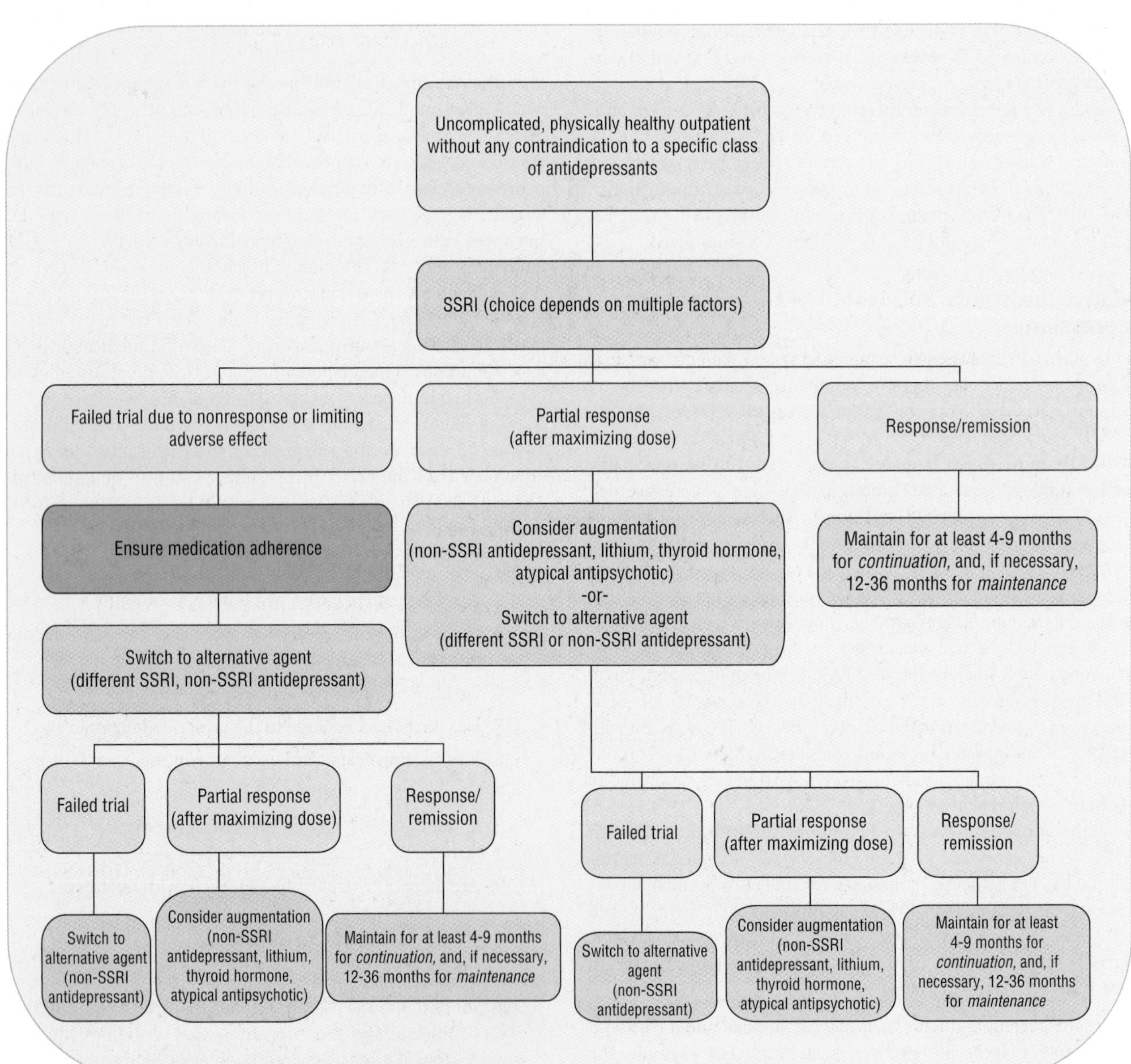

FIGURE 68-2 Suggested algorithm for treatment of uncomplicated MDD. (SSRI, selective serotonin reuptake inhibitor.) Note: both the BAP guidelines and the STAR*D trial suggest that switching and augmentation strategies are supported by stronger evidence compared to dose increases (among poor antidepressant responders).

is started at one half the initial dose that would be administered to younger adults, and the dose is increased at a slower rate.

Personalized Pharmacotherapy

7 Pharmacogenetic applications in psychiatry have been explored for some time. Pharmacogenetic tests (eg, the FDA-approved AmpliChip to evaluate CYP2D6 and CYP2C19 polymorphisms) are now available. However, there are no standard or well-accepted guidelines for the use of pharmacogenetic testing as it relates to antidepressant treatment. In contrast, PK parameters have long been one of the primary considerations when choosing among the antidepressants, particularly within a medication class.[2] For example, PK parameters help the clinician choose a particular SSRI (eg, longer fluoxetine half-life for partial nonadherence).

A clinician can use other aspects of a medication's pharmacological profile to tailor the treatment to a particular patient. For example, antidepressants can generally be classified as either activating or sedating based upon their mechanism of action, and this is often a major consideration in antidepressant choice. Medications that promote noradrenergic activity (eg, venlafaxine) or serotonin (eg, SSRIs) may be activating upon initiation and therefore poor choices for a patient suffering from significant insomnia. In contrast, medications with antihistaminergic properties (eg, mirtazapine) may be highly sedating and therefore appropriate for the depressed patient suffering from insomnia. Furthermore, trazodone has moderate antihistaminergic properties (ie, sedating), but also has antagonist properties at post-synaptic 5-HT receptors (ie, it may block activating effects of other serotonergic antidepressants). In fact, some antidepressants are so effective at helping patients to sleep, they have been studied (typically in lower doses compared to depressive disorders) as pharmacotherapy for primary insomnia.

EVALUATION OF THERAPEUTIC OUTCOMES

8 Several monitoring parameters, in addition to plasma concentrations, are useful in managing patients (Table 68-9).[2,39,40] Patients must be monitored for adverse effects, such as sedation and anticholinergic effects, and for remission of previously documented target symptoms. The presence of side effects does not necessarily indicate adequate dosage. In addition, changes in social and occupational functioning should be assessed. Patients receiving SNRIs should have their blood pressure monitored at regular intervals. Patients older than 40 years of age should receive a pretreatment ECG before starting TCA therapy, and followup ECGs should be performed periodically. Patients should be monitored for the emergence of suicidal ideation after initiation of any antidepressant, especially if other risk factors for suicidality (eg, sleep disturbances) are present. If significant activation or insomnia occurs upon antidepressant initiation, a short-term anxiolytic or hypnotic may be appropriate.[27] Weight gain and sexual dysfunction, common events associated with most

TABLE 68-9 Adverse Drug Reactions and Monitoring Parameters Associated with Select New-Generation Antidepressants

Drug	ADR(s)	Monitoring	Comments
Antidepressants from Each Pharmacologic Class			
Common to all antidepressants			
	Suicidality	Behavioral changes Mental status	(US boxed warning) for all antidepressants; caregivers should be alerted to monitor for acute changes in behavior (especially early in treatment)
Selective Serotonin Reuptake Inhibitors (SSRIs)			
Common to all SSRIs			
	Anxiety or nervousness	Assess severity and impact on patient functioning and quality of life	Most prominent on initial treatment; generally subsides over time as antidepressant causes neurochemical adaptations
	Insomnia	Sleep patterns	Among SSRI class: fluoxetine may be more activating; fluvoxamine and paroxetine may be more sedating
	Nausea	Frequency and severity	
	Serotonin syndrome	Autonomic function (eg, pulse, temperature); neuromuscular function	Criteria include mental status change, clonus, hyperthermia, diaphoresis, and tachycardia
	Sexual dysfunction	Assess severity and impact on patient functioning and quality of life	Spontaneous self-reporting may be low; clinician should assess symptoms; reversible on drug discontinuation
SSRI-Specific			
Citalopram (possibly escitalopram)	QT interval prolongation	Electrocardiogram; electrolytes (eg, potassium, magnesium)	Caution use in "at-risk" patients (eg, electrolyte disturbance); discontinue if QTc persistently >500 milliseconds
Fluoxetine	Anorexia	Weight (over time)	SSRIs are generally considered weight neutral
Fluvoxamine	Somnolence	Mental status	May be less tolerable than other SSRIs
Paroxetine	Anticholinergic effects	Symptoms: dry mouth, constipation, urinary retention, mental status	Paroxetine possesses relatively more anticholinergic effects than other SSRIs
Serotonin–Norepinephrine Reuptake Inhibitors (SNRIs)			
Common to all SNRIs			
	Cardiovascular changes	Increases in blood pressure; heart rate	Possibly less likely with duloxetine; may need to lower/discontinue dose
	Insomnia	Sleep patterns	Possibly less likely with duloxetine

(Continued)

TABLE 68-9 Adverse Drug Reactions and Monitoring Parameters Associated with Select New-Generation Antidepressants (*Continued*)

Drug	ADR(s)	Monitoring	Comments
	Nausea	Frequency and severity	
	Serotonin syndrome	Autonomic function (eg, pulse temperature); neuromuscular function	Criteria include mental status changes, clonus, hyperthermia, diaphoresis, and tachycardia
	Sexual dysfunction	Assess severity and impact on patient functioning and quality of life	Spontaneous self-reporting may be low; clinicians should assess symptoms; reversible on drug discontinuation
SNRI-Specific			
Desvenlafaxine	Dose-related hyperlipidemia	Lipid profile	Elevations in total cholesterol, low-density lipoproteins, and triglycerides
Duloxetine	Orthostatic hypotension	Blood pressure, pulse	Initial treatment or on dose increase
Venlafaxine	Dose-related hypertension	Blood pressure, pulse	May need to lower dose or discontinue
Mixed Serotonergic Effects (Mixed 5-HT)			
Nefazodone	Liver toxicity	Liver function tests	Nefazodone use is extremely limited in the United States due to concerns about liver toxicity
Trazodone	Orthostatic hypotension	Blood pressure, pulse	May be more severe as compared with other antidepressants; rate-limiting side effect
	Priapism	Patient report of sexual side effects, especially painful erection	Patient should seek medical attention for prolonged erection (ie, >4 hours)
Vilazodone	Serotonin syndrome	Autonomic function (eg, pulse temperature); neuromuscular function	Criteria include mental status changes, clonus, hyperthermia, diaphoresis, and tachycardia
Serotonin and α_2-Adrenergic Antagonist			
Mirtazapine	Weight gain	Body weight	Frequently occurring and significant (>7%) weight gain among adults
Norepinephrine and Dopamine Reuptake Inhibitor (NDRI)			
Bupropion	Seizure activity	Electroencephalogram	See text for proper dosing, which can help decrease seizure risk; caution use in patients with eating disorders or alcohol use disorders

Data from references 2, 39, 40, 46, 65.

antidepressants, are associated with nonadherence and should be monitored and discussed with the patient.

In addition to the clinical interview, psychometric rating instruments (such as those highlighted earlier in this chapter and in Chapter e62) allow for rapid and reliable measurement of the nature and severity of depressive and associated symptoms. It is helpful to administer the rating scales prior to treatment, 6 to 8 weeks after initiation of therapy, and periodically thereafter. Interviewing a family member or friend (with the patient's permission) regarding symptoms and daily functioning also can assist in assessment of progress. Patients should be monitored at more frequent intervals early in treatment, particularly for suicidality. Monitoring is then continued at regular intervals throughout the continuation and maintenance phases of treatment. Regular monitoring for reemergence of target symptoms should be continued for several months after antidepressant therapy is discontinued.

Finally, one useful set of criteria that can be used with a variety of psychometric scales was suggested by Mann.[34] Following these criteria, the following definitions are used: (a) *nonresponse* is less than 25% decrease in baseline symptoms, (b) *partial response* is a 26% to 49% decrease in baseline symptoms, and (c) *partial remission or response* is greater than a 50% decrease in baseline symptoms. Consistent with other recommendations, *remission* is a return to baseline functioning with no symptoms present.[2]

COLLABORATIVE PRACTICE

Significant evidence exists to show that depression is common and chronic and causes significant morbidity and mortality. Pharmacists, in conjunction with other healthcare providers, can play a crucial role in the screening, recognition, and treatment of this disorder. In fact, the US Preventive Services Task Force recommends screening adults for depression in clinical practices that have systems in place to ensure accurate diagnosis, effective treatment, and followup.[112] In addition, pharmacists and other healthcare clinicians play a crucial role in ensuring adherence to medication regimens through assessment of a patient's willingness and ability to take a medication, including an assessment of financial viability, and through patient education regarding dosing, side effects and drug interactions, and guidance regarding followup appointments with prescribing clinicians.

ACKNOWLEDGMENT

The authors would like to thank Brian Wells, PharmD Candidate, for his thoughtful review and comments on this book chapter.

ABBREVIATIONS

AHRQ	Agency for Healthcare Research and Quality
APA	American Psychiatric Association
BAP	British Association of Psychopharmacology
BDI	Beck Depression Inventory
BDNF	brain-derived neurotrophic factor
CAM	complementary and alternative medicine
DA	dopamine
DHA	docosahexaenoic acid
DSM-5	*Diagnostic and Statistical Manual of Mental Disorders, Fifth edition*
ECG	electrocardiogram
ECT	electroconvulsive therapy
EPA	eicosapentaenoic acid
5-HT	serotonin

GI	gastrointestinal
HAM-D	Hamilton Rating Scale for Depression
HPA	hypothalamic–pituitary–adrenal
KKW	kilocalories per kilogram per week
5-MTHF	5-methyltetrahydrofolate
MADRS	Montgomery-Åsberg Depression Rating Scale
MAOI	monoamine oxidase inhibitor
MDD	major depressive disorder
NDRI	norepinephrine and dopamine reuptake inhibitor
NE	norepinephrine
NIMH	National Institute of Mental Health
NT	neurotransmitter
PD	pharmacodynamic
PK	pharmacokinetic
rTMS	repetitive transcranial magnetic stimulation
SAMe	*S*-adenosyl-L-methionine
SNRI	serotonin–norepinephrine reuptake inhibitor
SS	serotonin syndrome
SSRI	selective serotonin reuptake inhibitor
STAR*D	Sequenced Treatment Alternatives to Relieve Depression
T_3	triiodothyronine
TCA	tricyclic antidepressant
TRD	treatment resistant depression
TREAD	Treatment with Exercise Augmentation for Depression

REFERENCES

1. American Psychiatric Association. *Diagnostic and Statistical Manual of Mental Disorders*. 5th ed. Arlington, VA: American Psychiatric Association, 2013.
2. American Psychiatric Association. *Practice Guideline for the Treatment of Patients With Major Depressive Disorder*. 3rd ed. Arlington, VA: American Psychiatric Association, 2010.
3. Cleare A, Pariante CM, Young AH, et al. Evidence-based guidelines for treating depressive disorders with antidepressants: A revision of the 2008 British Association for Psychopharmacology guidelines. *J Psychopharmacol* 2015;29(5):459-525.
4. Kessler RC, Berglund P, Demler O, et al. The epidemiology of major depressive disorder: Results from the National Comorbidity Survey Replication (NCS-R). *JAMA* 2003;289(23):3095-3105.
5. Burt VK, Stein K. Epidemiology of depression throughout the female life cycle. *J Clin Psychiatry* 2002;63(Suppl 7):S9-S15.
6. Steffens DC, Skoog I, Norton MC, et al. Prevalence of depression and its treatment in an elderly population: The Cache County study. *Arch Gen Psychiatry* 2000;57(6):601-607.
7. Kessler RC, Walters EE. Epidemiology of DSM-III-R major depression and minor depression among adolescents and young adults in the National Comorbidity Survey. *Depress Anxiety* 1998;7(1):3-14.
8. Larsson B, Ivarsson T. Clinical characteristics of adolescent psychiatric inpatients who have attempted suicide. *Eur Child Adolesc Psychiatry* 1998;7(4):201-208.
9. Weissman MM, Gershon ES, Kidd KK, et al. Psychiatric disorders in the relatives of probands with affective disorders. The Yale University—National Institute of Mental Health Collaborative Study. *Arch Gen Psychiatry* 1984;41(1):13-21.
10. Sullivan PF, Neale MC, Kendler KS. Genetic epidemiology of major depression: Review and meta-analysis. *Am J Psychiatry* 2000;157(10):1552-1562.
11. Stahl SM. Blue genes and the mechanism of action of antidepressants. *J Clin Psychiatry* 2000;61(3):164-165.
12. Hirschfield R. History and the evolution of the monoamine hypothesis of depression. *J Clin Psychiatry* 2000;61(Suppl 6):S4-S6.
13. Delgado PL, Moreno FA, Potter R, et al. Norepinephrine and serotonin in antidepressant action: Evidence from neurotransmitter depletion studies. In: Briley M, Montgomery S, eds. *Antidepressant Therapy at the Dawn of the Third Millennium*. London: Marin Dunitz, 1999:141-163.
14. Baldessarini RJ. Drugs and the treatment of psychiatric disorders: Depression and anxiety disorders. In: Hardman JG, Limbird LE, eds. *Goodman and Gilman's The Pharmacological Basis of Therapeutics*, 12th ed. New York: McGraw-Hill, 2016. Accesspharmacy.mhmedical.com/content.aspx?bookid=1613§ionid=102158640. (Accessed January 20, 2016)
15. Stahl SM. Blue genes and the monoamine hypothesis of depression. *J Clin Psychiatry* 2000;61(2):77-78.
16. Feighner JP. Mechanism of action of antidepressant medications. *J Clin Psychiatry* 1999;60(Suppl 4):S4-S11; discussion 12-13.
17. Stahl SM. Basic psychopharmacology of antidepressants, part 1: Antidepressants have seven distinct mechanisms of action. *J Clin Psychiatry* 1998;59(Suppl 4):S5-S14.
18. Siever LJ, Davis KL. Overview: Toward a dysregulation hypothesis of depression. *Am J Psychiatry* 1985;142(9):1017-1031.
19. Ordway GA, Klimek V, Mann JJ. Neurocircuitry of mood disorders. In: Davis KL, Charney D, Coyle JT, Nemeroff C, eds. *Neuropsychopharmacology: The Fifth Generation of Progress*. American College of Neuropsychopharmacology; 2002:1051-1064.
20. Berton O, Nestler EJ. New approaches to antidepressant drug discovery: Beyond monoamines. *Nat Rev Neurosci* 2006;7(2): 137-151.
21. Thase M. Mood disorders. In: Sadock BJ, Sadock VA, eds. *Neurobiology. Kaplan & Sadock's Comprehensive Textbook of Psychiatry*. Philadelphia, PA: Lippincott Williams & Wilkins, 2004.
22. Patten SB, Barbui C. Drug-induced depression: A systematic review to inform clinical practice. *Psychother Psychosom* 2004;73(4): 207-215.
23. Botts S, Ryan M. *Depression. Drug-Induced Diseases: Prevention, Detection, and Management*, 2nd ed. Bethesda, MD: American Society of Health-System Pharmacists, 2010.
24. Montgomery SA, Asberg M. A new depression scale designed to be sensitive to change. *Br J Psychiatry* 1979;134:382-389.
25. Beck AT, Ward CH, Mock J, Erbaugh J. An inventory for measuring depression. *Arch Gen Psychiatry* 1961;4:561-571.
26. McGirr A, Renaud J, Seguin M, et al. An examination of DSM-IV depressive symptoms and risk for suicide completion in major depressive disorder: A psychological autopsy study. *J Affect Disord* 2007;97(1-3):203-209.
27. Wichniak A, Wierzbicka A, Jernajczyk W. Sleep and antidepressant treatment. *Curr Pharm Des* 2012;18(36):5802-5817.
28. Lebowitz BD, Pearson JL, Schneider LS, et al. Diagnosis and treatment of depression in late life. Consensus statement update. *JAMA* 1997;278(14):1186-1190.
29. Trivedi MH. The link between depression and physical symptoms. *Prim Care Companion J Clin Psychiatry* 2004;6(Suppl 1):S12-S16.
30. Centers for Disease Control and Prevention, National Center for Injury Prevention and Control. Injury Prevention & Control: Data & Statistics (WISQARS™). Available at: http://www.cdc.gov/injury/wisqars/leadingcauses.html. (Accessed December 15, 2015)
31. Jacobs DG, Baldessarini RJ, Fawcett JA, et al. Practice guidelines for the assessment and treatment of patients with suicidal behaviors. *Am J Psychiatry* 2003;160(11 Suppl):S1-S60.
32. Fawcett JA, Baldessarini RJ, Coryell WH, et al. Defining and managing suicidal risk in patients taking psychotropic medications. *J Clin Psychiatry* 2009;70(6):782-789.
33. Gibbons RD, Brown CH, Hur K, et al. Suicidal thoughts and behavior with antidepressant treatment: Reanalysis of the randomized placebo-controlled studies of fluoxetine and venlafaxine. *Arch Gen Psychiatry* 2012;69(6):580-587.
34. Mann JJ. The medical management of depression. *N Engl J Med* 2005;353(17):1819-1834.
35. Blackburn IM, Moore RG. Controlled acute and follow-up trial of cognitive therapy and pharmacotherapy in out-patients with recurrent depression. *Br J Psychiatry* 1997;171:328-334.
36. Gaynes BN, Lux L, Lloyd S, et al. Nonpharmacologic Interventions for Treatment-Resistant Depression in Adults. Comparative Effectiveness Review No. 33. (Prepared by RTI International-University of North Carolina (RTI-UNC) Evidence based Practice Center under Contract No. 290-02-0016I.) AHRQ Publication No. 11-EHC056-EF. Rockville, MD: Agency for Healthcare Research and Quality, September 2011. Available at: http://www.effectivehealthcare.ahrq.gov. (Accessed December 15, 2015)
37. Patkar AA, Pae CU, Masand PS. Transdermal selegiline: The new generation of monoamine oxidase inhibitors. *CNS Spectr* 2006;11(5):363-375.
38. Watanabe MD, Winter ME. Tricyclic antidepressants: Amitriptyline, desipramine, imipramine, and nortriptyline. In: Winter ME, ed. *Basic Clinical Pharmacokinetics*, 4th ed. Baltimore, MD: Lippincott Williams & Wilkins, 2004:423-437.

39. Medscape Reference. WebMD, LLC (Copyright 1994-2016). Available at: reference.medscape.com. (Accessed December 15, 2015)
40. Lexicomp Online. Lexi-Comp, Inc (Copyright 1978-2016). Available at: http://online.lexi.com. (Accessed December 15, 2015)
41. Stahl SM, Grady MM, Moret C, Briley M. SNRIs: Their pharmacology, clinical efficacy, and tolerability in comparison with other classes of antidepressants. *CNS Spectr* 2005;10(9):732-747.
42. Horst WD, Preskorn SH. Mechanisms of action and clinical characteristics of three atypical antidepressants: Venlafaxine, nefazodone, bupropion. *J Affect Disord* 1998;51(3):237-254.
43. Walsh BT, Seidman SN, Sysko R, Gould M. Placebo response in studies of major depression: Variable, substantial, and growing. *JAMA* 2002;287(14):1840-1847.
44. Cipriani A, Furukawa TA, Salanti G, et al. Comparative efficacy and acceptability of 12 new-generation antidepressants: A multiple-treatments meta-analysis. *Lancet* 2009;373(9665):746-758.
45. Gartlehner GHR, Morgan LC, Thaler K, et al. Second-Generation Antidepressants in the Pharmacologic Treatment of Adult Depression: An Update of the 2007 Comparative Effectiveness Review. (Prepared by the RTI International–University of North Carolina Evidence-based Practice Center, Contract No. 290-2007-10056-I.) Available at: http://www.effectivehealthcare.ahrq.gov. (Accessed December 15, 2015)
46. FETZIMA (Levomilnacipran). Full Prescribing Information. Forest Pharmaceuticals, Inc. Subsidiary of Forest Laboratories, Inc. St. Louis, MO 63045 USA, July, 2014.
47. Citrome L. Vilazodone for major depressive disorder: A systematic review of the efficacy and safety profile for this newly approved antidepressant—what is the number needed to treat, number needed to harm and likelihood to be helped or harmed? *Int J Clin Pract* 2012;66(4):356-368.
48. Katona CL, Katona CP. New generation multi-modal antidepressants: Focus on vortioxetine for major depressive disorder. *Neuropsychiatr Dis Treat* 2014;10:349-354.
49. Elmaadawi AZ, Singh N, Reddy J, Nasr SJ. Prescriber's guide to using 3 new antidepressants. *Curr Psychiatry* 2015;14(2):28-36.
50. Gorman JM. Mirtazapine: Clinical overview. *J Clin Psychiatry* 1999;60(Suppl 17):S9-S13.
51. Bryant SG, Brown CS. Current concepts in clinical therapeutics: Major affective disorders, Part 2. *Clin Pharm* 1986;5(5):385-395.
52. Preskorn SH. Clinically relevant pharmacology of selective serotonin reuptake inhibitors. An overview with emphasis on pharmacokinetics and effects on oxidative drug metabolism. *Clin Pharmacokinet* 1997;32(Suppl 1):S1-S21.
53. Goldstein BJ, Goodnick PJ. Selective serotonin reuptake inhibitors in the treatment of affective disorders—III. Tolerability, safety and pharmacoeconomics. *J Psychopharmacol* 1998;12(3 Suppl B):S55-S87.
54. Masand PS, Gupta S. Long-term side effects of newer-generation antidepressants: SSRIs, venlafaxine, nefazodone, bupropion, and mirtazapine. *Ann Clin Psychiatry* 2002;14:175-182.
55. La Torre A, Giupponi G, Duffy D, Conca A. Sexual dysfunction related to psychotropic drugs: A critical review—part I: Antidepressants. *Pharmacopsychiatry* 2013;46(5):191-199.
56. Westenberg HG, Sander C. Tolerability and safety of fluvoxamine and other antidepressants. *Int J Clin Pract* 2006;60(4):482-491.
57. FDA Drug Safety Communication. Revised recommendations for Celexa (Citalopram hydrobromide) related to a potential risk of abnormal heart rhythms with high doses. Available at: http://www.fda.gov/Drugs/DrugSafety/ucm297391.htm. (Accessed December 15, 2015)
58. Castro VM, Clements CC, Murphy SN, et al. QT interval and antidepressant use: A cross sectional study of electronic health records. *BMJ* 2013;346:f288.
59. Bryant SG, Brown CS. Current concepts in clinical therapeutics: Major affective disorders, Part 1. *Clin Pharm* 1986;5(4):304-318.
60. Settle EC. Antidepressant drugs: Disturbing and potentially dangerous adverse effects. *J Clin Psychiatry* 1998;59(Suppl 16): S25-S30.
61. Nemeroff CB. The burden of severe depression: A review of diagnostic challenges and treatment alternatives. *J Psychiatr Res* 2007;41(3-4):189-206.
62. Feighner JP. Cardiovascular safety in depressed patients: Focus on venlafaxine. *J Clin Psychiatry* 1995;56(12):574-579.
63. Stimmel GL, Gutierrez MA. Counseling patients about sexual issues. *Pharmacotherapy* 2006;26(11):1608-1615.
64. VIIBRYD (vilazodone HCl) Full Prescribing Information. Forest Pharmaceuticals, Inc. Subsidiary of Forest Laboratories, Inc. St. Louis, MO 63045, USA, March, 2015.
65. BRINTELLIX (vortioxetine) Full Prescribing Information. Takeda Pharmaceuticals America, Inc. Deerfield, IL 60015, USA, July, 2014.
66. Johnston JA, Lineberry CG, Ascher JA, et al. A 102-center prospective study of seizure in association with bupropion. *J Clin Psychiatry* 1991;52(11):450-456.
67. Rabkin JG, Quitkin FM, McGrath P, et al. Adverse reactions to monoamine oxidase inhibitors. Part II. Treatment correlates and clinical management. *J Clin Psychopharmacol* 1985;5(1):2-9.
68. Varon J, Marik PE. The diagnosis and management of hypertensive crises. *Chest* 2000;118(1):214-227.
69. Boyer EW, Shannon M. The serotonin syndrome. *N Engl J Med* 2005;352(11):1112-1120.
70. Hemeryck A, Belpaire FM. Selective serotonin reuptake inhibitors and cytochrome P-450 mediated drug-drug interactions: An update. *Curr Drug Metab* 2002;3(1):13-37.
71. Kent JM. SNaRIs, NaSSAs, and NaRIs: New agents for the treatment of depression. *Lancet* 2000;355(9207):911-918.
72. DeVane CL. Differential pharmacology of newer antidepressants. *J Clin Psychiatry* 1998;59(Suppl 20):S85-S93.
73. DeVane CL. Metabolism and pharmacokinetics of selective serotonin reuptake inhibitors. *Cell Mol Neurobiol* 1999;19(4):443-466.
74. Wells BG. Tricyclic antidepressants. In: Taylor WJ, Caviness MHD, eds. A Textbook for the Clinical Application of Therapeutic Drug Monitoring. Irving, TX: Abbott Laboratories, 1986:449-465.
75. Rudorfer MV, Potter WZ. Metabolism of tricyclic antidepressants. *Cell Mol Neurobiol* 1999;19(3):373-409.
76. Olver JS, Burrows GD, Norman TR. The treatment of depression with different formulations of venlafaxine: A comparative analysis. *Hum Psychopharmacol* 2004;19(1):9-16.
77. Jefferson JW, Pradko JF, Muir KT. Bupropion for major depressive disorder: Pharmacokinetic and formulation considerations. *Clin Ther* 2005;27(11):1685-1695.
78. Dunner DL, Zisook S, Billow AA, et al. A prospective safety surveillance study for bupropion sustained-release in the treatment of depression. *J Clin Psychiatry* 1998;59(7):366-373.
79. Timmer CJ, Sitsen JM, Delbressine LP. Clinical pharmacokinetics of mirtazapine. *Clin Pharmacokinet* 2000;38(6):461-474.
80. Krastev Z, Terziivanov D, Vlahov V, et al. The pharmacokinetics of paroxetine in patients with liver cirrhosis. *Acta Psychiatr Scand Suppl* 1989;350:91-92.
81. Démolis JL, Angebaud P, Grangé JD, et al. Influence of liver cirrhosis on sertraline pharmacokinetics. *Br J Clin Pharmacol* 1996;42(3):394-397.
82. Loke YK, Trivedi AN, Singh S. Meta-analysis: Gastrointestinal bleeding due to interaction between selective serotonin uptake inhibitors and non-steroidal anti-inflammatory drugs. *Aliment Pharmacol Ther* 2008;27(1):31-40.
83. Shin JY, Park MJ, Lee SH, et al. Risk of intracranial haemorrhage in antidepressant users with concurrent use of non-steroidal anti-inflammatory drugs: Nationwide propensity score matched study. *BMJ* 2015;351:h3517.
84. Shelton RC. Does Concomitant Use of NSAIDs Reduce the Effectiveness of Antidepressants? *Am J Psychiatry* 2012;169(10): 1012-1015.
85. Freeman MP, Fava M, Lake J, et al. Complementary and alternative medicine in major depressive disorder: The American Psychiatric Association Task Force report. *J Clin Psychiatry* 2010;71(6): 669-681.
86. Trivedi MH, Greer TL, Church TS, et al. Exercise as an augmentation treatment for nonremitted major depressive disorder: A randomized, parallel dose comparison. *J Clin Psychiatry* 2011;72(5):677-684.
87. Turvey CL, Conwell Y, Jones MP, et al. Risk factors for late-life suicide: A prospective, community-based study. *Am J Geriatr Psychiatry* 2002;10(4):398-406.
88. Reynolds CF, Dew MA, Pollock BG, et al. Maintenance treatment of major depression in old age. *N Engl J Med* 2006;354(11):1130-1138.
89. Kohn R, Epstein-Lubow G. Course and outcomes of depression in the elderly. *Curr Psychiatry Rep* 2006;8(1):34-40.
90. Schatzberg AF, Kremer C, Rodrigues HE, et al. Double-blind, randomized comparison of mirtazapine and paroxetine in elderly depressed patients. *Am J Geriatr Psychiatry* 2002;10(5):541-550.
91. Cosgrave E, McGorry P, Allen N, Jackson H. Depression in young people. A growing challenge for primary care. *Aust Fam Physician* 2000;29(2):123-127.
92. Wagner KD, Ambrosini P, Rynn M, et al. Efficacy of sertraline in the treatment of children and adolescents with major depressive disorder: Two randomized controlled trials. *JAMA* 2003;290(8):1033-1041.

93. Olfson M, Marcus SC, Shaffer D. Antidepressant drug therapy and suicide in severely depressed children and adults: A case-control study. *Arch Gen Psychiatry* 2006;63(8):865-872.
94. Valuck RJ, Libby AM, Sills MR, et al. Antidepressant treatment and risk of suicide attempt by adolescents with major depressive disorder: A propensity-adjusted retrospective cohort study. *CNS Drugs* 2004;18(15):1119-1132.
95. Simon GE, Savarino J, Operskalski B, Wang PS. Suicide risk during antidepressant treatment. *Am J Psychiatry* 2006;163(1):41-47.
96. Hallfors DD, Waller MW, Ford CA, et al. Adolescent depression and suicide risk: Association with sex and drug behavior. *Am J Prev Med* 2004;27(3):224-231.
97. Haavisto A, Sourander A, Ellilä H, et al. Suicidal ideation and suicide attempts among child and adolescent psychiatric inpatients in Finland. *J Affect Disord* 2003;76(1-3):211-221.
98. Leonard HL, Meyer MC, Swedo SE, et al. Electrocardiographic changes during desipramine and clomipramine treatment in children and adolescents. *J Am Acad Child Adolesc Psychiatry* 1995;34(11):1460-1468.
99. Robinson GE. Controversies about the use of antidepressants in pregnancy. *J Nerv Ment Dis* 2015;203(3):159-163.
100. Oberlander TF, Warburton W, Misri S, et al. Neonatal outcomes after prenatal exposure to selective serotonin reuptake inhibitor antidepressants and maternal depression using population-based linked health data. *Arch Gen Psychiatry* 2006;63(8):898-906.
101. Chambers CD, Hernandez-Diaz S, Van Marter LJ, et al. Selective serotonin-reuptake inhibitors and risk of persistent pulmonary hypertension of the newborn. *N Engl J Med* 2006;354(6):579-587.
102. Cohen LS, Altshuler LL, Harlow BL, et al. Relapse of major depression during pregnancy in women who maintain or discontinue antidepressant treatment. *JAMA* 2006;295(5):499-507.
103. Rubinow DR. Antidepressant treatment during pregnancy: Between Scylla and Charybdis. *Am J Psychiatry* 2006;163(6):954-956.
104. Yonkers KA, Wisner KL, Stewart DE, et al. The management of depression during pregnancy: A report from the American Psychiatric Association and the American College of Obstetricians and Gynecologists. *Gen Hosp Psychiatry* 2009;31(5):403-413.
105. Hendrick V, Altshuler L. Management of major depression during pregnancy. *Am J Psychiatry* 2002;159(10):1667-1673.
106. Reefhuis J, Devine O, Friedman JM, et al. Specific SSRIs and birth defects: Bayesian analysis to interpret new data in the context of previous reports. *BMJ* 2015;351:h3190.
107. Freeman MP. Breastfeeding and antidepressants: Clinical dilemmas and expert perspectives. *J Clin Psychiatry* 2009;70(2):291-292.
108. Sequenced Treatment Alternatives to Relieve Depression (STAR*D). Available at: http://www.edc.gsph.pitt.edu/stard/. (Accessed December 15, 2015)
109. Rush AJ, Trivedi MH, Wisniewski SR, et al. Bupropion-SR, sertraline, or venlafaxine-XR after failure of SSRIs for depression. *N Engl J Med* 2006;354(12):1231-1242.
110. Nierenberg AA, Fava M, Trivedi MH, et al. A comparison of lithium and T(3) augmentation following two failed medication treatments for depression: A STAR*D report. *Am J Psychiatry* 2006;163(9):1519-1530.
111. Fava M, Rush AJ, Wisniewski SR, et al. A comparison of mirtazapine and nortriptyline following two consecutive failed medication treatments for depressed outpatients: A STAR*D report. *Am J Psychiatry* 2006;163(7):1161-1172.
112. U.S. Preventive Services Task Force. Screening for Depression. Rockville, MD: Agency for Healthcare Research and Quality (AHRQ). Available at: http://archive.ahrq.gov/research/jun02/0602RA30.htm. (Accessed December 15, 2015)
113. Tint A, Haddad PM, Anderson IM. The effect of rate of antidepressant tapering on the incidence of discontinuation symptoms: A randomised study. *J Psychopharmacol* 2008;22(3):330-332.
114. Karp JF, Butters MA, Begley AE, et al. Safety, tolerability, and clinical effect of low-dose buprenorphine for treatment-resistant depression in midlife and older adults. *J Clin Psychiatry* 2014;75(8):e785-e793.

69

Bipolar Disorder

Shannon J. Drayton and Christopher S. Fields

KEY CONCEPTS

1. Bipolar disorder is a cyclic mental illness with recurrent mood episodes that occur over a person's lifetime. The symptoms, course, severity, and response to treatment differ among individuals.
2. Bipolar disorder is likely caused by genetic factors, environmental triggers, and the dysregulation of neurotransmitters, neurohormones, and second messenger systems in the brain.
3. Clinicians should obtain a detailed history, including potential substance use and medical illness, to avoid a delay in the diagnosis and treatment of bipolar disorder.
4. The goal of therapy for bipolar disorder should be to improve patient functioning by reducing mood episodes. This is accomplished by maximizing adherence to therapy and limiting adverse effects.
5. Patients and family members should be educated about bipolar disorder and treatments. Long-term monitoring and adherence to treatment are major factors in achieving stabilization of the disorder.
6. Lithium and valproate are the mainstays of treatment for both acute mania and prophylaxis for recurrent manic and depressive episodes. Anticonvulsants (eg, lamotrigine, carbamazepine) and second-generation antipsychotics (eg, aripiprazole, quetiapine) are alternative or adjunctive treatments for bipolar disorder depending on the phase of illness (ie, mania, depression, maintenance). Anticonvulsants may be more effective than lithium in several mood subtypes (eg, mixed states and rapid cycling). The use of lithium, valproate, or quetiapine for acute bipolar depression should be considered a first-line treatment option.
7. Baseline and follow-up laboratory tests are required for most medications for bipolar disorder to monitor for adverse effects.
8. Some patients can be stabilized on one mood stabilizer, but others may require combination therapies or adjunctive agents during an acute mood episode. If possible, adjunctive agents should be tapered and discontinued when the acute mood episode remits and the patient is stabilized. Adjunctive agents may include benzodiazepines, additional mood stabilizers, antipsychotics, and/or antidepressants.

1 Bipolar disorder is a common, chronic, and often severe cyclic mood disorder characterized by recurrent fluctuations in mood, energy, and behavior.[1-3] It differs from recurrent major depression (or unipolar depression) in that a manic or hypomanic episode occurs during the course of the illness.[1] Bipolar disorder is a lifelong illness with a variable course and requires both nonpharmacologic and pharmacologic treatments for mood stabilization.[1,2]

EPIDEMIOLOGY

The overall prevalence of bipolar disorder was 4.5% in a U.S. comorbidity study: 1% meeting criteria for bipolar I, 1.1% for bipolar II, and 2.4% of patients with subthreshold bipolar disorder (ie, cyclothymia, unspecified bipolar disorder).[4] Symptom onset for depression, mania, or hypomania in bipolar disorder typically occurs in late adolescence or early adulthood, with greater than two-thirds of those affected developing symptoms before age 18 years.[5] Bipolar I disorder occurs equally in men and women, whereas bipolar II disorder is more common in women.[1,2] Depression and mixed presentations may occur more frequently in women.[6-8]

ETIOLOGY AND PATHOPHYSIOLOGY

2 The exact etiology of bipolar disorder is unknown. Bipolar disorder is thought to be a complex disease that is influenced by developmental, genetic, neurobiologic, and psychological factors.[9] Many theories have been proposed regarding the pathophysiology of mood disorders. Family, twin, and adoption studies report an increased lifetime prevalence risk of having mood disorders among first-degree relatives of patients with bipolar disorder.[10,11] Genetic linkage studies suggest multiple gene loci can be involved in the heredity of mood disorders.[12-14] Neuroimaging studies indicate that several anatomic regions (primarily the anterior paralimbic and adjacent prefrontal regions) may contribute to functional abnormalities in bipolar patients.[15] Many researchers suspect that altered synaptic and circuit functioning accounts for mood and cognitive changes seen in bipolar disorder, rather than dysfunction of individual neurotransmitters.[16] Environmental or psychosocial stressors, immunologic factors, and sleep dysregulation all have been associated with bipolar disorder and can negatively influence the course of illness.[17-21]

CLINICAL PRESENTATION AND DIAGNOSIS

1 The essential feature of bipolar spectrum disorders is a history of mania or hypomania that is not caused by any other medical condition, substance, or psychiatric disorder.[1,2] The *Diagnostic and Statistical Manual of Mental Disorders, Fifth Edition* (*DSM-5*) of the American Psychiatric Association (APA) details the present understanding of mood disorders.[1] Bipolar disorder is divided into five subtypes based on the identification of specific mood episodes: bipolar I, bipolar II, cyclothymic disorder, other specified bipolar and related disorder, and unspecified bipolar and related disorder.[1] Table 69-1 for a definition of mood disorders by type of episode. Specifiers can be added to bipolar I and II to reflect the most recent mood state (ie, hypomanic or major depressive episode). Table 69-2 for the evaluation and diagnostic criteria of mood episodes. Bipolar disorder is a cyclic mood

TABLE 69-1 Mood Disorders Defined by Episodes

Disorder Subtype	Episode(s)[a]
Major depressive disorder, single episode	Major depressive episode
Major depressive disorder, recurrent	Two or more major depressive episodes
Bipolar I disorder[b]	Manic episode ± major depressive or hypomanic episode
Bipolar II disorder[c]	Major depressive episode + hypomanic episode
Persistent depressive disorder (Dysthymia)	Depressed mood most days for at least 2 years (1 year in children and adolescents)
Cyclothymic disorder[d]	Chronic fluctuations between subsyndromal depressive and hypomanic episodes (2 years for adults and 1 year for children and adolescents)
Unspecified bipolar and related disorder	Mood states do not meet full criteria for any specific disorder in the bipolar and related disorders class

[a]The length and severity of a mood episode and the interval between episodes vary from patient to patient. Manic episodes are usually shorter and end more abruptly than major depressive episodes. The average length of untreated manic episodes ranges from 4 to 13 months. Episodes can occur regularly (at the same time or season of the year) and often cluster at 12-month intervals. Women have more depressive episodes than manic episodes, whereas men have a more even distribution of episodes.

[b]For bipolar I disorder, 90% of individuals who experience a manic episode later have multiple recurrent major depressive, manic, or hypomanic episodes alternating with a normal mood state.

[c]Approximately 5% to 15% of patients with bipolar II disorder will develop a manic episode over a 5-year period. If a manic episode develops in a patient with bipolar II disorder, the diagnosis is changed to bipolar I disorder.

[d]Patients with cyclothymic disorder have a 15% to 50% risk of later developing a bipolar I or II disorder.

Data from references 1 to 3.

disorder, and patients may sequentially experience different types of episodes with or without a period of normal mood (euthymia) between episodes. Individuals with bipolar disorder can have mood fluctuations that continue for months, or after one episode they can sometimes go years without recurrence of any type of mood episode. Comorbid conditions associated with bipolar disorder include, but are not limited to, substance abuse, personality disorders, anxiety disorders, eating disorders, and a higher incidence of several medical conditions.[1-3,22-26]

DIAGNOSTIC DIFFICULTY

Episodes of mania or depression may be induced or caused by medical illness, medications, or substance intoxication or withdrawal (refer to Table 69-3[27-36] for causes of mania and Chapter 68 for causes of depression).[1,2] A complete medical, psychiatric, and medication history; physical examination; and laboratory testing are important tools to rule out any organic causes of mania or depression.[2] An accurate diagnosis is critical because some psychiatric and neurologic disorders present with manic-like or depressive-like symptoms.[2,3] Bipolar disorder commonly co-occurs with substance use disorders and may be difficult to diagnose in the presence of cocaine use or other illicit substances (psychostimulants, bath salts, synthetic marijuana).[37] When making the diagnosis of new-onset bipolar disorder in a geriatric population, clinicians should be particularly aware of secondary causes of mania and depression that may impact treatment.[38]

Another disease state that has a similar presentation to bipolar disorder is schizoaffective disorder. This disease is essentially a mix between schizophrenia and bipolar disorder or unipolar depression. Patients with schizoaffective disorder have mood episodes, but the distinguishing factor from bipolar disorder is that these patients experience psychosis between mood episodes during

TABLE 69-2 Evaluation and Diagnosis of Mood Episodes

Diagnosis Episode	Impairment of Functioning or Need for Hospitalization[a]	*DSM-5* Criteria[b]
Major depressive	Yes	At least 2 week period of either depressed mood or loss of interest or pleasure in normal activities, associated with at least five of the following symptoms: • Depressed, sad mood (adults); can be irritable mood in children • Decreased interest and pleasure in normal activities • Decreased or increased appetite, weight loss or weight gain • Insomnia or hypersomnia • Psychomotor retardation or agitation • Decreased energy or fatigue • Feelings of excessive guilt or worthlessness • Impaired concentration or indecisiveness • Recurrent thoughts of death, suicidal thoughts or attempts
Manic	Yes	At least 1 week period of abnormally and persistently elevated mood (expansive or irritable) and energy, associated with at least three of the following symptoms (four if the mood is only irritable): • Inflated self-esteem (grandiosity) • Decreased need for sleep • Increased talking (pressure of speech) • Racing thoughts (flight of ideas) • Distractibility (poor attention) • Increased goal-directed activity (socially, at work, or sexually) or psychomotor agitation • Excessive involvement in activities that are pleasurable but have a high risk for serious consequences (buying sprees, sexual indiscretions, poor judgment in business ventures)
Hypomanic	No	At least 4 days of abnormally and persistently elevated mood (expansive or irritable) and energy, associated with at least three of the following symptoms (four if the mood is only irritable): • Inflated self-esteem (grandiosity) • Decreased need for sleep • Increased talking (pressure of speech) • Racing thoughts (flight of ideas) • Distractibility (poor attention) • Increased goal-directed activity (socially, at work, or sexually) or psychomotor agitation • Excessive involvement in activities that are pleasurable but have a high risk for serious consequences (buying sprees, sexual indiscretions, poor judgment in business ventures)

[a]Impairment in social or occupational functioning; may include need for hospitalization because of potential self-harm, harm to others, or psychotic symptoms.

[b]The disorder is not caused by a medical condition (eg, hypothyroidism) or substance-induced disorder (eg, antidepressant treatment, medications, drugs of abuse). Numerous specifiers are available to further characterize episodes (eg, with mixed features, with anxious distress, with rapid cycling, with melancholic features).

Data from reference 1.

TABLE 69-3 Secondary Causes of Mania

Medical conditions that induce mania
- CNS disorders (brain tumor, strokes, head injuries, subdural hematoma, multiple sclerosis, systemic lupus erythematosus, temporal lobe seizures, Huntington disease)
- Infections (encephalitis, neurosyphilis, sepsis, human immunodeficiency virus)
- Electrolyte or metabolic abnormalities (calcium or sodium fluctuations, hyperglycemia or hypoglycemia)
- Endocrine or hormonal dysregulation (Addison disease, Cushing disease, hyperthyroidism or hypothyroidism, menstrual-related or pregnancy-related or perimenopausal mood disorders)

Medications or drugs that induce mania
- Alcohol intoxication
- Drug withdrawal states (alcohol, α_2-adrenergic agonists, antidepressants, barbiturates, benzodiazepines, opiates)
- Antidepressants (MAOIs, TCAs, 5-HT and/or NE and/or DA reuptake inhibitors, 5-HT antagonists)
- DA-augmenting agents (CNS stimulants: amphetamines, cocaine, sympathomimetics; DA agonists, releasers, and reuptake inhibitors)
- Hallucinogens (LSD, PCP)
- Marijuana intoxication precipitates psychosis, paranoid thoughts, anxiety, and restlessness
- NE-augmenting agents (α_2-adrenergic antagonists, β-agonists, NE reuptake inhibitors)
- Steroids (anabolic, adrenocorticotropic hormone, corticosteroids)
- Thyroid preparations
- Xanthines (caffeine, theophylline)
- Nonprescription weight loss agents and decongestants (ephedra, pseudoephedrine)
- Herbal products (St. John wort)

Somatic therapies that induce mania
- Bright light therapy
- Deep brain stimulation
- Sleep deprivation

CNS, central nervous system; DA, dopamine; 5-HT, serotonin; LSD, lysergic acid diethylamide; MAOI, monoamine oxidase inhibitor; NE, norepinephrine; PCP, phencyclidine; TCA, tricyclic antidepressant.

Data from references 1, 27 to 36.

periods of euthymic mood. Clinicians must rely on the longitudinal history provided by collateral historians who know the patient well to determine if the patient is psychotic between mood episodes. It can be difficult for clinicians to obtain a full psychiatric history on patients presenting with manic or psychotic symptoms, thus making schizoaffective disorder difficult to differentiate from bipolar disorder. Schizoaffective disorder is best treated with mood stabilizers and antipsychotics as maintenance therapy.

COURSE OF ILLNESS

3 Bipolar disorder is frequently not recognized or treated for many years because of its fluctuating course and episodic mood states.[2,3] Patients may experience delays ranging from 8 to 13 years after the onset of the index mood episode until initiation of appropriate medications.[39] This delay confers a risk of poor social functioning, increased hospitalizations, and a greater likelihood of lifetime suicide attempts.[40] Onset of illness in early childhood tends to be associated with increased mood episodes, rapid cycling, and comorbid psychiatric conditions as well as a stronger family history of mood disorders.[41] Gender differences may influence a patient's course of illness, tolerability of medication, and response to treatment. Women are more likely to have increased depressive symptoms, older age of onset, better compliance, complex management in pregnancy, and higher association with physical illness such as thyroid abnormalities than men are. In men there may be increased incidence of mania and substance use.[42]

The kindling theory is used to explain why bipolar disorder progresses over one's life and why preventive treatment is imperative. Episodes can become more frequent, severe, and refractory to treatment with aging.[2,43] Usually there is a period of normal functioning between episodes, but approximately 20% to 30% of patients with bipolar I disorder and 15% with bipolar II disorder have no interepisode period of euthymia because of mood lability, residual mood symptoms, or a direct switch to the opposite polarity.[1]

Rapid cycling (more than four mood episodes per year) is more common in women and occurs in approximately 10% to 20% of bipolar I and II disorder patients.[2,3,44] Frequent and severe episodes of depression appear to be the most common hallmark of rapid cycling. Use of alcohol, stimulants, and antidepressants, as well as, sleep deprivation hypothyroidism, and seasonal changes can play a role in rapid cycling.[3,44,45] Seasonal patterns of mania in the summer and depression during the winter have been observed. Rapid-cycling patients have a poorer long-term prognosis and often require combination therapies.[3]

Fluctuations in hormones and neurotransmitters during the luteal phase of the menstrual cycle, postpartum period, and perimenopause (starting ~10 years before menopause) can precipitate mood changes and increase cycling.[1,46] Women with bipolar I disorder are at greater risk for relapse into mania or depression during the postpartum period.[2] If a severe mood episode occurs postpartum, there is an increased risk for recurrences during subsequent postpartum periods.[2]

Alcohol and substance abuse is common among patients with bipolar disorder and can have a significant impact on the age of onset, course of the illness, and response to treatment.[3,22,23] Alcohol and drug abuse or dependence has been reported in 46% and 41% of bipolar patients, respectively.[2,22] Patients with substance use disorders are more likely to have an earlier onset of their illness, mixed states, higher rates of relapse, a poorer response to treatment, comorbid personality disorders, increased suicide risk, and more psychiatric hospitalizations.[3] Bipolar patients often self-medicate with substances such as alcohol, marijuana, or cocaine during episodes, resulting in further impairment of judgment, poor impulse control, treatment nonadherence, and a worsening of the clinical course.[2,3,47]

More than one half (55%-65%) of bipolar I patients have some degree of functional disability after the onset of their illness, and approximately 10% to 20% of bipolar patients have severe impairment in their psychosocial and occupational functioning.[2,3,48] In a 1-year longitudinal study in 258 bipolar patients, two-thirds had four or more mood episodes a year despite comprehensive pharmacologic treatment, and approximately 33.2% of the year was spent being depressed compared with 10.8% of the time in a manic phase.[48]

Compared with the general population, individuals with bipolar disorder have a 2.3 times higher mortality rate. Suicide attempts occur in up to 50% of patients with bipolar disorder, and approximately 10% to 19% of individuals with bipolar I disorder commit suicide.[1-3,49] Studies suggest patients with bipolar II disorder have more suicide attempts than bipolar I patients.[49]

The best predictor for level of functioning during a person's lifetime is adherence with medication treatment. Medication discontinuation occurs in up to 50% of patients secondary to intolerance of drug-induced side effects.[50] Failure to recognize the disorder, reluctance to acknowledge it, or poor adherence with treatment are reasons an estimated two-thirds of patients with bipolar disorder do not receive appropriate treatment. Nonadherence with pharmacologic treatment and substance abuse are major factors in relapse and hospitalizations.[2,3]

TREATMENT

Desired Outcomes

4 The desired outcome in treating bipolar disorder is to effectively resolve acute manic, hypomanic, and depressive episodes, prevent further episodes, maintain good functioning, promote treatment

TABLE 69-4 General Principles for the Management of Bipolar Disorder

Goals of treatment
- Eliminate mood episode with complete remission of symptoms (ie, acute treatment)
- Prevent recurrences or relapses of mood episodes (ie, continuation phase treatment)
- Return to baseline psychosocial functioning
- Maximize adherence with therapy
- Minimize adverse effects
- Use medications with the best tolerability and fewest drug interactions
- Treat comorbid substance use and abuse
- Eliminate alcohol, marijuana, cocaine, amphetamines, and hallucinogens
- Minimize nicotine use and stop caffeine intake at least 8 hours prior to bedtime
- Avoidance of stressors or substances that precipitate an acute episode

Monitor for
- Mood episodes: Document symptoms on a daily mood chart (document life stressors, type of episode, length of episode, and treatment outcome); monthly and yearly life charts are valuable for documenting patterns of mood cycles
- Medication adherence (missing doses of medications is a primary reason for nonresponse and recurrence of episodes)
- Adverse effects, especially sedation and weight gain (manage rapidly and vigorously to avoid noncompliance)
- Suicidal ideation or attempts (suicide completion rates with bipolar I disorder are 10%-15%; suicide attempts are primarily associated with depressive episodes, mixed episodes with severe depression, or presence of psychosis)

Data from references 2, 22, and 51.

adherence, and minimize side effects.[2,3] The general principles and goals for the management of bipolar disorder are found in Table 69-4.

General Approach to Treatment

5 Treatment of bipolar disorder must be individualized because the clinical presentation, severity, and frequency of episodes vary widely among patients. Treatment approaches should include both nonpharmacologic and pharmacologic strategies.[3] Patients and family members should be educated about bipolar disorder (eg, symptoms, causes, and course) and treatment options. Long-term adherence to treatment is the most important factor in achieving stabilization of the disorder.

6 The treatment of bipolar disorder can vary depending on what type of episode the patient is experiencing. Once diagnosed with bipolar disorder, patients should remain on a mood stabilizer (eg, lithium, valproate) for their lifetime. During acute episodes, medications can be added and then tapered once the patient is stabilized and euthymic. For example, when treating a patient for mania with psychotic features, the patient should be on a mood stabilizer and an antipsychotic. If the antipsychotic is the patient's maintenance therapy, the dose should be increased or perhaps the medication should be changed altogether if the patient goes into a manic episode. If treating a patient for a severe depressive episode, a clinician may need to maximize the dose of the mood stabilizer or add another medication (eg, quetiapine).

Nonpharmacologic Therapy

The basics of nonpharmacologic approaches should address issues of adequate nutrition, sleep, exercise, and stress reduction.[3] Sleep deprivation, high stress, and deficiencies in dietary essential amino acids, fatty acids, vitamins, and minerals can exacerbate mood episodes and result in poorer outcomes.[3] Mood charting is an effective strategy in detecting early signs and symptoms of mania and depression. Another effective treatment is to combine medications with adjunctive psychoeducational programs, supportive counseling, insight-oriented psychotherapy (individual or group), couples or family therapy, cognitive behavioral therapy, and communication enhancement training.[2,3,22,51]

Pharmacologic Therapy

6 Pharmacotherapy is crucial for the acute and maintenance treatment of bipolar disorder and includes lithium, valproate, carbamazepine, lamotrigine, first-generation antipsychotics (FGAs) a second-generation antipsychotics (SGAs), and adjunctive agents such as antidepressants and benzodiazepines. General treatment guidelines for the acute treatment of mood episodes in patients with bipolar I disorder are found in Table 69-5.[52-53]

Product information, dosing, and administration of agents used in the treatment of bipolar disorder are found in Table 69-6.

6 The term *mood stabilizer* is often used to describe the class of medications used in the treatment of bipolar disorder, but this may not be accurate, as some medications are more effective for acute mania, some for the depressive episode, and others for the maintenance phase.[54] Lithium, valproate (or divalproex sodium), extended-release carbamazepine, aripiprazole, asenapine, cariprazine, olanzapine, quetiapine, risperidone, and ziprasidone are currently approved by the U.S. Food and Drug Administration (FDA) for the treatment of acute mania in bipolar disorder; only lithium, aripiprazole, olanzapine, and lamotrigine are approved for the maintenance treatment of bipolar disorder. Quetiapine and lurasidone are the only FDA-approved monotherapy antipsychotics for bipolar depression.

Combination therapies (eg, lithium plus valproate or carbamazepine; lithium or valproate plus an SGA) can provide better acute response and long-term prevention of relapse and recurrence than monotherapy in some bipolar patients.[55] The majority of patients hospitalized for an acute episode will be on combination therapy.

Several guidelines and algorithms have been published regarding the treatment of bipolar disorder, and these are generally based on the best available data and clinical consensus of experts. The Canadian Network for Mood and Anxiety Treatments (CANMAT) and International Society for Bipolar Disorders (ISBD) published updated treatment guidelines in 2013.[53] In addition, an international task force of the World Federation of Societies of Biological Psychiatry (WFSBP) has published guidelines for the treatment of bipolar disorder. The WFSBP mania, depression, and maintenance guidelines were updated in 2009, 2010, and 2013, respectively.[56,57,58]

Based on the CANMAT and ISBD guidelines and available research, an example treatment algorithm and guidelines for acute mood episodes in adult patients with bipolar I disorder are listed in Table 69-5. Selection of treatments for acute mood episodes (eg, mania, depression) and for maintenance treatment should be individualized. Treatment plans should be based on patient-specific characteristics, comorbid psychiatric and medical conditions, consideration of drug interactions, and avoidance of adverse effects.[2]

Specific Pharmacologic Therapies

Lithium Lithium was first used in 1949 as a treatment for mania and was approved in 1972 in the United States for the treatment of acute mania and for maintenance therapy. Despite numerous investigations into the biologic and clinical properties of lithium, there is no unified theory for its mechanism of action.[22,59] Chronic lithium administration may modulate gene expression and have neuroprotective effects. Lithium has unique pharmacokinetics because it is a monovalent cation. It is rapidly absorbed, is widely distributed with no protein binding, is not metabolized, and is excreted unchanged in the urine and in other body fluids.[60]

Efficacy Lithium is considered a first-line agent for acute mania, acute bipolar depression, and maintenance treatment of bipolar I and II disorders.[53] Early placebo-controlled studies with lithium reported up to a 78% response rate in aborting an acute manic or hypomanic episode, but more recent studies suggest a slower onset of action and a more moderate effectiveness when compared with other agents.[61] In placebo-controlled studies in bipolar depression,

TABLE 69-5 Algorithm and Guidelines for the Acute Treatment of Mood Episodes in Patients with Bipolar I Disorder

Acute Manic or Mixed Episode		**Acute Depressive Episode**	
General Guidelines		**General Guidelines**	
Assess for secondary causes of mania or mixed states (eg, alcohol or drug use) Discontinue antidepressants Taper off stimulants and caffeine if possible Treat substance abuse Encourage good nutrition (with regular protein and essential fatty acid intake), exercise, adequate sleep, stress reduction, and psychosocial therapy		Assess for secondary causes of depression (eg, alcohol or drug use) Taper off antipsychotics, benzodiazepines, or sedative–hypnotic agents if possible Treat substance abuse Encourage good nutrition (with regular protein and essential fatty acid intake), exercise, adequate sleep, stress reduction, and psychosocial therapy	
Hypomania	**Mania**	**Mild to Moderate Depressive Episode**	**Severe Depressive Episode**
First, optimize current mood stabilizer or initiate mood-stabilizing medication: lithium,[a] valproate,[a] carbamazepine,[a] or SGAs Consider adding a benzodiazepine (lorazepam or clonazepam) for short-term adjunctive treatment of agitation or insomnia if needed Alternative medication treatment options: oxcarbazepine **Second**, if response is inadequate, consider a two-drug combination: Lithium[a] **plus** an anticonvulsant or an SGA Anticonvulsant **plus** an anticonvulsant or SGA	**First**, two- or three-drug combinations (lithium,[a] valproate,[a] or SGA) **plus** a benzodiazepine (lorazepam or clonazepam) and/or antipsychotic for short-term adjunctive treatment of agitation or insomnia; lorazepam is recommended for catatonia Do not combine antipsychotics Alternative medication treatment options: carbamazepine[a]; if patient does not respond or tolerate, consider oxcarbazepine **Second**, if response is inadequate, consider a three-drug combination: Lithium[a] **plus** an anticonvulsant **plus** an antipsychotic Anticonvulsant **plus** an anticonvulsant **plus** an antipsychotic **Third**, if response is inadequate, consider ECT for mania with psychosis or catatonia,[d] or add clozapine for treatment-refractory illness	**First**, initiate and/or optimize mood-stabilizing medication: lithium,[a] quetiapine, lurasidone Alternative anticonvulsants: lamotrigine,[b] valproate[a]; antipsychotics: fluoxetine/olanzapine combination	**First**, optimize current mood stabilizer or initiate mood-stabilizing medication: lithium[a] or quetiapine or lurasidone Alternative fluoxetine/olanzapine combination If psychosis is present, initiate an antipsychotic in combination with above Do not combine antipsychotics Alternative anticonvulsants: lamotrigine,[b] valproate[a] **Second**, if response is inadequate, consider carbamazepine[a] or adding antidepressant **Third**, if response is inadequate, consider a three-drug combination: Lithium **plus** lamotrigine[b] **plus** an antidepressant Lithium **plus** quetiapine **plus** antidepressant[c] **Fourth**, if response is inadequate, consider ECT for treatment-refractory illness and depression with psychosis or catatonia[d]

ECT, electroconvulsive therapy; SGA, second-generation antipsychotic.

[a]Use standard therapeutic serum concentration ranges if clinically indicated; if partial response or breakthrough episode, adjust dose to achieve higher serum concentrations without causing intolerable adverse effects; valproate is preferred over lithium for mixed episodes and rapid cycling; lithium and/or lamotrigine is preferred over valproate for bipolar depression.

[b]Lamotrigine is not approved for the acute treatment of depression, and the dose must be started low and slowly titrated up to decrease adverse effects if used for maintenance therapy of bipolar I disorder. Lamotrigine may be initiated during acute treatment with plans to transition to this medication for long-term maintenance. A drug interaction and a severe dermatologic rash can occur when lamotrigine is combined with valproate (ie, lamotrigine doses must be halved from standard dosing titration).

[c]Controversy exists concerning the use of antidepressants, and they are often considered third line in treating acute bipolar depression, except in patients with no recent history of severe acute mania or potentially in bipolar II patients.

[d]ECT is used for severe mania or depression during pregnancy and for mixed episodes; prior to treatment, anticonvulsants, lithium, and benzodiazepines should be tapered off to maximize therapy and minimize adverse effects.

Data from references 2, 52, and 53.

lithium has been found to have efficacy, but there can be a 6- to 8-week delay for its antidepressant effects.[61] Lithium's role in the maintenance phase of bipolar disorder in preventing mania and depressive episodes is supported by numerous studies.[61] Lithium also produces a prophylactic response of reducing suicide in patients with bipolar disorder.[62] Relapse can be reduced with the combination of lithium and other medications such as divalproex sodium, carbamazepine, lamotrigine, and antipsychotics.[61] Abrupt discontinuation or noncompliance with lithium therapy can increase the risk of relapse.[61]

Adverse Effects Adverse effects related to lithium use can be divided into those that occur early in therapy but are generally innocuous and transient, those that are not dose-related occurring with long-term treatment, and toxic effects that occur with high serum concentrations.[60]

Initial gastrointestinal (GI) and central nervous system (CNS) side effects are often dose-related and are worse at peak serum concentrations (1-2 hours postdose). Standard approaches for minimizing adverse effects include lowering the dose, taking doses with food, using extended-release products, and trying once-daily dosing at bedtime. Diarrhea can sometimes be managed by switching from tablet or capsule formulation to liquid formulation. Diarrhea produced by lithium is commonly an osmotic diarrhea, and therefore switching to a formulation that clears the gut quickly can ameliorate symptoms. Muscle weakness and lethargy develop in about 40% to 50% of patients,[60] but these symptoms are usually transient. A benign fine hand tremor can be evident in up to 45% to 50% of patients and will usually resolve with continued treatment.[60] Strategies to reduce the tremor include standard approaches (eg, switch to long-acting preparation, lower dose if possible) or adding a β-adrenergic antagonist (eg, propranolol 20-120 mg/day).[60]

Polydipsia with polyuria associated with or without nephrogenic diabetes insipidus (DI) can occur in patients treated with lithium. About 30% to 50% of patients will develop nephrogenic DI soon after initiation of lithium treatment.[60] Nephrogenic DI will persist in about 10% to 25% of patients on continued treatment and typically is reversible with discontinuation of lithium.[60] Other nonspecific renal effects may be seen with lithium treatment, but no causality has been established for many of these findings.[60]

Hypothyroidism can occur in 1% to 4% of patients treated with lithium and does not require discontinuation of lithium.[60]

TABLE 69-6 Products, Dosage and Administration, and Clinical Use of Agents Used in the Treatment of Bipolar Disorder

Drug **"Brand name"**	Initial Dosing	Usual Dosing; Special Population Dosing	Comments
Lithium salts: FDA-approved for bipolar disorder			
Lithium carbonate[a,b] "Eskalith" "Eskalith CR" "Lithobid" Lithium citrate[a,b] "Cibalith-S"	300 mg twice daily	900-2,400 mg/day in two to four divided doses, preferably with meals Renal impairment: lower doses required with frequent serum monitoring There is wide variation in the dosage needed to achieve therapeutic response and trough serum lithium concentration (ie, 0.6-1.2 mEq/L [mmol/L] for maintenance therapy and 0.8-1.2 mEq/L [mmol/L] for acute mood episodes taken 12 hours after the last dose)	Use alone or in combination with other medications (eg, valproate, carbamazepine, antipsychotics) for the acute treatment of mania and for maintenance treatment
Anticonvulsants: FDA-approved for bipolar disorder			
Divalproex sodium[a] "Depakote" "Depakote ER" Valproic acid[a] "Stavzor"	250-500 mg twice daily A loading dose of divalproex (20-30 mg/kg/day) can be given	750-3,000 mg/day (20-60 mg/kg/day) given once daily or in divided doses Titrate to clinical response Dose adjustment needed with hepatic impairment	Use alone or in combination with other medications (eg, lithium, carbamazepine, antipsychotics) for the acute treatment of mania and for maintenance treatment Use caution when combining with lamotrigine because of potential drug interaction
Lamotrigine[b] "Lamictal"	25 mg daily	50-400 mg/day in divided doses. Dosage should be slowly increased (eg, 25 mg/day for 2 weeks, then 50 mg/day for weeks 3 and 4, and then 50-mg/day increments at weekly intervals up to 200 mg/day) Dose adjustment needed with hepatic impairment	Use alone or in combination with other medications (eg, lithium, carbamazepine) for long-term maintenance treatment for bipolar I disorder
Carbamazepine "Equetro"	200 mg twice daily	200-1,800 mg/day in two to four divided doses Titrate to clinical response Dose adjustment needed with hepatic impairment	Use alone or in combination with other medications (eg, lithium, valproate, antipsychotics) for the acute and long-term maintenance treatment of mania or mixed episodes for bipolar I disorder. APA guidelines recommend reserving it for patients unable to tolerate or who have inadequate response to lithium or valproate Extended-release tablets should be swallowed whole and not be broken or chewed
Anticonvulsants: not FDA-approved for bipolar disorder			
Carbamazepine "Tegretol" "Epitol" "Tegretol-XR" "Carbatrol"	200 mg twice daily	200-1,800 mg/day in two to four divided doses Titrate to clinical response Dose adjustment needed with hepatic impairment	"Carbatrol" capsules can be opened and contents sprinkled over food
Valproic acid "Depakene" Valproate sodium "Depacon"	250-500 mg twice daily A loading dose of divalproex (20-30 mg/kg/day) can be given	750-3,000 mg/day (20-60 mg/kg/day) given once daily or in divided doses Titrate to clinical response Dose adjustment needed with hepatic impairment	Use caution when combining with lamotrigine because of potential drug interaction
Oxcarbazepine "Trileptal"	300 mg twice daily	300-1,200 mg/day in two divided doses Titrate based on clinical response Dose adjustment required with severe renal impairment	Use after patients have failed treatment with carbamazepine or have intolerable side effects May have fewer adverse effects and be better tolerated than carbamazepine

(*Continued*)

TABLE 69-6 Products, Dosage and Administration, and Clinical Use of Agents Used in the Treatment of Bipolar Disorder (*Continued*)

Drug	Initial Dosing	Usual Dosing; Special Population Dosing	Comments
Atypical antipsychotics: FDA-approved for bipolar disorder			
Aripiprazole[a,b] "Abilify"	10-15 mg daily	10-30 mg/day once daily	
Asenapine[a] "Saphris"	5-10 mg twice daily sublingually	5-10 mg twice daily sublingually	
Cariprazine[a] "Vraylar"	1.5 mg daily	3-6 mg daily	
Lurasidone[c] "Latuda"	20 mg daily	20-120 mg daily with food	
Olanzapine[a,b] "Zyprexa" "Zyprexa Zydis"	2.5-5 mg twice daily	5-20 mg/day once daily or in divided doses	
Olanzapine and fluoxetine[c] "Symbyax"	6 mg olanzapine and 25 mg fluoxetine daily	6-12 mg olanzapine and 25-50 mg fluoxetine daily	
Quetiapine[a,c] "Seroquel"	50 mg twice daily	50-800 mg/day in divided doses or once daily when stabilized	
Risperidone[a] "Risperdal" "Risperdal M-Tab"	0.5-1 mg twice daily	0.5-6 mg/day once daily or in divided doses	
Ziprasidone[a] "Geodon"	40-60 mg twice daily	40-160 mg/day in divided doses	
Benzodiazepines	Dosage should be slowly adjusted up and down according to response and adverse effects		Use in combination with other medications (eg, antipsychotics, lithium, valproate) for the acute treatment of mania or mixed episodes Use as a short-term adjunctive sedative–hypnotic agent

FDA-approved agents may be used as monotherapy in various phases of the illness as noted in table footnotes.[a,b,c]

[a]FDA-approved for acute mania.

[b]FDA-approved for maintenance.

[c]FDA-approved for acute bipolar depression.

Data from references 2, 3, 22, and 53.

Supplemental exogenous thyroid hormone (ie, levothyroxine) can be added to the patients' regimen. If lithium is discontinued, the need for the exogenous thyroid hormone should be reassessed, because hypothyroidism can be reversible.

Lithium can cause a variety of benign and reversible cardiac effects, particularly T-wave flattening or inversion (in up to 30% of patients), atrioventricular block, and bradycardia.[60] If a patient has significant preexisting cardiac disease, consultation with a cardiologist and an electrocardiogram (ECG) is recommended at baseline and during lithium therapy.

Other adverse effects associated with the use of lithium include: acne and folliculitis (1%), reversible leukocytosis, and weight gain.[60] Weight gain is common (~20% of patients gain greater than 10 kg [22 lb]) and can be related to fluid retention, the consumption of high-calorie beverages as a result of polydipsia, or a decreased metabolic rate because of hypothyroidism.[22,63]

Lithium is an extremely toxic medication if accidentally or intentionally taken in overdose. Lithium toxicity usually occurs with blood levels greater than 1.5 mEq/L (mmol/L), but elderly patients may experience toxicity at lower levels.[2] Severe lithium intoxication occurs when concentrations are higher than 2 mEq/L (mmol/L), and there is a worsening in several key symptoms: *GI* (eg, vomiting, diarrhea, or incontinence), *coordination* (eg, severe fine to coarse hand tremor, unstable gait, slurred speech, and muscle twitching), and *cognition* (eg, poor concentration, drowsiness, disorientation, apathy, and coma).[2] There have been several reports of seizures, cardiac dysrhythmias, permanent neurologic impairments with ataxia and memory deficits, and kidney damage with reduced glomerular filtration rate after lithium intoxication.[2]

Situations that predispose patients to lithium toxicity include sodium restriction, dehydration, vomiting, diarrhea, age greater than 50, heart failure, cirrhosis, and drug interactions that decrease lithium clearance. Heavy exercise, sauna baths, hot weather, and fever can promote sodium loss. Patients should be cautioned to maintain adequate sodium and fluid intake (2.5-3 qt [~2.5-3 L] per day of fluids) and to avoid the excessive use of coffee, tea, cola, and other caffeine-containing beverages and alcohol.

If lithium toxicity is suspected, the person should go to an emergency room to be monitored, and lithium should be discontinued.[2] Gastric lavage and IV fluids may be needed, and the patient should be monitored for fluid balance, renal and electrolyte status, and neurologic changes. Under the following circumstances clinicians should consider hemodialysis and continue until the lithium concentration is below 1 mEq/L (mmol/L) when taken 8 hours after the last dialysis: in lithium-naïve patients when lithium concentrations equal or exceed 4 mEq/L (mmol/L) regardless of clinical status, in patients previously taking lithium when lithium concentrations are 2.5 mEq/L (mmol/L) or greater and moderate-to-severe neurologic toxicity, or as clinically indicated.[60]

Drug–Drug Interactions Thiazide diuretics, nonsteroidal anti-inflammatory drugs, cyclooxygenase-2 inhibitors, angiotensin-converting enzyme inhibitors, and salt-restricted diets can elevate lithium levels.[60] Neurotoxicity can occur when lithium is combined with antipsychotics, metronidazole, methyldopa, phenytoin, and verapamil.[2,60] Combining lithium with calcium channel blockers is not recommended because of reports of decreased lithium levels and neurotoxicity.[60] Analgesics such as acetaminophen or aspirin and loop diuretics are less likely to interfere with lithium clearance. Caffeine and theophylline can enhance the renal elimination of lithium. Because lithium has no effect on hepatic metabolizing enzymes, it has fewer drug–drug interactions compared with carbamazepine, oxcarbazepine, and valproate.

Dosing and Administration Lithium dosing depends on the patient's age and weight, tolerance to adverse effects, and the acuity of the illness. Lithium therapy is usually initiated with low to moderate doses (600 mg/day) for prophylaxis and higher doses (900-1,200 mg/day) for acute mania, using a two- to three-times daily dosing regimen.[2,60] The dose should be adjusted based on the steady-state serum concentration and clinical picture of the patient. Immediate-release lithium preparations should be given in two or three divided daily doses, whereas extended-release products can be given once or twice daily. In clinical practice many clinicians dose the immediate-release and extended-release preparations once daily. It can be best to initially begin a patient on divided dosing, but once stabilized many patients are able to switch to once-daily dosing without decompensating.

Lithium levels should be monitored for efficacy and to guide dosing. In general, lithium serum concentrations should be maintained between 0.6 and 1.0 mEq/L (mmol/L).[61] Lithium levels are considered to be at steady state at approximately day 5, and serum samples should be drawn 12 hours postdose. Once a desired serum concentration has been achieved, levels should be drawn in 2 weeks and then if stable every 3 to 6 months or as clinically indicated. Maintenance lithium serum concentrations are usually measured every 3 months, but can be adjusted to every 6 months for stabilized patients, and every 1 to 2 months for patients with frequent mood episodes.[2] Lithium clearance rates increase by 50% to 100% during pregnancy and return to normal postpartum; thus, lithium levels should be determined monthly during pregnancy and weekly the month before delivery. At delivery, rapid fluid changes can significantly increase lithium levels; thus, a reduction to prepregnancy lithium doses and adequate hydration are recommended.[2]

The recommended guidelines for baseline and routine laboratory testing for lithium are listed in Table 69-7.[65-68] A therapeutic trial for outpatients should last a minimum of 4 to 6 weeks with lithium serum concentrations of 0.6 to 1.2 mEq/L (mmol/L). Acutely manic patients can require serum concentrations of 1 to 1.2 mEq/L (mmol/L), and some need up to 1.5 mEq/L (mmol/L) to achieve a therapeutic response. Although serum concentrations less than 0.6 mEq/L (mmol/L) may be associated with higher rates of relapse, some patients can do well at 0.4 to 0.7 mEq/L (mmol/L).[61] For bipolar prophylaxis in elderly patients, serum concentrations of 0.4 to 0.6 mEq/L (mmol/L) are recommended because of increased sensitivity to adverse effects.[60]

Anticonvulsants

Divalproex sodium (also known as sodium valproate) was marketed in 1995, for the acute treatment of mania in adults and is now the most prescribed mood stabilizer in the United States. It is FDA-approved only for the treatment of acute manic or mixed episodes; however, it is commonly used in clinical practice as maintenance monotherapy for bipolar disorder. Limited data support its use in acute bipolar depression. Carbamazepine is commonly used for both acute and maintenance therapy. The only formulation approved in the United States for bipolar disorder is extended-release carbamazepine, although other formulations can be used. Some data support the use of oxcarbazepine, a 10-keto analogue of carbamazepine, in the treatment of bipolar disorder; however, it is not approved for the treatment of bipolar disorder in the United States. Valproate, carbamazepine, and oxcarbazepine all have a wide range of neurologic, GI, electrolyte, and hematologic adverse effects that require regular assessment and routine blood work. Lamotrigine is FDA-approved for the maintenance treatment of bipolar I disorder. This medication appears to be most effective in the prevention of relapse of depression and does not appear to have efficacy for treatment of acute depression or mania.[69]

Valproate Sodium and Valproic Acid Valproate has antimigraine, mood-stabilizing, and antiaggressive effects.[64] In 1995, the enteric-coated formulation divalproex sodium (sodium valproate) was approved for the acute treatment of mania. Several controlled studies have shown valproate to be as effective as lithium and olanzapine in patients with pure mania, and it can be more effective than lithium in certain subtypes of bipolar disorder (eg, rapid cycling, mixed features, comorbid substance abuse).[2,3,22,44,70] Placebo- and lithium-controlled and open studies report that valproate reduces or prevents recurrent manic, depressive, and mixed episodes.[2,3,22]

Giving lithium, carbamazepine, antipsychotics, or benzodiazepines with valproate can augment its antimanic effects. The addition of valproate to lithium can have synergistic effects in patients who are treatment-refractory and have specifiers of rapid cycling or mixed features, and the combination has demonstrated efficacy in maintenance therapy for bipolar I disorder. Combinations of valproate and carbamazepine can have synergistic effects, but the potential drug interactions make blood level monitoring of both agents essential.[22] Adding adjunctive SGAs to valproate can be effective for breakthrough mania or if there is incomplete or partial response to monotherapy. Clozapine, olanzapine, and quetiapine can increase the risk of sedation and weight gain when combined with valproate. The combination of valproate and lamotrigine can be effective, but there is an increased risk of rashes, ataxia, tremor, sedation, and fatigue.[64]

Adverse Effects The most frequent dose-related adverse effects with valproate are GI complaints (anorexia, nausea, indigestion, vomiting, mild diarrhea, and flatulence), fine hand tremors, and sedation.[2,22,64] The GI complaints are usually transient, but giving the medication with food, using lower initial doses with gradual increases in doses, or switching to divalproex sodium extended-release tablets can minimize them.[2,22] Reduction of the dose or the addition of a β-blocker can alleviate tremors, and giving the total daily dose at bedtime can minimize daytime sedation.[2,22]

Other adverse effects of valproate include ataxia, lethargy, alopecia, changes in the texture or color of hair, pruritus, prolonged bleeding because of inhibition of platelet aggregation, transient increases in liver enzymes, and hyperammonemia.[22,64] Increased appetite and weight gain occurs in approximately 50% of patients on long-term valproate therapy. Thrombocytopenia can occur at higher doses, and patients should be monitored for bleeding and bruising. Lowering the valproate dose can restore platelet counts to normal levels.[2] Fatal necrotizing hepatitis is a rare idiosyncratic, non–dose-related adverse effect that has occurred in children with epilepsy receiving multiple anticonvulsants.[22,64] A life-threatening hemorrhagic pancreatitis has been reported in both children and adults.[2,22,64] An in-depth discussion of adverse effects can be found in Chapter 56.

Drug–Drug Interactions A summary of drug–drug interactions for valproate can be found in Chapter 56.

Dosing and Administration For healthy inpatient adults with acute mania, the initial starting dosage of valproate is typically 20 mg/kg/day in divided doses over 12 hours. The daily dose is adjusted by 250 to 500 mg every 1 to 3 days based on clinical response and tolerability. Maximum recommended dosing is 60 mg/kg/day (see Table 69-6).[2,22,64] For outpatients who are hypomanic or euthymic, or for elderly patients, the initial starting dose is generally lower (5-10 mg/kg/day in divided doses) and gradually titrated to avoid adverse effects. Once an optimal dose has been achieved, the total daily dose can be divided into two doses or given at bedtime if tolerated.[2,22,64] Extended-release divalproex can be administered once daily, but bioavailability can be 15% lower than that of immediate-release products, thus requiring slightly higher doses.[2] In clinical practice, patients with bipolar disorder who are stable can be

TABLE 69-7 Guidelines for Baseline and Routine Laboratory Tests and Monitoring for Patients with Bipolar Disorder Taking Mood Stabilizers

	Baseline: Physical Examination and General Chemistry[a]	Hematologic Tests[b]		Metabolic Tests[c]		Liver Function Tests[d]		Renal Function Tests[e]		Thyroid Function Tests[f]		Serum Electrolytes[g]		Dermatologic[h]	
	Baseline	Baseline	6-12 months	Baseline	6-12 months	Baseline	6-12 months	Baseline	6-12 months	Baseline	6-12 months	Baseline	6-12 months	Baseline	6-12 months
SGAs[i]	X			X	X										
Carbamazepine[j]	X	X	X			X	X	X				X	X	X	X
Lamotrigine[k]	X													X	X
Lithium[l]	X	X	X	X	X			X	X	X	X	X	X	X	X
Oxcarbazepine[m]	X											X	X		
Valproate[n]	X	X	X	X	X	X	X							X	X

SGAs, second-generation antipsychotics.

[a]Screen for drug abuse and serum pregnancy.

[b]Complete blood cell count (CBC) with differential and platelets.

[c]Fasting glucose, serum lipids, and weight.

[d]Lactate dehydrogenase, aspartate aminotransferase, alanine aminotransferase, total bilirubin, and alkaline phosphatase.

[e]Serum creatinine, blood urea nitrogen, urinalysis, urine osmolality, and specific gravity.

[f]Triiodothyronine, total thyroxine, thyroxine uptake, and thyroid-stimulating hormone.

[g]Serum sodium.

[h]Rashes, hair thinning, and alopecia.

[i]Second-generation antipsychotics: Monitor for increased appetite with weight gain (primarily in patients with initial low or normal body mass index); monitor closely if rapid or significant weight gain occurs during early therapy; cases of hyperlipidemia and diabetes reported.

[j]Carbamazepine: Manufacturer recommends CBC and platelets (and possibly reticulocyte counts and serum iron) at baseline, and that subsequent monitoring be individualized by the clinician (eg, CBC, platelet counts, and liver function tests every 2 weeks during the first 2 months of treatment, and then every 3 months if normal). Monitor more closely if patient exhibits hematologic or hepatic abnormalities or if the patient is receiving a myelotoxic drug; discontinue if platelets are <100,000/mm^3 (<100 × 10^9/L), if white blood cell (WBC) count is <3,000/mm^3 (<3 × 10^9/L), or if there is evidence of bone marrow suppression or liver dysfunction. Serum electrolyte levels should be monitored in the elderly or those at risk for hyponatremia. Carbamazepine interferes with some pregnancy tests.

[k]Lamotrigine: If renal or hepatic impairment, monitor closely and adjust dosage according to manufacturer's guidelines. Serious dermatologic reactions have occurred within 2 to 8 weeks of initiating treatment and are more likely to occur in patients receiving concomitant valproate, with rapid dosage escalation, or using doses exceeding the recommended titration schedule.

[l]Lithium: Obtain baseline electrocardiogram for patients older than 40 years or if preexisting cardiac disease (benign, reversible T-wave depression can occur). Renal function tests should be obtained every 2 to 3 months during the first 6 months, and then every 6 to 12 months; if impaired renal function, monitor 24-hour urine volume and creatinine every 3 months; if urine volume >3 L/day, monitor urinalysis, osmolality, and specific gravity every 3 months. Thyroid function tests should be obtained once or twice during the first 6 months, and then every 6 to 12 months; monitor for signs and symptoms of hypothyroidism; if supplemental thyroid therapy is required, monitor thyroid function tests and adjust thyroid dose every 1 to 2 months until thyroid function indices are within normal range, and then monitor every 3 to 6 months.

[m]Oxcarbazepine: Hyponatremia (serum sodium concentrations <125 mEq/L [mmol/L]) has been reported and occurs more frequently during the first 3 months of therapy; serum sodium concentrations should be monitored in patients receiving drugs that lower serum sodium concentrations (eg, diuretics or drugs that cause inappropriate antidiuretic hormone secretion) or in patients with symptoms of hyponatremia (eg, confusion, headache, lethargy, and malaise). Hypersensitivity reactions have occurred in approximately 25% to 30% of patients with a history of carbamazepine hypersensitivity and require immediate discontinuation.

[n]Valproate: Weight gain reported in patients with low or normal body mass index. Monitor platelets and liver function during first 3 to 6 months if evidence of increased bruising or bleeding. Monitor closely if patients exhibit hematologic or hepatic abnormalities or in patients receiving drugs that affect coagulation, such as aspirin or warfarin; discontinue if platelets are <100,000/mm^3/L (<100 × 10^9/L) or if prolonged bleeding time. Pancreatitis, hyperammonemic encephalopathy, polycystic ovary syndrome, increased testosterone, and menstrual irregularities have been reported; not recommended during first trimester of pregnancy due to risk of neural tube defects.

Data from references 2, 22, 60, 64 to 68.

switched between formulations without having to change the dose. This is not the case for patients with seizure disorder.

Recommended baseline and routine laboratory tests for patients taking valproate are listed in Table 69-7. Although therapeutic serum concentrations of valproic acid have not been established in bipolar disorder, most clinicians use the anticonvulsant therapeutic serum range of 50 to 125 mcg/mL (347-866 μmol/L) taken 12 hours after the last dose.[2,22] In one study patients with valproate levels greater than 94.1 mcg/mL (652 μmol/L) had greater efficacy for bipolar mania.[71] Patients with cyclothymia or mild bipolar II disorder can have a therapeutic response to lower doses and blood levels, whereas some patients with a more severe form of bipolar disorder can require up to 150 mcg/mL (1,040 μmol/L). Serum valproic acid levels are most useful when assessing for compliance and toxicity.

Carbamazepine Carbamazepine, a iminostilbene derivative, is structurally related to tricyclic antidepressants (TCAs).[65] Carbamazepine is not a first-line agent for bipolar disorder, and is generally reserved for use after treatment failure with lithium or divalproex sodium. Carbamazepine is effective for the treatment of mania, but its use is generally reserved due to drug interactions.[56] Data supporting the use of carbamazepine for bipolar depression are lacking and are not strong for the use of carbamazepine in maintanence treatment.[57,58] The combination of carbamazepine with lithium, valproate, and antipsychotics is often used for treatment-resistant patients experiencing a manic episode.[22]

Adverse Effects A summary of adverse effects for carbamazepine can be found in Chapter 56. Acute overdoses of carbamazepine are potentially lethal, and serum levels above 15 mcg/mL (63 μmol/L) are associated with ataxia, choreiform movements, diplopia, nystagmus, cardiac conduction changes, seizures, and coma.[2] Gastric lavage, emesis, ECG, and symptomatic treatment are recommended for the management of carbamazepine toxicity.[65]

Drug–Drug Interactions There are numerous drug-drug interactions that clinicians must consider when prescribing carbamazepine. Carbamazepine significantly induces the hepatic cytochrome P450 isoenzyme 3A4 and to a lesser degree 1A2, 2C9/10, and 2D6, which increases the metabolism of many medications (eg, quetiapine, aripiprazole).[2,3,65] Women taking oral contraceptives who receive carbamazepine should be counseled to use a nonhormonal method of birth control.[65]

Carbamazepine is metabolized to an active 10,11-epoxide metabolite; thus, medications that inhibit 3A4 isoenzymes can result in carbamazepine toxicity (eg, diltiazem, fluconazole, ketoconazole, nefazodone, verapamil).[2,3,22,65] When carbamazepine is combined with valproate, the carbamazepine dose should be reduced because valproate displaces carbamazepine from protein-binding sites, thus increasing free levels.[3,22] Combining clozapine and carbamazepine is not recommended because of decreased clozapine concentrations and the possibility of bone marrow suppression with both agents.[65]

Dosing and Administration During an acute manic episode in most hospitalized patients, carbamazepine can be started at 400 to 600 mg/day in divided doses with meals and increased by 200 mg/day every 2 to 4 days up to 10 to 15 mg/kg/day. In outpatients the initial dose of carbamazepine should be lower and titrated gradually in order to avoid adverse effects. In clinical practice many patients are able to tolerate once-daily dosing of carbamazepine once their mood episode has stabilized. The dose of carbamazepine should be gradually increased until response is achieved or there is evidence of toxicity. During the first month of therapy, serum concentrations of carbamazepine may be affected due to autoinduction of cytochrome P450 3A4 enzymes.[65]

Carbamazepine serum levels are usually obtained every 1 to 2 weeks during the first 2 months, and then every 3 to 6 months during maintenance therapy. Serum levels should be drawn 10 to 12 hours after the dose (trough levels) and at least 4 to 7 days after a dosage change. Although there is no correlation between carbamazepine serum concentration and degree of antimanic or antidepressant response, most clinicians attempt to maintain levels between 6 and 10 mcg/mL (25 and 42 μmol/L) (although some treatment-resistant patients can require serum concentrations of 12-14 mcg/mL [51-59 μmol/L]). Recommended baseline and routine laboratory tests for carbamazepine are listed in Table 69-7.

Oxcarbazepine There are currently less data supporting the use of oxcarbazepine than carbamazepine in the treatment of bipolar disorder. Guidelines typically recommend oxcarbazepine as a third-line treatment option for bipolar mania, as a third- or fourth-line treatment option for maintenance treatment, and it is not recommended for the treatment of bipolar depression.[53]

Adverse Effects Severe dermatologic reactions (eg, Stevens-Johnson syndrome) have been reported at 3 to 10 times the rate of the general population, therefore oxcarbazepine should be discontinued at the first sign of a skin reaction.[66] Other adverse effects may include impaired cognitive or psychomotor performance, somnolence or fatigue, and coordination difficulties.[66] In one study, hyponatremia was reported to occur in patients taking oxcarbazepine and carbamazepine at rates of 29.9% and 13.5%, respectively.[72] Severe hyponatremia (sodium ≤128 mEq/L [mmol/L]) was reported by Dong et al. as 12.4% and 2.8% of patients for oxcarbazepine and carbamazepine, respectively.[72] An in-depth discussion of adverse effects can be found in Chapter 56.

Drug–Drug Interactions Oxcarbazepine, a cytochrome P450 2C19 enzyme inhibitor and a 3A3/4 enzyme inducer, has the potential for causing drug interactions.[66] It induces the metabolism of oral contraceptives; thus, alternative contraceptive measures are required.[3,73]

Dosing and Administration Initial dosing is usually 150 to 300 mg twice daily, and daily doses can be increased by 300 to 600 mg every 3 to 6 days up to 1,200 mg/day in divided doses (with or without food).[66]

Lamotrigine The effectiveness of lamotrigine for the maintenance treatment of bipolar I disorder in adult patients was established in two multicenter, double-blind, placebo-controlled studies.[2] Doses of 200 mg/day were more effective than lower doses, and there were no advantages to using 400 mg/day. Lamotrigine has mood-stabilizing effects; it may have augmenting properties when combined with lithium or valproate, and has low rates of switching patients to mania.[74] Although lamotrigine is not effective for acute mania compared with standard mood stabilizers, it may be beneficial as maintenance therapy of treatment-resistant bipolar I and II disorders.[2,3,58] Lamotrigine seems to be most effective for the prevention of bipolar depression; therefore, clinically it is often used in the treatment of patients with bipolar II. There are case reports of possible lamotrigine-induced mania when added to lithium, carbamazepine, and valproate.[75] In each of the cases reported, the patients had depressive mood symptoms or rapid mood changes requiring additional therapy.[75]

Adverse Effects Common adverse effects include headache, nausea, dizziness, ataxia, diplopia, drowsiness, tremor, rash, and pruritus.[67] Approximately 10% of patients in premarketing clinical trials developed a maculopapular rash and required discontinuation of therapy.[67] Although most rashes are self-limiting and resolve with continued treatment, some cases progressed to life-threatening conditions such as Stevens-Johnson syndrome. The incidence of rash appears to be greatest with coadministration of valproate, with higher than recommended initial doses, and with rapid dose escalation.[67] Patients should be warned about the rash, and the need for discontinuing lamotrigine if the rash is diffuse, involves mucosal membranes, and is accompanied by a fever or sore throat.

For an in-depth discussion of the adverse effects of lamotrigine, see Chapter 56.

Drug–Drug Interactions Valproate decreases the clearance of lamotrigine (ie, more than doubles the half-life), and lamotrigine must be administered at a reduced dosage (approximately half the standard dose).[67] For an in-depth discussion of drug–drug interactions with lamotrigine, see Chapter 56.

Dosing and Administration For the maintenance treatment of bipolar disorder, the usual dosage range of lamotrigine is 50 to 300 mg/day. The target dose is generally 200 mg/day (100 mg/day in combination with valproate and 400 mg/day in combination with carbamazepine).[67] For patients not taking medications that affect lamotrigine's clearance, the dose is 25 mg/day for the first 2 weeks of therapy, 50 mg/day for weeks 3 and 4, 100 mg/day for week 5, and 200 mg/day for week 6 and beyond.[2,67] Patients who stop lamotrigine therapy for more than a few days should be restarted on a low dose and titrated every 2 weeks back to their maintanence dose.

Antipsychotics

FGAs and SGAs such as aripiprazole, asenapine, haloperidol, olanzapine, quetiapine, risperidone, and ziprasidone are effective as monotherapy or adjunctive therapy in the treatment of acute mania.[76] Controlled studies in acute mania with lithium or valproate plus an antipsychotic suggest greater efficacy with combination therapies compared to any of these agents alone.[2,76] FGAs (eg, chlorpromazine and haloperidol) are effective in up to 70% of patients with acute mania, particularly those with psychosis and psychomotor agitation. SGAs have demonstrated similar efficacy for the treatment of acute mania associated with agitation, aggression, and psychosis.[2,76]

Treating acute bipolar depression is very challenging, and some antipsychotics may play a useful role. Multiple large randomized controlled trials support use of quetiapine and lurasidone as a monotherapy and adjunctive treatment options for bipolar depression.[77] Data also support use of combined fluoxetine/olanzapine in treating bipolar depression.[77]

Long-term safety of antipsychotics as monotherapy or as adjunctive therapy for bipolar maintenance treatment should be evaluated.[2,53,76] Risks versus benefits must be weighed due to the long-term adverse effects (eg, weight gain, type 2 diabetes, hyperlipidemia, hyperprolactinemia, and tardive dyskinesia) antipsychotics may cause.[76,78] Aripiprazole, olanzapine, quetiapine, and risperidone long-acting injection are effective monotherapy options for maintenance treatment in bipolar disorder.[53] First-generation depot antipsychotics (eg, haloperidol decanoate, fluphenazine decanoate) can have a place in maintenance treatment of bipolar disorder in patients who are noncompliant or treatment-resistant.[2]

Clozapine monotherapy has acute and long-term mood-stabilizing effects in refractory bipolar disorder, but requires regular white blood cell monitoring for agranulocytosis.[22,76]

Clinical **Controversy...**

What is the role of SGAs in bipolar disorder?

The desire to shorten hospital stays may contribute to increased use of SGAs added to a traditional mood stabilizer to return patients quickly to a baseline level of functioning. When and even whether to taper and discontinue the SGA once an acute manic episode has subsided is a complex decision. The risk of metabolic side effects including weight gain, hyperglycemia, and hyperlipidemia must be weighed against the potential benefits offered by the SGA. Often the longitudinal course of each patient's bipolar illness and each patient's response and relapse pattern with previous medications will inform decision making.

Adverse Effects A summary of adverse effects for antipsychotics can be found in Chapter 67.

Drug–Drug Interactions A summary of drug interactions with antipsychotics can be found in Chapter 67.

Dosing and Administration For acute mania, higher initial doses of antipsychotics can be required (eg, olanzapine 20 mg/day in hospitalized patients). Once acute mania is controlled (usually within 7-28 days), the antipsychotic can be gradually tapered and discontinued, and the patient maintained on the mood stabilizer monotherapy.

Monitoring (7) Recommendations for baseline and routine laboratory testing for patients receiving carbamazepine, lamotrigine, lithium, oxcarbazepine, SGAs, and valproate are found in Table 69-7.

Alternative Medication Treatments

(8) **Benzodiazepines** Weighing the risk-to-benefit ratio, high-potency benzodiazepines such as clonazepam and lorazepam are commonly used as an alternative to or in combination with antipsychotics when patients are experiencing acute mania, agitation, anxiety, panic, and insomnia, or cannot take mood stabilizers (eg, during the first trimester of pregnancy).[2,3,79,80] Lorazepam is available for intramuscular injection and is useful in the acute management of agitation. Benzodiazepines cause minimal adverse effects compared with antipsychotics, and at higher doses, rapidly sedate agitated patients.[3] They can cause CNS depression, sedation, cognitive and motor impairment, dependence, and withdrawal reactions. When no longer required, benzodiazepines should be gradually tapered and discontinued to avoid withdrawal symptoms.

Antidepressants For many years antidepressants were recommended as adjunctive therapy for acute bipolar depression. Data from the Systematic Treatment Enhancement Program for Bipolar Disorder (STEP-BD) suggest that adjunctive antidepressants may be no better than placebo for acute bipolar depression when combined with mood stabilizers.[81] Controversy exists concerning the use of antidepressants, and many clinicians consider them third line in treating acute bipolar depression, except in patients with no history of severe and/or recent mania or potentially in bipolar II patients.[82] The concern of mood switching (ie, rapidly switching from depression to mania or hypomania) with the use of antidepressants is valid, although not common. Data show that the rate of mood switch with selective serotonin reuptake inhibitors (SSRIs) is around 3.8%, similar to placebo, when combined with mood stabilizers. The rate of mood switch with dual-acting agents (eg, TCAs or venlafaxine) is higher, and thus these agents should be used with caution.[82,83] Before initiating therapy with an antidepressant it is very important to ensure that the patient is on a therapeutic dosage or blood level of a primary mood stabilizer.[2] Patients who have a history of mania after a depressive episode or who have frequent cycling should be treated cautiously with antidepressants.[2,3] In general, the antidepressant should be gradually withdrawn 2 to 6 months after remission, and the patient maintained on a mood-stabilizing agent.[84,85] For more information, see Chapter 68 for comparisons among antidepressants.

Calcium Channel Antagonists Verapamil, a nondihydropyridine, has demonstrated mood-stabilizing properties in some studies, but negative results were found in other trials.[3,22,86] Nimodipine, a dihydropyridine, can be more effective than verapamil for rapid-cycling bipolar disorder because of its anticonvulsant properties, high lipid solubility, and good penetration into the brain.[3,22,45,86] Calcium channel blockers are generally well tolerated, and the most common adverse effects are bradycardia and hypotension. These are seldom used in everyday clinical practice.

Newer Anticonvulsants Third-generation anticonvulsants have been investigated for treating bipolar disorder with the hope that a different mechanism of action would be beneficial for mood stabilization. Gabapentin, levetiracetam, tiagabine, topiramate, and zonisamide have negative or limited positive data supporting their use in bipolar disorder. Topiramate has been used as an add-on weight-reduction medication, but there are no randomized, controlled trials supporting its use in bipolar disorder.[87]

Special Populations

The approach for treating bipolar disorder in special populations (eg, comorbid medical or psychiatric disorders, pregnancy) can vary among clinicians. Patients with comorbid medical conditions or concomitant substance abuse, those older than 65 or younger than 18 years, and pregnant patients can require different treatment approaches.

Clinical **Controversy...**

What are the roles of traditional mood stabilizers, antipsychotics, and benzodiazepines in the pregnant female patient with acute mania?

Ebstein's anomaly, a congenital heart defect associated with first trimester exposure to lithium was once thought to be much more common than recent data suggest, leading some clinicians to consider treating pregnant patients with severe debilitating acute manic episodes with lithium, though this remains controversial. Valproic acid and carbamazepine remain contraindicated during the first trimester of pregnancy due to concerns about neural tube defects. Given the length of time haloperidol has been available, there is considerable safety data on this first-generation antipsychotic in treating the acutely manic patient. Safety data on SGAs are still limited. Short-acting benzodiazepines such as lorazepam are often considered during the first trimester of pregnancy for severe manic episodes in an effort to minimize exposure to traditional mood stabilizers. A risk benefit analysis of all psychotropic interventions during pregnancy is critical to maternal and fetal well-being.

Comprehensive management during pregnancy is important to decrease the risk of birth defects, perinatal complications and mortality, preterm birth, low birth weight, and low Apgar scores.[88] Pharmacotherapy during pregnancy is complicated, and the risk-to-benefit ratio must be weighed. Clinicians should always use the lowest effective dose of any medication during pregnancy. Monotherapy should also be considered in order to decrease risk to the mother and child.

When lithium is given during the first trimester the prevalence of Ebstein's anomaly is estimated between 1 and 10.78:1000 and the risk of neural tube defects is 13.4:1000.[88] Lithium freely crosses the placenta and is found in equal concentrations in maternal and fetal blood.[60] When lithium is used during pregnancy, it should be tapered down to the lowest effective dose necessary to decrease the risk of relapse. Lithium can cause perinatal complications such as hypotonia, jaundice, cyanosis, and lethargy.[88] Milk concentrations of lithium range from 30% to 50% of the mother's serum concentration, and serum concentrations in the nursing infant are 10% to 50% of the mother's; thus, breastfeeding is usually discouraged.[2,89] If using lithium during pregnancy, dose adjustments and close monitoring of serum levels will be needed due to changes in glomerular filtration rates and renal perfusion rates during pregnancy and immediately after delivery.[88]

Neural tube defects cause the most concern for clinicians treating pregnant patients during their first trimester. Data from the North American Antiepileptic Drug Pregnancy Registry show the risk of neural tube defects is about 0.12% for nonexposed babies.[90] Carbamazepine's risk of neural tube defects is estimated to be 3%.[90] Carbamazepine is excreted in breast milk (the milk-to-maternal plasma ratio of carbamazepine is ~0.4).[3] Craniofacial abnormalities, developmental delays, microcephaly, and other abnormalities are also of concern when using anticonvulsants. For pregnant patients treated with lamotrigine, the risk of neural tube defects is estimated to be 2%, but data for lamotrigine are limited compared with those for some older anticonvulsants.[90] Valproate is usually not recommended during the first trimester of pregnancy because the risk of neural tube defects is estimated to be 4%.[90] Australian registry data in patients with epilepsy show dose-related teratogenicity with doses greater than 1,100 mg/day of valproate.[91] Administration of folate can reduce the risk of neural tube defects; therefore, the risks versus benefits of using valproate during pregnancy must be discussed with the patient.[22] Women of childbearing age on valproic acid and pregnant women should receive folic acid supplementation. Valproic acid is excreted into human breast milk in low concentrations (less than 1%-10% of the mother's serum level), so is considered to be compatible with breastfeeding.[3] One case report of thrombocytopenia and anemia from valproate exposure has been reported in a nursing infant. If the mother receives valproate during breastfeeding, mother and infant should have identical laboratory monitoring.

Caution should be used when prescribing antipsychotics during pregnancy. FGAs have been prescribed for many years in pregnancy and data show little teratogenic risk, but the data are not without question.[92] Data on the SGAs are limited, and clinicians should consider the potential risk of gestational diabetes.[92] Extrapyramidal symptoms, neonatal withdrawal, and sedation should also be considered when prescribing both FGAs and SGAs. There is still a paucity of human data with antipsychotics, and therefore risk-to-benefit ratio must be weighed.

There are few controlled studies in children and adolescents with bipolar disorder; thus, little is known about the long-term efficacy and safety of specific agents or combination therapies in this population.[10,93] Lithium, valproic acid, and carbamazepine are all used in pediatric bipolar disorder though data are limited supporting their use. Lithium is the only medication approved as a mood stabilizer for children older than 12 years.[94] Aripiprazole and risperidone are FDA-approved for bipolar mania in patients aged 13 to 17 years.[95] Quetiapine is approved as monotherapy or adjunct to lithium or divalproex in patients aged 10 to 17 years during a manic episode.[95] It did not show efficacy in a small pilot study of adolescent bipolar depression.[96] Olanzapine is approved for use in patients with manic or mixed episodes aged 13 to 17 years.[95] Ziprasidone has supporting data for it's use in pediatric acute mania, but does not have FDA approval.[97] Long-term data are still needed for all of these agents. Recommendations on the treatment of pediatric bipolar depression and maintenance treatment are lacking due to insufficient data.[97] Published guidelines for treatment of bipolar disorder in children and adolescents include the *Practice Parameters for the Assessment and Treatment of Children and Adolescents with Bipolar Disorder* by the American Academy of Child and Adolescent Psychiatry.[10]

Patients with bipolar illness are more likely to have medical comorbidities than the general population (64.3% vs 48.3%).[98] As people age, medical comorbidities tend to increase, which complicates the management of bipolar disorder in elderly patients. Renal clearance decreases, and elimination half-life nearly doubles for lithium in elderly patients.[99] Half-life of valproate has been reported to increase with aging.[100] Patients with dementia can have increased sensitivity to the side effects of mood stabilizers and antipsychotics. No prospective, randomized, placebo-controlled trials have been published examining efficacy of lithium or valproate in elderly patients.[101]

Personalized Pharmacotherapy

New information is quickly evolving in the area of pharmacogenetics and pharmacogenomics that may help clinicians individualize treatment for patients with bipolar disorder. Genetic testing is available to determine if patients are poor or rapid metabolizers of cytochrome P450 2D6 and 2C19, thus helping predict potential response as well as adverse effects. It is recommended to obtain genetic testing for the human leukocyte antigen (HLA) allele, HLA-B 1502, in patients of Asian ancestry to help detect a higher risk of Stevens-Johnson syndrome and toxic epidermal necrolysis.[65]

EVALUATION OF THERAPEUTIC OUTCOMES

The establishment and maintenance of a therapeutic alliance between the patient and clinician is essential in monitoring a patient's psychiatric status and safety; enhancing treatment adherence; promoting good nutrition, sleep, and exercise; identifying stressors; recognizing new mood episodes; and minimizing adverse reactions and drug interactions.[2] Patients who have a partial response or nonresponse to established bipolar therapies should be reassessed for an accurate diagnosis, concomitant medical or psychiatric conditions, compliance with treatment (including blood levels if appropriate), and medications or substances that exacerbate mood symptoms. Nonadherence to medication treatment, delusional symptoms, alcohol or substance abuse, rapid cycling, or mixed states are often associated with poorer treatment outcomes.

ABBREVIATIONS

APA	American Psychiatric Association
CANMAT	Canadian Network for Mood and Anxiety Treatments
CNS	central nervous system
DI	diabetes insipidus
DSM-5	*Diagnostic and Statistical Manual of Mental Disorders, Fifth Edition*
ECG	electrocardiogram
ECT	electroconvulsive therapy
FDA	Food and Drug Administration
FGAs	first-generation antipsychotics
GI	gastrointestinal
HLA	human leukocyte antigen
ISBD	International Society for Bipolar Disorders
SGAs	second-generation antipsychotics
SSRI	selective serotonin reuptake inhibitor
STEP-BD	Systematic Treatment Enhancement Program for Bipolar Disorder
TCA	tricyclic antidepressant
WFSBP	World Federation of Societies of Biological Psychiatry

REFERENCES

1. American Psychiatric Association. *Diagnostic and Statistical Manual of Mental Disorders*, Fifth Edition. Arlington VA: American Psychiatric Association; 2013:123-169.
2. American Psychiatric Association. Practice guideline for the treatment of patients with bipolar disorder (revision). *Am J Psychiatry* 2002;159:1-50.
3. Goldberg JF, Harrow M, eds. Bipolar Disorders: Clinical Course and Outcome. Washington, DC: American Psychiatric Press, 1999.
4. Merikangas KE, Akiskal HS, Angst J, et al. Lifetime and 12-month prevalence of bipolar spectrum disorder in the National Comorbidity Survey replication. *Arch Gen Psychiatry* 2007;64:543-552.
5. Perlis RH, Dennehy EB, Miklowitz DJ, et al. Retrospective age-at-onset of bipolar disorder and outcome during two-year follow-up: Results from the STEP-BD study. *Bipolar Disorder* 2009 Jun; 11(4):391-400.
6. Nivoli AM, Pacchiarotti I, Rosa AR, et al. Gender differences in a cohort study of 604 bipolar patients: The role of predominant polarity. *J Affect Disord* 2011;133(3):443-449.
7. Suppes T, Mintz J, McElroy SL, et al. Mixed hypomania in 908 patients with bipolar disorder evaluated prospectively in the Stanley Foundation Bipolar Treatment Network: A sex-specific phenomenon. *Arch Gen Psychiatry* 2005;62(10):1089-1096.
8. Sherazi R, McKeon P, McDonough M, et al. What's new? The clinical epidemiology of bipolar I disorder. *Harv Rev Psychiatry* 2006;14(6):273-284.
9. Miklowitz DJ, Cicchetti D. Toward a life span developmental psychopathology perspective on bipolar disorder. *Dev Psychopathol* 2006;18(4):935-938.
10. McClellan J, Kowatch R, Findling RL; Work Group on Quality Issues. Practice parameters for the assessment and treatment of children and adolescents with bipolar disorder. *J Am Acad Child Adolesc Psychiatry* 2007;46:107-125.
11. Smoller JW, Finn CT. Family, twin, and adoption studies of bipolar disorder. *Am J Med Genet C Semin Med Genet* 2003;123:48-58.
12. Baum AE, Akula N, Cabanero M, et al. A genome wide association study implicates diacylglycerol kinase eta (DGKH) and several other genes in the etiology of bipolar disorder. *Mol Psychiatry* 2008;13:197-207.
13. Newberg AR, Catapano LA, Zarate CA, et al. Neurobiology of bipolar disorder. *Expert Rev Neurother* 2008;8:93-110.
14. Kato T. Molecular genetics of bipolar disorder and depression. *Psychiatry Clin Neurosci* 2007;61:3-19.
15. Hales RE, Yudofsky SC, Roberts LW, eds. *The American Psychiatric Publishing Textbook of Psychiatry,* Sixth Edition. Arlington, VA: Ameican Psychiatric Association; 2014.
16. Martinowich K, Schloesser RJ, Manji HK. Bipolar disorder: From genes to behavior pathway. *J Clin Invest* 2009;119:726-736.
17. Beyer JL, Kuchibhatla M, Cassidy F, Krishnan KR. Stressful life events in older bipolar patients. *Int J Geriatr Psychiatry* 2008;23(12):1271-1275.
18. Miklowitz DJ, Johnson SL. Social and familial factors in the course of bipolar disorder: Basic processes and relevant interventions. *Clin Psychol* (New York) 2009;16(2):281-296.
19. Goldstein BI, Kemp DE, Soczynska JK, et al. Inflammation and the phenomenology, pathophysiology, comorbidity, and treatment of bipolar disorder: A systematic review of the literature. *J Clin Psychiatry* 2009;70:1078-1090.
20. Drexhage RC, Kniijff EM, Padmos RC, et al. The mononuclear phagocyte system and its cytokine inflammatory networks in schizophrenia and bipolar disorder. *Expert Rev Neurother* 2010;10:59-76.
21. Gruber J, Miklowitz DJ, Harvey AG, et al. Sleep matters: Sleep functioning and course of illness in bipolar disorder. *J Affect Disord* 2011;134:416-429.
22. Goodnick PJ, ed. Mania: Clinical and Research Perspectives. Washington, DC: American Psychiatric Press; 1998.
23. Ostacher MJ, Perlis RH, Nierenberg AA, et al. Impact of substance use disorders on recovery from episodes of depression in bipolar disorder patients: Prospective data from the Systematic Treatment Enhancement Program for Bipolar Disorder (STEP-BD). *Am J Psychiatry* 2010;167:289-297.
24. Sala R, Goldstein BI, Morcillo C, et al. Course of comorbid anxiety disorders among adults with bipolar disorder in the U.S. population. *J Psychiatr Res* 2012 Jul;46(7):865-872.
25. McElroy SL, Guerdjikova A, Lavanier S, O'Melia A. Bipolar disorder with co-occurring eating disorders: Prevalence and pharmacotherapeutic indications. *FOCUS J Lifelong Learn Psychiatry* 2011;9(4):435-448.
26. Weber NS, Fisher JA, Cowan DN, Niebuhr DW. Psychiatric and general medical conditions comorbid with bipolar disorder in the National Hospital Discharge Survey. *Psychiatr Serv* 2011;62(10):1152-1158.
27. Ceïde ME, Rosenberg PB. Brief manic episode after rituximab treatment of limbic encephalitis. *J Neuropsychiatry Clin Neurosci* 2011;23(4):E8.
28. Chopra A, Tye SJ, Lee KH, et al. Underlying neurobiology and clinical correlates of mania status after subthalamic nucleus deep brain stimulation in Parkinson's disease: A review of the literature. *J Neuropsychiatry Clin Neurosci* 2012;24(1):102-110.
29. Dias RS, Lafer B, Russo C, et al. Longitudinal follow-up of bipolar disorder in women with premenstrual exacerbation: Findings from STEP-BD. *Am J Psychiatry* 2011;168(4):386-394.

30. Goldsmith M, Singh M, Chang K. Antidepressants and psychostimulants in pediatric populations: Is there an association with mania? *Pediatr Drugs* 2011;13(4):225-243.
31. Habek M, Brina M, Brina VV, et al. Psychiatric manifestations of multiple sclerosis and acute disseminated encephalomelitis. *Clin Neurol Neurosurg* 2006;108(3):290-294.
32. Navinés R, Castellví P, Solà R, Martín-Santos R. Peginterferon- and ribavirin-induced bipolar episode successfully treated with lamotrigine without discontinuation of antiviral therapy. *Gen Hosp Psychiatry* 2008;30(4):387-389.
33. Plante DT, Winkelman JW. Sleep disturbance in bipolar disorder: Therapeutic implications. *Am J Psychiatry* 2008;165(7):830-843.
34. Santos CO, Caeiro L, Ferro JM, Figueira ML. Mania and stroke: A systematic review. *Cerebrovasc Dis* 2011;32(1):11-21.
35. Spiegel DS, Weller AL, Pennell K, et al. The successful treatment of mania due to acquired immunodeficiency syndrome using ziprasidone: A case series. *J Neuropsychiatry Clin Neurosci* 2010;22(1):111-114.
36. Valentí M, Pacchiarotti I, Bonnín CM, et al. Risk factors for antidepressant-related switch to mania. *J Clin Psychiatry* 2012;73(2):e271-e276.
37. Goldberg JF, Garno JL, Callahan AM, et al. Overdiagnosis of bipolar disorder among substance use disorder inpatients with mood instability. *J Clin Psychiatry* 2008;69:1751-1757.
38. Brooks JO, Hoblyn JC. Secondary mania in older adults. *Am J Psychiatry* 2005;162(11):2033-2038.
39. Drancourt N, Etain B, Lajnef M, et al. Duration of untreated bipolar disorder: Missed opportunities on the long road to optimal treatment. *Acta Psychiatr Scand* 2013;127:136-144. doi:10.1111/j.1600-0447.2012.01917.x [Epub ahead of print]
40. Conus P, Macneil C, McGorry PD. Public health significance of bipolar disorder: implications for early intervention and prevention. *Bipolar Disord* 2014 Aug;16(5):548-555.
41. Frias A, Palma C, Farriols N. Comorbidity in pediatric bipolar disorder: prevalence, clinical impact, etiology and treatment. *J Affect Disord* 2015 Mar 15;174:378-389.
42. Vega P, Barbeito S, Ruiz de Azúa S. Bipolar disorder differences between genders: Special considerations for women. *Womens Health* 2011;7(6):663-676.
43. Post RM. Transduction of psychosocial stress into the neurobiology of recurrent affective disorder. *Am J Psychiatry* 1992;149:999-1010.
44. Carvalho AF, Dimellis D, Gonda X, et al. Rapid cycling in bipolar disorder: A systematic review. *J Clin Psychiatry* 2014 Jun;75(6):e578-e586.
45. Barrios C, Chaudhry TA, Goodnick PJ. Rapid cycling bipolar disorder. *Expert Opin Pharmacother* 2001;2:1963-1973.
46. Rasgon N, Bauer M, Glenn T, et al. Menstrual cycle related mood changes in women with bipolar disorder. *Bipolar Disord* 2003;5:48-52.
47. Sherwood Brown E, Suppes T, Adinoff B, Rajan Thomas N. Drug abuse and bipolar disorder: Comorbidity or misdiagnosis? *J Affect Disord* 2001;65:105-115.
48. Post RM, Denicoff KD, Leverich GS, et al. Morbidity in 258 bipolar outpatients followed for 1 year with daily prospective ratings on the NIMH life chart method. *J Clin Psychiatry* 2003;64:680-690.
49. Abreu LN, Lafer B, Baca-Garcia E, Oquendo MA. Suicidal ideation and suicide attempts in bipolar disorder type I: An update for the clinician. *Rev Bras Psiquiatr* 2009;31(3):271-280.
50. Lingam R, Scott J. Treatment non-adherence in affective disorders. *Acta Psychiatr Scand* 2002;105:164-172.
51. Suppes T, Dennehy EB, Hirschfeld RM, et al. The Texas implementation of medication algorithms: Update to the algorithms for treatment of bipolar I disorder. *J Clin Psychiatry* 2005;66:870-886.
52. Miklowitz DJ, Otto MW, Frank E, et al. Psychosocial treatments for bipolar depression; a 1-year randomized trail from the Systematic Treatment Enhancement Program. *Arch Gen Psychiatry* 2007;64:419-427.
53. Yatham LN, Kennedy SH, Parikh SV, et al. Canadian Network for Mood and Anxiety Treatments (CANMAT) and International Society for Bipolar Disorders (ISBD) collaborative update of CANMAT guidelines for the management of patients with bipolar disorder: Update 2013. *Bipolar Disord* 2013;15:1-44.
54. Bauer MS, Mitchner L. What is a "mood stabilizer"? An evidence-based response. *Am J Psychiatry* 2004;161:3-18.
55. Buoli M, Serati M, Altamura AC. Is the combination of a mood stabilizer plus an antipsychotic more effective than mono-therapies in long-term treatment of bipolar disorder? A systematic review. *J Aff Disorders* 2014 Jan;152-154:12-18.
56. Grunze H, Vieta E, Goodwin GM, et al. The World Federation of Societies of Biological Psychiatry (WFSBP) guidelines for the biological treatment of bipolar disorders: Update 2009 on the treatment of acute mania. *World J Biol Psychiatry* 2009;10:85-116.
57. Grunze H, Vieta E, Goodwin G, et al. World Federation of Societies of Biological Psychiatry (WFSBP) guidelines for biological treatment of bipolar disorders: Update 2010 on the treatment of acute bipolar depression. *World J Biol Psychiatry* 2010;11:81-109.
58. Grunze H, Vieta E, Goodwin GM, et al. The World Federation of Societies of Biological Psychiatry (WFSBP) guidelines for the biological treatment of bipolar disorders: Update 2012 on the long-term treatment of bipolar disorder. *World J Biol Psychiatry* 2013;14:154-219.
59. Shaldubina A, Agam G, Belmaker RH. The mechanism of lithium action: State of the art, ten years later. *Prog Neuropsychopharmacol Biol Psychiatry* 2001;25:855-866.
60. Lithium. In: AHFS Drug Information (via Lexicomp Online). @ 2015; Hudson (OH): Lexi-Comp, Inc.; [updated 01/01/06; accessed 09/2/15]. Available at: http://online.lexi.com/lco/action/home.
61. Curran G and Ravindran A. Lithium for bipolar disorder: A review of the recent literature. *Expert Rev Neurother* 2014;14(9):1079-1098.
62. Cipriani A, Hawton K, Stockton S, Geddes JR. Lithium in prevention of suicide in mood disorders: Updated systematic review and meta-analysis. *BMJ* 2013;346:f3646.
63. Goodwin FK. Rationale for long-term treatment of bipolar disorder and evidence for long-term lithium treatment. *J Clin Psychiatry* 2002;63(Suppl 10):5-12.
64. Valproate Sodium, Valproic Acid, Divalproex Sodium. In: AHFS Drug Information (via Lexicomp Online). @ 2015; Hudson (OH): Lexi-Comp, Inc.; [updated 11/12/13; accessed 09/2/15]. Available at: http://online.lexi.com/lco/action/home.
65. Carbamazepine. In: AHFS Drug Information (via Lexicomp Online). @ 2015; Hudson (OH): Lexi-Comp, Inc.; [updated 10/03/14; accessed 09/2/15]. Available at: http://online.lexi.com/lco/action/home.
66. Oxcarbazepine. In: AHFS Drug Information (via Lexicomp Online). @ 2015; Hudson (OH): Lexi-Comp, Inc.; [updated 10/03/14; accessed 09/2/15]. Available at: http://online.lexi.com/lco/action/home.
67. Lamotrigine. In: AHFS Drug Information (via Lexicomp Online). @ 2015; Hudson (OH): Lexi-Comp, Inc.; [updated 10/03/14; accessed 09/2/15]. Available at: http://online.lexi.com/lco/action/home.
68. American Diabetes Association, American Psychiatric Association, American Association of Clinical Endocrinologists, et al. Consensus development conference on antipsychotic drugs and obesity and diabetes. *Diabetes Care* 2004;27:596-601.
69. Amann B, Born C, Crespo JM, et al. Lamotrigine: When and where does it act in affective disorders? A systematic review. *J Psychopharmacol* 2011;25(10):1289-1294.
70. Macritchie K, Geddes JR, Scott J, et al. Valproate for acute mood episodes in bipolar disorder. *Cochrane Database Syst Rev* 2003;(1):CD004052.
71. Allen MH, Hirschfeld RM, Wozniak PJ, et al. Linear relationship of valproate serum concentration to response and optimal serum levels for acute mania. *Am J Psychiatry* 2006;163:272-275.
72. Dong X, Leppik IE, White J, Rarick J. Hyponatremia from oxcarbazepine and carbamazepine. *Neurology* 2005;65:1976-1978.
73. Perucca E. Clinically relevant drug interactions with antiepileptic drugs. *Br J Clin Pharmacol* 2005;61:246-255.
74. Malhi GS, Mitchell PB, Salim S. Bipolar depression: Management options. *CNS Drugs* 2003;17:9-25.
75. Raskin S, Teitelbaum A, Zislin J, Durst R. Adjunctive lamotrigine as a possible mania inducer in bipolar patients. *Am J Psychiatry* 2006;163:159-160.
76. Tohen M, Vieta E. Antipsychotic agents in the treatment of bipolar mania. *Bipolar Disord* 2009;11:45-54.
77. Citrome L. Treatment of bipolar depression: Making sensible decisions. *CNS Spectrum* 2014;19:4-12.
78. Marder SR, Essock SM, Miller AL, et al. Physical health monitoring of patients with schizophrenia. *Am J Psychiatry* 2004;161:1334-1349.
79. McEvoy GK, Miller J, Snow EK, et al. Benzodiazepines. AHFS Drug Information 2007. Bethesda, MD: American Society of Health-System Pharmacists, 2007:2508-2518.
80. Alderfer BS, Allen MH. Treatment of agitation in bipolar disorder across the life cycle. *J Clin Psychiatry* 2003;64(Suppl 4):3-9.
81. Sachs GS, Nierenberg AA, Calabrese JR, et al. Effectiveness of adjunctive antidepressant treatment for bipolar disorder. *N Engl J Med* 2007;356:1711-1722.
82. Gigsman HJ, Geddes JR, Rendell JM, et al. Antidepressants for bipolar depression: A systematic review of randomized, controlled trials. *Am J Psychiatry* 2004;161:1537-1547.

83. Post RM, Altshuler LL, Leverich GS, et al. Mood switch in bipolar depression: Comparison of adjunctive venlafaxine, bupropion, and sertraline. *Br J Psychiatry* 2006;189:124-131.
84. Sachs GS, Koslow CL, Ghaemi SN. The treatment of bipolar depression. *Bipolar Disord* 2000;2:256-260.
85. Sachs GS, Printz DJ, Kahn DA, et al. The expert consensus guideline series: Medication treatment of bipolar disorder 2000. *Postgrad Med* 2000;Spec No:1-104.
86. Levy NA, Janicak PG. Calcium channel antagonists for the treatment of bipolar disorder. *Bipolar Disord* 2000;2:108-119.
87. Aronne LJ, Segal KR. Weight gain in the treatment of mood disorders. *J Clin Psychiatry* 2003;64(Suppl 8):22-29.
88. Gentile S. Lithium in pregnancy: the need to treat, the duty to ensure safety. *Expert Opinion on Drug Safety* 2012;11(3):425-437.
89. Ernst CL, Goldberg JF. The reproductive safety profile of mood stabilizers, atypical antipsychotics, and broad-spectrum psychotropics. *J Clin Psychiatry* 2002;63(Suppl 4):42-55.
90. Hernadez-Diaz S, Smith DR, Shen A, et al. Comparative safety of antiepileptic drugs during pregnancy. *Neurology* 2012;78:1692-1699.
91. Vajda FJE, Hitchcock A, Graham J, et al. The Australian register of antiepileptic drugs in pregnancy: The first 1002 pregnancies. *Aust N Z J Obstet Gynaecol* 2007;47:468-474.
92. Galbally M, Snellen M and Power J. Antipsychotic drugs in pregnancy: A review of their maternal and fetal effects. *Ther Adv Drug Saf* 2014;5(2):100-109.
93. Chang KD, Ketter TA. Special issues in the treatment of pediatric bipolar disorder. *Expert Opin Pharmacother* 2001;2:613-622.
94. Madaan V, Chang KD. Pharmacotherapeutic strategies for pediatric bipolar disorder. *Expert Opin Pharmacother* 2007;8:1801-1819.
95. Gentile S. Clinical usefulness of second-generation antipsychotics in treating children and adolescents diagnosed with bipolar or schizophrenic disorders. *Pediatr Drugs* 2011;13(5):291-302.
96. Zuddas A, Zanni R, Usala T. Second generation antipsychotics (SGAs) for non-psychotic disorders in children and adolescents: A review of the randomized controlled studies. *Eur Neuropsychopharmacol* 2011;21:600-620.
97. Goldstein BI Sassi R, Diler RS. Pharmacologic treatment of bipolar disorder in children and adolescents. *Child Adolesc Psychiatric Clin N Am* 2012:911-939.
98. McIntyre RS, Konarski JZ, Soczynska JK, et al. Medical comorbidity in bipolar disorder: Implications for functional outcomes and health service utilization. *Psychaitr Serv* 2006;57(8):1140-1144.
99. Hardy BG, Shulman KI, Mackenzie SE. Pharmacokinetics of lithium therapy. *J Clin Psychopharmacol* 1987;4:201-205.
100. Bryson SM, Verma N, Scott PJW, et al. Pharmacokinetics of valproic acid in young and elderly subjects. *Br J Clin Psychiatry* 1983;16:104-105.
101. Young RC. Evidence-based pharmacological treatment of geriatric bipolar disorder. *Psychiatr Clin North Am* 2005;28:837-869.

Anxiety Disorders: Generalized Anxiety, Panic, and Social Anxiety Disorders

70

Sarah T. Melton and Cynthia K. Kirkwood

KEY CONCEPTS

1. Anxiety disorders are among the most common of mental disorders and are underdiagnosed and undertreated.
2. The long-term goal in treatment of generalized anxiety disorder (GAD) is remission with minimal or no anxiety symptoms and no functional impairment.
3. Antidepressants are the agents of choice for the management of GAD.
4. Antidepressants have a lag time of 2 to 4 weeks or longer before antianxiety effects occur in GAD.
5. When monitoring the effectiveness of antidepressants in panic disorder, it is important to allow an adequate amount of time (8-12 weeks) to achieve full therapeutic response.
6. The optimal duration of panic therapy is unknown; 12 to 24 months of pharmacotherapy is recommended before gradual drug discontinuation over 4 to 6 months is attempted.
7. Social anxiety disorder (SAD) is a chronic long-term illness requiring extended therapy. After improvement, at least a 6- to 12-month medication maintenance period is recommended.
8. The selective serotonin reuptake inhibitors or venlafaxine are considered first-line pharmacotherapy for social anxiety disorder.
9. An adequate trial of antidepressants in generalized SAD lasts at least 8 weeks, and maximal benefit may not be seen until 12 weeks.
10. The three principal domains in which improvement should be observed in generalized SAD are symptoms, functionality, and well-being.

Anxiety is an emotional state commonly caused by the perception of real or perceived danger that threatens the security of an individual. It allows a person to prepare for or react to environmental changes. Everyone experiences a certain amount of nervousness and apprehension when faced with a stressful situation. This is an adaptive response and is transient in nature.

Anxiety can produce uncomfortable and potentially debilitating psychological (eg, worry or feeling of threat) and physiologic arousal (eg, tachycardia or shortness of breath) if it becomes excessive. Some individuals experience persistent, severe anxiety symptoms and possess irrational fears that significantly impair normal daily functioning. These persons often suffer from an anxiety disorder.[1]

(1) Anxiety disorders are among the most frequent mental disorders encountered in clinical practice and are often underdiagnosed and undertreated.[2] Healthcare professionals often mistake anxiety disorders for physical illnesses, and only one quarter of patients receive appropriate treatment.[3] Failure to diagnose and manage anxiety disorders results in negative outcomes including overuse of healthcare resources, increased risk for suicide and substance abuse.[4] Individuals with anxiety disorders develop cardiovascular, cerebrovascular, gastrointestinal (GI), and respiratory disorders at a significantly higher rate than the general population.[4]

To treat anxiety appropriately, the clinician must make a reliable diagnosis. It is essential that the distinction between short-term symptoms of anxiety and anxiety disorders be understood. Common or situational anxiety is a normal response to a stressful circumstance. Although symptoms can be severe, they are temporary and usually last no more than 2 or 3 weeks. Although short-term, "as-needed" treatment with an anxiolytic agent such as a benzodiazepine is common and can provide some symptomatic relief, prolonged drug therapy is not recommended for situational anxiety.[5]

EPIDEMIOLOGY

Anxiety disorders, as a group, are the most commonly occurring psychiatric disorders. According to large population-based surveys, up to 33.7% of the population are affected by an anxiety disorder during their lifetime.[6] According to the National Comorbidity Survey Replication of the prevalence, severity, and comorbidity estimates of mental disorders in the United States, the most recent 1-year prevalence rate for anxiety disorders was 21.3% in persons aged 18 years and older. Specific phobias were the most common anxiety disorder, with a 12-month prevalence of 10.1%. The 1-year prevalence of generalized anxiety disorder (GAD) was 2.9%, that of panic disorder was 3.1%, and that of social anxiety disorder (SAD) was 8.0%.[6]

In general, anxiety disorders are a group of heterogeneous illnesses that develop before age 30 years and are more common in women, individuals with social issues, and those with a family history of anxiety and depression. Patients often develop another anxiety disorder, major depression, or substance abuse.[1-3] The clinical picture of mixed anxiety and depression is much more common than an isolated anxiety disorder.[7,8]

ETIOLOGY

The differential diagnosis of anxiety disorders includes medical and psychiatric illnesses and certain drugs.[7,8] Hypotheses on the etiology of anxiety disorders are based on interactions between a combination of factors including vulnerability (eg, genetic predisposition and early childhood adversity) and stress (eg, occupational and traumatic experience). The vulnerability may be associated with genetic factors and neurobiologic adaptations of the central nervous system (CNS).[9]

Medical Diseases Associated with Anxiety

Anxiety symptoms are an inherent part of the initial clinical presentation of several diseases, thus complicating the distinction between anxiety disorders and medical disorders.[5,8] Anxiety disorders are

TABLE 70-1 Common Medical Illnesses Associated with Anxiety Symptoms

Cardiovascular
Angina, arrhythmias, cardiomyopathy, congestive heart failure, hypertension, ischemic heart disease, mitral valve prolapse, myocardial infarction
Endocrine and metabolic
Cushing disease, diabetes, hyperparathyroidism, hyperthyroidism, hypothyroidism, hypoglycemia, hyponatremia, hyperkalemia, pheochromocytoma, vitamin B_{12} or folate deficiencies
Gastrointestinal
Crohn disease, irritable bowel syndrome, ulcerative colitis, peptic ulcer disease
Neurologic
Migraine, seizures, stroke, neoplasms, poor pain control
Respiratory system
Asthma, chronic obstructive pulmonary disease, pulmonary embolism, pneumonia
Others
Anemias, cancer, systemic lupus erythematosus, vestibular dysfunction

Data from references 4, 7, and 8.

TABLE 70-2 Drugs Associated with Anxiety Symptoms

Anticonvulsants: Carbamazepine, phenytoin
Antidepressants: Bupropion, selective serotonin reuptake inhibitors, serotonin–norepinephrine reuptake inhibitors
Antihypertensives: Clonidine, felodipine
Antibiotics: Quinolones, isoniazid
Bronchodilators: Albuterol, theophylline
Corticosteroids: Prednisone
Dopamine agonists: Amantadine, levodopa
Herbals: Ma huang, ginseng, ephedra
Illicit substances: Ecstasy, marijuana
Nonsteroidal antiinflammatory drugs: Ibuprofen, indomethacin
Stimulants: Amphetamines, caffeine, cocaine, methylphenidate, nicotine
Sympathomimetics: Pseudoephedrine, phenylephrine
Thyroid hormones: Levothyroxine
Toxicity: Anticholinergics, antihistamines, digoxin

Data from references 1 and 5.

associated with chronic medical illness, low levels of physical health-related quality of life (QOL), and physical disability.[2] If anxiety symptoms are secondary to a medical illness, they usually will subside as the medical situation stabilizes. However, the knowledge that one has a physical illness can trigger anxious feelings and further complicate therapy. Persistent anxiety subsequent to a physical illness requires further assessment for an anxiety disorder. Common somatic symptoms of anxiety that frequently present in medical disorders include abdominal pain, palpitations, tachycardia, sweating, flushing, tremor, chest pain or tightness, and shortness of breath. Although less specific, symptoms of muscle tension, headache, and fatigue are also common manifestations of anxiety. Medical disorders most closely associated with anxiety are listed in Table 70-1.

Psychiatric Diseases Associated with Anxiety

Anxiety can be a presenting feature of several major psychiatric illnesses. Anxiety symptoms are extremely common in patients with mood disorders, schizophrenia, dementia, and substance-use disorders. Most psychiatric patients will have two or more concurrent psychiatric disorders (comorbidity) within their lifetime.[6] It is important to diagnose and treat all comorbid psychiatric conditions in patients with anxiety disorders.

Drug-Induced Anxiety

Drugs are a common cause of anxiety symptoms (Table 70-2). Anxiety occurs during the use of CNS-stimulating drugs in a dose-dependent manner, but ingestion of minimal amounts can result in marked anxiety, including panic attacks, in some individuals. The onset of drug-induced anxiety is usually rapid after the initiation of therapy. A thorough medication history evaluating for a recent drug or dosage change is important to rule out a drug-induced etiology for the anxiety.

Anxiety occurs occasionally during the use of CNS depressants, especially in children and the elderly; however, anxiety complaints are more common as complications of drug withdrawal after the abrupt discontinuation of these agents.[7]

PATHOPHYSIOLOGY

Data from biochemical and neuroimaging studies indicate that the modulation of normal and pathologic anxiety states is associated with multiple regions of the brain and abnormal function in several neurotransmitter systems, including norepinephrine (NE), γ-aminobutyric acid (GABA), serotonin (5-HT), corticotropin-releasing factor (CRF), and cholecystokinin.[10] Current neuroanatomic models of fear (ie, the response to danger) and anxiety (ie, the feeling of fear that is disproportionate to the actual threat) include some key brain areas. The amygdala, a temporal lobe structure, plays a critical role in the assessment of fear stimuli and learned response to fear.[10,11] The locus ceruleus (LC), located in the brain stem, is the primary NE-containing site, with widespread projections to areas responsible for implementing fear responses (eg, vagus, lateral and paraventricular hypothalamus). The hippocampus is integral in the consolidation of traumatic memory and contextual fear conditioning. The hypothalamus is the principal area for integrating neuroendocrine and autonomic responses to a threat.[10,11]

Neurochemical Theories

Noradrenergic Model

The basic premise of the noradrenergic theory is that the autonomic nervous system of anxious patients is hypersensitive and overreacts to various stimuli. Many anxious patients clearly display symptoms of peripheral autonomic hyperactivity. In response to threat or fearful situations, the LC serves as an alarm center, activating NE release and stimulating the sympathetic and parasympathetic nervous systems. Chronic central noradrenergic overactivity downregulates α_2-adrenoreceptors in patients with GAD. This receptor is hypersensitive in some patients with panic disorder.[10] By administering drugs that have a relatively specific effect on the LC, researchers have further explored the NE theory of anxiety and panic disorder. Drugs with anxiogenic effects (eg, yohimbine [an α_2-adrenergic receptor antagonist]) stimulate LC firing and increase noradrenergic activity. NE in turn increases glutamate release (an excitatory neurotransmitter).[10] This produces subjective feelings of anxiety and can precipitate a panic attack in those with panic disorder, but not in normal volunteers.[10] Drugs with anxiolytic or antipanic effects (eg, benzodiazepines and antidepressants) inhibit LC firing, decrease noradrenergic activity, and block the effects of anxiogenic drugs.[10]

GABA-Receptor Model

There are two superfamilies of GABA-protein receptors: $GABA_A$ and $GABA_B$. Drugs that reduce anxiety and produce sedation target the $GABA_A$ receptor. The $GABA_B$ receptor is a G-protein–coupled receptor postulated to be involved in the presynaptic inhibition of GABA release.[10-12] $GABA_A$ receptors are ligand-gated ion channels composed of five protein subunits. Several classes of subunits (ie, α_{1-6}, β_{1-3}, γ_{1-3}, δ, ε, θ, π, ρ_{1-3}) surround a central pore, and the receptor is connected to the cytoskeleton.[12,13] Benzodiazepine ligands enhance the inhibitory effects of GABA.[12] GABA, the major inhibitory neurotransmitter in the CNS, has a strong regulatory or inhibitory effect on the 5-HT, NE, and dopamine (DA) systems. When GABA binds to the $GABA_A$ receptor, neuronal excitability is reduced.

The specific role of the GABA receptors in anxiety disorders has not been established. The number of $GABA_A$ receptors can change with alterations in the environment (eg, chronic stress), and the subunit expression can be altered by hormonal changes.[12,13]

Serotonin Model

Although there are data suggesting that the 5-HT system is dysregulated in patients with anxiety disorders, definitive evidence that shows a clear abnormality in 5-HT function is lacking. 5-HT is primarily an inhibitory neurotransmitter that is used by neurons originating in the raphe nuclei of the brain stem and projecting diffusely throughout the brain (eg, cortex, amygdala, hippocampus, and limbic system). Abnormalities in serotonergic functioning through release and uptake at the presynaptic autoreceptors ($5\text{-}HT_{1A/1D}$), the serotonin-reuptake transporter (SERT) site, or effect of 5-HT at the postsynaptic receptors (eg, $5\text{-}HT_{1A}$, $5\text{-}HT_{2A}$, and $5\text{-}HT_{2C}$) may play a role in anxiety disorders.[10] Preclinical models suggest that greater 5-HT function facilitates avoidance behavior; however, primate studies show that reducing 5-HT increases aggression.[10] It is postulated that greater 5-HT activity reduces NE activity in the LC, inhibits defense/escape response via the periaqueductal gray (PAG) region, and reduces hypothalamic release of CRF. The selective serotonin reuptake inhibitors (SSRIs) acutely increase 5-HT levels by blocking the SERT to increase the amount of 5-HT available postsynaptically, and are efficacious in blocking the manifestations of panic and anxiety.[10]

Low 5-HT activity may lead to a dysregulation of other neurotransmitters. NE and 5-HT systems are closely linked, and interactions between the two are reciprocal and vary. NE may act at presynaptic 5-HT terminals to decrease 5-HT release, and its activity at postsynaptic receptors can cause increased 5-HT release.

Buspirone is a selective $5\text{-}HT_{1A}$ partial agonist that is effective for GAD but not for panic disorder. Because the selective $5\text{-}HT_{1A}$ partial agonists reduce serotonergic activity, GAD symptoms may reflect excessive 5-HT transmission or overactivity of the stimulatory 5-HT pathways.[14] There is circumstantial evidence for the involvement of serotonergic and dopaminergic systems in the pathophysiology of generalized SAD.[15]

Neuroimaging Studies

Functional neuroimaging studies support the crucial role of the amygdala, anterior cingulate cortex (ACC), and insula in the pathophysiology of anxiety.[11] In GAD there is an abnormal increase in the brain's fear circuitry, as well as increased activity in the prefrontal cortex, which appears to have a compensatory role in reducing GAD symptoms.[16] Patients with panic have abnormalities of midbrain structures, including the PAG. Neuroimaging studies have shown activation of insula and upper brain stem (including the PAG), as well as deactivation of the ACC during experimental panic attacks.[10] Patients with SAD have greater activity than matched comparison subjects in the amygdala and insula, structures linked to negative emotional responses.[17] Both pharmacotherapy and psychotherapy decreased cerebral blood flow in the amygdala, hippocampus, and surrounding cortical areas in patients with SAD.[17]

CLINICAL PRESENTATION

The *Diagnostic and Statistical Manual of Mental Disorders, Fifth Edition* classifies anxiety disorders into categories including GAD, panic disorder, agoraphobia, SAD, specific phobia, and separation anxiety disorder.[1] The characteristic features of these illnesses are anxiety and avoidance behavior. Anxiety symptoms must cause significant distress and impairment in social, occupational, or other areas of functioning, and should not be secondary to a drug or illicit substance or a general medical disorder, or occur solely as part of another psychiatric disorder.[1] The anxiety-related syndromes posttraumatic stress disorder and obsessive-compulsive disorder are discussed in Chapter 71.

Generalized Anxiety Disorder

The diagnostic criteria for GAD require persistent symptoms for most days for at least 6 months.[1] The essential feature of GAD is unrealistic or excessive anxiety and worry about a number of events or activities.[1] The anxiety or apprehensive expectation is accompanied by at least three psychological or physiologic symptoms. Anxiety and worry are not confined to features of another psychiatric illness (eg, having a panic attack, being embarrassed in public).[1]

The onset, course of illness, and comorbid conditions of GAD are important considerations. GAD has a gradual onset with an average age of 21 years; however, there is a bimodal distribution. Onset occurs earlier when GAD is the primary presentation and later when GAD is secondary. GAD can be exacerbated or precipitated in later life by severe psychological stressors. Most patients present between the ages of 35 and 45 years, with women twice as likely to have GAD as men. The course of the illness is chronic (ie, episodes can last for a decade or longer); there is a high percentage of relapse and low rates of recovery.[1] Patients report substantial interference with their lives and have a high probability of seeking treatment. Lifetime comorbidity with another psychiatric disorder occurs in 90% of patients with GAD, with depression being found in over 60%.[18]

Panic Disorder

Panic disorder begins as a series of unexpected (spontaneous) panic attacks involving an abrupt surge of intense fear or intense discomfort. The unexpected panic attacks are followed by at least 1 month of persistent concern about having another panic attack, worry about the possible consequences of the panic attack, or a significant maladaptive change in behavior related to the attacks.[1] During an attack, patients describe at least four physiologic and physical symptoms.

CLINICAL PRESENTATION Generalized Anxiety Disorder

Psychological and Cognitive Symptoms

- Excessive anxiety
- Worries that are difficult to control
- Feeling keyed up or on edge
- Trouble concentrating or mind going blank

Physical Symptoms

- Restlessness
- Fatigue
- Muscle tension
- Sleep disturbance
- Irritability

Data from references 1, 2, and 4.

CLINICAL PRESENTATION Panic Attack

Psychological Symptoms

- Depersonalization (being detached from oneself)
- Derealization (feelings of being detached from one's environment)
- Fear of losing control, going crazy, or dying

Physical Symptoms

- Abdominal distress
- Chest pain or discomfort
- Chills
- Dizziness or light-headedness
- Feeling of choking
- Heat sensations
- Nausea
- Palpitations
- Paresthesias
- Sensations of shortness of breath or smothering
- Sweating
- Tachycardia
- Trembling or shaking

Data from references 1, 2, and 4.

Panic attacks usually last no more than 20 to 30 minutes, with the peak intensity of symptoms within the first 10 minutes. Often patients seek help at a physician's office or emergency department, only to have their symptoms resolve before or on arrival. Because panic symptoms mimic those present in several medical conditions, patients often are misdiagnosed, and multiple referrals are common.[1]

Secondary to the panic attacks, up to 50% of patients develop agoraphobia.[1] Agoraphobia is marked fear or anxiety about being in at least two situations in which escape might be difficult or where help might not be available in the event of developing panic-like symptoms.[1] As a result, patients often avoid specific situations (eg, using public transportation, being in open or enclosed places, being in a crowd or being outside of the home alone) in which they fear a panic attack might occur.[1]

Complications of panic disorder include depression (10%-65% have major depressive disorder), alcohol abuse, and high use of health services and emergency rooms.[1] Patients with panic disorder have a high lifetime risk for suicide attempts compared with the general population.[1] The usual course is chronic but waxing and waning.

Social Anxiety Disorder

SAD is characterized by marked fear about one or more social situations in which the individual is exposed to possible scrutiny by others. Exposure to the feared circumstance usually provokes an immediate situation-related panic attack. Blushing is the principal physical indicator and distinguishes SAD from other anxiety disorders. The fear and anxiety is out of proportion to the actual threat posed by the social situation and is persistent, typically lasting for 6 months or longer.[1] If the fear is restricted to speaking or performing in public, the SAD is specified as performance only.

The mean age of onset of SAD is during the mid-teens. Rates of SAD are slightly higher among women than men and more frequent in younger cohorts. It is a chronic disorder with a mean duration of 20 years.[1] People with SAD can be reluctant to seek professional help despite the existence of beneficial treatments because consultation with a clinician is perceived as a feared social interaction.[19]

Differentiating SAD from other anxiety disorders can be difficult. Panic attacks occur in both SAD and panic disorder, but the distinction between the two is the rationale behind fear; fear of anxiety symptoms is characteristic of panic disorder, whereas fear of embarrassment from social interaction typifies SAD.[1] A majority of SAD patients eventually develop a concurrent mood, anxiety, or substance abuse disorder.[19]

Specific Phobia

Specific phobia is marked and persistent fear of a circumscribed object or situation (eg, insects or heights). Apart from contact with the feared object or situation, the patient is usually free of symptoms. Most persons simply avoid the feared object and adjust to certain restrictions on their activities.[1]

CLINICAL PRESENTATION Social Anxiety Disorder

Fears of Being

- Scrutinized by others
- Negatively evaluated (ie, humiliated, embarrassed, or rejected)

Some Feared Situations

- Eating or writing in front of others
- Interacting with authority figures
- Speaking in public
- Talking with strangers
- Use of public toilets

Symptoms of Anxiety

- Blushing
- "Butterflies in the stomach"
- Diarrhea
- Stumbling over words
- Sweating
- Tachycardia
- Trembling

Specifier

Performance; Applies only if the fear is restricted to speaking or performing in public.

Data from references 1 and 19.

TREATMENT
Generalized Anxiety Disorder

Desired Outcomes

2 The goals of therapy in the acute management of GAD are to reduce the severity and duration of the anxiety symptoms and to improve overall functioning. The long-term goal in GAD is remission with minimal or no anxiety symptoms, no functional impairment, and increased QOL.[18] Prevention of recurrence is another long-term consideration.

General Approach

Once GAD is diagnosed, a patient-specific treatment plan, which usually consists of both psychotherapy and drug therapy, is developed. The plan depends on the severity and chronicity of symptoms, age, medication history, and comorbid medical and psychiatric conditions.[18] Factors such as anticipated adverse effects, history of prior response in the patient or family member, patient preference, and cost should be considered when treatment is initiated. Psychotherapy is the least invasive and safest treatment modality. Antianxiety medication is indicated for patients experiencing symptoms severe enough to produce functional disability. Table 70-3 lists drug choices for GAD, panic disorder, and SAD.

Nonpharmacologic Therapy

Nonpharmacologic treatment modalities in GAD include psychoeducation, short-term counseling, stress management, psychotherapy, meditation, or exercise. Psychoeducation includes information on the etiology and management of GAD. Anxious patients should be instructed to avoid caffeine, nicotine, nonprescription stimulants, diet pills, and excessive use of alcohol. Most patients with GAD require psychological therapy, alone or in combination with antianxiety drugs, to overcome fears and to learn to manage their anxiety and worry.[19] Cognitive behavioral therapy (CBT) is the most effective psychological therapy in GAD patients. CBT for GAD includes self-monitoring of worry, cognitive restructuring, relaxation training, and rehearsal of coping skills.[19] Psychotherapy or medication alone has comparable efficacy in acute treatment.[22] The relapse rate with CBT is less than with other types of psychological modalities.[22] Controlled trials comparing the efficacy of combining drug and psychotherapy over long-term treatment are lacking.[22] Advantages of CBT over pharmacotherapy include patient preference and lack of troubling adverse effects. However, CBT is not widely available, requires specialized training, and entails weekly sessions for an extended time period (ie, 12-20 weeks).[23]

TABLE 70-3 Drug Choices for Anxiety Disorders

Anxiety Disorder	First-Line Drugs	Second-Line Drugs	Alternatives
Generalized anxiety disorder	Duloxetine Escitalopram Paroxetine Sertraline Venlafaxine XR	Benzodiazepines Buspirone Imipramine Pregabalin	Hydroxyzine Quetiapine
Panic disorder	SSRIs Venlafaxine XR	Alprazolam Citalopram Clomipramine Clonazepam Imipramine	Phenelzine
Social anxiety disorder	Escitalopram Fluvoxamine CR Paroxetine Sertraline Venlafaxine XR	Clonazepam Citalopram	Gabapentin Phenelzine Pregabalin

CR, controlled-release; SSRI, selective serotonin reuptake inhibitor; XR, extended-release.

Data from references 2, 18, 20 to 23.

Pharmacologic Therapy

The benzodiazepines are the most effective and commonly prescribed drugs for the rapid relief of acute anxiety symptoms (Table 70-4). All benzodiazepines are equally effective anxiolytics, and consideration of pharmacokinetic properties and the patient's clinical situation will assist in the selection of the most appropriate agent.[23,24]

Because of the lack of dependency and tolerable adverse effect profile, antidepressants have emerged as the treatment of choice for the management of chronic anxiety, especially in the presence of comorbid depressive symptoms. Buspirone is an additional anxiolytic option (Table 70-5) in patients without comorbid depression or other anxiety disorders. Because of the high risk of adverse effects and toxicity, barbiturates, antipsychotics, antipsychotic–antidepressant combinations, and antihistamines generally are not indicated in the treatment of GAD.[4] The benzodiazepines are more effective in treating the somatic and autonomic symptoms of GAD as opposed to the psychic symptoms (eg, apprehension and worry), which are reduced by antidepressants.[4]

The most recent treatment guidelines from the World Federation of Societies of Biological Psychiatry, the National Institute for Health and Clinical Evidence, and British Association for Psychopharmacology are evidence-based.[4,21,22] A descriptive flowchart with recommendations based on levels of evidence from the International Psychopharmacology Algorithm Project for the psychosocial and pharmacologic management of GAD is shown in Fig. 70-1.[36]

Alternative Drug Treatments

Hydroxyzine, pregabalin, and atypical antipsychotics are alternatives.[18,22,28] The effectiveness of hydroxyzine as an antianxiety agent for long-term use (ie, more than 4 months) has not been assessed by systematic clinical studies.[35] Hydroxyzine is commonly used in the primary care setting, but it is considered be to be a second-line agent because of adverse effects and lack of efficacy for comorbid disorders.[4] Pregabalin, which binds to the $\alpha_2\delta$ subunit of voltage-gated calcium channels to reduce nerve terminal calcium influx, acts on "hyperexcited" neurons. Pregabalin produced anxiolytic effects similar to lorazepam, alprazolam, and venlafaxine in acute efficacy trials.[24] Quetiapine extended-release 150 mg/day monotherapy was superior to placebo in three studies, and as effective as paroxetine 20 mg/day and escitalopram 10 mg/day but with an earlier onset of action.[28] In a 52-week treatment of GAD, quetiapine extended-release was superior to placebo in the prevention of anxiety relapse.[28] Quetiapine is not FDA-approved for GAD, and the long-term risks and benefits of atypical antipsychotics in the treatment of GAD are unclear.[28] Despite some evidence of efficacy, support for the use of kava kava for GAD has been blunted by ongoing safety concerns following numerous reports of liver toxicity.[37] Although valerian, St. John's wort, and passionflower have been used to manage GAD, there is insufficient evidence of their effectiveness and safety.[37,38]

Clinical Controversy...

Atypical antipsychotics have been used as monotherapy and as add-on treatment for nonresponse to first-line pharmacotherapy of GAD in numerous trials. Adverse effects include sedation, orthostatic hypotension, metabolic syndrome, extrapyramidal effects, and others. Although effective in GAD, they are not approved for this indication and should probably be reserved for use by specialists.

TABLE 70-4 Benzodiazepine Antianxiety Agents

Drug	Brand Name	Approved Dosage Range (mg/day)	Maximum Dosage for Geriatric Patients (mg/day)	Approximate Equivalent Dose (mg)	Comments
Alprazolam[a]	Niravam,[b] Xanax Xanax XR	0.75-4 1-10[c]	2	0.5	Associated with interdose rebound anxiety
Chlordiazepoxide[a]	Librium	25-400	40	10	
Clonazepam[a]	Klonopin Klonopin Wafer[b]	1-4[c]	3	0.25-0.5	
Clorazepate[a]	Tranxene	7.5-60	30	7.5	
Diazepam[a]	Valium	2-40	20	5	
Lorazepam[a]	Ativan	0.5-10	3	1	Preferred in elderly
Oxazepam[a]	Serax	30-120	60	30	Preferred in elderly

XR, extended-release.

[a]Available generically.

[b]Orally disintegrating formulation.

[c]Panic disorder dose.

Dosing and equivalence data from references 25-27.

Antidepressant Therapy

3 Antidepressants are considered first-line agents in the management of GAD. Venlafaxine extended-release, duloxetine, paroxetine, and escitalopram are FDA-approved antidepressants for GAD (see Table 70-5). Imipramine is considered a second-line agent, despite its efficacy, because of higher toxicity and adverse effect rates.[4] 4 The antianxiety response of antidepressants is delayed by 2 to 4 weeks or longer.[4] The pharmacology, pharmacokinetics, and drug interactions of the antidepressants are reviewed in Chapter 68.

Efficacy Antidepressants are efficacious in the acute and long-term management of GAD. Data support the use of the SSRIs (eg, escitalopram, paroxetine, sertraline), and the serotonin–norepinephrine reuptake inhibitors (SNRIs) (eg, venlafaxine extended-release and duloxetine), for acute therapy (8- to 12-week trials) with response rates between 60% and 68%, and remission rates of 30%.[4,22] A recent meta-analysis indicated that fluoxetine was most likely to achieve remission of GAD symptoms, and sertraline was the best tolerated. In a subanalysis comparing duloxetine, escitalopram, paroxetine, venlafaxine, and pregabalin, duloxetine was most likely to produce a beneficial response, escitalopram most likely to establish a remission, and pregabalin was best tolerated.[39]

Mechanism of Action The mechanism of action of antidepressants in anxiety disorders is not fully understood. Research indicates that antidepressants modulate receptor activation of neuronal signal

TABLE 70-5 Nonbenzodiazepine Antianxiety Agents for Generalized Anxiety Disorder

Drug	Brand Name	Initial Dose	Usual Range (mg/day)[a]	Comments
Antidepressants				
Duloxetine	Cymbalta	30 or 60 mg/day	60-120	FDA-approved
Escitalopram	Lexapro	10 mg/day	10-20	FDA-approved, available generically
Imipramine	Tofranil	50 mg/day	75-200	Available generically
Paroxetine	Paxil Pexeva	20 mg/day	20-50	FDA-approved, available generically, avoid in pregnancy
Sertraline	Zoloft	50 mg/day	50-200	Available generically
Venlafaxine XR	Effexor XR	37.5 or 75 mg/day	75-225[b]	FDA-approved, available generically
Vilazodone	Viibryd	10 mg/day	20-40[b]	During concomitant use of a strong CYP3A4 inhibitor (eg, itraconazole, clarithromycin, voriconazole), dose should not exceed 20 mg once daily
Vortioxetine	Brintellix	5 mg/day	5-20	
Azapirone				
Buspirone	BuSpar	7.5 mg twice daily	15-60[b]	FDA-approved, available generically
Diphenylmethane				
Hydroxyzine	Vistaril	25 or 50 mg four times daily	200-400	FDA-approved, available generically, approved in children for anxiety and tension in divided daily doses of 50-100 mg
Anticonvulsant				
Pregabalin	Lyrica	50 mg three times daily	150-600	Dosage adjustment required in renal impairment
Atypical antipsychotic				
Quetiapine XR	Seroquel XR	50 mg at bedtime	150-300	

XR, extended-release.

[a]Elderly patients are usually treated with approximately one half of the dose listed.

[b]No dosage adjustment is required in elderly patients.

Data from references 4, 24, 28 to 35.

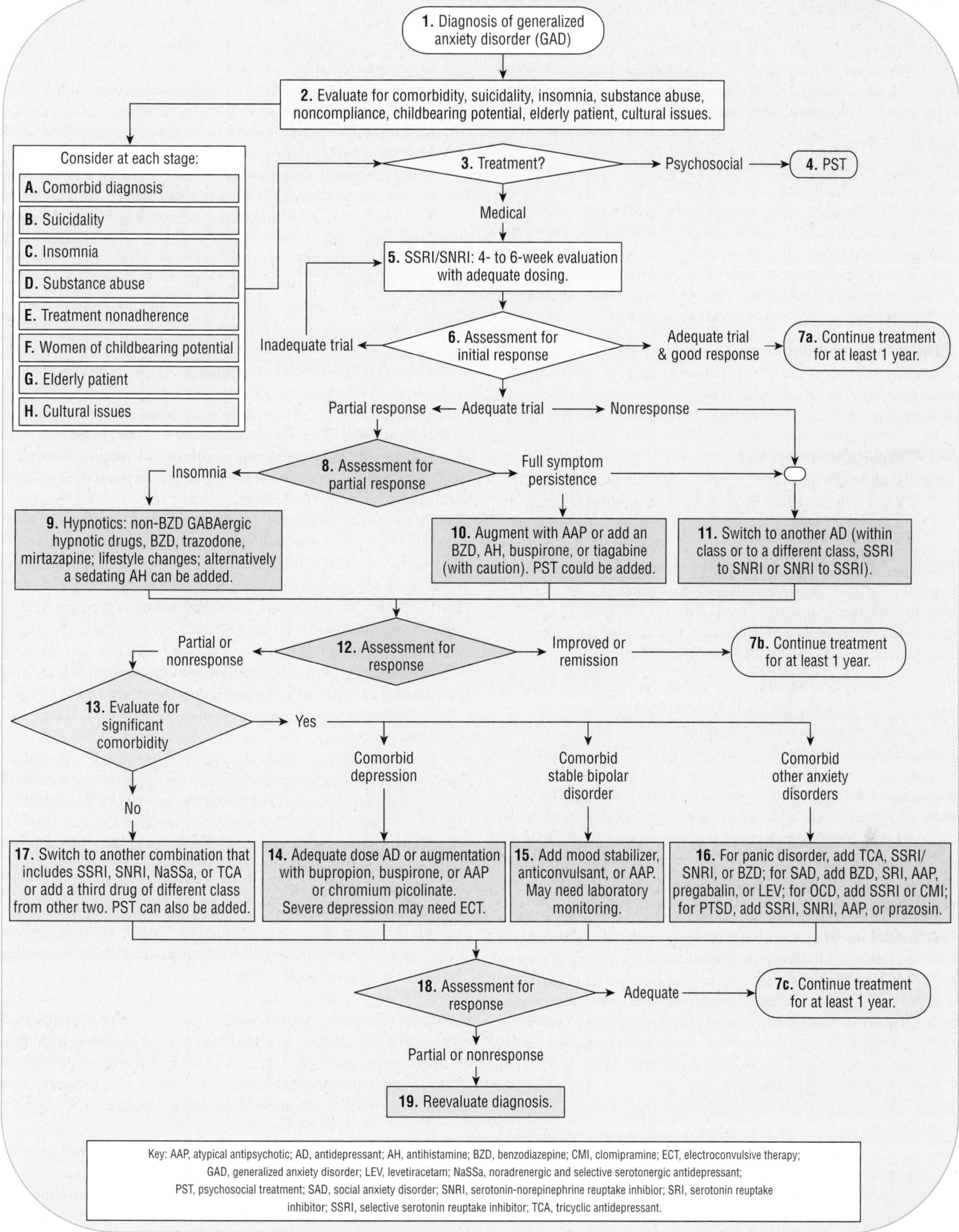

FIGURE 70-1 International Psychopharmacology Algorithm Project (IPAP) generalized anxiety disorder (GAD) algorithm flowchart. Yellow, first-line treatment (nodes 2, 3, 5, 6); green, second-line treatment (nodes 8-12); blue, third-line treatment, no comorbidity (nodes 13,17,18,19); orange, third-line treatment, with comorbidity (nodes 14-16); light green, assessment and evaluation. Levels of evidence used in development of the flowchart were: 1, more than one placebo-controlled trial with sample sizes over 30; 2, one placebo-controlled trial (or active vs active drug comparison) with sample size of 30 or greater; 3, one or small ($n < 30$) placebo-controlled trial; 4, case reports or open-label trials; and 5, expert consensus without published evidence. *(Used by permission of The International Psychopharmacology Algorithm Project. IPAP–Generalized Anxiety Disorder Algorithm. http://www.ipap.org/gad/index.php, accessed December 22, 2015.*

transduction pathways connected to the neurotransmitters 5-HT, DA, and NE. In an animal model of anxiety, a number of candidate genes were identified that were normalized by fluoxetine treatment selectively in the hypothalamus.[40] It is theorized that by activating stress-adapting pathways, SSRIs and SNRIs reduce the somatic anxiety symptoms and the general distress experienced by patients.

Adverse Effects The adverse effects of medications used to treat generalized anxiety are provided in Table 70-6. SSRIs and SNRIs are generally well tolerated, with GI adverse effects and sleep disturbances being the most commonly reported. Headaches and diaphoresis occur early in treatment and are often transient, whereas weight gain and sexual dysfunction may continue in long-term treatment. The use of tricyclic antidepressants (TCAs) is limited by troublesome adverse effects (eg, sedation, anticholinergic effects, and weight gain) in some patients and the risk of toxicity in overdose.

Dosing and Administration The antidepressants can be dosed once a day (see Table 70-5). Some patients require small initial daily doses for the first week of therapy to limit the development of transient increased anxiety, also known as jitteriness syndrome.

Benzodiazepine Therapy

Although all benzodiazepines possess anxiolytic properties, only 7 of the 14 currently marketed agents have FDA approval for the treatment of GAD (see Table 70-4). Estazolam, flurazepam, temazepam, quazepam, and triazolam are marketed as sedative–hypnotic agents. Clonazepam is marketed as an antipanic agent and anticonvulsant,[41] and midazolam is labeled for preoperative sedation. Alprazolam is indicated for the treatment of panic disorder with or without agoraphobia, as well as GAD.[42] Clobazam in indicated for adjunctive treatment of seizures in Lennox-Gastaut syndrome.[27]

Pharmacology and Mechanism of Action The GABA-receptor model of anxiety theorizes that benzodiazepines ameliorate anxiety through potentiation of the inhibitory activity of GABA.[43] Benzodiazepines bind on the $GABA_A$ receptor at the α_1, α_2, α_3, and α_5 subunits in combination with a β subunit and the γ_2 subunit.[43] The anxiolytic effects of benzodiazepines are mediated at the α_2 site, while sedative effects result from binding at the α_1 subunit. The binding sites of GABA and benzodiazepines are at the receptor interfaces of α/β and α/γ_2, respectively. The GABA receptor controls tonic inhibition to reduce neuronal excitability.[43] Other neurotransmitters (eg, 5-HT, NE, and DA) may also be involved in benzodiazepine activity.

Pharmacokinetics A wide difference in milligram potency exists between the benzodiazepine compounds; however, when appropriately dosed, all agents have similar anxiolytic and sedative–hypnotic activity. The variations in lipid solubility between compounds influence the pharmacokinetic properties of benzodiazepines. Knowledge of the different pharmacokinetic and pharmacodynamic properties can assist in choosing an appropriate anxiolytic (Table 70-7). After a single dose, the onset, intensity, and duration of pharmacologic effects are important factors to consider when using benzodiazepines for the short-term, intermittent, or as-needed treatment of anxiety.

The primary determinant of a drug's onset of effect after a single oral dose is the rate of drug absorption. Because of high lipophilicity, diazepam and clorazepate are absorbed rapidly and distributed quickly into the CNS. Therefore, the onset of anxiolytic effect occurs within 30 to 60 minutes, which results in a rapid and intense relief of anxiety. High lipophilicity also increases the extent of drug redistribution into the periphery, particularly adipose tissue, resulting in a shorter duration of effect after a single dose than is suggested by single-dose elimination half-life studies.[44] Clinically, patients perceive a rapid onset of action, but some experience an unpleasant feeling of drowsiness or loss of control. This "rush" can be euphoric and contribute to abuse.

Compared with diazepam, lorazepam and oxazepam are relatively less lipophilic and have a slower absorption and onset of effect. These benzodiazepines have smaller volumes of distribution and a resulting longer duration of action.[44]

Parenteral administration via the intramuscular route should be avoided with diazepam secondary to variability in the rate and extent of drug absorption. Intramuscular lorazepam provides rapid, reliable, and complete absorption.

After multiple dosing, the rate and extent of drug accumulation are functions of the drug's elimination half-life in relation to dosing intervals, clearance, and formation of active metabolites. Differences in clinical effects that occur during and after repeated dosages with the benzodiazepines are related in part to variability in metabolism and metabolite accumulation.[44]

The benzodiazepines undergo two primary metabolic processes, hepatic oxidation (catalyzed by cytochrome P450 3A4) and glucuronide conjugation. With the exception of lorazepam and oxazepam (which are conjugated only) and clonazepam (which undergoes nitroreduction), all benzodiazepines are oxidized first and then conjugated and excreted renally.[44] Diazepam's metabolism is also catalyzed by cytochrome P450 2C19. Oxidation can be impaired in patients with liver disease, in the elderly, and in those who simultaneously use drugs that inhibit oxidation resulting in higher levels of the parent drug and/or an active metabolite.

Many benzodiazepines are converted to desmethyldiazepam (DMDZ), an active metabolite with a long elimination half-life (see Table 70-7). DMDZ is further oxidized to oxazepam and then conjugated and excreted. After multiple dosing, accumulation of DMDZ is slow and extensive, providing a long-lasting antianxiety effect. If oxidation of DMDZ is impaired, the half-life is prolonged, and extensive drug accumulation can result with repeated dosing.

Clorazepate is a prodrug and possesses no anxiolytic effects until metabolized to DMDZ. Before absorption, clorazepate is metabolized rapidly in the stomach through a pH-dependent process under acidic conditions.

Benzodiazepines with shorter half-lives (eg, alprazolam, lorazepam, and oxazepam) reach steady-state plasma concentrations rapidly, and drug accumulation after repeated dosing is minimal. Oxazepam and lorazepam have no active metabolites.

Benzodiazepine protein binding is extensive, especially for the drugs with a long elimination half-life. After a single dose of a benzodiazepine with a long elimination half-life, the expected duration of clinical activity may not parallel the drug's pharmacokinetic half-life because of drug redistribution.[44] After multiple dosing, drugs with long elimination half-lives and active metabolites require 1 to 2 weeks to reach steady state.

Efficacy Clinical trials of benzodiazepines show that 65% to 75% of patients with GAD have a marked to moderate response, with most of the improvement occurring in the first 2 weeks of therapy.[21,22] Benzodiazepines are more effective on the somatic symptoms of anxiety and fail to obviate the cognitive or psychic symptoms (eg, worry).

Adverse Effects The most common adverse events associated with benzodiazepine therapy involve CNS depression (see Table 70-6). This is manifested clinically as drowsiness, sedation, psychomotor impairment, and ataxia.[45,46] A transient mild drowsiness is experienced commonly by patients during the first few days of treatment; however, tolerance often develops. Disorientation, depression, confusion, irritability, aggression, and excitement are reported.[45,46]

Impairment of memory and recall also can occur during benzodiazepine treatment. The memory loss induced by the benzodiazepines typically is limited to events occurring after drug ingestion (anterograde amnesia).[45,46] Anterograde amnesia is secondary to disordered consolidation processes that store information and is not impairment in the perception or retrieval of information.[3]

TABLE 70-6 Monitoring of Adverse Effects Associated with Medications Used for Anxiety Disorders

Medication Class/Drug	Adverse Drug Reaction	Monitoring Parameter	Comments
SSRIs			
	Jitteriness syndrome	Patient interview	
	Suicidality	Patient interview	Monitor weekly in first few weeks in patients with comorbid depression and patients under age 25
	Nausea, diarrhea	Patient interview	Typically transient
	Headache	Patient interview	Typically transient
	Weight gain	Body weight, BMI, waist circumference	Paroxetine may be more likely to cause weight gain
	Sexual dysfunction	Patient interview	Significant reason for nonadherence
	Hyponatremia	Basic metabolic panel	Monitor at baseline and periodically thereafter. More frequent monitoring required in high-risk groups, especially the elderly (>65 years)
	Thrombocytopenia	Complete blood count	Reported with citalopram
	Teratogenicity	Pregnancy test at baseline	Avoid paroxetine in pregnancy; Pregnancy Category D
	QT prolongation	ECG	Before starting citalopram, consider ECG and measurement of QT interval in patients with cardiac disease
	Discontinuation syndrome	Patient interview	Avoid abrupt discontinuation in all but fluoxetine
SNRIs			
	Jitteriness syndrome	Patient interview	
	Suicidality	Patient interview	Monitor weekly in first few weeks in patients with comorbid depression and patients under age 25
	Nausea, diarrhea	Patient interview	Typically transient
	Headache	Patient interview	Typically transient
	Elevated blood pressure	Blood pressure	Monitor blood pressure on initiation and regularly during treatment
	Sexual dysfunction	Patient interview	Significant reason for nonadherence
	Discontinuation syndrome	Patient interview	Avoid abrupt discontinuation
TCAs			
	Jitteriness syndrome	Patient interview	
	Suicidality	Patient interview	Monitor weekly in first few weeks in patients with comorbid depression and patients under age 25
	Anticholinergic effects	Patient interview	Contraindicated with narrow-angle glaucoma, prostatic hypertrophy, and urinary retention
	Weight gain	Body weight, BMI, waist circumference	
	Sexual dysfunction	Patient interview	Significant reason for nonadherence
	Sedation	Patient interview	Administer dosage at bedtime when feasible
	Arrhythmia	ECG	At baseline and periodically in children and patients >40 years of age
	Orthostatic hypotension	Blood pressure with position changes	
	Cholinergic rebound	Patient interview	Avoid abrupt discontinuation; taper doses
Benzodiazepines			
	Drowsiness, fatigue	Patient interview	Avoid operating large machinery; tolerance to sedation develops after repeated dosing
	Anterograde amnesia and memory impairment	Patient interview	Risk of anterograde amnesia is worsened with concomitant intake of alcohol
	Dependence	Patient interview; Prescription Monitoring Program	Monitor for early refills or escalation of dosage
	Withdrawal symptoms	Physical examination; patient interview	Taper doses on discontinuation
	Respiratory depression	Respiratory rate	Avoid administering with other CNS depressants (ie, opioids, alcohol)
	Psychomotor impairment	Physical examination	Increased risk of falls
	Paradoxical disinhibition	Physical examination; family report	Increase in anxiety, irritability, or agitation may be seen in the elderly or children
Other Drugs			
Buspirone	Nausea, abdominal pain	Patient interview	Typically transient
	Drowsiness, dizziness	Patient interview	Typically transient
Phenelzine	Jitteriness syndrome	Patient interview	
	Suicidality	Patient interview	Monitor weekly in first few weeks in patients with comorbid depression and patients under age 25
	Hypertensive crisis	Blood pressure	Tyramine-free diet and avoidance of drug interactions required
	Orthostatic hypotension	Blood pressure with position changes	Fasting labs at baseline and then periodically
Pregabalin	Dizziness, somnolence	Patient interview	
	Peripheral edema	Physical examination	
	Thrombocytopenia	Complete blood count	
	Weight gain	Body weight	
Quetiapine	Sedation	Patient interview	
	Metabolic syndrome	Body weight, BMI, waist circumference, fasting lipids and glucose	Fasting labs at baseline and then periodically
	Akathisia	Patient interview	
	Tardive dyskinesia	Abnormal Involuntary Movement Scale	
	Orthostatic hypotension	Blood pressure with position changes	

BMI, body mass index; ECG, electrocardiogram; SNRI, serotonin–norepinephrine reuptake inhibitor; SSRIs, selective serotonin reuptake inhibitors; TCAs, tricyclic antidepressants.

TABLE 70-7 Pharmacokinetics of Benzodiazepine Antianxiety Agents

Drug	Time to Peak Plasma Level (Hours)	Elimination Half-Life, Parent (Hours)	Metabolic Pathway	Clinically Significant Metabolites	Protein Binding (%)
Alprazolam	1-2	12-15	Oxidation	—	80
Chlordiazepoxide	1-4	5-30	*N*-Dealkylation Oxidation	Desmethyl chlordiazepoxide Demoxepam DMDZ[a]	96
Clonazepam	1-4	30-40	Nitroreduction	—	85
Clorazepate	1-2	Prodrug	Oxidation	DMDZ	97
Diazepam	0.5-2	20-80	Oxidation	DMDZ Oxazepam	98
Lorazepam	2-4	10-20	Conjugation	—	85
Oxazepam	2-4	5-20	Conjugation	—	97

[a]Desmethyldiazepam (DMDZ) half-life 50-100 hours.

Data from references 27 and 44.

Benzodiazepines with high affinity for binding to the benzodiazepine receptor (eg, alprazolam) appear to possess a higher potential for amnesia.[45,46]

Abuse, Dependence, Withdrawal, and Tolerance Two serious complications of benzodiazepine therapy are the potential for abuse and development of physical dependence. Benzodiazepine abuse is rare in the general population of users; however, individuals with a history of multiple drug abuse (eg, alcohol or sedatives) are at the greatest risk for becoming benzodiazepine abusers.[46]

Because of the chronicity of illness, persons with GAD and panic disorder are at high risk of developing benzodiazepine dependence. Benzodiazepine dependence is a physiologic phenomenon demonstrated by the appearance of a predictable abstinence syndrome (withdrawal symptoms) on abrupt discontinuation of therapy.[46,47] Withdrawal symptoms can result because of the sudden dissociation of a benzodiazepine from its receptor site. After abrupt discontinuation, an acute decrease in GABA neurotransmission results, producing a less inhibited CNS.

Benzodiazepine Discontinuation After benzodiazepine therapy is discontinued suddenly, several events can occur. Rebound anxiety represents an immediate but transient return of original symptoms having an increased intensity compared with baseline. Recurrence or relapse is the return of original symptoms with similar intensity as before treatment.

Withdrawal symptoms are the emergence of new symptoms and a worsening of preexisting symptoms after benzodiazepine discontinuation. Symptoms can persist for days to weeks and resolve gradually over months.

Common symptoms of benzodiazepine withdrawal include anxiety, insomnia, restlessness, muscle tension, and irritability. Less frequently occurring symptoms are nausea, malaise, coryza, blurred vision, diaphoresis, nightmares, depression, hyperreflexia, and ataxia. Tinnitus, confusion, paranoid delusions, hallucinations, and seizures occur rarely. Withdrawal seizures can occur with both therapeutic and high doses of benzodiazepines with a short elimination half-life, usually within 3 days of drug discontinuation. They can occur approximately 1 week after discontinuation of agents with a long elimination half-life. High benzodiazepine doses, a long duration of therapy, and concurrent ingestion of drugs that lower the seizure threshold are risk factors for withdrawal seizures.

The onset of withdrawal symptoms in patients ingesting benzodiazepines with short elimination half-lives occurs much earlier (within 24-48 hours) than in those taking benzodiazepines with long elimination half-lives (within 3-8 days). Other factors associated with an increased incidence and severity of benzodiazepine withdrawal include high doses and long-term benzodiazepine therapy.[46,47]

A strategy to minimize the severity of benzodiazepine withdrawal is a 25% per week reduction in dosage until 50% of the dose is reached, and then dosage reduction by one-eighth every 4 to 7 days.[47] If therapy exceeds 8 weeks, a slow dosage taper over 2 to 3 weeks is recommended; however, if the duration of treatment is 6 months, a taper over 4 to 8 weeks should ensue.[47] Long-term use of benzodiazepines (ie, 1 year or longer) requires a 2- to 4-month slow taper.[47] Tapering will not eliminate the emergence of withdrawal symptoms entirely but will prevent severe withdrawal. Slow drug taper is extremely important for the drugs with a short elimination half-life, because some individuals have greater difficulty with discontinuation. Withdrawal symptoms with short half-life benzodiazepines were no more severe than with longer half-life agents; therefore, switching from a short- to long-acting benzodiazepine before gradual taper is not supported.[47] Adjunctive use of pregabalin can help reduce withdrawal severity during the benzodiazepine taper.[48] A combination of psychotherapy interventions (including CBT) with tapering protocols resulted in superior discontinuation outcomes.[49] Patients should avoid the intake of alcohol and stimulants during the withdrawal process. Although tolerance develops to the sedative, muscle relaxant, and anticonvulsant activities, the benzodiazepines do not appear to lose anxiolytic or antipanic efficacy. However, the anxiolytic efficacy of benzodiazepines in long-term clinical trials (greater than 6-8 months of chronic use) has not been documented.[4,21,22,]

Drug Interactions Drug interactions with the benzodiazepines generally fall into two categories: pharmacodynamic and pharmacokinetic. Simultaneous use of alcohol and a benzodiazepine results in additive CNS depressant effects. In addition, concurrent use of a benzodiazepine and other drugs with CNS depressant properties (eg, opioids, antipsychotics, and antihistamines) can potentiate the adverse sedative effects. When ingested alone in an overdose attempt, benzodiazepines are rarely life-threatening; however, the combination of benzodiazepines with alcohol or other CNS depressant agents is potentially fatal.

Concurrent use of medications that inhibit cytochrome P450 3A4 (eg, ketoconazole, nefazodone, and ritonavir) can increase the blood levels of alprazolam and diazepam. Drugs that induce cytochrome P450 3A4 (eg, carbamazepine, St. John's wort) can reduce benzodiazepine levels. Consult a drug interaction Web site (http://www.factsandcomparisons.com/facts-comparisons-online.aspx) for further information.

Dosing and Administration Benzodiazepine dosage requirements vary widely among patients and must be individualized. Therapy should be initiated using low doses (eg, alprazolam 0.25 mg three times a day or equivalent doses of other benzodiazepines) and titrated upward to relieve anxiety symptoms and avoid adverse events.

After an initial treatment response is achieved, agents with long elimination half-lives can be dosed at bedtime. Dosage adjustments should be made weekly. Three to 4 weeks of a daily dose at the maximum dose constitutes an adequate clinical trial (see Table 70-4).[2,21,22]

The duration of benzodiazepine therapy for the acute management of anxiety should be limited to 2 to 4 weeks. In general, benzodiazepines should be used with a regular dosing regimen and not on an as-needed basis.[4,18] Only in the treatment of short-term distress (eg, air travel, dental phobia) as-needed use may be justified.[4] Individuals with persistent symptoms should be managed with antidepressants because of the risk of dependence with continued benzodiazepine therapy.

Patient education should include the anticipated length of drug therapy, potential side effects, and consequences of the ingestion of alcohol and other CNS depressants. Patients should understand that benzodiazepines provide symptomatic relief but do not solve underlying psychological problems. Patients should be instructed not to decrease or discontinue benzodiazepine usage without contacting their prescriber.

Buspirone Therapy

Buspirone is a nonbenzodiazepine anxiolytic that lacks anticonvulsant, muscle relaxant, hypnotic, motor impairment, and dependence properties. It is considered to be a second-line agent for GAD because of inconsistent reports of efficacy (particularly long-term), delayed onset of effect (ie, 2 weeks or longer), and lack of efficacy for other potential concurrent depressive and anxiety disorders.[2] Unlike benzodiazepines, buspirone is effective for the psychic symptoms of anxiety.[2]

Pharmacology and Mechanism of Action Buspirone's anxiolytic mechanism of action is unknown. It is thought to exert its anxiolytic effect through partial agonist activity at the 5-HT_{1A} presynaptic receptors, thus reducing the firing of 5-HT neurons.[44]

Pharmacokinetics After an oral dose, buspirone is absorbed rapidly and completely and undergoes extensive first-pass metabolism. The mean elimination half-life is 2.5 hours, and it must be dosed two to three times daily, which adversely affects adherence to the drug regimen.[44]

Adverse Effects Adverse events include dizziness, nausea, and headaches[44] (see Table 70-6).

Drug Interactions Drugs that inhibit cytochrome P450 3A4 (eg, verapamil, itraconazole, fluvoxamine) can increase buspirone levels. Rifampin caused a 10-fold reduction in buspirone levels. Buspirone reportedly elevates blood pressure in patients taking a monoamine oxidase inhibitor (MAOI).

Dosing and Administration The dose of buspirone can be titrated in increments of 5 mg/day every 2 to 3 days as needed.[44] The onset of improvement in psychic symptoms precedes the relief of somatic symptoms; maximum therapeutic benefit might not be evident for 4 to 6 weeks.

Buspirone is a treatment option for patients with GAD, particularly for patients with uncomplicated GAD, in patients who fail other anxiolytic therapies, or in patients with substance abuse. It is not useful in clinical situations requiring immediate anxiolysis or for situations requiring as-needed anxiolytic therapy.[44] Evidence suggests that buspirone may have less efficacy in patients who have previously used benzodiazepines.[2]

Special Populations

The management of anxiety in patients with substance abuse, pregnant women, children, elderly patients, and those patients with adherence problems requires special consideration in the choice of anxiolytic. Patients with GAD may misuse alcohol, cannabis, or other substances to manage anxiety. The symptoms of GAD are similar to those of withdrawal, and it is difficult to confirm the diagnosis of GAD until after abstinence is obtained. Benzodiazepine therapy should be avoided in this population.

There is evidence that maternal anxiety during pregnancy and the postpartum period potentially pose significant risk to the child. Clinical practice guidelines for anxiety disorders recommend use of fluoxetine, sertraline, or citalopram; however, jitteriness, myoclonus, and irritability in the neonate and premature infant have been reported.[50] Paroxetine (Pregnancy Category D) should be avoided in pregnant women because of risk of cardiovascular malformations.[31]

Cleft lip, cleft palate, and other teratogenic effects are associated with benzodiazepine use, but a causal relationship is inconclusive. Clinicians should avoid benzodiazepine use during the first trimester, use the lowest dosage for the shortest period of time, divide the total daily dosage into two or three doses to prevent high peak plasma levels, and use the agent as monotherapy.[18,50] Benzodiazepine risks during the third trimester include sedation, withdrawal symptoms, and "floppy baby syndrome" (eg, hypotonia, low Apgar scores, hypothermia). Alprazolam should be avoided during pregnancy because of neonatal withdrawal. Should benzodiazepines be required during pregnancy, the preferred agents are diazepam and chlordiazepoxide.[51] The antidepressants are favored for GAD during pregnancy based on safety considerations. Diazepam and clonazepam should not be used in nursing mothers because infants can experience sedation, lethargy, and weight loss.[18,50]

There are few controlled clinical trials of drugs in children and adolescents with GAD. CBT alone or in conjunction with antidepressants can have long-term benefits.[52] Randomized controlled trials of fluvoxamine, fluoxetine, sertraline, duloxetine, and venlafaxine extended-release indicate short-term efficacy[52]; however, irritability and oppotional behavior was reported with clonazepam.[52] No antidepressant is FDA-indicated for GAD in children or adolescents. Increased monitoring for behavioral changes with benzodiazepines and suicide-related adverse effects with antidepressants is necessary if these agents are prescribed.

Patients with hepatic disease are at risk for drug accumulation and subsequent complications. Duloxetine use should be avoided in patients with hepatic insufficiency.[29] Drug accumulation of benzodiazepines can result in the elderly secondary to a decreased capacity for oxidation and alterations in the volume of distribution. Therefore, intermediate- or short-acting benzodiazepines without active metabolites are preferred for chronic use. Elderly patients are also sensitive to the CNS adverse effects of benzodiazepines (regardless of half-life), and their use is associated with a high frequency of falls and hip fractures. Recent studies of buspirone, duloxetine, escitalopram, sertraline, venlafaxine, and pregabalin showed efficacy in elderly patients with GAD.[2,53-55]

Personalized Pharmacotherapy

The need for treatment is determined by patient-specific factors including severity and duration of symptoms, degree of disability, and the presence of coexisting disorders (ie, mood or other anxiety disorders). The patient should be assessed for response to or intolerance of previous treatment approaches. The selection of a specific treatment modality should be based on concurrent medical conditions, contraindications, patient's preference of treatment, and the availability of potential treatment options. The clinician should consider FDA warnings (eg, QTc prolongation for citalopram, teratogenicity with paroxetine) and potential for adverse events with medical disease (eg, anticholinergic effects and weight gain with paroxetine in patients with diabetes, obesity, or benign prostatic hyperplasia) when selecting an agent. Increased risk of suicidality should be considered in patients taking antidepressants who are younger than 25 years.

All patients should receive education that includes information about GAD, treatment choices, and resources for support in the community. The patient should be an integral part of decision making and should be informed about effectiveness, common adverse effects, duration of treatment, cost associated with treatment, and what to expect when treatment is discontinued.[2]

Evaluation of Therapeutic Outcomes

Initially, anxious patients should be monitored once every 2 weeks for a reduction in the frequency, duration, and severity of anxiety symptoms and improvement in functioning.[2] The clinician should assess the patient for response to treatment by asking about specific target symptoms of anxiety and emergence of adverse events. Ideally, the patient should have no or minimal anxiety or depressive symptoms and no functional impairment. Use of an objective measurement of remission of GAD (eg, Hamilton Rating Scale for Anxiety score less than or equal to 7 and a Sheehan Disability Scale score less than or equal to 1 on each item) can assist in the evaluation of drug response.[2,18] The definition of treatment resistance is defined as a poor, partial, or lack of response with at least two antidepressants from different classes. Treatment strategies for patients who do not achieve an appropriate response with a first-line agent include increasing the dose of the SSRI/SNRI, changing to a different agent in the same class, changing to a different agent of a different class, or augmentation of therapy. At any point of nonresponse or loss of previous response, the clinician should assess for (a) symptoms (eg, psychotic symptoms) that may suggest a need for additional medications or (b) reasons for treatment nonadherence (eg, adverse effects, cost of medications, limited understanding of the illness or treatments).[18] Patients should also be assessed for concurrent substance abuse, concurrent illnesses, and suicidal thoughts. Once a patient has responded to pharmacotherapy, the regimen should be continued for at least 1 year.[18] Early discontinuation is associated with a greater risk of relapse.[18]

TREATMENT
Panic Disorder

Desired Outcomes

The goal of therapy in panic disorder is remission. Patients should be free of panic attacks, have no or minimal anticipatory anxiety and agoraphobic avoidance, and have no functional impairment.[20]

General Approach

Therapeutic options include single or combined pharmacologic agents, concurrent psychotherapy, or psychotherapy followed by pharmacotherapy. Most patients without agoraphobic avoidance will improve with pharmacotherapy alone; however, if avoidance is present, CBT typically is initiated concurrently. With all effective drug therapies, resolution of agoraphobic avoidance tends to occur slowly. A meta-analysis comparing the use of SSRIs and venlafaxine in panic disorder showed response to be similar among treatments.[56] Adding psychosocial treatment to pharmacotherapy may improve long-term outcomes by reducing the likelihood of relapse when pharmacotherapy is stopped.[20]

Nonpharmacologic Therapy

Patients should be educated to avoid substances that can precipitate panic attacks, including caffeine, nicotine, alcohol, drugs of abuse, and nonprescription stimulants.[1,20] Epidemiologic data suggest that daily smoking increases risk for panic attacks and may be a causal or exacerbating factor in some individuals with panic disorder.[20] Preliminary evidence suggests that aerobic exercise (eg, walking for 60 minutes or running for 20-30 minutes 4 day/wk) may benefit patients with panic disorder.[21] CBT is associated with short-term improvement in 80% to 90% of patients and 6-month improvement in 75% of patients. A course of CBT for panic disorder is 16 to 20 hours in length conducted over a period of 4 months.[21] Bibliotherapy (the use of self-help books), exercise, and Internet-based CBT are other options.[20]

Pharmacologic Therapy

Panic disorder is treated effectively with several drugs including SSRIs, the SNRI venlafaxine, the TCA imipramine, and the benzodiazepines alprazolam and clonazepam[20,21] (Table 70-8). Alprazolam, clonazepam, fluoxetine, paroxetine, sertraline, and venlafaxine are approved for this indication. SSRIs are the first-line agents because of their tolerability and efficacy in acute and long-term studies[2,20]; however, the benzodiazepines are the most commonly used drugs for panic disorder.[20] In a meta-analysis of the pharmacotherapy of panic disorder, the following antidepressants were significantly superior to placebo with the following increasing order of effectiveness: citalopram, sertraline, paroxetine, fluoxetine, and venlafaxine for panic symptoms and paroxetine, fluoxetine, fluvoxamine, citalopram, venlafaxine, and mirtazapine for overall anxiety symptoms.[56] Imipramine is effective for panic disorder; however, it is considered to be a second-line agent because of the significant cardiovascular and anticholinergic effects associated with it. Five practice guidelines are published.[2,4,20-22] An algorithm for the pharmacologic therapy of panic disorder appears in Fig. 70-2.

Benzodiazepines are considered second-line agents. Because of the risk of dependency, benzodiazepines should be used only after several trials of antidepressants have failed.[2,20] Because of potential emergence of depressive symptoms during treatment, benzodiazepines should not be used as monotherapy in a patient who is clinically depressed or has a history of depression. In patients whose illness is complicated by a history of alcohol or drug abuse, benzodiazepine use should be avoided.[20] Controlled trials have established that the short-term (4-6 weeks) addition of alprazolam or clonazepam to antidepressants produces a more rapid therapeutic response, with discontinuation of the benzodiazepine by week 7 of therapy.[2]

Alternative Drug Treatments

Buspirone, trazodone, bupropion, antipsychotics, antihistamines, and β-blockers are ineffective in panic disorder.[2,4,20-22] The majority of studies assessing the efficacy of MAOIs in treating panic disorder were open-labeled, and lacked adequate sample sizes. MAOIs are reserved for the most refractory or difficult patients.[20]

Antidepressant Therapy

Tricyclic Antidepressants

Efficacy Imipramine is the most studied TCA, alleviating panic attacks in 75% of patients with panic disorder. Imipramine effectively blocks panic attacks within at least 4 weeks; however, maximal improvement (including antiphobic response) does not occur until 8 to 12 weeks.[20]

Adverse Effects The adverse effects of medications used to treat panic disorder are found in Table 70-6. Up to 40% of patients experience stimulant-like effects, including anxiety, insomnia, and jitteriness.[20] These adverse effects often affect patient adherence, prevent medication dosage increases, and interfere with the overall treatment outcome.

Other problems with TCA use in panic disorder are well documented and include anticholinergic effects, orthostatic hypotension, delayed onset of antipanic effects, and toxicity in overdose.[20] Approximately 25% of patients reportedly discontinue treatment because of side effects, especially weight gain.[20]

TABLE 70-8 Drugs Used in the Treatment of Panic Disorder

Class/Generic Name	Brand Name	Starting Dose	Antipanic Dosage Range (mg)	Comments
SSRIs				
Citalopram	Celexa	10 mg/day	20-40	Dosage used in clinical trials; maximum dose limited by QT prolongation; available generically
Escitalopram	Lexapro	5 mg/day	10-20	Dosage used in clinical trials; available generically
Fluoxetine	Prozac	5 mg/day	10-30	Available generically
Fluvoxamine	Luvox	25 mg/day	100-300	Available generically
Paroxetine	Paxil	10 mg/day	20-60	FDA-approved; available generically
	Pexeva			
	Paxil CR	12.5 mg/day	25-75	
Sertraline	Zoloft	25 mg/day	50-200	FDA-approved; available generically
SNRI				
Venlafaxine XR	Effexor XR	37.5 mg/day	75-225	FDA-approved; available generically
Benzodiazepines				
Alprazolam	Xanax	0.25 mg three times a day	4-10	FDA-approved; available generically
	Xanax XR	0.5-1 mg/day	1-10	
Clonazepam	Klonopin	0.25 mg once or twice per day	1-4	FDA-approved; available generically
Diazepam	Valium	2-5 mg three times a day	5-20	Dosage used in clinical trials; available generically
Lorazepam	Ativan	0.5-1 mg three times a day	2-8	Dosage used in clinical trials; available generically
TCA				
Imipramine	Tofranil	10 mg/day	75-250	Dosage used in clinical trials; available generically
MOI				
Phenelzine	Nardil	15 mg/day	45-90	Dosage used in clinical trials

CR, controlled release; MOI, monoamine oxidase inhibitor; SNRI, serotonin–norepinephrine reuptake inhibitor; SSRIs, selective serotonin reuptake inhibitors; TCA, tricyclic antidepressant; XR, extended release.

Data from references 4, 20, and 57.

Dosing and Administration When using imipramine, treatment should be slowly increased by 10 mg every 2 to 4 days as tolerated (Table 70-8).

Selective Serotonin Reuptake Inhibitors

Efficacy Clinical studies indicate that all SSRIs are effective in panic disorder.[20] The percentage of patients who become panic-free ranges between 60% and 80%.[20] 5 The antipanic effect of SSRIs is delayed for at least 4 weeks, and some patients do not respond for 8 to 12 weeks.[20]

Adverse Effects Typical antidepressant doses of SSRIs can cause side effects of insomnia, jitteriness, restlessness, and agitation, and lead to drug discontinuation in patients with panic disorder. Other adverse effects associated with SSRI use in panic disorder are listed in Table 70-6.

Dosing and Administration Low initial doses of SSRIs are recommended (see Table 70-8) to avoid stimulatory side effects (eg, insomnia or nervousness), and should be maintained for the first week of therapy. Doses at the upper end of the dosing range can be necessary to achieve response.[21,57]

Serotonin–Norepinephrine Reuptake Inhibitors

Efficacy Venlafaxine extended-release 75 to 150 mg/day was superior to placebo in the proportion of patients becoming free from full-symptom panic attacks. Other data support efficacy of venlafaxine in reducing the severity of anticipatory anxiety, fear, and avoidance.[57] Venlafaxine is similar in efficacy to paroxetine in patients with panic disorder and superior to placebo in a relapse prevention study.[57]

Adverse Effects The most common adverse effects of venlafaxine extended-release in panic trials were nausea, dry mouth, constipation, anorexia, insomnia, somnolence, tremors, sweating, and sexual dysfunction.[20]

Dosing and Administration The dosage of venlafaxine extended-release is 37.5 mg/day for the first 3 to 7 days, and then increased to a minimum of 75 mg/day (Table 70-8). Increasing the dose to 150 mg/day after initial nonresponse or partial response is recommended. A dose–response relationship was not evident in clinical trials.[32]

Benzodiazepines

Efficacy The high-potency benzodiazepines clonazepam and alprazolam are the preferred agents.[20,21] Diazepam and lorazepam are possibly effective in treating panic disorder when taken in sufficiently high doses.[20] Alprazolam provides rapid relief for patients in distress, but because of its short half-life, multiple daily dosing is required and often results in profound withdrawal symptoms with missed doses.[20] Therapeutic response to benzodiazepines occurs in 1 to 2 weeks. Relapse rates of 50% or higher are common despite slow drug tapering during discontinuation of therapy.[47]

Adverse Effects Patient acceptance of benzodiazepines usually is not a problem, and except for sedation, side effects are rarely reported (see Table 70-6).

Dosing and Administration Doses of clonazepam can be increased by 0.25 or 0.5 mg every 3 days to 4 mg/day if needed.[41] Alprazolam can be slowly increased over several weeks to reach an ideal dose. The duration of action of immediate-release alprazolam can be as little as 4 to 6 hours with resulting breakthrough symptoms; use of the extended-release alprazolam or clonazepam will avoid this problem. Most patients require 3 to 6 mg/day of alprazolam, and some need higher doses to obtain a full therapeutic (antipanic and antiphobic) response.

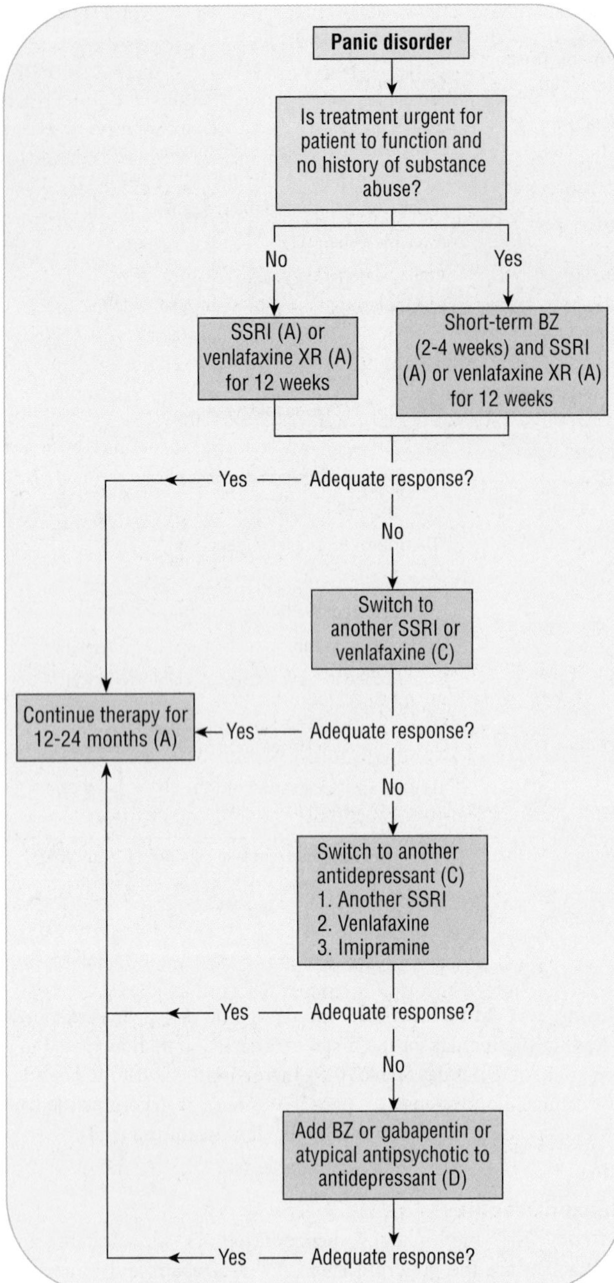

FIGURE 70-2 Algorithm for the pharmacotherapy of panic disorder. Strength of recommendations: A, directly based on category I evidence (ie, meta-analysis of randomized controlled trials [RCT] or at least one RCT); B, directly based on category II evidence (ie, at least one controlled study without randomization or one other type of quasi-experimental study); C, directly based on category III evidence (ie, nonexperimental descriptive studies); D, directly based on category IV evidence (ie, expert committee reports or opinions and/or clinical experience of respected authorities). (BZ, benzodiazepine; SSRI, selective serotonin reuptake inhibitor.) *(Adapted from references 20 and 21.)*

Clinical **Controversy...**

There is an ongoing controversy about the long-term use of benzodiazepines in the treatment of anxiety and related disorders. Most treatment guidelines recommend that use of benzodiazepines be limited to short-term use because of the risk for tolerance, dose escalation, dependence, and potential abuse. In addition, recent data highlight a potential increased risk for the development of dementia with long-term use of benzodiazepines.[58] Despite these concerns, benzodiazepines are commonly prescribed in practice, and some experts argue that the benefits of long-term benzodiazepine use outweigh the potential adverse effects for most patients.

Treatment Resistance

Common reasons for treatment failures are comorbid psychiatric disorders, rapid dosage increases with resulting intolerable side effects, and underdosage.[20] All standard treatments should be tried before using augmentation strategies. In patients with a partial response to one agent, a low dose of another antipanic agent (eg, a TCA, benzodiazepine, or an SSRI) can be added.[20]

Phases of Therapy

Acute Phase

The main goal of therapy in the acute phase is reduction of symptoms (eg, resolution of panic attacks, reduction in anxiety and phobic fears, resumption of the patient's usual activities).[20,22] The duration of this phase is generally 1 to 3 months depending on the choice of drug. Therapy should be altered if there is no response after 6 to 8 weeks of an adequate dose.

The guiding principle for SSRIs and SNRIs in panic disorder is to start with low doses (approximately one fourth to one-half of the starting doses for depression), use an adequate dose, and treat for about 12 weeks.[20,22] Adverse effects, often from too high an initial dose, can prevent achievement of an optimal dosage, compromise treatment response, and contribute to patient nonadherence.

The duration of the acute phase with benzodiazepines is approximately 1 month because response is rapid. A regular dosing schedule rather than an "as-needed" schedule is preferred for patients with panic disorder who are taking benzodiazepines, where the goal is to prevent panic attacks rather than reduce symptoms once an attack has already occurred.[20]

Maintenance Phase and Discontinuation

6 The optimal length of therapy is unknown; however, the total duration of therapy appears to be 12 to 24 months before drug discontinuation over 4 to 6 months is attempted.[20] The dose used in the acute phase is continued into the maintenance phase.[20] When drugs are discontinued too early, a high rate of relapse occurs; thus, longer periods of treatment are associated with a more sustained response. Reinstitution of drug usually results in renewed clinical response.[20] Pharmacotherapy, even of a long duration, might not prevent relapse, and many patients require long-term therapy.

The most important determinant of adherence with maintenance therapy is the tolerability of adverse events.[20] Some adverse events that are experienced short term become unbearable during long-term management (eg, sexual dysfunction and weight gain). TCAs, SSRIs (except fluoxetine), and venlafaxine can be associated with discontinuation symptoms.

The primary risk of long-term benzodiazepine use is the development of dependence and withdrawal symptoms upon discontinuation. Abuse of benzodiazepines usually is confined to patients with a personal or family history of substance or alcohol abuse.[45,46] The approach to benzodiazepine discontinuation involves a slow and gradual tapering of the dose because withdrawal symptoms and rebound anxiety may occur during discontinuation. Benzodiazepines should be tapered over 2 to 4 months at rates no higher than 10% of the dose per week.[20,47] Patients receiving benzodiazepines and antidepressants should be told not to decrease or discontinue therapy unless authorized by their clinician.[20]

Special Populations

Elderly patients with panic disorder have fewer, less intense symptoms and avoidant behavior than younger patients.[20] Youth often present with fear that they are dying or being smothered, and agoraphobia can be manifested as a fear of leaving home.[1] CBT is effective in both populations. If pharmacotherapy is used, antidepressants, especially the SSRIs, are preferred for management of panic disorder, and benzodiazepines are second-line agents because of potential problems with disinhibition in these two populations. Limited data suggest that the course of panic disorder is highly variable during pregnancy and the postpartum period. It is unclear whether uncontrolled symptoms of panic disorder affect the course or outcome of pregnancy.[20] Little evidence exists on the use of psychosocial interventions for women with panic disorder who are pregnant, breast-feeding, or planning to become pregnant. Nonpharmacologic interventions should be considered as first-line treatment in these patients. Pharmacotherapy may also be indicated but requires careful evaluation of the potential benefits and risks.[20]

Personalized Pharmacotherapy

Research is evolving regarding pharmacogenetic properties related to benzodiazepine agents. While all benzodiazepines bind to the $GABA_A$ receptor, they have different physiochemical properties, most notably lipid solubility, which influence their pharmacokinetics, including rate of absorption and diffusion. Pharmacogenomic studies of benzodiazepines have focused on metabolizing enzymes. In particular, benzodiazepines are biotransformed by different cytochrome P450 isoforms and also by different UDP-glucuronosyltransferase subtypes. Evaluation of these factors in patients with genetic alterations in metabolism is an important part of personalized therapy. The most recent data available regarding research on the effects of pharmacogenetic properties of the benzodiazepines can be located online at The Pharmacogenomics Knowledgebase.[59]

Considerations that guide selection of the treatment modality for panic disorder include patient preference, treatment history, the presence of co-occurring medical or other psychiatric conditions, cost, and treatment availability. Psychosocial treatment in the form of CBT is recommended for patients who prefer nonpharmacologic therapy and who are able to invest the effort and time to attend weekly sessions and between-session homework exercises. Pharmacotherapy with a first-line agent is recommended for patients who prefer medications or who do not have access to or resources to engage in CBT. Combination with psychotherapy and pharmacotherapy is appropriate for patients who have failed monotherapy with medication or CBT.

Providing education about the disorder may relieve some of the symptoms of panic by helping the patient to realize that the symptoms are neither life-threatening nor uncommon. Patients should be informed regarding the lag time before a therapeutic response will occur and any problematic side effects that might affect early adherence (eg, jitteriness syndrome). Many patients are reluctant to take drugs for fear that their illness will worsen or that they will become addicted. Adverse events are often perceived as a worsening of the illness and can contribute to nonadherence or prevent necessary dosage increases. A strong therapeutic alliance between the clinician and the patient is important in supporting the patient through the aspects of the treatment that may provoke anxiety.

Evaluation of Therapeutic Outcomes

During the first few weeks of the acute phase of therapy, patients with panic disorder should be seen every 1 to 2 weeks when starting a new medication, and then every 2 to 4 weeks to adjust drug dosages based on improvement in panic symptoms and to monitor for adverse events.[20,21] After the dose is stabilized and symptoms have decreased, visits every 2 months should suffice.[22] The patient should be counseled to maintain a diary to record the date, time, frequency, duration, and intensity of panic episodes, level of anticipatory anxiety or agoraphobic avoidance, and the severity of distress and impairment related to the panic disorder. Treatment outcomes can be assessed objectively by use of the Panic Disorder Severity Scale. Remission is defined as equal to or less than 3 with no or mild agoraphobic avoidance, anxiety, disability, or depressive symptoms. Treatment response is indicated by a 40% or greater reduction in overall score.[2]

At scheduled visits, the clinician can inquire about the level of disability experienced by the patient and have the patient complete the Sheehan Disability Scale (with a goal of less than or equal to 1 point on each item). During drug discontinuation, the frequency of appointments should be increased to evaluate for emergence of potential withdrawal symptoms and monitor for relapse.

TREATMENT
Social Anxiety Disorder

Desired Outcomes

The goals of therapy in the acute phase of treatment are to reduce physiologic symptoms of anxiety (eg, tachycardia, flushing, and sweating), social anxiety, and phobic avoidance. The duration of this phase is 4 to 12 weeks, depending on the drug therapy.

The goals of therapy in the continuation phase (3-6 months) are to extend the therapeutic benefits, especially the patient's ability to participate in social activities, and improve QOL. Although the primary goal of treatment is to reduce anxiety symptoms to manageable levels, even modest reductions in avoidance and discomfort can be highly valued by patients.[19]

7 At least a 6- to 12-month medication maintenance period is recommended to maintain improvement and decrease the rate of relapse.[2,4,22] Situations suggesting a possible need for long-term treatment include the presence of unresolved symptoms or comorbidity, an early onset of disease, and a prior history of relapse.[19] The long-term goal in the treatment of SAD is remission with the disappearance of the core symptoms of social anxiety, little or no anxiety, and no functional impairment or concurrent depressive symptoms.[19,61]

General Approach

Patients with SAD should be identified early and treated aggressively.[19] Obstacles to effective treatment include patient avoidance of therapy secondary to fear and shame, treatment directed toward somatic symptoms or concurrent conditions, and financial barriers.[19] Patients with SAD often respond more slowly and less completely than patients with other anxiety disorders. Therefore, it is important to set reasonable expectations for response to therapy. Consideration of current symptoms, prior treatments, concurrent conditions, and history of substance abuse guide treatment selection.

CBT and pharmacotherapy are effective in the treatment of SAD.[2,19,60,62] Pharmacotherapy is often the most practical choice because CBT might not be available in medically underserved areas. Acute treatment outcomes for CBT and pharmacotherapy are equivalent.[2,4,19] Drug therapy is superior in reducing subjective general anxiety acutely, although CBT has a greater likelihood of maintaining response after termination.[19,61,62]

There are no data to predict which patients will respond best to pharmacotherapy, CBT, or a combination, or maintain gains after discontinuing pharmacotherapy. The only significant indication of treatment response in pharmacotherapy is duration of treatment.[19,60-63] Some patients elect lifelong therapy, and many are reluctant to attempt drug discontinuation because of fear of relapse.

Nonpharmacologic Therapy

Patients should be educated about SAD and support groups. Self-help group programs that focus on effective communication can benefit people with anxiety involving public speaking.

CBT consists of exposure therapy, cognitive restructuring, relaxation training techniques, and social skills training.[2,4,19,22,62] Through CBT, patients learn to overcome anxiety in social situations and alter the beliefs and responses that maintain this anxiety. Therapy usually lasts several months and often is conducted in groups.[19,62]

Clinical Controversy...

It is controversial if pharmacotherapy or psychotherapy is better treatment for patients diagnosed with SAD. Some studies have directly compared pharmacotherapy and CBT for SAD, with mixed findings depending on whether short- or long-term results were examined and what types of outcome variables were studied.

Pharmacologic Therapy

Antidepressant Therapy

8 The SSRIs and venlafaxine are beneficial for concurrent depression, and are safe when used in patients with substance abuse. Paroxetine, sertraline, fluvoxamine extended-release, and venlafaxine extended-release are approved for the treatment of SAD, and are considered first-line agents because of efficacy and tolerability (Table 70-9). Controlled trials comparing different SSRIs, or SSRIs and an SNRI, demonstrated equivalent efficacy between agents.[19,60-62] TCAs are not effective in SAD.[2,22] Evidence-based guidelines for the treatment of SAD were published by the Canadian Psychiatric Association, World Federation of Societies of Biological Psychiatry, the National Institute for Health and Care Excellence, and the British Association for Psychopharmacology.[2,4,19,22] An algorithm for the pharmacotherapy of SAD appears in Fig. 70-3.

Selective Serotonin Reuptake Inhibitors

Efficacy Large trials of escitalopram, fluvoxamine (immediate- and controlled-release), paroxetine, sertraline, and venlafaxine extended-release have shown efficacy and tolerability. Results of studies with fluoxetine have been inconsistent. The onset of effect was delayed 4 to 8 weeks, and maximum benefit was often not observed until 12 weeks or longer. Large relapse prevention trials with escitalopram, paroxetine, and sertraline demonstrated relapse rates of 4% to 14% with continued drug treatment, compared with 36% to 39% with placebo.[60,62]

Dosing and Administration SSRIs should be initiated at doses similar to those used for the treatment of depression and administered as a single daily dose (see Table 70-9). If the patient suffers from comorbid panic disorder, the SSRI dose should be started at one-fourth or one-half of the dose. The dose–response curve for SSRIs tends to be relatively flat, but individual patients can require higher doses. Increase the dose as tolerated in patients who have not responded after 4 weeks of therapy.[19,60-63] When discontinuing an SSRI, the dosage should be tapered monthly (ie, decreasing sertraline by 50 mg or paroxetine by 10 mg) to reduce the risk of relapse and discontinuation symptoms.

Venlafaxine

Efficacy The efficacy of venlafaxine extended-release was established in four double-blind, parallel-group, 12-week, multicenter, placebo-controlled, flexible-dose studies and one double-blind, parallel-group, 6-month, placebo-controlled, fixed/flexible-dose study.[32] Efficacy was assessed with the Liebowitz Social Anxiety Scale (LSAS).

TABLE 70-9 Drugs Used in the Treatment of Social Anxiety Disorder

Drug	Brand Name	Initial Dose	Usual Range (mg/day)	Comments
SSRIs				
Citalopram	Celexa	20 mg/day	20-40	Dosage used in clinical trials; maximum dose of 40 mg limited by QT prolongation; available generically
Escitalopram	Lexapro	5 mg/day	10-20	Dosage used in clinical trials; available generically
Fluvoxamine CR	Luvox CR	100 mg	100-300	FDA-approved; available generically
Paroxetine	Paxil	10 mg/day	10-60	FDA-approved; available generically
Paroxetine CR	Paxil CR	12.5 mg/day	12.5-37.5	FDA-approved; available generically
Sertraline	Zoloft	25-50 mg/day	50-200	FDA-approved; available generically
SNRI				
Venlafaxine XR	Effexor XR	75 mg/day	75-225	FDA-approved; available generically
Benzodiazepine				
Clonazepam	Klonopin	0.25 mg/day	1-4	Dosage used in clinical trials; used as augmenting agent; available generically
MOI				
Phenelzine	Nardil	15 mg at bedtime	60-90	Dosage used in clinical trials
Alternative Agents				
Buspirone	BuSpar	10 mg twice per day	45-60	Dosage used in clinical trials; used as augmenting agent; available generically
Gabapentin	Neurontin	100 mg three times a day	900-3,600	Dosage used in clinical trials; dosage adjustment required in renal impairment
Pregabalin	Lyrica	100 mg three times a day	600	Dosage used in clinical trials; dosage adjustment required in renal impairment
Quetiapine	Seroquel	25 mg at bedtime	25-400	Dosage used in clinical trials

CR, controlled-release; MOI, monoamine oxidase inhibitor; SNRI, serotonin–norepinephrine reuptake inhibitor; SSRIs, selective serotonin reuptake inhibitors; XR, extended-release.

Data from references 2, 4, 22, and 60.

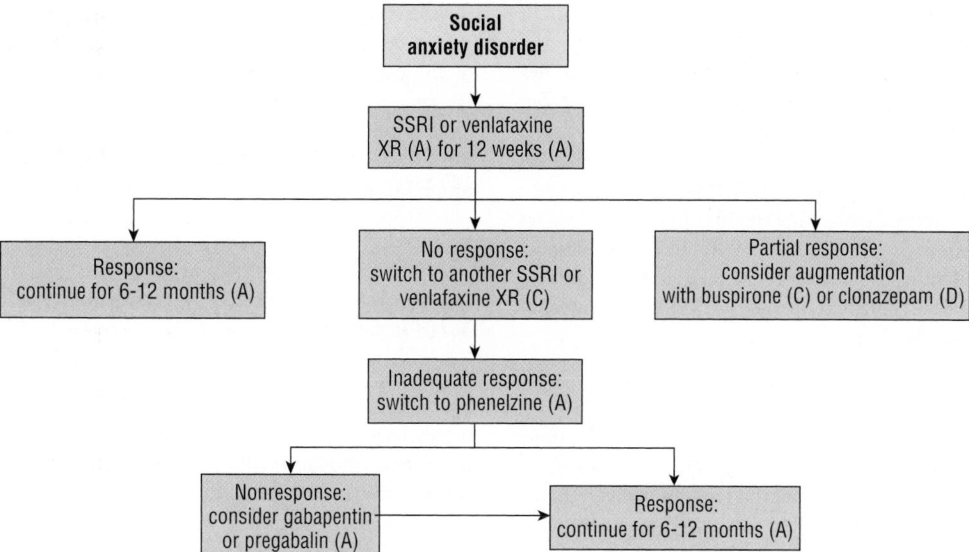

FIGURE 70-3 Algorithm for the pharmacotherapy of social anxiety disorder. Strength of recommendations: A, directly based on category I evidence (ie, meta-analysis of randomized controlled trials [RCT] or at least one RCT); B, directly based on category II evidence (ie, at least one controlled study without randomization or one other type of quasi-experimental study); C, directly based on category III evidence (ie, nonexperimental descriptive studies); D, directly based on category IV evidence (ie, expert committee reports or opinions and/or clinical experience of respected authorities); (SSRI, selective serotonin reuptake inhibitor). *(Adapted from references 2, 4, 22, and 60.)*

In these five trials, venlafaxine extended-release was significantly more effective than placebo on change from baseline to end point on the LSAS total score.[32]

Adverse Effects Adverse effects included anorexia, dry mouth, nausea, insomnia, and sexual dysfunction (see Table 70-6).

Dosing and Administration Additional therapeutic benefits of venlafaxine extended-release above 75 mg/day were not shown.[32] Venlafaxine should be tapered slowly (ie, decreasing by 37.5 mg/mo) to decrease the risk of relapse during discontinuation.

Alternative Agents

Benzodiazepines Benzodiazepines are commonly used in the treatment of patients who cannot tolerate or fail to respond to antidepressants. They are not considered first-line therapy for SAD because of concerns over the adverse effects, potential for dependence, the possibility of rebound anxiety, and ineffectiveness in the treatment of depression. Clonazepam is the most extensively studied benzodiazepine for the treatment of generalized SAD.[19,60-63]

If clonazepam is prescribed, the acute phase of therapy is about 1 month. Patients should be instructed not to decrease or discontinue clonazepam without consulting their clinician because of the risks of rebound anxiety and withdrawal symptoms. Clonazepam should be gradually tapered at a rate not to exceed 0.25 mg every 2 weeks.

Anticonvulsants Gabapentin and pregabalin were effective in controlled trials, whereas levetiracetam was ineffective.[60-64]

β-Blockers β-Blockers decrease the perception of anxiety by blunting the peripheral autonomic symptoms of arousal (eg, rapid heart rate, sweating, blushing, and tremor), and they are often used to decrease anxiety in performance-related situations.[60] For patients with performance anxiety, 10 to 80 mg of propranolol or 25 to 100 mg of atenolol can be taken 1 hour before a performance as needed. A test dose should be taken at home before the presentation to assure that β-blockade is sufficient and there are no adverse events. Controlled trials with β-blockers do not support daily use in SAD.[19]

Treatment Resistance

9 An adequate antidepressant trial usually consists of 8 to 12 weeks (at maximum dosages).[19,60-63] Subsequent options include a trial of a second SSRI or venlafaxine extended-release. Some patients experience clinical benefit during the first 4 weeks of therapy.[19,60-63] If nonresponsiveness continues, a trial of an alternative agent is warranted.

There are little data on the choice of treatments if there is a partial response to antidepressants therapy. Published studies offer preliminary support for the combination of an SSRI with a benzodiazepine, gabapentin, or pregabalin.[19,60-63]

Atypical antipsychotics and MAOIs are options in treatment-resistant SAD. Quetiapine monotherapy showed a large effect size on the Social Phobia Inventory when compared with placebo.[19,60-63] Although phenelzine is effective in 77% of patients with SAD,[2,19] dietary restrictions, potential drug interactions, and adverse effects (eg, weight gain and hypertensive crisis) have limited its use. If a patient is switched from another antidepressant to phenelzine, an appropriate washout period should be followed.

Special Populations

SAD can present in children of preschool to elementary school age. If the disorder is not treated, it can persist into adulthood and increase the risk of depression and substance abuse. CBT and social skills training are effective nonpharmacologic therapies in children.[19,60-63] Placebo-controlled and open-label trials have provided evidence of efficacy of pharmacotherapy with an SSRI or SNRI in children between ages 6 and 17 years.[2,19,60-63] Children and adolescents prescribed an SSRI or SNRI for social anxiety (or for other purposes) should be closely monitored for increased risk of suicidal ideation. Headache, nausea, drowsiness, insomnia, jitteriness, and stomachaches were reported in children receiving antidepressants.[19,60-63]

Benzodiazepines should be reserved as the last-line agents in children with SAD.[19,52] If prescribed, they should be used for the shortest time period possible. The adverse effects of benzodiazepines in children include drowsiness, oppositional behavior, disinhibition, and fatigue.

Approximately one-fifth of patients with SAD also suffer from an alcohol use disorder. Many people with SAD report that they use alcohol to cope with anxiety. Paroxetine significantly reduced social anxiety and the frequency and severity of alcohol use in patients with SAD and an alcohol use disorder.[65] MAOIs and benzodiazepines are not appropriate therapy for patients with SAD and alcohol use disorder. SSRIs are the drugs of choice.

Personalized Pharmacotherapy

Despite the availability of effective treatments for social anxiety, most adults in the United States with social anxiety do not receive mental healthcare for their symptoms. Often the symptoms that patients desire to relieve interfere with the ability to seek treatment. Patients often feel embarrassed of what others might think or say about them. It is important to develop an alliance with the patient and offer reassurance throughout the treatment process.

Certain complications may influence the choice of first-line pharmacotherapy. Comorbid depression or suicidal ideation requires careful evaluation and close monitoring. Patients with comorbid substance abuse on presentation may require postponing pharmacotherapy until after detoxification and avoidance of use of benzodiazepines as part of treatment.

Patient-specific education about treatment is important. Patients should be instructed about the gradual onset of effect, when to expect full therapeutic benefit, and that long-term therapy is required. When drug therapy is discontinued, the dosage needs to be gradually decreased over several months, and the patient should be seen more frequently to monitor for signs and symptoms of relapse or withdrawal.

It is important to remember that although pharmacotherapy usually leads to improvement in social and occupational functioning, most patients do not achieve a full remission. Many patients require additional treatment, often in the form of CBT.

There is little evidence available to predict response to pharmacotherapy for social anxiety. Variation in a functional polymorphism known to influence 5-HT reuptake is associated with SSRI response in patients with generalized SAD. In a trial that evaluated whether variation in the 5-HT transporter gene promoter (5HTTLPR) influences the efficacy of SSRIs, a trend was seen for a linear association between 5HTTLPR genotype and likelihood of response to SSRI.[66] Reduction in social anxiety symptoms during SSRI treatment was significantly associated with 5HTTLPR genotype using either the diallelic or triallelic classification.[66]

Evaluation of Therapeutic Outcomes

10 The pharmacotherapy of SAD can be monitored in three principal domains: SAD symptoms (eg, fears and physical symptoms), functionality, and well-being or overall improvement.[25,26,63] Response to pharmacotherapy in SAD is defined as a stable, clinically meaningful improvement; patients no longer have the full range of symptoms but typically continue to experience more than minimal symptoms.[25,26,63]

During the acute phase of treatment, patients should be seen weekly while the drug dosage is titrated. Once the patient responds and the dosage is stabilized, the patient can be seen monthly. Many patients report improvement during the first 4 weeks of therapy, but more than one-quarter of those who do not have a response at week 8 may have a response at 12 weeks. At each visit, the patient should be asked about adverse effects and improvement in symptoms. The patient should be instructed to keep a diary to record fear levels, physical symptoms, cognitions, and anxious behaviors in actual exposures to social situations. The LSAS is a clinician-rated scale of clinical severity and change in SAD for monitoring response.[29] Patients can use the Social Phobia Inventory for self-assessment of SAD symptoms.[29] Full remission is a complete resolution of symptoms across the three SAD domains that is maintained for 3 months or a LSAS score of less than or equal to 30 points.[29]

TREATMENT
Specific Phobia

Specific phobia is considered unresponsive to drug therapy, although highly responsive to CBT. The use of benzodiazepines or paroxetine in patients who failed CBT is supported by limited data. Benzodiazepines can be detrimental in patients with specific phobias treated with CBT.[22]

CONCLUSION

Anxiety disorders are common in the population and occur concurrently with other psychiatric disorders. The proper management of anxiety disorders begins with the correct diagnosis; not all patients should receive antianxiety agents. Nonpharmacologic interventions often are effective alone or when combined with drug therapy.

There are several subtypes of anxiety disorders, and the diagnosis determines the type of drug and nonpharmacologic intervention selected. Although benzodiazepines remain the drugs of choice for situational anxiety, antidepressants have emerged as first-line therapy for GAD, panic disorder, and SAD. Benzodiazepines are reserved for use in situations requiring immediate anxiety relief during the first 2 to 4 weeks of therapy with a long-term agent such as an antidepressant. Antidepressants, including the SSRIs and SNRIs, and the benzodiazepines clonazepam and alprazolam are used extensively in patients with GAD, panic disorder, and SAD.

The long-term goal of therapy for GAD, panic disorder, and SAD is remission of core anxiety symptoms with no impairment in functionality, minimal anxiety, and no depressive symptoms. Augmentation with anticonvulsants and atypical antipsychotics show some promise in treatment-resistant cases.

ABBREVIATIONS

ACC	anterior cingulate cortex
CBT	cognitive behavioral therapy
CNS	central nervous system
CRF	corticotropin-releasing factor
DA	dopamine
DMDZ	desmethyldiazepam
GABA	γ-aminobutyric acid
GAD	generalized anxiety disorder
GI	gastrointestinal
5-HT	serotonin
LC	locus ceruleus
LSAS	Liebowitz Social Anxiety Scale
MAOI	monoamine oxidase inhibitor
NE	norepinephrine
PAG	periaqueductal gray
QOL	quality of life
SAD	social anxiety disorder
SERT	serotonin reuptake transporter
SNRI	serotonin–norepinephrine reuptake inhibitor
SSRI	selective serotonin reuptake inhibitor
TCA	tricyclic antidepressant

REFERENCES

1. American Psychiatric Association. *Diagnostic and Statistical Manual of Mental Disorders*, Fifth Edition. Washington, DC: American Psychiatric Association, 2013:189-233.
2. Katzman MA, Bleau P, Blier P, et al. Canadian clinical practice guidelines for the management of anxiety, posttraumatic stress and obsessive-compulsive disorders. *BMC Psychiatry* 2014;14(Suppl 1):S1.
3. Craske MG, Roy-Byrne PP, Stein MB, et al. Treatment for anxiety disorders: Efficacy to effectiveness to implementation. *Behav Res Ther* 2009;47(11):931-937.
4. Bandelow B, Sher L, Bunevicius R, et al. Guidelines for the pharmacological treatment of anxiety disorders, obsessive-compulsive disorder and posttraumatic stress disorder in primary care. *Int J Psychiatry Clin Pract* 2012;16:77-84.
5. Roy-Byrne P. Treatment-refractory anxiety; definition, risk factors, and treatment challenges. *Dialogues Clin Neurosci* 2015;17(2):191-206.
6. Bandelow B, Michaelis S. Epidemiology of anxiety disorders in the 21st century. *Dialogues Clin Neurosci* 2015;17(3):327-335.
7. Brandish EK, Baldwin DS. Anxiety disorders. *Medicine* 2012;40(11): 599-606.
8. Niles AN, Dour H, Stanton AL, et al. Anxiety and depressive symptoms and medical illness among adults with anxiety disorders. *Psychosom Res* 2015;78(2):109-115.
9. Smoller JW, Block SR, Young MM. Genetics of anxiety disorders: The complex road from DSM to DNA. *Depress Anxiety* 2009;26(11):965-975.
10. Martin EI, Ressler KJ, Binder E, et al. The neurobiology of anxiety disorders: Brain imaging, genetics, and psychoneuroendocrinology. *Psychiatr Clin North Am* 2009;32:549-575.
11. Damsa C, Losel M, Moussally J. Current status of brain imaging in anxiety disorders. *Curr Opin Psychiatry* 2009;22(1):96-110.
12. Nuss P. Anxiety disorders and GABA neurotransmission: a disturbance of modulation. *Neuropsychiatr Dis Treat* 2015;11:165-175.
13. Uusi-Oukari M, Korpi ER. Regulation of $GABA_A$ receptor subunit expression by pharmacological agents. *Pharmacol Rev* 2010;62(1):97-135.
14. Akimova E, Lanzenberger R, Kasper S. The serotonin-1A receptor in anxiety disorders. *Biol Psychiatry* 2009;66(7):627-635.
15. Warwick JM, Carey PD, Cassimjee N, et al. Dopamine transporter binding in social anxiety disorder: the effect of treatment with escitalopram. *Metab Brain Dis* 2012;27(2):151-158.
16. Stein MB. Neurobiology of generalized anxiety disorder. *J Clin Psychiatry* 2009;70(Suppl 2):15-19.
17. Freitas-Ferrari MC, Hallak JE, Trzesniak C, et al. Neuroimaging in social anxiety disorder: A systematic review of the literature. *Prog Neuropsychopharmacol Biol Psychiatry* 2010;34(4):565-580.
18. Davidson JR, Zhang W, Connor KM, et al. A psychopharmacological treatment algorithm for generalized anxiety disorder (GAD). *J Psychopharm* 2010;24(1):3-26.
19. National Institute for Health and Care Excellence: Guidance. Social anxiety disorder: recognition, assessment and treatment. NICE Clinical Guideline 159. May 2013. Available at: http://www.nice.org.uk/guidance/cg159. Accessed December 22, 2015.
20. American Psychiatric Association. Practice guideline for the treatment of patients with panic disorder. Arlington, VA: American Psychiatric Association, 2009. Available at: http://www.psychiatryonline.com/pracGuide/pracGuideTopic_9.aspx. Accessed December 22, 2015.
21. National Institute for Health and Care Excellence. Generalised anxiety disorder and panic disorder (with or without agoraphobia) in adults. Management in primary, secondary, and community care. NICE Clinical Guideline 113. January 2011. Available at: http://www.nice.org.uk/guidance/cg113. Accessed December 22, 2015.
22. Baldwin DS, Anderson IM, Nutt DJ, et al. Evidence-based pharmacological treatment of anxiety disorders, post-traumatic stress disorder and obsessive-compulsive disorder: A revision of the 2005 guidelines from the British Association for Pharmacology. *J Psychopharmacol* 2014;28(5):403-439.
23. Katzman MA. Current considerations in the treatment of generalized anxiety disorder. *CNS Drugs* 2009;23(2):103-120.
24. Lydiard RB, Rickels K, Herman B, et al. Comparative efficacy of pregabalin and benzodiazepines in treating the psychic and somatic symptoms of generalized anxiety disorder. *Int J Neuropsychopharmacol* 2010;13:229-241.
25. Bostwick JR, Cusher MI, Yasugi S. Benzodiazepines: A versatile clinical tool. *Current Psychiatry* 2012;11(4):55-64.
26. PL Detail-Document, Benzodiazepine Toolbox. Pharmacist's Letter/Prescriber's Letter. August 2014.
27. Benzodiazepines. Facts and Comparisons® eAnswers (Online). Wolters Kluwer Health Inc., 2015. Available at: http://www.wolterskluwercdi.com/facts-comparisons-online/. Accessed December 22, 2015.
28. Hershenberg R, Gros DF, Brawman-Mintzer O. Role of atypical antipsychotics in the treatment of generalized anxiety disorder. *CNS Drugs* 2014;28(6):519-533.
29. Cymbalta [package insert]. Indianapolis, IN: Eli Lily and Company, June 2015.
30. Lexapro [package insert]. St. Louis, MO: Forest Pharmaceuticals Inc, June 2014.
31. Paxil [package insert]. Research Triangle Park, NC: GlaxoSmithKline, June 2014.
32. Effexor XR [package insert]. Philadelphia, PA: Wyeth Pharmaceuticals Inc, a subsidiary of Pfizer Inc., February 2015.
33. Gommoll C, Forero G, Mathews M, et al. Vilazodone in patients with generalized anxiety disorder: a double-blind, randomized, placebo-controlled, flexible-dose study. *Int Clin Psychopharmacol* 2015;30(6):297-306.
34. Pae CU, Wang SM, Han C, et al. Vortioxetine, a multimodal antidepressant for generalized anxiety disorder: A systematic review and meta-analysis. *J Psychiatr Res* 2015;64:88-98.
35. Vistaril [package insert]. New York: Pfizer Labs, May 2014.
36. The International Psychopharmacology Algorithm Project. IPAP—Generalized Anxiety Disorder Algorithm. http://www.ipap.org/gad/index.php, accessed December 22, 2015.
37. Sarris J, Moylan S, Camfield DA, et al. Complementary medicine, exercise, meditation, diet, and lifestyle modification for anxiety disorders: A review of current evidence. *Evid Based Complement Alternat Med* 2012;2012:809653.
38. Zoberti K, Pollard CA. Treating anxiety without SSRIs. *J Fam Pract* 2010;59(3):148-154.
39. Baldwin D, Woods R, Lawson R, Taylor D. Efficacy of drug treatments for generalized anxiety disorder: Systematic review and meta-analysis. *BMJ* 2011;342:d1199.
40. David DJ, Samuels BA, Rainer Q, et al. Neurogenesis-dependent and -independent effects of fluoxetine in an animal model of anxiety/depression. *Neuron* 2009;62(4):479-493.
41. Klonopin [package insert]. San Francisco, CA: Genentech, December 2013.
42. Xanax XR [package insert]. New York, NY: Pharmacia and Upjohn Company Inc, September 2013.
43. Möhler H. GABA (A) receptor diversity and pharmacology. *Cell Tissue Res* 2006;326:505-516.
44. Labbate LA, Fava M, Rosenbaum JF, Arana GW. *Handbook of Psychiatric Therapy*, 6th ed. Philadelphia, PA: Lippincott Williams & Wilkins, 2010:163-192.
45. Lader M. Benzodiazepines revisited—Will we ever learn? *Addiction* 2011;106:2086-2109.
46. Lader M. Benzodiazepine harm: how can it be reduced? *Br J Clin Pharmacol* 2014;77(2):295-301.
47. Lader M, Tylee A, Donoghue J. Withdrawing benzodiazepines in primary care. *CNS Drugs* 2009;23(1):19-34.
48. Hadley SJ, Mandel F, Schweitzer E. Switching from long-term benzodiazepine therapy to pregabalin in patients with generalized anxiety disorder: A double-blind, placebo-controlled trial. *J Psychopharmacol* 2012;26:461-470.
49. Canadian Agency for Drugs and Technologies in Health. Discontinuation strategies for patients with long-term benzodiazepine use: A review of clinical evidence and guidelines. Ottawa (ON): July 2015. Available at: http://www.ncbi.nlm.nih.gov/pubmedhealth/PMH0078914/pdf/PubMedHealth_PMH0078914.pdf. Accessed December 22, 2015.
50. Oyebode F, Rastogi A, Berrisford G, et al. Psychotropics in pregnancy: Safety and other considerations. *Pharmacocol Ther* 2012;135(1):71-77.
51. Bellantuono C, Tofani S, Di Sciascio G, Santone G. Benzodiazepine exposure in pregnancy and risk of major malformations: A critical overview. *Gen Hosp Psychiatry* 2013;35:3-8.
52. Wehry AW, Beesdo-Baum K, Hennelly MM, et al. Assessment and treatment of anxiety disorders in children and adolescents. *Curr Psychiatry Rep* 2015;17(7):52. doi:10.1007/s11920-015-0591-z.
53. Carter NJ, McCormack PL. Duloxetine: A review of its use in the treatment of generalized anxiety disorder. *CNS Drugs* 2009;23(6): 523-541.
54. Mokhber N, Azarpazhooh MR, Khajehdaluee M, et al. Randomized, single-blind, trial of sertraline and buspirone for treatment of elderly patients with generalized anxiety disorder. *Psychiatry Clin Neurosci* 2010;64(2):128-133.

55. Karaiskos D, Pappa D, Tzavellas E, et al. Pregabalin augmentation of antidepressants in older patients with comorbid depression and generalized anxiety disorder-an open-label study. *Int J Geriatr Psychiatry* 2013;28(1):100-105.
56. Andrisano C, Chiesa A, Serretti A. Newer antidepressants and panic disorder: A meta-analysis. *Int Clin Psychopharmacol* 2012;28:33-45.
57. Bandelow B, Baldwin DS, Zwanzger P. Pharmacological treatment of panic disorder. *Mod Trends Pharmacopsychiatry* 2013;29:128-143.
58. Billioti de Gage S, Moride Y, Ducruet T, et al. Benzodiazepine use and risk of Alzheimer's disease: case-control study. *BMJ* 2014;349:g5205.
59. PharmGKB: The Pharmacogenomic Database. Available at: http://www.pharmgkb.org/index.jsp. Accessed December 22, 2015.
60. Blanco C, Bragdon LB, Schneier FR, et al. The evidence-based pharmacotherapy of social anxiety disorder. *Int J Neuropsychopharmacol* 2013;16(1):235-249.
61. Jörstad-Stein EC, Heimberg RG. Social phobia: An update on treatment. *Psychiatr Clin North Am* 2009;32(3):641-663.
62. Canton J, Scott KM, Glue P. Optimal treatment of social phobia: Review and meta-analysis. *Neuropsychiatr Dis Treat* 2012;8:203-215.
63. Dalrymple KL. Issues and controversies surrounding the diagnosis and treatment of social anxiety disorder. *Expert Rev Neurother* 2012;2(8):993-1008.
64. Kawalec P, Cierniak A, Pilc A, et al. Pregabalin for the treatment of social anxiety disorder. *Expert Opin Investig Drugs* 2015;24(4):585-594.
65. Ipser JC, Wilson D, Akindipe TO, et al. Pharmacotherapy for anxiety and comorbid alcohol use disorders. *Cochrane Database Syst Rev* 2015 Jan 20;1:CD007505.
66. Klumpp H, Fitzgerald DA, Cook E, et al. Serotonin transporter gene alters insula activity to threat in social anxiety disorder. *Neuroreport* 2014;25(12):926-931.

Posttraumatic Stress Disorder and Obsessive-Compulsive Disorder

71

Cynthia K. Kirkwood, Sarah T. Melton, and Barbara G. Wells

KEY CONCEPTS

1. The short-term goal in posttraumatic stress disorder (PTSD) is reduction in core symptoms, while the long-term goal is remission.
2. Cognitive behavioral therapy and eye movement desensitization and reprocessing are the most effective nonpharmacologic methods to reduce symptoms of PTSD.
3. The selective serotonin reuptake inhibitors (SSRIs) and venlafaxine are considered first-line treatments for PTSD.
4. An adequate trial of SSRIs in PTSD requires appropriate dosing and duration of treatment.
5. Patients with PTSD who respond to pharmacotherapy should continue treatment for at least 12 months.
6. SSRIs are the drugs of choice for the treatment of obsessive-compulsive disorder (OCD).
7. Augmentation of SSRI treatment of OCD with low doses of antipsychotics may be helpful.
8. If an inadequate response to an SSRI for OCD occurs after 4 to 6 weeks at the maximum dose, switch to another SSRI.
9. Medication taper can be considered after 1 to 2 years of treatment in patients with OCD.

Traumatic or stressful events (eg, wars, terrorist attacks, torture, natural disasters, robbery, physical assault) can lead to development of posttraumatic stress disorder (PTSD). Initially diagnosed in veterans of war, PTSD is now acknowledged as a significant psychiatric illness in the civilian population and among deployed service personnel of the Afghanistan and Iraq campaigns in whom the suicide rate has escalated.[1,2] PTSD continues to be poorly recognized and diagnosed in clinical practice.[3,4] Because of its co-occurrence with anxiety disorders, depression, substance abuse, and traumatic brain injury, the overlapping symptoms can lead to diagnostic uncertainty. Advances in the science and treatment of PTSD can assist clinicians in all fields of healthcare to screen patients for a history of trauma and effectively manage PTSD if it is present.

Intrusive obsessive thoughts and compulsive ritualistic behaviors characterize obsessive-compulsive disorder (OCD). OCD can be severely debilitating and impair functioning in social, family, and work settings, with an overall decrease in quality of life (QOL). OCD is associated with an increased risk of suicide, with 15% of patients reporting a previous history of suicide attempt.[5] Increased understanding of symptom dimensions and treatment response can improve QOL in patients suffering from OCD.

EPIDEMIOLOGY

The estimated lifetime prevalence of PTSD is 8.7% in the US population.[1] Lifetime prevalence of OCD has been estimated at 2.3% in the general population.[6]

PTSD is associated with the incidence of trauma. It is estimated that approximately 60% of men and 50% of women are exposed to a life-threatening traumatic event.[7] Of these individuals 8.2% of men and 20% of women will develop PTSD. Previous exposure to a trauma and the intensity of response to the event increase the risk of PTSD. Men tend to be assaulted more frequently, but women are more likely to experience rape and sexual abuse.[7] Genetic factors can increase vulnerability to PTSD if an individual is exposed to a traumatic event. Veterans and those whose jobs increase the risk of traumatic exposure (eg, firefighters, police) have higher rates of PTSD.[1]

The epidemiology of OCD is influenced by age and gender. OCD typically begins early in life, with 25% of cases occurring by age 14.[1] Age of onset has a bimodal distribution with peaks around 10 and 21 years.[8] The onset of illness is earlier in men than in women.[6] Early age of onset has been associated with higher probabilities of comorbid anxiety disorders, oppositional defiant disorder, attention-deficit/hyperactivity disorder, and tic disorders.[9] Heredity is stronger when there is an early age of onset or comorbidity with tic disorder.[10]

ETIOLOGY

The exact etiologies of PTSD and OCD are not known. It is likely that abnormalities in several areas of brain functioning interact to cause these chronic disorders. Genetics may play a role in expression of PTSD and OCD, but environmental factors likely are also involved. A number of genetic markers for PTSD are under evaluation, including genes associated with the hypothalamic-pituitary adrenal axis and the serotonin transporter.[11,12] A genome-wide association study did not detect any single nucleotide polymorphisms (SNPs) associated with OCD, but there was a significant enrichment of methylation quantitative trait loci (mQTLs) and frontal lobe expression of quantitative trait loci (eQTLs) in the highest ranked autosomal SNPs, suggesting that these signals may influence gene expression and perhaps the etiology of OCD.[10] Genetic etiologies of both PTSD and OCD are current research areas.

Controversy exists over the existence of a subtype of OCD characterized as a pediatric autoimmune neuropsychiatric disorder associated with streptococcal infections (PANDAS). A relationship between the sudden onset of OCD and chronic tic disorder with an age of onset between 3 years and puberty with possible exacerbations and remissions, and a temporal association with streptococcal infection associated with symptoms of OCD or neurologic abnormalities has been proposed.[13] Although most patients with OCD do not have a streptococcal etiology, an accurate medical history regarding onset of illness is imperative because specific treatment strategies are indicated.

PATHOPHYSIOLOGY

Research findings in the areas of neuroendocrinology, neurobiology, and neuroimaging have advanced a number of theories on the pathophysiology of anxiety disorders, OCD, and PTSD. Neuroendocrine changes in the hypothalamic–pituitary–adrenal (HPA) axis are implicated in the pathophysiology of PTSD.[14] As reviewed in Chapter 70, data from neurochemical and neuroimaging studies indicate that the modulation of normal and pathologic anxiety states is associated with multiple regions of the brain (eg, amygdala, hippocampus, thalamus, and prefrontal cortex).[14,15] Abnormal function in several neurotransmitter systems, including norepinephrine (NE), γ-aminobutyric acid (GABA), glutamate, dopamine (DA), and serotonin (5-HT), may affect the manifestations of anxiety disorders, OCD and PTSD.[14,16]

Neuroendocrine Theories

Neuroendocrine studies provide data that abnormalities occurring pretrauma, during trauma, and posttrauma contribute to PTSD. Normally the immediate reaction to stress occurs as an automatic response from the amygdala to the sympathetic and parasympathetic systems and the HPA axis.[14] The release of corticotropin-releasing factor (CRF) stimulates cortisol secretion from the adrenal gland. Both catecholamines and cortisol levels rise in tandem. Cortisol reduces the stress response by tempering the sympathetic reaction through negative feedback on the pituitary and hypothalamus.[14] These systems return to normal after a few hours.

Recent data implicate a role for the neuropeptides CRF and neuropeptide Y (NPY) in PTSD. Patients with PTSD have a hypersecretion of CRF but demonstrate subnormal levels of cortisol at the time of trauma and chronically.[14] Lower plasma cortisol concentrations were associated with greater severity of PTSD symptoms in nonmilitary patients.[16] Dysregulation of the HPA axis is postulated to be a risk factor for eventual development of PTSD.[14] Higher plasma concentrations of NPY were found in combat-exposed men who did not develop PTSD and could play a role in resiliency.[16]

Neurochemical Theories

Several neurotransmitters may be involved in the pathophysiology of PTSD. 5-HT, NE, and glutamate are associated with the processing of emotional and somatic contents of memories in the amygdala. The cortex and hippocampus are involved in storing the facts and related cues of memory.[16] The noradrenergic theory posits that the autonomic nervous system of anxious patients is hypersensitive and overreacts to stimuli. The alarm center, the locus ceruleus, releases NE to stimulate the sympathetic and parasympathetic nervous systems. Hyperactive noradrenergic signaling in patients with PTSD is a consistent research finding and includes increased 24-hour catecholamine excretion.[16] Glutamate signaling abnormalities may result in distortion of amygdala-dependent emotional processing under stress.[14,16] Dysregulation of the processing of sensory input and memories may contribute to the dissociative and hypervigilant symptoms in PTSD. Abnormalities of GABA inhibition may lead to increased awareness or response to stress, as seen in PTSD.[16]

Both 5-HT and DA are implicated in the pathogenesis of OCD. Selective and potent serotonergic reuptake inhibitors have consistently been shown effective for symptoms of the illness.[17] A recent meta-analysis concluded that higher doses of selective serotonin reuptake inhibitors (SSRIs) were associated with improved efficacy in the treatment of OCD.[17] DA dysregulation may contribute to some forms of OCD. Neurologic symptoms (eg, tics) are part of the clinical presentation in some patients with OCD. Tourette's disorder, a disorder of DA function, is often a concurrent disease.[1] Augmentation with antipsychotic drugs may improve symptoms in patients with OCD who are partially responsive to SSRIs.[18]

Neuroimaging Studies

Neuroimaging studies suggest that certain areas of the brain are altered by psychological trauma. In PTSD most functional neuroimaging studies have involved the amygdala, ventromedial prefrontal cortex (vmPFC), dorsal anterior cingulate cortex (dACC), and hippocampus. Findings of increased activation of the amygdala after trauma-related imagery, sounds, or smells indicate that this structure plays a role in the persistence of traumatic memory.[15] Decreased amygdala activation is correlated with resilience to PTSD and response to cognitive behavioral therapy (CBT).[15] Hypofunctioning of the vmPFC is theorized to prevent extinction in patients with PTSD and is inversely correlated with severity of symptoms.[15] Hyperresponsivity of the dACC and the insular cortex may correlate with impaired response to emotional stimuli or those that predict threat. The most consistent findings are decreased hippocampus volumes and *N*-acetylaspartate levels in patients with PTSD.[14,15] In twin studies, the unaffected twin of patients with PTSD also demonstrated smaller hippocampi compared with twins without PTSD. These findings suggest that lower hippocampal volumes in patients with PTSD are likely a precursor associated with vulnerability for subsequent development of PTSD.[14]

Neuroimaging studies suggest that dysfunction in the cortical–striatal–thalamic circuits is responsible for impulsive behavior and inability to regulate socially acceptable behaviors.[19] Drugs that decrease hyperactivity in the cortical–striatal–thalamic circuits decrease symptoms of OCD.[10] Glutamate may play a role in OCD symptomatology.[20]

CLINICAL PRESENTATION

The *Diagnostic and Statistical Manual of Mental Disorders, Fifth Edition* (DSM-5) made several changes to the classification of anxiety and related disorders.[1] There are now individual chapters for anxiety disorders, trauma- and stress-related disorders, and obsessive-compulsive and related disorders. The movement of PTSD and acute stress disorder (ASD) from the DSM-5 anxiety disorders chapter was based on evidence that anxiety is just one of several reactions to trauma or other adverse events.[1] The DSM-5 OCD and related disorders chapter also includes hoarding disorder and trichotillomania (hair-pulling disorder). Generalized anxiety disorder, panic disorder, and social anxiety disorder are discussed in Chapter 70.

Posttraumatic Stress Disorder

Exposure to a traumatic event is required for a diagnosis of PTSD.[1] The person must have witnessed, experienced, or been confronted with a situation that involved definite or threatened death or serious injury, sexual violence, or possible harm to self or others.[1] Some examples of traumatic events include physical attacks by an intimate partner, severe traffic accidents, military combat, earthquakes, being held hostage, child sexual abuse, witnessing a murder or injury of another, and learning of a traumatic event that happened to a close family member or friend.

The resulting PTSD symptoms include persistent reexperiencing of the traumatic event, avoidance of stimuli associated with the trauma, numbing of general responsiveness, and persistent symptoms of hyperarousal. Patients must have at least one intrusion symptom, at least one symptom of avoidance of stimuli associated with the trauma, at least two symptoms of negative alterations in cognition and mood, and at least two symptoms of increased arousal.[1] Symptoms from each category need to be present for longer than 1 month and cause significant distress or impairment in functioning. Most persons diagnosed with PTSD also meet criteria for another mental disorder.[1,21]

Anxiety and dissociative symptoms (eg, absence of emotional responsiveness, derealization, inability to recall important features of the trauma) emerging within 1 month after exposure to a traumatic stressor are classified as ASD. Symptoms of ASD are experienced during or immediately after the trauma, last for at least 3 days, and resolve within 1 month.[1]

CLINICAL PRESENTATION Posttraumatic Stress Disorder

Intrusion Symptoms

- Recurrent, intrusive distressing memories of the trauma
- Recurrent, disturbing dreams of the event
- Feeling that the traumatic event is recurring (eg, dissociative flashbacks)
- Physiologic reaction to or psychological distress from reminders of the trauma

Avoidance Symptoms

- Avoidance of conversations, thoughts, or feelings about the trauma
- Avoidance of people, places, or activities that are reminders of the event

Persistent Negative Alterations in Thinking and Mood

- Inability to recall an important aspect of the trauma
- Anhedonia
- Estrangement from others
- Restricted affect
- Negative beliefs about oneself
- Distorted beliefs causing one to blame others or themselves for the trauma
- Negative mood state

Hyperarousal Symptoms

- Decreased concentration
- Easily startled
- Self-destructive behavior
- Hypervigilance
- Insomnia
- Irritability or anger outbursts

Specifiers

- Dissociative symptoms: depersonalization or derealization
- With delayed expression: full criteria are not met until at least 6 months posttrauma

Data from references 1 and 21.

The age of onset and course of PTSD are variable. PTSD can occur at any age. The presentation is not predictable, because symptoms are related to the duration and intensity of the trauma, the presence of other psychiatric disorders, and how the patient deals with the trauma. Symptoms emerge soon after a traumatic event and either dissipate or chronically persist in survivors.[22] About 95% of patients who recover do so within a year, and 40% have persistent symptoms 6 years later. PTSD co-occurs with mood, anxiety, and substance use disorders. The course of illness is fluctuating, worsening with life stressors.[22]

Obsessive-Compulsive Disorder

Patients with OCD exhibit a great variety of symptoms on presentation to clinicians. The diversity and oddity of symptoms that manifest can obscure accurate diagnosis and delay appropriate treatment of the disorder. Patients can be secretive about symptoms and purposefully refuse to report symptoms.[5] Patients can present in a seemingly incongruous manner to nonpsychiatrists for other complaints—dermatologists for eczema or chapped skin, pediatricians for parental concerns over a child's compulsive hand washing, neurologists for tics, or dentists for gum lesions from compulsive teeth brushing.

The diagnostic criteria for OCD require the presence of obsessions and/or compulsions (although most patients have both) that are severe enough to cause marked distress, to be time-consuming (occupy more than 1 h/day), or cause significant impairment in social or occupational functioning.[1] An obsession is a recurrent, persistent idea, thought, impulse, or image that is experienced as intrusive and inappropriate and produces marked anxiety. Common obsessions involve thoughts about contamination (eg, concern with germs or dirt) and repeated doubts.[1]

CLINICAL PRESENTATION Obssessive-Compulsive Disorder

Obsessions

- Repetitive thoughts (eg, feeling contaminated by germs, doubting whether the stove was turned off)
- Repetitive images (eg, recurrent sexually explicit pictures)
- Repetitive urges (eg, need for symmetry or putting things in specific order, impulse to shout out obscenities in a church)

Compulsions

- Repetitive activities (eg, hand washing, checking, arranging, need to ask, need to confess)
- Repetitive mental acts (eg, counting excessively, repeating words silently, praying)

Specifiers

- Insight
  - Good or fair insight
  - Poor insight
  - Absent insight/delusional beliefs
- Related to a tic disorder

Data from references 1 and 8.

A compulsion is defined as a repetitive behavior or mental act generally performed in response to an obsession. Diagnostically, compulsive behavior is not pleasurable and is designed to prevent discomfort or the occurrence of a dreaded event that is often unknown. For example, many patients are obsessed with feelings of doubt (eg, whether a window was left unlocked), causing them marked distress and leading to repetitive checking (or compulsive behaviors). These behaviors are usually performed according to certain rules or in a stereotyped fashion. Because patients recognize their compulsive behavior as silly or senseless, they become extremely adept at denying symptoms, disguising their rituals, and concealing their illness from friends and family.[1] Individuals vary widely in their insight into the irrationality of their obsessive-compulsive symptoms.

Patients with OCD often have concurrent depression, other anxiety disorders, and substance abuse. It is a chronic illness in most patients, with severity of symptoms varying in intensity over time. Many patients with OCD have significantly impaired QOL and ability to function.[5,23]

TREATMENT

Desired Outcomes

1 The short-term goal of therapy in the management of PTSD is reduction in core symptoms (ie, intrusive reexperiencing, avoidance, and hyperarousal). Patients should also have improvements in disability, concurrent psychiatric conditions, resilience, and QOL. The long-term goal in PTSD is remission.

General Approach to Treatment

In general, patients who seek treatment acutely after a trauma and are in intense distress should receive therapy based on their presenting symptoms (eg, a nonbenzodiazepine hypnotic for difficulty sleeping). Short courses of exposure-based, trauma-focused cognitive behavioral therapy (TFCBT) can be helpful to prevent chronic PTSD in patients with ASD or acute PTSD.[21] If symptoms (eg, hyperarousal, avoidance, dissociation, sleep difficulties, or depressed mood) persist for 3 to 4 weeks and the patient experiences marked social, occupational, and/or interpersonal impairment, they can be treated with pharmacotherapy, psychotherapy, or both. Many patients with PTSD will improve substantially with pharmacotherapy but retain some symptoms. Treatment regimens usually combine psychoeducation, psychosocial support and/or treatment, and pharmacotherapy.[21,22,24]

Nonpharmacologic Therapy

Psychotherapy can be used when a patient suffers from mild symptoms, in patients who prefer not to use medications, or in conjunction with drugs in patients with severe symptoms to improve response. Patients who have experienced trauma should be educated that they can experience anxiety, depression, nightmares, and even flashbacks as a reaction to the event. Brief courses of prolonged exposure, a form of CBT, in close proximity to the traumatic event resulted in lower rates of PTSD 3 and 6 months later.[4] Single-session critical incident stress debriefing was not shown to be effective in preventing development of PTSD and actually can cause harm.[21,24]

2 Psychotherapies for treating PTSD include stress management, TFCBT, eye movement desensitization and reprocessing (EMDR), and psychoeducation.[21] Short-term reductions in symptoms can be achieved with stress management, group therapy, hypnosis, or psychodynamic therapy.[21,24] The cognitive and behavioral approaches of TFCBT and EMDR are more effective than stress management or group therapy to reduce symptoms of PTSD.[21]

TABLE 71-1 Dosing of Antidepressants in the Treatment of PTSD

Drug	Brand Name	Initial Dose	Usual Range (mg/day)	Comments
SSRIs				
Fluoxetine[a]	Prozac®	10 mg/day	10-40[b]	
Paroxetine[a]	Paxil®, Pexeva®	10-20 mg/day	20-40	Maximum dose is 50 mg/day[c]
Sertraline[a]	Zoloft®	25 mg/day	50-100	Maximum dose is 200 mg/day[c]
Other Agents				
Amitriptyline[a]	Elavil®	25 or 50 mg/day	75-200[b]	
Imipramine[a]	Tofranil®	25 or 50 mg/day	75-200[b]	
Mirtazapine[a]	Remeron®	15 mg/night	30-60[b]	
Phenelzine[a]	Nardil®	15 or 30 mg every night	45-90[b]	
Venlafaxine extended-release[a]	Effexor XR®	37.5 mg/day	75-225[b]	

PTSD, posttraumatic stress disorder; SSRIs, selective serotonin reuptake inhibitors.

[a]Available generically.

[b]Dosage used in clinical trials but not FDA-approved.

[c]Dosage is FDA-approved.

Data from references 27, 29, and 30.

Psychoeducation includes information about the disease state, treatment options, and avoidance of excessive use of alcohol and other substances of abuse. Novel nonpharmacologic approaches (eg, interpersonal psychotherapy, narrative exposure therapy, imagery modification, transcranial magnetic stimulation) and delivery methods (eg, telemedicine, computer-delivered CBT) are under study.[25,26]

Pharmacologic Therapy

3 Antidepressants are the major pharmacotherapeutic treatment for PTSD. In addition to their efficacy in PTSD, these agents are also effective for concurrent depression and anxiety disorders. SSRIs and venlafaxine are the first-line pharmacotherapy of PTSD.[24,27,28] The tricyclic antidepressants (TCAs) and monoamine oxidase inhibitors (MAOIs) can also be effective, but they have less favorable side-effect profiles (Table 71-1). Both sertraline and paroxetine are approved for the acute treatment of PTSD,[29,30] and sertraline is approved for the long-term (ie, 52 weeks) management of PTSD.[30] A number of drugs can be used as augmentation agents (eg, antiadrenergic drugs and atypical antipsychotics).[27,28] Benzodiazepines are not effective for PTSD.[27,28] A number of treatment guidelines are published.[31] Table 71-2 provides a summary of key points from the treatment guidelines for PTSD. An algorithm for the treatment of PTSD appears in Fig. 71-1.

Antidepressant Therapy

Selective Serotonin Reuptake Inhibitors SSRIs act pharmacologically to enhance serotonergic functioning. Large prospective studies documented the efficacy of sertraline and paroxetine in the acute management of PTSD.[28] A recent meta-analysis found that SSRIs were significantly better than placebo, but the effect size was small.[32] Adverse reactions reported in patients with PTSD treated with SSRIs include gastrointestinal (GI) symptoms, sexual dysfunction, insomnia, and agitation. Long-term use of SSRIs (durations of 9-12 months) was effective in preventing relapse.[27]

TABLE 71-2 Summary of Key Points in Treatment Guidelines for PTSD

Recommendation	Level of Evidence	Comments
First-Line Treatments		
SSRIs: Fluoxetine, paroxetine, sertraline	I	At 4 weeks if there is partial response, continue for another 4 weeks. At 8 weeks, if no improvement, increase dose to maximum tolerated or switch to another first-line treatment
SNRIs: Venlafaxine	I	
Second-Line Treatments		
TCAs: Amitriptyline, imipramine	II	The risk of adverse effects and potential for fatalities in a TCA overdose are higher than with SSRIs or SNRIs
Other: Mirtazapine	II	
Augmentation with prazosin for sleep/nightmares	II[24]	Recommended in the VA guidelines[24]
Augmentation with risperidone	II[31]	The VA guidelines[24] recommend against using risperidone as an augmenting agent secondary to metabolic adverse effects. There is insufficient evidence to support use of other atypical antipsychotics
Third-Line treatments		
MAOIs: Phenelzine	IV[31]	The VA guidelines[24] recommend phenelzine to be used cautiously (Level III)

PTSD, posttraumatic stress disorder; SNRIs, serotonin–norepinephrine reuptake inhibitors; SSRIs, selective serotonin reuptake inhibitors; TCA, tricyclic antidepressant; VA, Veterans Affairs.

Levels of evidence: I, strong recommendation, full evidence from controlled trials; II, recommended, limited positive evidence from controlled trials; III, may be recommended, evidence from uncontrolled trials or case reports/expert opinion; IV, evidence is insufficient to recommend, inconsistent findings.

Data from references 24 and 27.

Other Antidepressants The serotonin–norepinephrine reuptake inhibitor (SNRI) venlafaxine has shown efficacy in PTSD. In a 12-week, placebo-controlled trial comparing venlafaxine extended-release and sertraline, venlafaxine was effective in reducing the avoidance/numbing and hyperarousal clusters of PTSD, whereas sertraline improved all PTSD symptom clusters.[33] The remission rates for venlafaxine extended-release were 30.2% after 12 weeks[33] and 50.1% after 6 months.[34]

Other antidepressants have been studied in controlled trials. Mirtazapine was effective on global ratings of symptoms in 64% of patients with PTSD in doses up to 45 mg/day and is considered a second-line agent.[24,27] Bupropion sustained-release was not effective in patients with chronic PTSD.[21]

The TCAs amitriptyline and imipramine are also considered second-line agents, and the MAOI phenelzine is considered a third-line antidepressant if therapeutic trials of SSRIs or venlafaxine have failed. TCAs are associated with a higher burden of adverse effects compared with SSRIs (eg, daytime drowsiness, toxicity in overdose, and poor compliance).[24,27]

Alternative Drug Treatments

Atypical antipsychotics, α_1-adrenergic antagonists, antidepressants, mood stabilizers, and anticonvulsants can be used as augmenting agents for persistent symptoms, in cases of partial response to SSRI therapy after 4 to 6 weeks, or for comorbidities.[35] Data on the efficacy of atypical antipsychotics are conflicting. Overall there is a modest positive effect of risperidone and quetiapine in double-blind trials with intrusive and hypervigilance symptoms showing the most improvement.[36] A large, 6-month trial failed to show improvement in PTSD symptoms with the adjunctive use of risperidone to antidepressant therapy in military service personnel.[37]

Prazosin can be useful in some patients with PTSD. It decreased nightmares and sleep disturbances and improved the core PTSD symptoms in daily doses of 1 to 4 mg. Its presumed mechanism of action is reduction of noradrenergic transmission.[38,39] Other options for persistent sleep disturbances with less evidence include trazodone, mirtazapine, eszopiclone, and atypical antipsychotics.[39,40]

Anticonvulsants can assist in reducing impulsive anger and can also be used in patients with comorbid bipolar disorder. Some data support efficacy of lamotrigine as an augmenting agent. Data with other anticonvulsants are inconsistent.[35] The use of an anticonvulsant is not recommended as monotherapy.[24]

Special Populations

Children who experience stress and trauma (eg, sexual or physical abuse or loss of a parent) are predisposed to develop mood and anxiety disorders. SSRIs are the initial pharmacologic agents of choice in this patient population.[41] Psychotherapy is also a treatment option (eg, TFCBT).[42]

Dosage and Administration

Acute Phase PTSD symptoms respond slowly to pharmacotherapy, and some patients never experience full resolution. SSRIs should be started 3 to 4 weeks after exposure to a trauma in patients with no improvement in their acute stress response. The initiation of an SSRI should be at a low dose with gradual titration upward toward antidepressant doses. (4) Eight to 12 weeks is an appropriate duration of antidepressant therapy to determine response.[21,24,27,43]

Continuation Phase Many patients are undergoing psychotherapy during the continuation phase of therapy, and dosages can vary as patients deal with past traumatic experiences. During this phase, symptoms continue to improve. Six-month relapse prevention trials in patients responsive to fluoxetine or sertraline indicate low rates of relapse with SSRI therapy compared with placebo.[43]

Maintenance and Discontinuation (5) Patients with PTSD who respond to pharmacotherapy should continue treatment for at least 12 months.[21,27,43] If residual symptoms persist, drug therapy should be continued. The decision about when to discontinue therapy is based on response to therapy, presence of ongoing stresses, and adverse effects. The patient must be confident in the discontinuation plan and can require extra support throughout the process. Drug therapy should be withdrawn and tapered slowly over a period of at least 1 month to reduce the potential for relapse.

Personalized Pharmacotherapy

The choice of pharmacotherapy should be individualized to the patient's presenting symptoms. Selection of an SSRI or venlafaxine monotherapy is based on the patient's history of prior response, safety, and side-effect tolerability. When selecting an agent, the clinician should consider the potential for adverse consequences in patients with comorbid conditions (eg, anticholinergic effects and weight gain with paroxetine in patients with diabetes, obesity, or benign prostatic hypertrophy) or adverse effects (eg, insomnia with fluoxetine in patients with sleep difficulties). Increased risk of suicidality should be considered in patients taking antidepressants who are younger than 25 years. If symptoms of insomnia or nightmares continue, prazosin can be added to provide relief. Risperidone or

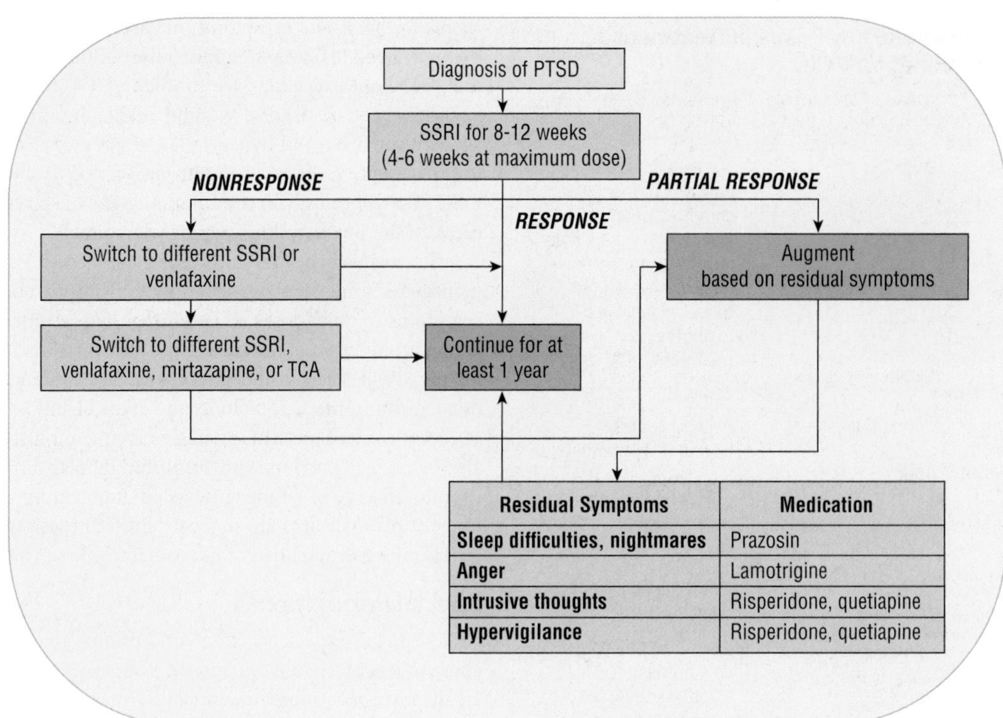

FIGURE 71-1 Algorithm for the pharmacotherapy of posttraumatic stress disorder (PTSD). *(Data from references 24 and 27.)*

quetiapine can be added for patients who fail to respond or have a partial response to antidepressant therapy.

Clinical **Controversy...**

When initiating treatment for PTSD it is unclear if pharmacotherapy should be initiated alone or in combination with psychotherapy. Currently there is insufficient evidence to guide clinicians.

Evaluation of Therapeutic Outcomes

During the acute phase of therapy, patients should be seen frequently. During months 3 to 6 of therapy, the patient can usually be seen monthly, and in months 6 to 12, visits can usually be extended to every 2 months. On each visit the patient should be asked about previously identified target symptoms of PTSD as well as other symptoms including insomnia, suicidal ideation, anger outbursts, irritability, psychosis, ongoing trauma, and disability. The Clinician-Administered PTSD Scale (CAPS) can be used by the clinician to assess symptom severity at visits.[24] A remission in patients with PTSD is defined as a 70% or greater reduction in symptoms. Patients who have a 50% response or greater reduction in symptoms are considered to have an adequate response, while those with a 25% to 50% reduction in symptoms are considered partial responders. Before deciding that a patient is not responsive to pharmacotherapy, the clinician should ensure that the medication trial has been adequate in both dose and duration.

Many patients with PTSD are sensitive to the adverse effects of drugs. They should be monitored carefully for adverse reactions that can delay the escalation of drug dosages or cause the patient distress. See Chapter 68 for details on monitoring antidepressants. Routine assessment of the metabolic profile is necessary if an atypical antipsychotic is used concurrently.[27] When pharmacotherapy is discontinued, patients should be seen more frequently and monitored carefully for signs of relapse or withdrawal.

TREATMENT

Desired Outcomes

Major goals of therapy for OCD include reduction in the frequency and severity of obsessive thoughts and time spent performing compulsive acts. Treatment for OCD generally does not completely eliminate obsessions or compulsions, but patients can feel remarkably improved with partial resolution of symptoms. Patients typically experience waxing and waning symptoms with only 20% achieving full remission.[44] Optimal treatment increases psychosocial and occupational functioning and improves overall QOL. Efforts should be made to minimize adverse drug events and prevent drug interactions.

General Approach to Treatment

It is important at the outset of therapy to identify and document the specific target symptoms for pharmacotherapy. Rating scales can be used to measure symptom severity at baseline and during treatment to ascertain the degree of improvement. The Yale-Brown Obsessive-Compulsive Scale (YBOCS) is the most widely used clinician-administered scale. A QOL scale can assist the clinician in identifying other areas to target for treatment (eg, depression and reduced physical well-being).[45,46]

The FDA has approved five antidepressants for the management of OCD: clomipramine, fluoxetine, fluvoxamine, paroxetine, and sertraline. CBT and SSRIs are considered effective first-line treatment modalities.[45,46] Initial therapy may include CBT alone, SSRI monotherapy, or the combination of CBT and an SSRI, and the choice is based on clinical judgment of symptom severity and patient preferences.[45] CBT alone can be used in cooperative patients who do not desire drug therapy or those with mild anxiety or depressive symptoms. Patients unable to participate in CBT or with a prior history of medication therapy response should be treated with SSRI monotherapy. Combined CBT and SSRIs is recommended in patients with failure on an SSRI alone or in those with severe OCD.

TABLE 71-3 Summary of Key Points in Treatment Guidelines for OCD

Recommendation	Level of Evidence	Comments
First-Line Treatments		
CBT alone	I	13-20 sessions
SSRI alone	I	8-12 weeks, at least 4-6 weeks at maximum tolerated dose
CBT + SSRI	I	13-20 CBT sessions and 8- to 12-week SSRI with 4-6 weeks at maximum tolerated dose If monotherapy with CBT or SSRI alone does not provide adequate response, combination therapy with CBT + SSRI should be tried before augmentation with another pharmacologic agent
Second-Line Treatments		
Switch to another SSRI or clomipramine	I	
Augmentation with antipsychotic	II	
Third-Line Treatments		
Switch to another antipsychotic augmenting agent	II	
Augmentation of SSRI with clomipramine	III	
Maintenance and Discontinuation Phase		
After 1-2 years, gradual taper over several months	I	
Periodic CBT booster sessions for 3-6 months	II	

CBT, cognitive behavioral therapy; OCD, obsessive-compulsive disorder; SSRI, selective serotonin reuptake inhibitor.

Levels of evidence: I, recommended with substantial clinical confidence; II, recommended with moderate clinical confidence; III, may be recommended on the basis of individual circumstances.

Data from reference 45.

If a combination of CBT and an SSRI is unsuccessful, another SSRI should be tried before augmentation therapy. If there is no response or partial response to combined CBT and three adequate antidepressant trials (one of which is clomipramine), augmentation with another drug and more intensive CBT can be tried.[45] Augmentation with antipsychotics has proven efficacious in some patients with partial response.[18,45]

Table 71-3 provides a summary of key points from the treatment guidelines for OCD. Although some OCD symptoms can improve over the first 4 to 6 weeks of therapy, an adequate trial of any medication is considered to be 8 to 12 weeks.

Nonpharmacologic Therapy

A number of nonpharmacologic treatments are effective for OCD. CBT with behavioral techniques (ie, exposure and response prevention [ERP]) is the most common initial nonpharmacologic treatment of choice. ERP is preferred for patients with mild symptoms, particularly children and adolescents, and in those without a psychiatric comorbidity or with a desire to avoid medications.[47] Clinicians can use motivational interviewing techniques to assist patients with treatment acceptance.[45]

Other options are deep brain stimulation (DBS) and ablative neurosurgery.[46,48] DBS is FDA-approved as a humanitarian device for severe, treatment-resistant OCD. It should not be used alone as first-line treatment but may be added to CBT or used in refractory patients. Surgery should be reserved for rare cases.[45,48] Data for the efficacy of transcranial magnetic stimulation are inconclusive.[46]

Pharmacologic Therapy

Practice guidelines for the treatment of patients with OCD were published by the American Psychiatric Association.[45,46]

6 SSRIs are considered to be the drugs of choice for patients with OCD.[45] While not FDA-approved, escitalopram has also shown efficacy in reduction of OCD symptoms.[49] Clomipramine, a TCA with strong 5-HT reuptake inhibition, has an active metabolite, desmethylclomipramine, which inhibits NE reuptake.[45,50] Meta-analytic findings of greater efficacy of clomipramine than SSRIs are not consistent with comparative trial data.[45]

Alternative Drug Treatments

Recent studies have examined novel augmentation approaches. Augmentation with the drugs that modulate the excitatory neurotransmitter glutamate (eg, riluzole, memantine, and topiramate) have shown initial promising results.[44,47] Ondansetron, dextroamphetamine, and D-cycloserine as possible augmentation agents in refractory OCD patients have had mixed results. These alternative augmenting treatments are reserved for refractory patients.[44,45]

Special Populations

Children and Adolescents OCD affecting children and adolescents is prevalent. There are symptom and treatment similarities and differences between OCD developing earlier in life and that which develops later. Younger patients exhibit poorer insight regarding obsessions, have more obsessions involving fear of harm and separation, and possess more rituals involving family members. CBT weekly or daily and including family members has also been effective.[47] ERP is preferred as the first-line treatment for children and adolescents with milder symptom severity and less comorbidity.[47] Effects of pediatric ERP have been reported to last up to 2 years.[47] CBT and SSRI treatment are considered first-line for pediatric patients.[51]

Clomipramine, fluvoxamine, sertraline, paroxetine, and fluoxetine are approved by the FDA for treatment of OCD in children and adolescents.[45] Childhood and adult OCD appear to respond similarly to drug therapy. SSRIs are effective (50%-56% respond to the initial agent) and well tolerated in the treatment of OCD and are generally considered first-line agents.[45,51] In children, the most commonly described side effects of SSRI therapy include sedation, nausea, diarrhea, insomnia, anorexia, tremor, and hyperstimulation.[51] The starting dose of clomipramine in children is 25 mg daily in divided doses. The dose can be increased over the first 2 weeks up to 3 mg/kg or 100 mg, whichever is smaller. Over the next several weeks, the dose can be increased up to 3 mg/kg with a maximum of 200 mg daily.[50] The risk of suicidality in youth is discussed in Chapter 68.

Hepatic and Renal Disease Clomipramine and the SSRIs are extensively metabolized in the liver, and patients with significant liver disease should be prescribed these drugs cautiously and in lower doses than those used in healthy subjects. The pharmacokinetics of sertraline is not altered in patients with significant renal dysfunction, and dosage adjustment is not necessary in these patients.[30] Increased plasma concentrations of paroxetine occur in subjects with renal impairment.[29] The initial dose of paroxetine should be reduced in patients with severe renal impairment, and upward titration should occur more slowly.[30] No dosage adjustment is necessary for patients with renal impairment receiving clomipramine.[50]

Elderly Little information is available on treating OCD in the elderly. Selection of medication for an elderly person with OCD should be based on history of response and adverse effect profile. Treatment should be initiated with low doses in elderly patients, and doses should be increased slowly, with vigilance for emergence of adverse effects.[27,45] Because of clomipramine's sedative and anticholinergic side effects, it is not usually chosen as first-line therapy for elderly OCD patients.[45] The use of SSRIs in elderly patients is discussed in Chapter 68.

Pregnancy Risk–benefit analysis should be made by practitioners when deciding to use pharmacotherapy options during pregnancy.[45] The use of SSRIs in pregnancy and lactation is discussed in Chapter 68.

Antidepressant Therapy

Serotonergic Antidepressants The only potent 5-HT reuptake inhibitors consistently demonstrating efficacy in controlled trials are the TCA clomipramine and the SSRIs fluoxetine, fluvoxamine, paroxetine, and sertraline.

Current evidence indicates that 5-HT is important for the antiobsessional effects of medication.[10] SSRIs and clomipramine inhibit 5-HT reuptake into the presynaptic neuron. Inhibiting reuptake of 5-HT makes more 5-HT available to postsynaptic receptors and reduces formation of the 5-HT metabolite 5-hydroxyindoleacetic acid. Although other antidepressants, such as imipramine and amitriptyline, inhibit 5-HT reuptake, they are less potent and selective than SSRIs. Prolonged exposure to increased amounts of 5-HT after chronic antidepressant treatment (2-3 weeks) leads to altered responsiveness of postsynaptic 5-HT receptors or presynaptic autoregulatory receptors that govern 5-HT release in specific brain regions. An improvement in obsessional symptoms may correlate with plasma concentrations of clomipramine but not desmethylclomipramine, the metabolite of clomipramine with less selectivity for 5-HT reuptake inhibition.

Most experts agree that SSRIs are better tolerated than clomipramine. SSRIs are less likely to cause cardiovascular, sedative, anticholinergic, and weight-gain side effects, and to reduce the seizure threshold. Clomipramine is less likely than SSRIs to cause insomnia, akathisia, nausea, and diarrhea. Antidepressant side effects can be more severe when larger doses are used and with faster dose escalation.

Pharmacokinetics Clomipramine is rapidly absorbed after oral administration. Maximum plasma concentrations occur within 2 to 6 hours. Clomipramine is highly protein-bound (97%) in the blood and has a half-life of 19 to 37 hours.[50] The drug is metabolized to desmethylclomipramine, which is pharmacologically active. The pharmacokinetics of SSRIs is discussed in Chapter 68.

Efficacy SSRIs are effective in the treatment of OCD. Well-designed trials comparing these medications with placebo, head-to-head comparative trials, and meta-analyses have established that fluoxetine, fluvoxamine, paroxetine, sertraline, citalopram, and escitalopram are equally effective and that clomipramine may be somewhat more effective.[23,49] Almost half (40%-60%) of patients with OCD respond to a serotonergic antidepressant, with remission occurring in 8% to 37% of patients. Most patients continue to have symptoms that limit their functioning.[52]

Other Antidepressants Venlafaxine, which acts as a 5-HT and NE reuptake inhibitor, may be effective for OCD.[21,47]

Augmentation with Antipsychotics (7) Augmentation of SSRI treatment with low doses of antipsychotics may be helpful. Typical antipsychotics are generally not recommended because of an increased risk for extrapyramidal symptoms.[44] One-third of treatment-refractory patients with OCD responded to antipsychotic augmentation.[44] Evidence supports augmentation with low-dose aripiprazole in a short-term efficacy trial.[53] Evidence supporting efficacy of risperidone is mixed and quetiapine is inconclusive.[46,54] The long-term use of second-generation antipsychotic augmentation resulted in modest improvement and higher rates of adverse effects (eg, sedation, weight gain, increased blood glucose).[55] The benefits and risks of using second-generation antipsychotic augmentation should be evaluated carefully.

Dosage and Administration Table 71-4 summarizes dosing guidelines for SSRIs and clomipramine. The dose to achieve response in OCD is often higher than doses used in other indications.[45,46] If there is inadequate response to an average dose, then it should be incrementally increased to the maximum dose within 5 to 9 weeks from the start of treatment. (8) If there is an inadequate response after 4 to 6 weeks at the maximum dose, then another SSRI should

TABLE 71-4 Dosing of Serotonin Reuptake Inhibitors in the Treatment of OCD

Drug	Brand Name	Initial Dose	Usual Range	Comments
Citalopram[a,b]	Celexa®	20 mg daily	20-40 mg daily	Maximum dose is 40 mg in adults daily to prevent QTc prolongation; maximum dose of 20 mg daily in elderly patients, CYP2C19 poor metabolizers, or use with concurrent moderate-to-strong CYP2C19 inhibitors (eg, cimetidine, omeprazole)
Clomipramine[a]	Anafranil®	25 mg daily	100-250 mg daily	Plasma levels (clomipramine and desmethylclomipramine) should be <500 ng/mL (mcg/L; ~1.7 μmol/L) (12 hours postdose to prevent conduction delays and seizures)
Escitalopram[a,b]	Lexapro®	10 mg daily	10-20 mg daily	Doses up to 40 mg may be needed in some patients
Fluoxetine[a]	Prozac®	20 mg daily	40-60 mg daily	Doses of 80 mg or higher may be needed in some patients
Fluvoxamine[a]	Luvox CR®	50 mg daily	50-200 mg daily	For initial doses use immediate-release. Doses up to 300 mg daily have been used in some patients
Paroxetine[a]	Paxil®, Pexeva®	20 mg daily	40-60 mg daily	Higher doses may be needed in some patients
Sertraline[a]	Zoloft®	50 mg daily	50-200 mg daily	Higher doses may be needed in some patients

OCD, obsessive-compulsive disorder.

[a]Available generically.

[b]Not FDA-approved for treatment of obsessive-compulsive disorder. Optimal dosing guidelines are not well established.

Data from references 29, 30, 44, and 50.

TABLE 71-5 Monitoring of Patients Being Treated for OCD

Drug	Adverse Drug Reaction	Monitoring Parameter	Comments
Clomipramine	Dry mouth, constipation, nausea, dyspepsia, anorexia, somnolence, tremors, dizziness, nervousness	Patient interview	Tolerance should occur in 2 weeks
	Seizures	Patient interview	
	Orthostatic hypotension, tachycardia, ECG changes	Vital signs, ECG	Obtain baseline ECG in patients >40 years and those with cardiovascular disease
	Suicidality	Patient interview	Highest risk is in patients <25 years
	Agranulocytosis, leukopenia	CBC with differential	Labs if patient complains of sore throat, fever
	Weight gain	Patient body weight	Assess at each visit
SSRIs	Nausea, vomiting, diarrhea, sexual dysfunction, headache, insomnia	Patient interview	Generally mild and short-lived
	Anxiety and agitation	Patient interview	May occur in some patients early in treatment
	Discontinuation syndrome	Patient interview	
	Suicidality	Patient interview	Highest risk is in patients <25 years
	QTc prolongation	ECG, electrolytes	Of most concern with citalopram doses over 40 mg daily in adults and 20 mg daily in elderly patients or in those with risk factors of patients >65 years, female sex, cardiovascular disease, hypokalemia, hypomagnesemia, or concurrent use of drugs that prolong QTc

CBC, complete blood count; ECG, electrocardiogram; OCD, obsessive-compulsive disorder; SSRI, selective serotonin reuptake inhibitor.

be tried.[45] Eight to 12 weeks is considered an adequate trial before changing to another agent.

Although the appropriate maintenance dose of antidepressants is unknown, gradual dose reduction can occur in some patients without loss of efficacy.[44]

Personalized Pharmacotherapy

The choice of an SSRI for treatment is based on history of prior response, safety, and side-effect tolerability of the patient. All SSRIs are considered to be equally efficacious, but a patient may respond better to one agent over another.[45] When selecting pharmacotherapy, the clinician should consider FDA warnings (eg, QTc prolongation for citalopram), potential for adverse consequences in patients with comorbid conditions (eg, anticholinergic effects and weight gain with paroxetine in patients with diabetes, obesity, or benign prostatic hypertrophy), or adverse effects (eg, insomnia with fluoxetine in patients with sleep difficulties). Increased risk of suicidality should be considered in patients taking SSRIs who are younger than 25 years. Drug interactions should be avoided—citalopram, escitalopram, and sertraline have the least potential for inhibition of CYP450 isoenzymes (see Chapter 68).

Risks to consider with clomipramine include lethality in overdose in patients with suicidal ideation, anticholinergic effects in patients with constipation, narrow-angle glaucoma, or urinary hesitancy, and potential for seizures in patients with epilepsy. Clomipramine use is associated with the risk of QTc prolongation when used alone and in combination with other agents that prolong the QTc interval.[50]

Clinical **Controversy...**

Data from fixed-dose studies indicate that higher SSRI doses are more efficacious than lower doses, although there is a higher adverse effect burden. However, there are no fixed-dose studies to guide clinicians on how high to increase the dose of clomipramine. Daily doses between 75 and 300 mg have been found to be effective, but doses exceeding 250 mg daily (the approved maximum dose) should be employed only with caution and close monitoring of plasma concentrations and QTc intervals.

Evaluation of Therapeutic Outcomes

Target symptoms of OCD should be monitored closely. The degree of response can indicate a need to modify dosage, change drug, or augment therapy. Rating scales can be used to monitor symptom response to therapy for OCD (eg, YBOCS) and changes in QOL. The clinician should inquire about and address problematic adverse effects (including the emergence of suicidal ideation) reported by the patient and the amount of time the patient spends obsessing and performing compulsions. Changes in social and occupational functioning should be assessed.

Table 71-5 details the monitoring of clomipramine pharmacotherapy in patients with OCD. Monitoring of SSRIs can be found in Chapter 68 and antipsychotics in Chapter 67. After patients have responded in the acute phase of treatment, treatment gains are maintained with maintenance-phase strategies.

9 Monthly follow-up visits are recommended for at least 3 to 6 months, and a medication taper can be considered after 1 to 2 years of treatment. Medication should not be rapidly discontinued, and booster CBT sessions can reduce the risk of relapse when medication is withdrawn. The drug dosage can be decreased by 10% to 25% every 1 to 2 months with careful observation for symptom relapse.[45] Some patients require lifelong medication therapy.

ABBREVIATIONS

ASD	acute stress disorder
CAPS	Clinician-Administered Posttraumatic Stress Disorder Scale
CBT	cognitive behavioral therapy
CRF	corticotropin-releasing factor
DA	dopamine
dACC	dorsal anterior cingulate cortex
DBS	deep brain stimulation
EMDR	eye movement desensitization and reprocessing
eQTLs	expression of quantitative trait loci
ERP	exposure and response prevention
GABA	γ-aminobutyric acid
5-HT	serotonin
HPA	hypothalamic–pituitary–adrenal
MAOI	monoamine oxidase inhibitor

mQTLs	methylation quantitative trait loci
NE	norepinephrine
NPY	neuropeptide Y
OCD	obsessive-compulsive disorder
PANDAS	pediatric autoimmune neuropsychiatric disorder associated with streptococcal infection
PTSD	posttraumatic stress disorder
QOL	quality of life
SNP	single nucleotide polymorphism
SNRI	serotonin–norepinephrine reuptake inhibitor
SSRI	selective serotonin reuptake inhibitor
TCA	tricyclic antidepressant
TFCBT	trauma-focused cognitive behavioral therapy
vmPFC	ventromedial prefrontal cortex
YBOCS	Yale-Brown Obsessive-Compulsive Scale

REFERENCES

1. American Psychiatric Association. *Diagnostic and Statistical Manual of Mental Disorders*, 5th ed. Arlington, VA: American Psychiatric Association, 2013.
2. Sher L, Braquehais M, Casas M. Posttraumatic stress disorder, depression, and suicide in veterans. *Cleve Clin J Med* 2012;79(2):92-97.
3. World Health Organization. Guidelines for the management of conditions specifically related to stress. Geneva: WHO. Available at: http://www.who.int/mental_health/emergencies/stress_guidelines/en/ed. Accessed, November 19, 2015.
4. Wisco BE, Marx BP, Keane TM. Screening, diagnosis and treatment of post-traumatic stress disorder. *Mil Med* 2012;177(Suppl 8):7-13.
5. Fenske JN, Schwenk TL. Obsessive-compulsive disorder: Diagnosis and management. *Am Fam Physician* 2009;80(3):239-245.
6. Ruscio AM, Stein DA, Chiu WT, Kessler RC. The epidemiology of obsessive-compulsive disorder in the National Comorbidity Survey Replication. *Mol Psychiatry* 2010;15(1):53-63.
7. Klein S, Alexander DA. Epidemiology and presentation of post-traumatic disorders. *Psychiatry* 2006;8:282-287.
8. Grant JE. Obsessive-compulsive disorder. *NEJM* 2014;371:646-653.
9. Skriner LC, Freeman J, Garcia A, et al. Characteristics of young children with obsessive-compulsive disorder: Baseline features from the POTS Jr. sample. *Child Psychiatry Hum Dev* 2015 Mar 28. [Epub ahead of print], pp.1-11. doi:10.1007/S10578-015-0546-y.
10. Nestadt G, Grados M, Samuels JF. Genetics of OCD. *Psychiatr Clin North Am* 2010;33(1):141-158.
11. Navarro-Mateu F, Escamez T, Koenen KC, et al. Meta-analysis of the 5-HTTLPR polymorphisms in post-traumatic stress disorder. *PLoS One* 2013;8:e66227.
12. Ressler KJ, Mercer KB, Bradley B, et al. Post-traumatic stress disorder is associated with PACAP and the PAC1 receptor. *Nature* 2011;470:492-497.
13. Mullen S. Review of pediatric autoimmune neuropsychiatric disorder associated with streptococcal infections. *Ment Health Clin* [Internet] 2015;5(4):184-188.
14. Sherin JE, Nemeroff CB. Posttraumatic stress disorder: The neurobiological impact of psychological trauma. *Dialogues Clin Neurosci* 2011;13:263-278.
15. Shin LM, Liberzon I. The neurobiology of fear, stress and anxiety disorders. *Neuropsychopharmacology* 2010;35:169-191.
16. Martin EI, Ressler KJ, Binder E, Nemeroff CB. The neurobiology of anxiety disorders: Brain imaging, genetics and psychoneuroendocrinology. *Psychiatr Clin North Am* 2009;32:549-575.
17. Bloch MH, McGuire J, Landeros-Weisenberger A, et al. Meta-analysis of the dose–response relationship of SSRIs in obsessive-compulsive disorder. *Mol Psychiatry* 2010;15:850-855.
18. Komossa K, Depping AM, Meyer M, et al. Second-generation antipsychotics for obsessive-compulsive disorder. *Cochrane Database Syst Rev* 2010;(12):CD008141. doi:10.1002/14651858.CD008141. pub 2.
19. Nakoa T, Okada K, Kanba S. Neurobiological model of obsessive-compulsive disorder: Evidence from recent neuropsychological and neuroimaging findings. *Psychiatry Clin Neurosci* 2014;68(8):587-605.
20. MacMaster FP. Translational neuroimaging research in pediatric obsessive-compulsive disorder. *Dialogues Clin Neurosci* 2010;12:165-174.
21. Katzman MA, Bleau P, Blier P, et al. Canadian clinical practice guidelines for the management of anxiety, posttraumatic stress and obsessive-compulsive disorders. *BMC Psychiatry* 2014;14(Suppl 1):S1.
22. Shalev AY. Posttraumatic stress disorder and stress-related disorders. *Psychiatr Clin North Am* 2009;32:687-704.
23. Feinberg N, Reghuneudanan S, Simpson HB, et al. Obsessive-compulsive disorder (OCD): Practice strategies for pharmacologic and somatic treatment in adults. *Psychiatry Res* 2015;227:114-125.
24. U.S. Department of Veterans Affairs. VA/DoD Clinical Practice Guideline: Management of Post-Traumatic Stress Disorder and Acute Stress Reaction: Guideline Summary, Version 2.0. Washington, DC, 2010. Available at: http://www.healthquality.va.gov/ptsd/CPG_Summary_FINAL_MgmtofPTSDfinal11612.pdf. Accessed, November 19, 2015.
25. Bomyea J, Lang AJ. Emerging interventions for PTSD: Future directions for clinical care and research. *Neuropharmacology* 2012;62:607-616.
26. Karsen EF, Watts BV, Holtzheimer PE. Review of the effectiveness of transcranial magnetic stimulation for post-traumatic stress disorder. *Brain Stimul* 2014;7:151-157.
27. Bandelow B, Sher L, Bunevicius R, et al. Guidelines for the pharmacological treatment of anxiety disorders, obsessive-compulsive disorder, and post-traumatic stress disorder in primary care. *Int J Psychiatry Clin Pract* 2012;16:77-84.
28. Ipser JC, Stein DJ. Evidence-based pharmacotherapy of post-traumatic stress disorder. *Int J Neuropsychopharmacol* 2012;15(6):825-840.
29. Paxil [package insert]. Research Triangle Park, NC: GlaxoSmithKline, June 2014.
30. Zoloft [package insert]. New York, NY: Pfizer Inc, August 2014.
31. Bajor LA, Ticlea AN, Osser DN. The Psychopharmacology Algorithm Project at the Harvard South Shore Program: An update on posttraumatic stress disorder. *Harv Rev Psychiatry* 2011;19:240-258.
32. Hoskins M, Pearce J, Bethell A, et al. Pharmacotherapy for posttraumatic stress disorder: Systematic review and meta-analysis. *BJP* 2015;206:93-100.
33. Davidson J, Rothbaum BO, Tucker P, et al. Venlafaxine extended release in posttraumatic stress disorder: A sertraline- and placebo-controlled study. *J Clin Psychopharmacol* 2006;26:259-267.
34. Davidson J, Baldwin D, Stein DJ, et al. Treatment of posttraumatic stress disorder with venlafaxine extended release: A 6-month randomized controlled trial. *Arch Gen Psychiatry* 2006;63:1158-1165.
35. Berger W, Mendlowicz MV, Marques-Portella C, et al. Pharmacologic alternatives to antidepressants in posttraumatic stress disorder: A systematic review. *Prog Neuropsychopharmacol Biol Psychiatry* 2009;33:169-180.
36. Ahern EP, Juergens T, Cordes T, et al. A review of atypical antipsychotic medications for posttraumatic stress disorder. *Int Clin Psychopharmacol* 2011;26:193-200.
37. Krystal JH, Rosenheck RA, Cramer JA, et al. Adjunctive risperidone treatment for antidepressant-resistant symptoms of chronic military service-related PTSD: A randomized trial. *JAMA* 2011;306:493-502.
38. Aurora RN, Zak RS, Auerbach SH, et al. Best practice guide for the treatment of nightmare disorder in adults. *J Clin Sleep Med* 2010;6(4):389-401.
39. Nappi CM, Drummond SPA, Hall JMH. Treating nightmares and insomnia in posttraumatic stress disorder: A review of current evidence. *Neuropharmacology* 2012;62:576-585.
40. Pollack MH, Hoge EA, Worthington JJ, et al. Eszopiclone for the treatment of posttraumatic stress disorder and associated insomnia: A randomized, double-blind, placebo-controlled trial. *J Clin Psychiatry* 2011;72:892-897.
41. Ipser JC, Stein DJ, Hawkridge S, Hoppe L. Pharmacotherapy for anxiety disorders in children and adolescents. Cochrane Database Syst Rev 2009;(3):CD005170. doi:10.1002/14651858.CD005170.pub2.
42. Keeshin BR, Strawn JR. Psychological and pharmacologic treatment of youth with posttraumatic stress disorder: An evidence-based review. *Child Adolesc Psychiatr Clin N Am* 2014;23:399-411.
43. Baldwin DS, Anderson IM, Nutt DJ, et al. Evidence-based pharmacological treatment of anxiety disorders, post-traumatic stress disorder and obsessive-compulsive disorder: A revision of the 2005 guidelines from the British Association of Psychopharmacology. *J Psychopharmacol* 2014;28(5):403-439.
44. Stein DJ, Koen N, Fineberg N, et al. A 2012 evidence-based algorithm for the pharmacotherapy for obsessive-compulsive disorder. *Curr Psychiatry Rep* 2012;14:211-219.

45. American Psychiatric Association. Practice Guideline for the Treatment of Patients with Obsessive-Compulsive Disorder. Arlington, VA: American Psychiatric Association, 2007. Available at: http://psychiatryonline.org/pb/assets/raw/sitewide/practice_guidelines/guidelines/ocd.pdf. Accessed, November 19, 2015.
46. American Psychiatric Association. Guideline Watch (2013): Practice Guideline for the Treatment of Patients with Obsessive-Compulsive Disorder. Available at: http://psychiatryonline.org/pb/assets/raw/sitewide/practice_guidelines/guidelines/ocd-watch.pdf. Accessed, November 19, 2015.
47. Walsh KH, McDougle CJ. Psychotherapy and medication management for obsessive-compulsive disorder. *Neuropsychiatr Dis Treat* 2011;7:485-494.
48. Greenberg BD, Rauch SL, Haber SN. Invasive circuitry-based neurotherapeutics: Stereotactic ablation and deep brain stimulation for OCD. *Neuropsychopharmacology* 2010;35:317-336.
49. Dougherty DD, Jameson M, Deckersbach T, et al. Open-label study of high (30 mg) and moderate (20 mg) dose escitalopram for the treatment of obsessive-compulsive disorder. *Int Clin Psychopharmacol* 2009;24:306-311.
50. Anafranil [package insert]. Hazelwood, MO: Mallinckrodt Inc, October 2014.
51. Kalra SK, Swedo SE. Children with obsessive-compulsive disorder: Are they just "little adults"? *J Clin Invest* 2009;119:737-746.
52. McGuire JF, Lewin AB, Horng B, et al. The nature, assessment, and treatment of obsessive-compulsive disorder. *Postgrad Med* 2012;124(1):152-165.
53. Muscatello MR, Bruno A, Pandolfo G, et al. Effect of aripiprazole augmentation of selective serotonin reuptake inhibitors or clomipramine in treatment-resistant obsessive-compulsive disorder: A double-blind, placebo-controlled study. *J Clin Psychopharmacol* 2011;31:174-179.
54. Diniz JB, Shavitt RG, Fossaluza V, et al. A double-blind, randomized, controlled trial of fluoxetine plus quetiapine or clomipramine versus fluoxetine plus placebo for obsessive-compulsive disorder. *J Clin Psychopharmacol* 2011;31:763-768.
55. Matsunga H, Nagata T, Hayashida K, et al. A long-term trial of the effectiveness and safety of atypical antipsychotic agents in augmenting SSRI-refractory obsessive-compulsive disorder. *J Clin Psychiatry* 2009;70(6):863-868.

Sleep–Wake Disorders

72

John M. Dopp and Bradley G. Phillips

KEY CONCEPTS

1. Common causes of insomnia include concomitant psychiatric disorders, significant psychosocial stressors, excessive alcohol use, caffeine intake, and nicotine use.
2. Good sleep hygiene, including relaxing before bedtime, exercising regularly, establishing a regular bedtime and wake-up time, and discontinuing alcohol, caffeine, and nicotine, alone and in combination with drug therapy, should be part of patient education and treatments for insomnia.
3. Long-acting benzodiazepines should be avoided in the elderly.
4. Benzodiazepine-receptor agonist tolerance and dependence are avoided by using low-dose therapy for the shortest possible duration.
5. Obstructive sleep apnea may be an independent risk factor for the development of hypertension. When hypertension is present, it is often refractory to drug therapy until sleep-disordered breathing is alleviated.
6. Nasal continuous positive airway pressure (PAP) is the first-line therapy for obstructive sleep apnea, and weight loss should be encouraged in all obese patients.
7. Pharmacologic management of narcolepsy is focused on two primary areas: treatment of excessive daytime sleepiness and rapid eye movement (REM) sleep abnormalities.
8. Short-acting benzodiazepine receptor agonists, ramelteon, or melatonin taken at appropriate target bedtimes for east or west travel reduce jet lag and shorten sleep latency.
9. Dopamine agonists are standard therapy for restless legs syndrome (RLS) but have adverse effects that require careful monitoring by patients and providers.

Approximately 70 million Americans suffer with a sleep-related problem, and as many as 60% of those experience a chronic disorder.[1] In a study by the National Institute on Aging, of 9,000 patients aged 65 years and older, more than 80% report a sleep-related disturbance.[1]

INTRODUCTION TO SLEEP

Sleep Cycles

Sleep is divided into two phases: nonrapid eye movement (NREM) sleep and rapid eye movement (REM) sleep. Each night humans typically experience four to six cycles of NREM and REM sleep, with each cycle lasting between 70 and 120 minutes.[2] There are four stages of NREM sleep. Healthy sleep will typically progress through the four stages of NREM sleep prior to the first REM period. From wakefulness, sleep typically progresses quickly through stages 1 and 2. Stage 1 of NREM sleep is the stage between wakefulness and sleep, and individuals describe this experience as being awake, being drowsy, or being asleep. During stages 3 and 4 NREM, both metabolic activity and brain waves slow. This slow-wave sleep occurs most frequently early in the sleep period. Stages 3 and 4 sleep are called *delta sleep*, as the sleep is characterized by high-amplitude slow activity known as delta waves (0.5-3 Hz) with no eye movements and low tonic muscle activity.

REM sleep involves a dramatic physiologic change from NREM sleep, to a state in which the brain becomes electrically and metabolically activated.[2] REM occurs in bursts and is accompanied by a 62% to 173% increase in cerebral blood flow, generalized muscle atonia, bursts of bilateral REMs, poikilothermia, dreaming, and fluctuations in respiratory and cardiac rate.[2] REM cycles tend to lengthen in the later stages of the sleep cycle.[2]

Circadian Rhythm

At birth human infants spend up to 20 hours a day sleeping. At 3 to 6 months of age there is a differentiation between REM and NREM sleep. By age 3 years the ultradian sleep–wake rhythm changes to a circadian pattern. The suprachiasmatic nucleus of the brain serves as the biologic clock and paces the circadian rhythm. Although the length of a day is 24 hours, in environments devoid of light cues, the sleep–wake cycle lasts about 25 hours.[3] In midlife, there is a gradual decline in sleep efficiency and sleep time.[2] The elderly have lighter and more fragmented sleep, with intermittent arousals, shifts in the sleep stages, and a gradual reduction of slow-wave sleep.

Neurochemistry

The neurochemistry of sleep is complex, as sleep cannot be localized to either a specific area of the brain or a neurotransmitter. NREM sleep appears to be controlled by the basal forebrain, the lower brain stem to the thalamus, and hypothalamus.[3] Numerous neurotransmitters mediate NREM sleep, including γ-aminobutyric acid (GABA) and adenosine.[3] REM sleep appears to be turned on by cholinergic cells in the mesencephalic, medullary, and pontine gigantocellular regions. REM sleep appears to be turned off by the dorsal raphe nucleus, the locus coeruleus, and the nucleus parabrachialis lateralis, the latter two of which are primarily noradrenergic. The ascending reticular activating system and the posterior hypothalamus facilitate arousal and wakefulness.[4] Dopamine has an alerting effect; decreases in dopamine promote sleepiness.[5] Neurochemicals involved in wakefulness include norepinephrine and acetylcholine in the cortex and histamine and neuropeptides such as substance P and corticotropin-releasing factor in the hypothalamus.[5,6]

Polysomnography

Sleep is typically measured and observed in sleep laboratories using an electroencephalogram (EEG), electrooculograms of each eye, electrocardiogram, electromyogram, air thermistors, abdominal and thoracic strain belts, and oxygen saturation monitor. This study is named polysomnography (PSG) and is used to assess and record variables that characterize sleep and aid in diagnosis of sleep disorders. Variables obtained during PSG include sleep onset, arousals, sleep stages, eye movements, leg and jaw movements, arrhythmias, airflow during sleep, respiratory effort, and oxygen desaturations. Home sleep monitoring that measures variables such as electrocardiogram, oxygen saturation, airflow, and respiratory effort is also increasingly used to diagnose sleep apnea.

CLASSIFICATION OF SLEEP DISORDERS

The *Diagnostic and Statistical Manual of Mental Disorders, Fifth Edition* (DSM-5) classifies sleep–wake disorders into 10 categories: (1) Insomnia disorder, (2) hypersomnolence disorder, (3) narcolepsy, (4) breathing-related sleep disorders, (5) circadian rhythm sleep disorders, (6) non-REM sleep arousal disorders, (7) nightmare disorder, (8) REM sleep behavior disorder, (9) restless legs syndrome (RLS), and (10) substance- or medication-induced sleep disorder.[7]

INSOMNIA

Insomnia is the most common complaint in general medical practice.[8] It causes distress, frequently because of a fear or a feeling of not being able to fall asleep at bedtime, and can impair work-related productivity because of daytime fatigue or drowsiness. Insomnia is subjectively characterized as a complaint of difficulty falling asleep, difficulty maintaining sleep, or experiencing nonrestorative sleep.[7,8,9] Insomnia lasting less than 3 months is considered short-term, while insomnia lasting longer than 3 months is considered to be chronic.[7,9]

Epidemiology

Primary insomnia usually begins in early or middle adulthood and is rare in childhood or adolescence. Symptoms of insomnia occur in 33% to 50% of the adult population.[8] A 1-year prevalence study of insomnia in the United States reports that one-third of the individuals surveyed complained of insomnia, and 17% reported that the symptoms were serious.[1] Conservative estimates of chronic insomnia range from 9% to 12% in adulthood and up to 20% in the elderly.[1,10] Although young adults are more likely to complain that they have difficulty falling asleep, middle-aged and elderly adults are more likely to complain that they have middle-of-the-night awakening or early morning awakening. Women complain of insomnia twice as frequently as men. Individuals who are elderly, unemployed, separated, or widowed, and those with a lower socioeconomic status report a significantly higher incidence of insomnia than the general population. Forty percent of individuals with insomnia also have a concurrent psychiatric disorder (anxiety, depression, or substance abuse).[11] A significant percentage of those with insomnia use nonprescription drugs or alcohol to self-treat.

Differential Diagnosis

Primary insomnia is considered to be an endogenous disorder caused by either a neurochemical or a structural disorder affecting the sleep–wake cycle. Individuals with primary insomnia can be light sleepers who are easily aroused by noise, temperature, or anxiety. Some studies suggest that primary insomnia is a "hyperarousal state," in that insomnia patients have increased metabolic rates compared with controls and thus take longer to fall asleep.[2] Comorbid or secondary insomnia is frequently a symptom or manifestation of another medical disorder. Evaluation of patients with a complaint of transient or short-term insomnia should focus on recent stressors, such as a separation, a death in the family, a job change, or college exams.

1 Chronic insomnia is frequently comorbid with psychiatric or medical conditions. A complete diagnostic examination should be completed in these individuals and should include routine laboratory tests, physical and mental status examinations, as well as ruling out any medication- or substance-related causes.[12] Special consideration should also be given to other sleep disorders that can have a similar presentation, including RLS, periodic limb movements of sleep (PLMS), and sleep apnea. Common causes of insomnia are listed in Table 72-1.

TABLE 72-1 Common Etiologies of Insomnia

Situational
• Work or financial stress, major life events, interpersonal conflicts
• Jet lag or shift work
Medical
• Cardiovascular (angina, arrhythmias, heart failure)
• Respiratory (asthma, sleep apnea)
• Chronic pain
• Endocrine disorders (diabetes, hyperthyroidism)
• Gastrointestinal (gastroesophageal reflux disease, ulcers)
• Neurologic (delirium, epilepsy, Parkinson disease)
• Pregnancy
Psychiatric
• Mood disorders (depression, mania)
• Anxiety disorders (eg, generalized anxiety disorder, obsessive-compulsive disorder)
• Substance abuse (alcohol or sedative–hypnotic withdrawal)
Pharmacologically induced
• Anticonvulsants
• Central adrenergic blockers
• Diuretics
• Selective serotonin reuptake inhibitors
• Steroids
• Stimulants

TREATMENT

Desired Outcomes

The goals of treatment of insomnia are to correct the underlying sleep complaint, consolidate sleep, improve daytime functioning and sleepiness, and avoid adverse effects from selected therapies. Drug therapy should be used in the lowest possible dose, for the shortest possible time period.

General Approach to Treatment

Therapeutic management of insomnia is initially based on whether the individual has experienced a transient, short-term, or chronic sleep disturbance. Clinical history should assess the onset, duration, and frequency of the symptoms; effect on daytime functioning; sleep hygiene habits; and history of previous symptoms or treatment.[13] Management of all patients with insomnia should include identifying the cause of the insomnia, patient education on sleep hygiene, and stress management. Any unnecessary pharmacotherapy should be eliminated.[10] Transient insomnia, which occurs as a result of an acute stressor, is expected to resolve quickly and should be treated with good sleep hygiene and careful use of sedative–hypnotics.[11] Short-term insomnia, associated with situational, personal, or medical stress, can be treated similarly.[13]

TABLE 72-2 Nonpharmacologic Recommendations for Management of Insomnia

Stimulus control procedures
1. Establish regular times to wake up and to go to sleep (including weekends).
2. Sleep only as much as necessary to feel rested.
3. Go to bed only when sleepy. Avoid long periods of wakefulness in bed. Use the bed only for sleep or intimacy; do not read or watch television in bed.
4. Avoid trying to force sleep; if you do not fall asleep within 20-30 minutes, leave the bed and perform a relaxing activity (eg, read, listen to music) until drowsy. Repeat this as often as necessary.
5. Avoid blue spectrum light from television, smart phones, tablets, and other mobile devices.
6. Avoid daytime naps.
7. Schedule worry time during the day. Do not take your troubles to bed.
Sleep hygiene recommendations
1. Exercise routinely (three to four times weekly) but not close to bedtime because this can increase wakefulness.
2. Create a comfortable sleep environment by avoiding temperature extremes, loud noises, and illuminated clocks in the bedroom.
3. Discontinue or reduce the use of alcohol, caffeine, and nicotine.
4. Avoid drinking large quantities of liquids in the evening to prevent nighttime trips to the restroom.
5. Do something relaxing and enjoyable before bedtime.

Chronic insomnia requires careful assessment for possible underlying medical causes, nonpharmacologic approaches, and careful use of sedative–hypnotics.[12]

Nonpharmacologic Therapy

2 In many cases insomnia can be treated without sedative–hypnotics. Education about normal sleep and habits for good sleep hygiene are important for all patients with insomnia. Nonpharmacologic interventions for insomnia frequently consist of short-term cognitive behavioral therapies, most commonly stimulus control therapy, sleep restriction, relaxation therapy, cognitive therapy, paradoxical intention, biofeedback, and education on good sleep hygiene (Table 72-2).[10,14] In patients aged 55 and older, research indicates that cognitive behavioral therapy may be more effective than pharmacologic therapy at improving certain measures of insomnia.[15,16]

Pharmacologic Therapy

Miscellaneous Agents Antihistamines exhibit sedating properties and are included in many nonprescription sleep agents. They are effective in the treatment of mild insomnia and are generally safe.[13] Diphenhydramine and doxylamine are more sedating than pyrilamine. Patients quickly experience tolerance to sedative effects, and increasing the dose of antihistamines will not produce a linear increase in response. Antihistamines are considered to be less effective than benzodiazepines, and they have the disadvantages of anticholinergic side effects, which are especially troublesome in the elderly.[13,17]

Antidepressants are alternatives for patients with nonrestorative sleep who should not receive benzodiazepines, especially those who have depression, pain, or a risk of substance abuse. Using antidepressants for insomnia without depression is common but not well-studied, and the doses used for treating insomnia are not effective antidepressant doses.[9,13,14] Sedating antidepressants such as amitriptyline, doxepin, and nortriptyline are effective for inducing sleep continuity, although daytime sedation and side effects can be significant.[9,13] Anticholinergic activity, adrenergic blockade, and cardiac conduction prolongation can be problematic, especially in the elderly and in overdose situations.[9] Low-dose doxepin (3-6 mg) was recently Food and Drug Administration (FDA)-approved for the treatment of sleep maintenance insomnia. Mirtazapine is a sedating antidepressant that may help patients sleep, but it may also cause daytime sedation and weight gain.

Trazodone in doses of 25 to 100 mg at bedtime is sedating and can improve sleep continuity.[11] Trazodone is popular for the treatment of insomnia in patients prone to substance abuse, as dependence is not a problem with trazodone, and in patients with selective serotonin reuptake inhibitor and bupropion-induced insomnia.[11] Other side effects include carryover sedation and α-adrenergic blockade. Orthostasis can occur at any age, but it is more dangerous in the elderly. Priapism is a rare but serious side effect.[18]

Suvorexant is a recently approved dual orexinA and orexin B receptor antagonist that instead of inducing sleepiness turns off wake signaling. Suvorexant doses of 10 to 20 mg at bedtime are indicated for difficulty initiating and maintaining sleep. The most commonly reported side effect with suvorexant use is somnolence, and patients should be counseled that sleep paralysis, cataplexy, and other narcolepsy-like symptoms may rarely occur.[19]

Ramelteon is a melatonin-receptor agonist approved for the treatment of sleep-onset insomnia. It is selective for the MT1 and MT2 melatonin receptors that are thought to regulate the circadian rhythm and sleep onset. The recommended dose is 8 mg taken at bedtime to induce sleep. Although generally well tolerated, the most common adverse events reported are headache, dizziness, and somnolence. Ramelteon is not a controlled substance and can be a viable option for patients with a history of substance abuse. It effectively treats sleep-onset difficulties in patients with chronic obstructive pulmonary disease and sleep apnea.[20,21]

Valerian is a herbal sleep remedy that has been studied for its sedative–hypnotic properties in patients with insomnia. The mechanism of action is not fully understood but may involve increasing concentrations of GABA. The recommended dose for insomnia ranges from 300 to 600 mg. An equivalent dose of dried herbal valerian root is 2 to 3 g soaked in one cup of hot water for 20 to 25 minutes.[22]

Benzodiazepine-Receptor Agonists The most commonly used treatments for insomnia have been the benzodiazepine-receptor agonists (BZDRAs). BZDRAs are effective as sedative–hypnotics and are FDA-labeled for the treatment of insomnia (Table 72-3). The FDA requires BZDRA labeling to include a caution regarding anaphylaxis, facial angioedema, and complex sleep behaviors (eg, sleep driving, phone calls, sleep eating, etc.). The BZDRAs consist of the newer nonbenzodiazepine $GABA_A$ agonists and the traditional benzodiazepines. All BZDRAs bind to $GABA_A$ receptors in the brain, resulting in agonist effects on GABAergic transmission and hyperpolarization of neuronal membranes. Traditional benzodiazepines have sedative, anxiolytic, muscle relaxant, and anticonvulsant properties; newer nonbenzodiazepine GABA agonists possess only sedative properties.

Benzodiazepine Hypnotics Benzodiazepines relieve insomnia by reducing sleep latency and increasing total sleep time. They increase stage 2 sleep while decreasing delta sleep.[11] Benzodiazepine hypnotics should not be prescribed for individuals who are pregnant or who have untreated sleep apnea or a history of substance abuse. Patients should be instructed to avoid alcohol and other central nervous system (CNS) depressants.

Adverse Effects Side effects are dose-dependent and vary according to the pharmacokinetics of the individual benzodiazepine. High doses with long or intermediate elimination half-lives have a greater potential for producing daytime sedation, psychomotor incoordination, and cognitive deficits. Most traditional benzodiazepines maintain hypnotic efficacy for 1 month. However, tolerance can develop with time.

TABLE 72-3 Pharmacokinetics of Benzodiazepine-Receptor Agonists

Generic Name (Brand Name)	t_{max} (hours)[a]	Half-Life[b] (hours)	Daily Dose Range (mg)	Metabolic Pathway	Clinically Significant Metabolites
Estazolam (ProSom)	2	12-15	1-2	Oxidation	–
Eszopiclone (Lunesta)	1-1.5	6	2-3	Oxidation	–
				Demethylation	
Flurazepam (Dalmane)	1	8	15-30	Oxidation	Hydroxyethylflurazepam, Flurazepam aldehyde
				N-dealkylation	*N*-desalkylflurazepam[c]
Quazepam (Doral)	2	39	7.5-15	Oxidation, *N*-dealkylation	2-Oxo-quazepam, *N*-desalkylflurazepam[c]
Temazepam (Restoril)	1.5	10-15	15-30	Conjugation	–
Triazolam (Halcion)	1	2	0.125-0.25	Oxidation	–
Zaleplon (Sonata)	1	1	5-10	Oxidation	–
Zolpidem (Ambien;Intermezzo)	1.6	2-2.6	1.75-10[d]	Oxidation	–

[a]Time to peak plasma concentration.

[b]Half-life of parent drug.

[c]*N*-desalkylflurazepam, mean half-life 47 to 100 hours.

[d]Oral and sublingual dosing 5 to 10 mg; sublingual tablets for middle-of-the night dosing 1.75 to 3.5 mg (1.75 for women, 3.5 mg for men).

Anterograde amnesia, an impairment of memory and recall of events occurring after the dose is taken, has been reported with most BZDRAs (it is more likely to occur with short-acting agents).[11] Rebound insomnia, characterized by increased wakefulness beyond baseline amounts that last for a few nights after abrupt discontinuation, occurs with BZDRAs. The lowest effective dosage should be used to minimize rebound insomnia and avoid adverse effects on memory.

3 Benzodiazepine half-lives are prolonged in older patients, increasing the potential for drug accumulation and the incidence of CNS side effects, including prolonged sedation and cognitive and psychomotor impairment. BZDRAs with long elimination half-lives (eg, flurazepam and quazepam) are generally not first-line agents in these patients. Benzodiazepine use is associated with increased risk of falls and hip fractures in the elderly, but since insomnia itself increases fall and fracture risk, it is unclear if benzodiazepines increase risk independent of sleep problems.[23]

Nonbenzodiazepine GABA$_A$ Agonists Zolpidem, zaleplon, and eszopiclone are nonbenzodiazepine hypnotics that selectively bind to GABA$_A$ receptors and effectively induce sleepiness. Zolpidem has a duration of action of 6 to 8 hours.[24] It is comparable in efficacy to benzodiazepine hypnotics and is effective for reducing sleep latency and nocturnal awakenings and increasing total sleep time. It does not appear to have significant effects on next-day psychomotor performance. Sustained-release, sublingual, and reduced-strength (1.75 and 3.5 mg) formulations of zolpidem are available and are used to increase total sleep time, to reduce sleep latency, and for middle-of-the night rescue dosing, respectively.

Zolpidem is less disruptive of sleep stages than benzodiazepines. Adverse effects are dose-related and can include drowsiness, amnesia, dizziness, headache, and gastrointestinal (GI) complaints.[24] Sleep eating during zolpidem therapy can result in significant weight gain. The recommended daily dose of zolpidem is 10 mg in male patients, or 5 mg in female patients, elderly patients and those with hepatic impairment. Because food decreases its absorption, zolpidem should be taken on an empty stomach.[25]

Zaleplon has a rapid onset of action and a half-life of 1 hour, and it is metabolized to inactive metabolites.[26] It is effective for decreasing time to sleep onset but not for reducing nighttime awakening or for increasing total sleep time.[27] Because of its short half-life, zaleplon has no effect on next-day psychomotor performance and can be used as a sleep aid for middle-of-the-night awakenings.[28] The recommended dose is 10 mg in adults and 5 mg in the elderly.[26] The most common adverse effects with zaleplon are dizziness, headache, and somnolence. There are two drug interactions of note: zaleplon plasma levels are increased when combined with cimetidine and decreased with rifampin.[24]

Eszopiclone is effective at reducing time to sleep onset, wake time after sleep onset, and number of awakenings, and increasing total sleep time and sleep quality. Eszopiclone's duration of action is up to 6 hours,[29] so it can be a good option for treatment of sleep maintenance insomnia or early morning awakenings. The most common adverse effects with eszopiclone are somnolence, unpleasant taste, headache, and dry mouth.[29] Eszopiclone is labeled for long-term use and may be taken nightly for up to 6 months.[29,30]

Other Considerations In general, the nonbenzodiazepine hypnotics seem to be associated with less withdrawal, tolerance, and rebound insomnia than the benzodiazepine hypnotics. None of the nonbenzodiazepine GABA$_A$ agonists have significant active metabolites.

Evaluation of Therapeutic Outcomes

An algorithm for the evaluation and treatment of dyssomnias is shown in Fig. 72-1.[31] Patients with short-term or chronic insomnia should be evaluated after 1 week of therapy to assess for drug efficacy, adverse effects, and adherence to nonpharmacologic recommendations.

Clinical **Controversy...**

Population studies suggest that use of sedative–hypnotics may be associated with increased mortality. Even though causality cannot be established based on the evidence to date, these studies raise important concerns. Although the evidence does not warrant discontinuation of hypnotics, it reemphasizes the importance of using sedative–hypnotics prudently at the lowest dose possible, for the shortest duration necessary.

Patients should be instructed to keep a sleep diary. The diary requires daily recording of bedtime, wake time, latency of sleep

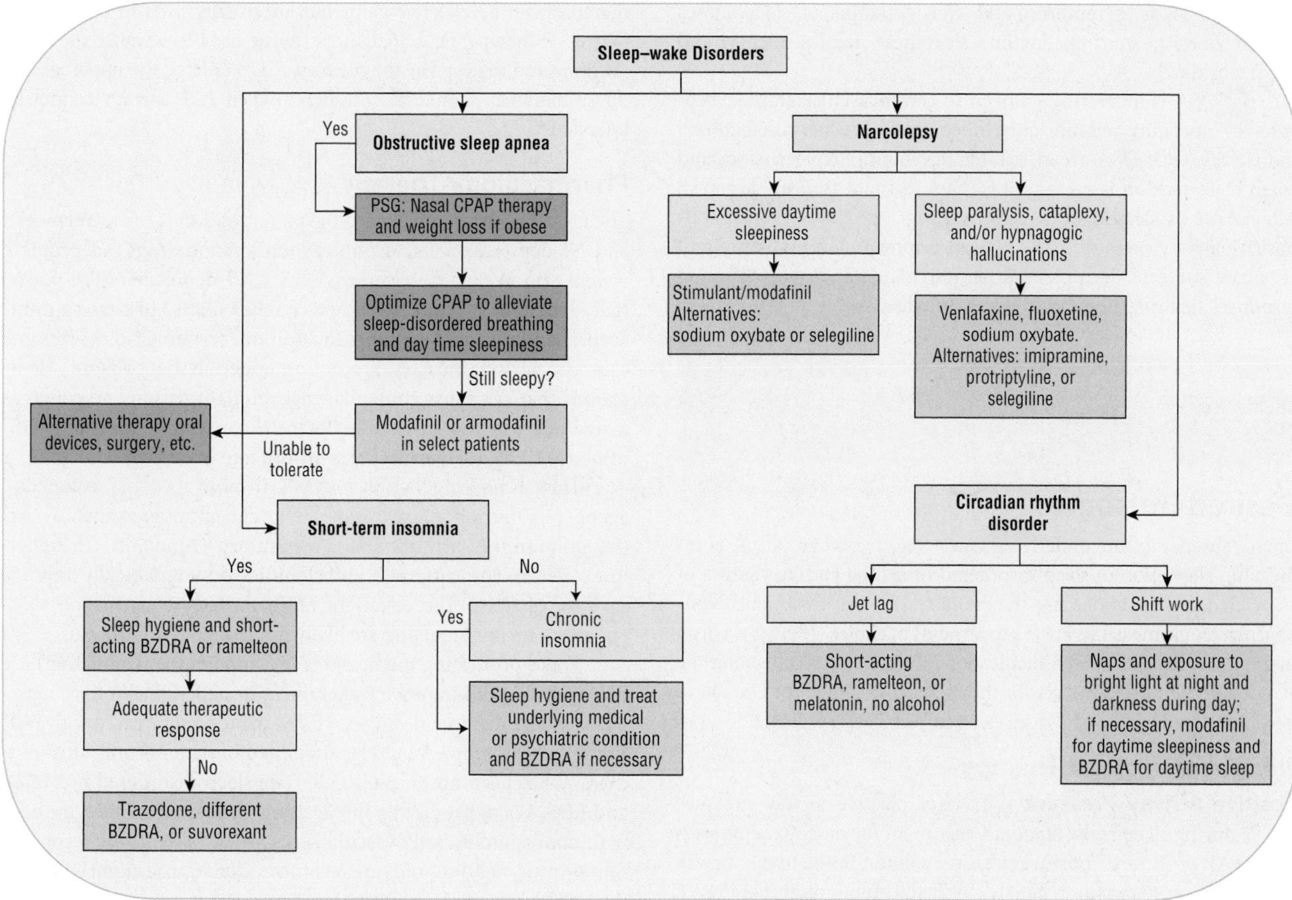

FIGURE 72-1 Algorithm for treatment of dyssomnias. (BZDRA, benzodiazepine-receptor agonist; CPAP, continuous positive airway pressure.) *(Reprinted with permission from Jermaine DM. Sleep disorders. In: Carter BL, Angaran DM, Lake KD, et al, eds.* Pharmacotherapy Self-Assessment Program, 2nd ed. *Neurology and Psychiatry. Kansas City, MO: American College of Clinical Pharmacy, 1995:146-7.)*

onset, number and duration of awakenings, medication ingestion, naps, and an index of sleep quality. For patients with chronic insomnia, possible medical, psychiatric, and pharmacologic causes should be identified and managed.[11] Patients with insomnia should receive education about possible medication side effects and their management.

4 Clinicians should educate patients about the concepts of tolerance, withdrawal, and rebound insomnia. Tolerance and dependence can be avoided by using hypnotics at the lowest possible dose, intermittently, and for the shortest duration possible. Patients should receive instruction about frequency of drug use and the expected duration of therapy, to help prevent development of dependence. Withdrawal symptoms can be diminished by tapering the dosage gradually.

SLEEP APNEA

Sleep apnea is a common disease, affecting 20 to 25 million Americans. It has a higher prevalence in men, particularly in African American and Hispanic populations.[32,33] Sleep apnea also occurs in children and adolescents. It is characterized by repetitive episodes of cessation of breathing during sleep followed by blood oxygen desaturation and brief arousal from sleep to restart breathing. As a result, individuals with sleep apnea experience fragmented sleep, poor sleep architecture, and periods of apnea and hypopnea. PSG is used to diagnose and quantify sleep apnea as central, obstructive, or mixed. Central sleep apnea (CSA) involves impairment of the respiratory drive, whereas OSA is caused by upper airway collapse and obstruction. Patients with mixed sleep apnea experience both CSA and OSA. Severity of sleep apnea is determined by the number of apnea (total cessation of airflow) and hypopnea (partial airway closure with blood oxygen desaturation) episodes documented by PSG, which is expressed as the respiratory disturbance index (RDI). Mild sleep apneics have an RDI of between 5 and 15 episodes/hour, moderate 15 to 30 episodes/hour, whereas individuals with severe OSA exhibit more than 30 episodes/hour.

OSA is associated with motor vehicle accidents, depression, increased cancer risk, stroke, and cardiovascular disease.[34-37] Alleviation of sleep-disordered breathing may improve patient outcomes, particularly those related to cardiovascular disease.[37]

Obstructive Sleep Apnea

OSA is characterized by partial or complete closure of the upper airway, posterior from the nasal septum to the epiglottis, during inspiration. The reason for the loss of upper airway patency is not fully understood and is likely caused by several competing factors. Anatomical factors including neck obesity, narrow airway, and fixed upper airway lesions (eg, polyps, enlarged tonsils) can narrow the upper airway. Intraluminal negative pressure generated during each inspiration also promotes collapse of the upper airway that competes with dilating forces, primarily the pharyngeal dilator muscle. Acromegaly, amyloidosis, and hypothyroidism as well as neurologic conditions that impair upper airway muscle tone may cause OSA. The hallmarks of OSA are witnessed apneas, gasping, or both. Other recognized signs, symptoms, and considerations of sleep apnea include obesity, snoring, daytime sleepiness, family history, and hypertension.

5 OSA is increasingly linked to cardiovascular and cerebrovascular morbidity and mortality, independent of other risk factors.[37] Individuals with OSA are at risk for developing hypertension, and when hypertension is present, it is often resistant to drug therapy.[38] Alleviation of sleep-disordered breathing (with nasal continuous positive airway pressure [CPAP]) can improve blood pressure and attenuate some of the potential hemodynamic and neurohumoral responses that may link OSA to systemic disease.[39,40]

TREATMENT: OSA

Desired Outcomes

In the absence of an underlying cause (eg, hypothyroidism, acromegaly), alleviation of sleep-disordered breathing and prevention of associated complications are the primary goals of treatment. Nonpharmacologic measures are the treatments of choice. There is no drug therapy for OSA. However, medications that worsen sleep should be avoided. Practice parameters for the medical treatment of OSA have been published by the American Academy of Sleep Medicine.[41]

Nonpharmacologic Therapy

Positive Airway Pressure 6 Nasal positive airway pressure (PAP) during sleep is the standard treatment for most patients with OSA. PAP produces a positive pressure column in the upper airway using room air to maintain patency. A flexible tube connects the PAP machine to a mask that covers the nose.

PAP delivery may be continuous (CPAP), bilevel (providing a reduced applied pressure during expiration), or auto titrating continuous positive airway pressure therapy (AutoPAP). AutoPAP machines may be programmed to a pressure range and the machine provides individualized pressure based on breath-to-breath analysis of the necessary pressure to keep the airway open. CPAP pressure may be determined during PSG, when the pressure setting is increased (up to 20 cm H_2O) until sleep-disordered breathing is eliminated or by determining which pressure the AutoPAP machine uses 90% to 95% of the time. Barriers to PAP adherence, such as ill-fitted mask and nasal dryness, can be managed. PAP nonadherence for one night results in a complete reversal of the gains made in daytime alertness.[42] In the clinical setting, poor PAP adherence may impact blood pressure control and management in patients with OSA and hypertension.

Weight Reduction Obesity can worsen sleep apnea, and weight management should be implemented for all overweight patients with OSA. OSA can predispose to weight gain, and in obese patients with mild OSA weight loss alone can be effective.[43] Individuals who are morbidly obese and have severe OSA can undergo bariatric surgery for weight loss.

Surgery Surgical therapy (uvulopalatopharyngoplasty) opens the upper airway by removing the tonsils, trimming and reorienting the posterior and anterior tonsillar pillars, and removing the uvula and posterior portion of the palate. This is not a first-line option because it is invasive. In very severe cases tracheostomy may be necessary. This procedure can be indicated for select individuals who are morbidly obese, have severe facial skeletal deformity, experience severe drops in oxygen saturation (eg, less than 70% [0.70]), or have significant cardiac arrhythmias associated with their OSA.

Other Therapies For individuals who experience OSA only during certain sleep positions (eg, when lying on their back), positional therapies can be effective alone but are usually used in conjunction with PAP therapy. Oral appliances can be used to advance the lower jawbone and to keep the tongue forward to enlarge the upper airway. These therapies should be considered when PAP therapy cannot be tolerated.[44]

Pharmacologic Therapy

The most important pharmacologic intervention is the avoidance of all CNS depressants (eg, alcohol, hypnotics) and drugs that promote weight gain. Weight gain worsens OSA. CNS-depressant use is potentially lethal, as it reduces the brain's reflex ability to cause a mini-arousal and resume breathing. In addition, certain CNS depressants can relax airway muscles, promoting upper airway collapse. Medications that can cause rhinopharyngeal inflammation and cough as a side effect of therapy (ie, angiotensin-converting enzyme [ACE] inhibitor) may also worsen sleep-disordered breathing.

There is no drug therapy for OSA. In clinical trials, serotonergic agents (eg, fluoxetine, paroxetine), tricyclic antidepressants (TCAs) (ie, imipramine, protriptyline), respiratory stimulants (theophylline), medroxyprogesterone, and clonidine do not clinically improve severity of OSA. The effects of antihypertensive agents on sleep apnea are inconsistent and are likely not clinically significant.

Wake-promoting medications (eg, modafinil, armodafinil) are FDA-approved to improve wakefulness in patients who have residual excessive daytime sleepiness (EDS) while being treated with PAP. Initiation of therapy should be attempted in patients only after PAP therapy has been optimized to alleviate sleep-disordered breathing and EDS. Wake-promoting medications should be avoided in those with concomitant cardiovascular disease. In patients with concurrent rhinitis, nasal steroids are recommended for use along with PAP therapy.[41]

Evaluation of Therapeutic Outcomes

Individuals with sleep apnea should be evaluated after 1 to 3 months of treatment for improvement in alertness and daytime symptoms (eg, sleepiness, impaired memory, and irritability) and weight reduction. Individuals experiencing symptoms (eg, daytime sleepiness, snoring, loss of blood pressure control) despite PAP therapy should have PSG repeated. Symptoms can recur if patients gain weight, requiring a higher pressure setting. Conversely, PAP pressure settings can be decreased if weight loss is achieved. Patient adherence to PAP therapy can be monitored by assessing the built-in compliance meter that measures the hours used at effective pressure.

Central Sleep Apnea

CSA causes fragmented sleep and consequent daytime somnolence. However, unlike OSA, arousals from sleep are not required to initiate airflow. During PSG, there is an absence of airflow out of the mouth and nose with no activation of the inspiratory muscles. The prevalence of CSA is not well established and is less than OSA. CSA can be idiopathic but more commonly is caused by underlying autonomic nervous system lesions (eg, cervical cordotomy), neurologic diseases (eg, poliomyelitis, encephalitis, and myasthenia gravis), high altitudes, opioid abuse, and congestive heart failure. For these reasons, potential underlying causes for CSA should be evaluated and treated. For example, worsening CSA in heart failure patients can signal the need to optimize heart failure therapies. Practice parameters for the treatment of CSA have been published by the American Academy of Sleep Medicine.[45]

Drug therapy for CSA is limited and is individualized for each patient, based on underlying etiology. Acetazolamide, which induces a metabolic acidosis that stimulates respiratory drive, and theophylline, which improves severity of CSA, have been studied but have minimal effects on clinical variables.[46,47]

CLINICAL PRESENTATION Narcolepsy

Symptoms

- Patients may complain of EDS and disrupted nighttime sleep; often they have some accompanying REM sleep abnormality, sleep paralysis, cataplexy, and/or hallucinations.

Laboratory Tests

- Although not routinely tested, there is a high incidence of human leukocyte antigen (HLA) haplotypes DR2 and HLA-DQ6/DQB1 in narcolepsy.
- Cerebrospinal fluid (CSF) concentrations of hypocretin-1 can be measured to confirm a diagnosis. CSF concentrations less than 110 pg/mL (110 ng/L) positively predict narcolepsy.

Other Diagnostic Tests

- Narcolepsy is diagnosed using the multiple sleep latency test (nap test). The patient takes four to five naps in a day, and narcolepsy is diagnosed if the patient falls asleep quickly (within less than 5 minutes) and goes into REM sleep in two of those nap periods.

NARCOLEPSY

Narcolepsy is a severely debilitating neurologic disease that affects between 0.03% and 0.06% of adult Americans.[48] Despite the debilitating nature of the disease, it can be undiagnosed or misdiagnosed for years. Prevalence is equal or somewhat higher in men compared with women. It is commonly recognized in the second decade of life and increases in severity through the third and fourth decades.[48] Individuals with narcolepsy complain of EDS, and in the sleep laboratory, individuals with narcolepsy exhibit impairment of both the onset and the offset of REM and NREM sleep and have arousals and disturbed sleep during the night.

Four characteristic symptoms differentiate narcolepsy from other sleep disorders and are known as the *narcolepsy tetrad*: EDS, cataplexy, hallucinations, and sleep paralysis. Cataplexy, a sudden bilateral loss of muscle tone of varying severity and duration without the loss of consciousness, occurs in 70% to 80% of people with narcolepsy.[48] Patients can suffer subtle changes, such as jaw or head slumping, or severe weakness, such as knee buckling or collapsing to the ground. Cataplexy is often precipitated by situations characterized by high emotion (eg, laughter, anger, excitement). Cataleptic episodes can be brief, lasting seconds, or can last for several minutes. Sleep paralysis is an episodic loss of voluntary muscle tone that occurs when the individual is falling asleep or waking. Individuals are conscious but not able to move or speak. Hallucinations while falling asleep (ie, hypnagogic) and on awakening (ie, hypnopompic) are brief, dream-like experiences that intrude into wakefulness and are experienced by nearly 70% of narcoleptics. Unfortunately, these symptoms sometimes lead to an incorrect diagnosis of mental illness.[48] Cataplexy, sleep paralysis, and hypnagogic hallucinations can be caused by REM sleep disturbances.[48]

Loss of normal function of the hypocretin-orexin neurotransmitter system appears to play a central role in the pathophysiology of narcolepsy. Neurons containing hypocretin-orexin are found in the lateral hypothalamus and project to various parts of the brain that are thought to regulate sleep. In 75% of narcoleptic patients, hypocretin-orexin is undetectable in CSF.[49,50] Because narcoleptic patients have deficiencies in hypocretin-orexin–producing neurons,[51] an autoimmune process may be responsible for the destruction of hypocretin-producing cells.[51,52] Onset of disease occurs in adolescence or adulthood, but not at birth, suggesting that environmental influences might also play a role. Molecular studies of HLA have found a high prevalence of the HLA-DR2 and HLA-DQ6/DQB1 haplotypes in narcoleptics.[53] However, the HLA-DR2 haplotype is also common in the nonnarcoleptic population and is not diagnostic.[52] There may also be a genetic component, as 3% of patients have a first-degree relative with the disorder.[49]

Clinical **Controversy...**

An increased risk of narcolepsy was associated with use of a 2009 H1N1 influenza vaccine used in Europe (containing a vaccine adjuvant) causing some individuals to forego influenza immunization. However, a study performed by the U.S. Centers for Disease Control and Prevention found that vaccines licensed in the United States (without adjuvants) are not associated with increased risk of narcolepsy.[54] Despite this evidence, some individuals still believe influenza immunization increases narcolepsy risk. As with autism and other disproven risks of immunization, clinicians should urge patients that narcolepsy is not a risk of influenza immunization.

TREATMENT: Narcolepsy

Desired Outcomes

The primary objective of pharmacologic treatment of narcolepsy is to reduce symptoms that adversely impact quality of life. The goal is to produce the fullest possible return of normal function for patients at work, school, home, and in social settings.

Nonpharmcologic Therapy

Nonpharmacologic management of narcolepsy includes counseling the patient and family concerning the illness to alleviate misconceptions around the individual's behavior. Good sleep hygiene should be encouraged as well as two or more scheduled daytime naps. Daytime naps lasting 15 minutes each can help the individual with narcolepsy feel refreshed.

Pharmacologic Therapy

7 Pharmacologic management of narcolepsy is focused on two primary areas: treatment of EDS and REM sleep abnormalities. Drug therapy for narcolepsy is summarized in Table 72-4.

Modafinil, a racemic compound unrelated to psychostimulants, is a recognized standard treatment for EDS.[55] Armodafinil is the active R-isomer of modafinil and is also FDA-approved for treatment of EDS in narcolepsy. The precise mechanism of action of modafinil and armodafinil is not fully understood. Common adverse effects are usually mild and include headache, nausea, nervousness, anxiety, and insomnia. The dose of modafinil is between 200 and 400 mg/day, and armodafinil doses are between 150 and 250 mg/day.[56] Although both of these agents are effective in treating EDS, they lack efficacy for the treatment of cataplectic symptoms.[57]

TABLE 72-4 Dosing of Drugs Used to Treat Narcolepsy

Generic Name	Brand Name	Initial Dose (mg)	Usual dose (mg)	Comments
Excessive Daytime Somnolence				
Dextroamphetamine	Dexedrine	5-10	5-60	Concurrent use of amphetamines and acidic foods may reduce amphetamine absorption
Dextroamphetamine/ Amphetamine salts[a]	Adderall	5-20	5-60	See above
Methamphetamine[b]	Desoxyn	5-15	5-15	See above
Lisdexamfetamine	Vyvanse	20-30	20-70	Prodrug of dextroamphetamine
Methylphenidate	Ritalin	10-40	30-80	May increase risk of bleeding with concomitant warfarin therapy
Modafinil	Provigil	100-200	200-400	May reduce effectiveness of hormonal contraceptives
Armodafinil	Nuvigil	150	150-250	May reduce effectiveness of hormonal contraceptives
Sodium oxybate[c]	Xyrem	4.5 grams/night	4.5-9 grams/night	Do not use with other CNS depressants
Agents for cataplexy				
Fluoxetine	Prozac	10-20	20-80	Will see cataplexy benefits sooner than antidepressant benefits
Imipramine	Tofranil	50-100	50-250	Anticholinergic side effects
Nortriptyline	Aventyl, Pamelor	50-100	50-200	Anticholinergic side effects
Protriptyline	Vivactil	5-10	5-30	
Venlafaxine	Effexor	37.5	37.5-225	May increase blood pressure
Selegiline	Eldepryl	5-10	20-40	Doses <10 mg per day do not require dietary tyramine restrictions

CNS, central nervous system.

[a]Dextroamphetamine sulfate, dextroamphetamine saccharate, amphetamine aspartate, and amphetamine sulfate.

[b]Not available in some states.

[c]Also is effective at treating cataplexy.

Data from references 52 and 55.

EDS can also be treated with stimulants to improve alertness and to increase daytime performance. Dextroamphetamine and methylphenidate also have FDA approval for the treatment of narcolepsy. Methamphetamine and mixed amphetamine salts have also been used on an off-label basis. Methylphenidate and amphetamines have a fast onset of action and durations of 6 to 10 and 3 to 4 hours, respectively. The doses of methylphenidate and amphetamine formulations can range from 5 to 60 mg daily.

Stimulants improve alertness and daytime performance, and they can elevate mood and prevent sleep. Side effects can include insomnia, hypertension, palpitations, and irritability. Tolerance to long-term stimulant therapy can occur, necessitating dosage increases. Amphetamine use is associated with more likelihood of abuse and tolerance, especially when prescribed in high doses. Lisdexamfetamine is a new amphetamine prodrug rapidly absorbed and converted in the body to dextroamphetamine. It has a longer duration of action and less risk of abuse since it is active only when taken orally.

The most commonly used treatments for cataplexy are TCAs, serotonin norepinephrine reuptake inhibitors (SNRIs), and selective serotonin reuptake inhibitors (SSRIs). The mechanism of antidepressants in relieving cataplexy, hypnagogic hallucinations, and sleep paralysis can be mediated through blockade of serotonin and norepinephrine reuptake in the locus coeruleus and raphe and subsequent suppression of REM sleep.[58] Imipramine, protriptyline, clomipramine, fluoxetine, and nortriptyline are effective in approximately 80% of patients. Selegiline improves hypersomnolence and cataplexy through REM suppression and an increase in REM latency. Methylphenidate and amphetamines alone are usually ineffective for complete relief of cataplexy.

Sodium oxybate (γ-hydroxybutyrate, Xyrem) improves symptoms of EDS and decreases episodes of sleep paralysis, cataplexy, and hypnagogic hallucinations. Nightly administration of sodium oxybate changes sleep architecture to resemble normal sleep. It increases slow-wave sleep, decreases nighttime awakenings, and increases REM efficiency.[59] Sodium oxybate is available only as a liquid and is taken as two doses; one is taken at bedtime and the second dose is taken 2.5 to 4 hours later. Sodium oxybate is a potent sedative–hypnotic and should not be used concomitantly with any other sedating medications. The most common side effects include nausea, somnolence, confusion, dizziness, and incontinence.

Evaluation of Therapeutic Outcomes

Patients with narcolepsy should keep a diary of the frequency and severity of cataplexy, sleep paralysis, and sleep hallucinations. Patients should be evaluated regularly during medication titrations and then every 6 to 12 months to assess for adverse drug effects (eg, sleep disturbances, hypertension, and cardiovascular abnormalities). The healthcare provider should consider the benefit-to-risk ratio for the individual patient, the cost of medication, the convenience of administration, and the cost of laboratory tests when selecting narcolepsy therapies.[54] One wake-promoting agent may work better than another in an individual patient. Thus, if one agent is not effective at adequate doses, a trial with another agent should be undertaken.

CIRCADIAN RHYTHM DISORDERS

The sleep–wake cycle is under the circadian control of oscillators and can be disrupted by misalignment between an individual's biologic clock and external demands on the sleep cycle. Circadian rhythm sleep disorders usually present with either insomnia or hypersomnia, depending on the individual's performance requirements. Two commonly occurring circadian rhythm sleep disorders are jet lag and shift work sleep problems.

Jet Lag

Jet lag occurs when a person travels across time zones, and the external environmental time is mismatched with the internal circadian clock. Sleep disturbances typically last for 2 to 3 days but can last as long as 7 to 10 days if the time zone changes are more than 8 hours. Compared with westward travel, eastward travel is associated with a longer duration of jet lag. Jet lag leads to increased incidence of GI disturbances and a decrease in alertness and performance.

8 Treatment of jet lag includes nonpharmacologic approaches alone or in combination with drug therapy. Jet lag can be minimized in coast-to-coast travel in the United States if the duration is less than 7 days and the normal sleep–wake cycle is observed. For travel lasting longer than 7 days, jet lag severity can be lessened by 1- to 2-hour adjustments in sleep and wake times prior to departure to the destination time zone. Short-acting BZDRAs, ramelteon, and 0.5 to 5 mg melatonin, taken at appropriate target bedtimes for east or west travel, reduce jet lag and shorten sleep latency.[60]

Shift Work Sleep Disorder

Shift workers comprise approximately 20% of the workforce.[61] Night shift work causes a misalignment in the sleep–wake cycle and circadian rhythm that is associated with a decrease in alertness, performance, and quality of daytime sleep. More than 65% of workers on rotating shifts complain of insomnia, compared with only 20% who work one shift.[62] Shift workers ultimately are at risk of developing shift work sleep disorder (SWSD). SWSD is a complaint of insomnia or excessive sleepiness that occurs because of circadian sleep disruption due to working shifts during normal sleep time.[9,61] Shift workers have a higher injury rate, divorce rate, occurrence of on-the-job sleepiness, and incidence of substance use. They may also be at increased risk of developing peptic ulcers, depression, breast cancer, and sleepiness-related accidents.[61-63] Night shift workers are usually in a state of permanent circadian misalignment because of the tendency to revert to conventional sleep schedules on nonwork days.[62]

Treatment for shift work sleep problems includes optimizing sleep hygiene, extending daytime sleep by sleeping in the afternoon, scheduling a 2- to 3-hour nap on days off from work, or switching to a day shift job. Short-acting BZDRAs, ramelteon, and melatonin can consolidate sleep during day sleep periods and reduce lost sleep time. Modafinil and armodafinil are FDA-approved to improve wakefulness in patients with EDS associated with SWSD. Scheduled exposure to bright lights at night and darkness in the daytime improves adaptation to night work and daytime sleep.[62]

Restless Legs Syndrome

RLS, or Ekbom syndrome, is characterized by paresthesias that are usually felt deep in the calf muscles but can also appear in the thighs and arms with the urge to keep limbs in motion. RLS occurs in both males and females, and it occurs more frequently in the elderly. It has been associated with chronic kidney disease, iron deficiency, and pregnancy. Caffeine, stress, alcohol, and fatigue can worsen symptoms. Data suggest that RLS can be caused by iron deficiency in the substantia nigra in the CNS.[64] The diagnosis of RLS is based on patient- or partner-reported symptoms and specific diagnostic criteria. Criteria required to diagnose RLS include (a) an urge to move the limbs that is usually associated with uncomfortable and unpleasant sensations, (b) symptoms that begin or worsen during rest or inactivity, (c) symptoms that are exclusively present or worse in the evening or night, and (d) symptoms that are temporarily relieved by movement.[65] The discomfort returns when the person tries to sleep, resulting in insomnia. Practice parameter recommendations for treatment of RLS are shown in Table 72-5.

9 Dopamine agonists are standard therapy for RLS but have adverse effects that require careful monitoring by patients and providers. Dopamine agonists ropinirole, pramipexole, and rotigotine are FDA-approved for RLS treatment.[66] Lower doses of dopamine agonists are used when treating RLS compared with Parkinson disease. Providers should caution patients that compulsive behaviors (eg, gambling, shopping, eating, etc) and sudden periods of extreme sleepiness may emerge during therapy with dopamine agonists. Levodopa therapy is associated with a high incidence of symptom augmentation and, because of a short half-life, might not provide relief over the entire night. Augmentation is a worsening in symptom severity, increase in symptom distribution, or emergence of symptoms earlier in the evening. Sedative–hypnotic agents can be effective in patients who have frequent awakenings from their RLS symptoms. Clonazepam at doses ranging from 0.5 to 2 mg has been most frequently studied; however, patients may experience carryover sedation because of its long duration of action. Shorter half-life sedative–hypnotics (eg, zolpidem, zaleplon) can improve sleep and reduce daytime sleepiness without carryover sedation. Opiates such as methadone 5 to 20 mg, codeine 30 to 120 mg, and oxycodone 2.5 mg are effective for patients with painful RLS. The potential for tolerance and dependence on opiate therapy should be considered. Gabapentin 300 to 900 mg near bedtime can also be considered for those with paresthetic or painful RLS symptoms.[67] Gabapentin enacarbil (Horizant) is a gabapentin prodrug that is now FDA-approved for the treatment of RLS at a dose of 600 mg taken at 5 PM. Iron studies should be completed in patients with RLS and iron supplementation initiated in those who are iron-deficient. In patients with ferritin concentrations below 50 to 75 ng/mL (mcg/L), iron supplementation improves RLS symptoms.[68] Patients with RLS or PLMS should be evaluated regularly to monitor for excessive daytime somnolence, tolerance, efficacy, and adverse effects of the medication. Therapy should be monitored for adverse effects found in Table 72-6.

TABLE 72-5 Evidence-Based Guidelines for Drug Therapy of RLS

Medication Recommendation[a] (Brand Name)	Strength of Recommendation[b]	Body of Evidence Level[c]
Pramipexole (Mirapex)	Standard	High
Ropinirole (Requip)	Standard	High
Levodopa and dopa decarboxylase inhibitor (Sinemet)	Guideline	High
Opioids (eg, codeine, oxycodone, hydrocodone, methadone)	Guideline	Low
Gabapentin enacarbil (Horizant)	Guideline	High
Gabapentin[d] (Neurontin)	Option	Low
Carbamazepine (Tegretol)	Option	Low
Clonidine (Catapres)	Option	Low
Supplemental iron[e]	Option	Very low

RLS, restless legs syndrome.

[a]At the time of publishing, rotigotine was not available in the United States, thus, no recommendations were made for rotigotine in the published practice parameters.

[b]"Standard" indicates recommendations for which there is high or moderate quality of evidence where the benefits clearly outweigh the harms; "Guideline" indicates low quality of evidence where benefits clearly outweigh the harms, or high or moderate quality of evidence when the benefits are closely balanced with harm/burden or there is uncertainty about the benefits/harms/burdens.

[c]Level of evidence: High, very confident in effect estimate of agent; Moderate, moderately confident in effect estimate; Low, limited confidence in effect estimate; Very low, very little confidence in effect estimate.

[d]Pregabalin is recommended similarly to gabapentin.

[e]In patients with low serum ferritin concentrations.

Data from reference 66.

TABLE 72-6 Monitoring Patients Taking Medications for RLS and PLMS

Drug or Drug Class	Adverse Drug Reaction	Monitoring Parameter	Comments
Dopamine agonists	Compulsive behaviors	Frequency and quantity of eating, gambling, shopping, other reward behaviors	May occur at any time during therapy
Levodopa/carbidopa	Symptom augmentation	Location and timing of RLS irsymptoms	Appearance of symptoms in other areas of body and earlier in day
Gabapentin/Pregabalin	Dizziness	Subjective dizziness, falls	—
Sedative hypnotics (clonazepam, temazepam, zolpidem, etc)	Carryover sedation	Morning sleepiness, grogginess	More likely to occur with longer duration agents
Opioids (oxycodone, codeine, hydrocodone, etc)	Tolerance, constipation	Patient RLS symptoms and response to ongoing therapy	—
Oral iron therapy (ferrous sulfate, etc)	GI upset, constipation	Monitor for constipation	Prophylactic stool softeners may be necessary to reduce risk of constipation

GI, gastrointestinal; PLMS, periodic limb movements of sleep; RLS, restless leg syndrome.

Periodic Limb Movements of Sleep

RLS patients commonly have PLMS, while approximately one-third of patients with PLMS have RLS.[65] PLMS are stereotypic, repetitive, periodic movements of the legs that occur during sleep every 20 to 40 seconds and last 10 minutes to several hours.[66] The movements usually involve the big toe, but the ankle, knee, and hip can also flex. They can be terminated by a violent kick or other body movement. Often patients will be unaware of these movements and only recognize consequent insufficient sleep and morning leg cramps. A bed partner can describe PLMS. PLMS is diagnosed in the sleep laboratory using electromyogram recordings.

PLMS can occur with RLS or alone because of systemic disease (eg, renal failure) or drug therapy.[69] TCAs, SSRIs, dopaminergic antagonists, xanthines, nicotine, alcohol, and caffeine can all worsen PLMS. The treatment approach for PLMS is similar to that of RLS. If PLMS do not cause disruptions for the patient or bed partner or daytime symptoms, they may not require treatment. Symptomatic or problematic PLMS should be treated with dopaminergic medications to suppress limb movements or sedative–hypnotics to reduce awakenings and consolidate sleep.

PARASOMNIAS

Parasomnias are abnormal behavior or physiologic events that either occur during sleep or are exaggerated by sleep. Many of these disorders are considered to be disorders of partial arousal from various sleep stages. Parasomnias can be categorized as disorders of arousal (sleepwalking, sleep terrors), sleep–wake transition disorders (sleeptalking), rhythmic movement disorder, REM parasomnias (REM behavior disorder, nightmares), and miscellaneous parasomnias (enuresis, bruxism). Sleepwalking, sleep terrors, and sleep-talking predominantly occur during NREM sleep, whereas others (REM behavior disorder) occur during REM sleep.

Sleepwalking and sleep terrors are found normally in children between the ages of 4 and 12 years and usually resolve in adolescence. These disorders are increasingly recognized to also occur in adulthood, and, contrary to previous beliefs, are not related to psychological or psychiatric pathology.[70] Sleep terrors can begin in adults between the ages of 20 and 30 years. Onset of sleepwalking in adults without a childhood history of sleepwalking should prompt a search for a neurologic or substance use condition.[71] Sleepwalking and sleep terror disorder involve intrusions of wakefulness into NREM sleep during the first third of the night. In sleepwalking, individuals become ambulatory, are difficult to awaken, and are amnestic for the event. Sleep terrors involve intense fear and autonomic arousal. Individuals are difficult to awaken, inconsolable, and amnestic for the event.[71] Patients with REM behavior disorder act out their dreams, often in a violent manner, and are at risk for injury.

Treatment of sleepwalking involves protecting the individual from harm by putting safety latches on doors and windows, removing hazardous objects from bedrooms, and covering glass doors with heavy curtains. In adult patients, benzodiazepines, SSRIs, or TCAs can be beneficial therapies for sleepwalking or other NREM disorders of arousal.[70] Benzodiazepines can also be helpful in curtailing sleep terrors in adults.[71] Nightmares are anxiety-provoking dreams characterized by vivid recall. Treatment is directed at reducing stress, anxiety, and sleep deprivation. In extreme cases, low-dose benzodiazepines can be indicated. Clonazepam is the treatment of choice for REM behavior disorder. Melatonin (3-12 mg at bedtime) and pramipexole can also be an effective therapy for REM behavior disorder.[72]

PERSONALIZATION OF THERAPY

For the treatment of insomnia, the choice of a particular BZDRA can be based on its pharmacokinetic profile. When used as a single dose, extent of distribution and elimination half-life are important in predicting the duration of action. However, after multiple doses, the elimination half-life and formation of active metabolites determine the extent of drug accumulation and resultant clinical effects.[11] Advanced age, liver dysfunction, and drug interactions can prolong drug effects. The pharmacokinetic profiles of BZDRAs are summarized in Table 72-3. To individualize treatment of narcolepsy many clinicians prescribe both immediate-release and sustained-release stimulants to increase alertness throughout the day. Sustained-release stimulants are prescribed with scheduled administration times, and immediate-release stimulants can be taken as needed when the patient requires alertness (eg, driving, etc).

ABBREVIATIONS

ACE	angiotensin-converting enzyme
AutoPAP	Auto-titrating positive airway pressure
BZDRA	benzodiazepine receptor agonist
CNS	central nervous system
CPAP	continuous positive airway pressure
CSA	central sleep apnea
CSF	cerebrospinal fluid
DSM-5	*Diagnostic and Statistical Manual of Mental Disorders,* Fifth Edition
EDS	excessive daytime sleepiness
EEG	electroencephalogram
FDA	Food and Drug Administration
GABA	γ-aminobutyric acid
GI	gastrointestinal
HLA	human leukocyte antigen

NREM	nonrapid eye movement
OSA	obstructive sleep apnea
PAP	positive airway pressure
PLMS	periodic limb movements of sleep
PSG	polysomnography
RDI	respiratory disturbance index
REM	rapid eye movement
RLS	restless legs syndrome
SWSD	shift work sleep disorder
SNRI	serotonin norepinephrine reuptake inhibitor
SSRI	Selective serotonin reuptake inhibitor
TCA	tricyclic antidepressant

REFERENCES

1. Walsh JK, Engelhardt CL. The direct economic costs of insomnia in the United States for 1995. *Sleep* 1999;22:S386-S393.
2. Neylan TC, Reynolds CF III, Kupfer DJ. Sleep disorders. In: Yudofsky SC, Hales RE, eds. *American Psychiatric Press Textbook of Neuropsychiatry*, 4th ed. Washington, DC: American Psychiatric Press; 2003:975-1000.
3. Benca RM, Cirelli C, Rattenborg NC, Tononi G. Basic science of sleep. In: Sadock BJ, Sadock VA, eds. *Kaplan and Sadock's Comprehensive Textbook of Psychiatry,* 8th ed. Philadelphia, PA: Lippincott Williams & Wilkins; 2005:280-294.
4. Dagan Y, Abadi J. Sleep–wake disorder disability: A lifelong untreatable pathology of the circadian time structure. *Chronobiol Int* 2001;18:1019-1027.
5. Franken P. Long-term versus short-term processes regulating REM sleep. *J Sleep Res* 2002;11:17-28.
6. Stickgold R, Hobson JA, Fosse R, Fosse M. Sleep, learning and dreams: Off-line memory reprocessing. *Science* 2001;294:1052-1058.
7. American Psychiatric Association. Sleep-wake disorders. In: *Diagnostic and Statistical Manual of Mental Disorders,* 5th ed. 2013. Available at: http://dx.doi.org/10.1176/appi.books.9780890425596.dsm12. Accessed November 1, 2015.
8. Schutte-Rodin S, Broch L, Buysse D, et al. Clinical guideline for the evaluation and management of chronic insomnia in adults. *J Clin Sleep Med* 2008;4:487-504.
9. American Academy of Sleep Medicine. *International Classification of Sleep Disorders: Diagnostic and Coding Manual*, 3rd ed. Westchester, Ill: American Academy of Sleep Medicine; 2014.
10. Chesson AL, Anderson WM, Littner M, et al. Practice parameters for the nonpharmacologic treatment of chronic insomnia. *Sleep* 1999;8:1-6.
11. Kirkwood CK. Management of insomnia. *J Am Pharm Assoc* 1999;39:688-696.
12. Sateia MJ, Doghramji K, Hauri PJ, et al. Evaluation of chronic insomnia. *Sleep* 2000;23:1-39.
13. Lippmann S, Mazour I, Shabab H. Insomnia: Therapeutic approach. *South Med J* 2001;94:866-874.
14. Vaughn-McCall W. A psychiatric perspective on insomnia. *J Clin Psychiatr* 2001;62(Suppl 10):27-32.
15. Morgenthaler TI, Kramer M, Alessi C, et al. Practice parameters for the psychological and behavioral treatment of insomnia: An update. An American Academy of Sleep Medicine report. *Sleep* 2006;29:1415-1419.
16. Sivertsen B, Omvik S, Pallesen S, et al. Cognitive behavioral therapy vs zopiclone for treatment of chronic primary insomnia in older adults: A randomized controlled trial. *JAMA* 2006;295:2851-2858.
17. Hauri PJ. Insomnia. *Clin Chest Med* 1998;19:157-168.
18. Trazodone [Product Information]. Weston, FL: Apotex Corp; 2014.
19. Belsomra, suvorexant [Product Information]. Whitehouse Station, NJ: Merck and Co., Inc.; 2014.
20. Kryger M, Roth T, Wang-Weigand S, et al. The effects of ramelteon on respiration during sleep in subjects with moderate to severe chronic obstructive pulmonary disease. *Sleep* Breath 2009;13:79-84.
21. Kryger M, Wang-Weigand S, Roth T. Safety of ramelteon in individuals with mild to moderate obstructive sleep apnea. *Sleep Breath* 2007;11:159-164.
22. Schulz V, Hansel R, Tyler VE. *Rational Phytotherapy: A Physician's Guide to Herbal Medicine*. Berlin: Springer; 1998:81.
23. Stone KL, Ensrud KE, Ancoli-Israel S. Sleep, insomnia and falls in elderly patients. *Sleep* Med 2008;9(Suppl 1):S18-S22.
24. Terzano MG, Rossi M, Palomba V, et al. New drugs for insomnia: Comparative tolerability of zopiclone, zolpidem and zaleplon. *Drug Saf* 2003;26:261-282.
25. Ambien, zolpidem [product information]. Bridgewater, NJ: Sanofi-Aventis; 2012.
26. Elie R, Ruteher E, Farr IK, et al. Sleep latency is shortened during 4 weeks of treatment with zaleplon, a novel nonbenzodiazepine hypnotic. *J Clin Psychiatry* 1999;60:536-544.
27. Walsh JK, Fry J, Erwin CS, et al. Efficacy and tolerability of 14-day administration of zaleplon 5 mg and 10 mg for the treatment of primary insomnia. *Clin Drug Investig* 1998;16:347-354.
28. Walsh JK, Pollack CP, Shark MMB, et al. Lack of residual sedation following middle-of-the-night zaleplon administration in sleep maintenance insomnia. *Clin Neuropharmacol* 2000;23:17-21.
29. Lunesta, eszopiclone [product information]. Marlborough, MA: Sunovion; 2010.
30. Krystal AD, Walsh JK, Laska E, et al. Sustained efficacy of eszopiclone over 6 months of nightly treatment: Results of a randomized, double-blind, placebo-controlled study in adults with chronic insomnia. *Sleep* 2003;26:793-797.
31. Jermaine DM. Sleep disorders. In: Carter BL, Angaran DM, Lake KD, Raebel MA, eds. *Pharmacotherapy Self-Assessment Program,* 2nd ed. Psychiatry Module. Kansas City: American College of Clinical Pharmacy; 1995:139-154.
32. Young T, Peppard PE, Gottlieb DJ. Epidemiology of obstructive sleep apnea: A population health perspective. *Am J Respir Crit Care Med* 2002;165:1217-1239.
33. Young T, Palta M, Dempsey J, et al. The occurrence of sleep-disordered breathing among middle-aged adults. *N Engl J Med* 1993;328:1230-1235.
34. Peppard PE, Szklo-Coxe M, Hla KM, Young T. Longitudinal association of sleep-related breathing disorder and depression. *Arch Intern Med* 2006;166:1709-1715.
35. Young T, Finn L, Peppard PE, et al. Sleep disordered breathing and mortality: Eighteen-year follow-up of the Wisconsin sleep cohort. *Sleep* 2008;31:1071-1078.
36. Terán-Santos J, Jimenez-Gomez A, Cordero-Guevara J. The association between sleep apnea and the risk of traffic accidents. *N Engl J Med* 1999;340:847-851.
37. Somers VK, White DP, Amin R, et al. Sleep apnea and cardiovascular disease: An American Heart Association/American College of Cardiology Foundation scientific statement from the American Heart Association Council for High Blood Pressure Research Professional Education Committee, Council on Clinical Cardiology, Stroke Council, and Council on Cardiovascular Nursing. *J Am Coll Cardiol* 2008;52:686-717.
38. Calhoun DA, Jones D, Textor S, et al. Resistant hypertension: Diagnosis, evaluation, and treatment: A scientific statement from the American Heart Association Professional Education Committee of the Council for High Blood Pressure Research. *Circulation* 2008;117:e510-e526.
39. Marin JM, Agusti A, Villar I, et al. Association between treated and untreated obstructive sleep apnea and risk of hypertension. *JAMA* 2012;307:2169-2176.
40. Kato M, Roberts-Thomson P, Phillips BG, et al. Impairment of endothelium dependent vasodilation of resistance vessels in patients with obstructive sleep apnea. *Circulation* 2000;102:2607-2610.
41. Morganthaler TI, Kapen S, Lee-Chiong T, et al. Practice parameters for the medical therapy of obstructive sleep apnea. *Sleep* 2006;29:1031-1035.
42. Kribbs NB, Pack AJ, Kline LR, et al. Effects of one night without nasal CPAP treatment on sleep and sleepiness in patients with obstructive sleep apnea. *Am Rev Respir Dis* 2003;147:1162-1168.
43. Peppard PE, Young T, Palta M, et al. Longitudinal study of moderate weight change and sleep-disordered breathing. *JAMA* 2000;284:3015-3021.
44. Ferguson KA, Cartwright R, Rogers R, et al. Oral appliances for snoring and obstructive sleep apnea: A review. *Sleep* 2006;29:244-262.
45. Aurora RN, Chowdhuri S, Ramar K, et al. The treatment of central sleep apnea syndromes in adults: Practice parameters with an evidence-based literature review and meta-analyses. *Sleep* 2012;35:17-40.
46. Javaheri S. Acetazolamide improves central sleep apnea in heart failure: A double-blind, prospective study. *Am J Respir Crit Care Med* 2006;173:234-237.
47. Javaheri S, Parker TJ, Wexler L, et al. Effect of theophylline on sleep-disordered breathing in heart failure. *N Engl J Med* 1996;335:562-567.
48. Mitler M, Hayduk R. Benefits and risks of pharmacotherapy for narcolepsy. *Drug Saf* 2002;25:791-809.
49. Nishino S, Ripley B, Overeem S, et al. Low cerebrospinal fluid hypocretin (orexin) and altered energy homeostasis in human narcolepsy. *Ann Neurol* 2001;50:381-388.
50. Thannicakal TC, Moore RY, Nienhuis R, et al. Reduced number of hypocretin neurons in human narcolepsy. *Neuron* 2000;27:469-474.

51. Lin L, Hungs M, Mignot E. Narcolepsy and the HLA region. *J Neuroimmunol* 2001;117:9-20.
52. Mignot E, Thorsby E. Narcolepsy and the HLA system [letter]. *N Engl J Med* 2001;344:692.
53. Nakayama J, Miura M, Honda M, et al. Linkage of human narcolepsy with HLA association to chromosome 4p-13-q21. *Genomics* 2000;65:84-86.
54. Duffy J, Weintraub E, Vellozzi C, DeStefano F, et al. Narcolepsy and influenza A (H1N1) pandemic 2009 vaccination in the United States. *Neurology* 2014;83:1823-1830.
55. Morgenthaler TI, Kapur VK, Brown T, et al. Practice parameters for the treatment of narcolepsy and other hypersomnias of central origin. *Sleep* 2007;30:1705-1711.
56. Robertson P, Hellriegel ET. Clinical pharmacokinetic profile of modafinil. *Clin Pharmacokinet* 2003;42:123-127.
57. Feldman N. Narcolepsy. *South Med J* 2003;96:277-287.
58. Rosenthal MS. Physiology and neurochemistry of sleep. *Am J Pharm Educ* 1998;62:204-208.
59. Mamelak M, Black J, Montplaisir J, et al. A pilot study of the effects of sodium oxybate on sleep architecture and daytime alertness in narcolepsy. *Sleep* 2004;27:1327-1334.
60. Herxheimer A, Petrie KJ. Cochrane Depression, Anxiety and Neurosis Group. Melatonin for the prevention and treatment of jet lag [systematic review]. *Cochrane Database Syst Rev* 2005;2.
61. Drake CL, Roehrs T, Richardson G, et al. Shift work sleep disorder: Prevalence and consequences beyond that of symptomatic day workers. *Sleep* 2004;27:1453-1462.
62. Garbarino S, Nobili L, Beelke, M, et al. Sleep disorders and daytime sleepiness in state police shiftworkers. *Arch Environ Health* 2002;57:167-175.
63. Knutsson A. Health disorders of shift workers. *Occup Med (Lond)* 2003;53:103-108.
64. Connor JR, Boyer PJ, Menzies SL, et al. Neuropathological examination suggests impaired brain iron acquisition in restless legs syndrome. *Neurology* 2003;61:304-309.
65. Allen RP, Picchietti D, Hening W, et al. Restless legs syndrome: Diagnostic criteria, special considerations and epidemiology: A report from the restless legs syndrome diagnosis and epidemiology workshop at the National Institutes of Health. *Sleep Med* 2003;4:101-119.
66. Aurora RN, Kristo DA, Bista SR, et al. The treatment of restless legs syndrome and periodic limb movement disorder in adults—An update for 2012: Practice parameters with an evidence-based systematic review and meta-analyses. *Sleep* 2012;35:1039-1062.
67. Garcia-Borreguero D, Larrosa O, de la Llave Y, et al. Treatment of restless legs syndrome with gabapentin: A double-blind, cross-over study. *Neurology* 2002;59:1573-1575.
68. Wang J, O'Reilly B, Venkataraman R, et al. Efficacy of oral iron in patients with restless legs syndrome and low-normal ferritin: A randomized, double-blind, placebo-controlled study. *Sleep Med* 2009;10:973-975.
69. Montplaisir J, Nicolas A, Denesle R, Gomez-Mancilla B. Restless legs syndrome improved by pramipexole: A double-blind randomized trial. *Neurology* 1999;52:938-943.
70. Mahowald MW, Cramer Bornemann MA. NREM arousal parasomnias. In: Kryger MH, Roth T, Dement WC, eds. *Principles and Practice of Sleep Medicine,* 5th ed. St. Louis: Elsevier Saunders, 2011:1075-1082.
71. Schenck CH, Mahowald MW. Parasomnias managing bizarre sleep-related behavior disorders. *Postgrad Med* 2000;107:145-156.
72. Mahowald MW, Schenck CH. REM sleep parasomnias. In: Kryger MH, Roth T, Dement WC, eds. *Principles and Practice of Sleep Medicine,* 5th ed. St. Louis: Elsevier Saunders, 2011:1083-1097.

Disorders Associated with Intellectual Disabilities

73

Nancy C. Brahm, Steven R. Erickson, and Douglas W. Stewart

KEY CONCEPTS

1. Persons diagnosed with Down syndrome (DS) can be at increased risk for medical and psychiatric comorbidities.
2. In persons with DS, a thorough evaluation is needed to differentiate between depression and Alzheimer disease.
3. Treatment plans for persons with autism spectrum disorder (ASD) focus on increasing social interactions, improving verbal and nonverbal communication, and minimizing the occurrence or impact of ritualistic, repetitive behaviors and other related mood and behavioral problems (eg, overactivity, irritability, and self-injury).
4. Many purported pharmacologic and nonpharmacologic treatments for ASD lack objective evidence-based support.
5. A structured teaching approach focusing on increasing social communication and integration with peers is needed when providing services to persons with ASD.
6. Nonpharmacologic interventions for sleep disturbances in children with a diagnosis of ASD should be implemented prior to pharmacotherapy considerations.
7. Psychopharmacologic treatment planning should include monitoring of objective, measurable, medication-responsive target behaviors, and assessment of potential adverse effects is of critical importance when treating behavioral symptoms of ASD, as the response of individuals to medication therapy is highly variable.
8. The use of Food and Drug Administration-approved medication for off-label indications is an acceptable clinical practice if founded on evidence-based research and informed consent.
9. The level of impairment in Rett syndrome (RTT) is increasingly associated with the particular genetic mutation involved.

INTRODUCTION

Intellectual disabilities (IDs) can be identified in childhood or adolescence. Current criteria for diagnosis are based on deficiencies in intellectual and adaptive functioning with an onset during the developmental period.[1] This diagnosis is made regardless of the presence or absence of concomitant medical or psychiatric disorders. In the case of mild ID, deficiencies may not be apparent in early life. Problems can be noted when the chronologic age of the child and the developmental milestones achieved by peers with similar backgrounds, cultures, socioeconomic status, and psychosocial settings differ significantly.[1] These gaps between developmental advances widen as the individual ages. Adaptive functioning deficits pose a number of challenges in treating those with an ID.

Whereas it has been estimated that a psychiatric disorder may beset approximately one-fifth of the general population in the United States,[2] the prevalence may range widely from approximately 7% to 97% for persons with an ID, largely a function of diagnostic criteria and study design.[3] Similarly, the impact of life events, the stress of these events, and limited coping skills may also contribute.[4] Underrecognition of the need for mental health services may be due to a lack of caregiver awareness of psychiatric disorders in persons with IDs and/or insufficient provider training and clinical experience with this population.[2] Additional barriers to accurate diagnosis may arise from deficits in adaptive functioning, a mechanism by which individuals effectively manage commonly encountered life demands and independence compared with nondevelopmentally disabled peers.[1] Communication deficits are a barrier-specific to this population. Furthermore, problematic behaviors that may arise limit opportunities for those with an ID to experience more social interactions and limit integration into the community.[3]

Another potential problem for the clinician assessing persons with an ID is a significant gap between receptive and expressive language skills. If not readily recognized, intellectual capabilities can be overestimated, resulting in incongruent expectations and/or abilities. In the general population, features of psychiatric illnesses are more readily identifiable, and the clinician is able to effectively interview and evaluate the patient. The term "diagnostic overshadowing" has been used to refer to clinician perceptions that behavioral problems are secondary to an ID and not the result of a psychiatric comorbidity.[5]

The term "mental retardation" is no longer used, replaced with "intellectual disability" (ID).[1] The American Association on Intellectual and Developmental Disabilities (AAIDD) supports this designation and has a definition on their Web site.[6] The change reinforces the concept that an intellectual disability is not "an absolute, invariate trait of the person" but recognizes the impart of the environment, individual supports, and personhood.[7] For this chapter, the designation "ID" will be applied to the population of individuals who require varying levels of support due to limitations in general mental abilities that result in impairment of adaptive functioning, with an onset during the developmental period, in more than one area and at home or in the community.[1] This chapter focuses on Down syndrome (DS), autism spectrum disorder (ASD), and Rett syndrome (RTT).

DOWN SYNDROME

1 DS is associated with common dysmorphic features and a wide range of medical and psychiatric concerns, including a number of developmental abnormalities. Congenital heart defects, seizures, orthopedic abnormalities, sensory defects, and disorders of the eye (eg, cataracts and glaucoma), gastrointestinal (GI) tract, immune system, skin, and thyroid gland are all associated with DS. Persons diagnosed with DS also have a high probability (30%) of early onset Alzheimer disease (AD).[8] This section will focus on DS and the comorbidities of AD and leukemia.

CLINICAL PRESENTATION Intellectual Disability

General

- Limitations in intellectual functioning and adaptive behavior.
- Onset before 18 years, which may also be referred to as the developmental period.

Specific Activities or Knowledge Impacted

- Limitations are considered within the framework of the individual's community, culture, and age.
- Problems in understanding and applying abstract relationships, such as problem solving, planning, and learning from experience. Standardized intelligence testing may be used to provide a numerical value and help determine limitations.
- Unable to meet developmental and sociocultural standards for personal independence and social responsibility when compared to peers of the same age and culture.
- Ongoing support(s) needed in one or more areas of daily life, such as communication and/or social participation and independent living.
- Independent living may require supports that may be needed in more than one setting: home, school/work or community and the use of long-term personalized supports will improve life functionality.
- Strengths and limitations are both present.
- The term "mental retardation" did not represent the scope of individual accomplishments of which each individual may be capable and was replaced with "ID."

Data from references 1, 6, and 7.

Epidemiology

DS is the most frequently occurring genetically based syndrome associated with an ID.[9] The incidence ranges from 1 in 650 to 1,000 births.[9]

Etiology and Pathophysiology

The etiology of DS is the presence of an extra chromosome 21. DS, also referred to as trisomy 21, represents one of the most studied abnormal chromosomal conditions. Nondisjunction of chromosome 21 accounts for the majority of the characteristics associated with DS. Chromosomes divide and separate in a process known as disjunction during meiotic division. Failure to fully separate at this stage can result in both chromosomes remaining in the same cell, creating an abnormal number of chromosomes on each strand. The nondisjunction at chromosome 21 is strongly linked to increased maternal age. For many years, advanced maternal age has been recognized to positively correlate with an increased risk for DS, particularly over age 35 years.[9] Consideration has been given to paternal age as a potential risk factor for DS. An analysis by Steiner and colleagues found that for couples with younger fathers, the odds of having a child with DS were increased almost twofold,[10] whereas Fisch and colleagues found that older fathers in combination with older mothers, when both were 35 years or older, significantly impacted the incidence of DS.[11]

It has been theorized that two variables, lack of maternal folic acid supplementation, and genetic variability that decreases enzymatic processes in folate pathways, may negatively impact meiotic nondisjunction of chromosome 21. Questionnaire data from the National Down Syndrome Project were analyzed. No association between supplementation use and nondisjunction was found based on maternal age and ethnicity, but an association was found between older maternal age and meiosis II nondisjunction. Hollis and colleagues opined that this could explain previously reported differences in findings; additional confirmation, controlling for maternal age, is needed.[12]

Clinical Presentation and Diagnosis

The consequences of this chromosomal variance include characteristic facial features, some degree of ID, hypotonia, an increased risk for congenital heart disease, and early onset AD.[13,14] The characteristic facial features make children with DS more readily identifiable at birth. IDs range from mild to severe.[13]

For the purpose of this chapter, the term *dual diagnosis* refers to an intellectually disabled person with a comorbid psychiatric disorder.[2] Psychiatric and/or behavioral disorders, such as depression and anxiety in persons with an ID, may result from environmental variables (relocation, change in caregivers), personal variables (age, level of disability, comorbid medical conditions), and the extent to which the individual can cope. The association between life events with depression and anxiety was researched in a community-based population receiving services from three organizations (n = 988, 509 male, 479 female, mean age 61 years). Variables assessed were age, sex, ID, residential setting, and history of depression or anxiety, using a 28-item checklist for life events. Depression and anxiety instruments included the Inventory of Depressive Symptomatology Self Reports and the Glasgow Anxiety Scale of people with an Intellectual Disability. Almost all of the study population (979 of 988, 99.1%) had been exposed to at least one life event during the prior 12-month period. As anticipated, the cohort of persons 65-years or older experienced more events.[4] The authors also found associations between major depression, generalized anxiety disorder, panic disorder, and the number of negative life events.[4]

This has implications for depression in persons with DS. A review of the literature found the majority of the information on pharmacotherapy was derived from case reports. Selective serotonin reuptake inhibitors (SSRIs) and amitriptyline have been used successfully, but desipramine was not effective.[15]

The differential diagnosis for mood disorders in all patients should include an evaluation of thyroid function. The risk of a thyroid disorder as a comorbidity in people with DS is estimated at 4% to 18%.[14] Because clinical signs and symptoms of hypothyroidism and dementia can mimic some of the features of depression, thyroid function and changes in cognition should be evaluated in patients with DS.[15]

TREATMENT
Down Syndrome

Desired Outcomes

Treatment goals in DS are to identify medical and psychiatric comorbidities, set realistic goals, and provide effective nonpharmacologic and pharmacologic interventions to improve the quality and length of life.

CLINICAL PRESENTATION Down Syndrome

General

- Individual may have the characteristic physical features described below.

Diagnostic Features

- Facial features can suggest DS, but an additional diagnostic evaluation is necessary.
- Degree of ID ranges from mild to severe.
- Growth delays are common.

Common Physical Characteristics

- Hypotonia can be evident at birth.
- Facial features include flat nasal bridge and profile, with upslanted eye folds.
- The palate can be narrow and the neck thick and broad.
- Hands are characteristically short and broad.

Other Clinical Concerns

- An increased risk for congenital heart problems; a cardiac evaluation is generally done shortly after birth with periodic follow-up.
- Congenital cataracts, hearing problems, and hypothyroidism are common.
- Leukemia is often diagnosed in early childhood.
- Features of AD can present by the third or fourth decade.
- Heart problems, conditions related to AD, and leukemia are common causes of death.

Data from references 13, 14, and 17.

General Approach

Medical screenings should assess for hypothyroidism, cardiac problems, sensory impairments (including hearing loss secondary to chronic otitis media with effusion or vision defects due to congenital cataracts or glaucoma), and GI problems (including constipation and celiac disease).[14] Guidelines for health supervision and anticipatory guidance in infants, children, and adolescents with DS are available through the American Academy of Pediatrics (AAP).[14] Routine screenings are also recommended throughout life to address psychosocial changes, potential residential or vocational stressors, and the consequences of aging.[14]

Nonpharmacologic Treatments

The use of social supports for both individuals with DS and their family is known to facilitate development of functional adaptive skills.[14] Family education and development of a support network assist caregivers by providing tools and resources necessary to enable persons with DS to achieve their full potential. In the treatment of psychiatric disorders, treatment modalities useful in the general population are also applicable to those with DS. Nonpharmacologic options for depression include psychotherapy and electroconvulsive therapy (ECT).[15] Information on the effectiveness of ECT in the DS population is limited to case reports. If communication skills are adequate, psychotherapy may also be an option, including psychodynamic psychotherapy and cognitive behavior therapy (CBT). A review of the literature found that psychotherapy applicability can vary with the level of ID. For persons with mild intellectual impairment and depression, this treatment modality may be beneficial. The current behavioral therapy models are more effective in addressing specific problematic behaviors rather than the underlying emotional problems of persons with ID. Usefulness of these strategies for persons with DS and more severe ID is not known.[15]

Pharmacologic Treatments

Pharmacotherapy for the treatment of depression in patients with DS follows guidelines used in the general population. For more information on the treatment of depression, see Chapter 68.

Features of depression commonly seen in persons with DS, in order of frequency, include apathy, disordered sleep, and changes in weight. Difficulty identifying depression in this population is impacted by the level of cognitive impairment, the ability to express abstract concepts (such as helplessness or hopelessness), and the level of adaptive functioning.[15] Clinical trials focused specifically on this population are few, and most information comes from small studies or case reports. Efficacy of SSRIs and amitriptyline is reported. If psychotic features (eg, delusions and hallucinations) are present, low-dose antipsychotic augmentation is recommended. In the studies reviewed, treatment duration was 2 to 3 years.[15]

As with treatment of depression in the general population, it is essential to ensure that the medication trial uses appropriate dose and duration of antidepressant or combination antidepressant/antipsychotic. Ruling out comorbid medical conditions that could contribute to depression is essential.

Personalized Pharmacotherapy

In addition to the chromosomal aberration and dysmorphic features associated with DS, one of the common presenting features of depression is disordered sleep. Obstructive sleep apnea rates are estimated at 50% to 75% in the DS population.[14] Daytime drowsiness and problematic behaviors may be indicative of both an affective disorder, such as depression, and a medical condition secondary to DS. A comprehensive evaluation, including the impact of obesity on sleep, is needed prior to the addition of pharmacotherapy. If pharmacotherapy is indicated, the medication list for each patient should be carefully reviewed for potential drug-drug interactions and drug-disease contraindications.

Evaluation of Therapeutic Outcomes

Assessment of therapeutic outcomes for those with DS starts with a thorough multidisciplinary evaluation to establish a baseline problem list, identification of clear therapeutic goals, and using valid pharmacotherapeutic rationale to guide medication dosing and adverse drug effect monitoring.

An in-depth list of treatment targets, both subjective and objective, is important in persons with DS to assist in evaluation of medication response. Careful monitoring for emergence of potential side effects should be regularly conducted and documented as part of ongoing assessment of medication effectiveness and to ensure that side effects are not a contributing factor to behavioral changes.

Down Syndrome and Alzheimer Disease

2 Persons with DS are at greater risk for AD, and the proportion of the population affected doubles every 5 years through age 60. By age 72, the prevalence is 67%.[16]

In adults with DS, challenging behaviors, such as aggression, stealing, loss of previous skills, and disinhibition, may be a prodromal presentation. Changes in mood and emotional stability may also present.[16] Assessing changes in functionality and cognition are problematic in this population, particularly in those with greater intellectual impairments. Early studies in this population did not specify the criteria used for diagnosing probable or possible AD. A well-delineated diagnosis of major or mild neurocognitive disorder due to AD requires a documented decline from baseline cognitive functioning. It is recommended that baseline status be documented once before 35 years of age with reassessment annually up to every 5 years.[17] To meet the diagnostic criteria, the following are needed: baseline functioning data to assess change, functionality changes not explained by general aging, and progressive decline.[1] Accurate diagnosis requires use of an appropriate assessment scale for those with DS. Specific tools include the Dementia Scale for Down's Syndrome and the Cambridge Examination for Mental Disorders of Older People with Down's Syndrome and Others with Intellectual Disabilities.[17]

Risk factors for AD in those with DS include age, genetics, gender, estrogen, and metabolic syndrome, although information is limited in some areas. In persons older than 40 years with DS, behavior changes, such as fear, sadness, and overall regression, are the primary features of the early stages of dementia. Mood and emotional dyscontrol are reported to occur at the same time as marked adaptive functioning declines.[16] Diagnostic criteria for AD include changes in memory, language skills, and activities of daily living (ADLs). In addition, major functional declines may include behavioral disinhibition, stereotypic or ritualistic behavior, and/or apathy.[1] Information on the natural progression of cognitive changes in those with DS and AD continues to emerge.

Pathophysiology

Neuritic plaques and neurofibrillary tangles are the hallmarks of AD. A gene for amyloid-β precursor protein is located on chromosome 21.[18] The severity of ID has been theorized to significantly impact the incidence of AD, but further study is needed to validate this theory. A study of DS (n = 405) with and without dementia identified specific amyloid-β precursor proteins that might be predictors of dementia in DS regardless of age, gender, and level of ID.[18] A more extensive discussion of the pathophysiology of AD is beyond the scope of this chapter. For more information about AD, see Chapter 54.

TREATMENT

Down Syndrome with Alzheimer Disease

Desired Outcomes

The therapeutic goal is to maintain functioning and quality of life as close to baseline as possible for as long as possible. Approaches to therapy for persons with DS combined with AD include nonpharmacologic and pharmacologic interventions.

Nonpharmacologic Treatments

Traditionally, this population receives some level of residential living supports in either the family home or a residential facility. Depending on the level of ID, a family member, other caregiver, or residential facility staff may provide information to the clinician regarding functional status.

Pharmacologic Treatments

Pharmacologic treatments neither cure nor stop the pathologic changes associated with AD. The goals of pharmacotherapy in persons with DS and AD, as in the general population of AD patients, are to slow the decline in cognitive function and help preserve ADLs to the greatest extent possible. The use of cholinesterase inhibitors and an *N*-methyl-D-aspartate (NMDA) receptor antagonist in the DS population has been studied. Limited trial data exist on the use of memantine in persons with DS over age 40. In one prospective randomized double-blind trial (n = 88), memantine was given for 52 weeks. Inclusion criteria were a diagnosis of DS, with or without dementia, and over 40 years. Both groups declined in cognition and functional abilities.[19]

Trials of cholinesterase inhibitors to enhance learning and memory in persons with DS have had small sample sizes. One trial with promising results is a 24-week, randomized, double-blind, placebo-controlled trial of donepezil in 21 females with DS with severe ID. Treatment arms were placebo or donepezil (3 mg). The assessment instrument was a modified International Classification of Functioning, Disability and Health (ICF) scaling system. The authors reported that the ICF score improvement was significant with donepezil, and it was well tolerated.[20] For more information about pharmacotherapy treatment guidelines in AD, see Chapter 54.

Preexisting medical comorbidities, such as congenital heart defects, or concomitant pharmacotherapy may limit use of cholinesterase inhibitors in persons with DS. Clinicians are encouraged to monitor patients receiving cholinesterase inhibitors for commonly reported adverse drug effects and the potential for drug interactions.

A potential neurologic comorbidity of concern in this population is seizures, and risk increases with age. Distribution of seizure onset is trimodal, with the first peak incidence appearing before 1 year of age (40%; predominantly infantile spasms). The second peak occurs between the ages 20 and 30 years (40%). The final peak corresponds to the onset of Alzheimer-related dementia (20%).[16] Advancing age and a diagnosis of DS are independent risk factors for seizures.[17] Monitoring for new-onset seizure activity and medicating with anticonvulsants, as appropriate, are essential. For more information about epilepsy and seizure disorders, see Chapter 56.

Evaluation of Therapeutic Outcomes

Baseline functioning must be established early in adult life prior to the onset of AD, which generally occurs during the third or fourth decade of life. This is particularly crucial in individuals without expressive language skills. Follow-up evaluations should be performed before age 35 years (at least once) then annually to every 5 years.[16] If cholinesterase inhibitors are used, evaluations every 2 to 4 months (after achieving a maintenance dose) are recommended to monitor for effectiveness. Monitoring for potential medication-related side effects, including diarrhea, nausea, vomiting, insomnia, and headache, is also essential.

Down Syndrome and the Immune System

Leukemia is frequently diagnosed in DS children. The two forms more commonly encountered in DS children are acute lymphoblastic leukemia (ALL) and acute myeloid leukemia (AML). The risk for ALL in a DS child is 10 times, up to 40 times, greater compared to peers in the general population and continues to be elevated until 30 years of age.[21,22] The rate of DS-AML is similarly elevated (150 times greater) in children younger than 5 years of age.[21] The most commonly identified form of DS-AML is acute megakaryoblastic leukemia (AMKL). The incidence of this disorder in DS has been identified as high as 500 times greater than in the non-DS pediatric population. Another myelodysplastic disorder almost unique to children with DS is transient abnormal myeloproliferative (TAM) disorder.

A mutation in the erythroid transcription factor or GATA-binding factor 1 (GATA-1) was suspected and found between TAM and DS-AML, as TAM precedes AML in this population.[21]

In the DS population, ALL survival rates are lower than in the general pediatric population. This may be a function of differences in treatment intensity between DS and non-DS patients[22] and more chemotherapy-related toxicities, such as mucositis and cardiotoxicity, compared with non-DS children with ALL.[23] Chemotherapy-induced cardiotoxicity is of particular concern in children with DS, as 50% may have a congenital heart defect.[14] In those treated with anthracyclines, rates of cardiomyopathy are inconsistently reported.[23]

Cardiotoxicity secondary to anthracyclines in pediatric patients with diagnoses of DS and AML has been inconsistently reported. Conventional anthracycline high-dose or high-intensity regimens are associated with increased rates of cardiomyopathy in this population compared to both without DS and AML. Similar findings have been reported for youth with DS and ALL.[23] Interpretation of the literature on cardiotoxicity and anthracycline-related toxicities requires several considerations, such as population demographics. Potential confounds include age, agent used, and assessment instruments and criteria to evaluate cardiotoxicity. For example, the pediatric populations under consideration have ranged from those approximately 1 year of age to those with an average age of 6 years. In addition, some studies used different assessment methodology, making comparisons problematic.[23]

AUTISM SPECTRUM DISORDER AND AUTISM

Autism was first described by Leo Kanner in 1943 and has been historically described as early infantile autism, childhood autism, and Kanner autism.[1] Autism is not a disease but a neurodevelopmental disorder with multiple possible etiologies.[24] The onset is typically before 3 years of age and is usually, but not always, associated with some degree of ID.[1] Originally autism, or autistic disorder, was one of five behaviorally defined pervasive developmental disorders (PDDs) that included Asperger disorder, Rett syndrome (RTT), childhood disintegrative disorder, and pervasive developmental disorder not otherwise specified (PDD-NOS). These disorders are now referred to under the single designation of ASD and are characterized by two underlying problems—impaired social interaction and communication (regarded as one conjoined problem) and restricted behavior. Further distinctions are made based on severity, which is based on the amount of support needed, challenges with social communication, restricted interests, and repetitive behaviors. Also included are specifications of with or without an accompanying intellectual impairment.[1] There are three levels of severity, Level 1, the least severe, though Level 3, the most severe. This section will focus specifically on autism, which is characterized by severe and sustained impairments in three behavioral domains: (a) reciprocal social interaction (withdrawal or lack of interest in peers), (b) language and communication skills (limitations in the use of speech and nonverbal skills), and (c) range of interests and activities (repetitive, restricted behaviors, stereotyped mannerisms).[1,25]

Epidemiology

There has been a recent sharp increase in the reported prevalence of autism. The most recent national estimate is 1:68 children identified with ASD.[26] It is suggested that the reported increased prevalence is primarily related to changing and broadening diagnostic criteria, along with an increased index of suspicion, rather than due to an actual increased incidence, as autism is behaviorally identified, and the diagnostic boundaries are not always clear.[27,28] In addition, inclusion of individuals with diagnoses of Asperger disorder and PDD-NOS in newer studies may contribute to the increase.[28] Some behaviors (eg, stereotypies) seen in persons with autism can also be seen in nonautistic individuals. One study found children with a history of early institutionalization demonstrated more stereotypical behaviors that markedly decreased following increased interactions postplacement.[29] There is a significant impact of intellectual ability on the expression of symptoms of autism,[30] resulting in a lack of homogeneity in clinical expression of the condition. Autism is between four and five times more prevalent in males.[24] When present, ID ranges from mild to severe. The heterogeneity and early onset represent two methodologic problems for large-scale research studies.[24]

Etiology and Pathophysiology

The etiology of autism is attributed to multiple causal factors, including gene mutations, abnormalities in brain development, and genetic–environment interactions.[25] Autism may occur concomitantly with other developmental disorders that have a known genetic basis, such as RTT and fragile X syndrome.[28] Current research primarily focuses on genetics and neuropathology. Although a single genetic mutation or variant leading to autism has yet to be identified, research findings indicate that structural alterations in the genome deoxyribonucleic acid (DNA), known as copy number variations (CNVs), may be involved in ASD. Research identified a number of CNVs associated with ASDs, as this appears to be a highly heritable disorder.[31]

These findings provide support for the heterogeneity of neurodevelopmental disorders, whereby disruption represents a critical period in the development of excitatory and inhibitory neuron development. A combination of genetic and/or environmental factors, in the absence of any compensatory mechanism, may interfere with brain plasticity.[30] A meta-analysis provided some support for the theory that ASD may arise from interference in the excitatory and inhibitory balance expression and/or timing during critical periods.[32] A review of the literature found persons with autism demonstrated what was termed "unusual sensory processing." Additional findings included (a) a diagnosis of autism was associated with greater sensory symptoms than in other developmental disorders, (b) increased age was associated with decreased symptoms, and (c) for children there was a positive correlation between social impairment and sensory symptoms.[33]

Siblings of affected children have a significantly greater risk of having autism (3%-18.7%) than those in the general population.[34] Results from a national volunteer registry (n = 2,920 children, 1,235 families, a minimum of 1 child meeting ASD diagnostic criteria, and a minimum of 1 full sibling) found that the sibling concordance rate was 10.9%. Overall an additional 8.9% of the siblings demonstrated language delay with autistic-like speech quality.

Further support for the high heritability of the disorder was shown by additional research in this area. Sibling risk varies based on the gender of the index child: 4% versus 7% for female compared with male. If a second child is diagnosed, the risk for concordance in subsequent siblings increases to between 25% and 30%, higher than previously reported. The risk for a monozygotic twin with autism ranges from 60% to 95% that both twins will be diagnosed with autism.[35] A study of over 14,000 children diagnosed with ASD in Sweden found that ASD heritability was estimated to be 0.50, and the autistic disorder heritability was estimated to be 0.54. Interpreted, this means the heritability of ASD was estimated to be approximately 50%.[36]

Parental age was investigated as a potential risk factor for autism. While results are far from conclusive, a number of intriguing results were found. A case–control study design of a cohort of age- and sex-matched pairs (n = 68) found a significant effect linking the age of both parents and a child with a diagnosis of autism.

Unadjusted parental ages were higher for both parents (paternal 4 years higher, maternal 4.8 years higher) compared with controls. After adjusting for variables, such as educational level and gestational age, the differences widened to 5.9 and 6.5 years, respectively.[37] Shelton et al found increasing paternal age was a risk factor if the mother was younger than 30 years.[38] Other work found that increasing paternal age was associated with greater risk.[39]

Environmental exposures, including toxic chemical exposure, teratogens, perinatal insults, prenatal infections,[28] and copper and zinc levels[40] are under investigation. Immunization with measles-mumps-rubella (MMR) vaccine has been investigated, and no causal association identified.[41]

Autism frequently occurs concomitantly with epilepsy[42] and may be associated with microdeletion gene defects that are also risk factors for schizophrenia and attention-deficit/hyperactivity disorder (ADHD). Examples include the association between autism, ID, schizophrenia, and seizures with microdeletions on the 15q13.3 and 1q21.1 regions.[43] Other sites also may be implicated. The two most common single gene abnormalities associated with autism are fragile X syndrome and tuberous sclerosis.[35]

The neurodevelopmental foundation of autism has sparked significant interest in early morphologic changes in brain development, particularly findings of early brain overgrowth. Head circumference at birth ranges from slightly below normal to within normal limits. This finding changes by 2 to 3 months of age when accelerated head growth occurs. The rate of growth may exceed 2 standard deviations above the average. Approximately 60% of infants diagnosed with autism compared with 6% of normal infants have this rate of accelerated head growth. The increase positively correlates to the increase in ID severity. Following this period of accelerated head growth, during which time the infant brain may achieve the size of the adult brain, deceleration or a complete cessation of head growth is noted.[24]

Accelerated brain growth may predispose the developing brain to increased vulnerability. This is consistent with the concept of plasticity, whereby development of cortical circuitry is established during critical postnatal periods. During this period of development, a balance of excitatory and inhibitory neurofunctionality occurs. It has been theorized that during this critical period if an imbalance occurs, this results in neurodevelopmental disorders, such as autism.[36] This theory is consistent with the diagnostic criteria of onset within the first 3 years, abnormalities in three major areas (socialization, communication, and repetitive behaviors[1]), and disruption in neurocircuitry development.

Dysfunction of virtually all neural systems in the brain has been proposed at some point as a potential basis of autism.[44] The neuropathologic changes noted in persons with autism are suggested to be of prenatal origin, primarily in the first 6 months of gestation.[24] Evidence has been published that suggests that autism affects a functionally diverse and widely distributed set of neural systems, making the disorder far broader in scope than a simple social interaction disorder.[44] Despite these findings, the pattern of brain abnormality appears somewhat discrete. Autism spares many perceptual and cognitive systems. A localized neural deficit can have more widespread neurofunctional implications through its influence on brain development.[44]

There is research to support abnormalities in cholinergic receptors and decreases in the nicotinic receptor binding in the cholinergic system, as well as dysfunction in the GABAergic system[42] in persons with autism. Nicotinic receptors enhance cognitive processing (ie, memory and attention) open the possibility of therapeutic intervention via cholinergic receptor modulation.[45] Approximately 25% to 60% of children with autism have elevated peripheral platelet concentrations of the neurotransmitter serotonin.[46] Studies of dopamine and catecholamine metabolites have failed to consistently show abnormalities.

Clinical **Controversy...**

Well-conducted case–control, cross-sectional, ecologic, and cohort studies investigating use of thimerosal, an organomercury compound previously used as a vaccine preservative, found no causal association between thimerosal-containing vaccines and the development of autism or deficits in neuropsychological function.[57] In a large sample of privately insured children with older siblings, receiving the MMR vaccine was not associated with increased risk of ASD, regardless of whether the older siblings had ASD.[58] Despite the lack of evidence, the neurotoxic effect of mercury exposure continues to be a hotly debated issue among many advocates for persons with autism. Clinicians must be well informed on this issue to educate parents and caregivers.

Clinical Presentation and Diagnosis

The differential diagnostic features of ASD are listed in Table 73-1. A multiple-step process has been suggested as a structured approach to diagnosis if ASD is suspected. As a spectrum disorder, the severity or level of impairment may be highly variable. This structured approach includes a determination of intellectual function and level of language development, followed by assessment of the child's behavior as it relates to chronologic age, mental age, and language age. It is important to identify relevant comorbid medical conditions and the presence of any related contributing psychosocial factors.[47]

Persons with autism are typically normal in physical appearance. Seizure rates among those with ASD are reported to be between 2% and 21%.[48,49] Patients with comorbid seizure disorders often have greater impairment in intellectual function.[1] Other medical comorbidities commonly reported in this population include sleep disturbances, food intolerances, and GI dysfunction.[50]

The cardinal features of autism are gross and sustained impairment of reciprocal social interaction; sustained abnormalities in verbal and nonverbal communication skills; and restricted, repetitive, and stereotypical patterns of behavior, interests, and activities.[1] These are primarily manifested as gaze aversion, little/no interest in making friends, preference for solitary activities, repetition of words/phrases, monotone voice, insistence on sameness, and a lack of awareness of other's feelings.[1,51] In most cases (approximately 75%),

TABLE 73-1 Comparison of Diagnostic Features of ASD and Rett Syndrome

Feature	ASD	Rett Syndrome
Age at recognition (months)	0-36	24-28
Sex ratio	M > F	F >> M
Loss of skills after initial mastery	Variable	A defining feature
Social skills	Very poor	Varies with stage
Communication skills	Usually poor	Very poor
Circumscribed interests	Variable (mechanical)	NA
Eye contact	Very poor	Varies with stage
Family history of similar problems	Sometimes	Rare
Seizure disorder	2.4%-26%	Frequent
Head growth decelerates	No	Yes
IQ range	Normal to severe ID	Severe ID
Outcome	Good to very poor	Very poor

ASD, autism spectrum disorder; F, female; IQ, intelligence quotient; M, male; NA, not applicable.

Data from references 1, 48, and 54.

there is an associated diagnosis of ID, ranging from mild to profound: approximately 30% function in the mild to moderate range of ID, whereas 45% to 50% have severe to profound impairment.[47] Epidemiologic data suggest that the risk for development of autism increases as the intelligence quotient (IQ) decreases.[47] A few individuals with autism have unusual abilities called splinter functions or islets of precocity. The most significant of these are evidenced in the autistic savant, in which the individuals can have precocity in mathematic calculations, art, music, or rote memory.[1,47]

In many instances, parents note that they were concerned about the child's lack of interest in social interactions since birth but were sure at least by 3 years of age.[1] In a controlled setting, use of an integrated model for screening was effective in diagnosing children before 36 months of age.[52] Original findings of behaviors suggesting the need for an intellectual evaluation included lack of babbling, pointing, or other gestures by 12 months, no single-word language development by 16 months, no two-word language development by 24 months of age, and loss of previously held language or social skills at any age.[28] Earlier intervention is recommended when the early signs and symptoms of autism are recognized. It is difficult to determine if autism is present in persons with severe to profound ID. A diagnosis is made in such cases when there are qualitative deficits in social and communicative skills and the specific behaviors characteristic of ASD are present.[1] A central difference is that persons with ID alone typically relate to adults in a manner consistent with their mental age, use their language to communicate with others, and present with a relatively even profile of impairments without splinter functions.[47]

Although there are no definitive biologic markers for identifying individuals with autism, a number of medical evaluations should occur at baseline, to assist in distinguishing the diagnosis as autism and to rule out other disorders. Table 73-2 delineates the parameters to be considered in a medical evaluation for persons suspected of having autism and the rationale for the assessment.

TABLE 73-2 Medical Screening for Individuals with ASD

Parameter	Rationale
Health, medical, behavioral, and developmental history	Perform initial screening or confirm diagnosis, identify underlying cause; assess strengths and weaknesses; identify comorbidities; measure head circumference; identify resources needed
Wood's light examination	Identify depigmented macules associated with tuberous sclerosis
Hearing and vision testing	Profound hearing loss can illicit symptoms mimicking autism (receptive language deficits); most are normal
Heavy metal testing	Perform if there is a history of malnutrition, recurrent vomiting, early onset seizures, dysmorphic features, presence of ID, or developmental delays
Genetic testing for karyotype, fragile X, Rett syndrome	Benefits family for genetic counseling purposes; evaluation of siblings, if applicable; review family history for three generations
Test for inborn errors of metabolism/ metabolic testing	Indicated in those with a history of lethargy, recurrent vomiting, early seizures, dysmorphic or coarse facial features, ID
CBC, thyroid function testing	CBC if anemia suspected; thyroid function tests to rule out baseline thyroid abnormality that can affect mood/activity level
EEG	Evaluate neurologic findings that cannot be explained by the diagnosis of autism alone or in the presence of developmental regression, particularly language
Neuroimaging	Evaluate neurologic findings that cannot be explained by the diagnosis of autism alone; identify specific neuropathologic changes associated with autism, including brain volume

ASD, autism spectrum disorder; CBC, complete blood count; EEG, electroencephalograph; ID, intellectual disability.

Data from references 28, 40, and 53.

Those individuals with autism and IQs above 70 who use communicative language by ages 5 to 7 have the best prognoses.[47] Conversely, low IQ scores and failure to develop communicative language by age 5 years correlate with a poorer long-term prognosis.[53] Outcome studies in persons with autism correlate IQ, particularly verbal IQ, with the ability to be employed and live independently.[44,54] Learning disabilities are an independent risk factor for development of behavioral problems, and 41% of children with mild, moderate, or severe learning difficulties have a significant emotional behavioral disturbance.[54] Studies indicate that high-IQ children with autism can make positive changes in communication and social domains more effectively over time. The areas less likely to improve are those related to ritualistic and repetitive behaviors.[50] Up to 80% of children diagnosed with ASD continued to experience marked impairment in social interactions as adults. Mild to moderate ID was reported for approximately 30%.[55]

In addition to the core symptoms of autism, many persons with this disorder exhibit other significant maladaptive behaviors, such as aggression to self and others. These behavioral issues can interfere with day-to-day activities and are challenging for the individual, families, and caregivers.[56]

Clinical **Controversy...**

Many families, clinicians, and advocates are concerned that the new diagnostic categorization will have the unintended consequence of eliminating some persons with previously diagnosed high-functioning autism (ie, formerly Asperger disorder) from eligibility for services by recognizing the essential shared features of the ASD while attempting to individualize diagnosis through dimensional descriptors. Additional study will clarify if these concerns are well founded.

TREATMENT
ASD

Desired Outcomes

Treatment goals in persons with a diagnosis of ASD are to address deficits in communication and social interaction using a structured approach, minimize the impact of restricted behaviors (eg, stereotypies or repetition), and facilitate behavior appropriate to the level of intellectual ability, language development, and chronologic age.

General Approach

3 The multimodal treatment plan should address (a) establishing realistic goals for educational efforts, (b) identifying the presence of behavioral target symptoms for intervention, (c) prioritizing target symptoms and comorbid conditions for intervention, (d) using specific methods of outcome monitoring of functional domains (behavioral, adaptive skills, academic skills, social interaction skills, communication skills), and (e) monitoring for efficacy and potential adverse effects of medication (if used). The National Institutes of Health (NIH) suggests that evidence-based treatment strategies include the use of both psychoeducational therapies and medications.[59] An effective, well-designed, multimodal treatment plan that is consistently executed has the most potential to positively shape the autistic individual's interaction with the environment and improve the quality of life of patients and their families.

After a thorough diagnostic evaluation, treatment planning for the individual with autism is critical to assure consistency and efficacy of interventions. With the often severe nature of the behavioral

CLINICAL PRESENTATION Autism Spectrum Disorder

General

- It is a behaviorally defined disorder.
- Multifactor causality is suspected. This includes gene mutations, abnormalities in brain development, and genetic–environment interactions.
- Individuals typically present with delays or abnormalities in six or more of the symptoms below, with at least two impairments in social interactions and one each in communication and restricted interests or repetitive behaviors.

Diagnostic Features

- Significant impairment in nonverbal communication.
- Unable to develop peer relationships.
- Lack of spontaneous interactions with people or the environment.
- Developmental delays in communication.
- Inability to use expressive language appropriate to developmental level.
- Lack of developmentally appropriate play.
- Limited scope of play or interest.
- Inability to tolerate change.
- Stereotypic or repetitive, nonfunctional motor movements.

Data from references 1, 28, and 54.

and adaptive problems, it is not surprising that many potential treatment modalities lacking an evidence basis have been proposed for persons with autism. 4 The two treatment approaches for autism with evidence-based support and clinical consensus are behavioral/psychoeducational therapies[28,60] and psychoactive medication intervention[25] as appropriate. All stakeholders (the patient, family, caregivers, educators, and clinical professionals) should be involved in the treatment planning process. Treatment decisions should be evidence-based and individualized to the specific identified needs of the individual. The potential for communication deficits often limit self-reporting of psychopathology. A multifaceted approach to information gathering should include direct observation; interviews with patient, parents, family, caregivers, and teachers; and review of the medical record, including any behavioral rating scale information.

4 Available evidence suggests that appropriately designed, consistently implemented educational services positively impact the acquisition of social, communicative, self-care, and cognitive skills, each of which facilitates the person's long-term success. Services, such as occupational therapy, physical therapy, and speech pathology, are often integral aspects of an overall educational plan. 5 Because of the pervasive need for sameness in routine, ongoing and consistent year-round educational programming is more effective than intermittent, episodic interventions. Effective language and communication training can lead to generalized improvements in social skills and repetitive behaviors, and thus positively impact other nonspecific, maladaptive, behavioral problems such as noncompliance, self-injury, and aggression.[61]

Nonpharmacologic Treatment

Intervention strategies, such as discrete trial training, have demonstrated improvement in challenging behaviors. Educational techniques include structuring the environment, family training, peer role modeling, and sensory integration to optimize environmental interactions.[60]

Pharmacologic Treatment

Many of the studies of psychopharmacologic interventions in persons with ASD have methodologic shortcomings, including problems in experimental design and sample size, loose or poorly defined diagnostic criteria, and many clinical outcomes that were limited in duration or of dubious clinical significance.

4 Among a number of scientifically unsupported treatments for autism is the use of complementary and alternative medicine (CAM). A study of 540 families of children with ASD found that the child/family had tried an average of seven CAM therapies.[62] Elimination diets in which casein (from dairy products) and/or gluten (from wheat products) are excluded from the diet have demonstrated no benefit. Other such purported therapies include omega-3 fatty acids and selected herbal remedies, specifically ginkgo biloba. The omega-3 trials demonstrated no significant differences between supplementation and placebo. Several of the trials reviewed had methodological problems identified. Again, utilization of ginkgo biloba or placebo as adjunctive therapy with risperidone did not show efficacy.[63]

Current research on the neurobiologic basis of autism is centered on the serotonergic, peptidergic, dopaminergic, and noradrenergic systems. This research has particular applications for insomnia in children with ASD, as the prevalence of sleep disorders has been reported to range from 44% to 83%.[64] 6 Parents commonly rate sleep disturbance as a significant clinical issue. As with nonautistic individuals, it is important to determine the underlying etiology of the sleep problem. Behavioral interventions (eg, improved sleep hygiene, eliminating maladaptive sleep habits, and parental education) should be undertaken prior to implementing pharmacotherapy. No medication has been FDA-approved for pediatric insomnia. While controlled trial data are limited, there is support for the use, safety, and effectiveness of melatonin. In a review of the literature for use of melatonin in ASD, 85% (n = 107) reported improved sleep, specifically shorter sleep onset latencies. Doses ranged from 0.75 to 6 mg. Adverse effects were mild (headaches, GI upset, dizziness).[65]

Aggression to self and others and severe tantrums are a concern, particularly with adults with ASD. In addition to inclusion of nonpharmacologic interventions, pharmacotherapy is frequently utilized. Despite limited evidence-based support, psychoactive medications have been widely used to minimize the frequency and intensity of these behaviors. 7 It is important that clinicians identify and carefully monitor specific behavioral target symptom response to avoid the practice of overprescribing psychoactive medications.

An association between dopamine dysregulation and increased aggression, including self-injury, consistent with animal models, has been proposed.[56] Such findings have led to the use of antipsychotic agents that act as dopaminergic antagonists to address aggression and self-injurious behavior. The first-generation antipsychotic agent with the most evidence for short- and long-term safety and efficacy is haloperidol. Target behaviors included impaired learning, anger, mood lability, hyperactivity, and social withdrawal. Although results for improvement in the target behaviors were greater in the antipsychotic treatment compared with the placebo group, the risk for the development of dyskinesias and the introduction of new antipsychotic medications have markedly limited haloperidol's use.[25]

As few psychopharmacologic agents have been well studied in this population, and even fewer have received FDA approval, current research is directed primarily toward the second-generation antipsychotics (SGAs). 8 Off-label use of FDA-approved medications (ie, use of an approved drug for an unapproved use) is an acceptable clinical practice when there is evidence-based support for the use of the medication and informed consent is obtained; however, there is a relative lack of robust research in this area at the present time.

Risperidone and aripiprazole are currently FDA-approved to treat the behavioral (irritability) symptoms associated with autism.[66,67] Risperidone has the most evidence-based support for treating behavioral problems associated with autism. It is FDA-approved for treatment of the following behaviors in children and adolescents with autism: aggression, self-injury, temper tantrums, and irritability.[25]

A review of the literature found both short- and long-term use (up to 1 year) of orally administered aripiprazole was effective for irritability in pediatric patients with ASD, aged 6 to 17 years. The dosage range was 2 to 15 mg/day. In this range, aripiprazole was well tolerated with moderate side effects that resolved with continued use.[68-71] Weight gain was reported during the first 3 to 6 months, and then it plateaued.[68] The use of olanzapine is supported by limited trial data in children and adolescents with autism. Trial durations were generally short (6-8 weeks) with small numbers of participants. Positive results are generally reported in global improvement scale assessment; however, the significant weight gain and sedation noted in olanzapine trials are important considerations in weighing risk versus potential benefit.[25] A post-hoc analysis of the health-related quality of life of pediatric patients receiving aripiprazole found improved scores compared to placebo in three of five subscales, including emotional, social, and cognitive functioning.[72]

At this time there is no FDA-approved medication for the core symptoms of autism. Prior to the inclusion of pharmacotherapy for behavior as a component of the plan, utilization of a multifaceted approach is recommended.[73]

The SGAs are less likely to elicit extrapyramidal side effects than first-generation agents due to more potency at serotonin$_{2A}$ (5-HT$_{2A}$) receptors versus dopamine receptors. However, the SGAs have been implicated in weight gain in some persons with autism.[25] The potential serum prolactin elevation related to risperidone use is of concern. Elevated serum prolactin may lead to amenorrhea, galactorrhea, and osteoporosis in females and gynecomastia and sexual dysfunction in males. The minimum degree of prolactin elevation that is clinically relevant is uncertain as are the implications for long-term use in a pediatric population. If detected, strategies include evaluating the risk–benefit with continued use, reducing doses, or changing to another agent with less impact on prolactin. It is recommended that clinicians monitor for the evidence of potential risperidone-mediated prolactin elevations regardless of whether a prolactin level is obtained.[74] Additional monitoring recommendations for antipsychotic use can be found in Chapter 67.

Serotonin synthesis differs between children diagnosed with ASD and children without this diagnosis. Compared with adults, 5-hydroxytryptamine (5-HT) synthesis may peak at twice the adult level in developmentally normal children by age 5 years, whereas children with ASD have a more gradual developmental arc with a lower peak.[75] The use of SSRIs is often associated with a decrease in some of the core behavioral symptoms such as stereotypies, social withdrawal, and rigid adherence to routine. A review of the literature for citalopram,[76] escitalopram, fluoxetine, and fluvoxamine[75] found limited support for use of SSRIs to address behaviors of ASD.

Oxytocin administration has been studied using intranasal or infusion routes of administration. Oxytocin is involved in regulating social behavior in humans, and has been the subject of a number of small studies of patients with ASD. At best, data demonstrate promising effects related to repetitive behaviors and social cognition (eye gaze and emotion recognition).[77] More research is needed with adequately powered studies.

Psychostimulants have been studied in persons with autism to address hyperactivity, impulsivity, and inattention. Psychostimulants block the reuptake of dopamine and norepinephrine. It is hypothesized that ADHD represents a dysfunction in regulation of these catecholamines.[78] Study design of methylphenidate trials in persons with ASD complicates interpretation of results. Some trials were uncontrolled, and some included children with various diagnoses. The largest and most rigorously controlled trial involved 72 participants, with 74% having a primary diagnosis of autism. In this placebo-controlled trial, methylphenidate was given in divided doses of 0.125, 0.25, and 0.5 mg/kg (morning and noon doses). In an analysis of the 66 youths completing the trial, 16 could not tolerate the 0.5 mg/kg dose phase. All three doses performed better than placebo on improving the core symptoms of ADHD according to parent and teacher ratings. Parent ratings for ADHD were better with the medium dose compared with the low dose. Teacher ratings for inattention were better with the medium dose compared with the low dose.[79] Overall, findings suggest that treatment response to psychostimulants varies and, in general, stimulants do not work as well in this population of children compared with normally developing peers.[80] The α_2-agonists, clonidine and guanfacine, have been used to treat hyperactivity and agitation in persons with autism because of their effects on inhibition of noradrenergic release and transmission. Both agents have FDA approval for treating symptoms associated with ADHD. However, as with many psychoactive medications used in the population with autism, there is a lack of methodologically sound studies supporting use of these agents. Two trials with guanfacine targeted symptoms that included inattentiveness and hyperactivity. Both reported positive outcomes. In the first (n = 80, average age of 7.7 years), guanfacine use was associated with statistically significant improvement in global functioning. In the second trial (n = 25, 20 completed), all subjects had not tolerated previous methylphenidate use. Improvement was noted on measures; some reached statistical significance.[80]

Limited data are available on the use of cholinesterase inhibitors for disruptive behaviors, such as hyperactivity and irritability. Use of donepezil for these or the core autism symptoms cannot be supported.[80] No benefit for ADHD or core symptoms was found for galantamine, and results for rivastigmine were unclear. Modification of glutamate activity in the brain may lead to improvement in various ASD-related outcomes. Use of the NMDA-receptor antagonist memantine was associated with hyperactivity. Combined with risperidone, memantine treated patients saw improvement in irritability, stereotyped behaviors, and hyperactivity.[81] Additional study is needed for this agent.

Limited support for anticonvulsants as interventions for hyperactivity and impulsivity in children with ASD was found despite the high comorbidity of seizures in this population.[80]

The current dearth of evidence-based psychopharmacologic and behavioral research in persons with autism is being addressed by a network of NIH-funded research centers, including the Research Units of Pediatric Psychopharmacology, Centers for Programs of Excellence in Autism, and Studies to Advance Autism Research and Treatment. The mission of these units is to foster well-controlled, multicenter, behavioral, and psychopharmacologic intervention studies targeting behavioral symptoms in persons with autism.

Personalized Pharmacotherapy

Aggression toward self and others and severe tantrums are a concern, particularly in adults with ASD. In addition to nonpharmacologic interventions, pharmacotherapy is frequently used. Despite limited evidence-based support, psychoactive medications have been widely used to minimize the frequency and intensity of these behaviors. Although pharmacogenomics to guide rational and targeted pharmacotherapy would be helpful, at present this information is not available.[82] This may be in part because of the heterogeneity of the ASD population.

Pharmacogenetic research has been limited by lack of sensitive outcome assessment tools to measure the effectiveness of treatments and the presence of multiple confounding factors in studies such as age, sex, medication dosage, and treatment duration, and whether or not the study subjects were drug naïve.[83] Studies that have been conducted (primarily with risperidone) are of limited clinical utility due to small sample size, and they need to be replicated in larger populations with more diverse makeup.[83,84] However, a small study in children with ASD found that genetic variation, focused on loci that influence monoaminergic signaling, may lead to variation in response to methylphenidate.[85] Until well-conducted, reproducible study results are available to confirm the early work that has been done, using the patient's genotype to algorithmically predict a medication and dose likely to be effective and safe for a given patient with autism remains elusive.

Evaluation of Therapeutic Outcomes

7 Monitoring the safety, efficacy, and tolerability of psychopharmacologic interventions in persons with autism is imperative to minimize adverse medication-related sequelae and optimize desired therapeutic outcomes. Clinical investigators have used a variety of psychometric assessment instruments in attempts to measure changes in core symptoms.

A variety of instruments have been developed and used in clinical trials to measure symptoms, such as communication impairment, restricted interests, and repetitive behavior. A comprehensive review of many of these instruments is beyond the scope of this chapter. Pharmacotherapy in autism is usually directed toward minimizing maladaptive behaviors, such as irritability, hyperactivity, compulsive, ritualistic, and perseverative behavior, and variants of self-injurious behavior. The Aberrant Behavior Checklist was designed for assessment of behavioral changes in institutionalized individuals enrolled in pharmacotherapy trials; however, a community-based version is also available.[86,87] The Aberrant Behavior Checklist consists of 54 items divided into 5 domains: irritability, hyperactivity, stereotypic behavior, lethargy, and inappropriate speech: the lower the score in each domain, the greater the behavioral improvement. The Children's Yale-Brown Obsessive Compulsive Scale modified for pervasive developmental disorders is a validated scale sensitive to changes in repetitive behavior severity pretreatment and posttreatment.[88]

Intensive medication-related side effects monitoring and assessment is important in this population, as self-reporting may be unreliable. An instrument that is caregiver-rated such as the Monitoring of Side Effects Scale can be useful for this purpose. The Monitoring of Side Effects Scale is a multisystem, quantitative, and qualitative caregiver assessment that rates the presence or absence and severity of a variety of potential medication-related adverse effects for clinician review.[89] Signs and symptoms are written in layperson language and are listed by body area or system. As such, it is a broad-based screening tool that can be enhanced by side effect–specific scales such as those for akathisia (Barnes Akathisia Scale [BAS]), extrapyramidal effects (Simpson-Angus Scale), or tardive dyskinesia (Dyskinesia Identification System: Condensed User Scale [DISCUS]).[90-92]

7 Use of SGAs has been associated with increased risk of developing metabolic syndrome. Children and adults receiving these agents should be monitored for hyperglycemia, dyslipidemia, and weight gain in a manner consistent with the consensus guidelines suggested by the American Diabetes Association and the American Psychiatric Association. For monitoring guidelines, see Chapter 67.

RETT SYNDROME

In 1966, Andreas Rett, an Austrian physician, published the first paper describing this disorder in a German language journal. He documented a sequence of developmental changes affecting young girls who initially achieved normal developmental milestones and then experienced regression. The significance of these findings and worldwide interest were not fully apparent until 1981, when similar findings were published in English.[93] Seizures, autonomic dysfunction, and cardiac dysfunction are frequent comorbidities with Rett syndrome (RTT). The primary goals of treatment are to optimize quality of life.

Epidemiology

The typical, or classic, presentation of RTT affects females almost exclusively. The worldwide prevalent is estimated to be 1:10,000 to 22,000.[94]

Etiology and Pathophysiology

RTT was originally identified as a neurodevelopmental disorder originating from an X-linked dominant mutation at the Xq28 site involving the methyl-CpG-binding protein 2 (MeCP2). This

CLINICAL PRESENTATION Rett Syndrome

General features

- RTT is diagnosed primarily in females.
- Previously acquired skills are lost following apparently normal prenatal and early development.
- Seizure disorders may occur in 50% to 90% of the RTT population.

Additional Features

- Sudden death secondary to cardiac dysfunction is greater than in the general population.
- Head growth slows.
- Scoliosis may develop.
- Sleep and respiration can be problematic.
- Motor skills may vary.
- Stereotypies may occur.
- General mood disorders and behaviors consistent with anxiety and fear are common.

Data from references 94, 98, 99, and 102.

represents the most commonly identified mutation in the majority (approximately 96%) of cases.[95] In-depth molecular studies found a variety of mutations on the *MECP2* gene that impact the presentation of the clinical phenotype. These mutations may provide an explanation for differences in severity, presentation, and onset and now lend credibility to RTT as a neuroprogressive disorder as well.[96]

The etiology of RTT has not been fully identified. It has been determine that the loss of genetic coding of the MeCP2 protein at the Xq28 site occurs.[94] Current research focuses on identification of specific gene mutations and location of those mutations on the gene. These are increasingly linked to the presentation, severity, and outcomes of the individual.[97,98] It was once thought the MeCP2 protein was specific to brain cells. Recent research with mice models found this protein present in non-neuronal brain cells where release of a neurotoxin is theorized.[98]

Clinical **Controversy...**

Redefining diagnostic criteria can have significant impact on applied epidemiology, enrollment for benefit eligibility, and clinical research. Such changes should not be taken lightly. As new knowledge is created through scientific study, it may be necessary to refine diagnostic criteria to make the diagnosis more precise, the prognosis more accurate, and the population-based information more valid due to better homogeneity. RTT is a still a clinical diagnosis. Molecular biology tests may be additive or confirmatory. These tests, however, do not supersede clinical decision-making.

Clinical Presentation and Diagnosis

The clinical criteria for RTT began with the description of this constellation of aberrant behaviors, neurodevelopmental trajectory, and clinical findings. The criteria have been refined over time in order to provide consistency in population-based data collection and for clinical research purposes. Specific mutations associated with RTT were discovered in 1999, and this led to revision of criteria in 2002. More recently, a consensus panel of international clinical experts produced a new set of diagnostic criteria and nomenclature.[99]

Genetic variations have been identified that are thought to moderate the symptoms and progression of RTT, the extent of which is not fully understood. What is known is that females are predominately affected by RTT, and no causal association has been identified. An uneventful pregnancy and birth are followed by seemingly normal development with acquisition of developmentally appropriate milestones. Growth, including head circumference, is within normal limits at birth. Developmental regression appears between 6 and 18 months with the loss of previously acquired skills. Additional developmentally regressive changes have been grouped into a series of stages associated with a range of ages during which these changes occur.[96]

9 The order of symptom appearance and regressive changes associated with RTT distinguish it from other developmental disorders. Increasingly, it is believed that the developmental changes and severity may be a function of the *MECP2* mutation (Table 73-3). Important features for include the onset that typically begins from approximately 6 months to 18 months of age, during which loss of previously acquired skills occur; seizures may appear. The growth rate declines, and head size decreases (microcephaly).[96] Between the ages of 1 and 4 years, developmental regression presents. During this period, indications of ID and loss of language are seen. Also noted are behavioral changes, such as loss of social interactions, and autistic-like features (eg, stereotypic hand movements). A period of pseudo-stability or a wake-up period, whereby previously lost skills, such as with communication, may partially reappear between 4 and 7 years. Scoliosis/respiratory problems, problematic sleep, and symptoms of mood changes continue. Losses in motor functionality that may be total, and autonomic fluctuations represent the final set of changes and may last for years or decades.[96] Presentations vary in terms of onset and severity. Increasingly, the specific genetic mutation and location may explain these variations.[97] Specific information was identified from a database of genotyped

TABLE 73-3 RTT Syndrome Features

	Onset Age	Duration	Suspected Gene Mutation[a]	Characteristics
Critical point for diagnosis	6-18 months, up to 48 months	Months to years	*MECP2* *FOXG1, and* *CKDL5* *p.Arg294X*	Found in 90% of patients Found in 10% of patients Head growth decreases or ceases
				Increased social withdrawal
			p.Arg133Cys *p.Arg306Cys*	Purposeful hand movements cease Hand use more preserved
Critical point for diagnosis	12-18 months to 4 years	Weeks to months		Onset of intellectual disability; may be severe
				Breathing irregularities
				Autistic features appear
			CDKL5 p.R133c	Early onset seizures Latest onset
	4-7 years	Years; may stabilize here	*R294X* *R294X, R168X*	Seizures increase Partial return of language skills Deterioration slows or ceases Variable ambulatory status
	>7 years old	Decades, if at all	*p.Arg306Cys* *p.Thr158Met*	Scoliosis Least severe Most severe Dystonias

CDKL5, cyclin-dependent kinase-like 5; *FOXG1*, forkhead box protein G1; MeCP2, methyl-CpG-binding protein 2; RTT, Rett syndrome.

[a]Unless otherwise indicated, specific mutations on the *MECP2* gene are associated with variability in the onset and/or severity of RTT developmental changes. No differentiations are made between typical and atypical RTT diagnostic criteria.

Data from references 94, 95, 96, 99, 102, and 103.

participations (n = 1052 with 4,940 unique contacts). Researchers isolated 16 mutation groups with 8 common point mutations.[95] Specific moderating influences for RTT features corresponded with age of onset, autonomic symptoms, seizures, and head growth.[95]

Prior to identification of specific genotypes linked to RTT features, the presence of stereotypic hand movements, social and environmental withdrawal, and irritability (including the inability to be soothed when crying) gave rise to investigating commonalities between RTT and autism. In patients with RTT, impairments in communication and environmental interactions, eye contact, and stereotypies vary and are linked to specific mutations,[95] whereas with autism, this level of genotypic specificity has not been identified.

TREATMENT
Rett Syndrome

Desired Outcomes

Treatment goals in RTT are to identify the characteristic developmental changes of each stage and provide effective nonpharmacologic and pharmacologic interventions as appropriate to improve quality of life.

General Approach

Treatment plans should address the physiologic changes of each stage, optimizing pharmacotherapy, as appropriate. Effective strategies require a systematic approach to (a) address the specific medical needs identified, (b) monitor the medications used as appropriate, and (c) reassess the need for continued pharmacotherapy.

Nonpharmacologic Therapy

Behavioral problems are not commonly encountered with RTT. Other considerations include evaluating for respiratory complications, such as obstructive sleep apnea with polysomnography and therapeutic interventions, if indicated.[100] Surgical intervention may be indicated to lessen the severity of scoliosis. A retrospective review of RTT patients who underwent surgery (n = 24, 29 surgical procedures) found preexisting RTT features, including seizure disorders, frequent upper respiratory infections, and cardiac conduction abnormalities required a high degree of intensive postoperative care.[101]

Pharmacologic Therapy

Information on pharmacotherapy for comorbidities associated with RTT comes primarily from case reports, case series, and small trials. There are currently no approved medications for the treatment of RTT.

One of the more problematic aspects of caring for RTT patients is seizures, both in terms of prevalence and treatment issues. Accurate data on the prevalence of seizure disorders are lacking, but it is estimated that up to 60% of those with RTT experience them.[102]

The International Rett Syndrome Database was used to determine if specific gene mutations influenced seizure onset and frequency. In addition to demographic data and specific health and developmental information, enrollees (n = 685) had a *MECP2* mutation. Researchers found the groups most affected by active seizures were between ages 7 and 12 years (49%) and 12 and 17 years (54%). Also identified were specific deletions and mutations associated with seizures activity. A large deletion was associated with the earliest onset where a *p.R133c* mutation was associated with the latest onset; active seizures were more commonly associated with either a large deletion or a *p.T158M* mutation.[103]

Antiepileptic medication usage was also extracted from the international database (n = 135). The most frequently used medications were valproate (47%), carbamazepine (39%), lamotrigine (30%), levetiracetam ((24%), and topiramate (19%) with 34% (n = 116) receiving at least one medication since seizures onset.[103] While some of the enrollees were seizure-free, 129 of 339 (38%) met criteria for drug-resistant epilepsy. Internationally, lamotrigine and valproate were more frequently used.[103]

Comorbidities, including seizures and cardiac problems, can impact drug selection. Cardiac mortality is significantly elevated in RTT. Patients with RTT have a 300-fold increase in sudden death from arrhythmias compared with the general population.[104] Causality has not been determined. Electrocardiogram (ECG) findings of QT prolongation and dyssynchronous innervations cannot account for the marked increase in mortality. Administration of medications that prolong the QT interval should be undertaken only with caution and ECG monitoring. Any pharmacotherapy should take into consideration cardiac implications and other potential adverse drug effects.

Personalized Pharmacotherapy

RTT is an X-linked dominant mutation at the Xq28 site. Mutations on this gene have been identified that may provide an explanation for differences in severity and onset for seizures and physiological variation, as well as developmental regression. Future advances in pharmacogenomics may help identify personalized pharmacotherapy for this population.

Evaluation of Therapeutic Outcomes

The most medication-responsive feature of RTT is seizure activity. Seizure frequency changes with age.[103] For more information about epilepsy and seizure disorders, see Chapter 56. Depending on the anticonvulsant used, laboratory monitoring may be needed. Seizure frequency and adverse effects should be monitored when medications are added or doses changed and at regular intervals thereafter. During the late teens and 20s, reassessing the need for continued anticonvulsant treatment is recommended, since seizures have been known to spontaneously abate in later phases of the disorder.

ABBREVIATIONS

AAIDD	American Association on Intellectual and Developmental Disabilities
AAP	American Academy of Pediatrics
AD	Alzheimer disease
ADHD	attention-deficit/hyperactivity disorder
ADL	activities of daily living
ALL	acute lymphoblastic leukemia
AMKL	acute megakaryoblastic leukemia
AML	acute myelogenous leukemia
ASD	autism spectrum disorder
BAS	Barnes Akathisia Scale
CAM	complementary and alternative medicine
CBT	cognitive behavior therapy
CNV	copy number variation
DISCUS	Dyskinesia Identification System Condensed User Scale
DMR	Dementia Questionnaire for Mentally Retarded Persons
DNA	deoxyribonucleic acid
DS	Down syndrome
ECG	electrocardiogram
ECT	electroconvulsive therapy
GABA	γ-aminobutyric acid

GATA-1	Erythroid transcription factor or GATA-binding factor 1
GI	gastrointestinal
5-HT	5-hydroxytryptamine
5-HT_{2A}	serotonin_{2A}
ICF	International Classification of Functioning, Disability and Health Scaling System
ID	intellectual disability
IQ	intelligence quotient
MeCP2	methyl-CpG-binding protein 2
MECP2	methyl-CpG-binding gene mutation
MMR	measles-mumps-rubella
NIH	National Institutes of Health
NMDA	*N*-methyl-D-aspartate
PDD	Pervasive Developmental Disorder
RTT	Rett syndrome
SGA	second-generation antipsychotic
SSRI	selective serotonin reuptake inhibitor
TAM	transient abnormal myeloproliferative

REFERENCES

1. American Psychiatric Association: *Diagnostic and Statistical Manual of Mental Disorders*, Fifth Edition. Arlington, VA, American Psychiatric Association, 2013.
2. Werner S, Stawski M. Mental health: knowledge, attitudes and training of professionals on dual diagnosis of intellectual disability and psychiatric disorder. *J Intellect Disabil Res* 2012;56:291-304.
3. Turygin N, Matson JL, Adams H. Prevalence of co-occurring disorders in a sample of adults with mild and moderate intellectual disabilities who reside in a residential treatment setting. *Res Dev Disabil* 2014;35:1802-1808.
4. Hermans H, Evenhuis HM. Life events and their associations with depression and anxiety in older people with intellectual disabilities: Results of the HA-ID study. *J Affect Disord* 2012;138:79-85.
5. Bishop KM, Robinson LM, VanLare S. Healthy aging for older adults with intellectual and development disabilities. *J Psychosoc Nurs Ment Health Serv* 2013;51:15-18.
6. AAIDD. American Association on Intellectual and Developmental Disabilities Web site. Available at: http://aaidd.org/intellectual-disability/definition#.VNkJbi7xVA8 Accessed August 6, 2015.
7. Schalock RL, Luckasson RA, Shogren KA, et al. The renaming of mental retardation: understanding the change to the term intellectual disability. *Intellect Dev Disabil* 2007;45:116-124.
8. Tsao R, Kindelberger C, Freminville B, et al. Variability of the aging process in dementia-free adults with Down syndrome. *Am J Intellect Dev Disabil* 2015;120:3-15.
9. Barca D, Tarta-Arsene O, Dica A, et al. Intellectual disability and epilepsy in down syndrome. *Maedica* 2014;9:344-350.
10. Steiner B, Masood R, Rufibach K, et al. An unexpected finding: younger fathers have a higher risk for offspring with chromosomal aneuploidies. *Eur J Hum Genet* 2014;4:466-472.
11. Fisch H, Hyun G, Golden R, et al. The influence of paternal age on Down syndrome. *J Urol* 2003;169:2275-2278.
12. Hollis ND, Allen EG, Oliver TR, et al. Preconception folic acid supplementation and risk for chromosome 21 nondisjunction: A report from the National Down Syndrome Project. *Am J Med Genet A* 2013;161A:438-444.
13. Bunt CW, Bunt SK. Role of the family physician in the care of children with down syndrome. *Am Fam Physician* 2014;90:851-858.
14. Bull MJ. Health supervision for children with Down syndrome. *Pediatrics* 2011;128:393-406.
15. Walker JC, Dosen A, Buitelaar JK, Janzing JG. Depression in Down syndrome: A review of the literature. *Res Dev Disabil* 2011;32:1432-1440.
16. Zigman WB. Atypical aging in Down syndrome. *Dev Disabil Res Rev* 2013;18:51-67.
17. Ross WT, Olsen M. Care of the adult patient with Down syndrome. *South Med J* 2014;107:715-721.
18. Coppus AMW, Schuur M, Vergeer J, et al. Plasma β amyloid and the risk of Alzheimer's disease in Down syndrome. *Neurobiol Aging* 2011;33:1988-1994.
19. Hanney M, Prasher V, Williams N, et al. Memantine for dementia in adults older than 40 years with Down's syndrome (MEADOWS): A randomised, double-blind, placebo-controlled trial. *Lancet* 2012;379:528-536.
20. Kondoh T, Kanno A, Itoh H, et al. Donepezil significantly improves abilities in daily lives of female Down syndrome patients with severe cognitive impairment: A 24-week randomized, double-blind, placebo-controlled trial. *Unt J Psychiatry Med* 2011;41:71-89.
21. O'Rafferty C, Kelly J, Storey L, et al. Child and adolescent Down syndrome-associated leukaemia: the Irish experience. *Ir J Med Sci* 2014;(1971-):1-6.
22. Bohnstedt C, Levinsen M, Rosthoj S, et al. Physicians compliance during maintenance therapy in children with Down syndrome and acute lymphoblastic leukemia. *Leukemia* 2013;27:866-870.
23. Hefti E, Blanco JG. Anthracycline-related cardiotoxicity in patients with acute myeloid leukemia and Down syndrome: A literature review. *Cardiovasc Toxicol* 2015:1-9. doi 10.1007/s12012-015-9307-1
24. Polsek D, Jagatic T, Cepanec M, et al. Recent Developments in neuropathology of autism spectrum disorders. *Transl Neurosci* 2011;2:256-264.
25. Malone RP, Waheed A. The role of antipsychotics in the management of behavioural symptoms in children and adolescents with autism. *Drugs* 2009;69:535-548.
26. Baoi J. Prevalence of autism spectrum disorder among children aged 8 years. *MMWR Morb Mortal Wkly Rep* 2014;63:1-21.
27. Muhle R, Trentacoste SV, Rapin I. The genetics of autism. *Pediatrics* 2004;113:e472-86.
28. Johnson CP, Myers SM. Disabilities CoCw. Identification and evaluation of children with autism spectrum disorders. *Pediatrics* 2007;120:1183-1215.
29. Bos KJ, Zeanah CH, Jr., Smyke AT, et al. Stereotypies in children with a history of early institutional care. *Arch Pediatr Adolesc Med* 2010;164:406-411.
30. LeBlanc JJ, Fagiolini M. Autism: A "critical period" disorder? *Neural Plast* 2011;2011:921680.
31. Salyakina D, Cukier HN, Lee JM, et al. Copy number variants in extended autism spectrum disorder families reveal candidates potentially involved in autism risk. *PLoS One* 2011;6:e26049.
32. Ben-Sasson A, Hen L, Fluss R, Cermak SA, Engel-Yeger B, Gal E. A meta-analysis of sensory modulation symptoms in individuals with autism spectrum disorders. *J Autism Dev Disord* 2009;39:1-11.
33. Simmons DR, Robertson AE, McKay LS, Toal E, McAleer P, Pollick FE. Vision in autism spectrum disorders. *Vision Res* 2009;49:2705-2739.
34. Ozonoff S, Young GS, Carter A, et al. Recurrence risk for autism spectrum disorders: A Baby Siblings Research Consortium Study. *Pediatrics* 2011;128:e488-e495.
35. Dhillon S, Hellings JA, Butler MG. Genetics and mitochondrial abnormalities in autism spectrum disorders: A review. *Curr Genomics* 2011;12:322-332.
36. Sandin S, Lichtenstein P, Kuja-Halkola R, et al. The familial risk of autism. *JAMA* 2014;311:1770-1777.
37. Rahbar MH, Samms-Vaughan M, Loveland KA, et al. Maternal and paternal age are jointly associated with childhood autism in Jamaica. *J Autism Dev Disord* 2012;42:1928-1938.
38. Shelton JF, Tancredi DJ, Hertz-Picciotto I. Independent and dependent contributions of advanced maternal and paternal ages to autism risk. *Autism Res* 2010;3:30-39.
39. Hultman CM, Sandin S, Levine SZ, et al. Advancing paternal age and risk of autism: new evidence from a population-based study and a meta-analysis of epidemiological studies. *Mol Psychiatry* 2011;16:1203-1212.
40. Russo AJ, Devito R. Analysis of copper and zinc plasma concentration and the efficacy of zinc therapy in individuals with Asperger's syndrome, Pervasive Developmental Disorder Not Otherwise Specified (PDD-NOS) and autism. *Biomarker Insights* 2011;6:127-133.
41. Hensley E, Briars L. Closer look at autism and the measles-mumps-rubella vaccine. *JAPhA* 2010;50:736-741.
42. Sgado P, Dunleavy M, Genovesi S, et al. The role of GABAergic system in neurodevelopmental disorders: a focus on autism and epilepsy. *Int J Physiol Pathophysiol Pharmacol* 2011;3:223-335.
43. Mefford HC, Batshaw ML, Hoffman EP. Genomics, intellectual disability, and autism. *N Engl J Med* 2012;366:733-743.
44. Costa e Silva JA. Autism, a brain developmental disorder: some new pathopysiologic and genetics findings. *Metabolism* 2008;57 (Suppl 2): S40-S43.
45. Deutsch SI, Urbano MR, Neumann SA, et al. Cholinergic abnormalities in autism: is there a rationale for selective nicotinic agonist interventions? *Clin Neuropharmacol* 2010;33:114-120.
46. Kazek B, Huzarska M, Grzybowska-Chlebowczyk U, et al. Platelet and intestinal 5-HT2A receptor mRNA in autistic spectrum disorders-results of a pilot study. *Acta Neurobiol Exp (Wars)* 2010;70:232-238.

47. Sadock BJ, Sadock VA. Pervasive Developmental Disorders. In: *Synopsis of Psychiatry*. 10th ed. Baltimore, MD: Williams and Wilkins; 2007:1191-1205.
48. El Achkar CM, Spence SJ. Clinical characteristics of children and young adults with co-occurring autism spectrum disorder and epilepsy. *Epilepsy Behav* 2015;47:183-190.
49. Amiet C, Gourfinkel-An I, Bouzamondo A, et al. Epilepsy in autism is associated with intellectual disability and gender: Evidence from a meta-analysis. *Biol Psychiatry* 2008;64:577-582.
50. Ming X, Brimacombe M, Chaaban J, Zimmerman-Bier B, Wagner GC. Autism spectrum disorders: Concurrent clinical disorders. *J Child Neurol* 2008;23:6-13.
51. Corsello CM. Early intervention in autism. *Infants & Young Children* 2005;18:74-85.
52. Oosterling IJ, Wensing M, Swinkels SH, et al. Advancing early detection of autism spectrum disorder by applying an integrated two-stage screening approach. *J Child Psychol Psychiatry* 2010;51:250-258.
53. Prater CD, Zylstra RG. Autism: a medical primer. *Am Fam Physician* 2002;66:1667-1674.
54. Baird G, Cass H, Slonims V. Diagnosis of autism. *BMJ* 2003;327: 488-493.
55. Vanbergeijk E, Klin A, Volkmar F. Supporting more able students on the autism spectrum: college and beyond. *J Autism Dev Disord* 2008;38:1359-1370.
56. Parikh MS, Kolevzon A, Hollander E. Psychopharmacology of aggression in children and adolescents with autism: A critical review of efficacy and tolerability. *J Child Adolesc Psychopharmacol* 2008;18:157-178.
57. Schultz ST. Does thimerosal or other mercury exposure increase the risk for autism? A review of current literature. *Acta Neurobiol Exp (Wars)* 2010;70:187-195.
58. Jain A, Marshall J, Buikema A, Bancroft T, Kelly JP, Newschaffer CJ. Autism occurrence by MMR vaccine status among US children with older siblings with and without autism. *JAMA* 2015;313: 1534-1540.
59. National Institute of Neurological Disorders and Stroke. Autism Fact Sheet (NIH Publication No. 06-1877). Available at: http://www.ninds.nih.gov/disorders/autism/detail_autism.htm#268313082 Accessed August 6, 2015.
60. Beversdorf D. Therapeutic interventions in autism: A review for primary care physicians. *Mo Med* 2008;105:390-395.
61. Bodfish JW. Treating the core features of autism: are we there yet? *Ment Retard Dev Disabil Res Rev* 2004;10:318-326.
62. Green VA, Pituch KA, Itchon J, et al. Internet survey of treatments used by parents of children with autism. *Res Dev Disabil* 2006;27: 70-84.
63. Brondino N, Fusar-Poli L, Rocchetti M, et al. Complementary and alternative therapies for Autism Spectrum Disorder. *Evid Based Complement Alternat Med* 2015;2015:258589.
64. Miano S, Ferri R. Epidemiology and management of insomnia in children with autistic spectrum disorders. *Paediatr Drugs* 2010;12:75-84.
65. Schwichtenberg AJ, Malow BA. Melatonin treatment in children with developmental disabilities. *Sleep Med Clin* 2015;10:181-187.
66. Baribeau DA, Anagnostou E. An update on medication management of behavioral disorders in autism. *Curr Psychiatry Rep* 2014;16:437.
67. Politte LC, McDougle CJ. Atypical antipsychotics in the treatment of children and adolescents with pervasive developmental disorders. *Psychopharmacology (Berl)* 2014;231:1023-1036.
68. Curran MP. Aripiprazole: in the treatment of irritability associated with autistic disorder in pediatric patients. *Paediatr Drugs* 2011;13: 197-204.
69. Aman MG, Kasper W, Manos G, et al. Line-item analysis of the Aberrant Behavior Checklist: results from two studies of aripiprazole in the treatment of irritability associated with autistic disorder. *J Child Adolesc Psychopharmacol* 2010;20:415-422.
70. Marcus RN, Owen R, Kamen L, et al. A placebo-controlled, fixed-dose study of aripiprazole in children and adolescents with irritability associated with autistic disorder. *J Am Acad Child Adolesc Psychiatry* 2009;48:1110-1119.
71. Marcus RN, Owen R, Manos G, et al. Aripiprazole in the treatment of irritability in pediatric patients (aged 6-17 years) with autistic disorder: Results from a 52-week, open-label study. *J Am Acad Child Adolesc Psychiatry* 2011;21:229-236.
72. Varni JW, Handen BL, Corey-Lisle PK, et al. Effect of aripiprazole 2 to 15 mg/d on health-related quality of life in the treatment of irritability associated with autistic disorder in children: A post hoc analysis of two controlled trials. *Clin Ther* 2012;34:980-992.
73. Canitano R, Scandurra V. Psychopharmacology in autism: An update. *Prog Neuropsychopharmacol Biol Psychiatry* 2011;35:18-28.
74. Anderson GM, Scahill L, McCracken JT, et al. Effects of short- and long-term risperidone treatment on prolactin levels in children with autism. *Biol Psychiatry* 2007;61:545-550.
75. West L, Brunssen SH, Waldrop J. Review of the evidence for treatment of children with autism with selective serotonin reuptake inhibitors. *J Spec Pediatr Nurs* 2009;14:183-191.
76. King BH, Hollander E, Sikich L, et al. Lack of efficacy of citalopram in children with autism spectrum disorders and high levels of repetitive behavior: Citalopram ineffective in children with autism. *Arch Gen Psychiatry* 2009;66:583-590.
77. Preti A, Melis M, Siddi S, Vellante M, Doneddu G, Fadda R. Oxytocin and autism: A systematic review of randomized controlled trials. *J Child Adolesc Psychopharmacol* 2014;24:54-68.
78. Handen BL, Taylor J, Tumuluru R. Psychopharmacological treatment of ADHD symptoms in children with autism spectrum disorder. *Int J Adolesc Med Health* 2011;23:167-173.
79. Posey DJ, Aman MG, McCracken JT, et al. Positive effects of methylphenidate on inattention and hyperactivity in pervasive developmental disorders: An analysis of secondary measures. *Biol Psychiatry* 2007;61:538-544.
80. Aman MG, Farmer CA, Hollway J, Arnold LE. Treatment of inattention, overactivity, and impulsiveness in autism spectrum disorders. *Child Adolesc Psychiatr Clin N Am* 2008;17:713-738.
81. Ghaleiha A, Asadabadi M, Mohammadi MR, et al. Memantine as adjunctive treatment to risperidone in children with autistic disorder: A randomized, double-blind, placebo-controlled trial. *Int J Neuropsychopharmacol* 2013;16:783-789.
82. Hu VW. A systems approach towards an understanding, diagnosis and personalized treatment of autism spectrum disorders. *Pharmacogenomics* 2011;12:1235-8.
83. Correia CT, Almeida JP, Santos PE, et al. Pharmacogenetics of risperidone therapy in autism: Association analysis of eight candidate genes with drug efficacy and adverse drug reactions. *Pharmacogenomics J* 2010;10:418-430.
84. Lit L, Sharp FR, Bertoglio K, et al. Gene expression in blood is associated with risperidone response in children with autism spectrum disorders. *Pharmacogenomics J* 2012;12:368-371.
85. McCracken JT, Badashova KK, Posey DJ, et al. Positive effects of methylphenidate on hyperactivity are moderated by monoaminergic gene variants in children with autism spectrum disorders. *Pharmacogenomics J* 2014;14:295-302.
86. Aman MG, Singh NN, Turbott SH. Reliability of the Aberrant Behavior Checklist and the effect of variations in instructions. *Am J Ment Defic* 1987;92:237-240.
87. Aman MG, Singh NN. *Aberrant Behavior Checklist–Community. Supplemental Manual*. East Aurora, NY: Slosson Educational Publications; 1994.
88. Scahill L, McDougle CJ, Williams SK, et al. Children's Yale-Brown Obsessive Compulsive Scale modified for pervasive developmental disorders. *J Am Acad Child Adolesc Psychiatry* 2006;45:1114-1123.
89. Kalachnik JE. Medication monitoring procedures: thou shall, here's how. In: Gadow KD, Poling, AG, ed. *Pharmacotherapy and Mental Retardation*. Boston, MA: College-Hill; 1985:231-268.
90. Barnes TR. A rating scale for drug-induced akathisia. *Br J Psychiatry* 1989;154:672-676.
91. Simpson GM, Angus JW. A rating scale for extrapyramidal side effects. *Acta Psychiatr Scand Suppl* 1970;212:11-19.
92. Kalachnik JE. Measuring side effects of psychopharmacologic medications in individuals with mental retardation and developmental disabilities. *Ment Retard Dev Disabil Res Rev* 1999;5:348-359.
93. Hagberg B, Aicardi J, Dias K, Ramos O. A progressive syndrome of autism, dementia, ataxia, and loss of purposeful hand use in girls: Rett's syndrome: Report of 35 cases. *Ann Neurol* 1983;14:471-479.
94. Dolce A, Ben-Zeev B, Naidu S, Kossoff EH. Rett syndrome and epilepsy: An update for child neurologists. *Pediatr Neurol* 2013;48:337-345.
95. Cuddapah VA, Pillai RB, Shekar KV, et al. Methyl-CpG-binding protein 2 (MECP2) mutation type is associated with disease severity in Rett syndrome. *J Med Genett* 2014;51:152-158.
96. Liyanage VR, Rastegar M. Rett syndrome and MeCP2. *Neuromolecular Med* 2014;16:231-264.
97. Anderson A, Wong K, Jacoby P, et al. Twenty years of surveillance in Rett syndrome: What does this tell us? *Orphanet J Rare Dis* 2014;9:87.

98. Chapleau CA, Lane J, Larimore J, et al. Recent progress in Rett syndrome and MeCP2 dysfunction: Assessment of potential treatment options. *Future Neurol* 2013;8:21-28.
99. Neul JL, Kaufmann WE, Glaze DG, et al. Rett syndrome: Revised diagnostic criteria and nomenclature. *Ann Neurol* 2010;68:944-950.
100. Hagebeuk EE, Bijlmer RP, Koelman JH, Poll-The BT. Respiratory disturbances in Rett syndrome: Don't forget to evaluate upper airway obstruction. *J Child Neurol* 2012;27:888-892.
101. Karmaniolou I, Krishnan R, Galtrey E, et al. Perioperative management and outcome of patients with Rett syndrome undergoing scoliosis surgery: S retrospective review. *J Anesth* 2015;29:492-498.
102. Chapleau CA, Lane J, Pozzo-Miller L, Percy AK. Evaluation of current pharmacological treatment options in the management of Rett syndrome: From the present to future therapeutic alternatives. *Curr Clin Pharmacol* 2013;8:358-369.
103. Bao X, Downs J, Wong K, Williams S, Leonard H. Using a large international sample to investigate epilepsy in Rett syndrome. *Dev Med Child Neurol* 2013;55:553-558.
104. De Felice C, Maffei S, Signorini C, et al. Subclinical myocardial dysfunction in Rett syndrome. *Eur Heart J Cardiovasc Imaging* 2012;13:339-345.

74 Diabetes Mellitus

Curtis L. Triplitt, Thomas Repas, and Carlos Alvarez

KEY CONCEPTS

1. Diabetes mellitus (DM) is a group of metabolic disorders characterized by high blood glucose as well as altered fat and protein metabolism that results from defects in insulin secretion, insulin action (sensitivity), or both.
2. The incidence of type 2 DM is increasing. This has been attributed to obesity, dietary habits, and increasing numbers of people who are sedentary and genetically susceptible.
3. The two major classifications of DM are type 1 (insulin deficient) and type 2 (insulin resistance combined with β-cell dysfunction). They differ in clinical presentation, onset, etiology, and disease progression. Both are associated with microvascular and macrovascular complications.
4. Diabetes can be diagnosed by one of four criteria: (1) fasting plasma glucose ≥ 126 mg/dL (≥ 7.0 mmol/L); (2) a 2-hour value from a 75-g oral glucose tolerance test (OGTT) ≥ 200 mg/dL (more than or equal to 11.1 mmol/L); a casual plasma glucose level ≥ 200 mg/dL (≥ 11.1 mmol/L) with symptoms of diabetes; or a hemoglobin A_{1c} (HbA_{1c}) ≥ 6.5% (≥ 0.065; ≥ 48 mmol/mol Hb). The diagnosis should be confirmed by repeat testing if obvious hyperglycemia is not present.
5. Goals of therapy in DM are directed toward attaining normoglycemia (or appropriate glycemic control based on the patient's comorbidities), reducing the onset and progression of diabetes-related complications, intensive therapy for associated cardiovascular risk factors, and improving quality and quantity of life.
6. Intensive glycemic control is paramount for reduction of microvascular complications (eg, neuropathy, retinopathy, and nephropathy). Good blood pressure control in patients with diabetes will not only reduce the risk of retinopathy and nephropathy, but also reduce cardiovascular risk.
7. Short-term (less than 5 years) intensive glycemic control does not lower the risk of macrovascular events—significant reductions in macrovascular complications may take 15 to 20 years. Excellent glycemic control from the time of diagnosis may result in a sustained reduction in microvascular and macrovascular risk, and has been coined metabolic memory or legacy effect.
8. Knowledge of the patient's quantitative and qualitative meal patterns, activity levels, pharmacokinetics of insulin preparations, and pharmacology of oral and injected antihyperglycemic agents are essential to individualize the treatment plan and optimize blood glucose control while minimizing risks for hypoglycemia and other adverse effects of pharmacologic therapies.
9. Insulin therapy is required in Type 1 DM. Intensive basal-bolus insulin therapy or pump therapy in motivated individuals is more likely to achieve optimal glycemic outcomes. Basal-bolus therapy includes a basal insulin for fasting and a rapid acting insulin for mealtime coverage. The addition of mealtime pramlintide in patients with uncontrolled or erratic postprandial glycemia may be warranted.
10. Metformin should be included in the regimen for most type 2 DM patients, if tolerated and not contraindicated, due to its effectiveness, low risk of hypoglycemia, positive or neutral effects on weight, potential impact on macrovascular risk cardiovascular risk, and low cost.
11. Type 2 DM treatment often requires multiple therapeutic agents (combination therapy), including oral and injected antihyperglycemics to attain glycemic goals. There is a persistent reduction in β-cell function over time. The thiazolidinediones (TZDs) and the GLP-1 receptor agonists have been shown to slow, but not arrest, β-cell failure.
12. Aggressive management of cardiovascular risk factors in type 2 DM is necessary to reduce the incidence of cardiovascular events and death. This includes smoking cessation, use of antiplatelet therapy as well as moderate or high potency statins in most patients with DM, and treatment of hypertension.
13. Strategies to prevent type 1 DM have not yet been successful. Prevention strategies for type 2 DM include dietary restriction of fat, aerobic exercise for a minimum of 30 minutes 5 times a week, weight loss, and increased fiber intake. These lifestyle habits can reduce the risk of type 2 DM by 60%. No medication is currently FDA approved for the prevention of diabetes, but several have been shown to delay diabetes onset in high-risk patients.
14. Patient education, self-care, and adherence to therapeutic lifestyle and pharmacologic interventions are crucial for optimal outcomes. Interprofessional teams including physicians (primary care, endocrinologists, ophthalmologists, and vascular surgeons), dietitians, nurses, pharmacists, podiatrists, social workers, behavioral health specialists, and certified diabetes educators (CDEs) working together can assist persons with DM achieve optimal health outcomes.

INTRODUCTION

Diabetes mellitus (DM) is a heterogeneous group of metabolic disorders characterized by hyperglycemia. It is associated with abnormalities in carbohydrate, fat, and protein metabolism and may result in chronic complications including microvascular, macrovascular, and neuropathic disorders. In 2012, an estimated 29 million Americans 20 years of age or older, roughly 12% to 14% of the population, have DM. Over one-fourth have not yet been diagnosed. An additional 86 million are at high risk for developing diabetes. The economic burden of DM approximated $245 billion in 2012. DM is the leading cause of blindness in adults aged 20 to 74 years and the leading cause of end-stage renal disease in the United States. It also resulted in approximately 73,000 lower extremity amputations in 2010. Finally, a cardiovascular event is responsible for two-thirds of deaths in individuals with type 2 DM and is the leading cause of death in type 1 DM of long-duration.[1]

Optimal management of the patient with DM will reduce or prevent complications, decrease morbidity and mortality, and improve quality of life. Research, clinical trials, and drug development efforts over the past several decades have not only improved health outcomes in patients with DM but also significantly expanded the available therapeutic options.

ETIOLOGY AND CLASSIFICATION[2]

Diabetes mellitus is a metabolic disorder characterized by resistance to the action of insulin, insufficient insulin secretion, or both. The clinical manifestation of these disorders is hyperglycemia. The vast majority of patients with DM are classified into one of two broad categories: type 1 DM caused by an absolute deficiency of insulin, or type 2 DM defined by the presence of insulin resistance and β-cell dysfunction. Women who develop diabetes during pregnancy are classified as having gestational diabetes. Finally, uncommon types of diabetes caused by infections, drugs, endocrinopathies, pancreatic destruction, and known genetic defects are classified separately (Table 74-1).

TABLE 74-1 Etiologic Classification of Diabetes Mellitus[a]

1. **Type 1 diabetes[b]** (β-cell destruction, usually leading to absolute insulin deficiency)
   Immune mediated
   Idiopathic
2. **Type 2 diabetes[a]** (may range from predominantly insulin resistance with relative insulin deficiency to a predominantly insulin secretory defect with insulin resistance)
3. **Other specific types**
   - Genetic defects of β-cell function
     - Chromosome 20q, HNF-4α (MODY1)
     - Chromosome 7p, glucokinase (MODY2)
     - Chromosome 12q, HNF-1α (MODY3)
     - *Other rare forms*
     - Chromosome 13q, insulin promoter factor-1 (MODY4)
     - Chromosome 17q, HNF-1β (MODY5)
     - Chromosome 2q, neurogenic differentiation 1/β-cell e-box transactivator 2 (MODY6)
     - Chromosome 9q, carboxyl ester lipase (MODY7)
     - Mitochondrial DNA
   - Genetic defects in insulin action
     - Type A insulin resistance
     - Leprechaunism
     - Rabson-Mendenhall syndrome
     - Lipoatrophic diabetes
   - Diseases of the exocrine pancreas
     - Pancreatitis
     - Trauma/pancreatectomy
     - Neoplasia
     - Cystic fibrosis
     - Hemochromatosis
     - Fibrocalculous pancreatopathy
   - Endocrinopathies
     - Acromegaly
     - Cushing syndrome
     - Glucagonoma
     - Pheochromocytoma
     - Hyperthyroidism
     - Somatostatinoma
     - Aldosteronoma
   - Drug or chemical induced
     - Pyriminil
     - Pentamidine
     - Nicotinic acid
     - Glucocorticoids
     - Thyroid hormone
     - Diazoxide
     - β-Adrenergic agonists
     - Thiazides
     - Phenytoin
     - γ-Interferon
     - Others
   - Infections
     - Congenital rubella
     - Cytomegalovirus
     - Others
   - Uncommon forms of immune-mediated diabetes
     - "Stiff-man" syndrome
     - Anti-insulin receptor antibodies
   - Other genetic syndromes sometimes associated with diabetes
     - Down syndrome
     - Klinefelter syndrome
     - Turner syndrome
     - Wolfram syndrome
     - Friedreich ataxia
     - Huntington chorea
     - Laurence-Moon-Bieldel syndrome
     - Myotonic dystrophy
     - Porphyria
     - Prader-Willi syndrome
4. **Gestational diabetes mellitus (GDM)**

[a]Other rare forms may exist for all categorizations.

[b]Patients with any form of diabetes may require insulin treatment at some stage of their disease. Such use of insulin does not itself classify the patient.

Data from reference 2.

Type 1 Diabetes[2-4]

This form of diabetes results from autoimmune destruction of the β-cells of the pancreas. Evidence of β-cell autoimmunity, including islet cell antibodies (ICA), antibodies to glutamic acid decarboxylase, islet protein tyrosine phosphatase-like molecule IA2, and/or antibodies to insulin are present at the time of diagnosis in 90% of individuals. Type 1 diabetes most commonly presents in children and adolescents; however, it can occur at any age. Younger individuals typically have a more rapid rate of β-cell destruction and often present with ketoacidosis. Adults may maintain sufficient insulin secretion to prevent ketoacidosis for many years; this is referred to as latent autoimmune diabetes in adults (LADA).

Type 2 Diabetes[2,5]

Type 2 DM is characterized by a combination of some degree of insulin resistance with a relative lack of insulin secretion that is insufficient to normalize plasma glucose levels, with a progressive loss of β-cell over time. Most individuals with type 2 diabetes exhibit abdominal obesity, which is the major contributor to insulin resistance. In addition, hypertension, dyslipidemia (high triglyceride levels and low HDL-cholesterol levels), and elevated plasminogen activator inhibitor-1 (PAI-1) levels, which contributes to a hypercoagulable state, are often present. Patients with type 2 diabetes are at increased risk of developing macrovascular complications in addition to microvascular complications. Type 2 diabetes has a strong genetic predisposition and is more common in all ethnic groups other than those of European ancestry.

Gestational Diabetes Mellitus[2]

Gestational diabetes mellitus (GDM) is defined as glucose intolerance which is first recognized during pregnancy. Hormone changes during pregnancy result in increased insulin resistance, and GDM may ensue when the mother cannot adequately compensate with increased insulin secretion to maintain normoglycemia. In most, glucose intolerance first appears near the beginning of the third trimester. However, risk assessment and intervention should begin from the first prenatal visit. If DM is diagnosed prior to pregnancy, this is not GDM, but rather pregnancy with preexisting DM. Detection is important, as therapy will reduce perinatal morbidity and mortality.

Other Specific Types of Diabetes (Less Than 5% of Diabetes)[2]

Maturity onset diabetes of youth (MODY) is characterized by impaired insulin secretion in respond to a glucose stimulus with minimal or no insulin resistance. Patients typically exhibit mild hyperglycemia at an early age, but diagnosis may be delayed. The disease is inherited in an autosomal dominant pattern with at least six different loci identified to date (MODY 2 and 3 are most common). The production of mutant insulin molecules has been identified in a few families and results in mild glucose intolerance.

Several genetic mutations have been described in the insulin receptor and are associated with insulin resistance. Type A insulin resistance is a clinical syndrome characterized by acanthosis nigricans, virilization in women, polycystic ovaries, and hyperinsulinemia. Anti-insulin receptor antibodies may block the binding of insulin. This was referred to in the past as type B insulin resistance. Endocrinopathies, pancreatic exocrine dysfunction, drugs, infections, among others may also result in hyperglycemia (see Table 74-1).

EPIDEMIOLOGY[1-5]

Type 1 DM accounts for 5% to 10% of all cases of DM and is most often due to autoimmune destruction of the pancreatic β-cells.[2] Type 1 DM is thought to be initiated by the exposure of a genetically susceptible individual to an environmental trigger. β-Cell autoimmunity develops in less than 10% of the genetically susceptible individuals and progresses to type 1 DM in less than 1%.[3] The prevalence of β-cell autoimmunity and the incidence of type 1 DM in various populations is directly related. Sweden, Sardinia, and Finland have the highest prevalence of islet cell antibody (ICA) (3%-4.5%) and this is associated with the highest incidence of type 1 DM; 22 to 35 per 100,000.[4] The prevalence of type 1 DM is increasing, but the cause of this increase is not fully understood.

Markers of β-cell autoimmunity are detected in 14% to 33% of persons with adult-onset diabetes. This type of DM is referred to as LADA. These patients often have a poor response to oral agents and require insulin therapy much sooner than most patients with type 2 DM.[4]

Idiopathic type 1 DM is a nonautoimmune form of diabetes frequently seen in patients of African and Asian descent. These patients have periods of profound hyperglycemia and intermittently require insulin therapy.[4]

Type 2 DM accounts for up to 90% of all cases of DM. Overall the prevalence of type 2 DM in the United States is about 11.3% in persons age 20 or older; this prevalence is increasing. It is estimated that for every four persons, who are diagnosed with DM, one person remains undiagnosed.[1]

There are multiple risk factors for the development of type 2 DM, including family history (ie, parents or siblings with diabetes); obesity (ie, ≥ 20% over ideal body weight, or body mass index [BMI] ≥ 25 kg/m^2); chronic physical inactivity; race or ethnicity (see list below); history of impaired glucose tolerance, impaired fasting glucose (IFG), or hemoglobin A_{1c} (HbA_{1c}) 5.7% to 6.4% (0.057-0.064; 39-46 mmol/mol Hb) (see diagnosis of diabetes section); hypertension (high than or equal to 140/90 mm Hg in adults); high-density lipoprotein (HDL) cholesterol ≤ 35 mg/dL (≤ 0.91 mmol/L) and/or a triglyceride level ≥ 250 mg/dL (≥ 2.83 mmol/L); history of GDM (see etiology and classification section) or delivery of a baby weighing more than 9 pounds (more than 4 kg); history of vascular disease; presence of acanthosis nigricans; and polycystic ovary disease.[5]

The prevalence of type 2 DM increases with age and varies widely among racial and ethnic populations. The prevalence of type 2 DM is especially high in Native Americans, Hispanic Americans, African Americans, Asian Americans, and Pacific Islanders. While the prevalence of type 2 DM increases with age, the disorder is increasingly being diagnosed in adolescence. The increased incidence of type DM in adolescence and young adults has been attributed to an increase in overweight/obesity and sedentary lifestyle, in addition to genetic predisposition.[2] Most cases of type 2 DM appear to be polygenetic.[2]

Gestational diabetes mellitus complicates approximately 9% of all pregnancies in the United States.[2] Most women become normoglycemic after pregnancy; however, 30% to 50% of these women develop type 2 DM later in life.

Secondary forms of DM occur due to a variety of causes.[2] MODY is due to one of six genetic defects. Endocrine disorders, such as acromegaly and Cushing syndrome, may also induce hyperglycemia. Any disease of the exocrine pancreas such as cystic fibrosis, pancreatitis, and hereditary hemochromatosis can damage β-cells and impair insulin secretion. Only 1% to 2% of all cases of DM are due to these secondary causes.

PATHOGENESIS[2-4,6-9]

Diabetes mellitus is caused by derangements in the secretion of insulin, glucagon, and other hormones and results in abnormal carbohydrate and fat metabolism. In the fasting state 75% of total body glucose disposal occurs in tissues, including the brain and peripheral nerves that do not require insulin. Brain glucose uptake occurs at the same rate during fed and fasting periods. The remaining 25% of glucose metabolism takes place in the liver and muscle, which is dependent on insulin. In the fasting state, approximately 85% of glucose production is derived from the liver, and the remaining amount is produced by the kidney. Glucagon, produced by pancreatic α cells, is secreted in the fasting state to oppose the action of insulin and stimulate hepatic glucose production and glycogenolysis. Glucagon and insulin secretion are closely linked. Appropriate secretion of both hormones is needed to keep plasma glucose levels normal. In the fed state, carbohydrate ingestion increases the plasma glucose concentration and stimulates insulin release from the pancreatic β-cells. The resultant hyperinsulinemia (1) suppresses hepatic glucose production, (2) stimulates glucose uptake by peripheral tissues, and (3) suppresses glucagon release (in conjunction with incretin hormones). The majority (approximately 80%-85%) of glucose is taken up by muscle. A small amount (approximately 4%-5%) is metabolized by adipocytes.[6-8]

Although fat tissue is responsible for only a small amount of total body glucose disposal, it plays a very important role in the maintenance of total body glucose homeostasis. Small increases in the plasma insulin concentration exert a potent antilipolytic effect, reducing plasma-free fatty acid levels. The decline in plasma-free fatty acid concentrations results in an increased glucose uptake in muscle and indirectly reduces hepatic glucose production.

Type 1 Diabetes Mellitus[2-4,9]

Type 1 DM results from pancreatic β-cell failure with "absolute" deficiency of insulin secretion. Most often this is due to immune-mediated destruction of pancreatic β-cells, but rare unknown or idiopathic processes may also contribute. There often is a long preclinical period of positive autoimmune markers which progress to immune-mediated β-cell destruction with resultant hyperglycemia when 80% to 90% of the β-cells have been destroyed. After the initial diagnosis there is occasionally a period of transient remission called the "honeymoon" phase before β-cell destruction requires lifelong insulin therapy (Fig. 74-1).

In order for type 1 DM to develop, a genetically susceptible individual must be exposed to a trigger that initiates the autoimmune process and destruction of pancreatic β-cell. However, it is unknown precisely what the inciting factors are. Several triggers have been implicated including cow's milk (or lack of breastfeeding), viruses, dietary, or other environmental exposures. Vitamin D deficiency has been observed to be more prevalent in patients who develop type 1 DM. However, further study is needed to confirm whether vitamin D deficiency causes type 1 DM or whether the relationship is merely an association.[10]

The autoimmune process is mediated by macrophages and T lymphocytes with circulating autoantibodies to various β-cell antigens. The most commonly detected antibody associated with type 1 DM is the ICA. Other autoantibodies may be formed to insulin, glutamic acid decarboxylase 65, tyrosine phosphatases IA-2 and IA-2β and ZnT8 (zinc transporter 8). These antibodies are generally considered markers of disease rather than mediators of β-cell destruction. They have been used to identify individuals at risk for type 1 DM and in evaluating disease prevention strategies.[3]

More than 90% of newly diagnosed persons with type 1 DM have one or more of these antibodies, as will up to 4% of unaffected first-degree relatives. β-Cell autoimmunity may precede the diagnosis of type 1 DM by up to 13 years. Autoimmunity may remit in some individuals, or progress to absolute β-cell failure in others. Other autoimmune disorders such as Hashimoto's thyroiditis, Graves' disease, Addison's disease, vitiligo and celiac sprue are more common in patients with type 1 DM. The extent of involvement can range from no associated autoimmune disorders to polyglandular failure.

There are strong genetic linkages to the *DQA* and *B* genes as well as certain human leukocyte antigens (HLAs). Genetic polymorphisms on chromosome 6 have been associated with a higher risk of developing type 1 DM (*DR3* and *DR4*) but others are protective

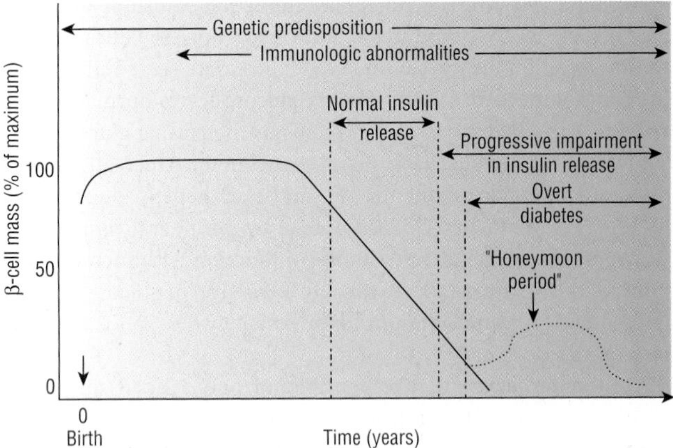

FIGURE 74-1 Scheme of the natural history of the β-cell defect in type 1 diabetes mellitus. *(Copyright© 2008 American Diabetes Association. From Medical Management of Type 1 Diabetes, Fifth Edition. Reprinted with permission from The American Diabetes Association.)*

(*DRB1*04008-DQB1*0302* and *DRB1*0411-DQB1*0302*).[9] Additional candidate gene regions have been identified on other chromosomes as well. Because twin studies do not show 100% concordance, environmental factors, such as infectious, chemical, or dietary exposures, likely contribute to the expression of the disease.

Insulin lowers blood glucose by a variety of mechanisms, including stimulation of tissue glucose uptake, suppression of glucose production by the liver, and suppression of free fatty acid (FFA) release from fat cells.[6] The suppression of FFAs plays an important role in glucose homeostasis. Increased levels of FFAs inhibit the uptake of glucose by muscle and stimulate hepatic gluconeogenesis.[7]

Amylin is a hormone that is cosecreted from the pancreatic β-cell with insulin. Amylin is also deficient in patients with type 1 DM secondary to the destruction of β-cells. Amylin suppresses inappropriate glucagon secretion, slows gastric emptying, and causes central satiety.

Type 2 Diabetes Mellitus[6-8]

Type 2 diabetes is caused by multiple defects including: (1) impaired insulin secretion; (2) deficiency and resistance to incretin hormones; (3) insulin resistance involving muscle, liver, and adipocytes; (4) excess glucagon secretion; and (5) sodium-glucose cotransporter upregulation in the kidney.

Impaired Insulin Secretion[6-8]

The pancreas in people with a normal-functioning β-cell is able to adjust its secretion of insulin to maintain normal plasma glucose levels. In nondiabetic individuals, insulin increases in proportion to the severity of the insulin resistance and plasma glucose remains normal. Impaired insulin secretion is a hallmark finding in type 2 DM. In early β-cell dysfunction, first-phase insulin, as seen with an IV bolus of glucose, is deficient. First phase insulin involves the release of stored insulin in the β-cell and acts to "prime" the liver to nutrient intake. Without appropriate first phase insulin release, second phase insulin must compensate for the ensuing postprandial hyperglycemia in order to normalize glucose levels. When the insulin released is no longer sufficient to normalize plasma glucose, dysglycemia, including prediabetes and diabetes can ensue. β-Cell mass and function in the pancreas are both reduced. β-Cell failure is progressive, and starts years prior to the diagnosis of diabetes. People with type 2 DM lose approximately 5% to 7% of β-cell function per year. The reasons are likely multifactorial including (1) glucose toxicity; (2) lipotoxicity; (3) insulin resistance; (4) age; (5) genetics; and (6) incretin deficiency. Age results in declining β-cell responsiveness and possibly mass. High-risk ethnicity/races are predisposed to β-cell failure. Glucotoxicity occurs when glucose levels chronically exceed 140 mg/dL (7.8 mmol/L). The β-cell is unable to maintain sufficient insulin secretion and, paradoxically, releases less insulin as glucose levels increase (Fig. 74-2).

Incretin Hormone Deficiency/Resistance[6-8]

In patients with type 2 DM, decreased postprandial insulin secretion is a result of both impaired pancreatic β-cell function and reduced stimulus from gut hormones to secrete insulin. The role gut hormones play in insulin secretion is best shown by comparing the insulin response to an oral glucose load versus an isoglycemic intravenous glucose infusion. In individuals who do not have diabetes, 73% more insulin is released in response to an oral glucose load compared to an intravenous (IV) glucose load given to mimic plasma glucose levels achieved during the oral glucose load. The increased insulin secretion in response to an oral glucose stimulus is referred to as "the incretin effect" and is the result of gut hormones, stimulated by oral intake of nutrients (glucose, fat, or protein), that promote pancreatic insulin secretion. In patients with type 2 patients, this "incretin effect" is blunted with the increase in insulin

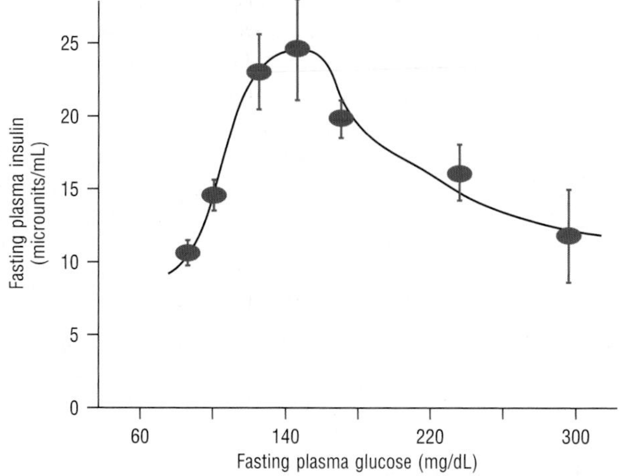

FIGURE 74-2 The relationship between fasting plasma insulin and fasting plasma glucose in 177 normal weight individuals. Plasma insulin and glucose increase together up to a fasting glucose of 140 mg/dL (7.8 mmol/L). When the fasting glucose exceeds 140 mg/dL (7.8 mmol/L), the β-cell makes progressively less insulin, which leads to an overproduction of glucose by the liver and results in a progressive increase in fasting glucose. *(Reprinted from DeFronzo RA. Pathogenesis of type 2 diabetes mellitus. Med Clin N Am 2004;88:787-835, Copyright © 2004, with permission from Elsevier.)*

secretion approximately half of that seen in nondiabetic individuals. It is now known that two hormones, glucagon-like peptide-1 (GLP-1) and glucose-dependent insulinotropic polypeptide (GIP), are responsible for over 90% of the increased insulin secretion seen in response to an oral glucose load. Patients with type 2 DM remain sensitive to GLP-1 but GIP levels are normal or elevated in type 2 DM, which suggests that some individuals may be resistant to its effect.

Glucagon-like peptide-1 is secreted from the L-cells, found in the distal intestinal and colon mucosa, in response to mixed meals. Since GLP-1 levels rise within minutes of food ingestion, neural signals and possibly proximal gastrointestinal tract receptors stimulate GLP-1 secretion. The insulinotropic action of GLP-1 is glucose dependent, enhancing insulin secretion only when glucose concentrations are higher than 90 mg/dL (5.0 mmol/L). In addition to stimulating insulin secretion, GLP-1 suppresses glucagon secretion, slows gastric emptying, and reduces food intake by increasing satiety. These effects of GLP-1 combine to limit postprandial glucose excursions. GIP is secreted by K-cells in the intestine and may have a role with insulin secretion when glucose levels are near normal. It may also act as an insulin sensitizer in adipocytes. However, GIP has no effect on glucagon secretion, gastric motility, or satiety. The half-life GLP-1 and GIP are short (less than 10 minutes). Both hormones are rapidly inactivated by dipeptidyl peptidase-4 (DPP-4), an enzyme that removes two N-terminal amino acids. As patients progress from normoglycemic to type 2 DM, GLP-1 levels decrease as glucose values increase. However, it is unlikely to be a primary defect that causes diabetes in the majority of patients with type 2 DM. A small percentage of patients have the transcription factor 7-like 2 (TCF7L2) gene defect, which is associated with decreased β-cell response to GLP-1 and likely contributes to their risk of diabetes.

Insulin Resistance[6-8]

Resistance to the actions of insulin in the liver contributes significantly to excess hepatic glucose production. In patients with type 2 DM with mild to moderate fasting hyperglycemia (140-200 mg/dL, 7.8-11.1 mmol/L), basal hepatic glucose production is increased by approximately 0.5 mg/kg/min. Consequently, during the overnight sleeping hours the liver of an 80-kg person with diabetes with modest fasting hyperglycemia adds an additional 35 g of glucose to the systemic circulation. This increase in fasting hepatic glucose production is the cause of fasting hyperglycemia. In the postprandial state, the liver inappropriately continues hepatic glucose output. Therefore, patients with type 2 DM have two sources of glucose in the postprandial state, one from the diet and one from continued glucose production from the liver. These sources of glucose may result in marked hyperglycemia.

Peripheral skeletal muscle is the major site of postprandial glucose disposal and approximately 80% of total body glucose uptake occurs in skeletal muscle. In response to a physiologic increase in plasma insulin concentration, muscle glucose uptake increases linearly, reaching a plateau value of 10 mg/kg/min. Even in lean type 2 DM, the onset of insulin action in muscle is delayed by approximately 40 minutes, and the ability of insulin to stimulate glucose uptake in leg muscle is reduced by 50%. Impaired intracellular insulin signaling (secondary messenger system) is a well established abnormality, with notable impairments at almost every step of activation due to insulin resistance, lipotoxicity, and glucotoxicity. The compensatory hyperinsulinemia required to overcome impaired insulin signaling can activate an alternative pathway through MAP kinase, which may be involved in atherosclerosis. Mitochondrial dysfunction may also play a role in muscle insulin resistance. Mitochondrial function and/or density appear to be lower in type 2 DM. This may result in less energy expenditure and an increased risk of dysfunction with high-fat diets.

In obese nondiabetic people as well as patients with type 2 DM, fasting plasma FFA levels are increased and fail to suppress after glucose ingestion. Chronically elevated plasma FFA concentrations can impair insulin secretion and lead to insulin resistance in muscle and liver. FFAs are stored as triglycerides in adipocytes and serve as an important energy source during conditions of fasting. Insulin is a potent inhibitor of lipolysis and restrains the release of FFAs from the adipocyte by inhibiting the hormone-sensitive lipase enzyme. In addition to FFAs that circulate in plasma in increased amounts, patients with type 2 DM have increased stores of intracellular fat products in muscle and liver. This increased fat content correlates closely with the presence of insulin resistance in these tissues. FFA products interfere with multiple steps in the insulin signaling cascade as well as increase β-cell apoptosis. Excess lipolysis from fat can also contribute to gluconeogenesis indirectly through glycerol and FFA substrate use as well as increase a number of proinflammatory cytokines.

Weight gain leads to insulin resistance in most individuals. Obese individuals who do not have diabetes often have the same degree of insulin resistance as lean type 2 DM patients. Obese but metabolically normal patients do exist (6%-30%) as well as patients who are not obese but metabolically abnormal. Thus, obesity does not automatically result in insulin resistance.

The term *visceral adipose tissue* (VAT) refers to fat cells located within the abdominal cavity and includes omental, mesenteric, retroperitoneal, and perinephric adipose tissue. VAT has been shown to correlate with insulin resistance and explain much of the variation in insulin resistance seen. VAT represents 20% of fat in men and 6% of fat in women. Central obesity can most easily be assessed using waist circumference, which is a good surrogate marker for VAT. VAT fat tissue has been shown to have a higher rate of lipolysis than subcutaneous fat, resulting in an increase in FFA production. These fatty acids are released into the portal circulation and drain into the liver, where they stimulate the production of very-low-density lipoproteins and decrease insulin sensitivity in peripheral tissues and increase the risk for nonalcoholic fatty liver disease.

Visceral adipose tissue also produces a number of adipocytokines, such as tissue necrosis factor-α, interleukin 6, angiotensinogen, plasminogen activator inhibitor-1, and resistin—all of which contribute to insulin resistance, hypertension, and hypercoagulability. These factors drain into the portal circulation and reduce insulin sensitivity in peripheral tissues. The fat cell also has the capability of producing at least one adipocytokine that improves insulin sensitivity: adiponectin. Unfortunately, adiponectin levels decline as an individual becomes more obese. Adiponectin decreases hepatic glucose production, improves hepatic insulin sensitivity, and increases fatty acid oxidation in muscle.

Excess Glucagon Secretion[6-8]

Type 2 DM patients fail to suppress glucagon in response to a meal and may even have a paradoxical rise in glucagon levels. Two main factors contribute: (1) GLP-1 resistance/deficiency; and (2) insulin resistance and/or deficiency, which directly suppress glucagon. Thus, hepatic insulin resistance, hyperglucagonemia, and GLP-1 deficiency result in excessive production of glucose by the liver.

Sodium-Glucose Cotransporters[8]

Ninety percent of the filtered glucose is reabsorbed by sodium glucose cotransporter-2 (SGLT2), a high-capacity, low-affinity transporter. The remaining approximately 10% is reabsorbed by SGLT1. In normal healthy people, the renal threshold for glucosuria is at a plasma glucose value of approximately 180 mg/dL (approximately 10.0 mmol/L). In chronic hyperglycemia, such as in diabetes, the renal threshold is increased to 220 to 240 mg/dL (12.2-13.3 mmol/L) before glucosuria appears. The reason for the increased reabsorption of glucose by proximal renal tubular cells is likely due to SGLT2 receptor over expression, as evidenced by SGLT2 mRNA and protein content regulated in renal proximal tubule cells. Excess reabsorption of this glucose may worsen hyperglycemia.

Metabolic Syndrome[11]

The metabolic syndrome is a constellation of metabolic abnormalities that includes insulin resistance and confers a higher risk for cardiovascular disease (CVD). Patients with the metabolic syndrome are 5-times more likely to develop type 2 DM, if they do not already have type 2 DM. The metabolic syndrome does not identify synergism among identified risk factors, but rather additive risk, leading many to question its relevance as a clinical identity beyond the identification of a cluster of risk factors commonly occurring together. It may be useful to "package" risk factors into the metabolic syndrome to encourage aggressive management. The most recent definition of the metabolic syndrome was adopted by multiple organizations in 2009 and involves having central obesity, which is ethnically defined, in combination with at least two abnormal values from glucose, lipid, and/or blood pressure values (See: www.idf.org/metabolic-syndrome).

CLINICAL PRESENTATION[2,3,5]

The clinical presentations of type 1 DM and type 2 DM are different. Most patients (75%) develop type 1 DM before age 20 years, but it can develop at any age. Individuals with type 1 DM are often thin and are prone to ketoacidosis if insulin is withheld or under conditions of severe physiological stress. Symptoms such as polyuria, polydipsia, polyphagia, weight loss, and lethargy are common at the time of initial presentation. In the outpatient setting, some patients present with vague complaints of weight loss and fatigue but other symptoms may not be apparent unless a comprehensive history is taken. Twenty percent to 40% of patients with type 1 DM present with diabetic ketoacidosis (DKA) after several days of polyuria, polydipsia, polyphagia, and weight loss. This presentation is more common in patients from disadvantaged socioeconomic backgrounds. Rarely, type 1 DM is diagnosed in an asymptomatic patient who has a first degree family member with type 1 DM and has been closely monitored, or by casual laboratory glucose value.

Patients with type 2 DM often present without symptoms, but the presence of microvascular complications at the time of diagnosis suggest that many patients have had hyperglycemia for years. Often patients with type 2 DM are diagnosed during routine blood testing or screening. Lethargy, polyuria, nocturia, and polydipsia can be seen at diagnosis in some patients with type 2 diabetes, but significant weight loss is less common. Most patients with type 2 DM are overweight or obese. Classical clinical presentation characteristics should be used in conjunction with laboratory data to properly classify patients (see also Classical Clinical Presentation of Diabetes Mellitus Table).

CLINICAL PRESENTATION Diabetes Mellitus[a]

Characteristic	Type 1 DM	Type 2 DM
Age	<30 years[b]	>30 years[b]
Onset	Abrupt	Gradual
Body habitus	Lean	Obese or history of obesity
Insulin resistance	Absent	Present
Autoantibodies	Often present	Rarely present
Symptoms	Symptomatic[c]	Often asymptomatic
Ketones at diagnosis	Present	Absent[d]
Need for insulin therapy	Immediate	Years after diagnosis
Acute complications	Diabetic ketoacidosis	Hyperosmolar hyperglycemic state
Microvascular complications at diagnosis	No	Common
Macrovascular complications at or before diagnosis	Rare	Common

[a]*Clinical presentation can vary widely.*

[b]*Age of onset for type 1 DM is generally <20 years of age, but can present at any age. The prevalence of type 2 DM in children, adolescents, and young adults is increasing. This is especially true in ethnic and minority children.*

[c]*Type 1 may present acutely with symptoms of polyuria, nocturia, polydipsia, polyphagia, and weight loss.*

[d]*Type 2 children and adolescents are more likely to present with ketones, but after the acute phase may be treated with oral agents. Prolonged fasting can also produce ketones in individuals.*

Screening[2]

Type 1 Diabetes Mellitus

The prevalence of type 1 DM is low in the general population. Due to the acute onset of symptoms in most individuals, screening for type 1 DM in the asymptomatic general population is not recommended. Screening for β-cell autoantibody status in high-risk family members may be appropriate. However, such screening is most often recommended in the context of clinical trials for the prevention of type 1 DM.

Type 2 Diabetes Mellitus[2,5]

The American Diabetes Association (ADA) recommends screening for type 2 DM in adults who are overweight (BMI more than 25 kg/m^2, Asian-American BMI more than 23 kg/m^2) and have at least one other risk factor for the development of type 2 DM. Risk factors include: physical inactivity, first degree relative with diabetes or high risk ethnicity/race, women who delivered a baby heavier than 9 lb (heavier than 4 kg) or have a history of GDM, hypertension, high triglycerides, low HDL, women with polycystic ovary syndrome, diagnosed with prediabetes, presence of acanthosis nigricans, or a history of CVD. Age is a risk factor for type 2 DM and adults without risk factors should be screened starting at age 45 years. The recommended screening tests are a fasting plasma glucose, HbA_{1c}, or 2-hour OGTT. The optimal time between screening tests is not known, and the index of suspicion for the presence of diabetes should guide the clinician. Repeat testing every 3 to 5 years is cost-effective.[5]

Children and Adolescents[2,5,12]

Despite a lack of clinical evidence to support widespread testing of children for type 2 DM, it is clear that more children and adolescents are developing type 2 DM. Based on expert opinion, the ADA recommends screening overweight (defined as BMI more than 85th percentile for age and sex, weight for height more than 85th percentile, or weight more than 120% of ideal) youths who have at least two of the following risk factors: a family history of type 2 diabetes in first- and second-degree relatives; Native Americans, African Americans, Hispanic Americans, and Asians/South Pacific Islanders; those with signs of insulin resistance or conditions associated with insulin resistance (acanthosis nigricans, hypertension, dyslipidemia, polycystic ovary syndrome, or small for gestational age birthweight); or maternal history of diabetes or GDM during the child's gestation be screened. Screening should be done every 3 years starting at 10 years of age or at the onset of puberty if it occurs at a younger age.

Gestational Diabetes[2,5,13]

Risk assessment for GDM should occur at the first prenatal visit. Due to the increasing incidence of obesity and undiagnosed DM, it is reasonable to screen women with risk factors for the development of diabetes as soon as feasible. If the initial screening is negative they should undergo retesting at 24 to 28 weeks of gestation. Screening for GDM may be done in one of two ways: (1) a standard 75-g OGTT or (2) a nonfasting 50-g glucose tolerance test. With the standard 75-g OGTT, the diagnosis of GDM is confirmed when fasting, 1-hour, 2-hour, and/or 3-hour glucose values are greater or equal to cut-off values. If a nonfasting 50-g glucose tolerance test is performed, a fasting 100-g glucose tolerance test must be performed if the 1-hour value is elevated. Different glycemic cut-offs and criteria identify more or fewer patients with GDM and this may influence outcomes (Table 74-2).

DIAGNOSIS OF DIABETES[2,5]

The diagnosis of diabetes requires the use of glycemic cut points that discriminate patients with normal glucose hemostasis from patients with diabetes. The cut points are meant to reflect the level of glucose above which microvascular complications have been shown to increase. Cross-sectional studies have shown a consistent increase in the risk of developing retinopathy at a fasting glucose level above 99 to 116 mg/dL (5.5-6.4 mmol/L), at a 2-hour postprandial level above

TABLE 74-2 Screening for and Diagnosis of Gestational Diabetes Mellitus (GDM)

Strategies for Diagnosis of Gestational Diabetes
1. **"One-step" 75-g OGTT**
2. **"Two-step" approach with a 50-g (nonfasting) screen followed by a 100-g OGTT for those who screen positive**

1. Screening for and Diagnosis of GDM with a 75-g glucose load[1]

One abnormal value = diagnostic of GDM

Time	Plasma Glucose
Fasting	≥92 mg/dL (≥5.1 mmol/L)
1 hour	≥180 mg/dL (≥10.0 mmol/L)
2 hours	≥153 mg/dL (≥8.5 mmol/L)

2. Two-Step Strategy: Screening for and Diagnosis of GDM

Step 1: Perform a 50-g glucose load test (nonfasting), with plasma glucose measurement at 1 h, at 24-28 weeks of gestation in women not previously diagnosed with overt diabetes.

1 hour values ≥140 mg/dL[2] (≥7.8 mmol/L)

Step 2: The 100-g OGTT should be performed when the patient is fasting.

The diagnosis of GDM is made if *at least two* of the following four plasma glucose levels (measured fasting and 1 h, 2 h, 3 h after the OGTT) are met or exceeded

Carpenter/Coustan		National Diabetes Data Group	
Time		**Time**	
Fasting	95 mg/dL (5.3 mmol/L)	Fasting	105 mg/dL (5.8 mmol/L)
1 hour	180 mg/dL (10.0 mmol/L)	1 hour	190 mg/dL (10.5 mmol/L)
2 hours	155 mg/dL (8.6 mmol/L)	2 hours	165 mg/dL (9.2 mmol/L
3 hours	140 mg/dL (7.8 mmol/L)	3 hours	145 mg/dL (8.0 mmol/L)

[1]Should be performed at 24-28 weeks gestation unless the patient has overt diabetes. The test should be done in the morning after an 8- to 14-hour fast.

[2]The ACOG recommends a lower threshold of 135 mg/dL (7.5 mmol/L) in high-risk ethnic populations with higher prevalence of GDM; some experts also recommend 130 mg/dL (7.2 mmol/L).

Adapted from American Diabetes Association. Diagnosis and Classification of Diabetes. *Diabetes Care* 2015;38(Suppl 1):S8-S16.

TABLE 74-3 Criteria for the Diagnosis of Diabetes Mellitus[a]

1. HbA_{1c} ≥6.5% (≥0.065; ≥48 mmol/mol Hb). The test should be performed in a laboratory using a method that is National Glycohemoglobin Standardization Program (NGSP) certified and standardized to the DCCT assay.[a]
2. Fasting plasma glucose ≥126 mg/dL (≥7.0 mmol/L). Fasting is defined as no caloric intake for at least 8 hours.[a]
3. Two-hour plasma glucose ≥200 mg/dL (≥11.1 mmol/L) during an OGTT. The test should be performed as described by the World Health Organization, using a glucose load containing the equivalent of 75 g anhydrous glucose dissolved in water.[a]
4. In a patient with classic symptoms of hyperglycemia or hyperglycemic crisis, a random plasma glucose concentration ≥200 mg/dL (≥11.1 mmol/L).

[a]In the absence of unequivocal hyperglycemia, criteria 1 to 3 should be confirmed by repeat testing.

125 to 185 mg/dL (6.9-10.3 mmol/L), and an HbA_{1c} above 5.9% to 6.0% (0.059-0.060; 41-42 mmol/mol Hb). Current diagnostic criteria are slightly above these cut points (Table 74-3).

If a National Glycohemoglobin Standardization Program method is used, the HbA_{1c} is the logical test for the diagnosis of diabetes as it measures glycemic exposure over the past 2 to 3 months, in contrast to a single-day, single-point glucose measurement. In addition, patients do not need to fast and the HbA_{1c} is easily monitored. An HbA_{1c} of 6.0% to 6.4% (0.06-0.064; 42-46 mmol/mol Hb) denotes a tenfold increase in risk of developing diabetes, but does not consistently identify patients with IFG or impaired glucose tolerance. There are slight racial differences in normal HbA_{1c} levels. One-third fewer individuals with diabetes are identified using the HbA_{1C} more than or equal to 6.5% (more than 0.065; more than 48 mmol/mol Hb) threshold versus an FPG more than or equal to 126 mg/dL (more than 7.0 mmol/L), yet providers may be more likely to diagnose diabetes from an HbA_{1C} than from an elevated FPG level. The ADA continues to recommend three other glucose criteria for the diagnosis of DM in nonpregnant adults (see Table 74-3). If the patient has symptomatic hyperglycemia, reconfirming the diagnosis by one of the above criteria is not required.

People at high risk of diabetes can be diagnosed by plasma glucose or HbA_{1c} criteria. As shown in Table 74-4, IFG is a plasma glucose of at least 100 mg/dL (5.6 mmol/L) but less than 126 mg/dL (7.0 mmol/L). Impaired glucose tolerance (IGT) is defined as a 2-hour glucose value more than or equal to 140 mg/dL (more than or equal to 7.8 mmol/L) but less than 200 mg/dL (11.1 mmol/L) during a 75 g-OGTT.

Serial measurements, at clinician-defined intervals, can help to identify patients moving toward diabetes, and those who are stable. Patients who have even minor increases in glucose or HbA_{1c} values

TABLE 74-4 Categorizations of Abnormal Glucose Status

Fasting plasma glucose (FPG)
Impaired fasting glucose (IFG)
- 100-125 mg/dL (5.6-6.9 mmol/L)

Diabetes mellitus[a]
- FPG ≥126 mg/dL (≥7.0 mmol/L)

Two-Hour postload plasma glucose (oral glucose tolerance test)
Impaired glucose tolerance (IGT)
- Two-hour postload glucose 140-199 mg/dL (7.8-11.0 mmol/L)

Diabetes mellitus[a]
- Two-hour postload glucose ≥200 mg/dL (≥11.1 mmol/L)

HbA_{1c}
Increased risk of diabetes mellitus
- HbA_{1c} 5.7%-6.4% (0.057-0.064; 39-46 mmol/mol Hb)

Diabetes mellitus[a]
- HbA_{1c} ≥6.5% (≥0.065; ≥48 mmol/mol Hb)

[a]Diagnosis to be confirmed if not unequivocal hyperglycemia (see Table 74-3).

over time should be followed closely as these are likely the patients who will progress to DM. The HbA_{1c} measurement can be affected by anemias and several hemoglobinopathies, which would necessitate the use of one of the plasma glucose criterion in these individuals. More information about HbA_{1c} assay interference can be found at: http://www.ngsp.org/interf.asp.

TREATMENT

Desired Outcome[14,15]

The primary goals of DM management are to reduce the risk for microvascular and macrovascular disease complications, to ameliorate symptoms, to reduce mortality, and to improve quality of life. Early diagnosis and treatment to near-normal glycemia reduces the risk for developing microvascular disease complications, but aggressive management of cardiovascular risk factors including smoking cessation, treatment of dyslipidemia, intensive blood pressure control, and antiplatelet therapy are needed to reduce the likelihood for developing macrovascular disease. Hyperglycemia also contributes to poor wound healing by compromising white blood cell function and altering capillary function. DKA and hyperosmolar hyperglycemic state (HHS) are severe manifestations of poor diabetes control, almost always requiring hospitalization. Minimizing weight gain and hypoglycemia, especially severe hypoglycemia, are also therapeutic goals and may necessitate altering glycemic goals. Evidence-based guidelines, published by the ADA, may help in the attainment of these goals (Table 74-5).

General Approach to Treatment[14]

Appropriate care requires setting goals for glycemia, blood pressure, and blood cholesterol; monitoring for complications; making appropriate food choices and maintaining a healthy weight; engaging in regular physical activity; selecting and using medications wisely; and performing self-monitoring of blood glucose (SMBG) with periodic laboratory assessment of the aforementioned parameters.[5] Glucose control alone is not sufficient.[15]

Initial Evaluation[14]

A thorough medical history and identification of the specific type and duration of diabetes, characteristics of onset (eg, DKA or asymptomatic), dietary and weight history, social history, medication history including current and past medications for DM, current regimen including medications, diet, physical activity, and adherence should be obtained. Hospitalization history, hypoglycemia (frequency, cause, and timing), and diabetes-related complications should be documented. Laboratory evaluation should include, at a minimum, an HbA_{1C}, lipid profile, liver function tests, thyroid stimulating hormone, serum creatinine and electrolytes, and a urine analysis for microalbuminuria. In type 1 DM, consider screening for celiac disease by measuring tissue transglutaminase or antiendomysial antibodies. A physical examination and pertinent data should include the measurement of all vital signs, weight or body mass index, blood pressure, thyroid palpation, cardiovascular and carotid auscultation, and a skin examination including assessment for acanthosis nigricans (type 2 DM) or vitiligo (type 1 DM). In addition, a foot examination, including screening for impaired sensation detection with a 10 gram-force monofilament, should be performed.

Nonpharmacologic Therapy[5,12,14]

Medical Nutrition Therapy

Medical nutrition therapy is a cornerstone of treatment for all patients with DM.[4] It is imperative that patients understand the interrelationships between carbohydrate intake, medications, and

TABLE 74-5 Selected American Diabetes Association Evidence-Based Recommendations[a]

Recommendation Area	Specific Recommendation	Evidence Level[b]
Screening for diabetes	Screen overweight or obese at any age; screen those without risk factors beginning at age 45 years.	B
	To screen for diabetes an FPG, 2-hour 75-g OGTT, or HbA_{1c} are appropriate.	B
	Interval between screenings should be individualized based on risk, or every 3 years.	C
Monitoring	Home blood glucose monitoring is recommended for patients on multidose insulin or pump therapy at least prior to meals and snacks, and before events such as driving.	B
	Patients on other therapeutic interventions, including oral agents may perform home blood glucose monitoring, but ongoing instruction to patient on how to adjust therapy based on monitoring must be in place.	E
	Quarterly HbA_{1c} in individuals not meeting glycemic goals, twice yearly in individuals meeting glycemic goals, should be performed.	E
	In adults, measure fasting lipid profile at least annually.	B
	At least once a year, quantitatively assess urinary albumin (eg, urine albumin-to-creatinine ratio [UACR]) and estimated glomerular filtration rate (eGFR) in patients with type 1 diabetes duration of ≥5 years and in all patients with type 2 diabetes.	B
	All patients should be screened for diabetic peripheral neuropathy (DPN) starting at diagnosis of type 2 diabetes and 5 years after the diagnosis of type 1 diabetes at least annually thereafter, using simple clinical tests, such as a 10-g monofilament.	B
	A dilated eye examination should be performed within 5 years of diagnosis in type 1 DM, and shortly after diagnosis in type 2 DM, with follow-up every year, or every 2-3 years as recommended by an eye specialist.	B
Glycemic goals	HbA_{1c} goal for nonpregnant adults in general is <7% (<0.07; <53 mmol/mol Hb).	B
	HbA_{1c} goal should be individualized, with <6.5% (<0.065; <48 mmol/mol Hb) if achieved without significant hypoglycemia or adverse effects in younger, long-life expectancy, and no CVD patients.	B
	Less stringent HbA_{1c} goal (<8% [<0.08; <64 mmol/mol Hb]) may be appropriate in patients with a history of severe hypoglycemia, limited life expectancy, advanced micro/macrovascular complications or comorbidities, or in difficult to reach goal patients despite adequate therapy.	B
	Hospital: Critically ill: 140-180 mg/dL (7.8-10.0 mmol/L) (A), or more stringent guidelines down to 110-140 mg/dL (6.1-7.8 mmol/L) if without hypoglycemia (C). Noncritically ill: No clear evidence but in general premeal BG <140 mg/dL (<7.8 mmol/L) and random BG <180 mg/dL (<10.0 mmol/L) (C). A basal plus correction insulin regimen is the preferred treatment for patients with poor oral intake or who are taking nothing by mouth (NPO). An insulin regimen with basal, nutritional, and correction components is the preferred treatment for patients with good nutritional intake (A).	See text
Treatment		
Prevention of type 2 diabetes	Patients with IGT (A), IFG (E), or an A_{1C} of 5.7%-6.4% (0.057-0.064; 39-46 mmol/mol Hb) (E) should be referred to an intensive diet and physical activity behavioral counseling program targeting loss of 7% of body weight and increasing moderate-intensity physical activity (such as brisk walking) to at least 150 min/wk.	See text
	Metformin may be considered with IGT (A), IFG (E), or an A_{1C} 5.7%-6.4% (0.057-0.064; 39-46 mmol/mol Hb) (E), especially in obese, <60-year-old patients, and women with prior GDM.	See text
Medical nutrition therapy	Weight loss is recommended for all insulin-resistant/overweight or obese individuals. Either low-carbohydrate, low-fat calorie restricted diets, or Mediterranean diets may work.	A
	In individuals with type 2 diabetes, ingested protein appears to increase insulin response without increasing plasma glucose concentrations. Therefore, carbohydrate sources high in protein should not be used to treat or prevent hypoglycemia.	B
	Saturated fat should be <7% (<0.07; <53 mmol/mol Hb) of total calories.	B
	Monitoring carbohydrate intake by carbohydrate counting, exchanges, or experienced estimation is recommended to achieve glycemic goals.	B
	Routine supplementation with antioxidants, such as vitamins E and C is not advised due to lack of efficacy	A
	A Mediterranean-style eating pattern, rich in monounsaturated fatty acids, may benefit glycemic control and CVD risk factors and can therefore be recommended as an effective alternative to a lower-fat, higher-carbohydrate eating pattern.	B
Physical activity	150 min/wk of moderate intensity exercise spread over at least 3 days and with no more than 2 days without exercise.	A
	Resistance training of large muscle groups should be ≥2 times/wk.	A
Blood pressure	Systolic blood pressure should be treated to <140 mm Hg.	A
	Diastolic blood pressure should be treated to <90 mm Hg. Lower goals systolic blood pressure <130 mm Hg and/or diastolic blood pressure <80 mm Hg may be appropriate for some, such as younger patients, if attained without undue treatment burden. Lifestyle intervention for elevated blood pressure consists of weight loss, if overweight or obese; a Dietary Approaches to Stop Hypertension (DASH)-style dietary pattern including reducing sodium and increasing potassium.	A B B
	Initial drug therapy should be with an ACEi or ARB; if intolerant to one, the other should be tried.	C
Nephropathy	In treatment of nonpregnant patients with modest (30-299 mg/day) (C), or higher levels (≥300 mg/day) (A) of urinary albumin excretion, either ACE inhibitors or ARBs are recommended.	See text

(continued)

TABLE 74-5 Selected American Diabetes Association Evidence-Based Recommendations[a] (Continued)

Recommendation Area	Specific Recommendation	Evidence Level[b]
Dyslipidemia	If lipids are abnormal, annual monitoring is reasonable, if the LDL-C ≤100 mg/dL (≤2.59 mmol/L) upon screening, recheck every 5 years at a minimum is reasonable	E
	Lifestyle modification focusing on the reduction of saturated fat, trans fat, and cholesterol intake; increase omega-3 acids, viscous fiber, and plant stanols/sterols; weight loss if indicated, and increase physical activity should be recommended	A
	For patients with diabetes aged <40 years with additional CVD risk factors, consider using moderate or high-intensity statin (C)	See text
	For patients with diabetes aged 40-75 years without additional CVD risk factors, consider using moderate-intensity statin (A) If with additional risk factors, high-intensity statin (B) For patients with diabetes aged 75 years without additional risk factors consider using moderate intensity statin (B) If with additional risk factors, high-intensity statin (B)	
Antiplatelet Therapy	Use aspirin (75-162 mg daily) for secondary cardioprotection.	A
	Use aspirin (75-162 mg) for primary prevention in type 1 or 2 DM if the 10-year risk of CVD is ≥10%, the patient is >50 (men) or >60 (women) with at least one additional major CVD risk factor is present.	C
Hospitalized Patients	Critically ill: By IV insulin protocol(E); Noncritically ill: scheduled subcutaneous insulin with basal, nutritional, and correction coverage (A)	See text
Psychosocial	Include assessment of the patient's psychological and social situation as an ongoing part of the medical management of diabetes.	B

[a]Based on American Diabetes Association Practice Recommendations. Other evidence-based recommendations available.[8]

[b]Evidence levels:

A = Clear evidence from well-conducted, generalizable, randomized controlled trials that are adequately powered.

B = Supportive evidence from well-conducted cohort studies or well-conducted case-control study.

C = Supportive evidence from poorly controlled or uncontrolled studies or conflicting evidence with weight of evidence supporting intervention.

E = Expert consensus or clinical experience.

glucose control. A healthy meal plan that is moderate in carbohydrates and low in saturated fat (less than 7% of total calories) with all of the essential vitamins and minerals is recommended. The amount (grams) and type of carbohydrates (using the glycemic index is controversial), whether accounted for by exchanges or carbohydrate counting, should be considered. All foods can be a part of a healthy meal plan. It is not appropriate to chastise patients for eating sweets. If a healthy weight and normal glucose goals can be maintained, there is no reason to deny food choices. For individuals with type 1 DM, the focus is on physiologically regulating insulin administration with a balanced diet to achieve and maintain a healthy body weight. Overweight or obese patients with type 2 DM often require caloric restriction to promote weight loss. Portion size and the frequency of food intake must be addressed. Helping the patient adopt healthier eating behaviors that leads to sustained weight loss over time is more important than a specific diet. Financial and cultural food issues must also be considered. Discourage bedtime and between-meal snacks, set realistic goals, determine what the patient is willing to change, and follow-up to see how and if those changes occurred. A diet lower in fat is recommended for patients with CVD and avoiding a high protein diet in patients with nephropathy may be appropriate.[14]

Physical Activity[14,16]

Most patients with DM benefit from regular physical activity. Aerobic exercise improves insulin sensitivity, modestly improves glycemic control in the majority of individuals, reduces cardiovascular risk, contributes to weight loss or maintenance, and improves well-being. Patients should choose activities that they enjoy and are likely to do at regular intervals. Start exercise slowly in previously sedentary patients. It is unclear if asymptomatic patients should be screened for CVD prior to beginning an exercise regimen. The ADA does not currently recommend screening asymptomatic individuals. Screening is reasonable in patients with long-standing disease (DM more than or equal to 10 years), multiple cardiovascular risk factors, microvascular disease (especially renal disease), or evidence of atherosclerotic disease. If the patient has uncontrolled hypertension, autonomic neuropathy, insensate feet, or proliferative retinopathy, restrictions on recommended activities are recommended. Physical activity goals include at least 150 min/wk of moderate (50%-70% maximal heart rate) intensity exercise spread over at least 3 days a week with no more than 2 days between activity. In addition, resistance/strength training is recommended at least 2 times a week so long as the patient does not have proliferative diabetic retinopathy (PDR).[16]

Patient Education[14,17]

It is not appropriate to give patients with DM brief instructions and a few pamphlets.[15,17] Diabetes education, not only at the time of initial diagnosis but also at ongoing intervals over a lifetime, is critical. The American Association of Diabetes Educators (AADE) has developed the AADE7 self-care behaviors. The behaviors include healthy eating, being active, monitoring, taking medication, problem solving, reducing risk, and healthy coping. The patient must be involved in the decision-making process and have a strong working knowledge of the disease and associated complications. Emphasize that complications can be prevented or minimized with good glycemic control and managing risk factors for CVD. Motivational interviewing techniques have been shown to be effective. Briefly, this involves asking open-ended questions that encourage patients to identify and acknowledge barriers that hinder achieving health goals, and then work to address them with the educator's guidance.

Health professionals with formal training and experience in diabetes education can become certified. Certified Diabetes Educators (CDEs) must document their experience providing patient education and pass a certification examination. An increasing number of nurses, pharmacists, dietitians, and physicians are becoming a CDE. Formal diabetes education programs often employ several health professionals including CDEs. Accredited diabetes education program can receive payment through Medicare and private health insurance plans. The AADE and ADA accredit diabetes education programs.

Pharmacological Therapy[18,19]

Although nonpharmacological therapy is the cornerstone of treatment for all patients with DM, insulin is required for type 1 DM and nonpharmacological therapy alone is rarely sufficient for type 2 DM. Until 1995, only two treatment options were available—insulin and sulfonylureas. Since 1995, a number of new oral and injectable antidiabetic therapies have become available. These medications are often used in combination. Selecting the most appropriate pharmacological treatment approach has become increasing complex and a number of factors must be considered.

In type 1 DM, the insulin regimen should be tailored to the patient's lifestyle. This almost always involves a basal-bolus treatment strategy based on SMBG readings. This can be accomplished by using either multiple daily injections (MDI) or a continuous subcutaneous insulin infusion (CSII), also known as an insulin pump. When MDI or insulin pump therapy does not fit into the patient's lifestyle or is too complicated, a twice daily regimen using premixed insulins can be used. Some patients may require glucagon suppression therapy, as the hormone amylin is also deficient in patients with type 1 DM.

Intensive lifestyle changes in patients with type 2 DM after 10 years of follow-up failed to improve cardiovascular outcomes in the The Look Action for Health in Diabetes (Look AHEAD) trial.[20] Moreover, intensive lifestyle changes alone failed to achieve good glycemic control in the majority of patients. These findings reiterate the need for early use of antihyperglycemic medications in conjunction with diet and exercise in patients with type 2 DM.

Currently, nine classes of oral agents are approved for the treatment of type 2 diabetes: α-glucosidase inhibitors, biguanides, meglitinides, peroxisome proliferator activated receptor γ agonists (commonly called thiazolidinediones [TZDs] or glitazones), DPP-4 inhibitors, SGLT2 inhibitors, dopamine agonists, bile acid sequestrants, and sulfonylureas. Oral antidiabetic agents are often grouped according to their glucose-lowering mechanism of action. Biguanides and TZDs are often categorized as insulin sensitizers due to their ability to reduce insulin resistance. Sulfonylureas and meglitinides are often categorized as insulin secretagogues because they enhance endogenous insulin release. Three classes of injectable agents are also available for the treatment of type 2 diabetes: human insulins and insulin analogs, GLP-1 receptor agonists, and amylinomimetics.

Drug Treatments of Choice[18,19]

Type 1 DM must be treated with insulin, though adjunct medications may improve glycemic control. The optimal regimen for the treatment of type 2 DM is undetermined. Most patients with type 2 DM are initially treated with metformin due its long track record of use in clinical practice, efficacy, weight neutrality, low risk of hypoglycemia, and low cost. Common alternatives to metformin if intolerance or contraindicated include sulfonylureas, DPP-4 inhibitor, GLP-1 receptor agonist, or SGLT2 inhibitor. If the HbA_{1c} is more than 1% to 1.5% (0.01-0.015; 11-16 mmol/mol Hb) above goal, early dual therapy may be warranted. A patient with type 2 DM experiencing symptomatic hyperglycemia at the time of diagnosis should initially be treated with insulin therapy and transitioned to oral therapy or a GLP-1 receptor agonist once good glycemic control has been achieved. Type 2 DM patients who are mildly symptomatic (ie, without significant weight loss), may be started on early dual therapy. When selecting a treatment regimen medication, several factors in addition to contraindications and potential side effects should be considered. The agent's mechanism of action and efficacy to lower blood glucose to goal as well as its impact on fasting versus postprandial blood glucose must be considered. Additionally, the medication's long-term safety, ease-of-use, and cost should be discussed with the patient. Non-glycemic effects on weight, lipids, cardiovascular outcomes and risk factors, and even the perceived β-cell preservation/effects may sway the treatment selection.

Type 1 Diabetes Mellitus[18]

All patients with type 1 DM require insulin. However, how insulin is delivered should be based on the patient's preferences and lifestyle behaviors as well as clinician preferences and available resources.

Historically, after the discovery of insulin by Banting and Best in 1921, frequent injections of regular insulin, the only insulin then available, were given to control the symptoms of hyperglycemia. Subsequently developed insulin formulations, including neutral protamine Hagedorn (NPH), lente, and ultra-lente, were suspensions of regular insulin that had a delayed onset and longer duration of action. These "long-acting" insulins enabled many patients to use only one or two injections each day. Prior to the 1980s, SMBG and HbA_{1c} testing were not available. Patients and practitioners had no idea how well the blood glucose was controlled. Treatment was based on symptoms of hyperglycemia and hypoglycemia, which are easily misinterpreted by patients, and by measuring glucose in the urine. Neither symptoms nor urine glucose provide an accurate picture of glycemia. Moreover, while the renal threshold for glucose is relatively predictable in young healthy subjects, it is highly variable in older patients, heart failure, and patients with renal disease. Urine glucose levels will vary with time above the renal threshold, and a significant temporal lag in appearance should be expected versus blood glucose values. The advent of SMBG and HbA_{1c} testing in the 1980s truly revolutionized the treatment of diabetes. SMBG enabled patients to rapidly determine their blood glucose and make ongoing adjustments in the insulin regimen. The HbA_{1c} provided a measure of glycemic control over the previous 3 months that correlated with the risk of long-term complications. Modern diabetes management would be impossible without these two tools.

Contemporary management of type 1 DM attempts to match carbohydrate intake with glucose-lowering processes, most commonly insulin, as well as with physical activity. The goal is to allow the patient to live as normal a life as possible.

Normal physiologic secretion of insulin can be divided into a relatively constant background level of insulin ("basal") during the fasting and postabsorptive period, with prandial spikes of insulin after eating ("bolus" or "prandial") (Fig. 74-3). Insulin sensitivity and insulin secretion are not constant throughout the day, however, which renders the concept of stable basal insulin requirements inaccurate. Attempting to emulate normal secretion of insulin is a useful paradigm for understanding and applying insulin treatment for the management of type 1 DM. The timing of insulin onset, peak, and duration of effect must match meal patterns and exercise schedules to achieve near-normal blood glucose values throughout the day. One or two injections daily of any one insulin formulation will in no way mimic normal physiology, and therefore is unacceptable.

The simplest regimens that can approximate physiologic insulin release use "split-mixed" injections consisting of a morning dose of an intermediate acting insulin such as NPH and a "bolus" rapid-acting insulin or regular insulin prior to the morning and evening meals. The morning intermediate-acting insulin dose provides basal insulin during the day and provides "prandial" coverage for the mid-day meal. The evening intermediate-acting insulin dose provides basal insulin throughout the evening and overnight. If patients are very compulsive about timing of meals and carbohydrate intake, such a strategy may be acceptable. However, the majority of patients are not sufficiently predictable in their schedule or food intake to achieve "tight" glucose control with this approach.

Moreover, achieving good glycemic control overnight without causing nocturnal hypoglycemia can be a challenge using a twice daily split-mixed insulin regimen. Moving the evening NPH dose to bedtime may improve glycemic control and reduce the risk of nocturnal hypoglycemia. This can be a useful approach in those who

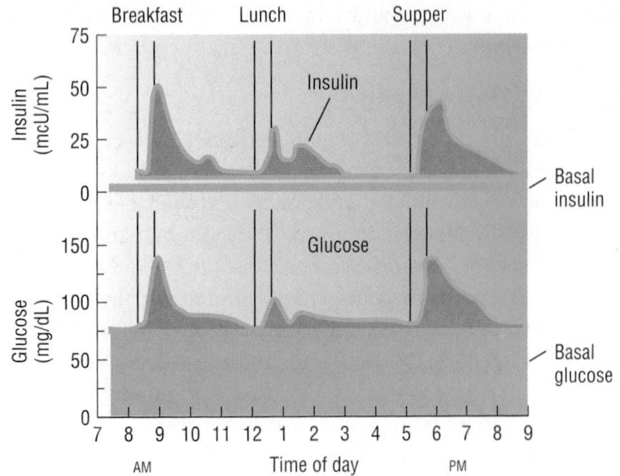

Intensive insulin therapy regimens

	7 AM (meal)	11 AM (meal)	5 PM (meal)	Bedtime
1. 2 doses,[a] R or rapid acting + N	R, L, A, GLU + N		R, L, A, GLU + N	
2. 3 doses, R or rapid acting + N	R, L, A, GLU + N	R, L, A, GLU	R, L, A, GLU + N	
3. 4 doses, R or rapid acting + N	R, L, A, GLU	R, L, A, GLU	R, L, A, GLU	N
4. 4 doses, R or rapid acting + N	R, L, A, GLU + N	R, L, A, GLU	R, L, A, GLU	N
5. 4 doses,[b] R or rapid acting + long acting	R, L, A, GLU	R, L, A, GLU	R, L, A, GLU	G or D[b] (G may be given anytime every 24 hours)
	←	Adjusted basal	→	
6. CS-II pump	Bolus	Bolus	Bolus	
7. 3 prandial doses pramlintide added to regimens above	P	P	P	

[a]Many clinicians may not consider this intensive insulin therapy.
[b]May be given twice a day in type 1 DM = 5 doses.

FIGURE 74-3 Relationship between insulin and glucose over the course of a day and how various insulin and amylinomimetic regimens could be given. (A, Afreeza; A, aspart; CS-II, continuous subcutaneous insulin infusion; D, detemir or degludec; G, glargine; GLU, glulisine; L, lispro; N, NPH; P, pramlintide; R, regular.)

decline or are unable to implement more intense insulin regimens. However, most patients with type 1 DM need an approach which also allows greater flexibility.

"Basal-bolus" regimens using MDI attempts to replicate normal insulin physiology with a combination of intermediate- or long-acting insulin to provide the basal component, and a rapid-acting insulin to provide prandial coverage. Several long-acting insulins can be used to provide the basal insulin component, including insulin detemir, glargine, or degludec. These long-acting insulin analogues are the most convenient means of providing basal coverage for most patients with type 1 DM. Bolus or prandial insulin can be provided by either regular insulin or one of the rapid-acting insulin analogs: lispro, aspart, or glulisine. The rapid onset and short duration of action of the rapid-acting insulin analogs more closely replicate normal physiology than does regular insulin. The patient reported convenience of injecting at a meal has made rapid acting insulins very popular, though trials comparing regular insulin to rapid acting insulins have found only modest improvements in glycemic control and the risk of hypoglycemia. When using a basal-bolus regimen, the patient determines the dose of the bolus insulin to be administered based on the preprandial SMBG, anticipated carbohydrate intake from the meal, and anticipated physical activity in the next 3 to 4 hours, as exercise may reduce insulin requirements. Many patients start with a fixed dose of insulin prior to meals and then learn how to adjust the insulin dose using an "adjusted insulin scale" or a "correction factor" based on the premeal glucose readings. Patients on more advanced regimens learn to adjust the bolus insulin dose based on anticipated carbohydrate intake and physical activity.

The "correction factor" is the approximate plasma glucose lowering effect of 1 unit of short-acting insulin in mg/dL. To calculate a patient's correct factor for regular insulin, 1,500 is divided by the total daily insulin dose in number of units that the patient currently uses. For rapid-acting insulin analogs, 1,700 or 1,800 is used when calculating the correction factor. For example, if a patient is currently taking 40 units of basal insulin and 12 units of rapid-acting insulin prior to three meals, the total daily insulin dose is 76 units. Using this calculation, 1,700 divided by 76 equals 22. Thus each unit of rapid acting insulin analog will lower the plasma glucose approximately 22 mg/dL (1.2 mmol/L). In order to make insulin dose calculations easier for the patient to determine, this would be rounded to either 20 mg/dL or 25 mg/dL per 1 unit of insulin (1.1 mmol/L or 1.4 mmol/L per 1 unit of insulin). Follow-up review of ongoing blood glucose data permits more precise individualization of the correction factor.

Carbohydrate counting is an effective tool for determining the amount of rapid acting insulin that should be injected for each meal. Instead of using a fixed dose of rapid acting insulin before meals, patients can self-adjust their dose based on either estimated grams of carbohydrates or carbohydrate "choices" that will be consumed. Patient who estimate the grams of carbohydrates in their meals commonly use the "insulin to carb ratio" to determine their bolus dose. One method of calculating the insulin to carb ratio is to use 500 divided by the total daily dose of insulin. For regular insulin, 450 may be used in this calculation. For example, if the patient's total daily insulin dose is 76 units, the calculation would be 500 divided by 76 which equals 7 g of carbohydrates. Thus 1 unit of rapid-acting insulin will cover approximately 7 g of carbohydrate. This is a starting point, and to make the calculation by the patient easier, the number may be rounded. Review of follow-up BG data before and 2 hours after meals will enable more precise determination of an individual's insulin to carbohydrate ratio. Although food charts give rough estimates of the amount of carbohydrate in different foods, patients often learn to adjust the mealtime insulin doses based on their own individual response to different food items.

In type 1 DM, approximately 50% of total daily insulin replacement should be in the form of basal insulin and the other 50% in the form of bolus insulin, divided between meals. If the patient's basal: bolus ratio is not close to this recommendation, the regimen should be reassessed. For patients with type 1 DM who are just starting insulin therapy, the initial total daily dose is usually between 0.5 and 0.6 units/kg/day. The basal insulin dose should be 50% of total dose and empirically the prandial insulin doses should be 20% of total dose prior to breakfast, 15% prior to lunch, and 15% prior to supper, though these doses should be adjusted based on the patient's eating habits. Most patients with type 1 DM patients require between 0.5 and 1 unit/kg of insulin each day. If the patient requires significantly higher amounts of insulin, this suggests the patient may be insulin resistance or have insulin antibodies.

Continuous subcutaneous insulin infusion or insulin pumps using a rapid-acting insulin analog is the most sophisticated and precise method for insulin delivery. In highly motivated patients, CSII is more likely to achieve excellent glycemic control than MDI. CSII can calculate recommended bolus doses of insulin based on carbohydrate intake. Insulin pump therapy may also be paired to continuous glucose monitoring (CGM), which allows calculation of a correction insulin dose, as well as alert the patient to hypoglycemia and hyperglycemia. The patient must still know if the pump calculations are correct. "Close-loop" CSII, where the pump automatically makes insulin-dosing decisions and appropriately adjusts the infusion to keep blood glucose values normalized, is currently in long-term trials. For now, patient's must still verify that the calculated bolus dose and basal infusion rates are appropriate. Another advantage of pump therapy is that the basal insulin infusion rate can be varied throughout the day. These features enable more precise insulin dosing and help patients to achieve better glycemic control.

Despite these advantages, insulin pumps require even greater attention to detail and more frequent SMBG than does a basal-bolus MDI regimen.[21] CSII is merely a tool. Thus if the patient is not well controlled or unwilling to actively adjust insulin dose when using injections, it is very unlikely that the patient will achieve superior control on a pump. CSII initiation and adjustment should be made by an experienced clinician. CSII requires a frank discussion with the patient about the demands of using CSII as well as setting appropriate expectations. Finally, patients need extensive training on how to use and maintain their pump.

All patients treated with insulin should be instructed how to recognize and treat hypoglycemia. Many patients experiencing hypoglycemia are tempted to over treat episodes of hypoglycemia resulting in rebound hyperglycemia. To minimize this problem, patients should be advised to follow the "rule of 15." If hypoglycemia is identified, the patient should consume 15 g of simple carbohydrate. Examples include consuming 8 oz (approximately 240 mL) orange juice, 8 oz (approximately 240 mL) of milk, 4 glucose tablets, or 1 tube of glucose gel and then retest their BG 15 minutes later. If the blood glucose remains less than 70 mg/dL (3.9 mmol/L), the patient should repeat the rule of 15 until their BG is has normalized.

At each visit, patients with type 1 DM should be questioned about hypoglycemia including the frequency and severity of hypoglycemic episodes. Any hypoglycemia requiring assistance of another person, a visit to an emergent or urgent care facility, or hospitalization should be documented and steps to prevent these episodes in the future should be taken.

Some patients with type 1 DM will develop hypoglycemic unawareness. Hypoglycemic unawareness may result from autonomic neuropathy or when the patient has frequent episodes of hypoglycemia. Patients who lose the warning signs of hypoglycemia appear to have a lower set point for the release of counterregulatory hormones. The loss of warning signs of hypoglycemia is a relative contraindication to continued intensive therapy. In such situations, hypoglycemic awareness may be restored by reducing or adjusting the insulin dose to scrupulously avoiding hypoglycemic episodes.

For children and pubescent adolescents, glycemic goals may need to be tempered with the risks of hypoglycemia. Table 74-6 lists glycemic goals.[22]

TABLE 74-6 Glycemic Goals of Therapy by Organization[8]

Biochemical Index	ADA		AACE/ACE	
Hemoglobin A_{1c}	<7% (<0.07; <53 mmol/mol Hb)[a]		≤6.5% (≤0.065; ≤48 mmol/mol Hb)	
Preprandial plasma glucose	80-130 mg/dL (4.4-7.2 mmol/L)		<110 mg/dL (<6.1 mmol/L)	
Postprandial plasma glucose	<180 mg/dL[b] (<10 mmol/L)		<140 mg/dL (<7.8 mmol/L)	
ADA Plasma Glucose and HbA_{1c} Goals for Adolescents and Children[c]				
	Plasma glucose goal		A_{1C}	
	Before meals	Bedtime/Overnight		
	90-130 (5.0-7.2 mmol/L)	90-150 (5.0-8.3 mmol/L)	<7.5% (<0.075; <58 mmol/mol Hb)[c]	
Framework for ADA Plasma Glucose and HbA_{1c} Goals in Older Adults				
Patient characteristics/ health status	**Rationale**	**Reasonable A_{1c} goal^**	**Fasting or preprandial glucose (mg/dL)**	**Bedtime glucose (mg/dL)**
Healthy (few coexisting chronic illnesses, intact cognitive and functional status)	Longer remaining life expectancy	<7.5% (<0.075; <58 mmol/mol Hb)	90-130 (5.0-7.2 mmol/L)	90-150 (5.0-8.3 mmol/L)
Complex/intermediate (multiple coexisting chronic illnesses* or 2+ instrumental ADL impairments or mild-to-moderate cognitive impairment)	Intermediate remaining life expectancy, high treatment burden, hypoglycemia vulnerability, fall risk	<8.0% (<0.08; <64 mmol/mol Hb)	90-150 (5.0-8.3 mmol/L)	100-180 (5.6-10.0 mmol/L)
Very complex/poor health (long-term care or end-stage chronic illnesses** or moderate-to-severe cognitive impairment or 2+ ADL dependencies)	Limited remaining life expectancy makes benefit uncertain	<8.5% (<0.085; <69 mmol/mol Hb)	100-180 (5.6-10.0 mmol/L)	110-200 (6.1-11.1 mmol/L)

AACE, American Association of Clinical Endocrinologists; ACE, American College of Endocrinology; ADA, American Diabetes Association; DCCT, Diabetes Control and Complications Trial.

[a]Assay should be National Glycohemoglobin Standardization Program (NGSP) certified measurement and DCCT standardized. More stringent glycemic control may be appropriate if accomplished without significant hypoglycemia or adverse effects. Less stringent HbA_{1c} goals may be appropriate in patients with a history of severe hypoglycemia, limited life expectancy, advanced micro/macrovascular complications or comorbidities, at-risk elderly, dementia, or in younger children.

[b]Postprandial glucose measurements should be made 1-2 hours after the beginning of the meal, generally the time of peak levels in patients with diabetes.

[c]Vulnerability to hypoglycemia and relatively low risk of complication prior to puberty considered. Adolescents and young adults may have adult goals if without developmental and psychological issues, and if without excessive hypoglycemia.

^A lower A_{1C} goal may be set for an individual if achievable without recurrent or severe hypoglycemia or undue treatment burden.

*Coexisting chronic illnesses are conditions serious enough to require medications or lifestyle management and may include arthritis, cancer, congestive heart failure, depression, emphysema, falls, hypertension, incontinence, stage 3 or worse chronic kidney disease, myocardial infarction, and stroke. By "multiple," we mean at least three, but many patients may have five or more (6).

**The presence of a single end-stage chronic illness, such as stage 3-4 congestive heart failure or oxygen-dependent lung disease, chronic kidney disease requiring dialysis, or uncontrolled metastatic cancer, may cause significant symptoms or impairment of functional status and significantly reduce life expectancy.

Insulin allergies are uncommon with human insulin. In most patients, local reactions will dissipate over time. If mild reactions at the site of injection occur, assess the patient's injection technique. Many times the patient is injecting cold insulin, which causes vasodilation around the injection site. For some patients a different type or source of insulin may alleviate the problem. If the allergic reaction does not improve or is systemic, insulin desensitization protocols are available.

Lipohypertrophy can occur in some patients with long-standing type 1 DM. Some patients give their insulin injections in the same site repeatedly to minimize discomfort; over time this can result in lipohypertrophy. Lipohypertrophy can sometimes be seen on physical examination and by palpating injection sites. Because insulin absorption from an area of lipohypertrophy is unpredictable, the patient must avoid insulin injections into these areas. Lipoatrophy, due to local adipocyte destruction, is uncommon but can be seen at injections sites as well.

When a patient taking insulin struggles to achieve good glycemic control, several issues should be explored including the overzealous use of insulin, injection site selection, and injection technique. The answer to all high blood glucose readings is not necessarily more insulin. Hyperglycemia can be due to too little insulin or it could be due to a "rebound" from low glucose and over treatment with excessive amounts of carbohydrate. Fastidious blood glucose testing or selected use of CGM can assist in differentiating the two problems. There is variability of insulin absorption from injection to injection and from site to site which may cause wide glucose swings. The most consistent absorption of insulin is from the abdominal wall. Patients are encouraged to take all their injections in the abdomen. If the patient is unable or unwilling to follow this advice, then systematic site rotation is the next preferable option. The patient should always give the insulin injection in the same region of the body and at the same time of the day each day. When in doubt, always re-evaluate the patient's injection technique including proper insulin dose, injecting the insulin dose, and testing blood glucose. Sometimes simple errors result in unpredictable glycemic control.

Asymptomatic erratic gastric emptying can severely hinder the ability to match the insulin to the meals. A gastric emptying study if suspected is appropriate. Type 1 DM patients who continue to have erratic postprandial glycemic control despite a careful evaluation for proper insulin use may benefit from addition of the amylinomimetic pramlintide. Pramlintide is taken prior to each meal and can modestly improve postprandial blood glucose control. It is not a substitute for bolus insulin, however. Moreover, pramlintide cannot be mixed with insulin requiring the patient to take an additional injection at each meal. When pramlintide is initiated, the dose of prandial insulin should be reduced by 30% to 50%, to prevent hypoglycemia. Pramlintide is then titrated based on gastrointestinal adverse effects and postprandial glycemic goals. Injecting pramlintide prior to the meal and the rapid acting insulin shortly after the meal may better match the postprandial increase in glucose due to delayed gastric emptying. The patient must be cognizant of the risk of hypoglycemia, gastrointestinal side effects, and how to minimize the risk of both.

Islet cell and whole pancreas transplantation is occasionally used in patients who require immunosuppressive therapy for other reasons, such as renal transplants. Many patients are able to stop insulin or only require a sulfonylurea or GLP-1 agonist to maintain good glycemic control. However, within 2 years following a pancreas transplant, 80% or more will need to reinitiate some form of insulin therapy.

Type 2 Diabetes Mellitus[19,22-24]

Pharmacotherapy for type 2 DM has changed dramatically in the last few years with the addition of several new drug classes and recommendations to achieve individualized glycemic control. Symptomatic patients may initially require treatment with insulin or combination therapy. All patients are treated with therapeutic lifestyle modification. Patients with HbA_{1c} of 7.5% (0.075; 58 mmol/mol Hb) or less are usually treated with an antihyperglycemic agent which is unlikely to cause hypoglycemia. Those with HbA_{1c} more than 7.5% but less than 8.5% (more than 0.075 but less than 0.085; more than 58 but less than 69 mmol/mol Hb) could be initially treated with a single agent, or combination therapy. Patients with higher initial HbA_{1c} will require two agents or insulin. All therapeutic decisions should consider the needs and preferences of the patient, if medically possible.[19,23]

The best oral therapy regimen for patients with type 2 DM is widely debated. Based on the results of the UKPDS and safety record, obese patients without contraindications are often started on metformin which is titrated to 2,000 mg/day. Metformin will also work in nonobese patients with type 2 DM; however, this population is more likely to be insulinopenic, necessitating medications that may increase insulin secretion. In the UKPDS, metformin use in obese type 2 DM patients reduced total mortality, but this study was before statin use, tight blood pressure control, and widespread recommendations on the use of antiplatelet therapy. The long-term durability of the glycemic response produced by metformin is suboptimal and patients will often require additional therapy over time. An insulin secretagogue, such as a sulfonylurea, is often added second. While sulfonylureas are less expensive than other add-on therapies, they have several potential drawbacks including weight gain and hypoglycemia. Moreover, the sulfonylureas do not produce a durable glycemic response. Better choices include DPP-4 inhibitors, GLP-1 receptor agonist and SGLT2 inhibitors but each has therapeutic and safety limitations as well. TZDs produce a more durable glycemic response and are unlikely to cause hypoglycemia, but weight gain, fluid retention and the risk of new onset heart failure as well as other long-term safe concerns have limited their use by many clinicians in recent years. Glycemic goal-oriented therapy meaning the intervention should be sufficient to achieve the glycemic goal. Figure 74-4 is a consensus algorithm by the ADA and the European Association for the Study of Diabetes.[23] Another commonly quoted type 2 DM treatment algorithm is published by the American Association of Clinical Endocrinologists/American College of Endocrinologists (AACE/ACE) (See: www.aace.com/publications). Both treatment guidelines recommend individualization of pharmacotherapy; however, the AACE/ACE algorithm directs clinicians to a specific medication based on level of evidence, glycemic lowering, hypoglycemia risk, side effects, and effects on weight. The ADA algorithm does not recommend one medication over another, but list these attributes next to the mediation for consideration by the clinician. One noted difference is that sulfonylureas are placed as a "last" choice in the AACE/ACE algorithm, whereas ADA places sulfonylureas as a potential second line agent.

Table 74-6 provides a framework for HbA_{1c} goal individualization. Treatment selection should be based on multiple factors. Consider some simple questions to guide therapy: (1) How long has the patient had diabetes? If the patient has had diabetes for several years, due to progress failure of β-cell function, the patient is more likely to require insulin therapy. (2) Comorbidities? If the patient has multiple comorbidities, CVD, dementia, life expectancy, depression, osteoporosis, heart failure, recurrent genitourinary (GU) infections, some medications may be poor choices based on their potential side effects. In addition, certain comorbidities should "loosen" the HbA_{1c} goal.[22] (3) What is the amount of glucose lowering required to achieve the goal? Each oral agent and GLP-1 receptor agonist has limits on HbA_{1c} reduction, though most medications produce a more robust reduction with a higher baseline HbA_{1c}. (4) Is the primary problem elevated post-prandial BG readings? Fasting BG readings? Or both? If the patient's postprandial BGs are the primary reason for poor control, pick a medication that addresses postprandial blood

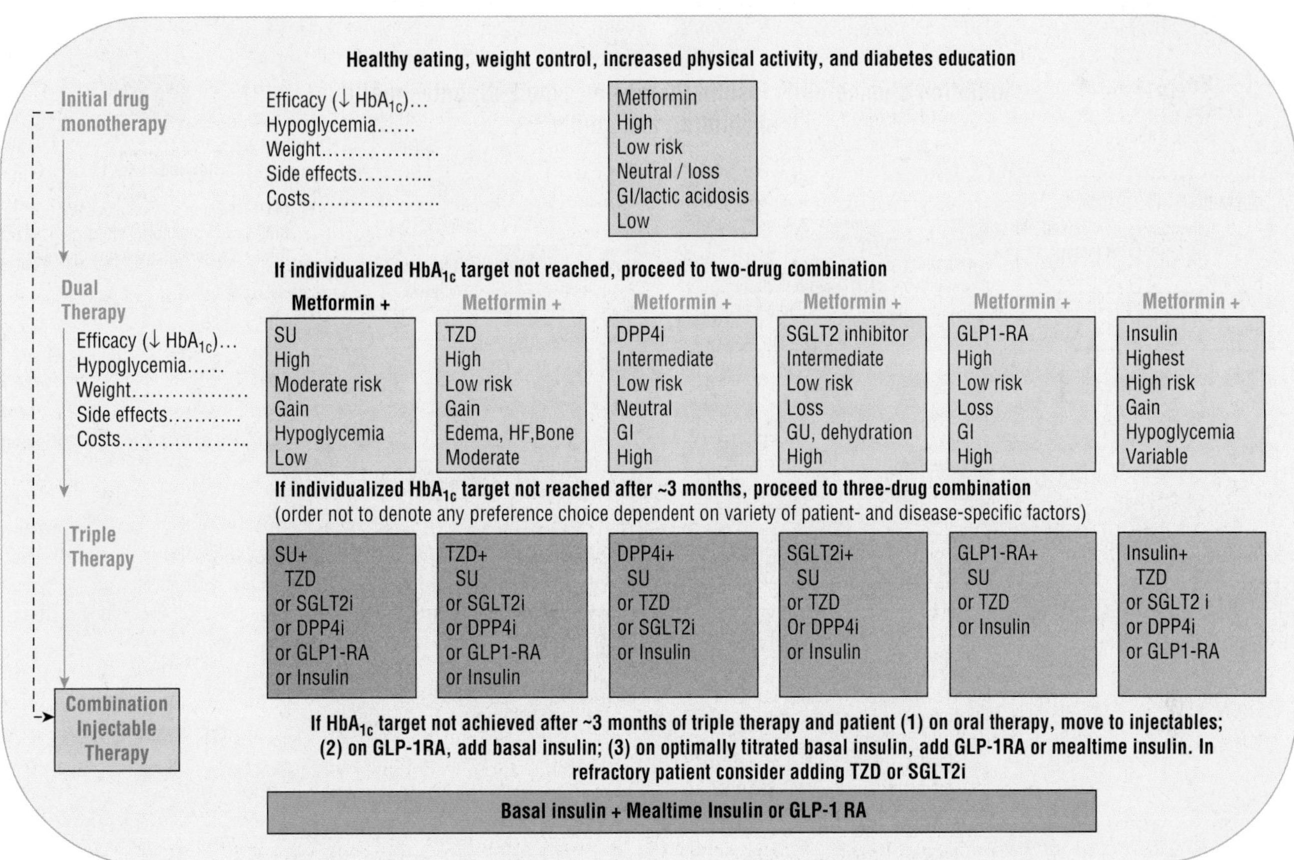

FIGURE 74-4 Antihyperglycemic Therapy Recommendations in Type 2 Diabetes. General Recommendations. *(Data from reference 20.)*

glucose excursions. Conversely, if the patient's fasting BG reading is consistent elevated, a medication that addresses fasting BG would be a better choice. (5) Adverse effect profile? Contraindications, hypoglycemia potential, and tolerability are based on the current status of the patient; (6) Motivation, resources, and potential difficulties with adherence should also influence treatment selection. (7) Age? If the patient is an older adult, the risk of hypoglycemia and other adverse effects increases and life expectancy diminishes. These factors should influence medication choices and HbA_{1c} goals. (8) Nonglycemic effects? CVD reduction with medications, lipid effects, blood pressure effects, weight, and durability of HbA_{1c} reduction may all influence the decision. See Table 74-6 for a framework for HbA_{1c} goal individualization.

β-Cell function is greatly diminished (by 50%-80%) by the time type 2 DM is diagnosed. Preserving β-cell function and arresting the progressive nature of type 2 DM would be a paradigm changing approach to treatment. However, the currently available medications slow, but do not arrest progression. It appears unlikely any one drug class will arrest β-cell failure, necessitating combination therapy. The combination of a TZD and GLP-1 receptor agonist is logical as TZDs reduce apoptosis of β-cells and GLP-1 receptor agonists augment pancreatic function. Two-year data in newly diagnosed patients given metformin, pioglitazone, and exenatide demonstrate near normal HbA_{1c} values.[25]

Nearly all patients with type 2 DM ultimately become relatively insulinopenic necessitating insulin therapy. Patients with type 2 DM often transition to insulin by using a bedtime injection of an intermediate- or long-acting basal insulin while continuing to use oral agents or GLP-1 receptor agonists for control during the day. This strategy is associated with less weight gain, equal efficacy, and lower risk of hypoglycemia when compared to starting prandial insulin or split-mix twice daily insulin regimens.[26] Patients who use a basal insulin should be monitored for hypoglycemia by asking about nocturnal sweating, poor sleep, nightmares, palpitations, and tremulousness as well as SMBG. Inadequate control with basal or bedtime insulin often presents with an HbA_{1c} above goal despite an FPG that is near goal. This is often due to rising postprandial glycemia throughout the day. Using a "basal plus" strategy, where a dose of bolus insulin is given prior to the largest meal of the day or the meal with the largest glucose excursion, may be simpler to implement than MDI. When prandial insulin is added to the evening meal, a reduction in the bedtime basal insulin dose may be warranted.[27] An alternative to starting a prandial insulin is to add a GLP-1 receptor agonist. If a biphasic mixed insulin is used, such as 70/30 NPH/Regular mix insulin, Humalog Mix 75/25 or Mix 50/50 or Novolog Mix 70/30, they should be given twice daily before the first and third meal. If adequate control is not achieved, a third dose of mix insulin may be given with the mid-day meal. This not only allows for better prandial coverage but also increases the risk of hypoglycemia. Premix insulins are not as flexible because the doses of the two insulin types cannot be independently changed.

Patients commonly adjust the wrong dose of insulin when high or low SMBG values are encountered. For a typical 2-injection regimen of premix insulin, if the pre-evening meal glucose is out of range, the morning insulin dose must be adjusted. Similarly, if the morning fasting glucose is out of range, the evening dose must be adjusted.[19]

Given that insulin resistance is commonplace in patients with type 2 DM, the insulin doses required to achieve good glycemic control are typically between 0.7 and 2.5 units/kg and sometimes more. Algorithms for insulin therapy in patients with type 2 diabetes have been developed by the Texas Diabetes Council (See: www.tdctoolkit.org/algorithms-guidelines), ADA[23], and AACE (See: www.aace.com/publications) **(Fig. 74-5)**.

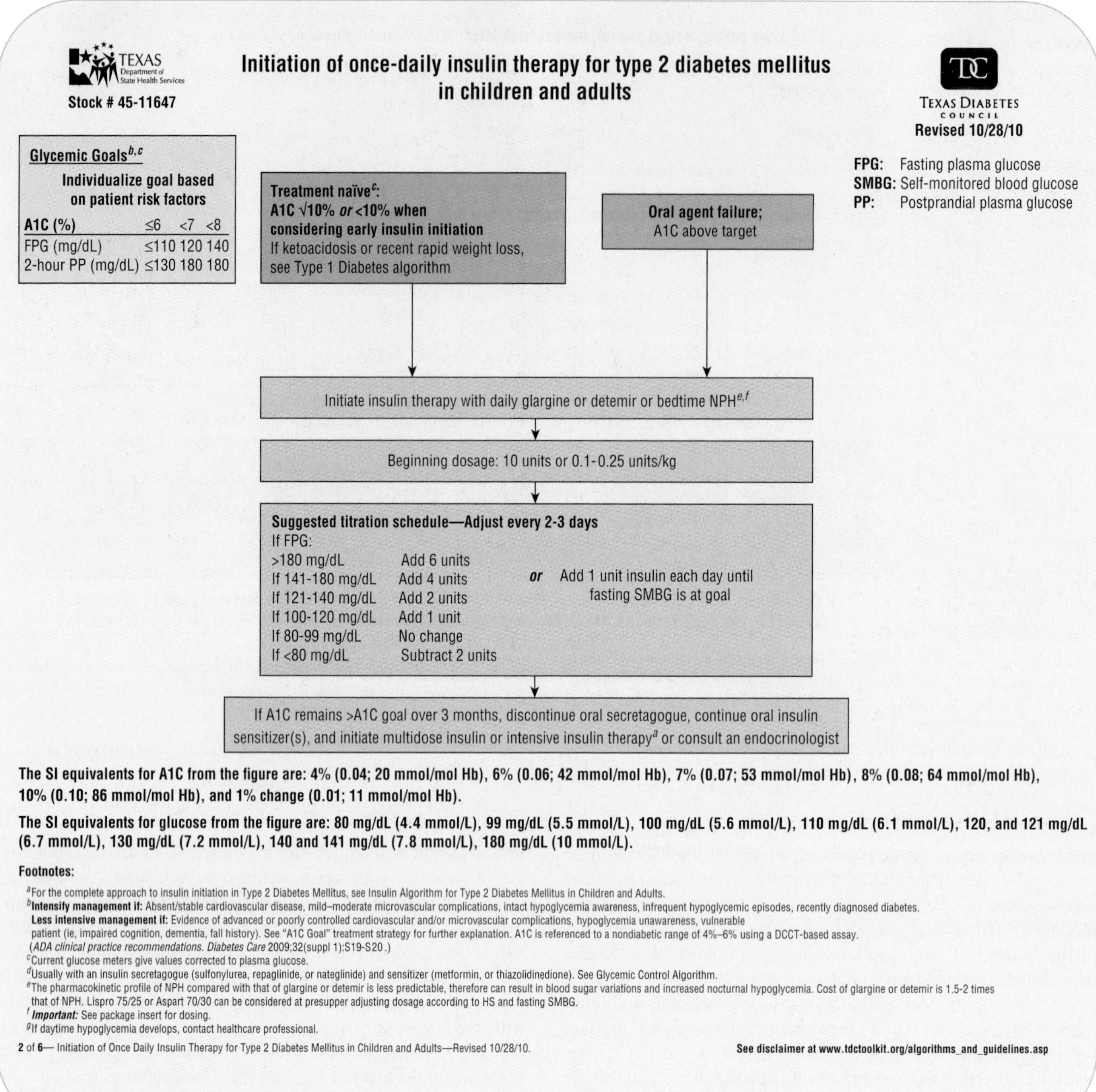

FIGURE 74-5 Simplified Insulin algorithm for type 2 DM in children and adults. See: *www.texasdiabetescouncil.org* for current algorithms. *(Reprinted from the Texas Diabetes Council.)*

Select Landmark DM Clinical Trials

In the Diabetes Complications and Control Trial (DCCT)[28] type 1 DM subjects were treated with intensive therapy—3+ injections of insulin daily or insulin pump, with frequent SMBG and alteration of insulin therapy based on SMBG results, plus frequent contact with a health professional or conventional therapy—one or two injections per day. After 6.5 years, retinopathy, neuropathy, and nephropathy were significantly reduced in the intensive group, though hypoglycemia was more common. In the United Kingdom Prospective Diabetes Study (UKPDS)[29] more than 5,000 patients with newly diagnosed type 2 DM were enrolled. Patients were followed for an average of 10 years. The study assessed "conventional therapy" (no drug therapy unless the patient was symptomatic or had FPG more than 270 mg/dL [more than 15.0 mmol/L]), versus intensive therapy starting with either sulfonylureas or insulin, aimed at keeping the fasting plasma glucose less than 108 mg/dL (less than 6.0 mmol/L). A subset of obese patients was studied using metformin as the primary therapeutic agent. Microvascular complications, primarily retinopathy, were reduced. At the conclusion of the DCCT and UKPDS trials, willing subjects in both trials continued to be followed over time to ascertain long-term micro- and macrovascular outcomes. In the follow-up of the DCCT, called the Epidemiology of Diabetes Interventions and Complications (EDIC),[31,32] continued micro- and new macrovascular benefit were seen despite similar HbA_{1c} values in the intensive and conventional treatment groups after study termination. Microvascular benefits were maintained for 10 to 15 years, and macrovascular events were significantly reduced. Similar results have been reported in the UKPDS follow-up trial in type 2 DM.[33] The ACCORD,[34] ADVANCE,[35] and VADT[36] were three trials that reported no benefit after 5 years of improved/intensive glycemic control for the reduction of macrovascular complications in patients with long-standing type 2 DM.

Special Populations

Children and Adolescents with Type 2 DM[12,37] Type 2 DM is increasing in adolescence.[1] Obesity and physical inactivity seem to be particular culprits in the pathogenesis of this disease. Given the many years that the patient will have to live with diabetes, and recent evidence that the timeline for microvascular complications may mimic that of older adults, extraordinary efforts should be expended on lifestyle modification measures in an attempt to normalize glucose levels. Failing that strategy, the only FDA approved oral agent for use in children (10-16 years of age) is metformin. Unfortunately, the durability of the response to metformin monotherapy is poor in many adolescents. Sulfonylureas are also commonly used. TZDs improved glycemic control when added to metformin therapy but are not currently FDA approved for use in children. DPP-4 inhibitors and the GLP-1 receptor agonists, while attractive options, have not been adequately studied in children. Insulin therapy continues to be the standard of care when glycemic goals cannot be achieved or maintained with metformin and sulfonylurea. In adolescent females, the possibility of future pregnancy should be considered. Screening and recommendations for treatment of hypertension, dyslipidemia, nephropathy, retinopathy, hypothyroidism, and celiac disease are available.

Older Adults with DM[38] Elderly patients with newly diagnosed with DM present a different therapeutic challenge. Consideration of the risks of hypoglycemia, the extent of comorbidities including severe microvascular disease, CVD, dexterity, self-care, nutritional status, social support, falls risk, mental status, and life expectancy should all influence glycemic goals and treatment selection (see Table 74-6). Avoidance of hypoglycemia, especially severe hypoglycemia is appropriate, but hyperglycemia that may exacerbate comorbidities should also be avoided.[22] Elderly patients may have an altered presentation of hypoglycemia as they lose adrenergic symptoms due to loss of autonomic nerve function as they age. This may cause neuroglycopenic symptoms to appear shortly after identification of hypoglycemia. DPP-4 inhibitors, shorter-acting insulin secretagogues, low-dose sulfonylureas, or α-glucosidase inhibitors may be used. Age-related decline in renal function may preclude metformin therapy, but lower doses may be used if the estimated glomerular filtration rate (eGFR) is consistently above 30 mL/min/1.73 m^2. SGLT2 inhibitor efficacy declines as renal function declines, thus most elderly patients may not have the same response as younger adults. SGLT2 inhibitors may also increase the frequency of voiding, cause possible orthostatic changes and increased falls risk. A higher risk of distal extremity fracture from falls with older adults has been documented with canagliflozin. Falls and fracture risk must be considered with TZDs which also tend to be extremity fractures from falls. DPP-4 inhibitors or α-glucosidase inhibitors are oral medications, which may be advantageous in older adults due to a low risk of hypoglycemia. Simple insulin regimens with daily basal insulin may be appropriate for glycemic control in elderly patients, especially if tight glycemic control is not the goal.

Clinical **Controversy...**

Glycemic Goal Setting in Older Adults.[38,88-90]

The US population continues to age. The ACCORD,[34] ADVANCE,[35] and VADT[36] enrolled older adults with multiple cardiovascular risk factors. All three studies failed to show a benefit in terms of CVD. Indeed, more people died in the ACCORD, resulting in early termination of the study. ADVANCE reported improvement in nephropathy outcomes. Diabetes in older adults is complicated by clinical and functional heterogeneity. Patients may be relatively healthy, independent living adults or, at the other end of the spectrum, require assistance with activities of daily living, have multiple comorbidities as well as cognitive impairments. What is the optimal goals and medication therapy for these individuals?

Clinical trial data in patient over 65 years of age for most medications are lacking. Many clinicians have decided that insulin, especially basal insulin, is a reasonable choice in this age group, and that metformin if not contraindicated is reasonable. In the new ADA guidelines, a patient-centered approach is recommended. It is unlikely that most patients would choose basal insulin as their initial intervention if asked. Also, the cost for basal insulin is significant, and one must ask if it is truly the most cost-effective choice. Severe hypoglycemia must be avoided in this population, as it has been associated with a higher risk of death 1 year following the incident. In addition, poor self-care behaviors, visual acuity, and dexterity may be of concern.

Medications that do not cause hypoglycemia may be advantageous in this population. Metformin, if not contraindicated, continues to be an excellent first choice. As renal function declines,[54] using metformin in a reduced dose is also reasonable. DPP-4 inhibitors are well tolerate and GLP-1 receptor agonist may help the patient lose weight. Both may be cost prohibitive and GLP-1 receptor agonists may be inappropriate for patients with GI symptoms or gastroparesis. Alpha glucosidase inhibitors are also very safe but gas and GI tolerability can be problematic. The optimal treatment goals and approaches for older adults remain elusive.

Gestational DM and Pregnancy with Preexisting Diabetes[2,5,13,22] Gestational DM is diagnosed during pregnancy. The adverse outcomes associated with GDM include birth defects, miscarriage, cesarean section delivery, maternal preeclampsia/eclampsia, preterm delivery, neonatal hypoglycemia, shoulder dystocia, birth injury, and hyperbilirubinemia. Medical nutritional therapy to minimize wide fluctuations in blood glucose is of paramount importance. Intensive educational efforts are usually necessary. Pregnant women without DM maintain plasma glucose concentrations between 50 and 130 mg/dL (2.8 and 7.2 mmol/L). Normoglycemia is the goal, and failure to maintain this despite dietary interventions often will necessitate medication use. Goals during therapy are *minimally* a preprandial goal of less than or equal to 90 mg/dL (less than or equal to 5.0 mmol/L), and either a 1-hour postprandial plasma glucose levels less than or equal to 120 mg/dL (less than or equal to 6.7 mmol/L) or 2-hour postprandial plasma glucose levels less than or equal to 110 mg/dL (less than or equal to 6.1 mmol/L). Ketosis should also be avoided as much as possible.

In patients who have preexisting type 1 or type 2 DM who become pregnant, premeal, bedtime, and overnight SMBG should be 60 to 90 mg/dL (3.3-5.0 mmol/L), with a peak postprandial SMBG of 100 to 120 mg/dL (5.6-6.7 mmol/L). HbA_{1c} during pregnancy should ideally be less than 6% (0.06; 42 mmol/mol Hb), but SMBG is the method of choice for monitoring glycemic control. Titration of insulin and switching to more complicated regimens that are guided by SMBG results is recommended. The safety of basal insulins other than NPH is still debated, but detemir has been rated pregnancy category B since 2012, and basal insulin use in GDM is increasing. Insulin pump therapy can be considered. In highly motivated patients, CSII can achieve excellent glycemic control and can be quickly adjusted.

Both metformin and glyburide have been studied as alternatives to insulin therapy. Glyburide was not detected in the cord serum of any infant in one study, whereas metformin crosses the placenta. Further study is needed prior to routinely recommending them in GDM, but in patients for whom the complexity of insulin is too difficult or refuses insulin, glyburide or metformin use is justified. Patients with gestational DM should be evaluated approximately 6 weeks after delivery to ensure that normal glucose tolerance has returned. The lifetime risk for the development of type 2 DM is 30% to 50%, making periodic reassessment of former GDM patients warranted.

Clinical **Controversy...**

Oral agents in Pregnancy

The use of oral antidiabetes agents for the management of gestational diabetes or type 2 DM during pregnancy continues to be controversial. For those patients who fail to maintain optimal glycemic control during pregnancy with diet and lifestyle modification, the next step has traditionally been to use insulin therapy. More recently, however, some clinicians have begun using oral agents including sulfonylureas and metformin in patients with GDM or type 2 DM during pregnancy.

A randomized, open-label, controlled trial evaluated the efficacy of glyburide compared to insulin initiated after 11 weeks of gestation.[81] The control of blood glucose compared to insulin therapy was similar, with less hypoglycemia in the glyburide group. There was not any evidence of significant difference in complications, including cord-serum insulin concentrations, incidence of macrosomia (birth weight more than or equal to 4,000 g), caesarean delivery, or neonatal hypoglycemia between regimens. Glyburide was not detected in the cord serum of any infant. However, this study limited enrollment of 11 weeks of gestation and beyond, therefore no conclusions can be made regarding teratogenicity from using glyburide in the first trimester of pregnancy.

A retrospective cohort study of 10,682 women with GDM who required medical therapy, however, revealed that babies born to women with GDM who were managed on glyburide were more likely have macrosomia and to be admitted to the intensive care unit compared to those treated with insulin therapy.[82] A more recently published large cohort evaluated 110,879 patients diagnosed with GDM in a US insurance claims database. Patients treated with glyburide had significantly more admissions to the NICU, respiratory distress, and macrosomia.[83]

A study of 751 women with GDM randomly assigned subjects at 20 to 33 weeks of gestation to open treatment with metformin and supplemental insulin, if required, or insulin therapy. This study did not find any increased rate of preeclampsia or other perinatal complications with metformin use compared with insulin.[84] Subsequently there have been a number of meta-analyses which revealed no differences in maternal or neonatal outcomes with the use of glyburide or metformin compared to the use of insulin in women with GDM.[85,86] Finally, a 2015 meta-analysis comparing metformin with glyburide found that metformin was associated with less maternal weight gain, lower birth weights, less macrosomia, and fewer large for gestational age infants. Failure rate was higher with metformin than glibenclamide.[87]

The current guidelines of the American Diabetes Association continue to recommend insulin therapy as the preferred treatment for managing women with gestational diabetes or type 2 DM in pregnancy who fail to achieve optimal control with diet and lifestyle modification alone.[39] Neither metformin or glyburide have formal FDA-approval for the management of diabetes in pregnancy.

Preconception Care for Women[13,39] An increasing prevalence of DM has been noted in reproductive-age women. Prepregnancy planning is mandatory. Organogenesis is largely completed within the first 8 weeks of pregnancy—well before good glycemic control can be achieved in the absence of preconception planning. Unfortunately, major congenital malformations due to poor glucose control in the first trimester of pregnancy remain the leading cause of mortality and serious morbidity in infants of mothers with type 1 or type 2 DM. For women with DM controlled by lifestyle measures alone, conversion to insulin as soon as the pregnancy is confirmed is appropriate. Patients previously treated with insulin may need intensification of their regimen to achieve therapeutic goals. Normal pregnancy is associated with a decrease in the BG concentration as glucose is diverted to the fetus. During precontraception planning, all drugs should be reviewed for safety. Drugs with known teratogenicity, such as ACE inhibitors and statins, should be stopped or substituted.

Sick Days Acute self-limited illness rarely presents a major problem for patients with type 2 DM, though following a reasonable sick day plan in severe illness may avoid urgent care visits from dehydration. Type 2 DM patients should perform SMBG more often, especially if medications that may cause hypoglycemia are administered. Sick day management for patients with type 1 DM is more challenging. While caloric intake generally declines, insulin sensitivity also decreases. Thus it often requires greater amounts of insulin to control BG during periods of acute illness. Patients need to increase the frequency of SMBG, check urine ketones, use of short-acting insulin, and should consume 120 to 150 g of carbohydrates per day. Patients should continue their usual insulin regimen and use supplemental rapid-acting insulin based on SMBG results. Additional insulin may be needed if ketonuria develops. Ketone testing should be done if two consecutive plasma glucose readings are above 250 mg/dL (13.9 mmol/L) or if vomiting occurs, as this may be a sign of ketosis. Sugar and electrolyte solutions, such as sports drinks, can be used to maintain hydration and provide electrolytes if there are significant gastrointestinal or urinary losses. They also provide glucose to keep the patient from developing hypoglycemia. However, if the patient BG remains consistently elevated, the patient should abstain from sugary drinks and increase intake of sugar-free liquids.

Diabetic Ketoacidosis and Hyperosmolar Hyperglycemic State[9,18,40] Diabetic ketoacidosis and hyperosmolar hyperglycemic state are true emergencies. In patients with type 1 diabetes, ketoacidosis is usually precipitated by the patient omitting insulin, or an acute illness with subsequent increase in counter-regulatory hormones such as cortisol, catecholamines, glucagon, and growth hormone. Infection is a common cause of DKA and should be thoroughly explored. Patients with DKA may be alert, stuporous, or comatose at presentation. The hallmark diagnostic laboratory values for DKA include hyperglycemia, anion gap acidosis, and large ketonemia or ketonuria. Patient with HHS present quite similarly but typically have much higher plasma glucose, elevated serum osmolality, and little to no ketonuria or ketonemia. HHS typically evolves over several days to weeks, whereas DKA evolves much quicker. Patients with DKA or HHS have fluid deficits of several liters as well as significant sodium and potassium deficits. Restoration of intravascular volume with normal saline, followed by hypotonic saline to replace free water, potassium supplements, and insulin given by continuous IV infusion to restore the patient's metabolic status are the cornerstones of therapy. Treatment with bicarbonate to correct the acidosis is generally not needed and may be harmful, especially in children. Treatment of the inciting medical condition is also vital. Hourly bedside monitoring of glucose and frequent monitoring (every 2-4 hours) of potassium is essential. A flow sheet is helpful in tracking the fluid and insulin therapies and laboratory parameters in these patients. Metabolic improvement is manifested by an increase in the serum bicarbonate or pH. Constant infusion of a fixed dose of insulin and the administration of IV glucose when the blood glucose level decreases to less than 250 mg/dL (less than 13.9 mmol/L) is preferable to titration of the insulin infusion based on the glucose level. The latter strategy may delay clearance of the ketosis and prolong treatment. Rapid correction of the glucose, a drop greater than 75 to 100 mg/dL/h (4.2-5.6 mmol/L/h), is not recommended because it has been associated with cerebral edema, especially in children. The insulin infusion should be continued until the urine ketones clear and the anion gap closes. Intramuscular regular insulin or subcutaneous insulin lispro or aspart given every 1 to 2 hours can be utilized rather than an insulin infusion in patients without hypoperfusion. Long-acting insulin should be given 1 to 3 hours prior to discontinuing the insulin infusion. Serum phosphorus usually starts high and plummets to lower-than-normal levels. Replacing phosphorus, while not unreasonable, is of questionable benefit. Fluid administration alone will reduce the glucose concentration, so a decrement in glucose values does not necessarily mean that the patient's metabolic status is improving. Patients may develop hyperchloremic metabolic acidosis with treatment if they have been given large volumes of normal saline in the course of their treatment. However, this does not require any specific treatment.

Hyperosmolar hyperglycemic state usually occurs in older patients with type 2 DM or in younger patients with prolonged hyperglycemia and dehydration or significant renal insufficiency. Occasionally patients with previously undiagnosed type 2 DM present with HHS. Large ketonemia is usually not seen because residual insulin secretion suppresses lipolysis. However, ketones from prolonged fasting may be present. Infection or another medical illness is the usual precipitant. Fluid deficits are often greater and BG concentrations higher—sometimes greater than 1,000 mg/dL (55.5 mmol/L)—in patients with HHS when compared to patients with DKA. Blood glucose should be lowered very gradually with hypotonic fluids and low-dose insulin infusions (1-2 units/h). Mortality is high with HHS.

Hospitalization for Intercurrent Medical Illness[41,42,44] Patients on oral agents may need transient therapy with insulin to achieve adequate glycemic control during a hospitalization. It is prudent to stop metformin in all patients who arrive in acute care settings as contraindications to metformin are prevalent in hospitalized patients. In patients requiring insulin, patients should receive scheduled doses of insulin with additional short-acting insulin. "Sliding-scale" insulin regimens which withhold insulin when the BG is lower than a predetermined threshold should be discouraged, as it is notorious for not controlling glucose and for sometimes resulting in therapeutic misadventures, with wide fluctuations of BG often recorded. In-hospital mortality is increased in many hyperglycemic conditions. At least one study documented a reduction in mortality in type 2 diabetes patients with acute MIs who receive constant IV insulin during the acute phase of the event to maintain near-normal glucose concentrations. Similar mortality improvements have been documented in some intensive care unit settings using IV insulin and tight glucose control. However, the Normoglycemia in Intensive Care Evaluation-Survival Using Glucose Algorithm Regulation (NICE-SUGAR) trial did not find a benefit from tight glycemic control in the ICU setting.[43] Thus, glycemic goals for hospitalized patients have been relaxed in recent years. The ADA and AACE released a joint consensus statement regarding inpatient glycemic control stating that glucose control measures should be implemented if the blood glucose is ≥ 180 mg/dL (10.0 mmol/L), and maintained between 140 and 180 mg/dL[4] (7.8 and 10.0 mmol/L). For noncritically ill patients there are no large outcome trials. Reasonable blood glucose goals for these patients are less than 140 mg/dL (7.8 mmol/L) premeal and less than 180 mg/dL (10.0 mmol/L) random.[22] Many protocols for IV insulin infusion are currently available and clinicians should use a well-established protocol. Point of care (POC) plasma glucose accuracy, especially in an ICU setting, has been controversial. The FDA has asked for improved accuracy from POC glucose meters to be approved for use in the hospital setting. Discharge planning is also important. Approximately one third of patients who develop hyperglycemia during a hospitalization will have newly diagnosed diabetes and another one third will likely have prediabetes. Obtaining an HbA_{1C} upon admission or prior to discharge can help determine who needs follow-up care.

Perioperative Management[22] Patients who require surgery may experience worsening of glycemia similar to those admitted to hospital for a medical illness. Acute stress increases counter-regulatory hormones. Therapy should be individualized based on the type of DM, nature of the surgical procedure, previous therapy, and metabolic control prior to the procedure. Patients on oral agents may need to be transiently switched to insulin to control blood glucose. In patients requiring insulin, scheduled doses of insulin or continuous insulin infusions are preferred. For patients who can eat soon after surgery, basal insulin continuation is warranted. The time-honored approach of giving one-half of the patient's usual morning NPH or basal insulin dose with dextrose 5% in water intravenously is acceptable, with resumption of scheduled insulin, perhaps at reduced doses, within the first day. Patients receiving basal-bolus insulin therapy can continue receiving their usual dose of long acting insulin while holding the premeal bolus doses until the patient eats. For patients requiring more prolonged periods without oral nutrition following major surgeries, such as coronary artery bypass grafting and major abdominal surgery, continuous IV infusion insulin is preferred. However, "tight" perioperative glucose control has not proven to improve outcomes. Use of IV insulin infusion has been shown to reduce postoperative deep sternal wound infections in patients following coronary artery bypass grafting. Metformin should be discontinued temporarily after any major surgery until it is clear that the patient is hemodynamically stable and normal renal function is documented.

Human Immunodeficiency Virus (HIV) Patients and Diabetes[45] Patients living with HIV are at higher risk for the development of type 2 DM. This risk may be related to HIV infection, concomitant infections such as hepatitis C, and medications often used to treat HIV and its comorbidities. Pentamidine, commonly used for *Pneumocystis Carinii* pneumonia infections, is a β-cell toxin and may cause some patients to develop hypoglycemia from insulin release followed by hyperglycemia. Megestrol, used as an appetite stimulant, can have glucocorticoid-like effects and cause hyperglycemia in some patients. Protease inhibitors, used to manage HIV, can worsen insulin sensitivity, decrease the ability of the β-cell to secrete insulin, and worsen lipotoxicity. Long-term use of stavudine also increases the risk of developing diabetes. Redistribution of fat from subcutaneous to the visceral compartment from medication or HIV infection caused by medications or HIV infection, also increases the risk of developing diabetes. Metformin is the drug of choice for HIV patients as weight gain can be minimized. Stavudine, zidovudine, and didanosine may cause lactemia, especially upon long-term use. It may be advisable to check lactate levels in patients taking this medications prior to metformin use. If lactate levels are greater than 2 times normal, alternative therapy should be considered. If excess visceral adiposity is noted, a TZD, which redistributes fat back to subcutaneous adipose tissue and causes visceral fat apoptosis may be considered. Drugs that promote weight loss should also be considered. Significant drug-drug interactions may also be present.

Prevention of Diabetes Mellitus[5] Efforts to prevent type 1 DM with niacinamide, injected insulin, or oral insulin therapy were all unsuccessful. Anti-CD3 and anti-CD20 monoclonal antibodies and a GAD vaccine delayed, but not stop β-cell destruction in type 1 DM. DiaPep277® development was halted as data from the full cohort analysis was negative. Low vitamin D levels has been associated with a higher the risk of developing type 1 DM and vitamin D supplementation in high risk patients continues to be of interest but has not yet been shown to be effective.

The "4 lifestyle pillars" for the prevention of type 2 diabetes are to decrease weight, increase aerobic exercise, increase fiber, and decrease fat intake. The Diabetes Prevention Program (DPP) confirmed that modest weight loss and regular physical activity can have a dramatic impact on insulin sensitivity and prevent the development of type 2 diabetes in patients with impaired glucose tolerance.[46] The study, which was originally planned to be ongoing for 5 years, was stopped early after 2.8 years. Patient assigned to the lifestyle arm of the study developed diabetes at a rate of 5% per year compared to an 11% per year rate in the usual care group, a 58% reduction. The exercise program involved walking 30 minutes 5 days each week. The mean weight loss was only 8 pounds (3.6 kg). A third arm of the DPP randomized subjects to metformin therapy 850 mg twice daily. Metformin therapy reduced the risk of developing type 2 DM by 31% when compared to usual care and resulted in a 4-pound (1.8 kg) weight loss. Interestingly, young and overweight individuals on metformin had a greater reduction in the risk of developing diabetes than normal weight and older study patients. Diet and exercise interventions were effective regardless of age or weight. The DREAM trial evaluated rosiglitazone and/or ramipril treatment for the delay or prevention of type 2 DM in impaired glucose tolerant subjects.[47] Rosiglitazone 8 mg daily, over approximately 3 years, reduced the incidence of type 2 diabetes by 60%. The ACT Now trial used pioglitazone 45 mg daily in patients with IGT and found a 72% reduction in the risk of development of diabetes over 2.4 years.[48] Low dose metformin and rosiglitazone combination have also shown to significantly reduce the risk of progression to diabetes. Acarbose reported a 25% reduction in the risk of type 2 DM in the STOP NIDDM study and may be most effective in populations who consume a diet high in whole grains such as rice. Liraglutide at 1.8 mg daily and at the obesity approved dose of 3.0 mg daily have been shown to decrease progression to type 2 DM.

All diabetes medications available for the prevention of diabetes, once discontinued, do not appear to have residual effects on β-cell function. Thus patients must continue the medication to "prevent" diabetes, thus raising the question about whether medications are merely early treatment. It should be noted that no pharmacologic agents are currently FDA approved for the prevention of type 2 diabetes. The ADA recommends metformin in conjunction with lifestyle changes in younger obese patients who have an HbA_{1c} more than 6% (0.06; 42 mmol/mol Hb) and dyslipidemia, hypertension, or a family history of diabetes.[5]

Drug Class Information

Insulin[18,19,49] Endogenously produced insulin is cleaved from the larger proinsulin peptide in the β-cell to the active peptide of insulin and inactive C-peptide. All commercially available insulin preparations contain only the active insulin peptide. Characteristics that are commonly used to categorize insulin preparations include source, strength, onset, and duration of action. Some insulin preparations, known as insulin analogs, have had amino acids substitutions in the insulin molecule that are designed to impart physiochemical and pharmacokinetic advantages. Table 74-7 summarizes available insulin preparations.

Insulin is available in several concentrations containing 100 units/mL (U-100), 200 units/mL (U-200), 300 units/mL (U-300), or 500 units/mL (U-500). The most commonly used insulin preparation is the U-100 concentration. Concentrated insulins containing more than 100 units/mL are generally reserved for individuals that require larger doses of insulin to control their diabetes. For some patients with type 1 diabetes who require extremely low doses of insulin, U-100 insulin may be diluted in order to accurately measure the necessary insulin doses. Diluents, instructions on dilution, and empty vials can be obtained from the manufacturers.

Historically, insulin was extracted from either beef or pork pancreases. Today recombinant DNA technology is exclusively used to manufacture insulin. Eli Lilly and Sanofi currently use a nonpathogenic strain of *Escherichia coli* to synthesize insulin; whereas Novo Nordisk uses *Saccharomyces cerevisiae*, or bakers' yeast.

Purity of insulin refers to the amount of proinsulin and other impurities present in the insulin product. Prior to 1980, most insulin products contained impurities (300-10,000 parts per million [ppm]) that sometimes caused local skin reactions as well as systemic antibody production. Today all recombinant DNA human insulin and insulin analogs contain less than 1 ppm of proinsulin.

When given by subcutaneous injection, regular crystalline insulin naturally associates into a hexameric (six insulin molecules) structure when zinc is present. Before absorption through a blood capillary can occur, the hexamer dissociates first into dimers and then monomers. This principle is the premise for additives such as protamine and extra zinc, which strengthen the hexamer interaction, prolonging onset, peak, and duration. Lispro, aspart, and glulisine insulin preparations dissociate more rapidly to monomers due to the substitution of amino acids on the β-chain of insulin resulting in a more rapid onset, peak, and duration of action when compared to regular insulin. Lispro (B-28 lysine and B-29 proline human insulin; monomeric) insulin has two amino acids transposed, aspart (B-28 aspartic acid human insulin; monomeric and dimeric) insulin has one amino acid substitution, and glulisine (B-3 lysine and B-29 glutamic acid) has two substitutions. Proteins are insoluble near their isoelectric point and the analog insulin glargine takes advantage of this property to prolong absorption. In comparison to human regular insulin, with an isoelectric point of 5.4, insulin glargine (A-21 glycine, B-30a-arginine, B-30a L-arginine, and B-30b L-arginine human insulin) has an isoelectric point of 6.8. In the vial, glargine is buffered to a pH of 4, a pH at which it is highly soluble, resulting in a clear colorless solution. When injected into the neutral pH of the body, it rapidly forms microprecipitates that slowly dissolve into dimers and monomers which can then be absorbed. The result is a long-acting insulin product with a duration of action of approximately 24-hours. The long-acting analog insulin detemir, in contrast, attaches a 14-carbon fatty acid at the B-29 position and removes the B-30 amino acid. This allows the fatty acid side chain to bind to interstitial albumin at the SQ injection site. In addition, stronger hexamer associations are form. Once detemir dissociates from albumin at the injection site and enters the blood, it is again binds to albumin, further prolonging its action. Insulin degludec, another long-acting insulin analog, has threonine at position B-30 removed and a 16-carbon fatty acid conjugated to lysine at position B-29 with a glutamic acid spacer. When injected, insulin degludec molecules reorganize from dihexamers to multihexamers that remain in solution at physiologic pH. Slow release of zinc ions from the multihexamers leads to a slow release of insulin degludec monomers.

The pharmacokinetics of insulin products given by subcutaneous injection are characterized by their onset, peak, and duration of action (Table 74-8). Absorption of insulin from a subcutaneous depot is dependent on several factors, including source of insulin, concentration of insulin, additives to the insulin preparations (eg, zinc and protamine), blood flow to the area (rubbing of injection area, increased skin temperature, and exercise in muscles near the injection site may enhance absorption), and injection site. The absorption of regular and NPH insulin is most rapid from abdominal fat, slower from posterior upper arms and lateral thigh area, and slowest from superior buttocks area. The abdomen provides the most consistent absorption for insulin. Insulin analogs appear

TABLE 74-7 Available Insulin Preparations and other Injectables

Generic Name	Manufacturer	Analog[a]	Administration Options	Room Temperature[b] Expiration
Rapid-acting insulins				
Humalog (insulin lispro)	Lilly	Yes	Insulin pen 3-mL, 3-mL and 10-mL vial, or 3-mL pen cartridge	28 days
NovoLog (insulin aspart)	Novo Nordisk	Yes	Insulin pen 3-mL, 10-mL vial, or 3-mL pen cartridge	28 days
Apidra (insulin glulisine)	Sanofi	Yes	Insulin pen 3-mL, 10-mL vial	28 days
Short-acting insulins				
Humulin R (regular) U-100	Lilly	No	10-mL vial, 3-mL vial	28 days
Novolin R (regular)	Novo Nordisk	No	10-mL vial	42 days
Intermediate-acting insulins				
NPH				
Humulin N	Lilly	No	3-mL and 10-mL vial, Insulin pen 3-mL	Vial: 31 days; pen: 14 days
Novolin N	Novo Nordisk	No	10-mL vial	42 days
Long-acting insulins				
Lantus (insulin glargine)	Sanofi	Yes	10-mL vial, Insulin pen 3-mL	28 days
Levemir (insulin detemir)	Novo Nordisk	Yes	10-mL vial, Insulin pen 3-mL	42 days
Tresiba (insulin degludec)	Novo Nordisk	Yes	Insulin pen 3-mL	56 days
Premixed insulins				
Premixed insulin analogs				
Humalog Mix 75/25 (75% neutral protamine lispro, 25% lispro)	Lilly	Yes	10-mLvial, Insulin pen 3-mL	Vial: 28 days; pen: 10 days
Novolog Mix 70/30 (70% aspart protamine suspension, 30% aspart)	Novo Nordisk	Yes	10-mL vial, Insulin pen 3-mL	Vial: 28 days; pen: 14 days
Humalog Mix 50/50 (50% neutral protamine lispro/50% lispro)	Lilly	Yes	10-mL vial, Insulin pen 3-mL	Vial: 28 days; pen:10 days
NPH-regular combinations				
Humulin 70/30	Lilly	No	3-mL and 10-mL vial, Insulin pen 3-mL	Vial: 31 days; pen: 10 days
Novolin 70/30	Novo Nordisk	No	10-mL vial	42 days
Concentrated insulins				
Regular insulin (U-500)	Lilly	No	20-mL vial, Insulin pen 3-mL	Vial: 40 days, pen: 28 days
Humalog (U-200 insulin lispro)	Lilly	Yes	Insulin pen 3-mL	28 days
Toujeo (U-300 insulin glargine)	Sanofi	Yes	Insulin pen 1.5-mL	42 days
Tresiba (U-200 insulin degludec)	Novo Nordisk	Yes	Insulin pen 3-mL	56 days
Inhaled insulin				
Afrezza (Technosphere insulin)	Mannkind	No	4 unit and 8 unit cartridges	Sealed-unopened blister card/ strip 10 days Opened- 3 days

[a]All diabetes injectables available in the US are now made by human recombinant DNA technology. An insulin analog is a modified human insulin molecule that imparts particular pharmacokinetic advantages.

[b]Room temperature defined as 59-86°F (15-30°C). All products are good until expiration date on product if unopened and stored correctly.

to retain their kinetic profile at all sites of injection. U-500 regular insulin has an onset similar to U-100 regular insulin, but a delayed peak and a longer duration of action when compared to U-100 regular insulin. The pharmacokinetic profile of U-500 is more similar to NPH. NPH insulin is a suspension. Variability in the absorption and dose due to improper mixing of the suspension by the patient or healthcare provider prior to administration can lead to a labile glucose response. NPH insulin and all suspension based insulin preparations should be inverted or rolled gently at least 20 times to fully suspend the insulin prior to each use. Detemir at low doses (less than 0.3 units/kg) should be dosed twice daily, whereas insulin glargine and insulin degludec are dosed daily. Technosphere insulin is a dry powder of human recombinant DNA regular insulin which is inhaled and absorbed through pulmonary tissue. Inhaled insulin has rapid absorption into the blood stream and reaches maximum concentrations in 12 to 15 minutes. The bioavailability is 21% to 30% compared to regular subcutaneous insulin. Patients with asthma, COPD, and smokers should not use technosphere insulin. There is also a higher risk of provoking bronchospasm with technosphere insulin.

The half-life of an IV injection of regular insulin is about 9 minutes. Changes in the IV insulin infusion rates will reach steady state in approximately 45 minutes. The pharmacokinetics of other soluble insulin preparations (lispro, aspart, glulisine, and glargine) given intravenously are similar to IV regular insulin. Thus they have no advantages over IV regular insulin but they are more expensive.

Insulin is degraded in the liver, muscle, and kidney. Liver deactivation is 20% to 50% in a single passage through the liver.

TABLE 74-8 Pharmacokinetics of Select Insulins Administered Subcutaneously

Type of Insulin	Onset (Hours)	Peak (Hours)	Duration (Hours)	Maximum Duration (Hours)	Appearance
Rapid acting					
Aspart	15-30 min	1-2	3-5	5-6	Clear
Lispro	15-30 min	1-2	3-4	4-6	Clear
Glulisine	15-30 min	1-2	3-4	5-6	Clear
Technosphere[a]	5-10 min	0.75-1	~3	~3	Powder
Short-acting					
Regular	0.5-1.0	2-3	4-6	6-8	Clear
Intermediate acting					
NPH	2-4	4-8	8-12	14-18	Cloudy
Long acting					
Detemir	~2 hours	—[b]	14-24	20-24	Clear
Glargine (U-100)	~2-3 hours	—[b]	22-24	24	Clear
Degludec	~2 hours	—[b]	30-36	36	Clear
Glargine (U-300)	~2 hours	—[b]	24-30	30	Clear

[a]Technosphere insulin is inhaled.

[b]Glargine is considered "flat" though there may be a slight peak in effect at 8-12 hours, and with detemir at ~8 hours, but both have exhibited peak effects during comparative testing, and these peak effects may necessitate changing therapy in a minority of type 1 DM patients. Degludec and U-300 insulin glargine appears to have less peak effect compared to U-100 insulin glargine.

Approximately 15% to 20% of insulin metabolism occurs in the kidney. This may explain the lower insulin dosage requirements and longer duration of activity observed in patients with endstage renal disease.

The connection between high insulin levels (hyperinsulinemia), insulin resistance, and cardiovascular events incorrectly leads some clinicians to believe that insulin therapy may cause macrovascular complications. Endogenous hyperinsulinemia in the setting of insulin resistance has been linked to increased cardiovascular events. However, hyperinsulinemia due to exogenous insulin use did not increase the risk of adverse macrovascular outcomes in the UKPDS or DCCT studies. Nor did basal insulin use in the Outcome Reduction with Initial Glargine Intervention trial increase cardiovascular risk.[50]

The most common adverse effects reported with insulin are hypoglycemia and weight gain. Hypoglycemia is more common in patients on intensive insulin therapy regimens. Patients with type 1 DM experience more hypoglycemic events when compared to type 2 DM patients who use insulin. In the UKPDS study, performed over 10 years in patients with type 2 DM, the percentage of patients that needed third party assistance due to a severe hypoglycemic reaction was 2.3%. In the DCCT study which enrolled patients with type 1 DM, tighter control increased the risk of severe hypoglycemia threefold when compared to conventional therapy. Moreover, insulin use is associated with an increased risk of hospitalizations in older adults based on public health surveillance data.[51]

Minimizing the risk of hypoglycemia for patients using insulin should include education about the signs and symptoms of hypoglycemia (tachycardia, tremulousness, and often, sweating), proper treatment of hypoglycemia, and blood glucose monitoring. Patient with neuroglycopenic symptoms may experience confusion, agitation, and eventually a loss of consciousness which may progress to coma. SMBG is essential for those on insulin, and is particularly important in patients with hypoglycemia unawareness. Patients with hypoglycemia unawareness should temporarily raise their glycemic goals and check their blood glucose level prior to any activities that require them to be alert and oriented (eg, driving and certain sports). Treatment of hypoglycemia dictates ingestion of carbohydrates. Glucose is preferred. If the patient is unconscious, IV glucose or glucagon injection should be given. Glucagon increases glycogenolysis in the liver and may be given in any situation in which IV glucose cannot be rapidly administered. A glucagon kit should be prescribed and readily available to all patients on insulin who have a history of severe hypoglycemia or at high risk for such events. Family and close friends of the patient should be educated regarding the reconstitution and injection of glucagon. It can take 10 to 15 minutes for the injection to start raising glucose levels and patients often vomit. It is important to position the patient on the side with the head tilted slightly downward to avoid aspiration.

Weight gain predominantly occurs in truncal fat and is dose dependent. Weight gain is undesirable in most type 2 DM patients, but may beneficial in underweight patients with type 1 DM. Weight gain can be minimized using physiologic insulin replacement strategies or combining insulin therapy with other medications that mitigate weight gain or promote weight loss (eg, metformin and GLP-1 receptor agonists).

The most common pulmonary adverse effect in patients receiving technosphere inhaled insulin was cough and upper respiratory infections. Technosphere insulin use in COPD and asthma is contraindicated due to bronchospasm risk. Technosphere insulin use has been associated with a small decline in pulmonary function. Specifically, the forced expiratory volume in 1 second declined by approximately 40 mL in clinical trials. This effect appears to be reversible after drug discontinuation. Technosphere insulin patients should have spirometry tests performed at baseline, 6 months, and annually thereafter. If a 20% reduction or greater in forced expiratory volume in 1 second is observed, technosphere insulin should be discontinued.

While much less common today in people using insulin, two forms of lipodystrophy still occur. Lipohypertrophy is caused by repeated injections into the same injection site. Due to insulin's anabolic actions, fat accumulates at the injection site and absorption at this site becomes variable. Lipoatrophy, in contrast, is due to insulin antibodies or allergic type-reactions that destroy the fat at the site of injection. Routinely rotating injection sites prevents these problems from developing and, when a lipodystrophy is detected, its use as an injection site should be avoided.

Several large studies using administrative data found an association between insulin glargine and cancer.[52] However, several other large database studies and meta-analysis have shown no such association. These conflicting results are likely due to patient selection. *In vivo* a metabolite of glargine is mostly present which has similar affinity for IGF-1 as regular insulin. In addition, the prospective, randomized Outcome Reduction with Initial Glargine Intervention trial reported no difference in cancer risk or cardiovascular events with low dose insulin glargine use over approximately 6 years.[50]

There are no significant drug-drug interactions with insulin but other medications may affect glucose control. Detemir theoretically could have albumin binding site interactions, but it occupies a very small percentage of total albumin binding sites. Table 74-9 lists common medications known to alter BG.

The dose of insulin must be individualized. In type 1 DM, the average daily requirement for insulin is 0.5 to 0.6 units/kg, with approximately 50% being delivered as basal insulin, and the remaining 50% dedicated to meal coverage. During the honeymoon phase, it may fall to 0.1 to 0.4 units/kg. During acute illness or with ketosis or states of relative insulin resistance, the need for higher dosages is common. In type 2 DM, a higher dosage is required for those patients with significant insulin resistance. Dosages vary widely depending on degree of insulin resistance and concomitant antihyperglycemic medication use. Patients initiating inhaled insulin and are insulin naïve should start with 4 units (4 unit cartridge) before each meal. Patients transitioning from a premixed formulation of subcutaneous insulin that includes both rapid-acting and intermediate or long-acting insulin should start with a dose that is 50% of the patient's previous total daily dose, divided across 3 meals.

TABLE 74-9 Medications That May Affect Glycemic Control[a]

Drug	Effect on Glucose	Mechanism/Comment
ACE inhibitors	Slight reduction	Improves insulin sensitivity
Alcohol	Reduction	Reduces hepatic glucose production
α-Interferon	Increase	Decreases insulin sensitivity/ induces counterregulatory hormones
Atypical antipsychotics	Increase	Decrease insulin sensitivity; weight gain
Calcineurin inhibitors	Increase	Decrease insulin secretion
Diazoxide	Increase	Decreases insulin secretion, decreases peripheral glucose use
Diuretics (thiazides)	Increase	May increase insulin resistance and/or decrease insulin secretion, K^+ change may be in part responsible
Glucocorticoids	Increase	Impairs insulin action
Fluoroquinolones	Increase/ Decrease	Unclear, potential drug interaction with sulfonylureas or change in insulin secretion
Nicotinic acid	Increase	Impairs insulin action, increases insulin resistance
Oral contraceptives	Increase	Unclear
Pentamidine	Decrease, then increase	Toxic to β-cells; initial release of stored insulin, then depletion
Phenytoin	Increase	Decreases insulin secretion
Protease inhibitors (PI)	Increase	Worsen insulin resistance/ decreases 1st phase insulin release or increases lipotoxicity. Dependent on PI
β-Blockers	May increase	Decreases insulin secretion
Ranolazine	Decrease	Improves oxidative glucose disposal
Salicylates	Decrease	Inhibition of I-κ-B kinase-β (IKK-beta) (only high doses, eg, 4-6 g/day)
Sympathomimetics	Slight increase	Increased glycogenolysis and gluconeogenesis

[a]This list is not inclusive of all medications reported to cause glucose changes.

U-500 regular insulin is reserved for use in patients with extreme insulin resistance. It is most often given two or three times a day. It is recommended to prescribe U-500 regular in a pen device. Extreme caution to avoid errors must be exercised when prescribing and dispensing U-500 regular in a vial. The prescription of U-500 should be written to include both the number of units and the volume (mL). For safety reasons, the dose should be administered using a tuberculin syringe. In an individual prescribed 120 units three times a day before meals, this prescription would be written as follows: "U-500 regular insulin inject 120 units (0.24 mL) subcutaneously three times daily before meals." The markings of one unit of a U-100 insulin syringe equals 5 units of U-500 regular. If an insulin syringe must be used, the same prescription as described above would be written as follows: "U-500 regular insulin: inject 120 units (24 units as measured by the unit markings of a U-100 syringe) subcutaneously three times daily before meals."

Table 74-7 outlines manufacturer-recommended expiration dates for insulin products when stored at room temperature (59-86°F [15-30°C]). For financial reasons, patients may attempt to use insulin preparations longer than the expiration dates. Careful attention must be paid to monitoring for deterioration of glycemic control and signs of clumping, precipitates, and discoloration in the insulin vial or pen cartridge.

Biguanides[19,23,53,54] Metformin is the only biguanide available in the United States. Metformin enhances insulin sensitivity in the liver and to a lesser degree in peripheral (muscle) tissues. This allows for an increased uptake of glucose into these insulin-sensitive tissues. All the mechanisms of how metformin accomplishes glucose reduction are still being investigated, though adenosine 5'-monophosphate–activated protein kinase activity, tyrosine kinase activity enhancement, increased adenosine 5'-monophosphate, and partial inhibition of the mitochondrial respiratory chain are involved. Metformin may also reduce glucagon dependent glucose release from the liver. Metformin has no direct effect on the β-cell, but insulin concentrations are reduced due to improved insulin sensitivity.

Metformin is often the drug of choice in patients with type 2 DM due to its efficacy, low cost, positive pleiotropic effects, and manageable side effect profile. Metformin consistently reduces HbA_{1c} levels by 1.5% to 2.0% (0.015-0.02; 16-22 mmol/mol Hb) and FPG levels by 60 to 80 mg/dL (3.3-4.4 mmol/L) in drug naïve patients with A_{1C} values approximately 9% (approximately 0.09; approximately 75 mmol/mol Hb), and can reduce FPG levels when they are extremely high (more than 300 mg/dL [more than 16.7 mmol/L]). Metformin may be useful in overweight or obese patients, causing a modest (2-3 kg) weight loss. Metformin also has positive effects on several components of the insulin resistance syndrome. Metformin decreases plasma triglycerides and low-density lipoprotein cholesterol (LDL-C) by approximately 8% to 15%, and modestly increases high-density lipoprotein cholesterol (HDL-C) (2%). Metformin reduces levels of PAI-1. Meta-analysis has shown that metformin may also lower the risk of pancreatic, colon, and breast cancer in type 2 DM patients.

The durability of A_{1C} reduction is fair—many patients will require additional antihyperglycemic therapy within 5 years. Early combination therapy, especially with medications that have a low risk of hypoglycemia, is recommended if the HbA_{1c} is > 8.5%. Metformin can be added to any other antihyperglycemic therapy, and is often continued when insulin therapy is initiated. This reduces the insulin dose requirements as well as the risk of hypoglycemia.

Metformin reduced macrovascular complications in obese subjects in the UKPDS.[30] Metformin significantly reduced all-cause mortality and risk of stroke versus intensive treatment with sulfonylureas or insulin. Metformin also reduced diabetes-related death and myocardial infarctions versus the conventional treatment arm of the UKPDS. Metformin causes gastrointestinal side effects, including abdominal discomfort, stomach upset, and/or diarrhea in approximately 30% of patients. These side effects are usually mild in nature and can be minimized with slow dose titration. Gastrointestinal side effects tend to be transient, lessening in severity over several weeks. Patients should take metformin with or immediately after meals. When initiating therapy, it is important to use a dose that is unlikely to cause gastrointestinal symptoms, typically 500 mg given with the largest meal. The dose is then increased in 500 mg increments over several weeks. Approximately 5% to 10% of patients cannot tolerate metformin despite the slow dose titration. Extended-release metformin may lessen some of the GI side effects.

The target dose for metformin is 1,000 mg BID or 2,000 mg daily if the extended release product is used. The minimal effective dose of metformin is 1,000 mg/day (Table 74-10). Approximately 80% of the glycemic-lowering effect may be seen at 1,500 mg daily.

Metallic taste, due to metformin in salivary secretions and hypoglycemia during intense exercise, has been documented. Metformin may cause vitamin B_{12} deficiency and B_{12} levels or methylmalonic acid should be measured if a deficiency is suspected. Peripheral neuropathy, a microvascular complication that is common in diabetes, could manifest or worsen with B_{12} deficiency. Vitamin B_{12} supplementation by sublingual, oral, or injection easily treats this deficiency.

Metformin partially blocks the mitochondrial respiratory chain, and has been associated with lactic acidosis. The risk of developing lactic acidosis with metformin use appears to be exceedingly small but moderate to severe renal insufficiency increases metformin serum concentrations and lactic acid production. Any disease state that increases lactic acid production or decreases lactic acid removal may predispose the patient to developing lactic acidosis. Tissue hypoperfusion states such as congestive heart failure, severe lung disease, shock, or septicemia, as well as severe liver disease or chronic alcohol abuse, all increase the risk of lactic acidosis. The clinical presentation of lactic acidosis is often nonspecific flu-like symptoms. The diagnosis is therefore made by laboratory confirmation of high lactic acid levels and acidosis.

Metformin is renally excreted and secreted and accumulates in patients with renal insufficiency. FDA product labeling for metformin in renal insufficiency has recently changed. Many organizations around the world, including the ADA, recommend that safe metformin use should be based on the patient's eGFR, rather than strict serum creatinine cut offs. When the eGFR is < 60 monitor renal function every 3 to 6 months, < 45 but ≥ 30 limit the dose to 50% of maximal dose and monitor renal function closely, and when eGFR < 30 mL/min/1.73 m^2 stop metformin.[54] Due to the risk of acute renal failure when IV contrast dye is used during imaging procedures, metformin therapy should be withheld starting the day of the procedure and resumed 2 to 3 days later, if normal renal function has been documented. It need not be withheld for days prior to the procedure.

Caution should be exercised in patients with hepatic impairment, which is poorly defined. It is unclear when lactic acid metabolism is impaired in liver dysfunction, but metabolism is normal at least until severe liver dysfunction. Most clinicians will inappropriately stop metformin with mildly elevated liver transaminases but it is reasonable to stop metformin when tests of liver function are affected such as bilirubin or the prothrombin time, or when liver transaminases are 5 to 10 times normal. Metformin use without lactic acidosis in patients with Child-Pugh C or Model for End-Stage Liver scores sufficient to require transplant have been reported. Survival may be prolonged in patients with advanced liver disease due to prevention of hepatocellular carcinoma.

Glucagon-Like Peptide 1 Receptor Agonists[19,23,53-56] All GLP-1 receptor agonists (GLP1-RAs) enhance insulin secretion in a glucose-dependent manner, suppress inappropriately high postprandial glucagon secretion resulting in decreased hepatic glucose production, increase satiety, slow gastric emptying, and promote weight loss. All GLP1-RAs result in pharmacologic levels of GLP-1 activity, which results in the gastric emptying effect, weight loss, and additional insulin/glucagon effect.

The average HbA_{1c} reduction observed with GLP1-RAs receptor agonists depend on baseline glycemic control and the product used. Once weekly extended release exenatide resulted in significantly greater reductions in HbA_{1c} compared to twice daily exenatide (–1.6% vs –0.9% [–0.016 vs –0.009; –18 vs –10 mmol/mol Hb]) as well as fasting plasma glucose (–35 mg/dL vs –12 mg/dL [–1.9 vs –0.7 mmol/L]).[57] Liraglutide and dulaglutide reduce HbA_{1c} approximately 0.4% (0.004; 4 mmol/mol Hb) greater than twice-daily exenatide. Albiglutide appeared to be slightly less effective than liraglutide.[58] Exenatide twice daily significantly decreases postprandial glucose excursions, but has only a modest effect on fasting plasma glucose values. Longer-acting GLP1-RAs lower fasting and postprandial plasma glucose levels similarly. Due to their longer half-life, they suppress glucagon overnight, which improves the fasting plasma glucose.

GLP-1 receptor agonists place in therapy is unclear. The ADA and AACE/ACE guidelines both recommend GLP1-RAs as second-line therapy. AACE/ACE emphasizes it as a drug that should be used in most patients as a second or third line drug. In contrast, ADA places it as a second-line drug, but does not emphasize it over other second-line medication choices. It is logical to use a GLP1-RA instead of basal insulin if the A_{1C} is less than 9% (0.09; 75 mmol/mol Hb), the patient is overweight or obese, and is not symptomatic from hyperglycemia.

These factors and favorable effects of long-term β-cell function lead many diabetologists to frequently use this class. Often cited issues are management of side effects, perceived risk of pancreatitis, injection device issues, and clinician comfort with basal insulin. GLP1-RAs increase satiety. The average weight loss with twice daily exenatide observed in clinical trials was 1 to 2 kg over 30 weeks without dietary advice being given to patients. Long-term, open-label follow-up studies of exenatide therapy show continued and sustained weight loss over 3 years. Exenatide extended release has similar weight reduction. Liraglutide produced slightly more weight loss than exenatide formulations in clinical trials. Albiglutide and dulaglutide resulted in less weight loss relative to other GLP1-RAs. It has been speculated this may be due to their molecular size, which may penetrate the CNS less efficiently.

Lixisenatide, approved in Europe, reported no cardiovascular benefit in a cardiovascular secondary prevention trial. There was no significant reduction in myocardial infarction, stroke, heart failure, or death.[59] Liraglutide was used in a large cardiovascular trial and reported positive results.

The most common adverse effects associated with GLP1-RAs are gastrointestinal. Adverse effects appear to be dose-related with all GLP1-RAs, so dose titration is recommended. Gastrointestinal adverse effects appear to decrease over time, though the incidence among agents will differ slightly. Withdraw rates in clinical trials of twice daily exenatide or liraglutide were 5% to 10%.

TABLE 74-10 Oral Agents for the Treatment of Type 2 Diabetes Mellitus

Drug Name (Generic Version Available? Y = yes, N = no)	Brand Name	Usual Dose (mg)	Recommended Starting Dosage (mg/day)		Maximal Dose (mg/day)	Pharmacokinetics/Drug Interactions	Major Adverse Events
			Nonelderly	*Elderly*			
Sulfonylureas							
Acetohexamide (Y)	Dymelor		250	125-250	1,500	Metabolized in liver; metabolite potency equal to parent compound; renally eliminated First-generation sulfonylureas, which bind to proteins ionically, are more likely to cause drug–drug interactions than second-generation sulfonylureas, which bind nonionically. Drugs that are inducers or inhibitors of CYP450 2C9 should be monitored carefully when used with a sulfonylurea[50]	Hypoglycemia: half-life directly related to risk of hypoglycemia. Longer half-life gives higher risk Hypoglycemia may be prolonged by alcohol intake Renal insufficiency, hepatic impairment, or elderly—start low dose Chlorpropamide should not be used in renal insufficiency or the elderly Hyponatremia—chlorpropamide and tolbutamide—especially at high doses Risk factors: >60 years old, female, on thiazide diuretics Weight gain: 1-2 kg Disulfiram reactions: reported with tolbutamide and chlorpropamide in patients consuming alcohol
Chlorpropamide (Y)	Diabinese	250/day	250	100	500	Metabolized in liver; also excreted unchanged renally	
Tolazamide (Y)	Tolinase	250/day	100-250	100	1,000	Metabolized in liver; metabolite less active than parent compound; renally eliminated	
Tolbutamide (Y)	Orinase	500-1,000 BID	1,000-2,000	500-1,000	3,000	Metabolized in liver to inactive metabolites that are renally excreted	
Glipizide (Y)	Glucotrol	5-10/day	5	2.5-5	40	Metabolized in liver to inactive metabolites. ALL: CYP2C9 strong inhibitors	Hypoglycemia: half-life directly related to risk of hypoglycemia. Longer half-life gives higher risk Renal insufficiency, hepatic impairment, or elderly—start low dose Weight gain: 1-2 kg Do Not use in LADA patients, may hasten need for insulin therapy
Glipizide (Y)	Glucotrol XL	5-10/day	5	2.5-5	20	Slow-release form; do not cut tablet	
Glyburide (Y)	DiaBeta Micronase	5-10/day	5	1.25-2.5	20	Metabolized in liver; elimination 1/2 renal, 1/2 feces. Two active metabolites. Low dose in renal insufficiency	
Glyburide, micronized (Y)	Glynase	6/day	3	1.5-3	12	Better absorption from micronized preparation	
Glimepiride (Y)	Amaryl	4/day	1-2	0.5-1	8	Metabolized in liver to inactive metabolites. Start lower dose in renal insufficiency	

(continued)

TABLE 74-10 Oral Agents for the Treatment of Type 2 Diabetes Mellitus (*Continued*)

Drug Name (Generic Version Available? Y = yes, N = no)	Brand Name	Usual Dose (mg)	Recommended Starting Dosage (mg/day)		Maximal Dose (mg/day)	Pharmacokinetics/Drug Interactions	Major Adverse Events
			Nonelderly	*Elderly*			
Glinides							
Nateglinide (Y)	Starlix	120 with meals	120 with meals	120 with meals	120 mg 3 times a day	Rapidly absorbed and short half-life (1-1.5 hours) Nateglinide is predominantly metabolized by CYP2C9 (70%) and CYP3A4 (30%) to less active metabolites. Glucuronide conjugation then allows rapid renal elimination. No dosage adjustment is needed in moderate to severe renal insufficiency	Dose is 120 mg with significant meals. (0-30 minutes prior). 60 mg dose has little efficacy Weight gain of 2-3 kg has been noted with repaglinide, whereas weight gain with nateglinide appears to be <1 kg
Repaglinide (Y)	Prandin	2-4 with meals	0.5-1 with meals	0.5-1 with meals	16	Caution with gemfibrozil with trimethoprim—Increased and prolonged hypoglycemic reactions are possible and have been documented Repaglinide is highly protein bound, and is mainly metabolized by oxidative metabolism and glucuronidation. The CYP3A4 and 2C8 system is involved with metabolism Moderate to severe renal insufficiency does not affect repaglinide, but moderate to severe hepatic impairment may	Repaglinide—may adjust dose based on size of carbohydrate in meal. Hypoglycemia is the main side effect. Consider starting a lower dose of repaglinide
Biguanides							
Metformin (Y)	Glucophage	2 g/day	500 mg twice a day	Assess renal function	2,550	Metformin is not metabolized and does not bind to plasma proteins. Metformin is eliminated by renal tubular secretion and glomerular filtration. Half-life of plasma metformin is 6 hours, but red blood cells are a second compartment of distribution for metformin, delivering an effective half-life of 17 hours. The main depot of metformin is in the splanchnic tissue, specifically the large intestine Cimetidine competes for renal tubular secretion May increase metformin levels	
Metformin ER (Y)	Glucophage XR	Sam as above	500-1,000 mg with evening meal	Assess renal function	2,550		Take full dose with evening meal or may split dose; may consider trial if intolerant to immediate release
Metformin solution	Riomet	Same as above	500 mg daily	Assess renal function	2,000		Metformin is indicated in >10 years olds

Thiazolidinediones							
Pioglitazone (Y)	Actos	15-30/day	15	15	45	Pioglitazone is primarily metabolized by CYP2C8, a lesser extent by CYP3A4 (17%), and by hydroxylation/oxidation. The majority of pioglitazone is eliminated in the feces with 15%-30% appearing in urine as metabolites. Two active metabolites (M-III and M-IV) are present which have longer half-lives than parent compound No dosage adjustment in moderate to severe renal disease, though edema must be monitored Pioglitazone dose is recommended to be limited to 15 mg daily in combination with gemfibrozil	Fluid retention effects: Peripheral edema, fluid overload, dilutional anemia, worsening macular edema, contribute to weight gain Weight gain: can be substantial in some patients—average is 1-4 kg- in general ½ is fluid, but other half is increase in fat Contraindicated in New York Heart Association Class 3 and 4 heart failure Fractures of distal extremities in postmenopausal women—fracture of wrists, fingers, ankles and toes may occur Bladder cancer: excess of 3 in 10,000 patient-year (from 7 to 10 in 10,000) risk of bladder cancer with pioglitazone at 5 years. Eight and ten year data showed no association Anovulatory women may resume ovulation if caused by insulin resistances
Rosiglitazone (N)	Avandia	2-4/day	2-4	2	8 mg/day or 4 mg twice a day	Rosiglitazone is metabolized by CYP2C8, and to a lesser extent by CYP2C9, and also by *N*-demethylation and hydroxylation. Two-thirds is found in urine and one-third in feces Highly (>99%) bound to albumin No dosage adjustment in moderate to severe renal disease, though edema must be monitored	
a-Glucosidase inhibitors							
Acarbose (Y)	Precose	50 with meals	25 mg 1-3 times a day	25 mg 1-3 times a day	25-100 mg 3 times a day	Acarbose-Metabolites absorbed and eliminated in bile. Slow titration key for tolerability. With meals Miglitol—Eliminated renally after absorption	Start 25 mg at one meal—preferably a low carbohydrate meal, increase dose as tolerated Only effective in complex carbohydrate diets Based on early, reversible ALT elevations, acarbose maximum dose of 50 mg 3 times a day for patients ≤60 kg or 100 mg 3 times a day for patients >60 kg Gastrointenstinal-urgency, diarrhea, flatulence, bloating, abdominal discomfort If hypoglycemia within 2 hours of ingestion—use glucose of high amounts of fructose—complex carbohydrate absorption will be delayed
Miglitol (Y)	Glyset	50 with meals	25 mg 1-3 times a day	25 mg 1-3 times a day	25-100 mg 3 times a day		

(*continued*)

TABLE 74-10 Oral Agents for the Treatment of Type 2 Diabetes Mellitus (*Continued*)

Drug Name (Generic Version Available? Y = yes, N = no)	Brand Name	Usual Dose (mg)	Recommended Starting Dosage (mg/day)		Maximal Dose (mg/day)	Pharmacokinetics/Drug Interactions	Major Adverse Events
			Nonelderly	*Elderly*			
Sodium Glucose Cotransporter-2 inhibitors							
Canagliflozin (N)	Ivokana	300/day	100-300 mg daily	100 mg daily	300 mg daily	Renal dosing—see text Glucuronidated into two inactive metabolites Systemic exposure to canagliflozin is increased in patients with renal impairment; however, the efficacy is reduced in patients with renal impairment due to the reduced filtered glucose load Canagliflozin—weak P-glycoprotein inhibitor—digoxin levels may need to be monitored. Rifampin—UGT inducer—significantly reduces canagliflozin levels. Use alternative drug	Adverse Effects Apply for the Class: Genital urinary infections—more common in women and men Women with recurrent history at highest risk Postural hypotension can occur due to the potential glucose-induced diuresis and hypovolemia If the patient is on loop diuretics, reduction or discontinuation will be necessary. Thiazide diuretics usually do not need adjustment unless on high doses for diuresis. Reduction in antihypertensives, if blood pressure is normal, may be necessary Rare cases of euglycemic diabetic ketoacidosis have been reported. Caution in severe, acute illness, in first 2 weeks of therapy, and in LADA or type 1 DM use, which is currently off-label
Dapagliflozin (N)	Farxiga	5/day	2.5-5 mg daily	2.5 mg daily	5 mg daily	Renal dosing—see text Dapagliflozin is highly protein bound (>90%) and only 2% is cleared by the kidneys. It is mostly glucuronidated by UGT in the liver to both an inactive (majority) and active (<1%) metabolites. The active metabolite is not produced in dapagliflozin doses below 50 mg	
Empagliflozin (N)	Jardiance	25/day	10-25 mg daily	10 mg daily	25 mg daily	Renal dosing—see text Empagliflozin is mostly glucuronidated Rifampin—UGT inducer significantly reduces empagliflozin levels—use alternative drug[59]	
Dipeptidyl Peptidase-4 inhibitors							
Sitagliptin (N)	Januvia	100/day	100 mg daily	25-100 mg daily based on renal function	100 mg daily	50 mg daily if estimated creatinine clearance >30 to <50 mL/min (>0.5 to <0.83 mL/s); 25 mg if creatinine clearance <30 mL/min (<0.5 mL/s) Sitagliptin is metabolized approximately 20% by CYP450 3A4 with some CYP450 2C8 Neither an inhibitor nor inducer, but is a p-glycoprotein substrate, but had negligible effects on digoxin and cyclosporine A, increasing the AUC by only 30%	Overall well tolerated medications Most common side effects include: Headache Nasopharyngitis Upper respiratory infection Urticaria/rash/facial edema—1% Rare cases of Stevens-Johnson syndrome have been reported Severe joint pain has also very rarely been reported. The mechanism is currently unknown Saxagliptin: Small reduction in absolute lymphocyte count (0.5%-1.5%). If prolonged infection is noted—consider stopping the medication[52] Saxagliptin and alogliptin: Increased risk of heart failure on package insert

Saxagliptin (N)	Onglyza	5/day	5 mg daily	2.5-5 mg daily based on renal function	5 mg daily	2.5 mg daily if creatinine clearance <50 mL/min (<0.83 mL/s) or if on strong inhibitors of CYP3A4/5 1 active metabolite 5 hydroxy saxagliptin—½ as potent as saxagliptin Metabolism by CYP3A4 and strong inhibitors/inducers will affect levels Saxagliptin is a substrate for p-glycoprotein substrate, but is neither an inhibitor nor inducer. Rifampin, an inducer, can decrease active levels by 50%	
Linagliptin (N)	Tradjenta	5/day	5 mg daily	5 mg daily	5 mg daily	Not substantially eliminated by renal, found in feces. Do not use with strong inducer of CYP3A4/p-glycoprotein Excreted unchanged, mostly through bile. Renal excretion less than 5% Linagliptin is a weak to moderate inhibitor of CYP3A4, and a substrate for p-glycoprotein	
Alogliptin (N)	Nesina	25 mg/day	25 mg daily	25 mg	25 mg	12.5 mg CrCl <60 mL/min (<1 mL/s), 6.25 mg <30 mL-15 mL/min (<0.5-0.25 mL/s) ~75% eliminated unchanged in urine No significant drug–drug interactions	
Bile Acid Sequestrants							
Colesevelam (N)	Welchol	3.75 g/day	6 tablets daily or 3 tablets BID 1.875 g BID or 3.75 g daily	6 tablets daily or 3 tablets BID 1.875 g BID or 3.75 g daily	3.75 g/day	Colesevelam binds bile in the gut Absorption drug–drug interactions: levothyroxine, glyburide, and oral contraceptives Phenytoin, warfarin, digoxin, and fat-soluble vitamins(A, E, D, K) have postmarketing reports of altered absorption. Any fat soluble drug may be affected Medications suspected of an interaction should be moved at least 4 hours prior to dosing the colesvelam	Dosing-six 625-mg tablets daily (total dose/day = 3.75 g), may be split into 3 tablets 2 times a day if desired or 3.75-g oral suspension packet, dosed daily, or a 1.875-g oral suspension packet dose twice daily Not recommended if triglycerides are ? 300 mg/dL (3.39 mmol/L)

(*continued*)

TABLE 74-10 Oral Agents for the Treatment of Type 2 Diabetes Mellitus (*Continued*)

Drug Name (Generic Version Available? Y = yes, N = no)	Brand Name	Usual Dose (mg)	Recommended Starting Dosage (mg/day)		Maximal Dose (mg/day)	Pharmacokinetics/Drug Interactions	Major Adverse Events
			Nonelderly	*Elderly*			
Dopamine Agonist							
Bromocriptine mesylate (N)	Cycloset	3.2-4/day	1.6-4.8 mg daily	1.6-4.8 mg daily	4.8 mg daily	Bromocriptine is a quick release formulation Bioavailability may be increased ~50% if given with a meal. Peak plasma concentration is about 1 hour if taken without food, but with food it is 90-120 minutes Only ~7% reaches the systemic circulation due to gastrointestinal-based metabolism and first-pass metabolism Bromocriptine is extensively metabolized by the CYP3A4 pathway, and the majority (~95%) is excreted in the bile. The half-life is approximately 6 hours. Plasma exposure is increased in females by approximately 18%-30%, but no dosage adjustment is currently recommended Drug–drug interactions: Bromocriptine is extensively metabolized by CYP3A4 and strong inhibitors or inducers may change bromocriptine levels. As bromocriptine is highly protein bound, it may increase the unbound fraction of other highly protein bound drugs Drug-disease interactions: Antipsychotics and psychotic disorders as they decrease dopamine activity, atypical antipsychotics, as they may decrease the effectiveness of bromocriptine, and ergot-based therapy for migraines as bromocriptine may increase migraine and ergot related nausea and vomiting Sympathomimetic drugs: case reports of hypertension and tachycardia when administered together	Bromocriptine is dosed with 0.8-mg tablets administered within 2 hours of waking from sleep daily with food. From 0.8 mg daily, the dose may be increased weekly based on response and side effects by 0.8-mg tablet increments, to a maximum of 4.8 mg daily (0.8 mg × 6 tablets) If miss window to administer in AM, skip dose. Nausea, vomiting, fatigue, headache, and dizziness, asthenia, dizziness, constipation, and constipation were all common side effects. 24% of patients eventually stopped therapy—most side effects "reappear" for a few days when the dose is increased Risk of orthostatic hypotension: blood pressure and symptoms of orthostasis should be closely monitored Somnolence can occur in about 5% of patients as well—caution with activities/driving

Discontinuation rates due to GI side effects with the longer-acting GLP1-RAs were 2% to 5%.

The nausea produced by the GLP1-RA is directly linked to their effect on gastric emptying. Tachyphylaxis occurs over time to this effect in most patients. Long-acting preparations tend to have less impact on gastric emptying, and thus a slightly lower risk of nausea, compared to twice daily exenatide. Patients should be instructed to eat slowly and stop eating when satiated otherwise nausea may worsen or cause vomiting. GLP1-RAs enhance insulin secretion in a glucose-dependent manner, thus hypoglycemia is uncommon when combined with metformin, DPP-4 inhibitors, SGLT2 inhibitors, or a TZD. However, when combined with a sulfonylurea or insulin, hypoglycemia may occur.

Antibody formation to GLP1-RAs may occur. Antibodies not reduce efficacy or increase side effects with most GLP1-Ras; however, neutralizing antibodies may attenuate the glycemic lowering effects of exenatide extended release in up to 6% of patients. Local injection site reactions were also more common in antibody positive patients. Hypersensitivity reactions, including anaphylaxis and angioedema, have been reported with most GLP1-RAs.

GLP-1 receptor agonist has been associated with cases of acute pancreatitis, but no causal relationship has been established. While additional study is needed, it should be noted that (1) patients with type 2 DM are at inherently higher risk for developing pancreatitis; (2) GLP1-RAs may mask the initial signs of pancreatitis, including nausea, vomiting, and abdominal pain; and (3) large database studies have not linked GLP1-RAs use to a higher incidence of acute pancreatitis. In a patient with a history of pancreatitis, the benefits must be weighed against the potential risks. A GLP1-RA should not be used in patients with chronic pancreatitis. If a patient reports abdominal pain, nausea, and repeated vomiting, it is best to discontinue therapy temporarily and confirm that the symptoms are not a sign of a more serious underlying problem.

Longer acting GLP1-RAs are contraindicated in patients with a history of medullary thyroid carcinoma or multiple endocrine neoplasia type 2 due to a risk of medullary thyroid carcinoma. This contraindication is based on rodent model data that reported a higher risk of C-cell tumors of the thyroid. Rodents may not be the ideal model to study this effect as they express a high number of GLP-1 receptors on thyroid C-cells. The expression of GLP-1 receptors in the thyroid of humans is minimal. Rodents also have a higher baseline prevalence of C-cell tumors compared to humans. Though there have been case reports of medullary thyroid carcinoma, no increased incidence has been reported and no causality has been established. There is no contraindication in patients with a history of other types of thyroid cancers such as papillary or follicular.

The injection device for each GLP1-RA product is different and patients must be instructed how to use the product. Dosing of twice daily exenatide (Byetta) should begin with 5 mcg BID, and titrated to 10 mcg BID in 1 month or when tolerability allows and if warranted for glycemic control. Twice daily exenatide should be injected subcutaneously up to 60 minutes before the morning and evening meals. If the patient does not eat breakfast, they may take the first injection of the day at lunch. The peak effect of twice daily exenatide is at approximately 2 hours, so anecdotally the patient may get better appetite suppression if injected an hour prior to the meal. Extended release exenatide (Bydureon) is a 2 mg suspension injected subcutaneously every 7 days without regard to meals. No dose titration is needed and steady state is attained at 6 to 8 weeks after treatment initiation. Extended release exenatide requires a multistep process to mix the powder in a diluent prior to injection.

The initial dose of liraglutide is 0.6 mg daily. This is a non-therapeutic dose used to minimize side effects. Liraglutide is then increased to 1.2 mg daily when GI side effects have dissipated. Patients may be continued on the 1.2-mg dose or increased to the maximum dose of 1.8 mg daily, which may provide some additional HbA_{1c} lowering and slightly more weight loss. Dosing should not be confused with liraglutide approved for weight loss. The maximum dose approved for weight loss is 3.0 mg daily whereas the maximum dose of 1.8 mg daily is approved for treatment of type 2 DM. Liraglutide comes in a pen device that can deliver all three doses.

Dulaglutide and albiglutide should be started at the lowest dose and increased to their maximum dose over time to improve gastrointestinal tolerability. For GLP1-RAs administered weekly, if a dose is missed it should be taken as soon as possible but not within 3 days of the next dose. If it is 3 days or less until the next dose, skip the dose and take the next dose on the regularly scheduled date. Caution should be used in moderate to severe renal impairment, as gastrointestinal side effects of all GLP1-RAs are more frequent, which can result in acute renal failure or injury.

Storage, pharmacokinetic and product information can be found in **Table 74-11**.

Sulfonylureas[19,23,53,54] Sulfonylureas enhancement insulin secretion by binding to a specific sulfonylurea receptor (SUR1) on pancreatic β-cells. Binding closes an adenosine triphosphate-dependent K^+ channel, leading to decreased potassium efflux and subsequent depolarization of the membrane. Voltage-dependent Ca^{+2} channels open and allow an inward flux of Ca^{+2}. Increases in intracellular Ca^{+2} bind to calmodulin on insulin secretory granules, causing translocation of secretory granules of insulin to the cell surface and resultant exocytosis of the granule of insulin. Elevated secretion of insulin from the pancreas travels via the portal vein and subsequently suppresses hepatic glucose production.

Sulfonylureas are classified as first-generation and second-generation agents. The classification schemes are based on relative potency. First-generation agents are lower in potency relative to the second-generation drugs: glimepiride, glipizide, and glyburide (see Table 74-10). When given in equipotent doses, all sulfonylureas are equally effective at lowering blood glucose. On average, HbA_{1c} will fall 1.5% to 2% (0.015-0.02; 17-22 mmol/mol Hb) in drug-naïve patients, with fasting plasma glucose reductions of 60 to 70 mg/dL (3.3-3.9 mmol/L), but is dependent on baseline values and duration of diabetes.

Sulfonylureas are the second most prescribed oral drugs for the treatment of type 2 DM. However, their place in therapy is controversial. Based on their extensive track record of safety and effectiveness, many clinicians feel comfortable using them in patients with type 2 DM. Diabetologists often avoid using sulfonylureas and instead use DPP-4 inhibitors or SGLT2 inhibitors. The ADA[23] and AACE/ACE[54] have very different stances on sulfonylurea use. The ADA algorithm recommends sulfonylurea use equally to other second line treatments. The AACE/ACE algorithm lists sulfonylureas as an option, but only after other medications with a low risk of hypoglycemia. Soon after sulfonylureas are taken, a robust reduction in HbA_{1c} is seen, but long-term durability is poor in most patients. Sulfonylureas cause a tachyphylaxis to their insulin secretion effect on the β-cell. *In vitro* testing of β-cells has reported depolarization of the cell, resulting in its inability to secrete insulin. Whether this effect is reversible is unclear. Clinically this is recognized by the deterioration of HbA_{1c}. Sulfonylureas are low cost medications.

Sulfonylureas have been showed to reduce the microvascular complications associated with type 2 DM in several studies.[29] Whether sulfonylureas reduce or increase macrovascular events is controversial. The UKPDS reported no significant benefit or harm in newly diagnosed type 2 DM patients given sulfonylureas over 10 years. However, the University Group Diabetes Program study documented higher rates of coronary artery disease in type 2 patients given tolbutamide, when compared with patients given insulin or placebo. This study has been widely criticized. Some sulfonylureas bind to the SUR-2A receptor that is found in cardiac tissue. Binding to the SUR-2A receptor has been implicated in blocking

TABLE 74-11 Available GLP-1 Receptor Agonists and Amylinomimetics

Generic Name	Administration Options	Room Temperature[b] Expiration	Pharmacokinetics/Drug Interactions[a]	Major Adverse Events
Glucagon like peptide-1 agonists				
Exenatide (Byetta)	5 mcg and 10 mcg pen, 60 doses/pen Dosed twice daily at or before meals	30 days (≤77°F [≤25°C])	Pharmacokinetics: 53% homology to GLP-1, t_{max} ~2 hours, and duration of action 4-6 hours Drug Interactions: Caution with warfarin: May increase INR Delayed Gastric Emptying may delay absorption of medication. Move 1 hour before or at least 3 hours after injection	Nausea >35% Vomiting/diarrhea 10%, respectively Start with 5 mcg BID Expect recurrence of GI with increase in dose to10 mcg BID. Inject closer to meals to limit nausea, but maximal satiety may be achieved by injecting 1-2 hours prior to food intake Drug Class Warning: -Pancreatitis
Exenatide (Bydureon)	2 mg single use pen device, 2 mg vial with separate diluent, single-use system Dosed weekly	30 days (≤77°F [≤25°C])	Pharmacokinetics: Exenatide embedded in microspheres slowly release over 10 weeks upon injection. Levels gradually increase with each weekly injection. 6-8 weeks to steady-state Attains therapeutic levels at week 2 Drug Interactions: See exenatide	Slightly less nausea and vomiting versus twice daily exenatide Drug Class Warning: -Pancreatitis -Long-acting GLP-1 agonist- do not use in medullary thyroid CA, MEN2
Liraglutide (Victoza)	3-mL pen, Delivers 0.6 mg, 1.2 mg, or 1.8 mg dose Dosed daily	30 days	Pharmacokinetics: 97% homology to GLP-1 A C-16 fatty acid (palmitic acid) self-associates into heptamers, prolonging half-life to 13 hours T_{max} is reached 8-12 hours after injection with steady state in 3 days Drug Interactions: Delay in gastric emptying may affect absorption of other medications	Nausea: 1.2 mg—10%-30% Nausea: 1.8 mg—15%-40% Vomiting: 5% Diarrhea: 8%-15% Stay on titration dose of 0.6 mg (nontherapeutic dose) daily until GI side effects dissipate. Then increase dose to 1.2 mg daily Drug Class Warning: -Pancreatitis -Long-acting GLP-1 agonist- do not use in medullary thyroid CA, MEN2
Albiglutide (Tanzeum)	30 mg and 50 mg single use pen Dosed weekly	4 weeks (≤86°F [≤30°C])	Pharmacokinetics: Recombinant fusion protein consists of two copies of a 30 amino acid sequence of a modified human GLP-1 (fragment 7-36) which is fused to human albumin. Fragment 97% homology to GLP-1, Half-life: 5 days. May not penetrate CNS Drug Interactions: Delay in Gastric Emptying may affect absorption of other medications	Nausea 9%-15% Vomiting 5%-12% Diarrhea 12% Drug Class Warning: -Pancreatitis -Long-acting GLP-1 agonist- do not use in medullary thyroid CA, MEN2
Dulaglutide (Trulicity)	0.75 mg and 1.5 mg single use pen (0.5 mL) 0.75 mg and 1.5 mg single use prefilled syringe (0.5 mL) Dosed weekly	14 days (≤86°F [≤30°C]))	Pharmacokinetics: Two identical disulfide-linked chains, each containing a modified human GLP-1 analog (90% homology to GLP-1) covalently linked to a modified human immunoglobulin G4 heavy chain fragment Half-life: 5 days Drug Interactions: Delay in Gastric Emptying may affect absorption of other medications	Nausea: 0.75 mg—8%-18% Nausea-1.5 mg—17%-28% Vomiting 3-5%, but as high as 17% with 1.5 mg dosing Diarrhea: 8%-17% Drug Class Warning: -Pancreatitis -Long-acting GLP-1 agonist- do not use in medullary thyroid CA, MEN2
Amylinomimetic				
Pramlintide (Symlin)	1.5 mL pen: delivers 15, 30, 45, or 60 mcg dose; 2.7 mL pen: delivers 60 or 120 mcg dose Dosed with each meal	30 days	Pharmacokinetics: The t_{max} is approximately 20 minutes. The $t_{1/2}$ is approximately 45 minutes, Metabolized by kidneys, One active metabolite (2-37 pramlintide) has a similar half-life as the parent compound. No accumulation seen in renal insufficiency. Injection into the arm—not recommended Drug Interactions: Pramlintide may delay gastric emptying	Dosing: type 1 DM start at 15 mcg before meals, may increase as tolerated, most can advance dose to 30-45 mcg before meals Type 2 DM- start with 60 mcg before meals, most advance to 120 mcg before meals Nausea: type 1 DM > type 2 DM Vomiting: type 1 DM > type 2 DM Severe hypoglycemia possible: decrease prandial insulin 30%-50% prior to initiation

CNS, central nervous system; GI, gastrointestinal; $t_{1/2}$, half-life of medication; t_{max}, time at maximum concentration.

[a]All diabetes injectables available in the US are now made by human recombinant DNA technology. An insulin analog is a modified human insulin molecule that imparts particular pharmacokinetic advantages.

[b]Room temperature defined as 59-86°F (15-30°C). All products are good until expiration date on product if unopened and stored correctly.

ischemic preconditioning via K^+ channel closure in the heart. Recent meta-analyses have conflicting conclusions. One analysis found that sulfonylureas increased CVD risk and another found a reduced risk.

The most common side effect of sulfonylureas is hypoglycemia. The pretreatment fasting plasma glucose is a strong predictor of hypoglycemic potential. The lower the FPG is upon initiation, the greater likelihood for hypoglycemia. Those who skip meals, exercise vigorously, or lose substantial amounts of weight are also more prone to experiencing hypoglycemia. A lower dose should initially be used in high-risk patients, in addition, hypoglycemia on low-dose sulfonylureas may dictate a switch to therapy with a low risk of hypoglycemia. Severe hypoglycemia on sulfonylureas would warrant the same intervention.

Weight gain is common with sulfonylureas—typically 1 to 2 kg. Many patients report having a sulfa allergy, but cross reactivity with sulfonylureas is very rare. However, if the patient has a history of anaphylaxis type reactions to sulfa, it may be best to use a different class of medication.

The usual starting dose and maximum dose of sulfonylureas are summarized in Table 74-10. The dosage can be titrated as soon as every 2 weeks based on fasting plasma glucose values (use a longer interval with chlorpropamide) to achieve glycemic goals. Immediate-release glipizide's maximal dose is 40 mg/day, but its maximal effective dose is about 10 to 15 mg per day. Indeed, the maximal effective dose of sulfonylureas is typically 60% to 75% of the stated maximum dose.

Dipeptidyl Peptidase 4 Inhibitors (DPP-4 Inhibitors)[19,23,53-55] Several DPP-4 inhibitors are approved by the FDA including sitagliptin, saxagliptin, linagliptin, and alogliptin. The DPP-4 inhibitors prolong the half-life of endogenously produced GLP-1 and GIP. GIP levels are normal in patients with type 2 DM and may play a role in stimulating insulin secretion. GIP has no effect on glucagon. However, levels of GLP-1 are deficient in patients with type 2 DM. As these agents block nearly 100% of the DPP-4 enzyme activity for at least 12 hours, normal physiologic, nondiabetic GLP-1 levels are achieved. DPP-4 inhibitors significantly reduce inappropriately elevated postprandial glucagon and improve β-cell response to hyperglycemia. This results in reduction of glucose levels without increase in hypoglycemia when used as monotherapy. These drugs do not alter gastric emptying and do not cause nausea or have significant effects on satiety. DPP-4 inhibitors have a neutral impact on weight.

The average reduction in HbA_{1c} seen with a DPP-4 inhibitor is 0.7% to 1% (0.007-0.01; 8-11 mmol/mol Hb) when used at maximum doses. DPP-4 inhibitors have a shallow dose-response curve. These drugs are well tolerated, and the dose not need to be titrated. DPP-4 inhibitors may have greater glucose lowering efficacy in patients of Asian descent.[60] DPP-4 inhibitors are considered second line therapy in ADA algorithm and fourth-line therapy in the AACE/ACE though they may be used sooner if other medications have intolerances. Potential advantages of the DPP-4 inhibitors include once daily dose, oral administration, weight neutrality, low risk of hypoglycemia, and they are well tolerated. They may be used in older adults with moderate to severe renal insufficiency and with CVD. However, their ability to lower BG is modest and they are expensive.

The DPP-4 enzymes metabolize a wide variety of peptides including neuropeptide Y, growth hormone-releasing hormone, vasoactive intestinal polypeptide, and others. DPP-4 plays an important role for T-cell activation. Theoretically the inhibition of DPP-4 could be associated with adverse immunologic reactions. To date, however, there has been no evidence of clinically relevant changes in immune function.[61] Reducing the dose of alogliptin, saxagliptin, or sitagliptin, based on renal function is appropriate, as only 100% of the enzyme can be inhibited, and long-term exposure to higher levels in humans has not been extensively studied.

Recent long-term cardiovascular outcome studies have found no increased in the risk of mortality, myocardial infarction, or other major CV events with alogliptin, saxagliptin, or sitagliptin.[62-64] However, the risk of hospitalization for heart failure was increased with saxagliptin and equivocal with alogliptin. A meta-analysis showed no increased risk of mortality, MI, or cerebrovascular events; however, the risk of heart failure was increased in patients treated long-term with DPP-4 inhibitors.[65] In April 2015, the US FDA advisory committee recommended making changes to labeling for both saxagliptin and alogliptin, to include information about increased risk of hospitalization for heart failure. See Table 74-10 for information about dosing DPP-4 inhibitors.

Sodium-Glucose Cotransporter-2 Inhibitors[19,23,53,54,66] Several SGLT2 inhibitors have been approved by the FDA including canagliflozin, dapagliflozin, and empagliflozin. The reabsorption of glucose in the proximal tubule of the kidney from the filtered urine into renal tubular epithelial cells is facilitated by a family of ATP-dependent proteins, the sodium-glucose cotransporters (SGLT). By inhibiting SGLT2, the renal tubular threshold for glucose reabsorption is lowered and glucosuria occurs at lower levels of plasma glucose concentrations. SGLT2 inhibition lowers blood glucose through an insulin-independent mechanism. Although SGLT2 inhibitors block the reabsorption of 90% of the filtered glucose load, which could theoretically result in up to 170 g loss of glucose/day in the urine, urinary glucose excretion (UGE) does not exceed 75 to 85 g per day or less than 50% of the filtered glucose load. The reason for this is that SGLT1 never has to work at its maximal capacity. When presented with the excess glucose, SGLT1 can reabsorb up to 30% to 40% of the filtered glucose load. Thus, when SGLT2 is inhibited, SGLT1 instantaneously can augment its reabsorption of glucose and blunt the glucosuric effect of the SGLT2 inhibitor. Since glucose reabsorption in the proximal tubule is coupled with sodium reabsorption, SGLT2 inhibitors promote mild sodium depletion (for 1-2 days after start of therapy) and intravascular water.

The SGLT2 inhibitors reduce the HbA_{1c} by 0.5% to 1% (0.005-0.01; 5-11 mmol/mol Hb) and can be used as either monotherapy or add-on therapy. They appear to be more efficacious if the patient has higher baseline HbA_{1c} values. In addition, increased UGE leads to the loss of 200 to 300 kcal/day (840-1,260 kJ/day), which may contribute to 1 to 5 kg of weight loss. Visceral fat loss is responsible for the weight reduction rather than muscle mass loss. SGLT2 inhibitors modestly reduce SBP by 3 to 4 mm Hg and DBP by 1 to 2 mm Hg. Modest changes in lipid profiles have been described in clinical trials of SGLT2 inhibitors. SGLT2 inhibitors' are unlikely to cause hypoglycemia unless combined with medications such as sulfonylureas, meglitinides, or insulin.

Empagliflozin has demonstrated CV risk reduction in a dedicated CV outcomes trial (EMPA-REG OUTCOME).[67] Empagliflozin, when added to standard of care, reduced a composite of CV death (including fatal stroke and fatal MI) (HR 0.86, 95.02% CI 0.74-0.99), all-cause mortality (HR 0.68 95% CI 0.57-0.82) and death from CV causes (HR 0.62 95% CI 0.49-0.77) after a follow-up of 5 years. Canagliflozin (CANVAS) and dapagliflozin (DECLARE-TIMI 58) are currently being studied in CV trials with results due in 2018 and 2019, respectively.

In the ADA algorithm, the SGLT2 inhibitors are considered a second-line therapy and in the AACE/ACE algorithm as third-line treatment choice. Older adults and patients with stage 4 or 5 chronic kidney disease are not optimal candidates for SGLT2 inhibitors. Older adults typically have diminished renal function and, because they may have poor thirst response, they are predisposed to dehydration. Concomitant diuretic use may cause orthostatic hypotension and electrolyte abnormalities. Renal impairment decreases the efficacy of the SGLT2 inhibitors. As GFR declines, the amount of glucose that reaches the proximal tubule declines. SGLT2 inhibitors lower HbA_{1c} approximately 0.4% to 0.5% (0.004-0.005; 4-5 mmol/mol Hb) when GFR is 30 to 45 mL/min/1.73 m^2 (0.29-0.43 mL/s/m^2).

The mechanism of action and osmotic diuresis with SGLT inhibitors may affect several laboratory tests. LDL-C and HDL-C increase slightly with SGLT2 inhibitors. Hemoconcentration from diuresis can result in a 2% to 3% increase in hematocrit. Urinary analysis will always be positive for glucose due to the mechanism of action. Additionally, the 1,5-anhydroglucitol (1,5-AG) assay, commonly known as Glycomark®, will give falsely lowered results, which may falsely indicate higher postprandial glycemia. Its use is not recommended during SGLT2 inhibitor therapy.

The most common adverse effect is GU infections. Yeast GU infections are most common, and there is a slight increase in urinary tract infections. GU infections occur more frequently in women and uncircumcised men, but led to discontinuation in less than 1% of patients in the clinical trials. Lowering the dose of a SGLT2 inhibitor will not decrease the risk of a GU infection. It is important to tell all patients, male and female, about the signs and symptoms of GU infections. Greater than 10% of people with diabetes will have asymptomatic bacteriuria at any given time, thus routine urinary analysis is not recommended. Pyelonephritis and urosepsis were not more common in SGLT2 inhibitors trials, but the FDA required SGLT2 inhibitors to add both risks to their labels based on postmarketing surveillance data. Symptomatic hypotension may occur more frequently in patients with an eGFR less than 60 mL/min/1.73 m^2. If the patient takes a loop diuretic, discontinuation will be necessary. If the patient has a compelling need for the loop diuretic, an alternate medication class may be necessary. Thiazide diuretics usually do not need adjustment unless on high doses for diuresis.

The SGLT2 inhibitor's mechanism is insulin independent and less likely to cause hypoglycemia unless combined with medications such as sulfonylureas, meglitinides, or insulin.

Cases of euglycemic DKA have been reported. Most cases have been in patients with type 1 diabetes, which is not a currently approved use by the FDA.[67] Risk factors include: dehydration, any insulinopenic patient including LADA, type 1 DM, or long-standing type 2 DM, or serious intercurrent illness. It is advisable to make sure the patient is well hydrated prior to treatment initiation, temporarily stop the drug if a serious illness is encountered, and to not decrease the insulin dose prospectively when it is initiated. Dapagliflozin has been associated with bladder tumors and patients with a prior or active history of bladder cancer should not use this medication. It is likely a chance finding, but surveillance continues. Canagliflozin has been associated with a 30% higher risk of bone fracture after more than 1 year usage. Canagliflozin trials enrolled an older population and these patients are at higher risk of developing orthostatic hypotension. Many of the fractures were distal fractures of the upper extremities after a fall. After 2 years of treatment, a 0.3% to 1% placebo-subtracted reduction in hip and lumbar at the hip and lumbar spine were noted on dual-energy x-ray absorptiometry. Mechanisms may involve changes in phosphorus reabsorption, increases in parathyroid hormone, or weight loss.

Canagliflozin should be initiated at 100 mg orally daily and may be titrated up to 300 mg daily. Patients with an eGFR between 45 and 60 mL/min/1.73 m^2 should receive no more than 100 mg of canagliflozin. Canagliflozin use is not recommended to start or continue therapy when the eGFR is consistently less than 45 mL/min/1.73 m^2. Dapagliflozin should be started at 5 mg daily and may be titrated to 10 mg orally daily in patients that require additional glycemic control. Renal function should be assessed and dapagliflozin should not be started or continued in patients with an eGFR consistently less than 60 mL/min/1.73 m^2. Empagliflozin may be started at 10 mg orally daily and titrated to 25 mg daily as tolerated. Therapy should not be started or it should be discontinued if patients have an eGFR consistently less than 45 mL/min/1.73 m^2 (see Table 74-10).

Clinical **Controversy...**

Diabetes Drugs and Regulatory Approval:

Diabetes mellitus (DM) is a major risk factor for cardiovascular disease (CVD) with 65% of people with DM dying of CVD. Prior to the EMPA-REG study there was no conclusive evidence that any glucose lowering therapy decreased CVD risk or death.[67] Most drugs were developed and approved based solely on their glucose lowering ability. HbA_{1c} has been used as the principal surrogate marker of DM treatment effectiveness, primarily because reducing hyperglycemia has demonstrated benefits on DM symptoms and on the incidence of microvascular complications.[77] The degree of hyperglycemia as reflected by HbA_{1c} is correlated with the incidence and prevalence of cardiovascular complications and death.[78] However, despite lowering HbA_{1c}, rosiglitazone was associated with an increased risk of myocardial infarction and death in a 2007 meta-analysis.[69] This led to restrictions put in place by the FDA on the use of rosiglitazone. Large, randomized clinical trials of "intensive" vs "standard" glucose control failed to demonstrate CVD benefit, further clouding the narrative that lower blood glucose using antihyperglycemic agents decrease CVD events.[34-36] Given the aggregate of these data that demonstrated either a neutral or increased effect on CVD events, the FDA issued a Guidance for Industry in 2008 recommending that new DM agents be assessed for CVD safety prior to approval. This approach has been criticized for its perceived increased burden to achieve approval for new drugs.[79] However, it has been noted that there has been an increase in novel DM agents over the last decade.[80] It is also important to note the invalidation of HbA_{1c} as a surrogate for CVD and the significance of investigating the CV effects of these drugs independent of their glucose lowering abilities.

Thiazolidinediones[19,23,53,54] Thiazolidinediones are also referred to as TZDs or glitazones. Pioglitazone and rosiglitazone are the two currently FDA approved TZDs for the treatment of type 2 DM (see Table 74-10). TZDs work by binding to the peroxisome proliferator activator receptor-γ (PPAR-γ), which are primarily located on fat cells and vascular cells. The concentration of these receptors in the muscle is very low, but improvement in mitochondrial function through changes in lipotoxicity, glucotoxicity, and possibly binding of mitochondrial membrane proteins occurs. TZDs enhance insulin sensitivity at muscle, liver, and fat tissues indirectly. TZDs cause preadipocytes to differentiate into mature fat cells in subcutaneous fat stores. Small fat cells are more sensitive to insulin and more able to store FFAs. This allows a flux of FFAs out of the plasma, visceral fat, and liver into subcutaneous fat, a less insulin-resistant storage tissue. Muscle intracellular fat products, which contribute to insulin resistance, also decline. TZDs also effect adipokines (eg, angiotensinogen, tissue necrosis factor-α, interleukin 6, plasminogen activator inhibitor-1), which can positively affect insulin sensitivity, endothelial function, and inflammation. Of particular note, adiponectin is reduced with obesity and diabetes, but is increased with TZD therapy, which improves endothelial function, insulin sensitivity, and has a potent antiinflammatory effect.

Pioglitazone and rosiglitazone reduce HbA_{1c} values approximately 1.0% to 1.5% (11-16 mmol/mol Hb) and reduce FPG levels by 60 to 70 mg/dL (3.3-3.9 mmol/L) at maximal doses. Glycemic-lowering onset is slow and maximal effects may not be seen until 3 to 4 months of therapy. It is important to inform patients of this fact and that they should not stop therapy even if minimal changes in SMBG are initially seen. Pioglitazone consistently decreases plasma triglyceride levels by 10% to 20%, whereas rosiglitazone tends to have a neutral effect. LDL-C concentrations tend to increase with rosiglitazone 5% to 15%, but do not significantly increase with pioglitazone. Both appear to convert small, dense LDL particles, which have been shown to be more atherogenic, to large, buoyant LDL particles, which may be less atherogenic. Any increase in LDL cholesterol, however, is of concern. Both drugs increase HDL, though pioglitazone may raise it more than rosiglitazone.

The ADA algorithm recommends the TZDs as a second-line treatment choice for type 2 DM. The AACE/ACE algorithm list them as a fifth line choice. Although the TZDs are very effective insulin sensitizers, they can cause edema, new onset or worsening of preexisting heart failure, and fractures. In addition, TZD use has been linked in the past to bladder cancer. Many clinicians, inappropriately, believe that the cardiovascular risk associated with rosiglitazone use also applies to pioglitazone. As all side effects with TZDs are dose related, starting with a low dose and seeing if a patient will respond is reasonable. This may be 3 to 6 months on pioglitazone 15 mg daily before a decision about efficacy is made. Low dose pioglitazone may be used when high dose insulin is necessary, though edema and weight gain must be followed carefully.

Macrovascular complications with TZDs are controversial. In the PROactive study, pioglitazone 45 mg was added to standard therapy in patients who had experienced a cardiovascular event or had peripheral vascular disease.[68] After 3 years of treatment, there was no difference in the primary endpoint but the secondary endpoint (all-cause mortality, nonfatal myocardial infarction, or stroke) was reduced 16% ($P = 0.027$). Pioglitazone has also been shown to decrease the risk of recurrent strokes, but this was in a nondiabetic population. Also of note, patients in the pioglitazone group were more likely to be hospitalized for heart failure, though this did not increase mortality. Several published meta-analysis of rosiglitazone reported higher myocardial infarction (MI) rates, but none have reported a higher risk of mortality.[69] A prospective, multicenter, open-label noninferiority trial in 4,447 patients of rosiglitazone added to background metformin or sulfonylurea versus the active comparator metformin plus sulfonylurea found that rosiglitazone was noninferior to the comparator for all CV outcomes except heart failure. A nonsignificant increase in risk for MI (HR, 1.14; 95% CI, 0.80-1.63) as well as a nonsignificant reduction in stroke (HR, 0.72; 95% CI, 0.49-1.05) were reported. On subset analysis, previous ischemic heart disease trended toward a higher risk (HR, 1.26; CI, 0.95-1.68; $P = 0.055$).[70] Most studies with rosiglitazone trend toward, but do not reach, statistically significant increases in ischemic events.

Retention of fluid leads to several possible side effects with TZDs. The etiology of the fluid retention has not been fully elucidated, but appears to include peripheral vasodilation and improved insulin sensitization at the kidney with a resultant increase in renal sodium and water retention. Resultant effects from water retention may include peripheral edema, heart failure, hemodilution of hemoglobin and hematocrit, and weight gain. Peripheral edema is reported in 4% to 5% of patients using TZD monotherapy but the incidence of edema is significantly increased (more than 15%) when a TZD is used in combination with insulin. TZDs are contraindicated in patients with New York Heart Association Class III and IV heart failure, and great caution should be exercised when given to patients with Class I and II heart failure. Edema is dose related and if not severe, a reduction in the dose as well as use of spironolactone, triamterene, or amiloride may allow the continuation of therapy in the majority of patients. Rarely, TZDs have been reported to worsen macular edema of the eye.

Weight gain, which is also dose related, can be seen with both rosiglitazone and pioglitazone. Mechanistically, both fluid retention and fat accumulation play a part in explaining the weight gain. Average weight gain varies but a 4-kg weight gain is not uncommon. Rarely, a patient will gain large amounts of weight in a short period of time, and this may necessitate discontinuation of therapy.

Thiazolidinediones have also been associated with an increased fracture rate in the upper and lower limbs of postmenopausal women. These fractures are not osteoporotic in the classic sense, and do not occur in common osteoporosis fracture sites such as spine or hip. Most occur in wrists, forearms, ankles, or feet. TZDs may increase the risk of a fracture by 25%. The underlying pathophysiology is speculative, but may relate to TZDs effect on the pluripotent stem cell and shunting of new cells to fat instead of osteocytes as well as altering osteoblasts/osteoclasts. It would be prudent to consider a patient's risk factors for fractures if a TZD is being considered.

The risk of bladder cancer is controversial. Bladder tumors have been noted in rodent models using TZDs, which prompted a10-year observational study with pioglitazone. The study reported an excess of 3 in 10,000 patient-year risk of bladder cancer after 5 years of pioglitazone use. Eight and ten year data using the same database showed no association. Excess risk, if present, appears to be mostly in men and smokers, and is dose and duration associated. Mechanisms are speculative, but may involve microcrystals of the drug in the bladder which cause chronic irritation.

Premenopausal anovulatory patients may resume ovulation on TZDs due to their insulin sensitizing effects. Adequate pregnancy and contraception precautions should be explained to all women capable of becoming pregnant.

The recommended starting dosages of pioglitazone is 15 to 30 mg once daily and for rosiglitazone it is 2 to 4 mg once daily. Dosages may be increased after 3 to 4 months based on the response to treatment and side effects. The maximum dose and maximum effective dose of pioglitazone is 45 mg and 8 mg once daily for rosiglitazone. To minimize side effects, the lowest effective dose should be used.

α-Glucosidase Inhibitors[19,23,53,54] Currently, there are two α-glucosidase inhibitors approved by the FDA, acarbose and miglitol. α-Glucosidase inhibitors competitively inhibit maltase, isomaltase, sucrase, and glucoamylase in the small intestine, delaying the breakdown of sucrose and complex carbohydrates. There is no malabsorption of these nutrients, but merely a delay their absorption. The net effect from this action is to reduce the postprandial blood glucose rise. Distal intestinal degradation of undigested carbohydrate by the gut flora results in gas, CO_2 and methane, as well as production of short-chain fatty acids, which may stimulate glucagon like peptide-1 release from intestinal L-cells.

Postprandial glucose concentrations are reduced by 40 to 50 mg/dL (2.2-2.8 mmol/L) while fasting glucose levels are relatively unchanged. The overall glucose lowering effect of the α-glucosidase inhibitors in terms of HbA_{1c} is 0.3% to 1% (0.003-0.01; 3-11 mmol/mol Hb). Patients near target HbA_{1c} levels with near-normal fasting plasma glucose levels but high postprandial SMBG are candidates for therapy. The ADA does not list the class on their treatment algorithm, but the AACE/ACE algorithm considers them an alternative medication that can be used when other medications may be contraindicated or the patient has intolerances. Data from China have reported that acarbose is as effective as metformin in patients consuming high carbohydrate diet from mostly rice. It has also been shown to prevent type 2 DM. The STOP-NIDDM study in subjects with impaired glucose tolerance documented a significant reduction in the risk of cardiovascular events, though the total number of events were very small.[71] No large cardiovascular study confirming these preliminary results has been completed. For information about dosing α-glucosidase inhibitors see Table 74-10.

Short-Acting Insulin Secretagogues[19,23,53,54]

By binding a site adjacent to sulfonylurea receptor, nateglinide and repaglinide stimulate insulin secretion from the β-cells of the pancreas. Repaglinide and nateglinide both require the presence of glucose to stimulate insulin secretion. As glucose levels diminish to normal, stimulated insulin secretion diminishes. As monotherapy, both nateglinide and repaglinide significantly reduce postprandial glucose excursions and reduce HbA_{1c} by approximately 0.8% to 1% (0.008-0.01; 9-11 mmol/mol Hb). This class of agents is not listed on the ADA algorithm but is consider a less favorable choice on the AACE/ACE treatment algorithm. DPP-4 inhibitors and SGLT2 inhibitors have largely taken the place of this class due to a low risk of hypoglycemia and daily dosing with similar or more robust glycemic reductions. Nateglinide or repaglinide may be used in patients with renal insufficiency, and may be a good option for those with erratic meal schedules. Multiple daily dosing may decrease adherence. For dosing and adverse reaction data see Table 74-10.

Amylinomimetics[19,23,53,54] Pramlintide is an antihyperglycemic agent used in patients currently treated with insulin. Pramlintide is a synthetic analog of amylin, a neurohormone cosecreted from the β-cells with insulin. Amylin is very low or absent in type 1 DM, and lower than normal in patients with a long duration of type 2 DM. Pramlintide suppresses inappropriately high postprandial glucagon secretion, increases satiety, and slows gastric emptying so that the rate of glucose appearance into the plasma better matches the glucose disposition.

The average HbA_{1c} reduction is approximately 0.6% (0.006; 7 mmol/mol Hb) in patients with type 2 DM. By improving satiety, pramlintide may reduce the number of calories a patient eats at a meal. The 120-mcg dose produced an average weight loss of 1.5-kg weight in patients with type 2 DM on insulin. In patients with type 1 DM, the average reduction in HbA_{1c} was 0.4% to 0.5% (0.004-0.005; 4-5 mmol/mol Hb). In type 2 DM patients on basal insulin, adding pramlintide instead of prandial insulin resulted in similar efficacy and no weight gain. When pramlintide is injected before the meal, gastric emptying may delay absorption of mealtime nutrients. This may necessitate delaying the rapid-acting insulin dose until the conclusion of the meal. Pramlintide is not considered on the AACE/ACE or ADA algorithm. GLP-1 RAs and DPP-4 inhibitors have become the classes of choice to decrease inappropriate glucagon.

The most common adverse effects associated with pramlintide are gastrointestinal. Nausea occurs in approximately 20% of patients with type 2 DM and 40% to 50% of patients with type 1 DM. The higher rate of nausea in patient with type 1 DM is likely related to the near absolute amylin deficiency, and thus sensitivity or perhaps number, of amylin receptors. Vomiting or anorexia occurs in approximately 10% of patients with type 1 and type 2 DM. Gastrointestinal adverse effects decrease over time and are dose related, thus starting with a low dose and slowly titrating as tolerated is recommended. Pramlintide alone does not cause hypoglycemia, but when used in patients on insulin hypoglycemia can occur. The risk of severe hypoglycemia early in therapy is highest in patients with type 1 DM, with a twofold increase in risk of severe hypoglycemic reactions. It is imperative that the prandial insulin dose, if used, be reduced 30% to 50% when pramlintide is initiated. This will minimize severe hypoglycemic reactions.

Pramlintide dosing is different in patient with type 1 and type 2 DM. In type 2 DM, the starting dose is 60 mcg prior to meals, and is titrated to the maximally recommended 120-mcg dose as tolerated and warranted based on postprandial plasma glucose concentrations. In type 1 DM, dosing starts at 15 mcg prior to meals, and can be titrated up in 15-mcg increments to a maximum of 60 mcg prior to each meal, if tolerated. Most type 1 DM patients are able to tolerate 30 to 45 mcg prior to meals. Snacks may also be covered with pramlintide. Storage information can be found in Table 74-11.

Bile Acid Sequestrants[19,23,53,54] Currently, the only bile acid sequestrant approved for the treatment of type 2 DM is colesevelam. Colesevelam acts in the intestinal lumen to bind bile acid, decreasing the bile acid pool for reabsorption. It is unclear how colesevelam reduces BG. Possible mechanisms include effects on the farnesoid X and TGR5 receptors within the intestine as well as effects on farnesoid X receptor within the liver. There is evidence that colesevelam may affect the secretion of GLP-1 and GIP.

Hemoglobin A_{1c} reductions from baseline were approximately 0.4% (0.004; 4 mmol/mol Hb) when a dose of 3.8 g/day is given as add-on therapy to metformin, sulfonylureas, or insulin. The fasting plasma glucose was modestly reduced about 5 to 10 mg/dL (0.3-0.6 mmol/L). Colesevelam is not mentioned on the ADA algorithm but is considered an alternative medication on the AACE/ACE algorithm. Colesevelam also reduces LDL-C cholesterol in patients with type 2 DM. A 12% to 16% reduction in LDL-C was reported from baseline LDL-C concentrations of approximately 105 mg/dL (approximately 2.72 mmol/L). Triglycerides increased when combined with sulfonylureas or insulin, but not with metformin. Colesevelam is weight neutral and has a low risk of hypoglycemia. Colesevelam has been used in pediatric patients (10-17 years of age) for cholesterol reduction, but not type 2 DM. Although colesevelam lowers plasma glucose and LDL-C, it has not been proven to prevent cardiovascular morbidity or mortality. Patients with type 2 DM patients who need a small reduction in A_{1C} as well as additional LDL-C lowering would be candidates for this agent. See Table 74-10 for dosing and adverse reactions.

Dopamine Agonists[19,23,53,54] Bromocriptine mesylate is FDA approved for the treatment of type 2 DM. Bromocriptine used for type 2 DM is a quick release formulation of the dopamine agonist. The exact mechanism by which bromocriptine improves glycemic control is unknown. Low hypothalamic dopamine levels, especially upon waking are augmented, which may decrease sympathetic tone and output. These effects are speculated to improve hepatic insulin sensitivity and decrease hepatic glucose output. In clinical trials, bromocriptine mesylate reduced HbA_{1c} by a 0.3% to 0.6% (0.003-0.006; 3-7 mmol/mol Hb). Bromocriptine's target population for use is unclear. The ADA algorithm does not mention bromocriptine but the AACE/ACE treatment algorithm lists bromocriptine as an alternative medication in combination with other agents.

The effects of bromocriptine on macrovascular events have been explored in a safety trial. Bromocriptine decreased a composite cardiovascular endpoint. After 1 year of treatment, the composite outcome occurred in 37 (1.8%) bromocriptine treated subjects versus 32 (3.2%) subjects who received usual care (HR 0.6; 95% CI 0.35-0.96). See Table 74-10 for adverse effects and dosing.

EVALUATION OF THERAPEUTIC OUTCOMES

Monitoring for Complications[14,22]

The ADA recommends screening for complications at the time of diagnosis of DM. Current recommendations continue to advocate yearly dilated eye examinations in type 2 DM and an initial dilated eye examination in the first 3 to 5 years in type 1 DM, then yearly thereafter. Less frequent eye examinations, every 2 to 3 years, may be appropriate if the patient has no evidence of retinopathy and is at low risk of developing eye disease. The patient's blood pressure should be assessed at each visit. The feet should be examined at each visit including palpation of distal pulses and a visual inspection for skin integrity, calluses, and deformities. Pedal sensory loss due to polyneuropathy should screened for annually using the 10-g force Semmes-Weinstein monofilament. Screening for nephropathy should done at the time diagnosis in patients type 2 DM and 5 years after diagnosis if the patient has type 1 DM with urine microalbumin. Yearly testing for lipid abnormalities is appropriate if the patient is on lipid lowering therapy. It is generally accepted that a thyroid stimulating hormone concentration be measured in patients with type 1 DM and LADA as thyroid abnormalities are more common in DM.

Glycemic Goals and HbA_{1C}[22]

Controlled clinical trials provide ample evidence that glycemic control is paramount in reducing microvascular complications in both type 1 DM[28] and type 2 DM.[29] HbA_{1c} measurements are the gold standard for following long-term glycemic control for the previous 2 to 3 months. Other strategies such as measurement of fructosamine, which measures all glycated plasma proteins, or a glycated albumin test may be necessary to assess diabetes control in patients with altered red blood cell lifespan. Fructosamine measures glucose control over 2 to 3 weeks. Unfortunately, fructosamine measures are not as reliable as the HbA_{1c} due to significant intra-patient variability. Moreover, the correlation between fructosamine measurements and the risk complications from diabetes is unknown—thus fructosamine goals have not been established.

The HbA_{1c} goal recommended by the ADA is < 7% (0.07; 53 mmol/mol Hb) in most adults. The AACE/ACE guidelines recommend < 6.5% (0.065; 48 mmol/mol Hb). Both guidelines recommend that treatment goals need to be individualized. Less stringent HbA_{1c} goals may be appropriate in patients with a history of severe hypoglycemia, limited life expectancy, advanced micro/macrovascular complications or comorbidities, and in patients who are frail, have dementia, or have limited social or financial resources. Less stringent goals should also be used for younger children (see Table 74-6). More aggressive glycemic goals should be considered in patients who are newly diagnosed and younger using treatments that are less likely to cause hypoglycemia, weight gain, and other adverse effects.

The estimated average glucose (eAG) is correlated with HbA_{1c} readings and now is regularly reported below HbA_{1c} value by most laboratories. For example, an HbA_{1c} of 7% (0.07; 53 mmol/mol Hb), correlates with an eAG of 154 mg/dL (8.5 mmol/L). Similarly, the International Federation of Clinical Chemistry (IFCC) recommends a standardize approach to report the HbA_{1c} using mmol/mol Hb. For example, an NGSP HbA_{1c} of 7.0% (0.07) is reported as 53 mmol/mol Hb.[22]

Self-Monitored Blood Glucose and Continuous Glucose Monitoring[14,22]

Self-monitored blood glucose is a tool that provides an opportunity to intervene when an SMBG value is obtained and increases patient safety by detecting hypoglycemia so that it can be treated. In general, SMBG frequency should match how frequently medication changes are needed to achieve glycemic control as well as the risk of hypoglycemia.

Frequent SMBG is necessary to achieve near-normal blood glucose concentrations if insulin is used. Assessment for hypoglycemia, hyperglycemia, adjustment of prandial doses of insulin, to administer corrective doses of insulin, to see how a change in diet, exercise or to check accuracy of continuous glucose monitors are but a few of the reasons a patient may need to perform SMBG. This is particularly true in patients with type 1 DM. The optimal frequency of SMBG for patients with type 2 DM on oral agents is unknown and its role controversial. What is clear is that patients must be empowered to change their therapeutic regimen in response to test results, or testing SMBG will not be useful.

Alternate site testing performed on the palm, forearm, or the thigh may improve adherence to SMBG recommendations, but only some BG test strips are designed for alternative site testing. Alternative sites tend to have less nerve endings than fingertips and may be more comfortable for a patient. However, glucose readings from alternative site testing will lag behind fingertip capillary blood by 20 to 30 minutes. Therefore, alternate site testing is discouraged in any situation where immediate action will be needed based on the glucose reading, such as testing for hypoglycemia or in patients with hypoglycemia unawareness, wide fluctuations in SMBG, or when the blood glucose is changing rapidly, such as after a meal.

Choosing an appropriate meter depends on the patient's dexterity, eye acuity, strip cost, and desired features. Insurance coverage often influences meter choice due to strip cost. Demonstrate to and then have the patient confirm SMBG technique. Each meter has specifications for hematocrit, elevation, and temperature tolerances for optimal operation.

Continuous glucose monitoring (CGM) is useful in select patients. CGM measures interstitial glucose, which lags behind capillary SMBG. CGM can be useful in patients with frequent episodes of hypoglycemia, hypoglycemic unawareness, and nocturnal hypoglycemia. CGM can be used to identify glucose patterns and evaluate patients with higher or lower than expected HbA_{1c} results. CGM must be calibrated after insertion of a new sensor and every 12 hours thereafter with SMBG readings. Alarms need to be properly set and a new sensor must be placed every 3 to 7 days. The ADA currently recommends that CGM can be considered in adults with type 1 DM who are at least 25 years of age and those younger than 25 years of age who can demonstrate adherence to its use.[5] CGM data can be transmitted to insulin pumps which can then make recommendations to the patient to adjust insulin doses.

Treatment of Concomitant Conditions and Complications

Retinopathy[72]

Patients with established retinopathy should see an ophthalmologist or optometrist trained in diabetic eye disease. A dilated eye examination is required to fully evaluate the retina. Early background retinopathy may reverse with improved glycemic control and optimal blood pressure control. More advanced retinopathy will not fully regress with improved glycemia. Aggressive reductions in blood glucose may acutely worsen retinopathy. Diabetic retinopathy is caused by microcirculation ischemia coupled with inappropriate growth factor release. Laser photocoagulation has markedly improved sight preservation in diabetic patients and is extensively used in patients with macular edema and proliferative retinopathy. Intravitreal anti-vascular endothelial growth factor (VEGF) therapy has also been shown to be highly effective for sight preservation. Both bevacizumab, used off-label, and ranibizumab are anti-VEGF monoclonal antibodies, and aflibercept is a VEGF decoy receptor. People with diabetes also have a higher rate of cataracts and open-angle glaucoma.

Neuropathy[72,73]

Neuropathy in diabetes can generally be placed into three categories: (1) peripheral neuropathy, (2) autonomic neuropathy, and (3) focal neuropathies. Distal, symmetrical, peripheral neuropathy is the most common complication seen in type 2 DM patients in outpatient clinics. Paresthesias, perceived hot or cold, numbness, or pain are the predominant symptoms. The feet are involved far more often than the hands as it affects longer nerves first and progresses proximally. Improved glycemic control is the primary treatment and may alleviate some of the symptoms. If neuropathy is painful, symptomatic pain treatment is indicated, though it will not change the course of the neuropathy. No medication has been shown to be superior to another for pain relief. Treatment with low-dose tricyclic antidepressants, gabapentin, pregabalin, carbamazepine, duloxetine, venlafaxine, topical capsaicin, tramadol, and nonsteroidal antiinflammatory drugs may be considered. If these are unsuccessful, patients often are sent to a pain clinic or neurologist for further evaluation. Duloxetine and pregabalin are FDA approved for this indication. The numb variant of peripheral neuropathy is not treated with medications, but may lead to pressure areas on the foot and subsequent ulceration.

Clinical manifestations of diabetic autonomic neuropathy may include resting tachycardia, exercise intolerance, orthostatic hypotension, constipation, gastroparesis, erectile dysfunction, anhidrosis, heat intolerance, gustatory sweating, dry skin, impaired neurovascular function, and hypoglycemic unawareness. Gastroparesis can be a severe and debilitating complication of DM. Improved glycemic control, discontinuation of medications that slow gastric motility, and the use of metoclopramide for only a few weeks at a time or low dose erythromycin may be helpful. Gastric pacemakers can be considered if symptoms are severe and persistent. Domperidone, though not FDA approved, is available outside of the United States and may be useful. The hallmark of diabetic diarrhea is its nocturnal occurrence. A differential versus celiac disease, exocrine insufficiency, and gut bacterial overgrowth should be considered. Diabetic diarrhea frequently responds to a 10- to 14-day course of an antibiotic such as doxycycline or metronidazole. In more unresponsive cases, octreotide may be useful. If a patient develops orthostatic hypotension, antihypertensive agents should be stopped and dietary sodium intake should be liberalized. Some patients may require pharmacologic treatment for orthostatic hypotension with mineralocorticoids or adrenergic agonist agents. In severe cases, supine hypertension may be extreme, mandating that the patient sleep in a sitting or semirecumbent position. Patients with cardiac autonomic neuropathy are at a higher risk for silent MI and sudden cardiac death. Erectile dysfunction is common in diabetes, and initial treatment should include a trial of one of the phosphodiesterase type 5 inhibitors prior to referral. People with diabetes often require the highest doses of these medications to have an adequate response. Sudomotor dysfunction may cause reduced sweating and dry, cracked skin. Use of hydrating creams and ointments is needed. Autonomic neuropathy may also result in gustatory sweating after eating, which may be treated with antiperspirants or anticholinergic drugs. Hypoglycemic unawareness requires the patient to avoid hypoglycemia, as the body will slowly increase the glycemic level at which it will signal the autonomic signals.

Focal neuropathies are uncommon, but occur more often in older patient with poorly controlled diabetes. Diabetic amyotrophy, which is characterized by a proximal thigh muscle pain and weakness, is one of the most debilitating. In addition, cranial nerve III, IV, and VI neuropathies, as well as Bell's palsy occur more frequently in patients with diabetes. The clinical presentation can be quite dramatic, but the course is usually self-limited, and partial or full recover occurs in a few weeks to months. Carpal tunnel syndrome, caused by radial nerve entrapment in wrist, is also more common in people with diabetes, and tarsal tunnel syndrome may cause foot paresthesias.

Microalbuminuria and Nephropathy[72,74]

Diabetes mellitus, particularly type 2 DM, is the biggest contributor statistically to the development of end-stage renal disease in the United States.[1] The ADA recommends a screening urinary analysis for albumin at the time of diagnosis in persons with type 2 DM. In type 1 DM, microalbuminuria rarely occurs before puberty. Screening individuals with type 1 DM should begin with puberty and after 5 years' disease duration. There are three methods for assessing microalbuminuria: (1) measurement of the urine albumin:creatinine ratio can be determined in a random spot collection, preferably the first morning void. (2) 24-hour timed collection—more cumbersome but more accurate; and (3) timed (eg, 4- or 10-hour overnight) collection. Microalbuminuria on a spot urine specimen is defined as a ratio of 30 to 300 mg/g (3.4-34 mg/mmol) albumin:creatinine. On timed collections, microalbuminuria is defined as 30 to 300 mg/24 h or an albumin excretion rate of 20 to 200 mcg/min. Due to day-to-day variability, microalbuminuria should be confirmed on at least two of three samples over 3 to 6 months unless the results are unequivocally positive. Additionally, when assessing urine protein or albumin, conditions that may cause transient elevations in urinary albumin excretion should be excluded. These conditions include intense exercise, recent urinary tract infections, hypertension, short-term hyperglycemia, heart failure, and acute febrile illness.

In type 2 DM, the presence of microalbuminuria is a strong risk factor for macrovascular disease and is frequently present at the time of diagnosis. Microalbuminuria is a weaker predictor for future end-stage kidney disease in type 2 versus type 1 DM. Glucose and blood pressure control are important for preventing and retarding the progression of nephropathy. ACE inhibitors and ARBs, considered first-line treatment modalities, have shown efficacy in preventing the clinical progression of renal disease in patients with diabetes. Using a combination of agents to block the renin-angiotensin aldosterone system—for example using an ACE inhibitor with an ARB, aldosterone receptor blockers, or direct renin inhibitors—has not been shown to improve outcomes and may increase adverse effects. Diuretics frequently are necessary due to the volume-expanded state of the patient and are recommended second-line therapy. The ADA currently recommends less than 140/90 mm Hg in patients with nephropathy but lower blood pressures values, if they can be safely obtained, may lower the risk further. Three or more antihypertensives are often needed to reach goal blood pressures.

Peripheral Arterial Disease and Foot Ulcers[72]

Claudication and nonhealing foot ulcers are common in patients with type 2 DM. Smoking cessation, correction of lipid abnormalities, good glycemic control, and antiplatelet therapy are important strategies in treating peripheral arterial disease. Cilostazol may be useful for reducing symptoms in select patients. Revascularization is successful in selected patients; however, small vessel disease that cannot be bypassed is common in diabetes. Local debridement and appropriate footwear are vitally important in the early treatment of foot lesions. In more advanced lesions, multiple treatments including grafts, topical wound healing, and hyperbaric treatments may be necessary. Foot examinations each visit and a yearly Semmes-Weinstein 10 gram-force monofilament test to assess for loss of protective sensation can be used to identify high-risk patients that need further podiatric evaluation.

Coronary Heart Disease[74,75]

The risk for coronary heart disease (CHD) is 2 to 4 times greater in diabetic patients than in nondiabetic individuals. CHD is the major source of mortality in patients with DM. Addressing multiple CV risk factor—lipids, hypertension, smoking cessation, and antiplatelet therapy—will reduce macrovascular events. The ADA recommends aspirin therapy in all patients who have established CV disease. If the patient is allergic to aspirin, clopidogrel may be used. The ADA currently recommends antiplatelet therapy for primary prevention of a CV event if the patient's 10-year risk of CVD is at least 10%, or in women and men at least 50 years old with an additional risk factor. β-Blocker therapy supplies an even greater protection from recurrent CHD events in patients with diabetes than in nondiabetic subjects. Therefore, β-blockers should not be avoided in patients with diabetes. Masking of hypoglycemic symptoms can be a problem in some patients with type 1 DM but this risk can be managed with proper glycemic control interventions (see also the Chapter on Ischemic Heart Disease).

The Collaborative Atorvastatin Diabetes Study (CARDS) randomized patients with diabetes and no documented CVD to atorvastatin 10 mg daily (n = 1,428) or placebo (n = 1,410). The trial was stopped early when the primary efficacy endpoint of major cardiovascular events was reduced by 37% (P = 0.001). All-cause death was reduced 27% (P = 0.059). The Heart Protection Study randomized 5,963 patients age more than 40 years with diabetes and total cholesterol more than 135 mg/dL (3.49 mmol/L). A significant 22% reduction (95% CI, 13-30) in the event rate for major cardiovascular events was seen with simvastatin 40 mg/day. This was evident even at lower LDL-C levels (less than 116 mg/dL [less than 3.00 mmol/L]), and suggests that approximately 30% to 40% reduction in LDL-C levels regardless of starting LDL-C levels may be appropriate. The ADA recommends statin therapy, regardless of baseline lipid or LDL-C levels in patients with overt CVD or without documented CVD who are over the age of 40 and have CVD risk factors besides diabetes.

Low-density lipoprotein cholesterol has been the primary target of therapy for years. However, more recently the AHA/ACC 2013 guidelines[76] recommend that rather than aiming for specific LDL-C targets, decision for treatment should be based on CV risk. In people with type 1 or type 2 diabetes who are ages 40-75 years, the decision whether to use moderate or high intensity statin should be based on risk. Those who have established CVD and/or an estimated 10-year risk of more than 7.5% (more than 0.075; more than 58 mmol/mol Hb) should be treated with high intensity statin; all others may be treated with moderate intensity statin (**Table 74-12**). High intensity statins include atorvastatin 40 to 80 mg day or rosuvastatin

TABLE 74-12 Recommendations for Statin Treatment in People with Diabetes

Age (Years)	Risk Factors	Recommended Statin Dose*	Monitoring with Lipid Panel
<40	None CVD risk factor(s)** Overt CVD ***	None Moderate to High High	Annually as needed to monitor for adherence
40-75	None CVD risk factor(s) ** Overt CVD***	Moderate High High	As needed to monitor for adherence
>75	None CVD risk factor(s)** Overt CVD***	Moderate Moderate to High High	As needed to monitor for adherence

*In addition to lifestyle therapy.

**CVD risk factors include LDL cholesterol ≥100 mg/dL (≥2.59 mmol/L), high blood pressure, smoking, and overweight and obesity.

***Overt CVD includes those with previous cardiovascular events or acute coronary syndromes.

American Diabetes Association 2015 Clinical Practice Recommendations. Cardiovascular disease and risk management. Diabetes Care 2015;38(Suppl. 1):S49 -S57. *Material from this publication has been used with the permission of American Diabetes Association.*

20 to 40 mg day. Moderate intensity statin therapy includes atorvastatin 10 to 20 mg; rosuvastatin 5 to 10 mg; simvastatin 20 to 40 mg; pravastatin 40 to 80 mg; lovastatin 40 mg; and fluvastatin XL 80 mg. Caution is advised when beginning statins in women of child bearing age because statins may cause birth defects.

After a statin is initiated for CV risk reduction, extremely elevated triglycerides may require additional pharmacological therapy. Improved glycemic control, weight loss, and exercise will also have a positive impact on serum triglycerides. Patients with marked hypertriglyceridemia (≥ 500 mg/dL [5.65 mmol/L]) are at risk for pancreatitis. Efforts to reduce triglycerides with improved glycemic control, elimination of other secondary causes (including medications), and the use of fibrates, omega-3 fatty acid, or niacin can be used.

The routine use of fibrates in patients with diabetes is controversial. The Fenofibrate Intervention and Event Lowering in Diabetes (FIELD) was conducted in patients with type 2 DM and failed to show a CV benefit from fenofibrate 200 mg daily when compared to placebo. In a subgroup analysis, subjects without CVD at baseline appeared to have a significant reduction in CVD events. The lipid arm of the ACCORD also randomized patient to fenofibrate or placebo. Fenofibrate did not significantly lower cardiovascular events. Niacin in combination with a statin failed to improved CVD outcomes in patients with diabetes as well.

Hypertension[74]

The role of hypertension in increasing microvascular and macrovascular risk in patients with DM has been confirmed in the UKPDS. The ADA has loosened their goals for blood pressure (less than 140/80 mm Hg) in patients with DM based the results of the ACCORD study. The ACCORD blood pressure arm studied type 2 DM patients, with a goal of achieving a systolic blood pressure of either less than 120 mm Hg (achieved 119 mm Hg) or less than 140 mm Hg (133 mm Hg achieved). The lower pressure group did not have lower CVD or renal outcomes, but did have a lower risk of stroke. A goal of less than 130 mm Hg can still be considered in younger patients, patients at high risk of a stroke or if renal disease is present. ACE inhibitors and ARBs are generally recommended for initial therapy, as they have shown to be cardioprotective, and likely have special renal protective effects. Many patients require multiple agents, on average three, to attain the BP goals. Diuretics and calcium channel blockers frequently are useful as second and third agents. African Americans receive renoprotection from ACE inhibitors or ARBs, but they lower blood pressure less than other agents in this population. For this reason, combination therapy with a diuretic or calcium channel blocker be considered as first-line therapy in African Americans. After initial therapy, which agent to add next remains controversial.

SUMMARY

A comprehensive care plan for the patient with DM will not only include strategies to achieve optimal glycemic control aimed at appropriate glycemic goals but will also screen, prevent, and manage microvascular and macrovascular complications. Current Health Plan Employer Data and Information Set (HEDIS), performance measures published by the National Committee for Quality Assurance (NCQA) recognize that quality care includes targets for glycemia, lipids, and hypertension. Publicly reported quality measures indicate that we are moving closer to these targets. Glycemic control is paramount in managing type 1 or type 2 DM. It requires frequent assessment and adjustments in diet, exercise, and pharmacologic therapies. The HbA_{1c} should be measured twice a year in patients meeting treatment goals on a stable therapeutic regimen.[14] Quarterly assessments are recommended for those whose therapy has changed or who are not meeting glycemic goals. A fasting lipid profile should be obtained as part of an initial assessment and to determine if statin therapy has reduced LDL cholesterol as expected. Documenting foot examinations (each visit), urine albumin (annually), dilated eye examinations (yearly or more frequently) are also important. People with diabetes should receive the influenza vaccine annually and the pneumococcal vaccines and the hepatitis B vaccine series. Screening and mitigating cardiovascular risks—including smoking cessation and antiplatelet therapy—are components of preventive medicine strategies. Utilizing an integrated electronic health record, standardized progress notes, and flow sheets can assist the clinician determine whether the patient has met these standards of care. As with many chronic diseases, adherence to dietary recommendation, physical activity, and medications is a challenge for most patients. Frequent follow-up, patient education, and simplification of medication regimens using combination products are helpful (Table 74-13). Many patients do not take medications due to side effects and perceived risks. Frequent monitoring and patient engagement in the decision-making process is needed (Table 74-14).

TABLE 74-13 Available Combination Antihyperglycemic Products[a]

Medication	Combined with:	Trade Name
Metformin and/or metformin extended release	Pioglitazone	Actoplus Met
	Rosiglitazone	Avandamet
	Sitagliptin	Janumet
	Saxagliptin	Kombiglyze XR
	Linagliptin	Jentadueto
	Alogliptin	Kazano
	Glyburide	Glucovance
	Glipizide	Metaglip
	Repaglinide	Prandimet
	Canagliflozin	Invokamet
	Dapagliflozin	Xigduo XR
	Empagliflozin	Synjardy
Linagliptin	Empagliflozin	Glyxambi
Glimepiride	Pioglitazone	Duetact
	Rosiglitazone	Avandaryl
Pioglitazone	Alogliptin	Oseni

[a]at time chapter written.

TABLE 74-14 Drug Monitoring for Diabetes Mellitus Medications[a]

Medication Class	Adverse Drug Reaction	Monitoring Parameters	Comments
Alpha-glucosidase inhibitors	Gastrointestinal (GI) upset	Gas, bloating, loose stools	Titrate, take in less carbohydrate
Bile Acid Sequestrants	Constipation	Bowel movement frequency	Drink H_2O, Don't use if history of bowel obstruction
	Raises triglycerides	Triglycerides	Not recommended TG >500 mg/dL (>5.65 mmol/L)
Biguanides	Gastrointestinal distress	Reflux, nausea, vomiting, stomach upset, loose stools	Take with food and titrate dose, split doses, consider extended release
	Lactic Acidosis	High anion gap on electrolyte panel, hypoxic states, renal function, impaired liver function	Lactate levels not measured, but can be if suspected toxicity
DPP-4 inhibitors	Hypersensitivity/ Angioedema and exfoliating dermatologic skin reactions	Skin rash, signs/symptoms of angioedema	Risk factors, such as history of angioedema, possibly ACE inhibitor use, and past history of severe dermal drug reactions should be explored
	Pancreatitis	Amylase, Lipase, abdominal pain with nausea/ vomiting	Discontinue, look for underlying causes
SGLT2 inhibitors	GU infections, Dehydration/Orthostatic UTI	Signs/symptoms Blood pressure, syncopal symptoms, eGFR Signs/symptoms	Monitor eGFR and blood pressure, adjust diuretics SE may be more pronounced over first 2 weeks
Dopamine agonists	Hypotension	Syncopal symptoms	Usually worse for first days of dosage change. Decrease/stop antihypertensives
	Worsening psychiatric issues	Signs/symptoms of underlying mental illness	Avoid use with antipsychotics
	CNS effects	Mental alertness/asthenia/fatigue/headache	Titrate slowly
	Gastrointestial side effects	Nausea	Titrate slowly
Thiazolidinediones	Heart failure/pulmonary edema	Signs/symptoms of heart failure, increased BNP, weight	Discontinue
	Peripheral edema	Peripheral edema measures	Limit dose, consider diuretic (see text), or discontinue
	Weight gain	Weight	Consider if weight is fluid or likely caloric intake
	Peripheral fractures	None except fracture	Avoid use in osteoporosis and osteopenia
Sulfonylureas	Hypoglycemia	Self-monitored blood glucose	Consider dosing
Meglitinides	Hypoglycemia	Self-monitored blood glucose	Adjustment
GLP-1 receptor agonists	Gastrointestinal	Nausea/vomiting	Titrate slowly, avoid in gastroparesis
	Pancreatitis	Amylase, Lipase, abdominal pain with nausea/ vomiting	Discontinue, look for underlying causes
	C-cell tumors of thyroid	None recommended, calcitonin	Do not use in at risk populations (MEN2 or MTC)
Amylinomimetic	Gastrointestinal upset	Nausea/vomiting	Titrate slowly, avoid in gastroparesis
Insulin	Hypoglycemia	Self-monitored blood glucose	

ABBREVIATIONS

AACE	American Association of Clinical Endocrinologists
AADE	American Association of Diabetes Educators
ACCORD	Action to Control Cardiovascular Risk in Diabetes
ACE	angiotensin-converting enzyme
ACE	American College of Endocrinologists
ADA	American Diabetes Association
ADVANCE	Action in Diabetes and Vascular Disease: Preterax and Diamicron MR Controlled Evaluation
AHEAD	Action for Health in Diabetes
ALT	alanine aminotransferase
ARB	angiotensin-receptor blockers
BG	blood glucose
BMI	body mass index
BNP	brain natriuretic peptide
CARDS	Collaborative Atorvastatin Diabetes Study
CDE	certified diabetes educator
CGM	continuous glucose monitoring
CHD	coronary heart disease
CVD	cardiovascular disease
CSII	continuous subcutaneous insulin infusion
CYP450	cytochrome P450
DCCT	Diabetes Control and Complications Trial
DKA	diabetic ketoacidosis
DM	diabetes mellitus
DPP-4	dipeptidyl peptidase-4
DPP	Diabetes Prevention Program
eAG	estimated average glucose
EDIC	Epidemiology of Diabetes Interventions and Complications
eGFR	estimated glomerular filtration rate
FDA	Food and Drug Administration
FFA	free fatty acid
FIELD	Fenofibrate Intervention and Event Lowering in Diabetes
GCT	glucose challenge test
GDM	gestational diabetes mellitus
GIP	glucose-dependent insulinotropic polypeptide
GLP-1	glucagon-like peptide-1
GLP1-RA	GLP-1 receptor agonist
GU	genitourinary

Hb	hemoglobin
HbA_{1c}	hemoglobin A_{1c}
HDL-C	high-density lipoprotein cholesterol
HHS	hyperosmolar hyperglycemic state
HLA	human leukocyte antigen
ICA	islet cell antibody
IFCC	International Federation of Clinical Chemistry
IFG	impaired fasting glucose
IGT	impaired glucose tolerance
INR	international normalized ratio
IV	intravenous
LADA	latent autoimmune diabetes in adults
LDL-C	low-density lipoprotein cholesterol
MAP	mitogen activated protein
MDI	multiple daily injections
MEN2	multiple endocrine neoplasia type 2
MODY	maturity onset diabetes of youth
NGSP	National Glycohemoglobin Standardization Program
NHANES III	The Third National Health and Nutrition Evaluation Survey
NPH	neutral protamine Hagedorn
OGTT	oral glucose tolerance test
PAI-1	activator-1 plasminogen-inhibitor
PDR	proliferative diabetic retinopathy
POC	Point of care
PPAR-γ	peroxisome proliferator activator receptor-γ
SGLT	sodium glucose cotransporter
SUR	sulfonylurea receptor
SMBG	self-monitoring of blood glucose
TZD	thiazolidinedione
UGE	urinary glucose excretion
UKPDS	United Kingdom Prospective Diabetes Study
VADT	Veterans Affairs Diabetes Trial
VAT	visceral adipose tissue
VEGF	vascular endothelial growth factor

REFERENCES

1. Centers for Disease Control and Prevention. National diabetes statistics report: Estimates of diabetes and its burden in the United States, 2014. Atlanta, GA: U.S. Department of Health and Human Services, Centers for Disease Control and Prevention; 2014.
2. American Diabetes Association. Clinical Practice Recommendations. Classification and diagnosis of diabetes mellitus. *Diabetes Care* 2016;39(Suppl 1):S13-S22.
3. Michels A, Gottlieb P, Pathogenesis of type 1A diabetes. In: De Groot LJ, Beck-Peccoz P, Chrousos G, Dungan K, Grossman A, Hershman JM, Koch C, McLachlan R, New M, Rebar R, Singer F, Vinik A, Weickert MO, eds. *Endotext [Internet]*. South Dartmouth (MA): MDText.com, Inc.; 2000-2015 (12/17/2015).
4. Steck AK, Rewers MJ. Epidemiology and risk factors for type 1 diabetes. In: DeFronzo RA, Ferrannini E, eds. *International Textbook of Diabetes*. 4th ed. Chichester West Sussex, UK: John Wiley & Sons; 2015:17-28.
5. American Diabetes Association. Prevention or delay of type 2 diabetes mellitus. *Diabetes Care* 2016;39(Suppl 1):S36-S38.
6. DeFronzo RA. Pathogenesis of type 2 diabetes mellitus: Metabolic and molecular implications for identifying diabetes genes. *Diabetes* 1997;5:117-269.
7. DeFronzo RA. Pathogenesis of type 2 diabetes mellitus. *Med Clin N Am* 2004;88:787-835.
8. DeFronzo RA. From the triumvirate to the ominous octet: A new paradigm for the treatment of type 2 diabetes mellitus. *Diabetes* 2009;58:773-795.
9. Atkinson MA, Eisenbarth GS, Michels AW. Type 1 Diabetes. *Lancet* 2014;389:69-82.
10. Zipitis CS, Akobeng AK. Vitamin D supplementation in early childhood and risk of type 1 diabetes: A systematic review and meta-analysis. *Arch Dis Child* 2008;93:512-517.
11. Alberti KGMM, Eckel RH, Grundy SM, et al. Harmonizing the metabolic syndrome: A joint interim statement of the International Diabetes Federation Task Force on Epidemiology and Prevention; National Heart, Lung, and Blood Institute; American Heart Association; World Heart Federation; International Atherosclerosis Society; and International Association for the Study of Obesity. *Circulation* 2009;120:1640-1645.
12. American Diabetes Association. Standards of Care. Children and Adolescents in: Clinical Practice Recommendations. *Diabetes Care* 2016;39(Suppl 1):S86-S93.
13. International association of diabetes and pregnancy study groups recommendations on the diagnosis and classification of hyperglycemia in pregnancy. *Diabetes Care* 2010;33:676-682.
14. American Diabetes Association. Clinical Practice Recommendations. Foundations of care and comprehensive medical evaluation. *Diabetes Care* 2016;39(Suppl 1):S23-S35.
15. Gaede P, Vedel P, Larsen N, et al. Multifactorial intervention and cardiovascular disease in patients with type 2 diabetes. *N Engl J Med* 2008;358:580-591.
16. Thent ZC, Das S, Henry LJ. Role of exercise in the management of diabetes mellitus: The global scenario. *PLoS ONE* 2013;8:e80436. doi:10.1371/journal.pone.0080436.
17. Haas L, Maryniuk M, Beck J, et al. National standards diabetes self-management education. *Diabetes Care* 2014;37(Suppl 1):S144-S153.
18. Hirsch IB, Skylar JS. The management of type 1 diabetes. In: De Groot LJ, Beck-Peccoz P, Chrousos G, Dungan K, Grossman A, Hershman JM, Koch C, McLachlan R, New M, Rebar R, Singer F, Vinik A, Weickert MO, eds. *Endotext [Internet]*. South Dartmouth (MA): MDText.com, Inc.; 2000-2015.
19. Juang PS, Henry RR. Treatment of type 2 diabetes. In: De Groot LJ, Beck-Peccoz P, Chrousos G, Dungan K, Grossman A, Hershman JM, Koch C, McLachlan R, New M, Rebar R, Singer F, Vinik A, Weickert MO, eds. *Endotext [Internet]*. South Dartmouth (MA): MDText.com, Inc.; 2000-2015.
20. The Look AHEAD research group. Cardiovascular effects of intensive lifestyle intervention in type 2 diabetes. *N Eng J Med* 2013;369:145-154.
21. Millstein R, Becerra NM, Shubrook JH. Insulin pumps: Beyond basal-bolus. *Cleve Clin J Med* 2015;82:835-842.
22. American Diabetes Association. Clinical Practice Recommendations. Glycemic targets. *Diabetes Care* 2016;39(Suppl 1):S39-S46.
23. Inzucchi SE, Bergenstal RM, Buse JB, et al. Management of hyperglycemia in type 2 diabetes: A patient-centered approach: Update to position statement of the American Diabetes Association (ADA) and the European Association for the Study of Diabetes (EASD). *Diabetes Care* 2015;38:140-149.
24. DeFronzo RA, Eldor R, Abdul-Ghani M. Pathophysiologic approach to therapy in patients with newly diagnosed type 2 diabetes. *Diabetes Care* 2013;36(Suppl 2):S127-S138.
25. Abdul-Ghani MA, Puckett C, Triplitt C, et al. Initial combination therapy with metformin, pioglitazone, and exenatide is more effective than sequential add-on therapy in subjects with new-onset diabetes. Results from the efficacy and durability of initial combination therapy for type 2 diabetes (EDICT): A randomized trial. *Diabetes Obes Metab* 2015;17:268-275.
26. Holman RR, Farmer AJ, Davies MJ, et al. Three-year efficacy of complex insulin regimens in type 2 diabetes. *N Engl J Med* 2009;361: 1736-1747.
27. Davidson MB, Insulin therapy: A personal approach. *Clin Diabetes* 2015;33:123-135.
28. Diabetes Control and Complications Trial Research Group. The effect of intensive treatment of diabetes on the development and progression of long-term complications in insulin-dependent diabetes mellitus. *N Engl J Med* 1993;329:977-986.
29. UK Prospective Diabetes Study Group. Intensive blood-glucose control with sulphonylureas or insulin compared with conventional treatment and risk of complications in patients with type 2 diabetes (UKPDS 33). *Lancet* 1998;352:837-853.
30. UK Prospective Diabetes Study (UKPDS) Group. Effect of intensive blood-glucose control with metformin on complications in overweight patients with type 2 diabetes (UKPDS 34). *Lancet* 1998;352:854-865.
31. Lachin JM, White NH, Hainsworth DP, et al. Effect of intensive diabetes therapy on the progression of diabetic retinopathy in patients with type 1 diabetes: 18 years of follow-up in the DCCT/EDIC. *Diabetes* 2015;64:631-642.
32. DCCT/EDIC Study Research Group. Intensive diabetes treatment and cardiovascular disease in patients with type 1 diabetes. *N Engl J Med* 2005;353:2643-2653.

33. Holman RR, Paul SK, Bethel MA, Mathews DR, Neil HAW. 10-year follow-up of intensive glucose control in type 2 diabetes. *N Engl J Med* 2008;359:1577-1589.
34. The Action to Control Cardiovascular Risk in Diabetes Study Group. Effects of intensive glucose lowering in type 2 diabetes. *N Engl J Med* 2008;358:2545-2559.
35. The ADVANCE Collaborative Group. Intensive blood glucose control and vascular outcomes in patients with type 2 diabetes. *N Engl J Med* 2008;358:2560-2572.
36. Duckworth W, Abraira C, Mortiz T, et al. Glucose control and vascular complications in veterans with type 2 diabetes. *N Engl J Med* 2009;360:1-11.
37. Onge ES, Miller SA, Motycha C, DeBerry A. A review of the treatment of type 2 diabetes in children. *J Pediatr Pharmacol Ther* 2015;20:4-16.
38. American Diabetes Association. Clinical Practice Recommendations. Older Adults. *Diabetes Care* 2016;39(Suppl 1):S81-S85.
39. American Diabetes Association. Clinical Practice Recommendations. Management of diabetes in pregnancy. *Diabetes Care* 2016;39(Suppl 1): S94-S98.
40. Kitabchi AE, Umpierrez GE, Miles JM, Fisher JN. Hyperglycemic crises in adult patients with diabetes. A consensus statement from the American Diabetes Association. *Diabetes Care* 2009;32:1335-1343.
41. Umpierrez GE, Hellman R, Korytkowski MT, et al. Management of hyperglycemia in hospitalized patients win non-critical care setting: An endocrine society clinical practice guideline. *J Clin Endocrinol Metab* 2012;97:16-38.
42. Moghissi ES, Korykowski MT, DiNardo M, et al. American Association of Clinical Endocrinologists and American Diabetes Association consensus statement on inpatient glycemic control. *Diabetes Care* 2009;32:1119-1131.
43. The NICE-SUGAR Study Investigators. Intensive versus conventional glycemic control in critically ill patients. *N Engl J Med* 2009;360: 1283-1297.
44. American Diabetes Association. Clinical Practice Recommendations. Diabetes care in the hospital. *Diabetes Care* 2016;39(Suppl 1):S99-S104.
45. Kulra S, Agrawai N. Diabetes and HIV. Current understand and future perspectives. *Curr Diabet Rep* 2013;13:419-427.
46. Diabetes Prevention Program Research Group. Long-term effects of lifestyle intervention or metformin on diabetes development and microvascular complications over 15-year follow-up: The diabetes prevention program outcomes study. *Lancet Diabetes Endocrinol* 2015;3:866-875.
47. The DREAM Trial Investigators. The effect of rosiglitazone on the frequency of diabetes in patients with impaired glucose tolerance or impaired fasting glucose. A randomised controlled trial. *Lancet* 2006;368:1096-1105.
48. DeFronzo R, Tripathy D, Schwenke D. et al. Pioglitazone for diabetes prevention in impaired glucose tolerance. *N Engl J Med* 2011;364: 1104-1115.
49. Donner T. Insulin-pharmacology, therapeutics regimens and principles of intensive therapy In: De Groot LJ, Beck-Peccoz P, Chrousos G, Dungan K, Grossman A, Hershman JM, Koch C, McLachlan R, New M, Rebar R, Singer F, Vinik A, Weickert MO, eds. *Endotext [Internet]*. South Dartmouth (MA): MDText.com, Inc.; 2000-2015 (03/05/2016).
50. The ORIGIN trial investigators. Basal insulin and cardiovascular and other outcomes in dysglycemia. *N Engl J Med* 2012;367:319-328.
51. Budnitz DS, Lovegrove MC, Shehab N, Richards CL. Emergency hospitalizations for adverse drug events in older Americans. *N Engl J Med* 2011;365:2002-2012.
52. Fagot J-P, Blotiere P-V, Ricordeau P, et al. Does insulin glargine increase the risk of cancer compared with other basal insulins? *Diabetes Care* 2013;36:294-301.
53. Evans JL, Balkan BB, Rushakoff RJ. Oral and injectable (non-insulin) pharmacological agents for type 2 diabetes. In: De Groot LJ, Beck-Peccoz P, Chrousos G, Dungan K, Grossman A, Hershman JM, Koch C, McLachlan R, New M, Rebar R, Singer F, Vinik A, Weickert MO, eds. *Endotext [Internet]*. South Dartmouth (MA): MDText.com, Inc.; 2000-2015 (03/05/2016).
54. Garber AJ, Abrahamson MJ, Barzilay JI, et al. Consensus statement by the American Association of Clinical Endocrinologists and American College of endocrinology on the comprehensive type 2 diabetes management algorithm-2015 executive summary. *Endo Prac* 2015;21:1403-14214.
55. Nauck M. Incretin therapies: Highlighting common features and differences in the modes of action of glucagon-like peptide-1 receptor agonists and dipeptidyl peptidase-4 inhibitors. *Diabetes Obes Metab* 2016;18:203-216.
56. Triplitt C, Solis-Herrera C. GLP-1 receptor agonists: Practical considerations for clinical practice. *Diabetes Educ* 2015;41(Suppl 1): 32S-46S.
57. Blevins T, Pullman J, Malloy J, et al. DURATION-5. Exenatide once weekly resulted in greater improvements in glycemic control compared to exenatide twice daily in patients with type 2 diabetes. *J Clin Endocrinol Metab* 2011;96:1301-1310.
58. Trujillo JM, Nuffer W, Ellis SL. GLP-1 receptor agonists: A review of head-to-head clinical studies. *Ther Adv Endocrinol Metab* 2015;6:19-28.
59. Pfeffer MA, Blaggett B, Diaz R, et al. Lixisenatide in patients with type 2 diabetes and acute coronary syndrome. *N Engl J Med* 2015;373:2247-2257.
60. Kim YG, Hahn S, Oh TJ, et al. Differences in glucose lowering efficacy of dipeptidyl peptidase-4 inhibitors between Asians and non-Asians. A systematic review and meta-analysis. *Diabetologia* 2013;56:696-708.
61. Anz D, Kruger S, Haubner S, Rapp M, Bourquin C, Endres S. The dipeptidyl peptidase-IV inhibitors sitagliptin, vildagliptin and saxagliptin do not impair innate and adaptive immune responses. *Diabetes Obes Metab* 2014;16:569-572.
62. White WB, Cannon CP, Heller SR. et al. Alogliptin after acute coronary syndrome in patients with type 2 diabetes. *N Engl J Med* 2013;369:1327-1335.
63. Scirica BM, Bhatt DL, Braunwald E, et al. Saxagliptin and cardiovascular outcomes in patients with type 2 diabetes mellitus. *N Engl J Med* 2013;369:1317-1326.
64. Green JB, Bethel MA, Armstrong PW, et al. Effect of sitagliptin on cardiovascular outcomes in type 2 diabetes. *N Engl J Med* 2015;373:232-242.
65. Savarese G, Perrone-Filardi P, D'Amore C, et al. Cardiovascular effects of dipeptidyl peptidase-4 inhibitors in diabetic patients: A meta-analysis. *Int J Cardiol* 2015;181:239-244.
66. Abdul-Ghani MA, Norton L, Defronzo RA. Role of sodium glucosecotransporter 2 (SGLT 2) inhibitors in the treatment of type 2 diabetes. *Endocr Rev* 2011;32:515-531.
67. Zinman B, Wanner C, Lachin JM, et al. Empagliflozin, cardiovascular outcomes, and mortality in type 2 diabetes. *N Eng J Med* 2015;373: 2117-2128.
68. Dormandy JA, Charbonnel B, Eckland DJA, et al. Secondary prevention of vascular events in patients with type 2 diabetes in the PROactive study prospective pioglitazone clinical trial in macrovascular events: A randomized controlled trial. *Lancet* 2005;366:1279-1289.
69. Mahaffey KW, Hafley G, Dickerson S, et al. Results of a reevaluation of cardiovascular outcomes in the RECORD trial. *Am Heart J* 2013;166:240-249.
70. Home PD, Pocock SJ, Beck-Nielsen H, et al. Rosiglitazone evaluated for cardiovascular outcomes in oral agent combination therapy for type 2 diabetes (RECORD): A multicentre, randomised, open-label trial. *Lancet* 2009;373:2125-2135.
71. Chiasson JL. Acarbose for the prevention of diabetes, hypertension, and cardiovascular disease in subjects with impaired glucose tolerance: The study to prevent non-insulin-dependent diabetes mellitus (STOP-NIDDM) trial. *Endocr Pract* 2006;12(Suppl 10):25-30.
72. American Diabetes Association. Clinical Practice Recommendations. Microvascular complications and foot care. *Diabetes Care* 2016;39(Suppl 1):S72-S80.
73. Boulton AJ, Malik RA, Arezzo JC, Sosenko JM. Diabetic somatic neuropathies. *Diabetes Care* 2004;27:1458-1486.
74. American Diabetes Association. Clinical Practice Recommendations. Cardiovascular disease and risk management. *Diabetes Care* 2016;39(Suppl 1):S60-S71.
75. Feingold KR, Grunfeld C. Diabetes and Dyslipidemia. In: De Groot LJ, Beck-Peccoz P, Chrousos G, Dungan K, Grossman A, Hershman JM, Koch C, McLachlan R, New M, Rebar R, Singer F, Vinik A, Weickert MO, eds. *Endotext [Internet]*. South Dartmouth (MA): MDText.com, Inc.; 2000-2015 (Accessed 12/17/2015).
76. Stone NJ, Robinson JG, Lichtenstein AH, et al. 2013 ACC/AHA guideline on the treatment of blood cholesterol to reduce atherosclerotic cardiovascular risk in adults: A report of the American College of Cardiology/American Heart Association task force on practice guidelines. *Circulation* 2014;129(25 Suppl 2):S1-S45.
77. Gore MO, McGuire DK. Cardiovascular disease and type 2 diabetes mellitus: Regulating glucose and regulating drugs. *Current Cardiology Reports* 2009;11:258-263.
78. Saydah S, Tao M, Imperatore G, Gregg E. GHb level and subsequent mortality among adults in the U.S. *Diabetes Care* 2009;32:1440-1446.
79. Rendell M. The path to approval of new drugs for diabetes. *Expert Opin Drug Saf* 2013;12:195-207.

80. Alvarez CA, Lingvay I, Vuylsteke V, et al. Cardiovascular risk in diabetes mellitus: Complication of the disease or of antihyperglycemic medications. *Clin Pharmacol Ther* 2015;98:145-161.
81. Langer O, Conway DL, Berkus MD, Xenakis EM, Gonzales O. A comparison of glyburide and insulin in women with gestational diabetes mellitus. *N Engl J Med* 2000;343:1134-1138.
82. Cheng YW, Chung JH, Block-Kurbisch I, Inturrisi M, Caughey AB. Treatment of gestational diabetes mellitus: Glyburide compared to subcutaneous insulin therapy and associated perinatal outcomes. *J Matern Fetal Neonatal Med* 2012;25(4):379-384.
83. Castillo WC, Boggess K, Sturmer T, Brookhart MA, Benjamen DK, Funk MJ. Association of adverse pregnancy outcomes with glyburide vs insulin in women with gestational diabetes. *JAMA Pediatr* 2015;169:452-458.
84. Rowan JA, Hague WM, Gao W, Battin MR, Moore MP. MiG Trial Investigators. Metformin versus insulin for the treatment of gestational diabetes. *N Engl J Med* 2008;358:2003-2015.
85. Nicholson W, Bolen S, Witkop CT, Neale D, Wilson L, Bass E. Benefits and risks of oral diabetes agents compared with insulin in women with gestational diabetes: A systematic review. *Obstet Gynecol* 2009;113:193-205.
86. Dhulkotia JS, Ola B, Fraser R, Farrell T. Oral hypoglycemic agents vs insulin in management of gestational diabetes: A systematic review and metaanalysis. *Am J Obstet Gynecol* 2010;203:457.
87. Balsells M, Garcia-Patterson A, Sola I, et al. Glibenclamide, metformin and insulin for the treatment of gestational diabetes: A systematic review and meta-analysis. *BMJ* 2015;350:h102. doi:10.1136/bmj.h102.
88. Araki A, Iimuro S, Sakurai T, et al. Japanese elderly diabetes intervention trial study group. Long-term multiple risk factor interventions in Japanese elderly diabetic patients: The Japanese elderly diabetes intervention trial: Study design, baseline characteristics and effects of intervention. *Geriatr Gerontol Int* 2012;12(Suppl 1):7-17.
89. Kirkman MS, Briscoe VJ, Clark N, et al. Diabetes in older adults. *Diabetes Care* 2012;35:2650-2664.
90. Sinclair AJ, Paolisso G, Castro M, et al. European diabetes working party for older people. European diabetes working party for older people 2011 clinical guidelines for type 2 diabetes mellitus. Executive summary. *Diabetes Metab* 2011;37(Suppl 3):S27-S38.

75

Thyroid Disorders

Jacqueline Jonklaas and Michael P. Kane

KEY CONCEPTS

1. Thyrotoxicosis is most commonly caused by Graves' disease, which is an autoimmune disorder in which thyroid-stimulating antibody (TSAb) directed against the thyrotropin receptor elicits the same biologic response as thyroid-stimulating hormone (TSH).
2. Hyperthyroidism may be treated with antithyroid drugs such as methimazole (MMI) or propylthiouracil (PTU), radioactive iodine (RAI: sodium iodide-131 [^{131}I]), or surgical removal of the thyroid gland; selection of the initial treatment approach is based on patient characteristics such as age, concurrent physiology (eg, pregnancy), comorbidities (eg, chronic obstructive lung disease), and convenience.
3. MMI and PTU reduce the synthesis of thyroid hormones and are similar in efficacy, although their dosing ranges differ by 10-fold. Overall, PTU may have a greater incidence of side effects.
4. Response to MMI and PTU is seen in 4 to 6 weeks and therefore β-blocker therapy may be concurrently initiated to reduce adrenergic symptoms. Maximal response is typically seen in 4 to 6 months; treatment usually continues for 1 to 2 years, and therapy is monitored by clinical signs and symptoms and by measuring the serum concentrations of TSH and free thyroxine (T_4).
5. Adjunctive therapy with β-blockers controls the adrenergic symptoms of thyrotoxicosis but does not correct the underlying disorder; iodine may also be used adjunctively in preparation for surgery and acutely for thyroid storm.
6. Many patients choose to have ablative therapy with ^{131}I rather than undergo repeated courses of MMI or PTU treatment; most patients receiving RAI eventually become hypothyroid and require thyroid hormone supplementation.
7. Hypothyroidism is most often due to an autoimmune disorder known as *Hashimoto's thyroiditis*.
8. The drug of choice for replacement therapy in hypothyroidism is levothyroxine.
9. Studies of combination therapy with levothyroxine and liothyronine have not shown reproducible benefits. This approach to treatment of hypothyroidism requires further study.
10. Monitoring of levothyroxine replacement therapy is achieved by observing clinical signs and symptoms and by measuring the serum TSH level. An elevated TSH indicates under-replacement; a suppressed TSH indicates over-replacement.

INTRODUCTION

Thyroid hormones affect the function of virtually every organ system. In a child, thyroid hormone is critical for normal growth and development. In an adult, the major role of thyroid hormone is to maintain metabolic stability. Substantial reservoirs of thyroid hormone in the thyroid gland and blood provide constant thyroid hormone availability. In addition, the hypothalamic–pituitary–thyroid axis is exquisitely sensitive to small changes in circulating thyroid hormone concentrations, and alterations in thyroid hormone secretion maintain peripheral free thyroid hormone levels within a narrow range. Patients seek medical attention for evaluation of symptoms due to abnormal thyroid hormone levels or because of diffuse or nodular thyroid enlargement.

Thyroid Hormone Synthesis

The thyroid hormones thyroxine (T_4) and triiodothyronine (T_3) (Fig. 75-1) are formed within thyroglobulin (TG), a large glycoprotein synthesized in the thyroid cell. Because of the unique tertiary structure of this glycoprotein, iodinated tyrosine residues present in TG are able to bind together to form active thyroid hormones.

Iodide is actively transported through the basolateral membrane via a Na^+/I^- symporter from the extracellular space into the thyroid follicular cell against an electrochemical gradient, driven by the coupled transport of sodium.[1] Structurally related anions such as thiocyanate (SCN^-), perchlorate (ClO_4^-), and pertechnetate (TcO_4^-) are competitive inhibitors of iodine transport.[1] In addition, bromine, fluorine, and, under certain circumstances, lithium block iodide transport into the thyroid (Table 75-1). Inorganic iodide that enters the thyroid follicular cell is ushered through the cell to the apical membrane, where it is transported into the follicular lumen by pendrin, and possibly other transport proteins.[1] Located on the luminal side of the apical membrane, thyroid peroxidase oxidizes iodide and covalently binds the organified iodide to tyrosine residues within TG (Fig. 75-2). It is interesting that although salivary glands and the gastric mucosa are able to actively transport iodide, they are unable to effectively incorporate iodide into proteins given the lack of similar oxidizing machinery.

The iodinated tyrosine residues monoiodotyrosine (MIT) and diiodotyrosine (DIT) combine to form iodothyronines (Fig. 75-3). Thus, two molecules of DIT combine to form T_4, whereas MIT and DIT constitute T_3. In addition to its role in iodine organification, the hemoprotein thyroid peroxidase also catalyzes the formation of iodothyronines (coupling).

Iodine deficiency causes an increase in the MIT:DIT ratio in TG and leads to a relative increase in the production of T_3.[2] Because T_3 is more potent than T_4, the increase in T_3 production in iodine-deficient areas may be beneficial. The thionamide drugs used to treat hyperthyroidism inhibit thyroid peroxidase and thus block thyroid hormone synthesis.

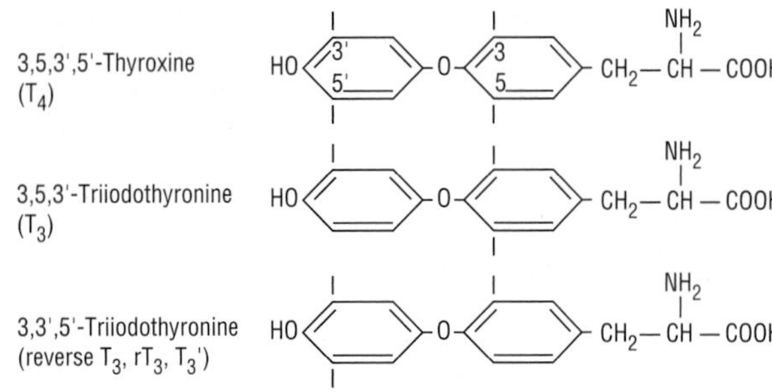

FIGURE 75-1 Structure of thyroid hormones.

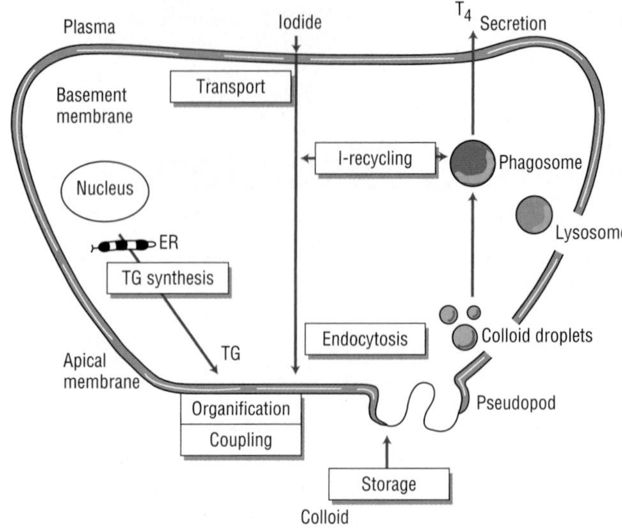

FIGURE 75-2 Thyroid hormone synthesis. Iodide is transported from the plasma, through the cell, to the apical membrane, where it is organified and coupled to the thyroglobulin (TG) synthesized within the thyroid cell. Hormone stored as colloid reenters the cell through endocytosis and moves back toward the basal membrane, where thyroxine (T_4) is secreted.

Thyroglobulin is stored in the follicular lumen and must reenter the cell, where the process of proteolysis liberates thyroid hormone into the bloodstream. Thyroid follicles active in hormone synthesis are identified histologically by columnar epithelial cells lining a follicular lumen, which is depleted of colloid. Inactive follicles are lined by cuboidal epithelial cells and are replete with colloid. Both iodide and lithium block the release of preformed thyroid hormone, through poorly understood mechanisms.

T_4 and T_3 are transported in the bloodstream primarily by three proteins: (1) thyroxine-binding globulin (TBG), (2) transthyretin (TTR), and (3) albumin. It is estimated that 99.96% of circulating T_4 and 99.5% of T_3 are bound to these proteins. However, only the unbound (free) thyroid hormone is able to diffuse into the cell, elicit a biologic effect, and regulate thyroid-stimulating hormone (TSH; also known as *thyrotropin*) secretion from the pituitary. Multiple functions have been ascribed to these transport proteins, including (a) assuring minimal urinary loss of iodide, (b) providing a mechanism for uniform tissue distribution of free hormone, and (c) transport of hormone into the central nervous system.

Whereas T_4 is secreted solely from the thyroid gland, less than 20% of T_3 is produced in the thyroid. The majority of T_3 is formed from the breakdown of T_4 catalyzed by the 5′-monodeiodinase enzymes found in extrathyroidal peripheral tissues. Because the binding affinity of nuclear thyroid hormone receptors (TRs) is 10 to 15 times higher for T_3 than for T_4, the deiodinase enzymes play a pivotal role in determining overall metabolic activity. Three different monodeiodinase enzymes are present in the body. Of the enzymes that catalyze 5′-monodeiodination, type I enzymes are present in peripheral tissues such as the liver and kidney, whereas type II enzymes are found in the CNS, pituitary, and thyroid. Type III enzymes, found in the placenta, skin, and developing brain, inactivate T_4 and T_3 by deiodinating the inner ring at the 5 position. The principal characteristics of these enzymes are listed in Table 75-2. T_4 may also be acted on by the enzyme 5′-monodeiodinase to form reverse T_3, but this accounts for a small component of hormone metabolism. Polymorphisms in the deiodinase genes may prove to be of clinical significance. For example, a polymorphism in the type I deiodinase leading to increased activity seems to be associated with an increased circulating ratio of free T_3 to free T_4.[3] Reverse T_3 has no known biologic activity. T_3 is removed from the body by deiodinative degradation and through the action of sulfotransferase enzyme systems converting to T_3 sulfate and 3,3-diiodothyronine sulfates, thus facilitating enterohepatic clearance. Thyronamines are derivatives of thyroid hormone that are present in low concentrations in human serum.[4] The most studied thyronamine, 3-iodothyronamine, can theoretically be made from T_4 by decarboxylation and deiodination. Administration of pharmacologic amounts of 3-iodothyronamine to animals has profound effects on temperature regulation and cardiac function, and shifts fuel metabolism from carbohydrates to lipids. However, a possible physiologic role for thyronamines has yet to be determined, although altered levels may be associated with some disease states.[4]

TABLE 75-1 Thyroid Hormone Synthesis and Secretion Inhibitors

Mechanism of Action	Substance
Blocks iodide transport into the thyroid	Bromine Fluorine Lithium (?)
Impairs organification and coupling of thyroid hormones	Thionamides Sulfonamide (?) Salicylamide (?) Antipyrine (?)
Inhibits thyroid hormone secretion	Iodide (large doses), lithium

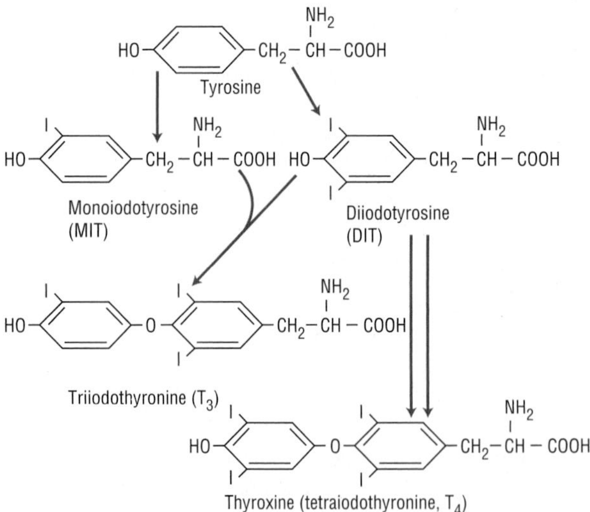

FIGURE 75-3 Scheme of coupling reactions. After tyrosine is iodinated to form monoiodotyrosine (MIT) or diiodotyrosine (DIT) (organification of the iodine), MIT and DIT combine to form triiodothyronine (T_3) or two molecules of DIT combine to form thyroxine T_4.

TABLE 75-2 Properties of Iodothyronine 5′-Deiodinase Isoforms

Property	Type I	Type II	Type III
Susceptibility to propylthiouracil	High	Low	Low
Tissue localization	Thyroid, liver, kidney	Pituitary, thyroid, CNS, brown adipose tissue	Placenta, developing brain, skin
Preferred substrate	rT_3 and T_3	T_4 and rT_3	T_3 and T_4
Physiologic or pathophysiologic role	Clearance of rT_3 and T_3, predominant extrathyroidal source of T_3 in hyperthyroidism	Intracellular T_3 production, especially for brain in hypothyroidism or iodine deficiency, and maintenance of plasma T_3	Clearance of T_3 and T_4
Developmental expression	Expressed latest in development; predominant deiodinase in adult	Expressed second; especially high in brain and brown adipose tissue	Expressed first; high in developing brain; may be important for fetal thyroid hormone metabolism

rT_3, reverse T_3; T_3, triiodothyronine; T_4, thyroxine.

Thyroid Hormone Regulation and Action

The growth and function of the thyroid are stimulated by activation of the thyrotropin receptor by TSH.[5] The receptor belongs to the family of G-protein–coupled receptors. The thyrotropin receptor is coupled to the α subunit of the stimulatory guanine-nucleotide–binding protein ($G_s\alpha$), activating adenylate cyclase and increasing the accumulation of cyclic adenosine monophosphate. Through this mechanism, TSH stimulates the expression of Na^+/I^- symporter, TG, and thyroid peroxidase genes as well as increases apical iodide efflux. Somatic activating mutations in the receptor are commonly seen in autonomously functioning thyroid nodules.[6] Rarely, germline-activating mutations of the TSH receptor have been reported in kindreds with Leclere's syndrome, and thyrotoxicosis can result from germline-activating mutations in G-protein signaling in McCune-Albright syndrome. Conversely, thyrotropin resistance results from point mutations that prevent TSH binding, leading to abnormalities in the thyrotropin receptor–adenylate cyclase system and congenital hypothyroidism.[5] Individuals with this abnormality have high levels of TSH but decreased TG levels and a normal or small gland.

Thyroid hormone nuclear receptors regulate the transcription of target genes in the presence of physiologic concentrations of T_3.[7] Unlike most other nuclear receptors, TRs also actively regulate gene expression in the absence of hormone, typically resulting in an opposite effect. TRs translocate from the cytoplasm to the nucleus, interact in the nucleus with T_3, and target genes and other proteins required for basal and T_3-dependent gene transcription. TRs exist in several isoforms, including TRβ1, TRβ2, and TRα1.[7] Thyroid hormone has different actions in different tissues based on tissue-specific expression of the different TR isoforms. There is interest in developing thyroid hormone analogs that selectively activate specific TR isoforms. Such agents could theoretically have targeted desirable effects such as stimulating energy expenditure without having adverse effects on other tissues.[8]

The production of thyroid hormone is regulated in two main ways. First, thyroid hormone is regulated by TSH secreted by the anterior pituitary. The secretion of TSH is itself under negative feedback control by the circulating level of free thyroid hormone and the positive influence of hypothalamic thyrotropin-releasing hormone (TRH). Second, extrathyroidal deiodination of T_4 to T_3 is regulated by a variety of factors including nutrition, nonthyroidal hormones, ambient temperatures, drugs, and illness.

EPIDEMIOLOGY—THYROTOXICOSIS

Thyrotoxicosis results when tissues are exposed to excessive levels of T_4, T_3, or both.[9] Hyperthyroidism, which is one cause of thyrotoxicosis, refers specifically to overproduction of thyroid hormone by the thyroid gland. In the National Health and Nutrition Examination Survey (NHANES) III, 0.7% of those surveyed who were not taking thyroid medications and had no history of thyroid disease had subclinical hyperthyroidism (TSH less than 0.1 milli-international unit/L, and T_4 normal), and 0.5% had "clinically significant" hyperthyroidism (TSH less than 0.1 milli-international unit/L, and T_4 more than 13.2 mcg/dL).[10] The prevalence of suppressed TSH values peaks in people aged 20 to 39, declines in those 40 to 79, and increases again in those 80 or older. Abnormal TSH levels were more common among women than among men.

ETIOLOGY/PATHOPHYSIOLOGY—THYROTOXICOSIS

If the clinical history and examination do not provide pathognomonic clues to the etiology of the patient's thyrotoxicosis, measurement of the radioactive iodine uptake (RAIU) is critical in the evaluation (Table 75-3). The normal 24-hour RAIU ranges from 10% to 30% with some regional variation that is due to differences in iodine intake. An elevated RAIU indicates endogenous hyperthyroidism, that is, the patient's thyroid gland is actively overproducing T_4, T_3, or both. Conversely, a low RAIU in the absence of iodine excess indicates that high levels of thyroid hormone are not a consequence of thyroid gland hyperfunction but are likely due to thyroiditis or hormone ingestion. The importance of differentiating endogenous hyperthyroidism from other causes of thyrotoxicosis lies in the widely different prognosis and treatment of the diseases in these two categories. Therapy of thyrotoxicosis associated with thyroid hyperfunction is mainly directed at decreasing the rate of thyroid hormone synthesis, secretion, or both. Such measures are ineffective in treating thyrotoxicosis that is not the result of endogenous hyperthyroidism, because hormone synthesis and regulated hormone secretion are already at a minimum.

TABLE 75-3 Differential Diagnosis of Thyrotoxicosis

Increased RAIU[a]	Decreased RAIU
TSH-induced hyperthyroidism	Inflammatory thyroid disease
TSH-secreting tumors	Subacute thyroiditis
Selective pituitary resistance to T_4	Painless thyroiditis
Thyroid stimulators other than TSH	Ectopic thyroid tissue
TSAb (Graves' disease)	Struma ovarii
hCG (trophoblastic diseases)	Metastatic follicular carcinoma
Thyroid autonomy	Exogenous sources of thyroid hormone
Toxic adenoma	Medications containing thyroid hormone or iodine
Multinodular goiter	Food sources containing thyroid gland

hCG, human chorionic gonadotropin; RAIU, radioactive iodine uptake; TSAb, thyroid-stimulating antibody; TSH, thyroid-stimulating hormone.

[a]The RAIU may be decreased if the patient has been recently exposed to excess iodine.

CLINICAL PRESENTATION Thyrotoxicosis

General

- Signs and symptoms of thyrotoxicosis affect multiple organ systems. Patients often have symptoms for an extended time period before the diagnosis of hyperthyroidism is made.

Symptoms

- The typical clinical manifestations of thyrotoxicosis include nervousness, anxiety, palpitations, emotional lability, easy fatigability, menstrual disturbances, and heat intolerance. A cardinal sign is loss of weight concurrent with an increased appetite.
- Elderly patients are more likely to develop atrial fibrillation with thyrotoxicosis than younger patients. The frequency of bowel movements may increase, but frank diarrhea is unusual. For the elderly patient and for the patient with very severe disease, anorexia may be present as well. Palpitations are a prominent and distressing symptom, particularly in the patient with preexisting heart disease. Proximal muscle weakness is common and is noted on climbing stairs or in getting up from a sitting position. Women may note their menses are becoming scanty and irregular. Extremely thyrotoxic patients may have tachycardia, heart failure, psychosis, hyperpyrexia, and coma, a presentation described as thyroid storm.[27]

Signs

- A variety of physical signs may be observed including warm, smooth, moist skin, exophthalmos (in Graves' disease only), pretibial myxedema (in Graves' disease only), and unusually fine hair. Separation of the end of the fingernails from the nail beds (onycholysis) may be noted. Ocular signs that result from thyrotoxicosis include retraction of the eyelids and lagging of the upper lid behind the globe when the patient looks downward (lid lag). Physical signs of a hyperdynamic circulatory state are common and include tachycardia at rest, a widened pulse pressure, and a systolic ejection murmur. Gynecomastia is sometimes noted in men. Neuromuscular examination often reveals a fine tremor of the protruded tongue and outstretched hands. Deep tendon reflexes are generally hyperactive. Thyromegaly is usually present.

Diagnosis

- Low TSH serum concentration. Elevated free and total T_4 and T_3 serum concentrations, particularly in more severe disease.
- Elevated radioactive iodine uptake (RAIU) by the thyroid gland when hormone is being overproduced; suppressed RAIU in thyrotoxicosis due to thyroid inflammation (thyroiditis).

Other Tests

- Thyroid-stimulating antibodies (TSAbs)
- TG
- Thyrotropin receptor antibodies

Causes of Thyrotoxicosis Associated with Elevated RAIU

TSH-Induced Hyperthyroidism

To better understand these syndromes, we must first review TSH biosynthesis and secretion. TSH is synthesized in the anterior pituitary as separate α- and β-subunit precursors. The α subunits from luteinizing hormone (LH), follicle-stimulating hormone (FSH), human chorionic gonadotropin (hCG), and TSH are similar, whereas the β subunits are unique and confer immunologic and biologic specificity. Free β subunits are devoid of receptor binding and biologic activity and require combination with an α subunit to express their activity. Criteria for the diagnosis of TSH-induced hyperthyroidism include (a) evidence of peripheral hypermetabolism, (b) diffuse thyroid gland enlargement, (c) elevated free thyroid hormone levels, and (d) elevated or inappropriately "normal" serum immunoreactive TSH concentrations. Because the pituitary gland is extremely sensitive to even minimal elevations of free T_4, a "normal" or elevated TSH level in any thyrotoxic patient indicates the inappropriate production of TSH.

TSH-Secreting Pituitary Adenomas

TSH-secreting pituitary tumors occur sporadically and release biologically active hormone that is unresponsive to normal feedback control.[11] The mean age at diagnosis is around 40 years, with women being diagnosed more than men (8:7). These tumors may co-secrete prolactin or growth hormone; therefore, the patients may present with amenorrhea/galactorrhea or signs of acromegaly. Most patients present with classic symptoms and signs of thyrotoxicosis. Visual field defects may be present due to impingement of the optic chiasm by the tumor. Tumor growth and worsening visual field defects have been reported following antithyroid therapy because lowering of thyroid hormone levels is associated with loss of feedback inhibition from high thyroid hormone levels.

Diagnosis of a TSH-secreting adenoma should be made by demonstrating lack of TSH response to TRH stimulation, inappropriate TSH levels, elevated α-subunit levels, and radiologic imaging; given the lack of routine availability of TRH, the other three criteria are essential. Note that some small tumors are not identified by MRI. Moreover, 10% of "normal" individuals may have incidental pituitary tumors or other benign focal lesions noted on pituitary imaging.

Transsphenoidal pituitary surgery is the treatment of choice for TSH-secreting adenomas. Pituitary gland irradiation is often given following surgery to prevent tumor recurrence. Dopamine agonists and octreotide have been used to treat tumors, especially those that co-secrete prolactin.

Pituitary Resistance to Thyroid Hormone

Resistance to thyroid hormone is a rare condition that can be due to a number of molecular defects, including mutations in the TRβ gene. Pituitary resistance to thyroid hormone (PRTH) refers to selective resistance of the pituitary thyrotrophs to thyroid hormone. As nonpituitary tissues respond normally to thyroid hormone, patients experience the toxic peripheral effects of thyroid hormone excess. About 90% of patients studied have an appropriate increase in TSH in response to TRH; conversely, the TSH will be suppressed by T_3 administration.

Patients with PRTH require treatment to reduce their elevated thyroid hormone levels. Determining the appropriate serum T_4 level is difficult because TSH cannot be used to evaluate adequacy of therapy. Any reduction in thyroid hormone carries the risk of inducing thyrotroph hyperplasia. Ideally, agents that suppress TSH secretion could be used to treat these individuals. Glucocorticoids, dopaminergic drugs, somatostatin and its analogs, and thyroid hormone analogs with reduced metabolic activity have all been tried, but with relatively little benefit. β-Blocker therapy can also be used. Triiodothyroacetic acid (TRIAC), an agent that is devoid of thyromimetic properties on peripheral tissues, but blocks the secretion of TSH, has been used to treat this condition. However, it is not available in the United States. Given the ability of retinoid X receptor ligands to inhibit TSH production, drugs such as bexarotene may have therapeutic benefit in PRTH.

Graves' Disease

1 Graves' disease is an autoimmune syndrome that usually includes hyperthyroidism, diffuse thyroid enlargement, exophthalmos, and, less commonly, pretibial myxedema and thyroid acropachy (Fig. 75-4).[9,12] Graves' disease is the most common cause of hyperthyroidism, with a prevalence estimated to be 3 per 1,000 population in the United States. Hyperthyroidism results from the action of thyroid-stimulating antibodies (TSAbs), which are directed against the thyrotropin receptor on the surface of the thyroid cell. When these immunoglobulins bind to the receptor, they activate downstream G-protein signaling and adenylate cyclase in the same manner as TSH. Autoantibodies that react with orbital muscle and fibroblast tissue in the skin are responsible for the extrathyroidal manifestations of Graves' disease, and these autoantibodies are encoded by the same germline genes that encode for other autoantibodies for striated muscle and thyroid peroxidase. Clinically, the extrathyroidal disorders may not appear at the same time that hyperthyroidism develops.

There is now compelling evidence that heredity predisposes the susceptible individual to development of clinically overt autoimmune thyroid disease in the setting of appropriate environmental and hormonal triggers. A role for gender in the emergence of Graves' disease is suggested by the fact that hyperthyroidism is approximately eight times more common in women than in men. Other lines of evidence support a role for heredity. First, there is a well-recognized clustering of Graves' disease within some families. Twin studies in Graves' disease have revealed that a monozygotic twin has a 35% likelihood of ultimately developing the disease compared with a 3% likelihood for a dizygotic twin, resulting in estimation that 79% of the predisposition to Graves' disease is genetic.[13] Second, the occurrence of other autoimmune diseases, including Hashimoto's thyroiditis, is also increased in families of patients with Graves' disease. Third, several studies have demonstrated an increased frequency of certain human leukocyte antigens (HLAs) in patients with Graves' disease. Differing HLA associations have been identified in the various ethnic groups studied. In whites, for example, the relative risk of Graves' disease in carriers of the HLA-DR3 haplotype is between 2.5 and 5, whereas lesser associations have been reported for HLA-B8 and the HLA-DQA*0501 allele.[14] Several gene loci have been associated with autoimmune thyroid diseases such as Graves' disease. It is thought that these susceptibility genes interact with environmental triggers to induce thyroid disease through epigenetic effects.[15]

The thyroid gland is diffusely enlarged in the majority of patients with Graves' disease and is commonly 40 to 60 g (two to three times the normal size). The surface of the gland is either smooth or bosselated, and the consistency varies from soft to firm. For patients

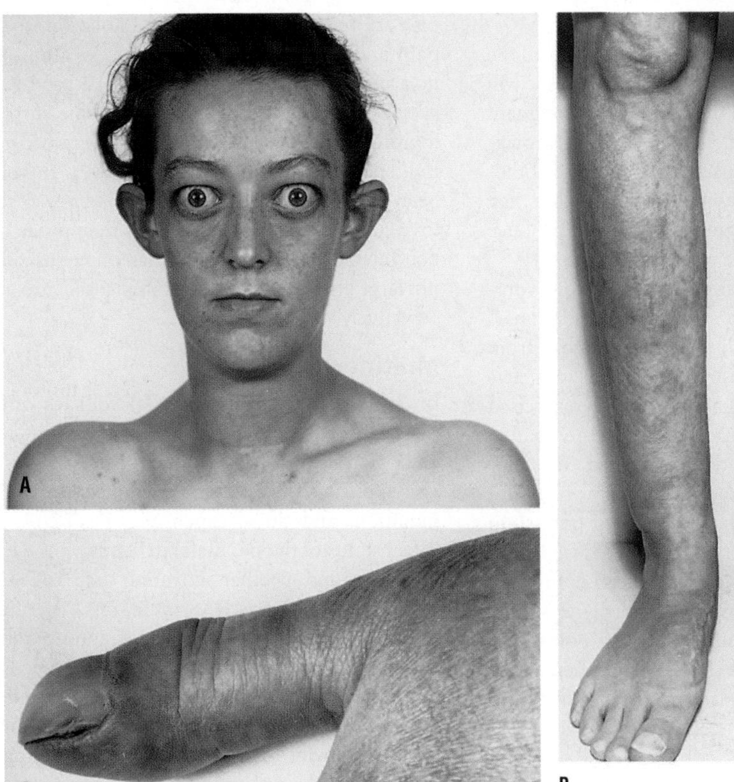

FIGURE 75-4 Features of Graves' disease. (*A*) Facial appearance in Graves' disease; lid retraction, periorbital edema, and proptosis are marked. (*B*) Thyroid dermopathy over the lateral aspects of the shins. (*C*) Thyroid acropachy. *Reproduced with permission from Fauci AS, Kasper DL, Longo DL, et al., eds. Harrison's Principles of Internal Medicine. 16th ed. New York: McGraw-Hill; 2005:2114.*

TABLE 75-4 Thyroid Function Tests in Different Thyroid Conditions

	Total T_4	Free T_4	Total T_3	TSH
Normal	4.5-10.9 mcg/dL	0.8-2.7 ng/dL	60-181 ng/dL	0.5-4.7 milli-international units/L
Hyperthyroid	↑↑	↑↑	↑↑↑	↓↓*
Hypothyroid	↓↓	↓↓	↓	↑↑*
Increased TBG	↑	Normal	↑	Normal

*primary thyroid disease.

with severe disease, a thrill may be felt and a systolic bruit may be heard over the gland, reflecting the increased intraglandular vascularity typical of hyperplasia. Whereas the presence of any of the extrathyroidal manifestations of this syndrome, including exophthalmos, thyroid acropachy, or pretibial myxedema, in a thyrotoxic patient is pathognomonic of Graves' disease, most patients can be diagnosed on the basis of their history and examination of their diffuse goiter (see Fig. 75-4). An important clinical feature of Graves' disease is the occurrence of spontaneous remissions, albeit uncommon. The abnormalities in TSAb production may decrease or disappear over time.

The results of laboratory tests in thyrotoxic Graves' disease include an increase in the overall hormone production rate with a disproportionate increase in T_3 relative to T_4 (Table 75-4). In an occasional patient, the disproportionate overproduction of T_3 is exaggerated, with the result that only the serum T_3 concentration is increased (T_3 toxicosis). The saturation of TBG is increased due to the elevated levels of serum T_4 and T_3. As a result, the concentrations of free T_4 and free T_3 are increased to an even greater extent than are the measured serum total T_4 and T_3 concentrations. The TSH level will be suppressed or undetectable due to negative feedback by elevated levels of thyroid hormone at the pituitary.

For the patient with symptomatic disease, measurement of the serum free T_4 concentration, total T_4, total T_3, and the TSH value will confirm the diagnosis of thyrotoxicosis. If the patient is not pregnant or lactating, a 24-hour RAIU should be obtained if there is any diagnostic uncertainty, for example, recent onset of symptoms or other factors suggestive of thyroiditis. An increased RAIU documents that the thyroid gland is inappropriately utilizing the iodine to produce more thyroid hormone at a time when the patient is thyrotoxic.

Thyrotoxic periodic paralysis is a rare complication of hyperthyroidism commonly observed in Asian and Hispanic populations.[16] It presents as recurrent proximal muscle flaccidity ranging from mild weakness to total paralysis. The paralysis may be asymmetric and usually involves muscle groups that are strenuously exercised before the attack. Cognition and sensory perception are spared, whereas deep tendon reflexes are markedly diminished. The condition is characterized by hypokalemia and low urinary potassium excretion. Hypokalemia results from a sudden shift of potassium from extracellular to intracellular sites rather than reduced total body potassium. High-carbohydrate loads and exercise provoke the attacks. Treatment includes correcting the hyperthyroid state, potassium administration, spironolactone to conserve potassium, and propranolol to minimize intracellular shifts. Some patients with this condition have a mutation in the inwardly rectifying potassium channel Kir2.6.[17]

Trophoblastic Diseases

Human chorionic gonadotropin is a stimulator of the TSH receptor and may cause hyperthyroidism. The basis for the thyrotropic effect of hCG is the structural similarity of hCG to TSH (similar α subunits and unique β subunits). For patients with hyperthyroidism caused by trophoblastic tumors, serum hCG levels usually exceed 300 units/mL and always exceed 100 units/mL. The mean peak hCG level in normal pregnancy is 50 units/mL. On a molar basis, hCG has only 1/10,000 the activity of pituitary TSH in mouse bioassays. Nevertheless, this thyrotropic activity may be very substantial for patients with trophoblastic tumors, whose serum hCG concentrations may reach 2,000 units/mL.

Toxic Adenoma

An autonomous thyroid nodule is a discrete thyroid mass whose function is independent of pituitary and TSH control. The prevalence of toxic adenoma ranges from about 2% to 9% of thyrotoxic patients, and depends on iodine availability and geographic location. Toxic adenomas are benign tumors that produce thyroid hormone. They arise from gain-of-function somatic mutations of the TSH receptor or, less commonly, the $G_s\alpha$ protein; more than a dozen TSH receptor mutations have been described.[6] These nodules may be referred to as *toxic adenomas*, or "hot" nodules, because of their persistent uptake on a radioiodine thyroid scan, despite suppressed uptake in the surrounding non-nodular gland (Fig. 75-5). The amount of thyroid hormone produced by an autonomous nodule is mass related. Therefore, hyperthyroidism usually occurs with larger nodules (ie, those more than 3 cm in diameter). Older patients (older than 60 years) are more likely (up to 60%) to be thyrotoxic from autonomous nodules than are younger patients (12%). There are many reports of isolated elevation of serum T_3 in patients with autonomously functioning nodules. Therefore, if the T_4 level is normal, a T_3 level must be measured to rule out T_3 toxicosis. If autonomous function is suspected but the TSH is normal, the diagnosis can be confirmed by a failure of the autonomous nodule to decrease its iodine uptake during exogenous T_3 administration sufficient to suppress TSH. Surgical resection, thionamides, percutaneous ethanol injection, and radioactive iodine (RAI) ablation are treatment options, but since thionamides do not halt the proliferative process in the nodule, definitive therapies are recommended. Ethanol ablation may be associated with pain and damage to surrounding extrathyroidal tissues, limiting its acceptance in the United States. It has been hypothesized that sublethal radiation doses received by the surrounding non-nodular thyroid tissue during RAI therapy of toxic nodules may lead to induction of thyroid cancer. However, thyroid cancer has rarely been associated with RAI therapy, and newer studies suggest hyperthyroidism itself, rather than RAI therapy, as being associated with non-thyroid malignancies.[18] An autonomously functioning nodule, if not large enough to cause thyrotoxicosis, can often be managed conservatively without therapy.

Multinodular Goiters

In multinodular goiters (MNGs), follicles with autonomous function coexist with normal or even nonfunctioning follicles. The pathogenesis of MNG is thought to be similar to that of toxic adenoma: diffuse hyperplasia caused by goitrogenic stimuli, leading to mutations and clonal expansion of benign neoplasms. The functional status of the nodule(s) depends on the nature of the underlying mutations, whether activating such as TSH receptor mutations or inhibitory such as RAS mutations. Thyrotoxicosis in an MNG occurs when a sufficient mass of autonomous follicles generates enough thyroid hormone to exceed the needs of the patient. It is not surprising that this type of hyperthyroidism develops insidiously over a period of several years and predominantly affects older individuals with long-standing goiters. The patient's complaints of weight loss, depression, anxiety, and insomnia may be attributed to old age. Any unexplained chronic illness in an elderly patient presenting with an MNG calls for the exclusion of hidden (silent) thyrotoxicosis.[19] Current third-generation TSH assays are able to detect subclinical hyperthyroidism.

A

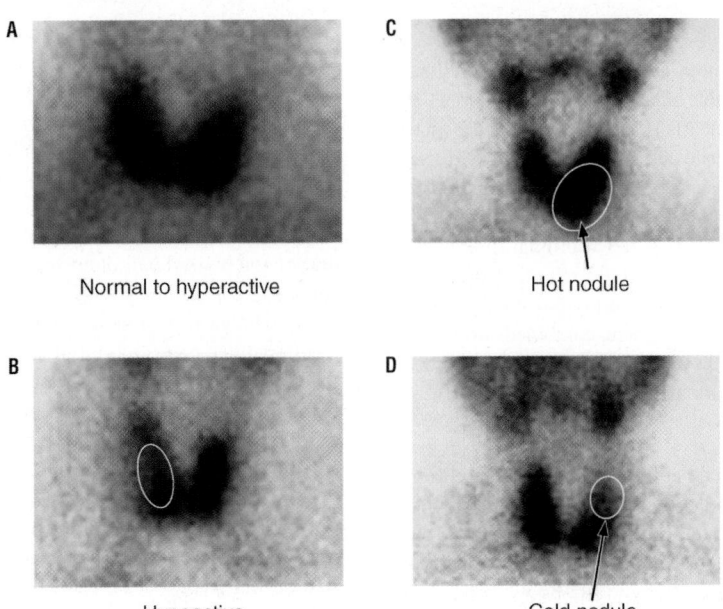

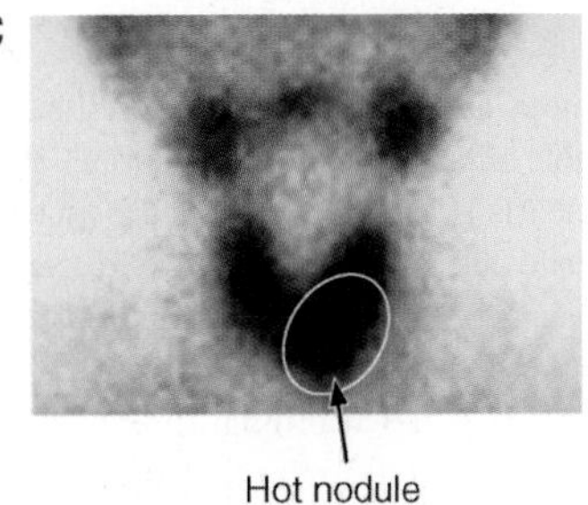

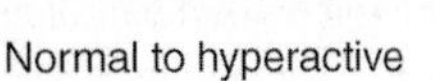

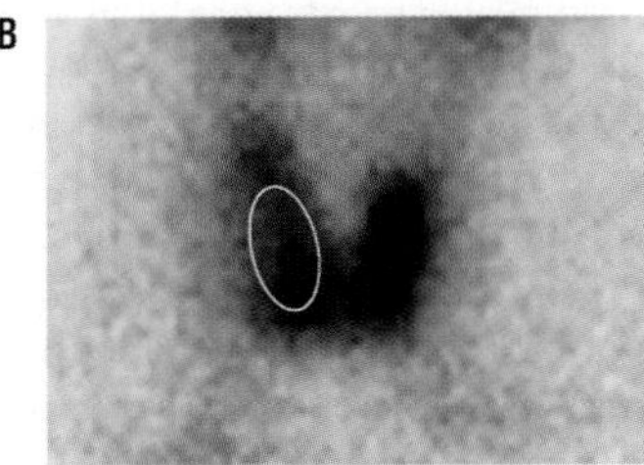

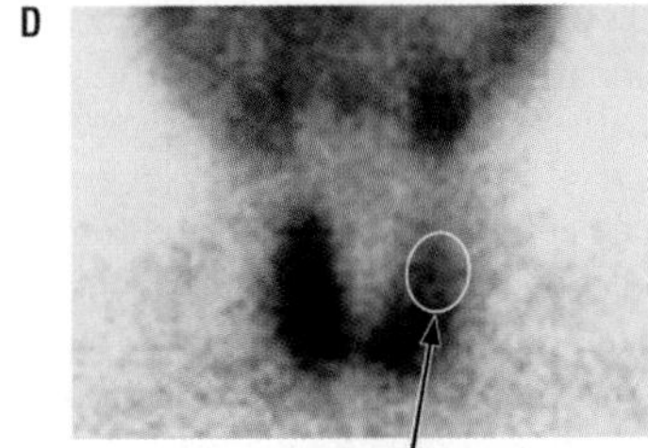

FIGURE 75-5 Radioiodine thyroid scans. (*A*) Normal or increased thyroid uptake of iodine-125 (^{125}I). (*B*) Thyroid with marked decrease in ^{125}I uptake in a large palpable mass. (*C*) Increased ^{125}I uptake isolated to a single nodule, the "hot nodule." (*D*) Decreased thyroid ^{125}I uptake in an isolated region, the "cold nodule." *Reproduced with permission from Molina PE. Endocrine Physiology. 2nd ed. New York: McGraw-Hill; 2006:90. Images courtesy of Dr. Luis Linares, Memorial Medical Center, New Orleans, LA.*

A thyroid scan will show patchy areas of autonomously functioning thyroid tissue intermixed with hypofunctioning areas. When the patient is euthyroid, therapy is based on the need to reduce goiter size due to mass-related symptoms such as dysphagia. Doses of thyroid hormone sufficient to suppress TSH levels may slow goiter growth or cause some degree of shrinkage, but, in general, suppression therapy for nodular disease is inadequate to address mass effect. The preferred treatment for toxic MNG is RAI or surgery. Surgery is usually selected for younger patients and patients in whom large goiters impinge on vital organs. Alternatively, percutaneous injection of 95% ethanol has also been used to destroy single or multinodular adenomas with a 5-year success rate approaching 80%.

Causes of Thyrotoxicosis Associated with Suppressed RAIU

Subacute Thyroiditis

Painful subacute (granulomatous or de Quervain) thyroiditis often develops after a viral syndrome, but rarely has a specific virus been identified in thyroid parenchyma.[20] A genetic predisposition exists, with markedly higher risk for developing subacute thyroiditis for patients with HLA-Bw35. Systemic symptoms often accompany the syndrome, including fever, malaise, and myalgia, in addition to those symptoms due to thyrotoxicosis. Typically, patients complain of severe pain in the thyroid region, which often extends to the ear on the affected side. With time, the pain may migrate from one side of the gland to the other. On physical examination, the thyroid gland is firm and exquisitely tender. Signs of thyrotoxicosis are present.

Thyroid function tests typically run a triphasic course. Initially, serum T_4 levels are elevated due to release of preformed thyroid hormone from disrupted follicles. The 24-hour RAIU during this time is less than 2% due to thyroid inflammation and TSH suppression by the elevated T_4 level. As the disease progresses, intrathyroidal hormone stores are depleted, and the patient may become mildly hypothyroid with an appropriately elevated TSH level. During the recovery phase, thyroid hormone stores are replenished, and serum TSH concentration gradually returns to normal. Recovery is generally complete within 2 to 6 months. Most patients remain euthyroid, and recurrences of painful thyroiditis are extremely rare. The patient with painful thyroiditis should be reassured that the disease is self-limited and is unlikely to recur. Thyrotoxic symptoms may be relieved with β-blockers. Nonsteroidal anti-inflammatory agents will usually relieve the pain. Occasionally, prednisone (30-40 mg daily) must be used to suppress the inflammatory process. Antithyroid drugs are not indicated because they will not be effective as they do not decrease the release of preformed thyroid hormone.

Painless Thyroiditis

Since its description in 1975, painless (silent and lymphocytic) thyroiditis has been recognized as a common cause of thyrotoxicosis and may represent up to 15% of cases of thyrotoxicosis in North America. In the setting of development of lymphocytic thyroiditis during the first 12 months after the end of pregnancy, the condition is also called *postpartum thyroiditis*. The etiology is not fully understood and may be heterogeneous, but evidence indicates that autoimmunity underlies most cases. There is an increased frequency of HLA-DR3 and DR5 in patients with painless thyroiditis; non-endocrine autoimmune diseases are also more common. Histologically, diffuse lymphocytic infiltration is generally identified. The triphasic course of this illness mimics that of subacute thyroiditis. Most patients present with mild thyrotoxic symptoms. Lid retraction and lid lag are present, but exophthalmos is absent. The thyroid gland may be diffusely enlarged, but thyroid tenderness is absent.

The 24-hour RAIU will typically be suppressed to less than 2% during the thyrotoxic phase of painless thyroiditis. Anti-TG and antithyroid peroxidase antibody (anti-TPOAb) levels are elevated in more than 50% of patients. Patients with mild hyperthyroidism and painless thyroiditis should be reassured that they have a self-limited disease, although patients with postpartum thyroiditis may experience recurrence of the disease with subsequent pregnancies. As with other thyrotoxic syndromes, adrenergic symptoms may be ameliorated with propranolol or metoprolol. Antithyroid drugs, which inhibit new hormone synthesis, are not indicated because they do not decrease the release of preformed thyroid hormone. A small proportion of patients may have recurrent episodes of thyroiditis, or may develop permanent hypothyroidism.[20]

Struma Ovarii

Struma ovarii is a teratoma of the ovary that contains differentiated thyroid follicular cells and is capable of making thyroid hormone. This extremely rare cause of thyrotoxicosis is suggested by the absence of thyroid enlargement in a thyrotoxic patient with a suppressed RAIU in the neck and no findings to suggest thyroiditis. The diagnosis is established by localizing functioning thyroid tissue in the ovary with whole-body RAI (sodium iodide-131 [^{131}I]) scanning. Interestingly, struma ovarii without associated hyperthyroidism is much more common than struma ovarii associated with hyperthyroidism. Because the tissue is neoplastic and potentially malignant, combined surgical and radioiodine treatment of malignant struma ovarii for both monitoring and therapy of relapse is the recommended treatment.

Thyroid Cancer

In widely metastatic differentiated papillary or follicular carcinomas with relatively well-preserved function, sufficient thyroid hormone can be synthesized and secreted to produce thyrotoxicosis. In most instances, a previous diagnosis of thyroid malignancy has been made. The diagnosis can be confirmed by whole-body ^{131}I scanning. Treatment with ^{131}I is generally effective at ablating functioning thyroid metastases.

Exogenous Thyroid Hormone

Thyrotoxicosis factitia was described in the recent American Thyroid Association guidelines on the management of hyperthyroidism as "all causes of hyperthyroidism due to ingestion of thyroid hormone."[9] This category includes hyperthyroidism produced by the intentional ingestion of exogenous thyroid hormone. Obesity is the most common non-thyroidal disorder for which thyroid hormone is inappropriately used, but thyroid hormone has been used for almost every conceivable problem from menstrual irregularities and infertility to hypercholesterolemia and baldness. There is little evidence to suggest that treatment with thyroid hormone is beneficial for such conditions in euthyroid individuals.[21] Obviously, thyrotoxicosis factitia can also occur when too large a dose of thyroid hormone is employed for conditions in which it is likely to be beneficial, such as differentiated thyroid carcinoma. In addition to this iatrogenic cause, accidental ingestion such as may occur with pediatric ingestion or pharmacy error. Rarely, thyrotoxicosis factitia is caused by the purposeful and secretive ingestion of thyroid hormone by patients (usually with a medical background) who wish to obtain attention or lose weight.

Thyroid hormone may also be accidentally ingested in food sources. Reports of thyrotoxicosis in Minnesota and Nebraska in 1980s were attributed to ingestion of ground beef contaminated by bovine thyroid glands.[22,23] More recently thyrotoxicosis due to porcine thyroid tissue in meat products has been reported in Spain and Uruguay.[24]

Thyrotoxicosis factitia should be suspected in a thyrotoxic patient without evidence of increased hormone production, thyroidal inflammation, or ectopic thyroid tissue. The RAIU uptake is at low levels because the patient's thyroid gland function is suppressed by the exogenous thyroid hormone. Measurement of plasma TG is a valuable laboratory aid in the diagnosis of thyrotoxicosis factitia. TG is normally secreted in small amounts by the thyroid gland; however, when thyroid hormone is taken orally, TG levels tend to be lower than the normal range. In other entities characterized by a low RAIU, such as thyroiditis, leakage of preformed thyroid hormone results in elevated TG levels. If a history of thyroid hormone ingestion is elicited or deduced, exogenous thyroid hormone should be withheld for between 4 and 6 weeks, and thyroid function tests repeated to document that the euthyroid state has been restored. Rarely, thyroid hormone analogs or metabolites may be the drug of abuse, detection of which may be difficult with standard thyroid hormone assays. For example, tiratricol (TRIAC), an endogenous metabolite of T_3 that has been used for weight loss and paradoxically by body builders, will suppress TSH at high enough doses and may cross-react in many T_3 immunoassays; thus, thyrotoxicosis factitia due to tiratricol abuse may be misinterpreted as T_3 toxicosis, and also lead to serious side effects.[25]

Medications Containing Iodine

Amiodarone may induce thyrotoxicosis (2%-3% of patients), overt hypothyroidism (5% of patients), subclinical hypothyroidism (25% of patients), or euthyroid hyperthyroxinemia, depending on the underlying thyroid pathology or lack thereof.[26] Because amiodarone contains 37% iodine by weight, approximately 6 mg/day of iodine is released for each 200 mg of amiodarone, 1,000 times greater than the recommended daily amount of iodine of 150 mcg/day. As a result of this iodine overload, iodine-exacerbated thyroid dysfunction commonly occurs among those patients with preexisting thyroid disease: thyrotoxicosis in patients with hyperthyroidism or euthyroid nodular autonomy and hypothyroidism in patients with autoimmune thyroid disease. In contrast to hyperthyroidism with increased synthesis of thyroid hormone induced by amiodarone (type I), destructive thyroiditis with leakage of TG and thyroid hormones also occurs (type II), typically among individuals with otherwise normal glands. The two types of amiodarone-induced thyrotoxicosis may be differentiated using color flow Doppler ultrasonography. Such distinction is critically important, given the therapeutic implications of the two syndromes: type I amiodarone-induced hyperthyroidism responds somewhat to thionamides, whereas type II may respond to glucocorticoids.[26] Obviously, RAI therapy is inappropriate in type I due to the drug-induced iodine excess, and in type II due to lack of increased hormone synthesis. The manifestations of amiodarone-induced thyrotoxicosis may be atypical symptoms such as ventricular tachycardia and exacerbation of underlying chronic obstructive pulmonary disease, both of which are significant given the severe underlying cardiac pathology that led to the use of amiodarone in the first place. Amiodarone also directly interferes with type I 5′-deiodinase, leading to reduced conversion of T_4 to T_3 and hyperthyroxinemia without thyrotoxicosis.[26]

TREATMENT

Thyrotoxicosis

2 Three common treatment modalities are used in the management of hyperthyroidism: surgery, antithyroid medications, and RAI (Table 75-5).

Desired Outcomes

The overall therapeutic objectives are to eliminate the excess thyroid hormone and minimize the symptoms and long-term consequences of hyperthyroidism.

General Approach to Treatment

Therapy must be individualized based on the type and severity of hyperthyroidism, patient age and gender, existence of nonthyroidal conditions, and response to previous therapy.[28,29] For example, patients with swallowing or breathing difficulties due to impingement of the esophagus or trachea are generally taken for surgical removal of the thyroid. Clinical guidelines for the treatment of hyperthyroidism have been published.[9] Selected recommendations from these guidelines are shown (Table 75-6).

Nonpharmacologic Therapy

Surgical removal of the hypersecreting thyroid gland became feasible in 1923 when Plummer discovered that iodine reduced the gland's vascularity, making this definitive procedure possible.

TABLE 75-5 Treatments for Hyperthyroidism Caused by Graves' Disease

Treatment	Advantages	Disadvantages	Comment
Methimazole (PTU second-line therapy)	Noninvasive Low initial cost Low risk of permanent hypothyroidism Possible remissions due to immune effects	Low cure rate (average 40%-50%) Adverse drug reactions Drug compliance	First-line treatment in children, adolescents, and pregnancy Initial treatment in severe cases or preoperative preparation
Radioactive iodine (^{131}I)	Cure of hyperthyroidism Lowest cost, before adjustment for quality of life	Permanent hypothyroidism almost inevitable Might worsen ophthalmopathy Pregnancy must be deferred for 6-12 months; no breast-feeding Small potential risk of exacerbation of hyperthyroidism	Best treatment for toxic nodules and toxic multinodular goiter
Surgery	Rapid, effective treatment, especially in patients with large goiters	Most invasive Least costly in long term after quality-of-life adjustment Permanent hypothyroidism Pain, scar	Potential choice in pregnancy if major side effect from antithyroid drugs Potential complications (recurrent laryngeal nerve damage, hypoparathyroidism) Useful when coexisting suspicious nodule present Option for patients who refuse radioiodine

Surgery should be considered for patients with a large thyroid gland (more than 80 g), severe ophthalmopathy, and a lack of remission on antithyroid drug treatment. In case of cosmetic issues or pressure symptoms, the choice in MNG stands between surgery, which is still the first choice, and radioiodine therapy if uptake is adequate. In addition to surgery, the solitary nodule, whether hot or cold, can be treated with percutaneous ethanol injection therapy. For hot nodules, radioiodine is the therapy of choice.[9] Appropriate preparation of the patient for thyroidectomy includes methimazole (MMI) until the patient is biochemically euthyroid (usually 6-8 weeks), followed by the addition of iodides (500 mg/day) for 10 to 14 days before surgery to decrease the vascularity of the gland. Propranolol for several weeks preoperatively and 7 to 10 days after surgery has also been used to maintain a pulse rate of less than 90 beats/min. Combined pretreatment with propranolol and 10 to 14 days of potassium iodide also has been advocated.

The overall complication rate when surgery is performed for MNG by an experienced endocrine surgeon is low.[30] If subtotal thyroidectomy, or an operation that attempts to maintain euthyroidism, is performed for Graves' disease, there is a risk of recurrence of hyperthyroidism that is directly related to remnant size. Near total thyroidectomy is generally recognized as the procedure of choice for patients with Graves' disease.[9] The complication rates of surgery for Graves' disease are low when surgery is performed by a high-volume thyroid surgeon. Surgical complications include hypoparathyroidism (up to 2%) and laryngeal nerve injury (up to 1%). Formal cost-effective

TABLE 75-6 Selected Recommendations from the American Thyroid Association Hyperthyroidism Guidelines[9]

Recommendation Number	Question	Recommendation	Grading
8	If ^{131}I therapy is chosen (*for GD*), how should it be accomplished?	Sufficient radiation should be administered in a single dose (typically 10-15 mCi) to render the patient with GD hypothyroid.	Strong recommendation; moderate quality
13	If antithyroid drugs are chosen as initial management of GD, how should the therapy be managed?	Methimazole should be used in virtually every patient who chooses antithyroid drug therapy for GD, except during the first trimester of pregnancy when propylthiouracil is preferred, in the treatment of thyroid storm, and in patients with minor reactions to methimazole who refuse radioactive iodine therapy or surgery.	Strong recommendation; moderate quality
24	If thyroidectomy is chosen for treatment of GD, how should it be accomplished?	If surgery is chosen as the primary therapy for GD, near-total or total thyroidectomy is the procedure of choice.	Strong recommendation; moderate quality
35	If ^{131}I therapy is chosen (*for TMNG*), how should it be accomplished?	For radioactive iodine treatment of TMNG, sufficient radiation should be administered in a single dose to alleviate hyperthyroidism.	Strong recommendation; moderate quality
36	If ^{131}I therapy is chosen (*for TA*), how should it be accomplished?	For radioactive iodine treatment of TA, sufficient radiation to alleviate hyperthyroidism should be administered in a single dose.	Strong recommendation; moderate quality
40	If surgery is chosen (*for TMNG*), how should it be accomplished?	If surgery is chosen as treatment for TMNG, near-total or total thyroidectomy should be performed.	Strong recommendation; moderate quality
42	If surgery is chosen (*for TA*), how should it be accomplished?	If surgery is chosen as the treatment for TA, an ipsilateral thyroid lobectomy, or isthmusectomy if the adenoma is in the thyroid isthmus, should be performed.	Strong recommendation; moderate quality
72	How should hyperthyroidism in pregnancy be managed?	GD during pregnancy should be treated with the lowest possible dose of antithyroid drugs needed to keep the mother's thyroid hormone levels slightly above the normal range for total T_4 and T_3 values in pregnancy and the TSH suppressed. Free T_4 estimates should be kept at or slightly above the upper limit of the nonpregnant reference range. Thyroid function should be assessed monthly, and the antithyroid drug dose adjusted as required.	Strong recommendation; low quality

GD, Graves' disease; ^{131}I, radioactive I-131; TMNG, toxic multinodular goiter; TA, toxic adenoma, SH = subclinical hyperthyroidism.

analysis indicates that a total thyroidectomy may be the most cost-effective method for managing hyperthyroidism when considering outcomes in quality-adjusted life-years.[31]

Pharmacologic Therapy

Antithyroid Medications

3 **Thionamide Drugs** Two drugs within this category, MMI and PTU, are approved for the treatment of hyperthyroidism in the United States.[32] They are classified as thioureylenes (thionamides), which incorporate an N–C–S=N group into their ring structures.

Mechanism of Action MMI and PTU share several mechanisms to inhibit the biosynthesis of thyroid hormone.[33] These drugs serve as preferential substrates for the iodinating intermediate of thyroid peroxidase and divert iodine away from potential iodination sites in TG. This prevents subsequent incorporation of iodine into iodotyrosines and ultimately iodothyronine ("organification"). Second, they inhibit coupling of MIT and DIT to form T_4 and T_3. The coupling reaction may be more sensitive to these drugs than the iodination reaction. Experimentally, these drugs exhibit immunosuppressive effects, although the clinical relevance of this finding is unclear. For patients with Graves' disease, antithyroid drug treatment has been associated with lower TSAb titers and restoration of normal suppressor T-cell function. However, perchlorate (ClO_4^-), which has a different mechanism of action, also decreases TSAbs, suggesting that normalization of the thyroid hormone level may itself improve the abnormal immune function. PTU inhibits the peripheral conversion of T_4 to T_3. This effect is dose related and occurs within hours of PTU administration. MMI does not have this effect. Over time, depletion of stored hormone and lack of continuing synthesis of thyroid hormone results in the clinical effects of these drugs.

Pharmacokinetics Both antithyroid drugs are well absorbed (80%-95%) from the gastrointestinal tract, with peak serum concentrations about 1 hour after ingestion. The plasma half-life ranges of PTU and MMI are 1 to 2.5 and 6 to 9 hours, respectively, and are not appreciably affected by thyroid status. Urinary excretion is about 35% for PTU and less than 10% for MMI. These drugs are actively concentrated in the thyroid gland, which may account for the disparity between their relatively short plasma half-lives and the effectiveness of once-daily dosing regimens even with PTU. Approximately 60% to 80% of PTU is bound to plasma albumin, whereas MMI is not protein bound. MMI readily crosses the placenta and appears in breast milk. Older studies suggested that PTU crosses the placental membranes only one tenth as well as MMI; however, these studies were done in the course of therapeutic abortion early in pregnancy. Newer studies show little difference between fetal concentrations of PTU and MMI, and both are associated with elevated TSH in about 20% and low T_4 in about 7% of fetuses.[34]

4 ***Dosing and Administration*** MMI is available as 5 and 10 mg tablets and PTU as 50 mg tablets. MMI is approximately 10 times more potent than PTU. Initial therapy with MMI is given in two or three divided doses totaling 30 to 60 mg/day. PTU is given in dose ranges from 300 to 600 mg daily, usually in three or four divided doses. Although the traditional recommendation is for divided doses, evidence exists that both drugs can be given as single daily doses. Patients with severe hyperthyroidism may require larger initial doses, and some may respond better at these larger doses if the dose is divided. The maximal blocking doses of MMI and PTU are 120 and 1,200 mg daily, respectively. Once the intrathyroidal pool of thyroid hormone is reduced and new hormone synthesis is sufficiently blocked, clinical improvement should ensue. Usually within 4 to 8 weeks of initiating therapy, symptoms will diminish and circulating thyroid hormone levels will return to normal. At this time the tapering regimen can be started. Changes in dose for each drug should be made on a monthly basis, because the endogenously produced T_4 will reach a new steady-state concentration in this interval. Typical ranges of daily maintenance doses for MMI and PTU are 5 to 30 mg and 50 to 300 mg, respectively.

If the objective of therapy is to induce a long-term remission, the patient should remain on continuous antithyroid drug therapy for 12 to 24 months. Antithyroid drug therapy induces permanent remission rates of 10% to 98%, with an overall average of about 40% to 50%.[35] This is much higher than the remission rate seen with propranolol alone (22%-36%). Patient characteristics for a favorable outcome include older patients (older than 40 years), low T_4:T_3 ratio (less than 20), a small goiter (less than 50 g), short duration of disease (less than 6 months), no previous history of relapse with antithyroid drugs, duration of therapy 1 to 2 years or longer, and low TSAb titers at baseline or a reduction with treatment.[33] A 2012 study provides preliminary evidence that a new assay that has better specificity for detection of antibodies that stimulate the TSH receptors, without detecting coexistent blocking antibodies, may be a useful predictor of remission of Graves' disease.[36]

It is important that patients be followed every 6 to 12 months after remission occurs. If a relapse occurs, alternate therapy with RAI is preferred to a second course of antithyroid drugs. Relapses seem to plateau after about 5 years and eventually 5% to 20% of patients will develop spontaneous hypothyroidism. There has been interest in whether concurrent administration of T_4 with thionamide therapy for thyrotoxicosis and subclinical hyperthyroidism can reduce autoantibodies directed toward the thyroid gland and improve remission rate. In a Japanese study, adjunctive treatment with T_4 was associated with a 20-fold reduction in the recurrence rate of Graves' disease compared with the recurrence rate seen for patients treated with antithyroid drugs alone.[37] Attempts to reproduce these results in American and European patients with Graves' disease have failed to show any delay or reduction in the recurrence of Graves' disease with T_4 administration, and this approach is generally not recommended because of the higher rates of side effects seen with the larger doses of antithyroid drugs needed with this regimen.[9]

Subclinical hyperthyroidism is defined as the finding of a serum TSH below the lower limit of the reference range combined with free T_4 and T_3 concentrations that are normal. Subclinical hyperthyroidism is associated with an increased risk of atrial fibrillation, and may be associated with increased all-cause mortality. Some studies show an increased risk of hip fractures in postmenopausal women with subclinical hyperthyroidism. Most practitioners agree that treatment of older patients (greater than 65 years) with TSH values below 0.1 milli-international unit/L is reasonable. In patients who are younger or have TSH values of 0.1 to 0.4 milli-international unit/L a decision whether to treat the patient for mild hyperthyroidism or to monitor thyroid function depend on the patient's cardiovascular risk factors and bone health.[9,38]

Adverse Effects Minor adverse reactions to MMI and PTU have an overall incidence of 5% to 25% depending on the dose and the drug, whereas major adverse effects occur in 1.5% to 4.6% of patients receiving these drugs.[32] Pruritic maculopapular rashes (sometimes associated with vasculitis based on skin biopsy), arthralgias, and fevers occur in up to 5% of patients and may occur at greater frequency with higher doses and in children. Rashes often disappear spontaneously but, if persistent, may be managed with antihistamines.

One of the most common side effects is a benign transient leukopenia characterized by a white blood cell (WBC) count of less than 4,000/mm^3. This condition occurs in up to 12% of adults and 25% of children, and sometimes can be confused with mild leukopenia seen in Graves' disease. This mild leukopenia is not a harbinger of the more serious adverse effect of agranulocytosis, so therapy can usually be continued. If a minor adverse reaction occurs with one antithyroid drug, the alternate thiourea may be tried, but cross-sensitivity occurs for about 50% of patients.[32]

Agranulocytosis is one of the serious adverse effects of thiourea drug therapy and is characterized by fever, malaise, gingivitis, oropharyngeal infection, and a granulocyte count less than 250/mm^3.[32] These drugs are concentrated in granulocytes, and this reaction may represent a direct toxic effect rather than hypersensitivity. This toxic reaction has occurred with both thioureas, and the incidence varies from 0.5% to 6%. It is higher for patients over age 40 receiving an MMI dose greater than 40 mg/day or the equivalent dose of PTU, is linked to HLA class II genes containing the DRB1*08032 allele, and is more frequent with initial MMI doses of 30 mg compared with 15 mg.[39] Agranulocytosis usually develops in the first 3 months of therapy. Because the onset is sudden, routine WBC count monitoring has not been recommended. Colony-stimulating factors have been used with some success to restore cell counts to normal, but it is unclear how effective this form of therapy is compared with routine supportive care. Peripheral lymphocytes obtained from patients with PTU-induced agranulocytosis undergo transformation in the presence of other thionamides, suggesting that these severe reactions are immunologically mediated and patients should not receive other thionamides. Aplastic anemia has been reported with MMI and may be associated with an inhibitor to colony-forming units. Once antithyroid drugs are discontinued, clinical improvement is seen over several days to weeks. Patients should be counseled to discontinue therapy and contact their physician when flu-like symptoms such as fever, malaise, or sore throat develop. In addition, many clinicians will concomitantly provide an order for a complete blood cell count (with WBC count differential) when prescribing MMI or PTU therapy. If the patient becomes ill and is unable to reach the provider, the patient can still visit the nearest laboratory to have potential agranulocytosis evaluated.

Arthralgias and a lupus-like syndrome (sometimes in the absence of antinuclear antibodies) have been reported in 4% to 5% of patients. This generally occurs after 6 months of therapy. Uncommonly, polymyositis, presenting as proximal muscle weakness and elevated creatine phosphokinase, has been reported with PTU administration. Gastrointestinal intolerance is also reported to occur in 4% to 5% of patients. Hypoprothrombinemia is a rare complication of thionamide therapy. Patients who have experienced a major adverse reaction to one thiourea drug should not be converted to the alternate drug because of cross-sensitivity.[9]

Older reports suggested that congenital skin defects (aplasia cutis) may be caused by MMI and carbimazole, although a registry review from the Netherlands could not find an association between maternal use of these drugs and skin defects. Several serious congenital malformations including tracheoesophageal fistulas and choanal atresia have been observed with MMI and carbimazole but not PTU use during pregnancy.[40,41] Thus, PTU has traditionally been considered the drug of choice throughout pregnancy for women with hyperthyroidism, because of concerns about the possible teratogenic effects of MMI. However, currently heightened concerns about the greater risk of hepatotoxicity with PTU when compared to MMI have led to the recommendation that PTU no longer be considered a first-line drug, except during the first trimester of pregnancy.[9] The issue of choice of antithyroidal agent during pregnancy has been further complicated by a recent study that suggested that fetuses exposed to either MMI or PTU during gestation may have increased risk of drug-induced fetal malformations.[42]

Hepatotoxicity can be seen with both MMI and PTU with a prevalence of approximately 1.3%. At moderate doses, some authors have found that initial hepatic enzyme elevations eventually normalize in most patients with continued therapy. PTU-induced subclinical liver injury is common and is usually transient and asymptomatic. Thus, it has generally been thought that therapy with PTU may be continued with caution in the absence of symptoms and hyperbilirubinemia. However, a 1997 literature review documented 49 cases of hepatotoxicity. Twenty-eight cases were associated with PTU use, and 21 cases were associated with MMI use. The hepatotoxicity was associated with seven deaths and three deaths in the PTU and MMI groups, respectively. There did not appear to be a relationship between the dose or duration of thionamide treatment and outcome. During the past 20 years of PTU use in the United States, 22 adults developed severe hepatotoxicity leading to 9 deaths and 5 liver transplants. The risk of this complication was greater in children (1:2,000) than in adults (1:10,000).[43] A recent reanalysis of data reported to the FDA from 1982 to 2008 found that toxicity in children was generally related to higher doses of PTU and that toxicity in both children and adults was associated with therapy lasting more than 4 months in duration.[44] In light of such evidence, it has been recommended by the American Thyroid Association and the FDA that PTU not be considered as first-line therapy in either adults or children.[9,45] One of three exceptions includes the first trimester of pregnancy, when the risk of MMI-induced embryopathy may exceed that of PTU-induced hepatotoxicity. Other exceptions include intolerance to MMI and thyroid storm.

Iodides Iodide was the first form of drug therapy for Graves' disease. Its mechanism of action is to acutely block thyroid hormone release, inhibit thyroid hormone biosynthesis by interfering with intrathyroidal iodide utilization (the Wolff-Chaikoff effect), and decrease the size and vascularity of the gland. This early inhibitory effect provides symptom improvement within 2 to 7 days of initiating therapy, and serum T_4 and T_3 concentrations may be reduced for a few weeks. Despite the reduced release of T_4 and T_3, thyroid hormone synthesis continues at an accelerated rate, resulting in a gland rich in stored hormones. The normal and hyperfunctioning thyroid soon escapes from this inhibitory effect within 1 to 2 weeks by decreasing the active transfer of iodide into the gland. Iodides are often used as adjunctive therapy to prepare a patient with Graves' disease for surgery, to acutely inhibit thyroid hormone release and quickly attain the euthyroid state in severely thyrotoxic patients with cardiac decompensation, or to inhibit thyroid hormone release following RAI therapy. However, large doses of iodine may exacerbate hyperthyroidism or indeed precipitate hyperthyroidism in some previously euthyroid individuals (Jod-Basedow disease). This Jod-Basedow phenomenon is most common in iodine-deficient areas, particularly for patients with preexisting nontoxic goiter. Iodide is contraindicated in toxic MNG.

Potassium iodide is available either as a saturated solution (SSKI), which contains 38 mg of iodide per drop, or as Lugol's solution, which contains 6.3 mg of iodide per drop. The typical starting dose of SSKI is 3 to 10 drops daily (120-400 mg) in water or juice. There is no documented advantage to using doses in excess of 6 to 8 mg/day. When used to prepare a patient for surgery, it should be administered 7 to 14 days preoperatively. As an adjunct to RAI, SSKI should not be used before, but rather 3 to 7 days after RAI treatment, so that the radioactive iodide can concentrate in the thyroid. The most frequent toxic effects with iodide therapy are hypersensitivity reactions (skin rashes, drug fever, rhinitis, and conjunctivitis), salivary gland swelling, "iodism" (metallic taste, burning mouth and throat, sore teeth and gums, symptoms of a head cold, and sometimes stomach upset and diarrhea), and gynecomastia.

Other compounds containing organic iodide have also been used therapeutically for hyperthyroidism. These include various radiologic contrast media that share a triiodoaminobenzene and monoaminobenzene ring with a propionic acid chain (eg, iopanoic acid and sodium ipodate). The effect of these compounds is a result of the iodine content inhibiting thyroid hormone release as well as competitive inhibition of 5′-monodeiodinase conversion related to their structures, which resemble thyroid analogs. Unfortunately, these extremely useful agents are no longer available in the United States.

5 **Adrenergic Blockers** Because many of the manifestations of hyperthyroidism are mediated by β-adrenergic receptors, β-blockers

(especially propranolol) have been used widely to ameliorate symptoms such as palpitations, anxiety, tremor, and heat intolerance. Although β-blockers are quite effective for symptom control, they have no effect on the urinary excretion of calcium, phosphorus, hydroxyproline, creatinine, or various amino acids, suggesting a lack of effect on peripheral thyrotoxicosis and protein metabolism. Furthermore, β-blockers neither reduce TSAb nor prevent thyroid storm. Propranolol and nadolol partially block the conversion of T_4 to T_3, but this contribution to the overall therapeutic effect is small in magnitude. Inhibition of conversion of T_4 to T_3 is mediated by D-propranolol, which is devoid of β-blocking activity, and L-propranolol, which is responsible for the antiadrenergic effects, has little effect on the conversion.

β-Blockers are usually used as adjunctive therapy with antithyroid drugs, RAI, or iodides when treating Graves' disease or toxic nodules; in preparation for surgery; or in thyroid storm. The only conditions for which β-blockers are primary therapy for thyrotoxicosis are those associated with thyroiditis. The dose of propranolol required to relieve adrenergic symptoms is variable, but an initial dose of 20 to 40 mg four times daily is effective (heart rate less than 90 beats/min) for most patients. Younger or more severely toxic patients may require as much as 240 to 480 mg/day because there seems to be an increased clearance rate for these patients. β-Blockers are contraindicated for patients with decompensated heart failure unless it is caused solely by tachycardia (high output). Nonselective agents and those lacking intrinsic sympathomimetic activity should be used with caution for patients with asthma and bronchospastic chronic obstructive lung disease. β-Blockers that are cardioselective and have intrinsic sympathomimetic activity may have a slight margin of safety in these situations. Other patients in whom contraindications exist are those with sinus bradycardia, those receiving monoamine oxidase inhibitors or tricyclic antidepressants, and those with spontaneous hypoglycemia. β-Blockers may also prolong gestation and labor during pregnancy. Other side effects include nausea, vomiting, anxiety, insomnia, lightheadedness, bradycardia, and hematologic disturbances.

Antiadrenergic agents such as centrally acting sympatholytics and calcium channel antagonists may have some role in the symptomatic treatment of hyperthyroidism. These drugs might be useful when contraindications to β-blockade exist. When compared with nadolol 40 mg twice daily, clonidine 150 mcg twice daily reduced plasma catecholamines, whereas nadolol increased both epinephrine and norepinephrine after 1 week of treatment. Diltiazem 120 mg given every 8 hours reduced heart rate by 17%; fewer ventricular extrasystoles were noted after 10 days of therapy, and diltiazem has been shown to be comparable to propranolol in lowering heart rate and blood pressure.

6 **Radioactive Iodine** Although other radioisotopes have been used to ablate thyroid tissue, ^{131}I is considered to be the agent of choice for Graves' disease, toxic autonomous nodules, and toxic MNGs.[9] RAI is administered as a colorless and tasteless liquid that is well absorbed and concentrates in the thyroid. ^{131}I is a β- and γ-emitter with a tissue penetration of 2 mm and a half-life of 8 days. Other organs take up ^{131}I, but the thyroid gland is the only organ in which organification of the absorbed iodine takes place. Initially, RAI disrupts hormone synthesis by incorporating into thyroid hormones and TG. Over a period of weeks, follicles that have taken up RAI and surrounding follicles develop evidence of cellular necrosis, breakdown of follicles, development of bizarre cell forms, nuclear pyknosis, and destruction of small vessels within the gland, leading to edema and fibrosis of the interstitial tissue. Pregnancy is an absolute contraindication to the use of RAI since radiation will be delivered to the fetal tissue, including the fetal thyroid.

β-Blockers may be given any time without compromising RAI therapy, accounting for their role as a mainstay of adjunctive therapy to RAI treatment. If iodides are administered, they should be given 3 to 7 days after RAI to prevent interference with the uptake of RAI in the thyroid gland. Because thyroid hormone levels will transiently increase following RAI treatment due to release of preformed thyroid hormone, patients with cardiac disease and elderly patients are often treated with thionamides prior to RAI ablation. For patients with underlying cardiac disease, it may be necessary to reinstitute antithyroid drug therapy following RAI ablation. The standard practice is to withdraw the thionamide 4 to 6 days prior to RAI treatment and to reinstitute it 4 days after therapy is concluded. Administering antithyroid drug therapy immediately following RAI treatment may result in a higher rate of post-treatment recurrence or persistent hyperthyroidism. Pretreatment with PTU may lead to higher rates of treatment failure, but this does not appear to be the case with MMI pretreatment. Use of lithium, as adjunctive therapy to RAI therapy, has multiple benefits of increasing the cure rate, shortening the time to cure, and preventing post-therapy increase in thyroid hormone levels.[46] Lithium is likely to achieve these effects by increasing RAI retention in the thyroid and inhibiting thyroid hormone release from the gland.

Corticosteroid administration will blunt and delay the rise in antibodies to the TSH receptor, TG, and thyroid peroxidase while reducing T_3 and T_4 concentrations following RAI. Bartalena et al. found no progression in ophthalmopathy for patients receiving prednisone after RAI (0% worsened) compared with 3% worsening in those receiving MMI, and 5% worsening in those receiving RAI alone.[47] Theoretically, if shared thyroidal and orbital antigen is involved in the pathogenesis of Graves' ophthalmopathy, antigen released with RAI treatment could aggravate preexisting eye disease. There is some disagreement as to what degree of ophthalmopathy should be considered a contraindication to RAI. However, in those with moderate or severe orbitopathy it seems reasonable to delay RAI until the patient's eye disease has been stable.

Destruction of the gland attenuates the hyperthyroid state, and hypothyroidism commonly occurs months to years following RAI.[9,33] The goal of therapy is to destroy overactive thyroid cells, and a single dose of 4,000 to 8,000 rad results in a euthyroid state in 60% of patients at 6 months or less. The remaining 40% become euthyroid within 1 year, requiring two or more doses. It is advisable that a second dose of RAI be given 6 months after the first RAI treatment if the patient remains hyperthyroid.[9] Variables that predict an unsuccessful outcome of RAI include gender (men are less likely to develop hypothyroidism), race, the size of the thyroid (euthyroidism is less likely in large glands), severity of disease, and perhaps a higher level of TSAb. In a recent study, predictors of successful treatment with RAI included higher ablative dose, female gender, lower free T_4 levels at diagnosis, and absence of a palpable goiter.[48] The acute, short-term side effects of ^{131}I therapy are minimal and include mild thyroidal tenderness and dysphagia. Concern over increased risk of mutations and congenital defects now appears to be unfounded because long-term follow-up studies have not revealed increased risk for these complications.[49] In some studies examining the risk of malignancies after RAI therapy, there seems to be a small but significant increase in the risk of cancer of the small bowel and thyroid.[49] Although RAI is very effective in the treatment of hyperthyroidism, long-term follow-up from Great Britain suggests that among patients with hyperthyroidism treated with RAI, mortality from all causes and mortality resulting from cardiovascular and cerebrovascular disease and fracture are increased.

A common approach to Graves' hyperthyroidism is to administer a single dose of 5 to 15 mCi (80-200 μCi/g of tissue). The optimal method for determining ^{131}I treatment doses for Graves' hyperthyroidism is unknown, and techniques have varied from a fixed dose to more elaborate calculations based on gland size, iodine uptake, and iodine turnover.[9] In a trial of 88 patients with Graves' disease, no difference in outcome was seen among high or low, fixed or adjusted doses. Thyroid glands estimated to weigh more than 80 g may require larger doses of RAI. Larger doses are likely to induce hypothyroidism and are seldom given outside the United States due to the imposition of stringent safety restrictions. For example, in the United Kingdom, a nursery school teacher is advised to stay out of school for 3 weeks following a 15 mCi dose of ^{131}I.

Thyrotoxicosis—**Controversy...**

When treating pregnant women with hyperthyroidism the recommendation has been to use PTU in the first trimester to avoid teratogenesis and to switch to MMI for the remainder of pregnancy to avoid hepatotoxicity. Recent data suggest that birth defects may have a similar incidence in fetuses exposed to PTU, compared with those who are exposed to MMI. Future studies will help to determine the drug of choice for treating hyperthyroidism during pregnancy, and whether one drug should be maintained for the duration of pregnancy.

Special Populations

Graves' Disease and Pregnancy

Inappropriate production of hCG is a cause of abnormal thyroid function tests during the first half of pregnancy, and hCG can cause either subclinical (normal T_4 and suppressed TSH) or overt hyperthyroidism. This is because the homology of hCG and TSH leads to hCG-mediated stimulation through the TSH receptor. A recent study showed that at hCG concentrations greater than 400 international units/mL, TSH levels were invariably suppressed and free T_4 levels were generally above the normal range. Most patients with hCG greater than 200 international units/mL did not have symptoms of hyperthyroidism. The variability of the thyrotropic potency of hCG is believed to depend on its carbohydrate composition.

Recently, two very comprehensive guidelines have been published by the American Thyroid Association and the Endocrine Society regarding the management of thyroid disease during pregnancy.[50,51] Hyperthyroidism during pregnancy is almost solely caused by Graves' disease, with approximately 0.1% to 0.4% of pregnancies affected. Although the increased metabolic rate is usually well tolerated in pregnant women, two symptoms suggestive of hyperthyroidism during pregnancy are failure to gain weight despite good appetite and persistent tachycardia. There is no increase in maternal mortality or morbidity in well-controlled patients; however, postpartum thyroid storm has been reported in about 20% of untreated individuals. Fetal loss is also more common, due to the facts that spontaneous abortion and premature delivery are more common in untreated pregnant women, as are low-birth-weight infants and eclampsia. Transplacental passage of TSAb may occur, causing fetal as well as neonatal hyperthyroidism. An uncommon cause of hyperthyroidism is molar pregnancy; women present with a large-for-dates uterus and evacuation of the uterus is the preferred management approach.

Because RAI is contraindicated in pregnancy and surgery is usually not recommended (especially during the first trimester), antithyroid drug therapy is usually the treatment of choice for hyperthyroidism. MMI readily crosses the placenta and appears in breast milk.

Propylthiouracil has been considered the drug of choice during the first trimester of pregnancy, with the lowest possible doses used to maintain the maternal T_4 level in the high-normal range.[43,45] During this period the risk of MMI-associated embryopathy is believed to outweigh that of PTU-associated hepatotoxicity. To prevent fetal goiter and suppression of fetal thyroid function, PTU is usually prescribed in daily doses of 300 mg or less and tapered to 50 to 150 mg daily after 4 to 6 weeks. PTU doses of less than 200 mg daily are unlikely to produce fetal goiter.[34] During the second and third trimesters, when the critical period of organogenesis is complete, MMI has been thought to be the drug of choice because of the greater risk of hepatotoxicity with PTU.[43,45] However, a recent study has raised the question of whether this strategy of switching thionamides, and thus exposing the fetus to both drugs, is the optimum approach.[42] Thionamide doses should be adjusted to maintain free T_4 within 10% of the upper normal limit of the nonpregnant reference range. During the last trimester, TSAbs fall spontaneously, and some patients will go into remission so that antithyroid drug doses may be reduced. A rebound in maternal hyperthyroidism occurs in about 10% of women postpartum and may require more intensive treatment than in the last trimester of pregnancy. For example, a study of patients who were euthyroid after thionamide discontinuation and subsequently became pregnant showed a relative risk of 4.26 for relapse of hyperthyroidism occurring 4 to 8 months after delivery.[52]

Neonatal and Pediatric Hyperthyroidism

Following delivery, some babies of hyperthyroid mothers will be hyperthyroid due to placental transfer of TSAbs, which stimulates thyroid hormone production in utero and postpartum. This is likely if the maternal TSAb titers were quite high. The disease is usually expressed 7 to 10 days postpartum and treatment with antithyroid drugs (PTU 5-10 mg/kg/day or MMI 0.5-1 mg/kg/day) may be needed for as long as 8 to 12 weeks until the antibody is cleared (immunoglobulin G half-life is about 2 weeks). Iodide (potassium iodide one drop per day or Lugol's solution one to three drops per day) and sodium ipodate may be used for the first few days to acutely inhibit hormone release.

Childhood hyperthyroidism has classically been managed with either MMI or PTU. Long-term follow-up studies suggest that this form of therapy is quite acceptable, with 25% of a cohort experiencing remission every 2 years.[53] Again, current recommendations suggest use of MMI as a first-line agent in both adults and children.[9]

Thyroid Storm

Thyroid storm is a life-threatening medical emergency characterized by decompensated thyrotoxicosis, high fever (often more than 39.4°C [more than 103°F]), tachycardia, tachypnea, dehydration, delirium, coma, nausea, vomiting, and diarrhea.[27] Although Graves' disease and less commonly toxic nodular goiter are usually the underlying thyrotoxic pathology,[54] at least two cases of subacute thyroiditis leading to thyroid storm have been reported.

Precipitating factors for thyroid storm include infection, trauma, surgery, RAI treatment, and withdrawal from antithyroid drugs. Although the duration of clinical decompensation lasts for an average duration of 72 hours, symptoms may persist up to 8 days. With aggressive treatment, the mortality rate has been lowered to 20%. The following therapeutic measures should be instituted promptly: (a) suppression of thyroid hormone formation and secretion, (b) antiadrenergic therapy, (c) administration of corticosteroids, and (d) treatment of associated complications or coexisting factors that may have precipitated the storm. Specific agents used in thyroid storm are outlined in Table 75-7. PTU in large doses may be the preferred thionamide because, in addition to interfering with the production of thyroid hormones, it also blocks the peripheral conversion of T_4 to T_3. However, β-blockers and corticosteroids will serve the same purpose. A theoretical advantage of MMI is that it has a longer duration of action. If patients are unable to take medications orally, the tablets can be crushed into suspension and instilled by gastric or rectal tube or given IV. Iodides, which rapidly block the release of preformed thyroid hormone, should be administered after thionamide is initiated to inhibit iodide utilization by the overactive gland. If iodide is administered first, it could theoretically provide substrate to produce even higher levels of thyroid hormone.

Antiadrenergic therapy with the short-acting agent esmolol is preferred, both because it may be used in the patient with pulmonary disease or at risk for cardiac failure and because its effects may

TABLE 75-7 Drug Dosages Used in the Management of Thyroid Storm

Drug	Regimen
Propylthiouracil	900-1,200 mg/day orally in four or six divided doses
Methimazole	90-120 mg/day orally in four or six divided doses
Sodium iodide	Up to 2 g/day IV in single or divided doses
Lugol's solution	5-10 drops three times a day in water or juice
Saturated solution of potassium iodide	1-2 drops three times a day in water or juice
Propranolol	40-80 mg every 6 hours
Dexamethasone	5-20 mg/day orally or IV in divided doses
Prednisone	25-100 mg/day orally in divided doses
Methylprednisolone	20-80 mg/day IV in divided doses
Hydrocortisone	100-400 mg/day IV in divided doses

be rapidly reversed.[55] Corticosteroids are generally recommended, although there is no convincing evidence of adrenocortical insufficiency in thyroid storm, and the benefits derived from steroids may be caused by their antipyretic action and their effect of stabilizing blood pressure.[27] General supportive measures, including acetaminophen as an antipyretic (do not use aspirin or other nonsteroidal anti-inflammatory agents because they may displace bound thyroid hormone), fluid and electrolyte replacement, sedatives, digitalis, antiarrhythmics, insulin, and antibiotics, should be given as indicated. Plasmapheresis and peritoneal dialysis have been used to remove excess hormone (and to remove thyroid-stimulating immunoglobulins in Graves' disease) when the patient has not responded to more conservative measures, although these measures do not always work.

An analysis was undertaken to identify cases of thyroid storm occurring in Japan during the period 2004 to 2008.[54] The mortality rate was approximately 10% in the group of 282 patients identified. The most common trigger of the thyrotoxicosis was discontinuation or irregular use of antithyroidal agents. The most common cause of death was either multiorgan failure or congestive heart failure.

EVALUATION OF THERAPEUTIC OUTCOMES—THYROTOXICOSIS

After therapy (surgery, thionamides, or RAI) for hyperthyroidism has been initiated, patients should be evaluated on a monthly basis until they reach a euthyroid condition. Clinical signs of continuing thyrotoxicosis (tachycardia, weight loss, and heat intolerance, among others) or the development of hypothyroidism (bradycardia, weight gain, and lethargy, among others) should be noted. β-Blockers may be used to control symptoms of thyrotoxicosis until the definitive treatment has returned the patient to a euthyroid state. If T_4 replacement is initiated, the goal is to maintain both the free T_4 level and the TSH concentration in the normal range. Once a stable dose of T_4 is identified, the patient may be followed up every 6 to 12 months.

A common, potentially confusing clinical situation should be mentioned. Some patients may have TSH concentrations that continue to be suppressed despite having free T_4 concentrations that become normal or low. For patients with long-standing hyperthyroidism, the pituitary thyrotrophs responsible for making TSH become atrophic. The average amount of time required for these cells to resume normal functioning is 6 to 8 weeks. Therefore, if a thyrotoxic patient has his or her free T_4 concentration lowered rapidly, before the thyrotrophs resume normal function, a period of "transient central hypothyroidism" will be observed. In addition, autoimmune mechanisms may also play a role, with a slower TSH recovery in patients with higher titers of thyroid-binding inhibitory immunoglobulins.

EPIDEMIOLOGY—HYPOTHYROIDISM

Hypothyroidism is defined as the clinical and biochemical syndrome resulting from decreased thyroid hormone production.[56] Overt hypothyroidism occurs in 1.5% to 2% of women and 0.2% of men, and its incidence increases with age. In the Third National Health and Nutrition Examination Survey (NHANES III), levels of serum TSH and total T_4 were measured in a representative sample of adolescents and adults (age 12 or older). Among 16,533 people who neither were taking thyroid medication nor reported histories of thyroid disease, 3.9% had subclinical hypothyroidism (serum TSH more than 4.5 milli-international units/L, and T_4 normal), and 0.2% had "clinically significant" hypothyroidism (TSH more than 4.5 milli-international units/L, and T_4 less than 4.5 mcg/dL).[10]

ETIOLOGY—HYPOTHYROIDISM

The vast majority of patients have primary hypothyroidism due to thyroid gland failure due to chronic autoimmune thyroiditis. Special populations with higher risk of developing hypothyroidism include postpartum women, individuals with a family history of autoimmune thyroid disorders and patients with previous head and neck or thyroid irradiation or surgery, other autoimmune endocrine conditions (eg, type 1 diabetes mellitus, adrenal insufficiency, and ovarian failure), some other nonendocrine autoimmune disorders (eg, celiac disease, vitiligo, pernicious anemia, Sjögren's syndrome, and multiple sclerosis), primary pulmonary hypertension, and Down's and Turner's syndromes. Secondary hypothyroidism due to pituitary failure is uncommon but should be suspected in a patient with decreased levels of T_4 and inappropriately normal or low TSH levels. Most patients with secondary hypothyroidism due to inadequate TSH production will have clinical signs of more generalized pituitary insufficiency, such as abnormal menses and decreased libido, or evidence of a pituitary adenoma, such as visual field defects, galactorrhea, or acromegaloid features, but isolated TSH deficiency can be congenital or acquired as a result of autoimmune hypophysitis.[57] Generalized (peripheral and central) resistance to thyroid hormone is extremely rare.

PATHOPHYSIOLOGY—HYPOTHYROIDISM

Table 75-8 outlines the causes of hypothyroidism. These causes fall into two broad categories involving dysfunction of the thyroid gland itself, or dysfunction at the level of the pituitary or hypothalamus.

Chronic Autoimmune Thyroiditis

7 Autoimmune thyroiditis (Hashimoto's disease) is the most common cause of spontaneous hypothyroidism in the adult.[56] Patients may present either with goitrous thyroid gland enlargement and mild hypothyroidism or with thyroid gland atrophy and more severe thyroid hormone deficiency. Both forms of autoimmune thyroiditis probably result from cell- and antibody-mediated thyroid injury. The bulk of evidence suggests that the presence of specific defects in suppressor T-lymphocyte function leads to the survival of a randomly mutating clone of helper T lymphocytes, which are directed against

TABLE 75-8 Causes of Hypothyroidism

Primary hypothyroidism
Hashimoto's disease
Iatrogenic hypothyroidism
Less Common:
- Iodine deficiency
- Enzyme defects
- Thyroid hypoplasia
- Goitrogens

Secondary hypothyroidism
Pituitary disease
Hypothalamic disease

normally occurring antigens on the thyroid membrane. Once these T lymphocytes interact with thyroid membrane antigen, B lymphocytes are stimulated to produce thyroid antibodies.[58]

Antithyroid peroxidase (antimicrosomal) antibodies are present in virtually all patients with Hashimoto's thyroiditis and appear to be directed against the enzyme thyroid peroxidase.[59] These antibodies are capable of fixing complement and inducing cytotoxic changes in thyroid cells. Antibodies that are capable of stimulating thyroid growth through interaction with the TSH receptor may occasionally be found particularly in goitrous hypothyroidism; conversely, antibodies that inhibit the trophic effects of TSH may be present in the atrophic type.

Iatrogenic Hypothyroidism

Iatrogenic hypothyroidism follows exposure to destructive amounts of radiation (radioiodine or external radiation) or surgery. Hypothyroidism occurs within 3 months to a year after ^{131}I therapy in most patients treated for Graves' disease. Thereafter, it occurs at a rate of approximately 2.5% each year. External radiation therapy to the region of the thyroid using doses of greater than 2,500 centigray (cGy) for therapy of neck carcinoma also causes hypothyroidism. This effect is dose dependent, and more than 50% of patients who receive more than 4,000 cGy to the thyroid bed develop hypothyroidism. Total thyroidectomy causes hypothyroidism within 1 month. Excessive doses of thionamides used to treat hyperthyroidism can also cause iatrogenic hypothyroidism.

Other Causes of Primary Hypothyroidism

Iodine deficiency, enzymatic defects within the thyroid gland, thyroid hypoplasia, and maternal ingestion of goitrogens during fetal development may cause cretinism. Early recognition and treatment of the resultant thyroid hormone deficiency is essential for optimal mental development.[60] Large-scale neonatal screening programs in North America, Europe, Japan, and Australia are now in place.[61] The frequency of congenital hypothyroidism in North America and Europe is 1 per 3,500 to 4,000 live births. In the United States, there are racial differences in the incidence of congenital hypothyroidism, with whites being affected seven times as frequently as blacks.

In the adult, hypothyroidism is rarely caused by iodine deficiency and goitrogens. Iodine ingestion in the form of expectorants can lead to hypothyroidism. In sensitive persons (particularly those with autoimmune thyroiditis), the iodide blocks the synthesis of thyroid hormone, leading to an increased secretion of TSH and thyroid enlargement. Thus, both iodine excess and iodine deficiency can cause decreased secretion of thyroid hormone. An example of a goitrogen that can induce hypothyroidism is raw bok choy.[62] Several medications can cause hypothyroidism, including lithium, amiodarone, interferon-alfa, interleukin-2, tyrosine kinase inhibitors, and perchlorate.

Pituitary Disease

Thyroid-stimulating hormone is required for normal thyroid secretion. Thyroid atrophy and decreased thyroid secretion follow pituitary failure. Pituitary insufficiency may be caused by destruction of thyrotrophs by either functioning or nonfunctioning pituitary tumors, surgical therapy, external pituitary radiation, postpartum pituitary necrosis (Sheehan's syndrome), trauma, and infiltrative processes of the pituitary such as metastatic tumors, tuberculosis, histiocytosis, and autoimmune mechanisms.[63,64] In all these situations, TSH deficiency most often occurs in association with other pituitary hormone deficiencies. The identification of secondary hypothyroidism due to bexarotene use has led to recognition of the role of rexinoids and retinoids to cause dysregulation of TSH production.[65,66]

Note that pituitary enlargement in hypothyroidism does not invariably indicate the presence of a primary pituitary tumor. Pituitary enlargement is seen in patients with severe primary hypothyroidism due to compensatory hyperplasia and hypertrophy of the thyrotrophs.[67] With thyroid hormone replacement therapy, serum TSH concentrations decline, indicating that the TSH secretion is not autonomous, and the pituitary resumes a more normal configuration. These patients are easily separated from patients with primary pituitary failure by measuring a TSH level.

Hypothalamic Hypothyroidism

Thyrotropin-releasing hormone deficiency also causes a rare form of central hypothyroidism. In both adults and children it may occur

CLINICAL PRESENTATION

General

- Hypothyroidism can lead to a variety of end-organ effects with a wide range of disease severity, from entirely asymptomatic individuals to patients in coma with multisystem failure. In the adult, manifestations of hypothyroidism are varied and nonspecific. In the child, thyroid hormone deficiency may manifest as growth or intellectual retardation.

Symptoms

- Common symptoms of hypothyroidism include dry skin, cold intolerance, weight gain, constipation, and weakness. Complaints of lethargy, depression, fatigue, exercise intolerance, or loss of ambition and energy are also common but are less specific. Muscle cramps, myalgia, and stiffness are frequent complaints of hypothyroid patients. Menorrhagia and infertility may present commonly in women.

Signs

- Objective weakness is common, with proximal muscles being affected more than distal muscles. Slow relaxation of deep tendon reflexes is common. The most common signs of decreased levels of thyroid hormone include coarse skin and hair, cold or dry skin, periorbital puffiness, and bradycardia. Speech is often slow and the voice may be hoarse. Reversible neurologic syndromes such as carpal tunnel syndrome, polyneuropathy, and cerebellar dysfunction may also occur. Galactorrhea may be found in women.

Diagnosis

- In primary hypothyroidism, TSH serum concentration should be elevated. In secondary hypothyroidism, TSH levels may be within or below the reference range; when TSH bioactivity is altered, the levels reported by immunoassay may even be elevated.
- Free and/or total T_4 and T_3 serum concentrations should be low.

Other Tests

- TPOAbs and anti-TG antibodies are likely to be elevated in autoimmune thyroiditis.

as a result of cranial irradiation, trauma, infiltrative diseases, or neoplastic diseases.

CLINICAL PRESENTATION—HYPOTHYROIDISM

Thyroid hormone is essential for normal growth and development during embryonic life. Uncorrected thyroid hormone deficiency during fetal and neonatal development results in mental retardation and/or cretinism. Both in children and adults, there is slowing of physical and mental activity, as well as of cardiovascular, gastrointestinal, and neuromuscular function.

A rise in the TSH level is the first evidence of primary hypothyroidism. Many patients will have a free T_4 level within the normal range (compensated or subclinical hypothyroidism) with few, if any, symptoms of hypothyroidism. As the disease progresses, the free T_4 concentration will drop below the normal level. Interestingly, because of TSH stimulation, thyroidal production will shift toward greater amounts of T_3, and thus T_3 concentrations will often be maintained in the normal range in spite of a low T_4. As the hypothyroidism continues to progress, the T_3 concentration will eventually become low too. The RAIU is not a useful test in the evaluation of a hypothyroid patient, as it may be low, normal, or even elevated. For most hypothyroid patients with pituitary disease, serum TSH concentrations are generally low or normal. A serum TSH concentration in the normal range is clearly inappropriate if the patient's T_4 is low.

TREATMENT
Hypothyroidism

Most cases of hypothyroidism result from progressive and permanent damage to the thyroid gland. Replacement of thyroid hormone is the cornerstone of treatment.

Desired Outcomes

The goals of therapy are to restore normal thyroid hormone concentrations in tissue, provide symptomatic relief, prevent neurologic deficits in newborns and children, and reverse the biochemical abnormalities of hypothyroidism.

General Approach to Treatment

8 Levothyroxine (L-thyroxine, T_4) is considered to be drug of choice for treatment of hypothyroidism (Table 75-9).[21,68] Other commercially available thyroid preparations can be obtained but are not considered preferred therapy. Available thyroid preparations are synthetic (L-thyroxine, liothyronine, and liotrix) or natural in origin (ie, desiccated thyroid). The preparations containing both T_4 and T_3 (liotrix, desiccated thyroid) have relatively high proportions of T_3 and may cause thyrotoxicosis.[21,69] Liothyronine is a short-acting preparation that requires dosing multiple times a day in order to achieve stable hormone concentrations.[70] The availability of sensitive and specific assays for total and free hormone levels as well as TSH now allows precise dose titration to allow adequate replacement without inadvertent overdose. The response of TSH to TRH had been advocated for use by some in order to "fine tune" thyroid replacement, but this is not necessary if the third-generation chemiluminometric assays for TSH, which have detection limits of about 0.01 milli-international unit/L, are used. Clinical guidelines for the management of hypothyroidism have been published by the American Thyroid Association and the American Association of Clinical Endocrinologists in 2012.[68] More recent guidelines (2014) sponsored by the American Thyroid Association provide specific treatment recommendations and critically examine the use of combination therapy with T_4 and T_3[21] (Table 75-10).

Pharmacologic Therapy

Levothyroxine is the drug of choice for thyroid replacement and suppressive therapy because it is chemically stable, relatively inexpensive, active when orally administered, free of antigenicity, and has uniform potency. Whereas T_3 is the biologically more active form of thyroid hormone, levothyroxine administration results in a pool of thyroid hormone that is readily and consistently converted to T_3; in this regard, levothyroxine may be thought of as a prohormone. The ability of levothyroxine to achieve normal T_3 concentrations was illustrated in a study of recently athyreotic patients in whom levothyroxine monotherapy produced similar T_3 levels to those documented prior to the patient's thyroidectomy.[71] Several other studies, however, suggest that athyreotic individuals taking T_4 may have low or low-normal T_3 levels.[72-74]

Liothyronine (T_3) is chemically pure with known potency and has a shorter half-life of 1.5 days. Although it can be used diagnostically in the T_3 suppression test, T_3 has some clinical disadvantages, including a higher incidence of cardiac adverse effects, higher cost, and difficulty in monitoring with conventional laboratory tests. If used, T_3 needs to be administered three times a day and it may take a prolonged period of adjustment to achieve stable euthyroidism.[70] Liotrix is a combination of synthetic T_4 and T_3 in a 4:1 ratio. It is chemically stable and pure and has a predictable potency. The major limitations to this product are high cost and lack of therapeutic rationale, because most T_3 is peripherally converted from T_4. In addition, the T_4:T_3 ratio is much higher than the 14:1 molar ratio produced by the thyroid gland in humans.

9 Trials comparing levothyroxine alone with a combination of levothyroxine plus partial replacement with liothyronine (T_3) have

TABLE 75-9 Thyroid Preparations Used in the Treatment of Hypothyroidism

Drug/Dosage Form	Content	Relative Dose	Comments/Equivalency
Thyroid USP Armour Thyroid, Nature-Throid, and Westhroid (T_4:T_3 ratio approximately 4.2:1); Armour, 1 grain = 60 mg; Nature-Throid and Westhroid, 1 grain = 65 mg. Doses include 1/4, 1/2, 1, 2, 3, 4, and 5 grain tablets	Desiccated pork thyroid gland	1 grain (equivalent to 74 mcg [~60-100] mcg of T_4)	High T_3:T_4 ratio; inexpensive
Levothyroxine Synthroid, Levothroid, Levoxyl, Levo-T, Unithroid, and other generics 25, 50, 75, 88, 100, 112, 125, 137, 150, 175, 200, 300 mcg tablets; Tirosint 13-150 mcg liquid in gelatin capsule; 200 and 500 mcg per vial injection	Synthetic T_4	100 mcg	Stable; predictable potency; generics may be bioequivalent; when switching from natural thyroid to L-thyroxine, lower dose by one half grain; variable absorption between products; half-life = 7 days, so daily dosing; considered to be drug of choice
Liothyronine Cytomel 5, 25, and 50 mcg tablets	Synthetic T_3	33 mcg (~equivalent to 100 mcg T_4)	Uniform absorption, rapid onset; half-life = 1.5 days, rapid peak and troughs
Liotrix Thyrolar 1/4-, 1/2-, 1-, 2-, and 3-grain tablets	Synthetic T_4:T_3 in 4:1 ratio	Thyrolar 1 = 50 mcg T_4 and 12.5 mcg T_3	Stable; predictable; expensive; risk of T_3 thyrotoxicosis because of high ratio of T_3 relative to T_4

TABLE 75-10 Selected Recommendations from the American Thyroid Association Hypothyroidism Guidelines[21]

Recommendation Number	Question	Synopsis or Paraphrase of Recommendation	Grading
1a	Is levothyroxine monotherapy considered to be the standard of care for hypothyroidism?	Levothyroxine is recommended as the preparation of choice for the treatment of hypothyroidism due to its efficacy in resolving the symptoms of hypothyroidism.	Strong recommendation, moderate quality
1b	What are the clinical and biochemical goals for levothyroxine replacement in primary hypothyroidism?	Levothyroxine replacement therapy has three main goals. These are (i) to provide resolution of the patients' symptoms and hypothyroid signs, (ii) to achieve normalization of serum thyrotropin and, (iii) to avoid overtreatment.	Strong recommendation, moderate quality
2b	Are there situations in which therapy with levothyroxine dissolved in glycerin and supplied in gelatin capsules may have advantages over standard levothyroxine?	Although there are preliminary small studies suggesting that levothyroxine dissolved in glycerin and supplied in gelatin capsules may be better absorbed than standard levothyroxine, the present lack of controlled long-term outcome studies does not support a recommendation for the use of such preparations in these circumstances.	Weak recommendation, low quality
4a	What factors determine the levothyroxine dose required by a hypothyroid patient for reaching the appropriate serum thyrotropin goal?	When deciding on a starting dose of levothyroxine, the patient's weight, lean body mass, pregnancy status, etiology of hypothyroidism, degree of thyrotropin elevation, age, and general clinical context, should all be considered.	Strong recommendation, moderate quality
4b	What is the best approach to initiating and adjusting levothyroxine therapy?	Thyroid hormone therapy should be initiated as an initial full replacement or as partial replacement with gradual increments in the dose titrated upward using serum thyrotropin as the goal. Dose adjustments should be made, with thyrotropin assessment 4-6 weeks after any dosage change.	Strong recommendation, moderate quality
9b	What approach should be taken in patients treated for hypothyroidism who have normal serum thyrotropin values but still have unresolved symptoms?	A minority of patients with hypothyroidism, but normal serum thyrotropin values, may perceive a suboptimal health status of unclear etiology. Acknowledgment of the patients' symptoms and evaluation for alternative causes is recommended in such cases.	Weak recommendation, low quality
12	In adults requiring thyroid hormone replacement treatment for primary hypothyroidism, is treatment with thyroid extracts superior to treatment with levothyroxine alone?	We recommend that levothyroxine be considered as routine care for patients with primary hypothyroidism, in preference to use of thyroid extracts. High-quality controlled long-term outcome data are lacking to document superiority of this treatment compared to levothyroxine therapy.	Strong recommendation, moderate quality
13b	In adults requiring thyroid hormone replacement treatment for primary hypothyroidism, is combination treatment including levothyroxine and liothyronine superior to the use of levothyroxine alone?	There is no consistently strong evidence of superiority of combination therapy over monotherapy with levothyroxine. Therefore, we recommend against the routine use of combination treatment with levothyroxine and liothyronine as a form of thyroid replacement therapy in patients with primary hypothyroidism.	Weak recommendation, moderate quality
13c	In adults requiring thyroid hormone replacement treatment for primary hypothyroidism who feel unwell while taking levothyroxine, is combination treatment including levothyroxine and liothyronine superior to the use of levothyroxine alone?	For patients with primary hypothyroidism who feel unwell on levothyroxine therapy alone, there is currently insufficient evidence to support the routine use of a trial of a combination of levothyroxine and liothyronine therapy outside a formal clinical trial or N- of-1 trial, due to uncertainty in long-term risk benefit ratio of the treatment.	Insufficient evidence
14	Are there data regarding therapy with triiodothyronine alone, either as standard liothyronine or as sustained release triiodothyronine, that support the use of triiodothyronine therapy alone for the treatment of hypothyroidism?	Although short-term outcome data in hypothyroid patients suggest that thrice-daily synthetic liothyronine may be associated with beneficial effects on parameters such as weight and lipids, longer-term controlled clinical trials are needed before considering synthetic liothyronine therapy for routine clinical use.	Strong recommendation, moderate quality

Strong recommendation: Benefits clearly outweigh risks and burden or risks and burden clearly outweigh benefits.

Weak recommendation: Benefits finely balanced with risks and burden.

Quality of evidence: High, moderate, or low.

generally shown that combinations of T_4 + T_3 are no better than T_4 alone. At least 13 such trials with varying designs have been performed to date.[21] Four of these trials have found that patients expressed a preference for combination therapy. By way of illustration, in one trial of combination therapy, Clyde et al.[75] compared levothyroxine alone for treatment of primary hypothyroidism with combination therapy using levothyroxine plus liothyronine. These investigators demonstrated no beneficial changes in body weight, serum lipid levels, hypothyroid symptoms as measured by a health-related quality-of-life questionnaire, and standard measures of cognitive performance.[75] As discussed in recent guidelines,[21] three meta-analyses and a systematic review have also suggested no benefits.[76-79] A secondary analysis, however, suggested that individuals harboring a specific deiodinase polymorphism may have a poorer psychological response to levothyroxine therapy and a better response to combination therapy with both T_4 and T_3. However, no prospective study investigating whether the presence of these polymorphisms affects satisfaction with replacement therapy has yet been reported.[80]

A recent study conducted in rats suggested impairment of type 2 deiodinase activity in the whole body during levothyroxine monotherapy due to deiodinase inactivation, compared with maintenance of deiodinase activity in the hypothalamus.[81] The lesser activation in the hypothalamus lead to efficient T_3 production in the hypothalamus and normalization of TSH before T_3 normalized in the rest of the body. Accompanying the inactivation of type 2 deiodinase in other tissues, lower serum T_3 and higher T_4/T_3 ratios were seen in rats during monotherapy with L-thyroxine, compared with combination therapy employing a subcutaneous slow release T_3 pellet. Clinical trials of a slow release T_3 preparation, other than a pharmacokinetic study of T_3 sulfate in profoundly hypothyroid individuals,[82] has yet to be conducted.

Desiccated thyroid has historically been derived from pig, beef, or sheep thyroid glands, although pigs are currently the usual source. The *United States Pharmacopeia*, requires thyroid USP to contain 38 mcg (±15%) of L-thyroxine and 9 mcg (±10%) of liothyronine for each 60 to 65 mg (one grain). Thyroid USP, as an animal protein-derived product, may be antigenic in allergic or sensitive patients. Even though desiccated thyroid is inexpensive, its limitations preclude it from being considered as a drug of choice for hypothyroid patients.

Hypothyroidism—**Controversy...**

A small percentage of patient taking levothyroxine do not feel well despite their treatment. Trials of combination therapy have generally not shown improved patient outcomes. Recent animal data examining inactivation of deiodinases in specific tissues suggest that sustained delivery of T_3 may have different tissue effects, compared with intermittent delivery of T_3. Future trials of a sustained release T_3 preparation are eagerly awaited.

Pharmacokinetics

The half-life of levothyroxine is approximately 7 days. This long half-life is responsible for a stable pool of prohormone and the need for only once-daily dosing with levothyroxine. Older studies with levothyroxine suggested that bioavailability was low and erratic; however, this product has been reformulated, and the average bioavailability improved to approximately 80%.[83] Different levothyroxine preparations contain different excipients such as dyes and fillers. The bioavailabilities of Synthroid, Levoxyl, and generic levothyroxine preparations were compared in a blinded, randomized, four-way crossover trial.[84] The study was sponsored by the manufacturers of Synthroid, who have challenged the authors' conclusions that the levothyroxine preparations are bioequivalent and should be interchangeable for the majority of patients. However, because the relationship between T_4 concentration and TSH is not linear, very small changes in T_4 concentration can lead to substantial changes in TSH, which is a more accurate reflection of hormone replacement status. Currently, the FDA mandates that L-thyroxine bioequivalency testing be done using normal volunteers (600 mcg in the fasted state) and three baseline free T_4 concentrations be used to correct for endogenous T_4 production. Bioequivalency is based on the area under the curve (AUC) and maximum concentration (C_{max}) of T_4 out to 48 hours. Approximately 70% of the AUC is derived from endogenous production. TSH is not considered, and it is now very clear that T_4 is too insensitive as a measure of bioequivalency.[85,86] To avoid overtreatment and undertreatment, once a product is selected, therapeutic interchange should be discouraged. Currently, there are several levothyroxine products available, and a number of permutations for interchange are available considering that there are AB1, AB2, AB3, and AB4 products available, and since no reference listed drug is mandated in bioequivalency testing.

Adverse Effects

Serious untoward effects are unusual if dosing is appropriate and the patient is carefully monitored during initial treatment. A cross-sectional study showed that of a population of 1,525 individuals taking levothyroxine, 40% actually had abnormal TSH values.[87] A recent study showed that 57% of individuals 65 years or older receiving thyroid hormone treatment had abnormal TSH values.[88] Both of these studies suggest failure to keep a patient's TSH at goal is common. Levothyroxine replacement in athyreotic hypothyroid patients restores systolic and diastolic left ventricular performance within 2 weeks, and the use of levothyroxine may increase the frequency of atrial premature beats but not necessarily ventricular premature beats. Excessive doses of thyroid hormone may lead to heart failure, angina pectoris, and myocardial infarction; rarely, the latter may be caused by coronary artery spasm. Allergic or idiosyncratic reactions can occur with the natural animal-derived products such as desiccated thyroid, but these are extremely rare with the synthetic products used today. The 0.05 mg (50 mcg) Synthroid tablet is the least allergenic (due to a lack of dye and few excipients) and should be tried for the patient suspected to be allergic to thyroid hormone tablets.

Hyperremodeling of cortical and trabecular bone due to hyperthyroidism leads to reduced bone density and may increase the risk of fracture. Compared with normal controls, excess exogenous thyroid hormone results in histomorphometric and biochemical changes similar to those observed in osteoporosis and untreated hyperthyroidism.[89,90] The risk for this complication seems to be related to the dose of levothyroxine, patient age, and gender. Markers for bone turnover include urinary *N*-telopeptides, pyridinoline crosslinks of type I collagen, osteocalcin, and bone-specific alkaline phosphatase. When doses of levothyroxine are used to suppress TSH concentrations to below-normal values (eg, less than 0.3 milli-international unit/L) in postmenopausal women, this adverse effect is more likely to be seen. Cortical bone is affected to a greater degree than trabecular bone at suppressive doses of L-thyroxine. In contrast, it appears to be much less likely in men and in premenopausal women. Maintaining the TSH between 0.7 and 1.5 milli-international units/L does not alter bone mineral density in premenopausal women. Although not all studies have shown consistent results, a recent cohort study suggests that there is no adverse effect on bone density with treatment with L-thyroxine to achieve a normal TSH.[91]

Drug-Drug and Drug-Food Interactions

The time to maximal absorption of levothyroxine is about 2 hours and this should be considered when T_4 concentrations are determined. Ingestion of L-thyroxine with food can impair its absorption.[21,92] This can potentially affect the TSH concentration achieved if levothyroxine timing with respect to food is varied.[93] Mucosal diseases, such as celiac sprue, diabetic diarrhea, and ileal bypass surgery, can also reduce absorption. Cholestyramine, calcium carbonate, sucralfate, aluminum hydroxide, ferrous sulfate, soybean formula, dietary fiber supplements, and espresso coffee may also impair the absorption of levothyroxine from the gastrointestinal tract (reviewed extensively in recent treatment of hypothyroidism guidelines[21]). Acid suppression with histamine blockers and proton pump inhibitors may also reduce levothyroxine absorption.[94] Drugs that increase nondeiodinative T_4 clearance include rifampin, carbamazepine, and possibly phenytoin. Selenium deficiency and amiodarone may block the conversion of T_4 to T_3.

Several non-randomized studies have suggested that liquid formulations of levothyroxine or formulations in which the levothyroxine is dissolved in glycerin and encased in a gelatin capsule may circumvent the impaired absorption of levothyroxine that may occur with tablet preparations. For patients receiving enteral feeding, liquid levothyroxine added directly to the feeding tube was associated with a similar serum TSH to that seen in another group of patients in whom the feeding was interrupted in order to administer crushed tablets.[95] The former procedure was found to be more convenient by providers. In a study of patients taking proton pump inhibitors, switching to an oral solution was associated with a decrease in serum TSH from a mean of 5.4 milli-international units/L to 1.7 milli-international units/L, suggesting better absorption of the liquid preparation in these patients.[96] A study of patients with gastritis who had a stable serum TSH while taking levothyroxine tablets and were then switched to a lower dose of levothyroxine gel capsules, showed that two-thirds of patients had a similar TSH on the lower dose, again suggesting better absorption of the gel capsule formulation.[97] Another study suggested that the serum TSH achieved by levothyroxine gel capsules was not affected by the timing with respect to breakfast.[98] If the findings of these studies are bolstered by randomized controlled studies in the future, these levothyroxine formulations may prove very convenient for hypothyroid patients.

10 Dosing and Administration

Recent studies suggest that the average maintenance dose of levothyroxine for most adults is about 125 mcg/day.[56] The replacement dose of levothyroxine is affected by body weight. Estimates of weight-based doses for replacement in hypothyroid patients include 1.6 and 1.7 mcg/kg/day.[21] There is, however, a wide range of replacement doses, necessitating individualized therapy and appropriate TSH monitoring to determine an adequate but not excessive dose.

In addition to alleviation of symptoms, the goal of treatment for patients with hypothyroidism is to maintain the patient's TSH within the normal range. Some clinicians are of the opinion that the traditional reference range of approximately 0.5 to 4.5 milli-international units/L includes at its upper end some individuals who have unrecognized thyroid disease.[99] Thus, some believe that the reference range should be modified downward to 0.5 to 3.5 milli-international units/L or even 0.5 to 2.5 milli-international units/L.[100] If this premise is accepted, both the TSH values that trigger L-thyroxine treatment and the TSH treatment goal could potentially be altered. There are cogent arguments on both sides of the issue. Those who suggest maintaining current reference ranges believe that lowering the upper limit of the reference range could result in treating many individuals with thyroid hormone who would not necessarily benefit from such treatment.[101] Those who favor narrowing the reference range suggest that additional patients would, in fact, derive benefit from thyroid hormone treatment.[100] TSH reference ranges also differ for different populations, such as those who are pregnant, specific ethnic groups, and older individuals.[21]

The required dose of levothyroxine is dependent on the patient's age[102] and the presence of associated disorders, as well as the severity and duration of hypothyroidism.[21] Most patients will require approximately 1.7 mcg/kg/day once they reach steady state for full replacement. Dose requirement may be better estimated based on ideal body weight, rather than actual body weight.[103] In patients with long-standing disease and older individuals without known cardiac disease, therapy should be initiated with 50 mcg daily of levothyroxine and increased after 1 month. The recommended initial daily dose for older patients with known cardiac disease is 25 mcg daily titrated upward in increments of 25 mcg at monthly intervals to prevent stress on the cardiovascular system. Some patients may experience an exacerbation of angina with higher doses of thyroid hormone. Although the TSH is an indicator of underreplacement or overreplacement, clinicians often fail to alter the dose based on TSH values clearly outside of the normal range.

Patients with subclinical or mild hypothyroidism (seen more commonly in the elderly and women) have no or few signs or symptoms, normal serum T_3 and T_4 concentrations, and an elevated basal TSH concentration.[38] The prevalence of this disorder in the NHANES III study was found to be 4.3%.[10] Untreated individuals with moderate degrees of subclinical hypothyroidism and negative TPOAb may revert to euthyroidism during followup.[104] Increased mortality may be associated with moderate, but not mild subclinical hypothyroidism.[105] Spontaneous recovery of thyroid function and uncertainties about which patient groups may benefit from therapy contribute to the debate about treatment of subclinical hypothyroidism. Although the treatment of subclinical hypothyroidism is controversial, patients presenting with marked elevations in TSH (more than 10 milli-international units/L) and high titers of TPOAb or prior treatment with ^{131}I may be most likely to benefit from treatment. It should be noted that some studies find that only one of four treated patients experienced improvement. Other patients who may improve with replacement include those with mild symptoms of hypothyroidism and depression. Reduction of events due to ischemic heart disease was only observed in younger patients in one study.[106] If treatment is pursued, reasonable goals in this situation would be to maintain serum T_4 and T_3 levels in the normal range and reduce TSH to a value of 0.5 to 2.5 milli-international units/L in younger patients and 4 to 6 milli-international units/L in older patients.[38]

Once euthyroidism is attained, the daily maintenance dose of levothyroxine does not fluctuate greatly. As patients age, the dosing requirement may be reduced.[21,102] Third-generation TSH assays improved the accuracy with which thyroid hormone replacement can be monitored. The TSH concentration is the most sensitive and specific monitoring parameter for adjustment of levothyroxine dose. Plasma TSH concentrations begin to fall within hours and are usually normalized within 2 weeks, but they may take up to 6 weeks for some patients, depending on the baseline value. Both TSH and T_4 concentrations are used to monitor therapy, and they should be checked every 6 weeks until a euthyroid state is achieved.[21,68] Laboratory assessment of thyroid function should be performed approximately 6 weeks after levothyroxine dose initiation or change. This time frame allows achievement of steady state, as the half-life of levothyroxine is approximately 1 week. Serum T_4 concentrations can be useful in detecting noncompliance, malabsorption, or changes in levothyroxine product bioequivalence. An elevated TSH concentration indicates insufficient replacement. The appropriate dose maintains the TSH concentration in the normal range. T_4 disposal is accelerated by nephrotic syndrome, other severe systemic illnesses, and several antiseizure medications (phenobarbital, phenytoin, and carbamazepine) and rifampin. Pregnancy increases the T_4 dose requirement for 75% of women, probably because of factors such as increased degradation by the placental deiodinase, increased T_4 pool size, and transfer of T_4 to the fetus. The etiology of hypothyroidism also affects the magnitude of the dosage increase.[107] Initiating postmenopausal hormone replacement therapy increases the dose needed in 35% of women, perhaps due to an increased circulating TBG level. Patient noncompliance with prescribed T_4, the most common cause of inadequate treatment, might be suspected for patients with a dose that is higher than expected, variable thyroid function test results that do not correlate well with prescribed doses, and an elevated serum TSH concentration with serum free T_4 at the upper end of the normal range, which can suggest improved compliance immediately before testing, with a lag in the thyrotropin response.

For patients with central hypothyroidism caused by hypothalamic or pituitary failure, the serum TSH cannot be used to assess adequacy of replacement. Alleviation of the clinical syndrome and restoration of serum T_4 to the normal range are the only criteria available for estimating the appropriate replacement dose of L-thyroxine. Keeping free T_4 values in the upper part of the normal laboratory reference range is a reasonable approach,[108] with modification of this goal to the middle of the normal range in older patients or patients with comorbidities. Concurrent use of dopamine, dopaminergic agents (bromocriptine), somatostatin or somatostatin analogs (octreotide), and corticosteroids suppresses TSH concentrations in individuals with primary hypothyroidism and may confound the interpretation of this monitoring parameter.[21,68]

TSH-suppressive levothyroxine therapy can be given to patients with nodular thyroid disease and diffuse goiter, and to patients with a history of thyroid irradiation. It is also usually given to patients with papillary or follicular thyroid cancer. The rationale for suppression therapy is to reduce TSH secretion, which promotes growth and function of abnormal thyroid tissue. However, such management, other than for patients with thyroid cancer or with elevated TSH levels, is quite controversial. Some clinicians rarely recommend or use such therapy; others will recommend a trial of levothyroxine as suppressive therapy in some patients. Three meta-analyses concluded that suppressive therapy for nodules was associated with a small decrease in nodule growth,[109] a statistically nonsignificant reduction in nodule growth,[110] and a significant reduction in nodule growth with longer-term treatment.[111] L-thyroxine may be given in nontoxic MNG to suppress the TSH to low-normal levels of 0.5 to 1 milli-international unit/L if the baseline TSH is more than 1 milli-international unit/L. Goiter size and thyroid volume may be reduced with suppression therapy. Diffuse goiter associated with autoimmune thyroiditis may also be treated with levothyroxine to reduce goiter size and thyroid volume. If suppressive therapy with levothyroxine is pursued, the age, gender, and menopausal status of the patient need to be considered, along with the risk of cardiac arrhythmias and reduced bone mineral density. Levothyroxine suppression therapy is of benefit to all but the lowest-risk thyroid cancer patients and is generally used in the management of patients with differentiated thyroid cancer, with the TSH goal being influenced by the patient's thyroid cancer stage and other risk factors.[112,113] Current guidelines from the American Thyroid Association suggest suppressing the TSH to below 0.1 milli-international unit/L in higher-risk patients, but keeping TSH around the lower limit of normal (0.1-0.5 milli-international unit/L) in low-risk patients.[114]

Hypothyroidism—**Controversy...**

There is currently controversy about when subclinical thyroid disease should be treated. This is based on uncertainty about benefits and risks with respect to symptom relief, cardiovascular outcomes, and mortality. Generally the decision to treat is affected by patient age, comorbidities, and degree of TSH elevation.

Special Populations

Myxedema Coma

Myxedema coma is a rare consequence of decompensated hypothyroidism.[27,115] Clinical features include hypothermia, advanced stages of hypothyroid symptoms, and altered sensorium ranging from delirium to coma. Mortality rates of 60% to 70% necessitate immediate and aggressive therapy. Traditionally, the initial treatment has been IV bolus levothyroxine 300 to 500 mcg.[21] However, as deiodinase activity is markedly reduced, impairing T_4 to T_3 conversion, initial treatment with IV T_3, or a combination of both hormones has also been advocated.[27] Glucocorticoid therapy with IV hydrocortisone 100 mg every 8 hours should be given until coexisting adrenal suppression is ruled out.[21] All therapies must be administered parenterally as cessation of gastrointestinal peristalsis occurs, preventing absorption of orally administered medications. Consciousness, lowered TSH concentrations, and improvement in vital signs are expected within 24 hours. Maintenance doses of levothyroxine are typically 75 to 100 mcg given IV until the patient stabilizes and oral therapy is begun. Supportive therapy must be instituted to maintain adequate ventilation, blood pressure, and body temperature, and ensure euglycemia. Any underlying disorder, such as sepsis or myocardial infarction, obviously must be diagnosed and treated.

Congenital Hypothyroidism

In congenital hypothyroidism, full maintenance therapy should be instituted early to improve the prognosis for mental and physical development.[116,117] The average maintenance dose in infants and children depends on the age and weight of the child. Several studies demonstrate that aggressive therapy with levothyroxine is important for normal development, and current recommendations are for initiation of therapy as soon as possible after birth at a dose of 10 to 15 mcg/kg/day.[61,118] This dose is used to keep T_4 concentrations at about 10 mcg/dL within 30 days of starting therapy and is associated with improved IQs in treated infants. The dose is progressively decreased to a typical adult dose as the child ages, the adult dose being given in the age range of 11 to 20 years.[118]

Hypothyroidism During Pregnancy

Hypothyroidism during pregnancy leads to an increased rate of stillbirths and possibly lower neuropsychological scores in infants born of women who received inadequate replacement during pregnancy.[50,119] Thyroid hormone is necessary for fetal growth and must come from the maternal side during the first 2 months of gestation. Although liothyronine may cross the placental membrane slightly better than levothyroxine, the latter is considered the drug of choice. The objective of treatment is to decrease TSH to normal, based on the normal reference range for pregnancy. Current guidelines suggest a TSH below 2.5 milli-international units/L during the first trimester and a TSH below 3 milli-international units/L during the remainder of pregnancy.[50,51] Based on elevated TSH levels during pregnancy, it was found in one study that the mean dose of levothyroxine had to be increased by 48% to decrease TSH into the normal range. However, in individual women the dosage increase needed may vary from approximately 10% to 80%. Increased production of binding proteins, a marginal decrease in free hormone concentration, modification of peripheral thyroid hormone metabolism, and increased T_4 metabolism by the fetal-placental unit all may contribute to increased thyroid hormone demand. As these changes regress after delivery the need for increased levothyroxine will decline.[50,51] Up to 60% of women need to have levothyroxine dose adjustment during pregnancy. Upward adjustment will usually be needed by the eighth week of pregnancy. The etiology of the hypothyroidism affects the magnitude of the required increase in levothyroxine dose.[107] After delivery the levothyroxine dose can be reduced based on T_4 concentrations and measurement of TSH, typically about 6 to 8 weeks after delivery. Many patients can return to their pre-pregnancy dose requirement.

EVALUATION OF THERAPEUTIC OUTCOMES—HYPOTHYROIDISM

Patients with idiopathic hypothyroidism and Hashimoto's thyroiditis on optimal thyroid hormone replacement therapy should have TSH and free T_4 serum concentrations in the normal range.[21] Those who are being treated for thyroid cancer should have TSH suppressed to low levels, with the appropriate TSH concentration being determined based on the patient's risk of recurrence or progression, and TG should be undetectable.[119] Given the half-life of T_4 of 7 days, the appropriate monitoring interval is no more often than 4 weeks. The signs and symptoms of hypothyroidism should be improved or absent (see Clinical Presentation of Hypothyroidism discussed earlier), although it may take several months for the full benefit of therapy to manifest.

CONCLUSION—HYPOTHYROIDISM

Untreated hypothyroidism is a devastating disease that if unrecognized eventually progresses into myxedema coma in the absence of any endogenous thyroid reserve. Levothyroxine is a readily available and efficacious hormone that rapidly reverses the biochemical and clinical abnormalities that characterize hypothyroidism. Serum TSH and thyroid hormone levels are useful measures for adjusting the levothyroxine dose during therapy. Until regeneration of thyroid cells from pluripotent stem cells has been fully realized, levothyroxine is the most effective treatment for this common disorder.

ABBREVIATIONS

AUC	area under the curve
cGy	centigray
C_{max}	maximum concentration
ClO_4^-	perchlorate
DIT	diiodotyrosine
FSH	follicle-stimulating hormone
$G_s\alpha$	the α subunit of the stimulatory guanine-nucleotide–binding protein
hCG	human chorionic gonadotropin
HLA	human leukocyte antigen
^{131}I	sodium iodide-131
L-thyroxine	levothyroxine
LH	luteinizing hormone
MIT	monoiodotyrosine
MMI	methimazole
MNG	multinodular goiter
NHANES III	Third National Health and Nutrition Examination Survey
PRTH	pituitary resistance to thyroid hormone
PTU	propylthiouracil
RAI	radioactive iodine
RAIU	radioactive iodine uptake
SCN^-	thiocyanate
SSKI	saturated solution of potassium iodide
T_3	triiodothyronine
T_4	thyroxine
TBG	thyroxine-binding globulin
TBPA	thyroid-binding prealbumin
TcO_4^-	pertechnetate
TG	thyroglobulin
TPOAb	thyroid peroxidase antibodies
TR	thyroid hormone receptor
TRH	thyrotropin-releasing hormone
TRIAC	triiodothyroacetic acid
TSAb	thyroid-stimulating antibody
TSH	thyroid-stimulating hormone
TTR	transthyretin
WBC	white blood cell

REFERENCES

1. Portulano C, Paroder-Belenitsky M, Carrasco N. The Na^+/I^- symporter (NIS): Mechanism and medical impact. *Endocr Rev* 2014;35(1):106-149.
2. Obregon MJ, Escobar del Rey F, Morreale de Escobar G. The effects of iodine deficiency on thyroid hormone deiodination. *Thyroid* 2005;15(8):917-929.
3. Verloop H, Dekkers OM, Peeters RP, Schoones JW, Smit JW. Genetics in endocrinology: Genetic variation in deiodinases: a systematic review of potential clinical effects in humans. *Eur J Endocrinol* 2014;171(3):R123-135.
4. Piehl S, Hoefig CS, Scanlan TS, Kohrle J. Thyronamines—past, present, and future. *Endocr Rev* 2011;32(1):64-80.
5. Kleinau G, Neumann S, Gruters A, Krude H, Biebermann H. Novel insights on thyroid-stimulating hormone receptor signal transduction. *Endocr Rev* 2013;34(5):691-724.
6. Kleinau G, Biebermann H. Constitutive activities in the thyrotropin receptor: Regulation and significance. *Adv Pharmacol* 2014;70: 81-119.
7. Brent GA. Mechanisms of thyroid hormone action. *J Clin Invest* 2012;122(9):3035-3043.
8. Malm J, Farnegardh M, Grover GJ, Ladenson PW. Thyroid hormone antagonists: Potential medical applications and structure activity relationships. *Curr Med Chem* 2009;16(25):3258-3266.
9. Bahn RS, Burch HB, Cooper DS, et al. Hyperthyroidism and other causes of thyrotoxicosis: Management guidelines of the American Thyroid Association and American Association of Clinical Endocrinologists. *Endocr Pract* 2011;17(3):456-520.
10. Hollowell JG, Staehling NW, Flanders WD, et al. Serum TSH, T(4), and thyroid antibodies in the United States population (1988 to 1994): National Health and Nutrition Examination Survey (NHANES III). *J Clin Endocrinol Metab* 2002;87(2):489-499.
11. Beck-Peccoz P, Persani L, Mannavola D, Campi I. Pituitary tumours: TSH-secreting adenomas. *Best Pract Res Clin Endocrinol Metab* 2009;23(5):597-606.
12. Burch HB, Cooper DS. A young woman with palpitations, goitre and low thyroid-stimulating hormone. *CMAJ* 2014;186(4):289-291.
13. Brix TH, Kyvik KO, Christensen K, Hegedus L. Evidence for a major role of heredity in Graves' disease: A population-based study of two Danish twin cohorts. *J Clin Endocrinol Metab* 2001;86(2): 930-934.
14. Ban Y, Concepcion ES, Villanueva R, Greenberg DA, Davies TF, Tomer Y. Analysis of immune regulatory genes in familial and sporadic Graves' disease. *J Clin Endocrinol Metab* 2004;89(9): 4562-4568.
15. Hasham A, Tomer Y. Genetic and epigenetic mechanisms in thyroid autoimmunity. *Immunol Res* 2012;54(1-3):204-213.
16. Vijayakumar A, Ashwath G, Thimmappa D. Thyrotoxic periodic paralysis: Clinical challenges. *J Thyroid Res* 2014;2014:649502.
17. Ryan DP, da Silva MR, Soong TW, et al. Mutations in potassium channel Kir2.6 cause susceptibility to thyrotoxic hypokalemic periodic paralysis. *Cell* 2010;140(1):88-98.
18. Ryodi E, Metso S, Jaatinen P, et al. Cancer incidence and mortality in patients treated with RAI or thyroidectomy for hyperthyroidism—a nation-wide cohort study with a long-term follow-up. *J Clin Endocrinol Metab* 2015;100(10):3710-3717.
19. Goichot B, Caron P, Landron F, Bouee S. Clinical presentation of hyperthyroidism in a large representative sample of outpatients in France: Relationships with age, aetiology and hormonal parameters. *Clin Endocrinol (Oxf)* 2016;84(3):445-451.
20. Samuels MH. Subacute, silent, and postpartum thyroiditis. *Med Clinics North Am* 2012;96(2):223-233.
21. Jonklaas J, Bianco AC, Bauer AJ, et al. Guidelines for the treatment of hypothyroidism: Prepared by the american thyroid association task force on thyroid hormone replacement. *Thyroid* 2014;24(12):1670-1751.
22. Hedberg CW, Fishbein DB, Janssen RS, et al. An outbreak of thyrotoxicosis caused by the consumption of bovine thyroid gland in ground beef. *N Engl J Med* 1987;316(16):993-998.
23. Kinney JS, Hurwitz ES, Fishbein DB, et al. Community outbreak of thyrotoxicosis: Epidemiology, immunogenetic characteristics, and long-term outcome. *Am J Med* 1988;84(1):10-18.
24. Conrey EJ, Lindner C, Estivariz C, et al. Thyrotoxicosis outbreak linked to consumption of minced beef and chorizo: Minas, Uruguay, 2003-2004. *Public Health* 2008;122(11):1264-1274.
25. Cohen-Lehman J, Charitou MM, Klein I. Tiratricol-induced periodic paralysis: A review of nutraceuticals affecting thyroid function. *Endocr Pract* 2011;17(4):610-615.
26. Basaria S, Cooper DS. Amiodarone and the thyroid. *Am J Med* 2005;118(7):706-714.
27. Klubo-Gwiezdzinska J, Wartofsky L. Thyroid emergencies. *Med Clin North Am* 2012;96(2):385-403.

28. Sundaresh V, Brito JP, Wang Z, et al. Comparative effectiveness of therapies for Graves' hyperthyroidism: A systematic review and network meta-analysis. *J Clin Endocrinol Metab* 2013;98(9): 3671-3677.
29. Abraham P, Avenell A, McGeoch SC, Clark LF, Bevan JS. Antithyroid drug regimen for treating Graves' hyperthyroidism. *Cochrane Database Syst Rev* 2010(1):CD003420.
30. Zambudio AR, Rodriguez J, Riquelme J, Soria T, Canteras M, Parrilla P. Prospective study of postoperative complications after total thyroidectomy for multinodular goiters by surgeons with experience in endocrine surgery (see comment). *Ann Surg* 2004;240(1):18-25.
31. In H, Pearce EN, Wong AK, Burgess JF, McAneny DB, Rosen JE. Treatment options for Graves disease: A cost-effectiveness analysis. *J Am Coll Surg* 2009;209(2):170-179.e1-2.
32. Cooper D. Drug therapy: Antithyroid drugs. *New Engl J Med* 2005;352(9):905-917.
33. Cooper DS. Hyperthyroidism. *Lancet* 2003;362(9382):459-468.
34. Momotani N, Noh JY, Ishikawa N, Ito K. Effects of propylthiouracil and methimazole on fetal thyroid status in mothers with Graves' hyperthyroidism. *J Endocrinol Metab* 1997;82(11):3633-3636.
35. Raber W, Kmen E, Waldhausl W, Vierhapper H. Medical therapy of Graves' disease: Effect on remission rates of methimazole alone and in combination with triiodothyronine. *Eur J Endocrinol* 2000;142(2):117-124.
36. Giuliani C, Cerrone D, Harii N, et al. A TSHR-LH/CGR chimera that measures functional thyroid-stimulating autoantibodies (TSAb) can predict remission or recurrence in Graves' patients undergoing antithyroid drug (ATD) treatment. *J Clin Endocrinol Metab* 2012;97(7):E1080-1087.
37. Hashizume K, Ichikawa K, Sakurai A, et al. Administration of thyroxine in treated Graves' disease. Effects on the level of antibodies to thyroid-stimulating hormone receptors and on the risk of recurrence of hyperthyroidism. *N Engl J Med* 1991;324(14):947-953.
38. Cooper DS, Biondi B. Subclinical thyroid disease. *Lancet* 2012;379(9821):1142-1154.
39. Takata K, Kubota S, Fukata S, et al. Methimazole-induced agranulocytosis in patients with Graves' disease is more frequent with an initial dose of 30 mg daily than with 15 mg daily. *Thyroid* 2009;19(6):559-63.
40. Foulds N, Walpole I, Elmslie F, Mansour S. Carbimazole embryopathy: An emerging phenotype. *Am J Med Genet Part A* 2005;132A(2):130-135.
41. Di Gianantonio E, Schaefer C, Mastroiacovo PP, et al. Adverse effects of prenatal methimazole exposure. *Teratology* 2001;64(5):262-266.
42. Andersen SL, Olsen J, Wu CS, Laurberg P. Birth defects after early pregnancy use of antithyroid drugs: A Danish nationwide study. *J Clin Endocrinol Metab* 2013;98(11):4373-4381.
43. Bahn RS, Burch HS, Cooper DS, et al. The Role of Propylthiouracil in the Management of Graves' Disease in Adults: Report of a meeting jointly sponsored by the American Thyroid Association and the Food and Drug Administration. *Thyroid* 2009;19(7):673-674.
44. Glinoer D, Cooper DS. The propylthiouracil dilemma. *Curr Opin Endocrinol Diabetes Obes* 2012;19(5):402-407.
45. Cooper DS, Rivkees SA. Putting propylthiouracil in perspective. *J Clin Endocrinol Metab* 2009;94(6):1881-1882.
46. Bogazzi F, Giovannetti C, Fessehatsion R, et al. Impact of lithium on efficacy of radioactive iodine therapy for Graves' disease: A cohort study on cure rate, time to cure, and frequency of increased serum thyroxine after antithyroid drug withdrawal. *J Clin Endocrinol Metab* 2010;95(1):201-208.
47. Bartalena L, Marcocci C, Bogazzi F, et al. Relation between therapy for hyperthyroidism and the course of Graves' ophthalmopathy. *N Engl J of Med* 1998;338(2):73-78.
48. Boelaert K, Syed AA, Manji N, et al. Prediction of cure and risk of hypothyroidism in patients receiving 131I for hyperthyroidism. *Clin Endocrinol* 2009;70(1):129-138.
49. Franklyn JA, Maisonneuve P, Sheppard M, Betteridge J, Boyle P. Cancer incidence and mortality after radioiodine treatment for hyperthyroidism: A population-based cohort study. *Lancet* 1999;353(9170):2111-2115.
50. Stagnaro-Green A, Abalovich M, Alexander E, et al. Guidelines of the American Thyroid Association for the diagnosis and management of thyroid disease during pregnancy and postpartum. *Thyroid* 2011;21(10):1081-1125.
51. De Groot L, Abalovich M, Alexander EK, et al. Management of thyroid dysfunction during pregnancy and postpartum: An Endocrine Society clinical practice guideline. *J Clin Endocrinol Metab* 2012;97(8):2543-2565.
52. Rotondi M, Cappelli C, Pirali B, et al. The effect of pregnancy on subsequent relapse from Graves' disease after a successful course of antithyroid drug therapy. *J Clin Endocrinol Metab* 2008;93(10):3985-3988.
53. Segni M, Leonardi E, Mazzoncini B, Pucarelli I, Pasquino AM. Special features of Graves' disease in early childhood. *Thyroid* 1999;9(9):871-877.
54. Akamizu T, Satoh T, Isozaki O, et al. Diagnostic criteria, clinical features, and incidence of thyroid storm based on nationwide surveys. *Thyroid* 2012;22(7):661-679.
55. Duggal J, Singh S, Kuchinic P, Butler P, Arora R. Utility of esmolol in thyroid crisis. *Can J Clin Pharmacol* 2006;13(3):e292-295.
56. Roberts CG, Ladenson PW. Hypothyroidism. *Lancet* 2004;363(9411):793-803.
57. LaFranchi S. Thyroid hormone in hypopituitarism, Graves' disease, congenital hypothyroidism, and maternal thyroid disease during pregnancy. *Growth Horm IGF Res* 2006;16(Suppl A):S20-24.
58. Sinclair D. Clinical and laboratory aspects of thyroid autoantibodies. *Ann Clin Biochem* 2006;43(Pt 3):173-183.
59. Stassi G, De Maria R. Autoimmune thyroid disease: New models of cell death in autoimmunity. *Nat Rev Immunol* 2002;2(3):195-204.
60. de Escobar GM, Obregon MJ, del Rey FE. Maternal thyroid hormones early in pregnancy and fetal brain development. *Best Pract Res Clin Endocrinol Metabol* 2004;18(2):225-248.
61. Buyukgebiz A. Newborn screening for congenital hypothyroidism. *J Pediatr Endocrinol Metab* 2006;19(11):1291-1298.
62. Chu M, Seltzer TF. Myxedema coma induced by ingestion of raw bok choy. *N Engl J Med* 2010;362(20):1945-1946.
63. Urban RJ. Hypopituitarism after acute brain injury. *Growth Horm IGF Res* 2006;16(Suppl A):S25-29. PubMed PMID: 16697673.
64. Prabhakar VK, Shalet SM. Aetiology, diagnosis, and management of hypopituitarism in adult life. *Postgrad Med J* 2006;82(966): 259-266.
65. Golden WM, Weber KB, Hernandez TL, Sherman SI, Woodmansee WW, Haugen BR. Single-dose rexinoid rapidly and specifically suppresses serum thyrotropin in normal subjects. *J Clin Endocrinol Metab* 2007;92(1):124-130.
66. Sherman SI, Gopal J, Haugen BR, et al. Central hypothyroidism associated with retinoid X receptor-selective ligands. *N Engl J Med* 1999;340(14):1075-1079.
67. Joshi AS, Woolf PD. Pituitary hyperplasia secondary to primary hypothyroidism: A case report and review of the literature. *Pituitary* 2005;8(2):99-103.
68. Garber JR, Cobin RH, Gharib H, et al. Clinical practice guidelines for hypothyroidism in adults: Cosponsored by the american association of clinical endocrinologists and the american thyroid association. *Thyroid* 2012;22(12):1200-1235.
69. Lev-Ran A. Part-of-the-day hypertriiodothyroninemia caused by desiccated thyroid. *JAMA* 1983;250(20):2790-2791.
70. Celi FS, Zemskova M, Linderman JD, et al. The pharmacodynamic equivalence of levothyroxine and liothyronine: A randomized, double blind, cross-over study in thyroidectomized patients. *Clin Endocrinol (Oxf)* 2010;72(5):709-715.
71. Jonklaas J, Davidson B, Bhagat S, Soldin SJ. Triiodothyronine levels in athyreotic individuals during levothyroxine therapy. *JAMA* 2008;299(7):769-777.
72. Ito M, Miyauchi A, Morita S, et al. TSH-suppressive doses of levothyroxine are required to achieve preoperative native serum triiodothyronine levels in patients who have undergone total thyroidectomy. *Eur J Endocrinol* 2012;167(3):373-378.
73. Gullo D, Latina A, Frasca F, Le Moli R, Pellegriti G, Vigneri R. Levothyroxine monotherapy cannot guarantee euthyroidism in all athyreotic patients. *PloS One* 2011;6(8):e22552.
74. Alevizaki M, Mantzou E, Cimponeriu AT, Alevizaki CC, Koutras DA. TSH may not be a good marker for adequate thyroid hormone replacement therapy. *Wiener Klinische Wochenschrift* 2005;117(18): 636-640.
75. Clyde PW, Harari AE, Getka EJ, Shakir KM. Combined levothyroxine plus liothyronine compared with levothyroxine alone in primary hypothyroidism: A randomized controlled trial (see comment). *JAMA* 2003;290(22):2952-2958.
76. Ma C, Xie J, Huang X, et al. Thyroxine alone or thyroxine plus triiodothyronine replacement therapy for hypothyroidism. *Nuc Med Comm* 2009;30(8):586-593.
77. Joffe RT, Brimacombe M, Levitt AJ, Stagnaro-Green A. Treatment of clinical hypothyroidism with thyroxine and triiodothyronine: A literature review and metaanalysis. *Psychosomatics* 2007;48(5): 379-384.

78. Grozinsky-Glasberg S, Fraser A, Nahshoni E, Weizman A, Leibovici L. Thyroxine-triiodothyronine combination therapy versus thyroxine monotherapy for clinical hypothyroidism: Meta-analysis of randomized controlled trials. *J Clin Endocrinol Metab* 2006;91(7):2592-2599.
79. Escobar-Morreale HF, Botella-Carretero JI, Escobar del Rey F, Morreale de Escobar G. REVIEW: Treatment of hypothyroidism with combinations of levothyroxine plus liothyronine. *J Clin Endocrinol Metabol* 2005;90(8):4946-4954.
80. Panicker V, Saravanan P, Vaidya B, et al. Common variation in the DIO2 gene predicts baseline psychological well-being and response to combination thyroxine plus triiodothyronine therapy in hypothyroid patients. *J Clin Endocrinol Metab* 2009;94(5):1623-1629.
81. Werneck de Castro JP, Fonseca TL, Ueta CB, et al. Differences in hypothalamic type 2 deiodinase ubiquitination explain localized sensitivity to thyroxine. *J Clin Invest* 2015;125(2):769-781.
82. Santini F, Giannetti M, Ricco I, et al. Steady-State Serum T3 Concentrations for 48 Hours Following the Oral Administration of a Single Dose of 3,5,3′-Triiodothyronine Sulfate (T3S). *Endocr Pract* 2014;20(7):680-689.
83. Berg JA, Mayor GH. A study in normal human volunteers to compare the rate and extent of levothyroxine absorption from Synthroid and Levoxine. *J Clin Pharmacol* 1992;32(12):1135-1140.
84. Dong BJ, Hauck WW, Gambertoglio JG, et al. Bioequivalence of generic and brand-name levothyroxine products in the treatment of hypothyroidism. *JAMA* 1997;277(15):1205-1213.
85. Blakesley V, Awni W, Locke C, Ludden T, Granneman GR, Braverman LE. Are bioequivalence studies of levothyroxine sodium formulations in euthyroid volunteers reliable? *Thyroid* 2004;14(3): 191-200.
86. Hennessey JV. Levothyroxine dosage and the limitations of current bioequivalence standards. *Nat Clin Pract Endocrinol Metab* 2006;2(9):474-475.
87. Canaris GJ, Manowitz NR, Mayor G, Ridgway EC. The Colorado thyroid disease prevalence study. *Arch Inter Med* 2000;160(4): 526-534.
88. Somwaru LL, Arnold AM, Joshi N, Fried LP, Cappola AR. High frequency of and factors associated with thyroid hormone over-replacement and under-replacement in men and women aged 65 and over. *J Clin Endocrinol Metab* 2009;94(4):1342-1345.
89. Vestergaard P, Mosekilde L. Hyperthyroidism, bone mineral, and fracture risk—a meta-analysis. *Thyroid* 2003;13(6):585-593.
90. Uzzan B, Campos J, Cucherat M, Nony P, Boissel JP, Perret GY. Effects on bone mass of long term treatment with thyroid hormones: A meta-analysis. *J Clin Endocrinol Metab* 1996;81(12):4278-4289.
91. Schneider R, Schneider M, Reiners C, Schneider P. Effects of levothyroxine on bone mineral density, muscle force, and bone turnover markers: A cohort study. *J Clin Endocrinol Metab* 2012;97(11):3926-3934.
92. Wenzel KW. Bioavailability of levothyroxine preparations. *Thyroid* 2003;13(7):665.
93. Bach-Huynh TG, Nayak B, Loh J, Soldin S, Jonklaas J. Timing of levothyroxine administration affects serum thyrotropin concentration. *J Clin Endocrinol Metab* 2009;94(10):3905-3912.
94. Sachmechi I, Reich DM, Aninyei M, Wibowo F, Gupta G, Kim PJ. Effect of proton pump inhibitors on serum thyroid-stimulating hormone level in euthyroid patients treated with levothyroxine for hypothyroidism. *Endocr Pract* 2007;13(4):345-349.
95. Pirola I, Daffini L, Gandossi E, et al. Comparison between liquid and tablet levothyroxine formulations in patients treated through enteral feeding tube. *J Endocrinol Invest* 2014;37(6):583-587.
96. Vita R, Saraceno G, Trimarchi F, Benvenga S. Switching levothyroxine from the tablet to the oral solution formulation corrects the impaired absorption of levothyroxine induced by proton-pump inhibitors. *J Clin Endocrinol Metab* 2014;99(12):4481-4486.
97. Santaguida MG, Virili C, Del Duca SC, et al. Thyroxine softgel capsule in patients with gastric-related T4 malabsorption. *Endocrine* 2015;49(1):51-57.
98. Cappelli C, Pirola I, Gandossi E, Formenti A, Castellano M. Oral liquid levothyroxine treatment at breakfast: A mistake? *Eur J Endocrinol* 2014;170(1):95-99.
99. Spencer CA, Hollowell JG, Kazarosyan M, Braverman LE. National Health and Nutrition Examination Survey III thyroid-stimulating hormone (TSH)-thyroperoxidase antibody relationships demonstrate that TSH upper reference limits may be skewed by occult thyroid dysfunction. *J Clin Endocrinol Metab* 2007;92(11):4236-4240.
100. Wartofsky L, Dickey RA. The evidence for a narrower thyrotropin reference range is compelling. *J Clin Endocrinol Metab* 2005;90(9): 5483-5488.
101. Surks MI, Goswami G, Daniels GH. The thyrotropin reference range should remain unchanged. *J Clin Endocrinol Metabol* 2005;90(9): 5489-5496.
102. Sawin CT, Herman T, Molitch ME, London MH, Kramer SM. Aging and the thyroid. Decreased requirement for thyroid hormone in older hypothyroid patients. *Am J Med* 1983;75(2):206-209.
103. Santini F, Pinchera A, Marsili A, et al. Lean body mass is a major determinant of levothyroxine dosage in the treatment of thyroid diseases. *J Clin Endocrinol Metab* 2005;90(1):124-127.
104. Somwaru LL, Rariy CM, Arnold AM, Cappola AR. The natural history of subclinical hypothyroidism in the elderly: The cardiovascular health study. *J Clin Endocrinol Metab* 2012;97(6):1962-1969.
105. McQuade C, Skugor M, Brennan DM, Hoar B, Stevenson C, Hoogwerf BJ. Hypothyroidism and moderate subclinical hypothyroidism are associated with increased all-cause mortality independent of coronary heart disease risk factors: A PreCIS database study. *Thyroid* 2011;21(8):837-843.
106. Razvi S, Weaver JU, Butler TJ, Pearce SH. Levothyroxine treatment of subclinical hypothyroidism, fatal and nonfatal cardiovascular events, and mortality. *Arch Intern Med* 2012;172(10):811-817.
107. Loh JA, Wartofsky L, Jonklaas J, Burman KD. The magnitude of increased levothyroxine requirements in hypothyroid pregnant women depends upon the etiology of the hypothyroidism. *Thyroid* 2009;19(3):269-275.
108. Slawik M, Klawitter B, Meiser E, et al. Thyroid hormone replacement for central hypothyroidism: A randomized controlled trial comparing two doses of thyroxine (T4) with a combination of T4 and triiodothyronine. *J Clin Endocrinol Metab* 2007;92(11):4115-4122.
109. Zelmanovitz F, Genro S, Gross JL. Suppressive therapy with levothyroxine for solitary thyroid nodules: A double-blind controlled clinical study and cumulative meta-analyses. *J Clin Endocrinol Metab* 1998;83:3881-3885.
110. Castro MR, Caraballo PJ, Morris JC. Effectiveness of thyroid hormone suppressive therapy in benign solitary thyroid nodules: A meta-analysis. *J Clin Endocrinol Metab* 2002;87(9):4154-4159.
111. Sdano MT, Falciglia M, Welge JA, Steward DL. Efficacy of thyroid hormone suppression for benign thyroid nodules: Meta-analysis of randomized trials. *Otolaryngol Head Neck Surg* 2005;133(3):391-396.
112. Jonklaas J, Sarlis NJ, Litofsky D, et al. Outcomes of patients with differentiated thyroid carcinoma following initial therapy. *Thyroid* 2006;16(12):1229-1242.
113. Carhill AA, Litofsky DR, Ross DS, et al. Long-Term Outcomes Following Therapy in Differentiated Thyroid Carcinoma: NTCTCS Registry Analysis 1987-2012. *J Clin Endocrinol Metab* 2015;100(9):3270-3279.
114. Cooper DS, Doherty GM, Haugen BR, et al. Revised American Thyroid Association management guidelines for patients with thyroid nodules and differentiated thyroid cancer. *Thyroid* 2009;19(11):1167-1214.
115. Popoveniuc G, Chandra T, Sud A, et al. A diagnostic scoring system for myxedema coma. *Endocr Pract* 2014;20(8):808-817.
116. Rovet J, Daneman D. Congenital hypothyroidism: A review of current diagnostic and treatment practices in relation to neuropsychologic outcome. *Paediatr Drugs* 2003;5(3):141-149.
117. Rose SR, Brown RS, Foley T, et al. Update of newborn screening and therapy for congenital hypothyroidism. *Pediatrics* 2006;117(6):2290-2303.
118. Leger J, Olivieri A, Donaldson M, et al. European Society for Paediatric Endocrinology consensus guidelines on screening, diagnosis, and management of congenital hypothyroidism. *Horm Res Paediatr* 2014; 81(2):80-103.
119. Haddow JE, Palomaki GE, Allan WC, et al. Maternal thyroid deficiency during pregnancy and subsequent neuropsychological development of the child (see comment). *N Engl J Med* 1999;341(8):549-555.

76

Adrenal Gland Disorders

Andrew Y. Hwang, Steven M. Smith, and John G. Gums

KEY CONCEPTS

1. Glucocorticoid secretion from the adrenal cortex is stimulated by adrenocorticotropic hormone (ACTH) or corticotropin that is released from the anterior pituitary in response to the hypothalamic-mediated release of corticotropin-releasing hormone (CRH).
2. To ensure the proper treatment of Cushing syndrome, diagnostic procedures should (a) establish the presence of hypercortisolism and (b) discover the underlying etiology of the disease.
3. The rationale for treating Cushing syndrome is to reduce the morbidity and mortality resulting from disorders such as diabetes mellitus, cardiovascular disease, and electrolyte abnormalities.
4. The treatment of choice for both ACTH-dependent and ACTH-independent Cushing syndrome is surgery, whereas pharmacologic agents are reserved for adjunctive therapy, refractory cases, or inoperable disease.
5. Pharmacologic agents that may be used to manage the patient with Cushing syndrome include steroidogenesis inhibitors, adrenolytic agents, neuromodulators of ACTH release, and glucocorticoid-receptor blocking agents.
6. Spironolactone, a competitive aldosterone-receptor antagonist, is the drug of choice in bilateral adrenal hyperplasia (BAH)–dependent hyperaldosteronism.
7. Addison disease (primary adrenal insufficiency) is a deficiency in cortisol, aldosterone, and various androgens resulting from the loss of function of all regions of the adrenal cortex.
8. Secondary adrenal insufficiency usually results from exogenous steroid use, leading to hypothalamic–pituitary–adrenal (HPA)–axis suppression followed by a decrease in ACTH release, and low levels of androgens and cortisol.
9. Virilism results from the excessive secretion of androgens from the adrenal gland and often manifests as hirsutism in females.

The adrenal glands were first characterized by Eustachius in 1563. After Addison identified a case of adrenal insufficiency in humans, adrenal anatomy and physiology flourished. Most of the work done in the early and mid-1900s centered on the glucocorticoid cortisol. With the discovery of aldosterone by Simpson and Tait in 1952, adrenal pharmacology turned toward the mineralocorticoid. Conn[1] followed with his classical description of primary aldosteronism (PA) in 1955, and numerous clinicians and investigators have continued to explore the variety of disease processes promoted through the adrenal gland.

PHYSIOLOGY, ANATOMY, AND BIOCHEMISTRY

The adrenal glands are located extraperitoneally to the upper poles of each kidney (Fig. 76-1). On average, each adrenal gland weighs 4 g and is 2 to 3 cm in width and 4 to 6 cm in length. The gland is fed by small arteries from the abdominal aorta and renal and phrenic arteries. Drainage of the adrenal gland occurs via the renal vein on the left and the inferior vena cava on the right.

The adrenal medulla occupies 10% of the total gland and is responsible for the secretion of catecholamines. The adrenal cortex accounts for the remaining 90% and is responsible for the secretion of three types of hormones (Fig. 76-2) from three separate zones.

The zona glomerulosa accounts for 15% of the total adrenal cortex and is responsible for mineralocorticoid production, of which aldosterone is the principal end product. Aldosterone maintains electrolyte and volume homeostasis by altering potassium and magnesium secretion and renal tubular sodium reabsorption. The zona fasciculata, the middle zone, makes up 60% of the cortex, is high in cholesterol, and is responsible for basal and stimulated glucocorticoid production. Glucocorticoids, mainly cortisol, are responsible for the regulation of fat, carbohydrate, and protein metabolism. The zona reticularis occupies 25% of the adrenal cortex, and is responsible for adrenal androgen production. The androgens, testosterone and estradiol, are the major end products and influence the reproductive system in addition to modulating primary and secondary sex characteristics.

Hormone Production and Metabolism

Adrenal steroid hormone synthesis begins with the conversion of cholesterol to pregnenolone by cytochrome P450 (CYP) enzymatic side-chain cleavage. Following this rate-limiting step, pregnenolone is converted to various 19- and 21-carbon steroids, depending on the enzymatic capabilities within each zone of the cortex. Androgenic properties predominate in the 19-carbon steroids, whereas mineralocorticoid and glucocorticoid properties manifest in the 21-carbon steroids.

Aldosterone production is initiated by the 21-hydroxylation of progesterone to form deoxycorticosterone. Subsequently, aldosterone synthase converts deoxycorticosterone to aldosterone through the intermediary, corticosterone. The zona glomerulosa preferentially produces aldosterone for three main reasons. First, the zona glomerulosa lacks 17α-hydroxylase activity and therefore can only convert pregnenolone to progesterone. Second, in contrast to the other zones, cells in the zona glomerulosa possess aldosterone synthase activity, which catalyzes the terminal steps in aldosterone synthesis. Lastly, cells of the zona glomerulosa display a greater number of angiotensin II receptors than cells of the other zones. Binding of angiotensin II to these receptors provides the stimulus for initiating the aldosterone biosynthesis cascade. Thus, aldosterone synthesis

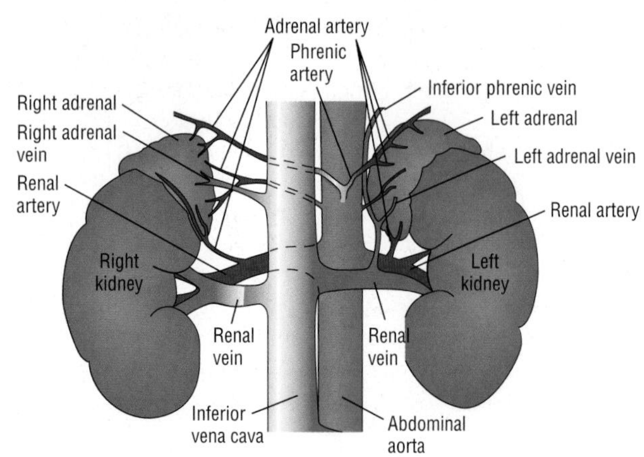

FIGURE 76-1 Anatomy of the adrenal gland.

is a unique feature of the zona glomerulosa, explaining why aldosterone is not affected during disease processes limited to the zona fasciculata or reticularis.

Cortisol is produced from pregnenolone via four successive hydroxylations. These hydroxylations occur primarily in the zona fasciculata, although the zona reticularis is also capable of producing glucocorticoids.

Androgens, produced primarily in the zona reticularis and less commonly in the zona fasciculata, have a 19-carbon structure and serve as precursors to more potent analogues produced in the periphery. The adrenal gland can synthesize estradiol and estrone from testosterone and androstenedione, respectively; however, these synthesized quantities are extremely small. The rates of production for the various steroids produced by the adrenal gland are listed in Table 76-1.

Glucocorticoid metabolism occurs in the liver and is responsible for converting inactive steroids to active metabolites, as well as modifying active steroids to less active or inactive metabolites. Most pharmaceutical steroid products are active; however, in the case of prednisone and cortisone, metabolism is necessary for conversion to the active prednisolone and cortisol, respectively.

Following metabolic conversion, glomerular filtration is primarily responsible for eliminating endogenously produced glucocorticoids. The half-life of cortisol is 70 to 120 minutes, whereas aldosterone exhibits extremely high intrinsic clearance and a corresponding half-life of only 15 minutes.

TABLE 76-1 Rates of Adrenal Production and Plasma Concentrations of Various Steroids

Steroid	24-Hour Secretion (mg)	Plasma Concentration
Aldosterone	0.15	2-9 ng/dL (supine, normal-sodium diet)
Androstenedione	2.2-2.5	50-250 ng/dL
Corticosterone	1-4	2.4 ± 1.5 ng/dL (female) 4.2 ± 2.2 ng/dL (male)
Cortisol	8-25	0-25 mcg/dL
11-Deoxycorticosterone	0.60	2-19 ng/dL
11-Deoxycortisol	0.40	12-158 ng/dL
Progesterone	0	<20 ng/dL (female)[a] 300-2,000 ng/dL (female)[b] <20-140 ng/dL (male)
Testosterone (total)	0.23 (female)	6-86 ng/dL (female) 270-1,070 ng/dL (male)

[a]Follicular phase of menstrual cycle.

[b]Luteal phase of menstrual cycle.

Data from Kratz A, Ferraro M, Sluss PM, Lewandrowski KB. Laboratory reference values. N Engl J Med *2004;351(15):1548–1563. Copyright © 2004 Massachusetts Medical Society. All rights reserved.*

Metabolism and conversion of the various steroids can be altered by a variety of disease states and medicinal compounds. Drugs known to enhance steroid clearance include phenytoin, phenobarbital, rifampin, and mitotane. Likewise, diseases such as hyperthyroidism and renal disease can enhance steroid clearance. In contrast, drugs such as estrogens and estrogen-containing oral contraceptives reduce steroid clearance. Similarly, liver disease, age, pregnancy, hypothyroidism, anorexia nervosa, protein–calorie malnutrition, and renal disease are associated with reduced steroid clearance.

Plasma glucocorticoids are bound to one of three plasma proteins in varying degrees. Corticosteroid-binding globulin (CBG), albumin, and α_1-glycoprotein are capable of binding glucocorticoids, with CBG being the principal binding protein. Steroid binding serves as a reservoir for steroids in their inactive state and more than 95% of cortisol is normally bound in this fashion. This binding prevents glucocorticoid activity at receptor-activating sites. Therefore, a

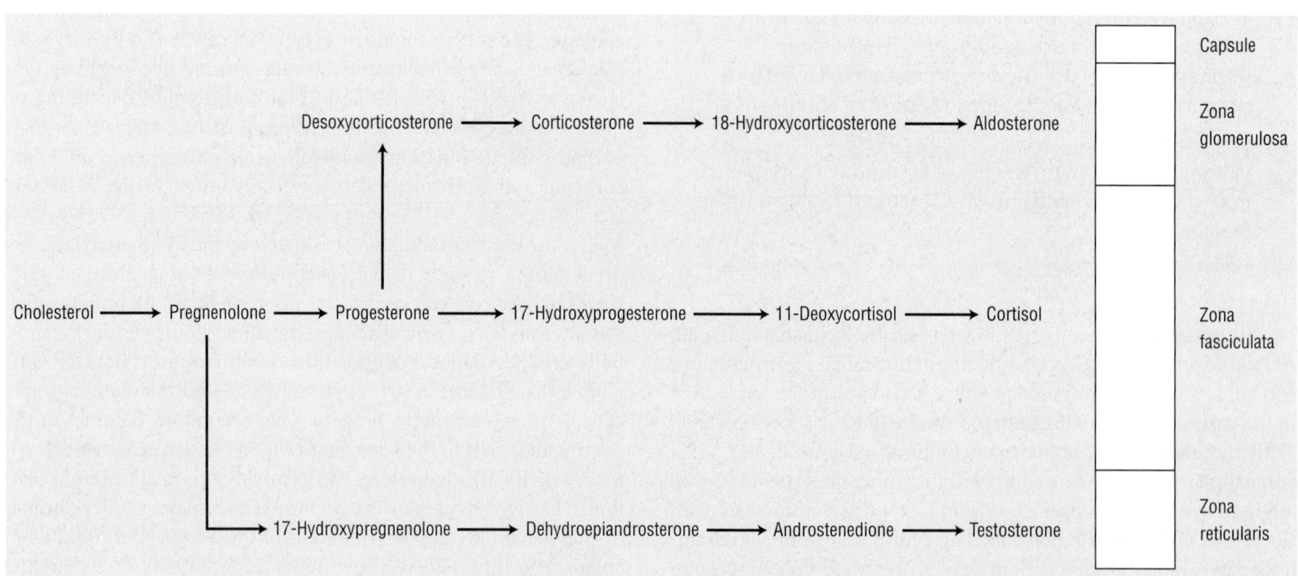

FIGURE 76-2 Hormone synthetic pathways in relation to the zones of the adrenal cortex.

final but important variable in altered plasma concentration of free (active) steroids is concentration of plasma proteins.

Regulation of Hormone Secretion

1 Glucocorticoid secretion is regulated by the pituitary hormone, adrenocorticotropic hormone (ACTH [also known as corticotropin]). Under normal conditions, ACTH is released from the anterior pituitary in response to corticotropin-releasing hormone (CRH), which is secreted by the median eminence of the hypothalamus (Fig. 76-3). Vasopressin and oxytocin have weak ACTH-releasing activity through binding to the inferior V_3 receptor. CRH, in combination with vasopressin and oxytocin, stimulates greater ACTH secretion than each hormone individually.

Additionally, histochemical studies have demonstrated that certain neurotransmitters, such as serotonin and norepinephrine, can stimulate production of CRH or ACTH directly. After release, ACTH stimulates the adrenal gland to release cortisol and, to a lesser extent, aldosterone and androgens. The rising cortisol concentration inhibits the secretion of CRH and ACTH through a negative feedback mechanism. In addition, leptin, an adipocyte hormone, can have an inhibitory effect on hypothalamic–pituitary–adrenal (HPA) activity.

Adrenal androgens are regulated in a similar fashion to cortisol. When plasma androgen reaches sufficient concentrations, production is terminated via a negative feedback loop. Androgen release is increased during puberty and in women with hirsutism. Adrenal androgen release decreases with age and in fasting states, including anorexia nervosa.

In contrast to cortisol and adrenal androgens, regulation of aldosterone secretion is considerably more complex. The renin–angiotensin system regulates aldosterone secretion through both intrarenal and extrarenal mechanisms. Renin production and subsequent aldosterone secretion is stimulated by blood pressure lowering (due to volume depletion), erect posture, salt depletion, β-adrenergic stimulation, and CNS excitation (see Chapter 13). Renin production is inhibited by salt loading, angiotensin II, vasopressin, potassium, calcium, blood pressure increases, and a variety of drugs. The renin-mediated production of angiotensin II is the initial stimulus for aldosterone synthesis. Additionally, angiotensin II can be acted on by aminopeptidase and converted to angiotensin III. Both angiotensin II and III are capable of stimulating the zona glomerulosa to secrete aldosterone. Following aldosterone secretion, increases in renal sodium and water retention as well as blood pressure occur, thereby turning off the stimulus for renin release.

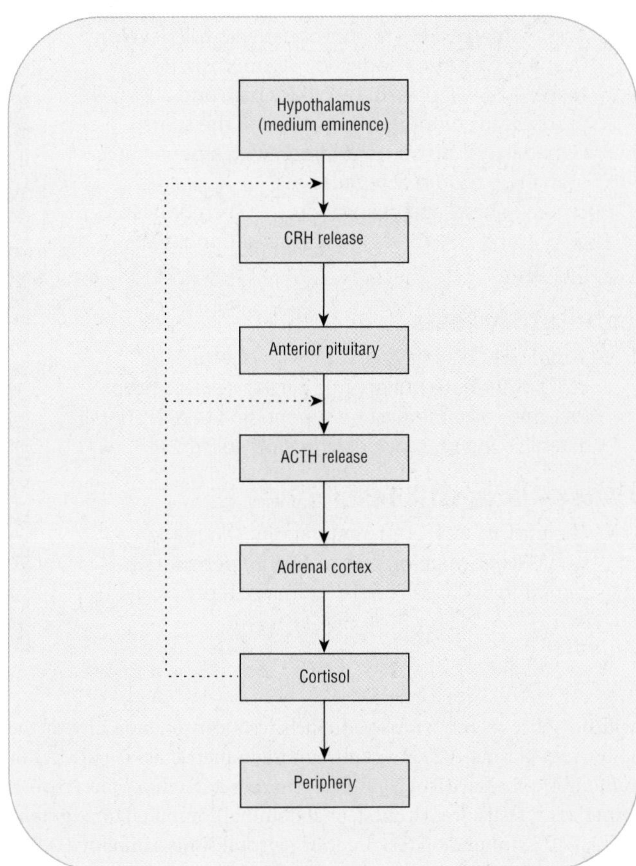

FIGURE 76-3 Negative feedback system involved in the regulation of cortisol secretion under normal conditions. (ACTH, adrenocorticotropic hormone; CRH, corticotropin-releasing hormone.)

HYPERFUNCTION OF THE ADRENAL GLAND

Adrenal disorders can be categorized as hyperfunction or hypofunction of the adrenal gland. Hyperfunction of the adrenal gland generally involves excess production of adrenal hormones, most notably cortisol, resulting in Cushing syndrome, or aldosterone, resulting in hyperaldosteronism.

Cushing Syndrome

In 1932, Cushing first described a syndrome of pituitary basophilism that attracted national attention. Until this time, no definitive diagnosis existed for patients with unexplained central obesity, cutaneous striae, osteoporosis, weakness, hypertension, diabetes mellitus, and congestion. Cushing emphasized that the disease was of a pituitary origin. Ten years later, Albright focused his attention on the "sugar hormone," which he believed originated from the adrenal cortex.[2]

After the development of a method for measuring urinary steroids, Daughaday discovered elevated steroids in the urine of patients with Cushing syndrome. Finally, the end product was identified, and Cushing syndrome was correctly explained as an excess of cortisol in the plasma (hypercortisolism).

Etiology

Cushing syndrome results from the effects of supraphysiologic levels of glucocorticoids originating either from exogenous administration or, less commonly, from endogenous overproduction by the adrenal glands. Excess glucocorticoids are produced in response to overproduction of ACTH (ACTH-dependent) or by abnormal adrenocortical tissues regardless of ACTH stimulation (ACTH-independent). ACTH-dependent Cushing syndrome (≈80% of all Cushing syndrome cases) usually originates from overproduction of ACTH by the pituitary gland, which chronically stimulates the adrenal glands causing bilateral adrenal hyperplasia (BAH). Approximately 85% of these cases are caused by pituitary adenomas (Cushing disease). Ectopic ACTH-secreting tumors and nonneoplastic corticotropin hypersecretion, possibly secondary to excess CRH production, account for the remainder of ACTH-dependent causes.[3] Ectopic ACTH syndrome refers to excessive ACTH production resulting from an endocrine or nonendocrine tumor, usually of the pancreas, thyroid, or lung. Small-cell carcinoma of the lung will lead to ectopic ACTH secretion in 0.5% to 2% of cases, whereas bronchial carcinoid tumors are usually the most common.[4] Distinguishing between the various etiologies requires a careful history and pertinent laboratory work (Table 76-2).

The remaining 20% of Cushing syndrome cases are ACTH-independent and divided almost equally between adrenal adenomas and adrenal carcinomas, with rare cases caused by macronodular hyperplasia, primary pigmented nodular adrenal disease, and

TABLE 76-2 Various Etiologies of Cushing Syndrome and Their Respective Differences

	Pituitary-Dependent	Ectopic ACTH Syndrome	Adrenal Adenoma	Adrenal Carcinoma
Course	Slow	Rapid	Slow	Rapid
Symptoms	Mild to moderate	Atypical	Mild to moderate	Severe
Dominant sex/age	Female/male	Male	None noted	Children
Virilization	+	+	+	+++
Abdominal mass	0	0	0	++
Plasma ACTH concentration	Slightly elevated	High	Low	Low
Dexamethasone suppression test	≥50% suppression	No suppression	No suppression	No suppression
Iodocholesterol scan	Bilateral uptake	Bilateral uptake	Unilateral	None

ACTH, adrenocorticotropic hormone.

McCune-Albright syndrome.[3,5] The majority of adrenal cortex tumors are benign adenomas. Adrenal carcinoma is found more often in children than in adults with Cushing syndrome.

Clinical Presentation

Patients with Cushing syndrome commonly present (>90% of patients) with central obesity and facial rounding. In addition, approximately 50% of patients will exhibit some peripheral obesity and fat accumulation. Fat accumulation in the dorsocervical area (buffalo hump) can be associated with major weight gain, whereas increased supraclavicular fat pads are more specific for Cushing syndrome. Striae are usually present along the lower abdomen and take on a red to purple color. Traditionally, hypertensive complications have been major contributors to the morbidity and mortality of Cushing syndrome. Hypertension is diagnosed in 75% to 85% of patients, with diastolic blood pressures greater than 119 mm Hg noted in over 20% of patients.[6] In addition, glucose intolerance is present in 60% of patients. Thus, many patients meet diagnostic criteria for the metabolic syndrome and have a corresponding increased risk of coronary heart disease (CHD) and stroke. Screening for Cushing syndrome in this population and in patients with uncontrolled diabetes mellitus has been suggested,[7,8] particularly when these conditions surface at an unusually early age.[9] However, screening all patients with type 2 diabetes is likely not cost-effective.[10]

CLINICAL PRESENTATION Cushing Syndrome

General

- The most common findings, which are present in 90% of patients, are central obesity and facial rounding.

Symptoms

- Approximately 65% and 58% of patients complain of myopathies and muscular weakness, respectively.

Signs

- Peripheral obesity and fat accumulation is found in 50% of patients.
- Facial plethora is caused by an underlying atrophy of the skin and connective tissue and is seen in approximately 84% of patients.
- Patients often are described as having moon faces with a buffalo hump.
- Hypertension is seen in 75% to 85% of patients.
- Psychiatric changes can occur in as many as 55% of patients.
- Approximately 50% to 60% of patients will develop Cushing syndrome–induced osteoporosis. Of these, 40% will present with back pain and 20% will progress to compression fractures of the spine.
- Gonadal dysfunction is common with amenorrhea seen in up to 75% of females.
- Excess adrenal and ovary androgen secretion is responsible for 80% of females presenting with hirsutism.

Laboratory Tests

- A midnight plasma cortisol, late-night salivary cortisol, 24-hour urinary free cortisol (UFC), and/or low-dose dexamethasone suppression test (DST) will establish the presence of hypercortisolism.

Other Diagnostic Tests

- The plasma ACTH test, metyrapone stimulation test, CRH stimulation test, or inferior petrosal sinus sampling (IPSS) will help determine the etiology.

Diagnosis

2 The diagnosis of Cushing syndrome involves two steps: (a) establishing the presence of hypercortisolism, which is relatively easy, and (b) differentiating between etiologies, which can be challenging (Fig. 76-4).[5,8,11] The presence of hypercortisolism can be established via one or more of the following tests: 24-hour UFC, midnight plasma cortisol, late-night salivary cortisol, or the low-dose DST (using 1 mg dexamethasone for the overnight test or 0.5 mg/6 h for the classic 2-day study). However, because these tests cannot determine the etiology of Cushing syndrome, other tests and procedures will be subsequently employed. Such tests can include any of the following: plasma ACTH via immunoradiometric assay (IRMA) or radioimmunoassay (RIA); adrenal vein catheterization; metyrapone stimulation test; adrenal, chest, or abdominal computed tomography (CT); CRH stimulation test; inferior petrosal sinus sampling (IPSS); jugular venous sampling (JVS); cavernous sinus sampling; and pituitary magnetic resonance imaging (MRI). High-dose DST has been used in the past, but is no longer recommended due to its poor specificity and limited diagnostic value. Other possible tests and procedures include insulin-induced hypoglycemia, somatostatin receptor

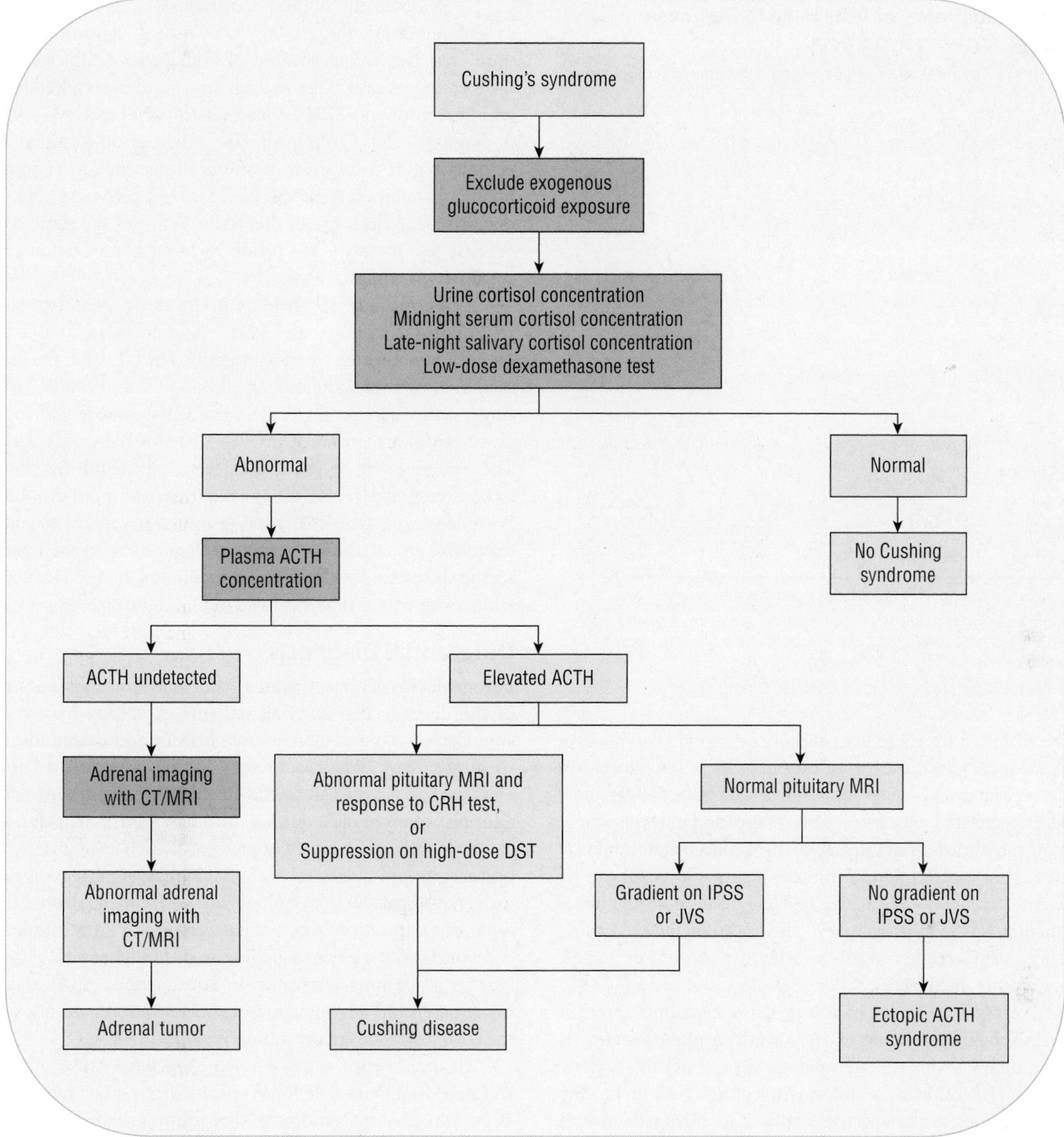

FIGURE 76-4 Algorithm for diagnosing Cushing syndrome. (ACTH, adrenocorticotropic hormone; CRH, corticotropin-releasing hormone; CT, computed tomography; DST, dexamethasone suppression test; IPSS, inferior petrosal sinus sampling; JVS, jugular venous sampling; MRI, magnetic resonance imaging.)

scintigraphy, the desmopressin stimulation test, the naloxone CRH stimulation test, the loperamide test, the hexarelin stimulation test, and radionuclide imaging.[5,6,8,11-16] Table 76-3 summarizes some of the tests used to diagnose Cushing syndrome.

Elevated UFC concentrations are highly suggestive of Cushing syndrome, especially values fourfold greater than the upper limit of normal.[3,13] In contrast to plasma measurements of cortisol, UFC measures only unbound cortisol. Consequently, the UFC test is unaffected by conditions and medications that alter CBG levels. Normal reference values for UFC are 20 to 90 mcg per 24-hour period. A twofold to threefold increase in urine cortisol is not uncommon in the patient with hyperfunction of the adrenal gland. Starvation, hydration from water loading (≥5 L/day), alcoholism, and acute stress are all capable of elevating urine cortisol concentrations. Likewise, elevated UFC results can occur during therapy with topical steroids, carbamazepine, and fenofibrate depending on the type of UFC test. Conversely, renal impairment (creatinine clearance [CrCl] of <60 mL/min) can falsely lower UFC concentrations. Because other pathologic conditions can increase the amount of free cortisol, additional tests may be warranted to confirm the diagnosis, or the diagnostic evaluation should be repeated when the acute stress has resolved. Of all urinary measures, UFC is the most useful assessment for patients with suspected Cushing syndrome.[8,13,15]

In healthy individuals, cortisol release follows a circadian rhythm whereby serum cortisol concentration peaks around 8:00 AM and thereafter declines by 60% to 80%, reaching a nadir between 3:00 and 4:00 AM. This rhythm is lost in the patient with Cushing syndrome. Although many patients with Cushing syndrome will have serum cortisol values in the high normal range if the serum is assayed in the morning, only 3.4% will have normal values if measured late at night.[17] Thus, a midnight serum cortisol greater than 7.5 mcg/dL (>1.8 mcg/dL if the patient is sleeping) is a highly sensitive assay for Cushing syndrome. However, this test is cumbersome and rarely recommended because it requires that

TABLE 76-3 Summary of Tests Used to Diagnose Cushing Syndrome

Test	Normal	Hyperplasia	Adenoma	Carcinoma
Plasma				
Cortisol (mcg/dL, AM/PM)	5-25/5-15	↑/↑↑	↑↑/↑↑	↑↑↑/↑↑↑
After low-dose DST	↓	↔	↔	↔
After high-dose DST	↓	↓/↔	↔	↔
ACTH (pg/mL)	6-76	↑↑	↓	↓
Urine				
Cortisol (mcg/24 hours)	20-90	↑↑	↑↑	↑↑↑
Saliva				
Cortisol (mcg/dL, PM)	Assay-dependent	↑↑	↑↑	↑↑↑

ACTH, adrenocorticotropic hormone; DST, dexamethasone suppression test.

Data from Kratz A, Ferraro M, Sluss PM, Lewandrowski KB. Laboratory reference values. N Engl J Med *2004;351(15):1548–1563. Copyright © 2004 Massachusetts Medical Society. All rights reserved.*

patients be admitted for more than 48 hours to avoid false-positive responses secondary to the stress of hospitalization. An alternative assay is the measurement of late-night salivary cortisol. Salivary cortisol is highly correlated with free serum cortisol and independent of salivary flow rates. Moreover, salivary cortisol concentration reflects changes in serum cortisol within minutes. Salivary cortisol can be considered an acceptable alternative to UFC because of its convenience, stability (1 week), accuracy, and reproducibility. Unfortunately, normal reference ranges are assay-dependent, and cutoff points vary among institutions.[18,19]

In the overnight DST, 1 mg of dexamethasone is administered at 11:00 PM. The following morning at 8:00 AM fasting plasma cortisol is obtained for analysis. This supraphysiologic dose of dexamethasone suppresses ACTH stimulation and cortisol production in healthy individuals. In contrast, the negative feedback loop is ineffective in patients with Cushing syndrome who generally exhibit a morning cortisol concentration above 5 mcg/dL. Some patients with Cushing syndrome administered the overnight DST can slightly suppress cortisol and using 1.8 mcg/dL as a cutoff can increase sensitivity, but at the expense of reduced specificity.[20] Therefore, the overnight DST is useful only as a screening tool for Cushing syndrome. Drugs that induce or inhibit CYP3A4 metabolism can significantly alter dexamethasone concentration, increasing the likelihood of false-positive and false-negative DSTs. Concurrent measurements of dexamethasone concentration with cortisol may improve the accuracy of testing for patients on CYP3A4-modifying drugs, although dexamethasone assays are not widely available. Also noteworthy, pregnancy and estrogen use (including oral contraceptives) increase CBG levels and frequently elicit false-positive results.[13] Consequently, UFC testing is preferred over DST in these patient populations.

The first test used to determine the etiology of Cushing syndrome is the plasma ACTH test. Plasma ACTH concentrations can be measured via RIA or IRMA.[12] In ACTH-dependent Cushing syndrome, ACTH can be normal or elevated. Very high levels of ACTH favor ectopic production. In contrast, ACTH values generally are low (<5 pg/mL) in ACTH-independent (adrenal) Cushing syndrome. Furthermore, ACTH levels can appear artificially low in some ectopic ACTH-producing tumors because ACTH can be secreted as an active prohormone that is not detected by the assay.

IPSS offers the highest sensitivity and specificity of any test in differentiating the etiology of Cushing syndrome. This technique requires catheterization of both petrosal sinuses with serial measurements of ACTH in each sinus and a peripheral vein after administration of CRH. A central-to-peripheral ACTH gradient is diagnostic for Cushing disease, whereas no gradient indicates ectopic ACTH production. Complications, such as venous thromboembolism, brain stem vascular damage, high cost, and technical expertise, can limit use of this test.[12] JVS uses the same concept as IPSS, is less invasive, and produces fewer complications; however, sensitivity is compromised.

Abnormal adrenal anatomy is effectively identified using high-resolution CT scanning and MRI.[21] Nodules as small as 1 to 1.5 cm on the adrenal cortex are easily identified by CT. With the use of thin-section scanning, nodules as small as 3 to 5 mm can be visualized.[22] Importantly, adrenal incidentalomas (masses observed incidentally on imaging) are prevalent in 5% to 10% of the general population. These masses may be functional (secreting), requiring intervention, or nonfunctional (nonsecreting), requiring only periodic observation. For this reason, abnormal imaging results are unable to conclusively diagnose adrenal disease when used alone. Nonadrenal imaging studies may be useful for identifying ectopic sources of ACTH secretion in patients for whom IPSS has ruled out Cushing disease.

Differential Diagnosis

Iatrogenic (exogenous) Cushing syndrome is the most common form of the disease. Therefore, all patients exhibiting hypercortisolism should undergo a comprehensive history and evaluation assessing medication use before laboratory testing is performed to identify endogenous causes. Iatrogenic Cushing syndrome can occur from administration of oral, inhaled, intranasal, intra-articular, and topical glucocorticoids, as well as progestins such as medroxyprogesterone acetate and megestrol acetate.[23] Disease severity correlates with exogenous glucocorticoid potency, dose, frequency, route, and treatment duration. Moreover, patients taking CYP3A4 inhibitors concomitantly with a glucocorticoid can be at higher risk of developing iatrogenic Cushing syndrome.[24,25] If exogenous glucocorticoids are being taken, the plasma cortisol concentration can increase, while the corticosterone concentration remains low.[17]

In the absence of any known exogenous causes, the clinician will need to differentiate the syndrome from other syndromes, such as pseudo-Cushing syndrome, that mimic true Cushing syndrome. Patients with obesity, chronic alcoholism, depression, and acute illness of any type can present with certain features of Cushing syndrome. However, these patients may lack true Cushing syndrome. For example, depressed patients, although mimicking the urinary steroid abnormalities of Cushing syndrome, will not resemble a cushingoid patient in appearance. In chronic alcoholism, steroid laboratory panels generally return to baseline after ceasing alcohol intake. And obese patients often will have normal cortisol concentrations on both serum and urinary screening. Thus, identifying true cases of Cushing syndrome requires a comprehensive history in combination with laboratory and possibly imaging assessment.

Treatment

Desired Outcomes 3 If left untreated, Cushing syndrome is associated with high morbidity and mortality due to associated disorders such as hypertension, diabetes mellitus, cardiovascular disease, and electrolyte abnormalities. These disorders limit the survival of the patient with Cushing syndrome to 4 to 5 years following initial diagnosis. The desired outcomes of treatment are to limit such detrimental outcomes and return the patient to a normal functional state by removing the source of hypercortisolism while minimizing pituitary or adrenal deficiencies.

4 The treatment of choice for both ACTH-dependent and ACTH-independent Cushing syndrome is surgical resection of

TABLE 76-4 Possible Treatment Options in Cushing Syndrome Based on Etiology

	Treatment	
Etiology	**Nondrug**	**Drug**
Ectopic ACTH syndrome	Surgery, chemotherapy, irradiation	Metyrapone Ketoconazole
Pituitary-dependent	Surgery, irradiation	Mitotane Metyrapone Mifepristone Cabergoline Pasireotide
Adrenal adenoma	Surgery, postoperative replacement	Ketoconazole
Adrenal carcinoma	Surgery	Mitotane

ACTH, adrenocorticotropic hormone.

any offending tumors.[3,11] However, several secondary pharmacologic treatment plans are available, depending on the etiology of the disease (Table 76-4).[3,26-29] These pharmacologic options are generally reserved as second-line treatment in patients who are not surgical candidates, and may also be used in preoperative patients, or as adjunctive therapy in postoperative patients awaiting response. Rarely, monotherapy is used as a palliative treatment when surgery is not indicated.

Pharmacologic Therapy 5 Pharmacotherapy of Cushing syndrome (dosing and monitoring parameters can be found in Tables 76-5 and 76-6, respectively)[3,28,29] can be divided into four categories based on the anatomic site of action of the agent: (1) steroidogenesis inhibitors, (2) adrenolytic agents, (3) neuromodulators of ACTH release, and (4) glucocorticoid-receptor blocking agents.[26,27]

Steroidogenesis Inhibitors As their name implies, steroidogenesis inhibitors block the production of cortisol. This class includes metyrapone, ketoconazole, and etomidate. Metyrapone inhibits 11β-hydroxylase, the enzyme responsible for converting 11-deoxycortisol to cortisol. Following administration, a sudden decrease in cortisol concentration occurs within hours and prompts a compensatory rise in plasma ACTH concentrations. As ACTH increases and blockage of cortisol synthesis persists, adrenal steroidogenesis efforts are shunted toward androgen production. Consequently, metyrapone is associated with significant androgenic side effects, including hirsutism and increased acne, making it less ideal for women. In addition, metyrapone blocks aldosterone synthesis and causes the accumulation of aldosterone precursors, which exhibit weak mineralocorticoid activity. Blood pressure and electrolyte perturbations can ensue, depending on the level of circulating 11-deoxycortisol and the degree of aldosterone inhibition. Additional adverse effects, including nausea, vomiting, vertigo, headache, dizziness, abdominal discomfort, and allergic rash, have been reported following administration, but are often signs of overtreatment.[26,27,30] Metyrapone is currently available through the manufacturer only for compassionate use.

The imidazole derivative antifungal, ketoconazole, effectively inhibits steroidogenesis via multiple mechanisms when used in large doses. In contrast to the quick onset of metyrapone, the benefits of ketoconazole therapy are achieved only after several weeks of therapy. In addition to lowering serum cortisol levels, ketoconazole exhibits antiandrogenic activity attributable to its inhibition of multiple CYP enzymes as well as 11β-hydroxylase and 17α-hydroxylase.[26] This activity may be beneficial in women with Cushing syndrome, but can cause gynecomastia and hypogonadism in men. Sustained therapy with ketoconazole also imparts beneficial effects on serum cholesterol profiles, including lowering total and low-density lipoprotein (LDL) cholesterol levels. Ketoconazole induces a reversible elevation of hepatic transaminases in approximately 10% of patients.[31] However, concerns have been raised over the risk of severe hepatotoxicity associated with ketoconazole use. In July 2013, the US Food and Drug Administration (FDA) significantly changed the labeling of oral ketoconazole, removing various indications for fungal infections and recommending that oral ketoconazole not be used as first-line therapy for fungal infections. Similarly, the European Medicines Agency has recently recommended complete removal of oral ketoconazole from European Union markets. These changes were based largely on data in patients with fungal infections, who require lower doses of ketoconazole. However, few data are available on the incidence of severe hepatotoxicity with ketoconazole at the higher doses used in Cushing

TABLE 76-5 Drug Dosing in the Treatment of Cushing Syndrome

Drug	Brand Name	Initial Dose	Usual Range	Special Populations	Comments
Cabergoline	Dostinex®, 0.5 mg tablets	0.5 mg once weekly	0.5-7 mg once weekly		Maximum: 7 mg/week
Etomidate	Amidate®, 2 mg/mL solution	0.03 mg/kg IV bolus	0.1-0.3 mg/kg/hr infusion		Maximum: 0.3 mg/kg/hr infusion; titrate based on serum cortisol concentration
Ketoconazole	Nizoral®, 200 mg tablets	200 mg once or twice a day	200-1,200 mg/day, divided twice a day	Contraindicated in patients with hepatic disease	Maximum: 1,600 mg/day; CYP3A4 substrate and inhibitor (strong)
Metyrapone	Metopirone®, 250 mg tablets	0.5-1 g/day, divided every 4-6 hours	1-2 g/day, divided every 4-6 hours		Maximum: 6 g/day; CYP3A4 inducer
Mifepristone	Korlym®	300 mg once daily, increased by 300 mg/day every 2-4 weeks	600-1,200 mg/day	Do not exceed 600 mg/day in mild to moderate hepatic impairment; avoid in severe hepatic impairment. Do not exceed 600 mg/day in renal impairment	Maximum: 1,200 mg/day not to exceed 20 mg/kg/day
Mitotane	Lysodren®, 500 mg tablets	0.5-1 g/day, increased by 0.5-1 g/day every 1-4 weeks	1-4 g/day		Maximum: 12 g/day (most patients unable to tolerate >8 g/day). Take with food to decrease GI effects
Pasireotide	Signifor®, 0.3, 0.6, 0.9 mg/mL solutions	0.6-0.9 mg twice daily	0.3-0.9 mg twice daily	Reduce dose in hepatic impairment	Maximum: 1.8 mg/day

CYP, cytochrome P450 enzyme; GI, gastrointestinal.

TABLE 76-6 Drug Monitoring in the Treatment of Cushing Syndrome

Drug	Adverse Drug Reaction	Monitoring Parameters	Comments
Cabergoline	Nausea, dizziness, headache, nasal congestion, constipation, psychiatric symptoms, valvulopathy	Echocardiogram	
Etomidate	Sedation, pain at injection site, hypotension, myoclonus, nausea, vomiting	Frequent sedation scoring initially, serum potassium, serum cortisol	
Ketoconazole	GI upset, dermatologic reactions; elevated hepatic transaminases, hepatotoxicity (rare)	Liver function tests, including ALT/AST, total bilirubin, ALP, prothrombin time, and INR testing	Approximately 10% will experience reversible LFT elevations; recent FDA restrictions on fungal infection indications
Metyrapone	Androgenic effects (hirsutism, acne, etc), blood pressure and electrolyte abnormalities, nausea, vomiting, vertigo, headache, dizziness, abdominal discomfort, allergic rash	Blood pressure, electrolytes	
Mifepristone	Hypokalemia, nausea, fatigue, headache, peripheral edema, dizziness, endometrial hyperplasia	Serum potassium, pregnancy testing, pelvic ultrasound	Abortifacient; rule out pregnancy in women of childbearing potential
Mitotane	GI upset, nausea, diarrhea, lethargy, somnolence, CNS disturbances	UFC and urinary steroid production, serum potassium	GI upset in up to 80%; GI and CNS effects appear to be dose-dependent
Pasireotide	Nausea, diarrhea, cholelithiasis, increased hepatic transaminases, hyperglycemia, sinus bradycardia, QT prolongation	Serum glucose, glycohemoglobin A1c, liver function tests	Only available as a subcutaneous injection; expensive

ALP, alkaline phosphatase; ALT, alanine aminotransferase; AST, aspartate aminotransferase; CNS, central nervous system; FDA, Food and Drug Administration; GI, gastrointestinal; INR, international normalized ratio; LFT, liver function tests; UFC, urinary free cortisol.

syndrome. Consequently, monitoring during treatment with ketoconazole should include liver function at baseline, including aspartate aminotransferase (AST), alanine aminotransferase (ALT), total bilirubin, alkaline phosphatase (ALP), prothrombin time, and international normalized ratio (INR) testing, according to FDA recommendations. In addition, weekly monitoring of serum ALT should be continued throughout therapy with ketoconazole. In general, ketoconazole should be avoided in patients with preexisting hepatic disease. Additional common adverse effects include gastrointestinal (GI) discomfort and dermatologic reactions.

Ketoconazole may be used concomitantly with metyrapone to achieve synergistic reductions in cortisol levels. Because these drugs differ in their onset of action, coadministration allows for more complete suppression of cortisol synthesis. Moreover, the antiandrogenic actions of ketoconazole therapy may offset the androgenic potential of metyrapone, thus attenuating a major limitation of metyrapone monotherapy.

The anesthetic etomidate is an imidazole derivative similar to ketoconazole that inhibits 11β-hydroxylase.[26] Inhibition of aldosterone synthase and antiproliferative effects on adrenal cortical cells may also play a role.[32] Etomidate is available only in a parenteral formulation and is therefore limited to patients with acute hypercortisolemia requiring emergency treatment or in preparation for surgery. Low doses of etomidate are often sufficient to suppress cortisol synthesis, thus potentially avoiding some of the adverse effects observed with higher doses used in anesthesia. However, close monitoring is recommended to avoid excess sedation with this agent.[32] Frequent monitoring of serum cortisol is also advised to prevent hypocortisolemia. Replacement corticosteroid doses may be necessary if complete blockade of cortisol is desired.

Adrenolytic Agents Mitotane is a cytotoxic drug that structurally resembles the insecticide dichlorodiphenyltrichloroethane (DDT). Mitotane inhibits the 11-hydroxylation of 11-desoxycortisol and 11-desoxycorticosterone in the adrenal cortex, resulting in a net inhibition of cortisol and corticosterone synthesis. Similar to ketoconazole, mitotane takes weeks to months to exert beneficial effects. Sustained cortisol suppression occurs in most patients (~80%) and may persist following discontinuation of therapy in up to one-third of patients. Because of its cytotoxic nature, mitotane degenerates cells within the zona fasciculata and reticularis, resulting in atrophy of the adrenal cortex. The zona glomerulosa is minimally affected during acute therapy but can be damaged during long-term treatment.[28,29]

Importantly, mitotane can induce significant neurologic and GI side effects and patients should be monitored carefully or hospitalized when initiating therapy. Nausea and diarrhea are common adverse effects that occur at doses greater than 2 g/day and can be avoided by gradually increasing the dose and/or administering the agent with food. Most patients are unable to tolerate doses exceeding 8 g/day. Approximately 80% of patients treated with mitotane develop lethargy and somnolence, and other central nervous system (CNS) adverse drug reactions occur in approximately 40% of patients. Furthermore, significant but reversible hypercholesterolemia and prolongation of bleeding times can result from mitotane use.[26,27] Mitotane increases production of CBG resulting in artifactually elevated plasma cortisol; thus, UFC and urinary steroid production should be monitored to assess response to therapy.[26] If necessary, steroid replacement therapy can be given. However, because mitotane also increases extra-adrenal metabolism of exogenously administered corticosteroids (especially hydrocortisone), higher steroid replacement doses may be required. In select patients, supplemental androgen therapy also may be necessary.

Neuromodulatory Agents Pituitary secretion of ACTH is normally mediated by various neurotransmitters, including serotonin, γ-aminobutyric acid (GABA), acetylcholine, and the catecholamines. Although ACTH-secreting pituitary tumors (Cushing disease) self-regulate ACTH production to some degree, these neurotransmitters are still capable of promoting pituitary ACTH production. Consequently, agents that target these neurotransmitters have been proposed for the treatment of Cushing disease. Such agents include cyproheptadine, ritanserin, ketanserin, bromocriptine, cabergoline, valproic acid, octreotide, lanreotide, pasireotide, rosiglitazone, and tretinoin. However, with the exception of pasireotide, none of these drugs have demonstrated consistent clinical efficacy in the treatment of Cushing disease.

Cyproheptadine, a nonselective serotonin-receptor antagonist and anticholinergic drug, can decrease ACTH secretion in some patients with Cushing disease. However, side effects, including sedation and weight gain, significantly limit the use of this drug. Likewise, selective serotonin type 2-receptor antagonists, including ritanserin and ketanserin, have demonstrated limited efficacy. Owing to their poor efficacy and high relapse rates, these drugs should be avoided except in nonsurgical candidates refractory to more conventional treatments.

Dopamine D_2-receptor agonists, including bromocriptine and cabergoline, initially reduce ACTH secretion in as many as half of all patients with Cushing disease. This action occurs through activation of inhibitory D_2 receptors that are expressed in approximately 80% of pituitary adenomas.[33] Reductions in ACTH levels are often minor and rarely sustained with long-term bromocriptine therapy. Cabergoline exhibits a higher specificity and affinity for D_2 receptors as well as a prolonged half-life compared with bromocriptine. These differences may explain the greater response rates observed with cabergoline monotherapy; however, a sustained response occurs in only 30% to 40% of patients.[34,35] Although generally well-tolerated, side effects associated with cabergoline include nausea, orthostasis, headache, nasal congestion, constipation, nightmares, vivid dreams, and psychosis. The risk of cabergoline-associated cardiac valvulopathy (observed with higher doses used to treat Parkinson disease) has not been well-studied in lower doses typically used for treatment of Cushing disease.[36]

The somatostatin analogues octreotide and lanreotide generally are ineffective in reducing ACTH secretion in Cushing disease. These two agents primarily target somatostatin receptor subtype 2 (sst_2), whereas pituitary adenomas predominantly express sst_5. Pasireotide, a recently approved somatostatin analogue, exhibits a high affinity for sst_1, sst_2, sst_3, and, especially, sst_5 receptor subtypes. In a phase 3 study of 162 adults with Cushing disease and an elevated UFC level, pasireotide administered at 600 or 900 mcg injected subcutaneously twice daily reduced the median UFC by 50% by month 2; levels remained stable for the duration of the 12-month study. Pasireotide was especially effective at normalizing UFC concentrations in patients whose baseline UFC was less than five times the upper limit of normal. Clinical signs and symptoms of Cushing disease were also improved as were blood pressure, weight, LDL cholesterol, and quality of life. Side effects were mostly GI in nature, although 73% of subjects experienced an adverse event related to hyperglycemia; preexisting diabetes mellitus or impaired glucose tolerance increased the risk for these events. Notably, glycated hemoglobin A1c increased by an average of 1.4%. Gallstones were also rarely seen with six subjects undergoing cholecystectomy.[37]

Since coexpression of D_2 and sst_5 receptors is common in adrenocorticotropin-secreting adenomas, the combination of pasireotide and cabergoline may produce synergistic effects in reducing cortisol levels.[3] Limited data suggest that step-wise addition of cabergoline and ketoconazole in patients unresponsive to pasireotide may achieve normalization of UFC in the majority of patients; however, additional studies are needed to confirm the efficacy of this combination therapy. Potential drug-drug interactions exist with the combination of pasireotide and ketoconazole, and thus, the combination should be used with caution.[38,39]

Glucocorticoid-Receptor Blocking Agents Mifepristone is a potent progesterone- and glucocorticoid-receptor antagonist that inhibits dexamethasone suppression and increases endogenous cortisol and ACTH levels in normal subjects.[26,30] Clinical experience and trial data in Cushing syndrome suggest that mifepristone is highly effective in reversing the manifestation of hypercortisolism, including hyperglycemia, hypertension, and weight gain.[40] Consequently, mifepristone has an FDA-approved indication for treatment of endogenous Cushing syndrome in patients who have type 2 diabetes or glucose intolerance, and who are not eligible for or have had poor response to surgery. However, because of its novel site of action, mifepristone induces a compensatory rise in ACTH and cortisol. Consequently, efficacy and toxicity monitoring must rely on clinical signs rather than laboratory assessments. Common adverse effects of mifepristone include fatigue, nausea, headache, arthralgia, peripheral edema, endometrial thickening (with or without vaginal bleeding), and significant reductions in serum potassium. Oral potassium supplementation or spironolactone can be effective in mitigating the latter adverse effect, although high doses may be required.[40]

Close monitoring of 24-hour UFC and serum cortisol is essential to detect treatment-induced adrenal insufficiency. Steroid secretion should be monitored with all of these drugs except mifepristone and steroid replacement given as needed. Whatever the choice, pharmacologic therapy in pituitary-dependent disease is mainly centered around patient stabilization prior to surgery or in patients waiting for potential response to other therapies.

Clinical **Controversy...**

The traditional strategy for suppressing hypercortisolism in Cushing disease consists of titrating medications to achieve normal cortisol levels. However, some clinicians advocate a "block and replace" strategy, whereby greater doses of medications are used to completely suppress endogenous cortisol production, followed by administration of physiologic doses of glucocorticoids to treat adrenal insufficiency.

Nonpharmacologic Therapy

Surgery The treatment of choice for Cushing disease is transsphenoidal resection of the pituitary tumor.[3,11,29,30,41] The advantages of this procedure include preservation of pituitary function, low complication rate, and high clinical improvement rate. The overall cure rate of histologically proven microadenomas (tumor diameter <10 mm) approaches 90%, whereas remission rates for macroadenomas (tumor diameter ≥10 mm) generally do not exceed 65%.

For persistent disease following transsphenoidal surgery or when tumor-specific surgery is not possible, several second-line treatment options are available and should be tailored toward the individual patient.[29] In the case of persistent disease following transsphenoidal surgery, repeat surgery may be performed, particularly in patients with evidence of incomplete resection or pituitary lesion on imaging.[29] Although overall remission rates are lower with subsequent procedures, remission can be achieved rapidly when compared to alternative second-line treatments.[29] Alternatively, radiotherapy may be preferred for tumors invading the dura or cavernous sinus because these tumors respond poorly to surgical intervention.[42] Radiotherapy provides clinical improvement in approximately 50% of patients within 3 to 5 years, but increases the risk for pituitary-dependent hormone deficiencies (hypopituitarism).

Laparoscopic adrenalectomy is often preferred in patients with unilateral adrenal adenomas for whom transsphenoidal surgery and pituitary radiotherapy have failed or cannot be used.[3,11,30] Bilateral adrenalectomy rapidly reverses hypercortisolism. However, patients can develop Nelson syndrome, an aggressive pituitary tumor that secretes high quantities of ACTH, which causes hyperpigmentation. Because Nelson syndrome occurs in as many as 30% of bilateral adrenalectomy cases, patients should undergo regular MRI scans and ACTH level assessments. Additionally, these patients require lifelong glucocorticoid and mineralocorticoid supplementation.

Adrenal Adenoma Surgical resection of benign adrenal adenoma is associated with relatively few side effects and a high cure rate (95%). The contralateral gland in the patient with adrenal adenoma is usually atrophic; therefore, steroid replacement is needed both perioperatively and postoperatively. Table 76-7 outlines an approach to steroid replacement for three separate routes of hydrocortisone. Therapy should be continued for 6 to 12 months following surgery. Before replacement therapy is discontinued, recovery of the adrenal

TABLE 76-7 Alternative Steroid Replacement Regimens in the Adrenal Adenoma Patient

	Hydrocortisone Dose (mg)		
Time	IV	IM	po
Operation day	300	50 before surgery and 50 after surgery	
Postoperative day 1	200	50 every 12 hours	
Postoperative day 2	150	50 every 12 hours	
Postoperative day 3	100	50 every 12 hours	
Postoperative day 4		50 every 12 hours	25 every 6 hours
Postoperative day 5		25 every 12 hours	25 every 6 hours[a]
Postoperative day 7			25 every 6 hours
Postoperative days 8-10			25 every 8 hours
Postoperative days 11-20			25 every 12 hours
Postoperative days 21+			20 at 8 AM
			10 at 4 PM

po, orally.

[a]Add fludrocortisone 0.05-2 mg orally once daily starting on postoperative day 5. Adjust dose based on blood pressure, body weight, and serum electrolytes.

axis can be assessed by measuring the morning (8 AM) cortisol concentration. The cortisol concentration should exceed 20 mcg/dL before discontinuing exogenous steroids.[23]

Adrenal Carcinoma Unlike the benign adenoma patient, those with adrenal carcinoma generally have an unfavorable outcome with surgical resection.[11] Often the complete tumor cannot be excised, leaving the patient with some degree of symptoms and extra-adrenal involvement. Radiotherapy can be used if metastases are discovered. In the patient with adrenal carcinoma who is not a surgical candidate, the focus of treatment is on palliative pharmacologic intervention.

Mitotane may be used in inoperable functional and nonfunctional adrenal carcinoma or as adjuvant therapy in surgical patients with a high risk of relapse and may prolong survival by 2 to 3 years.[43] However, mitotane induces tumor regression in fewer than 20% of patients.[44] Metyrapone and ketoconazole can be given as adjunctive treatment to attempt control of steroid hypersecretion. 5-Fluorouracil also has been used in combination therapy.

Ectopic Adrenocorticotropic Hormone Syndrome In ectopic ACTH syndrome, ACTH-secreting tumors may exist in a variety of sites, including thymic, pulmonary, appendiceal, pancreatic, and thyroid tissues. Locating these sites is often difficult, but essential for determining an appropriate treatment strategy. Surgical resection is the most effective treatment option for these patients, but only approximately 10% to 30% of patients are cured following surgery due to high rates of metastatic disease or occult tumors. The remaining 70% to 90% receive postoperative medication.

Pharmacologic management with steroidogenesis inhibitors is effective in patients with ectopic ACTH syndrome and may be used as primary treatment in patients with occult or metastatic ectopic ACTH syndrome.[29] Mitotane has been used in this setting; however, its side-effect profile generally limits its use. Mifepristone and somatostatin analogues also have been reported to reduce the clinical signs of ectopic ACTH syndrome.[45]

Additional tumor-directed therapy can include systemic chemotherapy, interferon α, chemoembolization, radiofrequency ablation, and radiation therapy.[42] If all else fails, bilateral adrenalectomy can prevent the downstream effects (eg, steroidogenesis) of high levels of tumor ACTH secretion.

Clinical **Controversy...**

Steroidogenesis inhibitors can be used as primary treatment of hypercortisolism due to ectopic ACTH-secreting tumors. However, a direct-targeted therapy has been suggested for the treatment of ectopic ACTH-secreting tumors given that these tumors may express functional sst_2 and D_2 receptors. Despite limited evidence indicating their efficacy, medications that target these receptors, such as pasireotide or cabergoline, may reduce ACTH secretion and, thus, normalize cortisol concentration. Limited evidence exists regarding their efficacy in these tumors and their role in therapy remains to be determined.

Personalized Pharmacotherapy

Several factors may limit the ability to personalize pharmacotherapy in patients with Cushing syndrome. First, few rigorous studies have compared the various pharmacologic options used in Cushing syndrome. Apart from the benefits seen with pasireotide in patients with modestly elevated UFC and the use of mifepristone in patients with concomitant hyperglycemia, data are limited in terms of clinical predictors of disease response to these agents. Second, virtually nothing is known of the pharmacogenomic predictors of individual patient response in these disease states. Finally, because most agents are used off-label, scarce data exist on agent-specific pharmacokinetic parameters in this patient population.

With these limitations in mind, drug selection is determined according to the etiology of Cushing syndrome, individual patient factors, and cost. Once the etiology has been correctly identified, gender should be considered since some pharmacologic options (steroidogenesis inhibitors in particular) used in Cushing syndrome affect the sex hormones. Specifically, metyrapone is a clear second choice in women due to a high incidence of hirsutism, whereas ketoconazole may be a secondary choice in men due to drug-induced gynecomastia and hypogonadism. During pregnancy, metyrapone is commonly used, while mifepristone must be avoided. Additionally, women desiring pregnancy within the next 5 years should avoid mitotane as this agent is stored in adipose tissue for up to several years following discontinuation. Preexisting medication profiles should be considered also, since many of the pharmacologic options can inhibit (eg, ketoconazole) or induce (eg, metyrapone) important CYP isoenzymes such as 3A4.

Ultimately, pharmacotherapy is guided by patient response and several agents may need to be tried sequentially to elicit a substantial response. Combination therapy may be more effective and better tolerated than monotherapy in some patients, but studies on what constitutes the most appropriate drug regimens are lacking.

Hyperaldosteronism

Excess aldosterone secretion is categorized as either primary or secondary hyperaldosteronism.[46-49] In PA, the stimulation for aldosterone secretion arises from within the adrenal gland. Conversely, extra-adrenal stimulation is classified as secondary aldosteronism.

Primary Aldosteronism

Etiology The most common causes of PA include BAH (65%) and aldosterone-producing adenoma (APA; otherwise known as Conn syndrome) (30%). Other rare causes include unilateral (primary) adrenal hyperplasia, adrenal cortex carcinoma, renin-responsive adrenocortical adenoma, and three forms of familial hyperaldosteronism (FH): FH type I, also known as glucocorticoid-remediable aldosteronism (GRA); FH type II, also known as familial occurrence of adenoma or hyperplasia type II; and FH type III.[46,48,49]

Clinical Presentation PA is present in approximately 10% of the general hypertensive population and is a leading cause of secondary hypertension and apparent resistant hypertension. The disease is more common in women than in men, and diagnosis usually occurs between the third and sixth decades of life. Signs and symptoms can include arterial hypertension, which is often moderate to severe and resistant to pharmacologic intervention, as well as hypokalemia (10%-40% of PA patients), muscle weakness, fatigue, and headache. These features are nonspecific for PA and many patients are asymptomatic. Historically, hypokalemia was considered a requisite feature for PA diagnosis; however, normokalemia exists frequently in patients and should not obviate concern for PA.

CLINICAL PRESENTATION Primary Aldosteronism

Symptoms

- Patients may complain of muscle weakness, fatigue, paresthesias, and headache.

Signs

- Hypertension
- Tetany/paralysis
- Polydipsia/nocturnal polyuria

Laboratory Tests

- A plasma-aldosterone-concentration–to–plasma-renin-activity (PAC–to–PRA) ratio, or aldosterone-to-renin ratio (ARR) greater than 30 and a PAC greater than 15 is suggestive of PA.
- Common laboratory findings include suppressed renin activity, elevated plasma aldosterone concentration (PAC), hypernatremia (>142 mEq/L), hypokalemia, hypomagnesemia, elevated bicarbonate concentration (>31 mEq/L), and glucose intolerance.

Confirmatory Tests

- Oral or IV saline loading, fludrocortisone suppression test (FST), and genetic testing

Diagnosis Diagnostic confirmation of PA is obtainable through screening, confirmatory tests, and subtype differentiation (Fig. 76-5). As in Cushing syndrome, discovery of the underlying etiology ensures proper treatment. Table 76-8 lists the various abnormalities that must be ruled out when suspicion of hyperaldosteronism is high.

Initial diagnosis is made through proper screening of patients with suspected PA. Such patients include those with blood pressure greater than 160/100 mm Hg, appreciating that the prevalence of PA increases with hypertensive severity, and those with resistant hypertension. Screening for PA is most often done by using the PAC-to-PRA ratio, otherwise known as the ARR. An elevated ARR is highly suggestive of PA; however, an optimal cutoff ratio remains elusive because testing conditions (posture, time, current drug therapy, recent dietary salt intake), patient characteristics, and variable levels of specificity and sensitivity among assays can significantly alter test results.[50] ARR cutoffs of 20 to 40 or 30 with an aldosterone concentration greater than 15 ng/dL are used most often.[47,50-52]

Following a positive ARR screening test, confirmatory testing must be performed to exclude any false-positive cases. Confirmatory tests include the oral sodium loading test, saline infusion test, FST, and the captopril challenge test. Although individual tests can vary in sensitivity, specificity, and reliability, any test can be used depending on patient- and institution-specific considerations. FST generally is considered the most reliable, but requires hospitalization. Prior to performing these tests, potassium must be normalized and renin–angiotensin–aldosterone system (RAAS) inhibitors should be temporarily discontinued, if possible. Positive tests indicate autonomous aldosterone secretion under inhibitory pressures and are diagnostic for PA. After diagnosis, patients with confirmed PA before age 20 or with a family history of PA or strokes before age 40 should undergo genetic testing for GRA.[50]

Differentiating between an APA and BAH is imperative to formulate a proper treatment plan. Most adenomas are singular and small (<1 cm) and occur more often in the left adrenal gland than the right. Patients with APA generally have more severe hypertension, more profound hypokalemia, and higher plasma and urinary aldosterone concentrations compared with patients with BAH. Adrenal venous sampling (AVS) provides the most accurate means of differentiating unilateral from bilateral forms of PA. However, AVS is expensive, invasive, and frequently unavailable. CT scanning can detect most adenomas, although an incidentaloma can occasionally cause confusion. If CT scanning is inconclusive, AVS is performed to characterize lateralization.[47,53-55]

The underlying abnormality in BAH remains a mystery, but some investigators believe that a hormone factor stimulates the zona glomerulosa, resulting in increased sensitivity to angiotensin II. In contrast to those with an APA, patients with BAH are able to maintain control of the renin–angiotensin system, with little effect following doses of ACTH.

Therapeutic Management

6 ***BAH-Dependent Aldosteronism*** Aldosterone-receptor antagonists are the treatment of choice in bilateral cases of PA (drug dosing and monitoring parameters can be found in Tables 76-9 and 76-10, respectively). Spironolactone, a nonselective aldosterone-receptor antagonist, competes with aldosterone for binding at the aldosterone receptor, thus preventing the negative downstream effects of aldosterone-receptor activation. Additionally, spironolactone is capable of inhibiting aldosterone synthesis within the adrenal gland; however, the magnitude of this inhibition is relatively small and the effect only occurs at doses above those recommended in the clinical setting.[56] Spironolactone is available in oral form, with most patients responding to doses between 25 and 400 mg/day. The clinician should wait 4 to 8 weeks before reassessing the patient for urinary electrolytes and blood pressure control. Adverse effects of spironolactone are dose-dependent and include GI discomfort, impotence, gynecomastia, menstrual irregularities, and hyperkalemia. Gynecomastia and menstrual irregularities observed with spironolactone therapy arise from activity at androgen and progesterone receptors and inhibition of testosterone biosynthesis. Additionally, because salicylates increase the renal secretion of canrenone, the active metabolite of spironolactone, patients should be advised to avoid concomitant therapy with salicylates. In patients intolerant of spironolactone, alternative options include eplerenone and amiloride.[48,49,57-59]

Eplerenone is a selective aldosterone-receptor antagonist with high affinity for the aldosterone receptor and low affinity for androgen and progesterone receptors. Consequently, eplerenone elicits fewer sex steroid–dependent effects than spironolactone. Recent data suggest that eplerenone reduces blood pressure less than spironolactone in patients with PA, although long-term data

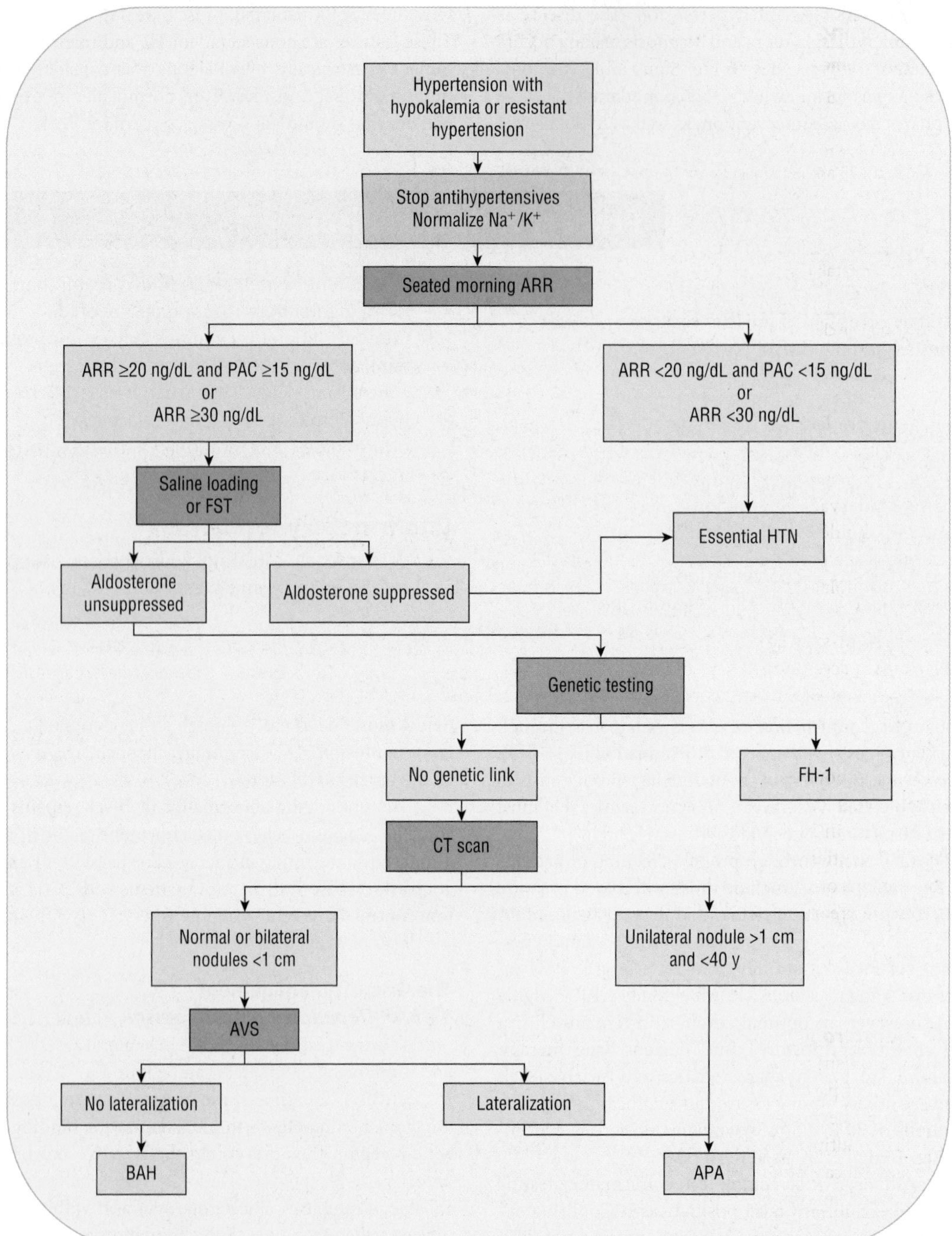

FIGURE 76-5 Algorithm for the diagnosis of primary aldosteronism. (ARR, aldosterone-to-renin ratio; APA, aldosterone-producing adenoma; AVS, adrenal venous sampling; BAH, bilateral adrenal hyperplasia; CT, computed tomography; FH-1, familial hyperaldosteronism type 1; FST, fludrocortisone suppression test; HTN, hypertension; PAC, plasma aldosterone concentration.)

TABLE 76-8 Differential Diagnosis of Primary Aldosteronism

Disease	Plasma Renin Activity	Plasma Aldosterone Concentration	Blood Pressure
Primary aldosteronism	Low	High	High
Edematous disorders	High	High	Normal
Malignant hypertension	High	High	High
Congenital adrenal hyperplasia	Low	Low	High
Cushing syndrome	Low to normal	Low to normal	High
Liddle syndrome	Low	Low	High
Bartter syndrome	High	High	Low to normal
Licorice ingestion	Low	Low	High
Low-renin essential hypertension	Low	Low to normal	High

TABLE 76-9 Drug Dosing in the Treatment of Hyperaldosteronism

Drug	Brand Name	Initial Dose	Usual Range	Special Populations	Comments
Amiloride	Midamor®, 5 mg tablets	5 mg twice daily	20 mg/day in two divided doses	CrCl 10-50 mL/min: reduce dose by 50%; CrCl <10 mL/min: CI	Maximum: 30 mg/day
Eplerenone	Inspra®, 25 and 50 mg tablets	50 mg once daily	100-300 mg/day in single or divided doses; titrate at 4- to 8-week intervals	CrCl <30 mL/min: CI	Maximum: 300 mg/day
Spironolactone	Aldactone®, 25, 50, and 100 mg tablets	25 mg once daily	100-400 mg/day in single or divided doses; titrate at 4- to 8-week intervals	CrCl 10-50 mL/min: extend dosing interval to once daily; CrCl <10 mL/min: CI	Maximum: 400 mg/day

CI, contraindicated; CrCl, creatinine clearance.

comparing these agents are lacking.[60] Eplerenone dosing starts at 50 mg daily, with titration to 50 mg twice a day; some patients may require total daily doses as high as 200 to 300 mg.[57] Titration should occur at 4- to 8-week intervals. In addition, eplerenone is a substrate of CYP3A4 and should not be taken with potent CYP3A4 inhibitors. Eplerenone is the preferred aldosterone antagonist during pregnancy since spironolactone can cause ambiguous genitalia in a male fetus.[61]

Amiloride, a potassium-sparing diuretic, is dosed at 5 mg twice a day up to 30 mg/day if necessary. Amiloride is less effective than spironolactone and patients often require additional therapy to adequately control blood pressure. Additional second-line options include calcium channel blockers, ACE inhibitors, and diuretics such as chlorthalidone, although all lack outcome data in PA.[55,58] However, some agents (eg, diuretics, calcium channel blockers) can promote a reactive rise in PRA, ultimately leading to increased aldosterone levels and potentially worsening PA. A prudent strategy would be to use these agents only in combination with RAAS inhibitors to mitigate the downstream aldosterone effects of any increase in PRA.

Aldosterone synthase inhibitors, currently under development, may offer additional therapeutic options in the future.

APA-Dependent Aldosteronism The treatment of choice for APA-dependent aldosteronism remains laparoscopic resection of the adenoma.[62] Nearly 100% of patients show blood pressure improvement while 30% to 72% are permanently cured.[59,63] Because APAs are small and often occur in multiples, resection should target the entire adrenal gland. In successful cases, blood pressure control is achieved in 1 to 3 months. Medical management can be efficacious in this population if surgery is contraindicated. However, medical management may be significantly more expensive than unilateral resection.

Glucocorticoid-Remediable Aldosteronism Glucocorticoids are very effective in treating GRA.[42] Low doses of long-acting glucocorticoids are used (0.125-0.5 mg/day of dexamethasone or 2.5-5 mg/day of prednisone) because complete suppression of ACTH-stimulated aldosterone release is unnecessary. Spironolactone, eplerenone, and amiloride are alternative treatment options.[47]

Secondary Aldosteronism

Secondary aldosteronism results from an appropriate response to excessive stimulation of the zona glomerulosa by an extra-adrenal factor, usually the renin–angiotensin system. Excessive potassium intake can promote aldosterone secretion, as can oral contraceptive use, pregnancy (aldosterone secretion 10 times normal by the third trimester), and menses. Congestive heart failure, cirrhosis, renal artery stenosis, and Bartter syndrome also can lead to elevated aldosterone concentrations.

Treatment of secondary aldosteronism is dictated by etiology. Control or correction of the extra-adrenal stimulation of aldosterone secretion should resolve the disorder. Medical therapy with spironolactone is the mainstay of treatment until an exact etiology can be located.

HYPOFUNCTION OF THE ADRENAL GLAND

Hypofunction of the adrenal gland can affect any or all adrenal hormones, depending on the etiology of the disorder. However, hypofunction does not always lead to insufficient production of adrenal hormones as might be expected. As described further, some types of adrenal hypofunction can lead to excess production of certain hormones.

Addison Disease

7 Primary adrenal insufficiency, or Addison disease, most often involves the destruction of all regions of the adrenal cortex. Deficiencies arise in cortisol, aldosterone, and the various androgens

TABLE 76-10 Drug Monitoring in the Treatment of Hyperaldosteronism

Drug	Adverse Drug Reaction	Monitoring Parameters	Comments
Amiloride	Electrolyte abnormalities (hyperkalemia), hypotension, nausea, vomiting, diarrhea, headache	Serum creatinine, serum potassium, blood pressure	Electrolyte abnormalities (hyperkalemia) more pronounced with reduced renal function
Eplerenone	Electrolyte abnormalities (hyperkalemia), hypotension, dizziness, headache; gynecomastia and menstrual irregularities are uncommon	Serum creatinine, serum potassium, blood pressure	Electrolyte abnormalities (hyperkalemia) more pronounced with reduced renal function. CYP3A4 substrate; avoid use with potent CYP3A4 inhibitors
Spironolactone	GI discomfort, impotence, gynecomastia, menstrual irregularities, electrolyte abnormalities (hyperkalemia), hypotension	Serum creatinine, serum potassium, blood pressure	Electrolyte abnormalities (hyperkalemia) more pronounced with reduced renal function

CYP, cytochrome P450 enzyme; GI, gastrointestinal.

and levels of CRH and ACTH increase in a compensatory manner. In developed countries, autoimmune dysfunction is responsible for most cases (80%-90%), whereas tuberculosis predominates as the cause in developing countries. Approximately 50% of patients with autoimmune etiologies present with one or more concomitant autoimmune disorders, usually involving other endocrine organs. Autoimmune thyroid disorders (eg, Hashimoto thyroiditis or Graves disease) are the most common, but the ovaries, pancreas, parathyroid gland, and organs of the GI system can also be affected. This polyglandular failure syndrome, termed autoimmune polyendocrine syndrome (APS), is associated with the idiopathic etiology only and has not been seen with adrenal insufficiency associated with tuberculosis or other invasive diseases. Medications that inhibit cortisol synthesis (ketoconazole) or accelerate cortisol metabolism (phenytoin, rifampin, phenobarbital) can also cause primary adrenal insufficiency.[64]

8 Secondary insufficiency is characterized by reduced glucocorticoid production secondary to decreased ACTH levels. Low levels of ACTH most commonly result from exogenous steroid use, leading to suppression of the HPA axis and decreased release of ACTH, resulting in impaired androgen and cortisol production. These effects occur with oral, inhaled, intranasal, and topical glucocorticoid administration.[65-67] Moreover, mirtazapine and progestins, such as medroxyprogesterone acetate and megestrol acetate, have been reported to induce secondary adrenal insufficiency.[68,69] Chronic suppression also can result in atrophy of the anterior pituitary and hypothalamus, impairing recovery of function if the exogenous steroid is reduced. Endogenous secondary insufficiency can occur with tumor development in the hypothalamic–pituitary region. Secondary disease classically presents with normal concentrations of mineralocorticoids since the zona glomerulosa is controlled by the renin–angiotensin system rather than ACTH levels.

Approximately 90% of the adrenal cortex must be destroyed before adrenal insufficiency symptoms will occur.[70] Specific etiologies for both primary and secondary insufficiency are listed in Table 76-11. Adrenal hemorrhage can result from multiple etiologies including traumatic shock, coagulopathies, ischemic disorders, and other situations of severe stress, but septicemia is the most common. Symptoms include truncal pain, fever, shaking, chills, hypotension preceding shock, anorexia, headache, vertigo, vomiting, rash, psychiatric symptoms, abdominal rigidity or rebound, and death in 6 to 48 hours if not treated. The most common organisms found on autopsy are *Neisseria meningitidis*, *Pseudomonas aeruginosa*, *Streptococcus pneumoniae*, Group A *Streptococcus*, and *Haemophilus influenzae*.[70,71]

TABLE 76-11 Etiologies of Primary and Secondary Adrenal Insufficiency

Primary Insufficiency	Secondary Insufficiency
Slow onset	Craniopharyngioma
Acquired immunodeficiency syndrome	Cure of Cushing syndrome
Adrenomyeloneuropathy	Empty sella syndrome
Adrenoleukodystrophy	Tumors of the third ventricle
Amyloidosis	Histiocytosis
Autoimmune adrenalitis[a]	Hypothalamic tumors
Bilateral adrenalectomy	Hypopituitarism
Congenital adrenal hypoplasia	Long-term corticosteroid administration
Hemochromatosis	Lymphocytic hypophysitis
Isolated glucocorticoid deficiency	Pituitary surgery, radiation, or tumor
Metastatic neoplasia	Sarcoidosis
Systemic fungal, bacterial, or viral infections, tuberculosis[b]	Medications—progestins and glucocorticoid discontinuation
Medications—ketoconazole, etomidate, rifampin, phenytoin, phenobarbital	Postpartum pituitary necrosis
	Necrotic or bleeding pituitary macroadenoma
Fast onset	
Adrenal thrombosis, hemorrhage, sepsis, trauma, or necrosis	Head trauma, lesions of the pituitary stalk, pituitary or adrenal surgery for Cushing syndrome

[a]Accounts for approximately 70% of cases.

[b]Accounts for approximately 20% of cases.

Diagnosis

Distinguishing Addison disease from secondary insufficiency is difficult; however, the following guidelines may be helpful:

1. Hyperpigmentation, commonly found in areas of skin exposed to increased friction, is seen only in Addison disease because of excess secretion of ACTH and other proopiomelanocortin (POMC) peptides that induce melanocyte-stimulating hormone production. Secondary adrenal insufficiency is fundamentally characterized by deficient ACTH and POMC peptide secretion and a corresponding low level of melanocyte-stimulating hormone production. In fact, some patients with secondary insufficiency may exhibit pale-colored skin secondary to hypopigmentation.
2. Aldosterone secretion usually is preserved in secondary insufficiency.
3. Weight loss, dehydration, hyponatremia, hyperkalemia, and elevated blood urea nitrogen are common in Addison disease.
4. Addison disease will have an abnormal response to the short corticotropin stimulation test. Plasma ACTH levels are usually elevated (400-2,000 pg/mL) in primary insufficiency, versus low to normal (5-50 pg/mL; see Table 76-3) in secondary insufficiency. A normal corticotropin stimulation test does not rule out secondary adrenal insufficiency, particularly in mild cases.

The short corticotropin stimulation test, also known as the cosyntropin stimulation test, can be used to assess patients suspected of hypocortisolism. Patients are given 250 mcg of synthetic ACTH IV or intramuscularly, with serum cortisol measured at baseline and 30 to 60 minutes after the injection. A resulting cortisol concentration ≥18 mcg/dL (500 nmol/L) rules out adrenal insufficiency.[72] Because 250 mcg represents a massive supraphysiologic dose, this test can elicit normal, elevated cortisol responses in some cases of mild secondary insufficiency. Thus, some suggest that higher cutoff values (≥22 mcg/dL [≥600 nmol/L]) should be used to prevent false-negative test results.[73] Alternatively, a low-dose corticotropin stimulation test, using 1 mcg of synthetic ACTH, can achieve equivalent results to the standard test and is more sensitive in establishing the diagnosis of secondary insufficiency.[74] Other tests include the insulin hypoglycemia test, the metyrapone test, and the CRH stimulation test.[75,76]

The standard cutoffs described above are of limited use in acutely ill patients.[77] Severe infection, trauma, burns, illnesses, or surgery can increase cortisol production by as much as a factor of 6, making the recognition of adrenal insufficiency in this population extremely difficult. In the critically ill, a random cortisol concentration below 15 mcg/dL (415 nmol/L) is suggestive of adrenal insufficiency, whereas a concentration greater than 34 mcg/dL (940 nmol/L) suggests that adrenal insufficiency is unlikely.[77] For patients who fall between these two values, a poor response to corticotropin (<9 mcg/dL [250 nmol/L] increase in plasma cortisol from baseline at 30 or 60 minutes) indicates the possibility of adrenal insufficiency and a need for corticosteroid supplementation.[77] A severe hypoproteinemic patient (albumin <2.5 g/L) will have markedly lower CBG, which can underestimate the actual free fraction of cortisol. These patients may benefit from measurement of free cortisol, although the assay may not be routinely available.[64,76]

Therapeutic Management

Treatment of Addison disease must include adequate patient education, so that the patient is aware of treatment complications, expected outcome, consequences of missed doses, and drug side effects. The agents of choice are hydrocortisone, cortisone, and prednisone, administered twice daily with the treatment objective being the establishment of the lowest effective dose while mimicking the normal diurnal adrenal rhythm.[72] Usually a twice-daily dosing schedule is adequate with the dose depending on the agent used.

Endogenous cortisol production varies between 5 and 10 mg/m^2/day.[78] Hence, the classic 12 to 15 mg/m^2/day rule for cortisol supplementation can be excessive in most patients. Recommended starting doses to properly mimic endogenous cortisol production are 15 to 25 mg of hydrocortisone daily, which is roughly equal to 25 to 37.5 mg of cortisone acetate or 2.5 mg of prednisone.[64,78] The majority of the dose (67%) is given in the morning, whereas the remainder (33%) is given 6 to 8 hours later to duplicate the normal circadian rhythm of cortisol production. Recent data also suggest that continuous infusion of glucocorticoids delivered via infusion pump may provide a more physiological circadian maintenance of ACTH and cortisol concentration when compared to conventional oral replacement.[79] Since no laboratory test adequately determines the appropriateness of dosing, the patient's symptoms should be monitored every 6 to 8 weeks to assess proper glucocorticoid replacement.

In primary insufficiency, fludrocortisone acetate can be used to supplement mineralocorticoid loss. For most patients, a dose of 0.05 to 0.2 mg by mouth once a day is adequate to maintain volume status. If parenteral therapy is needed, 2 to 5 mg of deoxycorticosterone trimethylacetate in oil intramuscularly every 3 to 4 weeks can be substituted. Mineralocorticoid replacement attenuates the development of hyperkalemia, but may be unnecessary in some primary cases because glucocorticoids, particularly at large doses, also bind to mineralocorticoid receptors. For example, a daily dose of hydrocortisone 40 to 50 mg has similar mineralocorticoid effects to 0.1 mg of fludrocortisone. Adverse effects must be monitored closely and include gastric upset, edema, hypertension, hypokalemia, insomnia, excitability, and diabetes mellitus. In addition, patient weight, blood pressure, and electrocardiogram should be monitored regularly.[75,76]

Clinical **Controversy...**

The primary source of dehydroepiandrosterone (DHEA) and androgens in women is the adrenal cortex. DHEA is converted to more potent androgens and estrogens in the periphery. Consequently, women with adrenal insufficiency can have decreased libido. DHEA, available as a dietary supplement, has been advocated as an option for female patients with adrenal insufficiency complaining of decreased libido and low energy. However, clinical trial data surrounding the benefits of DHEA are conflicting, and the general consensus on routine recommendation in clinical practice is currently lacking.

Most adrenal crises occur secondary to glucocorticoid dose reduction or lack of stress-related dose adjustments. Patients receiving corticosteroid replacement therapy should receive an additional 5 to 10 mg of hydrocortisone shortly before strenuous activities such as exercise.[75,76] Likewise, during times of severe physical stress such as febrile illnesses or injury, patients should be instructed to double their daily dose until recovery.[76,80] For major trauma, surgery, or in critically ill patients, larger doses—up to 10 times the usual daily dose—may be required.[76] Parenteral therapy should be used for patients experiencing diarrhea or vomiting. In patients with concomitant, newly diagnosed, or uncontrolled hypothyroidism, thyroid replacement should take place only after adequate glucocorticoid replacement as euthyroidism can trigger an adrenal crisis by accelerating cortisol metabolism.[72]

The end point of therapy is difficult to assess in most patients, but a reduction in excess pigmentation is a good clinical marker. The development of features of Cushing syndrome indicates excessive replacement. Treatment of secondary adrenal insufficiency is identical to primary disease treatment, except that mineralocorticoid replacement usually is unnecessary. Patient education is paramount with emphasis placed on the medication regimen and adrenal crisis prevention.

Acute Adrenal Insufficiency

Adrenal crisis, or Addisonian crisis, is characterized by an acute adrenocortical insufficiency and represents a true endocrine emergency. Anything that increases adrenal requirements dramatically can precipitate an adrenal crisis. Stressful situations, surgery, infection, and trauma all are potential triggering events, especially in the patient with some underlying adrenal or pituitary insufficiency. The most common cause of adrenal crisis is HPA-axis suppression brought on by abrupt withdrawal of chronic glucocorticoid use.

CLINICAL PRESENTATION Adrenal Insufficiency

Symptoms

- Patients commonly complain of weakness, weight loss, GI symptoms, craving for salt, headaches, memory impairment, depression, and postural dizziness.
- Early symptoms of acute adrenal insufficiency also include myalgias, malaise, and anorexia. As the situation progresses, vomiting, fever, hypotension, and shock will develop.

Signs

- Increased pigmentation
- Hypotension (postural)
- Fever
- Decreased body hair
- Vitiligo
- Features of hypopituitarism (amenorrhea and cold intolerance)

Laboratory Tests

- The short cosyntropin stimulation test can be used to assess patients suspected of hypercortisolism.

Other Diagnostic Tests

- Other tests include the insulin hypoglycemia test, the metyrapone test, and the CRH stimulation test.

Treatment of adrenal crisis involves the administration of parenteral glucocorticoids. Hydrocortisone is the agent of choice owing to its combined glucocorticoid and mineralocorticoid activity. Hydrocortisone is initially administered at a dose of 100 mg IV through rapid infusion, followed by a continuous infusion (usually 10 mg/h) or intermittent bolus of 100 to 200 mg every 24 hours.[64,76,81] Intravenous administration is continued for 24 to 48 hours, at which time if the patient is stable, oral hydrocortisone can be administered at a dose of 50 mg every 6 to 8 hours, followed by tapering to the individual's chronic replacement needs. Fluid replacement often is required and can be accomplished with dextrose 5% in normal saline solution (D_5NS) at a rate to support blood pressure. During initial treatment for adrenal crisis, mineralocorticoid replacement generally is unnecessary because of hydrocortisone's mineralocorticoid activity. If hyperkalemia is present after the hydrocortisone maintenance phase, additional mineralocorticoid supplementation can be achieved with 0.1 mg of fludrocortisone acetate daily.

Patients with adrenal insufficiency should be instructed to carry a card or wear a bracelet or necklace, such as MedicAlert, that contains information about their condition. Additionally, patients should have easy access to injectable hydrocortisone or glucocorticoid suppositories in case of an emergency or during times of physical stress, such as febrile illness or injury.[64]

Hypoaldosteronism

Hypoaldosteronism is rare and usually associated with low-renin status (hyporeninemic hypoaldosteronism), diabetes, complete heart block, or severe postural hypotension, or it can occur postoperatively following tumor removal. Hypoaldosteronism can be part of a larger adrenal insufficiency or a stand-alone defect. In nonselective hypoaldosteronism, generalized adrenocortical insufficiency is the most likely etiology (see Addison Disease). In selective hypoaldosteronism, insufficient aldosterone levels are precipitated by a specific defect in the stimulation of adrenal aldosterone secretion, with 21-hydroxylase deficiency being most common. Pseudohypoaldosteronism results from a defect in peripheral aldosterone action, whether from increased peripheral resistance or a reduced number of functional aldosterone receptors.

Laboratory analysis reveals hyponatremia, hyperkalemia, or both. Patients often will present with hyperchloremic metabolic acidosis. In most cases, the deficiency is in mineralocorticoid production and replacement with fludrocortisone in a dose of 0.1 to 0.3 mg is usually effective. Patients should be monitored for blood pressure response as well as electrolyte status.

Congenital Adrenal Hyperplasia

Because many enzyme systems are needed to complete the complex cholesterol-to-cortisol pathway, enzyme deficiencies can lead to disruptions of the normal cascade of events (see Fig. 76-2). This group of enzyme disorders is collectively referred to as congenital adrenal hyperplasia because of the resultant chronic adrenal gland stimulation that occurs following enzyme deficiency.[76,82,83] The most frequent cause of congenital adrenal hyperplasia is steroid 21-hydroxylase deficiency, accounting for more than 90% of cases. Any enzyme deficiency is capable of affecting any one or all three of the steroid pathways. Therefore, treatment focuses on replacement of the deficient hormone, psychological support, and surgical repair of the external genitalia in most female patients.[84] Six of the most common enzyme deficiencies are outlined briefly in Table 76-12.

Adrenal Virilism

9 Virilism, excessive secretion of androgens from the adrenal gland, commonly occurs as a result of congenital enzyme defects. Depending on the enzyme deficiency, patients accumulate excess levels of a variety of androgens, most notably testosterone. The condition affects women more often than men, with hirsutism being the dominant feature. Additional coexisting features can include voice deepening, acne, increased muscle mass, menstrual abnormalities, clitoral enlargement, redistribution of body fat and loss of female body contour, breast atrophy, and hair recession and crown balding.[85]

Treatment of virilism centers on suppression of the pituitary–adrenal axis with exogenous glucocorticoids. In adults, the usual steroids used are dexamethasone (0.25-0.5 mg), prednisone (2.5-5 mg), or hydrocortisone (10-20 mg).[86]

Hirsutism

Women presenting with hirsutism exhibit excess terminal hair growth in an androgen-dependent distribution. Such growth has obvious cosmetic consequences, but also can adversely affect quality

TABLE 76-12 Congenital Adrenal Hyperplasia

Enzyme Deficiency (Disorder)	Symptoms	Laboratory Tests	Comments
21-Hydroxylase (nonvirilizing CAH)	Enlarged female genitalia and adrenal gland (caused by cholesterol)	All steroids are low in blood and urine	Poor prognosis for infants
17-Hydroxylase (nonvirilizing CAH)	Hypertension usually present	Low concentrations of cortisol and estrogens	Mineralocorticoid replacement not necessary
21-Hydroxylase (virilizing CAH)	Pubertal irregularities (acne, early pubic hair, voice lowering, and increased muscularity); mature normally with replacement	High progesterone, renin, 17-hydroxyprogesterone, and ACTH; low cortisol, sodium, and aldosterone	Most common form of CAH (90% of total), incidence of 1:10,000; monitor growth velocity, bone age, renin, and 17-hydroxyprogesterone
11-Hydroxylase (virilizing CAH)	Hypertension secondary to high deoxycortisol and virilism from androgen excess; mistaken for Cushing, but no glucose intolerance	Low plasma cortisone and aldosterone; high ACTH and MSH concentrations	Second most common form of CAH (9% of total), incidence of 1:100,000; final step in biosynthesis of corticosterone and cortisol; found only in adrenal cortex
3-Hydroxysteroid dehydrogenase (mixed CAH)	Both cortisol and aldosterone deficiencies	Decreased aldosterone, cortisol, estrogens, and androgens; increased pregnenolone and cholesterol	Defect affects both adrenals and gonads
18-Hydroxysteroid dehydrogenase (corticosterone methyloxidase deficiency)	Hypotension	Restricted to zona glomerulosa; sole aldosterone defect; hyponatremia, hyperkalemia, increased renin	Mineralocorticoid replacement without glucocorticoid replacement

ACTH, adrenocorticotropic hormone; CAH, congenital adrenal hyperplasia; MSH, melanocyte-stimulating hormone.

of life and psychological well-being.[87] Most cases of hirsutism occur in women with some degree of excess androgen production. Androgen excess can be derived from either the ovaries or the adrenal glands, or rarely from pituitary disorders. Polycystic ovarian syndrome (PCOS) is responsible for most cases of ovarian excess and is the most common cause of hirsutism overall.[88] Congenital adrenal hyperplasia accounts for 5% of cases while adrenal and ovarian tumors cause hyperandrogenemia in 0.2% of women.

Cosmetic approaches generally are tried first, with repeated photoepilation offering the greatest long-term success.[89] If these approaches are unsuccessful, subsequent treatment should include pharmacologic intervention. Oral contraceptives are the treatment of choice in most hirsute women, particularly in those requiring concurrent contraception. If oral contraceptives are used, a progestin with low androgen activity (norethindrone, ethynodiol diacetate) or antiandrogenic activity (drospirenone) should be chosen. Other antiandrogens, including spironolactone and finasteride, can supplement or replace oral contraceptive therapy in women who cannot or choose not to conceive. Antiandrogens can take 6 to 12 months to alleviate hirsutism and treatment should be continued for 2 years, followed by a slow dose reduction.[90] Dexamethasone (and other glucocorticoids) can be modestly effective if the androgen source is adrenal, but can induce cushingoid symptoms even at doses of 0.5 mg/day.

Gonadotropin-releasing hormone can be an effective adjunct or alternative to oral contraceptives if the source of androgen is ovarian. However, these products generally are not recommended due to excessive costs, injectable-only routes of administration, and adverse effects resulting from estrogen deficiency. Additionally, insulin sensitizers, such as metformin or thiazolidinediones, can show modest improvement in women with PCOS, but their routine use is not recommended.[88]

Eflornithine hydrochloride, an irreversible ornithine decarboxylase inhibitor, moderately reduces the rate of hair growth but does not remove hair already present. The drug is available as a topical cream applied as a thin layer to the affected area twice daily, at least 8 hours apart. Reduction in unwanted hair can be noted within 6 to 8 weeks with a maximal effect at 8 to 24 weeks; therapy must be continued indefinitely to prevent hair regrowth.[86,90] Skin irritation can occur that resolves on discontinuation.

PRINCIPLES OF GLUCOCORTICOID ADMINISTRATION

Originally, the term *glucocorticoid* was given to these agents to describe their glucose-regulating properties. However, carbohydrate metabolism is only one of the myriad effects exhibited by steroids. The activity produced by these drugs is a function of the receptor activated (glucocorticoid vs mineralocorticoid), the location of the receptor, as well as the agent and dose prescribed.

The mechanism of action of glucocorticoids is complex and not fully known. The glucocorticoid enters the cell through passive diffusion and binds to its specific receptor. Between 5,000 and 100,000 receptors exist in each cell. Steroids exhibit various binding affinities to the vast number of receptors in almost every tissue and therefore elicit a wide variety of biologic effects.

Following receptor binding, a structural change occurs in the receptor, known as *activation*. After activation, the receptor–steroid complex binds to deoxyribonucleic acid sites in the cell called *glucocorticoid response elements* (GREs). This binding alters nearby gene expression and stimulates, or in some cases, inhibits transcription of specific mRNAs. Consequently, the resulting protein, which produces the stimulatory or inhibitory glucocorticoid action, varies according to the tissue and cell type in which the glucocorticoid receptor exists.

Pharmacokinetic properties of the glucocorticoids vary by agent and route of administration. In general, most orally administered steroids are well absorbed. Water-soluble agents are more rapidly absorbed following intramuscular injection than are lipid-soluble agents. Intravenous administration is recommended when a quick onset of action is needed. A summary of these agents is provided in Table 76-13.

In addition to causing iatrogenic Cushing syndrome, systemic steroids can lead to increased susceptibility to infection, osteoporosis, sodium retention with resultant edema, hypokalemia, hypomagnesemia, cataracts, peptic ulcer disease, seizures, and generalized suppression of the HPA axis. Long-term complications tend to be insidious and less likely to respond to steroid withdrawal.

Suppression of the HPA axis is a major concern whenever systemic steroids are tapered or withdrawn. Single doses of glucocorticoids can prevent the axis from responding to major stressors for several hours. In general, steroid administration at a high dose for long periods of time causes suppression of the axis. However, the possibility of suppression occurs any time the patient is exposed to supraphysiologic steroid doses.[23,91] Symptoms of steroid withdrawal resemble those seen in a patient with adrenocortical deficiency.

A variety of recommendations for steroid tapering are available.[23,92-94] In general, patients who have been on long-term steroid therapy will need to be gradually withdrawn toward physiologic doses over months. On average, the normal adult produces approximately 10 to 30 mg of cortisol per day with the peak concentration occurring around 8:00 AM. As the steroid or steroid-equivalent dose approaches the 20- to 30-mg level, the taper should be slowed and the patient checked for axis function. The primary modes to test HPA integrity are the ACTH test, either high or low dose, or a morning (8:00 AM) serum cortisol. A normal morning serum cortisol (>20 mcg/dL) or a normal ACTH test indicates that daily steroid maintenance therapy may be discontinued. If morning serum cortisol is between 3 and 20 mcg/dL, the ACTH or CRH stimulation test can be useful in the assessment of pituitary–adrenal function.[23]

TABLE 76-13 Relative Potencies of Glucocorticoids

Glucocorticoid	Antiinflammatory Potency	Equivalent Potency (mg)	Approximate Half-Life (min)	Sodium-Retaining Potency
Cortisone	0.8	25	30	2
Hydrocortisone	1	20	90	2
Prednisone	3.5	5	60	1
Prednisolone	4	5	200	1
Triamcinolone	5	4	300	0
Methylprednisolone	5	4	180	0
Betamethasone	25	0.6	100-300	0
Dexamethasone	30	0.75	100-300	0

A morning cortisol less than 3 mcg/dL indicates axis suppression and the need for continued replacement therapy. Suppression can persist for up to a year in some patients. Caution should be used to prevent disease exacerbation during the steroid taper and to avoid the need for another course of high-dose steroids.

Alternate-day therapy (ADT) regimens have been promoted as a means to lessen the impact of prolonged steroid administration.[23,94] ADT theoretically minimizes the hypothalamic–pituitary suppression as well as some of the adverse effects seen with once-daily therapy. This hypothetical advantage may be especially pertinent in treating children and young adults, in whom growth suppression is a major concern. ADT is not recommended for initial management, but rather in the management of the stabilized patient who needs long-term therapy. The patient is exposed to "on" and "off" days, with the "on" day dose gradually increased corresponding with a dose-reduction in the "off" day dose over a period of 14 days. After 2 weeks, no medication is taken on "off" days. Not all patients will have equivalent disease control on ADT, and it should be avoided in certain indications.[23,94]

EVALUATION OF THERAPEUTIC OUTCOMES

Successful glucocorticoid therapy involves counseling and monitoring the patient, as well as recognizing complications of therapy (Table 76-14). The risk-to-benefit ratio of glucocorticoid administration should always be considered, especially with concurrent disease states such as hypertension, diabetes mellitus, peptic ulcer disease, and uncontrolled systemic infections.

TABLE 76-14 Factors in Successful Glucocorticoid Therapy

Monitoring	Glucose concentrations (serum and urine) Electrolytes (serum and urine) Ophthalmologic examinations Stool tests for occult blood loss Growth and development (children and adolescents)
Counseling	Take with food to minimize GI discomfort Never discontinue medication on your own; check with your physician; gradual dose reduction is usually necessary Carry or wear medical identification indicating that you are on long-term glucocorticoid therapy Dosage increases can be necessary at times of increased stress (surgery or emergency treatments) Be aware of potential side effects (ie, visual disturbances, bruising, and delayed wound healing) What to do if you miss a dose: If your dosing schedule is: *Every other day*: Take as soon as possible if remembered that morning. If not remembered until later, skip that day. Take the next morning, and then skip the following day *Every day*: Take as soon as possible, but skip if almost time for the next dose. Never double doses
Recognizing complications	Early in therapy and essentially unavoidable: insomnia, enhanced appetite, weight gain Common in patients with underlying risk factors: hypertension, diabetes mellitus, peptic ulcer disease Long-term intense treatment: cushingoid habitus, hypothalamic pituitary–adrenal suppression, impaired wound healing Delayed and insidious: cataracts, atherosclerosis Rare and unpredictable: psychosis, glaucoma, pancreatitis

Data from references 95 and 96.

ABBREVIATIONS

ACTH	adrenocorticotropic hormone
ADT	alternate-day therapy
ALP	alkaline phosphatase
ALT	alanine aminotransferase
APA	aldosterone-producing adenoma
APS	autoimmune polyendocrine syndrome
ARR	aldosterone-to-renin ratio
AST	aspartate aminotransferase
AVS	adrenal venous sampling
BAH	bilateral adrenal hyperplasia
CBG	corticosteroid-binding globulin
CHD	coronary heart disease
CNS	central nervous system
CrCl	creatinine clearance
CRH	corticotropin-releasing hormone
CT	computed tomography
CYP	cytochrome P450
D_5NS	dextrose 5% in normal saline solution
DDT	dichlorodiphenyltrichloroethane
DHEA	dehydroepiandrosterone
DST	dexamethasone suppression test
FDA	Food and Drug Administration
FH	familial hyperaldosteronism
FST	fludrocortisone suppression test
GABA	γ-aminobutyric acid
GI	gastrointestinal
GRA	glucocorticoid-remediable aldosteronism
GRE	glucocorticoid response element
HPA	hypothalamic–pituitary–adrenal
INR	international normalized ratio
IPSS	inferior petrosal sinus sampling
IRMA	immunoradiometric assay
JVS	jugular venous sampling
LDL	low-density lipoprotein
MRI	magnetic resonance imaging
PA	primary aldosteronism
PAC	plasma aldosterone concentration
PAC-to-PRA	plasma-aldosterone-concentration–to–plasma-renin-activity
PCOS	polycystic ovarian syndrome
POMC	proopiomelanocortin
PRA	plasma renin activity
RAAS	renin–angiotensin–aldosterone system
RIA	radioimmunoassay
sst_2	somatostatin receptor subtype 2
UFC	urinary free cortisol

REFERENCES

1. Conn JW. Primary aldosteronism, a new clinical syndrome. *J Lab Clin Med* 1955;45:6-17.
2. Albright F. Cushing syndrome. *Harvey Lect* 1942–1943;38:123-186.
3. Lacroix A, Feelders RA, Stratakis CA, Nieman LK. Cushing syndrome. *Lancet* 2015;386(9996):913-927.
4. Isidori AM, Kaltsas GA, Pozza C, et al. The ectopic adrenocorticotropin syndrome: Clinical features, diagnosis, management, and long-term follow-up. *J Clin Endocrinol Metab* 2006;91:371-377.
5. Boscaro M, Barzon L, Sonino N. The diagnosis of Cushing syndrome: Atypical presentations and laboratory shortcomings. *Arch Intern Med* 2000;160:3045-3053.
6. Arlt W. Disorders of the adrenal cortex. In: Kasper D, Fauci A, Hauser S, Longo D, Jameson J, Loscalzo J., eds. *Harrison's Principles of Internal Medicine,* 19th ed. New York, NY: McGraw-Hill; 2015. http://accessmedicine.mhmedical.com/content.aspx?bookid=1130&Sectionid=79752055.

7. Catargi B, Rigalleau V, Poussin A, et al. Occult Cushing syndrome in type-2 diabetes. *J Clin Endocrinol Metab* 2003;88:5808-5813.
8. Findling JW, Raff H. Screening and diagnosis of Cushing syndrome. *Endocrinol Metab Clin North Am* 2005;34:385-402.
9. Nieman LK, Biller BMK, Findling JW, et al. The diagnosis of Cushing syndrome: An Endocrine Society clinical practice guideline. *J Clin Endocrinol Metab* 2008;93:1526-1540.
10. Terzolo M, Reimondo G, Chiodini I, et al. Screening of Cushing syndrome in outpatients with type 2 diabetes: Results of a prospective multicentric study in Italy. *J Clin Endocrinol Metab* 2012;97:3467-3475. doi:10.1210/jc.2012-1323.
11. Nieman LK, Ilias I. Evaluation and treatment of Cushing syndrome. *Am J Med* 2005;118:1340-1346.
12. Lindsay JR, Nieman LK. Differential diagnosis and imaging in Cushing syndrome. *Endocrinol Metab Clin North Am* 2005;34:403-421.
13. Arnaldi G, Angeli A, Atkinson AB, et al. Diagnosis and complications of Cushing syndrome: A consensus statement. *J Clin Endocrinol Metab* 2003;88:5593-5602.
14. Jackson RV, Hockings GI, Torpy DJ, et al. New diagnostic tests for Cushing syndrome: Uses of naloxone, vasopressin and alprazolam. *Clin Exp Pharmacol Physiol* 1996;23:579-581.
15. Ambrosi B, Bochicchio D, Colombo P, et al. Loperamide to diagnose Cushing syndrome. *JAMA* 1993;270:2301-2302.
16. Arvat E, Giordano R, Ramunni J, et al. Adrenocorticotropin and cortisol hyperresponsiveness to hexarelin in patients with Cushing disease bearing a pituitary microadenoma, but not in those with macroadenoma. *J Clin Endocrinol Metab* 1998;83:4207-4211.
17. Newell-Price J, Trainer P, Besser M, Grossman A. The diagnosis and differential diagnosis of Cushing syndrome and pseudo-Cushing states. *Endocr Rev* 1998;19:647-672.
18. Papanicolaou DA, Mullen N, Kyrou I, Nieman LK. Nighttime salivary cortisol: A useful test for the diagnosis of Cushing syndrome. *J Clin Endocrinol Metab* 2002;87:4515-4521.
19. Viardot A, Huber P, Puder JJ, et al. Reproducibility of nighttime salivary cortisol and its use in the diagnosis of hypercortisolism compared with urinary free cortisol and overnight dexamethasone suppression test. *J Clin Endocrinol Metab* 2005;90:5730-5736.
20. Findling JW, Raff H, Aron DC. The low-dose dexamethasone suppression test: A reevaluation in patients with Cushing syndrome. *J Clin Endocrinol Metab* 2004;89:1222-1226.
21. Rockall AG, Babar SA, Sohaib SA, et al. CT and MR imaging of the adrenal glands in ACTH-independent Cushing syndrome. *Radiographics* 2004;24:435-452.
22. Peppercorn PD, Reznek RH. State-of-the-art CT and MRI of the adrenal gland. *Eur Radiol* 1997;7:822-836.
23. Hopkins RL, Leinung MC. Exogenous Cushing syndrome and glucocorticoid withdrawal. *Endocrinol Metab Clin North Am* 2005;34:371-384.
24. Bolland MJ, Bagg W, Thomas MG, et al. Cushing syndrome due to interaction between inhaled corticosteroids and itraconazole. *Ann Pharmacother* 2004;38:46-49.
25. Samaras K, Pett S, Gowers A, et al. Iatrogenic Cushing syndrome with osteoporosis and secondary adrenal failure in human immunodeficiency virus-infected patients receiving inhaled corticosteroids and ritonavir-boosted protease inhibitors: Six cases. *J Clin Endocrinol Metab* 2005;90:4394-4398.
26. Nieman LK. Medical therapy of Cushing disease. *Pituitary* 2002;5:77-82.
27. Labeur M, Arzt E, Stalla GK, Paez-Pereda M. New perspectives in the treatment of Cushing syndrome. *Curr Drug Targets Immune Endocr Metabol Disord* 2004;4:335-342.
28. McEvoy GK, ed. American Hospital Formulary Service (AHFS) Drug Information. Bethesda, MD: American Society of Health-System Pharmacists; 2015.
29. Nieman LK, Biller BMK, Findling JW, et al. Treatment of Cushing Syndrome: An Endocrine Society Clinical Practice Guideline. *J Clin Endorcrinol Metab* 2015;100:2807-2831.
30. Utz AL, Swearingen B, Biller BM. Pituitary surgery and postoperative management in Cushing disease. *Endocrinol Metab Clin North Am* 2005;34:459-478.
31. Dang CN, Trainer P. Pharmacological management of Cushing syndrome: An update. *Arq Bras Endocrinol Metabol* 2007;51:1339-1348.
32. Preda VA, Sen J, Karavitaki N, Grossman AB. Etomidate in the management of hypercortiolaemia in Cushing syndrome: a review. *Eur J Endocronol* 2012;167:137-143.
33. Pivonello R, Ferone D, de Herder WW, et al. Dopamine receptor expression and function in corticotroph pituitary tumors. *J Clin Endocrinol Metab* 2004;89:2452-2462.
34. Godbout A, Manavela M, Danilowicz K, et al. Cabergoline monotherapy in the long-term treatment of Cushing disease. *Eur J Endocrinol* 2010;163:709-716.
35. Tritos NA, Biller BMK, Swearingen B. Management of Cushing disease. *Nat Rev Endocrinol* 2011;7:279-289.
36. Tritos NA, Biller BM. Medical management of Cushing disease. *J Neurooncol* 2014;117(3):407-414.
37. Colao A, Petersenn S, Newell-Price J, et al. A 12-month phase 3 study of pasireotide in Cushing disease. *N Engl J Med* 2012;366:914-924.
38. Feelders RA, de Bruin C, Pereira AM, et al. Pasireotide alone or with cabergoline and ketoconazole in Cushing disease. *N Engl J Med* 2010;362:1846-1848.
39. Nieman LK. Update in the medical therapy of Cushing disease. *Curr Opin Endocrinol Diabetes Obesm* 2013;20:330-334.
40. Fleseriu M, Biller BMK, Findling JW, et al. Mifepristone, a glucocorticoid receptor antagonist, produces clinical and metabolic benefits in patients with Cushing syndrome. *J Clin Endocrinol Metab* 2012;97:2039-2049.
41. Semple PL, Vance ML, Findling J, Laws ER. Transsphenoidal surgery for Cushing disease: Outcome in patients with a normal magnetic resonance imaging scan. *Neurosurgery* 2000;46:553-558.
42. Biller BMK, Grossman AB, Stewart PM, et al. Treatment of adrenocorticotropin-dependent Cushing syndrome: A consensus statement. *J Clin Endocrinol Metab* 2008;93:2454-2462.
43. Terzolo M, Angeli A, Fassnacht M, et al. Adjuvant mitotane treatment for adrenocortical carcinoma. *N Engl J Med* 2007;356:2372-2380.
44. Veytsman I, Nieman L, Fojo T. Management of endocrine manifestations and the use of mitotane as a chemotherapeutic agent for adrenocortical carcinoma. *J Clin Oncol* 2009;27:4619-4629.
45. Morris D, Grossman A. The medical management of Cushing syndrome. *Ann N Y Acad Sci* 2002;970:119-133.
46. Stowasser M, Gordon RD. Primary aldosteronism: From genesis to genetics. *Trends Endocrinol Metab* 2003;14:310-317.
47. Stowasser M, Gordon RD. Primary aldosteronism. *Best Pract Res Clin Endocrinol Metab* 2003;17:591-605.
48. Wu V, Chao C, Kuo C, et al. Diagnosis and Management of Primary Aldosternoism. *Acta Nephrologica* 2012;26(3):111-120.
49. Chao C, Wu V, Kuo C, et al. Diagnosis and management of primary aldosteronism: an updated review. *Ann Med* 2013;45:375-383.
50. Funder JW, Carey RM, Fardella C, et al. Case detection, diagnosis, and treatment of patients with primary aldosteronism: An Endocrine Society clinical practice guideline. *J Clin Endocrinol Metab* 2008;93:3266-3281.
51. Schwartz GL, Turner ST. Screening for primary aldosteronism in essential hypertension: Diagnostic accuracy of the ratio of plasma aldosterone concentration to plasma renin activity. *Clin Chem* 2005;51:386-394.
52. Kumar B, Swee M. Aldosterone-renin ratio in the assessment of primary aldosteronism. *JAMA* 2014;312(2):184-185.
53. Mulatero P, Dluhy RG, Giacchetti G, et al. Diagnosis of primary aldosteronism: From screening to subtype differentiation. *Trends Endocrinol Metab* 2005;16:114-119.
54. Young WF, Stanson AW, Thompson GB, et al. Role for adrenal venous sampling in primary aldosteronism. *Surgery* 2004;136: 1227-1235.
55. Nwariaku FE, Miller BS, Auchus R, et al. Primary hyperaldosteronism: Effect of adrenal vein sampling on surgical outcome. *Arch Surg* 2006;141:497-502.
56. Ye P, Yamashita T, Pollock DM, Rainey WE. Contrasting effects of eplerenone and spironolactone on adrenal cell steroidogenesis. *Horm Metab Res* 2009;41:35-39.
57. Nishizaka MK, Calhoun DA. Primary aldosteronism: Diagnostic and therapeutic considerations. *Curr Cardiol Rep* 2005;7:412-417.
58. Young WF Jr. Primary aldosteronism: Management issues. *Ann N Y Acad Sci* 2002;970:61-76.
59. Young WF. Primary aldosteronism—Treatment options. *Growth Horm IGF Res* 2003;13:S102-S108.
60. Parthasarathy HK, Menard J, White WB, et al. A double-blind, randomized study comparing the antihypertensive effect of eplerenone and spironolactone in patients with hypertension and evidence of primary aldosteronism. *J Hypertens* 2011;29:980-990.
61. Cabassi A, Rocco R, Berretta R, et al. Eplerenone use in primary aldosteronism during pregnancy. *Hypertension* 2012;49:e18-19.
62. Meria P, Kempf BF, Hermieu JF, et al. Laparoscopic management of primary aldosteronism: Clinical experience with 212 cases. *J Urol* 2003;169:32-35.
63. Meyer A, Brabant G, Behrend M. Long-term follow-up after adrenalectomy for primary aldosteronism. *World J Surg* 2005;29:155-159.

64. Banco I, Hahner S, Tomlinson J, Arlt W. Diagnosis and management of adrenal insufficiency. *Lancet Diabetes Endocrinol* 2015;3:216-226.
65. Levin C, Maibach HI. Topical corticosteroid-induced adrenocortical insufficiency: Clinical implications. *Am J Clin Dermatol* 2002;3:141-147.
66. Bello CE, Garrett SD. Therapeutic issues in oral glucocorticoid use. *Lippincotts Prim Care Pract* 1999;3:333-341.
67. Sizonenko PC. Effects of inhaled or nasal glucocorticosteroids on adrenal function and growth. *J Pediatr Endocrinol Metab* 2002;15:5-26.
68. Goodman A, Cagliero E. Megestrol-induced clinical adrenal insufficiency. *Eur J Gynaecol Oncol* 2000;21:117-118.
69. Schule C, Baghai T, Bidlingmaier M, et al. Endocrinological effects of mirtazapine in healthy volunteers. *Prog Neuropsychopharmacol Biol Psychiatry* 2002;26:1253-1261.
70. Alevritis EM, Sarubbi FA, Jordan RM, Peiris AN. Infectious cause of adrenal insufficiency. *South Med J* 2003;96:888-890.
71. Torrey SP. Recognition and management of adrenal emergencies. *Emerg Med Clin North Am* 2005;23:687-702.
72. Michels A, Michels N. Addison Disease: Early Detection and Treatment Principles. *Am Fam Physician* 2014;89(7):563-568.
73. Oelkers W. The role of high- and low-dose corticotropin tests in the diagnosis of secondary adrenal insufficiency. *Eur J Endocrinol* 1998;139:567-570.
74. Magnotti M, Shimshi M. Diagnosing adrenal insufficiency: Which test is best—The 1-mcg or the 250-mcg cosyntropin stimulation test? *Endocr Pract* 2008;14:233-238.
75. Arlt W, Allolio B. Adrenal insufficiency. Lancet 2003;361:1881-1893.
76. Charmandari E, Nicolaides NC, Chrousos GP. Adrenal insufficiency. *Lancet* 2014;383(9935):2152-67.
77. Cooper MS, Stewart PM. Corticosteroid insufficiency in acutely ill patients. *N Engl J Med* 2003;348:727-734.
78. Crown A, Lightman S. Why is the management of glucocorticoid deficiency still controversial: A review of the literature. *Clin Endocrinol (Oxf)* 2005;63:483-492.
79. Oksnes M, Bjornsdottir S, Isaksson M. Continuous subcutaneous hydrocortisone infusion versus oral hydrocortisone replacement for treatment of Addison disease: A randomized clinical trial. *J Clin Endocrinol Metab* 2014;99(5):1665-1674.
80. Nieman LK, Turner MC. Addison disease. *Clin Dermatol* 2006;24:276-280.
81. Jacobi J. Corticosteroid replacement in critically ill patients. *Crit Care Clin* 2006;22:245-253.
82. Speiser PW, White PC. Congenital adrenal hyperplasia. *N Engl J Med* 2003;349:776-788.
83. Forest MG. Recent advances in the diagnosis and management of congenital adrenal hyperplasia due to 21-hydroxylase deficiency. *Hum Reprod Update* 2004;10:469-485.
84. Merke DP, Bornstein SR. Congenital adrenal hyperplasia. Lancet 2005;365:2125-2136.
85. Yildiz BO. Diagnosis of hyperandrogenism: Clinical criteria. *Best Pract Res Clin Endocrinol Metab* 2006;20:167-176.
86. Rosenfield RL. Hirsutism. *N Engl J Med* 2005;353:2578-2588.
87. Koulouri O, Conway GS. Management of hirsutism. *BMJ* 2009;338:823-826.
88. Martin KA, Chang RJ, Ehrmann DA, et al. Evaluation and treatment of hirsutism in premenopausal women: An Endocrine Society clinical practice guideline. *J Clin Endocrinol Metab* 2008;93:1105-1120.
89. Azziz R. The evaluation and management of hirsutism. *Obstet Gynecol* 2003;101:995-1007.
90. Moghetti P. Treatment of hirsutism and acne in hyperandrogenism. *Best Pract Res Clin Endocrinol Metab* 2006;20:221-234.
91. Henzen C, Suter A, Lerch E, et al. Suppression and recovery of adrenal response after short-term, high-dose glucocorticoid treatment. *Lancet* 2000;355:542-545.
92. Krasner AS. Glucocorticoid-induced adrenal insufficiency. *JAMA* 1999;282:671-676.
93. Kountz DS, Clark CL. Safely withdrawing patients from chronic glucocorticoid therapy. *Am Fam Physician* 1997;55:521-552.
94. Baxter JD. Advances in glucocorticoid therapy. Adv Intern Med 2000;45:317-349.
95. United States Pharmacopeial Convention Inc. USPDI. *Advice for the Patient: Drug Information in Lay Language,* Vol. II, 19th ed. Taunton, MA: Rand-McNally; 1999:612-616.
96. Boumpas DT, Chrousos GP, Wilder RL, et al. Complications of therapy. In: Boumpas DT, moderator. Glucocorticoid therapy for immune-mediated diseases: Basic and clinical correlates. *Ann Intern Med* 1993;119:1198-1208.

Pituitary Gland Disorders

e77

Joseph K. Jordan, Amy Heck Sheehan, and Karim Anton Calis

KEY CONCEPTS

1. Pharmacologic therapy for acromegaly should be considered when surgery and irradiation are contraindicated, when there is poor likelihood of surgical success, when rapid control of symptoms is needed, or when other treatments have failed to normalize growth hormone (GH) and insulin-like growth factor-1 (IGF-1) serum concentrations.
2. Pharmacotherapy for acromegaly using dopamine agonists provides advantages of oral dosing and reduced cost compared to somatostatin analogs and pegvisomant. However, dopamine agonists effectively normalize IGF-1 serum concentrations in only 10% of patients. Therefore, somatostatin analogs remain the mainstay of therapy.
3. Blood glucose concentrations should be monitored frequently in the early stages of somatostatin analog therapy for acromegaly.
4. Pegvisomant appears to be the most effective agent for normalizing IGF-1 serum concentrations. However, further study is needed to determine the long-term safety and efficacy of this agent for the treatment of acromegaly.
5. Recombinant GH is currently considered the mainstay for treatment of children with growth hormone-deficient short stature. Prompt diagnosis of growth hormone deficiency (GHD) and initiation of replacement therapy with recombinant GH is crucial for optimizing final adult heights.
6. All GH products are generally considered to be equally effective. The recommended dose for treatment of GHD short stature in children is 0.3 mg/kg/wk.
7. Pharmacologic agents that antagonize dopamine or increase the release of prolactin can induce hyperprolactinemia. Discontinuation of the offending medication and initiation of an appropriate therapeutic alternative usually normalizes serum prolactin concentrations.
8. Cabergoline appears to be more effective than bromocriptine for the medical management of prolactinomas and offers the advantage of less-frequent dosing and fewer adverse effects.
9. Although preliminary data do not suggest cabergoline has significant teratogenic potential, cabergoline is not recommended for use during pregnancy, and patients receiving cabergoline who plan to become pregnant should discontinue the medication as soon as pregnancy is detected.
10. Pharmacologic treatment of panhypopituitarism includes the use of glucocorticoids, thyroid hormone, sex steroids, and recombinant GH, where appropriate, as lifelong replacement therapies.

INTRODUCTION

In the 1950s, Geoffrey Harris and his colleagues uncovered the physiologic importance of pituitary hormones and proposed the theory of neurohormonal regulation of the pituitary by the hypothalamus.[1] Today the pituitary gland is recognized for its essential role in body homeostasis, and for this reason it is often referred to as the *master gland.* The hypothalamus and the pituitary gland are closely connected, and together they provide a means of communication between the brain and many of the body's endocrine organs. The hypothalamus uses nervous input and metabolic signals from the body to control the secretion of pituitary hormones that regulate growth, thyroid function, adrenal activity, reproduction, lactation, and fluid balance.

ANATOMY AND PHYSIOLOGY

The hypothalamus (Fig. e77-1) is a small region at the base of the brain that receives autonomic nervous input from different areas of the body to regulate limbic functions, food and water intake, body temperature, cardiovascular function, respiratory function, and diurnal rhythms. In addition, the hypothalamus controls the release of hormones from the anterior and posterior regions of the pituitary gland. Neurons in the hypothalamus produce vasopressin and oxytocin and make many hormone-releasing factors that stimulate or inhibit the release of trophic hormones. At the base of the hypothalamus, a projection known as the *median eminence* is rich with nerve axons and blood vessels and provides both chemical and physical connections between the hypothalamus and the pituitary gland.

The pituitary gland, also referred to as the *hypophysis*, is located at the base of the brain in a cavity of the sphenoid bone known as the *sella turcica*. The pituitary is separated from the brain by an extension of the dura mater known as the *diaphragma sellae*. The pituitary is a very small gland, weighing between 0.4 and 1 g in adults. It is divided into two distinct regions: the anterior lobe, or adenohypophysis; and the posterior lobe, or the neurohypophysis (see Fig. e77-1).

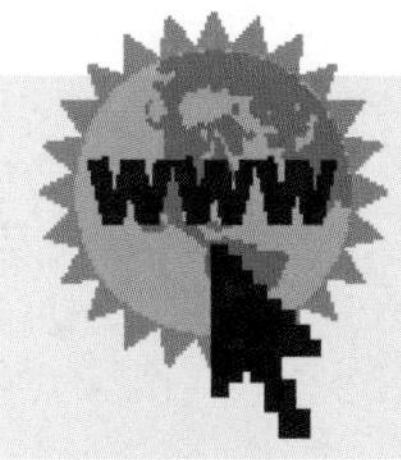

The complete chapter, learning objectives, and other resources can be found at **www.pharmacotherapyonline.com.**

Pregnancy and Lactation: Therapeutic Considerations

78

Kristina E. Ward

KEY CONCEPTS

1. Complex physiology surrounds the process of fertilization and pregnancy progression.
2. Drug characteristics and physiologic changes modify drug pharmacokinetics during pregnancy, including changes in absorption, protein binding, distribution, and elimination, requiring individualized drug selection and dosing.
3. Although drug-induced teratogenicity is a serious concern during pregnancy, most drugs required by pregnant women can be used safely. Informed selection of drug therapy is essential.
4. Healthcare practitioners must know where to find and how to evaluate evidence related to the safety of drugs used during pregnancy and lactation.
5. Health issues influenced by pregnancy, such as nausea and vomiting, can be treated safely and effectively with nonpharmacologic treatment or carefully selected drug therapy.
6. Some acute and chronic illnesses pose additional risks during pregnancy, requiring treatment with appropriately selected and monitored drug therapies to avoid harm to the woman and the fetus.
7. Management of the pregnant woman during the peripartum period not only can encompass uncomplicated pregnancies/deliveries, but can also include a wide variety of potential complications that require use of evidence-based treatments to maximize positive maternal and neonatal outcomes.
8. Understanding the physiology of lactation and pharmacokinetic factors affecting drug distribution, metabolism, and elimination can assist the clinician in selecting safe and effective medications during lactation.

A controversial and emotionally charged subject because of medicolegal and ethical implications, drug use in pregnancy and lactation is a topic often underemphasized in the education of health professionals. Clinicians are responsible for ensuring safe and effective therapy before conception, during pregnancy and parturition, and after delivery. Active patient participation is essential. Optimal treatments of illnesses during pregnancy sometimes differ from those used in the nonpregnant patient.

In many cases, medication dosing recommendations for acute or chronic illnesses in pregnant women are the same as for the general population. However, some cases require different dosing and selection of medications. Principles of drug use during lactation, although similar, are not the same as those applicable during pregnancy.

PHYSIOLOGY OF PREGNANCY

(1) Fertilization and progression of pregnancy are complex, resulting in survival of only approximately 50% of embryos.[1] Because most losses occur early, usually in the first 2 weeks after fertilization, many women do not realize they were pregnant. Spontaneous loss of pregnancy later in gestation occurs in about 15% of pregnancies that survive the first 2 weeks after fertilization.[2]

Fertilization occurs when a sperm attaches to the outer protein layer of the egg, the zona pellucida, and renders the egg nonresponsive to other sperm.[3] The attached sperm releases enzymes that allow the sperm to fully penetrate the zona pellucida and contact the egg's cell membrane. The membranes of the sperm and egg then combine to create a new, single cell called a zygote. Male and female chromosomes join in the zygote, fuse to create a single nucleus, and organize for cell division.

Fertilization usually occurs in the fallopian tube.[4] The fertilized egg travels down the fallopian tube over 2 days, with cell division taking place. By day 3, the fertilized egg reaches the uterus. Cell division continues for another 2 to 3 days in the uterine cavity before implantation. Approximately 6 days after fertilization, the cell mass is termed a *blastocyst*. Human chorionic gonadotropin (hCG) now is produced in amounts detectable by commercial laboratories. Implantation begins with the blastocyst sloughing the zona pellucida to rest directly on the endometrium allowing initiation of growth into the endometrial wall. By day 10 postfertilization, the blastocyst is implanted under the endometrial surface and receives nutrition from maternal blood. On the first day of the third week postfertilization it is called an *embryo*.[4,5]

After the embryonic period (between weeks 2 and 8 postfertilization), the embryo is renamed a *fetus*. Most body structures are formed during the embryonic period, and they continue to grow and mature during the fetal period. The fetal period continues until the pregnancy reaches term, approximately 40 weeks after the last menstrual period.[5]

Gravidity is the number of times that a woman has been pregnant. A multiple birth is counted as a single pregnancy. *Parity* refers to the number of pregnancies exceeding 20 weeks of gestation and relates information regarding the outcome of each pregnancy. In sequence, the numbers reflect (a) term deliveries, (b) premature deliveries, (c) aborted pregnancies, and (d) number of living children. A woman who has been pregnant four times; has experienced two term deliveries, one premature delivery, and one ectopic pregnancy; and has three living children would be designated G_4P_{2113}.[6,7]

Characteristics of Pregnancy

Pregnancy lasts approximately 280 days (about 40 weeks or 9 months); the time period is measured from the first day of the last menstrual period to birth. *Gestational age* refers to the age of the embryo or fetus beginning with the first day of the last menstrual period, which is about 2 weeks prior to fertilization. When calculating the estimated due date, add 7 days to the first day of the last menstrual period then subtract 3 months. Pregnancy is divided into three periods of 3 calendar months, each called a *trimester*.[6]

Early symptoms of pregnancy include fatigue and increased frequency of urination. After the first or second missed menstrual period, nausea and vomiting can occur. While commonly called *morning sickness*, it can happen at any time of the day. Nausea and vomiting usually resolve at 14 to 16 weeks of gestation. A pregnant woman can feel fetal movement in the lower abdomen at 14 to 20 weeks of gestation; multiparous women feel movement earlier than women who are primiparous. Signs of pregnancy include cessation of menses, change in cervical mucus consistency, bluish discoloration of the vaginal mucosa, increased skin pigmentation, and anatomic breast changes.[6,7]

Pharmacokinetic Changes During Pregnancy

2 Normal physiologic changes that occur during pregnancy may alter medication effects, resulting in the need to more closely monitor and, sometimes, adjust therapy. Physiologic changes begin in the first trimester and peak during the second trimester. For medications that can be monitored by blood or serum concentration measurements, monitoring should occur throughout pregnancy.

During pregnancy, maternal plasma volume, cardiac output, and glomerular filtration increase by 30% to 50% or higher, potentially lowering the concentration of renally cleared drugs.[8,9] As body fat increases during pregnancy, the volume of distribution of fat-soluble drugs may increase. Plasma albumin concentration decreases, which increases the volume of distribution of drugs that are highly protein bound. However, unbound drugs are more rapidly cleared by the liver and kidney during pregnancy, resulting in little change in concentration. Hepatic perfusion increases, which could theoretically increase the hepatic extraction of drugs. Nausea and vomiting, as well as delayed gastric emptying, may alter the absorption of drugs. Likewise, a pregnancy-induced increase in gastric pH may affect the absorption of weak acids and bases. Higher levels of estrogen and progesterone alter liver enzyme activity and increase the elimination of some drugs but result in accumulation of others.[8-10]

Transplacental Drug Transfer

2 Although once thought to be a barrier to drug transfer, the placenta is the organ of exchange for a number of substances, including drugs, between the mother and fetus. Most drugs move from the maternal circulation to the fetal circulation by diffusion.[11] Certain chemical properties, such as lipid solubility, electrical charge, molecular weight, and degree of protein binding of medications, may influence the rate of transfer across the placenta.

Drugs with molecular weights less than 500 Da readily cross the placenta, whereas larger molecules (600-1,000 Da) cross more slowly.[11] Drugs with molecular weights greater than 1,000 Da, such as insulin and heparin, do not cross the placenta in significant amounts. Lipophilic drugs, such as opioids and antibiotics, cross the placenta more easily than do water-soluble drugs. Maternal plasma albumin progressively decreases, while fetal albumin increases during the course of pregnancy, which may result in higher concentrations of certain protein-bound drugs in the fetus. Fetal pH is slightly more acidic than maternal pH, permitting weak bases to more easily cross the placenta. Once in the fetal circulation, the molecule becomes more ionized and less likely to diffuse back into the maternal circulation.[11]

DRUG SELECTION DURING PREGNANCY

3 Many misconceptions exist regarding the association of medications and birth defects. Although some drugs have the potential to cause teratogenic effects, most medications required by pregnant women can be used safely.

The baseline risk for congenital malformations is approximately 3% to 6%, with approximately 3% considered severe.[2,12] Medication exposure is estimated to account for less than 1% of all birth defects. Genetic causes are responsible for 15% to 25%, other environmental issues (eg, maternal conditions and infections) account for 10%, and the remaining 65% to 75% of congenital malformations result from unknown causes.[2,12]

Factors such as the stage of pregnancy during exposure, route of administration, and dose can affect outcomes.[12] In the first 2 weeks following conception, exposure to a teratogen may result in an "all-or-none" phenomenon, which could either destroy the embryo or cause no problems.[13] Organogenesis occurs during the embryonic period. As organ systems are developing, teratogenic exposures may result in structural anomalies. For the remainder of the pregnancy, exposure to teratogens may result in growth retardation, central nervous system (CNS) abnormalities, or death. Examples of medications associated with teratogenic effects in the period of organogenesis include chemotherapy drugs (eg, methotrexate and cyclophosphamide), sex hormones (eg, androgens and progestational drugs), lithium, retinoids, thalidomide, certain antiepileptic drugs, and coumarin derivatives. Other medications, such as nonsteroidal antiinflammatory drugs (NSAIDs) and tetracycline derivatives, are more likely to exhibit effects in the second or third trimester.

Medications are necessary during pregnancy for treatment of acute and chronic conditions. Identifying patterns of medication use before conception, eliminating nonessential medications and discouraging self-medication, minimizing exposure to medications known to be harmful, and adjusting medication doses are all strategies to optimize the health of the mother while minimizing the risk to the fetus. In summary, a small number of medications have the potential to cause congenital malformations, and many can be avoided during pregnancy. In situations where a drug may be teratogenic but is necessary for maternal care, considerations related to route of administration, dosage form, and dosing may lessen the risk.

Methods and Resources for Determining Drug Safety in Pregnancy

4 When assessing the safety of using medications during pregnancy, evaluation of the quality of the evidence is important. Ideally, safety data from randomized, controlled trials are most desirable, but pregnant women are not usually eligible for participation in clinical trials. Other types of data commonly used to estimate the risk associated with medication use during pregnancy include animal studies, case reports, case-control studies, prospective cohort studies, historical cohort studies, and voluntary reporting systems.

Animal studies are a required component of drug testing, but extrapolation of the results to humans is not always valid.[14] Thalidomide was found to be safe in some animal models, but proved to have teratogenic effects in human offspring. The value of case reports is limited because birth defects in the offspring of women who used medication during pregnancy may occur by chance.[14] Case-control studies identify an outcome (congenital anomaly), match subjects with or without that outcome, and report how often exposure to a suspected agent occurred. Recall bias is a concern, as women with an affected pregnancy may be more likely to remember drugs used during the pregnancy than those with a normal outcome.

Cohort studies evaluate the intervention (use of a particular drug) in a group of persons and compare outcomes in a similar group of subjects without the intervention.[14,15] Prospective studies eliminate some of the problems with recall bias, but require time and large numbers of participants. Despite these disadvantages, cohort studies are often used for evaluating the effects of a drug exposure on pregnancy outcomes.

Teratology information services provide pregnant women with information about potential exposures during pregnancy and follow these women throughout the pregnancy to assess the outcomes of the pregnancy.[14] Services may publish pooled data to facilitate information sharing about medications used during pregnancy. Some pharmaceutical companies have organized voluntary reporting systems (also called pregnancy registries) for drugs used during pregnancy.

4 Computerized databases (eg, *www.motherisk.org*, LactMed [*www.toxnet.nlm.nih.gov*]), tertiary compendia, and textbooks with information from large cohorts of treated women offer valuable assistance. New information regarding drug use in pregnancy and lactation can be obtained from searches of the primary literature for cohort and case-control studies.

The FDA developed risk categories (ie, A, B, C, D, X, with A considered safe and X considered teratogenic) to guide clinicians regarding medication risk during pregnancy. Very few drugs are ranked as safe during pregnancy (category A) because a controlled trial is required to establish safety; this implies that few drugs are safe. Because of multiple limitations of the risk categories, the FDA instituted new labeling requirements for drugs submitted for approval after June 30, 2015 to replace the pregnancy risk categories. Use of the new system will be phased in gradually for drugs approved after June 30, 2001. The new labeling requirements include a subsection for pregnancy that includes information about pregnancy exposure registries, a risk summary, clinical considerations, and supporting data. The lactation subsection provides information about drug use during lactation. A new subsection includes information for females and males of reproductive potential.[16]

In summary, determining drug safety during pregnancy is limited by the quality of data and the types of study designs that can be used. While information from product labeling may provide a rough estimate of risks for medication-related adverse fetal outcomes, careful evaluation of other available information sources is necessary to make decisions about medication use in pregnant women.

PRECONCEPTION PLANNING

Pregnancy outcomes are influenced by maternal health status, lifestyle, and history prior to conception. The goal of preconception care is health promotion, through modification of behavioral, biomedical, and social risks in all women of reproductive age to ensure optimal health and improve pregnancy outcomes.[17] Almost half of all pregnancies in the United States are unintended. Preconception planning is important, since some behaviors and exposures impart risk to the fetus during the first trimester, often before prenatal care is begun or even before pregnancy is detected. Table 78-1 lists selected preconception risk factors, the potential adverse pregnancy outcomes, and management or prevention options.

The most common major congenital abnormalities are neural tube defects (NTDs), cleft palate and lip, and cardiac anomalies. Each year in the United States approximately 1 in 1,000 infants are born with NTDs.[18] Folic acid supplementation of women substantially reduces the incidence of NTDs in their offspring. This is also true in women who have previously delivered babies with NTDs.[18] NTDs occur within the first month of conception because neural tube closure occurs during the first month of pregnancy. Folic acid supplementation between 0.4 and 0.9 mg daily is recommended throughout a woman's reproductive years, since many pregnancies are unplanned and may not be recognized until after the first month.

Use of alcohol and recreational drugs during pregnancy is associated with birth defects.[17] Of births in the United States in 2003, 10% were to mothers who smoked tobacco during pregnancy.[15] Smoking can cause preterm birth, low birth weight, and other adverse outcomes. In a systematic review of 72 trials of smoking cessation and perinatal outcomes, incidences of low birth weight and preterm birth were reduced, and birth weight increased by 54 g with smoking cessation.[19] Use of nicotine replacement during pregnancy is controversial, since its use is not supported by clinical trial data; however, nicotine replacement theoretically imparts less risk than exposure to the over 4,000 chemicals found in cigarettes.[20]

PREGNANCY-INFLUENCED ISSUES

Pregnancy causes or exacerbates conditions that pregnant women commonly experience, including constipation, gastroesophageal reflux, hemorrhoids, and nausea and vomiting. Women with pregnancy-influenced gastrointestinal (GI) issues can be treated safely with lifestyle modification or medications, many of them nonprescription. Gestational diabetes, gestational hypertension, and venous thromboembolism (VTE) have the potential to cause adverse pregnancy consequences. Gestational thyrotoxicosis (GTT) is usually self-limiting.

GI Tract

5 Constipation during pregnancy is prevalent, affecting up to 40% of women and may contribute to the development or exacerbation of hemorrhoids; hemorrhoids are more prevalent in pregnant women compared with the general population.[21,22] Moderate physical exercise and increased intake of dietary fiber and fluid should be instituted first for constipation.[22] If additional treatment is needed, supplemental fiber and/or a stool softener is appropriate. Bulk-forming agents (eg, psyllium, methylcellulose, and polycarbophil) are safe for long-term use because they are not absorbed. Osmotic laxatives (eg, polyethylene glycol, lactulose, and sorbitol) and stimulant laxatives (eg, senna and bisacodyl) can also be used. Use of magnesium and sodium salts may cause electrolyte imbalance. Castor oil and mineral oil should be avoided because they cause stimulation of uterine contractions and impairment of maternal fat-soluble vitamin absorption, respectively.[21-23] Data supporting other management options for hemorrhoids during pregnancy are limited. Conservative treatment (ie, high dietary fiber intake, adequate oral fluid intake, and use of sitz baths) should be tried first. Laxatives and stool softeners can be used if conservative management is inadequate for preventing or treating constipation. Topical anesthetics, skin protectants, and astringents (eg, witch hazel) can be used for anal irritation and pain. Hydrocortisone may reduce inflammation and pruritis.[22]

Between 30% and 80% of pregnant women experience gastroesophageal reflux disease. An algorithm starting with lifestyle and dietary modifications (eg, small, frequent meals; alcohol and tobacco avoidance; food avoidance before bedtime; elevation of the head of the bed) should be used.[21,24] If symptoms are not relieved, antacids (eg, aluminum, calcium, or magnesium preparations) or sucralfate are acceptable; however, sodium bicarbonate and magnesium trisilicate should be avoided. Histamine-2 (H_2) receptor blockers can be used for patients unresponsive to lifestyle changes and antacids; evidence supports the use of ranitidine and cimetidine. Literature evaluating the use of famotidine and nizatidine is limited, but they are likely safe.[24] The use of proton pump inhibitors (PPIs) during

TABLE 78-1 Selected Preconception Risk Factors for Adverse Pregnancy Outcomes

Preconception Risk Factor	Potential Adverse Pregnancy Outcomes	Management or Prevention Options
Use of known teratogens		
• Antiepileptic drugs	• Known teratogens; causes craniofacial, cardiac, and limb defects[a] • NTD • Fetal hydantoin syndrome	• Use lowest possible dose to maintain control • Folic acid 4 mg daily
• Isotretinoins	• Miscarriage • Known teratogen; causes CNS, craniofacial, and cardiac defects[a]	• Use effective pregnancy prevention
• Oral anticoagulants	• Fetal warfarin syndrome	• Switch to nonteratogenic anticoagulant (eg, LMWH) before becoming pregnant
Lifestyle factors		
• Alcohol misuse	• Fetal alcohol syndrome	• Cease alcohol intake before conception
• Obesity	• NTD • Preterm delivery • Diabetes, HTN, VTE • Cesarean section	• Weight loss with appropriate nutritional intake before pregnancy

• Tobacco use	• Preterm birth
	• Low birth weight
	• Spontaneous abortion
	• Increased perinatal mortality
		• Ideally, cease tobacco use before conception
		• Nonpharmacologic therapies (eg, CBT, counseling, hypnosis)
		• No consensus for NRT product, dosing, or frequency:
		  • Intermittent forms (eg, gum)
		  • Transdermal patch (limit to 16 h/day)
		• Bupropion risk may be less than risk posed by smoking; efficacy unclear
		• Varenicline safety unknown

CBT, cognitive behavioral therapy; CNS, central nervous system; HTN, hypertension; LMWH, low-molecular weight heparin; NRT, nicotine replacement therapy; NTD, neural tube defect; VTE, venous thromboembolism.

[a]List is not all-inclusive.

Data from references 17-20.

pregnancy does not appear to increase the risk of major birth defects; most data comes from use of omeprazole.[25] Since more data and clinical experience are available for H_2 antagonists, use of PPIs should be reserved for women with inadequate response to H_2 antagonists.

Nausea and vomiting of pregnancy (NVP) is estimated to affect up to 90% of pregnant women. NVP usually begins between weeks 4 and 6 of gestation and usually resolves by weeks 16 to 20; peak symptoms occur between weeks 8 and 12.[26,27] Hyperemesis gravidarum (HG; ie, unrelenting vomiting causing weight loss of more than 5% prepregnancy weight, dehydration, electrolyte imbalance, and ketonuria) occurs in 0.5% to 2% of women.[26] Dietary modifications, such as eating frequent, small, bland meals and avoiding fatty or spicy foods, may be helpful. Applying pressure at acupressure point P6 on the volar aspect of the wrist may be beneficial. Ginger has shown efficacy for hyperemesis in randomized, controlled trials and is probably safe. Pharmacotherapeutic approaches for NVP that have shown efficacy include pyridoxine (vitamin B_6), and antihistamines (including doxylamine). The American College of Obstetricians and Gynecologists (ACOG) considers pyridoxine alone or in combination with doxylamine first-line; the combination was approved by FDA in 2013.[26] Metoclopramide and phenothiazines are generally considered safe, but may cause sedation and extrapyramidal effects, including dystonia. Conflicting data exist regarding ondansetron use. While recent studies showed no increase in risk of congenital anomalies, a large case-control study found an increased risk of oral clefts. Some suggest using metoclopramide before ondansetron.[26,27] Corticosteroids may be effective for HG; use should be reserved until after the first trimester because of a small increase in the risk of oral clefts.

Gestational Diabetes

5 Gestational diabetes mellitus (GDM) is diabetes diagnosed in the second or third trimester that is not overt diabetes.[28] It develops in about 3% to 5% of pregnant women in the United States.[29] Risks of GDM are many and include fetal loss, increased risk of major malformations, and fetal macrosomia. The American Diabetes Association and a consensus panel of the International Association of Diabetes and Pregnancy Study Groups (IADPSG) recommends universal screening of pregnant women not previously diagnosed with diabetes.[28,30] At the first prenatal visit, all women considered high-risk for diabetes (eg, obesity, glycosuria, and strong family history of diabetes) should be screened for overt diabetes which would indicate pregestational origin. Overt diabetes occurs if the A1C is greater than or equal to 6.5% (0.065; 48 mmol/mol Hgb), fasting plasma glucose (FPG) is greater than or equal to 126 mg/dL (7.0 mmol/L), or 2-hour plasma glucose 200 mg/dL (11.1 mmol/L) or greater during an oral glucose tolerance test (OGTT), or if random plasma glucose (RPG) is greater than or equal to 200 mg/dL (11.1 mmol/L) in a patient with hyperglycemic crisis or classic hyperglycemic symptoms. If overt diabetes is not diagnosed or for women not at high-risk for diabetes, screening for GDM should occur at weeks 24 to 28 using either the one-step (75-g OGTT) or two-step (50-g, 1-hour glucose challenge test followed by a 100-g, 3-hour OGTT) method.[28] Table 78-2 summarizes screening and diagnosis of GDM.

Clinical **Controversy...**

Insulin has traditionally been the drug of choice to treat diabetes, including gestational diabetes, during pregnancy if drug therapy is indicated. Randomized, controlled trials of glyburide and metformin use in GDM have shown efficacy and short-term safety.[31] However, long-term safety data are limited, and both agents cross the placenta. ACOG considers oral medications (specifically, glyburide and metformin) and insulin equivalent in efficacy and lists all three as appropriate first-line drug treatment of GDM.[32]

Dietary modification (medical nutrition therapy), exercise, and blood glucose monitoring is considered first-line therapy for all women who have GDM, since as many as 85% of women can achieve control with these interventions alone.[31] Self-monitoring of blood glucose four times daily (fasting, and 1 or 2 hours after each meal) is recommended until normoglycemia at which time monitoring may be modified.[32] Drug therapy should be initiated if glycemic control

TABLE 78-2 Screening and Diagnosis of Gestational Diabetes Mellitus

One-Step Method		Two-Step Method	
Give:	75-g OGTT[a] *If any plasma glucose levels are met or exceeded, GDM is diagnosed*	***Step 1***:	Give 50-g GLT[b]
Fasting:	≥92 mg/dL (5.1 mmol/L)	1-hr:	≥140 mg/dL (7.8 mmol/L) *If plasma glucose level is met or exceeded, proceed to Step 2*
1-hr:	≥180 mg/dL (10 mmol/L)	***Step 2***:	Give 100-g OGTT *If two or more plasma glucose levels are met or exceeded, GDM is diagnosed*
2-hr:	≥153 mg/dL (8.5 mmol/L)		Carpenter/Coustan Method[c]
		Fasting	95 mg/dL (5.3 mmol/L)
		1-hr	180 mg/dL (10 mmol/L)
		2-hr	155 mg/dL (8.6 mmol/L)
		3-hr	140 mg/dL (7.8 mmol/L)

GLT, glucose load test; OGTT, oral glucose tolerance test.

[a]Perform with plasma glucose measurement in fasting state. Should be performed in the morning after at least 8-hours of fasting.

[b]Perform with plasma glucose measurement in nonfasting state.

[c]Carpenter and Coustan developed diagnostic criteria for gestational diabetes that lowered diagnostic plasma glucose levels compared to the National Diabetes Data Group.

Data from references 28 and 29.

is not achieved with lifestyle interventions. Glycemic control is preprandial capillary glucose concentrations at or below 95 mg/dL (5.3 mmol/L) along with one of the following: a 1-hour postprandial glucose at or below 140 mg/dL (7.8 mmol/L) or a 2-hour postprandial glucose of 120 mg/dL (6.7 mmol/L) or below.[31] Human insulin is the drug of choice for diabetes management during pregnancy because it does not cross the placenta. Glyburide and metformin are alternatives, but long-term safety data are limited.[31,32] The ACOG considers insulin and oral medications (specifically, glyburide and metformin) equivalent and supports either for first-line drug therapy.[32]

Evidence supporting dietary modification, self-monitored blood glucose, exercise, and pharmacologic interventions for women with GDM is largely based on one randomized clinical trial that showed reductions in perinatal morbidity (composite of death, nerve palsy, bone fracture, and shoulder dystocia) with nutritional education, blood glucose monitoring, and insulin treatment.[32,33]

Hypertensive Disorders of Pregnancy

5 Hypertensive disorders of pregnancy (HDP) complicate approximately 10% of pregnancies. Four categories of HDP are established: (1) preeclampsia-eclampsia, (2) chronic hypertension (HTN; preexisting hypertension or developing before 20 weeks of gestation), (3) chronic HTN with superimposed preeclampsia, and (4) gestational HTN (HTN without proteinuria developing after 20 weeks of gestation.[34,35] Hypertension in pregnancy is defined as either systolic blood pressure (sBP) above 140 mm Hg or diastolic blood pressure (dBP) above 90 mm Hg based upon two or more measurements at least 4 hours apart.[34] Nondrug managements of HDP center on activity restriction, stress reduction, and exercise; however, no evidence indicates that any of these approaches improves pregnancy outcome, and prolonged bed rest may increase the risk of complications (eg, venous thromboembolic disease).[36] Use of supplemental calcium 1 to 2 g/day decreases the risk of hypertension by 35% (95% CI; 19%-47%) and preeclampsia by 55% (95% CI, 35%-69%).[37] High-risk patients (those with the lowest initial calcium intake) benefited most. The ACOG states the findings are not applicable to populations with adequate calcium intake, such as in the United States.[35] Supplemental calcium may still be appropriate for some pregnant women.[36,37] Antihypertensive drug therapy is discussed under Chronic Illnesses in Pregnancy.

While preeclampsia usually develops after 20 weeks of gestation, up to 30% of chronic and gestational hypertension are complicated by preeclampsia. Preeclampsia is a multisystem syndrome that complicates 2% to 8% of pregnancies and can cause poorer outcomes, including renal failure, maternal morbidity/mortality, preterm delivery, and intrauterine growth restriction.[38,39] Risk factors for development of preeclampsia include nulliparity, previous personal or family history of preeclampsia, prepregnancy body mass index above 30 kg/m^2, tobacco use, underlying medical conditions (eg, chronic hypertension, diabetes, antiphospholipid antibodies, autoimmune disease, renal disease), multiple gestations, and ethnicity (black greater than white or Hispanic). Maternal age over 40 years is also a potential risk factor.[39,40] Diagnosis of preeclampsia includes elevated blood pressure as with HDP, and proteinuria (300 [or more] mg/24 hours, protein/creatinine ratio of at least 0.3 mg/mg (approximately 30 mg/mmol), or urine dipstick of 1+). If proteinuria is not present, new onset of any of the following with new onset HTN is indicative of preeclampsia: thrombocytopenia (count less than 100,000/μL [100×10^9/L]), serum creatinine above 1.1 mg/dL (97 μmol/L) or a doubling of serum creatinine, elevated liver transaminases, pulmonary edema, or cerebral or visual symptoms.[35] Signs of more severe preeclampsia include: persistent severe headache, vomiting; hyperreflexia, chest pain or dyspnea, and HELLP (hemolysis, elevated liver enzymes, low platelets).[40,41] Treatment of hypertension in women with preeclampsia depends upon the blood pressure measurement and follows the same principles discussed under Chronic Illnesses in Pregnancy. Low-dose aspirin (60-81 mg/day) beginning late in the first trimester in women at risk for preeclampsia decreases the risk of its development by 17%, which corresponds to prevention of one preeclampsia case for every 72 at-risk women treated. Decreased rates of preterm birth (8% reduction) and fetal or neonatal death (14% reduction) also result from low-dose aspirin use.[42] The only cure for preeclampsia is delivery of the placenta.[41]

Preeclampsia may progress rapidly to eclampsia, which is the occurrence of seizures superimposed on preeclampsia. Eclampsia is a medical emergency. In high-risk women (ie, previous severe preeclampsia, renal disease, autoimmune disease, diabetes, and chronic hypertension), use of low-dose aspirin prevents one case of preeclampsia for every 19 women treated.[42] Magnesium sulfate decreases the risk of progression to eclampsia by almost 60%; it is recommended to prevent eclampsia as well as treat eclamptic seizures. The usual dose of magnesium sulfate is 4 to 6 g IV over 15 to 20 minutes followed by a 2 g/h continuous infusion; duration of use varies, but the usual duration is 24 hours. Diazepam and phenytoin should be avoided.[43]

Thyroid Abnormalities

5 Pregnant women with overt hyperthyroidism should be treated with a thioamide (ie, methimazole and propylthiouracil [PTU]), and those with overt hypothyroidism should receive thyroid replacement (ie, levothyroxine).[44]

During pregnancy, stimulation of the thyroid gland may occur because of hCG's structural similarity to thyroid-stimulating hormone (TSH; thyrotropin). In some women, gestational transient thyrotoxicosis (GTT) may result. Occurrence of GTT is often associated with HG. By 20 weeks of gestation, GTT usually resolves as production of hCG declines. Treatment with antithyroid medication is not usually needed.[44] Nausea and vomiting can be treated as for patients without this pseudo-hyperthyroid state.

Although not all women experience postpartum thyroiditis (PPT) similarly, the typical presentation is characterized by transient hyperthyroidism during the first several months postpartum, a period of transient hypothyroidism between 4 and 8 months postpartum, and, finally, euthyroidism within 1 year. The initial hyperthyroid state usually does not require treatment; however, β-blockers (propranolol, starting at 10-20 mg daily as needed) can provide symptomatic relief of adrenergic symptoms. Because PTT is from a destructive inflammation process and not overproduction of thyroid hormone, antithyroid drugs are ineffective. Levothyroxine replacement is suggested for a total of 6 to 12 months.[44] Up to one-third of women affected by PPT develop permanent hypothyroidism.

Thromboembolism

5 The risk of VTE in pregnant women is increased by fivefold to tenfold over nonpregnant women.[45] Low-molecular-weight heparin (LMWH) is recommended over unfractionated heparin (UFH) and warfarin for treatment of acute thromboembolism during pregnancy. Treatment should be continued throughout pregnancy and for 6 weeks after delivery; the minimum total duration of therapy should not be less than 3 months. Fondaparinux and injectable direct thrombin inhibitors (eg, lepirudin and bivalirudin) should be avoided unless a severe allergy to heparin (eg, heparin-induced thrombocytopenia) is present. The novel oral anticoagulants (eg, dabigatran, rivaroxaban, and apixaban) are not recommended.[45] Warfarin is not used because it causes nasal hypoplasia, stippled epiphyses, limb hypoplasia, and eye abnormalities; the risk period appears to be between 6 and 12 weeks of gestation. CNS anomalies are associated with second- and third-trimester exposure.

Recurrent VTE is divided into three categories: low risk, intermediate risk, and high risk of recurrence. Antepartum monitoring is recommended for women with a single episode of VTE who have a low risk of recurrence (ie, one transient risk factor [eg, surgery, injury, lengthy travel, or immobility]). For intermediate risk (ie, hormone-related, pregnancy-related, or unprovoked VTE) and high risk (ie, more than one unprovoked VTE or continuous risk factors), antepartum prophylaxis with LMWH plus 6-week postpartum prophylaxis with either LMWH or warfarin is recommended. Specific recommendations for thrombophilias (eg, antiphospholipid antibodies, Factor V Leiden, protein C and S deficiencies) can be found in the American College of Chest Physicians clinical practice guidelines.[45]

Women with prosthetic heart valves should receive LMWH (twice daily) or UFH (every 12 hours) during pregnancy. LMWH should be adjusted to achieve a peak anti-Xa level at 4 hours post-subcutaneous dose, while UFH treatment should target a mid-interval aPTT at least twice the control value or an anti-Xa heparin level of 0.35 to 0.7 units/mL (0.35-0.7 kU/L).[45] After a discussion of potential risks, LMWH or UFH can be used until week 13 of gestation with subsequent substitution of warfarin until the middle of the third trimester when LMWH or UFH should be resumed. In women considered very high-risk for VTE (eg, older-generation prosthetic mitral valve, and history of thromboembolism), prevention of maternal complications, such as valve thrombosis exceeds the risk of fetal malformation; use of warfarin is appropriate until replacement with LMWH or UFH near the end of the third trimester. High-risk women with prosthetic heart valves may also receive low-dose aspirin (75-100 mg/day).[45]

ACUTE CARE ISSUES IN PREGNANCY

In some cases, the risks associated with the acute illness are magnified during pregnancy, and early screening and treatment become critical. In other cases, such as during treatment of certain sexually transmitted infections (STIs), the urgency regarding treatment comes from an increased likelihood of infection leading to preterm labor. Occasionally, common acute care issues, such as migraine headache, improve during pregnancy.

Urinary Tract Infection

6 The most common infections in pregnant and nonpregnant women are urinary tract infections (UTIs). Typically, UTIs are characterized as asymptomatic (eg, asymptomatic bacteriuria) or symptomatic (eg, lower [cystitis] or upper [pyelonephritis]). *Escherichia coli* is the primary cause of infection in 75% to 90% of cases.[46,47] Other gram-negative rods, such as *Proteus* and *Klebsiella*, as well as Group B *Streptococcus* (GBS) account for some infections. The presence of GBS in the urine indicates heavy colonization of the genitourinary tract, increasing the risk for GBS infection in the newborn.[47]

The incidence of asymptomatic bacteriuria ranges from 2% to 10%. Untreated, bacteriuria progresses to pyelonephritis in approximately 30% of pregnant women.[46,47] While no consensus regarding screening for asymptomatic bacteriuria exists, a urine culture obtained at the first prenatal visit is appropriate; some advocate a urine culture in each trimester. Use of rapid screening tests, such as dipsticks, should be avoided because of poor performance in pregnant women.[47] Acute cystitis occurs in about 1% to 3% of pregnant women. Signs and symptoms of acute cystitis include urgency, frequency, hematuria, pyuria, and dysuria.[46]

Treatment of asymptomatic bacteriuria is necessary to prevent pyelonephritis. For asymptomatic bacteriuria, the agents of choice and treatment duration are not well defined. Treatment of acute cystitis is similar to that of asymptomatic bacteriuria. Using outcomes of cure rates, recurrent infection, incidence of preterm delivery or rupture of membranes, admission to neonatal intensive care, need for change of antibiotic, or incidence of prolonged fever, antibiotic treatment has demonstrated effectiveness in treating symptomatic UTIs (including pyelonephritis) in pregnancy. No specific treatment appears superior to other commonly used treatments.[48] Treatment courses for asymptomatic bacteriuria and cystitis of 7 to 14 days are common, but shorter courses of therapy may be sufficient.

The most commonly used antibiotics to treat asymptomatic bacteriuria and cystitis are the β-lactams (including penicillins and cephalosporins) and nitrofurantoin.[48,49] β-Lactams are not known teratogens; however, the incidence of *E. coli* resistance to ampicillin and amoxicillin limits their use as single agents. Nitrofurantoin is not active against *Proteus* species and should not be used after week 37 in patients with glucose-6-phosphate dehydrogenase deficiency because of a theoretical risk for hemolytic anemia in the neonate. Sulfa-containing drugs can contribute to the development of newborn kernicterus; use should be avoided during the last weeks of gestation. Trimethoprim is a folate antagonist and is relatively contraindicated during the first trimester because of associations with cardiovascular malformations. Regionally, increased rates of *E. coli* resistance to trimethoprim-sulfa may limit its use. Fluoroquinolones and tetracyclines are contraindicated because of potential associations with impaired cartilage development and deciduous teeth discoloration (if given after 5 months of gestation), respectively.[49]

Patients with pyelonephritis usually present with bacteriuria and systemic symptoms of costovertebral angle tenderness, dysuria, fever, flank pain, nausea, and vomiting.[46] Complications of pyelonephritis include premature delivery, low infant birth weight, hypertension, anemia, bacteremia, and transient renal failure. Hospitalization is the standard of care for pregnant women with pyelonephritis.[46,49] Inpatient therapy has included parenteral administration of second- or third-generation cephalosporins (eg, cefuroxime and ceftriaxone), ampicillin plus gentamicin, or ampicillin-sulbactam. Switching to oral antibiotics can occur after the woman is afebrile for 48 hours; however, nitrofurantoin should be avoided because it does not achieve therapeutic levels outside of the urine. Outpatient antibiotic therapy can be considered after initial inpatient observation in women who are afebrile and less than 24 weeks of gestation. The total duration of antibiotic therapy for acute pyelonephritis is 10 to 14 days.[49] Suppression therapy with nitrofurantoin can be considered for use until week 37 of gestation.[46]

Sexually Transmitted Infections

6 Sexually transmitted infections in pregnant women range from infections that may be transmitted across the placenta and infect the infant prenatally (eg, syphilis) to organisms that may be transmitted during birth and cause neonatal infection (eg, *Chlamydia trachomatis, Neisseria gonorrhoeae*, or herpes simplex virus [HSV]) to infections that pose a threat for preterm labor (eg, bacterial vaginosis [BV]). Initial screening during the first prenatal visit is recommended for human immunodeficiency virus (HIV), hepatitis B surface antigen, and syphilis. Women younger than 25 years and older women with increased risk (eg, new sex partner, two or more sex partners, nonmonogamous sex partner, or sex partner with an STI) should be screened for *C. trachomatis* and gonorrhea; women at high risk for hepatitis C should also be screened during the first prenatal visit.[50] Treatment for select STIs is summarized in Table 78-3.

TABLE 78-3 Management of Sexually Transmitted Infections in Pregnancy

STI	Drug Name (Brand Name)	Usual Dose	Monitoring	Comments
Bacterial vaginosis	*Recommended:* Metronidazole (Flagyl) ***OR*** Metronidazole 0.75% gel *Alternatives[a]:* Clindamycin (Cleocin)	• 500 mg by mouth two times daily × 7 days • 5 g intravaginally once daily × 5 days	Follow-up testing not required if symptoms resolve	No link between intravaginal clindamycin and newborn complications Oral or vaginal preparations can be used
Chlamydia	*Recommended:* Azithromycin (Zithromax) *Alternatives[a]:* Amoxicillin (Amoxil) Erythromycin base Erythromycin ethylsuccinate	1 g by mouth × 1 dose	Test-of-cure at 3-4 weeks after therapy completion; retest all after 3 months	Gonorrheal coinfection common; both are treated concurrently Chlamydia is asymptomatic in men and women Women below age 25 years and those at high risk should be retested in the third trimester
Genital herpes	*Recommended:* Acyclovir (Zovirax) ***OR*** Valacyclovir	400 mg by mouth three times a day 500 mg by mouth twice a day	Routine serologic testing for HSV-2 is not recommended	Start treatment at 36 weeks of gestation
Gonorrhea	*Recommended:* Ceftriaxone (Rocephin) *PLUS* Azithromycin (Zithromax)	250 mg IM × 1 dose 1 g by mouth × 1 dose	Because of high reinfection rate, repeat testing for gonorrhea 3 months after treatment	Chlamydial coinfection common; both are treated concurrently Consult with infectious disease specialist if cephalosporin allergy
Syphilis[b]				
Primary, secondary, early latent	*Recommended:* Benzathine penicillin G (Bicillin L-A)	2.4 million units IM × 1 dose; a second dose can be given 1 week after initial dose	Nontreponemal serologic evaluation[c] at 6 and 12 months	For treatment failure or reinfection, use same drug and dose but increase to 3 weekly doses unless neurosyphilis is present
Tertiary, late latent	*Recommended:* Benzathine penicillin G (Bicillin L-A)	2.4 million units IM × 3 doses at 1-week intervals	Nontreponemal serologic evaluation[c] at 6, 12, and 24 months. CSF examination may be required	Use this regimen for late latent or latent syphilis of unknown duration
Neurosyphilis	*Recommended:* Aqueous penicillin G (Pfizerpen) *Alternative[a]:* Procaine penicillin (Wycillin, Pfizerpen-AS) *PLUS* Probenecid	3-4 million units IV every 4 hours or 18-24 million units IV continuously × 10-14 days 2.4 million units IM daily × 10-14 days 500 mg by mouth four times daily × 10-14 days	If initial elevation of leukocytes in CSF, repeat CSF examination every 6 months until normalization	Consider repeat treatment if CSF leukocytes or protein do not normalize after 2 years Use alternative regimen only if compliance can be ensured
Trichomoniasis	*Recommended:* Metronidazole	2 g by mouth × 1 dose	Rescreen HIV patients at 3 months after treatment	While tinidazole is an alternative for nonpregnant women, avoid during pregnancy

CSF, cerebrospinal fluid; IM, intramuscular; STI, sexually transmitted infection.

[a]Refer to reference 50 for specific dosing recommendations.

[b]Pregnant women with history of penicillin allergy should undergo penicillin desensitization as no proven alternatives exist.

[c]Nontreponemal evaluation consists of VDRL (Venereal Disease Research Laboratory) and RPR (rapid plasma regain).

Data from reference 50.

Syphilis

Syphilis is caused by *Treponema pallidum*; complications are many (eg, mucocutaneous lesions, altered mental status, visual and auditory abnormalities, gumma, cranial nerve palsies). For women who live in areas with a high prevalence of syphilis, are at high risk, have not been previously tested, or had positive serology in the first trimester, additional serologic testing early in the third trimester (around 28 weeks) and at delivery is recommended.[50] With the exception of neurosyphilis, which is treated with aqueous penicillin G, the drug of choice for all stages of syphilis is benzathine penicillin G. If a penicillin allergy is present, women with IgE-mediated hypersensitivity can undergo desensitization. Penicillin effectively prevents transmission to the fetus and treats the fetus, if already infected. Treatment during the second half of pregnancy may increase the risk for preterm labor and fetal distress because a Jarisch-Herxheimer reaction may occur; however, treatment should not be withheld or delayed.[50]

Chlamydia and Gonorrhea

Chlamydia is the most commonly reported STI in the United States; complications of *C. trachomatis* include pelvic inflammatory disease (PID), ectopic pregnancy, and infertility. *C. trachomatis* infects the newborn through exposure to the infected cervix during delivery. Perinatal infection most commonly causes conjunctivitis that develops 5 to 12 days postpartum. A subacute, afebrile pneumonia with an onset at ages 1 to 3 months may occur.[50]

Gonorrhea, an STI caused by *N. gonorrhoeae*, is the second-most commonly reported notifiable infection in the United States.[50] In women, recognizable symptoms may be absent initially, but gonorrheal infection can cause PID, a known risk for infertility. Perinatal gonococcal infection results from exposure to the infected cervix during birth. Symptoms usually manifest within 2 to 5 days after delivery. Milder manifestations include rhinitis, vaginitis, and urethritis. More severe presentations include ophthalmia neonatorum and sepsis.[50] Identification and treatment of the infection in neonates is crucial, as permanent sequelae such as blindness can occur.

Antimicrobial resistance rates among *N. gonorrhoeae* are increasing which has prompted the Centers for Disease Control and Prevention to remove oral cephalosporins as a preferred treatment option.[50] Coinfection with *C. trachomatis* is common; treatment of most *N. gonorrhoeae* infections includes treatment for *C. trachomatis*.[50]

Bacterial Vaginosis and Trichomoniasis

Bacterial vaginosis and trichomoniasis are STIs characterized by vaginal discharge. BV results from the lack of normal vaginal flora (ie, *Lactobacillus* species) and replacement with anaerobic bacteria, mycoplasmas, and *Gardnerella vaginalis*.[50] It is a risk factor for premature rupture of membranes, preterm labor, preterm birth, intraamniotic infection, and postpartum endometritis. In women at high or low risk for preterm delivery, data to support routine screening for asymptomatic BV at the first prenatal visit are equivocal.[50]

Trichomoniasis is caused by the protozoa, *Trichomonas vaginalis*. Infection with *T. vaginalis* is associated with an increased risk of premature rupture of the membranes, preterm delivery, and low birth weight. Treatment may prevent respiratory or genital infection in the neonate.[50]

Genital Herpes

Genital herpes is a chronic disease most frequently caused by herpes simplex virus-2 (HSV-2), although the number of anogenital herpes infections caused by HSV-1 is increasing. Neonatal herpes often occurs in infants born to women lacking histories of genital herpes. The risk of neonatal transmission is under 1% for women with a history of recurrent herpes at term or those who acquire herpes in the first half of pregnancy, but is 30% to 50% for women who initially acquire genital herpes near term.[50] However, because recurrent herpes occurs more commonly than new acquisition during pregnancy, it remains the cause for most cases of neonatal transmission. Prevention strategies include counseling uninfected women to avoid intercourse during the third trimester with partners having known or suspected genital herpes infection. Women with no history of orolabial herpes should avoid receptive oral sex during the third trimester with partners who have orolabial herpes. Prevention of genital herpes transmission to pregnant women using antiviral agents has not been studied.[50]

All women should be asked about symptoms of genital herpes at the time of delivery and should be examined for lesions. Women who have no symptoms (including prodromal symptoms) or lesions proceed with vaginal childbirth; however, those with evidence of an outbreak undergo cesarean section to decrease the risk of neonatal transmission.[50]

Maternal use of acyclovir during the first trimester has not demonstrated an increased risk for birth defects. Valacyclovir is an alternative, but is more expensive.[50] For initial or recurrent episodes, most women receive oral acyclovir therapy; IV acyclovir is reserved for severe infections. In women seropositive for HSV but who have not experienced an outbreak, no data suggest a treatment benefit.[50]

Headache

6 Primary headaches (eg, tension and migraine) in pregnant and nonpregnant women are the most common types of headache. Secondary headaches can also occur and include those caused by eclampsia, stroke, postdural puncture, cerebral angiopathy, and cerebral venous thrombosis.[51]

Migraine headaches are associated with estrogen fluctuations in women of childbearing age. Between 60% and 70% of pregnant women with a history of migraine headaches experience symptom improvement during pregnancy; 20% experience complete cessation. Improvement is more likely in women who have migraine without aura and in women with a history of menstrual migraine. Women with menstrual migraine are more likely to have postpartum recurrence.[51] Tension headaches are less studied. Most women report no change in the frequency or intensity of tension headaches, and remission is possible.

Relaxation, stress management, and biofeedback are all effective nonpharmacologic treatment methods that should be attempted in pregnant women with migraines and tension headaches because these interventions pose a minimal risk. For tension headache, acetaminophen or ibuprofen can be used if nonpharmacologic treatments fail. While ibuprofen is considered safe, all NSAIDs are contraindicated in the third trimester because of the potential for premature closure of the ductus arteriosus. Aspirin should be avoided in the third trimester because, in addition to its effects on the ductus arteriosis, it can cause maternal and fetal bleeding as well as decreased uterine contractility (hence, prolonged labor). Opioids are rarely used.[51]

Pharmacologic treatment for migraines involves use of analgesics (ie, acetaminophen and ibuprofen). Opioids have been used, but may contribute to migraine-associated nausea; long-term use near term can cause neonatal withdrawal. For migraines that are not responsive to other treatments, triptans may be used; sumatriptan is the triptan of choice because for other triptans, there is relatively little information about use in pregnancy. Ergotamine and dihydroergotamine are contraindicated because of effects on uterine tone. Promethazine, prochlorperazine, and metoclopramide can be used for patients who have migraine-associated nausea.[51]

Tension-type headaches do not usually require prophylaxis. Chronic, preventive treatment is reserved for women with severe headaches (usually migraines) that are not responsive to other treatments. The agent of choice is propranolol given at the lowest effective dose.

Alternatives include tricyclic antidepressants. Amitriptyline and nortriptyline (each dosed 10-25 mg by mouth daily) are preferred over the selective serotonin reuptake inhibitors (SSRI) or serotonin–norepinephrine reuptake inhibitors (SNRI) because data on safe use of these agents during pregnancy are conflicting.[51]

CHRONIC ILLNESSES IN PREGNANCY

For the majority of women and their healthcare providers, pregnancy is a new consideration for a previously diagnosed health condition. Medications used to treat the chronic illness can often be used throughout the pregnancy and during breastfeeding. See Table 78-4 for treatment of chronic illnesses during pregnancy.

Allergic Rhinitis and Asthma

6 Asthma and rhinitis are common chronic illnesses in pregnancy. Asthma affects approximately 8% of pregnancies.[52] During pregnancy, almost equal proportions of patients have symptoms that worsen, improve, or remain unchanged. Diagnosis and staging of asthma during pregnancy is the same as in nonpregnant women, although more frequent follow-up is necessary because of changes in disease severity.[53,54] Health consequences of untreated or poorly treated asthma include preterm labor, preeclampsia, intrauterine growth restriction, premature birth, low birth weight, and stillbirth; therefore, the treatment goal is to achieve and maintain control of asthma symptoms. Asthma is controlled when there are no daytime symptoms, limitations of activities, nocturnal symptoms, short-acting β_2-agonist use, or exacerbations, and there is normal pulmonary function.[54]

Risks of medication use to the fetus are lower than the risks of untreated asthma; therefore, use of medications to achieve and maintain control is warranted. Treatment recommendations are divided into multiple steps based on symptom control and follow a stepwise approach. Once control is achieved, the goal is maintenance of control at the lowest controlling step; however, stepping down may be delayed until after delivery because of the potential effects of exacerbation on pregnancy outcomes.[53,54]

TABLE 78-4 Treatment of Chronic Illnesses in Pregnancy

Chronic Illness	Treatment	Comments
Allergic rhinitis	Intranasal corticosteroids Intranasal cromolyn First generation antihistamines (chlorpheniramine, diphenhydramine, hydroxyzine)	Budesonide and beclomethasone most widely studied intranasal corticosteroids Second generation antihistamines do not appear to increase fetal risk, but are less extensively studied than first generation products Use of external nasal dilator, short-term topical oxymetazoline, or ICS may be preferable to oral decongestants
Asthma		Budesonide is the preferred ICS, but any may be used
Step 1 (intermittent)	SABA (albuterol)	Alternatives are cromolyn (less effective), leukotriene receptor antagonists (less experience in pregnancy), and theophylline (more potential toxicity)
Step 2 and above (persistent)	SABA (albuterol) Step-appropriate ICS LABA	Systemic corticosteroids recommended to gain control in patients with most severe disease
Epilepsy	Probably Safest AEDs • Carbamazepine • Lamotrigine • Levetiracetam • Phenytoin Lower risk than VPA • Gabapentin • Oxcarbazepine • Zonisamide Significant risk greater than other AEDs • Phenobarbital • Topiramate • VPA	Polytherapy carries higher risk of major malformations than monotherapy Rates of major malformation with probably safest AEDs clusters around 2-2.5% Phenytoin, lamotrigine, and carbamazepine may cause cleft palate Phenobarbital is associated with cardiac malformations Risk for most AED-associated malformations is dose-related Emerging evidence suggests risk of structural teratogenesis with levetiracetam is low
HIV	Currently receiving ART: Continue current regimen if viral load is suppressed AR -naïve, no evidence of resistance: • Dual NRTI backbone ***PLUS*** • Ritonavir-boosted PI ***OR*** • NNRTI ***OR*** • Integrase inhibitor	In women currently receiving ART, antiretroviral drug resistance testing should be performed to guide ART If efavirenz is part of current ART, continue use since NTDs usually occur through weeks 5-6 of gestation and pregnancy often is not recognized during that time period If ART-naïve, any regimen containing efavirenz should be initiated after first 8 weeks of pregnancy
Hypertension, chronic	Initial treatment: Labetalol Nifedipine Methyldopa	ACE inhibitors, ARBs, renin inhibitors, mineralocorticoid receptor antagonists are not recommended Atenolol has been associated with fetal growth restriction Thiazide diuretics theoretically lower the increase in plasma volume during pregnancy, but are considered second-line
Thyroid disorders	Hypothyroid Levothyroxine Hyperthyroid • PTU • Methimazole	For hypothyroidism, attain a TSH of 0.1-2.5, 0.2-3, and 0.3-3 milli-international units/L (mIU/L) in the first, second, and third trimester, respectively Use PTU in first trimester followed by switch to methimazole in second and third trimester to balance the risk of PTU-induced hepatotoxicity and methimazole embryopathy

ACE, angiotensin converting enzyme, AED, antiepileptic drug; ARB, angiotensin receptor blocker; ART, antiretroviral therapy; ICS, inhaled corticosteroid; LABA, long-acting beta agonist; NNRTI, non-nucleoside reverse transcriptase inhibitor; NRTI, nucleoside reverse transcriptase inhibitor; NTD, neural tube defects; PI, protease inhibitor; PTU, propylthiouracil; SABA, short-acting beta agonist; TSH, thyroid stimulating hormone; VPA, valproic acid.

[a]List is not all-inclusive.

Data from references 40, 44, 53-55, 61-64.

Approximately 20% of all pregnancies are impacted by allergic rhinitis. Notably, nasal congestion can be caused by pregnancy because of vascular engorgement in the nasal passages and hormonal effects on mucus secretion. Treatment strategies for allergic rhinitis during pregnancy are similar to those used in nonpregnant women and include avoidance of allergens, immunotherapy, and pharmacotherapy. Immunotherapy is not contraindicated in pregnancy, but dose increases during pregnancy are not advised in order to lessen the risk for anaphylaxis.[55,56]

Diabetes

6 Poorly controlled diabetes can cause fetal malformations, fetal loss, and maternal morbidity. Women with diabetes should use effective contraception until optimal glycemic control is achieved before attempting pregnancy. Additionally, diabetic retinopathy may worsen, hypertension may develop, and renal function may deteriorate during pregnancy, requiring enhanced monitoring for these target-organ problems.[31,57]

Glycemic control can change dramatically during pregnancy; frequent adjustment to management may be needed. Medical nutrition therapy and supervised physical activity programs should continue. Self-monitored blood glucose should occur before and after meals, with occasional early morning (ie, 2-4 am) measurement.[57] For patients with type 1 diabetes, human insulin may be continued. No data have shown the use of insulin detemir and insulin glargine to cause major safety concerns in pregnancy, but studies have been small and retrospective; the available evidence supports insulin detemir as the first-line long-acting insulin analogue.[58] Glyburide and metformin are now considered first-line treatments for GDM,[32] so they may be potential alternatives for treatment of type 2 diabetes during pregnancy.

Epilepsy

6 Seizure frequency does not change for most pregnant women with epilepsy. Studies have demonstrated no frequency change in 54% to 80% of women with epilepsy, while decreased frequency ranges between 3% and 24% and increased frequency ranges from 14% to 32%.[59] Seizures may become more frequent because of changes in maternal hormones, sleep deprivation, and medication adherence problems (because of perceived teratogenic risk). Another potential cause is changes in free serum concentrations of antiepileptic drugs resulting from increased maternal volume of distribution, decreased protein binding from hypoalbuminemia, increased hepatic drug metabolism, and increased renal drug clearance. A woman's clinical condition and her free serum concentrations of antiepileptic drug should be the basis for dose adjustments.

The risks of uncontrolled seizures, particularly tonic-clonic seizures, to the fetus are considered to be greater than those associated with the antiepileptic drugs. Major malformations are two to three times more likely to occur in children born to women taking antiepileptic drugs than to those who do not.[60] Major malformations with valproic acid are dose related and range from 6% to 9%; use of valproic acid should be avoided during pregnancy to minimize the risk of NTDs (eg, spina bifida), facial clefts, and cognitive teratogenicity.[61,62]

When possible, antiepileptic drug monotherapy is recommended with medication regimen optimization occurring before conception. If gradual drug withdrawal is attempted because of epilepsy remission, it should be fully completed and evaluated before trying to conceive. Medication change to avoid use of valproic acid and phenobarbital is suggested; if either is used during pregnancy because of treatment failure with other medications, the lowest effective dose should be used.[62] All women taking antiepileptic drugs should receive folic acid supplementation: 4 to 5 mg daily starting before pregnancy and continuing through at least the first trimester, but preferably through the entire pregnancy.[60,62]

Human Immunodeficiency Virus Infection

6 The rate of perinatal HIV transmission is below 2% as a result of national recommendations for universal prenatal HIV counseling and testing, antiretroviral therapy (ART) use, cesarean delivery, and breastfeeding avoidance. The primary goal for HIV-infected women who receive combination ART and desire pregnancy is to achieve sustained viral load suppression below the limits of detection before conception and throughout pregnancy. In women newly diagnosed with HIV or who have not previously received ART, ART should be initiated as soon as pregnancy is determined since risk of perinatal transmission is lower with earlier viral suppression. The treatment regimen should be selected from those suggested for nonpregnant adults, with special consideration given to the teratogenic profile of each drug. Women currently receiving ART should be continued on their regimen provided that viral suppression below the level of detection is documented.[63] For ART-naïve women, use of a three-drug combination regimen is recommended. Recommendations regarding combination ART change frequently as new data becomes available; the clinical guidelines provided at https://aidsinfo.nih.gov are the most up-to-date.

For pregnant women with HIV RNA levels above 1,000 copies/mL (1,000 × 10^3/L) approaching delivery, scheduled cesarean section at 38 weeks of gestation is recommended to reduce the risk of perinatal HIV transmission. Scheduled cesarean section is not recommended if HIV RNA levels are 1,000 copies/mL (1,000 × 10^3/L) or below because of risks for increased complications and the low rate of perinatal transmission. If maternal viral load is greater than 1,000 copies/mL (1000 × 10^3/L) or not known, IV zidovudine should be initiated with a 1-hour loading dose (2 mg/kg) followed by a continuous infusion (1 mg/kg) for 2 hours (cesarean) or until delivery (for vaginal delivery). Zidovudine IV should still be administered in the presence of resistance to oral zidovudine. Women with a viral load at or below 1,000 copies/mL (1,000 × 10^3/L or less) near delivery do not require zidovudine IV, but should continue their ART. Specific recommendations for different clinical scenarios during antepartum, intrapartum, and postpartum are provided in the clinical guidelines.[63]

Hypertension

6 Typically, a physiologic decrease in blood pressure occurs during the first part of pregnancy, reaching its lowest point between 16 and 18 weeks of gestation; this decrease may mask undiagnosed hypertension. By the third trimester, blood pressure usually returns to prepregnancy levels. Hypertension occurring before 20 weeks of gestation, the use of antihypertensive medications before pregnancy, or the persistence of hypertension beyond 12 weeks postpartum defines chronic hypertension in pregnancy. It is classified as mild/nonsevere (sBP 140-159 mm Hg or dBP 90-109 mm Hg) or severe (sBP 160 mm Hg or greater or dBP 110 mm Hg or greater).[64]

Chronic hypertension can cause fetal growth restriction, maternal complications, and hospital admission. Treatment of nonsevere hypertension reduces the risk of severe hypertension by 50% but does not substantially affect fetal outcomes.[65] According to ACOG, drug therapy is recommended for women with persistent chronic hypertension with a blood pressure of 160/105 mm Hg and above. If no evidence of end-organ damage is present and sBP is below 160 mm Hg and dBP is below 105 mm Hg, pharmacologic treatment is not suggested.[35] When antihypertensive medication is used, maintenance of sBP between 120 and 160 mm Hg and dBP between 80 and 105 mm Hg is recommended.[35] No international consensus on management of chronic hypertension exists; definitions and recommendations vary.

Sustained severe hypertension in pregnancy requires treatment as maternal end organ complications, such as stroke, can occur. Lowering of blood pressure should occur over a period of hours to prevent compromise of uteroplacental blood flow. Initial choice of pharmacologic agent varies, but recommended agents are parenteral labetalol and hydralazine; however, hydralazine is associated with more maternal and fetal adverse effects. Oral nifedipine may also be used. Although still commonly used, limited evidence supports the use of magnesium sulfate to lower blood pressure except when being used concomitantly for preeclampsia. Nitroprusside, diazoxide, and nitroglycerin should be reserved for refractory hypertension in an appropriately monitored environment.[38,40]

Mental Health Conditions

6 Psychiatric illness affects approximately 500,000 pregnancies each year according to a practice guideline reaffirmed by ACOG in 2014.[66] Anxiety disorders, including panic disorder, obsessive-compulsive disorder, generalized anxiety disorder, posttraumatic stress disorder, social anxiety disorder, and phobias, can cause adverse maternal and fetal outcomes such as spontaneous abortion, preterm delivery, prolonged labor, and fetal distress.[66]

Depression occurs in 14% to 23% of pregnant women. Maternal depression is associated with greater risk for premature birth, low birth weight, miscarriage, and fetal growth restriction.[67] In addition to the potential impact of maternal depression on obstetric complications, untreated depression may have long-term implications for normal infant development.[66] Up to 6.4% of Americans have bipolar disorder, with men and women equally affected; the incidence in pregnancy is unclear although perinatal episodes tend toward depressive manifestations. Schizophrenia occurs in 1% to 2% of women; however, the incidence in pregnancy is unknown. Maternal schizophrenia is associated with increased risk of perinatal death, low birth weight, small-for-gestational-age infants, cardiovascular malformations, preterm delivery, stillbirth, and infant death.[66]

Up to 70% of women with mental health conditions discontinue or refuse treatment because of concerns about teratogenicity, or because of paranoid or delusional thinking.[68] Therefore, the risks and benefits of psychotropic medication use during pregnancy must be discussed with the patient. Because most psychotropic medications are used to treat more than one condition, the reader should refer to other sources for information about treatment of specific mental health diagnoses. In general, monotherapy is preferred over polytherapy even if higher doses are required.[66]

Through 2005, the use of SSRIs was considered relatively safe. Conflicting studies about the risk of cardiac malformations with paroxetine are published in the literature; if absolute risk is increased, it appears small and clinically insignificant.[67,69] Despite this association, SSRIs are not considered major teratogens, as no consistent information supports an association with structural malformations.[67] Risks with SNRIs are less defined. Use of SSRIs and SNRIs in the latter part of pregnancy is associated with persistent pulmonary hypertension of the newborn and Prenatal Antidepressant Exposure Syndrome (encompasses cardiac, respiratory, neurological, GI, and metabolic complications from drug toxicity or withdrawal of drug therapy).[68] Tricyclic antidepressants were commonly used in pregnancy before the introduction of SSRIs and are not considered major teratogens, although they have also been associated with a neonatal withdrawal syndrome when used late in pregnancy.[66,68] Importantly, women who stop taking antidepressants are more likely to relapse, which can also have implications for the well-being of the fetus.

Studies completed over 30 years ago showed an increased risk of oral clefts with diazepam use during pregnancy; these findings were not confirmed in a meta-analysis that found the absolute risk of oral cleft changed from six cases to seven cases per 10,000 exposures (0.01%).[66] Benzodiazepine use in the third trimester can cause infant sedation and withdrawal symptoms (eg, restlessness, hypertonia, hyperreflexia, tremulousness, apnea, diarrhea, and vomiting). "Floppy baby syndrome," consisting of low Apgar scores, hypothermia, poor muscle tone, feeding difficulties, and poor temperature adaptation, has also been described.[66]

Mood stabilizers, such as lithium, lamotrigine, carbamazepine, and valproic acid, are often used to treat bipolar disorder.[66] The reader can find information related to the safety of seizure medications used for mood stabilization in the section on epilepsy. Lithium's place in the treatment of bipolar disorder during pregnancy is controversial because of concerns about cardiovascular anomalies, especially Ebstein's anomaly, in exposed infants.[66] A meta-analysis calculated that the risk ratio for cardiac malformations was between 1.2 and 7.7 and for all congenital malformations was between 1.5 and 3. Stated differently, the risk for Ebstein's anomaly after prenatal lithium exposure would rise from 1:20,000 to 1:1,000; it is no longer considered a major human teratogen, but careful monitoring of serum lithium concentrations along with renal and thyroid function during pregnancy is prudent.[69,70] Other reported neonatal side effects include floppy baby syndrome, nephrogenic diabetes insipidus, hypoglycemia, cardiac arrhythmias, thyroid dysfunction, polyhydramnios, and premature delivery. Lithium may cause lethargy, hypotonia, hypothermia, cyanosis, and changes in electrocardiogram in infants exposed through breastfeeding. If breastfeeding, the infant's lithium levels, thyroid function, and complete blood count should be monitored.[66]

While neither the typical nor atypical antipsychotics have been adequately studied for the risk of adverse pregnancy outcomes, the typical antipsychotics are considered to have minimum toxic or teratogenic potential. Chlorpromazine, haloperidol, and perphenazine have long histories of use during pregnancy, with no reported significant teratogenic effect.[66] Atypical antipsychotics are considered first-line treatment for schizophrenia because of their more favorable side-effect profiles and potential increased efficacy for treating negative symptoms compared with the older agents; use has increased during pregnancy. While one systematic review found no or minimal increases in risk of major malformations with atypical antipsychotics,[69] others have found a higher rate (10% vs 2%) of low-birth-weight infants with olanzapine, clozapine, quetiapine, and risperidone compared with non-exposed infants and an increased risk of cardiovascular defects.[66,69] Atypical antipsychotics can cause weight gain, gestational diabetes, and metabolic syndrome which have implications for poorer obstetric outcomes.[69]

Thyroid Disorders

6 Universal screening for thyroid disorders during pregnancy is not recommended.[44] Hypothyroidism is present in 2 to 10 per 1,000 pregnancies. Untreated hypothyroidism increases the risk of preeclampsia, premature birth, miscarriage, and growth restriction; impaired neurological development in the fetus may also occur. Causes of hypothyroidism include autoimmune diseases (eg, Hashimoto's thyroiditis), iodine deficiency (uncommon in the United States), and thyroid dysfunction following surgery or ablative therapy for previous hyperthyroidism. If hypothyroidism is present, thyroid replacement should occur. A reasonable levothyroxine starting dose is 0.1 mg/day.[44] Women receiving thyroid replacement therapy before pregnancy may have an increased dosage requirement during pregnancy. Laboratory follow-up of TSH should occur every 4 to 6 weeks during pregnancy to allow for dose titration according to TSH levels.[44]

Hyperthyroidism affects approximately 0.2% of pregnancies and is associated with fetal death, low birth weight, intrauterine growth restriction, and preeclampsia. Graves' disease accounts for 95% of hyperthyroidism in pregnancy.[44] Therapy includes the thioamides (ie, methimazole and PTU). The risks of uncontrolled hyperthyroidism outweigh the risks of the thioamides. The goal of therapy is to attain free thyroxine concentrations near the upper limit of normal to allow for dose minimization and to limit fetal or neonatal hypothyroidism.[44] Iodine-131 is contraindicated because of the risk of thyroid damage in the fetus.

LABOR AND DELIVERY

Management of the pregnant woman during the perinatal period often requires drug therapy for pain and for potential complications.

Preterm Labor

7 Preterm labor occurs between 20 and 37 weeks of gestation when changes in cervical dilation and/or effacement happen along with regular uterine contractions or when the initial presentation includes regular contractions and cervical dilation of at least 2 cm.[71] Preterm birth is the leading cause of infant morbidity and mortality with an incidence that peaked in 2006 at 12.8% in the United States. Rates decreased to 11.7% in 2011, but are still double the European rate. Risk factors for preterm delivery include previous preterm delivery, infections, multiple gestation, poverty, nonwhite race, maternal complication factors (eg, smoking and use of illicit drugs or alcohol), and uterine functional causes (eg, incompetent cervix); previous pregnancy with an adverse outcome, and prior second trimester loss confer a higher risk.[72]

No adequate tests are available for monitoring and preventing preterm labor. Monitoring of uterine activity along with intensive surveillance does not minimize risk.[71] The presence of fetal fibronectin, a glycoprotein found in cervicovaginal secretions, indicates a high risk of preterm birth. Cervical shortening is also associated with preterm delivery. Fetal fibronectin determinations and cervical ultrasound have not helped to prevent preterm labor but have been useful for their negative predictive value.[71] Bed rest and hydration do not decrease the risk of preterm birth and should not be recommended routinely; they carry risks of VTE, bone demineralization, and deconditioning.

Tocolytic Therapy

The purposes of tocolytic therapy are threefold: (a) postpone delivery long enough to allow for the maximum effect of antenatal corticosteroid administration; (b) allow for transportation of the mother to a facility equipped to deal with high-risk deliveries; and (c) prolongation of pregnancy when there are underlying, self-limited conditions that can cause labor, such as pyelonephritis or abdominal surgery, that are unlikely to cause recurrent preterm labor.[71] Tocolytics are generally not utilized beyond 34 weeks of gestation. Use of tocolytics has not reduced the number of premature deliveries. The criteria for starting tocolysis are regular uterine contractions with cervical change. Tocolytic therapy should not be used in cases of previability, intrauterine fetal demise, a lethal fetal anomaly, intrauterine infection, fetal distress, severe preeclampsia, vaginal bleeding, or maternal hemodynamic instability.[71]

Four classes of tocolytics are available in the United States: β-agonists, magnesium, calcium channel blockers, and prostaglandin inhibitors (ie, NSAIDs). All four therapies prolong pregnancy between 48 hours to 1 week; however, this prolongation is not associated with a statistically significant reduction in overall rates of respiratory distress syndrome, neonatal death, or preterm birth before 37 weeks of gestation.[73,74] Prostaglandin inhibitors and calcium channel blockers may be preferable based on the probability of delaying delivery and improving neonatal outcomes.[73]

The β-agonists terbutaline and ritodrine have been used for tocolytic therapy. Ritodrine is no longer available in the United States. Relative to other agents, β-agonists have a higher incidence of maternal side effects, including hyperkalemia, arrhythmias, hyperglycemia, hypotension, and pulmonary edema. Recommended terbutaline doses vary because its use as a tocolytic agent is off-label; a commonly used dose is 250 mcg subcutaneously which may be repeated in 15 to 30 minutes for inadequate response with a maximum of 500 mcg given in a 4-hour period.[74] A black box warning was issued in 2011 recommending against oral dosing or prolonged parenteral use (beyond 48-72 hours) because of maternal cardiotoxicity and death.[71,74]

Intravenous magnesium sulfate has been used for tocolysis; however, a Cochrane review does not support its effectiveness.[74,75] Heterogeneity of study designs and results along with small treatment arms in the included studies may partially explain this finding; however, its use remains unsupported by evidence. These findings should not affect the use of magnesium sulfate for neuroprotection. The incidence of cerebral palsy is increased in premature infants. Several studies evaluating the use of IV magnesium (6 g load followed by 2 g/h continuous infusion until delivery) during preterm labor (up to 34 weeks of gestation) found the occurrence of moderate or severe cerebral palsy was decreased by 45% to 50%.[74] Maternal side effects are rare but can include pulmonary edema. At toxic levels, hypotension, muscle paralysis, tetany, cardiac arrest, and respiratory depression may occur.[74] Magnesium undergoes renal excretion; dose adjustment is required in women with impaired renal function.

Nifedipine is associated with fewer side effects than magnesium or β-agonist therapy and decreases risk of delivery within 7 days compared to β-agonists.[73,74] One concern with the use of nifedipine is its hypotensive effect and corresponding change in uteroplacental blood flow. However, a meta-analysis showed reduced neonatal morbidity with calcium channel blocker use. With the initial diagnosis of preterm labor, nifedipine loading doses range between 10 and 40 mg with subsequent dosing of 10 and 20 mg every 4 to 6 hours with dose adjustment based on patterns of preterm contractions.[74]

Nonsteroidal antiinflammatory drugs, such as indomethacin, have been used effectively for tocolysis.[71,73,74] Oral or rectal doses of 50 to 100 mg initially, followed by an oral dose of 25 to 50 mg every 6 hours for 48 hours, have been used. An increased rate of premature constriction of the ductus arteriosus has been noted in infants with indomethacin use after 32 weeks of gestation and with use exceeding 48 hours.[74] Indomethacin may be used when tocolysis is needed despite treatment with magnesium for neuroprotection because other agents, such as calcium channel blockers and β-agonists, can cause hypotension when administered concurrently with magnesium.

Other Drug Therapies for Preterm Labor Prevention

Infection is a potential cause of preterm labor. Antibiotics have been used, in addition to tocolytics and corticosteroids, to improve the outcome of preterm labor; however, a Cochrane review showed no reduction in the incidence of preterm delivery, respiratory distress syndrome, or neonatal sepsis but a trend toward increased neonatal mortality.[71] Therefore, routine use of antibiotics is not recommended. However, if a patient experiences preterm premature rupture of membranes (PPROM) before 34 weeks of gestation, prophylactic antibiotics should be initiated because a reduction in major morbidities (ie, death, respiratory distress syndrome, early sepsis, severe intraventricular hemorrhage, and necrotizing enterocolitis) was demonstrated.[76,77] A 7-day course of broad-spectrum antibiotics should be used with the intent to prolong latency, which is the time from ruptured membranes to delivery. One recommended regimen is ampicillin (2 g IV every 6 hours) plus erythromycin (250 mg IV every 6 hours) for 48 hours, followed by amoxicillin (250 mg orally three times daily) and erythromycin base (333 mg orally every 8 hours), although multiple regimens have shown benefit.[76] Amoxicillin-clavulanate is not recommended since it causes increased rates of necrotizing enterocolitis.

Progesterone administration in the setting of prior preterm birth is based upon its effects to diminish cervical ripening (softening of the cervix necessary for cervical dilation before birth), reduce uterine wall contractility, and modulate inflammation.[72] Evidence supports progesterone supplementation to prevent spontaneous preterm birth. Use of intramuscular 17-α-hydroxyprogesterone weekly (250 mg) or vaginal progesterone suppositories (100 mg) starting between weeks 16 and 24 continued through week 36 in women with a previous spontaneous preterm birth is recommended.[78]

Clinical **Controversy...**

Women who present with PPROM receive, among other important interventions, antibiotic prophylaxis for 7 days to prevent chorioamnionitis and neonatal sepsis. The goal is to prolong pregnancy and reduce neonatal morbidity.[76,77] However, some evidence suggests that use of antibiotic prophylaxis may have a role in women with premature rupture of the membranes presenting at 36 weeks of gestation or more to reduce occurrence of chorioamnionitis and endometritis. Results should be interpreted cautiously since the outcomes measured were secondary endpoints and analyzed through meta-analysis of studies, all of which used different antibiotic regimens.[79]

Antenatal Corticosteroids

Use of antenatal corticosteroids for fetal lung maturation to prevent respiratory distress syndrome, intraventricular hemorrhage, and death in infants delivered prematurely is supported by a Cochrane review and recommended by ACOG.[71,80] The current clinical recommendation is to administer betamethasone 12 mg intramuscularly every 24 hours for two doses or dexamethasone 6 mg intramuscularly every 12 hours for four doses to pregnant women between 24 and 34 weeks of gestation who are at risk for preterm delivery within the next 7 days.[71] Benefits from antenatal corticosteroids are believed to begin within 24 hours.

Salvage ("rescue") treatment administered to women at risk of delivering within 7 days but who received a previous course of therapy is also supported by a Cochrane review. Risk of respiratory distress syndrome was lower with the administration of rescue steroids compared with placebo (risk ratio 0.83, 95% confidence interval 0.75-0.91).[81]

Group B *Streptococcus* Infection

7 Maternal infection with GBS is associated with invasive disease in the newborn.[82,83] Women colonized with GBS have an increased risk for pregnancy loss, premature delivery, and transmission of the bacteria to the infant during delivery. Between 10% and 30% of pregnant women are colonized with GBS. The rate of invasive infection (defined as isolation of GBS from blood or other sterile body site excluding urine) in pregnant women is 0.12 per 1,000 live births (range, 0.11-0.14 per 1,000 births). The incidence of early-onset disease in neonates, although higher than in pregnant women, has declined steadily from 1.5 per 1,000 live births in 1993 to approximately 0.24 cases per 1,000 live births in 2010. The consequences of neonatal infections include bacteremia, pneumonia, meningitis, and fatality in the newborn.[83] The case-fatality rate is approximately 4%.

Recommendations for prevention of GBS infection were last updated in 2010.[83] Universal prenatal screening for GBS colonization is recommended. Antibiotics are given if the woman previously gave birth to an infant with invasive GBS disease or in the presence of GBS bacteriuria. All other pregnant women should have a vaginal/rectal culture at 35 to 37 weeks of gestation. If negative, antibiotics are not indicated. If a woman presents in labor and no screening information is available, antibiotics are given for fever greater than 100.4°F (38°C), membrane rupture at least 18 hours prior, or gestation under 37 weeks.

Penicillin G 5 million units given IV, followed by 2.5 million units given every 4 hours until delivery is the recommended treatment regimen.[83] Alternatively, ampicillin 2 g can be given IV, followed by 1 g every 4 hours. For women with penicillin allergy but not at risk for anaphylaxis, cefazolin 2 g IV, followed by 1 g every 8 hours, is recommended. In women at high risk for anaphylaxis, clindamycin 900 mg IV every 8 hours or erythromycin 500 mg IV every 6 hours is recommended. For penicillin-allergic women, GBS cultures should be sent for sensitivities. If resistant to clindamycin or erythromycin, vancomycin 1 g IV every 12 hours until delivery is appropriate.

Cervical Ripening and Labor Induction

7 Throughout gestation, the cervix is closed and firm. During the last few weeks of pregnancy, the cervix softens and thins to facilitate labor. This process is mediated by hormonal changes, including final mediation by prostaglandins E_2 and $F_2\alpha$, which increase collagenase activity in the cervix leading to thinning and dilation.

The rate of pregnancy induction ranges from 9.5% to 33.5%; the most common indications for induction are postdatism (beyond 42 weeks) and pregnancy-induced hypertension, which account for 80% of inductions.[84-86] Other reasons for induction include suspected fetal growth retardation, maternal hypertension, premature rupture of membranes with no active onset of labor, and social factors. Contraindications include placenta previa, oblique or transverse lie, pelvic structure abnormality, prolapsed umbilical cord, and active herpes. Concerns with induction of labor are ineffective labor and side effects, such as uterine hyperstimulation, that may adversely affect the infant and increase the likelihood of cesarean section.

Scoring systems have been used to determine the likelihood of successful labor induction. The Bishop scoring system is most commonly used and is based on five parameters: cervical dilation, cervical effacement (thinning), station of the baby's head, consistency of the cervix, and position of the cervix.[84,86] A Bishop score under six indicates the need for cervical ripening while a score above eight corresponds to a likely successful vaginal delivery.

A number of nonpharmacologic methods are used for cervical ripening. Castor oil, hot baths, sexual intercourse, and nipple stimulation all have been suggested for labor induction.[87] Minimal evidence supports the efficacy of these methods. Use of a Foley catheter placed in an unfavorable cervix for ripening has been found as effective as prostaglandin E_2. Membrane stripping is safe and inexpensive.[86]

Prostaglandin E_2 analogs (eg, dinoprostone [Prepidil gel, Cervidil vaginal insert]) are commonly used for cervical ripening. Prepidil 500 mcg is administered intracervically. The dose may be repeated after 6 hours to a maximum of three doses in 24 hours.[86] After administration, the patient remains supine for 30 minutes. Cervidil contains 10 mg dinoprostone with a slower, more constant release of medication than the gel.[86] The insert is removed when labor begins or after 12 hours. Patients must be attached to a fetal heart rate monitor for the duration of Cervidil use and for 15 minutes after its removal.[87]

Misoprostol, a prostaglandin E_1 analog, is an effective and inexpensive drug for cervical ripening and labor induction. Intravaginal administration of 25 mcg misoprostol (oral tablets are split to obtain dose) given every 3 to 6 hours is at least as effective as other prostaglandin agents and results in a shorter time to delivery.[86] Oral misoprostol has been used successfully for cervical ripening and labor induction, but the evidence for safety is more extensive with intravaginal use. The most commonly encountered side effects are uterine hyperstimulation and meconium-stained amniotic fluid. Use of misoprostol is contraindicated in women with a previous uterine scar because of its association with uterine rupture, a catastrophic medical event.

Progesterone inhibits uterine contractions. Preliminary studies show that mifepristone, an antiprogesterone agent, compared with placebo results in a shorter time to delivery and fewer cesarean sections.[88] Limited information on fetal and maternal outcomes is available because of the small sample sizes.

Oxytocin is the most commonly used agent for labor induction after cervical ripening. By the end of pregnancy, the number of oxytocin receptors has increased by 300-fold.[85,87] A solution of 10 mU/mL (10 U/L) is used for infusion. Oxytocin is effective in both low-dose (physiologic) and high-dose (pharmacologic) regimens. Refer to the ACOG practice bulletin for detailed administration information.[86]

Labor Analgesia

7 The first phase of labor occurs from onset of labor to complete cervical dilation while the second phase of labor is the period of time between complete cervical dilation and delivery. During the first phase of labor, women perceive visceral pain caused by uterine contractions. Pain in the second phase of labor is associated with perineal stretching.[89]

Nonpharmacologic Approaches to Analgesia

Women who receive continuous support from nurses, midwives, childbirth educators, or doulas (lay women trained in labor support), have fewer operative vaginal deliveries, cesarean deliveries, and requests for pain medication.[90] Warm water baths provide temporary pain relief may decrease the use of pharmacologic pain treatments, but do not decrease the rate of assisted vaginal deliveries or cesarean sections; maternal and neonatal infection, and neonatal water aspiration are potential risks. Intradermal injections of sterile water in the sacral area provide short-term decreases in back pain during labor. However, requests for pain medication did not decrease in studies. Acupuncture has also been used for pain relief. Several randomized, controlled trials have shown that acupuncture decreases the need for analgesia, but more methodologically sound studies are needed. Use of audioanalgesia (music or white noise), relaxation and breathing techniques, application of heat and cold, aromatherapy, acupressure, transcutaneous electrical nerve stimulation (TENS), and hypnosis have little to no evidence of effectiveness derived from randomized, controlled trials.[89,90]

Pharmacologic Approaches to Labor Pain Management

Maternal request alone is a sufficient medical indication for labor analgesia.[91] The two main types of pharmacologic approaches in the United States are parenteral opioids and epidural analgesia.

Parenteral opioids are commonly used to alleviate labor pain.[91] In comparison with epidural analgesia, parenteral opioids have lower rates of oxytocin augmentation, result in shorter stages of labor, and require fewer instrumental deliveries and cesarean sections for fetal distress.[92]

Approximately 60% of women in the United States choose an epidural for pain relief during labor and report better pain relief than with other analgesic modalities.[92] With epidural analgesia, a catheter is introduced into the epidural space, and an opioid and/or an anesthetic (eg, fentanyl and/or bupivacaine) is administered. Combined spinal-epidural analgesia consists of injecting a single opioid bolus into the subarachnoid space to provide instant pain relief with additional use of a local anesthetic epidural; compared with traditional epidurals, combined spinal-epidural anesthesia has a slightly shorter mean time to onset of effective analgesia.[89] Patient-controlled epidural analgesia allows the patient to control the amount and timing of the anesthetic; it results in a lower total dose of local anesthetics used over the course of labor compared with continuous epidural infusions and allows a reduction in the time between onset of pain and administration of analgesia.[93]

Side effects of the regional anesthesia include hypotension, pruritus, and inability to void. Epidural analgesia is associated with prolongation of the first and second stages of labor, higher numbers of instrumental deliveries and cesarean sections (for fetal distress), and maternal fever.[89,92] A rare complication of epidural anesthesia is puncture of the subarachnoid space leading to a severe headache, which occurs in approximately 1% of women. Other complications include hypotension, nausea, vomiting, itching, and urinary retention.[92] Low back pain has not been associated with the use of epidural analgesia.

Postpartum Hemorrhage

7 The placenta is delivered after the delivery of the baby and is referred to as the third stage of labor. Postpartum hemorrhage (PPH) is an obstetrical emergency and is a major cause of morbidity and mortality worldwide.[94] The traditional definition of PPH is loss of more than 500 mL of blood within 24 hours of a vaginal delivery or 1,000 mL after a cesarean section; however, other definitions have also been suggested. Risk factors include retained placenta, failure to progress during the second stage of labor, placenta previa, placenta accreta, lacerations, instrumental delivery, large for gestational age newborn, hypertensive disorders, labor induction, augmentation of labor with oxytocin, prior history, maternal obesity, and preeclampsia.[94]

A stepwise approach to the treatment of PPH is advised. After the exclusion of retained products of conception and cervical and vaginal lacerations, attention should be turned to the management of uterine atony if present. The most common cause of PPH is uterine atony.[94,95] Initial management should include oxytocin. Controlled traction of the cord, which involves gently pulling on the cut umbilical cord to remove the placenta, may reduce minor PPHs but early clamping and cutting of the umbilical cord has no effect on rates of PPH.[95] Administration of a uterotonic medication (intramuscular oxytocin, ergonovine, or combination) before placental delivery and instituting active management of labor after all uncomplicated vaginal deliveries result in reduced maternal blood loss, fewer cases of PPH, and less prolongation of the third stage of labor.[95] Other uterotonic agents should be used if an inadequate response is attained with oxytocin alone. Methylergonovine, carboprost, misoprostol, and dinoprostone have all been used; less evidence is available for misoprostol and dinoprostone. Some limited evidence supports use of tranexamic acid, an antifibrinolytic agent. If uterotonic drug therapies fail to control the bleeding, uterine artery embolization, intrauterine balloon catheters, or a variety of different surgical techniques can be used.[94,95]

POSTPARTUM ISSUES

Drug Use During Lactation

8 A wide variety of benefits (eg, health, nutritional, immunologic, psychological, economic, developmental, and social) are imparted by breastfeeding to infants, mothers, and the family. Women should breastfeed exclusively for 6 months and continue until at least 12 months of age while other foods are introduced.[96] Healthy People 2020 increased targets for breastfeeding to 81.9% of neonates at the time of birth and to 60.5% for infants being breastfed at 6 months.[96]

Adequate milk removal from the breast by breastfeeding or pumping is necessary to maintain or increase milk production.[97] Relactation is the process of increasing the breast milk supply for women whose milk has not "come in," who have inadequate milk production despite appropriate breastfeeding frequency or pumping, or who have weaned or never breastfed after delivery. Metoclopramide can be used if nonpharmacologic measures are ineffective because of its stimulation of prolactin secretion. The most common dose is 10 mg orally three times daily for 7 to 14 days.[97] Breast milk production may decrease after metoclopramide therapy is stopped, but production will continue if lactation has been established successfully.

Most drugs transfer into breast milk, but breastfeeding may be continued in most circumstances. Healthcare providers should encourage breastfeeding women who require medications to continue breastfeeding whenever possible. Passive diffusion is the primary mechanism for drug transfer into breast milk, but other drug-related factors influence drug transfer from maternal circulation into breast milk, including (a) degree of protein binding in maternal plasma, (b) molecular weight, (c) lipid solubility (and corresponding fat content of milk), (d) maternal plasma concentration, (e) drug half-life, and (f) drug pH.[98] The degree of protein binding to maternal plasma proteins is one of the most significant factors affecting drug transfer to breast milk; highly bound medications transfer in low amounts. Low-molecular-weight drugs passively diffuse into breast milk, but larger molecules are not likely to transfer in large amounts. Higher lipid solubility of drugs also increases the likelihood of transfer. Colostrum is secreted in the first couple of days after birth and has high quantities of immunoglobulins, maternal lymphocytes, and maternal macrophages. While greater amounts of drugs are present in colostrum, the amount received by the nursing infant is minimal because of the limited volume of colostrum produced. A greater volume of mature milk is produced, but drug transfer into mature milk is lower because of tight cell-to-cell junctions. The higher the concentration of drug in the mother's serum, the higher the concentration will be in the breast milk. As the drug is metabolized and excreted by the mother, the mother's serum concentration drops, and the drug in the breast milk may redistribute back into the mother's bloodstream. Maternal plasma pH is 7.4, while the pH of breast milk ranges between 6.8 and 7. Weak bases are not ionized in the maternal circulation and easily transfer to breast milk.[98] In the lower pH of breast milk, molecules become ionized and are less likely to diffuse back into maternal circulation ("ion trapping"). Likewise, drugs with longer half-lives are more likely to maintain higher levels in breast milk, resulting in greater exposure to the infant.

Infant-related factors may also influence the amount of drug ingested through breastfeeding. Both the frequency of feedings and the amount of milk ingested are important considerations. Exclusively breastfed infants are more likely to ingest larger amounts of drugs than older infants who receive other foods. Drugs unstable in gastric acid (aminoglycosides, PPIs, heparin, and insulin) are less likely to be absorbed by infants.[98] Finally, infants may vary in their ability to metabolize and excrete ingested medication. Premature and full-term infants may not have full renal and liver function.

Strategies for reducing the risk to the infant include selection of medications that would be considered safe for use in the infant. Drugs with shorter half-lives accumulate less, and those that are more protein bound do not cross into breast milk as well as those that are less protein bound. Drugs with lower oral bioavailability and lower lipid solubility are good choices. If the mother is using a once-daily medication, administration before the infant's longest sleep period may be advised to increase the interval to the next feeding. For medications taken multiple times per day, administration immediately after breastfeeding provides the longest interval for back diffusion of drug from the breast milk to the mother's serum. During short-term drug therapy, the mother can pump and discard milk to preserve her milk-producing capability if the medication is not considered compatible with breastfeeding.[99,100]

Information regarding drug use during breastfeeding is available from expert committees (eg, American Academy of Pediatrics Committee on Drugs) and evidence-based textbooks or databases (eg, LactMed [*www.toxnet.nlm.nih.gov*]). All may be of assistance in determining safe and appropriate medications to use during breastfeeding.

Mastitis

8 Mastitis is inflammation of the breast that occurs in 3% to 20% in lactating women.[101] It can be infectious or noninfectious; the most common cause is milk stasis. Signs and symptoms include breast tenderness, redness, warmth, flulike symptoms, and fever (temperature 101.3°F [38.5°C] or greater). Risk factors for developing mastitis include breast engorgement, plugged milk ducts, oversupply of milk, and cracked nipples.[101]

Penicillin-resistant *Staphylococcus aureus* is the most common bacterial cause of mastitis; *E. coli* and *Streptococcus* have also been implicated.[101] A 10- to 14-day course of antibiotics is usually given for treatment of mastitis; penicillinase-resistant penicillins (eg, dicloxacillin, oxacillin) and cephalosporins (eg, cephalexin) are frequently prescribed. Antiinflammatory drugs, such as ibuprofen, may provide some pain relief. Application of heat may also be helpful. Affected women should be counseled to continue breastfeeding from both breasts throughout treatment and to pump if breasts are not emptied completely with feedings.[101]

Postpartum Depression

8 Mood disorders in the postpartum period may include postpartum blues, postpartum depression, and postpartum psychosis.[102] Postpartum blues ("baby blues") is common, usually affecting 15% to 85% of new mothers within the first 10 days of delivery, and generally does not require treatment. Symptoms include anxiety, anger, fatigue, insomnia, tearfulness, and sadness. Postpartum psychosis is more severe and can present as mania, psychotic depression, or schizophrenia but is rare, affecting less than 1% of new mothers; hospitalization is usually indicated.[102]

Postpartum depression affects up to 13% of women, with almost 5% experiencing major depression.[102] Symptoms may develop during pregnancy or up to 6 months after delivery, although the strict definition for major depressive disorder after delivery specifies symptom occurrence within 4 to 6 weeks. Psychotherapy, including interpersonal psychotherapy, cognitive behavioral therapy, and group/family therapy, has been shown effective for treatment of postpartum depression.[102]

Some evidence suggests that the benefits to the infant of breastfeeding exceed the risks of breastfeeding from an antidepressant-treated mother with postpartum depression. In cases where pharmacotherapy is warranted, selection of medication with low transfer to breast milk is desirable.[99] Sertraline, paroxetine, fluoxetine, and nortriptyline are the most studied in the postpartum period. A Cochrane review found that SSRIs are more likely to be effective than placebo for treatment of postpartum depression, but the evidence with tricyclic antidepressants is insufficient to assess outcome.[102]

ABBREVIATIONS

ACOG	American College of Obstetricians and Gynecologists
ART	antiretroviral therapy
BV	bacterial vaginosis
CNS	central nervous system
dBP	diastolic blood pressure
FPG	fasting plasma glucose
GBS	Group B *Streptococcus*
GDM	gestational diabetes mellitus
GI	gastrointestinal
GTT	gestational transient thyrotoxicosis
H_2	histamine-2
hCG	human chorionic gonadotropin
HDP	hypertensive disorders of pregnancy
HELLP	hemolysis, elevated liver enzymes, low platelets

HG	hyperemesis gravidarum
HIV	human immunodeficiency virus
HSV-1	herpes simplex virus 1
HSV-2	herpes simplex virus 2
HTN	hypertension
IADPSG	International Association of Diabetes and Pregnancy Study Groups
LMWH	low-molecular-weight heparin
NNRTI	nonnucleoside reverse transcriptase inhibitor
NRTI	nucleoside reverse transcriptase inhibitor
NSAID	nonsteroidal antiinflammatory drug
NTD	neural tube defect
NVP	nausea and vomiting of pregnancy
OGTT	oral glucose tolerance test
PID	pelvic inflammatory disease
PPH	postpartum hemorrhage
PPI	proton pump inhibitor
PPROM	preterm premature rupture of membranes
PPT	postpartum thyroiditis
PTU	propylthiouracil
RPG	random plasma glucose
sBP	systolic blood pressure
SNRI	serotonin–norepinephrine reuptake inhibitor
SSRI	selective serotonin reuptake inhibitor
STI	sexually transmitted infection
TENS	transcutaneous electrical nerve stimulation
TSH	thyroid-stimulating hormone
UFH	unfractionated heparin
UTI	urinary tract infection
VTE	venous thromboembolism

REFERENCES

1. Ord T. The scourge: Moral implications of natural embryo loss. *Am J Bioeth* 2008;8:12-19.
2. Brent RL. Environmental causes of human congenital malformations: The pediatrician's role in dealing with these complex clinical problems caused by a multiplicity of environmental and genetic factors. *Pediatrics* 2004;113(4 Suppl):957-968.
3. Gupta SK, Bansal P, Ganguly A, Bhandari B, Chakrabarti K. Human zona pellucida glycoproteins: Functional relevance during fertilization. *J Reprod Immunol* 2009;83(1-2):50-55.
4. Cunningham FJ, Leveno KJ, Bloom SL, et al. Implantation and placental development. In: Cunningham FJ, Leveno KJ, Bloom SL, et al., eds. *Williams Obstetrics*. 24th ed. [electronic version] 2014, *AccessMedicine*. Available at: *http://accessmedicine.mhmedical.com/content.aspx?bookid=1057§ionid=59789141*. (Accessed August 11, 2015.)
5. Cunningham FJ, Leveno KJ, Bloom SL, et al. Embryogenesis and fetal morphological development. In: Cunningham FJ, Leveno KJ, Bloom SL, et al., eds. *Williams Obstetrics*. 24th ed. [electronic version] 2014, *AccessMedicine*. Available at: *http://accessmedicine.mhmedical.com/content.aspx?bookid=1057§ionid=59789143*. (Accessed August 11, 2015.)
6. Cunningham FJ, Leveno KJ, Bloom SL, et al. Prenatal care. In: Cunningham FJ, Leveno KJ, Bloom SL, et al., eds. *Williams Obstetrics*. 24th ed. [electronic version] 2014, *AccessMedicine*. Available at: *http://accessmedicine.mhmedical.com/content.aspx?bookid=1057§ionid=59789146*. (Accessed August 11, 2015.)
7. Bernstein HB, VanBuren G. Normal pregnancy and prenatal care. In: DeCherney AH, Nathan L, Laufer N, et al., eds. *CURRENT Diagnosis & Treatment: Obstetrics & Gynecology*. 11th ed. [electronic version] 2013, *AccessMedicine*. Available at: *http://accessmedicine.mhmedical.com/content.aspx?bookid=498§ionid=41008595*. (Accessed August 11, 2015.)
8. Feghali MN, Mattison DR. Clinical therapeutics in pregnancy. *J Biomed Biotechnol.* 2011;2011:783528. doi: 10.1155/2011/783528.
9. Flick AA, Kahn DA. Maternal physiology during pregnancy & fetal & early neonatal physiology. In: DeCherney AH, Nathan L, Laufer N, et al., eds. *CURRENT Diagnosis & Treatment: Obstetrics & Gynecology*. 11th ed. [electronic version] 2013, *AccessMedicine*. Available at: *http://accessmedicine.mhmedical.com/content.aspx?bookid=498§ionid=41008597*. (Accessed August 11, 2015.)
10. Cunningham FJ, Leveno KJ, Bloom SL, et al. Embryogenesis and fetal morphological development. In: Cunningham FG, Leveno KJ, Bloom SL, et al., eds. *Williams Obstetrics*. 24th ed. [electronic version] 2014, *AccessMedicine*. Available at: *http://accessmedicine.mhmedical.com/content.aspx?bookid=1057§ionid=59789143*. (Accessed August 11, 2015.)
11. Syme MR, Paxton JW, Keelan JA. Drug transfer and metabolism by the human placenta. *Clin Pharmacokinet* 2004;43:487-514.
12. Brent RL. The role of the pediatrician in preventing congenital malformations. *Pediatr Rev* 2011;32:411-421.
13. Adam MP. The all-or-none phenomenon revisited. *Birth Defects Res A Clin Mol Teratol* 2012;94:664-669.
14. Kallen BA. Methodological issues in the epidemiological study of the teratogenicity of drugs. *Congenit Anom (Kyoto)* 2005;45:44-51.
15. Schaefer C, Ornoy A, Clementi M, et al. Using observational cohort data for studying drug effects on pregnancy outcome—methodological considerations. *Reprod Toxicol* 2008;26:36-41.
16. Food and Drug Administration. Content and Format of Labeling for Human Prescription Drug and Biological Products; Requirements for Pregnancy and Lactation Labeling (Final Rule). Federal Register 79:233 (December 4, 2014):72064-72103.
17. Berghella V, Buchanan E, Pereira L, Baxter JK. Preconception care. *Obstet Gynecol Surv* 2010;65:119-131.
18. U.S. Preventive Services Task Force. Folic acid for the prevention of neural tube defects: U.S. Preventive Services Task Force recommendation statement. *Ann Intern Med* 2009;150:626-631.
19. Lumley J, Chamberlain C, Dowswell T, et al. Interventions for promoting smoking cessation during pregnancy. *Cochrane Database Syst Rev* 2009(3):CD001055.
20. De Long NE, Barra NG, Hardy DB, Holloway AC. Is it safe to use smoking cessation therapeutics during pregnancy? *Expert Opin Drug Saf* 2014;13:1721-1731.
21. Boregowda G, Shehata HA. Gastrointestinal and liver disease in pregnancy. *Best Pract Res Clin Obstet Gynaecol* 2013;27:835-853.
22. Avsar AF, Keskin HL. Haemorrhoids during pregnancy. *J Obstet Gynaecol* 2010;30:231-237.
23. Trottier M, Erebara A, Bozzo P. Treating constipation during pregnancy. *Can Fam Physician* 2012;58:836-838.
24. van der Woude CJ, Metselaar HJ, Danese S. Management of gastrointestinal and liver diseases during pregnancy. *Gut* 2014;63:1014-1023.
25. Majithia R, Johnson DA. Are proton pump inhibitors safe during pregnancy and lactation? Evidence to date. *Drugs* 2012;72:171-179.
26. Maltepe C, Koren G. The management of nausea and vomiting of pregnancy and hyperemesis gravidarum—a 2013 update. *J Popul Ther Clin Pharmacol* 2013;20:e184-192.
27. Niebyl JR, Briggs GG. The pharmacologic management of nausea and vomiting of pregnancy. *J Fam Pract* 2014;63(2 Suppl):S31-37.
28. American Diabetes Association. Classification and diagnosis of diabetes. *Diabetes Care* 2015;38(Suppl 1):S8-16.
29. Klein J, Charach R, Sheiner E. Treating diabetes during pregnancy. *Expert Opin Pharmacother* 2015;16:357-368.
30. International Association of Diabetes and Pregnancy Study Groups Consensus Panel, Metzger BE, Gabbe SG, et al. International Association of Diabetes and Pregnancy Study Groups recommendations on the diagnosis and classification of hyperglycemia in pregnancy. *Diabetes Care* 2010;33:676-682.
31. American Diabetes Association. (12) Management of diabetes in pregnancy. *Diabetes Care* 2015;38(Suppl 1):S77-79.
32. Committeee on Practice Bulletins—Obstetrics. Practice Bulletin No. 137: Gestational diabetes mellitus. *Obstet Gynecol* 2013;122(2 Pt 1): 406-416.
33. Crowther CA, Hiller JE, Moss JR, et al. Effect of treatment of gestational diabetes mellitus on pregnancy outcomes. *N Engl J Med* 2005;352:2477-2486.
34. Vadhera RB, Simon M. Hypertensive emergencies in pregnancy. *Clin Obstet Gynecol* 2014;57:797-805.
35. American College of Obstetricians and Gynecologists; Task Force on Hypertension in Pregnancy. Report of the American College of Obstetricians and Gynecologists' Task Force on Hypertension in Pregnancy. *Obstet Gynecol* 2013;122:1122-1131.
36. Magee LA, Pels A, Helewa M, et al. Canadian Hypertensive Disorders of Pregnancy (HDP) Working Group. Diagnosis, evaluation, and management of the hypertensive disorders of pregnancy. *Pregnancy Hypertens* 2014;4:105-145.
37. Hofmeyr GJ, Lawrie TA, Atallah AN, et al. Calcium supplementation during pregnancy for preventing hypertensive disorders and related problems. *Cochrane Database Syst Rev* 2014;6:CD001059.

38. Magee LA, Abalos E, von Dadelszen P, et al. How to manage hypertension in pregnancy effectively. *Br J Clin Pharmacol* 2011;72:394-401.
39. Trogstad L, Magnus P, Stoltenberg C. Pre-eclampsia: Risk factors and causal models. *Best Pract Res Clin Obstet Gynaecol* 2011;25:329-342.
40. Moussa HN, Arian SE, Sibai BM. Management of hypertensive disorders in pregnancy. *Womens Health (Lond Engl)* 2014;10:385-404.
41. Payne B, Magee LA, von Dadelszen P. Assessment, surveillance and prognosis in pre-eclampsia. *Best Pract Res Clin Obstet Gynaecol* 2011;25:449-462.
42. Duley L, Henderson-Smart DJ, Meher S, King JF. Antiplatelet agents for preventing pre-eclampsia and its complications. *Cochrane Database Syst Rev* 2007(2):CD004659.
43. Duley L, Gulmezoglu AM, Henderson-Smart DJ, Chou D. Magnesium sulphate and other anticonvulsants for women with pre-eclampsia. *Cochrane Database Syst Rev* 2010(11):CD000025.
44. American College of Obstetricians and Gynecologists. Practice Bulletin No. 148: Thyroid disease in pregnancy. *Obstet Gynecol* 2015;125:996-1005.
45. Bates SM, Greer IA, Middeldorp S, et al. VTE, thrombophilia, antithrombotic therapy, and pregnancy: Antithrombotic therapy and prevention of thrombosis, 9th ed: American College of Chest Physicians Evidence-Based Clinical Practice Guidelines. *Chest* 2012;141(2 Suppl):e691S-736S.
46. Law H, Fiadjoe P. Urogynaecological problems in pregnancy. *J Obstet Gynaecol* 2012;32:109-112.
47. Smaill FM, Vazquez JC. Antibiotics for asymptomatic bacteriuria in pregnancy. *Cochrane Database Syst Rev* 2015;8:CD000490.
48. Vazquez JC, Abalos E. Treatments for symptomatic urinary tract infections during pregnancy. *Cochrane Database Syst Rev* 2011(1):CD002256.
49. O'Dell KK. Pharmacologic management of asymptomatic bacteriuria and urinary tract infections in women. *J Midwifery Womens Health* 2011;56:248-265.
50. Workowski KA, Bolan GA. Centers for Disease Control and Prevention (CDC). Sexually transmitted diseases treatment guidelines, 2015. *MMWR Recomm Rep* 2015;64(RR-03):1-137.
51. Macgregor EA. Headache in pregnancy. *Neurol Clin* 2012;30:835-866.
52. Vatti RR, Teuber SS. Asthma and pregnancy. *Clin Rev Allergy Immunol* 2012;43(1-2):45-56.
53. From the Global Strategy for Asthma Management and Prevention, Global Initiative for Asthma (GINA) 2015. Available at: *http://www.ginasthma.org*. (Accessed August 18, 2015.)
54. National Asthma Education and Prevention Program. Expert Panel Report 3 (EPR-3): Guidelines for the Diagnosis and Management of Asthma-Summary Report 2007. *J Allergy Clin Immunol* 2007; 120(5 Suppl):S94-138.
55. Piette V, Daures JP, Demoly P. Treating allergic rhinitis in pregnancy. *Curr Allergy Asthma Rep* 2006;6:232-238.
56. Gilbert C, Mazzotta P, Loebstein R, Koren G. Fetal safety of drugs used in the treatment of allergic rhinitis: A critical review. *Drug Saf* 2005;28:707-719.
57. Ballas J, Moore TR, Ramos GA. Management of diabetes in pregnancy. *Curr Diab Rep* 2012;12:33-42.
58. Lambert K, Holt RI. The use of insulin analogues in pregnancy. *Diabetes Obes Metab* 2013;15:888-900.
59. Harden CL, Hopp J, Ting TY, et al. Management issues for women with epilepsy-Focus on pregnancy (an evidence-based review): I. Obstetrical complications and change in seizure frequency: Report of the Quality Standards Subcommittee and Therapeutics and Technology Assessment Subcommittee of the American Academy of Neurology and the American Epilepsy Society. *Epilepsia* 2009;50:1229-1236.
60. Tomson T, Battino D. Pregnancy and epilepsy: What should we tell our patients? *J Neurol* 2009;256:856-862.
61. Harden CL, Meador KJ, Pennell PB, et al. Management issues for women with epilepsy-Focus on pregnancy (an evidence-based review): II. Teratogenesis and perinatal outcomes: Report of the Quality Standards Subcommittee and Therapeutics and Technology Subcommittee of the American Academy of Neurology and the American Epilepsy Society. *Epilepsia* 2009;50:1237-1246.
62. Harden CL. Pregnancy and epilepsy. *Continuum (Minneap Minn)* 2014;20(1 Neurology of Pregnancy):60-79.
63. Panel on Treatment of HIV-Infected Pregnant Women and Prevention of Perinatal Transmission. Recommendations for Use of Antiretroviral Drugs in Pregnant HIV-1-Infected Women for Maternal Health *and* Interventions to Reduce Perinatal HIV Transmission in the United States. Available at: *http://aidsinfo.nih.gov/contentfiles/lvguidelines/perinatalGL.pdf*. (Accessed August 19, 2015.)
64. American College of Obstetricians and Gynecologists. ACOG Practice Bulletin No. 125: Chronic hypertension in pregnancy. *Obstet Gynecol* 2012;119(2 Pt 1):396-407.
65. Mustafa R, Ahmed S, Gupta A, Venuto RC. A comprehensive review of hypertension in pregnancy. *J Pregnancy* 2012;2012:105918. doi: 10.1155/2012/105918.
66. ACOG Practice Bulletin: Clinical Management Guidelines for Obstetrician-Gynecologists number 92, April 2008 (replaces practice bulletin number 87, November 2007). Use of psychiatric medications during pregnancy and lactation. *Obstet Gynecol* 2008;111:1001-1020.
67. Yonkers KA, Wisner KL, Stewart DE, et al. The management of depression during pregnancy: A report from the American Psychiatric Association and the American College of Obstetricians and Gynecologists. *Obstet Gynecol* 2009;114:703-713.
68. Gentile S. Drug treatment for mood disorders in pregnancy. *Curr Opin Psychiatry* 2011;24:34-40.
69. Pearlstein T. Use of psychotropic medication during pregnancy and the postpartum period. *Womens Health (Lond Engl)* 2013;9:605-615.
70. Levey L, Ragan K, Hower-Hartley A, Newport DJ, Stowe ZN. Psychiatric disorders in pregnancy. *Neurol Clin* 2004;22:863-893.
71. American College of Obstetricians and Gynecologists; Committee on Practice Bulletins-Obstetrics. ACOG practice bulletin no. 127: Management of preterm labor. *Obstet Gynecol* 2012;119:1308-1317.
72. Iams JD. Clinical practice. Prevention of preterm parturition. *N Engl J Med* 2014;370:254-261.
73. Haas DM, Caldwell DM, Kirkpatrick P, et al. Tocolytic therapy for preterm delivery: Systematic review and network meta-analysis. *BMJ* 2012;345:e6226. doi: 10.1136/bmj.e6226.
74. Abramovici A, Cantu J, Jenkins SM. Tocolytic therapy for acute preterm labor. *Obstet Gynecol Clin North Am* 2012;39:77-87.
75. Crowther CA, Brown J, McKinlay CJ, Middleton P. Magnesium sulphate for preventing preterm birth in threatened preterm labour. *Cochrane Database Syst Rev* 2014;8:CD001060.
76. American College of Obstetricians and Gynecologists. ACOG Practice Bulletin No. 139: Premature rupture of membranes. *Obstet Gynecol* 2013;122:918-930.
77. American College of Obstetricians and Gynecologists. ACOG Practice Bulletin No. 120: Use of prophylactic antibiotics in labor and delivery. *Obstet Gynecol* 2011;117:1472-1483.
78. Committee on Practice Bulletins-Obstetrics, The American College of Obstetricians and Gynecologists. Practice bulletin no. 130: Prediction and prevention of preterm birth. *Obstet Gynecol* 2012;120: 964-973.
79. Sullivan SA, Soper D. Antibiotic prophylaxis in obstetrics. *Am J Obstet Gynecol* 2015;212:559-560.
80. Brownfoot FC, Gagliardi DI, Bain E, et al. Different corticosteroids and regimens for accelerating fetal lung maturation for women at risk of preterm birth. *Cochrane Database Syst Rev* 2013;8:CD006764.
81. Crowther CA, McKinlay CJ, Middleton P, Harding JE. Repeat doses of prenatal corticosteroids for women at risk of preterm birth for improving neonatal health outcomes. *Cochrane Database Syst Rev* 2011(6):CD003935.
82. Phares CR, Lynfield R, Farley MM, et al. Epidemiology of invasive group B streptococcal disease in the United States, 1999-2005. *JAMA* 2008;299:2056-2065.
83. Verani JR, McGee L, Schrag SJ, et al. Prevention of perinatal group B streptococcal disease—revised guidelines from CDC, 2010. *MMWR Recomm Rep* 2010;59(RR-10):1-36.
84. Swamy GK. Current methods of labor induction. *Semin Perinatol* 2012;36:348-352.
85. Sanchez-Ramos L. Induction of labor. *Obstet Gynecol Clin North Am* 2005;32:181-200.
86. Committee on Practice Bulletins-Obstetrics. ACOG Practice Bulletin No. 107: Induction of labor. *Obstet Gynecol* 2009;114(2 Pt 1): 386-397.
87. Tenore JL. Methods for cervical ripening and induction of labor. *Am Fam Physician* 2003;67:2123-2128.
88. Hapangama D, Neilson JP. Mifepristone for induction of labour. *Cochrane Database Syst Rev* 2009(3):CD002865.
89. Jones L, Othman M, Dowswell T, et al. Pain management for women in labour: An overview of systematic reviews. *Cochrane Database Syst Rev* 2012;3:CD009234.
90. Arendt KW, Tessmer-Tuck JA. Nonpharmacologic labor analgesia. *Clin Perinatol* 2013;40:351-371.
91. American College of Obstetricians and Gynecologists. Committee Opinion No. 295: Pain relief during labor. 2004, Reaffirmed 2008. Available at: *http://www.acog.org/Resources-And-Publications/Committee-Opinions-List*. (Accessed August 25, 2015.)

92. Anim-Somuah M, Smyth RM, Jones L. Epidural versus non-epidural or no analgesia in labour. *Cochrane Database Syst Rev* 2011(12):CD000331.
93. Heesen M, Bohmer J, Klohr S, et al. The effect of adding a background infusion to patient-controlled epidural labor analgesia on labor, maternal, and neonatal outcomes: A systematic review and meta-analysis. *Anesth Analg* 2015;121:149-158.
94. Mousa HA, Blum J, Abou El Senoun G, et al. Treatment for primary postpartum haemorrhage. *Cochrane Database Syst Rev* 2014;2:CD003249.
95. Weeks A. The prevention and treatment of postpartum haemorrhage: What do we know, and where do we go to next? *BJOG* 2015;122:202-210.
96. Section on Breastfeeding. Breastfeeding and the use of human milk. *Pediatrics* 2012;129:e827-841.
97. Academy of Breastfeeding Medicine Protocol Committeee. ABM Clinical Protocol #9: Use of galactogogues in initiating or augmenting the rate of maternal milk secretion (First Revision January 2011). *Breastfeed Med* 2011;6:41-49.
98. Rowe H, Baker T, Hale TW. Maternal medication, drug use, and breastfeeding. *Child Adolesc Psychiatr Clin N Am* 2015;24:1-20.
99. Sachs HC, Committee On Drugs. The transfer of drugs and therapeutics into human breast milk: An update on selected topics. *Pediatrics* 2013;132:e796-809.
100. Berlin CM Jr, van den Anker JN. Safety during breastfeeding: Drugs, foods, environmental chemicals, and maternal infections. *Semin Fetal Neonatal Med* 2013;18:13-18.
101. Amir LH, Academy of Breastfeeding Medicine Protocol C. ABM clinical protocol #4: Mastitis, revised March 2014. *Breastfeed Med* 2014;9:239-243.
102. Molyneaux E, Howard LM, McGeown HR, et al. Antidepressant treatment for postnatal depression. *Cochrane Database Syst Rev* 2014;9:CD002018.

79

Contraception

Sarah P. Shrader and Kelly R. Ragucci

KEY CONCEPTS

1. The attitude of the patient and sexual partner toward contraceptive methods, efficacy rate, the reliability of the patient in using the method correctly (which may affect the effectiveness of the method), noncontraceptive benefits, and the patient's ability to pay must be considered when selecting a contraceptive method.
2. Patient-specific factors (eg, frequency of intercourse, age, smoking status, and concomitant diseases or medications) must be evaluated when selecting a contraceptive method.
3. Adverse effects or difficulties using the chosen method should be monitored carefully and managed in consideration of patient-specific factors.
4. Accurate and timely counseling on the optimal use of the contraceptive method and strategies for minimizing sexually transmitted diseases (STDs) must be provided to all patients when contraceptives are initiated and on an ongoing basis.
5. Emergency contraception (EC) may prevent pregnancy after unprotected intercourse or when regular contraceptive methods have failed.

Unintended pregnancy is a significant public health problem. In the United States, approximately 6 million females become pregnant each year.[1] The most recent data reveal that 37% of pregnancies are unintended, with the highest rates occurring in women aged 20 to 34 years.[1] However, teen pregnancy rates are still an issue and slow to decline; teen births account for 11% of all the births in the United States.[1] About half of all unintended pregnancies end in abortion, and 40% occur in sexually active couples who claim they used some method of contraception.[1] If the goal of contraception—for pregnancies to be planned and desired—is to be realized, education on the use and efficacy of contraceptive methods must be improved.

ETIOLOGY AND PATHOPHYSIOLOGY

Comprehension of the hormonal regulation of the normal menstrual cycle is essential to understanding contraception in women (Fig. 79-1). The cycle of menstruation begins with menarche, usually around age 12 years, and continues to occur in nonpregnant women until menopause, usually around age 50 years. Factors such as race, body weight, medical conditions, and family history can affect the menstrual cycle.[2,3] The cycle includes the vaginal discharge of sloughed endometrium called *menses*. The menstrual cycle comprises three phases: (1) follicular (or preovulatory), (2) ovulatory, and (3) luteal (or postovulatory).

The Menstrual Cycle

The first day of menses is referred to as *day 1 of the menstrual cycle* and marks the beginning of the follicular phase.[2] The follicular phase continues until ovulation, which typically occurs on day 14. The time after ovulation is referred to as the *luteal phase*, which lasts until the beginning of the next menstrual cycle. The median menstrual cycle length is 28 days, but it can range from 21 to 40 days. Generally, variation in length is greatest in the follicular phase, particularly in the years immediately after menarche and before menopause.[2]

The menstrual cycle is influenced by the hormonal relationships among the hypothalamus, anterior pituitary, and ovaries.[2] The hypothalamus secretes gonadotropin-releasing hormone (GnRH) in a pulsatile fashion.[2] These GnRH bursts stimulate the anterior pituitary to secrete bursts of gonadotropins, follicle-stimulating hormone (FSH), and luteinizing hormone (LH). FSH and LH direct events in the ovarian follicles that result in the production of a fertile ovum.

Follicular Phase

In the first 4 days of the menstrual cycle, FSH levels rise and allow the recruitment of a small group of follicles for continued growth and development (see Fig. 79-1).[2] Between days 5 and 7, one follicle becomes dominant and later ruptures, releasing the oocyte. The dominant follicle develops increasing amounts of estradiol and inhibin, which cause a negative feedback on the hypothalamic secretion of GnRH and pituitary secretion of FSH, causing atresia of the remaining follicles recruited during the cycle.

Once the follicle has received FSH stimulation, it must receive continued FSH stimulation or it will die.[2] FSH allows the follicle to enlarge and synthesize estradiol, progesterone, and androgen. Estradiol stops the menstrual flow from the previous cycle, thickening the endometrial lining of the uterus to prepare it for embryonic implantation. Estrogen is responsible for increased production of thin, watery cervical mucus, which will enhance sperm transport during fertilization. FSH regulates the aromatase enzymes that convert androgens to estrogens in the follicle. If a follicle has insufficient aromatase, the follicle will not survive.

Ovulation

When estradiol levels remain elevated for a sustained period of time, the pituitary releases a midcycle LH surge (see Fig. 79-1).[2] This LH surge stimulates the final stages of follicular maturation and ovulation (follicular rupture and release of the oocyte). On average, ovulation occurs 24 to 36 hours after the estradiol peak and 10 to 16 hours after the LH peak. The LH surge, which occurs 28 to 32 hours before a follicle ruptures, is the most clinically useful predictor of approaching ovulation. After ovulation, the oocyte is released and travels to the fallopian tube, where it can be fertilized and transported to the uterus for embryonic implantation. Conception is most successful when intercourse takes place from 2 days before ovulation to the day of ovulation.

Luteal Phase

After rupture of the follicle and release of the ovum, the remaining luteinized follicles become the corpus luteum, which synthesizes androgen, estrogen, and progesterone (see Fig. 79-1).[2] Progesterone

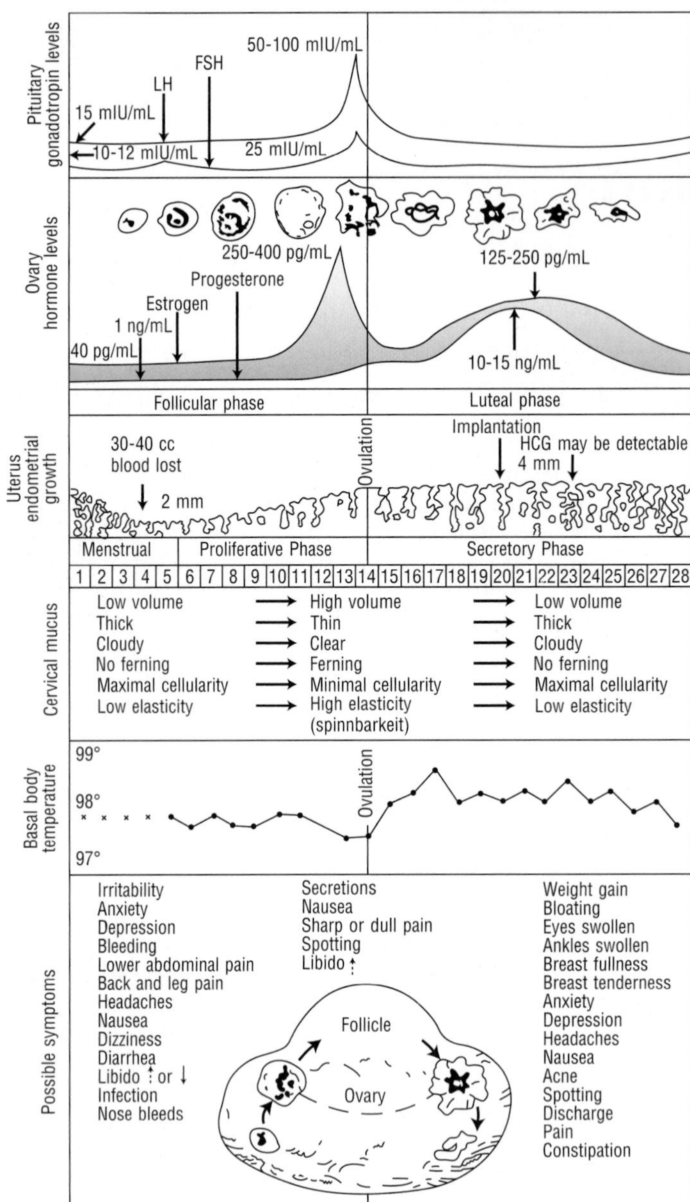

FIGURE 79-1 Menstrual cycle events, idealized 28-day cycle. (FSH, follicle-stimulating hormone; HCG, human chorionic gonadotropin, LH, luteinizing hormone.)

LH: 15 mIU/mL = 15 IU/L; 50-100 mIU/mL = 50-100 IU/L.

FSH: 10-12 mIU/mL = 10-12 IU/L; 25 mIU/mL = 25 IU/L.

Estrogen: 40 pg/mL = ~150 pmol/L; 250-400 pg/mL = ~920-1,470 pmol/L; 125-250 pg/mL = ~460-920 pmol/L.

Progesterone: 1 ng/mL = 3 nmol/L; 10-15 ng/mL = ~30-50 nmol/L.

Temperatures: 99°F = 37.2°C; 98°F = 36.7°C; 97°F = 36.1°C.

(From Hatcher et al.[2] This figure may be reproduced at no cost to the reader.)

helps to maintain the endometrial lining, which sustains the implanted embryo and maintains the pregnancy. It also inhibits GnRH and gonadotropin release, preventing the development of new follicles. If pregnancy occurs, human chorionic gonadotropin prevents regression of the corpus luteum and stimulates continued production of estrogen and progesterone secretion to maintain the pregnancy until the placenta is able to fulfill this role.

If fertilization or implantation does not occur, the corpus luteum degenerates, and progesterone production declines.[2] The life span of the corpus luteum depends on the continuous presence of small amounts of LH, and its average duration of function is 9 to 11 days. As progesterone levels decline, endometrial shedding (menstruation) occurs, and a new menstrual cycle begins. At the end of the luteal phase, when estrogen and progesterone levels are low, FSH levels start to rise, and follicular recruitment for the next cycle begins.

EPIDEMIOLOGY

Contraception implies the prevention of pregnancy following sexual intercourse by inhibiting viable sperm from coming into contact with a mature ovum (ie, methods that act as barriers or prevent ovulation) or by preventing a fertilized ovum from implanting successfully in the endometrium (ie, mechanisms that create an unfavorable uterine environment). These methods differ in their relative effectiveness, safety, and patient acceptability (Tables 79-1 and 79-2).[2,3]

TABLE 79-1 Pregnancy and Continuation Rates for Various Pharmacologic Contraceptive Methods

Method	Pregnancy Typical Use (%)	Pregnancy Ideal Use (%)	Continuation After 1 Year (%)
Combined oral contraceptive	9	<1	71
Combined hormonal transdermal contraceptive patch	9	<1	—
Combined hormonal vaginal contraceptive ring	9	<1	—
Depot medroxyprogesterone acetate	6	<1	70
Copper IUD	<1	<1	78
Levonorgestrel IUD	<1	<1	80
Progestin-only implant	<1	<1	88

Data from references 2 and 3.

The actual effectiveness of any contraceptive method is difficult to determine because many factors affect contraceptive failure. A failure in patients who use the contraceptive agent properly is considered a method failure or perfect-use failure. It is also important to consider user failure or typical-use failure rates, which are usually higher because they take into account the user's ability to follow directions correctly and consistently.[2,3]

CLINICAL PRESENTATION

Most health maintenance annual visits should include assessment of and counseling about reproductive health. Clinicians may use this opportunity to provide contraception and educate patients on prevention of sexually transmitted diseases (STDs). Traditionally, hormonal contraception is provided subsequent to breast and pelvic

TABLE 79-2 Comparison of Methods of Nonhormonal Contraception

Method	Absolute Contraindications	Advantages	Disadvantages	Percent of Women with Pregnancy[a]: Perfect Use	Percent of Women with Pregnancy[a]: Typical Use
Condoms, male	Allergy to latex or rubber	Inexpensive STD protection, including HIV (latex only)	High user failure rate Poor acceptance Possibility of breakage Efficacy decreased by oil-based lubricants Possible allergic reactions to latex in either partner	2	18
Condoms, female	Allergy to polyurethane History of TSS	Can be inserted just before intercourse or ahead of time STD protection, including HIV	High user failure rate Dislike ring hanging outside vagina Cumbersome	5	21
Diaphragm with spermicide	Allergy to latex, rubber, or spermicide Recurrent UTIs History of TSS Abnormal gynecologic anatomy	Low cost Decreased incidence of cervical neoplasia Some protection against STDs	High user failure rate Decreased efficacy with increased frequency of intercourse Increased incidence of vaginal yeast UTIs, TSS Efficacy decreased by oil-based lubricants Cervical irritation	6	12
Cervical cap (FemCap)	Allergy to spermicide History of TSS Abnormal gynecologic anatomy Abnormal papanicolaou smear	Low cost Latex-free Some protection against STDs FemCap reusable for up to 2 years	High user failure rate Decreased efficacy with parity Cannot be used during menses	9	16[b]
Spermicides alone	Allergy to spermicide	Inexpensive	High user failure rate Must be reapplied before each act of intercourse May enhance HIV transmission No protection against STDs	18	28
Sponge (Today)	Allergy to spermicide Recurrent UTIs History of TSS Abnormal gynecologic anatomy	Inexpensive	High user failure rate Decreased efficacy with parity Cannot be used during menses No protection against STDs	9[c]	12[d]

HIV, human immunodeficiency virus; STD, sexually transmitted disease; TSS, toxic shock syndrome; UTI, urinary tract infection.

[a]Failure rates in the United States during first year of use.

[b]Failure rate with FemCap reported to be 24% per package insert.

[c]Failure rate with Today sponge reported to be 20% in parous women.

[d]Failure rate with Today sponge reported to be 32% in parous women.

Data from reference 2.

examinations. However, the need for the physical examination may delay access to contraception and reinforces the incorrect perception that these methods of contraceptives are harmful. Therefore, the American Congress of Obstetrics and Gynecology (ACOG) allow provision of hormonal contraception after a simple medical history and blood pressure measurement.[4] Other preventive measures, such as pelvic and breast examinations, provision of the human papillomavirus vaccine, and screening for cervical neoplasia, can be accomplished during routine annual office visits.

TREATMENT

Desired Outcomes

The obvious goal of treatment with all methods of contraception is to prevent pregnancy. However, many health benefits are associated with contraceptive methods, including prevention of STDs (with condoms), improvements in menstrual cycle regularity (with hormonal contraceptives), improvements in certain health conditions (with hormonal contraceptives), and management of perimenopause.[2,5]

Nonpharmacologic Therapy

Periodic Abstinence

1 2 Motivated couples may use the abstinence (rhythm) method of contraception, avoiding sexual intercourse during the days of the menstrual cycle when conception is likely to occur. Physiologic changes, such as basal body temperature and cervical mucus, are used during each cycle to determine the fertile period. The major drawbacks are the relatively high pregnancy rates and avoidance of intercourse for several days during each menstrual cycle.[2]

Barrier Techniques

1 2 The effectiveness of barrier methods depends almost exclusively on motivation to use them consistently and correctly.[2] These methods include condoms, diaphragms, cervical caps, and sponges (see Table 79-2). A major disadvantage is higher failure rates than most hormonal contraceptives; thus, provision of counseling and an advanced prescription for emergency contraception (EC) are recommended for all patients using barrier methods as their primary means of contraception.

Male condoms create a mechanical barrier, preventing direct contact of the vagina with semen, genital lesions, and infectious secretions.[2] Most condoms in the United States are made of latex, which is impermeable to viruses. A small proportion are made from lamb intestine, which is not impermeable to viruses. Synthetic condoms manufactured from polyurethane are another option; these condoms are latex-free and do protect against viruses. Condoms are used worldwide as protection from STDs including human immunodeficiency virus (HIV). When condoms are used in conjunction with any other barrier method, their effectiveness theoretically approaches 98%. Spillage of semen or perforation and tearing of the condom can occur, but proper use minimizes these problems. Mineral oil-based vaginal drug formulations (eg, Cleocin, Premarin, and Monistat), lotions, or lubricants can decrease the barrier strength of latex, thus making water-soluble lubricants (eg, Astroglide and K-Y Jelly) preferable. Condoms with spermicides are no longer recommended because they provide no additional protection against pregnancy or STDs and may increase vulnerability to HIV.[2,6,7]

The female condom is a prelubricated, loose-fitting polyurethane sheath, closed at one end, with flexible rings at both ends.[2] Properly positioned, the ring at the closed end covers the cervix, and the sheath lines the walls of the vagina. The outer ring remains outside the vagina, covering the labia. The pregnancy rate is reported to be higher when compared to male condoms. Male and female condoms should not be used together, as slippage and device displacement may occur.

The diaphragm, a reusable dome-shaped rubber cap with a flexible rim that is inserted vaginally, fits over the cervix in order to decrease access of sperm to the ovum. The diaphragm requires a prescription from a clinician who has fitted the patient for the correct size.[2] Its efficacy is increased when it is used in conjunction with spermicidal cream or jelly. The diaphragm may be inserted up to 6 hours before intercourse and must be left in place for at least 6 hours afterward. However, leaving it in place for more than 24 hours is not recommended due to the potential for toxic shock syndrome (TSS). With subsequent acts of intercourse, the diaphragm should be left in place, and a condom should be used for additional protection.

The cervical cap (FemCap) is a soft, deep cup with a firm round rim that is smaller than a diaphragm and fits over the cervix like a thimble.[2] The cervical cap is available in three sizes and requires a prescription from a clinician who has fitted the patient for the correct size. It should be filled with spermicide prior to insertion. The cervical cap can be inserted 6 hours prior to intercourse and should not be removed for at least 6 hours after intercourse. It can remain in place for multiple episodes of intercourse without adding more spermicide but should not be worn for more than 48 hours at a time to reduce the risk of TSS. Failure rates are higher than with other methods. Diaphragms and cervical caps do not protect against some STDs including HIV, thus condoms should also be used.

Pharmacologic Therapy

Spermicides

1 2 Spermicides, most of which contain nonoxynol-9, are chemical surfactants that destroy sperm cell walls and act as barriers that prevent sperm from entering the cervical os.[2] They are available as creams, films, foams, gels, suppositories, sponges, and tablets. Spermicides offer no protection against STDs. In fact, when used frequently (more than two times per day), nonoxynol-9 may increase the risk of transmission of HIV by causing small disruptions in the vaginal epithelium.[2,6,7] The World Health Organization (WHO) and the Centers for Disease Control and Prevention (CDC) do not promote products containing nonoxynol-9 for protection against STDs.

Spermicide-Implanted Barrier Techniques

1 2 The vaginal contraceptive sponge (Today) contains 1 g of the spermicide nonoxynol-9.[2] It has a concave dimple on one side to fit over the cervix and a loop on the other side to facilitate removal. After being moistened with water, the sponge is inserted into the vagina up to 6 hours before intercourse. The sponge provides protection for 24 hours, regardless of the frequency of intercourse during this time. After intercourse, the sponge must be left in place for at least 6 hours before removal and should not be left in place for more than 24 to 30 hours to reduce the risk of TSS. Sponges should not be reused; after removal, they should be discarded. The sponge comes in one size and is available over the counter (OTC).

Hormonal Contraception

Hormonal contraceptives contain a combination of estrogen and progestin or a progestin alone. Oral contraceptive (OC) preparations first became available in the 1960s, but options have expanded to include a transdermal patch, a vaginal contraceptive ring, and long-acting injectable, implantable, and intrauterine contraceptives.

Combined hormonal contraceptives (CHCs) contain both estrogen and progestin and work primarily before fertilization to prevent conception. Progestins provide most of the contraceptive effect by thickening cervical mucus to prevent sperm penetration, slowing tubal motility, delaying sperm transport, and inducing endometrial atrophy. Progestins block the LH surge, therefore inhibiting ovulation. Estrogens suppress FSH release from the pituitary, which may contribute to blocking the LH surge and preventing ovulation. However, the primary role of estrogen in hormonal contraceptives is to stabilize the endometrial lining and provide cycle control.[2,3]

Estrogens Three synthetic estrogens found in hormonal contraceptives available in the United States are ethinyl estradiol (EE), mestranol, and estradiol valerate. Mestranol must be converted by the liver to EE before it is pharmacologically active and is 50% less potent than EE.[2,3] Most combined OCs, transdermal patch, and vaginal ring contain estrogen at doses of 20 to 50 mcg of EE.[3]

Progestins A variety of progestins are available in the United States, and they vary in their progestational activity and differ with respect to inherent estrogenic, antiestrogenic, and androgenic effects.[2,3] Estrogenic and antiestrogenic properties are secondary to the extent of progestins' metabolism to estrogenic substances. Androgenic activity depends on two variables: the presence of sex hormone (testosterone) binding globulin (SHBG-TBG) and the androgen-to-progesterone activity ratio. If the amount of SHBG-TBG is decreased, free testosterone levels increase, and androgenic side effects are more prominent.[3]

Considerations with Combined Hormonal Contraceptive Use

1 When selecting a CHC, clinicians are challenged by weighing the benefits and risks associated with the many formulations available. The clinician must determine if the form of contraception is appropriate based upon the patient's lifestyle and potential adherence. A complete medical examination and papanicolaou (Pap) smear are not necessary before a CHC is prescribed. A medical history and blood pressure measurement should be obtained before prescribing a CHC, along with a discussion of the benefits, risks, and adverse effects with each patient.[2,3,8,9] For example, OCs are associated with noncontraceptive benefits, including relief from menstruation-related problems (eg, decreased menstrual cramps, decreased ovulatory pain [mittelschmerz], and decreased menstrual blood loss), improvement in menstrual regularity, and decreased iron deficiency anemia.[5] Women who take combination OCs have a reduced risk of ovarian and endometrial cancer. There is a 50% reduction in risk in women who have used OCs for 5 years or more, and protection may persist for more than 10 years post-use. Combination OCs may also reduce the risk of ovarian cysts, ectopic pregnancy, pelvic inflammatory disease, endometriosis, uterine fibroids, and benign breast disease. The CHC transdermal patch and vaginal ring are other combined hormonal options that may be more convenient for women than taking a tablet each day.

2 3 Adverse effects may hinder adherence and therefore efficacy, so they should be discussed prior to initiating a hormonal contraceptive agent.[9] Excessive or deficient amounts of estrogen and progestin are related to the most common adverse effects.[2,3,9] An important concern regarding the use of CHCs is the lack of protection against STDs. Because of their high efficacy in preventing pregnancy, patients may choose not to use condoms. In addition to public health awareness, clinicians must encourage patients to use condoms for prevention of STDs. OCs have an extensive history of safety concerns, which traditionally were related to high dose estrogen tablets. Overall, the health risks associated with pregnancy, the specific health risks associated with CHCs, and the noncontraceptive benefits of CHCs should be factored into risk-to-benefit considerations. To replace the traditional absolute and relative contraindications to the use of OCs, the CDC developed a graded list of precautions for clinicians to consider when initiating CHCs (Table 79-3).[8,21]

Women Older Than 35 Years Use of CHC in women older than 35 is controversial. Older women, especially women in their 40s, retain a level of fertility even in the perimenopausal state and can use hormonal contraception to prevent pregnancy. Formulations with lower doses of estrogen (less than 30 mcg) have increased the use of CHCs in these women. In addition to the benefit of pregnancy prevention, they may improve or decrease the chance of developing perimenopausal and menopausal symptoms and increase bone mineral density (BMD). However, the benefits of using CHCs must be weighed against the risks in women older than 35. The increased risk of venous thromboembolism (VTE) should be considered especially in perimenopausal women older than 40. Older data suggest an increased risk of myocardial infarction (MI) in older women using CHCs, although many women in these studies were current smokers and used older formulations containing higher doses (greater than 50 mcg) of estrogen. More recent data do not support the increased risk of cardiovascular disease when low-dose formulations of CHCs are used in healthy, nonobese women. Other concerns include the increased risk of ischemic stroke in women with migraines and the increased risk of breast cancer in older women.[3,8]

The risks and benefits of using CHCs in women greater than 35 must be considered on an individual basis. It is recommended that use of CHCs (with less than 50 mcg of estrogen) may be considered in healthy nonsmoking women. CHCs should not be recommended in women older than 35 years with migraine (with or without aura), uncontrolled hypertension, smoking, or diabetes with vascular disease.[3,8]

Smoking In early studies, OCs with 50 mcg EE or more were associated with MI in women who smoked cigarettes.[2,3] The United States case-control studies have found that both nonsmoking and smoking women, regardless of age, taking OCs with less than 50 mcg EE did not have an increased risk of MI or stroke. However, these studies included few women older than 35 years who were smokers. European studies, with a higher population of older smoking women, demonstrated an increased risk of MI in this population. Therefore, practitioners should prescribe CHC with caution, if at all, to women older than 35 years who smoke. Smoking 15 or more cigarettes per day by women in this age group is a contraindication to CHC, and the risks generally outweigh the benefits of CHC in those who smoke fewer than 15 cigarettes per day.[8] Progestin-only contraceptive methods should be considered for women in this group.

Hypertension CHCs can cause small increases (ie, 6-8 mm Hg) in blood pressure, regardless of estrogen dosage.[3,8] This has been documented in both normotensive and mildly hypertensive women given a 30 mcg EE OC. In case-control studies of women with hypertension, OCs have been associated with an increased risk of MI and stroke. Use of low-dose CHC is acceptable in women younger than 35 years with well-controlled and frequently monitored hypertension. If a CHC-related increase in blood pressure occurs, discontinuing the CHC usually restores blood pressure to pretreatment values within 3 to 6 months.[3] Systolic blood pressure greater than or equal to 160 mm Hg or diastolic blood pressure greater than or equal to 100 mm Hg is considered a contraindication to the use of CHCs. Hypertensive women who have a systolic blood pressure 140 to 159 or diastolic blood pressure 90 to 99 mm Hg should also avoid CHCs as the risks generally outweigh the benefits. Women with hypertension who are taking potassium-sparing diuretics, angiotensin-converting enzyme inhibitors, angiotensin-receptor blockers, or aldosterone antagonists may have increased serum potassium concentrations if they are also using an OC-containing drospirenone, which has antialdosterone properties.[3]

Dyslipidemia Generally, synthetic progestins adversely affect lipid metabolism by decreasing high-density lipoprotein (HDL) and increasing low-density lipoprotein (LDL).[3,8] Estrogens tend to have more beneficial effects by enhancing removal of LDL and increasing HDL levels. Estrogens may moderately increase triglycerides. As a net result, most low-dose CHCs have no significant impact on HDL, LDL, triglycerides, or total cholesterol. CHCs containing

TABLE 79-3 US Medical Eligibility Criteria for Contraceptive Use: Classifications for Combined Hormonal Contraceptives

Category 4: Unacceptable health risk (method not to be used)
- Breastfeeding or nonbreastfeeding <21 days postpartum
- Current breast cancer
- Severe (decompensated) cirrhosis
- History/risk of or current deep venous thrombosis/pulmonary embolism (not on anticoagulant therapy); thrombogenic mutations
- Major surgery with prolonged immobilization
- Migraines with aura, any age
- Systolic blood pressure ≥160 mm Hg or diastolic ≥100 mm Hg
- Hypertension with vascular disease
- Current and history of ischemic heart disease
- Benign hepatocellular adenoma or malignant liver tumor
- Moderately or severely impaired cardiac function; normal or mildly impaired cardiac function <6 months
- Smoking ≥15 cigarettes per day and age ≥35
- Complicated solid organ transplantation
- History of cerebrovascular accident
- SLE; positive or unknown antiphospholipid antibodies
- Complicated valvular heart disease

Category 3: Theoretical or proven risks usually outweigh the advantages
- Breastfeeding 21-30 days postpartum with or without risk factors for VTE
- Nonbreastfeeding 21-42 days postpartum with other risk factors for VTE
- Past breast cancer and no evidence of disease for 5 years
- History of DVT/PE (not on anticoagulant therapy or established on anticoagulant therapy for at least 3 months), but lower risk for recurrent DVT/PE
- Current gallbladder disease, symptomatic and medically treated
- Migraines without aura, age ≥35 (*category 4 with continued use*)
- History of bariatric surgery; malabsorptive procedures
- History of cholestasis, past COC-related
- Hypertension; systolic blood pressure 140-159 mm Hg or diastolic 90-99 mm Hg
- Normal or mildly impaired cardiac function ≥6 months
- Postpartum 21-42 days with other risk factors for VTE
- Smoking <15 cigarettes per day and age ≥35
- Use of ritonavir-boosted protease inhibitors
- Use of certain anticonvulsants (phenytoin, carbamazepine, barbiturates, primidone, topiramate, oxcarbazepine, and lamotrigine)
- Use of rifampicin or rifabutin therapy
- Diabetes with vascular disease or >20 years duration (*possibly category 4 depending upon severity*)
- Multiple risk factors for arterial cardiovascular disease (older age, smoking, diabetes, and hypertension) (*possibly category 4 depending on category and severity*)

Category 2: Advantages generally outweigh theoretical or proven risks
- Age ≥40 (in the absence of other comorbid conditions that increase CVD risk)
- Sickle-cell disease
- Undiagnosed breast mass
- Cervical cancer and awaiting treatment; cervical intraepithelial neoplasia
- Family history (first-degree relatives) of DVT/PE
- Major surgery without prolonged immobilization
- Diabetes mellitus (type 1 or type 2), nonvascular disease
- Gallbladder disease; symptomatic and treated by cholecystectomy or asymptomatic
- Migraines without aura, age <35 (*category 3 with continued use*)
- History of pregnancy-related cholestasis
- History of high blood pressure during pregnancy
- Benign liver tumors; focal nodular hyperplasia
- Obesity
- Breastfeeding 30 days or more postpartum
- Postpartum 21-42 days without other risk factors
- Nonbreastfeeding 21-42 days postpartum without risk factors for VTE
- Rheumatoid arthritis on or off immunosuppressive therapy
- Smoking and <35 years old
- Uncomplicated sold organ transplantation
- Superficial thrombophlebitis
- Stable SLE without antiphospholipid antibodies
- Unexplained vaginal bleeding before evaluation
- Uncomplicated valvular heart disease
- Use of nonnucleoside reverse transcriptase inhibitors
- Hyperlipidemia (*possibly category 3 based upon type, severity, and other risk factors*)
- Inflammatory bowel disease (*possibly category 3 for those with increased risk of VTE*)

Category 1: No restriction (method can be used)
- Thalassemia, iron deficiency anemia
- Mild compensated cirrhosis
- Benign ovarian tumors
- Benign breast disease or family history of cancer
- Family history of cancer
- Schistosomiasis
- Viral hepatitis (carrier/chronic)
- Minor surgery without immobilization
- Depression
- Gestational diabetes mellitus
- Endometrial cancer/hyperplasia, endometriosis
- Epilepsy
- Gestational trophoblastic disease
- Nonmigrainous headaches (category 2 for continued use)
- History of bariatric surgery; restrictive procedures
- History of pelvic surgery
- HIV infected or high risk
- Malaria
- Ovarian cancer
- Past ectopic pregnancy
- PID
- Postabortion
- More than 42 days postpartum
- Severe dysmenorrhea
- Sexually transmitted infections
- Varicose veins
- Thyroid disorders
- Tuberculosis
- Uterine fibroids
- Use of nucleoside reverse transcriptase inhibitors
- Use of broad-spectrum antibiotics, antifungals, and antiparasitics

CHC, combined hormonal contraception; HIV, human immunodeficiency virus; VTE, venous thromboembolism; PE, pulmonary embolism; CVD, cardiovascular disease; PID, pelvic inflammatory disease.

Data from references 8 and 21.

more androgenic progestins (eg, levonorgestrel) may result in lower HDL levels in some patients. Although the lipid effects of CHCs theoretically can influence cardiovascular risk, the mechanism of increased cardiovascular disease in CHC users is believed to be due to thromboembolic and thrombotic changes, not atherosclerosis. Women with controlled dyslipidemia can use low-dose CHCs, although periodic fasting lipid profiles are recommended. Women with uncontrolled dyslipidemia (LDL greater than 160 mg/dL [4.14 mmol/L], HDL less than 35 mg/dL [0.91 mmol/L], triglycerides greater than 250 mg/dL [2.83 mmol/L]) and additional risk factors (eg, coronary artery disease, diabetes, hypertension, smoking, or positive family history) should consider an alternative method of contraception.

Diabetes Any effect of CHCs on carbohydrate metabolism is thought to be due to the progestin component.[3,8] However, with the exception of some levonorgestrel-containing products, formulations containing low doses of progestins do not significantly alter insulin, glucose, or glucagon release after a glucose load in healthy women or in those with a history of gestational diabetes. The new progestins are believed to have little, if any, effect on carbohydrate metabolism. CHCs do not appear to alter the hemoglobin A_{1C} values or accelerate the development of microvascular complications in women with diabetes. Therefore, nonsmoking women younger than 35 years with diabetes but no associated vascular disease can safely use CHCs. Diabetic women with vascular disease (eg, nephropathy, retinopathy, neuropathy, or other vascular disease) or diabetes of more than 20 years' duration should not use CHCs.[3,8]

Migraine Headaches Women with migraine headaches may experience a decreased or an increased frequency of migraine headaches when using CHCs.[3,8,10] Studies have demonstrated a higher risk of stroke in women experiencing migraine with aura compared to women with simple migraine. In population-based studies, the risk of stroke in women with migraines has been elevated twofold to threefold. However, given the low absolute risk of stroke in young women (age less than 35 years), CHCs in healthy, nonsmoking women with migraine headaches without aura may still be considered.[8] Likewise, women with nonmigrainous headaches may also use CHCs without restriction. Women of any age who have migraine with aura and women over the age of 35 with any type of migraine should not use CHC.[8] Women who develop migraines (with or without aura) while receiving CHC should discontinue use and consider a progestin-only option.

Breast Cancer Worldwide epidemiologic data from 54 studies in 25 countries (many of which studied high dose OCs) were collected to assess the relationship between OCs and breast cancer.[3] Overall, investigators noted a small increase in the relative risk of having breast cancer diagnosed while combined OCs are taken and for up to 10 years following discontinuance. There is no increased excess risk of diagnosis 10 years or more after OCs are discontinued. Cancers diagnosed in women who used combined OCs were less advanced clinically than cancers diagnosed in women who had not used OCs. Breast cancers diagnosed in ever-users were less clinically advanced than those diagnosed in never-users for up to 20 years after discontinuing OCs. Although some studies have found differences in risk of breast cancer based on the presence of *BRCA1* and *BRCA2* mutations, the most recent cohort study found no association with low-dose OCs and the presence of either mutation. The choice to use CHCs should not be affected by the presence of benign breast disease or a family history of breast cancer with either mutation. Women with current or past history of breast cancer should not use CHCs.[2,3,8]

Thromboembolism Estrogens increase hepatic production of factor VII, factor X, and fibrinogen in the coagulation cascade, therefore increasing the risk of thromboembolic events (eg, deep vein thrombosis and pulmonary embolism). These risks are increased in women who have underlying hypercoagulable states (eg, deficiencies in antithrombin III, protein C, and protein S; factor V Leiden mutations, prothrombin G2010 A mutations) or who have acquired conditions (eg, obesity, pregnancy, immobility, trauma, surgery, and certain malignancies) that predispose them to coagulation abnormalities.[3,8] The incidence of thromboembolism and mortality is increased threefold in current OC users compared to nonusers. However, this risk is still less than the risk of VTE incurred during pregnancy. OCs containing newer progestins, such as drospirenone, desogestrel, and norgestimate, are associated with a slightly increased risk of thrombosis.[2,3] Although the mechanism for this increased risk is unclear, it is thought that third- and fourth-generation progestins may have a greater effect on the procoagulant, anticoagulant, and fibrinolytic pathways.[2,11,12] These progestins may also be associated with increased resistance to protein C and may increase levels of sex hormone-binding globulin.[2,11,12] It is thought that continuous, higher exposure to estrogen seen with the transdermal patch or vaginal ring is the reason for an increased thromboembolic risk with these agents as well.[11] An advisory committee to the FDA decided to change the product labeling of the transdermal patch as well as products containing drospirenone to include additional information about the increased risk of thromboembolism.[13,14] In addition, the vaginal ring also has an additional precaution in the product labeling.[15] Therefore, for women who are at an increased risk of thromboembolism (eg, older than 35 years, obesity, smoking, personal or family history of venous thrombosis, prolonged immobilization), it would be prudent to first consider low-dose oral estrogen contraceptives containing older progestins or progestin-only contraceptive methods.

Clinical **Controversy...**

Weighing the risk versus benefit of using CHCs containing third- and fourth-generation progestins, transdermal patch, and vaginal ring to determine their place in therapy is controversial. Third-generation progestins (eg, desogestrel and norgestimate) and a fourth-generation progestin (eg, drospirenone) have been associated with a higher risk of thromboembolism. Mechanisms underlying this increased risk may include: (a) a greater effect on the procoagulant, anticoagulant, and fibrinolytic pathways than earlier generation progestins; (b) increased resistance to the anticoagulant effect of activated protein C; (c) increased levels of sex hormone-binding globulin; and (d) antiandrogenic effects of drospirenone make the CHC more estrogenic. The overall risk of VTE with older low-dose agents is 6 per 10,000 women per year (compared with 2-3 per 10,000 in nonusers). The risk increases to 10 to 15 per 10,000 women per year with drospirenone-containing OCs. Risk of VTE is also higher with the transdermal patch (10-15 per 10,000 women per year) and possibly with the vaginal ring (8 per 10,000 women per year). It is thought that continuous, higher exposure to estrogen seen with these formulations may be the cause of this increased risk. It is important to remember that regardless of contraceptive product, the risk is still lower than the risk of thromboembolism during pregnancy (17 per 10,000 women per year).

Obesity The prevalence of obesity continues to rise each year among all age groups including women of childbearing age. It has been hypothesized that women with increased body weight have increased basal metabolic rates and induction of hepatic enzymes, leading to increased hormonal clearance and decreased serum concentrations of hormonal contraceptives. In addition, women who are obese have more adipose tissue, increasing hormonal sequestration, and decreased free hormone serum concentrations resulting in lower efficacy.[2,3] It is estimated that there is an additional two to four pregnancies per 100 woman-years of use in overweight or obese users.[16,17] This decreased efficacy may be a particular issue with the low-dose OCs. In addition, the transdermal contraceptive patch should not be used as a first-line option in women weighing greater than 90 kg.[14] Increased pregnancy rates have not been demonstrated in obese women using depot medroxyprogesterone acetate (DMPA) or the levonorgestrel intrauterine device (IUD). It is important to note that the CDC recommends that the benefit outweighs the potential risk of decreased efficacy in obese women.[8]

Obese women are also at risk of VTE, although studies evaluating the incidence of thromboembolism in obese women taking hormonal contraceptives have produced conflicting results. With low-dose estrogen containing products, the incidence increases from 5 to 10 cases in nonusers to 15 to 30 cases in users per 10,000 women per year. At baseline, obesity doubles the risk of thromboembolism compared to someone with a normal body mass index (BMI). ACOG suggests that progestin-only hormonal contraception may be more appropriate for obese women over the age of 35 years, and women should be counseled on the risk and consider alternative contraceptive methods on an individual basis.[17] Again, it should be noted that the risk of thromboembolism during pregnancy and in the peripartum period is significantly greater than the risk with any hormonal contraceptive agent.

Systemic Lupus Erythematosus Contraception is important in women with systemic lupus erythematosus (SLE), because the risks associated with pregnancy are high in this population. Historically, clinicians have thought that CHCs exacerbated the symptoms of SLE. It is postulated that estrogen may cause cutaneous lupus to progress to systemic lupus by promoting B-cell hyper-responsiveness and inducing or increasing autoimmunity.[3] Trials have shown that OCs with less than 50 mcg ethinyl estradiol do not increase the risk of flare among women with stable SLE and without antiphospholipid/anticardiolipin antibodies. Because 25% of women with SLE who become pregnant choose to terminate the pregnancy, effective contraception is essential for these patients. CHCs should be avoided in women with SLE and antiphospholipid antibodies or vascular complications. Progestin-only contraceptives can be used in this situation.[8]

Oral Contraceptives 1 2 With perfect-use OCs have a 99% efficacy rate, but with typical-use up to 8% of users may become pregnant (see Table 79-1).[2,3] The OCs currently available are modifications of the original products introduced in the 1960s and contain significantly less estrogen and progestin. High-dose formulations were associated with vascular and embolic events, cancers, and significant side effects, but reductions in hormone doses have been associated with fewer complications.

Monophasic OCs contain the same amounts of estrogen and progestin for 21 days, followed by 7-day placebo phase. Multiphasic pills contain variable amounts of estrogen and progestin for 21 days, also followed by a 7-day placebo phase. There are no published data demonstrating increased safety or efficacy with the multiphasic tablets compared to monophasic tablets.[2,18,19] Extended-cycle tablets and continuous combination regimens may offer some benefits for patients in terms of side effects and convenience. With combination OCs, the types and doses of estrogen and progestin remain constant during the 21 to 24 days that active tablets are taken, though the doses and ratios of estrogens and progestins vary from one preparation to another. The inclusion of 3 additional days of active pills to shorten the pill-free interval has been shown to reduce hormone fluctuation between menstrual cycles. With extended use of OCs, active combination tablets are taken continuously for 84 days or longer followed by 7 days of inactive pills or estrogen only pills.[3] The claimed advantage of extended cycle regimens is that patients have fewer total menstrual cycles per year, which may be helpful in those with severe premenstrual syndrome. No significant differences have been found with regard to bleeding and spotting in those with extended use.[3] Table 79-4 lists available OC products by brand name and specifies hormonal composition.[20] Progestin-only "minipills" (28 days of active hormone per cycle) are also available options. Progestin-only OCs are less effective than combination OCs and are associated with irregular and unpredictable menstrual bleeding.[2,3] Minipills must be taken every day of the menstrual cycle at approximately the same time to maintain contraceptive efficacy. If a progestin-only OC is taken more than 3 hours late, patients should use a backup method of contraception for 48 hours.[3] Minipills may not block ovulation (nearly 40% of women continue to ovulate normally), so the risk of ectopic pregnancy is higher with their use than with other hormonal contraceptives.

Initiating an Oral Contraceptive 4 OCs may be initiated by several different methods, including on the first day of bleeding during the menstrual cycle, on the first Sunday after the menstrual cycle begins or on the fifth day after the menstrual cycle begins. The most popular "Sunday start" method is to begin pills on the first Sunday after the menstrual cycle begins, as this may provide for weekends free of menstrual periods.[2,3,9] Women should be instructed to use a second method of contraception (typically recommend condoms) for at least 7 days after initiation for maximum effectiveness. It may be preferable to have women use additional contraception for the entire first cycle, due to user failure in the first month. In the "quick start" method for initiating OCs, the patient takes the first tablet on the day of her office visit. Women should be instructed to use a second method of contraception for at least 7 days and informed that the menstrual period will be delayed until completion of the active tablets in the current OC pack. This method has been shown to be more successful in getting women to start OCs and to continue using OCs through the third cycle of use.

Postpartum Use of CHCs In the postpartum phase, there is concern about use of CHCs because of the mother's hypercoagulability and the effects on lactation. In the first 21 days postpartum (when the risk of thrombosis is higher), estrogen-containing hormonal contraceptives should be avoided (see Table 79-3).[8,21] If contraception is required during this period, progestin-only contraceptive methods may be acceptable alternatives. It is recommended that women who are breastfeeding avoid CHCs for the first 42 days postpartum in those with risk factors for VTE and for 30 days in those without risk factors. In those women who are not breastfeeding, CHCs should be avoided for up to 42 days postpartum in those with risk factors for VTE.[21] After 42 days postpartum, there is no restriction to the use of CHCs.

Choice of Oral Contraceptive 1 2 Because all combined OCs are similarly effective in preventing pregnancy (see Table 79-1), the initial choice is based on the hormonal content and dose, preferred formulation, and coexisting medical conditions (see Table 79-3).[3,8,20] In women without coexisting medical conditions, an OC containing 35 mcg or less of EE and less than 0.5 mg of norethindrone or an equivalent is recommended (see Table 79-4).[3] This strategy is based on evidence that complications and side effects from CHC (ie, VTE, stroke, or MI) result from excessive hormonal content. Adolescents, underweight women (less than 50 kg [110 lb]), women older than 35 years, and those who are perimenopausal may have fewer side effects with OCs containing 20 to 25 mcg of EE.[3] With nonadherence to OCs, the risk of pregnancy may be greater in women taking OCs containing less than 35 mcg of EE. Women with oily skin, acne, or hirsutism should be given low androgenic OCs.[3] Choice of agent based upon coexisting medical conditions have been previously addressed (see Table 79-3).[8,21]

It may be easier to identify/manage side effects and easier to manipulate to alter the timing of the menstrual cycle in patients taking monophasic OCs. They are preferred over multiphasic OCs upon initiation.[2,3] Extended-cycle OCs either eliminate or reduce the number of menstrual cycles per year, leading to less premenstrual symptoms and dysmenorrhea. Commercially available extended-cycle OCs are available, or monophasic 28 day OCs can be cycled by skipping the 7-day placebo phase. With continued use of extended-cycle OCs for 1 year, no significant changes in adverse effects have been noted. However, long-term studies have not been performed to assess the risk of cancer, VTE, or changes in fertility. Continuous combination regimens provide a shortened pill-free interval, from the traditional 7 days to 2 to 4 days. These various extended-cycle regimens may be beneficial for women with symptoms such as dysmenorrhea, severe premenstrual syndrome, or menstrual migraines.

Managing Oral Contraceptive Side Effects 3 Many symptoms occurring with early OC use (eg, nausea, bloating, breakthrough bleeding) improve spontaneously by the third cycle of use after adjusting to the altered hormone levels.[2,3] Women should be counseled to continue their OC for 2 to 3 months before a change is made to adjust the hormonal content unless a serious adverse effect is present. Despite the 2 to 3 month adjustment period, a large majority of women who discontinue OCs do so because of the side effects. Patient education and early reevaluation within 3 to 6 months are necessary to identify and manage adverse effects, in an effort to improve adherence. The most common adverse effect is irregular bleeding. Women on extended-cycle regimens should be counseled to expect this during the first 6 months. For women experiencing bleeding irregularities beyond the recommended time-frame, then

TABLE 79-4 Composition of Commonly Prescribed Oral Contraceptives[a]

Product	Estrogen	Micrograms[b]	Progestin	Milligrams[b]	Spotting and Breakthrough Bleeding
50 mcg Estrogen					
Ogestrel 0.5/50	Ethinyl estradiol	50	Norgestrel	0.5	4.5
Zovia 1/50	Ethinyl estradiol	50	Ethynodiol diacetate	1	13.9
Sub-50 mcg Estrogen Monophasic					
Aubra, Aviane, Falmina, Lessina, Lutera, Orsythia, Sronyx, levonorgestrel/EE	Ethinyl estradiol	20	Levonorgestrel	0.1	26.5
Brevicon, Modicon, Necon 0.5/35, Nortrel 0.5/35 Wera	Ethinyl estradiol	35	Norethindrone	0.5	24.6
Zovia 1/35, Kelnor 1/35	Ethinyl estradiol	35	Ethynodiol diacetate	1	37.4
Apri, Desogen, desogestrel/EE, Emoquette, Ortho-Cept, Reclipsen, Enskyce	Ethinyl estradiol	30	Desogestrel	0.15	13.1
Levora, ChatealPortia, Altavera, Kurvelo, Marlissa	Ethinyl estradiol	30	Levonorgestrel	0.15	14
Gildess Fe 1/20, Junel 1/20, Junel Fe 1/20, Loestrin 1/20; Fe 1/20, Microgestin 1/20; Fe 1/20, Trina Fe 1/20	Ethinyl estradiol	20	Norethindrone 1 mg	1	26.5
Gildess Fe 1.5/30, Junel 1.5/30, Junel Fe 1.5/30, Loestrin Fe 1.5/30, Microgestin 1.5/30, Microgestin Fe 1.5/30, Larin (Fe) 1.5/30	Ethinyl estradiol	30	Norethindrone acetate	1.5	25.2
Cryselle, Elinest, Lo-Ovral, Low-Ogestrel	Ethinyl estradiol	30	Norgestrel	0.3	9.6
Necon 1/35, Norinyl 1+35, Nortrel 1/35, Ortho-Novum 1/35, Alyacen 1/35, Cyclafem 1/35, Dasetta 1/35, Pirmella 1/35	Ethinyl estradiol	35	Norethindrone	1	14.7
Estarylla, Norgestimate/ethinyl estradiolOrtho-Cyclen, Mononessa, Mono-Linyah, Previfem, Sprintec	Ethinyl estradiol	35	Norgestimate	0.25	14.3
Balziva, Femcon Fe chewable, Zenchent, Briellyn, Gildagia, Philith, Wymzya chewable, Vyfemla	Ethinyl estradiol	35	Norethindrone	0.4	11
Yasmin, Ocella, Safyral, Syeda, Zarah, drospirenone/EE	Ethinyl estradiol	30	Drospirenone	3	14.5
Generess Fe chewable, Layolis Fe, norethindrone/EE	Ethinyl estradiol	25	Norethindrone	0.8	14.5
Sub-50 mcg Estrogen Monophasic Extended Cycle					
Lo Loestrin-24 FE[c]	Ethinyl estradiol	10	Norethindrone	1	50[e]
Larin (Fe) 1/20, Minastrin 24 Fe chewable	Ethinyl estradiol	20	Norethindrone	1	50[e]
Amethia Lo, Camrese Lo, levonorgestrel/EE, LoSeasonique	Ethinyl estradiol	20/10	Levonorgestrel	0.1	50[e]
Amethyst	Ethinyl estradiol	20	Levonorgestrel	0.09	52[e]
Introvale, levonorgestrel/EE, Jolessa, Quasense[d]	Ethinyl estradiol	30	Levonorgestrel	0.15	58.5[e]
Amethia, Ashlyna, Daysee, Seasonique	Ethinyl estradiol	30/10	Levonorgestrel	0.15	50[e]
Quartette	Ethinyl estradiol	20/25/30/10	Levonorgestrel	0.15	50[e]
Beyaz, Gianvi, Loryna, Nikki, Vestura, Yazc	Ethinyl estradiol	20	Drospirenone	3	52.5[e]
Sub-50 mcg Estrogen Multiphasic					
Caziant, Cyclessa, Velivet	Ethinyl estradiol	25 (7)	Desogestrel	0.1 (7)	11.1
		25 (7)		0.125 (7)	
		25 (7)		0.15 (7)	
Tilia Fe, Tri-Legest Fe	Ethinyl estradiol	20 (5)	Norethindrone acetate	1 (5)	21.7
	Ethinyl estradiol	30 (7)	Norethindrone acetate	1 (7)	
	Ethinyl estradiol	35 (9)	Norethindrone acetate	1 (9)	
Kariva, Mircette, Azurette, Viorele	Ethinyl estradiol	20 (21)	Desogestrel	0.15 (21)	19.7
	Ethinyl estradiol	10 (5)	Desogestrel		
Necon 10/11	Ethinyl estradiol	35 (10)	Norethindrone	0.5 (10)	17.6
	Ethinyl estradiol	35 (11)	Norethindrone	1 (11)	

(continued)

TABLE 79-4 Composition of Commonly Prescribed Oral Contraceptives[a] (*Continued*)

Product	Estrogen	Micrograms[b]	Progestin	Milligrams[b]	Spotting and Breakthrough Bleeding
Ortho-Novum 7/7/7, Nortrel 7/7/7, Necon 7/7/7, Alyacen 7/7/7, Cyclafem 7/7/7, Dasetta 7/7/7, Pirmella 7/7/7	Ethinyl estradiol	35 (7)	Norethindrone	0.5 (7)	14.5
	Ethinyl estradiol	35 (7)	Norethindrone	0.75 (7)	
	Ethinyl estradiol	35 (7)	Norethindrone	1 (7)	
Ortho Tri-Cyclen, Trinessa, Tri-Previfem, Tri-Sprintec, Tri-Estarylla, Tri-Linyah, Norgestimate/EE	Ethinyl estradiol	35 (7)	Norgestimate	0.18 (7)	17.7
	Ethinyl estradiol	35 (7)	Norgestimate	0.215 (7)	
	Ethinyl estradiol	35 (7)	Norgestimate	0.25 (7)	
Ortho Tri-Cyclen Lo, Norgestimate/EE	Ethinyl estradiol	25 (7)	Norgestimate	0.18 (7)	11.5
	Ethinyl estradiol	25 (7)	Norgestimate	0.215 (7)	
	Ethinyl estradiol	25 (7)	Norgestimate	0.25 (7)	
Aranelle, Leena, Tri-Norinyl	Ethinyl estradiol	35 (7)	Norethindrone	0.5 (7)	25.5
	Ethinyl estradiol	35 (9)	Norethindrone	1 (9)	
	Ethinyl estradiol	35 (5)	Norethindrone	0.5 (5)	
Enpresse, Trivora, Levonest Myzilra	Ethinyl estradiol	30 (6)	Levonorgestrel	0.05 (6)	
	Ethinyl estradiol	40 (5)	Levonorgestrel	0.075 (5)	
	Ethinyl estradiol	30 (10)	Levonorgestrel	0.125 (10)	
Natazia	Estradiol valerate	3 (2) 2 (22) 1 (2)	Dienogest	0 (2) 2 (5) 3 (17) 0 (4)	
Progestin Only					
Camila, Errin, Heather, JencyclaJolivette, Lyza, Ortho Micronor, Nor-QD, Nora-BE, norethindrone	Ethinyl estradiol	–	Norethindrone	0.35	42.3

[a]28-day regimen (21-day active pills, then 7-day pill-free interval) unless otherwise noted.

[b]Number in parentheses refers to the number of days the dose is received in multiphasic oral contraceptives.

[c]28-day regimen (24-day active pills, then 4-day pill-free interval).

[d]91-day regimen (84-day active pills, then 7-day pill-free interval).

[e]Percent reporting after 6 to 12 months of use.

Data from references 2, 3 and 20.

the estrogen or progestin content may need to be adjusted.[3,9] Serious adverse effects that may occur with the use of CHCs are listed in Table 79-5, and common side effects and recommended monitoring are reviewed in Table 79-6.[2,3,9] Patients should be instructed to immediately discontinue CHCs if they experience serious warning signs, described as ACHES (abdominal pain, chest pain, headaches, eye problems, and severe leg pain).[3]

Managing Oral Contraceptive Drug Interactions 3 The effectiveness of an OC is sometimes limited by drug interactions that interfere with GI absorption, increase intestinal motility by altering gut bacteriologic flora, and alter the metabolism, excretion, or binding of the OC.[2] The lower the dose of hormone in the OC, the greater the risk that a drug interaction will compromise its efficacy. Women should be instructed to use an additional method of contraception if there is a possibility of a drug interaction altering the efficacy of the OC.[3] Although less well documented, these recommendations generally apply to patients receiving transdermal and vaginal CHC products.

Of all antibiotics, rifampin is the one with a true documented pharmacokinetic interaction.[2,8,9] Pharmacokinetic studies of other antibiotics have not shown any consistent interaction, but case reports of individual patients have shown a reduction in EE levels when OCs are taken with tetracyclines and penicillin derivatives. Women may use their OC when also taking antimicrobials other than rifampin (or derivatives) without use of an additional nonhormonal form of contraception.[8] It is important to note the difference and always recommend that women receiving concomitant rifampin (or derivatives) and OCs be counseled on the possibility for decreased efficacy and to use an additional nonhormonal form of contraception while on the combination and for at least 7 days after the rifampin therapy has been discontinued.[8] Additional recommendations suggest using an additional nonhormonal form of contraception for up to 28 days after discontinuation.[22] Some clinicians may continue to inform women of the slight risk of decreased efficacy with other antimicrobials just to be conservative, but it is not required or supported with evidence. If a woman is going to be receiving the interacting medication for more than 2 months, it is suggested to switch oral contraception to DMPA or an IUD to avoid the interaction and eliminate the need for long-term additional nonhormonal contraception. Women receiving certain anticonvulsants for a seizure disorder should be offered another form of contraception such as DMPA or IUDs rather than OCs (see Table 79-3).[8] Some anticonvulsants (mainly phenobarbital, carbamazepine, phenytoin) induce the metabolism of estrogen and progestin, inducing breakthrough bleeding and potentially reducing contraceptive efficacy. In addition, some anticonvulsants (eg, phenytoin) are known teratogens. Use of combined OCs with lamotrigine may decrease the effectiveness of lamotrigine and increase the possibility of worsening the seizure disorder. Finally, use of certain antiretroviral therapies in combination with OCs may decrease the efficacy of the OC.[8]

TABLE 79-5 Symptoms of a Serious or Potentially Serious Nature of Combined Hormonal Contraception

Symptom	Possible Cause
SERIOUS: Stop immediately	
Loss of vision, proptosis, diplopia, papilledema	Retinal artery thrombosis
Unilateral numbness, weakness, or tingling	Hemorrhagic or thrombotic stroke
Severe pains in chest, left arm, or neck	Myocardial infarction
Hemoptysis	Pulmonary embolism
Severe pains, tenderness or swelling, warmth or palpable cord in legs	Thrombophlebitis or thrombosis
Slurring of speech	Hemorrhagic or thrombotic stroke
Hepatic mass or tenderness	Liver neoplasm
POTENTIALLY SERIOUS: May continue with caution while being evaluated	
Absence of menses	Pregnancy
Spotting or breakthrough bleeding	Cervical endometrial or vaginal cancer
Breast mass, pain or swelling	Breast cancer
Right upper-quadrant pain	Cholecystitis, cholelithiasis or liver neoplasm
Mid-epigastric pain	Thrombosis of abdominal artery or vein, MI or PE
Migraine headache	Vascular spasm which may precede thrombosis
Severe nonvascular headache	Hypertension, vascular spasm
Galactorrhea	Pituitary adenoma
Jaundice, pruritus	Cholestatic jaundice
Depression, sleepiness	B6 deficiency
Uterine size increase	Leiomyomata, adenomyosis, pregnancy

Data from references 2 and 3.

Patient Instructions with Oral Contraceptives 4 Many women who take OCs are not educated properly on the appropriate use of these medications. Women should be given the package insert that accompanies all estrogen products and instructed to read it. The written patient information should be supplemented with verbal information describing the mechanism of the medication, both common and serious side effects (ie, ACHES symptoms), and management of these side effects. Although several transient self-limiting side effects often occur, the patient should be aware of the danger signals that require immediate medical attention (see Table 79-5). The benefits and risks should be discussed, including the fact that OCs provide no physical barrier to the transmission of STDs, including HIV. Detailed instructions on when to start taking the OC should be provided. Patients should be told the importance of routine daily administration to ensure consistent plasma concentrations and improve adherence.

Missed Doses of Oral Contraceptives. Specific instructions should be given regarding what to do if a tablet is missed. The latest

TABLE 79-6 Monitoring Patients Taking Hormonal Contraceptives

Drug (or Drug Class)	Adverse Drug Reactions	Monitoring Parameter	Comments
Combined hormonal contraception	Nausea/vomiting	Patient symptoms	Typically improves after two to three cycles; consider changing to lower estrogenic
	Breast tenderness	Patient symptoms	
	Weight gain	Weight	
	Acne, oily skin	Visual inspection	Consider changing to lower androgenic
	Depression, fatigue	Depression screening	Data are limited and conflicting
	Breakthrough bleeding/spotting	Menstrual symptoms	Consider changing to higher estrogenic
	Application site reaction (transdermal)	Visual inspection	
	Vaginal irritation (vaginal ring)	Patient symptoms	
Depot medroxyprogesterone acetate	Menstrual irregularities	Menstrual symptoms	Typically improves after 6 months
	Weight gain	Weight	
	Acne	Visual inspection	
	Hirsutism	Visual inspection	
	Depression	Depression screening	Data are limited and conflicting
	Decreased bone density	BMD	Do not routinely screen with DXA
Levonorgestrel IUD	Menstrual irregularities	Menstrual symptoms	Typically spotting, amenorrhea
	Insertion-related complications	Cramping, pain	Prophylactic NSAIDs or local anesthetic may reduce occurrence
		Cramping, pain, spotting, dyspareunia, missing strings	
	Expulsion	Lower abdominal pain, unusual vaginal discharge, fever	IUD strings should be checked regularly by women to ensure IUD properly placed
	Pelvic inflammatory disease		Overall risk of developing is rare, but counseling on STD prevention is important
Copper IUD	See levonorgestrel IUD above	See levonorgestrel IUD above	Menstrual irregularities are typically heavier menses with copper IUD
Progestin-only implant	Menstrual irregularities	Menstrual symptoms	
	Insertion-site reactions	Pain, bruising, skin irritation, erythema, pus, fever	Typically well-tolerated and resolve without treatment, infection is rare

BMD, Bone Mineral Density; DXA, Dual Energy X-ray Absorptiometry; IUD, Intrauternine Device; STD, Sexually Transmitted Disease.

Data from references 2 and 9.

recommendations from the CDC strive to balance simplicity with the best evidence.[21] For women who routinely have difficulty with adhering to daily dosing, counseling regarding other options such as the vaginal ring, transdermal patch, DMPA, implants, or IUDs should be provided. If warranted, suggesting EC may also be necessary.

If one tablet is missed or late then take the tablet as soon as remembered and continue taking the rest of the tablets as prescribed (for most women that means two tablets taken on the same day). Typically no additional nonhormonal contraception methods are warranted. If two or more consecutive tablets are missed then take one missed tablet as soon as remembered and discard the remaining missed tablets. Continue taking the OC tablets as scheduled (this means two tablets may need to be taken on the same day—ie, one of the missed tablets and one of the regularly scheduled tablets). Counsel to use additional nonhormonal contraception until tablets have been taken for 7 consecutive days. If tablets were missed in the last week of hormonal tablets then omit the hormone-free interval by finishing tablets containing hormones and then starting a new pack. Counsel to use additional nonhormonal contraception until tablets have been taken for 7 consecutive days. For all scenarios when two or more consecutive tablets are missed, consider counseling on use of EC if warranted. Additional information regarding missed doses of OCs and vaginal rings or transdermal patches can be found on the CDC website.[21] It is important to remember that handling missed or late doses of progestin-only OCs are different. If a woman forgets a tablet or is more than 3 hours late then additional nonhormonal contraception should be used for 48 hours.[8]

Vomiting and Severe Diarrhea While on Oral Contraceptives

Efficacy of OCs may be decreased when vomiting or severe diarrhea occurs, and recommendations for dosing OCs in this situation have been developed.[21] The recommendations are based on theoretical concerns and are identical to missed tablet instructions. If vomiting or diarrhea occurs for less than 48 hours then no redosing of OCs is warranted. If vomiting or diarrhea persists greater than 48 hours then continue taking tablets and use additional nonhormonal contraception until tablets have been taken for 7 consecutive days after the vomiting or diarrhea subsides. If this scenario occurs during the last week of the hormonal tablets, then finish the tablets, skip the hormone-free tablets and begin a new pack. Additional nonhormonal contraception should be used until 7 consecutive days of tablets are taken without gastrointestinal symptoms. Counsel patients on use of EC if warranted.

Discontinuing Oral Contraceptives and Return of Fertility

There is no evidence that OC use decreases subsequent fertility; there are similar findings with the transdermal patch and vaginal ring.[2] The average delay in ovulation after discontinuing OCs is 1 to 2 weeks; however, delayed ovulation is more common in women with a history of irregular menses. If amenorrhea does continue beyond 6 months, women should be counseled to see a physician for further fertility work-up.[2,3] In the past, women were counseled to allow two to three normal menstrual periods before becoming pregnant to permit the reestablishment of menses and ovulation. However, in several large cohort and case-control studies, infants conceived in the first month after discontinuation of an OC had no greater chance of miscarriage or being born with a birth defect than those born in the general population.

Transdermal Contraceptives 1 2 A CHC is available as a transdermal patch (Ortho Evra), which includes 0.75 mg of EE and 6 mg of norelgestromin, the active metabolite of norgestimate.[2,3] Comparative trials have shown the transdermal patch to be as effective as combined OCs in patients weighing less than 90 kg. Of the 15 pregnancies reported in the clinical trials, five were among women weighing more than 90 kg; therefore, this product is not recommended as a first-line option for these women.[2,3,17] 3 Some patients experience application-site reactions, but other side effects are similar to those experienced with OCs (eg, breast discomfort, headache, and nausea).[3] A warning from the manufacturer states that women using the patch are exposed to approximately 60% more estrogen than from a typical OC containing 35 mcg of EE. Evidence suggests that higher exposure to estrogen may lead to increased thromboembolic risk, and the labeling for the contraceptive patch now contains a warning of this risk.[14] The patch should be applied to the abdomen, buttocks, upper torso, or upper arm at the beginning of the menstrual cycle and replaced every week for 3 weeks (the fourth week is patch-free).[2,3] The patch releases estrogen and progestin for 9 days. If there is delayed application for less than 48 hours since patch should have been applied or detachment less than 24 hours, a new patch should be applied immediately, or the detached patch can be reapplied, with no additional nonhormonal contraception necessary. If there is delayed application for 48 hours or more since the patch should have been applied or detachment for 24 hours or more, a new patch should be applied as soon as possible, and additional nonhormonal contraception should be utilized until the patch has been worn for 7 consecutive days. If the delayed application or detachment occurs in the third patch week, the hormone-free week should be omitted and a new patch should be applied immediately.[14,21] Users have demonstrated greater adherence with the patch than with an OC, but whether this results in reduced pregnancy rates remains to be seen. The benefits of adherence must be weighed against of the risk of increased estrogen exposure and possibility of VTE.

Vaginal Rings 1 2 The vaginal contraceptive ring contains EE and etonogestrel (NuvaRing).[15] It is a 54-mm flexible ring, 4 mm in thickness. Over a 3-week period, the ring releases approximately 15 mcg/day of EE and 120 mcg/day of etonogestrel. Comparative trials have shown the vaginal ring to be as effective as combined OCs. On the first cycle of use, the ring should be inserted on or before the fifth day of the menstrual cycle, remain in place for 3 weeks, then removed for 1 week to allow for withdrawal bleeding. The new ring should be inserted on the same day of the week as it was during the last cycle, similar to starting a new OC pack on the same day of the week. If the ring has been displaced for less than 3 hours, a new ring should be inserted as soon as possible and kept in until the scheduled removal day. No additional nonhormonal contraception is necessary. If there is a delay of 3 or more hours, a new ring should be inserted immediately and additional nonhormonal contraception should be utilized, or intercourse should be avoided until the ring has been in place for 7 consecutive days. If the delayed reinsertion occurs during the third week of ring use, a new ring can be reinserted right away to start the next 21 day cycle. There may be some spotting or vaginal bleeding. If a woman forgets to change the ring after the third week, she can simply reinsert a new ring during the fourth week and begin a new cycle. She will still be protected, and no back up protection will be necessary.[14]

3 Side effects, precautions, and contraindications for use of the hormonal ring are similar to those for all CHCs. The most commonly reported reasons for discontinuation of use were device-related issues, such as foreign-body sensation, device expulsion, and vaginal symptoms.[14] Cycle control with the vaginal ring appears to be equal or better than with combined OCs, with a low incidence of breakthrough bleeding and spotting after the second cycle of use. Patient acceptability of the delivery system has been studied, and the majority of women do not complain of discomfort in general or during intercourse.[3,14] A potential concern is the possibility of increased VTE (8 cases per 10,000 per year vs 6 cases with most CHCs) since etonogestrel is a metabolite of desogestrel which may be associated with increased risk.[23] The ring should be inserted vaginally. In contrast to diaphragms and cervical caps, precise placement is not an issue because the hormones are absorbed anywhere in the vagina. Women should be in a comfortable position, and compress the ring

between the thumb and index finger and push it into the vagina. There is no danger of inserting the ring too far because the cervix will prevent it from traveling up the genital tract. Removal of the ring is performed in a similar manner; pulling it out and discarding into the foil patch (the ring should not be flushed down the toilet).[14] Patients should be discouraged from douching, but other vaginal products, including antifungal creams and spermicides, can be used.[3,14]

Injectable Progestins Steroid hormones provide longer-term contraception when injected into the skin. Sustained progestin exposure blocks the LH surge, thus inhibiting ovulation. Should ovulation occur, progestins reduce ovum motility in the fallopian tubes. Even if fertilization occurs, progestins thin the endometrium, reducing the chance of implantation. Progestins also thicken the cervical mucus, producing a barrier to sperm penetration. This method of contraception does not provide any protection from STDs.[2,3]

1 2 Women who may benefit from injectable progestins are those who are breastfeeding, those who are intolerant to estrogens (ie, have a history of estrogen-related headache, breast tenderness, or nausea) or those with concomitant medical conditions in which estrogen is not recommended (see Table 79-3). Additionally, injectable progestins are beneficial for women with adherence issues; they have lower failure rates than CHC methods (see Table 79-1).[2,8,20]

Depot Medroxyprogesterone Acetate 1 2 It is similar in structure to naturally occurring progesterone. DMPA (Depo-Provera) is administered every 3 months either by deep intramuscular injection in the gluteal or deltoid muscle or subcutaneously in the abdomen or thigh within 5 days of onset of menstrual bleeding.[24,25] With perfect use, the efficacy of DMPA is more than 99%; however, with typical use, 3% of women experience unintended pregnancy.[2] Although these injections may inhibit ovulation for up to 14 weeks, the dose should be repeated every 3 months (12 weeks) to ensure continuous contraception. The manufacturer recommends excluding pregnancy in women with a lapse of 13 or more weeks between injections for the intramuscular formulation or 14 or more weeks between injections for the subcutaneous formulation. Depo-Provera is available as a 150 mg/mL injection vial or prefilled syringe for IM injection and Depo-SubQ Provera 104 is available as a prefilled syringe.[24,25] Administration of both formulations of DMPA requires a medical office visit; however, studies of patient self-administration of subcutaneous DMPA have demonstrated positive results.[26]

Although no adverse effects have been documented in infants exposed to DMPA through breast milk, the manufacturer recommends not initiating DMPA until 6 weeks postpartum in breastfeeding women.[24,25] However, the CDC cites a lack of evidence supporting this claim and classifies DMPA use during this timeframe as a category 1 or 2 suggesting that the benefit may outweigh the theoretical risk.[8] Women who are not breastfeeding but require contraception can receive DMPA immediately postpartum.[8] Women with sickle-cell disease are good candidates for DMPA, as studies have demonstrated a reduction in sickle cell pain crises in women using DMPA.[8] In addition, women with seizure disorders may experience fewer seizures when taking DMPA for contraception, and there is not a concern with anticonvulsants reducing the contraceptive efficacy of DMPA.[2,8] Because return of fertility may be delayed after discontinuation of DMPA, it should not be recommended to women desiring pregnancy in the near future. The median time to conception from the first omitted dose is 10 months. Sixty-eight percent of women will be able to conceive within 12 months, 83% within 15 months, and 93% within 18 months of the last injection.[2,24,25]

3 Menstrual irregularities are the most frequent adverse effects of both formulations of DMPA and are most common in the first year of use. These irregularities include spotting, prolonged bleeding, and amenorrhea; counseling women on these possibilities is important before initiation of the method.[8,9] Women who cannot tolerate prolonged bleeding may benefit from a short course of non-steroidal anti-inflammatory drugs (NSAIDs) (for 5-7 days) during the bleeding. In addition, a short course of estrogen (if no contraindications are present) for approximately 10 to 20 days. Examples of estrogen regimens to help prolonged bleeding during DMPA include one pack of low dose combined OCs, 1 mg of oral estradiol or 0.795 to 1.25 mg of oral conjugated equine estrogen.[9] The incidence of irregular bleeding decreases from 30% in the first year to 10% thereafter. After 12 months of therapy, 55% of women report amenorrhea, with the incidence increasing to 68% after 2 years.[24,25]

Other adverse effects, including breast tenderness and depression, occur less commonly. Weight gain is a concern for many women using DMPA, and the incidence and amount gained vary widely. It has been reported that weight gain averages 1 kg annually and may not resolve until 6 to 8 months after the last injection or patients gain 5 kg on average after using DMPA for 5 years.[2,3,24,25]

Depot medroxyprogesterone acetate has been associated with short-term bone loss in younger women of reproductive age. This potential side effect may be due to lower ovarian estrogen production that occurs when gonadotropin secretion is suppressed.[2,27] Because longitudinal studies demonstrated effects on BMD, the FDA issued a black box warning for DMPA in 2004.[24,25] It states that DMPA should be continued for more than 2 years only if other contraceptive methods are inadequate. It also states that the loss of BMD seems to be greater with increasing duration of use and may not be completely reversible. However, the majority of clinicians view the effects of DMPA on BMD (which in the majority of cases is reversible) as a surrogate marker and there are no clear data that demonstrate the effects of DMPA on fracture risk.[27,28] The ACOG and CDC continue to recommend that for most patients the benefits of DMPA outweigh the risks even when used beyond 2 years of use.[8,27] ACOG does not recommend the routine screening of BMD in most patients.[27] A discussion regarding the risks and benefits of this contraceptive option is recommended prior to initiation and with prolonged use.

Long-acting Reversible Contraception (LARC) It refers to a category of hormonal and nonhormonal contraceptives that include IUDs and implants. This type of contraception is highly efficacious in preventing pregnancy, but the effects are quickly reversible upon removal.[29] LARC does not require effort or adherence by the patient once they are inserted. Therefore, perfect-use and typical-use efficacy rates do not differ, and the efficacy rate is similar to that of surgical options such as tubal ligation (see Table 79-1).[2,29] When compared to other methods of hormonal contraception, especially OCs, LARC methods are not used as frequently in the United States. However, increased education campaigns are demonstrating effectiveness. The use of LARC increased to 7% of all women, and in women aged 25 to 34 their use is up to 11%.[30] All women should be considered potential candidates for this method.[29,31] In the past, many clinicians offered LARC only when adherence was an issue or in women with contraindications to estrogen. Due to the high efficacy rates of LARC methods, many advocates propose that increased use may decrease unintended pregnancy rates.[29]

Subdermal Progestin Implants 1 2 Nexplanon (formerly called Implanon in the United States) is a single 4-cm-long implant, containing 68 mg of etonogestrel that is placed under the skin of the upper arm using a preloaded inserter.[2,32] Clinicians must receive training from the manufacturer prior to insertion or removal of the device. The implant releases etonogestrel at a rate of 60 mcg daily for the first month, then decreases to an average of 30 mcg daily at the end of the 3 years of recommended use. The primary mechanism of action is suppression of ovulation. When ovulation is not suppressed, etonogestrel still is effective as the progestin thickens the cervical mucus and produces an atrophic endometrium. With both perfect and typical use, the efficacy rate is over 99%.[2,32] However, in overweight and obese women weighing more than 130% of their ideal body weight, the manufacturer states the possibility of decreased efficacy. However, it is noted that overweight women were excluded from studies, and recent small studies have not demonstrated any decreased effects.[31,32]

4 The etonogestrel implant should be inserted between days 1 and 5 of the menstrual cycle in women who have not previously used hormonal contraception.[32] If it is inserted at any other time of the menstrual cycle, then it is recommended to use an additional nonhormonal contraceptive method for 7 days. Women currently taking OCs can have the implant inserted within 7 days after taking the last active OC tablet. Women currently taking progestin-only OCs should have the implant inserted without skipping any days, on the same day that the progestin-only IUD is removed, or on the day that the DMPA injection is due. After removal, fertility returns within 30 days.

3 The major adverse effect associated with Nexplanon is irregular menstrual bleeding, which led to discontinuation of the implant in 11% of patients in clinical trials.[29,32] Women should be counseled about the risk of irregular bleeding patterns so that patients will not request early removal of Nexplanon. Some women (22%) became amenorrheic with continued use, but many continued to have prolonged bleeding and spotting (18% and 34%, respectively) and frequent bleeding (7%).[9,31,32] Women who cannot tolerate prolonged bleeding may benefit from a short course of NSAIDS (for 5-7 days) during the bleeding. In addition, a short course of estrogen (if no contraindications are present) for approximately 10 to 20 days.[9] Insertion and removal complications are rare (less than 2%).[31,32] Information from the manufacturer suggests using precaution when there is potential for drug interactions in the presence of potent CYP450 inducers (eg, rifampin, phenytoin, and carbamazepine).[32] This information conflicts with CDC recommendations; those recommendations classify combining those medications with Nexplanon as a category 2, suggesting that the benefits may outweigh the theoretical risks. However, the CDC does still recommend use of additional nonhormonal contraception or switching to DMPA or an IUD.[8]

Intrauterine Devices 1 2 There are currently four IUDs available, all are T-shaped and are medicated, one with copper (ParaGard) and three with levonorgestrel (Mirena, Skyla, and Liletta). Clinicians must receive training from the manufacturer prior to insertion or removal of the IUDs. These IUDs have several possible mechanisms of action including inhibition of sperm migration, damaging ovum or disrupting transport, and possibly damaging the fertilized ovum. Due to the presence of local progestin, the Mirena, Skyla, and Liletta IUDs have additional mechanisms of endometrial suppression and thickening cervical mucus. The most recent evidence regarding the mechanisms of action demonstrate that the contraceptive activity of IUDs occurs before implanatation.[2,29] Efficacy rates with IUDs are greater than 99% with both perfect and typical use.[2,29] IUDs should not be used in the presence of current pregnancy, current pelvic inflammatory disease, current STD, puerperal or postabortion sepsis, purulent cervicitis, undiagnosed abnormal vaginal bleeding, malignancy of genital tract, uterine anomalies or fibroids distorting uterine cavity, allergy to IUD component, or Wilson's disease (for copper IUD).[33,34] The risk of pelvic inflammatory disease among IUD users is low. There are no long-term effects on fertility, and average time to return of fertility is similar to oral contracpetives.[29,31]

3 ParaGard is a highly effective IUD that can be left in place for 10 years.[2,33] A disadvantage of ParaGard is increased menstrual blood flow and dysmenorrhea; average monthly blood loss among users increased by 35% in clinical trials. Mirena, Skyla, and Liletta are the more recently approved IUDs in the United States and contain the progestin levonorgestrel.[34-36] Mirena releases 20 mcg of levonorgestrel daily and can be used for 5 years.[2,34] Liletta and Skyla are the most recent IUDs to be approved and release 18 mcg and 14 mcg of levonorgestrel daily, respectively.[2,35,36] They can be left in place for 3 years. Systemically absorbed levonorgestrel is minimal and considerably less than with OCs. The levonorgestrel IUD produces its effects locally via suppression of the endometrium, causing a reduction in menstrual blood loss. In contrast to the copper IUD, menstrual flow in users of the levonorgestrel IUD is decreased, and development of amenorrhea has been observed in 20% of users in the first year and 60% in the fifth year. A disadvantage of the levonorgestrel IUD is increased spotting in the first 6 months of use; women should be counseled that the spotting will decline gradually over time.[2,34] Women who cannot tolerate prolonged bleeding may benefit from a short course of NSAIDS (for 5-7 days) during the bleeding. In addition, a short course of estrogen (if no contraindications are present) could be used for approximately 10 to 20 days.[9]

Due to the local effects on the endometrium and decrease in blood loss, Mirena has an additional indication for treatment of heavy menstrual bleeding (menorrhagia).[34] Return to fertility is rapid and typically occurs within 30 days after removal of the IUD.[29] Historically, use in nulliparous and adolescent women was considered a precaution to use of an IUD. However, recent evidence, clinical experience, and expert opinion do not preclude use in these populations. Risk versus benefits should be considered, and the woman must be counseled on the efficacy and potential adverse effects.[29,37] Strong consideration of an IUD is appropriate in this population due to high efficacy rates.[37] In addition, Skyla does not include nulliparous women as a precaution, and about 40% of patients in the clinical trials were nulliparous.[36] The influence of drug interactions on the efficacy of IUDs is not a primary concern based on manufacturer and CDC recommendations.[8,34-36]

Clinical **Controversy...**

Controversy exists regarding the potential for decreased efficacy of oral emergency contraception (both levonorgestrel and ulipristal) in overweight or obese women. No large scale studies have been designed to fully resolve the controversy. Meta-analyses of limited pooled data have suggested an association with increased body weight and decreased efficacy of oral EC.[38] The data demonstrate that there may be a decline in efficacy in women weighing greater than 75 kg. There is no effect of increased body weight on efficacy of a copper IUD. This issue is controversial because oral EC is the most widely used EC method due to its accessibility.

Emergency Contraception

5 Emergency contraception is used to prevent unwanted pregnancy after unprotected or inadequately protected sexual intercourse (eg, no contraception, condom breakage, OC nonadherence, sexual assault). Pregnancy occurs when the fertilized egg is implanted into the endometrial lining. After intercourse, implantation of the fertilized egg typically takes approximately 5 days.[39] Progestin-only and progesterone receptor modulator products are approved by the FDA and recommended as first-line EC options.[2,3,39] Insertion of the copper IUD or prescribing higher doses of combined OCs (Yuzpe method) are other options but are not widely used.

Currently, the progestin-only formulation containing levonorgestrel 1.5 mg tablet × 1 dose (currently marketed in a variety of products, including Next Choice One Dose and Plan B One Step) is approved specifically for EC in the United States.[20] Studies support that the primary mechanism of action of progestin-only EC is inhibiting or delaying ovulation, and there is no evidence that there is an effect on implantation or disrupt a fertilized egg after implantation has occurred.[39] The levonorgestrel-containing EC formulation is the regimen of choice due to availability, improved tolerability, and potentially increased efficacy rates. All formulations are now offered as one dose options, to be given within 72 hours (3 days) of unprotected intercourse. However, the earlier the medication is given, the greater the efficacy and less chance of a pregnancy. Notably, there is some evidence that this regimen may be effective for up to 5 days after unprotected intercourse; but consideration of ulipristal or a copper IUD may be a better option if a woman can get access in time.[39] Levonorgestrel-containing EC products are now available without a prescription to patients of all ages in the United States.[39]

5 Ulipristal (Ella) is the newest EC product and was approved for use by the FDA in 2010. Ulipristal is a selective progesterone receptor modulator with mixed progesterone agonist and antagonist properties.[39,40] Its mechanism of action depends on the timing of administration relative to the woman's menstrual cycle.[41] The primary mechanism of action appears to be delay of ovulation. Ulipristal is available by prescription only and is available as a single dose of 30 mg taken within 120 hours (5 days) after unprotected intercourse. Evidence supports that it maintains efficacy for the full 120-hour window.[39,40] Data exist to support noninferiority of ulipristal compared to levonorgestrel-containing EC.[42]

5 Determining the exact effectiveness rate of EC is difficult; however, the range has been reported to be between 59% and 94%.[39] Evidence reported that EC may prevent an average of 75% of expected pregnancies when taken appropriately. It is recommended that women have an advanced prescription on hand or access to an OTC formulation to maximize the effectiveness of EC.

3 Common adverse effects include nausea, vomiting, and irregular bleeding.[39] Nausea and vomiting occur significantly less when progestin-only and progesterone receptor modulator EC is administered. Many women will experience irregular bleeding regardless of which EC method is used, with the menstrual period usually occurring 1 week before or after the expected time. Routine screening prior to or after receiving progestin-only and progesterone receptor modulator EC is not recommended. If a pregnancy already exists, the EC will not disrupt or harm the embryo. Additionally, there are no contraindications to the use of these methods of EC (for the Yuzpe and copper IUD methods clinicians must adhere to their contraindications and precautions). No current data regarding the safety of repeated use EC are available, but current consensus suggests that the risks are low, and women can receive multiple regimens if warranted. Appropriate counseling should be provided regarding timing of the dose, common adverse effects, and use of a regular contraceptive method (additional nonhormonal contraceptive methods should be used after EC for at least 7 days).

Personalized Pharmacotherapy

Selecting a contraceptive method should involve the patient and clinician using a shared decision-making model. Contraceptive pharmacotherapy should be personalized for each patient, taking into account desired outcomes from a contraceptive and noncontraceptive perspective. Factors to consider include efficacy, presence of coexisting medical conditions or medications, safety, adverse effects, cost, and patient preference of the contraceptive method (eg, long-acting, short-acting, hormonal, oral, non-oral, barrier). In addition, access to timely contraception is important. The ACOG favors many strategies to improve comprehensive contraception including full coverage by the Affordable Care Act in the United States, over-the-counter access for certain hormonal contraceptives, and advanced provision or counseling regarding EC.[43] In addition, a few states have (or are in the process of obtaining) expanded scope of practice to include provision of hormonal contraception by a pharmacist working under a collaborative practice agreement.[44]

EVALUATION OF THERAPEUTIC OUTCOMES

4 Patients should receive both verbal and written instructions on the chosen method of contraception. Follow-up appointments can increase adherence and provide opportunities to address other health maintenance issues. The contraceptive outcome of pregnancy prevention can be assessed when needed by obtaining a serum or urine pregnancy test.

Monitoring of the Pharmaceutical Care Plan

Contraceptive users should receive an annual well woman exam that may include a cytologic screening (as appropriate), pelvic and breast examination. Consultation should provide routine health maintenance screening and to assess for clinical problems or adverse effects related to contraception (see Table 79-6). It is important to note that these annual screenings do not have to occur prior to prescribing hormonal contraception.

Annual blood pressure monitoring is recommended for all users of CHC. When a patient with a history of glucose intolerance or diabetes mellitus begins or discontinues the use of hormonal contraception, glucose levels must be monitored. Monitoring for the presence of adverse effects related to hormonal content or the presence of coexisting medical conditions is recommended for women using CHCs. Women using Nexplanon should be monitored annually for menstrual cycle disturbances, local inflammation, or infection at the implant site, acne, breast tenderness, headaches, and hair loss. Women using DMPA should be asked at 3-month follow-up visits about weight gain, menstrual cycle disturbances, and fractures. Women using IUDs should be asked at 1- to 3-month follow-up visits about IUD placement (checking for IUD strings to assure the IUD is still in the proper position), changes in menstrual bleeding patterns, and symptoms and protection against STDs. Clinicians should check for proper IUD positioning and symptoms of upper genital tract infection.

Finally, clinicians should monitor and when indicated screen for HIV and STDs. All women should receive counseling about healthy sexual practices including the use of condoms to prevent the transmission of STDs when necessary.

ABBREVIATIONS

ACOG	American Congress of Obstetrics and Gynecology
BMD	bone mineral density
BMI	body mass index
CDC	Centers for Disease Control and Prevention
CHC	combined hormonal contraception
DMPA	depot medroxyprogesterone acetate
EC	emergency contraception
EE	ethinyl estradiol
FDA	Food and Drug Administration
FSH	follicle-stimulating hormone
GnRH	gonadotropin-releasing hormone
HDL	high-density lipoprotein
HIV	human immunodeficiency virus
IUD	intrauterine device
LARC	long-acting reversible contraception
LDL	low-density lipoprotein
LH	luteinizing hormone
MI	myocardial infarction

NSAID	non-steroidal anti-inflammatory drug
OC	oral contraceptive
OTC	over the counter
Pap	papanicolaou (smear)
SHBG-TBG	sex hormone (testosterone) binding globulin
SLE	systemic lupus erythematosus
STD	sexually transmitted disease
TSS	toxic shock syndrome
VTE	venous thromboembolism
WHO	World Health Organization

REFERENCES

1. Mosher WD, Jones J, Abma JC. Intended and unintended births in the United States: 1982–2010. National Health Statistics Reports, No. 55. Hyattsville, MD: National Center for Health Statistics; 2012.
2. Hatcher RA, Trussell J, Nelson AL, et al. *Contraceptive Technology*. 21st ed. Ardent New York: Median, Inc.; 2015.
3. Dickey RP. *Managing Contraceptive Pill Patients*. 15th ed. Fort Collins, CO: Durant: EMIS Inc.; 2014.
4. American College of Obstetricians and Gynecologists. Screening for Cervical Cancer. Practice Bulletin No.131. *Obstet Gynecol* 2012;120:1239-1242.
5. American College of Obstetricians and Gynecologists. Noncontraceptive uses of hormonal contraceptives. Practice Bulletin No. 110. *Obstet Gynecol* 2010;115:206-218.
6. Grimes DA, Lopez LM, Raymond EG, et al. Spermicide used alone for contraception. *Cochrane Database of Systematic Reviews* 2013;(12):CD005218.
7. Wilkinson D, Ramjee G, Tholandi M, Rutherford GW. Nonoxynol-9 for preventing vaginal acquisition of HIV infection by women from men. *Cochrane Database of Systematic Reviews* 2002;(3):CD003936.
8. Centers for Disease Control and Prevention. U.S. Medical Eligibility Criteria for Contraceptive Use, 2010. *MMWR* 2010;59(RR04):1-85.
9. Centers for Disease Control and Prevention. U.S. Selected Practice Recommendations for Contraceptive Use, 2013. *MMWR* 2013;63(RR-5):1-60.
10. MacGregor EA. Contraception and headache. *Headache* 2013;53:247-276.
11. Lidegaard OM, Nielsen LH, Skovlund CW, Lokkegaard E. Venous thromboembolism in users of non-oral hormonal contraception: Follow-up study, Denmark 2001–2010. *BMJ* 2012;344:e2990.
12. Jick SS, Hernandez RK. Risk of non-fatal thromboembolism in women using oral contraceptives containing drospirenone compared with women using oral contraceptives containing levonorgestrel: Case-control study using United States claims data. *BMJ* 2011;342:d2151.
13. Yasmin/Yaz Package Insert, 2015. Bayer HealthCare Pharmaceuticals, Inc. Whippany, NJ. Available at: http://labeling.bayerhealthcare.com/html/products/pi/fhc/YAZ_PI.pdf.
14. Ortho Evra Package Insert, 2014. Jannsen Pharmaceuticals, Inc. Titusville, NJ. Available at: http://www.orthoevra.com/sites/default/files/assets/OrthoEvraPI.pdf.
15. NuvaRing Package Insert, 2014. Merck & Co., Inc. Whitehouse Station, NJ. Available at: http://www.merck.com/product/usa/pi_circulars/n/nuvaring/nuvaring_pi.pdf.
16. Dinger J, Minh TD, Buttmann N, Bardenheuer K. Effectiveness of oral contraceptive pills in a large U.S. cohort comparing progestogen and regimen. *Obstet Gynecol* 2011;117:33-40.
17. Artal R. ACOG Women and Obesity. Available at: http://www.acog.org/About-ACOG/ACOG-Districts/District-II/Women-and-Obesity. (Accessed August 7, 2015.)
18. Van Vliet HAAM, Grimes DA, Helmerhorst FM, Schulz KF. Biphasic versus monophasic oral contraceptives for contraception. *Cochrane Database Syst Rev* 2006;3:CD002032.
19. Van Vliet HAAM, Grimes DA, Helmerhorst FM, Schulz KF. Biphasic versus triphasic oral contraceptives for contraception. *Cochrane Database Syst Rev* 2006;3:CD003283.
20. PL Detail-Document, Comparison of Oral Contraceptives and Non-Oral Alternatives. Pharmacist's Letter/Prescriber's Letter. July 2015: Volume 31.
21. Centers for Disease Control and Prevention. Update to CDC's U.S. Medical Eligibility Criteria for Contraceptive Use, 2010: Revised Recommendations for the Use of Contraceptive Methods During the Postpartum Period. *MMWR* 2011;60:878-883.
22. Faculty of sexual and reproductive healthcare. Royal College of Obstetricians & Gynaecologists. Drug interactions with hormonal contraception. Clinical effectiveness unit. January 2011. (Updated January 2012). Available at: http://www.fsrh.org/pdfs/CEUGuidanceDrugInteractionsHormonal.pdf.
23. PL Detailed Document, Hormonal Contraceptives and the Risk of Thrombosis. Pharmacist's Letter/Prescriber's Letter. August 2012: Volume 28.
24. Depo-Provera Package Insert, 2002. Pfizer. New York, NY. Available at: http://www.accessdata.fda.gov/drugsatfda_docs/label/2003/20246scs019_Depo-provera_lbl.pdf.
25. Depo-SubQ Provera 104 Package Insert, 2015. Pfizer. New York, NY. Available at: http://labeling.pfizer.com/ShowLabeling.aspx?id=549.
26. Beasley A, White K, Cremers S, Westhoff C. Randomized clinical trial of self versus clinical administration of subcutaneous depot medroxyprogesterone acetate. *Contraception* 2014;89:352-356.
27. Depot medroxyprogesterone acetate and bone effects. Committee Opinion No. 602. American College of Obstetricians and Gynecologists. *Obstet Gynecol* 2014;123:1398-1402.
28. Lopez LM, Chen M, Mullins Long S, et al. Steroidal contraceptives and bone fractures in women: Evidence from observational studies. *Cochrane Database of Systematic Reviews* 2015;(7):CD009849. DOI: 10.1002/14651858.CD009849.pub3.
29. American College of Obstetricians and Gynecologists. Long-acting reversible contraception: Implants and intrauterine devices. Practice Bulletin No. 121. *Obstet Gynecol* 2011;118:184-196.
30. Branum AM, Jones T. Trends in long-acting reversible contraception use among U.S. women aged 15-44. NCHS data brief, no. 188. Hyattsville, MD: National Center for Health Statistics; 2015.
31. Espey E, Ogburn T. Long-acting reversible contraceptives. *Obstet Gynecol* 2011;117:705-719.
32. Nexplanon Package Insert, 2015. Merck & Co., Inc. Whitehouse Station, NJ. Available at: http://www.merck.com/product/usa/pi_circulars/n/nexplanon/nexplanon_pi.pdf.
33. ParaGard Package Insert, 2013. Teva Pharmaceuticals USA, Inc. Sellersville, PA. Available at: http://paragard.com/Pdf/ParaGard-PI.pdf.
34. Mirena Package Insert, 2014. BayerHealthcare Pharmaceuticals, Inc. Whippany, NJ. Available at: http://labeling.bayerhealthcare.com/html/products/pi/Mirena_PI.pdf.
35. Liletta Package Insert, 2015. Actavis Pharma, Inc. Parsippany, NJ. Available at: http://pi.actavis.com/data_stream.asp?product_group=1960&p=pi&language=E.
36. Skyla Package Insert, 2013. BayerHealthcare Pharmaceuticals, Inc. Whippany, NJ. Available at: http://labeling.bayerhealthcare.com/html/products/pi/Skyla_PI.pdf.
37. Adolescents and long-acting reversible contraception: implants and intrauterine devices. Committee Opinion No. 539. American College of Obstetricians and Gynecologists. *Obstet Gynecol* 2012;120:983-988.
38. Glasier A, Cameron ST, Blithe D, et al. Can we identify women at risk of pregnancy despite using emergency contraception? Data from randomized trials of ulipristal acetate and levonorgestrel. *Contraception* 2011;84:363-367.
39. Emergency contraception. Practice Bulletin No. 152. American College of Obstetricians and Gynecologists. *Obstet Gynecol* 2015;126:e1-11.
40. Shrader SP, Hall LN, Ragucci KR, Rafie S. Updates in hormonal emergency contraception. *Pharmacotherapy* 2011;31:887-895.
41. Brache V, Cochon L, Jesam C, et al. Immediate pre-ovulatory administration of 30 mg ulipristal acetate significantly delays follicular rupture. *Hum Reprod* 2010;25:2256-2263.
42. Glasier AF, Cameron ST, Fine PM, et al. Ulipristal acetate versus levonorgestrel for emergency contraception: A randomized non-inferiority trial and meta-analysis. *Lancet* 2010;375:555-579.
43. Access to contraception. Committee Opinion No. 615. American College of Obstetricians and Gynecologists. *Obstet Gynecol* 2015;125:250-255.
44. Pharmacist Prescribers Increase Access to Effective Contraceptives. Accessed September 20, 2015. Available at: http://sop.washington.edu/pharmacist-prescribers-increase-access-effective-contraceptives/.

80

Menstruation-Related Disorders

Elena M. Umland and Jacqueline Klootwyk

KEY CONCEPTS

1. While a urine pregnancy test should be one of the first steps in evaluating amenorrhea, the majority of primary amenorrhea case can be attributed to either physical anomalies of the gonads, outflow tract or anomalies of the hypothalamic–pituitary axis.
2. For hypoestrogenic conditions associated with primary and secondary amenorrhea, estrogen (with a progestin) is provided.
3. Heavy menstrual bleeding (HMB) is generally caused by either systemic disorders or specific uterine abnormalities.
4. Pregnancy, including intrauterine pregnancy, ectopic pregnancy, and miscarriage, must be at the top of the differential diagnosis for any woman presenting with heavy menses.
5. When compared to other conventional medical therapies used for HMB, the levonorgestrel intrauterine system is associated with a 61% lower discontinuation rate and 82% fewer treatment failures.
6. Intrauterine devices (IUDs) are considered therapeutic options in a variety of menstruation-related disorders. Guidelines from the American College of Obstetricians and Gynecologists (ACOG) indicate that both nulliparous and multiparous women at low risk of sexually transmitted diseases are good candidates for IUD use.
7. Abnormal uterine bleeding associated with ovulatory dysfunction (AUB-O) is a spectrum of disorders commonly associated with heavy or irregular bleeding from the endometrium which primarily results from a dysfunctioning menstrual system, specifically the effects of chronic unopposed estrogen.
8. Polycystic ovary syndrome (PCOS) can present as a variety of menstruation disorders, including amenorrhea, HMB, and anovulatory bleeding. Although its definition continues to evolve, it is generally considered a disorder of androgen excess that often includes polycystic ovarian morphology and ovulatory dysfunction.
9. Metformin use for anovulatory bleeding associated with PCOS is beneficial not only for managing AUB-O and positively affecting fertility but also for improving glucose tolerance and other metabolic parameters that contribute to cardiovascular risk.
10. The selective serotonin reuptake inhibitors (SSRIs) are first-line pharmacologic treatment options for premenstrual dysphoric disorder (PMDD).

Problems related to the menstrual cycle are exceedingly common in women of reproductive age. This chapter discusses the most frequently encountered menstruation-related difficulties: amenorrhea; heavy menstrual bleeding (HMB); abnormal uterine bleeding associated with ovulatory dysfunction (AUB-O), including polycystic ovary syndrome (PCOS); dysmenorrhea; and premenstrual syndrome (PMS) and premenstrual dysphoric disorder (PMDD). The need for effective treatments of these disorders stems from their negative impact on any or all of the following: quality of life, reproductive health, and long-term detrimental health effects, such as increased risk of osteoporosis with amenorrhea and cardiovascular disease with PCOS.

AMENORRHEA

Amenorrhea is described as either primary or secondary in nature. Primary amenorrhea is the absence of menses by age 16 years in the presence of normal secondary sexual development or the absence of menses by age 14 in the absence of normal secondary sexual development.[1] Secondary amenorrhea is the absence of menses for three cycles or for 6 months in a previously menstruating woman. There is a significant amount of overlap between the two. The initial evaluation of amenorrhea is often the same, regardless of age of onset, except in unusual clinical situations.[2,3]

Epidemiology

Primary amenorrhea occurs in less than 0.1% of the general population. Secondary amenorrhea, in comparison, has an incidence of 3% to 4% in the general population and occurs more frequently in women younger than 25 years with a history of menstrual irregularities and in those involved in competitive athletics.[3]

Etiology

(1) While a urine pregnancy test should be one of the first steps in evaluating amenorrhea, the majority of primary amenorrhea cases can be attributed to either anomalies of the gonads or outflow tract or anomalies of the hypothalamic–pituitary axis.[1] Similarly, greater than 50% of secondary amenorrhea cases are due to the impact of disturbances of the hypothalamic–pituitary–adrenal axis or the hypothalamic–pituitary–ovarian axis.[3] Specifically, hypothalamic suppression, chronic anovulation, hyperprolactinemia, ovarian failure, and uterine disorders.[4] Therefore, in organizing an approach to diagnosis and treatment, it is helpful to consider the organs involved in the menstrual cycle, which include the uterus, ovaries, anterior pituitary, and hypothalamus.

Pathophysiology

Each organ in the hypothalamic–pituitary–ovarian–uterine axis is of importance in determining amenorrhea's etiology and

TABLE 80-1 Pathophysiology of Selected Menstrual Bleeding Disorders

Organ System	Condition	Pathophysiology/Laboratory Findings
Amenorrhea		
Uterus	Asherman's syndrome	Postcurettage/postsurgical uterine adhesions
	Congenital uterine abnormalities	Abnormal uterine development
Ovaries	Turner's syndrome	Lack of ovarian follicles
	Gonadal dysgenesis	Other genetic abnormalities
	Premature ovarian failure	Early loss of follicles
	Chemotherapy/radiation	Gonadal toxins
Anterior pituitary	Pituitary prolactin-secreting adenoma	↑ Prolactin suppresses the HPO axis
	Hypothyroidism	TRH causes ↑ prolactin, other abnormalities
	Medication (antipsychotics, verapamil)	↑ Prolactin suppresses the HPO axis
Hypothalamus	FHA	↓ Pulsatile GnRH secretion in the absence of other abnormalities
	Eating disorder	↓ Pulsatile GnRH secretion, ↓ FSH and LH secondary to weight loss
	Exercise	↓ Pulsatile GnRH secretion, ↓ FSH and LH secondary to low body fat
	Anovulation/PCOS	Asynchronous gonadotropin and estrogen production, abnormal endometrial growth
Abnormal Uterine Bleeding Associated with Ovulatory Dysfunction (AUB-O)		
Physiologic causes	Adolescence	Immaturity of the HPO axis: no LH surge
	Perimenopause	Declining ovarian function
Pathologic causes	Hyperandrogenic anovulation (PCOS)	Hyperandrogenism: high testosterone, high LH, hyperinsulinemia, and insulin resistance
	Hypothalamic dysfunction (physical or emotional stress, exercise, weight loss)	Suppression of pulsatile GnRH secretion and estrogen deficiency: low LH, low FSH
	Hyperprolactinemia (pituitary gland tumor, psychiatric medications)	High prolactin
	Hypothyroidism	High TSH
	Premature ovarian failure	High FSH
Heavy Menstrual Bleeding (HMB)		
Hematologic	von Willebrand disease	Factor VII defect causing impaired platelet adhesion and increased bleeding time
	Idiopathic thrombocytopenic purpura	Decrease in circulating platelets, can be acute or chronic
Hepatic	Cirrhosis	Decreased estrogen metabolism, underlying coagulopathy
Endocrine	Hypothyroidism	Alterations in the HPO axis
Uterine	Fibroids	Alteration of endometrium, changes in uterine contractility
	Adenomyosis	Alteration of endometrium, changes in uterine contractility
	Endometrial polyps	Alteration of endometrium
	Gynecologic cancers	Various dysplastic alterations of endometrium, uterus, cervix

FHA, functional hypothalamic amenorrhea; FSH, follicle-stimulating hormone; GnRH, gonadotropin-releasing hormone; HPO, hypothalamic–pituitary–ovarian axis; LH, luteinizing hormone; PCOS, polycystic ovary syndrome; TSH, thyroid-stimulating hormone; TRH, thyrotropin-releasing hormone.

Data from references 1-9, 14, and 17.

pathophysiology. Beginning with the uterus/outflow tract and progressing caudally will result in a comprehensive differential diagnosis. Table 80-1 lists the pathophysiology of amenorrhea relative to the organ system(s) involved and the specific condition(s) that results in amenorrhea.

Uterus/Outflow Tract

For menstruation to occur, a uterus, functional endometrium, and patent vagina must be present. Several anatomic abnormalities may cause amenorrhea.[1] If primary amenorrhea is the presenting symptom, a congenital anomaly such as imperforate hymen or uterine agenesis may be present and often discovered by physical examination. An acquired condition of the genital tract, such as Asherman's syndrome or cervical stenosis, is more likely in secondary amenorrhea.

Ovaries

Normal ovarian function is critical for menstruation to occur. The ovaries must respond appropriately to follicle-stimulating hormone (FSH) and luteinizing hormone (LH) by secreting estrogen and progesterone in the proper sequence to influence endometrial growth and shedding (Fig. 80-1).

Premature ovarian failure occurs when no viable follicles remain in the ovaries. This is because estrogen production is insufficient to stimulate endometrial growth in the absence of follicles. In a woman younger than 30 years, amenorrhea due to premature ovarian failure may be the result of genetic anomalies.[2]

The ovaries may play a role in amenorrhea through anovulation. Ovulation is required for the follicle (an estrogen-secreting body) to become a corpus luteum (a progesterone-secreting body). Without ovulation, the proper sequence of estrogen production, progesterone

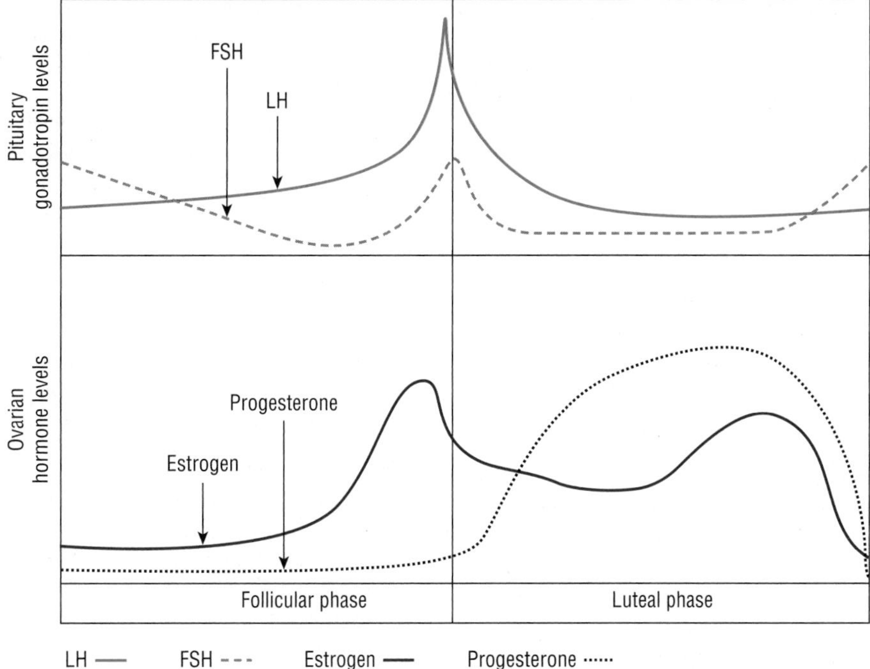

FIGURE 80-1 Hormonal fluctuations with the normal menstrual cycle. (FSH, follicle-stimulating hormone; LH, luteinizing hormone.)

production, and estrogen/progesterone withdrawal will not occur. This can result in amenorrhea. Anovulation can occur secondary to thyroid disease, androgen excess (as in PCOS), or chronic illness.

Pituitary Gland

The anterior pituitary gland secretes FSH and LH in sequential fashion in response to hypothalamic stimulation and a complex ovarian feedback mechanism. Normal secretion of FSH and LH is altered by several endocrinologic and iatrogenic conditions, including thyroid disease, hyperprolactinemia, and dopaminergic drug administration.

Hypothalamus

The hypothalamus secretes cyclic gonadotropin-releasing hormone (GnRH), which causes the pituitary to produce FSH and LH. Disrupting this cyclic process will interrupt the hormonal cascade that results in normal menstruation. Anorexia nervosa, bulimia, intense exercise, and stress may cause hypothalamic amenorrhea. Further, recent research has confirmed the role of leptin insufficiency in causing hypogonadotropic hypogonadism leading to hypothalamic amenorrhea.[10]

TREATMENT

The treatment options for amenorrhea are as varied as its causes.

Desired Outcome(s)

Therapeutic modalities for amenorrhea should ensure the occurrence of normal puberty and restore the menstrual cycle.

CLINICAL PRESENTATION Amenorrhea

General

- Although patients may be concerned about cessation of menses and implications for fertility, patients are generally not in acute distress.

Symptoms

- Patients will note cessation of menses.
- Patients may complain of infertility, vaginal dryness, or decreased libido.

Signs

- Cessation of menses for more than 6 months in women with established menstruation, absence of menses by age 16 in the presence of normal secondary sexual development, or absence of menses by age 14 in the absence of normal secondary sexual development.
- Recent significant weight loss or weight gain.
- Presence of acne, hirsutism, hair loss, or acanthosis nigrans may suggest androgen excess.

Laboratory Tests

- Pregnancy test
- Serum FSH and LH
- Thyroid-stimulating hormone
- Prolactin
- If hyperandrogenic state (ie, PCOS) is suspected, consider free and total testosterone, dehydroepiandrosterone, fasting glucose, fasting lipid panel

Other Diagnostic Tests

- Progesterone challenge to confirm functional anatomy and adequate estrogenization.
- Pelvic ultrasound to evaluate for polycystic ovaries, presence/absence of uterus, and/or structural abnormalities of the reproductive tract organs.

Treatment goals include bone density preservation, bone loss prevention, and ovulation restoration to improve fertility as desired. Amenorrhea from hypoestrogenism may affect quality of life via hot flash induction (premature ovarian failure), dyspareunia, and, in prepubertal females, lack of secondary sexual characteristics and absence of menarche. Treatment is targeted at reversing these effects.

General Approach to Treatment

The overall success of any intervention to treat amenorrhea depends on proper identification of the disorder's underlying cause(s). Once the cause is identified, the appropriate intervention(s) can be made. For patients experiencing amenorrhea secondary to hypoestrogenic states, a diet rich in calcium and vitamin D is essential to minimize any negative impact on bone health.

Nonpharmacologic Therapy

Nonpharmacologic therapy for amenorrhea varies depending upon the underlying cause. Amenorrhea secondary to anorexia may respond to weight gain. In young women for whom excessive exercise is an underlying cause, reduction of exercise quantity and intensity are important. Cognitive behavioral therapy has been shown to restore ovarian function in women with functional hypothalamic amenorrhea (FHA).[11]

Pharmacologic Therapy

2 For hypoestrogenic conditions associated with primary or secondary amenorrhea, estrogen (with a progestin) is provided. It can be administered as an oral contraceptive (OC), conjugated equine estrogen, or estradiol patch. Estrogen therapy in this patient population reduces osteoporosis risk[12] and improves quality of life. Table 80-2 lists therapeutic agents for amenorrhea treatment, including recommended doses. Figure 80-2 illustrates a treatment algorithm for management of amenorrhea.

When hyperprolactinemia is the cause of amenorrhea, dopamine agonists such as bromocriptine and cabergoline aid in reducing prolactin concentrations and the resumption of menses. Bromocriptine normalizes prolactin levels in 58% of affected women while cabergoline has the same effect in 85%.[16]

Amenorrhea related to PCOS-induced anovulation may respond to agents that reduce insulin resistance. Metformin for this purpose is discussed in the "abnormal uterine bleeding" section.

Progestins induce withdrawal bleeding in women with secondary amenorrhea, and several factors predict progesterone's efficacy for this purpose.[14] These factors include estrogen concentrations greater than or equal to 35 pg/mL (128 pmol/L) and endometrial thickness (greater initial thickness resulting in more withdrawal bleeding).

Progestin efficacy for secondary amenorrhea varies by formulation used. Progesterone in oil administered intramuscularly results in withdrawal bleeding in 70% of treated patients, whereas oral medroxyprogesterone acetate (MPA) induces withdrawal bleeding in 95% of treated patients.[14] Table 80-2 identifies the types and doses of progestins used for secondary amenorrhea treatment. Figure 80-2 illustrates when to consider progestin use for amenorrhea treatment.

Special Populations

Amenorrhea in the adolescent population is of concern because developmentally this is the time when peak bone mass is achieved. The cause of amenorrhea, whether primary or secondary, must be promptly identified, as amenorrhea and its related hypoestrogenism negatively affect bone development. In addition to treating or eliminating amenorrhea's underlying cause, ensuring that the patient is receiving adequate amounts of calcium and vitamin D is imperative. Estrogen replacement, typically via an OC, is important.

Drug Class Information

Table 80-3 identifies the significant pharmacologic properties of agents used for amenorrhea management which require monitoring.

Evaluation of Therapeutic Outcomes

Table 80-3 lists the expected outcomes and specific monitoring parameters for treatment modalities used in amenorrhea management.

HEAVY MENSTRUAL BLEEDING

Heavy menstrual bleeding is the term now used to in place of menorrhagia.[9] The classical definition, however, remains the same: menstrual blood loss greater than 80 mL per cycle or

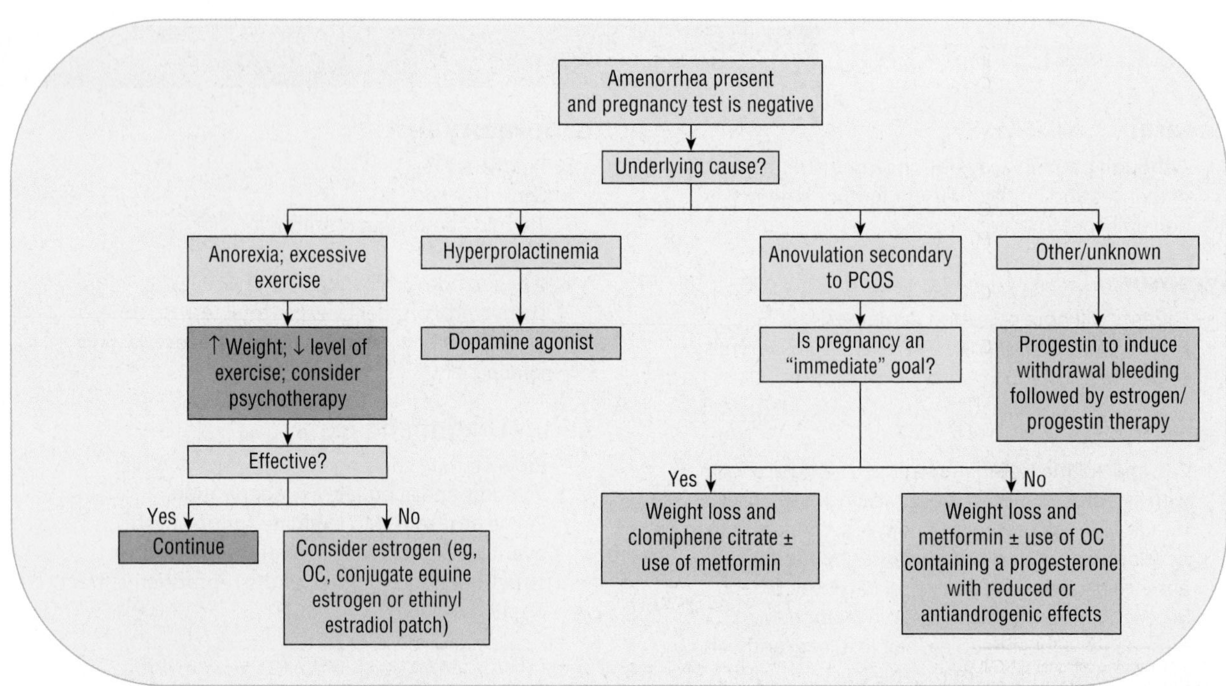

FIGURE 80-2 Treatment algorithm for amenorrhea. (OC, oral contraceptive; PCOS, polycystic ovary syndrome.)

TABLE 80-2 Therapeutic Agents for Selected Menstrual Disorders

Specific Menstrual Disorder(s)	Agent(s)	Brand Name(s)	Usual Recommended Dose
Amenorrhea (primary or secondary)[1,8,13,14]	CEE	Premarin®, Cenestin®, Enjuvia®	0.625-1.25 mg by mouth daily on days 1-25 of the cycle
	Ethinyl estradiol patch	Alora®, Climara®, Estraderm®, Vivelle-Dot®	50 mcg/24 hours
	Combination OC	Various	30-40 mcg formulations
Amenorrhea (secondary)[13,15]	Oral MPA	Provera®	5-10 mg by mouth on days 14-25 of the cycle
	Progesterone vaginal gel	Crinone®	1.125 g of 4% gel intravaginally every other day for 6 doses; if no response, increase to 8% gel for 6 doses
	Norethindrone	Aygestin®	5 mg by mouth daily for 7-10 days
	Micronized progesterone	Prometrium®	400 mg by mouth daily for 7-10 days
Amenorrhea related to hyperprolactinemia[4,16,17]	Bromocriptine	Parlodel®, Parlodel® SnapTabs	2.5-15mg daily in two to three divided doses
	Cabergoline	Dostinex®	0.25-2 mg by mouth once weekly or in two divided doses
Anovulatory bleeding	Combination OC	Desogen 28®, Ortho-Cept 28®, Yasmin 28®, Yaz®, Beyaz®, and others	≤35 mcg ethinyl estradiol
Dysmenorrhea[8,18-20]	Combination OC	Norgestrel containing: Cryselle 28®, Lo/Ovral 28® Levonorgestrel containing: Levora 28®, Nordette 28®, Aviane 28®, Lessina 28® Extended-cycle: Introvale®, Quasense®, Seasonale®, Seasonique®, LoSeasonique®, Lybrel®	<35 mcg formulations + norgestrel or levonorgestrel; use of extended-cycle formulations is beneficial for this indication
	Injectable MPA	Depo-Provera®, Depo-SubQ Provera 104®	150 mg intramuscularly or 104 mg subcutaneously every 12 weeks
	LNG-IUS	Mirena®	20 mcg released daily
	NSAIDs (any are acceptable); the most commonly studied/cited are included in this table	Diclofenac (Cataflam®); ibuprofen (Motrin®, Advil®), mefenamic acid (Ponstel®)	Diclofenac 50 mg by mouth three times daily; ibuprofen 800 mg by mouth three times daily; mefenamic acid 500 mg by mouth as a loading dose, then 250 mg by mouth up to four times daily as needed
		Naproxen (Naprosyn®)	Naproxen 550-mg loading dose by mouth started 1-2 days prior to menses followed by 275 mg by mouth every 6-12 hours as needed
	Celecoxib	Celebrex®	400 mg by mouth followed by 200 mg by mouth every 12 hours as needed during menses
Heavy Menstrual Bleeding[9,21-28]	Combination OC	Various	Optimal dose unknown
	LNG-IUS	Mirena®	20 mcg released daily
	Oral MPA	Provera®	5-10 mg by mouth on days 5-26 of the cycle or during the luteal phase
	Tranexamic acid	Lysteda®	1,300 mg by mouth every 8 hours once heavy bleeding begins; dose for 4-7 days as needed per cycle
PCOS-related amenorrhea and/or AUB-O[29,30]	Injectable MPA	Depo-Provera®, Depo-SubQ Provera 104®	150 mg intramuscularly or 104 mg subcutaneously every 12 weeks
	Combination OC[20,21]	Desogestrel containing: Desogen 28®, Ortho-Cept 28® Norgestimate containing: OrthoTri-Cyclen Lo® Drospirenone containing: Yasmin 28®, Yaz®, Beyaz®	≤30 mcg ethinyl estradiol with either desogestrel, norgestimate or drospirenone
	Oral MPA	Provera®	10 mg by mouth for 10 days[5]
	Metformin	Glucophage®, Fortamet®, Glucophage XR®, Glumetza®	1,500-2,000 mg by mouth daily[21]
PMDD[31-33]	Clomipramine	Anafranil®	25-75 mg by mouth daily taken either continuously or only during the luteal phase
	Drospirenone	Yasmin 28®, Yaz®, Beyaz®	3 mg (+ ≤30 mcg ethinyl estradiol) by mouth on days 1-21 of the menstrual cycle[23]
	Leuprolide	Lupron Depot®	3.75 mg intramuscularly[22]
	SSRIs	Citalopram = Celexa®; escitalopram = Lexapro®; fluoxetine = Prozac®, Sarafem®; paroxetine = Paxil®; sertraline = Zoloft®	Citalopram 10-30 mg; escitalopram 10-20 mg; fluoxetine 10-20 mg; fluvoxamine 50 mg; paroxetine 10-30 mg; sertraline 25-150 mg; all agents are given by mouth daily and can be dosed either continuously or during the luteal phase only
	SNRIs	Venlafaxine = Effexor®, Effexor XR®; duloxetine = Cymbalta®	Venlafaxine 50-200 mg, can be dosed continuously or during the luteal phase only; duloxetine 60 mg dosed continuously

CEE, conjugated equine estrogen; LNG-IUS, levonorgestrel intrauterine system; MPA, medroxyprogesterone acetate; NSAID, nonsteroidal anti-inflammatory drug; OC, oral contraceptive; PCOS, polycystic ovary syndrome; PMDD, premenstrual dysphoric disorder; SSRI, selective serotonin reuptake inhibitors; SNRI, serotonin norepinephrine reuptake inhibitors.

Data from references 1, 4, 8, 9, 13-33.

TABLE 80-3 Pharmacologic Properties and Monitoring Parameters for Select Agents Used in the Management of Menstrual Disorders

Therapeutic Agent/ Drug Class	Mechanism of Action/Role in Particular Menstrual Disorders	Adverse Drug Reactions	Monitoring for Expected Outcomes of Specific Menstrual Disorders	Comments
Dopamine agonists (bromocriptine and cabergoline)	Suppresses prolactin production from pituitary tumors such that resumption of normal FSH and LH production occurs	Hypotension, nausea, constipation, anorexia, Raynaud's phenomenon, fatigue, headache	Amenorrhea related to hyperprolactinemia: Baseline and weekly prolactin levels should be measured with dosage increases until resumption of menses is observed. Continue therapy for 6-12 months following return of menses and continued normalization of serum prolactin levels	Inhibits CYP3A4 and is metabolized by CYP3A4 St. John's Wort induces CP3A4; coadministration may lead to treatment failure
Clomipramine	PMDD: Exact mechanism unknown	Dry mouth, constipation, fatigue, vertigo, sweating	Reduction in or absence of initial symptoms and improved quality of life within 1-3 menstrual cycles of therapy	
Combination OCs	Exogenous estrogen and progesterone that suppresses FSH and LH production and thus inhibits ovulation Can be used to reduce menstrual flow (menorrhagia, dysmenorrhea), and control menstrual cycle (anovulatory bleeding secondary to hypoestrogenism)	Thromboembolism, breast enlargement, breast tenderness, bloating, nausea, GI upset, headache, peripheral edema	Amenorrhea: Resumption of menses within 1-2 months of therapy Anovulatory bleeding: Improvement in pattern of abnormal bleeding within 1-2 months of therapy Dysmenorrhea: Reduction in or absence of pelvic pain within 1-2 months of therapy Menorrhagia: Reduction in blood loss with menses over 1-2 months of therapy. Improvement in hemoglobin/ hematocrit after 3 months of therapy compared to baseline	St. John's Wort contributes to altered menstrual bleeding Rifampin induces estrogen metabolism, possibly contributing to treatment failure Sulfa-containing drugs may contribute to increased photosensitivity
CEE	Estrogen replacement for hypoestrogenic states leading to anovulatory bleeding	As noted for combination OC	Anovulatory bleeding: Improvement in pattern of abnormal bleeding within 1-2 months of therapy	Same as OCs
Drospirenone-containing OCs	Progesterone with antimineralocorticoid and antiandrogenic properties; decreases emotional lability associated with PMDD	As noted for combination OC; increased risk of hyperkalemia	PCOS-related amenorrhea or anovulatory bleeding: In addition to the improvement in the pattern of abnormal bleeding within 1-2 months of treatment, women should also experience an improvement in androgen-excess symptoms such as acne/oily skin and hirsutism	Same as OCs Coadministration of potassium-sparing diuretics or diets high in potassium may contribute to increased serum potassium concentrations, particularly in women with renal dysfunction
Ethinyl estradiol transdermal patch	Same as combination OCs and CEE	As noted for combination OC; however, lesser effects on serum cholesterol concentrations because patch avoids first-pass metabolism	Amenorrhea: Resumption of menses within 1-2 months of therapy	Same as OCs
Leuprolide	GnRH agent that contributes to suppression of FSH and LH and ultimately a reduction in estrogen and progesterone, inhibiting the normal menstrual cycle/hormonal fluctuations	Hot flashes, night sweats, headache, nausea	PMDD: Improvement in PMDD signs and symptoms within 1-2 months of therapy	
LNG-IUS	Suppresses FSH and LH and ultimately estrogen and progesterone, inhibiting the usual growth of the endometrium	Irregular menses, amenorrhea	Dysmenorrhea: Reduction in or absence of pelvic pain after 1-2 months of therapy Menorrhagia: Reduction in blood loss with menses over 1-2 months of therapy. Improvement in hemoglobin/ hematocrit after 3 months of therapy compared to baseline	

(continued)

TABLE 80-3 Pharmacologic Properties and Monitoring Parameters for Select Agents Used in the Management of Menstrual Disorders (*Continued*)

Therapeutic Agent/ Drug Class	Mechanism of Action/Role in Particular Menstrual Disorders	Adverse Drug Reactions	Monitoring for Expected Outcomes of Specific Menstrual Disorders	Comments
MPA (oral and injectable)	Suppresses FSH and LH and ultimately estrogen and progesterone, inhibiting the usual growth of the endometrium	Edema, anorexia, depression, insomnia, weight gain or loss, increase in serum total and LDL cholesterol, may reduce HDL cholesterol	Dysmenorrhea: Reduction in or absence of pelvic pain after 1-2 months of therapy Menorrhagia: Reduction in blood loss with menses over 1-2 months of therapy. Improvement in hemoglobin/hematocrit after 3 months of therapy compared to baseline PCOS-related amenorrhea and/or anovulatory bleeding: Resumption of menses over 1-2 courses of therapy	
Metformin	Inhibits hepatic glucose production and increases sensitivity of tissues to insulin, thus reducing insulin resistance	Anorexia, nausea, vomiting, diarrhea, flatulence, lactic acidosis (rare)	PCOS-related amenorrhea and/or anovulatory bleeding: If desired, monitor for ovulation after 3-6 months of therapy	IV contrast dye may increase the risk of lactic acidosis; stop metformin 1 day prior and restart when renal function is normal and stabilized following the IV dye
NSAIDs	Inhibits prostaglandin release that occurs with menses, thus reducing inflammatory response contributing to dysmenorrhea	GI upset, stomach ulcer, nausea, vomiting, heartburn, indigestion, rash, dizziness	Dysmenorrhea: Reduction in or absence of pelvic pain within hours of initiating. Menorrhagia: Reduction in blood loss with menses over 1-2 months of therapy	
SSRIs	Exact mechanism in PMDD unknown	Sexual dysfunction (reduced libido, anorgasmia), insomnia, sedation, hypersomnia, nausea, diarrhea	Improvement in PMDD signs and symptoms observed within 1-3 months of therapy	
Tranexamic acid	Antifibrinolytic effects by reversibly blocking lysine binding sites on plasminogen, preventing fibrin degradation and a reduction in menstrual blood loss	Nausea, vomiting, diarrhea, dyspepsia	Menorrhagia: Reduction in blood loss with menses should be noticeable with the first month of therapy. Improvement in hemoglobin/hematocrit after 3 months of therapy compared to baseline	
Venlafaxine	Exact mechanism in PMDD unknown		Improvement in PMDD signs and symptoms observed within 1-3 months of therapy	

CEE, conjugated equine estrogen; FSH, follicle-stimulating hormone; GnRH, gonadotropin-releasing hormone; HDL, high-density lipoprotein; LDL, low-density lipoprotein; LH, luteinizing hormone; LNG-IUS, levonorgestrel intrauterine system; MPA, medroxyprogesterone acetate; NSAID, nonsteroidal anti-inflammatory drug; OC, oral contraceptive; PMDD, premenstrual dysphoric disorder; SSRI, selective serotonin reuptake inhibitor.

Data from references 9, 16, 17, 19, 21-23, 28, 31-36.

menstrual bleeding lasting greater than 7 days per cycle.[9] This definition has been questioned because of difficulty quantifying menstrual loss in clinical practice. Additionally, many women with "heavy menses" but whose blood loss is less than 80 mL merit treatment consideration because of flow containment issues, unpredictably heavy flow days, or other associated symptoms.[19,37] More recently, diagnosis has also been considered based upon the impact of HMB on quality of life and social, professional, familial or sexual roles.

Epidemiology

Up to as many as 20% to 30% of women are affected by HMB,[9,21,28] and it is responsible for 12% to 15% of referrals to gynecologists.[9,21,22] In women with coagulation disorders such as von Willebrand disease or platelet dysfunction, the rates of HMB are as high as 100% and 98%, respectively.[6,38]

Etiology

While the specific cause of HMB may be unknown in up to 50% of patients, (3) HMB is generally caused by either systemic disorders or specific uterine abnormalities. (4) Pregnancy, including intrauterine pregnancy, ectopic pregnancy, and miscarriage, must be at the top of the differential diagnosis list for any woman presenting with heavy menses.[8] Bleeding disorders including von Willebrand disease, symptomatic hemophilia, platelet dysfunction, and Factory VII and XI deficiencies must also be considered as these were found to exist in 20% of women with HMB.[8] Hypothyroidism also may be associated with heavy menses.[9,39] Specific uterine causes of HMB are more common in older childbearing women and include fibroids, adenomyosis, endometrial polyps, and gynecologic malignancies.[9] Fibroids, specifically, have been identified in as many as 40% of women with HMB.[28]

Pathophysiology

Table 80-1 lists the pathophysiology of HMB relative to the organ system(s) involved and the specific conditions that may result in HMB.

TREATMENT

Effective medical treatments, as opposed to surgical interventions, are recommended as the initial treatment choice for women with HMB. Table 80-2 identifies the variety of pharmacologic treatment options and their recommended dosing for HMB management. Figure 80-3 presents an algorithm for HMB treatment.

Desired Outcome(s)

Therapy for HMB should reduce menstrual flow, improve the patient's quality of life, and defer the need for surgical intervention.

General Approach to Treatment

Several treatment options exist for HMB. Initial and subsequent treatment options should be thoughtfully chosen in an effort to avoid surgery.

Nonpharmacologic Therapy

Nonpharmacologic interventions for HMB include surgical procedures that are generally reserved for patients not responding to pharmacologic treatment. These interventions vary from conservative endometrial ablation to hysterectomy.[21,37]

Pharmacologic Therapy

Among the agents used to treat HMB, the nonsteroidal anti-inflammatory drugs (NSAIDs) have the advantage of administration only during menses and are associated with a 10% to 51% reduction in blood loss[34] For women desiring to avoid pregnancy, hormonal contraception (HC) use is beneficial for HMB and should be considered as a 40% to 50% reduction in menstrual blood loss has been observed in patients treated with cyclic combined HCs.[35] The best studied HC option for HMB, and the only OC approved by the FDA for the indication of HMB is the four-phasic formulation containing estradiol valerate and dienogest.[34,36]

Another HMB treatment option is the levonorgestrel-releasing intrauterine system (LNG-IUS). This is the most effective treatment to reduce menstrual flow.[23,34,40] In particular, a 79% to 97% reduction in blood loss has been observed with its use,[40] and its use has also resulted in postponing or cancelling scheduled endometrial ablation surgery or hysterectomy. Among women using this treatment option, only 9% eventually opted for surgery.[34] Further, its therapeutic efficacy is similar to endometrial ablation up to 2 years following treatment.[24]

Cyclic progesterone therapy for 21 days, starting on day 5 after onset of menses, results in a 37% to 87% reduction in menstrual blood loss.[28] While progesterone use provides no benefit in efficacy over other medical treatments,[28] its use may be considered in women with contraindications to estrogen.[34]

Tranexamic acid was recently approved in the United States for primary HMB treatment. Its use is associated with a significant 34% to 60% reduction in menstrual blood loss.[28,41] Compared to many of the other options, its use may be preferable among women desiring pregnancy or in whom hormonal therapy may not be appropriate.

Drug Treatments of First Choice For women in whom pregnancy is not an immediate goal, it is reasonable to start with either an OC or the LNG-IUS. While either choice is acceptable for both nulligravid and multiparous women who desire a long-term reversible form of contraception,[35,40] cost-effectiveness data suggest LNG-IUS is the best first-line choice for women desiring contraception.[28,37] Clinical trial data illustrate a higher failure rate with the OCs (32%) compared to the LNG-IUS (11%) as the primary treatment method.[28] 5 When compared to other conventional medical therapies used for HMB, the levonorgestrel intrauterine system is

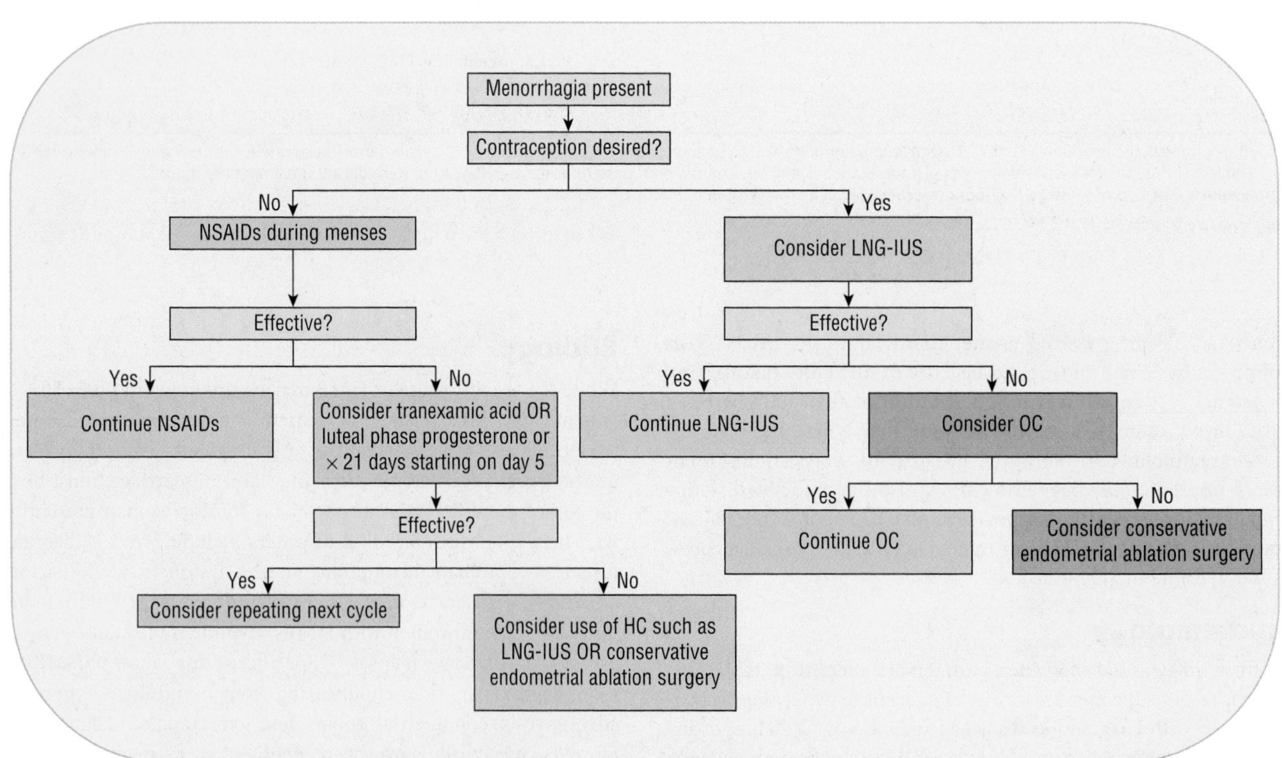

FIGURE 80-3 Treatment algorithm for HMB. (LNG-IUS, levonorgestrel-releasing intrauterine system; NSAIDs, nonsteroidal anti-inflammatory drugs; OC, oral contraceptive; HC, hormonal cotraceptive.)

CLINICAL PRESENTATION Heavy Menstrual Bleeding

General

- Patients may or may not be in acute distress.

Symptoms

- Patients may complain of heavy/prolonged menstrual flow. They also may have signs of fatigue and lightheadedness in cases of severe blood loss. These symptoms may or may not occur with dysmenorrhea.

Signs

- Orthostasis, tachycardia, and pallor may be noted, especially in cases of significant acute blood loss.

Laboratory Tests

- Complete blood count and ferritin levels; hemoglobin and hematocrit results may be low.
- If the history dictates, testing (eg, prothrombin time, activated partial thromboplastin time, international normalized ratio, von Willebrand factor antigen, Factor VIII) may be performed to identify coagulation disorder(s) as a cause.

Other Diagnostic Tests

- Pelvic ultrasound
- Pelvic magnetic resonance imaging
- Papanicolaou (Pap) smear
- Endometrial biopsy
- Hysteroscopy
- Sonohysterogram

associated with a 61% lower discontinuation rate and 82% fewer treatment failures.[23]

Alternative Drug Treatments For women who have HMB associated with ovulatory cycles and do not desire hormonal therapy and/or contraception, NSAIDs during menses is a reasonable choice in the absence of any contraindications or GI illnesses such as peptic ulcer disease or gastroesophageal reflux disease. This choice is convenient (only taken during menses) and comparatively inexpensive. Given their side effects, reduced efficacy compared to the first-line agents, and/or cost, use of oral progesterone and depot MPA should be reserved. Tranexamic acid is another treatment option which has been associated with a significant improvement in quality of life and high patient satisfaction following three cycles of use.[27,42]

Special Populations

Although historically it was believed that IUD use should be avoided in nulliparous women, 6 guidelines from the American College of Obstetricians and Gynecologists (ACOG) indicate that both nulliparous and multiparous women at low risk of sexually transmitted diseases are good candidates for IUD use.[40] Therefore, any of the treatments discussed (including the LNG IUS) are options in any female presenting with HMB.

Dosage adjustment for tranexamic acid is recommended for reduced renal function. Women with serum creatinine between 1.4 and 2.8 mg/dL (124 and 248 μmol/L) should receive only 1,300 mg by mouth twice daily; women with serum creatinine between 2.9 and 5.7 mg/dL (256 and 504 μmol/L) should receive 1,300 mg by mouth once daily; those with serum creatinine above 5.7 mg/dL (504 μmol/L) should receive 650 mg by mouth once daily. Additionally, due to its potential to increase the risk for venous thromboembolism, it should be used with extreme caution in women with a history of thrombosis and should not be combined with estrogen-containing contraceptives.

Drug Class Information

Table 80-3 identifies the significant pharmacologic properties of agents used for the management of HMB that require monitoring.

Evaluation of Therapeutic Outcomes

Table 80-3 illustrates the expected outcomes and specific monitoring parameters for the treatment modalities used in HMB management.

ABNORMAL UTERINE BLEEDING WITH OVULATORY DYSFUNCTION

7 Abnormal uterine bleeding associated with ovulatory dysfunction (AUB-O) is a spectrum of disorders commonly associated with heavy or irregular bleeding from the endometrium which primarily results from a dysfunctioning menstrual system, specifically the effects of chronic unopposed estrogen.[7] While it does encompass bleeding patterns such as HMB and amenorrhea, this section will focus specifically on AUB-O as it relates to oligo-anovulation.

Epidemiology

One of the most common causes of AUB-O is PCOS, for which the prevalence rates range from 6% to 25%.[30] In fact, PCOS is the most common endocrine abnormality among US women of reproductive age.[43] 8 PCOS can present as a variety of menstruation disorders, including amenorrhea, HMB, and/or AUB-O. Although its exact definition continues to evolve, it is a disorder of androgen excess that often includes polycystic ovarian morphology and ovulatory dysfunction. It is a significant risk factor for the metabolic syndrome, type 2 diabetes, dyslipidemia, hypertension, and possibly cardiovascular disease.[30] PCOS is a common cause of ovulation dysfunction in adult women, with other common causes including hyperprolactinemia, hypothalamic amenorrhea, also known as hypogonadotropic hypogonadism, premature ovarian failure, and thyroid dysfunction.[2,7]

Etiology

When considering the etiology of AUB-O, the patient's age must be taken into account. As previously discussed, all patients presenting with abnormal bleeding should be evaluated for pregnancy. It is common for adolescents to experience physiologic anovulatory cycles in the first few years following menarche because their hypothalamic–pituitary–gonadal axis is still maturing. However, if regular menstrual cycles have not been established within 5 years of menarche, further evaluation for the cause, such as PCOS, should be considered.[30] Anovulatory cycles may "unmask" an underlying bleeding disorder. When irregular menses is associated with significant bleeding, an inherited bleeding disorder should be a considered as a cause, especially in adolescence.[6] Women experiencing anovulation in their reproductive years should be evaluated for pathologic causes, including PCOS, thyroid dysfunction, hyperprolactinemia, primary pituitary disease, premature ovarian failure, hypothalamic dysfunction, disordered eating, adrenal disease, and androgen-producing tumors.[7] Women in their perimenopausal years may experience "physiologic" anovulatory cycles because of intermittently declining estrogen levels. Regardless of age, evaluation for endometrial hyperplasia and/or endometrial cancer should be considered when a woman experiences excessive bleeding with anovulatory cycles.[7,34] When considering the etiology of anovulation, it is common for several conditions to coexist (eg, PCOS and hypothyroidism), each contributing to the woman's constellation of symptoms.

Pathophysiology

Normal menstrual cycles occur through a complex interaction of the hypothalamus, pituitary gland, ovaries, and endometrium (see Fig. 80-1). In an ovulatory cycle, the ovary produces a mature, estrogen-secreting follicle in response to FSH release from the pituitary. The endometrium proliferates under the influence of this estrogen production. At a critical level of estrogen concentration, the pituitary responds by producing an "LH surge," which creates a cascade of ovarian events, culminating in ovulation. Upon oocyte release, the follicle becomes a progesterone-producing corpus luteum. The endometrium "organizes" into secretory endometrium in the presence of adequate progesterone. If conception and implantation do not occur, corpus luteum involution causes a decline in estrogen and progesterone leading to predictable, organized menstrual flow as the endometrium sloughs.

If ovulation does not occur, progesterone is not produced, and the endometrium will continue to proliferate in an "unorganized" fashion under the influence of continued estrogen production. Eventually the endometrium will become so thick that it can no longer be supported by continued estrogen production. This results in unorganized, sporadic sloughing of the endometrium, characteristic of the unpredictable and heavy bleeding associated with anovulation, which has several etiologies dependent on the patient's situation. In adolescence, hypothalamic–pituitary axis immaturity contributes to the absence of the LH surge required for ovulation. In the anorexic patient, the hypothalamus loses much of its pulsatile GnRH release, leading to low levels of FSH and LH, enough for estrogen production but not enough to induce ovulation. Oocyte decline and abnormal follicular development contribute to anovulatory cycles common among women in the perimenopause transition.[7]

Clinical **Controversy...**

DIAGNOSIS OF PCOS IN ADOLESCENTS[44]

The criteria for diagnosing PCOS in adolescents are controversial as the pathologic features used for the diagnosis in adults, specifically acne and irregular menses, may be normal pubertal occurrences. It is difficult to ascertain that adolescent hyperandrogenism (as opposed to adult hyperandrogenism) is not a consequence of the lack of synchronicity among the hypothalamic–pituitary–ovarian (HPO) axis during prolonged anovulatory cycles that are typical during puberty. In this patient population, obesity, increased insulin and increased androgens are common, and as such, should not be used in diagnosing PCOS. More research is needed to definitively identify the appropriate diagnosis of PCOS among adolescents so that appropriate treatment(s) can be recommended.

TREATMENT

Optimizing therapy for AUB-O depends on accurate identification of the disorder's cause(s). The treatment options for AUB-O are wide and varied.

Desired Outcome(s)

When applicable, control of excessive bleeding in the short-term is paramount. Longer-term goals of therapy include restoring the natural cycle of orderly endometrial growth and shedding,[7,45] decreasing anovulation complications (eg, osteopenia and infertility), and improving overall quality of life. Table 80-2 identifies the agents used to manage AUB-O and their recommended doses.

General Approach to Treatment

Although the appropriate primary treatment choice for AUB-O depends on the accurate diagnosis of its cause and identification of desired outcomes, additional treatment may be necessary to manage other signs and symptoms. Medical treatment, as opposed to surgical management, to resolve AUB-O should be initiated and any underlying HMB should be managed as AUB-O is primarily an endocrinologic abnormality.[7]

CLINICAL PRESENTATION Abnormal Uterine Bleeding with Ovulatory Dysfunction

General

- Patients may or may not be in acute distress.

Symptoms

- Irregular, heavy, or prolonged uterine bleeding, perimenopausal symptoms (eg, hot flashes, night sweats, and vaginal dryness).

Signs

- Acne, hirsutism, and obesity

Laboratory Tests

- Pregnancy testing
- If PCOS is suspected, consider free or total testosterone, fasting glucose, fasting lipid panel
- If perimenopause is suspected, measure FSH
- Thyroid-stimulating hormone

Other Diagnostic Tests

- Endometrial biopsy for women with risk factors for endometrial hyperplasia or malignancy
- Pelvic ultrasound to evaluate for polycystic ovaries
- If perimenopause is suspected, measure FSH

Nonpharmacologic Therapy

Nonpharmacologic treatment options for AUB-O depend on the underlying cause. In a woman of reproductive age with PCOS, moderate weight loss of 2% to 5% may result in improved menstrual regularity and ovulatory function, reduced hirsutism, increased insulin sensitivity, and improved response to fertility treatments.[46] Further, sustained weight loss has resulted in a return to ovulatory cycles in women without PCOS who experienced anovulatory cycles.[7] In women who have completed childbearing or who have not responded to medical management, endometrial ablation or resection and hysterectomy are surgical options. In the short term, ablation results in less morbidity and shorter recovery periods compared to other surgical interventions. Importantly, procedure choice involves shared decision-making with the patient.

Pharmacologic Therapy

Estrogen is the recommended treatment for managing acute severe bleeding episodes because it promotes endometrial stabilization.[47] Following its initial use to control acute bleeding episodes, therapy continuation may be necessary to prevent future occurrences. HC use fulfills this role and contributes to predictable menstrual cycles.

Hormonal contraceptives prevent recurrent AUB-O by providing a progestin and suppressing ovarian hormones and adrenal androgen production. They also, indirectly, increase sex hormone-binding globulin (SHBG) which binds androgens and reduces their circulating free concentrations. For women with high androgen levels and its related signs such as hirsutism (eg, those with PCOS), HCs containing less than or equal to 35 mcg of ethinyl estradiol and a progesterone that exhibits minimal androgenic side effects (eg, norgestimate and desogestrel) or with antiandrogenic effects (eg, drospirenone) may be desirable.[29]

Clinical **Controversy...**

PROGESTERONE IN PCOS

Hormonal contraceptives containing antiandrogenic progesterones are very effective for managing the acne and hirsutism that accompany PCOS; they also suppress ovarian androgen production and increase SHBG, thus reducing free testosterone concentrations. Controversy regarding their use in PCOS exists secondary to their potential adverse effects on insulin resistance, glucose tolerance, vascular reactivity, and coagulability.[29] An increase in high-sensitivity C-reactive protein (a predictor of cardiovascular disease) and an increase in homocysteine levels (indicating an increased risk of cardiovascular disease) have been observed with the use of such OCs.[48] Another trial found a reduction in brachial artery flow-mediated dilatation and an increase in carotid intima-media thickness, both indicators of endothelial dysfunction, following therapy with OCs containing ethinyl estradiol and cyproterone acetate in women with PCOS.[49] Additional, longer-term clinical trials will clarify whether the benefits of these agents outweigh the risks. It has been suggested that cardiovascular risk calculators be employed as an adjunct to guidelines suggesting the use of OCs in this patient population.[50]

In women with contraindication(s) to estrogen or in whom the side effects are unacceptable, progesterone-only products are an option. They should be strongly considered for women experiencing HMB associated with anovulatory cycles.[7] In women with PCOS, depot and intermittent oral MPA provide endometrial protection through endometrial shedding.[5] Another progesterone option is placement of the LNG-IUS,[7,51] particularly if pregnancy is not a desired outcome of treatment. Studied specifically in women over 30 years of age, use of the LNG-IUS resulted in a greater than 95% reduction in menstrual blood loss by 2 years[52] and patient satisfaction rates were greater than 80% with 74% agreeing to recommend it to other women.[52]

Metformin improves insulin sensitivity. In patients with PCOS, which contributes to reduced circulating androgen concentrations and increased ovulation rates.[30,45] These improvements occur due to the SHBG increase that occurs via increased insulin sensitivity.

9 Metformin use for AUB-O associated with PCOS is beneficial not only for managing the AUB-O and positively affecting fertility but also for improving glucose tolerance and other metabolic parameters that contribute to cardiovascular risk.[7,30]

If the treatment goal is improved fertility via ovulation induction, clomiphene citrate is another option. Treatment with 50 mg/day for 5 days can be initiated between menstrual cycle days 3 and 5. This often occurs after inducing withdrawal bleeding with a progesterone such as MPA 10 mg daily orally for 10 days. If ovulation does not occur with this dose of clomiphene, a dose of 100 mg/day is warranted. In rare instances, it may be increased by 50 mg increments up to 250 mg/day.

Drug Treatments of First Choice As with many menstruation-related disorders, there is not one universal treatment option of first choice for AUB-O. Rather, the treatment(s) chosen depends on accurate etiologic diagnosis as well as identification of the desired treatment outcome(s).

Hormonal contraceptives are the first-choice treatment in women with AUB-O who do not desire pregnancy.[7] The use of HCs containing ethinyl estradiol and a progesterone with minimal androgenic or antiandrogenic effects is effective for cycle control and minimizing the androgenic signs and symptoms of PCOS.[29,47]

Relative to anovulation in women with PCOS, insulin-sensitizing agents such as metformin may improve ovulatory frequency and metabolic parameters. Clomiphene use may further assist in achieving ovulation induction.

More recent data provide evidence for additional benefits of metformin's use compared to clomiphene for ovulation induction.[45] When used for ovulation induction[45] as well as its use throughout pregnancy[53] in women with PCOS, metformin has also been associated with reduced miscarriage rates in this patient population.

Clinical **Controversy...**

LETROZOLE USE FOR PCOS/AUB-O[54,55]

The use of letrozole, an aromatase inhibitor, for ovulation induction has recently been examined in obese patients with PCOS, but remains controversial. Letrozole has been shown to have statistically significant higher rates of live births (27.5% vs 19.1%) and ovulation rates (61.7% vs 48.3%) over clomiphene citrate. These patients had an average BMI of 35 kg/m^2.[54] Fetal teratogenicity is a concern with both letrozole and clomiphene. While clomiphene is FDA approved for ovulation induction in premenopausal women, letrozole is only approved for breast cancer in postmenopausal women. Additionally, a recent meta-analysis evaluating aromatase inhibitors for anovulatory bleeding in women with PCOS concluded that the evidence was of low quality and that further research is warranted.

Special Populations

Anovulatory cycles are fairly common in the perimenarchal reproductive years. Ovulation typically is established 1 year or more following menarche. AUB-O occurring in this population may be excessive. If excessive bleeding occurs, the patient should be evaluated for bleeding disorders, as the prevalence of bleeding disorders, including von Willebrand disease, prothrombin deficiency, and idiopathic thrombocytopenia purpura, in this population ranges from 5% to 24%.[6]

If identified, the specific bleeding disorders should be treated. Acute severe bleeding can be managed with high-dose estrogen. OCs containing less than or equal to 35 mcg of ethinyl estradiol is a first-line treatment in adolescents with chronic anovulation.[47]

Drug Class Information

Table 80-3 identifies the significant pharmacologic properties of agents used to treat AUB-O that require monitoring.

Personalized Pharmacotherapy

While not typically an issue among the relatively young population of patients treated with metformin for PCOS, one must be cognizant of the risk of lactic acidosis in metformin users with renal impairment. As such, this drug should be avoided in women with serum creatinine greater than 1.4 mg/dL (124 μmol/L).

Evaluation of Therapeutic Outcomes

Table 80-3 lists the expected outcomes and specific monitoring parameters for the treatment modalities used to manage AUB-O.

DYSMENORRHEA

Dysmenorrhea is one of the most commonly encountered gynecologic complaints. It is defined as crampy pelvic pain occurring with or just prior to menses. Primary dysmenorrhea implies pain in the setting of normal pelvic anatomy and physiology.[56] Secondary dysmenorrhea is associated with underlying pelvic pathology.[57]

Epidemiology

Dysmenorrhea prevalence rates range from 16% to 90%,[57-59] and its presence may be associated with significant interference in work and school attendance. In addition, significant reductions in quality of life and lower overall life satisfaction and contentment ratings have been observed in women with dysmenorrhea compared to controls.[56] Risk factors include menarche before the age of 12 years, current age less than 30 years, heavy menses, nulliparity, low body mass index, and a history of sexual abuse.[57]

Etiology

For most patients, dysmenorrhea is associated with normal ovulatory cycles and normal pelvic anatomy. This is referred to as primary, or functional, dysmenorrhea. However, in approximately 10% of the adolescents and young adults presenting with painful menses, an underlying anatomic or physiologic cause exists.[57] Comparatively, secondary dysmenorrhea associated with pelvic pathology should be suspected in women over 30 years of age without a history of dysmenorrhea.[57]

Pathophysiology

The most significant mechanism for primary dysmenorrhea is the release of prostaglandins and leukotrienes into the menstrual fluid, initiating an inflammatory response and possibly vasopressin-mediated vasoconstriction.[8,19] Causes of secondary dysmenorrhea include endometriosis, current or history of pelvic inflammatory disease, uterine fibroids, and adenomyosis leiomyomata.[57] Pregnancy and miscarriage must be considered in new onset dysmenorrhea.

TREATMENT

Initial treatment choice is influenced by whether or not the woman desires pregnancy. Nonpharmacologic options have been studied and observed to be as effective as some existing pharmacologic options.

Desired Outcome(s)

Medical management of dysmenorrhea should relieve the pelvic pain, result in reducing lost school and work days, and contribute to an improved quality of life. Table 80-2 identifies the agents used to manage dysmenorrhea and their recommended doses. Figure 80-4 shows a treatment algorithm for dysmenorrhea management.

General Approach to Treatment

A variety of effective treatment options for dysmenorrhea are available, including nonhormonal and hormonal pharmacologic options and noninvasive nonpharmacologic options. Treatment choice is influenced by the desire for contraception, the patient's level of sexual activity, potential for adverse effects, and cost.

CLINICAL PRESENTATION Dysmenorrhea

General

- Patients may or may not be in acute distress, depending on the level of menstrual pain experienced

Symptoms

- Patients complain of crampy pelvic pain beginning shortly before or at the onset of menses. Symptoms typically last from 8 to 72 hours.
- Associated symptoms may include low back pain, headache, diarrhea, fatigue, and/or nausea and vomiting.

Laboratory Tests

- Pelvic examination should be performed to screen for sexually transmitted diseases and/or pelvic inflammatory disease as a cause of the pain in sexually active females.
- Gonorrhea, Chlamydia cultures or polymerase chain reaction, wet mount.

Other Diagnostic Tests

- Transvaginal/pelvic ultrasound can be used to identify potential anatomic abnormalities such as masses/lesions or to detect ovarian cysts and endometriomas.

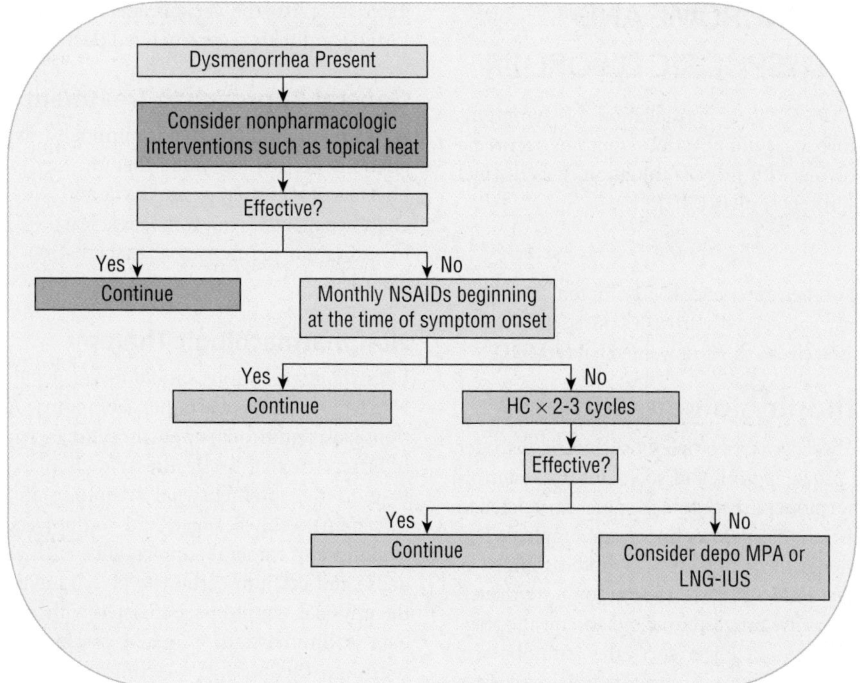

FIGURE 80-4 Treatment algorithm for dysmenorrhea. (LNG-IUS, levonorgestrel-releasing intrauterine system; MPA, medroxyprogesterone acetate; NSAIDs, nonsteroidal anti-inflammatory drugs; HC, hormonal contraceptive.)

Nonpharmacologic Therapy

Several nonpharmacologic interventions are used for managing dysmenorrhea. Among these, topical heat therapy, exercise, and a low-fat vegetarian diet have been shown to reduce dysmenorrhea intensity.[57,58,60] Dietary changes may shorten dysmenorrhea duration. Topical heat application via an abdominal patch is as effective as 400 mg of ibuprofen dosed three times daily.[60,61] Because topical heat, exercise, and dietary changes do not impart systemic effects, they are associated with little to no risk compared to the pharmacologic options. Recent data is suggestive of the benefits of powdered ginger (250 mg by mouth every 6 hours) in significantly reducing the pain associated with dysmenorrhea when begun at the onset of menses.[62,63] Nonpharmacologic options that are reserved for use following a failed trial of pharmacologic interventions include transcutaneous electric nerve stimulation, acupressure, and acupuncture.[58]

Pharmacologic Therapy

Given the role of prostaglandins in dysmenorrhea pathophysiology, NSAIDs are the initial treatment of choice. These agents do not differ in efficacy. The most commonly used agents are naproxen and ibuprofen.

All NSAIDs have a propensity for causing GI distress and ulceration; their administration with food or milk minimizes these effects. In women who have a history of NSAID-induced gastric effects, the use of celecoxib, a cyclo-oxygenase-2 (COX-2) inhibitor, is an alternative.[19,20] Choice of one agent over another may be based on cost, convenience, and patient preference. Some research suggests that NSAID therapy should begin at the onset of menses or perhaps even the day before and continued around the clock instead of waiting until symptom onset. The data substantiating this are weak.[58] Acetaminophen is inferior to NSAID in treatment of this disorder.[58] If an NSAID or celecoxib use is contraindicated or not desired, hormonal agents should be considered.

Hormonal contraceptives improve dysmenorrhea by inhibiting endometrial tissue proliferation which reduces endometrial-derived prostaglandins that cause the pelvic pain.[8,58] Significant improvements in mild, moderate, and severe dysmenorrhea have been noted with HCs. Evidence supporting monophasic versus multiphase OC regimens, however, is lacking. And while the use of extended-cycle OCs would be desirable for this purpose, data illustrating their superiority over traditional monthly OCs do not currently exist.

Long-acting progesterones, such as depot MPA and the LNG-IUS, can be considered for dysmenorrhea treatment. Their efficacy is secondary to their ability to render most patients amenorrheic within 6 to 12 months of use.[8,58] Because the pelvic pain of dysmenorrhea is related to the prostaglandins released during menses, in the setting of amenorrhea the underlying cause of dysmenorrhea is removed.

Drug Treatments of First Choice Several factors influence the choice of first-line treatment for dysmenorrhea. If contraception is desired, then a hormonal option may be considered taking into account cost, adherence issues, and side effects. If contraception is not desired, then NSAID use would be desirable from cost and convenience standpoints. If NSAIDs are not tolerated, celecoxib could be recommended. In patients for whom OCs, NSAIDs, or celecoxib is not an option, topical heat should be considered.

Special Populations

Dysmenorrhea is common in adolescent females. The treatment measures used for adult patients are also appropriate for adolescents. Although NSAIDs, topical heat, and OCs are among the top choices, use of the levonorgestrel IUD is also an option.[40]

Drug Class Information

Table 80-3 identifies the significant pharmacologic properties for agents used to treat dysmenorrhea that require monitoring.

Evaluation of Therapeutic Outcomes

Table 80-3 lists the expected outcomes and specific monitoring parameters for the treatment modalities used in the management of dysmenorrhea.

PREMENSTRUAL SYNDROME AND PREMENSTRUAL DYSPHORIC DISORDER

Premenstrual syndrome (PMS) is a constellation of symptoms including mild mood disturbances and physical symptoms occurring prior to menses and resolving with menses initiation. It is distinct from Premenstrual Dysphoric Disorder (PMDD).

Epidemiology

Up to 80% of menstruating women experience PMS symptoms.[64,65] However, a spectrum of premenstrual mood disturbances exists, and PMDD is the most severe. Approximately 3% to 9% of women have PMDD.[64-66]

Etiology and Pathophysiology

Premenstrual dysphoric disorder is a complex psychiatric disorder with multiple biological, psychological, and sociocultural determinants.[67] Although cyclic hormonal changes are in some way related to PMS and PMDD, the association is neither linear nor simple. When ovulation is suppressed medically or surgically, symptoms improve. Some evidence suggests that PMS and PMDD symptoms are related to low levels of the centrally active progesterone metabolite allopregnanolone in the luteal phase and/or lower cortical γ-aminobutyric acid levels in the follicular phase.[67] A number of studies suggest a link between PMS and PMDD and low serotonin levels.[67] Despite similar affective symptoms, hypothalamic–pituitary–adrenal (HPA) axis function in PMS and PMDD is distinct from that seen in major depressive disorder. Specifically, women with PMS show a decrease in stimulated HPA axis response, whereas this response is increased in women with major depressive disorder. Although several cross-cultural studies suggest that PMS physical symptoms are consistent across cultures, the negative affective symptoms are part of the negative "menstrual socialization" in western culture.[2,67]

TREATMENT

Women experiencing PMS and PMDD symptoms miss significantly more work and school than do controls. They also report significant impairment of their ability to participate in social activities and hobbies and in their relationships with others.[66] Given this, the need for effective treatment modalities is clear.

Desired Outcome

Premenstrual syndrome and PMDD interventions should alleviate the presenting symptoms and subsequently improve quality of life. Table 80-2 lists the various agents used in the managing PMS and PMDD and their recommended dosing.

General Approach to Treatment

A treatment modality that is minimally invasive or without systemic effects is desired for initial therapy. Key to the successful choice of pharmacologic therapy for PMS and PMDD is having the patient chart her specific symptoms for at least two menstrual cycles to assist in ruling out premenstrual exacerbation of underlying psychiatric disorders.

Nonpharmacologic Therapy

Lifestyle interventions should be started and followed for 2 months while the patient charts her symptoms. Although these interventions lack significant supporting clinical trial data, anecdotal reports of efficacy exist. Some lifestyle changes for women with mild-to-moderate premenstrual symptoms include minimizing intake of caffeine, refined sugar, and sodium and increasing exercise.[31,33] Vitamin and mineral supplements, such as vitamin B_6 (50-100 mg daily) and calcium carbonate (1,200 mg daily), may help to reduce the physical symptoms associated with PMS; however, clinical trial data is limited and/or mixed precluding a definitive conclusion regarding their use.[31,33] A clinical trial review concludes that the following options lack efficacy and safety data and should not be recommended: herbal medicines, homeopathic remedies, dietary supplements, relaxation, massage therapy, reflexology, chiropractic treatments, and biofeedback.[68,69]

Pharmacologic Therapy

If symptoms persist after 2 months of symptom charting and lifestyle modifications, pharmacologic therapy for PMDD management is warranted. Most recent investigations have focused on the selective serotonin reuptake inhibitors (SSRIs) for this disorder.[70] Studies have revealed very positive results relative to most symptoms associated with PMDD. Other agents that have been studied and are alternatives include the selective serotonin–norepinephrine reuptake inhibitor (SNRI) venlafaxine, as well as HCs and GnRH agonists.

Drug Treatments of First Choice 10 The first-line pharmacologic treatment options for PMDD are the SSRIs.[31,33,36,71] Among this class of agents, data support the use of citalopram, escitalopram, fluoxetine, fluvoxamine, paroxetine, and sertraline. Current research evaluating the dosing of these agents continuously or only during the luteal phase has illustrated similar efficacy between the two regimens such that one regimen cannot be recommended over another.[33,36,70,71] The optimal duration of treatment is still not

CLINICAL PRESENTATION PMDD

A summary of the American Psychiatric Association's criteria for PMDD is as follows:[2,36,67]

- Symptoms are temporally associated with the last week of the luteal phase and remit with onset of menses.
- At least five of the following symptoms are present: affective lability, anger or irritability often characterized by interpersonal conflicts, markedly depressed mood, anxiety, decreased interest in activities, fatigue, difficulty concentrating, changes in appetite, sleep disturbance, feelings of being overwhelmed, and physical symptoms, such as breast tenderness or bloating.
- One of the symptoms must be affective lability, irritability, markedly depressed mood, or anxiety.
- Symptoms interfere significantly with work and/or social relationships.
- Symptoms are not an exacerbation of another underlying psychiatric disorder.
- The criteria are confirmed prospectively by daily ratings over two menstrual cycles and must have occurred during most menstrual cycles in the past year.

evident as relapse within 6 to 8 months of therapy discontinuation has been observed in at least half of all treated patients.[71] The use of paroxetine, specifically, may be questioned, as this agent has been associated with an increased risk of congenital abnormalities when taken during the first trimester of pregnancy.[31] Paroxetine use should be avoided in women of childbearing age who do not use a reliable form of contraception.

The SSRIs are efficacious in approximately 60% of treated patients compared to less than 30% of those receiving placebo.[31,71] An adequate therapeutic trial is at least two menstrual cycles.[71]

Alternative Drug Treatments The SNRI, venlafaxine, has been studied for PMDD and, similar to the SSRIs, found to result in a 58% or greater improvement in symptoms in more than half of the treated patients.[31,33]

The use of a monophasic OC containing 20 mcg of ethinyl estradiol and 3 mg of drospirenone, a progesterone with antiandrogenic effects, improves premenstrual symptoms in women with PMDD.[32] The continuous cycle HC regimen delivering 90 mcg of levonorgestrel and 20 mcg of ethinyl estradiol daily has also been studied in controlled trials resulting in a 30% to 59% improvement in symptoms.[72] As with the SSRI and SNRI agents, optimal treatment duration is unknown, and superiority of one HC relative to another OC has not been established.

If treatment with the above options is unsuccessful, hormonal treatment with a GnRH agonist, such as leuprolide, can be considered.[31] Leuprolide improves premenstrual emotional symptoms as well as some physical symptoms, such as bloating and breast tenderness. However, its cost, the need for intramuscular administration, and its hypoestrogenism side effects (eg, vaginal dryness, hot flashes, and bone demineralization) severely limit its use.

Drug Class Information

Table 80-3 lists the significant pharmacologic properties for agents used to treat PMDD that require monitoring.

Personalized Pharmacotherapy

It is important that concomitant drug therapy of women prescribed any of the SSRIs or venlafaxine be evaluated closely for pharmacokinetic drug–drug interactions given the interface of these drugs with cytochrome P450 isoenzyme systems.

Evaluation of Therapeutic Outcomes

Table 80-3 lists the expected outcomes and specific monitoring parameters for the treatment modalities used in PMDD management.

ABBREVIATIONS

ACOG	American College of Obstetricians and Gynecologists
AUB-O	abnormal uterine bleeding with ovulatory dysfunction
COX-2	cyclo-oxygenase-2
FHA	functional hypothalamic amenorrhea
FSH	follicle-stimulating hormone
GnRH	gonadotropin-releasing hormone
HC	hormonal contraceptive
HMB	heavy menstrual bleeding
HPA	hypothalamic–pituitary–adrenal
HPO	hypothalamic–pituitary–ovarian
IUDs	Intrauterine devices
LH	luteinizing hormone
LNG-IUS	levonorgestrel-releasing intrauterine system
MPA	medroxyprogesterone acetate
NSAID	nonsteroidal anti-inflammatory drug
OC	oral contraceptive
PCOS	polycystic ovary syndrome
PMDD	premenstrual dysphoric disorder
PMS	premenstrual syndrome
SHBG	sex hormone-binding globulin
SNRI	serotonin–norepinephrine reuptake inhibitor
SSRI	selective serotonin reuptake inhibitor

REFERENCES

1. Marsh CA, Grimstad FW. Primary amenorrhea: Diagnosis and management. *Obstetrical & Gynecological Survey* 2014;69(10):603-612.
2. Fritz MA, Speroff L. *Clinical Gynecologic Endocrinology and Infertility*. 8th ed. Philadelphia: Lippincott Williams & Wilkins; 2010:435-493, 591-619.
3. Fourman LT, Fazeli PK. Neuroendocrine causes of amenorrhea—an update. *J Clin Endocrinol Metab* 2015;100(3):812-824.
4. Heiman DL. Amenorrhea. *Prim Care Clin Office Pract* 2009;36:1-17.
5. Klein DA, Poth MA. Amenorrhea: An approach to diagnosis and management. *Am Fam Physician* 2013;87(11):781-788.
6. James AH, Kouides PA, Abdul-Kadir R, et al. Von Willebrand disease and other bleeding disorders in women: Consensus on diagnosis and management from an international expert panel. *Am J Obstet Gynecol* 2009;201:12.e1-e8.
7. The American College of Obstetricians and Gynecologists. ACOG Practice Bulletin No. 136. Management of abnormal uterine bleeding associated with ovulatory dysfunction. *Obstet Gynecol* 2013;122(1):176-185.
8. Jamieson MA. Disorders of menstruation in adolescent girls. *Pediatr Clin N Amer* 2015;62:943-961.
9. Uhm S, Perriera L. Hormonal contraception as treatment for heavy menstrual bleeding: A systematic review. *Clin Obstet Gynecol* 2014;57(4):694-717.
10. Chou SH, Mantzoros C. 20 Years of leptin: Role of leptin in human reproductive disorders. *J Endocrinol* 2014;223:T49-T62.
11. Michopoulos V, Mancini F, Loucks TL, Berga S. Neuroendocrine recovery initiated by cognitive behavioral therapy in women with functional hypothalamic amenorrhea: A randomized controlled trial. *Fertil Steril* 2013;99(7):2084-2091.
12. Tolaymat LL, Kaunitz AM. Use of hormonal contraception in adolescents: Skeletal health issues. *Curr Opin Obstet Gynecol* 2009;21(5):396-401.
13. DeSouza MJ, Nattiv A, Joy E, et al. 2014 Female athlete triad coalition consensus statement on treatment and return to play of the Female Athlete Triad. *Clin J Sport Med* 2014;24(2):96-119.
14. Simon JA. Progestogens in the treatment of secondary amenorrhea. *J Reprod Med* 1999;44(2 Suppl):185-189.
15. Master-Hunter T, Heiman DL. Amenorrhea: Evaluation and treatment. *Am Fam Physician* 2006;73(8):1374-1382.
16. Faje A, Nachtigall L. Current treatment options for hyperprolactinemia. *Expert Opin Pharmacother* 2013;14(12):1611-1625.
17. Arduc A, Gokay F, Isik S, et al. Retrospective comparison of cabergoline and bromocriptine effects in hyperprolactinemia: A single center experience. *J Endocrinol Invest* 2015;38:447-453.
18. French L. Dysmenorrhea in adolescents—Diagnosis and treatment. *Pediatr Drugs* 2008;10(1):1-7.
19. Marjoribanks J, Ayeleke RO, Farquhar C, Proctor M. Nonsteroidal anti-inflammatory drugs for dysmenorrhea. *Cochrane Database Syst Rev* 2015(7):CD001751. doi:10.1002/146 51858.CD001751.pub3.
20. Daniels S, Robbins J, West CR, Nemeth MA. Celecoxib in the treatment of primary dysmenorrhea: Results from two randomized, double-blind, active- and placebo-controlled, crossover studies. *Clin Ther* 2009;31(6):1192-1208.
21. Bhattacharya S, Middleton LJ, Stourapas A, et al. Hysterectomy, endometrial ablation and Mirena® for heavy menstrual bleeding: A systematic review of clinical effectiveness and cost-effectiveness analysis. *Health Technol Assess* 2011;15(9):iii-xvi, 1-252.
22. Lethaby A, Hussain M, Rishworth JR, Rees MC. Progesterone or progestogen-releasing intrauterine systems for heavy menstrual bleeding. *Cochrane Database of Syst Rev* 2015(4):CD002126. doi: 10.1002/14651858. CD002126.pub3.
23. Qiu J, Cheng J, Wang Q, Hua J. Levonorgestrel-releasing intrauterine system versus medical therapy for HMB: A systematic review and meta-analysis. *Med Sci Monit* 2014;20:1700-1713.

24. Kaunitz AM, Meredith S, Inki P, et al. Levonorgestrel-releasing intrauterine system and endometrial ablation in heavy menstrual bleeding: A systematic review and meta-analysis. *Obstet Gynecol* 2009;113:1104-1116.
25. Tasci Y, Caglar GS, Kayikcioglu F, et al. Treatment of HMB with levonorgestrel releasing intrauterine system: Effects on ovarian function and uterus. *Arch Gynecol Obstet* 2009;280:39-42.
26. Desai RM. Efficacy of levonorgestrel releasing intrauterine system for the treatment of HMB due to benign uterine lesions in perimenopausal women. *J Midlife Health* 2012;3(1):20-23.
27. Naoulou B, Tsai MC. Efficacy of tranexamic acid in the treatment of idiopathic and non-functional heavy menstrual bleeding: A systematic review. *Acta Obstet Gynecol Scand* 2012;91(5):529-537.
28. Hashim HA. Medical treatment of idiopathic heavy menstrual bleeding. What is new? An evidence based approach. *Arch Gynecol Obstet* 2013;287:251-260.
29. Mathur R, Levin O, Azziz R. Use of ethinyl estradiol/drospirenone combination in patients with polycystic ovary syndrome. *Ther Clin Risk Manag* 2008;4(2):487-492.
30. Setji TL, Brown AJ. Polycystic ovary syndrome: Update on diagnosis and treatment. *Am J Med* 2014;127(10):912-919.
31. Biggs WS, Demuth RH. Premenstrual syndrome and premenstrual dysphoric disorder. *Am Fam Physician* 2011;84(8):918-924.
32. Lopez LM, Kaptein AA, Helmerhorst FM. Oral contraceptives containing drospirenone for premenstrual syndrome. *Cochrane Database Syst Rev* 2012(2):CD006586. doi:10.1002/14651858. CD006586.pub4.
33. Maharaj S, Trevino K. A comprehensive review of treatment options for premenstrual syndrome and premenstrual dysphoric disorder. *J Psychiatr Pract* 2015;21(5):334-350.
34. Bitzer J, Heikinheimo O, Nelson AL, Calaf-Alsina J, Fraser IS. Medical management of heavy menstrual bleeding: A comprehensive review of the literature. *Obstet Gynecol Surv* 2015;70(2):115-130.
35. The American College of Obstetricians and Gynecologists. ACOG Practice Bulletin No. 110. Noncontraceptive uses of hormonal contraceptives. *Obstet Gynecol* 2010;115(1):206-219.
36. Hantsoo L, Epperson CN. Premenstrual dysphoric disorder: Epidemiology and treatment. *Curr Psychiatry Rep* 2015;17:87.
37. Heliovaara-Peeipo S, Hurskainen R, Teperi J, et al. Quality of life and costs of levonorgestrel-releasing intrauterine system or hysterectomy in the treatment of HMB: A 10-year randomized trial. *Am J Obstet Gynecol* 2013;209:535.e1-14.
38. Von Mackensen S. Quality of life in women with bleeding disorders. *Haemophilia* 2011;17(Suppl 1):33-37.
39. Ray S, Ray A. Non-surgical interventions for treating heavy menstrual bleeding (HMB) in women with bleeding disorders. *Cochrane Database Syst Rev* 2014(11):CD010338. doi: 10.1002/14651858. CD010338.pub2.
40. The American College of Obstetricians and Gynecologists. ACOG Practice Bulletin No. 121. Long-acting reversible contraception: Implants and intrauterine devices. *Obstet Gynecol* 2011;118:184-196.
41. Leminen H, Hurskainen R. Tranexamic acid for the treatment of heavy menstrual bleeding: Efficacy and safety. *Int J Womens Health* 2012;4:413-421.
42. Kadir RA. HMB: Treatment options. *Thromb Res* 2009;123(Suppl 2): S21-S29.
43. Azziz R, Carmina E, Dewailley D, et al. Task force on the phenotype of the polycystic ovary syndrome of the androgen excess and PCOS society criteria for the polycystic ovary syndrome: The complete task force report. *Fertil Steril* 2009;91:456-488.
44. Witchel SF, Oberfield S, Rosenfield RL, et al. The diagnosis of polycystic overy syndrome during adolescence. *Horm Res Paediatr* 2015;83:376-389.
45. Palomba S, Pasquali R, Orio F, Nestler JE. Clomiphene citrate, metformin or both as first-step approaches in treating anovulatory infertile patients with polycystic ovary syndrome (PCOS): A systematic review of head-to-head randomized controlled studies and meta-analysis. *Clin Endocrinol* 2009;70(2):311-321.
46. Du Q, Yang S, Wang Y, et al. Effects of thiazolidinediones on polycystic ovary syndrome: A meta-analysis of randomized placebo-controlled trials. *Adv Ther* 2012;29(9):763-774.
47. Sweet MG, Schmidt-Dalton TA, Weiss PM, Madsen KP. Evaluation and management of abnormal uterine bleeding in premenopausal women. *Am Fam Phys* 2012;85(1):35-43.
48. Harmanci A, Cinar N, Bayraktar M, Yildiz BO. Oral contraceptive plus antiandrogen therapy and cardiometabolic risk in polycystic ovary syndrome. *Clin Endocrinol* 2013;78:120-125.
49. Gode F, Karagoz C, Posaci C, et al. Alteration of cardiovascular risk parameters in women with polycystic ovary syndrome who were prescribed ethinyl estradiol-cyproterone acetate. *Arch Gynecol Obstet* 2011;284:923-929.
50. Beller JP, McCartney CR. Cardiovascular risk and combined oral contraceptives: Clinical decisions in settings of uncertainty. *Am J Obstet Gynecol* 2013;208(1):39-41.
51. Dhamangaonkar PC, Anuradha K, Saxena A. Levonorgestrel intrauterine system (Mirena): An emerging tool for conservative treatment of abnormal uterine bleeding. *J Midlife Health* 2015;6(1):26-30.
52. Mansukhani N, Unni J, Dua M, et al. Are women satisfied when using levonorgestrel-releasing intrauterine system for treatment of abnormal uterine bleeding? *J Midlife Health* 2013;4(1):31-35.
53. Khattab S, Mohsen IA, Foutouh IA, et al. Metformin reduces abortion in pregnant women with polycystic ovary syndrome. *Gynecol Endocrinol* 2006;22:680-684.
54. Legro RS, Brzyski RG, Diamond MP, et al. Letrozole versus clomiphene for infertility in the polycystic ovary syndrome. *N Engl J Med* 2014;371:119-129.
55. Franik S, Kremer JAM, Nelen WLDM, Farquhar C. Aromatase inhibitors for subfertility treatement in women with polycystic ovary syndrome. *Cochrane Database Syst Rev* 2014(2):CD010287. doi: 10,1002.14651858.CD010287.pub2.
56. Iacovides S, Avidon I, Bentley A, Baker FC. Reduced quality of life when experiencing menstrual pain in women with primary dysmenorrhea. *Acta Obstet Gynecol Scand* 2014;93:213-217.
57. Osayande AS, Hehulic S. Diagnosis and initial management of dysmenorrhea. *Am Fam Physician* 2014;89(5):341-346.
58. Morrow C, Naumburg EH. Dysmenorrhea. *Prim Care* 2009;36(1):19-32.
59. Polat A, Celik H, Gurates B. Prevalence of primary dysmenorrhea in your adult female university students. *Arch Gynecol Obstet* 2009;279(4):527-532.
60. Potur DC, Komurcu N. The effects of local low-dose heat application on dysmenorrhea. *J Pediatr Adolesc Gynecol* 2014;27:216-221.
61. Navvabi-Rigi S, Kermansaravi F, Navidian A, et al. Comparing the analgesic effect of heat patch containing iron chip and ibuprofen for primary dysmenorrhea: A randomized clinical trial. *BMC Women's Health* 2012;12:25-31.
62. Shirvani MA, Motahari-Tabari N, Alipour A. The effect of mefenamic acid and ginger on pain relieve in primary dysmenorrhea: A randomized clinical trial. *Arch Gynecol Obstet* 2015;291:1277-1281.
63. Daily JW, Zhang X, Kim DS, Park S. Efficacy of ginger for alleviating the symptoms of primary dysmenorrhea: A systematic review and meta-analysis of randomized clinical trials. *Pain Med* 2015;16(12):2243-2255.
64. Rapkin AJ, Mikacich JA. Premenstrual dysphoric disorder and severe premenstrual syndrome in adolescents: Diagnosis and pharmacological treatment. *Pediatr Drugs* 2013;15:191-202.
65. Robinson LLL, Ismail KMK. Clinical epidemiology of premenstrual disorder: Informing optimized patient outcomes. *Int J Womens Health* 2015;7:811-818.
66. Dennerstein L, Lehert P, Heinemann K. Epidemiology of premenstrual symptoms and disorders. *Menopause Int* 2012;18(2):48-51.
67. Matsumoto T, Asakura H, Hayashi T. Biopsychosocial aspects of premenstrual syndrome and premenstrual dysphoric disorder. *Gynecol Endocrinol* 2013;29(1):67-73.
68. Deligiannidis KM, Freeman MP. Complementary and alternative medicine for the treatment of depressive disorders in women. *Psychiatr Clin North Am* 2010;33(2):441-463.
69. Dante G, Facchinetti F. Herbal treatments for alleviating premenstrual symptoms: A systematic review. *J Psychosom Obstet Gynecol* 2011;32(10):42-51.
70. Marjoribanks J, Brown J, O'Brien PMH, Wyant K. Selective serotonin reuptake inhibitors for premenstrual syndrome. *Cochrane Database of Syst Rev* 2013(6):CD001396. doi:10.1002/14651858. CD001396. pub3.
71. Freeman EW. Therapeutic management of premenstrual syndrome. *Expert Opin Pharmacother* 2010;11(17):2879-2889.
72. Freeman EW, Halbreich U, Grubb GS, et al. An overview of four studies of a continuous oral contraceptive (levonorgestrel 90 mcg/ethinyl estradiol 20 mcg) on premenstrual dysphoric disorder and premenstrual syndrome. *Contraception* 2012;85:437-445.

81

Endometriosis

Deborah A. Sturpe and Kathleen J. Pincus

KEY CONCEPTS

1. Endometriosis should be suspected in any woman of reproductive age with recurring cyclic or acyclic pelvic pain and/or subfertility, especially if pain does not improve with nonsteroidal anti-inflammatory drugs and hormonal contraceptives.
2. The etiology of endometriosis is likely multifactorial and requires a genetic or immunologic predisposition. Retrograde menstruation is the most widely accepted theory to account for displacement of endometrial tissue, although alternative theories have been proposed.
3. Treatment goals include improvement of painful symptoms and maintenance or improvement of fertility. Therapy is considered successful based on resolution of symptoms or achievement of pregnancy.
4. Both drug therapy and surgery may treat endometriosis-related pain, but infertility can be treated only with surgery or assisted reproductive techniques.
5. No medical therapy has been proven to be more effective than another; thus, the choice among agents is determined primarily by side-effect profile, cost, and individual patient response.
6. For endometriosis pain, surgical therapy is typically reserved for medical therapy failure.
7. Diagnosis of endometriosis can be made only via surgical visualization of lesions, not by physical examination or laboratory testing. Empiric treatment without confirmation of diagnosis is acceptable in most cases.
8. To help avoid loss of bone mineral density, add-back therapy should be used in any woman receiving a gonadotropin-releasing hormone agonist.

INTRODUCTION

1 Endometriosis causes secondary dysmenorrhea and is associated with infertility. Presence of endometrial tissue outside the uterus is chronic and relapsing. Endometriosis treatment targets pain relief and fertility improvement.

EPIDEMIOLOGY

Endometriosis has up to a 10% estimated prevalence in the general female population.[1-3] Though the prevalence is substantially higher in patients with pelvic pain or infertility. Only 4% of premenopausal women presenting to primary care for nongynecologic problems have endometriosis, whereas up to 80% of adult women and 50% of adolescents with chronic pelvic pain are diagnosed with the disorder.[3,4] The incidence is 10-fold higher in women with infertility (20%-50%) compared with that in fertile women (0.5%-5%).[1-5] A genetic predisposition for endometriosis has also been noted, with a sixfold higher risk in women with first-degree relatives with severe endometriosis.[2,3,6,7]

ETIOLOGY

Endometriosis is characterized by findings of endometrial tissue outside the normal uterine cavity. It may be diagnosed at any age, but is most commonly found during the reproductive years (range 12-80 years, average 28 years). Risk of developing endometriosis increases with early menarche (≤11 years), shorter menstrual cycles (less than 27 days), and heavy, prolonged menstruation.[4,6,8] Conversely, higher parity and increased duration of lactation decrease the risk of endometriosis.[4,6,8] Taller, thinner women are more likely to develop endometriosis than patients with higher body weights, body mass indexes, or waist-to-hip ratios potentially due to higher follicular-phase estradiol levels.[6,8] The woman's own birth history may also relate to the risk of developing endometriosis with lower birth weights (less than 5.5 pounds [2.5 kg]), multiple fetal gestations, and in utero exposure to diethylstilbesterol conferring higher risks of future development of endometriosis potentially due to alterations in gestational exposure to hormones including estrogen.[2,6] Altered pelvic anatomy, such as Müllerian duct anomalies and cervical or vaginal outlet obstruction, also increases risk of developing endometriosis.[2,6] Regular exercise (greater than 4 h/wk), diets high in fruits and vegetables, and cigarette smoking are associated with decreased risk of endometriosis, where alcohol use, caffeine consumption, and high polychlorinated biphenyl concentrations are associated with increased risk.[4,6] Comorbid autoimmune disorders, such as rheumatoid arthritis, systemic lupus erythematosus, and autoimmune thyroid disease, are more common in cohorts of patients with endometriosis than population controls.[6,7]

Gene mutation studies suggest genes regulating inflammation, sex steroid regulation, metabolism, biosynthesis, detoxification, vascular function, and tissue remodeling may contribute to endometriosis, but no validated associations have been confirmed.[9] Alterations on chromosomes 7 and 10 have been identified in clusters of women with endometriosis.[2] It is most likely that a multitude of genetic mutations are involved with the development of endometriosis.

PATHOPHYSIOLOGY

2 Multiple theories exist to explain why endometrial tissue is present outside the uterine cavity, and the true pathophysiology is likely multifactorial.[2,7] The most widely accepted theory proposes that endometrial tissue is deposited in the peritoneal cavity by retrograde menstruation through the fallopian tubes.[2,7] However, retrograde menstruation occurs in up to 90% of women while only approximately 10% develop endometriosis, indicating that additional factors are necessary for endometrial lesions to attach, survive, and proliferate.[7] Endometrial fragments are routinely cleared by the

immune system; there is currently much interest in researching the role immune deficiencies and alterations play in the development of endometriosis.[7] Endometrial tissue from women with endometriosis has been shown to be more resistant to natural killer cell lysis than endometrium from women without the disease, and women with endometriosis have been found to have impaired macrophage function.[7] Alternative theories include: inappropriate differentiation of mesothelial cells into endometrium-like tissue (coelomic metaplasia); hormonal or immunologic stimuli promoting differentiation of cells in the peritoneal lining to endometrial cells (induction theory); differentiation of stem cells from either bone marrow or the endometrial basalis layer into endometrial-like tissues (stem cell theory); and spread of menstrual tissue to distant sites through veins or lymphatic vessels (hematogenous or lymphatic spread).[2,7]

Endometriosis is a chronic inflammatory disorder that exhibits cellular proliferation, cellular invasion, and angiogenesis not unlike solid tumor malignancies.[7] Genetic alterations including upregulation of BCL-2, which inhibits cellular apoptosis, may predispose endometriotic lesion survival in certain women.[7] Endometriosis also demonstrates estrogen-dependency and progesterone resistance. Endometriotic tissue has a higher expression of aromatase enzymes and lower expression of 17-beta-hydroxysteriod dehydrogenase. Together these alterations result in increased concentrations of estrogen.[7] Endometriotic tissue also has decreased progesterone receptor expression, including an absence of certain receptor subtypes, which impairs progression from the luteal to secretory phase of menstruation.[7] Other noted genetic alterations demonstrated in patients with endometriosis included cytokines, matrix metalloproteinases, transcriptions factors, prostaglandins, and tumor suppressor genes.[2,7]

Pain associated with endometriosis results from increased concentrations of inflammatory markers, including prostaglandins and increased nerve density at lesion sites. Proinflammatory cytokines found in endometrial lesions, including tumor necrosis factor-α and interleukins 1, 6, and 8, promote lesion formation, adhesion, and infiltration and induce pain through pelvic nerve stimulation.[2,3,7,10] Prostaglandin $F_2\alpha$ induces vasoconstriction and can cause uterine contractions, a component of dysmenorrhea, while prostaglandin E_2 can induce pain through direct actions on nerves.[2] Overexpression of nerve growth factors promotes neuroangiogenesis in endometriotic tissue which leads to increased pain receptors expression; and it is hypothesized that endometriotic nerve fibers influence dorsal root neurons which increase the perception of pain.[7] Researchers have demonstrated that these nerve fibers are found significantly more often in patients with endometriosis than in those without endometriosis, in greater density in patients with higher pain scores ($\geq$3 vs $\leq$20), and in greater density in patients with deep infiltrating lesions.[11,12] The interplay between increased density of nerve fibers in endometrial lesions and increased concentrations of cytokines and prostaglandins in peritoneal fluid combines to confer significant pelvic pain in many patients. The location and depth of infiltration of endometriotic lesions impact the severity of pain symptoms.[10]

The pathophysiology for infertility in endometriosis is less well defined, especially in mild disease. In advanced endometriosis, inflammation and anatomic abnormalities such as ovarian cysts and adhesions may physically block fallopian tubes and decrease receptivity of the endometrium, thus hindering oocyte and embryo development.[2,3,13] The same inflammatory cytokines (macrophages, interlukins 1 and 6, and tumor necrosis factor-α) that lead to pain also create a hostile peritoneal environment leading to damage of sperm DNA and cell membranes.[13-15] Hormonal dysregulation resulting from the disease may also lead to altered endometrial receptivity and implantation, prolonged follicular phases, altered oocyte and embryo quality, or abnormal uterotubal transport which can adversely impact fertility.[13,15]

CLINICAL PRESENTATION Endometriosis

Symptoms

- Dysmenorrhea and infertility are the most common symptoms.
- Other symptoms include dyspareunia, menorrhagia, chronic pelvic pain (cyclic or acyclic), ovulation pain, sacral back pain, cyclic or perimenstrual bowel and bladder complaints (eg, GI disturbances, painful defecation, tenesmus dysuria, and/or hematuria), chronic fatigue, or rarely neuropathic pain.
- Some patients may be asymptomatic.

Signs

- Findings on physical examination are best observed during menstruation and may include pelvic or uterosacral ligament tenderness, enlarged ovaries, pelvic masses or nodules, or a fixed, retroverted uterus.
- Findings on laparoscopic examination may range from a few small lesions located on the ovaries, serosal surfaces, or peritoneum to large cysts called endometriomas. Lesions are often described as: "powder burn" or "gunshot" lesions; dark brown, black, or blue lesions, nodules, and cysts; and "chocolate cysts" (endometriomas containing blood).

Diagnosis

- Definitive diagnosis can be made only by direct surgical visualization of endometrial lesions; however, treatment guidelines allow for nondefinitive diagnosis in patients presenting with chronic pelvic pain provided that other causes of pain are ruled out and that pain responds to empiric therapies.
- Ultrasonography, magnetic resonance imaging, and computed tomography have much lower sensitivity for endometrial lesions, but have utility in assessing for pelvic or adnexal masses.

Disease Staging

- Severity of disease can be classified according to the American Society of Reproductive Medicine staging system (stage I [mild] to stage IV [severe]), but clinical utility of this staging system is limited because findings do not correlate with painful symptoms, nor does the staging system predict pregnancy rates. Staging may be useful in guiding decisions regarding prognosis and treatment for infertility.

Data from references 3 and 17.

TREATMENT

Endometriosis is a chronic, relapsing disease. Lifelong treatment plans must consider individual patient symptoms, goals for fertility, and impact on quality of life.[16] Various organizations, including the American College of Obstetricians and Gynecologists (ACOG), the American Society for Reproductive Medicine, the Society of Obstetricians and Gynaecologists of Canada, and the European Society of Human Reproduction and Embryology (ESHRE), have published evidence-based and/or expert opinion-based guidelines for treating endometriosis.[3,10,13,16,17] The ESHRE guideline, updated in 2014, uses structured methodology and grades recommendations based on the strength and quality of available evidence (Table 81-1).[17]

Desired Outcomes

Identification of endometriosis treatment goals depends on individual patient presentation and needs. 3 4 Typical goals include minimization of associated pain, improved quality of life, and correction of associated infertility. The first two outcomes can often be achieved through use of pharmacologic therapy and surgery.[3,10,15] Infertility is nonresponsive to medical therapies; thus, surgical intervention to remove endometrial lesions coupled with various assisted reproductive techniques must be employed.[3,13] Even with such efforts, not all women with endometriosis will be able to conceive, and exact success rates are unknown due to a paucity of well-designed clinical studies.

TABLE 81-1 Evidence-Based Recommendations for Treatment of Endometriosis-Related Pain

	Grade of Recommendation[a]
Treatment Options	
CHCs	
Oral	B
Transdermal	C
Vaginal	C
Progestins	
Oral	A
Depot	A
Danazol	A
LNG-IUS	B
GnRH agonists with immediate initiation of add-back therapy	A
Nonsteroidal anti-inflammatory drugs or other analgesics	GPP
Aromatase inhibitors in combination with oral CHC pills, progestins, or GnRH agonists	B
Surgical treatment	A
Considerations for Selecting Among Strategies	
Analgesics, CHCs, or progestins are acceptable to use as empiric therapy	GPP
CHCs may be dosed continuously	C
Aromatase inhibitors should be reserved for use in patients who are refractory to other medical and surgical treatments	B
CHCs and the LNG-IUS are preferred therapies for secondary prevention of dysmenorrhea postoperatively	A
Hysterectomy-oophorectomy may be considered in women finished with childbearing who have failed more conservative options	GPP

CHCs, combined hormonal contraceptives; GnRH, gonadotropin-releasing hormone; LNG-IUS, levonorgestrel-releasing intrauterine system.

[a]Strength of recommendations: A = meta-analysis or multiple randomized trials of high quality; B = meta-analysis or multiple randomized trials of moderate quality, or single randomized trial, large nonrandomized trial(s), or case control/cohort studies of high quality; C = single randomized trial, large nonrandomized trial(s) or case control/cohort studies of moderate quality; D = nonanalytic studies or case reports/case series of high or moderate quality; GPP = good practice point/expert opinion.

Data from reference 17.

General Approach to Treatment

Treatment of the asymptomatic patient with incidental findings of endometriosis is considered unnecessary.[17] For patients presenting with endometriosis-related pain, the foundation of therapy includes medical treatment, surgical treatment, or both. To date, no studies have directly compared medical and surgical treatment as first-line therapy. Furthermore, determining the optimal medical or surgical approach is difficult secondary to a paucity of well-designed, randomized, controlled trials comparing options. 5 All commonly prescribed medical therapies relieve endometriosis-related pain by regressing lesions via induction of a pseudopregnancy or pseudomenopausal state, but medications do not eradicate lesions or improve fertility. The choice of initial therapy thus depends on factors such as the patient's primary complaint, the location and extent of disease, desire for future fertility, cost of therapy, contraindications to therapy, and potential side effects.[3,10,16,17] Information regarding drugs commonly prescribed for endometriosis, their dosing, side effects, and special monitoring parameters are listed in Tables 81-2 and 81-3. No endometriosis treatments are guaranteed to provide full relief of symptoms; consequently, analgesics such as nonsteroidal anti-inflammatory drugs or opioids are often used as adjunctive therapy for pain relief.

Nonpharmacologic Therapy

Surgery, generally performed via laparoscopy, is used in endometriosis as both a diagnostic and a therapeutic tool.[13,17] 4 6 Due to lack of data supporting superiority of surgical versus medical therapies in relieving endometriosis pain, surgical therapy is typically reserved for patients experiencing medication failure or who suffer from infertility, although clinicians are encouraged to "see and treat" any symptomatic patient undergoing diagnostic surgery by removing visible lesions.[17] Women with continuing pain symptoms who do not desire pregnancy may be offered the option of hysterectomy with or without oophorectomy, although such radical surgery does not guarantee freedom from symptoms.[17]

Use of perioperative medical therapy is a source of treatment controversy. Although most experts agree that preoperative medication use does not improve surgical outcomes, the role of postoperative medical therapy is less certain.[17] The ESHRE guideline now clearly delineates between adjunctive medical therapy (used within 6 months of surgery) and secondary prevention (used later than 6 months postsurgery).[17] The guideline recommends against adjunctive therapy solely for further reduction of pain, but does acknowledge that medical therapies may be started immediately postsurgery for other indications such as contraception or menstrual cycle control.[17] For secondary prevention of dysmenorrhea after surgery, the levonorgestrel intrauterine system (LNG-IUS) or combined hormonal contraceptives (CHCs) are recommended due to equivalent efficacy and better tolerability than other therapeutic options.[17-19]

Clinical **Controversy...**

Many women seek relief of endometriosis pain through complementary and alternative methods such as electrical nerve stimulation, acupuncture, traditional Chinese medicine, and dietary therapy (particularly vitamins B_6, A, C, and E, mineral salts such as calcium, magnesium, selenium, zinc, and iron, lactic ferments, and omega-3 and omega-6 fatty acids). Reputable data to support such methods are often sparse to nonexistent, thus practice guidelines recommend against such use.[17] However, these same guidelines do recognize that such methods may be beneficial in some women. Unfortunately, it is difficult to determine who may benefit most (or least). Provided a treatment is unlikely to cause harm, it may be reasonable to support use of complementary and alternative therapies in women specifically interested in such options.

TABLE 82-2 Dosing of Drugs Used in Treatment of Endometriosis

Drug	Brand Name	Initial Dose	Usual Range	Other
CHCs				
CHC pill	Various (see Chapter 79)	One pill orally daily	One pill orally daily	Continuous dosing may improve efficacy
Etonogestrel/ethinyl estradiol (vaginal ring)	NuvaRing	Insert one ring monthly	Insert one ring monthly	Continuous dosing may improve efficacy
Norelgestromin/ethinyl estradiol (transdermal)	Ortho Evra	Apply one patch weekly	Apply one patch weekly	Continuous dosing may improve efficacy
Progestins				
Depot medroxyprogesterone acetate (IM or SubQ)	Depo-Provera Depo-SubQ Provera	150 mg IM every 13 weeks 104 mg SubQ every 12-14 weeks	150 mg IM every 13 weeks 104 mg SubQ every 12-14 weeks	
Oral medroxyprogesterone acetate	Provera	30 mg orally daily	30-60 mg orally daily	
LNG-IUS[a]	Mirena	Single insertion for up to 5 years	Single insertion for up to 5 years	
Norethindrone acetate	Aygestin	5 mg orally daily	Titrate as needed to maximum dose 20 mg orally daily	
GnRH Agonists				
Goserelin	Zoladex	3.6 mg monthly SubQ implant	3.6 mg monthly SubQ implant	Use add-back therapy
Leuprolide	Lupron Depot	3.75 mg IM monthly or 11.25 mg IM every 3 months	3.75 mg IM monthly or 11.25 mg IM every 3 months	Use add-back therapy
Nafarelin	Synarel	400 mcg intranasally daily, dosed as one spray in one nostril AM and one spray in opposite nostril PM	May titrate to maximum 800 mcg intranasally daily, dosed as one spray in each nostril twice daily	Use add-back therapy
Triptorelin	Trelstar Depot	3.75 mg IM monthly	3.75 mg IM monthly	Use add-back therapy
Androgens				
Danazol	Danocrine	100-200 mg orally twice daily	Titrate as needed to maximum 400 mg orally twice daily	
Aromatase Inhibitors				
Anastrozole	Arimidex	1 mg orally daily	1 mg orally daily	Use with CHC, progestin, or GnRH agonist
Letrozole	Femara	2.5 mg orally daily	2.5 mg orally daily	Use with CHC, progestin, or GnRH agonist

CHC, combined hormonal contraceptive; GnRH, gonadotropin-releasing hormone; IM, intramuscular; LNG-IUS, levonorgestrel-releasing intrauterine system; SubQ, subcutaneous.

[a]At this time, only Mirena has been studied in the endometriosis population. Other LNG-IUSs (Liletta and Skylar) should not be recommended until data are available to support their use.

Pharmacologic Therapy

6 Pharmacologic therapy is typically the first choice for treatment of endometriosis-related pain to minimize risks from multiple surgeries such as scarring and tissue adhesions.

Drug Treatments of First Choice

First-line therapy for endometriosis-associated pain typically includes oral CHCs, oral progestins (norethindrone acetate or medroxyprogesterone acetate) or the depot progestin medroxyprogesterone acetate (DMPA) since these drugs are considered as effective as, but less costly and toxic than, other pharmacologic options.[3,10,16,17] Choice among these classes and agents depends on patient characteristics such as the desire for contraception, pain pattern, contraindications, and potential side effects, as no direct comparisons are available in the literature. Long-term maintenance therapy with these agents should be considered for women achieving a good therapeutic response.[3] 7 These drugs may be used empirically for suspected endometriosis prior to laparoscopy in patients of any age.[3,10,16,17] Despite a clear lack of efficacy data in the endometriosis population, analgesics are also recommended as adjunctive therapy to these other first-line options.[17]

Alternative Drug Treatments

Alternative choices for endometriosis pain include the LNG-IUS, transdermal or vaginal CHC, a gonadotropin releasing hormone (GnRH) agonist, or danazol.[3,16,17,20] 7 Selection is again driven primarily by patient preference, patient-specific response, side-effect profile, available dosage forms, and medication costs, since no method has been proven superior to another.[3,10,16,17] Unlike the first-line agents, either the safety of long-term use is unknown or efficacy is less well defined for these alternative options. A major concern with long-term use (greater than 6 months) of GnRH agonist is bone mineral density loss, but add-back therapy with an estrogen and progestin combination minimizes this loss along with mitigation of other bothersome side effects and has been shown to be safe for up to 10 years of use.[21,22] 8 Consequently, it is recommended to start add-back therapy on immediate initiation of GnRH agonist treatment.[3,16,17]

A pharmacologic option for endometriosis pain refractory to the aforementioned drug and nondrug methods is an aromatase inhibitor in combination with a CHC, progestin, or GnRH agonist, particularly in women with rectovaginal endometriosis.[17] Because long-term studies of aromatase inhibitors are lacking, use is reserved for refractory patients due to concern over potential long-term side effects, especially in a premenopausal population

Special Populations

Treatment of the adolescent patient with endometriosis presents a unique challenge, as these patients often present with normal physical findings and laparoscopic findings that are atypical for

TABLE 81-3 Monitoring Drug Therapy for Endometriosis

Drug	Adverse Drug Reactions	Monitoring Parameters	Comments
CHC pills	Nausea, vomiting, breast tenderness, weight gain, acne, oily skin, depression, fatigue, breakthrough bleeding or spotting, elevated blood pressure	Blood pressure within 3 months of starting new method	Many symptoms improve after two to three cycles of use
Etonogestrel/ethinyl estradiol (vaginal ring)	Nausea, vomiting, breast tenderness, weight gain, acne, oily skin, depression, fatigue, breakthrough bleeding or spotting, vaginal irritation, elevated blood pressure	Blood pressure within 3 months of starting new method	Many symptoms improve after two to three cycles of use
Norelgestromin/ethinyl estradiol (transdermal)	Nausea, vomiting, breast tenderness, weight gain, acne, oily skin, depression, fatigue, breakthrough bleeding or spotting, application site reaction, elevated blood pressure	Blood pressure within 3 months of starting new method	Many symptoms improve after two to three cycles of use
Depot medroxyprogesterone acetate (IM or SubQ)	Menstrual irregularities, weight gain, acne, hirsutism, depression, decreased bone mineral density	None	Bone mineral density testing specifically not recommended at this time
Oral medroxyprogesterone acetate	Menstrual irregularities, nausea, peripheral edema Venous thromboembolism	None	
LNG-IUS	Menstrual irregularities, insertion-related complications, expulsion, pelvic inflammatory disease	None	Counsel on sexually transmitted infection prevention
Norethindrone acetate	Breast tenderness, nausea, peripheral edema Venous thromboembolism	None	
Goserelin	Acne, depression, hot flashes, mood swings, peripheral edema, vaginitis Bone mineral density loss	May consider bone mineral density testing every 1-2 years and serum lipid levels every 6 months if treatment extended beyond 12 months	Add-back therapy prevents many adverse reactions
Leuprolide	Acne, depression, dizziness, headache, hot flashes, mood swings, nausea/vomiting, triglyceride elevation, vaginitis Anaphylaxis, bone mineral density loss, venous thromboembolism	May consider bone mineral density testing every 1-2 years and serum lipid levels every 6 months if treatment extended beyond 12 months	Add-back therapy prevents many adverse reactions
Nafarelin	Acne, headache, hot flashes, mood swings, vaginal dryness Bone mineral density loss, venous thromboembolism	May consider bone mineral density testing every 1-2 years and serum lipid levels every 6 months if treatment extended beyond 12 months	Add-back therapy prevents many adverse reactions
Triptorelin	Headache, high blood pressure, hot flashes Anaphylaxis, angioedema	May consider bone mineral density testing every 1-2 years and serum lipid levels every 6 months if treatment extended beyond 12 months	Add-back therapy prevents many adverse reactions
Danazol	Acne, peripheral edema, hirsutism, lipid abnormalities, weight gain Hepatic dysfunction	Liver function tests and serum cholesterol every 3-6 months	
Anastrozole	Arthralgias, hot flashes, myalgias, nausea, diarrhea Decreased bone mineral density	May consider bone mineral density testing every 1-2 years if treatment extended beyond 12 months	Limited adverse reaction data in premenopausal women with endometriosis
Letrozole	Arthralgias, hot flashes, myalgias, nausea, diarreha Decreased bone mineral density	May consider bone mineral density testing every 1-2 years if treatment extended beyond 12 months	Limited adverse reaction data in premenopausal women with endometriosis

CHC, combined hormonal contraceptive; IM, intramuscular; LNG-IUS, levonorgestrel-releasing intrauterine system; SubQ, subcutaneous.

endometriosis; thus, endometriosis must be strongly suspected in any patient whose dysmenorrhea fails to respond to first-line agents.[16] Treatment recommendations for such patients are extrapolated from adult guidelines and generally follow the same recommendations as for adult patients.[16,20] Pertinent differences include preference for diagnostic laparoscopy after first-line medical treatment failure before initiation of alternative medical treatments and limitation of GnRH agonist therapy due to concern about drug-associated bone loss in a population that has not yet reached peak bone mineral density.[16,17,20] In at least one study, use of progestin-only add-back therapy during GnRH agonist treatment in adolescents did not fully prevent bone loss, possibly emphasizing the need to carefully consider selection of this drug class in the adolescent population and to consider routine monitoring of bone mineral density if prescribed.[23] Despite these limitations in treating adolescents, early recognition and treatment of endometriosis in this population may be critical for maintenance of quality of life and reduction of future disease-related complications.[24-26]

Clinical **Controversy...**

Treatment of vasomotor and urogenital symptoms in women with surgically induced menopause due to endometriosis may be problematic as the potential relief of menopausal symptoms must be weighed against the risk of disease reactivation upon administration of hormone therapy. Despite this risk, guidelines support use of hormone therapy in women after surgical hysterectomy-oophorectomy until the average age of menopause.[17] Although estrogen therapy alone would typically be prescribed for this patient population, endometriosis guidelines endorse use of estrogen-progestin combination therapy since risk of disease reactivation may be lowered by the addition of the progestin component. However, hormone therapy related risks are known to be greater with estrogen-progestin therapy versus estrogen therapy alone. Thus no clear guidance exists on how to best treat this patient population.

Drug Class Information

No single drug therapy has been shown to be superior to another for the treatment of endometriosis pain. Therefore, the choice of drug between and within classes is often dependent on patient factors and clinician experience.

Combined Hormonal Contraception Effectiveness of oral CHCs in treating endometriosis pain has been demonstrated in only a small number of observational, placebo-controlled, and active-comparator trials.[17,27] Despite this overall paucity of clinical trial data, the widespread use and effectiveness of oral CHCs for other dysmenorrheas, the secondary benefits of contraception and menstrual regulation, and the good safety record of these agents leads to oral CHCs being recommended as first-line therapy.[17] There is no evidence to suggest superiority of any particular oral CHC over another, although most studies used monophasic pills. Effectiveness of the CHC patch and vaginal ring has also been demonstrated in one study.[28] Overall, the choice between CHCs should be guided by patient preference, likelihood of adherence, and cost.

Administration of CHCs may be cyclic (includes a placebo or nondrug week) or continuous. Effectiveness of continuous dosing was first demonstrated in a prospective study in which patients with recurrent postoperative dysmenorrhea were switched from cyclic to continuous CHC dosing.[29] Severity of pain was significantly reduced after the switch, and more than 80% of patients reported satisfaction with the method. In a more recent randomized, placebo-controlled trial comparing cyclic and continuous dosing of a low-dose monophasic oral contraceptive pill after laparoscopy, the continuous dosing strategy provided statistically superior improvement in pain and disease recurrence compared with both the cyclic dosing and placebo groups at 6, 12, 18, and 24 months postoperatively, while the cyclic dosing group demonstrated superiority only over placebo after 12 months of therapy.[30] One theory that may explain these findings is prevention of retrograde menstruation through induction of an amenorrheic state with continuous dosing. Based on these findings, the ESHRE guidelines recommend continuous CHC dosing as an option for patients.[17]

Progestins Various studies have demonstrated the effectiveness of progestins in treating the pain of endometriosis. The largest body of data support use of oral norethindrone acetate, oral dienogest (not available in the United States), oral medroxyprogesterone acetate, and DMPA. As with all endometriosis treatments, active comparator studies (eg, progestin vs GnRH agonist, progestin vs danazol) have failed to demonstrate superiority of any one drug class over another.[31] There are no trials that directly compare the various progestins with one another; thus, selection of an agent must consider its dosage form, cost, and potential side effects.

One concern over use of DMPA is its potential to cause bone mineral density loss, and for this reason both the intramuscular and the subcutaneous products carry FDA black box warnings against use for more than 2 years. Despite this labeling, ACOG has stated that the concern over bone mineral density and potential fracture risk should not deter clinicians from prescribing and continuing DMPA in appropriate patients since bone loss appears to be almost completely reversible upon discontinuation of the drug.[32] Although this ACOG statement specifically addresses use of DMPA for contraception, one may surmise that the same may hold true in the endometriosis population. Prolonged delays in return to ovulation after cessation of therapy of DMPA is also concerning, thus it may not be optimal for use in women desiring future pregnancy.[16]

Levonorgestrel Intrauterine System The LNG-IUS is an intriguing option for treating endometriosis due to its ability to locally deliver progestin to the uterine cavity, causing atrophy and pseudodecidualization of the uterine lining and endometrial cell apoptosis, without significant systemic absorption.[33] To date, almost all studies demonstrating effectiveness of the LNG-IUS have been conducted in patients previously undergoing conservative surgery, with time to insertion of the LNG-IUS varying from immediately to 5 years after surgery.[34] Effectiveness has also been shown in adolescent patients after surgery.[33] Although three LNG-IUS products are now available in the United States, only Mirena has been studied in endometriosis patients. The three systems differ in the amount of daily drug delivered, thus it cannot be assumed that the other two products (Skyla and Liletta) will demonstrate similar benefits.

Disadvantages of the LNG-IUS include potential difficulty of inserting the device into nulliparous women, a 5% expulsion rate, and the potential for growth of ovarian endometriomas since the method does not inhibit ovulation.[16]

Gonadotropin-Releasing Hormone Agonists GnRH agonists create a functional oophorectomy via inhibition of follicle-stimulating hormone and luteinizing hormone secretion. For the first 2 to 3 weeks after initiation, GnRH agonists create a gonadotropin flare prior to receptor downregulation. This flare often causes a temporary increase in pain. Initiating therapy during the mid-luteal phase and/or overlapping the first 3 weeks of therapy with a CHC or progestin may minimize such effects, and use of analgesics during this time frame is also critical.[35] Of the four agents available for use in the United States (goserelin, leuprolide, nafarelin, and triptorelin), route of administration and cost is the primary distinguishing factor that determines choice of drug.

Pain relief with GnRH agonists is superior to placebo and comparable to other therapies such as danazol, CHCs, DMPA, and the LNG-IUS.[36] As previously noted, many clinicians now prescribe GnRH agonists indefinitely due to the fast recurrence of pain that occurs upon discontinuation and ability to avoid unwanted side effects through use of add-back therapy.

Side effects are the primary limitation of GnRH agonist use. The pharmacologically induced hypoestrogenic environment results in bone mineral density loss and vasomotor symptoms such as hot flashes, vaginal dryness, and insomnia. Without add-back therapy, loss of bone mineral density is estimated at 4% to 8% within a 6-month treatment course, and this loss continues progressively over time.[37,38]

Cost of the GnRH agonists is high. In one study, every 6-week dosing of intramuscular triptorelin was compared with its usual every 4-week dosing regimen.[39] Pain relief and serum hormone levels were equivalent between groups, suggesting that an extended interval strategy may be an option for cost savings.

Add-Back Therapy 8 Add-back therapy refers to use of pharmacologic agents in addition to GnRH agonists in order to minimize side effects (eg, hot flashes and decreased libido), improve adherence, and most importantly protect bone mineral density.[22,37] Regimens investigated for this purpose have generally included progestin monotherapy or estrogen-progestin combinations, with a recent meta-analysis and randomized, controlled trial concluding that only an estrogen-progestin combination is protective of bone mineral density loss.[38,40] Although it may seem counterintuitive to use such therapy in endometriosis patients, it appears that maintaining serum estrogen levels at less than 50 pg/mL (184 pmol/L) prevents GnRH agonist side effects while still preventing growth of new endometrial tissue.[16,22] For this reason, CHCs should not be used as add-back therapy as they will cause serum estrogen levels to exceed this threshold.[35] Instead, the estrogen and progestin doses typically used in menopausal women are more appropriate. Examples of regimens studied include oral conjungated equine estrogens 0.625 mg/day plus oral norethindrone acetate 5 mg/day, and transdermal estradiol 25 mcg twice weekly plus oral medroxyprogesterone acetate 5 mg/day, and oral estradiol 2 mg/day plus oral norethindrone acetate 1 mg/day.[40]

Danazol

Danazol has been shown to be effective both empirically and after surgery compared with placebo.[41] Formerly the "gold standard" of endometriosis treatment, the popularity of danazol has decreased with the development of agents with more favorable side-effect profiles. Danazol should not be initiated in women with hyperlipidemia or liver disease. It is teratogenic; thus, barrier forms of contraception must be used.

In an effort to diminish the high rate of androgenic side effects noted with danazol while maintaining effectiveness, vaginal danazol formulations (100-200 mg/day) have been investigated in three small studies.[42-44] Each study was a nonrandomized, prospective trial in women who had failed other therapies such as surgery, GnRH agonists, and the LNG-IUS. In each, improvements in dysmenorrhea, deep dyspareunia, and pelvic pain were noted without incidence of systemic side effects; thus, vaginal delivery of this drug may prove to be a viable method. Unfortunately, a vaginal formulation is not yet available in the United States.

Aromatase Inhibitors Aromatase inhibitors are the most recent drug class to be formally added as a treatment option in endometriosis guidelines.[17] Because aromatase is a key enzyme in the conversion of adrenal androgens to estrogens, the agents diminish endometrial lesions by lowering overall estrogen concentrations by 97% to 99%.[45] Numerous case reports and retrospective, nonrandomized and noncomparative, as well as randomized comparative studies support the effectiveness of both letrozole and anastrozole in decreasing pain, improving quality of life, and reducing postoperative recurrence of disease in women refractory to other treatment efforts.[17,45-50] In all cases, the aromatase inhibitor was used in combination with a progestin, a combined oral contraceptive, or a GnRH agonist. Because most safety information for the aromatase inhibitors is derived from use in postmenopausal women with cancer, it is unknown if similar issues will be experienced by premenopausal women using these agents for endometriosis. Of particular concern is the impact of use on bone mineral density. Based on available data, it does appear that use of progestins and combined oral contraceptives in combination with the aromatase inhibitors helps limit bone mineral density loss.[45,49]

Personalized Pharmacotherapy

At this point in time, no evidence exists to suggest how to select or dose therapy for endometriosis based on pharmacogenomic, pharmacogenetic, or pharmacokinetic differences between patients. As additional understanding of the pathogenesis of endometriosis emerges, such personalized pharmacotherapy options might be realized.

EVALUATION OF THERAPEUTIC OUTCOMES

Size, number, and distribution of endometrial lesions do not correlate with pain symptoms or fertility potential; thus, therapeutic outcome monitoring should focus solely on subjective relief of symptoms.[3] Although traditional measures such as visual pain scales and symptom diaries have been used to measure treatment effectiveness, such measures do not capture overall patient satisfaction with treatment, a factor which has been correlated to treatment adherence.[51] A patient-reported outcome instrument, the Endometriosis Treatment Satisfaction Questionnaire, has been developed and validated.[51] The tool includes six items (pain before and/or during periods, pain during and/or after sex, endometriosis pain, bleeding/spotting, tolerability, overall satisfaction) that are rated by patients on a 7-point Likert scale.[51] The SF-36 has also been validated in the endometriosis population.[52]

3 Endometriosis-related pain should be relieved within 2 months of initiating medical therapy. If symptoms persist, consideration should be given to different medical and/or surgical therapy. For endometriosis-related infertility, most experts recommend 6 months of watchful waiting after surgical intervention. If pregnancy is not achieved within that time, assisted reproductive techniques can be considered.

ABBREVIATIONS

ACOG	American College of Obstetricians and Gynecologists
ESHRE	European Society of Human Reproduction and Embryology
CHC	combined hormonal contraceptive
DMPA	depot medroxyprogesterone acetate
GnRH	gonadotropin-releasing hormone
LNG-IUS	levonorgestrel-releasing intrauterine system

REFERENCES

1. Brown J, Farquhar C. Endometriosis: an overview of Cochrane Reviews. *Cochrane Database Syst Rev* 2014;(3):CD009590.
2. Bulun SE. Endometriosis. *N Engl J Med* 2009;360(3):268-279.
3. Committee on Gynecologic Practice. ACOG Practice Bulletin No. 114: Management of endometriosis. *Obstet Gynecol* 2010;116(1):223-236.
4. Ferrero S, Arena E, Morando A, Remorgida V. Prevalence of newly diagnosed endometriosis in women attending the general practitioner. *Int J Gynaecol Obstet* 2010;110(3):203-207.
5. Meuleman C, Vandenabeele B, Fieuws S, et al. High prevalence of endometriosis in infertile women with normal ovulation and normospermic partners. *Fertil Steril* 2009;92(1):68-74.
6. McLeod BS, Retzloff MG. Epidemiology of endometriosis: An assessment of risk factors. *Clin Obstet Gynecol* 2010;53(2):389-396.
7. Burney RO, Guidice LC. Pathogenesis and pathophysiology of endometriosis. *Fertil Steril* 2012;98(3):511-519.
8. Peterson CM, Johnstone EB, Hammoud AO, et al. Risk factors associated with endometriosis: Importance of study population for characterizing disease in the ENDO study. *Am J Obstet Gynecol* 2013;208(6):451.e1-11.
9. Tempfer CB, Simoni M, Destenaves B, Fauser BC. Functional genetic polymorphisms and female reproductive disorders: Part II—Endometriosis. *Hum Reprod Update* 2009;15(1):97-118.
10. Practice Committee of the American Society for Reproductive Medicine. Treatment of pelvic pain associated with endometriosis: A committee opinion. *Fertil Steril* 2014;101(4):927-935.
11. Wang G, Tokushige N, Markham R, Fraser IS. Rich innervation of deep infiltrating endometriosis. *Hum Reprod* 2009;24(4):827-834.

12. Mechsner S, Kaiser A, Kopf A, et al. A pilot study to evaluate the clinical relevance of endometriosis-associated nerve fibers in peritoneal endometriotic lesions. *Fertil Steril* 2009;92(6):1856-1861.
13. Practice Committee of the American Society for Reproductive Medicine. Endometriosis and infertility: A committee opinion. *Fertil Steril* 2012;98(3):591-598.
14. Mansour G, Aziz N, Sharma R, et al. The impact of peritoneal fluid from healthy women and from women with endometriosis on sperm DNA and its relationship to the sperm deformity index. *Fertil Steril* 2009;92(1):61-67.
15. Ziegler D, Borghese B, Chapron C. Endometriosis and infertility: Pathophysiology and management. *Lancet* 2010;376(9742):730-738.
16. Leyland N, Casper R, Laberge P, Singh SS. Endometriosis: Diagnosis and management. *J Obstet Gynaecol Can* 2010;32(7 Suppl 2):S1-S32.
17. Dunselman GAJ, Vermeulen N, Becker C, et al. ESHRE guideline: Management of women with endometriosis. *Human Reprod* 2014;29(3):400-412.
18. Wu L, Wu Q, Liu L. Oral contraceptive pills for endometriosis after conservative surgery: A systematic review and meta-analysis. *Gynecol Endocrinol* 2013;29(10):883-890.
19. Tanmahasamut P, Rattanachaiyanont M, Angsuwathana S, et al. Postoperative levonorgestrel-releasing intrauterine system for pelvic endometriosis-related pain. *Obstet Gynecol* 2012;199(3):519-526.
20. Dovey S, Sanfilippo J. Endometriosis and the adolescent. *Clin Obstet Gynecol* 2010;53(2):420-428.
21. Bedaiwy MA, Casper RF. Treatment with leuprolide acetate and hormonal add-back for up to 10 years in stage IV endometriosis patients with chronic pelvic pain. *Fertil Steril* 2006;86(1):220-222.
22. Wu D, Hu M, Hong L, et al. Clinical efficacy of add-back therapy in treatment of endometriosis: a meta-analysis. *Arch Gynecol Obstet* 2014;290(3):513-523.
23. DiVasta AD, Laufer MR, Gordon CM. Bone density in adolescents treated with a GnRH agonist and add-back therapy for endometriosis. *J Pediatr Adolesc Gynecol* 2007;20(5):293-297.
24. Ballweg ML. Treating endometriosis in adolescents: Does it matter? *J Pediatr Adolesc Gynecol* 2011;24(5 Suppl):S2-S6.
25. Dun EC, Kho KA, Morozov VV, et al. Endometriosis in adolescents. *JSLS* 2015;19(2):pii.e2015.00019
26. Brosens I, Gordts S, Benagiano G. Endometriosis in adolescents is a hidden, progressive and severe disease that deserves attention, not just compassion. *Hum Reprod* 2013;28(8):2026-2031.
27. Davis LJ, Kennedy SS, Moore J, Prentice A. Oral contraceptives for pain associated with endometriosis. *Cochrane Database Syst Rev* 2007;(3):CD001019.
28. Vercellini P, Barbara G, Somigliana E, et al. Comparison of contraceptive ring and patch for the treatment of symptomatic endometriosis. *Fertil Steril* 2010;93(7):2150-2161.
29. Vercellini P, Frontino G, Giorgi OD, et al. Continuous use of an oral contraceptive for endometriosis-associated recurrent dysmenorrhea that does not respond to a cyclic pill regimen. *Fertil Steril* 2003; 80(3):560-563.
30. Seracchioli R, Mabrouk M, Frasca C, et al. Long-term oral contraceptive pills and postoperative pain management after laparoscopic excision of ovarian endometrioma: A randomized controlled trial. *Fertil Steril* 2010;94(2):464-471.
31. Brown J, Kives S, Akhtar M. Progestagens and anti-progestagens for pain associated with endometriosis. *Cochrane Database Syst Rev* 2012;(3):CD002122.
32. Committee on Adolescent Health Care, Committee on Gynecologic Practice. Committee Opinion No. 602: Depot medroxyprogesterone acetate and bone effects. *Obstet Gynecol* 2014;123(6):1398-1402.
33. Yoost J, LaJoie AS, Hertweck P, Loveless M. Use of levonorgestrel intrauterine system in adolescents with endometriosis. *Pediatr Adolesc Gynecol* 2013;26(2):120-124.
34. Abou-Setta AM, Houston B, Al-Inany HG, Farquhar C. Levonorgestrel-releasing intrauterine device (LNG-IUD) for symptomatic endometriosis following surgery. *Cochrane Database Syst Rev* 2013;(1):CD005072.
35. DiVasta AD, Laufer MR. The use of gonadotropin releasing hormone analogues in adolescent and young patients with endometriosis. *Curr Opin Obstet Gynecol* 2013;25(4):287-292.
36. Brown J, Pan A, Hart RJ. Gonadotrophin-releasing hormone analogues for pain associated with endometriosis. *Cochrane Database Syst Rev* 2010;(12):CD008475.
37. Surrey ES. Gonadotropin-releasing hormone agonist and add-back therapy: What do the data show? *Curr Opin Obstet Gynecol* 2010;22(4):283-288.
38. Divasta AD, Feldman HA, Gallagher JS, et al. Hormonal add-back therapy for females treated with gonadotropin-releasing hormone agonist for endometriosis. *Obstet Gynecol* 2015;126(3):617-627.
39. Kang JL, Wang XX, Nie ML, Huang XH. Efficacy of gonadotropin-releasing hormone agonist and an extended-interval dosing regimen in the treatment of patients with adenomyosis and endometriosis. *Gynecol Obstet Invest* 2010;69(2):73-77.
40. Farmer JE, Prentice A, Breeze A, et al. Gonadotrophin-releasing hormone analogues for endometriosis: bone mineral density. *Cochrane Database Syst Rev* 2003;(4):CD001297.
41. Farquhar C, Prentice A, Singla AA, Selak V. Danazol for pelvic pain associated with endometriosis. *Cochrane Database Syst Rev* 2007;(4):CD000068.
42. Razzi S, Luisi S, Calonaci F, et al. Efficacy of vaginal danazol treatment in women with recurrent deeply infiltrating endometriosis. *Fertil Steril* 2007;88(4):789-794.
43. Bhattacharya SM, Tolasaria A, Khan B. Vaginal danazol for the treatment of endometriosis-related pelvic pain. *Int J Gynaecol Obstet* 2011;115(3):294-295.
44. Ferrero S, Tramalloni D, Venturini PL, Remorgida V. Vaginal danazol for women with rectovaginal endometriosis and pain symptoms persisting after insertion of a levonorgestrel-releasing intrauterine device. *Int J Gynaecol Obstet* 2011;113(2):116-119.
45. Pavone ME, Bulun SE. Aromatase inhibitors for the treatment of endometriosis. *Fertil Steril* 2012;98(6):1370-1379.
46. Abushahin F, Goldman KN, Barbieri E, et al. Aromatase inhibition for refractory endometriosis-related chronic pelvic pain. *Fertil Steril* 2011;96(4):939-942.
47. Colette S, Donnez J. Are aromatase inhibitors effective in endometriosis treatment? *Expert Opin Investig Drugs* 2011;20(7):917-931.
48. Nothnick WB. The emerging use of aromatase inhibitors for endometriosis treatment. *Reprod Biol Endocrinol* 2011;9:87.
49. Ferrero S, Gillott DJ, Venturini PL, Remorgida V. Use of aromatase inhibitors to treat endometriosis-related pain symptoms: A systematic review. *Reprod Biol Endocrinol* 2011;9:89.
50. Alborzi S, Hamedi B, Omidvar A, et al. A comparison of the effect of short-term aromatase inhibitor (letrozole) and GnRH agonist (triptorelin) versus case control on pregnancy rate and symptom and sign recurrence after laparoscopic treatment of endometriosis. *Arch Gynecol Obstet* 2011;284(1):105-110.
51. Deal LS, Williams VS, DiBenedetti DB, Fehnel SE. Development and psychometric evaluation of the endometriosis treatment satisfaction questionnaire. *Qual Life Res* 2010;19(6):899-905.
52. Stull DE, Wasiak R, Kreif N, et al. Validation of the SF-36 in patients with endometriosis. *Qual Life Res* 2014;23(1):103-117.

82

Hormone Therapy in Women

Sophia N. Kalantaridou, Laura M. Borgelt, Devra K. Dang, and Karim Anton Calis

KEY CONCEPTS

1. The decision to use menopausal hormone therapy (MHT) and the type of formulation used must be individualized based on several factors, including the severity of menopausal symptoms and the risks of cardiovascular disease, breast cancer, osteoporotic fracture, and venous thromboembolic events (VTE).
2. Menopausal hormone therapy is the most effective treatment option for alleviating moderate to severe vasomotor symptoms.
3. Cardiovascular disease—including coronary artery disease, stroke, and peripheral vascular disease—is the leading cause of death among women, and MHT should not be used for reducing the risk of cardiovascular disease.
4. The risk of breast cancer associated with MHT appears to be associated with the addition of progestogen therapy to estrogen. Use of estrogen alone does not increase the risk of breast cancer.
5. In recently postmenopausal women who are at increased fracture risk, systemic estrogen therapy may be indicated for the prevention of osteoporotic fractures when alternate therapies are either contraindicated or cause excessive adverse effects.
6. Menopausal hormone therapy appears to improve depressive symptoms in symptomatic menopausal women.
7. Use of MHT at doses lower than those prescribed historically (ie, prior to the Women's Health Initiative [WHI] study) appears to be effective in reducing bone loss and managing menopausal symptoms.
8. Because of the increased risk of endometrial hyperplasia and endometrial cancer with estrogen monotherapy (ie, unopposed estrogen), use of systemic estrogen in women with an intact uterus must always be accompanied by a progestogen or an estrogen agonist antagonist for endometrial protection.
9. Premenopausal hormone therapy in young women with primary ovarian insufficiency (POI) differs markedly from MHT, and results of randomized trials conducted in menopausal women, including the WHI trial, cannot be extrapolated to premenopausal women with ovarian dysfunction.

MENOPAUSE AND MENOPAUSAL HORMONE THERAPY

All women undergo menopause, but every woman experiences it differently. Natural menopause occurs in stages including perimenopause (in the 5th decade), menopause, and postmenopause (1 year after menopause and beyond). Induced menopause can be experienced any time before natural menopause with bilateral oophorectomy (removal of both ovaries) or iatrogenic ablation of ovarian function (eg, chemotherapy, pelvic radiation). Symptoms of menopause can vary widely with induced menopause typically causing more severe symptoms. Due to the variability in duration, severity, and presence of menopausal symptoms among women, treatment should be individualized with treatment goals and decisions established in a shared decision making process.

Epidemiology

Menopause is the permanent cessation of menses following the loss of ovarian follicular activity. The median age at the onset of menopause in the United States is 51 years, but can vary widely from 40 to 58 years.[1] An estimated 6,000 women in the United States reach menopause each day, and will spend approximately 40% of their lives in postmenopause.[2] It is estimated that by 2025, the number of postmenopausal women will be 1.1 billion worldwide.[1] By definition, menopause is a normal physiologic event that occurs after 12 consecutive months of amenorrhea, so the time of the final menses is determined retrospectively. Women who have undergone hysterectomy (removal of the uterus) must rely on their symptoms to estimate the actual time of menopause, but typically occurs a few years earlier than natural menopause.

Etiology

A nomenclature and staging system for the female reproductive aging continuum was developed at the Stages of Reproductive Aging Workshop (STRAW) in 2001 and revised in 2011 with the STRAW + 10 staging system.[3] The menopause transition refers to the span of time including menstrual, endocrine, and symptom changes starting with variation in menstrual cycle length and ending with the final menstrual period (FMP). Postmenopause occurs for the years beyond the FMP with stabilization of hormone levels and limited endocrine changes.

Pathophysiology

A woman is born with approximately two million primordial follicles in her ovaries. During a normal reproductive life span, she ovulates fewer than 500 times. The vast majority of follicles undergo atresia.

The hypothalamic–pituitary–ovarian axis dynamically controls reproductive physiology throughout the reproductive years. The pituitary is regulated by pulsatile secretion of gonadotropin-releasing hormone (GnRH) from the hypothalamus. Follicle-stimulating hormone (FSH) and luteinizing hormone (LH), produced by the pituitary in response to GnRH, regulate ovarian function. These gonadotropins also are influenced by negative feedback from estradiol and progesterone. Ovarian follicular activity is reflected by the circulating concentrations of sex steroids and by peptide hormones including inhibin, activin, and anti-Mullerian hormone (AMH). AMH is a product of growing ovarian follicles, which appears to be independent of the hypothalamic–pituitary–gonadal axis. It is a principal regulator of early follicular recruitment from the primordial pool such that the concentration of AMH in blood may also reflect the nongrowing follicle population. AMH concentrations decline with age. While AMH levels may predict the median time to menopause, obtaining levels of AMH, FSH, and estradiol may be best reserved for women seeking fertility.[4] The sex steroids include estradiol, produced by the dominant follicle; progesterone, produced by the corpus luteum after maturation of the dominant ovarian follicle; and androgens, primarily testosterone and androstenedione, secreted by the ovarian stroma. Sex steroids are important for the healthy functioning of many organs, including the bones, brain, skin, and reproductive and urogenital tracts. They act primarily by regulating gene expression.

Pathophysiologic changes associated with menopause are caused by loss of ovarian follicular activity. Ovarian primordial follicle numbers decrease with advancing age, and at the time of menopause, few follicles remain in the ovary. Hence, the postmenopausal ovary is no longer the primary site of estradiol or progesterone synthesis. The postmenopausal ovary secretes primarily androstenedione. In contrast to the acute fall in circulating estrogen at the time of menopause, the decline in circulating androgens commences in the decade leading up to the average age of natural menopause and closely parallels increasing age. Whether the ovary continues to secrete testosterone after menopause remains controversial. Hypertrophy of the ovarian stroma may develop after menopause, probably secondary to high LH concentrations, thereby resulting in increased ovarian testosterone production. Alternatively, the ovaries may become fibrotic and a poor source of sex steroids. No endocrine event clearly signals the time just prior to final menses.[5]

As women age, a progressive rise in circulating FSH and a concomitant decline in ovarian inhibin-B and AMH are observed. In women who continue to experience menstrual bleeding, FSH determinations on day 2 or 3 of the menstrual cycle exceeding 10 to 12 International Units/L (10-12 IU/L) may indicate diminished ovarian reserve. Alternatively, low AMH concentrations, measured at any time in the cycle, predicts diminishing ovarian reserve. Clear elevations in serum FSH are seen in women approximately at age 40 years.[5] When ovarian function has ceased, serum FSH concentrations are greater than 40 IU/L. Menopause is characterized by a 10- to 15-fold increase in circulating FSH concentrations compared with concentrations of FSH in the follicular phase of the cycle, a fourfold to fivefold increase in LH, and a greater than 90% decrease in circulating estradiol concentrations.[5] During the perimenopause, FSH concentrations may rise to the postmenopausal range during some cycles but return to premenopausal levels during subsequent cycles. Thus, high concentrations of FSH should not be used to diagnose menopause in perimenopausal women.

Clinical Presentation

The perimenopause commences with the onset of menstrual irregularity and ends 12 months after the last menstrual period.[3] Approximately 90% of women have 4 to 8 years of menstrual cycle changes with heavier flow of longer duration before natural menopause occurs.[1] The menstrual cycle irregularity is most often caused by the increased frequency of anovulatory cycles, but may also be due to thyroid abnormalities, hyperprolactinemia, or polycystic ovary syndrome. Women commonly experience symptoms during the perimenopause, which substantially impact their health and daily function. Vasomotor symptoms (eg, hot flushes and night sweats) occur in up to 75% of women for 6 months to 2 years, and some women have bothersome symptoms for 10 years or longer.[1] Vasomotor symptoms persist for an average 7.4 years with moderate to severe vasomotor symptoms extending in 42% of women age 60 to 65 years.[6,7] Research has shown that 25% of women experience severe vasomotor symptoms, 30% experience severe psychological symptoms (eg, depression and anxiety), and 50% report moderate to severe symptoms of sleep disturbance, joint pain, or headache, and at least one in four women have sexual dysfunction.[8,9] Genitourinary syndrome of menopause (GSM) is a collection of symptoms associated with decreased estrogen and other sex steroids that create changes to the labia majora/minora, clitoris, vestibule/introitus, vagina, urethra, and bladder.[10] Resulting symptoms include genital dryness, burning, and irritation; sexual symptoms of lubrication difficulty, discomfort or pain, and impaired sexual function; and urinary symptoms of urgency, dysuria, and recurrent urinary tract infections. Vaginal symptoms occur in an estimated 45% of women, but only 4% can identify these symptoms as vulvovaginal atrophy related to menopause.[11]

Women who experience severe symptoms, either from early in the menopause transition or from their FMP, are likely to continue to experience severe symptoms for several years.[8] The perimenopause is associated with a higher vulnerability to depression with the risk increasing from early to late perimenopause and decreasing during postmenopause.[12] Women with a history of depression are nearly five times as likely to be diagnosed with depression during the perimenopause, whereas women with no history of depression are two to four times more likely to have a diagnosis compared with premenopausal women.[12]

In addition to the symptoms of menopause, loss of estrogen production results in significant metabolic changes including effects on body composition, cognition, lipids, vascular function, and bone metabolism. The menopause transition is associated with a significant increase in central abdominal fat leading to an average weight gain during the menopausal transition of 5 pounds; however this is likely to be related to aging and lifestyle rather than menopause.[1] Skin changes including decreased thickness and elasticity, loss of

CLINICAL PRESENTATION Perimenopause and Menopause

Signs

- Perimenopause: DUB as a result of anovulatory cycles (other gynecologic disorders should be excluded).
- Menopause: signs of GSM.

Symptoms

- Vasomotor symptoms (hot flushes and night sweats)
- Sleep disturbances
- Mood changes
- Problems with concentration and memory
- Vaginal dryness and dyspareunia
- Arthralgia

Laboratory Tests

- Perimenopause: FSH on day 2 or 3 of the menstrual cycle greater than 10 to 12 IU/L
- Menopause: FSH greater than 40 IU/L

Other Relevant Diagnostic Tests

- Thyroid function tests
- Iron stores
- Lipid profile

collagen, and wrinkling, and hair changes including alopecia and hirsutism are also associated with menopause. Poor concentration and memory are common during the menopause transition and early postmenopause.[1] Memory performance and processing speed slightly decline during the menopausal transition, but reach premenopausal levels after menopause. It is important to note that these cognitive symptoms can be affected by other symptoms of menopause including sleep disturbances, hot flushes, depressed mood, fatigue, and midlife stressors.

Dysfunctional uterine bleeding (DUB) may occur during the perimenopausal years because of anovulatory cycles; however, abnormal uterine bleeding always merits investigation when it cannot be simply explained by menopausal cyclical irregularity. Treatment options for DUB include insertion of an intrauterine progestin-only device, systemic progestogen therapy, or the combined oral contraceptive pill unless contraindicated.

Treatment: Menopause

Desired Outcomes

Menopause is a natural life event, not a disease. The primary goals of therapy for menopause are to relieve symptoms and improve quality of life while minimizing adverse effects. This can be best achieved by individualizing treatment based on medical, social, and family history as well as her symptoms and quality of life goals.

General Approach to Treatment

In women with mild vasomotor symptoms, nonpharmacologic therapy can be considered. In women with moderate to severe hot flushes and vulvovaginal symptoms, menopausal hormone therapy (MHT) is the treatment of choice unless contraindicated (Table 82-1). Treatment of mild vulvovaginal symptoms should include nonhormonal lubricants and moisturizers. However, for some women these treatments are not effective. Fig. 82-1 outlines an algorithm for the general management of menopausal women.

1 The decision to use MHT and the type of formulation used must be individualized based on several factors, including the severity of menopausal symptoms and the risks of cardiovascular disease, breast cancer, osteoporotic fracture, and venous thromboembolic events (VTE). Breast cancer risk is increased with concomitant progestogen use in menopausal women with an intact uterus.[13] VTE may also increase with higher estrogen doses and oral administration.[14,15]

The duration of therapy also needs to be individualized according to severity of symptoms, health status, and concerns regarding risks. Approved indications of MHT include treatment of moderate to severe vasomotor symptoms, moderate to severe vulvovaginal atrophy, and prevention of postmenopausal osteoporosis. For treatment of vasomotor symptoms, systemic MHT is the most effective pharmacologic intervention (see Fig. 82-1). For symptoms of vulvar and vaginal atrophy, such as vaginal dryness, intravaginal products should be considered.

Nonpharmacologic Therapy

Mild menopausal symptoms may be managed effectively with lifestyle modifications, including wearing layered clothing that can be removed or added as necessary, lowering room temperature, decreasing intake of hot spicy foods, caffeine, and hot beverages, exercise, and other good general health practices. Dietary supplements have been promoted as alternatives to MHT with conflicting results.[16]

Pharmacologic Therapy

Pharmacologic therapy is the mainstay of management of menopausal symptoms and includes both hormonal (estrogen with or without progestogen) and nonhormonal medications.

Drug Treatment of First Choice 2 Menopausal hormone therapy is the most effective treatment option for alleviating moderate to severe vasomotor symptoms. In women with an intact uterus, systemic MHT consists of an estrogen plus a progestogen or estrogen agonist/antagonist (eg, bazedoxifene) to prevent endometrial hyperplasia. In women who have undergone hysterectomy, estrogen therapy is given unopposed by a progestogen. Mild vulvovaginal symptoms may be adequately managed with nonhormonal lubricants and moisturizers.[17] However, vaginal estrogen therapy (cream, tablet, and ring) may be needed for moderate to severe vulvovaginal symptoms. Progestogen therapy for endometrial protection is not recommended with the use of low-dose vaginal estrogens (ie, those with minimal systemic exposure), but it should be noted that endometrial safety studies of vaginal estrogen therapy do not extend beyond 1 year.

Published Guidelines A number of national and international guidelines and consensus statements on the management of menopause are available.[1,18-23] The United States Preventive Services Task Force also provides a recommendation statement on the use of MHT for the prevention of chronic medical conditions in postmenopausal women.[24]

TABLE 82-1 FDA-Labeled Indications and Contraindications for Menopausal Hormone Therapy with Estrogens and Progestins

Indications	
For systemic use	Treatment of moderate to severe vasomotor symptoms (ie, moderate to severe hot flushes)
For intravaginal use (low systemic exposure)	Treatment of moderate to severe symptoms of vulvar and vaginal atrophy (ie, moderate to severe vaginal dryness, dyspareunia, and atrophic vaginitis)
Contraindications	
Absolute contraindications	Undiagnosed abnormal genital bleeding Known, suspected, or history of cancer of the breast Known or suspected estrogen- or progesterone-dependent neoplasia Active deep vein thrombosis, pulmonary embolism, or a history of these conditions Active or recent (eg, within the past year) arterial thromboembolic disease (eg, stroke, myocardial infarction) Liver dysfunction or disease
Relative contraindications	Elevated blood pressure Hypertriglyceridemia Impaired liver function and past history of cholestatic jaundice Hypothyroidism Fluid retention Severe hypocalcemia Ovarian cancer Exacerbation of endometriosis Exacerbation of asthma, diabetes mellitus, migraine, systemic lupus erythematosus, epilepsy, porphyria, and hepatic hemangioma

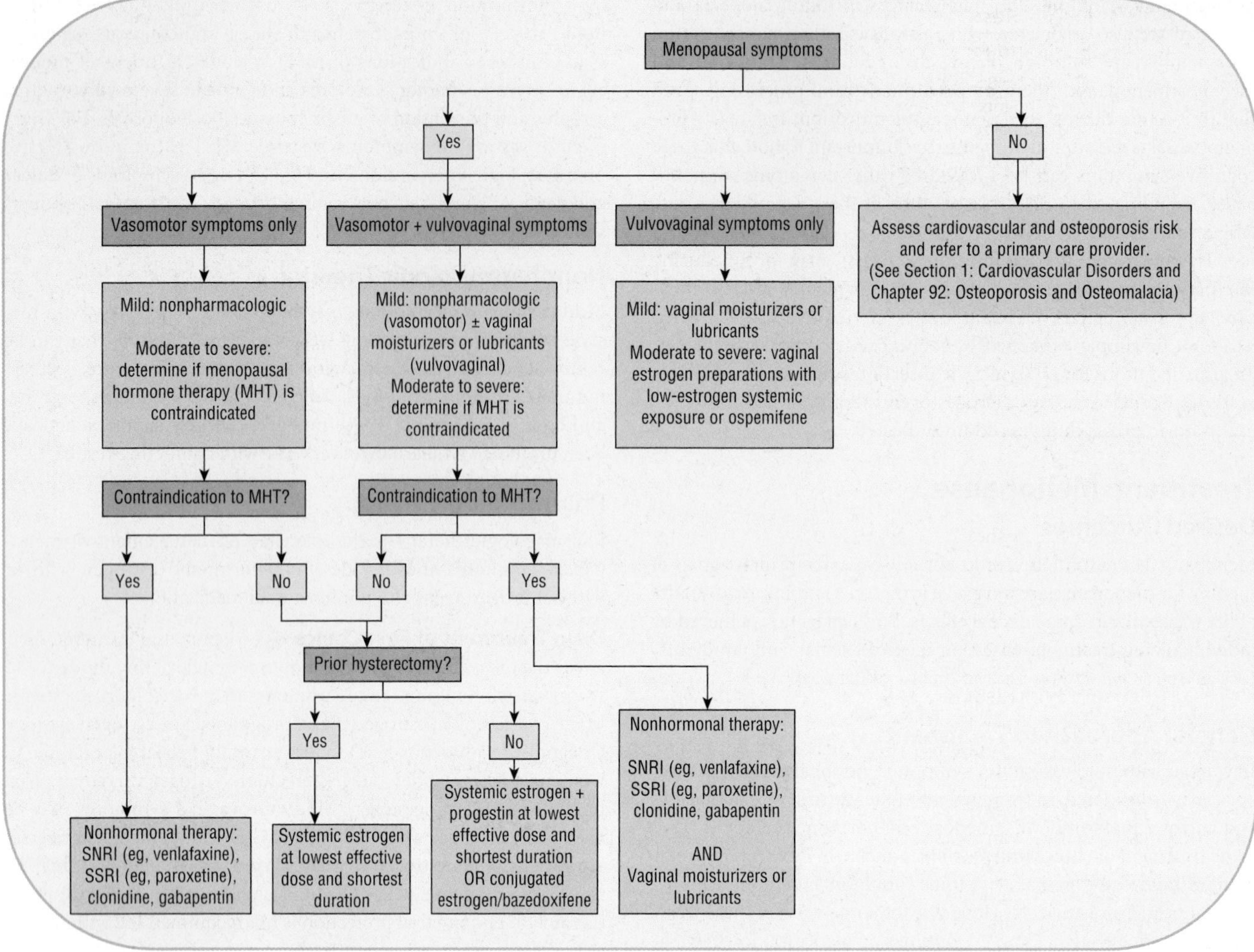

FIGURE 82-1 Algorithm for pharmacologic management of menopausal symptoms.

Therapy for Perimenopausal Women Despite a decline in fertility with age, sexually active women may become pregnant during the perimenopausal years. Furthermore, perimenopausal women can experience hot flushes despite having menstrual cycles. Combined hormonal contraceptives (containing low-dose estrogen and progestogen) provide contraception and vasomotor symptom relief. Perimenopausal women should not use estrogen-containing contraceptives if they smoke or have a history of estrogen-dependent cancer, heart disease, high blood pressure, diabetes, or thromboembolism. For perimenopausal women with DUB due to anovulatory cycles, a progestin-only intrauterine device may be a useful option. Combined hormonal contraceptives provide the additional benefit of reducing the risk of ovarian and endometrial cancer.

Menopausal Hormone Therapy for Vasomotor Symptoms and GSM Menopausal hormone therapy remains the most effective treatment for moderate and severe vasomotor symptoms, impaired sleep quality, and vulvovaginal symptoms of menopause.

Vasomotor Symptoms Fewer than 25% of women experience a menopausal transition without symptoms, whereas more than 25% suffer severe menopausal symptoms, most commonly hot flushes and night sweats. The average duration of vasomotor symptoms is 7.4 years with some women experiencing symptoms for more than 10 years.[6] Women with mild vasomotor symptoms can experience relief by lifestyle modification, and at least 25% of women in clinical trials reported significant improvement of vasomotor symptoms when taking placebo. The most effective treatment for vasomotor symptoms is MHT with 80% to 90% relief of symptoms. Benefits and risks of MHT should be weighed individually and assessed on an annual basis. The formulation, dose, and duration of therapy will also depend on patient symptoms and medical history.

Genitourinary Syndrome of Menopause Estrogen receptors have been demonstrated in the lower genitourinary tract, and up to 50% of postmenopausal women suffer symptoms of vulvovaginal atrophy caused by estrogen deficiency. Atrophy of the vaginal mucosa results in vaginal dryness, burning, irritation, discomfort, and dyspareunia. Lower urinary tract symptoms include urethritis, recurrent urinary tract infection, urinary urgency, and frequency.

Most women with moderate-to-severe vulvovaginal symptoms require local or systemic estrogen therapy for symptom relief. Local (vaginal) estrogen delivery is preferred when vaginal symptoms are the only menopausal symptom complaint, as it minimizes systemic absorption and is more effective than oral estrogen therapy with 80% to 90% symptom relief compared to 75% with oral estrogen.[17,20] Vaginal estrogen has also been shown to improve atrophic symptoms and vaginal mucosal appearance, decrease vaginal pH, improve vaginal and/or urethral cytology, and reduce the risk of lower urinary tract symptoms and recurrent urinary tract infections possibly by modifying the vaginal flora.[17,20,25] Moderate to severe vulvovaginal symptoms can be treated with a vaginal estrogen cream, tablet, or ring; or with the selective estrogen receptor modulator (SERM) ospemifene 60 mg orally per day.[26] Ospemifene has a nearly full estrogen agonist effect in the vaginal epithelium to improve dyspareunia and has been well tolerated without breast or endometrial concerns after 1 year of use.

Dose-related adverse effects of vaginal estrogen include vulvovaginal candidiasis, vaginal bleeding, breast pain, and nausea.[17] Concomitant progestogen therapy is unnecessary when low-dose

TABLE 82-2 Principal Results of the Women's Health Initiative Hormone Therapy Trial

	Estrogen + Progestogen Arm (Mean duration 5.2 years)			Estrogen-only Arm (Mean duration 6.8 years)		
Outcome	MHT (n = 8,506) No. Patients (annualized %)	Placebo (n = 8,102) No. Patients (annualized %)	Hazard Ratio (Nominal 95% CI)	MHT (n = 5,310) No. Patients (annualized %)	Placebo (n = 5,429) No. Patients (annualized %)	Hazard Ratio (Nominal 95% CI)
CHD	164 (0.37)	122 (0.30)	1.29 (1.02-1.63)	177 (0.49)	199 (0.54)	0.91 (0.75-1.12)
Stroke	127 (0.29)	85 (0.21)	1.41 (1.07-1.85)	158 (0.44)	118 (0.32)	1.39 (1.10-1.77)
VTE	151 (0.34)	67 (0.16)	2.11 (1.58-2.82)	101 (0.28)	78 (0.21)	1.33 (0.99-1.79)
Invasive Breast Cancer	166 (0.38)	124 (0.30)	1.26 (1.00-1.59)	94 (0.26)	124 (0.33)	0.77 (0.59-1.01)
Colorectal Cancer	45 (0.10)	67 (0.16)	0.63 (0.43-0.92)	61 (0.17)	58 (0.16)	1.08 (0.75-1.55)
Hip Fracture	44 (0.10)	62 (0.15)	0.66 (0.45-0.98)	38 (0.11)	64 (0.17)	0.61 (0.41-0.91)
Death	231 (0.52)	218 (0.53)	0.98 (0.82-1.18)	291 (0.81)	289 (0.78)	1.04 (0.88-1.22)
Global Index	751 (1.70)	623 (1.51)	1.15 (1.03-1.28)	692 (1.92)	705 (1.90)	1.01 (0.91-1.12)

Data from references 16 and 44.

vaginal estrogen is used. It should be noted that one vaginal ring (Femring®) is known to deliver a systemic dose of estrogen.

Therapeutic response is typically attained after 2 weeks of daily estrogen use. For maintenance therapy, the frequency of administration is generally decreased to 2 to 3 times weekly.

Assessing Benefits and Risks of Systemic Menopausal Hormone Therapy The Women's Health Initiative (WHI) was a randomized, double-blind, placebo-controlled trial launched in 1991 to evaluate the effects of MHT on heart disease, osteoporosis, and cancer. The WHI trial had two arms: the estrogen-plus-progestin arm involving women with an intact uterus and the estrogen-alone arm involving women with a history of hysterectomy.[13,27] The combined estrogen and progestin arm included 16,608 women aged 50 to 79 years (mean age 63 years), and the estrogen-only arm enrolled 10,739 women aged 50 to 79 years (mean age 64 years). The primary outcome was incidence of coronary heart disease (CHD) (nonfatal myocardial infarction or CHD death), and the primary safety outcome was invasive breast cancer. A global index was used to summarize the balance of risks and benefits, which included the two primary outcomes plus stroke, pulmonary embolism, endometrial cancer, colorectal cancer, hip fracture, and death due to other causes. The estrogen-plus-progestin arm was terminated prematurely after only 5.2 years (the planned duration was 8.5 years) because the global index statistic supported risks exceeding benefits on the major clinical outcomes. The estrogen-only arm also was terminated early (after 6.8 years) because of excess risk of stroke. Results of the WHI trial are shown in Table 82-2. Upon discontinuation of the trial, participants were asked to discontinue study medication and invited to participate in a follow-up phase of the study that has resulted in multiple ancillary analyses.[28-41]

More than a decade later, use of MHT has greatly evolved to recognize the need to individualize therapy for women based on patient specific factors (eg, age, risk factors, and goals of therapy). A summary of various clinical considerations described in the 2012 Hormone Therapy Position Statement of the North American Menopause Society is provided in Table 82-3.

Clinical **Controversy...**

Some authorities recommend that the duration of MHT should not exceed 5 years when estrogen and progestogen are used together because of the increased risk of breast cancer. However, in some women, vasomotor symptoms may persist for many years after menopause, and therapy for longer durations may be warranted.

TABLE 82-3 Summary of North American Menopause Society Position Statement on Menopausal Hormone Therapy

Symptom/Condition	Summary statement(s)
Vasomotor symptoms	Estrogen therapy (+/- progestogen) is the most effective therapy, including consequences of vasomotor symptoms such as sleep quality, irritability, difficulty concentrating, and quality of life
Vulvovaginal symptoms	Estrogen therapy is the most effective treatment for moderate to several vulvovaginal symptoms. Local therapy is recommended for sole vaginal symptoms; progestogen generally not indicated (data for up to 1 year)
Sexual function	Low-dose local estrogen therapy may improve lubrication, blood flow and vaginal sensation; however MHT is not recommended as treatment for other problems of sexual function (eg, libido, orgasmic response)
Osteoporosis	Standard-dose MHT reduces postmenopausal osteoporotic fractures (hip, vertebral, and nonvertebral) and many systemic MHT products are approved for prevention of osteoporosis. MHT is not indicated for treatment. Benefits of MHT dissipate when discontinued
Coronary heart disease	Observational and randomized control data are conflicting. Estrogen only therapy may reduce CHD risk when initiated in newly menopausal women (age 50-59 years). Estrogen + progestogen therapy initiated between ages 50 and 59 years or within 10 years of menopause does not appear to increase CHD risk. Women initiating therapy after 10 years since menopause have an increased risk of CHD. MHT is not recommended any time for coronary protection
Stroke	Increased risk of ischemic stroke (not hemorrhagic) exists with estrogen only and estrogen + progestogen use. Risk dissipates upon discontinuation
Venous thromboembolism (VTE)	Increased risk of VTE with oral MHT, but risk is rare when used between ages of 50 and 59 years. Risk increases with personal risk factors including obesity, previous history of VTE, presence of Factor V Leiden mutation. Risk dissipates upon discontinuation. The type of progestogen may impact risk. Transdermal formulations appear to have lower VTE risk than oral formulations

Data from reference 23.

Furthermore, several national and international organizations have published guidelines or position statements to outline points of consensus regarding the safe and effective use of MHT.[20,23] Overall, consensus recommendations regarding the use of MHT include:

- Menopausal hormone therapy is the most effective treatment for vasomotor symptoms in recently menopausal women (before age 60 years or within 10 years of menopause).
- Menopausal hormone therapy is effective and appropriate for prevention of osteoporosis-related fractures in recently menopausal women at risk.
- Estrogen-only therapy may decrease heart disease and all-cause mortality in 50 to 59 year-old-women with a history of hysterectomy. In this age group, combined estrogen and progestogen therapy shows similar trends for mortality, but no significant difference in CHD.
- Estrogen alone is appropriate for women after hysterectomy; additional progestogen is required when a uterus is present.
- Use of MHT should be individualized based on the severity of menopausal symptoms and personal risk factors (eg, age, time since menopause, history of VTE, stroke, ischemic heart disease, and breast cancer).
- Risk of VTE and stroke increases with oral MHT containing estrogen, but the absolute risk is low in women below 60 years of age. Based on observational studies, transdermal MHT and low-dose oral estrogen therapy appear to have a lower risk of VTE and stroke compared to standard-dose oral estrogen regimens.
- Menopausal hormone therapy is contraindicated in women with a personal history of breast cancer. The risk of MHT-related breast cancer appears to be associated with the addition of progestogen to estrogen and increases after 5 or more years of continuous combined use. However, use of estrogen alone appears to decrease rather than increase breast cancer risk.
- The lowest dose of hormone therapy should be used for the shortest possible duration to adequately manage menopausal symptoms.

Cardiovascular Disease 3 Cardiovascular disease—including coronary artery disease, stroke, and peripheral vascular disease—is the leading cause of death among women, and MHT should not be used for reducing the risk of cardiovascular disease. Menopause is associated with the development of a more adverse lipid profile, thereby increasing the risk for cardiovascular disease.

In the decade prior to the publication of the WHI results in 2002, an expectation of coronary benefit had been a major reason for use of postmenopausal hormones because observational studies indicated that women who use MHT have a 35% to 50% lower risk of CHD than nonusers. In addition, previous studies had shown that estrogen exerts protective effects on the cardiovascular system, including lipid-lowering, antioxidant, and vasodilating effects.[42] However, in the 2000s, published results of several randomized clinical trials provided no evidence of cardiovascular disease protection and even some evidence of harm with MHT.[13,43,44]

The primary findings of the estrogen plus progestogen arm of the WHI trial showed an overall increase in the risk of CHD (HR 1.29, 95% CI 1.02-1.63) among healthy postmenopausal women receiving combined estrogen–progestogen MHT compared with those receiving placebo.[13,27] The primary findings of the estrogen-only arm of the WHI trial show no effect (either increase or decrease) on the risk of CHD in women taking estrogen alone.[27] Subgroup analyses performed in the years after the WHI was first published in 2002 revealed that women who initiated MHT 10 or more years after the time of menopause tended to have increased CHD risk compared with women who initiated therapy within 10 years of menopause.[45,46] Neither estrogen alone nor estrogen plus progestogen was associated with a statistically significant effect on CHD in women aged 50 to 59 years, and MHT was associated with reduced overall mortality, although this decrease was not statistically significant.[45] More recently, subgroup analyses from the WHI that included only adherent study participants found that the risk of CHD with estrogen plus progestogen use is increased in the first 2 years of treatment, even in women aged 50 to 59 years at study entry. However, the risk of CHD in women who initiated therapy within 10 years of menopause appears to decrease after 6 years of treatment.[46] Most women who commence estrogen or estrogen plus progestogen therapy do so within the first few years of becoming menopausal.

A randomized controlled study of 1,006 recently menopausal women revealed that 10-year MHT was associated with a significantly reduced risk of cardiovascular disease.[47] In addition, studies of recently menopausal women showed that the presence and severity of hot flushes are associated with vascular endothelial dysfunction and vascular inflammation (markers of increased risk for CHD); MHT improved both of these parameters.[48-50]

In an attempt to resolve some of the controversy, the Kronos Early Estrogen Prevention Study (KEEPS) randomized 727 recently menopausal women (mean age 52 years and less than 3 years since FMP) to cyclic progestogen and either oral estrogen (conjugated estrogen 0.45 mg/day), transdermal estrogen (estradiol 50 mcg/day), or placebo to examine the rate of atherosclerosis.[51] During 4 years of treatment, there was no difference among the study arms on atherosclerotic progression as evidenced by carotid intima-media thickness and coronary artery calcium.

Menopausal hormone therapy should not be initiated or continued solely for the prevention of cardiovascular disease. Adherence to a healthful lifestyle (cessation of smoking, regular exercise, healthy diet, and body mass index less than 25 kg/m^2) may prevent the onset of cardiovascular disease in postmenopausal women.

In the estrogen plus progestogen arm of the WHI study, the increased risk for stroke and venous thromboembolism continued throughout the 5 years of therapy.[13] Increased risk was observed only for ischemic stroke and not for hemorrhagic stroke.[30] In the estrogen-alone arm of the study, a similar increased risk for stroke was observed.[27] After the cessation of treatment, there is no increased risk for stroke.[52,53]

Clinical **Controversy ...**

Data are conflicting regarding the risk of cardiovascular disease with MHT. In older women, MHT appears to increase cardiovascular disease risk, whereas in recently menopausal women with vasomotor symptoms, MHT may have a beneficial effect.

Venous Thromboembolism Venous thromboembolism, including thrombosis of the deep veins of the legs and embolism to the pulmonary arteries, is uncommon in the general population. Women taking oral estrogen therapy have a twofold increased risk for thromboembolic events, with the highest risk occurring in the first year of use.[13,27] However, women with certain risk factors for venous thromboembolism including those with a Factor V Leiden mutation, obesity, and history of previous thromboembolic events, are at increased risk with MHT.[20] Lower doses of estrogen are associated with a decreased risk for thromboembolism as compared with higher doses. Oral administration of estrogen increases the risk of venous thromboembolism compared to the transdermal route.[14] In addition, the norpregnane progestogens, unlike micronized progesterone, appear to be thrombogenic. Currently, there is no indication for thrombophilia screening before initiating MHT. However, MHT should be avoided in women at high risk for thromboembolic events.

Breast cancer 4 The risk of breast cancer associated with MHT appears to be associated with the addition of progestogen therapy to estrogen. Use of estrogen alone does not increase the risk of breast cancer. The WHI trial found that combined estrogen plus progestogen oral therapy has an increased risk of invasive breast cancer (HR 1.26, 95% CI: 1.0-1.59) and a trend toward increasing risk with increasing duration of therapy.[13] This risk does not persist after discontinuation of hormone treatment.[52] The estrogen-only arm of the WHI trial found a decreased risk for breast cancer during the 7-year follow-up period, which persisted after discontinuation of treatment.[27,53]

In the estrogen plus progestogen arm of the WHI, the increased breast cancer risk did not appear until after 3 years of study participation.[13] The risk was seen only in women who initiated therapy within 5 years of the start of menopause but not in those who started therapy more than 5 years after menopause.[54] The breast cancers diagnosed in women in the MHT group had similar histology and grade but were more likely to be in an advanced stage compared with women in the placebo group.[29] The risk of breast cancer returns to baseline rapidly after discontinuation of MHT.[52,54] In an unselected postmenopausal population, the Million Women Study found that current use of MHT increased breast cancer risk and breast cancer mortality (relative risk 1.66 and 1.22, respectively).[55] Increased incidence was observed for estrogen-only use (relative risk 1.30), for estrogen plus progestogen (relative risk 2), and for tibolone (relative risk 1.45). The risk for estrogen only and estrogen plus progestin therapy were higher for those who initiated treatment within 5 years of menopause compared to those who started therapy 5 or more years after menopause.[56]

For women in the United States, the lifetime risk of developing breast cancer is approximately one in eight, and the greatest incidence occurs in women older than 60 years (Chapter 129).[57] In a collaborative re-analysis of data from 51 studies evaluating 52,705 women with breast cancer and 108,411 controls, less than 5 years of combined estrogen–progestogen therapy was associated with a 15% increase in breast cancer risk, and the risk increased with longer duration (relative risk 1.35 with 5 or more years of use).[58] However, 5 years after discontinuation of MHT, the risk of breast cancer was no longer increased.[58]

Addition of progestogens to estrogen may increase breast cancer risk beyond that observed with estrogen alone.[59]

Sex-steroid deficiency during the menopause results in lipomatous involution of the breast, which is seen as decreased mammographic breast density and markedly improved radiotransparency of breast tissue. Thus, mammographic changes indicating breast cancer can be recognized more easily and earlier after the menopause. Conversely, use of MHT results in increased mammographic breast density, and increased density on mammography has been associated with higher breast cancer risk.[60]

Endometrial Cancer The WHI trial suggests that combined oral MHT does not increase endometrial cancer risk compared with placebo (HR 0.81, 95% CI: 0.48-1.36).[35] However, estrogen alone given to women with an intact uterus significantly increases uterine cancer risk.[61] The excess risk increases with dose and duration of estrogen (10 years of unopposed estrogen increases the risk 10-fold), is apparent within 2 years of the start of treatment, and persists for many years after estrogen replacement is discontinued.[61] Estrogen-induced endometrial cancer usually is of a low stage and grade at the time of diagnosis, and it can be prevented almost entirely by progestogen coadministration.[35] The sequential addition of progestogen to estrogen for at least 10 days of the treatment cycle or continuous combined estrogen–progestogen does not increase the risk of endometrial cancer.

Lower doses of estrogen may be associated with a lower risk of endometrial hyperplasia.[62] SERMs do not result in endometrial hyperplasia. A 4-year trial of raloxifene in women with osteoporosis showed no increased risk of endometrial cancer.[63]

Ovarian Cancer Lifetime risk of ovarian cancer is low (1.7%). The WHI trial suggested that orally administered combined MHT does not increase the risk of ovarian cancer (HR 1.58, 95% CI: 0.77-3.24).[35] An observational study reported an increased risk of ovarian cancer in women taking postmenopausal estrogen-only therapy for more than 10 years (relative risk 1.8, 95% CI: 1.1-3.0 and 3.2, 95% CI: 1.7-5.7 for 10-19 years and 20 or more years, respectively), but no increased risk of ovarian cancer among women receiving combination estrogen–progestogen therapy.[64] A recent analysis of 52 epidemiological studies suggests that ovarian cancer risk is increased in current users of MHT, even with less than 5 years of use. The increased risk appears to decrease but not completely disappear a decade after discontinuation of MHT.[65]

Lung Cancer The WHI trial found that combined oral estrogen–progestogen therapy did not increase lung cancer incidence, but significantly increased deaths from lung cancer, mainly from nonsmall cell lung cancers (HR 1.87, 95% CI: 1.22-2.88).[66] The estrogen-only arm of the WHI trial found no increased risk for lung cancer death.[67] It should be noted that the WHI was not designed to assess lung cancer.

Osteoporosis Postmenopausal osteoporosis is a serious age-related disease that affects millions of women throughout the world. Menopause is accompanied by accelerated bone loss, and the central role of estrogen deficiency in postmenopausal osteoporosis is well established (Chapter 93).

The WHI was the first randomized trial to demonstrate that MHT reduces the risk of fractures at the hip, spine, and wrist.[13,34] These findings are in agreement with observational data and several meta-analyses of the efficacy of MHT for reducing fractures in postmenopausal women.

Estrogen therapy reduces bone turnover and increases bone density in postmenopausal women of all ages. The protective effect persists as long as the treatment is maintained. With cessation of therapy, postmenopausal bone loss resumes at the same rate as in untreated women.[52,53] The standard bone-sparing daily estrogen dose is equivalent to 0.625 mg conjugated equine estrogen (CEE). However, lower doses of estrogen have been shown to increase bone mass to the same extent as standard-dose estrogen therapy.[68,69] Whether lower doses of estrogen are safer (eg, lower incidence of venous thromboembolism and breast cancer) remains to be proven.

5 In younger postmenopausal women who are at increased fracture risk, systemic estrogen therapy may be indicated for the prevention of osteoporotic fractures when alternate therapies are either contraindicated or cause excessive adverse effects. General protective health measures, such as regular weight-bearing exercise and avoidance of detrimental lifestyle habits such as smoking and alcohol abuse, are appropriate for all women. Some women require calcium supplementation to their usual dietary intake. Adequate vitamin D intake and/or supplementation are also needed. Appropriate risk assessment and evaluation is needed to determine appropriate treatment strategies in menopausal women. See Chapter 93 for a full discussion of osteoporosis prevention and treatment.

Mood, Cognition, and Dementia 6 Menopausal hormone therapy appears to improve depressive symptoms in symptomatic menopausal women, most likely by relieving flushing and improving sleep. Women with vasomotor symptoms receiving MHT have improved mental health and fewer depressive symptoms compared with women receiving placebo; however, MHT may worsen quality of life in women without flushes.[70]

Clinical **Controversy...**

Conflicting data exist regarding the effect of MHT on well-being and quality of life. Some experts believe well-being and quality of life may be improved as a direct result of menopausal symptom relief (eg, vasomotor, vulvovaginal) while others believe there is no change in overall well-being or quality of life with MHT.

More than 33% of women 65 years and older will develop dementia during their lifetime.[71] Several observational studies have suggested that estrogen therapy may be protective against Alzheimer disease (see Chapter 54). The WHI Memory Study (WHIMS, an ancillary study of the WHI trial) evaluated the effect of MHT on dementia and cognition in 4,532 women 65 to 79 years old.[32] The study found that postmenopausal women 65 years and older taking estrogen plus progestogen therapy had twice the rate of dementia, including Alzheimer disease, than women taking placebo (HR 2.05, 95% CI: 1.21-3.48).[32] In addition, estrogen plus progestogen therapy in these women did not prevent mild cognitive impairment, a cognitive and functional state between normal aging and dementia that frequently progresses to dementia.[32] The estrogen alone arm of the WHI trial showed similar findings.[36,41]

In contrast, the Women's Health Initiative Memory Study of Younger Women (WHIMSY) found that neither estrogen plus progestogen or estrogen therapy alone confer any risk or benefit to cognitive function when taken by postmenopausal women aged 50 to 55 years old.[72] In another study, the ancillary Cognitive and Affective Study (KEEPS-Cog) of the Kronos Early Estrogen Prevention Cognitive Study (KEEPS) evaluated the effects of up to four years of MHT on cognition and mood in recently menopausal women (mean age 52.6 years and 1.4 years past FMP) with low cardiovascular risk.[73] Specifically, 693 women participated with 220 women randomized to receive 0.45 mg/day oral conjugated equine estrogens (o-CEE) plus 200 mg/day micronized progesterone (m-P) for the first 12 days of each month, 211 women randomized to receive 50 mcg/day transdermal estradiol (t-E2) plus 200 mg/day m-P for the first 12 days of each month, and 262 women randomized to receive placebo pills and patches. After a mean length of follow-up of 2.85 years for cognition outcomes, no treatment-related benefits were observed. After a mean length of follow-up for 2.76 years regarding mood outcomes, model estimates indicated that women treated with o-CEE showed improvements in depression and anxiety symptoms over the 48 months of treatment, compared to women on placebo.

Diabetes In healthy postmenopausal women, hormone therapy appears to have a beneficial effect on fasting glucose levels in women with elevated fasting insulin concentrations.[74] Also, in women with coronary artery disease, hormone therapy reduces the incidence of diabetes by 35%.[75] Women who received estrogen plus progestogen in the WHI trial had a statistically significant 21% reduction (HR, 0.79; 95% CI, 0.67-0.93) in the incidence of type 2 diabetes requiring treatment.[76] These findings provide important insights into the metabolic effects of hormone therapy but are insufficient to recommend the long-term use of hormone therapy in women with diabetes.

Body Weight A meta-analysis of randomized controlled trials showed that unopposed estrogen or estrogen combined with a progestogen has no effect on body weight, suggesting that hormone therapy does not cause weight gain in excess of that normally observed at the time of menopause.[77]

Gallbladder Disease Gallbladder disease is a commonly cited complication of oral estrogen use. The WHI studies reported an increased risk for cholecystitis, cholelithiasis, and cholecystectomy among women taking oral estrogen or estrogen–progestogen therapy.[78] Transdermal estrogen is an alternative to oral therapy for women at high risk for cholelithiasis.

Estrogens Estrogens are naturally occurring hormones or synthetic steroidal or nonsteroidal compounds with estrogenic activity. The primary indication for systemic estrogen-based MHT is the relief of moderate and severe vasomotor and vulvovaginal symptoms, and the initial dose should be the lowest effective dose for symptom control.

Adverse Effects Common adverse effects of estrogen include nausea, headache, breast tenderness, and heavy bleeding. More serious adverse effects include increased risk for CHD, stroke, venous thromboembolism, breast cancer, and gallbladder disease. Transdermal estradiol is associated with a lower incidence of breast tenderness and deep vein thrombosis than is oral estrogen.[14,15,47]

Dosage and Administration 7 Use of MHT at doses lower than those prescribed historically (ie, prior to the WHI study) appears to be effective in reducing bone loss and managing menopausal symptoms (see Table 82-1).[68,69,79,80] Low-dose estrogen regimens include 0.3 to 0.45 mg conjugated estrogens, 0.5 mg micronized 17β-estradiol, and 0.014 to 0.0375 mg transdermal 17β-estradiol patch.[20] Topical gels, sprays, and creams are also available in low doses. Lower doses typically have fewer adverse effects and may have better overall benefit-risk profiles than standard doses. The lowest effective dose of estrogen, consistent with individualized patient treatment goals and assessment of safety and effectiveness, should be used.

Various systemically administered estrogens (typically oral and transdermal) are equally effective for replacement therapy (Table 82-4). Estrogens can be administered orally, percutaneously (transdermal patches and topical products), intravaginally (creams, tablets, or rings), intramuscularly, and even subcutaneously in the form of implanted pellets. The choice of estrogen delivery (product, route, and method) should be determined in consultation with the patient to ensure acceptability and enhance adherence. In general, the oral and transdermal routes are used most frequently.

Oral Estrogen Oral conjugated equine estrogen has been available for more than 50 years. CEE is prepared from the urine of pregnant mares and is composed of estrone sulfate (50%-60%) and multiple other equine estrogens such as equilin and 17α-dihydroequilin.

Estradiol is the predominant and most active form of endogenous estrogens. A micronized form of estradiol (produced by a technique that yields extremely small particles of the pure hormone) is readily absorbed from the small intestines. When given orally, estradiol is metabolized by the intestinal mucosa and the liver during the first hepatic passage, and only 10% reaches circulation as free estradiol. Metabolism of estrogen is partly mediated by the cytochrome P450 3A4 isoenzyme. Gut and liver metabolism converts a large proportion of estradiol to the less potent estrone. Thus, measurement of serum estradiol is not useful for monitoring oral estrogen replacement. The principal metabolites of micronized estradiol are estrone and estrone sulfate. Administration of estradiol via the oral route results in estrone concentrations that are three to six times those of estradiol. Ethinyl estradiol is a highly potent semisynthetic estrogen that has similar activity following administration by the oral or nonoral route.

Orally administered estrogens stimulate the synthesis of hepatic proteins and increase the circulating concentrations of sex hormone-binding globulin, which, in turn, may compromise the bioavailability of androgens and estrogens.

TABLE 82-4 FDA-Approved Estrogen Products for Menopausal Hormone Therapy

Drug	Brand Name[a]	Initial Dose/Low Dose	Usual Dose Range	Comments
Systemic Estrogen Products (for the treatment of moderate and severe vasomotor symptoms ± urogenital symptoms)				
Oral estrogens[b]				
Conjugated equine estrogens	Premarin	0.3 or 0.45 mg once daily	0.3-1.25 mg once daily	Dosage form available as 0.3, 0.45, 0.625, 0.9, 1.25 mg
Synthetic conjugated estrogens	Cenestin, Enjuvia	0.3 mg once daily	0.3-1.25 mg once daily	Dosage form available as 0.3, 0.45, 0.625, 0.9, 1.25 mg
Esterified estrogens (75%-85% estrone + 6%-15% equilin)	Menest	0.3 mg once daily	0.3-2.5 mg once daily	Administer 3 weeks on and 1 week off Dosage form available as 0.3, 0.625, 1.25, 2.5 mg
Estropipate (piperazine estrone sulfate)	Ogen, Ortho-Est, Generics	0.75 mg once daily	0.75-6 mg once daily	Dosage form available as 0.75, 1, 5, 3, 6 mg
Estradiol acetate	Femtrace	0.45 mg once daily	0.45-1.8 mg once daily	Dosage form available as 0.45, 0.9, 1.8 mg
Micronized 17β-estradiol	Estrace Generics	1 mg once daily	1 or 2 mg once daily	Administer 3 weeks on and 1 week off Dosage form available as 1, 2 mg
Transdermal estrogens patches				
17β-estradiol	Alora	0.025 mg/day (patch applied twice weekly)[c]	0.025-0.1 mg/day (patch applied twice weekly)[c]	Dosage form available as 0.025, 0.05, 0.075, 0.1 mg/day
	Climara	0.025 mg/day (patch applied twice weekly)[c]	0.025-0.1 mg/day (patch applied twice weekly)[c]	Dosage form available as 0.025, 0.0375, 0.05, 0.06, 0.075, 0.1 mg/day
	Menostar	0.014 mg/day (patch applied once weekly)[c,d]	0.014 mg/day (patch applied once weekly)[c,d]	Dosage form available as 0.014 mg/day
	Estraderm	-	0.05 or 0.1 mg/day (patch applied twice weekly)[c]	Dosage form available as 0.05, 0.1 mg/day
	Minivelle, Vivelle, Vivelle Dot	0.025 mg/day (patch applied twice weekly)[c]	0.025-0.1 mg/day, 0.05 is standard dose (patch applied twice weekly)[c]	Dosage form available as 0.025, 0.0375, 0.05 (standard dose), 0.075, 0.1 mg/day
Other topical forms of estrogen				
17β-estradiol topical emulsion	Estrasorb 0.25% emulsion	–	Two pouches once daily (which delivers 0.05 mg of estradiol per day)	Apply to legs
17β-estradiol topical gel	EstroGel 0.06% metered-dose pump	–	1.25 g/day once daily (contains 0.75 mg estradiol)	Apply from wrist to shoulder
	Elestrin 0.06% metered-dose pump		1-2 unit doses once daily (1 unit dose: 0.87 g, which contains 0.52 mg estradiol)	Apply to upper arm
	Divigel 0.1% (topical once daily)	0.25 g once daily	0.25-1 g (provides 0.25-1 mg of estradiol)	Apply to upper thigh. Dosage form available as 0.25, 0.5, 1 g
17β-estradiol transdermal spray	Evamist	1 spray once daily	2-3 sprays once daily (1.53 mg of estradiol per spray)	Apply to inner surface of forearm
Implanted estrogens[e]				
Implanted 17β-estradiol	Estradiol pellets	25 mg implanted subcutaneously every 6 months	50-100 mg implanted subcutaneously every 6 months	
Vaginal estrogens				
Estradiol acetate vaginal ring	Femring	12.4 mg every 3 months	12.4, 24.8 mg ring (delivers 0.05 or 0.1 mg estradiol/day)	
Intravaginal Estrogen Products (for the treatment of urogenital symptoms only/low systemic exposure)				
Conjugated equine estrogens (CEE) vaginal cream	Premarin		0.5-2 g/day (contains 0.625 mg CEE per g)	
17β-estradiol vaginal cream	Estrace		1 g/day (contains 0.1 mg estradiol per g)	
17β-estradiol vaginal ring	Estring	2 mg replaced every 90 days	2 mg ring (delivers 0.0075 mg/day) replaced every 90 days	
Estradiol hemihydrate vaginal tablet	Vagifem	10 mcg twice weekly	10 or 25 mcg twice weekly	

[a]United States brand names.

[b]Orally administered estrogens stimulate synthesis of hepatic proteins and increase circulating concentrations of sex hormone-binding globulin, which in turn may compromise the bioavailability of androgens and estrogens. Women with elevated triglyceride concentrations or significant liver function abnormalities are candidates for non-oral estrogen therapy.

[c]Do not apply estrogen patches on or near breasts. Avoid waistline as patch may rub off with tight-fitting clothing.

[d]FDA-approved for prevention of postmenopausal osteoporosis only.

[e]Not available in the United States.

Other Routes of Estrogen Administration Nonoral routes of estrogen administration may offer both advantages and disadvantages compared with the oral route, but long-term data are not available. Nonoral forms of estrogens bypass the GI tract and thereby avoid first-pass liver metabolism. These routes of estradiol delivery result in a more physiologic estradiol-to-estrone ratio (estradiol concentrations greater than estrone concentrations), as seen in the normal premenopausal state.

When compared with standard oral estrogen doses, transdermal therapy appears to offer no significant increase in triglycerides, C-reactive protein, sex hormone binding globulin, and blood pressure.[20,81] Transdermal estrogen has also been associated with a lower risk of deep vein thrombosis, stroke, and MI. Transdermal estrogen patches share the advantages of other nonoral estrogen routes and have the added advantage of delivering estradiol to the general venous circulation at a continuous rate. The matrix transdermal systems (estrogen in adhesive) generally are well tolerated, and fewer than 5% of women experience skin reactions. The incidence of skin irritation diminishes when the application site is rotated. Topical anti-inflammatory products (eg, hydrocortisone cream) can be applied for managing the rashes, and switching to another transdermal patch is often a viable option.

Topical gels, sprays, and emulsions are convenient forms of systemic estrogen therapy, but variability in drug absorption has been noted with some formulations. Intravaginal creams, tablets, and rings are used for treatment of urogenital (vulvar and vaginal) atrophy. Intravaginal tablets and rings are sustained-release delivery systems that can maintain adequate estradiol concentrations. While most tablets and rings provide local estrogen, one intravaginal ring product (Femring®) is designed to achieve systemic concentrations of estrogen and is also indicated for treatment of moderate to severe vasomotor symptoms. Estradiol pellets (for subcutaneous implantation), containing pure crystalline 17β-estradiol, have been available for more than 50 years. They are inserted subcutaneously into the anterior abdominal wall or buttock. Pellets are difficult to remove and may continue to release estradiol for a long time after insertion. Implantation should not be repeated until serum estradiol concentrations have fallen to values similar to those at the midfollicular phase of the menstrual cycle. Estradiol pellets are not available in the United States.

Progestogens 8 Because of the increased risk of endometrial hyperplasia and endometrial cancer with estrogen monotherapy (ie, unopposed estrogen), use of systemic estrogen in women with an intact uterus must always be accompanied by a progestogen or an estrogen agonist antagonist (eg, bazedoxifene) for endometrial protection.[82] Some data suggest that progestins may also improve vasomotor symptoms, but their use for this purpose is not considered first line or standard therapy.[83]

Progestogens reduce nuclear estradiol receptor concentrations, suppress DNA synthesis, and decrease estrogen bioavailability by increasing the activity of endometrial 17-hydroxysteroid dehydrogenase, an enzyme responsible for converting estradiol to estrone.[61]

The first generation of progestogens included the C-19 androgenic progestogens norethindrone (also known as norethisterone), norgestrel, and levonorgestrel. More recent preparations have included the C-21 progestogens dydrogesterone and medroxyprogesterone acetate (MPA), which are less androgenic. Drospirenone, a synthetic progestogen analog of the potassium-sparing diuretic spironolactone, has both antiandrogenic and antialdosterone properties. Micronized progesterone also has become available for use in postmenopausal women. The most commonly used oral progestogens are MPA, micronized progesterone, and norethindrone acetate. The latter can be administered transdermally in the form of a combined estrogen–progestogen patch.

Adverse Effects Common adverse effects of progestogens include irritability, weight gain, bloating, and headache. Changing from a cyclic to a continuous-combined regimen or changing from one progestogen to another may decrease the incidence or severity of untoward effects. Adverse effects of progestogens are difficult to evaluate and can vary with the agent administered. Some women experience "premenstrual-like" symptoms, such as mood swings, bloating, fluid retention, and sleep disturbance. Newer methods and routes of progestogen delivery (eg, locally by an intrauterine device that releases levonorgestrel or a progesterone-containing bioadhesive vaginal gel) may be associated with fewer adverse effects.

Dosage and Administration Several progestogen regimens designed to prevent endometrial hyperplasia are available for use in women with an intact uterus (Table 82-5). Progestogens can be used continuously (resulting in endometrial atrophy) or cyclically (resulting in monthly withdrawal bleeding). For cyclic use, the progestogen must be taken for a sufficient period of time during each cycle. In general, a minimum of 12 to 14 days of progestogen therapy per month is required for complete protection against estrogen-induced endometrial hyperplasia. For women with a history of hysterectomy, use of progestogens is not indicated. However, in women with endometriosis who have had a hysterectomy, the use of a progestogen along with estrogen may minimize endometriosis exacerbations.

Menopausal Hormone Therapy Regimens Many products have been used for MHT, and most include an estrogen and a progestogen in various regimens, routes, and administration schedules. Additionally, products that combine estrogen with an estrogen agonist/antagonist are also available for once-daily dosing. Common combination MHT regimens are described in Table 82-6.

Continuous Cyclic Estrogen–Progestogen (Sequential) Treatment Estrogen typically is administered continuously (daily). A progestogen is coadministered with the estrogen for at least 12 to 14 days of a 28-day cycle.[84] The progestogen causes scheduled withdrawal bleeding in approximately 90% of women. With this regimen, bleeding usually begins 1 to 2 days after the last progestogen dose. Occasionally, bleeding begins during the latter phase of progestogen administration.

Continuous Combined Estrogen–Progestogen Treatment Continuous combined estrogen–progestogen administration results in endometrial atrophy and the absence of vaginal bleeding. Continuous combined MHT is more acceptable than traditional cyclic therapy. This method of treatment can be achieved by using either

TABLE 82-5 Progestogen Dosing for Endometrial Protection (Cyclic Administration)

Progestogen	Brand Name	Dosage
Dydrogesterone[a]	Duphaston	10-20 mg/day for 12-14 days per calendar month (oral dosage form available as 10 mg tablets)
Medroxyprogesterone acetate	Provera	5-10 mg/day for 12-14 days per calendar month (oral dosage form available as 2.5, 5, 10 mg tablets)
Micronized progesterone	Prometrium	200 mg/day for 12-14 days per calendar month (oral dosage form available as 100 and 200 mg tablets)
Norethindrone acetate	Aygestin[b]	5 mg/day for 12-14 days per calendar month (oral dosage form available as 2.5, 5 mg tablets)

[a]Not available in the United States.

[b]Not approved for postmenopausal hormone therapy in the United States.

TABLE 82-6 Common Combination Menopausal Hormone Therapy Regimens

Regimen	Brand name	Dosage
Oral Regimens		
Conjugated equine estrogen (CEE) + medroxyprogesterone acetate (MPA)	Prempro (continuous)	0.625 mg/2.5 MPA, 0.625 mg/5 mg daily Low dose: 0.3 mg/1.5 mg, 0.45 mg/1.5 mg daily
	Premphase (continuous sequential)	0.625 mg CEE daily only in the first 2 weeks of a 4-week cycle then 0.625 mg daily CEE + 5 mg MPA daily in the last 2 weeks of a 4-week cycle
Conjugated equine estrogen (CEE) + bazedoxifene	Duavee (continuous)	0.45 mg/20 mg daily
Ethinyl estradiol (EE) + norethindrone acetate (NETA)	Generic, Femhrt (continuous)	5 mcg EE/1 mg NETA daily Low dose (Femhrt only): 2.5 mcg EE/0.5 mg NETA daily
Estradiol (E) + drospirenone (DRSP)	Angeliq (continuous)	1 mg E/5 mg DRSP daily Low dose: 0.5 mg E/0.25 mg DRSP daily
Estradiol (E) + norgestimate	Prefest (estrogen/intermittent progestogen)	1 mg E daily for first 3 days then 1 mg E/0.09 mg norgestimate daily for next 3 days; this pattern is repeated continuously
Estradiol (E) + norethindrone acetate (NETA)	Activella (continuous) Mimvey (continuous)	1 mg E/0.5 mg NETA daily Low-dose: 0.5 mg E/0.1 mg NETA daily 1 mg E/0.5 mg NETA daily
Transdermal Regimens		
Estradiol + norethindrone acetate patch	CombiPatch (continuous) CombiPatch (continuous sequential)	Continuous: 0.05/0.14 mg, 0.05/0.25 mg (apply 1 patch twice weekly) Continuous sequential: 0.05 mg of an estradiol only patch (apply 1 patch twice weekly) in the first 2 weeks of a 4-week cycle then either dose of the CombiPatch (apply 1 patch twice weekly) in the last 2 weeks of a 4-week cycle
Estradiol (E) + levonorgestrel patch	Climara Pro (continuous)	0.045 mg E/0.015 mg/day(apply 1 patch once weekly)

CEE, conjugated equine estrogen; DRSP, drospirenone; E, estradiol; EE, ethinyl estradiol; NETA, norethindrone acetate; MPA, medroxyprogesterone acetate.

commercially available oral and transdermal preparations or by administering systemic estrogen along with the use of the levonorgestrel-releasing intrauterine system.

Continuous Long-Cycle Estrogen–Progestogen Treatment This modified sequential regimen was developed to decrease the incidence of uterine bleeding. In the continuous long-cycle (or cyclic withdrawal) estrogen–progestogen regimen, estrogen is given daily, and progestogen is given six times per year, every other month for 12 to 14 days, resulting in six periods per year. Bleeding episodes may be heavier and last for more days than withdrawal bleeding with continuous cyclic regimens. The effect of continuous long-cycle estrogen–progestogen treatment on endometrial protection is unclear.

Intermittent Combined Estrogen–Progestogen Treatment The intermittent combined estrogen–progestogen regimen, also called *continuous-pulsed estrogen–progestogen* or *pulsed-progestogen*, consists of 3 days of estrogen therapy alone, followed by 3 days of combined estrogen and progestogen, which is then repeated without interruption. This regimen is designed to lower the incidence of uterine bleeding. It is based on the assumption that pulsed-progestogen administration will prevent downregulation of progesterone receptors that can be produced by continuous combined regimens. The lower progestogen dose induces fewer side effects and can be better tolerated. The long-term effect of intermittent combined regimens in endometrial protection is undetermined.

Bioidentical Hormones Bioidentical hormone therapy is terminology used to describe hormone therapy formulations that are custom-prepared (ie, compounded) for individual patients.[85] Commonly compounded formulations include estrone, estradiol, estriol, progesterone, testosterone, and dehydroepiandrosterone. Although claims have been made to suggest that bioidentical hormones are safer and more "natural" alternatives to commercially available preparations, there is a paucity of evidence regarding the efficacy, safety, and pharmaceutical quality of these products.[86,87] Furthermore, saliva testing is often used to adjust hormone levels, and there is no scientific evidence to support this practice. Bioidentical hormones appear to carry the same risks as traditional hormone therapy products. Several major medical organizations, along with the FDA, have released statements to dissuade patients and clinicians from using this treatment approach.[85,86,88]

Other Treatments for Menopause-Related Symptoms In women who have contraindications to MHT use, prefer not to take estrogen and/or progestogen, or cannot tolerate estrogen and/or progestogen administration, a number of other medications may be considered, depending on the goals of therapy.[89,90] These include the prescription medications testosterone, SERMs, and tibolone (not currently available in the United States) as well as nonhormonal prescription medications (eg, selective serotonin reuptake inhibitors).

Alternatives to estrogen for treatment of hot flushes include tibolone, selective serotonin reuptake inhibitors (eg, paroxetine and fluoxetine), dual serotonin and norepinephrine reuptake inhibitors (eg, venlafaxine), MPA, megestrol acetate, clonidine, and gabapentin (Table 82-7). Progestogens alone may be an option for some women (eg, those with a history of venous thrombosis), but weight gain, vaginal bleeding, and other adverse effects often limit their use. Tibolone and progestogens cannot be considered nonhormonal agents for treatment of hot flushes in women for whom MHT is contraindicated. For this group of patients, selective serotonin reuptake inhibitors such as paroxetine mesylate and serotonin-norepinephrine reuptake inhibitors such as venlafaxine are considered by some to be a first-line therapy.[91-93] Furthermore, in breast cancer patients, evidence suggests that selective serotonin reuptake inhibitors could interfere with metabolism of endocrine therapies, such as tamoxifen via cytochrome P450 2D6 inhibition.[94] Clonidine is often effective for symptom control, but its side effects (eg, sedation, dry mouth, and hypotension) are not always well tolerated by women.

Androgens Androgens have important biologic effects in women, acting both directly via androgen receptors in tissues, such as bone,

TABLE 82-7 Alternatives to Estrogen for Treatment of Hot Flushes[a]

Drug	Brand Name[b]	Initial Dose	Usual Dose Range	Comments
Tibolone[c]	Livial (not available in the United States)	2.5 mg	2.5 mg/day	Tibolone is not recommended during the perimenopause period because it may cause irregular bleeding
Venlafaxine	Effexor, Effexor XR	37.5 mg	37.5-150 mg/day	Adverse effects include nausea, headache, somnolence, dizziness, insomnia, nervousness, xerostomia, anorexia, constipation, diaphoresis, weakness, and hypertension
Desvenlafaxine	Pristiq	100-150 mg	100-150 mg/day	Adverse effects include nausea, headache, somnolence, dizziness, insomnia, xerostomia, anorexia, constipation, diaphoresis, and weakness
Paroxetine, paroxetine CR[d]	Brisdelle,[e] Paxil, Paxil CR, Pexeva	17.5 mg/day (paroxetine),[e] 10 mg/day (paroxetine), or 12.5 mg/day (paroxetine CR)	7.5 mg/day,[e] 10-20 mg/day or 12.5–25 mg/day	Adverse effects include nausea, somnolence, insomnia, headache, dizziness, xerostomia, constipation, diarrhea, weakness, and diaphoresis
Megestrol acetate	Megace	20 mg/day	20-40 mg/day	Progesterone may be linked to breast cancer etiology; also, there is concern regarding the safety of progestational agents in women with preexisting breast cancer
Clonidine	Catapres and generic tablets (oral) Catapres-TTS (transdermal) Kapvay tablets (extended release; oral)	0.1 mg/day	0.1 mg/day	Adverse effects include drowsiness, dizziness, hypotension, and dry mouth, especially with higher doses
Gabapentin	Gralise, Neurontin	300 mg at bedtime	900 mg/day (divided in three daily doses), doses up to 2,400 mg/day (divided in three daily doses) have been studied	Adverse effects include somnolence and dizziness; these symptoms often can be obviated with a gradual increase in dosing

CR, controlled release.

[a]Treatment of postmenopausal hot flushes is an off-label indication in the United States for all medications listed except for one formulation of paroxetine (paroxetine mesylate).

[b]United States brand names.

[c]Not available in the United States.

[d]Other selective serotonin reuptake inhibitors (eg, citalopram, escitalopram, fluoxetine, and sertraline) have also been studied and may be used for the treatment of hot flushes.

[e]The brand Brisdelle contains 7.5 mg of paroxetine and is FDA-approved to treat moderate to severe vasomotor symptoms of menopause. This specific product is not FDA-approved for treating psychiatric conditions.

Data from references 131-135.

skin fibroblasts, hair follicles, and sebaceous glands, and indirectly via the aromatization of testosterone to estrogen in the ovaries, bone, brain, adipose tissue, and other tissues. There is a natural decline in androgen production with aging, and pathophysiologic states affecting ovarian and adrenal function have been associated with androgen deficiency in women. The therapeutic use of testosterone in women is controversial.

A cluster of symptoms that characterizes androgen insufficiency in women, manifested as diminished sense of well-being, persistent or unexplained fatigue, and sexual function changes such as decreased libido, decreased sexual receptivity, and decreased pleasure has been reported. However, studies designed to evaluate this have shown no relationships between serum total and free testosterone levels and either sexual function or well-being in women.[95,96] Thus, as data supporting an androgen deficiency syndrome are lacking, in 2014 the American Endocrine Society reaffirmed their recommendation against making a diagnosis of androgen deficiency in women.[95,97] However, large randomized placebo-controlled clinical trials involving naturally[98,99] and surgically[100] postmenopausal women presenting with low libido demonstrate that testosterone therapy, with and without concurrent estrogen therapy, may improve the quality of the sexual experience, with additional preliminary data in premenopausal women.[101]

Androgens should not be used during pregnancy or lactation or in women with suspected androgen-dependent neoplasia. Adverse effects from excessive dosage include virilization, fluid retention, and potentially adverse lipoprotein lipid effects, which are more likely with oral administration. There is no evidence that systemic transdermal testosterone is associated with increased cardiovascular morbidity or mortality[102] or of a significant change in the risk of invasive breast cancer.[103] However, further studies are required to determine the long-term safety of testosterone in women.

Most of the earlier studies showing clinical improvement with testosterone therapy reported supraphysiologic concentrations. Other studies have used transdermal patch therapy to achieve free testosterone concentrations in the upper normal range for young women.[100,104] Evidence regarding efficacy and safety of testosterone in women is lacking, and the generalized use of testosterone is currently not recommended.[97] In the United States, there are no testosterone products approved for use in women.

Selective Estrogen Receptor Modulators (SERMs) Selective estrogen receptor modulators are a group of nonsteroidal compounds that are chemically distinct from estradiol. They act as estrogen agonists in some tissues, such as bone, and as estrogen antagonists in other tissues, such as breast and endometrial tissue, through specific, high-affinity binding to the estrogen receptor. Individual SERMs differ in their activity and tissue specificity resulting in varying patterns of estrogen-receptor agonism in some tissues and estrogen-receptor antagonism in others.[105]

Efficacy The ideal SERM would protect against osteoporosis and decrease the incidence of breast, endometrial, and colorectal cancer and CHD without exacerbating menopausal symptoms or increasing the risk of venous thromboembolism or gallbladder disease. To date, no SERM meets these ideals. Tamoxifen, the first-generation SERM (a nonsteroidal triphenylethylene derivative), has estrogen antagonist activity on the breast and estrogen-like agonist activity on bone and endometrium. The second-generation SERM raloxifene, a nonsteroidal benzothiophene derivative, is used to reduce the risk of postmenopausal osteoporosis and invasive breast cancer, and also for treatment of postmenopausal osteoporosis. Raloxifene, however, has an increased incidence of hot flushes compared to placebo.[106]

The third generation SERM, bazedoxifene, in conjunction with conjugated estrogens forms a tissue-selective estrogen complex (TSEC) and is FDA-approved for use in moderate to severe vasomotor symptoms and prevention of osteoporosis.[105,107] This agent appears to have a favorable breast, endometrial, and ovarian safety profile, even after prolonged use.[108] While this TSEC has demonstrated high effectiveness for vasomotor symptoms (approximately 75% reduction),[108,109] SERMs alone do not alleviate, and may even exacerbate vasomotor symptoms, and also increase the risk for venous thromboembolism.

Ospemifene is an orally administered third generation SERM approved by the FDA for the treatment of moderate-to-severe dyspareunia from menopausal vulvar and vaginal atrophy. Ospemifene's labeling carries a boxed warning about its estrogenic effect on the endometrium: there is an increased risk of endometrial hyperplasia and endometrial cancer in a woman with a uterus who takes unopposed estrogen therapy. Ospemifene labeling includes a boxed warning about the possible risk of stroke and venous thromboembolism, and this drug has a 7.5% incidence of hot flushes.

Adverse Effects Depending on the tissue selectivity, several SERMs are associated with hot flushes and less often with leg cramps. SERMs can increase the risk of venous thromboembolism and fatal stroke to a degree similar to that of oral estrogen, but the degree of risk is product specific.[63] Common adverse effects (greater than or equal to 5%) of bazedoxifene include muscle spasms, nausea, diarrhea, dyspepsia, upper abdominal pain, oropharyngeal pain, dizziness, and neck pain. Adverse effects of ospemifene include hot flushes, vaginal discharge, muscle spasm, genital discharge, and hyperhidrosis.

Dose and Administration Conjugated estrogens/bazedoxifene is supplied as 0.45 mg/20 mg tablets and is taken once daily. Ospemifene is a 60 mg tablet taken once daily with food. Other available SERMs are also dosed orally once daily.

Tibolone Tibolone is a gonadomimetic synthetic steroid in the norpregnane family with combined estrogenic, progestogenic, and androgenic activity. Tibolone has been used for three decades in Europe for treatment of menopausal symptoms and prevention of osteoporosis but is currently not approved in the United States. The hormonal effects of this synthetic steroid depend on its metabolism and activation in peripheral tissues. The parent compound has been described as a prodrug that is metabolized quickly in the gastrointestinal (GI) tract. It has several active metabolites, including a $\Delta 4$-isomer and 3α-OH and 3β-OH compounds. The $\Delta 4$-isomer metabolite confers significant progestogenic and androgenic properties.

Efficacy Tibolone has beneficial effects on mood and libido and improves menopausal symptoms and vaginal atrophy. Tibolone protects against bone loss and significantly reduces the risk of vertebral fractures in postmenopausal women with osteoporosis.[110] It has also been shown to decrease the risk of breast cancer and colon cancer in healthy women aged 60 to 85 years.[110] It also appears to be more effective than conventional MHT for management of sexual dysfunction.[111]

Adverse Effects Tibolone use in elderly women has been reported to be associated with an increased risk of stroke.[110] Tibolone use is associated with breast cancer recurrence in breast cancer patients with vasomotor symptoms.[112] Tibolone lowers concentrations of total cholesterol, triglycerides, and lipoprotein (a) but may decrease high-density lipoprotein (HDL) cholesterol.[113] The Million Women Study, an observational cohort study, found a greater risk of endometrial cancer (adjusted relative risk 1.79, 95% CI: 1.43-2.25).[114] However, other randomized placebo-controlled studies have not shown an increased risk of endometrial cancer with tibolone and suggest that tibolone has an endometrial safety profile similar to continuous combined CEE and MPA.[115] The most commonly reported adverse effects of tibolone include weight gain and bloating.

Complementary and Alternative Medicine Some women prefer to use natural remedies due to a belief that they are safer. Randomized, placebo-controlled trials of complementary and alternative therapies have been equivocal and have not established the safety and efficacy of herbal remedies, homeopathic treatments, or acupuncture for the prevention or treatment of hot flushes.

Phytoestrogens Phytoestrogens have physiologic effects in humans.[116] They are plant compounds with estrogen-like biologic activity and relatively weak estrogen receptor-binding properties. Epidemiologic studies suggest that consumption of a phytoestrogen-rich diet, which is common in traditional Asian societies, is associated with a lower risk of breast cancer.[116]

The biologic potencies of phytoestrogens vary. Most of these compounds are nonsteroidal and are less potent than synthetic estrogens. The three main classes of phytoestrogens are isoflavones, lignans, and coumestans, all of which are found in plants or their seeds.[116] The most commonly studied phytoestrogen is the isoflavone class. Genistein and daidzein are the most abundant active components of isoflavones. The concentration of isoflavones per gram of soy protein varies considerably among preparations. Also, a single plant often contains more than one class of phytoestrogen. Common food sources of phytoestrogens include soybeans (isoflavones), cereals, oilseeds such as flaxseed (lignans), and alfalfa sprouts (coumestans).

Mild estrogenic effects have been seen in postmenopausal women.[116] An early study suggested that phytoestrogen supplementation is no more effective than placebo in relieving hot flushes or other symptoms of menopause in postmenopausal women. However, a systematic review indicated that high levels of genistein extracts appear to reduce the number of daily hot flushes compared with placebo without harmful endometrial effects.[117,118] A limitation of this review is that many of the studies included were of poor quality and short duration but it is worth.

Phytoestrogens decrease low-density lipoprotein (LDL) cholesterol and triglyceride concentrations with no significant change in HDL cholesterol concentrations.[119] Furthermore, phytoestrogens have the ability to inhibit LDL oxidation and normalize vascular reactivity in estrogen-deprived primates.[119] In addition, bone mineral density (BMD) may be improved by phytoestrogens.[116] Common adverse effects include constipation, bloating, and nausea.[120]

A recent meta-analysis reported that phytoestrogen use is not associated with increased rates of endometrial cancer, vaginal bleeding, and breast cancer.[120] Large, long-term studies are needed to further document the effects of phytoestrogens on the breast, bone, and endometrium. Furthermore, before phytoestrogens can be considered an alternative to conventional MHT in postmenopausal women, additional data are needed to clarify differences among classes of phytoestrogens, including dosing, biologic activity, safety, and efficacy.

Other Herbal Products Black cohosh (*Cimicifuga racemosa* or *Actaea racemosa*), a widely used herbal supplement, may not offer substantial benefits for relief of vasomotor symptoms.[121] A systematic review of 16 studies involving 2,027 women found insufficient evidence to support the use of black cohosh for menopausal symptoms, but further research is warranted.[122] This substance does not appear to have strong intrinsic estrogenic properties but may act through the serotonergic system. Black cohosh appears to be generally well tolerated, although hepatotoxicity has been reported. It is unclear if this is due to the herb itself or is a result of adulteration of the commercially available products.[123] The long-term effects of black cohosh are unknown. Other herbals and alternative treatments that may be used by women include dong quai, red clover leaf (contains phytoestrogens), kava, and dehydroepiandrosterone. These have not been shown to be effective in the treatment of menopausal symptoms and may carry the risk of adverse events.[124] Complementary and alternative therapies should not be recommended to treat menopausal symptoms.

Personalized Pharmacotherapy

The severity of menopausal symptoms varies widely from woman to woman. The decision to use MHT must be individualized and based on several parameters, including vasomotor and vulvovaginal symptoms, age, fracture risk, cardiovascular disease risk, breast cancer risk, and thromboembolism risk. MHT is not indicated for prevention of chronic diseases of aging. The initiation of MHT should be considered for healthy symptomatic women who are within 10 years of menopause or age younger than 60 years and who do not have contraindications to therapy.[23] The duration of estrogen–progestogen therapy is limited by the risk of breast cancer at 3 to 5 years of use; estrogen-only therapy allows for more flexibility up to 7 years.[20] It is recommended that treatment be individualized and used at the lowest effective dose for the shortest duration that is needed to relieve vasomotor symptoms.

Long-term use of MHT or initiation in older women is associated with greater risks. Once advised of increased risks associated with continuing MHT beyond age 60 years, extending therapy may be acceptable under close medical supervision. For example, in women with severe and persistent menopausal symptoms, use should not discontinued based solely on age but rather individualized based on assessment of potential risks and benefits.[22]

Estrogen therapy is the most effective treatment for moderate and severe vasomotor symptoms, impaired sleep quality, and vulvovaginal symptoms of menopause (see Fig. 82-1). A thorough discussion of the risks and benefits of MHT should be completed with the patient so that she can weigh the risks and benefits versus alternatives and make a rational decision about whether to use MHT. For a healthy recently menopausal woman who has vasomotor symptoms, the benefits of hormonal therapy generally outweigh the risks. These benefits include the control of vasomotor symptoms, treatment of urogenital atrophy, and prevention of postmenopausal bone loss. Nonetheless, VTE and stroke are concerning short-term risks.

Menopausal hormone therapy should be tailored for optimal formulation, dose, route of delivery, and counseling should be based on age, years since menopause, and hysterectomy status. All types and routes of administration of estrogen are equally effective in relieving vasomotor symptoms and vulvovaginal atrophy.[20] A dose-dependent relationship between estrogen administration and suppression of hot flushes is well established. Some women, especially younger women, may require a higher than average dose of estrogen to suppress symptoms. On the other hand, many women with hot flushes at the time of menopause require lower doses of estrogen.[125] Initiation of therapy with low doses of estrogen often will minimize adverse effects, such as breast tenderness and unscheduled bleeding. Transdermal estradiol is less likely than oral estrogen to cause nausea and headache. In many cases changing from one estrogen regimen to another can alleviate certain adverse effects.

Prior to initiating pharmacologic therapy, a complete medical history and physical examination should be performed. Medical history should include a personal and family history of cardiovascular disease and thrombotic problems. The physical examination should include a complete cardiovascular examination, clinical assessment of thyroid status, and breast and pelvic examinations. Papanicolaou cervical cytologic examination and screening mammography negative for malignancy are required before initiating MHT. Thyroid function tests and lipoprotein lipid profile also are performed at the discretion of the clinician. Oral estrogen should be avoided in women with hypertriglyceridemia, liver disease, and gallbladder disease. For these women, transdermal administration is a safer approach. Sequential estrogen/progestogen therapy results in scheduled vaginal withdrawal bleeding but often is scant or completely absent in older women. For many women, scheduled withdrawal bleeding is one of the main reasons for avoiding or discontinuing MHT. Because there is no physiologic need for bleeding, new MHT regimens that reduce monthly bleeding (eg, continuous long-cycle regimens) or prevent monthly bleeding (eg, continuous combined and intermittent combined regimens) were developed. Continuous combined estrogen–progestogen administration results in endometrial atrophy and the absence of vaginal bleeding. Initially, it causes unpredictable spotting or bleeding, which usually resolves within 6 to 12 months. Decreasing the estrogen dose or increasing the progestogen dose usually decreases or stops the spotting. Occasionally, a drug-free period of 1 or 2 weeks is useful to stop the bleeding. Women who recently have undergone menopause have a higher risk for excessive, unpredictable bleeding while receiving continuous therapy; thus, this regimen is best reserved for women who are at least 2 years postmenopause.

If MHT is to be initiated, the selection of the drug should also take into account the potential for drug interactions, including those involving the cytochrome P450 (CYP450) microsomal enzyme system. Estrogen is metabolized partly by the CYP 450 isoenzymes 1A2 and 3A4, and the progestin medroxyprogesterone is metabolized by CYP450 3A4. Inducers or inhibitors of these enzymes may either decrease or increase, respectively, the therapeutic effects or result in side effects. Similarly, selection of nonhormonal drug therapy options should take into account the potential for interactions with other prescription and nonprescription medications the patient may be taking. Selective serotonin reuptake inhibitors and serotonin norepinephrine reuptake inhibitors can have major interactions with other drugs also affecting CYP450 2D6 and 3A4 (Chapter 68). Patients using vaginal estrogen creams or nonestrogen vaginal moisturizers should be warned that products with oil-based lubricants or vehicles can weaken latex condoms, which can decrease protection against sexually transmitted infections. Pharmacodynamic drug interactions (eg, additive side effects) should also be considered.

Evaluation of Therapeutic Outcomes

The relief of moderate and severe hot flushes is the primary goal of MHT. In order to adequately assess treatment effect, women should be encouraged to continue their MHT regimen for at least 1 month. The main reasons for discontinuing MHT are side effects such as bleeding, breast tenderness, bloating, and "premenstrual-like symptoms." Reducing the dose or changing the regimen or the route of administration can minimize these effects. Alternatively, if vasomotor symptoms are not controlled adequately with a lower-dose regimen, increasing the estrogen dose may be a reasonable option. Therefore, after the menopausal woman begins MHT, a brief follow-up visit 6 weeks later may be useful to discuss patient concerns about MHT and to evaluate the patient for symptom relief, adverse effects, and patterns of withdrawal bleeding. Women receiving MHT should be seen by the clinician for annual monitoring (Table 82-8).

TABLE 82-8 Management of Patients Taking Hormone Therapy Regimens

Drug	Adverse Drug Reaction	Monitoring Parameter	Suggested Change
Initiation of Hormone Therapy			
Hormone therapy should be used only as long as vasomotor symptom control is necessary (usually 2-3 years)			
6-Week Follow-up Visit			
• To discuss patient concerns about hormone therapy • To evaluate the patient for symptom relief, adverse effects, and patterns of withdrawal bleeding (if continuous sequential hormone therapy is given)			
Drug	**Adverse Drug Reaction**	**Monitoring Parameter**	**Suggested Change**
Estrogen		Persistence of hot flushes	Increase estrogen dose
Estrogen	Breast tenderness		Reduce estrogen dose; switch to a transdermal regimen
Progestogen	Bloating Premenstrual-like symptoms		Switch to another progestogen
Annual Follow-up Visit			
Annual monitoring: medical history, physical examination (including pelvic examination), blood pressure measurement, and routine endometrial cancer surveillance (as indicated). Additional follow-up is determined based on the patient's initial response to therapy and the need for any modification of the regimen			
Breast examinations: annual mammograms (scheduled based on patient's age and risk factors)			
Osteoporosis prevention: BMD should be measured in women 65 years and older and in women younger than 65 years with risk factors for osteoporosis. Repeat testing should be performed as clinically indicated.			
In women taking sequential hormone therapy	Transvaginal ultrasound, and where indicated an endometrial biopsy should be performed if vaginal bleeding occurs at any time other than the expected time of withdrawal bleeding or when heavier or more prolonged withdrawal bleeding occurs (if endometrial pathology cannot be excluded by endovaginal ultrasonography, further evaluation may be required, such as hysteroscopy)		
In women taking continuous combined hormone therapy	Endometrial evaluation should be considered when irregular bleeding persists for more than 6 months after initiating therapy		

BMD, bone mineral density.

The main indication for MHT is relief of menopausal symptoms. If combined estrogen/progestogen treatment is stopped within 5 years, no evidence of increased risk of breast cancer is observed.[13] Estrogen-alone treatment is not associated with an increased risk of breast cancer.[35]

Many women have no difficulty abruptly stopping MHT; others develop vasomotor symptoms after discontinuation. Although these symptoms may be mild and resolve over a few months, in some women the symptoms are severe and intolerable. There is no evidence that gradual discontinuation of MHT reduces the recurrence of hot flushes compared with sudden discontinuation.[126]

CONCLUSION

Menopause is a natural life event—not a disease. Therefore, the decision to use MHT must be individualized based on the severity of menopausal symptoms and the risk for cardiovascular disease, breast cancer, thromboembolism, and osteoporotic fracture (Table 82-9).

The WHI trial reported increased risk of cardiovascular disease, breast cancer, stroke, and thromboembolic disease among women using continuous combined therapy with CEE plus MPA compared with placebo. In the estrogen-alone arm of the study, CEE had no effect on cardiovascular disease or breast cancer risk compared to placebo, but an increased risk of stroke and thromboembolic disease was noted in those who received estrogen. The WHI trial also demonstrated that quality of life and cognition were no better in the group receiving MHT than in the placebo group, and that MHT increases dementia risk in women 65 years or older. Recent studies suggest dose, duration, and timing (early or late menopause) of therapy may alter the benefit-risk profile and should be considered for individual patients.

In the absence of contraindications, MHT is the most effective treatment for managing postmenopausal symptoms, such as hot flushes, night sweats, and vaginal dryness. For many women, the benefits of short-term use of MHT for the relief of menopausal symptoms, far outweighs any risks. For symptoms of genital atrophy alone, the use of local, nonsystemic estrogen, nonhormonal lubricants and moisturizers, or ospemifene should be considered.

Long-term use of MHT cannot be recommended routinely for osteoporosis prevention given the availability of alternative therapies, such as bisphosphonates and raloxifene. For long-term MHT use, the potential harm (cardiovascular disease, breast cancer, and thromboembolism) outweighs the potential benefits. MHT should not be used for prevention of CHD. Women with cardiovascular risk factors (eg, hypertension and lipid abnormalities) can benefit from reduction of these risk factors through interventions such as weight loss, lipid-lowering therapy, use of aspirin, and physical activity.

PRIMARY OVARIAN INSUFFICIENCY AND PREMENOPAUSAL HORMONE REPLACEMENT THERAPY

Primary ovarian insufficiency (POI) is a condition characterized by sex-steroid deficiency, amenorrhea, and infertility in women younger than 40 years.[127] POI was once considered irreversible and was described as "premature menopause," and the condition is still referred to as *premature ovarian failure*. However, POI is not an early, natural menopause. Normal menopause results from ovarian follicle depletion, whereas POI is characterized by intermittent ovarian function in half of affected women.[127] These women produce estrogen intermittently and may ovulate despite the presence of high gonadotropin concentrations. Pregnancies have occurred in 5% to 10% of women after the diagnosis of POI, even in women with no follicles observed on ovarian biopsy.

Epidemiology

The prevalence of POI increases with increasing age, reaching approximately 1% of women by age 40 years.[128]

Etiology

A number of physiologic or metabolic abnormalities can lead to POI (Table 82-10). In most cases, the etiology cannot be identified.

TABLE 82-9 Evidence-Based Hormone Therapy Guidelines for Menopausal Symptom Management

Recommendation	Recommendation Grade[a]
In the absence of contraindications, estrogen-based postmenopausal hormone therapy should be used for treatment of moderate to severe vasomotor symptoms	A1
Systemic or vaginal estrogen therapy should be used for treatment of urogenital symptoms and vaginal atrophy	A1
Postmenopausal women taking estrogen-based therapy should be followed up every year, taking into account findings from new clinical trials	A1
Postmenopausal women taking estrogen-based therapy should be informed about potential risks	A1
Safety and tolerability may vary substantially with the type and regimen of hormone therapy	B2
Breast cancer risk increases after use of continuous combined hormone therapy for longer than 5 years	A1
Breast cancer risk does not increase after long-term estrogen-only therapy (6.8 years) in postmenopausal women with hysterectomy	A1
Hormone therapy should not be used for primary or secondary prevention of coronary heart disease	A1
Oral hormone therapy increases risk of venous thromboembolism	A1
Non-oral hormone therapy may be safer for postmenopausal women at risk for venous thromboembolism who choose to take hormone therapy	B2
Oral hormone therapy increases risk of ischemic stroke	A1
Although hormone therapy decreases risk of osteoporotic fractures, it cannot be recommended as a first-line therapy for the treatment of osteoporosis	A1
Potential harm (cardiovascular disease, breast cancer, and thromboembolism) from long-term hormone therapy (use greater than 5 years) outweighs potential benefits	A1
Young women with primary ovarian insufficiency have severe menopausal symptoms and increased risk for osteoporosis and cardiovascular disease. Decisions on whether and how these young women must be treated should not be based on studies of hormone therapy in women older than 50 years	B3

Quality of evidence: 1, evidence from more than one properly randomized controlled trial; 2, evidence from more than one well-designed clinical trial with randomization from cohort or case-controlled analytic studies or multiple time series, or dramatic results from uncontrolled experiments; 3, evidence from opinions of respected authorities based on clinical experience, descriptive studies, or reports of expert communities.

[a]*Strength of recommendations:* A, good evidence to support recommendation; B, moderate evidence to support recommendation; C, poor evidence to support recommendation.

Pathophysiology

Primary ovarian insufficiency may occur as a result of ovarian follicle dysfunction or ovarian follicle depletion and may present as either primary amenorrhea (absence of menses in a girl who has reached age 16 years) or secondary amenorrhea (cessation of menses in a woman previously menstruating for at least 6 months). Approximately 50% of women with POI have documented ovarian follicle function.[127]

Clinical Presentation

No characteristic menstrual pattern or history precedes POI. Approximately 50% of patients with this condition have a history of oligomenorrhea or DUB (prodromal POI), and approximately 25% develop amenorrhea acutely. Some patients develop amenorrhea postpartum, whereas others experience amenorrhea after discontinuing oral contraceptives. Primary amenorrhea is not associated with symptoms of estrogen deficiency. In cases of secondary amenorrhea, symptoms may include hot flushes, night sweats, fatigue, and mood changes. Prodromal POI may present with hot flushes even in women who menstruate regularly. Incomplete development of secondary sex characteristics may occur in women with primary amenorrhea, whereas these characteristics typically are normal in women with secondary amenorrhea. In general, women with POI have normal fertility before the disorder develops.

Primary ovarian insufficiency is defined by the presence of at least 4 months of amenorrhea and at least two serum FSH concentrations measuring greater than 40 IU/L (obtained at least 1 month apart) in women younger than 40 years. A complete history should be taken, considering other factors that can affect ovarian function such as prior ovarian surgery, chemotherapy, radiation, and autoimmune disorders. In patients with primary amenorrhea, particular attention should be paid to breast and pubic hair development according to

TABLE 82-10 Etiology of Primary Ovarian Insufficiency

Idiopathic or karyotypically normal spontaneous primary ovarian insufficiency
Autoimmunity:
(A) Isolated autoimmune primary ovarian insufficiency
(B) As a component of an autoimmune polyglandular syndrome in association with Addison's disease, hypothyroidism, hypoparathyroidism, or mucocutaneous candidiasis (*AIRE* gene mutations; 21q22.3)
Ovarian insufficiency due to chemotherapy, radiation, and extensive ovarian surgery
Chromosomal abnormalities:
(A) X-chromosome defects (X-monosomy; X-mosaicism; X-chromosome translocations or partial deletions; *FMR1* gene permutations, Xq27,3; *FMR2* gene permutations, Xq28; *BMP15* gene mutation, Xp11.2)
(B) Autosomal chromosome abnormalities
Gonadotropin-receptor abnormalities affecting ovarian function (FSH-receptor gene mutations, 2p21-p16; LH-receptor gene mutations, 2p21)
Enzyme deficiencies affecting ovarian function
(A) Cholesterol desmolase deficiency
(B) 17α-hydroxylase deficiency
(C) 17-20 desmolase deficiency
Galactosemia (galactose-1-phosphate uridyl transferase, *GALT* gene mutations, 9p13)
Blepharophimosis, ptosis, and epicanthus in versus syndrome type 1 (autosomal dominant syndrome, in which primary ovarian insufficiency is the predominant syndrome)
Perrault's syndrome (familial autosomal recessive primary ovarian insufficiency in association with deafness)

Tanner stages. Short stature, stigmata of Turner syndrome, and other dysmorphic features of gonadal dysgenesis should be considered. Ideally, a pelvic examination is performed but is not always clinically appropriate. Alternatively, transabdominal ultrasonography can be performed in patients with primary amenorrhea to confirm the presence of normal anatomic structures. In the majority of cases, physical examination is completely normal. A karyotype should be performed in all patients experiencing POI. Women with ovarian insufficiency and a karyotype containing a Y chromosome should undergo bilateral gonadectomy because of substantial risk for gonadal germ cell neoplasia.[127] Ovarian biopsy and antiovarian antibody testing are investigational procedures with no proven clinical benefit in POI. As clinically indicated, the workup should include tests for the diagnosis of other possible associated autoimmune disorders, such as hypothyroidism, diabetes mellitus, and Addison's disease.

In the majority of patients, ovarian insufficiency develops after the establishment of regular menses. Young women with POI who develop ovarian dysfunction before they achieve peak adult bone mass sustain sex steroid deficiency for more years than do naturally menopausal women. This deficiency can result in a significantly higher risk for osteoporosis[129] and cardiovascular disease.[130,131] Importantly, a survey of more than 19,000 women between the ages of 25 and 100 years suggests that ovarian insufficiency occurring before age 40 years is associated with significantly increased mortality, with an age-adjusted odds ratio for all-cause mortality of 2.14 (95% CI: 1.15-3.99).[132]

Young women find the diagnosis of POI particularly traumatic and frequently need extensive emotional and psychological support. Although most of these women will, in fact, be infertile, it is important to emphasize that POI can be transient and that spontaneous pregnancies have occurred even years after diagnosis.

Treatment: Primary Ovarian Insufficiency

Women with POI require hormone replacement, and long-term follow-up is necessary. Optimal hormone therapy depends on whether the patient has primary or secondary amenorrhea. Young women with primary amenorrhea in whom secondary sex characteristics have failed to develop initially should be given very low doses of estrogen in an attempt to mimic the gradual pubertal maturation process. A typical regimen is 0.3 mg CEE unopposed (ie, no progestogen) daily for 6 months, with incremental dose increases at 6-month intervals until the required maintenance dose is achieved. Gradual dose escalation often results in optimal breast development and allows time for the young woman to adjust psychologically to her physical maturation. Cyclic progestogen therapy, given 12 to 14 days per month, should be instituted toward the end of the second year of treatment.

Women with secondary amenorrhea who have been estrogen deficient for 12 months or longer also should be given low-dose estrogen replacement initially to avoid adverse effects such as mastalgia and nausea. However, the dose can be titrated up to maintenance levels over a 6-month period, and progestogen therapy can be instituted with the initiation of estrogen therapy. Women with a brief history of secondary amenorrhea are less likely to experience undesired effects from hormone therapy if they are given a reduced dose for the first month of therapy, followed by a full dose from the second month onward.

An estrogen dose equivalent to at least 1.25 mg CEE (or 100 mcg transdermal estradiol) is needed to achieve adequate estrogen replacement in young women. A progestogen should be given for 12 to 14 days per calendar month to prevent endometrial hyperplasia (Table 82-11). Estrogens given in usual replacement doses do not suppress spontaneous follicular activity or ovulation. Because women with POI can have spontaneous pregnancies, hormone therapy should produce regular, predictable menstrual flow patterns (ie, only cyclic regimens should be used). Patients who miss an expected menses should be tested for pregnancy and should discontinue hormone therapy if the result is positive. Because most young women negatively associate MHT with menopause in older women, some clinicians prefer to prescribe oral contraceptives for hormone replacement in premenopausal women with hypogonadism. However, oral contraceptives may not inhibit ovulation or effectively prevent pregnancy in young women with elevated gonadotropin levels.

Women with POI have testosterone deficiency.[133] In these young women, testosterone replacement, in addition to estrogen, was considered potentially important.[104,133] However, a prospective, randomized, placebo-controlled study conducted at the National Institutes of Health showed that long-term "physiologic" testosterone supplementation (150 mcg/day), in addition to standard hormone replacement, did not significantly improve BMD and sexual function in these young women.[134,135] More importantly, however, this study provided evidence that treatment with a physiological dose of estradiol (delivered via a transdermal patch) combined with oral medroxyprogesterone not only reduced the decline in lower hip and spine BMD in women with POI but actually restored it to normal levels.[134]

TABLE 82-11 Premenopausal Hormone Replacement Therapy in Primary Ovarian Insufficiency *(Continuous Sequential Therapy)*

Regimen[a]	Brand Name	Dosage
Estrogen Therapy		
Conjugated equine estrogens	Premarin	1.25 mg (oral; daily)
Estropipate (piperazine estrone sulfate)	Ogen Ortho-Est	2.5 mg (oral; daily)
Micronized 17β-estradiol	Estrace	4 mg (oral; daily)
Transdermal estrogen system (estradiol)	Alora Climara Vivelle, Vivelle Dot	0.1 mg, apply patch twice weekly 0.1 mg, apply patch twice weekly 0.1 mg, apply patch twice weekly
Progestogen Therapy		
Dydrogesterone[b]	Duphaston	10-20 mg/day for 12-14 days per calendar month (oral dosage form available as 10 mg tablets)
Medroxyprogesterone acetate	Provera Generic MPA	5-10 mg/day for 12-14 days per calendar month (oral dosage form available as 2.5, 5, 10 mg tablets)
Micronized progesterone	Prometrium	200 mg/day for 12-14 days per calendar month (oral dosage form available as 100 and 200 mg tablets)
Norethindrone acetate	Norethindrone acetate	5 mg/day for 12-14 days per calendar month (oral dosage form available as 5 mg tablets)
	Aygestin	5 mg/day for 12-14 days per calendar month (oral dosage form available as 2.5, 5 mg tablets)

[a]Off-label indication in the United States.

[b]Not available in the United States.

CLINICAL PRESENTATION Primary Ovarian Insufficiency

Symptoms

- Primary amenorrhea: no symptoms of estrogen deficiency.
- Secondary amenorrhea: vasomotor symptoms (hot flushes and night sweats), sleep disturbances, mood changes, sexual dysfunction, problems with concentration and memory, vaginal dryness, and dyspareunia.

Signs

- Primary amenorrhea: incomplete development of secondary sex characteristics.
- Secondary amenorrhea: normal development of secondary sex characteristics, signs of urogenital atrophy.

Laboratory Tests

- FSH greater than 40 IU/L.
- Other relevant diagnostic tests (eg, bone mineral density, ultrasound of the ovaries).
- Thyroid function tests, fasting glucose level, and adrenocorticotropic hormone stimulation test.

Desired Outcome

The goal of therapy in young women with POI is to provide a hormone replacement regimen that maintains sex steroid status as effectively as the normally functioning ovary.

General Approach to Treatment

9 Premenopausal hormone therapy in young women with POI differs markedly from MHT, and results of randomized trials conducted in menopausal women, including the WHI trial, cannot be extrapolated to premenopausal women with ovarian dysfunction. In POI, hormone replacement therapy with estrogen and a progestogen is aimed at mimicking the normal age-specific physiology and should generally be continued until the average age of natural menopause. Unlike postmenopausal women who have a natural decline in estrogen with aging and in whom MHT prolongs exposure to estrogen well beyond completion of the normal span of reproductive life, those with POI require exogenous sex steroids to compensate for an abnormal decrease in production by their ovaries. The observation that nearly half of young women with POI have significantly reduced BMD within 1.5 years of their diagnosis despite taking "standard" hormone therapy,[129] emphasizes the importance of providing optimal hormone therapy using dosing regimens that provide true physiologic replacement.[134]

Personalized Pharmacotherapy

Despite the heterogeneous nature of POI, efforts are ongoing to identify genetic factors that may influence the development and manifestation of this condition. However, the use of personalized pharmacotherapy to treat POI has not been described, and recommendations regarding how currently available therapies can be individualized to maximize benefit or reduce risk are not yet available.

Evaluation of Therapeutic Outcomes

Similar to the treatment of menopause, an assessment of the efficacy of hormone therapy, and its accompanying risks, should be performed on a regular basis. Young women with POI should be monitored annually for their response to treatment, and their adherence with hormone therapy should be assessed regularly. Patients should be evaluated continuously for the presence of signs and symptoms of associated autoimmune endocrine disorders, such as hypothyroidism, adrenal insufficiency, and diabetes mellitus. Baseline BMD testing should be performed in all women with POI. Mammography should be performed annually after age 45 years in accordance with accepted guidelines. Additional mammography screening in premenopausal women younger than 45 years who are receiving physiologic hormone therapy is not warranted. Other tests should be performed as clinically indicated.

CONCLUSION

Approximately 1% of women spontaneously develop ovarian insufficiency before age 40 years. POI is not an early natural menopause. Most affected women produce estrogen intermittently and may ovulate despite the presence of high gonadotropin concentrations. However, these women sustain sex steroid deficiency for more years than do naturally menopausal women, resulting in a significantly higher risk for osteoporosis and cardiovascular disease.

Women with POI need exogenous sex steroids to compensate for the decreased production by their ovaries. Thus, premenopausal hormone therapy is required at least until these women reach the age of natural menopause.

The goal of therapy is to provide a hormone replacement regimen that maintains sex steroid status as effectively as the normally functioning ovary.[131] This usually requires the administration of estrogen at a higher dose than the standard dose given to older women experiencing natural menopause.[131]

Because women with POI can have spontaneous pregnancies, hormone therapy should produce regular, predictable menstrual flow patterns. Patients who miss an expected menses should be tested for pregnancy and, if positive, the hormone therapy should be promptly discontinued.

Annual follow-up should include assessment of adherence with the prescribed hormone therapy regimen and evaluation for signs and symptoms of associated endocrine disorders.

ACKNOWLEDGMENT

This research was supported in part by the Intramural Research Program of the National Institute of Child Health and Human Development, National Institutes of Health.

ABBREVIATIONS

AMH	anti-Mullerian hormone
BMD	bone mineral density
CEE	conjugated equine estrogens
CHD	coronary heart disease
DUB	dysfunctional uterine bleeding
FMP	final menstrual period
FSH	follicle-stimulating hormone
GI	gastrointestinal
GnRH	gonadotropin-releasing hormone
GSM	genitourinary syndrome of menopause

HDL	high-density lipoprotein
HR	hazard ratio
LDL	low-density lipoprotein
LH	luteinizing hormone
MHT	menopausal hormone therapy
MPA	medroxyprogesterone acetate
NETA	norethindrone acetate
o-CEE	oral conjugated equine estrogens
POI	primary ovarian insufficiency
SERM	selective estrogen receptor modulator
STRAW	Stages of Reproductive Aging Workshop
TSEC	tissue-selective estrogen complex
VTE	venous thromboembolism
WHI	Women's Health Initiative
WHIMSY	Women's Health Initiative Memory Study of Younger Women

REFERENCES

1. Shifren JL, Gass ML. NAMS recommendations for Clinical Care of Midlife Women Working Group. The North American Menopause Society recommendations for clinical care of midlife women. *Menopause* 2014;21:1038-1062.
2. Takahashi TA, Johnson KM. Menopause. *Med Clin North Am* 2015;99:521-534.
3. Harlow SD, Gass M, Hall JE, et al. Executive summary of the Stages of Reproductive Aging Workshop + 10: Addressing the unfinished agenda of staging reproductive aging. *J Clin Endocrinol Metab* 2012;97:1159-1168.
4. Freeman EW, Sammel MD, Lin H, Gracia CR. Anti-mullerian hormone as a predictor of time to menopause in late reproductive age women. *J Clin Endocrinol Metab* 2012;97:1673-1680.
5. Burger HG. The endocrinology of the menopause. *J Steroid Biochem Mol Biol* 1999;69:31-35.
6. Avis NE, Crawford SL, Greendale G, et al. Duration of menopausal vasomotor symptoms over the menopause transition. *JAMA Intern Med* 2015;175:531-539.
7. Gartoulla P, Worsley R, Bell RJ, Davis SR. Moderate to severe vasomotor and sexual symptoms remain problematic for women aged 60 to 65 years. *Menopause* 2015;22:694-701.
8. Mishra GD, Kuh D. Health symptoms during midlife in relation to menopausal transition: British prospective cohort study. *BMJ* 2012;344:e402.
9. Avis NE, Brockwell S, Randolph JF Jr, et al. Longitudinal changes in sexual functioning as women transition through menopause: Results from the Study of Women's Health Across the Nation. *Menopause* 2009;16:442-452.
10. Portman DJ, Gass ML. Vulvovaginal Atrophy Terminology Consensus Conference Panel. Genitourinary syndrome of menopause: New terminology for vulvovaginal atrophy from the International Society for the Study of Women's Sexual Health and the North American Menopause Society. *Menopause* 2014;21:1063-1068.
11. Nappi RE, Kokot-Kierepa M. Vaginal Health: Insights, Views & Attitudes (VIVA)—results from an international survey. *Climacteric* 2012;15:36-44.
12. Freeman EW, Sammel MD, Lin H. Temporal associations of hot flashes and depression in the transition to menopause. *Menopause* 2009;16:728-734.
13. Rossouw JE, Anderson GL, Prentice RL, et al. Risks and benefits of estrogen plus progestin in healthy postmenopausal women: Principal results From the Women's Health Initiative randomized controlled trial. *JAMA* 2002;288:321-333.
14. Canonico M, Oger E, Plu-Bureau G, et al. Hormone therapy and venous thromboembolism among postmenopausal women: Impact of the route of estrogen administration and progestogens: The ESTHER study. *Circulation* 2007;115:840-845.
15. Canonico M, Plu-Bureau G, Lowe GD, Scarabin PY. Hormone replacement therapy and risk of venous thromboembolism in postmenopausal women: Systematic review and meta-analysis. *BMJ* 2008;336:1227-1231.
16. Chen MN, Lin CC, Liu CF. Efficacy of phytoestrogens for menopausal symptoms: A meta-analysis and systematic review. *Climacteric* 2015;18:260-269.
17. North American Menopause Society. Management of symptomatic vulvovaginal atrophy: 2013 position statement of The North American Menopause Society. *Menopause* 2013;20:888-902.
18. Stuenkel CA, Davis SR, Gompel A, et al. Treatment of symptoms of the menopause: An Endocrine Society clinical practice guideline. *J Clin Endocrinol Metab* 2015:jc20152236.
19. North American Menopause Society. Management of osteoporosis in postmenopausal women: 2010 position statement of The North American Menopause Society. *Menopause* 2010;17:25-54; quiz 5-6.
20. North American Menopause Society. The 2012 hormone therapy position statement of: The North American Menopause Society. *Menopause* 2012;19:257-271.
21. Goodman NF, Cobin RH, Ginzburg SB, et al. American Association of Clinical Endocrinologists medical guidelines for clinical practice for the diagnosis and treatment of menopause. *Endocr Pract* 2011;17 Suppl 6:1-25.
22. American College of Obstetricians and Gynecology. ACOG Practice Bulletin No. 141: Management of menopausal symptoms. *Obstet Gynecol* 2014;123:202-216.
23. North American Menopause Society. The North American Menopause Society Statement on Continuing Use of Systemic Hormone Therapy After Age 65. *Menopause* 2015;22:693.
24. Moyer VA, U.S. Preventive Services Task Force. Menopausal hormone therapy for the primary prevention of chronic conditions: U.S. Preventive Services Task Force recommendation statement. *Ann Intern Med* 2013;158:47-54.
25. Grady D, Brown JS, Vittinghoff E, et al. Postmenopausal hormones and incontinence: The Heart and Estrogen/Progestin Replacement Study. *Obstet Gynecol* 2001;97:116-120.
26. Wurz GT, Kao CJ, DeGregorio MW. Safety and efficacy of ospemifene for the treatment of dyspareunia associated with vulvar and vaginal atrophy due to menopause. *Clin Interv Aging* 2014;9:1939-1950.
27. Anderson GL, Limacher M, Assaf AR, et al. Effects of conjugated equine estrogen in postmenopausal women with hysterectomy: The Women's Health Initiative randomized controlled trial. *JAMA* 2004;291:1701-1712.
28. Manson JE, Hsia J, Johnson KC, et al. Estrogen plus progestin and the risk of coronary heart disease. *N Engl J Med* 2003;349:523-534.
29. Chlebowski RT, Hendrix SL, Langer RD, et al. Influence of estrogen plus progestin on breast cancer and mammography in healthy postmenopausal women: The Women's Health Initiative Randomized Trial. *JAMA* 2003;289:3243-3253.
30. Wassertheil-Smoller S, Hendrix SL, Limacher M, et al. Effect of estrogen plus progestin on stroke in postmenopausal women: The Women's Health Initiative: A randomized trial. *JAMA* 2003;289:2673-2684.
31. Shumaker SA, Legault C, Rapp SR, et al. Estrogen plus progestin and the incidence of dementia and mild cognitive impairment in postmenopausal women: The Women's Health Initiative Memory Study: A randomized controlled trial. *JAMA* 2003;289:2651-2662.
32. Rapp SR, Espeland MA, Shumaker SA, et al. Effect of estrogen plus progestin on global cognitive function in postmenopausal women: The Women's Health Initiative Memory Study: A randomized controlled trial. *JAMA* 2003;289:2663-2672.
33. Hays J, Ockene JK, Brunner RL, et al. Effects of estrogen plus progestin on health-related quality of life. *N Engl J Med* 2003;348:1839-1854.
34. Cauley JA, Robbins J, Chen Z, et al. Effects of estrogen plus progestin on risk of fracture and bone mineral density: The Women's Health Initiative randomized trial. *JAMA* 2003;290:1729-1738.
35. Anderson GL, Judd HL, Kaunitz AM, et al. Effects of estrogen plus progestin on gynecologic cancers and associated diagnostic procedures: The Women's Health Initiative randomized trial. *JAMA* 2003;290:1739-1748.
36. Espeland MA, Rapp SR, Shumaker SA, et al. Conjugated equine estrogens and global cognitive function in postmenopausal women: Women's Health Initiative Memory Study. *JAMA* 2004;291:2959-2968.

37. Hsia J, Langer RD, Manson JE, et al. Conjugated equine estrogens and coronary heart disease: The Women's Health Initiative. *Arch Intern Med* 2006;166:357-365.
38. Curb JD, Prentice RL, Bray PF, et al. Venous thrombosis and conjugated equine estrogen in women without a uterus. *Arch Intern Med* 2006;166:772-780.
39. Stefanick ML, Anderson GL, Margolis KL, et al. Effects of conjugated equine estrogens on breast cancer and mammography screening in postmenopausal women with hysterectomy. *JAMA* 2006;295:1647-1657.
40. Manson JE, Allison MA, Rossouw JE, et al. Estrogen therapy and coronary-artery calcification. *N Engl J Med* 2007;356:2591-2602.
41. Shumaker SA, Legault C, Kuller L, et al. Conjugated equine estrogens and incidence of probable dementia and mild cognitive impairment in postmenopausal women: Women's Health Initiative Memory Study. *JAMA* 2004;291:2947-2958.
42. Koh KK, Jin DK, Yang SH, et al. Vascular effects of synthetic or natural progestagen combined with conjugated equine estrogen in healthy postmenopausal women. *Circulation* 2001;103:1961-1966.
43. Viscoli CM, Brass LM, Kernan WN, et al. A clinical trial of estrogen-replacement therapy after ischemic stroke. *N Engl J Med* 2001;345:1243-1249.
44. Herrington DM, Reboussin DM, Brosnihan KB, et al. Effects of estrogen replacement on the progression of coronary-artery atherosclerosis. *N Engl J Med* 2000;343:522-529.
45. Rossouw JE, Prentice RL, Manson JE, et al. Postmenopausal hormone therapy and risk of cardiovascular disease by age and years since menopause. *JAMA* 2007;297:1465-1477.
46. Toh S, Hernandez-Diaz S, Logan R, et al. Coronary heart disease in postmenopausal recipients of estrogen plus progestin therapy: Does the increased risk ever disappear? A randomized trial. *Ann Intern Med* 2010;152:211-217.
47. Schierbeck LL, Rejnmark L, Tofteng CL, et al. Effect of hormone replacement therapy on cardiovascular events in recently postmenopausal women: Randomised trial. *BMJ* 2012;345:e6409.
48. Bechlioulis A, Kalantaridou SN, Naka KK, et al. Endothelial function, but not carotid intima-media thickness, is affected early in menopause and is associated with severity of hot flushes. *J Clin Endocrinol Metab* 2010;95:1199-1206.
49. Bechlioulis A, Naka KK, Kalantaridou SN, et al. Increased vascular inflammation in early menopausal women is associated with hot flush severity. *J Clin Endocrinol Metab* 2012;97:E760-E764.
50. Bechlioulis A, Naka KK, Kalantaridou SN, et al. Short-term hormone therapy improves sCD40L and endothelial function in early menopausal women: Potential role of estrogen receptor polymorphisms. *Maturitas* 2012;71:389-395.
51. Harman SM, Black DM, Naftolin F, et al. Arterial imaging outcomes and cardiovascular risk factors in recently menopausal women: A randomized trial. *Ann Intern Med* 2014;161:249-260.
52. Heiss G, Wallace R, Anderson GL, et al. Health risks and benefits 3 years after stopping randomized treatment with estrogen and progestin. *JAMA* 2008;299:1036-1045.
53. LaCroix AZ, Chlebowski RT, Manson JE, et al. Health outcomes after stopping conjugated equine estrogens among postmenopausal women with prior hysterectomy: A randomized controlled trial. *JAMA* 2011;305:1305-1314.
54. Chlebowski RT, Kuller LH, Prentice RL, et al. Breast cancer after use of estrogen plus progestin in postmenopausal women. *N Engl J Med* 2009;360:573-587.
55. Beral V. Million Women Study Collaborators. Breast cancer and hormone-replacement therapy in the Million Women Study. *Lancet* 2003;362:419-427.
56. Beral V, Reeves G, Bull D, et al. Breast cancer risk in relation to the interval between menopause and starting hormone therapy. *J Natl Cancer Inst* 2011;103:296-305.
57. Swanson GM. Breast cancer risk estimation: A translational statistic for communication to the public. *J Natl Cancer Inst* 1993;85:848-849.
58. Collaborative Group on Hormonal Factors in Breast Cancer. Breast cancer and hormone replacement therapy: Collaborative reanalysis of data from 51 epidemiological studies of 52,705 women with breast cancer and 108,411 women without breast cancer. Collaborative Group on Hormonal Factors in Breast Cancer. *Lancet* 1997;350:1047-1059.
59. Schairer C, Lubin J, Troisi R, et al. Menopausal estrogen and estrogen-progestin replacement therapy and breast cancer risk. *JAMA* 2000;283:485-491.
60. McTiernan A, Martin CF, Peck JD, et al. Estrogen-plus-progestin use and mammographic density in postmenopausal women: Women's Health Initiative randomized trial. *J Natl Cancer Inst* 2005;97:1366-1376.
61. Casper RF. Estrogen with interrupted progestin HRT: A review of experimental and clinical studies. *Maturitas* 2000;34:97-108.
62. Pickar JH, Yeh I, Wheeler JE, et al. Endometrial effects of lower doses of conjugated equine estrogens and medroxyprogesterone acetate. *Fertil Steril* 2001;76:25-31.
63. Barrett-Connor E, Mosca L, Collins P, et al. Effects of raloxifene on cardiovascular events and breast cancer in postmenopausal women. *N Engl J Med* 2006;355:125-137.
64. Lacey JV Jr, Mink PJ, Lubin JH, et al. Menopausal hormone replacement therapy and risk of ovarian cancer. *JAMA* 2002;288:334-341.
65. Collaborative Group On Epidemiological Studies of Ovarian Cancer, Beral V, Gaitskell K, et al. Menopausal hormone use and ovarian cancer risk: Individual participant meta-analysis of 52 epidemiological studies. *Lancet* 2015;380:1835-1842.
66. Chlebowski RT, Schwartz AG, Wakelee H, et al. Oestrogen plus progestin and lung cancer in postmenopausal women (Women's Health Initiative trial): A post-hoc analysis of a randomised controlled trial. *Lancet* 2009;374:1243-1251.
67. Chlebowski RT, Anderson GL, Manson JE, et al. Lung cancer among postmenopausal women treated with estrogen alone in the women's health initiative randomized trial. *J Natl Cancer Inst* 2010;102:1413-1421.
68. Lindsay R, Gallagher JC, Kleerekoper M, Pickar JH. Effect of lower doses of conjugated equine estrogens with and without medroxyprogesterone acetate on bone in early postmenopausal women. *JAMA* 2002;287:2668-2676.
69. Lindsay R, Gallagher JC, Kleerekoper M, Pickar JH. Bone response to treatment with lower doses of conjugated estrogens with and without medroxyprogesterone acetate in early postmenopausal women. *Osteoporos Int* 2005;16:372-379.
70. Hlatky MA, Boothroyd D, Vittinghoff E, et al. Quality-of-life and depressive symptoms in postmenopausal women after receiving hormone therapy: Results from the Heart and Estrogen/Progestin Replacement Study (HERS) trial. *JAMA* 2002;287:591-597.
71. Ott A, Breteler MM, van Harskamp F, et al. Incidence and risk of dementia. The Rotterdam Study. *Am J Epidemiol* 1998;147:574-580.
72. Espeland MA, Shumaker SA, Leng I, et al. Long-term effects on cognitive function of postmenopausal hormone therapy prescribed to women aged 50 to 55 years. *JAMA Intern Med* 2013;173:1429-1436.
73. Gleason CE, Dowling NM, Wharton W, et al. Effects of Hormone Therapy on Cognition and Mood in Recently Postmenopausal Women: Findings from the Randomized, Controlled KEEPS-Cognitive and Affective Study. *PLoS Med* 2015;12:e1001833; discussion e1001833.
74. Espeland MA, Hogan PE, Fineberg SE, et al. Effect of postmenopausal hormone therapy on glucose and insulin concentrations. PEPI Investigators. Postmenopausal Estrogen/Progestin Interventions. *Diabetes Care* 1998;21:1589-1595.
75. Kanaya AM, Herrington D, Vittinghoff E, et al. Glycemic effects of postmenopausal hormone therapy: The Heart and Estrogen/progestin Replacement Study. A randomized, double-blind, placebo-controlled trial. *Ann Intern Med* 2003;138:1-9.
76. Margolis KL, Bonds DE, Rodabough RJ, et al. Effect of oestrogen plus progestin on the incidence of diabetes in postmenopausal women: Results from the Women's Health Initiative Hormone Trial. *Diabetologia* 2004;47:1175-1187.
77. Norman RJ, Flight IH, Rees MC. Oestrogen and progestogen hormone replacement therapy for peri-menopausal and post-menopausal women: Weight and body fat distribution. *Cochrane Database Syst Rev* 2000:CD001018.
78. Cirillo DJ, Wallace RB, Rodabough RJ, et al. Effect of estrogen therapy on gallbladder disease. *JAMA* 2005;293:330-339.
79. Bachmann GA, Schaefers M, Uddin A, Utian WH. Lowest effective transdermal 17beta-estradiol dose for relief of hot flushes in postmenopausal women: A randomized controlled trial. *Obstet Gynecol* 2007;110:771-779.
80. Haines C, Yu SL, Hiemeyer F, Schaefers M. Micro-dose transdermal estradiol for relief of hot flushes in postmenopausal Asian women: A randomized controlled trial. *Climacteric* 2009;12:419-426.
81. Lowe GD, Upton MN, Rumley A, et al. Different effects of oral and transdermal hormone replacement therapies on factor IX, APC

resistance, t-PA, PAI and C-reactive protein—A cross-sectional population survey. *Thromb Haemost* 2001;86:550-556.

82. Furness S, Roberts H, Marjoribanks J, Lethaby A. Hormone therapy in postmenopausal women and risk of endometrial hyperplasia. *Cochrane Database Syst Rev* 2012;8:CD000402.
83. Loprinzi CL, Levitt R, Barton D, et al. Phase III comparison of depomedroxyprogesterone acetate to venlafaxine for managing hot flashes: North Central Cancer Treatment Group Trial N99C7. *J Clin Oncol* 2006;24:1409-1414.
84. The Writing Group for the PEPI Trial. Effects of hormone replacement therapy on endometrial histology in postmenopausal women. The Postmenopausal Estrogen/Progestin Interventions (PEPI) Trial. The Writing Group for the PEPI Trial. *JAMA* 1996;275:370-375.
85. McBane SE, Borgelt LM, Barnes KN, et al. Use of compounded bioidentical hormone therapy in menopausal women: An opinion statement of the Women's Health Practice and Research Network of the American College of Clinical Pharmacy. *Pharmacotherapy* 2014;34:410-423.
86. American College of Obstetrics and Gynecologists Committee on Gynecologic Practice, American Society for Reproductive Medicine Practice Committee. Compounded bioidentical menopausal hormone therapy. *Fertil Steril* 2012;98:308-312.
87. Committee on Gynecologic Practice and the American Society for Reproductive Medicine Practice Committee. Committee opinion No. 532: Compounded bioidentical menopausal hormone therapy. *Obstet Gynecol* 2012;120:411-415.
88. Food and Drug Administration. Bio-identicals: Sorting myths from facts. 2008. *http://www.fda.gov/ForConsumers/ConsumerUpdates/ucm049311.htm*. (Accessed August 30, 2015).
89. Sturdee DW, Pines A. International Menopause Society Writing Group, et al. Updated IMS recommendations on postmenopausal hormone therapy and preventive strategies for midlife health. *Climacteric* 2011;14:302-320.
90. North American Menopause Society. Nonhormonal management of menopause-associated vasomotor symptoms: 2015 position statement of The North American Menopause Society. *Menopause* 2015.
91. Loprinzi CL, Kugler JW, Sloan JA, et al. Venlafaxine in management of hot flashes in survivors of breast cancer: A randomised controlled trial. *Lancet* 2000;356:2059-2063.
92. Evans ML, Pritts E, Vittinghoff E, et al. Management of postmenopausal hot flushes with venlafaxine hydrochloride: A randomized, controlled trial. *Obstet Gynecol* 2005;105:161-166.
93. Simon JA, Portman DJ, Kaunitz AM, et al. Low-dose paroxetine 7.5 mg for menopausal vasomotor symptoms: Two randomized controlled trials. *Menopause* 2013;20:1027-1035.
94. Stearns V, Johnson MD, Rae JM, et al. Active tamoxifen metabolite plasma concentrations after coadministration of tamoxifen and the selective serotonin reuptake inhibitor paroxetine. *J Natl Cancer Inst* 2003;95:1758-1764.
95. Davis SR, Davison SL, Donath S, Bell RJ. Circulating androgen levels and self-reported sexual function in women. *JAMA* 2005;294:91-96.
96. Bell RJ, Donath S, Davison SL, Davis SR. Endogenous androgen levels and well-being: Differences between premenopausal and postmenopausal women. *Menopause* 2006;13:65-71.
97. Wierman ME, Arlt W, Basson R, et al. Androgen therapy in women: A reappraisal: An Endocrine Society clinical practice guideline. *J Clin Endocrinol Metab* 2014;99:3489-3510.
98. Shifren JL, Davis SR, Moreau M, et al. Testosterone patch for the treatment of hypoactive sexual desire disorder in naturally menopausal women: Results from the INTIMATE NM1 Study. *Menopause* 2006;13:770-779.
99. Davis SR, Moreau M, Kroll R, et al. Testosterone for low libido in postmenopausal women not taking estrogen. *N Engl J Med* 2008;359:2005-2017.
100. Shifren JL, Braunstein GD, Simon JA, et al. Transdermal testosterone treatment in women with impaired sexual function after oophorectomy. *N Engl J Med* 2000;343:682-688.
101. Davis S, Papalia MA, Norman RJ, et al. Safety and efficacy of a testosterone metered-dose transdermal spray for treating decreased sexual satisfaction in premenopausal women: A randomized trial. *Ann Intern Med* 2008;148:569-577.
102. van Staa TP, Sprafka JM. Study of adverse outcomes in women using testosterone therapy. *Maturitas* 2009;62:76-80.
103. Davis SR, Wolfe R, Farrugia H, et al. The incidence of invasive breast cancer among women prescribed testosterone for low libido. *J Sex Med* 2009;6:1850-1856.
104. Kalantaridou SN, Calis KA, Mazer NA, et al. A pilot study of an investigational testosterone transdermal patch system in young women with spontaneous premature ovarian failure. *J Clin Endocrinol Metab* 2005;90:6549-6552.
105. Santen RJ, Kagan R, Altomare CJ, et al. Current and evolving approaches to individualizing estrogen receptor-based therapy for menopausal women. *J Clin Endocrinol Metab* 2014;99:733-747.
106. Glusman JE, Huster WJ, Paul S. Raloxifene effects on vasomotor and other climacteric symptoms in postmenopausal women. *Prim Care Update Ob Gyns* 1998;5:166.
107. Palacios S, Mejia Rios A. Bazedoxifene/conjugated estrogens combination for the treatment of the vasomotor symptoms associated with menopause and for prevention of osteoporosis in postmenopausal women. *Drugs Today (Barc)* 2015;51:107-116.
108. Mirkin S, Komm B, Pickar JH. Conjugated estrogen/bazedoxifene tablets for the treatment of moderate-to-severe vasomotor symptoms associated with menopause. *Womens Health (Lond Engl)* 2014;10:135-146.
109. Pinkerton JV, Abraham L, Bushmakin AG, et al. Evaluation of the efficacy and safety of bazedoxifene/conjugated estrogens for secondary outcomes including vasomotor symptoms in postmenopausal women by years since menopause in the Selective estrogens, Menopause and Response to Therapy (SMART) trials. *J Womens Health (Larchmt)* 2014;23:18-28.
110. Cummings SR, Ettinger B, Delmas PD, et al. The effects of tibolone in older postmenopausal women. *N Engl J Med* 2008;359:697-708.
111. Nijland EA, Weijmar Schultz WC, Nathorst-Boos J, et al. Tibolone and transdermal E2/NETA for the treatment of female sexual dysfunction in naturally menopausal women: Results of a randomized active-controlled trial. *J Sex Med* 2008;5:646-656.
112. Kenemans P, Bundred NJ, Foidart JM, et al. Safety and efficacy of tibolone in breast-cancer patients with vasomotor symptoms: a double-blind, randomised, non-inferiority trial. *Lancet Oncol* 2009;10:135-146.
113. Christodoulakos GE, Lambrinoudaki IV, Panoulis CP, et al. Effect of hormone replacement therapy, tibolone and raloxifene on serum lipids, apolipoprotein A1, apolipoprotein B and lipoprotein(a) in Greek postmenopausal women. *Gynecol Endocrinol* 2004;18:244-257.
114. Beral V, Bull D, Reeves G, Million Women Study Collaborators. Endometrial cancer and hormone-replacement therapy in the Million Women Study. *Lancet* 2005;365:1543-1551.
115. Langer RD, Landgren BM, Rymer J, et al. Effects of tibolone and continuous combined conjugated equine estrogen/medroxyprogesterone acetate on the endometrium and vaginal bleeding: Results of the OPAL study. *Am J Obstet Gynecol* 2006;195:1320-1327.
116. Murkies AL, Wilcox G, Davis SR. Clinical review 92: Phytoestrogens. *J Clin Endocrinol Metab* 1998;83:297-303.
117. Tice JA, Ettinger B, Ensrud K, et al. Phytoestrogen supplements for the treatment of hot flashes: The Isoflavone Clover Extract (ICE) Study: A randomized controlled trial. *JAMA* 2003;290:207-214.
118. Lethaby A, Marjoribanks J, Kronenberg F, et al. Phytoestrogens for menopausal vasomotor symptoms. *Cochrane Database Syst Rev* 2013;12:CD001395.
119. Lissin LW, Cooke JP. Phytoestrogens and cardiovascular health. *J Am Coll Cardiol* 2000;35:1403-1410.
120. Tempfer CB, Froese G, Heinze G, et al. Side effects of phytoestrogens: A meta-analysis of randomized trials. *Am J Med* 2009;122:939-946.e9.
121. Newton KM, Reed SD, LaCroix AZ, et al. Treatment of vasomotor symptoms of menopause with black cohosh, multibotanicals, soy, hormone therapy, or placebo: A randomized trial. *Ann Intern Med* 2006;145:869-879.
122. Leach MJ, Moore V. Black cohosh (Cimicifuga spp.) for menopausal symptoms. *Cochrane Database Syst Rev* 2012;9:CD007244.
123. National Institutes of Health Office of Dietary Supplements. Dietary supplements fact sheet: Black cohosh. 2008. *http://ods.od.nih.gov/factsheets/BlackCohosh_pf.asp*. (Accessed August 30, 2015)
124. Nedrow A, Miller J, Walker M, et al. Complementary and alternative therapies for the management of menopause-related symptoms: A systematic evidence review. *Arch Intern Med* 2006;166:1453-1465.
125. Ettinger B. Vasomotor symptom relief versus unwanted effects: role of estrogen dosage. *Am J Med* 2005;118 Suppl 12B:74-78.
126. Cunha EP, Azevedo LH, Pompei LM, et al. Effect of abrupt discontinuation versus gradual dose reduction of postmenopausal hormone therapy on hot flushes. *Climacteric* 2010;13:362-367.
127. Kalantaridou SN, Davis SR, Nelson LM. Premature ovarian failure. *Endocrinol Metab Clin North Am* 1998;27:989-1006.

128. Coulam CB, Adamson SC, Annegers JF. Incidence of premature ovarian failure. *Obstet Gynecol* 1986;67:604-606.
129. Anasti JN, Kalantaridou SN, Kimzey LM, et al. Bone loss in young women with karyotypically normal spontaneous premature ovarian failure. *Obstet Gynecol* 1998;91:12-15.
130. Kalantaridou SN, Naka KK, Papanikolaou E, et al. Impaired endothelial function in young women with premature ovarian failure: Normalization with hormone therapy. *J Clin Endocrinol Metab* 2004;89:3907-3913.
131. van der Schouw YT, van der Graaf Y, Steyerberg EW, et al. Age at menopause as a risk factor for cardiovascular mortality. *Lancet* 1996;347:714-718.
132. Snowdon DA, Kane RL, Beeson WL, et al. Is early natural menopause a biologic marker of health and aging? *Am J Public Health* 1989;79:709-714.
133. Kalantaridou SN, Calis KA, Vanderhoof VH, et al. Testosterone deficiency in young women with 46,XX spontaneous premature ovarian failure. *Fertil Steril* 2006;86:1475-1482.
134. Popat VB, Calis KA, Kalantaridou SN, et al. Bone mineral density in young women with primary ovarian insufficiency: Results of a three-year randomized controlled trial of physiological transdermal estradiol and testosterone replacement. *J Clin Endocrinol Metab* 2014;99:3418-3426.
135. Kalantaridou SN, Vanderhoof VH, Calis KA, et al. Physiologic transdermal testosterone replacement (150 mcg/day) does not significantly improve sexual function in women with 46,XX spontaneous premature ovarian failure: A placebo-controlled randomized study, OR27-4. Abstract presented at the Annual Meeting of the Endocrine Society, June 2–5; 2007, Toronto, Canada.

Erectile Dysfunction

83

Mary Lee and Roohollah Sharifi

KEY CONCEPTS

1. The incidence of erectile dysfunction is low in men younger than 40 years of age. The incidence increases as men age likely as a result of concurrent medical conditions that impair the vascular, neurologic, psychogenic, and hormonal systems necessary for a normal penile erection.
2. Many commonly used drugs have sympatholytic, anticholinergic, sedative, or antiandrogenic effects that may exacerbate or contribute to the development of erectile dysfunction. Clinicians should be familiar with these agents and be prepared to make adjustments in drug regimens to minimize adverse effects of these drugs on a patient's erectile function.
3. The first step in clinical management of erectile dysfunction is to identify and, if possible, reverse the underlying causes. Risk factors for erectile dysfunction, including hypertension, diabetes mellitus, smoking, and chronic ethanol abuse, should be addressed and minimized.
4. Specific treatments for erectile dysfunction include vacuum erection devices (VEDs), pharmacologic treatments, psychotherapy, and surgery. Of these, phosphodiesterase type 5 inhibitors are the medications of first choice.
5. The ideal treatment of erectile dysfunction should have a fast onset, be effective, be convenient to administer, be cost effective, have a low incidence of serious adverse effects, and be free of serious drug interactions.
6. Specific treatment is first initiated with the least invasive forms of treatment, including VEDs or oral phosphodiesterase type 5 inhibitors, followed by intracavernosal injections or intraurethral inserts, and finally by surgical insertion of a penile prosthesis.
7. Vacuum erection devices can have a slow onset of action (up to 20 minutes) during initial use and are not discreet; therefore, they are most effective for a couple in a stable relationship.
8. Although phosphodiesterase type 5 inhibitors are convenient and effective regardless of the etiology of erectile dysfunction, they fail in 30% to 40% of patients. Also, phosphodiesterase type 5 inhibitors are contraindicated in patients taking any dosage formulation of nitrate.
9. Testosterone supplementation should be reserved for patients with primary, secondary, or mixed hypogonadism who have erectile dysfunction as a consequence of a decreased libido. Testosterone supplementation should not be used by patients with erectile dysfunction who have normal serum testosterone levels.
10. Although intracavernosal injections and intraurethral pellets of alprostadil are effective independent of the etiology of erectile dysfunction, they fail in up to one third of patients. To self-administer medication by these routes, patients require training to minimize administration-related adverse effects.

The National Institutes of Health Consensus Development Panel on Impotence defines erectile dysfunction as the persistent failure to achieve a penile erection to allow for satisfactory sexual intercourse.[1] A persistent failure refers to erectile dysfunction for a minimum of 3 months.[2] Patients may refer to it as impotence.

Erectile dysfunction must be distinguished from disorders of libido or ejaculation, and infertility, which are caused by different pathophysiologic mechanisms and are treated with alternative agents (Table 83-1). A patient may suffer from one or more disorders of sexual dysfunction. For example, an elderly man with primary hypogonadism may suffer from decreased libido and erectile dysfunction. Diagnosis of the type of sexual disorder that a patient has is key to initiating the most appropriate treatment.

EPIDEMIOLOGY

1 The incidence of erectile dysfunction is low in men younger than 40 years of age but increases as men age. The Massachusetts Male Aging Study, a cross-sectional survey of a random sample of 1,290 men in the Boston area, was conducted during the period from 1987 to 1989. The study reported an overall prevalence of 52% for any degree of erectile dysfunction in men aged 40 to 70 years, with an age-related increase in incidence ranging from 12.4% in men aged 40 to 49 years, up to 46.4% in men aged 60 to 69 years.[3] In men older than 70 years, the prevalence of erectile dysfunction increases and has been reported to be as high as 80%, depending on the population studied.[4] In the more recent Health Professional Follow-Up Study of more than 31,000 male health professionals aged 53 to 90 years, the prevalence of erectile dysfunction was 33%.[5] Interestingly, although the prevalence of erectile dysfunction increases with patient age, many patients fail to seek medical treatment.[6,7]

Erectile dysfunction is sometimes assumed to be a symptom of the aging process in men. However, more likely it results from concurrent medical conditions of the patient (eg, hypertension, arteriosclerosis, hyperlipidemia, diabetes mellitus, metabolic syndrome, or psychiatric disorders) or from medications that patients may be taking for these diseases.[8] For example, up to 50% of patients with diabetes mellitus develop erectile dysfunction, and medications such as diuretics are associated with a high incidence of erectile dysfunction.

TABLE 83-1 Types of Sexual Dysfunction in Men

Type of Dysfunction	Definition
Decreased libido	Decreased sexual drive or desire
Increased libido	Inappropriate and excessive sexual drive or desire
Erectile dysfunction (impotence)	Failure to achieve a penile erection suitable for satisfactory sexual intercourse
Delayed ejaculation	Commonly referred to as "dry sex"; ejaculation is delayed or absent
Retrograde ejaculation	Ejaculate passes retrograde into the bladder, instead of toward the anterior urethra (antegrade) and out of the penis
Infertility	Sperm are insufficient in number, have abnormal morphology, or have inadequate motility, and fail to fertilize the ovum

PHYSIOLOGY OF A NORMAL PENILE ERECTION

A normal penile erection requires full functioning of several physiologic systems: vascular, nervous, and hormonal. The patient also must be psychologically receptive to sexual stimuli.[9,10]

Vascular System

The penis comprises two corpora cavernosa on the dorsal side and one corpus spongiosum on the ventral side. The corpus spongiosum surrounds the urethra and forms the glans penis. The corpora are composed of multiple interconnected sinuses, which can fill with blood to produce an erection. The corpora cavernosa are encased by the tunica albuginea, a fibrous tissue membrane, which has limited distensibility. In the flaccid state, arterial flow into and venous outflow from the corpora are balanced. During the erectile phase, arterial blood flow increases and blood fills the sinusoids within the corpora, which causes penile swelling and elongation. The erection is prolonged by a decrease in venous outflow from the corpora, which is caused by compression of subtunical venules against the tunica albuginea by the swollen corpora (Fig. 83-1).

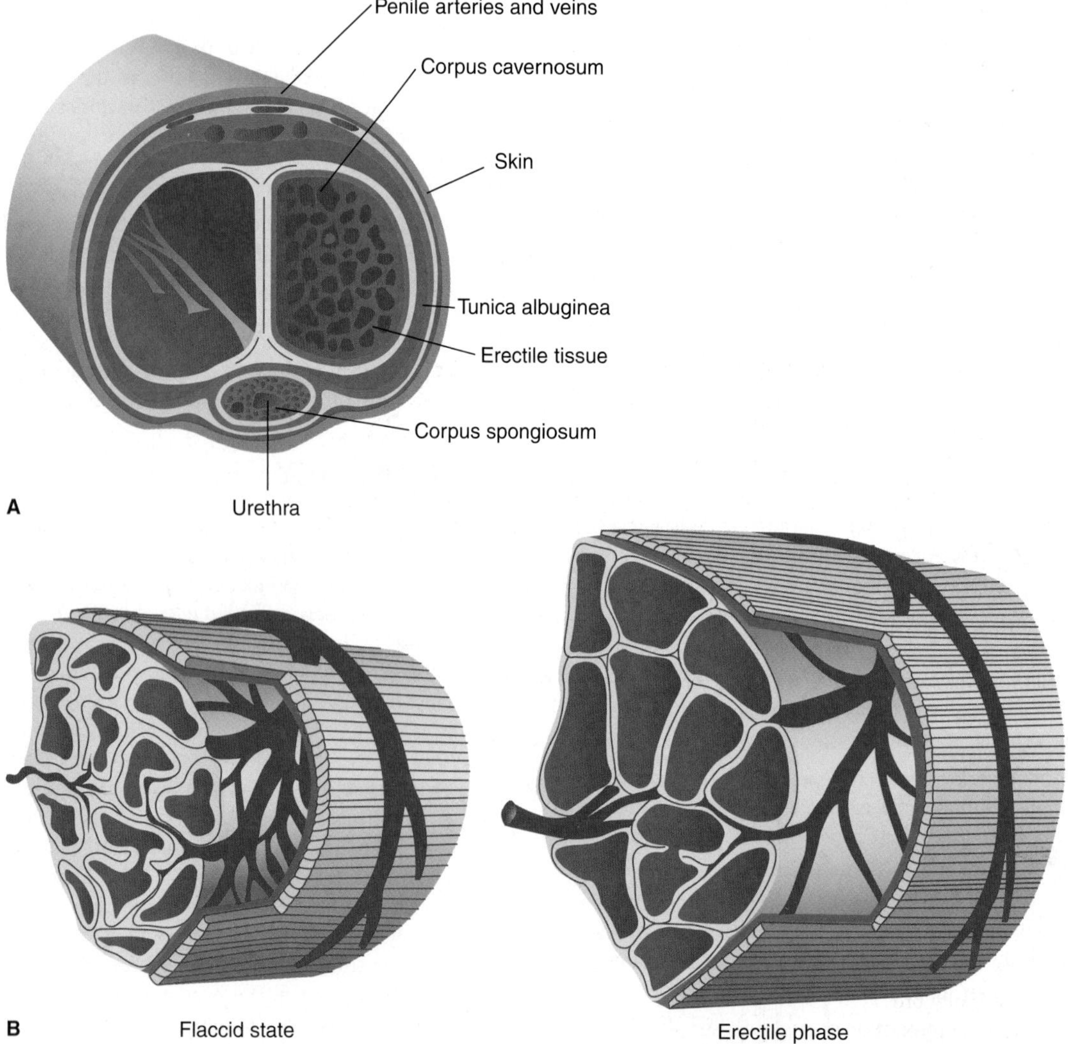

FIGURE 83-1 Microanatomy of and vascular changes in the penis in flaccid and erect states. In the flaccid state, arterial flow into and venous outflow from the corpora are balanced. During the erectile phase, arterial blood flow increases and blood fills the sinusoids within the corpora, causing penile swelling and elongation. The erection is prolonged by a decrease in venous outflow from the corpora, which is caused by compression of subtunical venules by the swollen corpora. *(Reprinted with permission from Walsh PC, ed. Campbell's Urology, 8th ed. Philadelphia, PA: WB Saunders; 2002:1595, 1697. Copyright © 2002 with permission from Elsevier.)*

Arterial flow into the corpora is enhanced by acetylcholine-mediated vasodilation. Acetylcholine indirectly enhances arterial flow to the corpora and increases sinusoidal filling of the corporal tissue. That is, acetylcholine is a co-neurotransmitter, which works along with other nonpeptidergic intracellular neurotransmitters—including cyclic guanosine monophosphate (cGMP), cyclic adenosine monophosphate (cAMP), or vasoactive intestinal polypeptide—to produce vasodilation. In effect, cGMP and cAMP are secondary messengers that direct desired effects in target tissues.

Specifically, acetylcholine produces an erection probably through two different pathways. Through one pathway, in the presence of sexual stimulation to genital tissue, acetylcholine enhances the production of nitric oxide by endothelial cells and nonadrenergic–noncholinergic neurons. Nitric oxide enhances the activity of guanylate cyclase, which increases the conversion of cyclic guanosine triphosphate to cGMP. cGMP activates a cGMP-dependent kinase, which decreases intracellular calcium concentrations in smooth muscle cells of penile arteries and cavernosal sinuses. As a result, smooth muscle relaxation occurs, which enhances arterial blood flow to and blood filling of the corpora.[10] An erection results.

In an alternative pathway, acetylcholine or prostaglandin E enhances the activity of adenyl cyclase, which increases the conversion of cyclic adenosine triphosphate to cAMP, a potent muscle relaxant. Similar to cGMP, cAMP decreases intracellular calcium concentrations to produce smooth muscle relaxation in cells of the arteries and cavernosal sinuses. Arterial blood flow to and blood filling of the corpora are enhanced, and a penile erection results.[10]

Nervous System and Psychogenic Stimuli

Some erections are mediated by a sacral nerve reflex arc (eg, erections can occur while the patient is sleeping). However, in the conscious patient, sensory sexual stimulation mediates erections via the CNS. That is, when a patient sees an attractive partner, hears sweet words, smells a particular scent, or tastes or touches a pleasant object, these situations can result in an erection. In this case, the patient's brain processes this information and the nervous impulse is carried down the spinal cord to peripheral cholinergic nerves that innervate the vascular supply to the corpora, resulting in an erection.

The medial preoptic area of the hypothalamus is thought to be that portion of the brain responsible for integrating external stimuli. Here dopamine exerts a proerectogenic effect, whereas, α_2-adrenergic stimulation causes the penis to become and/or remain flaccid. After moving down the spinal cord, stimulatory nerve impulses travel to the penis by efferent peripheral nerves, including inhibitory sympathetic neurons (T11-L2), proerectogenic parasympathetic neurons (S2-S4), and proerectogenic somatic neurons (S2-S4).

In summary, acetylcholine produces an erection by working along with other coneurotransmitters, including cGMP and cAMP. Thus, an erection is mediated neurologically, maintained by arterial blood filling of the corpora, and sustained by occlusion of venous outflow from the corpora.

Detumescence, or the progression of an erect penis to a flaccid state, results from the actions of norepinephrine, which contracts vascular smooth muscle to decrease arterial inflow to the corpora and contracts sinusoidal tissue in the corpora. As a result, venous outflow from the corpora increases.

Hormonal System

Testosterone is principally produced by the testes at a daily rate of 4 to 8 mg and a normal physiologic serum concentration is 300 to 1,100 ng/dL (10.4-38.2 nmol/L). Production follows a circadian pattern with highest blood levels in the morning and lowest levels in the evening. Physiologically active (free) testosterone comprises only 2% of circulating blood levels. About 44% of testosterone in the bloodstream is tightly bound to sex hormone-binding globulin and is inactive. Approximately 50% is reversibly bound to albumin and 4% is reversibly bound to corticosteroid-binding globulin; both of these portions of testosterone are in equilibrium with the 2% of testosterone that is free. Thus, the bioavailable portion of testosterone is normally 56% and comprises that which is bound to albumin and corticosteroid-binding globulin, and that which is free.[11] However, the bioavailable percentage of testosterone can vary considerably with changes in sex hormone-binding globulin. Sex hormone-binding globulin increases with aging, hyperthyroidism, human immunodeficiency virus disease, and hepatic cirrhosis; and decreases with obesity, diabetes mellitus, hypothyroidism, nephrotic syndrome, and corticosteroid use.[11]

Testosterone stimulates libido (sexual drive) and increases muscle mass in males. In addition, androgen receptors have been identified in the penile arterial endothelium and are thought to increase cavernosal levels of nitric oxide and cGMP, thereby enhancing vascular processes essential for a penile erection.[10,12] In some target cells with 5-α reductase, testosterone is activated to dihydrotestosterone. Dihydrotestosterone, which is more potent than testosterone, stimulates prostate gland growth, increases facial and body hair, induces baldness, and causes acne. In adipose tissue, a small portion of testosterone is converted to estradiol which can lead to gynecomastia.

Beginning at age 40 years, men experience a gradual decrease in testicular production of testosterone, with an associated decrease in muscle mass and sexual function.[10] The Massachusetts Male Aging Study reported that 6% to 12% of elderly males had symptoms of hypogonadism.[3] The European Male Aging Study described three cardinal symptoms of low serum testosterone levels: decreased libido, erectile dysfunction, and loss of spontaneous morning erections.[11] Other symptoms include fatigue, malaise, depressed mood, decreased bone density, increased fat:muscle ratio, gynecomastia, anemia, and insulin resistance.[12]

Within the normal physiologic serum total testosterone concentration, sexual drive is usually normal. However, because of variability in circulating levels of sex hormone-binding globulin and the lack of precision of available assays,[13,14] a patient's serum concentration of testosterone should always be interpreted in the context of the patient's symptoms and physical exam findings. To confirm hypogonadism when the serum total testosterone concentration is equivocal, the clinician should repeat the serum level measurement or obtain a serum-free (bioavailable) testosterone level.[15,16]

The relationship between erectile dysfunction and serum testosterone levels is complicated. Patients with normal serum testosterone levels may have erectile dysfunction, and patients with subnormal serum testosterone levels may have normal sexual function.[15] When a patient has hypogonadism and libido is decreased, a patient may not develop erections. In this case, erectile dysfunction is considered secondary to a decreased libido.

As a result, although the Food and Drug Administration defines hypogonadism as when the serum testosterone concentration is less than 300 ng/dL (10.4 nmol/L) in an adult man, treatment is indicated only in patients who are symptomatic or have signs of hypogonadism. Similarly, the European Association of Urology and the American Society of Andrology guidelines state that a serum testosterone greater than 350 ng/dL (12.2 nmol/L) requires no treatment, a serum testosterone of 230 to 350 ng/dL (8.0-12.2 nmol/L) requires treatment if the patient is symptomatic, and a serum testosterone below 230 ng/dL (8.0 nmol/L) generally should be treated.[13]

PATHOPHYSIOLOGY

Erectile dysfunction can result from any single abnormality or combination of abnormalities of the four systems necessary for a normal penile erection. Vascular, neurologic, or hormonal etiologies of erectile dysfunction are collectively referred to as *organic erectile dysfunction*. Approximately 80% of patients with erectile dysfunction have the organic type. Patients who do not respond to psychogenic stimuli and have no organic cause for dysfunction have *psychogenic erectile dysfunction*.[8,15,16]

Diseases that compromise vascular flow to the corpora cavernosum (eg, peripheral vascular disease, arteriosclerosis, and essential hypertension) are associated with an increased incidence of erectile dysfunction. Diseases that impair nerve conduction to the brain (eg, spinal cord injury or stroke) or conditions that impair peripheral nerve conduction to the penile vasculature (eg, diabetes mellitus) can result in erectile dysfunction.[17]

Diseases associated with hypogonadism, primary, secondary, or mixed, result in subphysiologic levels of testosterone, which cause diminished sexual drive (decreased libido) and secondary erectile dysfunction. Primary hypogonadism occurs with surgical removal of the testes for treatment of prostate or testicular cancer, or with testicular injury or disease. Secondary hypogonadism may result from hypothalamic or pituitary disorders of luteinizing hormone–releasing hormone or luteinizing hormone, respectively; or elevated prolactin levels, which can be associated with pituitary tumors or can occur in patients with chronic renal failure. In aging males, the etiology of hypogonadism is mixed. In addition to decreased Leydig cell function in the testes, the release of gonadotropin from the hypothalamus is reduced, the circadian pattern of luteinizing hormone release from the pituitary gland is impaired, and sex hormone-binding globulin production increases.[14]

Patients must be in the proper mental frame of mind to be receptive to sexual stimuli. Patients who suffer from malaise, have reactive depression or performance anxiety, are sedated, or have Alzheimer disease, hypothyroidism, or mental disorders commonly complain of erectile dysfunction. In most studies, patients with psychogenic erectile dysfunction generally exhibit a higher response rate to various interventions than do patients with organic erectile dysfunction because the former have less severe disease.

Social habits of patients have been linked to erectile dysfunction. The vasoconstrictor effect of cigarette smoking may compromise blood flow to the corpora and decrease cavernosal filling. Excessive ethanol intake may lead to androgen deficiency, peripheral neuropathy, or chronic liver disease, all of which can contribute to erectile dysfunction.

2 Medications may cause erectile dysfunction through similar pathophysiologic mechanisms (Table 83-2).[18-20] Medications are responsible for approximately 10% to 25% of cases of erectile dysfunction.

TABLE 83-2 Medication Classes That Can Cause Erectile Dysfunction

Drug Class	Proposed Mechanism by Which Drug Causes Erectile Dysfunction	Special Notes
Anticholinergic agents (antihistamines, antiparkinsonian agents, tricyclic antidepressants, phenothiazines)	Anticholinergic activity	• Second-generation nonsedating antihistamines (eg, loratadine, fexofenadine, or cetirizine) are associated with less erectile dysfunction than first-generation agents • Selective serotonin reuptake inhibitor (SSRI) and multiple receptor reuptake inhibitor antidepressants cause less erectile dysfunction than tricyclic antidepressants. Of the SSRIs, paroxetine, sertraline, fluvoxamine, and fluoxetine cause erectile dysfunction more commonly than venlafaxine, nefazodone, trazodone, bupropion, duloxetine, mirtazapine, escitalopram, or vilazodone • Phenothiazines with less anticholinergic effect (eg, chlorpromazine) can be substituted in some patients if erectile dysfunction is a problem
Dopamine antagonists (eg, metoclopramide, phenothiazines)	Inhibit prolactin inhibitory factor, thereby increasing prolactin levels	• Increased prolactin levels inhibit testicular testosterone production; depressed libido results
Estrogens or drugs with antiandrogenic effects (eg, luteinizing hormone-releasing hormone superagonists, digoxin, spironolactone, ketoconazole, cimetidine)	Suppress testosterone-mediated stimulation of libido	• In the face of a decreased libido, a secondary erectile dysfunction develops because of diminished sexual drive
CNS depressants (eg, barbiturates, narcotics, benzodiazepines, short-term use of large doses of alcohol, anticonvulsants)	Suppress perception of psychogenic stimuli	
Agents that decrease penile blood flow (eg, diuretics, peripheral β-adrenergic antagonists, or central sympatholytics [methyldopa, clonidine, guanethidine])	Reduce arteriolar flow to corpora	• Any diuretic that produces a significant decrease in intravascular volume can decrease penile arteriolar flow • Safer antihypertensives include angiotensin-converting enzyme inhibitors, postsynaptic α_1-adrenergic antagonists (terazosin, doxazosin), calcium channel blockers, and angiotensin II receptor antagonists[9]
Miscellaneous • Finasteride, dutasteride • Lithium carbonate • Gemfibrozil • Interferon • Clofibrate • Monoamine oxidase inhibitors (eg, phenelzine, isocarboxazid, tranylcypromine) Opiates	Unknown mechanism	

Data from references 17, 18, 19 and 20.

DIAGNOSIS

With the availability in the late 1990s of effective medications for erectile dysfunction independent of the etiology, diagnostic evaluation of erectile dysfunction became streamlined. Key assessments include a description of the severity of erectile dysfunction, complete medical, psychosocial, and surgical histories, review of concurrent medications, physical examination, and selected clinical laboratory tests.[9,21]

To assess the severity of erectile dysfunction, the patient should be asked about the quality of sexual intercourse for the past 4 weeks to 6 months. A self-administered standardized questionnaire, such as the International Index of Erectile Function (IIEF), is often used. It is administered before initiation of any treatment and repeated at regular intervals during treatment. It includes 15 questions about the quality of sexual function and satisfactoriness of sexual intercourse.[22] Questions include the following: How often were you able to maintain an erection? How difficult was it to sustain an erection? How satisfied are you with your sexual life? The physician should carefully assess the expectations for erectile function of the patient and the partner to ensure that expectations are reasonable. Shorter versions of the IIEF and other self-reporting questionnaires are also used in clinical practice. For example, the IIEF-EF comprises the six questions from the IIEF that focus on erectile function. The patient responds to each question, each response is scored on a range of 1 to 5. A score of 26 to 30 is considered normal function, 22 to 25 is mild erectile dysfunction, 17 to 21 is mild-to-moderate erectile dysfunction, 11 to 16 is moderate erectile dysfunction, and 10 or less is severe erectile dysfunction.

A medical history should be obtained to identify concurrent medical illnesses (eg, hypertension, atherosclerosis, hyperlipidemia, diabetes mellitus, and depression) or surgical procedures (eg, perineal or pelvic) that are risk factors for or are associated with organic or psychogenic erectile dysfunction. Underlying diseases that do not optimally respond to treatment should be addressed before specific treatment for erectile dysfunction is initiated. If the patient smokes cigarettes, drinks excessive amounts of ethanol, or uses recreational drugs, these social habits should be discontinued before specific treatment for erectile dysfunction is started.

A complete listing of the patient's prescription and nonprescription medications and dietary supplements should be reviewed by the clinician, who should identify drugs that may be contributing to erectile dysfunction. If possible, causative agents should be discontinued or the dose should be reduced.

A physical examination of the patient should include a check for hypogonadism (ie, signs of gynecomastia, small testicles, and decreased beard or body hair). The penis should be evaluated for diseases associated with abnormal penile curvature (eg, Peyronie's disease), which are associated with erectile dysfunction. Femoral and lower extremity pulses should be assessed to provide an indication of vascular supply to the genital area. Anal sphincter tone and other genital reflexes should be checked for the integrity of the nerve supply to the penis. A digital rectal examination in patients 50 years or older is needed to rule out benign prostatic hyperplasia, which may contribute to erectile dysfunction.

Selected laboratory tests should be obtained to identify the presence of underlying diseases that could cause erectile dysfunction. They include a fasting serum blood glucose and lipid profile. Serum testosterone levels should be checked in patients older than 50 years and in younger patients who complain of decreased libido and erectile dysfunction. At least two early morning serum testosterone levels on different days are needed to confirm the presence of hypogonadism.[23]

CLINICAL PRESENTATION Erectile Dysfunction

General

- Men are affected emotionally in many different ways
- Depression
- Performance anxiety
- Marital difficulties and avoidance of sexual intimacy (patients are often brought to a physician by their partners).
- Nonadherence to medications patient believes are causing erectile dysfunction.

Symptoms

- Erectile dysfunction or inability to have sexual intercourse, which may or may not be associated with decreased libido and ejaculatory disorders.

Signs

- If completing an IIEF survey, results are consistent with low satisfaction with the quality of erectile function.
- Medical history may identify concurrent medical illnesses or past surgical procedures that interfere with good vascular flow to the penis, damaged nerve function to the corpora, or mental disorders associated with decreased reception of sexual stimuli.
- Medication history may reveal prescription or nonprescription medications that could cause or contribute to erectile dysfunction.
- Physical examination may reveal signs of hypogonadism (eg, gynecomastia, small testicles, decreased body hair or beard, and decreased muscle mass), which may contribute to erectile dysfunction. The patient may have an abnormally curved penis when erect, decreased pulses in the pelvic region (suggesting impaired vascular flow to the penis), or decreased anal sphincter tone (suggesting impaired nerve function to the corpora). Men older than 50 years should undergo a digital rectal examination to determine whether an enlarged prostate is contributing to the patient's erectile dysfunction.

Laboratory Tests

- If the patient has signs of hypogonadism and complains of decreased libido, a serum testosterone concentration may be below the normal range, which would be consistent with a hormonal cause of erectile dysfunction. A low serum testosterone level should always be confirmed with a repeat blood level.
- If the patient has an enlarged prostate noted on digital rectal examination, a blood sample for prostate-specific antigen should be obtained. If elevated, the patient should be evaluated for a prostate disorder, which could contribute to erectile dysfunction.

TABLE 83-3 Recommendations of the Third Princeton Consensus Conference for Cardiovascular Risk Stratification of Patients Being Considered for Phosphodiesterase Inhibitor Therapy

Risk Category	Description of Patient's Condition	Management Approach
Low risk	Has asymptomatic cardiovascular disease with <3 risk factors for cardiovascular disease Has well-controlled hypertension Has mild congestive heart failure (NYHA class I or II) Has mild valvular heart disease Had a myocardial infarction >8 weeks ago	Patient can be started on phosphodiesterase inhibitor
Intermediate risk	Has ≥3 risk factors for cardiovascular disease Has mild or moderate, stable angina Had a recent myocardial infarction or stroke within the past 2-8 weeks Has moderate congestive heart failure (NYHA class III) History of stroke, transient ischemic attack, or peripheral artery disease	Patient should undergo complete cardiovascular workup and treadmill stress test to determine tolerance to increased myocardial energy consumption associated with increased sexual activity. Reclassify in low or high risk category
High risk	Has unstable or refractory angina, despite treatment Has uncontrolled hypertension Has severe congestive heart failure (NYHA class IV) Had a recent myocardial infarction or stroke within past 2 weeks Has moderate or severe valvular heart disease Has high-risk cardiac arrhythmias Has obstructive hypertrophic cardiomyopathy	Phosphodiesterase inhibitor is contraindicated; sexual intercourse should be deferred

NYHA, New York Heart Association.

Data from references 17, 18, 19 and 20.

Finally, erectile dysfunction is a potential marker for arteriosclerosis. Therefore, older patients and those at intermediate and high risk for cardiovascular disease should undergo a cardiovascular risk assessment before starting on drug treatment for erectile dysfunction. By doing so, patients will be categorized into low-, intermediate-, or high-risk groups for cardiovascular morbidity related to sexual intercourse. Patients in the intermediate-risk group should undergo additional testing to reclassify them into the low- or high-risk group. The high-risk group should defer sexual activity and drug treatment for erectile dysfunction. Patients in the low-risk group may start specific treatment for erectile dysfunction.[9,24-26] The risk assessment is described in Table 83-3 and detailed in the Third Princeton Consensus Panel recommendations.[26]

TREATMENT

Erectile Dysfunction

Desired Outcomes

The goal of treatment is improvement in the quantity and quality of penile erections suitable for intercourse and considered satisfactory by the patient and his partner. Simple as this may sound, healthcare providers must ensure that patients and their partners have reasonable expectations for any therapies that are initiated. Furthermore, only patients with erectile dysfunction should be treated. Patients who have normal sexual function should not seek—or be encouraged to seek—treatment in an effort to enhance sexual function or enable increased activity. In addition, treatment should be well tolerated and be of reasonable cost.

General Approach to Treatment

3 The Third Princeton Consensus Conference recommendations are a widely accepted multidisciplinary approach to managing erectile dysfunction that maps out a stepwise treatment plan.[26] This approach is based on the knowledge that erectile dysfunction and cardiovascular disease and its risk factors co-exist in many patients, and that sexual intercourse can precipitate serious cardiovascular consequences in high-risk patients. The first step in clinical management of erectile dysfunction is to identify and, if possible, reverse underlying causes. Risk factors for erectile dysfunction, including hypertension, coronary artery disease, dyslipidemia, diabetes mellitus, smoking, or chronic ethanol abuse, should be addressed and minimized. Patients should follow a heart-healthy lifestyle, which includes physical fitness, weight loss to achieve a normal body mass index, low cholesterol diet, no excessive ethanol intake, and no smoking.[27] In some cases, these types of interventions are sufficient to restore erectile function.[28,29] However, if erectile dysfunction does not respond to these measures, specific treatment is indicated.

For patients with psychogenic erectile dysfunction, psychotherapy can be used as monotherapy or as an adjunct to specific treatments for the disorder. To enhance the relevance of psychotherapy, both the patient and the partner should be included in the counseling sessions. Treatment should be individualized and should address immediate factors that may be causing performance anxiety or depression. The effectiveness of psychotherapy is generally low, and long-term psychotherapy is often necessary.

4 5 6 Specific treatments of erectile dysfunction include vacuum erection devices (VEDs), pharmacologic treatments, and surgery. The ideal treatment of this disorder should have a fast onset, be effective, be convenient to administer, be cost-effective, have a low incidence of serious adverse effects, and be free of serious drug interactions (Table 83-4). Generally, when choosing from among treatment approaches, those that are least invasive are selected first; more invasive therapies are reserved for patients who do not respond to first-line agents.

The American Urological Association Guideline on the Management of Erectile Dysfunction,[21] the 2009 International Consultation of Sexual Medicine,[30] the 2010 European Urology Association guideline,[31] and the American College of Physicians[2] clearly identify oral phosphodiesterase type 5 inhibitors for first-line treatment. VEDs, intracavernosal injection of erectogenic agents, or intraurethral prostaglandin inserts are second-line treatments. Prescribing of a particular agent for a patient should be individualized. Surgical intervention should be reserved for patients who fail to respond to

TABLE 83-4 Dosing Regimens for Selected Drug Treatments for Erectile Dysfunction

Drug	Brand Name	Initial Dose	Usual Range	Special Population Dose	Other
Phosphodiesterase Inhibitor					
Sildenafil	Viagra	50 mg orally 1 hour before intercourse	25-100 mg 1 hour before intercourse. Limit to one dose per day	In patients age 65 years and older, start with 25 mg dose. In patients with creatinine clearance less than 30 mL/min (0.5 mL/s) or severe hepatic impairment, limit starting dose to 25 mg. In patients taking potent P450 CYP3A4 inhibitors, limit starting dose to 25 mg every 48 hours.	Titrate dose so that erection lasts no more than 1 hour. Food decreases absorption by 1 hour. Contraindicated with nitrates by any route of administration.
Vardenafil	Levitra	5-10 mg orally 1 hour before intercourse	5-20 mg 1 hour before intercourse. Limit to one dose per day	In patients age 65 years and older, start with 5 mg Levitra. No dosage adjustment is required in patients with decreased creatinine clearance. In patients with moderate hepatic impairment, start with 5 mg Levitra. In patients taking potent P450 CYP3A4 inhibitors, limit starting dose to 2.5-5 mg every 24-72 hours. Not recommended in patients with congenital prolonged QT interval or in patients taking Type 1A or Type 3 antiarrhythmics.	Titrate dose so that erection lasts no more than 1 hour. Food decreases absorption by 1 hour. Contraindicated with nitrates by any route of administration.
	Staxyn	10 mg tablet to dissolve on the tongue 1 hour before intercourse	10 mg tablet to dissolve on the tongue 1 hour before intercourse. Limit to one dose per day.	Dose of Staxyn requires no adjustment in patients 65 years or older or in patients with creatinine clearance less than 30 mL/min (0.5 mL/s). Do not use in patients with moderate or severe hepatic impairment or those taking moderately or highly potent P450 CYP3A4 inhibitors. Do not initiate Staxyn in patients taking α-adrenergic antagonists.	Staxyn should be taken without any liquid or food. The tablet should be placed on the tongue where it will dissolve. No up-titration of dose is recommended. Do not substitute Staxyn for Levitra, or vice versa.
Tadalafil	Cialis	5-10 mg orally at least 30 minutes before intercourse OR 2.5-5 mg orally once daily	10-20 mg at least 30 minutes before intercourse. Limit to one dose per day; the drug improves erectile function for up to 36 hours 2.5-5 mg once daily. Limit to one dose per day	Dose of tadalafil requires no dosage adjustment in patients 65 years or older. In patients with creatinine clearance of 30-50 mL/min (0.5-0.83 mL/s), limit starting dose to 10 mg every 48 hours; if less than 30 mL/min (0.5 mL/s), limit starting dose to 5 mg every 72 hours. In patients with mild-moderate hepatic impairment, limit starting dose to 10 mg every 24 hours. Do not use in patients with severe hepatic impairment. In patients taking potent P450 CYP3A4 inhibitors, limit starting dose to 10 mg every 72 hours (if using it on demand) or 2.5 mg daily (if using a continuous daily regimen).	Titrate dose so that erection lasts not more than 1 hour. Food does not affect rate or extent of drug absorption. Contraindicated with nitrates by any route of administration. When taken with large amounts of ethanol, tadalafil may cause orthostatic hypotension.
Avanafil	Stendra	100 mg orally 15-30 minutes before intercourse	50-200 mg orally 15-30 minutes before intercourse	In patients with creatinine clearance of 30-89 mL/min (0.5-1.49 mL/s), no dosage adjustment is needed. Do not use if creatinine clearance is less than 30 mL/min (0.5 mL/s), if the patient has severe hepatic disease, or if the patient is taking P450 CYP3A4 inhibitors.	May be taken with food. When taken with large amounts of ethanol, avanafil may cause orthostatic hypotension.
Prostaglandin E1					
Alprostadil intracavernosal injection	Caverject, Edex	2.5 mcg intracavernosally 5-10 minutes before intercourse	10-20 mcg 5-10 minutes before intercourse. Maximum recommended dose is 60 mcg. Limit to not more than one injection per day and not more than three injections per week with a 24 hour interval between doses.	None	Titrate dose to achieve an erection that lasts 1 hour Patient will require training on aseptic intracavernosal injection technique. Avoid intracavernosal injections in patients with sickle cell anemia, multiple myeloma, leukemia, severe coagulopathy, schizophrenia, poor manual dexterity, severe venous incompetence, severe cardiovascular disease, or Peyronie's disease.

(continued)

TABLE 83-4 Dosing Regimens for Selected Drug Treatments for Erectile Dysfunction (*Continued*)

Drug	Brand Name	Initial Dose	Usual Range	Special Population Dose	Other
Alprostadil intraurethral pellet	Muse	125-250 mcg intraurethrally 5-10 minutes before intercourse	250-1,000 mcg just before intercourse. Limit to not more than two doses per day	None	Patient will require training on proper intraurethral administration techniques. Use applicator provided to administer medications to avoid urethral injury.
Testosterone Supplements					
Methyltestosterone	Android, Testred, Methitest	10 mg once daily	10-50 mg once daily	Will likely cause fluid retention in patients with renal or hepatic disease	Not recommended for use due to extensive first-pass hepatic catabolism and because it is associated with hepatotoxicity.
Fluoxymesterone	Androxy	5 mg once daily	5-20 mg once daily	Contraindicated in patients with severe renal or hepatic impairment	Not recommended because it is associated with hepatotoxicity. This is a 17α-alkylated androgen.
Testosterone buccal system	Striant	30 mg every 12 hours, morning and evening	30 mg every 12 hours, morning and evening		Time the dose so that buccal system is removed before every morning and evening toothbrushing. Place buccal system just above incisor tooth on both sides of the mouth, and hold in place for 30 seconds to adhere. To remove, slide buccal system down toward the tooth. Buccal tablet may become detached during eating. If this occurs, discard and replace with new buccal system. Do not chew or swallow buccal system.
Testosterone cypionate intramuscular injection	Depo-Testosterone	200-400 mg every 2-4 weeks	200-400 mg every 2-4 weeks (up to 6 weeks)	Contraindicated in patients with severe hepatic or renal impairment	During the dosing interval, supraphysiologic serum concentrations of testosterone are produced during a portion of the dosing interval. This has been linked to mood swings.
Testosterone enanthate intramuscular injection	Delatestryl	200-400 mg every 2-4 weeks	200-400 mg every 2-4 weeks (up to 6 weeks)	Although not so labeled, it should probably not be used in patients with severe hepatic or renal impairment	During the dosing interval, supraphysiologic serum concentrations of testosterone are produced during a portion of the dosing interval. This has been linked to mood swings.
Testosterone undecanoate intramuscular injection	Aveed	750 mg as a single dose	750 mg as a single dose on day 0, week 4, and then 750 mg every 10 weeks		Only available in facilities certified through a Risk Evaluation and Mitigation Strategy Program.
Testosterone transdermal patch	Androderm	4 mg as a single dose at bedtime	2-6 mg as a single dose at bedtime	Safety in patients with hepatic or renal dysfunction has not been evaluated	When administered at bedtime, serum concentrations of testosterone in the usual circadian pattern are produced. Apply to those sites recommended in the package labeling: upper arm, back, abdomen, and thigh. Rotate application sites every 7 days. May have to apply multiple patches at one time to achieve appropriate serum testosterone level. Avoid swimming, showering, or washing administration site for 3 hours after patch application.

(*continued*)

TABLE 83-4 Dosing Regimens for Selected Drug Treatments for Erectile Dysfunction (*Continued*)

Drug	Brand Name	Initial Dose	Usual Range	Special Population Dose	Other
Testosterone gel	Androgel 1%, Testim 1%	5-10 g of gel (equivalent to 50-100 mg testosterone, respectively) as a single dose in the morning	5-10 g of gel (equivalent to 50-100 mg testosterone, respectively) as a single dose in the morning. Titrate dose up at 14-day intervals	None	Cover application site to avoid inadvertent transfer to others. Avoid swimming, showering, or washing administration site for 2 hours after gel application. Apply to those sites recommended in the product labeling: shoulders, upper arms, or abdomen. Children and women should avoid contact with unclothed or unwashed application sites. Patients should wash hands with soap and water after administration of transdermal testosterone product. For patients who have difficulty measuring the appropriate dose using tubes of gel, it is also available in premeasured dose packets or from a pump dispenser.
	Androgel 1.6%	2 pumps (equivalent to 40.5 mg testosterone) as a single dose in the morning	2-4 pumps (equivalent to 40.5-81 mg) as a single dose in the morning		Apply to shoulders and upper arms. Avoid swimming, showering, or washing administration site for 2 hours after application. Titrate dose 14-28 days after starting treatment.
Testosterone transdermal spray	Fortesta	Four sprays (equivalent to 40 mg testosterone) once daily	Four to seven sprays (equivalent to 40-70 mg testosterone) once daily. Titrate dose up at 14- to 35-day intervals.		Cover application site to avoid inadvertent transfer to others. Avoid swimming, showering, or washing administration site for 2 hours after spray application. Apply to those sites recommended in the product labeling: front and inner thighs. Children and women should avoid contact with unclothed or unwashed application sites. Patients should wash hands with soap and water after administration of transdermal testosterone product.
Testosterone transdermal solution	Axiron	Two pump sprays (equivalent to 60 mg testosterone) to left or right axilla daily	One to four pump sprays (equivalent to 30-120 mg testosterone, respectively) to left or right axilla daily. Titrate dose up at 14- to 35-day intervals		Limit application to axilla. Apply antiperspirant or deodorant before Axiron. Avoid swimming, showering, or washing administration site for 2 hours after application.
Testosterone subcutaneous implant pellet	Testopel	150-450 (equivalent to 2-6 pellets) mg as a single dose every 3-6 months. Administration of the dose requires a forearm incision and subcutaneous dose implant under local anesthesia	150-450 mg as a single dose every 3-6 months		Trained health professional is required to administer the dose. Should use sterile implanter kit. Clinical onset is delayed for 3-4 months after initial dose. Generic formulations are available in higher strengths: 100 mg or 200 mg per pellet.

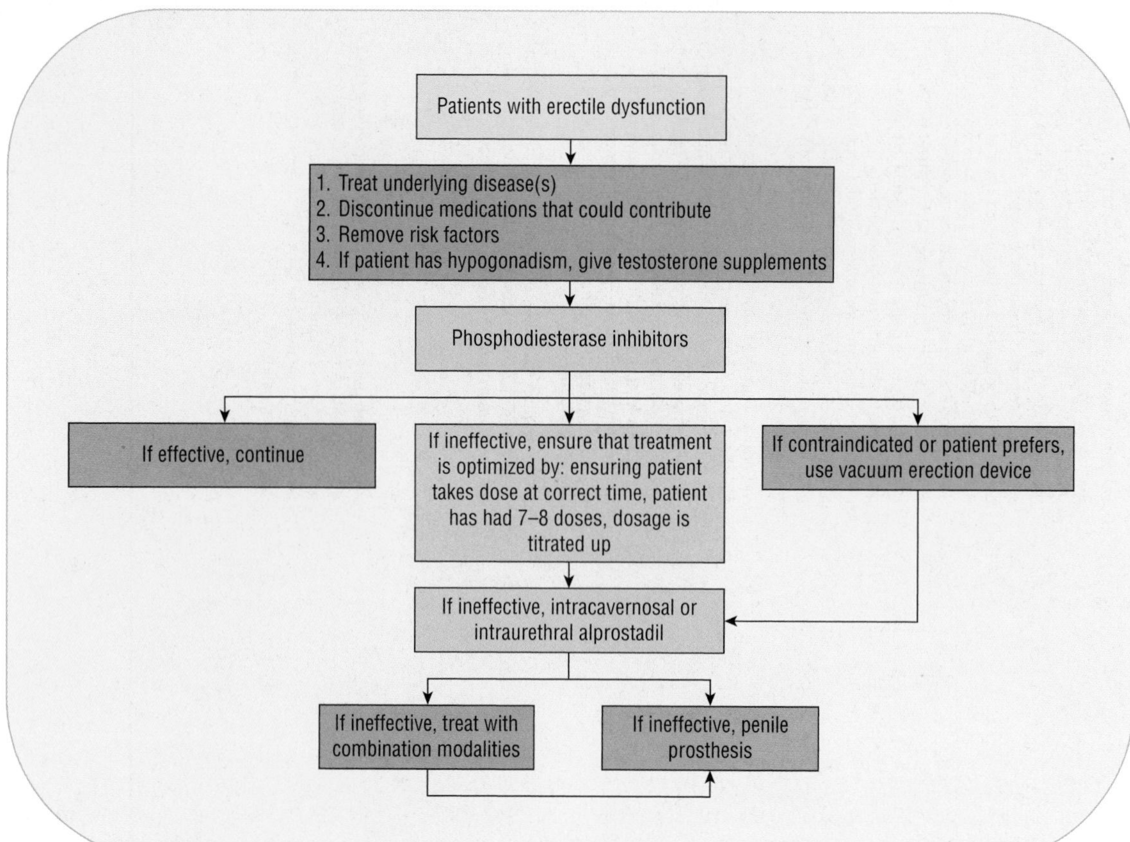

FIGURE 83-2 Algorithm for selecting treatment for erectile dysfunction.

first- and second-line treatments. A sample algorithm that guides selection of treatment is shown in Fig. 83-2.

Vacuum Erection Device

A VED is a noninvasive medical device with few contraindications to use. A patient makes a one-time purchase and the device can be used repeatedly.

A VED has two parts: a pump, which generates a negative vacuum pressure; and a cylinder, which is closed at one end and into which the penis is inserted. The patient inserts his penis into the open end of the cylinder, which is then pushed up flush against his lower abdomen to create a vacuum chamber. Then the patient activates the pump to produce a vacuum pressure, which draws arteriolar blood into the corpora cavernosa. To prolong the erection, the patient can use constriction bands or tension rings, which are placed at the base of the penis, to keep the arteriolar blood in and reduce venous outflow from the penis. With the assistance of loading cones to protect the glans, these bands or rings can be rolled over the glans penis and up the erect penile shaft. Alternatively, they can be first threaded onto the plastic cylinder before the penis is inserted. Once the penis is erect, the band or ring can be rolled off the cylinder onto the base of the penis (Fig. 83-3). However, some patients prefer to apply the band or ring before the penis is erect.[32,33]

7 The onset of action of the VED is 3 to 20 minutes; a faster onset of 2 to 3 minutes is associated with continued, more experienced use.[32] VEDs are not discreet. That is, a patient's use of a VED is evident to the partner. For this reason, VEDs appear to work best in older patients who are married or who have stable sexual relationships. In this group, VEDs could be considered first-line therapy, and the overall satisfaction rate can be as high as 60% to 80% (range, 27%-94%).[32,33] VEDs may be used as second-line therapy in patients who do not respond to oral phosphodiesterase type 5 inhibitors, which includes patients who have had radical prostatectomy[34] or those who do not respond to injectable drug treatments for erectile dysfunction. The combination of a VED with intracavernosal or intraurethral alprostadil[32] or a phosphodiesterase type 5 inhibitor[34] is associated with a higher efficacy rate than use of the VED alone. As a result, combination therapy sometimes is attempted before penile prosthesis surgery is considered in the patient who fails to respond to a VED alone.

Patients may discontinue using VEDs because they are inconvenient and not discreet. It has been reported that the dropout rate is as high as 56% during the first year of use.[32,33] Also, 6% to 11% of partners complain that the penis is cool to the touch or is discolored (bluish) in appearance, particularly when constriction bands are used.

Vacuum erection devices are available with battery-operated pumps, which offer convenience, particularly in patients with arthritis of the hands. The American Urological Association recommends the use of commercially available VEDs by prescription only. These have safety mechanisms that minimize the likelihood of excessively high vacuum pressures which can cause penile discomfort and injury.[21]

Penile pain, bruising, or injury from VEDs most often is caused by the constriction bands used to sustain an erection. Because these rings trap blood in the corpora and reduce arteriolar flow into the penis, the penile shaft may feel cold and numb. If the constriction bands are applied for longer than 30 minutes, the penile shaft may turn blue and hurt. Patients may complain that a hinge-like erection is produced in that the penis pivots on the rubber ring or tension band. Patients sometimes fail to ejaculate.

Vacuum erection devices are contraindicated in patients with sickle cell disease or patients with a history of prolonged erections. These patients are prone to priapism, which can be exacerbated by the use of constriction bands with VEDs. The devices also should be used cautiously by patients taking oral anticoagulants because warfarin, through a poorly understood and idiosyncratic mechanism, can cause priapism. Finally, VEDs are contraindicated in patients with severe penile curvature.

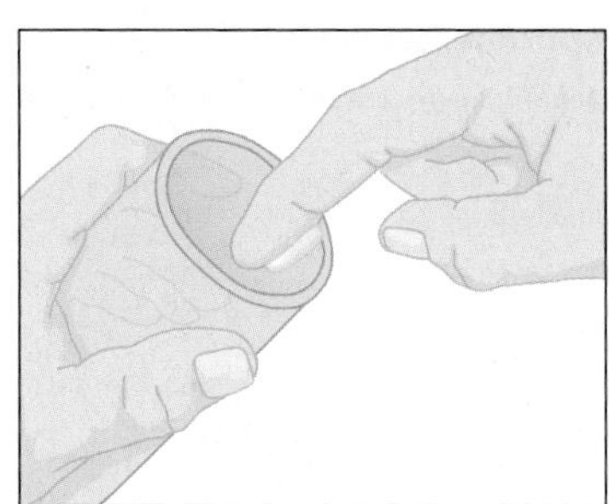

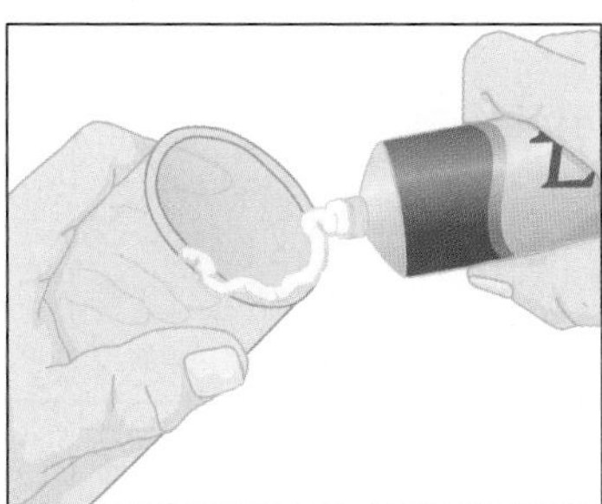

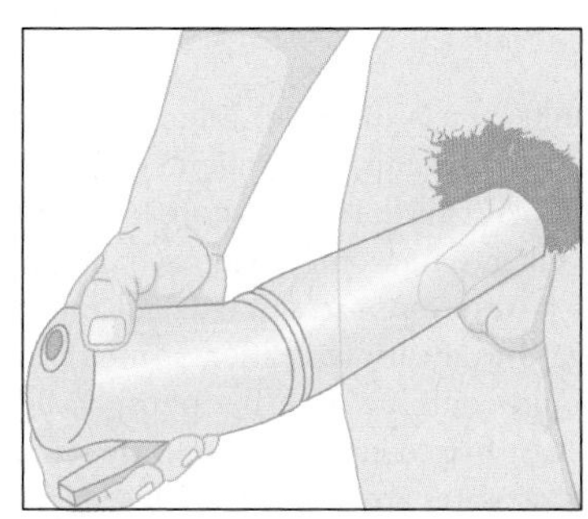

Assemble your system according to the two-step procedure.

Step 1

Apply Osbon Personal Lubricant™ to the following:

1. two inches inside the open end of the cylinder;
2. the rim of the cylinder that meets the body to form the vacuum seal; and
3. the entire head of the penis.

Applying lubricant properly will help you achieve the best erection possible.

Tip: Trimming the pubic hair around the base of the penis with a pair of scissors may also prove helpful in creating an airtight seal.

Step 2

It is recommended that you stand for this step (the system can also be used when you are sitting or lying down).

Place the lubricated penis inside the cylinder with the label on the cylinder facing up. With one hand, hold the cylinder at a downward 45° angle with the open end snugly against the body.

Tip: Rotate cylinder slightly back and forth to make an airtight seal against the body, make sure the testicles are not drawn into the cylinder.

FIGURE 83-3 Technique for using a vacuum erection device. *(From Osbon Erec Aid Esteem Vacuum Therapy System User Guide. Eden Prairie, MN: TIMM Medical Technologies.)*

Phosphodiesterase Type 5 Inhibitors

Mechanism

In the presence of sexual stimulation, nitric oxide is released by neurons and endothelial cells in cavernosal tissue, thereby enhancing the activity of guanylate cyclase, the enzyme responsible for conversion of guanylate triphosphate to cGMP (Fig. 83-4).[35] cGMP is a vasodilatory secondary messenger that upregulates the response to nitric oxide by activating protein kinase G. This decreases intracellular calcium levels, resulting in smooth muscle relaxation, enhanced arterial flow to the corpora cavernosa, and enhanced blood filling of cavernosal sinuses.[35] Catabolism of cGMP in cavernosal tissue is mediated by phosphodiesterase isoenzyme type 5.

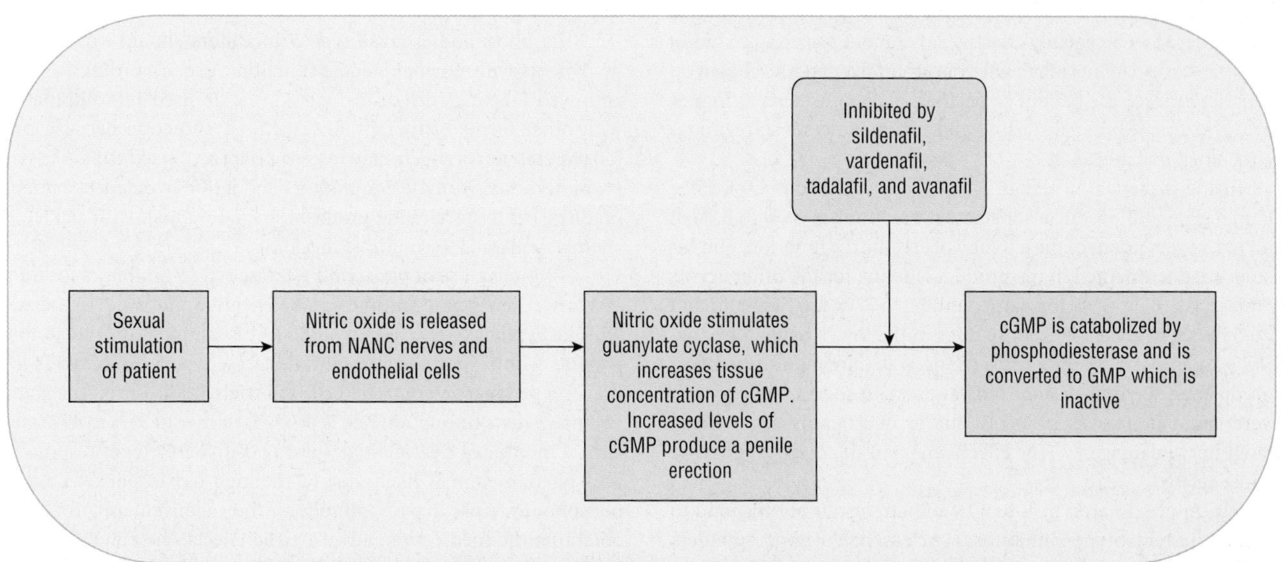

FIGURE 83-4 Mechanism of action of phosphodiesterase type 5 inhibitors. All inhibit catabolism of cGMP, a vasodilatory secondary messenger. (cGMP, cyclic guanosine monophosphate; NANC, nonadrenergic noncholinergic.)

TABLE 83-5 Pharmacodynamics and Pharmacokinetics of Phosphodiesterase Inhibitors

	Sildenafil (Viagra)	Vardenafil (Levitra/Staxyn)	Tadalafil (Cialis)	Avanafil (Stendra)
Inhibits PDE-5	Yes	Yes	Yes	Yes
Inhibits PDE-6	Yes	Minimally	No	Minimally
Inhibits PDE-11	No	No	Yes	Minimally
Time to peak plasma level (hours)	0.5-1	0.7-0.9/1.5	2	0.5-0.8
Oral bioavailability (%)	40	15/21-44	36	15
Fatty meal decreases rate of oral absorption?	Yes	Yes/No[a]	No	No
Mean plasma half-life (hours)	3.7	4.4-4.8/4-6	18	4-5
Active metabolite	Yes	Yes/Yes	No	Yes
Is CYP 3A4 principally responsible for metabolism?	Yes	Yes	Yes	Yes
Other CYP enzymes responsible for metabolism	CYP 2C9	CYP 3A5, CYP 2C9		CYP 2C
Percentage of dose excreted in feces	80	91-95/91-95	61	62
Percentage of dose excreted in urine	13	2-6/2-6	36	21
Clinical onset (minutes)	30	30/60	45	25-40
Duration (hours)	4	4-5/4-6	24-36	6+

PDE, phosphodiesterase.

[a]When Staxyn is taken with water, the area under the curve decreases by 29%.

Used with permission from Nehra A, Jackson G, Miner M, et al. The Princeton III Consensus Recommendations for the Management of Erectile Dysfunction and Cardiovascular Disease. Mayo Clin Proc 2012;87(8):766-778.

Four competitive, reversible inhibitors of the phosphodiesterase isoenzyme type 5 found in genital tissue are marketed for erectile dysfunction in the United States (Table 83-5). Chemically, they are nonhydrolyzable analogs of cGMP and they act by decreasing catabolism of cGMP. However, phosphodiesterase isoenzyme type 5 is also found in peripheral vascular tissue, tracheal smooth muscle, and platelets. Inhibition of phosphodiesterase in these nongenital tissues can produce unwanted effects.[35]

The four marketed phosphodiesterase type 5 inhibitors differ in their degree of selectivity in inhibiting phosphodiesterase isoenzyme type 5 and other phosphodiesterase isoenzymes, pharmacokinetic profiles, drug–food interactions, and adverse effects (see Table 83-4).

Efficacy

Because of their apparent effectiveness, convenient route of administration, and comparatively low incidence of serious adverse effects, phosphodiesterase type 5 inhibitors are considered first-line therapy for erectile dysfunction, particularly in younger patients. They allow for discreet use. Although not based on direct comparison trials, all four commercially available phosphodiesterase type 5 inhibitors are considered to be equally effective.[35,36] Patient preference studies show that some patients may prefer one agent over another based on the preferences of the patient or partner; or the onset, duration, or cost of treatment.[37] Usual starting and maintenance dose regimens are included in Table 83-4.

In the presence of sexual stimulation and in doses of 25 to 100 mg, sildenafil produces satisfactory erections in 56% to 82% of patients, independent of the etiology of erectile dysfunction. Similar results are documented in the product labeling for the other agents in this class (65%-80% for vardenafil, 62%-77% for tadalafil, and 50%-55% for avanafil). Response rates in the lower range for phosphodiesterase type 5 inhibitors have been documented in patients with diabetes mellitus or after radical prostatectomy, or those with severe vascular disease, probably due to neuropathy, or surgery-related nerve damage.[21,38] The effectiveness of the drugs appears to be dose related.

8 Approximately 30% to 40% of patients do not respond to phosphodiesterase type 5 inhibitors.[21] At least half of nonresponders can benefit from education on proper use of the drugs.[39] Therefore, follow-up is always recommended after a phosphodiesterase type 5 inhibitor is initiated. Education of patients should include the following points: (a) patients must engage in sexual stimulation (foreplay) for the best response; (b) sildenafil and vardenafil should be taken on an empty stomach, at least 2 hours before meals, for the fastest response, but tadalafil and avanafil can be taken without regard to meals; (c) patients who do not respond to the first dose should continue with the phosphodiesterase type 5 inhibitor for at least five to eight doses before failure is declared, as increasing success rates are reported with sequential dose administration; (d) some patients require dosage titration up to 100 mg sildenafil, 20 mg vardenafil, 20 mg tadalafil, or 200 mg avanafil for a response; (e) patients should avoid excessive alcohol intake, which can cause drowsiness and hypotension and worsen erectile dysfunction; (f) involvement of the sexual partner can help improve the patient's response to treatment; (g) treatment of concomitant medical illnesses which contribute to erectile dysfunction (eg, diabetes mellitus, hypertension, and hypogonadism) should be optimized (if the patient has depression because of divorce or loss of a sexual partner, or has performance anxiety, psychologic counseling may be helpful); (h) if applicable, the patient should stop smoking and reduce weight if obese.[28,29]

The phosphodiesterase type 5 inhibitors should not be used by patients with normal erectile function. Also, according to FDA-approved labeling, the drugs should not be used in combination with other forms of therapy for erectile dysfunction because prolonged erections (which may lead to priapism) may result.[21,40] Also, phosphodiesterase type 5 inhibitors should be avoided in patients predisposed to developing priapism, including men with sickle cell anemia, leukemia, or multiple myeloma.

Long-term use of phosphodiesterase type 5 inhibitors for up to 10 consecutive years continues to be effective and is not associated with tachyphylaxis.[4,40-42] The voluntary discontinuation rate among patients who respond to phosphodiesterase type 5 inhibitors is less than 2% per year in controlled clinical trials;[40,41] however, the actual voluntary discontinuation rate is probably closer to 35% to 47% after 6 to 24 months of treatment, despite a positive treatment response.[36] This phenomenon is likely due to the high out-of-pocket costs of phosphodiesterase type 5 inhibitors, the inconvenient process of obtaining the medication, adverse drug effects, the patient's loss of interest in sexual intercourse, or the efficacy of the medication being below the patient's expectations.[43]

Clinical **Controversy...**

Whether tachyphylaxis—a rapid decrease in drug response—develops with long-term use of phosphodiesterase type 5 inhibitors is unclear. Some patients continue to respond to the medication even after many years of regular use, although they may require increasing doses over time. Other patients eventually become nonresponsive to treatment. This change in response could be due to upregulation of phosphodiesterase type 5 enzymes.[42]

Despite the initial effectiveness of phosphodiesterase type 5 inhibitors and the measures to salvage patients with re-education, some patients with severe vascular or neurologic disease will show minimal or no response to maximum doses of a phosphodiesterase type 5 inhibitor. Various strategies have been attempted in this subgroup of patients, including the following:

1. The effectiveness of switching from one phosphodiesterase type 5 inhibitor to another when the patient does not respond to an initial agent is controversial. In one study, vardenafil was beneficial in 12% of patients who did not respond to sildenafil.[44] Controlled clinical trials in larger patient groups are needed before this strategy is used as routine treatment.
2. Switching the patient from an as-needed to an everyday regimen of tadalafil may be reasonable in a patient who has difficulty coordinating the timing of tadalafil before meals or sexual intercourse.
3. High-dose phosphodiesterase type 5 inhibitor treatment (eg, sildenafil 200 mg) has been used anecdotally. However, such doses are also associated with a higher frequency of adverse effects.[45]
4. In older patients (age greater than or equal to 65 years) with late-onset hypogonadism and erectile dysfunction, correcting the former with testosterone supplementation improves the response to a phosphodiesterase type 5 inhibitor.[46]
5. Phosphodiesterase type 5 inhibitors have been combined with intracavernosal or intraurethral alprostadil in selected patients.[4,47,48]

Clinical **Controversy...**

For patients who fail to respond to a particular phosphodiesterase type 5 inhibitor, a common strategy employed is to increase the dose of the medication above the FDA-labeled dosage range. The maximum effective and safe dosage is not known.

Selectivity of Other Phosphodiesterase Isoenzymes

More than 25 different phosphodiesterase isoenzymes have been identified; however, the physiologic effects of stimulation and inhibition of some of these isoenzymes remain to be elucidated. Of note, phosphodiesterase isoenzyme type 6 is localized to the rods and cones of the eye. Inhibition of this isoenzyme has been associated with blurred vision and cyanopsia. Sildenafil is the most potent inhibitor of phosphodiesterase isoenzyme type 6, vardenafil and avanafil are intermediate inhibitors, and tadalafil is the least potent inhibitor.[35] Likewise, phosphodiesterase isoenzyme type 11 is localized to striated muscle. Inhibition of this isoenzyme has been associated with myalgia and muscle pain. Tadalafil exerts the greatest inhibitory activity against phosphodiesterase type 11.[35]

Pharmacokinetics and Drug–Food Interactions

Pharmacokinetic parameters of the phosphodiesterase type 5 inhibitors are listed in Table 83-4.[49]

Sildenafil and the conventional oral formulation of vardenafil have similar pharmacokinetic profiles. Both drugs have a 1-hour onset of action and short duration of action. Oral absorption is significantly delayed by 1 hour when either drug is taken within 2 hours of a fatty meal. In contrast, tadalafil has a slower onset of action of 2 hours, has a prolonged duration of action up to 36 hours, and food does not affect its rate of absorption. Thus, tadalafil offers greater spontaneity for patients, as one dose can last through an entire weekend and allows for multiple acts of sexual intercourse over multiple days with a single dose.[36] An oral disintegrating tablet formulation of vardenafil, which dissolves on the tongue, has 1.2- to 1.4-fold higher bioavailability than the conventional oral tablet; however its clinical efficacy appears comparable to the conventional tablet. The oral disintegrating tablet formulation is not susceptible to the drug–food interaction of the conventional oral tablet, which is an advantage for some patients.[50] Avanafil has a slightly faster onset than, but similar duration to, sildenafil and vardenafil. Food does not significantly affect the rate or extent of absorption of avanafil.

The onset of action of these agents has undergone reexamination to assess how soon after drug administration patients can expect to have an erection suitable for intercourse. Although up to 50% of patients may develop an erection within 20 to 30 minutes of sildenafil 100 mg, vardenafil 20 mg, tadalafil 20 mg, or avanafil 200 mg, the rest of the patients may require a full hour to achieve an adequate erectile response.[51] Therefore, patients should be instructed to allow adequate time for the drug to work. In addition, sildenafil and vardenafil have been reported to be effective in some patients up to 12 hours after dosing, which is long after plasma concentrations have declined. It has been hypothesized that this may be due to the continued intracellular action of the phosphodiesterase type 5 inhibitor.[52]

Concomitant ingestion of ethanol with phosphodiesterase type 5 inhibitors can result in orthostatic hypotension and drowsiness. Therefore, the manufacturer recommends that patients avoid ethanol when taking these medications.

All four phosphodiesterase type 5 inhibitors are hepatically catabolized principally by the cytochrome P450 3A4 microsomal isoenzyme, and other P450 isoenzymes (minor routes) and/or other hepatic enzymes (see Table 83-5). Sildenafil has an active metabolite, which is excreted primarily in the urine. Tadalafil has a clinically insignificant active metabolite; however, 36% of the parent drug is renally eliminated. Thus, both sildenafil and tadalafil doses should be reduced in patients with significant renal impairment. Vardenafil and avanafil have active metabolites that are largely excreted in feces. No specific dosage reduction of these medications is recommended in patients with reduced renal function because of the intermittent nature of the dosing schedule. Avanafil is not recommended when the creatinine clearance is less than 30 mL/min (0.5 mL/s) (see Table 83-4).

Dosing

The usual oral doses of the phosphodiesterase type 5 inhibitors are listed in Table 83-4. Sildenafil, vardenafil, and avanafil should be taken on demand at least 30 to 60 minutes before sexual intercourse. Tadalafil should be taken at least 2 hours before sexual intercourse. The durations of action for sildenafil, vardenafil, and avanafil are 4 to 5 hours, whereas the effects of tadalafil last for 36 hours. The agents vary as to whether doses must be adjusted for patients 65 years and older and those with compromised hepatic or renal function. Patients should be advised to take not more than the amount prescribed and not more than one dose per day. Doses higher than those recommended have been described in the published literature (eg, sildenafil 200 mg[45]); however, such dosing regimens have not consistently produced improved erectile responses.

For patients who do not respond to an adequate course of on-demand phosphodiesterase type 5 inhibitors for erectile dysfunction, daily low dosing of tadalafil may improve endothelial function in cavernosal tissue. That is, regular use of phosphodiesterase type 5 inhibitors may activate endothelial nitric oxide synthase, increase local concentrations of cGMP, which may lead to increased oxygen tension, improved blood flow, and reduced endothelial damage and cavernosal fibrosis.[53] A preliminary clinical trial of daily dosing of tadalafil 5 mg showed a 86% frequency of successful sexual intercourse compared with conventional on-demand use of tadalafil 20 mg, which produced 95% global efficacy.[54,55] Other potential advantages of daily low dosing regimens include a lower potential for dose-related adverse effects and increased spontaneity of sexual intercourse.[52] However, disadvantages of the daily low-dose regimen are the high cost of treatment and patients with more severe erectile dysfunction, who may require higher doses of a phosphodiesterase type 5 inhibitor, may not respond.[52] Although clinical trials of daily dosing of tadalafil 10 and 20 mg,[54,55] and sildenafil 50 and 100 mg[56,57] have been published, the only FDA-approved labeling is for daily dosing of tadalafil 2.5 or 5 mg.

Clinical **Controversy...**

It is not known if short-term phosphodiesterase type 5 inhibitor use can cure erectile dysfunction. Some have theorized that such a regimen can permanently increase cavernosal tissue levels of cGMP.[58]

Adverse Effects

Most adverse effects of the phosphodiesterase type 5 inhibitors are mild or moderate and are self-limited, and patients often become tolerant to them with continued use.[59,60] The rates of drug discontinuation caused by adverse effects are low, ranging from 2.1% to 25%, and are similar for all four agents. In usual doses, the most common adverse effects are headache (11%), facial flushing (12%), dyspepsia (5%), nasal congestion (3.4%), and dizziness (3%),[61] all of which are dose-related and result from vasodilation or smooth muscle relaxation secondary to inhibition of phosphodiesterase isoenzyme type 5 in extragenital tissues.

Sildenafil and vardenafil produce an 8- to 10-mm Hg decrease in systolic and a 5- to 6-mm Hg decrease in diastolic blood pressure starting approximately 1 hour after a dose is taken and lasting for 4 hours. Most patients are asymptomatic as a result of these blood pressure changes, but some patients, particularly those taking multiple antihypertensives or nitrates or those with baseline hypotension, may develop clinical symptoms as a consequence of these peripheral vascular effects. Avanafil can produce similar decreases in blood pressure, especially when used along with other antihypertensives or α-adrenergic antagonists. Tadalafil does not produce decreases in blood pressure but must be used with caution in patients with cardiovascular disease because of the cardiac risk inherent to sexual activity. The management approach for such patients, developed based on an analysis of deaths in men who were using sildenafil and commonly referred to as the recommendations of the Princeton Consensus Guideline Conference III,[26] should be applied to all the phosphodiesterase type 5 inhibitors (see Table 83-3).

Sildenafil, vardenafil, and avanafil cause increased sensitivity to light, blurred vision, or loss of blue–green color discrimination in 2% to 3% of patients. The adverse effect is dose-related with the incidence increasing to 40% to 50% in patients taking sildenafil 200 mg.[62] These effects result from inhibition of phosphodiesterase type 6 in the photoreceptor cells of retinal rods and cones. Visual adverse effects commonly occur at the time of peak serum concentrations. Although visual adverse effects are mild and reversible, caution regarding use is recommended for airplane pilots, who rely on seeing green and blue lights for landing planes. Avanafil has moderate and tadalafil has minimal to no inhibitory activity against phosphodiesterase type 6, and a lower incidence of visual adverse effects (less than 1%) has been reported.[63] Nevertheless, according to current product labeling, all phosphodiesterase type 5 inhibitors should be used cautiously in patients at risk for retinitis pigmentosa, a genetic disease associated with retinal phosphodiesterase deficiency.

Nonarteritic anterior ischemic optic neuropathy (NAION) is a sudden, unilateral, painless blindness, which may be irreversible. Isolated cases of NAION have been associated with phosphodiesterase type 5 inhibitor use.[62] NAION has developed at variable and unpredictable times after starting a phosphodiesterase type 5 inhibitor, ranging from 6 hours to months or years after the first dose.[62] Although a cause-and-effect relationship has not been established,[64] the blood pressure-lowering effects of these medications may decrease blood flow to the optic nerve and lead to a sudden unilateral decrease in vision. Because NAION may lead to permanent vision loss, the FDA has required inclusion of warnings on the product labeling of phosphodiesterase type 5 inhibitors. Specifically, before receiving these agents, patients at risk for NAION should be evaluated by an ophthalmologist, risk factors for NAION should be addressed, and the patient should be cautioned against using a phosphodiesterase type 5 inhibitor.

Patients at risk of NAION include a wide variety of patients: those with glaucoma, macular degeneration, diabetic retinopathy, dyslipidemia, or hypertension, those who have undergone eye surgery or have experienced eye trauma, patients who are age 50 years or more, or smokers. A patient who experiences sudden vision loss in one eye while taking a phosphodiesterase type 5 inhibitor should be evaluated for NAION before continuing treatment. If NAION is present, the phosphodiesterase type 5 inhibitor should be discontinued as there is a 15% to 25% risk of developing NAION in the other eye in the ensuing 5 to 10 years.[62]

Tadalafil produces lower back and limb muscle pain, which occurs in a dose-related fashion in 7% to 30% of patients treated with doses of 10 to 100 mg.[35] The mechanism for this is not known. It may be linked to inhibition of type 11 phosphodiesterase, a unique characteristic of tadalafil.

Acute unilateral hearing loss has also been reported after use of a phosphodiesterase type 5 inhibitor. A cause–effect relationship has not been established. In the cases reported, the hearing loss occurred within 1 day of starting treatment; it was variably accompanied by tinnitus or vertigo, and often resulted in residual hearing loss despite discontinuation of the phosphodiesterase type 5 inhibitor.[65,66] The product labeling now includes a warning that a phosphodiesterase type 5 inhibitor should be immediately stopped and the patient should see a physician if sudden hearing loss develops.

Priapism is a rare adverse effect of phosphodiesterase type 5 inhibitors, particularly sildenafil and vardenafil, which have shorter plasma half-lives than tadalafil. Priapism has been associated with excessive doses of the phosphodiesterase type 5 inhibitor or concomitant use with other erectogenic drugs.

Recently, sildenafil use has been associated with an increased risk of melanoma. The proposed mechanism theorized is that phosphodiesterase type 5 inhibition activates *BRAF*, a human gene that produces a protein that causes proliferation of melanoma cells. However, a cause-effect relationship has not been established.[67,68]

Recommendations for adverse effect monitoring are included in Table 83-6.

Drug Interactions

Approximately 8% of patients taking organic nitrates may develop sudden, severe hypotension if these agents are taken with phosphodiesterase type 5 inhibitors as a result of two major factors: (a)

TABLE 83-6 Drug Monitoring Table

Drug	Adverse Drug Reaction	Monitoring Parameter	Comments
Phosphodiesterase Inhibitor			
Sildenafil	Headache Flushing Gastroesophageal reflux Nasal congestion Cyanopsia NAION Hypotension Priapism Hearing loss	Clinical symptoms Visual complaints, loss of vision Blood pressure Pulse	Discontinue sildenafil if the patient has any visual or hearing loss and refer the patient to a physician If the patient is taking any antihypertensives, stabilize the blood pressure before starting sildenafil If the patient develops priapism, he should proceed to the emergency department
Vardenafil	Headache Flushing Gastroesophageal reflux Nasal congestion Cyanopsia NAION Hypotension QT interval prolongation on EKG Priapism Hearing loss	Clinical symptoms Visual complaints, loss of vision Blood pressure Pulse Palpitations or dizziness	Discontinue vardenafil if the patient has any visual or hearing loss and refer the patient to a physician If the patient is taking any antihypertensives, stabilize their blood pressure before starting vardenafil If the patient has palpitations or dizziness, check EKG. If QT prolongation is present, refer the patient for appropriate medical care If the patient develops priapism, he should proceed to the emergency department
Tadalafil	Headache Flushing Gastroesophageal reflux Nasal congestion Cyanopsia Hearing loss NAION Hypotension Low back or muscle pain Priapism	Clinical symptoms Visual complaints, loss of vision Blood pressure Pulse Palpitations or dizziness Hearing loss	Discontinue tadalafil if the patient has any visual or hearing loss and refer the patient to a physician If the patient is taking any antihypertensives, stabilize their blood pressure before starting tadalafil If the patient develops priapism, he should proceed to the emergency department
Avanafil	Headache Flushing Gastroesophageal reflux Nasal congestion Cyanopsia Hearing loss NAION Hypotension Low back or muscle pain Priapism	Clinical symptoms Visual complaints, loss of vision Blood pressure Pulse Palpitations or dizziness Hearing loss	Discontinue avanafil if the patient has any visual or hearing loss and refer the patient to a physician If the patient is taking any antihypertensives, stabilize their blood pressure before starting avanafil If the patient develops priapism, he should proceed to the emergency department
Prostaglandin E_1			
Alprostadil, intracavernosal	Penile pain Hematoma at injection site Priapism Hypotension Fibrotic nodules along penile shaft Decreased blood pressure Dizziness	Clinical symptoms Presence of hematoma or fibrotic nodules Blood pressure Pulse	Penile pain responds to acetaminophen To avoid hematoma, apply pressure to injection site for 510 minutes after injection If the patient develops priapism, he should proceed to the emergency department Fibrotic nodules are rare but may occur after repeated injections. These may cause curvature of the penis during an erection and this requires assessment by a urologist Hypotension and dizziness are uncommon and are associated with inadvertent venous injection of the drug
Alprostadil, intraurethral	Aching pain in penis, testicles, legs, and perineum Urethral burning, bleeding, or tearing Decreased blood pressure Dizziness Female partner may experience vaginal pain and burning sensation	Clinical symptoms Urethral injury as evidenced by pain, bleeding, or tissue damage Blood pressure Pulse	Burning pain usually resolves spontaneously. If urethral injury is suspected, this requires assessment by a urologist. Pain experienced by the female partner is due to leakage of medication from male urethra into vagina. Pain will usually resolve spontaneously If the patient develops priapism, he should proceed to the emergency department Hypotension and dizziness are uncommon, occurring in only 3% of patients, and are associated with systemic absorption of the drugs Alprostadil is embryotoxic and contact should be avoided if the female sex partner is pregnant

(continued)

TABLE 83-6 Drug Monitoring Table (*Continued*)

Drug	Adverse Drug Reaction	Monitoring Parameter	Comments
Testosterone Supplements			
Methyltestosterone	Sodium and water retention Hyperlipidemia Increased hematocrit Gynecomastia Sleep apnea Increased libido Mood swings Oligospermia Hepatotoxicity Prostate enlargement	Physical exam for edema Blood pressure Serum lipids, hematocrit, hepatic transaminases, prostate specific antigen	Discontinue if the patient has signs of hepatoxicity. If hematocrit exceeds 55%, methyltestosterone should be discontinued. Testosterone supplements may worsen LUTS in patients with BPH. It is contraindicated in patients with untreated prostate cancer or men with breast cancer
Fluoxymesterone	Sodium and water retention Hyperlipidemia Increased hematocrit Gynecomastia Sleep apnea Increased libido Mood swings Oligospermia Hepatotoxicity Prostate enlargement	Physical exam for edema Blood pressure Serum lipids, hematocrit, hepatic transaminases, prostate-specific antigen	Discontinue if the patient has signs of hepatoxicity. If hematocrit exceeds 55%, fluoxymesterone should be discontinued. Testosterone supplements may worsen LUTS in patients with BPH. It is contraindicated in patients with untreated prostate cancer or men with breast cancer
Testosterone buccal system	Sodium and water retention Hyperlipidemia Increased hematocrit Gynecomastia Sleep apnea Increased libido Mood swings Oligospermia Hepatotoxicity Gum irritation and pain Bitter taste Prostate enlargement	Physical exam for edema Blood pressure Serum lipids, hematocrit, hepatic transaminases, prostate-specific antigen	Discontinue if the patient has signs of hepatoxicity. If hematocrit exceeds 55%, testosterone buccal system should be discontinued. Testosterone supplements may worsen LUTS in patients with BPH. It is contraindicated in patients with untreated prostate cancer or men with breast cancer
Testosterone cypionate or enanthate	Sodium and water retention Hyperlipidemia Increased hematocrit Gynecomastia Sleep apnea Increased libido Oligospermia Mood swings Hepatotoxicity Prostate enlargement	Clinical symptoms Physical exam for edema Blood pressure Serum lipids, hematocrit, hepatic transaminases, prostate-specific antigen	Discontinue if the patient has signs of hepatoxicity. If hematocrit exceeds 55%, testosterone supplement should be discontinued. Testosterone supplements may worsen LUTS in patients with BPH. It is contraindicated in patients with untreated prostate cancer or men with breast cancer. These formulations produce supraphysiologic serum concentrations of testosterone. Mood swings have been reported with these agents
Testosterone undecanoate	Acne Injection site pain Pulmonary oil microembolism (POME) Anaphylactic reactions Prostate enlargement Sodium and water retention Increased hematocrit Gynecomastia	Clinical symptoms Physical exam for edema Blood pressure Serum lipids, hematocrit, hepatic transaminases, prostate-specific antigen	Discontinue if the patient has signs of hepatoxicity. If hematocrit exceeds 55%, testosterone supplement should be discontinued. Testosterone supplements may worsen LUTS in patients with BPH. It is contraindicated in patients with untreated prostate cancer or men with breast cancer. These formulations produce supraphysiologic serum concentrations of testosterone. Mood swings have been reported with these agents. Signs of POME include cough, dyspnea, chest pain, and syncope. This medication should only be administered by a health care provider or setting which is certified through a Risk Evaluation and Mitigaton Strategy program
Testosterone patch	Sodium and water retention Hyperlipidemia Gynecomastia Sleep apnea Increased libido Contact dermatitis Erythema Pruritus Prostate enlargement	Clinical symptoms Physical exam for edema Blood pressure Serum lipids, hematocrit, hepatic transaminases, prostate-specific antigen	Testosterone supplements may worsen LUTS in patients with BPH. It is contraindicated in patients with untreated prostate cancer or men with breast cancer. Contact dermatitis has been associated with the alcohol-based agent used to enhance transdermal drug absorption. It responds to topical corticosteroids. Of significance, hepatotoxicity has not been reported with transdermal patches

(*continued*)

TABLE 83-6 Drug Monitoring Table (*Continued*)

Drug	Adverse Drug Reaction	Monitoring Parameter	Comments
Testosterone gel/spray/ axillary solution	Sodium and water retention Hyperlipidemia Gynecomastia Sleep apnea Increased libido Dermatitis Erythema Pruritis Prostate enlargement	Clinical symptoms Physical exam for edema Blood pressure Serum lipids, hematocrit, hepatic transaminases, prostate specific antigen	Testosterone supplements may worsen LUTS in patients with BPH. It is contraindicated in patients with untreated prostate cancer or men with breast cancer
Testosterone subcutaneous implant	Sodium and water retention Hyperlipidemia Increased hematocrit Gynecomastia Sleep apnea Increased libido Mood swings Oligospermia Hepatotoxicity Prostate enlargement Pain and infection at the implant site	Clinical symptoms Physical exam for edema Blood pressure Serum lipids	Subcutaneous implant pellet may be extruded with loss of the dose. Androgen-related adverse effects may persist for a long time after drug administration unless the implant is removed. If hematocrit exceeds 55%, testosterone supplement should be discontinued. Testosterone supplements may worsen LUTS in patients with BPH. It is contraindicated in patients with untreated prostate cancer or men with breast cancer

LUTS, lower urinary tract symptoms.

organic nitrates on their own produce hypotension, and (b) organic nitrates are nitric oxide donors, which can stimulate the activity of guanylate cyclase and increase tissue levels of cGMP.[49] For this reason, use of phosphodiesterase type 5 inhibitors is contraindicated in patients taking nitrates given by any route at scheduled times or intermittently.[26,69] Furthermore, nitrates should be withheld for 24 hours after sildenafil or vardenafil administration and for 48 hours after tadalafil administration.[26,69] Finally, if a patient who has taken a phosphodiesterase type 5 inhibitor requires medical treatment of angina, non-nitrate-containing agents (eg, calcium channel blocker, β-adrenergic antagonist, and morphine) should be used.

If severe hypotension occurs after exposure to nitrates and a phosphodiesterase type 5 inhibitor, the patient should be placed in a Trendelenburg position and aggressive fluid administration initiated. If severe hypotension continues, parenteral β-adrenergic agonists (eg, dopamine) should be administered cautiously.

Interestingly, dietary sources of nitrates, nitrites, or L-arginine (a precursor for nitrates) do not interact with phosphodiesterase type 5 inhibitors. This is because dietary sources do not increase circulating levels of nitric oxide in humans.

The phosphodiesterase type 5 inhibitors have a low potential to interact with antihypertensive medications.[70] In a retrospective analysis of patients taking sildenafil in combination with α-adrenergic antagonists, β-adrenergic antagonists, diuretics, angiotensin—converting enzyme inhibitors, angiotensin receptor blockers, or calcium channel blockers, the incidence of hypotension was similar to that reported in patients taking sildenafil alone.[71] This finding was confirmed by a retrospective analysis of pooled data on more than 4,800 patients in 35 clinical trials.[70]

Small decreases in blood pressure with clinically symptomatic orthostatic hypotension have been described in some patients taking phosphodiesterase type 5 inhibitors and α-adrenergic antagonists. The degree of hypotension that develops is dependent on several factors: (a) stability of patient's blood pressure prior to taking both drugs; (b) dose of the α-adrenergic antagonist used; (c) particular α-adrenergic antagonist used; (d) particular phosphodiesterase type 5 inhibitor used; and (e) timing of administration of both drugs. The drug interaction produces less hypotension when the patient has stable blood pressure prior to taking both drugs; a low dose of α-adrenergic antagonist is taken; a uroselective (eg, tamsulosin or silodosin) or extended-release formulation of an α-adrenergic antagonist (eg, alfuzosin, or modified-release doxazosin) is used; tadalafil is preferentially prescribed over sildenafil, vardenafil, or avanafil; and when there is an interval of 4 to 6 hours between the dosing of the α-adrenergic antagonist and phosphodiesterase type 5 inhibitor.[70,72-75]

Hepatic metabolism of all three phosphodiesterase type 5 inhibitors can be inhibited by enzyme inhibitors of CYP 3A4, including fluvoxamine, fluoxetine, nefazodone, verapamil, diltiazem, cimetidine, erythromycin, clarithromycin, ketoconazole, fluconazole itraconazole, ritonavir, saquinavir, and grapefruit juice.[70] Potent CYP 3A4 inhibitors may increase plasma levels of phosphodiesterase type 5 inhibitors by 3-fold or more.[4,75] Lower starting doses of the phosphodiesterase type 5 inhibitor should be used in these patients to minimize dose-related adverse effects, including cyanopsia, hypotension, flushing, nasal congestion, and priapism (see Table 83-4). Similarly CYP 3A4 inducers, including carbamazepine, phenytoin, and phenobarbital, can decrease plasma levels of phosphodiesterase type 5 inhibitors.

If used with type 1A antiarrhythmics (eg, quinidine or procainamide) or type 3 antiarrhythmics (eg, sotalol, amiodarone), vardenafil can prolong the QT interval. This is a unique drug interaction of vardenafil and not a pharmacologic class effect.

Testosterone Replacement Regimens

Mechanism

9 Testosterone replacement regimens supply exogenous testosterone and restore serum testosterone levels to the normal range (300-1,100 ng/dL; 10.4-38.2 nmol/L). In so doing, testosterone replacement regimens correct symptoms of hypogonadism, which include malaise, loss of muscle strength, depressed mood, and decreased libido. Testosterone can directly stimulate androgen receptors in the CNS and is thought to be responsible for maintaining normal sexual drive. In addition, testosterone may stimulate nitric oxide synthase, thereby increasing cavernosal concentrations of nitric oxide, and enhancing the effects of phosphodiesterase type 5 in cavernosal tissue.[76]

Indications

Testosterone replacement regimens are indicated in symptomatic patients with primary, secondary, or mixed hypogonadism, as confirmed by both the presence of a decreased libido and low serum concentrations of testosterone.[2] Mixed hypogonadism is characteristic of aging men who undergo andropause, in which the Leydig cells of the testes slowly and progressively decrease testosterone production, and hypothalamic and pituitary production of gonadotropin and luteinizing hormone, respectively, are altered.[77] Serum testosterone levels decrease starting at age 40 years by approximately 10% per decade of life. This is often referred to as late-onset hypogonadism, symptomatic late-onset hypogonadism andropause, or the male menopause. Symptoms include decreased libido, erectile dysfunction, gynecomastia, small testes, reduced growth of body hair and beard, decreased muscle mass, and increased body fat. If left untreated, patients develop anemia and osteoporosis.

Serum testosterone concentrations typically are measured in the early morning (approximately 8 am) because the secretion pattern of this hormone follows a circadian pattern, with highest serum concentrations in the morning hours and the lowest level at night (approximately 10 pm). A low measured serum testosterone level is confirmed with a repeat measurement on a separate day. Confirmation of a low serum testosterone level is essential because of an approximate 10% intra-individual variation of measured levels and variable performance characteristics of various testosterone assays.[77] Simultaneous serum luteinizing hormone levels help to distinguish patients with primary hypogonadism, who have elevated luteinizing hormone levels, from those with secondary hypogonadism, who have decreased luteinizing hormone levels.[2,78]

Testosterone replacement regimens should never be administered to men with normal serum testosterone levels, patients who are asymptomatic with hypogonadism, or in patients with isolated erectile dysfunction as the only sign of hypogonadism.[2,76,78]

Efficacy

Testosterone replacement regimens restore muscle strength and sexual drive and improve mood in patients with hypogonadism. Improvements are generally observed within days or weeks of the start of testosterone replacement. Administration of testosterone will correct the serum testosterone level to the normal range. No additional benefit has been demonstrated for large doses of testosterone, which increase the serum testosterone level from the low end to the upper end of the normal range or to the above-normal range.[79] Testosterone replacement regimens do not directly correct erectile dysfunction; instead, they improve libido, thereby correcting secondary erectile dysfunction.[79]

Testosterone replacement regimens can be administered parenterally, orally, buccally, or transdermally (see Tables 83-4). Intramuscular injections of testosterone enanthate and cypionate are the preferred treatment for symptomatic patients with primary or secondary hypogonadism because they are effective, inexpensive, and not associated with the bioavailability problems or hepatotoxic adverse effects of oral androgens.[2,77,78] Patients generally require dosing every 2 to 4 weeks. A longer-acting depot intramuscular formulation of testosterone undecanoate, which can be dosed every 10 weeks, offers greater convenience but is more expensive than testosterone enanthate or cypionate. A subcutaneous implant of testosterone pellets lasts 3 to 6 months, but it requires a surgical incision in the forearm and is expensive. Although convenient for the patient, testosterone patches, gels, and sprays are much more expensive than testosterone enanthate or cypionate; therefore, they should be reserved for patients who refuse injectable testosterone. Oral formulations are associated with hepatotoxicity and are not recommended; and the buccal formulation must be dosed twice a day and is expensive.

In the ideal testosterone replacement regimen, the medication would mimic the normal circadian pattern of serum testosterone concentrations such that peak and trough concentrations occur in the early morning and late afternoon, respectively; produce serum concentrations in the normal range; produce serum concentrations of dihydrotestosterone and estradiol, which are (metabolites of testosterone) that mimic the normal physiologic pattern; and produce minimal adverse effects.[79] The ideal replacement regimen should be inexpensive and be convenient for the patient to use. Table 83-4 compares commercially available testosterone replacement regimens for these characteristics and shows that an ideal regimen has yet to be identified.

Pharmacokinetics

Natural testosterone has poor oral bioavailability because of extensive first-pass hepatic metabolism; therefore, large doses must be taken. To improve oral bioavailability, alkylated derivatives were formulated. Of these derivatives, methyltestosterone and fluoxymesterone are more resistant to hepatic catabolism and can be taken in smaller daily doses, which are theoretically safer. However, oral alkylated derivatives of testosterone are not metabolized to dihydrotestosterone or estradiol, are associated with a higher incidence of serious hepatotoxicity, and therefore are not preferred for management of hypogonadism.

An alternative to oral administration is the testosterone buccal system (Striant), which is applied to the gum above the upper incisor teeth twice per day. Over time it forms a gel from which testosterone is absorbed. One advantage of this route of administration is that the drug bypasses first-pass hepatic catabolism, which allows for increased bioavailability of testosterone. Serum testosterone levels are maintained in the normal range for approximately 80% of the day.[80]

Several testosterone esters have been formulated for intramuscular injection, with different durations of action (see Table 83-4). The shorter-acting testosterone propionate, which requires dosing three times per week, has been replaced with testosterone cypionate or enanthate, which can be dosed every 2, 4, or 6 weeks in most patients. These testosterone formulations produce supraphysiologic serum testosterone levels 2 to 4 days after each dose; these have been linked to mood swings and polycythemia in some patients. After the first and second dose, which are given 4 weeks apart, intramuscular injections of testosterone undecanoate generally last 10 weeks. Although this can be convenient for the patient, testosterone undecanoate has been associated with pulmonary oil microembolism or anaphylactic reactions that can necessitate hospitalization. For this reason, testosterone undecanoate is restricted to settings certified through a Risk Evaluation and Mitigation Strategy Program.[81] An even longer-acting parenteral testosterone is available as a subcutaneous implant for dosing every 3 to 6 months. Although this schedule minimizes repeat visits to the clinician's office for dosing, the implant must be administered by a physician, and the implanted pellet may be extruded after administration. Extrusion has been reported in up to 8.5% of treated patients and results in loss of drug effect.

Transdermal testosterone replacement regimens can be delivered as once-daily patches or gel. For convenience, the gel is available in premeasured dose packets or in a pump dispenser. Testosterone patches increase serum testosterone levels into the normal range in 2 to 6 hours. Serum testosterone levels return to baseline 24 hours after patch or gel administration. However, unlike oral or injectable supplements, transdermal testosterone patches applied at bedtime or testosterone gel applied each morning produce physiologic patterns of serum testosterone levels throughout the day. Although these formulations are often described as producing more "natural" hormone levels, the clinical importance of this biochemical effect is unknown.[76]

The original Testoderm brand patch was formulated for scrotal application. Scrotal skin is thinner and has a richer vascular supply than does the skin on the arms or thighs. Therefore, application of Testoderm patches produced excellent absorption of the hormone. However, the patch could detach when the scrotum became damp or moist, when the patient exercised, or if the scrotum was excessively hairy.[81] Due to its inconvenient site of application, the scrotal patch is no longer commercially available in the United States.

For improved convenience, Androderm patches were formulated for application to the upper arms, back, abdomen, or thighs. The addition of absorption enhancers and adhesives has been linked to a higher incidence of contact dermatitis with Androderm patches compared with the original Testoderm scrotal patch or to gel formulations.[77]

Testosterone gel 1% formulation (AndroGel) is applied in much larger doses (5 or 10 g each day) to the skin of the shoulders, upper arms, or abdomen. The hormone is absorbed quickly, within 30 minutes, but several hours may be required for complete absorption of the dose. For this reason, the patient should be reminded to wait at least 2 hours after application before showering. To prevent inadvertent transfer of testosterone gel to others, the patient should thoroughly wash his hands with soap and water after administration of a dose, allow the application site to dry undisturbed for several minutes before dressing or covering it, and ensure that there is no contact with clothing contaminated with the gel by children and female members of the household.

A high-strength testosterone gel (1.6%) formulation is also available. It allows administration of a daily dose with a smaller amount of gel. It should be applied to the shoulder or upper arms.

Dosing

Table 83-4 lists the usual doses for testosterone replacement regimens. Three months is considered as an adequate treatment trial with a particular dose.[11,77,78] Thus, a dose should not be increased until the patient has used one particular dose for at least this time period. The serum testosterone level should return to the normal range and symptoms of androgen deficiency should be relieved with appropriate dosing. Repeated serum testosterone levels that exceed the normal range require a dosage reduction or increased interval between drug doses. Table 83-7 provides guidance on the timeline for monitoring serum testosterone levels based on the particular testosterone replacement regimen. After starting treatment, patients should be reassessed in 1 to 3 months. The patient's libido, mood, and quality of life may improve in 3 to 4 weeks, erectile function may improve in 6 months, but other symptoms of hypogonadism (eg, bone density) may take longer to resolve. If the patient is responding to treatment and serum testosterone levels have returned to normal, the patient can be followed up annually. At each visit, the use of a validated self-assessment tool (eg, Androgen Deficiency in Aging Men Questionnaire) can assist the physician in gauging the patient's response to treatment.[82]

Before initiating any testosterone replacement regimen in patients 40 years and older, patients should be screened for breast cancer, benign prostatic hyperplasia, and prostate cancer. All are testosterone-dependent conditions and theoretically could be worsened by exogenous administration of testosterone. However, no confirmed cases of prostate cancer caused by testosterone supplementation in a hypogonadal patient have been documented.[83-85] Nevertheless, untreated prostate cancer is a contraindication to androgen supplementation. To screen for prostate disorders, a prostate-specific antigen serum concentration should be obtained and a digital rectal examination of the prostate performed. These tests are generally repeated at 1-year intervals after treatment is started. Other baseline tests that are recommended include hematocrit and liver function tests. These should be repeated 3 and 6 months after the start of a testosterone replacement regimen. If normal, these tests can be repeated annually thereafter. If the hematocrit exceeds 55% (0.55), the testosterone replacement regimen should be withheld to avoid polycythemia and its consequences.

The dropout rate with testosterone supplementation is high. Approximately 30% and 85% of patients stop testosterone replacement after 6 and 12 months, respectively. The reasons for this include the cost of the medication, slow onset of response, and inadequate perceived benefit.[86]

TABLE 83-7 Timing of Serum Testosterone Level Monitoring in Patients on Testosterone Replacement Regimens

When to Monitor Serum Testosterone Levels	
Oral testosterone tablets/capsules	2-3 hours after dose
Intramuscular testosterone cypionate or enanthate	Midpoint of dosing interval
Intramuscular testosterone undecanoate	Right before the 4th dose
Transdermal gel	Anytime after the first 1-2 weeks of continuous use
Transdermal patch	3-12 hours after patch application
Testosterone subcutaneous implant	1-4 months after implantation
Buccal system	Before a dose

Adverse Effects

Testosterone replacement regimens can cause sodium retention, which can lead to weight gain, or exacerbate hypertension, congestive heart failure, and edema (Table 83-6). Although serum lipoprotein perturbations may occur, testosterone replacement regimens have a neutral effect in that they decrease both total cholesterol and high-density lipoprotein cholesterol levels. Two recent retrospective studies have associated testosterone supplementation with an increased risk of myocardial infarction and stroke.[87,88] However, these studies did not prove a cause-effect relationship and are considered inconclusive. Nevertheless, the Food and Drug Administration has posted a warning that testosterone supplementation may lead to cardiovascular disease and physicians should discuss this potential risk with patients before initiating treatment. This was prompted by the significant increase in testosterone use in the United States, inadequate monitoring of serum testosterone levels prior to and during testosterone supplementation, and the potential hazards of using testosterone supplementation in elderly patients with cardiovascular risk factors.[89]

Gynecomastia can occur as a result of conversion of testosterone to estrogen in peripheral tissues. This has been reported most often in patients with liver cirrhosis or those who are obese.

Oral alkylated testosterone replacement regimens have caused hepatotoxicity, ranging from mild elevations of hepatic transaminases to serious liver diseases, including peliosis hepatis (hemorrhagic liver cysts), hepatocellular and intrahepatic cholestasis, and benign or malignant tumors. For this reason, parenteral testosterone replacement regimens are preferred.

Transdermal testosterone patches may cause contact dermatitis, which responds well to topical corticosteroids. This adverse effect has been associated with the presence of permeation enhancers, which are added to patch formulations. If the dermatitis becomes problematic, an alternative is testosterone gel formulations, which are associated with a lower incidence of contact dermatitis compared with patches.

Polycythemia occurs most often in patients receiving parenteral testosterone formulations. If this occurs, testosterone injections should be stopped and can be replaced with a transdermal testosterone product.[78]

Alprostadil

Mechanism

Alprostadil, also known as prostaglandin E_1, stimulates adenyl cyclase, resulting in increased production of cAMP, a secondary messenger that decreases the intracellular calcium concentration and causes smooth muscle relaxation of the arterial blood vessels and sinusoidal tissues in the corpora. This results in enhanced blood flow to and blood filling of the corpora. Because it does not require nitric oxide to produce its clinical effects, patients with erectile dysfunction due to diseases that are associated with an impaired nitric oxide pathway (eg, diabetes mellitus, postradical prostatectomy, and who have failed phosphodiesterase type 5 treatment) may respond to alprostadil.[90] In one study, 88% of men who failed to respond to sildenafil responded to intracavernosal alprostadil.[91]

Alprostadil is commercially available as an intracavernosal injection (Caverject and Edex) and as an intraurethral insert (medicated urethral system for erection [MUSE]).

Indications

Both commercially available formulations of alprostadil are FDA approved as monotherapy for management of erectile dysfunction. Alprostadil is more effective by the intracavernosal route than the intraurethral route.

The enhanced efficacy of the intracavernosal injection may be related to the excellent bioavailability of the drug when injected directly into the corpora cavernosum. In contrast, intraurethral alprostadil doses generally are several hundred times larger than intracavernosal doses. This is because intraurethral alprostadil must be absorbed from the urethra, through the corpus spongiosum, and into the corpus cavernosum, where it exerts its full proerectogenic effect.

Although several other agents, including papaverine and phentolamine, have been used off-label for intracavernosal therapy, alprostadil is preferentially prescribed. This is because intracavernosal alprostadil has been FDA approved for erectile dysfunction, it does not require extemporaneous compounding, and it has a low potential for causing prolonged erections and priapism.

Both formulations of alprostadil are considered more invasive than VEDs or phosphodiesterase type 5 inhibitors. For this reason, intracavernosal alprostadil is generally prescribed after patients do not respond to or cannot use less invasive interventions. Intracavernosal alprostadil is preferred over intraurethral alprostadil because of its greater effectiveness. Intracavernosal alprostadil may be preferred in patients with diabetes mellitus, who are accustomed to injectable drug therapy and may have peripheral neuropathies, which decrease the patient's perception of pain upon injection. Intraurethral alprostadil is generally reserved as a treatment of last resort for patients who do not respond to other less invasive and more effective forms of therapy, and who refuse surgery.

Intracavernosal Alprostadil

Efficacy

The overall efficacy of intracavernosal alprostadil is 70% to 90%.[92] Three characteristics of intracavernosal alprostadil include the following:

1. The effectiveness of alprostadil is dose related. The mean duration of erection is directly related to the dose of alprostadil administered and ranges from 12 to 44 minutes.
2. A higher percentage of patients with psychogenic and neurogenic erectile dysfunction respond to alprostadil at a lower dose compared to patients with vasculogenic erectile dysfunction.
3. Tolerance does not appear to develop with continued use of intracavernosal alprostadil at home.

(10) Although 70% to 75% of patients respond to intracavernosal alprostadil, a high proportion of patients elect to discontinue its use over time. Depending on the study and the length of observation, 30% to 50% of patients voluntarily discontinue therapy, usually during the first 6 to 12 months, and this increases to 54% and 67% after 2 to 4 years, respectively.[4] Common reasons for discontinuation include lack of perceived effectiveness; inconvenience of administration; an unnatural, nonspontaneous erection; needle phobia; loss of interest; or cost of therapy.[92]

Approximately one third of patients do not respond to usual doses of intracavernosal alprostadil. In these patients, intracavernosal alprostadil has been used successfully along with VEDs. Such combination therapy can be attempted by patients before transitioning to more invasive surgical procedures.[32,76] Alternatively, intracavernosal injections of synergistic combinations of vasoactive agents that act by different mechanisms have been used. Intracavernosal drug combinations typically produce an erection that lasts longer than an erection produced by any one of the agents in the mixture. In addition, because of the low dosage of each agent in the combination, fewer systemic and local fibrotic adverse effects develop compared with high-dose monotherapy. For example, when used in low-dose combination regimens, papaverine is less likely to induce hypotension and liver dysfunction, and phentolamine is less likely to induce tachycardia and hypotension.[4,92,93] However, as previously mentioned, such intracavernosal drug combinations are not commercially available and must be extemporaneously compounded.

Pharmacokinetics

Intracavernosal injection should be administered into only one corpus cavernosum. From this injection site, the drug will reach the other corpus cavernosum through vascular communications between the two corpora. Alprostadil acts rapidly, with an onset of 5 to 15 minutes. The duration is directly related to the dose. Within the usual dosage range of 2.5 to 20 mcg, the duration of erection is not more than 1 hour. Higher doses are expected to exhibit a longer duration of action. Local 15-hydroxy dehydrogenase in the corpora cavernosum quickly converts alprostadil to inactive metabolites. Any alprostadil that escapes into the systemic circulation is deactivated on first pass through the lungs. Hence, the plasma half-life of alprostadil is approximately 5-10 minutes, and the potential for systemic adverse effects is negligible. Dose modification is not necessary in patients with renal or hepatic disease.

Dosing

The usual dose of intracavernosal alprostadil is 10 to 20 mcg, with a maximum recommended dose of 60 mcg. Doses greater than 60 mcg have not produced any greater improvement in penile erection, but may cause hypotension or prolonged erections lasting more than 1 hour.[78] The dose should be administered 5 to 10 minutes before intercourse. The manufacturer recommends that patients be slowly titrated up to the minimally effective dosage to minimize the likelihood of hypotension. Under a physician's supervision, patients should be started with a 1.25-mcg dose, which can be increased in increments of 1.25 to 2.50 mcg at 30-minute intervals up to the lowest dose that produces a firm erection for 1 hour and does not produce adverse effects. In clinical practice, this process is rarely done because it is time consuming. Thus, many physicians start the patient on 10 mcg and move quickly up the dosage range to identify the best dose for the patient. To avoid adverse effects, patients should receive not more than one injection per day and not more than three injections per week with a 24-hour interval between doses (see Table 83-3).

Intracavernosal injections should be performed using a 0.5-inch (1.3 cm), 27- or 30-gauge needle. A tuberculin syringe or a syringe prefilled with diluent as supplied by the manufacturer should be used to ensure precise measurement of doses. Patients with needle phobia, poor vision, or poor manual dexterity can use commercially available autoinjectors to facilitate administration of intracavernosal alprostadil.

Intracavernosal injections require that the patient or the sexual partner practice good aseptic techniques (to avoid infection), have good manual skills and visual ability, and be comfortable with injection techniques. When practicing self-injection, the patient should use one hand to firmly hold the glans penis against his thigh to

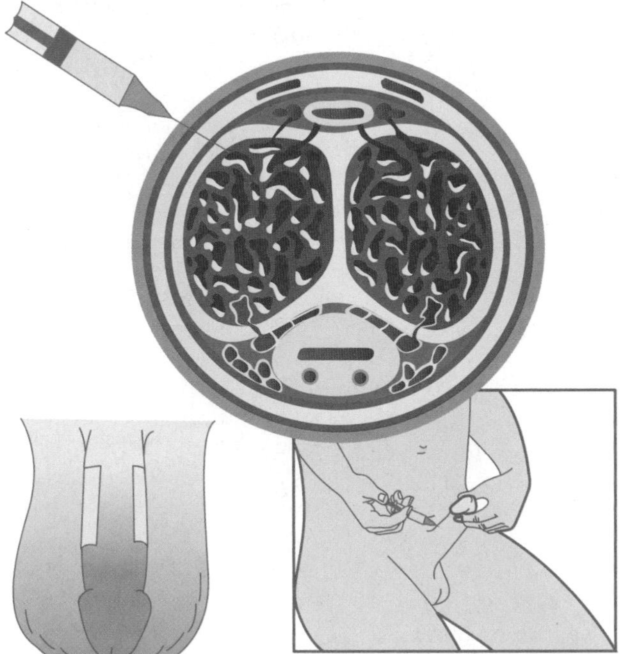

FIGURE 83-5 Technique for administration of intracavernosal injections. *(From Caverject [package insert]. New York, NY: Pfizer Inc.; 1999. Data from http://media.pfizer.com/files/products/uspi_caverject_powder.pdf.)*

expose the lateral surface of the shaft. The injection should be made at right angles into one of the lateral surfaces of the proximal third of the penis. The injection should never be made into the dorsal or ventral surface of the penis. This will prevent inadvertent injection of the drug into arteries on the dorsal surface or the urethra on the ventral surface. After the injection, the penis should be massaged to help distribute the drug into the opposite corpus cavernosum. Injection sites should be rotated with each dose. Finally, manual pressure should be applied to the injection site for 5 minutes to reduce the likelihood of hematoma formation (Fig. 83-5).

Once the optimal dosage of intracavernosal alprostadil is established, the patient should return for routine medical follow-up every 3 to 6 months. Some patients subsequently require dosage adjustment, largely attributed to worsening of the underlying disease that is contributing to the erectile dysfunction.

Adverse Effects

Intracavernosal alprostadil is most commonly associated with local adverse effects. Hematoma and bruising at the injection site occurs most often during the first year of therapy. These effects are largely the result of poor injection technique. To minimize the risk of injection site hematomas, patients should apply pressure to the injection site for 5 minutes after each dose. Similarly, infection at the injection site has been reported. Meticulous aseptic technique is necessary to prevent this complication.

Cavernosal plaques or areas of fibrosis at injection sites form in approximately 2% to 12% of patients. When they occur, the patient should suspend further injections for 2 to 4 months or until the plaques resolve. These plaques may cause penile curvature, similar to Peyronie's disease, which makes sexual intercourse difficult or impossible. The cause of corporal fibrosis and plaque formation is unknown. This adverse effect may be caused by poor injection technique or by alprostadil itself. Although patients have developed corporal fibrosis, alprostadil may be less likely to cause this adverse effect compared to other intracavernosal drug combinations, such as phentolamine or papaverine. Unlike cavernosal fibrosis associated with large doses and repeated administration of papaverine, penile scarring secondary to alprostadil appears to be unpredictable.

Alprostadil causes penile pain in approximately 10% to 44% of patients. The pain has been described as a burning discomfort or dull pain near the injection site or during the erection, which generally does not persist after the penis becomes flaccid. The pain usually is mild, generally does not require discontinuation of therapy, and often abates even with continued treatment. However, 2% to 5% of patients discontinue taking alprostadil because of severe pain. The pain can be managed by oral analgesics (eg, acetaminophen), if necessary. One investigator has recommended adding procaine to intracavernosal alprostadil, but this may mask the signs of more serious adverse effects of the drug or of penile injury during intercourse and is not recommended.[79] The mechanism of this adverse reaction is poorly understood. Alprostadil may intrinsically produce pain. In addition, the pain may be a result of the pH of the parenteral solution. Alprostadil is acidic, and the commercially available Caverject formulation is buffered with sodium citrate, a weak base, to reduce pain on injection.

Priapism, a prolonged, painful erection lasting more than 1 hour, occurs in 1% to 15% of treated patients. It occurs most often during the dose titration period and is rare thereafter. Blood sludging in the corpora can lead to tissue hypoxia and irreversible cavernosal fibrosis and scarring. The risk for this complication is greatest for erections that persist beyond 4 to 6 hours. Patients are advised to seek medical attention immediately when drug-induced erections last more than 4 hours, as this may progress to a urologic emergency. Its management includes supportive care, including analgesics for pain and sedatives for anxiety. In addition, needle aspiration of sludged blood in the corpora or intracavernosal injection of α-adrenergic agonists (eg, phenylephrine) has been used. These procedures facilitate venous drainage of the corpora, allowing venous outflow to "catch up" with arterial inflow.

The likelihood of prolonged erections with intracavernosal alprostadil is dose related. Therefore, to prevent this adverse effect, the lowest effective dose should be used, and the dose should be titrated to ensure that the duration of the erection is not more than 1 hour.

Intracavernosal alprostadil rarely causes systemic adverse effects, owing to the agent's local catabolism in cavernosal tissue and rapid deactivation in pulmonary tissue (if any of the drug escapes into the systemic circulation). However, large doses greater than 20 mcg are associated with dizziness and hypotension in some patients and is one reason why such large doses are not commonly used.

Intracavernosal injection therapy should be used cautiously by patients at risk for priapism, including patients with sickle cell disease, leukemia, or multiple myeloma. It should be used cautiously by patients who may develop bleeding complications secondary to injections, including patients with thrombocytopenia or those taking anticoagulants. It also should be used cautiously by patients who use poor-quality injection technique, including patients with psychiatric disorders, obese patients (who may not be able to reach or see the penile injection site), patients who are blind, patients with severe arthritis, or patients with abnormal penile anatomy.

Intraurethral alprostadil should be avoided in patients with urethral stricture or urethritis, or if the female partner is pregnant.

Intraurethral Alprostadil

Efficacy

10 Intraurethral alprostadil inserts are marketed as MUSE, which contains a medication pellet inside a prefilled urethral applicator. Multiple studies show this product has an overall effectiveness rate of 43% to 65%[92,93] compared with 70% to 90% for intracavernosal alprostadil. Its decreased effectiveness and inconvenient administration method have resulted in this product being considered a

third-line treatment option for patients with erectile dysfunction. However, some patients have responded to intraurethral alprostadil even though they did not respond to intracavernosal alprostadil[94] or sildenafil.[95]

Intraurethral alprostadil has been combined with a VED to improve treatment response.[96]

The voluntary dropout rate is high and has been reported to be 57% and 75% after 3 and 15 months, respectively.[95]

Pharmacokinetics

Following intraurethral instillation, alprostadil is absorbed quickly through the urethra, into the corpus spongiosum, and then into the corpora cavernosum. As much as 80% of each dose is absorbed by the urethra and corpus spongiosum in less than 10 minutes, with peak absorption occurring in 20 to 25 minutes. An estimated 20% of each dose is delivered to the corpora cavernosum. As with intracavernosal injections of alprostadil, any drug absorbed into the systemic circulation is rapidly metabolized on first pass through the lungs.

The onset after intraurethral insertion is similar to that of intracavernosal injection, 5 to 10 minutes, and the duration is 30 to 60 minutes.

Dosing

The usual dose of intraurethral alprostadil is 125 to 1,000 mcg. The dose should be administered 5 to 10 minutes before sexual intercourse. Not more than two doses per day are recommended. Before administration, the patient should be advised to empty his bladder, voiding completely (see Table 83-3).

Similar to intracavernosal injection treatments, intraurethral insertion of alprostadil requires good manual and visual skills to minimize the risk of urethral injuries. Intraurethral alprostadil is supplied in a prefilled intraurethral applicator. The patient should void first to moisten the urethra. With one hand the patient holds the glans penis, and with the other hand the patient inserts the intraurethral applicator 0.5 inch (1.3 cm) into the urethra. The drug pellet is then pushed into the urethra. The penis should be massaged to enhance drug dissolution in the urethral fluids and drug absorption (Fig. 83-6).

Adverse Effects

The urethra can be injured because of an improper administration technique. Injuries can lead to urethral stricture and difficulty voiding. Patients should receive complete education about optimal administration procedures before starting treatment.

Urethral pain has been reported in 24% to 32% of patients. Usually it is mild and does not require discontinuation of treatment. Female sexual partners may experience vaginal burning, itching, or pain, which probably is related to transfer of alprostadil from the man's urethra to the woman's vagina during intercourse.

Prolonged painful erections (priapism) have been rarely reported. Syncope and dizziness have been reported rarely (only 2%-3% of patients) and likely are related to use of excessively large doses.

Clinical **Controversy...**

Although not recommended by the manufacturer, combinations of erectogenic medications or use of erectogenic medications with VEDs is a common practice. Published clinical trials of good research design are often lacking. Use of such combinations must take into consideration the published data available to support the use, potential adverse effects of the combination, and cost.

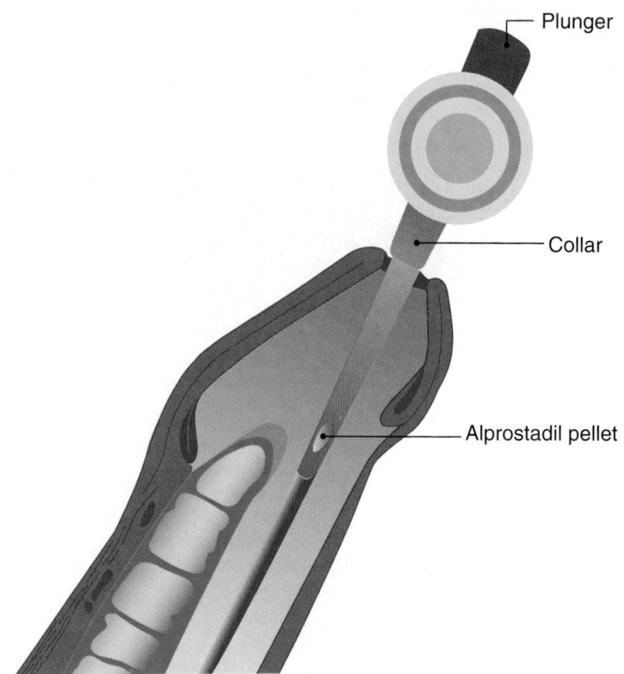

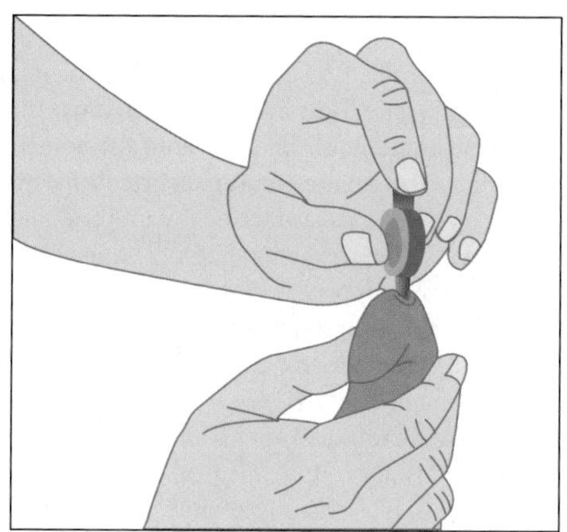

FIGURE 83-6 Technique for administration of intraurethral alprostadil with a medicated urethral system for erection applicator. *(From Muse [package insert]. Mountain View, CA: Vivus, Inc.; 2003.)*

Unapproved Agents

A variety of other commercially available and investigational agents have been used for management of erectile dysfunction. Although it is beyond the scope of this chapter to discuss all of them, some of the more commonly used agents are discussed here.

Yohimbine

Yohimbine, a tree-bark derivative also known as *yohimbe*, is widely used as an aphrodisiac. Yohimbine is a central α_2-adrenergic antagonistic that increases catecholamines and improves mood. Some investigators believe that yohimbine has peripheral proerectogenic effects. Yohimbine may reduce peripheral α-adrenergic tone, thereby permitting a predominant cholinergic tone, which could result in a vasodilatory response.[21,96] The usual oral dose is 6 mg three times per day.

Based on a meta-analysis of published studies that concluded that yohimbine is only mildly efficacious for psychogenic erectile dysfunction,[96] the American Urological Association has cautioned against the use of yohimbine.[21] In addition, yohimbine can cause many systemic adverse effects, including anxiety, insomnia, tachycardia, and hypertension.

Papaverine

Papaverine is a nonspecific phosphodiesterase type 5 inhibitor that decreases metabolic catabolism of cAMP in cavernosal tissue. As a result of enhanced tissue levels of cAMP, smooth muscle relaxation occurs. Cavernosal sinusoids fill with blood, and a penile erection results.

Papaverine is not FDA approved for erectile dysfunction. Intracavernosal papaverine alone is not commonly used for management of erectile dysfunction because the large doses required produce dose-related adverse effects, such as priapism, corporal fibrosis, hypotension, and hepatotoxicity.[21,97] Papaverine is more often administered in lower doses combined with phentolamine and/or alprostadil. A variety of formulas have been used, but no one mixture has been proven better than other mixtures. Combination formulations are considered safer and are associated with the potential for fewer serious adverse effects than high doses of any one of these agents.

A portion of each papaverine dose is systemically absorbed, and its prolonged plasma half-life of 1 hour contributes to adverse effects. The usual dose of papaverine is 7.5 to 60 mg when used as a single agent for intracavernosal injection. When used in combination, the dose decreases to 0.5 to 20 mg.

If treated with papaverine, patients with a history of underlying liver disease or alcohol abuse should undergo liver function testing at baseline and every 6 to 12 months during continued treatment.

Phentolamine

Phentolamine is a competitive nonselective α-adrenergic blocking agent. It reduces peripheral adrenergic tone and enhances cholinergic tone. As a result, it improves cavernosal filling and is proerectogenic.[21]

Phentolamine has most often been administered as an intracavernosal injection. Monotherapy is avoided because large doses are required for an erection, and at these large doses systemic hypotensive adverse effects would be prevalent. Most often, phentolamine has been used in combination with other vasoactive agents for intracavernosal administration. A ratio of 30 mg papaverine to 0.5 to 1 mg phentolamine is typical, and the usual dose ranges from 0.1 to 1 mL of the mixture. Such a mixture promotes local effects of phentolamine and minimizes systemic hypotensive adverse effects.

Hypotension is the most common adverse effect of intracavernosal phentolamine. It is more common and more severe with large doses or in patients with a poor injection technique who have injected into a vein (rather than the cavernosa). Prolonged erections have been reported in patients who used excessive doses of intracavernosal medications in combination.

Penile Prostheses

Surgical insertion of a penile prosthesis is the most invasive treatment of erectile dysfunction. It is reserved for patients who do not respond to or who are not candidates for less invasive oral or injectable treatments.

Prosthesis insertion requires anesthesia and skilled urologists. Two prostheses are widely used: malleable and inflatable. Malleable or semirigid prostheses consist of two bendable rods that are inserted into the corpora cavernosa. The patient appears to have a permanent erection after the procedure; the patient is able to bend the penis into position at the time of intercourse.

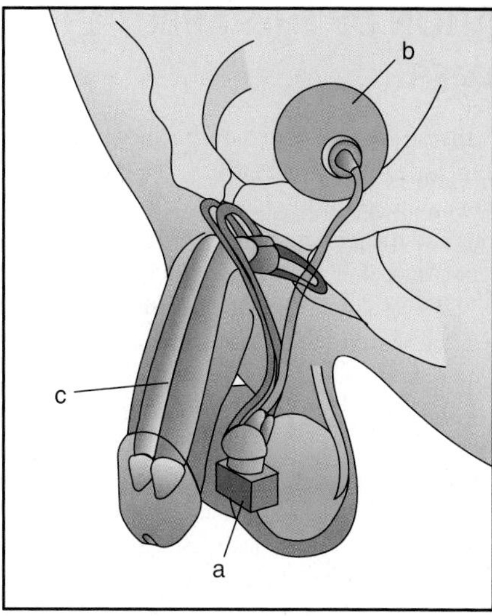

FIGURE 83-7 Example of surgically implanted penile prosthesis. (a, activation mechanism; b, reservoir with fluid for inflating prosthesis; c, inflatable rods in corpora.) *(From http://kidney.niddk.nih.gov/kudiseases/pubs/impotence.)*

The inflatable prosthesis has several mechanical parts. The inflatable prosthesis produces a more natural erection. The patient develops an erection only when the device is activated. Some newer advances in inflatable prosthesis technology have resulted in devices with fewer mechanical parts. These devices can be placed during shorter surgical procedures and have a low 5-year mechanical failure rate (6%-10%) as compared with the original inflatable prostheses (Fig. 83-7).[21,98]

Penile prostheses provide penile rigidity suitable for vaginal intercourse and are associated with a greater than 90% patient satisfaction rate, which is generally higher than that observed with any other drug treatment or VED.[99] The surgical success rate after insertion is 82% to 98%.[21]

Adverse effects of prosthesis insertion can occur early or late after the surgical procedure. The most common early complication is infection. Late complications include mechanical failure of the prosthesis, particularly when an inflatable prosthesis has been inserted. With improved technology, the mechanical failure rate has decreased to 5%.[99] Other late complications include erosion of the rods through the penis or late-onset infection. Although some salvage procedures have been devised, in many cases the prosthesis requires removal.

Personalized Pharmacotherapy

For the management of erectile dysfunction, treatment selection must be individualized based on the patient's preferences for and perception of the effectiveness of various treatment options, out-of-pocket costs for treatment, and potential adverse effects.

In general, patients prefer a discreet form of treatment that is not obvious to the sexual partner and that does not require careful attention to timing of administration relative to sexual intercourse. Because treatment for erectile dysfunction is not included as a covered item on many insurance plans, the cost of treatment is likely to be a consideration for most patients.

For patients with both moderately symptomatic benign prostatic hyperplasia and erectile dysfunction, a reasonable approach is the use of daily tadalafil, which should be effective for both conditions.

For patients who fail treatment with a single medication, a VED, a combination drug regimen, or surgical intervention are options.

EVALUATION OF THERAPEUTIC OUTCOMES

The primary therapeutic outcomes of specific treatments for erectile dysfunction include (a) improvement in the quantity and quality of penile erections suitable for intercourse and (b) avoidance of adverse drug reactions and drug interactions.

At baseline and after the patient has completed a clinical trial period of several weeks with a specific treatment for erectile dysfunction, the physician should conduct assessments to determine whether the quality and quantity of penile erections has improved. A patient's level of satisfaction is highly individualized, depending on his lifestyle and expectations. Therefore, a patient who has successful intercourse once per week might be completely satisfied, whereas another patient might judge this to be unsatisfactory. Patients with unrealistic expectations in this regard must be identified and counseled by clinicians to avoid adverse effects of excessive use of erectogenic agents.

Failure to improve the quality and quantity of penile erections suitable for intercourse after an appropriate clinical trial period with a specific treatment for erectile dysfunction occurs in a significant percentage of patients. In this case, physicians generally take the following steps in order:

1. Ensure that the patient has been prescribed a maximum tolerated dose and has an adequate clinical trial of a specific treatment before discarding it as ineffective.
2. Switch to another drug (see Fig. 83-2).
3. Reserve surgical treatment for patients who do not respond to drug treatment.

CONCLUSION

Erectile dysfunction is a common disorder of aging men. Its incidence is higher in patients with underlying medical disorders that compromise the vascular, neurologic, hormonal, or psychogenic systems necessary for a normal penile erection. Medications are common causes of erectile dysfunction. By correcting the underlying etiology, erectile dysfunction can often be reversed without the use of specific treatments.

When treatment of erectile dysfunction is needed, the least invasive options should be used first because they produce the lowest incidence of serious adverse effects. Phosphodiesterase type 5 inhibitors are first-line treatment. If this fails or if the patient cannot use a phosphodiesterase type 5 inhibitor, a VED or intracavernosal alprostadil injection therapy can be initiated. If this treatment fails, the patient can attempt a combination of intracavernosal alprostadil plus VED, combination intracavernosal therapy, or intraurethral alprostadil. If this treatment fails, the patient may require insertion of a penile prosthesis.

Some insurance companies do not reimburse for drug treatments for erectile dysfunction, so cost is an important issue for patients.

Clinicians should provide clear and simple advice. Patient confidentiality and privacy, which are extremely important to men with erectile dysfunction, should be maintained at all times.

ABBREVIATIONS

cAMP	cyclic adenosine monophosphate
cGMP	cyclic guanosine monophosphate
CNS	central nervous system
IIEF	International Index of Erectile Function
LUTS	lower urinary tract symptoms
NAION	nonarteritic anterior ischemic optic neuropathy
VED	vacuum erection device

REFERENCES

1. NIH Consensus Conference. NIH Consensus Development Panel on Impotence. Impotence. *JAMA* 1993;270:83-90.
2. Qaseem A, Snow V, Denberg TD, et al. Clinical efficacy assessment subcommittee of the American College of Physicians: Hormonal testing and pharmacologic treatment of erectile dysfunction: A clinical practice guideline from the American College of Physicians. *Ann Intern Med* 2009;151:639-649.
3. Johannes CB, Aranjo AB, Feldman HA, et al. Incidence of erectile dysfunction in men 40–69 years old: Longitudinal results from the Massachusetts Male Aging Study. *J Urol* 2000;163:460-463.
4. Porst H. Burnett A, Brock G, et al. SOP conservative (medical and mechanical treatment of erectile dysfunction. *J Sex Med* 2013;10:130-171.
5. Bacon CG, Mittleman MA, Kawach I, et al. Sexual function in men older than 50 years of age: Results from the Health Professionals Follow-up Study. *Ann Intern Med* 2003;139:161-168.
6. Kim SC, Seo KK, Kim TH. Reasons and predictive factors for discontinuation of PDE-5 inhibitors despite successful intercourse in erectile dysfunction patients. *Int J Impot Res* 2013;26:87-93.
7. Frederick LR, Cakir OO, Arora H, et al. Undertreatment of erectile dysfunction: Claims analysis of 6.2 million patients. *J Sex Med* 2014;11:2546-2553.
8. Ludwig W, Phillips M. Organic causes of erectile dysfunction in men under 40. *Urol Int* 2014;92:1-6.
9. Albersen M, Mwamukonda KB, Shindel AW, Lue TF. Evaluation and treatment of erectile dysfunction. *Med Clin North Am* 2011;95:201-212.
10. Andersson KE. Mechanisms of penile erection and basis for pharmacological treatment of erectile dysfunction. *Pharmacol Rev* 2011;63(4):811-859.
11. Pye SR, Huhtaniemi IT, Finn JD, et al. Late-onset hypogonadism and mortality in aging men. *J Clin Endocrinol Metab* 2014;99:1357-1366.
12. Tajar A, Huhtaniemi IT, O'Neill TW, et al. Characteristics of androgen deficiency in late-onset hypogonadism: Results from the European Male Aging Study. *J Clin Endocrinol Metab* 2012;97(5):1508-1516.
13. Paduch DA, Brannigan RE, Fuchs EF, et al. The laboratory diagnosis of testosterone deficiency. *Urology* 2014;83:980-988.
14. Wang C, Nieschlag E, Swerdloff R, et al. Investigation, treatment and monitoring of late onset hypogonadism in males. *Int J Androl* 2009;32:1-10.
15. Greenspan MB, Barkin J. Erectile dysfunction and testosterone deficiency syndrome: The portal to men's health. *Can J Urol* 2012;19(Suppl 1):18-27.
16. Luenfeld B, Mskhalaya G, Kalinchenko S, et al. Recommendations on the diagnosis, treatment, and monitoring of late onset hypogonadism in men-a suggested update. *Aging Male* 2013;16:153-150.
17. Berookhim BM, Bar-Chama N. Medical implications of erectile dysfunction. *Med Clin North Am* 2011;95:213-221.
18. Clayton AH, Croft HA, Handiwala L. Antidepressants and sexual function: Mechanisms and clinical implications. *Postgrad Med* 2014;126:91-99.
19. Kennedy SH, Rizvi S. Sexual dysfunction, depression, and the impact of antidepressants. *J Clin Psychopharmacol* 2009;29(2):157-164.
20. Handler J. Managing erectile dysfunction in hypertensive patients. *J Clin Hypertens* 2011;13:450-454.
21. American Urological Association Guideline on the Management of Erectile Dysfunction: Diagnosis and Treatment Recommendations; updated 2006, confirmed 2011. http://www.auanet.org/content/guidelines-and-quality-care/clinical-guidelines.cfm?sub=ed. (Accessed August 19, 2015)
22. Rosen RC, Riley A, Wagner G, et al. The International Index of Erectile Function (IIEF): A multidimensional scale for assessment of erectile dysfunction. *Urology* 1997;49:822-830.
23. Bhasin S, Cunningham GR, Hayes FJ. Testosterone therapy in men with androgen deficiency syndromes: An Endocrine Society Clinical Practice Guideline. *J Clin Endocrinol Metab* 2010;95(6):2536-2559.
24. Inman BA, St. Souver JL, Jacobson DJ, et al. A population-based longitudinal study of erectile dysfunction and future coronary artery disease. *Mayo Clin Proc* 2009;84:108-113.
25. Nehra A. Erectile dysfunction and cardiovascular disease: Efficacy and safety of phosphodiesterase type 5 inhibitors in men with both conditions. *Mayo Clin Proc* 2009;84:139-148.
26. Nehra A, Jackson G, Miner M, et al. The Princeton III Consensus recommendations for the management of erectile dysfunction and cardiovascular disease. *Mayo Clin Proc* 2012;87(8):766-778.

27. Miner M, Rosenberg MT, Barkin J. Erectile dysfunction in primary care: A focus on cardiometabolic risk evaluation and stratification for future cardiovascular events. *Can J Urol* 2014;21:25-38.
28. Gupta BP, Murad H, Clifton MM, et al. The effect of lifestyle modification and cardiovascular risk factor reduction on erectile dysfunction. *Arch Intern Med* 2011;171:1797-1803.
29. Kovac JR, Labbate C, Ramasamy R, et al. Effects of cigarette smoking on erectile dysfunction. *Andrologia* 2015;47(10):1087-1092. Doi:10.1111/and.12393.
30. Montorsi F, Adaikan G, Becher E, et al. Summary of the recommendations on sexual dysfunction in men. *J Sex Med* 2010;7:3572-3588.
31. Hatzimouratidis K, Amar E, Eardley I, et al. Guidelines on male sexual dysfunction, erectile dysfunction and premature ejaculation. *Eur Urol* 2010;57:804-814.
32. Pahlajani G, Raina R, Jones S, et al. Vacuum erection devices revisited: Its emerging role in the treatment of erectile dysfunction and early penile rehabilitation following prostate cancer therapy. *J Sex Med* 2012;9:1182-1189.
33. Hoyland K, Vasdev N, Adshead J. The use of vacuum erection devices in erectile dysfunction after radical prostatectomy. *Rev Urol* 2013;15:67-71.
34. Sun L, Peng FL, Yu ZL, et al. Combined sildenafil with vacuum erection device therapy in the management of diabetic men with erectile dysfunction after failure of first-line sildenafil monotherapy. *Int J Urol* 2014;21:1263-1267.
35. Uckert S, Kuczyk MA, Oelke M. Phosphodiesterase inhibitors in clinical urology. *Expert Rev Clin Pharmacol* 2013;6:323-332.
36. Bruzziches R, Francomano D, Gareri P, et al. An update on pharmacological treatment of erectile dysfunction with phosphodiesterase type 5 inhibitors. *Expert Opin Pharmacother* 2013;14:1333-1344.
37. Mirone V, Fusco F, Rossi A, et al. Tadalafil and vardenafil vs sildenafil: A review of patient preference studies. *BJU Int* 2009;103:1212-1217.
38. Albersen M, Orabi H, Lue TF. Evaluation and treatment of erectile dysfunction in the aging male: A mini-review. *Gerontology* 2012;58:3-14.
39. Hatzichristou D, Moysidis K, Apostolidis A, et al. Sildenafil failures may be due to inadequate patient instructions and follow-up: A study of 100 non-responders. *Eur Urol* 2005;47:518-523.
40. Carson CC. Long-term use of sildenafil. *Expert Opin Pharmacother* 2003;4:397-405.
41. Lombardi G, Macchiarella A, Cecconi F, Del Popolo G. Ten-year follow-up of sildenafil use in spinal cord-injured patients with erectile dysfunction. *J Sex Med* 2009;6(12):3449-3457.
42. Vernet D, Magee T, Qian A, et al. Phosphodiesterase type 5 is not upregulated by tadalafil in cultures of human penile cells. *J Sex Med* 2006;3:84-94.
43. Carvalheira A, Forjaz V, Pereira NM. Adherence to phosphodiesterase type 5 inhibitors in the treatment of erectile dysfunction in long–term users: How do men use the inhibitors. *Sex Med* 2014;2(2):96-102.
44. Brisson TE, Broderick GA, Thiel DD, et al. Vardenafil rescue rates of sildenafil nonresponders: Objective assessment of 327 patients with erectile dysfunction. *Urology* 2006;68:397-401.
45. McMahon CG. High dose sildenafil as a salvage therapy for severe erectile dysfunction. *Int J Impot Res* 2002;14:533-538.
46. Aversa A, Francomano D, Lenzi A. Does testosterone supplementation increase PDE5-inhibitor responses in difficult-to-treat erectile dysfunction patients? *Expert Opin Pharmacother* 2015;16(5):625-628.
47. Dhir RR, Lin H-C, Canfield SE, Wang R. Combination therapy for erectile dysfunction: An update review. *Asian J Androl* 2011;13:382-390.
48. Mydlo JH, Viterbo R, Crispen P. Use of combined intracorporal injection and a phosphodiesterase-5 inhibitor therapy for men with a suboptimal response to sildenafil and/or vardenafil monotherapy after radical retropubic prostatectomy. *BJU Int* 2005;95:843-846.
49. Tsertsvadze A, Fink HA, Yazdi F, et al. Oral phosphodiesterase-5 inhibitors and hormonal treatments for erectile dysfunction: A systematic review and meta-analysis. *Ann Intern Med* 2009;151:650-661.
50. Sperling H, Gittelman M, Norenberg C, et al. Efficacy and safety of an orodispersible vardenafil formulation for the treatment of erectile dysfunction in elderly men and those with underlying conditions: An integrated analysis of two pivotal trials. *J Sex Med* 2011;8:261-271.
51. Shabsigh R, Seftel AD, Rosen RC, et al. Review of time of onset and duration of clinical efficacy of phosphodiesterase type 5 inhibitors in treatment of erectile dysfunction. *Urology* 2006;68:689-696.
52. Eardley I, Donatucci C, Corbin J, et al. Pharmacotherapy for erectile dysfunction. *J Sex Med* 2010;7:524-540.
53. Fusco F, Razzoli F, Imbimbo C, et al. A new era in the treatment of erectile dysfunction: Chronic phosphodiesterase type 5 inhibition. *BJU Int* 2010:105:1634-1639.
54. Ricardi U, Gontero P, Ciammella P, et al. Efficacy and safety of tadalafil 20 mg on demand vs tadalafil 5 mg once-a-day in the treatment of post-radiotherapy erectile dysfunction in prostate cancer men: A randomized phase II trial. *J Sex Med* 2010;7:2851-2859.
55. Porst H, Giuliano F, Glina S, et al. Evaluation of the efficacy and safety of once-a-day dosing of tadalafil 5 mg and 10 mg in the treatment of erectile dysfunction: Results of a multicenter, randomized, double-blind, placebo-controlled trial. *Eur Urol* 2006;50:351-359.
56. Lee KCJ, Brock GB. Daily dosing of PDE5 inhibitors: Where does it fit in? *Curr Urol Rep* 2013;14:269-278.
57. El-Sakka AI. Alleviation of post-radical prostatectomy cavernosal fibrosis: Future directions and potential utility for PDE5 inhibitors. *Expert Opin Investig Drugs* 2011;20(1):1305-1309.
58. Montorsi F, Briganti A, Salonia A, et al. Can phosphodiesterase inhibitors cure erectile dysfunction? *Eur Urol* 2006;49:979-986.
59. Taylor J, Baldo OB, Storey A, et al. Differences in side effect, duration and related bother levels between phosphodiesterase type 5 inhibitors. *BJU Int* 2009;103:1392-1395.
60. Giuliano F, Jackson G, Montorsi F, et al. Safety of sildenafil citrate: Review of 67 double-blind placebo-controlled trials and the postmarketing safety database. *Int J Clin Pract* 2010;64:240-255.
61. Jannini EA, Isidori AM, Gravina GL, et al. The Endotrial Study: A spontaneous, open label, randomized, multicenter cross-over study on the efficacy of sildenafil, tadalafil, and vardenafil in the treatment of erectile dysfunction. *J Sex Med* 2009;6:2547-2560.
62. Laties A. Vision disorders and phosphodiesterase type 5 inhibitors. *Drug Saf* 2009;32:1-18.
63. Katz EG, Tan RB, Rittenberg D, et al. Avanafil for erectile dysfunction in elderly and young adults: Differential pharmacology and clinical utility. *Ther Clin Risk Manag* 2014;10:701-711.
64. Nathoo NA, Etminan M, Mikelberg FS. Association between phosphodiesterase-5-inhibitors and nonarteritic anterior ischemic optic neuropathy. *J Neuroophthalmol* 2015;35:12-15.
65. Maddox Pt, Saunders J, Chandrasekhar SS. Sudden hearing loss from PDE-5 inhibitors: A possible cellular stress etiology. *Laryngoscope* 2009;119:1586-1589.
66. Okuyucu S, Guven OE, Akoglu E, et al. Effect of phosphodiesterase-5 inhibitor on hearing. *J Laryngol Otol* 2009;123:718-722.
67. Li WQ, Qureshi AA, Robinson KC. Sildenafil use and increased risk of incident melanoma. *JAMA Intern Med* 204;174 (6):964-970.
68. Loeb S, Folkvalijon Y, Lambe M, et al. Use of phosphodiesterase type 5 inhibitors for erectile dysfunction and risk of malignant melanoma. *JAMA* 2015;313:2449-2455.
69. Levine GN, Steinke EE, Bakaeen FG, et al. Sexual activity and cardiovascular disease: A scientific statement from the American Heart Association. *Circulation* 2012;125:1058-1072.
70. Schwartz BG, Kloner RA. Drug interactions with phosphodiesterase-5 inhibitors used for the treatment of erectile dysfunction or pulmonary hypertension. *Circulation* 2010;122(1):88-95.
71. Kloner RA. Pharmacology and drug interaction effects of the phosphodiesterase 5 inhibitors: Focus on α blocker interactions. *Am J Cardiol* 2005;96(Suppl):42M-46M.
72. Reffelmann T, Kieback A, Kloner RA. The cardiovascular safety of tadalafil. *Expert Opin Drug Saf* 2008;7:43-52.
73. Giuliano F, Kaplan SA, Cabanis MJ, Astruc B. Hemodynamic interaction study between the $alpha_1$ blocker alfuzosin and the phosphodiesterase-5 inhibitor tadalafil in middle-aged healthy male subjects. *Urology* 2006;67:1199-1204.
74. Ng CF, Wong A, Cheng CW, et al. Effect of vardenafil on blood pressure profile of patients with erectile dysfunction concomitantly treated with doxazosin gastrointestinal therapeutic system for benign prostatic hyperplasia. *J Urol* 2008;180:1042-1046.
75. Corona G, Razzoli E, Forti G, Maggi M. The use of phosphodiesterase 5 inhibitors with concomitant medications. *J Endocrinol Invest* 2008;31(9):799-808.
76. Barkin J. Erectile dysfunction and hypogonadism. *Can J Urol* 2011;18(Suppl 1):2-7.

77. Afiadata A, Ellsworth P. Testosterone replacement therapy: Who to evaluate, what to use, how to follow and who is at risk? *Hosp Pract* 2014;41:69-82.
78. Conners WP, Morgentaler A. The evaluation and management of testosterone deficiency: The new frontier in urology and men's health. *Curr Urol Rep* 2013;14:557-564.
79. Matsumoto AM. Testosterone administration in older men. *Endocrinol Metab Clin North Am* 2013;42:271-286.
80. Wang C, Swerdloff R, Kipnes M, et al. New testosterone buccal system (Striant) delivers physiological testosterone levels: Pharmacokinetics study in hypogonadal men. *J Clin Endocrinol Metab* 2004;89:3821-3829.
81. Corona G, Maseroli E, Maggi M. Injectable testosterone undecanoate for the treatment of hypogonadism. *Expert Opin Pharmacother* 2014;15:1903-1926.
81. Ullah MI, Riche DM, Koch CA. Transdermal testosterone replacement therapy in men. *Drug Des Dev Ther* 2014;8:101-112.
82. Morely JE, Charlton E, Patrick P, et al. Validation of a screening questionnaire for androgen deficiency in aging males. *Metabolism* 2000;49:1239-1242.
83. Kang DY, Li HJ. The effect of testosterone replacement therapy on prostate-specific antigen levels in men being treated for hypogonadism: A systematic review and meta-analysis. *Medicine* 2015;94:e410.
84. Morgentaler A, Benesh JA, Denes BS, et al. Factors influencing prostate specific antigen response among men treated with testosterone therapy for 6 months. *J Sex Med* 2014;11:2818-2825.
85. Dupree JM, Langille GM, Kkhera M, et al. The safety of testosterone supplementation therapy in prostate cancer. *Nat Rev Urol* 2014;11:526-530.
86. Schoenfeld MJ, Shortridge E, Cui Z, et al. Medication adherence and treatment patterns for hypogonadal patients treated with topical testosterone therapy: A retrospective medical claims analysis. *J Sex Med* 2013;10:1401-1409.
87. Vigen R, O'Donnell CI, Baron AE, et al. Association of testosterone therapy with mortality, myocardial infarction, and stroke in men with low testosterone levels. *JAMA* 2013;310:1829-1836.
88. Finkle WD, Greenland S, Ridgeway GK, et al. Increased risk of nonfatal myocardial infarction following testosterone therapy prescription in men. *PLoS One* 2014;9(1);e85805.
89. Garnick MB. Testosterone replacement therapy faces FDA scrutiny. *JAMA* 2015;313:563-564.
90. Kendirci M, Tanriverdi O, Trost L, et al. Management of sildenafil treatment failures. *Curr Opin Urol* 2006;16:449-459.
91. Jakubczyk T. Intracavernosal injections in the diagnosis and treatment of PDE-5 resistant erectile dysfunction. *Cent European J Urol* 2013;66:215-216.
92. Albersen M, Orabi H, Lue TF. Evaluation and treatment of erectile dysfunction in the aging male: A mini-review. *Gerontology* 2012;58:3-14.
93. Khera M, Goldstein I. Erectile dysfunction. *BMJ Clin Evid* 2011;2011. pii 1803.
94. Engel JD, McVary KT. Transurethral alprostadil as therapy for patients who withdrew from or failed prior intracavernous injection therapy. *Urology* 1998;51:687-692.
95. Costa P, Potempa AJ. Intraurethral alprostadil for erectile dysfunction: A review of the literature. *Drugs* 2012;72:2243-2254.
96. Ernst E, Pittler MH. Yohimbine for erectile dysfunction: A systematic review and meta-analysis of randomized clinical trials. *J Urol* 1998;159:422-426.
97. Brown SL, Haas CA, Koehler M, et al. Hepatotoxicity related to intracavernous pharmacotherapy with papaverine. *Urology* 1998;52:844-847.
98. Trost LW, McCaslin R, Linder B, et al. Long-term outcomes of penile prostheses for the treatment of erectile dysfunction. *Expert Rev Med Devices* 2013;10:353-366.
99. Mulcahy JJ, Kramer A, Brant WO, et al. Current management of penile implant infections, device reliability, and optimizing cosmetic outcome. *Curr Urol Rep* 2014;15(6):413. Doi: 10.107/s11934-014-0413-6.

Benign Prostatic Hyperplasia

Mary Lee and Roohollah Sharifi

84

KEY CONCEPTS

1 Although symptomatic benign prostatic hyperplasia (BPH) is rare in men younger than 50 years, it is common in men 60 years and older. Prostate growth is androgen-dependent. Symptoms commonly result from both static and dynamic factors.

2 BPH symptoms may be exacerbated by medications, including antihistamines, phenothiazines, tricyclic antidepressants, and anticholinergic agents. In these cases, discontinuing the causative agent can relieve symptoms.

3 For patients with mild disease who are asymptomatic or have mildly bothersome symptoms and no complications of BPH disease, watchful waiting is indicated. Watchful waiting includes behavior modification, lifestyle modification, discontinuation of medications that contribute to voiding symptoms, and return visits to the physician at 6- or 12-month intervals for assessment of worsening symptoms or signs of bladder outlet obstruction.

4 If symptoms progress to a moderate or severe level, drug therapy or surgery is indicated. α_1-Adrenergic antagonists quickly relieve voiding symptoms, but do not prevent disease progression. 5α-Reductase inhibitors delay symptom progression and reduce the incidence of BPH-related complications in patients with prostates of at least 30 to 40 g, but may not reduce voiding symptoms for 3 to 6 months.

5 All α_1-adrenergic antagonists are equally effective in relieving BPH symptoms. Older second-generation immediate-release formulations of α_1-adrenergic antagonists (eg, terazosin, doxazosin) can cause adverse cardiovascular effects, mainly first-dose syncope, orthostatic hypotension, and dizziness. For patients who cannot tolerate these hypotensive adverse effects, the third-generation, pharmacologically uroselective agents α_{1A}-adrenergic antagonists (eg, tamsulosin, silodosin) or an extended-release formulation of alfuzosin, a second-generation, functionally uroselective agent, are good alternatives.

6 5α-Reductase inhibitors are useful primarily for patients with large prostates greater than 30 to 40 g who wish to avoid surgery and cannot tolerate the side effects of α_1-adrenergic antagonists. 5α-Reductase inhibitors have a slow onset of action, taking up to 6 months to exert maximal clinical effects, which is a disadvantage of their use, especially when used as single drug therapy for BPH. In addition, decreased libido, erectile dysfunction, and ejaculation disorders are common adverse effects, which may be troublesome problems in sexually active patients.

7 Phosphodiesterase inhibitors can be used in patients with moderate to severe BPH and erectile dysfunction. They improve irritative voiding symptoms, but do not produce significant increases in urinary flow rate or reductions in postvoid residual (PVR) urine volume. Hence, a phosphodiesterase inhibitor is considered less effective than an α-adrenergic antagonist for BPH. A phosphodiesterase inhibitor may be used alone; however, symptom improvement and an increase in peak urinary flow rate has been demonstrated when the phosphodiesterase inhibitor is used along with an α-adrenergic antagonist or a 5α-reductase inhibitor.

8 Anticholinergic agents are indicated in patients with moderate to severe lower urinary tract symptoms (LUTS) with a predominance of irritative voiding symptoms. In this case, the drugs are commonly added on to an existing regimen of an α_1-adrenergic antagonist or a 5α-reductase inhibitor. Because older patients are at high risk of systemic and central nervous system anticholinergic adverse effects, uroselective anticholinergic agents may be preferred over nonuroselective agents. To minimize the risk of acute urinary retention, anticholinergics should be used cautiously in patients when the PVR urine volume is greater than 100 to 150 mL before initiating treatment with an anticholinergic agent. In addition, the potential anticholinergic medication burden should be assessed before starting an anticholinergic agent.

9 Mirabegron is a β_3-adrenergic agonist that relaxes the detrusor muscle to increase the bladder's storage capacity and prolong the interval between voidings. Although not FDA-approved for management of BPH, it is indicated for treatment of overactive bladder symptoms, including urgency and nocturia. These symptoms mimic irritative lower urinary tract voiding symptoms. Thus, mirabegron is used as an alternative to anticholinergic agents in patients with irritative voiding symptoms that do not respond to α_1-adrenergic antagonists or in patients who cannot tolerate anticholinergic adverse effects.

10 Surgery is indicated for moderate to severe symptoms of BPH for patients who do not respond to or do not tolerate drug therapy, or for patients with complications of BPH. It is the most effective mode of treatment because it relieves symptoms and increases peak urinary flow rate in the greatest number of men with BPH. However, the two standard techniques, transurethral resection of the prostate (TURP) and open prostatectomy, are associated with the highest rates of complications, including retrograde ejaculation and erectile dysfunction. Therefore, minimally invasive surgical procedures are often desired by patients. These relieve symptoms and are associated with a lower rate of adverse effects and do not require hospitalization, but they have higher reoperation rates than the standard procedures.

Benign prostatic hyperplasia (BPH) is the most common benign neoplasm of American men. A nearly ubiquitous condition among elderly men, BPH is of major societal concern, given the large number of men affected, the progressive nature of the condition, and the healthcare costs associated with it.

This chapter discusses BPH and its available treatments: watchful waiting, α_1-adrenergic antagonists, 5α-reductase inhibitors, phosphodiesterase inhibitors, anticholinergic agents, mirabegron, and surgery. The limitations of phytotherapy are described.

EPIDEMIOLOGY

According to the results of autopsy studies, approximately 80% of older men develop histologic evidence of BPH. About half of the patients with microscopic changes develop an enlarged prostate gland, and as a result, they may develop symptoms including difficulty emptying urine from the urinary bladder. Approximately half of symptomatic patients eventually require treatment. Thus, the disease can be characterized by three stages: BPH, benign prostatic enlargement (BPE), and benign prostatic obstruction (BPO). While BPH itself may not require treatment, some patients with BPE, depending on the size of the prostate, will be at risk of developing complications of BPH. In these patients, 5α-reductase inhibitors can reduce disease complications and delay the need for prostate surgery. In patients with moderate to severe BPO, bothersome voiding symptoms require medical or surgical treatment.

1 The peak incidence of clinical BPH occurs between ages 63 and 65 years. Symptomatic disease is uncommon in men younger than 50 years, but some urinary voiding symptoms are present by the time men turn 60 years. The Boston Area Normative Aging Study estimated that the cumulative incidence of clinical BPH was 78% for patients at age 80 years.[1] Similarly, the Baltimore Longitudinal Study of Aging projected that approximately 60% of men at least 60 years old develop clinical BPH.[2]

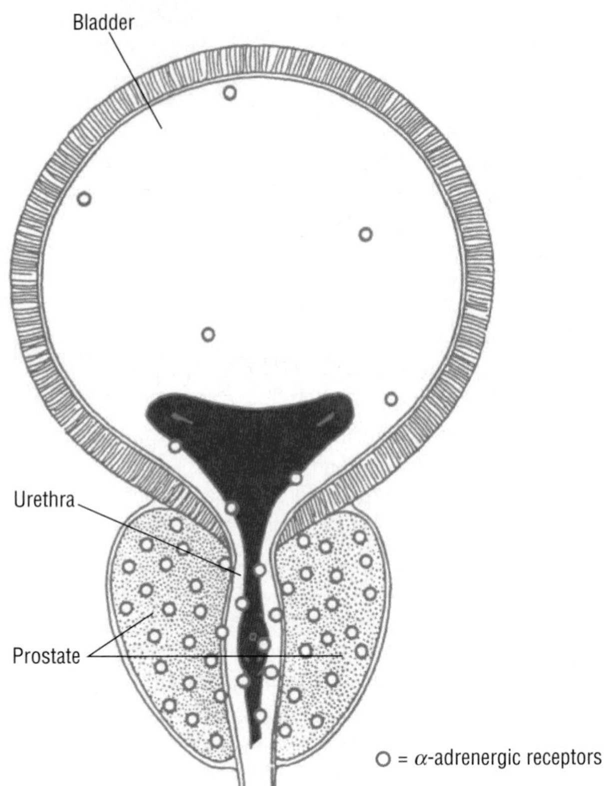

FIGURE 84-1 Representation of the anatomy of and α-adrenergic receptor distribution in the prostate, urethra, and bladder. *(Narayan P, Indudhara R. Pharmacotherapy for benign prostatic hyperplasia. Western Journal of Medicine. 1994;161(5):495-506. Copyright © 1994 with permission from BMJ Publishing Group Ltd.)*

NORMAL PROSTATE PHYSIOLOGY

Located anterior to the rectum, the prostate is a small heart-shaped, chestnut-sized gland located below the urinary bladder. It surrounds the proximal urethra like a doughnut.

Soft, symmetric, and mobile on palpation, a normal prostate gland in an adult man weighs 15 to 20 g. Physical examination of the prostate must be done by digital rectal examination (ie, the prostate is manually palpated by inserting a finger into the rectum). Thus, the prostate is examined through the rectal wall.

The prostate has two major functions: (a) to secrete fluids that make up a portion (20%-40%) of the ejaculate volume and (b) to provide secretions with antibacterial effect possibly related to its high concentration of zinc.[2]

At birth, the prostate is the size of a pea and weighs approximately 1 g. The prostate remains that size until the boy reaches puberty. At that time, the prostate undergoes its first growth spurt, growing to its normal adult size of 15 to 20 g by the time the young man is 25 to 30 years old. The prostate remains this size until the patient reaches age 40 years, when a second growth spurt begins and continues for the rest of his lifetime. During this period, the prostate can quadruple in size or grow even larger.

The prostate gland comprises three types of tissue: epithelial tissue, stromal tissue, and the capsule. Epithelial tissue, also known as *glandular tissue*, produces prostatic secretions. These secretions are delivered into the urethra during ejaculation and contribute to the total ejaculate volume. Androgens stimulate epithelial tissue growth. Stromal tissue, also known as *smooth muscle tissue*, is embedded predominantly with α_1-adrenergic receptors. Of the α_1-adrenergic receptors, 65% to 75% of them are of the α_{1A} subtype.[3] Stimulation of these receptors by norepinephrine causes smooth muscle contraction, which results in an extrinsic compression of the urethra, reduction of the urethral lumen, and decreased urinary bladder emptying. The normal prostate is composed of a higher amount of stromal tissue than epithelial tissue, as reflected by a stromal-to-epithelial tissue ratio of 2:1. This ratio is exaggerated to 5:1 for patients with BPH, which explains why α_1-adrenergic antagonists are quickly effective in symptomatic management and why 5α-reductase inhibitors reduce an enlarged prostate gland by only 25%.[2,4] The capsule, or outer shell of the prostate, is composed of fibrous connective tissue and smooth muscle, which also is embedded with α_1-adrenergic receptors. When stimulated with norepinephrine, the capsule contracts around the prostatic urethra (Fig. 84-1).

Testosterone is the principal testicular androgen in males, whereas androstenedione is the principal adrenal androgen. These two hormones are responsible for penile and scrotal enlargement, increased muscle mass, and maintenance of the normal male libido. These androgens are converted by 5α-reductase in target cells to dihydrotestosterone (DHT), an active metabolite. Two types of 5α-reductase exist. Type I enzyme is localized to sebaceous glands in the frontal scalp, liver, and skin, although a small amount is in the prostate. DHT produced at these target tissues causes acne and increased body and facial hair. Type II enzyme is localized to the prostate, genital tissue, and hair follicles of the scalp. In the prostate, DHT induces growth and enlargement of the gland.[3]

In prostate cells, DHT has greater affinity for intraprostatic androgen receptors than testosterone, and DHT forms a more stable complex with the androgen receptor. Thus, DHT is considered a more potent androgen than testosterone in the prostate. Of note, despite the decrease in testicular androgen production in the aging male, intracellular DHT levels in the prostate remain normal, probably due to increased activity of intraprostatic 5α-reductase.[3]

Estrogen, a product of peripheral metabolism of androgens, is believed to stimulate the growth of the stromal portion of the prostate gland. Estrogens are produced when testosterone and androstenedione are converted by aromatase enzymes in peripheral adipose tissues. In addition, estrogens may induce the androgen receptor.[2] As men age, the ratio of serum levels of testosterone to estrogen decreases as a result of a decline in testosterone production by the testes and increased adipose tissue conversion of androgen to estrogen.

PATHOPHYSIOLOGY

Although the precise pathophysiologic mechanisms causing BPH remain unclear, the role of intraprostatic DHT and type II 5α-reductase in the development of BPH is evidenced by several observations:

1. BPH does not develop in men who are castrated before puberty.
2. Patients with type II 5α-reductase enzyme deficiency do not develop BPH.
3. Castration causes an enlarged prostate to shrink.
4. Administration of testosterone to orchiectomized dogs of advanced age produces BPH.

The pathogenesis of BPH is often described as resulting from both static and dynamic factors. Static factors relate to anatomic enlargement of the prostate gland, which produces a physical block at the bladder neck and thereby obstructs urinary outflow. Enlargement of the gland depends on androgen stimulation of epithelial tissue and estrogen stimulation of stromal tissue in the prostate. Dynamic factors relate to excessive α-adrenergic tone of the stromal component of the prostate gland, bladder neck, and posterior urethra, which results in contraction of the prostate gland around the urethra and narrowing of the urethral lumen.

Symptoms of BPH disease may result from static and/or dynamic factors, and this must be recognized when drug therapy is considered. For instance, some patients may present with obstructive voiding symptoms, but have prostates of normal size. In these patients, dynamic factors likely are responsible for the symptoms. However, for patients with enlarged prostate glands, static and dynamic factors likely are working in concert to produce the observed symptoms. Moreover, the likelihood of developing moderate to severe obstructive voiding symptoms is directly related to the increasing size of the prostate gland.[5]

Static factors may be accentuated if the patient becomes stressed or is in pain. In these situations, increased α-adrenergic tone may precipitate excessive contraction of prostatic stromal tissue. When the stressful event resolves, voiding symptoms often improve.[2]

MEDICATION-RELATED SYMPTOMS

2 Medications in several pharmacologic categories should be avoided for patients with BPH because they may exacerbate symptoms.[6] Testosterone replacement regimens, used to treat primary or secondary hypogonadism, deliver additional substrate that can be metabolized to DHT by the prostate. Although no cases of BPH have been reported because of exogenous testosterone administration, cautious use is advised for older patients with prostatic enlargement. α-Adrenergic agonists, used as oral or intranasal decongestants (eg, pseudoephedrine, ephedrine, or phenylephrine), can stimulate α-adrenergic receptors in the prostate, resulting in muscle contraction. By decreasing the caliber of the urethral lumen, bladder emptying may be compromised. β-Adrenergic agonists (eg, terbutaline) may cause relaxation of the bladder detrusor muscle, which prevents bladder emptying.[7] Drugs with significant anticholinergic adverse effects (eg, antihistamines, phenothiazines, tricyclic antidepressants, or anticholinergic drugs used as antispasmodics or to treat Parkinson disease) may decrease contractility of the urinary bladder detrusor muscle. For patients with BPH who have a narrowed urethral lumen, loss of effective detrusor contraction could result in acute urinary retention, particularly for patients with significantly enlarged prostate glands and a PVR urine volume greater than 150 mL. Diuretics, particularly in large doses, can produce polyuria, which may present as urinary frequency, similar to that experienced by patients with BPH.

CLINICAL PRESENTATION

Patients with BPH can present with a variety of symptoms and signs of disease. All symptoms of BPH can be divided into two categories: obstructive and irritative.

Obstructive symptoms, also known as *prostatism* or *bladder outlet obstruction*, result when dynamic and/or static factors reduce bladder emptying. The force of the urinary stream becomes diminished, urinary flow rate decreases, and bladder emptying is incomplete and slow. Patients report urinary hesitancy and straining and a weak urine stream. Urine dribbles out of the penis, and the urinary bladder always feels full, even after patients have voided. Some patients state that they need to press on their bladder to force out the urine. In severe cases, patients may go into urinary retention when bladder emptying is not possible. In these cases, suprapubic pain can result from bladder overdistension.

Approximately 50% to 80% of patients have irritative voiding symptoms, which typically occur late in the disease course. Irritative voiding symptoms result from long-standing obstruction of the bladder neck. The detrusor muscle cholinergic receptors become supersensitive to small volumes of urine in the bladder. Involuntary bladder contractions are triggered resulting in urinary urgency and frequency.[8] Patients report waking up every 1 to 2 hours at night to void (nocturia), which significantly reduces quality of life. As BPH progresses, the bladder muscle undergoes hypertrophy so that it can generate a greater contractile force to empty urine past the anatomic obstruction at the bladder neck. Decompensation eventually occurs, and the hypertrophied bladder muscle is no longer able to generate adequate contractile force; the bladder becomes ineffective in emptying urine. Acute urinary retention and recurrent urinary tract infections, and renal failure complicate progressive, untreated disease.

Other factors implicated in the pathophysiology of BPH include chronic prostatic inflammation, advanced atherosclerosis of the blood supply to the pelvis, and decreased release of nitric oxide and decreased production of cyclic guanosine monophosphate (cGMP) at the bladder neck and in the prostate.[9]

Symptoms of BPH vary over time. Symptoms may improve, remain stable, or worsen spontaneously. Thus, BPH is not necessarily a progressive disease; approximately 85% of patients with BPH have stable symptoms when evaluated 4 years after initial diagnosis.[10] Between one and two-thirds of men with mild disease stabilize or improve without treatment over 2.5 to 5 years.[2,6] However, worsening symptoms and complications of BPH develop in patients, particularly those with a prostate gland size 30 to 40 mL or PSA of 1.4 ng/mL (mcg/L) or greater.[2,6]

Collectively, obstructive and irritative voiding symptoms and their negative impact on a patient's quality of life are referred to as *lower urinary tract symptoms* (LUTS). However, LUTS is not pathognomonic for BPH and may be caused by other diseases, such as neurogenic bladder and urinary tract infection.[2]

Another presentation of BPH is silent prostatism. Patients have LUTS, but adapt to the symptoms and do not voluntarily complain about them. Such patients do not present for medical treatment until

CLINICAL PRESENTATION Benign Prostatic Hyperplasia

General

- A patient is in no acute distress unless he has moderate to severe symptoms or complications of BPH.

Symptoms

- Obstructive symptoms: Slow urinary stream, intermittency, hesitancy, straining to urinate, incomplete emptying, dribbling
- Irritative symptoms: Urgency, frequency, nocturia

Signs

- Digital rectal examination reveals an enlarged prostate (>20 g) with no nodules or indurations; prostate is soft, symmetric, and mobile.

Laboratory Tests

- Increased blood urea nitrogen (BUN) and serum creatinine with long-standing, untreated bladder outlet obstruction, elevated prostate-specific antigen (PSA) level.

Other Diagnostic Tests

- Increased American Urological Association (AUA) Symptom Score, decreased urinary flow rate (<10 mL/s), and increased PVR urine volume

complications of BPH disease arise or a spouse brings in the symptomatic patient for medical care.

When BPH progresses, it can produce complications that include the following:

1. Acute, painful urinary retention, which can lead to acute renal failure.
2. Persistent or intermittent gross hematuria when tissue growth exceeds its blood supply.
3. Overflow urinary incontinence or unstable bladder.
4. Recurrent urinary tract infection that results from urinary stasis.
5. Bladder diverticula.
6. Bladder stones.
7. Chronic renal failure from long-standing bladder outlet obstruction.

Approximately 17% to 20% of patients with symptomatic BPH require treatment because of disease complications.[11] Men older than 70 years with large prostates greater than 40 g and a PVR urine volume greater than 100 mL are three times more likely to have severe symptoms or suffer from acute urinary retention and to require prostatectomy than patients with smaller prostates.[12] Thus, a serum PSA level of 1.4 ng/mL (mcg/L) has been used as a surrogate marker for an enlarged prostate gland to identify patients at risk for developing complications of BPH disease and has been used to guide selection of the most appropriate treatment modality in some patients.[12,13]

DIAGNOSTIC EVALUATION

Because the obstructive and irritative voiding symptoms associated with BPH are not unique to the disease and can be presenting symptoms of other genitourinary tract disorders, including prostate or bladder cancer, neurogenic bladder, prostatic calculi, or urinary tract infection, the patient presenting with signs and symptoms of BPH must be thoroughly evaluated.

A careful medical history should be taken to ensure that a complete listing of symptoms is collected to identify concomitant disorders that may be contributing to voiding symptoms. The medical history should be followed by a thorough medication history, including all prescription and nonprescription medications and dietary supplements that the patient is taking. Any drugs that could be causing or exacerbating the patient's symptoms should be identified. If possible, the suspected drugs should be discontinued or the dosing regimen modified to ameliorate the voiding symptoms.

The patient should undergo a physical examination, including a digital rectal examination, although the size of the prostate gland may not correspond to symptoms. BPH usually presents as an enlarged, soft, smooth, symmetric gland, greater than 20 g in size. Some patients have only a slightly enlarged gland and yet have bothersome or even serious voiding difficulties. Other patients have intravesical enlargement of the prostate gland (ie, the gland grows into the urinary bladder and produces a ball-valve blockage of the bladder neck). This type of prostate enlargement is not palpable on digital examination.

The patient's perception of the severity of BPH symptoms guides selection of a particular treatment modality in a patient. To evaluate the patient's perceptions objectively, validated instruments, such as the AUA Symptom Score (Table 84-1), are commonly used. Using the AUA Symptom Score, the patient rates the "bothersomeness" of seven obstructive and irritative voiding symptoms.[14] Each item is rated for severity on a scale from 0 to 5, such that 35 is the maximum score and is consistent with the most severe symptoms. Patients usually are stratified into the three groups shown in the

TABLE 84-1 Categories of BPH Disease Severity Based on Symptoms and Signs

Disease Severity	AUA Symptom Score	Typical Symptoms and Signs
Mild	≤7	Asymptomatic Peak urinary flow rate <10 mL/s PVR urine volume >25-50 mL
Moderate	8-19	All of the above signs plus obstructive voiding symptoms and irritative voiding symptoms (signs of detrusor instability)
Severe	≥20	All of the above plus one or more complications of BPH

AUA, American Urological Association; BPH, benign prostatic hyperplasia; BUN, blood urea nitrogen; PVR, postvoid residual.

table based on disease severity for the purposes of deciding a treatment approach.

In addition, the patient can complete a voiding diary in which he records the number of voids, the volume of each void, and voiding symptoms for several days. This information is used to evaluate symptom severity and tailor recommendations for lifestyle modifications that may ameliorate symptoms.

The only clinical laboratory test that must be performed is a urinalysis. Because many of the voiding symptoms of BPH could be caused by other urologic disorders, a urinalysis can help screen for hematuria, urolithiasis, and infection. To screen for prostate cancer, another common cause of glandular enlargement, a PSA test should be performed for patients aged 40 years or more, with at least a 10-year life expectancy in whom the potential benefit of diagnosing the disorder will be outweighed by the cost of the test.[14]

Objective measures of bladder emptying include peak and average urinary flow rate (normal is at least 10 mL/s). These measures are determined using an uroflowmeter, which checks the rate of urine flow out of the bladder. This is a quick noninvasive outpatient procedure in which the patient is instructed to drink water until his bladder feels full and then the patient's urinary flow is clocked during voiding. A low urinary flow rate (<10-12 mL/s) implies failure of bladder emptying due to obstruction or a functional disorder of the detrusor muscle. Thus, the degree of bladder outlet obstruction may not correlate with peak urinary flow rate.[14]

Another objective measure is PVR urine volume (normal is 0 mL), which is assessed using a transabdominal ultrasound. A high PVR urine volume (>25-50 mL) implies failure of bladder emptying and a predisposition for urinary tract infections. Because of a weak correlation among voiding symptoms, prostate size, and urinary flow rate, most physicians use a combination of measures, including the patient's assessment of symptoms along with objective evaluation of urinary outflow, PVR, and presence of complications of BPH to determine the need for treatment.

Many other tests can be performed if additional information is needed to assess the severity of BPH disease and its complications, to assist in the preoperative assessment of the patient, or to distinguish prostate enlargement due to BPH from that caused by prostate cancer. Tests include a serum BUN and creatinine, voiding cystometrogram, transrectal ultrasound of the prostate, IV pyelogram, renal ultrasound, and prostate biopsy.

TREATMENT

The goals of treatment are to control symptoms, as evidenced by a minimum of a 3-point decrease in the AUA symptom index, prevent progression of BPH disease by reducing the risk of developing complications, and delay the need for surgical intervention

As a disease of symptoms, BPH is treated by relieving bothersome symptoms. However, selection of a single best treatment for a patient must consider the variable costs and adverse effects of treatment options, the inability to predict the course of the disease in an individual patient, and the potential benefit that may occur in a comparatively small number of treated patients.

The AUA Guidelines on Management of Benign Prostatic Hyperplasia is the principal tool used in the United States[14] and is similar to the European Guidelines[15] (Fig. 84-2) with the exception that the European Guidelines recommend tadalafil for moderate to severe LUTS in younger male patients (who are likely to be sexually active) who are physically trim and that 5α-reductase inhibitors are recommended for long-term treatment of patients with BPH who have a prostate volume greater than 40 mL and a PSA greater than 1.4 ng/mL (mcg/L). The AUA Guidelines were originally published in 2010, and although reaffirmed in 2014, were not revised. The European Guidelines were updated and published in 2013.

All patients should be encouraged to initiate and maintain a heart healthy lifestyle, including a low-fat diet, high intake of plenty of fresh fruits and vegetables, regular physical exercise, and no smoking.[16,17] If the patient is overweight, he should be encouraged to lose weight. If the patient has diabetes mellitus, dyslipidemia, or hypertension, he should be advised to optimize management of those disorders.

Specific treatment options include watchful waiting, pharmacologic therapy, and surgical intervention. Although phytotherapy is used by some patients alone or along with conventional medications for BPH, head-to-head comparisons with FDA-approved treatments are lacking; consequently, such herbals cannot be recommended at this time.[14]

3 Patients with mild disease are asymptomatic or have mildly bothersome symptoms and have no complications of BPH disease. These patients can be managed with watchful waiting, which entails having the patient return for reassessment at intervals of 6 to

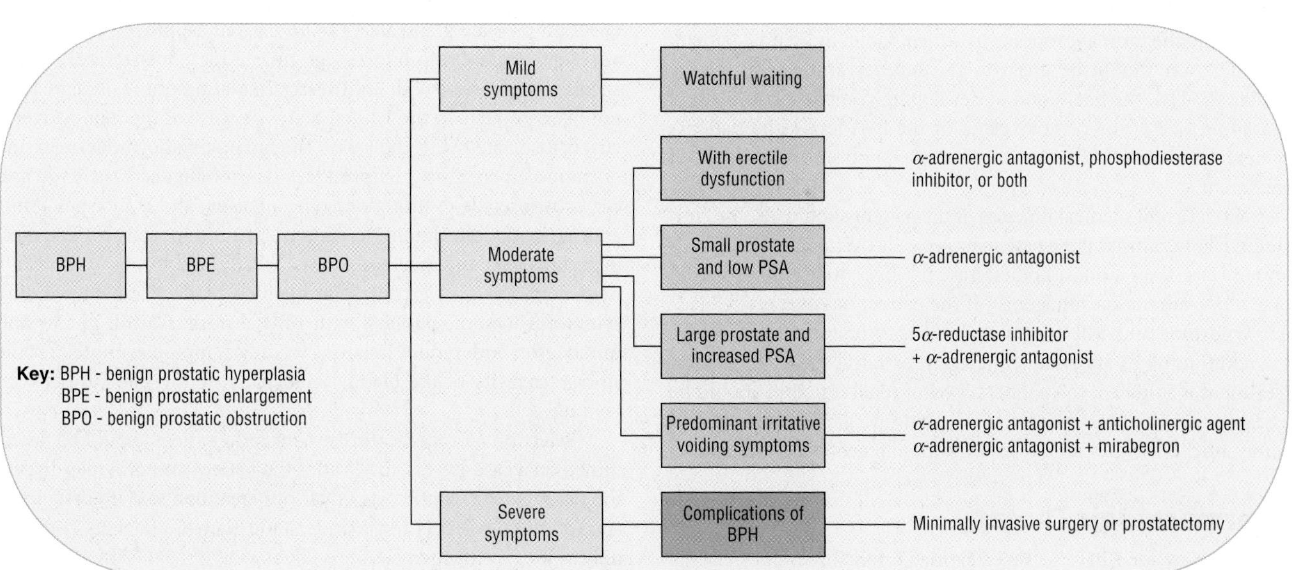

FIGURE 84-2 Management algorithm for benign prostatic hyperplasia (BPH).

12 months. At each return visit, the patient should complete a standardized, validated survey tool to assess severity of symptoms and objective signs of disease should be assessed using measurement of urinary flow rate and PVR urine volume. Watchful waiting should be accompanied by patient education about the disease and behavior modification to avoid practices that exacerbate voiding symptoms. Behavior modification includes restricting fluids close to bedtime, minimizing caffeine and alcohol intake, frequent emptying of the bladder during waking hours or before long trips (to avoid overflow incontinence and urgency), and avoiding drugs that could exacerbate voiding symptoms.[17] At each visit, physicians should assess the patient's risk of developing acute urinary retention by evaluating the patient's prostate size or using PSA as a surrogate marker of prostate enlargement.[14]

4 If symptoms progress to the moderate or severe level, or the patient perceives his symptoms to be bothersome, the patient should be offered specific treatment. In these patients, watchful waiting delays—but does not decrease—the need for prostatectomy. In symptomatic patients, watchful waiting can lead to intractable urinary retention, increased PVR urine volumes, and significant voiding symptoms.[18,19] Recommended treatment options include drug therapy with an α_1-adrenergic antagonist or 5α-reductase inhibitor, a combination of an α_1-adrenergic antagonist and a 5α-reductase inhibitor, a phosphodiesterase inhibitor alone or combined with an α_1-adrenergic antagonist or 5α-reductase inhibitor, or the addition of an anticholinergic agent to an α_1-adrenergic antagonist or 5α-reductase inhibitor; or surgery.

Patients with serious complications of BPH should be offered surgical correction (transurethral or open prostatectomy, or a minimally invasive surgical procedure). Drug therapy is considered an interim measure for such patients because it only delays worsening of complications and the need for surgical intervention.[6,14,18]

TABLE 84-2 Medical Treatment Options for Benign Prostatic Hyperplasia

Category	Mechanism	Drug (Brand Name)
Reduces dynamic factor	Blocks α_1-adrenergic receptors in prostatic stromal tissue	Prazosin (Minipress) Alfuzosin (Uroxatral) Terazosin (Hytrin) Doxazosin (Cardura)
	Blocks α_{1A}-receptors in the prostate	Tamsulosin (Flomax) Silodosin (Rapaflo)
	Causes smooth muscle relaxation of prostate, bladder neck, and prostatic urethra	Tadalafil (Cialis)
Reduce static factor	Blocks 5α-reductase enzyme	Finasteride (Proscar) Dutasteride (Avodart)
	Blocks dihydrotestosterone at its intracellular receptor	Bicalutamide (Casodex)[a] Flutamide (Eulexin)[a]
	Blocks pituitary release of luteinizing hormone	Leuprolide (Lupron)[a] Goserelin (Zoladex)[a]
	Blocks pituitary release of luteinizing hormone and blocks androgen receptor	Megestrol acetate (Megace)[a]
Other	Relaxes detrusor muscle of bladder	Tolterodine (Detrol) Oxybutynin (Ditropan) Trospium (Sanctura) Solifenacin (Vesicare) Darifenacin (Enablex) Fesoterodine (Toviaz) Tadalafil (Cialis) Mirabegron (Myrbetriq)

[a]Not FDA approved for treatment of benign prostatic hyperplasia.

Desired Outcomes

The desired outcomes of treatment include reducing LUTS as evidenced by an improvement of AUA Symptom Score by at least three points, an increase in the peak urinary flow rate, and a normalization of PVR to less than 50 mL. In addition, treatment should prevent the development of disease complications and reduce the need for surgical intervention. Treatment should be well tolerated and be cost-effective.

Personalized Pharmacotherapy

In selecting the most appropriate treatment for an individual patient, consideration should be given to the severity and quality of the patient's LUTS, the likelihood of developing complications of BPH (based on size of the prostate gland or the PSA level), the patient's preference for medical versus surgical intervention, and the cost of treatment.

Concurrent medical illnesses of the patient should also be considered. For example, if the patient has erectile dysfunction and moderate LUTS, then a phosphodiesterase inhibitor might be preferred over an α_1-adrenergic antagonist. If the patient has overactive bladder syndrome and BPH, irritative voiding symptoms may require the addition of an anticholinergic agent or mirabegron. If medical treatment is initiated, the patient's level of renal function should be assessed, as the daily dose of some α-adrenergic antagonists and some anticholinergics require modification to avoid accumulation.

Pharmacologic Therapy

Drug therapy for BPH can be categorized into three types: agents that relax prostatic smooth muscle (reducing the dynamic factor), agents that interfere with testosterone's stimulatory effect on prostate gland enlargement (reducing the static factor), and agents that relax bladder detrusor muscle (improving the urine storage capacity of the bladder) (Tables 84-2 and 84-3). Of the agents that relax prostatic smooth muscle, second- and third-generation α_1-adrenergic antagonists have been most widely used. These agents relax the intrinsic urethral sphincter and prostatic smooth muscle, thereby enhancing urinary outflow from the bladder. Phosphodiesterase inhibitors also relax bladder neck and prostatic smooth muscle. α_1-Adrenergic antagonists and phosphodiesterase inhibitors do not reduce prostate size. Of the agents that interfere with testosterone's stimulatory effect on prostate gland size, the only agents approved by the FDA are 5α-reductase inhibitors (eg, finasteride, dutasteride). Other agents that interfere with androgen stimulation of the prostate have not been popular in the United States because of the many adverse effects associated with their use. The luteinizing hormone-releasing hormone superagonists leuprolide and goserelin decrease libido and can cause erectile dysfunction, gynecomastia, and hot flashes. Antiandrogens (eg, bicalutamide, flutamide) produce nausea, diarrhea, gynecomastia, and hepatotoxicity. Finally, antimuscarinic agents relax detrusor muscle contraction, which reduces irritable voiding symptoms in some patients with BPH. Antimuscarinic agents and mirabegron both reduce irritative voiding symptoms, improve urine storage capacity of the bladder, and increase the interval between voidings.[18,19]

Selection of a medical treatment for a patient should be determined on a case-by-case basis after the patient and provider discuss the risks, benefits, and costs of various treatments. With drug therapy for BPH, patients must understand that the benefits continue only as long as the medication is taken.

If possible, drug therapy should be initiated with a single agent, usually an α_1-adrenergic antagonist, which is faster acting and more effective than a 5α-reductase inhibitor. In addition, α_1-adrenergic

TABLE 84-3 Comparison of α_1-Adrenergic Antagonists, 5α-Reductase Inhibitors, Phosphodiesterase Inhibitors, and Anticholinergic Agents for Benign Prostatic Hyperplasia

	α_1-Adrenergic Antagonists	5α-Reductase Inhibitors
Relaxes prostatic smooth muscle	Yes	No
Decreases prostate size	No	Yes
Halts disease progression	No	Yes
Peak onset	1-6 weeks	3-6 months
Efficacy in relieving BOO	++	++ (for patients with enlarged prostates)
Frequency of dosing	One to two times per day, depending on the agent and dosage formulation	Once per day
Decreases PSA	No	Yes
Sexual dysfunction adverse effects	EJD	Decreased libido, ED, EJD
Cardiovascular adverse effects	Yes	No
	Phosphodiesterase Inhibitors	**Anticholinergic Agents**
Relaxes prostatic smooth muscle	Yes	No
Decreases prostate size	No	No
Halts disease progression	No	No
Peak onset	4 weeks	1-2 weeks
Efficacy in relieving BOO	+	0 (irritative symptoms only)
Frequency of dosing	Once per day	Once per day
Decreases prostate-specific antigen	No	No
Sexual dysfunction adverse effects	No	ED
Cardiovascular adverse effects	Yes (mild hypotension)	Yes (tachycardia)
	β_3-Adrenergic Agonists	
Relaxes prostatic smooth muscle	No	
Decreases prostate size	No	
Halts disease progression	No	
Peak onset	2 weeks, but may take up to 8 weeks	
Efficacy in relieving BOO	0 (irritative symptoms only)	
Frequency of dosing	Once per day	
Decreases prostate-specific antigen	No	
Sexual dysfunction adverse effects	No	
Cardiovascular adverse effects	Yes (hypertension)	

BPH, benign prostatic hyperplasia; ED, erectile dysfunction; EJD, ejaculation disorder; PSA, prostate-specific antigen.

+Notation is a quantitative assessment.

antagonists are effective in reducing LUTS independent of prostate size, have no effect on PSA, and are associated with less sexual dysfunction than are 5α-reductase inhibitors. A 5α-reductase inhibitor is a good first-choice agent for a symptomatic patient with a significantly enlarged prostate (>40 g) who cannot tolerate the cardiovascular adverse effects of α_1-adrenergic antagonists.

For patients at risk for developing complications of BPH, specifically patients with an enlarged prostate gland greater than 40 g,[11] and an elevated PSA greater than or equal to 1.4 ng/mL (mcg/L), combination drug therapy with an α_1-adrenergic antagonist and a 5α-reductase inhibitor is more beneficial than single drug therapy. The pharmacologic rationale for such a combination is that using two drugs with different mechanisms of action can be more effective than either drug alone. The clinical benefit of combination drug therapy is that it quickly relieves symptoms, delays disease progression, and reduces the need for surgical intervention. Since combination drug therapy is expensive and associated with more adverse effects than single drug therapy, it should be reserved for those patients who will benefit the most from it.

For patients with both erectile dysfunction and BPH, a phosphodiesterase inhibitor alone or in combination with an α-adrenergic antagonist may be used. However, it should be noted that a phosphodiesterase inhibitor alone will only relieve LUTS, and will produce a clinically insignificant urinary flow rate increase or postvoid urine volume decrease. Therefore, a phosphodiesterase inhibitor is generally considered less effective than an α-adrenergic antagonist.

For patients with LUTS with a predominance of irritative voiding symptoms, an anticholinergic agent could be added to an existing drug regimen for BPH. To reduce the risk of developing systemic anticholinergic adverse effects, an uroselective anticholinergic agent or mirabegron may be prescribed. To avoid the risk of developing acute urinary retention with an anticholinergic agent, anticholinergics should be used cautiously when the patient's PVR volume is greater than 250 to 300 mL.

α-Adrenergic Antagonists

Three generations of α-adrenergic antagonists have been used to treat BPH. They all relax smooth muscle in the prostate and bladder neck. Because of their antagonism of presynaptic α_2-adrenergic receptors that results in tachycardia and arrhythmias, first-generation agents such as phenoxybenzamine have been replaced by the second-generation postsynaptic α_1-adrenergic antagonists and third-generation uroselective postsynaptic α_{1A}-adrenergic antagonists.

5 The second- and third-generation α_1-adrenergic antagonists are considered equally effective for treatment of BPH.[14,19,20] These agents generally improve the AUA Symptom Score by 30% to 40%, decreasing the AUA Symptom Index by three to six points, within 2 to 6 weeks, depending on the need for dose titration; increase urinary flow rate by 2 to 3 mL/s in 60% to 70% of treated patients; and reduce PVR urine volume. With continued use, durable clinical benefit has been demonstrated for years.[20] Their effectiveness in reducing BPH symptoms and the severity of adverse effects appear to be dose-dependent.[20] They have no effect on prostate volume. α_1-Adrenergic antagonists do not reduce PSA levels, preserving the utility of this prostate cancer marker in this high-risk population.[14]

α-Adrenergic antagonists differ in their propensity to cause hypotensive adverse effects and ejaculation disorders. Modified- or extended-release formulations and third-generation α_{1A}-adrenergic antagonists produce a lower prevalence of hypotension than immediate-release, second-generation agents. α_{1A}-Adrenergic antagonists are more likely to produce ejaculation disorders than α_1-adrenergic antagonists. Finally, older, immediate-release, second-generation α-adrenergic antagonists and tamsulosin are available as inexpensive generic formulations, which may be desirable in selected patients.[14,20,21]

Second-generation agents include prazosin, terazosin, doxazosin, and alfuzosin. At the usual doses used to treat BPH, immediate-release formulations of prazosin, terazosin, and doxazosin antagonize peripheral vascular α_1-adrenergic receptors in addition to those in the prostate. As a result, first-dose syncope, orthostatic hypotension, and dizziness are characteristic adverse effects. To improve tolerance to these adverse effects, therapy should start with a low dose of 1 mg daily and then should be slowly titrated up to a full therapeutic dose over several weeks.[19-21] Additive blood-pressure-lowering effects commonly occur when these agents are used with antihypertensive agents, which limit the use of these agents for some patients.[14] These agents differ in terms of duration of action and dosage formulation. Whereas prazosin requires dosing two to three times per day, terazosin, doxazosin, and alfuzosin offer more convenient once-daily dosing. Because prazosin requires twice- to thrice-daily dosing and has significant cardiovascular adverse effects, it is not recommended in the current AUA guidelines for treatment of BPH.[14] Extended-release dosage formulations are available for doxazosin and alfuzosin. These offer the convenience of once-daily dosing, treatment initiation with a full therapeutic dose, and decreased dose-related hypotension as the formulation produces lower peak serum concentrations than immediate-release products. An α_1-adrenergic antagonist is not preferred as single-drug therapy for treatment of both BPH and hypertension in a patient. In the Antihypertensive and Lipid-Lowering Treatment to Prevent Heart Attack Trial (ALLHAT) of 24,000 patients with hypertension, doxazosin produced more congestive heart failure than amlodipine, lisinopril, or chlorthalidone.[22] Thus, both the AUA and the Joint National Committee on Prevention, Detection, Evaluation and Treatment of High Blood Pressure[14,23] recommend that patients with BPH and hypertension be treated with separate and appropriate drug treatment for each medical condition.

Alfuzosin is considered functionally and clinically uroselective in that usual doses used to treat BPH are less likely than other second-generation agents to cause cardiovascular adverse effects in animal or human models.[24] This clinical observation has been observed more often with the once-daily, extended-release formulation of alfuzosin, which is the only commercially available formulation in the United States, as compared with the immediate-release formulation that is dosed three times per day, which is available in Europe.[24] Its clinical uroselectivity has been postulated to be due to higher concentrations of alfuzosin achieved in the prostate versus serum after usual doses,[25] absence of high peak serum levels with the extended-release formulation, and the fixed dosing schedule of the extended-release formulation. The extended-release alfuzosin dosing is FDA approved for 10 mg daily, with no dose titration increase. This formulation is particularly convenient for patients who are starting to take the medication.

Tamsulosin and silodosin are the only third-generation α_1-adrenergic antagonists available in the United States. They are pharmacologically selective for prostatic α_{1A}-adrenergic receptors, which comprise approximately 70% to 75% of the adrenergic receptors in the prostate gland, prostatic urethra, and bladder neck.[20,21,26] Blockade of these receptors relaxes smooth muscle of the prostate and bladder neck and improves bladder emptying in patients with BPH. In addition, both of these agents have low affinity for vascular α_{1B}-adrenergic receptors, which explains why hypotension is not as frequent with usual daily doses as compared with second-generation agents.[26,27]

Silodosin has 50-fold greater selectivity for the α_{1A}-adrenergic receptor than the α_{1D}-adrenergic receptor and has 100-fold greater selectivity for the α_{1A}-adrenergic receptor than the α_{1B}-adrenergic receptor.[28] Silodosin demonstrates greater pharmacologic uroselectivity than tamsulosin, which has a 10-fold greater selectivity for the α_{1A}-adrenergic receptor than the α_{1D}-adrenergic receptor and has 2.5-fold greater selectivity for the α_{1A}-adrenergic receptor than the α_{1B}-adrenergic receptor.[28] However, these pharmacologic differences are not associated with a clinically significant difference in efficacy or adverse effects, as reported in one direct comparison clinical trial.[29]

The uroselectivity of α_{1A}-adrenergic receptors has multiple implications. Dose titration is minimal; therefore, patients can begin tamsulosin 0.4 mg daily or silodosin 8 mg daily. Patients can be instructed to take the dose anytime during the day, unlike immediate-release formulations of terazosin and doxazosin, which should be taken at bedtime so that patients can sleep through the time when peak cardiovascular adverse effects are most likely to occur. Tamsulosin and silodosin should be taken 30 minutes after the same meal every day because food decreases their bioavailability, reduces the peak serum concentration of the drug, and lowers the risk of hypotensive adverse effects. The onset of peak action is quick, in the range of 1 week. Increasing the daily dose of tamsulosin to 0.8 mg daily produces inconsistent improvements in effectiveness, but does increase adverse effects.[30] These agents are well tolerated in patients with well-controlled hypertension; and the addition of tamsulosin to furosemide, enalapril, nifedipine, and atenolol does result in hypotension.[31]

As compared with tamsulosin, silodosin requires dosage reduction in patients with hepatic impairment or when the creatinine clearance is 30 to 50 mL/min (0.5-0.83 mL/s), is contraindicated in patients with severe hepatic insufficiency or a creatinine clearance less than 30 mL/min (0.5 mL/s), and has the potential to produce more adverse effects because of elevated plasma concentrations if used concurrently with potent CYP 3A4 inhibitors (eg, clarithromycin, itraconazole, ketoconazole, ritonavir) or P-glycoprotein inhibitors (eg, cyclosporine). Silodosin also causes more ejaculatory dysfunction than tamsulosin.[27] Finally, silodosin is commercially available from only one source, whereas tamsulosin is available as a generic formulation.

The usual doses of α_1-adrenergic antagonists are summarized in Table 84-4.

When using immediate-release formulations of the second-generation α_1-adrenergic antagonists terazosin and doxazosin, slow titration up to a therapeutic maintenance dose is necessary to minimize orthostatic hypotension and first-dose syncope. Conservatively, dosages should be increased in an orderly stepwise process, at 2- to 7-day intervals, depending on the patient's response to the medication. A faster titration schedule can be used as long as the patient does not develop orthostatic hypotension or dizziness. Two sample titration schedules for terazosin are as follows:

1. Schedule 1: Slow titration
   - Days 4 to 14: 2 mg at bedtime
   - Weeks 2 to 6: 5 mg at bedtime
   - Weeks 7 and on: 10 mg at bedtime
2. Schedule 2: Quicker titration
   - Days 1 to 3: 1 mg at bedtime
   - Days 4 to 14: 2 mg at bedtime
   - Weeks 2 to 3: 5 mg at bedtime
   - Weeks 4 and on: 10 mg at bedtime

Patients should continue taking the drug as long as they continue to respond to it. Durable responses for 6 and 10 years have been reported for tamsulosin[32] and doxazosin,[33] respectively.

With the exception of silodosin and alfuzosin, no dosage adjustments are recommended for α_1-adrenergic antagonists for patients with renal failure. A reduced starting dose of 4 mg daily of silodosin is recommended for patients with moderate renal impairment (creatinine clearance 30-50 mL/min [0.5-0.83 mL/s]). Alfuzosin should be avoided when the creatinine clearance is less than 30 mL/min (0.5 mL/s).

Because these drugs are hepatically catabolized, the lowest effective dose should be used for patients with hepatic dysfunction, and patients should be monitored carefully for adverse effects.

TABLE 84-4 Dosing of Drugs Used in Treatment of Benign Prostatic Hyperplasia

Drug	Brand Name	Initial Dose	Usual Dose	Special Population Dose
***α*-Adrenergic Antagonists**				
Prazosin	Minipress	0.5 mg twice a day orally	1-5 mg twice a day orally	For uptitrating the dose, double the dose every 2 weeks
Terazosin	Hytrin	1 mg at bedtime orally	10-20 mg daily orally	For uptitrating the dose, increase slowly to 2 mg, 5 mg, and then 10 mg daily in a stepwise fashion. Take extra care if the patient is taking other drugs that lower blood pressure
Doxazosin	Cardura Cardura XL	1 mg daily orally 4 mg daily orally	8 mg daily orally 4-8 mg daily	For the immediate-release formulation, doses of 16 mg daily have been used for hypertension. For the XL formulation, increase from 4 to 8 mg daily after a 3- to 4-week interval. When switching from the immediate- to the extended-release formulation, start at 4 mg of the extended-release formulation no matter what maintenance dose of immediate-release doxazosin the patient is taking
Alfuzosin	Uroxatral	10 mg daily orally	10 mg daily orally (no dose titration)	This is an extended-release formulation, and it should not be chewed or crushed. The drug should be taken after meals and used cautiously in patients with creatinine clearance is less than 30 mL/min (0.5 mL/s)
Tamsulosin	Flomax	0.4 mg daily orally	0.4-0.8 mg daily orally	This is an extended-release formulation, and it should not be chewed or crushed. The drug should be taken after meals. No dosage adjustment is needed in patients with renal or liver dysfunction. Allow several weeks after starting a dose before increasing to a higher dose
Silodosin	Rapaflo	8 mg daily orally	8 mg daily orally (no dose titration)	This drug is contraindicated when creatinine clearance is less than 30 mL/min (0.5 mL/s). If creatinine clearance is 30-50 mL/min (0.5-0.83 mL/s), use 4 mg daily orally, preferably after the same meal each day. Should not be given to patients on potent CYP 3A4 inhibitors or to patients known to be poor metabolizers of CYP 2D6.
5*α*-Reductase Inhibitors				
Finasteride	Proscar	5 mg daily orally	5 mg daily orally	No dosage adjustment in patients with renal impairment. Use cautiously in patients with hepatic impairment
Dutasteride	Avodart	0.5 mg daily orally	0.5 mg daily orally	No dosage adjustment in patients with renal impairment. Use cautiously in patients with hepatic impairment
Dutasteride + tamsulosin	Jalyn	1 tablet (equivalent to 0.5 mg dutasteride + 0.4 mg tamsulosin) daily orally	1 tablet daily orally	No dosage adjustment needed in patients with renal or hepatic impairment
Phosphodiesterase Inhibitor				
Tadalafil	Cialis	5 mg daily orally	5 mg daily orally	If creatinine clearance is 30-50 mL/min (0.5-0.83 mL/s), use 2.5 mg daily orally. Do not use if creatinine clearance is less than 30 mL/min (0.5 mL/s)
Anticholinergic Agents				
Darifenacin	Enablex	7.5 mg daily orally	7.5-15 mg daily orally	For uptitrating the dose, double the dose after 2 weeks. If the patient is taking a potent CYP3A4 inhibitor (eg, ketoconazole, itraconazole, ritonavir, nelfinavir, and clarithromycin), do not exceed 7.5 mg daily orally
Fesoterodine	Toviaz	4 mg daily orally	4-8 mg daily orally	This is an extended-release formulation, and it should not be chewed or crushed. If the patient is taking a potent CYP3A4 inhibitor (eg, ketoconazole, itraconazole, ritonavir, nelfinavir, and clarithromycin), do not exceed 4 mg daily orally. If the creatinine clearance is less than 30 mL/min (0.5 mL/s), do not exceed 4 mg daily orally
Oxybutynin	Ditropan	5 mg two to three times a day orally	5-10 mg two to three times a day orally	Increase daily dose at 5-mg increments at weekly intervals. No specific dosing modifications available for patients with renal impairment, however use cautiously in these patients.
	Ditropan XL	5 mg daily orally	5-30 mg daily orally	This is an extended release formulation, and it should not be crushed or chewed. Increase daily dose at 5-mg increments at weekly intervals. No specific dosing modifications available for patients with renal impairment, but use cautiously in these patients.
	Oxytrol TDS	1 patch (3.9 mg oxybutynin) twice weekly	1 patch (3.9 mg) twice weekly	This is a transdermal patch. Apply to abdomen, hip, or buttock. Rotate application site. Do not expose patch to sunlight. No specific dosing modifications available for patients with renal impairment, however use cautiously in these patients.
	Gelnique 10% gel	1 g gel (100 mg oxybutynin) daily	1 g gel (100 mg oxybutynin) daily	This is available as premeasured dose packets. Apply to abdomen, thighs, upper arms or shoulders. Wash hands after application. Do not bathe, shower, or swim for 1 hour after application. Cover application site with clothing until medication dries on skin. Rotate application site daily. No specific dosing modifications available for patients with renal impairment, but use cautiously in these patients.

(continued)

TABLE 84-4 Dosing of Drugs Used in Treatment of Benign Prostatic Hyperplasia (*Continued*)

Drug	Brand Name	Initial Dose	Usual Dose	Special Population Dose
Solifenacin	Vesicare	5 mg daily orally	5-10 mg daily orally	If the creatinine clearance is less than 30 mL/min (0.5 mL/s) or the patient has moderate hepatic impairment, do not exceed 5 mg daily orally. If the patient is taking a potent CYP3A4 inhibitor (eg, ketoconazole, itraconazole, ritonavir, nelfinavir, and clarithromycin), do not exceed 5 mg daily orally
Tolterodine	Detrol	2 mg twice daily orally	2 mg twice daily orally	If the patient has significant renal impairment, limit dose to 1 mg twice a day
	Detrol LA	4 mg daily orally	4 mg daily orally	The LA formulation is an extended-release formulation, and it should not be chewed or crushed. If the creatinine clearance is 10-30 mL/min (0.17-0.5 mL/s) or the patient has mild/moderate hepatic impairment, do not exceed 2 mg daily orally. If the creatinine clearance is less than 10 mL/min (0.17 mL/s), do not use Detrol LA
Trospium	Sanctura	20 mg twice daily orally	20 mg twice daily orally	Avoid alcohol ingestion for 2 hours after a dose. Use cautiously in patients with moderate or severe hepatic impairment. In patients older than 75 years, use the immediate-release formulation and start with 20 mg daily orally. If the creatinine clearance is less than 30 mL/min (0.5 mL/s), use 20-mg immediate-release formulation
	Sanctura XR	60 mg daily orally	60 mg daily orally	The XR is an extended-release formulation, and it should not be chewed or crushed. This is not recommended in patients with creatinine clearance less than 30 mL/min (0.5 mL/s)
β_3-Adrenergic Agonist				
Mirabegron	Myrbetriq	25 mg daily orally	25-50 mg daily orally	This is an extended-release formulation. Do not chew, crush, or divide tablet. In patients with a creatinine clearance of 15-29 mL/min (0.25-0.48 mL/s) or those with moderate hepatic impairment, the maximum daily dose should be 25 mg daily. This drug is not recommended in patients with creatinine clearance less than 15 mL/min (0.25 mL/s).

Approximately 10% to 12% of patients discontinue taking second-generation α_1-adrenergic antagonists because of adverse effects, especially those that affect the cardiovascular system (eg, syncope, dizziness, hypotension).[34] Patients who tolerate hypotension poorly should avoid immediate-release formulations of second-generation α_1-adrenergic antagonists. This includes patients with poorly controlled angina, serious cardiac arrhythmias, patients with reduced circulating volume, patients with untreated hypertension, and patients taking multiple antihypertensives.[21,34] These patients are candidates for a third-generation α_1-adrenergic antagonists or alfuzosin.

Tiredness and asthenia, anejaculation, flu-like symptoms, and nasal congestion are the most common dose-related adverse effects of tamsulosin and silodosin. These adverse effects are extensions of their α-adrenergic antagonist activity and are dose-related, but with proper education patients likely will not discontinue treatment.[34,35]

Floppy iris syndrome has been associated with doxazosin, silodosin, and tamsulosin use, although the number of reported cases is highest with tamsulosin.[36] The mechanism for this adverse reaction is related to blockade of α_{1A}-adrenergic receptors in iris dilator muscles. As a result, during cataract surgery, pupillary constriction occurs despite the use of mydriatic agents and the iris billows out (floppy iris), both of which complicate the procedure or can increase the likelihood of postoperative complications, including posterior capsular rupture, retinal detachment, residual retained lens material, or endophthalmitis.[37,38] Permanent loss of vision can result.

Patients who are taking α_1-adrenergic antagonists and who plan to undergo cataract surgery should inform their ophthalmologist that they are taking this medication so that appropriate measures can be taken during eye surgery, for example, use of iris retractors, pupillary expansion rings, or potent mydriatic agents.[36-38] No benefit has been demonstrated with holding the α_1-adrenergic antagonist preoperatively.

For patients who are scheduled to have cataract surgery, and who have not yet started an α_1-adrenergic antagonist, they should be advised to delay the start of the α_1-adrenergic antagonist until surgery has been completed. Patients with severe sulfa allergy should avoid tamsulosin.

Caution is needed when CYP 3A4 inhibitors, for example cimetidine and diltiazem, are used with α_1-adrenergic antagonists because a drug–drug interaction could lead to decreased metabolism of the latter agents. In contrast, concurrent use of potent CYP 3A4 stimulators, for example carbamazepine and phenytoin, may increase hepatic catabolism of α_1-adrenergic antagonists.

Phosphodiesterase inhibitors (eg, sildenafil, vardenafil, tadalafil) may produce hypotension if used in large doses along with α_1-adrenergic antagonists. The mechanisms for this interaction are related to the intrinsic vasodilatory effects of phosphodiesterase inhibitors and the higher susceptibility of elderly patients to venous pooling because of autonomic incompetence.[24,39] The prevalence of hypotension depends on the specific phosphodiesterase inhibitor and α_1-adrenergic antagonist agent, specifically the combination of tadalafil and tamsulosin is least likely to produce a clinically significant drug interaction, as compared with other combinations.[39] Therefore, a patient's blood pressure should be stabilized on the α_1-adrenergic antagonist before starting a phosphodiesterase inhibitor. In addition, patients who are taking phosphodiesterase inhibitors with α_1-adrenergic antagonists should have their blood pressure monitored closely when initiating combined drug use.

Clinical **Controversy...**

Among the α_1-adrenergic antagonists, agents that are pharmacologically or clinically uroselective appear to have a lower potential to cause hypotension than nonuroselective agents. However, it is unclear if there is any distinct clinical advantage of using alfuzosin, over tamsulosin or silodosin.

5α-Reductase Inhibitors

6 Finasteride competitively inhibits type II 5α-reductase, the predominant isoform of the enzyme in the prostate, suppresses intraprostatic DHT by 80% to 90%, and decreases serum DHT levels by 70%.[14,40] Dutasteride is a nonselective inhibitor of type I and II 5α-reductase. It more quickly and completely suppresses

intraprostatic DHT production and decreases serum DHT levels by 90%.[41] However, direct comparison clinical trials show no advantages of these pharmacodynamic actions of dutasteride when compared with finasteride.[41] These agents are indicated for management of moderate to severe BPH disease for patients with enlarged prostate glands of at least 40 g.[14,15,41] For such patients, 5α-reductase inhibitors may slow disease progression and decrease the risk of disease complications, thereby decreasing the ultimate need for surgical intervention. When taken continuously for 4 years or 6 years, dutasteride or finasteride, respectively, has been shown to decrease the risk of acute urinary retention and prostatectomy.[43,44] For patients with severe disease, these agents generally can be used with a 6-month short course of an α_1-adrenergic antagonist, which will provide fast symptom relief until the 5α-reductase inhibitor starts to work. 5α-Reductase inhibitors may be preferred for patients with BPH and an enlarged prostate gland who have uncontrolled arrhythmias, have poorly controlled angina, are taking multiple antihypertensive agents, or are unable to tolerate hypotensive adverse effects of α_1-adrenergic antagonists.

5α-Reductase inhibitors also reduce or stop prostate-related bleeding by inhibiting prostatic vascular endothelial growth factor. Thus, the prevalence of gross hematuria in patients with BPH may be reduced with treatment of 5α-reductase inhibitors.[14]

5α-Reductase inhibitors reduce prostate size by 25%, increase peak urinary flow rate by 1.6 to 2.0 mL/s, improve voiding symptoms in approximately 30% of treated patients, and produce few serious adverse effects. Compared with α_1-adrenergic antagonists, 5α-reductase inhibitors have several disadvantages. 5α-Reductase inhibitors have a delayed peak onset of clinical effect, which is undesirable for patients with bothersome symptoms, and an adequate clinical trial is 6 to 12 months. In addition, patients experience less objective improvement of the AUA Symptom Score and urinary flow rate with 5α-reductase inhibitors than with α_1-adrenergic antagonists.[14] 5α-Reductase inhibitors cause more sexual dysfunction than α_1-adrenergic receptor antagonists; therefore, physicians consider 5α-reductase inhibitors to be the second-line agents for treatment of BPH in sexually active males (Tables 84-3 and 84-5).[14,44]

In the Prostate Cancer Prevention Trial, patients with BPH who had large prostate glands and a PSA level less than 3 ng/mL (mcg/L) were prescribed finasteride 5 mg daily for up to 7 years. Finasteride reduced the 7-year prevalence of prostate cancer by 25%.[45] However, finasteride was associated with a 27% increase in the number of patients who developed high-grade prostate cancer, which usually is invasive. Although originally thought to be a disadvantage of finasteride use, it is now thought that the higher incidence of prostate cancer was due to biopsy sampling bias. That is, since finasteride

TABLE 84-5 Monitoring of Drugs Used in Treatment of Benign Prostatic Hyperplasia

Drug	Adverse Reaction	Monitoring Parameter	Comment
α-Adrenergic antagonists	Syncope Lightheadedness Orthostatic hypotension Tachycardia Nasal congestion Ejaculatory dysfunction Priapism Floppy iris syndrome	Blood pressure Heart rate	If prescribing an immediate-release formulation, start the patient on the lowest possible dose and instruct the patient to take the first dose at bedtime. Slowly uptitrate the dose over several weeks. Stabilize the patient's blood pressure on the α-adrenergic antagonist before adding any other hypotensive agent. If the patient needs cataract surgery, instruct the patient to inform the ophthalmologist so that appropriate measures can be taken during the procedure to prevent intraoperative complications. If the patient has a painful erection lasting longer than 4 hours, the patient should seek immediate medical attention
5α-Reductase inhibitors	ED Decreased libido Ejaculatory dysfunction Gynecomastia	PSA	The patient's PSA level should decrease by 50% if he is adherent to therapy
Phosphodiesterase inhibitor	Headache Dizziness Nasal congestion Dyspepsia Back pain Myalgia Hearing loss	Blood pressure Pulse Hearing loss	If the patient experiences hearing loss, discontinue tadalafil
Anticholinergic agents	Dry mouth Constipation Headache Tachycardia Blurry vision Acute urinary retention Drowsiness Confusion Angioedema Anaphylaxis ED	Mental status Bowel habits Ability to urinate	Adverse effects are dose-related and generally reversible. Patients with signs of severe allergic reaction need immediate medical attention
β_3-adrenergic agonist	Hypertension Tachycardia Dry mouth Nausa Constipation Diarrhea Headache Nasopharyngitis Impaired cognition	Blood pressure Bowel habits	Adverse effects are dose-related and generally reversible.

ED, erectile dysfunction; PSA, prostate-specific antigen.

reduces the size of the prostate gland, this results in increased sensitivity of sampling biopsies to detect prostate cancer.[46]

Another clinical trial produced similar results. The Reduction by Dutasteride in Prostate Cancer Events (REDUCE) study compared the effect of 4 years of continuous use of dutasteride versus placebo on reducing the incidence of prostate cancer in more than 6,700 men at high risk for developing prostate cancer. At the end of the study, dutasteride-treated patients had a 22.8% decreased relative risk of prostate cancer. Of the patients with biopsy-positive prostate cancer, a similar number of patients in each treatment group developed high grade tumors of Gleason grade 7 to 10 with no statistical difference between the groups.[47]

Thus, when finasteride is administered long-term to patients with BPH, it could be useful as chemoprophylaxis in patients with a family history of prostate cancer or in men of African descent who have an increased risk of developing prostate cancer. The possibility of developing a high-grade prostate cancer should be discussed with the patient before treatment is initiated with a 5α-reductase inhibitor for prevention of prostate cancer.[45,48]

Finasteride is well absorbed from the gastrointestinal (GI) tract (95%), and its absorption is unaffected by food. Peak serum concentrations are reached 1 to 2 hours after the dose. Finasteride is highly protein bound. The liver extensively metabolizes finasteride to inactive metabolites, which are largely excreted in stool. The plasma half-life is 4.7 to 7.1 hours, but its biologic half-life probably is longer, as decreased serum DHT levels persist for up to 2 weeks after finasteride dosing is stopped.

For BPH, finasteride is given in doses of 5 mg by mouth daily. The dose can be taken with meals or on an empty stomach. No dosage adjustment is needed for patients with renal dysfunction. Although no dosage reduction is recommended for patients with hepatic insufficiency, patients should be monitored carefully. Maximal reductions in prostate volume or symptom improvement may not be evident for 12 months, but noticeable changes from baseline should occur after 6 months of continuous treatment. No clinically relevant drug interactions have been reported with 5α-reductase inhibitors.

Patients must continue to take 5α-reductase inhibitors as long as they respond. Durable responses to finasteride and dutasteride have been reported with continued treatment for 6 years[43] and 4 years,[41] respectively. Upon discontinuation of the drug, prostate size and voiding symptoms generally return to baseline.

5α-Reductase inhibitors can produce sexual dysfunction, and this has led to discontinuation of therapy in up to 12% of treated patients in one pooled analysis.[41] Ejaculation disorders (dry sex or delayed ejaculation) have been reported in 3% to 8% of treated patients.[44] These disorders, which are possible results of decreased prostatic secretion, are reversible with drug discontinuation.

Erectile dysfunction has been reported in 3% to 16% of patients.[41,44] It may be secondary to ejaculation disorders or may be due to drug-induced inhibition of nitric oxide synthase (which is needed to produce nitric oxide, a vasodilatory substance) in cavernosal tissue. The role of 5α-reductase inhibitors in causing erectile dysfunction is not clear, as elderly men with BPH commonly develop erectile dysfunction as they age or have concurrent medical illnesses or concomitant drug therapies that may predispose to the development of sexual dysfunction.[49] Decreased libido has been reported in 2% to 10% of treated patients.[44]

Other minor adverse effects include nausea, abdominal pain, asthenia, dizziness, flatulence, headache, rash, muscle weakness, and gynecomastia.

5α-Reductase inhibitors are in FDA pregnancy category X, which means that they are contraindicated in pregnant females. Exposure of the male fetus to finasteride may produce pseudohermaphroditic offspring with ambiguous genitalia, similar to those of patients with a rare genetic deficiency of type II 5α-reductase. Because of this teratogenic effect, women who are pregnant or seeking to become pregnant should not handle 5α-reductase inhibitor tablets and should not have contact with semen from men being treated with 5α-reductase inhibitors. Women health professionals of childbearing age should handle this product with protective gloves if there is any chance that they are pregnant.

Usual doses of 5α-reductase inhibitors produce a median reduction of serum PSA levels by 50% at months 6 to 12 after the start of treatment. To interpret a PSA level in a patient being treated with a 5α-reductase inhibitor, it is generally recommended that the actual measured level be doubled to get an estimate of the true level.[14] For this reason, PSA levels must be measured before treatment begins, and the patient should have a digital rectal examination. After 6 months of therapy, the patient should have a repeat PSA. This PSA level can be used as the new baseline for the patient.[50] Alternatively, when compared to the pretreatment PSA, if the during treatment level does not decline by 50% and the patient has been adherent to the 5α-reductase inhibitor regimen, he should be evaluated for prostate cancer. Annually thereafter, the patient should have a PSA assay and digital rectal examination. Patients with an increase in PSA level of 0.3 ng/mL (mcg/L) or more above the baseline nadir level should be evaluated for prostate cancer[50] or noncompliance to the prescribed regimen.

Clinical **Controversy...**

Whether or not a 5α-reductase inhibitor should be initiated in an asymptomatic patient with BPH who has risk factors for disease complications is unclear. Treatment would shrink an enlarged prostate, however, it is also costly and associated with sexual dysfunction, gynecomastia, and other adverse effects.[51]

Phosphodiesterase Type 5 Inhibitors

7 Several observations led to the use of phosphodiesterase type 5 inhibitors for management of BPH. BPH and erectile dysfunction are often present concurrently in the same patient.[35,52] The pathophysiology of BPH and erectile dysfunction may be common in so far as both disorders may be associated with increased smooth muscle contraction and pelvic atherosclerosis.[49,52] Improvement of BPH symptoms has been reported to ameliorate erectile dysfunction; and vice versa.[35,52] Adverse effects of α-adrenergic antagonists and 5α-reductase inhibitors include erectile dysfunction, which responds to a phosphodiesterase type 5 inhibitor.[35]

Phosphodiesterase type 5 inhibitors relax smooth muscle in the prostate and bladder neck, probably by increasing cGMP. By so doing, phosphodiesterase type 5 inhibitors interrupt the Rho-protein kinase pathway, which normally regulates smooth muscle contraction mediated by endothelin and α-adrenergic stimulation, and reduces LUTS.[35,54-56]

In multiple clinical trials of patients with moderate LUTS, tadalafil caused significant improvements in voiding symptoms as measured by the AUA Symptom Index score or International Prostate Symptom Score (IPSS), with the level of improvement similar to that observed with α-adrenergic antagonists.[56,57] However, no or minimal increase in urinary flow rate or reduction in PVR urine volume occurred with tadalafil alone.[58-60] Tadalafil 2.5 mg was inferior to 5 mg, and doses of 10 mg or 20 mg were not superior to 5 mg.[53-61] This is the basis of the current product labeling dose of tadalafil 5 mg daily for BPH. The onset of clinical symptom improvement is within 4 weeks.[56,62]

The most common adverse effects observed are headache, flushing, gastroesophageal reflux, sinusitis, visual disturbances, and back pain, which are generally reversible and do not require discontinuation of therapy. When tadalafil was combined with an α-adrenergic antagonist, patients experienced significant improvements in LUTS, increased urinary flow rates, and decreased PVR volume[59]; however, the improvement was similar to that observed with an α-adrenergic antagonist alone.[63]

A few other BPH studies have employed sildenafil 50 mg or 100 mg daily or vardenafil 10 mg twice a day.[59,63] However, most of the clinical trials have evaluated tadalafil for treatment of BPH. This is probably because BPH is viewed as a chronic disease; tadalafil has been FDA-approved for once-daily dosing; and tadalafil has the longest half-life and duration of action among the phosphodiesterase inhibitors.[64] The recommended tadalafil dose is 5 mg daily. Based on the limited clinical benefit, cost, and potential adverse effects of tadalafil, it would be prudent to reserve its use for patients with both BPH and erectile dysfunction.[58,59,64] Patients with known cardiovascular disease should be assessed and stratified according to the Princeton Consensus Panel guidelines[65] to identify those patients who can safely use tadalafil. If used in combination with an α-adrenergic antagonist, precautions should be taken to minimize hypotension, specifically, stabilize the patient's blood pressure on the α-adrenergic antagonist before adding tadalafil.[39] If used in combination with a 5α-reductase inhibitor, tadalafil may be used instead of an α-adrenergic antagonist, and the combination may be associated with less sexual dysfunction, particularly in younger, sexually active patients.

Anticholinergic Agents

8 Treatment with an α_1-adrenergic antagonist, 5α-reductase inhibitor, or surgery may improve urinary flow rate and bladder emptying; however, the patient may still complain of irritative voiding symptoms (eg, urinary frequency, urgency, and nocturia), which mimic those of overactive bladder syndrome. A variety of anticholinergic agents, including oxybutynin or tolterodine, have been added to an α-adrenergic antagonist regimen to relieve these symptoms.[66]

By blocking muscarinic receptors in the detrusor muscle, anticholinergic agents can reduce uninhibited detrusor contractions, a sequela of prolonged bladder outlet obstruction. Thus, irritative voiding symptoms are reduced. The peak clinical effect is observable in several weeks. It is recommended that a patient should be reevaluated 4 to 6 weeks after starting an anticholinergic agent for BPH. Because older patients are sensitive to the central nervous system adverse effects and dry mouth, such patients should be started on the lowest effective dose and then slowly titrated up.[66,67] Anticholinergic agents are contraindicated in patients with narrow angle glaucoma, urinary or gastric retention, or severely decreased intestinal motility. The total anticholinergic burden should be considered prior to making the decision to initiate an anticholinergic agent if the patient is already taking other anticholinergic agents (eg, antipsychotic, antidepressant, antihistamine, antiparkinsonian agents). When multiple anticholinergic agents are taken concurrently, anticholinergic adverse effects, including dry mouth, nausea, constipation, blurred vision, and confusion, will more likely occur and be more severe.

Uroselective anticholinergic agents, which preferentially inhibit M_3 receptors (eg, darifenacin or solifenacin), or transdermal (oxybutynin), or extended-release formulations of anticholinergic agents (eg, tolterodine) are recommended for patients who poorly tolerate systemic adverse effects of other anticholinergic agents. In the presence of BPH, anticholinergic agents can cause acute urinary retention in patients with poor detrusor contractility. Therefore, before prescribing an anticholinergic agent, a PVR urine volume should be measured and should be 150 mL or less[14,67]

Mirabegron

Approximately 95% of the β-adrenergic receptors in the urinary bladder are of the β_3 subtype. When stimulated, β_3-adrenergic receptors increase production of cyclic adenosine monophosphate (cAMP), which relaxes the detrusor muscle.[68]

9 Mirabegron is a β_3-adrenergic agonist. As a result of relaxing the detrusor muscle during the storage phase of the micturition cycle, mirabegron reduces irritative voiding symptoms, increases urinary bladder capacity, and increases the interval between voidings. Mirabegron does not inhibit voiding or reduce urinary flow rate, nor does it increase PVR urine volume or cause acute urinary retention.[8,69,70] The clinical effect of mirabegron for LUTS is similar to that of anticholinergic agents, but mirabegron is better tolerated.[8,70] Mirabegron does not produce anticholinergic adverse effects, nor does it cause acute urinary retention.

Mirabegron is indicated for symptomatic management of overactive bladder syndrome. Its symptoms overlap with the irritative component of LUTS. For this reason, mirabegron is used as an alternative to anticholinergic agents in patients with LUTS, when irritative symptoms persist despite treatment with an α_1-adrenergic antagonist or 5α-reductase inhibitors.[8] The usual starting dose of mirabegron is 25 mg daily, increasing to 50 mg daily if needed. A usual daily dose of 25 mg daily is recommended for patients with impaired renal function (creatinine clearance of 15-20 mL/min [0.25-0.33 mL/s]) or mild hepatic impairment. Mirabegron should not be used in patients with moderate to severe hepatic dysfunction or a creatinine clearance less than 15 mL/min (0.25 mL/s). Adverse effects include increased blood pressure, headache, dry mouth, constipation, and nasopharyngitis.

Combination Drug Therapy

Many drug combinations have been used for BPH. With an α_1-adrenergic antagonist as initial therapy, medications are often added when the patient's symptoms are still bothersome. For example, α_1-adrenergic antagonists seem to be more effective in reducing obstructive voiding symptoms than irritative symptoms. To reduce irritative symptoms, an anticholinergic agent[71,72] mirabegron, or a phosphodiesterase type 5 inhibitor[59] may be added. Similarly, a 5α-reductase inhibitors has a slow onset of action. To achieve faster symptom relief, an α_1-adrenergic antagonist, mirabegron,[70] or a phosphodiesterase inhibitor[73] has been added on. These combinations do not reduce the need for prostate surgery or reduce the risk of disease progression. When such combinations are used, the benefit of reducing bothersome symptoms must be balanced by the increased risk of adverse effects and drug interactions and the higher cost of treatment.

However, the combination of an α_1-adrenergic antagonist and a 5α-reductase inhibitor is ideal for patients with both severe symptoms and an enlarged prostate gland of at least 40 g and PSA of at least 1.4 ng/mL (mcg/L), a surrogate marker for an enlarged prostate gland.[11,14] Such patients appear to be at high risk for disease progression, as evidenced by symptom worsening and development of disease complications, including acute urinary retention, recurrent urinary tract infection, or need for surgical intervention.[11]

In the landmark Multiple Treatment of Prostate Symptoms Study (MTOPS), a regimen of finasteride and doxazosin for 5 years was shown to prevent symptom progression by 66%, decrease the risk of developing acute urinary retention by 81%, and decrease the need for prostate surgery by 67%. Moreover, urinary symptom improvement and higher urinary flow rates at 15 to 18 months were observed in patients treated with combination therapy, as compared with monotherapy with finasteride alone or doxazosin alone.[11] In another key clinical trial, the Combination of Avodart and Tamsulosin (COMBAT) study, dutasteride versus tamsulosin versus a combination of dutasteride and tamsulosin were evaluated in patients with large prostate glands and a mean PSA of 4 ng/mL (mcg/L). The combination regimen was more effective in reducing symptoms 9 months after the start of treatment than dutasteride alone or tamsulosin alone. Whether the combination of dutasteride and tamsulosin prevents disease progression after 4 years awaits long-term study results, although preliminary subgroup analysis has shown that combination therapy reduces the percentage of patients who develop disease progression.[74,75]

Although not proven by direct comparison trials, any combination of 5α-reductase inhibitor and α_1-adrenergic antagonist probably is similarly effective for patients with the aforementioned characteristics.[76] The disadvantages of a combination regimen include increased medication cost to the patient and an increased incidence of adverse drug effects (ie, 18%-27% of patients discontinued treatment because of hypotension).

Clinical **Controversy...**

The combination of an α_1-adrenergic antagonist and 5α-reductase inhibitor can relieve LUTS, slow progression of BPH, and reduce the need for prostate surgery for patients with moderate to severe symptoms and a prostate of 40 g or larger. It may be possible to discontinue the α_1-adrenergic antagonist after 6 to 9 months; however, this potentially cost-saving measure requires further clinical study. A preliminary clinical trial showed BPH disease progression when either drug was discontinued after 2 years of continuous use.[77,78]

Surgical Intervention

10 The gold standard for treatment of patients with complications of BPH is prostatectomy performed either transurethrally or as an open surgical procedure.[14,15] Surgical intervention is also used for patients with moderate to severe symptoms, who are not responsive to drug therapy, who are noncompliant with drug therapy, or who prefer surgical intervention. Surgical intervention is always indicated for patients with complications of BPH, including acute urinary retention not responsive to drug treatment, chronic urinary retention associated with decreased renal function or overflow urinary incontinence, urolithiasis, or recurrent hematuria.[79] Surgical removal of the prostatic adenoma offers the highest rate of symptom improvement, but it also has the highest complication rate.

With TURP, an endoscopic resectoscope inserted through the urethra is used to remove the inside core of the prostatic adenoma. This enlarges the opening at the bladder neck and prostatic urethra. Often performed as outpatient surgery, this procedure produces on average a peak urinary flow rate increase of 125%, improves the AUA Symptom Score by 10 to 18 points, and improves voiding symptoms by almost 90% in approximately 90% of patients.[6] A common complication of TURP is retrograde ejaculation, occurring in up to 75% of patients. Bleeding, urinary incontinence, and erectile dysfunction occur in smaller, but significant numbers of patients (2%-15%).[79] Approximately 2% to 10% and 12% to 15% of patients require second surgeries within 5 and 8 years, respectively.[79]

Alternatively, an open surgical procedure (open prostatectomy) can be performed retropubically or suprapubically. This procedure is usually reserved for men with prostate glands larger than 80 mL. This necessitates hospitalization for at least a few days, anesthesia, and a longer recuperation time. Adverse effects of open prostatectomy include bleeding, urinary and soft-tissue infection, retrograde ejaculation in 77% of patients, erectile dysfunction in 16% to 33% of patients, and urinary incontinence in 2% of patients. The reoperation rate is 3% to 5% at 10 years.[14]

Transurethral incision of the prostate (TUIP) is an alternative surgical procedure for patients with moderate to severe voiding symptoms who have an enlarged prostate gland less than 30 g in size. In the short term TUIP is as effective as TURP but requires less operation time, causes less blood loss, and produces fewer adverse effects.[14] TUIP involves using an endoscopic resectoscope to make one or two incisions at the bladder neck to widen the opening. In limited long-term studies, the reoperation rate for TUIP is slightly higher than with TURP.

Minimally invasive surgical procedures are highly desirable by patients. The procedures do not require hospitalization, are associated with less blood loss, have a lower potential to produce adverse effects, are less expensive than continuous drug therapy regimens lasting years, and may be particularly useful for debilitated patients with moderate to severe voiding symptoms and smaller-sized prostate glands, or for patients who are taking anticoagulants. These procedures typically use heat energy from microwaves, water, or laser (holmium, potassium titanyl phosphate, or thulium) to destroy prostate tissue.[14,15] Commonly used procedures include transurethral needle ablation of the prostate, green light laser ablation, and transurethral microwave thermotherapy of the prostate.[80-82] A disadvantage of all minimally invasive surgical procedures is the high percentage of patients who may develop acute urinary retention in the immediate postoperative period. In addition, patients who undergo minimally invasive procedures generally experience smaller improvements in voiding symptoms and urinary flow rates, and are more likely to require reoperation after an initial improvement in symptoms than patients who undergo TURP or open prostatectomy.[80-82]

Phytotherapy

Although phytotherapy is widely used in Europe for the management of BPH, the published data on herbal agents are largely inconclusive and conflicting. Studies often lack placebo controls, which are essential for assessing treatments for BPH because spontaneous regression of mild symptoms can occur. Furthermore, because these agents are marketed under the Dietary Supplements Health and Education Act, their efficacy, safety, and quality are not regulated by the FDA. For these reasons, herbal products—including saw palmetto berry (*Serenoa repens*), stinging nettle (*Urtica dioica*), South African star grass (*Hypoxis rooperi*), pumpkin seed (*Cucurbita pepo*), and African plum (*Pygeum africanum*)—are not recommended for treatment of BPH.[14] Excellent reviews on phytotherapy for BPH have been published.[83,84]

EVALUATION OF THERAPEUTIC OUTCOMES

The primary therapeutic outcome of BPH therapy is improvement of voiding symptoms with minimal treatment-related adverse effects. As a disease for which therapy is directed at the voiding symptoms that the patient finds most bothersome, assessment of outcomes depends on the patient's perceptions of the effectiveness of therapy. Use of a validated, standardized instrument, such as the AUA Symptom Score, for assessing patient's voiding symptoms is important in this process.[14]

For patients being considered for surgical treatment, objective measures of bladder emptying are useful and include the urinary flow rate and PVR urine volume (see "Diagnostic Evaluation").

Because this patient population is at high risk for prostate cancer, PSA should be measured and a digital rectal examination performed annually if the patient has a life expectancy of at least 10 years. For patients taking 5α-reductase inhibitors, a second PSA taken after 6 months of treatment should be compared with baseline measurements. If the patient is suspected of having developed renal impairment as a consequence of long-standing bladder outlet obstruction, then BUN and serum creatinine should be evaluated at regular intervals.

SUMMARY

A ubiquitous disease of aging men, symptomatic BPH requires medical attention to preserve the patient's quality of life and to prevent disease complications, many of which can be life-threatening in this patient population. In men who have no or mildly bothersome symptoms, watchful waiting and behavior modification are the best treatment approach, as BPH remains stable or even regresses in approximately half of these men.

For patients with voiding symptoms that are moderate to severely bothersome, pharmacotherapy is indicated. An α_1-adrenergic antagonist is the agent of first choice. Second-generation agents include terazosin, doxazosin, and alfuzosin, and third-generation agents include tamsulosin and silodosin. Immediate-release formulations of terazosin and doxazosin cause more cardiovascular adverse effects than do extended-release formulations (eg, doxazosin or alfuzosin), or uroselective α_{1A}-adrenergic agents (eg, tamsulosin, silodosin, or alfuzosin). 5α-Reductase inhibitors are preferred drug treatment for patients with enlarged prostates who poorly tolerate the hypotensive adverse effects of α_1-adrenergic antagonists. However, 5α-reductase inhibitors have a slow onset of action. For patients who do not respond to monotherapy, combination drug therapy could be attempted. Such regimens have been found to be most effective for patients with enlarged prostates greater than 40 g. Alternatively, surgery is an option.

For patients with both moderate to severe BPH and erectile dysfunction, a phosphodiesterase inhibitor alone or combined with an α-adrenergic antagonist may be prescribed. For patients with moderate to severe BPH with a predominance of irritative voiding symptoms, an anticholinergic agent, mirabegron, or a phosphodiesterase inhibitor may be added to an existing drug treatment regimen for BPH. Before starting an anticholinergic agent in a patient with BPH, the patient's PVR should be documented at less than 150 mL.

For patients who have complications of BPH, surgery is required. Although it has more adverse complications than does pharmacotherapy or watchful waiting, TURP is considered the gold standard.

ABBREVIATIONS

ALLHAT	Antihypertensive and Lipid-Lowering Treatment to Prevent Heart Attack Trial
AUA	American Urological Association
BPE	benign prostatic enlargement
BPO	benign prostatic obstruction
BPH	benign prostatic hyperplasia
BUN	blood urea nitrogen
cAMP	cyclic adenosine monophosphate
cGMP	cyclic guanosine monophosphate
COMBAT	Combination of Avodart and Tamsulosin (Study)
CYP	cytochrome P-450
DHT	dihydrotestosterone
GI	gastrointestinal
IPSS	International Prostate Symptom Score
LUTS	lower urinary tract symptoms
MTOPS	Multiple Treatment of Prostate Symptoms (Study)
PSA	prostate-specific antigen
PVR	postvoid residual (pertains to urine volume)
REDUCE	Reduction by Dutasteride in Prostate Cancer Events
TURP	transurethral resection of the prostate
TUIP	transurethral incision of the prostate

REFERENCES

1. Glynn RJ, Campion EW, Bouchard GR, Silbert JE. The development of benign prostatic hyperplasia among volunteers in the normative aging study. *Am J Epidemiol* 1985;131:79-90.
2. Thorpe A, Neal D. Benign prostatic hyperplasia. *Lancet* 2003;361: 1359-1367.
3. Lepor H, Hill LA. Silodosin for the treatment of benign prostatic hyperplasia: Pharmacology and cardiovascular tolerability. *Pharmacotherapy* 2010;30:1303-1312.
4. Roehrborn CG. Pathology of benign prostatic hyperplasia. *Int J Impot Res* 2008;20:S11-S18.
5. St. Sauver JL, Jacobson DJ, Girman CJ, et al. Tracking of longitudinal changes in measures of benign prostatic hyperplasia in a population based cohort. *J Urol* 2006;175:1918-1922.
6. Wasson JH, Reda DJ, Bruskewitz RC, et al. for the Veterans Affairs Cooperative Study Group on Transurethral Resection of the Prostate. A comparison of transurethral surgery with watchful waiting for moderate symptoms of benign prostatic hyperplasia. *N Engl J Med* 1995;332:75-79.
7. Wuerstle MC, Van Den Eede SK, Poon KT, et al. for the Urologic Diseases in American Project. Contribution of common medications to lower urinary tract symptoms in men. *Arch Intern Med* 2011;171: 1680-1682.
8. Suarez O, Osborn D, Kaufman M, et al. Mirabegron for male lower urinary tract symptoms. *Curr Urol Rep* 2013;14:580-584.
9. Lythgoe C, McVary K. The use of PDE-5 inhibitors in the treatment of lower urinary tract symptoms due to benign prostatic hyperplasia. *Curr Urol Rep* 2013;14:585-594.
10. de la Rosette JJ, Alivizatos G, Madersbacher S, et al. EAU guidelines on benign prostatic hyperplasia. *Eur Urol* 2001;40:256-265.
11. McConnell JD, Roehrborn CG, Bautista OM, et al. The long term effect of doxazosin, finasteride, and combination therapy on the clinical progression of benign prostatic hyperplasia. *N Engl J Med* 2003;349:2387-2398.
12. Roehrborn CG. Male lower urinary tract symptoms (LUTS) and benign prostatic hyperplasia (BPH). *Med Clin North Am* 2011;95: 87-100.
13. Rosenberg MT, Witt ES, Miner M, et al. A practical primary care approach to lower urinary tract symptoms caused by benign prostatic hyperplasia. *Can J Urol* 2014;21(supplement 2):12-24.
14. McVary KT, Roehrborn CG, Avins AL, et al. American Urological Association Guideline: Management of Benign Prostatic Hyperplasia (BPH). 2010, reviewed and validity confirmed 2014. Available at: http://www.auanet.org/education/guidelines/benign-prostatic-hyperplasia.cfm. Last Accessed Aug. 15, 2015.
15. Oelke M, Bachmann A, Descazeaud A, et al. EAU guidelines on the treatment and follow-up of non-neurogenic male lower urinary tract symptoms including benign prostatic obstruction. *Eur Urol* 2013;64:118-140.
16. Parsons JK. Lifestyle factors, benign prostatic hyperplasia, and lower urinary tract symptoms. *Curr Opin Urol* 2011;21:1-4.
17. Newman DK, Guzzo T, Lee D, et al. An evidence-based strategy for the conservative management of the male patient with incontinence. *Curr Opin Urol* 2014;24:553-559.
18. Sarma AV, Wei JT. Benign prostatic hyperplasia and lower urinary tract symptoms. *N Engl J Med* 2012;367:248-257.
19. Strittmatter F, Gratzke C, Stief CG. Current pharmacological treatment options for male lower urinary tract symptoms. *Expert Opin Pharmacother* 2013;14:1043-1054.
20. Lepor H, Kazzazi A, Djavan B. α-Blockers for benign prostatic hyperplasia: The new era. *Curr Opin Urol* 2012;22:7-15.
21. Nickel JC, Sander S, Moon TD. A meta-analysis of the vascular-related safety profile and efficacy of alpha-adrenergic blockers for symptoms related to benign prostatic hyperplasia. *Int J Clin Pract* 2008;62:1547-1559.
22. ALLHAT Collaborative Research Group. Major cardiovascular events in hypertensive patients randomized to doxazosin vs chlorthalidone: The Antihypertensive and Lipid-Lowering Treatment to Prevent Heart Attack Trial (ALLHAT) [erratum appear in JAMA 2002;288:2976]. *JAMA* 2000;283:1967-1975.
23. James PA, Oparil S, Carter BL, et al. Evidence-based guideline for the management of high blood pressure in adults. Report from the panel members appointed to the Eighth Joint National Committeee (JNC 8). *JAMA* 2014;311:507-520.
24. Zhang LT, Lee SW, Park K, et al. Multicenter, prospective, comparative cohort study evaluating the efficacy and safety of alfuzosin 10 mg with regard to blood pressure in men with lower urinary tract symptoms suggestive of benign prostatic hyperplasia with or without antihypertensive medications. *Clin Interv Aging* 2015;10:277-286.
25. Mottet N, Bressolle F, Delmas V, et al. Prostatic tissue distribution of alfuzosin in patients with benign prostatic hyperplasia following repeated oral administration. *Eur Urol* 2003;44:101-105.

26. Osman NI, Chapple CR, Cruz F. Silodosin: A new subtype selective alpha-1-antagonist for the treatment of lower urinary tract symptoms in patients with benign prostatic hyperplasia. *Expert Opin Pharmacother* 2012;13:2085-2096,
27. Capitanio U, Salonia A, Briganti A, et al. Silodosin in the management of lower urinary tract symptoms as a result of benign prostatic hyperplasia: Who are the best candidates. *Int J Clin Pract* 2013;67:544-551.
28. Curran MP. Silodosin. *Drugs* 2011;71:897-907.
29. Chapple CR, Montorsi F, Tammela TL, et al. European Silodosin Study Group. Silodosin therapy for lower urinary tract symptoms in men with suspected benign prostatic hyperplasia: Results of an international randomized, double-blind, placebo and active-controlled clinical trial performed in Europe. *Eur Urol* 2011;59:342-352.
30. Aharony S, Lam O, Corcos J. Is there a demonstrated advantage to increase tamsulosin dosage in patients with benign prostatic hyperplasia? *Urology* 2014;84:493-494.
31. Bird ST, Delaney JA, Brophy JM. Tamsulosin treatment for benign prostatic hyperplasia and risk of severe hypotension in men aged 40-85 years in the United States: Risk window analyses using between and within patient methodology. *BMJ* 2013;347:f6320. doi.10.7136/bmj.f6320.
32. Narayan P, Evans CP, Moon T. Long-term safety and efficacy of tamsulosin for the treatment of lower urinary tract symptoms associated with benign prostatic hyperplasia. *J Urol* 2003;170: 498-502.
33. Dutkiewicz S. Long term treatment with doxazosin in men with benign prostatic hyperplasia: 10 year follow-up. *Int Urol Nephrol* 2004;36:169-173.
34. Michel MC. The forefront for novel therapeutic agents based on the pathophysiology of lower urinary tract dysfunction: Alpha-blockers in the treatment of male voiding dysfunction—How do they work and why do they differ in tolerability? *J Pharmacol Sci* 2010;112(2):151-157. Epub 2010 Feb 4. Review. PubMed PMID: 20134112.
35. Mirone V, Sessa A, Giuliano F, et al. Current benign prostatic hyperplasia treatment: Impact on sexual function and management of related sexual adverse effects. *Int J Clin Pract* 2011;10005-11013.
36. Friedman AH. Tamsulosin and the intraoperative floppy iris syndrome. *JAMA* 2009;301:2044-2045.
37. Bell CM, Hatch WV, Fischer HD, et al. Association between tamsulosin and serious ophthalmic adverse events in older men following cataract surgery. *JAMA* 2009;301:1991-1996.
38. Yaycioglu O, Altan-Yaycioglu RA. Intraoperative floppy iris syndrome: Facts for the urologist. *Urology* 2010;76:272-276.
39. Goldfischer E, Kowalczyk JJ, Clark WR, et al. Hemodynamic effects of once-daily tadalafil in men with signs and symptoms of benign prostatic hyperplasia on concomitant α_1-adrenergic antagonist therapy: Results of a multicenter randomized, double-blind, placebo-controlled trial. *Urology* 2012;79:875-882.
40. Wu C, Kapoor A. Dutasteride for the treatment of benign prostatic hyperplasia. *Expert Opin Pharmacother* 2013;14:1399-1408.
41. Nickel JC, Gilling P, Tammela TL, et al. Comparison of dutasteride and finasteride for treating benign prostatic hyperplasia: The Enlarged Prostate International Comparator Study (EPICS). *BJU Int* 2011;108:388-394.
42. Roehrborn CG, Nickel JC, Andriole GL, et al. Dutasteride improves outcomes of benign prostatic hyperplasia when evaluated for prostate cancer risk reduction: Secondary analysis of the Reduction by Dutasteride of Prostate Cancer Events (REDUCE) trial. *Urology* 2011;78:641-647.
43. Roehrborn CG, Bruskewitz R, Nickel JC, et al. Sustained decrease in incidence of acute urinary retention and surgery with finasteride for 6 years in men with benign prostatic hyperplasia. *J Urol* 2004; 171:1194-1198.
44. Welliver C, Butcher M, Potini Y. Impact of alpha blockers, t-alpha reductase inhibitors and combination therapy on sexual function. *Curr Urol Rep* 2014;15:441-448.
45. Thompson IM, Goodman PJ, Tangen CM, et al. The influence of finasteride on the development of prostate cancer. *N Engl J Med* 2003;349:215-249.
46. Thompson IM, Tangen CM, Goodman PJ, et al. Finasteride improves the sensitivity of digital rectal examination for prostate cancer detection. *J Urol* 2007;177:1749-1752.
47. Andriole GL, Bostwick DG, Brawley OW, et al. for the REDUCE Study Group. Effect of dutasteride on the risk of prostate cancer. *N Engl J Med* 2010;362:1192-1202.
48. Theoret MR, Ning YM, Zhang JJ, et al. The risks and benefits of 5α-reductase inhibitors for prostate cancer prevention. *N Engl J Med* 2011;365:97-99.
49. Kirby M, Chapple C, Jackson G. Erectile dysfunction and lower urinary tract symptoms: A consensus on the importance of co-diagnosis. *Int J Clin Pract* 2013;67:606-618.
50. Keating GM. Dutasteride/Tamsulosin in benign prostatic hyperplasia. *Drugs Aging* 2012;29:405-419.
51. Toren P, Margel D, Kulkarni G, et al. Effect of dutasteride on clinical progression of benign prostatic hyperplasia in asymptomatic men with enlarged prostate: A post hoc analysis of the Reduce Study. *BMJ* 2013;346:f2109. doi:10.1136/bmj.f2109.
52. Shelbaia A, Elsaied WM, Elghamrawy H, et al. Effect of selective alpha-blocker tamsulosin on erectile function in patients with lower urinary tract symptoms due to benign prostatic hyperplasia. *Urology* 2013;82:130-135.
53. Laydner HK, Oliveira P, Oliveira RA, et al. Phosphodiesterase 5 inhibitors for lower urinary tract symptoms secondary to benign prostatic hyperplasia: A systematic review. *BJU Int* 2010;107: 1104-1109.
54. Porst H, Dim ED, Casabe AR, et al. for the LVHJ study team. Efficacy and safety of tadalafil once daily in the treatment of men with lower urinary tract symptoms suggestive of benign prostatic hyperplasia: Results of an international randomized, double-blind, placebo-controlled trial. *Eur Urol* 2011;60:1105-1113.
55. Sciarra A. Lower urinary tract symptoms (LUTS) and sexual dysfunction (SD): New targets for new combination therapies? *Eur Urol* 2007;51:1485-1487.
56. Oelke M, Stunghal R, Sontag A, et al. Time to onset of clinically meaningful improvement with tadalafil 5 mg once daily for lower urinary tract symptoms secondary to benign prostatic hyperplasia: Analysis of data pooled from 4 pivotal, double-blind placebo-controlled studies. *J Urol* 2015;193:1581-1589.
57. Oelke M, Giuliano F, Mirone V, et al. Monotherapy with tadalafil or tamsulosin similarly improved lower urinary tract symptoms suggestive of benign prostatic hyperplasia in an international, randomized, parallel, placebo-controlled clinical trial. *Eur Urol* 2012;61:917-925.
58. Lee KCJ, Brock GB. Daily dosing of PDE 5 inhibitors: Where does it fit in? *Curr Urol Rep* 2013;14:269-278.
59. Gacci M, Corona G, Salvi M, et al. A systematic review and meta-analysis on the use of phosphodiesterase 5 inhibitors alone or in combination with α-blockers for lower urinary tract symptoms due to benign prostatic hyperplasia. *Eur Urol* 2012;61:994-1003.
60. Roehrborn CG, Chapple C, Oelke M, et al. Effects of tadalafil once daily on maximum urinary flow rate in men with lower urinary tract symptoms suggestive of benign prostatic hyperplasia. *J Urol* 2014;191:1045-1050.
61. Egerdie RB, Auerbach S, Roehrborn CG, et al. Tadalafil 2.5 mg or 5 mg administered once daily for 12 weeks in men with both erectile dysfunction and signs and symptoms of benign prostatic hyperplasia: Results of a randomized, placebo-controlled, double-blind study. *J Sex Med* 2012;9:271-281.
62. Carson CC, Rosenberg M, Kissel J, et al. Tadalafil-a therapeutic option in the management of BPH-LUTS. *Int J Clin Pract* 2014;68:94-103.
63. Yan H, Zong H, Cui Y, et al. The efficacy of PDE5 inhibitors alone or in combination with alpha-blockers for the treatment of erectile dysfunction and lower urinary tract symptoms due to benign prostatic hyperplasia: A systematic review and meta-analysis. *J Sex Med* 2014;11:1539-1545.
64. Kaplan SA, Gonzalez RR, Te AE. Combination of alfuzosin and sildenafil is superior to monotherapy in treating lower urinary tract symptoms and erectile dysfunction. *Eur Urol* 2007;51:1717-1723.
65. Nehra A, Jackson G, Miner M, et al. The Princeton III Consensus Recommendations for the management of erectile dysfunction and cardiovascular disease. *Mayo Clin Proc* 2012;87:766-778.
66. Kaplan SA, Roehrborn CG, Abrams P, et al. Antimuscarinics for treatment of storage lower urinary tract symptoms in men: A systematic review. *Int J Clin Pract* 2011;65:487-507.
67. Liao CH, Kuo YC, Kuo HC. Predictors of successful first-line antimuscarinic monotherapy in men with e-nlarged prostate and predominant storage symptoms. *Urology* 2013;81:1030-1033.
68. Nitti VW, Rosenberg S, Mitcheson DH, et al. Urodynamics and safety of the β_3-adrenoceptor agonist mirabegron in males with lower tract symptoms and bladder outlet obstruction. *J Urol* 2013;190:1320-1327.
69. Yamaguchi O. Latest treatment for lower urinary tract dysfunction: Therapeutic agents and mechanism of action. *Int J Urol* 2013;20:28-39.
70. Maeda T, Kikuchi E, Hasegawa M, et al. Solifenacin or mirabegron could improve persistent overactive bladder symptoms after dutasteride treatment in patients with benign prostatic hyperplasia. *Urology* 2015;85:1151-5. http://dx.doi.org/10.1016/j.urology. 2015.01.028. Epub 2015 March 12.

71. Kaplan SA, Roehrborn CG, Rovner ES, et al. Tolterodine and tamsulosin for treatment of men with lower urinary tract symptoms and overactive bladder: A randomized controlled trial. *JAMA* 2006; 296:2319-2328.
72. Hao N, Tian Y, Liu W, et al. Antimuscarinics and α-blockers or α-blocker monotherapy on lower urinary tract symptoms—a meta-analysis. *Urology* 2014;83:556-562.
73. Casabe A, Roehrborn CG, DaPozzo LF, et al. Efficacy and safety of the coadministration of tadalafil once daily with finasteride for 6 months in men with lower urinary tract symptoms and prostatic enlargement secondary to benign prostatic hyperplasia. *J Urol* 2014;191:727-733.
74. Roehrborn CG, Siami P, Barkin J, et al. for CombAT Study Group. The effects of combination therapy with dutasteride and tamsulosin on clinical outcomes in men with symptomatic benign prostatic hyperplasia: 4 year results from the COMBAT study. *Eur Urol* 2010;57: 123-131.
75. Haillot O, Fraga Am, Maciukiewicz P, et al. The effects of combination therapy with dutasteride plus tamsulosin on clinical outcomes in men with symptomatic BPH: 4 year post hoc analysis of European men in the CombAT study. *Prostate Cancer Prostatic Dis* 2011;14:302-306.
76. Wilt TJ, Dow JN. Benign prostatic hyperplasia. Part 1—Diagnosis. *BMJ* 2008:336:146-149.
77. Gravas S, Oelke M. Current status of 5α-reductase inhibitors in the management of lower urinary tract symptoms and BPH. *World J Urol* 2010;28:9-15.
78. Lin VC, Liao CH, Kuo HC. Progression of lower urinary tract symptoms after discontinuation of 1 medication form 2-year combined alpha-blocker and 5 alpha reductase inhibitor therapy for benign prostatic hyperplasia in men—a randomized multicenter study. *Urology* 2014:83:416-421. doi:10.1016/j.urology.2013.09.036. Epub 2013 Dec 12.
79. Smith RD, Patel A. Transurethral resection of the prostate revisited and updated. *Curr Opin Urol* 2011;21:36-41.
80. Lourenco T, Pickard R, Vale L, et al. Minimally invasive treatments for benign prostatic enlargement: Systematic review of randomized controlled trials. *Br Med J* 2009;2008:337. doi:10.1136/bmj.a1662.
81. Djavan B, Eckersberger E, Handl MJ, et al. Durability and retreatment rates of minimal invasive treatments of benign prostatic hyperplasia: A cross-analysis of the literature. *Can J Urol* 2010;17:5249-5254.
82. Hollingsworth JM, Wilt TJ. Lower urinary tract symptoms in men. *BMJ* 2014;349:g4474. doi:10.1136/bmj.g4474.
83. Pagano E, Laudato M, Griffo M, et al. Phytotherapy of benign prostatic hyperplasia. A mini review. *Phytother Res* 2014;28:949-955.
84. Cheetam PJ. Role of complimentary therapy for male LUTS. *Curr Urol Rep* 2013;14:606-613.

85

Urinary Incontinence

Eric S. Rovner, Jean Wyman, and Sum Lam

KEY CONCEPTS

1. In evaluating urinary incontinence (UI), drug-induced or drug-aggravated etiologies must be ruled out.
2. Accurate diagnosis and classification of UI type are critical to the selection of appropriate pharmacotherapy.
3. Goals of treatment for UI are reduction of symptoms, minimization of adverse effects, and improvement in quality of life.
4. Nonpharmacologic, nonsurgical treatment is the first-line treatment for several types of UI, and should be continued even when drug therapy is initiated.
5. Antimuscarinic agents are second-line treatments for urge incontinence. Choice of agent should be based on patient characteristics (eg, age, comorbidities, concurrent medications, and ability to adhere to the prescribed regimen).
6. Mirabegron, a β_3-adrenergic agonist, is another second-line treatment for urge incontinence, and can be considered in patients who failed to achieve optimal efficacy or cannot tolerate adverse effects of antimuscarinic agents.
7. Duloxetine (approved in Europe only), α-adrenergic receptor agonists, and topical (vaginal) estrogens (alone or together) are the drugs of choice for urethral underactivity (stress incontinence).
8. Assessment of patient outcomes should include efficacy, adverse effects, adherence, and quality of life.
9. Management of UI should target individualized goals, which may change over time. If therapeutic goals are not achieved with a given agent at optimal dosage for an adequate duration of trial, consider switching to an alternative agent.

Urinary incontinence (UI) is defined as involuntary leakage of urine.[1] It is frequently accompanied by other bothersome lower urinary tract symptoms, such as urgency, increased daytime frequency, and nocturia. It is among the most common medical condition occurring in humans and yet it is an underdetected and underreported health problem that can significantly affect quality of life. Patients with UI may have depression as a result of the perceived lack of self-control, loss of independence, and lack of self-esteem, and they often curtail their activities for fear of an "accident." UI may also have serious medical and economic ramifications for untreated or undertreated patients, including perineal dermatitis, worsening of pressure ulcers, urinary tract infections, and falls.

This chapter highlights the epidemiology, etiology, pathophysiology, treatment of stress, urge, mixed, and overflow UI in men and women.

EPIDEMIOLOGY

UI is highly prevalent, and the impact of this condition is substantial, crossing all racial, ethnic, and geographic boundaries. In addition, lower urinary tract symptoms (eg, urgency, urinary frequency, and nocturia) associated with overactive bladder (OAB) are also quite debilitating.[2] Several studies have objectively shown that UI is associated with reduced levels of social and personal activities, increased psychological distress, and overall decreased quality of life as measured by numerous indices.[3] The condition can affect people of all age groups, but the peak incidence of UI, at least in women, appears to occur around the age of menopause, with a slight decrease in the age group 55 to 60 years, and then a steadily increasing prevalence after age 65 years.

Determining the true prevalence of UI is difficult because of problems with definition, reporting bias, and other methodological issues. The Medical, Epidemiologic, and Social Aspects of Aging survey found that the prevalence of UI in noninstitutionalized women at age 60 years and older was approximately 38%. Almost one-third of those surveyed noted urine loss at least once weekly, and 16% noted UI daily. A publication from a National Institutes of Health working group conference estimated the median level of UI prevalence to be approximately 20% to 30% during young adult life, with a broad peak around middle age (30%-40% prevalence) and an increase in the elderly (30%-50% prevalence).[4]

In the United States, chronic UI is one of the most common reasons cited for institutionalization of the elderly, and the condition is frequently encountered in the nursing home setting. Little is known about the basic differences in clinical and epidemiologic characteristics of incontinence across racial or ethnic groups. Some studies report a higher incidence of UI overall in white populations as compared with African Americans, but differences in access to healthcare as well as cultural attitudes and mores may contribute to these differences.[5,6]

Consistent across all studies of unselected, noninstitutionalized populations is that UI is at least half as common in men as in women.[7] Overall, the prevalence of UI in men has been estimated to be approximately 9%.[8] The prevalence of UI in men increases steadily with age across most studies, with the highest prevalence recorded in the oldest patient cohorts.[9]

ETIOLOGY AND PATHOPHYSIOLOGY

Anatomy

The lower urinary tract consists of the bladder, urethra, urinary or urethral sphincter, and surrounding musculofascial structures, including connective tissue, nerves, and blood vessels. The urinary bladder is a hollow organ composed of smooth muscle and connective tissue located deep in the bony pelvis in men and women.

The urethra is a hollow tube that acts as a conduit for urine flow out of the bladder. An epithelial cell layer termed the *urothelium*, which is in constant contact with urine, lines the interior surface of both the bladder and the urethra. Previously considered inert and inactive, the urothelium may play an active role in the pathophysiology of many lower urinary tract disorders, including interstitial cystitis/bladder pain syndrome and UI[8] and may be a targeted location for future pharmacologic therapeutic interventions for some types of lower urinary tract dysfunction.[10] The urinary or urethral sphincter is a combination of smooth and striated muscle within and surrounding the proximal portion of the urethra adjacent to the bladder. In the male, the prostate gland lies just beyond the bladder outlet and is intimately associated with the urethral sphincter. Its location accounts for both the favorable effects of pharmacological manipulation on male lower symptoms as well as the risk of UI in males following some types of prostate surgery.

To understand the principles of pharmacotherapy for UI, an understanding of the neuroanatomy and neurophysiology of the bladder and urethra is needed. The primary motor (efferent) input to the detrusor muscle of the bladder is parasympathetic and travels along the pelvic nerves emanating from spinal cord segments S2 to S4. Acetylcholine appears to be the primary neurotransmitter at the neuromuscular junction in the human lower urinary tract. Both volitional and involuntary detrusor contractions are mediated by activation of postsynaptic muscarinic receptors by acetylcholine. Of the five known subtypes of muscarinic receptors, the majority of bladder smooth muscle cholinergic receptors are of the M_2 variety. In humans, the ratio of M_2/M_3 receptor numbers is approximately 3:1. However, M_3 receptors are the subtype responsible for both emptying contractions of normal micturition as well as involuntary bladder contractions that may result in UI.[8] Thus, most pharmacologic antimuscarinic therapy is primarily anti-M_3 based. Administration of such agents results in detrusor smooth muscle relaxation and a reduction of bladder overactivity.

Beta-3-adrenergic receptors are found in the lower urinary tract at the level of the detrusor muscle and the urothelium.[8] Although found elsewhere, stimulation of these receptors in the detrusor results in smooth muscle relaxation. Clinically, administration of β_3-agonists is associated with attenuation of bladder contractility and, similarly to antimuscarinics, is used clinically to treat overactive bladder and related urge incontinence. β-Receptors are also located on the urethra but their clinical significance is considered to be negligible.

Clinically relevant α-adrenergic receptors are located at the level of the bladder outlet on the smooth and striated muscle of the urethra.[8] Stimulation of these receptors with α-adrenergic agonists results in increased urethral closure pressure. Such effects are usually not pronounced enough to treat stress urinary incontinence; however, use of these agents may result in unwanted adverse effects such as aggravation of bladder outlet obstruction and result in poor bladder emptying (urinary retention).

Other potentially relevant motor and sensory pathways, neurotransmitters, and receptors have been identified in the lower urinary tract (eg, transient receptor potential channels, E-series prostaglandin receptors). However, the exact role of such targets, as well as ways of modulating their activity pharmacologically in humans has yet to be elucidated and further discussion is beyond the scope of this chapter.

Urinary Continence

To prevent incontinence during the bladder filling and storage phase of the micturition cycle, the urethra, or more accurately the urethral sphincter, must maintain adequate closure in order to resist the flow of urine from the bladder at all times until voluntary voiding is initiated. Urethral closure or resistance to flow is maintained to a large degree by the proximal (under involuntary control) and distal (under both voluntary and involuntary control) urinary sphincters. Variable contributions to urethral closure may also come from the urethral mucosa, submucosal spongy tissue, and the overall length of the urethra. During bladder filling and urinary storage, the bladder accommodates to increasing volumes of urine flowing in from the upper urinary tract without a significant increase in bladder (intravesical) pressure. The maintenance of a low intravesical pressure despite increasing volumes of urine is a unique property of the bladder and is termed *compliance*. In addition, bladder or detrusor smooth muscle activity is normally suppressed during the filling phase by centrally mediated neural reflexes. Normal bladder emptying occurs with opening of the urethral sphincters concomitant with a volitional bladder contraction. Bladder contraction occurs in a coordinated fashion, resulting in a rise in intravesical pressure. The rise in intravesical pressure is ideally of adequate magnitude and duration to empty the bladder to completion. Opening and funneling of the bladder outlet results in urine flow into the urethra until the bladder is emptied to near completion.

The bladder and urethra normally operate in unison during the bladder filling and storage phase, as well as the bladder emptying phase of the micturition cycle. The smooth and striated muscles of the bladder and urethra are organized during the micturition cycle by a number of reflexes coordinated at the pontine micturition center in the midbrain. Disturbances in the neural regulation of micturition at any level (brain, spinal cord, or pelvic nerves) often lead to characteristic changes in lower urinary tract function that may result in UI.[11,12]

Mechanisms of Urinary Incontinence

Simply stated, UI may occur as a result of abnormalities of only the urethra (including the bladder outlet and urinary sphincter) or only the bladder or as a combination of abnormalities in both. Abnormalities may result in either overactivity or underactivity of the bladder and/or urethra, with resulting development of UI. Although this simple classification scheme excludes extremely rare causes of UI such as congenital ectopic ureters and urinary fistulas, it is useful for gaining a working understanding of the condition and understanding the basis for therapeutic intervention including pharmacotherapy of various lower urinary tract disorders.

Urethral Underactivity (Stress Urinary Incontinence) This type of incontinence is characterized by brief bursts of UI concomitant with exertional activities such as exercise, running, lifting, coughing, and sneezing. The pathophysiology of *stress urinary incontinence* (SUI) is related to decreased or inadequate urethral closure forces. In individuals with SUI, the muscular tissues surrounding the urethra that form the urethral sphincter are compromised and thus not able to resist the expulsive forces resulting from transient increases in intra-abdominal pressure during physical activity. Such forces are transmitted to the bladder (an intra-abdominal organ), compressing it to such an extent as to cause the egress of urine through the urethra. SUI is characterized by episodic, usually low volume urinary leakage but is clearly proportional to the amount of physical exertion or other increases in abdominal pressure such as that related to coughing and sneezing as well as the ambient urethral closure forces.

Risk factors for SUI in the woman include pregnancy, childbirth, menopause, cognitive impairment, obesity, and aging.[13,14] In men, SUI is most commonly the result of prior lower urinary tract surgery and injury to the sphincter mechanism within and external to the urethra. Radical prostatectomy for treatment of adenocarcinoma of the prostate and transurethral resection of the prostate (TURP) are probably the most common proximate causes of SUI in the man. Notably, compared with its prevalence in women, SUI in men is actually quite rare.

SUI may be caused or aggravated by some pharmacologic agents such as α-antagonists and angiotensin-converting enzyme (ACE) inhibitors.[15] α-Antagonists may relax the smooth muscle at the level of the urethral sphincter, resulting in a weakened closure mechanism and the onset of SUI. Alternatively, some α-agonists, such as those used clinically for nasal congestion or weight loss, may improve SUI in some individuals, and may even potentially aggravate some types of voiding problems such as those related to bladder outlet obstruction from an enlarged prostate. An adverse effect of some ACE inhibitors is chronic cough, which can also aggravate existing SUI.

Bladder Overactivity (Urge Urinary Incontinence) Urge incontinence is defined as the leakage of urine associated with urgency, a compelling desire to void.[1] This is most often related to detrusor (bladder) overactivity due to involuntary bladder contractions. Bladder overactivity describes the condition in which the detrusor muscle contracts inappropriately during urinary storage that, in the neurologically normal individual, results in a sense of urinary urgency. The terms *overactive bladder* and *detrusor (bladder) overactivity* are distinct and should not be used interchangeably.

The International Continence Society defines OAB as a symptom syndrome characterized by urinary urgency, with frequency and nocturia, with/without associated UI in the absence of a known pathologic condition that may result in similar symptoms (eg, urinary tract infection, bladder cancer).[8] *Frequency* is defined as micturition more than eight times per day. *Urgency* is described as a sudden compelling desire to urinate that is difficult to delay.[1] People suffering from OAB typically have to empty their bladder frequently, and, when they experience a sensation of urgency, they may leak urine if they are unable to reach the toilet quickly. Many patients have associated nocturia (>1 micturition per night) and/or nocturnal incontinence (enuresis). Patients with urge urinary incontinence (UUI) often, but invariably experience high-volume urine leakage when it occurs. Although detrusor overactivity may be related to OAB, the former diagnosis requires urodynamic testing while the latter is symptomatically defined.

Most patients with OAB and UUI have no identifiable underlying etiology and thus are classified as "idiopathic." Patients with a relevant neurologic condition and with UI related to involuntary bladder contractions demonstrated on urodynamic testing are classified as having neurogenic detrusor overactivity. Clearly identifiable risk factors for UUI include normal aging, neurologic disease (including stroke, Parkinson disease, multiple sclerosis, and spinal cord injury), and bladder outlet obstruction (eg, due to benign prostatic hyperplasia [BPH] or prostate cancer).

The pathophysiology of OAB and UUI is not well understood but is likely related to either neurogenic or myogenic factors or combination of both.[16] A full discussion of these differences is complex and beyond the scope of this chapter. However, in practice, although the cause of UUI is difficult to define, the treatment is identical regardless of etiology and pathophysiology.

Some pharmacologic agents may cause or aggravate UUI. Diuretics will cause the rapid accumulation of urine in the bladder with resulting urinary urgency and frequency that can result in UUI. Alcohol will have similar effects. Anticholinesterase inhibitors may also produce urgency and frequency.

Urethral Overactivity and/or Bladder Underactivity (Overflow Incontinence) Overflow incontinence is urinary leakage resulting from an overfilled and distended bladder that is unable to empty. This type of UI occurs when the bladder is filled to capacity at all times but is unable to empty, causing urine to leak from a distended bladder past a normal or even overactive sphincter. Another term related to overflow incontinence is *chronic urinary retention*.[16]

Overflow incontinence is the result of urethral overactivity, bladder underactivity, or a variable combination of both. Clinically and practically, the most common causes of urethral overactivity in men are anatomic urethral obstruction, including that due to BPH and prostate cancer. In women, urethral overactivity is rare but may result from cystocele formation (with resultant kinking or obstruction of the urethra) or surgical overcorrection following surgery for the repair of SUI (iatrogenic obstruction). In both men and women, overflow UI may be associated with systemic neurologic dysfunction or diseases, such as spinal cord injury or multiple sclerosis.

Bladder underactivity occurs as a result of the detrusor muscle of the bladder becoming progressively weakened and eventually losing the ability to voluntarily contract and expel urine during voiding. In the absence of adequate contractility, the bladder is unable to empty completely, and large volumes of residual urine are left after voiding. Both myogenic and neurogenic factors have been implicated in producing the impaired contractility seen in this condition. Clinically, overflow incontinence is most commonly seen in the setting of long-term chronic bladder outlet obstruction in men, such as that due to BPH or prostate cancer, diabetes mellitus, or denervation due to radical pelvic surgery, such as abdominopelvic resection or radical hysterectomy.

There are numerous pharmacologic agents that can result in urinary retention and overflow incontinence. Agents that increase urethral resistance or closure pressure include α-agonists and tricyclic antidepressants. Over-the-counter cold and cough remedies as well as diet pills may contain agents with α-adrenergic properties and/or antihistaminic properties that can result in voiding dysfunction and urinary retentions. Agents that can decrease bladder contractility include anticholinergics, tricyclic antidepressants, calcium channel blockers, narcotic analgesics, and antipsychotics.

Mixed Incontinence and Other Types of Urinary Incontinence Various types of UI may coexist in the same patient. The combination of bladder overactivity resulting in urinary incontinence (UUI or urinary urge incontinence) and urethral underactivity resulting in urinary incontinence (SUI or stress urinary incontinence) is termed *mixed incontinence*. The diagnosis is often difficult because of the confusing array of presenting symptoms. Bladder overactivity may also coexist with impaired bladder contractility. This occurs most commonly in the elderly and is termed *detrusor hyperactivity with impaired contractility*.[17]

Functional incontinence is not caused by bladder- or urethra-specific factors. Rather, in patients with conditions such as dementia or cognitive or mobility deficits, the UI is linked to the primary disease process more than any extrinsic or intrinsic deficit of the lower urinary tract. An example of functional incontinence occurs in the postoperative orthopedic surgery patient. Following extensive orthopedic reconstructions such as total hip arthroplasty, patients are often immobile secondary to pain or traction. Therefore, patients may be unable to access toileting facilities in a reasonable amount of time and may become incontinent as a result. Treatment of this type of UI may involve simple interventions such as placing a urinal or commode at the bedside that allows for uncomplicated access to toileting. Pharmacologically, functional incontinence can be induced by sedative-hypnotics, narcotic analgesics, and other medications with cognitive adverse effects.

Many localized or systemic illnesses may result in UI because of their effects on the lower urinary tract or the surrounding structures:

1. Dementia/delirium
2. Depression
3. Urinary tract infection (cystitis)
4. Postmenopausal atrophic urethritis or vaginitis
5. Diabetes mellitus
6. Neurologic disease (eg, stroke, Parkinson disease, multiple sclerosis, spinal cord injury)
7. Pelvic malignancy

TABLE 85-1 Medications That Influence Lower Urinary Tract Function

Medication	Effect
Diuretics, acetylcholinesterase inhibitors	Polyuria resulting in urinary frequency, urgency
α-Receptor antagonists	Urethral muscle relaxation and stress urinary incontinence
α-Receptor agonists	Urethral muscle contraction (increased urethral closure forces) resulting in urinary retention (more common in men)
Calcium channel blockers	Urinary retention due to reduced bladder contractility
Narcotic analgesics	Urinary retention due to reduced bladder contractility
Sedative hypnotics	Functional incontinence caused by delirium, immobility
Antipsychotic agents	Anticholinergic effects resulting in reduced bladder contractility and urinary retention
Anticholinergics	Urinary retention due to reduced bladder contractility
Antidepressants, tricyclic	Anticholinergic effects resulting in reduced bladder contractility, and α-antagonist effects resulting in urethral smooth muscle contraction (increased urethral closure forces) both contributing to urinary retention
Alcohol	Polyuria resulting in urinary frequency, urgency
ACEIs	Cough as a result of ACEIs may aggravate stress urinary incontinence

ACEIs, angiotensin-converting enzyme inhibitors.

8. Constipation
9. Congenital malformations of the urinary tract

1 As noted above, many commonly used medications may precipitate or aggravate existing voiding dysfunction and UI (Table 85-1).[18]

Generally, SUI is considered the most common type of UI and probably accounts for at least a portion of UI in more than half of all incontinent women. Some studies have found that mixed UI (SUI plus UUI) is the most common type of UI. However, the proportions of SUI, UUI, and mixed UI vary considerably with age group and gender of patients studied, study methodology, and a variety of other factors.

CLINICAL PRESENTATION

2 UI may present in a number of ways, depending on the underlying pathophysiology. A complete medical and medication history, including an assessment of symptoms and a physical examination, is essential for correctly classifying the type of incontinence and thereby assuring appropriate therapy.

Urine Leakage

UI represents a spectrum of severity in terms of both volume of leakage and degree of bother to the patient. It is important to carefully consider the level of patient discomfort and bother when discussing urine leakage as each individual may or may not desire therapy. A careful and complete history during the patient interview is essential to accurately determine the precise nature of the problem. The onset, nature, timing, and volume of incontinence are recorded as is the use of pads. Use of absorbent products, such as panty liners, pads, or briefs, is an important point of discussion, but the clinician must keep in mind that use of these products varies among patients. The number and type of pads may not relate to the amount or type of incontinence, as their use is a function of personal preference and hygiene. A high number of absorbent pads may be used every day by a patient with severe, high-volume UI or, alternatively, by a fastidiously hygienic patient with low-volume leakage who simply changes pads often to prevent wetness or odor. Nevertheless, a large number of pads that are described by the patient as "soaked" is indicative of high-volume urine loss.

Regardless of the volume of urine loss, the desire to seek evaluation for UI in the majority of patients is most commonly elective and therapy is often contingent on the degree of bother to the individual patient. As with the use of absorbent products, patients differ with regard to the amount of urine loss they will tolerate before considering the condition bothersome enough to seek assistance. However, it is critically important that in some individuals new-onset UI may be the first manifestation of an undiagnosed illness (eg, diabetes, multiple sclerosis), or may occur as a result of treatment or drug therapy of an unrelated condition. It is these individuals who mandate a full evaluation and treatment.

Symptoms

Under the best of circumstances, UI is difficult to categorize based on symptoms alone (Table 85-2).[19] In a study of patients who appeared to have SUI based on symptoms and patient history, urodynamics showed that only 72% of patients had SUI as the sole cause of incontinence.[20]

CLINICAL PRESENTATION Urinary Incontinence Related to Urethral Underactivity (SUI)

General

- The patient usually notes UI during activities such as exercise, running, lifting, coughing, and sneezing. Occurs much more commonly in women (generally seen only in men with prior lower urinary tract surgery, neurologic disease, or other injury compromising the sphincter).

Symptoms

- Urine leakage with physical activity (volume is proportional to activity level). No UI with physical inactivity, especially when supine (minimal or no nocturia). May develop urgency and frequency as a compensatory mechanism (or as a separate component of bladder overactivity).

Diagnostic Tests

- Observation of urethral meatus while patient coughs or strains.

TABLE 85-2 Differentiating Bladder Overactivity-Related UI (Urge Urinary Incontinence) from Urethral Underactivity Related UI (Stress Urinary Incontinence)

Symptoms	Bladder Overactivity (UUI)	Urethral Underactivity (SUI)
Urgency (strong, sudden desire to void)	Yes	Not common
Frequency with urgency	Yes	Rarely
Leaking during physical activity (eg, coughing, sneezing, lifting)	No	Yes
Amount of urinary leakage with each episode of incontinence	Large if present	Usually small
Ability to reach the toilet in time following an urge to void	No or just barely	Yes
Nocturnal incontinence (presence of wet pads or undergarments in bed)	Yes	Rare
Nocturia (waking to pass urine at night)	Usually	Seldom

Patients with SUI characteristically complain of urinary leakage with physical activity. Volume of leakage is proportional to the level of activity. They will often leak urine during periods of exercise, coughing, sneezing, lifting, or even when rising from a seated to a standing position. Patients with pure SUI will not have leakage when physically inactive, especially when they are supine. Often they will have little or no UI at night, will not awaken to void during the night (nocturia), will not wet the bed, and often do not even wear absorbent products during the night. Urinary urgency and frequency may be associated with SUI, either as a separate component caused by bladder overactivity (mixed incontinence) or as a compensatory mechanism wherein the patient with SUI learns to toilet frequently to prevent large-volume urine loss during physical activity.

Typical symptoms of UUI and bladder overactivity include frequency, urgency, and high-volume incontinence. Nocturia and nocturnal incontinence are often present. Urine leakage is unpredictable, and the volume loss may be quite large. Patients often wear protection both day and night. Urinary frequency can be affected by a number of factors unrelated to bladder overactivity, including excessive fluid intake (polydipsia) and bladder hypersensitivity states such as interstitial cystitis and urinary tract infection. In some patients, bladder overactivity manifests as UI without awareness in the absence of a sense of urinary urgency or frequency. *Urinary urgency*, a sensation of impending micturition, requires intact sensory input from the lower urinary tract. In patients with spinal cord injury, sensory neuropathies, and other neurologic diseases, a diminished ability to perceive or process sensory input from the lower urinary tract may result in bladder overactivity and UI without urgency or urinary frequency. When bladder contraction occurs without warning and sensation is absent, the condition is referred to as *reflex incontinence*.

Patients with overflow incontinence may present with lower abdominal fullness as well as considerable obstructive urinary symptoms, including hesitancy, straining to void, decreased force of urinary stream, interrupted stream, and a vague sense of incomplete bladder emptying. These patients may also have a significant component of urinary frequency and urgency. In patients with acute urinary retention and overflow incontinence, lower abdominal pain may be present. Although these symptoms are not specific for overflow incontinence, they may warrant further investigation, including an assessment of postvoid residual urine volume.

Signs

A presenting complaint of UI mandates a directed physical examination and a brief neurologic assessment. The workup ideally includes an abdominal examination to exclude a distended bladder, neurologic assessment of the perineum and lower extremities, pelvic examination in women (looking especially for evidence of prolapse or hormonal deficiency), and genital and prostate examination in men. Perineal skin maceration, erythema, breakdown, and ulceration may be indicative of chronic, severe UI. Patients with chronic incontinence may also manifest fungal infections of the skin of the perineum and upper thighs.

SUI can usually be objectively demonstrated by having the patient cough or strain during the examination and observing the urethral meatus for a sudden spurt of urine. In women, SUI may be associated with varying degrees of vaginal prolapse, including cystourethrocele (bladder and urethral prolapse).

In both men and women, digital rectal examination provides an opportunity to check ambient rectal tone and the integrity of the sacral reflex arc (eg, anal wink) as well as assess the patient's ability to perform a voluntary pelvic floor muscle contraction (ie, Kegel exercise), which may be an important factor in deciding on appropriate therapy. In men, a digital examination of the prostate assesses for the presence of prostate cancer, inflammation, and BPH.

A targeted neurologic examination includes assessment of reflexes, rectal tone, and sensory or motor deficits in the lower extremities, which might be indicative of systemic or localized neurologic disease. Neurologic diseases have the potential to affect bladder and sphincter function and thus may have significant implications in the incontinent patient.

CLINICAL PRESENTATION Urinary Incontinence Related to Bladder Overactivity (UUI)

General

- Can have bladder overactivity and UI without urgency if sensory input from the lower urinary tract is absent.

Symptoms

- Urinary frequency (>8 micturitions per day), urgency with or without UI; nocturia (≥1 micturition per night) and enuresis may be present.

Diagnostic Tests

- Urodynamic studies are the gold standard for diagnosis for the diagnosis of detrusor overactivity. Urinalysis and urine culture should be negative (rule out urinary tract infection as the cause of frequency).

CLINICAL PRESENTATION Overflow Incontinence (Chronic Urinary Retention)

General

- Important but uncommon type of UI in both men and women. Urethral overactivity is usually due to prostatic enlargement (men) or cystocele formation or surgical overcorrection following stress incontinence surgery in women. Bladder underactivity resulting in overflow incontinence can result from many causes including neurogenic disease, diabetes, and postoperatively from pelvic surgery (eg, radical hysterectomy).

Symptoms

- Lower abdominal fullness, hesitancy, straining to void, decreased force of stream, interrupted stream, sense of incomplete bladder emptying. May have urinary frequency and urgency. Abdominal pain if acute urinary retention is present.

Signs

- Increased postvoid residual urine volume.

Diagnostic Tests

- Assessment of postvoid residual urine either by imaging (ultrasound, etc) or catheterization. Renal function tests to rule out renal failure due to chronic urinary retention.

Prior Medical or Surgical Illness

UI may present in the setting of concurrent, seemingly unrelated illnesses. New-onset UI may be the initial manifestation of systemic illnesses such as diabetes mellitus, metastatic malignancies, and neurologic diseases such as Parkinson disease, brain tumors, and multiple sclerosis. Central nervous system (CNS) disease, or injury above the level of the pons, generally results in symptoms of bladder overactivity and UUI. Spinal cord injury or disease may manifest as bladder overactivity and UUI or as overflow incontinence, depending on the spinal level and completeness of the injury or disease.

Medications may have wide-ranging effects on lower urinary tract function (see Table 85-1). A thorough inquiry into the use of new medications in the setting of recent-onset UI may show a relationship.

Acute UI manifesting in the immediate postoperative setting may be secondary to a number of factors, including surgical manipulation and immobility, and to a number of medications, especially opioid analgesics and sedative-hypnotics.

Prior surgery may have effects on lower urinary tract function. UI following prostate surgery in men is highly suggestive of injury to the sphincter and resultant SUI. Pelvic surgery for benign and malignant conditions may result in denervation or injury to the lower urinary tract. This includes bowel surgery and gynecologic procedures. For example, new-onset total UI following gynecologic surgery suggests intraoperative bladder injury and subsequent development of a postoperative vesicovaginal fistula. Radiation therapy to the pelvis for malignant disease (eg, prostate cancer or cervical cancer) may result in injury to the bladder or urethra and subsequent UI.

In women, UI may be related to several gynecologic factors, including childbirth, hormonal status, and prior gynecologic surgery although recently the relationship of some of these factors to UI has come under debate.[21] Pregnancy and childbirth, particularly vaginal delivery, are associated with SUI and pelvic prolapse. Significant SUI in the nulliparous woman is uncommon. UI that becomes progressive at or around menopause suggests a hormonal component that may be responsive to estrogen or hormone replacement therapy.

UI may present in the setting of other significant pelvic floor disorders, signs, and symptoms. Constipation, diarrhea, fecal incontinence, dyspareunia, sexual dysfunction, and pelvic pain may be related to UI. A history of gross hematuria in the setting of UI mandates further urologic investigation, including radiologic imaging of the upper urinary tract and cystoscopy. Acute dysuria with or without hematuria in the setting of UI suggests cystitis. Urinalysis and urine culture should be performed in these patients.

TREATMENT

Desired Outcomes

3 The efficacy goals for the management of UI include restoration of continence, reduction of the number of UI episodes, and prevention of complications (pressure ulcers, nursing home placement, etc). Other desired outcomes are minimization of adverse treatment consequences and cost, as well as improvement in the patient's quality of life.

General Approach to Treatment

Nonsurgical, nonpharmacologic intervention is the first-line treatment for UI. Drug therapy may be considered in patients whose UI is not adequately controlled by nonpharmacologic therapies and in those who have no major contraindications to drug treatment. In general, pharmacotherapy provides a better response when combined with behavioral interventions. Selection of agent should be based on the type of UI, and patient characteristics (eg, age, comorbidities, concurrent drug therapies, ability to maintain medication adherence). Surgery can be considered when the degree of bother or lifestyle compromise is sufficient and other nonsurgical interventions are undesired or ineffective.

Antimuscarinic agents have been the mainstay of pharmacotherapy for OAB and UUI. According to the American Urological Association (AUA) guideline,[22] clinicians should avoid antimuscarinic agents in patients with narrow-angle glaucoma unless approved by the treating ophthalmologist. Antimuscarinic agents should be cautiously used in patients with frailty, impaired gastric emptying, or a history of urinary retention, or in those who are taking other drugs with anticholinergic properties. When one agent offers inadequate symptom control and/or unacceptable adverse drug events, consider a dose modification or switching to another agent. Before initiating antimuscarinic therapy, patients should be informed of adverse effects and strategies to minimize them. Before abandoning effective antimuscarinic therapy, clinicians should manage constipation and dry mouth (bowel regimen, fluid management, dose modification, or alternative antimuscarinics).[22]

Nonpharmacologic Therapy

Nonsurgical Treatment

4 Nonpharmacologic, nonsurgical treatment of UI is recommended as the first-line treatment at a primary care level. It is the

only option for patients in whom pharmacologic and/or surgical management is inappropriate or undesired. Examples of patients who fulfill these criteria for nonpharmacologic treatment include those with mild to moderate symptoms and who do not want to take medication; those with comorbid conditions that place them at high risk for adverse effects from drug therapy; those who are not medically fit for surgery; those who plan future pregnancies (which may adversely affect long-term surgical outcomes); those with overflow incontinence whose condition is not amenable to surgery or drug therapy; and those who are delaying surgery or do not want to undergo surgery.[23,24]

Nondrug interventions for UI include behavioral interventions, external neuromodulation, anti-incontinence devices, and supportive interventions (Table 85-3).[23,24] Behavioral interventions are generally the first-line treatment for SUI, UUI, and mixed UI. Interventions include lifestyle modifications, voiding schedule regimens, and pelvic floor muscle rehabilitation. Because the key to success with any type of behavioral intervention is motivation of patients or caregivers, these individuals must be active participants in developing a treatment plan. Regular follow-up is needed to help motivate patients and caregivers, provide reassurance and support, and monitor treatment outcomes.

External neuromodulation may include nonimplantable electrical stimulation (EStim), percutaneous tibial nerve stimulation (PTNS), or extracorporeal magnetic stimulation (MStim). Neuromodulation is typically prescribed when traditional pelvic floor muscle rehabilitation has failed. Anti-incontinence devices such as bed alarms, catheters, pessaries, penile clamps, and external collection devices are reserved for special situations depending on patients' UI symptoms, cognitive and mobility status, and overall health status. Supportive interventions such as physical therapy may be beneficial for patients with muscle weakness and slow gait to reach the toilet in a timelier manner, and absorbent products will provide greater confidence in dealing with unpredictable urine loss.

Surgical Treatment

Only rarely does surgery play a role in the initial management of UI. In the absence of secondary complications from UI (eg, skin breakdown or infection), the decision to surgically treat symptomatic UI should be based on the premise that the degree of bother or lifestyle compromise to the patient is great enough to warrant an elective operation, and that nonsurgical therapy either is undesired or has been ineffective.

Successful application of surgery depends mostly on defining the underlying abnormalities responsible for UI (bladder vs urethra, underactivity vs overactivity). Once the underlying factors are determined, other considerations include renal function, sexual function, severity of leakage, history of abdominal or pelvic surgery, presence of concurrent abdominal or pelvic pathology requiring surgical correction, and finally the patient's suitability for the procedure and willingness to accept the risks of surgery.

If patients with uncomplicated SUI become dissatisfied with the initial management approaches of pelvic floor exercises, medications, and/or behavioral modification, surgical treatment assumes the primary role.

Surgical correction of female SUI (urethral underactivity) is directed toward either (a) repositioning the urethra and/or creating a backboard of support, or otherwise stabilizing the urethra and bladder neck in a well-supported retropubic (intra-abdominal) position that is receptive to changes in intra-abdominal pressure; or (b) improving the sealing mechanism and/or creating compression or otherwise augmenting the urethral resistance provided by the intrinsic sphincteric unit, with (ie, sling) or without (ie, periurethral injectable bulking agents) urethral and bladder neck support.

Bulking agents are injected into the urethra at the level of the urinary sphincter as an office-based procedure and are generally considered quite safe. However, their durability and efficacy are likely inferior to other options.[25]

Midurethral synthetic slings have become the most common approach to the treatment of SUI in women in the United States.[26] These can be inserted as outpatient procedures that have shorter convalescence periods and allow faster return to usual activities compared with many of the older procedures. These procedures are generally felt to be highly durable and efficacious. However, safety concerns have been expressed regarding the implantation of surgical mesh in some patients, the implications of which are yet to be fully clarified.[27]

SUI in men is very rare in the absence of prior pelvic surgery, injury, or neurologic disease. When it occurs, SUI in men can be treated in a number of ways.[28] Bulking agents can be injected periurethrally and submucosally into the region of the external urinary sphincter. This approach is less effective and far less durable than alternative surgical procedures, although it can be performed in the office setting without the need for general anesthesia.

The artificial urinary sphincter is generally considered to be the gold standard for treatment of male SUI.[28] Placement of this manually operated silicone device has been associated with very high long-term success and satisfaction rates.[29] Male slings placed through a perineal incision are an alternative to the artificial urinary sphincter. However, long-term efficacy and safety data are lacking.[30]

Most patients with UUI are managed nonsurgically with a combination of behavioral modification, pelvic floor exercises, and pharmacologic therapy. However, for patients refractory to such measures, invasive therapy can be beneficial. Posterior tibial nerve stimulation is an office-based percutaneous treatment for UUI or OAB. Therapy consists of weekly 30-minute treatments with a needle placed posteriorly to the medial malleolus of the ankle for 3 months. Efficacy appears similar to or slightly better than oral pharmacotherapy.[31] However, long-term efficacy and safety data are lacking.[32]

Surgery for the treatment of UUI generally consists of implantation of a sacral nerve stimulator (neuromodulation) or endoscopic office-based injection of botulinum toxin directly into the detrusor muscle.[33,34] Neuromodulation is a staged surgical procedure in which a neurostimulator lead is placed transforaminally at the level of sacral spinal cord root S3. Its exact mechanism is unknown, but the device may exert its favorable effects on urination and UUI by rebalancing the afferent and efferent nerve impulses to the lower urinary tract and pelvic floor. The injection of botulinum toxin is performed in the office generally with local anesthesia. Following transurethral injection directly into the detrusor muscle using a small needle in a template fashion, the toxin is taken up by the local neurons. The intracellular toxin cleaves SNAP-25, a cystoplasmic protein critical for the attachment of neurotransmitter containing vesicles to the cell membrane at the nerve terminal. As the vesicles containing neurotransmitter are unable to fuse to the cell membrane and release its contents into the synaptic cleft, neural transmission to the postsynaptic muscle fascicle is interrupted. This results in a graded, initially irreversible but transient weakness and paralysis of the affected muscle. The duration of effect of the toxin is about 4 to 8 months, after which repeat injection is necessary to maintain effect. The therapeutic algorithm involving these two choices for treatment of refractory UUI is evolving and is determined largely by patient preference.[35]

Few surgical treatments for bladder underactivity are effective. After an appropriate evaluation for reversible causes, the most effective management of this condition is intermittent self-catheterization performed by the patient or a caregiver three or four times per day. Sacral nerve stimulation (neuromodulation) has shown some efficacy in this patient population, but success rates for detrusor underactivity (nonobstructive urinary retention) are inferior to those seen with urinary frequency and urgency.[36] Proper patient selection for this therapy remains poorly defined. Alternative methods

TABLE 85-3 Nonpharmacologic Management of Urinary Incontinence

Intervention	Description	Patient Characteristics
Lifestyle Modifications		
Behavioral changes (eg, fluid and caffeine modifications, smoking cessation, weight loss, constipation prevention)	Self-management strategies targeted toward reducing or eliminating risk factors that cause or exacerbate UI	Used as first-line therapies or in combination with pharmacological treatment in patients with stress, urgency, and mixed incontinence
Scheduling Regimens		
Timed voiding	Toileting on a fixed schedule where interval does not change, typically every 2 hours during waking hours	Used for patients with cognitive or physical impairments
Habit retraining	Scheduled toiletings with adjustments of voiding intervals (longer or shorter) based on patient's voiding pattern	Used for institutionalized or homebound patients with cognitive or physical impairments
Prompted voiding	Scheduled toiletings that require prompts to void from a caregiver, typically every 2 hours; patient assisted in toileting only if response is positive; used in conjunction with operant conditioning techniques for rewarding patients for maintaining continence and appropriate toileting	Used for patients who are functionally able to use toilet or toilet substitute, able to feel urge sensation, and able to request toileting assistance appropriately; primarily used in institutional settings or in homebound patients with an available caregiver
Bladder training	Scheduled toiletings with progressive voiding intervals; includes teaching urgency suppression strategies using relaxation and distraction techniques, self-monitoring, and use of reinforcement techniques; sometimes combined with drug therapy	Used for stress, urgency, and mixed incontinence in patients who are cognitively intact, able to toilet, and motivated to comply with training program
Pelvic Floor Muscle Rehabilitation		
Pelvic floor muscle exercises (eg, Kegel exercises)	Regular practice of pelvic floor muscle contractions; may involve use of pelvic floor muscle contraction for prevention of stress leakage and urge inhibition	Used for stress, urgency, and mixed incontinence in patients who can isolate and correctly contract pelvic floor muscles; requires cognitively intact and highly motivated patient
Biofeedback	Use of electronic or mechanical instruments to display visual or auditory information about neuromuscular or bladder activity; used to teach correct pelvic floor muscle contraction or urge inhibition; home trainers available	Used for stress, urgency, and mixed incontinence in patients who have the capability to learn voluntary control through observation and are motivated; used in conjunction with pelvic floor muscle exercises
Vaginal weight training	Active retention of increasing vaginal weights; typically used in combination with pelvic floor muscle exercises at least twice per day	Women with stress incontinence who are cognitively intact, can correctly contract pelvic floor muscles, able to stand, and have sufficient vaginal vault and introitus to retain cone, and are highly motivated; contraindicated in patients with moderate to severe pelvic organ prolapse
External Neuromodulation		
Nonimplantable electrical stimulation	Application of electrical current through vaginal, anal, surface, or fine needle electrodes; used to inhibit bladder overactivity and improve awareness, contractility, and efficacy of pelvic floor muscle contraction; handheld stimulators for home use are available	Used for stress, urgency, and mixed incontinence in patients who are highly motivated; contraindicated in patients with diminished sensory perception; urinary retention, history of cardiac arrhythmia, cardiac pacemakers, implantable defibrillators, pregnant or attempting pregnancy; vaginal or anal electrodes are contraindicated in moderate or severe pelvic organ prolapse
Percutaneous tibial nerve stimulation	Application of a pulsed electrical current through a fine needle electrode placed externally near the tibial nerve	Used for treatment of overactive bladder with urinary urgency, frequency, and urgency incontinence; contraindicated in patients with pacemakers or implantable defibrillators, prone to excessive bleeding, or women who are pregnant
Extracorporeal magnetic electrical stimulation	Pulsed magnetic stimulation to pelvic floor musculature causing depolarization of motor neurons, thus inducing pelvic floor muscle contraction; stimulation is provided through a specially designed chair that contains a device for producing a pulsing magnetic field	Used for treatment of stress, urgency, and mixed incontinence; contraindicated in patients with demand cardiac pacemakers or metallic joint replacements; may be useful treatment option when other approaches fail or are not feasible
Alternative Medicine Therapies		
Acupuncture	Involves insertion of disposable sterile fine stainless steel needles into points on the skin that are thought to suppress or stimulate spinal and/or supraspinal reflexes to the bladder and/or urethra	Used for stress, urgency, and mixed incontinence and UI due to spinal cord injury
Anti-Incontinence Devices		
Bed or pant alarms	Sensor devices that respond to wetness; used to awaken or alert individuals via noise or vibrating mechanism	Primarily used for nocturnal enuresis in children; system available for monitoring incontinence in home care and institutional environments

(continued)

TABLE 85-3 Nonpharmacologic Management of Urinary Incontinence (*Continued*)

Intervention	Description	Patient Characteristics
Pessaries	Intravaginal devices designed to support the bladder neck, relieve minor to moderate pelvic organ prolapse, and change pressure transmission to the urethra	Used for female stress incontinence and mild to moderate pelvic organ prolapse; in postmenopausal women, topical estrogen therapy is typically prescribed to prevent ulceration and breakdown of vaginal tissue; requires good manual dexterity to manipulate device
Urethral insert (women only)	Intraurethral device	Used in female stress incontinence with stress incontinence who are cognitively intact and have good manual dexterity
Urethral compression device (men only)	Penile clamp	Used in men patients with stress incontinence who are cognitively intact and have good manual dexterity
External collection devices (men only)	Condom catheter with leg bag	Used in men with urgency, stress, and overflow incontinence and in those with functional impairments
Catheters	Disposable, intermittent urethral catheters and indwelling urethral and suprapubic catheters	Used for overflow incontinence; used in patients who are bed-bound or with significant mobility impairments and severe incontinence; those with terminal illness; those with sacral pressure ulcers until healing occurs
Supportive Interventions		
Toileting substitutes and other environmental modifications	Female and male urinals, bedside commodes, elevated toilet seats	Used for patients with mobility impairments that make reaching toilet in timely fashion difficult
Absorbent products	Variety of reusable and disposable liners, pads, male drip collectors, male guard, collector undergarment, fitted brief, and pant systems; some products contain a polymer that absorbs and wicks urine away from the body	Used for all types of incontinence
Physical therapy	Gait and/or strength training	Used for older patients with mobility impairments that make reaching a toilet in timely fashion difficult

of management that are less satisfactory or more invasive include indwelling urethral or suprapubic catheters and urinary diversion.

Urethral overactivity is most commonly caused by anatomic obstruction. Anatomic obstruction in men is most often caused by benign prostatic enlargement. Treatments may include transurethral surgical resection of the prostate (see Chapter 84).

Rarely, bladder outlet obstruction is caused by a functional obstruction at the level of the bladder neck or external sphincter. Hypertrophy of the smooth muscle fibers at the level of the bladder neck in men and women may result in obstruction to the flow of urine. In patients who do not respond to pharmacologic therapy with α-adrenergic receptor antagonists, endoscopic incision using the cystoscope is highly effective in treating this very uncommon condition.

Pharmacologic Therapy

Urge Urinary Incontinence

5 Antimuscarinic agents and β_3-adrenergic agonist (mirabegron) are the second-line drug treatments for relieving UUI symptoms and preventing its complications. Table 85-4 summarizes AUA recommendations for treating OAB in adults.[22] Table 85-5 lists the usual dosage for approved agents for OAB or UUI. Table 85-6 suggests common monitoring parameters for these agents.

Antimuscarinic agents (see Table 85-5) antagonize muscarinic receptors and suppress premature detrusor contractions, thereby enhance bladder storage. They have similar contraindications, precautions, and side-effect profiles, with incidence/severity varies with each individual agent.[37] Choice of therapy should be based on patient characteristics (eg, age, comorbidities, concurrent medications, and ability to adhere to the prescribed regimen). These agents improve quality of life in patients with UUI, and are considered equally effective based on statistical superiority over placebo or active controls. In clinical trials, major efficacy outcomes for these agents in the management of UI are reduction of the mean number of UI episodes, decrease in the number of micturitions per day, and increase of urine volume voided per micturition.[38]

TABLE 85-4 AUA Guideline for Treatment of Overactive Bladder in Adults

Recommendation	Evidence Strength Grade[b]
First-Line Treatments	
Behavioral therapies (eg, bladder training, bladder control strategies, pelvic floor muscle training, fluid management)	B
Behavioral therapies may be combined with antimuscarinic therapies	C
Second-Line Treatments	
Oral antimuscarinics or β_3-adrenergic agonist as second-line therapy	B
If an IR and an ER formulation are available, prefer ER formulations because of lower rates of dry mouth	B
Transdermal oxybutynin (patch or gel) may be offered	C
Third-Line Treatments	
Intradetrusor onabotulinum toxin A (100 units) in carefully selected patients who have been refractory to first- and second-line OAB treatments[a]	B/C
Peripheral tibial nerve stimulation in a carefully selected patient population	C
Sacral neuromodulation in carefully selected patients with severe refractory OAB symptoms or in those who are not candidates for second-line therapy and are willing to undergo a surgical procedure	C

AUA, American Urological Association; ER, extended-release; IR, immediate-release; OAB, overactive bladder.

[a]The patient must be able and willing to return for frequent postvoid residual evaluation and able and willing to perform self-catheterization if necessary.

[b]When sufficient evidence existed, the body of evidence for a particular treatment was assigned a strength rating of A (high), B (moderate), or C (low). Both B and C indicate that benefits outweigh risks/burdens.

TABLE 85-5 Dosing of Medications Approved for OAB or UUI

Drug	Brand Name	Initial Dose	Usual Range	Special Population Dose	Comments
Anticholinergics/Antimuscarinics					
Oxybutynin IR	Ditropan	2.5 mg twice daily	2.5-5 mg two to four times daily		Titrate in increments of 2.5 mg/day every 1-2 months; available in oral solution
Oxybutynin XL	Ditropan XL	5-10 mg once daily	5-30 mg once daily		Adjust dose in 5-mg increments at weekly interval; swallow whole
Oxybutynin TDS	Oxytrol Oxytrol for Women (OTC)		3.9 mg/day apply one patch twice weekly		Apply every 3-4 days; rotate application site
Oxybutynin gel 10%	Gelnique		One sachet (100 mg) topically daily		Apply to clean and dry, intact skin on abdomen, thighs or upper arms/shoulders; contains alcohol
Oxybutynin gel 3%	Gelnique 3%		Three pumps (84 mg) topically daily		Same as above
Tolterodine IR	Detrol		1-2 mg twice daily	1 mg twice daily if patient is taking CYP3A4 inhibitors, or with renal/hepatic impairment	
Tolterodine LA	Detrol LA		2-4 mg once daily	2 mg once daily in those who are taking CYP3A4 inhibitors or with renal/hepatic impairment	Swallow whole; avoid in patients with creatinine clearance ≤10 mL/min (≤0.17 mL/s)
Trospium chloride IR	Sanctura		20 mg twice daily	20 mg once daily in patient age ≥75 years or creatinine clearance ≤30 mL/min (≤0.5 mL/s)	Take 1 hour before meals or on empty stomach; patient age ≥75 years should take at bedtime
Trospium chloride ER	Sanctura XR		60 mg once daily	Avoid in patient age ≥75 years or creatinine clearance ≤30 mL/min (≤0.5 mL/s)	Take 1 hour before meals or on empty stomach; swallow whole
Solifenacin	VESIcare	5 mg daily	5-10 mg once daily	5 mg daily if patient is taking CYP3A4 inhibitors or with creatinine clearance ≤30 mL/min (≤0.5 mL/s) or moderate hepatic impairment; avoid in severe hepatic impairment	Swallow whole
Darifenacin ER	Enablex	7.5 mg once daily	7.5-15 mg once daily	7.5 mg daily if patient is taking potent CYP3A4 inhibitors or with moderate hepatic impairment; avoid in severe hepatic impairment	Titrate dose after at least 2 weeks; swallow whole
Fesoterodine ER	Toviaz	4 mg once daily	4-8 mg once daily	4 mg daily if patient is taking potent CYP3A4 inhibitors or with creatinine clearance ≤30 mL/min (≤0.5 mL/s); avoid in severe hepatic impairment	Prodrug (metabolized to 5-hydroxymethyl tolterodine); swallow whole
β_3-Adrenergic Agonist					
Mirabegron ER	Myrbetriq	25 mg once daily	25-50 mg once daily	25 mg once daily if creatinine clearance 15-29 mL/min (0.25-0.49 mL/s) or moderate hepatic impairment; avoid in patients with ESRD or severe hepatic impairment	Swallow whole

CYP, cytochrome P450 enzyme; ER, extended-release; ESRD, end-stage renal disease; IR, immediate release; LA, long acting; OAB, overactive bladder; OTC, over-the-counter; TDS, transdermal system; UUI, urge urinary incontinence; XL, extended release.

Oxybutynin Immediate Release Oxybutynin immediate release (IR) is the oldest and least expensive treatment for UUI. It has the disadvantage of giving substantial nonurinary antimuscarinic effects (see Table 85-6). It also causes orthostatic hypotension, and sedation/weight gain, due to the blockage of α-adrenergic-, and histamine H_1-receptors, respectively.[39] Overall, significant adverse effects of this agent jeopardize medication adherence and can prevent dose escalation to achieve optimal benefit. Its multiple daily dosing may be too complicated for patients with cognitive impairment or those who are taking multiple medications. Oral solution formulation may be easier to administer to patients who have difficulty in swallowing.

To optimize tolerability, initiate dose at no more than 2.5 mg twice daily, increase to 2.5 mg three times daily after 1 month, then titrate in increments of 2.5 mg/day every 1 to 2 months until the desired response or the maximum recommended dosage. Side effects may be managed by dose reduction. Dry mouth may be relieved by use of sugarless hard candy, gum, or a saliva substitute. Constipation can be minimized by increasing the intake of water, dietary fiber, physical activity, or laxative therapy.

Oxybutynin Extended-Release An extended-release (XL) formulation of oxybutynin can be considered an alternative therapy

TABLE 85-6 Monitoring of Medications Approved for OAB or UUI

Drug	Adverse Drug Reaction	Monitoring Parameters	Comments
Antimuscarinic			
Oxybutynin IR Oxybutynin XL Oxybutynin TDS Oxybutynin gel 10% Oxybutynin gel 3% Tolterodine IR Tolterodine LA Trospium chloride IR Trospium chloride ER Solifenacin Darifenacin ER Fesoterodine ER	Anticholinergic adverse effects: dry mouth, constipation, headache, dyspepsia, dry eyes, blurred vision, cognitive impairment, tachycardia, sedation, orthostatic hypotension Application site reactions (topical agents): pruritus, erythema	Contraindications and precautions: urinary retention, gastric retention, severely decreased GI motility, angioedema, myasthenia gravis, uncontrolled narrow-angle glaucoma Worsening of renal/hepatic condition or concomitant drug therapy, which may necessitate dosage reduction or drug cessation Mental status change or risk for falls in elderly or frail patients	In general, ER, LA, XL, and topical products are associated with fewer anticholinergic adverse effects, particularly dry mouth Possible transference of drug from topical application Avoid open fire or smoke until alcohol-based gel has dried
β_3-Adrenergic Agonist			
Mirabegron ER	Hypertension, nasopharyngitis, urinary tract infection, headache	Precautions: urinary retention, severe uncontrolled hypertension Worsening of renal/hepatic condition, which may necessitate dosage reduction or drug cessation Increased effect of narrow therapeutic index drugs that are CYP2D6 substrates QT prolongation	Mirabegron is a CYP2D6 inhibitor

CYP, cytochrome P450 enzyme; ER, extended-release; IR, immediate release; LA, long acting; OAB, overactive bladder; TDS, transdermal system; UUI, urge urinary incontinence; XL, extended release.

in patients who cannot tolerate IR formulation. It delivers a controlled amount of oxybutynin over a 24-hour period, and has a reduced first-pass metabolism. The lower plasma concentration of active metabolite, *N*-desethyloxybutynin, due to reduced first-pass metabolism, may explain the lower dry mouth incidence associated with the XL product.[40] In short-term studies of up to 12 weeks' duration, oxybutynin XL was better tolerated than oxybutynin IR, with approximately 7% of patients discontinuing treatment because of adverse effects (compared with approximately 27% of those taking oxybutynin IR).[40]

In short-term studies, oxybutynin XL was at least as effective as tolterodine IR or long acting (LA) in managing urinary symptoms. Pooled results of two open-label studies suggested that oxybutynin XL was inferior in patient-perceived improvement in bladder control and adverse effects profile to tolterodine LA. However, both agents provided similar patients' or physicians' perception of benefit over baseline and proportions of withdrawals due to lack of efficacy. A major limitation of this study was lack of blinding, which may lead to patient and observer bias.[41]

Oxybutynin XL should be administered once daily, and should not be crushed or chewed. Elderly patients should start with a dose of 5 mg once daily and titrate gradually to desired effects, which may take at least 4 weeks after dose initiation or escalation. Drug interactions may occur when oxybutynin is used with other anticholinergic drugs, potent CYP3A4 inhibitors (eg, itraconazole, miconazole, erythromycin, and clarithromycin), and acetylcholinesterase inhibitors via pharmacodynamic antagonism.[40]

Transdermal Oxybutynin The oxybutynin transdermal system (TDS) is another option for patients who cannot tolerate IR oxybutynin or who prefer topical drug delivery route. In 2013, the US Food and Drug Administration (FDA) approved the oxybutynin TDS as the first over-the-counter treatment for OAB in women aged 18 years and over. The patch allows oxybutynin to bypass first-pass hepatic and gut metabolism, and gives a more tolerable adverse effect profile compared with oral formulations.[42] It is as effective as oxybutynin IR in reducing the frequency of UUI episodes and improving patient-perceived urinary leakage.[42,43] Compared with tolterodine LA, oxybutynin TDS provided similar efficacy outcomes, including attaining complete continence and improving quality of life.[41] A large multicenter trial reported improved quality of life and good tolerability in patients 65 years or older; increase in work productivity was noted among younger patients.[44,45]

Patients should apply oxybutynin TDS to dry, intact skin on the abdomen, hip, or buttocks every 3 to 4 days (twice weekly). Rotating application site at least weekly may help minimize local side effects. The most common adverse effects are pruritus (14%-17%) and erythema (6%-9%) at the application site, dry mouth (5%-10%), constipation (3%), and abnormal vision (2.5%).[42]

Oxybutynin Topical Gel This formulation (available in 10% or in 3%) causes significantly less dry mouth than oxybutynin (6.1% vs 73.1%).[46-48] In short-term studies, it is more effective than placebo, but gives dry mouth and application site reactions as the most common adverse effects.[49] Although it did not cause cognitive impairment in older adults in short-term studies, clinicians should monitor for anticholinergic effects during long-term therapy, particularly in frail patients.[50]

The most common adverse events include dry mouth (8%-12%), application site reactions (5%-11%), and dizziness (3%).[46,47] Clinicians should counsel patients to avoid applying sunscreen within half an hour before or after application and to avoid showering within 1 hour after application. The transfer of gel between individuals may occur if vigorous skin contact is made at the application site; patients should avoid open fires or exposure to smoking until this alcohol-based gel has dried.[46,47]

Tolterodine Immediate Release Tolterodine is a competitive muscarinic receptor antagonist that is as effective as oxybutynin IR, and is associated with lower drug discontinuation rates (8% vs 27% oxybutynin IR).[41,51] It may have better medication adherence than oxybutynin due to better tolerability.[52]

Tolterodine is predominantly eliminated by hepatic metabolism, which is partially under the control of genetic polymorphism.[51] The principal metabolic pathway in extensive metabolizers involves oxidation of the parent drug by CYP isoenzyme 2D6 to the active 5-hydroxymethyl metabolite (DD01). In CYP2D6 poor metabolizers (approximately 7% of the US population), the principal metabolic pathway involves CYP3A4. Because tolterodine is principally metabolized by CYP3A4 in this case, its elimination may be impaired by CYP3A4 inhibitors (eg, fluoxetine, sertraline, fluvoxamine, macrolide antibiotics, azole antifungals, and grapefruit juice). For example, fluoxetine, an inhibitor of CYP2D6 and 3A4, decreases the metabolism of tolterodine to DD01, and results in significant increase of drug exposure to tolterodine.[51] Whether tolterodine significantly alters the pharmacokinetics of drugs metabolized by CYP2D6 is unknown, so caution is advised with concurrent use with agents metabolized by CYP2D6.[51]

Tolterodine IR can be given 1 to 2 mg twice daily with or without food. It is not recommended in patients with creatinine clearance less than 10 mL/min (<0.17 mL/s) or severe hepatic impairment. The dose should be reduced to 2 mg in patients with mild to moderate hepatic impairment, or creatinine clearance 10 to 30 mL/min (0.17-0.5 mL/s), or in those taking potent CYP3A4 inhibitors. The maximum benefit from tolterodine may take up to 8 weeks after therapy initiation or dose escalation.[51]

The most common adverse effects of tolterodine are dry mouth, dyspepsia, headache, constipation, and dry eyes. Of note, patients who have known hypersensitivity to fesoterodine fumarate should not receive tolterodine because both agents are metabolized to DD01. Monitoring of QT prolongation is advisable in patients who are also taking Class IA (eg, quinidine, procainamide) or Class III (eg, amiodarone, sotalol) antiarrhythmic medications.[51]

Tolterodine Long Acting Tolterodine LA offers a convenient once-daily dosing, and causes less dry mouth than taking IR products. It is better than placebo in efficacy outcomes, including ability to complete tasks before voiding and patient perception of benefit.[53] It also improves OAB symptoms in men who were taking α-adrenergic blockers.[54]

Tolterodine LA should be given once daily, and should not be crushed or chewed. The dose should be limited to 2 mg once daily in patients with mild to moderate hepatic impairment (Child-Pugh class A or B), severe renal impairment creatinine clearance 10 to 30 mL/min (0.17-0.50 mL/s), or taking drugs that are potent CYP3A4 inhibitors (ketoconazole, itraconazole, clarithromycin, or ritonavir). Patients with creatinine clearance less than 10 mL/min (<0.17 mL/s) or severe hepatic impairment (Child-Pugh class C) should avoid taking the drug. Patients should be counseled that it takes up to 8 weeks to see maximum benefit after starting therapy or dose escalation. Common adverse effects and monitoring parameters for tolterodine LA are similar to its IR product.[53]

Fesoterodine Fumarate Fesoterodine fumarate is also indicated for symptoms of urinary frequency, urgency, or urge incontinence. It is a prodrug that is metabolized to its active metabolite, 5-hydroxymethyl tolterodine (also a metabolite of tolterodine), by nonspecific plasma esterases.[55]

In a short-term study, fesoterodine was better than tolterodine ER 4 mg and placebo on reducing UUI episodes, micturitions, urgency and improving health-related quality of life. However, fesoterodine caused more dry mouth (28% vs 13%), and constipation (4% vs 3%) than tolterodine ER. It has been associated with higher discontinuation rates due to adverse events (5% vs 3%).[56]

The usual starting dose is 4 mg daily, increasing to 8 mg daily, as needed and tolerated. The dose of fesoterodine should not exceed 4 mg daily in the presence of severe renal impairment (creatinine clearance <30 mL/min [≤0.50 mL/s]) or in patients also taking potent CYP3A4 inhibitors. Fesoterodine is not recommended in patients with severe hepatic impairment. It is available in XL tablets, which should be swallowed whole; patients should not chew, crush, or divide the product.[55]

The most common adverse effects of fesoterodine are dry mouth (27%), constipation (5.1%), dyspepsia (2%), and dry eyes (1.6%). Anticholinergic adverse effects associated with fesoterodine are dose-related.[55]

Trospium Chloride Immediate Release Trospium chloride, a quaternary ammonium anticholinergic, is a second-generation antimuscarinic agent for UUI. Trospium chloride is poorly absorbed after oral administration (<10%), and food reduces bioavailability by 70% to 80%. It is principally cleared by the renal route (60%). Metabolites account for approximately 40% of the excreted dose following oral administration. The major metabolic pathway is hypothesized as ester hydrolysis with subsequent conjugation. CYP is not expected to contribute significantly to the elimination of trospium. The plasma half-life is approximately 20 hours; with renal clearance about 30 L/h. Active tubular secretion is a major route of elimination for trospium. When creatinine clearance is less than 30 mL/min (0.50 mL/s), drug exposure and drug concentration are significantly increased.[57]

In a study involving a large proportion of elders (mean age, 63 years), trospium chloride was better than placebo in efficacy outcomes of UUI. In a 12-week, controlled study, trospium chloride IR was noninferior to oxybutynin IR in managing UUI, but was associated with less dry mouth.[58]

The frequency of anticholinergic side effects of trospium was higher in patients 75 years and older than younger subjects. This occurrence is believed to be pharmacodynamic (ie, increased sensitivity). No data at present support the hypothesis that trospium chloride is less neurotoxic than nonquaternary ammonium anticholinergics (based on the hypothesis of reduced transit across the blood–brain barrier of trospium chloride due to its positive electrical charge on the quaternary nitrogen). Trospium may interact with other drugs that are eliminated by active tubular secretion via competition (eg, procainamide, pancuronium, morphine, vancomycin, and tenofovir).[57] Trospium IR is dosed 20 mg twice daily, and should be taken on an empty stomach. Dosage reduction (by 50% of the daily dose) is recommended when creatinine clearance is less than 30 mL/min (0.50 mL/s). In older patients (75 years and older), dose reduction to 20 mg once daily should be considered based upon tolerability.[57]

Trospium Chloride Extended-Release Trospium chloride ER offers once-daily dosing. Its efficacy and safety have been demonstrated in patients with OAB, including those who are older and taking multiple medications.[59,60]

Trospium is eliminated primarily unchanged in the urine. It is not recommended in patients with severe renal impairment (creatinine clearance <30 mL/min [≤0.50 mL/s]). Alcohol should not be consumed within 2 hours of trospium ER administration. Coadministration with antacid may increase or decrease trospium exposure, but the clinical relevance of these findings is unknown. In addition, coadministration of immediate-release (IR) metformin 500 mg twice daily reduced the steady-state systemic exposure of trospium by approximately 29% and peak concentration by 34%.[60]

The usual dosage of trospium ER is 60 mg daily. Because food decreases the bioavailability by 35% to 60%, XL trospium chloride must be taken on an empty stomach (1 hour before or 2 hours after meals).[60] Common adverse effects with trospium chloride ER have been dry mouth (11%), constipation (9%), dizziness (2%), dry eyes (1.6%), flatulence (1.6%), nausea (1.4%), and abdominal pain (1.4%). Patients should be informed that alcohol may enhance the drowsiness caused by anticholinergic agents.[60]

Solifenacin Succinate Solifenacin succinate is a second-generation antimuscarinic agent indicated for the treatment of OAB with urge incontinence, urgency, and urinary frequency.[61] Solifenacin was better than tolterodine ER in terms of reducing the number of UUI episodes and pad usage and in improving patients' perception of their bladder condition.[62] Clinical data showed that solifenacin recipients had significant improvement in 5 of 10 quality-of-life domains from baseline compared with placebo recipients.[63] Compared with oxybutynin IR, solifenacin was associated with fewer episodes (35% vs 83%) and lower severity of dry mouth.[64,65]

Solifenacin is well absorbed (mean absolute bioavailability, 88%), and food has no clinically relevant effect on absorption. It is principally eliminated via metabolism and renal excretion of metabolites, with renal excretion of parent compound less than 10% of the dose. With a mean terminal disposition half-life of 50 to 60 hours, the drug can be dosed once daily.[61] The primary pathway for elimination of solifenacin is via CYP3A4. Adverse effects, including dry mouth, occurred similarly between younger and older patients.[64]

The recommended dose of solifenacin is 5 mg once daily. If the drug is well tolerated but the effectiveness is not optimal, the dose can be increased to 10 mg once daily. Little additional benefit is generally achieved with doses exceeding 5 mg daily. Solifenacin can be administered with or without food. For patients with creatinine clearance rates less than 30 mL/min (0.50 mL/s) or with moderate hepatic impairment (Child-Pugh class B), the daily dosage should not exceed 5 mg. Patients who have severe hepatic impairment (Child-Pugh class C) should avoid using this drug. If the patient is receiving concurrent therapy with one or more potent CYP3A4 inhibitors, the daily dose should not exceed 5 mg.

The most common adverse reactions of solifenacin are dry mouth (11%-28%), constipation (5%-13%), urinary tract infection (4%-5%), and blurred vision (3%-5%). It interacts with CYP3A4 inhibitors and inducers; close patient monitoring is required. Prolonged corrected QT intervals have been reported with high-dose solifenacin.[61]

Darifenacin Darifenacin is another second-generation antimuscarinic for the management of OAB or UUI. It improves urinary symptoms, and quality of life.[66,67] It may be considered in patients who are dissatisfied with previous antimuscarinic treatments.

The mean absolute bioavailabilities of the 7.5-, 15-, and 30-mg extended-release (ER) formulations are 15%, 19%, and 25%, respectively. Bioavailability is affected by formulation, CYP2D6 genotype, dose, and race. Bioavailability is enhanced using an ER formulation (70%-110% higher than IR), in heterozygous CYP2D6 extensive metabolizers and poor metabolizers (40%-90% higher than homozygous extensive metabolizers), and white race (56% higher than Japanese). Darifenacin is extensively metabolized, with cumulative urinary excretion of the parent compound less than 10%. The 2D6 and 3A4 isoenzymes of CYP are responsible for darifenacin metabolism. With a mean terminal disposition half-life of 3 to 5 hours (depending on CYP2D6 metabolizer status), an ER formulation is needed to allow once-daily dosing.[68]

Darifenacin ER should be initiated at 7.5 mg once daily, and may be increased to 15 mg once daily after 2 weeks to target clinical response. The dosage should be limited to 7.5 mg daily in patients with moderate hepatic impairment (Child-Pugh B), taking potent CYP3A4 inhibitors. It should be avoided in patients with severe hepatic impairment (Child-Pugh C). It must be swallowed whole without chewing, dividing, or crushing. The most frequently reported adverse reactions are constipation (21%), dry mouth (19%), headache (7%), dyspepsia (5%), and nausea (4%). Darifenacin may interact with substrates of CYP2D6 (flecainide, thioridazine, and tricyclic antidepressants).[68]

Clinical **Controversy...**

Should antimuscarinic pharmacotherapy be used to treat UUI in patients with mild cognitive impairment or dementia? Antimuscarinic agents may worsen cognitive function, especially in older adults. Caution should be exercised as these agents may antagonize the therapeutic effects of acetylcholine esterase inhibitors indicated for dementia.

Mirabegron Mirabegron has been approved by FDA in June 2012 for the treatment of OAB with symptoms of UUI, urgency, and urinary frequency.

6 Mirabegron is another second-line treatment for managing UUI. It increases bladder capacity by relaxing the detrusor smooth muscle during the storage phase of the urinary bladder fill-void cycle by the activation of β_3-adrenergic receptors. Similar to antimuscarinic agents, it is only modestly effective and reduces urinary frequency and incontinence episodes by less than one per day. It is associated with nonsignificant improvements in UUI, urgency episodes, and quality-of-life measures. It has been shown to have similar efficacy as with tolterodine ER.[22,69] It reduces mean number of incontinence episodes per 24 hours, mean number of micturitions per 24 hours, and increased mean volume voided per micturition. The efficacy is usually seen during 4 to 8 weeks of therapy.[69]

Mirabegron reaches its peak plasma concentrations at approximately 3.5 hours, and has an oral bioavailability of 29% to 35%. It achieves steady state within 7 days of therapy. It can be taken with or without food. Mirabegron is extensively distributed in the body, with a volume of distribution of approximately 1,670 L. It has protein binding of approximately 71% to both albumin and α_1-acid glycoprotein. Mirabegron is metabolized via multiple pathways involving dealkylation, oxidation, glucuronidation, and amide hydrolysis. It has two inactive metabolites (16% and 11% of total exposure), respectively. Isoenzymes CYP2D6 and 3A4 play a limited role in its elimination. Poor metabolizers of CYP2D6 had an increased mean peak concentration and drug exposure compared to extensive metabolizers of CYP2D6 (16% and 17%, respectively). Other enzymes that are involved in mirabegron metabolism include butylcholinesterase, uridine diphospho-glucuronosyltransferases (UGT), and possibly alcohol dehydrogenase.

Total body clearance of mirabegron is about 57 L/h, with a terminal elimination half-life of 50 hours. Renal clearance equals approximately 13 L/h, primarily through active tubular secretion along with glomerular filtration. The urinary elimination of unchanged mirabegron is dose-dependent and ranges from 6% to 12% after a daily dose of 25 to 100 mg.[69]

Mirabegron should be initiated at 25 mg once daily, and may titrate upward to 50 mg once daily after 8 weeks, based on individual efficacy and tolerability; limit dose to 25 mg once daily in patients with severe renal impairment or moderate hepatic disease. Mirabegron is available in ER tablets, and should be swallowed whole with water without chewing, dividing, or crushing. It should be avoided in patients with end-stage renal disease, severe hepatic impairment, or severe uncontrolled hypertension (≥180/110 mm Hg). Most commonly reported adverse reactions were hypertension (7%-11%), nasopharyngitis (4%), urinary tract infection (3%-6%), and headache (3%-4%). Patient should be monitored for increased blood pressure and urinary retention, particularly in patients with bladder outlet obstruction or those who are taking anticholinergic drugs.[69] Mirabegron has similar adverse effects (except less dry mouth) when compared with tolterodine ER. Blood pressure and heart rate changes were minimal (<1 mm Hg and <2 beats per minutes, respectively).[22] Mirabegron is a moderate inhibitor of CYP2D6, and may affect the dosage requirement for some 2D6 substrates (eg, metoprolol and desipramine). Thus, drug level monitoring for certain medications with a narrow therapeutic range, such as thioridazine, flecainide, and propafenone, is advised. When initiating a combination of mirabegron and digoxin, start with the lowest possible dose of digoxin and titrate based on drug level and clinical effect.[69]

Other Anticholinergics and Antimuscarinics Other drugs for treatment of UUI are less effective, are not safer, or have not been adequately studied.[23] Tricyclic antidepressants are generally no more effective than oxybutynin IR, and give bothersome and potentially serious adverse effects (eg, orthostatic hypotension, cardiac conduction abnormalities, dizziness, and confusion). They are also potentially life-threatening in overdose. Therefore, their use should be limited to individuals who have one or more additional medical indications for these agents (eg, depression or neuropathic pain); patients with mixed UI (because of their effect of decreasing bladder contractility and increasing outlet resistance); and possibly those with nocturnal incontinence associated with altered sleep patterns. Because of the lower incidence of adverse effects, desipramine and nortriptyline may be preferred over imipramine and doxepin. However, due to their lower anticholinergic activity, they may not be as effective. Other agents that are not recommended for UUI include propantheline, flavoxate, dicyclomine and hyoscyamine.

Clinical **Controversy...**

Which approved agent should be used as first-line pharmacotherapy of UUI (oxybutynin, tolterodine, trospium chloride, solifenacin, darifenacin, fesoterodine, or mirabegron)? Financial considerations currently favor generic oxybutynin IR. Choice of an initial agent should be individualized based on tolerability, affordability, and adherence issues. Patient comorbidities may favor the use of more expensive branded agents.

Comparative Data Several systematic reviews with meta-analyses have examined the comparative effectiveness and adverse effects of antimuscarinic drugs for UI and OAB.[37,70,71] In general, higher doses of a particular drug were associated with greater adverse effects, particularly dry mouth. LA products (oxybutynin and tolterodine) had less dry mouth as compared to IR formulations.

In one meta-analysis of 86 randomized controlled trials, clinical effects of different doses of muscarinic drugs (tolterodine, solifenacin, fesoterodine) were compared.[70] For tolterodine, daily regimens of 1 mg, 2 mg, and 4 mg had similar effects for UI episodes and micturitions in 24 hours. For solifenacin, frequency and urgency were better with 10 mg when compared with 5 mg. For fesoterodine, some outcomes (patient-reported cure, UI episodes, micturitions per 24 hours) were better for 8 mg versus 4 mg; however, there were no differences in efficacy between 4 mg and 12 mg, although dry mouth was significantly higher with 12 mg. Comparing of the IR products of oxybutynin and tolterodine found similar in efficacy. Oxybutynin IR was associated with lower tolerability, particularly dry mouth, than tolterodine IR or LA. Oxybutynin IR, TDS (patch), and tolterodine LA produced similar reductions in the number of incontinence episodes. However, the oral agents were associated with higher frequencies of dry mouth and constipation. In contrast, the patch formulation was associated with higher frequencies of local (application site) reactions.[70]

Solifenacin had greater clinical efficacy (patient-reported cure or improvement, UI episodes, urgency episodes, and quality of life) than did tolterodine, although constipation was more common. Darifenacin 15 mg daily dose had similar efficacy to oxybutynin in reducing OAB symptoms but a lower occurrence of dry mouth. When comparing darifenacin 30 mg with oxybutynin 30 mg, dry mouth rates were similar, but constipation was more frequent in patients treated with darifenacin 30 mg.[70,71]

In a systematic review of 94 randomized controlled trials involving drugs for UUI, all drugs showed similar small benefits.[37] Per 1,000 treated women, continence was restored in this decreasing order: fesoterodine, oxybutynin or trospium, solifenacin, and tolterodine. Rates of treatment discontinuation due to adverse effects in this decreasing order: oxybutynin, fesoterodine, trospium, and solifenacin.[37] Tolterodine was found to be better tolerated than fesoterodine or oxybutynin. More data are needed to assess long-term adherence and drug safety, quality-of-life improvements, and comparative effectiveness among drugs.[37]

Currently, there is no direct comparison between antimuscarinics and mirabegron. In a meta-analysis of 44 trials examining the effects of mirabegron 50 mg versus antimuscarinics in patients with OAB, mirabegron and antimuscarinics had similar efficacy in reducing UI and UUI, with the exception of solifenacin 10 mg that was more efficacious in improving micturition frequency and frequency of UUI. However, mirabegron had a similar incidence of dry mouth as placebo, and significantly lower incidence than antimuscarinics.[38] Selection of an initial drug therapy most likely depends on side-effect profile, comorbidities, concurrent drug therapy, and patient preference in drug delivery methods. Table 85-7 lists the frequencies for the most common adverse events for all approved treatment agents based on manufacturers' product information.

Botulinum Toxin A Enthusiasm is considerable for the application of botulinum toxin A for treatment of voiding dysfunction. Botulinum toxin is a naturally occurring powerful muscle relaxant produced by *Clostridium botulinum*.

Injected into smooth or striated muscle, botulinum toxin acts as a neurotoxin by temporarily paralyzing the muscle. The mechanism of action of the paralytic effect is generally ascribed to prevention of the release of the neurotransmitter acetylcholine into the synapse at the neuromuscular junction, although other pathways in neurotransduction may also be affected.

This compound is commercially produced for medical use in a number of conditions such as muscle spasticity, hyperhidrosis, and cosmetic reduction of skin wrinkles. It is currently indicated for the treatment of detrusor overactivity associated with neurologic condition and OAB.[72-74] Intradetrusor onabotulinumtoxin A is recommended by AUA as the third-line treatment in adult patients with refractory OAB.[22] In the lower urinary tract, it has also been used to treat external urethral sphincter spasticity by direct injection into the external urethral sphincter.

Botulinum toxin is delivered into the detrusor muscle (intravesical injection) using a cystoscope equipped with a needle. The usual dosage is between 100 and 300 units per session. It is injected through the needle directly into the bladder muscle in 10 to 30 injections spaced over 5 to 10 minutes. The procedure is carried out as an outpatient procedure without general anesthesia. The duration of therapeutic effect varies, lasting usually from 4 to 8 months. Repeat injections are necessary to maintain the beneficial effects.[74]

The adverse effects of botulinum toxin A when used in the urinary tract most frequently include dysuria, hematuria, urinary tract infection, and urinary retention. Urinary retention occurs in up to 20% of treated individuals and persists until the paralytic effects have worn off (up to 6-8 months). Therapeutic and adverse effects may not become evident for 3 to 7 days, presumably because this period of time is required for uptake of the toxin following injection.[73,74]

Intravesical (ie, bladder) injection of botulinum toxin A in patients with refractory OAB resulted in increased bladder capacity, increased bladder compliance, and improved quality of life.[73,74] Adverse effects include urinary tract infection and urinary retention.[73] Comparative data with placebo and other interventions, long-term safety and efficacy outcomes, and data regarding the optimal dose of botulinum toxin for idiopathic OAB are needed.

An alternative mechanism of delivery other than intravesical injection would greatly improve the appeal of this agent as needle injection can be painful in some individuals. Results of an open-label trial of intravesical botulinum toxin A in dimethylsulfoxide in 21 women with refractory idiopathic detrusor overactivity demonstrated a significant reduction in the frequency of incontinence episodes without any effect on postvoid residual urine volumes.[75] Further studies are needed in this regard.

Catheterization Combined with Medications Patients with UUI and an elevated postvoid residual urine volume due to retention may require intermittent self-catheterization along with frequent

TABLE 85-7 Adverse Event Incidence Rates with Approved Drugs for Bladder Overactivity[a]

Drug	Dry Mouth	Constipation	Dizziness	Vision Disturbance
Oxybutynin IR	71	15	17	10
Oxybutynin XL	61	13	6	14
Oxybutynin TDS	7	3	NR	3
Oxybutynin gel	10	1	3	3
Tolterodine	35	7	5	3
Tolterodine LA	23	6	2	4
Trospium chloride IR	20	10	NR	1
Trospium chloride XR	11	9	NR	2
Solifenacin	20	9	2	5
Darifenacin ER	24	18	2	2
Fesoterodine ER	27	5	NR	3
Mirabegron ER	3	3	3	NR

IR, immediate release; LA, long acting; TDS, transdermal system; XL, extended release; XR/ER, extended release; NR, not reported.

[a]All values constitute mean data, predominantly using product information from the manufacturers.

voiding between catheterizations. If intermittent catheterization is not possible, surgical placement of a suprapubic catheter may be necessary. Use of a chronic indwelling catheter should be avoided because of the increased occurrence of urinary tract infections and nephrolithiasis.

Regardless of catheterization status, patients may experience symptom relief with judicious use of oxybutynin (IR, XL, or TDS formulations), tolterodine (IR or LA formulations), trospium chloride, solifenacin, fesoterodine, darifenacin, or mirabegron, as these agents relax the detrusor muscle and enhance bladder storage. Patients with UUI and symptoms of urinary retention may also benefit from an α-adrenergic receptor antagonist that relaxes the internal bladder sphincter (eg, prazosin, terazosin, doxazosin, tamsulosin, silodosin, and alfuzosin). Although theoretically of benefit, bethanechol, a cholinergic agonist, has not been demonstrated effective in improving bladder emptying in well-done trials. In addition, it causes numerous bothersome (eg, muscle and abdominal cramping and diarrhea) and potentially life-threatening adverse effects and should not be used in patients with asthma or heart disease.[23]

Urethral Underactivity

7 Urethral underactivity, or SUI, may be aggravated by agents with α-adrenergic receptor blocking activity, including prazosin, terazosin, doxazosin, tamsulosin, alfuzosin, silodosin, methyldopa, clonidine, guanfacine, guanadrel, and labetalol. The goal of therapy for SUI is to improve the urethral closure mechanism by stimulating α-adrenergic receptors in the smooth muscle of the bladder neck and proximal urethra, enhancing the supportive structures underlying the urethral epithelium, or enhancing the positive effects of serotonin and norepinephrine in the afferent and efferent pathways of the micturition reflex.[76]

Estrogens Local and systemic estrogens have been used extensively for the pharmacologic management of SUI since the 1940s. Estrogens are believed to work via several mechanisms, including enhancement of the proliferation of urethral epithelium, local circulation, and numbers and/or sensitivity of urogenital α-adrenergic receptors. However, a trial has questioned whether estrogens exert a stimulatory effect on vaginal collagen production, at least over the short-term.[77]

A meta-analysis of 34 trials evaluating the use of local or systemic estrogen therapy on UI in postmenopausal women found that systematic administration of estrogen alone or in combination with progesterone resulted in UI worsening.[78] In fact, observational studies have documented that oral or systemic estrogen use is associated with an increased risk of UI compared with that in nonusers.[79] There was some evidence that vaginal estrogen (vaginal cream or pessaries) may improve UI, and reduce urgency and frequency. The long-term effects of this therapy in older women are unknown. A recent meta-analysis of 17 trials of local estrogen compared to placebo or no treatment found beneficial effects on UI and OAB symptoms and some urodynamic parameters.[80] Different forms of vaginal estrogen (ring, pessary) appear to have similar improvements in urinary symptoms (SUI, UUI, frequency, urgency). Studies comparing vaginal estrogen alone or in combination with antimuscarinic drugs (tolterodine or oxybutynin) or pelvic floor muscle exercises found greater improvement in subjective measures of UI in the combination approach. If estrogens are to be used for treatment of UI or OAB in postmenopausal women, only topical products should be administered, potentially combined with other treatment modalities such as pelvic floor muscle exercises or antimuscarinic drugs.

α-Adrenergic Receptor Agonists Numerous open trials have supported the use of a variety of α-adrenergic receptor agonists in SUI, including ephedrine, norfenefrine, phenylpropanolamine, and midodrine. Phenylpropanolamine was withdrawn from the US market in 2000 because of a risk for stroke in women using the agent.[80] Some patients may have left over supplies of this agent or may obtain it from international sources. If so, individuals with the contraindications listed later in the chapter (especially coronary artery disease and/or cardiac arrhythmias) should be warned against self-treatment with this or other α-adrenergic receptor agonists.

Placebo-controlled comparative trials with phenylpropanolamine, norfenefrine, and norephedrine support the modest efficacy of these agents for treatment of mild or moderate SUI.[81,82] These agents have been found to variably affect maximum urethral closure pressure and functional urethral length.

Adverse effects include hypertension, headache, dry mouth, nausea, insomnia, and restlessness. Contraindications to the use of these agents include the presence of hypertension, tachyarrhythmias, coronary artery disease, myocardial infarction, cor pulmonale, hyperthyroidism, renal failure, and narrow-angle glaucoma.

Several studies have evaluated whether the clinical and urodynamic effects of a combination of estrogen and an α-adrenergic receptor agonist exceed those of the individual therapies in SUI.[82] In general, combination therapy has resulted in somewhat superior clinical and urodynamic responses compared with monotherapy, including severity of complaints, amount of urine lost per episode, number of daily voluntary micturitions, number of leakage episodes per day, patient preference, pad use, maximum urethral closure pressure, functional urethral length, and pressure transmission ratio.

Duloxetine Duloxetine, a dual inhibitor of serotonin and norepinephrine reuptake (SNRI), was approved in 2004 for treatment of depression and painful diabetic neuropathy in the United States.[83] It is approved for SUI in Europe only. It is believed to affect central serotoninergic and noradrenergic regions, which are involved in ascending and descending control of urethral smooth muscle and the external urethral sphincter. These mechanisms facilitate the bladder-to-sympathetic reflex pathway, increasing urethral and external urethral sphincter muscle tone during the storage phase.

The mean terminal disposition half-life, clearance, and volume of distribution of duloxetine in healthy volunteers are 10 to 12 hours, 114 to 119 L/h, and 1,787 to 1,943 L, respectively. Duloxetine is metabolized by CYP2D6 and 1A2 enzymes to form multiple metabolites and then eliminated in the urine. Duloxetine may increase the concentrations, drug exposure and half-lives of CYP2D6 substrates (eg, desipramine). Meanwhile, the drug concentration of duloxetine can be increased by CYP2D6 inhibitors (eg, paroxetine) and CYP1A2 inhibitors (eg, fluvoxamine).[83]

Moderate hepatic dysfunction (Child-Pugh class B) significantly increases mean AUC and terminal disposition half-life of duloxetine. Mild or moderate renal impairment (creatinine clearance 30-80 mL/min [0.50-1.33 mL/s]) does not affect drug disposition. In severe renal impairment (hemodialysis patients), mean peak plasma concentration and AUC are both increased 100%, whereas metabolite concentrations are increased up to 900%.[83]

In six large double-blinded, randomized, placebo-controlled clinical trials that evaluated duloxetine for SUI, duloxetine therapy produced significant reductions in UI episode frequency and number of micturitions per day, improvement in incontinence quality-of-life questionnaire scores and patient self-assessment, and increase in mean micturition interval. Results were independent of baseline UI severity (severity based on incontinent episode frequency). Significant intergroup differences were seen by week 4. However, cure rates were generally not improved by duloxetine. When evaluating the absolute differences between treatments, the actual benefit of duloxetine was generally quite modest.[83] Duloxetine also reduced incontinence episodes and improved quality of life in men with SUI after radical prostatectomy.[84]

A randomized, placebo-controlled clinical trial evaluated the effects of duloxetine (80 mg daily), pelvic floor muscle training (PFMT), and the combination of both modalities on incontinent episode frequency, incontinence-related quality of life, pad use, and patient global impression of change. Sham PFMT was used in the placebo group. Results indicated that duloxetine plus PFMT were probably additive in effect and that combination therapy afforded greater improvement than either monotherapy.[85]

The adverse events associated with duloxetine may make adherence problematic. In the SUI trials, treatment-emergent adverse events occurred in 68% to 93% of duloxetine and 50% to 72% of placebo recipients. Premature study withdrawal rates (due to adverse events) were as high as up to 33%. The most common adverse events reported with duloxetine were nausea (≤46%), headache (≤27%), constipation (≤27%), dry mouth (≤22%), and insomnia (≤14%). Of interest, the drug may be associated with small increases in blood pressure (such as venlafaxine, another SNRI) and withdrawal symptoms (sleep disturbances). Unfortunately, adherence to long-term therapy is quite poor due to a combination of adverse events and lack of efficacy.[86]

Despite these negatives, duloxetine is the first drug approved by a regulatory agency for treating SUI in Europe. Based on studies conducted to date, a dosage regimen of 40 to 80 mg/day (in one or two doses) appears reasonable. Gradual dose titration (40 mg daily for 2 weeks, then 80 mg daily) helps reduce the risks of nausea, dizziness, and premature drug discontinuation. If cessation of duloxetine is desired, consider tapering the dosage by 50% for 2 weeks before discontinuation to avoid withdrawal symptoms.

Venlafaxine Venalfaxine is another SNRI. A double-blind, randomized, placebo-controlled clinical trial has demonstrated the benefit of venlafaxine 75 mg once daily for 12 weeks over placebo in terms of incontinence episode frequency, voiding interval, quality of life, and patient global impression of improvement. Nausea occurred in 40% of the venlafaxine group compared with 15% of the placebo group.[87]

Overflow Incontinence

Overflow incontinence secondary to benign or malignant prostatic hyperplasia may be amenable to pharmacotherapy. For management of malignant prostatic disease, see Chapter 131. The pharmacotherapy of BPH is discussed in Chapter 84.

Clinical **Controversy...**

The optimal approach to pharmacotherapy of SUI is unclear. Although not supported by evidence-based medicine, many clinicians initiate a trial of topical estrogen, followed by addition of an α-adrenergic receptor agonist in estrogen nonresponders unless contraindicated. No drugs, except duloxetine in Europe, have been approved for the management of SUI. However, long-term tolerability issues may hinder chronic use.

PERSONALIZED PHARMACOTHERAPY

Patient factors (age, comorbidities, concurrent drug therapies, ability to adhere to prescribed regimen, etc) should be considered when selecting pharmacotherapy for patients with UI.

All anticholinergic/antimuscarinic drugs have similar contraindications and precautions, including urinary retention, gastric retention, uncontrolled narrow-angle glaucoma, CNS effects, angioedema, and myasthenia gravis. IR formulations of older agents (oxybutynin and tolterodine) have been associated with higher rates of anticholinergic adverse effects (dry mouth, constipation, headache, dyspepsia, dry eyes, cognitive impairment, tachycardia, and urinary retention). Older patients are particularly susceptible to these adverse events, thus require close monitoring. Significant dry mouth may lead to dental caries, ill-fitting dentures, and swallowing difficulty. Orthostatic hypotension and sedation may lead to falls in patients with baseline cognitive or cardiac conditions. Constipation is prevalent among the older patients because of polypharmacy and age-related physiologic changes.

All patients on anticholinergics should be warned about risk of somnolence and advised not to drive or operate heavy machinery until they know how the drugs affect them. Women with mixed UI or UUI plus urethritis or vaginitis may benefit from a topical estrogen (alone or in combination with an anticholinergic drug). Men with irritative symptoms of BPH that are nonresponsive to drug therapy may benefit from anticholinergic therapy while being closely monitored for the risk of precipitating acute urinary retention.

Antimuscarnic drugs should be considered for the management of UUI as monotherapy or in combination with nonpharmacologic interventions. None of the currently available antimuscarnic agents appears to have a clear advantage in efficacy over others. Selection of an agent should be based on drug tolerability, dosing convenience, cost considerations, and patient preference. In general, LA or ER products given once daily are preferable over IR ones because of better tolerability. Dose escalation of IR formulations may result in improved efficacy, albeit limited, at the cost of an increase in adverse event frequency and severity. Newer antimuscarnic agents and mirabegron may be good choices for patients who are intolerable of CNS adverse effects associated with older agents. Topical formulations, such as oxybutynin TDS or gel, may offer favorable systemic adverse effect profiles and convenient dosing. Selection of an agent should also be based on patient factors, such as renal/hepatic function, concomitant diseases, concurrent drug therapy, and medication adherence. It is advisable to review concomitant medications for any possibility of additive, synergistic, antagonistic drug interactions in cholinergic system and liver enzymes (CYP3A4 and 2D6).

EVALUATION OF THERAPEUTIC OUTCOMES

8 Assessment of patient outcomes should include efficacy, side effects, adherence, and quality of life. During long-term management of UI, patient-specific clinical signs and symptoms of most distress ("bother") to the individual must be monitored. A daily diary may be useful in this regard. Some of the short-form instruments used in incontinence research for measuring symptom impact and condition-specific quality of life can be used in clinical monitoring. In addition, quantitating the use of ancillary supplies, such as pads, may be useful.

9 The main goal of therapy is to minimize the signs and symptoms most bothersome to the patient, as well as the use of pads and other ancillary supplies or devices. Total elimination of UI signs and symptoms may not be possible, and patients and practitioners need to mutually establish realistic goals of therapy. Because the therapies for UI frequently have nuisance adverse effects (eg, anticholinergic effects such as dry mouth, constipation, sedation, etc) that may compromise regimen adherence, the presence and severity of adverse effects must be carefully elicited at each visit to the health-care practitioner. Queries of the patient and caregiver regarding CNS effects are important in elderly or frail patient as these effects can be severe enough to cause loss of independent living skills. Emergence of adverse effects may necessitate drug dosage adjustment or use of alternative strategies (eg, chewing sugarless gum, sucking on hard sugarless candy, or use of saliva substitutes in xerostomia) or even drug discontinuation. Patient should be encouraged to persist with a particular treatment for 4 to 8 weeks before declaring treatment failure. Nonresponders to an antimuscarinic should be offered at least one other antimuscarinic and/or dose modification attempted to obtain a better balance between efficacy and side effects.

ABBREVIATIONS

ACE	angiotensin-converting enzyme
AUA	American Urological Association
AUC	area under the plasma or serum concentration-versus-time curve
BPH	benign prostatic hyperplasia
CYP	cytochrome P450
DD01	5-hydroxymethyl metabolite
ER	extended-release
EStim	electrical stimulation
FDA	Food and Drug Administration
IR	immediate release
LA	long acting
MStim	magnetic stimulation
OAB	overactive bladder
PFMT	pelvic floor muscle training
PTNS	peripheral tibial nerve stimulation
SNRI	serotonin and norepinephrine reuptake
SUI	stress urinary incontinence
TDS	transdermal system
UI	urinary incontinence
UGT	uridine diphospho-glucuronosyltransferases
UUI	urge urinary incontinence
XL	extended release

REFERENCES

1. Milsom I, Altman D, Cartwright, R, et al. Epidemiology of urinary incontinence (UI) and other lower rrinary tract symptoms (LUTS), pelvic organ prolapse (POP) and anal incontinence (AI). In: Abrams P, Cardozo L, Khoury S, Wein A, eds. *Incontinence*, 5th ed. International Consultation on Urological Disease - European Association of Urology (ICUD-EAU), 2013:15-108.
2. Milsom I, Kaplan SA, Coyne KS, et al. Effect of bothersome overactive bladder symptoms on health-related quality of life, anxiety, depression, and treatment seeking in the United States: Results from EpiLUTS. *Urology* 2012;80(1):90-96.
3. Simeonova Z, Milsom I, Kullendorff AM, et al. The prevalence of urinary incontinence and its influence on the quality of life in women from an urban Swedish population. *Acta Obstet Gynecol Scand* 1999; 78:546-551.
4. Brown JS, Nyberg LM, Kusek JW, et al. Proceedings of the National Institute of Diabetes, Digestive and Kidney Diseases International Symposium on epidemiologic issues in urinary incontinence in women. *Am J Obstet Gynecol* 2003;188:S77-S88.
5. Bump RC. Racial comparisons and contrasts in urinary incontinence and pelvic organ prolapse. *Obstet Gynecol* 1993;81:421-425.
6. Burgio KL, Matthews KA, Engel BT. Prevalence, incidence and correlates of urinary incontinence in healthy, middle-aged women. *J Urol* 1991;146:1255-1259.
7. Breakwell SL, Walker SN. Differences in physical health, social interaction and personal adjustment between continent and incontinent homebound aged women. *J Community Health Nurs* 1988;5:19-31.
8. Andersson KE, Chapple C, Cardozo L, et al. Pharmacological treatment of urinary incontinence. In: Abrams P, Cardozo L, Khoury S, Wein A, eds. *Incontinence*, 5th ed. International Consultation on Urological Disease - European Association of Urology (ICUD-EAU) 2013:623-672.
9. Malmsten UG, Milsom I, Molander U, Norlen LJ. Urinary incontinence and lower urinary tract symptoms: An epidemiological study of men aged 45–99 years. *J Urol* 1997;158:1733-1737.
10. Kanai A, Wyndaele JJ, Andersson KE, et al. Researching bladder afferents-determining the effects of $\beta(3)$-adrenergic receptor agonists and botulinum toxin type-A. *Neurourol Urodyn* 2011;30(5):684-691.
11. Fowler C. Integrated control of the lower urinary tract—Clinical perspective. *Br J Pharmacol* 2006;147(Suppl 2):s14-s24.
12. Blok BF. Brain control of the lower urinary tract. *Scand J Urol Nephrol Suppl* 2002;(210):11-15.
13. Kuh D, Cardozo L, Hardy R. Urinary incontinence in middle-aged women: Childhood enuresis and other lifetime risk factors in a British prospective cohort. *J Epidemiol Community Health* 1999;53:453-458.
14. Groutz A, Gordon D, Keidar R, et al. Stress urinary incontinence: Prevalence among nulliparous compared with primiparous and grand multiparous premenopausal women. *Neurourol Urodyn* 1999; 18:419-425.
15. Ruby CM, Hanlon JT, Boudreau RM, et al. Health, aging and body composition study. The effect of medication use on urinary incontinence in community-dwelling elderly women. *J Am Geriatr Soc* 2010;58(9):1715-1720.
16. Haylen BT, de Ridder D, Freeman RM, et al. An International Urogynecological Association (IUGA)/International Continence Society (ICS) joint report on the terminology for female pelvic floor dysfunction. *Int Urogynecol J* 2010;21:5-26.
17. Resnick NM, Yalla S. Detrusor hyperactivity with impaired contractile function. An unrecognized but common cause of incontinence in the elderly patient. *JAMA* 1987;257:3076-3081.
18. Hall SA, Yang M, Gates MA, et al. Associations of commonly used medications with urinary incontinence in a community based sample. *J Urol* 2012;188(1):183-189.
19. Rovner ES, Wein AJ. Today's treatment of overactive bladder and urge incontinence. *Womens Health Prim Care* 2000;3:179-192.
20. James M, Jackson S, Shepard A, Abrams P. Pure stress leakage symptomatology: Is it safe to discount detrusor instability? *Br J Obstet Gynaecol* 1999;106:1255-1258.
21. Fritel X, Ringa V, Quiboeuf E, Fauconnier A. Female urinary incontinence, from pregnancy to menopause: A review of epidemiological and pathophysiological findings. *Acta Obstet Gynecol Scand* 2012;91(8):901-910.
22. Gormley EA, Lightner DJ, Burgio KL, Chai TC, et al. Diagnosis and treatment of overactive bladder (non-neurogenic) in adults: AUA/SUFU guideline amendment. 2014. Available at: http://www.auanet.org/common/pdf/education/clinical-guidance/Overactive-Bladder.pdf. Accessed June 3, 2016.
23. Cottenden A, Bliss DZ, Buckley B, et al. Management using continence products. In: Abrams P, Cardozo L, Khoury S, Wein A,

eds. *Incontinence,* 5th ed. International Consultation on Incontinence-European Urological Association. 2013:1651-1786.

24. Shamliyan T, Wyman J, Bliss DZ, Kane RL, Wilt TJ. Prevention of Urinary and Fecal Incontinence. Prepared by the Minnesota Evidence-based Practice Center under Contract 290-02-0009. Publication No. 08-E003. Rockville, MD: Agency for Healthcare Policy and Research; 2007.
25. Kirchin V, Page T, Keegan PE, Atiemo K, Cody JD, McClinton S. Urethral injection therapy for urinary incontinence in women. *Cochrane Database Syst Rev* 201215;2:CD003881.
26. Suskind AM, Kaufman SR, Dunn RL, et al. Population-based trends in ambulatory surgery for urinary incontinence. *Int Urogynecol J* 2013;24:207-211.
27. Koski ME, Rovner ES. Implications of the FDA statement on transvaginal placement of mesh: The aftermath. *Curr Urol Rep* 2014;15(2):380.
28. Sandhu JS. Treatment options for male stress urinary incontinence. *Nat Rev Urol* 2010;7(4):222-228.
29. Wilson LC, Gilling PJ. Post-prostatectomy urinary incontinence: A review of surgical treatment options. *BJU Int* 2011;107(Suppl 3): 7-10.
30. Welk BK, Herschorn S. The male sling for post-prostatectomy urinary incontinence: A review of contemporary sling designs and outcomes. *BJU Int* 2012;109(3):328-344.
31. Peters KM, Macdiarmid SA, Wooldridge LS, et al. Randomized trial of percutaneous tibial nerve stimulation versus extended-release tolterodine: Results from the overactive bladder innovative therapy trial. *J Urol* 2009;182(3):1055-1061.
32. Abrams P, Cardozo L, Khoury S, Wein A, eds. Recommendations of the International Scientific Committee: Evaluation and treatment of urinary incontinence, pelvic organ prolapse, and faecal incontinence. In: *Incontinence,* 3rd ed. Plymouth, UK: Health Publications Ltd., 2005:1589-1630.
33. Van Kerrebroeck PE, Marcelissen TA. Sacral neuromodulation for lower urinary tract dysfunction. *World J Urol* 2012;30(4):445-450.
34. Rovner E, Kennelly M, Schulte-Baukloh H, et al. Urodynamic results and clinical outcomes with intradetrusor injections of onabotulinum toxin A in a randomized, placebo-controlled dose-finding study in idiopathic overactive bladder. *Neurourol Urodyn* 2011;30(4):556-562.
35. Shepherd JP, Lowder JL, Leng WW, Smith KJ. InterStim sacral neuromodulation and botox botulinum—A toxin intradetrusor injections for refractory urge urinary incontinence: A decision analysis comparing outcomes including efficacy and complications. *Female Pelvic Med Reconstr Surg* 2011;17(4):199-203.
36. van Kerrebroeck PE, van Voskuilen AC, Heesakkers JP, et al. Results of sacral neuromodulation therapy for urinary voiding dysfunction: Outcomes of a prospective, worldwide clinical study. *J Urol* 2007; 178(5):2029-2034.
37. Shamliyan T, Wyman JF, Ramakrishnan R, Sainfort F, Kane RL. Benefits and harms of pharmacologic treatment for urinary incontinence in women: A systematic review. *Ann Intern Med* 2012;156(12):861-874, W301-W310.
38. Maman K, Aballea S, Nazir J, et al. Comparative efficacy and safety of medical treatments for the management of overactive bladder: A systematic review and mixed treatment comparison. *Eur Urol* 2014;65:755-765.
39. Ortho-McNeil-Janssen Pharmaceuticals. Ditropan (Oxybutynin) Package Insert. Raritan, NJ: Ortho-McNeil-Janssen; 2012.
40. Janssen Pharmaceuticals. Ditropan XL (Oxybutynin Chloride) Extended-Release Tablets Package Insert. Titusville, NJ: Janssen Pharmaceuticals; 2015.
41. Lam S, Hilas O. Pharmacologic management of overactive bladder. *Clin Intervent Aging* 2007;2:337-345.
42. Activis Pharma. Oxytrol (Oxybutynin Transdermal System) Package Insert. Parsippany, NJ: Activis Pharma; 2015.
43. Cartwright R, Srikrishna S, Cardozo L, Robinson D. Patient-selected goals in overactive bladder: A placebo controlled randomized double-blind trial of transdermal oxybutynin for the treatment of urgency and urge incontinence. *BJU Int* 2011;107(1):70-76.
44. Pizzi LT, Talati A, Gemmen E, et al. Impact of transdermal oxybutynin on work productivity in patients with overactive bladder: Results from the MATRIX study. *Pharmacoeconomics* 2009;27(4):329-339.
45. Newman DK. The MATRIX study: Evaluating the data in older adults. *Director* 2008;16(2):21-24.
46. Activis Pharma. Gelnique 3% (Oxybutynin Chloride 3% Gel) Package Insert. Parsippany, NJ: Activis Pharma; 2015.
47. Activis Pharma. Gelnique (Oxybutynin Chloride 10% Gel) Package Insert. Corona, CA: Activis Pharma; 2015.
48. Sand PK, Davila GW, Lucente VR, et al. Efficacy and safety of oxybutynin chloride topical gel for women with overactive bladder syndrome. *Am J Obstet Gynecol* 2012;206(2):168.e1-e6.
49. Staskin DR, Dmochowski RR, Sand PK, et al. Efficacy and safety of oxybutynin chloride topical gel for overactive bladder: A randomized, double-blind, placebo controlled, multicenter study. *J Urol* 2009;181: 1764-1772.
50. Esin E, Ergen A, Cankurtaran M, et al. Influence of antimuscarinic therapy on cognitive functions and quality of life in geriatric patients treated for overactive bladder. *Aging Ment Health* 2015;19:217-223.
51. Pharmacia & Upjohn. Detrol (Tolterodine) Package Insert. New York, NY: Pharmacia & Upjohn; 2008.
52. Gomes T, Juurlink DN, Mamdani MM. Comparative adherence to oxybutynin or tolterodine among older patients. *Eur J Clin Pharmacol* 2012;68(1):97-99.
53. Pharmacia & Upjohn. Detrol LA (Tolterodine Tartrate Extended Release Capsule). New York, NY: Pharmacia & Upjohn; 2011.
54. Chapple CR, Herschorn S, Abrams P, et al. Efficacy and safety of tolterodine extended-release in men with overactive bladder symptoms treated with an α-blocker: Effect of baseline prostate-specific antigen concentration. *BJU Int* 2010;106(9):1332-1338.
55. Pfizer Laboratories, Toviaz (Fesoterodine Fumarate Extended-Release Tablets) Package Insert. New York, NY: Pfizer; 2014.
56. Kaplan SA, Schneider T, Foote JE, et al. Superior efficacy of fesoterodine over tolterodine extended release with rapid onset: A prospective, head-to-head, placebo-controlled trial. *BJU Int* 2011;107(9):1432-1440.
57. Allergan. Sanctura (Trospium Chloride) Tablets Package Insert. Irvine, CA: Allergan; 2012.
58. Zellner M, Madersbacher H, Palmtag H, et al. Trospium chloride and oxybutynin hydrochloride in a German study of adults with urinary urge incontinence: Results of a 12-week, multicenter, randomized, double-blind, parallel-group, flexible-dose noninferiority trial. *Clin Ther* 2009;31(11):2519-2539.
59. Sand PK, Rovner ES, Watanabe JH, Oefelein MG. Once-daily trospium chloride 60 mg extended release in subjects with overactive bladder syndrome who use multiple concomitant medications: Post hoc analysis of pooled data from two randomized, placebo-controlled trials. *Drugs Aging* 2011;28(2):151-160.
60. Allergan, Sanctura XR (Trospium Chloride Extended-Release Capsules) Package Insert. Irvine, CA: Allergan; 2012.
61. Astellas Pharma Technologies. Vesicare (Solifenacin Succinate) Package Insert. Norman, Oklahoma: Stellas Pharma Technologies; 2013.
62. Chapple CR, Martinez-Garcia R, Selvaggi L, et al. A comparison of the efficacy and tolerability of solifenacin succinate and extended release tolterodine at treating overactive bladder syndrome: Results of the STAR trial. *Eur Urol* 2005;48:464-470.
63. Kelleher CJ, Cardozo L, Chapple CR, Haab F, Ridder AM. Improved quality of life in patients with overactive bladder symptoms treated with solifenacin. *BJU Int* 2005;95:81-85.
64. Herschorn S, Pommerville P, Stothers L, et al. Tolerability of solifenacin and oxybutynin immediate release in older (>65 years) and younger (≤65 years) patients with overactive bladder: Sub-analysis from a Canadian, randomized, double-blind study. *Curr Med Res Opin* 2011;27(2):375-382.
65. Herschorn S, Stothers L, Carlson K, et al. Tolerability of 5 mg solifenacin once daily versus 5 mg oxybutynin immediate release 3 times daily: Results of the VECTOR trial. *J Urol* 2010 May; 183(5):1892-1898.
66. Dwyer P, Kelleher C, Young J, et al. Long-term benefits of darifenacin treatment for patient quality of life: Results from a 2-year extension study. *Neurourol Urodyn* 2008;27(6):540-547.
67. Abrams P, Kelleher C, Huels J, et al. Clinical relevance of health-related quality of life outcomes with darifenacin. *BJU Int* 2008;102(2):208-213.
68. Warner Chilcott. Enablex (Darifenacin Extended Release) Package Insert. Rockaway, NJ: Warner Chilcott; 2013.
69. Astellas Pharma Technologies. Myrbetriq (Mirabegron) Package Insert. Norman, OK: Astellas Pharma Technologies; 2015.
70. Madhuvrata P, Cody JD, Ellis G, Herbison GP, Hay-Smith EJ. Which anticholinergic drug for overactive bladder symptoms in adults. *Cochrane Database Sys Rev* 2012 Jan 18;1:CD005429.
71. Novara G, Galfano A, Secco S, et al. A systematic review and meta-analysis of randomized controlled trials with antimuscarinic drugs for overactive bladder. *Eur Urol* 2008;54:740-764.
72. Anger JT, Weinberg A, Suttorp MJ, et al. Outcomes of intravesical botulinum toxin for idiopathic overactive bladder symptoms: A systematic review of the literature. *J Urol* 2010;183(6):2258-2264.
73. Dmochowski R, Chapple C, Nitti VW, et al. Efficacy and safety of onabotulinum toxin A for idiopathic overactive bladder: A

double-blind, placebo controlled, randomized, dose ranging trial. *J Urol* 2010;184(6):2416-2422.
74. Duthie JB, Vincent M, Herbison GP, Wilson DI, Wilson D. Botulinum toxin injections for adults with overactive bladder syndrome. *Cochrane Database Syst Rev* 2011;(12):CD005493.
75. Petrou SP, Parker AS, Crook JE, et al. Botulinum A toxin/ dimethylsulfoxide bladder instillations for women with refractory idiopathic detrusor overactivity: A phase I/II study. *Mayo Clin Proc* 2009;84:702-706.
76. Tsakiris P, de la Rosette JJ, Michel MC, et al. Pharmacologic treatment of male stress urinary incontinence: Systematic review of the literature and levels of evidence. *Eur Urol* 2008;53:53-59.
77. Jackson S, James M, Abrams P. The effect of oestradiol on vaginal collagen metabolism in postmenopausal women with genuine stress incontinence. *BJOG* 2002;109:339-344.
78. Cody JD, Jacobs ML, Richardson K, et al. Oestrogen therapy for urinary incontinence in post-menopausal women. Cochrane Database Syst Rev. 2012. Issue 10, Art. No.: CD001405. DOI: 10.1002/14651858.CD001405.pub2.
79. Grady D, Brown JS, Vittinghoff E, et al. Postmenopausal hormones and incontinence: The Heart & Estrogen/Progestin Replacement Study. *Obstet Gynecol* 2001;97:116-120.
80. Weber MA, Kleijn MH, Langendam M, et al. Local oestrogen for pelvic floor disorders: A systematic review. *PLOS One* 2015 Sep 18; 10(9):e013625.
81. Kernan WN, Viscoli CM, Brass LM, et al. Phenylpropanolamine and the risk of hemorrhagic stroke. *N Engl J Med* 2000:343:1826-1832.
82. Alhasso A, Glazener CM, Pickard R, N'dow J. Adrenergic drugs for urinary incontinence in adults. *Cochrane Database Syst Rev* 2005;3: CD001842.
83. Guay DRP. Duloxetine in the management of stress urinary incontinence. *Am J Geriatr Pharmacother* 2005;3:25-38.
84. Cornu JN, Merlet B, Ciofu C, et al. Duloxetine for mild to moderate postprostatectomy incontinence: Preliminary results of a randomised, placebo-controlled trial. *Eur Urol* 2011;59(1):148-154.
85. Ghoneim GM, VanLeeuwen JS, Elser DM, et al. A randomized controlled trial of duloxetine alone, pelvic floor muscle training alone, combined treatment and no active treatment in women with stress urinary incontinence. *J Urol* 2005;173:1647-1653.
86. Bump RC, Voss S, Beardsworth A, et al. Long-term efficacy of duloxetine in women with stress urinary incontinence. *Br J Urol Int* 2008;102:214-218.
87. Erdinc B, Gurates B, Celik H, et al. The efficacy of venlafaxine in the treatment of women with stress urinary incontinence. *Arch Gynecol Obstet* 2009;279:343-348.

Function and Evaluation of the Immune System

e86

Daniel A. Zlott, Nicole Weimert Pilch, and Geoffrey M. Thiele

KEY CONCEPTS

1. Cells of the immune system are derived from the pluripotent stem cell. Hematopoiesis is closely regulated to assure adequate numbers of different cell types. The development of these different cells or cell lineages depends on cell-to-cell interactions and hematopoietic growth factors.
2. Upon activation, dendritic cells (DCs) express higher concentrations of major histocompatibility complex class II molecules, B7-1, B7-2, CD40, ICAM-1, and LFA-3 molecules than other antigen-presenting cells (APCs). They also produce more IL-12. These differences may explain why, in vitro, DCs are the most efficient APC.
3. A T lymphocyte expresses hundreds of T-cell receptors (TCRs). All the TCRs expressed on the surface of an individual T lymphocyte have the same antigen specificity.
4. An immature B lymphocyte expresses thousands of membrane-bound surface immunoglobulin (sIg) as IgM (monomeric) or IgD, all with the same specificity (ie, antigen-binding site). Upon antigen stimulation and T cell help, the immature B lymphocyte matures (proliferates, class-switches and becomes a plasma cell) to secrete different isotypes (eg, IgM [pentamer], IgA, immunoglobulin G [IgG], and IgE) with the same specificity as the original membrane-bound sIg.
5. Serum protein electrophoresis determines the total concentration of all circulating proteins, including the immunoglobulins (ie, IgG, IgA, IgM, IgD, and IgE). The concentration of the individual isotypes can be determined with isotype-specific quantification methods. Most clinical laboratories quantitate only IgG, IgM, and IgA because they are the most prevalent isotypes in the bloodstream. In patients with allergic disorders, quantification of IgE is rarely useful.
6. An understanding of the mechanism of action of immunomodulators allows a clinician to anticipate potential adverse effects. The benefit of manipulating immune responses must be balanced with the potential consequences and long-term sequela (eg, tumor growth, infections, etc) of such manipulation.

The immune system is a complex network of barriers, organs, cellular elements, and molecules that interact to defend the body against invading pathogens. The *immune system* is actually composed of two distinct systems of immunity: innate immunity and adaptive immunity. In brief, innate immunity includes a series of nonspecific barriers (physical and chemical), along with cellular and molecular elements strategically deployed and positioned to prevent or quickly neutralize infection. Adaptive immunity works in concert with the innate immune system. In contrast to innate immunity, adaptive immunity constantly evolves and adapts to the invading pathogens. The hallmarks of the adaptive immune response are; *diversity*, *memory*, *mobility*, *self-versus nonself-discrimination*, *redundancy*, *replication*, and *specificity*.[1] *Diversity* indicates the capability of the immune system to respond to many different pathogens or strains of pathogens. Immunological *memory* ensures a quicker and more vigorous response to a subsequent encounter with the same pathogen. If an individual has seen something before, the odds are good that he or she will see it again. So the individual will make more of these cells and have them ready. *Mobility* of components of the immune system enables local reactions to provide systemic protection. *Discrimination of self versus nonself* helps prevent the immune response from responding to ourselves, and thus results in tolerance to our own materials. *Redundancy* refers to the ability of the immune system to produce components with similar biological effects from multiple cells lines, such as inflammatory cytokines. *Replication* of the cellular components of the immune system amplifies the immune response. *Specificity* describes the ability of the immune system to distinguish between dissimilar antigens.

MAJOR TISSUES AND ORGANS OF THE IMMUNE SYSTEM

While numerous cells of the immune system have the ability to migrate to most body tissues, some tissues and organs serve as key members of the immune system. These include primary and secondary lymphoid tissues and organs. *Primary lymphoid tissues and organs*, the bone marrow and thymus, provide an environment for the development and maturation of select cells of the immune system. It is here that these select cells of the immune system mature and become tolerant of self and competent to respond to foreign antigens. Importantly, no immune response occurs in these sites. *Secondary lymphoid organs* provide an environment where various cells of the immune system interact with and respond to antigens.[2]

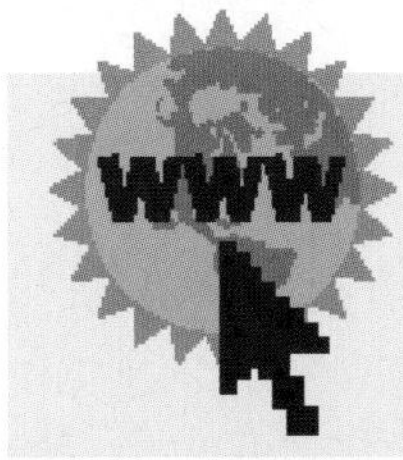

The complete chapter, learning objectives, and other resources can be found at **www.pharmacotherapyonline.com.**

87

Systemic Lupus Erythematosus

Beth H. Resman-Targoff

KEY CONCEPTS

1. Systemic lupus erythematosus (SLE) is considered a disease primarily of young women, but can occur in anyone. The prevalence and severity vary with sex, race, ethnicity, and socioeconomic factors.
2. Understanding the etiology of SLE and environmental factors that can initiate or exacerbate the disease may make it possible to avoid those triggers.
3. SLE is an autoimmune disease characterized by the presence of autoantibodies, some of which may play a role in the pathogenesis of the disease. An understanding of disease mechanisms can lead to targeted drug therapy.
4. SLE is a multisystem disease that can involve almost any organ and may present in many different ways. Therapy is determined by the manifestations in each patient. These may change and fluctuate in severity over time.
5. Lifestyle changes can modify risk factors for SLE flares and complications.
6. The overall goals of therapy are to prevent disease flares and involvement of other organs, decrease disease activity and prevent damage, maintain remission, reduce use of corticosteroids, and improve quality of life, while minimizing adverse effects and costs. Most patients with SLE should receive hydroxychloroquine alone or in combination with other therapy appropriate for the disease manifestations.
7. Pregnancy planning is essential for good outcomes. Pregnancy outcomes are best when the disease is controlled before conception. Drugs used to treat SLE may adversely affect fertility and the fetus.
8. Antiphospholipid antibodies are associated with arterial and venous thrombosis and obstetric complications.
9. Many drugs can induce a lupus-like syndrome. The manifestations and laboratory findings may be different between the traditional drug-induced lupus and that seen with use of tumor necrosis factor-alpha inhibitors.
10. Since SLE can present in many different ways, it is difficult to design standard response criteria. Development of appropriate criteria is essential for getting new drugs approved.

Systemic lupus erythematosus (SLE) is an autoimmune disease associated with autoantibody production. The term "lupus" was first used to describe a skin disease in medieval times. The name may have been selected since the lesions looked like skin that had been gnawed by a wolf. In the mid-1800s, it was recognized that other organs may be affected and we now know that SLE is a multisystem disease. The common finding in SLE is production of antibodies to self-constituents.[1] This is an exciting time in the management of SLE because better understanding of disease mechanisms has led to the development of new drugs. In addition, new response criteria are being developed to show efficacy of drugs, even with the background of standard therapy. This has led to the first approval of a drug for treatment of SLE in over 50 years. Despite these advances, management of this disease remains a challenge. It has a myriad of manifestations and many of the drugs used to treat it are not approved for this indication. As a result, dosing of many of the drugs considered to be standard-of-care therapy must be personalized.

EPIDEMIOLOGY

(1) Systemic lupus erythematosus is generally considered to occur most frequently in women of reproductive age (15-50 years old).[2] This is especially characteristic of the disease in nonwhite women. Statistics regarding SLE depend on the population studied and sampling and recruitment criteria. These have profound effects on estimates of incidence and prevalence, disease activity and severity, and mortality. The incidence is 1 to 10 per 100,000 person-years and the prevalence is 20 to more than 200 per 100,000 persons.[2,3] Rates are 9 times higher in women than in men so overall population statistics can be rather misleading.[2] It is affected by ethnicity, which includes genetic, geographic, cultural, social, and other aspects within a group. Rates are two to four times higher in nonwhites than in the white population.[3] It is most common in those of African origin, but is also more common in people of Asian, Arab, and Chaldean background, Hispanics, and Native Americans (called First Nations in Canada) than in whites.[3,4] Most people are of mixed race, so race by itself can be difficult to analyze. Nonwhites tend to have an earlier onset, more severe disease, and a higher mortality rate, but it can be difficult to separate out the influence of socioeconomic factors and access to medical care.[5] The disease tends to be more severe in men, children, and those with onset at a later age (over 50 years).[3]

Survival rates have improved recently with better therapy and earlier diagnosis and initiation of treatment. Overall SLE survival is 95% at 5 years and 92% at 10 years after diagnosis. This is reduced to about 88% at 10 years with lupus nephritis and even less than that in African Americans with lupus nephritis.[6] The survival rate may be lower in men, but the small number of males in most studies makes this difficult to determine.[3]

ETIOLOGY

(2) The exact etiology for SLE is unknown but many abnormal factors have been identified that appear to play a role in the disease. Some are predisposing factors and others are involved in the disease mechanisms. Categories of these elements include genetic influences, epigenetic regulation of gene expression, environmental factors, hormones, and abnormalities in immune cells and cytokines.[4]

The incidence of SLE is increased in affected families. First-degree relatives of patients with SLE are 20 times more likely to develop the disease than those in a general population.[7] Ten percent of patients with SLE have relatives with the disease.[8] The concordance rate is 25% for identical twins and 2% for fraternal twins.[2] The genetic predisposition to SLE is a result of the interplay of a combination of genes. In rare cases, it is thought to result primarily from a single abnormal gene.[4] The major histocompatibility complex (MHC) class II alleles HLA-DR2 and HLA-DR3 are known to be linked to SLE. An increasing number of other gene loci are being identified as having associations with the disease.[2] Gene expression is regulated by deoxyribonucleic acid (DNA) methylation and histone modifications. These epigenetic changes can cause alterations that may influence SLE. Interestingly, hydralazine and procainamide, two drugs that may induce lupus, inhibit DNA methylation.[9]

In a genetically susceptible individual, environmental triggers can initiate the disease. It is possible that the type of trigger may influence the specific organ involvement. Cigarette smoke has many components, such as hydrazine, that may affect the immune system. Chronic smokers and former smokers are more likely to have elevated titers of anti-double-stranded DNA (anti-dsDNA) antibodies. Cigarette smoking is phototoxic and associated with cutaneous lupus.[10] Ultraviolet light can cause keratinocytes in the skin to release nuclear material that can further stimulate the immune system and autoantibody production by B cells.[9,10] Viruses may trigger SLE. Several studies have suggested a potential role for the Epstein–Barr virus.[11] Other implicated triggers include infections, medications (including vaccines and biologics), psychological stress, silica dust, hydrazines, petroleum, solvents (such as nail polish and metal cleaners), dyes, and pesticides.[10]

The higher prevalence in women suggests that hormones such as estrogens and progesterones may play a role in SLE, but the presence of the X chromosome may also contribute. The incidence of SLE is increased tenfold in men with Klinefelter (XXY) syndrome and decreased in women with Turner (XO) syndrome.[2]

PATHOPHYSIOLOGY

3 Systemic lupus erythematosus is a multisystem disease characterized by disorders of the immune system (Fig. 87-1). T and B lymphocyte activation and signaling are altered in SLE and there is abnormal clearance of apoptotic debris.[2] The number of plasma cells is increased in active SLE and these cells produce autoantibodies, which can cause tissue damage.[9] Antibodies directed at dsDNA are seen in about 60% to 70% of patients with SLE and less than 0.5% of patients without the disease.[2] The titers of anti-dsDNA may fluctuate with disease activity and may predict disease flare. Some autoantibodies may play a role in the pathogenesis of clinical features of SLE; these autoantibodies may target Ro/SSA (antigen Ro/Sjögren syndrome A, ribonucleoprotein complex), La/SSB (antigen La/Sjögren syndrome antigen B, RNA-binding protein), C1q (subunit of the C1 complement component), Sm (nuclear particles), *N*-methyl-D-aspartate (NMDA) receptor (amino acid released by neurons), phospholipids, nucleosomes (from apoptotic cellular debris), and

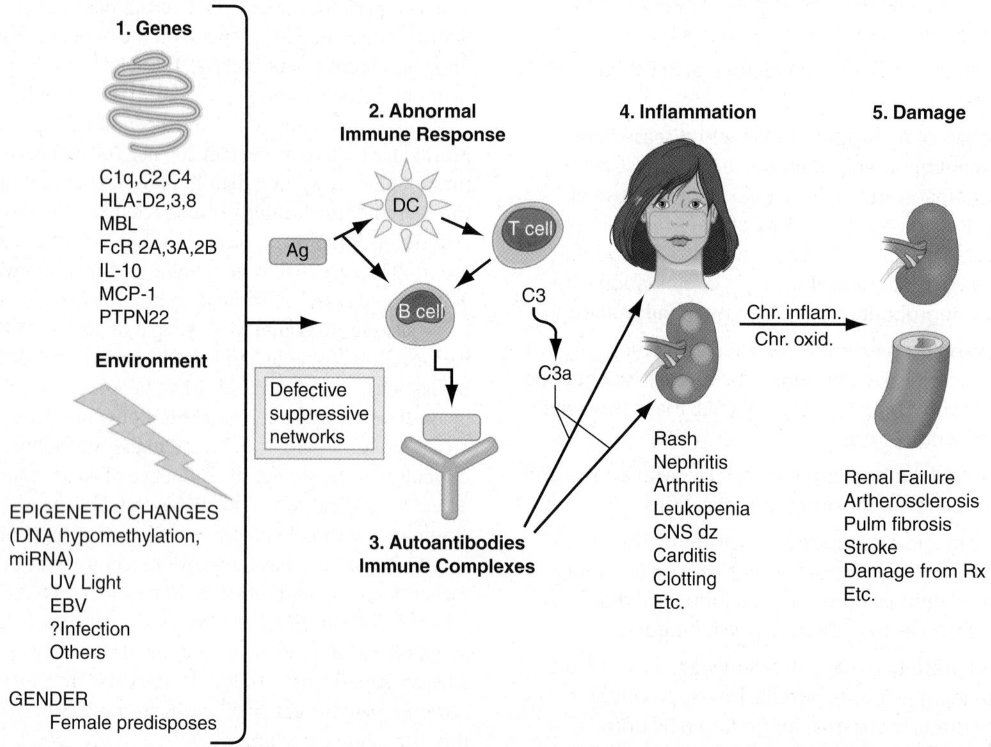

FIGURE 87-1 Pathogenesis of systemic lupus erythematosus (SLE). Genes confirmed in more than one genome-wide association analysis in northern European whites (several confirmed in Asians as well) as increasing susceptibility to SLE or lupus nephritis are listed (reviewed in SG Guerra et al. *Arthritis Res Ther* 2012;14:211). Gene-environment interactions (reviewed in KH Costenbader et al. *Autoimmune Rev* 2012;11:604) result in abnormal immune responses that generate pathogenic autoantibodies and immune complexes that deposit in tissue, activate complement, cause inflammation, and over time lead to irreversible organ damage (reviewed in GC Tsokos. *N Engl J Med* 2011;365:2110 and BH Hahn, in DJ Wallace, BH Hahn, eds. Dubois' Lupus Erythematosus and Related Syndromes, 8th ed. New York, Elsevier, 2013). Ag, antigen; C1q, complement system; C3, complement component; CNS, central nervous system; DC, dendritic cell; EBV, Epstein-Barr virus; HLA, human leukocyte antigen; FcR, immunoglobulin Fc-binding receptor; IL, interleukin; MCP, monocyte chemotactic protein; PTPN, phosphotyrosine phosphatase; UV, ultraviolet. *(Reproduced with permission from Hahn BH. Systemic lupus erythematosus. In: Kasper DL, Fauci AS, Hauser SL, et al., eds. Harrison's Principles of Internal Medicine. 19th ed. 2015.)*

histones (protein core of nucleosome). The autoantibodies can be present for many years before SLE is clinically apparent and they may be associated with specific organ involvement, such as anti-dsDNA with lupus nephritis.[2]

Immune complexes form when antinuclear antibodies (ANA) bind to nuclear material in blood and tissues, and they can accumulate in the kidneys, skin, CNS, and other sites. They activate the complement cascade, leading to an influx of inflammatory cells and tissue injury. Antibodies to blood cells can cause cytopenias. Antibodies against phospholipids can lead to thrombosis and fetal loss. These antiphospholipid antibodies interfere with protein C and endothelial cell function, inducing tissue factor that leads to thrombus formation. They also cause platelet aggregation. The antiphospholipid antibodies bind to placental trophoblast cells and activate complement, which can lead to fetal loss.[9]

T cell abnormalities contribute to the immune disorders observed in SLE. There are increased T helper cells type 2 and 17 and diminished number and function of T regulatory cells. Cytokines, such as tumor necrosis factor-alpha (TNF-α), interferon-gamma, and interleukin-10, produced by activated T cells can stimulate B cells.[2]

Cytokines play multiple roles in SLE. Anti-T-cell antibodies decrease interleukin-2 production, which can increase the risk for infections by decreasing the activity of cytotoxic T cells and increasing the lifespan of autoreactive T cells. Increased T cell production of interkeukin-17 and expression of adhesion molecule CD44 may contribute to kidney and other organ damage. Plasmacytoid dendritic cells accumulate in skin and kidneys and secrete interferon-α. B-lymphocyte stimulator (BLyS), also known as B cell activating factor of the TNF family (BAFF), increases survival of B cells. Interleukin-6 promotes production of antibodies.[9] The role of TNF-α in SLE is unclear. In some patients it appears to be harmful, and in others, protective.[2]

CLINICAL PRESENTATION

4 Systemic lupus erythematosus is an autoimmune disease that can involve almost any organ and may present in many different ways. This can make it difficult to establish a diagnosis and an extensive work-up may be needed to determine the full extent of involvement and to exclude other possible etiologies for the manifestations. More common features include involvement of the skin and mucus membranes, joints, kidneys, CNS, serous membranes, cardiovascular system, and hematologic cell lines. Fatigue and depression are frequent symptoms and can adversely affect quality of life.[12] Arthritis or arthralgias are experienced by 83% to 95% of patients with SLE.[8] SLE may present differently in men and women. For example, men tend to get SLE at an older age and are more likely to have renal and hematologic involvement, but have fewer dermatologic features. Race and ethnicity may also affect the specific manifestations.[13]

Disease manifestations fluctuate with periods of remission, flares, and progression.[14] The presence of ANA may be used as a screening test for SLE. Most patients with SLE have these antibodies, but they are not specific for the disease.[15]

An international group of SLE researchers developed and validated new criteria for classification of SLE in 2012. These are referred to as the Systemic Lupus International Collaborating Clinics (SLICC) classification criteria and were developed to identify patients with the disease for clinical studies. They are not intended for establishing a diagnosis in an individual patient, but may be helpful in assessing the likelihood that a patient has SLE. The widely used American College of Rheumatology (ACR) criteria were developed in 1982 and revised in 1997. The 1997 version was not validated. The SLICC criteria are more clinically relevant and sensitive than the ACR criteria. When validated, the SLICC criteria had a sensitivity of 97% and specificity of 84% compared to 83% and 96% for the ACR criteria. The number of criteria was expanded from 11 to 17 and, unlike the ACR criteria, they are divided into clinical and immunologic parameters. The ACR criteria required 4 of the 11 elements to be present, serially or simultaneously. To satisfy the SLICC criteria, a patient must still meet at least four of the elements, but now these must include at least one clinical and one immunologic criterion or the patient must have biopsy-proven lupus nephritis with positive ANA or anti-dsDNA antibodies. An abbreviated version of the SLICC criteria, with comparison to the ACR criteria, is shown in Table 87-1.[16-18] It may be possible to classify patients earlier in their disease course as having SLE with the SLICC criteria.[19]

An international working group of SLE experts devised a consensus definition of SLE flare: "A flare is a measurable increase in disease activity in one or more organ systems involving new or worse clinical signs and symptoms and/or laboratory measurements. It must be considered clinically significant by the assessor and usually there would be at least consideration of a change or an increase in treatment."[20]

Some skin involvement is seen in about 75% of patients with SLE.[21] This can be disfiguring and affect a patient's feelings of self-esteem.[22] Three main types of cutaneous lupus erythematosus have been observed. They may occur with or without SLE. Acute cutaneous lupus erythematosus is typically seen in patients with SLE and is characterized by a photosensitive malar rash over the cheeks and nose with sparing of the nasolabial folds. The malar rash is present in 52% of patients with SLE at the time of diagnosis. The arms and trunk may be involved. The manifestations usually wax and wane without scarring.[23] Severe SLE is less common with the other forms of cutaneous lupus. Subacute cutaneous lupus erythematosus is highly photosensitive and is manifested by annular or psoriasiform plaques that usually heal without scarring. It can be accompanied by musculoskeletal complaints and patients usually have anti-Ro/SSA autoantibodies.[24] It is more common than other types of cutaneous lupus erythematosus in patients with drug-induced lupus. About half of patients with subacute cutaneous lupus erythematosus meet criteria for SLE.[23] Many

CLINICAL PRESENTATION

Symptoms

- Fatigue, depression, photosensitivity, joint pain, headache, weight loss, nausea/abdominal pain

Signs

- Rash, alopecia, fever, oral and nasal ulcers, arthritis, renal dysfunction, seizure, psychosis, pleuritis, pleural effusion, cardiovascular disease, pericarditis/myocarditis, heart murmur, hypertension, anemia, leukopenia, thrombocytopenia, lymphadenopathy, Raynaud's phenomenon, vasculitis

Diagnostic Tests

- Serology: autoantibodies, antiphospholipid antibodies, complement; inflammatory markers: C-reactive protein, erythrocyte sedimentation rate; blood chemistries; complete blood count; urinalysis; lumbar puncture; renal biopsy

TABLE 87-1 2012 Systemic Lupus International Collaborating Clinics Classification Criteria for Systemic Lupus Erythematosus (SLICC)

Clinical Criteria

1. Acute/subacute cutaneous lupus/malar rash[a]/photosensitive rash[a]
2. Chronic cutaneous lupus/discoid rash
3. Oral OR nasal ulcers
4. Nonscarring alopecia
5. Arthritis/synovitis or tenderness
6. Serositis (pleuritis, pericarditis)
7. Renal (urine protein-to-creatinine ratio [or 24-hour urine protein] representing 500 mg protein/24 h OR red blood cell casts)
8. Neurologic (seizure, psychosis, mononeuritis multiplex, myelitis, peripheral or cranial neuropathy, acute confusional state)
9. Hemolytic anemia[b]
10. Leukopenia (<4,000/mm^3 [<4 × 10^9/L]) OR lymphopenia (<1,000/mm^3 [<1 × 10^9/L])[b]
11. Thrombocytopenia (<100,000/mm^3 [<100 × 10^9/L])[b]

Immunologic Criteria

1. Antinuclear antibody (ANA)
2. Anti-double-stranded DNA (dsDNA)[c]
3. Anti-Sm[c]
4. Antiphospholipid antibody (lupus anticoagulant, anticardiolipin, anti-β_2-glycoprotein I, false positive rapid plasma reagin test for syphilis)[c]
5. Low complement (C3, C4, CH50)
6. Direct Coomb's test (without hemolytic anemia)

At least four criteria, including at least one clinical and one immunologic criterion OR biopsy-proven lupus nephritis with positive ANA or anti-dsDNA required for diagnosis.

[a]In the ACR Criteria, malar rash, and photosensitivity are two separate criteria.

[b] In the ACR Criteria, hemolytic anemia, leukopenia, lymphopenia, and thrombocytopenia count as one criterion.

[c]In the ACR Criteria, anti-dsDNA, anti-Sm, and antiphospholipid antibody count as one criterion.

Data from Petri M, Orbai AM, Alarcón GS, et al. Derivation and validation of the Systemic Lupus International Collaborating Clinics classification criteria for systemic lupus erythematosus. *Arthritis Rheum* 2012;64:2677-2686; Tan EM, Cohen AS, Fries JF, et al. The 1982 revised criteria for the classification of systemic lupus erythematosus. *Arthritis Rheum* 1982;25:1271-1277; and Hochberg MC. Updating the American College of Rheumatology revised criteria for the classification of systemic lupus erythematosus. *Arthritis Rheum* 1997;40:1725.

subtypes of chronic cutaneous lupus erythematosus have been identified. The most common is discoid lupus, which is confined to the head and neck in about two-thirds of patients, but it can be generalized.[25] Chronic discoid lupus is the first manifestation of SLE in up to 10% of cases. Discoid lupus progresses to SLE in about 5% to 10% of patients. It is more common in smokers and African Americans. It may be associated with scarring, scarring alopecia, malar rash, photosensitivity, oral ulcers, leukopenia, vasculitis, and chronic seizures. Chronic discoid lupus is associated with a lower incidence of arthritis, end-stage renal disease, and immunologic markers such as ANA, anti-dsDNA, and antiphospholipid antibodies.[26]

Lupus nephritis is present at the time of SLE diagnosis in about 35% of adult patients and 50% to 60% of patients develop it by 10 years. It is more common in African American and Hispanic patients than in whites and more prevalent in men than in women. The International Society of Nephrology/Renal Pathology Society devised a classification system for lupus nephritis based on histologic findings: Class I: minimal mesangial, Class II: mesangial proliferative; Class III: focal (less than 50% of glomeruli involved); Class IV: diffuse (50% or more of glomeruli involved); Class V: membranous; and Class VI: advanced sclerosing (at least 90% globally sclerosed glomeruli without residual activity). Patients with nephritis may also have hypertension and atherosclerosis.[6]

The central and peripheral nervous systems can be involved in SLE. The frequency of this involvement is around 30% to 40%, but can range from 12% to 95% depending on the population studied and methods for detecting the occurrence.[27,28] About 50% to 60% of neuropsychiatric events appear within the first year after the diagnosis of SLE, usually during times of generalized disease activity. Mild nonspecific neuropsychiatric findings such as headache, mood disorders, anxiety, and mild cognitive dysfunction are common in SLE but may not reflect overt CNS disease activity. Findings more indicative of neuropsychiatric lupus include cerebrovascular disease (ischemic stroke and/or transient ischemic attack) and seizures in 5% to 15% of patients; severe cognitive dysfunction, major depression, acute confusional state, and peripheral nervous disorders (eg, polyneuropathy and mononeuropathy) in 1% to 5%; and psychosis, myelitis, chorea, cranial neuropathies, and aseptic meningitis in less than 1% of patients. Risk factors include general SLE disease activity, prior neuropsychiatric events, and presence of moderate-to-high titers of antiphospholipid antibodies.[27] It is important to assess contributing factors and to rule out other possible etiologies of these manifestations such as corticosteroid use.[29] The diagnostic approach will vary depending on the clinical presentation and preliminary findings, but can include a thorough history and physical, lumbar puncture with cerebrospinal fluid analysis (mostly to exclude infection), electroencephalogram, serology, complete blood count, blood chemistries, neuropsychological assessment of cognitive function, nerve conduction studies, and magnetic resonance imaging.[27]

Cardiovascular disease is a leading cause of death in patients with SLE. Not only are there cardiac manifestations of SLE, such as pericarditis and myocarditis, but patients with SLE are also at increased risk for accelerated atherosclerosis. This is probably related to the chronic inflammation associated with the disease and adverse effects of the drugs (eg, high-dose corticosteroids) used to treat it. Antiphospholipid antibodies and type I interferons may play a role in the pathogenesis. Drugs such as hydroxychloroquine and mycophenolate mofetil may have a cardioprotective effect.[30]

TREATMENT
Systemic Lupus Erythematosus

Treatment of SLE is determined by the patient's symptoms and organ involvement.

Desired Outcomes

The overall goals of therapy are to prevent disease flares and involvement of other organs, decrease disease activity and prevent damage, maintain remission, reduce use of corticosteroids, and improve quality of life, while minimizing adverse effects and costs. Success in achieving these outcomes depends on disease severity and the type and extent of organ impairment. In general, the prognosis is better if lupus is limited to skin and musculoskeletal findings. The worst prognosis is seen with renal or CNS involvement.[8] Many of the desired outcomes have been observed with antimalarials, although most patients require additional therapy.[31] Survival and quality of life have improved with better understanding of disease mechanisms and new therapeutic options. Mortality is affected by SLE disease activity, cardiovascular risks, and infections.

General Approach

Patients with SLE should be counseled about the importance of lifestyle modifications such as protection from the sun, smoking cessation, exercise, and weight control. The need for immunizations should be assessed with consideration of appropriate timing with respect to immunosuppressive drug use. The effects of disease activity and treatment on pregnancy outcomes should be discussed. Patients should be evaluated and treated for any comorbidities such as hypertension, hyperlipidemia, and depression. Mild symptoms can be managed with nonsteroidal antiinflammatory drugs (NSAIDs) with or without other analgesics.[32] Antimalarial drugs have numerous beneficial effects in SLE and many experts feel that most patients with the disease should always receive one of these drugs.[31] Corticosteroids are used to treat most forms of SLE and up to 80% of patients receive low doses indefinitely as maintenance therapy. The need for osteoporosis prevention should be assessed.[33] If the above therapy is ineffective or major organs are involved, immunosuppressive or immunomodulatory drugs are added.[32] The specific treatment is determined by the organs involved and severity of the disease. It is summarized in Fig. 87-2.[14]

Nonpharmacologic Therapy

5 Patient perceptions of well-being and quality of life are affected not only by disease activity, but also by social support, coping mechanisms, feelings of helplessness, and abnormal illness-related behaviors.[32] Good social support can improve outcomes, in part by making it easier for patients and their families to navigate the healthcare system and utilize resources. Counseling and support groups may help patients' mental well-being and coping mechanisms, but do not affect SLE disease activity. Aerobic cardiovascular exercise may help decrease patients' risk for cardiovascular events and osteoporosis and may also improve fatigue and sleep disturbances, which are frequently experienced in SLE.[34]

Since photosensitivity is common in SLE, patients should wear protective clothing and hats and use sunscreens to protect themselves from the sun. They should avoid tanning salons.[25] The FDA issued regulations for testing and labeling of sunscreens that took effect in 2012. Sunscreens labeled as broad spectrum protect against ultraviolet A and B radiation. They have sun protection factors (SPFs) of 15 to 50+.[35] Patients with SLE should use sunscreens with high SPF values and apply them every 2 hours while in the sun.[25]

Patients should be counseled to stop smoking. Smoking cessation is important, not only because it decreases cardiovascular risk, but because smoking can exacerbate SLE and diminish the effectiveness of antimalarials.[36] Smokers also have a higher incidence of active rashes with skin damage and scarring.[37]

Pharmacotherapy

6 Treatment is personalized based on the manifestations of SLE in the patient. It consists of a combination of immunosuppression and symptomatic and supportive therapies. The only drugs approved by the FDA for treatment of SLE are aspirin, prednisone, hydroxychloroquine, and belimumab. The use of other drugs for SLE, even those considered "standard of care," is considered to be "off-label" use. For many of these drugs, the optimal doses and duration of therapy for induction and maintenance of response in SLE have not been determined.

Organization or expert task force treatment recommendations have been published for lupus nephritis, neuropsychiatric lupus, and antiphospholipid antibody carriers.[6,27,38] A committee of the ACR developed guidelines for screening, treatment, and management of lupus nephritis. All patients with nephritis should receive hydroxychloroquine to reduce damage and flares. An angiotensin-converting enzyme inhibitor or angiotensin receptor blocker can reduce proteinuria by about 30% in those with proteinuria of 0.5 g/day or more, and delay progression of renal disease. Blood pressure should be maintained at no more than 130/80 mm Hg. Patients with a low-density lipoprotein cholesterol greater than 100 mg/dL (2.59 mmol/L) should receive a statin to prevent accelerated atherosclerosis. More specific treatment is based on the type of nephritis. The first two classes, minimal mesangial and mesangial proliferative lupus nephritis do not usually need immunosuppressive therapy. Focal and diffuse lupus nephritis (Classes III and IV) are treated similarly with aggressive

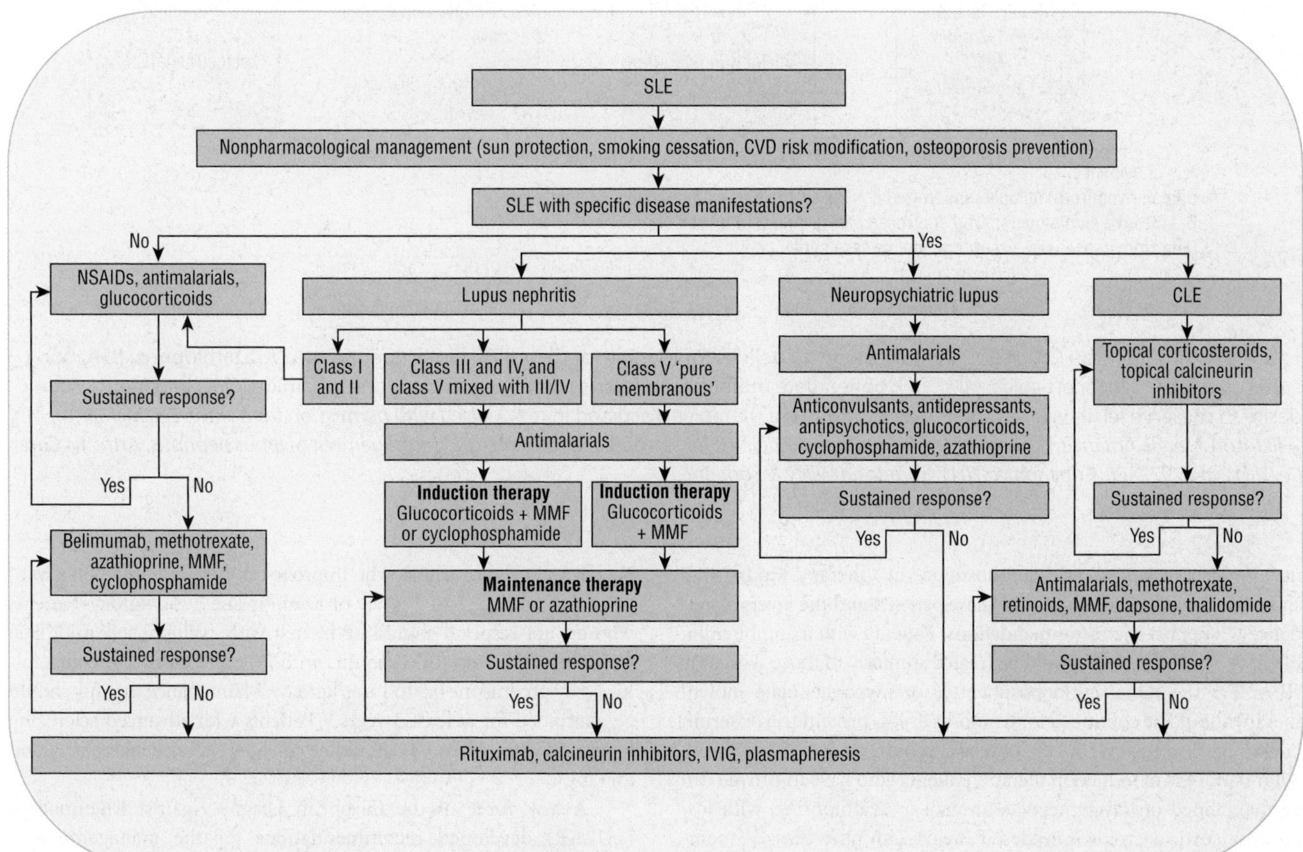

FIGURE 87-2 Algorithm for the treatment of SLE. Abbreviations: CLE, cutaneous lupus erythematosus; CVD, cardiovascular disease; IVIG, intravenous immunoglobulin; MMF, mycophenolate mofetil; SLE, systemic lupus erythematosus. (*Used with permission from Xiong W, Lahita RG. Pragmatic approaches to therapy for systemic lupus erythematosus. Nat Rev Rheumatol 2014;10:97-107.*)

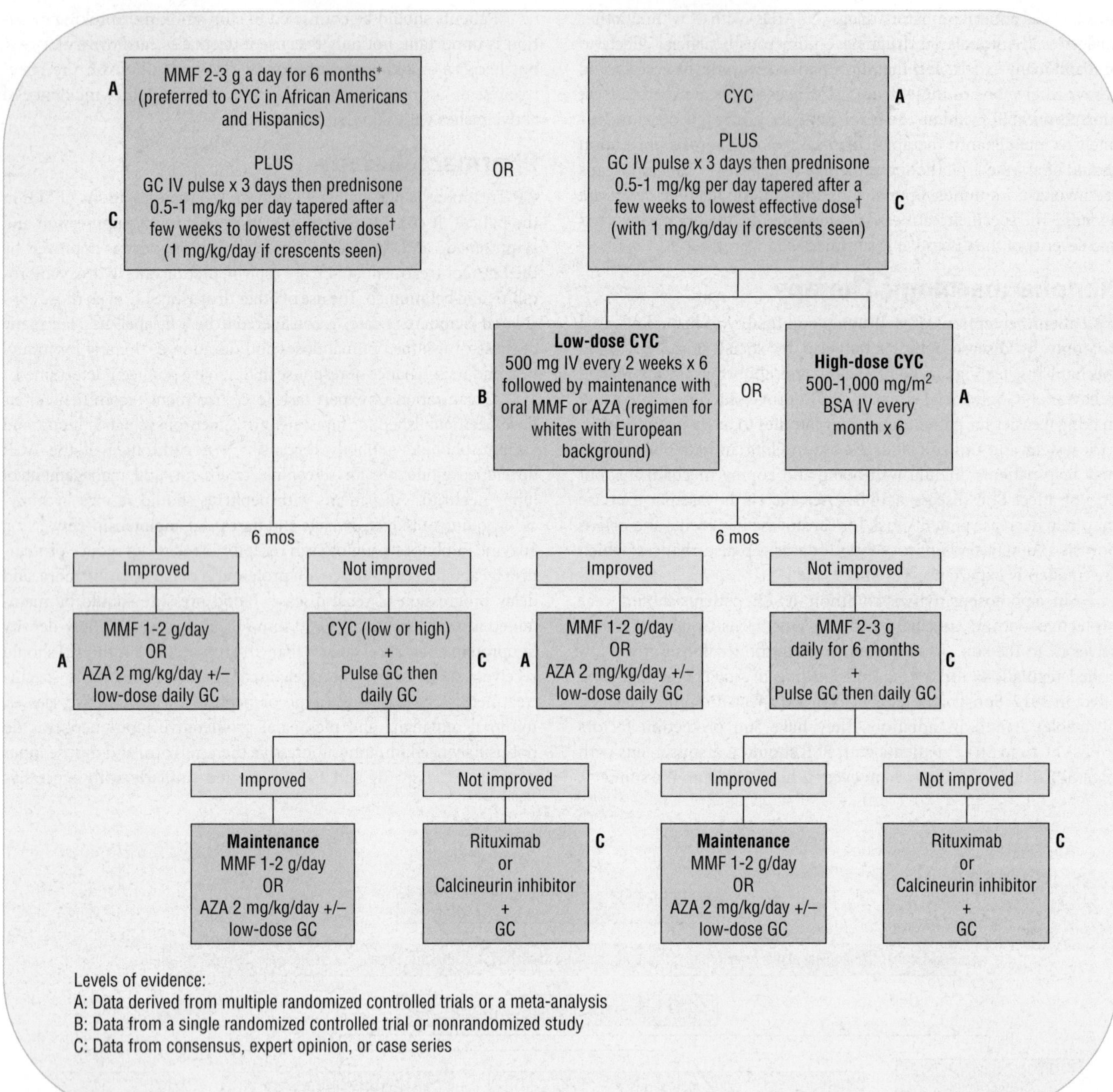

FIGURE 87-3 American College of Rheumatology guidelines for therapy for Class III/IV lupus nephritis. (AZA, azathioprine; BSA, body surface area; GC, glucocorticoids; MMF, mycophenolate mofetil; *, preference of MMF over cyclophosphamide (CYC) in patients who desire to preserve fertility; †, recommended background therapies discussed in text.) *(Used with permission from Hahn BH, McMahon MA, Wilkinson A, et al. American College of Rheumatology guidelines for screening, treatment, and management of lupus nephritis. Arthritis Care Res 2012; 64:797 -808. Copyright © 2012 from John Wiley & Sons, Inc.)*

use of glucocorticoids and immunosuppressive therapy. Figure 87-3 shows the induction regimens for these patients and the levels of evidence to support the recommendations. Patients with a combination of Class V with III or IV would be treated similarly to those with only III or IV. The initial cyclophosphamide or mycophenolate mofetil therapy should be continued for 6 months unless proteinuria or serum creatinine worsens by 50% or more at 3 months (Level A evidence). After 6 months of induction therapy, patients who have improved can be maintained on mycophenolate mofetil or azathioprine, with low doses of corticosteroids if needed. Patients with pure Class V, membranous lupus nephritis, and nephrotic range proteinuria of more than 3 g/day should receive induction therapy with mycophenolate mofetil 2 to 3 g/day with prednisone 0.5 mg/kg/day for 6 months (Level A evidence). Those who improve can be maintained on mycophenolate mofetil 1 to 2 g/day or azathioprine 2 mg/kg/day. Patients who do not respond should be treated with cyclophosphamide 500 to 1,000 mg/m^2/mo for 6 months with IV pulse glucocorticoids, followed by prednisone 0.5 to 1 mg/kg/day.[6] Maintenance therapy should be continued for at least 3 years.[39] Patients with advanced sclerosing lupus nephritis (Class VI) should be considered for renal replacement therapy.[6]

A task force of the European League Against Rheumatism (EULAR) developed recommendations for the management of neuropsychiatric lupus. Treatment depends on the manifestations. Symptomatic therapy (eg, anticonvulsants and antidepressants) should be given as needed. More specific treatment depends on whether the problem is determined to be inflammatory or thrombotic or both. If there is inflammation or neurotoxic damage in the presence of generalized SLE activity, glucocorticoids alone or in conjunction with immunosuppressive drugs such as azathioprine or cyclophosphamide should be given (Strong evidence). If the condition does not respond, other treatments such as plasma exchange, IV immunoglobulin, or rituximab can be tried. If the problem is related to moderate-to-high titers of antiphospholipid antibodies and/or thrombosis, anticoagulants and/or inhibitors of platelet aggregation should be used (Sufficient evidence).[27]

For patients with intermittent joint pain associated with SLE, NSAIDs are good initial therapy. If the pain is more severe or persistent, prednisone in a dose of 10 mg/day or less in combination with hydroxychloroquine should be instituted. Intra-articular corticosteroid injections can be used for localized joint pain. If this therapy is inadequate, methotrexate can be added to hydroxychloroquine therapy. For patients who fail or are intolerant of these therapies, mycophenolate mofetil or azathioprine can be tried. If alternative treatment is needed, leflunomide, belimumab, rituximab, abatacept, or TNF-α inhibitors may be considered.[40]

The first step in management of cutaneous lupus erythematosus is counseling patients to protect themselves from ultraviolet light as described above.[25] Drug treatment is personalized based on the extent and severity of involvement. Topical corticosteroids are commonly used and may relieve symptoms such as itching or burning, but may not provide adequate clearing of lesions when used alone.[25] The choice of corticosteroid depends on the location of application. Low potency corticosteroids (eg, fluocinolone acetonide 0.01% and hydrocortisone 1%) should be used on areas with thin skin such as the face and groin, mid-potency (eg, triamcinolone acetonide) for trunk and extremities, and high potency (eg, clobetasol propionate) for thick-skin areas such as scalp, soles, and palms. Creams or, for more severe disease, ointments are used on the body, and foams or solutions on the scalp.[23] Intralesional corticosteroids may be used in discoid lupus, but should not be repeated more often than every 4 to 6 weeks.[25] To avoid the adverse effects of topical corticosteroids, such as skin atrophy, telangiectasias, and steroid-induced dermatitis, the lowest effective potency and duration of therapy should be used.[23] Alternatively, topical calcineurin inhibitors may be given instead. Pimecrolimus is more lipophilic than tacrolimus and has greater affinity for the skin. Antimalarials have photoprotective effects and are commonly used as first line systemic therapy in the management of cutaneous lupus. If hydroxychloroquine alone is ineffective, quinacrine, available from compounding pharmacies, may be added.[25] For refractory disease, systemic immunosuppressive drugs (eg, corticosteroids, methotrexate, mycophenolate mofetil, or azathioprine), immunomodulatory drugs (eg, dapsone, thalidomide, or lenalidomide), biologics (eg, rituximab or belimumab), or oral retinoids may be added. The evidence to support their use in management of cutaneous lupus is mainly from case reports rather than controlled studies. The choice of agents may be guided by other organ involvement.[23]

Dosing information for selected drugs is shown in Table 87-2. Since most of the drugs used to treat SLE are not FDA-approved for that indication, the doses given are based on other uses for those drugs. Table 87-3 lists adverse effects and drug monitoring parameters. Selected issues concerning the drugs are discussed below.

Nonsteroidal Antiinflammatory Drugs

Nonsteroidal antiinflammatory drugs are used as first-line treatment for arthritis, musculoskeletal complaints, fever, and serositis.[14] Low-dose aspirin is used in patients with antiphospholipid antibodies.[41] One concern with use of NSAIDs is that they can decrease renal function, which can complicate evaluation of lupus nephritis. They have the potential to increase cardiac events in patients who already are at elevated risk. Other adverse effects include hepatotoxicity, GI bleeding, and aseptic meningitis.[14]

Corticosteroids

Corticosteroids as monotherapy or as adjuncts to other treatment can control flares and maintain low disease activity in SLE. Their effects have a rapid onset, whereas other therapies may take months or over a year to achieve their maximum benefits. The corticosteroids can be used topically or systemically.

Clinical **Controversy...**

Corticosteroids are commonly used to treat SLE and their adverse effects are well known, but optimal dosing is still unclear. What constitutes an appropriate dose in different situations? How long should therapy be continued? How should it be tapered?

Although corticosteroids have been used in the management of SLE since the 1950s, optimal doses have not been determined. High doses given in a pulse IV administration regimen are used to treat flares and quickly reduce inflammation. Doses should slowly be tapered down to the lowest effective dose. Corticosteroids are the foundation for treatment of most forms of SLE.[33]

High doses of systemic corticosteroids are associated with infections, myopathy, psychological disturbances, osteonecrosis, and stroke.[33] Psychiatric disease, mostly mood disorder, occurs in 10% of patients receiving prednisone doses of 1 mg/kg or higher.[27] Common side effects of low (less than 7.5 mg prednisone/day) to moderate (7.5-30 mg/day) doses are shown in Table 87-3. Although higher doses may be divided, single morning doses may be associated with fewer adverse effects and less adrenal suppression. Chronic use of any dose is associated with coronary artery disease, cataracts, diabetes mellitus, and osteoporosis.[33] Corticosteroids increase catabolism of 25(OH) vitamin D and 1,25$(OH)_2$ vitamin D. Osteoporosis prophylaxis is often found to be inadequate.[42] To avoid adrenal insufficiency, patients on chronic corticosteroid therapy should not have treatment stopped abruptly and they may need increased doses at times of stress such as surgery.[43] Prolonged use of topical corticosteroids can lead to atrophy of the skin and telangiectasias (small dilated blood vessels).[23]

Antimalarials

The antimalarials chloroquine and hydroxychloroquine have long been used in rheumatology practice. Hydroxychloroquine is thought to have fewer adverse reactions and is the preferred drug. In the past, hydroxychloroquine was primarily used for skin and joint manifestations of SLE, but many experts believe that all patients with SLE should receive hydroxychloroquine. There is high quality evidence that it decreases disease activity and improves survival; moderate quality evidence that it increases bone mineral density and has protective effects against thrombosis and irreversible organ damage; and low quality evidence that it reduces severe flares, enhances the response to other drugs in patients with nephritis, has a beneficial effect on lipids, and protects against cancer. It can allow corticosteroid doses to be decreased. When given to patients with some findings consistent with SLE, it can delay the time for them to fully meet criteria for the disease.[44] Patients receiving hydroxychloroquine often have disease flares when the drug is discontinued.[31]

Hydroxychloroquine has antiinflammatory, immunomodulatory, and antithrombotic effects. It reduces concentrations of inflammatory cytokines such as interleukins 1, 2, 6, 17, and 22, interferon

TABLE 87-2 Dosing of Drugs Used to Treat Systemic Lupus Erythematosus

Drug	Brand Name	Initial or Starting Dose	Usual Range or Maintenance Dose	Special Population Doses	Comments (adverse drug reactions, special populations)
NSAIDs/salicylates	Various drugs				Caution in patients with renal insufficiency, cardiovascular disease, gastrointestinal problems
Glucocorticoids	Deltasone (prednisone), Medrol (prednisolone)	0.1-1.5 mg/kg/day PO	Prefer <10 mg/day PO		Dose depends on organ involvement and severity; initial dose may be given for 4-6 weeks, then tapered down for maintenance; no standard dose
	Solu-Medrol (methylprednisolone)	100-1,000 mg IV daily × 3			Severe disease; later, dose tapered and changed to PO
Hydroxychloroquine	Plaquenil	400 mg PO daily or twice daily	200-400 mg PO daily	Dosing adjustment may be needed with renal or hepatic dysfunction	Dose should not exceed 6.5 mg/kg/day to minimize retinopathy risk
Belimumab	Benlysta	10 mg/kg IV every 2 weeks × 3	10 mg/kg IV every 4 weeks	Use with caution in African Americans; no data on use in hepatic impairment; no adjustment for renal impairment if CrCl ≥15 mL/min (≥0.25 mL/s); pregnancy category C; no studies in pregnant or breastfeeding women	IV infusion over 1 h; consider premedication to prevent infusion and hypersensitivity reactions; hypersensitivity reactions up to 4 hours after administration; most common with first two infusions
Cyclophosphamide	Cytoxan	500-1,000 mg/m² BSA IV every month × 6 or 500 mg IV every 2 weeks × 6		Dosing adjustment might be needed with renal dysfunction; low and high doses may have equivalent efficacy in white patients with European background	Infertility in women and men, teratogenicity of concern
Mycophenolate mofetil	Cellcept Myfortic (enteric coated mycophenolate sodium)	2-3 g/day PO	0.5-3 g/day PO	Lower doses may be needed in Asians than non-Asians; may be more effective than cyclophosphamide in African Americans and Hispanics	Contraindicated in pregnancy
Azathioprine	Imuran	2 mg/kg/day PO	1.5-2 mg/kg/day PO		Lower dose if thiopurine methyltransferase (TPMT) deficient
Methotrexate	Rheumatrex, Trexall, Otrexup, Rasuvo		15-25 mg PO or SC weekly		Decrease toxicity by giving with folic acid
Rituximab	Rituxan	375 mg/m² BSA IV weekly × 4 or 500-1,000 mg IV on days 1 and 15		Variable doses have been used	Alternative for patients refractory to other treatments; may be more effective in African Americans

BSA, body surface area; CrCl, creatinine clearance; IV, intravenously; NSAIDs, nonsteroidal anti-inflammatory drugs; PO, orally.

alpha and gamma, and TNF-α. It alters antigen presentation and T cell proliferative responses. Its key activity may be decreasing activation of toll-like receptors, which are important in innate immunity and autoimmune diseases. It reduces platelet aggregation and thrombosis.[31] It also delays ultraviolet light absorption and may decrease the number of skin antigen-presenting cells.[22] Finally, it may reduce cardiovascular risk factors such as hyperlipidemia and diabetes mellitus and improve survival.[31] The LUMINA (LUpus in MInorities, NAture vs nurture) database was initiated in 1994 to look at differences in SLE outcomes based on ethnic backgrounds. It included African Americans, Hispanics, and Caucasians. Some findings based on study of this cohort are that hydroxychloroquine

TABLE 87-3 Monitoring of Drugs Used to Treat Systemic Lupus Erythematosus

Drug	Adverse Drug Reaction	Monitoring Parameter	Comments
NSAIDs/salicylates	Gastrointestinal bleeding, hepatic toxicity, renal toxicity, hypertension, cardiovascular events, aseptic meningitis	CBC[a], platelets[a], creatinine[a], urinalysis, AST/ALT[a], blood pressure[a]	Antihypertensive effects of calcium channel blockers affected less than other classes
Glucocorticoids, systemic	Osteoporosis, cataracts, glaucoma, hyperglycemia/diabetes, hypertension, dyslipidemia, thinning of the skin, weight gain, fat redistribution	Blood pressure[a], serum glucose[a], lipid panel[a], bone densitometry, ophthalmic examinations	Patients should receive osteoporosis preventive therapy; high doses of systemic corticosteroids are associated with infections, myopathy, psychological disturbances, osteonecrosis, and stroke
Glucocorticoids, topical	Skin atrophy, telangiectasias	Skin appearance	Avoid prolonged use, especially of high-potency steroids
Hydroxychloroquine	Retinal toxicity	Funduscopic and visual field examinations, consider electroretinogram, spectral domain optical coherence tomography, or fundus autofluorescence (frequency depends on level of risk), CBC, AST/ALT, albumin, chemistry panel, creatinine	Risk for retinal toxicity increased with doses >6.5 mg/kg/day ideal body weight, more than 5 years therapy, or age over 60 years
Belimumab	Infusion reactions, hypersensitivity, nausea, diarrhea, fever, nasopharyngitis, bronchitis, insomnia, pain in extremity, depression, migraine	Monitor for serious infections, hypersensitivity/infusion reactions, worsening depression, mood changes, or suicidal thoughts	No live vaccines 30 days before or during belimumab therapy; not recommended with other biologics or IV cyclophosphamide; consider premedication with acetaminophen and diphenhydramine
Cyclophosphamide	Myelosuppression, opportunistic infections, hemorrhagic cystitis, bladder malignancy, infertility	CBC[b], platelets[b], creatinine, AST/ALT, urinalysis[b], urine cytology[a], PAP test[a]	Greater risk for cystitis with oral form than IV; decrease with hydration and mesna
Mycophenolate mofetil	Myelosuppression, nausea, vomiting, diarrhea	CBC[c], platelets[c], creatinine, chemistry panel, AST/ALT, chest x-ray	Gastrointestinal side effects may limit use and compliance; these symptoms may be less with use of an enteric-coated form
Azathioprine	Myelosuppression, hepatotoxicity	CBC[c,d], platelets[c,d], creatinine[e], AST/ALT[c,f], chemistry panel[e], albumin, TPMT assay, PAP test	Test thiopurine methyltransferase (TPMT) before starting; toxicity greatly increased if deficient
Methotrexate	Hepatic, hematologic, pulmonary toxicity; stomatitis	CBC[c,g], platelets[c,g], creatinine[c,g], AST/ALT[c,g], albumin[c,g], bilirubin, chemistry panel[h], alkaline phosphatase[c], chest x-ray	Check hepatitis B and C serologies before starting if at risk
Rituximab	Infusion reactions, infections, neutropenia, mucocutaneous reactions, fever, fatigue, progressive multifocal leukoencephalopathy	CBC[i], platelets[i], creatinine, vital signs, human antichimeric antibody (HACA) titers	Consider pretreatment with acetaminophen, diphenhydramine, corticosteroid to decrease infusion reactions

Monitoring parameters should be checked at baseline and at interval noted: [a]52 weeks, [b]4 weeks, [c]12 weeks, [d]every 1-2 weeks after dose change, [e]26 weeks, [f]every 2 weeks after dose change, [g]2-4 weeks during 3 months after dose change, [h]8 weeks, [i]8-16 weeks.

Data from Schmajuk G, Yazdany J. Drug monitoring in systemic lupus erythematosus: A systematic review. *Semin Arthritis Rheum* 2011;40:559-575; Yazdany J, Panopalis P, Gillis JZ, et al. Systemic Lupus Erythematosus Quality Indicators Project Expert Panels. A quality indicator set for systemic lupus erythematosus. *Arthritis Rheum* 2009;61:370-377; Dennis GJ. Belimumab: A BLyS-specific inhibitor for the treatment of systemic lupus erythematosus. *Clin Pharmacol Ther* 2012;91:143-149; online.lexi.com. (Accessed December 11, 2015).

may delay the occurrence of integument damage (severe skin damage including scarring, ulcers, and scarring alopecia) and decrease accrual of damage.[22]

Clinical **Controversy...**

Should whole blood hydroxychloroquine concentrations be monitored? Some studies show a correlation between concentration and SLE disease control while others do not. Should blood hydroxychloroquine concentrations be used to monitor adherence but not for dosage adjustment?

Although some studies showed reduced disease activity and flares with hydroxychloroquine whole blood concentrations over 1,000 ng/mL (mcg/L; 2,977 nmol/L), other studies where doses were adjusted to achieve that concentration did not shown better disease control. It has been suggested that hydroxychloroquine concentration monitoring be used as a measure of adherence to therapy. The drug has a long elimination half-life of at least 5 days with a terminal half-life of about 40 days. Low concentrations may therefore be an indicator of consistent nonadherence or abnormal metabolism.[45] It may take 2 to 8 weeks to see the therapeutic effects of hydroxychloroquine.[31]

Adverse effects with hydroxychloroquine are usually mild. Most common are GI and skin reactions and they usually improve with dose reduction. The main concern is retinal toxicity, but the incidence is low and less than that seen with chloroquine.[31] The incidence increases to 1% in patients receiving the drug for more than 5 years or who have received a cumulative dose of 1,000 g. Other risk factors are daily doses more than 400 mg or 6.5 mg/kg ideal body weight, advanced age, or patients with kidney or liver dysfunction or preexisting retinal or macular disease. The retinal damage has a characteristic bull's-eye appearance on funduscopic examination and is irreversible. Early recognition of damage may minimize vision loss. The current American Academy of Ophthalmology monitoring recommendations are to have several baseline screening tests including visual acuity, dilated examination of the cornea and retina, visual fields, and at least one newer, more sensitive test such as electroretinogram, spectral domain optical coherence tomography, or fundus autofluorescence. After 5 years, patients should begin annual examinations unless the patient is considered to be at high risk, in which case yearly testing would begin earlier. If there are changes suspicious for toxicity, the drug should be stopped, or, after consultation with the patient about risks of blindness, examinations should be repeated every 3 to 6 months until the diagnosis is confirmed.[46]

Biologic Agents

Since autoantibody formation is an important feature of SLE, B cells make a logical target for SLE therapy. B-lymphocyte stimulator (BLyS) is a cytokine that is important for B cell survival, maturation, and differentiation. Belimumab is a fully human IgG1-λ monoclonal antibody that binds to soluble BLyS, which prevents BLyS from binding to receptors on B cells and promotes apoptosis of B lymphocytes. Belimumab is FDA-approved for treatment of autoantibody-positive active SLE in addition to standard therapy. It is the first drug approved by the FDA in over 50 years for management of SLE.[47] Approval of belimumab was based on two international phase III trials: BLISS-76, conducted primarily in Western Europe and North America, and BLISS-52, which was carried out in Eastern Europe, Latin America, and the Asia-Pacific region. These trials had strict entry criteria and used the new SLE Responder Index (SRI) assessment criteria. For both studies, the primary efficacy endpoint was the SRI at 52 weeks. Entry requirements included age of at least 18 years old, positive ANA or anti-dsDNA, and active SLE (SELENA-SLEDAI [measure of disease activity] score of 6 or greater) while receiving standard treatment (prednisone, NSAIDs, antimalarials, and/or immunosuppressive drugs [but not cyclophosphamide or other biologics]). Patients had to be on stable therapy for at least 30 days. The most common organ systems involved were musculoskeletal and mucocutaneous. Patients with severe active lupus nephritis or CNS lupus were excluded. Patients received belimumab 1 mg/kg, 10 mg/kg, or placebo by IV infusion every 2 weeks for two doses, then every 4 weeks, in addition to their standard therapy. There were restrictions on concomitant medications, and those became stricter as the studies progressed. The response rate was significantly higher in the group receiving belimumab 10 mg/kg as compared to placebo in both studies.[48] Patients receiving belimumab also had greater improvement in health-related quality of life.[49] A posthoc analysis of SRI response in patients of African descent showed that they did not benefit from belimumab and actually had lower SRI scores than those receiving placebo.[50] Subsequent experience from academic clinical practice found favorable responses to belimumab in all racial and ethnic groups.[51]

Rituximab is a chimeric monoclonal antibody directed at the CD20 antigen on B cells.[14] Although many case reports and open-label trials have reported beneficial effects of rituximab in SLE, randomized, placebo-controlled trials of rituximab have not demonstrated efficacy in SLE. The largest of these were the EXPLORER (Efficacy and Safety of Rituximab in Moderately-to-Severely Active Systemic Lupus Erythematosus) trial which evaluated patients with extrarenal involvement treated with rituximab and immunosuppressive drugs and the LUNAR (LUpus Nephritis Assessment with Rituximab) trial that examined use of rituximab with mycophenolate mofetil and corticosteroids in patients with lupus nephritis. Failure to show significant benefit could be due to the short duration of the trials or the choice of endpoints. Further improvement has been observed in the second year of therapy. Exploratory analyses of specific patient subgroups or use of different response criteria suggested some benefit. Rituximab may be more effective in patients of African descent with lupus nephritis than those of other races, or in combination with cyclophosphamide instead of mycophenolate mofetil.[52,53] It may serve as an alternative therapy in treatment of refractory lupus nephritis, severe hematological lupus, and some CNS manifestations of the disease. It may also prove useful for maintenance therapy, as a steroid-sparing agent, or when preservation of fertility is desired.[53]

Other drugs targeting B cells are being investigated in SLE. Examples of these are blisibimod, which inhibits BLyS, and atacicept which blocks both BLyS- and APRIL (a proliferation-inducing ligand)-mediated B cell stimulation. Sifalimumab blocks interferon alpha. Other biologic agents have been tried in SLE with varying degrees of success, such as tocilizumab, which inhibits interleukin-6, and abatacept, which inhibits T cell costimulation.[54] The observed efficacy of drugs may depend on the definition of response used. Interestingly, a study of abatacept for lupus nephritis failed to show efficacy, but when other investigators applied endpoint criteria used in different studies of the disease to that data, very different results were observed.[55]

As discussed later, there is concern about TNF-α inhibitors inducing lupus. However, short term induction therapy with infliximab may confer long-lasting benefits in patients with lupus nephritis. When TNF-α inhibitors are used to treat lupus arthritis, patients respond but relapse within a few months after the drug is stopped.[56] Good results have been observed with etanercept as long term treatment of refractory lupus arthritis.[57] Biologic drugs should not be combined.

Immunosuppressive Drugs

Cyclophosphamide has long been used to treat severe organ involvement in SLE such as lupus nephritis, neuropsychiatric lupus, and severe systemic vasculitis.[14] Its role in therapy is being redefined because of the availability of newer drugs, as discussed elsewhere in this chapter. Response rate and dosing requirements may vary with patient race. Cyclophosphamide is an alkylating agent that causes cross-linkage of DNA leading to cell death. It may also suppress B cells and IgG production, and decrease production of adhesion molecules and cytokines. Cyclophosphamide has an oral bioavailability of 75% to 100%. It is a prodrug that is metabolized to active and inactive metabolites via the cytochrome P450 enzyme system. Cyclophosphamide is primarily cleared by the liver, but its active metabolites may persist in renal failure.[58]

Cyclophosphamide can potentially cause hemorrhagic cystitis and bladder cancer due to acrolein, a metabolite of the drug that concentrates in the bladder. The risk appears to be greater with oral administration, higher cumulative doses, and in smokers. The association with intermittent pulse IV doses in SLE patients is less clear. Hydration and frequent voiding may decrease the risk of these adverse effects. With oral administration, patients are advised to take the drug in the morning and to drink fluids for several hours. Adherence is not good with this regimen. With IV administration, IV fluids are begun before administration of the cyclophosphamide and continued for several hours after. Patients are encouraged to maintain oral hydration for 72 hours. Another method to decrease bladder toxicity is to use sodium-2-mercaptoethane sulfonate (Mesna), which binds acrolein and prevents its harmful effects on the bladder. Although mesna is sometimes used with high-dose cyclophosphamide, it is only FDA-approved for use with ifosfamide. Use of mesna with daily oral cyclophosphamide is expensive and inconvenient based on available dosage forms. The recommended mesna regimen with IV pulse doses of cyclophosphamide is to give IV doses, each equivalent to 20% of the cyclophosphamide dose, 15 to 30 minutes before the cyclophosphamide, then 4 and 8 hours after. Since oral mesna is about 50% bioavailable, the 4- and 8-hour mesna doses after cyclophosphamide may be given orally, each in doses equivalent to 40% of the administered dose of cyclophosphamide.[58] In practice, a variety of mesna regimens are used.

Mycophenolic acid (MPA) reversibly inhibits the enzyme inosine 5-monophosphate dehydrogenase (IMPDH), which is important for de novo synthesis of purine (guanosine) nucleotides. This inhibits proliferation and differentiation of lymphocytes. The drug also has other immunomodulating effects such as induction of activated T cell apoptosis, inhibition of adhesion molecule expression, and antifibrotic and antiproliferative effects on cells such as fibroblasts, dendritic cells, and vascular smooth muscle cells.[59]

Mycophenolate mofetil is hydrolyzed to MPA, its active form. The mofetil salt has greater bioavailability. MPA is bound to albumin, so unbound drug concentrations can be affected by changes in albumin. MPA is glucuronidated in the liver to an inactive metabolite, mycophenolic glucuronide. The metabolite undergoes enterohepatic recycling, with conversion back to the active form.[59]

Mycophenolate mofetil has been most studied in treatment of lupus nephritis. It has been shown to be at least as effective as cyclophosphamide for induction therapy and as azathioprine for maintenance treatment.[60,61] The Aspreva Lupus Management Study (ALMS) was a multinational study of lupus nephritis in 370 patients. The 6-month induction phase showed mycophenolate mofetil to be equivalent in efficacy to monthly IV pulse doses of cyclophosphamide, including in a small group of patients with an estimated glomerular filtration rate (eGFR) less than 30 mL/min (0.5 mL/s).[59] The response to therapy at 6 months correlated with the baseline complement C4 concentration, time since diagnosis of lupus nephritis, and eGFR. Normalization of complement C3 and/or C4 and reduction in proteinuria of at least 25% at 8 weeks also predicted renal improvement at 6 months.[62] In the 36-month maintenance phase, mycophenolate mofetil was superior to azathioprine in maintaining renal response to treatment and preventing disease relapse. Although adverse events occurred in more than 97% of patients in both groups, more patients receiving azathioprine withdrew from the study due to toxicity than those receiving mycophenolate mofetil.[63] The MAINTAIN trial did not find a difference in the rate of renal flare with mycophenolate mofetil compared to azathioprine 5 years after induction with IV cyclophosphamide. The difference in these results compared to the ALMS trial may be due to the difference in populations studied. The MAINTAIN trial studied 105 predominantly white European patients, whereas the larger ALMS trial included a more racially diverse population.[59]

Mycophenolate mofetil may also be useful for other manifestations of SLE such as arthritis, cutaneous lupus, and hematologic involvement, including hemolytic anemia and thrombocytopenia.[59]

The most common adverse effects observed with mycophenolate mofetil are GI, including nausea, vomiting, and diarrhea. These may be severe enough to require discontinuation of therapy. Hematologic effects such as red cell aplasia may also be seen. The side effects may be diminished with a reduction in dose. Use of an enteric-coated form may decrease GI symptoms. Numerous congenital malformations have been reported with mycophenolate mofetil and it is contraindicated in pregnancy.[59]

Azathioprine is a purine analog that is metabolized to mercaptopurine. It inhibits DNA synthesis and prevents immune cell proliferation.[64] Mercaptopurine is inactivated by thiopurine methyltransferase (TPMT). If activity of that enzyme is low, patients may experience more severe toxicity. Myelosuppression and gastrointestinal adverse effects correlate with TPMT polymorphism, but hepatotoxicity may not. Other metabolic pathways are also involved in the elimination of azathioprine.[65] The metabolism of azathioprine and mercaptopurine is inhibited by allopurinol and febuxostat. If the combination of these drugs is to be used, a reduction in dose is required.[64] Azathioprine is less effective than cyclophosphamide for induction therapy in lupus nephritis, but it can be useful as an alternative to mycophenolate mofetil for maintenance treatment.[6] Azathioprine may also be used for SLE-related arthritis, serositis, and mucocutaneous manifestations. It has steroid-sparing effects, allowing use of lower doses of corticosteroids.[14]

Methotrexate is an inhibitor of dihydrofolate reductase, which is needed for DNA synthesis and cell proliferation.[32] Its toxicities are reduced by administration of folic acid. It is important to note that it is dosed once weekly in the management of SLE. It is used for arthritis and skin disease and as a steroid-sparing drug.[14]

Numerous other immunosuppressive drugs have been used in SLE, especially in patients who have contraindications to use of the agents already discussed or who cannot tolerate them, or those whose disease is refractory to conventional treatment.

Alternative Treatments

Studies have shown that SLE patients receiving conventional treatment frequently feel they have unmet needs. Often these are psychosocial and may include anxiety or depression. These needs can lead patients to try alternative therapies. It is important for healthcare providers to have an open dialogue with patients about these therapies so that patients will report them. This allows practitioners to monitor for interactions with other treatments and to guide patients to therapies with greater potential for benefit and less for harm.[66]

Complementary and alternative medicine includes health systems, products, and practices that are outside the realm of conventional medicine. In general, these have not been evaluated in randomized controlled trials involving SLE patients.[66]

Concentrations of dehydroepiandrosterone (DHEA), a weak adrenal androgen, are typically decreased in SLE. Some small studies have suggested that DHEA supplementation may offer some limited benefit for patients' assessment of disease activity, steroid effects on bone mineral density, and time to flares in SLE.[66]

Vitamin D concentrations are decreased in SLE, especially in patients with high disease activity and those with darker skin pigmentation (eg, African Americans). A contributing factor to the deficiency is that patients are told to protect themselves from sunlight because of the photosensitivity that accompanies SLE.[42] This can not only affect bone health, but some studies show that low concentrations of vitamin D may also be associated with greater SLE disease activity, flares, and fatigue.[67] Low concentrations also correlate with increased cardiovascular risk factors such as hypertension and hyperlipidemia.[68] B and T lymphocytes, dendritic cells, macrophages, and neutrophils have vitamin D receptors, which suggests a role for vitamin D in both innate and adaptive immune processes.[67] Some experts suggest that most patients with SLE should receive vitamin D supplements of at least 400 IU/day of vitamin D3.[25] One recommendation is to check a baseline 25(OH) vitamin D concentration with a current goal of 30 ng/mL (75 nmol/L). An optimal goal has not yet been determined. The concentration should be rechecked 3 months after a change in vitamin D dosing since that is the time required to reach steady state.[42]

Special Populations

Pregnancy and Contraception

7 Pregnancy planning with assessment of risk factors is key for achieving good outcomes for women with SLE and healthy babies. Timing of pregnancies with respect to disease activity and use of teratogenic medications make contraception counseling very important.[69] Cyclophosphamide therapy is associated with ovarian failure and infertility. This is especially of concern in older women who wish to conceive.[6] Estrogen-containing oral contraceptives are associated with thrombosis, especially in women with antiphospholipid antibodies.[70] Estrogen replacement may increase the risk of thrombosis in postmenopausal women.[10] Although SLE flares have been a concern with use of hormonal contraceptives, recent studies in mild-to-moderate disease did not show such an association, but the results may be influenced by study inclusion and exclusion criteria.[70] Progesterone-only contraceptives may be used but the adverse effects of acne and hirsutism may make them less desirable and the risk of osteoporosis increases after 2 years of use. Intrauterine devices may be better choices for contraception.[71,72]

Pregnancy during SLE is considered to be high risk. The risk of maternal mortality, cesarean delivery, preterm labor, and preeclampsia and the risk of thrombotic, infectious, and hematologic complications are increased.[73,74] Fetal loss, intrauterine growth restriction, and early preeclampsia may relate to uterine-placental insufficiency with poor placental blood flow.[75] Preeclampsia occurs in 10% to 30% of women with SLE and is defined as hypertension (BP greater than 140/90) and proteinuria (greater than 300 mg/24 h) that develop for the first time after 20 weeks of gestation.[73,76] This can be difficult to distinguish from lupus nephritis. The risk for preterm preeclampsia may be decreased by 90% with daily use of low-dose aspirin begun before 16 weeks' gestation.[75] Flares during pregnancy may be difficult to identify since they may share characteristics of a normal pregnancy.[72] The complications are more likely in patients with active disease, especially lupus nephritis. If the mother has anti-Ro/SSA or anti-La/SSB antibodies, the fetus is at risk for neonatal lupus with rash and cardiac abnormalities including heart block. These risks are significantly decreased with continued use of hydroxychloroquine.[73] Treatment of pregnant women with antiphospholipid antibodies is discussed below. Pregnancy should be discouraged in patients with severe pulmonary hypertension, advanced renal insufficiency, severe restrictive lung disease, heart failure, or a history of severe preeclampsia. It also is not advised within 6 months of a severe SLE flare, active lupus nephritis, or a stroke. The best pregnancy outcomes are observed in patients who have had inactive disease for at least 6 months prior to the pregnancy. Drugs used to control the SLE should be those such as hydroxychloroquine, which can be continued throughout the pregnancy and may decrease the incidence of flares.[73] Any potentially teratogenic drugs (eg, methotrexate, leflunomide, mycophenolate, cyclophosphamide, and thalidomide) should be stopped at least 3 months before attempting pregnancy. Leflunomide should be removed through the oral cholestyramine elimination procedure (8 g three times a day for 11 days with confirmation of undetectable serum concentrations) prior to conception. Close monitoring and disease management of the mothers and fetuses are essential during pregnancy. The risks of drug use and harmful effects of disease flare both need to be considered.[72] If a flare occurs and an immunosuppressive drug is required during the pregnancy, azathioprine may be considered, since the fetal liver is unable to metabolize it to its active form. The dose should not exceed 2 mg/kg/day.[77] If corticosteroids are needed, maintenance doses should be kept at the equivalent of prednisone 10 mg daily or less to decrease the risk of gestational diabetes mellitus, infections, and premature rupture of membranes.[33,72] Patients on long-term steroid therapy may need stress doses at the time of delivery. Fluorinated corticosteroids (such as dexamethasone or betamethasone) should be avoided unless they are being used to treat the fetus, since they cross the placenta.[73] Cyclophosphamide should only be used during pregnancy if alternatives failed and the mother's life is in danger.[72] If treatment of hypertension is needed, methyldopa and labetalol are preferred, with nifedipine or hydralazine considered as alternatives.[72,73] Angiotensin-converting enzyme inhibitors and angiotensin receptor blockers may cause fetal malformations and neonatal renal failure and death.[73] Diuretics are generally avoided but if one is needed, furosemide is preferred.[72] NSAIDs should be used with caution during early pregnancy. Congenital malformations have been reported with use in the first trimester and impaired fetal renal function after 20 weeks. They should not be used after 32 weeks of gestation because they increase the risk of premature closure of the ductus arteriosus by almost 15-fold.[73]

SLE–Antiphospholipid Syndrome Overlap

8 The antiphospholipid antibodies consist of anticardiolipin, anti-β-2-glycoprotein I, and lupus anticoagulant and they can promote clotting and inflammation.[78] Complement also plays a key role in antiphospholipid syndrome (APS) pathogenesis.[41] The diagnosis of APS requires at least one clinical and one laboratory feature. The clinical aspects are vascular events such as venous or arterial thrombi and/or obstetric complications. The obstetric complications meeting the criteria are three or more unexplained consecutive miscarriages before the 10th week of gestation, one or more unexplained deaths of fetuses at or beyond the 10th week of gestation, and one or more births of infants before the 34th week of gestation associated with eclampsia or severe preeclampsia or features of placental insufficiency.[79] Adverse pregnancy outcomes after 12 weeks of gestation are especially associated with the presence of lupus anticoagulant.[80] Laboratory criteria are the presence of antiphospholipid antibodies on two separate occasions, 12 weeks apart.[79] Antiphospholipid antibodies are found in about 40% of patients with SLE, but less than 40% of those experience thrombotic events.[81] Patients with lupus anticoagulant or persistently positive anticardiolipin at medium-high titers are at high risk for thrombosis, and those with all three antibodies (triple positivity) are at highest risk. Patients with isolated, intermittently positive anticardiolipin or anti-β_2-glycoprotein I at low-medium titers are considered to be at low risk. Patients with thrombosis often have other cardiovascular risk factors (such as hypertension, hyperlipidemia, smoking, or use of estrogen-containing medications) or an underlying autoimmune disease such as SLE. It is recommended that any modifiable factors be controlled. In deciding choice, intensity, and duration of treatment, the clinician should balance benefits with the patient's risk of bleeding. Consideration should also be given to whether thrombotic events are associated with identified transient precipitating factors. An international group of physicians who had clinical and research experience with APS reviewed the literature and developed consensus guidelines for management of thrombosis in patients with antiphospholipid antibodies (Table 87-4).[38]

Patients with antiphospholipid antibodies may also have a false-positive test for syphilis (rapid plasma reagin).[15] Other common manifestations of APS are cognitive impairment, thrombocytopenia, stroke or transient ischemic attack, chorea, migraine, heart valve lesions, and livedo reticularis.[78,79]

It is not clear how to treat pregnant women with antiphospholipid antibodies. Those with no history of thrombosis who have experienced early fetal loss may be treated with low-dose aspirin (81 mg) alone or in combination with prophylactic doses of heparin or low-molecular-weight heparin.[78] Not only does heparin have anticoagulant effects, but it also has anti-inflammatory and immunomodulating properties and can inhibit complement activation.[81] Those

TABLE 87-4 Recommendations for Thromboprophylaxis in Patients with Systemic Lupus Erythematosus and Antiphospholipid Antibodies

Recommendation	Grade of Recommendation
1. General measures for aPL carriers	
Control cardiovascular risk factors if high-risk aPL profile	Nongraded
Thromboprophylaxis with low molecular weight heparin in high risk situations such as surgery, prolonged immobilization, and after childbirth	1C
2. Primary thromboprophylaxis	
Regularly assess patients for presence of aPL	Nongraded
Thromboprophylaxis with hydroxychloroquine (1) and low-dose aspirin (2) for patients with positive LA or persistent aCL at medium-high titers	1B (1) 2B (2)
3. Secondary thromboprophylaxis	
Treat patients with arterial or venous thrombosis and aPL who do not meet APS criteria with standard thrombosis treatment	1C
Treat patients with definite APS and first venous event with warfarin to target INR 2-3	1B
Treat patients with definite APS and arterial thrombosis with warfarin at INR greater than 3 or combined antiaggregant-warfarin (INR 2-3) therapy	Nongraded
Assess bleeding risk before high-intensity warfarin or combined antiaggregant-warfarin therapy	Nongraded
4. Duration of treatment	
Indefinite antithrombotic therapy in patients with definite APS and thrombosis	1C
For first venous event, low-risk APS profile and known transient precipitating factor, anticoagulate for 3-6 months	Nongraded
5. Refractory and difficult cases	
If recurrent thrombosis, fluctuating INR, major bleeding or high risk for major bleeding, consider alternative such as low molecular weight heparin, hydroxychloroquine, or statins	Nongraded

aPL, antiphospholipid antibodies; LA, lupus anticoagulant; aCL, anticardiolipin; APS, antiphospholipid syndrome; INR, international normalized ratio.

Grades of recommendation: 1B: Strong recommendation, moderate quality evidence, 1C: Strong recommendation, low or very low-quality evidence; 2B: Weak recommendation, moderate quality evidence; 2C: Weak recommendation, low or very low-quality evidence

Used with permission from Ruiz-Irastorza G, Cuadrado MJ, Ruiz-Arruza I, et al. Evidence-based recommendations for the prevention and long-term management of thrombosis in antiphospholipid antibody-positive patients: Report of a Task Force at the 13th International Congress on Antiphospholipid Antibodies. Lupus. 2011;20:206-218.

without thrombosis who have had later miscarriages or premature births associated with preeclampsia or placental insufficiency may receive low dose aspirin plus prophylactic or intermediate doses of heparin or prophylactic doses of low-molecular-weight heparin. Pregnant patients with APS and a history of thrombosis should receive low-dose aspirin with therapeutic doses of heparin or low-molecular-weight heparin. Warfarin should be avoided during pregnancy; it is teratogenic between 6 and 12 weeks gestation and increases the risk of fetal bleeding after 12 weeks.[78] If low-molecular-weight heparin is used, it should be switched to unfractionated heparin 4 weeks before the anticipated delivery date. The heparin should be stopped at the start of labor or 8 hours before a planned cesarean delivery.[72] All women with APS should receive anticoagulation with prophylactic doses of heparin, low-molecular-weight heparin, or warfarin for 4 to 6 weeks postpartum. Both heparin and warfarin are safe during breastfeeding.[78]

Better control of APS can be achieved by adding hydroxychloroquine, statins, and vitamin D to standard therapy. For patients who do not respond to conventional APS treatment or for whom it is contraindicated, alternative therapies include other platelet inhibitors, new oral anticoagulants, rituximab, and the complement inhibitor, eculizumab.[41,78]

Clinical **Controversy...**

Can new oral anticoagulants be used to treat APS? Some evidence suggests that they are effective, but thrombotic events have been reported when patients are switched to them from warfarin. Large ongoing controlled studies may provide answers.

The most severe form of APS is called catastrophic and is associated with widespread thrombosis, multiorgan failure, and 50% mortality.[78,79]

Drug-Induced Lupus

9 About 10% to 15% of cases of SLE can be attributed to drugs.[82] These are idiosyncratic reactions precipitated by the interplay of genetic predisposition, concurrent illnesses, environmental factors, and other drugs or foods. Various pathophysiologic mechanisms have been proposed for different drugs in inducing lupus. Most drugs are small molecules that can induce an immune response by binding to larger molecules such as proteins, a process called haptenization. Another proposed mechanism is interfering with macrophage uptake of apoptotic or necrotic cells, leading to accumulation of nucleosomes that can be targets for anti-DNA antibodies.[83] Other proposed mechanisms are altered T cell function due to DNA hypomethylation and interference with T cell maturation.[82]

Because the manifestations of drug-induced lupus are so diverse, there are no standard diagnostic criteria. The diagnosis is based on lupus-like findings in a patient with no history of the disease and the temporal relationship with the drug, including onset at least 1 month after initiation and improvement in symptoms within days to months after the drug is discontinued. The time-frame, however, can be variable. The patient will often have laboratory findings such as a positive ANA or anti-histone antibodies, but usually not anti-dsDNA or anti-Sm antibodies.[82]

Many drugs of varied classes have been implicated. The drugs considered to have the highest risk for inducing traditional symptomatic drug-induced lupus are procainamide (20%) and hydralazine (5%-8%), especially with hydralazine doses over 200 mg per day or a cumulative dose of more than 100 g. The incidence of positive ANAs with these drugs is 80% to 90% and 50% respectively.[82] Common manifestations include arthralgias, arthritis, and myalgias. Constitutional symptoms such as fever, fatigue, and weight loss are common, but the incidence is about one-half that seen with idiopathic SLE. Other clinical features include rash, serositis (pleuritis, pericarditis), hematologic abnormalities, and hepatosplenomegaly. Glomerulonephritis and neuropsychiatric symptoms are rare in drug-induced lupus. The incidence and types of reactions vary depending on the offending drug. Laboratory abnormalities associated with drug-induced lupus include positive ANA (99%) and antibodies to histones (96%). Other antibodies such as anticardiolipin (5%-20%), anti-dsDNA (less than 5%), and antineutrophil cytoplasmic antibodies (ANCA) may be seen with some drugs. A drug with moderate risk for lupus is quinidine. The incidence of quinidine- and procainamide-induced lupus is declining because of decreased prescribing of the drugs and use of lower doses. The other almost 100 drugs of many different classes that have been implicated are considered to be of low risk. One that affects younger patients, including children, is minocycline.[83] Other drugs with well-established links to lupus are isoniazid, methyldopa, and chlorpromazine.[82] A variant of the syndrome is drug-induced subacute cutaneous lupus, which has been associated with calcium channel antagonists, thiazide diuretics, angiotensin-converting enzyme inhibitors, interferon, ticlopidine, leflunomide, and terbinafine. The mean age for this syndrome is 59 years; most patients are women, and positive ANA, anti-Ro/SSA, and anti-La/SSB are common. It may occur after weeks to years of therapy.[82,83] Chronic cutaneous lupus has been reported with fluorouracil and NSAIDs.[83] It can take months for skin lesions to resolve after the offending drug has been stopped.[10]

A separate category of drug-induced lupus is that involving TNF-α inhibitors, such as infliximab, etanercept, adalimumab, and certolizumab pegol. This is called TAILS or TNF-α inhibitor-induced lupus syndrome. These drugs, especially chimeric infliximab, are known to induce autoantibodies. Other theories explaining the mechanism for TNF-α inhibitor-induced lupus are that they cause a shift into other pathways of cytokine production, induce cell apoptosis, increase the risk for bacterial infection, or suppress T-helper 1 immune response and favor T-helper 2 response. It is common for patients receiving these drugs to develop positive ANAs and anti-dsDNA of the IgM subtype. Antihistone antibodies are less commonly seen than with other drug-induced lupus (17%-57%). As with traditional drug-induced lupus, the incidence of clinical lupus is low compared to the numbers that develop autoantibodies.[82,83] Rashes, hypocomplementemia, leukopenia, and thrombocytopenia are more common features with TNF-α inhibitors than traditional drug-induced lupus, and arthralgias, arthritis, and myalgias are less common. Renal and neurological disorders are rare. The underlying diseases being treated with these drugs may be a factor in development of the observed reactions. Autoimmune diseases have also been reported following use of interferon therapy.[83]

The primary treatment for drug-induced lupus is stopping the implicated drug. Some patients require treatment with corticosteroids. If patients do not improve, a diagnosis of idiopathic SLE should be considered.[83]

Immunizations

Patients with SLE are at increased risk for infections because of immune dysfunction caused by the disease itself and the immunosuppressive therapy the patients receive. It is important to try to protect patients against these infections, but there are areas of concern regarding the safety and efficacy of vaccines in patients with SLE. SLE cases developing or flaring after vaccine administration have been reported, but the actual risk appears low when considering how many people receive immunizations.[84] These reactions may be a response to adjuvants added to increase the immunogenicity of vaccines and could be part of the syndrome called "ASIA—Autoimmune/inflammatory Syndrome Induced by Adjuvants."[85] Another concern is that immunosuppressed patients may have an impaired response to vaccines as compared with healthy individuals. This can be assessed by checking titers after immunization. In some cases revaccination may be needed. Whenever possible, to achieve the best response, vaccines should be administered when SLE is stable and prior to initiating immunosuppressive medications. Killed vaccines are considered safe in immunosuppressed patients. It is recommended that SLE patients receive pneumococcal vaccine, since they are particularly susceptible to *Streptococcus pneumoniae* infections. They should also receive annual influenza vaccines. Hydroxychloroquine may improve the response to vaccines and decrease the risk of infections. Patients with splenectomy should receive Haemophilus influenzae and meningococcal vaccines. Those considered to be at risk should be immunized against hepatitis B.[84] Live-attenuated virus vaccines, such as measles–mumps–rubella, varicella, zoster, intranasal influenza, and yellow fever, are contraindicated in patients receiving biologic agents. They should be avoided with consideration of risks versus benefits in patients taking high doses of other immunosuppressive drugs.[86] Doses of corticosteroids equivalent to prednisone 20 mg/day or more given for at least 2 weeks are considered immunosuppressive.[87] Live vaccines should be given at least 4 weeks before starting immunosuppressive drugs or 1 month after stopping them, depending on the duration of drug effects.[86,87]

PERSONALIZED PHARMACOTHERAPY

Pharmacotherapy is determined by disease manifestations and patient-specific factors. Primary goals should be remission of symptoms and organ manifestations or low disease activity and prevention of flares. Hydroxychloroquine should be considered for all patients with SLE. Corticosteroids should be used in the lowest effective dose or discontinued. Symptoms affecting quality of life such as fatigue, pain, and depression should be managed.[39] Organ function should be considered in selection of therapy. Leading causes of mortality in SLE are infections, cardiovascular disease, malignancy, and renal complications related to the disease and treatment. Therapy to prevent and manage these conditions should be individualized based on comorbidities present.[88]

Race appears to influence response to treatment, but many people are of mixed race. Genetic testing may provide a better guide in the future. In studies of lupus nephritis, whites with Western or Southern European backgrounds respond as well to low-dose IV cyclophosphamide ("Euro-Lupus" regimen of 500 mg every 2 weeks for six doses) as to high-dose regimens (500-1,000 mg/m^2 body surface area once a month for six doses) (Level B evidence). African Americans and Hispanics respond less well to IV cyclophosphamide than do whites or Asians. Patients of African or Hispanic origin may respond better to mycophenolate mofetil than to cyclophosphamide. Asians require lower doses of mycophenolate mofetil (Level C evidence).[6] African Americans and Hispanics may respond to rituximab better than whites.[54] Patients of African descent did not respond to belimumab in the BLISS studies, but favorable results were seen in later studies.[50,51]

Blood concentrations of drugs are not usually measured in SLE management, even for drugs that are monitored that way when used for other diseases. Hydroxychloroquine blood concentrations may correlate with efficacy or adherence, but they are not routinely monitored.[45] Although therapeutic mycophenolate drug concentration monitoring is used in transplant patients, it is not yet standard practice in SLE patients. Preliminary studies have shown that MPA area under the plasma concentration–time curve and trough concentrations correlate with SLE disease activity but only weakly with adverse effects or daily doses.[89] Patients should have TPMT testing before receiving azathioprine[89] and be screened for glucose-6-phosphate dehydrogenase (G6PD) deficiency before getting dapsone.[24]

Pregnancy plans should be considered in choosing therapy. Attention must be given to the effects of drugs on fertility and on the fetus, as well as the adverse effects of active disease on pregnancy outcomes.

EVALUATION OF THERAPEUTIC OUTCOMES

Patients must be assessed for the activity and extent of lupus and monitored for adverse drug effects. Monitoring for specific drugs is listed in Table 87-3. (10) Many instruments have been developed and modified over the years to assess SLE therapy in trials. It is difficult to assess SLE therapy because milder forms of the disease may fluctuate, regardless of therapy. Examples of measures of disease activity include the Safety of Estrogens in Lupus Erythematosus National Assessment-Systemic Lupus Erythematosus Disease Activity Index (SELENA-SLEDAI), and British Isles Lupus Assessment Group (BILAG). The SELENA-SLEDAI is a measure of disease activity that scores severity of 24 manifestations. BILAG measures clinical disease activity in eight organ systems compared to the prior month. The organ domains are given scores based on severity: A (severe disease activity flare that requires additional treatment), B (moderate disease activity), C (mild, stable disease), D (previously affected but no current disease activity), and E (never been involved). Updates of these instruments are the SLEDAI-2K and the BILAG-2004. Individually, these indices were inadequate for showing superiority of new drugs over standard therapy. To overcome this problem, belimumab investigators developed the SRI assessment criteria. The SRI has three components: (a) Reduction in disease activity by SELENA-SLEDAI by at least 4 points; (b) No worsening of disease activity (BILAG A) and no more than one new BILAG B score; and (c) less than 0.3 point increase (worsening) in physician global assessment (PGA). The PGA assesses patients' general health status. Another important assessment of therapy is health-related quality of life (HRQoL), which may use a tool such as the generic Medical Outcomes Survey Short Form-36 (SF-36).[90]

A EULAR panel developed recommendations for the monitoring of patients with SLE in clinical practice and observational studies. Patients should be evaluated for SLE disease activity and organ involvement, cardiovascular risk factors, comorbidities, and risk for infection. Clinical and laboratory assessments should be performed every 6 to 12 months in patients with inactive disease and no organ damage, and more frequently if abnormalities are found.[91]

The Cutaneous Lupus Erythematosus Disease Area and Severity Index (CLASI) may be used to assess disease activity and damage in cutaneous lupus erythematosus and response to therapy.[92]

ABBREVIATIONS

ACR	American College of Rheumatology
ALMS	Aspreva Lupus Management Study
ANA	antinuclear antibody
ANCA	antineutrophil cytoplasmic antibodies
Anti-dsDNA	anti-double-stranded DNA
APRIL	a proliferation-inducing ligand
APS	antiphospholipid syndrome
BAFF	B cell activating factor of the TNF family
BILAG	British Isles Lupus Assessment Group
BLyS	B-lymphocyte stimulator
CLASI	Cutaneous Lupus Erythematosus Disease Area and Severity Index
DHEA	dehydroepiandrosterone
DNA	deoxyribonucleic acid
eGFR	estimated glomerular filtration rate
EULAR	European League Against Rheumatism
G6PD	glucose-6-phosphate dehydrogenase
HRQoL	health-related quality of life
IMPDH	inosine 5-monophosphate dehydrogenase
La/SSB	antigen La/Sjögren syndrome antigen B
Mesna	sodium-2-mercaptoethane sulfonate
MHC	major histocompatibility complex
MPA	mycophenolic acid
NMDA	*N*-methyl-D-aspartate
NSAID	nonsteroidal antiinflammatory drug
PGA	physician global assessment
Ro/SSA	antigen Ro/Sjögren syndrome A
SELENA-SLEDAI	Safety of Estrogens in Lupus Erythematosus: National Assessment-Systemic Lupus Erythematosus Disease Activity Index
SF-36	Medical Outcomes Survey Short Form-36
SLE	systemic lupus erythematosus
SLICC	Systemic Lupus International Collaborating Clinics
SPF	sun protection factor
SRI	SLE Responder Index
TAILS	TNF-α inhibitor-induced lupus syndrome
TNF-α	tumor necrosis factor-alpha
TPMT	thiopurine methyltransferase

REFERENCES

1. Scofield RH, Oates J. The place of William Osler in the description of systemic lupus erythematosus. *Am J Med Sci* 2009;338:409-412.
2. Azevedo PC, Murphy G, Isenberg DA. Pathology of systemic lupus erythematosus: The challenges ahead. *Methods Mol Biol* 2014;1134:1-16.
3. Pons-Estel GJ, Alarcón GS, Scofield L, et al. Understanding the epidemiology and progression of systemic lupus erythematosus. *Semin Arthritis Rheum* 2010;39:257-268.
4. Lim SS, Drenkard C. Epidemiology of lupus: An update. *Curr Opin Rheumatol* 2015;27:427-432.
5. Sánchez E, Rasmussen A, Riba L, et al. Impact of genetic ancestry and sociodemographic status on the clinical expression of systemic lupus erythematosus in American Indian-European populations. *Arthritis Rheum* 2012;64:3687-3694.
6. Hahn BH, McMahon MA, Wilkinson A, et al. American College of Rheumatology guidelines for screening, treatment, and management of lupus nephritis. *Arthritis Care Res* 2012;64:797-808.
7. Niewold TB. Advances in lupus genetics. *Curr Opin Rheumatol* 2015;27:440-447.
8. Robinson M, Cook SS, Currie LM. Systemic lupus erythematosus: A genetic review for advanced practice nurses. *J Am Acad Nurse Pract* 2011;23:629-637.
9. Tsokos GC. Systemic lupus erythematosus. *N Engl J Med* 2011;365:2110-2121.
10. Zandman-Goddard G, Solomon M, Rosman Z, et al. Environment and lupus-related diseases. *Lupus* 2012;21:241-250.
11. Hanlon P, Avenell A, Aucott L, Vickers MA. Systematic review and meta-analysis of the sero-epidemiological association between Epstein-Barr virus and systemic lupus erythematosus. *Arthritis Res Ther* 2014;16:R3.
12. Choi ST, Kang JI, Park IH, et al. Subscale analysis of quality of life in patients with systemic lupus erythematosus: Association with depression, fatigue, disease activity and damage. *Clin Exp Rheumatol* 2012;30:665-672.
13. Tan TC, Fang H, Magder LS, Petri MA. Differences between male and female systemic lupus erythematosus in a multiethnic population. *J Rheumatol* 2012;39:759-769.
14. Xiong W, Lahita RG. Pragmatic approaches to therapy for systemic lupus erythematosus. *Nat Rev Rheumatol* 2014;10:97-107.
15. Petri M, Orbai AM, Alarcón GS, et al. Derivation and validation of the Systemic Lupus International Collaborating Clinics classification criteria for systemic lupus erythematosus. *Arthritis Rheum* 2012;64:2677-2686.
16. Adrianto I, Wang S, Wiley GB, et al. Association of two independent functional risk haplotypes in TNIP1 with systemic lupus erythematosus. *Arthritis Rheum* 2012;64:3695-3705.

17. Tan EM, Cohen AS, Fries JF, et al. The 1982 revised criteria for the classification of systemic lupus erythematosus. *Arthritis Rheum* 1982;25:1271-1277.
18. Hochberg MC. Updating the American College of Rheumatology revised criteria for the classification of systemic lupus erythematosus. *Arthritis Rheum* 1997;40:1725.
19. Inês L, Silva C, Galindo M, et al. Classification of systemic lupus erythematosus: Systemic Lupus International Collaborating Clinics versus American College of Rheumatology criteria. A comparative study of 2,055 patients from a real-life, international systemic lupus erythematosus cohort. *Arthritis Care Res* 2015;67:1180-1185.
20. Ruperto N, Hanrahan LM, Alarcón GS, et al. International consensus for a definition of disease flare in lupus. *Lupus* 2011;20:453-462.
21. Kuhn A, Bonsmann G, Anders HJ, et al. The diagnosis and treatment of systemic lupus erythematosus. *Dtsch Arztebl Int* 2015;112:423-432.
22. Pons-Estel GJ, Alarcón GS, González LA, et al. Possible protective effect of hydroxychloroquine on delaying the occurrence of integument damage in lupus: LXXI, data from a multiethnic cohort. *Arthritis Care Res* 2010;62:393-400.
23. Okon LG, Werth VP. Cutaneous lupus erythematosus: Diagnosis and treatment. *Baillieres Best Pract Res Clin Rheumatol* 2013;27:391-404.
24. Chang AY, Werth VP. Treatment of cutaneous lupus. *Curr Rheumatol Rep* 2011;13:300-307.
25. Hansen CB, Dahle KW. Cutaneous lupus erythematosus. *Dermatol Ther* 2012;25:99-111.
26. Santiago-Casas Y, Vilá LM, McGwin G Jr, et al. Association of discoid lupus erythematosus with clinical manifestations and damage accrual in a multiethnic lupus cohort. *Arthritis Care Res* 2012;64:704-712.
27. Bertsias GK, Ioannidis JP, Aringer M, et al. EULAR recommendations for the management of systemic lupus erythematosus with neuropsychiatric manifestations: Report of a task force of the EULAR standing committee for clinical affairs. *Ann Rheum Dis* 2010;69:2074-2082.
28. Jeltsch-David H, Muller S. Neuropsychiatric systemic lupus erythematosus: Pathogenesis and biomarkers. *Nat Rev Neurol* 2014;10:579-596.
29. Bhangle SD, Kramer N, Rosenstein ED. Corticosteroid-induced neuropsychiatric disorders: Review and contrast with neuropsychiatric lupus. *Rheumatol Int* 2013;33:1923-1932.
30. Knight JS, Kaplan MJ. Cardiovascular disease in lupus: Insights and updates. *Curr Opin Rheumatol* 2013;25:597-605.
31. Costedoat-Chalumeau N, Dunogue B, Morel N, et al. Hydroxychloroquine: A multifaceted treatment in lupus. *Presse Med* 2014;43:e167-e180.
32. Lisnevskaia L, Murphy G, Isenberg D. Systemic lupus erythematosus. *Lancet* 2014;384:1878-1888.
33. Mosca M, Tani C, Carli L, Bombardieri S. Glucocorticoids in systemic lupus erythematosus. *Clin Exp Rheumatol* 2011;29:S126-S129.
34. Haija AJ, Schulz SW. The role and effect of complementary and alternative medicine in systemic lupus erythematosus. *Rheum Dis Clin North Am* 2011;37:47-62.
35. Food, Drug Administration HHS. Labeling and effectiveness testing; sunscreen drug products for over-the-counter human use. Final rule. *Fed Regist* 2011;76:35620-35665.
36. Chasset F, Francès C, Barete S, et al. Influence of smoking on the efficacy of antimalarials in cutaneous lupus: a meta-analysis of the literature. *J Am Acad Dermatol* 2015;72:634-639.
37. Kuhn A, Sigges J, Biazar C, et al. Influence of smoking on disease severity and antimalarial therapy in cutaneous lupus erythematosus: Analysis of 1002 patients from the EUSCLE database. *Br J Dermatol* 2014;171:571-579.
38. Ruiz-Irastorza G, Cuadrado MJ, Ruiz-Arruza I, et al. Evidence-based recommendations for the prevention and long-term management of thrombosis in antiphospholipid antibody-positive patients: Report of a Task Force at the 13th International Congress on Antiphospholipid Antibodies. *Lupus* 2011;20:206-218.
39. van Vollenhoven RF, Mosca M, Bertsias G, et al. Treat-to-target in systemic lupus erythematosus: Recommendations from an international task force. *Ann Rheum Dis* 2014;73:958-967.
40. Artifoni M, Puechal X. How to treat refractory arthritis in lupus? *Joint Bone Spine* 2012;79:347-350.
41. Chighizola CB, Raschi E, Borghi MO, Meroni PL. Update on the pathogenesis and treatment of the antiphospholipid syndrome. *Curr Opin Rheumatol* 2015;27:476-482.
42. Kamen DL. Vitamin D in lupus—new kid on the block? *Bull NYU Hosp Jt Dis* 2010;68:218-222.
43. Duru N, van der Goes MC, Jacobs JW, et al. EULAR evidence-based and consensus-based recommendations on the management of medium to high-dose glucocorticoid therapy in rheumatic diseases. *Ann Rheum Dis* 2013;72:1905-1913.
44. Ruiz-Irastorza G, Ramos-Casals M, Brito-Zeron P, Khamashta MA. Clinical efficacy and side effects of antimalarials in systemic lupus erythematosus: A systematic review. *Ann Rheum Dis* 2010;69:20-28.
45. Costedoat-Chalumeau N, Le Guern V, Piette JC. Routine hydroxychloroquine blood concentration measurement in systemic lupus erythematosus reaches adulthood. *J Rheumatol* 2015;42:1997-1999.
46. Marmor MF, Kellner U, Lai TY, et al. Revised recommendations on screening for chloroquine and hydroxychloroquine retinopathy. *Ophthalmology* 2011;118:415-422.
47. Dennis GJ. Belimumab: A BLyS-specific inhibitor for the treatment of systemic lupus erythematosus. *Clin Pharmacol Ther* 2012;91:143-149.
48. Chan RW, Jiang P, Peng X, et al. Plasma DNA aberrations in systemic lupus erythematosus revealed by genomic and methylomic sequencing. *Proc Natl Acad Sci U S A* 2014;111:E5302-E5311.
49. Strand V, Levy RA, Cervera R, et al. Improvements in health-related quality of life with belimumab, a B-lymphocyte stimulator-specific inhibitor, in patients with autoantibody-positive systemic lupus erythematosus from the randomised controlled BLISS trials. *Ann Rheum Dis* 2014;73:838-844.
50. Burness CB, McCormack PL. Belimumab: In systemic lupus erythematosus. *Drugs* 2011;71:2435-2444.
51. Hui-Yuen JS, Reddy A, Taylor J, et al. Safety and efficacy of belimumab to treat systemic lupus erythematosus in academic clinical practices. *J Rheumatol* 2015;42:2288-2295.
52. Coca A, Sanz I. Updates on B-cell immunotherapies for systemic lupus erythematosus and Sjogren's syndrome. *Curr Opin Rheumatol* 2012;24:451-456.
53. Eko SL, van Vollenhoven RF. Rituximab and lupus—a promising pair? *Curr Rheumatol Rep* 2014;16:444.
54. Fattah Z, Isenberg DA. Recent developments in the treatment of patients with systemic lupus erythematosus: Focusing on biologic therapies. *Expert Opin Biol Ther* 2014;14:311-326.
55. Wofsy D, Hillson JL, Diamond B. Abatacept for lupus nephritis: Alternative definitions of complete response support conflicting conclusions. *Arthritis Rheum* 2012;64:3660-3665.
56. Aringer M, Smolen JS. Therapeutic blockade of TNF in patients with SLE-promising or crazy? *Autoimmun Rev* 2012;11:321-325.
57. Cortés-Hernández J, Egri N, Vilardell-Tarrés M, Ordi-Ros J. Etanercept in refractory lupus arthritis: An observational study. *Semin Arthritis Rheum* 2015;44:672-679.
58. Monach PA, Arnold LM, Merkel PA. Incidence and prevention of bladder toxicity from cyclophosphamide in the treatment of rheumatic diseases: a data-driven review. *Arthritis Rheum* 2010;62:9-21.
59. Dall'Era M. Mycophenolate mofetil in the treatment of systemic lupus erythematosus. *Curr Opin Rheumatol* 2011;23:454-458.
60. Liu LL, Jiang Y, Wang LN, et al. Efficacy and safety of mycophenolate mofetil versus cyclophosphamide for induction therapy of lupus nephritis: A meta-analysis of randomized controlled trials. *Drugs* 2012;72:1521-1533.
61. Maneiro JR, Lopez-Canoa N, Salgado E, Gomez-Reino JJ. Maintenance therapy of lupus nephritis with mycophenolate or azathioprine: Systematic review and meta-analysis. *Rheumatology* 2014;53:834-838.
62. Dall'Era M, Stone D, Levesque V, et al. Identification of biomarkers that predict response to treatment of lupus nephritis with mycophenolate mofetil or pulse cyclophosphamide. *Arthritis Care Res* 2011;63:351-357.
63. Dooley MA, Jayne D, Ginzler EM, et al. Mycophenolate versus azathioprine as maintenance therapy for lupus nephritis. *N Engl J Med* 2011;365:1886-1895.
64. Schmajuk G, Yazdany J. Drug monitoring in systemic lupus erythematosus: A systematic review. *Semin Arthritis Rheum* 2011;40:559-575.
65. Liu YP, Xu HQ, Li M, et al. Association between thiopurine S-methyltransferase polymorphisms and azathioprine-induced adverse drug reactions in patients with autoimmune diseases: A meta-analysis. *PLoS ONE* 2015;10:e0144234.
66. Greco CM, Nakajima C, Manzi S. Updated review of complementary and alternative medicine treatments for systemic lupus erythematosus. *Curr Rheumatol Rep* 2013;15:378.

67. Gatenby P, Lucas R, Swaminathan A. Vitamin D deficiency and risk for rheumatic diseases: An update. *Curr Opin Rheumatol* 2013;25:184-191.
68. Lertratanakul A, Wu P, Dyer A, et al. 25-hydroxyvitamin D and cardiovascular disease in patients with systemic lupus erythematosus: Data from a large international inception cohort. *Arthritis Care Res* 2014;66:1167-1176.
69. Hahn BH. Pregnancy in women with systemic lupus erythematosus: Messages for the clinician. *Ann Intern Med* 2015;163:232-233.
70. Culwell KR, Curtis KM. Contraception for women with systemic lupus erythematosus. *J Fam Plann Reprod Health Care* 2013;39:9-11.
71. Cravioto MD, Jiménez-Santana L, Mayorga J, Seuc AH. Side effects unrelated to disease activity and acceptability of highly effective contraceptive methods in women with systemic lupus erythematosus: A randomized, clinical trial. *Contraception* 2014;90:147-153.
72. Baer AN, Witter FR, Petri M. Lupus and pregnancy. *Obstet Gynecol Surv* 2011;66:639-653.
73. Lateef A, Petri M. Managing lupus patients during pregnancy. *Baillieres Best Pract Res Clin Rheumatol* 2013;27:435-447.
74. Peart E, Clowse ME. Systemic lupus erythematosus and pregnancy outcomes: An update and review of the literature. *Curr Opin Rheumatol* 2014;26:118-123.
75. Ostensen M, Clowse M. Pathogenesis of pregnancy complications in systemic lupus erythematosus. *Curr Opin Rheumatol* 2013;25:591-596.
76. Clowse ME. Managing contraception and pregnancy in the rheumatologic diseases. *Baillieres Best Pract Res Clin Rheumatol* 2010;24:373-385.
77. Saavedra MA, Sánchez A, Morales S, et al. Azathioprine during pregnancy in systemic lupus erythematosus patients is not associated with poor fetal outcome. *Clin Rheumatol* 2015;34:1211-1216.
78. Ruiz-Irastorza G, Crowther M, Branch W, Khamashta MA. Antiphospholipid syndrome. *Lancet* 2010;376:1498-1509.
79. Gómez-Puerta JA, Cervera R. Diagnosis and classification of the antiphospholipid syndrome. *J Autoimmun* 2014;48-49:20-25.
80. Lockshin MD, Kim M, Laskin CA, et al. Prediction of adverse pregnancy outcome by the presence of lupus anticoagulant, but not anticardiolipin antibody, in patients with antiphospholipid antibodies. *Arthritis Rheum* 2012;64:2311-2318.
81. Alijotas-Reig J. Treatment of refractory obstetric antiphospholipid syndrome: The state of the art and new trends in the therapeutic management. *Lupus* 2013;22:6-17.
82. Araújo-Fernández S, Ahijón-Lana M, Isenberg DA. Drug-induced lupus: including anti-tumour necrosis factor and interferon induced. *Lupus* 2014;23:545-553.
83. Chang C, Gershwin ME. Drug-induced lupus erythematosus: Incidence, management and prevention. *Drug Saf* 2011;34:357-374.
84. Pasoto SG, Ribeiro AC, Bonfa E. Update on infections and vaccinations in systemic lupus erythematosus and Sjögren's syndrome. *Curr Opin Rheumatol* 2014;26:528-537.
85. Pellegrino P, Clementi E, Radice S. On vaccine's adjuvants and autoimmunity: Current evidence and future perspectives. *Autoimmun Rev* 2015;14:880-888.
86. Rubin LG, Levin MJ, Ljungman P, et al. 2013 IDSA clinical practice guideline for vaccination of the immunocompromised host. *Clin Infect Dis* 2014;58:e44-e100.
87. Kim DK, Bridges CB, Harriman KH. Advisory Committee on Immunization Practices recommended immunization schedule for adults aged 19 years or older: United States, 2015. *Ann Intern Med* 2015;162:214-223.
88. Bichile T, Petri M. Prevention and management of co-morbidities in SLE. *Presse Med* 2014;43:e187-195.
89. Croyle L, Morand EF. Optimizing the use of existing therapies in lupus. *Int J Rheum Dis* 2015;18:129-137.
90. Strand V, Chu AD. Measuring outcomes in systemic lupus erythematosus clinical trials. *Expert Rev Pharmacoecon Outcomes Res* 2011;11:455-468.
91. Mosca M, Tani C, Aringer M, et al. European League Against Rheumatism recommendations for monitoring patients with systemic lupus erythematosus in clinical practice and in observational studies. *Ann Rheum Dis* 2010;69:1269-1274.
92. Thanou A, Merrill JT. Top 10 things to know about lupus activity measures. *Curr Rheumatol Rep* 2013;15:334.

e88

Drug Allergy

Lynne M. Sylvia

KEY CONCEPTS

1. Drug allergy is responsible for 6% to 10% of adverse reactions to medications. Most of these immune events are mediated by IgE or activated T cells.
2. Two theories—the prohapten/hapten concept and the p-i concept—have been proposed to explain how drugs stimulate the immune response.
3. Anaphylaxis is an acute, life-threatening allergic reaction involving multiple organ systems that generally begins within 1 hour but almost always within 2 hours after exposure to the inciting allergen. Anaphylaxis requires prompt treatment to restore respiratory and cardiovascular functions. Epinephrine is the drug of first choice and should be administered to counteract bronchoconstriction and peripheral vasodilation. IV fluids should be administered aggressively to restore intravascular volume.
4. Factors that influence the likelihood of drug allergy are the chemical composition of the drug, whether the drug contains proteins of nonhuman origin, the route of drug administration, and the sensitivity of the individual as determined by genetics or environmental factors. For some drugs, genetic predisposition to specific human leukocyte antigen alleles has been identified as a risk factor for allergic-mediated skin reactions.
5. Ideally, cephalosporins should be avoided in patients with history of an immediate penicillin allergy but, most studies suggest there is little risk of an allergic response to a cephalosporin even in a person with a positive penicillin skin test result. Similarities in the R1 side chain of the agents should be considered when assessing the risk of cross-reactivity.
6. Fewer than 1% of patients receiving nonionic radiocontrast agents experience some type of adverse reaction. Of the variety of reactions reported, about 90% are nonimmediate and mostly urticarial, with severe immediate reactions occurring as infrequently as 0.02%.
7. Aspirin and other nonsteroidal anti-inflammatory drugs (NSAIDs) can produce two general types of reactions, urticaria/angioedema and rhinosinusitis/asthma, in susceptible patients. Most patients with aspirin sensitivity requiring aspirin for prevention of cardiovascular disease can safely undergo and complete a graded challenge or desensitization.
8. Cross-reactivity between sulfonamide antibiotics and nonantibiotics is low. The low cross-reactive rate may be explained by differences in the chemical structures and reactive metabolites of the sulfonamide antibiotics and nonantibiotics.
9. The basic principles of management of allergic reactions to drugs or biologic agents include (a) discontinuation of the medication or agent when possible; (b) treatment of the adverse clinical signs and symptoms; and (c) substitution, if necessary, of another agent.
10. The gold standard for evaluating the risk of an immediate allergy to penicillin is the skin test. Skin testing can demonstrate the presence of penicillin-specific immunoglobulin E and predict a relatively high risk of immediate reactions. Skin testing does not predict the risk of delayed reactions or most dermatologic reactions.
11. When an allergenic drug is considered medically necessary, no adequate therapeutic alternative exists, and there is no reliable skin testing method, two options are available to the clinician: induction of drug tolerance (previously known as desensitization) and graded challenge.

INTRODUCTION

1 *Drug allergy*, as defined by the World Health Organization, is an immunologically mediated drug hypersensitivity reaction.[1] The hyperresponse of the immune system to the antigenic drug leads to host tissue damage manifesting as an organ-specific or generalized systemic reaction. The International CONsensus (ICON) on Drug Allergy has recently proposed that the term *drug allergy* should be used for drug reactions in which a definite immune mechanism (either antibody- or T cell-mediated) has been proven.[2] *Drug hypersensitivity reaction (DHR)* is the term that should be used for more heterogenous reactions that clinically resemble allergy but may or may not be mediated via an immune response.[2] The expert panel has recommended that the term *pseudoallergy* be abandoned. Examples of drug allergies are anaphylaxis from β-lactam antibiotics, halothane hepatitis, Stevens–Johnson's syndrome (SJS) from carbamazepine, heparin-induced thrombocytopenia, allopurinol hypersensitivity syndrome, and serum sickness from phenytoin. Examples of drug hypersensitivity reactions are isolated urticaria after radiocontrast media, aspirin-induced asthma, opiate-related urticaria, and flushing after vancomycin infusion.

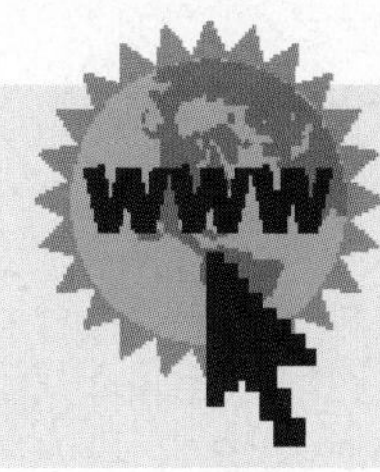

The complete chapter, learning objectives, and other resources can be found at **www.pharmacotherapyonline.com.**

89

Solid-Organ Transplantation

Heather J. Johnson and Kristine S. Schonder

KEY CONCEPTS

1. Generally patients receive a combination of two to four immunosuppressive drugs in order to minimize individual drug toxicities as well as block different aspects of the immune response.
2. While the calcineurin inhibitors (CI) tacrolimus and cyclosporine, inhibitors of interleukin (IL)-2 and thus T-cell activation, are the backbone of immunosuppressive regimens, they are associated with serious adverse effects, primarily, nephrotoxicity, and neurotoxicity.
3. Calcineurin inhibitor-induced nephrotoxicity is one of the most common adverse effects observed in renal and nonrenal transplant recipients. Therapeutic drug monitoring is used in an attempt to optimize the use of calcineurin inhibitors and prevent toxicity.
4. Corticosteroids are a key component of most immunosuppressive strategies because they block the initial steps in allograft rejection. Their significant adverse effects have led to steroid-minimizing and steroid-free imunosuppressive protocols. Corticosteroids, however, remain first-line treatment for allograft rejection.
5. Azathioprine and mycophenolic acid derivatives inhibit T-cell proliferation by altering purine synthesis. Bone marrow suppression is the most significant adverse effect associated with these agents.
6. Sirolimus and everolimus inhibit the mTOR (mammalian target of rapamycin) receptor, which alters T-cell response to IL-2. The adverse effects associated with these agents include leukopenia, thrombocytopenia, anemia, and hyperlipidemia.
7. Antibody preparations that target specific receptors on T cells are classified based on their ability to deplete lymphocyte counts. Most lymphocyte-depleting antibodies are associated with significant infusion-related reactions, where as nondepleting agents are generally better tolerated.
8. Long-term allograft and patient survival is limited by chronic rejection, cardiovascular disease, infection, and long-term immunosuppressive complications such as malignancy.

INTRODUCTION

Solid-organ transplantation provides a lifesaving treatment for patients with end-stage cardiac, kidney, liver, lung, and intestinal disease. Over 300 U.S. hospitals offer transplant services, and pharmacists are often an integral part of the transplant team.[1] In 2009, over 250 pharmacists were members of the American College of Clinical Pharmacy's Transplant Interest Group and more that 65% of responding centers reported a pharmacist on their transplant teams.[2] The Centers for Medicare and Medicaid Services regulations require that transplant programs have a multidisciplinary team including individuals with experience in pharmacology. While the regulations do not specifically state that each center must have a pharmacist, a pharmacist could provide the desired expertise in transplant pharmacotherapy that the regulations mandate.[1]

Since 1980 over 630,000 transplants have been performed, with over half being kidney transplants. A recent analysis estimated that since 1987 over 2.27 million life years have been saved by transplantation, with an average of 4.3 years per patient.[3] In 2014, 29,532 solid-organ transplants were performed and over half of these in were for patients over 50 years of age. Kidneys remain the most commonly transplanted organs; 11,570 from cadaveric donors and 5,536 from living donors in 2014. The next most frequently transplanted organ was the liver, with 6,449 from cadaveric donors and 280 from living donors. Heart and pancreas (or combined kidney–pancreas) transplants account for over 2,600 and 700 transplants, respectively while 1,900 lung transplants were performed during 2014.[1] While the demand for transplantation continues to grow, the number of cadaveric donors has remained relatively stable during the past decade. In 2014, more than 122,000 persons in the United States were waiting for a transplant (over 101,000 people were awaiting a kidney, 15,000 a liver, 4,100 and 1,500 respectively were on the list for a heart or lung). Median waiting time for a cadaveric kidney is more than 4 years. The median waiting time for a liver or heart transplant is about 1 year and approximately 6 months, respectively. For heart, liver, and lung transplantation clinical status is an important factor affecting waiting times, with the sickest patients receiving priority for available organs.[1]

To increase the number of organs available for transplantation, several strategies have been employed in the past several years. Living donors account for one third of all renal transplants, more than any other organ. Living-donor transplantation is also becoming increasingly important for those with end-stage liver and lung disease. Efforts to expand the cadaveric donor pool have included relaxation of age restrictions, development of better preservation solutions, use of "extended-criteria" and nonheart-beating donors, and, in the case of liver transplants, the transplantation of one liver to more than one recipient or implantation of only a segment of a liver. Although very controversial, some have advocated the creation of a regulated system for compensating individuals (paying them) for the "donation" of a kidney.[4]

Clinical **Controversy...**

Given the availability of non-interferon-based highly effective oral therapies for hepatitis c virus infection, some clinicians believe the donor pool could be expanded to include previously excluded donors with evidence of HCV infection.

Despite these efforts, more than 8,000 people who were on transplantation waiting lists died in 2012. Efforts to improve organ allocation have included allocation primarily on "medical necessity"

TABLE 89-1 Organ-Specific Patient and Graft Survival Rates[1]

	Patient Survival (%)		Graft Survival (%)	
Organ	1 year	5 years	1 year	5 years
Kidney				
Living donor	97.9	89.4	95.1	79.8
Deceased donor	94.3	80.4	89.0	66.6
Liver				
Living donor	90.1	77.6	82.5	65.9
Deceased donor	86.2	71.9	82.0	95.1
Heart	88.0	75.0	88.3	73.9
Lung				
Living donor	85.8	35.8	83.7	34.0
Deceased donor	83.3	47.3	82.5	46.0

versus time on the waiting list. Although dialysis can be used for an extended period of time to partially replace the function of the kidneys, such options are not readily available for most liver and heart transplantation candidates. Left ventricular assist devices are now used commonly as a bridge to transplantation for many heart transplantation candidates however, hepatocyte transplantation and artificial liver support remain investigational alternatives or bridges to liver transplantation.[5]

Patient and graft survival rates following transplantation have improved significantly over the past 30 years as a result of advances in pharmacotherapy, surgical techniques, organ preservation, and the postoperative management of patients (Table 89-1). The half-life of transplanted kidneys has continued to improve, but is lower for kidneys from deceased donors compared to living donors, 14.7 versus 26.6 years, respectively. Similarly, the half-life of transplanted livers and hearts from deceased donors has improved to 10 years for livers and 14.9 years for hearts.[1] In this chapter the epidemiology of end-stage kidney, liver, lung, and heart disease is briefly reviewed, the pathophysiology of organ rejection is presented, the pharmacotherapeutic options for individualized immunosuppressive regimens are critiqued, and the unique complications of these regimens along with the therapeutic challenges they present are discussed.

EPIDEMIOLOGY AND ETIOLOGY

The epidemiology and etiology associated with solid organ transplant is specific to the type of organ transplant.

Kidney

Kidney transplantation is the preferred long-term therapeutic option for most patients with end-stage renal disease because it provides the greatest potential improvement in quality of life. Dialysis catheter-related infections, peritoneal dialysis-associated peritonitis, and scheduled dialysis treatments are avoided, and dietary restrictions are fewer. Patients who receive a kidney transplant before the initiation of dialysis have markedly improved quality of life and prolonged life expectancy compared to those who were sustained on dialysis prior to their transplant.[6] The expanded use of living-donor transplantation has made this increasingly possible. Although the analysis of quality of life is complex, patients generally report improved quality of life following transplantation as compared with patients on maintenance dialysis.[7]

Diabetes mellitus, hypertension, and glomerulonephritis are the three leading causes of end-stage renal disease and account for more than 70% of patients (see Chapter 44).[1] Patients with medical conditions such as unstable cardiac disease or recently diagnosed malignancy, for whom the risk of surgery or chronic immunosuppression would be greater than the risks associated with chronic dialysis, are generally excluded from consideration for transplantation.

Liver

Noncholestatic cirrhosis (hepatitis C, alcoholic cirrhosis, hepatitis B, nonalcoholic steatohepatitis, and autoimmune hepatitis) is the primary cause of end-stage liver disease and more than 70% of liver transplant recipients have been diagnosed with one of these conditions.[1] Other indications for transplantation include acute liver failure, primary biliary cirrhosis, primary sclerosing cholangitis, as well as hepatocellular carcinoma. Livers are allocated based on a United Network for Organ Sharing-adapted, Model for End-stage Liver Disease (MELD) score.[8] This score, calculated from the patient's serum creatinine concentration, total serum bilirubin concentration, international normalized ratio, and etiology of cirrhosis, has been demonstrated to be a useful tool to predict impending mortality.

In general, active substance abuse is a contraindication to liver transplantation, but given the high mortality for acute alcoholic hepatitis and the current lack of viable treatments, some non-US centers have explored transplantation in this patient population.[9] Although hepatitis B and C can recur in the transplanted liver, these are not absolute contraindications to liver transplantation.[5,10]

Clinical Controversy...

While liver transplant recipients with alcoholic hepatitis must generally be substance abuse free, some clinicians believe the 6-month waiting period before transplant eligibility should be waived given the high mortality without transplantation.

Heart

Cardiac transplant candidates are typically patients with New York Heart Association class III or IV signs and symptoms despite maximal medical management and have an expected 1-year mortality risk of 50% or greater without a transplant.[11] Idiopathic cardiomyopathy and ischemic heart disease account for heart failure in more than 90% of heart transplantation recipients.[1] Other etiologies include valvular disease, retransplantation for graft atherosclerosis or dysfunction, and congenital heart disease. The role of heart transplantation as a therapeutic option for patients with heart failure is discussed in Chapter 14.

Absolute contraindications to orthotopic cardiac transplantation include the presence of an active infection (except in the case of an infected ventricular assist device, which is an indication for urgent transplantation) or the presence of other diseases (eg, malignancy) that may limit survival and/or rehabilitation and severe, irreversible pulmonary hypertension.

Lung

Lung transplantation is becoming an increasing viable life-saving option for patients with end-stage pulmonary failure not amenable to other treatment. The primary indications for lung transplantation are chronic obstructive lung disease/emphysema, idiopathic pulmonary arterial hypertension, cystic fibrosis, and idiopathic pulmonary fibrosis. The vast majority of lung transplants are cadaveric (greater than 99%) and bilateral lung transplants accounted for 67% of lung transplants in 2012. Lungs are allocated on the basis of the complex lung allocation score (LAS) which is used to prioritize candidates based on medical need and expected posttransplant survival given patient specific characteristics such as antecedent disease, age, body mass index, renal function, diabetes as well as measures of current functional status.[1,12]

PHYSIOLOGIC CONSEQUENCES OF TRANSPLANTATION

Transplantation is truly lifesaving for heart, liver, and lung transplantation recipients, whereas kidney transplantation is associated with improved quality of life and survival when compared with dialysis.[13] Although not all heart transplant recipients return to work, 89.9% of patients consider themselves to have no activity limitations at 1-year follow-up.[14] The specific physiologic consequences of kidney, liver, and heart transplantation are discussed below.

Kidney Transplantation

The glomerular filtration rate of a successfully transplanted kidney may be near normal almost immediately after transplantation. In some patients, however, the concentration of standard biochemical indicators of renal function, such as serum creatinine and blood urea nitrogen, may remain elevated for several days. Standard formulas used to predict drug dosing rely on a stable serum creatinine and may be inaccurate immediately following transplantation (see Chapter e42).

Although the allograft is able to remove uremic toxins from the body, it may take several weeks for other physiologic complications of ESRD, such as anemia, calcium and phosphate imbalance, and altered lipid profiles, to resolve. The renal production of erythropoietin and 1-hydroxylation of vitamin D may return toward normal early in the postoperative period. Because the onset of physiologic effects may be delayed, continuation of the patient's pretransplantation vitamin D, calcium supplementation, and/or phosphate binders may be warranted. Patients should be monitored for hypophosphatemia and hypercalcemia for the first few days to weeks after kidney transplantation.

Primary nonfunction of a renal allograft or delayed graft function (DGF) is characterized by the need for dialysis in the first postop week or the failure of the serum creatinine to fall by 30% of the pretransplantation value. The incidence of DGF in cadaveric kidney transplantation ranges from 8% to 50% and results in a slower return of the kidney's excretory, metabolic, and synthetic functions. DGF is associated with prolonged hospital stays, higher costs, difficult management of immunosuppressive therapy, slower patient rehabilitation, and poor graft survival.[15] Other early causes of renal dysfunction such as urethral obstruction or arterial or venous stenosis or thrombosis should be distinguished from DGF.

The primary cause of DGF is acute tubular necrosis (ATN). The incidence of ATN is higher when kidneys are harvested from donors who recently experienced a cardiac arrest, those who were hypotensive or on vasopressors, or older donors (age greater than 55 years). While cyclosporine and tacrolimus have been implicated in the prolongation of ATN, a clear cause-and-effect relationship has not been established. Nonetheless, most clinicians will decrease calcineurin inhibitor doses in patients with ATN. DGF predisposes patients to acute rejection, possibly as a consequence of decreased calcineurin inhibitor concentrations and a resultant reduction in the level of immunosuppression.[16]

Liver Transplantation

The physiologic consequences of liver transplantation are complex, involving changes in both its metabolic and synthetic function. Postoperatively, the liver transplant recipient will likely have many fluid, electrolyte, and nutritional abnormalities. Biliary tract dysfunction may alter the absorption of fats and fat-soluble drugs.[17] Poor absorption of the lipid-soluble drug cyclosporine improves after successful liver transplantation and reestablishment of bile flow. Vitamin E deficiency and its neurologic complications are usually reversed after successful liver transplantation. In stable adult liver transplant patients, the concentrations of retinol and tocopherol are similar to those seen in normal healthy subjects, indicating recovery of liver production and excretion of bile salts needed for fat-soluble vitamin absorption. Table 89-2 summarizes the effects of liver transplantation on metabolism and renal elimination that are seen in the immediate postoperative period. Most of these changes resolve as liver function normalizes.

TABLE 89-2 Perioperative Changes in Drug Disposition and Elimination Following Liver Transplantation

	Result	Comment
Serum proteins		
↓ Albumin	↑ Free fraction of drugs usually bound to albumin	Diazepam, salicylic acid binding greater in liver transplant than chronic liver disease because of endogenous binding inhibitors (up to 45 days post-transplant)
↑ Alpha-1-acid glycoprotein	Lower unbound fraction of drugs	Lidocaine
Metabolism/elimination		
Microsomal enzymes	↑ CYP2E1 activity	Increased drug metabolism (induction)
	↔ CYP2D6	Unaffected
	↓ CYP activity	Decreased drug elimination (inhibition)
Oxidation	Stable	
Conjugation	Normalizes after transplant	
Biliary function	↓ Absorption of lipophilic compounds	
	↑ Cyclosporine metabolites in blood	
Renal elimination	Elimination of gentamicin, vancomycin, cephalosporins less than predicted by serum creatinine	Renal elimination of metabolites limited

Data from reference 12.

Failure of the newly transplanted liver to function occurs in 10% to 15% of recipients. Early graft failure can result from preexisting disease in the donor, and even coagulation defects have been acquired through donor organs. The technical complexity of the operation can produce flaws in revascularization that also lead to graft nonfunction. Surgical complications include portal vein or hepatic artery thrombosis and bile duct leaks. Ischemic injury can also result in early graft dysfunction. While hyperacute rejection in liver transplantation rarely occurs, graft failure in the first 2 postoperative weeks may indicate antibody-mediated graft destruction.

Heart Transplantation

The orthotopically transplanted heart is denervated and no longer responds to physiologic stimuli and pharmacologic agents in a normal manner (Table 89-3).[13] In situations requiring an increased heart rate such as exercise or hypotension, the denervated heart is unable to increase heart rate but instead relies on increasing the stroke volume. Later in the course of exercise or hypotension, heart rate increases in response to circulating catecholamines. While the maximum exercise capacity of heart transplant recipients is below normal, most patients are able to resume normal lifestyles and participate in reasonably vigorous activities.[14] Partial reinnervation may occur over time, thereby facilitating more normal physiologic and pharmacologic responses and better exercise capacity.[14]

TABLE 89-3 Altered Responses to Cardiac Drugs in the Denervated Transplanted Heart

Drug	Effect	Mechanism	Comment
Digitalis	Normal inotropic effect; minimal effect on AV node	Direct myocardial effect; denervation	
Atropine	No effect on AV node	Denervation	
Adrenaline/noradrenaline	Increased contractility; increased chronotropy	Denervation; hypersensitivity	Increased cardiac output mediated by increased heart rate
Isoproterenol	Normal increase in contractility; normal increase in chronotropy	No neuronal uptake	
Quinidine	No vagolytic effect	Denervation	
Verapamil	AV block	Direct effect	
Nifedipine	No reflex tachycardia	Denervation	
Hydralazine	No reflex tachycardia	Denervation	
β-Blocker	Increased antagonist effect	Denervation	Impaired heart rate response, use sparingly
Adenosine	Negative chronotropic effect	Hypersensitivity; effect on sinus node of denervated heart	Life-threatening asystole (>0.5 minute) may occur if used to treat supraventricular arrhythmia or stress testing
Acetylcholine	Negative chronotropic effect	Hypersensitivity; effect on sinus node of denervated heart	

AV, atrioventricular.

Reproduced from Deng MC. Heart failure: Cardiac transplantation. Heart 2002;87:177–184 with permission from the BMJ Publishing Group Ltd.

A number of autoregulatory and physiologic responses present in the normal heart are interrupted or blunted for the first 6 weeks after transplantation. The donor sinus node function may be impaired as the result of the preservation regimen, direct surgical trauma at excision, the presence of long-acting antiarrhythmics (eg, amiodarone) taken prior to transplant by the recipient, and a lack of "conditioning" responsiveness to catecholamines.[14] Consequently, the transplanted heart generally requires chronotropic support with either milrinone or pacing in the perioperative period to maintain a heart rate greater than 90 beats minute and satisfactory hemodynamics (ie, blood pressure, urine output, and tissue perfusion).[18] Approximately 10% to 20% of transplant patients will have persistent chronotropic incompetence requiring either short courses of medications, such as terbutaline or theophylline, or permanent cardiac pacing.

Right ventricular function is frequently impaired, presumably as a result of preservation regimen injury and elevated pulmonary vascular resistance. A "restrictive" hemodynamic pattern may be present initially but usually improves in 6 weeks following transplantation. Donor–recipient size mismatch may contribute to early posttransplantation hemodynamic abnormalities characterized by higher right and left ventricular end-diastolic pressures. Supraventricular arrhythmias are usually transient and may result from over vigorous use of catecholamines or milrinone.

Myocardial depression frequently occurs and generally requires inotropic support with agents such as dobutamine, milrinone, and epinephrine. On occasion, intra- or postoperative administration of vasodilators, including nitric oxide, and inotropic agents may be necessary to treat right-sided failure in the transplant patient; milrinone and isoproterenol are preferred in this setting.[18]

Persistent abnormalities of diastolic function are often noted in the transplanted heart such that intracardiac pressures increase in an exaggerated fashion in response to exercise and/or volume infusion.[14] These abnormalities are due in part to denervation, but also to acute rejection or to the scarring secondary to previously treated rejection episodes, hypertension, or cardiac allograft vasculopathy.

Hypertension may occur following surgery secondary to the effect of elevated catecholamine levels and systemic vascular resistance as the residual effects of end-stage heart failure on the healthy heart. Systolic blood pressure should be maintained at 110 to 120 mm Hg to enhance cardiac function. In the acute post-transplantation period, intravenous nitroprusside or nitroglycerin may be needed, whereas oral angiotensin-converting enzyme inhibitors (ACEIs) and/or amlodipine are commonly used once the patient can ingest oral medications.

Lung Transplantation

Lung transplant recipients experience more complications than other solid organ transplant recipients as evidenced by a higher rate of posttransplant re-hospitalization. Primary graft dysfunction with a mortality of 30% to 40% occurs within 72 hours of transplant in up to 20% of recipients. It presents as noncardiogenic pulmonary edema and is thought to be a manifestation of ischemia-reperfusion injury and may be associated with prolonged cold ischemia (greater than 6 hours) as well as a number of other factors including female gender. Airway complications include ischemia and associated anastomotic dehiscence, bronchial stenosis and bronchiolitis obliterans. Dehiscence may result in mediastinitis, pneumothorax or hemorrhage. Bronchial stenosis which may occur in up to 24% of patients results in a narrowing the bronchus that is usually managed by bronchoscopy and balloon dilation. Respiratory infections are especially problematic in lung transplant recipients as their newly transplanted organ is in direct contact with the outside environment. Additionally, the absence of a cough reflex as well as a reduction in mucociliary clearance as the result of denervation and lymphatic interruption also contribute to the risk of pulmonary infections. Patients with cystic fibrosis are susceptible to the pathogens with which they were colonized before transplant.[1,12,19]

PATHOPHYSIOLOGY OF REJECTION

Rejection of a transplanted organ can take place at any time following surgery and is classified clinically as hyperacute, acute cellular, and/or humoral or chronic rejection.

General Concepts

Rejection is primarily mediated by activation of alloreactive T cells and antigen-presenting cells such as B lymphocytes, macrophages, and dendritic cells. Acute allograft rejection is caused primarily by the infiltration of T cells into the allograft, which triggers inflammatory

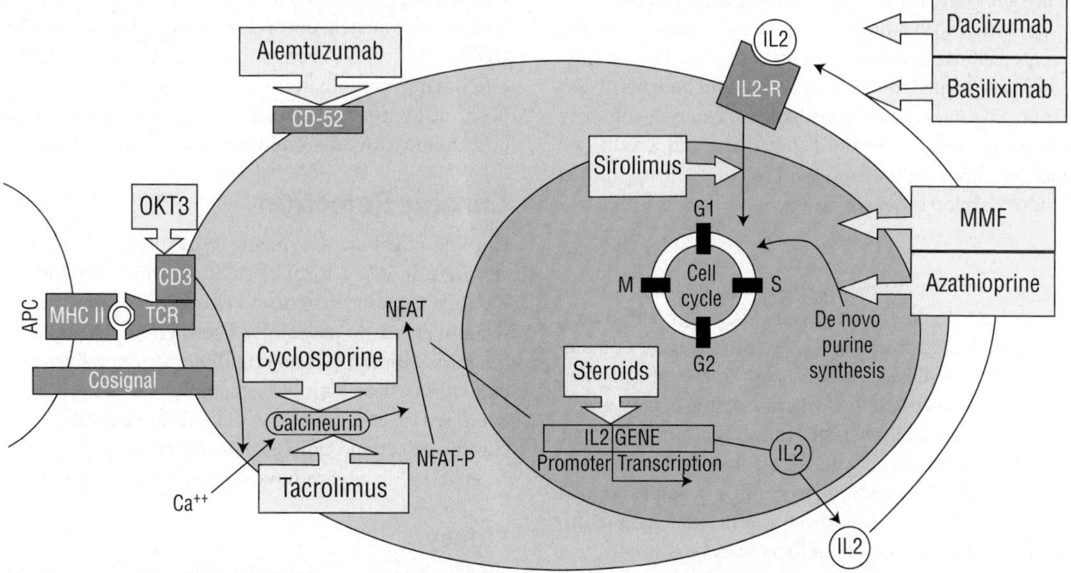

FIGURE 89-1 Stages of CD4 T-cell activation and cytokine production with identification of the sites of action of different immunosuppressive agents. Antigen major histocompatibility complex (MHC) II molecule complexes are responsible for initiating the activation of CD4 T cells. These MHC-peptide complexes are recognized by the T-cell recognition complex (TCR). A costimulatory signal initiates signal transduction with activation of second messengers, one of which is calcineurin. Calcineurin removes phosphates from the nuclear factors (NFAT-P) allowing them to enter the nucleus. These nuclear factors specifically bind to an interleukin (IL)-2 promoter gene facilitating IL-2 gene transcription. Interaction of IL-2 with the IL-2 receptor (IL-2R) on the cell membrane surface induces cell proliferation and production of cytokines specific to the T cell. (APC, antigen-presenting cells; MMF, mycophenolate mofetil.) *(Reprinted from Ann Thorac Surg, Vol. 77, Mueller XM, Drug immunosuppressive therapy for adult heart transplantation. Part I. Immune response to allograft and mechanism of action of immunosuppressants, pages 354–362, Copyright © 2004, with permission from Elsevier.)*

and cytotoxic effects on the graft. Complex interactions between the allograft and cellular cytokines, cell-to-cell interactions, CD4+ and CD8+ T cells, and B cells ultimately lead to chronic rejection and graft loss if adequate immunosuppression is not maintained.[20]

The sequence of events that underlies graft rejection is recognition, via MHC class I and II antigens, of the donor's histocompatibility differences by the recipient's immune system, recruitment of activated lymphocytes, initiation of immune effector mechanisms, and finally graft destruction. The specifics of this immune cascade of organ rejection are discussed in Chapter e86. The complex nature of cytokine interactions makes it very difficult to design drugs with exclusive actions (Fig. 89-1).

Efforts to allocate well-matched kidneys, according to human leukocyte antigens (HLA)-A, -B, and -DR, are foundational to minimize rejection and enhance survival. However, the benefit of having no recipient donor mismatches may be negated by excessive cold ischemia time (greater than 36 hours) and donor age older than 60 years. HLA tissue matching is not performed routinely before transplantation for livers and hearts because organ availability is more limited and the optimal cold ischemia time is shorter.[21] However, if the potential recipient's blood is reactive against a panel of random donor blood samples (ie, panel reactive antibody [PRA] greater than 10% to 20%), a negative T-cell crossmatch is required prior to transplantation. Transplanted organs must be matched for ABO blood group compatibility with the recipient. Liver transplantation may be carried out in emergency situations across ABO blood groups, but survival is lower.

Hyperacute Rejection

Hyperacute rejection may be evident within minutes of the transplantation procedure when preformed donor-specific antibodies are present in the recipient at the time of the transplant. It can also be induced by immunoglobulin G antibodies that bind to antigens on the vascular endothelium, such as class I MHC, ABO, and vascular endothelial cell antigens. Tissue damage can be mediated through antibody-dependent, cell-mediated cytotoxicity or through activation of the complement cascade. If present the ischemic damage to the microvasculature rapidly results in tissue necrosis.

Hyperacute rejection has become uncommon in kidney and heart transplants. A positive crossmatch presents a serious risk for graft failure even if hyperacute rejection does not occur. A negative lymphocytotoxicity crossmatch does not entirely rule out the possibility of hyperacute rejection because non-MHC antigens on the vascular endothelium can serve as targets of donor-specific antibodies. Early graft dysfunction is treated with supportive care and retransplantation if possible. The reason for the rarity of hyperacute rejection in liver transplantation is not fully understood, but the local release of cytokines may alter the immunologic reaction in the liver.[22]

Acute Cellular Rejection

Acute rejection is most common in the first few months following transplantation but can occur at any time during the life of the allograft. It is mediated by alloreactive T-lymphocytes that appear in the circulation and infiltrate the allograft through the vascular endothelium. After the graft is infiltrated by lymphocytes, the cytotoxic cells specifically target and kill the functioning cells in the allograft. At the same time, local release of lymphokines attracts and stimulates macrophages to produce tissue damage through a delayed hypersensitivity-like mechanism. These immunologic and inflammatory events lead to nonspecific signs and symptoms including pain and tenderness over the graft site, fever, and lethargy.

Kidney

Acute rejection, which may affect up to 20% of patients during the first 6 months following transplantation, is evidenced by an abrupt rise in serum creatinine concentration of greater than or equal to 30% over baseline. A specific histologic diagnosis can be obtained via biopsy of the allograft and is often used to guide rejection therapy. A biopsy specimen with a diffuse lymphocytic infiltrate is consistent with acute cellular rejection (ACR). After the diagnosis of rejection has been confirmed, the potential risks and benefits of specific antirejection therapies must be evaluated. Hypertension often worsens during an episode of rejection, and edema and weight gain are common as a result of sodium and fluid retention. Symptomatic azotemia may also develop in severe cases.

Liver

Approximately 18% of liver transplantation recipients will experience a rejection episode in the first post-transplant year. The clinical signs of ACR include leukocytosis and a change in the color or quantity of bile for those who still have an external drainage tube in place. A serum bilirubin 50% over baseline or increases in hepatic transaminases to values more than three times the upper limit of normal, are sensitive markers of rejection. Although a liver biopsy provides definitive evidence of the diagnosis of rejection, a prompt response to antirejection medication has also proven useful as a means to differentiate rejection from other causes of hepatic dysfunction.

Heart

Approximately 16% of heart transplantation recipients will experience at least one episode of acute rejection during the first year.[23] Because rejection of the cardiac allograft is not necessarily accompanied by overt clinical signs or symptoms and because the incidence of acute rejection is highest during the first year post-transplant, endomyocardial biopsies are often performed at regularly scheduled intervals following transplantation.[18] A typical biopsy schedule would be weekly for the first postoperative month, biweekly for the next 2 months, and monthly to bimonthly through the remainder of the first post-transplant year. Nonspecific symptoms, including low-grade fever, malaise, mild reduction in exercise capacity, heart failure, or atrial arrhythmias may also be evident and if present are reflective of a more severe rejection episode.

Lung

Up to 36% of lung transplant recipients will experience acute rejection in the first year.[19] Patients with acute rejection often present with nonspecific symptoms including fatigue, fever, cough, dyspnea, hypoxemia, mucus as well as a diminished FEV1 Because spirometry and radiography cannot delineate the cause of these nonspecific symptoms, bronchoscopy and transbronchial biopsy are the standard for establishing a diagnosis of rejection. Eosinophilia, lymphocyte proliferation, and infiltration are hallmark signs of rejections. Routine assessment after transplantation includes pulmonary functions tests as well as clinical and radiologic evaluations.[12,19]

Antibody-Mediated Rejection

Antibody-mediated rejection (AMR), sometimes referred to as vascular or humoral rejection, is characterized by the presence of antibodies directed against HLA antigens present on the donor vascular endothelium. The antibodies activate complement, which creates a membrane attack complex that directly damages the organ and further attracts inflammatory cells to the allograft. The resultant damage is histologically distinct from cellular rejection and involves microvascular injury, often to the peritubular capillaries.[24] Definitive diagnosis of AMR is based on the presence of three criteria: presence of donor-specific antibodies, immunofluorescence staining of C4d deposits in the peritubular capillaries, and evidence of allograft dysfunction.[25] Circulating immune complexes often precede humoral rejection. This form of rejection is less common than cellular rejection and generally occurs in the first 3 months after transplantation. It is associated with an increased fatality rate and appears to be more common when antilymphocyte antibodies are used for rejection prophylaxis. An increased risk of humoral rejection is associated with female gender, elevated PRA, cytomegalovirus seropositivity, a positive crossmatch, and prior sensitization to OKT3 (muromonab CD3).[26] Strategies to reverse humoral rejection include plasmapheresis, often in combination with intravenous immunoglobulin, high-dose intravenous corticosteroids, antithymocyte globulin (ATG), bortezomib, rituximab, and mycophenolate mofetil.

Chronic Rejection

Chronic rejection is a major cause of graft loss. It presents as a slow and indolent form of ACR, in which the involvement of the humoral immune system and antibodies against the vascular endothelium appear to play a role. Persistent perivascular and interstitial inflammation is a common finding in kidney, liver, and heart transplantation. As a result of the complex interaction of multiple drugs and diseases over time, it is difficult to delineate the true nature of chronic rejection. Unlike acute rejection, chronic rejection is not reversible with any immunosuppressive agents currently available.

Kidney

While advances in immunosuppression have reduced the rates of acute rejection in the first year post-transplant from over 50% to about 10%, chronic allograft nephropathy remains the most common cause of graft loss in the late post-transplantation period (greater than 1 year).[25] The syndrome is characterized in histological terms as interstitial fibrosis and tubular atrophy (IFTA) of unknown etiology. As many as two-thirds of allografts will be affected 5 years after transplantation.[27] Hypertension, proteinuria, and a progressive decline in kidney function represent the classic clinical triad of chronic allograft nephropathy. Factors that contribute to the development of chronic allograft nephropathy include calcineurin inhibitor nephrotoxicity, polyomavirus infection, hypertension, donor-related factors including ischemia time and undetected kidney disease in the donor kidney, and recurrence of the primary kidney disease in the recipient.

Liver

Approximately 3% to 5% of transplant livers are affected by chronic rejection, which is characterized by an obliterative arteriopathy and the gradual loss of bile ducts, often referred to as the vanishing bile duct syndrome. Initially patients experience an asymptomatic rise in the alkaline phosphatase and γ-glutamyl transpeptidase. As levels of bilirubin increase, patients become jaundiced and may experience itching.

Heart

Cardiac allograft vasculopathy, characterized by accelerated intimal thickening or development of atherosclerotic plaques, is the leading cause of graft failure and death in heart transplant recipients.[28] Endothelial injury, caused by both cell-mediated and humoral responses, is the first step in the process. Vasculopathy is restricted to the transplanted allograft. Routine surveillance with coronary angiography, intravascular ultrasound, or other procedures can aid in the diagnosis of vasculopathy. Evidence of cardiac allograft vasculopathy can be seen in as many as 14% of patients within 1 year of transplantation and up to 50% of patients within 5 years.[28] While chronic rejection of the kidney or liver allograft is generally not amenable to treatment, 3-hydroxy-3-methylglutaryl-coenzyme A (HMGCoA) reductase inhibitors and ACEIs have been used to decrease the incidence of vasculopathy in the heart allograft recepient.[28] Recently, sirolimus and everolimus have been shown to reduce the incidence and slow progression of cardiac allograft vasculopathy.[28] Percutaneous transluminal coronary angioplasty and coronary artery bypass grafting have been used in severe cases of vasculopathy; these procedures, however, are of limited value because of their association with increased mortality compared with the general population.[28]

Lung

Chronic rejection in the lung is known as bronchiolitis obliterans syndrome, a fibroproliferative disease which impacts the small airways. It is characterized by a reduction of FEV1 greater than 20% and occurs in up to 50% of patients in the first 5 years post-transplant. The long term prognosis is poor and survival is limited. Treatments are lacking, but chronic use of the azithromycin has shown some promise.[12,19]

TREATMENT OF REJECTION

Immunosuppression achieved with a variety of agents is the cornerstone to rejection management and the accepted regimens for most solid organs are usually comprised of two or more agents.

Desired Outcomes

Immediately following surgery, the primary goal of therapy is to prevent hyperacute and acute rejection. The high doses of immunosuppressants required to achieve this goal, if maintained long term, may result in serious complications such as nephrotoxicity, infection, thrombocytopenia, and drug-induced diabetes. Therefore rapid dosage reductions are frequently used to minimize these effects. Transplant immunosuppression must be balanced to optimize both graft and patient survival.

General Approach to Treatment

1 A multidrug approach is rational from an immunomechanistic viewpoint because the many agents have overlapping and potentially synergistic mechanisms of action. Furthermore, the use of a multidrug immunosuppression regimen may allow the use of lower doses of individual agents, thus reducing the severity of dose-related adverse effects (Fig. 89-2). The protocols and individual drug regimens tend to be medical center specific.[18,22,29] Although induction therapy may not be uniformly used, in almost every setting, patients receive IV methylprednisolone intraoperatively. Patients may also receive a descending dose of methylprednisolone over the first 5 to 7 postoperative days before beginning oral prednisone. Protocols generally combine a drug from two or three of the following classes: calcineurin inhibitors, antimetabolites or proliferation signal inhibitors, and corticosteroids.

If rejection is suspected, a biopsy can be done to ascertain the definitive diagnosis or the patient may be empirically treated for rejection. Empiric treatment generally involves administration of high-dose corticosteroids, usually 500 to 1,000 mg of methylprednisolone intravenously for one to three doses.[12,18,22,29] If signs and symptoms of rejection are resolved with empiric therapy, the maintenance immunosuppressive regimen is generally modified to provide a greater level of overall immunosuppression. If rejection is confirmed by biopsy, treatment may be based on the severity of rejection with polyclonal and monoclonal antibodies being reserved for moderate to severe rejections for those patients that have not responded to a course of corticosteroids.

Induction Therapy

Induction therapy provides a high level of immunosuppression, at the time of transplantation, with or without the immediate introduction of cyclosporine or tacrolimus (see Fig. 89-2). Two perioperative immunosuppressive strategies have been predominantly utilized to achieve this goal: (a) the provision of a highly intense immunosuppression, often on the basis of patient-specific risk factors such as age and race, or (b) the use of antibody therapy to provide enough immunosuppression to delay the initiation of therapy with the potentially nephrotoxic calcineurin inhibitors. The rationale for delayed calcineurin inhibitor administration varies slightly depending on the type of transplant. In renal transplantation, the newly transplanted kidney is very susceptible to nephrotoxic injury, whereas in liver and heart transplantation, the idea is to protect patients with preexisting renal insufficiency from further insults during the perioperative period. Additionally, calcineurin inhibitor dosage adjustment to maintain target concentrations may be difficult in the perioperative period secondary to fluctuations in gastrointestinal (GI) absorption and enteral intake.[22,29,30]

Acute Rejection

The primary goal of acute rejection therapy is to minimize the intensity of the immune response and prevent irreversible injury to the allograft. The available options include (a) increasing the doses of current immunosuppressive drugs, (b) starting "pulse" corticosteroids with subsequent dosage taper, (c) addition of another immunosuppressant indefinitely, or (d) short-term treatment with a polyclonal or monoclonal antibody. The treatment of acute rejection almost always begins with "pulse" corticosteroid therapy for several days (oral or intravenously). However, African American kidney transplant recipients may not respond as well to corticosteroids; thus ATG may be preferable for this patient population.[31]

Cytolytic agents are often reserved for those with corticosteroid-resistant rejection, signs of hemodynamic compromise (heart), or more severe rejections. Other innovative forms of therapy for persistent or intractable rejection have been investigated, including mycophenolate mofetil, tacrolimus, low-dose methotrexate, sirolimus, total lymphoid irradiation, and plasmapheresis and intravenous immunoglobulin. Prophylactic agents such as valganciclovir, nystatin, trimethoprim-sulfamethoxazole, H_2-receptor antagonists or proton-pump inhibitors, and/or antacids may be added to minimize adverse effects associated with these intensive immunosuppression regimens.[32]

Maintenance Therapy

The goal of maintenance immunosuppression is to prevent acute and chronic rejection while minimizing drug-related toxicity. As patients progress through the post-transplant course, the risk of acute rejection decreases, thus allowing the clinician to gradually reduce the doses of immunosuppressants or in some cases totally withdraw them over a period of 6 to 12 months. Transplant organ and type (cadaveric vs living-donor), the degree of HLA mismatch, time after transplantation, post-transplantation complications (including the number of acute rejections), previous immunosuppressive adverse reactions, compliance, and financial considerations are among the patient-specific factors considered in individualizing maintenance immunosuppression. Calcineurin inhibitors are generally a central component in most maintenance regimens, although calcineurin inhibitor-free immunosuppression remains a future goal because of the significant nephrotoxicity associated with these agents. Ideally, immunosuppression should be optimized to prevent acute rejection episodes, minimize the occurrence of chronic rejection, and prevent long-term toxicities.

Calcineurin Inhibitors

2 Cyclosporine and tacrolimus are the two calcineurin inhibitors (CIs) currently used for most solid-organ transplant recipients. More than 80% of transplant recipients receive tacrolimus as part of their immunosuppressive regimen.[1]

Pharmacology/Mechanism of Action Calcineurin inhibitors block T-cell proliferation by inhibiting the production of IL-2 and other cytokines by T cells (see Fig. 89-1). Cyclosporine and tacrolimus bind to unique cytoplasmic immunophilins: cyclophilin and FK-binding protein-12 (FKBP12), respectively. The drug–immunophilin complex inhibits the action of calcineurin, an enzyme that activates the nuclear factor of activated T cells, which is, in turn, responsible for the transcription of several key cytokines necessary

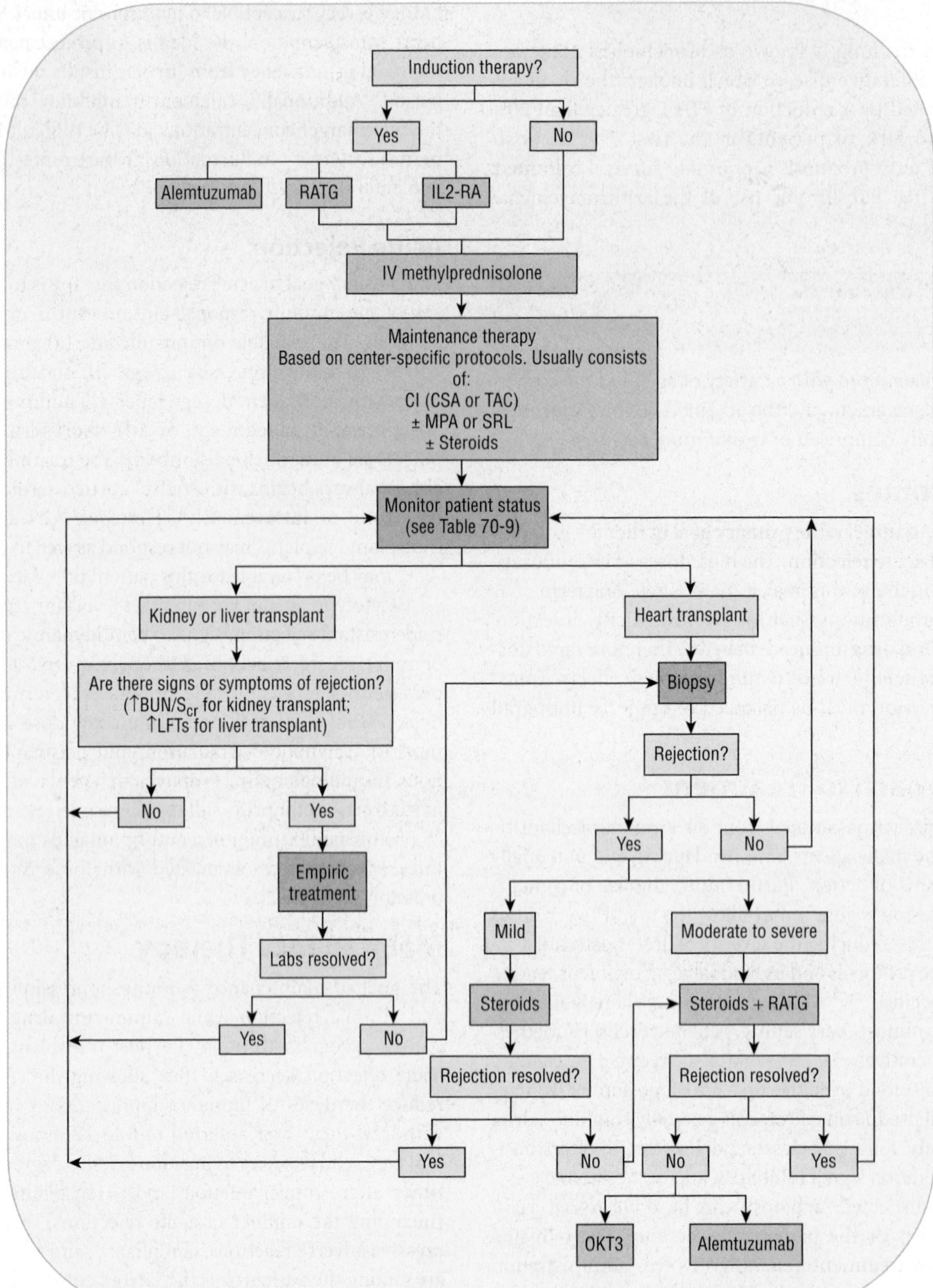

FIGURE 89-2 General approach to solid-organ transplant immunosuppression. (BUN, blood urea nitrogen; CI, calcineurin inhibitor; CSA, cyclosporine; IL2RA, interleukin-2 receptor antagonist; LFTs, liver function tests; MPA, mycophenolic acid; OKT3, muromonab CD3; RATG, rabbit antithymocyte immunoglobulin; S_{cr}, serum creatinine; SRL, sirolimus; TAC, tacrolimus.)

for T-cell activity, including IL-2. IL-2 is a potent T-cell growth factor and ultimately is responsible for activation and clonal expansion.

Pharmacokinetics The calcineurin inhibitors are highly lipophilic compounds, with variable but generally low bioavailability of approximately 30% (range: 5%-60%). Unlike tacrolimus, cyclosporine depends on bile for intestinal absorption, which lends to more interpatient and intrapatient variability. Liver recipients with a T-tube for diversion of bile may thus experience incomplete and erratic absorption of cyclosporine.[30]

Because of the significant variability in absorption of cyclosporine, and its associated pharmacokinetic problems, a microemulsion formulation was developed. Both forms are available commercially in the United States and are referred to as "cyclosporine, USP" and "cyclosporine, USP [MODIFIED]." The two formulations are not bioequivalent and should not be used interchangeably. The microemulsion formulation is self-emulsifying and forms a microemulsion spontaneously with aqueous fluids in the gastrointestinal tract, making it less dependent on bile for absorption. The result is a significantly greater rate and extent of absorption and decreased intraindividual variability in pharmacokinetic parameters. The relative bioavailability of the microemulsion formulation is 60% and peak concentrations are generally reached within 1.5 to 2 hours after oral administration. Tacrolimus, on the other hand, has a more predictable absorption pattern, reaching peak concentrations within 1 to 3 hours but still with a variable bioavailability ranging from 4% to 93% (average 20%).[30]

Following oral absorption, both cyclosporine and tacrolimus are highly protein bound. Ninety percent of cyclosporine is bound to lipoproteins in the blood while 99% of tacrolimus is bound primarily to albumin and α_1-acid glycoprotein. Cyclosporine is distributed widely into tissue and body fluids, resulting in a large and variable volume of distribution, ranging from 3 to 5 L/kg. Because of the high concentration of FKBP12 that is found in red blood cells, tacrolimus is distributed primarily in the vasculature, with a volume of distribution of 0.8 to 1.9 L/kg. Both drugs are extensively metabolized by the cytochrome P450 3A4 (CYP3A4) in both the gut and the liver, which accounts for both the poor bioavailability and numerous drug interactions which are highlighted in this is the first mention of this table so it should be highlighted in blue. Also it should be changed to be Table 89-4.[30,33-35]

Efficacy Both cyclosporine and tacrolimus are currently approved for prophylaxis of organ rejection in kidney, liver, and heart transplantation. The microemulsion formulation of cyclosporine has demonstrated equivalent or superior efficacy in kidney, liver, and heart transplantation recipients. Studies comparing tacrolimus with either formulation of cyclosporine as primary immunosuppression demonstrate equivalent efficacy between the two agents in all transplantation situations.

Adverse Effects Table 89-5 summarizes the adverse effects of calcineurin inhibitors, cyclosporine and tacrolimus, and other immunosuppressants. The nephrotoxic potential of both drugs is equal and is often related to the dose and duration of exposure. Neurotoxicity typically manifests as tremors, headache, and peripheral neuropathy; occasionally, however, seizures have been observed. Tacrolimus may be associated with an increased occurrence of neurologic complications compared with cyclosporine.

Cyclosporine appears to have a greater propensity to cause or worsen hypertension and hyperlipidemia compared with tacrolimus.[36,37] On the other hand, hyperglycemia is more common with tacrolimus than with cyclosporine but is often reversible when doses of tacrolimus and/or corticosteroids are reduced.[37] Cyclosporine is associated with cosmetic effects, such as hirsutism and

TABLE 89-4 The Impact of Medications on Immunosuppressive Concentrations

Medications	TAC	CSA	MPA	PSI
Anti-Infectives				
Clotrimazole	↑	↑		↑
Fluconazole	↑	↑		↑
Ketoconazole	↑	↑		↑
Voriconazole	↑	↑		↑
Itraconazole	↑	↑		↑
Posaconazole	↑	↑		↑
Erythromycin	↑	↑		↑
Clarithromycin	↑	↑		↑
Azithromycin	↑	↑		↑
Levofloxacin	↑	↑		
Ofloxacin	↑	↑		
Norfloxacin			↓	
Metronidazole			↓	
Selective gut decontamination			↓	
Nafcillin	↓	↓	↓	↓
Rifampin	↓	↓	↓	↓
Lopinavir/Ritonavir	↑	↑		
Nelfinavir				
Saquinavir				
Efavirenz	↓	↓		
Simeprevir		↑		
Ombitasvir/paritaprevir/ritonavir +dasabuvir	↑	↑		
Cardiovascular				
Verapamil	↑	↑		↑
Diltiazem	↑	↑		↑
CNS				
Nefazodone	↑	↑		
Carbamazepine	↓	↓		↓
Phenytoin	↓	↓		↓
Phenobarbital	↓	↓		↓
Immunosuppressants				
Cyclosporine			↓	↑
Tacrolimus				
Sirolimus		↑		
Everolimus		↑		
Mycophenolic acid		↓		

Data from references 26-28.

TABLE 89-5 Comparison of Common Adverse Effects of Maintenance Immunosuppressants

System/Adverse Effect	AZA	MPA	CI	Steroids	PSI	Bela
Neurologic						
Headache			X			
Tremors			X			
Seizures			X			
Mood changes				X		
Cardiovascular						
Hypertension			X	X		
Hyperlipidemia			X	X	X	
Peripheral edema						X
Gastrointestinal						
Nausea	X	X	TAC	X		
Diarrhea		X	TAC			X
Vomiting	X					
Bleeding				X		
Hepatotoxicity	X		TAC			
Renal						
Nephrotoxicity			X		X	
Hyperkalemia			X			
Hypomagnesemia			X			
Urinary tract infection						X
Hematologic						
Anemia						X
Leukocytosis						
Leukopenia	X	X			X	
Neutropenia						X
Thrombocytopenia	X	X			X	
Cosmetic						
Acne				X		
Alopecia			TAC			
Gingival hyperplasia			CSA			
Hirsutism			CSA			
Weight gain				X		
Endocrine						
Hyperglycemia			X	X		
Osteoporosis				X		

AZA, azathioprine; Bela, belatacept; CI, calcineurin inhibitor; CSA, cyclosporine; MPA, mycophenolic acid; PSI, proliferation signal inhibitor; TAC, tacrolimus.

gingival hyperplasia, which may be managed by converting from cyclosporine to tacrolimus or by improving hygiene in patients who cannot be switched to tacrolimus. Tacrolimus, in contrast, has been reported to cause alopecia, which is usually self-limiting and reversible.

Calcineurin Inhibitor Nephrotoxicity 3 Two types of nephrotoxicity can occur with calcineurin inhibitors. Acute nephrotoxicity is frequently seen early and is dose dependent and reversible, but chronic nephropathy is more common. Clinical manifestations of calcineurin inhibitor nephrotoxicity include elevated serum creatinine and blood urea nitrogen concentrations, hyperkalemia, hyperuricemia, mild proteinuria, and a decreased fractional excretion of sodium. Calcineurin inhibitor nephrotoxicity is the leading cause of renal dysfunction following nonrenal solid-organ transplant.

The predominant mechanism for calcineurin inhibitor nephrotoxicity is renal vasoconstriction, primarily of the afferent arteriole, resulting in increased renal vascular resistance, decreased renal blood flow by up to 40%, reduced glomerular filtration rate by up to 30%, and increased proximal tubular sodium reabsorption with a reduction in urinary sodium and potassium excretion. A number of other mechanisms have been implicated, including changes in the renin–angiotensin–aldosterone system, prostaglandin synthesis, nitrous oxide production, sympathetic nervous system activation, and calcium handling.[38]

Several approaches have been proposed to reduce calcineurin inhibitor nephrotoxicity including delaying administration immediately postoperatively in patients at high risk for nephrotoxicity (using alternative induction protocols including an IL-2 receptor antagonist or antilymphocyte globulin), monitoring calcineurin inhibitor trough blood concentrations, reducing the calcineurin inhibitor dosage if the vasoconstrictive effects are problematic, and avoiding other nephrotoxins (eg, aminoglycosides, amphotericin B, and nonsteroidal antiinflammatory agents) when possible[15,38] Currently, no proven therapies consistently prevent or reverse the nephrotoxic effects of calcineurin inhibitors.

In patients who have received a kidney transplant, it is often difficult to differentiate calcineurin inhibitor nephrotoxicity from renal allograft rejection. Because the clinical features of acute renal allograft rejection and calcineurin inhibitor nephrotoxicity overlap considerably, a renal biopsy is often necessary to differentiate the two (Table 89-6). However, differentiating between chronic renal allograft rejection and calcineurin inhibitor nephrotoxicity may be more difficult because, in addition to clinical signs and symptoms, biopsy findings may also be similar.

Drug–Drug and Drug–Food Interactions Drug interactions occur frequently with the calcineurin inhibitors because they are substrates for CYP3A4 and P-glycoprotein.[33-35] The most commonly administered drugs that are known to significantly alter cyclosporine and tacrolimus levels are highlighted in Table 89-4. Inhibitors of CYP3A4, such as diltiazem or erythromycin, can increase drug concentrations up to 82%, whereas drugs that induce CYP3A4 activity, such as phenytoin or rifampin, can decrease drug concentrations by 50%.[35] While in vitro data suggest that drugs that increase the pH of the GI tract, such as magnesium-, aluminum-, or calcium-containing antacids, sodium bicarbonate, and magnesium oxide, can cause a pH-mediated degradation of tacrolimus by physically adsorbing tacrolimus in the GI tract, this has not been borne out in clinical studies.[39] Some clinicians suggest separating such compounds from tacrolimus administration by at least 2 hours to avoid any potential interaction.

Cyclosporine, and to a lesser extent, tacrolimus, are inhibitors of CYP3A4 and P-glycoprotein.[30,40] The inhibitory effects of cyclosporine and tacrolimus on CYP3A4 can be seen with weaker substrates, such as the HMG-CoA reductase inhibitors ("statins"). Concomitant administration of a calcineurin inhibitor with an HMG-CoA reductase inhibitor results in an increase in the HMG-CoA reductase inhibitor levels, which increases the risk of HMG-CoA reductase inhibitor adverse effects, most notably myopathy.[41] Patients should be monitored for clinical signs of myopathy when receiving HMG-CoA reductase inhibitors in combination with cyclosporine and tacrolimus. The interaction appears to be more pronounced between cyclosporine and HMG-CoA reductase inhibitors due to inhibition of organic anion-transporter proteins (OATP) by cyclosporine.[42]

Consistency in administration of the calcineurin inhibitors with regard to meals and food intake is important to sustain an effective concentration time profile. High-fat meals can enhance both plasma clearance and the volume of distribution of cyclosporine by more than 60%.[43] Food reduces the rate and extent of tacrolimus absorption, and a high-fat meal may further delay gastric emptying and reduce the maximum achieved serum concentration (C_{max}), and the area under the concentration–time curve (AUC).[30] Furocoumarins, such as quercetin, naringin, and bergamottin, found in grapefruit juice, are potent inhibitors of CYP3A4 and have been reported to increase both cyclosporine and tacrolimus concentrations significantly. The AUC and C_{max} of cyclosporine have been reported to be increased by more than 55% and 35%, respectively. In addition the components of green tea as well as tumeric and ginger have been noted to increase calcineurin exposure.[30]

Dosing and Administration Initial oral cyclosporine doses range from 8 to 18 mg/kg per day administered every 12 hours. Higher doses of cyclosporine are used more commonly in two-drug regimens, whereas lower doses are part of triple-drug regimens. Oral tacrolimus doses usually are in the range of 0.1 to 0.3 mg/kg per day given every 12 hours. A recently-approved tacrolimus extended-release tablet (Envarsus®) has greater bioavailability than the immediate

TABLE 89-6 Differential Diagnosis of Acute Rejection and Cyclosporine or Tacrolimus Nephrotoxicity

	Nephrotoxicity in Renal Transplant Recipients	
	Acute Rejection	**CSA or TAC Nephrotoxicity**
History	Often <4 weeks postoperatively	Often >6 weeks postoperatively
Clinical presentation	Fever	Afebrile
	Hypertension	Hypertension
	Weight gain	Graft nontender
	Graft swelling/tenderness	Good urine output
	Decreased daily urine volume	
Laboratory biopsy	Rapid rise in serum Cr (0.3 mg/dL/day [27 μmol/L/day])	Gradual rise in serum Cr (>0.15 mg/dL/day [>13 μmol/L/day])
	Normal CSA or TAC concentration	Elevated CSA or TAC concentration
	Interstitial lymphocytic infiltrates	Interstitial fibrosis, tubular atrophy, glomerular thrombosis, arterial inflammation

Cr, creatinine; CSA, cyclosporine; TAC, tacrolimus.

release formulation and thus a lower recommended daily starting dose range of (0.11-0.17 mg/kg/day).[44] Children require higher doses to maintain therapeutic drug concentrations, up to 14 to 18 mg/kg per day for cyclosporine and 0.3 mg/kg per day for tacrolimus. The two once-daily formulations of tacrolimus are not interchangeable. Astagraf XL® or Advagraf® (tacrolimus extended-release capsule) is generally converted from standard tacrolimus formulations on a mg:mg basis whereas the more recently developed extended release form of tacrolimus, Envarsus® XR (tacrolimus prolonged release tablets) has greater bioavailability than the immediate release tacrolimus and the recommended conversion factor is 1 mg immediate release to 0.8 mg prolonged release, that is, a 20% reduction in total daily dose.[30,44,45] When patients were converted from immediate release tacrolimus to extended AstagrafXL® on a mg:mg conversion based on total daily dose, about one third of patients required downward dose adjustments to maintain the same 24-trough serum concentrations.[45] If oral administration is not possible, both CSA and TAC can be administered intravenously at approximately one third the oral dosage, since administration by this route avoids first-pass metabolism. The usual intravenous dose of cyclosporine is 2 to 5 mg/kg per day, given as a continuous infusion or as single or twice-daily injection. Intravenous tacrolimus doses range from 0.05 to 0.1 mg/kg per day and must be administered by continuous infusion.

Therapeutic Drug Monitoring Calcineurin inhibitor trough blood concentrations should be measured routinely to optimize therapy (Table 89-7). Radioimmunoassay (RIA) and fluorescence polarization immunoassay are among the methods to measure cyclosporine concentrations. Tacrolimus concentrations are most commonly measured by microparticle enzyme immunoassays or enzyme-linked immunoassays. Both drugs can be measured by high-performance liquid chromatography (HPLC), which is recognized as the reference procedure.[43] Therapeutic target ranges are assay specific because some quantitate parent plus metabolite concentration, while others only measure the parent compound. Thus, the target concentrations will be lower for the specific assays (LC-MS/MS) compared with nonspecific assays (RIA and microparticle enzyme immunoassays) by approximately 20% to 25%. The specific goal level for both drugs is dependent on transplant type, time after transplantation, concomitant immunosuppression, and transplantation center. One review of the role of tacrolimus in renal transplantation suggests that target 12-hour whole blood concentrations for tacrolimus should be 15 to 20 ng/mL (mcg/L; 18.6 to 24.8 nmol/L) 0 to 1 month after transplantation, 10 to 15 ng/mL (mcg/L; 12.4 to 18.6 nmol/L) 1 to 3 months after transplantation, and 5 to 12 ng/mL (mcg/L; 6.2 to 14.9 nmol/L) greater than 3 months after transplantation.[36] Blood drug concentrations should be measured frequently (daily or three times per week) following initiation of the drug and during the stabilization period after transplantation. With time, blood concentrations can be measured less frequently.

Studies have revealed lack of predictive value of trough cyclosporine concentrations and rejection.[46] Alternative strategies, including AUC and peak concentration determination, have been suggested to better correlate with rejection.[43,46] Limited sampling techniques using two to five blood samples within the first 4 hours after an oral dose have been used to determine AUC and it was observed that AUC levels greater than 4,400 ng/mL (mcg/L; greater than 3,361 nmol/L) per hour correlated with a reduction in rejection.[43,46] Cyclosporine peak concentration (C_{peak}) has also been found to correlate with rejection and toxicity. Some transplantation centers have adopted this strategy to manage cyclosporine concentrations because of the convenience and reduced cost associated with the measurement of a single blood concentration. The suggested therapeutic range for C_{peak} cyclosporine levels is 1,500 to 2,000 ng/mL (mcg/L; 1,248-1,664 nmol/L) for the first few months after transplant and 700 to 900 ng/mL (mcg/L; 582-749 nmol/L) after 6 to 12 months.[46]

Corticosteroids

4 Corticosteroids have been used since the beginning of the modern transplantation era. Despite their many adverse events, they continue to be a cornerstone of immunosuppression regimens in many transplant centers, with 30% and 60% of liver and kidney transplant patients, respectively, receiving corticosteroids for at least the first year after transplantation.[1] The most commonly used corticosteroids are methylprednisolone and prednisone.

Pharmacology/Mechanism of Action Corticosteroids block cytokine activation by binding to corticosteroid response elements, thereby inhibiting IL-1, IL-2, IL-3, IL-6, γ-interferon, and tumor necrosis factor-α synthesis (see Fig. 89-1). Additionally, corticosteroids interfere with cell migration, recognition, and cytotoxic effector mechanisms.[47]

Pharmacokinetics Prednisone is converted to prednisolone, its active moiety, in the liver and has multiple effects on the immune system. Prednisone is rapidly absorbed from the GI tract, achieving peak concentrations in 1 to 3 hours in transplant recipients. Bioavailability is greater than 90%. In kidney transplant recipients the pharmacokinetic half-life is short, 2 to 4 hours, but the pharmacodynamic effects extend beyond the time that concentrations are measurable, permitting daily administration.[47]

Efficacy Their efficacy is irrefutable based on the decades of clinical experience. Systematic studies comparing corticosteroid-free immunosuppressive agent combinations with conventional therapy are difficult to perform because of the hundreds of potential combinations that now exist. However, recent studies of corticosteroid-free immunosuppressive agent combinations with newer, more specific immunosuppressants suggest that corticosteroids may in the future have less of a role in maintenance immunosuppression.[48]

TABLE 89-7 Therapeutic Concentrations of Immunosuppressants

		Concentrations (ng/mL or mcg/L)	
Drug	Sampling medium	HPLC	RIA
Cyclosporine	Whole blood	100-300	375-400
	Plasma	75-100	150-250
Tacrolimus	Whole blood	8-13	5-20
	Plasma		0.2-0.8
Sirolimus (with CIs)	Whole blood	10-15	15-20
Sirolimus (without CIs)	Whole blood	15-25	20-30
Everolimus (with CIs)	Whole blood	3-8	

CIs, calcineurin inhibitors; HPLC, high performance liquid chromatography; RIA, radioimmunoassay. For expression of immunosuppressant drugs in SI units of nmol/L multiply levels in ng/mL(or mcg/L) by 0.832 for cyclosporine, 1.24 for tacrolimus, 1.094 for sirolimus, and 1.044 for everolimus.

Adverse Effects Adverse effects of prednisone that occur in more than 10% of patients include increased appetite, insomnia, indigestion (bitter taste), and mood changes. Side effects that occur less often but which are seen with high doses or prolonged therapy include cataracts, hyperglycemia, hirsutism, bruising, acne, sodium and water retention, hypertension, bone growth suppression, and ulcerative esophagitis. The adverse effects of corticosteroids are summarized in Table 89-5.

Drug–Drug and Drug–Food Interactions Barbiturates, phenytoin, and rifampin induce hepatic metabolism of prednisolone and thus may decrease the effectiveness of prednisone. Prednisone decreases the effectiveness of vaccines and toxoids.[47]

Dosing and Administration An intravenous corticosteroid, commonly high-dose methylprednisolone (250-1,000 mg), is given at the time of transplantation. The dose of methylprednisolone is tapered rapidly and usually discontinued within 3 to 5 days when oral prednisone is initiated. Prednisone doses are tapered progressively over several weeks to months, depending on the type of additional immunosuppression and organ function. It is preferable to administer corticosteroids between 7 AM and 8 AM to mimic the body's diurnal release of cortisol. While conversion to alternate-day regimens or complete withdrawal of prednisone in patients with stable post-transplantation courses has been used with success in some transplantation centers, corticosteroids are often continued for the entire life of the functional graft.[47]

The first-line therapy for the treatment of acute graft rejection is high-dose intravenous methylprednisolone (250-1,000 mg) daily for 3 days or oral prednisone (200 mg) daily for 3 days. Doses of oral prednisone are then tapered over 5 days to 20 mg/day. Prednisone should be taken with food to minimize GI upset. Corticosteroids should never be discontinued abruptly; tapering should be gradual because of suppression of the hypothalamic–pituitary–adrenal axis. Corticosteroids slow the growth rate of children, prompting clinicians to use alternate-day dosing or to withhold corticosteroids until rejection occurs.

Antimetabolites

5 Antimetabolites have been used since the early days of transplantation because they prevent proliferation of lymphocytes. Azathioprine, long considered a part of the "gold standard" regimen with cyclosporine and corticosteroids, has largely been supplanted by mycophenolic acid derivatives which are more specific in their effects on lymphocytes and have fewer side effects.

Mycophenolatic Acid Derivatives Two formulations of mycophenolic acid (MPA) are currently available in the United States: mycophenolate mofetil, the morpholinoethyl ester of MPA, and mycophenolate sodium, which is available as an enteric-coated formulation of the sodium salt of MPA.

Pharmacology/Mechanism of Action The immunosuppressive effect of MPA is exerted through noncompetitive binding to inosine monophosphate dehydrogenase (IMPDH), the key enzyme responsible for guanosine nucleotide synthesis via the de novo pathway. Inhibition of IMPDH results in decreased nucleotide synthesis and diminished DNA polymerase activity, ultimately reducing lymphocyte proliferation.[49] Although MPA inhibits both types of IMPDH: IMPDH I, expressed by all cells in the body, and IMPDH II, which is expressed only in T and B lymphocytes, it is more specific for IMPDH II.[49] In addition to this, T and B lymphocytes only use the de novo pathway for nucleotide synthesis (see Fig. 89-1), making MPA very specific for these cells. Other cells within the body have a salvage pathway by which they can synthesize nucleotides, making them less susceptible to the actions of MPA and thereby reducing, but not eliminating, the potential for the hematologic adverse effects seen with azathioprine. In addition to decreasing lymphocyte proliferation, MPA may also downregulate activation of lymphocytes.[50]

Pharmacokinetics Because MPA is unstable in an acidic environment, mycophenolate mofetil acts as a prodrug that is readily absorbed from the GI tract, after which it is rapidly and completely converted to MPA in the liver. The enteric coating of mycophenolate sodium protects MPA from the acidic gastric pH and allows MPA to be released directly into the small intestine for absorption. The absolute bioavailability of mycophenolate mofetil and mycophenolate sodium is 94% and 72% of the active moiety, respectively. Peak concentrations of mycophenolate mofetil are reached within 1 to 2 hours following oral administration, while the enteric coating of mycophenolate sodium delays absorption and peak concentrations are not reached until 4 hours after administration.[50]

MPA is extensively bound (97%) to albumin and is eliminated by the kidney and also undergoes glucuronidation in the liver to an inactive glucuronide metabolite (MPAG) that is subsequently excreted in the bile and urine. Enterohepatic cycling of MPAG can lead to deconjugation, thereby recirculating MPA into the bloodstream. This can account for 10% to 60% of total MPA exposure and results in a second peak 6 to 12 hours after oral administration.[50] The half-life of MPA is 18 hours.

Efficacy Currently, mycophenolate mofetil is approved for use in kidney, liver, and heart transplantation and is recommended as a component of maintenance immunosuppression regimens for most kidney and heart transplant recipients.[18,29] Early studies comparing mycophenolate to azathioprine in patients receiving cyclosporine and corticosteroids demonstrated a statistically significant improvement with MPA in patient and graft survival at 1 and 3 years.[50] Subsequent studies have confirmed the efficacy of mycophenolate combined with tacrolimus. Mycophenolate has also demonstrated efficacy in the treatment of acute rejection.[50]

Mycophenolic acid derivatives are a key component of calcineurin inhibitor–sparing protocols. MPA monotherapy has been associated with an unacceptable rejection rate. Combination of MPA with sirolimus, on the other hand, resulted in improved renal function with no change in acute rejection incidence or and patient and graft survival.[50]

Adverse Effects Unlike cyclosporine and tacrolimus, MPA is not associated with nephrotoxicity, neurotoxicity, or hypertension. The most common side effects are related to the GI tract, including nausea, vomiting, diarrhea, and abdominal pain (see Table 89-5), which occur with similar frequency during intravenous and oral therapy. Strategies to reduce GI symptoms are not well studied. Changing formulation may or may not improve symptoms and it is clear that dose reduction and discontinuation increase the risk of rejections.[50] Mycophenolic acid also has hematologic effects, such as leukopenia and anemia, particularly with higher doses. Recently, the rare but serious adverse event of progressive multifocal leukoencephalopathy (PML) has been reported, but could not substantiated in further analyses.[50] Because peripheral intravenous mycophenolate administration is associated with local edema and inflammation, central venous administration may be the preferred route.

Drug–Drug and Drug–Food Interactions Food has no effect on MPA AUC, but it delays the absorption and decreases MPA C_{max} by 40% and 33% when mycophenolate mofetil and mycophenolate sodium, respectively, are administered. Concomitant administration with aluminum- and magnesium-containing antacids or cholestyramine significantly decreases the AUC of MPA and should be avoided.[50] It has been suggested that administration of iron may produce similar results, but this has not been tested. Concomitant administration of mycophenolate mofetil with pantoprazole has been reported to decrease MPA levels by 57% and AUC by 12% in healthy volunteers. The same effect was not observed with mycophenolate sodium.[51]

Acyclovir, commonly used in renal transplant recipients for the treatment and prevention of viral infections, competes with MPAG for renal tubular secretion. AUCs of both entities are increased during concomitant acyclovir and MPA administration. No pharmacokinetic interaction with other antiviral agents has been demonstrated, but, there is potential for additive pharmacodynamic effects such as bone marrow suppression.

Decreased MPA trough concentrations have been reported when MPA is administered with cyclosporine compared with those achieved when MPA is given with tacrolimus or sirolimus.[50] This interaction is most likely a result of cyclosporine inhibition of multidrug-resistance-associated protein 2 (MRP2), which inhibits the enterohepatic recycling of MPAG, resulting in decreased MPA concentrations.[50] Cyclosporine decreases MPA levels by approximately 40% to 50% compared to tacrolimus.[34] To achieve equivalent MPA and MPAG serum concentrations, it may be necessary to administer higher doses of MPA with cyclosporine compared to tacrolimus. Antibiotics may also interfere with enterohepatic recycling of MPAG by decreasing bacterial-mediated deglucuronidation in the colon.[50]

Dosing and Administration Mycophenolate mofetil is currently available in both oral and intravenous formulations. Although intravenous administration of equal doses closely mimics oral administration, the two cannot be considered bioequivalent. Mycophenolate sodium is only available as an oral formulation. To optimize immunosuppression and minimize adverse effects, MPA is administered in two divided doses given every 12 hours. The total daily dose for kidney and liver transplants is typically 2 g/day for mycophenolate mofetil and 1.44 g/day for mycophenolate sodium. Higher doses may be required in heart transplant recipients if targeting a trough concentration of greater than 1.5 mcg/mL (mg/L; greater than 4.7 μmol/L) in select patients.[18] The recommended pediatric dose is 600 mg/m² for mycophenolate mofetil and 400 mg/m² for mycophenolate sodium, in two divided doses.

While an increasing body of literature suggests that therapeutic drug monitoring of MPA is of value it remains controversial.[51-53] Plasma appears to be the most appropriate medium in which to measure MPA for therapeutic drug monitoring. Numerous studies have demonstrated a relationship between plasma MPA concentrations and improved clinical outcomes in patients receiving concomitant CIs and corticosteroids. Patients with trough MPA levels between 1.0 and 3.5 mcg/mL (mg/L; 3.1-10.9 μmol/L) experienced fewer significant complications. Unbound concentrations as opposed to total MPA concentrations have been suggested as the most relevant to measure, especially in patients with liver disease, hypoalbuminemia, and severe infection.[50] Trough concentrations may not be accurate in predicting total drug exposure during a 12-hour interval and thus AUC monitoring has been proposed as the most appropriate measure of MPA drug exposure to guide therapy.[50] Better outcomes are associated with MPA AUC concentrations of greater than 42.8 mcg/mL (mg/L; 134 μmol/L) per hour (by HPLC),[52] although a reference range of 30 to 60 mcg/mL (mg/L; 94 to 188 μmol/L) has been proposed. The correlation between MPA AUC levels and adverse effects is low. Further studies are required to determine the best means to evaluate MPA concentrations, the acceptable targets for each, and the appropriate strategy to monitor MPA concentrations.[52]

Clinical **Controversy...**

Therapeutic drug monitoring of mycophenolic acid is controversial. Its ability to diminish adverse effects or predict long-term survival remains unknown.

Azathioprine Azathioprine, a prodrug for 6-mercaptopurine (6-MP), has been used as an immunosuppressant in combination with corticosteroids since the earliest days of the modern transplantation era. Its use has dramatically declined with the availability of newer immunosuppressants, but it remains an option for patients intolerant of other medications.[18,29]

Pharmacology/Mechanism of Action Azathioprine is an inactive compound that is converted rapidly to 6-MP in the blood and is subsequently metabolized by three different enzymes. Xanthine oxidase, found in the liver and GI tract, converts 6-MP to the inactive final end product, 6-thiouric acid. Thiopurine *S*-methyltransferase (TPMT), found in hematopoietic tissues and red blood cells, methylates 6-MP to an inactive metabolite, 6-methylmercaptopurine. Finally, hypoxanthine-guanine phosphoribosyltransferase is the first step responsible for converting 6-MP to 6-thioguanine nucleotides (6-TGNs), the active metabolites, which are incorporated into nucleic acids, ultimately disrupting both the salvage and de novo pathways of DNA, RNA, and protein synthesis. This process is toxic to the cell and renders the cell unable to proliferate (see Fig. 89-1). Eventually, 6-TGNs are catabolized by xanthine oxidase and thiopurine *S*-methyltransferase to inactive products.[53]

Pharmacokinetics Oral bioavailability of azathioprine is approximately 40%. Metabolism of 6-MP is primarily by xanthine oxidase to inactive metabolites, which are excreted by the kidneys. The half-life of azathioprine, the parent compound, is very short, approximately 12 minutes. The half-life of 6-MP is longer, ranging from 0.7 to 3 hours. However, it is the activity of the 6-TGNs that determines the pharmacodynamic half-life of the drug which has been estimated to be 9 days.[54]

Adverse Effects Dose-limiting adverse effects of azathioprine are often hematologic (see Table 89-5). Leukopenia, anemia, and thrombocytopenia can occur within the first few weeks of therapy and can be managed by dose reduction or discontinuation of azathioprine. Other common adverse effects include nausea and vomiting, which can be minimized by taking azathioprine with food. Alopecia, hepatotoxicity, and pancreatitis are less common adverse effects of azathioprine and are reversible on dose reduction or discontinuation. Activity of TPMT can affect the occurrence of adverse effects with azathioprine. Approximately 10% of the population has intermediate TPMT activity and 0.3% has low activity of the enzyme. In both scenarios, the incidence of leukopenia and hepatotoxicity is increased. As a result, TPMT genotyping may be useful to guide dosing of azathioprine to minimize adverse effects.[53]

Drug–Drug and Drug–Food Interactions The xanthine oxidase inhibitors allopurinol and febuxostat can increase azathioprine and 6-MP concentrations by as much as fourfold.[54] The metabolic pathways shift to favor production of 6-TGNs, which ultimately results in increased bone marrow suppression and pancytopenia. Doses of azathioprine should be reduced by 50% to 75% when allopurinol is added to a patient's drug regimen.

Dosing and Administration Usual initial doses of azathioprine range from 3 to 5 mg/kg per day intravenously or orally. Individualization to maintain the white blood cell count between 3,500 and 6,000 cells/mm³ (3.5 and 6.0 × 10^9/L) may be accomplished in some patients with doses as low as 0.25 mg/kg per day. Patients are often instructed to take azathioprine in the evening when initiating or titrating therapy to allow for dose adjustments based on morning determinations of their white blood cell count.

Proliferation Signal Inhibitors

6 Two proliferation signal inhibitors (PSI) have been approved in the United States for use in transplantation. Sirolimus, also known as rapamycin, is an immunosuppressive macrolide antibiotic that is structurally similar to tacrolimus, and is effective in reducing the risk of acute rejection. Everolimus, a synthetic derivative of sirolimus, was developed to improve upon the pharmacokinetics of sirolimus. Everolimus was approved in the United States in 2009 and has a significantly shorter half-life than sirolimus.

Pharmacology/Mechanism of Action Sirolimus and everolimus both bind to FKBP12, forming a complex that binds to the mammalian target of rapamycin (mTOR), which inhibits the body's response to cytokines (see Fig. 89-1). As such, the drugs are commonly referred to as mTOR inhibitors. IL-2 stimulates mTOR to activate kinases that ultimately advance the cell cycle from G1 to the S phase. Thus these drugs reduce T-cell proliferation by inhibiting the cellular response to IL-2 and progression of the cell cycle.[55,56]

Pharmacokinetics Bioavailability after oral administration is low for both, only 14% to 20%, with peak concentrations being reached within 1 to 2 hours.[55,56] Both have large volumes of distribution, 5.6 to 16.7 L/kg for sirolimus and approximately 110 L (about 1.5 L/kg for a 70 kg individual) for everolimus. Both are metabolized primarily by CYP3A4 in the gut and the liver. Likewise, both are also substrates for P-glycoprotein. The half-life for sirolimus is reported to be 60 hours but can be as long as 110 hours in patients with liver dysfunction, while that of everolimus is much shorter, 18 to 35 hours.[55,56]

Efficacy Sirolimus is only approved for the prevention of rejection in kidney transplant recipients when given in combination with corticosteroids and cyclosporine or after withdrawal of cyclosporine in patients with low to moderate immunologic risk. Because of the risks of delayed wound healing sirolimus is usually not started until 3 months after transplantation or once the surgical wound has healed. Sirolimus has also been demonstrated to be effective in combination with tacrolimus or mycophenolate in kidney transplants, with patient survival rates greater than 99% and graft survival rates greater than 96%.[47] Combination therapy with sirolimus and mycophenolate can be used to avoid the use of calcineurin inhibitors and decrease the risk of nephrotoxicity. Everolimus is approved for use in both kidney and liver transplantation. In kidney transplant recipients it was studied in combination with basiliximab, cyclosporine, and corticosteroids, whereas in liver transplant recipients it was initiated at least 30 days after transplantation in combination with reduced-dose tacrolimus and corticosteroids. Everolimus has also been used with tacrolimus with similar results as sirolimus.[57] Everolimus appears to have less of an effect on wound healing and thus may potentially be used earlier after transplantation.

Early cyclosporine withdrawal has been studied in patients receiving sirolimus-based immunosuppressive protocols. Ideal candidates are patients who have not had a recent or severe rejection episode and have adequate renal function 3 months after transplant. Rejection occurred in 5.6% of patients after discontinuation of cyclosporine and no difference in graft survival was noted. Long-term follow-up (2 years) showed improved renal function and blood pressure without an increase in acute rejection or graft loss in patients who discontinued cyclosporine.[47] Similar results have been demonstrated with everolimus.[57]

PSIs have demonstrated efficacy to reduce CI use and nephrotoxicity in liver,[58] heart,[55] and lung transplant patients.[56] PSIs are also being investigated in liver transplant patients as a means to reduce the recurrence of hepatitis C and hepatocellular carcinoma.[58] They may also reduce the incidence of chronic rejection and prolong long-term patient survival after heart transplantation.[28]

Clinical **Controversy...**

The benefits of PSIs after liver and lung transplant include decreased CI-induced nephrotoxicity, anti-cancer properties, and anti-CMV and anti-HCV activity. Early introduction in these patients has demonstrated increased hepatic artery thrombosis and bronchial anastamotic dehiscence. The optimal timing of initiation of PSIs in these populations is controversial to minimize potential benefits while minimizing serious complications.

Adverse Effects Both everolimus and sirolimus are associated with dose-related myelosuppression. Thrombocytopenia is usually seen within the first 2 weeks of sirolimus therapy but generally improves with continued treatment; leukopenia and anemia are also typically transient.[55,56] Sirolimus trough serum concentrations greater than 15 ng/mL (mcg/L; 16 nmol/L) have been correlated with thrombocytopenia and leukopenia.[55] Hypercholesterolemia and hypertriglyceridemia are also common in patients receiving everolimus or sirolimus. It is postulated that the mechanism of this adverse effect is related to an overproduction of lipoproteins or inhibition of lipoprotein lipase. Peak cholesterol and triglyceride levels are often seen within 3 months of sirolimus initiation but usually decrease after 1 year of therapy and can be managed by reducing the dose, discontinuing sirolimus, or initiating therapy with an HMG-CoA reductase inhibitor or fibric acid derivative. One study suggested that the dyslipidemia associated with sirolimus is not a major risk factor for early cardiovascular complications following kidney transplantation.[55] Delayed wound healing and dehiscence could be a result of inhibition of smooth muscle proliferation and intimal thickening.[55] Mouth ulcers are reported in as many as 60% of patients treated with sirolimus and appear to be dose-related.[55] Reversible interstitial pneumonitis has been described in kidney, liver, and heart–lung transplantation recipients.[47] Other adverse effects reported with sirolimus include increased liver enzymes, hypertension, rash, acne, diarrhea, and arthralgia (see Table 89-4).

Drug–Drug and Drug–Food Interactions The major metabolic pathway for everolimus and sirolimus is CYP3A4; thus, the drug interactions mediated by induction or inhibition of the CYP3A4 enzyme system are similar to those seen with cyclosporine and tacrolimus (see Table 89-4). Administration of the microemulsion formulation of cyclosporine with sirolimus significantly increases the AUC and trough sirolimus serum concentrations: this has not been observed with the standard formulation of cyclosporine. Conversely, cyclosporine concentrations and AUC are increased when it is given concomitantly with sirolimus. The mechanism is proposed to be competitive binding to CYP3A4 and P-glycoprotein.[55,56] It is recommended that patients separate the dose of sirolimus and cyclosporine by 4 hours to minimize the interaction.[55] Concomitant administration of tacrolimus does not affect sirolimus levels.[55] Although everolimus AUC was increased by the administration of a single dose of the microemulsion cyclosporine formulation, no specific recommendations for dose timing are given. It should be expected, however, that any changes in CSA dose may also necessitate a modification of everolimus dose and increased attention to therapeutic drug monitoring.[56]

As with cyclosporine and tacrolimus, grapefruit juice increases sirolimus levels. Administration of sirolimus with a high-fat meal is associated with a delayed rate of absorption, decreased C_{max}, and increased AUC, indicating an increased drug exposure, whereas the half-life remains unchanged.[55] Conversely, administration of everolimus with a high-fat meal was associated with decreases in both C_{max} and AUC.[56]

Dosing and Administration The fixed sirolimus dosing regimen, approved for concomitant use with cyclosporine includes a loading dose of 6 to 15 mg followed by 2 or 5 mg daily, respectively. Therapeutic monitoring of sirolimus is advocated using whole-blood concentrations measured by HPLC, which is specific for the parent compound (see Table 89-7). For everolimus a starting dose of 0.75 mg twice daily is indicated in regimens that contain cyclosporine, corticosteroids, and basiliximab. Target serum concentrations are 3 to 8 ng/mL (mcg/L; 3-8 nmol/L).

Co-Stimulatory Signal Inhibitor

Belatacept, derived from abatacept, is the only drug currently approved in this class of immunosuppressive agents. Belatacept may ultimately replace calcineurin inhibitors in the majority of immunosuppressive regimens, since its use has not been associated with toxicities seen with CIs, namely nephrotoxicity.[59] As of the fall of 2016, belatacept is only approved for kidney transplantation.

Pharmacology/Mechanism of Action Belatacept is a selective costimulation blocker that binds costimulatory ligands (CD80 and CD86) on antigen presenting cells, preventing interaction with CD28 on T cells. The interaction of CD80 and CD86 with CD28 is required for the initiation of "signal 2," the co-stimulatory signal that produces calcineurin, protein kinases, and nuclear factor-κ β that lead to activation and proliferation of T-cells. Thus, blockade of CD80 and CD86 prevents T-cell activation.[60]

Pharmacokinetics Belatacept which is only available as an intravenous formulation has a volume of distribution of 0.11 L/kg, half-life of approximately 11 days and is not effected by reduced kidney or liver function.[59]

Efficacy A phase III clinical trial comparing belatacept to cyclosporine in first time kidney transplant patients demonstrated similar efficacy in terms of both patient and graft survival. In the trial, the cyclosporine group experienced more chronic allograft nephropathy at month 12. However, the belatacept group experienced more frequent and more severe ACR. Despite this, the measured GFR was 13 to 15mL/min (0.22-0.25 mL/s) higher in the belatacept group compared to the cyclosporine group, a trend that persisted for 7 years.[59]

Additionally, belatacept-treated patients had better blood pressure control and lower lipid levels as well as less diabetes than CI-treated patients. Whether this translates long term to less cardiovascular mortality remains to be demonstrated.[60]

Studies have also evaluated conversion from CI-based regimens to belatacept in kidney transplant recipients with stable kidney function. The results show improved GFR from baseline in those converted to belatacept compared to patients who remained on CIs. However, the difference was not statistically significant as the study was not adequately powered.[61] Acute rejection occurred more frequently in patients who switched to belatacept, compared with no acute rejection in the patients who remained on CIs.[59]

Early studies with belatacept in liver transplant patients were associated with increased graft loss and death which lead to the subsequent termination of ongoing studies.[62] There is limited postmarketing experience with belatacept in liver transplant recipients with poor kidney function as a bridge to future calcineurin therapy.[63]

Adverse Effects The most common adverse effects of belatacept include anemia, neutropenia, diarrhea, urinary tract infections, headache, and peripheral edema.[59] In the clinical trials, patients who were Epstein Barr virus (EBV) naïve experienced a significantly higher incidence of post-transplant lymphoproliferative disease (PTLD). Most of the cases of PTLD occurred within the first 18 months of treatment and the majority occurred in the central nervous system. There was no increase in incidence of PTLD in patients who were EBV-seropositive. As a result, belatacept carries a black box warning for PTLD and is contraindicated in patients who are EBV-seronegative. Progressive multifocal leukoencephalopathy (PML) was also reported with belatacept.[59]

Drug-Drug and Drug-Food Interactions No drug or food interactions have been reported with belatacept.

Dosing and Administration Patients for whom belatacept is being considered must be screened for EBV-serostatus prior to initiation of therapy. Only patients who are EBV-seropositive should receive belatacept due to the increased risk of PTLD in EBV-seronegative patients. The risk evaluation and mitigation strategy (REMS) for belatacept involves screening for symptoms of PTLD and PML with counseling and education. As a primary immunosuppressant for first time kidney transplants, belatacept is administered as 10 mg/kg intravenously over 30 minutes on days 0, 4, 14, 28, and at the end of weeks 8 and 12. Thereafter, the dose is reduced to the maintenance dose of 5 mg/kg administered IV over 30 minutes every 4 weeks beginning at week 16.

When converting to belatacept from a CI-based regimen, the proposed dosing schedule is 5 mg/kg IV administered every 2 weeks for 5 doses on days 0, 14, 28, 42, and 56, then every 4 weeks thereafter. The CI dose should be decreased by 50% after the second dose of belatacept and then discontinued after the fourth dose.[59]

Antibody Agents

7 Both polyclonal and monoclonal antibody preparations are used in transplantation. These agents can be differentiated by their level of specificity, that is, particular receptor(s) they effect, or their downstream effects.

Depleting Antibodies

Antithymocyte Globulin Two ATG formulations are available in the United States: ATG (Atgam, Pfizer, New York, NY), an equine polyclonal antibody, and RATG (Thymoglobulin, Genzyme, Cambridge, MA), a rabbit polyclonal antibody. The rabbit preparation is less immunogenic and may have other advantages over the equine preparation. Both ATG and RATG are often used as induction therapy to prevent acute rejection. In 2012, over 60% of kidney transplant recipients received RATG induction whereas fewer than 20% of liver transplant recipients did.[1]

Pharmacology/Mechanism of Action Because of their polyclonal antibody nature, both ATG and RATG exert their immunosuppressive effect by binding to a wide array of lymphocyte receptors such as CD2, CD3, CD4, CD8, CD25, and CD45. Binding of ATG or RATG to the various receptors results in complement-mediated lysis and subsequent lymphocyte depletion. While T cells are the major lymphocytic target for the compounds, other blood cell components such as B cells and other leukocytes are also affected (see Fig. 89-1). Damaged T cells are subsequently removed by the spleen, liver, and lungs.

Pharmacokinetics ATG is poorly distributed into lymphoid tissue and binds primarily to circulating lymphocytes, granulocytes, and platelets. The terminal half-life of ATG is 5.7 days. RATG has a volume of distribution of 0.12 L/kg, and its terminal half-life in renal transplant recipients is significantly longer than ATG at 30 days.[32] Peak plasma concentrations are reached after 5 to 7 days of ATG or RATG infusions. Antiequine antibodies have been noted in up to 78% of patients who are receiving ATG therapy. Similarly, antirabbit antibodies have been reported in up to 68% of patients who are receiving RATG therapy. The effects of preformed antibodies on the efficacy and safety of these preparations have not been well studied.

Efficacy ATG and RATG are used most commonly for the treatment of acute allograft rejection or as induction therapy to prevent acute rejection. ATG is currently approved for both indications in kidney transplants. RATG is approved only for the treatment of acute allograft rejection in kidney transplantations. Both drugs have been studied extensively for both indications.[26,32]

Use of RATG as part of quadruple therapy in liver transplantation is associated with similar rates of patient and graft survival and acute rejection compared with dual therapy. In kidney transplant RATG was associated with improved graft survival at 5 years as compared with equine ATG. Quadruple-drug therapy results in similar rates of patient and graft survival and malignancy in heart transplantations, but a significantly lower rate of acute rejection and infection episodes is seen at 1 year compared with triple-drug therapy. Cytomegalovirus (CMV) is an adverse effect of this strategy, but recent data indicate that routine prophylaxis is successful in preventing its development.[56]

Adverse Effects Most adverse effects reported with ATG and RATG are related to the lack of specificity for T cells. Dose-limiting myelosuppression (leukopenia, anemia, and thrombocytopenia) occurs frequently. Other adverse effects include anaphylaxis, hypotension, hypertension, tachycardia, dyspnea, urticaria, and rash. Serum sickness is seen more frequently with ATG than with RATG. Nephrotoxicity has been reported but is rare in the absence of serum sickness. Infusion-related febrile reactions are common with the first few doses and can be managed by premedicating the patient with acetaminophen, diphenhydramine, and corticosteroids. Finally, as with any immunosuppressive agent, ATG and RATG are associated with an increased risk of infections, particularly viral infections, and malignancy.

Drug–Drug and Drug–Food Interactions No drug or food interactions have been reported with ATG or RATG.

Dosing and Administration ATG doses range from 10 to 30 mg/kg per day as a single dose for 7 to 14 days. RATG is a more potent compound and is administered at doses of 1 to 1.5 mg/kg per day as a single daily dose for 7 to 14 days for acute rejection or for 5 to 10 days for induction of immunosuppression. It is recommended that both ATG and RATG be administered through a central line or through a high-flow vein with an in-line 0.22-micron filter over at least 4 hours to minimize phlebitis and thrombosis.[32] Heparin and hydrocortisone are commonly added to the infusion to minimize phlebitis and thrombosis.[32]

Alemtuzumab Alemtuzumab is approved for use in B-cell chronic lymphocytic leukemia.[64] However, its effects on depleting both T and B lymphocytes make it useful in solid-organ transplants. While alemtuzumab is not FDA approved for solid organ transplantation, it is increasingly recognized as a viable therapeutic option for induction or treatment of acute rejection. In 2012, commercial distribution of alemtuzumab ceased for transplantation and leukemia, requiring centers to enroll in the manufacturer's distribution program for these indications.[65]

Pharmacology/Mechanism of Action Alemtuzumab is a humanized monoclonal antibody against the CD52 surface antigen found on both T and B lymphocytes, as well as macrophages, monocytes, eosinophils, and natural killer cells. When alemtuzumab binds to the CD52 surface antigen, antibody-dependent lysis occurs, which removes both T and B lymphocytes from the blood, bone marrow, and organs, resulting in complete lymphocyte depletion.[64]

Pharmacokinetics The pharmacokinetics of alemtuzumab in solid-organ transplantation patients have not been investigated. Data from patients with B-cell chronic lymphocytic leukemia indicate that the volume of distribution of alemtuzumab after repeated dosing is 0.18 L/kg. The mean half-life after the first 30 mg dose was 11 hours, but increased to 6 days after 12 weeks of therapy. The extrapolation of these data to solid-organ transplantation is difficult because of the differences in dosing strategies (single or multiple 30-mg doses in solid-organ transplantation vs weekly to thrice weekly dosing in B-cell chronic lymphocytic leukemia). One or two doses of alemtuzumab result in complete and prolonged lymphocyte depletion. Following administration, B lymphocyte counts return to normal within 3 to 12 months. T lymphocytes, however, remain depressed for as long as 3 years following administration.[34,64]

Efficacy Alemtuzumab is effective as induction therapy for the prevention of acute rejection in kidney, liver, pancreas, intestinal, and lung transplants.[56] Additionally, alemtuzumab has been used to successfully treat acute rejection following transplantation and is effective for corticosteroid- and antibody-resistant rejection.[26]

Adverse Effects Adverse effects of alemtuzumab are primarily infusion related, hematologic, and infectious. Because alemtuzumab causes complete lymphocyte depletion and associated cytokine release, infusion-related reactions include rigors, hypotension, fever, shortness of breath, bronchospasms, and chills. The potential for developing these reactions can be reduced by administering premedications such as acetaminophen, corticosteroids and diphenhydramine or by administering smaller doses and escalating the dose gradually. Hematologic effects include pancytopenia, neutropenia, thrombocytopenia, and lymphopenia.

Drug–Drug and Drug–Food Interactions No drug or food interactions have been reported with alemtuzumab.

Dosing and Administration Several dosing regimens have been proposed for alemtuzumab in solid-organ transplantation. The most common dosing strategy is 30 mg as a single dose; some centers administer a second dose 1 to 5 days after transplantation.[64] Other studied dosing strategies include 0.3 mg/kg per dose, as a single- or multiple-dose regimen, and, finally, two 20-mg doses given on the day of transplantation and the first postoperative day.[64]

Nondepleting Antibodies

Interleukin-2 Receptor Antagonists Basiliximab, a chimeric monoclonal antibody (25% murine) is the only available IL-2 receptor antagonist currently marketed in the United States. It is approved for use in kidney transplantation, but is also extensively used in other organ transplants as well.[66]

Pharmacology/Mechanism of Action Basiliximab exerts its immunosuppressive effect by specifically binding with high affinity to the α-chain (CD25) on the surface of activated T lymphocytes (see Fig. 89-1). Binding of basiliximab to the IL-2 receptor prevents IL-2-mediated activation and proliferation of T cells, a critical step in clonal expansion of T cells and the development of allograft rejection. Saturation of the IL-2 receptor occurs rapidly and confers an immunosuppressive effect that lasts for 4 to 6 weeks after administration.[66]

Pharmacokinetics Most of the pharmacokinetic data available for basiliximab was derived following administration to renal transplantation patients. Caution must be used when extrapolating these data to nonrenal transplantation recipients. The volume of distribution is approximately 8 L and it has a half-life of approximately 7 days. Clearance is increased in patients who have received a liver transplant, and therefore it is recommended that patients with greater than 10 L of ascites receive an additional dose of basiliximab on postoperative day 8.[67]

Efficacy Basiliximab is approved for use in kidney transplantation in combination with cyclosporine and corticosteroids, although induction therapy has also been studied extensively in liver and heart transplantation recipients. In 2012, over 20% of kidney, liver and heart transplant recipients received an IL-2 receptor antagonist at the time of transplant.[1] Use of basiliximab in liver transplant recipients has been increasing as a means of delaying CI initiation in the setting of acute kidney injury. A meta-analysis of basiliximab efficacy in renal transplantation concluded that IL-2 receptor antagonists reduced the risk of rejection significantly with no increases in graft loss, infectious complications, malignancy, or death.[66] Similar results were seen in liver and heart transplantation patients.[67]

IL-2 receptor antagonists offer a reasonable addition to calcineurin inhibitor—or corticosteroid-sparing protocols. While CI therapy cannot be completely avoided in most cases, IL-2 receptor antagonists allow for delayed use or reduced doses of CIs, thus minimizing the risk of nephrotoxicity in the early post-transplantation period. Similar rates of rejection and corticosteroid-resistant rejection were seen in patients with DGF who received an IL-2 receptor antagonist in conjunction with lower tacrolimus doses compared with patients without DGF who received standard tacrolimus doses and no IL-2 receptor inhibitor induction.[67]

Adverse Effects Few adverse effects have been reported with basiliximab. In contrast to lymphocyte-depleting agents, basiliximab has

TABLE 89-8 Factors Negatively Effecting Allograft and Patient Survival

	Kidney	Liver	Heart
Donor factors	Decreased HLA matching	Size mismatch	Size mismatch
		Age (youngest, oldest)	Increased age
	Increased age		Prolonged ischemia time
	Increased serum creatinine		
	Cardiac instability		
	Prolonged ischemia time		
	History of hypertension		
Recipient factors	Age <15, >50 years	Increased age	Age <5, >60 years
	Retransplantation	Retransplantation	ICU pretransplant
	African race	African race	Mechanical ventilation
	Elevated PRA	ICU pretransplant	
	Multiparous women	ABO blood type	LVAD
	Poor drug compliance	Poor drug compliance	IABP
			Poor drug compliance

HLA, human leukocyte antigens; IABP, intraaortic balloon pump; LVAD, left ventricular assist device; PRA, panel of reactive antibodies.

not been associated with infusion-related reactions. However, since the marketing of basiliximab, an increased number of hypersensitivity reactions have been reported. Of note, only one patient developed anti-idiotypic antibodies to the murine portion during clinical trials.[67] No increased risk of malignancy has been reported.

Drug–Drug and Drug–Food Interactions Reports of increased cyclosporine and tacrolimus levels in patients receiving concomitant basiliximab were recently published.[66]

Dosing and Administration Basiliximab is usually administered as two 20-mg intravenous doses, intraoperatively and again on postoperative day 4. Basiliximab is compatible with both 0.9% sodium chloride and 5% dextrose and can be administered either centrally or peripherally over 20 to 30 minutes in a volume of 50 mL. This regimen results in saturation of the IL-2 receptor for 30 to 45 days.

Investigational Agents

Rituximab Rituximab is a chimeric monoclonal antibody against the CD20 receptor found on B cells. While it is FDA approved for non-Hodgkin lymphoma and rheumatoid arthritis, it has also been used for the treatment of antibody mediated rejection and post-transplant lymphoproliferative disorder as well as suppression of alloantibodies prior to transplantation.[68] Rituximab has been shown to improve graft survival when given in combination with plasmapheresis and IVIG in patients with AMR.[26] In highly sensitized patients, rituximab administration prior to transplantation has been shown to suppress alloantibodies and even allow transplantation across ABO-incompatibility.[68] In PTLD, rituximab is most effective in patients with CD20 positive malignancies.[68] The optimal dose of rituximab in transplantation has not been defined.

Bortezomib Bortezomib, a proteosomal inhibitor that is FDA approved for the treatment of multiple myeloma, has been used in the treatment of AMR. In one series, 20 patients with AMR received 4 doses of bortezomib 1.3 mg/m^2 on days 1, 4, 7, and 11 with plasmapheresis. Bortezomib was effective in lowering donor specific antibodies by 50%.[26] Another series showed benefit of bortezomib over rituximab.[26] However, bortezomib is associated with a high incidence of side effects (up to 33% required hospitalization)that primarily effect the GI tract; diarrhea that leads to dehydration, nausea, edema, vomiting, and infections.[26]

Janus Kinase Inhibitors Janus kinases are important for transduction of intracellular signals in lymphocytes to stimulate proliferation and lymphocyte activity. Tofacitinib is a Janus Kinase 3 (JAK3) inhibitor that has been compared to cyclosporine in combination with mycophenolate mofetil and steroids. Tofacitinib showed similar efficacy to cyclosporine, but was associated with an increased incidence of cytomegalovirus and BK virus infections.[69] Clinical trials continue to evaluate long-term efficacy and safety of JAK3 inhibitors.

EVALUATION OF THERAPEUTIC OUTCOMES

8 The success of transplantation can be measured in terms of length of graft and patient survival as well as improvements in quality of life. Several donor and recipient factors that have an impact on graft and patient survival have been identified (Table 89-8). The greatest risk to short-term graft survival is acute rejection. Routine surveillance of appropriate biochemical markers and serum drug concentrations are essential to minimize the potential for acute rejection. These parameters should be assessed daily to weekly for the first 1 to 3 months after transplantation. Monitoring should include complete blood counts, serum electrolyte concentrations, serum creatinine and blood urea nitrogen concentrations, and the appropriate serum drug concentrations. Liver function tests should also be evaluated using the same schedule in liver transplantation recipients. Routine biopsies are necessary to monitor for acute rejection in heart transplantation recipients. As the time after transplantation increases, the frequency of monitoring decreases. Once 3 months have elapsed after transplantation, monitoring of these parameters can be reduced to biweekly or monthly for most patients. Table 89-9 depicts a typical post-transplantation laboratory monitoring plan.

Long-term graft survival is limited by chronic rejection. Overall survival rates for solid-organ transplantations are described in terms of half-life, or the time after transplantation at which only 50% of transplanted organs are still functioning. Estimated half-lives for kidneys are 26.9 years for HLA-identical grafts and 12.2 and 10.8 years, respectively, for grafts from a sibling or parent who are 1-haplotype matches. The estimated half-life for HLA-matched grafts was 17.3 years while a markedly lower value of 7.8 years has been noted with mismatched kidneys.[1] The overall median patient survival time for heart transplantation recipients is 9.8 years, but in these patients surviving the first year after transplantation, the median survival increases to 12 years.[1] The highest rate of mortality occurs within the first year after liver transplantation due to the risks of surgery and early postoperative complications.

TABLE 89-9 Laboratory Monitoring after Transplantation

	1-2 Weeks	1 Month	2-4 Months	4-12 Months	>12 Months
SCr/BUN	Daily	1-2 times per week	Every 1-2 weeks	Monthly	Every 1-2 months
Chemistries[a]	Daily	1-2 times per week	Every 1-2 weeks	Monthly	Every 1-2 months
Liver function tests[b]					
Kidney or heart recipient	Once	Once	Monthly	Every 1-3 months	Every 1-3 months
Liver recipient	Daily	1-3 times per week	Every 1-2 weeks	Monthly	Every 1-2 months
Immunosuppressant level	Daily	1-2 times per week	Every 1-2 weeks	Monthly	Every 1-2 months
Complete blood count[c]	Daily	1-2 times per week	Every 1–2 weeks	Monthly	Every 1-2 months
Lipid panel[d]	Once	Every 3 months	Every 3 months	Every 3 months	Every 3 months
HbA_{1c}	Once	Every 3 months	Every 3 months	Every 3 months	Every 3 months

BUN, blood urea nitrogen; HbA_{1c}, hemoglobin A1c; SCr infusion, serum creatinine.

[a]Chemistries include sodium, potassium, chloride, CO_2 content, magnesium, calcium, phosphorus, and blood glucose.

[b]Liver function tests include total bilirubin, aspartate transaminase (AST), alanine transaminase (ALT), gamma glutamyl transpeptidase (GGTP), alkaline phosphatase.

[c]Complete blood count includes white blood cells (WBC), red blood cells (RBC), platelets, and/or differential.

[d]Lipid panel includes total cholesterol, low-density lipoprotein (LDL), high-density lipoprotein (HDL), triglyceride, and/or very low-density lipoprotein (VLDL).

PERSONALIZED PHARMACOTHERAPY

Individualization of immunosuppression therapy starts with identifying the patient's risk of rejection prior to transplantation. Most clinicians will use induction therapy with a lymphocyte depleting agent for patients at high risk of rejection, including those patients who are sensitized to more HLA antigens due to previous exposure to blood products or previous transplant, younger patients and African Americans. Similarly, organs associated with a higher risk of rejection, including heart and lung transplants, require higher doses of immunosuppressants as maintenance therapy.

Therapeutic drug monitoring is a key component of individualizing the immunosuppressant regimen to ensure adequate immunosuppression is achieved while minimizing drug-related toxicities. Blood concentrations are routinely monitored for CIs and PSIs throughout the duration of therapy. Studies are ongoing to determine the correlation between blood concentrations and MPA. Consensus guidelines suggest that MPA monitoring may be warranted when MPA is used as the primary immunosuppressant, CI doses are reduced or discontinued, the patient has altered liver or kidney function, or medications that interact with MPA are administered concomitantly.[52]

Other patient-specific factors can influence CI pharmacokinetics and thus dosing requirements. Children require significantly higher CI doses on a mg/kg basis than do their adult counterparts, up to 3-fold higher in the youngest of patients. Advancing age appears to decrease CI requirements, presumably through increased absorption and decreased metabolic activity. Patients greater than 64 years required lower doses than younger recipients.[30] Beyond these factors, some transplant dependent factors can also impact immunosuppressant exposure. Ischemic reperfusion injury in the setting of liver transplantation has been shown to increase p-gP expression and thus decrease CI absorption whereas uremia seen in the setting of delayed graft function in renal transplantation is associated with decreased p-gP and thus higher CI levels.[30]

Pharmacogenetic assessment to optimize immunosuppressive therapy regimens is slowly emerging. Cytochrome P450 genetic polymorphisms are important for CI metabolism. Both cyclosporine and tacrolimus are metabolized by CYP3A5, which contributes to the interpatient variability associated with CIs. It is estimated that 30% of Caucasians and 50% of African Americans express high levels of CYP3A5 enzymes. Patients who express CYP3A5 require significantly higher doses of CIs to achieve therapeutic levels.[70] There are ethnic differences in CYP3A5 expressions that impact tacrolimus exposure as well as ultimate graft outcome. Up to 73% of patients of African descent express CYP3A5*1 which is associated with a 2-fold reduction in dose normalized tacrolimus levels, that is, patients require higher doses to achieve the same target as nonexpressers.[30] In African Americans who do not achieve target tacrolimus trough concentrations, the risks of antibody mediated rejection and ACR are significantly elevated.[71] Furthermore, one study suggests that African Americans may require monitoring of MPA levels due to more rapid clearance of MPA compared to Caucasians.[72] CYP3A5 genotyping may help to identify patients who require higher doses of CIs to optimize immunosuppressive therapy earlier after transplantation and potentially decrease the risk of rejection. However, larger studies are needed to determine the effectiveness of this strategy.

Pharmacodynamic monitoring of immunosuppressants of the specific targets of immunosuppressants rather than blood concentrations is in its infancy. Research is ongoing to determine the value of monitoring calcineurin activity for CIs[73] and IMPDH activity for MPA.[50]

Generic Substitution

In recent years a number of generic versions of immunosuppressants have entered the market. While generic versions of corticosteroids and azathioprine have long been available, there are now generic versions of cyclosporine, USP [MODIFIED], tacrolimus, and mycophenolate mofetil. While these formulations have demonstrated bioequivalence to the innovator product in healthy individuals, bioequivalence testing in transplant patients is not required for approval.[74]

Several potential factors including the complexity of the regimens and the impact of end organ disease could alter absorption and result in PK variability not seen in healthy volunteers. The presence of diabetes may delay gastric emptying, whereas cystic fibrosis may lead to differences in tacrolimus or cyclosporine secondary to fat malabsorption. Finally, none of the available generic formulations have been studied in pediatric patients.[75]

As generic medications may offer a significant cost advantage compared with the innovator product, their use will increase over time. Much of the concern with generic substitution for immunosuppressant and other narrow therapeutic index medications relates to the potential for increased or decreased systemic exposure that although within the "acceptable" regulatory range may put patients at risk because of inadequate maintenance of the desired serum concentrations. Systems that alert patients and prescribers to changes in formulation (eg, labels on medications, direct notification to physicians) could trigger clinicians to more closely monitor patients for efficacy and toxicity as well as heighten therapeutic drug monitoring during a switch. However, the extent to which increased monitoring could offset cost savings associated with generic substitution has not been fully delineated.

IMMUNOSUPPRESSION-RELATED COMPLICATIONS

Comorbidities such as cardiovascular disease and malignancy, recurrent disease, drug toxicities (namely nephrotoxicity), and chronic rejection are the primary causes of mortality in patients who have a functioning graft for 5 or more years after transplantation.[1]

Cardiovascular Disease

Cardiovascular disease is a leading cause of morbidity and mortality in transplant patients.[76] Hypertension, hyperlipidemia, and diabetes are common complications in transplantation recipients and are independent risk factors for cardiovascular disease. Chronic rejection has been linked to hypertension and hyperlipidemia.[37,76]

Hypertension

Corticosteroids, cyclosporine, tacrolimus, and impaired kidney graft function may cause post-transplantation hypertension. Calcineurin inhibitor-associated hypertension may be due to increased endothelin production as well as stimulation of the sympathetic and renin angiotensin systems.[77] In addition to the propensity to cause peripheral vasoconstriction, CIs promote sodium retention, resulting in extracellular fluid volume expansion. Tacrolimus appears to have less potential to induce hypertension following transplantation than cyclosporine.[36,78]

Calcium channel blockers have traditionally been the first-line agents to treat hypertension after transplantation.[29,79] They may ameliorate the nephrotoxic effects of cyclosporine, improve renal hemodynamics, decrease the incidence of DGF and the development of allograft atherosclerosis, and enhance the degree of immunosuppression.

ACEIs and angiotensin II receptor blockers have traditionally been avoided in kidney transplantation recipients, especially in the perioperative period, because of the potential for hyperkalemia and negative influence on glomerular filtration rate. They are now however, considered to be an equivalent alternative to calcium channel blockers for the treatment of hypertension in all transplant recipients, and are preferred in patients with proteinuria.[29] When ACEIs or angiotensin II receptor blockers are used in patients after transplantation, serum creatinine and potassium levels should be monitored closely. If the increase in serum creatinine is greater than 30% within 1 to 2 weeks after initiating ACEIs or angiotensin II receptor blockers, other alternatives must be considered (see Chapter 46).

Multiple antihypertensive agents are usually necessary to achieve the goal blood pressure in transplant recipients; consequently, the addition of a β-blocker, diuretic, or centrally acting antihypertensive may also be necessary. Beta-blockers are generally considered to be second-line therapy in solid-organ transplantation recipients because of the potential to worsen metabolic disturbances caused by immunosuppressants, such as hyperkalemia and dyslipidemia. Calcineurin inhibitor-induced hypertension is often salt-sensitive, making it very responsive to diuretics. Central-acting agents (eg, clonidine) are used often as adjunctive therapy in transplantation recipients who are unable to achieve blood pressure control with calcium channel blockers or ACEIs.

Hyperlipidemia

Hyperlipidemia may be exacerbated by corticosteroids, calcineurin inhibitors, sirolimus, diuretics, and β-blockers.[22,29] Corticosteroids promote insulin resistance and a decrease in lipoprotein lipase activity, as well as excessive triglyceride production. The mechanism of CIs may decrease the activity of the low-density lipoprotein (LDL) receptor or lipoprotein lipase, altering LDL catabolism.[22] Tacrolimus appears to have less potential than cyclosporine to induce hyperlipidemia.[36] It is controversial whether the management of hyperlipidemia in transplant recipients should be more aggressive than current guidelines for the general population.[29,79] (see Chapter 21) Aggressive lipid lowering may not only arrest the progress or prevent the complications of atherosclerosis but may also promote graft survival in kidney and heart transplant recipients. Current recommendations suggest monitoring lipid panels 2 to 3 months after transplantation and annually thereafter.[18,29]

HMG-CoA reductase inhibitors should be used with caution in transplantation recipients because of several reports of rhabdomyolysis when these agents are combined with calcineurin inhibitors.[41] However, beyond their impact on hyperlipidemia, HMG-CoA reductase inhibitors also have immunomodulatory effects on MHC expression and T-cell activation and reduce cardiac allograft rejection.[41]

Concurrent use of simvastatin and cyclosporine is contraindicated, due to the increased risk of rhabdomyolysis.[80] The concurrent use of medications known to increase the risk of myopathy (such as gemfibrozil) should be avoided.[41] Baseline and follow-up creatinine phosphokinase measurements (every 6 months) have proven useful to identify patients with subclinical rhabdomyolysis. Pravastatin may be preferred as a result of its lower interactive potential with CIs because it is not metabolized by CYP3A4. The potential for hepatotoxicity from HMG-CoA reductase inhibitors warrants close monitoring of liver function in all transplant recipients.[29,79]

Bile acid-binding resins may be used to lower cholesterol in transplant patients, but adequate doses are difficult to achieve without the development of GI adverse effects. Because the absorption of cyclosporine is dependent on the presence of bile in the GI tract, patients should be instructed to separate dosing of bile acid-binding resins and cyclosporine and most other immunosuppressants by at least 2 hours. For transplant patients who have hypertriglyceridemia refractory to dietary intervention, fish oil and fibric acid derivatives are well-tolerated, effective alternatives (see Chapter 21). Fibric acid derivatives are most effective in lowering serum triglyceride concentrations.

New-Onset Diabetes after Transplantation

Corticosteroids and CIs can impair glucose control in previously diabetic patients, as well as cause new-onset diabetes after transplantation (NODAT) in 5% to 30% of patients.[24,29] Corticosteroids induce insulin resistance and impair peripheral glucose uptake, whereas CIs appear to inhibit insulin production.[22] Tacrolimus seems to be more diabetogenic than cyclosporine, although recent studies have failed to show a statistical difference.[36] Other possible risk factors that have been identified for NODAT include African American or Hispanic ethnicity, age greater than 40 years at time of transplant, family history, and weight, as well as CMV and Hepatitis C virus infection.[22]

Up to 40% of patients with NODAT will require insulin therapy.[22] In diabetic patients who can be managed with an oral hypoglycemic agent, glipizide, which is metabolized extensively by the liver, may be preferred over renally eliminated agents such as glyburide. Metformin should be used with extreme caution because of the risk of lactic acidosis in those with moderate renal impairment. Frequent blood glucose monitoring is imperative in the early postoperative phase to improve glucose control and to identify those with NODAT. Changes in renal function secondary to CI nephrotoxicity or DGF or acute rejection in kidney transplant recipients affects the elimination of many hypoglycemic agents, including insulin, and may result in hyper- or hypoglycemia. Dose changes of immunosuppressant drugs also affect glycemic control. Tapering of immunosuppressive medications may result in reduced insulin requirements, whereas corticosteroid pulses for the treatment of rejection may result in increased insulin requirements.

Infection

Increased risk of infection is a natural consequence of therapeutic immunosuppression. Many infections, including cytomegalovirus and fungal infections, in solid organ transplant recipients are reviewed in Chapter 122.[81]

Polyomavirus-associated nephropathy (PVAN) is an important cause of renal dysfunction in kidney transplant recipients. Primary infection with BK virus occurs in childhood as an asymptomatic infection in 50% to 90% of the general population. The precise mechanism of transmission is not clear but is suspected to be via the oral or respiratory routes. The virus may remain latent primarily in the genitourinary tract until reactivation as the result of compromised immune function and is common in kidney transplant recipients. Reactivation can be detected by measuring the presence of BK virus in the urine, a finding that is seen in approximately 30% to 40% of kidney transplant recipients, although it does not progress to nephropathy in the majority of patients. However, BK viremia if it develops has been noted to progress to allograft nephropathy in 50% of patients.[80] The development of BK virus nephropathy results in graft loss in about 46% of effected patients.[81]

It has been recommended that all kidney transplant recipients be screened for urinary BK virus replication monthly for the first 3 to 6 months after transplant and every 3 months thereafter for the first year.[29,81] Screening for BK virus presence in serum should also occur any time the serum creatinine is elevated without known cause and after treatment of acute rejection.[29] Treatment of BK virus should be initiated when plasma concentrations persist above 10,000 copies/mL (10×10^6/L).[29,81,82] The first line of treatment is to reduce immunosuppressive medications. Other treatment strategies include the addition of cidofovir, leflunomide, or fluoroquinolones, although studies with these agents are limited.[82]

Hepatitis C virus (HCV) recurs almost universally following liver transplantation and the course of the disease is accelerated. Within 5 years, 10% to 20% of liver transplant recipients with HCV recurrence will progress to cirrhosis requiring retransplantation, compared to the general population where 20% to 30% will develop cirrhosis over 20 to 30 years. Recipient risk factors for recurrence include HCV viremia either before or in the first 3 month post-transplant, interleukin-28B TT genotype, and female sex. Advanced donor age and the presence of graft steatosis have also been associated with HCV progression.[10,84] Recommendations for the treatment of HCV were developed in 2014 by the American Association for the Study of Liver Diseases and the Infectious Disease Society of America and continue to rapidly evolve. [85] Additionally pretransplant antiviral therapy may reduce the risk of recurrent HCV post-liver transplant.[83] First generation direct acting antivirals (DAA) boceprevir and telaprevir have significant drug interactions with both CIs and PSIs, and have largely been replaced by the latter generation DAAs. Management of drug–drug interactions with immunosuppressants and the DAAs is an important consideration for clinicians. The ritonavir-boosted combination of ombitasvir/paritaprevir and dasabuvir (Viekira Pak) resulted in a 57-fold increase is tacrolimus AUC, whereas the same combination caused a 5.8-fold increase in cyclosporine AUC. Simeprevir, an intestinal CYP3A4 and p-glycoprotein inhibitor, is contraindicated with cyclosporine-based regimens due to a 6-fold increase in simeprevir exposure when coadministered with cyclosporine. Conversely, ledipasvir, sofosbuvir and daclatasvir do not appear to significantly impact immunosuppressant concentrations. Ribavirin does not have any direct pharmacokinetic interactions with immunosuppressants, however, clinicians should note the overlapping toxicities, especially anemia as well as the need to adjust doses of ribavirin in patients with reduced kidney function. The DAAs have been generally well-tolerated, but simeprevir and ombitasvir/paritaprevir/ritonavir should be used in patients with Child-Pugh class B or C liver disease.[85]

In the absence of preventative therapy, hepatitis B recurs in approximately 80% of patients after transplantation. Initial studies with short-term intravenous administration of hepatitis B immunoglobulin (HBIg) showed equally high rates of recurrence upon discontinuation of therapy. However, strategies that employ the long-term administration of HBIg with or without antiviral therapy report much lower recurrence rates, 15% to 30% and 20% to 40%, for nonreplicative and replicative hepatitis B virus, respectively.[87] Common strategies include intravenous HBIg 10,000 units during the anhepatic phase followed by 10,000 units daily for 6 days. Antihepatitis B surface titer should be monitored weekly to ensure adequate levels for protection as well as to optimize HBIg use. HBIg has been typically dosed to maintain titers greater than 100 to 500 international units/L. Long-term HBIg therapy is extremely costly, estimated at $100,000 for the first postoperative year and $50,000 for each subsequent year. Combination therapy with antiviral agents appears to be synergistic and is the current standard. Lamivudine resistance is a concern with long-term utilization both pre- and post-transplant. The role of newer antiviral agents, including adefovir, entecavir, and tenofovir, remains to be defined. Treatment for active hepatitis B virus graft infection should include HBIg, antiviral therapy, and concomitant reduction in immunosuppression.[87]

Malignancy

Although advances in immunosuppression have decreased the incidence of acute rejection and increased patient survival, they have also increased the patient's lifetime exposure to immunosuppression. While the precise mechanism is unclear, post-transplantation malignancy seems to be related to the overall level of immunosuppression, as evidenced by a difference in the rates of malignancy associated with quadruple versus triple versus dual immunosuppressant regimens. The risk of de novo malignancy in transplantation recipients is increased threefold to fivefold over the general population.[50] The risk of lung and colon cancers may be as much as doubled in renal transplant recipients.[88] A number of cancers that are uncommon in the general population occur with much higher prevalence in transplantation recipients: post-transplantation lymphomas and lymphoproliferative disorders (PTLDs), Kaposi sarcoma, renal carcinoma, in situ carcinomas of the uterine cervix, hepatobiliary tumors, and anogenital carcinoma are a few examples.[88] Skin cancers are the most common tumors. Factors that may predispose transplant recipients to skin cancers include copious sun exposure and therapy with azathioprine.[50] While too early to definitively assess the impact of MPA derivatives on malignancy, one analysis showed a lower risk of PTLD with MMF compared with AZA.[50] Proliferation signal inhibitors have a theoretical benefit in terms of the development of malignancy. In addition to immunosuppressive properties, PSIs also have antiproliferative effects. In fact, a decreased incidence of malignancy was reported in patients receiving PSIs versus CIs, and conversion to PSIs from CIs can result in regression of Kaposi sarcoma.[88]

PTLD encompasses a broad spectrum of disorders, ranging from benign polyclonal hyperplasia to malignant monoclonal lymphomas. Factors that predispose patients to PTLD include Epstein-Barr virus seronegativity at transplantation and intense immunosuppression, particularly with lymphocyte depleting agents. Nonrenal transplantation recipients are more likely to develop PTLD secondary to the intensive immunosuppression used to reverse rejection. Administration of ganciclovir or acyclovir preemptively during antilymphocyte therapy may decrease the risk of EBV seroconversion and infection, reducing the eventual risk of PTLD. Treatment of life-threatening PTLD generally includes severe reduction or cessation of immunosuppression. Other options include systemic chemotherapy or rituximab.[88]

Post-transplantation malignancies appear an average of 5 years after transplantation and increase with the length of follow-up. As many as 72% of patients surviving greater than 20 years may be effected. Malignancy accounts for 11.8% of deaths after cardiac transplantation and is the single most common cause of death in the 6th to the 10th post-transplant years.[88]

CLINICAL BOTTOM LINE

Transplantation is a lifesaving therapy for several types of end-organ failure. Advances in the understanding of transplant immunology have produced an unprecedented number of choices in terms of immunosuppression. The increasing number of effective immunosuppressive therapies offers clinicians diverse ways to prevent allograft rejection.

However, the vast array of currently available immunosuppressive agents make it increasingly difficult to evaluate their long-term efficacy. Clinicians must be keenly aware of the adverse effects of immunosuppressive medications and their management in order to optimize the care of the transplanted patient.

ABBREVIATIONS

ACEI	angiotensin-converting enzyme inhibitor
ACR	acute cellular rejection
AMR	antibody-mediated rejection
ATG	antithymocyte globulin
ATN	acute tubular necrosis
AUC	area under the concentration curve
C_2	concentration 2 hours after dose
C_{peak}	peak concentration
CI	calcineurin inhibitors
CMV	cytomegalovirus
CYP	cytochrome P450 liver enzyme system
DAA	direct acting antivirals
DGF	delayed graft function
EBV	Epstein Barr virus
FKBP	FK-binding protein
GI	gastrointestinal
HBIg	hepatitis B immunoglobulin
HLA	human leukocyte antigen
HMGCoA	hydroxy-3-methylglutaryl-coenzyme A
HPLC	high-performance liquid chromatography
IFTA	interstitial fibrosis and tubular atrophy
IL	interleukin
IMPDH	inosine monophosphate dehydrogenase
LAS	lung allocation score
LDL	low-density lipoprotein
MELD	model for end-stage liver disease
MHC	major histocompatibility complex
6-MP	6-mercaptopurine
MPA	mycophenolic acid
MPAG	mycophenolic acid glucuronide
MRP2	multidrug-resistance-associated protein 2
mTOR	mammalian target of rapamycin
NODAT	new-onset diabetes after transplantation
OATP	organic anion-transporter proteins
OKT3	muromonab-CD3
PML	progressive multifocal leukoencephalopathy
PRA	panel of reactive antibodies
PSI	proliferation signal inhibitor
PTLD	post-transplantation lymphoproliferative disorder
PVAN	polyomavirus associated nephropathy
RIA	radioimmunoassay
REMS	risk evaluation and mitigation strategy
TPMT	thiopurine S-methyltransferase

REFERENCES

1. Organ Procurement and Transplantation Network (OPTN) and Scientific Registry of Transplant Recipients (SRTR). OPTN/SRTR 2012 Annual Data Report. Rockville, MD: Department of Health and Human Services, Health Resources and Services Administration, Healthcare Systems Bureau, Division of Transplantation; 2014.
2. Alloway RR, Dupuis R, Gabardi A. Evolution of the role of the transplant pharmacist on the multidisciplinary transplant team. *Am J Transplant* 2011;11:1576-1583.
3. Rana A, Gruessner A, Agopian VG, et al. Survival benefit of solid-organ transplant in the United States. *JAMA Surg* 2015;150:252-259.
4. Working Group on Incentives for Living Donation. Incentives for organ donation: Proposed standards for an internationally acceptable system. *Am J Transplant* 2012;12:306-312.
5. Tritto G, Davies NA, Jalan R. Liver replacement therapy. *Semin Respir Crit Care Med* 2012;33(1):70-79.
6. U.S. Renal Data System, USRDS 2012 Annual Data Report: Atlas of Chronic Kidney Disease and End-Stage Renal Disease in the United States. Bethesda, MD: National Institutes of Health, National Institute of Diabetes and Digestive and Kidney Diseases; 2012.
7. Kovacs AZ, Molnar MZ, Szeifert L, et al. Sleep disorders, depressive symptoms and health-related quality of life—A cross-sectional comparison between kidney transplant recipients and waitlisted patients on maintenance dialysis. *Nephrol Dial Transplant* 2011;26:1058-65.
8. Quante M, Benckert C, Thelen A, Jonas S. Experience since MELD implementation: How does the new system deliver? *Int J Hepatol* 2012;2012:264015. PubMed PMID: 23091734.
9. Mathurin P, Moren C, Samuel D, et al. Early liver transplantation for sever alcoholic hepatitis. *New Engl J Med* 2011;365:1790-1800.
10. Sheiner P, Rochon C. Recurrent hepatitis C after liver transplantation. *Mt Sinai J Med* 2012;79:190-198.
11. McCalmont V, Ohler L. Cardiac transplantation: Candidate identification, evaluation, and management. *Crit Care Nurs* 2008;31(3):216-229.
12. Hartert M, Senbaklavaci O, Gohrbandt B, et al. Lung transplantation: A treatment option in end-stage lung disease. *Dtsch Artebl Int* 2014;11:107-116.
13. Deng MC. Heart failure: Cardiac transplantation. *Heart* 2002;87:177-184.
14. Braith RW, Edwards DG. Exercise following heart transplantation. *Sports Med* 2000;30:171-192.
15. Wagner SJ and Brennan DC. Induction therapy in renal transplant recipients: How convincing is the current evidence. *Drugs* 2012;72:671-683.
16. Siedlecki A, Irish W, and Brennan DC. Delayed graft function in the kidney transplant. *Am J Transplant* 2011;11:2279-2296.
17. Venkataramanan R, Habucky K, Burckart GJ, et al. Clinical pharmacokinetics in organ transplant patients. *Clin Pharmacokinet* 1989;16:134-161.
18. Costanzo MR, Dipchand A, Starling R, et al. The International Society of Heart and Lung Transplantation guidelines for the care of heart transplant recipients. *J Heart Lung Transplant* 2010;29(8):914-956.
19. Thompson ML, Flynn JD, Clifford TM. Pharmacotherapy of lung transplantation: An overview. *J Pharm Pract* 2012;26:5-13.
20. Ingulli E. Mechanism of cellular rejection in transplantation. *Pediatr Nephrol* 2010;25(1):61-74.
21. http://optn.transplant.hrsa.gov/learn/about-transplantation/how-organ-allocation-works. (Accessed November 10, 2015)
22. Lucey MR, Terrault N, Ojo L, et al. Long-term management of the successful adult liver transplant: 2012 Practice guideline by the American Association for the Study of Liver Diseases and the American Society of Transplantation. *Liver Transplant* 2013;19:3-26.
23. Stehlik J, Edwards LB, Kucheryavaya AY, et al. Registry of the international society for heart and lung transplantation: 29th official adult heart transplant report—2012. *J Heart Lung Transplant* 2012;31(10):1052-1064.
24. Haas M. Pathologic features of antibody-mediated rejection in renal allografts: An expanding spectrum. *Curr Opin Nephrol Hypertens* 2012;21(3):264-271.
25. Fehr T, Gaspert A. Antibody-mediated kidney allograft rejection: Therapeutic options and their experimental rationale. *Transplant Internat* 2012;25:623-632.
26. Kim M, Martin ST, Townsend KR, and Gabardi S. Antibody-mediated rejection in kidney transplantation: A review of

pathophysiology, diagnosis, and treatment options. *Pharmacotherapy* 2014;34:733-744.

27. Birnbaum LM, Lipman M, Paraskevas S, et al. Management of chronic allograft neprhropathy: A systematic review. *Clin J Am Soc Nephr* 2009;4:800-865.
28. Schmauss D, Weis M. Cardiac allograft vasculopathy: Recent developments. *Circulation* 2008;117;2131-2141.
29. Kasiske BL, Zeier MG, Chapman JR, et al. KDIGO clinical practice guideline for the care of kidney transplant recipients. *Kidney Internat* 2009;9(Suppl 3):S1-S155.
30. Knops N, Levtchenko E, van den Heuvel B, and Kuypers D. From gut to kidney: Transporting and metabolizing calcineurin-inhibitors in solid organ transplantation. *Int J Pharmaceutics* 2013;452:14-35.
31. Malat GE, Culkin C, Palya A, Panganna K, Anil Kumar MS. African American kidney transplantation survival: The ability of immunosuppression to balance the inherent pre- and post-transplant risk factors. *Drugs* 2009;69(15):2045-2062.
32. Deeks ED and Keating GM. Rabbit antithymocyte globulin: A review of its use in the prevention and treatment of acute renal allograft rejection. *Drugs* 2009;69:1483-1512.
33. Spriet I, Meersseman W, deHoon J, von Winckelmann S, Wilmer A, Willems L. Mini-series, II: Clinical aspects. Clinically relevant CYP450-mediated drug interactions in the ICU. *Intensive Care Med* 2009;35:603-612.
34. Kuypers DRJ. Immunotherapy in elderly transplant recipients: A guide to clinically significant drug interactions. *Drugs Aging* 2009;26:715-737.
35. Effect of Concomitant Drug Administration on Immunosuppressant Agents, Trofe-Clark J, Lemonovich TL, and The AST Infectious Diseases Community of Practice. Interaction between anti-infective agents and immunosuppressants in solid organ transplantation. *Am J Transplant* 2013;13:318-326.
36. Lee RA and Gabardi S. Current trends in immunosuppressive therapies for renal transplant recipients. *Am J Health-Syst Pharm* 2012;69:1961-1975.
37. Lane JT and Dogogo-Jack S. Approach to the patient with new-onset diabetes after transplant (NODAT). *J Clin Endocrinol Metab* 2011;96:3289-3297.
38. Naesans M, Kuypers DR, Sarwal M. Calcineurin inhibitor nephrotoxicity. *Clin J Am Soc Nephrol* 2009;2:481-508.
39. Chisholm MA, Mulloy LL, Jagadeesan M, et al. Coadministration of tacrolimus with anti-acid drugs. *Transplantation* 2003;76:665-666.
40. Amundsen R, Asberg A, Ohm IK, Christensen H. Cyclosporine A- and tacrolimus-mediated inhibition of CYP3A4 and CYP3A5 in vitro. *Drug Metab Disp* 2012;40(4):665-661.
41. Olyaei A, Greer E, Santos RD, Rueda J. The efficacy and safety of 3-hydrocy-3-methylglutarul-CoA reductase inhibitors in chronic kidney disease, dialysis, and transplant patients. *Clin J Am Soc Nephrol* 2011;6(3):664-678.
42. Amundsen R, Christensen H, Zagihyan B, Åsberg A. Cyclosporine A, but not tacrolimus, shows relevant inhibition of organic anion-transporting protein 1B1-mediated transport of atorvastatin. *Drug Metab Disp* 2010;38(9):1499-1504.
43. Schiff J, Cole E, Cantarovich M. Therapeutic monitoring of calcineurin inhibitors for the nephrologist. *Clin J Am Soc Nephrol* 2007;2:374-384.
44. Kuypers DRJ. Immunosuppressive drug monitoring—What to use in clinical practice today to improve renal graft outcome. *Transpl Intl* 2005;18:140-150.
45. Envarsus XR® (tacrolimus extended-release tablets) [product information]. Edison, NJ: Veloxis Pharmaceuticals Inc.; 2015.
46. Cross SA and Perry CM. Tacrolimus once-daily formulation: In the prophylaxis of transplant rejection in renal or liver allograft recipients. *Drugs* 2007;67:1931-1943.
47. Bergmann TK, Barraclough KA, Lee KJ, and Staatz CE. Clinical pharmacokinetics and pharmacodynamics of prednisolone and prednisone in solid organ transplantation. *Clin Pharmacokinet* 2012;51:711-741.
48. Pascual J, Rouuela A, Galeano C, Crespo M, Zamora J. Very early steroid withdrawal or complete avoidance for kidney transplant recipients: A systematic review. *Nephrol Dial Transplant* 2012;27:825-832.
49. de Jonge H, Naesense M, Kuypers DRJ. New insights into the pharmacokinetics and pharmacodynamics of the calcineurin inhibitors and mycophenolic acid: Possible consequences for therapeutic drug monitoring in solid organ transplantation. *Ther Drug Monit* 2009;31(4):416-435.
50. Staatz CE and Tett SE. Pharmacology and toxicology of mycophenolate in organ transplant recipients: An update. *Arch Toxicol* 2014;88:1351-1389.
51. Rupprecht K, Schmidt C, Raspe A, et al. Bioavailability of mycophenolate mofetil and enteric-coated mycophenolate sodium is differently affected by pantoprazole in healthy volunteers. *J Clin Pharmacol* 2009;49(10):1196-1201.
52. Kuypers DRJ, Le Meur Y, Cantarovich M, et al. Consensus report on therapeutic drug monitoring of mycophenolic acid in solid organ transplantation. *Clin J Am Soc Nephrol* 2010;5:341-358.
53. Van Gelder T, van Schaik RH, and Hesselink DA. Pharmacogentetics and immunosuppressive drugs in solid organ transplantation. *Nat Rev Nephrol* 2014;10:725-731.
54. Imuran® (azathioprine) [product information]. San Diego, CA: Prometheus Laboratories Inc; 2011.
55. Shihab F, Christians U, Smith L, et al. Focus on mTor inhibitors and tacrolimus in renal transplantation: Pharmacokinetics, exposure-response relationships, and clinical outcomes. *Transplant Immunol* 2014;31:22-32.
56. Monchaud C, Marquet P. Pharmacokinetic optimization of immunosuppressive therapy in thoracic transplantation: Part II. *Clin Pharmacokinet* 2009;48:489-516.
57. Dantal J. Everolimus: Preventing organ rejection in adult kidney transplant recipients. *Expert Opin Pharmacother* 2012;13(5):767-778.
58. Kawahara T, Asthana S, Kneteman NM. m-TOR inhibitors: What role in liver transplantation? *J Hepatol* 2011;55:1441-1451.
59. Vincenti F, Rostaint L, Grinyo J, et al. Belatacept and long-term outcomes in kidney transplantation. N Engl J Med 2016;374:333-343.
60. Masson P, Jenderson I, Chapman JR, et al. Belatacept for kidney transplant recipients. *Cochrane Database Syst Rev* 2014;11:1-65.
61. Rostaing L, Massari P, Garcia VD, et al. Switching from calcineurin inhibitor-based regimens to a belatacept-based regimen in renal transplant recipients: A randomized phase II study. *Clin J Am Soc Nephrol* 2011;6:430-39.
62. Nulojix® (belatacept) [product information]. Princeton, NJ: Bristol-Myers Squibb Company; 2011.
63. LaMattina JC, Jason MP, Hanish SI, et al. Safety of belatacept bridging immunosuppression in hepatitis C-positive liver transplant recipients with renal dysfunction. *Transplantation* 2014;97:133-137.
64. Morgan RD, O'Callaghan JM, Knight SR, and Morris PJ. Alemtuzumab induction therapy in kidney transplantation: A systematic review and meta-analysis. *Transplantation* 2012;93:1179-1188.
65. www.campath.com. (Accessed November 2015)
66. McKeage K, McCormack PL. Basiliximab: A review of its use as induction therapy in renal transplantation. *Drugs* 2010;24(1):55-76.
67. Ramirez CB, Bozdin A, Frank A, et al. Optimizing use of basiliximab in liver transplantation. *Tranplant Res Risk Manage* 2010;2:1-10.
68. Ramanath V, Nistala R, Chaudhary K. Update on the role of rituximab in kidney diseases and transplant. *Expert Opin Biol Ther* 2012;12(2):223-233.
69. Wojciechowski D, Vincenti F. Tofacitinib in kidney transplantation. *Expert Opin Investig Drugs* 2013;22:1193-1199.
70. Barry A, Levine M. A systematic review of the effect of CYP3A5 genotype on the apparent oral clearance of tacrolimus in renal transplant recipients. *Ther Drug Monit* 2010;32(6):708-714.
71. Taber DJ, Gebregziabher MG, Srinivas TR, et al. African American Race modifies the influence of tacrolimus concentration on acute rejection and toxicity in kidney transplant recipients. *Pharmacotherapy*, 2015;35:569-577.
72. Tornatore KM, Sudchada P, Dole K, et al. Mycophenolic acid pharmacokinetics during maintenance immmunosuprpession in African American and Caucasian renal transplant patients. *J Clin Pharmacol* 2011;51:1213-1222.
73. van Rossum HH, de Fijter JW, van Pelt J. Pharmacodynamic monitoring of calcineurin inhibition therapy: Principles, performance, and perspectives. *Ther Drug Monit* 2010;32(1):3-10.
74. Christians U, Klawitter J, Clavijo CF. Bioequivalence testing of immunosuppressants: Concepts and misconceptions. *Kidney Int* 2010;77:S1-S7.
75. Uber PA, Ross HJ, Zuckermann AO, et al. Generic drug immunosuppression in thoracic transplantation: An ISHLT educational advisory. *J Heart Lung Transplant* 2009;28:655-660.
76. Webber A, Hirose R, Vincenti F. Novel strategies in immunosuppression: Issues in perspective. *Transplantation* 2011;91:1057-1064.
77. Weir MR and Salzberg DJ. Management of hypertension in the transplant patient. *J Am Soc Hypertension* 2011;5:425-432.

78. James PA, Oparil S, Carter BL, et al. 2014 Evidence-based guideline for the management of high blood pressure in adults: Report from the panel members appointed to the eighth joint national committee (JNC 8). *JAMA* 2014;311:507-520.
79. Florentin M, Elisaf MS. Simvastatin interactions with other drugs. *Expert Opin Drug Safety* 2012;11(3):439-444.
80. Grim SA and Clark. Management of infectious complications in solid-organ transplant recipients. *Clin Phar Ther* 2011:90:333-342.
81. Hirsch HH, Randhawa P, and The AST Infectious Diseases Community of Practice. BK virus in solid organ transplant recipients. *Am J Transplant* 2009;9:S136-S146.
82. Dharnidharka VR, Abdulnour HA, Araya CE. The BK virus in renal transplant recipients—Review of pathogenesis, diagnosis, and treatment. *Pediatr Nephrol* 2011;26:1763-1774.
83. Martin P, DiMartini A, Feng S, et al. Evaluation for liver transplantation in adults: 2013 Practice guideline by the AASLD and the American Society of Transplantation. *Hepatology* 2014;59:1144-1165.
84. Mitchell O and Gurakar A. Management of hepatitis C post-liver transplantation: A comprehensive review. *J Clin Translat Hepatol* 2015;3:140-148.
85. www.hcvguidelines.org. (Accessed November 2015)
86. Marino Z, Londono MC, and Forns X. Hepatitis C treatment for patients post liver transplant. *Curr Opin Organ Transplant* 2015;20:251-258.
87. Cholangitas E, Goulis J, Akriviadis E, Papatheodoridis GV. Hepatitis B immunoglobulin and/or nucleos(t)ide analogues for prophylaxis against hepatitis b virus recurrence after liver transplantation: A systematic review. *Liver Transplant* 2011;17(10):1176-1190.
88. Bottomley MJ and Harden PN. Update on the long-term complications of renal transplantation. *Br Med Bull* 2013;106:117-134.

90 Osteoarthritis

Lucinda M. Buys and Sara A. Wiedenfeld

KEY CONCEPTS

1. Millions of Americans have osteoarthritis (OA). OA prevalence increases with age and number of other chronic conditions, with women more commonly affected than men.
2. Contributors to OA are systemic (age, genetics, hormonal status, obesity, occupational, or recreational activity) and/or local (injury, overloading of joints, muscle weakness, or joint deformity).
3. OA is primarily a disease of cartilage that reflects a failure of the chondrocyte to maintain proper balance between cartilage formation and destruction. This leads to loss of cartilage in the joint, local inflammation, pathologic changes in underlying bone, and further damage to cartilage triggered by the affected bone.
4. The most common symptom associated with OA is pain, which leads to decreased function and motion. Pain relief is the primary objective of medication therapy.
5. Manifestations of OA are local, affecting one or a few joints; the knees are most commonly affected, as well as the hips and hands. Osteophytes (bony proliferation of affected joints) are often found, in contrast to the soft tissue swelling of rheumatoid arthritis.
6. Nonpharmacologic therapy is the foundation of the treatment plan for all patients with OA. Nonpharmacologic therapy should be initiated before or concurrently with pharmacologic therapy.
7. Based upon efficacy, safety, and cost considerations, scheduled acetaminophen, up to 4 g/day, should be tried initially for pain relief in knee and hip OA. If this fails, topical or oral nonsteroidal anti-inflammatory drugs (NSAIDs) are recommended, if there are no contraindications.
8. To decrease the risks of systemic toxicity, topical NSAIDs are recommended for patients older than 75 years.
9. Strategies to reduce NSAID-induced gastrointestinal (GI) toxicity include the use of nonacetylated salicylates, cyclooxygenase-2 (COX-2) selective inhibitors, or the addition of misoprostol or a proton pump inhibitor (PPI).
10. Other agents useful in treating knee OA include tramadol, intra-articular injections of corticosteroids, or duloxetine.

Osteoarthritis (OA) is the most common joint disease and is one of the leading causes of disability in the United States.[1,2] Knee OA alone is as important a contributor to disability as cardiovascular disease and more important than other comorbidities. OA is a common co-occurrence with other chronic health conditions that adversely affect quality of life.[1]

The progressive destruction of articular cartilage has long been appreciated in OA, but OA involves the entire diarthrodial joint, including articular cartilage, synovium, capsule, and subchondral bone, with surrounding ligaments and muscles also playing important roles. Changes in structure and function of these tissues produce clinical OA, characterized by joint pain and tenderness, with decreased range of motion, weakness, joint instability, and disability.

This chapter will review the epidemiology, etiology, pathogenesis, and diagnosis of OA. It will then focus on nonpharmacologic and pharmacologic treatments for OA. As millions of persons take medications for OA, the overall risks posed by these medications require careful consideration, particularly by clinicians who treat or advise patients on drug therapy for OA. This chapter examines the risks and benefits of OA treatments, with emphasis on those individuals who have the highest risk for adverse events, to help clinicians maximize benefit and minimize risks to their patients with OA.

EPIDEMIOLOGY

1 In 2010-2012, an estimated 52.5 million adults in the United States reported physician-diagnosed arthritis (OA, rheumatoid arthritis, gout, lupus or fibromyalgia) with 22.7 million reporting arthritis-attributable activity limitation (AAAL).[3] This represents an increase from 49.9 million adults in 2007-2009.[3] These rates are more than doubled from 21 million adults in 1995.[4] Prevalence of AAAL is expected to increase to 22 million in the United States by 2020, and an estimated 67 million persons will have OA by 2030.[2,3] OA imposes a tremendous cost burden, with total hospital costs in 2011 for care associated with a diagnosis of OA reaching approximately $15 billion and nearly 1 million OA-related hospital discharges.[5] The vast majority of these costs are related to knee- and hip-replacement surgery.[5] In 2012, medical expenses for treatment of OA and other nontraumatic joint disorders totaled $73.8 billion.[6] It is estimated that each individual with knee OA will use nearly $130,000 on total direct medical costs with 10% of the total attributable to OA over their lifetime.[7]

Prevalence By Age, Gender, and Race

Prevalence estimates for OA vary depending on the age group of interest, gender, ethnic group, and the specific joint involved. Estimates also depend on the specific means by which OA is assessed and documented. Clinical OA is based on physical examination and patient history, whereas radiographic OA is determined by x-ray or other imaging, and symptomatic OA is based on history and physical examination plus x-ray OA is more prevalent with increasing age.[2]

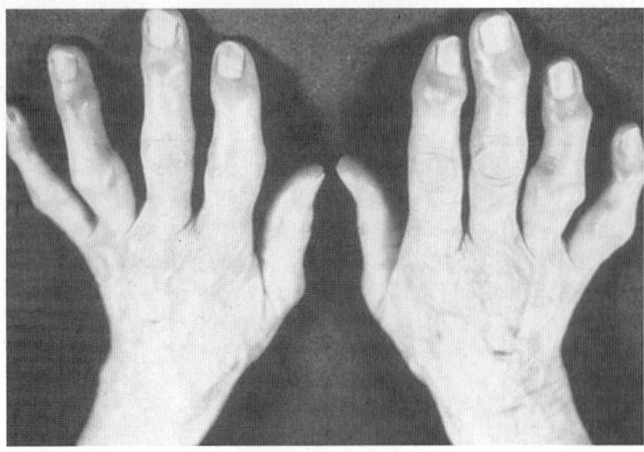

FIGURE 90-1 Heberden nodes (distal interphalangeal joint) noted on all fingers and Bouchard nodes (proximal interphalangeal joint) noted on most fingers. *(Reproduced with permission from Johnson BE. Chapter 23. Arthritis: Osteoarthritis, Gout, & Rheumatoid Arthritis. In: South-Paul JE, Matheny SC, Lewis EL. eds. CURRENT Diagnosis & Treatment in Family Medicine, 3e. New York, NY: McGraw-Hill; 2011.)*

In the United States, prevalence of self-reported doctor-diagnosed arthritis in the 2012 National Health Interview Survey (NHIS) is 22.7% for all persons over age 18, but 49.7% for persons age 65 and older.[3] Prevalence for AAAL among persons with doctor-diagnosed arthritis is 43.2% for all persons over age 18, and 44.4% for persons age 65 and older.[3] Radiologically confirmed hip OA shows clear trends through all age groups, affecting 1.6% of those between ages 30 to 39, up to a prevalence of 14% in those older than 85 years.[8] Radiographic hand OA is found in 5% of those aged 40, but in 65% of those older than 80 years.[9]

Prevalence of doctor-diagnosed arthritis is 25.9% in white populations, and ranges from 4.9% for Asian populations to 21.3% for black populations.[3] African-American men are approximately 35% more likely to have radiographic knee OA and twice as likely to have more severe knee OA than Caucasian men.[10] No significant differences were found between the prevalence of knee OA in African-American women and Caucasian women, but African-American women were 50% more likely than Caucasian women to have more severe involvement.[10] Before age 50, men are more likely to have OA than women, attributed to higher rates of sports and other injuries. Women exhibit a higher prevalence of hip and knee OA than men, and are at especially greater risk for hand OA, with 26% of women and 12% of men over age 70 affected.[9] Women are also more likely to have inflammatory OA of the proximal and distal interphalangeal joints of the hands, giving rise to the formation of Bouchard and Heberden nodes, respectively (Fig. 90–1).

Incidence

The incidence of symptomatic OA determined in a large HMO was 100 per 100,000 patient years for hand OA, 88 per 100,000 patient years for hip OA, and 240 per 100,000 patient years for knee OA.[8] As the incidence of a disease describes the number of newly diagnosed cases each year, OA poses a challenging situation for determining disease incidence. These reasons include: (1) not all patients with OA seek medical treatment, (2) OA is very common within the population, (3) not all radiographically diagnosed OA is symptomatic, and (4) many patients have multiple affected joints.

ETIOLOGY

2 The etiology of OA is multifactorial and complex, with development of OA depending on interplay between factors such as genetic predisposition and joint injury.[11,12] Many patients have more than one risk factor for the development of OA. The most common risk factors for the development of OA include age, obesity, sex, occupation, participation in certain sports, history of joint injury or surgery, and genetic predisposition.

Obesity

Obesity is the most important preventable risk factor for OA. This linkage is strongest for knee OA, although hip OA and even hand and wrist OA may be linked with obesity. As the epidemic of obesity spreads in the United States and in other developed countries, so will the burdens imposed by OA will continue to increase. Obesity often precedes OA and contributes to its development, rather than occurring as a result of inactivity from joint pain.[13] In an 11-year study of approximately 30,000 Norwegian men and women, obesity significantly increased the risk of developing OA.[14] Men who were obese at baseline had a 2.8-fold increase in developing knee OA compared with the non-obese men, whereas women who were obese at baseline had a 4.4-fold increased risk in developing knee OA compared with non-obese women. Also, there was an increased risk for severe knee OA in obese subjects. In addition to being a risk factor for OA, obesity is also a predictor for eventual prosthetic joint replacement. In a US study, women who were obese at age 18 were at increased risk of undergoing hip replacement surgery in later life.[2] The risk of developing OA increases by approximately 10% with each additional kilogram of weight, and in obese persons without OA, weight loss of even 5 kg (11 lbs) decreases the risk of future knee OA by half.[13]

Occupation, Sports, and Trauma

OA risk is increased for people in occupations involving excessive mechanical stress. Work that involves prolonged standing, kneeling, squatting, lifting, or moving of heavy objects increases risk of OA. Such occupations include construction, mining, healthcare assistance, factory work, carpentry, and farming.[2,11] Repetitive motion also contributes to hand OA, with the dominant hand usually affected.[9] Risk for OA depends on the type and intensity of physical activity and whether injury is incurred in the activity. Increased risk of OA is associated with participation in activities such as wrestling, boxing, baseball pitching, cycling, and football, although recreational participants do not have the increased risk seen in the professional athlete.[2,11] In a study of 30,000 Norwegians, exercise intensity was not associated with any increased risk in the obese subjects compared with those of normal weight.[14]

Traumatic injury to articular cartilage during sports and other activities or in accidents greatly increases OA risk.[2,15] Meniscal damage increases the risk of knee OA because of the loss of proper load bearing and shock absorption, increased focal load on cartilage and on subchondral bone. Knee injury in young persons is also an important risk factor for knee OA in old age.[11] Quadriceps muscle weakness is also recognized to increase the risk for knee OA, as these muscles are important in maintaining joint stability.[13] Whether knee malalignment increases risk of developing OA remains unsettled.[11] In the person who already has OA, knee malalignment is strongly associated with faster progression of OA.[11]

Genetic Factors

OA is a complex, polygenic disease. Identification of the genes involved may promote development of agents to prevent OA or to slow or halt its progression. Genetic influences on OA have been appreciated for many years. Heberden nodes are 10 times more prevalent in women than in men, for example, with a twofold higher risk if the woman's mother had them. Genetic links have been shown with OA of the first metatarsophalangeal joint and with generalized OA. Twin studies indicate that OA can be attributed substantially to genetic factors.[16] In other twin studies of OA progression, radiographic measurements over 2 years showed that the increased risk for a sibling having radiographic progression if the proband had progression was threefold for joint space narrowing and 1.5-fold for osteophyte progression.[17]

One approach OA researchers have used is the candidate gene approach which is hypothesis-based and focuses on genes with known function that could be plausibly linked with the disease. Genome-wide association studies (GWAS) associating OA with a specific region out of the total human genome, using cases versus controls, offers a powerful approach in seeking the genetic basis for OA.[18] Using GWA studies and candidate gene approaches, possible genetic associations to OA have been found, and some of these appear to code for known proteins which have intriguing connections.[18-20] These genes include *Col11A1* (extracellular matrix), *Chrom 19* (cartilage morphogenesis), *MCFL* (pain perception), *CHST11* (cartilage morphogenesis), *GDF5* (TGF-beta signaling), and *Chrom7Q22*. A meta-analysis of GWA studies with 6,709 knee OA cases and 44,439 controls revealed that the *Chrom7Q22* locus was very highly significantly associated with knee OA. The locus also included six genes that code for proteins known to be expressed in joint tissues.[19]

For most genes that appear to be linked to OA, the associations have been weak or modest, even if replicable.[21] It is quite likely that the genetic risk of developing OA, like many other diseases, may be substantially determined by a combination of modest genetic differences, and this underscores the point that understanding of the genetics and pathology of OA is in its infancy.

PATHOPHYSIOLOGY

OA falls into two major etiologic classes. *Primary (idiopathic) OA*, the more common type, has no identifiable cause. *Secondary OA* is associated with a known cause such as rheumatoid or another inflammatory arthritis, trauma, metabolic or endocrine disorders, and congenital factors.[22]

The old view of OA as a "wear-and-tear" or degenerative disease, largely focused on joint cartilage, has long been superseded by an appreciation of the dynamic nature of OA and that it represents a failure of the joint and surrounding tissues.[23] Some changes in the OA joint may reflect compensatory processes to maintain function in the face of ongoing joint destruction. Not only biomechanical forces but also inflammatory, biochemical, and immunologic factors are involved. An appreciation of the biology and function of normal cartilage can aid in understanding osteoarthritic cartilage and is summarized below.

Normal Cartilage

Function, Structure, and Composition of Cartilage

Articular cartilage possesses viscoelastic properties that provide lubrication with motion, shock absorbency during rapid movements, and load support. In synovial joints, articular cartilage is found between the synovial cavity on one side and a narrow layer of calcified tissue overlying subchondral bone on the other side (Fig. 90-2).[24] The layer of cartilage is narrow, with human medial femoral articular cartilage being approximately 2 to 3 mm thick. Despite this, healthy articular cartilage in weight-bearing joints withstands millions of cycles of loading and unloading each year. Cartilage is easily compressed, losing up to 40% of its original height when a load is applied. Compression increases the area of contact and disperses force more evenly to underlying bone, tendons, ligaments, and muscles. In addition, cartilage is almost frictionless, and together with its compressibility, this enables smooth movement in the joint, distributes load across joint tissues to prevent damage, and stabilizes the joint.

Strength, a low coefficient of friction, and compressibility of cartilage derive from its unique structure. Cartilage is a complex, hydrophilic, extracellular matrix (ECM). It is approximately 75% to 85% water and contains 2% to 5% chondrocytes collagen and other proteins, proteoglycans, and long hyaluronic acid (HA) molecules.[24] The two major structural components in articular cartilage

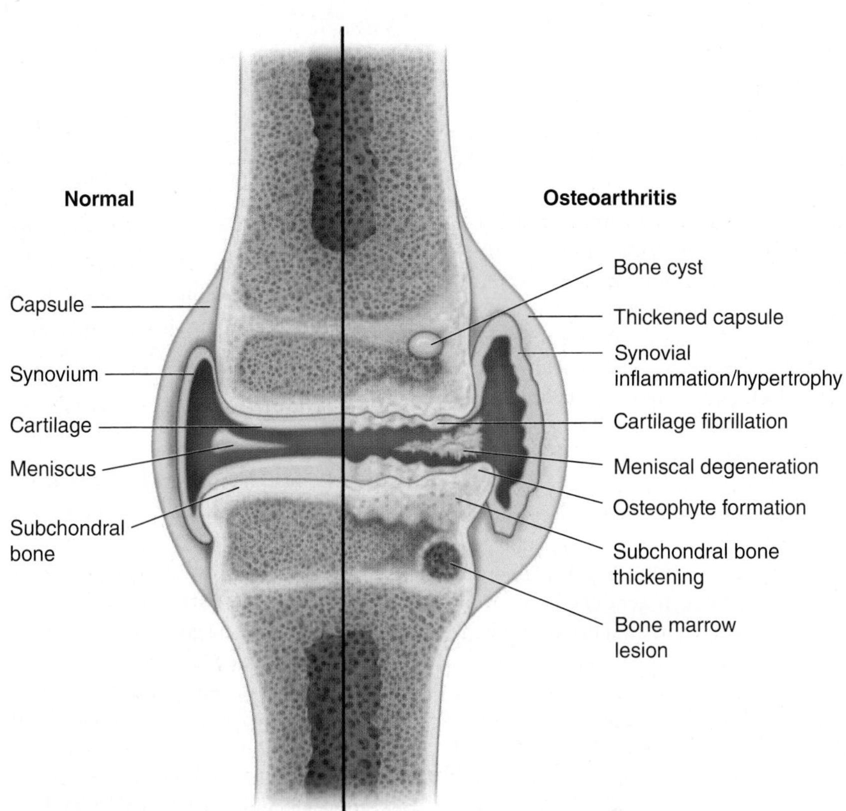

FIGURE 90-2 Characteristics of osteoarthritis in the diarthrodial joint. (*Used with permission from Loeser RF. Age-related changes in the musculoskeletal system and the development of osteoarthritis. Clin Geriatr Med. 2010;26(3):371-386.*)

are type II collagen and aggrecans.[25] Type II collagen has a tightly woven triple helical structure, which provides the tensile strength of cartilage. Aggrecan is a proteoglycan linked with HA, providing the long aggrecan molecules a high negative charge. These are squeezed together by surrounding fibrils of type II collagen. The strong electrostatic repulsion of proteoglycans held in close proximity gives cartilage the ability to withstand further compression. Within the cartilage ECM are the chondrocytes, the only cells in cartilage, responsible for laying down all the components of cartilage.

Normal cartilage turnover helps repair and restore cartilage in response to demands of joint loading and during physical activity. In adults, cartilage chondrocyte metabolism is slow and is regulated by growth factors, including bone morphogenetic protein 2, insulin-like growth factor-1, and transforming growth factor, and by catabolism and proteolysis stimulated by matrix metalloproteinases (MMPs), tumor necrosis factor-α (TNF-α), interleukin-1, and other cytokines. Tissue inhibitors of metalloproteinase (TIMP) also contribute to the balance by restraining the catabolic actions of MMPs. If cartilage is injured, chondrocytes react by removing the damaged areas and increasing synthesis of matrix constituents to repair and restore cartilage.[25,26]

Another component supporting healthy joints are the joint protective mechanisms, such as muscles bridging the joint, sensory receptors in feedback loops to regulate muscle and tendon function, supporting ligaments, and subchondral bone that has shock-absorbent properties.

Finally, it is important to note that adult articular cartilage is avascular, with chondrocytes nourished by synovial fluid. With movement and cyclic loading and unloading of joints, nutrients flow into the cartilage, whereas immobilization reduces nutrient supply. This is one of the reasons that normal physical activity is beneficial for joint health.

Osteoarthritic Cartilage

3 Important contributors to the development of OA are local mechanical influences, genetic factors, inflammation, and aberrant chondrocyte function leading to loss of articular cartilage.[25,26] At a molecular level, OA pathophysiology involves the interplay of dozens, if not hundreds, of extracellular and intracellular molecules with roles including chondrocyte regulation, phenotypic changes, proteolytic degradation of cartilage components, and interactions between articular cartilage, underlying subchondral bone, and the joint synovium.[25-28]

OA most commonly begins with damage to articular cartilage, through trauma or other injury, excess joint loading from obesity or other reasons, or instability or injury of the joint that causes abnormal loading. In response to cartilage damage, chondrocyte activity increases in an attempt to remove and repair the damage. Depending on the degree of damage, the balance between breakdown and resynthesis of cartilage can be lost, and a vicious cycle of increasing breakdown can lead to further cartilage loss and apoptosis of chondrocytes.[25-27,29] Recent studies have revealed several aspects of the very complex nature of OA. For example, expression of hundreds of specific genes are affected by acute experimental injury of human cartilage tissue, that is, injury alters the chondrocyte phenotype.[30] Researchers have also shown that within different regions of human OA cartilage obtained at surgery, chondrocyte gene expression from the most damaged areas of cartilage is different from that of less damaged or normal areas.[31] Another exciting discovery is that comparative proteomics of articular cartilage from normal persons compared with cartilage from those with OA showed different expression.[32]

There is an increased appreciation of the role of tissues beyond cartilage, within the joint and surrounding it, subchondral bone.[26] Subchondral bone undergoes pathologic changes that may precede, coincide with, or follow damage to the articular cartilage. In OA, subchondral bone releases vasoactive peptides and MMPs, and damage to subchondral bone may trigger further damage to articular cartilage.[33] Neovascularization and subsequent increased permeability of the adjacent cartilage occur and contributes further to cartilage loss.

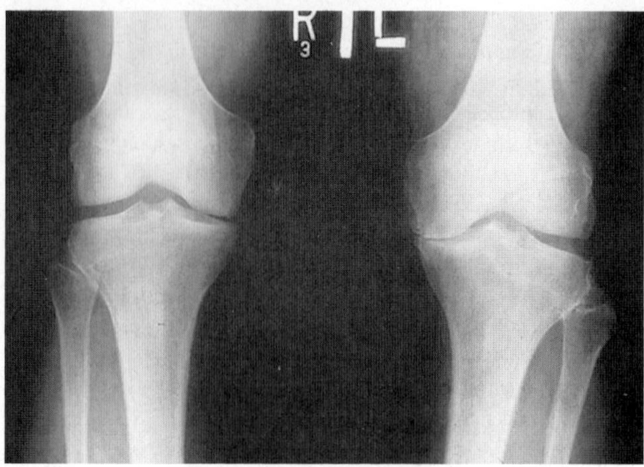

FIGURE 90-3 Plain x-ray films of the knee demonstrating joint space narrowing. (*Reproduced with permission from Johnson BE. Chapter 23. Arthritis: Osteoarthritis, Gout, & Rheumatoid Arthritis. In: South-Paul JE, Matheny SC, Lewis EL. eds. CURRENT Diagnosis & Treatment in Family Medicine, 3e. New York, NY: McGraw-Hill; 2011.*)

Joint space narrowing resulting from loss of cartilage can lead to a painful and deformed joint (Fig. 90-3). Remaining cartilage softens and develops fibrillations (vertical clefts into the cartilage), followed by splitting off more cartilage and exposure of underlying bone.[34] During this time, adjacent subchondral bone undergoes further pathologic changes, cartilage is eroded completely, leaving denuded subchondral bone, which becomes dense, smooth, and glistening (eburnation). A more brittle, stiffer bone results, with decreased weight-bearing ability and development of sclerosis and microfractures. New bone formations, or osteophytes, also appear at joint margins, distant from cartilage destruction and are thought to arise from local and humoral factors. There is direct evidence that osteophytes can help stabilize osteoarthritic joints.[35]

In the joint capsule and synovium, inflammatory changes and pathologic changes can occur.[24,26-28] Contributors to inflammation may include crystals or cartilage shards in synovial fluid. Other possible players are interleukin-1, prostaglandin E_2, TNF-α, and nitric oxide which are found in synovial fluid. With inflammatory changes in the synovium, effusions and synovial thickening occur.

4 The pain of OA is not related to the destruction of cartilage but arises from the activation of nociceptive nerve endings within the joint by mechanical and chemical irritants.[29] OA pain may result from distension of the synovial capsule by increased joint fluid, microfracture, periosteal irritation, or damage to ligaments, synovium, or the meniscus.

CLINICAL PRESENTATION

Diagnosis

5 The diagnosis of OA is made through history, physical examination, characteristic radiographic findings, and laboratory testing.[36] The major diagnostic goals are (1) to discriminate between primary and secondary OA and (2) to clarify the joints involved, severity of joint involvement, and response to prior therapies, providing a basis for a treatment plan. The American College of Rheumatology has published traditional diagnostic criteria and "decision trees" for OA diagnosis.[36] As with all guidelines, the authors stress these are for assisting the clinician rather than replacing clinical judgment. For example, traditional criteria are as follows: (1) For hip OA, a patient must have pain in the hip and at least two of the following three: an erythrocyte sedimentation rate less than 20 mm/h (<5.6 μm/s),

CLINICAL PRESENTATION Osteoarthritis

Age

- Usually older

Gender

- Age < 45 more common in men
- Age > 45 more common in women

Symptoms

- Pain
- Deep, aching character
- Pain on motion
- Stiffness in affected joints
- Resolves with motion, recurs with rest ("gelling phenomenon")
- Usually duration <30 minutes
- Often related to weather
- Limited joint motion
- May result in limitations of activities of daily living
- Instability of weight-bearing joints

Signs, history, and physical examination

- Monoarticular or oligoarticular, asymmetrical involvement
- Hands
  - Distal interphalangeal joints
    - Herberden nodes (osteophytes or bony enlargements) (Fig. 90-1)
  - Proximal interphalangeal joints
    - Bouchard's nodes (osteophytes)
  - First metacarpal joint
    - Osteophytes give characteristic square appearance to hands
- Knee
  - Pain related to climbing stairs
  - Transient joint effusion
  - Genu varum ("bow-legged")
- Hips
  - Groin pain during weight bearing exercises
  - Stiffness, especially after activity
  - Limited joint movement
- Spine
  - Lumbar involvement is most common at L3 and L4
  - Paresthesias
  - Loss of reflexes
- Feet
  - Typically involves the first metatarsalphalangeal joint
  - Shoulder, elbow, acromioclavicular, sternoclavicular, tempomandibular joints may also be affected
- Observation on joint examination
  - Bony proliferation or occasional synovitis
  - Local tenderness
  - Crepitus
  - Limited motion with passive/active movement
  - Deformity
- Radiologic Evaluation
  - Early Mild OA
    - Radiographic changes often absent
  - Progressive OA
  - Joint space narrowing (Fig. 90-3)
  - Subchondral bone sclerosis
  - Marginal osteophytes
- Late OA
  - Abnormal alignment of joints
  - Effusions

femoral or acetabular osteophytes on radiography, or joint space narrowing on radiography. This provides a sensitivity of 89% and a specificity of 91%.[2] For a clinical diagnosis of knee OA, a patient must have pain at the knee and osteophytes on radiography plus one of the following: age older than 50 years, morning stiffness not more than 30 minutes, crepitus on motion, bony enlargement, bony tenderness, or palpable warmth. This provides a sensitivity of 95% and a specificity of 69%. The addition of laboratory or radiographic data further improves accuracy of diagnosis. Criteria for hand OA have also been published.[37]

Prognosis

The prognosis for patients with primary OA is variable and depends on the joint involved. If a weight-bearing joint or the spine is involved, considerable morbidity and disability are possible. In the case of secondary OA, the prognosis depends on the underlying cause. Treatment of OA may relieve pain or improve function but does not reverse preexisting damage to the joint.

TREATMENT

Desired Outcome

Management of the patient with OA begins with a diagnosis based on a careful history, physical examination, radiographic findings, and an assessment of the extent of joint involvement. Treatment should be tailored to each individual. Goals are (1) to educate the patient, family members, and caregivers; (2) to relieve pain and stiffness; (3) to maintain or improve joint mobility; (4) to limit functional impairment; and (5) to maintain or improve quality of life.[38-40]

General Approach to Treatment

Treatment for each OA patient depends on the distribution and severity of joint involvement, comorbid disease states, concomitant medications, and allergies. Management for all individuals with OA should begin with both oral and written patient education, a customized activity and exercise program, and weight loss, if the patient is overweight or obese.[38-40]

The primary objective of medication is to alleviate pain.[38-40] Scheduled acetaminophen, up to 4 g/day, should be tried initially (knee, hip), if contraindications are not present. Application of topical NSAIDs over specific joints (knee, hands) and topical capsaicin (hands) is recommended as initial therapy. NSAIDs or possibly a cyclooxygenase-2 (COX-2)–selective inhibitor (celecoxib) can be prescribed after careful risk assessment if additional pain control is needed. Intra-articular corticosteroid injections (knee or hip) can relieve pain and are offered concomitantly with oral analgesics or after failed trials of first-line medications, depending on the practitioner's preference. With centrally acting serotonin reuptake inhibition and analgesic properties, tramadol can also be considered if acetaminophen or topical treatment is ineffective or not tolerated.

Opioid analgesics may be considered if first-line medications are ineffective or pose significant safety concerns in an individual patient. Consideration can also be given to duloxetine or less likely, HA injections when additional pain control is needed for knee OA. When symptoms are intractable or there is significant loss of function, joint replacement can be appropriate if the patient is a surgical candidate.

There is general agreement that glucosamine and/or chondroitin and topical rubefacients lack uniform efficacy in the treatment of hip and knee OA pain and are not preferred treatment options.

Nonpharmacologic Therapy

6 Nonpharmacologic therapy is an integral part of the treatment plan for all patients with OA.[38,40,41] Nonpharmacologic therapy is the only available treatment that has been shown to delay the progression of OA.[42] Delaying the progression of OA through active participation in nonpharmacologic therapy is critical to prevent future functional impairment. Patient-specific characteristics such as (1) number and location of affected joints, (2) degree of functional impairment, (3) body mass index (BMI), (4) motivation, and (5) overall health status determine which nonpharmacologic therapies should be offered. Nonpharmacologic therapy should be ongoing treatment for all patients, even those who require pharmacologic therapy for pain control (Table 90-1).

Patient Education

The first step in OA treatment is patient education about the disease process, the extent of OA, the prognosis, and treatment options. Education is paramount because OA is often seen as a wear-and-tear disease, an inevitable consequence of aging for which nothing helps. Even worse, patients may resort to the use of alternative but unproven medications or treatments. Organizations such as the Arthritis Foundation provide a wealth of educational information for patients regarding OA, OA medications, information about local clinics, and agencies offering physical and economic assistance. Exercise, weight loss, and nutritional information are also available. Most educational information is readily available online for patient use. Several mobile applications are available to provide education, track symptoms and exercise, and encourage better self-management of OA.

The benefits of patient education have been documented in a variety of programs.[43] These programs are provided across a wide spectrum of delivery methods: from trained volunteers using telephone calls to group sessions for patient support to one-on-one educational sessions with physical therapists or nurse educators. While nearly all of these delivery methods are effective, cost of delivery is highly variable. Long-term cost-effectiveness is very important for sustainability of these patient education programs.

TABLE 90-1 Nonpharmacologic Interventions in the Treatment of OA[37-39]

Type of Nonpharmacologic Intervention	Strength of Recommendation
Exercise	Strong
Weight loss (if overweight)	Strong
Patient education	Strong
Use of assistive device (ie, cane)	Moderate
Use of shoe insoles	Moderate
Application of heat	Moderate
Use of fitted knee braces	Minimal
Lateral patellar taping	Minimal
Passive exercise alone	Minimal

Strength of recommendation: Strong—fully supported by evidence-based guidelines, moderate—supported by evidence-based guidelines, minimal—little support by evidence-based guidelines.

Weight Loss

The association between OA and obesity has been well established. Studies also indicate a strong association between increasing BMI and surgical replacement of the hip and knee joints.[44] Weight loss of amounts as small as 4% body weight can lessen OA pain in the knee.[45] Greater amounts of weight loss, especially when associated with regular exercise improve joint function and substantially lessen pain.[45] Modest weight loss (5%) has been shown to provide some relief in obese patients with OA, but the goal weight loss should be an initial decrease in body weight of at least 10% to provide significant reductions in pain.[44] Patients with appropriate indications for bariatric surgery have significant improvement in joint function and pain associated with the subsequent weight loss.[46] The Intensive Diet and Exercise for Arthritis (IDEA) trial found that after 18 months, overweight and obese adults with knee OA who participated in the diet and exercise treatment group had less inflammation, less pain, better function, and better quality of life.[47] Weight loss requires a motivated patient, but it should be encouraged and supported for all obese and overweight patients with OA. Effective behavior change strategies should be employed to promote weight loss in patients with OA.[42]

Exercise

Exercise programs can improve joint function and can decrease disability, pain, and analgesic use by OA patients.[48,49] Low-impact aerobic exercise including both land- and water-based methods are preferred.[50] Exercises can be taught and then observed before the patient exercises at home. The frequency, types of exercise and setting of exercise are still uncertain, but patients who exercise at least two to three times per week with a variety of exercises (>8 types) have improved outcomes.[51] The patient should be instructed to decrease the number of repetitions if severe pain develops with exercise.

Some regular exercise should be encouraged for all patients with OA.[40] With weak or deconditioned muscles, the load is transmitted excessively to the joints; so weight-bearing activities can exacerbate symptoms. Many patients fear that exercise will promote further joint damage and avoid exercise as a means to protect the joint. However, avoidance of regular exercise by those with hip or knee OA leads to further deconditioning and/or weight gain. Further weight gain and deconditioning leads to more pain and impaired joint function, promoting a downward spiral of disability. Exercise therapy in addition to patient education has been shown to decrease or postpone the need for hip replacement surgery in patients with hip OA.[52]

Referral to the physical and/or occupational therapist is especially helpful for developing a customized exercise plan for patients with functional disabilities. The therapist can assess muscle strength and joint stability and recommend exercises and assistive and orthotic devices, such as canes, walkers, braces, heel cups, splints, or insoles for use during exercise or daily activities. Heat or cold treatments help maintain and restore joint range of motion and to reduce pain and muscle spasms. Warm baths or warm water soaks may decrease pain and stiffness. Heating pads should be used with caution, especially in the elderly. Patients should be warned not to fall asleep on the heat source or to lie on it for more than brief periods to avoid burns.

Surgery

Surgery can be recommended for OA patients with functional disability and/or severe pain unresponsive to medical therapy. Criteria for total joint replacement (arthroplasty) of the knee and hip have been developed although there is substantial overlap in eligibility criteria.[53] Total joint replacement surgeries are quite common and expected to increase. By 2030, projections estimate that 3.5 million total knee replacements will occur annually.[54] Although total knee arthroplasty can decrease pain and improve function for many patients, about 20% experience little or no improvement in pain, disability, and/or quality of life.[55]

Total joint arthroplasty is responsible for a large portion of the direct medical costs associated with OA in the United States. The cost-effectiveness of total knee arthroplasty has been evaluated for a Medicare-age population.[56] Calculations were based on Medicare claims data and costs and outcomes data. Cost projections were calculated for lifetime costs as well as quality-adjusted life expectancy (QALE) for different risk populations and across low-volume to high-volume hospitals. Although total knee arthroplasty was found to be cost-effective across hospital settings and patient risk categories, the procedure was found to be most cost-effective when performed in high-volume centers. Compared with nonsurgical management, knee arthroplasty is cost-effective at both low and high levels of improvement in pain and function in patients with severe knee OA.[54]

Other surgical options are also available. Arthrodesis (joint fusion) can reduce pain but will restrict motion and may be appropriate for smaller joints that are causing intractable pain. For patients with mild knee OA, an osteotomy (removal of bony tissue) may correct the misalignment of genu varum ("bowlegged" knees) or genu valgum ("knock-knees"). In addition, osteotomies of the pelvis or femur can ameliorate joint misalignment in hip OA, subsequently slowing progression of disease. Knee arthroscopy or lavage is not recommended.[38,50]

Pharmacologic Therapy

Drug therapy in OA is targeted at relief of pain. OA is commonly seen in older individuals who have other medical conditions, and OA treatment is often long-term. As such, a conservative and patient-centered approach to drug treatment is warranted.[38-41] **(Figs. 90-4 and 90-5)** Even when pharmacologic therapy is initiated, appropriate nondrug therapies should be continued and reinforced. Specific drug therapy recommendations depend on which joint(s) are affected, response to previous trials of medication, and patient comorbidities.

Knee and Hip OA

First-Line Treatments

Acetaminophen 7 The American College of Rheumatology, as well as others, recommend acetaminophen as a first-line treatment for knee and hip OA (Fig. 90-4).[38,40,57] Acetaminophen has been extensively studied in the treatment of knee and hip OA and is more effective than placebo in controlling OA pain.[58] Compared with oral NSAIDs, acetaminophen may be modestly less effective, but it has a lower risk of serious GI and cardiovascular adverse events and as a consequence is preferred as first-line treatment.[57] The significantly lower risks of both minor and major adverse events associated with acetaminophen in the treatment of knee and hip OA favors a trial of acetaminophen in all patients without underlying hepatic disease.[57]

Oral NSAIDs If the patient fails acetaminophen, the American College of Rheumatology and other key groups recommend nonspecific or COX-2 selective NSAIDs, depending on patient risk factors, as a first-line option for knee and hip OA.[38,40,57] NSAIDs have a consistent record of providing superior pain relief in comparison to acetaminophen, but no NSAID has proven superior to another.[57] Nonselective and COX-2 selective NSAIDs pose higher risks for GI, renal, and cardiovascular adverse events compared with acetaminophen. COX-2 inhibitors carry less risk for both minor and serious GI adverse events in comparison to nonselective NSAIDs (with the exception of diclofenac). It is unclear whether the reduced GI risk seen with COX-2 selectivity persists past 3 to 6 months, and this advantage is substantially diminished for patients taking aspirin.[57] PPIs and misoprostol significantly reduce the occurrence of GI adverse events in those taking NSAIDs.[57]

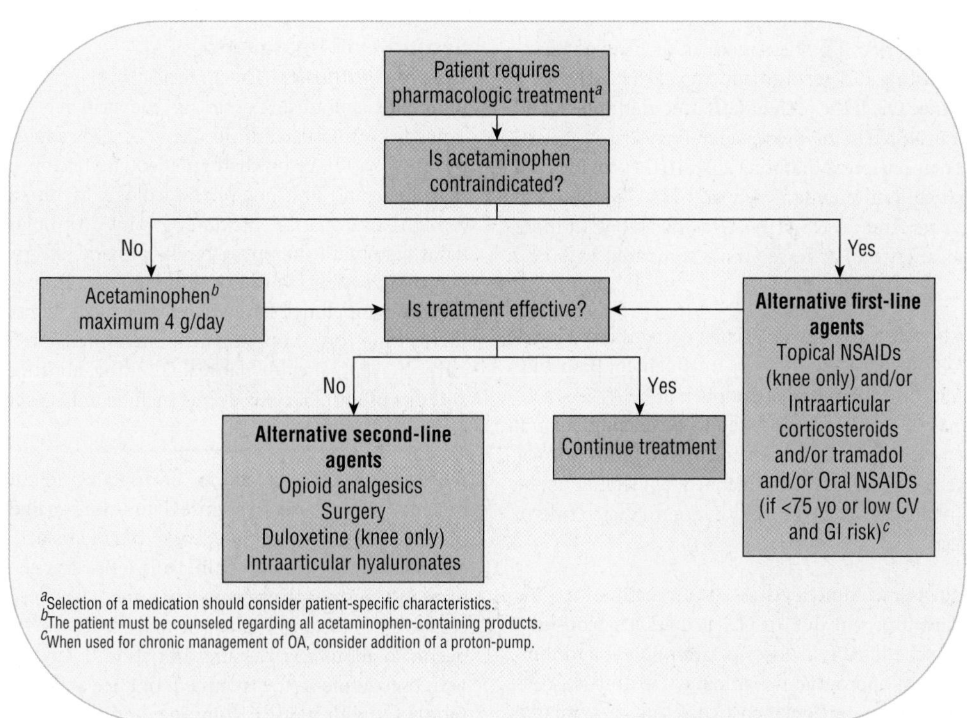

FIGURE 90-4 Treatment recommendations for knee and hip osteoarthritis. (CV, cardiovascular; GI, gastrointestinal; NSAIDs, nonsteroidal anti-inflammatory drugs.)

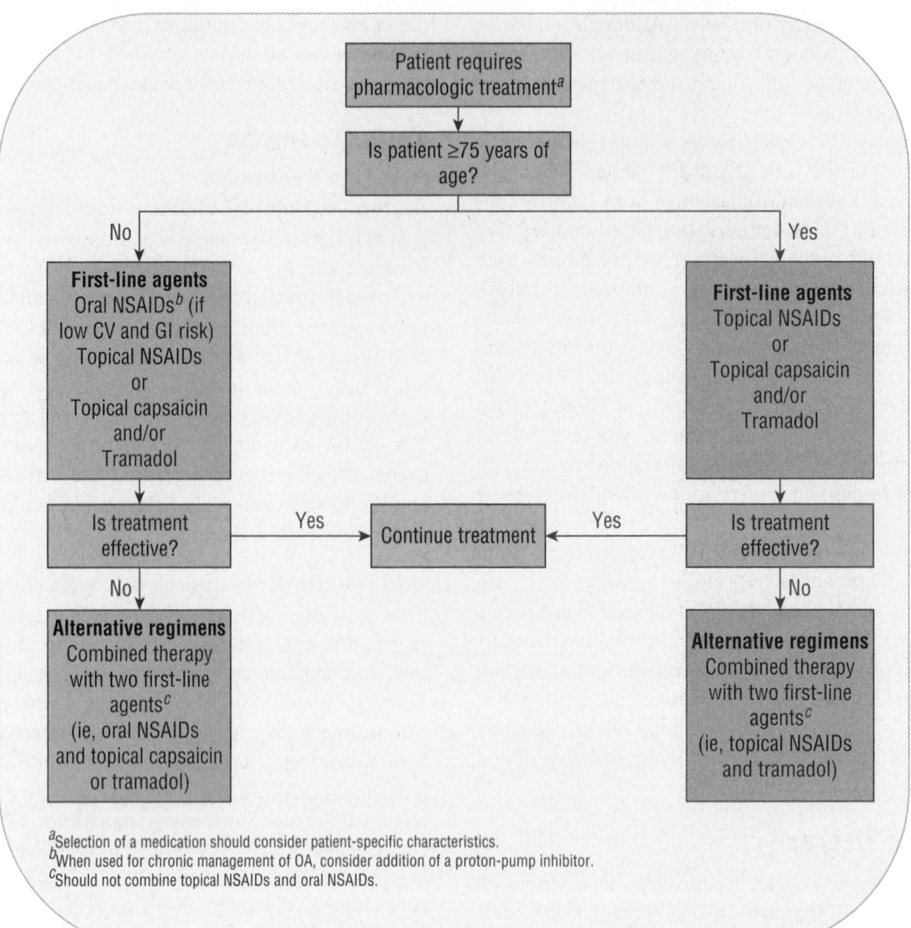

FIGURE 90-5 Treatment recommendations for hand osteoarthritis. (CV, cardiovascular; GI, gastrointestinal; NSAIDs, nonsteroidal anti-inflammatory drugs.)

Topical NSAIDs–Knee Only 8 The American College of Rheumatology and other authorities recommend topical NSAIDs as a first-line option for knee OA if the patient fails acetaminophen, and is preferred over oral NSAIDs for those older than 75.[38,40,57] Randomized trials have demonstrated that topical NSAIDs provide pain relief for OA similar to that obtained with oral NSAIDs but with fewer GI adverse events. Topical NSAIDs are associated with more frequent local (application site) adverse events compared with oral NSAIDs.[57]

Intra-Articular Corticosteroids Intra-articular corticosteroid injections are recommended as alternative first-line treatment for both knee and hip OA when pain control with acetaminophen or NSAIDs is suboptimal.[38,40] Injections can also be administered with concomitant oral analgesic therapy as needed for additional pain control. Intra-articular corticosteroids are generally safe and well tolerated, but should not be administered more frequently than once every 3 months due to risks of systemic adverse effects.

Tramadol Tramadol is recommended as an alternative first-line treatment of knee and hip pain due to OA in patients who have failed treatment with scheduled full-dose acetaminophen and topical NSAIDs, who are not appropriate candidates for oral NSAIDs and are not able to receive intra-articular corticosteroids.[40] Tramadol can also safely be added to partially effective acetaminophen or oral NSAID therapy. Fewer data support the use of tramadol as monotherapy for OA pain.

Second-Line Treatments

Opioid Analgesics The American College of Rheumatology recommends opioid analgesics as the primary second-line medication for both knee and hip OA.[40] Opioids should be considered in patients who have not had an adequate response to both nonpharmacologic and first-line pharmacologic therapies. Patients who are at high surgical risk, precluding joint arthroplasty are also candidates for opioid therapy. Opioids provide effective short-term pain control in patients with OA, although data from long-term use trials are less compelling.[59] Adverse effects, including serious events, limit the routine use of opioids in the treatment of OA pain. Common adverse events include nausea, vomiting, constipation, somnolence, and dry mouth. Serious events include falls, respiratory depression, and addiction.[59]

Duloxetine Duloxetine can be used as adjunctive treatment in patients with a partial response to first-line analgesics.[38,40] It may be a preferred second-line medication in patients with both neuropathic and musculoskeletal OA pain. Duloxetine has demonstrated efficacy primarily as add-on therapy when there has been less than optimal response to acetaminophen or oral NSAIDs.[60,61] Reduction in pain occurs at about 4 weeks after initiation.[62] Adverse events associated with duloxetine in the treatment of knee and hip OA are most commonly GI with nausea, vomiting, and constipation being the most common. The recommended dose is 60 mg once daily. However, some patients may benefit from higher doses; up to a maximum dose of 120 mg daily.[62] Adverse events have not been reported in OA trials

TABLE 90-2 Drug Dosing Table

Drug	Brand Name	Starting Dose	Usual Range	Special Population Dose	Other
Oral Analgesics					
Acetaminophen	Tylenol	325-500 mg three times a day	325-650 mg every 4-6 hours or 1 g three to four times a day	Chronic alcohol intake, hepatic disease	Contained in many combination analgesics
Tramadol	Ultram	25 mg in the morning	Titrate dose in 25 mg increments to reach a maintenance dose of 50-100 mg three times a day	Creatinine clearance <30 mL/min (<0.5 mL/s)—maximum dose is 200 mg daily	May need to taper dose upon discontinuation to prevent withdrawal symptoms
Tramadol ER	Ultram ER	100 mg daily	Titrate to 200-300 mg daily	Do not use if creatinine clearance <30 mL/min (<0.5 mL/s)	
Hydrocodone/ acetaminophen	Lortab, Vicodin	5 mg/325 mg three times daily	2.5-10 mg/325-650 mg three to five times daily	Titrate dose slowly in older patients	Maximum dose limited by total daily dose of acetaminophen
Oxycodone/ acetaminophen	Percocet	5 mg/325 mg three times daily	2.5-10 mg/325-650 mg three to five times daily	Titrate dose slowly in older patients	Maximum dose limited by total daily dose of acetaminophen
Topical Analgesics					
Capsaicin 0.025% or 0.075%	Capzasin-HP		Apply to affected joint three to four times per day		—
Diclofenac 1% gel	Voltaren		Apply 2 or 4 g per site as prescribed, four times daily		
Diclofenac 1.3% patch	Flector		Apply one patch twice daily to the site to be treated, as directed. Apply 40 drops to the affected knee, applying and rubbing in 10 drops		
Diclofenac 1.5% solution	Pennsaid		Apply 40 drops to the affected knee, applying and rubbing in 10 drops at a time. Repeat for a total of four times daily		
Diclofenac 2% solution	Pennsaid		Apply 40 mg (2 pump actuations) twice daily		
Intra-articular Corticosteroids					
Triamcinolone	Kenalog	5-15 mg per joint	10-40 mg per large joint (knee, hip, shoulder)	If multiple joints injected, maximum total dose is usually 80 mg	Often administered concomitantly with a local anesthetic
Methylprednisolone acetate	Depo-Medrol	10-20 mg per joint	20-80 mg per large joint (knee, hip, shoulder)	10-40 mg for medium joints (elbows, wrists)	
Nonsteroidal Antiinflammatory Drugs (NSAIDs)					
Aspirin, plain, buffered, or enteric-coated	Bayer, Ecotrin, Bufferin	325 mg three times a day	325-650 mg four times a day		Doses of 3,600 mg/day are needed for anti-inflammatory activity
Celecoxib	Celebrex	100 mg daily	100 mg twice daily or 200 mg daily		
Diclofenac XR	Voltaren-XR	100 mg daily	100-200 mg daily		
Diclofenac IR	Cataflam	50 mg twice a day	50-75 mg twice a day		
Diflunisal	Dolobid	250 mg twice a day	500-750 mg twice a day		
Etodolac	Lodine	300 mg twice a day	400-500 mg twice a day		
Fenoprofen	Nalfon	400 mg three times a day	400-600 mg three to four times a day		
Flurbiprofen	Ansaid	100 mg twice a day	200-300 mg/day in two to four divided doses		
Ibuprofen	Motrin, Advil	200 mg three times a day	1,200-3,200 mg/day in three to four divided doses		Available OTC and Rx
Indomethacin	Indocin	25 mg twice a day	Titrate dose by 25-50 mg/day until pain controlled or maximum dose of 50 mg three times a day		
Indomethacin SR	Indocin SR	75 mg SR once daily	Can titrate to 75 mg SR twice daily if needed		

(continued)

TABLE 90-2 Drug Dosing Table (*Continued*)

Drug	Brand Name	Starting Dose	Usual Range	Special Population Dose	Other
Ketoprofen	Orudis	50 mg three times a day	50-75 mg three to four times a day		
Meclofenamate	Meclomen	50 mg three times a day	50-100 mg three to four times a day		
Mefenamic acid	Ponstel	250 mg three times a day	250 mg four times a day		FDA approval for 1 week of therapy
Meloxicam	Mobic	7.5 mg daily	15 mg daily		
Nabumetone	Relafen	500 mg daily	500-1,000 mg one to two times a day		
Naproxen	Naprosyn	250 mg twice a day	500 mg twice a day		Available OTC and Rx
Naproxen sodium	Anaprox, Aleve	220 mg twice a day	220-550 mg twice a day		
Naproxen sodium controlled-release tablets	Naprelan		375-750 mg twice a day		
Oxaprozin	Daypro	600 mg daily	600-1,200 mg daily		
Piroxicam	Feldene	10 mg daily	20 mg daily		
Salsalate	Disalcid	500 mg twice a day	500-1,000 mg two to three times a day		

that most commonly used doses of 60 mg per day. A higher dose is associated with an increased risk of adverse reactions.

Intra-Articular Hyaluronic Acid The American College of Rheumatology, NICE, and others do not routinely recommend the use of intra-articular HA injections for knee OA pain.[38,40,41] HA injections do not appear to provide clinically meaningful improvement in pain and/or function scores, although some studies may report statistical differences in scores. These agents may be associated with serious adverse events such as increased pain, joint swelling, and stiffness. Limited efficacy and risks of serious events limit the routine use of these agents.

Hand Osteoarthritis

First-Line Treatments

Nonsteroidal Anti-inflammatory Drugs The American College of Rheumatology and NICE recommend topical NSAIDs as a first-line option for hand OA (**Fig. 90-5**).[41] Application of diclofenac gel compared with vehicle for hand OA provided significant relief, with mild application-site paresthesia as the only treatment-related adverse effect.[63] Topical diclofenac showed similar efficacy as oral ibuprofen and oral diclofenac, but with fewer GI adverse events.[64,65] Topical diclofenac was associated with more frequent local (application site) events compared with oral NSAIDs. In all of these studies, topical diclofenac had fewer GI adverse events.[57,64,65]

Oral NSAIDs are recommended as an alternative first-line treatment for hand OA by the American College of Rheumatology and as second-line therapy in the NICE guidelines.[40,41] For hand OA, there has long been a focus toward topical treatment, perhaps due to reluctance to undergo systemic exposure to strong treatment in patients without pain in a weight-bearing joint.[65] For the person who cannot tolerate local skin reactions or who received inadequate relief from topical NSAIDs, oral NSAIDs can offer relief, but the patient then faces increased risk for GI, renal, and cardiovascular adverse events.

Topical Capsaicin Capsaicin cream is recommended as an alternative first-line treatment for hand OA.[40] Clinical trial data supporting the use of capsaicin for the treatment of hand OA are limited to small studies, but the agent demonstrates modest benefits in improvement of pain scores.[64] Adverse effects associated with capsaicin are primarily skin irritation and burning, therefore it is a reasonable therapeutic alternative for patients not able to take oral NSAIDs.

Tramadol Tramadol is recommended by the American College of Rheumatology as an alternative first-line treatment for OA of the hand.[40] In clinical practice, tramadol is a therapeutic option for patients who do not respond to topical therapy and are not candidates for oral NSAID treatment because of high GI, cardiovascular, or renal risks. Tramadol may also be used in combination with partially effective acetaminophen, topical therapy, or oral NSAIDs.

Drug Class Information

Highlighted drug information will be reviewed further. This section is not intended to be all inclusive, but aims to provide pertinent drug information to facilitate the safe and effective use of these medications in patients with OA (**Table 90-2**).

First-Line Treatments

Acetaminophen

Pharmacology and Mechanism of Action Acetaminophen is understood to act within the central nervous system (CNS) by inhibiting synthesis of prostaglandins—agents that enhance pain sensations. Acetaminophen prevents prostaglandin synthesis by blocking the action of central cyclooxygenase (COX). Acetaminophen is well absorbed after oral administration, with a bioavailability of 60% to 98%. It achieves peak concentrations within 1 to 2 hours, it is inactivated in the liver by conjugation with sulfate or glucuronide, and its metabolites are renally excreted.

Adverse Effects Although acetaminophen is one of the safest analgesics, its use carries some risks, primarily hepatotoxicity.[66] Serious hepatotoxicity, including fatalities, have been well documented with acetaminophen overdose (see Chapter e9, for information on treatment of acetaminophen overdose). Continued reports of serious hepatotoxicity, including fatalities from unintentional overdose, have led to labeling revisions of all nonprescription acetaminophen containing analgesics.[67] Unintentional overdoses of acetaminophen are due to a variety of circumstances including narrow therapeutic window at the maximum dose (4 g/day), interpatient differences in sensitivity to liver injury from acetaminophen, a wide array of nonprescription and prescription products that contain acetaminophen, which may be hard for patients to identify on the label, and consumers' lack knowledge about the association of acetaminophen and serious liver injury.

Acetaminophen-related hepatotoxicity is dose-dependent. Even at therapeutic doses, acetaminophen may cause transient liver enzyme elevations and is potentially hepatotoxic.[68] Acetaminophen should be used cautiously for patients with liver disease or for those who abuse alcohol.[69] The most common risk factor for liver failure for these patients was chronic alcohol intake.[70] The FDA has recommended that chronic alcohol users (three or more drinks daily) avoid acetaminophen intake as it increases the risk of liver damage or GI bleeding. Other individuals do not appear to be at increased risk of GI bleeding.

Drug–Drug Interactions and Drug–Food Interactions Drug interactions with acetaminophen can occur; for example, isoniazid can increase the risk of hepatotoxicity. Chronic ingestion of maximal doses of acetaminophen may intensify the anticoagulant effect for patients taking warfarin; such individuals may need closer monitoring. Although food decreases the maximum serum concentration of acetaminophen by approximately half, the overall efficacy is unchanged.

Dosing and Administration When used for chronic OA, acetaminophen should be administered in a scheduled manner. It may be taken with or without food. Acetaminophen can be taken at 325 to 650 mg every 4 to 6 hours, but the total dose must not exceed 4 g daily (see "Adverse Effects" under "Acetaminophen"). FDA labeling requirements warn patients about potential liver toxicity if they inadvertently ingest more than the recommended dose when using multiple products containing acetaminophen. Additionally, prescription analgesics containing acetaminophen are limited to 325 mg per tablet to further decrease the opportunity for inadvertent overdose. Acetaminophen should be avoided in the setting of chronic alcohol intake or in those with underlying liver disease.

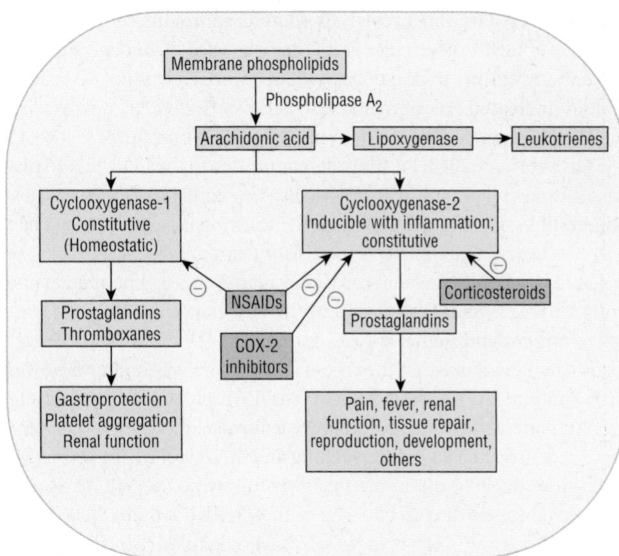

FIGURE 90-6 Pathway of synthesis for prostaglandins and leukotrienes. COX-1 and COX-2 are cyclooxygenase-1 and cyclooxygenase-2 enzymes, respectively. The minus (–) sign indicates inhibitory influence. Prostaglandins include PGE_2 and PGI_2; the latter is also known as prostacyclin.

Oral Nonsteroidal Anti-inflammatory Drugs

Pharmacology and Mechanism of Action NSAIDs reduce pain, inflammation, and fever by preventing synthesis of tissue prostaglandins and related prostanoids, which play a role in triggering these symptoms. All NSAIDs bind (reversibly) to the COX-2 enzyme, blocking its action and thus prostanoid production. Blockade of prostaglandin synthesis by inhibiting COX enzymes (mainly COX-2) is thought to account for NSAIDs' ability to relieve pain and inflammation (Fig. 90-6).[71] Nonselective NSAIDs were developed prior to extensive knowledge of COX enzymes, but in fact they block both COX-2 and COX-1. COX-1 has required "housekeeping" functions such as gastroprotection. COX-2 inhibitors selectively block COX-2 but not COX-1 activity.

The various NSAIDs exhibit several pharmacokinetic similarities, including high oral availability, high protein binding, and absorption as active drugs (except for sulindac and nabumetone, which require hepatic conversion for activity). There is a broad range of serum half-lives for different NSAIDs, which influence dosing frequency, and potentially, compliance with therapy.[72] Elimination of NSAIDs largely depends on hepatic inactivation, with a small fraction of active drug being renally excreted. NSAIDs penetrate joint fluid, reaching approximately 60% of blood levels.

Adverse Effects

GI Effects of Nonselective NSAIDs The most common adverse effects of NSAIDs involve the GI tract, contributing to many treatment failures.[73,74] Minor complaints such as nausea, dyspepsia, anorexia, abdominal pain, heartburn, and diarrhea affect 10% to 60% of patients. All NSAIDs increase ulcer risk, but the serious GI complications associated with NSAIDs include perforations, gastric outlet obstruction, and bleeding. These important GI complications occur in 1.5% to 4% of patients per year. NSAIDs are so widely used that these small percentages translate into substantial morbidity and mortality. Moreover, the risk increases substantially for patients with risk factors including a longer duration of NSAID usage, higher dosage, age older than 60, history of peptic ulcer disease of any cause, history of alcohol use, and concomitant use of glucocorticoids and/or anticoagulants.[71] A patient treated with NSAIDs has a three- to five-time higher risk of developing GI complications than a patient not treated with these medications.[75]

9 Options are available to reduce the GI risk of traditional NSAIDs. (1) Take the lowest dose possible, and take only when needed. (2) Take with the prostaglandin analog misoprostol four times daily to reduce the rate of ulcers and serious GI complications. However, many patients cannot tolerate the GI adverse events of misoprostol, especially diarrhea. (3) Take with a PPI daily.[75] Take with a full-dose H2 blocker daily. The PPI and the H2 blocker reduce minor GI complaints and the risk of ulcers, but they are not rigorously proven to decrease the serious complications, possibly because of lack of power to detect rare events in clinical trials.

Another choice that is available to reduce risk of GI events with an NSAID is to take a COX-2 selective inhibitor ("coxib").[72-74] Celecoxib is the only coxib available in the United States. Because this drug does not block the "housekeeping" gene, it may not have the same GI risks, but it is important to note it is not without GI risk.[70] A meta-analysis showed that COX-2 selective inhibitors were associated with significantly fewer gastroduodenal ulcers and clinically important ulcer complications. Celecoxib has been shown to be as safe to the upper GI tract as a nonselective NSAID plus a PPI.[76] Another concern is the risk associated with NSAID use in patients taking aspirin for cardioprotection. It appears that the GI risk is lower in patients taking a coxib medication and low-dose aspirin than a nonselective NSAID. However, in patients with high GI risk the combination may still be harmful and gastroprotection is appropriate.[76]

Cardiovascular Risk of COX-2 Inhibitors and Traditional NSAIDs Both nonselective and selective NSAIDs are associated with an increased risk for hypertension, stroke, myocardial infarction (MI), and death. NSAIDs should be avoided in patients with known active ischemic heart disease, cerebrovascular disease, and moderate-to-severe heart failure.[71] It is not entirely clear the mechanism for the cardiovascular effects of NSAIDs.[75] NSAIDs are associated with hypertension, increased preload, volume expansion, and reduced sodium excretion.[77] A large meta-analysis showed some differences among NSAIDs in terms of vascular risk. The risks with diclofenac and ibuprofen were similar to that of coxibs, but naproxen was not associated with an increased risk of major vascular events. Overall, coxibs were found to increase vascular risk by approximately one-third.[78]

In February 2014, an advisory committee to the FDA met to discuss the data relating the cardiovascular risk and NSAIDs. After their review, FDA decided to strengthen the warning label for non-aspirin NSAIDs, warning patients on the risk of heart attack and stroke. The updated labeling warns that cardiovascular events can happen at any point during NSAID therapy, and the risk may increase with longer treatment and higher doses. The FDA concluded that there was insufficient evidence that the risk of any NSAID was higher or lower than another. An increased risk for cardiovascular events is present even in patients with no underlying cardiovascular disease. The data reviewed also showed patients taking an NSAID following a first MI were more likely to die in the first year following the MI.[79,80] Strategies to reduce cardiovascular risk with NSAIDs are not well documented. Naproxen may present less cardiovascular risk than coxibs and diclofenac at higher doses; its use therefore seems prudent to consider when choosing a specific NSAID.[75,76,79]

Other Toxicities Associated with NSAIDs NSAIDs may cause kidney diseases, including acute renal insufficiency, sodium retention, acute interstitial nephritis, renal papillary necrosis, and accelerated chronic kidney disease. Sodium retention has been reported to occur in up to 25% of NSAID-treated patients and can be a cause of exacerbations of congestive heart failure.[77] Clinical features of these NSAID-induced renal syndromes include increased serum creatinine and blood urea nitrogen, hyperkalemia, elevated blood pressure, peripheral edema, and weight gain. Patients at high risk are those with conditions associated with decreased renal blood flow or taking certain medications. Examples are those with chronic renal insufficiency, congestive heart failure, severe hepatic disease, and nephrotic syndrome, those of advanced age, or those taking diuretics, angiotensin-converting enzyme inhibitors, cyclosporine, or aminoglycosides (**Fig. 90-7**).

Close monitoring is advisable for high-risk patients taking an NSAID, with monitoring of serum creatinine at baseline and within 3 to 7 days of drug initiation. For those with impaired renal function, the National Kidney Foundation recommends acetaminophen

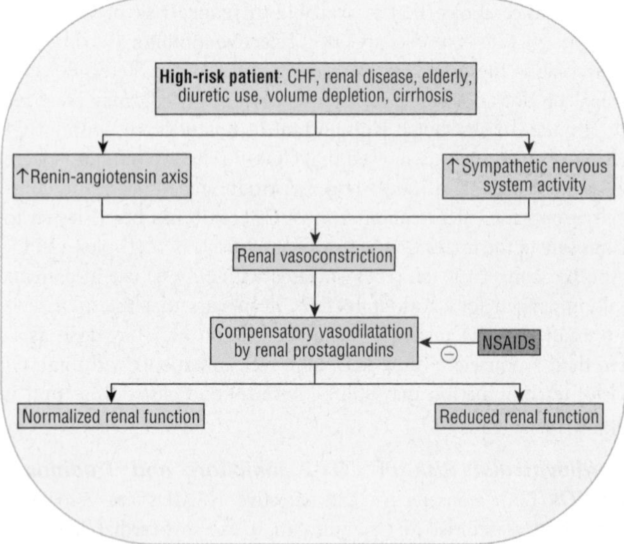

FIGURE 90-7 Mechanisms implicated in NSAID-induced renal injury. The minus (–) sign indicates inhibitory influence (CHF, congestive heart failure; NSAIDs, nonsteroidal anti-inflammatory drugs).

over NSAIDs, although acetaminophen may pose risks, as discussed earlier.

Coxibs and NSAIDs uncommonly cause drug-induced hepatitis; the two NSAIDs most frequently implicated are diclofenac and sulindac. Patient monitoring should include periodic liver enzymes (aspartate aminotransferase and alanine aminotransferase), with cessation of therapy if these values exceed two to three times the upper limit of normal. In a pooled analysis of 41 studies including celecoxib, there was a low rate of serious, hepatic-related adverse events with celecoxib (1.11%), with no significant difference from naproxen or ibuprofen, but a significantly higher incidence with diclofenac (4.24%).[81]

Other toxic effects of NSAIDs include hypersensitivity reactions, rash, and CNS complaints of drowsiness, dizziness, headaches, depression, confusion, and tinnitus.[72] It is also recommended that NSAIDs be avoided for patients with asthma who are aspirin-intolerant.

All nonspecific NSAIDs inhibit COX-1–dependent thromboxane production in platelets and thus increase bleeding risk. Unlike aspirin, celecoxib and nonspecific NSAIDs inhibit thromboxane formation reversibly, with normalization of platelet function 1 to 3 days after the drug is stopped. Warfarin and celecoxib are metabolized by the cytochrome P450 isoenzyme CYP2C9; patients receiving warfarin and COX-2 inhibitors should be followed closely.

Finally, if misoprostol is taken for GI protection, great care is indicated. Because of its abortifacient properties, misoprostol is contraindicated in pregnancy and in women of childbearing age who are not maintaining adequate contraception. It must be dispensed in its original container, which carries a warning for these individuals. Misoprostol is also available in a combination product with diclofenac, which bears the same restrictions as misoprostol alone.

Drug–Drug Interactions Avoidance of concomitant use, or anticipation and careful monitoring, can often prevent serious events with potentially interacting drugs. The most potentially serious interactions include the use of NSAIDs with lithium, warfarin, other agents that increase bleeding risk, oral hypoglycemics, methotrexate, antihypertensives, angiotensin-converting enzyme inhibitors, β-blockers, and diuretics.[72] In addition, there are probable drug interactions with tacrolimus for ibuprofen, naproxen, diclofenac, and possibly other NSAIDs.

Specific drug interactions are also seen with celecoxib.[82] Celecoxib metabolism is primarily via CYP2C9.[82] Cytochrome P450 inducers such as rifampin, carbamazepine, and phenytoin have the potential to reduce celecoxib levels. Concomitant administration of celecoxib with fluconazole can increase plasma concentrations of celecoxib, due to fluconazole inhibition of the CYP2C9 isoenzyme. Because warfarin and celecoxib are both metabolized by CYP2C9, patients receiving warfarin and COX-2 inhibitors should be followed closely. Because celecoxib inhibits CYP2D6, it has the potential to increase concentrations of a variety of agents, including antidepressants. Celecoxib is a sulfonamide and is thus noted to be contraindicated for those with sulfa allergies.[82]

Another drug interaction has been noted for those taking some NSAIDs and cardioprotective doses of aspirin. Ibuprofen, used at doses of 400 mg or more, may block aspirin's antiplatelet effect if it is taken before aspirin. Patients taking ibuprofen have been advised to take a single dose of ibuprofen at least 30 minutes after taking aspirin, or to take their aspirin at least 8 hours after taking ibuprofen. Other nonselective NSAIDs, such as naproxen, also may cause such interactions. Currently, the ACR recommends that patients who need an oral NSAID for OA choose an NSAID other than ibuprofen or COX-2 selective inhibitors.[40] Acetaminophen does not appear to interfere with the antiplatelet effect of aspirin.

Dosing and Administration Administration of NSAIDs must be tailored to the individual patient with OA. Selection of an NSAID depends on the prescriber's experience, medication cost, patient preference, allergies, toxicities, and adherence issues. Individual patient response differs among NSAIDs, so if an inadequate response is obtained with one NSAID, another NSAID may yet provide benefit.[40,41]

Topical Nonsteroidal Anti-inflammatory Drugs

Pharmacology and Mechanism of Action The mechanism of action of topical NSAIDs is considered to be through inhibition of the COX-2 enzyme in tissues near the site of application. Studies show significant placebo effects that could result from rubbing the product into the skin, which may have a counterirritant effect. Topical NSAIDs are significantly more efficacious compared with placebo vehicle in reducing pain due to musculoskeletal conditions, including OA. Most trials have shown topical diclofenac to be as effective as oral NSAIDs, including both oral diclofenac and other comparators.[57,65,83] Diclofenac 1% gel as well as the newer diclofenac solution, and diclofenac patches are currently approved in the United States for OA.

Adverse Effects Compared with oral NSAIDs, topical NSAIDs are associated with many fewer GI adverse events and fewer adverse events overall, except for local application site reactions. In comparison with placebo or oral NSAIDs, topical NSAID use is associated with more local adverse events, most often mild skin reactions such as itching or rash, but with very few serious adverse effects. In a comparison of oral (n=311) and topical diclofenac (n=311), significantly more persons receiving topical diclofenac developed dry skin, rash, and itching, but none was considered serious. However, significantly more persons receiving oral diclofenac had severe GI effects, asthma, dizziness, dyspnea, change from normal to abnormal hemoglobin, alanine aminotransferase increase to more than three times upper the limit of normal, and creatinine clearance changing from normal to abnormal.[57]

A nested case–control study from the United Kingdom revealed no significant association between topical NSAID use and renal failure, whereas oral NSAID use was significantly associated with a doubling of risk.[57] An estimated 1% to 15% of topical NSAID enters the systemic circulation; this is usually less than 5%, which contributes to its greater safety profile.[39,83]

Drug–Drug Interactions Interactions listed for topical diclofenac are the same as for oral NSAIDs, which are listed for oral NSAIDs. The most potentially serious interactions include the use of NSAIDs with lithium, warfarin, and other agents that increase bleeding risk, oral hypoglycemics, methotrexate, antihypertensives, angiotensin-converting enzyme inhibitors, β-blockers, and diuretics. Other topical agents have not been studied with topical diclofenac and changes in tolerability and absorption are possible. For all of these interactions, as there is only a small percentage of diclofenac absorbed, the risks are likely significantly less than with oral drug, but the patient and provider would have to be wise to monitor appropriately for these interactions with any of these drugs the patient is taking. Patients should avoid oral NSAIDs while using topical products to minimize potential for additive adverse effects. Care should be taken to avoid contact with the eyes or open wounds and to wash hands after application (except when treating hand OA).

Dosing and Administration Diclofenac 1% gel (Voltaren) can be used for hand or knee OA or other joints amenable to topical application (eg, not the hip). It is applied four times daily using the dose measuring cards provided by the manufacturer. The gel (4 g) is recommended for application to the affected area in the lower limb four times daily, and for upper extremities, the dose is 2 g four times daily. Diclofenac solution (Pennsaid®), only approved for knee OA, is available in 1.5% and 2% solution. Forty drops of the 1.5% solution are to be applied four times a day to each affected knee. The solution should be applied to the back, front, and sides of the knee. For each dose, the patient is advised to place 10 drops at a time directly onto the painful knee (or first into the hands and then immediately spread onto the knee) and rub the solution in. The patient is advised to repeats this process three more times until 40 drops have been applied to the painful knee for that particular dose. The 2% diclofenac solution is available in a meter-dose pump. Two actuations or 40 mg are applied twice daily to the affected knee(s). The entire dose should be pumped into the palm of the hand then applied evenly to the knee. The diclofenac patch (diclofenac epolamine 180 mg) is applied twice daily. If the patch does not stick well, the patient can secure the edges using first-aid tape. Patient counseling is important to carefully explain how to apply the topical products and how long to wait before dressing, putting on gloves, showering, and so forth.

Intra-Articular Corticosteroids

Pharmacology and Mechanism of Action The anti-inflammatory properties of corticosteroids as a class are the primary mechanism of pain relief in the treatment of OA. These properties decrease the formation and release of prostaglandins, kinins, liposomal enzymes, and histamine. These actions decrease erythema, swelling, heat, and tenderness of the inflamed joints.[40,84] Aspiration of the effusion and injection of glucocorticoid are carried out aseptically, with examination of the aspirate recommended to exclude crystalline arthritis or infection. Several randomized, placebo-controlled, double-blind studies have shown that intra-articular corticosteroids are superior to placebo in alleviating knee pain and stiffness caused by OA but with a relatively short duration.[84] The most commonly used corticosteroids for intra-articular use are triamcinolone acetonide and methylprednisolone acetate. The branched esters of triamcinolone and methylprednisolone are preferred by practitioners because of the reduced solubility that allows the agents to remain in the joint space longer.[85,86]

Adverse Events Adverse events associated with intra-articular injection of corticosteroids can be local or systemic in nature. Systemic adverse events are the same as with any other systemic corticosteroid and can include hyperglycemia, edema, elevated blood pressure, flushing, dyspepsia, and hypercortisolism. Evidence shows an acute (2- to 3-day) rise in blood glucose in patients with diabetes following a single corticosteroid injection. The risk of systemic adverse effects can be lessened by limiting the dose of the corticosteroid since doses greater than 40 mg for triamcinolone or methylprednisolone have not been shown to provide any additional benefit.[86] Local adverse effects can include infection in the affected joint, osteonecrosis, tendon rupture, and skin atrophy at the injection site. Systemic corticosteroid therapy is not recommended in OA, given the lack of proven benefit and the well-known adverse effects with long-term use.

Dosing and Administration Doses for injection of triamcinolone and methylprednisolone acetate into large joints in adults are shown in Table 90-2. Local anesthetics such as lidocaine or bupivacaine are commonly combined with corticosteroids to provide rapid pain relief.[86] This therapy is generally limited to three or four injections per year due to the potential systemic effects of corticosteroids and because the need for more frequent injections indicates little response to the therapy.

After injection, the patient should minimize activity and stress on the joint for several days. Initial pain relief may be seen within 24 to 72 hours after injection, with peak pain relief about 7 to 10 days after injection and lasting up to 4 to 8 weeks.

Capsaicin

Pharmacology and Mechanism of Action Capsaicin, isolated from hot peppers, releases and ultimately depletes substance P from afferent nociceptive nerve fibers. Substance P has been implicated in the transmission of pain in arthritis, and capsaicin cream has been shown in four placebo-controlled studies to provide pain relief in knee and hand OA when applied over affected joints.[65] Due to the larger surface area and distance from the site of application to the joint, it is not expected that application of capsaicin would provide efficacy in the treatment of hip OA.

Adverse Effects Adverse events associated with capsaicin are primarily local, with one in three patients experiencing burning, stinging, and/or erythema that usually subsides with repeated application. The FDA has issued a public drug safety communication notifying consumers that rare cases of severe burns have been reported.[87] Some patients may experience coughing associated with application.

Dosing and Administration To be effective, capsaicin must be used regularly, and it may take up to 2 weeks to take effect. Although use is recommended four times a day, a twice-daily application may enhance long-term adherence and still provide adequate pain relief.[65] Patients should be counseled not to get the cream in their eyes or mouth. Patients should also notify their healthcare provider immediately if they experience pain, swelling, or blistering skin at the site of application.

Capsaicin is a nonprescription product available as a cream, gel, solution, lotion, or patch in concentrations ranging from 0.025% to 0.15%.

Tramadol

Pharmacology and Mechanism of Action (10) Tramadol, an analgesic with affinity for the μ-opioid receptor, as well as weak inhibition of the reuptake of norepinephrine and serotonin neurotransmitter, has shown moderate pain improvement for patients with OA when compared with placebo.[88,89] Tramadol is also modestly effective as add-on therapy for patients taking concomitant acetaminophen, NSAIDs, or COX-2–selective inhibitors. Tramadol may be helpful for patients who cannot take NSAIDs or COX-2–selective inhibitors.

Adverse Events Opioid-like adverse effects such as nausea, vomiting, dizziness, constipation, headache, and somnolence are common with tramadol. These occur in 45% to 84% of treated patients.[90] Although the frequency of adverse effects is high, the severity of adverse effects is less than with NSAIDs, as tramadol use is not associated with life-threatening GI bleeding, cardiovascular events, or renal failure. The most notable serious adverse event associated with tramadol use is seizures. Withdrawal symptoms can occur if tramadol is stopped abruptly. Patients older than 65 are significantly more likely to experience adverse events.[90] Tramadol was initially not classified as a controlled substance but has been rescheduled as a class IV controlled substance due to its potential for dependence, addiction, and diversion.[91]

Drug–Drug Interaction Medications that lower the seizure threshold should be used with caution in patients taking tramadol. These include tricyclic antidepressants, first-generation antipsychotic medications, and cyclobenzaprine, as well as others. There is also an increased risk of serotonin syndrome (see Chapter e9, for information on this condition) when tramadol is used concomitantly with other serotonergic medications, including duloxetine.

Dosing and Administration Tramadol should be initiated at a lower dose (100 mg per day) and may be titrated as needed for pain control to a dose of 200 mg per day, with a maximum dose of 400 mg per day. Tramadol is available in a combination tablet with acetaminophen and as an extended-release tablet or capsule.

Second-Line Treatments

Opioid Analgesics

Opioid analgesics may be useful for patients who experience limited pain relief with acetaminophen, oral NSAIDs, intra-articular injections, or topical therapy or who cannot tolerate the adverse effects of these agents.[70] For patients with underlying conditions that limit the use of first-line analgesics, opioid analgesics can effectively relieve acute OA pain. A common clinical scenario may include the patient who cannot take oral NSAIDs because of renal failure or cardiovascular disease. Patients in whom all other treatment options have failed and who are at high surgical risk, precluding joint arthroplasty are also candidates for opioid therapy. It is important to carefully use opioids to promote safety. The CDC recommends the best practice for prescribing opioid include using the lowest effective dose and the smallest quantity needed, providing patients with information on how to use, store, and dispose of opioid medications, and avoiding combinations of opioids and sedating medications unless there is a specific indication to do so.[92]

Sustained-release (SR) compounds usually offer better pain control throughout the day, and are used when immediate-release (IR) opioids do not provide a sufficient duration of pain control. A variety of immediate and sustained-release opioid compounds have been studied including oxycodone IR and SR, morphine IR and SR, hydromorphone, and fentanyl transdermal patch.[59]

Adverse effects are common in opioid-treated OA patients. More than 75% of patients in clinical trials experience at least one typical opioid-related (ie, nausea, somnolence, constipation, dry mouth, and dizziness) adverse effect. Although this is not an unexpected finding, it serves as a reminder to use opioids cautiously in elderly patients who may be more susceptible to adverse effects.

Opioid dependence, addiction, tolerance, hyperalgesia, and issues surrounding drug diversion are more serious adverse effects associated with long-term treatment. Prescription opioid misuse/abuse/addiction is a major public health concern with the CDC reporting more than 16,000 deaths in 2013. In 2011, there were 420,000 emergency department visits attributed to the misuse and abuse of prescription opioids.[93] Patients should be educated on the risks of taking opioids including addiction, overdose, and death.[93,94]

If pain is intolerable and limits activities of daily living, and the patient has sufficiently good cardiopulmonary health to undergo major surgery, joint replacement may be preferable to continued reliance on opioids.

Duloxetine

Duloxetine is a centrally acting dual-reuptake inhibitor of both serotonin and norepinephrine, although norepinephrine reuptake inhibition does not occur until doses reach 60 mg per day. While the most common pain target in OA is peripheral nociceptive pain, there is some evidence that chronic nociceptive pain leads to central pain sensitization thereby lowering the pain threshold.[61] Duloxetine provides pain relief through the blocking of central pain transmitters, including serotonin and norepinephrine.

Adverse effects commonly associated with duloxetine therapy include nausea, dry mouth, constipation, and anorexia. Expected neurologic adverse effects include fatigue, somnolence, and dizziness. Rare, but serious adverse events associated with duloxetine include Stevens-Johnson syndrome and liver failure. Patients should be notified to contact their healthcare provider immediately if they develop a rash while taking duloxetine.

Particular care should be taken to avoid the use of duloxetine with other serotonergic medications including tramadol. As tramadol is a first-line treatment recommendation for OA, the likelihood of encountering this combination is high. Concomitant use of duloxetine with other medications that increase serotonin concentrations increases the risk of serotonin-syndrome.

Hyaluronic Acid Injections

Hyaluronate is a naturally occurring component of cartilage and synovial fluid. Exogenous intra-articular hyaluronate is available as a treatment for the symptoms of knee OA. The goal of intra-articular HA is to provide and maintain intra-articular lubrication. HA may also have anti-inflammatory, analgesic, and chondroprotective effects on the articular cartilage and joint synovium.[95] The efficacy of HA injections remains debated and uncertain after many trials and meta-analyses.[95] Many trials show a large placebo effect. Most HA products are injected once weekly for either 3 or 5 weeks, depending on the specific agent administered. Patients are generally advised to repeat the injection schedule by 6 months if they are satisfied with the previous course.[84] Strenuous or prolonged weight-bearing activities should be avoided for 48 hours after treatment. Routinely, the most improvement is expected from 5 to 13 weeks after injection with some effect still occurring at 24 weeks.[95] Injections are generally well tolerated, although acute joint swelling, effusion, and stiffness can occur as well as local skin reactions, including rash, ecchymosis, and pruritus have been reported. Local adverse effects are more frequent in products from animal origin.[96] Rarely, systemic adverse events including hypersensitivity reactions have occurred. Joint infections are rare but have been reported.

The effect of HA injections on knee OA appears to be modest at best.[95] HA products have not been shown to benefit patients with hip OA.[97] These agents are expensive because the treatment includes both drug costs and administration costs. Patient expectations and cost-effectiveness must be considered before choosing HA injection.[84]

Glucosamine and Chondroitin

Interest in chondroitin and glucosamine was spurred initially by anecdotal reports of benefit in animals and humans and by the ability of these substances to stimulate proteoglycan synthesis from articular cartilage in vitro. Enthusiasm for these agents has waned recently as additional efficacy data have become available to the point that the American College of Rheumatology conditionally recommends against the use of glucosamine and chondroitin.[40] Glucosamine, alone or in combination, has not been shown to provide uniform improvements in pain control or functional status in patients with OA of the knee or hip.[98]

Numerous trials have examined the safety and efficacy of glucosamine and chondroitin, but the duration of these studies has been relatively short. The efficacy of glucosamine and chondroitin was evaluated after 2 years and found not to be statistically superior than placebo.[99] The combination of glucosamine and chondroitin was well tolerated. There has previously been some concern that glucosamine may worsen diabetes or asthma; however, a 2-year follow-up trial did not substantiate this.[99] When the combination of glucosamine and chondroitin was compared with celecoxib in patients with knee OA, it was found to be noninferior in the reduction of pain at 6 months. The combination was well tolerated and the authors suggest glucosamine and chondroitin as a potential safe alternative for patients with cardiovascular or GI conditions.[100]

Because glucosamine and chondroitin are marketed in the United States as dietary supplements, neither the products nor their purity is adequately regulated by the FDA. The potential consequences related to the lack of regulatory oversight for these products can affect both efficacy and safety. Products containing less than labeled doses can compromise efficacy, while those containing ingredients not included on the labeling can compromise safety. A variety of brand name and generic products are available in various doses and formulations.

Clinical **Controversy...**

Vitamin D is hypothesized to play a role in many diseases including OA. Vitamin D is known to play a role in bone health and frequently vitamin D deficiency is found to coexist in older patients with OA. Studies have found conflicting evidence on whether vitamin D deficiency leads to an increased risk of development or progression of OA.

Considerations for Future Therapeutic Options

Strategies aimed at expanding therapeutic options for OA include an array of disease-modifying drugs, new drug classes to provide symptomatic relief of OA pain, and behavior modification strategies to improve patient participation in nonpharmacologic therapies.[101] Disease-modifying drugs are targeted at preventing, retarding, or reversing damage to articular cartilage. Currently, OA is a progressive disease. Current approaches to slow progression of OA are directed at three different tissue specific targets: (1) cartilage, (2) synovial membrane and associated inflammation, and (3) subchondral bone. Therapies directed at preserving cartilage include enzyme inhibitors of MMPs, inhibitors of inducible nitric oxide synthase, cathepsin K inhibitors, and nerve growth factor inhibitors.[101] Several of these investigational agents are in Phase I and Phase II clinical trials in humans.[102]

Several anti-inflammatory agents targeting symptom improvement as well as structure-modifying properties at the synovial membrane are in clinical trials. The agents include interleukin-1 inhibitors, the antitumor necrosis factor inhibitor, adalimumab, and adenosine A2 and A3 receptor agonists.[101] Current animal research supports these receptor targets to prevent ongoing joint destruction and early results for some of these agents, particularly adalimumab are encouraging.

Slowing the progression of OA may also be achieved by attempts to modify or repair bony changes associated with OA. Current strategies being evaluated in humans include the use of bisphosphonates, calcitonin, cholecalciferol, selective estrogen receptor modulators, parathyroid hormone, strontium, and MMP-13 inhibitors. The definitive role of these agents in modifying bone resorption as a strategy to delay the progression of bone damage associated with OA is yet to be determined.

Additionally, attempts to find new agents or methods to treat symptoms of OA are being made. Current research is exploring the utility of nerve growth factor inhibitors, cannabinoid receptor agonists, bradykinin receptor antagonists, kainate receptor antagonists, transient receptor potential ion channel agonists (TRVP-1).[101] Although many of these compounds are years away from potential market approval, the extensive nature of the work is encouraging.

In addition to pharmacologic agents, acupuncture has been examined in OA. In a systematic analysis of 18 randomized, controlled trials of manual or electroacupuncture, 10 showed positive effects for acupuncture.[103] However, in a recent, large, randomized, and well-controlled study, acupuncture was not seen to be any more effective than sham controls.[104]

Clinical **Controversy...**

The use of stem-cell therapy for the treatment of OA lacks efficacy and safety data from large, randomized, placebo controlled trials. Additionally, stem clinics in the United States are unlicensed and as such, their services are not covered by health insurance. The regulatory language authorizing stem cell clinics is ambiguous, allowing the proliferation of these entities, potentially exposing patients to risks without any known benefits.

PERSONALIZED PHARMACOTHERAPY

There is substantial negative impact on the quality of life for individual patients with OA. It is also clear that OA is associated with a negative impact on society as the disease is extremely common, and OA ranks second in causes of disability in the United States.[3,40]

Most OA patients use a multidisciplinary approach to their treatment.[40] Treatments include nonpharmacologic and pharmacologic therapy, in addition to surgical options in some patients. Unfortunately, many patients have less than optimal response to treatment and commonly require a change in therapy or augmentation of partially effective therapy. Achieving adequate pain control and minimizing functional impairment in OA patients requires careful assessment of comorbid conditions in each patient to safely provide effective pharmacotherapy treatments. Nonpharmacologic interventions may also require regular reinforcement and modifications.

It is becoming more important to consider OA as significant contributor to quality-of-life measures in the patients with multiple chronic conditions. About one-half of the US population has 1 chronic health condition, and 25% have 2 or more conditions.[1] Of those with at least 1 chronic health condition, 6.1% had arthritis only and 16.6% had arthritis with at least one other condition.[1] With nearly 25% of US adults with a least one chronic health condition having arthritis, comprehensive patient-centered medication management must be provided to these patients to maximize treatment goals for OA and other chronic conditions, while minimizing medication-related adverse outcomes.

A multidisciplinary intervention for knee OA initiated by pharmacists has been shown to improve adherence to OA guideline recommendations, decrease pain scores, and improve functional assessment scores.[105] These types of multidisciplinary disease state management programs that implement strategies to provide comprehensive care should be offered to all OA patients to maximize outcomes.

Total indirect and direct medical costs for OA patients are high. Direct medical costs associated with joint replacement continue to increase at higher than predicted rates due to increasing willingness of patients to undergo joint replacement surgery.[6] The highest costs associated with the pharmacotherapy of OA are hospitalization for treatment of NSAID-related complications, particularly serious GI adverse events. Historically, gastroprotective therapy or the use of COX-2–selective inhibitors for low-risk patients has not been cost-effective because of the large number needed to treat to prevent serious events, but most currently available PPIs are generic, multisource products, making concomitant treatment with PPIs cost-effective.[106] Pharmacoeconomic considerations for OA involve the selection of therapy for the initial treatment of patients with OA. Use of the nonprescription analgesic acetaminophen as initial therapy has greatly reduced medication costs in comparison with the use of NSAIDs, many of which are by prescription only. Oral NSAID costs vary considerably, depending on the medication, daily dose, and regimen selected. As oral NSAIDs as a class are therapeutically similar, the use of a less-expensive agent such as nonprescription ibuprofen or naproxen or a multisource generic product, may minimize the cost. More-expensive NSAIDs can be prescribed if neither of these offers benefit after a 2-week trial at sufficient doses. Topical NSAIDs are significantly more costly than oral agents, although may still be cost-effective in patients at high-risk for costly complications associated with oral NSAID therapy.

EVALUATION OF THERAPEUTIC OUTCOMES

For the person with OA, treatment decisions and pharmacotherapy monitoring (Table 90-3) is patient-specific. The patient's situation and individual needs should be considered when devising a treatment plan. Is the patient bothered primarily by pain, by limitations in activity, or with concerns about side effects from medications? Does the patient understand what OA is and why certain treatments are useful?

When the patient is first being assessed for the possibility of OA, the diagnosis is often straightforward, including history and physical examination, plain films of the affected joint(s), and laboratory tests. The older patient with unilateral knee pain, limited range of motion, no palpable warmth, crepitus, without prolonged morning stiffness, and without other suspicious findings, is highly likely to have knee OA. It is still reasonable to obtain x-ray films, which may help follow disease over time (although joint space narrowing often does not correlate with the extent of pain or difficulty walking). Basic laboratory tests can help decide what pharmacologic therapy is possible (eg, NSAIDs should not be used in patients with poor renal function), assessment of pain using a visual analog scale, range of motion for affected joints. Additional tests of OA severity may include measurement of grip strength, 50 ft walking time, patient and physician global assessment of OA severity, and assessment of ability to perform activities of daily living. Once the patient is assessed and diagnosed, patient and family education is essential.

TABLE 90-3 Drug Monitoring Table

Drug	Adverse Drug Reactions	Monitoring Parameters	Comments
Oral Analgesics			
Acetaminophen	Hepatotoxicity	Total daily dose limits	Use caution with multiple acetaminophen-containing products—total 4 g limit
Tramadol	Nausea, vomiting, somnolence	No routine laboratory tests recommended	Drug–drug interaction with other serotonergic medications
Opioids	Sedation, constipation, nausea, dry mouth, hormonal changes	No routine laboratory tests recommended	Risks of addiction, dependence, and drug diversion
NSAIDs	Dyspepsia, cardiovascular events, GI bleeding, renal impairment	BUN/creatinine, hemoglobin/hematocrit, blood pressure	Risks higher in those older than 75 years of age
Topical Analgesics			
Capsaicin	Skin irritation and burning	Inspection of areas of application	Wash hands thoroughly after application
NSAIDs	Skin itching, rash, irritation, dyspepsia, cardiovascular events, GI bleeding, renal impairment	Inspection of areas of application As needed: blood urea nitrogen/creatinine, hemoglobin/hematocrit, blood pressure	Wash hands thoroughly after application. Avoid oral NSAID or aspirin other than cardioprotective dose. Ensure patient applying gel, solution, or patch correctly
Injectable Drugs			
Intraarticular corticosteroids	Hypertension, hyperglycemia	Glucose, blood pressure	Hypothalamic–pituitary–adrenal axis suppression if used too frequently
Intraarticular hyaluronates	Local joint swelling, stiffness, pain	No routine laboratory tests recommended	Less effective than intraarticular corticosteroids; expensive

Nondrug therapy may include a referral for physical and/or occupational therapy services, where the therapists can help maintain and improve range of motion. Referral for nutritional counseling and weight loss may also be necessary if the patient is overweight or obese. These interventions may decrease pain and facilitate improved activity for OA patients.

Although all patients must be provided with nonpharmacologic therapies, these interventions usually require weeks to months to assess for efficacy. In the meantime, the patient needs pain relief. First-line therapy continues to be acetaminophen. Adverse events with acetaminophen are uncommon, although it is important that the patient understands the maximum daily dose limits and all possible sources of acetaminophen containing products. Although some do well on acetaminophen, many do not achieve sufficient pain relief. A step up to oral NSAIDs or opioid therapy might be necessary but poses significant risks beyond acetaminophen. A switch to NSAIDs requires careful consideration of the patient's age and comorbidities, renal function, history of GI problems, hypertension, and cardiovascular health. Periodic monitoring would include open-ended questions followed by direct questions relating to the commonest adverse effects associated with the respective medication. For an oral NSAID, symptoms of abdominal pain, heartburn, nausea, or change in stool color provide valuable clues to the presence of GI complications, although serious GI complications can occur without warning. Patients should be monitored for the development of hypertension, weight gain, edema, skin rash, and CNS adverse effects such as headaches and drowsiness. Baseline serum creatinine, complete blood count, and serum transaminases are repeated at 6- to 12-month intervals to identify GI, renal, and hepatic toxicities.

Topical NSAIDs have demonstrated efficacy in OA of the hand and knee and are as effective as oral NSAIDs. Although they carry the same cardiovascular, renal, and GI warnings, their AUC for a typical dose is only a few percent of the AUC from an equivalent dose of oral NSAID. Topical NSAIDs' most common side effects are local, with irritated skin, rash, or itching, usually mild, and with many fewer adverse effects of cardiovascular, GI, or renal nature. These agents are a welcome addition to the limited treatment modalities for the very common, costly, painful, and often disabling disease of OA. It is important that the patient apply the topical products appropriately to achieve maximum benefit and avoiding adverse events.

For patients receiving intra-articular corticosteroids, pain relief should begin with 2 to 3 days and last 4 to 8 weeks. Patients should be advised about possible injection site reactions, as well as possible systemic effects, especially for those with hypertension or diabetes, as there is a potential for increased blood pressure or blood glucose. For patients receiving opioids or tramadol, relief from pain should occur rapidly. Frail or elderly patients should be monitored carefully and cautioned about sedation, dysphoria, nausea, risk of falls, and constipation. Additional monitoring should include strategies to assess development of opioid tolerance and addiction.

CONCLUSION

OA is a very common, slowly progressive disorder that affects diarthrodial joints and is characterized by progressive deterioration of articular cartilage, subchondral sclerosis, and osteophyte production. Clinical manifestations include gradual onset of joint pain, stiffness, and limitation of motion. The primary treatment goals are to reduce pain, maintain function, and prevent further destruction. An individualized approach based on education, rest, exercise, weight loss as needed, and analgesic medication can succeed in meeting these goals. Recommended drug treatment starts with acetaminophen less than or equal to 4 g/day and topical analgesics as needed. If acetaminophen is ineffective, oral NSAIDs may be used in appropriately selected patients, often providing satisfactory relief of pain and stiffness. Individuals at increased risk for toxicity from NSAIDs, especially for GI, cardiovascular, or renal events, deserve special attention. Celecoxib may have safety advantages in some OA patients, but its safety relative to other NSAIDs and its role in OA remains poorly defined. Adjunctive therapy with tramadol, intra-articular corticosteroids and opioid analgesics may be helpful in patients with poorly controlled pain. Experimental therapy aimed at preventing the progression of OA requires further clinical investigation before entering widespread clinical use.

ABBREVIATIONS

AAAL	Arthritis-Attributable Activities Limitations
BMI	body mass index
CNS	central nervous system
COX	cyclooxygenase
ECM	extracellular matrix
FDA	Food and Drug Administration
GI	gastrointestinal
GWAS	genome-wide linkage studies
HA	hyaluronic acid
IDEA	Intensive Diet and Exercise for Arthritis
IR	immediate release
LOX	lipoxygenase
MI	Myocardial infarction
MMP	matrix metalloproteinase
NICE	National Institute for Health and Clinical Excellence
NSAID	nonsteroidal anti-inflammatory drug
OA	osteoarthritis
OARSI	Osteoarthritis Research International
PPI	proton pump inhibitor
QALE	quality-adjusted life expectancy
SR	sustained release
TIMP	tissue inhibitors of metalloproteinase

REFERENCES

1. Qin J, Theis KA, Barbour KE, et al. Impact of arthritis and multiple chronic conditions on selected life domains—United States, 2013. *MMWR Morb Mortal Wkly Rep* 2015;64(21):578-582.
2. Murphy L, Helmick CG. The impact of osteoarthritis in the United States: A population-health perspective. *Am J Nurs* 2012; 112(3 Suppl 1):S13-S19.
3. Centers for Disease Control and Prevention (CDC). Prevalence of doctor-diagnosed arthritis and arthritis-attributable activity limitation-united states, 2010-2012. *MMWR Morb Mortal Wkly Rep* 2013;62(44):869-873.
4. Lawrence RC, Felson DT, Helmick CG, et al. Estimates of the prevalence of arthritis and other rheumatic conditions in the United States. part II. *Arthritis Rheum* 2008;58(1):26-35.
5. Torio CM (AHRQ), Andrew RM (AHRQ). National inpatient hospital costs: The most expensive conditions by payer, 2011. *Agency for Healthcare Research and Quality* August 2013;HCUP Statistical Brief #160:09/15/2015.
6. Agency for Healthcare Research and Quality. Total expenses and percent distribution for selected conditions by type of service: United states, 2012. Medical Expenditure Panel Survey Household Component Data. Available at: http://meps.ahrq.gov/mepsweb/data_stats/tables_compendia_hh_interactive.jsp?_SERVICE=MEPSSocket0&_PROGRAM=MEPSPGM.TC.SAS&File=HCFY2012&Table=HCFY2012%5FCNDXP%5FC&_Debug= Last accessed 09/15, 2015.
7. Losina E, Paltiel AD, Weinstein AM, et al. Lifetime medical costs of knee osteoarthritis management in the United States: Impact of extending indications for total knee arthroplasty. *Arthritis Care Res (Hoboken)* 2015;67(2):203-215.
8. Dagenais S, Garbedian S, Wai EK. Systematic review of the prevalence of radiographic primary hip osteoarthritis. *Clin Orthop Relat Res* 2009;467(3):623-637.
9. Feydy A, Pluot E, Guerini H, Drape JL. Osteoarthritis of the wrist and hand, and spine. *Radiol Clin North Am* 2009;47(4):723-759.

10. Jordan JM. An ongoing assessment of osteoarthritis in African Americans and Caucasians in North Carolina: The Johnston county osteoarthritis project. *Trans Am Clin Climatol Assoc* 2015;126:77-86.
11. Zhang Y, Jordan JM. Epidemiology of osteoarthritis. *Clin Geriatr Med* 2010;26(3):355-369.
12. Kotlarz H, Gunnarsson CL, Fang H, Rizzo JA. Osteoarthritis and absenteeism costs: Evidence from US national survey data. *J Occup Environ Med* 2010;52(3):263-268.
13. Garstang SV, Stitik TP. Osteoarthritis: Epidemiology, risk factors, and pathophysiology. *Am J Phys Med Rehabil* 2006;85(11 Suppl):S2-11; quiz S12-4.
14. Mork PJ, Holtermann A, Nilsen TI. Effect of body mass index and physical exercise on risk of knee and hip osteoarthritis: Longitudinal data from the Norwegian HUNT study. *J Epidemiol Community Health* 2012;66(8):678-683.
15. Andersen S, Thygesen LC, Davidsen M, Helweg-Larsen K. Cumulative years in occupation and the risk of hip or knee osteoarthritis in men and women: A register-based follow-up study. *Occup Environ Med* 2012;69(5):325-330.
16. Munk HL, Svendsen AJ, Hjelmborg J, Sorensen GL, Kyvik KO, Junker P. Heritability assessment of cartilage metabolism. A twin study on circulating procollagen IIA N-terminal propeptide (PIIANP). *Osteoarthritis Cartilage* 2014;22(8):1142-1147.
17. Botha-Scheepers SA, Watt I, Slagboom E, et al. Influence of familial factors on radiologic disease progression over two years in siblings with osteoarthritis at multiple sites: A prospective longitudinal cohort study. *Arthritis Rheum* 2007;57(4):626-632.
18. Valdes AM, Spector TD. Genetic epidemiology of hip and knee osteoarthritis. *Nat Rev Rheumatol* 2011;7(1):23-32.
19. Evangelou E, Valdes AM, Kerkhof HJ, et al. Meta-analysis of genome-wide association studies confirms a susceptibility locus for knee osteoarthritis on chromosome 7q22. *Ann Rheum Dis* 2011;70(2):349-355.
20. Meulenbelt I. Osteoarthritis year 2011 in review: Genetics. *Osteoarthritis Cartilage* 2012;20(3):218-222.
21. Valdes AM, Spector TD. The contribution of genes to osteoarthritis. *Med Clin North Am* 2009;93(1):45-66, x.
22. Cisternas MG, Murphy L, Sacks JJ, Solomon DH, Pasta DJ, Helmick CG. Alternative methods for defining osteoarthritis and the impact on estimating prevalence in a US population-based survey. *Arthritis Care Res (Hoboken)* 2015.
23. Dieppe P. Developments in osteoarthritis. *Rheumatology (Oxford)* 2011;50(2):245-247.
24. Sandell LJ, Heinegdard D, Hering TH. Cell biology, biochemistry, and molecular biology of articular cartilage in osteoarthritis. In: Moscowitz RW, Altman RD, Hochberg MC, Buckwalter JA, Goldberg VM, eds, ed. *Osteoarthritis: Diagnosis and medical/surgical management.* 4th edition ed. Phildelphia, PA: Lippincott, Williams, & Wilkins; 2007:73-106
25. Felson D.T. Osteoarthritis. In: Fauci AS, Braunwald E, Kaspar DL, Hauser DL, Longo DLJ, Loscalzo J, eds, ed. *Harrison's principles of internal medicine.* New York, NY: McGraw-Hill; 2009:2158-2165.
26. Loeser RF, Goldring SR, Scanzello CR, Goldring MB. Osteoarthritis: A disease of the joint as an organ. *Arthritis Rheum* 2012;64(6):1697-1707.
27. Bijlsma JW, Berenbaum F, Lafeber FP. Osteoarthritis: An update with relevance for clinical practice. *Lancet* 2011;377(9783):2115-2126.
28. Goldring MB, Marcu KB. Cartilage homeostasis in health and rheumatic diseases. *Arthritis Res Ther* 2009;11(3):224.
29. Hunter DJ. Insights from imaging on the epidemiology and pathophysiology of osteoarthritis. *Radiol Clin North Am* 2009;47(4): 539-551.
30. Dell'accio F, De Bari C, Eltawil NM, Vanhummelen P, Pitzalis C. Identification of the molecular response of articular cartilage to injury, by microarray screening: Wnt-16 expression and signaling after injury and in osteoarthritis. *Arthritis Rheum* 2008;58(5):1410-1421.
31. Fukui N, Ikeda Y, Ohnuki T, et al. Regional differences in chondrocyte metabolism in osteoarthritis: A detailed analysis by laser capture microdissection. *Arthritis Rheum* 2008;58(1):154-163.
32. Wu J, Liu W, Bemis A, et al. Comparative proteomic characterization of articular cartilage tissue from normal donors and patients with osteoarthritis. *Arthritis Rheum* 2007;56(11):3675-3684.
33. Karsdal MA, Leeming DJ, Dam EB, et al. Should subchondral bone turnover be targeted when treating osteoarthritis? *Osteoarthritis Cartilage* 2008;16(6):638-646.
34. Rosenberg AE. Bones, joints and soft tissue tumors. In: Kumar V, Abbas AK, Fausto N, Aster J, eds., ed. *Robbins and cotran pathologic basis of disease, professional edition.* 8th ed ed. Philadelphia, PA: W.B. Saunders; 2009:1235-1236.
35. Altman RD. Laboratory diagnosis of osteoarthritis. In: Moscowitz RW, Altman RD, Hochberg MC, Buckwalter JA, Goldberg VM, eds. *Osteoarthritis: Diagnosis and Medical/Surgical Management.* 4th ed. Philadelphia, PA: Lippincott, Williams, & Wilkins; 2007:201-214.
36. American College of Rheumatology. Http://Www.rheumatology.org/publications/.
37. Zhang W, Doherty M, Leeb BF, et al. EULAR evidence based recommendations for the management of hand osteoarthritis: Report of a task force of the EULAR standing committee for international clinical studies including therapeutics (ESCISIT). *Ann Rheum Dis* 2007;66(3):377-388.
38. Bennell KL, Hunter DJ, Hinman RS. Management of osteoarthritis of the knee. *BMJ* 2012;345:e4934.
39. Conaghan PG, Dickson J, Grant RL, Guideline Development Group. Care and management of osteoarthritis in adults: Summary of NICE guidance. *BMJ* 2008;336(7642):502-503.
40. Hochberg MC, Altman RD, April KT, et al. American college of rheumatology 2012 recommendations for the use of nonpharmacologic and pharmacologic therapies in osteoarthritis of the hand, hip, and knee. *Arthritis Care Res (Hoboken)* 2012;64(4):455-474.
41. National Institute for Health and Care Excellence. Osteoarthritis care and management in adults. Available at: https://www.nice.org.uk/guidance/cg177. Updated 2014. Last accessed 08/25, 2015.
42. Knittle K, De Gucht V, Maes S. Lifestyle- and behaviour-change interventions in musculoskeletal conditions. *Best Pract Res Clin Rheumatol* 2012;26(3):293-304.
43. Hawker GA, Mian S, Bednis K, Stanaitis I. Osteoarthritis year 2010 in review: Non-pharmacologic therapy. *Osteoarthritis Cartilage* 2011; 19(4):366-374.
44. Bliddal H, Leeds AR, Christensen R. Osteoarthritis, obesity and weight loss: Evidence, hypotheses and horizons - A scoping review. *Obes Rev* 2014;15(7):578-586.
45. Vincent HK, DeJong G, Mascarenas D, Vincent KR. The effect of body mass index and hip abductor brace use on inpatient rehabilitation outcomes after total hip arthroplasty. *Am J Phys Med Rehabil* 2009; 88(3):201-209.
46. Josbeno DA, Kalarchian M, Sparto PJ, Otto AD, Jakicic JM. Physical activity and physical function in individuals post-bariatric surgery. *Obes Surg* 2011;21(8):1243-1249.
47. Messier SP, Mihalko SL, Legault C, et al. Effects of intensive diet and exercise on knee joint loads, inflammation, and clinical outcomes among overweight and obese adults with knee osteoarthritis: The IDEA randomized clinical trial. *JAMA* 2013;310(12):1263-1273.
48. Knittle K, De Gucht V, Maes S. Lifestyle- and behaviour-change interventions in musculoskeletal conditions. *Best Pract Res Clin Rheumatol* 2012;26(3):293-304.
49. Jenkinson CM, Doherty M, Avery AJ, et al. Effects of dietary intervention and quadriceps strengthening exercises on pain and function in overweight people with knee pain: Randomised controlled trial. *BMJ* 2009;339:b3170.
50. Nelson AE, Allen KD, Golightly YM, Goode AP, Jordan JM. A systematic review of recommendations and guidelines for the management of osteoarthritis: The chronic osteoarthritis management initiative of the U.S. bone and joint initiative. *Semin Arthritis Rheum* 2014;43(6):701-712.
51. Fernandes L, Storheim K, Nordsletten L, Risberg MA. Development of a therapeutic exercise program for patients with osteoarthritis of the hip. *Phys Ther* 2010;90(4):592-601.
52. Svege I, Nordsletten L, Fernandes L, Risberg MA. Exercise therapy may postpone total hip replacement surgery in patients with hip osteoarthritis: A long-term follow-up of a randomised trial. *Ann Rheum Dis* 2015;74(1):164-169.
53. Gossec L, Paternotte S, Maillefert JF, et al. The role of pain and functional impairment in the decision to recommend total joint replacement in hip and knee osteoarthritis: An international cross-sectional study of 1909 patients. Report of the OARSI-OMERACT task force on total joint replacement. *Osteoarthritis Cartilage* 2011;19(2):147-154.
54. Waimann CA, Fernandez-Mazarambroz RJ, Cantor SB, et al. Cost-effectiveness of total knee replacement: A prospective cohort study. *Arthritis Care Res (Hoboken)* 2014;66(4):592-599.
55. Skou ST, Roos EM, Laursen MB, et al. Total knee replacement plus physical and medical therapy or treatment with physical and medical therapy alone: A randomised controlled trial in patients with knee osteoarthritis (the MEDIC-study). *BMC Musculoskelet Disord* 2012;13:67.
56. Losina E, Walensky RP, Kessler CL, et al. Cost-effectiveness of total knee arthroplasty in the united states: Patient risk and hospital volume. *Arch Intern Med* 2009;169(12):1113-1121; discussion 1121-1122.

57. Chou R.McDonagh M.S. Nakamoto E, Griffin J. Analgesics for osteoarthritis: An update of the 2006 comparative effectiveness review. comparative effectiveness review no. 38. (prepared by the oregon evidence-based practice center under contract HHSA 290 2007 10057 I). *Agency for Healthcare Research and Quality.* 2011;No. 11(12)-EHC076-EF.
58. Bannuru RR, Schmid CH, Kent DM, Vaysbrot EE, Wong JB, McAlindon TE. Comparative effectiveness of pharmacologic interventions for knee osteoarthritis: A systematic review and network meta-analysis. *Ann Intern Med* 2015;162(1):46-54.
59. Nuesch E, Rutjes AW, Husni E, Welch V, Juni P. Oral or transdermal opioids for osteoarthritis of the knee or hip. *Cochrane Database Syst Rev* 2009;(4)(4):CD003115.
60. Frakes EP, Risser RC, Ball TD, Hochberg MC, Wohlreich MM. Duloxetine added to oral nonsteroidal anti-inflammatory drugs for treatment of knee pain due to osteoarthritis: Results of a randomized, double-blind, placebo-controlled trial. *Curr Med Res Opin* 2011; 27(12):2361-2372.
61. Hochberg MC, Wohlreich M, Gaynor P, Hanna S, Risser R. Clinically relevant outcomes based on analysis of pooled data from 2 trials of duloxetine in patients with knee osteoarthritis. *J Rheumatol* 2012;39(2):352-358.
62. Brown JP, Boulay LJ. Clinical experience with duloxetine in the management of chronic musculoskeletal pain. A focus on osteoarthritis of the knee. *Ther Adv Musculoskelet Dis* 2013;5(6):291-304.
63. Altman RD, Dreiser RL, Fisher CL, Chase WF, Dreher DS, Zacher J. Diclofenac sodium gel in patients with primary hand osteoarthritis: A randomized, double-blind, placebo-controlled trial. *J Rheumatol* 2009;36(9):1991-1999.
64. Altman RD. Pharmacological therapies for osteoarthritis of the hand: A review of the evidence. *Drugs Aging* 2010;27(9):729-745.
65. Altman RD, Barthel HR. Topical therapies for osteoarthritis. *Drugs* 2011;71(10):1259-1279.
66. Kuo HW, Tsai SS, Tiao MM, Liu YC, Lee IM, Yang CY. Analgesic use and the risk for progression of chronic kidney disease. *Pharmacoepidemiol Drug Saf* 2010;19(7):745-751.
67. Department of Health and Human Services. *Federal Register* 2009;81.
68. Watkins PB, Kaplowitz N, Slattery JT, et al. Aminotransferase elevations in healthy adults receiving 4 grams of acetaminophen daily: A randomized controlled trial. *JAMA* 2006;296(1):87-93.
69. Larson AM, Polson J, Fontana RJ, et al. Acetaminophen-induced acute liver failure: Results of a united states multicenter, prospective study. *Hepatology* 2005;42(6):1364-1372.
70. O'Neil CK, Hanlon JT, Marcum ZA. Adverse effects of analgesics commonly used by older adults with osteoarthritis: Focus on non-opioid and opioid analgesics. *Am J Geriatr Pharmacother* 2012;10(6):331-342.
71. Meara AS, Simon LS. Advice from professional societies: Appropriate use of NSAIDs. *Pain Med* 2013;14 Suppl 1:S3-10.
72. McEvoy GK, ed. AHFS drug information. ISBN 978-1-58528-247-0 ed. Bethesda, MD: *American Society of Health-System Pharmacists,* INC.; 2012.
73. Lanas A. Nonsteroidal antiinflammatory drugs and cyclooxygenase inhibition in the gastrointestinal tract: A trip from peptic ulcer to colon cancer. *Am J Med Sci* 2009;338(2):96-106.
74. Rostom A, Moayyedi P, Hunt R, Canadian Association of Gastroenterology Consensus Group. Canadian consensus guidelines on long-term nonsteroidal anti-inflammatory drug therapy and the need for gastroprotection: Benefits versus risks. *Aliment Pharmacol Ther* 2009;29(5):481-496.
75. Patricio JP, Barbosa JP, Ramos RM, Antunes NF, de Melo PC. Relative cardiovascular and gastrointestinal safety of non-selective non-steroidal anti-inflammatory drugs versus cyclo-oxygenase-2 inhibitors: Implications for clinical practice. *Clin Drug Investig* 2013;33(3):167-183.
76. Scarpignato C, Lanas A, Blandizzi C, et al. Safe prescribing of non-steroidal anti-inflammatory drugs in patients with osteoarthritis-an expert consensus addressing benefits as well as gastrointestinal and cardiovascular risks. *BMC Med* 2015;13:55-015-0285-0288.
77. Crofford LJ. Use of NSAIDs in treating patients with arthritis. *Arthritis Res Ther* 2013;15 Suppl 3:S2.
78. Coxib and traditional NSAID Trialists' (CNT) Collaboration, Bhala N, Emberson J, et al. Vascular and upper gastrointestinal effects of non-steroidal anti-inflammatory drugs: Meta-analyses of individual participant data from randomised trials. *Lancet* 2013;382(9894):769-779.
79. Bello AE, Holt RJ. Cardiovascular risk with non-steroidal anti-inflammatory drugs: Clinical implications. *Drug Saf* 2014;37(11): 897-902.
80. U.S. Food and Drug Administration. FDA drug safety communication: FDA strengthens warning that non-aspirin nonsteroidal anti-inflammatory drugs (NSAIDs) can cause heart attacks or strokes. Available at: http://www.fda.gov/Drugs/DrugSafety/ucm451800.htm. Updated 2015. Last accessed 09/13, 2015.
81. Soni P, Shell B, Cawkwell G, Li C, Ma H. The hepatic safety and tolerability of the cyclooxygenase-2 selective NSAID celecoxib: Pooled analysis of 41 randomized controlled trials. *Curr Med Res Opin* 2009;25(8):1841-1851.
82. Celebrex®[Package Insert]. Pfizer, Inc., NY, NY; May 2016. http://labeling.pfizer.com/ShowLabeling.aspx?id=793. Accessed June 9, 2016.
83. Derry S, Moore RA, Rabbie R. Topical NSAIDs for chronic musculoskeletal pain in adults. *Cochrane Database Syst Rev* 2012;9: CD007400.
84. Ayhan E, Kesmezacar H, Akgun I. Intraarticular injections (corticosteroid, hyaluronic acid, platelet rich plasma) for the knee osteoarthritis. *World J Orthop* 2014;5(3):351-361.
85. Pyne D, Ioannou Y, Mootoo R, Bhanji A. Intra-articular steroids in knee osteoarthritis: A comparative study of triamcinolone hexacetonide and methylprednisolone acetate. *Clin Rheumatol* 2004;23(2):116-120.
86. Law TY, Nguyen C, Frank RM, Rosas S, McCormick F. Current concepts on the use of corticosteroid injections for knee osteoarthritis. *Phys Sportsmed* 2015;43(3):269-273.
87. FDA Drug Safety Communication, Sept. 13, 2012. http://www.fda.gov/Drugs/DrugSafety/ucm318858.htm. Accessed August 14, 2015.
88. Cepeda MS, Camargo F, Zea C, Valencia L. Tramadol for osteoarthritis: A systematic review and metaanalysis. *J Rheumatol* 2007;34(3): 543-555.
89. Howes F, Buchbinder R, Winzenberg TB. Opioids for osteoarthritis? weighing benefits and risks: A cochrane musculoskeletal group review. *J Fam Pract* 2011;60(4):206-212.
90. Langley PC, Patkar AD, Boswell KA, Benson CJ, Schein JR. Adverse event profile of tramadol in recent clinical studies of chronic osteoarthritis pain. *Curr Med Res Opin* 2010;26(1):239-251.
91. Drug Enforcement Administration office of Diversion Control. Tramadol. Available at: http://www.deadiversion.usdoj.gov/drug_chem_info/tramadol.pdf. Updated 2014. Last accessed 09/10, 2015.
92. Centers for Disease Control and Prevention. What health care providers need to know about the epidemic. Available at: http://www.cdc.gov/drugoverdose/epidemic/providers.html. Updated 2015. Last accessed 09/11, 2015.
93. Centers for Disease Control and Prevention. Prescription drug overdose data. Available at: http://www.cdc.gov/drugoverdose/data/overdose.html. Updated 2015. Last accessed 09/11, 2015.
94. Chou R. 2009 clinical guidelines from the American pain society and the American academy of pain medicine on the use of chronic opioid therapy in chronic noncancer pain: What are the key messages for clinical practice? *Pol Arch Med Wewn* 2009;119(7-8):469-477.
95. Hunter DJ. Viscosupplementation for osteoarthritis of the knee. *N Engl J Med* 2015;372(11):1040-1047.
96. Henrotin Y, Raman R, Richette P, et al. Consensus statement on viscosupplementation with hyaluronic acid for the management of osteoarthritis. *Semin Arthritis Rheum* 2015;45(2):140-149.
97. Hunter DJ. Osteoarthritis: Hyaluronic acid is not effective in symptomatic hip OA. *Nat Rev Rheumatol* 2009;5(7):359-360.
98. Wandel S, Juni P, Tendal B, et al. Effects of glucosamine, chondroitin, or placebo in patients with osteoarthritis of hip or knee: Network meta-analysis. *BMJ* 2010;341:c4675.
99. Sawitzke AD, Shi H, Finco MF, et al. Clinical efficacy and safety of glucosamine, chondroitin sulphate, their combination, celecoxib or placebo taken to treat osteoarthritis of the knee: 2-year results from GAIT. *Ann Rheum Dis* 2010;69(8):1459-1464.
100. Hochberg MC, Martel-Pelletier J, Monfort J, et al. Combined chondroitin sulfate and glucosamine for painful knee osteoarthritis: A multicentre, randomised, double-blind, non-inferiority trial versus celecoxib. *Ann Rheum Dis* 2015.
101. Berenbaum F. Targeted therapies in osteoarthritis: A systematic review of the trials on www.clinicaltrials.gov. *Best Pract Res Clin Rheumatol* 2010;24(1):107-119.
102. Brandt KD, Mazzuca SA, Katz BP, et al. Effects of doxycycline on progression of osteoarthritis: Results of a randomized, placebo-controlled, double-blind trial. *Arthritis Rheum* 2005;52(7): 2015-2025.
103. Kwon YD, Pittler MH, Ernst E. Acupuncture for peripheral joint osteoarthritis: A systematic review and meta-analysis. *Rheumatology (Oxford)* 2006;45(11):1331-1337.

104. Scharf HP, Mansmann U, Streitberger K, et al. Acupuncture and knee osteoarthritis: A three-armed randomized trial. *Ann Intern Med* 2006;145(1):12-20.
105. Marra C, Cibere J, Grubisic M, et al. Pharmacist initiated intervention trial in osteoarthritis (PhIT-OA): A multidisciplinary intervention for knee osteoarthritis. *Arthritis Care Res (Hoboken)* 2012 Dec;64(12): 1837-45. doi: 10.1002/acr.21763.
106. Latimer N, Lord J, Grant RL, et al. Cost effectiveness of COX 2 selective inhibitors and traditional NSAIDs alone or in combination with a proton pump inhibitor for people with osteoarthritis. *BMJ* 2009;339:b2538.

Rheumatoid Arthritis

Kimberly Wahl and Arthur A. Schuna

91

KEY CONCEPTS

1. Rheumatoid arthritis (RA) is a systemic disease characterized by symmetrical inflammation of joints, yet may involve other organ systems.
2. Control of inflammation is the key to slowing or preventing disease progression as well as managing symptoms.
3. Drug therapy should be only part of a comprehensive program for patient management, which would also include physical therapy, exercise, and rest. Assistive devices and orthopedic surgery may be necessary in some patients.
4. Patients should be treated to target of low disease activity or remission.
5. Traditional or conventional synthetic disease-modifying antirheumatic drugs (referred to as DMARDs) should be started as soon as possible after diagnosis of RA.
6. Nonsteroidal anti-inflammatory drugs (NSAIDs) and/or corticosteroids should be considered adjunctive therapy early in the course of treatment and as needed if symptoms are not adequately controlled with DMARDs or biologic DMARDs (referred to as biologics).
7. When DMARDs used alone are ineffective or not adequately effective, other monotherapies or combination therapy with two or more DMARDs or a DMARD plus biologic agent may be used to induce a response.
8. Patients require careful monitoring for toxicity and therapeutic benefit for the duration of treatment.

Rheumatoid arthritis (RA) is the most common systemic inflammatory disease characterized by symmetrical joint involvement. Extra-articular involvement, including rheumatoid nodules, vasculitis, eye inflammation, neurologic dysfunction, cardiopulmonary disease, lymphadenopathy, and splenomegaly, can be manifestations of the disease. Although the usual disease course is chronic, some patients will enter a remission spontaneously.

EPIDEMIOLOGY

RA is estimated to have a prevalence of 1% and does not have any racial predilections. It can occur at any age, with increasing prevalence up to the seventh decade of life. The disease is three times more common in women. In people aged 15 to 45 years, women predominate by a ratio of 6:1; the sex ratio is approximately equal among patients in the first decade of life and in those older than 60 years.

Epidemiologic data suggest that a genetic predisposition and exposure to unknown environmental factors may be necessary for expression of the disease. The major histocompatibility complex molecules, located on T lymphocytes, appear to have an important role in most patients with RA. These molecules can be characterized using human lymphocyte antigen (HLA) typing. A majority of patients with RA have HLA-DR4, HLA-DR1, or both antigens in the major histocompatibility complex region. Patients with HLA-DR4 antigen are 3.5 times more likely to develop RA than those patients who have other HLA-DR antigens.[1] Although the major histocompatibility complex region is important, it is not the sole determinant as patients can have the disease without these HLA types. RA is six times more common among dizygotic twins and nontwin children of parents with rheumatoid factor-positive, erosive RA when compared with children whose parents do not have the disease. If one of a pair of monozygotic twins is affected, the other twin has a 30 times greater risk of developing the disease.[2,3]

PATHOPHYSIOLOGY

1 Chronic inflammation of the synovial tissue lining the joint capsule results in the proliferation of this tissue. The inflamed, proliferating synovium characteristic of RA is called *pannus*. This pannus invades the cartilage and eventually the bone surface, producing erosions of bone and cartilage and leading to destruction of the joint. The factors that initiate the inflammatory process are unknown.

The immune system is a complex network of checks and balances designed to discriminate self from nonself (foreign) tissues. It helps rid the body of infectious agents, tumor cells, and products associated with the breakdown of cells. In RA, this system is no longer able to differentiate self from nonself tissues and attacks the synovial and other connective tissues.

In addition to the genetic factors mentioned above, environmental factors play a role. It is known that smoking and pulmonary disease may increase risk. Infectious agents (eg, Epstein-Barr virus, *Escherichia coli*) and periodontal disease (*Porphyromonas gingivalis*) have been associated with RA.

The immune system has both humoral and cell-mediated functions (Fig. 91-1). The humoral component is necessary for the formation of antibodies. These antibodies are produced by plasma cells, which are derived from B lymphocytes. Most patients with RA form antibodies called *rheumatoid factors*. Rheumatoid factors have not been identified as pathogenic, nor does the quantity of these circulating antibodies always correlate with disease activity. Seropositive patients tend to have a more aggressive course of their illness than do seronegative patients. Anticitrullinated protein antibody (ACPA) is another antibody identified, which is produced in most patients with RA and has become an important diagnostic tool. Patients may develop ACPA long before they develop symptoms of RA, and those with positive antibodies have a poorer prognosis than those without.

The invasion of the synovium and joint by leukocytes results in synovitis. These leukocytes migrate to the region directed by chemokines and adhesion molecules. Early in the inflammatory process, increased vascularity aids in cell trafficking. The synovium

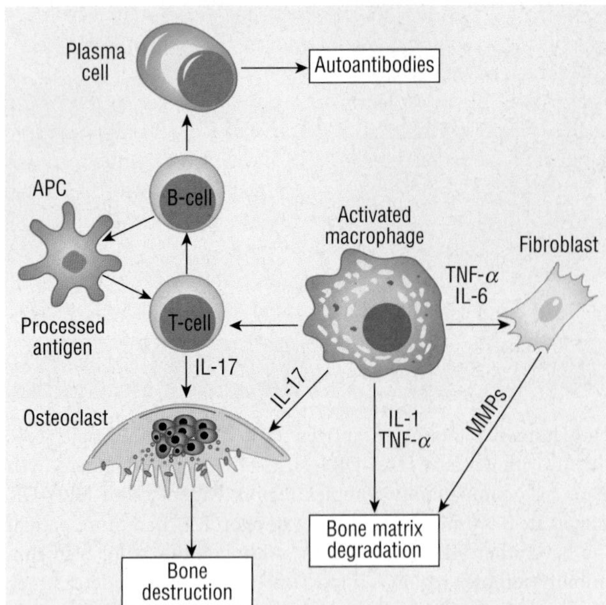

FIGURE 91-1 Pathogenesis of the inflammatory response. Antigen-presenting cells process and present antigens to T cells, which may stimulate B cells to produce antibodies and osteoclasts to destroy and remove bone. Macrophages stimulated by the immune response can stimulate T cells and osteoclasts to promote inflammation. They also can stimulate fibroblasts, which produce matrix metalloproteinases to degrade the bone matrix and produce proinflammatory cytokines. Activated T cells and macrophages release factors that promote tissue destruction, increase blood flow, and result in cellular invasion of synovial tissue and joint fluid. (APC, antigen-presenting cell; IL, interleukin; MMP, matrix metalloproteinase; TNF-*α*, tumor necrosis factor *α*.)

proliferates and fibroblasts are activated, and this promotes bone and connective tissue destruction.

Immunoglobulins can activate the complement system. The complement system amplifies the immune response by encouraging chemotaxis, phagocytosis, and the release of lymphokines by mononuclear cells, which are then presented to T lymphocytes. The processed antigen is recognized by major histocompatibility complex proteins on the lymphocyte, which activates it to stimulate the production of T and B cells. The proinflammatory cytokines tumor necrosis factor (TNF), interleukin (IL)-1 and IL-6 are key substances in the initiation and continuance of rheumatoid inflammation. IL-17 can induce proinflammatory cytokines in fibroblasts and synoviocytes and stimulate the release of matrix metalloproteinases and other cytotoxic substances, which leads to cartilage destruction. Activated T cells produce cytotoxins, which are directly toxic to tissues, and cytokines, which stimulate further activation of inflammatory processes and attract cells to areas of inflammation. Macrophages are stimulated to release prostaglandins and cytotoxins.[4-6] T-cell activation requires both stimulation by proinflammatory cytokines as well as interaction between cell surface receptors, called *costimulation*. One of these costimulation interactions is between CD28 and CD80/86. The binding of the CD80/86 receptor by the drug abatacept has proved to be an effective treatment for RA by preventing costimulation interactions between T cells.[7]

Although it has been suggested that T cells play a key role in the pathogenesis of RA, B cells clearly have an equally important role. Evidence for this importance may be found in the effectiveness of B-cell depletion using the drug rituximab in controlling rheumatoid inflammation. Activated B cells produce plasma cells, which form antibodies. These antibodies in combination with the complement system result in the accumulation of polymorphonuclear leukocytes, which release cytotoxins, oxygen-free radicals, and hydroxyl radicals that promote cellular damage to synovium and bone. The benefits of B-cell depletion occur even though antibody formation is not suppressed with rituximab therapy; this suggests that other mechanisms play a role in reducing RA activity. B cells produce cytokines that may alter the function of other immune cells, and they also have the ability to process antigens and act as antigen-presenting cells, which interact with T cells to activate the immune process.[8-11]

In the synovial membrane, $CD4^+$ T cells are abundant and communicate with macrophages, osteoclasts, fibroblasts, and chondrocytes either through direct cell–cell interactions using cell surface receptors or through proinflammatory cytokines such as TNF-*α*, IL-1, and IL-6. These cells produce metalloproteinases and other cytotoxic substances, which lead to the erosion of bone and cartilage. They also release substances promoting growth of blood vessels and adhesion molecules, which assists in proinflammatory cell trafficking

CLINICAL PRESENTATION Arthiritis

Symptoms

- Joint pain and stiffness of more than 6 weeks' duration. May also experience fatigue, weakness, low-grade fever, loss of appetite. Muscle pain and afternoon fatigue may also be present. Joint deformity is generally seen late in the disease.

Signs

- Tenderness with warmth and swelling over affected joints usually involving hands and feet. Distribution of joint involvement is frequently symmetrical. Rheumatoid nodules may also be present.

Laboratory Tests

- Rheumatoid factor (RF) detectable in 60% to 70%.
- Anticyclic citrullinated peptide (anti-CCP) antibodies have similar sensitivity to RF (50%-85%) but are more specific (90%-95%) and are present earlier in the disease.
- Elevated ESR and CRP are markers for inflammation.
- Normocytic normochromic anemia is common as is thrombocytosis.

Other Diagnostic Tests

- Joint fluid aspiration may show increased white blood cell counts without infection, crystals.
- Joint radiographs may show periarticular osteoporosis, joint space narrowing, or erosions.

and attachment of fibroblasts to cartilage and eventual synovial invasion and destruction.[12-15] TNF inhibitors are widely used to treat RA. Although anakinra inhibits IL-1 by attaching to receptors on cell surface, the benefits of this approach have not been as great as expected. Tocilizumab has proven effective as an inhibitor of IL-6 activity.

There are also a number of signaling molecules that are important for activating and maintaining inflammation. One of these is Janus kinase (JAK), which is a tyrosine kinase responsible for regulating leukocyte maturation and activation. JAK also has effects on the production of cytokines and immunoglobulins. Tofacitinib, an oral JAK inhibiting drug, has proven to be very effective in RA and appears to inhibit IL-6 activity as the major mechanism of action.

Vasoactive substances also play a role in the inflammatory process. Histamine, kinins, and prostaglandins are released at the site of inflammation. These substances increase both blood flow to the site of inflammation and the permeability of blood vessels. These substances cause the edema, warmth, erythema, and pain associated with joint inflammation and make it easier for granulocytes to pass from blood vessels to the site of inflammation.

The end results of the chronic inflammatory changes are variable. Loss of cartilage may result in a loss of the joint space. The formation of chronic granulation or scar tissue can lead to loss of joint motion or bony fusion (called *ankylosis*). Laxity of tendon structures can result in a loss of support to the affected joint, leading to instability or subluxation. Tendon contractures also may occur, leading to chronic deformity.[12,16]

The symptoms of RA usually develop insidiously over the course of several weeks to months. Prodromal symptoms include fatigue, weakness, low-grade fever, loss of appetite, and joint pain. Stiffness and muscle aches (myalgias) may precede the development of joint swelling (synovitis). Fatigue may be more of a problem in the afternoon. During disease flares, the onset of fatigue begins earlier in the day and subsides as disease activity lessens. Most commonly, joint involvement tends to be symmetrical; however, early in the disease some patients present with an asymmetrical pattern involving one or a few joints that eventually develops into the more classic presentation. Approximately 20% of patients develop an abrupt onset of their illness with fevers, polyarthritis, and constitutional symptoms (eg, depression, anxiety, fatigue, anorexia, and weight loss).[2,3]

No single test or physical finding can be used to make the diagnosis of RA. In early disease, the diagnosis can be particularly challenging given that radiographic findings are usually absent and rheumatoid factor (RF) test can be undetectable. Duration of joint pain and swelling, morning stiffness lasting more than 1 hour, and involvement of three or more joints are important early predictors of the development of persistent erosive RA.[17]

JOINT INVOLVEMENT

The joints affected most frequently by RA are the small joints of the hands, wrists, and feet (Fig. 91-2). In addition, elbows, shoulders, hips, knees, and ankles may be involved. Patients usually experience joint stiffness that typically is worse in the morning. The duration of stiffness tends to be correlated directly with disease activity, usually exceeds 30 minutes, and may persist all day. Chronic inflammation with lack of an adequate exercise program results in loss of range of motion, atrophy of muscles, weakness, and deformity (Figs. 91-3 and 91-4).

On examination, the swelling of the joints may be visible or may be apparent only by palpation. The swelling feels soft and spongy because it is caused by proliferation of soft tissues or fluid accumulation within the joint capsule. The swollen joint may appear erythematous and feel warmer than nearby skin surfaces, especially early in the course of the disease. In contrast, the swelling associated with osteoarthritis usually is bony (caused by osteophytes) and infrequently is associated with signs of inflammation.

Involvement of the hands and wrists is common in RA. Hand involvement is manifested by pain, swelling, tenderness, and grip weakness during the acute phase and by subluxation, instability, deformity, and muscle atrophy in the chronic phase of the disease. Functional difficulties with clasp, grasp, and pinch alter both strength and fine motor movement.

Deformity of the hand may be seen with chronic inflammation. These changes may alter the mechanics of hand function, reducing grip strength and making it difficult to perform usual daily activity.

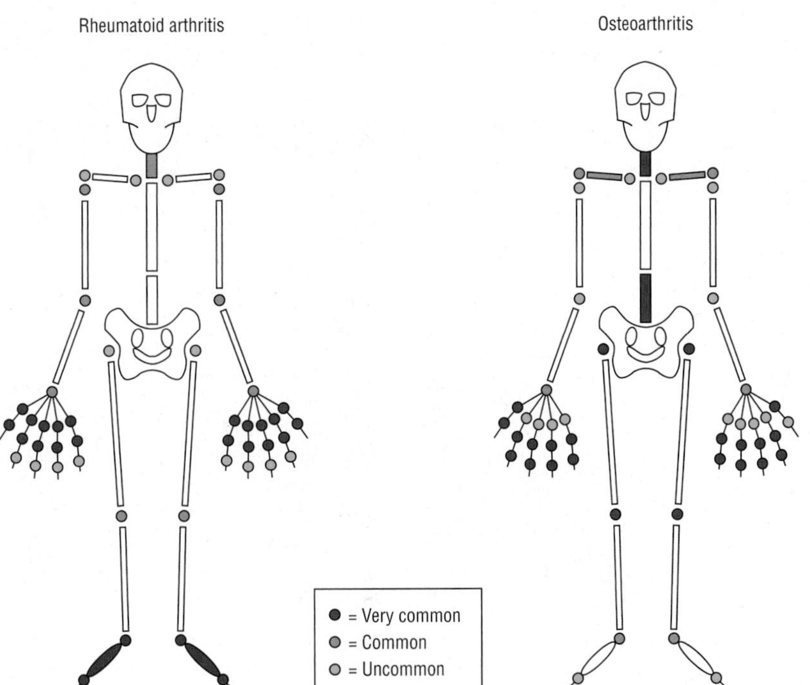

FIGURE 91-2 Patterns of joint involvement in rheumatoid arthritis and osteoarthritis.

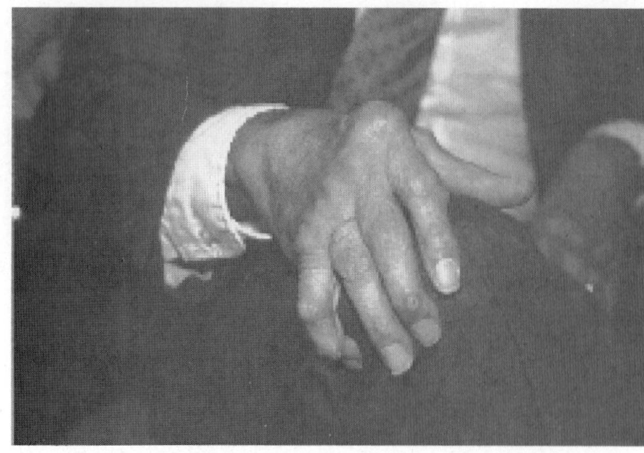

FIGURE 91-3 Deformities of rheumatoid arthritis, with marked ulnar deviation, swan-neck deformity, active synovitis, and nodules. *(Reproduced with permission from Brunicardi FC, Anderson DK, Billiar TR, et al.* Schwartz's Principles of Surgery, *8th ed. New York, NY: McGraw-Hill, 2005.)*

Pain in the elbow and shoulder may be the result of true joint inflammation or inflammation of soft-tissue structures such as tendons (tendonitis) or the bursa (bursitis). The knee also can be involved, with loss of cartilage, instability, and joint pain. Synovitis of the knee may cause the formation of a cyst behind the knee called a *popliteal* or *Baker's cyst*. These cysts may become painful as they get tense, or they may rupture, producing a clinical picture similar to thrombophlebitis secondary to the release of inflammatory components into the area of the calf muscle (pseudothrombophlebitis syndrome). Chronic joint pain leads to muscle atrophy, which can result in a laxity of the ligamentous structures that support the knee, causing instability. Maintenance of an adequate range of motion of the knee is essential to normal gait.

Foot and ankle involvement in RA is common. The metatarsophalangeal joints are involved frequently in RA, making walking difficult. Subluxation of the metatarsal heads leads to "cock-up" or hammer toe deformities. Subluxation also may cause a flexion deformity at the proximal interphalangeal joint of the toe, leading to pressure necrosis of the skin over the joint secondary to irritation caused by shoes. Hallux valgus (lateral deviation of the digit) and bunion or callus formation may occur at the great toe. A widening of the foot occurs commonly with long-standing disease.

Involvement of the spine usually occurs in the cervical vertebrae; lumbar vertebral involvement is rare. Involvement of the first and second cervical vertebrae (C1 to C2) can lead to instability of this joint. Patients with this problem are at a greater risk for spinal cord compression, although this complication is rare.

The temporomandibular joint (jaw) can be affected, resulting in malocclusion and difficulty in chewing food. Inflammation of cartilage in the chest can lead to chest wall pain. Hip pain may occur as a result of destructive changes in the hip joint, soft-tissue inflammation (eg, bursitis), or referred pain from nerve entrapment at the lumbar vertebrae.

EXTRA-ARTICULAR INVOLVEMENT

Although joint involvement in RA is a hallmark finding in RA, it is important to recognize that, as a systemic disease, other organ systems are often involved.

Rheumatoid Nodules

Rheumatoid nodules occur in 20% of patients with RA. These nodules are seen most commonly on the extensor surfaces of the elbows, forearms, and hands but also may be seen on the feet and at other

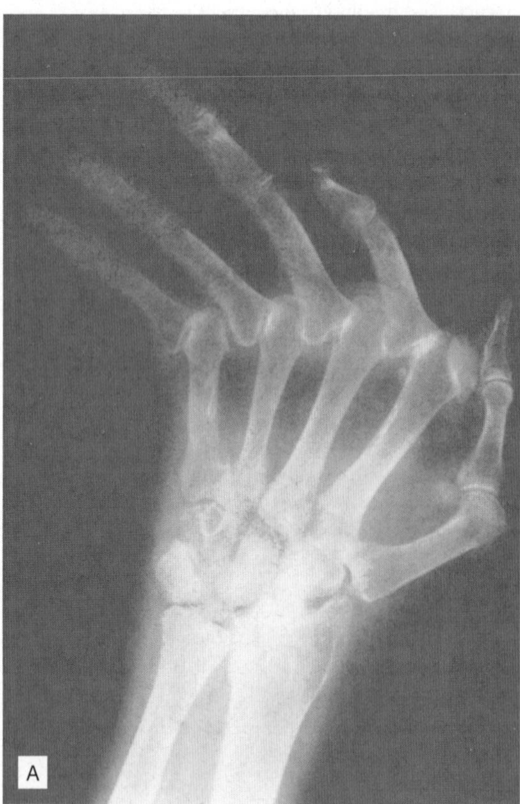

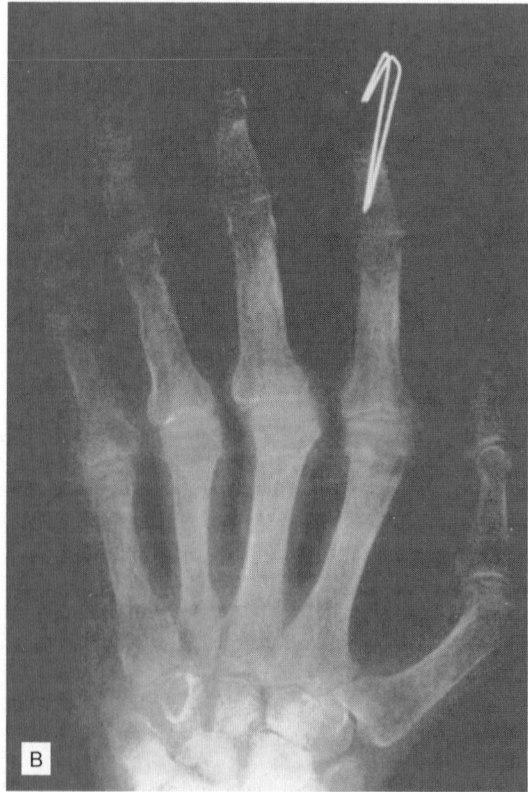

FIGURE 91-4 *A.* Preoperative view of metacarpophalangeal joints in rheumatoid arthritis. *B.* Following resection arthroplasty. *(Reproduced with permission from Skinner H., ed.* Current Diagnosis & Treatment in Orthopedics, *4th ed. New York, NY: McGraw-Hill, 2006:592.)*

pressure points. They also may develop in the lung or pleural lining of the lung and, rarely, in the meninges. Rheumatoid nodules usually are asymptomatic and do not require any special intervention. Nodules are observed more commonly in patients with erosive disease.[18]

Vasculitis

Vasculitis usually is seen in patients with long-standing RA. Vasculitis may result in a wide variety of clinical presentations. Invasion of blood vessel walls by inflammatory cells results in an obliteration of the vessel, producing infarction of tissue distal to the area of involvement. Most commonly, small-vessel vasculitis produces infarcts near the ends of the fingers or toes, especially around the nail beds. These infarcts are usually of little consequence.

Vasculitis also may cause the breakdown of skin, especially in the lower extremities, producing ulcers that may be indistinguishable in appearance from stasis ulcers. However, these ulcers do not heal with the usual modes of treatment used for stasis ulcers. Involvement of larger vessels with vasculitis can result in life-threatening complications. Infarction of vessels supplying blood to nerves can cause irreversible motor deficits. Involvement of vessels supplying other organ systems can lead to visceral involvement and a polyarteritis nodosa-like illness. Aggressive treatment of the inflammatory process is necessary in these patients. Fortunately, vasculitis has become much less frequently seen since the advent of methotrexate and biologic therapy.

Pulmonary Complications

RA may involve the pleura of the lung, which is often asymptomatic, although pleural effusions may result. Pulmonary fibrosis also may develop as a result of rheumatoid involvement; smoking appears to increase the risk of this complication. Rheumatoid nodules may develop in lung tissue and appear similar to neoplasms on chest radiographs. Interstitial pneumonitis and arteritis are rare, potentially life-threatening complications of RA.

Ocular Manifestations

Ocular manifestations include keratoconjunctivitis sicca and inflammation of the sclera, episclera, and cornea. Atrophy of the lacrimal duct may result in a decrease in tear formation, causing dry and itchy eyes, termed *keratoconjunctivitis sicca*. When this is observed in association with RA, it is referred to as *Sjögren syndrome*. Artificial tears may be used to relieve symptoms. The salivary glands may also be involved in Sjögren syndrome, resulting in dry mouth (xerostomia). Inflammation of the superficial layers of the sclera (episcleritis) is generally self-limiting. Involvement of deeper tissues (scleritis) usually results in a more serious, painful, and chronic inflammation. Rheumatoid nodules may develop on the sclera.

Cardiac Involvement

The heart is sometimes affected by RA. RA is associated with an increased risk of cardiovascular mortality. This risk appears to be higher in those with more active inflammation and is reduced with treatment, particularly with methotrexate.[19,20] Pericarditis may occur, resulting in the accumulation of fluid. Although many patients show evidence of previous pericarditis at autopsy, the development of clinically evident pericarditis with tamponade is a rare complication. Cardiac conduction abnormalities and aortic valve incompetence, caused by aortic root dilation, may occur. Myocarditis is a rare complication of RA.

Felty Syndrome

RA in association with splenomegaly and neutropenia is known as *Felty syndrome*. Thrombocytopenia also may be a manifestation of the syndrome. Patients with Felty syndrome and severe leukopenia are more susceptible to infection. The decrease in granulocytes appears to be mediated by the immune system because splenectomy does not result in improvement of the patient.[18]

Other Complications

Lymphadenopathy may occur in patients with RA, particularly in nodes proximal to more actively involved joints. Renal involvement is rare but can be associated with treatment, including nonsteroidal anti-inflammatory drugs (NSAIDs). Amyloidosis is a rare complication of longstanding RA. It appears to be more common in Europe than in the United States.

LABORATORY FINDINGS

Hematologic tests often reveal a mild-to-moderate anemia with normocytic, normochromic indices. The hematocrit may fall as low as 30% [0.30]. The anemia is usually inversely related to inflammatory disease activity and is referred to as an *anemia of chronic disease*. This type of anemia does not respond to iron therapy and can present a diagnostic dilemma because NSAIDs may induce gastritis and chronic blood loss, leading to iron-deficiency anemia. Laboratory tests useful in differentiating these anemias include stool guaiac (or other stool tests for occult blood), serum iron-to-iron-binding capacity ratio (decreased in iron deficiency), ferritin (decreased in iron deficiency), and mean corpuscular volume (more likely to be decreased in iron deficiency). Other causes of anemia also must be considered in the differential diagnosis (see Chapters 100 and 102).

Thrombocytosis is another common hematologic finding with active RA. Platelet counts rise and fall in direct correlation with disease activity in many patients. Thrombocytopenia may result from toxicity of immunosuppressive therapy. Thrombocytopenia also may be observed in Felty syndrome or vasculitis.

Although leukopenia is associated with Felty syndrome, it also may result from toxicity of methotrexate, gold, sulfasalazine, penicillamine, and immunosuppressive drugs. Leukocytosis is seen commonly as a result of corticosteroid treatment.

The erythrocyte sedimentation rate (ESR) is usually elevated in patients with RA and other inflammatory diseases. This test is very nonspecific, and although the ESR usually falls as patients respond to therapy, there is a large variability among patients in response to treatment. C-reactive protein (CRP) is another nonspecific marker for inflammatory arthritis when it is elevated. This protein is produced by the liver in response to certain cytokines.

RF is present in 60% to 70% of patients with RA. The usual laboratory test for RF is an antibody specific for immunoglobulin (Ig) M RF. Patients with RA and a negative test for RF may have IgG or IgA RFs, but tests for these are not routinely available. RF tests may be reported positive at a specific serum dilution. Serum is diluted to a standard series of dilutions; the greatest dilution that yields a positive test result will be reported (eg, RF positive at 1:640). Some laboratories quantify RF rather than using titers. Higher dilutional titers or serum concentrations of RFs usually indicate a more severe disease, but like the ESR, the large interpatient variability makes this test unreliable as a means of assessing patient progress. RF may be positive in patients without RA (Table 91-1).

ACPA has similar sensitivity for RA, being found in 50% to 85% of patients with the disease, but is more specific (90%-95%) and is detectable very early in the disease. Many rheumatologists will do both tests in evaluating new patients.

Antinuclear antibodies (ANAs) are detected in 25% of patients with RA. These antibodies usually have a diffuse pattern of immunofluorescence. Tests for antibodies to double-stranded DNA (usually

TABLE 91-1 Diseases Associated with a Positive Rheumatoid Factor

Rheumatic diseases
Rheumatoid arthritis
Sjögren syndrome (with or without arthritis)
Systemic lupus erythematosus
Progressive systemic sclerosis
Polymyositis/dermatomyositis
Infectious diseases
Bacterial endocarditis
Tuberculosis
Syphilis
Infectious mononucleosis
Infectious hepatitis
Leprosy
Other causes
Aging
Interstitial pulmonary fibrosis
Cirrhosis of the liver
Chronic active hepatitis
Sarcoidosis

positive in systemic lupus erythematosus) are negative. Serum complement is usually normal, although complement concentrations of joint fluid often are depressed from consumption secondary to the inflammatory process. In patients with vasculitis, serum complement concentrations may be low.[21,22]

Synovial fluid usually is turbid because of the large number of leukocytes in inflammatory fluid. White cell counts of 5,000 to 50,000/mm^3 (5×10^9 to 50×10^9/L) are not uncommon in inflamed joints. The fluid is usually less viscous than that in normal joints or fluid associated with osteoarthritis. Glucose concentrations of joint fluid are normal or low compared with those in serum drawn at the same time as synovial aspirates. The decrease is not as profound as the decrease associated with joint infection or systemic lupus erythematosus.

Early radiographic manifestations of RA include soft-tissue swelling and osteoporosis near the joint (periarticular osteoporosis). Joint space narrowing occurs as a result of cartilage degradation. Erosions tend to occur later in the course of the disease and usually are seen first in the metacarpophalangeal and proximal interphalangeal joints of the hands and the metatarsophalangeal joints of the feet. Periodic joint radiographs are a useful way of evaluating disease progression.

Diagnostic Criteria

The American College of Rheumatology and European League Against Rheumatism (ACR/EULAR) revised criteria for the diagnosis of RA.[23] These criteria were developed to be used for patients early in their disease; they, therefore, emphasize early manifestations of the disease. Late manifestations of RA such as erosive disease or nodules are no longer in the diagnostic criteria, but these patients would have previously met these criteria based on retrospective data.

Patients with synovitis of at least one joint and no other explanation for the finding are candidates for these criteria. The criteria use a scoring system with a score of more than 6 out of a possible total score of 10 as being diagnostic for RA. More points are given for patients presenting with more actively involved joints. Positive laboratory tests including RF, ACPA, CRP, and ESR result in additional points.

Duration of symptoms more than or equal to 6 weeks results in an additional point. It is important to note that not all patients with RA may have a score more than 6 initially, particularly if seen very early in their disease but may evolve to higher scores over time. Reassessment should be considered for those with ongoing symptoms.

Seronegative Inflammatory Arthritis

Although RA may have a negative RF titer, a number of other systemic inflammatory arthritic conditions exist including psoriatic arthritis, reactive arthritis, ankylosing spondylitis, and arthritis associated with inflammatory bowel disease. These conditions often tend to be less aggressive than what is typically seen with RA. Detailed discussion about these conditions is beyond the scope of this chapter, but further information may be found elsewhere.[2] Management principles are similar to those for RA.

TREATMENT

Desired Outcomes

2 The primary objective in the treatment of RA is to achieve remission or low disease activity which is referred to as "Treat to Target."[24] This goal is largely achieved by reducing inflammation using drugs known to alter disease progression. See Table 91-2 for a list of commonly used tools to assess RA disease activity with definitions for remission and low disease activity. While achieving complete clinical remission is the ideal target, it may not be possible to achieve in some patients; in this subset of patients, especially those with longstanding disease, achieving low-disease activity may be an appropriate alternative. It is important to recognize that no therapy will reverse joint damage which has already occurred.

General Approach to Treatment

The multifaceted treatment approach includes pharmacologic and nonpharmacologic therapies with recent emphasis being placed on aggressive treatment early in the disease course. Early aggressive treatment may prevent irreversible joint damage and disability. The current guideline recommends intial treatment with a conventional synthetic disease-modifying antirheumatic drug, preferably methotrexate, for most patients regardless of clinical disease activity.[25-27] Those who continue to have moderate-to-severe disease activity despite initial treatment should be switched to alternative therapies (another disease-modifying antirheumatic drug [DMARD] or biologic agent) or combination DMARD therapy. Patients who achieve remission can be considered for tapering, though not discontinuance of all RA therapies. Though remission is the target for treatment, patients who achieve low disease activity should continue RA treatment.

Clinical Controversy...

Currently there are no known predictors of which therapies are likely to be effective in a given patient. Once therapy is begun, some patients who achieve excellent response may taper and in some cases discontinue some drugs if they are on combination therapy. It is not clear which patients would benefit from this approach.

Nonpharmacologic Therapy

3 Rest, occupational therapy, physical therapy, use of assistive devices, weight reduction, and surgery are the most useful types of nonpharmacologic therapy used in patients with RA. Rest is an essential component of a nonpharmacologic treatment plan.[27,28] It relieves stress on inflamed joints and prevents further joint destruction. Rest also aids in alleviation of pain. Too much rest and immobility, however, may lead to decreased range of motion and, ultimately, muscle atrophy, and contractures.

Occupational and physical therapy can provide the patient with skills and exercises necessary to increase or maintain mobility. These disciplines may also supply patients with supportive and adaptive devices such as canes, walkers, and splints.

Other nonpharmacologic therapeutic options include weight loss and surgery. Weight reduction helps alleviate stress on inflamed joints. Tenosynovectomy, tendon repair, and joint replacements are surgical options for patients with RA. Such management is reserved for patients with severe disease.

Pharmacologic Therapy

4 5 Pharmacologic agents that reduce RA symptoms and impede radiographic joint damage can be categorized as either conventional synthetic DMARDs, biologic DMARDs (referred to as *biologics*) which include TNF-α inhibitor (TNFi) biologics or non-TNF biologics, and tofacitinib, which is considered different from DMARDs in the ACR 2015 RA treatment guidelines. DMARDs are a treatment cornerstone; they should be started as soon as possible after disease onset as early introduction results in more favorable outcomes,[29] including reducing mortality rates comparable to patients without the disease.[19] Nonsteroidal anti-inflammatory drugs (NSAIDs) and/or corticosteroids may be used for symptomatic relief if needed.[28] They provide relatively rapid improvement in symptoms compared with DMARDs, which may take weeks to months to take effect; however, NSAIDs have no impact on disease progression and the long-term complication risks of corticosteroids make them less desirable. NSAIDs and DMARDs have steroid-sparing properties that permit corticosteroid dose reductions.

DMARDs, biologics, and tofacitinib slow RA disease progression. DMARDs commonly used include methotrexate, hydroxychloroquine, sulfasalazine, and leflunomide. The biologic agents with disease-modifying activity include the TNFi drugs (adalimumab, certolizaumab, etanercept, golimumab, infliximab), the costimulation modulator abatacept, the IL-6 receptor antagonist tocilizumab, and rituximab, which depletes peripheral B cells. Tofacitinib, a newer agent, is a synthetic small molecule similar to DMARDs but with a very specific mechanism of action. Agents less frequently used because of reduced efficacy and/or greater toxicity include the IL-1 receptor antagonist anakinra, azathioprine, D-penicillamine, gold (including auranofin), minocycline, cyclosporine, and cyclophosphamide.

Clinical **Controversy...**

Though the current guideline recommends methotrexate as initial therapy for most patients with RA, the order in which DMARDs or biologic agents are choosen or the choice of monotherapy with an alternative agent versus combination therapy is not clearly defined. No direct comparative studies exist for biologics to guide in the determination of optimal treatment order.

DMARD monotherapy, preferably with methotrexate, is first-line therapy for patients with early (<6 months duration of disease symptoms) or established (≥6 months duration of disease symptoms) RA.[27] Methotrexate is recommended initially because long-term data suggest superior outcomes with methotrexate than with other DMARDs. There is also good documentation for better outcomes with methotrexate in combination therapy if methotrexate monotherapy does not achieve an adequate response. Leflunomide appears to have similar long-term efficacy as that of methotrexate.[30]

6 Monotherapy with nonmethotrexate DMARDs or combination therapy with two or more DMARDs may be effective when the initial DMARD treatment is unsuccessful.[27] For patients with moderate-to-high disease activity, dual DMARD combinations (methotrexate plus hydroxychloroquine, methotrexate plus leflunomide, or methotrexate plus sulfasalazine) or triple DMARDs (sulfasalazine, hydroxychloroquine, and methotrexate) are recommended as initial therapy.[25,27] Initial combination therapy with either methotrexate plus etanercept or methotrexate plus sulfasalazine plus hydroxychloroquine has been found to be more effective at 24 weeks of therapy than methotrexate monotherapy for most patients; however, stepwise therapy to dual or triple therapy may have similar efficacy later in the course of treatment.[31]

The biologic agents have proven effective for patients who fail treatment with DMARDs. However, the ACR now endorses use of anti-TNF biologics as monotherapy or as combination with DMARDs in patients who have moderate-to-high disease activity after treatment with previous DMARD.[25,27] Furthermore, use of biologics in combination with methotrexate is more effective than biologic monotherapy.[25] Infliximab, specifically, should be given in combination with methotrexate to prevent development of antibodies that may reduce infliximab drug efficacy or induce allergic reactions.

The ACR published recommendations for use of DMARDs, biologics, and tofacitinib in 2008 and updated them in 2012 and 2015. These recommendations are not intended to be prescriptive but provide guidance for treatment choice. Recommendations are given based on disease duration and degree of disease activity. The recommendations take into account barriers to treatment, including cost and insurance restrictions, by suggesting treatment options with and without expensive biologic agents. Simplified algorithms summarizing these treatment recommendations are provided in Fig. 91-5. For more details, see the published recommendations.[25,26,27]

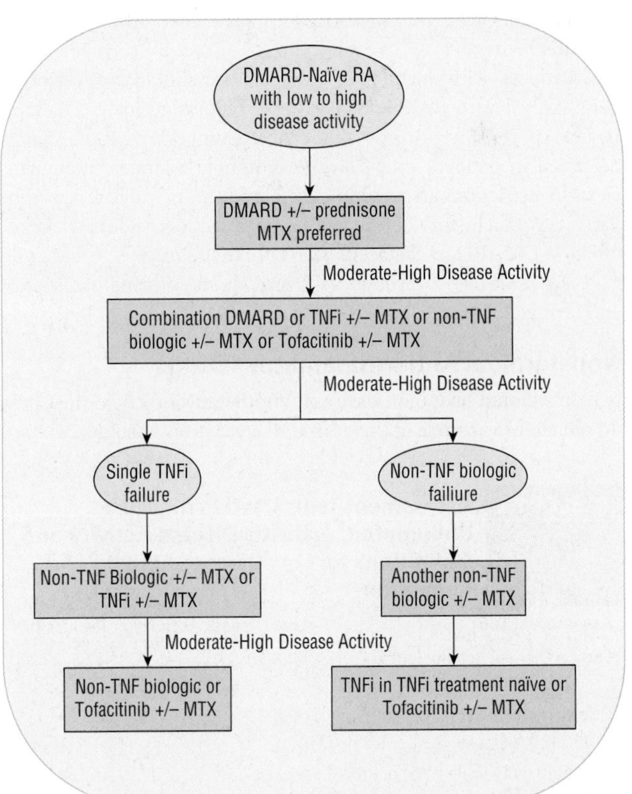

FIGURE 91-5 Algorithm for treatment of rheumatoid arthritis (RA) in early (<6 months) or established (≥6 months) RA with low to high disease activity. (DMARD, disease-modifying antirheumatic drug; MTX, methotrexate.)

Therapy with DMARDs and biologics result in immunosuppression. Additionally, prednisolone doses of 20 mg/day or more for 2 weeks is also generally accepted to produce a state of immunosuppression. Therefore, vaccination status should be assessed and updated before therapy is initiated to protect against vaccine-preventable infections. Corticosteroids significantly increase the risk for mild (relative risk 1.15) and serious infections (relative risk 1.9).[33] The use of corticosteroids in addition to DMARDs has been shown to produce a similar elevated risk of infection as corticosteroid monotherapy. Biologic agents are associated with an increased risk of serious infections as compared with DMARD therapy, increasing by 6 per 1000 patient–years for standard dosing and 17 per 1000 patient–years for high dosing.[34] When using a DMARD and biologic as combination therapy, the risk of serious infection increased by 55 per 1000 patient–years. Dual biologic use is not recommended due to the risk of infection.

While the ACR recommends vaccination before start of DMARD or biologic therapy when possible, killed (pneumococcal, intramuscular influenza, hepatitis B) and recombinant (human papillomavirus) vaccines can be given during therapy.[27] Live vaccines can be administered to patients already on DMARD therapy; however, they are not recommended for patients already taking biologics. For those patients who will be starting a biologic or tofacitinib, the ACR recommends administering the herpes zoster vaccine to patients who have reached 50 years of age instead of waiting until after the general-population recommended age of 60 years.

Some biologic agents are contraindicated in the setting of hepatitis C or malignancies because of immunosuppression. Conventional synthetic DMARDs are preferred for treatment of RA in patients with hepatitis C virus who have not been treated or are requiring treatment.[27] However, the 2015 ACR notes that for patients with hepatitis C virus who have completed or are currently undergoing treatment for hepatitis be treated no differently than other patients with RA. No restrictions are needed for patients with hepatitis B virus.

Patients with history of skin cancer should be preferentially treated with DMARDs. For those requiring biologic therapy, regular surveillance for new skin cancer is important. Rituximab is preferred in patients with previous lymphoproliferative malignancies. No restrictions are recommended for patients with solid tumors. Patients with a history of previous severe infections should use combination DMARD or abatacept over TNF inhibitors.[27]

7 Tables 91-2 through 91-4 provide monitoring parameters and dosing guidelines for DMARDs and NSAIDs used in RA.

Nonsteroidal Anti-inflammatory Drugs

NSAIDs should seldom be used as monotherapy for RA because they do not alter the course of the disease; instead, they should be viewed as adjuncts to DMARD treatment. NSAIDs possess both analgesic and antiinflammatory properties and reduce stiffness associated with RA. These agents mainly inhibit prostaglandin synthesis, which is only a small portion of the inflammatory cascade. For details on these agents see Chap. 90, Osteoarthritis.

TABLE 91-2 Assessment Tools Used to Measure Rheumatoid Arthritis Disease Activity and Definitions for Low Disease Activity and Remission

Assessment Tool	Low Disease Activity	Remission
Clinical Disease Activity Index (CDAI) (range 0-76)	>2.8-10	<2.8
Disease Activity Score (DAS28) (range 0-9.4)	>2.6-3.2	<2.6
Patient Activity Scale (PAS) or PASII (range 0-10)	>2.5-3.7	0-2.5
Routine Assessment of Patient Index Data 3 (RAPID-3) (range 0-10)	>1.0-2.0	0-1.0
Simplified Disease Activity Index (SDAI) (range 0-86)	>3.3-<11.0	<3.3

Corticosteroids

Corticosteroids are used in RA for their anti-inflammatory and immunosuppressive properties but should not be used as monotherapy.[35] They interfere with antigen presentation to T lymphocytes, inhibit prostaglandin and leukotriene synthesis, and inhibit neutrophil and monocyte superoxide radical generation. Corticosteroids also impair cell migration and cause redistribution of monocytes, lymphocytes, and neutrophils, thus blunting the inflammatory and autoimmune responses.

Corticosteroids may be injected into joints and soft tissues to control local inflammation or taken orally for a more systemic effect. Oral corticosteroids are absorbed rapidly and completely from the gastrointestinal tract. They are metabolized and inactivated primarily by the liver and excreted in the urine. The elimination half-life of most corticosteroids is sufficiently long that once-daily dosing is possible.

Oral corticosteroids can be used in several ways. They can be used in bridging therapy, continuous low-dose therapy, and short-term, high-dose bursts to control flares. Oral steroids (eg, prednisone, methylprednisolone) can be used to control pain and synovitis while DMARDs are taking effect. This is termed *bridging therapy* and is often used in patients with debilitating symptoms when DMARD therapy is initiated. Patients with difficult-to-control disease may be placed on low-dose, long-term corticosteroid therapy to control their symptoms. Prednisone doses below 7.5 mg daily are well tolerated but are not devoid of the long-term adverse effects associated with corticosteroids. The lowest dose of corticosteroid that controls symptoms should be used to reduce adverse effects. Alternate-day dosing of low-dose oral corticosteroids usually is ineffective in RA; symptoms usually flare on days without medication. High-dose corticosteroid bursts often are used to suppress disease flares. High doses are sustained for several days until symptoms are controlled, followed by a taper to the lowest effective dose.

Corticosteroids also may be delivered by injection. The intramuscular route may be preferable in patients with adherence problems for short-term therapy. Long-acting depot forms of corticosteroids include triamcinolone acetonide, triamcinolone hexacetonide, and methylprednisolone acetate. This provides the patient with 2 to 6 weeks of symptomatic control. The depot effect provides a physiologic taper, avoiding withdrawal reaction associated with hypothalamic–pituitary axis suppression. IV corticosteroids may be used to provide the patient with large amounts of drug during a steroid burst to control severe symptoms. Intra-articular injections of depot forms of corticosteroids can be useful in treating synovitis and pain when a small number of joints are affected. The onset and duration of symptomatic relief are similar to those of intramuscular injection. The intra-articular route often is preferred because it is associated with the fewest number of systemic adverse effects. If efficacious, intraarticular injections may be repeated every 3 months. No one joint should be injected more than two to three times per year because of the risk of accelerated joint destruction and atrophy of tendons. Soft tissues such as tendons and bursae also may be injected. This may help control the pain and inflammation associated with these structures. The onset and duration of symptomatic relief are similar to those of intramuscular and intra-articular injections.

The major limitation to the long-term use of corticosteroids is adverse effects. They include hypothalamic-pituitary–adrenal suppression, Cushing syndrome, osteoporosis, myopathies, glaucoma, cataracts, gastritis, hypertension, hirsutism, electrolyte imbalances, glucose intolerance, skin atrophy, and increased susceptibility to

TABLE 91-3 Usual Doses for Antirheumatic Drugs

Drug	Brand Name	Starting Dose	Usual Range or Maintenance Dose	Comments
Nonsteroidal anti-inflammatory drugs			See Table 90-2 in Chapter 90	
Methotrexate	Rasuvo Trexall Otrexup (SC)	Oral: 7.5 mg once weekly or 2.5 mg q 12 h for 3 days/wk or 10-15 mg once weekly SC or IM	Oral SC or IM: 7.5-15 mg q wk	May be given with folic acid 1-5 mg/day to reduce adverse reactions
Leflunomide	Arava	Oral: loading dose: 100 mg daily for 3 days, then 20 mg/day or 10-20 mg daily without loading dose	Oral: 10-20 mg daily	Not recommended in liver disease (ALT >2 times ULN)
Hydroxychloroquine	Plaquenil	Oral: 200-300 mg BID	Oral: After 1-2 mo may decrease to 200 mg daily or 200 mg BID	Take with food or milk; use with caution in renal or hepatic impairment
Sulfasalazine	Azulfidine	Oral: 0.5-1 g/day	Oral: Increase weekly to 1 g BID (max. dose is 3 g/day if inadequate response after 12 weeks of 2 g/day)	Not recommended in renal or hepatic impairment
Etanercept	Enbrel		50 mg SubQ once weekly or 25 mg twice weekly	
Infliximab	Remicade	3 mg/kg IV at 0, 2, 6 weeks then 3 q 8 weeks	3-10 mg/kg IV q 4-8 weeks	Given in combination with methotrexate therapy
Adalimumab	Humira		40 mg SubQ q 2 weeks (may increase to 40 mg once weekly if not taking methotrexate)	
Certolizumab	Cimzia	400 mg SubQ at 0, 2, 4 weeks	200 mg SubQ every other week	
Golimumab	Simponi		50 mg SubQ once monthly	
Rituximab	Rituxan	1,000 mg IV twice, 2 weeks apart	Initial dose may be repeated every 16-24 weeks based on response	
Abatacept	Orencia	IV: <60 kg: 500 mg 60-100 kg: 750 mg >100 kg: 1,000 mg at 0, 2, and 4 weeks or initial IV dose followed by 125 mg SubQ within 24 hours	IV: dose based on weight q 4 weeks SubQ: 125 mg once weekly	
Tocilizumab	Actemra	4 mg/kg IV q 4 weeks	4-8 mg/kg q 4 weeks (max 800 mg/infusion)	
Tofacitinib	Xeljanz		5 mg BID	5 mg once daily in moderate-to-severe renal insufficiency, moderate hepatic impairment, or concomitant CYP3A4 or CYP2C19 inhibitors
Minocycline	Dynacin Minocin		Oral: 100-200 mg daily	Use with caution in renal impairment
Anakinra	Kineret		100 mg SC once daily	
Auranofin	Ridaura		Oral: 3 mg daily to BID	
Gold thiomalate	Myochrysine	IM: 10 mg test dose first week, then 25 mg second week; then 25-50 mg/wk until toxicity or cumulative 1 g dose given	IM: 25-50 mg every other week for 2-20 weeks then every 3-4 weeks	CL_{cr} 50-80 mL/min (0.83-1.33 mL/s): give 50% recommended dose; CL_{cr} <50 mL/min (<0.83 mL/s) avoid use
Azathioprine	Imuran Azasan	Oral: 1 mg/kg/day (50-100 mg) for 6-8 weeks. May increase by 0.5 mg/kg q 4 weeks to 2.5 mg/kg/day	Oral: 50-150 mg daily	
D–Penicillamine	Cuprimine Depen	Oral: 125-250 mg daily	Oral: may ↑ by 125-250 mg q 1-2 months, max. 750 mg daily	Caution with renal impairment
Cyclophosphamide			Oral: 1-2 mg/kg/day	
Cyclosporine	Gengraf Neoral Sandimmune	Oral: 2.5 mg/kg/day divided twice daily	Oral: may ↑ by 0.5-0.75 mg/kg/day at 8 and 12 weeks to max dose 4 mg/kg/day	
Corticosteroids			Oral, IV, IM, IA, and soft-tissue injections: variable	

ALT, alanine aminotransferase; BID, twice daily; CL_{cr}, creatinine clearance; CYP, cytochrome P450; IA, intra-articular; IM, intramuscular; IV, intravenous; q, every; SC, subcutaneous; ULN, upper limits of normal.

infections. To minimize these effects, use the lowest effective corticosteroid dose and limit the duration of use. Prednisolone 7.5 mg daily results in an average of 9.5% loss of bone density from the spine. Corticosteroids double the risk for osteoporosis in patients.[36] Patients on long-term therapy should be given calcium and vitamin D to minimize bone loss. Alendronate is effective in preventing bone loss in corticosteroid-treated patients and should be considered prophylactically for patients when long-term corticosteroid therapy is anticipated, particularly for patients who are at high risk of bone loss (eg, postmenopausal women, patients >65 years).[37-40] There is

TABLE 91-4 Clinical Monitoring of Drug Therapy in Rheumatoid Arthritis

Drug	Adverse Drug Reaction	Initial Monitoring	Maintenance Monitoring	Symptoms to Inquire About[a]
NSAIDs and salicylates	GI ulceration and bleeding, renal damage	sCr or BUN, CBC q 2-4 wk p starting therapy × 1-2 mo salicylates: serum salicylate levels if therapeutic dose and no response	Same as initial plus stool guaiac q 6-12 mo	Blood in stool, black stool, dyspepsia, nausea/vomiting, weakness, dizziness, abdominal pain, edema, weight gain, SOB
Corticosteroids	Hypertension, hyperglycemia, osteoporosis[b]	Glucose, blood pressure q 3-6 mo	Same as initial	Blood pressure if available, polyuria, polydipsia, edema, SOB, visual changes, weight gain, headaches, broken bones or bone pain
Gold (intramuscular or oral)	Myelosuppression, proteinuria, rash, stomatitis	Baseline & until stable: UA, CBC w/plt preinjection	Same as initial—every other dose	Symptoms of myelosuppression, edema, rash, oral ulcers, diarrhea
Hydroxychloroquine	Macular damage, rash, diarrhea	Baseline: color fundus photography and automated central perimetric analysis	Ophthalmoscopy q 9-12 mo and Amsler grid at home q 2 wk	Visual changes including a decrease in night or peripheral vision, rash, diarrhea
Methotrexate	Myelosuppression, hepatic fibrosis, cirrhosis, pulmonary infiltrates or fibrosis, stomatitis, rash	Baseline: AST, ALT, alk phos, alb, t. bili, hep B and C studies, CBC w/plt, S_{cr}	CBC w/plt, AST, alb q 1-2 mo	Symptoms of myelosuppression, SOB, nausea/vomiting, lymph node swelling, coughing, mouth sores, diarrhea, jaundice
Leflunomide	Hepatitis, GI distress, alopecia	Baseline: ALT, CBC with platelets	CBC with platelets and ALT monthly initially and then every 6-8 wk	Nausea/vomiting, gastritis, diarrhea, hair loss, jaundice
Penicillamine	Myelosuppression, proteinuria, stomatitis, rash, dysgeusia	Baseline: UA, CBC w/plt, then q week × 1 month	Same as initial—q 1-2 mo, but q 2 wk if dose change	Symptoms of myelosuppression, edema, rash, diarrhea, altered taste perception, oral ulcers
Cyclophosphamide	Alopecia, infertility, GI distress, hemorrhagic cystitis, myelosuppression, nephrotoxicity, cardiotoxicity	UA, CBC w/plt q week × 1 month	Same as initial—q 2-4 wk	Nausea/vomiting, gastritis, diarrhea, hair loss, urination difficulties, chest pain, rash, respiratory difficulties
Cyclosporine	Hepatotoxicity, nephrotoxicity, hypertension, headache, malignancy, infections, GI distress	S_{cr}, blood pressure q month	Same as initial	Nausea/vomiting, diarrhea, symptoms of infection, symptoms of elevated blood pressure
Sulfasalazine	Myelosuppression, rash	Baseline: CBC w/plt, then q week × 1 month	Same as initial—q 1-2 mo	Symptoms of myelosuppression, photosensitivity, rash, nausea/vomiting
Tocilizumab	Local injection-site reactions, infection	AST/ALT, CBC w/plt, lipids	AST/ALT, CBC w/plt, lipids q 4-8 weeks	Symptoms of infection
Anakinra	Local injection-site reactions, infection	Neutrophil count	Neutrophil count monthly for 3 months then quarterly up to 1 year	Symptoms of infection
Etanercept, adalimumab, golimumab, certolizumab	Local injection-site reactions, infection	Tuberculin skin test hepatitis C screening	None	Symptoms of infection
Infliximab, rituximab, abatacept	Immune reactions, infection	Tuberculin skin test hepatitis C screening	None	Postinfusion reactions, symptoms of infection
Tofacitinib	Infection, malignancy, GI perforations, upper respiratory tract infections, headache, diarrhea, nasopharyngitis	Tuberculin skin test, hepatitis C screening, neutrophil count, lymphocytes, Hgb, AST/ALT	Neutrophils, Hgb, FLP at 4-8 weeks after treatment start, then lymphocytes, neutrophils, and Hgb q 3 months	Symptoms of infection or myelosuppression, SOB, blood in stool, black stool, dyspepsia

alb, albumin; alk phos, alkaline phosphatase; ALT, alanine aminotransferase; AST, aspartate aminotransferase; BUN, blood urea nitrogen; CBC, complete blood count; FLP, fasting lipid panel; GI, gastrointestinal; hep, hepatitis; Hgb, hemoglobin; p, after; plt, platelet; q, every; S_{cr}, serum creatinine; t. bili, total bilirubin; UA, urinalysis; NSAIDs, nonsteroidal anti-inflammatory drugs; SOB, shortness of breath.

[a]Altered immune function increases infection; this should be considered particularly in those patients taking azathioprine, methotrexate, and corticosteroids or other drugs as a symptom of myelosuppression.

[b]Osteoporosis is unlikely to manifest itself early in treatment, but all patients should be taking appropriate steps to prevent bone loss.

no evidence that corticosteroids alone increase the risk of gastrointestinal ulcerations, although they often have been implicated. Consequently, gastrointestinal protective measures usually are not indicated.[41,42]

Methotrexate

Methotrexate is now considered the DMARD of choice for initial therapy of most patients with RA. It inhibits cytokine production, inhibits purine biosynthesis, and may stimulate release of adenosine, all of which may lead to its anti-inflammatory properties. The drug has a fairly rapid onset of action; results may be seen as early as 2 to 3 weeks after starting therapy. Some 45% to 67% of patients remain on methotrexate therapy in studies ranging from 5 to 7 years.[43]

Absorption of methotrexate is variable and averages approximately 70% of an oral dose. Methotrexate is 35% to 50% bound to albumin; it may be displaced by highly protein-bound drugs such as

NSAIDs, but the clinical importance of this interaction in the relatively low doses of methotrexate used in RA is unknown. Methotrexate is extensively metabolized intracellularly to polyglutamated derivatives. It is excreted by the kidney, 80% unchanged, by glomerular filtration and active transport. Some methotrexate may be reabsorbed, but this transport process may be saturated even with low doses, resulting in increased renal clearance.

Methotrexate is contraindicated in pregnant and nursing women as it is teratogenic. Patients should use contraception to avoid pregnancy and discontinue the drug if conception is planned. It is also contraindicated in patients with chronic liver disease, immunodeficiency, pleural or peritoneal effusions, leukopenia, thrombocytopenia, preexisting blood disorders, and a creatinine clearance of less than 40 mL/min (0.67 mL/s).

The toxicities of methotrexate therapy are mainly gastrointestinal, hematologic, pulmonary, and hepatic. Stomatitis occurs in 3% to 10% of patients and may be painful or painless. Diarrhea, nausea, and vomiting may occur in up to 10% of patients. The most common hematologic toxicity is thrombocytopenia in 1% to 3% of patients. Leukopenia also may occur, but in a smaller number of patients. Although pulmonary fibrosis and pneumonitis can be severe adverse effects, they are rare.

Elevated liver enzymes may occur in up to 15% of patients; cirrhosis is rare. Liver function tests, aspartate aminotransferase or alanine aminotransferase, should be performed periodically. Methotrexate should be discontinued if these test values show sustained results greater than twice the upper limits of normal. Albumin should also be checked periodically as a sign of liver toxicity because some patients may not have liver inflammation manifested by aspartate aminotransferase or alanine aminotransferase elevation. Liver biopsy is now recommended before beginning methotrexate therapy only for patients with a history of excessive alcohol use, ongoing hepatitis B or C infections, or recurring elevation of aspartate aminotransferase. Biopsies during methotrexate therapy are recommended only for patients who develop consistently abnormal liver function tests.[27]

Because it is a folic acid antagonist, methotrexate can induce a folic acid deficiency. This deficiency is thought to be partly responsible for methotrexate toxicity, and supplementation with folic acid does alleviate some adverse effects. Addition of folic acid to a methotrexate regimen for RA does not compromise drug efficacy.[25,27,44]

Methotrexate may be given intramuscularly, subcutaneously, or orally. Doses greater than 15 mg per week generally are given parenterally because of decreased oral bioavailability of larger doses.

Leflunomide

Leflunomide is a DMARD that inhibits pyrimidine synthesis, leading to a decrease in lymphocyte proliferation and modulation of inflammation. It has efficacy similar to methotrexate for treating RA. The drug may cause liver toxicity and is contraindicated in patients with preexisting liver disease. Patients taking the drug should have alanine aminotransferase monitored monthly initially and periodically thereafter as long as they continue treatment. Leflunomide may cause bone marrow toxicity and complete blood count with platelets is recommended monthly for 6 months and then every 6 to 8 weeks thereafter.

The drug is teratogenic, and appropriate contraceptive measures are recommended to avoid pregnancy for all sexually active male and female patients who are taking leflunomide. If conception is desired, leflunomide must be discontinued. Because leflunomide undergoes enterohepatic circulation, the drug takes many months to drop to a plasma concentration considered safe during pregnancy (<0.02 mcg/mL [mg/L; <74 nmol/L]). Cholestyramine may be used to rapidly clear the drug from plasma. In addition to pregnancy, cholestyramine use may be warranted to rapidly clear the drug in the event of severe toxicity.

Leflunomide may be given as a loading dose of 100 mg daily for 3 days, followed by a maintenance dose of 20 mg daily. Lower doses may be used if patients have gastrointestinal intolerance, complain of hair loss, or have other signs of dose-related toxicity. The loading dose allows the patient to achieve a more rapid therapeutic response, usually within the first month. The long elimination half-life of the drug (14-16 days) would require the patient to take the drug for several months to achieve steady state without a loading dose. Some rheumatologists prefer to begin with maintenance dosing as the loading dose may put the patient at increased risk for toxicity.[30,45,46]

Hydroxychloroquine

Hydroxychloroquine is often used in mild RA or as an adjuvant in combination DMARD therapy in more progressive disease. The pharmacokinetics and mechanism of action of this drug are poorly understood, but it is thought to dampen antigen–antibody reactions at sites of inflammation.[28] It is well absorbed orally and widely distributed to body tissues. Hydroxychloroquine is partially metabolized in the liver and is excreted by the kidney. The onset of action of hydroxychloroquine may be delayed up to 6 weeks, but the drug is considered a therapeutic failure only when 6 months of therapy without a response has elapsed.

The main advantage of hydroxychloroquine is the lack of myelosuppressive, hepatic, and renal toxicities that may be seen with other DMARDs, which simplifies monitoring. Short-term toxicities of hydroxychloroquine include gastrointestinal effects such as nausea, vomiting, and diarrhea, which can be managed by taking doses with food. Ocular toxicity includes accommodation defects, benign corneal deposits, blurred vision, scotomas (small areas of decreased or absent vision in the visual field), and night blindness. Although the risk of true retinopathy with hydroxychloroquine approaches zero, preretinopathy may occur in 2.7% of patients. All patients must understand the importance of adhering to hydroxychloroquine monitoring guidelines, as delineated in Table 91-2. Any visual change must be reported immediately. Dermatologic toxicities include rash, alopecia, and increased skin pigmentation; neurologic adverse effects such as headache, vertigo, and insomnia usually are mild.[47,48]

Sulfasalazine

Sulfasalazine, a prodrug, is cleaved by bacteria in the colon into sulfapyridine and 5-aminosalicylic acid.[49] It is believed that the sulfapyridine moiety is responsible for the agent's antirheumatic properties, although the exact mechanism of action is unknown. Once the colonic bacteria have cleaved sulfasalazine, sulfapyridine and 5-aminosalicylic acid are absorbed rapidly from the gastrointestinal tract. Sulfapyridine distributes rapidly throughout the body, but higher concentrations are found in certain tissues such as serous fluid, liver, and intestines. Both sulfasalazine and its metabolites are excreted in the urine. Antirheumatic effects should be seen in 2 months.

Use of sulfasalazine is often limited by its adverse effects. Gastrointestinal adverse effects such as nausea, vomiting, diarrhea, and anorexia are the most common. These can be minimized by initiating therapy with low doses and titrating gradually to higher doses, dividing the dose more evenly throughout the day, or using enteric-coated preparations. Rash, urticaria, and serum sickness-like reactions can be managed with antihistamines and, if indicated, corticosteroids. If a hypersensitivity reaction occurs, therapy should be stopped immediately and another DMARD substituted. Sulfasalazine is associated with leukopenia, alopecia, stomatitis, and elevated hepatic enzymes. It also may cause the patient's urine and skin to turn a yellow-orange color, which is of no clinical consequence however; patients should be educated about this to avoid premature discontinuance.

Sulfasalazine's absorption can be decreased when antibiotics are used that destroy the colonic bacteria. Sulfasalazine also binds iron supplements in the gastrointestinal tract that can lead to a decreased absorption of sulfasalazine. The administration of these two agents should be separated temporally to avoid this interaction. Sulfasalazine can potentiate warfarin's effects by displacing it from protein-binding sites. Close monitoring of the patient's international normalized ratio is indicated.

In a meta-analysis of 15 randomized controlled trials, sulfasalazine was found to be superior in various rating scales compared with placebo, hydroxychloroquine, D-penicillamine, and gold.[50]

Other Disease-Modifying Antirheumatic Drugs

Gold salts, azathioprine, D-penicillamine, cyclosporine, minocycline, anakinra, and cyclophosphamide have all been used to treat RA. Although these drugs can be effective and they may be of value in certain clinical settings, they are used less frequently today because of toxicity, lack of long-term benefit, or both. Tables 91-2 and 91-3 provide dosing information and toxicity information.

Tofacitinib

Tofacitinib (Xeljanz) is a JAK inhibitor for use in patients with moderate to severe RA who have failed, or have intolerance to methotrexate.[51] JAK is a tyrosine kinase protein that facilitates the phosphorylation of the signal transducers and activators of transcription (STATs) proteins. These proteins in turn regulate inflammatory gene transcription. Thus, inhibition of JAK by tofacitinib results in modulation and suppression of the immune system through preventing activation of STATs.

In clinical trials, oral doses of tofacitinib 5 mg twice daily resulted in a statistically higher percentage of patients achieving at least a 20% improvement in RA symptoms at 3 months compared with placebo. An improvement in symptoms of 50% occurred in approximately 30% of patients.[52] In a comparison trial including adalimumab 40 mg every other week, tofacitinib showed similar ACR20 responses and both treatment arms achieved a greater ACR20 response compared with placebo.[53]

The FDA-approved dosing of tofacitinib is 5 mg twice daily as monotherapy or in combination with other nonbiologic DMARDs; tofacitinib should not be given with biologics. A dose reduction of 5 mg once daily should be used in patients with moderate or severe renal dysfunction, moderate hepatic dysfunction, concurrent therapy with potent CYP3A4 inhibitors such as rifampin or moderate CYP3A4 inhibitors, and potent CYP2C19 inhibitors such as fluconazole.[51]

Initiation of tofacitinib should be avoided in patients with severe hepatic impairment, lymphocyte count less than 500 cells/mm^3 ($<0.5 \times 10^9$/L), ANC less than 1000 cells/mm^3 ($<1 \times 10^9$/L), or hemoglobin less than 9 g/dL (<90 g/L; 5.59 mmol/L). Concurrent use of a potent CYP3A4 inducer may lead to a reduced effect from tofacitinib.

Risks, for which black box warnings exist, include serious infections, lymphomas, and other malignancies. Patients should be tested and treated for latent tuberculosis before therapy with tofacitinib. Monitoring for reductions in lymphocytes, neutrophils, and hemoglobin should be completed at baseline and periodically throughout therapy at 4 to 8 weeks postinitiation and every 3 months thereafter.

Tofacitinib therapy has been associated with elevated plasma liver enzymes and lipids. Gastrointestinal perforations have also been reported. Live vaccinations should not be given during treatment. Though tofacitinib is similar to DMARDs in that it is a synthetic, small molecule that is orally absorbed, it is considered to be in a different category than other synthetic DMARDs in the ACR 2015 RA treatment guidelines.[27] It is recommended for use after DMARDs and biologics due to lack of long-term efficacy and safety data. It may be a convenient oral alternative to other biologic agents; however, this must be considered along with the monitoring schedule required due to safety concerns.

Biologic Agents

Biologic agents are genetically engineered protein molecules that block the proinflammatory cytokines TNF-α (infliximab, etanercept, adalimumab, golimumab, and certolizumab), IL-1 (anakinra), and IL-6 (tocilizumab), deplete peripheral B cells (rituximab), or bind to CD80/86 on T cells to prevent the costimulation needed to fully activate T cells (abatacept). These drugs may be effective when DMARDs fail to achieve adequate responses but are considerably more expensive to use. These agents have no toxicities requiring laboratory monitoring, but they do carry a small increased risk for infection. There is an increased incidence of tuberculosis in patients treated with these agents. Tuberculin skin testing or interferon gamma release assay (IGRA) blood test is recommended prior to treatment with biologic agents so that latent tuberculosis can be detected.[26] Patients with a history of significant tuberculosis exposure or recurrent infection may not be good candidates for these drugs. Those who develop infections while on biologic agents should at least temporarily discontinue them until the infection is cured. Live vaccines should not be given to patients taking biologic agents.

TNF-*α* Inhibitors

While the TNFi biologics have differing structures, pharmacokinetics, and dosing, their side effects and contraindications are similar in that they all block TNF. Chronic heart failure (CHF) is a relative contraindication for all TNFi agents. Increased cardiac mortality has been seen in patients treated with infliximab and etanercept-associated heart failure exacerbations have been documented.[46,54] Patients with New York Heart Association class III or IV and an ejection fraction of 50% or less should not use TNFi therapy. Additionally, patients whose CHF worsens while taking TNFi therapy should discontinue the drug.[25] In the subset of patients with CHF or whose CHF worsens on TNFi therapy, combination DMARDs, non-TNF biologics, or tofacitinib are recommended.[27]

TNFi therapy has also been reported to induce a multiple sclerosis-like illness or exacerbate multiple sclerosis in patients with the disease. Patients with neurologic symptoms suggestive of multiple sclerosis should discontinue therapy. TNFi may predispose patients to increased cancer risk, especially lymphoproliferative cancer, as TNF plays a role in ridding the body of cancer cells. The US Food and Drug Administration (FDA) added a black box warning to product labeling for TNFi drugs alerting prescribers of increased lymphoproliferative and other cancers in children and adolescents treated with these drugs.[55]

Etanercept Etanercept is a fusion protein consisting of two p75-soluble TNF receptors linked to an Fc fragment of human IgG_1. The drug binds to TNF, making it biologically inactive and preventing it from interacting with the cell-surface TNF receptors that would lead to cell activation.

The drug is given by subcutaneous injection, 50 mg once weekly or 25 mg twice weekly, usually through self-injections or administration by a caregiver. Aside from local injection-site reactions, adverse effects are rare. There are case reports of pancytopenia and neurologic demyelinating syndromes such as multiple sclerosis associated with use of etanercept, but these are rare. No laboratory monitoring is required. Clinical trials have used etanercept in patients who failed DMARDs. Response was seen in 60% to 75% of patients. The drug has also been FDA approved for the treatment of juvenile RA, ankylosing spondylitis, psoriatic arthritis, and moderate-to-severe psoriasis. Clinical trials have shown that it slows erosive disease progression to a greater degree than oral methotrexate therapy.[56-58]

Infliximab Infliximab is a chimeric antibody combining portions of mouse and human IgG_1. Approximately 25% of the antibody is derived from mouse amino acids. This antibody, when injected in humans, binds to TNF and prevents its interaction with TNF receptors on inflammatory cells.

Infliximab is given by IV infusion at a dose of 3 mg/kg at 0, 2, and 6 weeks and then every 8 weeks. To prevent the formation of an antibody response to this foreign protein, oral methotrexate should be given concurrently in doses typically used to treat RA for as long as the patient continues on infliximab. Antibodies develop in 14% to 40% of patients, which results in a greater risk of infusion reactions and also may reduce the efficacy of the drug. Loss of response may be seen in patients with RA who have good initial response requiring increased doses or shorter intervals between doses to maintain response. Infusion reactions may occur in any patient treated with the drug. Both acute (within 24 hours of infusion) and delayed (24 hours to 14 days) reactions following infusion have been identified. An acute infusion reaction with symptoms including fever, chills, pruritus, and rash may occur during infusion or within 1 to 2 hours after giving the drug. Treatment includes slowing infusion rates and administering acetaminophen, diphenhydramine, or corticosteroids, depending on the severity of symptoms. Fortunately these reactions are rarely severe or anaphylactic in nature.[59] The drug may increase the risk of infection. Autoantibodies and lupus-like syndrome also have been reported. In addition to RA, infliximab is indicated for the treatment of psoriatic arthritis and ankylosing spondylitis.[60,61]

Adalimumab Adalimumab is a human IgG_1 antibody to TNF. Because it has no foreign protein components, it is less antigenic than infliximab. The drug is provided as either premixed syringes or injection pens containing 40 mg, which is administered by subcutaneous injection every 14 days. It has similar response rates to those seen with the other TNFi. Local injection-site reactions were the most common adverse reactions noted in clinical trials. It has the same precautions regarding tuberculosis and other infections as the other biologics.[62-64]

Golimumab Golimumab is a human antibody to TNF-α. In addition to RA, this agent is also indicated for treatment of psoriatic arthritis and ankylosing spondylitis. The drug is available as an injection pen, through which a dose of 50 mg is given monthly by subcutaneous injection. Precautions are similar to other TNFi.[65]

Certolizumab Certolizumab is a humanized antibody specific for human TNF-α. For RA, dosing recommendations are for 400 mg (2 doses of 200 mg) given by subcutaneous injection at weeks 0, 2, and 4 followed by 200 mg every 2 weeks. Precautions and side effects are similar to other TNFi.[66]

Clinical **Controversy...**

After failure of an initial anti-tumor necrosis factor (TNF) agent, subsequent treatment may include trials of an alternative anti-TNF agent or a change to a non-TNF biologic. It is not clear which of these strategies is more likely to be effective as randomized trials in anti-TNF treatment failures are lacking.

Non-TNF Biologics

Abatacept Abatacept is a costimulation modulator approved for the treatment of RA in patients with moderate to severe disease who fail to achieve an adequate response from one or more DMARDs. In patients who failed to achieve adequate responses with TNFi, one-half had a clinical response to abatacept.[67] Additionally, in the first head-to-head trial with biologic agents, the addition of abatacept to a stable methotrexate dose showed similar efficacy and adverse effects to adalimumab plus methotrexate in biologic-naive patients with an inadequate response to methotrexate monotherapy.[68]

By binding to CD80/CD86 receptors on antigen-presenting cells, abatacept inhibits interactions between the antigen-presenting cells and T cells. This prevents T-cell activation to promote the inflammatory process, thus resulting in reductions in cytokines, T-cell proliferation, and other consequences of T-cell activation.

Abatacept is a fusion protein made using the extracellular domain of human cytotoxic T lymphocyte antigen 4 (the binding portion of the drug) and a fragment of the Fc domain of human IgG modified to prevent complement fixation. The drug is given by IV infusion based on patient weight (<60 kg [<132 lb]: 500 mg; 60 to 100 kg [132-220 lb]: 750 mg; >100 kg [>220 lb]: 1,000 mg) every 2 weeks for two doses after the initial dose and then every 4 weeks. Alternatively, the drug may be given by subcutaneous injection with the first dose of 125 mg given within 24 hours of a single IV infusion and every 7 days after that. Abatacept may be used as monotherapy or in combination with DMARDs.

The adverse effects include headache, nasopharyngitis, dizziness, cough, back pain, hypertension, dyspepsia, urinary tract infection, rash, and extremity pain reported more frequently than placebo in clinical trials. Infusion reactions were 50% more likely with abatacept than with placebo and there was a slightly higher rate of serious infections with active treatment.[67,69,70] Live vaccines should not be given to patients during and for 3 months after the completion of abatacept therapy.[71]

Rituximab Rituximab is a monoclonal chimeric antibody consisting of mostly human protein with the antigen-binding region derived from a mouse antibody to CD20 protein found on the cell surface of mature B lymphocytes. The binding of rituximab to B cells results in nearly complete depletion of peripheral B cells. Although its mechanism of action in RA is not completely known, it is thought that this depletion in B cells decreases antigen presentation to T cells, thus decreasing symptoms and delaying structural damage. After administration of rituximab, it takes several months for B-cell recovery. This prolonged effect on B cells results in a variable duration of action that allows for intermittent therapy based on reactivation of arthritis symptoms.

Rituximab is useful in patients who failed methotrexate or TNFi.[72-76] Two infusions of 1,000 mg are given 2 weeks apart. Methylprednisolone 100 mg should be given 30 minutes prior to rituximab to reduce the incidence and severity of infusion reactions. Acetaminophen and antihistamines may also be of benefit in patients who have a history of reactions. Methotrexate should be given concurrently in the usual doses used for RA, as the combination has proved to provide the best therapeutic outcomes. Duration of benefit is variable after a course of rituximab and patients will need retreatment with reactivation of their disease. Live vaccines should not be given to patients given rituximab.

Tocilizumab IL-6 is a major cytokine believed to have a role in promoting inflammation in RA. Tocilizumab is a humanized monoclonal antibody that attaches to IL-6 receptors, preventing the cytokine from interacting with the IL-6 receptor.[77] It is FDA approved for use in adults with moderately to severely active RA who have failed to respond to one or more DMARDs. It is used as either monotherapy or in combination with methotrexate or another DMARD. A recent study completed in patients with severe RA unable to use methotrexate found tocilizumab monotherapy more efficacious in symptom improvement than adalimumab monotherapy.[78]

The initial starting dose is 4 mg/kg given IV every 4 weeks with dose escalation to 8 mg/kg IV every 4 weeks based on clinical response and tolerance.[77] The rates of adverse events are generally low but higher with combination therapy as compared to monotherapy. The most serious adverse effects reported include infusion reactions, increased infection risk, elevated plasma lipids, elevated liver enzymes, and gastrointestinal perforation. Tocilizumab use may also lead to increased metabolism of concomitant cytochrome P450 (CYP)3A4 substrate medications. It is recommended to monitor agents with narrow therapeutic window such as warfarin. Oral contraceptives and CYP3A4 statins may also be affected.

Anakinra Anakinra is a naturally occurring IL-1 receptor antagonist. Results of clinical trials suggest it to be less effective than other biologics.[79] The ACR did not include anakinra in their RA treatment recommendations because of limited use of this drug, but select patients with refractory disease could benefit from treatment with this drug.[25]

Treatment Strategies for Patients with Suboptimal Response to Biologics

TNFi are generally the first biologic agents chosen for most patients with RA. Approximately 30% of patients discontinue treatment with these drugs because of lack of efficacy or adverse effects. Lack of efficacy can further be defined as a primary failure (failure to see a treatment response 3 to 6 months after therapy initiation) or secondary failure (loss of response after an initial improvement is observed).

In such situations, addition of a DMARD may be beneficial if the patient is not already taking one. Dose escalation or decreased interval between infusions may be useful for those patients taking infliximab; higher doses of other TNFi have not been demonstrated to be effective. Choosing an alternative TNFi after failure of the initial TNFi agent may be beneficial for some patients[80]; however, no randomized controlled trials have compared the effectiveness of cycling among agents in this class. Treatment with rituximab, abatacept, tocilizumab or tofacitinib may also prove to be effective in TNFi treatment failures.[63,72,80]

Clinical **Controversy...**

As biologics lose patent protection, generic formulations of these products, called biosimilars, will be marketed. It remains to be seen whether these biosimilars will be as safe and effective as currently used biologics that they may replace.

PERSONALIZED PHARMACOTHERAPY

With various pathways involved leading to inflammation in RA and an increasing number of agents available, it is important to consider patient-specific factors when making therapeutic decisions. Disease activity and the presence of poor prognostic guide treatment and lead to early aggressive therapy in patients with more severe disease.

Therapy must be tailored for various comorbidities the patient may have (Table 91-6). Hepatitis and other liver diseases, heart failure, renal failure, and history of cancer are among the comorbidities that influence treatment choice. Individual patients may also significantly differ in their response to a specific agent; currently, there are no clear predictors of response to therapeutic interventions.

Pharmacokinetic parameters should be taken into consideration when determining therapeutic options for specific patients. NSAIDs should be avoided in patients with renal impairment or in patients at high risk for NSAID-induced renal injury including the elderly, those with congestive heart failure or cirrhosis, or patients at risk for volume depletion such as those using diuretics.[81] Dose adjustments are recommended in patients with renal dysfunction for methotrexate and anakinra. Dose reductions are also recommended

TABLE 91-5 Dosage Regimens for NSAIDs

Drug	Adult	Children	Dosing Schedule
		Recommended Anti-inflammatory Total Daily Dosage	
Aspirin	2.6-5.2 g	60-100 mg/kg	Four times daily
Celecoxib	200-400 mg	—	Daily to twice daily
Diclofenac	150-200 mg		Three times per day to four times daily Extended release twice daily
Diflunisal	0.5-1.5 g	—	Twice daily
Etodolac	0.2-1.2 g (max. 20 mg/kg)	—	Twice daily to four times daily
Fenoprofen	0.9-3.0 g	—	Four times daily
Flurbiprofen	200-300 mg	—	Twice daily to four times daily
Ibuprofen	1.2-3.2 g	20-40 mg/kg	Three times per day to four times daily
Indomethacin	50-200 mg	2-4 mg/kg (max. 200 mg)	Twice daily to four times daily Extended release daily
Meclofenamate	200-400 mg	—	Three times per day to four times per day
Meloxicam	7.5-15 mg	—	Daily
Nabumetone	1-2 g	—	Daily to twice daily
Naproxen	0.5-1.0 g	10 mg/kg	Twice daily Extended release–daily
Naproxen sodium	0.55-1.1 g	—	Twice daily
Nonacetylated salicylates	1.2-4.8 g	—	Twice daily to six times per day
Oxaprozin	0.6-1.8 g (max. 26 mg/kg)	—	Daily to three times a day
Piroxicam	10-20 mg	—	Daily
Sulindac	300-400 mg	—	Twice daily
Tolmetin	0.6-1.8 g	15-30 mg/kg	Twice daily to four times daily

NSAIDs, nonsteroidal anti-inflammatory drugs.

TABLE 91-6 Treatment of Rheumatoid Arthritis in Patients with High-Risk Conditions

Comorbidity	Recommendation
Latent TB	Use biologic, tofacitinib after 1 month treatment for latent TB
Active TB	Use biologic, tofacitinib only after completion of treatment for active TB
Pregnant/breastfeeding	Avoid methotrexate, leflunomide, minocycline
CHF	Prefer non-TNF inhibitor therapy
Skin cancer (melanoma or nonmelanoma	Use DMARDs preferably over biologics or tofacitinib
Previously treated lymphoproliferative disorder	Use rituximab, combination DMARD, abatacept or tocilizumab over TNF inhibitor
• Hepatitis B	No restrictions
• Hepatitis C infection not receiving or requiring treatment	Use DMARD over TNF inhibitor
• Hepatitis C infection treated or receiving treatment	No restrictions
• Previous serious infections	Use combination DMARD or abatacept over TNF inhibitor

CHF, chronic heart failure; DMARD, disease-modifying antirheumatic drug; TB, tuberculosis; TNF, tumor necrosis factor.

with tofacitinib in patients with moderate or severe renal impairment, moderate hepatic dysfunction, or patients treated concomitantly with CYP3A4 inhibitors.

While azathioprine is now used less frequently for RA, genetic testing for null or decreased thiopurine *S*-methyltransferase (TPMT) activity is available to help predict those patients with a higher risk of myelosuppression due to reduced metabolism of the drug, and dosage reductions may be made in those patients.[82]

EVALUATION OF THERAPEUTIC OUTCOMES

The evaluation of therapeutic outcomes is based primarily on improvements of clinical signs and symptoms of RA. Clinical signs of improvement include a reduction in joint swelling, decreased warmth over actively involved joints, and decreased tenderness to joint palpation. Improvement in RA symptoms includes reduction in perceived joint pain and morning stiffness, longer time to onset of afternoon fatigue, and improvement in ability to perform activities of daily living. Improvement of activities of daily living may be assessed objectively using a health assessment questionnaire score. Joint radiographs may be of some benefit in assessing the progression of the disease and should show little or no evidence of disease progression if treatment is effective.

Laboratory monitoring is of little value in monitoring individual patient response to therapy. Tables 91-2 and 91-3 provide monitoring of drug toxicity information. Routine monitoring of patients is essential to the safe use of these drugs. In addition, patients should be questioned about symptoms of the adverse effects outlined in the drug section of this chapter.

CONCLUSION

RA is the most common inflammatory arthritis, affecting approximately 1% of the population. The disease is characterized by symmetrical swelling and stiffness of the involved joints. The stiffness is usually more prominent in the morning. Extraarticular features of RA include rheumatoid nodules, vasculitis, and ocular, cardiac, and pulmonary complications. The course of the disease is highly variable. Treatment is aimed at reaching remission or low disease activity, which will result in relief of pain and inflammation and maintain and preserve joint function. Nondrug therapy, including exercise and adequate rest periods, should also be used early in the course of treatment. Early use of a DMARD or biologic agent results in better patient outcomes. Methotrexate should be considered for initial therapy in most patients. Patients who fail to achieve at least low disease activity with initial therapy could be considered for other DMARDs, combination DMARDs or biologics agent. These approaches have been shown to be effective in patients who fail to achieve adequate response from initial DMARD monotherapy. Corticosteroids and NSAIDs may be useful adjuncts for treatment, but because of adverse effects and limited impact on long-term outcomes, they should not be considered as sole treatment for most patients.

ABBREVIATIONS

ACPA	anticitrullinated protein antibody
ACR	American College of Rheumatology
ANA	antinuclear antibody
CHF	chronic heart failure
CRP	C-reactive protein
CYP	cytochrome P450
DMARD	disease-modifying antirheumatic drug
ESR	erythrocyte sedimentation rate
EULAR	European League Against Rheumatism
FDA	Food and Drug Administration
HLA	human lymphocyte antigen
Ig	immunoglobulin
IGRA	interferon gamma release assay
IL	interleukin
JAK	Janus kinase
NSAID	nonsteroidal antiinflammatory drug
RA	rheumatoid arthritis
RF	rheumatoid factor
TNF	tumor necrosis factor
TPMT	thiopurine *S*-methyltransferase

REFERENCES

1. Smith JB, Haynes MK. Rheumatoid arthritis—A molecular understanding. *Ann Intern Med* 2002;136(12):908-922.
2. Klippel JH CL, Stone JH, Crofford LJ, White PH, eds. *Primer on the Rheumatic Diseases*, 13th ed. Atlanta, GA: Arthritis Foundation, 2008.
3. Harris ED, Firestein GS. The clinical features of rheumatoid arthritis. In: Firestein GS, Budd RC, Harris ED, et al., eds. *Kelley's Textbook of Rheumatology*, 8th ed. St. Louis, MO: Saunders, 2008. *http://www.mdconsult.com.*
4. Jiang H, Chess L. Regulation of immune response by T cells. *N Engl J Med* 2006;354:1166-1176.
5. Brennan FM, McInnes IB. Evidence that cytokines play a role in rheumatoid arthritis. *J Clin Invest* 2008;118:3537-3545.
6. Moissec P, Korn T, Kuchroo VK. Interleukin-17 and type 17 helper T cells. *N Engl J Med* 2009;361:888-898.
7. Isaacs JD. Therapeutic T-cell manipulation in rheumatoid arthritis: Past, present and future. *Rheumatology* 2008;49:1461-1468.
8. Tsokos GC. B cells, be gone—B-cell depletion in the treatment of rheumatoid arthritis. *N Engl J Med* 2004;350(25):2546-2548.
9. Weinstein E, Peeva E, Putterman C, Diamond B. B-cell biology. *Rheum Dis Clin North Am* 2004;30(1):159-174.
10. Carter RH. B cells in health and disease. *Mayo Clin Proc* 2006;81: 377-384.
11. Youinou P, Taher TE, Pers J-O, et al. B lymphocyte cytokines and rheumatoid autoimmune disease. *Arthritis Rheum* 2009;60:1873-1880.
12. Choy EH, Panayi GS. Cytokine pathways and joint inflammation in rheumatoid arthritis. *N Engl J Med* 2001;344(12):907-916.
13. McInnes IB, Schett G. The pathogenesis of rheumatoid arthritis. *N Engl J Med* 2011;365:2205-2219.

14. Arend WP. Physiology of cytokine pathways in rheumatoid arthritis. *Arthritis Care Res* 2001;45:101-106.
15. Huber LC, Distler O, Tarner I, et al. Synovial fibroblasts: Key players in rheumatoid arthritis. *Rheumatology* 2006;45:669-675.
16. Firestein GS. Etiology and pathogenesis of rheumatoid arthritis. In: Firestein GS, Budd RC, Harris ED, et al., eds. *Kelley's Textbook of Rheumatology,* 8th ed. St. Louis, MO: Saunders, 2008. *http://www.mdconsult.com.*
17. Visser H. Early diagnosis of rheumatoid arthritis. *Best Pract Res Clin Rheumatol* 2005;19(1):55-72.
18. Hard ER. Extraarticular manifestations of rheumatoid arthritis. *Semin Arthritis Rheum* 1979;8:151-176.
19. Choi HK, Hernan MA, Seeger JD, et al. Methotrexate and mortality in patients with rheumatoid arthritis: A prospective study. *Lancet* 2002;359:1173-1177.
20. Wallberg-Jonsson S, Johansson H, Ohman ML, Rantapaa-Dahlqvist S. Extent of inflammation predicts cardiovascular disease and overall mortality in seropositive rheumatoid arthritis. A retrospective cohort study from disease onset. *J Rheumatol* 1999;26(12):2562-2571.
21. Colglazier CL, Sutej PG. Laboratory testing in rheumatic diseases: A practical review. *South Med J* 2005;98(2):185-191.
22. Shmerling RH. Diagnostic tests for rheumatic disease: Clinical utility revisited. *South Med J* 2005;98(7):704-711.
23. Aletaha D, Neogi T, Silman AJ, Fuovits J, et al. 2010 Rheumatoid arthritis classification criteria: An American College of Rheumatology/European League Against Rheumatism collaborative initiative. *Arthritis Rheum* 2010;62:2569-2581.
24. Smolen JS, Breedveld FC, Burmester GR, et al. Treating rheumatoid arthritis to target: 2014 update of the recommendations of an international task force. *Ann Rheum Dis* Published online first: 5 December 2015 doi:10.1136/annrheumdis-2015-207524.
25. Saag KG, Teng GG, Patkar NM, et al. American College of Rheumatology 2008 recommendations for the use of nonbiologic and biologic disease-modifying antirheumatic drugs in rheumatoid arthritis. *Arthritis Rheum* 2008;59:762-784.
26. Singh JA, Furst DE, Bharat A, et al. 2012 Update of the 2008 American College of Rheumatology recommendations for the use of disease-modifying antirheumatic drugs and biologic agents in the treatment of rheumatoid arthritis. *Arthritis Care Res* 2012;64(5):625-639.
27. Singh JA, Saag KG, Bridges SL, et al. 2015 American College of Rheumatology Guideline for the treatment of rheumatoid arthritis. *Arthritis Care Res* 2015: DOI 10.1002/acr.22783. Available at: http://www.rheumatology.org/Portals/0/Files/ACR%202015%20RA%20Guideline.pdf Last accessed November 18, 2015.
28. Genovese MC. The treatment of rheumatoid arthritis. In: Firestein GS, Budd RC, Harris ED, et al., eds. *Kelley's Textbook of Rheumatology,* 8th ed. St. Louis, MO: Saunders, 2008.
29. O'Dell JR. Therapeutic strategies for rheumatoid arthritis. *N Engl J Med* 2004;350(25):2591-2602.
30. Kalden JR, Schattenkirchner M, Sorensen H, et al. The efficacy and safety of leflunomide in patients with active rheumatoid arthritis: A five-year followup study. *Arthritis Rheum* 2003;48(6):1513-1520.
31. Moreland LW, O'Dell JR, Paulus HE, et al. A randomized comparative effectiveness study of oral triple therapy versus etanercept plus methotrexate in early, aggressive rheumatoid arthritis. *Arthritis Rheum* 2012;64(9):2824-2835.
32. Smolen JS, Emery P, Fleischmann R, et al. Adjustment of therapy in rheumatoid arthritis on the basis of achievement of stable low disease activity with adalimumab plus methotrexate or methotrexate alone: the randomised controlled OPTIMA trial. *Lancet* 2014;383:321-332.
33. Rahier JF, Moutschen M, Van Gompel A, et al. Vaccinations in patients with immune-mediated inflammatory diseases. *Rheumatology (Oxford)* 2010;49(10):1815-1827.
34. Singh JA, Cameron C, Noorbaloochi S, et al. Risk of serious infection in biological treatment of patients with rheumatoid arthritis: a systemic review and meta-analysis. *Lancet* 2015;386(9990):258-265.
35. Kavanaugh A, Wells AF. Benefits and risks of low-dose glucocorticoid treatment in the patient with rheumatoid arthritis. *Rheumatology* 2014;53:1742-1751.
36. DaSilva JAP, Jacogs JWG, Kirwan JR, et al. Safety of low dose glucocorticoid treatment in rheumatoid arthritis: Published evidence and prospective trial data. *Ann Rheum Dis* 2006;65:285-293.
37. Adachi JD, Saag KG, Delmas PD, et al. Two-year effects of alendronate on bone mineral density and vertebral fracture in patients receiving glucocorticoids: A randomized, double-blind, placebo-controlled extension trial. *Arthritis Rheum* 2001;44(1):202-211.
38. McIlwain HH. Glucocorticoid-induced osteoporosis: Pathogenesis, diagnosis, and management. *Prev Med* 2003;36(2):243-249.
39. da Silva JAP, Jacobs JWG, Kirwan JR, Boers M, et al. Safety of low dose glucocorticoid treatment in rheumatoid arthritis: published evidence and prospective trial data. *Ann Rheum Dis* 2006;65:285-293.
40. American College of Rheumatology Ad Hoc Committee on Glucocorticoid-Induced Osteoporosis. Recommendations for the prevention and treatment of glucocorticoid-induced osteoporosis. *Arthritis Rheum* 2001;44:1496-1503.
41. Morand EF. Corticosteroids in the treatment of rheumatologic diseases. *Curr Opin Rheumatol* 1998;10(3):179-183.
42. Bijlsma JWJ, Saag KG, Buttgereit F, da Silva JAP. Developments in glucocorticoid therapy. *Rheum Dis Clin North Am* 2005;31:1-17.
43. Pincus T, Ferraccioli G, Sokka T, et al. Evidence from clinical trials and long-term observational studies that disease-modifying anti-rheumatic drugs slow radiographic progression in rheumatoid arthritis: Updating a 1983 review. *Rheumatology* 2002;41(12):1346-1356.
44. Borchers AT, Keen CL, Cheema GS, Gershwin ME. The use of methotrexate in rheumatoid arthritis. *Semin Arthritis Rheum* 2004; 34(1):465-483.
45. Osiri M, Shea BJ, Robinson V, et al. Leflunomide for treating rheumatoid arthritis. *Cochrane Database Syst Rev* 2003(1):CD002047.
46. Cush JJ. Safety overview of new disease-modifying antirheumatic drugs. *Rheum Dis Clin North Am* 2004;30(2):237-255, v.
47. Maturi RK, Folk JC, Nichols B, Oetting TT, Kardon RH. Hydroxy-chloroquine retinopathy. *Arch Ophthalmol* 1999;117(9):1262-1263.
48. Suarez-Almazor ME, Belseck E, Shea B, et al. Antimalarials for treating rheumatoid arthritis. *Cochrane Database Syst Rev* 2000(4):CD000959.
49. Rains CP, Noble S, Faulds D. Sulfasalazine: A review of its pharmacological properties and therapeutic efficacy in the treatment of rheumatoid arthritis. *Drugs* 1995;50:137-156.
50. Weinblatt ME, Reda D, Henderson W, et al. Sulfasalazine treatment for rheumatoid arthritis: A meta-analysis of 15 randomized trials. *J Rheumatol* 1999;26(10):2123-2130.
51. Xeljanz (tofacitinib) Prescribing Information. Pfizer Labs; New York, NY; November 2012.
52. Fleischmann R, Kremer J, Cush J, et al. Placebo-controlled trial of tofacitinib monotherapy in rheumatoid arthritis. *N Engl J Med* 2012;367(6):495-507.
53. van Vollenhoven RF, Fleischmann R, Cohen S, et al. Tofacitinib or adalimumab versus placebo in rheumatoid arthritis. *N Engl J Med* 2012;367(6):508-519.
54. Scott DL, Kingsley MB. Tumor necrosis factor inhibitors for rheumatoid arthritis. *N Engl J Med* 2006;355:704-712.
55. Food and Drug Administration. Information for Healthcare Professionals: Tumor Necrosis Factor (TNF) Blockers (marketed as Remicade, Enbrel, Humira, Cimzia, and Simponi). FDA Alert August 4, 2009. Available at: http://www.fda.gov/Drugs/DrugSafety/PostmarketDrugSafetyInformationforPatientsandProviders/DrugSafetyInformationforHeathcareProfessionals/ucm174474.htm.
56. Genovese MC, Kremer JM. Treatment of rheumatoid arthritis with etanercept. *Rheum Dis Clin North Am* 2004;30(2):311-328, vi-vii.
57. Nanda S, Bathon JM. Etanercept: A clinical review of current and emerging indications. *Expert Opin Pharmacother* 2004;5(5):1175-1186.
58. Blumenauer B, Judd MG, Cranney A, et al. Etanercept for the treatment of rheumatoid arthritis. *Cochrane Database Syst Rev* 2003(3): CD004525.
59. Cheifitz A, Mayer L. Monoclonal antibodies, immunogenicity, and associated infusion reactions. *Mt Sinai J Med* 2005;72:250-256.
60. Blumenauer B, Judd M, Wells G, et al. Infliximab for the treatment of rheumatoid arthritis. *Cochrane Database Syst Rev* 2002(3):CD003785.
61. Maini SR. Infliximab treatment of rheumatoid arthritis. *Rheum Dis Clin North Am* 2004;30(2):329-347, vii.
62. Navarro-Sarabia F, Ariza-Ariza R, Hernandez-Cruz B, Villanueva I. Adalimumab for treating rheumatoid arthritis. *J Rheumatol* 2006;(6):1075-1081.
63. den Broeder A, van de Putte L, Rau R, et al. A single dose, placebo controlled study of the fully human anti-tumor necrosis factor-alpha antibody adalimumab (D2E7) in patients with rheumatoid arthritis. *J Rheumatol* 2002;29(11):2288-2298.
64. Keystone E, Haraoui B. Adalimumab therapy in rheumatoid arthritis. *Rheum Dis Clin North Am* 2004;30(2):349-364, vii.
65. Singh JA, Noorbaloochi S, Singh G. Golimumab for rheumatoid arthritis. *Cochrane Database Syst Rev* 2010(1):CD008341.
66. Mease PJ. Certolizumab pegol in the treatment of rheumatoid arthritis: A comprehensive review of its clinical efficacy and safety. *Rheumatology (Oxford)* 2011;50(2):261-270.
67. Genovese MC, Becker JC, Schiff M, et al. Abatacept for rheumatoid arthritis refractory to tumor necrosis factor alpha inhibition. *N Engl J Med* 2005;353(11):1114-1123.

68. Schiff M, Weinblatt, ME, Valante R, et al. Head-to-head comparison of subcutaneous abatacept versus adalimumab for rheumatoid arthritis: two-year efficacy and safety findings from AMPLE trial. *Ann Rheum Dis* 2014;73:86-94.
69. Maxwell L, Singh JA. Abatacept for rheumatoid arthritis. *Cochrane Database Syst Rev* 2009(4):CD007277.
70. Hervey PS, Keam SJ. Abatacept. BioDrugs 2006;20(1):53-61; discussion 62.
71. Orencia [package insert]. Princeton, NJ: Bristol-Meyers Squibb; August 2009, *http://packageinserts.bms.com/pi/pi_orencia.pdf.*
72. Cohen SB, Emery P, Greenwald MW, et al. Rituximab for rheumatoid arthritis refractory to anti-tumor necrosis factor therapy: Results of a multicenter, randomized, double-blind, placebo-controlled, phase III trial evaluating primary efficacy and safety at twenty-four weeks. *Arthritis Rheum* 2006;54(9):2793-2806.
73. De Vita S, Quartuccio L. Treatment of rheumatoid arthritis with rituximab: An update and possible indications. *Autoimmun Rev* 2006; 5(7):443-448.
74. Emery P, Fleischmann R, Filipowicz-Sosnowska A, et al. The efficacy and safety of rituximab in patients with active rheumatoid arthritis despite methotrexate treatment: Results of a phase IIB randomized, double-blind, placebo-controlled, dose-ranging trial. *Arthritis Rheum* 2006;54(5):1390-1400.
75. Smolen JS, Emery P, Keystone EC, et al. Consensus statement on the use of rituximab in patients with rheumatoid arthritis. *Ann Rheum Dis* 2007;66:143-150.
76. Schuna AA. Rituximab for the treatment of rheumatoid arthritis. *Pharmacotherapy* 2007;27:1702-1710.
77. Navarro-Millan I, Singh JA, Curtis JR. Systematic review of tocilizumab for rheumatoid arthritis: A new biologic agent targeting the interleukin-6 receptor. *Clin Ther* 2012;34(4):788-802.
78. Gabay C, Emery P, van Vollenhoven R, et al. Tocilizumab monotherapy versus adalimumab monotherapy for treatment of rheumatoid arthritis (ADACTA): A randomized, double-blind, controlled phase 4 trial. *Lancet* 2013;381:1541-1550.
79. Mertens M, Singh JA. Anakinra for rheumatoid arthritis. *Cochrane Database Syst Rev* 2009(1):CD005121.
80. Moots RJ, Naisbett-Groet B. The efficacy of biologic agents in patients with rheumatoid arthritis and an inadequate response to tumour necrosis factor inhibitors: A systematic review. *Rheumatology* 2012;51: 2252-2261.
81. Epstein M. Non-steroidal anti-inflammatory drugs and the continuum of renal dysfunction. *J Hypertens* 2002;20(suppl):S17-S23.
82. Ford LT, Berg JD. Thiopurine S-methyltransferase (TPMT) assessment prior to starting thiopurine drug treatment; a pharmacogenetic test whose time has come. *J Clin Pathol* 2010;63(4):288-295.

92

Osteoporosis and Osteomalacia

Mary Beth O'Connell and Jill S. Borchert

KEY CONCEPTS

1 Osteoporosis is a public health epidemic that affects all ages, genders, races, and ethnicities. Lifestyle behaviors, diseases, and medications should be reviewed to identify risk factors for developing osteoporosis and osteoporotic fractures. Healthcare providers should identify and resolve reversible risks. Patients with early onset or severe osteoporosis should be evaluated for secondary causes of bone loss.

2 Bone physiology and pathophysiology are complex, involving many different cell lines, pathways, and biofeedback systems. As these processes become more delineated, additional drug targets exist creating new investigational agents.

3 Ten-year probabilities for a major osteoporotic and hip fracture can be estimated for women (postmenopausal to age 90 years old) and men (50-90 years old) with the FRAX tool. This tool is a questionnaire that can be used in any setting, including a pharmacy, health fair, or clinic. Central bone densitometry can determine bone mass, predict fracture risk, and influence patient and provider treatment decisions.

4 Throughout life, everyone should practice a bone healthy lifestyle, which emphasizes regular exercise, nutritious diet, tobacco avoidance, minimal alcohol use, and fall prevention to prevent and treat osteoporosis.

5 Treatment should be considered for postmenopausal women and men older than 50 years who have a low-trauma hip or vertebral fracture, T-score of –2.5 or less at the femoral neck, total hip, or spine or low bone mass (T-score between –1.0 and –2.5) and a FRAX 10-year probability of major osteoporotic fracture of 20% or more or hip fracture of 3% or more.

6 The recommended dietary intake for calcium for American adults is 1,000 to 1,200 mg of elemental calcium daily with diet as the preferred source. Supplements are added only when diet is insufficient.

7 The recommended daily dietary intake for vitamin D for American adults is 600 units and for older adults 800 units, with some organizations and guidelines recommending higher doses of at least 800 to 1,000 units daily. The daily target is achieved through sun exposure, fortified foods, and supplements. Vitamin D insufficiency and deficiency, defined as 25(OH) vitamin D concentrations of less than 30 ng/mL [mcg/L; less than 75 nmol/L]) and less than 20 ng/mL [mcg/L; less than 50 nmol/L] respectively, are common in Americans.

8 Alendronate, risedronate, zoledronic acid, and denosumab decrease vertebral, hip, and nonvertebral fractures and are considered first-line osteoporosis treatments. Ibandronate, raloxifene, and teriparatide are alternatives and calcitonin is an agent of last resort.

9 Adherence to osteoporosis medications is frequently suboptimal, and poor adherence is associated with less fracture prevention. Healthcare providers should assess medication administration technique and adherence at each visit and provide needed education and medication problem solving.

10 The most common causes of medication-induced osteoporosis are long-term oral glucocorticoids and certain chemotherapeutic agents. All patients taking medications known to increase bone loss should practice a bone healthy lifestyle, be evaluated for a switch to a safer alternative medication, and be considered for osteoporosis therapy.

INTRODUCTION

1 Osteoporosis is a bone disorder characterized by low bone density, impaired bone architecture, and compromised bone strength that predisposes a person to increased fracture risk.[1] Osteoporosis is a major public health threat, especially with 55% of the people 50 years of age and older expected to have this disease. In the United States, 10.2 million Americans are estimated to have osteoporosis.[2] An additional 43.4 million Americans are estimated to have low bone density (sometimes referred to as osteopenia) and are at risk for osteoporosis. Attention to bone health is a requirement for all ages. Osteoporosis and osteoporotic fractures are multifactorial conditions, beginning at birth with genetics and then throughout life related to health behaviors that influence bone growth and maintenance, skeletal factors that lead to compromised bone strength, and nonskeletal factors that lead to falls (Fig. 92–1). Healthcare providers should educate patients about bone healthy lifestyles and encourage them to practice these health behaviors. Monitoring bone health in patients at risk and providing optimal treatment for patients with osteoporosis are also important.

EPIDEMIOLOGY

1 Low bone density, osteoporosis, and osteoporotic fractures are very common and affect all races and ethnic groups. Low bone density is estimated to occur in 53% of non-Hispanic white, 48% of Mexican American, and 36% of non-Hispanic Black women age 50 and older.[2] Osteoporosis affects 16% of non-Hispanic White, 20% of Mexican American, and 8% of non-Hispanic Black women age 50 and older. Disease prevalence greatly increases with age; from 7% in women 50 to 59 years of age to 35% in women 80 years of age and older. White and Hispanic women have the highest fragility fracture rate followed by Native American, African American, and Asian women when the data are adjusted for weight, bone mineral

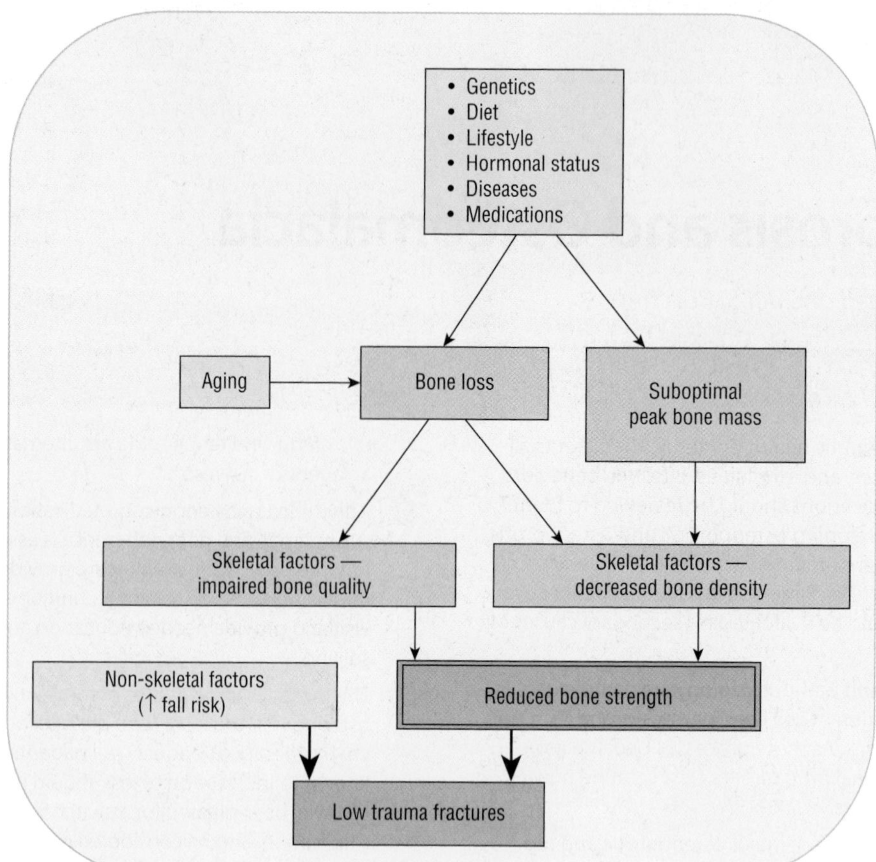

FIGURE 92–1 Etiology of osteoporosis and osteoporotic fractures.

density (BMD), and other factors.[3] Approximately 35% of men aged 50 years and older have low bone density rising to 53% in men 80 years and older. Osteoporosis prevalence in non-Hispanic White men is 4%, Mexican American men is 6%, non-Hispanic Black men is 1%. Osteoporosis prevalence rises to 11% in men 80 years and older. Although osteoporosis is a common finding in older adults with fractures, in one study up to 50% of fragility fractures occurred in patients with normal or low bone mass.[3]

Fragility wrist and vertebral fractures are common throughout adulthood, and hip fractures are more common in older adults. While women experience the majority of fractures, approximately 30% to 40% of fractures due to osteoporosis occur in men.[4] Forecasting predicts osteoporosis care to cost $25 billion by 2025.[1] Because of associated morbidity, hip fractures are the most costly accounting for almost 75% of fracture costs.[1,5] In a woman's lifetime, she has a 17% likelihood of a hip fracture, 15.6% likelihood of a vertebral fracture and 16% likelihood of a forearm fracture. In a man's lifetime, osteoporotic fracture risk is 13% to 30%.[4] The incidences of hip fracture and associated mortality are decreasing for both sexes,[5] possibly due to better efforts at osteoporosis prevention (eg, bone-healthy lifestyle) and use of bisphosphonates. However, rates in the United States remain higher than those in other countries and comorbidities are increasing[1] suggesting a need for continued focus on bone health.

ETIOLOGY

1 Figure 92–1 depicts a model describing the etiology of osteoporosis and fractures. The major risk factors (see Tables 92–1 to 92–3) influencing bone loss are hormonal status, genetics, exercise, aging, nutrition, lifestyle, concomitant diseases, and medications. [1,3,4,6-14] Nonhormonal risk factors are similar between women and men.

Low Bone Density

BMD is a major predictor of fracture risk. Every standard deviation decrease in BMD in women represents a 10% to 12% decrease in bone mass and a 1.5- to 2.6-fold increase in fracture risk.[3] Low BMD

TABLE 92-1 Risk Factors for Osteoporosis and Osteoporotic Fractures

Low bone mineral density[a]
Female sex[a]
Advanced age[a]
Race/ethnicity[a]
History of a previous fragility (low-trauma) fracture as an adult[a] (especially clinical vertebral fracture or hip fracture)
Osteoporotic fracture in a first-degree relative (especially parental hip fracture[a])
Low body weight or body mass index[a]
Premature menopause (before 45 years old)
Secondary osteoporosis (especially rheumatoid arthritis[a,b])
Past or present systemic oral glucocorticoid therapy[a,c]
Current cigarette smoking[a,c]
Alcohol intake of 3 or more drinks/day[a,c]
Low calcium intake
Low physical activity or immobilization
Vitamin D insufficiency and deficiency
Recent falls
Cognitive impairment
Impaired vision

[a]Factors included in World Health Organization fracture risk assessment tool (FRAX).

[b]Secondary causes included in the FRAX tool are type 1 diabetes, osteogenesis imperfecta as an adult, long-standing untreated hyperthyroidism, hypogonadism, premature menopause (<45 years old), chronic malnutrition, malabsorption, and chronic liver disease.

[c]Risk is larger with greater exposure.

Data from references 1, 3, 4, and 6-13.

TABLE 92-2 Select Medical Conditions Associated with Osteoporosis in Children and Adults

Endocrine/Hormonal
Primary or secondary ovarian failure
Testosterone deficiency
Hyperthyroidism
Cushing's syndrome
Growth hormone deficiency (in children)
Primary hyperparathyroidism
Diabetes, type 1 and type 2
Gastrointestinal
Nutritional disorders (eg, anorexia nervosa)
Malabsorptive states (eg, Crohn disease, celiac disease, gastrectomy, and bariatric surgery)
Chronic liver disease (eg, primary biliary cirrhosis)
Disorders of Calcium Balance
Hypercalciuria
Vitamin D deficiency
Inflammatory Disorders
Rheumatoid arthritis
Chronic Illness
Chronic kidney disease
Malignancies (eg, multiple myeloma, lymphoma, and leukemia)
Human immunodeficiency virus infection/acquired immunodeficiency syndrome
Organ transplant
Disuse/Immobility
Muscular dystrophy
Multiple sclerosis
Stroke/cerebrovascular accident
Genetic
Osteogenesis imperfecta
Cystic fibrosis
Hemochromatosis
Hypophosphatasia

Data from references 3, 4, 6-9, 12, and 32.

can occur as a result of failure to reach a normal peak bone mass, bone loss or both. Genetics accounts for 60% to 80% of peak bone mass variability.[3,12] Bone loss occurs when bone resorption exceeds bone formation, which also can result from high bone turnover when the number or depth of bone resorption sites greatly exceeds the rate and ability of osteoblasts to form new bone. Women and men begin to lose a small amount of bone mass starting in the third to fourth decade of life.[3,15] During perimenopause and menopause, bone loss occurs predominantly due to increases in bone resorption. By age 70 to 80, 30% to 40% of bone mass is lost. Older adults steadily lose bone mass as a consequence of an accelerated rate of bone remodeling combined with reduced bone formation.

Impaired Bone Quality

Bone strength is highly affected by the quality of the bone's composition and its structure, and a better predictor of fracture than BMD. Changes in bone mass do not fully reflect changes in bone thinning and decreased connectivity, both related to strength. BMD explains only 70% of femur and 44% of spine bone strength. Accelerated bone turnover can increase the amount of immature bone that is not adequately mineralized. Sex differences exist with thinning of trabeculae with aging in men causing less bone quality damage and impaired bone strength than in women.[15] With aging, fracture risk increases for a given T-score, partly related to bone quality changes.

Falls

One third to one half of older adults fall each year.[16] In older adults, 87% of fractures resulted from a fall. In 2013, 2.5 million older adults were treated in the emergency department for falls resulting in 734,000 hospitalizations, incurring costs of about $30 billion. The risk factors for falls overlap with the risk factors for osteoporosis and osteoporotic fractures.[1]

TABLE 92-3 Select Medications Associated with Increased Bone Loss and/or Fracture Risk

Medications	Comments
Anticonvulsant therapy (phenytoin, carbamazepine, phenobarbital, and valproic acid)	↓ BMD and ↑ fracture risk; increased vitamin D metabolism leading to low 25(OH) vitamin D concentrations
Antiretroviral therapy (ART) Nucleoside/nucleotide reverse transcriptase inhibitors (NRTIs) (zidovudine, didanosine, lamivudine, and tenofovir) Protease inhibitors (PI) (nelfinavir, indinivir, saquinavir, ritonavir, and lopinavir)	↓ BMD (NRTIs > PI), no fracture data; increased osteoclast activity and decreased osteoblast activity
Aromatase inhibitors (eg, letrozole and anastrozole)	↓ BMD and ↑ fracture risk; reduced estrogen concentrations
Canagliflozin	↓ BMD and ↑ fracture risk (FDA reviewing SLGT2 inhibitor class of medications)
Furosemide	↑ fracture risk; increased calcium renal elimination
Glucocorticoids (long-term oral therapy)	↓ BMD and ↑ fracture risk; increased bone resorption and decreased bone formation; dose and duration dependent; see special populations section
Gonadotropin-releasing hormone agonists or analogs (eg, leuprolide and goserelin)	↓ BMD and ↑ fracture risk; decreased sex hormone production
Heparin (unfractionated, UFH) or low molecular weight heparin (LMWH)	↓ BMD and ↑ fracture risk (UFH >>> LMWH) with long-term use (eg > 6 months); decreased osteoblast replication and increased osteoclast function
Medroxyprogesterone acetate depot administration	↓ BMD, no fracture data; possible BMD recovery with discontinuation; decreased estrogen concentrations
Proton pump inhibitor therapy (long-term therapy)	↓ BMD and ↑ fracture risk; possible calcium malabsorption secondary to acid suppression for carbonate salts
Selective serotonin reuptake inhibitors	↓ BMD and ↑ fracture risk; decreased osteoblast activity
Thiazolidinediones (pioglitazone and rosiglitazone)	↓ BMD and ↑ fracture risk; decreased osteoblast function
Thyroid—excessive supplementation	↓ BMD and ↑ fracture risk; risk increases with TSH concentration < 0.1 mIU/L; possible increase in bone resorption
Vitamin A—excessive intake (> 1.5 mg of retinol form)	↓ BMD and ↑fracture risk; decreased osteoblast activity and increased osteoclast activity

BMD, bone mineral density; TSH, thyroid-stimulating hormone; DXA, dual-energy X-ray absorptiometry.

Data from references 7, 8, and 10-14.

PATHOPHYSIOLOGY

Bone Physiology

The skeleton has two types of bone. Cortical bone makes up the majority of the skeleton (80%) and is found mostly in the long bones (eg, forearm and hip).[17] Trabecular bone is found mostly in the vertebrae and ends of long bones. This bone type is metabolically more active compared with cortical bone due to a much higher bone turnover rate because of its large surface area and honeycomb-like shape.

Bone is made of collagen and mineral components.[17] The collagen component gives bone its flexibility and energy-absorbing capability. The mineral component gives bone its stiffness and strength. The correct balance of these substances is needed for bone to adequately accommodate stress and strain and resist fractures. Imbalances can impair bone quality and lead to reduced bone strength.[18]

Bone strength reflects the integration of bone mass and bone quality (composition and microarchitecture). Bone mass increases rapidly throughout childhood and adolescence. Peak bone mass is attained by age 18 to 25 years.[1] Peak bone mass is highly dependent on genetic factors, which accounts for 60% to 80% of the variability.[6] The remaining 20% to 40% is influenced by modifiable factors such as nutritional intake (eg, calcium, vitamin D, and protein), exercise, adverse lifestyle practices (eg, smoking), hormonal status, and certain diseases and medications. Optimizing peak bone mass is important for preventing osteoporosis. The higher the peak bone mass, the more bone one can lose before being at an increased fracture risk. As the microarchitecture of bone deteriorates, the bone strength greatly decreases. Women lose more structure than men.[4]

2 Bone remodeling is a dynamic process that occurs continuously throughout life (see Fig. 92–2A-C).[19-22] One to two million tiny sections of bone are in the process of remodeling at any given time. Within these sections, the bone remodeling activities of bone resorption and bone formation are coupled and balanced. Bone remodeling is triggered to repair microdamage to the skeleton and serves to support calcium homeostasis through maintaining normal serum calcium by releasing calcium from the bone. Within an active bone remodeling unit, osteoclasts (bone resorbing cells) work to resorb bone during the resorptive phase then this process reverses and osteoblasts (bone-forming cells) work to form bone during the formation phase. Osteoblasts then become incorporated into the bone matrix as osteocytes (bone-communication cells). The unit then becomes inactive and enters a quiescent phase. If remodeling becomes unbalanced and bone resorption surpasses bone formation or if the phases become uncoupled and bone resorption occurs without adequate formation, a decrease in BMD is the result. Osteocytes play a key role in the process and can trigger a new remodeling cycle.

The signaling of the bone remodeling cycle through the steps from resorption through quiescence is highly complex; many cytokines, growth factors, and hormones influence each step.[19-21] The complete physiology of bone remodeling is not fully known, but appears to begin with signals from lining cells or osteocytes that are triggered by stress, microfractures, biofeedback systems responsive to cytokines and growth factors, and potentially certain diseases and medications (see Fig. 92–2B, step 1). A major stimulus for hematopoietic stem cell differentiation to become mature osteoclasts is the receptor activator of nuclear factor kappa β ligand (RANKL), which is a cytokine emitted from osteoblasts or osteocytes in step 2. Interleukin 1 and 6, macrophage colony stimulating factor (m-CSF), parathyroid hormone (PTH), parathyroid-releasing protein (PTHrP), 1,25(OH) vitamin D, tissue growth factor-β (TGF-β), prostaglandin E_2, and tumor necrosis factor-α (TNF-α) stimulate RANKL release whereas estrogen and calcitonin inhibit RANKL release. The RANKL then binds to its receptor RANK on the surface of osteoclast precursors initiating differentiation. The RANKL also stimulates mature osteoclast activation and bone adherence via $\alpha_v\beta_3$ integrins to resorb bone (step 3). This step is influenced by TGF-β, insulin-like growth factor-1 and 2 (IGF), platelet derived growth factor, bone morphometric protein, and fibroblast growth factor (FGF). After bone attachment, the osteoclasts secrete proteinases, such as cathepsin K, collagenase, gelatinase, tartrate-resistant acid phosphate, and matrix metalloproteases, and hydrogen ions to dissolve the mineralized bone. The hydrogen ion production is under src kinase control, which needs to be bound to other compounds such as Cbl, Fak, and phosphatidylinositol 3-kinase (Pl3K).

After bone is resorbed and a cavity is created, osteoclasts produce cytokines and growth factors to elicit osteoblast differentiation from mesenchymal stem cells, maturation and activity (step 4).[19,20] PTH and PTHrP also directly increase osteoblast differentiation and activity. Osteoblast differentiation can be inhibited by leptin and PPARγ, which direct mesenchymal cell maturation to adipocytes instead of osteoblasts. Mature osteoblasts and osteocytes produce osteoprotegerin (OPG) that binds to RANKL, thereby stopping bone resorption.

Bone formation occurs over two phases—formation then mineralization of bone (see Fig. 92–2C).[19-21,23] First wingless tail ligands (Wnt) bind to low-density lipoprotein receptor related protein 5 or 6 (LRP5/6) and a frizzled coreceptor. Wnt function is also influenced by PTH and PTHrP, which fit into the same receptor. Next LRP5/6 binds to axin, which then cannot bind to glycogen synthase kinase-3β (GSK-3β), thus preventing degradation of β-catenin (step 5). Accumulated β-catenin then enters the nucleus and signals target genes to create proteins to fill the resorption cavity with osteoid. Growth hormone and IGF-1 also increase bone collagen production. Next mineralization of bone with calcium, magnesium, and phosphorus follows to give the new matrix strength.

Once the cavity is mineralized, bone formation can be stopped through multiple signaling processes.[19-21] Both sclerostin and Dickkopf-1 (Dkk-1) are secreted from osteocytes and bind to LRP5/6 or secreted frizzled–related proteins, which can bind to Wnt to prevent Wnt signaling. Axin can then bind to GSK-3β, which then can cause β-catenin degradation, osteoblast apoptosis, and the end of osteoblastic activity (step 6). The mature osteoblasts can become lining cells or osteocytes. Quiescence is the phase when bone is at rest until another remodeling cycle is initiated. Later, osteocytes may trigger initiation of a new remodeling cycle through secretion of sclerostin or RANKL to stimulate osteoclasts and bone resorption.

Hormones can influence the remodeling steps. Estrogen has many positive effects in both sexes on the bone remodeling process, with most of its actions helping to maintain a normal bone resorption rate.[15,24] Estrogen suppresses the proliferation and differentiation of osteoclasts and increases osteoclast apoptosis. Estrogen decreases the production of several cytokines that are potent stimulators of osteoclasts, including interleukins 1 and 6, TNF-*α*, and m-CSF, and increases TGF-*α*, which increases osteoclast apoptosis. Estrogen also decreases the production of RANKL to reduce osteoclastogenesis.

Testosterone's role in bone health is becoming more apparent with recent identification of some direct effects on bone resorption and osteoblasts.[24] Most of testosterone's bone effects relate to its metabolism to estradiol and the above estrogen bone effects. Testosterone can also increase OPG production, which will inhibit bone resorption. Increased osteoblast proliferation and differentiation are direct effects. These effects might be from increasing TGF- β, TGF mRNA, FGF, and IGF-2, and decreasing IL-6.

CALCIUM HOMEOSTASIS, VITAMIN D, AND PARATHYROID HORMONE

Calcium homeostasis is maintained by vitamin D and PTH, which influence calcium gastrointestinal (GI) absorption and renal reabsorption.[18] Calcium absorption under normal conditions is approximately 30% to 35%, decreasing to 10% to 15% with low vitamin D concentrations.[22] Calcium absorption is thus lower in the winter due to decreased exposure to required ultraviolet light converting less vitamin D in the skin. It is reported to be higher in obesity, which is associated with greater vitamin D storage. Calcium absorption is predominantly an active rate-limited process in the duodenum and jejunum, which is controlled by many hormones, such as 1,25-dihydroxyvitamin D

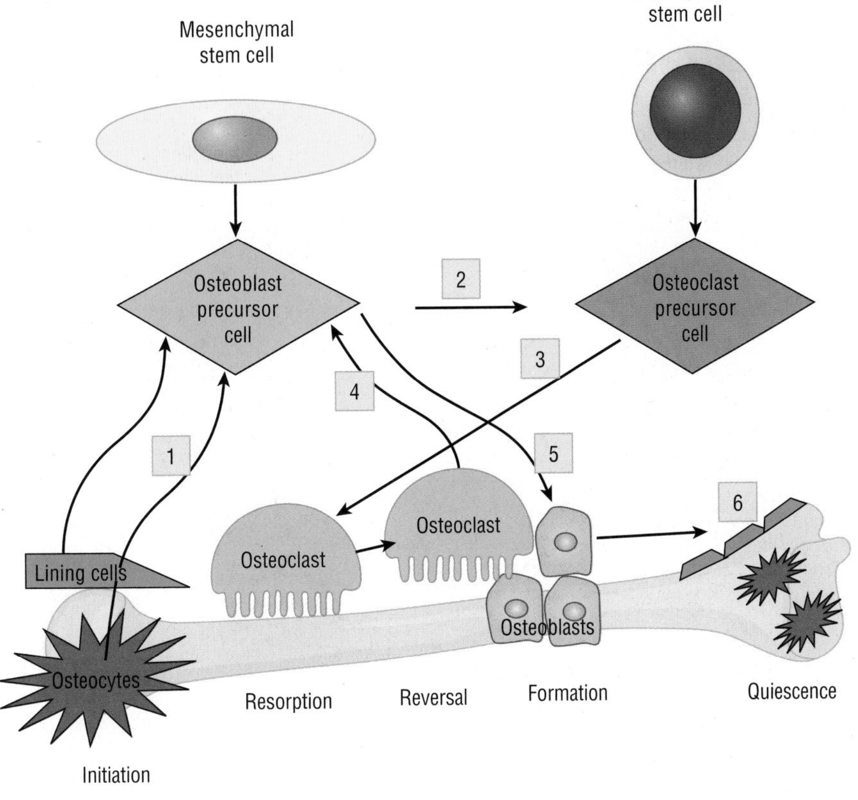

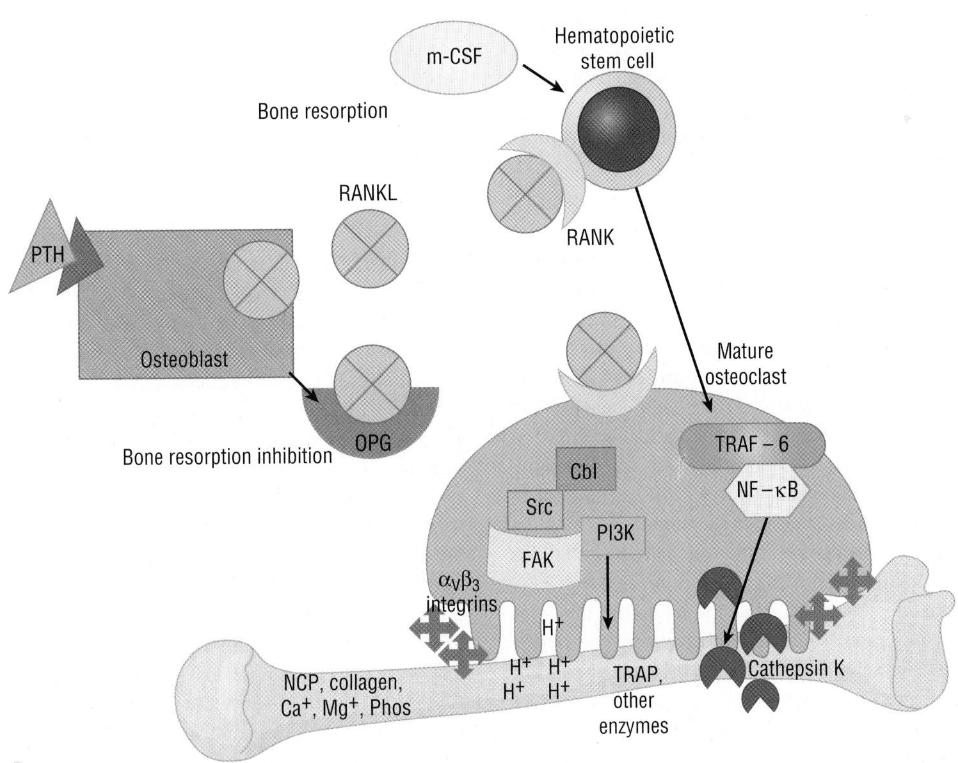

FIGURE 92–2 Bone remodeling cycle. (A) Overview of remodeling process, Step 1 = initiation, Step 2 and 3 = resorption, Step 4 = reversal, Step 5 = formation, and Step 6 = quiescence; (B) = molecular level detail of major pathways during bone resorption steps 2 and 3, which also showcase drug targets for approved and investigational agents;

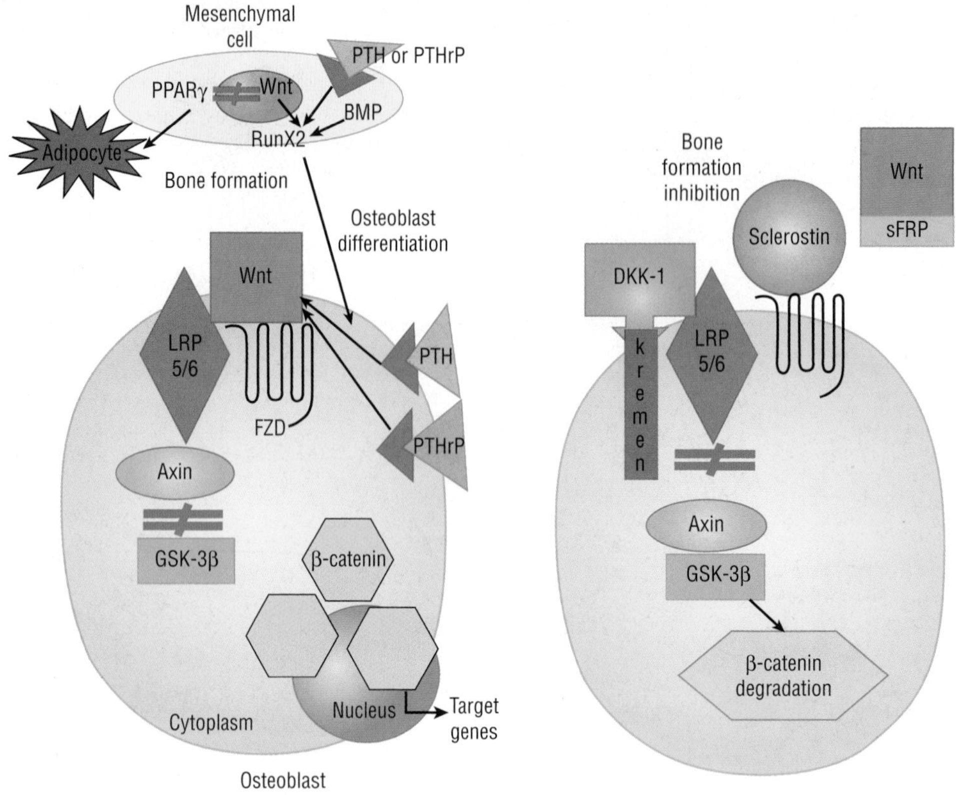

FIGURE 92–2 (*Continued*) (C) = molecular level detail of major pathways during bone formation steps 4 and 5, which also showcase drug targets for approved and investigational agents; BMP, bone morphogenetic protein; Ca+, calcium; m-CSF, macrophage-colony-stimulating factors; DKK-1, Dickkoff1; FAK, focal adhesion kinase, GSK-3β, glycogen synthase kinase-3β; H+, hydrogen ion; LRP5/6, lipoprotein-receptor related protein; Mg, magnesium; NF-KB, nuclear factor kappa B; NCP, noncollagenous proteins; OPG, osteoprotegerin; Phos, phosphorous; PI3K, phosphatidylinositol 3-kinase; PPARγ, peroxisome proliferator-activated receptor; PTH, parathyroid hormone; PTHrP, parathyroid hormone-related protein; RANK, receptor activator of nuclear factor-kb; RANKL, receptor activator of nuclear factor-kb; runX2, runt-related transcription factor; Scr; tyrosine scr kinase; TRAF-6, tumor necrosis factor receptor associated factor 6; TRAP, tartrate-resistant acid phosphate; Wnt, wingless tail. *(Data from references 19 to 21.)*

[1,25(OH) vitamin D], estrogen, and TRPV6, which is under genomic control and responsive to dietary calcium intake. A calcium transporter (calmodulin or calbindin) is required to bring calcium from the gut into the tissue wall and then across the enterocyte. Calcium is extruded into the circulation via Ca^{2+} adenosine triphosphatase (ATPase) and the sodium/calcium exchanger, high-energy steps. Throughout the intestine, paracellular passive calcium diffusion occurs. This diffusion accounts for less than 15% of absorbed calcium, is not rate limited, and possibility is sensitive to 1,25(OH) vitamin D. Solvent drag plays a minor role in calcium absorption.

When the calcium-sensing receptor on parathyroid cells detects low serum calcium, PTH production increases.[18,22] PTH then directly (minimal effect) and indirectly (predominant effect via increasing calcitriol production) cause calcium reabsorption by the kidney. Calcium reabsorption increases as 25(OH) vitamin D concentrations increases, plateauing around 10 to 15 ng/mL (mcg/L; 25-37 nmol/L).[25] Furosemide decreases and thiazide diuretics increase calcium resorption in the kidney.

Sometimes the increased fractional calcium absorption is insufficient to maintain normal serum calcium, requiring bone resorption for correction.[22] Consistent and high concentrations of PTH and calcitriol increase RANKL and decrease OPG resulting in increased osteoclast activity, which releases calcium from bone to restore calcium homeostasis. Of note, low PTH concentrations for a short time (eg, teriparatide) increase bone formation.

Active 1,25(OH) vitamin D concentrations depend on skin conversion, dietary and supplemental intake, and PTH control.[18,22,26] The sun's ultraviolet B rays convert 7-dehydrocholesterol in the skin to cholecalciferol (vitamin D_3), which is the most abundant vitamin D source. Few foods contain ergocalciferol (vitamin D_2). Supplements and multivitamins include cholecalciferol or ergocalciferol. Subsequent conversion of cholecalciferol and ergocalciferol to 25-hydroxyvitamin D [25(OH) vitamin D; calcidiol] occurs in the liver, and then PTH stimulates conversion of 25(OH) vitamin D via 25(OH) vitamin D-1α-hydroxylase (CYP27B1) to its final active form, 1α,25-dihydroxyvitamin D (calcitriol), in the kidney. Calcitriol binds to the intestinal vitamin D receptor (VDR) and then increases calcium-binding proteins calmodulin and calbindin. As a result, calcium and phosphorous intestinal absorption are increased. The feedback system is completed with CYP27B1 activity inhibited by adequate calcium and phosphorus, and FGF23 inhibiting PTH synthesis. Vitamin D receptors and CYP27B1 are found in many other tissues, such as bone, muscle, brain, breast, colon, heart, stomach, pancreas, lymphocytes, skin, and gonads.[26-28] Vitamin D is increasingly recognized as contributing to many nonbone benefits.

POSTMENOPAUSAL OSTEOPOROSIS

Estrogen deficiency causes significant bone density loss and compromises bone architecture. Estrogen deficiency increases proliferation, differentiation, and activation of new osteoclasts and prolongs survival of mature osteoclasts.[3,15] Interleukins, prostaglandin E_2, TNF-α, and interferon γ also increase resulting in more RANKL and less OPG. Loss of estrogen also increases calcium excretion and decreases calcium gut absorption through decreases in TRPV6 activity and 1,25(OH) vitamin D binding proteins. Estrogen deficiency can also be seen in other settings such as anorexia nervosa and during lactation, and from medications, such as prolonged depot medroxyprogesterone acetate implants, aromatase inhibitors, and gonadotropin releasing hormone agonists.[10,12]

Accelerated bone loss begins during perimenopause and continues up to 8 years after menopause due to increased bone resorption that exceeds bone formation.[3,15] During this time bone loss can be as high as 2% per year, with total BMD loss due to menopause about 10%. The number of remodeling sites increases and resorption pits are deeper and inadequately filled by normal osteoblastic function. During menopause, trabecular bone is most susceptible, leading predominantly to vertebral and wrist fractures.[3,15,29] Initially, women with early menopause (ie, before age 40) due to natural or induced causes have lower BMD than matched premenopausal women but risk for fractures and low bone density become the same after age 70.[3]

MALE OSTEOPOROSIS

Men are at a lower risk for developing osteoporosis and osteoporotic fractures because of larger bone size, greater peak bone mass, increase in bone width with aging, fewer falls, and shorter life expectancy.[4,30] However, the mortality rate after a fracture is greater for men than women. Male osteoporosis results from aging or secondary causes (see Tables 92–2 and 92–3). With aging sex hormone binding globulin increases, which results in less free testosterone and thereby less testosterone available for conversion to estrogen. Estrogen also inhibits bone resorption in men. The most common risk factors for men are smoking, alcohol abuse, low body weight, weight loss, age, long-term glucocorticoid use, androgen deprivation therapy, and low testosterone concentrations. Medical conditions and medications that cause hypogonadism increase bone loss.

AGE-RELATED OSTEOPOROSIS

Age-related bone loss begins after peak bone mass reached. About 0.5% BMD is loss each year after age 30 years, increasing to 1.6% after 80 years.[16,29] Age-related osteoporosis occurs in older adults because of accelerated bone turnover rate and reduced osteoblast bone formation, with a greater effect on cortical bone. These bone changes occur from hormone deficiencies; calcium and vitamin D deficiencies due to changes in intake, absorption, and metabolism; decreased production or function of cytokines or other bone biochemicals; increase in redox status and free radical formation, increase adipocytes, telomere shortening, and less exercise.[29,31] Fracture risk for a given BMD value increases with aging.[3,15] Hip-fracture risk rises dramatically in older adults as a consequence of the cumulative loss of cortical and trabecular bone and an increased risk for falls. Aging is associated with muscle changes as well, resulting in weakness, balance instability, and greater likelihood of falls.

SECONDARY CAUSES OF OSTEOPOROSIS

1 A secondary cause of osteoporosis is common (see Tables 92–2[3,4,6-9,12,32] and 92–3).[7,8,10-12] Symptoms, initial screening laboratory test results, medication profile review, and or a decreased Z-score from a dual-energy absorptiometry (DXA) test can suggest a secondary cause, warranting a more comprehensive work-up.

CLINICAL PRESENTATION

Table 92–4 outlines the clinical presentation of osteoporosis.[3,4,6,32-35] Osteoporosis is a silent disease, frequently not detected until a fracture is experienced or noticed on X-ray. Many vertebral fractures are asymptomatic, with patients sometimes attributing mild back pain to "old age." Some new vertebral fractures present with moderate to severe back pain that can radiate down the leg. The pain usually subsides after 2 to 4 weeks; however, residual chronic back pain can persist. Multiple vertebral fractures decrease height and sometimes curve the spine (kyphosis or lordosis). Patients with a nonvertebral fracture frequently present with severe pain, swelling, and reduced function and mobility at the fracture site.

TABLE 92-4 Clinical Presentation of Osteoporosis

General
- Many patients are unaware they have osteoporosis until testing or fracture
- Fractures can occur after bending, lifting, or falling, or independent of any activity

Symptoms
- Frequently asymptomatic
- Pain
- Immobility
- Depression, fear, and low self-esteem from physical limitations and deformities

Signs
- Shortened stature (>1.5" [>4 cm] loss from maximum height; > 0.8" [> 2 cm] in 1 year), kyphosis, or lordosis
- Fragility (low-trauma) vertebral, hip, wrist, or forearm fracture

Laboratory tests
- Routine tests: comprehensive metabolic profile (creatinine, calcium, phosphorous, electrolytes, alkaline phosphatase, and albumin), 25(OH) vitamin D, thyroid-stimulating hormone, complete blood count, total testosterone (for men), and 24-hour urine concentrations of calcium and creatinine
- Bone turnover markers (eg, urinary or serum NTX, serum CTX, and serum PINP) are sometimes used, especially to determine if high bone turnover exists
- Additional testing if the patient's history, physical examination, or initial laboratory and or diagnostic tests suggest a specific secondary cause (eg, intact parathyroid hormone, free testosterone, serum protein electrophoresis, serum parathyroid, and celiac panel)

Other diagnostic tests
- Spine and hip bone density measurement using central dual-energy X-ray absorptiometry (DXA)
- Vertebral fracture assessment (VFA) with DXA technology
- Radiograph ordered for other reasons that shows low bone density
- Radiograph to confirm fracture
- Balance and mobility tests

CTX, C-terminal crosslinking telopeptide of type 1 collagen; NTX, N-terminal crosslinking telopeptide of type 1 collagen; PINP, procollagen type 1 N-terminal propeptide.

Data from references 3, 4, 6, and 32-35.

CONSEQUENCES OF OSTEOPOROSIS

Osteoporosis can lead to fragility/low-trauma fractures, defined as fracture that occurs as a result of a fall from standing height or less or with minimal to no trauma.[1] Fractures of the vertebrae, hip, forearm, and humerus are considered major osteoporotic fractures whereas other fractures are generally not considered osteoporosis-related. Osteoporotic fractures can lead to increased morbidity and mortality and decreased quality of life. Pain and physical deformity are common, and these changes can lead to other health consequences, for example, severe kyphosis can lead to respiratory problems as a result of compression of the thoracic region and GI complications such as poor nutrition, from intra-abdominal compression. Depression is common because of fear, pain, loss of self-esteem from physical deformity, and loss of independence and mobility.

Hip fractures are associated with the greatest increase in morbidity and mortality. After a hip fracture, only 40% of patients regain their prefracture level of independence, while 20% require long-term care.[1] Following a hip fracture, almost one quarter of patients die within 1 year either from complications of the hip fracture or other comorbid disease processes.[1,3] Men have a higher 1-year mortality rate after hip fracture than women.

Wrist fractures occur more commonly in younger postmenopausal women and are frequently a result of a fall on an outstretched hand.[1] Though they cause less disability than other fracture sites, negative outcomes include prolonged pain and weakness, and decreased activities of daily living such as cooking and shopping.

Once a low-trauma fracture has occurred, the risk for subsequent fractures goes up exponentially.[1] Vertebral fractures, even if asymptomatic, are a major predictor of a future fracture with up to a 5-fold increase in future vertebral fractures and a doubling of the risk at other sites. Hip fractures are associated with a 2-fold or greater increase in risk for future fracture.

PATIENT ASSESSMENT

Bone pain, postural changes (ie, kyphosis or lordosis), and loss of height are simple useful physical examination findings. A measured height loss of greater than 0.8 inches (2 cm) or historic height loss (ie, from the tallest height recalled by the patient) of 1.5 inches (4 cm) warrants further investigation.[6,32] Height should be measured annually using a wall-mounted stadiometer.[32] A spine radiograph can be obtained to confirm the presence of vertebral fractures. Low bone density or osteopenia reported on routine radiographs is a sign of significant bone loss and requires further evaluation for osteoporosis. In addition to physical examination and laboratory studies (see Table 92–4), patients can be assessed with risk factor assessments tools, osteoporosis quality-of-life questionnaires, peripheral and central DXA, ultrasonography, and bone turnover biomarkers.

RISK FACTOR ASSESSMENT

The aim of an initial osteoporosis risk assessment screening (see Table 92–1) is to identify those patients who are at risk for osteoporosis and osteoporotic fractures, and or would benefit from further evaluation or pharmacologic intervention. The most commonly used questionnaire is the fracture risk assessment (FRAX) tool, with the Garvan tool as another option.[36]

3 The FRAX tool was created for the World Health Organization to be used with or without BMD data. This model uses 11 risk factors: age, race/ethnicity, sex, previous fragility fracture, parent history of hip fracture, body mass index, glucocorticoid use (current use or past use for 3 or more months of prednisolone 5 mg daily or equivalent doses of other glucocorticoids), current smoking, alcohol use of 3 or more drinks per day, rheumatoid arthritis, and select secondary causes; with femoral neck or total hip BMD data optional. The FRAX tool calculates an individual's percent probability of any major osteoporotic and hip fracture in the next 10 years. Each country establishes cut-off points for fracture risk treatment decisions. Some important risk factors for fracture, for example, falls, multiple fractures, or recent fracture, are not accommodated in the FRAX model.

The Garvan calculator uses 4 risk factors (age, sex, low-trauma fracture, and falls) with the option to also use BMD.[36,37] It calculates 5- and 10-year risk estimates of any major osteoporotic and hip fracture. This tool corrects some disadvantages of the FRAX tool since it includes falls and number of previous fractures, but it does not use as many other risk factors.

SCREENING USING PERIPHERAL BONE MINERAL DENSITY DEVICES

Peripheral bone density devices that use DXA (pDXA) or quantitative ultrasonography are helpful as screening tools to determine which patients require further evaluation with central DXA or for decision making if central DXA testing is not available.[1,34] Peripheral DXA of the forearm, heel, and finger uses a low amount of radiation and requires personnel with special training. Heel quantitative ultrasonography uses sound waves without radiation or need for specially trained personnel. Heel ultrasonography has better fracture predictive value than pDXA. The specific peripheral T-score threshold for referral is not universally defined and varies by device. These tests should not be used for diagnosis or for monitoring response to therapy.

Peripheral devices are considerably less expensive than central DXA, easy to use, portable, fast (less than 5 minutes), and can predict general fracture risk. They are popular for screening postmenopausal women at health fairs and community pharmacies. Because evidence is lacking to show fracture prediction in men, other assessments should be used for men.[1] Patients already identified as being at high risk for osteoporosis based on risk factors, fragility fracture, or secondary causes for osteoporosis should be referred for central DXA testing.

CENTRAL DUAL-ENERGY X-RAY ABSORPTIOMETRY

3 BMD measurements at the hip or spine can be used to assess fracture risk, establish the diagnosis and severity of osteoporosis, and sometimes confirm osteoporosis as causative for low-trauma fractures.[1,4,6,34] Central DXA is considered the gold standard for measuring BMD because of its high precision, short scan times, low radiation dose (comparable to the average daily dose from natural background), and stable calibration. Measurements of lumbar spine, femoral neck, and total hip BMD are recommended with the lowest BMD value used for diagnosis. The forearm (distal third of the radius) can be used as an alternative if these above areas cannot be scanned. Newer technologies available on some densitometers, such as the trabecular bone score, can provide measurements of bone quality and microarchitecture to better identify those at risk for fracture.[1]

Several consensus guidelines and position statements are consistent in recommending central BMD testing for all women aged 65 years or older, men aged 70 years or older, postmenopausal women younger than 65 years of age and men 50 to 69 years old with risk factors for fracture, and patients with an identified secondary cause for bone loss.[1,3,4,6,34] The United States Preventive Services Task Force (USPSTF) agrees with these recommendations for women 65 years and older, but for women between 50 to 65 years old, they recommend only ordering a DXA for those women with a FRAX score of 9.3% or more.[38] This group feels data are inadequate to make recommendations for men. Patients with a fragility fracture do not need a DXA for an osteoporosis diagnosis, but the results are helpful for determining the severity of osteoporosis and as a baseline for monitoring response to therapy. The DXA results can also help patients make decisions about the need for lifestyle changes and prescription osteoporosis medications. In the absence of a suspected or known secondary cause for osteoporosis or a history of a low-trauma fracture, central BMD testing is not recommended for children, premenopausal women, or men younger than 50 years of age.

A central DXA BMD report provides the actual bone density value, T-score, and Z-score.[33,34] The actual bone density value (g/cm^2) is most useful for serial monitoring of therapy response, which is typically performed 2 years after medication initiation. The T-score is used for diagnosis and is a comparison of the patient's BMD to the mean BMD of a healthy, young (20- to 29-year-old), sex-matched White reference population; no adjustments for race or ethnicity. The T-score is the number of standard deviations from the mean of the reference population. The Z-score is similar but compares the patient's BMD to the mean BMD for a healthy sex- and age-matched population. Patient-reported ethnicity should be used for the Z-score if available. The Z-score is sometimes helpful in determining whether a secondary cause for osteoporosis is present and is used for diagnosis (value ≤ −2.0) in children, premenopausal women, and men younger than 50 years of age. Follow-up monitoring for patients has not been clearly defined but in general recommendations are to repeat BMD testing every 2 years.[1] For patients with normal bone density or those in the upper range of low bone mass, time between screenings can be lengthened with some recommending repeat in 15 years.[1,6,15]

Using the spine DXA image, an assessment of morphometric vertebral fractures, the vertebral fracture assessment (VFA), can be calculated.[34] Each vertebra is assessed for compression (wedge, biconcave, and crush) and described as normal or mild (20%-25%), moderate (25%-40%), or severe (greater than 40%) compression.[3] This result becomes important for treatment decisions in patients with low bone mass. Because many vertebral fractures are asymptomatic, VFA is recommended in those who most likely have an undiagnosed vertebral fracture. For example, women 70 years or older or men 80 years or older with a T-score of −1.0 or less, postmenopausal women or men age 50 and older who have lost more than 1.5 inches (4 cm) in height, and those on glucocorticoids (≥ 5 mg prednisone or equivalent daily for 3 months or more.[1,3,4,34]

LABORATORY TESTS

Routine laboratory testing (see Table 92–4) is used for initial bone health assessment. To evaluate secondary causes, additional testing is conducted, which will be specific to the suspected secondary cause.

BONE TURNOVER MARKERS

Bone turnover markers are commonly used in clinical trials and sometimes in clinical practice.[1,35] They can be used to assess bone pathophysiology, predict fracture risk, and monitor response to osteoporosis medications. Markers of bone formation are bone-specific alkaline phosphatase, osteocalcin, and procollagen type 1 propeptides. Markers of bone resorption are hydroxypyridinium crosslinks of collagen pyridinoline and deoxypyridinoline, C-terminal crosslinking telopeptide of type 1 collagen, and N-terminal crosslinking telopeptide of type 1 collagen. Response to osteoporosis therapy can be measured as early as 2 to 3 months. Circadian variability, seasonal variations, food intake, recent exercise, some diseases and conditions, and assay variability can affect results and decrease utility in clinical practice. For serum markers, fasting morning samples should be obtained with repeat tests done at the same facility with the same assay. Coverage for these tests varies by health insurance.

DIAGNOSIS OF OSTEOPOROSIS

The diagnosis of osteoporosis is based on a low-trauma fracture or femoral neck, total hip and/or spine DXA using WHO T-score thresholds. Low bone mass (preferred term) or osteopenia is a T-score between −1 and −2.5, and osteoporosis is a T-score at or below −2.5.[1,4,6,34] Although these definitions are based on data from postmenopausal white women, they are also applied to perimenopausal women, men age 50 years and older, and adults from different races and ethnicities. The diagnosis of osteoporosis in children, premenopausal women, and men under 50 years of age should be based on a Z-score at or less than −2.0 in combination with other risk factors or fracture.[4,33,34] Without a history of clinically significant fracture, children and premenopausal women are given a diagnosis of bone mass below the expected range for age.

PREVENTION AND TREATMENT

Osteoporosis

Osteoporosis prevention and treatment begins with a bone healthy lifestyle starting at birth and continuing throughout life. Supplements and medications are used when lifestyle habits are suboptimal, osteoporosis has developed, or after a low-trauma fracture.

DESIRED OUTCOMES

The primary goal of osteoporosis care should be prevention. Optimizing skeletal development and peak bone mass accrual in childhood, adolescence, and early adulthood will ultimately reduce the future incidence of osteoporosis. Once low bone mass or osteoporosis develops, the objective is to stabilize or improve bone mass and strength and prevent fractures. In patients who have already suffered osteoporotic fractures, reducing pain and deformity, improving functional capacity, improving quality of life, and reducing future falls and fractures are the main goals.

GENERAL APPROACH TO PREVENTION AND TREATMENT

4 5 A bone-healthy lifestyle should begin at birth and continue throughout life. Insuring adequate intake of calcium and vitamin D along with other bone-healthy lifestyle practices are the first steps in prevention and treatment. Guidelines and position statements recommend considering prescription therapy in any postmenopausal woman or man age 50 years and older presenting with one of the following scenarios: a hip or vertebral fracture; T-score of −2.5 or lower at the femoral neck, total hip, or spine; or low bone mass (T-score between −1.0 and −2.5 at the femoral neck, total hip, or spine) with a 10-year probability of hip fracture of 3% or more, or a 10-year probability of any major osteoporosis-related fracture of 20% or more.[1,3,4,6] Figure 92–3 provides an osteoporosis management algorithm for postmenopausal women and men 50 years and older that incorporates both nonpharmacologic and pharmacologic approaches.

NONPHARMACOLOGIC THERAPY

4 Nonpharmacologic therapy, referred to as a bone-healthy lifestyle, includes proper nutrition, moderation of alcohol intake, smoking cessation, exercise, and fall prevention. A bone healthy lifestyle that is employed early in life will help to optimize peak bone mass and if continued throughout life it will minimize bone loss over time. Not only does a bone healthy lifestyle target BMD, but it also contributes to decreasing the risk of falls and fragility fractures.

Diet

Overall, a diet well balanced in nutrients and minerals without excessive protein and limited use of salt, alcohol and caffeine are important for bone health.[1,3,4,39] Adequate amounts of calcium, vitamin D, and protein have documented impacts on bone health.[25-27,39-44] Magnesium, boron, and vitamin K have a physiologic role in bone development and maintenance but either no or insufficient data exist to establish them independently as supplemental agents for prevention and treatment of osteoporosis.[40] Some of these agents are included in calcium combination products and are found in multivitamins. Strontium ranelate has documented positive bone effects and is marketed in Europe for prevention of osteoporosis.

Eating disorders are associated with increased bone loss and fractures. Being thin or having anorexia nervosa are well known to decrease bone mass.[12,45] In the past, obesity was thought protective

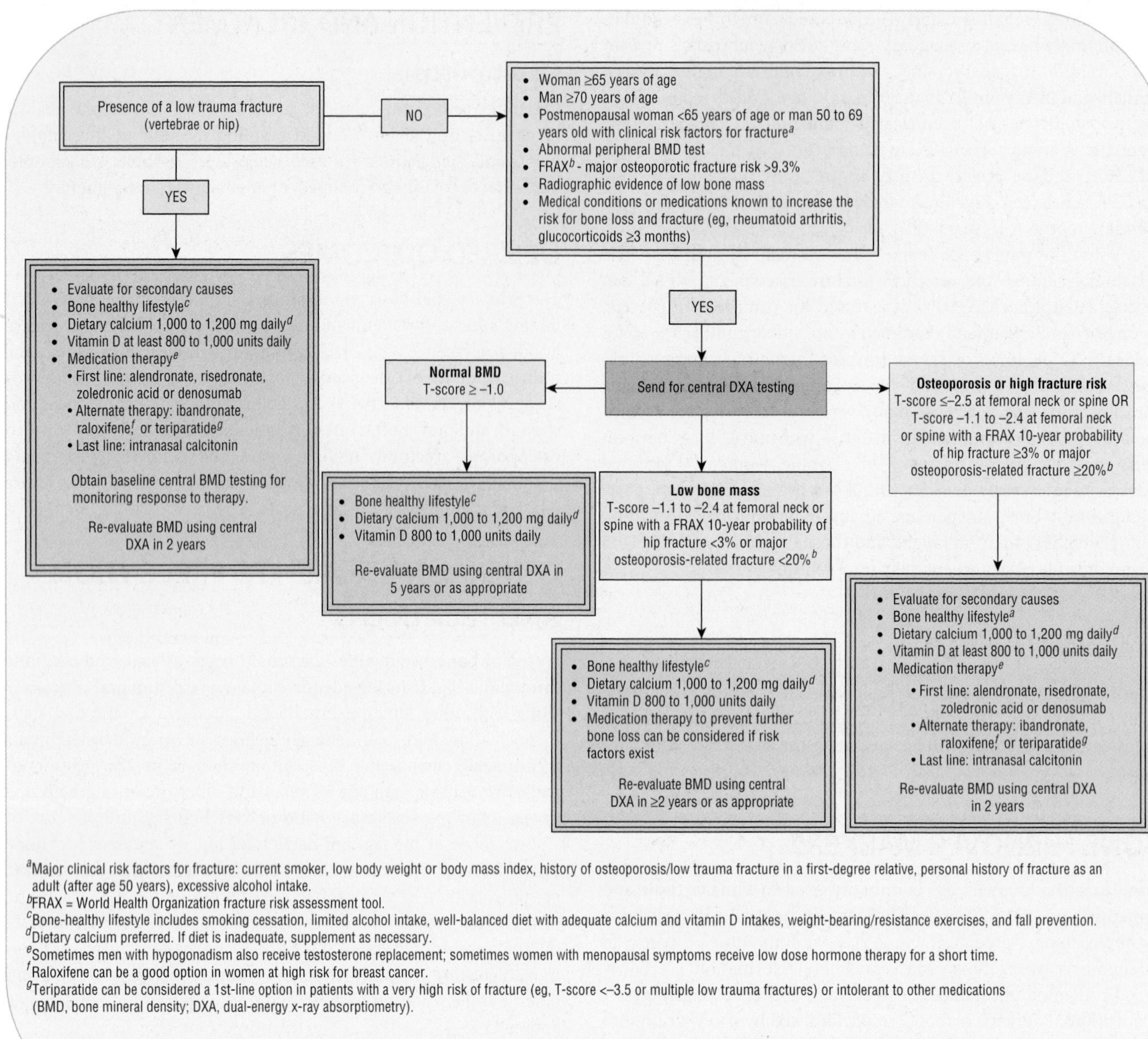

FIGURE 92–3 Algorithm for the management of osteoporosis in postmenopausal women and men aged 50 and older. *Data from references* 1, 3, 4, and 6.

due to increased estrogen production and stimulation of bone remodeling due to weight bearing; however, emerging literature suggests leptin and adipose have negative impacts on bone health.

Calcium

6 Adequate calcium intake is necessary for calcium homeostasis throughout life, bone development during growth, and bone maintenance.[46] The Institute of Medicine (IOM) recommended calcium intakes are based on age and gender (Table 92–5).[47] This value represents the amount needed for 97.5% of the population. Higher intakes might be needed when concomitant diseases and medications known to negatively affect calcium and vitamin D homeostasis exist. Using calcium-containing or fortified foods and beverages, which also contain other essential nutrients, is the preferred method to achieve daily calcium requirements. Dairy products have the highest amount of calcium per serving and are available in low-fat options. Some food sources are absorbed well but have low elemental calcium content (eg, broccoli). Carbohydrates, fat, and lactose increase calcium absorption whereas fiber, wheat bran, phytates (eg, beans), oxylates (eg, spinach and rhubarb), high-protein diets, caffeine, and smoking decrease absorption.

People should be encouraged to evaluate their food and beverage intake to determine if they are receiving adequate amounts of calcium. To calculate the amount of calcium in a serving of food, consumers can add a zero to the percentage of the daily value listed on food labels. For example, a serving of milk (8 oz. [~240 mL]) has 30% of the daily value of calcium. This translates to 300 mg calcium per serving. Websites can be used to calculate calcium content and identify foods and beverages high in calcium.[47,48]

Although many foods and beverages are high in calcium, the average calcium dietary intake is insufficient. Adult women consumed 590 to 730 mg and adult men consumed 725 to 970 mg calcium daily with amounts decreasing with advancing age for both sexes. Lactose intolerance limits dietary calcium intake. Approximately 25% of the US population has some level of lactose intolerance, with the incidence in Asian (85%) and African American (50%) populations higher than in whites (10%).[46,49] Lactose-intolerant patients have several options, including products containing lactase

TABLE 92-5 Calcium and Vitamin D Recommended Dietary Allowances and Upper Limits

Group and Ages	Elemental Calcium (mg)	Calcium Upper Limit (mg)	Vitamin D (Units)[a]	Vitamin D Upper Limit (Units)
Infants				
Birth to 6 months	200	1,000	400	1,000
6-12 months	260	1,500	400	1,500
Children				
1-3 years	700	2,500	600	2,500
4-8 years	1,000	2,500	600	3,000
9-18 years	1,300	3,000	600	4,000
Adults				
19–50 years	1,000	2,500	600[b]	4,000
51-70 years (men)	1,000	2,000	600[b]	4,000
51-70 years (women)	1,200	2,000	600[b]	4,000
>70 years	1,200	2,000	800[b]	4,000

[a]Other guidelines recommend intake to achieve a 25(OH) vitamin D concentration of more than 30 ng/mL (mcg/L; > 75 nmol/L),[1,4,6] which is higher than the Institute of Medicine goal of more than 20 ng/mL (mcg/L; > 50 nmol/L).[47]

[b]2014 National Osteoporosis Foundation Guidelines recommend 400 to 800 units for adults under 50 years old and 800 to 1,000 units for adults 50 years and older.[1]

Data from reference 47.

(Lactaid), lactose-reduced milk, lactose-free milk, calcium-fortified milk alternatives (eg, soy and almond), certain aged cheeses, or yogurt with active cultures along with other nondairy calcium-fortified products (eg, orange juice, breakfast cereals, and energy bars). Vegan diets sometimes have insufficient calcium intake, but products, such as tofu, calcium-fortified milk alternatives, and juices can be used. When diet cannot be enhanced to achieve adequate intakes, calcium supplements will be required.

Vitamin D

7 Table 92–5 lists the IOM recommended adequate intakes for Vitamin D.[47] The 3 main sources of vitamin D are sunlight (cholecalciferol and vitamin D3), diet, and supplements.[26] Vitamin D3 comes from oily fish, eggs, and fortified dairy products. Vitamin D2 comes from fungi and eggs (chickens given vitamin D2 in their diet). Websites can be used to identify the few foods high in vitamin D.[50] To calculate the amount of vitamin D in a serving of food, multiply the % daily value of vitamin D listed on the food label by 4 (eg, 20% vitamin D = 80 units).

Inadequate concentrations of 25(OH) vitamin D are common in all age groups, especially in older adults, minorities, malnutrition, obesity, institutional living (eg, nursing home), and northern latitude residences. Overall prevalence of hypovitaminosis D (≤ 20 ng/mL[mcg/L; ≤ 50 nmol/L]) was 42% in adults; similar between sexes but greater in minorities (ie, Blacks 82%, Hispanics 69%, and Whites 30%).[51] Low vitamin D concentrations result from insufficient intake, dietary fat malabsorption, decreased sun exposure, decreased skin production, or decreased liver and renal metabolism. Endogenous synthesis of vitamin D can be decreased by factors that affect exposure to or decrease skin penetration of ultraviolet B light rays. Sunscreen use, full body coverage with clothing (eg, women wearing veiled and full-length dresses), and darkly pigmented skin can all decrease vitamin D production. Seasonal variations in vitamin D concentrations are also seen with nadirs in late winter and peaks in late summer. Because few foods are naturally high or fortified with vitamin D, most people, especially older adults, require supplementation. Based on the NHANES 2007-2010 data, only 1% to 4% of adults ingested recommended vitamin D daily allowances from diet alone.[52]

Isoflavones

Phytoestrogens (isoflavones, lignans, and coumestans) are plant-derived compounds that possess weak estrogenic agonist and antagonist effects throughout the body. Isoflavones are found in soy products, lignans in seeds, berries, and grains and coumestans in broccoli and sprouts. Genistein is the most abundant and biologically active isoflavone in soybeans. Isoflavones, genistein and daidzein are also available as single agent or combination supplements. The evidence supporting a positive bone benefit from phytoestrogen intake is conflicting with most studies showing no effects[1,3,53]; however, a meta-analysis of randomized placebo controlled studies have found foods and supplements with at least 75 mg isoflavones increased spine but not hip BMD when compared to placebo.[54] Isoflavones from soy foods appear safe; however, more information is needed, especially in women with breast cancer and for isoflavone supplements.

Alcohol

4 Excessive but not moderate alcohol consumption is associated with an increased risk for osteoporosis and fractures.[1,3,4,39,40,46] Alcohol increases bone resorption by increasing RANKL and decreases bone formation by inhibiting Wnt signaling pathway and increasing oxidative stress that results in osteoblast apoptosis. Patients with alcohol problems might also have poor nutrition, decreased calcium absorption, altered vitamin D metabolism, and have balance impairments resulting in more falls and fractures. Alcohol consumption should not exceed 1 to 2 drinks per day for women and 2 to 3 drinks per day for men.

Caffeine

4 Although results are conflicting, excessive caffeine consumption is associated with increased calcium excretion, increased rates of bone loss, and a modestly increased risk for fracture.[39,46] Ideally, caffeine consumption should be limited to two servings or less per day. For those with greater intakes, the increased calcium excretion might be compensated by additional calcium intake.

Smoking

4 Counseling patients of all ages on smoking cessation can help to optimize peak bone mass, minimize bone loss, and ultimately reduce fracture risk.[39,40,55] Cigarette smoking is an independent risk factor for osteoporosis and is associated with an increased relative risk for fracture at all sites. The effect is dose and duration dependent, but even passive smoking shows adverse effects on BMD. The negative bone effects are associated with reduced intestinal calcium absorption, lower 25(OH) vitamin D concentrations possibly due to increased hepatic metabolism, an increase in bone resorption from a decrease in production and increase in metabolism of estradiol, increase in RANKL and decrease in OPG, decrease in osteoblasts and bone formation secondary to increase in cortisol and dehydroepiandrosterone sulfate, and impairment of osteoid production and mineralization. The detrimental effects of smoking on physical function and balance can contribute to an increased risk of falls.

Exercise

4 Physical activity or exercise is an important nonpharmacologic approach to preventing osteoporotic fractures. Exercise can decrease the risk of falls and fractures by stabilizing bone density and improving muscle strength, coordination, balance, and mobility.[1,39] Physical activity is especially important early in life as lack of exercise during growth can lead to suboptimal loading/straining, decreased stimulation of bone deposition, and a subsequently reduced peak bone

mass. All patients who are medically fit should be encouraged to perform a moderate-intensity weight-bearing activity (eg, walking, jogging, golf, and stair climbing) daily and a resistance activity (eg, weight machines, free weights, or elastic bands) at all ages. For men, guidelines specifically suggest men at risk of osteoporosis participate in weight-bearing activities three to four times weekly for 30 to 40 minutes per session.[4]

Fall Prevention

4 Risk of falling increases with advanced age predominantly as a result of balance, gait, and mobility problems, poor vision, reduced muscle strength, impaired cognition, multiple medical conditions (eg, arrhythmias, postural hypotension, Alzheimer's disease, and Parkinson disease), and polypharmacy (especially psychoactive, cardiovascular, diabetes, seizure, and pain medications).[16,56,57] The ability to adapt to falls also decreases with aging. Older adults are more likely to sustain a hip or pelvic fracture because they tend to fall backward or sideways instead of forward.[16]

Because of the link between falls and fractures, all older adults should be asked at least annually if they have fallen.[16,56] The Centers for Disease Control and Prevention have created an assessment tool; if an older adult scores 4 or more, a comprehensive falls assessment should be conducted. Patients with low (no falls) or moderate fall risk (1 fall per year and no injury) should have adequate vitamin D and calcium intake and increase exercise to improve gait and balance. Patients at high fall risk (≥2 falls or 1 fall with injury) should do the above plus have blood pressure, vision, foot, and medication assessments to resolve any problems, and have home optimized to prevent falls.

Generally, intervention programs that are multifactorial have greater effects on decreasing falls, fractures, other injuries, and nursing home and hospital admissions than single interventions.[1,16,39,56,57] Medication profiles should also be reviewed for any unnecessary medications that can affect cognition and balance and potentially increase fall risk. Consideration should be given to replacing high-risk medications with safer alternatives. Vitamin D supplementation has been associated with reduced falls. Maintenance of a regular individualized exercise program, such as tai chi, should be recommended to improve body strength, balance, and agility. Other recommendations include resolving vision, low blood pressure, heart rate/rhythm, and foot problems and using proper footwear. External hip protectors are specialized undergarments designed to pad the area surrounding the hip, decreasing the force of impact from a sideways fall. Conflicting results and poor adherence limit their use.

VERTEBROPLASTY AND KYPHOPLASTY

During a vertebroplasty and kyphoplasty cement is injected into fractured vertebra(e) for patients with debilitating pain from vertebral compression fractures.[58] In some studies the procedure stabilized the damaged vertebrae, reduced pain, and decreased opioid intake; however in other studies, the effects are similar to sham interventions, are short-term, and or are associated with vertebral fracturing around the cement, cement leakage into the spinal column, and rarely nerve damage.

PHARMACOLOGIC THERAPY

Because nonpharmacologic interventions alone are frequently insufficient to prevent or treat osteoporosis, medication therapy is often necessary. Table 92–6[1,3,15,59,60] describes fracture and BMD effects, Table 92–7 describes dosing and Table 92–8 outlines adverse effects and monitoring of osteoporosis medications. These medications should always be combined with a bone-healthy lifestyle.

MEDICATION

Drug Treatments of First Choice

8 Combined with adequate calcium and vitamin D intake, alendronate, risedronate, zoledronic acid, or denosumab are the prescription medications of choice based on evidence to reduce the risk of hip and vertebral fractures.[6] Ibandronate, teriparatide or raloxifene are alternatives and calcitonin is last-line therapy. The algorithm (see Fig. 92–3)[1,3,4,6] helps determine for whom medication

TABLE 92-6 Fracture and Bone Mineral Density Effects of Osteoporosis Medications from Pivotal Fracture Trials[a] in Postmenopausal Women

Medication	Vertebral Fracture	Nonvertebral Fracture	Hip Fracture	% Change in Spine BMD[b]	% Change in Hip BMD[b,c]
Bazedoxifene	35-40%↓	↔[d]	↔	2.2%↑	0.5%↑
Bazedoxifene with conjugated equine estrogens	ND	ND	ND	0.24%-1.6%↑	0.2%-1.5%↑
Bisphosphonates	41%-70%↓	25%-39%↓[e]	40%-51%↓[f]	4.3%-6.7%↑	2.8%-6.0%↑
Calcitonin	33%↓	↔	↔	3%↑	↔
Denosumab	68%↓	20%↓	40%↓	9.2%↑	6.0%↑
Estrogen with or without a progestogen	33%- 40%↓	13%-27%↓	30%-50%↓	3.5%-7%↑[f]	1.7%-5%↑[g]
Raloxifene	30%-68%↓[h]	↔	↔	2.6%↑	2.1%↑
Teriparatide	35%-65%↓	47%-53%↓	↔	8.6%-9.7%↑	3.5%↑

%, percent; BMD, bone mineral density; ↓, decrease; ↑, increase; ↔, no significant change; ND = no data.

[a]Fracture reductions are relative risk reductions, no head to head fracture studies except for raloxifene and bazedoxifene, data should only be used for relative between class comparisons, clinical trials with different patient samples and study designs, most pivotal fracture trials 3 years duration except for teriparatide studies (18 months).

[b]Relative to placebo; may vary based on duration of therapy and timing relative to menopause.

[c]Total hip (alendronate, ibandronate, zoledronic acid, bazedoxifene, denosumab, estrogen, and teriparatide) or femoral neck (calcitonin, estrogen, risedronate, and raloxifene).

[d]50% decreases in nonvertebral fractures in subgroup of high-risk postmenopausal women (very low BMD and or previous fractures).

[e]Risedronate and zoledronic acid only; nonvertebral fracture reductions with ibandronate and alendronate were not significant.

[f]Alendronate, risedronate, and zoledronic acid only; hip fracture data not reported with ibandronate.

[g]Data obtained from nonpivotal fracture trials.

[h]Plus data from a pivotal bazedoxifene trial with raloxifene as one of the comparators.

Data from references 1, 3, 15, 59, and 60.

TABLE 92-7 Drug Dosing Table

Drug	Brand Name	Dose	Comments
Antiresorptive Medications—Nutritional Supplements			
Calcium	Various	*Adequate daily intake:* IOM: 200-1,200 mg/day, varies per age; see Table 93–5); Supplement dose is difference between required adequate intake and dietary intake. Immediate-release doses should be <500-600 mg.	Recommend food first to achieve goal intake. Available in different salts including carbonate and citrate, absorption of other salts not fully quantified. Different formulations including chewable, liquid, gummy, softgel, drink, and wafer; different combination products. Review package to determine number of units to create a serving size and desired amount of elemental calcium. Give calcium carbonate with meals to improve absorption.
Vitamin D D3 (cholecalciferol) D_2 (ergocalciferol)	Over the counter, Tablets, 400, 1,000, and 2,000 units Capsule, 400, 1,000, 2,000, 5,000, and 10,000 units Gummies, 300, 500, 1,000 units Drops 300, 400, 1,000 and 2,000 units/mL or drop Solution, 400 and 5,000 units/mL Spray 1,000 and 5,000 units/spray Creams and lotions 500 and 1,000 units per ¼ teaspoonful. Prescription, Capsule, 50,000 units Solution, 8,000 units/mL	Adequate daily intake: IOM: 400-800 units/day to achieve adequate intake (see Table 93-5); NOF: 800-1,000 units orally daily; If low 25(OH) vitamin D concentrations, malabsorption, or altered metabolism higher doses (>2,000 units daily) might be required. *Vitamin D deficiency*: 50,000 units orally once to twice weekly for 8-12 weeks; repeat as needed until therapeutic concentrations.	Vegetarians and vegans need to read label to determine if a plant-based product. Slight advantage of D3 over D2 for increasing serum 25(OH) vitamin D concentrations. For drops, make sure measurement is correct for desired dose. Ability of sprays, lotions, and creams to resolve deficiencies or maintain adequate intakes is unknown.
Antiresorptive Prescription Medications			
Bisphosphonates			
Alendronate	Fosamax Fosamax Plus D Binosto (effervescent tab)	Treatment: 10 mg orally daily or 70 mg orally weekly Prevention: 5 mg orally daily or 35 mg orally weekly	Generic available for weekly tablet product. 70 mg dose is available as a tablet, effervescent tablet, oral liquid or combination tablet with 2,800 or 5,600 units of vitamin D3. Administered in the morning on an empty stomach with 6 to 8 ounces of plain water. Do not eat and remain upright for at least 30 minutes following administration. Do not co-administer with any other medication or supplements, including calcium and vitamin D.
Ibandronate	Boniva	Treatment: 150 mg orally monthly, 3 mg intravenous quarterly Prevention: 150 mg orally monthly	Generic available for oral product. Administration instructions same as for alendronate, except must delay eating and remain upright for at least 60 minutes.
Risedronate	Actonel Atelvia (delayed-release)	Treatment and Prevention: 5 mg orally daily, 35 mg orally weekly, 150 mg orally monthly	Generic available for immediate-release product. 35 mg dose is also available as a delayed-release product. Administration instructions same as for alendronate, except delayed-release product is taken immediately following breakfast.
Zoledronic acid	Reclast	Treatment: 5 mg intravenous infusion yearly Prevention: 5 mg intravenous infusion every 2 years	Can premedicate with acetaminophen to decrease infusion reactions. Contraindicated if CrCl <35 mL/min Also marketed under the brand name Zometa (4 mg) for treatment of hypercalcemia and prevention of skeletal-related events from bone metastases from solid tumors with different dosing.
RANK Ligand Inhibitor			
Denosumab	Prolia	Treatment: 60 mg subcutaneously every 6 months	Administered by a healthcare practitioner. Correct hypocalcemia before administration. Also marketed under the brand name Xgeva (70 mg/mL) for treatment of hypercalcemia and prevention of skeletal-related events from bone metastases from solid tumors with different dosing.
Estrogen Agonist/Antagonist and Tissue Selective Estrogen Complex			
Raloxifene	Evista	60 mg daily	Generic available
Bazedoxifene with conjugated equine estrogens (CEE)	Duavee	20 mg plus 0.45 mg CEE daily	For postmenopausal women with an uterus; no progestogen needed. Bazedoxifene monotherapy available in some countries.
Calcitonin			
Calcitonin (salmon)	Fortical	200 units (1 spray) intranasally daily, alternating nares every other day. 100 units subcutaneously daily	Generic available. Refrigerate nasal spray until opened for daily use, then room temperature. Prime with first use.

(continued)

TABLE 92-7 Drug Dosing Table (*Continued*)

Drug	Brand Name	Dose	Comments
Formation Medications			
Recombinant human parathyroid hormone (PTH 1-34 units)			
Teriparatide	Forteo	20 mcg subcutaneously daily for up to 2 years	First dose at night. Refrigerate before and after each use. Use new needle with each dose. Inject thigh or stomach. Discard after 28 days or if cloudy.

IOM, Institute of Medicine; NOF, National Osteoporosis Foundation; NSAID, nonsteroidal anti-inflammatory drug.

therapy should be used. In general, prescription therapy should be considered in any postmenopausal woman or man age 50 years and older presenting with osteoporosis or low bone mass combined with a 10-year probability of hip fracture of 3% or more or a 10-year probability of any major osteoporosis-related fracture of 20% or more. The use of osteoporosis prescription medications in children, pre- and perimenopausal women, and men younger than 50 years old is undergoing further investigation. Universal use of calcium and vitamin D to achieve adequate intakes (see Table 92–5) is controversial; however, guidelines recommend adequate intake.

The National Osteoporosis Foundation's clinician's guide,[1] the North American Menopause Society's position statement,[3] the

TABLE 92-8 Drug Monitoring Table

Drug	Adverse Drug Reaction	Monitoring Parameter	Comments
Antiresorptive Medications—Nutritional Supplements			
Calcium	Constipation, gas, upset stomach, kidney stones	Dietary calcium intake, constipation	Education about a bowel healthy lifestyle (eg, adequate water, fiber, and exercise)
Vitamin D	Hypercalcemia, hypercalciuria, weakness, headache, somnolence, nausea. Rare: cardiac rhythm disturbance	Serum 25(OH) vitamin D concentration, symptoms	Adverse effects usually not experienced until 25(OH) vitamin D concentrations more than 100-150 ng/mL (mcg/L; > 250-375 nmol/L), which are generally not achieved with recommended therapeutic doses
Antiresorptive Prescription Medications			
Bisphosphonates			
Bisphosphonates	Dyspepsia (oral), transient or chronic musculoskeletal pain, nausea, transient flu-like illness (injectable) Rare: GI perforation, ulceration, and/or bleeding (oral); osteonecrosis of the jaw; atypical femoral shaft fracture, severe musculoskeletal pain	Bone density, fractures, GI symptoms, muscle aches Serum calcium for zoledronic acid	Pregnancy category C for alendronate, risedronate, and ibandronate. Pregnancy category D for zoledronic acid. Adherence is suboptimal, thus should be frequently assessed Assess correct use of products with refills.
RANK Ligand Inhibitor			
Denosumab	Back pain, arthralgia, eczema, cellulitis, and infection; Rare: osteonecrosis of the jaw, atypical femoral shaft fracture	Serum calcium, bone density, fractures	Pregnancy category X. REMS: Medication guide and monitoring plan due to risks of serious infections, dermatologic adverse reactions, and suppression of bone turnover
Estrogen Agonist/Antagonist and Tissue Selective Estrogen Complex			
Raloxifene	Hot flushes, leg pain, spasms, or cramps, peripheral edema, venous thromboembolism (warm swollen leg, chest pain, shortness of breath, coughing up blood, and change in vision)	Bone density, fractures, hot flushes, leg cramps, and blood clots	Pregnancy category X. Warning for fatal stroke-rare events predominantly seen in women at high risk for stroke
Bazedoxifene with conjugated equine estrogens	Similar to raloxifene and estrogens	Bone density, fractures, leg cramps, blood clots	Pregnancy category X.
Calcitonin			
Calcitonin (salmon)	Nasal: rhinitis, epistaxis Injection: nausea, flushing, local inflammation	Bone density, fractures, nasal symptoms	Pregnancy category C.
Formation Medications			
Recombinant human parathyroid hormone (PTH 1-34 units)			
Teriparatide	Orthostasis with first few injections, pain at injection site, nausea, headache, dizziness, leg cramps, rare increase in uric acid, slightly increased calcium stays with regular adverse effects	Bone density, fractures, trough serum calcium concentration 1 month after therapy initiation	Pregnancy category C. If serum calcium is high (>10.6 mg/dL [>2.65 mmol/L]), calcium intake should be decreased. Warning about osteosarcoma in rats and therefore contraindicated in patients at high risk for this adverse event. REMS: Medication guide and communication plan due to the increased risk of osteosarcoma and to inform healthcare providers of the 2 year maximum lifetime treatment

REMS, Risk Evaluation and Mitigation Strategies.

American Association of Clinical Endocrinologists' guidelines for women,[6] the Endocrine Society's guidelines for men,[4] and the Agency for Healthcare Research and Quality update[61] provide guidance on osteoporosis prevention and treatment strategies.

Drug Class Information

Antiresorptive Therapies

Antiresorptive therapies include calcium, vitamin D, bisphosphonates, estrogen agonists antagonists (known previously as selective estrogen receptor modulators or SERMs), tissue selective estrogen complexes, calcitonin, denosumab, estrogen, and testosterone.

Calcium Supplementation 6 Calcium imbalance can result from inadequate dietary intake, decreased fractional calcium absorption, enhanced calcium excretion, and diseases and medications altering these processes. Adequate calcium intake (see Table 92–5) is considered a foundation for osteoporosis prevention and treatment in the guidelines and should be combined with vitamin D, especially when osteoporosis medications are taken.[1,3,4,6,46,47] In contrast, the USPSTF states low doses of calcium (ie, ≤1000 mg) for adults are ineffective and insufficient data existed to recommend higher doses to prevent osteoporotic fractures.[62] If dietary intake cannot be increased to achieve adequate intake, calcium supplements can be used. Dietary calcium intake needs to be quantified via calculators, questionnaires, or estimates to determine supplement dose. The National Osteoporosis Foundation has a calcium calculator,[1] the CaQ questionnaire assesses 23 food and beverage groups,[63]and age and gender estimates exist from the NHANES study.[41,49]

Efficacy Calcium generally maintains BMD although small BMD increases (0.6%-1.8%) have been documented. These BMD effects are less than other osteoporosis medications. Calcium alone does not prevent fractures, but when combined with vitamin D, it decreases fractures by 11% to 15%, vertebral fractures by 16%, and hip fractures by up to 30%.[42-44] Higher-than-recommended calcium intakes are not associated with any clinical advantages.

Adverse Events Calcium's most common adverse reaction, constipation, can first be treated with increased water intake, dietary fiber, and exercise. If still unresolved, smaller and more frequent administration or a lower total daily dose can be tried. Calcium carbonate can create gas and cause stomach upset, which might resolve with calcium citrate, a product with fewer GI side effects.

Clinical trials of calcium show no effect to a 17% increase in kidney stones.[64] In some cases, calcium binds to oxalate in the gut, which decreases oxalate urinary excretion thereby decreasing kidney stones. Increased fluid intake and decreased salt intake might be warranted to prevent kidney stones.

In 2008, an analysis revealed that calcium was associated with a 30% in myocardial infarction.[65] Since then multiple meta-analyses, reanalysis of trial data, and secondary analyses of studies that had diet, calcium supplements, cardiovascular disease, and mortality data have been conducted showing outcomes from no effect to a small negative effect depending on the methodology, studies included, control of confounders, and various other study design issues.[64,66,67] Recent studies do not find calcium causing coronary artery calcifications. Furthermore, coronary artery calcifications can result from other causes such as coronary inflammation.

The most recent osteoporosis guideline and expert consensus indicate calcium intake to meet IOM requirements is safe, but intakes should remain less than 1500 mg daily (less than the IOM upper limit) and preferably achieved through diet.

Drug Interactions Since calcium carbonate requires acid for disintegration, drugs such as the proton pump inhibitors can decrease absorption from the carbonate product. Fiber laxatives can decrease the absorption of calcium if given concomitantly. Calcium can decrease the oral absorption of some drugs including iron, tetracyclines, quinolones, bisphosphonates, and thyroid supplements.

Administration Most children and adults of all race and ethnic backgrounds do not ingest sufficient dietary calcium and therefore require supplements. To ensure adequate calcium absorption, 25(OH) vitamin D concentrations should be at least 10 to 15 ng/mL (mcg/L; 25-37 nmol/L). Because fractional calcium absorption is dose limited, maximum single doses of 500 to 600 mg or less of elemental calcium are recommended.[25] Since peaks in serum calcium concentrations after supplementation are hypothesized as a reason for negative cardiovascular effects, using lower doses more frequently has been proposed.[66] Calcium carbonate is the salt of choice as it contains the highest amount of elemental calcium (40%) and is the least expensive. Calcium carbonate should be taken with meals, which increases gastric acidity resulting in product dissolution and disintegration. Calcium citrate (21% calcium) has acid-independent absorption and does not need to be administered with meals. A 24-hour sustained-release calcium citrate product was designed to deliver 1,200 mg throughout the day; however, concern with intakes more than IOM recommended intakes, which potentially increases cardiovascular disease, limits its use. Although tricalcium phosphate contains 38% calcium, calcium-phosphate complexes could limit overall calcium absorption. This product might be helpful in patients with hypophosphatemia that cannot be resolved with increased dietary intake.

Disintegration and dissolution rates vary significantly between products and lots. Products labeled "USP Verified" for United States Pharmacopeia, which guarantees the identity, strength, purity, and quality of the product, or products from a reputable company, should be recommended. Products from unrefined oyster shell or coral calcium should not be recommended because of concerns for high concentrations of lead and other heavy metals. Some calcium products come in alternative dosage forms (eg, chews, dissolvable tablet, and liquid), which can be beneficial for select patients (eg, swallowing problems). For all products, encourage patients to read the labeling carefully as multiple tablets per day can be needed to obtain adequate calcium intake.

Some commercial calcium supplements contain other nutrients associated with bone physiology such as magnesium, vitamin K, "natural estrogens," or isoflavones. Minimal BMD and no fracture data exist for these combination products. These products are also more expensive. Combining too many vitamins and supplements might exceed upper-tolerable nutrient limits and increase toxicities.

Vitamin D Supplementation 7 Vitamin D intake is critical for intestinal calcium absorption and when combined with calcium can prevent bone loss and decrease osteoporotic fractures.[25-27] The IOM recommends adequate intakes of vitamin D from diet and or supplementation for all ages (see Table 92–5).[47] Osteoporosis guidelines recommend higher vitamin D maintenances doses (800-2,000 units daily).[1,3,4] The USPSTF states low doses of vitamin D (ie, ≤ 400 units) are not effective, but in 2014 they stated insufficient data existed to recommend higher doses to prevent osteoporotic fractures.[62]

The desired therapeutic range for vitamin D is controversial. The IOM defines 20 ng/mL (50 nmol/L; 1 ng/mL = 2.5 nmol/L) as the cut point for normal 25(OH) vitamin D,[47] below which a patient would be considered deficient. However, some experts and guidelines state the goal 25(OH) vitamin D concentration should be 30 to 60 ng/mL (mcg/L; 75-150 nmol/L) or 30 to 100 ng/mL (mcg/L; 75-250 nmol/L) with concentrations between 20 and 29 ng/mL (mcg/L; 50-72 nmol/L) considered insufficient and those less than 20 ng/mL (mcg/L; 50 nmol/L) considered deficient.

Current evidence suggests that the major effects of vitamin D are achieved with 25(OH) vitamin D concentrations between

6 and 20 ng/mL (mcg/L; 15-50 nmol/L), including increasing calcium absorption (10-15 ng/mL [mcg/L; 25-37 nmol/L]) and decreasing BMD loss (up to 20 ng/mL [mcg/L; 50 nmol/L]).[25] Daily vitamin D doses of 500 to 700 units generally are sufficient to achieve vitamin D concentrations more than 20 ng/mL (mcg/L; greater than 50 nmol/L), leading some experts to suggest the higher daily doses recommended in guidelines are not warranted. Other experts point out that not everyone achieves a 25(OH) vitamin D greater than 30 ng/mL (mcg/L; 75 nmol/L), and because the product is inexpensive and safe, the higher recommended doses are appropriate.

Serum 25(OH) vitamin D is the best indicator of total body vitamin D status.[1] Interassay variability exists; thus, the same laboratory should be used for repeat testing. Measurement of 25(OH) vitamin D concentration could be considered in anyone with high risk for low vitamin D (eg, older, obese, minimal sun exposure, insufficient vitamin D intake, dark pigmented skin, certain medical conditions especially liver and kidney disease or medications known to affect vitamin D metabolism), low bone density, history of a low-trauma fracture, frequent falls, unexplained muscle weakness, and/or bone pain.

Clinical **Controversy...**

A clinical question is should all older adults be supplemented with guideline recommended vitamin D doses or should a 25(OH) vitamin D level be drawn first to assess need and/or determine appropriate supplementation. Universal supplementation is supported by the fact vitamin D supplementation is safe and inexpensive. Treating 1,000 high-risk patients, defined as living in an institution, with vitamin D and calcium would prevent 9 hip fractures, which are associated with significant morbidity, mortality, and cost.[68] The vitamin D dose to prevent falls has been around 800 units; with studies based on dose and not on serum concentrations.[25-27]Adverse effects from vitamin D therapy are usually not seen until concentrations are greater than 100 ng/mL (mcg/L; 250 nmol/L); concentrations generally not achieved with guideline recommended vitamin D doses.[25,26] Because adequate intakes do not always result in vitamin D sufficiency, a vitamin D level could then be ordered after initiation to assess impact of vitamin D supplementation, saving the health system the cost of one vitamin D level. On the other hand, in 2014, the USPSTF stated insufficient evidence exists to support universal vitamin D screening in asymptomatic patients.[62] Results from a cost savings simulation showed population screening to determine need for vitamin D supplementation was significantly more cost beneficial than universal supplementation ($224 vs $189 savings, respectively), assuming the cost of a vitamin D level is $45.[69] In women and men around 65 years old, the difference is statistically significant but only a savings of $6 to $12. However, in 80-year-olds the cost savings from vitamin D screening is $132 to $135. Additional levels would be needed to assess impact of vitamin D replacement or maintenance doses. Vitamin D screening would identify vitamin D deficiency and insufficiency sooner allowing replacement therapy to begin sooner. Another vitamin D level would still be required for assessment of vitamin D doses but in this case, only for those that needed supplementation.

Efficacy Data show that higher-dose vitamin D supplementation (≥800 units) combined with calcium can decrease hip (16%-21%), nonvertebral (12%), and overall (8%-13%) fracture rates and increase BMD. However, these effects are generally not seen with vitamin D alone.[25-28,70] Megadose studies (greater than 300,000 units/year) demonstrated an increased fracture rate, and thus should be avoided.

Most studies and meta-analyses support vitamin D increasing muscle strength and balance, increasing to no change in gait, decreasing numbers of people falling, and decreasing the rate of falls. These findings are consistent with the USPSTF recommendations advocating vitamin D to prevent falls in community-dwelling older adults. Low vitamin D concentrations are associated with many diseases, but data supporting supplementation to prevent or treat these conditions are minimal. At this time, vitamin D supplementation is advocated in older adults with falls or at high risk for falls, and combined with calcium and vitamin D to decrease bone loss and fractures.

Drug Interactions Some medications can induce vitamin D metabolism including rifampin, phenytoin, barbiturates, valproic acid, and carbamazepine. Vitamin D absorption can be decreased by cholestyramine, colestipol, orlistat, and mineral oil. Vitamin D can enhance the absorption of aluminum; therefore aluminum-containing products should be avoided to prevent aluminum toxicity.

Administration The vitamin D dose is based on IOM adequate intakes (see Table 92–5), osteoporosis guideline recommendations or to achieve a 25(OH) vitamin D concentration ≥20-30 ng/mL (mcg/L; ≥50-75 nmol/L).[1,3,6,71] About 40% of older adults have hypovitaminosis D (≤ 20 ng/mL [mcg/L; ≤50 nmol/L]), which is higher in blacks (82%) and Hispanics (69%). Replacement doses will first be required in these patients before recommended maintenance doses.[51]

Vitamin D can be taken as a single agent or combination product. Supplements and multivitamins contain vitamin D3 or D2. Synthesized vitamin D3 can be made from irradiated sheep's wool and vitamin D2 from irradiated mushrooms. Although some data support slight differences between vitamin D3 and D2 absorption,[26] guidelines suggest either for prevention and treatment of vitamin D deficiency. Based on a meta-analysis, vitamin D3 was more efficient than vitamin D2 at raising 25(OH) vitamin D concentrations, and produced greater BMD changes with bolus dosing but not with maintenance doses.[72] The differences could be related to greater metabolism of vitamin D2 to inactive metabolites. The vitamin D3 dose to increase 25(OH) vitamin D concentration varies from 40 units to increase concentration by 0.8 ng/mL(mcg/L; 2 nmol/L) to 100 units to increase concentration by 1 ng/mL (mcg/L; 2.5 nmol/L),[71,73] with higher vitamin D doses needed to raise concentrations in obese patients. Higher-dose prescription vitamin D regimens administered weekly, monthly, or quarterly can be used for replacement therapy.[26] More than one multivitamin or large doses of cod liver oil daily are no longer advocated because of the risk of hypervitaminosis A, which can increase bone loss. Because the half-life of vitamin D is about 1 month, approximately 3 months of therapy are required before a new steady state is achieved and a repeat 25(OH) vitamin D concentration can be obtained.

Individuals with deficient concentrations of vitamin D are at risk for osteomalacia. Their management is discussed later in the chapter. In patients who are pregnant, obese, or with disorders (eg, celiac disease, cystic fibrosis, or Crohn's disease), or medications (eg, anticonvulsants, glucocorticoids, antifungals, and AIDS medications) affecting vitamin D absorption, higher doses and more frequent monitoring are required. In patients with severe hepatic or renal disease, the activated form of vitamin D (calcitriol) might be needed, however, newer research suggests adequate amounts of 25(OH)vitamin D are important for total body health creating a need for both cholecalciferol and calcitriol co-administration for these disease conditions.[74]

Bisphosphonates 8 9 Alendronate, risedronate, and intravenous zoledronic acid are FDA-indicated for postmenopausal, male, and glucocorticoid-induced osteoporosis. Intravenous and oral ibandronate and some specialized oral formulations of other bisphosphonates are indicated only for postmenopausal osteoporosis.

Pharmacology Bisphosphonates mimic pyrophosphate, an endogenous bone resorption inhibitor.[75,76] Bisphosphonate antiresorptive activity results from blocking prenylation and inhibiting guanosine triphosphatase-signaling proteins, which lead to decreased osteoclast maturation, number, recruitment, bone adhesion, and life span. Their various R2 side chains produce different bone binding, persistence, and affinities; however, the resulting clinical significances are not known.

Pharmacokinetics Oral bisphosphonate bioavailability is less than 1%; and is greatly decreased with concomitant food and beverages.[75-77] Within 24 hours of administration, bisphosphonates undergo rapid skeletal uptake and any drug not incorporated into bone is renally excreted. Incorporation into bone gives bisphosphonates long biologic half-lives of up to 10 years. Absorbed bisphosphonates are renally eliminated and elimination decreases linearly with declining renal function. Bisphosphonates differ in the strength of binding to bone (zoledronic acid greater than alendronate greater than ibandronate greater than risedronate) with zoledronic acid having greater bone absorption, longer bone retention times (less desorption), and more reattachment after bone release.

Efficacy Of the antiresorptive agents, bisphosphonates consistently provide some of the higher fracture risk reductions and BMD increases (see Table 92–6). Fracture clinical trial data are from daily oral bisphosphonate or annual intravenous therapy, not weekly, monthly, or quarterly regimens. Hip-fracture reduction has not been demonstrated with daily oral ibandronate; however, the study might have been underpowered. Because of the lack of hip-fracture reduction data, ibandronate is not a first-line therapy (see Fig. 92–3). Comparative fracture prevention trials do not exist. Annual intravenous zoledronic acid has documented secondary fracture prevention and a decrease in mortality in the treated group.[3,61]

BMD increases with bisphosphonates are dose dependent and greatest in the first 12 months of therapy.[44,78] Small increases in hip BMD continue for at least 3 years before plateauing, with the exact timing of the plateau varying by agent. For all bisphosphonates, increases in BMD are typically greater at the spine than at the hip. Weekly alendronate, weekly and monthly risedronate, and monthly oral and quarterly intravenous ibandronate therapy produce equivalent BMD changes to their respective daily regimens.[3,78] Alendronate and ibandronate therapy increases lumbar spine BMD more than risedronate therapy[78]; however, no evidence indicates that this difference would equate to greater fracture efficacy. After discontinuation, the increased BMD is sustained for a prolonged period of time that varies per bisphosphonate.[44]

The BMD increases with alendronate, risedronate, zoledronic acid, and oral ibandronate in men are similar to those in postmenopausal women.[4] Because of a lack of fracture data from pivotal trials in men, bisphosphonates are only FDA indicated to increase BMD, not to reduce fracture risk in men. A meta-analysis combining data from published randomized controlled trials showed reductions in vertebral and nonvertebral fractures in men.[79]

Adverse Events (see Table 92–8) Oral bisphosphonates are well tolerated if patients are selected for therapy appropriately and the patient takes them correctly.[1,6] Patients with creatinine clearances less than 30 to 35 mL/min (0.50–0.58 mL/s), who have serious GI conditions (abnormalities of the esophagus that delay emptying, such as stricture or achalasia), or who are pregnant should not take bisphosphonates. Some experts suggest bisphosphonates can be used in select patients with decreased renal function.[80]

GI complaints, including heartburn and dyspepsia, are one of the most common reasons cited by patients for discontinuing therapy.[6,76] While these mild GI effects are common, bisphosphonates are also associated with rare severe GI events, such as esophageal erosion, ulcer, or GI bleeding. If GI adverse events occur, switching to a different bisphosphonate or less frequent administration schedule might resolve the problem. Patients should be encouraged to discuss GI complaints with a healthcare provider. Intravenous ibandronate and zoledronic acid can be used for patients with GI contraindications or intolerances to oral bisphosphonates. Other common bisphosphonate adverse effects include injection reactions and musculoskeletal pain. If severe musculoskeletal pain occurs, the medication can be discontinued temporarily or permanently. Acute phase reactions (eg, fever, flulike symptoms, myalgias, and arthralgias) are typically associated with intravenous administration, but rarely have been reported with daily, weekly or monthly oral bisphosphonates. This reaction usually diminishes with subsequent administration.

Rare adverse effects include osteonecrosis of the jaw (ONJ) and subtrochanteric femoral (atypical) fractures.[76,81] ONJ occurs more commonly in patients with cancer, receiving higher-dose intravenous bisphosphonate therapy and other risk factors including glucocorticoid therapy and diabetes mellitus. In osteoporosis, the incidence of ONJ is 0.001% to 0.01%, which is similar to the incidence in the general population. Maxillary or mandibular bone surgery and poor oral hygiene are dental-specific risk factors for development of ONJ. When possible, major dental work should be completed before bisphosphonate initiation. For patients already on therapy, some practitioners withhold bisphosphonate therapy during and after major dental procedures, but no data exist to support any benefit of such practice. Atypical femoral shaft fractures are rare; some evidence suggests the risk may increase with longer duration of bisphosphonate use.[76] Since some patients with atypical fracture experience prodromal thigh or hip pain, any such pain should be evaluated.

Drug Interactions Because of poor bioavailability, oral bisphosphonates should not be administered at the same time as other medications. The administration instructions described below should be followed.

Dosing and Administration (see Table 92–7) Because bioavailability is very poor for bisphosphonates (less than 1%) and to minimize GI side effects, each oral tablet should be taken with at least 6 ounces (~180 mL) of plain water (not coffee, juice, mineral water, or milk) at least 30 minutes (60 minutes for ibandronate) before consuming any food, supplements (including calcium and vitamin D), or medications. The patient should also remain upright (ie, either sitting or standing) for at least 30 minutes after alendronate and risedronate and 1 hour after ibandronate administration. For patients with swallowing difficulties (eg, stroke and tube feeding), a buffered, strawberry-flavored effervescent tablet form of alendronate, which is dissolved in 4 ounces (~120 mL) of room temperature water, could be used. This formulation has the same food restrictions as traditional oral tablets. In contrast, delayed-release risedronate is available and it is administered immediately following breakfast with at least 4 ounces (~120 mL) of plain water. A patient who misses a weekly dose can take it the next day. If more than 1 day has lapsed, that dose is skipped until the next scheduled ingestion. If a patient misses a monthly dose, it can be taken up to 7 days before the next administration.

Before intravenous bisphosphonates are used, the patient's serum calcium concentration must be normal. Creatinine clearance should be monitored before each dose of zoledronic acid. The intravenous products need to be administered by a healthcare provider. The quarterly ibandronate injection comes as a prefilled syringe (3 mg/mL) kit with a butterfly needle. The injection is given intravenously over 15 to 30 seconds. The injection can also be diluted with dextrose 5% in water or normal saline and used with a syringe pump. Once-yearly administration of zoledronic acid should be infused over at least 15 minutes with a pump. Acetaminophen can be given to decrease acute phase reactions.

Although these medications are effective, adherence is poor and results in decreased effectiveness.[82] Although adherence is improved with once-weekly bisphosphonate administration over daily therapy, it is unclear if once-monthly therapy improves adherence more. While dosing frequency is a common barrier to adherence, adverse effects (eg, GI complaints) and concerns about adverse effects remain important predictors of adherence and persistence. Even after a hip fracture, bisphosphonate persistence is suboptimal.[61,82] To help overcome the barrier associated with dosing frequency, intravenous ibandronate and zoledronic acid could be used as replacements if cost is not an issue. Weekly alendronate plus vitamin D can potentially help to ensure better adherence with vitamin D intake, but at an increased cost over generic alendronate.

Clinical **Controversy...**

The ideal duration of bisphosphonate therapy is not known. Bisphosphonates are deposited into the bone and continue to suppress bone turnover after discontinuation, and some adverse effects, such as atypical fracture, are associated with duration of therapy.[83] To balance risk and benefit, some clinicians recommend a 'drug holiday,' defined as disruption of therapy during which medication effects exist with a plan for reinstitution. Two randomized, double-blind studies with a drug holiday after therapy with alendronate for 5 years or zoledronic acid for 3 years show a continued fracture benefit with discontinuing therapy. Because a beneficial response was predicted by hip T-score, experts recommend that a drug holiday could be considered in postmenopausal women after 5 years of oral bisphosphonates or 3 years of intravenous bisphosphonates if no significant fracture history, hip BMD T-score is above −2.5, and fracture risk is not high. In women with a high fracture risk or lower hip BMD T-scores, continuing oral bisphosphonates for 10 years or intravenous bisphosphonates for 6 years should be considered. These recommendations are based on limited data and questions remain regarding the applicability of this approach for patients with glucocorticoid-induced osteoporosis and men.

Denosumab (8) Denosumab is FDA approved for treatment of osteoporosis in women and men at high risk for fracture. It is also approved to increase bone mass in men receiving androgen deprivation therapy for nonmetastatic prostate cancer and in women receiving adjuvant aromatase inhibitor therapy for breast cancer who are at high risk for fracture.

Pharmacology Denosumab is a fully human monoclonal antibody that binds to RANKL, blocking its ability to bind to its RANK receptor on the surface of osteoclast precursor cells and mature osteoclasts. Denosumab inhibits osteoclastogenesis and increases osteoclast apoptosis.

Pharmacokinetics Following subcutaneous injection, rapid suppression of bone turnover occurs within 12 hours. Denosumab achieves peak concentration in approximately 10 days. The half-life is approximately 25 days and the concentration slowly declines over a period of 4 to 5 months.[84] The drug does not accumulate with repeated dosing at 6-month intervals. No dosage adjustment is necessary in renal impairment; however, hypocalcemia is more common in severe renal impairment. No studies have been conducted in hepatic impairment.

Efficacy Over 3 years, denosumab significantly decreased vertebral fractures, nonvertebral fractures, and hip fractures in postmenopausal women with low bone density (see Table 92–6).[84] The BMD effects are at least similar to weekly alendronate and can increase BMD in patients with prior alendronate therapy. Activity appears to dissipate upon medication discontinuation.

Adverse Events (see Table 92–8) In trials up to 8 years in duration, denosumab was generally well tolerated.[84] Dermatologic reactions not specific to the injection site such as dermatitis, eczema, and rashes were more common than with placebo.

Rare, serious adverse effects of denosumab include bone turnover suppression and serious infections including skin infections. If any signs of skin infection such as cellulitis appear, patients should be advised to seek medical attention. Since ONJ has been reported, major dental work should be completed before use when possible. As with the bisphosphonates, muscle, bone, and joint pain and atypical fractures have been reported with this antiresorptive agent. Since hypocalcemia can occur, any existing hypocalcemia should be corrected prior to use and adequate calcium and vitamin D intakes ensured. Severe hypocalcemia is more common in patients with underlying kidney dysfunction and the manufacturer recommends monitoring of serum calcium, magnesium, and phosphorus within 14 days of administration in those with a CrCl less than 30 mL/min (0.50 mL/s).

Drug Interactions No drug–drug interactions have been identified with denosumab.

Dosing and Administration (see Table 92–7) Denosumab is administered subcutaneously by a healthcare professional in the upper arm, upper thigh, or abdomen. The product is available as a refrigerated prefilled syringe that can be at room temperature up to 14 days before administration.

Mixed Estrogen Agonists/Antagonists and Tissue Selective Estrogen Complexes (8) Raloxifene is a second-generation mixed estrogen agonist/antagonist (EAA) approved for prevention and treatment of postmenopausal osteoporosis and for reducing the risk of invasive breast cancer in postmenopausal women with and without osteoporosis. Bazedoxifene is a third-generation EAA combined with conjugated equine estrogens (CEE) making it a tissue selective estrogen complex approved for prevention of postmenopausal osteoporosis and vasomotor menopausal symptoms. Raloxifene's breast cancer–prevention benefits make this medication desirable for younger postmenopausal women at risk for or with osteoporosis and breast cancer. Bazedoxifene with CEE is a good choice for younger postmenopausal women at risk for osteoporosis with menopausal symptoms.

Pharmacology EAAs bind with α- and β-estrogen receptors and various coactivators or corepressors to cause varying agonist or antagonist effects at different tissue sites.[59] Raloxifene is an agonist at bone receptors and antagonist at breast receptors; it has minimal effect on the uterus. Bazedoxifene is an agonist at bone, and antagonist at the uterus and breast, however it has no breast cancer prevention effects.

Pharmacokinetics Food has a nonsignificant effect on absorption, which is about 2% for raloxifene and 6%[85] for bazedoxifene due to extensive presystemic glucuronidation.[86] Raloxifene is 95% protein bound. The half-life of raloxifene is 28 hours and of bazedoxifene is 30 hours. EAAs are predominantly metabolized via glucuronidation and eliminated in the feces.

Efficacy Raloxifene and bazedoxifene decrease vertebral, but not hip fractures.[3,15,59,60] In a subgroup of high-risk postmenopausal women, bazedoxifene decreased nonvertebral fractures. The fracture prevention effects of bazedoxifene combined with CEE are unknown. EAAs increase spine and hip BMD, but to a lesser extent than bisphosphonates (see Table 92–6). Raloxifene's vertebral fracture prevention is greater in women without previous fracture. Bazedoxifene's BMD increases are greater than raloxifene but vertebral fracture prevention rates are similar. Bazedoxifene with CEE produced significantly greater increases in spine and hip BMD than raloxifene and placebo.[60] Raloxifene 7- and 8-year data and bazedoxifene 5- and 7-year data support long-term effects.[6,59] After raloxifene discontinuation, the medication effect is lost, with bone loss returning to age- or disease-related rates. EAAs cause some positive lipid effects (decreased total and low-density lipoprotein cholesterol, neutral to increased high-density lipoprotein cholesterol); however, triglycerides can increase slightly.[59] No benefit of raloxifene on cardiovascular disease was demonstrated in the RUTH (Raloxifene Use for the Heart) or MORE-CORE (Multiple Outcomes with Raloxifene study and its continuation) trials.

Adverse Events (see Table 92–8) Hot flushes are common (less than 28%) with raloxifene but decreased with bazedoxifene with CEE.[59,60] Raloxifene rarely causes endometrial thickening and bleeding; bazedoxifene decreases these adverse events making progestogen therapy not needed when combined with CEE. Leg cramps and muscle spasms are also common. Thromboembolic events are uncommon (less than 1.5%), but can be fatal. In large trials, no change in overall death, cardiovascular death, or overall stroke incidence was seen with raloxifene; however, a slight increase in fatal stroke (0.7/1,000 women–year difference) was documented, resulting in a boxed warning for raloxifene.[3,59] Fatal stroke with raloxifene occurred most frequently in women with a Framingham stroke risk score of 13 or more. Bazedoxifene with CEE also has all the adverse effects listed for estrogens as a class including increased thromboembolic events.

Drug Interactions Because of raloxifene's highly protein bound nature (95%), when given concomitantly with other highly protein bound medications, like warfarin, a potential for binding interactions exist therefore monitoring of both medications is suggested.[85] Cholestyramine can decrease raloxifene absorption. Rifampin, phenytoin, carbamazepine, and phenobarbital can decrease bazedoxifene intestinal and liver uridine diphosphate glucuronosyltransferase metabolism.[86] Estrogen metabolism is decreased with CYP3A4 inhibitors.

Dosing and Administration (see Table 92–7) Although once daily administration is easy, adherence and persistence problems exist. EAAs are contraindicated for women with an active or past history of venous thromboembolic disease, pregnancy, or childbearing potential.[85,86] Therapy should be stopped if a patient anticipates extended immobility. Women at high risk for a stroke (eg, Framingham stroke risk score ≥13) or coronary events and those with known coronary artery disease, peripheral vascular disease, atrial fibrillation, or a prior history of cerebrovascular events might not be good candidates for EAAs. These medications should be used with caution in patients with severe liver impairment or moderate to severe renal impairment, due to a lack of data. Bazedoxifene with CEE has all the contraindications and precautions for estrogens as a class.

Calcitonin 8 Calcitonin is FDA indicated for osteoporosis treatment for women who are at least 5 years past menopause. An FDA Advisory Committee Panel voted against calcitonin use for postmenopausal osteoporosis; however, it can be used if alternative therapies are not appropriate.[87] Other countries have discontinued the product.

Pharmacology Calcitonin is an endogenous hormone released from the thyroid gland when serum calcium is elevated. The prescription product contains salmon calcitonin, which is more potent and longer lasting than the mammalian form.

Pharmacokinetics Availability is 3% to 5%; and half-life is 18 minutes with nasal administration.[88]

Efficacy Only vertebral fractures have been documented to decrease with intranasal calcitonin therapy (see Table 92–6).[1,3,4,6,15] Calcitonin does not consistently affect hip BMD. No data exist for men. Intranasal calcitonin might provide some short-term pain relief to some patients with acute vertebral fractures.[3]

Adverse Events (see Table 92–8) Recent meta-analyses have revealed a weak relationship between calcitonin and cancer with no consistency in dose–response relationship or cancer cell line.[87,88] Risk–benefit ratio needs to be assessed before use.

Drug Interactions Lithium doses might need reduction.[88]

Dosing and Administration (see Table 92–7) Some patients do not like to administer medications intranasally. In clinical trials of calcitonin, a high dropout rate exists. Subcutaneous administration with 100 units daily is available, but rarely used because of more adverse effects and cost.[3] If the nasal product is used for vertebral fracture pain, calcitonin should be prescribed for short-term (4 weeks) treatment and should not be used in place of other more effective and less-expensive analgesics nor should it preclude the use of more appropriate osteoporosis therapy.

Hormone Therapies Hormone therapies are not recommended solely for osteoporosis but have positive bone effects when used for other indications. Estrogens are FDA indicated for prevention of osteoporosis for women at significant risk and for whom other osteoporosis medications cannot be used. Estrogens can be a good choice for women going through early menopause when positive bone effects are needs in addition to vasomotor symptom reduction.[89]

Testosterone is used to treat hypogonadism in men, but an osteoporosis medication should be added in men when risk for osteoporotic fracture is high.[4] A complete discussion of adverse events, drug interactions, dosing, and administration for estrogen and testosterone products for women can be found in Chapter 82, Hormone Therapy in Women, and for testosterone products for men in Chapter 84, Erectile Dysfunction.

Estrogen In women estrogens with or without a progestogen significantly decrease fracture risk and bone loss (see Table 92–6).[3,6,15,89] Oral and transdermal estrogens at equivalent doses and continuous or cyclic HT regimens have similar BMD effects. Effect on BMD is dose dependent, with some benefit seen with lower estrogen doses; however, fracture risk reduction has not been demonstrated with the lower doses. When estrogen therapy is discontinued, bone loss accelerates and fracture protection is lost.

Testosterone No fracture data are available, but some data support minor bone loss prevention for testosterone use in men and women.

Anabolic Therapies

Teriparatide 8 Teriparatide is FDA indicated for postmenopausal women who are at high risk for fracture, for men with idiopathic or hypogonadal osteoporosis who are at high risk for fracture, men or women intolerant to other osteoporosis medications, and patients with glucocorticoid-induced osteoporosis. Patients who have a history of osteoporotic fracture, multiple risk factors for fracture, very low bone density (eg, T-score less than −3.5), or have failed or are intolerant of previous bisphosphonate therapy could be candidates for teriparatide therapy.

Pharmacology Teriparatide is a recombinant human product representing the first 34 amino acids in human PTH. Teriparatide increases bone formation, the bone remodeling rate, and osteoblast number and activity. Its actions result from activation of Wnt signaling, induction of runx2 (transcription factor), increased IGF-1 production, and inhibition of osteoblast apoptosis and sclerostin.[3,15,19,21] Both bone mass and architecture are improved. PTH (1-84) is marketed in Europe.

Pharmacokinetics Bioavailability is 95%.[90] The peptide is cleared through hepatic and extrahepatic pathways, with a half-life of 60 minutes. No pharmacokinetic changes are noted with decreasing renal function. No studies have been performed in hepatic impairment. Alternative delivery formulations and once weekly administration are being investigated.[19]

Efficacy Two years of teriparatide reduces vertebral and nonvertebral fracture risk in postmenopausal women (see Table 92–6)[3,6,15]; however, no fracture data are available in men or patients taking glucocorticoids. Lumbar spine BMD increases are greater than other osteoporosis medications. Although wrist BMD is decreased, wrist fractures are not increased. Discontinuation of teriparatide therapy results in a decrease in BMD, which can be alleviated with subsequent antiresorptive therapy.[1]

Adverse Events Transient hypercalcemia rarely occurs with teriparatide (see Table 92–8). Because of an increased incidence of osteosarcoma in rats, teriparatide contains a box warning against use in patients at increased baseline risk for osteosarcoma (eg, Paget's bone disease, unexplained elevations of alkaline phosphatase, pediatric patients, young adults with open epiphyses, or patients with prior radiation therapy involving the skeleton). This adverse effect has not been seen in people.

Drug Interactions An increased calcium concentration could be a concern if on digoxin therapy.

Dosing and Administration Teriparatide is commercially available as a prefilled "pen" delivery device (see Table 92–7). The pen must be kept refrigerated and can be used immediately after removing from the refrigerator. The daily subcutaneous injection is delivered to the thigh or abdominal area with site rotation. The administration of the first dose should take place with the patient either sitting or lying down in case orthostatic hypotension occurs. The pen must be discarded 28 days after the initial injection. Duration of therapy is 18 to 24 months. The patient should receive patient education with each pen refill. Suboptimal adherence is documented to decrease efficacy. Besides the conditions listed above, teriparatide should not be used in patients with hypercalcemia, metabolic bone diseases other than osteoporosis, metastatic or skeletal cancers, or premenopausal women of child-bearing potential. Teriparatide should not be used in men with previous radiation therapy.[4]

Teriparatide is the most expensive osteoporosis therapy. Prior authorization might be required. Special arrangements need to be made when patients travel especially on airplanes.

Sequential and Combination Therapy

In the most recent guideline, sequential therapy is recommended but reserved for patients with severe osteoporosis because of cost.[1,91] In sequential therapy, the anabolic agent teriparatide is used for up to 2 years and then followed by an antiresorptive agent (eg, alendronate or denosumab). Starting with an antiresorptive first and then switching to teriparatide results in lower BMD increases.

Clinical **Controversy...**

The most recent osteoporosis guidelines[1] and some experts[32] recommend considering combination anabolic (teriparatide continuous or 3 months on and 3 months off) and antiresorptive (bisphosphonate or denosumab) therapy for very severe osteoporosis, especially when additional increases in hip BMD are necessary. These combinations improved hip BMD more than teriparatide alone, but generally did not improve spine BMD over monotherapy.[6,32,91,92] Of note, these results are not seen if the combination includes alendronate. Combination therapy produces greater BMD effects within the first 2.5 to 3 years; however, after 4 years the BMD effects are similar to sequential therapy with teriparatide followed by denosumab.[91] Because of no documented fracture benefit, increased cost, concern for dual suppression of bone turnover and decreased bone strength, and potential for more adverse effects with combination therapy, others feel combination therapy should not be used. Some experts feel sequential therapy with teriparatide followed by an antiresorptive is preferred over concurrent combination therapy for severe osteoporosis.[32] This controversy does not refer to multiple antiresorptive agents used together for multiple uses, for example bisphosphonate for osteoporosis and estrogens for menopause or raloxifene for breast cancer prevention.

Investigational Therapies

2 Besides the aforementioned investigational products, additional new classes of medications are beginning to show promise in phase II and III studies.[15,19,93] Investigational antiresorptive agents inhibit bone matrix degradation (cathepsin K inhibitors, eg, odanacatib) or block osteoclast activation (c-src kinase inhibitor, eg, saracatinib). Anabolic therapies under investigation include subcutaneously administered neutralizing antibodies against sclerostin (eg, romosozumab and blosozumab) or Dickkopf-1. These potential agents would allow for stimulation of bone formation through the Wnt-β-catenin signaling pathway. Other potential anabolic agents include novel parathyroid hormone–based drugs including a synthetic parathyroid hormone–related protein (PTHrP) analog (abaloparatide). Clinical trials of these new antiresorptive and anabolic agents will be carefully reviewed for antifracture efficacy and safety to determine potential place in therapy.

SPECIAL POPULATIONS

Osteoporosis is a particular threat in some subgroups because of age, genetic abnormalities, diseases, and medications.

Children

Although rare, osteoporosis in children and adolescents can lead to significant pain, deformity, and chronic disability. Secondary causes are the main contributors to osteoporosis in children (see Tables 92–2 and 92–3),[1,3,4,6-11] but genetic disorders and idiopathic juvenile osteoporosis can be the origin of bone disease.

The diagnosis and treatment of osteoporosis in children and adolescents are challenging.[9] No guidelines or consensus recommendations exist. The diagnosis of osteoporosis in children (less than 20 years of age) requires the presence of a clinically significant fracture history (vertebral compression fracture or two or more long bone fractures by age 10 or three or more long bone fractures by age 19) in combination with low bone mass.[33] Low bone mass is defined as a Z-score of –2.0 or less (adjusted for gender, age, and race/ethnicity) using central DXA of the spine or total body.

After correcting any underlying causes and instituting a bone-healthy lifestyle, pharmacologic treatment should be considered for children with low bone mass and fragility fractures.[9] Several small studies, mostly evaluating the intravenous bisphosphonate pamidronate or oral alendronate, have demonstrated increases in BMD. One study evaluating oral risedronate demonstrated increased spine BMD and a reduced risk of nonvertebral fracture. The optimal medication, dose, and duration of therapy are unknown, and more safety data are needed. A major concern with bisphosphonates is their effect on longitudinal bone growth and modeling; however, fracture healing, skeletal growth/maturation, or the appearance of growth plates does not appear to be impaired. Because bisphosphonates are released from bone for many years and cross the placenta, teratogenic effects are also a concern. Teriparatide cannot be used in children as it has a box warning indicating an increased risk for osteosarcoma. Pediatric experience with denosumab is limited.

Premenopausal Women

Clinically significant bone loss and fractures in healthy premenopausal women are rare. Risk factors are similar between premenopausal and postmenopausal osteoporosis.[12,94] Common risk factors in this group are anorexia nervosa, glucocorticoid use, and celiac disease. Bone loss during pregnancy is usually gained back after delivery and breastfeeding. Fifty percent to 90% of premenopausal women with osteoporosis have a secondary cause (see Tables 92–2 and 92–3) for the bone loss. Low-trauma fractures occurred in 28% of premenopausal women with normal BMD. Premenopausal fractures predict postmenopausal osteoporotic fractures.

Routine bone density screening and testing are not cost effective and should not be performed in healthy premenopausal women. Premenopausal women with known osteoporosis risk factors and low-trauma fractures can undergo central DXA examinations. In this case, the Z-score is used with Z-scores of –2.0 or less listed as bone mass below the expected range for age.[34]

Pharmacologic therapy for osteoporosis should be used with caution in premenopausal women as efficacy and safety have not been adequately demonstrated.[12,94] All premenopausal women should practice a bone healthy lifestyle. Secondary causes of bone loss should be resolved. For example, gaining weight and resumed menses are more effective in correcting bone loss secondary to anorexia nervosa than oral contraceptives. If the contributing factor cannot be eliminated, for example, chemotherapy or glucocorticoids, pharmacological therapy can be considered. Women with an unidentified cause for osteoporosis and no history of fracture should be treated with a bone-healthy lifestyle and watchful waiting.

Osteoporosis medication safety during pregnancy (medication pregnancy categories in Table 92–8) and breastfeeding have not been determined. Because of this, osteoporosis medications are generally not used in childbearing women, although they sometimes are prescribed along with contraceptive agents. A theoretical concern is risk for fetal harm with pregnancies that occur during and after bisphosphonate therapy due to the long half-lives of these agents and the potential for fetal exposure after therapy discontinued.

The Older Adult

Although osteoporosis, osteoporotic fractures, and postfracture morbidity and mortality increase with age, osteoporosis is underdiagnosed and undertreated in older adults. In a multinational study, only 17% of older adults received osteoporosis medications after a fracture.[95] Only 33% of nursing home residents with an osteoporosis diagnosis or past fracture received an osteoporosis medication, even though 89% of them were considered at high risk for a fracture.[96] When diagnosed with osteoporosis or after a low-trauma fracture, many older adults do not receive osteoporosis medications.

Guidelines recommend DXA for people 65 and older, however all older adults are not evaluated for osteoporosis.[1,3,4,34] Universal screening of older women was found to be cost effective, with more cost savings generated with greater age.[97] Reference standards for osteoporosis assessment tools are generally not available for the oldest older adults (eg, maximum age for FRAX is 90 years). In clinical practice, estimates for a 90-year-old person are applied to those adults older than 90 years. FRAX slightly overestimated whereas ultrasound underestimated osteoporosis in nursing home residents.[98] In an older adult with falls, the Garvan calculator might be better as falls are not included in FRAX.[99] Sarcopenia and decreased muscle mass and function are prevalent in older adults and can increase falls. Sarcopenia increased from 9% in 45 to 54 year olds to 33% to 46% in those 85 years and older.[27] After a hip fracture, 22% of women and 87% of men were found to have sarcopenia. Vitamin D 800 to 1,000 units daily has been associated with increasing muscle strength and balance and decreasing falls.

Older adults should practice a bone-healthy lifestyle, ingest adequate calcium and vitamin D,[1,3,4,29] and implement measures to prevent falls.[1,3,16,39,56,57] Exercise might be difficult in older adults due to osteoarthritis, and or limited by underlying cardiac and respiratory diseases. However, walking and lifting light weights can still stimulate bone remodeling. Lactose intolerance and hypercholesterolemia increase with aging; and can lower calcium intake from dairy products, which can increase the need for calcium supplements. Limited sun exposure due to frailty and institutional residence can increase the need for vitamin D supplementation for bone and muscle health. Encouraging older adults to do a home safety evaluation for falls can assist with fracture prevention. Multidisciplinary fall prevention programs with multiple interventions generally have greater impact on fall prevention than single discipline or single intervention. Many fall prevention materials are free on the Internet.

Osteoporosis medication efficacy and safety data are limited in the oldest older adults.[29] When deciding whether or not to use prescription medications in older adults, the following factors need to be taken into consideration: remaining life span, ability to take and afford medications, cognitive function, swallowing ability, GI disorders, polypharmacy, desire to avoid additional medications, and regimen complexity. Challenges with oral bisphosphonate administration requirements exist for older adults who are bed bound, have difficulties swallowing, have fluid restrictions for cardiovascular or kidney diseases, or forget to drink adequate amounts of fluid or stay upright for the given time. Sometimes not initiating or stopping osteoporosis medications might be warranted for older adults with conditions such as severe Alzheimer disease or during palliative or hospice care. Osteoporosis medications can put an older adult into the Medicare Part D medication insurance plan "donut hole," or timeframe older adult pays most of the medication expenses out of pocket, which might create adherence problems.

Chronic Kidney Disease

Fractures in patients with chronic kidney disease (CKD; glomerular filtration rate (GFR) less than 60 mL/min/1.73 m^2 [less than 1 mL/s/1.73 m^2] can stem from osteoporosis alone or in combination with chronic kidney disease-mineral and bone disorder (CKD-MBD) or renal osteodystrophy (see Chapters 50, Calcium and Phosphorus Homeostasis, and 44, Chronic Kidney Disease).[100] CKD, especially stages 4 and 5, is a risk factor for fracture, stemming from abnormalities in mineral and bone metabolism that result from progressive kidney disease. Bone turnover markers or sometimes bone biopsy might be necessary to differentiate the different types of bone diseases from osteoporosis in this population.

Vitamin D deficiency exists in 70% of patients with CKD stage 3 (GFR 30-59 mL/min [0.5-0.99 mL/s]) and 83% of patients with CKD stage 4 (GFR 15-29 mL/min [0.25-0.49 mL/s]) disease warranting 25(OH) vitamin D monitoring and replacement when needed. Adequate 25(OH) vitamin D concentrations should be achieved in end stage renal disease patients (CKD 5 – GFR less than 15 mL/min [less than 0.25 mL/s] and CKD5D – dialysis) as well; however, the strength of data are not yet strong.

Antiresorptive therapies would be appropriate for the management of osteoporosis; however, they are contraindicated in patients with osteomalacia or adynamic bone disease and might be ineffective for osteitis fibrosa cystica. In patients with osteoporosis and a CrCl more than 30 mL/min (>0.50 mL/s), routine management can be used (see Fig. 92–3). For patients with osteoporosis and a CrCl less than 30 or 35 mL/min (0.50 or 0.58 mL/s), bisphosphonates are not FDA indicated because of potential drug accumulation. However, limited data suggest oral bisphosphonates appear safe and efficacious in the low numbers of patients studied with CrCl as low as 15 mL/min (0.25 mL/s).[100] Some experts recommend decreasing the bisphosphonate dose by 50% and using the agent for less than 3 years.[80] Bisphosphonates have been associated with nephrotoxicity. Oral bisphosphonates have not been shown to cause renal damage, while zoledronic acid has been associated with an acute tubular necrosis-like reduction in GFR.[100] For this reason, assessment of renal function prior to infusion and proper hydration are important. Denosumab is not renally eliminated and one post-hoc analysis demonstrated reductions in vertebral fractures in patients with a GFR as low as 15 mL/min (0.25 mL/s). Hypocalcemia including severe hypocalcemia is more common in CKD.[84] Kidney and or bone specialists usually provide care to patients with significant kidney disease and osteoporosis.

Drug-Induced Disease

Glucocorticoid-Induced Osteoporosis

(10) Current and prior glucocorticoid use is the most common cause of drug-induced osteoporosis.[101-103] Approximately 30% to 50% of adult patients taking chronic oral glucocorticoids will experience a fracture, with annual fracture rates of 5.1% for vertebral fractures and 2.5% for nonvertebral fractures within the first year of use, changing to 3% for both fracture types for long-term users.[104] All doses and formulations have been associated with increased bone loss and fractures; however, risk is much greater with prednisone doses of 5 mg or more daily or equivalent and oral therapy. Fracture risk is not increased for patients receiving glucocorticoids for adrenal insufficiency. Although a well-documented risk, many patients receiving glucocorticoids are not evaluated and or treated for glucocorticoid-induced osteoporosis (GIO).[105] Various strategies have been tried to increase GIO prevention, assessment and treatment, but suboptimal patient care still existed warranting greater vigilance by all healthcare providers.

Bone losses with glucocorticoids are rapid with up to 12% to 15% loss over the first year, with the greatest decrease occurring in the first 6 months of therapy. Afterward bone loss is about 2% to 3% per year. Trabecular bone is affected more than cortical bone. The pathophysiology of glucocorticoid bone loss is multifactorial. Glucocorticoids decrease bone formation through decreased proliferation and differentiation and enhanced apoptosis of osteoblasts. They can interfere with the bone's natural repair mechanism through increased apoptosis of osteocytes. Glucocorticoids increase bone resorption by increasing RANKL and decreasing OPG. They can reduce estrogen and testosterone concentrations. A negative calcium balance is created from decreased calcium absorption and increased urinary calcium excretion via alterations in calcium transporters. The underlying disease requiring this medication also can affect bone metabolism negatively.

FRAX and central DXA can be used for BMD evaluation.[101-103] Based on FRAX estimates of the 10 year risk of major osteoporotic fracture, the patients are risk stratified; low: less than 10%, medium: 10% to 20%, and high: more than 20%.[103] Since FRAX does not account for specific dose, duration or accumulation, FRAX major osteoporotic fracture risk predictions are decreased by 20% if dose is less than 2.5 mg and increased by 15% if dose is more than 7.5 mg. For hip fracture risk predictions, the adjustments are decreased by 35% and increased by 20%, respectively. Patients are also classified as high risk if DXA T-score of −2.5 or less or a history of fragility fracture. A baseline central DXA is recommended before glucocorticoid initiation. Because of the rapid loss of bone that can occur with oral glucocorticoid therapy, central DXA can be repeated yearly thereafter or more often if needed. A VFA is suggested for patients with significant height loss, pain consistent with a vertebral fracture or spine, or receiving 5 or more mg prednisone or equivalent daily.

All patients using glucocorticoids should practice a bone-healthy lifestyle (described above) and minimize glucocorticoid exposure when possible.[101-103] All patients starting or receiving glucocorticoid therapy (any dose or duration) should ingest 1,200 to 1,500 mg elemental calcium and 800 to 1,200 units of vitamin D daily or more to achieve therapeutic 25 (OH) vitamin D concentrations. Minimizing fall risk is important. Counseling should occur for all patients using this medication for 3 months or more regardless of dose. Glucocorticoids should be used at the lowest dose and for the shortest duration possible. After discontinuation, fracture risk is still higher than never users.[101]

Revisions of the 2010 American GIO guidelines are expected in 2017. The current guidelines divide recommendations for prescription osteoporosis medication use by fracture risk, age, menopause and childbearing status, glucocorticoid dose and duration, and fragility fracture (see Tables 92–9 and 92–10).[103] Alendronate, risedronate, zoledronic acid, and teriparatide have FDA indications for GIO.[101,103] They decrease bone loss with a few studies showing decreased fracture rate with some agents. Raloxifene and denosumab do not have FDA indications, but have some clinical data documenting decreasing bone loss from glucocorticoids. Based on a database analysis, osteoporosis medications have been documented to decrease fracture rates by 48% at 1 year and 32% at 3 years in patients taking glucortiocoids.[105] Standard osteoporosis therapy doses are used. Patients receiving glucocorticoids are considered high risk, and therefore, a bisphosphonate drug holiday is generally not considered. Usually osteoporosis medications are not used in women with childbearing potential or pregnant. For

TABLE 93-9 Therapy to Prevent or Treat Glucocorticoid-Induced Osteoporosis in Postmenopausal Women and Men of More Than 50 Years Old

	Low Risk FRAX <10%	Medium Risk FRAX 10% to 20%	High Risk FRAX >20%, DXA T-score < −2.5, or fragility fracture
Prednisone dose*	<7.5 mg daily for ≥3 months	<7.5 mg daily for ≥3 months	<5 mg daily for ≤1 month
Medication options	No therapy	Alendronate, risedronate	Alendronate, risedronate, zoledronic acid
Prednisone dose[a]	≥7.5 mg daily for ≥3 months	≥7.5 mg daily for ≥3 months	≥5 mg daily for ≤1 month or any dose ≥1 month
Medication options	Alendronate, risedronate, zoledronic acid	Alendronate, risedronate, zoledronic acid	Alendronate, risedronate, zoledronic acid, teriparatide

[a]Or glucocorticoid equivalent.

Data from reference 103.

TABLE 93-10 Therapy to Prevent or Treat Glucocorticoid-Induced Osteoporosis in Premenopausal Women and Men of Less Than 50 Years Old With a Fragility Fracture

Patient	Prednisone 5-7.4 mg Daily for 1-3 Months	Prednisone More Than 7.5 mg Daily for 1-3 Months	Prednisone Less Than 7.5 mg Daily for More Than 3 Months	Prednisone More Than 7.5 mg Daily for More Than 3 Months
Nonchildbearing premenopausal women and men <50 years old	Alendronate and risedronate	Alendronate, risedronate, and zoledronic acid	Alendronate, risedronate, zoledronic acid, and teriparatide	Alendronate, risedronate, zoledronic acid, and teriparatide
Childbearing women	No consensus	No consensus	No consensus	Alendronate, risedronate, and teriparatide

Data from reference 103.

premenopausal and younger men (less than 50 years old) who have already experienced a fragility fracture, osteoporosis medications could be used after explaining risks and paucity of data to drive decisions.

Since glucocorticoids can cause hypogonadism, sometimes hormone therapy will be prescribed. The hormonal therapy for correcting hypogonadism symptoms most likely will have some positive bone effects as well.

Cancer-Treatment–Related Bone Loss

10 Cancers, metastases, and chemotherapies, such as antiandrogen and antiestrogen agents, can cause bone loss and osteoporosis.[106] Chemotherapy-induced ovarian failure can enhance bone loss. Glucocorticoids used as chemotherapy, chemotherapy premedication, and/or treatment for chemotherapy-induced nausea and vomiting also increase bone loss in patients with cancer.

DXA screening is advocated for patients at high risk for osteoporosis, which would include certain chemotherapies and cancers. When using FRAX, secondary osteoporosis can be checked "yes" when premature menopause and hypogonadism caused by chemotherapy and cancer are present.

Certain osteoporosis medications are used to prevent bone loss or treat osteoporosis due to chemotherapy, cancer, and metastases.[106] Bisphosphonates and denosumab decrease chemotherapy-induced bone loss and in some trials fractures.[106-111] These agents might also decrease cancer progression. Most research has been conducted in women with breast cancer and men with prostate cancer. Raloxifene decreases the risk of invasive breast cancer in high-risk women. Teriparatide might be used sometimes but it is contraindicated in patients with prior radiation to the skeleton because of risk for osteosarcoma. Zoledronic acid and denosumab are used for cancer-related hypercalcemia and skeletal-related events and are marketed with different product names since dosages are much higher than for osteoporosis.

Personalized Pharmacotherapy

Bone physiology and pathophysiology are under many genomic and genetic influences, thus isolating one or a few genes for correction will unlikely resolve the osteoporosis public epidemic. Heredity is important since family history, especially of a hip fracture in a parent, is a strong risk factor for osteoporosis development.[3,12] So far, 56 loci have been identified that influence BMD and 14 loci for fracture risk, ranging from impacts on bone resorption (RANKL, OPG) to formation (Wnt, LRP5, and sclerostin).[112] Calcium, vitamin D, and estrogen receptors are also under genetic influence. Studies investigating whether there is an association between response to currently available antifracture drugs and genetic profile have been conflicting. Genetic modulation is in its infancy for osteoporosis prevention and treatment but might lead to new medications and/or the ability to tailor medication choices to an individual's genetic profile.

EVALUATION OF THERAPEUTIC OUTCOMES

Monitoring of the Pharmaceutical Care Plan

Assessment of adherence and tolerability of medication should be performed at each visit. Having a patient repeat back instructions for medication administration will help identify administration problems and enable timely correction. Assessment of fracture, back pain, and height loss can help identify worsening osteoporosis.

To evaluate efficacy, a central DXA BMD measurement can be obtained after 2 years of initiating a medication to monitor response. To minimize test variability, BMD testing should be performed on the same DXA machine. A statistical change needs to be greater than the least significant change for that specific piece of equipment generally more than 2% to 3% for the lumbar spine and 5% to 6% for the femoral neck.[15] Since BMD continues to decrease with aging, no change from baseline can be an acceptable response. Because changes in BMD do not entirely explain changes in fracture risk, many experts believe that decisions on whether or not to continue a particular therapy should not be based solely on BMD response. Central DXAs are repeated every 2 years until BMD is stable, at which time the interval for reassessment could be lengthened. In patients with conditions associated with higher rates of bone loss (eg, glucocorticoid use and certain chemotherapy agents), more frequent monitoring might be warranted.

Bone turnover markers have been used to determine response to an osteoporosis prescription medication.[1,3,35] The patient either provides a first or second morning voiding sample or has blood drawn after an overnight fast to measure the markers 3 to 6 months after therapy initiation. The results are compared to baseline values. Significant changes need to be greater than the least significant change for that test, beyond that no specific guidelines for interpretation exist. Because no consensus on result interpretation and high-test variability exists, these tests are not routinely ordered.

Osteoporosis Services

9 Even with guidelines, many patients are not being evaluated or do not receive appropriate osteoporosis therapy.[1] Following a fracture less than one-quarter of women receive BMD testing or start osteoporosis therapy within 6 months of fracture.[113] Community pharmacies and health fairs can provide osteoporosis screenings using the FRAX tool to estimate fracture risk or ultrasonography to measure heel BMD. Osteoporosis prevention and treatment services have been clinically successful and financially sustainable in the community pharmacy setting[114,115] and as part of pharmacy services in a patient-centered medical home.[116] All healthcare providers should identify and resolve barriers to optimal medication adherence. Some pharmacists are beginning to administer denosumab in community pharmacies to improve adherence and ease of administration. Databases can be

used to identify patients after a low-trauma fracture who have not had a DXA exam or osteoporosis medication started. Many institutions are developing a fracture liaison service, which is generally a multidisciplinary, multifaceted program to increase treated patient numbers and improve osteoporosis treatment outcomes.[113]

To improve patient care, the Centers for Medicare and Medicaid Services have established quality measures centering on improving clinical processes related to screening for or treatment of osteoprososis.[117] Financial incentives tied to these measures could help bridge the gap in quality of care.

Osteomalacia

Osteomalacia is a condition of defective or delayed bone mineralization in adults, known as rickets in children.[118,119] The most common cause of osteomalacia is nutritional deficiency in vitamin D and or calcium intake. Other causes include chronic hypophosphatemia and diseases or medications that alter vitamin D metabolism (eg, long-term anticonvulsants) and certain rare diseases. Patients with osteomalacia present with pathologic fractures and/or deep bone pain, proximal muscle weakness, or no obvious symptoms besides low BMD. Children can present with additional symptoms. Patients with osteomalacia have a low 25(OH) vitamin D concentration (less than 12 ng/mL [mcg/L; less than 30 nmol/L]) and might have an elevated bone-specific alkaline phosphate, hypophosphatemia, and hypocalcemia.

Preventive vitamin D therapy can be considered for those with a history of symptomatic vitamin D deficiency, have conditions or take medications reducing metabolism or intake of vitamin D, and for pregnant women (600 units per day) and infants under 12 months (400 units per day).[119]

For patients with nutritional osteomalacia, high-dose vitamin D–replacement therapy was preferred therapy in the past but now high dose daily oral therapy is being used more frequently.[118,119] Prescription oral vitamin D3 50,000 units once to thrice weekly for at least 10 weeks is a commonly used high dose regimen for adults, which has a longer duration than vitamin D2. Depending on age, 2,000 to 6,000 units of vitamin D3 or D2 daily for 3 months is recommended for children with rickets. Other high-dose oral and intramuscular vitamin D regimens are less common. Adequate daily intake of calcium is also recommended. Once 25(OH) vitamin D concentrations are greater than 30 ng/mL (mcg/L; 75 nmol/L), chronic vitamin D maintenance therapy can be instituted. Oral ergocalciferol 50,000 units once or twice a month or nonprescription cholecalciferol 1,000 to 2,000 units once daily are reasonable maintenance options. For hypophosphatemic osteomalacia, phosphate therapy, and calcitriol are recommended. For secondary osteomalacia, the underlying condition should be treated.

CONCLUSION

Osteoporosis prevention begins at birth and continues throughout life by practicing a bone-healthy lifestyle (adequate calcium and vitamin D intake, exercise, no smoking, minimal alcohol use, and fall prevention). Generally, osteoporosis occurs in postmenopausal women and older men; however, the disease can occur in all ages as a result of secondary causes such as genetics, diseases, and medications. Central DXA can be used for screening, diagnosis, and monitoring and the FRAX tool can be used for screening and to assist in identifying patients at high risk for fracture requiring treatment.

Alendronate, risedronate, zoledronic acid, and denosumab are first-line therapies since these medications decrease hip, nonvertebral, and vertebral fractures. Teriparatide is the only medication that can build bone; however, cost and subcutaneous administration limit its use. Although medications decrease fracture risk, prescribing of osteoporosis medications and patient adherence to such therapy is suboptimal. All healthcare providers need to be actively involved in osteoporosis education, counseling, and prevention across the lifespan and attentive to treatment and medication adherence to prevent osteoporotic fractures in patients with osteoporosis.

DESIRED OUTCOMES

The primary goal of osteoporosis care should be prevention. Optimizing skeletal development and peak bone mass accrual in childhood, adolescence, and early adulthood will ultimately reduce the future incidence of osteoporosis. Once low bone mass or osteoporosis develops, the objective is to stabilize or improve bone mass and strength and prevent fractures. In patients who have already suffered osteoporotic fractures, reducing pain and deformity, improving functional capacity, improving quality of life, and reducing future falls and fractures are the main goals.

ABBREVIATIONS

25(OH) vitamin D	25-hydroxyvitamin D/calcidiol
BMD	bone mineral density
CEE	conjugated equine estrogens
CKD-MBD	chronic kidney disease-mineral and bone disorder
DKK-1	Dickkoff-1
DXA	dual-energy X-ray absorptiometry
EAA	estrogen agonist antagonist
FAK	focal adhesion kinase
FRAX	World Health Organization fracture risk assessment tool
GFR	glomerular filtration rate
GI	gastrointestinal
GIO	glucocorticoid-induced osteoporosis
GSK-3β	glycogen synthase kinase-3β
IOM	Institute of Medicine
LRP5/6	lipoprotein-receptor related protein
NF-κβ	nuclear factor kappa β
OPG	osteoprotegerin
PINP	procollagen type 1 N-terminal propeptide
PPARγ	peroxisome proliferator-activated receptor γ
PTH	parathyroid hormone
PTHrP	parathyroid hormone-related protein
RANK	receptor activator of nuclear factor-κβ
RANKL	receptor activator of nuclear factor-kappa β ligand
runX2	runt-related transcription factor
Scr	tyrosine scr kinase
TRAF-6	tumor necrosis factor receptor associated factor 6
USPSTF	United States Preventive Services Task Force
WHO	World Health Organization
Wnt	wingless tail

REFERENCES

1. Cosman F, de Beur SJ, LeBoff MS, et al. Clinician's guide to prevention and treatment of osteoporosis. *Osteoporos Int* 2014;25:2359-2381.
2. Wright NC, Looker AC, Saag KG, et al. The recent prevalence of osteoporosis and low bone mass in the United States based on bone mineral density at the femoral neck or lumbar spine. *J Bone Miner Res* 2014;29:2520-2526.
3. Management of osteoporosis in postmenopausal women: 2010 position statement of The North American Menopause Society. *Menopause* 2010;17:25-54; quiz 55-26.
4. Watts NB, Adler RA, Bilezikian JP, et al. Osteoporosis in men: an Endocrine Society clinical practice guideline. *J Clin Endocrinol Metab* 2012;97:1802-1822.

5. Brauer CA, Coca-Perraillon M, Cutler DM, Rosen AB. Incidence and mortality of hip fractures in the United States. *JAMA* 2009;302:1573-1579.
6. Watts NB, Bilezikian JP, Camacho PM, et al. American Association of Clinical Endocrinologists medical guidelines for clinical practice for the diagnosis and treatment of postmenopausal osteoporosis. *Endocr Pract* 2010;16(Suppl 3):1-37.
7. Miller PD. Unrecognized and unappreciated secondary causes of osteoporosis. *Endocrinol Metab Clin North Am* 2012;41:613-628.
8. Mirza F, Canalis E. Management of endocrine disease: secondary osteoporosis: pathophysiology and management. *Eur J Endocrinol* 2015;173:R131-R151.
9. Ward LM, Konji VN, MaJ. The management of osteoporosis in children. *Osteoporos Int* 2016;27:2147-2179.
10. Borgelt LM, Vondracek SF. Osteoporosis and osteomalacia. In: Tisdale JE, Miller DA, eds. *Drug-induced Diseases Prevention, Detection, and Management*. 2nd ed. Bethesda, MD: American Society of Health-System Pharmacists. 2010:991-1004.
11. Mazziotti G, Canalis E, Giustina A. Drug-induced osteoporosis: mechanisms and clinical implications. *Am J Med* 2010;123:877-884.
12. McLendon AN, Woodis CB. A review of osteoporosis management in younger premenopausal women. *Womens Health* 2014;10:59-77.
13. O'Sullivan S, Grey A. Adverse skeletal effects of drugs—beyond glucocorticoids. *Clin Endocrinol* 2015;82:12-22.
14. United States Food and Drug Administration. Invokana and invokamet (canagliflozin): drug safety communication—new information on bone fracture risk and decreased bone mineral density. 2015; *http://www.fda.gov/Safety/MedWatch/SafetyInformation/SafetyAlertsforHumanMedicalProducts/ucm461876.htm*. Last accessed, January 19, 2016.
15. Tella SH, Gallagher JC. Prevention and treatment of postmenopausal osteoporosis. *J Steroid Biochem Mol Biol* 2014;142:155-170.
16. Ambrose AF, Cruz L, Paul G. Falls and fractures: a systematic approach to screening and prevention. *Maturitas* 2015;82:85-93.
17. Walsh JS. Normal bone physiology, remodelling and its hormonal regulation. *Surgery* 2015;33:1-6.
18. Stewart AF. Normal physiology of bone and mineral homeostasis. In: Benjamin IJ, Briggs RC, Wing EJ, Fitz JG, eds. *Andreoli and Carpenter's Cecil Essentials of Medicine*. Philadelphia, PA: Saunders. 2016:732-740.
19. Baron R, Hesse E. Update on bone anabolics in osteoporosis treatment: rationale, current status, and perspectives. *J Clin Endocrinol Metab* 2012;97:311-325.
20. Thompson WR, Rubin CT, Rubin J. Mechanical regulation of signaling pathways in bone. *Gene* 2012;503:179-193.
21. Iñiguez-Ariza NM, Clarke BL. Bone biology, signaling pathways, and therapeutic targets for osteoporosis. *Maturitas* 2015;82:245-255.
22. Bringhurst FR, Demay MB, Krane SM, Kronenberg HM. Bone and mineral metabolism in health and disease. In: Kasper DL, Fauci AS, Hauser SL, et al., eds. *Harrison's Principles of Internal Medicine*. 19th ed. McGraw-Hill Companies, Inc. 2015.
23. Xiong J, O'Brien CA. Osteocyte RANKL: new insights into the control of bone remodeling. *J Bone Miner Res* 2012;27:499-505.
24. Oury F. A crosstalk between bone and gonads. *Ann N Y Acad Sci* 2012;1260:1-7.
25. Bouillon R, Van Schoor NM, Gielen E, et al. Optimal vitamin D status: a critical analysis on the basis of evidence-based medicine. *J Clin Endocrinol Metab* 2013;98:E1283-1304.
26. Haines ST, Park SK. Vitamin D supplementation: what's known, what to do, and what's needed. *Pharmacotherapy* 2012;32:354-382.
27. Anagnostis P, Dimopoulou C, Karras S, et al. Sarcopenia in post-menopausal women: is there any role for vitamin D? *Maturitas* 2015;82:56-64.
28. Theodoratou E, Tzoulaki I, Zgaga L, Ioannidis JP. Vitamin D and multiple health outcomes: umbrella review of systematic reviews and meta-analyses of observational studies and randomised trials. *BMJ* 2014;348:g2035.
29. Duque G. Osteoporosis in older persons: current pharmacotherapy and future directions. *Expert Opin Pharmacother* 2013;14:1949-1958.
30. Korpi-Steiner N, Milhorn D, Hammett-Stabler C. Osteoporosis in men. *Clin Biochem* 2014;47:950-959.
31. Syed FA, Ng AC. The pathophysiology of the aging skeleton. *Curr Osteoporos Rep* 2010;8:235-240.
32. Cosman F. Combination therapy for osteoporosis: a reappraisal. *Bonekey Rep* 2014;3:518.
33. Gordon CM, Leonard MB, Zemel BS, Densitometry ISfC. 2013 Pediatric Position Development Conference: executive summary and reflections. *J Clin Densitom* 2014;17:219-224.
34. The International Society for Clinical Densitometry. 2015 ISCD official positions – adult. 2015; *http://www.iscd.org/official-positions/2015-iscd-official-positions-adult/*. Last accessed, January 19, 2016.
35. Morris HA, Eastell R, Jorgensen NR, et al. Clinical usefulness of bone turnover marker concentrations in osteoporosis. *Clinica Chimica Acta* 2016: doi: 10.1016/j.cca.2016.06.036.
36. Marques A, Ferreira RJ, Santos E, et al. The accuracy of osteoporotic fracture risk prediction tools: a systematic review and meta-analysis. *Ann Rheum Dis* 2015;74:1958-1967.
37. Garvan Institute. Fracture risk calculator. *http://www.garvan.org.au/promotions/bone-fracture-risk/calculator/*. Last accessed, January 19, 2016.
38. United States Preventive Services Task Force. Screening for osteoporosis: U.S. Preventive Services Task Force recommendation statement. *Ann Intern Med* 2011;154:356-364.
39. Body JJ, Bergmann P, Boonen S, et al. Non-pharmacological management of osteoporosis: a consensus of the Belgian Bone Club. *Osteoporos Int* 2011;22:2769-2788.
40. Zhu K, Prince RL. Lifestyle and osteoporosis. *Curr Osteoporos Rep* 2015;13:52-59.
41. Tai V, Leung W, Grey A, et al. Calcium intake and bone mineral density: systematic review and meta-analysis. *BMJ* 2015;351:h4183.
42. Weaver CM, Alexander DD, Boushey CJ, et al. Calcium plus vitamin D supplementation and risk of fractures: an updated meta-analysis from the National Osteoporosis Foundation. *Osteoporos Int* 2016;27:367-376.
43. Bolland MJ, Leung W, Tai V, et al. Calcium intake and risk of fracture: systematic review. *BMJ* 2015;351:h4580.
44. Reid IR. Short-term and long-term effects of osteoporosis therapies. *Nat Rev Endocrinol* 2015;11:418-428.
45. Bialo SR, Gordon CM. Underweight, overweight, and pediatric bone fragility: impact and management. *Curr Osteoporos Rep* 2014;12:319-328.
46. National Institutes of Health Office of Dietary Supplements. Calcium dietary supplement fact sheet. 2013; *https://ods.od.nih.gov/factsheets/Calcium-HealthProfessional/*. Last accessed, January 19, 2016.
47. Institute of Medicine. Dietary reference intakes for adequacy: calcium and vitamin D. Dietary reference intakes for calcium and vitamin D. Washington, DC: The National Academies Press; 2011:345-401.
48. USDA national nutrient database for standard reference release 27 nutrients: calcium, Ca (mg). 2015;1-230. *https://ods.od.nih.gov/pubs/usdandb/Calcium-Content.pdf*. Last accessed, January 19, 2016.
49. Mangano KM, Walsh SJ, Insogna KL, et al. Calcium intake in the United States from dietary and supplemental sources across adult age groups: new estimates from the National Health and Nutrition Examination Survey 2003-2006. *J Am Diet Assoc* 2011;111:687-695.
50. USDA national nutrient database for standard reference release 27 nutrients: vitamin D (IU) 2014;1-149. *https://ods.od.nih.gov/pubs/usdandb/VitaminD-Content.pdf*. Last accessed, January 19, 2016.
51. Forrest KY, Stuhldreher WL. Prevalence and correlates of vitamin D deficiency in US adults. *Nutr Res* 2011;31:48-54.
52. Moore CE, Radcliffe JD, Liu Y. Vitamin D intakes of adults differ by income, gender and race/ethnicity in the U.S.A., 2007 to 2010. *Public Health Nutr* 2014;17:756-763.
53. Nieves JW. Skeletal effects of nutrients and nutraceuticals, beyond calcium and vitamin D. *Osteoporos Int* 2013;24:771-786.
54. Wei P, Liu M, Chen Y, Chen DC. Systematic review of soy isoflavone supplements on osteoporosis in women. *Asian Pac J Trop Med* 2012;5:243-248.
55. Yoon V, Maalouf NM, Sakhaee K. The effects of smoking on bone metabolism. *Osteoporos Int* 2012;23:2081-2092.
56. Panel on Prevention of Falls in Older Person American Geriatrics Society, British Geriatrics Society. Summary of the updated American Geriatrics Society/British Geriatrics Society clinical practice guideline for prevention of falls in older persons. *J Am Geriatr Soc* 2011;59:148-157.
57. Enderlin C, Rooker J, Ball S, et al. Summary of factors contributing to falls in older adults and nursing implications. *Geriatr Nurs* 2015;36:397-406.
58. Savage JW, Schroeder GD, Anderson PA. Vertebroplasty and kyphoplasty for the treatment of osteoporotic vertebral compression fractures. *J Am Acad Orthop Surg* 2014;22:653-664.
59. Pinkerton JV, Thomas S. Use of SERMs for treatment in postmenopausal women. *J Steroid Biochem Mol Biol* 2014;142:142-154.
60. Umland EM, Karel L, Santoro N. Bazedoxifene and conjugated equine estrogen: A combination product for the management of

vasomotor symptoms and osteoporosis prevention associated with menopause. Pharmacotherapy. 2016;36:548-561.
61. Effective Heath Care Program Agency for Healthcare Research and Quality. Treatment to prevent osteoporotic fractures: an update. 2012;1-7. *http://effectivehealthcare.ahrq.gov/ehc/products/160/1048/lbd_clin_fin_to_post.pdf.* Last accessed, January 19, 2016.
62. Moyer VA, Force* USPST. Vitamin D and calcium supplementation to prevent fractures in adults: U.S. Preventive Services Task Force recommendation statement. *Ann Intern Med* 2013;158:691-696.
63. Macdonald HM, Garland A, Burr J, et al. Validation of a short questionnaire for estimating dietary calcium intakes. *Osteoporos Int* 2014;25:1765-1773.
64. Wilczynski C, Camacho P. Calcium use in the management of osteoporosis: continuing questions and controversies. *Curr Osteoporos Rep* 2014;12:396-402.
65. Bolland MJ, Barber PA, Doughty RN, et al. Vascular events in healthy older women receiving calcium supplementation: randomised controlled trial. *BMJ* 2008;336:262-266.
66. Weaver CM. Calcium supplementation: is protecting against osteoporosis counter to protecting against cardiovascular disease? *Curr Osteoporos Rep* 2014;12:211-218.
67. Reid IR, Bolland MJ. Calcium risk-benefit updated—new WHI analyses. *Maturitas* 2014;77:1-3.
68. Avenell A, Mak JC, O'Connell D. Vitamin D and vitamin D analogues for preventing fractures in post-menopausal women and older men. *Cochrane Database Syst Rev* 2014;4:CD000227.
69. Lee RH, Weber T, Colon-Emeric C. Comparison of cost-effectiveness of vitamin D screening with that of universal supplementation in preventing falls in community-dwelling older adults. *J Am Geriatr Soc* 2013;61:707-714.
70. Reid IR, Bolland MJ, Grey A. Effects of vitamin D supplements on bone mineral density: a systematic review and meta-analysis. *Lancet* 2014;383:146-155.
71. Holick MF, Binkley NC, Bischoff-Ferrari HA, et al. Evaluation, treatment, and prevention of vitamin D deficiency: an Endocrine Society clinical practice guideline. *J Clin Endocrinol Metab* 2011;96:1911-1930.
72. Tripkovic L, Lambert H, Hart K, et al. Comparison of vitamin D2 and vitamin D3 supplementation in raising serum 25-hydroxyvitamin D status: a systematic review and meta-analysis. *Am J Clin Nutr* 2012;95:1357-1364.
73. Autier P, Gandini S, Mullie P. A systematic review: influence of vitamin D supplementation on serum 25-hydroxyvitamin D concentration. *J Clin Endocrinol Metab* 2012;97:2606-2613.
74. Nigwekar SU, Bhan I, Thadhani R. Ergocalciferol and cholecalciferol in CKD. *Am J Kidney Dis* 2012;60:139-156.
75. Watts NB, Diab DL. Long-term use of bisphosphonates in osteoporosis. *J Clin Endocrinol Metab* 2010;95:1555-1565.
76. Maraka S, Kennel KA. Bisphosphonates for the prevention and treatment of osteoporosis. *BMJ* 2015;351:h3783.
77. Cremers S, Papapoulos S. Pharmacology of bisphosphonates. *Bone* 2011;49:42-49.
78. Eastell R, Walsh JS, Watts NB, Siris E. Bisphosphonates for postmenopausal osteoporosis. *Bone* 2011;49:82-88.
79. Chen L, Wang G, Zheng F, et al. Efficacy of bisphosphonates against osteoporosis in adult men: a meta-analysis of randomized controlled trials. *Osteoporos Int* 2015;26:2355-2363.
80. Miller PD. The kidney and bisphosphonates. *Bone* 2011;49:77-81.
81. Khan AA, Morrison A, Hanley DA, et al. Diagnosis and management of osteonecrosis of the jaw: a systematic review and international consensus. *J Bone Miner Res* 2015;30:3-23.
82. Imaz I, Zegarra P, González-Enríquez J, et al. Poor bisphosphonate adherence for treatment of osteoporosis increases fracture risk: systematic review and meta-analysis. *Osteoporos Int* 2010;21:1943-1951.
83. Adler RA, Fuleihan GE, Bauer DC, et al. Managing osteoporosis in patients on long-term bisphosphonate treatment: report of a task force of the American Society for Bone and Mineral Research. *J Bone Miner Res* 2016;31:1-35.
84. Zaheer S, LeBoff M, Lewiecki EM. Denosumab for the treatment of osteoporosis. *Expert Opin Drug Metab Toxicol* 2015;11:461-470.
85. Eli Lilly Pharmaceuticals Inc. Evista prescribing information. 2011;1-18. *http://pi.lilly.com/us/evista-pi.pdf.* Last accessed, January 19, 2016.
86. Wyeth Pharmaceuticals Inc. Duavee prescribing information. 2015; *http://labeling.pfizer.com/ShowLabeling.aspx?id=1174.* Last accessed, January 16, 2016.
87. United States Food and Drug Administration. Questions and answers: changes to the indicated population for Miacalcin (calcitonin-salmon). 2015; *http://www.fda.gov/Drugs/DrugSafety/PostmarketDrugSafetyInformationforPatientsandProviders/ucm388641.htm.* Last accessed, January 19, 2016.
88. Upsher-Smith Laboratories Inc. Fortical prescribing information. 1-4. *http://www.upsher-smith.com/wp-content/uploads/Calcitonin-Salmon-PI.pdf.* Last accessed, January 19. 2016.
89. North American Menopause Society. The 2012 hormone therapy position statement of The North American Menopause Society. *Menopause* 2012;19:257-271.
90. Eli Lilly Pharmaceuticals Inc. Forteo prescribing information. In: Book Forteo prescribing information. 2015. *http://uspl.lilly.com/forteo/forteo.html#pi.* Last accessed, January 19, 2016.
91. Leder BZ, Tsai JN, Uihlein AV, et al. Denosumab and teriparatide transitions in postmenopausal osteoporosis (the DATA-Switch study): extension of a randomised controlled trial. *Lancet* 2015;386:1147-1155.
92. Lewiecki EM. Combination therapy: the Holy Grail for the treatment of postmenopausal osteoporosis? *Curr Med Res Opin* 2011;27:1493-1497.
93. Ferrari S. Future directions for new medical entities in osteoporosis. *Best Pract Res Clin Endocrinol Metab* 2014;28:859-870.
94. Cohen A, Shane E. Evaluation and management of the premenopausal woman with low BMD. *Curr Osteoporos Rep* 2013;11:276-285.
95. Greenspan SL, Wyman A, Hooven FH, et al. Predictors of treatment with osteoporosis medications after recent fragility fractures in a multinational cohort of postmenopausal women. *J Am Geriatr Soc* 2012;60:455-461.
96. Zarowitz BJ, Cheng LI, Allen C, et al. Osteoporosis prevalence and characteristics of treated and untreated nursing home residents with osteoporosis. *J Am Med Dir Assoc* 2015;16:341-348.
97. Schousboe JT, Ensrud KE, Nyman JA, et al. Universal bone densitometry screening combined with alendronate therapy for those diagnosed with osteoporosis is highly cost-effective for elderly women. *J Am Geriatr Soc* 2005;53:1697-1704.
98. Greenspan SL, Perera S, Nace D, et al. FRAX or fiction: determining optimal screening strategies for treatment of osteoporosis in residents in long-term care facilities. *J Am Geriatr Soc* 2012;60:684-690.
99. Curtis JR, Safford MM. Management of osteoporosis among the elderly with other chronic medical conditions. *Drugs Aging* 2012;29:549-564.
100. Miller PD. Chronic kidney disease and the skeleton. *Bone Res* 2014;2:14044.
101. Whittier X, Saag KG. Glucocorticoid-induced osteoporosis. *Rheum Dis Clin North Am* 2016;42:177-189.
102. Seibel MJ, Cooper MS, Zhou H. Glucocorticoid-induced osteoporosis: mechanisms, management, and future perspectives. *Lancet Diabetes Endocrinol* 2013;1:59-70.
103. Grossman JM, Gordon R, Ranganath VK, et al. American College of Rheumatology 2010 recommendations for the prevention and treatment of glucocorticoid-induced osteoporosis. *Arthritis Care Res (Hoboken)* 2010;62:1515-1526.
104. Amiche MA, Albaum JM, Tadrous M, et al. Fracture risk in oral glucocorticoid users: a Bayesian meta-regression leveraging control arms of osteoporosis clinical trials. *Osteoporos Int* 2015;27:1709-1718.
105. Overman RA, Gourlay ML, Deal CL, et al. Fracture rate associated with quality metric-based anti-osteoporosis treatment in glucocorticoid-induced osteoporosis. *Osteoporos Int* 2015;26:1515-1524.
106. Rizzoli R, Body JJ, Brandi ML, et al. Cancer-associated bone disease. *Osteoporos Int* 2013;24:2929-2953.
107. Early Breast Cancer Trialists' Collaborative Group. Adjuvant bisphosphonate treatment in early breast cancer: meta-analyses of individual patient data from randomised trials. *Lancet* 2015;386:1353-1361.
108. Gnant M, Pfeiler G, Dubsky PC, et al. Adjuvant denosumab in breast cancer (ABCSG-18): a multicentre, randomised, double-blind, placebo-controlled trial. *Lancet* 2015;386:433-443.
109. Butoescu V, Tombal B. Practical guide to bone health in the spectrum of advanced prostate cancer. *Can J Urol* 2014;21:84-92.
110. Mathew A, Brufsky A. Bisphosphonates in breast cancer. *Int J Cancer* 2015;137:753-764.
111. Skolarus TA, Caram MV, Shahinian VB. Androgen-deprivation-associated bone disease. *Curr Opin Urol* 2014;24:601-607.
112. Marini F, Brandi ML. Pharmacogenetics of osteoporosis. *Best Pract Res Clin Endocrinol Metab* 2014;28:783-793.

113. Aizer J, Bolster MB. Fracture liaison services: promoting enhanced bone health care. *Curr Rheumatol Rep* 2014;16:455.
114. Liu Y, Nevins JC, Carruthers KM, et al. Osteoporosis risk screening for women in a community pharmacy. *J Am Pharm Assoc (2003)* 2007;47:521-526.
115. Elias MN, Burden AM, Cadarette SM. The impact of pharmacist interventions on osteoporosis management: a systematic review. *Osteoporos Int* 2011;22:2587-2596.
116. Scott MA, Hitch WJ, Wilson CG, Lugo AM. Billing for pharmacists' cognitive services in physicians' offices: multiple methods of reimbursement. *J Am Pharm Assoc* 2012;52:175-180.
117. Centers for Medicare and Medicaid Services. 2015 physician quality reporting system (PQRS): implementation guide. 2015;1-53. *https://www.cms.gov/apps/ama/license.asp?file=/PQRS/Downloads/PQRS_2015_Measure-List_111014.zip*. Last accessed, January 19, 2016.
118. Weinstein RS. Osteomalacia and rickets. In: Goldman L, Schafer AI, eds. *Goldman-Cecil Medicine*. 25th ed. Philadelphia, PA: Elsevier Saunders. 2016:1645-1649.
119. Munns CF, Shaw N, Kiely M, et al. Global consensus recommendations on prevention and management of nutritional rickets. *J Clin Endocrinol Metab* 2016:jc20152175.

93

Gout and Hyperuricemia

Michelle A. Fravel and Michael E. Ernst

KEY CONCEPTS

1. In the absence of a history of gout, asymptomatic hyperuricemia may not require treatment.
2. Acute gouty arthritis may be treated effectively with short courses of high-dose nonsteroidal anti-inflammatory drugs (NSAIDs), corticosteroids, or colchicine.
3. Low-dose colchicine is highly effective at relieving acute attacks of gout; dose titration leads to more adverse effects but does not improve efficacy.
4. Treatment with urate-lowering drugs to reduce risk of recurrent attacks of gouty arthritis is considered cost-effective for patients having two or more attacks of gout per year.
5. Xanthine oxidase inhibitors are efficacious for the prophylaxis of recurrent gout attacks in both underexcreters and overproducers of uric acid. Either allopurinol or febuxostat should be initiated in patients with one of the following indications for urate-lowering therapy (ULT): (a) two or more gout attacks per year, (b) the presence of one or more tophus, (c) chronic kidney disease (stage 2 or worse), or (d) a history of urolithiasis. The dose of the xanthine oxidase inhibitor should be titrated to a goal serum urate concentration of less than 6 mg/dL (less than 357 μmol/L) (or less than 5 mg/dL [less than 297 μmol/L] if signs of gout persist at a level of 6 mg/dL [357 μmol/L]).
6. Uricosuric agents should be avoided for patients with renal impairment (a creatinine clearance below 50 mL/min [0.83 mL/s]), a history of renal calculi, or overproduction of uric acid.
7. Low-dose colchicine, NSAID, or corticosteroid therapy should be administered during the first 3 to 6 months of urate-lowering therapy (ULT) to minimize the risk of acute gout attacks that may occur during this initiation period.
8. Uric acid nephrolithiasis should be treated with adequate hydration (2-3 L/day), a daytime urine-alkalinizing agent, and 60 to 80 mEq/day (mmol/day) of potassium bicarbonate or potassium citrate.
9. Patients with hyperuricemia or gout should undergo comprehensive evaluation for signs and symptoms of cardiovascular disease, and aggressive management of cardiovascular risk factors (ie, weight loss, reduction of alcohol intake, control of blood pressure, glucose, and lipids) should be undertaken as indicated.

The term *gout* describes a heterogeneous clinical spectrum of diseases including elevated serum urate concentration (hyperuricemia), recurrent attacks of acute arthritis associated with monosodium urate (MSU) crystals in synovial fluid leukocytes, deposits of monosodium urate crystals (tophi) in tissues in and around joints, interstitial renal disease, and uric acid nephrolithiasis.[1]

The underlying metabolic disorder of gout is hyperuricemia, defined physiochemically as serum that is supersaturated with monosodium urate. At 37°C (98.6°F), serum urate concentrations above (or around) 7 mg/dL (416 μmol/L) begin to exceed the limit of solubility for monosodium urate.[1] For determination of the risk of gout, hyperuricemia is defined statistically as serum urate concentrations greater than two standard deviations above the population means for age- and sex-matched healthy populations, usually 7 mg/dL (416 μmol/L) for men and 6 mg/dL (357 μmol/L) for women.[1,2] Although hyperuricemia is fundamental to the development of gout, the mere presence of hyperuricemia itself is often an asymptomatic condition.

EPIDEMIOLOGY

Historically, gout has been referred to as the "disease of kings" since it was often associated with affluent societies and lifestyles of over-indulgence, gluttony, and intemperance.[1] Gout continues to occur more commonly in developed countries (eg, United States, Japan, United Kingdom, and Australia) as compared to developing countries (eg, China).[3] In the United States, the prevalence of gout is increasing. According to data from the 2007 to 2008 National Health and Nutrition Examination Survey (NHANES), the prevalence of gout in US adults is 3.9%, which corresponds to an estimated 8.3 million people. This represents a 1.2% increase in prevalence compared with NHANES-III survey data from 1988 to 1994.[4]

Elevated serum urate levels are the single most important risk factor for the development of gout, and the relationship between the risk of an attack of acute gouty arthritis and serum urate levels is linearly correlated. The 5-year cumulative risk of gout for patients with serum urate concentrations less than 7 mg/dL (less than 416 μmol/L) is 0.6%, compared with a risk of 30.5% for those with urate levels more than 10 mg/dL (more than 595 μmol/L).[5] Sustained elevation of serum urate is virtually essential for the development of gout; however, hyperuricemia does not always lead to gout, and many patients with hyperuricemia remain asymptomatic.[2] Although unusual, acute gouty arthritis has been reported to occur in the presence of normal serum uric acid concentrations.[6] The prevalence of hyperuricemia in the United States mirrors the trend seen with gout, affecting 21.4% of adults (43.3 million people) in 2007 to 2008 compared to just 18.2% in 1998 to 1994.[4]

The increased prevalence of gout and hyperuricemia may be partly explained by the aging of the population. Gout and hyperuricemia occur more commonly in the older adult with the highest prevalence, 12.6%, in those 80 years and older compared with just 0.4% in those between ages 20 and 29 years.[4] Another major contributor to the increased prevalence of gout in the United States is the obesity epidemic. Obese persons are twice as likely to have gout as nonobese counterparts.[7] Dietary and lifestyle factors linked to obesity have also been independently associated with gout. These include consumption of alcohol, sugary beverages, and red meat along with a sedentary lifestyle.[8]

Regarding sex distribution, gout affects men about three times more often than women.[4] The lowest rates of gout are observed in women younger than 45 years, approximately 0.6 cases per 1,000 person-years.[9] Serum uric acid levels in women approach those of men once menopause has occurred; thus, in older age groups the gender gap narrows, and approximately half of newly diagnosed cases of gout are found in women.[10,11] Gout in men younger than 30 years or in premenopausal women may indicate an inherited enzyme defect or the presence of renal disease. Although no genetic marker has been isolated for gout, the familial nature of gout strongly suggests an interaction between genetic and environmental factors.

ETIOLOGY AND PATHOPHYSIOLOGY

In humans, the production of uric acid is the terminal step in the degradation of purines. Uric acid serves no known physiologic purpose and is regarded as a waste product. Normal uric acid levels are near the limits of urate solubility, because of the delicate balance that exists between the amount of urate produced and excreted.[2] Humans have higher uric acid levels than other mammals because they do not express the enzyme uricase, which converts uric acid into the more soluble allantoin.[10]

Gout occurs exclusively in humans in whom a miscible pool of uric acid exists. Under normal conditions, the amount of accumulated uric acid is about 1,200 mg in men and about 600 mg in women. The size of the urate pool is increased several fold in individuals with gout. This excess accumulation may result from either overproduction or underexcretion of uric acid. Several conditions are associated with either decreased renal clearance or an overproduction of uric acid, leading to hyperuricemia. Table 93-1 lists some of these conditions.

Overproduction of Uric Acid

The purines from which uric acid is produced originate from three sources: dietary purine, conversion of tissue nucleic acid into purine nucleotides, and de novo synthesis of purine bases. The purines derived from these three sources enter a common metabolic pathway leading to the production of either nucleic acid or uric acid. Under normal circumstances, uric acid may accumulate excessively if production exceeds excretion. The average human produces about 600 to 800 mg of uric acid each day. Dietary purines play an unimportant role in the generation of hyperuricemia in the absence of some derangement in purine metabolism or elimination. However, diet modifications are important for patients with such problems who develop symptomatic hyperuricemia.

TABLE 93-1 Conditions Associated with Hyperuricemia

Primary gout	Obesity
Diabetic ketoacidosis	Sarcoidosis
Myeloproliferative disorders	Congestive heart failure
Lactic acidosis	Renal dysfunction
Lymphoproliferative disorders	Down syndrome
Starvation	Lead toxicity
Chronic hemolytic anemia	Hyperparathyroidism
Toxemia of pregnancy	Acute alcoholism
Pernicious anemia	Hypoparathyroidism
Glycogen storage disease type 1	Acromegaly
Psoriasis	Hypothyroidism
Hypoxanthine-guanine phosphoribosyltransferase deficiency	Phosphoribosylpyrophosphate synthetase overactivity
Polycythemia vera	Berylliosis
Renal transplantation	

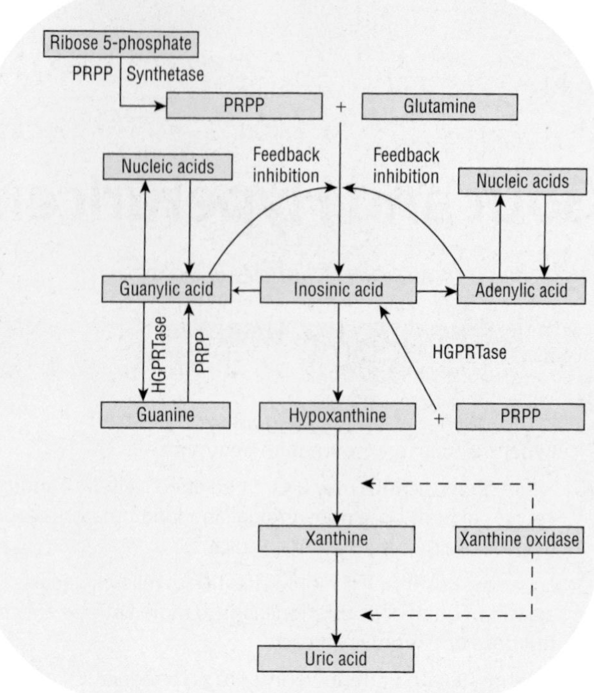

FIGURE 93-1 Purine metabolism. (HGPRT, hypoxanthine-guanine phosphoribosyltransferase; PRPP, phosphoribosyl pyrophosphate.)

Several enzyme systems regulate purine metabolism. Abnormalities in these regulatory systems can result in overproduction of uric acid. Uric acid may also be overproduced as a consequence of increased breakdown of tissue nucleic acids and excessive rates of cell turnover, as observed with myeloproliferative and lymphoproliferative disorders, polycythemia vera, psoriasis, and some types of anemias. Cytotoxic medications used to treat these disorders can result in overproduction of uric acid secondary to lysis and breakdown of cellular matter.

Two enzyme abnormalities resulting in an overproduction of uric acid have been well described (Fig. 93-1). The first is an increase in the activity of phosphoribosyl pyrophosphate (PRPP) synthetase, which leads to an increased concentration of PRPP. PRPP is a key determinant of purine synthesis and uric acid production. The second is a deficiency of hypoxanthine-guanine phosphoribosyltransferase (HGPRT). HGPRT is responsible for the conversion of guanine to guanylic acid and hypoxanthine to inosinic acid. These two conversions require PRPP as the cosubstrate and are important reactions involved in the synthesis of nucleic acids. A deficiency in the HGPRT enzyme leads to increased metabolism of guanine and hypoxanthine to uric acid and to more PRPP to interact with glutamine in the first step of the purine pathway.[12] Complete absence of HGPRT results in the childhood Lesch–Nyhan syndrome, characterized by choreoathetosis, spasticity, intellectual disability, and markedly excessive production of uric acid. A partial deficiency of the enzyme may be responsible for marked hyperuricemia in otherwise normal, healthy individuals.

Underexcretion of Uric Acid

Normally, uric acid does not accumulate as long as production is balanced with elimination. About two-thirds of the daily uric acid production is excreted in the urine and the remainder is eliminated

CLINICAL PRESENTATION Acute Gouty Arthritis

General

- Gout classically presents as an acute inflammatory monoarthritis. The first metatarsophalangeal joint is often involved ("podagra"), but any joint of the lower extremity can be affected and occasionally gout will present as a monoarthritis of the wrist or finger. The spectrum of gout also includes nephrolithiasis, gouty nephropathy, and aggregated deposits of sodium urate (tophi) in cartilage, tendons, synovial membranes, and elsewhere.

Signs and Symptoms

- Fever, intense pain, erythema, warmth, swelling, and inflammation of involved joints.

Laboratory Tests

- Elevated serum uric acid levels; leukocytosis.

Other Diagnostic Tests

- Observation of MSUs in synovial fluid or a tophus.
- For patients with long-standing gout, radiographs may show asymmetric swelling within a joint on or subcortical cysts without erosions.

through the gastrointestinal (GI) tract after enzymatic degradation by colonic bacteria. The vast majority of patients (90%) with gout have a relative decrease in the renal excretion of uric acid for an unknown reason (primary idiopathic hyperuricemia).[2]

A decline in the urinary excretion of uric acid to a level below the rate of production leads to hyperuricemia and an increased miscible pool of sodium urate. Almost all the urate in plasma is freely filtered across the glomerulus. The concentration of uric acid appearing in the urine is determined by multiple renal tubular transport processes in addition to the filtered load. Evidence favors a four-component model including glomerular filtration, tubular reabsorption, tubular secretion, and postsecretory reabsorption.

Approximately 90% of filtered uric acid is reabsorbed in the proximal tubule, probably by both active and passive transport mechanisms. There is a close linkage between proximal tubular sodium reabsorption and uric acid reabsorption, so conditions that enhance sodium reabsorption (eg, dehydration) also lead to increased uric acid reabsorption. The exact site of tubular secretion of uric acid has not been determined; this too appears to involve an active transport process. Postsecretory reabsorption occurs somewhere distal to the secretory site. Table 93-2 lists the drugs that decrease renal clearance of uric acid through modification of filtered load or one of the tubular transport processes. By enhancing renal urate reabsorption, insulin resistance is also associated with gout.

The pathophysiologic approach to the evaluation of hyperuricemia requires determining whether the patient is overproducing or underexcreting uric acid. This can be accomplished by placing the patient on a purine-free diet for 3 to 5 days and then measuring the amount of uric acid excreted in the urine in 24 hours. As it is very difficult to maintain a purine-free diet for several days, this test is done infrequently in clinical practice. Nevertheless, when it is performed, individuals who excrete more than 600 mg on a purine-free diet may be considered overproducers. Hyperuricemic individuals who excrete less than 600 mg of uric acid per 24 hours on a purine-free diet may be classified as underexcreters of uric acid.

TABLE 93-2 Drugs Capable of Inducing Hyperuricemia and Gout

Diuretics	Ethanol	Ethambutol
Nicotinic acid	Pyrazinamide	Cytotoxic drugs
Salicylates (<2 g/day)	Levodopa	Cyclosporine

On a regular diet, excretion of more than 1,000 mg per 24 hours reflects overproduction; less than this is probably normal.

CLINICAL PRESENTATION

1 Gout is diagnosed clinically by symptoms rather than laboratory tests of uric acid. In fact, asymptomatic hyperuricemia discovered incidentally generally requires no therapy because many individuals with hyperuricemia will never experience an attack of gout. These patients should still be encouraged to implement lifestyle measures to reduce serum urate concentrations.

Acute Gouty Arthritis

A classic acute attack of gouty arthritis is characterized by rapid and localized onset of excruciating pain, swelling, and inflammation. The attack is typically monoarticular at first, most often affecting the first metatarsophalangeal joint (great toe) and then, in order of frequency, the insteps, ankles, heels, knees, wrists, fingers, and elbows. In one half of initial attacks, the first metatarsophalangeal joint is affected, a condition commonly referred to as *podagra* (Fig. 93-2). Up to 90% of patients with gout will experience podagra at some point in the course of their disease.[2]

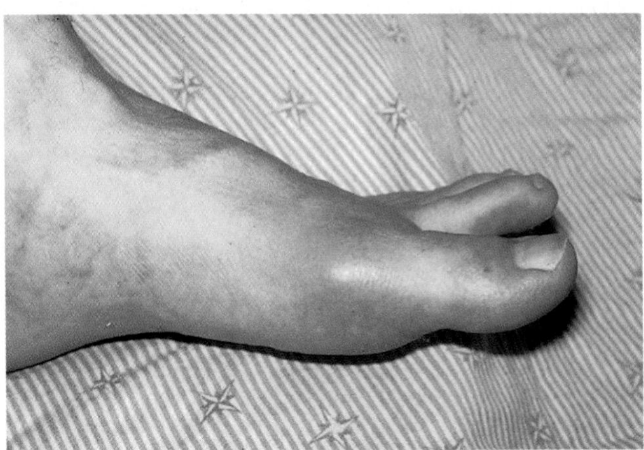

FIGURE 93-2 Acute gout attack of the first metatarsophalangeal joint. *(Reproduced with permission from Imboden J, Hellmann DB, Stone JH. Current Rheumatology Diagnosis and Treatment, 2nd ed. New York: McGraw-Hill, 2004:316.)*

TABLE 93-3 Clinical Manifestations of Gout

Classic acute gout ("podagra")	Monoarticular arthritis Frequently attacks the first metatarsophalangeal joint, although other joints of the lower extremities are also frequently involved Affected joint is swollen, erythematous, and tender
Interval gout	Asymptomatic period between attacks
Tophaceous gout	Deposits of monosodium urate crystals in soft tissues Complications include soft tissue damage, deformity, joint destruction, and nerve compression syndromes such as carpal tunnel syndrome
Atypical gout	Polyarthritis affecting any joint, upper or lower extremity May be confused with rheumatoid arthritis or osteoarthritis
Gouty nephropathy	Nephrolithiasis Acute and chronic renal impairment

Atypical presentations of gout also occur. For elderly patients, gout can present as a chronic polyarticular arthritis that can be confused with rheumatoid arthritis or osteoarthritis. Additionally, the onset of gout may be less dramatic than the typical acute attack and have fewer clinical findings.[13] Multiple small joints in the hands may be involved, especially in elderly women.[10] Table 93-3 summarizes the different clinical manifestations of gout.

The predilection of acute gout for peripheral joints of the lower extremity is probably related to the low temperature of these joints combined with high intra-articular urate concentration. Synovial effusions are likely to occur transiently in weight-bearing joints during the course of a day with routine activity. At night, water is reabsorbed from the joint space, leaving behind a supersaturated solution of monosodium urate, which can precipitate attacks of acute arthritis. Attacks generally begin at night with the patient awakened from sleep by excruciating pain.

The development of crystal-induced inflammation involves a number of chemical mediators causing vasodilation, increased vascular permeability, complement activation, and chemotactic activity for polymorphonuclear leukocytes.[14] Phagocytosis of urate crystals by the leukocytes results in rapid lysis of cells and a discharge of lysosomal and proteolytic enzymes into the cytoplasm. The ensuing inflammatory reaction is associated with intense joint pain, erythema, warmth, and swelling. Fever is common, as is leukocytosis. Untreated attacks may last from 3 to 14 days before spontaneous recovery.

Although acute attacks of gouty arthritis may occur without apparent provocation, a number of conditions may precipitate an attack. These include stress, trauma, alcohol ingestion, infection, surgery, rapid lowering of serum uric acid by ingestion of uric acid-lowering agents, and ingestion of certain drugs known to elevate serum uric acid concentrations (see Table 93-2). Other crystal-induced arthropathies that may resemble gout on clinical presentation are caused by calcium pyrophosphate dihydrate crystals (pseudogout) and calcium hydroxyapatite crystals, which are associated with calcific periarthritis, tendinitis, and arthritis.[14-17] Acute flares of gouty arthritis may occur infrequently, but over time the interval between attacks may shorten if appropriate measures to correct hyperuricemia are not undertaken. Later in the disease, tophaceous deposits of MSUs in the skin or subcutaneous tissues may be found. These tophi can be anywhere but are often found on the hands, wrists, elbows, or knees. It is estimated to take 10 or more years for tophi to develop.

TABLE 93-4 Differential Diagnosis of Acute Monoarthritis

1. Pseudogout (pyrophosphate crystal-related arthritis)
2. Palindromic rheumatism
3. Seronegative inflammatory arthritis
4. Trauma or hemarthrosis
5. Septic arthritis
6. Cellulitis
7. Type II dyslipidemia
8. Unrelated hyperuricemia (as in psoriasis, hypertension) when joint pain is not caused by gout

Diagnostic Evaluation

Table 93-4 lists the differential diagnosis of an acute monoarthritis.[18,19] A definitive diagnosis of gout requires aspiration of synovial fluid from the affected joint and identification of intracellular crystals of monosodium urate monohydrate in synovial fluid leukocytes.[2] Identification of MSUs is highly dependent on the experience of the observer. Crystals are needle-shaped, and when examined under polarizing light microscopy, they are strongly negatively birefringent (Fig. 93-3). Crystals can be observed in synovial fluid during asymptomatic periods.[20] If an affected joint is tapped, the resulting synovial fluid may have white cells and appear purulent. Such findings should always raise the question of infection. If any clinical features of infection are present, such as high fever, elevated white blood cell count, multiple joints affected, or an identified source of infection, proper diagnosis and treatment are critical. Patients with gout can have septic arthritis. Diabetes, alcohol abuse, and advanced age increase the likelihood of septic arthritis.

In lieu of obtaining a synovial fluid sample from an affected joint to inspect for urate crystals, the clinical triad of inflammatory monoarthritis, elevated serum uric acid level, and response to colchicine can be used to diagnose gout. However, this approach has limitations, including a failure to recognize atypical gout presentations and the fact that serum uric acid levels can be normal or even low during an acute gout attack.[2,5,21] In addition, use of colchicine as a diagnostic tool for gout is limited by lack of sensitivity and specificity for the disease. Other conditions such as psoriatic arthritis, sarcoidosis, and Mediterranean fever can respond to colchicine therapy. For patients with long-standing gout, radiographs may show punched-out marginal erosions and secondary osteoarthritic

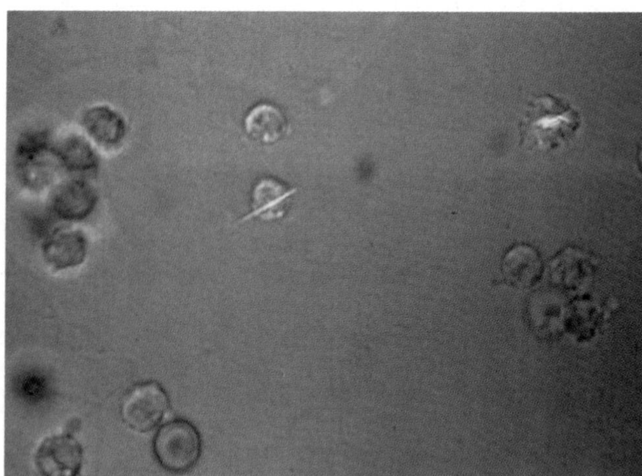

FIGURE 93-3 Urate crystal ingested by a polymorphonuclear leukocyte in synovial fluid. *(Reproduced with permission from Imboden J, Hellmann DB, Stone JH. Current Rheumatology Diagnosis and Treatment, 2nd ed. New York: McGraw-Hill, 2004:317.)*

TABLE 93-5 EULAR Evidence-Based Recommendations for Gout: Diagnostic Principles

1. In acute attacks the rapid development of severe pain, swelling, and tenderness that reaches its maximum within just 6-12 hours, especially with overlying erythema, is highly suggestive of crystal inflammation though not specific for gout
2. For typical presentations of gout (such as recurrent podagra with hyperuricemia), a clinical diagnosis alone is reasonably accurate but not definitive without crystal confirmation
3. Demonstration of MSU crystals in synovial fluid or tophus aspirates permits a definitive diagnosis of gout
4. A routine search for MSU crystals is recommended in all synovial fluid samples obtained from undiagnosed inflamed joints
5. Identification of MSU crystals from asymptomatic joints may allow definite diagnosis in intercritical periods
6. Gout and sepsis may coexist. When septic arthritis is suspected, gram staining and culture of synovial fluid should still be performed, even if MSU crystals are identified
7. While the most important risk factor for gout, serum uric acid levels do not confirm or exclude gout, as many people with hyperuricemia do not develop gout, and during acute attacks serum levels may be normal
8. Renal uric acid excretion should be determined in selected gout patients, especially those with a family history of young onset gout, onset of gout under age 25 years, or with renal calculi
9. Although radiographs may be useful for differential diagnosis and may show typical features in chronic gout, they are not useful in confirming the diagnosis of early or acute gout
10. Risk factors for gout and associated comorbidity should be assessed, including features of the metabolic syndrome (obesity, hyperglycemia, hyperlipidemia, hypertension)

EULAR, The European League Against Rheumatism; MSU, monosodium urate.
Data from Reference 22.

changes; however, in an acute first attack radiographs will be unremarkable.[19,22] The presence of chondrocalcinosis on radiographs may indicate pseudogout. Some studies have recently examined the use of magnetic resonance imaging and computed tomography to obtain images for patients with gout; however, this is not currently considered part of normal practice. Table 93-5 shows the European League Against Rheumatism (EULAR) evidence-based diagnostic principles.[22]

Recently, the American College of Rheumatology (ACR) and EULAR jointly developed recommendations for the classification of gout for the purpose of assisting in identifying subjects potentially eligible for enrollment into clinical trials of gout treatments.[23] Although they specifically state the recommendations should not be used clinically to diagnose gout, the classification system may be a useful reference when evaluating a patient presenting with symptoms suggestive of gout. The recommendations include a point-based system that includes clinical, laboratory, and imaging information, which can be used when a patient presents with at least one episode of swelling, pain, or tenderness in a peripheral joint or bursa but has no evidence of MSU crystals. An online calculator is available at http://goutclassificationcalculator.auckland.ac.nz/.

Uric Acid Nephrolithiasis

Clinicians should be suspicious of hyperuricemic states for patients who present with kidney stones, as nephrolithiasis occurs in approximately 15% of patients with gout.[24] The frequency of urolithiasis depends on serum uric acid concentrations, acidity of the urine, and urinary uric acid concentration. Typically, patients with uric acid nephrolithiasis have a urinary pH of less than 6. Uric acid has a negative logarithm of the acid ionization constant of 5.5. Therefore, when the urine is acidic, uric acid exists primarily in the unionized, less soluble form. At a urine pH of 5, urine is saturated at a uric acid level of 15 mg/dL (0.89 mmol/L). When the urine pH is 7, the solubility of uric acid in urine is increased to 200 mg/dL (11.9 mmol/L).[1] For patients with uric acid nephrolithiasis, urinary pH typically is less than 6 and frequently less than 5.5. When acidic urine is saturated with uric acid, spontaneous precipitation of stones may occur.

Other factors that predispose individuals to uric acid nephrolithiasis include excessive urinary excretion of uric acid and highly concentrated urine. The risk of renal calculi approaches 50% in individuals whose renal excretion of uric acid exceeds 1,100 mg/day (6.5 mmol/day). In addition to pure uric acid stones, hyperuricosuric individuals are at increased risk for mixed uric acid–calcium oxalate stones and pure calcium oxalate stones. Uric acid stones are usually small, round, and radiolucent. Uric acid stones containing calcium are radiopaque.[25]

Gouty Nephropathy

There are two types of gouty nephropathy: acute uric acid nephropathy and chronic urate nephropathy.[2] In acute uric acid nephropathy, acute renal failure occurs as a result of blockage of urine flow secondary to massive precipitation of uric acid crystals in the collecting ducts and ureters. This syndrome is a well-recognized complication for patients with myeloproliferative or lymphoproliferative disorders and is a result of massive malignant cell turnover, particularly after initiation of chemotherapy.

Chronic urate nephropathy is caused by the long-term deposition of urate crystals in the renal parenchyma. Microtophi may form, with a surrounding giant-cell inflammatory reaction. A decrease in the kidneys' ability to concentrate urine and the presence of proteinuria may be the earliest pathophysiologic disturbances. Hypertension and nephrosclerosis are common associated findings. Although renal failure occurs in a higher percentage of gouty patients than expected, it is not clear if hyperuricemia per se has a harmful effect on the kidneys. The chronic renal impairment seen in individuals with gout may result largely from the coexistence of hypertension, diabetes mellitus, and atherosclerosis.

Tophaceous Gout

Tophi (urate deposits) are uncommon in the general population of gouty subjects and are a late complication of hyperuricemia. The most common sites of tophaceous deposits for patients with recurrent acute gouty arthritis are the base of the fingers, olecranon bursae, ulnar aspect of the forearm, Achilles tendon, knees, wrists, and hands (Fig. 93-4).[2] Eventually, even the hips, shoulders, and spine may be affected. In addition to causing obvious deformities, tophi may damage surrounding soft tissue, cause joint destruction and pain, and even lead to nerve compression syndromes including carpal tunnel syndrome.

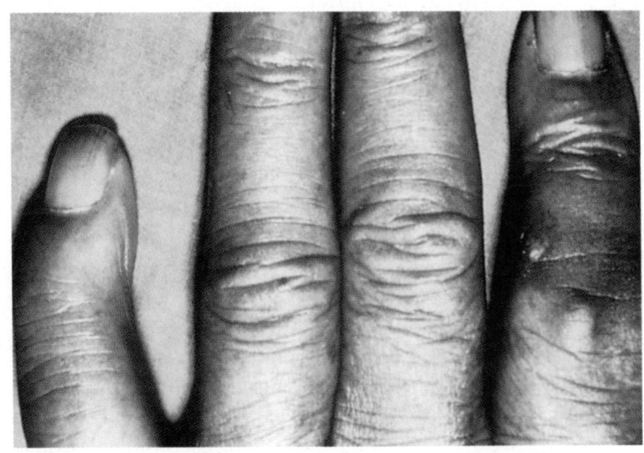

FIGURE 93-4 Tophaceous gout with subcutaneous nodule almost breaking through the skin. *(Reproduced with permission from South-Paul JE, Matheny SC, Lewis EL. Current Diagnosis and Treatment in Family Medicine. New York: McGraw-Hill, 2004:275.)*

TREATMENT

Desired Outcomes

The goals in the treatment of gout are to terminate the acute attack, prevent recurrent attacks of gouty arthritis, and prevent complications associated with chronic deposition of urate crystals in tissues. These can be accomplished through a combination of pharmacologic and nonpharmacologic methods, including focused patient education efforts. The first-ever ACR evidence- and consensus-based guidelines for the management of gout were published in 2012.[26,27] These guidelines provide specific recommendations for treatment of acute gout attacks, management of hyperuricemia in gout, and anti-inflammatory prophylaxis of acute gout during initiation of urate-lowering therapy (ULT). These guidelines will be discussed throughout the remainder of the treatment section of this chapter. Tables 93-6 and 93-7 summarize dosing and monitoring information for available pharmacotherapy used in management and prevention of gout.

Acute Gouty Arthritis

Nonpharmacologic Therapy

There are limited effective nonpharmacologic therapies for an acute gout attack; therefore, they are recommended strictly as adjunctive treatment.

Local ice application is the most effective.[27] In one small study, adjunctive ice application resulted in significantly greater pain reduction in those receiving the therapy compared with those not treated with ice (difference of 3.33 cm on a 10-cm visual analog pain scale, $P = 0.021$).[28] Complementary and alternative medicines, including flaxseed and celery root, are not recommended in ACR guidelines.[27]

Pharmacologic Therapy

2 For most patients, acute attacks of gouty arthritis may be treated successfully with nonsteroidal anti-inflammatory drugs (NSAIDs), corticosteroids, or colchicine. The ACR guidelines recognize these three modalities as first-line monotherapy for the treatment of acute gout. Treatment should commence within 24 hours of the onset of an attack. In more severe cases, those affecting multiple joints or causing higher intensity pain, combination or investigational drug therapy may be indicated (Fig. 93-5).[27]

Nonsteroidal Anti-Inflammatory Drugs NSAIDs are a mainstay of therapy for acute attacks of gouty arthritis because of their excellent efficacy and minimal toxicity with short-term use. Indomethacin has been historically favored as the NSAID of choice for acute gout flares, but there is little evidence to support one NSAID as being more efficacious than another. Three agents (indomethacin, naproxen, and sulindac) have US Food and Drug Administration (FDA)-approved labeling for the treatment of gout, although several others are likely to be effective.[27] Although choice of NSAID is not an important determinant of therapeutic success, timing of pharmacotherapy is. It is critical that therapy is initiated within 24 hours of acute gout attack onset and continued until complete resolution.[27] Following resolution of the attack, tapering of NSAID therapy may be considered, especially in patients with comorbidities such as hepatic or renal insufficiency where prolonged therapy would be undesirable.[27] Resolution of an acute attack for most patients generally occurs within 5 to 8 days after initiating therapy.

All NSAIDs have the potential to cause similar adverse effects. The most common areas affected include the GI system (gastritis, bleeding, perforation), kidneys (renal papillary necrosis, reduced creatinine clearance), cardiovascular system (sodium and fluid retention, increased blood pressure), and central nervous system (CNS) (impaired cognitive function, headache, dizziness). Caution should be exercised when using NSAIDs for individuals with a history of peptic ulcer disease, congestive heart failure, uncontrolled hypertension, renal insufficiency, coronary artery disease, or who are concurrently receiving anticoagulants or antiplatelets. Patients with active peptic ulcer disease, uncompensated congestive heart failure, severe renal impairment, or a history of hypersensitivity to aspirin or other NSAIDs should not be prescribed an NSAID.

Selective cyclooxygenase-2 (COX-2) inhibitors present a potentially better tolerated alternative to nonselective NSAIDs in patients with GI issues.[29] Specific COX-2 inhibitors, etoricoxib and lumiracoxib, have demonstrated efficacy in the treatment of acute gout in numerous controlled trials; however, these agents are not available in the United States. One study has established effectiveness of high-dose celecoxib (1,200 mg on day 1 followed by 400 mg twice daily thereafter) in the treatment of acute gout, but concerns regarding the cardiovascular risk of COX-2 inhibitors must be considered when using these agents (see Chapter 90, Osteoarthritis, for further discussion of COX-2 inhibitors).[30,31] The ACR guidelines recommend celecoxib as an option for patients unable to take NSAIDs but note that the risk-to-benefit ratio of celecoxib use in acute gout is unclear.[27]

Corticosteroids Corticosteroids have historically been reserved for treatment of acute gout flares when contraindications to other therapies exist, largely due to lack of evidence from controlled clinical trials. However, more recent evidence indicates that corticosteroids are equivalent to NSAIDs in the treatment of acute gout flares.[32,33] They can be used either systemically or by intra-articular injection. The ACR guidelines recommend that the number of joints involved be considered when choosing the route of corticosteroid administration. If only one or two joints are involved, either intraarticular or oral corticosteroids are recommended. If an attack is polyarticular, systemic therapy is necessary.[27] A hypothetical risk for a rebound attack upon steroid withdrawal exists; therefore, gradual tapering is often employed when discontinuing steroid therapy. The ACR guidelines suggest two different dosing strategies for oral corticosteroid therapy (prednisone or prednisolone) in the treatment of acute gout: (a) 0.5 mg/kg daily for 5 to 10 days followed by abrupt discontinuation or (b) 0.5 mg/kg daily for 2 to 5 days followed by tapering for 7 to 10 days. The guidelines also support the use of a methylprednisolone dose pack for acute treatment of gout, a 6-day regimen that starts with 24 mg on day 1 and decreases by 4 mg each day.[27] Intra-articular administration of triamcinolone acetonide in a dose of 20 to 40 mg may be useful in treating acute gout limited to one or two joints. Injection should be done under an aseptic technique in a joint determined not to be infected. Per ACR guideline recommendations, intra-articular corticosteroid therapy should be used in conjunction with either an NSAID, colchicine, or oral corticosteroid therapy; however, case reports suggest that this therapeutic approach may be as effective as monotherapy.[27,34] A single intramuscular injection of a long-acting corticosteroid, such as methylprednisolone, followed by oral corticosteroid therapy is recognized as a reasonable therapeutic approach to the treatment of acute gout by the ACR guidelines.[27] Alternatively, intramuscular corticosteroid monotherapy may be considered in patients with multiple affected joints who are unable to take oral therapy.

The adverse effects of corticosteroids are generally dose and duration dependent. Short-term use for treatment of acute attacks is generally well tolerated. Corticosteroids should be used with caution for patients with diabetes as they can increase blood sugar. In addition, patients with a history of GI problems, bleeding disorders, cardiovascular disease, and psychiatric disorders should be monitored closely. Long-term corticosteroid use should be avoided because of the risk for osteoporosis, hypothalamic–pituitary axis

TABLE 93-6 Pharmacotherapy of Acute Gout, Anti-Inflammatory Prophylaxis during Initiation of Urate-Lowering Therapy and Hyperuricemia in Gout[a]

Drug	Brand Name	Initial Dose	Usual Range	Special Population Dose	Other
Acute Gout					
NSAIDs					In general, not recommended in patients with advanced renal disease as NSAID use may decrease renal function; Use with caution in patients with mild to moderate renal impairment
Etodolac	Lodine, various	300 mg twice daily	300-500 mg twice daily		
Fenoprofen	Nalfon, various	400 mg three times daily	400-600 mg three to four times daily		
Ibuprofen	Advil, various	400 mg three times daily	400-800 mg three to four times daily		
Indomethacin	Indocin	50 mg three times daily	50 mg three times daily initially until pain is tolerable then rapidly reduce to complete cessation		
Ketoprofen	Orudis, various	75 mg three times daily or 50 mg four times daily	50-75 mg three to four times daily	Severe renal impairment (GFR <25 mL/min [0.42 mL/s]): 100 mg maximum daily dose Mildly impaired renal function: 150 mg maximum daily dose Impaired liver function with serum albumin <3.5 g/dL (<35 g/L): 100 mg maximum daily dose	
Naproxen	Naprosyn, various	750 mg followed by 250 mg every 8 hours until the attack has subsided		Not recommended in severe renal impairment (creatinine clearance <30 mL/min [<0.5 mL/s])	
Piroxicam	Feldene	20 mg once daily or divided twice daily			
Sulindac	Clinoril	200 mg twice a day	150-200 mg twice daily for 7-10 days		
Celecoxib	Celebrex	800 mg followed by 400 mg on day one then 400 mg twice daily for 1 week			Option for patients with GI contraindications to nonselective NSAIDs; unclear risk-to-benefit ratio at this time due to cardiovascular concerns
Oral colchicine	Colcrys	1.2 mg initially, followed by 0.6 mg 1 hour later		See Table 94-8	Dose adjustment recommended when used with selected CYP3A4 and P-glycoprotein inhibitors
Corticosteroids					
Oral		0.5 mg/kg prednisone equivalent daily for 5-10 days followed by discontinuation or 0.5 mg/kg daily for 2-5 days followed by tapering for 7-10 days	30-60 mg prednisone equivalent once daily for 3-5 days, then taper in 5-mg decrements spread over 10-14 days until discontinuation		The use of an oral methylprednisolone dose pack may be considered
Intramuscular		Triamcinolone acetonide 60 mg IM once; methylprednisolone 100 mg IM once	Triamcinolone acetonide 60 mg IM once; methylprednisolone 100-150 mg IM daily for 1-2 days		Administration of intramuscular triamcinolone is to be followed by oral prednisone or prednisolone
Intra-articular	Kenalog	Triamcinolone acetonide 10 mg (large joints), 5 mg (small joints)	Triamcinolone acetonide 10-40 mg (large joints), 5-20 mg (small joints)		Intraarticular administration is acceptable when only one to two joints involved and should be used in combination with NSAIDs, colchicine, or oral corticosteroids
Corticotropin	H.P. Acthar Gel	40 units IM or SC every 72 hours	40-80 units IM or SC every 24-72 hours		Contraindicated for IV administration
Interleukin-1 inhibitors					Reserve use for refractory cases
Anakinra	Kineret	100 mg SC daily for 3 days			
Canakinumab	Ilaris	Single dose 150 mg SC			

(*continued*)

TABLE 93-6 Pharmacotherapy of Acute Gout, Anti-Inflammatory Prophylaxis during Initiation of Urate-Lowering Therapy and Hyperuricemia in Gout[a] (*Continued*)

Drug	Brand Name	Initial Dose	Usual Range	Special Population Dose	Other
Anti-Inflammatory Prophylaxis during Initiation of Urate-Lowering Therapy					
NSAIDs			Lowest effective dosage		
Oral colchicine	Colcrys	0.6 mg daily	0.6 mg once or twice daily	See Table 93-8	
Prednisone or prednisolone		≤10 mg daily			Second-line therapy; recommended only if colchicine and NSAIDs are both contraindicated, ineffective or not tolerated
Interleukin-1 inhibitors					Reserve use for refractory cases Studied for 16-week duration
Rilonacept	Arcalyst	320 mg loading dose followed by 160 mg weekly (SC)			
Canakinumab	Ilaris	Single SC dose (50 mg-300 mg) or four times weekly SC dosing (50 mg—50 mg—25 mg—25 mg)			
Hyperuricemia in Gout					
Xanthine oxidase inhibitors					
Allopurinol	Lopurin, Zyloprim	100 mg daily	100-800 mg daily to achieve serum urate concentration <6 mg/dL (<357 μmol/L)	Start at dose of 50 mg daily for patients with a glomerular filtration rate <30 mL/min/1.73 m² (<0.29 mL/s/m²)	
Febuxostat	Uloric	40 mg daily	40-80 mg/daily	No dosage adjustment necessary for patients with mild-moderate renal dysfunction (creatinine clearance 30-89 mL/min [0.5-1.49 mL/s]) Insufficient data in patients with creatinine clearance <30 mL/min (<0.5 mL/s)	
Uricosurics					
Probenecid	Probalan	250 mg twice daily for 1 week	500-2,000 mg/day (target serum urate concentration <6 mg/dL [<357 mol/L])	Not recommended if creatinine clearance <50 mL/min (<0.83 mL/s)	
Other					
Pegloticase	Krystexxa	8 mg IV every 2 weeks			Optimal treatment duration has not been established
Lesinurad	Zurampic	200 mg once daily in combination with a xanthine oxidase inhibitor		Not recommended if creatinine clearance <45 mL/min (<0.75 mL/s) Not studied in patients with severe hepatic disease Contraindicated in tumor lysis syndrome and Lesch-Nyhan Syndrome	Should be used in combination with a xanthine oxidase inhibitor due to increased risk of acute renal failure with lesinurad monotherapy Use is not recommended in patients taking allopurinol doses <300 mg daily (normal renal function) or <200 mg daily (creatinine clearance <60 mL/min)

CYP, cytochrome P; GFR, glomerular filtration rate; IM, intramuscular; IV, intravenous; NSAID, nonsteroidal anti-inflammatory drug; SC, subcutaneous.

[a]Agents available in the United States.

suppression, cataracts, and muscle deconditioning that can occur with their use.

Corticotropin, or adrenocorticotropic hormone (ACTH), which stimulates the adrenal cortex to produce cortisol and corticosterone, can be administered in acute gout. Doses of 40 to 80 United States Pharmacopeia (USP) units are given intramuscularly every 6 to 8 hours for 2 to 3 days, and then discontinued. Studies with ACTH are limited, but it appears to provide similar efficacy to systemic antiinflammatory doses of corticosteroids.[35] When administered alone or in combination with colchicine, ACTH may provide earlier efficacy compared with indomethacin but with fewer adverse effects.[36] Because the studies have several limitations, the regimen should be considered only as an alternative, especially for patients with comorbidities where other regimens are contraindicated.[37] Examples of patients where ACTH has been used safely when other first-line gout therapies were contraindicated include those

TABLE 93-7 Drug Monitoring

Drug	Adverse Drug Reaction	Monitoring Parameter	Comments
NSAIDs	Renal dysfunction, gastritis (worse with concurrent aspirin), fluid retention, blood pressure elevation	Therapeutic Resolution of pain Avoidance of gout attacks when used for prophylaxis Toxic Blood pressure Renal function Edema Dark stools	Avoid for patients with peptic ulcer disease, active bleeding Use caution in congestive heart failure, dehydration, renal impairment Consider coadministration with a proton-pump inhibitor when used long term for patients at risk for GI bleeding
Systemic corticosteroids	GI upset, increased appetite, nervousness/restlessness, transient glucose intolerance, fluid retention, blood pressure elevation	Therapeutic Resolution of pain Avoidance of gout attacks when used for prophylaxis Toxic Glucose levels in patients with diabetes	Limit duration of therapy in patients with diabetes
Intra-articular corticosteroids	Injection pain, rebound arthritis	Therapeutic Resolution of pain Toxic Signs of rebound arthritis (pain relief followed by reemergence of pain)	Avoid if joint sepsis cannot be ruled out
Corticotropin	Increased appetite, nervousness/restlessness, transient glucose intolerance, fluid retention, blood pressure elevation	Therapeutic Resolution of pain	Requires intact pituitary–adrenal axis Less effective for patients receiving long-term oral corticosteroid therapy
Colchicine	Dose-dependent GI adverse effects (diarrhea, nausea, vomiting), rare myelosuppression, and reversible neuromyopathy	Therapeutic Resolution of pain Avoidance of gout attacks when used for prophylaxis Toxic GI symptoms Complete blood count	
Interleukin-1 inhibitors	Injection site reaction, neutropenia, immune hypersensitivity reaction, infectious disease, malignancy	Therapeutic Resolution of pain Avoidance of gout attacks when used for prophylaxis Toxic Neutrophil count (prior to initiation, monthly for the first 3 months of therapy then after 6, 9, and 12 months of therapy) Temperature (periodically to detect infection)	Safety for use in acute gout and gout prophylaxis during initiation of urate-lowering therapy has not yet been established; not FDA approved for use in gout
Allopurinol	Rash, potential for fatal hypersensitivity syndrome	Therapeutic Serum urate level Reduced frequency of gout attacks Toxic Rash Renal function	Can be used in both urate overproduction and urate underexcretion
Febuxostat	Liver enzyme elevation, nausea, arthralgias, and rash	Therapeutic Serum urate level Reduced frequency of gout attacks Toxic Liver function tests Renal function	Can be used in both urate overproduction and urate underexcretion
Probenecid	Urolithiasis	Therapeutic Serum urate level Reduced frequency of gout attacks Toxic Renal function	Useful in urate underexcretion Avoid for patients with history of urolithiasis
Pegloticase	Acute gout attack during treatment initiation, anaphylaxis, GI symptoms (constipation, nausea, vomiting), chest pain, nasopharyngitis	Therapeutic Serum urate levels Reduced frequency of gout attacks Toxic Signs/symptoms of anaphylaxis following infusion	Reserved for patients with gout refractory to conventional therapies Can be used in both urate overproduction and urate underexcretion
Lesinurad	Acute gout attack during treatment initiation, headache, GERD, major adverse cardiovascular events have been observed although a causal relationship has not been established	Therapeutic Serum urate levels Reduced frequency of gout attacks Toxic Renal function	Reserved for patients with hyperuricemia associated with gout who do not achieve target serum uric acid levels with conventional therapies Can be used in both urate overproduction and urate underexcretion Must be used in combination with a xanthine oxidase inhibitor due to increased risk of acute renal failure with monotherapy

FDA, Food and Drug Administration; GERD, gastroesophageal reflux disease; GI, gastrointestinal; NSAID, nonsteroidal anti-inflammatory drug.

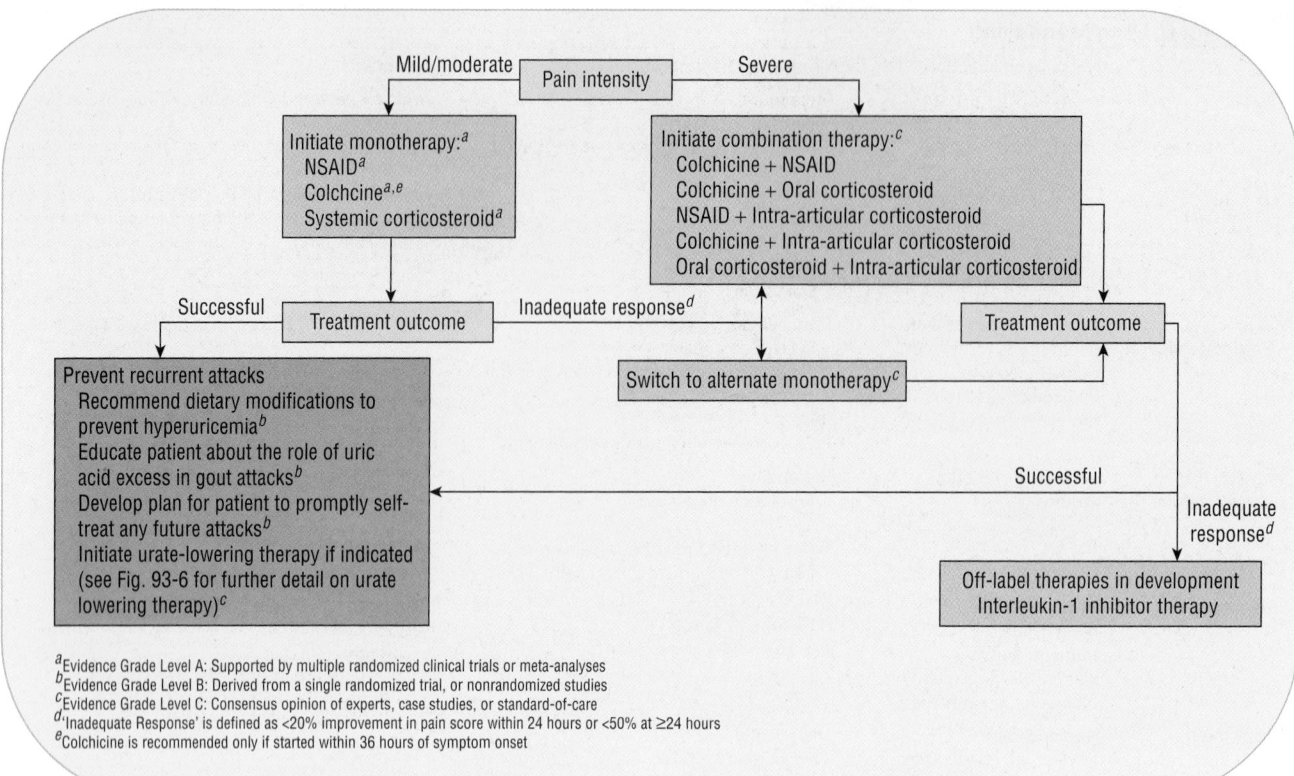

FIGURE 93-5 Algorithm for management of an acute gout attack.

with congestive heart failure, chronic renal failure, and history of GI bleeding.[38] The ACR guidelines support the use of ACTH in the treatment of acute gout in patients unable to take oral medications.[27]

Colchicine 3 Colchicine is an antimitotic drug that is highly effective at relieving acute attacks of gout.[39] When begun within the first 24 hours of an acute attack, colchicine produces a response in two-thirds of patients within hours of administration.[40] If the initiation of colchicine is delayed; however, the probability of success with the drug diminishes substantially. For this reason, the ACR guidelines advocate use of colchicine for treatment of acute gout only if started within 36 hours of attack onset.[27]

Although it is a highly effective therapy, oral colchicine can cause dose-dependent GI adverse effects, including nausea, vomiting, and diarrhea. Other important non-GI adverse effects include neutropenia and axonal neuromyopathy, which may be worsened for patients taking other myopathic drugs such as β-hydroxy-β-methylglutaryl-coenzyme A reductase inhibitors (statins) or for those with renal insufficiency.

Colchicine was used for many years as an unapproved drug with no FDA-approved prescribing information, dosage recommendations, or drug interaction warnings. More recently, the FDA approved a 0.6-mg tablet of colchicine (Colcrys®) for oral use. Data submitted in support of the safety and efficacy of colchicine in acute gout flares demonstrated that a substantially lower dose of colchicine (1.2 mg initially, followed by 0.6 mg 1 hour later) was as effective as higher doses traditionally used (continued hourly dosing until symptoms subside or GI symptoms become intolerable).[41] These findings suggest that prior use of high-dose colchicine regimens, may unnecessarily expose patients to increased toxicity with no additional efficacy.[42] In addition to the new low-dose regimen, the ACR guidelines also suggest that colchicine 0.6 mg once or twice daily can be started 12 hours following the initial 1.2 mg dose and continued until the acute attack resolves.[27] This off-label dosing recommendation is based upon pharmacokinetic data that suggest that colchicine levels begin to decline 12 hours after administration.[41]

Comprehensive review of postmarketing safety data revealed an increased risk of adverse events for patients receiving colchicine administered concurrently with P-glycoprotein or cytochrome P450 3A4 inhibitors (eg, clarithromycin or cyclosporine) (Table 93-8).[43-46] These interactions are thought to result in an increased colchicine concentration. Colchicine should also be used carefully for patients with renal and hepatic insufficiency. Refer to Table 93-8 for colchicine dosing recommendations in these special situations.

IV colchicine has resulted in fatalities and is no longer available.[47]

Hyperuricemia in Gout

Nonpharmacologic Therapy

Following treatment and resolution of the intense pain associated with an acute gout attack, the focus shifts to the prevention of future episodes. Recurrent gout attacks can be prevented by maintaining low uric acid levels. Although both nonpharmacologic and pharmacologic efforts to maintain low uric acid levels are critical in the management of gout, trials have shown high rates of nonadherence with ULT.[48] A likely explanation for this lack in patient adherence is the silent nature of intercritical gout (the period of time between two gout attacks). Patient education, therefore, is a critical first step in the management of hyperuricemia.[26,49] Education should address the recurrent nature of the disease and reinforce the objective of each lifestyle/dietary modification and medication therapy recommended.

Weight loss through caloric restriction and exercise should be promoted in all patients with gout and hyperuricemia, as this may enhance renal excretion of urate.[50] Restriction of alcohol intake is of great importance, as this is closely correlated with gout attacks.[51,52] Acute ingestions of alcohol cause lactic acidemia, which reduces renal urate excretion, and long-term alcohol

TABLE 93-8 Colchicine Dosing in Special Situations/ Colchicine Drug Interactions

	Treatment of Acute Gout Flares	Prophylaxis of Gout Flares
Renal Impairment[a]		
Mild/moderate (creatinine clearance = 30-80 mL/min [0.5-1.33 mL/s])	Dose adjustment not required	Dose adjustment not required
Severe (creatinine clearance <30 mL/min [<0.5 mL/s])	Dose adjustment not required; treatment course should be repeated no more than once every 2 weeks	0.3 mg daily (starting dose)
Dialysis	Single 0.6 mg dose; treatment course should not be repeated more than once every 2 weeks	0.3 mg twice weekly (starting dose)
Hepatic Impairment[b]		
Mild/moderate	Dose adjustment not required	Dose adjustment not required
Severe	Dose adjustment not required; treatment course should be repeated no more than once every 2 weeks	Dose reduction should be considered
Colchicine Drug Interactions		
Strong CYP3A4 inhibitors • Atazanavir • Clarithromycin • Darunavir/ritonavir • Indinavir • Itraconazole • Ketoconazole • Lopinavir/ritonavir • Nefazodone • Nelfinavir • Ritonavir • Saquinavir • Telithromycin • Tipranavir/ritonavir	Single 0.6 mg dose followed by 0.3 mg 1 hour later; dose to be repeated no earlier than 3 days	0.3 mg once every other day to 0.3 mg once daily
Moderate CYP3A4 inhibitors • Amprenavir • Aprepitant • Diltiazem • Erythromycin • Fluconazole • Fosamprenavir • Grapefruit juice and related citrus products • Verapamil	Single 1.2 mg dose; dose to be repeated no earlier than 3 days	0.3 mg-0.6 mg daily (0.6 mg dose may be given as 0.3 mg twice daily)
P-glycoprotein inhibitors • Cyclosporine Ranolazine	Single 0.6 mg dose; dose to be repeated no earlier than 3 days	0.3 mg once every other day to 0.3 mg once daily

[a]Treatment of gout flares with colchicine is not recommended in patients with renal impairment who are receiving colchicine for prophylaxis.

[b]Treatment of gout flares with colchicine is not recommended in patients with hepatic impairment who are receiving colchicine for prophylaxis.

intake promotes production of purines as a by-product of the conversion of acetate to acetyl coenzyme A in the metabolism of alcohol.[53] The ACR guidelines recommend limiting alcohol use in all gout patients and avoidance of any alcohol during periods of frequent gout attacks and in those with advanced gout under poor control.[26] The ACR guidelines also recommend limiting consumption of high-fructose corn syrup and purine-rich foods (organ meats and some seafood), which have been linked to uric acid elevation, and encourage the consumption of vegetables and low-fat dairy products, which have been shown to have urate-lowering effects.[26,54-59]

Another strategy to lower uric acid before initiating urate-lowering pharmacotherapy is to evaluate a patient's medication list for potentially unnecessary drugs that may elevate uric acid levels (see Table 93-2). These include thiazide and loop diuretics, calcineurin inhibitors, niacin, and low-dose aspirin. The ACR guidelines consider the potential elimination of uric acid-elevating medications as a baseline recommendation for all gout patients with hyperuricemia; however, the benefit of thiazide diuretics in the treatment of hypertension and of low-dose aspirin in cardiovascular disease prevention is specifically noted.[26]

The presence of gout should not be a contraindication to the use of thiazide diuretics in hypertensive patients, although clinicians should be aware that diuretics are independent risk factors for gout and can increase serum uric acid levels.[9] It may be important to avoid using diuretics if other agents can be used to control blood pressure, particularly if the patient has had frequent gout attacks or continues to have an elevated serum uric acid level despite appropriate therapy for gout. The ACR guidelines specifically recommend against discontinuing low-dose aspirin used for cardiovascular prevention in patients with gout, since aspirin's effect on elevating serum uric acid is negligible.[26]

Pharmacologic Therapy

4 After the first attack of acute gouty arthritis, a decision to institute prophylactic urate-lowering pharmacotherapy must be considered. This decision should carefully balance risk and benefit. Prophylactic pharmacotherapy has been found to be cost-effective if patients have two or more attacks per year, even if the serum uric acid concentration is normal or only minimally elevated.[60,61]

5 Consistent with this finding, the ACR guidelines recognize the occurrence of two or more gout attacks per year as an indication for pharmacologic ULT.[26] Other indications include the presence of one or more tophus, chronic kidney disease (stage 2 or worse), and a history of urolithiasis.[26]

Pharmacologic ULT can be started during an acute gout attack if appropriate antiinflammatory prophylaxis has been initiated[26] (see "Anti-inflammatory Gout Prophylaxis during Initiation of Pharmacologic Urate-Lowering Therapy" section and Fig. 93-6 for more detail). The goal of initiating ULTs is to achieve and maintain a serum uric acid concentration of less than 6 mg/dL (357 μmol/L), and preferably below 5 mg/dL (297 μmol/L) if signs and symptoms of gout persist.[26,62] Urate lowering should be prescribed for long-term use, as intermittent administration has been less effective in controlling gouty attacks.[26,63] Reduction of serum urate concentrations can be accomplished pharmacologically by decreasing the synthesis of uric acid (xanthine oxidase inhibitors) or by increasing the renal excretion of uric acid (uricosurics).

The ACR guidelines provide a step-wise approach in the treatment of hyperuricemia in gout[26] (see Fig. 93-6). Within this strategy, xanthine oxidase inhibitors are recommended as first-line therapy. Probenecid, a potent uricosuric therapy, is recommended as an alternative first-line therapy in patients with a contraindication or intolerance to xanthine oxidase inhibitor therapy. In refractory cases, combination therapy including a xanthine oxidase inhibitor plus an agent with uricosuric properties (probenecid, losartan, or fenofibrate) is suggested. Finally, in severe cases in which the patient cannot tolerate or is not responding to other therapies, pegloticase is recommended.

Xanthine Oxidase Inhibitors Xanthine oxidase inhibitors reduce uric acid by impairing the ability of xanthine oxidase to

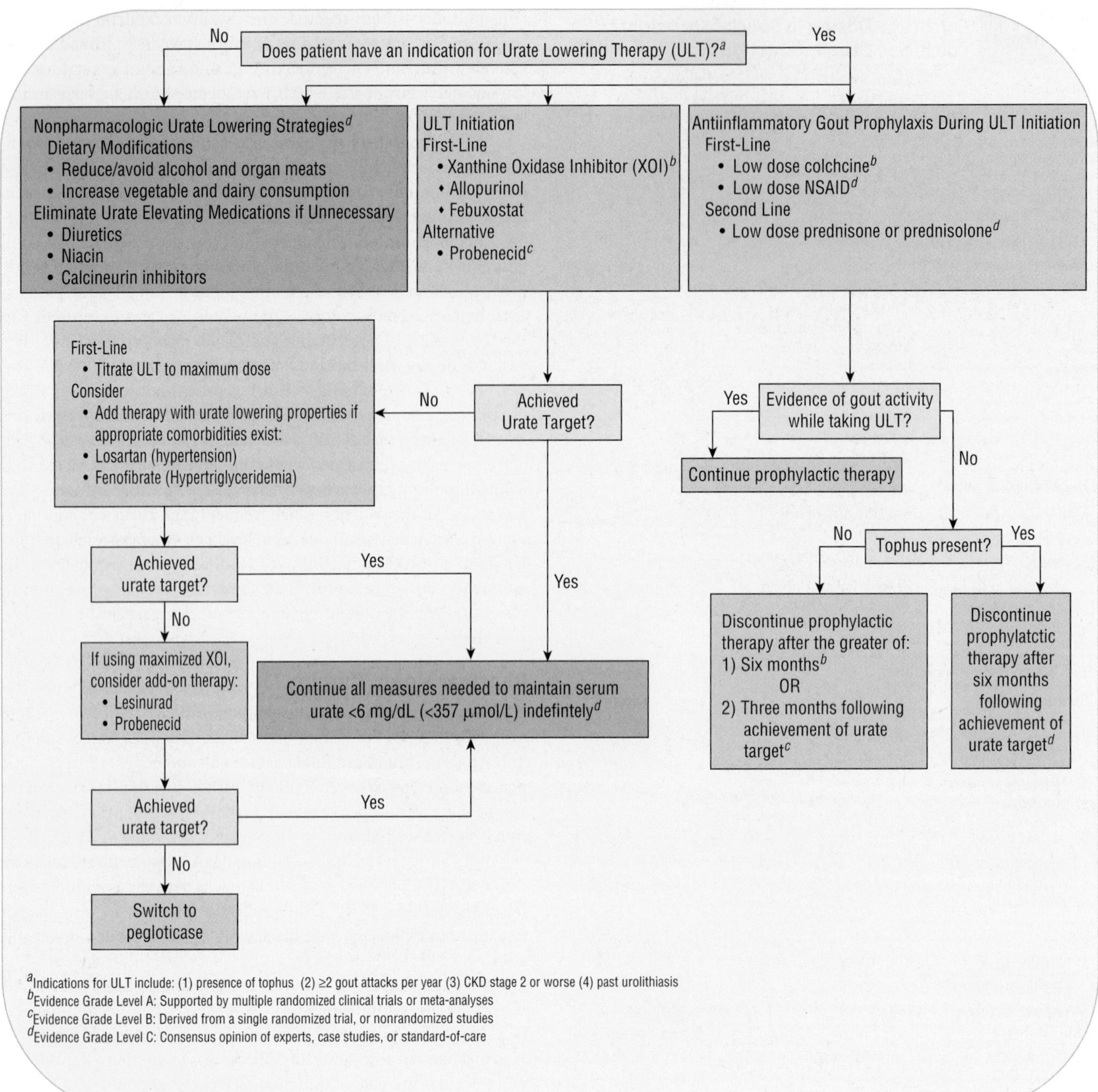

FIGURE 93-6 Algorithm for management of hyperuricemia in gout.

convert hypoxanthine to xanthine and xanthine to uric acid. Because they are efficacious for prophylaxis in both underexcreters and overproducers of uric acid, xanthine oxidase inhibitors are the most widely prescribed agents for the long-term prevention of recurrent attacks of gout. For nearly 40 years, allopurinol was the only agent available in the United States; a second xanthine oxidase inhibitor (febuxostat; Uloric) reached the US market in 2009.

Allopurinol is an effective urate-lowering agent,[64] but up to 5% of patients are unable to tolerate it because of adverse effects and long-term adherence with allopurinol is low.[48,65] Mild adverse effects such as skin rash, leukopenia, GI problems, headache, and urticaria can occur with allopurinol administration. More severe adverse reactions including severe rash (toxic epidermal necrolysis, erythema multiforme, or exfoliative dermatitis), hepatitis, interstitial nephritis, and eosinophilia reportedly occur in approximately 1:1,000 patients and are associated with a 20% to 25% mortality.[26] In a large population-based study in Taiwan, including almost 500,000 patients using allopurinol for the first time, the annual incidence rate of allopurinol hypersensitivity was 4.68 per 1,000 patients. Risk factors associated with the development of allopurinol hypersensitivity included female gender, age above 60 years, initial starting dose of allopurinol exceeding 100 mg/d, renal disease, cardiovascular disease, and use of allopurinol for treatment of asymptomatic hyperuricemia.[66]

As evidence has linked higher starting doses of allopurinol with an increased incidence of allopurinol hypersensitivity syndrome, conservative initial dosing is important.[67] ACR guidelines recommend that allopurinol be started at a dose no greater than 100 mg daily in patients with normal renal function and at a dose no greater than 50 mg daily in patients with chronic kidney disease (stage 4 or worse).[26] This conservative initial dosing strategy is intended to avoid allopurinol hypersensitivity syndrome and also prevent acute gout attacks common during initiation of ULT.

In clinical practice, allopurinol is often arbitrarily capped at a dose of 300 mg/d, resulting in achieving serum urate target concentration of less than 6.0 mg/dL (less than 357 μmol/L) in fewer than

50% of patients.[68,69,70] In patients with renal impairment, the maximum daily dose of allopurinol is typically reduced even further; however, this recommendation comes from a non-evidence-based algorithm and is therefore not supported by the ACR guidelines.[26,71] Ideally, the dose of allopurinol should be gradually titrated every 2 to 5 weeks up to a maximum dose of 800 mg/day until the serum urate target is met, in patients with and without renal impairment.[26] When the dose of allopurinol is maximized beyond 300 mg/day, patients should be educated about the signs and symptoms of a serious reaction, including pruritus and rash. These patients should also undergo routine monitoring for elevation of hepatic enzymes and signs of eosinophilia.[26]

Similar to allopurinol, febuxostat lowers serum urate concentrations in a dose-dependent manner.[72,73] In clinical trials, 40 mg/day of febuxostat was noninferior to conventionally dosed allopurinol (300 mg/day) in achieving the primary endpoint of serum urate concentration less than 6 mg/dL (less than 357 μmol/L), while 80 mg/day of febuxostat was more effective. The incidence of gout flares occurring during long-term follow-up is similar for both drugs.[74] Febuxostat is well tolerated, with adverse events mostly limited to nausea, arthralgias, and minor liver transaminase elevations.

One criticism of the studies comparing allopurinol and febuxostat is that a fixed dose of allopurinol was used, rather than titrating the dose to achieve the targeted serum urate level. An advantage of febuxostat is that it has been studied in patients with mild-to-moderate hepatic and renal impairment (creatinine clearances of 30-89 mL/min [0.50-1.49 mL/s]) and does not require dose adjustment in these patients.

Uricosuric Drugs Uricosuric drugs increase the renal clearance of uric acid by inhibiting postsecretory renal proximal tubular reabsorption of uric acid. The drug used most widely to increase uric acid excretion is probenecid. Several other uricosuric drugs are available in Europe, but not in the United States.

Uricosuric therapies, through their action to increase the elimination of uric acid, cause marked uricosuria and may cause stone formation. Probenecid, specifically, has been associated with a 9% to 11% risk of urolithiasis.[26,69,75] For this reason, patients with a history or urolithiasis should not use potent uricosuric drugs, such as probenecid.[26] The maintenance of adequate urine flow and alkalinization of the urine during the first several days of uricosuric therapy may help diminish the possibility of uric acid stone formation.[26]

Probenecid is given initially at a dose of 250 mg twice a day for 1 to 2 weeks and then 500 mg twice a day for 2 weeks. Thereafter, the daily dose is increased by 500 mg increments every 1 to 2 weeks until satisfactory control is achieved or a maximum dose of 2 g is reached. In addition to urolithiasis, major adverse effects associated with uricosuric therapy include GI irritation, rash and hypersensitivity, and precipitation of acute gouty arthritis. A disadvantage of uricosurics is that salicylates may interfere with this mechanism and result in treatment failure; however, low doses (325 mg/day or less) of enteric-coated aspirin may be used cautiously. In addition, probenecid can inhibit the tubular secretion of other organic acids; thus, increased plasma concentrations of penicillins, cephalosporins, sulfonamides, and indomethacin can occur.

6 Uricosuric drugs are contraindicated for patients who are allergic to them, for patients with impaired renal function [a creatinine clearance less than 50 mL/min (less than 0.83 mL/s)], and for patients who are overproducers of uric acid; for such patients, a xanthine oxidase inhibitor should be used.

Lesinurad Lesinurad (Zurampic) is the first FDA-approved selective uric acid reabsorption inhibitor (SURI). It works by inhibiting urate transporter 1 (URAT1), a transporter found in the proximal renal tubule. Inhibition of URAT1 results in uric acid excretion.

In one 4-week randomized controlled trial, the addition of lesinurad 200 mg, 400 mg, or 600 mg to daily allopurinol therapy (200-600 mg) demonstrated efficacy in reducing serum uric acid in patients with gout and an inadequate response to allopurinol therapy (defined as serum uric acid more than or equal to 6 mg/dL on more than or equal to 2 occasions more than or equal to 2 weeks apart while on allopurinol 200-600 mg daily for more than or equal to 6 weeks).[76] Patients taking 200 mg, 400 mg, and 600 mg of lesinurad achieved serum uric acid reduction of 16%, 22% and 30%, respectively, compared to 3% with placebo ($P < 0.0001$ for all comparisons).[76] Adverse effects noted with lesinurad therapy included serum creatinine elevation, elevated lipase, increased creatinine kinase, and urticaria.[76]

Lesinurad is approved as combination therapy with a xanthine oxidase inhibitor (including allopurinol and febuxostat) for treatment of hyperuricemia associated with gout in patients who have not achieved target serum uric acid levels with xanthine oxidase inhibitor monotherapy. Because lesinurad works by increasing renal uric acid secretion, it has been associated with adverse renal events, particularly when used as monotherapy.[77] Lesinurad carries a black box warning which highlights the increased risk of acute renal failure when used in the absence of xanthine oxidase inhibitor therapy. Lesinurad has been studied in combination with xanthine oxidase inhibitor therapy in three placebo-controlled trials for up to 12 months.[77] Although other doses have been studied, the only approved dose of lesinurad is 200 mg daily due to increased risk of renal events when used at higher doses.[77] Lesinurad should not be used in patients with creatinine clearance less than 45 mL/min.[77]

Because the ACR gout guidelines were published prior to the approval of a URAT1 inhibitor, lesinurad's place in therapy is not well established. Given lesinurad's ease of use (once daily oral tablet) and, thus far, reasonable safety profile, the medication may serve as first-line add-on therapy for the treatment of hyperuricemia in patients with gout who are unable to achieve target serum uric acid levels despite maximization of xanthine oxidase inhibitor therapy.[77] Limitations to widespread use may include high cost, given market exclusivity until patent expiration, and renal adverse events. Given the lack safety data beyond 12 months of use, postmarketing surveillance will also be important in guiding future use.

Pegloticase Pegloticase (Krystexxa) is a pegylated recombinant uricase that works to reduce serum uric acid by converting uric acid to allantoin, a water-soluble and easily excreted substance.

In two 6-month randomized controlled trials, biweekly pegloticase therapy demonstrated efficacy in reducing serum uric acid and resolving tophi in patients with severe gout and hyperuricemia (uric acid more than or equal to 8 mg/dL [more than or equal to 476 μmol/L]) who failed or had a contraindication to allopurinol therapy.[78] Severe gout referred to patients who met at least one of the following criteria: (a) three or more gout flares within the most recent 18 months, (b) one or more tophi, or (c) joint damage due to gout. Far more patients receiving pegloticase therapy compared with placebo achieved the primary outcome, maintenance of uric acid less than 6 mg/dL (less than 357 μmol/L) for at least 80% of the time during months 3 and 6 of the trial (42% vs 0%; $P < 0.001$).

Although clearly efficacious, pegloticase has several drawbacks that limit widespread use. One is the route of administration. The biweekly IV infusions of pegloticase must be given over no less than 2 hours, a potential inconvenience to many patients. Furthermore, given potential infusion-related allergic reactions, patients must be treated with antihistamines and corticosteroids before therapy. Cost is another major consideration. Pegloticase is estimated to cost more than $5,000 per month, not including administration costs associated with an IV infusion.[79] This represents a significantly greater cost burden compared with other ULT.[79]

The ideal duration of pegloticase therapy is currently unknown. Other ULTs, xanthine oxidase inhibitors for example, are typically used indefinitely in patients with gout and hyperuricemia. Immunogenicity issues associated with pegloticase therapy may limit the duration with which pegloticase therapy may be used effectively. In the previously cited 6-month pegloticase trials, 134 of 150 patients developed pegloticase antibodies that, for most patients, resulted in a loss of efficacy by month 4.[78]

Given these many limitations and the narrow patient population in which the drug has been studied, pegloticase is an agent of last resort that should be reserved for patients with refractory gout who are unable to take or have failed all other ULTs.

Miscellaneous Urate-Lowering Agents Lipid-lowering agents, in particular fenofibrate, can also be prescribed for patients with gout. Although dyslipidemia is common in gout patients, the fibrates are believed to exert their effects as an ancillary benefit by increasing the clearance of hypoxanthine and xanthine, leading to a sustained reduction in serum urate concentrations. Reductions of 20% to 30% in urate levels are observed with fenofibrate use.[80,81] Importantly, fenofibrate does not appear to not cause an acute gout flare when initiated and is well tolerated overall.[82,83]

Losartan, an angiotensin II receptor antagonist, has also demonstrated benefit in reducing serum urate concentrations independent of angiotensin receptor antagonism.[84] Losartan inhibits renal tubular reabsorption of uric acid and increases urinary excretion, and this effect seems to be a unique property of losartan that is not shared with other angiotensin II receptor antagonists.[85] In addition, it alkalinizes the urine, which helps reduce the risk for stone formation.

The ACR guidelines support the use of fenofibrate or losartan in combination with a xanthine oxidase inhibitor in patients with refractory disease.[26]

Anti-Inflammatory Gout Prophylaxis during Initiation of Pharmacologic Urate-Lowering Therapy

7 Initiation of ULT can prompt an acute attack of gout due to remodeling of urate crystal deposits in joints as a result of rapid lowering of urate concentrations.[27] The frequency of this phenomenon is inconsistently reported in clinical trials and may occur in as many of 75% of patients initiating ULT or as few as 25%.[86] Prophylactic antiinflammatory pharmacotherapy is often recommended to prevent gout attacks and, secondarily, to assist in ensuring patient acceptance of and adherence with ULT. The ACR guidelines recommend low-dose oral colchicine (0.6 mg twice daily) and low-dose NSAIDs (eg, naproxen 250 mg twice/day) as first-line prophylactic therapies, with stronger evidence supporting use of colchicine.[27] Low-dose corticosteroid therapy (eg, less than or equal to 10 mg/day prednisone) is recommended as an alternative in patients with intolerance, contraindication, or lack of response to first-line therapy.[27] Continuation of pharmacologic prophylaxis is recommended for at least 3 months after achieving target serum uric acid or 6 months total, whichever is longer. For patients with one or more tophi, prophylactic therapy should be continued for 6 months following achievement of serum urate target[27] (see Fig. 93-6).

Given the considerable duration of therapy required for acute gout prophylaxis during initiation of ULT, adverse effects of the pharmacologic agents employed must be seriously considered. Although the risk for gastric ulceration and bleeding is relatively small with short-term NASID therapy normally employed when treating acute gout flares, administration of a proton-pump inhibitor or other acid-suppressing therapy is indicated to protect from NSAID-induced gastric problems for patients on long-term prophylactic therapy.[27] Prolonged corticosteroid therapy is clearly linked to many severe adverse effects (ie, hyperglycemia, cushing syndrome, fluid retention, hypertension, osteoporosis, glaucoma, depression/euphoria) and, as suggested above, is not appropriate for first-line therapy for this reason.

Cost is another major consideration when selecting prophylactic pharmacotherapy given the need for an extended duration of therapy (6 months of therapy compared to approximately 1 week for acute gout treatment). While improved dosing recommendations resulted from the recent availability of an FDA-approved colchicine product, the research efforts that provided this additional information have come with a price. Market exclusivity rights were granted to the manufacturer of Colcrys and the resulting lack of competition has caused the price of the medication to increase from approximately $0.09 per tablet to more than $5 per tablet.[87] The cost of this brand name colchicine, if not covered by insurance, is a potential challenge to therapy for certain patients. To date there have been no formal pharmacoeconomic studies evaluating colchicine in comparison to other therapies for antiinflammatory prophylaxis during ULT initiation; however, NSAIDs and corticosteroids may present more affordable options for patients.

Clinical **Controversy...**

It is unclear if the benefit of long-term anti-inflammatory prophylaxis during initiation of ULT outweighs the risk in patients with gout and multiple comorbidities. Harms of extended-course NSAIDs in patients with renal impairment or GI disease, for example, may preclude use of the therapy, leaving only low-dose, daily colchicine as a costly alternative. Patients and providers must balance the risk of gout recurrence against the risk and/or cost of prophylactic therapy.

Investigational Drugs

Prior to the release of febuxostat in 2009 and pegloticase in 2010, several decades passed without the release of a new pharmacotherapeutic agent for the treatment of gout. Given the increased prevalence of gout and the presence of both treatment intolerance and treatment refractory cases, several new agents are currently under investigation.[88]

Interleukin-1 Inhibitors

During acute gout attacks, urate crystals elicit an inflammatory response that triggers the production of interleukin-1 (IL-1).[89] This finding has led to the investigational use of IL-1 inhibitors in the treatment and prevention of acute gout.

In small trials, two IL-1 inhibitors, anakinra and canakinumab, have demonstrated efficacy in the treatment of acute gout.[90-94] Neither is approved for treatment of acute gout by the FDA, and their use remains off-label. The ACR guidelines suggest that anakinra 100 mg subcutaneously daily for 3 days or single-dose canakinumab 150 mg subcutaneously can be considered for treatment of severe acute gout attacks refractory to other treatments. However, due to a lack of randomized controlled trials and an uncertain risk-to-benefit ratio, the guidelines note that the role of IL-1 inhibitors in the treatment of acute gout is unclear.[27]

Limited evidence also suggests efficacy of IL-1 inhibitors in the prevention of acute gout during the first 16 weeks of ULT initiation (subcutaneous rilonacept 320 mg loading dose followed by 160 mg weekly and subcutaneous canakinumab single dose [50-300 mg] or four times weekly dosing [50 mg—50 mg—25 mg—25 mg]).[95-97]

Given the limited evidence and lack of FDA approval for this indication, the ACR guidelines do not provide a recommendation for the use of IL-1 inhibitors for anti-inflammatory prophylaxis during initiation of ULT.

Clinical **Controversy...**

IL-1 inhibitors have demonstrated efficacy in treating and preventing acute gout. Given limited clinical trial data, however, these agents currently lack FDA approval for use in the management of gout. They may serve as safe and effective treatment options for patients with intolerances to traditional gout medications or in patients with treatment refractory disease. More evidence is needed to determine exactly where these agents fit in the armamentarium available for gout management.

Other Investigational Agents

Several investigational agents intended to be used for the management of gout are at various stages of development. Additional URAT1 inhibitors, to follow lesinurad, are currently in development (RDEA3170, levotofisopam, arhalofenate).[98] Arhalofenate also suppresses the production of IL-1β which may potentially lead to a reduction in gout flares in addition to urate lowering.[98,99] Other novel mechanisms of action include purine nucleoside phosphorylase (PNP) inhibition (ulodesine) and glucose transporter 9 (GLUT9) inhibition (tranilast).[96,97] Continued research will ultimately define the role of these agents in the management of gout and hyperuricemia.

Nephrolithiasis

8 The medical management of uric acid nephrolithiasis includes hydration sufficient to maintain a urine volume of 2 to 3 L/day, alkalinization of urine, avoidance of pne-rich foods, moderation of protein intake, and reduction of urinary uric acid excretion.

Maintenance of a 24-hour urine volume of 2 to 3 L with an adequate intake of fluids is desirable for all gout patients, but especially for those with excessive uric acid excretion (more than 1 g/day [more than 6 mmol/day]). Alkalinizing agents should be used with the objective of making the urine less acidic. Urine pH should be maintained at 6 to 6.5. In this pH range, up to 85% of uric acid will be in the form of the soluble urate ion.

Reduction of urine acidity is usually accomplished by the administration of potassium bicarbonate or potassium citrate 60 to 80 mEq/day (mmol/day).[100,101] Administration of alkali via sodium salts is a less desirable option for two reasons. First, the sodium-induced volume expansion will increase sodium excretion and can secondarily cause hypercalcemia because calcium passively follows the reabsorption of sodium in the proximal tubule and loop of Henle. In the presence of uric acid, the resultant hypercalcemia can lead to calcium oxalate stone formation. Second, older patients with uric acid kidney stones may also have hypertension, congestive heart failure, or renal insufficiency. Because of these conditions, they should not be overloaded with alkalinizing sodium salts or unlimited fluid intake, as these can worsen these conditions.

Acetazolamide, a carbonic anhydrase inhibitor, produces rapid and effective urinary alkalinization and sometimes is used in conjunction with alkali therapy. When a 250-mg dose of acetazolamide is given at bedtime, the excretion of acidic urine in the early morning hours is avoided. The usual tachyphylaxis (rapid tolerance) to this drug is obviated by a daily repletion dose of bicarbonate.

Since the advent of xanthine oxidase inhibitors, a low-purine, low-protein diet for the patient with uric acid nephrolithiasis is no longer as critical as it once was; however, it is still advisable to instruct the patient to avoid foods rich in purine and to limit protein to no more than 90 g/day. Such a diet is still palatable and reduces appreciably the amount of uric acid in the urine.

The mainstay of drug therapy for recurrent uric acid nephrolithiasis is xanthine oxidase inhibitors. They are effective in reducing both serum and urinary uric acid levels, thus preventing the formation of calculi. Xanthine oxidase inhibitors are recommended as prophylactic treatment for patients who will receive cytotoxic agents for the treatment of lymphoma or leukemia. The marked increase in uric acid production associated with cytolysis of a neoplasm predisposes a patient to the development of uric acid nephrolithiasis.

Uric Acid Lowering in the Absence of Gout

Asymptomatic Hyperuricemia

Questions are often raised regarding the indication for drug therapy for asymptomatic hyperuricemia. The purported benefits include prevention of acute gouty arthritis, tophi formation, nephrolithiasis, and chronic urate nephropathy. The first three complications are easily controlled should they develop; therefore, antihyperuricemic therapy is not warranted to prevent these conditions. The prevention of urate nephropathy might be a stronger indication because it is irreversible even with proper treatment. Available data indicate, however, that gouty nephropathy is extremely rare in the absence of clinical gout, and evidence that elevation of uric acid by itself may cause renal disease is weak and inconclusive. As discussed previously, renal impairment associated with hyperuricemia is very rare in the absence of concurrent hypertension and atherosclerosis. In addition, it is unclear whether uric acid-lowering therapy protects renal function in such individuals. Thus, the routine treatment of asymptomatic hyperuricemia on the grounds of reducing renal complications is presently not recommended.

Uric Acid and Cardiovascular Risk

The relationship between elevated serum urate concentrations and cardiovascular disease is controversial. In observational studies, hyperuricemia has been shown to be a risk factor for ischemic heart disease.[102-105] However, hyperuricemia is also associated with other known risk factors for cardiovascular disease, such as diabetes mellitus, dyslipidemia, and hypertension, and the individual contribution of hyperuricemia on the risk for cardiovascular disease is difficult to separate from these associated factors. Recently, a 12-year follow-up of the Health Professionals Study revealed a 28% higher risk of death from all causes, 38% higher risk of cardiovascular disease death, 55% higher risk of death from coronary heart disease, and a 59% higher risk of nonfatal myocardial infarction for men with a self-reported history of gout compared with those without this reported history.[106] These associations remained significant even after adjusting for age, body mass index, smoking, family history of myocardial infarction, and comorbidities such as diabetes and hypertension. To date, this study is the only one providing prospective data that implicate gout as an independent risk for coronary heart disease.

Given the epidemiologic relationship between uric acid and cardiovascular risk, the potential effects of urate lowering on various cardiovascular parameters have been investigated in a number of small trials. Effects on blood pressure and vasculature are one of the mechanisms studied. In one recent trial, the addition of allopurinol in blacks receiving chlorthalidone further improved clinic blood pressure control (4.3 mm Hg mean decrease in systolic blood pressure after 4 weeks of therapy).[107] Similar effects on blood pressure have been demonstrated with allopurinol in other clinical studies.[108-110] The mechanism by which allopurinol may decrease blood pressure is not clear but may be mediated through decreases in oxidative stress brought on as a result of inhibiting oxidant generation during the reaction between hypoxanthine and xanthine with xanthine oxidase.[107] Of note, febuxostat has also been shown to decrease oxidative stress in small clinical trials.[111,112]

While empirically initiating ULT in patients with asymptomatic hyperuricemia and elevated cardiovascular risk may seem attractive on the basis of epidemiologic studies and small prospective trials using surrogate markers, no studies have provided clear evidence that drug treatment of asymptomatic hyperuricemia or gout reduces cardiovascular morbidity and mortality. At this time, it is premature to implement therapy for patients with asymptomatic hyperuricemia in the absence of a history of gout. Risks of therapy must also be considered, such as the increased incidence of allopurinol hypersensitivity syndrome when allopurinol is used for the treatment of asymptomatic hyperuricemia. Whether or not ULT is implemented, efforts should be directed toward aggressive management of cardiovascular risk factors in all patients with hyperuricemia.

Clinical **Controversy...**

While asymptomatic hyperuricemia is not generally treated, some clinicians choose to initiate treatment on the basis that it may reduce the risks of vascular disease, including hypertension, cerebrovascular disease, and kidney disease. Allopurinol has been associated with decreases in blood pressure in recent trials; however, a defined mechanism has not been established. Given the lack of randomized controlled trials demonstrating improved cardiovascular outcomes with allopurinol use in patients with asymptomatic hyperuricemia, the benefit of treatment in this setting is unclear. Furthermore, adverse effects must be considered, such as the increased risk of allopurinol hypersensitivity syndrome.

Personalized Pharmacotherapy

While the ACR guidelines provide clear recommendations regarding use of pharmacotherapy in the management of gout and hyperuricemia, application of these recommendations requires personalization to fit the needs of a specific patient. When making therapeutic choices for an individual, it is critical to evaluate the adverse effect profile of a particular pharmacotherapeutic agent while considering a patient's baseline risk for those unwanted effects. This involves an analysis of patient demographics and comorbidities.[13]

Allopurinol hypersensitivity syndrome is perhaps the most concerning adverse effect of all potential side effects associated with gout therapies, given the high mortality rate associated with this reaction. As such, it would be ideal if patients at high risk for developing this syndrome could be screened for and, consequently, guided to alternative therapy. Recent research has identified a genetic link in certain populations that increases risk for the development of allopurinol hypersensitivity syndrome. Korean patients with chronic kidney disease (stage 3 or worse), Han Chinese patients, and Thai patients have been identified as being at increased risk for allopurinol hypersensitivity syndrome if found to have a specific genotype (HLA-B*5801 positive).[112-114] The ACR guidelines recommend that HLA-B*5801 testing be considered before allopurinol initiation in these specific subpopulations; for those found to be positive, alternative therapy should be used.[26]

Certain comorbidities may warrant dose adjustment of some gout therapies or, in certain instances, complete avoidance of certain medications. For example, patients with renal impairment should, in general, avoid NSAID therapy and must receive colchicine at reduced doses. Patients with GI disease should also avoid NSAID therapy and may not be able to tolerate colchicine therapy and, therefore, may find most success with corticosteroid therapy. In addition to comorbidities, polypharmacy and cost considerations may affect treatment decisions in an individual patient. Refer to Table 93-9 for an overview of important factors to consider when personalizing pharmacotherapy for an individual patient with gout.

Evaluation of Therapeutic Outcomes

Follow-up of patients with gout depends on the frequency of attacks and on the medications used to treat symptoms. For a patient who is experiencing a first attack of gout, long-term therapy is generally not indicated. As previously mentioned, the ACR guidelines recommend that urate-lowering pharmacotherapy be started only after two or more attacks of gout in 1 year, because the treatment is long-term and relatively expensive, the drugs used are potentially toxic, and adherence for patients without symptoms is generally poor.[26,61,65] Patients having a first attack should be educated about the likelihood of recurrence and what to do if another attack occurs. Approximately 60% of patients have a second attack within the first year, and 78% have a second attack within 2 years. Only 7% of patients do not have a recurrence within a 10-year period.[115]

Baseline blood work for patients receiving hypouricemic medications chronically should include renal function (serum creatinine, blood urea nitrogen), liver enzymes (aspartate aminotransferase, alanine aminotransferase), complete blood count, and electrolytes. There is generally no need to recheck these laboratory parameters for patients undergoing acute therapy with an NSAID or colchicine of limited duration. However, for patients requiring long-term therapy or prophylaxis, they should be rechecked every 6 to 12 months or as clinically indicated. For patients suspected of having an acute attack of gouty arthritis, it is reasonable to check a serum uric acid level, particularly if it is not the first attack and a decision is to be made regarding initiation of prophylactic therapy. However, clinicians should be mindful that acute gouty arthritis can occur in the presence of normal serum uric acid concentrations.[6] During titration of ULT, uric acid should be monitored every 2 to 5 weeks; once the urate target is achieved, uric acid should be monitored every 6 months.[26] This monitoring regimen is recommended not only to ensure appropriate dosing of ULT, but also to serve as an assessment of patient adherence given the known adherence issues with ULTs. (9) Because of the high rates of comorbidities associated with gout, including diabetes mellitus, chronic kidney disease, hypertension, obesity, myocardial infarction, heart failure, and stroke, elevated uric acid levels or gout should prompt evaluations for signs of cardiovascular disease and the need for appropriate risk reduction measures.[116] Additionally, clinicians should look for a possible correctable cause of hyperuricemia, such as medications (eg, thiazide and loop diuretics, niacin, calcineurin inhibitors), obesity, malignancy, and alcohol abuse. Patients should be encouraged to exercise, lose weight, reduce alcohol intake, reduce consumption of syrup-sweetened sodas and increase consumption of low-fat dairy foods and vegetables, and have periodic follow-up to address progress on these goals.

CONCLUSION

Hyperuricemia may lead to acute arthritis, chronic gout, or kidney stones or to no sequelae at all. Asymptomatic hyperuricemia may not need to be treated, although lifestyle modifications (eg, weight loss, reduction of alcohol intake, control of blood pressure) should be encouraged to help reduce serum urate and overall cardiovascular health.

TABLE 93-9 Personalized Pharmacotherapy in Gout

Conditions and Situations	Limitations to Pharmacotherapy	Alternative Therapies
Renal insufficiency	NSAIDs may lead to exacerbation of renal insufficiency	Consider reduced-dose colchicine or corticosteroids for short-term treatment of acute gout Consider reduced-dose colchicine for prophylaxis during initiation of urate-lowering therapy
	Uricosuric therapy is ineffective in patients with renal insufficiency	Consider allopurinol or febuxostat
	Lesiurad is not indicated in patients with renal insufficiency	Consider allopurinol or febuxostat for first-line urate lowering therapy; consider pegloticase for refractory cases
GI disease	Colchicine may cause GI upset and diarrhea	Consider corticosteroids for treatment of acute gout If monoarticular, consider joint injection
	NSAIDs may cause GI bleeding or ulceration	Consider gastroprotection with coadministration of proton-pump inhibitor when NSAID therapy is used Consider colchicine or corticosteroids for treatment of acute gout Consider low-dose colchicine for prophylaxis during initiation of urate-lowering therapy
Congestive heart failure	NSAIDs may cause a congestive heart failure exacerbation	Consider colchicine for treatment of acute gout Consider colchicine for prophylaxis during initiation of urate-lowering therapy
	Concurrent use of diuretic may increase serum urate	If diuretic remains necessary, consider initiating urate-lowering therapy Consider losartan as a therapy for congestive heart failure given its uricosuric properties
Hypertension	Diuretics may increase uric acid	Consider losartan as alternative or additional antihypertensive therapy given its uricosuric properties Consider addition of urate-lowering therapy if diuretic remains necessary
	NSAIDs may worsen blood pressure control	Consider colchicine or corticosteroids for treatment of acute gout Consider colchicine for prophylaxis during initiation of urate-lowering therapy
Polypharmacy	CYP3A4 inhibitors and P-glycoprotein inhibitors interact with colchicine leading to elevated colchicine levels	Reduce the dose of colchicine used for the treatment and prophylaxis of acute gout Consider NSAIDs or corticosteroids for treatment of acute gout Consider NSAIDs for prophylaxis during initiation of urate-lowering therapy
	Added pharmacotherapy may be undesirable in a patient with a large medication burden	Consider losartan as urate-lowering therapy in patients with comorbid hypertension Consider fenofibrate as urate-lowering therapy in patients with hypertriglyceridemia
Financial limitations	Febuxostat and colchicine are considerably more costly compared with other gout treatments	Consider allopurinol as urate-lowering therapy Consider NSAIDs or corticosteroids for treatment of acute gout Consider NSAIDs for prophylaxis of gout during initiation of urate-lowering therapy

CYP, cytochrome P; GI, gastrointestinal; NSAID, nonsteroidal anti-inflammatory drug.

Acute gouty arthritis responds well to short courses of NSAIDs, colchicine, or corticosteroids to treat the underlying inflammatory condition. The management of uric acid nephrolithiasis includes hydration and alkalinization of the urine. Prevention of recurrent gouty arthritis or recurrent nephrolithiasis and treatment of chronic gout require hypouricemic therapy with either a uricosuric drug or xanthine oxidase inhibitor. Xanthine oxidase inhibitors are effective in both underexcreters and overproducers of uric acid, making them the hypouricemic drugs of choice for most patients with gout. Finally, anti-inflammatory prophylaxis with low-dose colchicine or NSAID therapy is indicated during the initiation of ULT to prevent the development of acute gout due to rapid mobilization or urate.

ABBREVIATIONS

ACR	American College of Rheumatology
ACTH	adrenocorticotropic hormone
CNS	central nervous system
COX-2	cyclooxygenase-2
EULAR	European League Against Rheumatism
FDA	Food and Drug Administration
GI	gastrointestinal
GLUT9	glucose transporter 9
HGPRT	hypoxanthine-guanine phosphoribosyltransferase
IL-1	interleukin-1
MSU	monosodium urate
NSAID	nonsteroidal anti-inflammatory drug
PNP	purine nucleoside phosphorylase
PRPP	phosphoribosyl pyrophosphate (synthetase)
SURI	selective uric acid reabsorption inhibitor
ULT	urate-lowering therapy
URAT1	urate transporter 1
USP	United States Pharmacopeia

REFERENCES

1. Wortmann RL. Chapter 87: Gout and hyperuricemia. In: Firestein GS, Budd RC, Harris ED Jr, et al, eds. *Kelley's Textbook of Rheumatology*, 8th ed. Philadelphia, PA: WB Saunders, 2008.
2. Edwards NL, Choi HK, Terkeltaub RA. Chapter 12: Gout. In: Klippel JH, Stone SH, Crofford LJ, et al, eds. *Primer on the Rheumatic Diseases*, 13th ed. New York, NY: Springer Scientce+Business Media, 2008.
3. Li R, Sun J, Ren L, et al. Epidemiology of eight common rheumatic disease in China: A large-scale cross-sectional survey in Beijing. *Rheumatology* 2012;51:721-729.
4. Zhu Y, Pandya BJ, Choi HK. Prevalence of gout and hyperuricemia in the US general population: The National Health And Nutrition Examination Survey 2007–2008. *Arthritis Rheum* 2011;63:3136-3141.
5. Campion EW, Glynn RJ, DeLabry LO. Asymptomatic hyperuricemia. Risks and consequences in the Normative Aging Study. *Am J Med* 1987;82:421-426.
6. McCarty DJ. Gout without hyperuricemia. *JAMA* 1994;271:302-303.
7. Juraschek SP, Miller ER, Gelber AC. Body mass index, obesity, and prevalent gout in the United States in 1988–1944 and 2007–2010. *Arthritis Care Res* 2013;65:127-132.
8. Choi HK. A prescription for lifestyle change in patients with hyperuricemia and gout. *Curr Opin Rheumatol* 2010;22:165-172.

9. Hak AE, Curhan GC, Grodstein F, et al. Menopause, postmenopausal hormone use and risk of incident gout. *Ann Rheum Dis* 2010;69:1305-1309.
10. Neogi T. Gout. *NEJM* 2011;364:443-452.
11. Wallace KL, Riedel AA, Joseph-Ridge N, Wortmann R. Increasing prevalence of gout and hyperuricemia over 10 years among older adults in a managed care population. *J Rheumatol* 2004;31:1582-1587.
12. Wilson JM, Young AB, Kelley WN. Hypoxanthine-guanine phosphoribosyltransferase deficiency. *N Engl J Med* 1983;309:900-910.
13. Fravel MA, Ernst ME. Management of gout in the older adult. *Am J Geriatr Pharmacother* 2011;9:271-285.
14. Busso N, Ea HK. The mechanisms of inflammation in gout and pseudogout (CPP-induced arthritis). *Reumatismo* 2011;63:230-237.
15. McGill NW. Gout and other crystal arthropathies. *Med J Aust* 1997;166:33-38.
16. Schumacher HR. Crystal-reduced arthritis: An overview. *Am J Med* 1996;100(Suppl 2A):46S-52S.
17. MacMullan P, McCarthy G. Treatment and management of pseudogout: Insights for the clinician. *Ther Adv Musculoskel Dis* 2012;4:121-131.
18. Pal B, Foxall M, Dysart T, et al. How is gout managed in primary care? A review of current practice and proposed guidelines. *Clin Rheumatol* 2000;19:21-25.
19. Eggebeen AT. Gout: an update. *Am Fam Physician* 2007;76:801-808.
20. Agudelo CA, Weinberger A, Schumacher HR, et al. Definitive diagnosis of gout by identification of urate crystals in asymptomatic metatarsophalangeal joints. *Arthritis Rheum* 1979;22:559-560.
21. Logan JA, Morrison E, McGill PE. Serum uric acid in acute gout. *Ann Rheum Dis* 1997;56:696-697.
22. Zhang W, Doherty M, Pascual E, et al. EULAR evidence based recommendations for gout. Part I. Diagnosis. Report of a task force of the Standing Committee for International Clinical Studies Including Therapeutics (ESCISIT). *Ann Rheum Dis* 2006;65:1301-1311.
23. Neogi T, Jansen T, Dalbeth N, et al. 2015 Gout classification criteria: An American College of Rheumatology/European League Against Rheumatism collaborative initiative. *Ann Rheum Dis* 2015;74:1789-1798.
24. Kramer HM, Curhan G. The association between gout and nephrolithiasis: The National Health and Nutrition Examination Survey III, 1988–1994. *Am J Kid Dis* 2002;40:37-42.
25. Yu T. Nephrolithiasis in patients with gout. *Postgrad Med* 1978;63:164-170.
26. Khanna D, Fitzgerald JD, Khanna PP, et al. 2012 American College of Rheumatology guidelines for management of gout. Part 1: Systematic nonpharmacologic and pharmacologic therapeutic approaches to hyperuricemia. *Arthritis Care Res* 2012;64:1431-1446.
27. Khanna D, Khanna PP, Fitzgerald JD, et al. 2012 American College of Rheumatology guidelines for management of gout. Part 2: Therapy and anti-inflammatory prophylaxis of acute gouty arthritis. *Arthritis Care Res* 2012;64:1447-1461.
28. Schlesinger N, Detry MA, Holland BK, et al. Local ice therapy during bouts of acute gouty arthritis. *J Rheumatol* 2002;29:331-334.
29. van Durme CMPG, Wechalekar MD, Buchbinder R, et al. Non-steroidal anti-inflammatory drugs for acute gout. *Cochrane Database of Systematic Reviews* 2014, Issue 9. Art. No.: CD010120.
30. Schumacher HR, Berger MF, Li-Yu J, et al. Efficacy and tolerability of celecoxib in the treatment of acute gouty arthritis: A randomized controlled trial. *J Rheumatol* 2012;39:1859-1866.
31. Mukherjee D, Nissen SE, Topol EJ. Risk of cardiovascular events associated with selective COX-2 inhibitors. *JAMA* 2001;286: 954-959.
32. Janssens HJ, Janssen M, van de Lisdonk EH, et al. Use of oral prednisolone or naproxen for the treatment of gout arthritis: A double-blind, randomised equivalence trial. *Lancet* 2008;371:1854-1860.
33. Zhang Y, Yang H, Zhang J, et al. Comparison of intramuscular compound betamethasone and oral diclofenac sodium in the treatment of acute attacks of gout. *Int J Clin Pract* 2014;68:633-638.
34. Fernandez D, Noguera R, Gonzalez JA, et al. Treatment of acute attacks of gout with a small dose of intraarticular triamcinolone acetonide. *J Rheumatol* 1999;26:2285-2286.
35. Siegel LB, Alloway JA, Nashel DJ. Comparison of adrenocorticotropic hormone and triamcinolone acetonide in the treatment of acute gouty arthritis. *J Rheumatol* 1994;21:1325-1327.
36. Axelrod D, Preston S. Comparison of parenteral adrenocorticotropic hormone with oral indomethacin in the treatment of acute gout. *Arthritis Rheum* 1988;31:803-805.
37. Taylor CT, Brooks NC, Kelley KW. Corticotropin for acute management of gout. *Ann Pharmacother* 2001;35:365-368.
38. Ritter J, Kerr LD, Valeriano-Marcet J, Spiera H. ACTH revisited: Effective treatment for acute crystal induced synovitis in patients with multiple medical problems. *J Rheumatol* 1994;21:696-699.
39. Schlesinger N, Schumacher R, Catton M, Maxwell L. Colchicine for acute gout. *Cochrane Database Syst Rev* 2006;4:CD006190.
40. Ahern MJ, Reid C, Gordon TP, et al. Does colchicine work? The results of the first controlled study in acute gout. *Aust NZ J Med* 1987;17:301-304.
41. Terkeltaub RA, Furst DE, Bennett K, et al. High versus low dosing of oral colchicine for early acute gout flare: Twenty-four-hour outcome of the first multicenter, randomized, double-blind, placebo-controlled, parallel-group, dose-comparison colchicine study. *Arthritis Rheum* 2010;62:1060-1068.
42. van Echteld I, Wechalekar MD, Schlesinger N, et al. Colchicine for acute gout. *Cochrane Database of Systematic Reviews* 2014, Issue 8. Art. No.: CD006190.
43. Dogukan A, Oymak FS, Taskapan H, et al. Acute fatal colchicine intoxication in a patient on continuous ambulatory peritoneal dialysis (CAPD). Possible role of clarithromycin administration. *Clin Nephrol* 2001;55:181-182.
44. Rollot F, Pajot O, Chauvelot-Moachon L, et al. Acute colchicine intoxication during clarithromycin administration. *Ann Pharmacother* 2004;38:2074-2077.
45. Hung IF, Wu AK, Cheng VC, et al. Fatal interaction between clarithromycin and colchicine in patients with renal insufficiency: A retrospective study. *Clin Infect Dis* 2005;41:291-300.
46. Cheng VC, Ho PL, Yuen KY. Two probable cases of serious drug interaction between clarithromycin and colchicine. *South Med J* 2005;98:811-813.
47. Bonnel RA, Villalba ML, Karwoski CB, Beitz J. Deaths associated with inappropriate intravenous colchicine administration. *J Emerg Med* 2002;22:385-387.
48. Harrold LR, Andrade SE, Briesacher BA, et al. Adherence with urate-lowering therapies for the treatment of gout. *Arthritis Res Ther* 2009;11:R46.
49. Rees F, Jenkins W, Doherty M. Patients with gout adhere to curative treatment if informed appropriately: Proof-of concept observational study. *Ann Rheum Dis* 2012. Epub ahead of print.
50. Dessein PH, Shipton EA, Stanwix AE, et al. Beneficial effects of weight loss associated with moderate calorie/carbohydrate restriction, and increased proportional intake of protein and unsaturated fat on serum urate and lipoprotein levels in gout: A pilot study. *Ann Rheum Dis* 2000;59:539-543.
51. Choi HK, Atkinson K, Karlson EW, et al. Alcohol intake and risk of incident gout in men: A prospective study. *Lancet* 2004;363:1277-1281.
52. Zhang Y, Woods R, Chaisson CE, et al. Alcohol consumption as a trigger of recurrent gout attacks. *Am J Med* 2006;119: 800.e13-18.
53. Schlesinger N. Management of acute and chronic gouty arthritis: Present state-of-the-art. *Drugs* 2004;64:2399-2416.
54. Choi HK, Atkinson K, Karlson EW, et al. Purine-rich foods, dairy and protein intake, and the risk of gout in men. *N Engl J Med* 2004;350:1093-1103.
55. Choi HK, Willett W, Curhan G. Fructose-rich beverages and the risk of gout in women. *JAMA* 2010;304:2270-2278.
56. Choi HK, Curhan G. Soft drinks, fructose consumption, and ACR Guidelines for Gout Management: Part 1. 1445 the risk of gout in men: Prospective cohort study. *BMJ* 2008;36:309-312.
57. Singh JA, Reddy SG, Kundukulam J. Risk factors for gout and prevention: A systematic review of the literature. *Curr Opin Rheumatol* 2011;23:192-202.
58. Zhang Y, Chen C, Choi H, et al. Purine-rich foods intake and recurrent gout attacks. *Ann Rheum Dis* 2012;71:1448-1453.
59. Tsai YT, Liu JP, Tu YK, et al. Relationship between dietary patterns and serum uric acid concentrations among ethnic Chinese adults in Taiwan. *Asia Pac J Clin Nutr* 2012;21:263-270.
60. Ferraz MB, O'Brien B. A cost effectiveness analysis of urate lowering drugs in nontophaceous recurrent gouty arthritis. *J Rheumatol* 1995;22:908-914.
61. Dincer HE, Dincer AP, Levinson DJ. Asymptomatic hyperuricemia: To treat or not to treat. *Cleve Clin J Med* 2002;69:594-602.

62. Shoji A, Yamanaka H, Kamatani N. A retrospective study of the relationship between serum urate level and recurrent attacks of gouty arthritis: Evidence for reduction of recurrent gouty arthritis with antihyperuricemic therapy. *Arthritis Rheum* 2004;51:321-325.
63. Bull PW, Scott JT. Intermittent control of hyperuricemia in the treatment of gout. *J Rheumatol* 1989;16:1246-1248.
64. Seth R, Kydd ASR, Buchbinder R, et al. Allopurinol for chronic gout. *Cochrane Database of Systematic Reviews* 2014, Issue 10. Art. No.: CD006077.
65. Riedel AA, Nelson M, Joseph-Ridge N, et al. Compliance with allopurinol therapy among managed care enrollees with gout: A retrospective analysis of administrative claims. *J Rheumatol* 2004;31:1575-1581.
66. Yang C, Chen C, Deng S, et al. Allopurinol use and risk of fatal hypersensitivity reactions. A nationwide population-based study in Tawain. *JAMA* 2015;175:1550-1557.
67. Stamp LK, Taylor WJ, Jones PB, et al. Starting dose is a risk factor for allopurinol hypersensitivity syndrome: A proposed safe starting dose of allopurinol. *Arthritis Rheum* 2012;64:2529-2536.
68. Chao J, Terkeltaub R. A critical reappraisal of allopurinol dosing, safety, and efficacy for hyperuricemia in gout. *Curr Rheumatol Rep* 2009;11:135-140.
69. Perez-Ruiz F, Hernandez-Baldizon S, Herrero-Beites AM, et al. Risk factors associated with renal lithiasis during uricosuric treatment of hyperuricemia in patients with gout. *Arthritis Care Res (Hoboken)* 2010;62:1299-1305.
70. Saima C, Becker M. Update on emerging urate-lowering therapies. *Curr Opin Rheumatol* 2009;21:143-149.
71. Hande KR, Noone RM, Stone WJ. Severe allopurinol toxicity. Description and guidelines for prevention in patients with renal insufficiency. *Am J Med* 1984;76:47-56.
72. Ernst ME, Fravel MA. Febuxostat: A selective xanthine-oxidase/xanthine-dehydrogenase inhibitor for the management of hyperuricemia in adults with gout. *Clin Ther* 2009;31:2503-2518.
73. Becker MA, Schumacher HR, Wortmann RL, et al. Febuxostat compared with allopurinol in patients with hyperuricemia and gout. *N Engl J Med* 2005;353:2450-2461.
74. Tayar JH, Lopez-Olivo MA, Suarez-Almazor ME. Febuxostat for treating chronic gout. *Cochrane Database of Systematic Reviews* 2012, Issue 11. Art. No.: CD008653.
75. Thompson GR, Duff IF, Robinson WD, et al. Long term uricosuric therapy in gout. *Arthritis Rheum* 1962;5:384-396.
76. ZURAMPIC. Lesinurad. Wilmington, DE: AstraZeneca Pharmaceuticals, 2015.
77. Perez-Ruiz F, Sundy JS, Miner JN, et al. Lesinurad in combination with allopurinol: results of a phase 2, randomised, double-blind study in patients with gout with an inadequate response to allopurinol. Ann Rheum Dis Published Online First: [31 January 2016].
78. Sundy JS, Baraf HS, Yood RA, et al. Efficacy and tolerability of pegloticase for the treatment of chronic gout in patients refractory to conventional treatment: Two randomized controlled trials. *JAMA* 2011;306:711-720.
79. Shannon JA, Cole SW. Pegloticase: A novel agent for treatment-refractory gout. *Ann Pharmacother* 2012;46:368-376.
80. de la Serna G, Cadarso C. Fenofibrate decreases plasma fibrinogen, improves lipid profile, and reduces uricemia. *Clin Pharmacol Ther* 1999;66:166-172.
81. Feher MD, Hepburn AL, Hogarth MB, et al. Fenofibrate enhances urate reduction in men treated with allopurinol for hyperuricaemia and gout. *Rheumatol* 2003;42:321-325.
82. Hepburn AL, Kaye SA, Feher MD. Long-term remission from gout associated with fenofibrate therapy. *Clin Rheumatol* 2003;22:73-76.
83. Hepburn AL, Kaye SA, Feher MD. Fenofibrate: A new treatment for hyperuricaemia and gout? *Ann Rheum Dis* 2001;60:984-986.
84. Wurzner G, Gerster JC, Chiolero A, et al. Comparative effects of losartan and irbesartan on serum uric acid in hypertensive patients with hyperuricaemia and gout. *J Hypertens* 2001;19:1855-1860.
85. Shahinfar S, Simpson RL, Carides AD, et al. Safety of losartan in hypertensive patients with thiazide-induced hyperuricemia. *Kidney Int* 1999;56:1879-1885.
86. Borstad G, Bryant L, Abel M, et al. Colchicine for prophylaxis of acute flares when initiating allopurinol for chronic gouty arthritis. *J Rheumatol* 2004;31:2429-2432.
87. Kesselheim AS, Solomon DH. Incentives for drug development—The curious case of colchicine. *NEJM* 2010;362:2045-2047.
88. Kotz J. The gout pipeline crystallizes. *Nat Rev Drug Discov* 2012;11:425-426.
89. Tran T, Pham J, Shafeeq H, et al. Role of Interleukin-1 Inhibitors in the management of gout. *Pharmacotherapy* 2013;33:744-753.
90. Sivera F, Wechalekar MD, Andrés M, et al. Interleukin-1 inhibitors for acute gout. *Cochrane Database of Systematic Reviews* 2014, Issue 9. Art. No.: CD009993.
91. So A, De Meulemeester M, Pikhlak A, et al. Canakinumab for the treatment of acute flares in difficult-to-treat gouty arthritis. *Arthritis Rheum* 2010;62:3064-3076.
92. So A, De Smedt T, Revaz S, et al. A pilot study of IL-1 inhibition by anakinra in acute gout. *Arthritis Res Ther* 2007;9:R28.
93. Schlesinger N, De Meulemeester M, Pikhlak A, et al. Canakinumab relieves symptoms of acute flares and improves health-related quality of life in patients with difficult-to-treat gouty arthritis by suppressing inflammation: Results of a randomized, dose-ranging study. *Arthritis Res Ther* 2011;13:R53.
94. Chen K, Fields T, Mancuso C, et al. Anakinra's efficacy is variable in refractory gout: Report of ten cases. *Semin Arthritis Rheum* 2010;40:210-214.
95. Schumacher HR, Sundy JS, Terkeltaub R, et al. Rilonacept (interleukin-1 trap) in the prevention of acute gout flares during initiation of urate-lowering therapy: Results of a phase II randomized, double-blind, placebo-controlled trial. *Arthritis Rheum* 2012;64:876-884.
96. Schlesinger N, Mysler E, Lin HY, et al. Canakinumab reduces the risk of acute gouty arthritis flares during initiation of allopurinol treatment: Results of a double-blind, randomised study. *Ann Rheum Dis* 2011;70:1264-1271.
97. Sundy J, Schumacher R, Kivitz A, et al. Rilonacept for gout flare prevention in patients receiving uric acid-lowering therapy: results of RESURGE, a phase III, international safety study. *J Rheumatol* 2014;41:1703-1711.
98. Shahid H, Singh J. Investigational drugs for hyperuricemia. *Expert Opin Investig Drugs* 2015;24:1013-1030.
99. Diaz-Torne C, Perez-Herrero N, Perez-Ruiz F. New medications in development for the treatment of hyperuricemia of gout. *Curr Opin Rheumatol* 2015;27:164-169.
100. Riese RJ, Sakhaee K. Uric acid nephrolithiasis: Pathogenesis and treatment. *J Urol* 1992;148:765-771.
101. Pak CY, Sakhaee K, Fuller C. Successful management of uric acid nephrolithiasis with potassium citrate. *Kidney Int* 1986;30: 422-428.
102. Abbott RD, Brand FN, Kannel WB, et al. Gout and coronary heart disease: The Framingham Study. *J Clin Epidemiol* 1988;41: 237-242.
103. Freedman DS, Williamson DF, Gunter EW, et al. Relation of serum uric acid to mortality and ischemic heart disease. The NHANES I Epidemiologic Follow-up Study. *Am J Epidemiol* 1995;141:637-644.
104. Langford HG, Blaufox MD, Borhani NO, et al. Is thiazide-produced uric acid elevation harmful? Analysis of data from the Hypertension Detection and Follow-up Program. *Arch Intern Med* 1987;147:645-649.
105. Bengtsson C, Lapidus L, Stendahl C, Waldenstrom J. Hyperuricaemia and risk of cardiovascular disease and overall death. A 12-year follow-up of participants in the population study of women in Gothenburg, Sweden. *Acta Med Scand* 1988;224:549-555.
106. Choi HK, Curhan G. Independent impact of gout on mortality and risk for coronary heart disease. *Circulation* 2007;116:894-900.
107. Segal M, Srinivas T, Mohandas R, et al. The effect of the addition of allopurinol on blood pressure control in African Americans treated with a thiazide-like diuretic. *J Am Soc Hypertens* 2015;9: 610-619.
108. Beattie C, Fulton R, Higgins P, et al. Allopurinol initiation and change in blood pressure in odler adults with hypertension. *Hypertension* 2014:64:1102-1107.
109. Agarwal V, Hans N, Messerli F. Effect of allopurinol on blood pressure: A systematic review and met-analysis. *J Clin Hypertens* 2013;15:435-442.
110. Tausche A, Christoph M, Forkmann M, et al. As compared to allopurinol, urate-lowering therapy with febuxostat has superior effects on oxidative stress and pulse wave velocity in patients with sever chronic tophaceous gout. *Rheumatol Int* 2014;34:101-109.
111. Tsuruta Y, Kikuchi K, Tsuruta Y, et al. Febuxostat improves endothelial function in hemodialysis patient with hyperuricemia: A randomized controlled study. *Hemodial Int* 2015 May 21. [epub ahead of print]
112. Jung JW, Song WJ, Kim YS, et al. HLA-B58 can help the clinical decision on starting allopurinol in patients with chronic renal insufficiency. *Nephrol Dial Transplant* 2011;26:3567-3572.

113. Hung SI, Chung WH, Liou LB, et al. HLA-B*5801 allele as a genetic marker for severe cutaneous adverse reactions caused by allopurinol. *Proc Natl Acad Sci USA* 2005;102:4134-4139.
114. Tassaneeyakul W, Jantararoungtong T, Chen P, et al. Strong association between HLA-B*5801 and allopurinol-induced Stevens–Johnson syndrome and toxic epidermal necrolysis in a Thai population. *Pharmacogenet Genomics* 2009;19:704-709.
115. Gutman AB. The past four decades of progress in the knowledge of gout, with an assessment of the present status. *Arthritis Rheum* 1973;16:431-445.
116. Zhu Y, Pandya BJ, Choi HK. Comorbidities of gout and hyperuricemia in the US general population: NHANES 2007–2008. *Am J Med* 2012;125:679-687.

94 Glaucoma

Richard G. Fiscella, Timothy S. Lesar, Ohoud A. Owaidhah, and Deepak P. Edward

KEY CONCEPTS

1. Primary open-angle glaucoma (POAG) or ocular hypertension (OHT) is more prevalent outside Asia than primary angle closure glaucoma (PACG).
2. In any form of glaucoma, reduction of intraocular pressure (IOP) is essential.
3. IOP is a very important risk factor for glaucoma, but the most important considerations are progression of glaucomatous changes in the back of the eye (optic disk and nerve fiber layer) and visual field changes when diagnosing and monitoring for POAG or OHT.
4. Optic nerve changes often occur before visual field changes are exhibited.
5. Recent studies demonstrate that reduction in IOP prevents progression or even onset of glaucoma.
6. Newer medications simplify treatment regimens for patients. Prostaglandin analogs are considered the most potent topical medications for reducing IOP and flattening diurnal variations in IOP.
7. Local adverse events are common with topical glaucoma medications, but patient education and reinforcing adherence are essential to prevent glaucoma progression.

The glaucomas are a group of ocular disorders that lead to an optic neuropathy characterized by changes in the optic nerve head (optic disk) that is associated with loss of visual sensitivity and field. Increased intraocular pressure (IOP) is thought to play an important role in the pathogenesis of glaucoma, but it is not a diagnostic criterion for glaucoma. Consistently high IOP without signs or symptoms of glaucoma is called ocular hypertension (OHT).

Two major types of glaucoma have been identified: open angle and closed angle. Open-angle glaucoma (OAG) accounts for the great majority of cases in North America, while primary angle closure glaucoma (PACG) is more prevalent in Asia. Either type can be a primary inherited disorder, congenital, or secondary to disease, trauma, or drugs and can lead to serious complications. Both primary and secondary glaucomas may be caused by a combination of open-angle and closed-angle mechanisms (Table 94-1). Patients with consistently high IOP, or patients with clinical findings suspicious of early glaucomatous changes are called "glaucoma suspects."[1-6]

BASIC CONCEPTS

Aqueous Humor Dynamics and Intraocular Pressure

An understanding of IOP and aqueous humor dynamics will assist the reader in understanding the drug therapy of glaucoma.[1-3]

Aqueous humor is formed in the ciliary body and its epithelium (Figs. 94-1 and 94-2) through both filtration and secretion. Because ultrafiltration depends on pressure gradients, blood pressure and IOP changes influence aqueous humor formation. Osmotic gradients produced by active secretion of sodium and bicarbonate and possibly by other solutes such as ascorbate from the ciliary body epithelial cells into the aqueous humor result in movement of water from the pool of ciliary stromal ultrafiltrate into the posterior chamber, forming aqueous humor. Carbonic anhydrase (primarily isoenzyme type II), α- and β-adrenergic receptors, and sodium- and potassium-activated adenosine triphosphatases are found on the ciliary epithelium and appear to be involved in this secretion of the solutes sodium and bicarbonate.

Receptor systems controlling aqueous inflow have not been elucidated fully. Pharmacologic studies suggest that β-adrenergic agents increase inflow, whereas α_2-adrenergic blocking, β-adrenergic blocking, dopamine-blocking, carbonic anhydrase-inhibiting, melatonin-1 agonist, and adenylate cyclase-stimulating agents decrease aqueous inflow. Aqueous humor produced by the ciliary body is secreted into the posterior chamber at a rate of approximately 2 to 3 μL/min. The pressure in the posterior chamber produced by the constant inflow pushes the aqueous humor between the iris and lens and through the pupil into the anterior chamber of the eye (see Fig. 94-2).[1,3,7-9]

Aqueous humor in the anterior chamber leaves the eye by two routes: (a) filtration through the trabecular meshwork (conventional outflow) to the Schlemm's canal (80% to 85%) and (b) through the ciliary body and the suprachoroidal space (uveoscleral outflow or unconventional outflow). Cholinergic agents such as pilocarpine appear to increase outflow by physically opening the meshwork pores secondary to ciliary muscle contraction. Prostaglandins are thought to result in remodeling of extracellular matrix in the meshwork, thereby increasing outflow. The uveoscleral outflow of aqueous humor is increased by prostaglandin analogs and β- and α_2-adrenergic agonists. Constant inflow of aqueous humor from the ciliary body and resistance to outflow result in an IOP great enough to produce an outflow rate equal to the inflow rate (see Fig. 94-2). Novel adenosine receptor agonists, cannabinoids, serotonin agents, and dopamine agonists also increase aqueous humor outflow and reduce IOP.[1-4,7-9]

TABLE 94-1 General Classification of Glaucoma

I. Primary glaucoma
  A. Open angle
  B. Angle closure
    1. With pupillary block
    2. Without pupillary block
II. Secondary glaucoma
  A. Open angle
    1. Pretrabecular
    2. Trabecular
    3. Post-trabecular
  B. Angle closure
    1. Without pupillary block
    2. With pupillary block
III. Congenital glaucoma

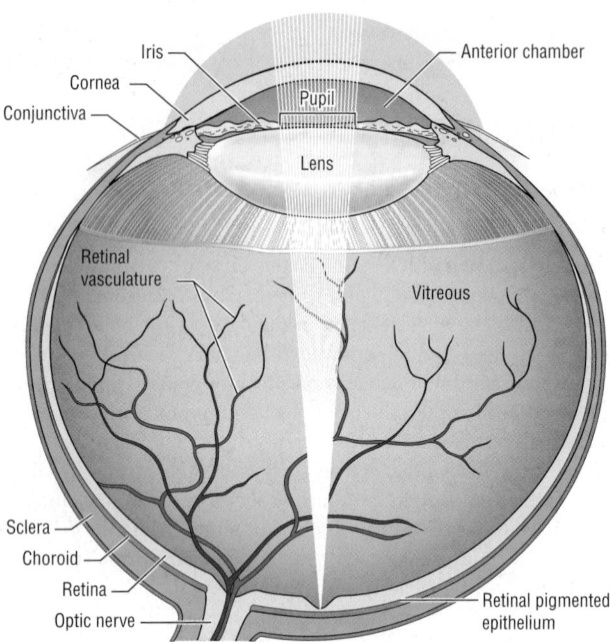

FIGURE 94-1 Anatomy of the eye.

The median IOP measured in large populations is 15.5 ± 2.5 mm Hg (2.1 ± 0.3 kPa); however, the distribution of pressures around the mean is skewed to the right (toward higher readings). IOP is not constant and changes with pulse, blood pressure, forced expiration or coughing, neck compression, and posture. Gender, general health, and lifestyle (eg, smoking) are some of the factors that may have a long-term effect on IOP.[1-6] The amount of caffeine in 1 cup of caffeinated coffee (182 mg) increases IOP by about 1 mm Hg (0.1 kPa) after 90 minutes, this increase in IOP is not clinically relevant. Patients who have thinner corneas have had laser refractory eye surgery (LASIK), or have had cataract surgery demonstrate falsely low IOP readings. IOP is measured by tonometry: indentation tonometry, applanation tonometry, or a noncontact method using an air pulse. Newer methods of tonometery include the Pascal tonometer, Icare™ rebound tonometer, and a contact lens-based investigational device that can remotely monitor 24-hour IOP changes from baseline.[10-12] These methods may result in slightly different pressure readings. IOPs consistently greater than 21 mm Hg (2.8 kPa) are found in 5% to 8% of the general population. The incidence increases with age, such that "abnormal" (ie, >22 mm Hg [>2.9 kPa]) IOP is found in 15% of those 70 to 75 years of age. Intermittently very high IOP (>40 mm Hg [>5.3 kPa]) is found in patients with PACG.[5] The increased IOP in all types of glaucoma results from the decreased facility for aqueous humor outflow. Aqueous humor production in primary open-angle glaucoma (POAG) is normal.[1-6]

Intraocular pressure demonstrates considerable circadian variation (often referred to as *diurnal* IOP or the IOP during the daily 24-hour cycle) primarily because of changes in the rate of aqueous humor formation. This circadian variation results in a minimum IOP at approximately 6 PM and a maximum IOP at awakening, although some studies suggest that both healthy and glaucoma patients may have their highest IOP at night after falling asleep.[1-3] Low systemic blood pressure in conjunction with high IOPs (decreased ocular perfusion pressure) at night can result in optic nerve head damage. Generally, the circadian IOP variation is less than 3 to 4 mm Hg (0.4 to 0.5 kPa); however, it may be greater for patients with glaucoma. This circadian variation and the poor relationship of IOP with visual loss make measurement of IOP a poor screening test for glaucoma. Controlling circadian increases in IOP is thought to be important in prevention of disease progression. Prostaglandin

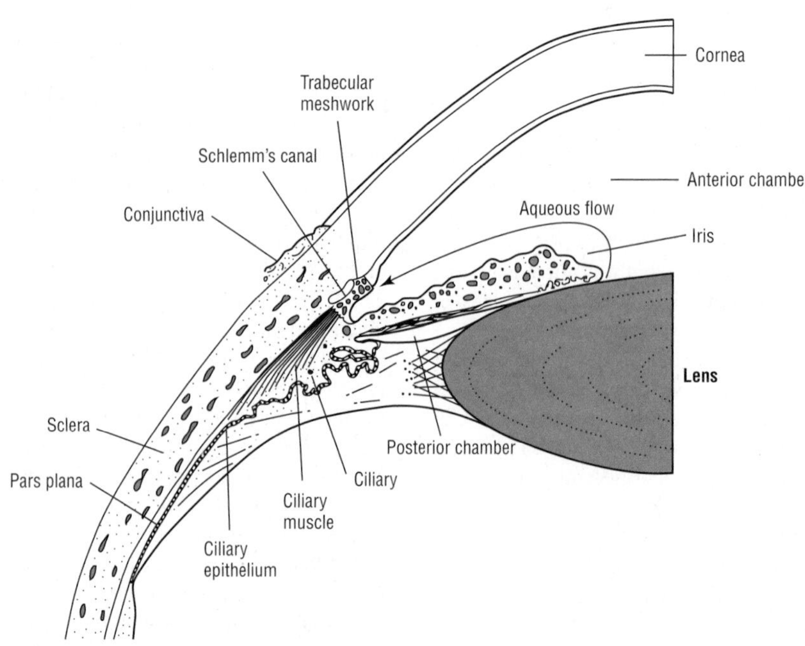

FIGURE 94-2 Anterior chamber of the eye and aqueous humor flow.

analogs and carbonic anhydrase inhibitors (CAIs) reduce nocturnal IOP, whereas β-blockers and alpha-2 adrenergic agents have minimal effects.[1,3,13]

Although increased IOP within any range is associated with a higher risk of glaucomatous damage, it is both an insensitive and nonspecific diagnostic and monitoring tool. Of individuals with IOP between 21 and 30 mm Hg (2.8 and 4.0 kPa), only 0.5% to 1% per year will develop optic disk changes and visual field loss (ie, glaucoma) over 5 to 15 years. However, more subtle retinal damage, such as alteration of color vision or decreased contrast sensitivity, occurs in a higher percentage of patients with IOPs greater than 21 mm Hg (2.8 kPa), and the incidence of visual field defects increases to as high as 28% in individuals with IOPs above 30 mm Hg (4.0 kPa). The risk of developing glaucoma increases with older age, family history of glaucoma, lower ocular perfusion pressure, lower blood pressure, thinner central cornea, optic disk hemorrhage, larger cup-to-disk ratio, and specific visual fields findings. For patients with preexisting optic nerve damage, the worse the existing damage, the more sensitive the eye is to a given IOP. As many as 20% to 30% of patients with glaucomatous visual field loss have an IOP of less than 21 mm Hg (2.8 kPa) (called *normal-tension glaucoma*, referring to the normal IOP). Thus the absolute IOP is a less-precise predictor of optic nerve damage. More direct measurements of therapeutic outcome, such as optic disk examination and visual field evaluation, also must be used as monitors of disease progression. Taking the above factors into consideration, glaucoma medications that provide maximal reduction of IOP over 24 hours and have minimal influence on blood pressure may be advantageous in treating glaucoma patients.[1-5,14-18]

Optic Disk and Visual Fields

The optic disk is the portion of the optic nerve ophthalmoscopically visible as it leaves the eye. It consists of approximately 1 million retinal ganglion nerve cell axons, blood vessels, and supporting connective tissue structures (lamina cribrosa). The small depression within the disk is termed the *cup* (Fig. 94-3). A normal physiologic cup does not extend beyond the optic nerve rim and has a varying diameter of less than one-third to one-half that of the disk (cup-to-disk ratio: 0.33 to 0.5). Table 94-2 lists the common alterations of the optic disk found in glaucoma. These disk changes result from optic nerve axonal degeneration and remodeling of the supporting structures. As the nerve axons die, the cup becomes larger in relation to the whole disk. A loss of retinal nerve fiber layer might be visualized in glaucoma patients with detectable visual field loss. This pattern of changes is consistent with visual field losses and loss of visual sensitivity seen in glaucoma.[1-4] Damage to the optic nerve can be documented by optic disk photographs, and disease stability or progression may be monitored by examining sequential photographs. Newer methods of assessing damage to the retinal nerve fiber layer and optic disk have been described. These include scanning laser polarimetry (GDX), confocal laser ophthalmoscopy (Heidelberg retinal tomography, or HRT), and optical coherence tomography (OCT). These methods offer the ability to assess the damage to the optic nerve quantitatively.

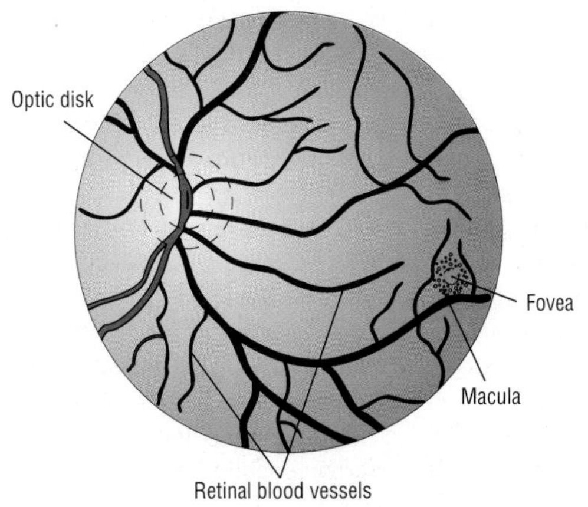

FIGURE 94-3 Normal fundus of the eye and optic disk and cup.

TABLE 94-2 Optic Disk and Visual Field Findings

Optic disk
Cup-to-disk ratio >0.5
Progressive increase in cup size
Cup-to-disk ratio asymmetry >0.2
Vertical elongation of the cup
Excavation of the cup
Increased exposure of lamina cribrosa
Pallor of the cup
Splinter hemorrhages
Cupping to edge of disk
Notching of the cup (usually superior or inferior)
Nerve fiber defects
Visual field findings
General peripheral field constriction
Isolated scotomas (blind spots)
Nasal visual field depression ("nasal step")
Enlargement of blind spot
Large arc-like scotomas
Reduced contrast sensitivity
Reduced peripheral acuity
Altered color vision

Determination of the visual field allows assessment of optic nerve damage and is an important monitoring parameter in treatment. However, visual field changes typically lag behind optic disk changes, and a loss of 25% to 35% of retinal ganglion cells is usually required before detectable visual field defects are noted. The peripheral visual field is measured using a visual field instrument called a *perimeter*. Characteristic visual field loss occurs in glaucoma (Fig. 94-4; see also Table 94-2), but loss of central visual acuity usually does not occur until late in the disease. Other indicators, such as color vision changes and contrast sensitivity, may allow earlier and more sensitive detection of glaucomatous changes.[1-4]

Genetics

Glaucoma is often inherited as a complex multifactorial disease, but it can also be inherited as a Mendelian autosomal-dominant or autosomal-recessive trait form. The common age-related adult-onset glaucoma, like POAG, although containing heritability of some significance, is more complex and is influenced by environmental factors. Genetic studies have more clearly defined the underlying molecular events responsible for the Mendelian forms of the disease. However, the chromosome locations identified may play some factor in the more complex forms. A number of major gene loci associated with POAG have been identified. The molecular mechanism of how mutations in any of these genes result in increased IOP with loss of visual field has not been elucidated. The future of genetic studies in glaucoma will include discovery of new glaucoma genes, determination of clinical phenotypes associated with these genes and mutations, understanding how environmental factors interact, and developing a database that can be used for further testing.

Genome-wide association studies have identified new loci that are associated with clinically relevant optic disk parameters, including the optic disk area and vertical cup-disk ratio. Genes associated with chronic angle closure glaucoma (ACG) have also been identified. Improved understanding of the genetic origins of POAG may lead to new diagnostic tools and therapies that target the underlying causes of the disease.[1-4,19-21]

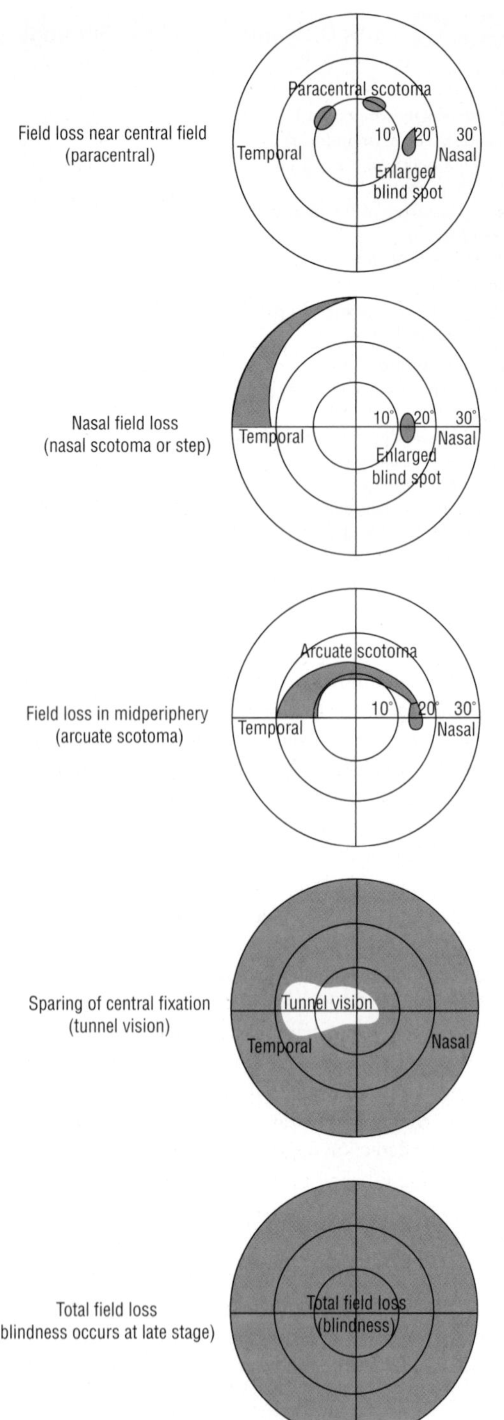

FIGURE 94-4 Schematic of the progression of visual field loss in glaucoma.

Epidemiology of Ocular Hypertension, Glaucoma Suspects, and Open-Angle Glaucoma

1 Overall, OHT occurs in 4.5% of non-Hispanic whites in the United States. The frequency increases to 7.7% of those older than 79 years.[22-25] The number of glaucoma suspects (ie, those with consistently high IOP or suspicious eye findings) is thought to be 3-6 million individuals in the United States. Left untreated, approximately 2% of glaucoma suspects will progress to glaucoma each year.[1-4,14-18,24,25]

Open-angle glaucoma is the second leading cause of blindness, affecting up to 4 million individuals in the United States and up to 70 million individuals worldwide. It is estimated that more than 135,000 persons in the United States and about 6-7 million in the world have glaucoma-related bilateral blindness. The prevalence rate varies with age, race, diagnostic criteria, and other factors. In the United States, OAG occurs in 1.5% of the population older than 30 years of age, 1.3% of whites and 3.5% of blacks. Recent study data have also suggested that the prevalence of OAG and OHT is also high among Latinos of Mexican ancestry, with approximately 4.74% and 3.56% of people affected, respectively.[20]

The incidence of OAG increases with increasing age. The incidence of the disease for patients 80 years of age is 3% in whites and 5% to 8% in blacks. In addition to increased IOP, older age, and ethnicity, the risk of glaucoma increases with family history, thinner central corneal thickness, lower ocular perfusion pressure, type 2 diabetes, myopia, and certain genetic mutations.[1-5,21-25]

Etiology of Open-Angle Glaucoma

2 The specific cause of glaucomatous optic neuropathy is presently unknown. Previously, increased IOP was considered to be the sole cause of the damage; however, it is now recognized that IOP is only one of many factors associated with the development and progression of glaucoma. Increased susceptibility of the optic nerve to ischemia (a reduced or dysregulated blood flow), excitotoxicity, autoimmune reactions, and other abnormal physiologic processes are likely additional contributory factors. The final outcome of these processes is believed to be apoptosis of the retinal ganglion cells, which results in axonal degeneration and finally permanent loss of vision. POAG may represent a number of distinct diseases or conditions that simply manifest the same symptoms. Susceptibility to visual loss at a given IOP varies considerably; some patients do not demonstrate damage at high IOPs, whereas other patients have progressive visual field loss despite an IOP in the normal range (normal-tension glaucoma).[1-4,6]

Although IOP poorly predicts which patients will have visual field loss, the risk of visual field loss clearly increases with increasing IOP within any range. In fact, recent studies demonstrate that lowering IOP, no matter what the pretreatment IOP, reduces the risk of glaucomatous progression or may even prevent the onset to early glaucoma in patients with OHT.[1-4,6,14-18]

The mechanism by which a certain level of IOP increases the susceptibility of a given eye to nerve damage remains controversial. Multiple mechanisms are likely to be operative in a spectrum of combinations to produce the death of retinal ganglion cells and their axons in glaucoma. Pressure-sensitive astrocytes and other cells in the optic disk supportive matrix may produce changes and remodeling of the disk, resulting in axonal death. Vasogenic theories suggest that optic nerve damage results from insufficient blood flow to the retina secondary to the increased perfusion pressure required in the eye, dysregulated perfusion, or vessel wall abnormalities, and results in degeneration of axonal fibers of the retina. Another theory suggests that the IOP may disrupt axoplasmal flow at the optic disk.[1-3]

Recently, focus on the mechanisms of the retinal ganglion cell apoptosis and the role of excessive glutamate and nitric oxide found in glaucoma patients has broadened the focus of drug therapy research to include evaluation of agents that act as neuroprotectants. Such agents may be particularly useful for patients with normal-pressure glaucoma, in whom pressure-independent factors may play a relatively larger role in disease progression. These agents would target risk factors and underlying pathophysiologic mechanisms of disease other than IOP.[2,8,13-15,26-29]

CLINICAL PRESENTATION Glaucoma

General

- Glaucoma can be detected in otherwise asymptomatic patients, or patients can present with characteristic symptoms, especially vision loss. POAG is a chronic, slowly progressive disease found primarily in patients older than 50 years of age, whereas PACG is more typically associated with symptomatic acute episodes or may be slowly progressive as with POAG

Symptoms

- POAG: None until substantial visual field loss occurs
- PACG: Nonsymptomatic or prodromal symptoms (blurred or hazy vision with halos around lights that is caused by a hazy, edematous cornea, and occasionally headache) may be present. Acute episodes produce symptoms associated with a cloudy, edematous cornea, ocular pain, or discomfort, nausea, vomiting, abdominal pain, and diaphoresis

Signs

- POAG: Disk changes and visual field loss (see Table 94-2); IOP can be normal or elevated (>21 mm Hg [>2.8 kPa])

  Mild: Optic disk abnormalities with normal visual field with standard perimetry
  Moderate: Optic disk changes plus visual field abnormalities in one hemifield that are not within 5 degrees of central visual fixation
  Severe: Optic disk changes with visual field loss in both hemifields and loss within 5 degrees of central fixation and abnormalities in at least one hemifield
- Acute ACG: Acute hyperemic conjunctiva, cloudy cornea, shallow anterior chamber, and occasionally an edematous and hyperemic optic disk; IOP is generally elevated markedly (40 to 90 mm Hg [5.3 to 12.0 kPa]) when symptoms are present
- Chronic ACG (CACG): Disk changes and visual field loss (see Table 94-2); IOP can be normal or elevated (>21 mm Hg [>2.8 kPa])

Laboratory Tests

- None

Other Diagnostic Tests

- Emerging tests include OCT, retinal nerve fiber analyzers, and confocal scanning laser tomography of the optic nerve

Pathophysiology of Open-Angle Glaucoma

3 As stated previously, optic nerve damage in POAG can occur at a wide range of IOPs, and the rate of progression is highly variable. Patients may exhibit pressures in the 20 to 30 mm Hg (2.7 to 4.0 kPa) range for years before any disease progression is noticed in the optic disk or visual fields. That is why POAG is often referred to as the "sneak thief of sight."

Clinical Presentation of Open-Angle Glaucoma

Primary open-angle glaucoma is a bilateral, often asymmetric, genetically determined disorder constituting 60% to 70% of all glaucomas and 90% to 95% of primary glaucomas in the United States (see Clinical Presentation of Glaucoma above). An increased IOP is not required for diagnosis of POAG. Symptoms do not present until substantial visual field constriction occurs. Central visual acuity typically is maintained even in the late stages of the disease. Even though POAG is a bilateral disease, it may have greater IOP and progression and severity in one eye. As such, each eye is treated individually.[1-4,6]

4 Detection and diagnosis involve evaluation of the optic disk and retinal nerve fiber layer, assessment of the visual fields, and measurement of IOP. The presence of characteristic disk changes and visual field loss with or without increased IOP confirms the diagnosis of glaucoma. Typical disk changes and field loss occurring at an IOP of less than 21 mm Hg (2.8 kPa) account for 20% to 30% of patients and are referred to as *normal-tension glaucoma*. Elevated IOP (>21 mm Hg [>2.8 kPa]) without disk changes or visual field loss is observed in 5% to 7% of individuals (*glaucoma suspects*) and is referred to as *OHT*. New technologies, such as OCT, retinal nerve fiber analyzers, or confocal scanning laser tomography of the optic nerve head, may allow early identification of signs of glaucomatous retinal changes in ocular hypertensives, thus allowing for earlier initiation of therapy.[1-5]

Secondary OAG has many causes, including exfoliation syndrome, pigmentary glaucoma, systemic diseases, trauma, surgery, ocular inflammatory diseases, and medications. A system for classifying secondary glaucomas into pretrabecular, trabecular, and post-trabecular forms has been proposed. This classification allows drug therapy to be chosen on the basis of the pathogenic mechanism involved. In pretrabecular forms, a normal meshwork is covered and does not permit aqueous humor outflow. Trabecular forms of secondary glaucoma result from either an alteration of meshwork or an accumulation of material in the intertrabecular spaces. The post-trabecular forms result primarily from disorders causing increased episcleral venous blood pressure.[1]

Prognosis of Open Angle Glaucoma

5 In most cases of POAG, the overall prognosis is excellent when it is discovered early and treated adequately. Even patients with advanced visual field loss can have continued visual field loss reduced if the IOP is maintained at low enough pressures (often <10 to 12 mm Hg [<1.3 to 1.6 kPa]). Medications will control IOP successfully in 60% to 80% of patients over a 5-year period. Progression of visual field loss still occurs in 8% to 20% of patients despite reaching standard therapy IOP goals. However, for untreated patients and for those who fail to achieve target IOP reduction, up to 80% have continued visual field loss. Estimates of progression to bilateral blindness in treated patients range from 4% to 22%. Compared with placebo, each 1 mm Hg (0.1 kPa) in IOP reduction reduces risk of disease progression by at least 10%.[1-4,14-18] After 2 years, visual field loss occurred in 25.6% of placebo patients compared with 15.2% of those treated with latanoprost.[18] Thus, the keys to medical treatment of POAG are an effective, well-tolerated drug regimen, close monitoring of therapy, and adherence.[1-4]

Epidemiology of Primary Angle Closure Glaucoma

The incidence of PACG varies by the ethnic group, with a higher incidence in individuals of Inuit, Chinese, and Asian-Indian descent. Incidence rates of 1% to 4% have been reported in these populations.[1,2] Because of the high frequency of PACG in populous Asia, PACG accounts for approximately one-third of glaucoma worldwide. PACG accounts for a disproportionately high proportion of blindness (estimated at up to 50%) worldwide.[1-3,5,30]

Etiology of Primary Angle Closure Glaucoma

In North America, PACG accounts for a minority of primary glaucomas. When severe ACG occurs, it may need to be treated as an emergency to avoid visual loss. PACG results from mechanical blockage of the (usually normal) trabecular meshwork by the peripheral iris. Partial or complete blockage of the meshwork occurs intermittently, potentially resulting in extreme fluctuations between normal IOP with no symptoms and very high IOP with symptoms of acute PACG. Between attacks of PACG, the IOP is usually normal unless the patient has concomitant POAG or nonreversible blockage of the meshwork with synechiae ("creeping" angle closure) that develops over time in the narrow-angle eye. PACG occurs in patients with inherited shallow anterior chambers (often seen in small eyes), which produce a narrow angle between the cornea and iris or tight contact between the iris and lens (pupillary block). The presence of a narrow angle is determined mainly by visualization of the angle by gonioscopy. Other tests for PACG involve provocation of an angle-closure-induced IOP increase. These tests, which attempt to produce angle closure through mydriasis (darkroom test or mydriasis test) or gravity (prone test), are rarely performed in the clinical setting.

Two major types of classic, reversible PACG have been described: PACG with pupillary block and PACG without pupillary block. PACG with pupillary block results when the iris is in firm contact with the lens. This produces a relative block of aqueous flow through the pupil to the anterior chamber (pupillary block), resulting in a bowing forward of the iris, which blocks the trabecular meshwork. PACG with pupillary block occurs most commonly when the pupil is in mid-dilation. In this position, the combination of pupillary block and relaxed iris allows the greatest bowing of the iris; however, angle closure may occur during miosis or mydriasis.

Primary angle closure glaucoma can occur without significant pupillary block for patients with an abnormality called a *plateau iris*. The ciliary processes in these cases are situated anteriorly, which indent the iris forward and cause closure of the trabecular meshwork, especially during mydriasis. The mydriasis produced by anticholinergic drugs or any other drug results in precipitation of both types of PACG glaucoma, whereas drug-induced miosis may produce pupillary block.[1-3,5,30]

Pathophysiology of Primary Angle Closure Glaucoma

The mechanism of IOP elevation in PACG is more clear than that of POAG. In PACG, a physical blockage of trabecular meshwork is present. In many cases, single or multiple episodes of high IOP that in some patients may exceed 40 mm Hg (5.3 kPa) and result in optic nerve damage. Very high IOP (>60 mm Hg [>8.0 kPa]) may result in permanent loss of visual field within a matter of hours to days.

One type of CAG, known as "creeping" angle closure, occurs in patients with narrow angles in which the iris adheres to the trabecular meshwork and may result in continuously increased IOP in ranges more similar to those of POAG, and the clinical behavior is similar to POAG, with individuals differing in the degree and rapidity of visual loss from any given elevated IOP.[1,30]

Clinical Presentation of Angle Closure Glaucoma

Most patients with untreated PACG typically experience intermittent nonsymptomatic or prodromal symptoms brought on by precipitating events (see Clinical Presentation of Glaucoma above). Increased IOP during such prodromal episodes is not great enough or long enough to produce the other symptoms of a full-blown attack. Such prodromal attacks last 1 to 2 hours, at which time pupillary block is broken by further mydriasis or miosis, or when miosis or mydriasis occurs in patients with plateau iris. The rate at which IOP increases may be a determinant of when full-blown symptoms occur. Visual fields demonstrate generalized constriction or typical glaucomatous defects as seen in POAG. In approximately 25% of patients, severe attacks may occur and if prolonged, total loss of vision may occur if the IOP is high enough. Tonometry reveals IOPs as high as 40 to 90 mm Hg (5.3 to 12.0 kPa). Patients who have developed adhesions between the iris and meshwork (anterior synechiae) may have chronic IOP elevation with intermittent spikes of high IOP when angle closure occurs.[1-2,30]

Drug-Induced Glaucoma

A number of medications are associated with increased IOP or carry labeling that cautions against use of the medication in glaucoma patients. The potential for a medication to produce or worsen glaucoma depends on the type of glaucoma and whether the patient is treated adequately.[1-4,31] Patients with treated, controlled POAG are at minimal risk of induction of an increase in IOP by systemic medications with anticholinergic properties or vasodilators; however, for patients with untreated glaucoma or uncontrolled POAG, the potential of these medications to increase IOP should be considered. Topical anticholinergic agents used to produce mydriasis may result in an increase in IOP. Potent anticholinergic agents such as atropine or homatropine are most likely to increase IOP. Weaker anticholinergics, such as tropicamide, that produce less cycloplegia are less likely to increase IOP and are favored, along with phenylephrine, when mydriasis is desired for POAG patients. Inhaled, nasal, topical, or systemic glucocorticoids may increase IOP for both normal individuals and patients with POAG.

Patients with POAG appear to be particularly susceptible to glucocorticoid-induced increases in IOP. Glucocorticoids reduce the facility of aqueous humor outflow through the trabecular meshwork. The decreased facility of outflow appears to result from the accumulation of extracellular material blocking the trabecular channels. The potential of a glucocorticoid to increase IOP is related to its anti-inflammatory potency and intraocular penetration. Thus, patients should be treated with the lowest potency and dose and for the shortest time possible when steroids are indicated.

For patients predisposed to CAG (ie, narrow anterior chambers), angle closure may be produced by any drug that causes mydriasis (eg, anticholinergics). A wide range of sulfa compounds causes idiosyncratic reactions that result in anterior choroidal effusions with anterior movement of the iris and lens, resulting in angle closure. The topical use of anticholinergics or sympathomimetic agents most likely will result in angle closure. Systemic and inhaled anticholinergic and sympathomimetic agents also must be used with caution in such patients. As discussed previously, potent miotic agents such as echothiophate may produce angle closure by increasing pupillary block. Table 94-3 lists the drugs associated with potentiation of glaucoma.

TABLE 94-3 Drugs That May Induce or Potentiate Increased Intraocular Pressure

Open-angle glaucoma
Ophthalmic corticosteroids (high risk)
Systemic corticosteroids
Nasal/inhaled corticosteroids
Fenoldopam
Ophthalmic anticholinergics
Succinylcholine
Vasodilators (low risk)
Cimetidine (low risk)
Closed-angle glaucoma
Topical anticholinergics
Topical sympathomimetics
Systemic anticholinergics
Heterocyclic antidepressants
Low-potency phenothiazines
Antihistamines
Ipratropium
Benzodiazepines (low risk)
Theophylline (low risk)
Vasodilators (low risk)
Systemic sympathomimetics (low risk)
CNS stimulants (low risk)
Serotonin-selective reuptake inhibitors
Imipramine
Venlafaxine
Topiramate
Tetracyclines (low risk)
Carbonic anhydrase inhibitors (low risk)
Monoamine oxidase inhibitors (low risk)
Topical cholinergics (low risk)

TREATMENT

Glaucoma Suspects and Ocular Hypertension

Treatment of the patient with possible glaucoma (OHT; ie, patients with IOP >22 mm Hg [>2.9 kPa]) is less controversial with the recent results of the Ocular Hypertensive Treatment Study (OHTS) than it was in the past.[14] The OHTS helped to identify risk factors for treatment. Patients with IOPs higher than 25 mm Hg (3.3 kPa), vertical cup-to-disk ratio of more than 0.5, and central corneal thickness of less than 555 μm are at greater risk for developing glaucoma. Risk factors such as family history of glaucoma, black, Latino/Hispanic ethnicity, severe myopia, and patients with only one eye must also be taken into consideration when deciding which individuals need treatment.

Patients without risk factors typically are not treated and are monitored for the development of glaucomatous changes. The use of risk calculators has been suggested as a means of determining who are at greatest risk in developing glaucoma. It is hoped that with future improvement in such calculators, one would be able to tailor treatment to those at greatest risk for developing glaucoma.

Patients with significant risk factors usually are treated with a well-tolerated topical agent such as a prostaglandin analog or β-blocking agent. Other options include a α_2-agonist (brimonidine) or a topical CAI, depending on individual patient characteristics. Therapy may be initiated in one eye to assess tolerance and efficacy; however, because each eye may respond differently to medications as well as possible contralateral effects, IOP response may be compared with baseline in individual eyes.

The goal of therapy is to lower the IOP to a level associated with a decreased risk of optic nerve damage, usually at least a 20%, if not a 25% to 30% decrease from the baseline IOP. Greater decreases may be required in high-risk patients or those with higher initial IOPs. Drug therapy should be monitored by measurement of IOP, examination of the optic disk, assessment of the visual fields, and evaluation of the patient for drug adverse effects and compliance with therapy. Patients who are unresponsive to or intolerant of a drug should be switched to an alternative agent rather than given an additional drug. Partial responders may be treated with combinations of well-tolerated topical medications (prostaglandins, β-blockers, brimonidine or a CAI). Use of multiple combinations of topical agents or when first-line agents fail to reduce IOP depends on the risk-to-benefit assessment of each patient. Some clinicians prefer to discontinue all medications for patients who fail to respond adequately to simple topical therapy, closely monitor for development of disk changes or visual field loss, and treat again when such changes occur.[6] The cost, inconvenience of frequent adverse effects of multiple-combination therapies, pilocarpine, dipivefrin, cholinesterase inhibitors, and oral CAIs generally result in an unfavorable risk-to-benefit ratio for glaucoma suspect patients.[1-4,6,32-35]

TREATMENT

Open-Angle Glaucoma

All patients with elevated IOP and characteristic optic disk changes and/or visual field defects not caused by other factors (ie, glaucoma by definition) should be treated. Recent findings that one in five patients with "normal" IOP and glaucomatous retinal nerve findings (ie, normal-tension glaucoma) do not have progression of visual field loss if left untreated have prompted recommendations to monitor normal-tension glaucoma patients without immediate threat of loss of central vision and to treat only when progression is documented. Some controversy exists as to whether the initial therapy of glaucoma should be surgical trabeculectomy (filtering procedure), argon or selective laser trabeculectomy, or medical therapy.[1-4,32-44] Presently, drug therapy remains the most common initial treatment modality. Drug therapy of patients with documented glaucomatous change with either elevated or normal IOP is initiated in a stepwise manner (Fig. 94-5), starting with a single, well-tolerated topical agent. The goal of therapy is to prevent further visual loss. A "target" IOP is chosen based on a patient baseline IOP and the amount of existing visual field loss. Typically, an initial target IOP reduction of 25-30% is desired. Greater reductions may be desired for patients with very high baseline IOPs or advanced visual field loss. Patients with normal baseline IOPs (normal-tension glaucoma) may have target IOPs of less than 10 to 12 mm Hg (1.3 to 1.6 kPa).[1-4]

Clinical **Controversy...**

How much should the IOP be reduced for patients who may have POAG? Although the major clinical trial (OHTS[3]) required a 20% reduction in IOP for patients with OHT, many clinicians believe a further lowering of IOP may be more beneficial in preventing the progression of OHT to glaucoma. The American Academy of Ophthalmology Preferred Practice Guidelines suggest 20% to 30% IOP lowering. It remains to be seen if a more aggressive approach earlier in the treatment of the POAG suspect would be more beneficial.

Pharmacotherapeutic Approach

6 Medications most commonly used to treat glaucoma are the prostaglandin analogs, nonselective β-blockers, brimonidine (a α_2-agonist), the topical CAIs, and the fixed combination products of timolol/dorzolamide, timolol/brimonidine, brimonidine/

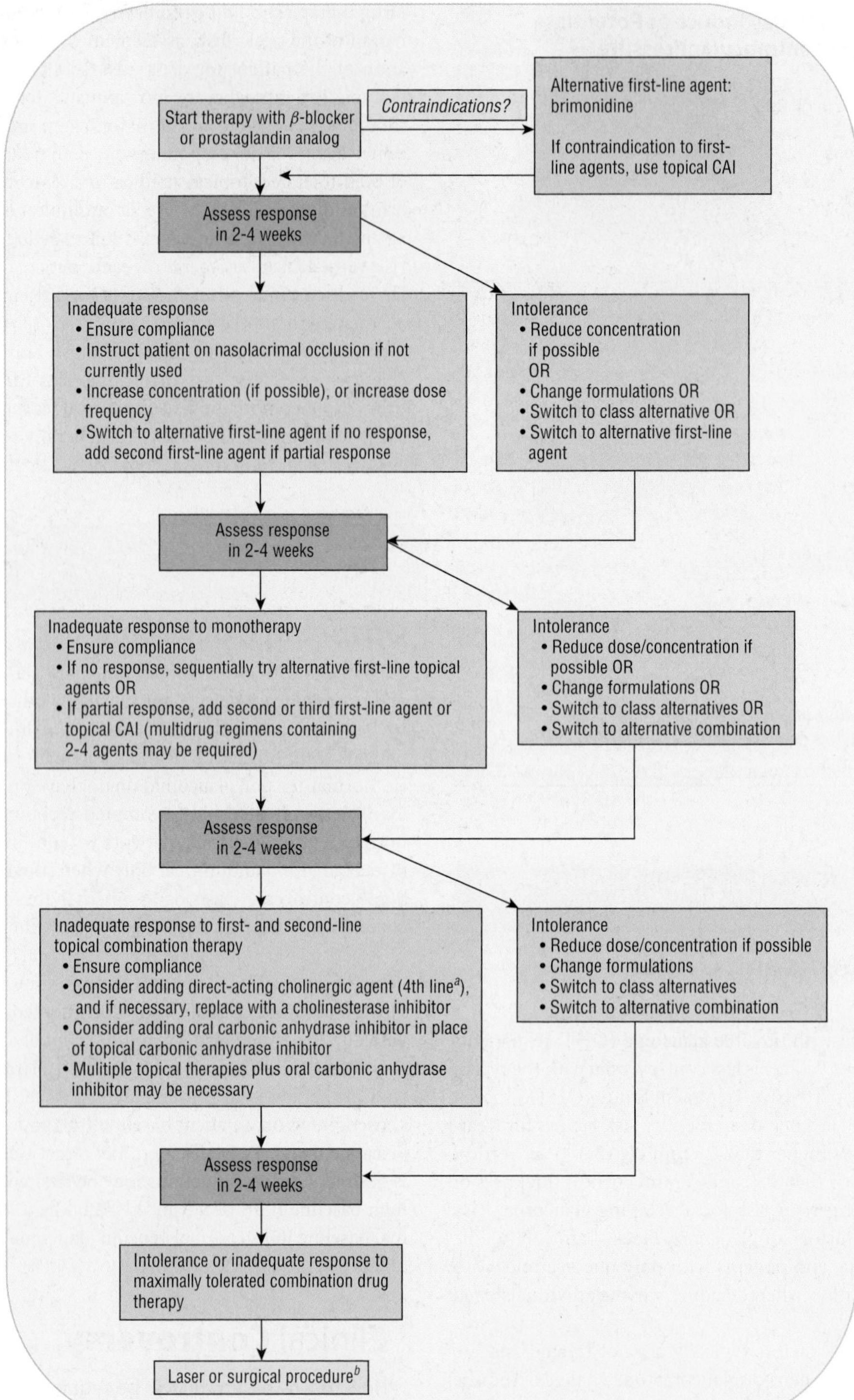

FIGURE 94-5 Algorithm for the pharmacotherapy of open-angle glaucoma. [a]Fourth-line agents not commonly used any longer or commercially unavailable. [b]Most clinicians believe the laser procedure should be performed earlier (eg, after three-drug maximum, poorly adherent patient). (CAI, carbonic anhydrase inhibitor.)

brinzolamide, or timolol/prostaglandins (marketed outside the United States).[1-4,32-35]

The prostaglandin analogs are often recommended as first-line therapy. They offer once-daily dosing, better IOP reduction, better 24-hour IOP control, good tolerance, and availability of lower-cost generics (see Fig. 94-5). The topical β-blockers have a long history of successful use, providing a combination of clinical efficacy and general tolerability. Brimonidine and topical CAIs are also well tolerated and effective agents, but often considered second-line agents (to prostaglandins and β-blockers).[1-4] Therapy optimally is started as a single agent, and may be started in one eye (except for patients with very high IOP or advanced visual field loss) to evaluate drug efficacy and tolerance, although response may differ between contralateral eyes. Monitoring of therapy should be individualized. Initial check for IOP response to therapy is typically done 4 to 6 weeks after the medication is started. Once IOPs reach acceptable levels, the IOP is monitored every 3 to 4 months or longer if there is prolonged control (over 6-12 months) without progression. More frequent monitoring is necessary if the IOP target is not achieved, disease progression is noted, and after any change in drug therapy.[1-4,6]

Clinical **Controversy...**

The American Academy of Ophthalmology has not designated any agent as the drug of choice for initiation of glaucoma treatment. In recent years, many clinicians have used the prostaglandin analogs because they are dosed once daily and achieve the best pressure reduction and are available as less expensive generic products.

Visual fields and disk changes are typically monitored every 6-12 months or earlier if the glaucoma is unstable or there is suspicion of disease worsening. Patients should always be questioned regarding adherence to and tolerance of prescribed therapy. Initial IOP response does not predict long-term IOP control, as tachyphylaxis to IOP reduction and or disease progression may occur.

The value of an agent with which the patient has shown a drop in IOP following an initial response can be measured by discontinuing the medication completely and determining if an increase in IOP occurs. Patients responding to but intolerant of initial therapy may be switched to another drug. For patients failing to respond to an initial drug, a switch to an alternative agent should be considered. If only a partial response occurs, addition of another topical drug to be used in combination is a possibility. A number of drugs or drug combinations may need to be tried before an effective and well-tolerated regimen is identified.

Prostaglandin agonists, β-blockers, brimonidine, CAIs, and pilocarpine may be used in various combinations. Adding a second drug generally results in a less-than-additive reduction in IOP. Using more than one drop per dose does not improve response but rather increases the likelihood of adverse effects and the cost of therapy. When using more than one medication, separation of drop instillation of each agent by at least 5 minutes is suggested to provide optimal ocular absorption.

Combination products reduce the number of daily doses, possibly improving adherence and preventing washout effect seen when a second medication is administered too soon after the initial medication. Use of combination products also reduces exposure to ophthalmic preservatives. Ocular surface disease (OSD) secondary to glaucoma therapy will often manifest as superficial punctate keratitis, tear-film instability or allergy.[45] In-vivo and animal studies have demonstrated the toxic effects of preservatives—benzalkonium chloride in particular—through various mechanisms. However, extrapolating these results to clinical use is difficult because these studies must control for effects such as blinking, tear dilution and turnover, and buffering capabilities of the human eye. While many crossover clinical trials show benefit to preservative-free therapies, many other studies demonstrate no improvement. Patients with medication-related OSD may try treatment with artificial tears, anti-inflammatory therapy, or possibly preservative-free therapy if feasible.

The IOP response to ocular hypotensive medication may vary with corneal thickness. The response might be better in those with normal or thin corneas than in those with thicker structures.

Because of the frequency of adverse effects, dipivefrin, carbachol, topical cholinesterase inhibitors, and oral CAIs are considered last-line agents to be used for patients who fail less-toxic combination topical therapy.

Nonpharmacologic Therapy: Laser and Surgical Procedures

When drug therapy fails, is not tolerated, or is excessively complicated, surgical procedures such as laser trabeculoplasty (argon or selective) or a surgical trabeculectomy (filtering procedure) may be performed to improve outflow. Laser trabeculoplasty is usually an intermediate step between drug therapy and trabeculectomy. The newer selective laser trabeculoplasty (SLT) procedure has demonstrated similar IOP reduction as argon laser trabeculoplasty (ALT) and may be repeatable. Recent studies have demonstrated good efficacy for this procedure in comparison with medical treatment options for POAG. Procedures with higher complication rates, such as those involving placement of draining tubes or destruction of the ciliary body (cyclodestruction), may be required when other methods fail (see Fig. 94-2).[1-4]

Surgical methods for reduction of IOP involve the creation of a channel through which aqueous humor can flow from the anterior chamber to the subconjunctival space (filtering bleb), where it is reabsorbed by the vasculature. A major reason for failure of the procedure is healing and scarring of the site. The use of aqueous shunts or valves to manage glaucoma has been increasing, and the results of a recent study have demonstrated improved safety and efficacy of these devices. However, glaucoma surgery is still plagued with the shortcomings despite modifications and improvements over the past century, including potentially vision-threatening complications such as hypotony, wound leaks, and infections.[38,39,46] Minimally invasive glaucoma surgery (MIGS) uses microincisions and implants that reduce IOP by targeting various areas of the outflow pathway.[46] These can either be approached from inside the eye (ab-interno) (eg, iStent, Hydrus, Trabectome, suprachoroidal shunts) or outside the eye (ab-externo) (eg, canaloplasty, Gold micro shunt, and Stegman Canal Expander).[46]

Modification of the healing process to maintain patency is possible with the use of antiproliferative agents. The antiproliferative agents 5-fluorouracil and mitomycin C are used for patients undergoing glaucoma-filtering surgery to improve success rates by reducing fibroblast proliferation and consequent scarring. Although used most commonly for patients with increased risk for suboptimal surgical outcome (after cataract surgery and a previous failed filtering procedure), use of these agents also improves success in low-risk patients.[38,39,46] A standardized formulation of mitomycin C (MMC) that is prepacked in a kit with a fixed dose and concentration was approved by FDA in 2012 and is commercially available under the name "Mitosol."

TREATMENT

Acute Angle Closure Crisis (AACC)

The goal of initial therapy for acute acute angle closure crisis (AACC) with high IOP is rapid reduction of the IOP to preserve vision and to avoid surgical or laser iridectomy on a hypertensive, congested eye. Iridectomy (laser or surgical) is the definitive treatment of PACG; it produces a hole in the iris that permits aqueous humor flow to move directly from the posterior chamber to the anterior chamber, opening up the block at the trabecular meshwork. Drug therapy of an AACC typically involves administration one or more topical antiglaucoma medications including miotics (eg, pilocarpine), secretory inhibitors (β-blockers, α_2-agonist, or topical/systemic CAIs), or a prostaglandin agonist.[5,30] The miosis produced by pilocarpine pulls the peripheral iris away from the meshwork. However, miotics may worsen angle closure by increasing pupillary block and producing anterior movement of the lens because of drug-induced accommodation. The aqueous secretory inhibitors and pilocarpine may not be effective due to ischemia of the ciliary body and pupillary sphincter, respectively. During this time, the urge to use excessive amounts of topical agents must be resisted. A hyperosmotic agent such as mannitol or glycerin may be needed to temporarily reduce IOP and restore response to the topical agents.

An osmotic agent also is commonly administered because these drugs produce the most rapid decrease in IOP. Oral glycerin 1 to 2 g/kg can be used if an oral agent is tolerated; if not, IV mannitol 1 to 2 g/kg should be used. Osmotic agents reduce IOP by withdrawing water from the eye secondary to the osmotic gradient between the blood and the eye. These drugs are among the first-line agents in the short-term treatment of an AACC or other forms of acute very high IOP elevations. Topical corticosteroids often are used to reduce the ocular inflammation and reduce the development of synechiae in PACG eyes. Patients failing therapy altogether will require an emergency iridectomy. Once the IOP is controlled, iridectomy is performed on the affected eye as well as the contralateral eye (if narrow angles are present).

Peripheral iridectomy essentially "cures" primary PACG without significant synechiae. Long-term drug therapy is not used unless IOP remains high because of the presence of synechiae blocking the trabecular meshwork or concurrent POAG. In such cases, the pharmacotherapeutic approach is essentially identical to that for the POAG patient, or laser or surgical procedures are performed.[1,2,5,30]

PHARMACOLOGIC AGENTS USED IN GLAUCOMA

Prostaglandin Analogs

The prostaglandin analogs, including latanoprost, travoprost, bimatoprost, and tafluprost, reduce IOP by increasing the uveoscleral and, to a lesser extent, trabecular outflow of aqueous humor. Some differences in receptor sites and mechanisms of action may exist between the two prostaglandins (latanoprost and travoprost) and the prostamide (bimatoprost). However, both classes appear to produce collagen changes matrix in the ciliary body and trabecular meshwork. Bimatoprost may be slightly more effective in lowering IOP, getting a larger percentage of patients to lower IOPs, and for patients unresponsive to latanoprost. If the patient does not respond to one prostaglandin agonist, a switch to another may be beneficial.[37,40,41] Generic forms of some prostaglandin analogs are now available, reducing the cost to patients for these agents. Tafluprost is available as a preservative-free solution, which may be useful in patients intolerant of common ophthalmic preservatives or those with corneal surface disorders.

Reduction in IOP with once-daily doses of prostaglandin analogs (a 25% to 35% reduction) is often greater than that seen with timolol 0.5% twice daily. In addition, nocturnal control of IOP is improved compared with timolol.[2,40,41] Interestingly, administration of prostaglandin analogs twice daily may reduce the IOP similarly to once-daily dosing. The drugs are administered at nighttime, although they are probably as effective if given in the morning.

Prostaglandin analogs are well tolerated and produce fewer systemic adverse effects than timolol. Local ocular tolerance generally is good, but ocular reactions such as punctate corneal erosions and conjunctival hyperemia do occur. Local intolerance occurs in 10% to 25% of patients with these agents.[1-3,9,33-35]

With prostaglandin analogs, altered iris pigmentation occurs in 15% to 30% of patients, particularly those with mixed-color irises (blue-brown, green-brown, blue-gray-brown, or yellow-brown eyes), which become browner in color over 3 to 12 months. The change in iris pigmentation will often appear within 2 years, and long-term consequences of this pigment change appear to be mostly cosmetic but irreversible upon discontinuation. Hypertrichosis is common and reverses upon discontinuation of the drug. Hyperpigmentation around the lids and lashes has also been reported and appears to reverse upon discontinuation. Loss of periorbital fat has been reported; this may lead to apparent enophthalmos and sunken eye especially when agents are used unilaterally.

Topical prostaglandin analogs may produce rates of corneal thinning that are slightly higher than ongoing age-related changes. This effect is unlikely to be clinically relevant.[7-9,33-35]

These agents have occasionally been associated with uveitis, and caution is recommended for patients with ocular inflammatory conditions. Cases of cystoid macular edema and worsening of herpetic keratitis have been reported.

Prostaglandin analogs can be used in combination with other antiglaucoma agents for additional IOP control because of their unique mechanism of action. Given their excellent efficacy and side-effect profile, prostaglandin analogs provide effective monotherapy or adjunctive therapy for patients who are not responding to or tolerating other agents. Long-term studies demonstrate these agents are safe, efficacious, and well tolerated in glaucoma therapy.[4,7-9,33-35] Various fixed combination prostaglandin products, often with timolol, are available in Canada and other countries.

β-Blocking Drugs

The topical β-blocking agents are one of the most commonly used antiglaucoma medications (Table 94-4). β-Blockers lower IOP by 20% to 30% with a minimum of local ocular adverse effects. β-blockers have minimal effects on nocturnal IOP. These are commonly one of the agents of first choice—along with prostaglandin analogs—in treating POAG if no contraindications exist.[1-4,9,33-35]

The β-blocking agents produce ocular hypotensive effects by decreasing the production of aqueous humor by the ciliary body without producing substantial effects on aqueous humor outflow facility. The mechanism by which β-blockers decrease aqueous humor inflow remains controversial, but it is most frequently attributed to β_2-adrenergic receptor blockade in the ciliary body.

Five ophthalmic β-blockers are presently available: timolol, levobunolol, metipranolol, carteolol, and betaxolol. Timolol, levobunolol, and metipranolol are nonspecific β-blocking agents, whereas betaxolol is a relatively β_1-selective agent. Carteolol is a nonspecific blocker with intrinsic sympathomimetic activity. Despite differences in potency, selectivity, lipophilicity, and intrinsic sympathomimetic activity, the five agents reduce IOP to a similar degree, although betaxolol has been reported to produce somewhat less lowering of IOP than timolol and levobunolol. Levobunolol, which possesses α-adrenergic effects, may be more effective than timolol and betaxolol in reducing IOP elevations after cataract surgery and may be more effective in controlling IOP than other agents when given as aqueous solutions on a once-daily schedule (up to 70% of patients). Timolol in the form of a gel-forming solution (Timoptic-XE) provides equivalent IOP control with once-daily administration when compared with the same concentration of the aqueous solution administered twice daily. The choice of a specific β-blocking agent generally is based on differences in adverse effect potential, individual patient response, and cost. Treatment with topical β-blockers may result in tachyphylaxis (short-term escape and long-term drift) in 20% to 25% of patients. The mean IOP reduction from baseline may be smaller for patients receiving topical β-blockers with concurrent systemic β-blockers.[9,33-35]

Local adverse effects with β-blockers usually are tolerable, although stinging on application occurs commonly, particularly with betaxolol solution (less with betaxolol suspension) and metipranolol. Other local effects include dry eyes, corneal anesthesia, blepharitis, blurred vision, and, rarely, conjunctivitis, uveitis, and keratitis. Some local reactions may be a result of preservatives used in the commercially available products. Switching from one agent to another or switching the type of formulation may improve tolerance in patients experiencing local adverse effects.

Systemic effects are the most important adverse effects of β-blockers. Drug absorbed systematically may produce decreased heart rate, reduced blood pressure, negative inotropic effects, conduction defects, bronchospasm, CNS effects, and alteration of serum

TABLE 94-4 Topical Drugs Used in the Treatment of Open-Angle Glaucoma

Drug	Pharmacologic Properties	Common Brand Names	Dose Form	Strength (%)	Usual Dose[a]	Mechanism of Action
β-Adrenergic Blocking Agents						
Betaxolol	Relative β_1-selective	Generic	Solution	0.5	One drop twice a day	All reduce aqueous production of ciliary body
		Betoptic-S	Suspension	0.25	One drop twice a day	
Carteolol	Nonselective, intrinsic sympathomimetic activity	Generic	Solution	1	One drop twice a day	
Levobunolol	Nonselective	Betagan	Solution	0.25, 0.5	One drop twice a day	
Metipranolol	Nonselective	OptiPranolol	Solution	0.3	One drop twice a day	
Timolol	Nonselective	Timoptic, Betimol, Istalol	Solution	0.25, 0.5	One drop every day—one to two times a day	
		Timoptic-XE	Gelling solution	0.25, 0.5	One drop every day[a]	
Adrenergic Agonists						
Non-specific Adrenergic Agent						
Dipivefrin**	Epinephrine prodrug	Propine	Solution	0.1	One drop twice a day	Increased aqueous humor outflow
α_2-Adrenergic Agonists						
Apraclonidine	Specific α_2-agonists	Iopidine	Solution	0.5 (U.D.), 1	One drop two to three times a day	Both reduce aqueous humor production; brimonidine known to also increase uveoscleral outflow; only brimonidine has primary indication
Brimonidine		Alphagan P	Solution	0.2 (generic) 0.15 (brand/generic), 0.1	One drop two to three times a day	
Cholinergic Agonists Direct Acting						
Carbachol**	Irreversible	Carboptic, Isopto Carbachol	Solution	1.5, 3	One drop two to three times a day	All increase aqueous humor outflow through trabecular meshwork
Pilocarpine	Irreversible	Isopto Carpine, Pilocar	Solution	0.5, 1, 2, 4, 6	One drop two to three times a day One drop four times a day	
		Pilopine HS**	Gel	4	Every 24 hours at bedtime	
Cholinesterase Inhibitors						
Echothiophate**		Phospholine Iodide	Solution	0.125	Once or twice a day	
Carbonic Anhydrase Inhibitors						
Topical						
Brinzolamide	All carbonic anhydrase inhibition	Azopt	Suspension	1	Two to three times a day	All reduce aqueous humor production of ciliary body
Dorzolamide		Trusopt Generic	Solution	2	Two to three times a day	
Systemic						
Acetazolamide		Generic	Tablet	125 mg, 250 mg	125-250 mg two to four times a day	
		Injection	500 mg/vial	250-500 mg		
		Diamox Sequels	Capsule	500 mg	500 mg twice a day	
Methazolamide		Generic	Tablet	25 mg, 50 mg	25-50 mg two to three times a day	

(continued)

TABLE 94-4 Topical Drugs Used in the Treatment of Open-Angle Glaucoma (*Continued*)

Drug	Pharmacologic Properties	Common Brand Names	Dose Form	Strength (%)	Usual Dose[a]	Mechanism of Action
Prostaglandin Analogs						
Latanoprost	Prostanoid agonist	Xalatan	Solution	0.005	One drop every night	Increases aqueous uveoscleral outflow and to a lesser extent trabecular outflow
Bimatoprost	Prostamide agonist	Lumigan	Solution	0.01, 0.03	One drop every night	
Travoprost	Prostanoid agonist	Travatan Z	Solution	0.004	One drop every night	
Tafluprost	Prostanoid agonist	Zioptan	Preservative free solution	0.0015	One drop every night	
Combinations						
Timolol–dorzolamide		Cosopt Generic	Solution	Timolol 0.5 dorzolamide 2	One drop twice daily	Reduce aqueous production
Timolol–brimonidine		Combigan	Solution	Timolol 0.5 brimonidine 0.2	One drop twice daily	Reduce aqueous production and increase uveoscleral outflow
Brinzolamide–brimonidine		Simbrinza		Brinzolamide 1 brimonidine 0.2	One drop three times daily	Reduce aqueous production and increase uveoscleral outflow
Timolol-latanoprost***		Xalacom	Solution	Timolol 0.5 latanoprost 0.005	One drop every night	All reduce aqueous production and increase uveoscleral outflow
Timolo-travoprost***		Duotrav	Solution	Timolol 0.5 travoprost 0.004	One drop every night	
Timolol-bimatoprost***		Ganfort	Solution	Timolol 0.5 Bimatoprost 0.03	One drop every night	

[a]Use of eyelid closure (ELC) technique for 5 minutes will increase the drug availability and reduce potential for local and systemic side effects.

**Often used as fourth-line agents; limited or no commerical availability.

***Not available in U.S.

lipids and may block the symptoms of hypoglycemia. The β_1-specific agents' betaxolol and possibly carteolol (as a consequence of intrinsic sympathomimetic activity) are less likely to produce the systemic adverse effects caused by β-adrenergic blockade, such as the cardiac effects and bronchospasm, but a real risk still exists. The use of timolol as a gel-forming liquid or betaxolol as a suspension allows for administration of fewer drugs per day and, therefore, reduces the chance for systemic adverse effects compared with the aqueous solutions.

Because of their systemic adverse effects, all ophthalmic β-blockers should be used with caution for patients with pulmonary diseases, sinus bradycardia, second- or third-degree heart block, congestive heart failure, atherosclerosis, diabetes, and myasthenia gravis, as well as for patients receiving oral β-blocker therapy. Use of the nasolacrimal occlusion (ELC; see Patient Education below for description) technique during administration reduces the risk or severity of systemic adverse effects, as well as optimizes response. Overall, β-adrenergic blocking agents are well tolerated by most patients, and most potential problems can be avoided by appropriate patient evaluation, drug choice, and monitoring of drug therapy. For patients failing or having an inadequate response to single-drug therapy with a β-blocking agent, the addition of a topical CAI, prostaglandin analog, or the α_2-adrenergic receptor agonist brimonidine usually will result in additional IOP reduction.[1-5,9,33-35]

α_2-Adrenergic Agonists

Brimonidine and the less lipid-soluble and less receptor-selective apraclonidine are α_2-adrenergic agonists structurally similar to clonidine. Apraclonidine is indicated and brimonidine is effective for prevention or control of postoperative or postlaser treatment increases in IOP. Brimonidine has a primary indication in OAG and is considered a second-line agent (often after a prostaglandin or β-blocker) or adjunctive agent. Apraclonidine is generally used only over the short term after ocular surgery due to high incidence of loss of control of IOP (tachyphylaxis) and a more severe and prevalent ocular allergy rate.

α_2-Agonists reduce IOP by decreasing the rate of aqueous humor production (some increase in uveoscleral outflow also occurs with brimonidine). The drugs reduce IOP by 18% to 27% at peak (2 to 5 hours) and by 10% at 8 to 12 hours. Comparative trials demonstrate a reduction in IOP similar to that obtained with 0.5% timolol. Use of brimonidine 0.2% every 8 to 12 hours appears to provide maximum IOP-lowering effects in long-term use. Use of ELC (see Patient Education below) may improve response and allow the longer dosing frequency (ie, every 12 hours). These agents have minimal effects on nocturnal IOP. Combinations of α_2-agonists with β-blockers, prostaglandin analogs, or CAIs produce additional IOP reduction.

An allergic-type reaction characterized by lid edema, eye discomfort, foreign-object sensation, itching, and hyperemia occurs in approximately 30% of patients with apraclonidine. Brimonidine produces this adverse effect in up to 8% of patients. This reaction commonly necessitates drug discontinuation. Systemic adverse effects with brimonidine include dizziness, fatigue, somnolence, dry mouth, and possibly a slight reduction in blood pressure and pulse. α_2-Agonists should be used with caution for patients with cardiovascular diseases, renal compromise, cerebrovascular disease, and diabetes, as well as in those taking antihypertensives and other cardiovascular drugs, monoamine oxidase inhibitors, and tricyclic antidepressants.

Brimonidine is also contraindicated in infants because of apneic spells and hypotensive reactions. In terms of overall efficacy and tolerability, brimonidine approximates that achieved with β-blockers.[1-4,9,33-35]

Brimonidine Purite 0.15% or 0.1% is a formulation of brimonidine in a lower concentration than the original product that contains a less corneal-toxic preservative than the commonly employed benzalkonium chloride. The newer formulations are as effective as the original because the more neutral pH of brimonidine Purite (0.15% pH 7.2; 0.1% pH 7.7) allows for higher concentrations of brimonidine in the aqueous humor with a similar reduction in IOP and a reduced incidence of ocular allergy.

A randomized clinical trial of topical brimonidine 0.2% twice daily preserved visual field better than treatment with topical timolol maleate 0.5% in patients with OAG and statistically normal IOP.[26] The IOP-lowering efficacy was similar between the two medications, suggesting that this finding was consistent with a non-IOP-related mechanism, possibly a neuroprotective action. However, validation of a neuroprotective role for brimonidine requires further research to confirm these results.[26-27] The combination product timolol 0.5% and brimonidine 0.2% (Combigan) may provide additional IOP lowering than either agent alone.[42]

Clinical **Controversy...**

Many animal trials demonstrate that brimonidine has excellent neuroprotective properties. Some clinicians believe that one of the major advantages of using brimonidine lies in its potential neuroprotective properties. However, neuroprotection has not been demonstrated in human trials, although a recent study produced the most clinically relevant data to date.[26,43]

Carbonic Anhydrase Inhibitors

Topical Agents

Carbonic anhydrase inhibitors reduce IOP by decreasing ciliary body aqueous humor secretion. CAIs appear to inhibit aqueous production by blocking active secretion of sodium and bicarbonate ions from the ciliary body to the aqueous humor.[1,2,9,33] The topical CAIs dorzolamide and brinzolamide, are well tolerated and are considered second line (after prostaglandins and β-lockers) for monotherapy or adjunctive therapy of POAG and OHT. These drugs reduce IOP by 15% to 26%.

Topical CAIs generally are well tolerated. Local adverse effects include transient burning and stinging, ocular discomfort and transient blurred vision, tearing, and, rarely, conjunctivitis, lid reactions, and photophobia. A superficial punctate keratitis occurs in 10% to 15% of patients. Brinzolamide produces more blurry vision but is less stinging than dorzolamide. Systemic adverse effects are unusual despite the accumulation of drug in red blood cells. Because of their favorable adverse-effect profile, topical CAIs provide a useful alternative agent for monotherapy or adjunctive therapy for patients with inadequate response to or who are unable to use other agents. The drugs may add additional IOP reduction for patients using other single or multiple topical agents. The usual dose of a topical CAI is one drop every 8 to 12 hours. Administration every 12 hours produces somewhat less IOP reduction than administration every 8 hours. Use of ELC should optimize response to CAI given at any interval.[1-3,9,33] The combination product timolol 0.5% and dorzolamide 2% (Cosopt) is dosed twice daily and produces equivalent IOP lowering to each product dosed separately. Both dorzolamide and timolol/dorzolamide (Cosopt) are now available as generic formulations. The combination product brimonidine 0.2% and brinzolamide 1% (Simbrinza) is dosed three times daily.

Systemic CAI Agents

Systemic CAIs are indicated for patients failing to respond to or tolerate maximum topical therapy. Systemic and topical CAIs should not be used in combination because no data exist concerning improved IOP reduction, and the risk for systemic adverse effects is increased. Oral CAIs reduce aqueous humor inflow by 40% to 60% and IOP by 25% to 40%. The available systemic CAIs (see Table 94-4) produce equivalent IOP reduction but differ for potency, adverse effects, dosage forms, and duration of action. Despite their excellent effects on elevated IOP of any etiology, the systemic CAIs frequently produce intolerable adverse effects. As a result, CAIs are considered third-line agents in the treatment of POAG and often used for short-term administration to lower IOP.

On average, only 30% to 60% of patients are able to tolerate oral CAI therapy for prolonged periods. Intolerance to CAI therapy results most commonly from a symptom complex attributable to systemic acidosis and including malaise, fatigue, anorexia, nausea, weight loss, altered taste, depression, and decreased libido. Other adverse effects include renal calculi, increased uric acid, blood dyscrasias, diuresis, and myopia. Elderly patients do not tolerate CAIs as well as younger patients. The available CAIs produce the same spectrum of adverse effects; however, the drugs differ in the frequency and severity of the adverse effects listed.

Carbonic anhydrase inhibitors should be used with some caution in patients with sulfa allergies (all CAIs, topical or systemic, contain sulfonamide moieties, although cross-sensitivity is thought to be very low), sickle cell disease, respiratory acidosis, pulmonary disorders, renal calculi, electrolyte imbalance, hepatic disease, renal disease, diabetes mellitus, or Addison's disease. Concurrent use of a CAI and a diuretic may rapidly produce hypokalemia. High-dose salicylate therapy may increase the acidosis produced by CAIs, whereas the acidosis produced by CAIs may increase the toxicity of salicylates.[1-4,9,33-35]

Parasympathomimetic Agents

The parasympathomimetic (cholinergic) agents reduce IOP by increasing aqueous humor trabecular outflow. The increase in outflow is a thought to be a result of physically pulling open the trabecular meshwork secondary to ciliary muscle contraction, thereby reducing resistance to outflow. These agents may actually reduce uveoscleral outflow. Their use as primary or even adjunctive agents in the treatment of glaucoma has decreased significantly because of local ocular adverse effects and/or frequent dosing requirements.

Pilocarpine, the parasympathomimetic agent of choice in POAG, is available as an ophthalmic solution and a hydrophilic polymer gel (see Table 94-4). Pilocarpine produces similar (20% to 30%) reductions in IOP as those seen with β-blocking agents. Pilocarpine in POAG is initiated as 1% solution, one drop three to four times daily. The use of ELC improves response and reduces the need for an every-6-hour dosing frequency. The use of one drop of 2% pilocarpine every 6 to 12 hours and ELC provides optimal response in many patients. Both drug concentration and frequency may be increased if IOP reduction is inadequate. Patients with darkly pigmented eyes frequently require higher concentrations of pilocarpine than do patients with lightly pigmented eyes. Concentrations of pilocarpine above 4% rarely improve IOP control in patients.

Pilocarpine 4% gel (Pilopine HS) once daily is equivalent to treatment with pilocarpine solution 4% four times daily or timolol 0.5% twice daily. Ocular adverse effects of pilocarpine include miosis, which decreases night vision and vision in patients with central cataracts. Visual field constriction may be seen secondary to miosis and should be considered when evaluating visual field changes in a glaucoma patient. Pilocarpine ciliary muscle contraction produces accommodative spasm, particularly in young patients still able to accommodate (prepresbyopic). Pilocarpine may also produce frontal headache, brow ache, periorbital pain, eyelid twitching, and conjunctival irritation or injection early in therapy, which tends to decrease in severity over 3 to 5 weeks of continued therapy.

Cholinergics produce a breakdown of the blood-aqueous humor barrier and may result in a worsening of an ocular inflammatory reaction or condition. Systemic cholinergic adverse effects of pilocarpine—such as diaphoresis, nausea, vomiting, diarrhea, cramping, urinary frequency, bronchospasm, and heart block—may be seen. Other adverse effects associated with direct-acting miotics include retinal tears or detachment, allergic reaction, permanent miosis, cataracts, precipitation of CAG, and, rarely, miotic cysts of the pupillary margin.

Carbachol is a potent direct-acting miotic agent; its duration of action is longer than that of pilocarpine (8 to 10 hours) because of resistance to hydrolysis by cholinesterases. This drug also may act as a weak inhibitor of cholinesterase. Patients with an inadequate response to or intolerance of pilocarpine as a result of ocular irritation or allergy frequently do well on carbachol. The ocular and systemic adverse effects of carbachol are similar to but more frequent, constant, and severe than those of pilocarpine.[33] Clinical use of carbachol is limited.

Echothiophate is a cholinesterase inhibitor, is used in the treatment of POAG. It is a long-acting, relatively irreversible agent (limited commercial availability; see Table 94-4). This agent is a potent inhibitor of pseudocholinesterase, but also inhibits true cholinesterase. Because of the serious ocular and systemic toxic effects of echothiophate, it is reserved primarily for patients who are either not responding to or are intolerant of other therapy. Because of its cataractogenic properties, most ophthalmologists use this agent only for patients without lenses (aphakia) and for patients with artificial lenses (pseudophakia). The ocular and periocular parasympathomimetic adverse effects are more common and more severe than with pilocarpine or carbachol.

In addition to the parasympathomimetic effects, echothiophate may produce severe fibrinous iritis (particularly with the irreversible inhibitors), synechiae, iris cysts, conjunctival thickening, occlusion of the nasolacrimal ducts, and cataracts. The inhibition of systemic pseudocholinesterase by echothiophate decreases the rate of succinylcholine hydrolysis, resulting in prolonged muscle paralysis. Echothiophate should be discontinued at least 2 weeks before procedures in which succinylcholine is used.

The role of echothiophate in glaucoma is limited by its frequency and potential toxicity. For phakic patients, cholinesterase inhibitors should be administered only if intolerance or failure results with other antiglaucoma medications. Echothiophate has been shown to provide additional IOP-lowering effects when used with β-blockers, CAIs, and sympathomimetic (adrenergic) agents. As with all agents for glaucoma, therapy should be initiated with lower concentrations of these agents. A once-daily administration frequency should be used for most patients unless very high IOP is present.

Use of ELC likely improves response, reduces systemic adverse effects, and should be performed by all patients administering echothiophate. The drug should be used with caution for patients with asthma, retinal detachments, narrow angles, bradycardia, hypotension, heart failure, Down's syndrome, epilepsy, parkinsonism, peptic ulcer, and ocular inflammation, as well as in those receiving cholinesterase inhibitor therapy for myasthenia gravis or exposure to carbamate or organophosphate insecticides and pesticides.

Dipivefrin

The mechanism of action by which dipivefrin (an epinephrine prodrug) lowers IOP has not been fully elucidated; however, a β_2-receptor–mediated increase in outflow facility through the trabecular meshwork and the uveoscleral route appears to be the primary mechanism. Compared with β-blockers or miotics, dipivefrin is less effective for reducing IOP. With the advent of the better-tolerated and more-efficacious agents to treat glaucoma, the clinical use of epinephrines has decreased dramatically and commercial availability discontinued.

A factor limiting the usefulness of dipivefrin is the high frequency of local ocular adverse effects. Tearing, burning, ocular discomfort, brow ache, conjunctival hyperemia, punctate keratopathy, allergic blepharoconjunctivitis, rare loss of eyelashes, stenosis of the nasolacrimal duct, and blurred vision may occur. Prolonged use (>1 year) may result in deposition of pigment (adrenochrome) in the conjunctiva and cornea. Pigment also may deposit in soft contact lenses, turning them black. Dipivefrin may produce mydriasis (particularly when combined with a β-blocker) and may precipitate acute CAG in patients with narrow anterior chambers. A transient increase in IOP may occur with initial therapy, particularly for patients not using other antiglaucoma medications. A relative contraindication to the use of dipivefrin is aphakia (ie, after cataract removal) or lens dislocation because of the development of swelling of the macular portion of the retina. The edema is dose dependent and disappears with drug discontinuation.

Systemic adverse effects of dipivefrin include headache, faintness, increased blood pressure, tachycardia, arrhythmias, tremor, pallor, anxiety, and increased perspiration. Dipivefrin should be used with caution for patients with cardiovascular diseases, cerebrovascular diseases, aphakia, CAG, hyperthyroidism, and diabetes mellitus, as well as for patients undergoing anesthesia with halogenated hydrocarbon anesthetics. Using ELC with dipivefrin will improve therapeutic response and reduce the risk of systemic adverse effects.[9,33-35]

Future Drug Therapies

It is hoped that new agents, improved formulations, and novel approaches to the reduction of IOP and other methods of prevention of glaucomatous visual field loss will provide more effective and better-tolerated therapies. Most areas of glaucoma development continue to focus on drugs that reduce IOP by either reducing aqueous production or increasing outflow. Classes of medication in development include the Rho kinase inhibitors (ROCK), which induce changes in the trabecular meshwork and thereby reduce impedance to aqueous outflow. These agents may also possess neuroprotective effects and produce an increase in ocular blood flow. Other classes of drugs in development include adenosine-1 receptor agonists, cannabinoids, serotonin agonists, dopamine agonists, nitric oxide/carbon dioxide modulators, and hydroxysteroid dehydrogenase inhibitors. Agents with dual ROCK inhibition and norepinephrine transport inhibition are in later clinical phase trials. Agents that are neuroprotective and act through mechanisms other than IOP reduction are also in development and are likely to be part of glaucoma therapy in the future.[7,8,27]

EVALUATION OF THERAPEUTIC OUTCOMES

The ultimate goal of drug therapy for the patient with glaucoma is to preserve visual function through reduction of IOP to a level at which no further optic nerve damage occurs. Because of the poor relationship between IOP and optic nerve damage, no specific target IOP exists. Indeed, drugs used to treat glaucoma may act in part to halt visual field loss through mechanisms separate from or in addition to IOP reduction, such as improvements in retinal or choroidal blood flow. Often a 25% to 30% reduction is desired, but greater reductions (40% to 50%) may be desired for patients with initially high IOPs. For patients with glaucoma, an IOP of less than 21 mm Hg (2.8 kPa) generally is desired, with progressively lower target pressures needed for greater levels of glaucomatous damage. Even lower IOPs (possibly even below 10 mm Hg [1.3 kPa]) are required for patients with very advanced disease, those showing continued damage at higher IOPs, and those with normal-tension glaucoma and pretreatment pressures in the low to middle teens. The IOP considered acceptable for a patient is often a balance of desired IOP and acceptable treatment-related toxicity and of patient quality of life.

PATIENT EDUCATION

7 An important consideration for patients failing to respond to drug therapy is adherence. Poor adherence or nonadherence occurs in 25% to 60% of glaucoma patients.

A large percentage of patients also fail to use topical ophthalmic drugs correctly. Patients should be taught the following procedure:

1. Wash and dry the hands; shake the bottle if it contains a suspension.
2. With a forefinger, pull down the outer portion of the lower eyelid to form a "pocket" to receive the drop.
3. Grasp the dropper bottle between the thumb and fingers with the hand braced against the cheek or nose and the head held upward.
4. Place the dropper over the eye while looking at the tip of the bottle; then look up and place a single drop in the eye.
5. The lids should be closed (but not squeezed or rubbed) for 5 minutes after instillation. This increases the ocular availability of the drug and reduces systemic absorption.
6. Recap bottle and store as instructed.

Note that many patients are physically unable to administer their own eye drops without assistance. ELC also should be used to improve ocular bioavailability and reduce systemic absorption.[1-4] The patient induces ELC for 5 minutes by gently closing the eyes. ELC decreases nasolacrimal drainage of drug, thereby decreasing the amount of drug available for systemic absorption by the nasopharyngeal mucosa. The use of ELC may improve drug response significantly, reduce adverse effects, and allow less-frequent dosing intervals and the use of lower drug concentrations.

Use of more than one drop per dose increases costs, does not improve response significantly, and may increase adverse effects. When two drugs are to be administered, instillations should be separated by at least 5 minutes (preferably 10 minutes) to prevent the drug administered first from being washed out. The patient should be taught not to touch the dropper bottle tip with eye, hands, or any surface.

Adherence to glaucoma therapy usually is inadequate, and it always should be considered as a possible cause of drug therapy failure. Assessment of adherence by healthcare providers generally is poor; so all patients should be encouraged continually to administer prescribed therapy diligently as instructed. To improve adherence, the patient, family, and care providers should be fully informed of the expectations of therapy and the need to continue therapy despite a lack of symptoms. Possible adverse effects of the medication and ways to reduce them should be discussed. Adherence will be improved by good communication, simplified and well tolerated dosing regimens, reminder devices, education, close monitoring, and individualized care planning.[1-4,6,44]

CONCLUSION

The glaucomas are a group of primary and secondary diseases whose management presents a considerable challenge to the clinician. Successful therapy requires rational use of antiglaucoma medications and patient adherence to the selected regimen, combined with conscientious monitoring for adverse effects and disease progression. The reward for successful therapy is considerable—the maintenance of vision. The overview of the clinical findings, pathology, and drug therapy presented in this chapter provides the clinician with the fundamentals necessary to understand and treat glaucoma.

ABBREVIATIONS

AACC	acute angle closure crisis
ACG	angle closure glaucoma
ALT	argon laser trabeculoplasty
CAG	closed-angle glaucoma
CAI	carbonic anhydrase inhibitor
ELC	eyelid closure
HRT	Heidelberg retinal tomography
IOP	intraocular pressure
MIGS	minimally invasive glaucoma surgery
OAG	open-angle glaucoma
OCT	optical coherence tomography
OHT	ocular hypertension
OHTS	Ocular Hypertensive Treatment Study
OSD	ocular surface disease
PACG	primary angle closure glaucoma
POAG	primary open-angle glaucoma
SLT	selective laser trabeculoplasty

REFERENCES

1. Quigley HA. Glaucoma. *Lancet* 2011;377:1367-1377.
2. Weinreb RN, Aung T, Madeiros FA. The pathophysiology and treatment of glaucoma. *JAMA* 2014;311:1901-1911.
3. Kwon YH, Fingert JH, Kuehn MH, Alward WLM. Primary open-angle glaucoma. *N Engl J Med* 2009;360:1113-1124.
4. American Academy of Ophthalmology Glaucoma Panel. Preferred Practice Pattern Guidelines. Primary open angle glaucoma. San Francisco, CA. American Academy of Ophthalmology. 2010. Available at: www.aao.org/ppp
5. American Academy of Ophthalmology Glaucoma Panel. Preferred Practice Pattern Guidelines. Primary angle closure. San Francisco, CA. American Academy of Ophthalmology. 2010. Available at: www.aao.org/ppp
6. American Academy of Ophthalmology Glaucoma Panel. Preferred Practice Pattern Guidelines. Primary open angle glaucoma suspect. San Francisco, CA. American Academy of Ophthalmology. 2010. Available at: www.aao.org/ppp
7. Bucolo C, Salomone S, Drago F, Reibaldi M, Longo A, Uva MG. Pharmacological management of ocular hypertension: Current approaches and future perspective. *Curr Opin Pharmacol* 2013;13:50-55.
8. Kolko M. Present and new treatment strategies in the management of glaucoma. *The Open Ophthalmol J* 2015;9(Suppl 1:M5):89-100.
9. Marquis RE, Whitson JT. Management of glaucoma: Focus on pharmacological therapy. *Drugs Aging* 2005;22:1-21.

10. Kotecha A, White E, Schlottmann PG, Garway-Heath DF. Intraocular pressure measurement precision with the Goldmann applanation, dynamic contour, and ocular response analyzer tonometers. *Ophthalmology* 2010;117:730-737 (Epub 2010 Feb 1).
11. Hsiao YC, Dzau JR, Flemmons MS, et al. Home assessment of diurnal intraocular pressure in healthy children using the Icare rebound tonometer. *JAAPOS* 2012;16(1):58-60.
12. Mansouri K, Medeiros FA, Tafreshi A, Weinreb RN. Continuous 24-hour monitoring of intraocular pressure patterns with a contact lens sensor: Safety, tolerability, and reproducibility in patients with glaucoma. *Arch Ophthalmol* 2012;13:1-6. doi:10.1001/archophthalmol.2012.2280.
13. Wax MB, Camras CB, Fiscella RG, et al. Emerging perspectives in glaucoma: Optimizing 24-hour control of intraocular pressure. *Am J Ophthalmol* 2002;133:S1-S10.
14. Kass MA, Heuer DK, Higginbotham EJ, et al. The ocular hypertension treatment study: A randomized trial determines that topical ocular hypotensive medication delays or prevents the onset of primary open-angle glaucoma. *Arch Ophthalmol* 2002;120:701-713, discussion 829, 830.
15. Leske MC, Heijl A, Hussein M, et al. Factors for glaucoma progression and the effect of treatment: The early manifest glaucoma trial. *Arch Ophthalmol* 2003;121:48-56.
16. Van Veldhuisen PC, Schwartz AL, Gaasterland DE, et al. The advanced glaucoma intervention study (AGIS): 7. The relationship between control of intraocular pressure and visual field deterioration. *Am J Ophthalmol* 2000;130:429-440.
17. Collaborative Normal-Tension Glaucoma Study Group. Comparison of glaucomatous progression between untreated patients with normal-tension glaucoma and patients with therapeutically reduced intraocular pressures. *Am J Ophthalmol* 1998;126:487-497.
18. Garway-Heath DF, Crabb DP, Bunce C, et al. Latanoprost for open angle glaucoma (UKGTS): A randomized, multicenter, placebo controlled trial. *Lancet* 2015;385:1295-2015.
19. Ramdas WD, van Koolwijk LM, Lemij HG, et al. Common genetic variants associated with open-angle glaucoma. *Hum Mol Genet* 2011;20(12):2464-2471.
20. Vithana EN, Khor CC, Qiao C, et al. Genome-wide association analyses identify three new susceptibility loci for primary angle closure glaucoma. *Nat Genet* 2012;44:1142-1146. doi:10.1038/ng.2390.
21. Wiggs JL. Genetic etiologies of glaucoma. *Arch Ophthalmol* 2007;125: 30-37.
22. Brandt JD, Beiser JA, Gordon MO, et al. Ocular Hypertension Treatment Study (OHTS) Group. Central corneal thickness and measured IOP response to topical ocular hypotensive medication in the Ocular Hypertension Treatment Study. *Am J Ophthalmol* 2004;138:717-722.
23. Ocular Hypertension Treatment Study Group; European Glaucoma Prevention Study Group; Gordon MO, Torri V, Miglior S, et al. Validated prediction model for the development of primary open-angle glaucoma in individuals with ocular hypertension. *Ophthalmology* 2007;114:10-19.
24. Quigley HA, Broman AT. The number of people with glaucoma worldwide in 2010 and 2020. *Br J Ophthalmol* 2006;90:262-267.
25. Brandt JD, Gordon MO, Beiser JA, et al. Ocular Hypertension Treatment Study Group. Changes in central corneal thickness over time: The ocular hypertension treatment study. *Ophthalmology* 2008; 115:1550-1556.
26. Krupin T, Liebmann JM, Greenfield DS, et al. A randomized trial of brimonidine versus timolol in preserving visual function: Results from the Low-pressure Glaucoma Treatment Study. *Am J Ophthalmol* 2011;151:671-681.
27. Quigley HA. Clinical trials for glaucoma neuroprotection are not impossible. *Curr Opin Ophthalmol* 2012;23:144-154.
28. Tanna AP, Rademake AW, Stewart WC, Feldman RM. Meta-analysis of the efficacy and safety of beta-2-adrenergic agonists, adrenergic antagonists, and topical carbonic anhydrase inhibitors with prostaglandin analogs. *Arch Ophthalmol* 2010;128(7):825-833.
29. Hoyng PF, van Beek LM. Pharmacological therapy for glaucoma: A review. *Drugs* 2000;59:411-434.
30. Wright C, Tawfik MA, Waisbourd M, Katz LJ. Primary angle-closure glaucoma: an update. *Acta Ophthalmologica* 2015; June 27. doi:1010.1111/aos12784 e-publication ahead of print.
31. Tripathi RC, Tripathi BJ, Haggerty C. Drug-induced glaucomas. *Drug Saf* 2003;26:749-767.
32. Grover DS, Smith O. Recent clinical pearls from clinical trials in glaucoma. *Curr Opin Ophthalmol* 2012;23:127-134.
33. Schuman JS. Antiglaucoma medications: A review of safety and tolerability issues related to their use. *Clin Ther* 2000;22:167-208.
34. Kanner E, Tsai JC. Glaucoma medications. Use and safety in the elderly population. *Drugs Aging* 2006;23:321-332.
35. Han JA, Frishman WH, Sun SW, et al. Cardiovascular and respiratory considerations with pharmacotherapy of glaucoma and ocular hypertension. *Cardiol Rev* 2008;16:95-108.
36. Katz LJ, Steinmann WC, Kabir A, et al. Selective laser trabeculoplasty versus medical therapy as initial treatment of glaucoma: A prospective, randomized trial. *J Glaucoma* 2012;21:460-468.
37. Law SK. Switching within glaucoma medication class. *Curr Opin Ophthalmol* 111:1439-1448.
38. Mearza AA, Aslanides IM. Uses and complications of mitomycin C in ophthalmology. *Expert Opin Drug Saf* 2007;6:27-32.
39. Loon SC, Chew PT. A major review of antimetabolites in glaucoma therapy. *Ophthalmologica* 1999;213:234-245.
40. van der Valk R, Webers CA, Schouten JSAG, et al. Intraocular pressure-lowering effects of all commonly used glaucoma drugs. A meta-analysis of randomized clinical trials. *Ophthalmology* 2005;112:1177-1185.
41. Cantor L. Achieving low target pressures with today's glaucoma medications. *Surv Ophthalmol* 2003;48(Suppl 1):S8-S16.
42. Sherwood MB, Craven ER, Chou C, et al. Twice-daily 0.2% brimonidine–0.5% timolol fixed-combination therapy vs monotherapy with timolol or brimonidine in patients with glaucoma or ocular hypertension. *Arch Ophthalmol* 2006;124:1230-1238.
43. Krupin T, Liebmann JM, Greenfield DS, et al. A randomized trial of brimonidine versus timolol in preserving visual function: Results from the Low-pressure Glaucoma Treatment Study. *Am J Ophthalmol* 2011;151:671-681.
44. Gray TA, Orton LC, Henson D, et al. Interventions for improving adherence to ocular hypotensive therapy. *Cochrane Database Syst Rev* 2009;2:CD006132. doi:10.1002/14651858.CD006132.pub2.
45. Anwar Z, Wellik SR, Galor A. Glaucoma therapy and ocular surface disease: Current literature and recommendations. *Curr Opin Ophthalmol* 2013;24:136-143.
46. Kahook MY, Salim S, Seibold LK. MIGS, Advances in Glaucoma Surgery. First edition. 2014 Slack Incorporated, Thorofare, NJ 08086, USA.

95

Allergic Rhinitis

J. Russell May

KEY CONCEPTS

1. Allergic rhinitis is a common disease. Prevention measures and treatment are justified in most cases because of the potential for complications.
2. Because an immune response to allergens results in release of inflammatory mediators that cause allergic rhinitis symptoms, patients must understand the rationale for proper timing and administration of prophylactic regimens.
3. Avoidance of allergens is difficult and it may be impractical to expect full success.
4. Antihistamines offer an effective option for treating both seasonal and persistent allergic rhinitis.
5. Intranasal steroids are highly effective in patients who use them properly.
6. While immunotherapy is the only disease-modifying treatment of allergic rhinitis, expense, potential risks, and the major time commitment required make patient selection critical.

Allergic rhinitis involves inflammation of the nasal mucous membrane. In a sensitized individual, allergic rhinitis occurs when inhaled allergenic particles contact mucous membranes and elicit a specific response mediated by immunoglobulin E (IgE). This acute response involves the release of inflammatory mediators and is characterized by sneezing, nasal itching, and watery rhinorrhea, often associated with nasal congestion. Itching of the throat, eyes, and ears frequently accompanies allergic rhinitis.

Allergic rhinitis may be regarded as seasonal allergic rhinitis, commonly known as *hay fever*, or persistent allergic rhinitis (formerly known as perennial rhinitis). Seasonal rhinitis occurs in response to specific allergens usually present at predictable times of the year, during plants' pollination (typically the spring or fall). Seasonal allergens include pollen from trees, grasses, and weeds. Persistent allergic rhinitis is a year-round disease caused by nonseasonal allergens, such as house dust mites, animal dander, and molds, or multiple allergic sensitivities. It typically results in less variable, chronic symptoms. Many patients have a combination of these two types of allergic rhinitis, with symptoms year-round and seasonal exacerbations.

EPIDEMIOLOGY

1 Allergic rhinitis is one of the most common diseases affecting adults and is the most common chronic disease in children in the United States, generating \$2 to \$5 billion in direct healthcare cost each year.[1] Sensitization to inhaled allergens is increasing with a prevalence of 15% to 30% in the United States.[2] Patients may be limited in their ability to carry out normal daily functions; higher levels of general fatigue, mental fatigue, anxiety, depressive disorders, and learning disabilities (secondary to sleep loss and fatigue) are possible.

In addition, the impact of allergic rhinitis goes well beyond these CNS issues. Allergic rhinitis is associated with several other serious medical conditions, including asthma, chronic rhinosinusitis, otitis media, nasal polyposis, respiratory infections, and orthodontic malocclusions.

ETIOLOGY

The development of allergic rhinitis is determined by genetics, allergen exposure, and the presence of other risk factors. A family history of allergic rhinitis, atopic dermatitis, or asthma suggests that rhinitis is allergic. The risk of developing allergic disease appears to increase if one parent is atopic and further increases if two are allergic; however, small sample sizes and the lack of reproducibility prevent generalization.[3]

Allergen exposure is another necessary factor. For allergic rhinitis to occur, an individual must be exposed over time to a protein that elicits the allergic response in that individual. Many potential sufferers never develop symptoms because they do not come into contact with the allergen that would produce symptoms in them.

Evidence suggests microbial exposure in the first years of life could help prevent allergic disease by stimulating a nonatopic immune response.[4] Farm children are exposed to higher concentrations of endotoxin, derived from cell walls of gram-negative bacteria, in barns and dust around the farmhouse. Consumption of nonpasteurized farm milk may cause further exposure. These observations have led to the idea that allergic disease could be prevented by proactively increasing exposure to harmless bacteria early in life (see Alternative Treatment Options below). This could explain why positive skin tests indicating allergen sensitization have been observed more frequently for people in higher socioeconomic classes and for people who live in suburban areas.

Other predisposing factors include an elevated serum IgE (>100 international units/mL [kIU/L]) before the age of 6 years, eczema, and heavy exposure to secondhand cigarette smoke.[5]

Allergens

Allergens that produce seasonal rhinitis include protein components of airborne pollen grains, often enzymes, from a variety of trees, grasses, and weeds. Ragweed and grass pollen are the most common offenders in the United States; however, this varies with the geographic region. In general, tree pollens cause symptoms in the spring, grass pollens cause symptoms in the late spring and summer, and weed pollens are the culprits from late summer through fall. Patients who are hypersensitive to all three may have overlapping problem periods and may be described as having perennial rhinitis when they are actually experiencing prolonged seasonal rhinitis. For this reason and the fact that most patients with seasonal problems are sensitive to at least some of the perennial allergens, there is little practical difference between the two types of allergic rhinitis. To complicate matters further, the antigenic components of many grasses—including fescue, Kentucky bluegrass, orchard, redtop, and timothy—cross-react extensively. By contrast, most tree allergens are antigenically distinct. Trees with allergenic pollen include ash, beech, birch, cedar, hickory, maple, oak, poplar, and sycamore. Flowering plants that depend on insect pollination do not cause allergic rhinitis because their pollen is too heavy and sticky and is not carried in the air.

Smaller mold spores are also important but cause allergy much less frequently. Various spores are present year-round; however, mold growth on decaying vegetation increases seasonally. Just walking through uncut fields or raking leaves can increase exposure. Thus, mold spores can be responsible for both perennial and seasonal allergies.

Indoor allergens are always present. Most important among these are house-dust mite fecal proteins, animal dander, cockroaches, and certain mold species. Dust mite levels are on the rise, possibly because of the construction of energy-efficient homes and offices with reduced ventilation and increased humidity, use of wall-to-wall carpeting, and the popularity of cool-water detergents and cold-water washing.[3]

PATHOPHYSIOLOGY

Knowledge of nasal physiology aids in the understanding of allergic rhinitis. The nose performs three "air conditioning" functions to prepare incoming gases for the lungs. During the fraction of a second that air is in the nose, it is heated, humidified, and cleaned. The cleaning process plays a role in the development of allergic rhinitis. As the air passes through the nose, the turbulence throws particulate matter against a mucous blanket. The rhythmic movements of the nasal cilia cause the mucous blanket to move posteriorly at approximately 9 mm/min, where it is eventually swallowed; thus, trapped foreign particles are removed via the GI tract and do not reach the lungs. It also concentrates foreign protein material into the posterior nasopharynx, where lymph tissues identify them and produce most of the allergic antibody that drives allergic rhinitis.

The vascular tissue in the nose is erectile. Stimulation of sympathetic fibers causes vasoconstriction, reduction in erectile tissue size and the size of the membranes and turbinates, and airway widening. Parasympathetic stimulation causes opposite effects.

Mast cells, in the nasal membranes, participate in the regulation of nasal patency by releasing mediators such as histamine. These are described below.

Immune Response to Allergens

2 Allergic reactions in the nose are mediated by antigen–antibody responses when allergens interact with specific IgE molecules bound to nasal mast cells and basophils. In allergic people, these cells are increased in both number and reactivity. During inhalation, airborne allergens enter the nose and are processed by lymphocytes, which produce antigen-specific IgE, thereby sensitizing genetically predisposed hosts to those agents. Upon nasal re-exposure, IgE bound to mast cells interacts with airborne allergen, triggering release of inflammatory mediators in vastly increased quantities (Fig. 95-1).[6]

Both immediate and late-phase reactions are observed after allergen exposure. The immediate reaction occurs within seconds to minutes, resulting in the rapid release of preformed mediators and newly generated mediators from the arachidonic acid cascade as the mast cell membrane is disturbed (Table 95-1). These mediators of immediate hypersensitivity include histamine, some leukotrienes, prostaglandin D_2, tryptase, and kinins.[6] In addition, the mast cell has been found to be a source of several cytokines that probably are relevant to the chronicity of the mucosal inflammation that

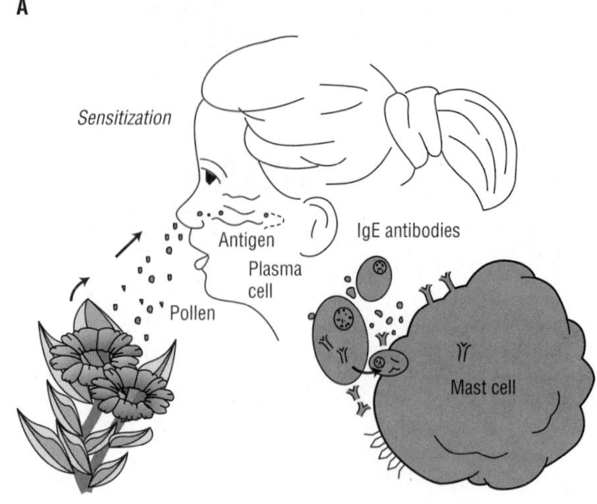

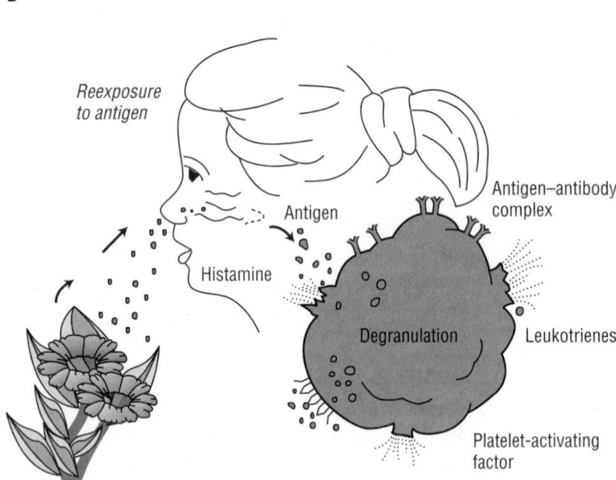

FIGURE 95-1 Allergen sensitization and the allergic response. *A.* Exposure to antigen stimulates IgE production and sensitization of mast cells with antigen-specific IgE antibodies. *B.* Subsequent exposure to the same antigen produces an allergic reaction when mast cell mediators are released.

characterizes allergic rhinitis.[7] Sensory nerve stimulation produces itching, and sneezing occurs via reflex stimulation of efferent vagal pathways. Neuropeptides substance P and calcitonin gene-related peptide from nonadrenergic, noncholinergic nerves affect vascular engorgement directly and via modulation of sympathetic tone. Histamine produces rhinorrhea, itching, sneezing, and obstruction, with the obstruction only partially blocked by H_1- or H_2-blocking agents.[8] Nasal obstruction is also caused by kinins, prostaglandin D_2, and leukotrienes C_4/D_4. Kinins, when directly administered, produce pain rather than itching.[9] These inflammatory mediators also produce vasodilation, increased vascular permeability, and production of increased nasal secretions.[10]

Four to eight hours after the initial exposure to an allergen, a late-phase reaction occurs symptomatically in 50% of allergic rhinitis patients.[11] This response, thought to be caused by cytokines released primarily by mast cells and thymus-derived helper lymphocytes, is characterized by profound infiltration and activation of migrating cells. This inflammatory response likely is responsible for the persistent, chronic symptoms of allergic rhinitis, including nasal congestion. The inflamed mucosa becomes hyperresponsive, a state characterized by exacerbation of nasal reactions to nonspecific or irritant triggers. In this state, the patient also reacts to increasingly

TABLE 95-1 Mast Cell Mediators

Mediators	Effects
Preformed and rapidly released	
Histamine	Stimulates irritant receptors
	Pruritus
	Vascular permeability
	Mucosal permeability
	Smooth muscle contraction
Neutrophil chemotactic factor	Influx of inflammatory cells
Eosinophil chemotactic factor	Influx of inflammatory cells
Kinins	Vascular permeability
N-α-tosyl L-arginine methyl esterase	Vascular permeability
Newly generated	
Leukotrienes	Smooth muscle contraction
	Vascular permeability
	Mucus secretion
	Chemotaxis
	Neutrophil chemotaxis
Thromboxanes	Smooth muscle spasm
Platelet-activating factor	Mucus secretion
	Airway permeability
	Chemotaxis
	Vascular permeability
Granule matrix contents	
Heparin	Antiinflammatory
Tryptase	Protein hydrolysis
Kallikrein	Protein hydrolysis

lower amounts of the same allergen.[12] The process also causes significant increases in nonspecific irritability (as seen in asthma) and the notion among patients that they have become "allergic to everything."

CLINICAL PRESENTATION

The patient with allergic rhinitis typically complains of clear rhinorrhea, paroxysms of sneezing, nasal congestion, postnasal drip, and pruritic eyes, ears, nose, or palate. Symptoms of allergic conjunctivitis are associated more frequently with seasonal than perennial allergic rhinitis, because a majority of the perennial allergens, such as dust mites and molds, are indoors, where air velocity is too low for substantial deposition of allergenic particles on the conjunctivae. However, with heavy exposure from animal or mold allergens, allergic conjunctivitis can be pronounced.

Symptoms secondary to the late-phase reaction, predominantly nasal congestion, begin 3 to 5 hours after antigen exposure and peak at 12 to 24 hours. Subsequent symptoms, both allergic and irritant, are elicited more easily because of the priming effect. For instance, a ragweed-sensitive patient, when exposed to ragweed pollen out of season, responds with modest symptoms and may be very tolerant of irritants such as air pollution or tobacco smoke. During the ragweed season, however, when the nasal mucosa is already inflamed, exposure to small doses of pollen or to irritants to which the patient is usually tolerant elicits a response clinically indistinguishable from the patient's allergy.

Diagnostic Considerations

Allergic rhinitis is distinguished from other causes of rhinitis by a thorough history, physical examination, and certain diagnostic tests. The medical history consists of a careful description of symptoms, environmental factors and exposures, results of previous therapy, use of other medications, previous nasal injuries, previous nasal or sinus surgery, family history, and the presence of other medical problems and medications. Historical identification of specific causative allergens may be difficult. For example, a reaction induced by mowing the lawn may not be caused by grass pollens but may be caused by the disturbance of various weeds, molds, or other plants in the lawn. With perennial allergic rhinitis, the cause-effect and temporal relationships are less clear, making the diagnosis of specific causes more difficult, especially with such covert allergens as house dust mites and molds.

In children, physical examination may reveal allergic shiners—a transverse nasal crease caused by repeated rubbing of the nose—and adenoidal breathing. Pale, bluish, edematous nasal turbinates coated with thin, clear secretions are characteristic of a purely allergic reaction. Tearing, conjunctival injection and edema, and periorbital swelling may be present. Physical findings are generally less clear-cut for adults.

Nasal scrapings will provide a representative sample of cells infiltrating the nasal mucosa and can be helpful in supporting the diagnosis.[13] Microscopic examination of the nasal smear from an allergic individual typically will show numerous eosinophils. The blood eosinophil count may be elevated in allergic rhinitis, but it is nonspecific and has limited usefulness.[14]

Allergy testing can help determine whether a patient's rhinitis is caused by an allergen. Immediate-type hypersensitivity skin tests are used for the diagnosis of allergic rhinitis. These include skin tests performed by the percutaneous route, where the diluted allergen is pricked or scratched into the skin surface, or by the intradermal route, where a small volume (0.01 to 0.05 mL) of diluted allergen is injected between the layers of skin. Percutaneous tests are more commonly performed and are safer and more generally accepted, with intradermal tests reserved for patients requiring confirmation in special circumstances.

In all allergy testing, a positive control (histamine) and a negative control are essential for correct interpretation. After 15 minutes of the application of the allergen, the site is examined for a positive reaction (defined as a wheal-and-flare reaction). Because correct testing is done with extremely minute doses, undetectable by nonsensitized individuals, this reaction is evidence of the presence of mast cell-bound IgE specific to the allergen tested. Many, but not all, common allergens are available as standardized allergenic extracts.

Antihistamines and a few other medications interfere with the wheal-and-flare reaction. First-generation antihistamines should be stopped at least 3 to 5 days before testing, and second-generation, nonsedating antihistamines should be stopped for 10 days before testing.[15] Medications with antihistamine properties (eg, sympathomimetic agents, phenothiazines, and tricyclic antidepressants) should be discontinued if possible before skin testing.

The radioallergosorbent test (RAST) was the first commonly used method for detecting IgE antibodies in the blood that are specific for a given allergen. Several other quantitative assays that include a reference curve calculated against standardized IgE are available. These tests are highly specific but may be slightly less sensitive than percutaneous tests.

Complications

Not only is allergic rhinitis aggravating, it frequently leads to further complications, particularly if the patient does not receive adequate treatment. Symptoms of untreated rhinitis may lead to disturbed sleep, chronic malaise, fatigue, and poor work or school performance. Patients often are plagued by loss of smell or taste, with sinusitis or polyps underlying many cases of allergy-related hyposmia. Postnasal drip with cough, hoarseness, and even vocal polyps also can be bothersome.

The role of allergic rhinitis in the development of acute otitis media or chronic middle ear effusion is often less clear. Children with allergic rhinitis appear to be at greater risk of these conditions because of nasal obstruction and negative middle ear pressure. Hearing problems in children related to middle ear effusion may lead to delayed development of language in young children or to school problems in older children.

Permanent facial disfigurement can result from chronic allergic rhinitis.[16] The chronic edema and venous stasis may contribute to the development of a high-arched, V-shaped palate. Mouth breathing caused by nasal obstruction can be responsible for dental malocclusion and orthodontic problems. Constant upward rubbing of the nose (allergic salute) can cause a transverse crease across the lower nose; nasal congestion often leads to venous pooling and dark circles under the eyes known as *allergic shiners*.

Allergic rhinitis is clearly associated with asthma. The prevalence of asthma in patients without rhinitis is less than 2%, while the prevalence of asthma in patients with rhinitis is 10% to 40%.[17] It is not known if allergic rhinitis is an early clinical manifestation of asthma or if the nasal disease itself is causative for asthma.

Recurrent sinusitis and chronic sinusitis are relatively common complications of allergic rhinitis. The structure of the mucus blanket breaks down, with decreased water production by serous glands, leaving hair cells trapped in the thicker mucus layer. This greatly reduces the clearance of trapped bacteria and offers ideal breeding grounds for the bacteria. Nasal polyps are less common but nonetheless bothersome; they require specific therapy but may improve with management of the underlying allergic state. Epistaxis also can be a problem; it is related to mucosal hyperemia and inflammation.

TREATMENT

A number of options exist for the treatment of allergic rhinitis, both nonpharmacologic and pharmacologic. Many of the pharmacologic options are available over-the-counter requiring that patients receive guidance in the selection process by a healthcare professional to obtain the most appropriate therapy. Both over-the-counter and prescription choices must be guided by patient-specific symptomatology and patient characteristics as described in this chapter.

Desired Outcomes

The therapeutic goal for patients with allergic rhinitis is to minimize or prevent symptoms and prevent long-term complications. This goal should be accomplished with no or minimal adverse medication effects and reasonable medication expenses. The patient should be able to maintain a normal lifestyle, including participating in outdoor activities, yard work, and playing with pets as desired.

General Approach to Treatment

Once the causative allergens and the specific symptoms are identified, management consists of three possible approaches: (a) allergen avoidance, (b) pharmacotherapy for prevention or treatment of symptoms, and (c) specific immunotherapy. The pharmacotherapy for symptoms approach includes several options that are based on patient-specific information (Table 95-2). Figure 95-2 depicts an algorithm for treatment options.

Nonpharmacologic Therapy

3 Avoidance of offending allergens is the most direct method of preventing allergic rhinitis, but it is often the most difficult to accomplish, especially for perennial allergens. Mold growth can be reduced by maintaining household humidity below 50% and removing obvious growth with bleach or disinfectant. Patients sensitive to animals will benefit most by removing pets from the home;[18] however, most animal lovers are reluctant to comply with this approach. Dog and cat allergens may produce symptoms in sensitized individuals.[7] After removing a cat from the home, it may take as long as 20 weeks for the home to reach allergen levels of a pet-free home. Washing cats weekly may reduce allergens but studies are inconclusive.[7] Some dogs display antigens more profusely than do others; clinically, a sensitized person may tolerate one animal better than another.

TABLE 95-2 Pharmacotherapeutic Options for Allergic Rhinitis

Medication Classes	Symptoms Controlled	Comments
Antihistamines		
Systemic	Sneezing, rhinorrhea, itching, conjunctivitis	For seasonal allergic rhinitis, begin treatment before allergen exposure. Nonsedating agents should be tried first. If ineffective or too expensive for the patient, the older agents may be used. For perennial allergic rhinitis, use an intranasal steroid as an alternative to or in combination with systemic antihistamines
Ophthalmic	Conjunctivitis	Logical addition to nasal steroids if ocular symptoms are present
Intranasal	Sneezing, rhinorrhea, nasal pruritus	Option for seasonal allergic rhinitis. Warn patients of potential drowsiness
Decongestants		
Systemic	Nasal congestion	Only needed when nasal congestion is present
Topical	Nasal congestion	Only needed when nasal congestion is present. Do not exceed 3-5 days
Intranasal corticosteroids	Sneezing, rhinorrhea, itching, nasal congestion	For seasonal allergic rhinitis, an option when congestion is present. Must begin therapy before allergen exposure. Excellent choice for perennial rhinitis
Mast cell stabilizers	See comments	Prevents symptoms; therefore, for seasonal allergic rhinitis, use before offending allergen's season starts. For perennial rhinitis, improvement may not be seen for up to 1 month
Intranasal anticholinergics	Rhinorrhea	Reserve for use when above therapies fail or cannot be tolerated
Leukotriene receptor antagonists	See comments	When combined with antihistamines, more effective than antihistamines alone. May be used as monotherapy in children with asthma and coexisting allergic rhinitis

Evidence to support avoidance measures for house dust mites suggests that accepted notions for reducing exposure have little practical effect.[18] While some evidence shows allergen levels can be reduced by washing bedding on a hot cycle, replacing carpets with hard flooring and using vacuum cleaners with HEPA filters, there is no documented evidence for a clinical benefit. Only encasing bedding in impermeable covers has some clinical benefit in children but not adults. Future studies are needed to determine if environmental control of allergens may be helpful in forestalling further rhinitis and preventing later asthma.

General recommendations have been made to prevent poor air quality in homes.[19] Steps include avoiding wall-to-wall carpeting, using moisture control to prevent the accumulation of molds, and controlling sources of pollution such as cigarette smoke. Patients with seasonal allergic rhinitis should keep windows closed and

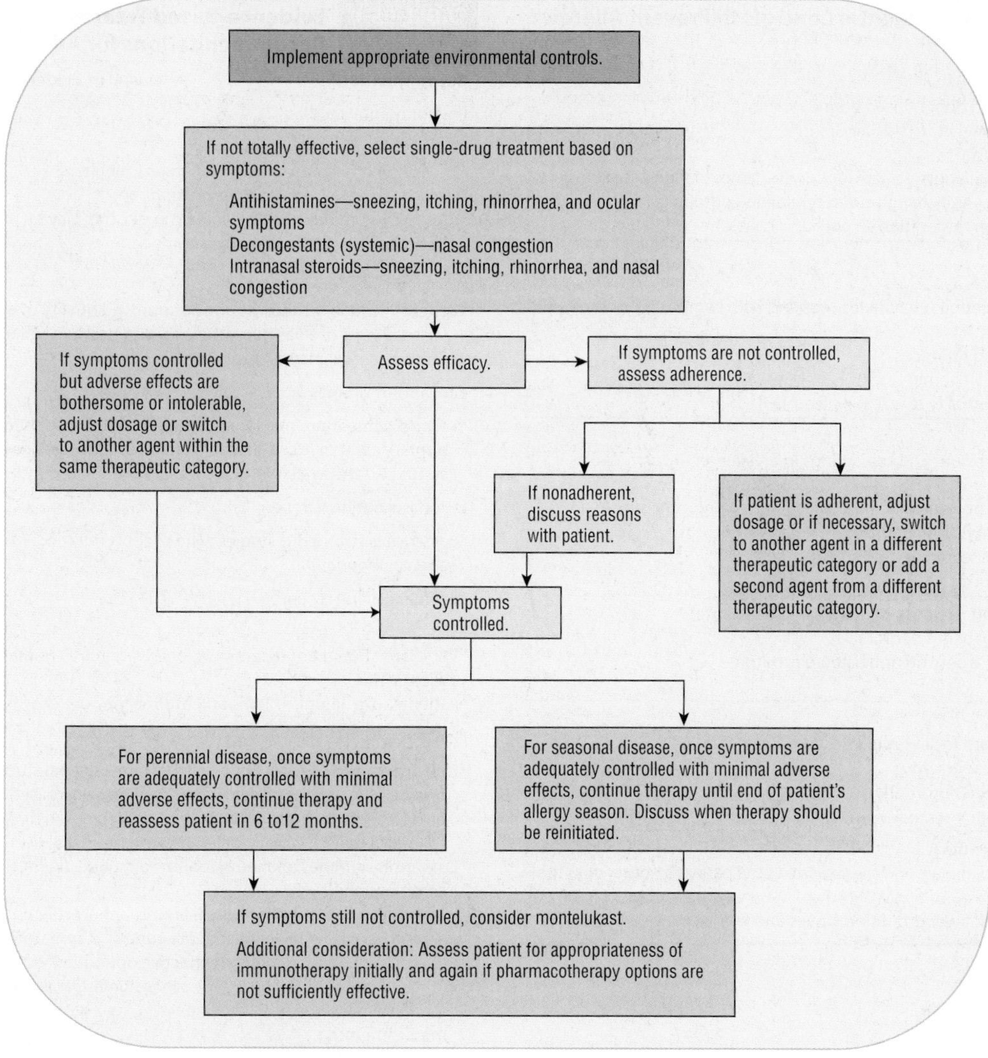

FIGURE 95-2 Treatment algorithm for allergic rhinitis.

minimize time spent outdoors during pollen seasons. Immediate hair washing and change of clothes are recommended upon returning indoors. Use of fans that direct outside air into the house should be avoided. Filter masks can be worn while gardening or mowing the lawn. Avoidance of upholstery and stuffed toys in the bedroom are easy steps to accomplish. Table 95-3 summarizes recommendations for environmental control. These measures are intended to be a part of a comprehensive treatment strategy that will likely include pharmacotherapy and, in selected cases, immunotherapy.

Clinical **Controversy...**

While avoidance steps are logical, there is little existing evidence that environmental control measures provide clinical benefit. Controlled trials that identify the efficacy of environmental controls on measurable allergic rhinitis endpoints need to be performed.

Other suggested measures for preventing allergic rhinitis include breastfeeding infants and avoidance of exposure to tobacco smoke.[18] Exclusive breastfeeding for the first 3 months of life may help prevent allergies. Avoidance of environmental tobacco smoke (ie, passive smoking) by children and pregnant woman may also reduce the development of allergies and has been strongly recommended. However, the evidence for both these recommendations is minimal.

Pharmacologic Therapy

Table 95-4 summarizes the most recent guidelines for treatment of allergic rhinitis with levels of evidence for each treatment strategy.[1] Therapeutic modalities for treating allergic rhinitis are generally directed at relief of symptoms as previously described in Table 95-2. Antihistamines and decongestants (both oral and topical) generally are used first in treating allergic rhinitis with medications. Several options in these two categories are available without a prescription, but patients will need sound advice to make appropriate choices. Knowledge of pathophysiology and the inflammatory state has led to prophylactic therapy for those with more severe disease using agents such topical steroids. However, in attempting to assess the evidence supporting any particular therapy, clinicians have difficulty interpreting the medical literature for a variety of reasons, including lack of uniformity in the research methodologies, inappropriate drug controls, and failure to identify types of rhinitis in study subjects (perennial vs seasonal and allergic vs nonallergic).

Antihistamines

4 Histamine (H_1)-receptor antagonists are competitive antagonists to histamine. They bind to H_1 receptors without activating them, preventing histamine binding and action. Second-generation antihistamines may also affect components of the inflammatory response such as histamine release, generation of adhesion molecules, and influx of inflammatory cells. Although it was once thought that the

TABLE 95-3 Environmental Controls to Prevent Allergic Rhinitis

Pollens
- Keep windows and doors closed during pollen season
- Avoid fans that draw in outside air
- Use air conditioning
- If possible, eliminate outside activities during times of high pollen counts
- Shower, shampoo, and change clothes following outdoor activity
- Use a vented dryer rather than an outside clothesline

Molds
- Use similar controls as above
- Avoid walking through uncut fields, working with compost or dry soil, and raking leaves
- Clean indoor moldy surfaces
- Fix all water leaks in home
- Reduce indoor humidity to <50% if possible

House dust mites
- Encase mattress, pillow, and box springs in an allergen-impermeable cover
- Wash bedding in hot water weekly
- Remove stuffed toys from bedroom
- Minimize carpet use and upholstered furniture
- Reduce indoor humidity to <50%, if possible

Animal allergens (if removal of pet is not acceptable)
- Keep pet out of patient's bedroom
- Isolate pet from carpet and upholstered furniture
- Wash pet weekly

Cockroaches
- Keep food and garbage in tightly closed containers
- Take out garbage regularly
- Clean up dirty dishes promptly
- Use roach traps

Other recommendations
- Do not allow smoking around the patient, in the patient's house, or in the family car
- Minimize the use of wood-burning stoves and fireplaces

Data from reference 3.

older antihistamines had no antiinflammatory action, some were shown to have these effects as early as the 1950s.[20] Antihistamines are available in oral, ophthalmic, and intranasal dosage forms.

The oral antihistamines are the most commonly used and can be divided into two major categories: nonselective (first generation) and peripherally selective (second generation). Nonselective agents are commonly referred to as *sedating antihistamines*, and peripherally selective agents are referred to as *nonsedating antihistamines*. These generalizing terms can be misleading. Individual agents should be judged on their specific characteristics because variation within these broad categories exists. Also, the nonsedating claim is only valid when the agents are used at recommended doses.[21] This is of particular concern as some of these antihistamines are available without a prescription. The mechanism for sedation is not well understood, but its central effect depends on the drugs' ability to cross the blood–brain barrier. Most older antihistamines are lipid soluble and cross this barrier easily. The peripherally selective agents have little or no central or autonomic nervous system effects. Table 95-5 lists common antihistamines, their chemical classifications, their relative potential for causing sedation, and their relative anticholinergic effects.

Antihistamines are much more effective in preventing the actions of histamines and essentially do not reverse these actions once they have taken place. Reversal of symptoms is largely caused by the anticholinergic properties of these drugs. This activity is responsible for the drying effect of antihistamines, which reduces the problem of nasal, salivary, and lacrimal gland hypersecretion. Antihistamines antagonize increased capillary permeability, wheal-and-flare formation, and itching.

TABLE 95-4 Evidence-Based Treatment Recommendations for Allergic Rhinitis

Recommendation	Level of Evidence[a]
Environmental factors	B
*Avoidance of known allergens *Environmental controls (removal of pets, air filters) *May consider this approach as *optional*. Note: Even though good evidence exists, this may be hard to achieve. See text for limitations of this approach.	
Nasal steroids	A
*Benefits include symptom control, improved quality of life, better sleep, cost-saving if used as monotherapy, targeted local effect. Patient preference will play a large role.	
Oral antihistamines	A
*Second generation (nonsedating) agents should be used in patients with primary complaints of sneezing and itching. Relief of eye symptoms, OTC status and the availability of lower cost generics may be advantages.	
Intranasal antihistamines	A
*Evidence is strong but studies were of short duration. May consider these agents as *optional*.	
Oral leukotriene receptor antagonists	D
*Clinicians should not recommend these agents as primary therapy for allergic rhinitis *Patients with allergic rhinitis and asthma may benefit from this therapy	
Combination therapy	Variable
*Oral antihistamines and oral decongestants: several studies show benefit but must be weighed against potential risks: increased insomnia, headache, dry mouth, nervousness, and increased blood pressure. Tolerance may develop with long-term use of oral decongestants. *Oral antihistamines and intranasal steroids: no evidence to support the combination. *Intranasal steroids and intranasal antihistamines: For patients who tolerate a nasal agent but have inadequate control of symptoms with a single agent, this combination is an effective option. *Intranasal steroids and topical decongestants: Combination more effective than intranasal therapy alone however, see text regarding risk of rhinitis medicamentosa.	
Immunotherapy	A
*Recommended in patients who have inadequate response to with pharmacologic therapy with or without environmental controls	

*See text for information on sublingual versus subcutaneous therapy

[a]Levels of evidence: A, a strong recommendation or recommendation based on excellent evidence where benefits clearly outweigh harms. B, a strong recommendation or recommendation based on good evidence that benefits outweighs harms. C, recommendation where evidence is not as strong or high quality evidence is impossible to obtain. D, an optional therapy for some patients but quality of evidence is suspect, or no recommendation because there is a lack of pertinent evidence and an unclear balance between benefits and harm. For each level of evidence, see comments for further clarification of recommendations.

In general, the antihistamines are well absorbed, have large volumes of distribution, and are metabolized by the liver. Serum half-lives vary considerably between patients. In addition, the therapeutic effects of these agents are more prolonged than might be predicted by their half-lives.

Drowsiness is usually the chief complaint of patients who take antihistamines. It can interfere with a patient's ability to drive a car or operate machinery and may interfere with the patient's ability to function adequately at the workplace. Remember that these problems can also be a reflection of the disease itself. For this reason, many recommend the use of peripherally selective agents as first-line treatment for any patient who is at high risk for the development of adverse events. This includes patients with renal or hepatic impairment, those with small weights (for whom adult doses may provide larger-than-recommended doses on a milligram-per-kilogram basis), patients with preexisting CNS or cardiac disorders,

TABLE 95-5 Relative Adverse-Effect Profiles of Antihistamines

Medications	Relative Sedative Effects	Relative Anticholinergic Effects
Alkylamine class, nonselective		
Brompheniramine maleate	Low	Moderate
Chlorpheniramine maleate	Low	Moderate
Dexchlorpheniramine maleate	Low	Moderate
Ethanolamine class, nonselective		
Carbinoxamine maleate	High	High
Clemastine fumarate	Moderate	High
Diphenhydramine hydrochloride	High	High
Phenothiazine class, nonselective		
Promethazine hydrochloride	High	High
Piperidine class, nonselective		
Cyproheptadine hydrochloride	Low	Moderate
Phthalazinone class, peripherally selective		
Azelastine (nasal only)	Low to none	Low to none
Bepotastine (ophthalmic only)	Low to none	Low to none
Piperazine class, peripherally selective		
Cetirizine	Low to moderate	Low to none
Levocetirizine	Low to moderate	Low to none
Piperidine class, peripherally selective		
Desloratadine	Low to none	Low to none
Fexofenadine	Low to none	Low to none
Loratadine	Low to none	Low to none
Olopatadine (nasal only)	Low to none	Low to none

patients who require higher doses, and patients who have shown a tendency to overuse nonprescription or prescription medications.[20]

The sedative effects of antihistamines can be useful for patients who suffer from sleeplessness caused by the symptoms of allergic rhinitis. In these patients, a bedtime dose may prove beneficial. However, they may cause residual daytime sedation, decreased alertness, and performance impairment.

The logic of preferentially using the second-generation agents is not clear-cut. A meta-analysis of performance-impairment trials did not show a clear and consistent distinction between diphenhydramine and the peripherally selective agents.[22] Another study showed that tolerance to sedation secondary to diphenhydramine developed by day 4 of treatment, becoming indistinguishable from placebo,[23] but sedation must be distinguished from impairment since the two are not equivalent. Despite this evidence, guidelines recommend the nonsedating agents.[1,18]

Anticholinergic (drying) effects contribute to the agents' therapeutic efficacy, but they also cause most adverse effects. Dry mouth, difficulty in voiding urine, constipation, and potential cardiovascular effects may be troublesome. Keep in mind that the differences may be small. Patients with a predisposition to urinary retention (eg, older men and those on concurrent anticholinergic therapy) should use antihistamines with caution. Caution also should be used for patients with increased intraocular pressure, hyperthyroidism, and cardiovascular disease.

Other adverse effects of oral antihistamines include loss of appetite (and paradoxically, weight gain with increased appetite), nausea, vomiting, and epigastric distress.

Antihistamines are only fully effective when taken approximately 1 to 2 hours before anticipated exposure to the offending allergen. This must be discussed with patients who face exposure daily during a pollen season and with those who have indoor perennial allergens where daily scheduled use is necessary. If tolerance develops to the therapeutic effect, a change to an agent in a different chemical class is usually effective.

Patients should be counseled about the proper use of antihistamines. Adverse effects, especially drowsiness, should be emphasized. Patients should be warned against taking other CNS depressants, including the use of alcohol. Patients should be told not to take a double dose when a dose is missed. Taking the antihistamine with meals or at least a full glass of water will help prevent GI adverse effects such as nausea, vomiting, and epigastric distress. Patients should check with their healthcare professional and read labels before taking nonprescription medications. Many cold products and sleep aids contain antihistamines. Patients should be instructed not to use more than one antihistamine at a time. Table 95-6 lists the recommended dosages of the commonly used agents with their prescription status.

Many patients respond to and tolerate the older agents quite well. Because many of the older agents are available generically, they are much less expensive. Patient cost for many of the older nonprescription agents is less than $5 for a 30-day supply, compared with more than $20 for some of the nonprescription selective agents and more than $70 for the selective prescription-only products. Although cost is a concern, patient safety should be the first consideration.

The selective agents have moved ahead of the nonselective choices in a recent survey of pharmacist recommended over-the-counter antihistamines.[24] Among the 2 million antihistamine recommendations, the top three were loratadine (41%), cetirizine (33%), and fexofenadine (15%) followed by the nonselective agents diphenhydramine (9%) and chlorpheniramine (2%).

For seasonal and persistent allergic rhinitis, the intranasal antihistamine azelastine is available. The 0.1% product can be used in children for seasonal allergies, while the 0.15% product is labeled for adults only for either type of allergic rhinitis. Despite this labeling, recent guidelines favor the use of the intranasal route for seasonal but not persistent allergic rhinitis.[18] Azelastine has been used successfully for patients who did not respond to loratadine.[25] Using the nasal route offers an alternative to switching to another oral antihistamine. Patient satisfaction has been varied because while the product produces rapid symptom relief, patients complain of drying effects, headache, and diminished effectiveness over time. Patients should be warned of the medication's potential to produce drowsiness, as its systemic availability is approximately 40%.[26,27] Olopatadine, another intranasal antihistamine, may cause less drowsiness as it is a selective H_1-receptor antagonist.

Allergic conjunctivitis, often associated with allergic rhinitis, can be treated with ophthalmic antihistamines such as levocabastine or bepotastine. Because systemic antihistamines usually are also effective for allergic conjunctivitis, one of these ophthalmic agents is a logical addition to nasal steroids when ocular symptoms occur, and it is an acceptable approach for patients whose only symptoms involve the eyes or to add for those whose symptoms persist on oral treatment.

Decongestants

Topical and systemic decongestants are sympathomimetic agents that act on adrenergic receptors in the nasal mucosa, producing vasoconstriction. Decongestants shrink swollen mucosa and improve ventilation. When nasal congestion occurs with allergic rhinitis, decongestants work well in combination with antihistamines.

TABLE 95-6 Medication Dosing for Allergic Rhinitis

Drugs	Brand Names	Dosages	Special Population Doses	Other
Antihistamines				
Oral				
Nonselective:				
Chlorpheniramine maleate	Various	Plain: 4 mg every 6 hours	Pediatrics: 6-12 years: 2 mg every 6 hours 2-5 years: 1 mg every 6 hours	OTC Available as liquid
		Sustained release: 12 mg every 12 hours	Pediatrics: 6-12 years: 0.67 mg every 12 hours	OTC
Clemastine fumarate	Tavist	1.34 mg every 8 hours	Pediatrics: 5 mg/kg per day divided every 8 hours (up to 25 mg per dose)	OTC Available as liquid
Diphenhydramine hydrochloride	Benadryl and others	25-50 mg every 8 hours	Pediatrics: 6-12 years: 10 mg once daily 2-5 years: 5 mg once daily	OTC Available as liquid
Peripherally selective:				
Loratadine	Alavert/Claritin	10 mg once daily	Pediatrics: 2-11 years: 30 mg twice daily	OTC Available as liquid
Fexofenadine	Allegra	60 mg twice daily or 180 mg once daily	Pediatrics: 1-5 years: 2.5 mg daily may increase to twice daily	OTC Available as liquid
Cetirizine	Zyrtec	5-10 mg once daily	6-12 months: 2.5 mg once daily Pediatrics: 6-11 years: 2.5 mg in the evening 6 months to 5 years: 1.25 mg in the evening	OTC Available as liquid
Levocetirizine	Xyzal	5 mg at bedtime		
Nasal				
Azelastine	Astopro	One to two sprays twice daily	Pediatrics: 5-11 years one spray twice daily	
Olopatadine	Patanase	Two sprays twice daily	Pediatrics: 6-11 years: one spray twice daily	
Ophthalmic				
Bepotastine	Bepreve	One drop twice daily		
Decongestants				
Oral				
Pseudoephedrine	Various	60 mg every 4-6 hours	Pediatrics: 6-12 years: 30 mg every 4-6 hours	OTC Available as liquid
		Sustained release: 120 mg every 12 hours	4-5 years: 15 mg every 4-6 hours	
		Controlled release: 240 mg once daily		
Phenylephrine	Various	10-20 mg every 4 hours	Pediatrics: 6-12 years: 5 mg every 4 hours 4-6 years: 2.5 mg every 4 hours	OTC Available as liquid
Nasal				
Oxymetazoline	Various	Two to three sprays twice daily		OTC
Phenylephrine	Various	Two to three sprays every 4 hours	Pediatrics: >12 years: use 0.25-0.5% two to three sprays every 4 hours 6-12 years: use 0.25% two to three sprays every 4 hours 2-6 years: use 0.125% one drop every 2-4 hours	OTC
Nasal steroids				
Beclomethasone	Beconase AQ Qnasl	One to two inhalations in each nostril twice daily (Beconase AQ) Two inhalations (160 mcg) in each nostril once daily (Qnasl)	Pediatric: Beconase AQ: 6-11 years: one inhalation in each nostril twice daily Qnasl: 4-11 years: one inhalation (40 mcg) in each nostril once daily	
Budesonide	Rhinocort Aqua	One spray each nostril daily (up to maximum of four sprays each nostril daily)		
Flunisolide	Various	Two sprays in each nostril twice daily	Pediatrics: 6-14 years: two sprays in each nostril twice daily	
Fluticasone	Flonase Veramyst	Two sprays in each nostril once daily	Pediatrics: >4 years: one spray in each nostril daily (Flonase) 2-11 years: one spray in each nostril daily (Veramyst)	OTC
Mometasone	Nasonex	Two sprays in each nostril daily	Pediatrics: 2-11 years: one spray in each nostril daily	
Triamcinolone	Nasacort	Two sprays in each nostril daily (reduce to one spray when symptoms controlled)	Pediatrics: 2-11 years: one spray in each nostril once daily	OTC
Other nasal medications				
Cromolyn	Nasalcrom	One spray in each nostril three to four times a day	Pediatrics: >2 years, same as adult dose	OTC
Ipratropium	Atrovent	Two sprays in each nostril two to four times per day	Pediatrics: 5-11 years: two sprays in each nostril two to three times a day	
Montelukast	Singulair	Oral: 10 mg once daily	Pediatrics: 6-23 months: 4 mg (oral granules) once daily 2-5 years: 4 mg once daily (chewable or granules) 6-14 years: 5 mg once daily (chewable)	

TABLE 95-7 Duration of Action of Topical Decongestants

Medications	Durations of Action (hours)
Short acting	
Phenylephrine hydrochloride	Up to 4
Intermediate acting	
Naphazoline hydrochloride	2-6
Tetrahydrozoline hydrochloride	
Long acting	
Oxymetazoline hydrochloride	Up to 12
Xylometazoline hydrochloride	

Topical Decongestants Topical decongestants are applied directly to swollen nasal mucosa via drops or sprays. Table 95-7 lists the common topical decongestants and their durations of action. The use of these agents results in little or no systemic absorption.

Because these agents are extremely effective and are available to patients without a prescription, they are widely used. However, prolonged use of these agents (for more than 3 to 5 days) can result in a condition known as *rhinitis medicamentosa*, or *rebound vasodilation*, with even more severe congestion. Patients who develop this condition use increasingly more spray more often with less response. Although the methods used to treat this "addiction" have not been studied formally, several are used commonly. Abrupt cessation works, but it is difficult because of rebound congestion that may leave the patient congested for several days or weeks. Sleeping may become difficult. Nasal steroids have been used successfully, but they take several days to work. Weaning the patient off topical decongestants can be accomplished by decreasing the dosing frequency or the concentration over several weeks. Combining the weaning process with nasal steroids may prove useful. Ultimately, the success of any plan depends on the patient's resolve and clear understanding of the importance of stopping the drug to end the problem.

Other adverse effects of topical decongestants include burning, stinging, sneezing, and dryness of the nasal mucosa.

Patients should be counseled on the use of topical decongestants to prevent rhinitis medicamentosa. Patients should be instructed to use as small a dose as possible as infrequently as possible and only when absolutely necessary (eg, at bedtime to aid in falling asleep). Duration of therapy always should be limited to 5 days or less.

Systemic Decongestants Oral decongestants are not as effective on an immediate basis as the topical agents, but their effects sometimes last longer and they cause less local irritation. In addition, rhinitis medicamentosa is not a problem with oral agents. The most commonly used agent is pseudoephedrine. Table 95-6 lists the usual doses for the regular and sustained-release versions. The use of phenylephrine is increasing because of regulations related to pseudoephedrine described below.

Concerns of safety have greatly limited the systemic decongestant options. Legal requirements for the sale of pseudoephedrine were put into place to combat the misuse of the drug as a component in making methamphetamine. Pseudoephedrine must now be sold behind the counter, and the monthly amount a patient can purchase is limited. Until this requirement, pseudoephedrine was the most frequently used systemic decongestant, and it was considered the safest. Doses of 180 mg have been shown to produce no measurable change in blood pressure or heart rate.[28] In higher doses (210 to 240 mg), pseudoephedrine has raised both blood pressure and heart rate.[29] Pseudoephedrine can cause mild CNS stimulation, even at therapeutic doses. Stroke, related to use of oral decongestants such as pseudoephedrine, can occur in patients with hypertension and/or vasospasm.[30] Although stroke complications seem to be associated with higher-than-recommended doses, there is also a stroke risk when these agents are taken properly. Severe hypertensive reactions can occur when pseudoephedrine is given concomitantly with monoamine oxidase inhibitors. Hypertensive patients should, unless necessary, avoid systemic decongestants.

Combination Products

Numerous products combine an antihistamine with a decongestant. While the combination may be rational because of the different mechanisms of action, remember that antihistamines must be taken on a regular schedule, but decongestants should only be used when needed. Both nonselective and peripherally selective antihistamines are available in such combinations. As mentioned previously, patients should read labels to avoid therapeutic duplication. Consideration should be given to how often and how severely the patient is congested before recommending these combinations. Only a short course of a combination product should be used.

Nasal Steroids

6 Nasal steroids are an excellent choice for treating perennial rhinitis, and can be useful in seasonal rhinitis, especially if begun in advance of symptoms. Nasal steroids appear to be effective with minimal adverse effects. Some believe that nasal steroids should be recommended as initial therapy over antihistamines because of their high level of efficacy when used properly and along with avoidance of allergens.[18] Multiple mechanisms are involved with the effects of nasal steroids on the nasal mucosa: reducing inflammation by reducing mediator release, suppressing neutrophil chemotaxis, reducing intracellular edema, causing mild vasoconstriction, and inhibiting mast cell-mediated late-phase reactions. Table 95-6 lists the available nasal steroids and their usual doses.

Topical steroids produce only minor adverse effects, most commonly sneezing, stinging, headache, and epistaxis. Despite concerns about safety of systemic steroids, nasal steroids have been found to have no significant association with hypothalamic–pituitary axis suppression, cataract formation, glaucoma, or bone mineral density changes in the doses used for allergic rhinitis. Growth suppression remains a question with some evidence showing that nasal steroids with higher bioavailability (eg, beclomethasone) may have a greater growth-suppression effect than less bioavailable agents.[31] These findings require more study. Most likely, all currently available nasal steroids are safe in the majority of patients, and their clinical benefits outweigh any small growth suppressive effect. Other concerns include local infections with *Candida albicans*, which occur rarely.

The therapeutic benefits of topical steroids are not immediate, and they are not decongestants. Patients need to understand this to ensure cooperation and continuation of therapy. Some patients notice improvement in a few days, but peak responses may not be observed for 2 to 3 weeks. Once a response is achieved, the dosage may be reduced. Blocked nasal passages should be cleared with a decongestant or saline irrigation before administration to ensure adequate penetration of the spray. Patients should be advised to avoid sneezing or blowing their noses for at least 10 minutes after administration. Topical steroids should not be used for patients with nasal septum ulcers or recent nasal surgery or trauma.

One additional benefit of nasal steroids in treating allergic rhinitis in individuals with asthma and upper airway conditions is that they may confer some protection against exacerbations of asthma, leading to fewer emergency room visits. The overall relative risk for an emergency visit among asthma patients who received intranasal steroids was 0.7.[32] No effect was seen for patients receiving antihistamines.

Other Inhalant Medications

Cromolyn sodium and ipratropium bromide offer two additional approaches for treating allergic rhinitis. While neither of these agents appears in the latest treatment guidelines, they are mentioned here for completeness. Cromolyn sodium is a mast cell stabilizer. Increased interest in this product has resulted from it becoming available without a prescription. Ipratropium bromide is an anticholinergic agent that may be useful in perennial allergic rhinitis.

Cromolyn sodium nasal spray is used for the symptomatic prevention and treatment of allergic rhinitis. It curtails antigen-triggered mast cell degranulation and release of the mediators of allergic reactions, including histamine. Cromolyn sodium has no direct antihistaminic, anticholinergic, or antiinflammatory properties. Similarly to topical steroids, the most common adverse effects—sneezing and nasal stinging—result from local irritation. Dosing information is given in Table 95-6. Cromolyn sodium must cover the entire nasal lining; therefore, patients should be instructed to clear nasal passages before administration. Inhaling gently through the nose during administration aids in this process. Dosing must be repeated at 6-hour intervals to maintain the effect.

For seasonal rhinitis, treatment with cromolyn sodium should be initiated just before the usual start of the offending allergen's season and continued throughout the season. In perennial rhinitis, the effects may not be seen for 2 to 4 weeks; therefore, antihistamines or decongestants may be needed during this initial phase of therapy. As cromolyn sodium begins to work, the need for these medications should decrease.

Ipratropium nasal spray is an anticholinergic agent that exhibits antisecretory properties when applied locally. It provides symptomatic relief of rhinorrhea associated with allergic and other forms of chronic rhinitis. Dosing information is given in Table 95-6. The optimal dose should be determined based on the specific patient's symptoms and response. Adverse effects are mild, with the most common being headache, nosebleeds, and nasal dryness.

Immunotherapy

6 Experience with immunotherapy has reached the one-century mark, as the first report of the successful use of grass pollen extract injections to treat allergic rhinitis was published in 1911.[33] Until recently, immunotherapy was only available for subcutaneous injection. Sublingual dosage forms for a very limited number of allergens are now available in the United States. The therapy was first called *desensitization*; however, this did not seem appropriate because skin reactivity sometimes remained. The name was later changed to *hyposensitization*. Although this term is still used today, *immunotherapy* is used more commonly and is less confusing.

Immunotherapy is the process of administering doses of antigens responsible for eliciting allergic symptoms into a patient with the hope of inducing tolerance to the allergen when natural exposure occurs. Several mechanisms have been proposed to explain the beneficial effects of immunotherapy, including induction of IgG-blocking antibodies, reduction in specific IgE (long-term), reduced recruitment of effector cells, altered T-cell cytokine balance (a shift from T-helper type 1 to T-helper type 2), T-cell anergy, and alteration of regulatory T-cell actvitiy.[34]

Immunotherapy is moderately expensive, has significant potential risks, and requires a major time commitment from the patient. However, the cost of immunotherapy may be covered by insurance, including Medicaid. Long-term savings can be realized since decades of treatment with medication can be averted through successful immunotherapy. Candidates for immunotherapy should have significant symptoms unsuccessfully controlled by avoidance and pharmacotherapy or should stand to benefit in other significant ways, such as with asthma. Immunotherapy may postpone the onset of asthma or possibly even prevent it.[35] Patients who are unable to tolerate the adverse effects of properly managed drug therapy also should be considered. Patients must be committed to the necessary regular office visits required to complete a course of subcutaneous therapy over several years.

The effectiveness of immunotherapy for seasonal allergic rhinitis appears to be better than that seen with perennial rhinitis, in part because it is more difficult to determine which allergen is responsible for perennial symptoms, and it is more often due to multiple sensitizations. Effectiveness has been shown in a number of clinical studies using a variety of pollen extracts, even for patients with severe disease resistant to pharmacotherapy.[35] Specific immunotherapy for house dust mites has had good results in appropriately selected patients, but more study is needed. Data indicate that for some patients 3 years of immunotherapy may be sufficient to give lasting benefit;[36] however, many require longer treatment. Sublingual and local nasal specific immunotherapy may offer acceptable alternatives to the traditional subcutaneous route in some patients.[18]

The selection of antigens should be based on patient history and skin test results. Numerous regimens for administration of selected allergens have been suggested. In the beginning of subcutaneous immunotherapy, very dilute solutions are given initially one to two times per week. The concentration is increased until the maximum tolerated or highest planned or effective dose is achieved. This maintenance dose is continued in slowly increasing intervals over several years, depending on clinical response. In light of the present understanding of the immunologic results of immunotherapy, it should be given year-round rather than seasonally.

Sublingual immunotherapy is available for ragweed and certain grass allergies. Because the types of allergens are limited, patient selection should be done carefully to ensure that those receiving this route of immunotherapy are the most likely to benefit. The products are started 12 weeks before the allergen season and continued throughout the season. The first dose is administered in the physician's office to allow observation of the patient for 30 minutes for hypersensitivity reactions. The patient places the tablet under the tongue where it dissolves. Patients should not swallow for at least 1 minute. After the first dose is administered without incident, patients can take immunotherapy at home. However, patients must be prescribed an autoinjectable epinephrine.

Adverse reactions can occur with subcutaneous immunotherapy and range from mild to life threatening. Among the most common are mild local reactions, consisting of induration and swelling at the site of the injection. These may be immediate or delayed. Other more serious reactions (eg, generalized urticaria, bronchospasm, laryngospasm, and vascular collapse) occur rarely; deaths can result from anaphylactic reactions. Severe reactions are treated with epinephrine as well as other modalities recommended for anaphylaxis. Because of this potential risk, subcutaneous immunotherapy must not be given without adequate direct observation in a medical facility. With sublingual immunotherapy, the most common reactions are pruritus of the mouth, ears, and tongue, throat irritation, and mouth edema.

Several patient types are poor candidates for immunotherapy, including patients with any medical condition that would compromise the ability to tolerate an anaphylactic-type reaction, patients with impaired immune systems, and patients with a history of nonadherence to therapy.

Clinical **Controversy...**

Since few patients suffer from hypersensitivity to a single allergen type, will the sublingual immunotherapy be helpful to patients with allergies to other grass or weed pollens than those contained in the currently available products?

Leukotriene Receptor Antagonists

Leukotriene receptor antagonists inhibit the cysteinyl leukotriene receptor. The cysteinyl leukotrienes are one type of inflammatory mediators released from mast cells in allergy. Montelukast is approved for the treatment of perennial allergic rhinitis in children as young as 6 months and for seasonal allergic rhinitis in children as young as 2 years. Montelukast is considered a third choice behind antihistamines and nasal steroids.[18]

Studies published to date show leukotriene receptor antagonists to be no more effective than peripherally selective antihistamines and less effective than intranasal steroids. However, when combined with antihistamines, they are more effective than the antihistamine alone.[37] In children with mild persistent asthma and coexisting allergic rhinitis, montelukast as monotherapy has been recommended.[1] Table 95-6 lists dosage regimens.

Alternative Treatment Options

A few other alternative options have been suggested for treatment of allergic rhinitis. As mentioned earlier in this chapter, microbial exposure in the early years of life could help prevent allergic disease by favoring a nonatopic immune response.[4] However, the use of probiotics may be limited to treatment or prevention of childhood eczema as available evidence shows little benefit in allergic airway diseases.[41] Butterbur, with the active ingredient petasin that exhibits antileukotriene and antihistamine activity, has shown some success but is not recommended for most patients.[18,42] Acupuncture is listed as an optional therapy in the latest guidelines, but high-quality evidence supporting the intervention is not available.[1]

Personalized Pharmacotherapy

The two primary pharmacotherapy options for the treatment of allergic rhinitis in adults and children are antihistamines and intranasal steroids. Patient preference should play a role when selecting between these two options. While limited evidence supports intranasal steroids over antihistamines, some patients may prefer simple oral therapy. Either choice requires clear patient counseling to ensure appropriate timing of therapy and expectations of effect.

For patients (both adults and children) who are not immunocompromised, have a high likelihood for adherence, and have adequate insurance and/or financial resources, subcutaneous specific immunotherapy is an excellent choice for treatment of seasonal allergic rhinitis and allergic rhinitis secondary to house dust mites. In some children, immunotherapy may prevent development of asthma. Sublingual immunotherapy may be beneficial to patients who are sensitive only to ragweed or certain types of grasses.

For patients experiencing an exacerbation of nasal congestion as part of their allergic rhinitis picture, decongestants can be used short term.

Leukotriene receptor antagonists should not be recommended as primary therapy for allergic rhinitis; however, patients with allergic rhinitis and asthma may benefit from this therapy.

Cromolyn is another alternative that is effective, but many patients may find its frequent daily dosing (up to six times daily) difficult.

A drug monitoring summary is shown in Table 95-8. Intranasal and ophthalmic antihistamines may be helpful for specific symptoms not relieved by first-line choices. An intranasal anticholinergic such as ipratropium is specifically useful for rhinorrhea.

TABLE 95-8 Monitoring of Medications for Allergic Rhinitis

Drug	Adverse Reaction	Monitoring Parameter	Comments
Antihistamines	Drowsiness	Caution patient about the potential for drowsiness, even with nonsedating and intranasal products	Do not mix with alcohol or other CNS depressants
	Gastrointestinal effects	Counsel patient to take with a meal or full glass of water	
	Anticholinergic effects	Watch for dry mouth and difficulty with urination. Caution patient about other medications with anticholinergic effects	Switching to an antihistamine with less anticholinergic effects may be necessary
Decongestants			
Topical	Rebound vasodilation	Watch for decreased response to topical agent	Avoid prolonged use (>3-5 days)
	Local irritation	Watching for burning, stinging, sneezing, and dryness of mucosa	Self-limiting due to short-term use. May try nasal saline for dryness.
Systemic	Hypertension	If used in a patient with hypertension, monitor blood pressure regularly and discontinue if the pressure increases	Usually not an issue for patients without preexisting hypertension. Use lowest effective dose
	CNS stimulation	Usually mild but discuss with patient	Use lowest effective dose
Nasal steroids	Local effects such as sneezing, stinging, and epistaxis	These effects may vary among products	
Other intranasal agents			
Cromolyn	Local effects such as sneezing, burning, or coughing	Usually mild but tell patient to report bothersome symptoms	If patient cannot tolerate local reactions, choose an alternative agent
Ipratropium	Headache, nosebleeds, and nasal dryness	Usually mild, tell patient to report bothersome symptoms	If patient cannot tolerate local reactions, choose an alternative agent
Montelukast	Behavioral changes	Monitor for mood and behavioral changes including suicidal ideation	Rare but should be monitored
Immunotherapy, SC	Local reactions	Watch for induration or swelling at site of injection	Anaphylaxis rare, but should only be given under direct medical supervision with epinephrine available
	Allergic reactions	Monitor for signs of anaphylaxis	
Immunotherapy, SL	Pruritis of ear, oral itching, mouth edema, throat irritation	Caution patient about these reactions as they are fairly common.	First dose giving in physician's office so patient can be observed for 30 minutes. Prescription must be accompanied by a prescription for an epinephrine autoinjector.

More supportive evidence is needed to determine which patients, if any, would benefit from the other alternative options mentioned earlier.

Evaluation of Therapeutic Outcomes

With allergic rhinitis, major outcomes include the effect of the disease on a patient's life, the efficacy and tolerability of treatment, and patient satisfaction. Consideration must be given to how the condition is affecting the patient's job or school performance, family and social interactions, and other aspects of quality of life. Drug therapy should prevent or minimize symptoms with few adverse effects. The patient should not have difficulty obtaining needed medication for financial or other reasons. Patients should be questioned about their satisfaction with the management of their allergic rhinitis. The management should result in minimal disruption to their lives.

Methods for assessing patient-reported outcomes and health-related quality of life in clinical trials related to allergy have been recommended.[43] These tools go beyond measuring improvement in symptoms and include such items as sleep quality, nonallergic symptoms (eg, fatigue, poor concentration, and others), emotions, and participation in a variety of activities. How well each of the current treatment modalities performs and how they compare in improving patient outcomes remain to be determined.

Clinicians caring for allergic rhinitis patients should develop a comprehensive pharmaceutical care plan that addresses several areas. Discuss and agree on therapeutic end points for allergic rhinitis, including the patient's acceptable level of symptom relief, onset of symptom relief expectations, and seasonal starts and stops. Discuss adverse drug reaction self-monitoring and prevention based on treatment selection. Assess patient attitude toward adherence to and persistence with oral, ocular, intranasal, or immunologic therapies. Ensure proper matching of treatment to symptoms and intervene with the prescriber if necessary. Conduct seasonal or annual review with patient.

The therapeutic goal for all patients with allergic rhinitis is to minimize or prevent symptoms. Evaluation of success is accomplished primarily through the discussions with the patient, in whom both relief of symptoms and tolerance of drug therapy must be discussed.

CONCLUSION

Allergic rhinitis is a common disease with symptoms ranging from mild to severe. If avoidance measures are unsuccessful, allergic rhinitis should be treated to improve quality of life and prevent long-term complications. Timing of treating is essential. Treatment regimens should be individualized based on patient symptoms and response. Care should be taken to correctly identify allergy as the cause of the patient's rhinitis before committing them to chromic treatment.

ABBREVIATIONS

IgE	immunoglobulin E
RAST	radioallergosorbent test

REFERENCES

1. Seidman MD, Gurgel RK, Lin, SY, et al. Clinical practice guidelines: Allergic rhinitis. *Otolaryngology—Head and Neck* 2015;152(1S): S1-S43.
2. Wheatley LM, Togias A. Allergic rhinitis. *N Engl J Med* 2015;372: 456-463.
3. Bousquet J, Khaltaev N, Cruz AA, et al. Allergic rhinitis and its impact on asthma (ARIA) 2008. *Allergy* 2008;63(Suppl 86):8-160.
4. von Mutius E, Radon K. Living on a farm: Impact on asthma induction and clinical course. *Immunol Allergy Clin North Am* 2008;28:631-647.
5. Wallace DV, Dykewicz MS, Bernstein DI, et al. The diagnosis and management of rhinitis: An updated practice parameter. *J Allergy Clin Immunol* 2008;122:S1-S83.
6. Wilson SJ, Shute JK, Holgate ST, et al. Localization of interleukin (IL)-4 but not 5 to human mast cell secretory granules by immunoelectron microscopy. *Clin Exp Allergy* 2000;30:493-500.
7. Riccio AAM, Tosco MA, Cosentino C, et al. Cytokine pattern in allergic and nonallergic chronic rhinosinusitis in asthmatic children. *Clin Exp Allergy* 2002;32:422-426.
8. Wood-Baker R, Lau L, Howarth PH. Histamine and the nasal vasculature: The influence of H1 and H2-histamine receptor antagonism. *Clin Otolaryngol* 1996;21:348-352.
9. Howarth PH. Mediators of nasal blockage in allergic rhinitis. *Allergy* 1997;52(40 Suppl):12-18.
10. Howarth PH. Leukotrienes in rhinitis. *Am J Respir Crit Care Med* 2000;161:S133-S136.
11. Clark RR, Baroody FM. What drives the symptoms of allergic rhinitis? *J Respir Dis* 1998;19:S6-S15.
12. Gerth van Wijk R. Perennial allergic rhinitis and nasal hyperreactivity. *Am J Rhinol* 1998;12:33-35.
13. Klaewsongkram J, Ruxrungtham K, Wannakrairot P, et al. Eosinophil count in nasal mucosa is more suitable than the number of ICAM-1-positive nasal epithelial cells to evaluate the severity of house dust mite-sensitive allergic rhinitis: A clinical correlation study. *Int Arch Allergy Immunol* 2003;132:68-75.
14. Braunstahl GJ, Fokkens WJ, Overbeek SE, et al. Mucosal and systemic inflammatory changes in allergic rhinitis and asthma: A comparison between upper and lower airways. *Clin Exp Allergy* 2003;33:579-587.
15. Hill SL, Krouse JH. The effects of montelukast on intradermal wheal and flare. *Otolarygol Head Neck Surg* 2003;129:199-203.
16. Scadding G. Optimal management of nasal congestion caused my allergic rhinitis in children. *Pediatr Drugs* 2008;10(3):151-162.
17. Bousquet J, Schunemann HJ, Zuberbier T, et al. Development and implementation of guidelines in allergic rhinitis—An ARIA-GA²LEN paper. *Allergy* 2012;65:1212-1221.
18. Brozek JL, Bousquet J, Baena-Cagnani CE, et al. Allergic rhinitis and its impact on asthma (ARIA) guidelines: 2010 revision. *J Allergy Clin Immunol* 2010;126:466-476.
19. Franchi M, Carrier P, Kotzias D, et al. Working toward healthy air in dwellings in Europe. *Allergy* 2006;61:864-868.
20. Casale TB, Blaiss MS, Gelfand E, et al. First do no harm: Managing antihistamine impairment in patients with allergic rhinitis. *J Allergy Clin Immunol* 2003;111:S835-S842.
21. Sansgiry SS, Shringarpure GS. Springtime confusion: Are consumers getting the right information on how to treat seasonal allergies? *J Allergy Clin Immunol* 2003;112:627-628.
22. Bender BG, Berning S, Dudden R, et al. Sedation and performance impairment of diphenhydramine and second-generation antihistamines: A meta-analysis. *J Allergy Clin Immunol* 2003;111:770-776.
23. Richardson GS, Roehrs TA, Rosenthal L, et al. Tolerance to daytime sedative effects of H1 antihistamines. *J Clin Psychopharmacol* 2002;22:511-515.
24. Pharmacy Times OTC Guide 2015. Available at: http://www.otcguide.net/recommendations/antihistamines-oral.
25. Berger WE, White MV. Efficacy of azelastine nasal spray in patients with an unsatisfactory response to loratadine. *Ann Allergy Asthma Immunol* 2003;91:205-211.
26. Astelin. Product Information. Somerset, NJ: Meda Pharmaceuticals, 2011.
27. Astepro. Product Information. Somerset, NJ: Meda Pharmaceuticals, 2010.
28. Empey DE, Young GA, Letley E, et al. Dose response study of the nasal decongestant and cardiovascular effects of pseudoephedrine. *Br J Clin Pharmacol* 1980;9:351-358.
29. Drew CDM, Knight GT, Hughes DTD, et al. Comparison of the effects of D-(−)-ephedrine and L-(+)-pseudoephedrine on the cardiovascular and respiratory systems in man. *Br J Clin Pharmacol* 1978;6:221-225.
30. Cantu C, Arauz A, Murilla-Bonilla LM, et al. Stroke associated with sympathomimetics contained in over-the-counter cough and cold drugs. *Stroke* 2003;34:1667-1673.
31. Mehle ME. Are nasal steroids safe? *Curr Opin Otolaryngol Head Neck Surg* 2003;11:201-205.
32. Adams RJ, Fuhlbrigge AL, Finkelstein JA, Weiss ST. Intranasal steroids and the risk of emergency department visits for asthma. *J Allergy Clin Immunol* 2002;109:636-642.
33. Noon L. Prophylactic inoculation against hay fever. *Lancet* 1911;1:1572-1573.

34. Valenta R, Campana R, Marth K, van Hage M. Allergen-specific immunotherapy: From vaccines to prophylactic approaches. *J Intern Med* 2012;272:144-157.
35. Incorvaia C, Frati F. One century of allergen-specific immunotherapy for respiratory allergy. *Immunotherapy* 2011;3(5):629-635.
36. Durham SR, Walker SM, Varga EM, et al. Long-term clinical efficacy of grass pollen immunotherapy. *N Engl J Med* 1999;341:468-475.
37. Rodrigo GT, Yanez A. The role of antileukotriene therapy in seasonal allergic rhinitis: A systematic review randomized trials. *Ann Allergy Asthma Immunol* 2006;96:779-786.
38. Polos PG. Montelukast is an effective monotherapy for mild asthma and for asthma with co-morbid allergic rhinitis. *Prim Care Respir J* 2006;15:310-311.
39. Casale TB, Condemi J, LaForce C, et al. Effect of omalizumab on symptoms of seasonal allergic rhinitis. *JAMA* 2001;286:2956-2967.
40. Frew AJ. Anti-IgE and asthma. *Ann Allergy Asthma Immunol* 2003;91:117-118.
41. Boyle RJ, Tang ML. The role of probiotics in the management of allergic disease. *Clin Exp Allergy* 2006;36:568-576.
42. Gray RD, Haggart K, Lee DK, et al. Effects of butterbur treatment in intermittent allergic rhinitis: A placebo-controlled evaluation. *Ann Allergy Asthma Immunol* 2004;93(1):56-60.
43. Baiardini I, Bousquet PJ, Brzoza Z, et al. Recommendations for assessing patient reported outcomes and health-related quality of life in clinical trials on allergy: A GA^{2}LEN taskforce position paper. *Allergy* 2010;65:290-295.

96 Acne Vulgaris

Debra Sibbald

KEY CONCEPTS

1. Acne is a highly prevalent disorder affecting many adolescents and adults.
2. The etiology of this complex disease originates from multiple causative and contributory factors. The diagnosis is based on the patient's history and clinical presentation.
3. Elements of pathogenesis involve defects in epidermal keratinization, androgen secretion, sebaceous function, bacterial growth, inflammation, and immunity.
4. Acne vulgaris is a chronic disorder which cannot be "cured." Goals of treatment and prevention include control and alleviation of symptoms by reducing the number and severity of lesions, slowing progression, limiting disease duration and recurrence, prevention of long-term disfigurement associated with scarring and hyperpigmentation and avoidance of psychologic suffering. Targeting goals may increase patient adherence to therapy.
5. The most critical target for treatment is the microcomedone. Minimizing or reversing follicular occlusion will arrest the pathogenic acne cascade and involves combining treatment measures to target all pathogenic elements.
6. Nondrug measures are aimed at long-term prevention and treatment. Patients should eliminate aggravating factors, maintain a balanced, low-glycemic load diet, and control stress. Cleanse twice daily with mild soap or soapless cleanser, and use only oil-free cosmetics. Comedone extraction in approximately 10% of patients produces immediate cosmetic improvement. Shave infrequently as possible, using a sharp blade or electric razor.
7. First-, second-, and third-line therapies should be appropriate for the severity and staging of the clinical presentation and directed toward control and prevention.
8. Treatment regimens should be tapered over time, adjusting to response. Combine the smallest number of agents at the lowest possible dosages to ensure efficacy, safety, avoidance of resistance, and patient adherence.
9. Once control is achieved, maintenance regimens should be simplified to continue with some suppressive therapy. Therapy must be continued beyond 8 weeks: efficacy is assessed through comedonal and inflammatory lesion (IL) count, control or progression of severity, and management of associated anxiety or depression. Safety end points include monitoring for treatment adverse effects.
10. Motivate the patient to continue long-term therapy through empathic and informative counseling.

In this chapter, I review the latest developments in understanding acne vulgaris and its treatment. The contents provide an analysis of the physiology of the pilosebaceous unit; the epidemiology, etiology, and pathophysiology of acne; relevant treatment with nondrug measures; and comparisons of pharmacologic agents, including drugs of choice recommended in best-practice guidelines. Options include a variety of alternatives such as retinoids, antimicrobial agents, hormones, and light therapy. Formulation principles are discussed in relation to drug delivery. Patient assessment, general approaches to individualized therapy plans, and monitoring evaluation strategies are presented.

EPIDEMIOLOGY

1 Acne vulgaris is a chronic disease and the most common one treated by dermatologists. The lifetime prevalence of acne approaches 90%, with the highest incidence in adolescents. Prevalence data available from the European Union, United States, Australia, and New Zealand show that acne affects 80% of individuals between puberty and 30 years of age, depending on the method of lesion counting (50%-95% prevalence range reported for adolescents and 20%-30% prevalence range for ages 20-40).[1] Other studies have reported acne in 28% to 61% of school children aged 10 to 12 years; 79% to 95% of those 16 to 18 years of age; and even in children aged 4 to 7 years. If mild manifestations were excluded and only moderate or severe manifestations were considered, the frequency in epidemiological studies in Western industrialized countries was still 20% to 35%.[2-5]

The onset of acne vulgaris during puberty occurs at a younger chronologic age in girls than boys (12% age 25-58 vs 3% in males of the same age) and periodic premenstrual flares may continue until menopause. It is triggered in children by the initiation of androgen production by the adrenal glands and gonads, and it usually subsides after the end of growth. However, to some degree, most patients continue to have symptoms into their mid-20s, and there is evidence that the duration of acne may last into middle age for most women, recorded in 54% of women and 40% of men older than 25 years of age.[6] In puberty, acne is often more severe in boys in about 15% of cases, which is tenfold greater than in girls. Women often have more severe forms during adulthood. When untreated, acne usually lasts for several years until it spontaneously remits. After the disease has ended, scars and dyspigmentation are not uncommon permanent negative outcomes.

Genetic factors have been recognized; there is a high concordance among identical twins, and there is also a tendency toward severe acne in patients with a positive family history of acne.

There are believed to be no gender differences in acne prevalence, although such differences are often reported and may represent social biases. In urban clinics, there is a clear preponderance of girls seeking treatment. There is also a perception that acne is less prevalent in rural populations. This is supported by the data from Varanasi, India, where 21.35% of boys (13-18 years) from rural areas had acne versus 37.5% of those from the urban areas.[7]

An international group of epidemiologists, community medicine specialists, and anthropologists have questioned whether acne might be predominantly a disease of Western civilization.[8] They assert that since acne vulgaris is nearly universal in westernized societies (afflicting 79%-95% of the adolescent population), one causative factor might be the Western glycemic diet. While this hypothesis is based on the observation that primitive societies subsisting on traditional (low glycemic) diets have no acne, the theory awaits validation and acceptance by the dermatologic community.

ETIOLOGY

2 Acne is a multifactorial disease. Genetic, racial, hormonal, dietary, and environmental factors have been implicated in its development. Its psychologic impact can be severe.

Four major etiologic factors are involved in the development of acne: increased sebum production, due to hormonal influences; alteration in the keratinization process and hyperproliferation of ductal epidermis; bacterial colonization of the duct with *Propionibacterium acnes*; and production of inflammation with release of inflammatory mediators in acne sites. These are reviewed in the Pathophysiology section later in this chapter.

The role of heredity in acne has not been clearly defined; however, there is a significant tendency toward more serious involvement if one or both parents had severe acne during their youth.

Environmental factors play a major role in determining the severity and extent of acne and may influence the choice of topical treatments. Heat and humidity may induce comedones; pressure or friction caused by protective devices such as helmets, shoulder pads, or pillows, and excessive scrubbing or washing can exacerbate existing acne by causing microcomedones to rupture. Pressure may cause acne lesions to form in patients who do not have acne vulgaris: this variant is called *mechanical acne*. Friction, wool, or other rough textured fabrics and occlusive clothing may also be mechanical irritants. Hair styles that are low on the forehead or neck may cause excessive sweating and occlusion, exacerbating acne. In most cases acne is worse in winter and improves during the summer, suggesting a salutary effect of sunlight. However, in some cases, exposure to sunlight worsens the disease.[9] Studies examining the relationship between tobacco smoking and acne show inconsistent results; however, dermatologists have begun to counsel people to quit tobacco smoking as a potential auxiliary treatment for acne.

The importance of psychologic factors in this prolonged and capricious condition has been repeatedly stressed. Two-thirds of affected teenagers wish that they could speak with their physician their healthcare provider about acne, but only one-third actually do. Emotions, such as intense anger and stress, can exacerbate acne, causing flares or increasing mechanical manipulation: picking, excoriating, or pinching lesions sometimes subconsciously or in sleep. This is probably the result of increased glucocorticoid secretion by the adrenal glands, which appears to potentiate the effects of androgens.[10]

Dietary influences are the focus of current investigations. In the past, acne was not felt to be influenced by diet, but patients could restrict certain foods they perceived exacerbate acne (chocolate, cola drinks, milk and milk products).[11,12] These recommendations, which still persist in some guidelines, are based on one or two poorly designed studies conducted more than 40 years ago. They have largely been discounted by well-designed current studies. A discussion of the issues surrounding dietary influences is elaborated in the Clinical Controversy on Diet box.

Clinical **Controversy...**

Diet and Acne

The role of dietary influences in acne continues to be disputed in the literature with increasing attention and vigor. Evidentiary studies are currently in progress to elaborate associations between various dietary influences and presentation of acne, following the dismissal of over-interpreted 40-year-old, poorly designed studies that disavowed potential effects of dietary ingestions on acne.[162,163] Researchers are examining nutritional factors both as factors in acne development as well as potential treatment modalities.

Beginning in 2005, a series of studies have linked consumption of dairy products with acne, perhaps due to natural hormonal components and/or other bioactive molecules in milk.[164,165] Acne has been positively associated with the reported quantity of milk ingested, particularly skim milk.[166] The Nurses Health Study, which included 47,355 women, used retrospective data on diet during high school and found an association between acne and the intake of milk. The authors suggest that natural hormonal components of milk and/or other bioactive molecules in milk could exacerbate acne.[167]

Other studies suggest that insulin-like growth factor (IGF), increased by ingestion of high glycemic loads, may play a role in acne.[168,169] Lactoferrin-enriched fermented milk ameliorates acne vulgaris with a selective decrease of triacylglycerols in skin surface lipids.[167] Lactoferrin is a whey milk protein that has a prominent activity against inflammation. When administered as a dietary supplement on a twice-daily regimen in mild-to-moderate acne vulgaris, it may lead to an overall improvement in acne lesion counts in the majority of affected adolescents and young adults.[170]

The strongest evidence points to a high glycemic load (HGL) diet as a significant factor in acne. In a well-designed randomized controlled trial, a significant reduction in acne was seen in patients who eliminated high glycemic index foods. Patients who consumed a low-glycemic-load diet, compared with a conventional HGL diet, had improvements of facial acne after 12 weeks. Accompanying changes in physical and endocrinologic parameters suggest that decreases in total energy intake, body weight, and indices of androgenicity and insulin resistance may also be associated with observed improvements in acne.[171] Other studies showed correlations between increases in the ratio of saturated to monounsaturated fatty acids and acne lesion counts and increased sebum outflow. This suggests a possible role of desaturase enzymes in sebaceous lipogenesis and the clinical manifestation of acne; these require further investigation.[172] Another study reported an improvement in acne and insulin sensitivity in low-glycemic-load diets compared with controls, suggesting nutrition-related lifestyle factors play a role in the etiology of acne. Independent effects of weight loss versus dietary intervention need to be isolated.[173] In an Australian study, no cases of acne were reported in participants who consumed low glycemic load diets.[166]

In 2015, a survey reported results of a French questionnaire of individuals (age 15-24) reporting or not reporting acne with associated epidemiological variables using univariate and multivariate analysis. Daily consumption of chocolate and sweets was independently and highly associated with acne (odds ratio 2.38), as was regular use of cannabis (odds ratio 2.88) whereas smoking tobacco (>10 cigarettes daily) was highly protective. Respective roles of sugar, lipids, and milk were not investigated.[174]

A systematic review of dietary influences on acne suggests that a possible role of dietary factors cannot be dismissed, as studies to date have not been sufficiently large or robust. While still controversial, diet is thought to play a role in the development or progression of acne vulgaris and further studies are ongoing. Investigations reviewing antioxidants from nutritional and topical sources and probiotics, as potential acne-fighting agents are now proceeding in early stages.[166]

PATHOPHYSIOLOGY

3 The pathogenesis of acne progresses through the following four major stages:

1. Increased sebum production by the sebaceous gland
2. *P. acnes* follicular colonization (and bacterial lipolysis of sebum triglycerides to free fatty acids)
3. Release of inflammatory mediators
4. Increased follicular keratinization

Improved understanding of acne development on a molecular level suggests that acne is a disease that involves both innate and adaptive immune systems and inflammatory events. Receptors that regulate sebaceous lipid metabolism work in concert with receptors regulating epidermal growth and differentiation. Acne can be considered as a model of immune-mediated chronic inflammatory skin disease: an innate immune response that is not able to control *P. acnes* followed by a Th1-mediated adaptive immune response that becomes self-maintaining independently from *P. acnes* itself.[13]

Acne usually begins in the prepubertal period, when the adrenal glands mature, and progresses as androgen production and sebaceous gland activity increase with gonad development.

As shown in Fig. 96-1, acne results from the development of an obstructed sebaceous follicle, called a *microcomedone*. Sebaceous glands increase their size and activity in response to circulating androgens. Most patients with acne do not overproduce androgens (with some exceptions); instead, they have sebaceous glands that are hyperresponsive to androgens.[14] Patients with acne have a significantly greater number of lobules per gland compared with unaffected individuals.

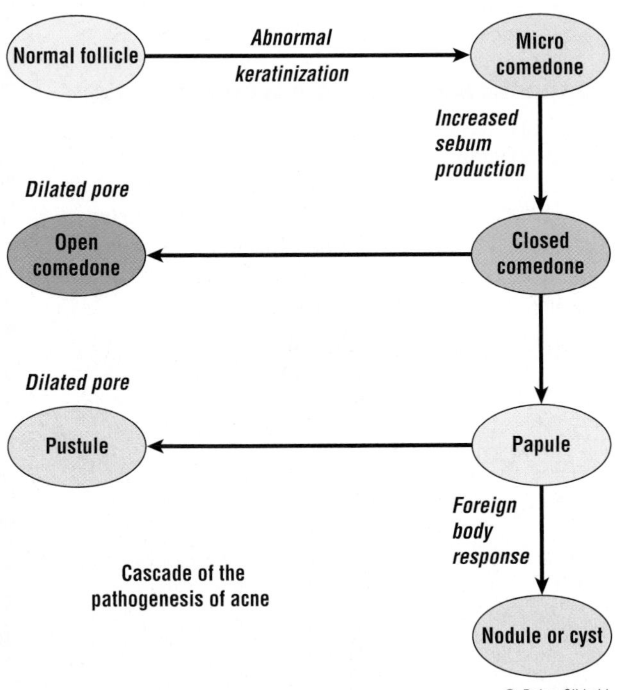

FIGURE 96-1 Cascade of the pathogenesis of acne. (*Used with permission from Mills OH, Kligman AM. Comedogenicity of sunscreens. experimental observations in rabbits. Arch Dermatol 1982;18(6):417-419.*)

Sebaceous lipids are regulated by peroxisome proliferator-activated receptors, which act in concert with retinoid X receptors to regulate epidermal growth and differentiation as well as lipid metabolism. Sterol response element-binding proteins mediate the increase in sebaceous lipids formation induced by insulin-like growth factor-1. Substance P receptors, neuropeptidases, α-melanocyte stimulating hormone, insulin-like growth factor (IGF)-1R and corticotropin-releasing hormone (CRH)-R1 are also involved in regulating sebocyte activity as are ectopeptidases. The sebaceous gland also acts as an endocrine organ in response to changes in androgens and other hormones. Oxidized squalene can stimulate hyperproliferative behavior of keratinocytes, and lipoperoxides produce leukotriene B4, a powerful chemoattractant.[14] The composition of sebum is changed, with a reduction in linoleic acid. The growth of keratinocytes changes. The infrainfundibulum increases its keratinization of cells with hypercornification and development of the microcomedone, the primary lesion of both noninflammatory and inflammatory acne.[13] Cells adhere to each other in an expanding mass, which forms a dense keratinous plug. In particular androgens, hormones could be a stimulus to pilosebaceous duct hypercornification. Sebum, produced in increasing amounts by the active gland, becomes trapped behind the keratin plug and solidifies, contributing to open or closed comedone formation.

Interleukin-1-α upregulation contributes to the development of comedones independently of colonization with *P. acnes*. A relative linoleic acid deficiency has also been described.[14]

A prominent role is played by the follicular colonization by *P. acnes*. *P. acnes* displays several activities which promote the development of acne lesions, including the promotion of follicular hyperkeratinization; the induction of sebogenesis; and the stimulation of an inflammatory response by the secretion of proinflammatory molecules and by the activation of innate immunity, followed by a *P. acnes*-specific adaptive immune response. In addition, *P. acnes*-independent inflammation mediated by androgens or by a neurogenic activation, followed by the secretion in the skin of proinflammatory neuropeptides, can occur in acne lesions.[13]

The pooling of sebum in the follicle provides ideal substrate conditions for proliferation of the anaerobic bacterium *P. acnes*, generating a T cell response, which results in inflammation.[15] *P. acnes* produces a lipase that hydrolyzes sebum triglycerides into free fatty acids. These free fatty acids may trigger the changes that lead to an increase in keratinization and microcomedone formation.[16,17] This closed comedone, or whitehead, is the first clinically visible lesion of acne. It takes approximately 5 months to develop. The closed comedone is almost completely obstructed to drainage and has a tendency to rupture.[18-20]

As the plug extends to the upper canal and dilates its opening, an open comedone, or blackhead, is formed. Its dark color is not due to dirt but to either oxidized lipid and melanin or to the impacted mass of horny cells. The cylindrically shaped, open comedone is very stable and may persist for a long time as soluble substances and liquid sebum escape more easily. Acne that is characterized by open and closed comedones is termed *noninflammatory acne*.

Acne produces chemotactic factors and promotes the synthesis of tumor factor-α and interleukin-1β. Cytokine induction by *P. acnes* occurs. Both recruitment of polymorphs into the follicle during the inflammatory process and release of *P. acnes*-generated chemokines lead to pus formation. The pus eventually bursts on the surface with resolution of the inflammation or into the dermis. *P. acnes* also produces enzymes that increase the permeability of the follicular wall, causing it to rupture, releasing keratin, hair, and lipids and irritating free fatty acids into the dermis. Several different types of inflammatory lesions (ILs) may form, including pustules, nodules, and cysts and may lead to scarring.

Hyperpigmentation and scarring are two sequelae of acne. A time delay of up to 3 years between acne onset and adequate treatment correlates to degree of scarring and emphasizes the need for early therapy.[11,12]

CLINICAL PRESENTATION Signs and Symptoms

Lesion Type: Acne Vulgaris Can be Noninflammatory or Inflammatory

- Noninflammatory acne is characterized by open and closed comedones that develop from the subclinical microcomedo
- The closed comedo is visible as a 1-2 mm whitehead most easily seen when the skin is stretched. It is often inconspicuous with no visible follicular opening
  - Is the first clinical sign of acne
  - Has a tendency to rupture
- The open comedo, or blackhead, is larger, approximately 2-5 mm and is dark-topped with contents extruding
  - Is relatively stable
- Inflammatory acne is traditionally characterized as having papulopustular and/or nodular lesions which may arise from the microcomedo or from noninflammatory clinically apparent lesions
  - A pustule is formed from a superficial aggregation of neutrophils
    - Appears as a raised white lesion filled with pus, usually less than 5 mm in diameter
    - Superficial pustules usually resolve within a few days without scarring
- A nodule is produced through deeper, dermal, inflammatory infiltration
  - Is the most severe variant of acne
  - Appears as warm, tender, firm lesions, with a diameter of 5 mm or greater
  - May be suppurative or hemorrhagic within the dermis, may involve adjacent follicles and sometimes extend down to fat
- Cysts are suppurative nodules named because they resemble inflamed epidermal cysts
  - Cystic acne may show double comedones, resulting from prior inflammation and fistulous links between neighboring sebaceous units
- Progression of ILs:
  - Pustules and cysts often rupture spontaneously and drain a purulent or bloody but odorless discharge[21]
  - Inflammatory lesions may itch as they erupt and can be tender or painful. Nodules may develop exudative sinus tracts resulting in tissue destruction
  - Often resolution of these lesions leaves erythematous or pigmented macules that can persist for months or longer, especially in dark-skinned individuals
  - Nodules and deep lesions may result in scarring

Regions of Involvement

- Acne lesions can occur anywhere on the body apart from the palms and soles
  - Are usually located on the face, back, neck, shoulders, and chest
  - May extend to buttocks or extremities
  - One or more anatomic areas may be involved in any given patient
  - The pattern of involvement, once present, tends to remain constant
  - Comedones frequently have a midfacial distribution in childhood and when evident early, are indicative of a poor prognosis
- Skin, scalp, and hair are frequently oily

Severity Grading Taxonomies

FDA Investigator Global Assessment 2005[22,24]

Type 1	Almost clear: rare noninflammatory lesions (NIL) with no more than 1 papule
Type 2	Mild, some NIL but no more than a few papules/pustules
Type 3	Moderate: many NIL, some ILs, no more than 1 nodule
Type 4	Severe: up to many NIL and IL, but no more than a few nodular lesions

European Union Guidelines Clinical Classification:[14]

I	Comedonal acne
II	Mild-moderate papulopustular (MMPP) acne
III	Severe papulopustular acne, moderate nodular acne (*this level combines FDA types 3 and 4, above*)
IV	Severe nodular acne, conglobate acne (*this is an additional level cf. the FDA types above*)

Diagnostic and Assessment Considerations

Palliating factors	Sunlight
Provoking factors	Premenstrual flares, humid environments, excessive sweating; exposure to chemicals; occlusive clothing; friction; oily cosmetics; manual manipulation; stress
Associated symptoms	Itch, pain, fever
Medical conditions	May contribute to or coexist with acne, including endocrine factors (eg, irregular menses, hirsutism, alopecia), pregnancy, atopy
Allergies	May cause acne symptoms, or present a contraindication to therapy
Medication history	Products may cause or interact with acne signs and symptoms
Social habits	Diet, or smoking (see clinical controversies)
Family history	Genetic predisposition to acne
Psychosocial issues	Assess global and disease specific quality of life (QOL) indicators or health-state utilities

CLINICAL PRESENTATION AND DIAGNOSTIC CONSIDERATIONS

To correctly diagnose acne vulgaris, the clinician considers patient assessment, which includes distinguishing all the presenting signs and symptoms of the clinical presentation, reviewing diagnostic and assessment considerations (see Clinical Presentation box), as well as considering psychosocial issues, differential diagnosis, and the possibility of drug-induced acne.

Psychosocial Issues

Assessment of acne's impact on QOL is an important consideration in clinical decision-making. The negative impact of facial acne is one of the primary motivators for patients to seek and to adhere to treatment.[23] Specific QOL indicators represent patients' perceptions of and reactions to their health. Assessing QOL impairment in patients with acne may aid in management by evaluating psychologic impact, which may not correlate with clinical severity; aid in detection of depression or need for psychologic care; and improve therapeutic outcomes.

Acne adversely affects all aspects of QOL. In addition to documentation regarding acne-specific QOL impairment, acne impact on general health and psychologic status has been assessed for relationship between sociodemographic variables, disease severity and mental status on QOL of acne sufferers. In a report of 195 cases, acne impact on health status was worse compared to other chronic diseases. Authors concluded acne is not a minor disease in comparison with other chronic conditions. Age of onset is capable to influence general health quality (GHQ status) which in turn affects QOL.[25]

Examples of global scales that have been used to evaluate acne include Skindex[26] and Dermatology QOL Index[27] examples of acne specific scales include the Acne-specific QOL questionnaire[28] and the Acne QOL Scale.[29] The Acne QOL Scale was developed to measure the impact of facial acne across four domains (acne symptoms, role-emotional, self-perception, and role-social) of health-related QOL. Health-state utilities (such as time trade-off [TTO]) are quantitative measures of patient preferences of health outcomes ranging from 0 (death) to 1 (perfect health) and can be used in clinical trials as outcome measures of treatment effects. TTO utilities for acne in the range of 0.94 to 0.96 can be compared with those of other diseases (eg, 0.92 for epilepsy, 0.94 for myopia), and help to identify the impact of acne on self-perception and psychologic functioning.[30]

Differential Diagnosis

Acne vulgaris is rarely misdiagnosed. The conditions most commonly mistaken for acne vulgaris include rosacea, perioral dermatitis, gram-negative folliculitis, and drug-induced acne.[31]

Acne rosacea (adult acne) is a chronic, progressive relapsing condition occurring after age 30 years in fair-complexioned persons. The diagnosis is clinical and based on history and physical findings. There are four subtypes: erythemato-telangietactic changes (erythema, flushing, telangiectasia [spider veins], stinging and burning); progressing to papular-pustular changes (ILs, with edema, papules, and pustules on central facial areas such as nose, cheeks, chin, and forehead); phymatous changes (thickened skin and prominent pores on nose, ears, chin, and eyelids; and ocular changes (foreign body sensation, dryness, burning, eyelid erythema).

Rosacea has key differences from acne vulgaris. Onset is not linked to androgens or endocrine changes; and comedones are not usually present. Aggravating factors include endogenous triggers: ingestion of alcohol, spicy foods, or hot drinks (especially those containing caffeine); smoking; and exogenous triggers: overexposure to sunlight; exposure to temperature extremes, heat and humidity, friction, irritating cosmetics, and steroids. Treatment may include antibiotics, particularly doxycycline (low, antiinflammatory dose) or erythromycin, topical metronidazole, pimecrolimus or azelaic acid as well as agents to reduce erythema (alpha adrenergics).[32]

Perioral dermatitis occurs primarily in young women and adolescents and is characterized by erythema, scaling, and papulopustular lesions commonly clustered around the nasolabial folds, mouth, and chin. The cause is unknown.[33]

Gram-negative folliculitis (*Proteus, Pseudomonas, Klebsiella*) may complicate acne, with a sudden change to pustules or large inflammatory cysts occurring after long-term treatment of acne with oral antibiotics. Folliculitis may be caused by staphylococci. There is a sudden onset of superficial pustules around the nose, chin, and cheeks. Patients with suspected folliculitis should be referred.[34]

Several conditions include acne vulgaris as a characteristic component, and understanding the mechanisms involved in these syndromes provides insight into the pathogenesis of acne. These include polycystic ovary syndrome (elevated androgen levels); PAPA syndrome (pyogenic arthritis, pyoderma gangrenosum, acne; early onset arthritis with increased inflammatory activity), and SAPHO syndrome (synovitis, acne, pustulosis, hyperostosis, osteitis syndrome; sterile inflammatory arthro-osteitis, with *P. acnes* as a possible trigger).[15]

Drug-Induced Acne

In addition to the conditions induced by drugs that were presented in Chapter 23, acneiform eruptions can also be caused by medications. Systemic corticosteroids can cause a pustular inflammatory form of acne, especially on the trunk. Onset is abrupt at 2 to 6 weeks after initiation of therapy. Acne has also been associated with most of the potent topical steroids, but not with hydrocortisone, which lacks the ability to inhibit protein synthesis. Discontinuation of the steroid results in an initial worsening of appearance due to removal of the anti-inflammatory action of the steroid itself. Caution patients about this reaction, which can be subdued through judicious use of topical hydrocortisone.[33-36]

Antiepileptics and tuberculostatics are the most commonly implicated in drug-induced acne, followed by lithium. Other heavy metals inducing acne include cobalt (in vitamin B_{12}).[37] Halogens, especially an excess of iodide in seafood, salt, and health foods, can exacerbate acne. In addition, halogens can provoke de novo acne lesions in individuals who have increased external exposure often due to occupational contact, or pool or hot tub disinfection; this variant is called *chloracne*.

In addition, certain minor ingredients in cosmetics have been implicated in cosmetic acne, including isopropyl myristate, cocoa butter, and fatty acids.

TREATMENT

The first step in determining a safe and efficacious treatment regimen for acne vulgaris is to establish desired outcomes for the patient, regarding both short- and long-term goals.

Desired Outcomes (Goals of Treatment)

4 Acne vulgaris is treated as a chronic disease, as it demonstrates typical chronicity characteristics: manifests as either acute outbreaks or slow onset; patterns of recurrence or relapse; a prolonged course; and psychologic and social impact. There are two governing principles: the chronic nature warrants early and aggressive treatment, and maintenance therapy is often needed for optimal outcomes.

Acne requires long-term control. This must be stressed with the patient to encourage adherence to lengthy treatment regimens, which address management of current symptoms and signs and preventive measures.

Basic goals of treatment include alleviation of symptoms by reducing the number and severity of lesions (objective and subjective grading) and improving appearance, slowing progression, limiting duration and recurrence, prevention of long-term disfigurement associated with scarring and hyperpigmentation, and avoidance of psychologic suffering.

A significant percentage change in lesion counts is desirable: most patients empirically validate a margin of 10% to 15% reduction in facial lesion counts as appropriate. Patient global self-assessment of acne improvement is a primary outcome.

General Approach to Treatment

5 The most critical treatment target is the microcomedone. Eliminating follicular occlusion will arrest the whole acne cascade. Nondrug and pharmacologic treatment and preventive measures should be directed toward cleansing, reducing triggers and combination therapy targeting all four pathogenic mechanisms. Combination therapy is often more effective than single therapy, and may decrease side effects and minimize resistance or tolerance to individual treatments.

The approach to acne management is largely determined by:

1. Severity index
2. Lesion type: predominantly noninflammatory or inflammatory
3. Treatment preferences including patient choices
4. Cost implications
5. Skin type and/or ethnic group
6. Patient age
7. Adherence
8. Response to previous therapy
9. Presence of scarring
10. Psychologic effects
11. Family history of persistent acne

Topical therapy is the standard of care for mild-to-moderate acne. Those with moderate-to-severe acne will require systemic therapy.

Topical treatments only work where applied. To reduce new lesion development, they require application to the whole affected area rather than individual spots. Most cause initial skin irritation, which may result in nonadherence or discontinuation. Irritation can be minimized by starting with lower strengths and gradually increasing frequency or dose. Where irritation persists, changing formulation from alcoholic solutions to washes, gels, or more moisturizing creams or lotions might help.

6 7 First-line, second-line, and third-line therapies should be selected and altered as appropriate for the severity and staging of the clinical presentation. Treatment is directed at control, not cure. Regimens should be tapered over time, adjusting to response. Combine the smallest number of agents at the lowest possible dosages to ensure efficacy, safety, avoidance of resistance, and patient adherence. Once control is achieved, simplify the regimen but continue with some suppressive therapy. As it takes 8 weeks for a microcomedone to mature, therapy must be continued beyond this duration to assess efficacy.[35] Most topical preparations may be used for years as needed.

Lesions typically recur for years. Microcomedones significantly decrease during therapy but rebound almost immediately after therapy is discontinued. The strategy for treating acne includes an induction phase followed by a maintenance phase, further supported by adjunctive treatments and/or cosmetic routines. Routine maintenance therapy involves regular use of appropriate agents to ensure remission and reduce potential for recurrence of visible lesions.

For successful long-term treatment, maintenance therapy must be tolerable, appropriate for the patient's lifestyle and convenient, continuing months to years, depending on age. Education about pathophysiology of acne and the psychosocial benefits of clearer skin are compelling reasons for patient adherence to consistent therapy to sustain remission.

Nonpharmacologic Therapy

8 9 Encourage patients with acne to discontinue or avoid aggravating factors, maintain a balanced, low-glycemic-load diet and control stress. Evidence shows that by being empathic and informative during counseling, the health professional may motivate the patient to continue long-term therapy.[8,9,32] One of the first approaches to nondrug management of acne is attention to cleansing techniques. Shaving recommendations, comedone extraction, dietary considerations, issues relating to ultraviolet light, and prevention of cosmetic acne should be reviewed with patients.

Cleansing

Cleansers are indicated in all patients with acne. However, washing too frequently in an attempt to remove surface oils is not likely helpful, as surface lipids do not affect acne. Contributory lipids are deep in the follicle and are not removed through washing. Antiseptic cleansers, while producing a clean, refreshed feeling, remove only surface dirt, oil, and aerobic bacteria. They do not affect *P. acnes*. Patients should wash no more than twice daily with a mild, nonfragranced opaque or glycerin soap or a soapless cleanser.

Soapless cleansers are an alternative to soaps.[38] Soaps are the most widely used cleansing products, but do not lend themselves to efficient delivery of active drug. Two main disadvantages exist. As soaps are rinsed off, the deposit of active agent is small, and the high pH required in soaps may degrade some active ingredients and be less tolerable on sensitive skin. Soaps produce a drying effect on the skin due to detergent action. As medicated cleansers require increased contact time, this drying action is pronounced, especially with peeling agents.

Cleansers often contain surfactant systems to remove fat from the skin surface. The oil is dispersed from the skin into the surfactant system; however, the active ingredient is sometimes trapped and removed upon rinsing. The balance between cleanliness and drying or irritation should also be taken into account. Most patients prefer products with foaming action, and these must contain additional secondary surfactants to enhance the foam and condition the skin.

There is no evidence that any particular washing regimen is superior. Evidence-based studies on the use of cleanser or medicated cleansers are lacking or poorly designed with small numbers of patients.[39] Avoid cream-based cleansers. Scrubbing should be minimized to prevent follicular rupture.

Because the acid pH of skin has an antimicrobial effect, it has been proposed that lowering lesional surface pH (with products such as Herpifix, marketed in Europe) may be correlated to the number of acne lesions. Studies are planned.

Synthetic polyester cleansing sponges abrade the skin surface, removing superficial debris. Considering the structure of comedones, they are unlikely to unseat these lesions. Sponges are available in soft or coarse textures, with or without soap. Circular or rubbing motions will increase irritation. Instruct patients to use single, gentle, continuous strokes on each side of the face, from the midline out toward the ears.

Cationic-bond strips are activated by water. As the strip dries, the cationic-bond binds the anionic dirt and oil in the pores and removes it when the strip is peeled off.

Shaving

Males should try electric and safety razors to determine which is more comfortable for shaving. When using a safety razor, the beard should be softened with soap and warm water or shaving gel. Shaving should be done as lightly and infrequently as possible, using a sharp blade and being careful to avoid nicking lesions. Strokes should be in the direction of hair growth, shaving each area only once.

Comedone Extraction

Comedone extraction has not been widely tested in clinical trials despite long-standing clinical use; however, it is painless and results in immediate cosmetic improvement. Pretreatment with a peeler for 4 to 6 weeks often facilitates the procedure.[36] Following cleansing with hot water, a comedone extractor is placed over the lesion and gentle pressure applied until the contents are expressed. This removes unsightly lesions, preventing progression to inflammation. A correctly sized extractor allows the central keratin plug to extrude through the opening. The small end of a plastic eye dropper, with bulb removed, may also be used. These instruments should be cleaned with alcohol after each use. Some initial reddening may be apparent. If the contents are not expressed with modest pressure, patients should not continue since improper extraction may further irritate the skin. A physician should be consulted if this technique is too difficult for the patient to manage. Since the follicle is difficult to remove completely, comedones may recur between 25 and 50 days following expression. Fewer than 10% of comedone extractions are a complete success, but the process is useful when done properly.[21]

Comedo removal may be helpful in the management of comedones resistant to other therapies. While the procedure cannot affect the clinical course of the disease, it can improve the patient's appearance, which may encourage adherence with the treatment program.

Ultraviolet Light

Although ultraviolet light was recommended in the past for desquamation, the practice is no longer advisable because of the well-established carcinogenic and photoaging effects of ultraviolet exposure. Moreover, inflamed skin is more susceptible to the damaging effects of ultraviolet light. Patients taking tretinoin may show heightened sensitivity.[40]

Before exposure to sunlight, patients with acne should apply sunscreens (sun protection factor [SPF] 15) in alcohol or oil-free bases and avoid using the acnegenic benzophenones. Sunscreen should be applied as the first product.

Prevention of Cosmetic Acne

Persistent low-grade acne is frequently caused by heavy cosmetic use in women after their mid-20s. Adolescent acne in younger women may be exacerbated with makeup overuse. The problem is perpetuated when resultant blemishes are concealed with more cosmetics.

Patients should be advised to discontinue oil-containing cosmetics and avoid cosmetic multistep regimens applying various cream-based cleansers and cover-ups. These are commercially advertised and often available with promotional bonuses through Internet shopping. Three-step basic systems usually combine medicated and nonmedicated ingredients. Their cosmetic names may not make apparent therapeutic agents are included. Initial steps usually involve cleansers, in lotions or creams, which may contain a multitude of unnecessary ingredients, including medicated peelers, oils, fragrances, and preservatives. Active ingredients including salicylic acid, sulfur, or benzoyl peroxide are often included in subtherapeutic or low doses. The second step is generally a water- or alcohol-based "toner" or "refresher" which might contain medicated mild comedolytic agents such as α-hydroxy acids (eg, glycolic acid), or even a humectant such as glycerin. The final product, often called intensive or repairing solutions, usually contains the lowest strength of peelers such as benzoyl peroxide, sulfur, or salicylic acid; plus potentially sensitizing fragrances and preservatives; or oil-soluble sunscreens not identified on the label. Bases may have significant oil content. There may be additional products such as masks or spot treatments that supplement the base routine of three steps. Multiple-step cosmetic programs are often costly, and should be avoided in favor of simple cleansers and more effective single-ingredient peelers at optimal concentrations.

The term *noncomedogenic* may refer to either water-based vehicles or products that are free of substances known to induce comedones. They are not necessarily oil-free. Water-based cosmetics may contain significant amounts of oil in the form of undiluted vegetable oils, lanolin, fatty acid esters (butyl stearate, isopropyl myristate), fatty acids (stearic acid), fatty acid alcohols, cocoa butter, coconut oil, red veterinary petrolatum, and sunscreens containing benzophenones. Water-based products are more likely to contribute to pore blockage than oil-free products.

Oil-free makeups are well-tolerated and lipstick, eye shadow, eyeliner, eyebrow pencils, and loose face powders are relatively innocuous. Heavier, oil-based preparations, particularly moisturizers and hairsprays, clog pores and accelerate comedone formation.[41]

Patients should restrict cosmetic use including makeup, moisturizers, or sunscreens to products labeled oil-free rather than water-based. Cover-up cosmetics for acne are available in several skin tones and in lotion and cream forms. They often contain peeling agents, antibacterial agents, or hydroquinone. Most contain sulfur. They may be applied as cosmetics two or three times daily, over the entire face or to individual lesions. Because the spread time of oil-free makeup is decreased, best results are achieved if applied to one-quarter of the face at a time. Topical medication should be applied after gentle cleansing and a foundation lotion may be used sparingly as a concealer.[42-44]

Because the action of most therapeutic acne agents is to dry the skin, the use of nonspecific moisturizers is counterproductive. Active agents, such as α-hydroxy acids (glycolic, lactic, pyruvic, and citric acids), may be present in a cosmetic formulation, since they reduce corneocyte adhesion.[45] Patients with acne should be restricted to oil-free α-hydroxy acid products unless absolutely necessary because of treatment with strong drying agents or isotretinoin.

Cosmetics, if correctly prescribed, may improve the performance of the therapy, whereas wrong procedures and/or inadequate cosmetics may worsen acne. Clinicians should make informed decisions about the role of various cosmetics and to identify the appropriate indications and precautions. The choice of the most effective product should take into consideration the ongoing pharmacologic therapy and acne type/severity as well.[46]

Vehicles

The formulation of an acne vehicle must consider the technical characteristics of maintaining and delivering the drug in an active state together with the need for an elegant product that the patient will enjoy using, so that it is more likely to be applied as required and deliver the full benefit. Physically and chemically, the vehicle will be used with one or more of the following goals: reduce excess oil, control bacteria associated with acne, reduce the effects of hyperkeratinization, and unclog pores. Performance, safety, and stability should be maximized while addressing technical and commercial factors.

Immiscible liquids might be delivered in oil-in-water or water-in-oil emulsions. In addition to having undesirable oil content, these vehicles also contain humectants, thickeners, preservatives, and fragrance, all of which may be problematic.

Solutions are simpler formulations. They are often used as the soaking liquid for fibrous cloth wipe products. The shelf-life depends upon whether multiple wipe packages are resealable, and whether the solvent volatility will affect storage, active agent availability or cause crystallization. Solutions are used mainly with topical antibiotics, which are often dissolved in specific types of alcohol. Although some antibiotics are only soluble in ethyl alcohol, isopropyl alcohol is generally better able to remove oil from the skin surface and is preferred for nonmedicated vehicles. Solutions and washes can be more easily applied to large areas such as the back.[47]

Non-greasy solutions, gels, lotions, and creams should be selected as bases for topical acne preparations. Lotions and creams will contain some oil-phase ingredients. Discourage moisturizers and oil-based products. Lotions are slightly less drying than gels, and creams are more emollient. Gels are very useful as they are mixtures of water or alcohol and totally oil free. Many gels contain ethanol or isopropyl alcohol. Propylene glycol is sometimes present in small amounts to add viscosity and lessen the drying effects of strong peeling agents. Gels are drying but may cause a burning irritation in some patients and may prevent certain kinds of cosmetics from adhering to the skin.[41] Propylene glycol gels are easy to apply and dry without a visible or sticky film. Nonalcoholic gels may be so effective and less drying than alcoholic solutions. Alcoholic or acetone gels are usually more drying and provide better penetration of the active ingredient.

Consider the patient's skin type and preferences in the choice of vehicle for topical agents. Patients with oily skin often prefer vehicles with higher proportions of alcohol (solutions and gels), while those with dry or sensitive skin prefer nonirritating lotions and creams. Hydrating and emollient products are often recommended to patients using drying treatment therapies, such as isotretinoin, to control adverse effects and improve adherence to treatment. Lotions can be used with any skin type and can be easily spread over hair-bearing skin, but will cause burning or dryness if they contain propylene glycol. Compatibility of vehicles and agents with cosmetics should also be considered.

The importance of vehicle effects in topical therapy has been demonstrated in placebo effect literature.[48] The percent contribution of vehicle (placebo) toward efficacy of reduction of lesions counts of eight commonly prescribed topical preparations at the end of 10 to 12 weeks of daily administration has been reported as a mean value of 55% (range 35%-82%).

How to Use Topical Preparations

Topical preparations should not be applied to individual lesions but to the whole area affected by acne to prevent new lesions from developing. Care should be advised in applying around the eyelid, mouth, and neck (to avoid chafing). Lotions should be applied with a cotton swab once or twice a day after washing or at bedtime if they leave a visible residue. Skincare products may cause skin dryness and redness particularly at the early stages of the treatment. Should this occur, the product should be applied more infrequently, the treatment should be stopped for a while or another topical product tried. To reduce irritation a topical vehicle with high water content may be applied over the medicinal product after a few minutes; the irritation usually subsides as the skin becomes accustomed to the topical skincare product.

Psychologic Approaches, Hypnosis, and Biofeedback

The psychologic effects of acne may be profound. The American Academy of Dermatology expert workgroup unanimously concluded that effective acne treatment can improve the emotional outlook of patients.[49] There is weak evidence of the possible benefit of biofeedback-assisted relaxation and cognitive imagery.[50,51]

Dressings

A pilot double-blind, randomized study of 20 patients has shown some benefit of treatment with a hydrocolloid acne dressing when compared with tape dressings for improving mild-to-moderate inflammatory acne vulgaris. Results showed greater reduction over 3 to 7 days in the overall severity of acne and inflammation, along with greater improvement in redness, oiliness, dark pigmentation, and sebum casual level. Less ultraviolet B light reaches the skin surface with the hydrocolloid dressing in place.[52,53]

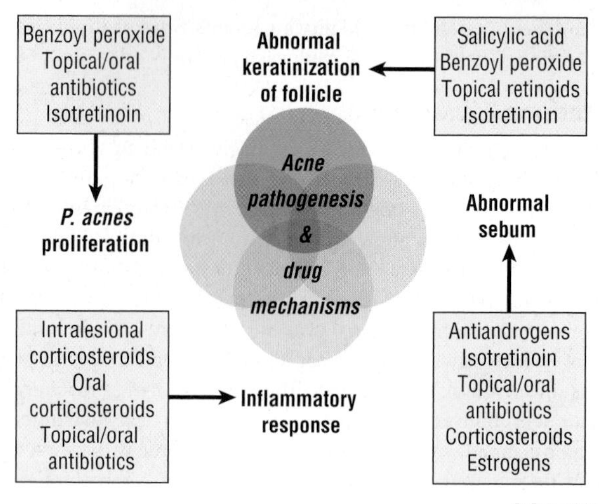

FIGURE 96-2 Acne pathogenesis and drug mechanisms.

Pharmacologic Therapy

Successful pharmacologic therapy must address one of the four mechanisms involved in the pathogenesis of acne. There are numerous agents available that prove one or more of these actions and are therefore effective (Table 96-2). However, the choice of active pharmacologic therapy depends on severity.

Mechanisms of drug action relating to acne pathogenesis are illustrated in Fig. 96-2.

Drug Treatments of First Choice

There is concordance among key opinion leaders in different settings regarding recommendations for drugs of choice for management of acne (the Global Alliance,[54] European Guidelines[14]).

For comedonal, noninflammatory acne, active agents of first choice include those that correct the defect in keratinization by producing exfoliation most efficaciously. Topical retinoids, in particular, adapalene, can be recommended as drugs of choice.[14,54] Benzoyl peroxide or azelaic acid can be considered, as alternatives (lower strength recommendation)[14,54] or a change could be made to an alternate topical retinoid. Limitations can apply that may necessitate the use of a treatment with a lower strength of recommendation as a first-line therapy (eg, financial resources and reimbursement limitations, legal restrictions, availability, drug licensing). Because the comedone is the initial lesion even in inflammatory acne, these agents are used to correct the defect in keratinization in all cases of acne.

For mild-to-moderate papulopustular inflammatory acne, it is important to reduce the population of *P. acnes* in the follicle and the generation of its extracellular products and inflammatory effects. Either the fixed-dose combination adapalene and benzoyl peroxide or the fixed-dose combination of clindamycin and benzoyl peroxide are strongly recommended as first choice therapy (high strength recommendation).[14,54] As alternatives, a different topical retinoid used with a different topical antimicrobial agent could be advised, with or without benzoyl peroxide. Azelaic acid or benzoyl peroxide can also be recommended (medium strength recommendation). In case of more widespread disease, a combination of a systemic antibiotic with adapalene can be recommended for the treatment of moderate papulopustular acne.

Low-strength recommendations are offered as considerations for treatment in the event of limitations that apply in selecting a first-choice agent. The choices would be blue light monotherapy, fixed-dose combination of erythromycin and tretinoin, fixed-dose combination of isotretinoin and erythromycin, or oral zinc. In case of more widespread disease, a combination of a systemic antibiotic with either benzoyl peroxide or with adapalene in fixed combination with benzoyl peroxide can be considered.[14]

For severe papulopustular or moderate nodular acne, oral isotretinoin monotherapy is strongly recommended as the drug of first choice (high strength recommendation). As alternatives, medium strength recommendations can be given for systemic antibiotics in combination with adapalene, with the fixed-dose combination of adapalene and benzoyl peroxide or in combination with azelaic acid.[14,54] In the event of limitations to use of these agents, considerations could be given to oral antiandrogens in combination with oral antibiotics or topical treatments, or systemic antibiotics in combination with benzoyl peroxide (low strength recommendation).

For nodular or conglobate acne, monotherapy with oral isotretinoin is strongly recommended as the drug of first choice (high strength recommendation).[14] As alternative agents, systemic antibiotics in combination with azelaic acid can be recommended (medium strength recommendation). If limitations exist to use of these agents, consideration could be given to oral antiandrogens in combination with oral antibiotics, systemic antibiotics in combination with adapalene, benzoyl peroxide, or the adapalene-benzoyl peroxide fixed-dose combination (low strength recommendation).[14]

For maintenance therapy for acne, the most recommended agents are topical retinoids. The most extensively studied maintenance treatment (four controlled trials) has been adapalene regimens.[14] Other published options include tazarotene or tretinoin. In general, maintenance therapy is begun after a 12-week induction and continues for 3 to 4 months. Continuing improvement using this schema is achieved, with relapse occurring when patients stop treatment, suggesting a longer duration of maintenance therapy is likely to be beneficial. Topical azelaic acid is an alternative to topical retinoids for acne maintenance therapy, with advantageous efficacy and safety profiles for long-term therapy. To minimize antibiotic resistance, long-term therapy with antibiotics is not recommended as an alternative to topical retinoids. If an antimicrobial effect is desired, the addition of benzoyl peroxide to topical retinoid therapy is preferred.

Published Guidelines

In general, recommendations should be based on critical appraisal and interpretation of the literature combined with clinical experience. There is considerable heterogeneity in the acne literature. The large number of products and product combinations, and the scarcity of comparative studies, has led to disparate opinions and few recommendations are evidence-based. Various evidence-based guidelines, available from multiple American, Canadian, European, Scandinavian, and South African sources from 2005 to 2015, do not provide concordance or clarity on all issues.

The 2012 European Guidelines for the Treatment of Acne focus primarily on major treatments, include use of light and laser therapy (see Clinical Controversy on Light Therapy box), but do not review general management issues such as psychologic determinants, scarring, diet, and so forth.[14] Where relevant, specific information from multiple sources will be integrated into the therapy section that follows.

Clinical **Controversy...**

Light Therapy

Increasingly, "diverse" light therapies (using various wavelengths) as convenient acne treatments with few[147] or temporary[148,149] adverse effects are reported. Conclusions based on outcomes with light therapy are contradictory.

Light therapies for acne are believed to work by killing *P. acnes* and by damaging and shrinking sebaceous glands, reducing sebum output. Light therapies may be used once or twice weekly as a course of 6 to 10 treatments, with each irradiation lasting 10 to 20 minutes.[149] *P. acnes* produce endogenous porphyrins that absorb light to form highly reactive singlet oxygen, which destroys the bacteria.[149] Since porphyrins have peak absorption at blue light wavelengths, blue light is often used to treat acne. Red light is also absorbed by porphyrins and can penetrate deeper into the skin,[150] where it may directly affect inflammatory mediators. Other light therapies attempt to selectively target and damage sebaceous glands directly, reducing their size and thus sebum output.[151] These include infrared lasers, low-energy pulsed dye lasers, and radiofrequency devices.[149]

Photodynamic therapy (PDT) uses specific light-activating creams, which are absorbed into the skin and amplify the response to light therapy but tend to produce more severe adverse effects. There are concerns that PDT may interfere with the skin's natural immune mechanisms[152,153] and cause long-term skin damage.

Previously, treatment was not available universally, but accessed privately via dermatologists or clinics, and expensive. Light therapies are increasingly popular among consumers and home-use blue light therapy is now available. Patients find it easier to comply with light treatments because of their short duration.

Medical science continues to debate whether light of different wavelengths is effective.[149] To date, very few trials compare light therapy with conventional acne treatments. The European evidence-based guidelines for the treatment of acne evaluated existing light therapies and concluded published evidence is still very scarce and standardized treatment protocols and widespread experience are still lacking. They were unable to make a recommendation for or against treatment of comedonal, MMPP or severe papulopustular/nodular acne with monotherapy visible light, visible or infrared wavelength lasers, or intense pulsed light or PDT, due to lack of or conflicting or insufficient evidence. Blue light has a low strength recommendation as a consideration for MMPP.[14]

An ongoing Cochrane review protocol continues to investigate the current state of evidence for use of light therapy in acne.[154]

In 2015, a summary report on light-based intervention therapies for acne rosacea was published.[155] In 106 studies, of 8-12 weeks, in 13,631 people age 40-50 with moderate to severe rosacea, there was low quality evidence for laser and intense pulsed light therapy. Laser therapy and intense pulsed light therapy were both effective for the treatment of telangiectasia, but only limited data was reported. Pulsed dye laser was more effective than yttrium-aluminium-garnet (Nd:YAG) laser based on one study, and it appeared to be as effective as intense pulsed light therapy (both low quality evidence).

An expert committee of the American Academy of Dermatology convened in 2007 to define guidelines for acne therapy and identify nine clinical questions to structure the primary issues in diagnosis and management (Table 96-1).[49] These guidelines address the management of adolescent and adult patients presenting with acne but not

TABLE 96-1 Guidelines for Managing Acne Vulgaris

Clinical Question Issues	Recommendation	Strength of Recommendation[a]	Level of Evidence[a]
I Systems for the grading and classification of acne	Use a grading/classification system	B	II
IIa Role of microbiologic testing	Do microbiologic testing	B	II
IIb Role of endocrinologic testing	Do endocrinologic testing	A	I
III Use of specific agents for topical therapy	Retinoids Benzoyl peroxide Antibiotics Other agents	A A A A	I I I I
IV Efficacy and safety of systemic antibiotics	Tetracyclines Macrolides Trimethoprim-sulfamethoxazole	A A A	I I I
V Efficacy and safety of hormonal agents	Contraceptive agents Spironolactone Antiandrogens Oral corticosteroids	A B B B	I II II II
VI Efficacy and safety of isotretinoin	Isotretinoin	A	I
VII Efficacy and safety of miscellaneous therapy	Intralesional steroids Chemical peels Comedo removal	C C C	III III III
VIII Efficacy and safety of complementary therapy	Herbal agents Psychologic approaches Hypnosis/biofeedback	B C B	I III II
IX Efficacy and safety of dietary restrictions[b]	Effect of diet	B	II

[a]An expert panel of the American Academy of Dermatology developed these clinical recommendations using the best available evidence. The panel rated evidence using the Strength of Recommendation Taxonomy (SORT), which uses this three-point scale:

I. Good quality patient-oriented evidence.

II. Limited quality patient-oriented evidence.

III. Other evidence including consensus guidelines, extrapolations from bench research, opinion, or case studies.

Similarly, recommendations were ranked as follows:

A. Recommendation based on consistent and good quality patient-oriented evidence.

B. Recommendation based on inconsistent or limited quality patient-oriented evidence.

C. Recommendation based on consensus, opinion, or case studies.

[b]See Clinical Controversy: Dietary Influences

Used with permission from Mills OH, Kligman AM. Comedogenicity of sunscreens. experimental observations in rabbits. Arch Dermatol *1982;18(6):417-419.*

the consequences of disease, including the scarring, postinflammatory erythema, or postinflammatory hyperpigmentation. The use of light and laser therapy was not addressed in the guidelines. In 2009, The Global Alliance to Improve Outcomes in Acne updated their 2003 recommendations to review new information about pathophysiology and treatment and included current published data on relevant issues. They provided seven summary statements, most of which are based primarily on expert opinion (level V evidence) because of a lack of studies or different designs and methodologies of existing studies (evidence from published studies constitute levels I to IV).[54]

The Alliance consensus statements were as follows:[54]

1. Acne should be approached as a chronic disease.
2. Strategies to limit antibiotic resistance are important in acne management.
3. Combination retinoid-based therapy is first-line therapy for acne.
4. More data are needed to define the role of laser and light therapy in acne.
5. Topical retinoids should be first-line agents in acne maintenance therapy.
6. Early, appropriate treatment is best to minimize potential for acne scars.
7. Assess adherence via verbal interview or use of a simple tool.

General Information Regarding Efficacy and Safety

The guidelines and recommendations of the American Academy of Dermatology considered the efficacy and safety of various treatments, such as topical agents, systemic antibacterial agents, hormonal agents, isotretinoin, miscellaneous therapies, complementary and alternative therapies, and dietary restriction, based on levels of evidence and best clinical practice.[49] More specific information about the efficacy and safety of each of these specific modalities is outlined below in sections on each individual agent.

Alternative Drug Treatments

Complementary and Alternative Medications People with acne often turn to complementary and alternative medicine (CAM), such as herbal medicine, acupuncture, and dietary modifications, because of their concerns about the adverse effects of conventional medicines. Although these products might be well tolerated, very limited data exist regarding their safety and efficacy.

A systematic review of CAM treatments for acne in 2006 identified 15 randomized controlled trials covering diverse approaches such as *Aloe vera*, pyridoxine, fruit-derived acids, kampo (Japanese herbal medicine), and ayurvedic herbal treatments.[55] Although mechanisms of potential benefit for some were biologically plausible, the included studies were of poor quality and inconclusive.

Another systematic review of seventeen traditional Chinese medicine randomized controlled trials found some benefit for acupuncture with moxibustion that was better than Western medicines, but the quality of included studies was limited.[55,56]

A review of studies published from 2007 to 2010 showed most studies were level of evidence grade D. Two studies of grade A concluded that topical tea tree oil 5% gel and gluconolactone are efficacious in mild-to-moderate acne, with the latter agent comparable with benzoyl peroxide 5%. No data supported these claims, and one study predated the review dimensions (published in 1992). Tea tree oil contains terpinen-4-ol, which appears to have some antimicrobial activity. One grade B study compared tea tree oil 5% against benzoyl peroxide 5% without placebo and concluded tea tree oil provided slower relief but less discomfort.[57]

A systematic review of four randomized controlled trials of tea tree oil in 2000 did not find conclusive evidence of benefit.[58] Tea tree oil continues to be studied for its efficacy and safety in acne.[59,60]

There is increasing interest in the use of CAM as adjuvant or single therapies: in America, 7% or people report using a complementary medicine, and 2% report seeing a complementary medicine practitioner.[61] Traditional Chinese medicine has been widely used to treat acne for many years, based on a diagnosis from a traditional Chinese medicine perspective according to the different syndromes of acne.

The Cochrane collaboration undertook a systematic review to assess the effectiveness and safety of any CAM in the management of acne vulgaris, reported in 2015.[60] This included 35 studies, with a total of 3,227 participants in parallel-group randomized controlled trials (or the first phase data of randomized cross-over trials) of any kind of CAM, compared with no treatment, placebo, or other active therapies, in people with a diagnosis of acne vulgaris. The primary outcome was improvement of clinical signs assessed through skin lesion counts. Some evidence from single studies showed low-glycemic load diet, tea tree oil, and pollen bee venom (PBV) may have an effect on reducing total skin lesion counts and acne severity scores. However, small sample sizes and poor methodological quality limited the strength of the evidence. Evidence from other existing randomized controlled trials does not support the use of herbal medicine, acupuncture, or wet-cupping therapy for the treatment of acne vulgaris. The evidence for a secondary outcome (number of participants with remission) for herbal medicine versus antibiotic was uncertain. Two trials reported QOL showed the benefit of herbal medicine compared with western drugs. The Cochrane review cautioned that there is a lack of evidence from the review of 31 studies to support the use of other CAMs, such as aloe vera, copaiba essential oil, dried fruit of Berberis vulgaris, or seaweed oligosaccharides for the treatment of this condition. Most studies were done in a traditional Chinese medicine context; therefore, results might be less generalizable to western medicine.

The review highlights potential adverse effects from herbal medicine (dizziness, dry mouth, nausea, diarrhea, or stomach upset); acupuncture (pain, itchiness, or redness) and tea tree oil gel (pruritus, dryness, burning sensations, and skin flaking).

The use of botanical preparations which are nonstandardized should be discouraged in favor of traditional quality-controlled preparations that have evidence of efficacy. The lack of appropriate data, absence of quality assessment, and inconsistencies in search methodology suggest that CAM cannot be recommended for acne therapy at this time.

Glycolic Acid Another agent considered as an alternative therapy for acne vulgaris is glycolic acid. The efficacy and tolerability of a 0.1% retinaldehyde/6% glycolic acid combination (Diacneal) has been evaluated for mild-to-moderate acne vulgaris.[62] Physician and patient ratings of acne symptom severity and tolerance performed at baseline and months 1, 2, and 3 showed mean numbers of papules, pustules, and comedones were significantly reduced from month 1 on, demonstrating that glycolic acid is effective and well tolerated in mild-to-moderate acne vulgaris.

Both glycolic acid-based, salicylic acid or salicylic acid derivative-based, (eg, lipohydroxyacid) and amino fruit acid-peeling preparations have been used in the treatment of acne. There is very little evidence from clinical trials published in peer-reviewed literature supporting the efficacy of peeling regimens.[49] Topical corneolytics, including retinaldehyde/glycolic acid or lactic acid, induce a comedolytic effect and may also facilitate skin absorption of topical drugs.[46] Further research on the use of peeling in the treatment of acne needs to be conducted to establish best practices for this modality.

Hydroquinone To control pigmentation, hydroquinone, which reversibly damages melanocytes, has been used as a hypopigmenting agent in concentrations of 2% to 4%, in preparations of clear or tinted gels, which are more drying, and as vanishing or opaque, flesh-tinted creams, with or without α-hydroxy acids or sunscreens. Hydroquinone causes fading of epidermal but not dermal pigmentation. Onset of response is usually 3 to 4 weeks, and the depigmentation lasts for 2 to 6 months but is reversible. While effective in the removal of melanin, hydroquinone has been clinically found to be a possible carcinogen and causes a blue-black discoloration known as ochronosis.[63]

After considering new data and information on the safety of hydroquinone, the U.S. Food and Drug Administration (FDA) issued a proposed ruling in 2006 about hydroquinone products. The FDA proposed reversing earlier rules that hydroquinone is generally recognized as safe and effective. The FDA has not yet issued a final ruling on the status of nonprescription hydroquinone, and many physicians consider a ban unnecessary, given the lack of convincing evidence of carcinogenic risk to humans and the rarity of ochronosis occurrence.

Treatment of Scarring Drug and nonmeasures for scar resolution are important in acne vulgaris because many patients are scarred despite adequate treatment. For patients with mild scarring, nonprescription α-hydroxy acids may be used, while severe scarring may be corrected with other treatment modalities that require consultation with a dermatologist. Dermabrasion, local or subcuticular excision, collagen implants, chemical peels (eg, 70% glycolic acid, trichloroacetic acid) and laser therapy have been used to improve scarring. Atrophic scars can be treated with laser resurfacing. Usually the scar is not completely removed, but a more cosmetically acceptable result is achieved. Keloids and hypertrophic scars can be treated with intralesional triamcinolone, cryotherapy, topical steroids, and silicone sheeting. Surgical options for scars include excision, augmentation with collagen or fat, chemical peels, subcision, and injection of autologous fibroblasts.

Special Populations

About 20% of young infants (2-3 months of age) develop papules, pustules, and less commonly closed or open comedones, primarily on the cheeks, due to placental transfer of maternal androgens (neonatal acne). The acne subsides within a few months with regular maturation. Boys are affected more often than girls because of a transient increase in testosterone secretion during the third and fourth month of intrauterine life. *Malassezia* spp. may be involved in pathogenesis.[21] Resolution occurs without therapy.[64] Infants with neonatal acne may have more severe teenage acne.[21]

The treatment of acne in children is similar to that in adults. Because topical therapies may be more irritating in children, initiation with low concentrations is preferred. Systemic treatments should be reserved for more extensive cases. Erythromycin is preferred over tetracyclines for children younger than 9 years of age because tetracyclines can affect growing cartilage and teeth.

Although treatment is with isotretinoin has numerous potential minor adverse effects in patients of all ages, an uncommon complication in young patients is premature epiphyseal closure. This generally occurs when isotretinoin is administered in high doses, thus limiting long-term therapy.

Selecting appropriate treatment in pregnant women can be challenging because many acne therapies are teratogenic; all topical and especially oral retinoids should be avoided. Oral therapies, such as tetracyclines and antiandrogens, are also contraindicated in pregnancy. Topical and oral treatment with erythromycin may be considered.

Acne in skin of color is an increasing problem, presenting unique challenges. Although combination therapy is now the standard of care in acne, concerns exist with the increased potential irritation and dryness in skin of color. Although individual medications can be titrated or applied at different times of day to avoid irritation, this is not always practical or desirable. There is a paucity of clinical studies that evaluate the safety and efficacy of acne medications in skin of color. One study has examined susceptibility to irritation in Fitzpatrick skin types I to III versus types IV to VI and found subjects with darker skin were not more susceptible and tolerability was comparable across the two groups. Hispanic subjects were not more susceptible to irritation compared with total study groups.[65]

Drug Class Information

This section reviews the pharmacology and mechanisms as related to pathophysiology for pharmacologic options recommended in the guidelines for mild, moderate, and severe acne. It will also review evidence of efficacy and safety as well as kinetics, interactions, dosing, and administration when relevant.

Exfoliants (Peeling Agents) Exfoliants induce continuous mild drying and peeling by primary irritation, damaging the superficial layers of the skin, and inciting inflammation. This stimulates mitosis, thickening the epidermis, and increasing horny cells, scaling, and erythema. A decrease in sweating results in a dry, less oily surface and may superficially resolve pustular lesions.

In the past, a rabbit model was used to study the efficacy of topical exfoliants in retarding tar-induced comedone formation and accelerating their loss (comedolysis). In this animal model, retinoic acid (tretinoin) was most active, compared with benzoyl peroxide and salicylic acid, which were respectively less active. Data from peer-reviewed literature regarding the efficacy of sulfur, resorcinol, sodium sulfacetamide, aluminum chloride, and zinc are limited. Traditional nonprescription exfoliants, including phenol, resorcinol, beta-naphthol, sulfur, Vleminckx solution, and sodium thiosulfate, are weak or ineffective. These agents are not comedolytic given that they affect the superficial epidermis rather than the hair canal. They have been supplanted by superior effective agents. Linoleic acid-rich phosphatidylcholine combined with 4% nicotinamide is suggested as an emulsion treatment that may be effective in normalization of follicular hyperkeratinization, and also provide anti-inflammatory effects.[66,67]

Resorcinol This phenol derivative is less keratolytic than salicylic acid. It is noted to be both bactericidal and fungicidal. Products containing resorcinol 1% to 2% have been used for acne, often in combination with other peeling agents such as sulfur or salicylic acid. The FDA considers resorcinol 2% and resorcinol monoacetate 3%, in combination with sulfur 3% to 8%, to be safe and effective and that the combination may enhance the activity of sulfur. However, the FDA is not convinced that resorcinol and resorcinol acetate are safe and effective when used as single ingredients, and has placed such products in category II (not generally recognized as safe and effective, or misbranded).[67]

Resorcinol is an irritant and sensitizer and should not be applied to large areas of the skin or on broken skin. It produces a reversible, dark brown scale on some dark-skinned individuals.

Protective packaging is important as resorcinol is reactive to light and oxygen. It has good solubility in both water and alcohol and is heat stabile Thus, it is incorporated into a variety of products, including emulsions.[68]

Salicylic Acid Salicylic acid, a β-hydroxy acid, has been used for many years for the treatment of acne, although few well-designed trials of its safety and efficacy exist. It is a natural ingredient in many plants such as willow tree or willow bark, and penetrates the pilosebaceous unit. It has comedolytic activity, although the concentrations in commercial preparations (<2%-3%) are generally low. While concentrations less than 2% may actually increase keratinization, concentrations between 3% and 6% are keratolytic, softening the horny layer and producing shedding of scales. Its mechanism remains unresolved, attributed to either reduced cohesion of corneocytes or shedding of epidermal cells, rather than breakdown of keratin.

Salicylic acid has no effect on the mitotic activity of normal epidermis and does not influence disordered cornification.[69] It may also provide mild antibacterial value, as it is active against *P. acnes*. It also offers slight anti-inflammatory activity at concentrations ranging from 0.5% to 5%. Its efficacy against comedones helps to prevent development of inflamed lesions, thus providing a delayed efficacy.[70]

Salicylic acid is effective. As a peeling agent, its relative strength compared with others in this class varies according to the model used in measurement. It is slightly *less* potent than equal-strength benzoyl peroxide when measured with the rabbit ear animal model, and slightly *more* potent when measured with a biologic microcomedone model.[70] Its anti-inflammatory properties may help dry ILs.[68] Its comedolytic properties are considered less potent than topical retinoids. It is often used when patients cannot tolerate a topical retinoid because of skin irritation.[71]

Its keratolytic effect may enhance the absorption of other agents. Salicylic acid is a mild irritant and may cause some degree of local skin peeling and discomfort (burning or reddening). It is not a sensitizer. Although the FDA recognizes salicylic acid as safe and effective, the compound offers no advantages over more modern topical agents such as benzoyl peroxide.[67,69,71]

Salicylic acid products are often used as first-line therapy for mild acne because of their widespread availability without a prescription. They are often available in alcohol–detergent impregnated pads as well as washes, bars, and semisolid vehicles. Lower concentrations are sometimes combined with sulfur to produce an additive keratolytic effect. Concentrations up to 5% to 10% can be used for acne, beginning with a low concentration and increasing as tolerance to the irritation develops. However, the maximum strength allowed in nonprescription acne products is 2%. In high concentrations of 20% to 30% in hydroethanolic vehicles, salicylic acid, either alone or in combination, can be used as a peeling agent for comedonal acne and hyperpigmentation. It has been shown to extrude closed and open comedones several days after peel, but it must be applied under strict control to offer this adjunctive benefit when treating acne vulgaris.[72]

Sulfur Sulfur medications often lessen the severity of acne, presumably because of keratolytic and antibacterial action. Sulfur helps to resolve comedones by an exfoliant action. Its popularity is due to its ability to quickly resolve pustules and papules, mask and conceal lesions (similar to a thick foundation lotion), and produce irritation leading to skin peeling and mild antibacterial action. Sulfur is used in the precipitated or colloidal form in concentrations of

2% to 10%, because it is practically insoluble in water and must be well dispersed. Its stability depends on effective maintenance of the dispersion.[68] Sulfur compounds (eg, sulfides, thioglycolates, sulfites, thiols, cysteines, and thioacetates) are also available and somewhat weaker. Sulfur can cause slight ophthalmic and dermatologic irritation, and patients should be cautioned to avoid eye contact. Use should be discontinued if excessive irritation results. Although it is often combined with salicylic acid or resorcinol to increase its effect, its use is limited by its offensive odor and the availability of more effective agents.[73]

Sulfur has met the criteria of the FDA Advisory Review Panel for nonprescription topical acne products and is considered safe and effective when used alone, although its antibacterial effects were not recognized by this panel. Sodium thiosulfate, zinc sulfate, and zinc sulfide were not considered safe and effective.

Topical Retinoids Normal epithelial cell differentiation is a vitamin A-dependent process, and currently, the most powerful peeling agents are related retinoid compounds. The effectiveness of topical retinoids in the treatment of acne is well documented. There is no consensus about the relative efficacy of currently available topical retinoids (tretinoin, adapalene, tazarotene) and oral isotretinoin. The rationale for the use of topical retinoids is based on their ability to target key stages in the development of the disease; the agents act by binding to specific nuclear receptors, reducing inflammation, and inhibiting sebocyte proliferation and differentiation, which reduces sebum production.

These agents act to reduce obstruction within the follicle and therefore are useful in the management of both comedonal and inflammatory acne. As a group, the retinoids are highly active peelers as they reverse abnormal keratinocyte desquamation.[74] They improve acne vulgaris by inhibiting microcomedone formation, diminishing the number of mature comedones and subsequently, ILs. They also normalize follicular epithelium maturation and desquamation. The third-generation retinoids (ie, adapalene and tazarotene) are receptor specific. Topical retinoids, unlike isotretinoin, do not decrease production of sebum, but primarily decrease inflammation, normalize keratinocyte differentiation, and increase keratinocyte proliferation and migration.[74]

Retinoids facilitate acne clearance through secondary effects of loosening and decreasing corneocytes. This increases skin permeability, facilitates absorption of other agents, such as antimicrobials or benzoyl peroxide, and increases penetration of oral antibiotics into the follicular canal. As a result, the overall duration of antibiotic treatment decreases, and the possibility of resistance lessens. Therefore, combination products with oral or topical antimicrobials are available for increased efficacy, faster onset of effects, decreased total antibiotic use and risk of resistance, and shorter duration of treatment.[74] Retinoids may also improve and prevent postinflammatory hyperpigmentation often seen in people with darker complexions who have acne.

Retinoic acid (vitamin A acid or tretinoin) is a powerful exfoliant that slows the desquamation process, reducing numbers of both microcomedones and comedones.[16] It is not to be used in pregnant women because of risk to the fetus. Gels and creams are less irritating than solutions.

Adapalene is a stable, fast-acting, antiacne treatment that has significant anti-inflammatory and comedolytic properties.[74-78] It causes epidermal and follicular epithelium hyperplasia, increased desquamation, keratinocyte differentiation, and loosening of corneocyte connections. Its anti-inflammatory effect is due to the inhibition of oxidative metabolism of arachidonic acid and inhibition of chemotactic reponses.[78] It is better at reducing ILs and total lesion count[78] and causes less local irritation because of its mechanisms and receptor specificity than tretinoin or tazarotene.[74-81] Release from lotions and hydroalcoholic gels is more effective than from creams and aqueous gels and a microsphere gel formulation may be less irritating.[74,80] It is a good first-line therapy for colder climates or in patients with sensitive skin.[63]

Adapalene is generally regarded as the topical retinoid of first choice for both treatment and maintenance therapy, as it is as effective but less irritating than other topical retinoids.[42,54] It is available in fixed-dose combinations in specialized gel vehicles with benzoyl peroxide to increase the efficacy in comparison with monotherapies. This strategy allows for the synergy of adapalene effects on normalizing desquamation with reduction of inflammation due to benzoyl peroxide action against *P. acnes*.

Tazarotene is also a specific agent with superior efficacy to parent retinoids, reducing both noninflammatory and ILs.[74] While its exact mechanism is unknown, it is thought to activate retinoid receptors and thereby affect keratinocyte differentiation, and inhibit proinflammatory transcription factors to decrease cell proliferation and inflammation.[74] It penetrates skin but accumulates in the upper dermis. It is as effective as adapalene in reducing noninflammatory and IL counts when applied half as frequently. Compared with tretinoin, it is as effective for comedonal and more effective for ILs when applied once daily.[82-84] Tazarotene foam, 0.1% has been studied as an alternative vehicle to the gel with less systemic absorption and is a safe and effective formulation.[85,86] Tazarotene is not degraded by sunlight.[16]

The retinoid class includes the systemic agent isotretinoin, which has effects on comedogenesis and sebum control, and is reviewed below under Anti-sebum Agents.

Retinoids tend to produce remissions that are maintained for extended periods of time, provided the accompanying irritation does not impede patient adherence. However, such adverse effects including erythema, xerosis, burning, and desquamation are issues for many patients. The concentration and/or vehicle of any particular retinoid may decrease tolerability.[75,76] Most retinoids are unstable and insoluble in water.

Topical retinoids are not teratogenic; however, tretinoin should be used cautiously in pregnancy and tazarotene is contraindicated. Tretinoin and adapalene are in FDA category C, while tazarotene, based on large-surface-area use in psoriasis (see Chapter 78), is in FDA category X.[21]

Skin type and age may influence tolerability in addition to choice of vehicle. Oily skin may be more resistant, and darker skin is more prone to postinflammatory hyperpigmentation due to retinoid dermatitis. To decrease irritation, start with the lowest concentration and increase as tolerated. Application of retinoids should be at night, a half hour after cleansing, starting with every other night for 1 to 2 weeks to adjust to irritation. Short contact time starting with 2 minutes and adding 30 seconds per dose can be advised for patients with sensitive skin or in the winter, discontinuing and resuming after a 3-day rest if undue irritation results. Doses can be increased only after beginning with 4 to 6 weeks of the lowest concentration and least irritating vehicle. Gels and creams are less irritating than solutions. Adapalene and tazarotene are photoirritants (not photosensitizers), and sun avoidance and sunscreen use are imperative.[74]

Overall, topical retinoids are the cornerstone of acne treatment and provide safe, effective, and economical means of treating all but the most severe cases of acne vulgaris. They should be the first step in moderate acne, alone or in combination with antibiotics and benzoyl peroxide, reverting to retinoids alone for maintenance once adequate results are achieved. Their lack of effect in inducing bacterial resistance enables long-term maintenance of remission.

A Cochrane systematic evidence-based assessment of all issues regarding acne treatment with topical retinoids is planned to establish optimal treatment regimens, compare efficacy and tolerability of combination therapy, assess effect on *P. acnes* resistance, and evaluate safety.[84]

Antibacterial Agents Choices for antibacterial therapy include benzoyl peroxide, prescription topical and systemic antibiotics, and combination products. These drugs kill *P. acnes* and inhibit the production of proinflammatory mediators by organisms that are not killed.[16]

Benzoyl Peroxide Benzoyl peroxide is a bactericidal agent that has proven effective in the treatment of acne. Because of concerns of resistance, it is often used in the management of patients treated with oral or topical antibiotics. It has the ability to prevent or eliminate the development of *P. acnes* resistance.

Benzoyl peroxide is a derivative of coal tar and was first used for acne vulgaris in the mid-1960s, becoming popular once stable formulations aimed at its heat-lability were developed in the mid-1970s.[79] These preparations are the single most useful group of topical nonprescription drugs. Used alone or in combination, benzoyl peroxide is the standard of care for mild-to-moderate papular-pustular acne.[14,54] It is an agent of first choice when combined with adapalene for most patients with mild-to-moderate inflammatory acne vulgaris and a second choice alternative for patients with non-inflammatory comedonal acne.[14,54] A systematic review of 22 trials using benzoyl peroxide for acne vulgaris provided evidence that it reduces acne-lesion count, although high quality evidence is not robust enough for firm conclusions.[87]

Benzoyl peroxide is well absorbed through the stratum corneum and concentrates in the pilosebaceous unit.[88] It has three principle actions useful in both noninflammatory and inflammatory acne. It produces powerful anaerobic antibacterial activity due to slow release of oxygen, thereby acting against gram-positive and gram-negative bacteria, yeasts, and fungi. This nonspecific antibacterial mechanism does not induce resistance with long-term use.[88] It has a rapid (within 2 hours) bactericidal effect that lasts at least 48 hours. As a result, it may decrease the number of inflamed lesions within 5 days. As an indirect effect, it induces suppression of sebum production; it does not reduce skin surface lipids, but is effective in reducing free fatty acids, which are comedogenic agents and triggers of inflammation.[88] Topical benzoyl peroxide 5% lowers free fatty acids 50% to 60% after daily application for 14 days, and decreases aerobic bacteria by 84% and anaerobic bacteria (primarily *P. acnes*) by 98%.

It also produces comedolysis. While earlier rabbit model studies showed a benzoyl peroxide effect greater than that of salicylic acid, these animal comedones were not physiologic but induced by tar. More recent studies using native microcomedones show an anti-comedogenic effect that is only comparatively slight, compared with tretinoin or salicylic acid.[89-91]

Finally, a supplementary benefit of benzoyl peroxide is an indirect anti-inflammatory action, which is due either to its antibacterial or oxidizing effects. This has been reported in several studies and thus can be used to support treatment of predominantly inflamed lesions.[88] The drug's antiacne effect is augmented by increased blood flow, dermal irritation, local anesthetic properties, and promotion of healing.[92-95] Because the primary effect of benzoyl peroxide is antibacterial, it is most effective for inflammatory acne. Many patients with noninflammatory comedonal acne will respond to its peeling action.

Benzoyl peroxide is available in a variety of preparations including gel, washes, lotions, and creams. There is no clear superiority of different preparations in terms of effectiveness. Newer delivery systems to enhance efficacy and tolerability are also being investigated.

Cleansers containing benzoyl peroxide are available as nonprescription liquid washes and solid bars of various strengths. The desquamative and antibacterial effectiveness in a soap or wash is minimized by limited contact time and removal with proper rinsing. Stable lotions are available in 2.5%, 5%, and 10%. Alcohol and acetone gels facilitate bioavailability and may be more effective, while water-based vehicles are less irritating and better tolerated. Paste vehicles are stiffer and more drying than ointments or creams, which facilitate absorption and allow the active ingredients to stay localized.

Concentrations of 2.5%, 5%, and 10% in a water-based gel have been compared with the vehicle alone. The 2.5% formulation is equivalent to the 5% and 10% formulation in reducing the number of ILs. The lower strength may not be as effective a peeler compared to higher strengths, which is due to an irritancy reaction. Thus, irritant side effects with the 2.5% gel are less frequent than with the 10% gel but are equivalent to the 5% gel. The lowest concentration of benzoyl peroxide should be used for treating patients with easily irritated skin and may lessen irritation when used in combination topical therapy with comedolytic agents.

Benzoyl peroxide may bleach hair, bedsheets, and clothing. It produces a mild primary irritant dermatitis that subsides with continued use and is more likely to occur in those with fair complexions, a tendency to irritancy, or propensity to sunburn. This irritation is dependent on the concentration and the vehicle, being higher with alcoholic gels compared with emulsion bases.[88] There are rare reports of contact allergic dermatitis. Cross-reactions with other sensitizers, notably Peruvian balsam and cinnamon, are well established. It may cross-sensitize to other benzoic acid derivatives such as topical anesthetics. Concomitant use of an abrasive cleanser may initiate or enhance sensitization.[96]

Another side effect is body odor from breakdown of the benzoyl peroxide that remains on clothing and bedsheets.

There is no indication that the normal use of benzoyl peroxide in the treatment of acne is associated with an increased risk of facial skin cancer. Although links have been made in experiments with mice, human relevance has not been established. The weak in vitro genotoxic potential is not manifested in vivo based on a lack of initiating or complete carcinogenic activity.[88] Overall, the cutaneous use of benzoyl peroxide is relatively safe, and is recognized by the FDA as category III, which means that more information is required to make a final determination of safety and efficacy for nonprescription use.[97-100] Safety is also confirmed by the American Academy of Dermatology and the German Best Guideline Acne (BGA) Monograph.[88]

Benzoyl peroxide has been used in combination with other antiacne medications, such as sulfur and chlorhydroxyquinoline, or in formulations with urea to facilitate drug delivery. No significant improvement has been demonstrated.

Benzoyl peroxide has also been combined with prescription agents to improve efficacy, reduce dosing strengths, decrease irritation, and reduce resistance of antibiotics.[101-104]

Benzoyl peroxide is often combined with topical retinoid for an antimicrobial effect or used in conjunction with an antimicrobial. It reduces the likelihood of antibiotic resistance. For long-term maintenance therapy, it is recommended as a highly efficient bactericidal agent to be added to a topical retinoid.[54]

The benefits in efficacy and tolerability of combining topical antibiotics with benzoyl peroxide over using either as monotherapy have been demonstrated in several trials, most in combination with clindamycin. Combination with erythromycin show advantages over oral tetracycline monotherapy.[105]

The adjunctive use of clindamycin/benzoyl peroxide gel with tazarotene cream promotes greater efficacy and may also enhance tolerability. Increased tolerability might be attributed to emollients in the clindamycin/benzoyl peroxide gel formulation.[106] A patented gel formulation of benzoyl peroxide 5%/clindamycin phosphate 1% (clindamycin) containing dimethicone and glycerin was studied both as a monotherapy and in combination with topical retinoid use. Certain additives, such as silicates and specific humectants, reduced irritation by maintaining barrier integrity.[107]

All single-agent preparations of benzoyl peroxide are now available without prescription. Recommend the weakest concentration (2.5%) in a water-based formulation, for anyone with a history of skin irritation, or who must use combination therapy.[107] There are many suggested routines to initiate therapy. One is to gently cleanse the skin and apply the preparation for 15 minutes the first evening, avoiding the eyes and mucous membranes. A mild stinging and reddening will appear. Each evening the time should be doubled until the product is left on for 4 hours and subsequently all night. Dryness and peeling will appear after a few days. Once tolerance is achieved, the strength may be increased to 5% or the base changed to the acetone or alcohol gels, or to paste. Alternatively, benzoyl peroxide can be applied for 2 hours for four nights, 4 hours for four nights, and then left on all night. It is important to wash the product off in the morning. Other drying agents should be discontinued. Patients with very sensitive skin or demonstrated sensitivity to benzoyl peroxide should not use the product, and it should be discontinued if irritation becomes severe upon use. Contact with eyes, lips, or mouth should be avoided.

A sunscreen is recommended if benzoyl peroxide is used. To avoid interactions, apply the sunscreen during the day and the benzoyl peroxide at night.

Comparison of Salicylic Acid and Benzoyl Peroxide Although both salicylic acid and benzoyl peroxide are used for mild-to-moderate acne, their mechanisms differ and therefore different types of acne respond to each. Benzoyl peroxide is a strong antibacterial agent, while salicylic acid acts primarily through keratolysis.

Studies have shown salicylic acid to be equal or slightly superior to benzoyl peroxide in reducing number of comedones and subsequently number of ILs. Any superiority salicylic acid demonstrates is likely because it interferes with an earlier step in pathogenesis—formation of the primary lesion of acne, the microcomedone.[69,71] However, studies of the compound did not use identical formulations. Instead, they compared salicylic acid cleansers to benzoyl peroxide washes and salicylic acid solutions to benzoyl peroxide creams. The effect of different bases is critical in determining differences in efficacy and therefore comparability of action since the base itself has an effect and influences penetration and duration of action.

In summary, the two products have similar efficacy, with salicylic acid noted as stronger in terms of retarding comedone formation. Benzoyl peroxide, as an antibacterial with some peeling effects, is considered the nonprescription and cosmetic gold standard for milder versions of the condition, used alone or in combination to increase efficacy and improve tolerability; however, salicylic acid is included in many of these products because of the perception of efficacy and safety for comedonal acne of type 1 or milder presentation.[70]

Topical Antibacterials The value of topical antibiotics in the treatment of acne has been investigated in many clinical trials. In addition to reduction of *P. acnes* as the primary mechanism for efficacy in acne, certain antibiotic drugs are also potent anti-inflammatory agents via other mechanisms.

Macrolides, including topical erythromycin and topical clindamycin, have been demonstrated to be effective and are well-tolerated, well-established acne treatments. However, they have become less effective since the early 1990s because of resistance by *P. acnes*.[108] Decreased sensitivity of *P. acnes* to these antibiotics can limit the use of either drug as a single therapeutic agent. Resistant strains are usually resistant to all of the macrolides. Addition of benzoyl peroxide or topical retinoids to the macrolide antibiotic regimen is more effective than monotherapy and mitigates against survival of resistant *P. acnes* populations.

Clindamycin is the preferred macrolide because of potent action, lack of absorption, and its limited systemic use because it can cause pseudomembranous colitis when given orally or by injection. It is available as a single ingredient topical preparation and can also be combined with benzoyl peroxide. A topical fixed-dose clindamycin phosphate 12% and benzoyl peroxide 30% combination gel once daily was more effective and twice daily at least as effective as clindamycin alone twice daily, with an early onset of action and an acceptable safety and tolerability profile.[109] Erythromycin is available alone and in combination with retinoic acid or benzoyl peroxide. Some topical antibiotic–benzoyl peroxide combinations require refrigeration.[49] Other topical antibiotics that are being studied include fluoroquinolones, such as 1% nadifloxacin cream, but are not available in the American market. Research approaches for developing new antibiotics against *P. acnes* include combining ribosomal effects of aminoglycosides molecules with bacteria-selective membrane-permeabilizing abilities in one drug.[110]

Oral Antibacterials Systemic antibiotics are a standard of care in the management of moderate and severe acne and treatment-resistant forms of inflammatory acne. There is evidence to support the use of tetracycline, doxycycline, minocycline, erythromycin, trimethoprim–sulfamethoxazole, trimethoprim, and azithromycin. Studies do not exist for the use of ampicillin, amoxicillin, or cephalexin. However, any antibiotic that can reduce the *P. acnes* population in vivo and interfere with the organism's ability to generate inflammatory agents should be effective.[49] Although erythromycin is effective, use should be limited to those who cannot use one of the tetracyclines (ie, pregnant women or children under 8 years of age because of the potential for damage to the skeleton or teeth). Ciprofloxacin, trimethoprim-sulfamethoxazole, and trimethoprim alone are also effective in instances where other antibiotics cannot be used or for patients who do not respond to conventional treatment.[67,111] A comparison of azithromycin with doxycycline reported doxycycline is a better option for treatment of acne vulgaris.[112]

The tetracycline antibiotic family has multiple modes of action, well-understood antibacterial effects, and anti-inflammatory effects that target an additional aspect of pathogenesis.[108,111,113] Agents, such as tetracycline, minocycline, and doxycycline, are used only as systemic agents. Through calcium chelation, they inhibit neutrophil and monocyte chemotaxis. Concentrations below the antibiotic threshold still inhibit inflammation, and improve both acne vulgaris and acne rosacea.

Tetracycline is no longer the drug of choice in this family; its disadvantages include diet-related effects on absorption and the drug's lower anti-inflammatory and antibacterial activity.

The incidence of significant adverse effects with oral antibiotic use is low. However, adverse effect profiles may be helpful for each systemic antibiotic used in the treatment of acne. Vaginal candidiasis may complicate the use of all oral antibiotics.[49] Doxycycline is very commonly a photosensitizer especially at higher doses.

Minocycline has been associated with pigment deposition in the skin, mucous membranes, and teeth, particularly among patients receiving long-term therapy and/or higher doses of the medication. In some cases this is irreversible. Pigmentation occurs most often in acne scars, anterior shins, and mucous membranes. Minocycline may cause dose-related dizziness, which resolves with dose titration; urticaria; hypersensitivity syndrome, autoimmune hepatitis, a systemic lupus erythematosus-like syndrome; and serum sickness-like reactions.[49,108]

The Cochrane collaboration has conducted a review into the efficacy and safety of minocycline, examining 39 randomized controlled trials. These studies show that minocycline is an effective treatment for moderate to severe inflammatory acne but present no evidence to support the first-line use of minocycline in acne treatment. The drug is more lipophilic, may act more quickly, and can be taken once daily. However, people treated with minocycline are at a significantly greater risk of developing an autoimmune syndrome than those given tetracycline or no treatment.[114]

The majority of oral antibiotic course durations follow guidelines. Costs of antibiotic therapy are reported lower for shorter courses and those using generic medications.[115]

Bacterial resistance to antibiotics is an increasing problem particularly because therapy is directed at control over a long period of time.[108] The development of strains with unidentified mutations suggest new mechanisms of resistance are evolving. Combined resistance to clindamycin and erythromycin is much more common than resistance to tetracycline.[14] Use of topical antibiotics can lead to resistance largely confined to the skin of treated sites, whereas oral antibiotics can lead to resistance in commensal flora at all body sites. Resistance is more common in patients with moderate-to-severe acne and in countries with high outpatient antibiotic sales. Resistance is disseminated primarily by person-to-person contact, and thus the spread occurs frequently.

There have been an increasing number of reports of systemic infections caused by resistant *P. acnes* in non-acne patients after surgery. A transmission of factors conferring resistance to bacteria other than *P. acnes* has been described.

The most likely effect of resistance is to reduce the clinical efficacy of antibiotic-based treatment regimens to a level below that in patients with fully susceptible flora. This has been shown as a decreased clinical efficacy of topical erythromycin in clinical trials; there is no evidence to date of this effect in treatments with oral tetracycline or topical clindamycin.

Studies on *P. acnes* resistance have highlighted the need for treatment guidelines to restrict the use of antibiotics to limit the emergence of resistant strains. Patients with less severe forms of acne should not be treated with oral antibiotics, and where possible such therapy should be limited to the shortest feasible duration (eg, 6-8 weeks). Local patterns of resistance should be considered.[105] The use of systemic antibiotics should be limited (both indication and duration) and topical antibiotic monotherapy should be avoided.

There should be early use of combination therapy with retinoids. Often, when oral antibiotics are combined with topical agents, the antibiotic may be discontinued after 6 months of therapy.[116] Nearly 70% of patients with acne require antibiotics for 12 weeks or less if aggressive retinoid therapy is used during that time.[108]

Another potential strategy that had been suggested is to eliminate the use of antibiotics and combine other topical agents. Neither retinoids nor benzoyl peroxide creates selective pressure for resistance and is one combination option. Although this approach has been evaluated for efficacy and safety, there is limited evidence of its effect on microbial resistance. In one open label study of adapalene and benzoyl peroxide, baseline counts of antibiotic resistant strains of *P. acnes* were reduced by week 4.[54,105]

The high sensitivity of *P. acnes* to acidified nitrite suggests a useful role in the treatment of antibiotic resistant acne. Nitric oxide and its intermediates diffuse as well as oxygen, and would be expected to penetrate the ILs well. The newly developed topical nitric oxide-releasing agent holds potential in limiting antibiotic resistance.[117] Further work to optimize the pharmacokinetic delivery of nitric oxide releasers could increase bactericidal effectiveness.[118]

Stricter cross-infection control measures are recommended when assessing acne. Any topical or systemic antibiotic therapy should be combined when possible with broad-spectrum antibacterial agents such as benzoyl peroxide. In addition, isotretinoin use should be initiated earlier in indicated patients, rather than prolonging antibiotic courses.[14]

Azelaic Acid Azelaic acid possesses activity against all four pathogenic factors that produce acne. It has anti-inflammatory and antibacterial activities. Azelaic acid also normalizes keratinization, which accounts for its anticomedogenic effect. It is a competitive inhibitor of mitochondrial oxidoreductases and of 5-α-reductase, inhibiting the conversion of testosterone to 5-dehydrotestosterone. It also possesses bacteriostatic activity to both aerobic and anaerobic bacteria including *P. acnes*. Azelaic acid is an antikeratinizing agent, displaying antiproliferative cytostatic effects on keratinocytes and modulating the early and terminal phases of epidermal differentiation.[119] It may produce hypopigmentation. Inhibition of thioredoxin reductase by azelaic acid provides a rationale for its depigmenting property.

Azelaic acid 20% cream is used in the treatment of mild-to-moderate inflammatory acne, has an excellent safety profile with minimal adverse effects, and is well-tolerated in comparison with other acne treatments. The most common adverse effects, occurring in approximately 1% to 5% of patients, are pruritus, burning, stinging, and tingling. Adverse reactions are generally transient and mild in nature. Other adverse reactions, such as erythema, dryness, rash, peeling, irritation, dermatitis, and contact dermatitis, have been reported in less than 1% of patients.[119]

Azelaic acid has been shown effective in clinical trials studied with topical 2% erythromycin, topical 5% benzoyl peroxide gel, and topical 0.05% tretinoin cream in the treatment of mild-to-moderate inflammatory acne. However, the agent has limited efficacy, compared with other antiacne therapies.[49] It is an alternative to first choice therapy for comedonal and all types inflammatory acne, particularly in combination.[14] It is an alternative to topical retinoids for maintenance therapy as its efficacy and safety profile are advantageous for long-term therapy.[14]

Azelaic acid should be applied twice a day, in the morning and evening. A majority of patients with ILs may experience an improvement in their acne within 4 weeks of beginning treatment. However, treatment may be continued over several months, if necessary.

Azelaic acid is in a pregnancy category B and should only be used in pregnant women if medically necessary. Patients with dark complexions should be monitored for early signs of hypopigmentation.

Dapsone Topical dapsone 5%, a synthetic sulfone, is a recently introduced treatment for acne available as a topical gel. Sulfones have both anti-inflammatory and antibacterial properties, and may be used in sulfonamide-allergic patients.

Dapsone's utility is attributable to its anti-inflammatory and antimicrobial properties that improve both inflammatory and non-inflammatory acne, with more prominent effects occurring in ILs. Short- and long-term safety and efficacy have been demonstrated.[120,121]

Topical dapsone gel 5% was shown to be safe, minimally irritating, and effective after 12 weeks in the treatment of mild-to-moderate inflammatory facial acne in 101 adult women with sensitive skin.[122] The response to dapsone 5% gel appears to be influenced by gender, with female patients experiencing a significantly greater reduction in acne lesion counts and a significantly higher clinical success rate following 12 weeks of treatment.[123]

Topical dapsone is a novel addition to the treatment armamentarium, especially for patients exhibiting sensitivities or intolerance to conventional antiacne agents.[124]

Topical dapsone 5%, alone or in combination, with adapalene 0.1% or benzoyl peroxide 4% has been shown to be safe and efficacious, but may be more irritating than other topical agents.[125,126]

Intralesional Steroids Intralesional corticosteroid injections are effective in the treatment of individual inflammatory acne nodules. The effect of intralesional injection with corticosteroids is a well-established and recognized treatment for large ILs. Cystic acne improved in patients receiving intralesional steroids.[49]

Systemic absorption of steroids may occur with intralesional injections. Adrenal suppression was observed in one study. The injection of intralesional steroids may be associated with local atrophy. Lowering the concentration and/or volume of steroid may minimize these complications.

Anti-sebum Agents No topical agents directly influence the production of sebum. Systemic drugs that influence sebum production include high-dose estrogens, antiandrogens (cyproterone acetate), spironolactone, and the retinoid isotretinoin. Antioxidants, such as sodium l-ascorbyl-2-phosphate 5%, may act to prevent the oxidation of sebum and studies are in preliminary stages.

Oral antiandrogens, such as spironolactone and cyproterone acetate, can also be useful in the treatment of acne. While flutamide can be effective, hepatotoxicity limits its use. There is no evidence to support the use of finasteride. There are limited data to support the effectiveness of oral corticosteroids in the treatment of acne. Oral corticosteroid therapy is of temporary benefit in patients who have severe inflammatory acne. In patients who have well-documented adrenal hyperandrogenism, low-dose oral corticosteroids may be useful in treatment of acne.[49]

Oral Contraceptives Estrogen-containing oral contraceptives can be useful in the treatment of acne in some women. Those currently approved by the FDA for the management of acne contain norgestimate with ethinyl estradiol and norethindrone acetate with ethinyl estradiol. There is good evidence and consensus opinion that other estrogen-containing oral contraceptives are also equally effective.[49]

The Cochrane collaboration conducted a review in 2012 to determine the effectiveness of combination oral contraceptives (COCs) for the treatment of facial acne compared with placebo or other active therapies. Thirty-one trials with a total of 12,579 women were reviewed.[126]

Combination oral contraceptive use reduced inflammatory and noninflammatory facial lesion counts, severity grades, and self-assessed acne in nine placebo comparison trials, according to the review. Progestins included levonorgestrel, norethindrone acetate, norgestimate, drospirenone, dienogest, and chlormadinone acetate. There were fewer clear differences in trials that compared varying progestin types, showing no superiority, little differences, or conflicting results. No conclusions could be reached regarding the effect of a COC compared with an antibiotic because there was only one underpowered trial.[126]

Most studies assessed women over six treatment cycles, which might not be adequate for a chronic condition like acne. In two trials, patients were more likely to discontinue because of adverse events. Thus even if COCs improve acne, women might not be willing to accept long-term use for acne because of other side effects.

The review concluded that COCs should be considered for women with acne who also want an oral contraceptive.

A meta-analysis review of 32 randomized controlled trials comparing use of antibiotics to oral contraceptive agents for acne compared with placebo, concluded that although antibiotics may be superior at 3 months, oral contraceptive agents are equivalent to antibiotics at 6 months in reducing acne lesions and, may be a better first-line alternative to systemic antibiotics for long-term acne management in women.[127]

There is a need for more research into comparative effectiveness of COCs in randomized control trials, and into the acceptability and need for long-term use of COCs for acne.[126]

Spironolactone At higher doses, spironolactone is an antiandrogenic compound. Dosages of 50 mg to 200 mg have been shown to be effective in acne. Spironolactone may cause hyperkalemia, particularly when higher doses are prescribed or when there is cardiac or renal compromise. It occasionally causes menstrual irregularity. A 5% spironolactone gel, studied in patients with increased sebum secretion, resulted in a decrease in the total acne lesions with no significant efficacy under the acne severity index.[128]

Cyproterone Acetate Cyproterone combined with ethinyl estradiol (in the form of an oral contraceptive) has been found effective in the treatment of acne in females. Higher doses have been found more effective than lower doses. No cyproterone/estrogen-containing oral contraceptives are approved for use in the United States.[126]

Oral Corticosteroids Oral corticosteroids have two potential modes of activity in the treatment of acne. One study demonstrated that low-dose corticosteroids suppress adrenal activity in patients who have proven adrenal hyperactivity.[129] Expert opinion is that short courses of higher dose oral corticosteroids may be beneficial in patients with highly inflammatory disease.

Oral Isotretinoin Isotretinoin revolutionized the treatment of acne, yet its use and availability are increasingly complex. The risk of potential adverse effects must be weighed against its ability to prevent lifelong and permanent physical and psychologic scarring.[130]

A good understanding of this agent's mechanisms and adverse effects is important. Oral isotretinoin is a natural metabolite of vitamin A. Its mechanism is elusive, as it does not bind to retinoid receptors. It has been shown to reduce sebogenesis and may also inhibit sebaceous gland activity, growth of *P. acnes*, inflammation, and improve follicular epithelial differentiation.[131] Systemic isotretinoin exerts a primary effect on comedogenesis, causing a decrease in size and reduction in formation of new comedones.[16] Isotretinoin is the only drug treatment for acne that produces prolonged remission.

Oral isotretinoin is approved for the treatment of severe recalcitrant nodular acne. Oral isotretinoin is also useful for the management of less severe acne that is treatment-resistant (unresponsive to adequate treatment, reasonable courses of antibiotic, or combination peelers and antibiotics administered for 6 weeks to 3 months) or that is producing either physical or psychologic scarring.[49]

The teratogenic effects of oral retinoid therapy are well documented. Because of its teratogenicity and the potential for many other adverse effects, this drug should be prescribed only by those physicians knowledgeable in its appropriate administration and monitoring. Female patients of child-bearing potential must only be treated with oral isotretinoin if they are participating in the approved pregnancy prevention and management program (ie, iPLEDGE). Two different forms of contraception must be started 1 month before and continue at least 1 month (but normally 4 months) after therapy and pregnancy monitoring undertaken before, during, and after therapy.[130]

The efficacy of conventional isotretinoin treatment (0.5-1.0 mg/kg/day for 16-32 weeks, reaching a cumulative dose of 120 mg/kg) for acne has been well established. The approved dosage of isotretinoin is 0.5 to 2.0 mg/kg/day. The drug is usually given over a 20-week course.

Initial flaring can be minimized with a beginning isotretinoin dose of 0.5 mg/kg/day or less. There are many reports regarding the efficacy of low-dose and intermittent isotretinoin treatment. Lower doses can be used for longer time periods, with a total cumulative dose of 120 to 150 mg/kg or the dose can be lowered to 20 mg on alternate days after an initial 2 months of therapy with higher dosage.[132-134] Reports suggest that low-dose regimens are superior to other regimens (conventional or intermittent) in terms of patient satisfaction, tolerability, and efficacy for patients with moderate acne. In patients with severely inflamed acne, an even greater initial dose reduction may be required. In the most severe cases of acne, consideration of pretreatment with oral corticosteroids may also be appropriate. Some patients experience a relapse of acne after the first course of treatment with isotretinoin. Relapses are more common in younger adults or when lower doses are used.

Drug absorption is greater when the drug is taken with food. One novel formulation is less dependent on the presence of fat in the gut for absorption.[135] When used, drying agents must be discontinued and replaced with moisturizers.

Because isotretinoin is a vitamin A derivative, it interacts with many of the biologic systems of the body, and consequently has a significant pattern of adverse effects. The pattern is similar to that seen in hypervitaminosis A. Side effects include those of the mucocutaneous (most common), musculoskeletal, and ophthalmic systems, as well as headaches and central nervous system effects. Most of the adverse effects, such as cheilitis, and dry nose, eyes, and mouth, are temporary and resolve after the drug is discontinued.[130] Laboratory monitoring during therapy should include triglycerides, cholesterol, transaminases, and complete blood counts.

Mood disorders, depression, suicidal ideation, and suicides have been reported sporadically in patients taking this drug. A causal relationship has not been established. These symptoms are quite common in adolescents and young adults, the age range of patients who are likely to receive isotretinoin. This issue and other key unresolved considerations regarding isotretinoin continue to be the subject of investigations and are discussed as a Clinical Controversy in this chapter.

Clinical **Controversy...**

Accutane Considerations

After almost three decades of experience with oral isotretinoin, the published data and opinion of experts still differ with respect to its use as first-line or reserve therapy, optimal dosing, and risk of depression. The 2012 European Guidelines for the treatment of acne noted conflicting viewpoints from major opinion leaders.[14] It is important to put into perspective issues surround its responsible and informed use.[130]

Some directives persist in reserving isotretinoin use only for severe acne, nodular or conglobate acne that has not responded to appropriate antibiotics and topical therapy.[156] For many reasons, other experts recommend that isotretinoin should be considered the first-choice therapy for severe acne, given its clinical effectiveness, prevention of scarring, and quick improvement of a patient's QOL, including minimizing depression. This position suggesting delaying the use of oral isotretinoin, the most effective choice, poses an ethical problem. Although comparative trials are missing, clinical experience confirms relapse rates after isotretinoin treatment are the lowest among available therapies.[14,157,158]

Evidence on best dosage, including cumulative dosage, is rare and partly conflicting for isotretinoin. In most trials, the higher doses associated with better response rates have less favorable safety/tolerability profiles. Attempts to determine the cumulative dose necessary to obtain an optimal treatment response and low relapse rate have not yet yielded sufficient evidence for a strong recommendation. Current expert opinion recommends for severe cases, a starting dosage of 0.3 to 0.5 mg/kg daily and for conglobate acne, a dose of 0.5 mg/kg daily or higher. Duration of therapy should be until a recommended cumulative dose of 120 mg/kg is reached, or at least 6 months. For insufficient response, prolong treatment. Opinions vary on whether or not to restrict use to patients under 12 years and whether to avoid lasers, peelers or wax epilation for at least 6 months after discontinuation of therapy.[14,159]

The causal relationship between the use of isotretinoin and risk of depression continues to be scrutinized with no consensus. The issue is complex as depression and suicidal ideation occur with severe acne in the absence of isotretinoin.

There are instances in which withdrawal of isotretinoin has resulted in improved mood, and reintroduction of isotretinoin has resulted in the return of mood changes. Treatment of severe acne with isotretinoin is often associated with mood improvement.[49] There is epidemiologic evidence that the incidence of these events is less in patients treated with isotretinoin than in an age-matched general population. There is also evidence that the risk of depressed mood is no greater during isotretinoin therapy than during therapy of an age-matched acne group treated with conservative therapy.[49]

A systematic review published in 2005 did not find any evidence to support worsening of depression after use, and some depressive scores improved with use, but nine of these studies had limitations.[160] A retrospective cohort study in Sweden found attempted suicide increased in users, but an increased risk was present before treatment. An increased risk of attempted suicide was present 6 months after isotretinoin, suggesting patients should be monitored for suicidal behavior after treatment discontinuation.[161]

The current literature is insufficient to support a meaningful causative association, but important study limitations exist. In the absence of definitive evidence, an idiosyncratic effect cannot be excluded. Prescribers of isotretinoin are advised to note prior psychiatric symptoms, monitor patients at each visit for early recognition, and advise patients about a possible risk of depression and suicidal behavior.[14,160,161]

This disputed association remains an important area for future research.

Pharmacologic Cleansing Options

Medicated Soaps and Washes Medicated soaps, washes, and foams may contain topical antiseptics such as triclosan; peeling agents such as salicylic acid, sulfur; antimicrobials such as benzoyl peroxide, clindamycin, or azelaic acid, alone or in combination in low concentrations. They may be nonprescription or prescription status.[136] Most washes should remain on the skin from 15 seconds to 5 minutes followed by thorough rinsing. This limits the amount of time the active ingredient is in contact with the skin. Other cleansers are applied after washing and left on the skin without rinsing.

Quaternary ammonium compounds are cationic detergents that are inactivated quickly in the presence of organic material such as sebum. The duration of action of these products is short.

Bacteriostatic soaps, such as hexachlorophene, carbanilides, and salicylanilides (halogenated hydroxyphenols), may alter normal flora or be acnegenic. Few ordinary soaps induce acne. However, acne patients are particularly susceptible to comedogenic contactants, and if these soaps are applied several times daily for long periods, they may become troublesome.

Soaps containing coal tar, which can induce folliculitis, are not indicated for acne.

In a very small group of patients in an 8-week, double-blind, randomized clinical trial, a combination cleanser containing triclosan, azelaic acid, and salicylic acid produced a greater histopathologic decrease in inflammatory response compared with a nonmedicated cleanser, but there was no significant difference in NILs in either group.[136] A rebound tendency was noted for the nonmedicated cleanser with respect to ILs at 4 weeks. Authors concluded that nonmedicated cleansers were an easier and cheaper way of managing patients with mild acne.

Chlorhexidine inhibits in vitro growth of *P. acnes*.[137] A 4% chlorhexidine gluconate preparation in a detergent base has been shown to be as effective as benzoyl peroxide washes in patients with mild acne, and both preparations reduced the number of inflammatory and NILs after 8 and 12 weeks, compared with vehicle alone.[138]

Alcohol-detergent medicated pads, impregnated with salicylic acid 0.5%, have reduced ILs and open comedones in mild-to-moderate acne. This type of medication is less abrasive, not rinsed off, and convenient.[139]

Alcohol-detergent wipes, swabs, or "pledgets" impregnated with antibiotics, such as clindamycin or lincomycin, are available. The antibiotic is deposited in low concentrations on the surface of the skin, and may not penetrate to the depths of the pilosebaceous duct. Although patients may like the convenience and perception of using an active agent, they should not be recommended over simple cleansing.

Abrasives consist of finely divided particles of fused aluminum or plastic together with cleansing and wetting agents. Abrasives peel and remove surface debris and may assist resorption of papules and pustules. Despite vigorous rubbing, removal of comedones is not accomplished. Particles containing active agents, such as sodium tetraborate decahydrate, dissolve on use, and their abrasiveness is therefore limited.[139] The effectiveness of an abrasive cleanser with and without polyethylene granules showed no difference in results in patients with mild-to-moderate acne. These products are not indicated in most cases but may be used in a patient who responds empirically.[140]

Personalized Pharmacotherapy

The individualized treatment of certain patient groups, including infants, children, pregnant women, and persons of color, is described under Special Populations.

Providers and patients must also weigh costs and drug availability in choosing a treatment regimen. One study showed that the average total cost of treatment per episode across all age groups is US $689.06.[141] Topical retinoids and fixed-dose combination therapies are in general more expensive than benzoyl peroxide preparations. A retrospective analysis investigated adherence to oral antibiotic guideline recommendations and opportunities for cost-savings. Of 17,448 courses, 84.5% aligned with duration guidelines, although 69.0% of courses did not include concomitant topical retinoid therapy. Costs of antibiotic therapy were lower for shorter courses and those using generic medications. Mean savings of $592.26 per person could result if prolonged courses met guidelines.[142]

Laser treatments and cosmetic procedures are also very costly. The economics of long-term maintenance therapy should be borne in mind when selecting a regimen. Patients should not spend large amounts on herbals and botanicals, as well as home remedies, given the lack of current good evidence to support their use. As acne is a chronic disease extending over many years, total cost implications are important and affect adherence and response.

Other practical considerations include the need for refrigeration of some products such as antibiotics. Local patterns of resistance should be kept in mind in choosing antibiotics. Extent and area of lesion involvement when large or inaccessible (eg, the back or trunk) as well as ease of application may determine the choice of route between topical and systemic therapy. The natural skin predilection toward oiliness versus dryness may dictate the choice of vehicle. Dietary interactions should be born in mind with certain drugs such as oral tetracycline. Sunscreens will need to be used with photosensitizers, and applied as the first topical agent.

Regimens that may require more frequency of application may be difficult for students or patients whose occupation limits flexibility. The frequency of primary nonadherence to acne treatment has been characterized in terms of the complexity of multidrug acne regimens. Overall, 27% of patients did not fill all their prescriptions: with 1, 2, or 3 or more treatments, 9%, 40%, and 31%, respectively, did not fill all their prescriptions. Authors concluded some patients may not complete acne treatment because 1 or more of their medications were never obtained. Primary adherence to an acne treatment regimen is better when only 1 treatment is prescribed.[143] History of poor adherence because of intolerance of topical treatments may be countered by reducing the strength of treatment, using a different preparation of the drug, or switching to an alternative topical agent that causes less irritation.

EVALUATION OF THERAPEUTIC OUTCOMES

10 Provide a monitoring framework for patients with acne. Parameters should be monitored by the patient and recorded in a diary. Therapy should be appropriately tapered in response to improvement or resolution. The healthcare professional should be responsible for ensuring that the treatment plan remains on schedule and is effective with no adverse effects. The patient should be contacted within 2 to 3 weeks to determine progress.

Acne is poorly understood by adolescents. These patients often lack knowledge of the cause of the disorder and aggravating factors, indications for self-care versus prescription treatment, expected onset of effect, sequence of the healing process, duration of treatment, appropriate application of topical agents, maximal achievable effects, expected adverse effects, safety concerns, and the benefit to QOL. Clinicians should review patient understanding of each of these important factors to ensure patient adherence. There is often a need to supplement counseling sessions with written materials to which the patient can refer at home.

Good adherence is the key to treatment success. Other strategies to increase adherence include use of once-daily regimens, online follow-up visits, and remote digital imaging for ongoing lesion assessment.[141,144,145] A randomized controlled trial compared the effectiveness of automated online counseling to standard web-based education on improving acne knowledge. While both models had a significant increase in knowledge from baseline, after 12 weeks, mean improvement in knowledge was higher in the automated counseling group than in the standard website group. The automated counseling website group rated their educational material more useful and more enjoyable to view than did the standard website group. Internet-based patient education appears to be an effective method of improving acne knowledge among adolescents.[146]

Monitoring of the Pharmaceutical Care Plan

Tables 96-2 to 96-4 provide a guide for monitoring patients with acne. Table 96-2 outlines individual drugs, their most common adverse effects, parameters to monitor, and issues to note. Table 96-3 outlines general effectiveness and safety end points, monitoring parameters, and degree of change and timeframes for short- and long-term outcomes. Table 96-4 is a guide for monitoring acne patients with consideration to the severity grading of acne types I through IV.

TABLE 96-2 Monitoring of Medications Used in Acne Treatment and Maintenance Therapy

Drug	Adverse Drug Reaction	Monitoring Parameter	Comments
Exfoliants			
Resorcinol	Irritant and sensitizer	Degree and/or changes in signs or symptoms of irritancy (redness, discomfort, peeling, skin breakdown, or dermatitis).	Should not be applied to large areas of the skin or on broken skin.
Sulfur	Avoid eye contact—slight ophthalmic and skin irritation	Degree and/or changes in signs or symptoms of irritancy (redness, discomfort, peeling, skin breakdown, or dermatitis). Use should be discontinued if excessive irritation results.	
Salicylic acid	Mild irritant—burning and reddening, local skin peeling	Degree and/or changes in signs or symptoms of irritancy (redness, discomfort, peeling, skin breakdown, or dermatitis).	Begin with a low concentration and increase as tolerance develops. Not a sensitizer.
Retinoids			
Isotretinoin	Side effects: mucocutaneous (most common), musculoskeletal, and ophthalmic systems. Common: dryness of mucus membranes (lips, mouth, eyes, nose) dry skin, itching, hair loss, thirst, back pain, myalgia, headaches, and central nervous system effects. Increased cholesterol. Teratogenic. Sun sensitivity. Depression and suicide—controversial.	Test for pregnancy twice before starting. Contraceptive measures must be started 1 month prior, continued during the 2 months of treatment and for at least 1 month after stopping treatment (but normally 4 months). Laboratory monitoring during therapy should include triglycerides, cholesterol, transaminases, and complete blood counts (before, during and after treatment). Degree and/or changes in signs or symptoms of irritancy to skin (redness, discomfort, peeling, skin breakdown, or dermatitis). Degree and/or changes in signs or symptoms of irritancy to mucous membranes (mouth, nose, eyes). Instances of headache or central nervous system symptoms. Note prior psychiatric symptoms, monitor patients at each visit for early recognition of changes in mood or psychological well-being (before, during, and after treatment).	Drying agents must be discontinued. Sun avoidance strategies and sunscreen use recommended. Vitamin A supplementation. Use moisturizers (lip balm, nasal moisturizers, eye lubricants, temp removal of contacts). Most adverse effects, such as cheilitis, and dry nose, eyes and mouth, are temporary and resolve after the drug is discontinued. Advise patients about a possible risk of depression and suicidal behavior.
Tretinoin/Retinoic acid	Common: erythema, dryness, burning, photosensitization. Rare: true contact allergy. Use cautiously in pregnancy. (Irritation: tazarotene > retinoic acid > adapalene)	Degree and/or changes in signs or symptoms of irritancy to skin (redness, discomfort, peeling, skin breakdown, or dermatitis). Skin changes in areas of sun exposure—dermatitis or hives.	Additive effects with concomitant topical drying medications; products with high concentrations of alcohol, astringents, abrasive soaps, etc. Gels and creams are less irritating than solutions. Sun avoidance strategies and sunscreen use recommended.
Adapalene	Side effects include erythema, xerosis, burning and desquamation. Less irritation than other retinoids. Photoirritation or sensitization.	Degree and/or changes in signs or symptoms of irritancy to skin (redness, discomfort, peeling, skin breakdown, or dermatitis). Skin changes in areas of sun exposure—dermatitis or hives.	Less photosensitivity than other agents. Sun avoidance strategies and sunscreen use recommended.
Tazarotene	Side effects include irritation, erythema, xerosis, burning and desquamation.	Skin changes in areas of sun exposure—dermatitis or hives.	Contraindicated in pregnancy due to the large surface area. Short contact therapy, 1-5 minutes every other night, gradually increasing to overnight advocated for dosing in patients with sensitive skin. Oily complexions may tolerate twice daily, short contact time.
Topical Antimicrobial Agents			
Benzoyl peroxide	Dryness and peeling appear after a few days; erythema; burning; pruritus. Rare reports of contact allergic dermatitis. May bleach hair and clothing. Body odor, odor on clothes and bedsheets. Irritation is concentration dependent—most frequent with 10% gel. Irritation from gels used as vehicles—water-based < alcohol = acetone	Once tolerance is achieved, the strength may be increased to 5% or the base changed to the acetone or alcohol gels, or to paste. Degree and/or changes in signs or symptoms of irritancy to skin (redness, discomfort, peeling, skin breakdown, or dermatitis). Hives.	Increased skin irritation or drying effect with other medications, soaps, and cosmetics with strong drying effect. Chemically incompatible with retinoic acid. Cross-reactions with other sensitizers, such as Peruvian balsam, cinnamon, and other benzoic acid derivatives (topical anesthetics).
Clindamycin	Erythema, peeling, itching, dryness and burning	Signs or symptoms of irritancy to skin (redness, discomfort, peeling, skin breakdown, or dermatitis).	

(continued)

TABLE 96-2 Monitoring of Medications Used in Acne Treatment and Maintenance Therapy (*Continued*)

Drug	Adverse Drug Reaction	Monitoring Parameter	Comments
Oral Antibiotics			
Erythromycin	Gastrointestinal upset (nausea, vomiting, diarrhea) Vaginal candidiasis	If gastrointestinal adverse effects occur, monitor hydration Vaginal discharge	Drug interactions: Inhibits CYP1A2 and CYP3A4: carbamazepine, cyclosporine, theophylline, and warfarin. Safe in pregnant women and children.
Tetracyclines	Gastrointestinal intolerance: (tetracycline > erythromycin > doxycycline = minocycline) Vaginal candidiasis Photosensitivity is dose-dependent (doxycycline > tetracycline).	Vaginal discharge. Skin changes in areas of sun exposure—dermatitis or hives.	Contraindicated in pregnant women or in children younger than 9 years of age. Absorption decreased by food, chelated by antacids and milk. To be taken on an empty stomach.
Minocycline	Drug-induced lupus. Pigment changes in skin, mucous membranes, and teeth. Hepatitis. Urticaria. Dose-related dizziness (resolves with dose titration). Autoimmune hepatitis and hypersensitivity syndrome.	Vaginal discharge. Skin changes in areas of sun exposure—dermatitis or hives. Changes or discoloration of skin, teeth, or mucous membranes. Monitor degree of dizziness as dose is titrated. Signs of hypersensitivity syndrome: fever, dermatitis, blistering reactions; systemic symptoms such as malaise, changes in blood pressure, or renal function.	Contraindicated in pregnant women or in children younger than 9 years of age. Decreased gastrointestinal absorption with Fe, Ca, Mg, Al. Sun avoidance strategies and sunscreen use recommended.
Doxycycline	Gastrointestinal upset. Photosensitizer (especially at higher doses).	If gastrointestinal side effects occur, monitor hydration. Skin changes in areas of sun exposure—dermatitis or hives.	Contraindicated in pregnant women or in children younger than 9 years of age. Sun avoidance strategies and sunscreen use recommended.
Antisebum			
Combination oral contraceptives	Breakthrough bleeding, headache. Serious: venous thromboembolism, hepatotoxicity.	Spotting or bleeding.	Oral antibiotics may decrease contraceptive efficacy—(significance controversial).
Spironolactone	Common: hyperkalemia, menstrual irregularity, gynecomastia, breast tenderness	Menstrual signs. Breast changes.	
Antiinflammatory			
Azelaic acid	Primary: pruritus, burning, stinging, and tingling Other: erythema, dryness, rash, peeling, irritation, dermatitis, and contact dermatitis in less than 1% of patients	Skin changes in areas of sun exposure—dermatitis or hives	Adverse reactions are generally transient and mild in nature.
Dapsone	Short- and long-term safety and efficacy demonstrated. Peeling, dryness, and erythema.	Skin changes in areas of sun exposure—dermatitis or hives	Does not induce phototoxicity or photoallergy in human dermal safety studies. Medications such as rifampin, anticonvulsants, trimethoprim/sulfamethoxazole, and St. John's wort may increase formation of dapsone hydroxylamine (toxicity).

Al, aluminum; Ca, calcium; Fe, iron; Mg, magnesium.

TABLE 96-3 Monitoring Therapy for Acne: Parameters and Frequency

Person Responsible and Frequencies for Monitoring:

Patient: daily while on drug therapy; Pharmacist: every 4-8 wk of therapy or next pharmacy visit

Parameter	Time Frame/Degree of Change	Actions
Short-Term Effectiveness End Points (Acne Resolution/Control)		
Lesion count	Decrease by 10-25% within 4-8 wk, with control, or more than a 50% decrease within 2-4 mo	If end points not achieved, refer to a physician for further therapy.
Comedones	Resolve by 3-4 mo	
Inflammatory lesions	Resolve within a few weeks	
Anxiety, depression	Achieve control or improvement within 2-4 mo	
Long Term		
Progression of severity	No progression of severity	If end points not achieved, refer to a physician for further therapy.
Recurrent episodes	Lengthening of acne-free periods throughout therapy	
Scarring or pigmentation	No further scarring or pigmentation throughout therapy	
Safety End Points (Treatment Side Effects)		
Dermatitis, increased dryness, gastrointestinal upset, photosensitivity	No adverse effects	Refer to a physician for alternate therapy, dose reduction, discontinuation or additive palliative treatment or preventative measures for adverse effects.

TABLE 96-4 Monitoring Care Plans for Acne Types I through IV

Acne Type	Description	Suggested Options	Follow-up Action If Patient Responds	Follow-up Action If Patient Does Not Respond in 3 Months	Adjustment in Therapy If Patient Does Not Respond Adequately to Previous Action
Type I	Mainly comedones with an occasional small inflamed papule or pustule; no scarring present	Topical retinoid is the drug of choice; can also consider benzoyl peroxide or salicylic acid	Continue until lesions are completely cleared and then stop or taper therapy	Treat as Type II acne	
Type II	Comedones and more numerous papules and pustules (mainly facial); mild scarring	Topical retinoid plus benzoyl peroxide, topical or antibiotic	Continue until lesions are completely cleared and then stop or taper therapy	Treat as Type III acne	
Type III	Numerous comedones, papules and pustules, spreading to the back, chest and shoulders, with an occasional cyst or nodule; moderate scarring	Systemic antibiotic plus topical retinoid, or benzoyl peroxide *Or*	Oral antibiotics typically are prescribed for daily use over 4-6 mo, with subsequent tapering and discontinuation as acne improves. Other agents can also be stopped or tapered at this time	Add oral contraceptive or antiandrogen (women only)	Oral isotretinoin (except in women who are or who may become pregnant); consider safety end points (potential adverse effects) before initiating therapy
Type IV	Numerous large cyst on the face, neck and upper trunk; severe scarring	Systemic antibiotic plus topical retinoid, and benzoyl peroxide ± oral contraceptive or antiandrogen (females only)	Oral antibiotics typically are prescribed for daily use over 4-6 mo, with subsequent tapering and discontinuation as acne improves Other agents can also be stopped or tapered at this time	If no response after 3-6 mo, oral isotretinoin (except in women who are or who may become pregnant). Consider safety end points (potential adverse effects) before initiating therapy	

CONCLUSION

Considerable gaps remain in the understanding of acne, despite all that is known about the pathogenesis of acne and the mechanisms of effective drugs for controlling its symptoms, progression, and complications at structural, biochemical, and physiologic levels. It is still not possible to precisely define the cause of one of the most common skin diseases, nor is it possible to identify a cure for a condition that affects a very large proportion of the global population.

ABBREVIATIONS

BGA	best guideline acne
CAM	complementary and alternative medicine
COC	combination oral contraceptive
CRH	corticotropin-releasing hormone
FDA	U.S. Food and Drug Administration
GHQ	general health quality
HGL	high glycemic load
IGF	insulin-like growth factor
IL	inflammatory lesions
MMPP	mild-to-moderate papulopustular
NIL	noninflammatory lesions
P. acnes	*Propionibacterium acnes*
PAPA	pyogenic arthritis, pyoderma gangrenosum, acne
PBV	pollen bee venom
PDT	photodynamic therapy
QOL	quality of life
SAPHO	synovitis, acne, pustulosis, hyperostosis, osteitis syndrome
SPF	sun protection factor
TTO	time trade-off

REFERENCES

1. Cunliffe WJ, Gould DJ. Prevalence of facial acne vulgaris in late adolescence and in adults. *Br Med J* 1979;1:1109-1110.
2. Rademaker M, Garioch JJ, Simpson NB. Acne in schoolchildren: No longer a concern for dermatologists. *BMJ* 1989;298:1217-1219.
3. Kilkenny M, Merlin K, Plunkett A, Marks R. The prevalence of common skin conditions in Australian school children, III: Acne vulgaris. *Br J Dermatol* 1998;139:840-845.
4. Nijsten T, Rombouts S, Lambert J. Acne is prevalent but use of its treatments is infrequent among adolescents from the general population. *J Eur Acad Dermatolog Venereol* 2007;21:163-168.
5. Bhate K, Williams HC. Epidemiology of acne vulgaris. [Review] *British Journal of Dermatology* 2013;168(3):474-485.
6. Smithard A, Glazebrook C, Williams HC. Acne prevalence, knowledge about acne and psychological morbidity in mid-adolescence: A community-based study. *Br J Dermatol* 2001;41:577-580.
7. Pandey SS. Epidemiology of acne vulgaris. *Indian J Dermatol* 1983;28:109-110.
8. Kubba R, Bajaj AK, Thappa DM, et al. Acne in India: Guidelines for management—IAA Consensus Document: Epidemiology of acne. *Indian J Dermatol Venereol Leprol* 2009;75(suppl 1):S3.
9. Shalita AR. Acne vulgaris: Pathogenesis and treatment. *Cosmet Toiletries* 1983;98:57-60.
10. Malus M, LaChance PA, Lamy L, Macaulay A, Vanasse M. Priorities in adolescent health care: The teenagers' viewpoint. *J Fam Pract* 1987;25:159-162.
11. Rosenberg EW. Acne diet reconsidered. *Arch Dermatol* 1981;117(4):193-195.
12. Fulton JE, Plewig G, Kligman AM. Effect of chocolate on acne vulgaris. *JAMA* 1969;210:2071-2074.
13. Antiga E, Verdelli A, Bonciani D, et al. Acne: A new model of immune-mediated chronic inflammatory skin disease. [Review] *Giornale Italiano di Dermatologia e Venereologia* 2015;150(2):247-54.
14. Nast A, Dreno B, Bettoli V, et al. Guidelines for the treatment of acne. *Journal of the European Academy of Dermatology and Venereology* 2012;26(suppl 1):1-29.
15. Chu A. Acne vulgaris. In: Lebwohl MG, Heyman WR, Berth-Jones J, Couslon I, eds. Treatment of Skin Diseases, 2nd ed. Philadelphia, PA: Mosby Elsevier, 2006:6-12.

16. Dreno B, Poli F. Epidemiology of acne. *Dermatology* 2003;206:7-10.
17. Tucker SB, Rogers S, Winkleman RK. Inflammation in acne vulgaris: Leukocyte attraction and cytotoxicity by comedonal material. *J Invest Dermatol* 1985;74:21-25.
18. Winston MH, Shalita AR. Acne vulgaris. *Pediatr Clin North Am* 1991;38(4):889-903.
19. Plewig G, Kligman AM. The dynamics of primary comedo formation. In: Plewig G, Kligman AM, eds. Acne: Morpho-genesis and Treatment. New York: Springer-Verlag, 1975:58-107.
20. Puissegur-Lupo M. Acne vulgaris, treatments and their rationale. *Postgrad Med* 1985;78(7):76-88.
21. Batra RS. Acne. In: Arndt KA, Tsu JTS, eds. Manual of Dermatologic Therapeutics, 7th ed. Philadelphia, PA: Lippincott, Williams and Wilkins, 2007:3-18.
22. U.S. Department of Health and Human Services Food and Drug Administration Center for Drug Evaluation and Research (CDER). Guidance for Industry. Acne vulgaris: developing drugs for treatment. 2005. Available at: http://www.fda.gov/dowloads/Drugs/GuidanceComplianceRegulatory Information/GuideancesCM071292.pdf.
23. Harrison-Atlas R, Bernhard JD, O'Connor RC, Weinraub LF. What to do when typical teenage acne strikes. *JCOM* 1996;3:9.
24. Pochi PE, Shalita AR, Straus JC, et al. Report of the consensus conference on acne classification. *J Am Acad Dermatol* 1991;24(3): 495-500.
25. Pagliarello C, Di Pietro C, Tabolli S. A comprehensive health impact assessment and determinants of quality of life, health and psychological status in acne patients. *Giornale Italiano di Dermatologia e Venereologia* 2015;150(3):303-308.
26. Chren MM, Lasek RJ, Quinn LM, et al. Skindex, a quality-of-life measure for patients with skin disease. Reliability, validity and responsiveness. *J Invest Dermatol* 1996;107(5):707-713.
27. Finlay AY, Khan GK. Dermatology Quality of Life Index (DLQI): A simple practical measure for routine clinical use. Clin Exp Dermatol. 1994;19(3):210-106.
28. Girman CJ, Hartmaier S, Thiboutot D, et al. Evaluating health-related quality of life in patients with facial acne: Development of a self-administered questionnaire for clinical trials. *Qual Life Res* 1996;5(5):481-490.
29. Gupta MA, Johnson AM, Gupta AK. The development of an acne quality of life scale: Reliability, validity and relationship to subjective acne severity in mild to moderate acne vulgaris. Acta Derm Venereol. 1998;78(6):451-456.
30. Wang KC, Zane LT. Recent advances in acne vulgaris research: Insights and clinical implications. In: James, WD, ed. Advances in Dermatology. Philadelphia, PA: Elsevier, 2008:197-209.
31. Johnson BA, Nunley JR. Topical therapy for acne vulgaris: How do you choose the best drug for each patient? *Postgrad Med J* 2000; 107(3):69-80.
32. Steinhoff M, Schauber J, Leyden JJ. New insights into rosacea pathophysiology: A review of recent findings. *J Am Acad Dermatol* 2013;69:S15-S26.
33. Habif TP. Acne, rosacea, and related disorders. In: Klein EA, Menczer BS, eds. Clinical Dermatology. Toronto: Mosby, 1990:756.
34. Kelly AP. Acne and related disorders. In: Sams WM, Lynch PJ, eds. Principles and Practice of Dermatology. New York: Churchill Livingstone, 1990:1014.
35. MacDonald Hull S, Sunliffe WJ. The use of a corticosteroid cream for immediate reduction in the clinical signs of acne vulgaris. *Acta Derm Venereol* 1989;69(5):452-453.
36. Brodell RT, O'Brien MR. Topical corticosteroid-induced acne: three treatment strategies to break the "addiction cycle." *Postgrad Med* 1999;106(6):225-229.
37. Hitch JM. Acneform eruption induced by drugs and chemicals. *JAMA* 1969;200:879.
38. Boothroyd S. Topical therapy and formulation principles. In: Webster GF, Rawlings AV, eds. Acne and Its Therapy. New York: Informa Healthcare USA, 2007:253-274.
39. Choi YS, Suh HS, Yoon MY, et al. A study of the efficacy of cleansers for acne vulgaris. *J Dermatol Treat* 2010;21(3):201-205.
40. Food and Drug Administration. Non-prescription drugs. 2009. Available at: http://www.fda.gov/OHRMS/DOCKETS/98fr/78n-0065-npr0003.pdf.
41. Russell JJ. Topical therapy for acne. *Am Fam Physician* 2000;61(2): 357-365.
42. Epinette WW, Gresit MC, Osols II. The role of cosmetics in postadolescent acne. *Cutis* 1982;29(5):500-514.
43. Plewig G, Kligman AM. Acne cosmetica. In: Plewig G, Kligman AM, eds. Acne: Morphogenesis and Treatment. New York: Springer-Verlag, 1975;226-229.
44. Mills OH, Kligman AM. Comedogenicity of sunscreens. experimental observations in rabbits. *Arch Dermatol* 1982;18(6):417-419.
45. Cappel M, Mauger D, Thiboutet D. Correlation between serum levels of insulin-like growth factor 1, dehydroepiandrosterone sulfate, and dihydrotestosterone and acne lesion counts in adult women. *Arch Dermatol* 2005;141:333-338.
46. Dall'oglio F, Tedeschi A, Fabbrocini G. Cosmetics for acne: Indications and recommendations for an evidence-based approach. [Review] *Giornale Italiano di Dermatologia e Venereologia* 2015;150(1):1-11.
47. Thiboutot DM. New treatments and therapeutic strategies for acne. *Arch Fam Med* 2000;9(2):179-187.
48. Chiou WL. Low intrinsic drug activity and dominant vehicle (Placebo) effect in the topical treatment of acne vulgaris. *Int J Clin Pharmacol Therapeut* 2012;50(6):434-437.
49. Strauss JS, Kowchk DP, Leyden JJ, et al. Guidelines of care for acne vulgaris management. *J Am Acad Dermatol* 2007;56:651-663.
50. Ellerbroek WC. Hypotheses toward a unified field theory of human behavior with clinical application to acne vulgaris. *Perspect Biol Med* 1973;16:240-262.
51. Hughes H, Brown BW, Lawlis GF, Fulton JE Jr. Treatment of acne vulgaris by biofeedback relaxation and cognitive imagery. *J Psychosom Res* 1983;27:185-191.
52. Chao CM, Lai WY, Wu BY, Chang HC, Huang WS, Chen YF. A pilot study on efficacy treatment of acne vulgaris using a new method: Results of a randomized double-blind trial with Acne Dressing. *J Cosmet Sci* 2006;57(2):95-105.
53. Rhei LD, Zatz JL, Motwani MR. Targeted delivery of actives from topical treatment products to the pilosebaceous unit. In: Webster GF, Rawlings AV, eds. Acne and Its Therapy. New York: Informa Healthcare USA, 2007:223-252.
54. Thiboutot D, Gollnick H, Bettoli V, et al. New Insights into the management of acne: an update from the Global Alliance to Improve Outcomes in Acne Group. *J Am Acad Dermatolog* 2009;60:S1-S50.
55. Magin PJ, Adams J, Pond CD, et al. Topical and oral CAM in acne: A review of the empirical evidence and a consideration of its context. *Complement Ther Med* 2006;14:62-76.
56. Li B, Chair H, Du YH, Xiao L, Xiong J. Evaluation of therapeutic effect and safety for clinical randomized and controlled trials of treatment of acne with acupuncture and moxibustion. *Zhongguo Zhen Jiu* 2009; 29(3):247-251.
57. Reuter J, Merfort I, Schempp CM. Botanicals in dermatology: an evidence-based review. *Am J Clin Dermatol* 2010;11:247-67.
58. Ernst E, Huntley A. Tea-tree oil: A systematic review of randomized clinical trials. *Forsch Komplementarmed Klass Natureheilkd* 2000;7: 17-20.
59. Hammer KA. Treatment of acne with tea tree oil (melaleuca) products: A review of efficacy, tolerability and potential modes of action. [Review] *International Journal of Antimicrobial Agents* 2015;45(2):106-110.
60. Cae H, Liu JP, Smith CA, et al. Complementary therapies for acne vulgaris (Review). The Cochrane collaboration, issue 1. New York: Wiley, 2015. Available at: http://www.thecochranelibrary.com.
61. Eisenberg DM, Davis RB, Ettner SL, et al. Trends in alternative medicine use in the United States, 1990–1997: Results of a follow-up national survey. *JAMA* 1998;280(18):1569-1575.
62. Poli F, Ribet V, Lauze C, Adhoute H, Morinet P. Efficacy and safety of 0.1% retinaldehyde/6% glycolic acid (Diacneal) for mild to moderate acne vulgaris. A multicentre, double-blind, randomized, vehicle-controlled trial. *Dermatol* 2005;210(suppl 1):14-21.
63. Food and Drug Administration. Non-prescription drugs. 2009. Available at: http://www.fda.gov/OHRMS/DOCKETS/98fr/78n-0065-npr0003.pdf.
64. Katsambas AD, Katoulis AC, Stavropoulos P. Acne neonatorum: A study of 22 cases. *Int J Dermatol* 1999;38(2):128-130.
65. Callender VD. Fitzpatrick skin types and clindamycin phosphate 1.2%/benzoyl peroxide gel: Efficacy and tolerability of treatment in moderate to severe acne. *J Drugs Dermatol* 2012;11(5):643-648.
66. Brown S. Therapeutic potpourri. *Dermatol Clin* 1989;7(1):71-74.
67. Sykes NL, Webster GF. Acne: A review of optimum treatment. *Drugs* 1994;48(1):59-70.
68. Zouboulis CC. Moderne aknetherapie. *Akt Dermatol* 2003;29:49-57.
69. Zander E, Weisman S. Treatment of acne vulgaris with salicylic acid pads. *Clin Ther* 1992;14:247-253.
70. Gross G. Benzoyl peroxide and salicylic acid therapy. In: Webster GF, Rawlings AV, eds. Acne and Its Therapy. New York: Informa Healthcare USA, 2007:117-136.
71. Shalita AR. Treatment of mild and moderate acne vulgaris with salicylic acid in an alcohol-detergent vehicle. *Cutis* 1981;28:556-561.

72. Kligman D, Kligman AM. Salicylic acid as a peeling agent for the treatment of acne. *Cosmetic Dermatol* 1997;10:44-47.
73. Lin AN, Reimer RJ, Carter DM. Sulfur revisited. *J Am Acad Dermatol* 1988;18:553-558.
74. Kroshinsky D, Shalita AR, Topical retinoids. In: Webster GF, Rawlings AV, eds. Acne and Its Therapy. New York: Informa Healthcare USA, 2007:103-112.
75. Galvin SA, Gilbert R, Baker M, Guibal F, Tuley MR. Comparative tolerance of adapalene 0.1% gel and six different tretinoin formulations. *Br J Dermatol* 1998;139(suppl 52):34-40.
76. Mills OH Jr., Berger RS. Irritation potential of a new topical tretinoin formulation and a commercially-available tretinoin formulation as measured by patch testing in human subjects. *J Am Acad Dermatol* 1998;38:S11-S16.
77. Jeremy AHT, Holland DB, Roberts SG, et al. Inflammatory events are involved in acne lesion initiation. *J Invest Dermatol* 2003;139:897-900.
78. Shroot B, Michel S. Pharmacology and chemistry of adapalene. *J Am Acad Dermatol* 1997;36(6):S96-S103.
79. Weiss JS, Shavin JS. Adapalene for the treatment of acne vulgaris. *J Am Acad Dermatol* 1998;39(2):50-54.
80. Brogden R, Goa K. Adapalene: A review of its pharmacological properties and clinical potential in the management of mild to moderate acne. *Drugs* 1997;53(3):511-519.
81. Verschoore M, Langner A, Wolska M, Jablonska S, Czernielewski J, Schaefer H. Vehicle controlled study of CD 271 lotion in the topical treatment of acne vulgaris. *J Invest Dermatol* 1993;100:221.
82. Russell JJ. Topical therapy for acne. *Am Fam Physician* 2000;61(2): 357-365.
83. Kakita L. Tazarotene versus tretinoin or adapalene in the treatment of acne vulgaris. *J Am Acad Dermatol* 2000;43(2 pt 3):851-854.
84. Tzellos T, Toulis KA, Dessinioti C, et al. Topical retinoids for the treatment of acne vulgaris (protocol). The Cochrane collaboration, issue 12. New York: Wiley, 2011. Available at: http://www.thecochranelibrary.com.
85. Jarratt M, Werner CP, Alio Saenz AB. Tazarotene foam versus tazarotene gel: A randomized relative bioavailability study in acne vulgaris. *Clinical Drug Investigation* 2013;33(4):283-289.
86. Feldman SR, Werner CP, Alio Saenz AB. The efficacy and tolerability of tazarotene foam, 0.1%, in the treatment of acne vulgaris in 2 multicenter, randomized, vehicle-controlled, double-blind studies. *Journal of Drugs in Dermatology: JDD* 2013;12(4):438-446.
87. Mohd Nor NH, Aziz Z. A systematic review of benzoyl peroxide for acne vulgaris. [Review] *Journal of Dermatological Treatment* 2013;24(5):397-386.
88. Gross G. Benzoyl peroxide and salicylic acid therapy. In: Webster GF, Rawlings AV, eds. Acne and Its Therapy. New York: Informa Healthcare USA, 2007:117-136.
89. Zander E, Weisman S. Treatment of acne vulgaris with salicylic acid pads. *Clin Ther* 1992;14:247-253.
90. Zouboulis CC. Moderne aknetherapie. *Akt Dermatol* 2003;29:49-57.
91. Gollnick H, Schramm M. Topical drug treatments in acne. *Dermatol* 1998;196:119-125.
92. Cotterill JA. Benzoyl peroxide. *Acta Derm Venereol* 1980;89(suppl): 57-63.
93. Cunliffe WJ, Holland KT. The effect of benzoyl peroxide on acne. *Acta Derm Venereol* 1981;61(3):267-269.
94. Lassus A. Local treatment of acne. A clinical study and evaluation of the effect of different concentrations of benzoyl peroxide gel. *Curr Med Res Opin* 1981;7(6):370-373.
95. Cunliffe WJ, Dodman B, Eady R. Benzoyl peroxide in acne. *Practitioner* 1978;220(3):470-482.
96. Maddin S. Benzoyl peroxide. *Can J Dermatol* 1989;1(4):92.
97. Report of the Expert Advisory Committee on Dermatology. The carcinogenic activity of benzoyl peroxide. Information Letter Ottawa: Health Protection Branch (Canada) 1987;711:1-9.
98. Cunliffe WJ, Burke B. Benzoyl peroxide: Lack of sensitization. *Acta Derm Venereol* 1982;62(5):458-459.
99. Tkach JR. Allergic contact urticaria to benzoyl peroxide. *Cutis* 1982;29(2):187-188.
100. Rietschel RL, Duncan SH. Benzoyl peroxide reactions in an acne study group. *Contact Dermatitis* 1982;8:323-326.
101. Bowman S, Gold M, Nasir A, Vamvakias G. Comparison of clindamycin/benzoyl peroxide, tretinoin plus clindamycin, and the combination of clindamycin/benzoyl peroxide and tretinoin plus clindamycin in the treatment of acne vulgaris: A randomized, blinded study. *J Drug Dermatol* 2005;4(5):611-618.
102. Korkut C, Piskin S. Benzoyl peroxide, adapalene, and their combination in the treatment of acne vulgaris. *J Dermatol* 2005;2(3):169-173.
103. Bikowski JB. Clinical experience results with clindamycin 1% benzoyl peroxide 5% gel (Duac) as monotherapy and in combination. *J Drug Dermatol* 2005;4(2):164-171.
104. Burkhart CG, Burkhart CN. Treatment of acne vulgaris without antibiotics: Tertiary amine-benzoyl peroxide combination vs. benzoyl peroxide alone (Proactiv Solution). *Int J Dermatol* 2007;46(1):89-93.
105. Gamble R, Dunn J, Dawson A, et al. Topical antimicrobial treatment of acne vulgaris: An evidence-based review. Am J Clin Dermatol. 2012;13(3):141-152.
106. Tanghetti E, Abramovits W, Solomon B, Loven K, Shalita A. Tazarotene versus tazarotene plus clindamycin/benzoyl peroxide in the treatment of acne vulgaris: A multicenter, double-blind, randomized parallel-group trial. *J Drugs Dermatol* 2006;5(3):256-261.
107. Del Rosso JQ, Tanghetti E. The clinical impact of vehicle technology using a patented formulation of 5%/clindamycin 1% gel: Comparative assessments of skin tolerability and evaluation of combination use with a topical retinoid. *J Drug Dermatol* 2006;5(2):160-164.
108. Webster G. Antimicrobial therapy in acne. In: Webster GF, Rawlings AV, eds. Acne and Its Therapy. New York: Informa Healthcare USA, 2007:97-102.
109. Kawashima M, Hashimoto H, Alio Saenz AB, et al. Clindamycin phosphate 12%-benzoyl peroxide 30% fixed-dose combination gel has an effective and acceptable safety and tolerability profile for the treatment of acne vulgaris in Japanese patients: a phase III, multicentre, randomised, single-blinded, active-controlled, parallel-group study. *British Journal of Dermatology* 2015;172(2):494-503.
110. Schmidt NW, Agak GW, Deshayes S, et al. Pentobra: A potent antibiotic with multiple layers of selective antimicrobial mechanisms against propionibacterium acnes. *Journal of Investigative Dermatology* 2015;135(6):1581-1589.
111. Bottomly WW, Cunliffe WJ. Oral trimethoprim as a third line antibiotic in the management of acne vulgaris. *Dermatol* 1993; 187:193-196.
112. Ullah G, Noor SM, Bhatti Z, et al. Comparison of oral azithromycin with oral doxycycline in the treatment of acne vulgaris. *Journal of Ayub Medical College, Abbottabad: JAMC* 2014;26(1):64-67.
113. Dalzeil K, Dykes PJ, Marks R. The effect of tetracycline and erythromycin in a model of acne-type inflammation. *Br J Exp Pathol* 1987;68:67-70.
114. Garner SE, Eady A, Bennett C, et al. Minocycline for acne vulgaris: Efficacy and safety (review). The Cochrane Collaboration, Issue 9. New York: Wiley, 2012. Available at: http://www.thecochranelibrary.com.
115. Straight CE, Lee YH, Liu G, et al. Duration of oral antibiotic therapy for the treatment of adult acne: A retrospective analysis investigating adherence to guideline recommendations and opportunities for cost-savings. *Journal of the American Academy of Dermatology* 2015;72(5):822-827.
116. Hughes BR, Murphy CE, Barnett J, Cunliffe WJ. Strategy of acne therapy with long-term antibiotics. *Br J Dermatol* 1989;121:623-628.
117. Aslam I, Fleischer A, Feldman S. Emerging drugs for the treatment of acne. [Review] *Expert Opinion on Emerging Drugs* 2015;20(1):91-101.
118. Weller R, Price RJ, Ormerod AD, et al. Antimicrobial effect of acidified nitrite on dermatophyte fungi, Candida and bacterial skin pathogens. *Journal of Applied Microbiology* 2001;90(4):648-652.
119. Passi S, Picardo M, De Luca C, Nazzaro-Porro M. Mechanism of azelaic acid action in acne. *G Ital Dermatol Venereol* 1989;10:455-463.
120. Draelos ZD, Carter E, Maloney JM, et al. Two randomized studies demonstrate the efficacy and safety of dapsone gel, 5% for the treatment of acne vulgaris. *J Am Acad Dermatol* 2007;56(3):439.e1-10.
121. Tan J. Dapsone 5% gel: A new option in topical therapy for acne. *Skin Therapy Letter* 2012;17(8):1-3.
122. Lynde CW, Andriessen A. Cohort study on the treatment with dapsone 5% gel of mild to moderate inflammatory acne of the face in women. *SKINmed* 2014;12(1):15-21.
123. Tanghetti E, Harper JC, Oefelein MG. The efficacy and tolerability of dapsone 5% gel in female vs male patients with facial acne vulgaris: Gender as a clinically relevant outcome variable. *Journal of Drugs in Dermatology: JDD* 2012;11(12):1417-1421.
124. Fleischer AB Jr., Shalita A, Eichenfield LF, et al. Dapsone gel 5% in combination with adapalene gel 0.1%, benzoyl peroxide gel 4% or moisturizer for the treatment of acne vulgaris: A 12-week, randomized, double-blind study. *J Drugs Dermatol* 2010;9(1):33-40.
125. Gamble R, Dunn J, Dawson A, et al. Topical antimicrobial treatment of acne vulgaris: An evidence-based review. *Am J Clin Dermatolgol* 2012;13(3):141-152.
126. Arowojolu AO, Gall MR, Lopez LM, et al. Combined oral contraceptive pills for treatment of acne. The Cochrane Collaboration, Issue 7. New York: Wiley, 2012. Available at: http://www.thecochranelibrary.com.

127. Koo EB, Petersen TD, Kimball AB. Meta-analysis comparing efficacy of antibiotics versus oral contraceptives in acne vulgaris. *Journal of the American Academy of Dermatology* 2014;71(3):450-9.
128. Afzli BM, Yaghoobi E, Yaghoobi R, et al. Comparison of the efficacy of 5% topical spironolactone gel and placebo in the treatment of mild and moderate acne vulgaris: A randomized controlled trial. *J Dermatol Treat* 2012;23(1):21-25.
129. Nader S, Rodriguez-Rigau LJ, Smith KD, Steinberger E. Acne and hyperandrogenism: Impact of lowering androgen levels with glucocorticoid treatment. *J Am Acad Dermatol* 1984;11:256-259.
130. Lowenstein EB, Lowenstein EJ. Isotretinoin systemic therapy and the shadow cast upon dermatology's downtrodden hero. *Clin Dermatol* 2011;29:652-661.
131. Rawlings AV. The molecular biology of retinoids and their receptors. In: Webster GF, Rawlings AV, eds. Acne and Its Therapy. New York: Informa Healthcare USA, 2007:45-53.
132. Agarwal US, Besarwal RK, Bhola K. Oral isotretinoin in different dose regimens for acne vulgaris: A randomized comparative trial. *Indian Journal of Dermatology, Venereology & Leprology* 2011;77(6):688-94.
133. Lee JW, Yoo KH, Park KY, et al. Effectiveness of conventional, low-dose and intermittent oral isotretinoin in the treatment of acne: A randomized, controlled comparative study. *British Journal of Dermatology* 2011;164(6):1369-1375.
134. Berk DR. Effectiveness of conventional, low-dose and intermittent oral isotretinoin in the treatment of acne: A randomized, controlled comparative study: comment. *British Journal of Dermatology* 2011; 165(1):205.
135. Webster GF, Leyden JJ, Gross JA. Results of a Phase III, double-blind, randomized, parallel-group, non-inferiority study evaluating the safety and efficacy of isotretinoin-Lidose in patients with severe recalcitrant nodular acne. *Journal of Drugs in Dermatology: JDD* 2014; 13(6):665-670.
136. Choi YS, Suh HS, Yoon MY, et al. A study of the efficacy of cleansers for acne vulgaris. *J Dermatol Treat* 2010;21(3):201-205.
137. Stoughton RB, Leyden JJ. Efficacy of 4 percent chlorhexidine gluconate skin cleanser in the treatment of acne vulgaris. *Cutis* 1987;39(6):551-553.
138. Shalita AR. Treatment of mild and moderate acne vulgaris with salicylic acid in an alcohol-detergent vehicle. *Cutis* 1982;28(11): 556-568.
139. Arndt KA. Acne. In: Arndt KA, ed. Manual of Dermatologic Therapeutics, 4th ed. Toronto: Little Brown, 1989:3-13.
140. Fulgha CC, Caltalano PM, Childers RC, et al. Abrasive cleansing in the management of acne vulgaris. *Arch Dermatol* 1982;118(9):658-659.
141. Yentzer BA, Ade RA, Fountain JM, et al. Simplifying regimens promotes greater adherence and outcomes with topical acne medications: A randomized controlled trial. *Cutis* 2012;86(2):103-108.
142. Straight CE, Lee YH, Liu G, et al. Duration of oral antibiotic therapy for the treatment of adult acne: A retrospective analysis investigating adherence to guideline recommendations and opportunities for cost-savings. *Journal of the American Academy of Dermatology* 2015;72(5): 822-827.
143. Anderson KL, Dothard EH, Huang KE, et al. Frequency of primary nonadherence to acne treatment. *JAMA Dermatology* 2015;151(6): 623-626.
144. Watson AJ, Bergman H, Williams CM, et al. A randomized trial to evaluate the efficacy of online follow-up visits in the management of acne. *Arch Dermatol* 2010;146(4):406-411.
145. Bergman H, Tsai KY, Seo SJ, et al. Remote assessment of acne: the use of acne grading tools to evaluate digital skin images. *Telemed J E Health* 2009;15(5):426-430.
146. Tuong W, Wang AS, Armstrong AW. Comparing the effectiveness of automated online counseling to standard web-based education on improving acne knowledge: A randomized controlled trial. *American Journal of Clinical Dermatology* 2015;16(1):55-60.
147. Elman M, Slatkine M, Harth Y. The effective treatment of acne vulgaris by a high-intensity, narrow band 405–420 nm light source. *J Cosmet Laser Ther* 2003;5:111-117.
148. Friedman PM, Jih MH, Kimyai-Asadi A, Goldberg LH. Treatment of inflammatory facial acne vulgaris with the 1450-nm diode laser: A pilot study. *Dermatol Surg* 2004;30:147-151.
149. Mariwalla K, Rohrer TE. Use of lasers and light-based therapies for treatment of acne vulgaris. *Lasers Surg Med* 2005;37(5):333-342.
150. Ross EV. Optical treatments for acne. *Dermatol Ther* 2005;18(3): 253-266.
151. Lloyd JR, Mirkov M. Selective photothermolysis of the sebaceous glands for acne treatment. *Lasers Surg Med* 2002;31(2):115-120.
152. Böhm M, Luger TA. The pilosebaceous unit is part of the skin immune system. *Dermatol* 1998;196(1):75-79.
153. Seaton E, Mouser PE, Charakida A, Alam S, Seldon PM, Chu AC. Investigation of the mechanism of action of nonablative pulsed-dye laser therapy in photorejuvenation and inflammatory acne vulgaris. *Brit J Dermatol* 2006;155(4):748-755.
154. Car J, Car M, Hamilton F, et al. Light therapies for acne (protocol). The Cochrane Collaboration, Issue 4. New York: Wiley, 2009. Available at: http://www.thecochranelibrary.com.
155. van Zuuren E, Fedorowicz Z, Carter B, et al. Interventions for Rosacea Cochrane Database Online Publication Date: April 2015. Available at: http://www.thecochranelibrary.com.
156. European Directive for systemic isotretinoin prescription. EMEA—Committee for Proprietary Medicinal Products (CPMP). 2012. Available at: http://www.ema.europa.eu/docs/en_GB/document_library/Referrals_document/Isotretinoin_29?WC500010882.pdf.
157. Ganceviciene R, Zouboulis CC. Isotretinoin: State of the art treatment for acne vulgaris. *J Dtsch Dermatol Ges* 2010;8(suppl 1):S47-S59.
158. Strauss JS, Krowchuk DP, Leyden JJ, et al. Guidelines for optimal use of isotretinoin in acne. *J Am Acad Dermatol* 2007;56:651-663.
159. Layton AM, Dreno B, Gollnick HPM, et al. A review of the European Directive for prescribing systemic isotretinoin for acne vulgaris. *J Eur Acad Dermatol Venereol* 2006;20:773-776.
160. Marqueling AL, Zane LT. Depression and suicidal behavior in acne patients treated with isotretinoin: A systematic review. *Semin Cutan Med Surg* 2005;24:92-102.
161. Sundstrom A, Alfredsson L, Sjolin-Forsberg G, Gerdén B, Bergman U, Jokinen J. Association of suicide attempts with acne and treatment with isotretinoin: retrospective Swedish cohort study. *Br Med J* 2010; 341:c5812.
162. Anderson PC. Foods as the cause of acne. *Am Fam Physician* 1971;3(3): n102-n103.
163. Fulton JE, Plewig G, Kligman AM. Effect of chocolate on acne vulgaris. *JAMA* 1969;210(11):2071-2074.
164. Adebamowo CA, Spiegelman D, Danby FW, Frazier AL, Willett WC, Holmes MD. High school dietary dairy intake and teenage acne. *J Am Acad Dermatol* 2005;52(2):207-214.
165. Danby FW. Acne and milk, the diet myth, and beyond. *J Am Acad Dermatol* 2005;52(2):360-362.
166. Bowers J. Diet and acne. Dermatology World 2011:31-34.
167. Kim J, Ko Y, Park YK, et al. Dietary effect of lactoferrin-enriched fermented milk on skin surface lipid and clinical improvement of acne vulgaris. *Nutrition* 2010;26(9):902-909.
168. Thiboutot D. Acne: Hormonal concepts and therapy. *Clin Dermatol* 2004;22:419-428.
169. Cappel M, Mauger D, Thiboutet D. Correlation between serum levels of insulin-like growth factor 1, dehydroepiandrosterone sulfate, and dihydrotestosterone and acne lesion counts in adult women. *Arch Dermatol* 2005;141(3):333-338.
170. Mueller EA, Trapp S, Frentzel A, et al. Efficacy and tolerability of oral lactoferrin supplementation in mild to moderate acne vulgaris: an exploratory study. *Curr Med Res Opin* 2011;27(4):793-797.
171. Smith RN, Mann NJ, Braue A, et al. The effect of a high protein, low-glycemic load diet versus a conventional high-glycemic load diet on biochemical parameters associated with acne vulgaris: A randomized, investigator-masked controlled trial. *J Am Acad Dermatol* 2007;57(2):247-256.
172. Smith RN, Braue A, Varigos GA, Mann NJ. The effect of a low glycemic load diet on acne vulgaris and the fatty acid composition of skin surface triglycerides. *J Dermatol Sci* 2008;50(1):41-52.
173. Smith RN, Mann NJ, Braue A, Makelainen H, Varigos GA. A low-glycemic-load diet improves symptoms in acne vulgaris patients: A randomized controlled trial. *Am J Clin Nutr* 2007; 86(1):107-115.
174. Wolkenstein P, Misery L, Amici JM, et al. Smoking and dietary factors associated with moderate-to-severe acne in French adolescents and young adults: Results of a survey using a representative sample. *Dermatology* 2015;230(1):34-39.

97

Psoriasis

Rebecca M. Law and Wayne P. Gulliver

KEY CONCEPTS[1]

1. Patients with psoriasis have a lifelong illness that may be very visible and emotionally distressing. There is a strong need for empathy and a caring attitude in interactions with these patients.
2. Psoriasis is a progressive T-lymphocyte–mediated systemic inflammatory disease that results from a complex interplay between multiple genetic factors and environmental influences. Genetic predisposition and precipitating "trigger" factors play a role in the "march of psoriasis." This march of innate and adaptive immune responses results in clinical expressions (eg, keratinocyte proliferation) and is possibly responsible for psoriatic comorbidities.
3. Diagnosis of psoriasis is usually based on recognition of the characteristic psoriatic lesion and not based on laboratory tests.
4. Treatment goals for patients with psoriasis are to minimize signs such as plaques and scales, alleviate symptoms such as pruritus, reduce the frequency of flare-ups, ensure appropriate treatment of associated comorbid conditions such as psoriatic arthritis (PsA) or clinical depression, and minimize treatment-related morbidity.
5. Management of patients with psoriasis generally involves both nonpharmacologic and pharmacologic therapies.
6. Nonpharmacologic alternatives such as stress reduction and the liberal use of moisturizers may be very beneficial and should always be considered and initiated when appropriate.
7. Pharmacologic alternatives for psoriasis include topical agents, phototherapy, and systemic agents (both traditional agents and newer biologic response modifiers).
8. Pharmacologic therapy is generally guided by the severity of disease, advancing from topical agents to phototherapy to systemic agents as needed.
9. Rotational therapy (ie, rotating systemic drug interventions) is a means to minimize drug-associated toxicities. However, continuous treatment has replaced rotational or sequential therapy and is now the standard of care for many dermatologists.
10. Some biologic response modifiers (BRMs) have proven efficacy for psoriasis; however, there are differences among these agents, including mechanism of action, duration of remission, and adverse-effect profile. BRMS are often used for moderate-to-severe psoriasis and may be first-line therapy especially if comorbidities exist.

Psoriasis is a chronic disease that waxes and wanes. It is never cured, and it is now known to be associated with multiple comorbidities including heart disease, diabetes, and the metabolic syndrome. The signs and symptoms of psoriasis may subside totally (go into remission) and then flare-up again (exacerbation). Triggers include stress, seasonal changes, and some drugs. Disease severity may vary from mild to disabling. Psoriasis imposes a burden of disease that extends beyond the physical dermatologic manifestations.

(1) Patients with psoriasis have a lifelong illness that may be very visible and emotionally distressing. There is a strong need for empathy and a caring attitude in interactions with these patients. Thus, management of this condition is necessarily long-term and multifaceted, and management modalities may change according to the severity of illness at the time.[1]

EPIDEMIOLOGY

Psoriasis is likely the most common immune-modulated inflammatory disease in North America and Europe, as it is thought to affect 17 million people, or approximately 2% of the population.[2,3] Worldwide prevalences vary between 0.1% and 3%, with reasons for variation ranging from racial to geographic and environmental.[3] Climate, sun exposure, and ethnicity are thought to affect prevalence, but correlation between latitude and prevalence is weak.[4] Prevalences higher than 3% have been reported occasionally in Canada and the United States. Lower frequencies of between 0.4% and 0.7% are seen for people of African and Asian descent.[4,5] Of interest is the fact that psoriasis is seldom seen in North and South American aboriginal Indians. It affects males and females equally.[3,6] The majority of patients (approximately 75%) have onset before the age of 40,[3] but psoriasis has been observed at birth and as late as the ninth decade of life.[3] Prevalence increases are roughly linear over the life course (about 0.12% at age 1 to 1.2% at age 18).[4] Many studies report two peak ages of onset: at 20 to 30 and 50 to 60 years.[3,5]

ETIOLOGY

(2) Psoriasis is a T-lymphocyte–mediated systemic inflammatory disease that results from a complex interplay between multiple genetic factors and environmental influences. Genetic predisposition coupled with some precipitating factor triggers an abnormal immune response, resulting in the initial psoriatic skin lesions. This has been called the "march of psoraisis"[2,6] to reflect the innate and adaptive immune responses that are present. This march leads to expressions of psoriasis with keratinocyte proliferation being central to the clinical presentation of psoriasis, and is likely responsible for various comorbidities as a consequence of the chronic inflammation associated with psoriasis.[2,4] For example, there is an association between psoriasis and cardiovascular disease, which appears to be an ongoing, two-way interplay.[2,6] The concept is that systemic inflammation enhances insulin resistance, causing endothelial dysfunction, leading to atherosclerosis and coronary events.[7]

Genetics

Dermatologists have recognized the familial tendencies of psoriasis for many years. Monozygotic twins have a concordance rate in the 80% range. Rates of family history in a psoriasis family range between 36% and 91%.[8,9] A study using the founder population of Newfoundland and Labrador noted that more than 80% of the patients had a positive family history.

There are psoriasis susceptibility genes and variants that reside on various chromosomes. The psoriasis susceptibility locus 1 (*PSORS1*) on chromosome 6p is a key gene locus, accounting for up to 50% of disease heritability.[4] In 2009, studies of the Newfoundland and Labrador population confirmed that major histocompatibility complex antigen (HLA)-Cw6 and tumor necrosis factor (TNF)-α as major psoriasis susceptibility genes, along with interleukin (IL)-23 loci that had previously been reported.[3,10] The findings have been confirmed in multiple populations worldwide.[11] Currently, roughly 40 additional loci are thought to be associated with psoriasis.[4] Corresponding genes to these loci are involved in pathogenesis pathways in the immune system (adaptive and innate). There appears to be a general role for T cells and a specific role for TH17 lymphocytes in psoriasis pathogenesis and as indicators of psoriasis risk.[4]

Predisposing Factors and Precipitating Factors

Injury to the skin, infection, drugs, smoking, alcohol consumption, obesity, and psychogenic stress have been implicated in the development of psoriasis. Examples of these precipitating factors include a horsefly bite causing skin trauma (known as the *Koebner phenomenon*),[12] a viral or streptococcal infection, or the use of β-adrenergic blockers.[13] Factors exacerbating preexisting psoriasis include drugs[13] (eg, lithium, nonsteroidal anti-inflammatory drugs [NSAIDs], antimalarials such as chloroquine, β-adrenergic blockers, fluoxetine, and withdrawal of corticosteroids), and psoriatic patients commonly have exacerbations during times of stress.[1,4,13] Smoking cigarettes has been shown in two international studies to be a risk factor for psoriasis.[14] Lifestyle intervention to mitigate risk factors has been recommended.[15]

PATHOPHYSIOLOGY

Psoriasis is a common chronic inflammatory disease that involves both adaptive and innate immunity.[4] The interaction between dermal dendritic cells, activated T cells of the TH-1, TH-17 lineage in concert with a multitude of cytokines and growth factors are responsible for the epidermal hyperplasia and dermal inflammation that is seen in the skin of patients with psoriasis. Cross-talk between the innate and adaptive immune systems mediated by cytokines including TNF-α, interferon gamma, and IL-1 is a major research focus.[4]

Comorbidities

It is well documented that psoriasis patients have significant associated comorbidities.[2,4,6] Psoriatic arthritis (PsA) is one of the most common and well-known extracutaneous manifestations of disease. Other associated comorbidities include the metabolic syndrome, other immune-mediated disorders such as Crohn disease, multiple sclerosis, and some psychological illnesses (anxiety, depression, and alcoholism).[16] Also, malignancies such as cutaneous T-cell lymphoma are associated with psoriasis, and melanoma and nonmelanoma skin cancer are associated with psoriasis treatments.

The National Psoriasis Foundation published a clinical consensus on psoriasis comorbidities with recommendations for screening and addressing issues such as cardiovascular risk, metabolic syndrome, and obesity.[17] The importance of screening for comorbidities in psoriasis patients cannot be overemphasized: Nearly half of the psoriatic patients older than age 65 have at least three comorbidities, (with two-thirds of this patient population having two or more comorbidities).[18] The presence of a specific comorbidity in a patient with psoriasis may influence the choice of pharmacotherapy.

PsA usually develops after the onset of psoriasis,[3] typically 10 years later.[16] However, 10% to 15% of patients report that the PsA appeared first.[3] The prevalence of PsA in psoriatic patients is about 30% but varies by disease severity.[16] In one US study, the prevalences were 14% for patients with mild psoriasis, 18% for those with moderate psoriasis, and 56% for patients with severe psoriasis.[19] TNF-α and HLA-Cw6 are linked to both PsA and psoriasis.[20] Although immunomodulating treatments for psoriasis (such as methotrexate [MTX] or TNF-α inhibitors) are useful for PsA, NSAIDs effective for joint symptoms of PsA may exacerbate psoriasis.

The metabolic syndrome is a cluster of risk factors including abdominal obesity, atherogenic dyslipidemia, hypertension, insulin resistance or glucose intolerance, prothrombotic state, and proinflammatory state.[17] Patients with psoriasis are at increased risk of developing the metabolic syndrome.[4,17] The syndrome is a strong predictor of cardiovascular diseases, stroke, and diabetes.[17,21,22] Patients with this syndrome are three times as likely to have a myocardial infarction (MI) or stroke, twice as likely to die from the MI or stroke, and five times as likely to develop type 2 diabetes.[17] A 2010 retrospective analysis of pooled data from three clinical trials (M02-528, CHAMPION, and REVEAL) showed that patients with psoriasis have a 28% and 12% increased 10-year risks of coronary heart disease (CHD) and stroke, respectively.[22]

Patients with psoriasis also have a decreased life expectancy and increased rates of mortality. Psoriasis is an independent risk factor for atherosclerosis, especially for younger patients with severe disease.[17] A 2006 study found that a relative risk (RR) of death for a 30-year-old person with severe psoriasis was 3.10, after controlling for traditional cardiovascular risk factors (eg, age, gender, hypertension, dyslipidemia, diabetes mellitus, smoking, body mass index [BMI], C-reactive protein [CRP], and family history of cardiovascular disease).[17,23] Three epidemiologic meta-analyses identified increased cardiovascular mortality risk (RR: 1.39, 1.37, 1.2) and stroke (RR 1.56, 1.59, and 1.21) for psoriatic patients.[4]

Types of Psoriasis

Plaque psoriasis, also known as *psoriasis vulgaris*, is the most common type of psoriasis (Table 97-1) and is seen in about 90% of psoriasis patients. Clinical presentation of plaque psoriasis is given in Table 97-2.

Up to 30% of patients with psoriasis have associated PsA.[4] Although nail involvement (psoriatic onychodystrophy) can occur with any type of psoriasis, it is seen in up to 90% of patients with PsA.[14] Fingernails are involved in about 50% of all patients with psoriasis and toenails are involved in 35% of patients.[14]

TABLE 97-1 Phenotypic Classifications of Psoriasis

Plaque (also known as psoriasis vulgaris)
Flexural and/or intertriginous (also known as inverse psoriasis)
Seborrheic
Scalp
Acrodermatitis of Hallopeau
Palm and/or soles (also known as palmar/plantar psoriasis)
Generalized pustular psoriasis
Guttate
Erythrodermic

TABLE 97-2 Clinical Presentation of Plaque Psoriasis

Signs and Symptoms of Plaque Psoriasis	
Lesions (plaques)	Erythematous Red-violet in color At least 0.5 cm in diameter Well demarcated—clearly distinguished from normal skin Typically covered by silver, flaking scales
Skin involvement	Either as single lesions at predisposed areas (eg, knees, elbows) or generalized over a wide BSA Mild psoriasis: ≤5% BSA involvement Moderate psoriasis: PASI ≥8 (higher in trials of biologics) Severe psoriasis: The rule of tens: PASI ≥10 or DLQI ≥10 or BSA ≥10% (in some phototherapy trials, BSA ≥20% used as lower limit) Categories in the European consensus: Mild psoriasis: BSA ≤10 and PASI ≤10 and DLQI ≤10. Moderate-to-severe psoriasis: (BSA >10 or PASI >10) and DLQI >10
Pruritus	More than 50% of patients with psoriasis have associated pruritus May be severe in some patients and may require treatment to minimize excoriations from constant scratching
Other associated concerns	Lesions may also be physically debilitating or socially isolating. Potential comorbidities: PsA, depression, hypertension, obesity, diabetes mellitus, Crohn disease, anxiety, alcoholism

BSA, body surface area; DLQI, Dermatology Life Quality Index; PASI, Psoriasis Area and Severity Index; PsA, psoriatic arthritis.

Data from reference 14.

DIAGNOSTIC CONSIDERATIONS

3 The diagnosis of psoriasis is a diagnosis based on recognition of the characteristic psoriatic lesion and not on laboratory tests. Diagnostic testing is rarely performed as a biopsy may be suggestive but is not diagnostic of psoriasis.

Psoriasis is traditionally classified into mild, moderate, or severe disease. In 2011, a European consensus (19 countries) formalized the definition of disease severity and treatment goals and defined plaque psoriasis severity as two main categories: mild versus moderate-to-severe. This became the basis for defining treatment goals in the 2015 European guidelines.[24,25] Both classification systems are in use today. In clinical practice, assessment of the severity of disease includes both an objective evaluation of the extent and symptoms as well as a subjective evaluation of the impact of disease on the patient's quality of life.[14] Assessment typically includes measures of symptom and involvement such as body surface area (BSA), Psoriasis Area and Severity Index (PASI), or Physician's Global Assessment (static PGA), as well as quality-of-life measures such as the Dermatology Life Quality Index (DLQI) or the Short Form (SF-36) Health Survey.[14]

Classification of psoriasis as mild, moderate, or severe disease is generally based on BSA or PASI measurements (see Table 97-2). Practically, to give a rough estimate of BSA involvement, palm size is approximately 1% BSA, head and neck involvement is approximately 10% BSA, both upper limbs approximately 20% BSA, trunk involvement (front and back) approximately 30% BSA, and both lower limbs approximately 40% BSA.

TREATMENT

Treatment of psoriasis is based on managing the underlying pathophysiology. Agents that modulate the abnormal immune response, such as topical corticosteroids (TCS) and biologic response modifiers (BRMs), are important treatment strategies for psoriasis. Topical therapies that affect cell turnover, such as retinoids, are also effective for psoriasis. In addition, nonpharmacologic therapies are effective adjuncts and should be considered for all patients with psoriasis. A treatment regimen should always be individualized, taking into consideration severity of disease, patient responses, and tolerability to various interventions. Furthermore, if comorbidities exist, they must be taken into treatment considerations and managed early. Optimal psoriasis care needs to maintain a focus on the patient's overall health-related quality of life.

Desired Outcomes

4 Goals of treatment for the patient with plaque psoriasis include the following[1]:

- Minimizing or eliminating the visible signs of psoriasis, such as plaques and scales
- Alleviating pruritus and minimizing excoriations
- Reducing the frequency of flare-ups
- Ensuring appropriate treatment of associated comorbid conditions such as PsA, hypertension, dyslipidemia, diabetes, or clinical depression
- Screening for and managing lifestyle factors that may trigger exacerbations (eg, stress, smoking, obesity)[26]
- Minimizing nonspecific triggers such as mild trauma (scratching, piercings, tattoos), sunburn, chemical irritants, environmental/work place factors[4]
- Providing guidance or counseling as needed (eg, stress-reduction techniques, smoking cessation programs)
- Avoiding or minimizing adverse effects from treatments used (topical, phototherapy, and/or systemic)
- Providing cost-effective therapy
- Maintaining or improving the patient's quality of life

Evaluation of Therapeutic Outcomes

Successful management of psoriasis should include not only clearance of skin lesions, which may take weeks to months depending on the severity of disease, but also control of associated conditions such as itching, and, importantly, comorbidities, including dyslipidemia, hypertension, PsA, and clinical depression. The ultimate goal is to provide enough control of this chronic disease and its comorbidities, (if present) so that the patient's quality of life (QOL) is minimally affected.

The 2011 European consensus defined induction and maintenance phases and provided separate treatment goals for induction and maintenance.[24,25] The induction phase is defined as the first 16 weeks of treatment for drugs with a rapid induction to remission (such as adalimumab or infliximab), extending the phase to 24 weeks of treatment for less rapidly effective drugs (such as MTX or etanercept).[25] To be considered successful therapy, a treatment regimen should result in a reduction of PASI greater than or equal to 75%, or PASI of 50% to 75% coupled with a DLQI less than 5.[25] Otherwise, treatment modifications should be considered. Treatment goals should be assessed at 10 to 16 weeks and then every 8 weeks thereafter.[25] It is important to treat beyond clearing visible skin lesions. In fact, a European consensus lead author writes, "Psoriasis is the first dermatological inflammatory disorder where the goal is to manage skin lesions and associated diseases."[26] Comorbidities and trigger factors must be managed as early as possible.

General Approach

5 Management of patients with psoriasis generally involves both nonpharmacologic and pharmacologic therapies. Nonpharmacologic

management strategies are important and should be used for all patients with psoriasis, regardless of the severity of disease. Pharmacologic therapies are always tailored to the individual patient with psoriasis, and different treatment strategies would be used depending on psoriatic disease severity, presence or absence of comorbid illnesses, and any special considerations such as hepatic or renal dysfunction.

Nonpharmacologic Therapy

6 Nonpharmacologic alternatives may be very beneficial and should always be considered and initiated when appropriate.[1] These include stress-reduction strategies, moisturizers, oatmeal baths, and skin protection using sunscreens.[27]

In particular, stress reduction has been shown to improve both the extent and severity of psoriasis, and includes methods such as guided imagery and stress-management clinics. Liberal use of nonmedicated moisturizers, applied ad lib, helps maintain skin moisture, reduces skin shedding, controls associated scaling, and may reduce pruritus. Oatmeal baths further reduce pruritus and with regular use may minimize the need for systemic antipruritic drugs.

Sunscreens, preferably with a sun protection factor (SPF) of 30 or more, should be regularly used because sunburns can trigger an exacerbation of psoriasis. Irritation to the skin should be minimized—harsh soaps or detergents should not be used. Cleansing should be done with tepid water and preferably with lipid-free and fragrance-free cleansers.[1,27]

For patients with comorbidities such as dyslipidemia, obesity, or cardiovascular disease, cessation of nicotine and alcohol consumption, diet control, and increasing physical activity are all important interventions.[2,26]

Pharmacologic Therapy

7 Pharmacologic alternatives for psoriasis are topical agents, phototherapy, and systemic agents, including biologic response modifiers (BRMs).

Drug Treatments of First Choice

8 For limited or mild to moderately severe disease, topical treatments are the usual standard of care, with phototherapy and photochemotherapy used in moderate-to-severe cases. For patients presenting with extensive or moderate-to-severe disease, systemic therapies with or without the use of topical treatments are the usual standard of care. Newer systemic treatments such as BRMs may be the treatments of choice, especially for patients with comorbidities such as PsA or if traditional systemic treatments (such as MTX or cyclosporine) are contraindicated. Once the disease is under control, it would be important to step down to the least potent, least toxic agent(s) that maintain control. 9 Sequential therapy and rotational therapy may minimize drug-associated toxicities; however, continuous treatment is now the standard of care for many dermatologists. Different treatment algorithms are used, depending on the severity of the plaque psoriasis (Figs. 97-1 and 97-2).[1]

Published Guidelines or Treatment Protocols There are treatment guidelines for both Canada and the United States.[14,28-35] All US guidelines are endorsed by the American Academy of Dermatology or the National Psoriasis Foundation, and Canadian guidelines are endorsed by the Canadian Dermatology Association. In Europe, guidelines from the British Association of Dermatologists[36] and a European 19-country consensus have been published.[24,25] These guidelines represent the current standards of care.

Topical Therapies

Approximately 80% of patients with psoriasis have mild-to-moderate disease,[30] and the majority of these patients can be treated with topical therapies alone.[30] Individualized approaches are essential because of the wide variation in patients' presentations, their psychosocial health, and their personal opinions as to what would be acceptable treatment.[14] Topical therapies include corticosteroids, vitamin D_3 analogs, retinoids, anthralin, and coal tar. In addition, topical calcineurin inhibitors may be useful for difficult-to-treat sites such as the intertriginous areas or the face.[4] These are generally efficacious and safe for this patient population. Topical agents are also used as adjunctive therapy for patients with more extensive disease who are being treated concurrently with phototherapy or systemic agents.

To determine the quantity of topical agents required, the fingertip unit[37] can be used. One fingertip unit is approximately 500 mg,[30,37] which is sufficient to cover one hand (front and back) or about 2% BSA.[38] The trunk (front and back) is about 30% BSA; to cover the entire trunk once, about 15 fingertip units, or 7,500 mg (7.5 g), would be required.

In a 2012 systematic review of topical and phototherapies for psoriasis by dermatologists in France, nine recommendations based on evidence and expert opinion are offered. However, quality

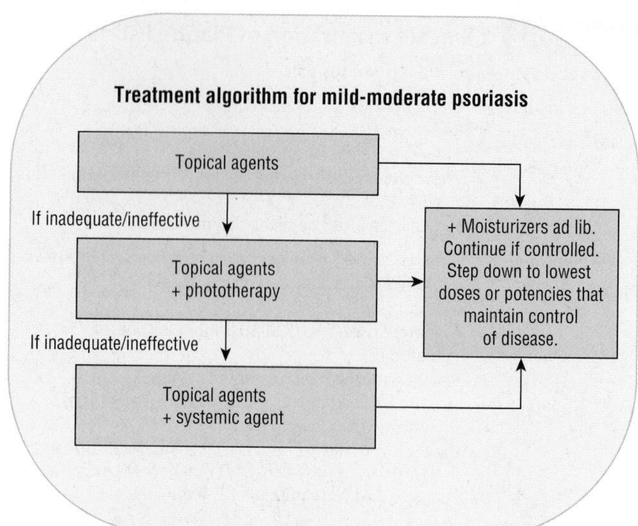

FIGURE 97-1 Treatment algorithm for mild-to-moderate psoriasis. *Reproduced with permission from Law RM. Chapter 64: Psoriasis. In: Chisholm-Burns M, ed. Pharmacotherapy Principles and Practice, 3rd ed. New York: McGraw-Hill, 2013:1127-1141.*

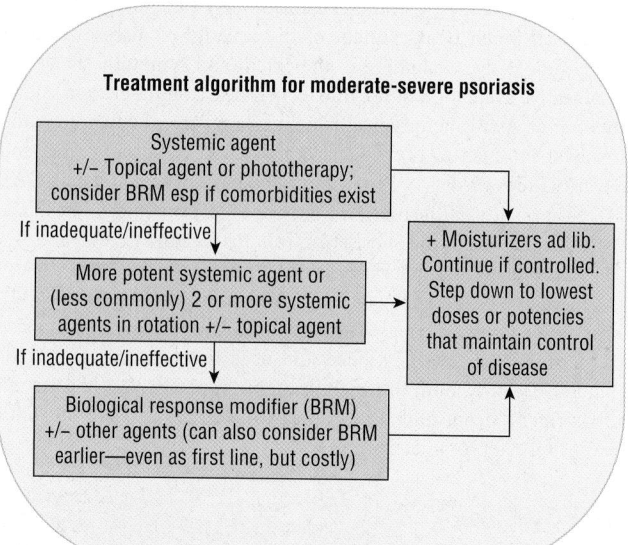

FIGURE 97-2 Treatment algorithm for moderate-to-severe psoriasis. *Reproduced with permission from Law RM. Chapter 64: Psoriasis. In: Chisholm-Burns M, ed. Pharmacotherapy Principles and Practice, 3rd ed. New York: McGraw-Hill, 2013:1127-1141.*

literature was limited, and the recommendations relating to optimal steroid use and optimal first-line treatment for psoriasis did not reach 80% consensus.[37]

Corticosteroids Topical corticosteroids have been the mainstay of therapy for the majority of patients with psoriasis for over half a century. They are generally well tolerated, although adverse effects can occur, including systemic ones on occasion. Table 97-3 provides a summary of topical corticosteroid formulations—including ointments, creams, gels, foams, lotions, sprays, shampoos, tape, and solutions[30]—and potencies.

The choice of vehicle affects corticosteroid potency: Ointments, being the most occlusive, enhance drug penetration and provide the most potent formulations. However, patients may prefer a

TABLE 97-3 Topical Corticosteroid Potency Chart

Potency Rating	Corticosteroid—Topical Preparations
Class 1: Superpotent	Betamethasone dipropionate 0.05% ointment (Diprolene and Diprosone ointment)
	Clobetasol propionate 0.05% lotion/spray/shampoo/foam (Clobex lotion/spray/shampoo, OLUX-E foam)
	Clobetasol propionate 0.05% cream and ointment (Cormax, Temovate, Dermovate)
	Desoximetasone 0.25% spray (Topicort)
	Fluocinonide 0.1% cream (Vanos)
	Halobetasol propionate 0.05% cream, lotion, and ointment (Ultravate)
	Flurandrenolide tape 4 mcg/cm² (Cordran)
Class 2: Potent	Amcinonide 0.1% ointment (Cyclocort ointment)
	Betamethasone dipropionate 0.05% cream/gel (Diprolene cream, gel, and Diprosone cream)
	Desoximetasone 0.25% cream, ointment (Topicort)
	Diflorasone diacetate 0.05% ointment (Florone, Psorcon)
	Fluocinonide 0.05% cream, gel, ointment (Lidex)
	Halcinonide 0.1% cream (Halog)
Class 3: Upper mid-strength	Amcinonide 0.1% cream (Cyclocort cream)
	Betamethasone valerate 0.1% ointment (Betnovate/Valisone ointment)
	Diflorasone diacetate 0.05% cream (Psorcon cream)
	Fluticasone propionate 0.005% ointment (Cutivate ointment)
	Mometasone furoate 0.1% ointment (Elocon ointment)
	Triamcinolone acetonide 0.5% cream and ointment (Aristocort)
Class 4: Mid-strength	Betamethasone valerate 0.12% foam (Luxiq)
	Clocortolone pivalate 0.1% cream (Cloderm)
	Desoximetasone 0.05% cream, ointment, and gel (Topicort LP)
	Fluocinolone acetonide 0.025% ointment (Synalar ointment)
	Fluocinolone acetonide 0.2% cream (Synalar-HP)
	Flurandrenolide 0.05% ointment (Cordran)
	Hydrocortisone valerate 0.2% ointment (Westcort ointment)
	Mometasone furoate 0.1% cream (Elocon cream)
	Triamcinolone acetonide 0.1% ointment (Kenalog)
Class 5: Lower mid-strength	Betamethasone dipropionate 0.05% lotion (Diprosone lotion)
	Betamethasone valerate 0.1% cream and lotion (Betnovate/Valisone cream & lotion)
	Desonide 0.05% lotion (DesOwen)
	Fluocinolone acetonide 0.01% shampoo (Capex shampoo)
	Fluocinolone acetonide 0.025%, 0.03% cream (Synalar cream)
	Flurandrenolide 0.05% cream and lotion (Cordran)
	Fluticasone propionate 0.05% cream and lotion (Cutivate cream and lotion)
	Hydrocortisone butyrate 0.1% cream (Locoid)
	Hydrocortisone valerate 0.2% cream (Westcort cream)
	Prednicarbate 0.1% cream (Dermatop)
	Triamcinolone acetonide 0.1% cream and lotion (Kenalog cream and lotion)
Class 6: Mild	Alclometasone dipropionate 0.05% cream and ointment (Aclovate)
	Betamethasone valerate 0.05% cream and ointment
	Desonide 0.05% cream, ointment, gel (DesOwen, Desonate, Tridesilon)
	Desonide 0.05% foam (Verdeso)
	Fluocinolone acetonide 0.01% cream and solution (Synalar)
	Fluocinolone acetonide 0.01% FS oil (Derma-Smoothe)
Class 7: Least Potent	Hydrocortisone 0.5%, 1%, 2%, 2.5% cream, lotion, spray, and ointment (various brands)

Data from The National Psoriasis Foundation—Mild Psoriasis: Steroid potency chart, http://www.psoriasis.org/netcommunity/sublearn03_mild_potency. Rosso JD, Friedlander SF. Corticosteroids: Options in the era of steroid-sparing therapy. J Am Acad Dermatol 2005;53:S50-S58; Leung DYM, Nicklas RA, Li JT, et al. Disease management of atopic dermatitis: An updated practice parameter. Ann Allergy Asthma Immunol 2004;93:S1-S17.

less greasy formulation, such as a cream or lotion for daytime use, although they may be willing to apply the more effective ointment-based corticosteroid during the night.[30] Providing additional occlusion will increase drug penetration of a topical preparation, resulting in enhanced potency. For example, flurandrenolide cream and lotion are potency class 5, but flurandrenolide tape was found to have higher efficacy than diflorasone diacetate ointment (potency class 1).[30,39,40]

Despite their widespread use, there have been few large-scale, randomized placebo-controlled corticosteroid trials and even fewer head-to-head comparisons with other therapies. The most comprehensive review to date is the analysis of topical psoriasis therapies done in 2002 but recent studies aren't included so this review was already somewhat out of date when published.[14,41] This systematic review found that all topical corticosteroid treatments considered were efficacious and significantly better than placebo; and that the highest potency corticosteroids were the most efficacious, followed by vitamin D_3 analogs.[14] The French group in 2012 found variable efficacy in their systematic review, noting that recommendations about topical steroid use should be mostly based on expert opinion, and that maintenance intermittent treatment may prolong remission.[42]

Corticosteroids have anti-inflammatory, antiproliferative, immunosuppressive, and vasoconstrictive effects.[30] These are mediated through a variety of mechanisms. Mechanisms of action include binding to intracellular corticosteroid receptors and regulation of gene transcription (in particular those which code for proinflammatory cytokines).[30]

Appropriate use of topical corticosteroids should include an assessment of disease severity and disease location as well as knowledge of the patient's preference and age. Lower potency corticosteroids should be used for infants and for lesions on the face, intertriginous areas, and areas with thin skin. For other areas of the body in adults, mid- to high-potency agents are generally recommended as initial therapy.[30] The highest potency corticosteroids are generally reserved for patients with very thick plaques or recalcitrant disease, such as plaques on palms and soles. The use of potency class 1 corticosteroids should be limited to a duration of 2 to 4 weeks,[30] recognizing that the risk of cutaneous and systemic side effects increases with continued use.

Cutaneous adverse effects include skin atrophy, acne, contact dermatitis, hypertrichosis, folliculitis, hypopigmentation, perioral dermatitis, striae, telangiectases, and traumatic purpura.[14,30] Systemic adverse effects have been reported not only with superpotent corticosteroids but also with extended or widespread use of mid-potency agents.[30] Systemic adverse effects include hypothalamic–pituitary–adrenal (HPA) axis suppression and less commonly Cushing syndrome, osteonecrosis of the femoral head, cataracts, and glaucoma.[30] All topical corticosteroids are pregnancy category C.[30]

Tachyphylaxis can occur with prolonged use, although its clinical significance is difficult to verify.[14] It is recommended that the frequency of use be gradually reduced once clinical response is seen, although there are no established tapering regimens.[30] The French group recommended twice-weekly maintenance therapy.[37] Other approaches include transitioning to weaker potency agents or combination with other nonsteroidal topical therapies.[30] Pulse dosing has also been used to minimize tachyphylaxis and adverse effects.[43]

Vitamin D_3 Analogs Topical vitamin D_3 analogs include calcipotriol (calcipotriene), calcitriol (the active metabolite of vitamin D), and tacalcitol. Only calcipotriol is currently available in the United States[30] and Canada.[14] Other analogs currently under study include maxacalcitol and becocalcidiol.[30] Their mechanisms of action include binding to vitamin D receptors, which results in inhibition of keratinocyte proliferation and enhancement of keratinocyte differentiation.[14,30] They also inhibit T-lymphocyte activity.[14]

The efficacy of calcipotriol for patients with mild psoriasis is well established in randomized double-blind placebo-controlled (DBPC) trials. In head-to-head comparison studies with other topical agents, calcipotriol was found to be more effective than anthralin (dithranol)[44] and comparable or slightly more effective than potency class 3 (upper mid-strength) topical corticosteroid ointments such as betamethasone valerate 0.1% ointment.[14,45,46] In an analysis of topical psoriasis therapies done in 2002,[41] calcipotriol was found to be as effective as all but the most potent topical corticosteroids.[14] Combination therapy with a topical steroid is particularly effective[47] and is discussed later in the chapter.

Vitamin D_3 analogs are generally well tolerated and have a good safety profile in comparison with other topical therapies.[47] They are considered the safest long-term topical treatments.[4] Cutaneous adverse effects most commonly include a mild irritant contact dermatitis; others include burning, pruritus, edema, peeling, dryness, and erythema.[14,30] These adverse effects may be mitigated with continued use.[30] Systemic adverse effects, including hypercalcemia and parathyroid hormone suppression, are rare unless patients are using more than the recommended maximum of 5 mg calcipotriol (100 g of calcipotriol 50 mcg/g cream or ointment) per week[14,30] or if there is underlying renal disease or impaired calcium metabolism.[30] When applied sparingly over a BSA of less than 30%, the risk of hypercalcemia is remote.[37]

Calcipotriol is pregnancy category C. It is inactivated by ultraviolet A (UVA) light thus it should be applied after rather than before UVA light exposure.[30]

Retinoids Tazarotene is a topical retinoid that acts through the following mechanisms: normalizing abnormal keratinocyte differentiation, diminishing keratinocyte hyperproliferation, and clearing the inflammatory infiltrate in the psoriatic plaque.[14,30] It is effective in clearing psoriatic plaque lesions and achieving remission.

In a placebo-controlled trial of tazarotene 0.1% and 0.05% gels for patients with plaque psoriasis, tazarotene provided a 50% or greater improvement in 63% (0.1% gel) and 50% (0.05% gel) of patients, respectively, after 12 weeks of use.[48] The therapeutic benefit appears to be maintained for 12 weeks after cessation of therapy.[48] Later clinical trials with tazarotene 0.1% and 0.05% creams versus a placebo vehicle provided similar findings.[49] The 2012 systematic review similarly found that about 50% of patients experienced a 50% or more improvement with no difference in formulations.[37]

Adverse effects of tazarotene include a high incidence of irritation at the site of application, a dose-dependent effect.[14] This results in burning, itching, and erythema, which can occur in lesional and perilesional skin.[30] Irritation may be reduced by using the cream formulation, lower concentration, alternate-day application, or short-contact (30-60 minutes) treatment.[30] Ad lib use of moisturizers is also beneficial. Tazarotene is also potentially photosensitizing, due to thinning of the epidermis that can occur with continued use.[30]

Tazarotene is pregnancy category X and should not be used in women of childbearing age unless effective contraception is being used.

Anthralin Anthralin is not as commonly used as other topical therapies currently available for psoriasis; however, there are situations where its use is appropriate and efficacious. It has a direct antiproliferative effect on epidermal keratinocytes,[1,14] normalizing keratinocyte differentiation.[30] Although the exact mechanism of action is unknown, it may have a direct effect on mitochondria[30,50] and reduce the mitotic activity. It also prevents T-lymphocyte activation.[30] Small placebo-controlled studies demonstrated efficacy for anthralin used continuously or as very short contact (1 minute of treatment).[30]

Currently, short-contact anthralin therapy (SCAT) is usually the preferred regimen, where the anthralin ointment is applied only to the thick plaque lesions for 2 hours or less and then wiped off.[1,30] Because lesions are generally well demarcated, zinc oxide ointment or a nonmedicated stiff paste should be applied to the surrounding normal skin to protect it from irritation and burning. Anthralin should be used with caution, if at all, on the face and intertriginous areas because of the risk of severe skin irritation.[30]

Concentrations for SCAT range from 1% to 4% or as tolerated; concentrations for continuous anthralin therapy vary from 0.05% to 0.4%. Note the 10-fold concentration differences. Aside from significant and often severe skin irritation, other adverse effects include folliculitis and allergic contact dermatitis, but these are uncommon.

Anthralin is pregnancy category C. People who handle the dry anthralin powder should avoid skin contact (eg, by wearing gloves while compounding).[1]

Coal Tar Coal tar was one of the earliest agents used to treat psoriasis. It is keratolytic and may have antiproliferative and anti-inflammatory effects.[1] Coal tar formulations include crude coal tar and tar distillates (liquor carbonis detergens) in ointments, creams, and shampoos. Because of limited efficacy coupled with patient acceptance and compliance issues, coal tar preparations are less commonly used today, especially in North American and European[37] countries.

A 2007 comparative study in Thailand reported that betamethasone valerate was significantly more effective than coal tar.[14,51] Although coal tar may have similar efficacy as calcipotriol, it has a slower onset of action.[14] In addition, coal tar has an unpleasant odor and will stain clothing; thus, it may be cosmetically unappealing to patients.

Adverse effects include folliculitis, acne, local irritation, and phototoxicity.[14] It is carcinogenic in animals, but for humans no convincing data have emerged regarding carcinogenicity with topical use.[30]

Coal tar concentrations as used in psoriasis treatments (0.5%-5%) are considered safe by the Food and Drug Administration (FDA).[33] However, occupational exposure to coal tar, especially in very high concentrations such as coal tar used in industrial paving,[33] was reported to increase the risk of lung cancer, scrotal cancer, and skin cancer.[30,33] The risk of teratogenicity when used in pregnancy is likely to be small, if it exists.[30]

Salicylic Acid Salicylic acid has keratolytic properties and has been used in various formulations including shampoos or bath oils for patients with scalp psoriasis. In combination with topical corticosteroids, it enhances steroid penetration thus increasing efficacy. It should not be used in combination with ultraviolet B (UVB) light phototherapy because of a filtering effect that may reduce efficacy. Systemic absorption and toxicity can occur, especially when applied to more than 20% BSA or when used in patients with renal impairment.

Avoid the use of salicylic acid in children. However, it may be used for limited and localized plaque psoriasis in pregnancy.[30]

Calcineurin Inhibitors Topical calcineurin inhibitors such as pimecrolimus 1% cream (Elidel) are used for the treatment of inflammatory skin diseases such as atopic dermatitis.[52-54] Pimecrolimus was found to be effective for plaque psoriasis when used under occlusion[53] and also effective for patients with moderate-to-severe inverse psoriasis (intertriginous areas are affected).[54] Because this cream is less irritating than calcipotriol and also avoids steroid adverse effects such as skin atrophy, it may be a useful alternative for patients with lesions in intertriginous areas or on the face.[4]

Phototherapies and Photochemotherapy

Phototherapy has been used for treating psoriasis for years and is still an important treatment modality today. It has been known for centuries that some skin diseases improve with sun exposure, and clinical studies with phototherapies have been reported since the late 19th century.[28] Phototherapy consists of using nonionizing electromagnetic radiation, either UVA or UVB, as light therapy to treat psoriatic lesions.[55]

UVB is given alone as either broadband or narrowband UVB (NB-UVB), currently with NB-UVB being the preferred method. UVB is also given as photochemotherapy with topical agents such as crude coal tar (Goeckerman regimen)[55] or anthralin (Ingram regimen) for enhanced efficacy.[28]

UVA is generally given with a photosensitizer, such as an oral psoralens, to enhance efficacy—this regimen is known as PUVA (photochemotherapy with oral methoxypsoralen and ultraviolet A light).[55]

With respect to comparative efficacy, NB-UVB is more efficacious than broadband UVB, but may be slightly less effective than PUVA.[28,56] PUVA is very effective in the majority of patients, with the potential for long remissions.[28] A meta-analysis showed that more patients are still clear at 6 months with PUVA versus with NB-UVB.[56] However, because of greater availability of UVB treatment centers, more evidence available now of the efficacy of UVB treatments for psoriasis (in particular, NB-UVB), and especially the increasing concerns about PUVA toxicities (including skin cancers), phototherapy for psoriasis currently uses UVB or NB-UVB where available. Failure of NB-UVB may justify PUVA therapy.[55]

UVB interferes with protein and nucleic acid synthesis, leading to decreased proliferation of epidermal keratinocytes.[28] UVA has similar effects on epidermal keratinocytes. However, because of deeper penetration into the dermis, it also has effects on dermal dendritic cells, fibroblasts, endothelial cells, mast cells, and skin-infiltrating inflammatory cells including granulocytes and T lymphocytes.[28]

Adverse effects of phototherapy include erythema, pruritus, xerosis, hyperpigmentation, and blistering, especially with higher dosages. It should be used with caution for patients with photosensitivity concerns, and drug interactions include photosensitizing medications such as tetracyclines. Patients must be provided with eye protection during UVB, NB-UVB, or PUVA treatments, and for 24 hours[55] or the remainder of the day[28] after PUVA treatments. In addition, patients receiving PUVA therapy may experience gastrointestinal symptoms such as nausea or vomiting, which may be minimized by taking the oral psoralens with food or milk.[28] For patients also receiving oral retinoids plus PUVA (RE-PUVA), the UVA dose should be reduced by one-third.[28] Long-term PUVA use can lead to photoaging and the development of PUVA lentigines. Psoralens bind to proteins in the lens of the eye; thus, there is a potential for increased cataract formation.

Furthermore, although UVB has a theoretical risk of photocarcinogenesis, the risk is significantly higher with PUVA and is dose related.[28,55] A meta-analysis reported a 14-fold increase in the incidence of squamous cell carcinoma (SCC) in patients receiving high-dose PUVA when compared with low-dose PUVA, with SCC of the male genitalia particularly elevated.[28,57] PUVA may also increase the risk of basal cell carcinoma and possibly melanoma,[28] which may occur 15 years after the first treatment.[55] Thus, the use of phototherapy or photochemotherapy is contraindicated in patients with a history of melanoma or multiple nonmelanoma skin cancers.

Targeted phototherapy using excimer lasers that selectively target psoriatic lesions without affecting normal skin is an option being studied and early results appear promising, although blistering and burning of treated lesions are more common, and long-term safety has not been established.[28]

Systemic Therapies

Systemic therapies are the mainstay of treatment for patients with moderate-to-severe psoriasis, with topical therapies remaining as useful adjuncts. However, as discussed below under combination therapies, topical calcipotriol and betamethasone dipropionate ointment may provide sufficient disease control for some patients.[14,58] Conversely, a subset of patients with limited disease may have debilitating symptoms, and the use of systemic therapies would be warranted.[29] Systemic therapies include the following traditional agents: acitretin, cyclosporine, MTX, mycophenolate mofetil (MMF), and hydroxyurea; as well as the newer BRMs, specifically adalimumab, alefacept, etanercept, infliximab, ustekinumab, and secukinumab.

Acitretin In the 1980s, etretinate became the first oral retinoid, or vitamin A acid derivative, available for the treatment of psoriasis. It has since been replaced by acitretin, its active metabolite.

Retinoids may be less effective than MTX or cyclosporine when used as monotherapy,[4] although the initial response may be more rapid than MTX for patients with severe inflammatory forms of psoriasis. Currently, acitretin is more commonly used in combination with topical calcipotriol or phototherapy.[14,29] Its efficacy appears to be dose dependent.[29] Although low-dose acitretin (25 mg/day) is safer and better tolerated than higher-dose (50 mg/day) therapy,[14] low-dose acitretin is not recommended as monotherapy.[4]

Common adverse effects of acitretin include hypertriglyceridemia and mucocutaneous adverse effects such as dryness of the eyes, nasal and oral mucosa, chapped lips, cheilitis, epistaxis, xerosis, brittle nails, and burning or sticky skin.[14,29] Less commonly, "retinoid dermatitis" may occur. Ophthalmologic changes include photosensitivity, decreased color vision and impaired night vision.[24] GI adverse effects including hepatitis and jaundice are rare with liver enzyme elevations usually being transient.[24] Periungual pyogenic granulomas are sometimes seen after long-term use of acitretin.[29] Rarely, skeletal abnormalities—such as disseminated idiopathic skeletal hyperostosis (DISH) syndrome—may occur.[14]

All retinoids are teratogenic and are pregnancy category X, including topical retinoids. Acitretin should not be used for women of childbearing age unless they are able and willing to use effective birth control not only for the duration of acitretin therapy but also for at least 2 years after discontinuing the agent.[14,24,29] Blood donation (men and women) is not permitted during and for at least 1 year after treatment.[24] Ethanol should be avoided during therapy and for 2 months after drug discontinuation because it causes the transesterification of acitretin to etretinate, which has a much longer elimination half-life.

Cyclosporine Cyclosporine is a systemic calcineurin inhibitor. The more bioavailable microemulsion formulation, Neoral, was approved by the FDA in 1997 for the treatment of psoriasis and rheumatoid arthritis.[32]

Cyclosporine is efficacious for both inducing remission and as maintenance therapy for patients with moderate-to-severe plaque psoriasis. It is also effective in treating pustular, erythrodermic, and nail psoriasis.[32] The 2009 Canadian Guidelines recommended that cyclosporine be normally reserved for intermittent use in periods up to 12 weeks for most patients with psoriasis,[14] although other recommendations are for periods of 1 year or up to 2 years.[32] Risk of toxicity increases with treatment duration: intermittent short-course therapy (less than 12 weeks) is preferable since this appears to significantly reduce the risk of nephrotoxicity as compared with continuous therapy.[14,24,32]

In comparative randomized controlled trials (RCTs), cyclosporine was significantly more effective than etretinate[59] and similar or slightly better in efficacy than MTX.[14,32,60] After inducing remission, maintenance therapy using low doses (1.25-3.0 mg/kg/day) may prevent relapse.[32] The dose should always be titrated to the lowest effective dose for maintenance. In one placebo-controlled study, the relapse rate was 42% for patients on 3.0 mg/kg/day versus 84% for patients on placebo.[61] For patients discontinuing cyclosporine, a gradual taper of 1 mg/kg/day each week may prolong the time before relapse, as compared with abrupt discontinuation.[29,32] Abrupt discontinuation resulted in a dramatic rebound of psoriasis in a few cases.[14] Because more than half of patients discontinuing cyclosporine will relapse within 4 months, patients should be provided with appropriate alternative treatments shortly before or after discontinuing cyclosporine therapy.[32]

Adverse effects of cyclosporine include cumulative renal toxicity, hypertension, and hypertriglyceridemia. The latter two are particularly significant for patients with prior elevation of diastolic blood pressure or triglycerides.[14] Hypertriglyceridemia can occur in up to 15% of patients with psoriasis who are treated with cyclosporine, although this effect is generally reversible upon cessation of therapy.[29]

The risk of SCC and other nonmelanoma skin cancers increases with duration of treatment[14] and with prior PUVA treatments.[29] Thus, although continuous therapy for up to 2 years may be efficacious,[32] it should be used only in a subset of patients[14] in whom renal function is monitored with annual determinations of glomerular filtration rate (GFR) and monthly measurements of blood pressure and creatinine clearance, with more frequent measurements during the initial 6 weeks of treatment.[14]

Baseline blood pressure, serum creatinine, serum urea nitrogen, triglycerides, complete blood count (CBC), uric acid, potassium, and magnesium should be obtained before initiating therapy, every 2 weeks for the first 12 weeks of therapy, and monitored monthly thereafter during therapy.[14,32] If the serum creatinine increases to 25% above the patient's baseline on 2 occasions (2 weeks apart), the cyclosporine dosage needs to be decreased by 25% to 50% and serum creatinine rechecked as often as every other week for 1 month. If the serum creatinine does not return to within 10% of the patient's baseline value, a further dose decrease of 25% to 50% should be considered. If the value continues to be greater than10% above the patient's baseline value, consider discontinuing cyclosporine therapy.[32] (Note: A 25% above-baseline cutoff for dosage reduction is the manufacturer's recommendation; the National Psoriasis Foundation consensus guidelines continue to recommend a 30% cutoff).[32] Age-appropriate malignancy screens should also be done, and patients should be seen for dental examinations at least yearly because of the risk of gingival hyperplasia.[32]

As a cytochrome P450 isoenzyme 3A4 (CYP3A4) substrate, cyclosporine has significant drug interactions. Serum concentration monitoring is not routinely needed for patients with psoriasis because doses used are lower than in transplant recipients, although monitoring may be advisable for patients taking interacting drugs.

Drugs that can increase cyclosporine concentrations include calcium channel blockers (verapamil, diltiazem, and nicardipine), amiodarone, thiazide diuretics, macrolide antibiotics, allopurinol, oral contraceptives, ezetimibe, selective serotonin reuptake inhibitors (fluoxetine, sertraline), fluoroquinolones (ciprofloxacin, norfloxacin), antifungals (ketoconazole, itraconazole, fluconazole, voriconazole), and cimetidine.[32] Grapefruit juice will also increase cyclosporine concentrations.

Drugs that can reduce cyclosporine concentrations include anticonvulsants (carbamazepine, oxcarbazepine, phenobarbital, phenytoin, valproic acid), rifampin, efavirenz, and St. John's wort.[32]

Conversely, cyclosporine may also affect the drug levels of some drugs. Concurrent use of potentially interacting drugs should be avoided when possible.

Methotrexate For decades, MTX has been the mainstay of systemic therapy for patients with moderate-to-severe psoriasis. It has direct anti-inflammatory benefits due to its effects on T-cell gene expression and also has cytostatic effects.[14] It is more efficacious than acitretin and similar or slightly less efficacious than cyclosporine.[14,34]

Although it also has a significant adverse effects profile, MTX is generally considered a safer alternative than cyclosporine unless there are preexisting contraindications such as liver disease. In some head-to-head clinical studies more patients dropped out of the cyclosporine treatment arms due to adverse effects.[29,34] While BRMs are undoubtedly more efficacious, they are much more costly, and some insurance companies require an inadequate response or intolerance to MTX (the gold standard) as a prerequisite for approving their use.[34] In a recent placebo-controlled comparative study with adalimumab (CHAMPION), the efficacy of MTX was 36% versus 80% for adalimumab and 19% for placebo.[62] Adalimumab also provided a more rapid response; however, the duration of remission is unclear.

Initial doses of 7.5 to 15 mg/week may be increased to 20 to 25 mg/week if the response is inadequate at 8 to 12 weeks, with appropriate adverse effect monitoring. MTX can be used continuously for years or decades with sustained benefits.[14] MTX inhibits folate biosynthesis; and the use of folate supplementation during prolonged MTX therapy as seen in dermatology remains controversial.[29,34]

Clinical **Controversy...**

FOLATE SUPPLEMENTATION FOR MTX THERAPY

Although some experts recommend folate supplementation for all patients receiving MTX for psoriasis, others add folate only when patient issues occur, such as gastrointestinal adverse effects or early bone marrow toxicity (as manifested by an increased mean corpuscular volume) that can be caused by megaloblastic anemia. Lack of folate supplementation has also been listed as a risk factor for hepatotoxicity from MTX use. One small 2006 placebo-controlled study in patients with psoriasis suggested that folate supplementation may result in a slight decrease in efficacy of treatment, but the study methodology has been questioned. A 2013 Cochrane review of folic acid and folinic acid for patients with rheumatoid arthritis who were on MTX also addressed this concern but found that supplementation did not appear to affect MTX efficacy while reducing some MTX side effects such as GI symptoms. (Available at: http://onlinelibrary.wiley.com/doi/10.1002/14651858.CD000951.pub2/full)

The most significant adverse effect is cumulative liver toxicity; and total lifetime dose of MTX must be monitored. Traditionally, patients received a pretreatment liver biopsy and subsequent biopsies when a cumulative dose of 1.5 g is reached. Liver biopsy is the gold standard for assessing histological changes and provides an invasive marker of liver fibrosis. Currently, it is recognized that pretreatment liver biopsies may not be practical or appropriate in all cases[14,34] and that baseline liver biopsies only be considered for patients with a history of significant liver disease.[34] It has also been recommended that a baseline liver biopsy be delayed for 2 to 6 months so that medication efficacy and tolerability can first be established[34] (ie, intention to continue with MTX use). Risk factors for hepatotoxicity from MTX include the following: a history of or current alcohol consumption, persistent abnormal liver chemistry studies, history of liver disease including chronic hepatitis B or C, family history of inheritable liver disease, history of significant exposure to hepatotoxic drugs or chemicals, diabetes mellitus, obesity, and hyperlipidemia.[29,34] For patients without preexisting risk factors for hepatotoxicity, it is recognized that they would likely have a low risk of fibrosis and would not require a baseline liver biopsy; furthermore, consideration can be made to continue MTX treatment for these patients without biopsies at all, to perform a liver biopsy after 3.5 to 4.0 g total cumulative dose, or to switch therapy to an alternate drug at that point.[29,34]

There are noninvasive markers of liver fibrosis, in particular the procollagen type III N-terminal peptide (P3NP or PIIINP) serum level, and the 2015 European recommendation for MTX monitoring is PIIINP determination before starting MTX and every 3 months thereafter.[24] However, a systematic review and meta-analysis of the diagnostic accuracy of non-invasive markers of liver fibrosis in patients with psoriasis taking MTX reported that: (1) the likelihood ratios for P3NP were suboptimal for it to be considered a "good test" and (2) liver function tests (LFTs) demonstrate low diagnostic accuracy for the detection of fibrosis; and the conclusion was that the clinical utility of LFTs, P3NP and liver ultrasound is poor, and that if these tests are used in isolation, a significant proportion of patients with liver fibrosis may remain unidentified.[63] Thus MTX monitoring recommendations currently differ between continents.

Other adverse effects include significant nausea, pulmonary toxicity, pancytopenia, acute myelosuppression, megaloblastic anemia, and a small but significant increase in lymphoma.[14] Although rare, pancytopenia can occur anytime with the use of low-dose weekly MTX and even after single doses of MTX.[29] Informing patients about the early symptoms of pancytopenia (dry cough, nausea, fever, dyspnea, cyanosis, stomatitis/oral symptoms, and bleeding) may aid early detection.[24] MTX is an abortifacient and is teratogenic (pregnancy category X) and should not be used in pregnancy. After MTX therapy is discontinued, it is recommended that men continue an effective birth control for 3 months (as one cycle of spermatogenesis is 74 days), and women should be on effective birth control for at least one ovulatory cycle.[14,29]

Significant drug interactions include serum albumin binding interactions with salicylates, phenytoin, sulfonamides/trimethoprim, ciprofloxacin, and thiazide diuretics, potentially increasing toxicity. Drugs that can reduce MTX renal elimination (such as acidic drugs, including salicylates or vitamin C) will also increase serum MTX levels and hence increase toxicity. In addition, drugs with hepatotoxic potential may pose an additive risk with MTX use.[29]

Systemic Therapy with Biologic Response Modifiers

10 Some BRMs have proven efficacy for psoriasis; however, there are differences among these agents, including mechanism of action, duration of remission, and adverse-effect profile. In general, because of their immunomodulatory effects, there is an increased risk of infection with most of these agents, including serious infections such as sepsis, new-onset or reactivation of tuberculosis (TB), and opportunistic infections such as histoplasmosis, cryptococcosis, aspergillosis, candidiasis, and pneumocystis. The use of live or live-attenuated vaccines during therapy is generally contraindicated. Currently, BRMs are often considered for patients with moderate-to-severe psoriasis when other systemic agents are inadequate or relatively contraindicated. BRMs are sometimes recommended for first-line therapy, alongside conventional systemic agents, for patients with moderate-to-severe psoriasis; however, in practice, drug access due to cost considerations may be a limiting factor. BRMs may be appropriate/preferred as first-line therapy if comorbidities exist. For example, BRMs such as infliximab or adalimumab would be an appropriate treatment option for patients with both plaque psoriasis and active PsA. BRMs currently available for treatment of psoriasis include adalimumab, alefacept, etanercept, infliximab, ustekinumab, and secukinumab.[64,65]

Currently, a number of RCTs describe short-term efficacy of various BRMs for psoriasis but few long-term studies are available. A recent 3-year open-label extension of a 1-year adalimumab phase 3 trial (REVEAL) has demonstrated sustained response with continuous use in initial PASI 75 responders, as discussed below.[66] More clinical evidence has enabled the development of guidelines in an attempt to optimize BRM therapies for psoriasis.[24,25,31,65] The current European consensus recommends either adalimumab or infliximab with etanercept as a suggested alternative,[24] but these guidelines are incomplete as newer BRMs such as secukinumab have not been included.[25,31]

Tumor Necrosis Factor-α Inhibitors Dysregulation of TNF-α production is associated with various inflammatory conditions, including rheumatoid arthritis, inflammatory bowel disease, ankylosing spondylitis, PsA, and psoriasis.[66-68] Elevated TNF-α levels are seen in both the affected skin and serum of patients with psoriasis; and these elevated levels have a significant correlation with psoriasis severity.[31] The biologic agents etanercept, adalimumab, and infliximab are TNF-α inhibitors which are effective for psoriasis and PsA.[41]

There are safety concerns common to TNF-α inhibitors, mainly from observations made through their use in rheumatoid arthritis and inflammatory bowel disease and more recently psoriasis.[66-68] One concern is an increased risk of infections, most commonly upper respiratory tract infections, and less commonly serious infections including sepsis, new-onset or reactivation TB, and opportunistic infections such as histoplasmosis, cryptococcosis, aspergillosis, candidiasis, and pneumocystis.[14,31,66-68] There have been reports of serious pulmonary and disseminated histoplasmosis, coccidioidomycosis, and blastomycosis infections,[69,70] sometimes with fatal outcomes when these infections were not consistently recognized and promptly treated in the patients taking TNF-α inhibitors.[69]

A second concern is the development or worsening of autoimmune diseases such as peripheral and central demyelinating disorders including multiple sclerosis and drug-induced lupus-like syndromes.[14,31] A third concern is the potential increased risk of malignancies such as lymphoma,[14,31] melanoma, and nonmelanoma skin cancer.[31] A fourth concern is the potential for other cutaneous adverse effects including vasculitis, granulomatous reactions, cutaneous infections, psoriasiform eruptions, and infusion or injection site reactions.[67] Flares of pustular psoriasis have been reported primarily for patients undergoing treatment for nondermatologic conditions such as rheumatoid arthritis.[14]

There is also a concern about chronic heart failure (CHF): there have been rare reports of worsening congestive heart failure (CHF) and new-onset CHF; TNF inhibitors are contraindicated in patients with preexisting moderate-to-severe CHF (NYHA class III/IV),[24,31] and those with milder CHF should have their TNF-α inhibitors withdrawn at the onset of new symptoms or worsening of preexisting CHF.[31]

Although the above are safety concerns common to etanercept, adalimumab, and infliximab, their safety profiles are not identical. For example, the risk for TB appears lowest with etanercept and highest with infliximab.[14] Nonetheless, they are contraindicated in patients with active TB.[24] Patients should be evaluated for active or latent TB before therapy and considered for a yearly PPD.[14,31] CBC and LFTs are also recommended before and periodically during therapy.[24] In addition, pretreatment C-reactive protein (CRP), hepatitis serology (HBV, HCV), and HIV testing have been recommended.[24] They are pregnancy category B and safe to use in pregnancy.[31] (Some manufacturers have cautioned that, since these drugs cross the placenta, infants exposed in utero may be at higher risk of infections and live vaccines would be contraindicated for several months after birth.[70])

Adalimumab is a human monoclonal antibody that provides rapid and efficacious control of psoriasis.[31] Clinical trials in patients with moderate-to-severe psoriasis have shown dramatic results. A 2006 12-week RCT with open-label extension to 52 weeks showed significant improvement within 1 week of therapy, with complete or nearly complete clearance in some patients, and clinical benefits were maintained for at least 1 year with continuous therapy for most patients.[14,71]

A 2008 52-week RCT (REVEAL) with an initial 16-week double-blind placebo-controlled (DBPC; period A) phase followed by a 17-week open-label phase (period B) followed by a 19-week DBPC phase (period C) showed a 71% PASI 75 response for adalimumab treated patients versus 7% for placebo-treated patients at week 16. All patients received open-label adalimumab from weeks 17 through 32. At week 33, patients achieving PASI 75 were rerandomized to adalimumab or placebo; patients achieving PASI 50 but less than 75 were continued on open-label adalimumab; and therapy for patients with PASI less than 50 was discontinued. At week 52, 5% of patients rerandomized to adalimumab lost adequate response versus 28% of patients rerandomized to placebo. Adalimumab was continued at 40 mg every other week. The study showed that adalimumab can produce rapid and dramatic results which can be sustained on continued use, in patients with moderate-to-severe psoriasis.[72]

Additional 3-year open-label extension study for patients in REVEAL showed that in patients with sustained initial PASI 75 responses, adalimumab efficacy was maintained for more than 3 years of continuous therapy and maintenance was best at PASI 100. Some patients with PASI less than 75 in REVEAL also achieved long-term PASI 75 responses.[66]

For comparative studies, as discussed in the MTX section, a head-to-head study showed that adalimumab was significantly more efficacious than MTX.[62]

Adalimumab is given as 80 mg subcutaneously in the first week, then 40 mg the following week, and thereafter 40 mg every other week continuously.[14,24,31,70] More frequent dosing has been explored.[14]

Adverse effects in adalimumab clinical trials including the 3-year extension were similar to those already described for this class of BRMs (ie, TB and other opportunistic infections such as candidiasis, CHF, malignancies including nonmelanoma skin cancer that may be related to psoriasis, and allergic reactions).[66,70-72]

Etanercept was one of the earliest BRMs available on the market for use in inflammatory diseases. It has demonstrated efficacy for rheumatoid arthritis. It was approved for use in PsA in the United States in June 2002 and approved in 2004 for use in moderate-to-severe psoriasis. It is also approved for treatment of juvenile rheumatoid arthritis and ankylosing spondylitis. Thus, as opposed to some of the other BRMs approved for psoriasis, etanercept has been extensively used in rheumatology both for adults and children.

The dosing of etanercept in psoriasis differs from its other indications, reflective of the dosing regimens found to be effective for psoriasis in clinical trials. Etanercept is used continuously, given as 50 mg subcutaneously twice weekly for the first 12 weeks, followed by 25 mg twice weekly[14] or 50 mg once weekly.[24,31] Significant improvement was seen in about 50% of patients in clinical trials by week 12 and more than 50% of participants by week 24; with continuing therapy, weaker responders continued to improve for up to 1 year.[14,29,73] Continuing therapy using 50 mg twice weekly regimens are being explored and may provide greater benefit.[14] Etanercept was efficacious in children and adolescents (aged 4-17 years) with plaque psoriasis dosed at 0.8 mg/kg (maximum 50 mg) once weekly.[74]

Infliximab also received approval for rheumatologic diseases before psoriasis and was on the market before adalimumab. Infliximab may be more efficacious than etanercept. A 2011 open-label study showed that psoriatic patients with an inadequate response to etanercept had rapid and sustained improvement when switched to infliximab.[75] Unlike etanercept or adalimumab, infliximab is a chimeric antibody with both murine and human components; thus, antibodies to the drug can develop, resulting in infusion reactions.[31] Regular therapy rather than intermittent dosing on an as-needed basis may minimize this occurrence.[31] The standard dosing regimen is three IV infusions of 5 mg/kg given over a 6-week induction period, followed by regular infusions every 8 weeks.[31]

Clinical response is seen rapidly. In a randomized controlled phase III trial, 80% of patients responded by week 10 (after three doses of infliximab); however, the response dropped to about 50% by week 50.[76,77] Rare reports of serious adverse events, including fatal cases of hepatosplenic T-cell lymphomas, have been associated with infliximab use.[28] Other rare instances of cholecystitis and autoimmune hepatitis, which may be a class effect for TNF-α inhibitors, have also been reported.[14]

Alefacept Alefacept was the first BRM to receive approval for the treatment of psoriasis, in January 2003 in the United States and in October 2004 in Canada. Over the years, it has accumulated an extensive and reassuring safety record, with no evidence of increased incidence of infections, cancers, or any other serious adverse events beyond background levels. The exception is that CD4 T lymphocytes can be depleted, and CD4 cell counts must be monitored.[14,78]

In comparison with other BRMs, alefacept monotherapy provides only limited control of psoriasis, and as discussed later, it is often explored in combination regimens to enhance response.[14] However, even with monotherapy, long periods of near-complete remission can be seen occasionally.[14]

Dosing is intended to be intermittent. Alefacept is given for a 12-week course, then repeated only when the loss of control becomes unacceptable (up to two more courses per year may be given).[14] Maximal response was generally seen by 6 to 8 weeks in responders, and currently there is no measure to predict which patients will respond.[31]

Ustekinumab This is an IL-12/23 monoclonal antibody approved for the treatment of psoriasis in adults 18 years or older with moderate-to-severe plaque psoriasis.[24] It selectively targets IL-12 and IL-23, two cytokines that play a role in the pathogenesis of psoriasis.[4,24] It binds to their shared p40 protein subunit thus preventing interaction with their cell surface IL-12Rβ 1receptor.[79] This shared binding may allow ustekinumab to exert its clinical effects in both psoriasis and PsA through interruption of the TH1 and TH17 cytokine pathways, central to both disease conditions.[79] Clinical response appears to be related to serum ustekinumab levels achieved.[79] In a comparison with etanercept, ustekinumab was significantly more efficacious (ACCEPT clinical trial).[79]

Ustekinumab can provide a rapid response that is seen within 2 weeks of initiating treatment.[79-81] Two large randomized placebo-controlled trials (PHOENIX 1 and PHOENIX 2) demonstrated clinical efficacy of ustekinumab, with approximately 70% of patients achieving 75% skin clearance after two doses and maintaining the response for 1 year with continued treatment.[79-81] The improvements were dramatic. Ustekinumab was also significantly more efficacious than etanercept (ACCEPT clinical trial).[79]

The impact of ustekinumab on patients' health-related QOL was evaluated in the PHOENIX 2 trial.[82] Patients showed a significant improvement not only in skin-related QOL, but also in symptoms of anxiety and depression (as assessed by the Hospital Anxiety and Depression Scale).[82] The subset of patients with PsA in PHOENIX 1 and PHOENIX 2 also showed significant improvement in QOL, anxiety, and depression.[83]

Weight-based dosing rather than fixed-dose was found to be clinically significant for efficacy in PHOENIX 1 and PHOENIX 2—heavier patients required a higher dose.[84] Serum ustekinumab concentrations were also affected by weight.[84] Dosing is 45 mg for patients weighing 100 kg (220 lb) or less, and 90 mg for those of higher weights. Ustekinumab is administered subcutaneously at weeks 0 and 4, then every 12 weeks as maintenance therapy.[79]

Cumulative 3-year safety data from PHOENIX 1 and 2, and ACCEPT have also been published.[85,86] Common adverse effects include upper respiratory infections, headache, fatigue, pruritus, back pain, injection site reactions, and arthralgia, with the most common events being headache and nasopharyngitis.[85] Ustekinumab does not appear to exacerbate atopic diseases.[85] Serious adverse effects include those seen with other BRMs, including serious tubercular, fungal, viral infections, and cancers. No evidence of a dose-response to infection rates was seen.[86] Serious infections and malignancy rates did not increase with long-term ustekinumab treatment up to 3 years.[85,86] In addition, a reversible posterior leukoencephalopathy syndrome (RPLS) has been reported.[67]

Secukinumab This is a fully human immunoglobulin (IgG)1κ monoclonal antibody that selectively binds and inhibits IL-17A, a proinflammatory cytokine, thus inhibiting the release of chemokines and other proinflammatory mediators. It was approved in the United States in January 2015 and in Canada in May 2015 for treatment of moderate-to-severe plaque psoriasis in adult patients who are candidates for systemic therapy or phototherapy.[87]

The approval was based on the results of four RCTs evaluating a total of more than 2,000 patients. Secukinumab was shown to induce a rapid response with clinically significant greater PASI rates by week 12, and with continued treatment was associated with sustained high responses through week 52.[88] Recommended dosing regimen is 300 mg (as two subcutaneous injections of 150 mg) at weeks 0, 1, 2, 3 followed by maintenance dosing starting at week 4.[87] Adverse effects from clinical trials commonly included nasopharyngitis, headache, upper respiratory tract infection, diarrhea, and uncommonly included neutropenia and detection of anti-secukinumab antibodies.[87,88]

Other BRMs are being investigated. BRMs with promising clinical trial results include ixekizumab and brodalumab (two other BRMs targeting IL-17) and tofacitinib (an oral agent that inhibits Janus kinase and currently used in treatment of rheumatoid arthritis). Thus there appears to be many more *needed* biologics in the near future for this disease.

Combination Therapies

Combination therapies may be beneficial in the management of plaque psoriasis: generally to either enhance efficacy or minimize toxicity. As shown in Figs. 97-1 and 97-2, combinations can include two topical agents, a topical agents plus phototherapy, a systemic agent plus topical therapy, a systemic agent plus phototherapy, two systemic agents used in rotation, or a systemic agent and a BRM. Rotational therapy is not commonly used in practice, and the use of a BRM added to a systemic agent is still under investigation.

The combination of a topical corticosteroid and a topical vitamin D_3 analog is particularly useful. This was shown in several studies to be efficacious and safe, with less skin irritation than monotherapy with either agent, and the combination product containing calcipotriol and betamethasone dipropionate ointment has demonstrated efficacy in RCTs for patients with relatively severe psoriasis.[14,30] The combination may also be steroid sparing.[30]

The combination of retinoids with phototherapy has also been shown to increase efficacy. Because retinoids may be photosensitizing and increase the risk of burning after ultraviolet (UV) light exposure, doses of phototherapy should be reduced to minimize adverse effects. An RCT with tazarotene and broadband UVB not only showed significant enhancement of UVB efficacy but also reduced the number of UVB treatment sessions needed for response.[28,30,89] The combination of acitretin and broadband UVB reduced the number of needed treatments, compared with UVB alone.[14,90] Acitretin with NB-UVB (RE-UVB) was highly effective for patients with difficult-to-control psoriasis.[30,91] The combination of acitretin and PUVA (RE-PUVA) also showed greater efficacy than monotherapy with either agent.[28,92] RE-PUVA can be used to achieve clearance with up to a twofold reduction in total UV exposure.[14] Phototherapy has also been used with other topical agents, such as UVB with coal tar (Goeckerman regimen)[55] to increase treatment response, because coal tar is also photosensitizing.

Cyclosporine and calcipotriol/betamethasone dipropionate in combination is superior to cyclosporine alone.[24] Cyclosporine may also be successfully used with SCAT; however, it should not be used with PUVA due to reduced efficacy and the potential increase risk of cutaneous malignancies.[32]

The combination of MTX and UVB appears to be synergistic.[29,34] There is also consensus/evidence that MTX in combination with a BRM such as etanercept may be beneficial.[24]

BRMs used in combination with other therapies are being explored. Some beneficial combinations have been found. Alefacept and NB-UVB in combination significantly reduced the number of UVB treatments needed with clearance seen in 43% of patients within 12 weeks.[14,93] Infliximab given concurrently with immunosuppressive agents such as MTX or azathioprine may result in a lower incidence of infusion reactions to infliximab.[31] MTX in combination with adalimumab or infliximab is widely used in rheumatology and low-dose MTX (eg, 7.5-10 mg once per week) is likely sufficient to reduce formation of anti-drug-antibodies and increase the respective trough levels of adalimumab or infliximab.[24]

Alternative Drug Treatments

Mycophenolate Mofetil (MMF) is a systemic agent occasionally used for patients with resistant cases of moderate-to-severe psoriasis.[14] This is currently not an approved indication in either Canada or the United States.

A few reports and small studies are available describing the efficacy of MMF when used as monotherapy or adjuvant therapy.[94] In addition, one small study evaluated the switch for eight patients with severe psoriasis from cyclosporine to MMF after a washout period of 2 to 4 weeks. On cyclosporine, seven of these patients had deteriorating renal function and hypertension, and one experienced loss of efficacy.[95] After the switch to MMF, there was significant loss of psoriasis control in five of the eight patients but also significant improvement in renal function for six patients.[94,95]

Conversely, another small study evaluated the sequential use of MMF followed by cyclosporine in eight patients with moderate-to-severe psoriasis.[96] There was significant improvement with MMF in all patients, and all patients further improved when switched to cyclosporine.[96]

MMF has some uncommon but significant adverse effects, including increased incidence of opportunistic infections such as cytomegalovirus, cryptococcosis, candidiasis, and *Pneumocystis jirovecii*.[94] Cases of progressive multifocal leukoencephalopathy have also been reported.[92] There may be an associated risk of malignancy.[97]

Hydroxyurea Hydroxyurea is an antimetabolite usually used for cancer treatments, but it has also been used in the systemic treatment of psoriasis for more than 30 years.[14,29] It is still occasionally tried for patients with recalcitrant severe psoriasis, although BRMs may be a better option for these patients.

Hydroxyurea has been compared with MTX for patients with moderate-to-severe psoriasis.[98] Weekly regimens showed greater efficacy for MTX with a faster clearance rate, although hydroxyurea was also efficacious. The authors concluded that weekly doses of hydroxyurea may be an alternative to MTX for patients experiencing intolerable MTX side effects or have reached the recommended cumulative dose.[98]

Adverse effects of hydroxyurea include significant bone marrow suppression, lesional erythema, localized tenderness, and reversible hyperpigmentation.[14,98]

Complementary and Alternative Medicines The use of complementary and alternative medicine (CAM) among patients with psoriasis is common, with a prevalence of 43% to 69% in various studies.[99] Most of these patients use herbs, special diets, or dietary supplements in conjunction with their usual antipsoriatic medications and not as replacements. Most patients do not discuss CAM use with their physicians.[99]

A 2009 systematic review of RCTs found that, although there is a large body of literature on CAM use in psoriasis, the quality of most studies was relatively low.[99] CAM agents and interventions with documented clinical efficacy in psoriasis include *Mahonia aquifolium*, fish oil, climatotherapy (Dead Sea salts), and stress reduction techniques.

Mahonia aquafolium (Oregon grape, Mountain grape, or barberry but *not* European barberry) is an evergreen native to southern British Columbia, western Oregon, and northern Idaho. The rhizome and root contain berberine as the primary active constituent. Berberine is an alkaloid that inhibits keratinocyte growth and reduces keratinocyte proliferation, and it also has antibacterial and antifungal activities. In at least two clinical trials *Mahonia aquifolium* was efficacious in reducing disease severity: In one randomized placebo-controlled study a *Mahonia aquifolium* 10% preparation applied topically twice daily resulted in a significant improvement in the PASI score and the Quality of Life Index (QLI), compared with placebo.[100] Adverse effects in clinical trials included rash, burning sensation, redness, and itching.

Fish oil contains two important long-chain polyunsaturated fatty acids—eicosapentaenoic acid (EPA) and docosahexaenoic acid (DHA). EPA and DHA are omega-3 fatty acids. They act as substrates competing with arachidonic acid for cyclooxygenase and lipoxygenase, thus reducing the production of proinflammatory molecules in psoriatic plaques.[99] Several randomized placebo-controlled and/or comparative trials for patients with psoriasis have demonstrated efficacy of fish oils. One study comparing EPA plus etretinate to etretinate monotherapy found significantly greater efficacy with the combination of EPA plus etretinate.[101]

Climatotherapy refers to the practice of traveling to the Dead Sea and sunbathing and/or bathing in the sea—the beneficial effects are likely from the high salinity of the sea and UV rays.[99] Several studies have demonstrated efficacy, including two studies using saline spa baths. One study used highly concentrated (25%-27%) saline spa baths plus UVB compared with UVB alone, and the other used low concentrated (4.5%-12%) saline spa bath plus UVB again compared with UVB alone. In both studies the clinical response was significantly better with the saline spa bath plus UVB combination.[99,102,103]

Stress-reduction techniques have inconsistently shown some benefit. One randomized study demonstrated that both meditation or meditation and imagery were efficacious as adjunctive treatments for patients with scalp psoriasis.[104] A second randomized study for patients with psoriasis receiving either UVB or PUVA therapy showed that the addition of a mindfulness-based stress-reduction audiotape played during light treatments reduced response times for patients receiving UVB but not PUVA therapy.[105] This confirmed the belief that psychological stress plays a role in psoriasis. More recently, in a case-control study of risk factors during the year before the onset of psoriasis, stressful life events were found to be significant.[106,107]

Personalized Pharmacotherapy

Despite the availability of good quality evidence and clinical practice guidelines, patients with psoriasis are still often undertreated or inappropriately managed.[25] A 2007 study in the United States involving 1,657 patients from National Psoriasis Foundation surveys found that 40% of patients with psoriasis were receiving no current treatment; of those, 27% had psoriasis involving greater than 10% BSA.[108] In addition, those receiving care may be undertreated.[108] Early access to care and adherence may also be issues.

Patient-specific therapies that take into consideration comorbid illnesses, adherence, and pharmacoeconomic issues in addition to the patient's psoriatic manifestations and responses to treatments are important, and will ultimately improve the quality of care. Treatment goals need to be defined for both short-term and long-term management time frames.[25] Without optimizing patient care, the concern is that patients with poorly managed psoriasis may follow a "diminished" life course compared with the course they might have taken if they did not have psoriasis, as the disease has significant psychological, social, and economic impacts in addition to its physical manifestations.[109]

To this end, a current focus is defining frameworks[109] and specific treatment goals[24,25] for implementation of practice guidelines, as described earlier in this chapter. The reader is encouraged to review the noted references for further information.

Special Populations

Psoriasis in Children Pediatric psoriasis is more often attributable to direct precipitating factors such as skin trauma, infections, drugs, or stress.[14,110] Compared with adults, plaque lesions in children are often smaller, thinner, and less scaly, which can make diagnosis more difficult. Face and flexures are more commonly involved than for adults. Psoriatic diaper rash can occur up to age 2. PsA is rare.[14]

Topical treatment is the standard of care for children with psoriasis, with topical corticosteroids often the treatment of first choice.[14] Other useful pharmacologic therapies include calcipotriol and anthralin; calcipotriol with or without topical corticosteroids has also been recommended as treatment of first choice[111] because it produces minimal adverse effects.[14] Since children's skin is thinner and better hydrated than that of adults, they are at higher risk of drug absorption leading to systemic adverse effects. The lowest potency corticosteroid that provides control should be used, and it should be tapered as the lesions improve. If long-term calcipotriol is used, monitoring of ionized calcium is recommended because of the risk of hypercalcemia.[14]

Systemic therapies are reserved for children with severe and recalcitrant psoriasis.[14,111] MTX can provide near to complete clearance[111] and has been safely used to control severe childhood psoriatic episodes and then withdrawn as lesions improve.[14] Regular monitoring for liver and blood toxicity is required.[14] The BRM etanercept was studied in a randomized placebo-controlled trial of 211 children and adolescents (4-17 years) with moderate-to-severe plaque psoriasis. It significantly reduced disease severity; however, four serious adverse events occurred (ovarian cyst requiring removal, gastroenteritis, gastroenteritis-associated dehydration, and left basilar pneumonia).[112] Etanercept has been studied in children with polyarticular juvenile rheumatoid arthritis without new safety concerns emerging.[14]

Phototherapy should be used with caution, especially for younger children, because of long-term carcinogenic risks and phototoxicities. For older children and adolescents with severe, extensive, or treatment-resistant disease, UVB may be a treatment option.[14]

Psoriasis in Pregnancy Hormonal changes in pregnancy can improve symptoms for patients with plaque psoriasis. In one study, 55% of patients showed improvements during pregnancy.[14,113] For patients with more than 10% BSA involvement who reported improvement, lesions decreased by more than 80% during pregnancy.[113] This appeared to correlate with high estrogen but not progesterone levels.[113] Thus, some pregnant women may require minimal treatment for their psoriasis.

Some antipsoriatic drugs have significant teratogenic risks, placing them in pregnancy category X. Thus, women of childbearing potential must use effective birth control during therapy, and may need to continue effective contraception after discontinuing therapy for a period of time, as discussed in detail throughout this chapter. In addition, drugs listed as pregnancy category C may carry known teratogenic risks in animal studies or have limited available data for use in pregnancy.

UVB has been considered the safest treatment for extensive psoriasis during pregnancy. It is recommended for patients with widespread disease not controlled by topical agents. One problem with this therapy is an increased potential for reactivation of herpes simplex, which may be transmitted to the infant at delivery.[14]

For more detailed information about antipsoriatic drugs in pregnancy, a systematic, drug-by-drug review of case reports and case-control studies is available.[114] The 2009 Canadian Guidelines provides a drug-by-drug summary of recommendations for topical agents, phototherapy, and systemic agents in pregnancy.[14] The 2015 European S3 Guidelines provides a discussion about most appropriate treatments for women with a wish for pregnancy in the near future, and which treatments to avoid.[24]

Psoriasis in the Elderly Age-related changes in organ function/drug clearance and greater drug sensitivity increase the risk of adverse drug events for elderly patients with psoriasis.

MTX is hepatotoxic and should be used with caution in the elderly. Cyclosporine has nephrotoxic potential and may also increase blood pressure. Both drugs have significant drug interactions, and polypharmacy, common in older patients, make management of interactions challenging.

In addition, older patients may have preexisting comorbidities, such as hyperlipidemia and metabolic syndrome, and this may further limit drug use. Adalimumab appears equally efficacious in older patients (older than 65 years) who may have higher incidences of hypertension, hyperlipidemia, depression, obesity, and diabetes.[115] Adverse effects profiles were similar between subgroups (various weights and comorbidities) with no significant differences in serious adverse events.[115] Topical psoriasis treatments are often prescribed for elderly patients as first-line therapy[14]; however, even with topicals, adverse effects—including systemic ones—can occur with greater frequency in these patients.[14]

Psoriasis in Patients with a History of Solid Tumors As discussed throughout this chapter, many antipsoriatic therapies carry significant cancer risks. PUVA, systemic therapies such as cyclosporine, and some BRMs are associated with increased risks of oncologic disorders.

A systematic review of the risk of malignancy associated with therapies for moderate-to-severe psoriasis confirmed the following[97]: PUVA is associated with an increased risk of cutaneous SCC and malignant melanoma; UVB is a much safer therapeutic modality than PUVA; cyclosporine increases risks of lymphoma, internal malignancies, and skin cancers; MTX may be associated with increased melanoma and Epstein–Barr virus–associated lymphomas; MMF may be associated with lymphoproliferative disorders; and the malignancy risk may be increased for biologic agents, especially the TNF-α inhibitors.[97]

The 2009 Canadian guidelines recommend that TNF-α inhibitors be used with caution for patients with a history of malignancy or existing malignancies, and the T-cell modulator alefacept is contraindicated for these patients.[14]

Pharmacoeconomic Considerations

(10) The wide gap in costs of agents for psoriasis makes economics and availability of insurance or other coverage important considerations in formulating a therapeutic plan.

Currently, the expensive BRMs are often considered for patients with moderate-to-severe psoriasis when less expensive systemic agents are inadequate or relatively contraindicated. BRMs have also been recommended as first-line therapy, alongside conventional systemic agents, for patients with moderate-to-severe psoriasis; however, in practice, drug access secondary to cost considerations can limit use. These agents may be needed early, though, for some patients with comorbidities.

A recent pharmacoeconomic analysis of BRMs in the treatment of psoriasis suggests that the cost-to-benefit ratio for BRMs may be favorable.[68] There are also cost differences among the BRMs. Of the TNF-α inhibitors, etanercept is the least costly, followed by adalimumab than infliximab.[116] However, etanercept is less efficacious.

Adalimumab (at doses of 40 mg every other week) is significantly less costly than ustekinumab, with similar efficacies, in patients with suboptimal response to etanercept.[117]

CONCLUSION

Psoriasis is a lifelong illness with no known cure. Significant comorbidities may coexist. Treatment should be patient-specific, with consideration given to disease severity, patient risk factors, age, and comorbidities. Newer treatment modalities, including numerous BRMs, are now parts of the armamentarium available in the management of this disease.

ABBREVIATIONS

BMI	body mass index
BRM	biologic response modifier
BSA	body surface area
CAM	complementary and alternative medicine
CBC	complete blood count
CHD	coronary heart disease
CHF	chronic heart failure
CRP	C-reactive protein
CYP3A4	cytochrome P450 isoenzyme 3A4
DBPC	double-blind placebo-controlled
DHA	docosahexaenoic acid
DISH	disseminated (or diffuse) idiopathic skeletal hyperostosis
DLQI	Dermatology Life Quality Index
EPA	eicosapentaenoic acid
FDA	Food and Drug Administration
GFR	glomerular filtration rate
HLA-C	major histocompatibility complex antigen
HPA	hypothalamic–pituitary–adrenal
IL	interleukin
LFT	liver function test
MI	myocardial infarction
MMF	mycophenolate mofetil
MTX	methotrexate
NSAIDs	nonsteroidal antiinflammatory drugs
NB-UVB	narrowband ultraviolet B (311 nm ultraviolet B light)
PASI	Psoriasis Area and Severity Index
PGA	Physician's Global Assessment
PsA	psoriatic arthritis
PUVA	psoralens with ultraviolet A light
QLI	Quality of Life Index
QOL	quality of life
RCT	randomized controlled trial
RE-PUVA	retinoid plus PUVA (as combination therapy)
RE-UVB	retinoid plus NBUVB (as combination therapy)
RPLS	reversible posterior leukoencephalopathy syndrome
RR	relative risk
SCAT	short-contact anthralin therapy
SCC	squamous cell carcinoma
SF-36	Short Form Health Survey
SPF	sun protection factor
TB	tuberculosis
TNF-α	Tumor necrosis factor-α
UV	ultraviolet
UVA	ultraviolet A (315 to 400 nm ultraviolet A light)
UVB	ultraviolet B, or broadband UVB (28 to 315 nm ultraviolet B light)

REFERENCES

1. Law RM. Chapter 64: Psoriasis. In: Chisholm-Burns M, ed. *Pharmacotherapy Principles and Practice,* 3rd ed. New York, NY: McGraw-Hill, 2013:1127-1141.
2. Reich K. The concept of psoriasis as a systemic inflammation: Implications for disease management. *J Eur Acad Dermatol Venereol* 2012;26(suppl 2):3-11.
3. Gulliver WP, Pirzada SM. Psoriasis: More than skin deep. In: Saeland S, ed. *Recent Advances in Skin Immunology*. Kevala, India: Research Signpost, 2008:167-179.
4. Boehncke WH, Schon MP. Psoriasis. *Lancet* 2015; 386:983-994.
5. Lowes, MA, Bowcock AM, Krueger JG. Pathogenesis and therapy of psoriasis. *Nature* 2007;445(7130):866-873.
6. Boehncke WH, Boehncke S, Tobin AM, Kirby B. The 'psoriatic march': A concept of how severe psoriasis may drive cardiovascular comorbidity. *Exp Dermatol* 2011;147:1031-1039.
7. Grozdev I, Korman N, Tsankov N. Psoriasis as a systemic disease. *Clin Dermatol* 2014;32:343-350.
8. Farber E, Bright R, Nall M. Psoriasis: A questionnaire survey of 2144 patients. *Arch Dermatol* 1974;98:248-259.
9. Farber EM, Nall ML, Watson W. Natural history of psoriasis in 61 twin pairs. *Arch Dermatol* 1974;109:207-211.
10. Nall L, Gulliver WP, Charmley P, et al. Search for the psoriasis susceptibility gene: The Newfoundland Study. *Cutis* 1999;64: 323-329.
11. Nair RP, Duffin KC, Helms C, et al. Genome-wide scan reveals association of psoriasis with IL-23 and NF-κB pathways. *Nat Genet* 2009;41:199-204.
12. Raychaudhuri SP, Jiang W-Y, Raychaudhuri SK. Revisiting the Koebner phenomenon. *Am J Pathol* 2008;172:961-971.
13. Basavaraj KH, Ashok NM, Rashmi R, Praveen TK. The role of drugs in the induction and/or exacerbation of psoriasis. *Int J Dermatol* 2010;49:1351-1361.
14. Papp KA, Gulliver W, Lynde CW, Poulin Y (Steering Committee). Canadian Guidelines for the Management of Plaque Psoriasis, 1st ed., June 2009. Available at: http://www.dermatology.ca/wp-content/uploads/2012/01/cdnpsoriasisguidelines.pdf. Accessed Oct. 31, 2015.
15. Boehncke S, Boehncke WH. 'Upgrading' psoriasis responsibly. *Exp Dermatol* 2014;23:710-711.
16. Guenther L, Gulliver W. Psoriasis comorbidities. *J Cutan Med Surg* 2009;13(suppl 2):S77-S87.
17. Kimball AB, Gladman D, Gelfand JM, et al. National Psoriasis Foundation clinical consensus on psoriasis comorbidities and recommendations for screening. *J Am Acad Dermatol* 2008;58:1031-1042.
18. Gulliver WP. Importance of screening for comorbidities in psoriasis patients. *Expert Rev Dermatol* 2008;3:133-135.
19. Gelfand JM, Gladman Dd, Mease PJ, et al. Epidemiology of psoriatic arthritis in the population of the United States. *J Am Acad Dermatol* 2005;53:573-577.
20. Rahman P, O'Reilly DD. Psoriatic arthritis genetic susceptibility and pharmacogenetics. *Pharmacogenomics* 2008;9:195-205.
21. Wilson PW, D'Agostino RB, Parise H, et al. Metabolic syndrome as a precursor of cardiovascular disease and type 2 diabetes mellitus. *Circulation* 2005;112:3066-3072.
22. Kimball AB, Guerin A, Latremouille-Viau D, et al. Coronary heart disease and stroke risk in patients with psoriasis: Retrospective analysis. *Am J Med* 2010;123:350-357.
23. Gelfand JM, Neimann AL, Shin DB, et al. Risk of myocardial infarction in patients with psoriasis. *JAMA* 2006;296:1735-1741.
24. European S3-Guidelines on the systemic treatment of psoriasis vulgaris. Updated 2015. EDF in cooperation with EADV and IPC. Available at: http://www.psoriasis-guideline.com/ To download or view follow the link to: http://www.euroderm.org/edf/index.php/

edf-guidelines/category/5-guidelines-miscellaneous. Accessed September 9, 2016.
25. Mrowietz U. Implementing treatment goals for successful long-term management of psoriasis. *J Eur Acad Dermatol Venereol* 2012; 26(suppl 2):12-20.
26. Mrowietz U, Steinz K, Gerdes S. Psoriasis: To treat or to manage? *Exp Dermatol* 2014;23:705-709.
27. Law RMT, Gulliver WP. Chapter 110: Psoriasis. In: Schwinghammer TL, Koehler JM, eds. *Pharmacotherapy Casebook and Instructor's Guide: A Patient-Focused Approach,* 10th ed. New York, NY: McGraw-Hill, 2017, in press.
28. Menter A, Korman NJ, Elmets CA, et al. 2009 guidelines of care for the management of psoriasis and psoriatic arthritis—section 5. Guidelines of care for the treatment of psoriasis with phototherapy and photochemotherapy. *J Am Acad Dermatol* 2010;62:114-135.
29. Menter A, Korman NJ, Elmets CA, et al. 2009 Guidelines of care for the management of psoriasis and psoriatic arthritis—section 4. Guidelines of care for the management and treatment of psoriasis with traditional systemic agents. *J Am Acad Dermatol* 2009;61: 451-485.
30. Menter A, Korman NJ, Elmets CA, et al. 2009 Guidelines of care for the management of psoriasis and psoriatic arthritis—section 3. Guidelines of care for the management and treatment of psoriasis with topical therapies. *J Am Acad Dermatol* 2009;60:643-659.
31. Menter A. Gottlieb A, Feldman SR, et al. Guidelines of care for the management of psoriasis and psoriatic arthritis—section 1. Overview of psoriasis and guidelines of care for the treatment of psoriasis with biologics. *J Am Acad Dermatol* 2008;58:826-850.
32. Rosmarin DM, Lebwohl M, Elewski BE, et al. Cyclosporine and psoriasis: 2008 National psoriasis Foundation Consensus Conference. *J Am Acad Dermatol* 2010;62:838-853.
33. National Psoriasis Foundation. National Psoriasis Foundation. Psoriatic Treatments. Available at: https://www.psoriasis.org/about-psoriasis/treatments. Accessed September 9, 2016.
34. Kalb RE, Strober B, Weinstein G, Lebwohl M. Methotrexate and psoriasis: 2009 National Psoriasis Foundation Consensus Conference. *J Am Acad Dermatol* 2009;60:824-837.
35. Guenther L, Langley RG, Shear NH, et al. Integrating biologic agents into management of moderate-to-severe psoriasis: A consensus of the Canadian Psoriasis Expert Panel. *J Cutan Med Surg* 2004;8:321-337.
36. Cohen SN, Baron SE, Archer CB. Guidance on the diagnosis and clinical management of psoriasis. *Clin Exp Dermatol* 2012;37(suppl 1): 13-18.
37. Paul C, Gallini A, Archier E, et al. Evidence-based recommendations on topical treatment and phototherapy of psoriasis: Systematic review and expert opinion of a panel of dermatologists. *J Eur Acad Dermatol Venereol* 2012;26(suppl 3):1-10.
38. Long CC, Finlay AY. The finger-tip unit—a new practical measure. *Clin Exp Dermatol* 1991;16:444-447.
39. Menter Kamili. Topical treatment of psoriasis. In: Yawalkar N, ed. *Current Problems in Dermatology*. Basel, Switzerland: S. Karger AG; 2009.
40. Krueger GG, O'Reilly MA, Weidner M, et al. Comparative efficacy of once-daily flurandrenolide tape versus twice-daily diflorasone diacetate ointment in the treatment of psoriasis. *J Am Acad Dermatol* 1998;38:186-190.
41. Mason J, Mason AR, Cork MJ. Topical preparations for the treatment of psoriasis: A systemic review. *Br J Dermatol* 2002;146:351-364.
42. Castela E, Archier E, Devaux S, et al. Topical corticosteroids in plaque psoriasis: A systematic review of efficacy and treatment modalities. *J Euro Acad Dermatol Venereol* 2012;26(suppl 3):36-46.
43. Katz HI, Prawer SE, Medansky RS, et al. Intermittent corticosteroid maintenance treatment of psoriasis: A double-blind multicenter trial of augmented betamethasone dipropionate ointment in a pulse dose treatment regimen. *Dermatologica* 1991;183:269-274.
44. Wall ARJ, Poyner TF, Menday AP. A comparison of treatment with dithranol and calcipotriol on the clinical severity and quality of life in patients with psoriasis. *Br J Dermatol* 1998;139:1005-1011.
45. Cunliffe WJ, Berth-Jones J, Claudy A, et al. Comparative study of calcipotriol (MC 903) ointment and betamethasone 17-valerate ointment in patients with psoriasis vulgaris. *J Am Acad Dermatol* 1992;26:736-743.
46. Kragballe K, Gjertsen BT, De Hoop D, et al. Double-blind, right/left comparison of calcipotriol and betamethasone valerate in treatment of psoriasis vulgaris. *Lancet* 1991;337:193-196.
47. Devaux S, Castela A, Archier E, et al. Topical vitamin D analogues alone or in association with topical steroids for psoriasis: A systematic review. *J Euro Acad Dermatol Venereol* 2012;26(suppl 3):52-60.
48. Weinstein GD, Krueger GG, Lowe NJ, et al. Tazarotene gel, a new retinoid, for topical therapy of psoriasis: Vehicle-controlled study of safety, efficacy, and duration of therapeutic effect. *J Am Acad Dermatol* 1997;37:85-92.
49. Weinstein GD, Koo JY, Krueger GG, et al. Tazarotene cream in the treatment of psoriasis: Two multicenter, double-blind, randomized, vehicle-controlled studies of the safety and efficacy of tazarotene cream 0.05% and 0.1% applied once daily for 12 weeks. *J Am Acad Dermatol* 2003;48:760-767.
50. McGill A, Frank A, Emmett N, et al. The anti-psoriatic drug anthralin accumulates in keratinocyte mitochondria, dissipates mitochondrial membrane potential, and induces apoptosis through a pathway dependent on respiratory competent mitochondria. *FASEB J* 2005;19:1012-1014.
51. Thawornchaisit P, Harncharoen K. A comparative study of tar and betamethasone valerate in chronic plaque psoriasis: A study in Thailand. *J Med Assoc Thai* 2007;90:1997-2002.
52. Stuetz A, Grassberger M, Meingassner JG. Pimecrolimus (Elidel, SDZ ASM 981)—preclinical pharmacologic profile and skin selectivity. *Semin Cutan Med Surg* 2001;20:233-241.
53. Mrowietz U, Graeber M, Brautigam M, et al. The novel azomycin derivative SDZ ASM 981 is effective for psoriasis when used topically under occlusion. *Br J Dermatol* 1998;139:992-996.
54. Gribetz C, Ling M, Lebwohl M, et al. Pimecrolimus cream 1% in the treatment of intertriginous psoriasis: A double-blind, randomized study. *J Am Acad Dermatol* 2004;51:731-738.
55. Matz H. Phototherapy for psoriasis: What to choose and how to use: Facts and controversies. *Clin Dermatol* 2010;28:73-80.
56. Archier E, Devaux S, Castela E, et al. Efficacy of Psoralen UV-A therapy vs. narrowband UV-B therapy in chronic plaque psoriasis: A systematic literature review. *J Euro Acad Dermatol Venereol* 2012;26(suppl 3):11-21.
57. Stern RS. Genital tumors among men with psoriasis exposed to psoralens and ultraviolet A radiation (PUVA) and ultraviolet B radiation: The photochemotherapy follow-up study. *N Engl J Med* 1990;322:1093-1097.
58. Anstey AV, Kragballe K. Retrospective assessment of PASI 50 and PASI 75 attainment with a calcipotriol/betamethasone dipropionate ointment. *Int J Dermatol* 2006;45:970-975.
59. Mahrie G, Schulze HJ, Farber L, et al. Low-dose short-term cyclosporine versus etretinate in psoriasis: Improvement of skin, nail, and joint involvement. *J Am Acad Dermatol* 1995;32:78-88.
60. Heydendael VM, Spuls POL, Opmeer BC, et al. Methotrexate versus cyclosporine in moderate-to-severe chronic plaque psoriasis. *N Engl J Med* 2003;349:658-665.
61. Shupack J, Abel E, Bauer E, et al. Cyclosporine as maintenance therapy in patients with severe psoriasis. *J Am Acad Dermatol* 1997;36: 423-432.
62. Saurat JH, Stingl G, Dubertret L, et al. Efficacy and safety results from the randomized controlled comparative study of adalimumab vs. methotrexate vs. placebo in patients with psoriasis (CHAMPION). *Br J Dermatol* 2008;158:558-566.
63. Maybury CM, Samarasekera E, Douriri A et al. Diagnostic accuracy of noninvasive markers of liver fibrosis in patients with psoriasis taking methotrexate: A systematic review and meta-analysis. *Br J Dermatol* 2014;170(6):1237-1247.DOI 10.1111/bjd.12905 .
64. Ferrandiz C, Carrascosa JM, Boada A. A new era in the management of psoriasis? The biologics: Facts and controversies. *Clin Dermatol* 2010;28:81-87.
65. Langley RG. Effective and sustainable biologic treatment of psoriasis: What can we learn from new clinical data? *J Euro Acad Dermatol Venereol* 2012;26(suppl 2):21-29.
66. Gordon K, Papp K, Poulin Y, et al. Long-term efficacy and safety of adalimumab in patients with moderate-to-severe psoriasis treated continuously over 3 years: Results from an open-label extension study for patients from REVEAL. *J Am Acad Dermatol* 2012;66: 241-251.
67. Moustou A-E, Matekovits A, Dessinioti C, et al. Cutaneous side effects of anti-tumor necrosis factor biologic therapy: A clinical review. *J Am Acad Dermatol* 2009;61:486-504.
68. Poulin Y, Langley R, Teiseira HD, et al. Biologics in the treatment of psoriasis: Clinical and economic overview. *J Cutan Med Surg* 2009;13(suppl 2):S49-S57.
69. Health Canada. Association of Enbrel (etanercept) with Histoplasmosis and Other Invasive Fungal Infections—For Health Professionals. 2009, Available at: http://www.healthycanadians.gc.ca/recall-alert-rappel-avis/hc-sc/2009/14545a-eng.php. Accessed September 9, 2016.

70. Adalimumab (Humura) product monograph. Date of Revision: April 6, 2016 and Control No. 190512. Available at: http://www.abbvie.ca/content/dam/abbviecorp/ca/english/docs/HUMIRA_PM_EN.pdf. Accessed September 9, 2016.
71. Gordon KB, Langley RG, Leonard C, et al. Clinical response to adalimumab treatment in patients with moderate-to-severe psoriasis: Double-blind, randomized controlled trial and open-label extension study. *J Am Acad Dermatol* 2006;55:598-606.
72. Menter A, Tyring SK, Gordon K, et al. Adalimumab therapy for moderate to severe psoriasis: A randomized, controlled phase III trial. *J Am Acad Dermatol* 2008;58:106-15.
73. Leonardi CL, Powers JL, Matheson RT, et al. Etanercept as monotherapy in patients with psoriasis. *N Engl J Med* 2003;349:2014-2022.
74. Paller AS, Siegfried EC, Langley RG, et al. Etanercept treatment for children and adolescents with plaque psoriasis. *N Engl J Med* 2008;358:241-251.
75. Gottlieb AB, Kalb RE, Blauvelt A, et al. The efficacy and safety of infliximab in patients with plaque psoriasis who had an inadequate response to etanercept: Results of a prospective, multicenter, open-label study. *J Am Acad Dermatol* 2011;67:642-650.
76. Reich K, Nestle FO, Papp K, et al. Infliximab induction and maintenance therapy for moderate-to-severe psoriasis: A phase III, multicenter, double-blind trial. *Lancet* 2005;366:1367-1374.
77. Menter A, Feldman SR, Weinstein GD, et al. A randomized comparison of continuous vs intermittent infliximab maintenance regimens over 1 year in the treatment of moderate-to-severe plaque psoriasis. *J Am Acad Dermatol* 2007;56:e1-e15.
78. Goffe B, Papp K, Gratton D, et al. An integrated analysis of thirteen trials summarizing the long-term safety of alefacept in psoriasis patients who have received up to nine courses of therapy. *Clin Ther* 2005;27:1912-1921.
79. Stelara (ustekinumab injection) product monograph. January 2014. Available at: https://www.cadth.ca/sites/default/files/cdr/monograph/Stelara_Product_Monograph.pdf and at www.janssen.ca and at http://www.stelarainfo.com/pdf/PrescribingInformation.pdf. Accessed October 31, 2015.
80. Leonardi C, Kimball AB, Papp K, et al. Efficacy and safety of ustekinumab, a human interleukin-12/23 monoclonal antibody, in patients with psoriasis: 76-Week results from a randomized, double-blind, placebo-controlled trial (PHOENIX 1). *Lancet* 2008;371:1665-1674.
81. Papp KA, Langley RG, Lebwohl M, et al. Efficacy and safety of ustekinumab, a human interleukin-12/23 monoclonal antibody, in patients with psoriasis: 52-Week results from a randomized, double-blind, placebo-controlled trial (PHOENIX 2). *Lancet* 2008;371:1675-1684.
82. Langley RG, Feldman SR, Han C, et al. Ustekinumab significantly improves symptoms of anxiety, depression, and skin-related quality of life in patients with moderate-to-severe psoriasis: Results from a randomized, double-blind, placebo-controlled phase III trial. *J Am Acad Dermatol* 2010;63:457-465.
83. Sofen H, Wasel N, Yeilding N, et al. Ustekinumab improves overall skin response and health-related quality of life, in a subset of moderate-to-severe psoriasis patients with psoriatic arthritis: Analysis of PHOENIX 1 and 2. *J Am Acad Dermatol* 2011 Feb;64(2 suppl 1): AB156.
84. Lebwohl M, Yeilding N, Szapary P, et al. Impact of weight on the efficacy and safety of ustekinumab in patients with moderate to severe psoriasis: Rationale for dosing recommendations. *J Am Acad Dermatol* 2010;63:571-579.
85. Lebwohl M, Leonardi C, Griffiths CEM, et al. Long-term safety experience of ustekinumab in patients with moderate-to-severe psoriasis (part I of II): Results from analyses of general safety parameters from pooled phase 2 and 3 clinical trials. *J Am Acad Dermatol* 2012;66:731-741.
86. Gordon KB, Papp KA, Langley RG, et al. Long-term safety experience of ustekinumab in patients with moderate-to-severe psoriasis (part II of II): Results from analyses of infections and malignancy from pooled phase II and III clinical trials. *J Am Acad Dermatol* 2012;66: 742-751.
87. Secukinumab (Cosentyx) product monograph. Novartis revised 1/2016. Available at: https://www.pharma.us.novartis.com/sites/www.pharma.us.novartis.com/files/cosentyx.pdf. Accessed September 9, 2016.
88. Langley RG, Elewski BE, Lebwohl M et al. Secukinumab in plaque psoriasis – results of two Phase 3 trials. *New Engl J Med* 2014; 371:4 Available at: http://www.nejm.org/doi/pdf/10.1056/NEJMoa1314258. Accessed September 9, 2016
89. Koo JY, Lowe NJ, Lew-Kaya DA, et al. Tazarotene plus UVB phototherapy in the treatment of psoriasis. *J Am Acad Dermatol* 2000;43:821-828.
90. Lowe NJ, Prystowsky JH, Bourget T, et al. Acitretin plus UVB therapy for psoriasis: Comparisons with placebo plus UVB and acitretin alone. *J Am Acad Dermatol* 1991;24:591-594.
91. Spuls PI, Rozenblit M, Lebwohl M. Retrospective study of the efficacy of narrowband UVB and acitretin. *J Dermatol Treat* 2003;14(suppl):17-20.
92. Tanew A, Guggenbichler A, Honigsmann H, et al. Photochemotherapy for severe psoriasis without or in combination with acitretin: A randomized, double-blind comparison study. *J Am Acad Dermatol* 1991;25:682-684.
93. Legat FJ, Hofer A, Wackernagel A, et al. Narrowband UV-B phototherapy, alefacept, and clearance of psoriasis. *Arch Dermatol* 2007;143:1016-1022.
94. Orvis AK, Wesson SK, Breza TS, et al. Mycophenolate mofetil in dermatology. *J Am Acad Dermatol* 2009;60:183-199.
95. Davidson SC, Morris-Jones R, Powles AV, et al. Change of treatment from cyclosporin to mycophenolate mofetil in severe psoriasis. *Br J Dermatol* 2000;143:405-407.
96. Pedraz J, Dauden E, Delgado-Jimenez Y, et al. Sequential study on the treatment of moderate-to-severe chronic plaque psoriasis with mycophenolate mofetil and cyclosporin. *J Eur Acad Dermatol Venereol* 2006;20:702-706.
97. Patel RV, Clark LN, Lebwohl M, et al. Treatments for psoriasis and the risk of malignancy. *J Am Acad Dermatol* 2009;60:1001-1017.
98. Ranjan N, Sharma NL, Shanker V, et al. Methotrexate versus hydroxycarbamide (hydroxyurea) as a weekly dose to treat moderate-to-severe chronic plaque psoriasis: A comparative study. *J Dermatol Treat* 2007;18:295-300.
99. Smith N, Weymann A, Tausk FA, et al. Complementary and alternative medicine for psoriasis: A qualitative review of the clinical trial literature. *J Am Acad Dermatol* 2009;61:841-856.
100. Bernstein S, Donsky H, Gulliver W, et al. Treatment of mild to moderate psoriasis with Relieva, a Mahonia aquifolium extract—A double-blind, placebo-controlled study. *Am J Ther* 2006;13:121-126.
101. Danno K, Sugie N. Combination therapy with low-dose etretinate and eicosapentaenoic acid for psoriasis vulgaris. *J Dermatol* 1998;25:703-705.
102. Brochow T, Schiener R, Franke A, et al. A pragmatic randomized controlled trial on the effectiveness of highly concentrated saline spa water baths followed by UVB compared to UVB only in moderate to severe psoriasis. *J Altern Complement Med* 2007;13:725-732.
103. Brochow T, Schiener R, Franke A, et al. A pragmatic randomized controlled trial on the effectiveness of low concentrated saline spa water baths followed by ultraviolet B (UVB) compared to UVB only in moderate-to-severe psoriasis. *J Eur Acad Dermatol Venereol* 2007;21:1027-1037.
104. Gaston L, Crombez J, Lassonde M, et al. Psychological stress and psoriasis: Experimental and prospective correlational studies. *Acta Derm Venereol* 1991;156:37-43.
105. Kabat-Zinn J, Wheeler E, Light T, et al. Influence of a mindfulness meditation-based stress reduction intervention on rates of skin clearing in patients with moderate to severe psoriasis undergoing phototherapy (UVB) and photochemotherapy (PUVA). *Psychosom Med* 1998;60:625-632.
106. Treloar V. Integrative dermatology for psoriasis: Facts and controversies. *Clin Dermatol* 2010;28:93-99.
107. Naldi L, Chatenoud L, Linder D, et al. Cigarette smoking, body mass index, and stressful life events as risk factors for psoriasis: Results from an Italian case-control study. *J Invest Dermatol* 2005;125:61-67.
108. Horn EJ, Fox KM, Patel V, et al. Are patients with psoriasis undertreated? Results of National Psoriasis Foundation survey. *J Am Acad Dermatol* 2007;57:957-962.
109. Augustin M, Alvaro-Gracia JM, Bagot M, et al. A framework for improving the quality of care for people with psoriasis. *J Euro Acad Dermatol Venereol* 2012;26(suppl 4):1-16.
110. Benoit S, Hamm H. Childhood psoriasis. *Clin Dermatol* 2007;25:555-562.
111. De Jager MEA, de Jong EMG, van de Kerkhof PCM, et al. Efficacy and safety of treatments for childhood psoriasis: A systemic literature review. *J Am Acad Dermatol* 2010;62:1013-1030.
112. Paller AS, Siegfried EC, Langley RG, et al. Etanercept treatment for children and adolescents with plaque psoriasis. *N Engl J Med* 2008;358:241-251.
113. Murase JE, Chan KK, Garite TJ, et al. Hormonal effect on psoriasis in pregnancy and post partum. *Arch Dermatol* 2005;141:601-606.

114. Lam J, Polifka JE, Dohil MA. Safety of dermatologic drugs used in pregnant patients with psoriasis and other inflammatory skin diseases. *J Am Acad Dermatol* 2008;59:295-315.
115. Menter A, Gordon KB, Leonardi CL, et al. Efficacy and safety of adalimumab across subgroups of patients with moderate to severe psoriasis. *J Am Acad Dermatol* 2010;63:448-456.
116. Bonafede M, Watson C, Fox K. Cost of tumor necrosis factor blocker per treated psoriatic arthritis patient using drug utilization data from a US managed care population. *J Am Acad Dermatol* 2012 Apr: 66(4)suppl 1: AB189 (poster reference no 5165. Poster abstracts. American Academy of Dermatology 70th Annual Meeting, San Diego, California, March 15-20, 2012).
117. Augustin M, Sundaram M, Mulani PM, et al. Cost per responder with adalimumab versus ustekinumab treatment for moderate-to-severe psoriasis with suboptimal response to etanercept. *J Am Acad Dermatol* 2012 Apr: 66(4)suppl 1: AB189 (poster reference no. 5056. Poster abstracts. American Academy of Dermatology 70th Annual Meeting, San Diego, California, March 15-20, 2012).

98

Atopic Dermatitis

Rebecca M. Law and Po Gin Kwa

KEY CONCEPTS

1. Atopic dermatitis (AD) is a chronic skin disorder involving inflammation associated with intense pruritus, a hallmark symptom. Management of AD must always include appropriate management of the associated pruritus.
2. AD is associated with other atopic diseases such as asthma and allergic rhinitis in the same patient or family. The three conditions are known as the *atopic triad*.
3. The prevalence of AD appears to have increased two- to threefold in many developed and developing countries during the last three decades. Recent data indicate age and country or regional differences, with some countries showing no change or even a decrease. Rural areas appear to have lower prevalence rates.
4. There are genetic and environmental factors in the pathogenesis and pathophysiologic manifestations of AD. The inheritance pattern is not straightforward. More than one gene may be involved in the disease, with the filaggrin gene (*FLG*) being a key player. Other genes coding for specific cytokines are also involved.
5. AD usually presents in infants and young children. The clinical presentation differs somewhat depending on the age of the patient.
6. Secondary bacterial skin infections are common in patients with AD and must be promptly treated.
7. Management of AD must always include appropriate nonpharmacologic management of any controllable environmental factors, such as avoidance of identified triggers. These may include aeroallergens (eg, mold, grass, pollen), foods (eg, peanuts, eggs, tomatoes), chemicals (eg, detergents, soaps), clothing material (eg, wool, polyester), temperature (eg, excessive heat), and humidity (eg, low humidity).
8. Nonpharmacologic management of AD entails managing the symptoms associated with pruritus and encouraging appropriate skin care habits such as proper bathing techniques and the copious use of moisturizers, which is a standard of care.
9. Topical corticosteroids (TCS) are the drugs of first choice for AD.
10. Topical calcineurin inhibitors (tacrolimus and pimecrolimus) are alternate treatment options for adults and children older than 2 years.
11. Phototherapy is a second-line treatment when TCS and topical calcineurin inhibitors fail.
12. This chronic illness has substantial socioeconomic impact. The cost may be magnified by undertreatment.

(1) Atopic dermatitis (AD) is a chronic, pruritic inflammatory skin disease. It is often referred to as *eczema*, which is a general term for several types of skin inflammation. AD is the most common type of eczema (Table 98-1).[1] Pruritus is the hallmark symptom and presentation and is responsible for much of the disease burden borne by patients and their families.[2]

(2) This form of dermatitis is commonly associated with a personal or family history of other atopic disorders, such as allergic rhinitis and asthma[2] (collectively known as the *atopic triad*). AD has been considered the start of the "atopic march"[2]; however, the association with other atopic conditions is multifactorial and complex, since this progression does not happen in all cases.[2] The disease can have periods of exacerbation, or flare-ups, followed by periods of remission. These flare-ups may be disruptive to the patient's quality of life and may affect the entire family. Disease flare-ups are difficult to manage and may be complicated by secondary infections. About one-half (estimate up to 65%) of cases in children first manifest before age 1 year[1-4]; these cases are termed *early onset atopic dermatitis*.[5] Onset of AD is most common between 3 and 6 months of age.[2] Approximately 85% to 90% of patients develop symptoms before age 5 years.[2]

Among children with AD, 10%-30% will have the skin condition in adulthood.[2] However, onset after age 30 years is much less common and is often caused by exposure to harsh or wet conditions[1] such as repeated skin trauma or exposure to harsh chemicals.

EPIDEMIOLOGY

(3) The prevalence of AD is generally said to have increased two- to threefold in developed and developing countries during the past three decades.[5] In developed countries, an estimated 15% to 30% of children and 2% to 10% of adults are affected.[5,6] The prevalence appears to be increasing worldwide, as earlier prevalence rates were estimated at 10% to 15% in children.[4]

(3) The largest international study of the prevalence of AD found both age and country differences in prevalence rates.[7] This international study was the International Study of Asthma and Allergies in Childhood (ISAAC), which was conducted in three phases.[8] The strength of this study was the use of a uniformly validated methodology which allowed a direct comparison of results from pediatric populations worldwide.[9] ISAAC Phase One included 700,000 children from 156 centers in 56 countries between 1992 and 1998. ISAAC Phase Two studied allergic causes from 30 centers in 22 countries. ISAAC Phase Three repeated a multicountry cross-sectional survey (1999-2004) and included 187,943 children between ages 6 and 7 years from 64 centers in 35 countries and 302,159 adolescents between ages 13 and 14 years from 105 centers in 55 countries. For children aged 6 to 7 years, most countries showed an increase of two standard deviations (SDs) in mean annual prevalence over a 5- to 10-year period. In contrast, for adolescents aged 13 to 14 years, the

TABLE 98-1 Types of Eczema (Dermatitis)[1]

- **Allergic contact eczema (dermatitis):** A red, itchy, weepy reaction where the skin has come into contact with a substance that the immune system recognizes as foreign, such as poison ivy or certain preservatives in creams and lotions.
- **Atopic dermatitis:** A chronic skin disease characterized by itchy, inflamed skin.
- **Contact eczema (dermatitis):** A localized reaction that includes redness, itching, and burning where the skin has come into contact with an allergen (an allergy-causing substance) or with an irritant such as an acid, cleaning agent, or other chemical.
- **Dyshidrotic eczema:** Irritation of the skin on the palms of hands and soles of the feet characterized by clear, deep blisters that itch and burn.
- **Neurodermatitis:** Scaly patches of the skin on the head, lower legs, wrists, or forearms caused by a localized itch (such as an insect bite) that become intensely irritated when scratched.
- **Nummular eczema:** Coin-shaped patches of irritated skin—most common on the arms, back, buttocks, and lower legs—that may be crusted, scaling, and extremely itchy.
- **Seborrheic eczema:** Yellowish, oily, scaly patches of skin on the scalp, face, and occasionally other parts of the body.
- **Stasis dermatitis:** A skin irritation on the lower legs, generally related to circulatory problems.

trends differ from country to country. Large increases in prevalence were seen in developing countries (eg, Mexico, Chile, Kenya, and Algeria, and seven countries in Southeast Asia). But in other countries with formerly very high prevalences, the mean annual prevalence in eczema symptoms has either leveled off or decreased. Most of the largest decreases (SD more than or equal to 2) in prevalence were reported from developed countries in northwest Europe, (eg, the United Kingdom, Ireland, Sweden, Germany) and New Zealand.[7] The ISAAC study has suggested that a maximum prevalence plateau of approximately 20% has emerged.[7,8]

There were no differences according to the sex of the study participant, or with gross national income at a country level.[7] This is consistent with other reports that AD affects men and women at approximately the same rate.[1] There appears to be a lower prevalence of AD in rural areas when compared with urban areas,[2] suggesting a link to the *hygiene hypothesis*,[10-11] which postulates that the absence of early childhood exposure to infectious agents increases susceptibility to allergic diseases.[10-12] In contrast, children attending daycare centers before 3 months of age have less atopy and asthma in later childhood,[11,12] and areas with diffuse and chronic helminth infestations have a low prevalence of allergic diseases.[12] In addition, a European birth cohort study involving 1,133 newborns showed that children born to farm families had a lower prevalence of sensitization to seasonal inhaled allergens such as grass pollen.[11,13] Maternal exposure during pregnancy (ie, prenatal exposure) to animal sheds correlated with the lower prevalence rate in the farm children. However, there were no differences in prevalence related to inhaled perennial allergens. Parasitic infections decreased the risk of allergen sensitization.[11] A recent systematic review reported that exposures to endotoxin, farm animals, and dogs may protect against AD.[14]

Although reported risk factors associated with higher prevalence include urban environment, higher socioeconomic status, higher level of family education, a family history of AD, female gender (after age 6 years), and smaller family size.[8] However, more recent studies are conflicting. There are no consistent findings that higher socioeconomic status or male/female gender affect the risk of AD.[2] Urban living does appear to increase the risk of AD, but studies attempting to identify causative environmental agents have been inconclusive.[2] Strongly associated risk factors include a family history of AD, and the loss of function mutations in the *FLG* gene.[2]

ETIOLOGY

(4) AD is a complex genetic disease that arises from gene–gene and gene–environment interactions. There are two major groups of genes involved. First, there are the genes encoding for epidermal or other epithelial structural proteins. Second, there are genes encoding for the major elements of the immune system.[5]

The inheritance pattern is not straightforward. More than one gene is likely involved in the disease. There is an increased risk for a child to have AD if there is a family history of other atopic diseases, such as hay fever or asthma. The risk of AD is two- to threefold higher in children with one atopic parent and three- to fivefold higher if both parents are atopic.[2] Studies of identical twins show that a person whose identical twin has AD is seven times more likely to have AD than someone in the general population.[1] And a person whose fraternal twin has AD is three times more likely to have AD than someone in the general population.[1] Another estimate is 80% concordance in monozygous twins and 20% in heterozygous twins.[10]

Thus, genetic predispositions to developing AD exist. Specifically, there are several possible genes on the chromosomes 3q21, 1q21, 16q, 17q25, 20p, and 3p26. Of these chromosomes, 1q21 has the highest linkage region. This region has a family of epithelium-related genes called the epidermal differentiation complex.[5] One of these genes, the filaggrin gene (*FLG*), on chromosome 1q21.3, encodes for profilaggrin which degrades to filaggrin proteins.[2] Filaggrin proteins playkey roless in epidermal differentiation, including terminal differentiation of the epidermis and formation of the skin barrier (including the stratum corneum).[2,15] Filaggrin breakdown products are natural moisturizers and contribute to epidermal hydration and barrier function.[2] Mutations or deficiency of *FLG* results in an abnormality in permeability barrier function.[15] Patients with AD who carry *FLG* mutations have more persistent disease, a higher incidence of skin infections with herpes virus (eczema herpeticum) and a greater risk for multiple allergies.[15] However, many patients with AD have no known *FLG* mutations, and conversely, about 40% of people with *FLG* null alleles do not develop AD.[2,15]

Epidermal barrier dysfunction is a prerequisite for the penetration of high-molecular-weight allergens in pollens, house dust mite products, microbes, and food.[5] In mice studies, this barrier abnormality lowers irritability thresholds, and enhanced cutaneous allergen penetration.[15] In humans, two common *FLG* variants (*R501X* and *2282del4*) with an estimated combined allele frequency of about 6% have been identified in individuals of European descent.[16] Eighteen other less common variants have also been identified in Europeans, with an additional 17 mutations restricted to individuals of Asian descent.[16] Each of these variants leads to nonsense mutations which either prevent or severely diminish the production of filaggrin in the epidermis.[16] Mutations of *FLG* seem to occur mainly in early onset AD patients and may be associated with the development of asthma in patients with AD.[5,16] However, *FLG* mutations are identified in only 30% of European patients with AD; implying that other genetic mutations affecting other epidermal structures may be important (eg, changes in the cornified envelope proteins involucrin and loricrin, or lipid composition).[5]

(4) There are other genes encoding for the immune system that may be associated with AD, especially those found on chromosome 5q31-33.[5] These genes code for cytokines that regulate IgE synthesis. Cytokines are produced by helper T cells (TH_0, TH_1, TH_2, TH_3).[11] T-helper type 1 (TH_1) cells produce cytokines that suppress immunoglobulin E (IgE) production (eg, interferon-γ and interleukin-12 [IL-12]).[5] T-helper type 2 (TH_2) cells produce cytokines that increase IgE production (eg, IL-5 and IL-13).[5,17] In patients with AD, there is an imbalance between TH_1 and TH_2 immune responses. These patients are genetically predisposed to TH_2 predominance, seen as increased TH_2 cell activity.[2,5,9,17] Increased TH_2 activity causes the release of IL-3, IL-4, IL-5, IL-10, and IL-13, resulting in blood

eosinophilia, increased total serum IgE, and increased growth and development of mast cells.[2,5,11,17,18] This is seen in the initial and acute phase of AD.[9] In addition, these cytokines affect the maturation of B cells and cause a genomic rearrangement in these cells that favors isotype class switching from immunoglobulin M (IgM) to IgE.[5] As discussed below, epidermal Langerhans cells (LC) and dendritic cells (DC) with high-affinity IgE receptors uptake allergens and mediate the inflammatory response.[11]

In summary, *FLG* deficiency alone can provoke a barrier abnormality in the epidermis and predispose to the development of dermatitis by enhancing allergen absorption through the skin.[19] Furthermore, there appears to be complex relationships, including genetic and nongenetic risk factors, that modify an individual's susceptibility to allergic disease.[20] Complex genetic factors contribute to the increased susceptibility to AD (*FLG* mutations and gene–gene interactions). These, along with environmental factors such as food allergens[21] (gene–environment interactions), result in the pathophysiologic changes and clinical presentations associated with AD.

PATHOPHYSIOLOGY

The initial mechanisms that trigger inflammatory changes in the skin in patients with AD are unknown. Neuropeptides, irritation, or pruritus-induced scratching may be causing the release of proinflammatory cytokines from keratinocytes. Alternatively, allergens in the epidermal barrier or in food[21] may cause T-cell mediated but IgE-independent reactions. Allergen-specific IgE is not a prerequisite.[5] Characteristic features in pathophysiology are skin barrier dysfunction, and immune deviation toward TH_2 with subsequent increased IgE.[10] The disease is further complicated by microbial colonization with pathologic organisms resulting in increased susceptibility for skin infections.[10]

As discussed above, skin barrier dysfunction plays a critical role in the development of AD,[10,11,15,,22] with loss of function mutations in *FLG* being a major risk factor.[15,22] Other factors may include a deficiency of skin barrier proteins, increased peptidase activity, lack of certain protease inhibitors, and lipid abnormalities.[22] There must be epidermal barrier dysfunction for high-molecular-weight allergens in pollens, house dust mite particles, microbes, and foods to penetrate the skin barrier. Atopic skin has reduced antimicrobial peptides (AMPs). AMPs are normally produced by keratinocytes, sebocytes, and mast cells, and they form a chemical shield on the surface of the skin. Reduced AMPs result in a diminished antimicrobial barrier, which correlates with increased susceptibility to infections and superinfections seen in these patients.[23]

On penetration of the epidermal barrier, allergens are met by DCs. DCs are antigen-presenting cells populating the skin, respiratory tract, and mucosa of the gastrointestinal (GI) tract (ie, at the front line of pathogen entry).[24] DCs then enhance TH_2 polarization, resulting in increased production of IgE. Keratinocytes in the skin of patients with AD also produce high levels of an IL-7–like protein, which again drives dendritic cells to enhance TH_2 polarization. Epidermal DCs in patients with AD bear IgE and express its high-affinity receptor (FcεRI).[25-27] Total serum IgE is often elevated in patients with AD,[1,2,18] especially during an exacerbation.

However, on initial presentation, patients with early onset AD generally do not have increased total serum IgE levels (ie, there is no detectable IgE-mediated allergic sensitization). IgE-mediated allergic sensitization may occur several weeks or months after the initial AD lesions appear. Although in some children—mostly girls—this sensitization never occurs.[5] Furthermore, elevated total serum IgE is not specific to AD and can be associated even with nonatopic conditions.[2]

Other potential biomarkers currently discovered include serum CD30, macrophage-derived chemoattractant (MDC), IL-12, -16, -18, and -31, and thymus and activation-regulated chemokine (TARC); however, to date none of them have shown reliable sensitivity nor specificity for clinical use.[2]

Predisposing Factors

Several factors can predispose patients to development of AD. These include climate, infection, genetics, environmental aeroallergens, and food.

Hot and extremely cold climates are both poorly tolerated by patients with this condition. Dry weather, common in the winter, causes increased skin dryness. Hot weather causes increased sweating, resulting in pruritus.

Patients with AD are commonly colonized by *Staphylococcus aureus* bacteria. Clinical infections with *S aureus* frequently cause flare-ups of AD.

As discussed previously, genetics plays a role in AD. Family history of AD is a strong risk factor.

Exposure to environmental aeroallergens is another risk factor. Dust mites, pollens, molds, cigarette smoke, and dander from animal hair or skin may worsen the symptoms of AD.[1,18]

The role of food as antigens in the pathogenesis of AD is still not fully understood.[15,21] Preliminary results (mostly animal studies) indicate that defects in the skin and gut barrier function may facilitate sensitization to food allergens.[21] Small amounts of environmental foods (low-dose exposure from foods on tabletops, hands, dust) may penetrate the skin barrier and be taken up by LCs, leading to TH_2 responses and IgE production.[28] However, early high-dose oral food consumption induces oral tolerance. The timing and balance of cutaneous and oral exposure determines whether a child will have allergy or tolerance.[28] Increased serum IgE antibodies to a particular food is evidence of sensitization to a food and is consistent with although not proof of a food allergy.[1,29] Eczema may frequently be a manifestation of food allergy,[28] and patients with AD have a higher prevalence of food allergy than those in the general population.[1] Conversely, there is a belief that food allergy may be caused by AD, and in most patients with coexisting AD and food allergy, AD precedes the food allergy. (The assumption is that AD is a causal risk factor for asthma and systemic allergen sensitization in the context of *FLG* mutations.[15]) Regardless, the two conditions coexist, and the likelihood of an infant or child with AD also having food allergy or allergies must be kept in mind.[29]

There is a known epidermal barrier dysfunction in AD, allowing for increased low-level skin permeability to allergenic foods. Certain foods may trigger acute reactions, including urticaria and anaphylaxis. The most commonly reported allergenic foods are eggs, milk, peanuts, wheat, soy, tree nuts, shellfish, and fish.[1] Individual food allergies, such as peanut allergy, have increased in prevalence in the past decade;[28,29] new food allergies may also be increasing in prevalence, particularly kiwi allergy[28,30] and sesame seed allergy.[28,31] Allergies to seafood, peanuts, and nuts are more likely to persist into adulthood, while allergies to milk, eggs, wheat, and soy generally resolve by late-childhood.[21] Consistent with the oral tolerance concept, early results from recent studies using sublingual and oral immunotherapy to specific food allergens (eg, milk or peanut) appear to indicate that it may be possible to induce oral tolerance, and that it may be possible to desensitize children to some allergenic foods.[32] Nine to 12 months of immunotherapy was needed to observe the beneficial effect and "the present evidence does not warrant routine recommendation" by the AAD.[33] Injectable allergen-specific immunotherapy is also being studied.[33] National Institute of Allergy and Infectious Diseases (NIAID) suggests limited food allergy testing (ie, cow's milk, eggs, wheat, soy, peanut) if a child younger than 5 years has moderate to severe AD and persistent disease despite optimal therapy.[29,33] For more information about management of food allergies the reader is directed to the 2010 NIAID-sponsored expert panel's report, available at www.niaid.nih.gov.[29]

TABLE 98-2 Skin Features Associated with Atopic Dermatitis[1]

- **Atopic pleat (Dennie-Morgan fold):** An extra fold of skin that develops under the eye.
- **Cheilitis:** Inflammation of the skin on and around the lips.
- **Hyperlinear palms:** Increased number of skin creases on the palms.
- **Hyperpigmented eyelids:** Eyelids that have become darker in color from inflammation or hay fever.
- **Ichthyosis:** Dry, rectangular scales on the skin.
- **Keratosis pilaris:** Small, rough bumps, generally on the face, upper arms, and thighs.
- **Lichenification:** Thick, leathery skin resulting from constant scratching and rubbing.
- **Papules:** Small raised bumps that may open when scratched and become crusty and infected.
- **Urticaria:** Hives (red, raised bumps) that may occur after exposure to an allergen, at the beginning of flares, or after exercise or a hot bath.

CLINICAL PRESENTATION

Diagnosis of AD is generally based on clinical presentation (Table 98-2).[1] There is currently no objective diagnostic test or reliable biomarker for the clinical confirmation of AD.[1,2] On occasion, skin biopsy specimens or other tests (eg, total and/or allergen-specific serum IgE, potassium hydroxide preparation, patch testing, and/or genetic testing) may be used to rule out other diseases or associated skin conditions.[2] *FLG* gene mutations may be associated with persistent and more severe AD as well as early onset cases.[22]

Clinical **Controversy...**

Although it has traditionally been thought that food allergies are a predisposing factor for the development of AD, some clinicians are now thinking that AD may be the predisposing factor for the development of food allergies in an individual. Often the signs and symptoms of AD appear before the food allergies.

5 AD follows a relapsing course.[33,34] Studies reviewing the natural course of the disease usually describe the disease pattern as persistent, intermittent, or in remission.[8] A 2004 study found that 43% were in complete remission after age 2 years, with 19% having persistent disease and 38% an intermittent pattern.[8]

The clinical presentation of AD differs depending on the age of the patient. In infancy, the earliest onset of AD usually occurs between 3 and 6 months of age, with 60% of patients develop symptoms within the first year of life, and 85% to 90% will have developed symptoms before the age of 5 years.[1,2] The initial presentation in infancy is an erythematous, papular skin rash that may first appear on the cheeks and chin as a patchy facial and that can then progress to red, scaling, oozing skin.[1] The rash shows a centrifugal distribution affecting the malar region of the cheeks, forehead, scalp, chin, and behind the ears while sparing the central areas (ie, the nose and paranasal creases). Lesions occur in the flexor surfaces, such as antecubital and popliteal fossae. Over the next few weeks and as the infant becomes more mobile and begins crawling, the lesions spread to the extensors of the lower legs, and eventually the entire body may be involved, with sparing of the groin, axillary region, and the nose.[1,2,34] These lesions are associated with uncontrollable itchiness, and the infant will become irritable and may try to rub his or her face to relieve the itch. Scratching may occur quite early, and infants with AD may scratch themselves continuously, even during sleep.[2] Sleep disruption occurs in up to 60% of children with AD, increasing to 80% or more during exacerbations.[2] Excessive rubbing or scratching may result in excoriation and development of secondary infections.

In childhood, the skin often appears dry, flaky, rough, cracked, and may bleed because of scratching. With repeated scratching and rubbing the skin becomes lichenified. Lichenification, usually localized to the flexural folds of the extremities, is characteristic of childhood AD in older children and in adults.[34] Lichenification signifies repeated rubbing of the skin and is seen mostly over the folds, bony protuberances, and forehead.[34] Excoriations and crusting are also commonly seen, along with secondary infections. Sometimes increased folds are seen underneath the eyes (so-called Dennie–Morgan folds).[34] Lesions are still most commonly seen in the flexor surfaces of the body, particularly the flexural creases of the antecubital and popliteal fossae.[34]

Sleep disturbances also occur. One study reported that there are both brief and longer awakenings associated with scratching episodes that affect sleep efficiency in school-age children with AD.[35]

In adulthood, lesions are more diffuse with underlying erythema. The face is commonly involved and may be dry and scaly. Lichenification may again be seen. A brown macular ring around the neck, representing a localized deposit of amyloid, is typical but not always present.[34]

Although no objective diagnostic test confirms the presence of AD,[1,2] some signs, symptoms, and other factors are commonly used in its diagnosis. These include pruritus, early age of onset, eczematous skin lesions that vary with age, chronic and relapsing courses, dry and flaky skin, IgE reactivity, family or personal history of asthma or hay fever, or other atopic diseases (Tables 98-3 and 98-4).[2,34] In addition, allergy skin testing may be helpful in identifying factors that trigger flares of AD.[1] Negative results may help rule out certain substances as triggers; however, positive results may be unrelated to disease activity, and false positives are common.[1]

1 Pruritus is a quintessential feature of AD, and a diagnosis cannot be made if there is no history of itching.[1-4,34] Scratching and rubbing itchy atopic skin further irritates the skin, increases inflammation, and exacerbates itchiness.[3] Atopic skin can itch during sleep. This nighttime itching is a problem for many infants and children with the disease, since there is no conscious control of scratching during sleep.[1,2,18] Pruritus is the symptom that most affects the health-related quality of life for most patients with AD. In studies, more than 50% of patients rated their pruritus as very bothersome or extremely bothersome, and reported that they often or always experienced intolerable symptoms.[34]

Pruritus can be triggered by a variety of factors. The most common triggers of itch have been reported as heat and perspiration (96%), wool (91%), emotional stress (81%), certain (usually vasodilatory) foods (49%), alcohol (44%), upper respiratory infections (36%), and house dust mites (more than 35%).[34,35]

TABLE 98-3 Clinical Features in the Diagnosis of Atopic Dermatitis[2]

Essential Features (Must Be Present):
- Pruritus
- Eczema (acute, subacute, chronic)
  - Typical morphology and age-specific patterns
    - Facial, neck, external involvement (infants, children)
    - Flexural lesions (any age group)
    - Sparing of groin and axillary regions
  - Chronic or relapsing history

Important Features (Seen in Most Cases, Supports the Diagnosis of AD):
- Early age of onset
- Atopy
  - Personal/family history
  - IgE reactivity
- Xerosis

TABLE 98-4 Major and Minor Signs and Symptoms of Atopic Dermatitis[1]

Major Indicators

- Pruritus (intense itching)
- Characteristic rash in locations typical of the disease
- Chronic or repeatedly occurring symptoms
- Personal or family history of atopic disorders (eczema, hay fever, asthma)

Selected Minor Indicators

- Early age of onset
- Dry skin that may also have patchy scales or rough bumps
- Increased serum IgE
- Numerous skin creases on the palms
- Hand or foot involvement
- Inflammation around the lips
- Nipple eczema
- Susceptibility to skin infection
- Positive allergy skin tests

Once pruritus occurs, the surrounding normally nonpruritic skin area (whether inflamed or noninflamed) may be very sensitive and react to light stimuli and begin itching (allokinesis). Allokinesis is typical of AD.[34,35] As a result of allokinesis, patients with AD may experience pruritic attacks when their skin is touched accidentally by mechanical factors such as clothing, especially wool products.[35]

Elevated serum IgE may be seen, consistent with the genetically predetermined dominance of TH_2 cytokines causing increased IgE. In addition, increased serum IgE antibodies to a particular food, consistent with a food allergy, is common in patients with AD. Serum-based tests for allergen-specific IgE (formerly a radioallergosorbent test referred to as RAST) are used to screen for allergy to a specific substance or substances.[33] (Currently, most laboratories use large autoanalyzers that rely on fluorescent or chemiluminesent labels rather than radiolabels to identify reactions, so RAST does not describe the technique used). In some cases, allergen-specific IgE tests may be used to monitor immunotherapy or to see if a child has outgrown a specific allergy. The negative predictive value is high (greater than 95%) but the specificity and positive predictive value are low (40%-60%).[33] Negative results help rule out a food allergy, whereas positive (elevated) allergen-specific IgE test results only signify sensitization and require clinical correlation and confirmation.[33] The level of IgE may not correlate with the severity of an allergic reaction, and the IgE level may remain elevated for years after an allergy has been outgrown.

A clinically useful set of criteria for the diagnosis of AD is as follows: atopy, pruritus, eczema, and altered vascular reactivity.[18,35]

COMPLICATIONS

6 Patients with AD are prone to skin infections. Atopic skin is drier and the stratum corneum has weakened protective abilities; combined with the abnormal skin barrier function and immune defense, there is an increased risk of secondary bacterial skin infections with staphylococci or streptococci, and viral infections such as herpes simplex or even fungal infections.[1,2] Constant scratching to relieve pruritus may cause excoriations, further compromising the integrity of the skin barrier. *S. aureus* is a common cause of secondary bacterial infections in AD.[10] Binding of *S aureus* is enhanced by skin inflammation as seen in AD. Many patients with AD are colonized with *S. aureus* and may have exacerbations after skin infections of this organism.[10] Secondary bacterial infections may present as yellowish crusty lesions and should be promptly treated. Oral (systemic) antibiotics are generally more effective than topical treatment.[1]

Patients with AD are also more prone to disseminated infections with herpes simplex or vaccinia virus. Severe viral infections such as eczema herpeticum or eczema vaccinatum might be linked to the severity of atopy. Smallpox vaccination is contraindicated in patients with AD.

TREATMENT

Desired Outcomes

In treating patients with AD, clinicians generally have the following clinical goals in mind:

1. Provide symptomatic relief—control the itching.
2. Control the AD.
3. Identify and, when possible, eliminate triggers and environmental aeroallergens.
4. Identify and minimize predisposing factors for exacerbations including any stressors.
5. Prevent future exacerbations.
6. Provide any social and psychological support needed for the patient, family, and caregivers.
7. Minimize or prevent adverse events from medications and other treatment modalities.
8. Treat to cure any secondary skin infections, if present.

Successful management of AD should include not only clearance of skin lesions, which may take days to weeks depending on the severity of disease, but also control of the itch, minimizing or eliminating triggers, monitoring the patient to minimize or prevent adverse events from medications or other treatment modalities, and providing adequate social and psychological support for the patient, family, and caregivers.

The ultimate goal is to provide enough control of this chronic disease so that future exacerbations are prevented, thus ensuring that the patient's quality of life is minimally affected by AD. Because the course of the disease evolves over time, management strategies may change.

7 Both nonpharmacologic and pharmacologic therapies are important in managing the signs and symptoms of AD. Nonpharmacologic strategies include identifying and minimizing or eliminating preventable risk factors, such as known triggers and allergens, as well as appropriate skin care.

Treatment guidelines and protocols for AD are available. These are listed in Table 98-5.

Nonpharmacologic Therapy

8 Nonpharmacologic approaches to the treatment of infants and children with AD include the following[1,36]:

1. Apply moisturizers frequently throughout the day. Moisturizers are a standard of care for AD and there is strong evidence that their use can reduce disease severity and the need for pharmacologic intervention.[36]
2. Give lukewarm baths. Currently there is insufficient evidence for AD patients to recommend the addition of oils, emollients, or most other additives to bath water, or the use of acidic spring water.[36]
3. Apply moisturizer immediately after bathing. Currently there is no standard for the frequency or duration of bathing appropriate for those with AD.[36]
4. Use nonsoap cleansers (which are neutral to low pH, hypoallergenic, fragrance free). Limited use.[36]
5. Use wet-wrap therapy (with or without topical corticosteroid) during flare-ups for patients with moderate to severe

TABLE 98-5 Useful Sources of Information about Treatment of Atopic Dermatitis

Published Guidelines or Treatment Protocols

- Eichenfield LF, Tom WL, Chamlin SL, et al. Guidelines of care for the management of atopic dermatitis. Section 1. Diagnosis and assessment of atopic dermatitis. *J Am Acad Dermatol* 2014;70:338-351.
- Eichenfield LF, Tom WL, Berger TG, et al. Guidelines of care for the management of atopic dermatitis. Section 2. Management and treatment of atopic dermatitis with topical therapies. *J Am Acad Dermatol* 2014;71:116-132.
- Sidbury R, Davis DM, Cohen DE, et al. Guidelines of care for the management of atopic dermatitis. Section 3. Management and treatment with phototherapy and systemic agents. *J Am Acad Dermatol* 2014;71:327-349.
- Sidbury R, Tom WL, Bergman JN, et al. Guidelines of care for the management of atopic dermatitis. Section 4. Prevention of disease flares and use of adjunctive therapies and approaches. *J Am Acad Dermatol* 2014; published online September 25, 2014. http://dx.doi.org/10.1016/j.jaad.2014.08.038.
- Eichenfield LF, Boguniewicz M, Simpson E, et al. Translating atopic dermatitis management guidelines into practice for primary care providers. *Pediatrics* 2015;136(3). http://www.pediatrics.org/cgi/doi/10.1542/peds.2014-3678.
- Ring J, Alomar A, Bieber M, et al. Guidelines for treatment of atopic eczema (atopic dermatitis) parts 1 and II. *J Eur Acad Dermatol Venereol* 2012;26:1045-1060, 1176-1193.
- Rubel D, Thirumoorthy T, Soebaryo W, et al. Consensus guidelines for the management of atopic dermatitis: An Asia-Pacific perspective. *J Dermatol* 2013;40:160-171.
- Baron SE, Cohen SN, Archer CB. British Association of Dermatologists and Royal College of General Practitioners. Guidance on the diagnosis and clinical management of atopic eczema. *Clin Exp Dermatol* 2012;37(suppl 1):7-12.
- Simpson EL. Atopic dermatitis: A review of topical treatment options. *Curr Med Res Opin* 2010;26(3):633-640.
- Carbone A, Siu A, Patel R. Pediatric atopic dermatitis: A review of the medical management. *Ann Pharmacother* 2010;44:1448-1458.
- National Institute of Arthritis and Musculoskeletal and Skin Diseases. Handout on Health: Atopic Dermatitis. US Department of Health and Human Services. NIH Publication No. 09-4272. May 2013, www.niams.nih.gov/Health_Info/Atopic_Dermatitis/default.asp.
- Lynde C, Barber K, Claveau J, et al. Canadian practical guide for the treatment and management of atopic dermatitis. *J Cutan Med Surg* 2005;8 (suppl 5):1-9. http://www.springerlink.com/content/r5432000056r2748/fulltext.html.

Useful Web sites

- National Institute of Arthritis and Musculoskeletal and Skin Diseases (NIAMS), U.S. National Institutes of Health: http://www.niams.nih.gov/Health_Info/Atopic_Dermatitis/default.asp
- American Academy of Allergy Asthma & Immunology (AAAAI): http://www.aaaai.org/conditions-and-treatments/allergies/Skin-Allergy
- American Academy of Dermatology: https://www.aad.org/education/clinical-guidelines, http://www.jaad.org/article/S0190-9622(13)01095-5/fulltext.
- DermNet NZ: http://dermnetnz.org/dermatitis/atopic.html.

AD. "Wet wrap" is applying damp tubular elasticized bandages and occlusive dressing to the limbs—this promotes skin hydration and absorption of emollients and TCS,[11] reducing disease severity and water loss.[11,36]

6. Keep child's fingernails filed short.
7. Select clothing made of soft cotton fabrics, not polyester.
8. Consider using sedating antihistamines at bedtime to reduce scratching at night.
9. Keep the child cool; avoid situations in which overheating occurs.
10. Learn to recognize skin infections and seek treatment promptly.
11. Attempt to distract the child with activities to keep him or her from scratching during the day.
12. Identify and remove irritants and allergens.

Hydration is crucial, and adequate skin hydration is a fundamental part of managing AD.[3,36] Transepidermal water loss is greater in atopic skin than in normal skin. Thus, any measures to improve skin moisturization, such as liberal use of moisturizers, would be beneficial. Moisturizers are a standard of care and may be steroid-sparing.[10,36-40] They are useful for both prevention and maintenance therapy.[10,36,39,40] They can be categorized based on their specific effects on the skin:

1. Occlusives: These agents provide an oily layer on the skin surface to slow transepidermal water loss, increasing the moisture content of the stratum corneum. These are the best moisturizers for patients with AD.[3]
2. Humectants: In the stratum corneum, these agents increase the water-holding capacity. However, they are not useful in patients with AD because they have a stinging effect on open skin.[3]
3. Emollients: These agents smooth out the surface of the skin by filling the spaces with droplets of oil. These are the least effective moisturizers.[3]

Note that the term "emollients" is sometimes more broadly used to mean all nonmedicated moisturizers, including occlusives.[37,38] Usual active ingredients in moisturizers include mineral oil, petrolatum, ceramide, and urea. Ceramide was shown to improve pruritus and sleep in pediatric patients with AD.[38] Ceramide-containing over-the-counter (OTC) moisturizers and prescription emollient devices (PEDs) with distinct ratios of lipids mimic endogenous compositions. However, to date these have not shown superiority in AD.[36]

The humidity in the home should be kept at or above 50% and the room temperature kept on the cool side.[18]

Appropriate skin care is crucial in preventing flare-ups.[1] A daily skin care routine should include the following[18]:

1. Using scent-free moisturizers liberally as needed each day. Large quantities can be used.
2. Bathing in lukewarm water (never hot) for 5 to 10 minutes.[36] once or twice daily.[3,36,37] Adding a capful of emulsifying oil[10] may help the body retain moisture; baths are better than showers. Bathing daily for 10 to 20 minutes may be desirable as long as a thick moisturizer is applied afterward.[37] A 20-minute soak followed by immediate application of topical anti-inflammatory agents (eg, TCS) without towel drying is known as the "soak and smear" technique and is useful when the topical anti-inflammatory agent alone is inadequate.[36] Bathing twice daily during disease flares may also be a useful method for enhancing skin penetration of topical therapies and for debridement of crusting and staphylococcal colonization.[37] The skin should be lightly towel dried (pat to dry, avoid rubbing or brisk drying).[1,37,38]
3. A scent-free moisturizer should then be applied while the skin is still moist or slightly damp (eg, within 3 minutes of towel drying).[3,37] Some fragrance-free moisturizers include Aveeno Baby Soothing Relief Moisture Cream, Cetaphil, Neutrogena Hand Cream, and Vanicream products. Lotions may be used on the scalp and other hairy areas and for mild dryness on the face, trunk, and limbs; creams are more occlusive than lotions; ointments are the most occlusive and

can be used for drier, thicker, or more scaly areas.[3] Occlusive moisturizers are best.[3]

4. Using nonsoap skin cleansers[1] may cause less skin irritation. Lipid- and fragrance-free skin cleansers may be particularly advantageous (eg, Cetaphil Gentle Skin Cleanser, Free and Clear Liquid Cleanser, Spectro Derm Cleanser). Aquanil, Dove, Neutrogena, and pHisoderm sensitive skin products have also been recommended as low-irritant products, and some are lipid free.
5. Avoiding alcohol-containing topical products including lotions, swabs, and wipes, as they may be drying.
6. Clothing should be double-rinsed. Mild detergents should be used to wash clothing, with no bleach or fabric softener.[3]

Pharmacologic Therapy

Topical Corticosteroids

9 *Topical corticosteroids* (TCS) are the standard of care to which other treatments are compared.[10,11,36-40] They remain the drug treatment of choice for AD. However, despite their extensive use, supporting data are limited regarding optimal corticosteroid concentrations, duration and frequency of therapy, and quantity of application.[10,36] The use of long-term intermittent application of TCS was beneficial and safe in two randomized controlled trials (RCTs); however, independent studies of other formulations are needed.

To maximize the anti-inflammatory benefit and minimize adverse effects, the choice of TCS should be matched with the severity and site of disease.[3] Low-potency TCS, such as hydrocortisone 1%, are suitable for the face, and medium-potency TCS, such as betamethasone valerate 0.1%, may be used for the body.[3] For longer-duration maintenance therapy, low-potency TCS are recommended.[36] Mid-strength and high-potency TCS should be used for short-term management of exacerbations.[36] Currently there is no established optimum regimen for controlling flare-ups—starting with a short burst of high-potency TCS to rapidly control active disease followed by a rapid taper in potency is equally acceptable as using the lowest-potency agent thought to be needed then adjusting upward if treatment fails.[36] Although twice-daily application is the usual clinical practice, there is some evidence of efficacy with once-daily use of some potent TCS.[36] Daily TCS applications are recommended until the inflammatory lesions are significantly improved—which may take up to several weeks at a time. Once control is achieved, either (a) stop the TCS and use moisturizers alone until the next flare-up, or (b) apply a TCS once or twice weekly to areas of the patient's body where frequent/repeated flare-ups occur—this method has reduced rates of relapse for those patients who experience frequent flare-ups at the same body sites.[36] Ultrahigh- and high-potency TCS, such as betamethasone dipropionate 0.05% or clobetasone propionate 0.05%, are typically reserved for short-term treatment of lichenified areas in adults.[39] Short-term treatments mean brief periods of 1 to 2 weeks.[37,38] After the lesions have cleared or significantly improved, a lower-potency agent (the least potent TCS that is effective)[36] should be used for maintenance when necessary.[39] Potent fluorinated TCS should be avoided not only on the face, but also the genitalia and the intertriginous areas, and in young infants. (For a corticosteroid potency comparison chart, see Table 97-2 in Chapter 97, or visit the National Psoriasis Foundation Web site at https://www.psoriasis.org/about-psoriasis/treatments/topicals/steroids/potency-chart.)

It is also important to remember that altering the local environment through hydration and/or occlusion (eg, wet-wrap therapy)[11] as well as changing the vehicle[41] may alter the absorption and effectiveness of the TCS.[10] Some vehicles are better suited for certain body areas,[41] such as a lotion for the scalp and hairy areas. Foams may be more cosmetically pleasing to some patients, as they easily disappear into the skin. The surface area of the skin involved and the skin thickness also play a role. In addition, tachyphylaxis is a clinical concern, but there is little experimental documentation.

Adverse effects of TCS may be systemic in nature, and they are directly related to the steroid potency, duration of use, and other factors as discussed above. Local adverse effects include striae and skin atrophy, perioral dermatitis, acne, rosacea, telangiectasias, purpura, focal hypertrichosis, and allergic contact dermatitis (often related to the vehicle).[36,42] The potential for systemic adverse effects is related to the potency of the TCS, the site of application, the occlusiveness of the preparation, the percentage of body surface area covered, and the duration of use. Potential systemic effects include hypothalamic-pituitary-adrenal (HPA) axis suppression, infections, hyperglycemia, cataracts, glaucoma, and growth retardation (in children).[1,18,36-38,42] However, growth retardation may also be related to the chronicity of the illness rather than to TCS use or dietary factors.[3] Although less likely, systemic adverse effects can occur with low-potency TCS. For example, a phase II study of a mild-potency corticosteroid (desonide 0.05% foam) in children and adolescents 3 months to 17 years showed that 4% (3 of 75) of patients experienced mild reversible HPA-axis suppression after a 4-week treatment period.[43]

When TCS therapy has failed for efficacy or safety reasons, numerous agents and interventions can be used as alternative or add-on therapy in patients with AD.

Topical Calcineurin Inhibitors

10 Topical immunomodulators such as the calcineurin inhibitors tacrolimus ointment (Protopic) and pimecrolimus cream (Elidel) have been shown to reduce the extent, severity, and symptoms of AD in adults and children.[10,36,39,40] Calcineurin inhibitors inhibit the activation of key cells involved in AD, including T cells and mast cells, blocking the production of proinflammatory cytokines and mediators.[36] Tacrolimus also decreases the number and costimulatory ability of epidermal dendritic cells.[36] Pimecrolimus has more favorable lipophilic characteristics and, in animal studies, appears to preferentially distribute to the skin as opposed to the systemic circulation.[44] Both tacrolimus ointment and pimecrolimus cream are approved for AD in adults and children older than 2 years.[10,36,39,40,44] Although clinical trials conducted in younger infants (eg, 2 to 23 months old) also showed significant efficacy without appreciable adverse effects, use in children younger than 2 years is not FDA-approved.[45] Tacrolimus 0.03% ointment is approved for moderate to severe AD for ages 2 years and older, with the 0.1% ointment limited to ages 16 years and older; pimecrolimus 1% cream is approved for mild-to-moderate AD for ages 2 years and older.[45] There is limited data comparing TCS with tacrolimus or pimecrolimus.

Because of continuing concerns regarding a possible risk of cancer with tacrolimus and pimecrolimus,[45] both drugs are recommended for use as second-line treatments for short-term and noncontinous chronic use in AD,[10,36-40] when the continued use of TCS is ineffective or inadvisable.[36,37] They may be appropriate in patients with corticosteroid-related adverse effects, patients with large body-surface areas of disease, patients unresponsive to TCS, or other reasons where treatment with TCS is inadvisable.[3] Children and adults with a weakened or compromised immune system should not be treated with these agents.[36] Unlike TCS, calcineurin inhibitors can be used on all body locations for prolonged periods,[3,10,11] although episodic use is recommended. They may be used as twice-weekly long-term therapy for maintenance.[11] Skin atrophy does not occur.[11,36] They may be used as steroid-sparing agents (sequentially or concomitantly with TCS) although clinical trial data are limited.[36]

The most common adverse effect of topical calcineurin inhibitors is transient discomfort (burning sensation) at the application site.[3,36] There is a potential for local skin carcinogenesis as seen in animal studies, or for systemic effects if high blood levels are reached (eg, increased susceptibility to infections due to immunosuppressive effects).[45]

Because there is a possible risk of cutaneous malignancy,[3,36,37] sun protection is recommended.[3,11,18,37,45] Patients should be encouraged to apply a high sun protection factor (SPF) broad-spectrum sunblock daily to all exposed skin (eg, SPF 30 or higher); and this counseling should especially be emphasized for those patients with the highest risk of developing skin cancer, including patients with red hair and/or Fitzpatrick skin types I and II, and patients receiving phototherapy or using tanning beds.[45]

Topical calcineurin inhibitors are very effective in relieving the associated pruritus. Both tacrolimus and pimecrolimus significantly relieve pruritus even after the first few days of treatment in both children and adults (studies report relief after just 3 days).[10]

Clinical **Controversy...**

With topical calcineurin inhibitors, there is a potential for local skin carcinogenesis as seen in animal and in vitro studies. In addition, pigmented melanocytic lesions have been seen in treated areas, raising concern about melanoma.[43] The FDA has a black box warning for both tacrolimus ointment and pimecrolimus cream about their potential cancer risk, but no causal relationship has been proven between use of a topical calcineurin inhibitor and the development of lymphoma or nonmelanoma skin cancer.[43]

Phototherapy

11 Phototherapy is effective for AD and is recommended[10,11,37-40] as second-line treatment when the disease is not controlled by TCS and/or tacrolimus or pimecrolimus ointment.[46,47] Phototherapy may be steroid-sparing, allowing for the use of lower-potency TCS, or even eliminating the need for maintenance TCS in some cases. Phototherapy can be used for acute or maintenance therapy in children and adults with AD.[47] Phototherapy may also help prevent secondary bacterial skin infections, commonly seen in patients with AD. However, in a few patients, phototherapy may worsen the AD; it is not recommended in patients whose disease flares up when exposed to sunlight. Relapse following cessation of therapy frequently occurs.[10]

Phototherapy may consist of either ultraviolet light therapy alone, or ultraviolet light therapy alongside drug or topical ointment (commonly called photochemotherapy). Psoralens plus ultraviolet A light (PUVA) is one type of photochemotherapy. The photosensitizer (psoralens) is administered either orally or in a bath immediately prior to ultraviolet A (UVA) light therapy. Topical ointments (such as crude coal tar) may also be used concomitantly with ultraviolet light therapy (eg, crude coal tar + ultraviolet B [UVB] light).

Ultraviolet lamps include UVA (315-400 nm), UVA1 (340-400 nm), broadband UVB (BB-UVB) (280-315 nm), and narrowband UVB (NB-UVB) (311 nm). Phototherapies used for AD have included PUVA, high- or medium-dose UVA1, BB-UVB, and NB-UVB.[10,46] Currently, no definitive recommendation can be made to differentiate between the various phototherapies.[47] NB-UVB is more effective than BB-UVB therapy and is generally the most commonly recommended light treatment and it has a better side-effects profile than UVA or PUVA.[10,47] BB-UVB may not effectively treat the scalp and skinfold areas. Medium-dose UVA1 is very effective for patients with an acute exacerbation of severe AD; however, the effect may be relatively short-lived and symptoms may recur within 3 months of stopping therapy.[46] Currently, medium-dose UVA1 is considered similar in efficacy as NB-UVB; and high-dose UVA1 is preferred in severe cases when available.[10] There is weaker evidence supporting the use of PUVA in AD[46] and it is not first choice.[10]

Patients need to wear eye protection during ultraviolet (UV) light therapy to prevent damage to the retina. Short-term adverse effects include erythema, skin pain, skin burning or sunburn, pruritus, and pigmentation.[47] Long-term adverse effects include premature aging of the skin (photoaging), lentigines, photosensitive eruptions, folliculitis, photo-onycholysis, herpes simplex virus (HSV) reactivation, facial hypertrichosis, and skin cancer.[46,47] For example, PUVA has been associated with squamous cell carcinoma and possibly melanoma, which may occur years after PUVA therapy has ceased.[46] UVA therapy may also cause cataract formation.[47]

Coal Tar

Although tar preparations had been widely used for AD and have been recommended as alternative topical therapy, few RCTs support their efficacy.[36] Their anti-inflammatory properties are not well characterized, and part of the improvement with the agent may be the result of a placebo effect, which can be significant in AD.

Coal tar products are also staining and malodorous, although newer products may be more cosmetically acceptable. They are not recommended on acutely inflamed skin, since this may result in additional skin irritation.

The use of coal tar in pregnancy has not been studied. Few data are available about tar excretion into breast milk; in addition, safety in children has not been established.[48] Adverse effects include tar folliculitis, acneiform eruptions, irritant dermatitis, burning, stinging, photosensitivity, and a risk of tar intoxication if used extensively in a young child.[48] Although animal studies showed that tar components can be converted to carcinogenic and mutagenic entities, there is inconclusive epidemiologic evidence supporting the claim that human use of topical tar preparations in dermatology leads to skin cancer.[48]

Clinical **Controversy...**

Animal studies showed that coal tar components can be converted to carcinogenic/mutagenic entities, and tar keratoses (small nodules that develop from cutaneous tar exposure) have the potential to regress, fall off, or develop into a squamous cell carcinoma. However, there is inconclusive epidemiologic evidence supporting the claim that human use of topical tar preparations in dermatology leads to skin or internal cancers such as bladder cancer or lymphoma.[48]

Other Topical Therapies

Patients with moderate to severe AD who have frequent bacterial infections may benefit from dilute bleach baths with intranasal mupirocin—one study showed enhanced clinical improvement.[36]

Systemic Therapies

Systemic therapies for the treatment of AD are generally not well-studied. Small case series or open studies are available for some agents, but few well-conducted RCTs exist. Agents described in published papers have included systemic corticosteroids, cyclosporine, interferon-γ, azathioprine, methotrexate, mycophenolate mofetil, intravenous immunoglobulin (IVIG), and biologic response modifiers.[10,47] Systemic therapies are indicated in AD care only for the subset of adult and pediatric patients in whom optimized topical regimens and/or phototherapy do not adequately control the disease, or where the quality of life is substantially affected.[47]

Systemic corticosteroids although often used for rapid disease suppression, are generally not recommended due to an unfavorable risk-benefit profile.[11,37-40,47] Short courses of oral corticosteroids may lead to atopic flares/rebound.[11,47] *Cyclosporine* is effective for severe, recalcitrant AD,[10,11,47] but its usefulness is limited by significant side effects, including hypertension and nephrotoxicity. There is also the potential for significant drug–drug and drug–food (eg, grapefruit juice) interactions. It should be reserved for short-term use in adults or children with severe refractory disease.[11,47] Maximal benefit is usually seen after 2 to 6 weeks of use and relapse may occur quickly after cessation of therapy.[10,11,46,47] Treatment durations currently recommended are 6 to 9 months[11] and up to 1 year—this is off label use.[47] In a meta-analysis of eight RCTs, cyclosporine was more efficacious than placebo, with reduced body surface area, erythema, sleep loss, and glucocorticoid use. However, all scores were back to pretreatment levels 8 weeks after ending cyclosporine therapy.[10]

Recombinant interferon-γ may be effective in a subset of patients with AD.[10] It may be an alternative for refractory AD (adults and children).[47] Two randomized placebo-controlled trials in patients with severe AD demonstrated significant improvement in symptoms.[49,50] Short-term adverse effects, such as headache, myalgias, and chills, occurred in substantial proportions of study patients. Transient liver transaminase elevations and granulocytopenia have also occurred.[51] There is no recommended optimal dose[47]; some recommend that a higher dose of this agent be used initially followed by a lower dosage during maintenance therapy.[46]

Azathioprine,[47,52] *methotrexate*,[47,53] *mycophenolate mofetil*,[47] and *IVIG* have shown efficacy in small case series or open-label studies primarily in adults with recalcitrant AD. There are two RCTs with azathioprine as monotherapy which showed efficacy, improving both quality of life and AD.[47,52] Additional RCTs are needed. Oral methotrexate, with a long history of pediatric use for various inflammatory conditions, appeared to be effective in a case series of children (aged 2-16 years) with severe AD[53] and has also shown efficacy in adults.[47]

Biologic response modifiers, unlike for psoriasis, are currently not approved for AD. The safety and efficacy of various biologic response modifiers in patients with AD have been studied,[51] mostly in case reports, small case series, or open-label studies with a limited number of patients. Theoretically, using protein-based therapies is inherently risky in a patient population more prone to developing IgE sensitization to protein antigens than the general population. Type 1 immediate hypersensitivity reactions such as anaphylaxis could result, and patients with severe disease are potentially the patients at greatest risk of anaphylaxis. None has been reported in the published literature, which detail 261 patients with AD treated with various biologics,[51] but these numbers are too small to generalize their findings to larger numbers of people or specific populations.

More specifically, the tumor necrosis factor (TNF)-α inhibitors infliximab and etanercept appeared effective in a few patients but not others, and adverse events have included infusion reactions with flushing and dyspnea, urticaria, and recurrent skin infections of methicillin-resistant *S aureus*. Similarly, omalizumab, rituximab, and alefacept have been shown in a few case reports and small case series to be somewhat effective. A case report series of omalizumab plus IVIG showed significant clinical improvement.[54] However, an RCT with omalizumab showed no clinical improvement in AD despite reducing IgE levels.[47]

Additional research is needed to determine the therapeutic potential and safety of biologics in patients with AD.[47,51]

Oral antihistamines are used widely, however, there is mixed evidence of efficacy in AD control.[47] There is some evidence that oral sedating antihistamines used at night may benefit patients with poor sleep due to pruritus.[11,47]

Complementary and Alternative Therapies

Traditional Chinese herbal therapy has been studied in placebo-controlled trials and appeared to provide temporary benefit for patients with severe AD. However, the effectiveness may wear off despite continued treatment, and long-term toxicity is unknown.[10,55]

Probiotics of various types have been studied in several RCTs with mixed results. One study group reported that prenatal and postnatal exposure for 6 months to *Lactobacillus rhamnosus GG* halved the frequency of AD at 2, 4, and 7 years but had no effect on atopic sensitization. Other study groups also administered lactobacilli, including *L rhamnosus GG*, but with mixed results. A recent placebo-controlled study comparing *Bifidobacterium lactis* and *L rhamnosus HN001* found that *L rhamnosus HN001* may be effective in preventing the development of AD in high-risk infants, but not *Bifidobacterium*. However, one study showed that *Lactobacillus acidophilus* supplementation actually increased the sensitization rate (40% vs 24%) and led to more IgE-associated AD.[56] More research is needed about the role of probiotics in prevention and treatment of AD.[56] Because of inconsistent evidence probiotic use is not recommended at this time.[33]

Immunotherapy using allergen-specific desensitization techniques in controlled settings for patients with AD may also be beneficial, and much research is ongoing including RCTs. A recent review and meta-analysis of immunotherapy in AD patients showed significant efficacy.[11,57] More research is also needed to adequately assess the role of homeopathy, hypnotherapy, acupuncture, massage therapy, and biofeedback therapy in the treatment of AD.

PERSONALIZED PHARMACOTHERAPY

12 AD may have significant implications not only for the patients themselves, but also their families and caregivers.

In 2006, an international study of 2,002 patients and caregivers from eight countries addressed the effect of AD on the lives of patients and society.[58] This European study found that, on average, patients experienced nine flares per year, with those having severe disease experiencing more flares and taking significantly longer to clear. The flares were associated with disturbed sleep, and 86% of patients avoided at least one type of everyday activity. Schoolwork performance and productivity were negatively affected. Patients missed an average of 2.5 days of school or work per year, and an analysis of adult patient performance at work and occupational absence showed that the social cost of lost productivity could amount to more than 2 billion Euros per year across the European Union. There were also emotional consequences; half of the patients experienced depression or unhappiness about their condition, and one-third reported that AD had eroded their self-confidence. In addition, concern about adverse effects from topical corticosteroid treatments resulted in poor adherence to therapy. On average, patients endured the symptoms of AD without initiating specific treatment 47% of the time they had an exacerbation. Approximately one-half of the respondents were concerned about using TCS, and 58% restricted them to particular sites, 39% used them less frequently or for shorter time periods than prescribed, and 66% used them as a last resort. The study concluded that AD is "an undertreated disease that has a significant, yet mostly avoidable, negative effect on patients, their caregivers, and society."[58]

Thus, healthcare professionals play an integral role in providing patient and caregiver education about this disease and specific treatment plans. The importance of adequate and appropriate education for the patient, family, and caregivers about AD and its management cannot be overemphasized. Patients should be involved in their own care whenever possible.

CONCLUSION

AD is a chronic skin condition that generally presents at an early age. It affects the patient, family, and caregivers. Nonpharmacologic management strategies are important in treatment; these include appropriate skin care, hydration, avoidance of triggers, and psychosocial support. Pharmacologic treatment emphasizes topical corticosteroids as the standard of care. Patient and caregiver education about AD and treatment strategies is critical to minimize nonadherence. Successful outcomes result when patients and caregivers are partners with healthcare professionals in the management of this chronic disease.

ACKNOWLEDGMENT

Portions of this chapter have been adapted with permission from reference 18.

ABBREVIATIONS

AD	atopic dermatitis
AMP	antimicrobial peptide
BB-UVB	broadband ultraviolet B light (280-315 nm)
DC	dendritic cell
FcεRI	high-affinity receptor
FDA	Food and Drug Administration
FLG	filaggrin gene
GI	gastrointestinal
HPA	hypothalamic-pituitary-adrenal
IgE	immunoglobulin E
IgM	immunoglobulin M
IL	interleukin
ISAAC	International Study of Asthma and Allergies in Childhood
IVIG	intravenous immunoglobulin
NB-UVB	Narrowband ultraviolet B light (311 nm)
NIAID	National Institute of Allergy and Infectious Diseases
PUVA	psoralens plus ultraviolet A light
RAST	radioallergosorbent test
RCT	randomized controlled trial
SD	standard deviation
SPF	sun protection factor
TCS	topical corticosteroids
TH_1	T-helper type 1
TH_2	T-helper type 2
TNF	tumor necrosis factor
UV	ultraviolet
UVA	ultraviolet A
UVB	ultraviolet B

REFERENCES

1. National Institute of Arthritis and Musculoskeletal and Skin Diseases. Handout on Health: Atopic Dermatitis. US Department of Health and Human Services. 2013. Available at: http://www.niams.nih.gov/Health_Info/Atopic_Dermatitis/default.asp. Accessed August 31, 2016.
2. Eichenfield LE, Tom WL, Chamlin SI, et al. Guidelines of care for the management of atopic dermatitis. Section 1. Diagnosis and assessment of atopic dermatitis. *J Am Acad Dermatol* 2014;70:338-351.
3. Lynde C, Barber K, Claveau J, et al. Canadian practical guide for the treatment and management of atopic dermatitis. *J Cutan Med Surg* 2005;8(suppl 5):1-9. Available at: http://www.springerlink.com/content/r5432000056r2748/fulltext.html. Accessed August 31, 2016.
4. Hanifin JM. Epidemiology of atopic dermatitis. *Immunol Allergy Clin North Am* 2002;22:1-24.
5. Bieber T. Mechanisms of disease: Atopic dermatitis. *N Engl J Med* 2008;358:1483-494.
6. Williams H, Flohr C. How epidemiology has challenged 3 prevailing concepts about atopic dermatitis. *J Allergy Clin Immunol* 2006;118:209-213.
7. Williams H, Stewart A, von Mutius E, et al. Is eczema really on the increase worldwide? *J Allergy Clin Immunol* 2008;121:947-954.
8. DaVeiga SP. Epidemiology of atopic dermatitis: A review. *Allergy Asthma Proc* 2012;23:227-234.
9. Nutten S. Atopic dermatitis: global epidemiology and risk factors. *Ann Nutr Metab* 2015;66(suppl 1):8-16.
10. Ring J, Alomar A, Bieber M, et al. Guidelines for treatment of atopic eczema (atopic dermatitis) parts 1 and II. *J Eur Acad Dermatol Venereol* 2012;26:1045-1060, 1176-1193.
11. Plotz SG, Wiesender M, Todorova A, Ring J. What is new in atopic dermatitis/eczema? *Expert Opin Emerging Drugs* 2014;19(4):441-458.
12. Akdis CA. New insights into mechanisms of immunoregulation in 2007. *J Allergy Clin Immunol* 2008;122:700-709.
13. Ege MJ, Herzum I, Buchele G, et al. Prenatal exposure to a farm environment modifies atopic sensitization at birth. *J Allergy Clin Immunol* 2008;122:407-412.
14. Flohr C, Yeo L. Atopic dermatitis and the hygiene hypothesis revisited. *Curr Probl Dermatol* 2011;41:1-34.
15. Irvine AD, McLean WH, Leung DY. *Filaggrin* mutations associated with skin and allergic diseases. *N Eng J Med* 2011;365(4):1315-1327.
16. Rodriguez E, Baurecht H, Herberich E, et al. Meta-analysis of filaggrin polymorphisms in eczema and asthma: Robust rick factors in atopic disease. *J Allergy Clin Immunol* 2009;123:1361-1370.
17. Honey B, Steinhoff M, Ruzicka T, Leung DYM. Cytokines and chemokines orchestrate atopic skin inflammation. *J Allergy Clin Immunol* 2006;118:178-189.
18. Law RM, Kwa PG. Chapter 111: Atopic dermatitis: The itch that erupts when scratched. In: Schwinghammer TL, Koehler JM, eds. *Instructor's Guide: Pharmacotherapy Casebook: A Patient-Focused Approach*, 8th ed. New York, NY: McGraw-Hill; 2011:111-1-111-5.
19. Leung DYM. Our evolving understanding of the functional role of filaggrin in atopic dermatitis. *J Allergy Clin Immunol* 2009;124:494-495.
20. Steinke JW, Rich SS, Borish L. Genetics of allergic disease. *J Allergy Clin Immunol* 2008;121(suppl):S384-S387.
21. Heratizadeh A, Wichmann K, Werfel T. Food allergy and atopic dermatitis: How are they connected? *Curr Allergy Asthma Rep* 2011;11:284-291.
22. Sicherer SC, Leung DYM. Advances in allergic skin disease, anaphylaxis and hypersensitivity reactions to foods, drugs, and insects in 2008. *J Allergy Clin Immunol* 2009;123:319-327.
23. Schauber J, Gallo RL. Antimicrobial pep tides and the skin immune defense system. *J Allergy Clin Immunol* 2008;122:261-266.
24. Novak N, Bieber T. Dendritic cells as regulators of immunity and tolerance. *J Allergy Clin Immunol* 2008;121(suppl):S370-S374.
25. Biebe T, de la Salle H, Wollenberg A, et al. Human epidermal Langerhans cells express the high affinity receptor for immunoglobulin E (Fc epsilon RI). *J Exp Med* 1992;175:1285-1290.
26. Wang B, Rieger A, Kilgus O, et al. Epidermal Langerhans cells from normal human skin bind monomeric IgE via Fc epsilon RI. *J Exp Med* 1992;175:1353-1365.
27. Novak N, Bieber T. The role of dendritic cell subtypes in the pathophysiology of atopic dermatitis. *J Am Acad Dermatol* 2005;53(suppl 2):S171-S176.
28. Lack G. Epidemiologic risks for food allergy. *J Allergy Clin Immunol* 2008;121:1331-1336.
29. Boyce JA, Assa'ad AH, Burks AW, et al. Guidelines for the diagnosis and management of food allergy in the United States. Report of the NIAID-sponsored expert panel. *J Allergy Clin Immunol* 2010; 126(6 suppl):S1-S58. Available at: http://www.niaid.nih.gov/topics/foodAllergy/clinical/Pages/default.aspx. Accessed August 31, 2016.
30. Lucas JSA, Lewis SA, Jourihane JO'B. Kiwi fruit allergy: A review. *Pediatr Allergy Immunol* 2003;14:420-428.
31. Cohen A, Goldberg M, Levy B, et al. Sesame food allergy and sensitization in children: The natural history and long-term follow-up. *Pediatr Allergy Immunol* 2007;18:217-223.
32. Burks AW, Laubach S, Jones SM. Oral tolerance, food allergy, and immunotherapy: Implications for future treatment. *J Allergy Clin Immunol* 2008;121:1344-1350.
33. Sidbury R, Tom WL, Bergman JN, et al. Guidelines of care for the management of atopic dermatitis. Section 4. Prevention of disease flares and use of adjunctive therapies and approaches. *J Am Acad Dermatol* 2014; published online September 25, 2014. Available at: http://dx.doi.org/10.1016/j.jaad.2014.08.038. Accessed August 31, 2016.
34. Kim BS. Atopic Dermatitis. eMedicine.Medscape Updated July 1, 2015. Available at: http://emedicine.medscape.com/article/1049085. Accessed August 31, 2016.
35. Beltrani VS, Boguneiwicz M. Atopic dermatitis. Dermatology Online Journal. 2003, Available at: http://dermatology.cdlib.org/92/reviews/atopy/beltrani.html. Accessed August 31, 2016.
36. Eichenfield LF, Tom WL, Berger TG, et al. Guidelines of care for the management of atopic dermatitis. Section 2. Management and treatment of atopic dermatitis with topical therapies. *J Am Acad Dermatol* 2014;71:116-132.
37. Simpson EL. Atopic dermatitis: A review of topical treatment options. *Curr Med Res Opin* 2010;26(3):633-640.
38. Carbone A, Siu A, Patel R. Pediatric atopic dermatitis: A review of the medical management. *Ann Pharmacother* 2010;44:1448-1458.

39. Rubel D, Thirumoorthy T, Soebaryo W, et al. Consensus guidelines for the management of atopic dermatitis: An Asia-Pacific perspective. *J Dermatol* 2013;40:160-171.
40. Baron SE, Cohen SN, Archer CB. British Association of Dermatologists and Royal College of General Practitioners. Guidance on the diagnosis and clinical management of atopic eczema. *Clin Exp Dermatol* 2012;37(suppl 1):7-12.
41. Rosso JD, Friedlander SF. Corticosteroids: Options in the era of steroid-sparing therapy. *J Am Acad Dermatol* 2005;53:S50-S58.
42. Hengge UR, Ruzicka T, Schwartz RA, et al. Adverse effects of topical glucocorticosteroids. *J Am Acad Dermatol* 2006;54:1-15.
43. Hebert AA. Desonide Foam Phase III Clinical Study Group. Desonide foam 0.05%: Safety in children as young as 3 months. *J Am Acad Dermatol* 2008;59:334-340.
44. Stuetz A, Grassberger M, Meingassner JG. Pimecrolimus (Elidel, SDZ ASM 981)—Preclinical pharmacologic profile and skin selectivity. *Semin Cutan Med Surg* 2001;20:233-241.
45. Berger TG, Duvic M, Van Voorhees AS, Frieden IJ. The use of topical calcineurin inhibitors in dermatology: Safety concerns. *J Am Acad Dermatol* 2006;54:818-823.
46. Abramovits W. A clinician's paradigm in the treatment of atopic dermatitis. *J Am Acad Dermatol* 2005;53:S70-S77.
47. Sidbury R, Davis DM, Cohen DE, et al. Guidelines of care for the management of atopic dermatitis. Section 3. Management and treatment with phototherapy and systemic agents. *J Am Acad Dermatol* 2014;71:327-349.
48. Pughdal KV, Schwartz RA. Topical tar: Back to the future. *J Am Acad Dermatol* 2009;61:294-302.
49. Hanifin JM, Schneider LC, Leung DY, et al. Recombinant interferon gamma therapy for atopic dermatitis. *J Am Acad Dermatol* 1993;28:189-197.
50. Jang IG, Yang JK, Lee HJ, et al. Clinical improvement and immunohistochemical findings in severe atopic dermatitis treated with interferon gamma. *J Am Acad Dermatol* 2000;42:1033-1040.
51. Bremmer MS, Bremmer SF, Baig-Lewis S, et al. Are biologics safe in the treatment of atopic dermatitis? A review with a focus on immediate hypersensitivity reactions. *J Am Acad Dermatol* 2009;61:666-676.
52. Meggitt SJ, Gray JC, Reynolds NJ. Azathioprine doses by thiopurine methyltransferase activity for moderate-to-severe atopic eczema: a double-blind, randomized controlled trial. *Lancet* 2006;367:839-846.
53. Rouse C, Siegfried E. Methotrexate for atopic dermatitis in children. *J Am Acad Dermatol* 2008;58(2 suppl 2):AB7, abstract P608.
54. Toledo F, Silvestre JF, Munoz C. Combined therapy with low-dose omalizumab and intravenous immunoglobulin for severe atopic dermatitis. Report of four cases. *J Eur Acad Dermatol Venereol* 2012;26:1325-1327.
55. Koo J, Arain S. Traditional Chinese medicine for the treatment of dermatologic disorders. *Arch Dermatol* 1998;134:1388-1393.
56. van der Aa LB, Heymans HAS, van Aalderen WMC, et al. Probiotics and prebiotics in atopic dermatitis: Review of the theoretical background and clinical evidence. *Pediatr Allergy Immunol* 2010;21:e355-e367.
57. Bae JM, Choi YY, Park CO, et al. Efficacy of allergen-specific immunotherapy for atopic dermatitis: a systematic review and meta-analysis of randomized controlled trials. *J Allergy Clin Immunol* 2013;132:110-117.
58. Zuberbier T, Orlow SJ, Paller AS, et al. Patient perspectives on the management of atopic dermatitis. *J Allergy Clin Immunol* 2006;118:226-232.

Dermatologic Drug Reactions and Common Skin Conditions

e99

Rebecca M. Law and David T. S. Law

KEY CONCEPTS

1. The skin is the largest organ of the human body. It performs many vital functions such as (a) protecting the body against injury, physical agents, and ultraviolet radiation; (b) regulating body temperature; (c) preventing dehydration, thus helping to maintain fluid balance; (d) acting as a sense organ; and (e) acting as an outpost for immune surveillance. Skin also has a role in vitamin D production and absorption.
2. Age-related factors affect the epidermis and dermis. Pediatric skin is thinner and better hydrated, which enhances topical drug absorption and potential drug toxicities. Elderly skin is drier, thinner, and more friable, which may predispose to external insults.
3. Patients presenting with a skin condition should be interviewed thoroughly regarding signs and symptoms, urgency, other subjective complaints, and medication history. The skin eruption should be carefully assessed to help distinguish between a disease condition and a drug-induced skin reaction.
4. Drug-induced skin reactions can be irritant or allergic in nature.
5. Allergic drug reactions can be classified into exanthematous, urticarial, blistering, and pustular eruptions. Exanthematous reactions include maculopapular rashes and drug hypersensitivity syndrome. Urticarial reactions include urticaria, angioedema, and serum sickness-like reactions. Blistering reactions include fixed drug eruptions, Stevens-Johnson's syndrome, and toxic epidermal necrolysis. Pustular eruptions include acneiform drug reactions and acute generalized exanthematous pustulosis. Other drug-induced skin reactions include hyperpigmentation and photosensitivity.
6. Not all skin reactions are drug induced.
7. Contact dermatitis is a common skin disorder caused either by an irritant or an allergic sensitizer.
8. The first goals of therapy in the management of contact dermatitis involve identification, withdrawal, and avoidance of the offending agent. A thorough history, including work history, must be carefully reviewed for potential contactants.
9. Other goals of therapy for contact dermatitis include providing symptomatic relief, implementing preventative measures, and providing coping strategies and other information for patients and caregivers.
10. Diaper dermatitis is most often seen in infants, although the condition may also be seen in older adults who wear diapers for incontinence. Management includes frequent diaper changes, air drying, gentle cleansing, and using barriers.
11. Skin cancers include squamous cell carcinoma, basal cell carcinoma, and malignant melanoma.

INTRODUCTION

1 Skin is an essential part of the body. Although it is not commonly thought of as such, skin is an organ. In fact, it is the human body's largest organ, with an average surface area of about 1.8 m^2.[1] The organ system that includes the skin is known as *the integumentary system.*

The human skin consists of an outer epidermis and an inner dermis. The epidermis primarily provides protection from the environment and performs a critical barrier function—keeping in water and other vital substances and keeping out foreign elements. The dermis is a connective tissue layer that primarily provides resiliency and support for various skin structures and appendages such as sweat glands, sebaceous glands, hair, and nails.

Because the skin surface is such a visible part of the body, changes that are slow or subtle often go unnoticed. Slowly enlarging and evolving moles or dry skin conditions can go undetected even though such changes can be life threatening in some cases (eg, malignancy). Health professionals who have direct contact with patients should be able to distinguish between common self-treatable skin lesions and common skin lesions that must be seen and treated professionally, such as melanoma and squamous cell carcinoma.

Skin infections and infestations are not covered in this chapter but are discussed in Chapter 110. Acne, psoriasis, and atopic dermatitis are discussed in Chapters 96 to 98.

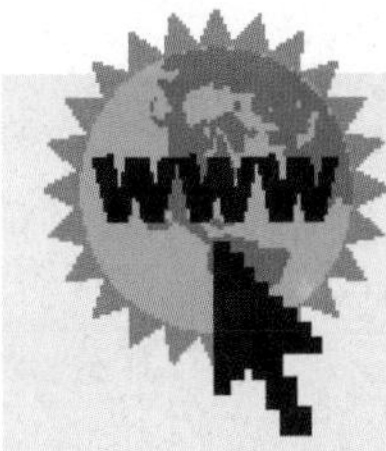

The complete chapter, learning objectives, and other resources can be found at **www.pharmacotherapyonline.com.**

100 Anemias

Kristen Cook

KEY CONCEPTS

1. Anemia is a group of diseases characterized by a decrease in either hemoglobin (Hb) or the volume of red blood cells (RBCs), which results in decreased oxygen-carrying capacity of the blood. Anemia is defined by the World Health Organization (WHO) as Hb less than 13 g/dL (less than 130 g/L; less than 8.07 mmol/L) in men and less than 12 g/dL (less than 120 g/L; less than 7.45 mmol/L) in women.
2. Acute-onset anemias are most likely to present with tachycardia, lightheadedness, and dyspnea. Chronic anemia often presents with weakness, fatigue, headache, vertigo, and pallor.
3. Iron-deficiency anemia (IDA) is characterized by decreased levels of ferritin (most sensitive marker) and serum iron, as well as decreased transferrin saturation. Hb and hematocrit decrease later. RBC morphology includes hypochromia and microcytosis. Most patients are adequately treated with oral iron therapy, although parenteral iron therapy is necessary in selected patient populations.
4. Vitamin B_{12} deficiency, a macrocytic anemia, can be due to inadequate intake, malabsorption syndromes, and inadequate utilization. Anemia caused by lack of intrinsic factor, resulting in decreased vitamin B_{12} absorption, is called *pernicious anemia*. Neurologic symptoms can be present and can become irreversible if the vitamin B_{12} deficiency is not treated promptly. Oral or parenteral therapy can be used for replacement.
5. Folic acid deficiency, a macrocytic anemia, results from inadequate intake, decreased absorption, and increased folate requirements. Treatment consists of oral administration of folic acid, even for patients with absorption problems. Adequate folic acid intake is essential in women of childbearing age to decrease the risk of neural tube defects in their children.
6. Anemia of inflammation (AI) is a newer term used to describe both anemia of chronic disease and anemia of critical illness. AI is a diagnosis of exclusion. It results from chronic inflammation, infection, or malignancy and can occur as early as 1 to 2 months after the onset of the disease. The serum iron level usually is decreased, but in contrast to IDA, the serum ferritin concentration is normal or increased. Treatment is aimed at correcting the underlying pathology. Anemia of critical illness occurs within days of acute illness.
7. Anemia is one of the most prevalent clinical problems in the elderly, although not an inevitable complication of aging. Low Hb concentrations are not "normal" in the elderly. Anemia is associated with an increased risk of hospitalization and mortality, reduced quality of life, and decreased physical functioning in the elderly.
8. IDA is a leading cause of infant morbidity and mortality. Age- and sex-adjusted norms must be used in the interpretation of laboratory results for pediatric patients. Primary prevention of IDA is the goal. A therapeutic trial of oral iron is the standard of care.

Anemia affects a large part of the world's population. According to the World Health Organization (WHO), almost 1.6 billion people (25% of the world's population) are anemic. Anemia is defined by the WHO as hemoglobin (Hb) less than 13 g/dL (less than 130 g/L; less than 8.07 mmol/L) in men or less than 12 g/dL (less than 120 g/L; less than 7.45 mmol/L) in women. In the United States, about 3.5 million Americans have anemia based on self-reported data from the National Center for Health Statistics. It is estimated that millions of people are unaware they have anemia, making it one of the most underdiagnosed conditions in the United States. Iron deficiency is the leading cause of anemia worldwide, accounting for as many as 50% of cases.[1] Recent data show that the overall prevalence of anemia has declined in the United States in preschool-aged children and women of childbearing age over the past 20 years, but the prevalence of iron deficiency anemia (IDA) did not change significantly in these same groups. The reasons for these changes remain unclear.[2] Although nutritional deficiencies occur less often in the United States, obesity surgery, which can cause deficiencies, is becoming increasingly common. Gastric bypass may result in folate, vitamin B_{12}, and iron deficiencies. Prevalence data are confounded by the lack of a standardized definition of anemia and lack of screening guidelines for most populations. The United States Preventive Services Task Force (USPSTF) guidelines for pregnant women recommend routine screening for IDA.

Anemia is not an innocent bystander because it can affect both length and quality of life. Retrospective observational studies of hemodialysis patients and heart failure patients suggest that anemia is an independent risk factor for mortality.[3] In addition, anemia significantly influences morbidity in patients with end-stage renal disease, chronic kidney disease, and heart failure.[4] Anemia is associated with psychomotor and cognitive abnormalities in children. Similarly, anemia is associated with cognitive dysfunction in patients with renal failure or cancer, and among community-dwelling elders.[5] Anemia during pregnancy is associated with increased risk for low birth weights, preterm delivery, and perinatal mortality.[6] Maternal

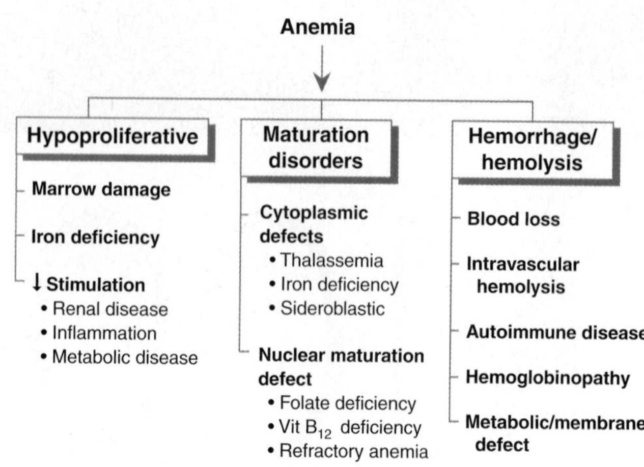

FIGURE 100-1 Functional classification of anemia. Each of the major categories of anemia (hypoproliferative, maturation disorders, and hemorrhage/hemolysis) can be further subclassified according to the functional defect in the several components of normal erythropoiesis.

IDA may be associated with postpartum depression in mothers and poor performance by offspring on mental and psychomotor tests. Global goals of treatment in anemic patients are to alleviate signs and symptoms, correct the underlying etiology, and prevent recurrence of anemia.

1 Anemia is a group of diseases characterized by a decrease in either Hb or circulating red blood cells (RBCs), resulting in reduced oxygen-carrying capacity of the blood. Anemia can result from inadequate RBC production, increased RBC destruction, or blood loss. It can be a manifestation of a host of systemic disorders, such as infection, chronic renal disease, or malignancy. Because anemia is a sign of underlying pathology, rapid diagnosis of the cause may be essential.

The functional classification of anemia is shown in Fig. 100-1. This chapter focuses on the most common causes of anemia—IDA, anemia associated with vitamin B_{12} or folic acid deficiency, and anemia of inflammation (AI) (eg, anemia of chronic disease [ACD]). Some of the other causes of anemia are addressed in other chapters.

Characteristic changes in the size of RBCs seen in erythrocyte indices can be the first step in the morphologic classification and understanding of the anemia. Anemia can be classified by RBC size as macrocytic, normocytic, or microcytic. Vitamin B_{12} deficiency and folic acid deficiency both are macrocytic anemias. An example of a microcytic anemia is iron deficiency, whereas a normocytic anemia may be associated with recent blood loss or chronic disease. More than one etiology of anemia can occur concurrently. Inclusion of the underlying cause of the anemia makes diagnostic terminology easier to understand (eg, microcytic anemia secondary to iron deficiency).

Microcytic anemias are a result of a quantitative deficiency in Hb synthesis, usually due to iron deficiency or impaired iron utilization. As a result, erythrocytes containing insufficient Hb are formed. Microcytosis and hypochromia are the morphologic abnormalities that provide evidence of impaired Hb synthesis.

Macrocytic anemias can be divided into megaloblastic and nonmegaloblastic anemias. The type of macrocytic anemia can be distinguished microscopically by peripheral blood smear examination. Megaloblasts are distinctive cells that express a biochemical abnormality of retarded DNA synthesis, resulting in unbalanced cell growth. Megaloblastic anemias may affect all hematopoietic cell lines. The most common causes of megaloblastic anemia are vitamin B_{12} and folate deficiency. Nonmegaloblastic macrocytic anemias may arise from liver disease, hypothyroidism, hemolytic processes, and alcoholism. Hemolytic anemias often are macrocytic, reflecting the increased numbers of circulating reticulocytes, which are larger on average than mature red cells.

MATURATION AND DEVELOPMENT OF RED BLOOD CELLS

In adults, RBCs are formed in the marrow of the vertebrae, ribs, sternum, clavicle, pelvic (iliac) crest, and proximal epiphyses of the long bones. In children, most bone marrow space is hematopoietically active to meet increased RBC requirements.

In normal RBC formation, a pluripotent stem cell yields an erythroid burst-forming unit. Erythropoietin (EPO) and cytokines such as interleukin-3 and granulocyte–macrophage colony-stimulating factor stimulate this cell to form an erythroid colony-forming unit in the marrow (Fig. 100-2). During this process, the nucleus becomes smaller with each division, finally disappearing in the normal erythrocyte. Hb and iron are incorporated into the gradually maturing RBC, which eventually is released from the marrow into the circulating blood as a reticulocyte. The maturation process usually takes about 1 week. The reticulocyte loses its nucleus and becomes an erythrocyte within several days. The circulating erythrocyte is a nonnucleated, nondividing cell. More than 90% of the protein content of the erythrocyte consists of the oxygen-carrying molecule Hb. Erythrocytes have a normal survival time of 120 days.[7]

Stimulation of Erythropoiesis

The hormone EPO, 90% of which is produced by the kidneys, initiates and stimulates the production of RBCs. Erythropoiesis is regulated by a feedback loop. The main mechanism of action of EPO is to prevent apoptosis, or programmed cell death, of erythroid precursor cells and allow their proliferation and subsequent maturation. A decrease in tissue oxygen concentration signals the kidneys to increase the production and release of EPO into the plasma, which increases

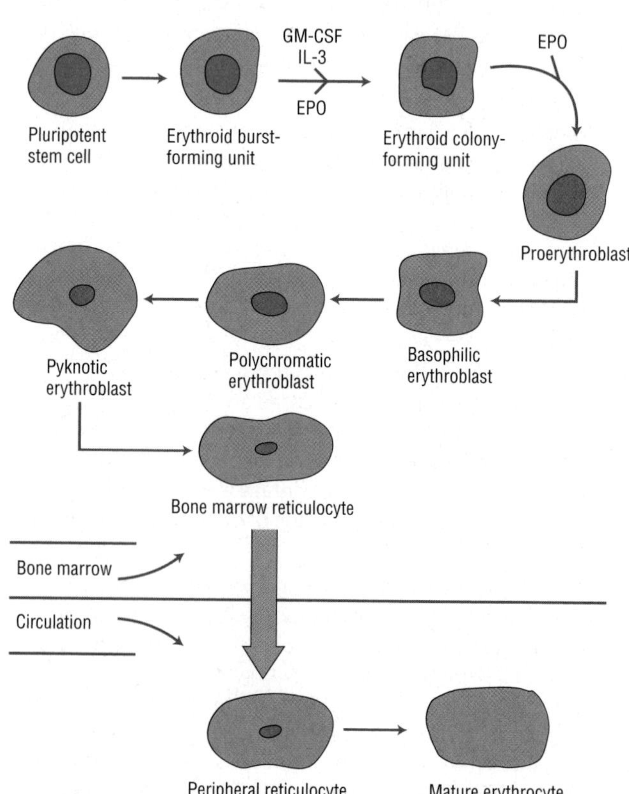

FIGURE 100-2 Erythrocyte maturation sequence (EPO, erythropoietin; GM-CSF, granulocyte-macrophage colony-stimulating factor; IL-3, interleukin-3).

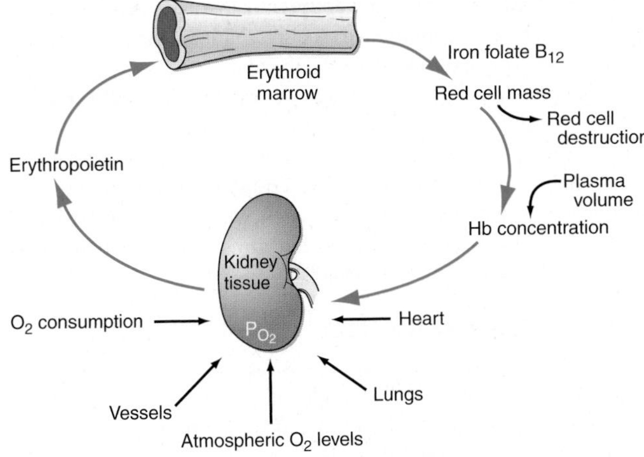

FIGURE 100-3 Physiologic regulation of red cell production by tissue oxygen tension. *(Reproduced with permission from Adamson JW, Longo DL. Anemia and polycythemia. In: Longo DL, Fauci AS, Kasper DL, et al., eds. Harrison's Principles of Internal Medicine. 18th ed. New York: Copyright © McGraw-Hill; 2012.)*

production and maturation of RBCs. Under normal circumstances, the RBC mass is kept at an almost constant level by EPO matching new erythrocyte production to the natural rate of loss of RBCs. A summary of erythropoiesis is shown in Fig. 100-3. Early appearance of large quantities of reticulocytes in the peripheral circulation (reticulocytosis) is an indication of increased RBC production.[7]

Synthesis of Hemoglobin

Hb contains a protein component with two α-chains and two β-chains. Each chain is linked to a heme group consisting of a porphyrin ring structure with an iron atom chelated at its center, which is capable of binding oxygen. The initial step in the synthesis of heme from the substrate succinyl CoA and glycine requires the presence of pyridoxine phosphate (vitamin B_6) as a catalyst. Following its synthesis in the cytoplasmic mitochondria of the RBC, heme diffuses into the extramitochondrial space, where it combines with the completed α- and β-chains and forms Hb. When hemolytic destruction of RBCs exceeds marrow production capacity and anemia develops, the Hb value decreases to a steady-state level at which production is equal to destruction.

Incorporation of Iron into Heme

Iron is an essential part of Hb. The specific plasma transport protein transferrin delivers iron to the bone marrow for incorporation into the Hb molecule. Transferrin enters cells by binding to transferrin receptors, which circulate and then attach to cells needing iron. Fewer transferrin receptors are present on the surface of cells that do not need iron, thus preventing iron-replete cells from receiving excess iron.[8]

Circulating transferrin normally is about 30% saturated with iron. Transferrin delivers extra iron to other body storage sites, such as the liver, marrow, and spleen, for later use. This iron is stored within macrophages as ferritin or hemosiderin. Ferritin consists of a Fe^{3+} hydroxyphosphate core surrounded by a protein shell called *apoferritin*. Hemosiderin can be described as compacted ferritin molecules with an even greater iron-to-protein shell ratio. Physiologically it is a more stable, but less available, form of storage iron. Since total body iron storage is generally reflected by ferritin levels, low serum levels of ferritin provide strong evidence of IDA.[9]

Normal Destruction of Red Blood Cells

Phagocytic breakdown destroys older blood cells, primarily in the spleen but also in the marrow (Fig. 100-4). Amino acids from the globin chains return to an amino acid pool; heme oxygenase acts on

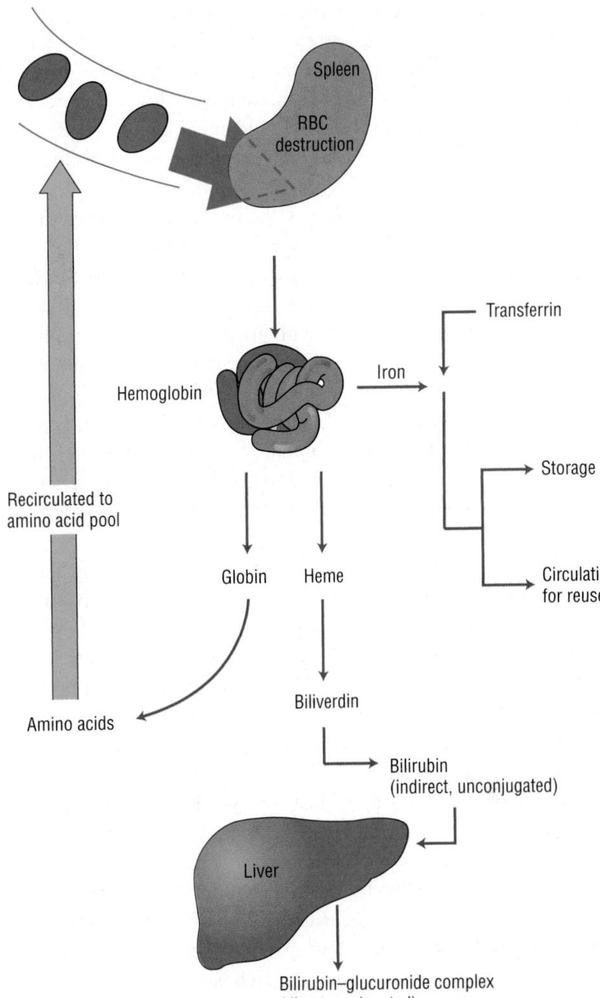

FIGURE 100-4 Destruction of red blood cells (RBCs).

the porphyrin heme structure to form biliverdin and to release its iron. Iron returns to the iron pool to be reused, although biliverdin is further catabolized to bilirubin. The bilirubin is released into the plasma, where it binds to albumin and is transported to the liver for glucuronide conjugation and excretion via bile. If the liver is unable to perform the conjugation, as occurs with intrinsic liver disease or oversaturation of conjugation enzymes by excessive cell hemolysis, the result is an elevated *indirect* (unconjugated) bilirubin. If the biliary excretion pathway for conjugated bilirubin is obstructed, an elevated *direct* bilirubin results. Comparison of direct and indirect bilirubin values helps to determine if the defect in bilirubin clearance occurs before or after bilirubin enters the liver. The Hb in RBCs destroyed by intravascular hemolysis becomes attached to haptoglobin and is carried back to the marrow for processing in the normal manner.[10]

DIAGNOSIS OF ANEMIA

General Presentation

History, physical examination, and laboratory testing are used in the evaluation of the patient with anemia. The workup determines if the patient is bleeding and investigates potential causes of the anemia, such as increased RBC destruction, bone marrow suppression, or iron deficiency. Diet can also be important in identifying causes of anemia. Additionally, information about concurrent nonhematologic disease states and a drug history are essential when evaluating the cause of the anemia (Chapter e103). History of blood transfusions and exposure to toxic chemicals also should be obtained.

Presenting signs and symptoms of anemia depend on its rate of development and the age and cardiovascular status of the patient. Severity of symptoms does not always correlate with the degree of anemia. Healthy patients may acclimate to very low Hb concentrations if the anemia develops slowly. Mild anemia often is associated with no clinical symptoms and may be found incidentally upon obtaining a complete blood count (CBC) for other reasons. The signs and symptoms in elderly patients with anemia may be attributed to their age or concomitant disease states. The elderly may not tolerate levels of Hb in the same way that younger persons do. Similarly, patients with cardiac or pulmonary disease may be less tolerant of mild anemia. Premature infants with anemia may be asymptomatic or have tachycardia, poor weight gain, increased supplemental oxygen needs, or episodes of apnea or bradycardia.

2 Anemia of rapid onset is most likely to present with cardiorespiratory symptoms such as palpitations, angina, orthostatic lightheadedness, and breathlessness due to decreased oxygen delivery to tissues or hypovolemia in those with acute bleeding. The patient also may have tachycardia and hypotension.

If onset is more chronic, presenting symptoms may include fatigue, weakness, headache, orthopnea, dyspnea on exertion, vertigo, faintness, sensitivity to cold, pallor, and loss of skin tone. Traditional signs of anemia, such as pallor, have limited sensitivity and specificity and may be misinterpreted. With chronic bleeding, there is time for equilibration within the extravascular space, so faintness and lightheadedness are less common.

Possible manifestations of IDA include glossal pain, smooth tongue, reduced salivary flow, pica (compulsive eating of nonfood items), and pagophagia (compulsive eating of ice). These symptoms are not likely to appear unless the anemia is severe.

Neurologic findings in vitamin B_{12} deficiency may precede hematologic changes. Early neurologic findings may include numbness and paraesthesias. Ataxia, spasticity, diminished vibratory sense, decreased proprioception, and imbalance may occur later as demyelination of the dorsal columns and corticospinal tract develop. Vision changes may result from optic nerve involvement. Psychiatric findings include irritability, personality changes, memory impairment, depression, and infrequently, psychosis.

Anemia associated with folate deficiency is typically macrocytic but, unlike B_{12} deficiency, occurs without neurological symptoms. Although the symptoms of anemia will improve with folate replacement and a partial hematologic response will occur, the neurologic manifestations of vitamin B_{12} deficiency will not be reversed with folic acid replacement therapy and consequently may progress or become irreversible if not treated appropriately.

Laboratory Evaluation

The initial evaluation of anemia involves a CBC (including RBC indices), reticulocyte index, and possibly an examination of a stool sample for occult blood. The results of the preliminary evaluation determine the need for other studies, such as examination of a peripheral blood smear. Based on laboratory test results, anemia can be categorized into three functional defects: RBC production failure (hypoproliferative), cell maturation ineffectiveness, or increased RBC destruction or loss (see Fig. 100-1).

Figure 100-5 shows a broad, general algorithm for the diagnosis of anemia based on laboratory data. There are many exceptions and additions to this algorithm, but it can serve as a guide to the typical presentation of common types and causes of anemia. The algorithm is less useful in the presence of more than one cause of anemia.

Hemoglobin

Values given for Hb represent the amount of Hb per volume of whole blood. The higher values seen in males are due to stimulation of RBC production by androgenic steroids, whereas the lower values in females reflect the decrease in Hb as a result of blood loss during menstruation. The Hb level can be used as a very rough estimate of the oxygen-carrying capacity of blood. Hb levels may be diminished because of a decreased quantity of Hb per RBC or because of a decrease in the actual number of RBCs.

CLINICAL PRESENTATION Anemia

General

- Patients may be asymptomatic or have vague complaints
- Patients with vitamin B_{12} deficiency may develop neurologic consequences
- In AI, signs and symptoms of the underlying disorder often overshadow those of the anemia

Symptoms

- Decreased exercise tolerance
- Fatigue
- Dizziness
- Irritability
- Weakness
- Palpitations
- Vertigo
- Shortness of breath
- Chest pain
- Neurologic symptoms in vitamin B_{12} deficiency

Signs

- Tachycardia
- Pale appearance (most prominent in conjunctivae)
- Decreased mental acuity
- Increased intensity of some cardiac valvular murmurs
- Diminished vibratory sense or gait abnormality in vitamin B_{12} deficiency

Laboratory Tests

- Hemoglobin, hematocrit, and RBC indices may remain normal early in the disease and then decrease as the anemia progresses
- Serum iron is low in IDA and AI
- Ferritin levels are low in IDA and normal to increased in AI
- Total iron binding capacity is high in IDA and is low or normal in AI
- Mean cell volume is elevated in vitamin B_{12} deficiency and folate deficiency
- Vitamin B_{12} and folate levels are low in their respective types of anemia
- Homocysteine is elevated in vitamin B_{12} deficiency and folate deficiency
- Methylmalonic acid is elevated in vitamin B_{12} deficiency

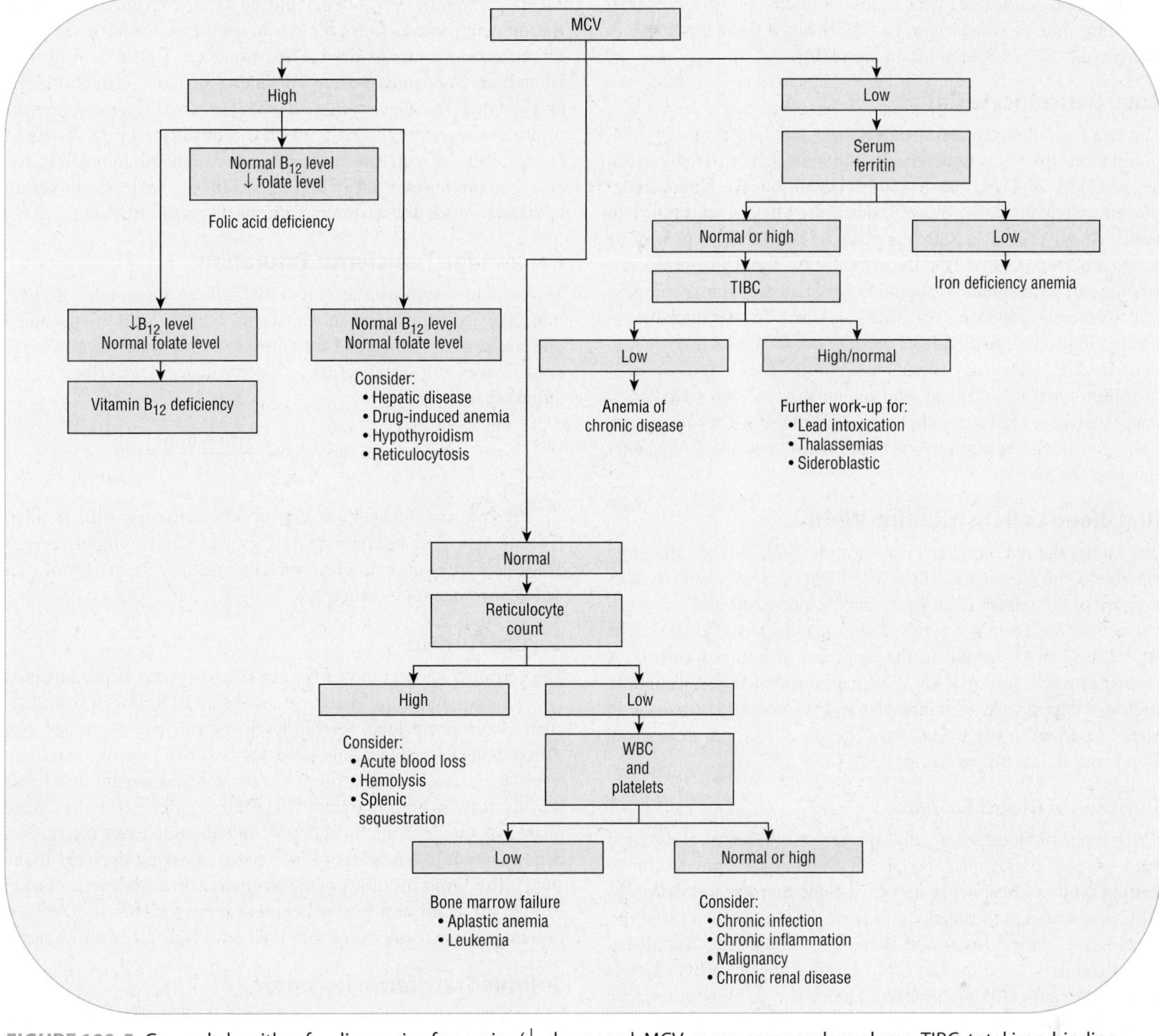

FIGURE 100-5 General algorithm for diagnosis of anemias (↓, decreased; MCV, mean corpuscular volume; TIBC, total iron-binding capacity; and WBC, white blood cells).

Hematocrit

Expressed as a percentage, hematocrit (Hct) is the actual volume of RBCs in a unit volume of whole blood. In general, it is about three times the Hb value (when Hb is expressed in g/dL). An alteration in this ratio may occur with abnormal cell size or shape and often indicates pathology. A low Hct indicates a reduction in either the number or the size of RBCs or an increase in plasma volume.

Red Blood Cell Count

The RBC count is an indirect estimate of the Hb content of the blood; it is an actual count of RBCs per unit of blood.

Red Blood Cell Indices

Wintrobe indices describe the size and Hb content of the RBCs and are calculated from the Hb, Hct, and RBC count. RBC indices, such as mean corpuscular volume (MCV) and mean corpuscular hemoglobin (MCH), are single mean values that do not express the variation that can occur in cells.

Mean Cell Volume MCV represents the average volume of RBCs. It may reflect changes in MCH. Cells are considered macrocytic if they are larger than normal, microcytic if they are smaller than normal, and normocytic if their size falls within normal limits. Folic acid and vitamin B_{12} deficiency anemias yield macrocytic cells, whereas iron deficiency and thalassemia are examples of microcytic anemias. When IDA (decreased MCV) is accompanied by folate deficiency (increased MCV), the overall MCV may be normal. Failure to understand that the MCV represents an average RBC size creates the potential for overlooking some causes of the anemia.

Mean Cell Hemoglobin MCH is the amount of Hb in a RBC, and usually increases or decreases with the MCV. Two morphologic changes, microcytosis and hypochromia, can reduce MCH. A microcytic cell contains less Hb because it is a smaller cell, while a hypochromic cell has a low MCH because of the decreased concentration of Hb present in the cell. Cells can be both microcytic and hypochromic, as seen with IDA. The MCH alone cannot distinguish between microcytosis and hypochromia. The most common cause of an elevated MCH is macrocytosis (eg, vitamin B_{12} or folate deficiency).

Mean Cell Hemoglobin Concentration The concentration of Hb per volume of cells is the mean cell Hb concentration (MCHC). Because MCHC is independent of cell size, it is more useful than MCH in distinguishing between microcytosis and hypochromia.

A low MCHC indicates hypochromia; a microcyte with a normal Hb concentration will have a low MCH but a normal MCHC. A decreased MCHC is seen most often in IDA.

Total Reticulocyte Count

The total reticulocyte count is an indirect assessment of new RBC production. It reflects how quickly immature RBCs (reticulocytes) are produced by bone marrow and released into the blood. Reticulocytes circulate in the blood about 2 days before maturing into RBCs. About 1% of RBCs are normally replaced daily, representing a reticulocyte count of 1%. The reticulocyte count in normocytic anemia can differentiate hypoproliferative marrow from a compensatory marrow response to an anemia. A lack of reticulocytosis in anemia indicates impaired RBC production. Examples include iron deficiency, B_{12} deficiency, anemia of chronic disease (ACD), malnutrition, renal insufficiency, and malignancy. A high reticulocyte count may be seen in acute blood loss or hemolysis. The reticulocyte index can aid in determining the functional classification of an anemia (see Fig. 100-5).

Red Blood Cell Distribution Width

The higher the red blood cell distribution width (RDW), the more variable is the size of the RBCs. The RDW increases in early IDA because of the release of large, immature, nucleated RBCs to compensate for the anemia, but this change is not specific for IDA. The RDW also can be helpful in the diagnosis of a mixed anemia. A patient can have a normal MCV yet have a wide RDW. This finding indicates the presence of microcytes and macrocytes, which would yield a "normal" average RBC size. The use of RDW to distinguish IDA from ACD is not recommended.

Peripheral Blood Smear

The peripheral blood smear can supplement other clinical data and help establish a diagnosis. Peripheral blood smears provide information on the functional status of the bone marrow and defects in RBC production. Additionally, it provides information on variations in cell size (anisocytosis) and shape (poikilocytosis). Automated blood counters, used for the CBC, can flag specific RBC changes that can be confirmed by a peripheral blood smear. Blood smears are placed on a microscope slide and stained as appropriate. Morphologic examination includes assessment of size, shape, and color. The extent of anisocytosis correlates with increased range of cell sizes. Poikilocytosis can suggest a defect in the maturation of RBC precursors in the bone marrow or the presence of hemolysis.

Serum Iron

The level of serum iron is the concentration of iron bound to transferrin. Transferrin is normally about one-third bound (saturated) to iron. The serum iron level of many patients with IDA may remain within the lower limits of normal because a considerable amount of time is required to deplete iron stores. Serum iron levels show diurnal variation (higher in the morning, lower in the afternoon), but this variation is probably not clinically significant in timing of levels.[9] Since serum iron levels are decreased by infection and inflammation, serum iron levels are best interpreted in conjunction with the total iron binding capacity. The serum iron level decreases with IDA and ACD and increases with hemolytic anemias and iron overload.

Total Iron-Binding Capacity

An indirect measurement of the iron-binding capacity of serum transferrin, total iron-binding capacity (TIBC) evaluation is performed by adding an excess of iron to plasma to saturate all transferrin with iron. Each transferrin molecule can carry two iron atoms. Normally, about 30% of available iron-binding sites are filled. With this laboratory test, all binding sites are filled to measure TIBC; the excess (unbound) iron is then removed and the serum iron concentration determined. Unlike the serum iron level, the TIBC does not fluctuate over hours or days. TIBC usually is higher than normal when body iron stores are low. The finding of a low serum iron level and a high TIBC suggests IDA. The TIBC is actually a measurement of protein serum transferrin, which can be affected by a variety of factors. Patients with infection, malignancy, inflammation, liver disease, and uremia may have a decreased TIBC and a decreased serum iron level, which are consistent with the diagnosis of ACD.

Percentage Transferrin Saturation

The ratio of serum iron level to TIBC indicates transferrin saturation. It reflects the extent to which iron-binding sites are occupied on transferrin and indicates the amount of iron readily available for erythropoiesis. It is expressed as a percentage, as described in the following formula:

$$\text{Transferrin saturation} = \frac{\text{serum iron}}{\text{TIBC}} \times 100$$

Transferrin normally is 20% to 50% saturated with iron. In IDA, transferrin saturation of 15% or lower is commonly seen.[10] Transferrin saturation is a less sensitive and specific marker of iron deficiency than are ferritin levels.

Serum Ferritin

The serum concentration of ferritin (storage iron) is proportional to total iron stores and therefore is the best indicator of iron deficiency or iron overload. Ferritin levels indicate the amount of iron stored in the liver, spleen, and bone marrow cells. Low serum ferritin levels are virtually diagnostic of IDA. In contrast, serum iron levels may decrease in both IDA and ACD. Since serum ferritin is an acute phase reactant, chronic infection or inflammation can increase its concentration independent of iron status, masking depleted tissue stores. This limits the utility of the serum ferritin if the level is normal or high for a chronically ill patient. For these patients, iron, even if present in these tissue stores, may not be available for erythropoiesis.

Soluble Transferrin Receptor

The soluble transferrin receptor (sTfR) assay is a laboratory test considered a sensitive, early, highly quantitative marker of iron depletion. The sTfR concentration is inversely correlated with tissue iron stores, and elevated levels are predictive of iron deficiency. Unlike ferritin, the sTfR is not an acute phase reactant; so its level remains normal for patients with chronic disease. It may be a useful test for distinguishing ACD from IDA.[9] The major limitation of this test is that it is not widely available in many laboratories.

Folic Acid

The results of folic acid measurements vary depending on the assay method used. Decreased serum folic acid levels (less than 4 ng/mL [less than 9 nmol/L]) indicate a folate deficiency megaloblastic anemia that may coexist with a vitamin B_{12} deficiency anemia. Erythrocyte folic acid levels are less variable than serum levels because they are slow to decrease in an acute process such as drug-induced folic acid deficiency and slow to increase with oral folic acid replacement. In addition, erythrocyte folic acid levels have the theoretical advantage of less susceptibility to rapid changes in diet and alcohol intake. Limitations with sensitivity and specificity do exist with measurements of erythrocyte folate. If the serum folate concentration is normal for a patient with suspected folate deficiency, then the erythrocyte folate level should be measured.[11]

Vitamin B_{12}

Low levels (less than 200 pg/mL [less than 148 pmol/L]) of vitamin B_{12} (cyanocobalamin or cobalamin) indicate deficiency. However, a deficiency may exist prior to the recognition of low serum levels. Serum values are maintained at the expense of vitamin B_{12} tissue stores. Vitamin B_{12} and folate deficiency may overlap, thus serum levels of both vitamins should be determined. Vitamin B_{12} levels may be falsely low with folate deficiency and pregnancy.[12]

Schilling Test

This test used to be the "gold standard" for assessing vitamin B_{12} absorption. Due to its cost, unavailable test components, and complexity, the test is rarely used today. Tests to replace it are under investigation.[13]

Homocysteine

Vitamin B_{12} and folate both are required for conversion of homocysteine to methionine. Increased serum homocysteine may suggest vitamin B_{12} or folate deficiency. Homocysteine levels also can be elevated in patients with vitamin B_6 deficiency, renal failure, hypothyroidism, or a genetic defect in cystathionine β-synthase.[14]

Methylmalonic Acid

A vitamin B_{12} coenzyme is needed to convert methylmalonyl coenzyme A to succinyl coenzyme A. Patients with vitamin B_{12} deficiency have increased concentrations of serum methylmalonic acid (MMA), which is a more specific marker for vitamin B_{12} deficiency than homocysteine. MMA levels are not elevated in folate deficiency because folate does not participate in MMA metabolism. Levels of both MMA and homocysteine usually are elevated prior to the development of hematologic abnormalities and reductions in serum vitamin B_{12} levels.[12] MMA levels must be interpreted cautiously for patients with renal disease and hypovolemia because the levels may be elevated due to decreased urinary excretion.

IRON-DEFICIENCY ANEMIA

Epidemiology

Iron deficiency is the most common nutritional deficiency in developing and developed countries. Data from the National Health and Nutrition Examination Survey (NHANES) indicate the prevalence of IDA in young children and women of childbearing age is 1.2% and 4.5%, respectively.[2] The normal ranges for Hb and Hct are so wide that a patient may lose up to 15% of RBC mass and still have a Hct within the normal range. Therefore, iron deficiency may precede the appearance of anemia.

Iron Balance

The normal iron content of the body is about 3 to 4 g. Iron is a component of Hb, myoglobin, and cytochromes. About 2 g of the iron exists in the form of Hb, and about 130 mg exists as iron-containing proteins such as myoglobin. About 3 mg of iron is bound to transferrin in plasma, and 1,000 mg of iron exists as storage iron in the form of ferritin or hemosiderin. The rest of the iron is stored in other tissues such as cytochromes.[9] Due to the toxicity of inorganic iron, the body has an intricate system for iron absorption, transport, storage, assimilation, and elimination. Hepcidin is a regulator of intestinal iron absorption, iron recycling, and iron mobilization from hepatic stores. It is a peptide hormone made in the liver, distributed in plasma, and excreted in urine. Hepcidin inhibits efflux of iron through ferroportin. Hepcidin synthesis is increased by iron loading and inflammation and decreased by iron deficiency and erythropoietic activity. Hepcidin is induced during infections and inflammation, which allows iron to sequester in macrophages, hepatocytes, and enterocytes.[15] As a result, hepcidin is likely an important mediator of AI. Hepcidin is usually suppressed in IDA.[16] Hepcidin testing is not routinely available.[17]

Most people lose about 1 mg of iron daily. Menstruating women can lose up to 0.6% to 2.5% more per day. Pregnancy requires an additional 700 mg of iron and a blood donation can result in as much as 250 mg of iron loss[18]; these patients are at higher risk for deficiency.

Iron is best absorbed in its ferrous (Fe^{2+}) form. The normal daily Western diet contains mainly the ferric (Fe^{3+}) nonabsorbed form. After iron is ionized by stomach acid and then reduced to the Fe^{2+} state, it is absorbed primarily in the duodenum, and to a smaller extent in the jejunum, via intestinal mucosal cell uptake. Subsequently, it is transferred across the cell into the plasma. Iron absorption is not directly proportional to iron intake. Rather as physiologic iron levels decrease, GI absorption of iron increases.

The daily recommended dietary allowance for iron is 8 mg in adult males and postmenopausal females and 18 mg in menstruating females. Children require more iron because of growth-related increases in blood volume, and pregnant women have an increased iron demand brought about by fetal development. In the absence of hemochromatosis, iron overload does not occur, because only the amount of iron lost per day is absorbed. The amount of iron absorbed from food depends on the body stores, the rate of RBC production, the type of iron provided in the diet, and the presence of any substances that may enhance or inhibit iron absorption.

Heme iron, which is found in meat, fish, and poultry, is about three times more absorbable than the nonheme iron found in vegetables, fruits, dried beans, nuts, grain products, and dietary supplements. Gastric acid and other dietary components such as ascorbic acid increase the absorption of nonheme iron. Dietary components that form insoluble complexes with iron (phytates, tannates, and phosphates) decrease absorption. Phytates, a natural component of grains, brans, and some vegetables, can form poorly absorbed complexes and partially explain the increased prevalence of IDA in poorer countries, where grains and vegetables compose a disproportionate amount of the normal diet. Polyphenols bind iron and decrease nonheme iron absorption when large amounts of tea or coffee are consumed with a meal. Although the mechanism is unknown, calcium inhibits absorption of both heme and nonheme iron. Finally, because gastric acid improves iron absorption, patients who have undergone a gastrectomy or have achlorhydria have decreased iron absorption.[19]

Etiology

Iron deficiency results from prolonged negative iron balance, which can occur due to increased iron demand or hematopoiesis, increased loss, or decreased intake/absorption. The onset of iron deficiency depends on an individual's initial iron stores and the imbalance between iron absorption and loss. Multiple etiologic factors usually are involved. Certain groups at higher risk for iron deficiency include children younger than 2 years, adolescent girls, pregnant/lactating females, and those older than 65 years. Patients older than 65 years of age with IDA should be considered for testing for occult GI bleeding.[18] Blood loss must initially be considered a cause of IDA in adults. Blood loss may occur as a result of many disorders, including trauma, hemorrhoids, peptic ulcers, gastritis, GI malignancies, arteriovenous malformations, diverticular disease, copious menstrual flow, nosebleeds, and postpartum bleeding. In less industrialized nations, the risk of IDA is largely related to dietary factors.

The USPSTF recommends routine screening for IDA in all pregnant women.[20] The USPSTF has concluded that evidence is insufficient to recommend for or against routine iron supplementation for nonanemic pregnant women.[18] However, iron deficiency in pregnant women is so common that the Centers for Disease Control and Prevention (CDC) guidelines recommend initiation of low-dose iron supplements or prenatal vitamins with 30 mg/day of iron at each woman's first prenatal visit.

Medication history, specifically regarding recent or past use of iron, alcohol, corticosteroids, warfarin or other anticoagulants, aspirin, and nonsteroidal anti-inflammatory drugs (NSAIDs), is a vital part of the history to assess bleeding risk. Other possible causes of hypochromic microcytic anemia include AI, thalassemia, sideroblastic anemia, and heavy metal (mostly lead) poisoning (see Fig. 100-4).

Pathophysiology

Iron is vital to the function of all cells. Without iron, cells lose their capacity for electron transport and energy metabolism. Iron deficiency usually is the result of a long period of negative iron balance. Manifestations of iron deficiency occur in three stages. In the initial stage, iron stores are reduced without reduced serum iron levels and can be assessed with serum ferritin measurement. The stores allow iron to be utilized when there is an increased need for Hb synthesis. Once stores are depleted, there still is adequate iron from daily RBC turnover for Hb synthesis. Further iron losses would make the patient vulnerable to anemia development. In the second stage, iron deficiency occurs when iron stores are depleted, and Hb is above the lower limit of normal for the population but may be reduced for a given patient. This can be determined by serial CBC measurements. Findings include reduced transferrin saturation and increased TIBC. The third stage occurs when the Hb falls to less than normal values.

Laboratory Findings

3 Abnormal laboratory findings for patients with IDA generally include low serum iron and ferritin levels and high TIBC. In the early stages of IDA, RBC size is not changed. Low ferritin concentration is the earliest and most sensitive indicator of iron deficiency. However, ferritin may not correlate with iron stores in the bone marrow because renal or hepatic disease, malignancies, infection, or inflammatory processes may increase ferritin values.[9] Hb, Hct, and RBC indices usually remain normal in early stages. In the later stages of IDA, Hb and Hct fall below normal values, and a microcytic hypochromic anemia develops. Microcytosis may precede hypochromia, as erythropoiesis is programmed to maintain normal Hb concentration in preference to cell size. As a result, even slightly abnormal Hb and Hct levels may indicate significant depletion of iron stores and should not be ignored. In terms of RBC indices, MCV is reduced earlier in IDA than Hb concentration.

Transferrin saturation (ie, serum iron level divided by the TIBC) is useful for assessing IDA. Low values may indicate IDA, although low serum transferrin saturation values also may be present in inflammatory disorders. The TIBC may help to differentiate the diagnosis in these patients: TIBC levels that are elevated can suggest IDA, while values that are low represent inflammatory disease.

TREATMENT

Iron Deficiency Anemia (Desired Outcomes)

The outcomes for all types of anemia in this chapter include: reversal of hematologic parameters to normal, return of normal function and quality of life, and prevention or reversal of long-term complications such as neurologic complications of vitamin B_{12} deficiency.

Dietary Supplementation and Oral Iron Preparations

The severity and cause of IDA determine the approach to treatment. Treatment is focused on replenishing iron stores. Because iron deficiency can be an early sign of other illnesses, treatment of the underlying disease may aid in the correction of iron deficiency.

Treatment of IDA usually consists of dietary supplementation and administration of oral iron preparations. Foods high in iron are listed in Table 100-1. Iron is best absorbed from meat, fish, and poultry. These foods as well as certain iron-fortified cereals can help treat IDA. Orange juice and other ascorbic acid-rich foods can be included with meals to increase absorption. Milk and tea reduce absorption and should be consumed in moderation. In most cases of IDA, oral administration of iron therapy with soluble Fe^{2+} iron salts is appropriate.

Fe^{2+} sulfate, succinate, lactate, fumarate, glutamate, and gluconate are absorbed similarly. The addition of copper, cobalt, molybdenum, or other minerals provides no advantage but increases cost of the product. Iron is best absorbed in the reduced Fe^{2+} form, with maximal absorption occurring in the duodenum, primarily due to the acidic medium of the stomach. Slow-release, sustained-release, or enteric coated iron preparations do not undergo sufficient dissolution until they reach the small intestine. In the alkaline environment of the small intestine, iron tends to form insoluble complexes, which significantly reduces absorption. The dose of iron replacement therapy depends on the patient's ability to tolerate the administered iron. Tolerance of iron salts improves with a small initial dose and gradual escalation to the full dose. For patients with IDA, the generally recommended dose is about 150 to 200 mg of elemental iron daily, usually in two or three divided doses to maximize tolerability. If patients cannot tolerate this daily dose of elemental iron, smaller amounts of elemental iron (eg, single 325 mg tablet of Fe^{2+} sulfate) usually are sufficient to replace iron stores, although at a slower rate. Table 100-2 lists the percentage of elemental iron of commonly available iron salts. Iron preferably is administered at least 1 hour before meals because food can interfere with iron absorption. Many patients must take iron with food because they experience GI upset when iron is administered on an empty stomach.

TABLE 100-1 Good Sources of Iron

Food	Serving Size	Amount (mg)
Ready to eat cereal, 100% fortified	3/4 cup (180 mL)	18
Instant plain oatmeal, fortified	1 cup (240 mL)	11
Wheat germ	1 oz (28g)	2.6
Broccoli	1 medium stalk	2.1
Baked potato	1 medium	2.7
Raw tofu	1/2 cup (120 mL)	4
Lentils	1/2 cup (120 mL)	3.3
Beef chuck	3 oz (85g)	3.2

TABLE 100-2 Oral Iron Products

Iron Salt	Percent Elemental Iron	Common: Formulations and Elemental Iron Provided
Ferrous sulfate	20	60-65 mg/324-325 mg tablet 60 mg/5 mL syrup 44 mg/ 5 mL elixir 15 mg/1 mL
Ferrous sulfate (exsiccated)	30	65 mg/200 mg tablet 50 mg/160 mg tablet
Ferrous gluconate	12	38 mg/325 mg tablet 28-29 mg/240-246 mg tablet
Ferrous fumarate	33	66 mg/200 mg tablet 106 mg/324-325 mg tablet

Clinical Controversy...

The treatment of patients who are found to be iron deficient, but do not have anemia, can improve fatigue or physical performance. Ferritin is typically used to measure deficiency in these studies. It is currently unknown whether these deficient patients should have a trial of iron therapy to improve symptoms.

Adverse reactions to therapeutic doses of iron are primarily GI in nature and consist of dark discoloration of feces, constipation or diarrhea, nausea, and vomiting. GI side effects usually are dose related and are similar among iron salts when equivalent amounts of elemental iron are administered. Dark stools do not interfere with testing for occult blood in the GI tract. Administration of smaller amounts of iron with each dose or administration with meals may minimize these adverse effects. Histamine-2 blockers or proton-pump inhibitors reduce gastric acidity and may impair iron absorption. Table 100-3 lists drug interactions with iron.

Failure to respond to appropriate treatment regimens necessitates reevaluation of the patient's condition. A "therapeutic trial of iron" approach will occasionally be used to confirm a presumptive diagnosis of IDA. Common causes of treatment failure include poor patient adherence, inability to absorb iron, incorrect diagnosis, continued bleeding, or a concurrent condition that impairs full reticulocyte response. Even when iron deficiency is present, response may be impaired when a coexisting cause for anemia exists. Rarely a patient has diminished ability to absorb iron, most often due to previous gastrectomy, such as gastric bypass surgery, or celiac disease. Regardless of the form of oral therapy used, treatment should continue for 3 to 6 months after the anemia is resolved to allow for repletion of iron stores and to prevent relapse. Patients should be instructed to store oral iron out of reach of children and pets as small amounts can result in a fatal overdose. Products containing more than 30 mg of elemental iron are required to be packaged as individual dosage units to prevent toxicity. Treatment for acute iron poisoning is discussed in Chapter e9.

Parenteral Iron Therapy

Indications for parenteral iron therapy include intolerance to oral, malabsorption, and nonadherence. Patients with significant blood loss who refuse transfusions and cannot take oral iron therapy also may require parenteral iron therapy. Parenteral iron therapy should also be considered, possibly first line, in patients with inflammatory bowel disease and those with gastric bypass/gastric resection due to poor oral absorption.[21] Parenteral iron therapy is also used for patients with chronic kidney disease (see Chapter 44), especially those undergoing hemodialysis, and for some cancer patients receiving chemotherapy on erythropoiesis-stimulating agents (ESAs; Chapter 127). Five different parenteral iron preparations currently available in the United States are iron dextran, sodium ferric gluconate, iron sucrose, ferumoxytol, and ferric carboxymaltose (Table 44-10). They differ in their molecular size, pharmacokinetics, bioavailability, and adverse effect profiles. Although toxicity profiles of these agents differ, clinical studies indicate that each is efficacious. Iron dextran parenteral preparations have been associated with more anaphylactic reactions and this product requires a test dose prior to full dose administration. Fatal reactions have also occurred in patients who tolerated the test dose. Iron dextran and ferumoxytol products have black box warnings in their labeling regarding severe allergic reactions. The safety profile of parenteral iron is largely assessed by spontaneous reports to the FDA and observational studies. All parenteral iron preparations carry a risk for anaphylactic reactions but likely to a lesser extent than iron dextran.[22,23] The FDA recommends that resuscitation equipment and trained staff be available during administration of all iron dextran preparations. A concern with parenteral iron is that iron may be released too quickly and overload the ability of transferrin to bind it, leading to free iron reactions that can interfere with neutrophil function. The following formula can be used to estimate the total dose of parenteral iron needed to correct anemia:

$$\text{Dose of iron (mg)} = \text{whole blood hemoglobin deficit (g/dL)} \times \text{body weight (lb) or}$$

$$\text{Dose of iron (mg)} = \text{whole blood hemoglobin deficit (g/L)} \times \text{body weight (kg)} \times 0.22$$

An additional quantity of iron to replenish stores should be added (about 600 mg for women and 1,000 mg for men).[9]

Iron dextran, a complex of Fe^{3+} hydroxide and the carbohydrate dextran, contains 50 mg of iron per milliliter and can be given via the intramuscular or IV route. Different brands of iron dextran are available and differ in their molecular weight. They are not interchangeable. The intramuscular route is no longer used routinely and requires Z-tract injection technique.[24]

Methods of IV administration include multiple slow injections of undiluted iron dextran solution or an infusion of a diluted preparation. This latter method often is referred to as total dose infusion.

Total replacement doses of IV iron dextran have been given as a single dose, but this method of administration is not FDA approved. A test dose still is required. Patients who receive total dose infusions are at higher risk for adverse reactions, such as arthralgias, myalgias, flushing, malaise, and fever. Other adverse reactions of iron dextran include staining of the skin, pain at the injection site, allergic reactions, and rarely anaphylaxis. Patients with preexisting immune-mediated diseases, such as active rheumatoid arthritis or systemic lupus erythematosus, are considered at high risk for adverse reactions because of their hyperreactive immune response.

Sodium ferric gluconate is a complex of iron bound to one gluconate and four sucrose molecules in a repeating pattern. Its molecular weight is 289 to 440 kDa. Sodium ferric gluconate is available in an aqueous solution. No direct transfer of iron from the Fe^{3+} gluconate to transferrin occurs. The complex is taken up quickly by the mononuclear phagocytic system and has a half-life of about 1 hour in the bloodstream. Sodium ferric gluconate appears to produce fewer anaphylactic reactions than iron dextran does. Adverse effects of sodium ferric gluconate include cramps, nausea, vomiting, flushing, hypotension, intense upper gastric pain, rash, and pruritus.[26]

Iron sucrose is a polynuclear iron (III) hydroxide in sucrose complex with a molecular weight of 34 to 60 kDa. Following IV administration of iron sucrose, the iron is released directly from the circulating iron sucrose to transferrin and is taken up by the mononuclear phagocytic system and metabolized. The half-life is about 6 hours, with a volume of distribution similar to that of iron dextran.

TABLE 100-3 Iron Salt–Drug Interactions

Drugs That Decrease Iron Absorption	Object Drugs Affected by Iron
Al-, Mg-, and Ca^{2+}-containing antacids	Levodopa ↓ (chelates with iron)
Tetracycline and doxycycline	Methyldopa ↓ (decreases efficacy of methyldopa)
$Histamine_2$ antagonists	Levothyroxine ↓ (decreased efficacy of levothyroxine)
Proton-pump inhibitors	Penicillamine ↓ (chelates with iron)
Cholestyramine	Fluoroquinolones ↓ (forms ferric ion quinolone complex)
	Tetracycline and doxycycline ↓ (when administered within 2 hours of iron salt)
	Mycophenolate ↓ (decreases absorption)

Iron sucrose injection should not be administered concomitantly with oral iron preparations because it will reduce the absorption of oral iron.[27] Adverse effects include leg cramps and hypotension.

Ferumoxytol was FDA-approved in 2009 to treat iron deficiency in adults with chronic kidney disease who are on or off dialysis. Typical dosing is 510 mg IV dose followed by a second 510 mg dose 3 to 8 days later. The dose can be readministered after 1 month if anemia persists. No test dose is required but anaphylaxis can occur and patients should be observed for at least 30 minutes after each dose. A black box warning was also added in 2015 due to case reports of fatal and nonfatal anaphylactic reactions to the product. It should not be used in patients who previously had an allergic reaction to other iron preparations.[28]

Ferric carboxymaltose is the newest approved parenteral iron product, receiving FDA approval in 2013. The approval of this product was delayed due to hypophosphatemia seen in clinical trials. No additional warnings were required and no clinical issues related to hypophosphatemia have been reported. This product received approval for treatment of IDA in those who have failed oral iron therapy or who have intolerance for oral therapy. It is also approved for chronic kidney disease patients not on hemodialysis.[29]

Increased risk for infection is a concern with parenteral iron preparations because iron is a growth factor for some bacteria, but a recently published meta-analysis concluded that IV iron does not increase risk for infection.[30] Parenteral iron products are discussed in more detail in Chapter 44.

MEGALOBLASTIC ANEMIAS

Macrocytic anemias are divided into megaloblastic and nonmegaloblastic anemias. Macrocytosis, as seen in megaloblastic anemias, is caused by abnormal DNA metabolism resulting from vitamin B_{12} or folate deficiency. It also can be caused by administration of various drugs, such as hydroxyurea, zidovudine, cytarabine, methotrexate, azathioprine, 6-mercaptopurine, and cladribine. In vitamin B_{12}- or folate-deficiency anemia, megaloblastosis results from interference with folic acid- and vitamin B_{12}-interdependent nucleic acid synthesis in the immature erythrocyte. The rate of RNA and cytoplasm production exceeds the rate of DNA production. The maturation process is impaired, resulting in immature large RBCs (macrocytosis). RNA and DNA synthesis depend on a series of reactions catalyzed by vitamin B_{12} and folic acid because of their role in the conversion of uridine to thymidine. As shown in Fig. 100-6, dietary folates are absorbed in this process and converted to 5-methyl-tetrahydrofolate (A), which then is converted via a B_{12}-dependent reaction (B) to tetrahydrofolate (C). After gaining a carbon, tetrahydrofolate is converted to 5,10-methyl-tetrahydrofolate (D), a folate cofactor used by thymidylate synthetase (E) in the biosynthesis of nucleic acids. The 5,10-methyl-tetrahydrofolate cofactor is converted to dihydrofolate (F) during biosynthesis. Dihydrofolate reductase normally reduces dihydrofolate back to tetrahydrofolate (C), which can again pick up a carbon and be recycled to produce more 5,10-methyl-tetrahydrofolate (D).

Although vitamin B_{12} and folate deficiency are common causes of macrocytosis, other possible causes must be considered if these deficiencies are not found. Other causes of macrocytosis include (1) a shift to immature or stressed RBCs as seen in reticulocytosis, aplastic anemia, and pure RBC aplasia; (2) a primary bone marrow disorder such as myelodysplastic syndromes, congenital dyserythropoietic anemias, and large granular lymphocyte leukemia; (3) lipid abnormalities as seen with liver disease, hypothyroidism, or hyperlipidemia; and (4) unknown mechanisms resulting from alcohol abuse and multiple myeloma. Macrocytosis is the most typical morphologic abnormality associated with excessive alcohol consumption. Even with adequate folate and vitamin B_{12} levels and the absence of liver disease, patients with high alcohol intake may present with an alcohol-induced macrocytosis. Cessation of alcohol ingestion results in resolution of the macrocytosis within a couple of months.

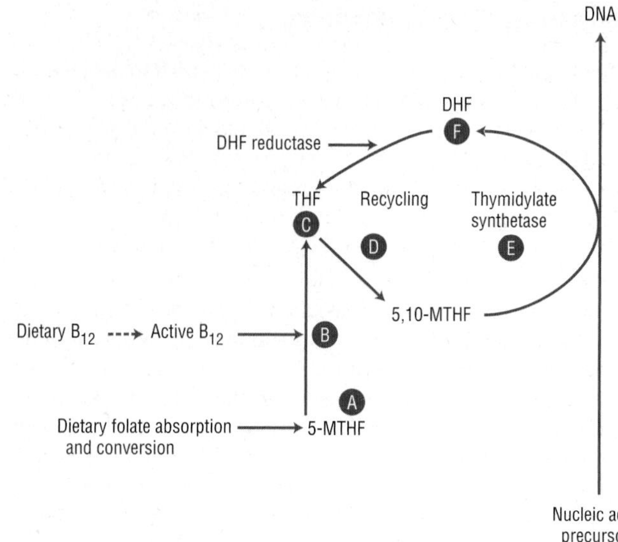

FIGURE 100-6 Drug-induced megaloblastosis (DHF, dihydrofolate; 5-MTHF, 5-methyl-tetrahydrofolate; 5,10-MTHF, 5,10-methyl-tetrahydrofolate; THF, tetrahydrofolate).

Vitamin B_{12} Deficiency Anemia

The prevalence of vitamin B_{12} deficiency anemia in the United States is unknown. Risk increases with age.[31] The use of gastric acid-suppressing agents, which may inhibit cobalamin release from food, is associated with an increased risk. Older adults in the United States have a high prevalence (up to 15%) of elevated MMA levels and associated low or low-normal vitamin B_{12} levels, likely due to atrophic gastritis and malabsorption of food-bound vitamin B_{12}.[31]

Etiology

4 The three major causes of vitamin B_{12} deficiency are inadequate intake, malabsorption syndromes, and inadequate utilization. Inadequate dietary consumption of vitamin B_{12} is rare. It usually occurs only in patients who are strict vegans and their breast-fed infants, chronic alcoholics, and elderly patients who consume a "tea and toast" diet because of financial limitations or poor dentition. Decreased vitamin B_{12} absorption can occur with loss of intrinsic factor by autoimmune mechanisms (such as pernicious anemia, in which gastric parietal cells are selectively damaged), chronic atrophic gastritis, or stomach surgery. One of the most frequent causes of low serum B_{12} levels results from the inability of vitamin B_{12} to be cleaved and released from proteins in food because of inadequate gastric acid production. Treatment of *Helicobacter pylori* may improve vitamin B_{12} status because this bacterial infection is a cause of chronic gastritis.[32] Vitamin B_{12} deficiency may occasionally result from overgrowth of bacteria in the bowel that use vitamin B_{12} or from injury or removal (from Crohn's disease or small bowel surgery, respectively) of ileal receptor sites where vitamin B_{12} and the intrinsic factor complex are absorbed. Blind loop syndrome, Whipple disease, Zollinger–Ellison syndrome, tapeworm infestations, intestinal resections, tropical sprue, surgical resection of the ileus, pancreatic insufficiency, inflammatory bowel disease, advanced liver disease, tuberculosis, and Crohn's disease may contribute to the development of vitamin B_{12} deficiency.[31] Metformin may reversibly decrease B_{12} absorption, likely due to its effects on the intestinal mucosa in the ileum. It rarely causes anemia on its own but can contribute to deficiency. Proton pump inhibitors and histamine 2 receptor antagonists may also contribute to vitamin B_{12} deficiency because an acidic

environment is needed for vitamin B_{12} to be absorbed in the GI tract from food.[33] A recent study suggested that these medications have a greater effect on deficiency in those who have taken them for 2 or more years.[33]

Pathophysiology

Vitamin B_{12} works closely with folate in the synthesis of building blocks for DNA and RNA, is essential in maintaining the integrity of the neurologic system, and plays a role in fatty acid biosynthesis and energy production. It is a water-soluble vitamin obtained exogenously by ingestion of meat, fish, poultry, dairy products, and fortified cereals. The body stores several years of vitamin B_{12}, of which about 50% is in the liver. The recommended daily allowance is 2 mcg in adults and 2.6 mcg in pregnant or breast-feeding women. The average western diet provides 5 to 15 mcg of vitamin B_{12} daily, of which 1 to 5 mcg is absorbed.[31] Vitamin B_{12} deficiency usually takes several years to develop following vitamin deprivation.

Once dietary cobalamin enters the stomach, pepsin and hydrochloric acid release the cobalamin from animal proteins. The free cobalamin then binds to R-protein, which is released from parietal and salivary cells. In the duodenum, the cobalamin-R-protein complex is degraded, releasing free cobalamin. The cobalamin then binds with intrinsic factor that serves as a cell-directed carrier protein similar to transferrin for iron. This complex attaches to mucosal cell receptors in the distal ileum, the intrinsic factor is discarded, and the cobalamin is bound to transport proteins (transcobalamin I, II, and III). The cobalamin bound to transcobalamin II is secreted into the circulation and is taken up by the liver, bone marrow, and other cells. Most circulating cobalamin is bound to transcobalamin I and transcobalamin III. Passive diffusion is an alternate pathway for vitamin B_{12} absorption independent of intrinsic factor or an intact terminal ileum and accounts for about 1% of vitamin B_{12} absorption.[31]

Vitamin B_{12} deficiency can cause neurologic and hematologic complications. These usually start with bilateral paraesthesia in extremities; deficits in proprioception and vibration can also be present. If not treated, this can progress to ataxia, dementia-like symptoms, psychosis, and vision loss. In children prolonged deficiency can lead to poor brain development.[13,34] Patients with unexplained neuropathies should be evaluated for vitamin B_{12} deficiency.

Laboratory Findings

In macrocytic anemias, MCV is elevated greater than 100 fL, but some patients deficient in vitamin B_{12} may have a normal MCV. If there is a coexisting cause of microcytosis, the MCV may not be elevated.[30] Mild leukopenia and thrombocytopenia are often present because abnormal DNA synthesis can affect all blood cell lines. A peripheral blood smear demonstrates macrocytosis accompanied by hypersegmented polymorphonuclear leukocytes (one of the earliest and most specific indications of this disease), oval macrocytes, anisocytosis, and poikilocytosis. Serum lactate dehydrogenase and indirect bilirubin levels may be elevated as a result of hemolysis or ineffective erythropoiesis.[13] Other laboratory findings include a low reticulocyte count, low serum vitamin B_{12} level (less than 200 pg/mL [less than 148 pmol/L]), and low Hct.

In the early stages of vitamin B_{12} deficiency, classic signs and symptoms of megaloblastic anemia may not be evident, and serum levels of vitamin B_{12} may be within normal limits. Therefore, measurement of MMA and homocysteine may be useful because these parameters are typically the first to change. Because MMA and homocysteine are involved in enzymatic reactions that depend on vitamin B_{12}, a deficiency in vitamin B_{12} leads to accumulation of these metabolites. Elevations in MMA are more specific for vitamin B_{12} deficiency. Homocysteine is also elevated in several other situations including folate deficiency, chronic renal disease, alcoholism, smoking, use of steroid or cyclosporine therapy, and smoking.[34] Low levels of vitamin B_{12} result in hyperhomocysteinemia, which some studies have reported to be an independent risk factor for cerebrovascular, peripheral vascular, coronary, and venous thromboembolic disease.[35]

Blood levels of vitamin B_{12} should be drawn for all patients with suspected vitamin B_{12} deficiency. Vitamin B_{12} values less than 200 pg/mL (less than 148 pmol/L) are suggestive of B_{12} deficiency. Some patients with clinical B_{12} deficiency manifesting as neurological disease may have normal hematological parameters.

Clinical **Controversy...**

Subclinical vitamin B_{12} deficiency is sometimes used with vitamin B_{12} levels 200 to 300 pg/mL (148-221 pmol/L).[36] A general multivitamin does not typically contain enough vitamin B_{12} to normalize levels in deficient persons. Whether to treat patients in this range is not clear in the absence of neurologic symptoms.

A Schilling test may theoretically be performed to diagnose pernicious anemia, but the usefulness of this test is questionable and rarely alters the clinical management of the vitamin B_{12} deficiency. The Schilling test was once performed to determine whether replacement of vitamin B_{12} should occur via an oral or parenteral route, but evidence now shows that oral replacement is as efficacious as parenteral supplementation because of the vitamin B_{12} absorption pathway independent of intrinsic factor.[31,37]

TREATMENT
Vitamin B_{12} Deficiency Anemia

The goals of treatment for vitamin B_{12} deficiency include reversal of hematologic manifestations, replacement of body stores, and prevention or resolution of neurologic manifestations. Early treatment is of paramount importance because neurologic damage may be irreversible if the deficiency is not detected and corrected within months. In addition to replacement therapy, any underlying etiology that is treatable, such as bacterial overgrowth, should be corrected. Indications for starting oral or parenteral therapy include megaloblastic anemia or other hematologic abnormalities and neurologic disease from deficiency.[34] Those with borderline low levels of B_{12} but no hematologic abnormalities should be followed at yearly intervals.[34] Patients should be counseled on the types of foods high in vitamin B_{12} content such as fortified cereals as seen in Table 100-4. Orally administered vitamin B_{12} can be used effectively to treat pernicious anemia because of the previously discussed alternate pathway of passive absorption, independent of intrinsic factor.[14] Daily

TABLE 100-4 Good Sources of Vitamin B_{12}

Food	Serving Size	Amount (mcg)
Beef liver, cooked	3 oz (85g)	70
Breakfast cereal, fortified (100%)	3/4 cup (180 mL)	6
Rainbow trout, cooked	3 oz (85g)	3.5
Sockeye salmon, cooked	3 oz (85g)	4.9
Beef, cooked	3 oz (85g)	2.1
Breakfast cereal, fortified (25%)	¾ cup (180 mL)	1.5
Clams, cooked	3 oz (85g)	84.1
Oysters, breaded and fried	6 pieces	1
Tuna, canned in water	3 oz (85g)	2.5
Milk	1 cup (240 mL)	1.2
Yogurt	8 oz (230g)	1.1

oral doses (1,000-2,000 mcg) of vitamin B_{12} is as effective as intramuscular administration in achieving hematologic and neurologic responses.[31,37] If vitamin B_{12} levels are marginally low and either MMA or both MMA and homocysteine levels are elevated, administration of 1,000 mcg of oral vitamin B_{12} daily should be strongly considered.[38] Timed-release preparations of oral cobalamin should be avoided.[39] Nonprescription 1,000 mcg cobalamin tablets are available, among several other strengths. A commonly used initial parenteral vitamin B_{12} regimen consists of daily injections of 1,000 mcg of cyanocobalamin for 1 week to saturate vitamin B_{12} stores in the body and resolve clinical manifestations of the deficiency. Thereafter, it can be given weekly for 1 month and monthly thereafter for maintenance. The series of daily parenteral injections may be omitted if administration is difficult or inconvenient. In this case the parenteral injection is then given weekly, sometimes for a longer than 1 month. Parenteral therapy is preferred for patients exhibiting neurologic symptoms until resolution of symptoms and normalization of hematologic indices because the most rapid-acting therapy is necessary.[40] When patients are converted from the parenteral to the oral form of cobalamin, 1,000 mcg of oral cobalamin daily can be initiated on the due date of the next injection. Vitamin B_{12} should be continued for life in patients with pernicious anemia.

In addition to the oral and parenteral forms, vitamin B_{12} is available as a nasal spray for patients in remission following intramuscular vitamin B_{12} therapy who have no nervous system involvement. The nasal spray is administered once weekly. Intranasal administration should be avoided for patients with nasal diseases or those receiving medications intranasally in the same nostril. Patients should not administer the spray 1 hour before or after ingestion of hot foods or beverages, which can impair cobalamin absorption. The efficacy of the nasal spray formulation has not been well studied, and it should be used for maintenance therapy only after hematologic parameters have normalized.

Potential adverse effects with vitamin B_{12} replacement therapy are rare. Uncommon side effects include hyperuricemia and hypokalemia due to marked increase in potassium utilization during production of new hematopoietic cells.

Folic Acid Deficiency Anemia

Epidemiology

Folic acid deficiency is one of the most common vitamin deficiencies occurring in the United States, largely because of its association with excessive alcohol intake and pregnancy.

Etiology

5 Major causes of folic acid deficiency include inadequate intake, decreased absorption, and increased folate requirements. Poor eating habits make this deficiency more common in elderly patients, teenagers whose diets consist of "junk food," alcoholics, food faddists, the impoverished, and those who are chronically ill or demented. Folic acid absorption may decrease for patients who have malabsorption syndromes or those who have received certain drugs. In alcoholics with poor dietary habits, alcohol interferes with folic acid absorption, interferes with folic acid utilization at the cellular level, and decreases hepatic stores of folic acid.

Increased folate requirements may occur when the rate of cellular division is increased, as seen in pregnant women; patients with hemolytic anemia, myelofibrosis, malignancy, chronic inflammatory disorders such as Crohn's disease, rheumatoid arthritis, or psoriasis; patients undergoing long-term dialysis; burn patients; and adolescents and infants during their growth spurts. This hyperutilization eventually can lead to anemia, particularly when the daily intake of folate is borderline, resulting in inadequate replacement of folate stores.

Several drugs have been reported to cause a folic acid deficiency. Some drugs (eg, azathioprine, 6-mercaptopurine, 5-fluorouracil, hydroxyurea, and zidovudine) directly inhibit DNA synthesis. Other drugs are folate antagonists; the most toxic is methotrexate (other examples include pentamidine, trimethoprim, and triamterene). A number of drugs (eg, phenytoin, phenobarbital, and primidone) antagonize folate via poorly understood mechanisms but are thought to reduce vitamin absorption by the intestine (see Chapter e103). Since folic acid doses as low as 1 mg/day may affect serum phenytoin levels, routine folic acid supplementation is not generally recommended. The decline in phenytoin concentration usually occurs within the first 10 days and may decrease phenytoin levels by 15% to 50%.[41] Alcohol can also interfere with folic acid and vitamin B_{12} absorption likely through its effects on the intestinal mucosa.[33]

Pathophysiology

Folic acid is a water-soluble vitamin readily destroyed by cooking or processing. It is necessary for the production of DNA and RNA. It acts as a methyl donor to form methylcobalamin, which is used in the remethylation of homocysteine to methionine. Because humans are unable to synthesize sufficient folate to meet total daily requirements, they depend on dietary sources. Major dietary sources of folate include fresh, green leafy vegetables, citrus fruits, yeast, mushrooms, dairy products, and animal organs such as liver and kidney. Most folate in food is present in the polyglutamate form, which must be broken down into the monoglutamate form prior to absorption in the small intestine. Once absorbed, dietary folate must be converted to the active form tetrahydrofolate through a cobalamin-dependent reaction. In 1997, the United States mandated that grain products be fortified with folic acid in an attempt to increase the dietary intake of folate. This amount of supplementation was chosen to decrease the incidence of neural tube defects without masking occult vitamin B_{12} deficiency.

As a result of grain product fortification, neural tube defect frequency has decreased by 25% to 30%.[42] Although body demands for folate are high because of high rates of RBC synthesis and turnover, the minimum daily requirement is 50 to 100 mcg. In the general population, the recommended daily allowance for folate is 400 mcg in nonpregnant females, 600 mcg for pregnant females, and 500 mcg for lactating females.[38] Because the body stores about 5 to 10 mg of folate, primarily in the liver, cessation of dietary folate intake can result in deficiency within 3 to 4 months.

Laboratory Findings

It is of paramount importance to rule out vitamin B_{12} deficiency when folate deficiency is suspected. Laboratory changes associated with folate deficiency are similar to those seen in vitamin B_{12} deficiency, except vitamin B_{12} and MMA levels are normal. Serum folate levels decrease to less than 3 ng/mL (7 nmol/L) within a few days of reduced dietary folate intake. The RBC folate level (less than150 ng/mL [less than 340 nmol/L]) also declines, and levels remain constant throughout the life span of the erythrocyte.[12] If serum or erythrocyte folate levels are borderline, serum homocysteine usually is increased with a folic acid deficiency. If serum MMA levels also are elevated, vitamin B_{12} deficiency must be ruled out given that folate does not participate in MMA metabolism.

TREATMENT

Folic Acid Deficiency Anemia

Therapy for folic acid deficiency consists of administration of exogenous folic acid to induce hematologic remission, replace body stores, and resolve signs and symptoms. In most cases, 1 mg daily is sufficient to replace stores, except in cases of deficiency due to malabsorption, in which case doses of 1 to 5 mg daily may be necessary. Parenteral folic acid is available but rarely necessary. Synthetic folic acid is

TABLE 100-5 Good Sources of Folate

Food	Serving	Amount (mcg)
Beef liver	3 oz (85g)	215
Cereal, 25% fortified	½-1½ cups (120-360 mL)	100-400
Lentils, cooked	1/2 cup (120 mL)	180
Chickpeas	1/2 cup (120 mL)	141
Asparagus	1/2 cup (120 mL)	132
Spinach, cooked	1/2 cup (120 mL)	131
Pasta, enriched	1/2 cup (120 mL)	83
Kidney beans	1/2 cup (120 mL)	46
White rice, cooked	1/2 cup (120 mL)	90
Tomato juice	1 cup (240 mL)	48
Brussels sprouts	1/2 cup (120 mL)	78
Orange	1 medium	47

almost completely absorbed by the GI tract and is converted to tetrahydrofolate without cobalamin. Therapy should continue for about 4 months if the underlying cause of the deficiency can be identified and corrected to allow for clearance of all folate-deficient RBCs from the circulation. Foods high in folic acid should also be encouraged in the diet as seen in Table 100-5. Long-term folate administration may be necessary in chronic conditions associated with increased folate requirements. Low-dose folate therapy (500 mcg daily) can be administered when anticonvulsant drugs produce a megaloblastic anemia so that discontinuation of anticonvulsant therapy may not be necessary. Adverse effects have not been reported with folic acid doses used for replacement therapy. It is considered nontoxic at high doses and is rapidly excreted in the urine.

Although megaloblastic anemia during pregnancy is rare, the most common cause is folate deficiency. The condition usually manifests as an underweight premature infant and suboptimal health of the mother. Periconceptional folic acid supplementation is recommended to decrease the occurrence and recurrence of neural tube defects, specifically anencephaly and spinal bifida. Folic acid supplementation at a dose of 400 mcg daily is recommended for all women. Women who have previously given birth to offspring with neural tube defects or those with a family history of neural tube defects should ingest 4 mg daily of folic acid.[41-43] Higher levels of folic acid supplementation should not be attained via ingestion of excess multivitamins because of the risk for fat soluble vitamin toxicity.[43] Prenatal vitamins usually have a higher amount of folic acid as compared with general multivitamins to ensure adequate supplementation is attained. It is essential that women in their childbearing years maintain adequate folic acid intake.

ANEMIA OF INFLAMMATION

Epidemiology

6 AI is a newer term used to describe both ACD and anemia of critical illness. This new term was developed to reflect the inflammatory process that underlies both of those types of anemia. The onset of anemia of critical illness is quicker, over days, and typically occurs in a hospital setting. ACD has a similar mechanism, but it develops over months to years from a chronic condition. AI is one of the most common forms of anemia seen clinically, particularly among the elderly. It is especially important in the differential diagnosis of iron deficiency. ACD is associated with common disease states that may mimic the symptoms of anemia, which causes the diagnosis of ACD to sometimes be overlooked in the outpatient setting. Anemia of critical illness is a common complication in critically ill patients and is found almost universally in this patient population.[44]

TABLE 100-6 Diseases Causing Anemia of Inflammation

Common causes
- Chronic infections
  - Tuberculosis
  - Other chronic lung infections (eg, lung abscess, bronchiectasis)
  - Human immunodeficiency virus
  - Subacute bacterial endocarditis
  - Osteomyelitis
  - Chronic urinary tract infections
- Chronic inflammation
  - Rheumatoid arthritis
  - Systemic lupus erythematosus
  - Inflammatory bowel disease
  - Inflammatory osteoarthritis
  - Gout
  - Other (collagen vascular) diseases
  - Chronic inflammatory liver diseases
- Malignancies
  - Carcinoma
  - Lymphoma
  - Leukemia
  - Multiple myeloma

Less common causes
- Alcoholic liver disease
- Congestive heart failure
- Thrombophlebitis
- Chronic obstructive pulmonary disease
- Ischemic heart disease

Etiology

The diagnosis of AI usually is one of exclusion. It is important to exclude IDA as the true or competing etiology. Various conditions associated with ACD may predispose patients to blood loss (malignancy, GI blood loss from treatments with aspirin, NSAIDs, or corticosteroids). ACD is often observed in patients with diseases that last longer than 1-2 months, although it can occur in conditions with a more rapid onset of several weeks, such as pneumonia. ACD tends to be a mild (Hb greater than 9.5 g/dL [greater than 95 g/L; greater than 5.90 mmol/L]) or moderate (Hb greater than 8 g/dL [greater than 80 g/L; greater than 4.97 mmol/L]) anemia.[45] Anemia associated with human immunodeficiency virus (HIV), autoimmune conditions, cancer, and heart failure are common forms of ACD. The degree of anemia in ACD is generally reflects the severity of underlying disease. Table 100-6 lists common diseases associated with ACD.

Factors that may contribute to anemia in critically ill patients include sepsis, frequent blood sampling, surgical blood loss, immune-mediated functional iron deficiency, decreased production of endogenous EPO, reduced RBC life span, and active bleeding, especially in the GI tract. A combination of these factors often exists, creating an anemic state over days. Additional comorbid factors include coagulopathies and nutritional deficits such as poor oral intake and altered absorption of vitamins and minerals, including iron, vitamin B_{12}, and folate.[46] Deleterious effects of anemia include an increased risk of cardiac-related morbidity and mortality, especially for patients with known cardiovascular disease. Persistent tissue hypoxia can result in cerebral ischemia, myocardial ischemia, multiple organ deterioration, lactic acidosis, and death. Consequences of anemia in critically ill patients may be enhanced because of the increased metabolic demands of critical illness. Weaning anemic patients from mechanical ventilation may be more difficult.[47]

Pathophysiology

AI is a response to stimulation of the cellular immune system by various underlying disease processes. AI is an anemia that traditionally has been associated with infectious or inflammatory processes, tissue injury, and conditions associated with release of proinflammatory cytokines. The pathogenesis of AI is multifactorial and is characterized by a blunted EPO response to anemia, an impaired proliferation of erythroid progenitor cells, and a disturbance of iron homeostasis. Increased iron uptake and retention occur within cells. The RBCs have a shortened life span, and the bone marrow's capacity to respond to EPO is inadequate to maintain normal Hb concentration. The cause of this defect is uncertain but appears to involve blocked release of iron from cells in the bone marrow. Iron availability to erythroid progenitor cells then is limited. Various cytokines, such as interleukin-1, interferon-γ, interleukin-6, and tumor necrosis factor released during illness may inhibit the production or action of EPO or the production of RBCs.[45] These cytokines also upregulate hepcidin, which blocks iron release from storage cells.[48] Hepcidin also decreases duodenal absorption of iron.[45]

Laboratory Findings

No definitive test can confirm the diagnosis of AI. The practitioner should maintain a high index of suspicion for any patient with a chronic inflammatory or neoplastic disease. AI may coexist with IDA and folic acid deficiency because many patients with these conditions have poor dietary intake or GI blood loss. Examination of the bone marrow reveals an abundance of iron, suggesting that the release mechanism for iron is the central defect. Patients with AI usually have a decreased serum iron level, but unlike patients with IDA, their serum ferritin level is normal or increased and their TIBC is decreased. Transferrin saturation is typically decreased. AI usually is normocytic and normochromic with mildly depressed Hb. Patients with concurrent AI and IDA usually have microcytes and a more severe anemia. Table 100-7 shows lab values seen in AI and IDA. Erythrocyte survival may be reduced for patients with AI, but a compensatory erythropoietic response does not occur. A low reticulocyte count indicates underproduction of RBCs.[45] As discussed in the IDA section, hepcidin levels are not routinely used for diagnosis but would likely be elevated in a patient with ACD.[49]

TREATMENT
Anemia of Inflammation

Treatment of AI depends somewhat on the underlying etiology. Guidelines exist for management of anemia for patients with cancer or chronic kidney disease (see Chaps. 44 and 127). Although the goals of therapy should include treating the underlying disorder and correcting reversible causes of anemia, accomplishment of these goals may not totally reverse hematologic and physiologic abnormalities. Iron is effective only if iron deficiency is present. During inflammation, oral or parenteral iron therapy may not be as effective. Absorption is impaired because of downregulation of ferroportin and iron diversion mediated by cytokines.[45] Because iron is a required nutrient for proliferating microorganisms, supplementation may theoretically increase the risk of infections. Iron therapy should be reserved for those patients with an established iron deficiency.[45]

RBC transfusions are effective but should be limited to situations in which oxygen transport is inadequate due to concomitant medical problems. Transfusions are typically considered for those with severe anemia (Hb less than 7 to 8 g/dL [less than 70 to 80 g/L; less than 4.34 to 4.97 mmol/L]). Transfusion risks may include transmission of blood-borne infections, development of autoantibodies, transfusion reactions, and iron overload.

ESAs have been used to stimulate erythropoiesis for patients with AI since a relative EPO deficiency exists for the degree of anemia. Two agents are available: recombinant epoetin alfa and recombinant darbepoetin alfa. Although both agents share the same mechanism of action, darbepoetin alfa has a longer half-life and can be administered less frequently. Although these agents are sometimes used to treat AI, they are not FDA-approved for this indication. Patients with chronic disease may have a relatively impaired response to ESAs. The initial dosage of epoetin alfa and darbepoetin alfa are typically 50 to 100 units per kilogram three times per week and 0.45 mcg per kilogram once weekly, respectively. These doses are typical starting doses for those with chronic kidney disease. Response to ESAs varies depending on dose and cause of the anemia. Higher doses may be needed to overcome hyporesponsiveness. ESA treatment is effective when the marrow has an adequate supply of iron, cobalamin, and folic acid.

Iron deficiency can occur in patients treated with ESAs; so close monitoring of iron levels is necessary. Some patients develop "functional" iron deficiency, in which the iron stores are normal but the supply of iron to the erythroid marrow is less than necessary to support the demand for RBC production. Therefore, many practitioners routinely supplement ESA therapy with oral or IV iron therapy. Potential toxicities of exogenous ESA administration include increases in blood pressure, nausea, headache, fever, bone pain, and fatigue. Less common adverse effects include seizures, thrombotic events, and allergic reactions such as rashes and local reactions at the injection site. If ESAs are used, the practitioner must monitor to ensure the patient's Hb does not exceed 12 g/dL (120 g/L; 7.45 mmol/L) with treatment or that Hb does not rise greater than 1 g/dL (greater than 10 g/L; greater than 0.62 mmol/L) every 2 weeks since both of these events have been associated with increased mortality and cardiovascular events.[50] Tumor progression with these agents can also occur and is discussed in Chapter 127. Further discussion of dosing guidelines and potential adverse outcomes of ESA treatment in populations for which treatment is FDA approved are discussed in Chapters 44 and 127.

Patients who are critically ill require the necessary substrates of iron, folic acid, and vitamin B_{12} for RBC production. Parenteral iron is generally preferred in this population because patients often are undergoing enteral therapy or because of concerns regarding inadequate iron absorption. The disadvantage of parenteral therapy is the theoretical risk of infection.

Pharmacologic doses of ESAs have been used to treat the anemia of critical illness. Few randomized controlled trials have evaluated the role of ESAs in critically ill patients, and the results of these trials have not consistently shown a decrease in transfusion requirements in ESA-treated patients.[51] Further investigation is necessary to determine the effectiveness of ESAs in critically ill patients. These agents are not FDA approved in this setting.

Many critically ill patients receive RBC transfusions despite the inherent risks associated with transfusions. Stored RBCs may not function as well as endogenous blood. Although RBC transfusions may increase oxygen delivery to tissues, cellular oxygen may not increase.[52] Transfusion practices in ICUs vary, and clinicians use different Hb concentrations as thresholds for administering transfusions. The decision to use transfusions must consider the risks,

TABLE 100-7 Laboratory Value Differences between Anemia of Inflammation and Iron-Deficiency Anemia

	Anemia of Inflammation	Iron-Deficiency Anemia
Iron	↓	↓
Transferrin	↓ or nl	↑
Transferrin saturation	↓	↓
Ferritin	↑ or nl	↓
Soluble transferrin receptor	Nl	↑

nl, normal limits.

including transmission of infections; volume overload, especially for patients with renal or heart failure; iron overload; and immune-mediated reactions such as febrile reactions, hemolysis, and anaphylaxis. The clinician also must consider administrative, logistic, and economic factors, including the shortage of blood supplies.

The recognition of hepcidin in the regulation of iron homeostasis and its role in ACD has led to interest in new agents targeted at hepcidin, including direct hepcidin antagonists and other novel agents.[49]

ANEMIA IN THE ELDERLY

Epidemiology

7 One of the most common clinical problems observed in the elderly is anemia. Anemia is a prevalent and increasing problem in the elderly, with about 20% of people 85 years and older affected.[53] Elderly patients with the highest incidence of anemia are those who are hospitalized, followed by residents of nursing homes and other institutions, with an estimated rate of 31% to 40%.[54] Although the incidence of anemia is high in the elderly, anemia should not be regarded as an inevitable outcome of aging. The body's set point of Hb does not fall with age. An underlying cause can be identified in about two-thirds of older patients. Undiagnosed and untreated anemia has been associated with adverse outcomes, including all-cause hospitalization, hospitalization secondary to cardiovascular disease, and all-cause mortality.[55] Anemia is an independent predictor of death and major clinical adverse events in elderly patients with stable symptomatic coronary artery disease.[56] Anemia can exacerbate neurologic and cognitive conditions and can adversely influence quality of life and physical performance in the elderly.[57] Anemia may be an indication of serious diseases such as cancer.

Pathophysiology

Aging is associated with a progressive reduction in hematopoietic reserve, which makes individuals more susceptible to developing anemia in times of hematopoietic stress.[58] Dysregulation of pro-inflammatory cytokines, most notably interleukin-6, may inhibit EPO production or interact with EPO receptors.[59] Although Hb levels may remain normal, the diminished marrow reserve leaves the elderly patient more susceptible to other causes of anemia. Renal insufficiency, which also is common in elderly patients, may reduce the ability of the kidneys to produce EPO. Older patients often have a normal creatinine level but a diminished glomerular filtration rate. Myelodysplastic syndromes are another common cause of anemia in the elderly, but most anemia cases in the elderly are multifactorial.

Etiology

In the acute care setting, the top three causes of anemia in the elderly are chronic disease (35%), unexplained cause (17%), and iron deficiency (15%), whereas in community-based outpatient clinics, the most common causes are unexplained (36%), infection (23%), and chronic disease (17%).[60] Another common problem in the elderly is vitamin B_{12} deficiency. The most common causes of clinically overt vitamin B_{12} deficiency are food/cobalamin malabsorption (more than 60% of cases) and pernicious anemia (15%-20% of cases).[61]

One often-overlooked major factor that may contribute to anemia in the older population is nutritional status. Cognitive and functional impairments in the older population may create barriers for patients to obtain and prepare a nutritious diet. Nutritional deficiencies that are not severe enough to affect the hematopoietic system in the younger population may contribute to anemia in the elderly. Edentulous or infirm elderly who may be too ill to prepare their meals are at risk for nutritional folate deficiency. Risk factors for inadequate folate intake in the elderly include low caloric intake, inadequate consumption of fortified cereals, and failure to take a vitamin/mineral supplement. However, unlike cobalamin levels, folate levels often increase rather than decline with age. High folic acid intake can occur if the elderly patient regularly uses a supplement and consumes fortified cereals.[62,63]

Bleeding with resultant iron deficiency in the elderly may be due to carcinoma, peptic ulcer, atrophic gastritis, drug-induced gastritis, postmenopausal vaginal bleeding, or bleeding hemorrhoids. Elderly women have a much lower incidence of IDA compared with younger, menstruating women. Until proven otherwise, iron deficiency in the elderly should be considered a sign of chronic blood loss. Steps should be taken to rule out bleeding, especially from the GI or female reproductive tract. AI is more common in the elderly, as diseases that contribute to AI such as cancer, infection, and rheumatoid arthritis are more prevalent in this population.

Laboratory Findings

For practical purposes, it is best to use usual adult reference values and WHO criteria for laboratory tests in the elderly. Anemia in elderly persons usually is normocytic and mild, with Hb values ranging between 10 and 12 g/dL (100-120 g/L; 6.21-7.45 mmol/L) in most anemic patients.[53] Evaluation of an elderly patient should be similar to strategies described previously for younger adults, perhaps with more emphasis on identifying occult blood loss and vitamin B_{12} deficiency. Vitamin B_{12} deficiency may be present even when plasma levels of vitamin B_{12} are within the normal range, but elevated MMA levels will reveal the deficiency. A refractory macrocytic anemia in the elderly should raise suspicion of a myelodysplastic syndrome.

TREATMENT
Anemia in the Elderly

Treatment of anemia in the elderly is the same as that described for each type of anemia discussed in this chapter. With IDA it is essential to treat the underlying cause, if known (ie, bleeding), and administer iron supplementation. Lower doses of iron supplementation are often recommended in the elderly (eg, 325 mg of ferrous sulfate once daily) to decrease the incidence of GI adverse effects, which can lead to additional morbidity and poor adherence. The goal of treatment of AI is resolution of the underlying cause, although curing the underlying chronic illness for elderly patients can be difficult. Routine treatment with ESAs is not currently standard of care for AI in the elderly.

ANEMIA IN PEDIATRIC POPULATIONS

Epidemiology

7 IDA is a leading cause of infant morbidity and mortality around the world.[64] Data from NHANES III indicated that 9% of children ages 12 to 36 months in the United States had iron deficiency and 3% had IDA.[65,66] Lack of a normal Hb at birth directly affects non-storage iron and increases the risk of IDA in the first 3 to 6 months of life. African American or Hispanic-American children have a higher incidence of anemia.[67] Requirements for iron absorption peak during puberty. An anemia of prematurity can occur 3 to 12 weeks after birth in infants younger than 32 weeks' gestation and spontaneously resolves by 3 to 6 months. The prevalence of vitamin B_{12} deficiency has been identified as 1 in 1,255 for levels less than 100 pg/mL (less than 74 pmol/L) and 1 in 200 for levels less than 200 pg/mL (less than 148 pmol/L), with the lowest levels in non-Hispanic whites.[68]

Pathophysiology

In contrast to anemias in adults, which tend to be manifestations of a broader underlying pathology, anemias in the pediatric population are more often due to a primary hematologic abnormality. The amount of iron present at birth depends on gestational length and weight. A decrease in EPO production results in a physiologic anemia peaking at 2 months.[69] Iron stores from birth are mostly depleted by 6 months of age.

Etiology

The age of the child can yield some clues regarding the etiology of the anemia. The optimal amount of nutritional iron and folate required varies among individuals based on life-cycle stages. Two peak periods place children at risk of developing IDA. The first peak occurs during late infancy and early childhood, when children undergo rapid body growth, have low levels of dietary iron, and exhaust stores accumulated during gestation. The second peak occurs during adolescence, which is associated with rapid growth, poor diets, and onset of menses in girls. Some studies suggest that overweight children are at significantly higher risk for IDA. Proposed factors include genetic influences; physical inactivity, leading to decreased myoglobin breakdown and lower amounts of released iron into the blood; and inadequate diet with limited intake of iron-rich foods.[70]

Conditions in the newborn period that can lead to IDA include prematurity and insufficient dietary intake. Premature infants are at increased risk for IDA because of their smaller total blood volume, increased blood loss through phlebotomy, and poor GI absorption. Factors leading to unbalanced iron metabolism in infants include insufficient iron intake, early introduction of cow's milk, intolerance of cow's milk, medications, and malabsorption. Dietary deficiency of iron in the first 6 to 12 months of life is less common today because of the increased use of iron supplementation during breast-feeding and use of iron-fortified formulas. Iron deficiency becomes more common when children change to regular diets.

When screening for iron deficiency in young children, a careful dietary history can help identify children at risk. High iron needs and the tendency to eat fewer iron-containing foods contribute to the etiology of iron deficiency during adolescence.

Other causes of microcytic anemia include thalassemia, lead poisoning, and sideroblastic anemia. Use of homeopathic or herbal medications and exposure to paint or certain cooking materials may place children at risk for lead exposure. Normocytic anemias in children include infection with human parvovirus B19 and glucose-6-phosphate dehydrogenase (G6PD) deficiency. Macrocytic anemias are caused by deficiencies in vitamin B_{12} and folate, chronic liver disease, hypothyroidism, and myelodysplastic disorders. Folic acid deficiency usually is due to inadequate dietary intake, but human milk and cow's milk provide adequate sources. Folic acid deficiency may be seen in infants and children who primarily consume goat's milk or health food milk alternatives, or in children with insufficient intake of green leafy vegetables. Vitamin B_{12} deficiency due to nutritional reasons is rare but may occur due to a congenital pernicious anemia.

Laboratory Findings

When evaluating laboratory values for pediatric patients, the clinician must use age- and sex-adjusted norms. It is important to know that many blood samples are capillary samples, such as heel or finger sticks, which may have slightly different results than venous samples. The USPSTF has concluded that evidence is insufficient to recommend for or against routine screening for IDA in asymptomatic, low risk, children aged 6 to 12 months. Hb is a sensitive test for iron deficiency, but it has low specificity in childhood anemias. If an abnormality is found, a CBC should be ordered to evaluate MCV and determine whether the anemia is microcytic, normocytic, or macrocytic. A peripheral blood smear and reticulocyte count also may be helpful. The peripheral blood smear can indicate the etiology based on RBC morphology, and the reticulocyte count helps differentiate between decreased RBC production and increased RBC destruction or loss. Other laboratory tests include serum iron, ferritin, TIBC, and transferrin saturation. Mild hereditary anemias may produce a mild hypochromic microcytic anemia that can be confused with IDAs. The RDW may be high with iron deficiency and is more likely to be normal with thalassemia. Laboratory features of anemia of prematurity include normocytic normochromic cells, low reticulocyte count, low serum EPO concentrations, and decreased RBC precursors in bone marrow. Laboratory diagnosis of vitamin B_{12} and folate deficiency in children is similar to that of adults.

TREATMENT
Anemia in Pediatric Populations

Primary prevention of IDA in infants, children, and adolescents is the most appropriate goal because delays in mental and motor development are potentially irreversible. In 2006, the USPSTF published revised recommendations to screen and supplement iron deficiency in the United States, focusing on children and pregnant women.[17] The USPSTF recommends routine iron supplementation for asymptomatic children aged 6 to 12 months who are at increased risk for IDA. Fair evidence was found that iron supplementation (eg, iron-fortified formula or iron supplements) might improve neurodevelopmental outcomes in children at risk for IDA. The quality of evidence of benefit for children 6 to 12 months of age not at risk for IDA was poor.

Interventions likely to prevent anemia include diverse foods with bioavailable forms of iron, food fortification for infants and children, and individual supplementation. Routine screening for iron deficiency in nonpregnant adolescents is recommended only for those with risk factors, which include vegetarian diets, malnutrition, low body weight, chronic illness, or history of heavy menstrual blood loss.

For infants aged 9 to 12 months with a mild microcytic anemia, the most cost-effective treatment is a therapeutic trial of iron. Fe^{2+} sulfate at a dose of 3 to 6 mg/kg/day of elemental iron divided once or twice daily between meals for 4 weeks is recommended. In children who respond, iron should be continued for two more months to replace storage iron pools, along with dietary intervention and patient education.[71] Parenteral iron therapy has a limited role and is rarely necessary.

For the macrocytic anemias in children, folate can be administered in a dose of 1 mg daily. However, vitamin B_{12} deficiency due to congenital pernicious anemia requires lifelong vitamin B_{12} supplementation. Dose and frequency should be titrated according to clinical response and laboratory values. No data regarding the use of oral vitamin B_{12} supplementation in children are available.

PERSONALIZED PHARMACOTHERAPY

In the treatment of the anemias discussed in this chapter, personalized pharmacotherapy is important in a few populations. When treating IDA, the elderly should be treated with lower doses of oral iron therapy. This typically is once daily dosing with ferrous sulfate 325 mg. Patients with immune-mediated disease are at higher risk for having hypersensitivity reactions to parenteral iron therapy. Patients who have neurologic symptoms upon diagnosis of vitamin B_{12} deficiency should strongly be considered for parenteral B_{12} supplementation. If ESAs are used to treat AI, iron status should be closely monitored to ensure efficacy of these agents as functional iron deficiency can develop.

EVALUATION OF THERAPEUTIC OUTCOMES

For IDA, a positive response to a trial of oral iron therapy is characterized by a modest reticulocytosis in days, with an increase in Hb starting after about 2 weeks with continued rapid rise in Hb. As the Hb level approaches normal, the rate of increase slows progressively. Hb should reach a normal level after about 2 months of therapy and often sooner.[9] If the patient does not develop reticulocytosis, reevaluation of the diagnosis or iron replacement therapy is necessary. Iron therapy should continue for a period sufficient for complete restoration of iron stores. Serum ferritin concentrations should return to the normal range prior to discontinuation of iron. The time interval required to accomplish this goal varies, although at least 6 to 12 months of therapy usually is warranted.

When large amounts of parenteral iron are administered, by either total dose infusion or multiple intramuscular or IV doses, the patient's iron status should be closely monitored. Patients receiving regular IV iron should be monitored for clinical or laboratory evidence of iron toxicity or overload. Iron overload may be indicated by abnormal hepatic function tests, serum ferritin greater than 800 ng/mL (greater than 800 mcg/L [1800 pmol/L]), or transferrin saturation greater than 50%. Serum ferritin and transferrin saturation should be measured in the first week after larger IV iron doses. Hb and Hct should be measured weekly, and serum iron and ferritin levels should be measured at least monthly.

In the treatment of vitamin B_{12} deficiency anemia, most patients respond rapidly to vitamin B_{12} therapy. The typical patient will experience an improvement in strength and well-being within a few days of treatment initiation. Reticulocytosis is evident in 3 to 5 days. Hb begins to rise after the first week and should normalize in 1-2 months. CBC count and serum cobalamin levels usually are drawn one to 2 months after initiation of therapy and 3 to 6 months thereafter for surveillance monitoring. Homocysteine and MMA levels can be repeated 2-3 months after initiation of replacement therapy to evaluate for normalization of levels, although levels begin to decrease in 1-2 weeks. Neuropsychiatric signs and symptoms can be reversible if treated early. If permanent neurologic damage has resulted, progression should cease with replacement therapy. Slow response to therapy or failure to observe normalization of laboratory results may suggest the presence of an additional abnormality such as iron deficiency, thalassemia trait, infection, malignancy, nonadherence, or misdiagnosis.

In folic acid deficiency anemia, symptomatic improvement, as evidenced by increased alertness and appetite, often occurs early during the course of treatment. Reticulocytosis begins in the first week. Hct begins to rise within 2 weeks and should reach normal levels within 2 months. MCV initially increases because of an increase in reticulocytes but gradually decreases to normal.

One of the earliest responses with ESA use is an increase in blood reticulocyte count, which usually occurs in the first few days. Baseline iron status should be checked before and during treatment, as many patients receiving ESAs require supplemental iron therapy. The optimal form and schedule of iron supplementation are not known. Hb levels should be monitored twice a week until stabilized. Hb should also be monitored twice weekly for 2 to 6 weeks after a dose adjustment.[46] A fall in Hb during ESA therapy may indicate a need for iron supplementation or signal occult blood loss. Baseline and periodic monitoring of iron, TIBC, transferrin saturation, or ferritin levels may be useful in optimizing iron repletion and limiting the need for ESAs. Patients who do not respond to 8 weeks of optimal dosage should not continue taking ESAs. Target Hb levels should be 11 to 12 g/dL (110-120 g/L; 6.83-7.45 mmol/L). Cost is an issue with ESA therapy; therefore, drug cost must be weighed against the effects on transfusions and hospitalizations.

Responses and monitoring of treatment are similar in the elderly as described for the general adult population described earlier in the chapter. If the reticulocyte count rises but the anemia does not improve, inadequate absorption of iron or continued blood loss should be suspected. As with any form of anemia, symptomatic improvement should be evident shortly after starting therapy and Hb/Hct should begin to rise within a few weeks of initiating therapy. A key component of symptom assessment among older adults is the functional domain. Patients should be asked about changes in self-care abilities, mobility, and stamina.

Therapeutic outcomes are assessed in children by monitoring Hb, Hct, and RBC indices 4 to 8 weeks after initiation of iron therapy. For premature infants, Hb or Hct should be monitored weekly.

ABBREVIATIONS

ACD	anemia of chronic disease
AI	anemia of inflammation
CBC	complete blood count
CDC	Centers for Disease Control and Prevention
EPO	erythropoietin
ESA	erythropoiesis-stimulating agent
Fe^{2+}	ferrous iron
Fe^{3+}	ferric iron
G6PD	glucose-6-phosphate dehydrogenase
Hb	hemoglobin
Hct	hematocrit
HIV	human immunodeficiency virus
IDA	iron-deficiency anemia
MCH	mean corpuscular hemoglobin
MCHC	mean corpuscular hemoglobin concentration
MCV	mean corpuscular volume
MMA	methylmalonic acid
NHANES	National Health and Nutrition Examination Survey
NSAID	nonsteroidal anti-inflammatory drugs
RBC	red blood cell
RDW	red blood cell distribution width
TIBC	total iron-binding capacity
USPSTF	United States Preventive Services Task Force
WHO	World Health Organization

REFERENCES

1. Benoist B, McLean E, Egli M, et al. *Worldwide Prevalence of Anaemia 1993-2005: WHO Global Database on Anaemia*. World Health Organization; 2008.
2. Cusick SE, Mei Z, Freedman DS, et al. Unexplained decline in the prevalence of anemia among US children and women between 1988-1994 and 1999-2002. *Am J Clin Nutr* 2008;88:1611-1617.
3. Nissenson A. Anemia not just an innocent bystander. *Arch Intern Med* 2003;163:1400-1404.
4. Mozaffarian D. Anemia predicts mortality in severe heart failure: The prospective randomized amlodipine survival evaluation (PRAISE). *J Am Coll Cardiol* 2003;41:1933-1939.
5. Chaves PHM, Carlson MC, Ferrucci L, et al. Association between mild anemia and executive function impairment in community-dwelling older women: The Women's Health and Aging Study II. *J Am Geriatr Soc* 2006;54:1429-1435.
6. Anemia in pregnancy. ACOG Practice Bulletin No. 95. American College of Obst and Gynecologists. *Obstet Gynecol* 2008;112:201-207.
7. Prchal JT, Thiagarajan P. Erythropoiesis. In: Kaushansky K, Lichtman MA, Beutler E, et al., eds. *Williams Hematology*, 8th ed. New York: McGraw Hill; 2010:453-458.
8. Wians FH, Urban JE, Keffer JH, Kroft SH. Discriminating between iron deficiency anemia and anemia of chronic disease using traditional indices of iron status vs. transferrin receptor concentration. *Am J Clin Pathol* 2001;115:112-118.
9. Beutler E. Disorders of iron metabolism. In: Kaushansky K, Lichtman MA, Beutler E, et al., eds. *Williams Hematology*, 8th ed. New York: McGraw-Hill; 2010:565-606.

10. Beutler E. Destruction of erythrocytes. In: Kaushansky K, Lichtman MA, Beutler E, et al., eds. *Williams Hematology*, 8th ed. New York: McGraw-Hill; 2010:449-454.
11. Galloway M, Rushworth L. Red cell or serum folate? Results from the National Pathology Alliance benchmarking review. *J Clin Pathol* 2003;56:924-926.
12. Snow CF. Laboratory diagnosis of vitamin B_{12} and folate deficiency. *Arch Intern Med* 1999;159:1289-1298.
13. Green R. Folate, cobalamin, and megaloblastic anemias. In: Kaushansky K, Lichtman MA, Beutler E, et al., eds. *Williams Hematology*, 8th ed. New York: McGraw-Hill; 2010:533-564.
14. Dharmarajan TS, Norkus EP. Approaches to vitamin B_{12} deficiency. Early treatment may prevent devastating complications. *Postgrad Med* 2001;110:99-105.
15. Ganz T. Hepcidin—A regulator of intestinal iron absorption and iron recycling by macrophages. *Best Pract Res Clin Haematol* 2005;18:171-182.
16. Goodnough LT, Nemeth E, Gan T. Detection, evaluation, and management of iron restricted erythropoiesis. *Blood* 2010;116:4754-4761.
17. Camaschella C. Iron-deficiency anemia. *N Engl J Med* 2015;372:1832-43.
18. Killip S, Bennett J, Chambers M. Iron deficiency anemia. *Am Fam Physician* 2007;75:671-678.
19. Hershko C, Ianculovich M, Souroujon M. A hematologist's view of unexplained iron deficiency anemia in males: Impact of *Helicobacter pylori* eradication. *Blood Cells Mol Dis* 2007;38:45-53.
20. U.S. Preventive Services Task Force (USPSTF). Screening for Iron Deficiency Anemia—Including Iron Supplementation for Children and Pregnant Women. Rockville, MD: Agency for Healthcare Research and Quality (AHRQ); 2006.
21. Gasche C, Berstad A, Befrits R, et al. Guidelines on the diagnosis and management of iron deficiency and anemia in inflammatory bowel diseases. *Inflamm Bowel Dis* 2007;13:1545-1553.
22. Faich G, Strobos J. Sodium Fe^{3+} gluconate complex in sucrose: Safer IV iron therapy than iron dextrans. *Am J Kidney Dis* 1999;33:464-470.
23. Chandler G, Harchowal J, Macdougall IC. Intravenous iron sucrose: Establishing a safe dose. *Am J Kidney Dis* 2001;38:988-991.
24. Silverstein SB, Gilreath JA, Rodgers GM. Intravenous iron therapy: A summary of treatment options and review of guidelines. *J Pharm Practice* 2008;21:431-443.
25. Munoz M, Garcia-Erce JA, Remacha AF. Disorders of iron metabolism: Part II: Iron deficiency and iron overload. *J Clin Pathol* 2011;64:287-296.
26. Ferrlecit [package insert]. Morristown, NJ: Watson Pharma; 2015.
27. Venofer [package insert]. Shirley, NY: American Regent; 2015.
28. Feraheme [package insert]. Lexington, MA: AMAG Pharmaceuticals; 2015.
29. Injectafer [package insert]. Shirley, NY: Amiercan Regent; 2013.
30. Avni T, Bieber A, Grossman A, et al. The safety of intravenous iron preparations: systematic review and meta-analysis. *Mayo Clin Proc* 2015;90:12-23.
31. Oh RC, Brown DL. Vitamin B_{12} deficiency. *Am Fam Physician* 2003;67:979-986, 993-994.
32. Kaptan K, Beyan C, Ural AU, et al. *Helicobacter pylori*—Is it a novel causative agent in vitamin B_{12} deficiency? *Arch Intern Med* 2000;160:1349-1353.
33. Hesdorffer CS, Longo DL. Drug-induced megaloblastic anemia. *NEJM* 2015;373:1649-58.
34. Hoffbrand AV. Chapter 105. Megaloblastic Anemias. In: Longo DL, Fauci AS, Kasper DL, Hauser SL, Jameson JL, Loscalzo J, eds. *Harrison's Principles of Internal Medicine*, 18th ed. New York: McGraw-Hill; 2012.
35. Aronow WS. Homocysteine. The association with atherosclerotic vascular disease in older persons. *Geriatrics* 2003;58:22-28.
36. Green R. Indicators for assessing folate and vitamin b-12 status and for monitoring the efficacy of intervention strategies. *Am J Clin Nutr* 2011;94(Suppl):666S-672S.
37. Vidal-Alaball J, Butler CC, Cannings-John R, et al. Oral vitamin B_{12} versus intramuscular vitamin B_{12} for vitamin B_{12} deficiency. *Cochrane Database Syst Rev* 2005;3:CD004655.
38. Cravens DD, Nashelsky J, Oh RC. How do we evaluate a marginally low B_{12} level? *J Fam Pract* 2007;56:62-63.
39. Solomon LR. Oral vitamin B_{12} therapy: A cautionary note. *Blood* 2004;103:2863.
40. Lane LA, Rojas-Fernandez. Treatment of vitamin B_{12}-deficiency anemia: Oral versus parenteral therapy. *Ann Pharmacother* 2002;36:1268-1272.
41. Yerby MS. Clinical care of pregnant women with epilepsy: Neural tube defects and folic acid supplementation. *Epilepsia* 2003;44(Suppl 3):33-40.
42. Pitkin RM. Folate and neural tube defects. *Am J Clin Nutr* 2007;85:285S-288S.
43. American College of Obstetricians and Gynecologists (ACOG). Neural Tube Defects. ACOG Practice Bulletin No. 44. Washington, DC: American College of Obstetricians and Gynecologists, 2003.
44. Corwin HL, Gettinger A, Pearl RG, et al. The CRIT Study: Anemia and blood transfusion in the critically ill—Current clinical practice in the United States. *Crit Care Med* 2004;32:39-52.
45. Weiss GW, Goodnough LT. Anemia of chronic disease. *N Engl J Med* 2005;352:1011-1023.
46. Rodriguez RM, Corwin HL, Gettinger A, et al. Nutritional deficiencies and blunted erythropoietin response as cause of anemia of critical illness. *J Crit Care* 2001;16:36-41.
47. Silver MR. Anemia in the long-term ventilator-dependent patient with respiratory failure. *Chest* 2005;128(Suppl):568S-575S.
48. Adamson J. The anemia of inflammation/malignancy: Mechanisms and management. *Hematol Am Soc Hematol Educ Program* 2008;159-165.
49. Poggiali E, Migone De Amicis M, Motta I. Anemia of chronic disease: A unique defect of iron recycling for many different chronic diseases. *Eur J Intern Med* 2014;25:12-17.
50. Procrit [package insert]. Thousand Oaks, CA: Amgen, 2009.
51. Rudis M, Jacobi J, Hassan E, et al. Managing anemia in the critically ill patient. *Pharmacotherapy* 2004;24:229-247.
52. Hébert PC, Wells G, Martin C, et al. Do blood transfusions improve outcomes related to mechanical ventilation? *Chest* 2001;119:1850-1857.
53. Guralnik JM, Eisenstaedt RS, Ferrucci L, et al. Prevalence of anemia in person 65 years and older in the United States: Evidence for a high rate of unexplained anemia. *Blood* 2004;104:2263-2268.
54. Carmel R. Anemia and aging: An overview of clinical, diagnostic, and biological issues. *Blood Rev* 2001;15:9-18.
55. Culleton BF, Manns BJ, Zhang J, et al. Impact of anemia on hospitalization and mortality in older adults. *Blood* 2006;107:3841-3846.
56. Muzzarelli S, Pfisterer M, TIME Investigators. Anemia as independent predictor of major events in elderly patients with chronic angina. *Am Heart J* 2006;152:991-996.
57. Woodman R, Ferrucci L, Guralnik J. Anemia in older adults. *Curr Opin Hematol* 2005;12:123-128.
58. Balducci L, Hardy CL, Lyman GH. Hematopoietic growth factors in the older cancer patient. *Curr Opin Hematol* 2001;8:170-187.
59. Eisenstaedt R, Penninx BW, Woodman RC. Anemia in the elderly: Current understanding and emerging concepts. *Blood Rev* 2006;20:213-226.
60. Balducci L. Epidemiology of anemia in the elderly: Information on diagnostic evaluation. *J Am Geriatr Soc* 2003;51(Suppl):S2-S9.
61. Andres E, Loukili N, Noel E, et al. Vitamin B_{12} (cobalamin) deficiency in elderly patients. *CMAJ* 2004;171:251-259.
62. Mulligan JE, Greene GW, Caldwell M. Sources of folate and serum folate levels in older adults. *J Am Diet Assoc* 2007;107:495-499.
63. Ford ES, Bowman BA. Serum and red blood cell folate concentrations, race, and education: Findings from the third National Health and Nutrition Examination Survey. *Am J Clin Nutr* 1999;69:476-481.
64. Milman N. Iron prophylaxis in pregnancy—General or individual and in which dose? *Ann Hematol* 2006;85:821-828.
65. Recommendations to prevent and control iron deficiency in the United States. *Morb Mortal Wkly Rep* 1998;47:1-36.
66. Moy RJ. Prevalence, consequences and prevention of childhood nutritional iron. *Clin Lab Haematol* 2006;28:291-298.
67. Coyer S. Anemia: Diagnosis and management. *J Pediatr Health Care* 2005;19:380-385.
68. Wright JD, Bialostosky K, Gunter EW, et al. Blood folate and vitamin B_{12}: United States, 1988-94. *Vital Health Stat* 1998;11:1-78.
69. Palis J, Segel GB. Chapter 6. Hematology of the fetus and newborn. In: Prchal JT, Kaushansky K, Lichtman MA, Kipps TJ, Seligsohn U, eds. *Williams Hematology*. 8th ed. New York: McGraw-Hill, 2010.
70. Nead KG, Halterman JS, Kaczorowski JM, et al. Overweight children and adolescents: A risk group for iron deficiency. *Pediatrics* 2004;114:104-108.
71. Kazal LA. Prevention of iron deficiency in infants and toddlers. *Am Fam Physician* 2002;66:1217-1224.

101

Coagulation Disorders

Heidi Trinkman, Donald Beam, and Tracy Hagemann

KEY CONCEPTS

1. Hemophilia is an inherited bleeding disorder resulting from a congenital deficiency in factor VIII or IX.
2. The goal of therapy for hemophilia is to prevent bleeding episodes, and as a result their long-term complications, and to arrest bleeding if it occurs.
3. Recombinant factor concentrates usually are first-line treatment of hemophilia as they have the lowest risk of infection.
4. Inhibitor formation is the most significant treatment complication in hemophilia. It is associated with significant morbidity and decreased quality of life.
5. Recombinant factor VIIa is effective for the treatment of acute bleeds in patients with hemophilia A or B that has developed inhibitors.
6. The goal of therapy for von Willebrand disease (vWD) is to increase von Willebrand factor (vWF) and factor VIII levels to prevent bleeding during surgery or arrest bleeding when it occurs.
7. Factor VIII concentrates that contain vWF are the agents of choice for treatment of type 3 vWD and some type 2 von Willebrand disease, and for serious bleeding in type 1 von Willebrand disease.
8. Desmopressin acetate often is effective for treatment of type 1 vWD. It also may be effective for treatment of some forms of type 2 vWD in addition to mild to moderate hemophilia A.

The coagulation system is intricately balanced and designed to stop bleeding at the site of vascular injury through complex interactions between the vascular endothelium, platelets, procoagulant proteins, anticoagulant proteins, and fibrinolytic proteins. Hemostasis stops bleeding at the site of vascular injury through the formation of an impermeable platelet and fibrin plug. Three key mechanisms facilitate hemostasis including vascular constriction, primary platelet plug formation (primary hemostasis), and clot propagation through fibrin formation (secondary hemostasis). Derangements in this system can lead to either bleeding or thrombosis. Bleeding disorders are the result of a coagulation factor defect, a quantitative or qualitative platelet defect or enhanced fibrinolytic activity.

COAGULATION FACTORS

Secondary hemostasis facilitates propagation and stabilization of the initial platelet plug formed in primary hemostasis through the formation of fibrin on the activated platelet surface. This step is initiated via the tissue factor pathway and is vital for adequate hemostasis. Coagulation factors circulate as inactive precursors (zymogens). Activation of these coagulation proteins leads to a cascading series of proteolytic reactions (Fig. 19-2). At each step, a clotting factor undergoes limited proteolysis and becomes an active protease (designated by a lowercase "a," as in Xa).

The coagulation factors can be divided into three groups on the basis of biochemical properties: vitamin K-dependent factors (II, VII, IX, and X), contact activation factors (XI and XII, prekallikrein, and high-molecular-weight kininogen), and thrombin-sensitive factors (V, VIII, XIII, and fibrinogen). Biologic half-life and blood product source varies by coagulation factor (Table 101-1).

CLINICAL MANIFESTATIONS AND DIAGNOSIS

The diagnosis of coagulation disorders can be established from a detailed clinical history, physical examination, and laboratory test results. The clinical history should ascertain if there is a family history of bleeding or known bleeding disorders. Laboratory testing can distinguish bleeding disorders caused by defects in the coagulation pathways (Fig. 19-4), fibrinolytic pathways, or alterations in the number or function of platelets. Table 101-2 describes common coagulation tests.

HEMOPHILIA

1 Hemophilia is a bleeding disorder that results from a congenital deficiency in a plasma coagulation protein. Hemophilia A (classic hemophilia) is caused by a deficiency of factor VIII, while hemophilia B (Christmas disease) is caused by a deficiency of factor IX. Hemophilia affects about 400,000 males worldwide.[1,2] The incidence of hemophilia A is about 1 in 5,000 male births and hemophilia B occurring in 1 in 30,000 male births.[2] Hemophilia A constitutes 80% to 85% of all patients with hemophilia with the other 15% to 20% being hemophilia B.[1] There are no significant racial differences in the incidence of hemophilia.

About one-third of patients with hemophilia have a negative family history, presumably representing a spontaneous mutation.[1] Both hemophilia A and hemophilia B are recessive X-linked diseases, which mean that the defective gene is located on the X chromosome. The disease primarily affects only males while females are carriers. Since affected males have the abnormal allele on their X chromosome and no matching allele on their Y chromosome, their sons would be normal (assuming the mother is not a carrier) and their daughters would be obligatory carriers. Female carriers have one normal allele and therefore do not usually have a bleeding tendency, although female carriers have lower factor VIII levels than females who are not carriers.[3] Sons of a female carrier and a normal male have a 50% chance of having hemophilia and daughters have a 50% chance of being carriers. Thus, there is a "skipped generation" mode of inheritance in which the female carriers do not express the disease but can pass it on to the next male generation. Hemophilia has been observed in a small number of females. It

TABLE 101-1 Blood Coagulation Factors

Factor[a]	Synonym	Biologic Half-Life (h)	Blood Product Source
I	Fibrinogen	100-150	Cryoprecipitate (200-300 mg/bag)
II	Prothrombin	50-80	FFP, PCC
V	Proaccelerin	12-36	FFP
VII	Proconvertin	4-6	Recombinant VIIa, FFP, PCC
VIII	Antihemophilic factor	12-15	FFP, factor concentrates, cryoprecipitate
IX	Christmas factor	18-30	FFP, PCC, factor concentrates
X	Stuart-Power factor	25-60	FFP, PCC
XI	Plasma thromboplastin antecedent	40-80	FFP
XII	Hageman factor	50-70	Not associated with bleeding diathesis
XIII	Fibrin-stabilizing factor	150	FFP, cryoprecipitate, factor concentrate
VWF	von Willebrand factor	8-12	FFP, cryoprecipitate, factor concentrate

FFP, fresh-frozen plasma; PCC, prothrombin complex concentrate.

[a]Coagulation factors are numbered with roman numerals in order of their discovery. The most common synonyms are listed. Factor III (tissue factor) and factor IV (calcium ions) have been omitted. There is no factor VI.

TABLE 101-2 Laboratory Procedures

Procedure	Identifies	Coagulation Cause of Abnormal Value	Clinical Manifestations
Prothrombin time (PT)	Factors I, II, V, VII, X	Newborn Vitamin K deficiency Inherited factor deficiencies[a] Warfarin therapy Liver disease Lupus anticoagulant (rare) Afibrinogenemia Dysfibrinogenemia	Bleeding following surgery, trauma, etc. Easy bruising
Activated partial thromboplastin time (aPTT)	Factors I, II, V, VIII, IX, X	Inherited factor deficiencies[a] Lupus anticoagulant Heparin therapy Liver disease Afibrinogenemia Dysfibrinogenemia	Joint and muscle bleeding Bleeding after surgery, trauma, etc.
	HMWK, prekallikrein		No bleeding manifestations
	Factor XII		Increased incidence of thrombotic disease possible with severe factor XII deficiency
	Factor XI		Variable bleeding tendency Bleeding following surgery, trauma, etc.
Thrombin time (TT)	Fibrinogen Inhibitors of fibrin aggregation	Afibrinogenemia Dysfibrinogenemia Heparin therapy	Lifelong hemorrhagic disease Variable clinical symptoms from asymptomatic to either a bleeding diathesis or prothrombotic
Platelet count	Thrombocytopenia	Quantitative platelet disorder, type 2B von Willebrand disease, immune thrombocytopenia, other cause of thrombocytopenia	Mucocutaneous bleeding
Platelet function analyzer	Platelet function	Qualitative platelet defects, von Willebrand disease, antiplatelet therapy Also prolonged in anemia and thrombocytopenia **Insensitive to mild platelet defects and has fallen out of favor as a screening test*	Mucocutaneous bleeding
Platelet aggregation	Gold standard to assess platelet function	Qualitative platelet defects, antiplatelet medications	Mucocutaneous bleeding
Euglobulin clot lysis time (ECLT)	Fibrinolytic defect	A decreased ECLT indicates hyperfibrinolysis, which indicates an abnormality in the fibrinolytic pathway including: plasminogen activator inhibitor 1 deficiency, α_2-plasminogen inhibitor deficiency Hypofibrinogenemia	Bleeding after trauma or surgical procedures especially in oral and urogenital areas

HMWK, high-molecular-weight kininogen.

[a]Bleeding manifestations depend on factor levels.

CLINICAL PRESENTATION Hemophilia

Signs and Symptoms

- Ecchymoses (palpable/raised)
- Hemarthroses (especially knee, ankle, and elbow)
- Joint pain
- Joint swelling and erythema
- Decreased range of motion
- Muscle hemorrhage
- Swelling at the site of muscle bleeding
- Pain with motion of affected muscle
- Signs of nerve compression
- Significant anemia from an iliopsoas or thigh bleed
- Oral bleeding with dental extractions or trauma
- Hematuria
- Intracranial hemorrhage (spontaneous or following trauma)
- Excessive bleeding with surgery

Laboratory Testing

- Prolonged activated partial thromboplastin time (aPTT)
- Decreased factor VIII or factor IX level
- Normal prothrombin time (PT)
- Normal platelet count
- Normal von Willebrand factor antigen and activity
- Normal bleeding time

can occur if both factor VIII and IX genes are defective or if a female patient has only one X chromosome as in Turner syndrome.[4]

In 1984, researchers isolated and cloned the human factor VIII gene. It is a large gene, consisting of 186 kilobases (kb).[5] More than 2,000 unique mutations in the factor VIII gene, including point mutations, deletions, and insertions, have been reported.[6] Deletions and nonsense mutations are often associated with the more severe forms of factor VIII deficiency because functional factor VIII is not produced. In 1993, researchers identified an inversion in the factor VIII gene at intron 22 that accounts for almost 50% of severe hemophilia A gene abnormalities.[7] That discovery has greatly simplified carrier detection and prenatal diagnosis in families with this gene mutation.

The factor IX gene, cloned and sequenced in 1982, consists of only 34 kb and is significantly smaller than the factor VIII gene.[5] Unlike the factor VIII gene in patients with severe hemophilia A, the factor IX gene in patients with hemophilia B has no predominant mutation. Direct gene mutation analysis is simpler in hemophilia B because of the smaller gene size, and to date more than 1,000 different mutations have been reported.[8] Most of these mutations are single base-pair substitutions. About 3% of factor IX gene mutations are deletions or complex rearrangements, and the presence of these mutations is associated with a severe phenotype.[7]

Hemophilia B Leyden is a rare variant in which factor IX levels initially are low but rise at puberty.[7] The mechanism of this disorder is controversial. Some propose that the binding of the androgen receptor and other transcription factors are responsible. Other molecular mechanisms for age-related gene regulation have been recently discovered and implicated in factor IX Leyden.[9] Identification of this genotype is clinically important because it confers a better prognosis.

Clinical Manifestations

The characteristic bleeding manifestations of hemophilia include palpable ecchymosis, bleeding into joint spaces (hemarthroses), muscle hemorrhages, and excessive bleeding after surgery or trauma. The severity of clinical bleeding generally correlates with the degree of deficiency of either factor VIII or factor IX. Factor VIII and factor IX activity levels are measured in units per milliliter, with 1 unit/mL representing 100% of the factor found in 1 mL of normal plasma.[10] Normal plasma levels range from 0.5 to 1.5 units/mL. Patients with less than 0.01 units/mL (1%) of either factor are classified as having severe hemophilia, those with between 0.01 and 0.05 units/mL (1%-5%) are moderate, and those with 0.05 units/mL and 0.4 units/mL (5%-40%) have mild hemophilia (Table 101-3).

Patients with severe disease experience frequent spontaneous hemorrhages, while those with moderate disease have excessive bleeding following mild trauma and rarely experience spontaneous hemarthroses. Patients with mild hemophilia may have few symptoms that their condition can be undetected for many years and they usually have excessive bleeding only after significant trauma or surgery. Disease severity does not always correlate with disease manifestations. Those with severe disease (<1% factor activity) may occasionally not display a severe phenotype, while some with milder forms of the disease may have more severe bleeding. Prolonged bleeding after circumcision is a common presenting sign. Most patients

TABLE 101-3 Laboratory and Clinical Manifestations of Hemophilia

	Severe (<0.01 units/mL)	Moderate (0.01-0.05 units/mL)	Mild (>0.05 units/mL)
Age at diagnosis	≤1 year	1-2 years	2 years to adult
Neonatal symptoms			
PCB	Usually	Usually	Rarely
ICH	Occasionally	Uncommonly	Rarely
Muscle/joint hemorrhage	Spontaneous	Minor trauma	Minor to major trauma
CNS hemorrhage	High risk	Moderate risk	Uncommon
Postsurgical hemorrhage (without prophylaxis)	Frank bleeding, severe	Wound bleeding, common	Wound bleeding
Oral hemorrhage following trauma, tooth extraction	Usually	Common	Common

CNS, central nervous system; ICH, intracranial hemorrhage; PCB, postcircumcisional bleeding.

Normal range of factor VIII/IX activity level is 0.5-1.5 units/mL (50%-150%). A value of 1 unit/mL corresponds to 100% of the factor found in 1 mL of normal plasma.

will have some manifestation of the disease sometime after their first year of life, when they begin to walk and increase their risk of bleeding due to falling.[1,7]

Diagnosis

The diagnosis of hemophilia should be considered in any male with unusual bleeding. A family history of bleeding is helpful in the diagnosis but is absent in up to 50% of patients with about one-third representing spontaneous mutations and the remaining secondary to an unrecognized family history.[5] Brothers of patients with hemophilia should be screened; sisters should consider undergoing carrier testing. Laboratory testing in patients with hemophilia will usually reveal an isolated prolonged partial thromboplastin time (PTT) and they will have a decreased factor VIII or factor IX level.

Patients with severe hemophilia A should be tested for the common factor VIII gene inversions. In patients with severe hemophilia A that lack an inversion mutation or in patients with moderate or mild hemophilia A, the gene can be sequenced to determine the exact mutation if needed. The exact mutation can determine carrier status but is not done routinely in everyone since it is very costly and does not change therapy. Techniques to determine the genetic mutation in patients with hemophilia B are similar, but no predominant mutation like the factor VIII inversion has been found. The smaller size of the factor IX gene facilitates direct DNA mutational analysis.[7]

Hemophilia can be diagnosed prenatally, if desired, by chorionic villus sampling in gestational weeks 9 to 14 or by amniocentesis after 15 to 17 weeks of gestation.[1,11] These are invasive procedures with a 0.5% to 1% chance for pregnancy loss so it is not routinely done.[11] A new noninvasive method uses cell-free fetal DNA in maternal circulation to determine the sex of the fetus; more invasive testing is required for a male fetus.[11] This method was used to successfully identify hemophilia mutations in 12 subjects,[12] but is still experimental and requires further validation.

TREATMENT

The comprehensive care of hemophilia requires an interprofessional team approach. The patient is best managed in specialized centers with trained personnel and appropriate laboratory, radiologic and pharmaceutical services.[1] The healthcare team includes hematologists, orthopedic surgeons, nurses, physical therapists, dentists, genetic counselors, psychologists, pharmacists, case managers, and social workers who have experience in caring for patients with bleeding disorders. The goal for comprehensive hemophilia care is to prevent bleeding episodes and their long-term sequelae so that patients with hemophilia can live full, active, and productive lives.

2 IV factor replacement therapy for the treatment or prevention of bleeding is the mainstay of treatment for hemophilia. Parents of children with hemophilia usually learn how to infuse factor concentrate to facilitate home treatment peripherally or via central venous access device. Older children and adult patients learn self-administration. Home healthcare nursing support may be helpful, particularly for the youngest patients in whom venous access may be difficult. In the setting of poor venous access, venous access devices may be indicated. Administration of factor at home is more convenient for families and allows for earlier treatment of acute bleeding episodes. However, serious bleeding episodes always require evaluation by medical personnel.

Patients with hemophilia should receive routine immunizations, including immunization against hepatitis B. Hepatitis A vaccine is also recommended for patients with hemophilia because of the risk (albeit small) of transmitting the causative agent through factor concentrates.[1,13] Administration of vaccines is preferred subcutaneously in patients with severe disease.[1] If intramuscular administration is required, use of a small-gauge needle with cold compresses and pressure to the site can prevent excessive bleeding.

A few special considerations apply to the perinatal care of male infants of hemophilia carriers. Intracranial or extracranial hemorrhage has been estimated to occur in 1% to 2% of newborns with hemophilia.[7] Vacuum extraction and forceps delivery increase the risk of cranial bleeding. Elective cesarean section has not been shown to prevent intracranial bleeding. The optimal mode of delivery or the use of prophylactic factor replacement in male infants of hemophilia carriers is controversial.[1] Circumcision should be postponed until a diagnosis of hemophilia is excluded. Factor levels can be assayed from cord blood samples or from peripheral venipuncture. Arterial puncture should be avoided because of the risk of hematoma formation. If an infant has hemophilia, many clinicians recommend a screening head ultrasound to rule out an intracranial hemorrhage prior to discharge from the nursery.

History of Hemophilia Treatment

Therapy for hemophilia has undergone dramatic advances over the past few decades. Fifty years ago, administration of fresh-frozen plasma was the only available treatment. The introduction of cryoprecipitate in the early 1960s allowed more specific therapy for hemophilia A.[14] Intermediate-purity factor VIII and IX plasma-derived concentrates became available in the 1970s.[14] Plasma-derived factor concentrates are made from the donations of thousands of people. Contamination of plasma pools with hepatitis B, hepatitis C, and the human immunodeficiency virus (HIV) during the late 1970s and early 1980s resulted in transmission to a large portion of patients with hemophilia. Since the mid-1980s, plasma-derived concentrates have been manufactured with a variety of virus-inactivating techniques, including dry heat, pasteurization, and treatment with chemicals (eg, solvent detergent mixtures).[5] Since 1986, no transmission of HIV through factor concentrates to patients with hemophilia in the United States has been reported.[5] Protein purification techniques, introduced in the 1990s, led to the production of high-purity plasma-derived concentrates with increased amounts of factor VIII or factor IX relative to the product's total protein content. Recombinant factor VIII and then factor IX also became available in the 1990s.[14] Significant improvements have been made with recombinant products in limiting the risk of infectious transmission from albumin used to stabilize some of the products. Like plasma-derived products, these products use viral inactivation steps. With each subsequent generation of recombinant factor VIII products, the use of human proteins has been reduced.[14]

More recently, several novel long-acting factor VIII or IX products have been developed. Different methods have been utilized to prolong the half-life of either factor VIII or IX including pegylation, polysialic acid, albumin fusion, and Fc fusion.[15-17] Two of these improved factor products were recently approved by FDA; both attach the factor to IgG1 which then binds to the neonatal Fc receptor (FcRn) present in the acidified endosomes of the endothelial cells. This binding protects the factor fusion product from targeted lysosomal degradation and facilitates recycling of the FcRn ligands at the endothelial surface resulting in a prolonged systemic half-life of the factor.[18,19] Currently these products are only approved for routine prophylaxis and their role in acute bleeds or surgical management of hemophilia patients has yet to be defined. Clinical trials for factor VIII and factor IX with improved pharmacokinetic properties are ongoing.

Hemophilia A

Table 101-4 summarizes most of the factor VIII products currently available in the United States. Most patients are treated with high-purity products, which generally have the lowest risk of transmitting infectious disease and are therefore recommended as first line

TABLE 101-4 Factor Concentrates

Brand Name	Product Type	Viral Inactivation or Exclusion Method	Other Contents
Factor VIII Concentrates			
Alphanate AHF/VWF complex	Plasma	Solvent detergent, dry heat	Albumin, heparin, vWF
Hemofil M AHF	Plasma	Solvent detergent, monoclonal antibody, ion-exchange chromatography	Albumin
Humate-P AHF/VWF complex	Plasma	Pasteurization	Albumin, vWF
Koāte-DVI	Plasma	Solvent detergent, dry heat, gel permeation chromatography	Albumin
Monarc-M	Plasma	Solvent detergent, monoclonal antibody	Albumin
Monoclate P	Plasma	Pasteurization, monoclonal antibody	Albumin
Wilate VWF/FVIII Complex	Plasma	Solvent detergent, dry heat	Sodium citrate, sucrose, vWF
Advate	Recombinant	Solvent detergent, column chromatography, monoclonal antibody	Trehalose
Eloctate B domain deleted, Fc Fusion	Recombinant	Solvent detergent, chromatography, nanofiltration	Sucrose, IgG_1
Helixate FS	Recombinant	Solvent detergent, ion-exchange chromatography, monoclonal antibody	Human plasma protein solution (fermentation only); sucrose
Kogenate FS	Recombinant	Solvent detergent, ion-exchange chromatography, monoclonal antibody	Human plasma protein solution (fermentation only); sucrose
Novoeight B domain deleted	Recombinant	Solvent detergent, chromatography, immunoaffinity column, monoclonal antibody, nanofiltration	Sucrose, Polysorbate 80
Nuwiq Bdomain deleted	Recombinant	Solvent detergent, nanofiltration	Sucrose, sodium citrate, L-arginine hydrochloride
Recombinate	Recombinant	Immunoaffinity, chromatography, monoclonal antibody	Albumin
ReFacto B domain deleted	Recombinant	Chromatography	Albumin (fermentation only); sucrose
Xyntha B domain deleted	Recombinant	Chromatography, solvent detergent, nanofiltration	Sucrose
Factor IX Concentrates			
AlphaNine SD	Plasma	Solvent detergent, nanofiltration	Heparin
Mononine	Plasma	Sodium thiocyanate, dual ultrafiltration	Heparin, mannitol
Alprolix Fc Fusion	Recombinant	Nanofiltration, chromatography	Sucrose, mannitol, IgG_1
BeneFix	Recombinant	Chromatography, nanofiltration	Sucrose, Polysorbate 80
Rixubis	Recombinant	Chromatography, solvent detergent, nanofiltration	Sucrose, mannitol
aPCC			
Feiba VH Immuno	Plasma	Vapor heat	IIa, VIIa, VIIIa, IXa, Xa
PCC			
Bebulin VH	Plasma	Vapor heat	Heparin, II, IX, X
Profilnine S/D	Plasma	Solvent detergent	II, IX, X
Other			
Corifact	Plasma	Heat, precipitation/adsorption, ion exchange chromatography	XIII, albumin
NovoSeven	Recombinant	Solvent detergent	VII

aPCC, activated prothrombin complex concentrate; PCC, prothrombin complex concentrate; vWF, von Willebrand factor.

agents.[1] Recombinant products, when available, are generally used rather than plasma-derived products.

Recombinant Factor VIII

3 Recombinant factor VIII is produced with recombinant DNA technology and is derived from cultured Chinese hamster ovary cells or baby hamster kidney cells transfected with the human factor VIII gene.[5] Since these products are not derived from blood donations, the risk of transmitting infections through administration of recombinant factor VIII is low and recombinant products are generally favored over plasma-derived products. A very small risk of viral infection of the cell lines used to produce the clotting factor still remains. Furthermore, human or animal proteins are used in the production process of some recombinant products.[14] Therefore, these products have a theoretical risk of transmitting infection, although hepatitis and HIV infection have never been reported with their use.[5] First-generation recombinant factor VIII products contain human albumin as a stabilizing protein.[5] Second-generation recombinant factor VIII products add sugar instead of human albumin as a stabilizer, but human albumin is used in the culture process. One second-generation product (ReFacto®) and one third-generation product (Xynitha®) delete the B domain of the factor VIII gene, yielding a smaller protein product.[5,20] This B domain does not appear to be necessary for coagulation function. Third-generation recombinant factor VIII products do not contain human protein either in the culture or in the stabilization processes.[14]

Plasma-Derived Factor VIII Products

Clinical trials have demonstrated that recombinant factor VIII products are comparable in effectiveness to plasma-derived products.[5]

Several different plasma-derived factor VIII products are available (Table 101-4). These products are derived from the pooled plasma of thousands of donors and therefore have the potential to transmit infection. Donor screening, testing of plasma pools for evidence of infection, viral reduction through purification steps, and viral inactivation procedures (eg, dry heat, pasteurization, and solvent detergent treatment) have resulted in a safer product. No cases of HIV transmission from factor concentrates have been reported since 1986.[5] However, isolated cases of hepatitis C infection with use of plasma-derived products have been reported.[5] Additionally, outbreaks of hepatitis A viral infections associated with plasma-derived products have been reported, likely because solvent detergent treatment does not inactivate this non-enveloped virus. Finally, possible infection with as yet unidentified viruses not inactivated by currently used methods remains a concern. In addition, Prion disease may be present in plasma-derived factor products.[21]

Factor VIII concentrates can be classified according to their level of purity, which refers to the specific activity of factor VIII in the product. Cryoprecipitate is a low-purity product that also contains vWF, fibrinogen, and factor XIII. Current American Association of Blood Banks standards call for a minimum of 80 international units of factor VIII per cryoprecipitate pack.[5] This product is no longer considered a primary treatment of factor VIII deficiency in countries where factor VIII concentrates are available because cryoprecipitate does not undergo a viral inactivation process. Intermediate-purity products have a specific factor VIII activity of 5 units/mg of protein and high-purity products have up to 2,000 units/mg of protein.[5] Ultrahigh-purity plasma-derived products are prepared with monoclonal antibody purification steps and have a specific activity of 3,000 units/mg of protein prior to addition of albumin as a stabilizer.

Factor VIII Concentrate Replacement

Appropriate dosing of factor VIII concentrate depends on the half-life of the infused factor, the patient's body weight, and the location and severity of the bleed. The presence or absence of an inhibitory antibody to factor VIII and the titer of this antibody also influence treatment. Recovery studies, which measure the immediate post-infusion factor level, and survival studies, which assess the half-life of the factor, can establish patient-specific pharmacokinetics. The location and magnitude of the bleeding episode determine the percent correction to target as well as the duration of treatment.[7] Serious or life-threatening bleeding requires peak factor levels of greater than 0.75 to 1 units/mL (75%-100%); less severe bleeding may be treated with a goal of 0.3 to 0.5 units/mL (30%-50%) peak plasma levels. Table 101-5 provides general guidelines for the management of bleeding in different locations.

Factor VIII is a large molecule that remains in the intravascular space. Therefore, the plasma volume (about 50 mL/kg) can be used to estimate the volume of distribution. In general, each unit of factor VIII concentrate infused per kilogram of actual body weight results in a 2% rise in plasma factor VIII levels.[7] The following equation can be used to calculate an initial dose of factor VIII:

$$\text{Factor VIII (units)} = (\text{Desired level - Baseline level}) \times 0.5 \times (\text{Weight [in kilograms]})$$

The baseline level usually is omitted from the equation when it is negligible compared to the desired level. The half-life of factor VIII ranges from 8 to 15 hours. It is generally necessary to administer 50% of the initial dose about every 12 hours to sustain the desired level of factor VIII. A single treatment may be adequate for minor bleeding such as oral bleeding or slight muscle hemorrhages. However, because of the potential for long-term joint damage with hemarthroses, 2 or 3 days of treatment is often recommended for these bleeds. Serious bleeding episodes may require maintenance of 70% to 100% factor activity for 1 week or longer. As previously mentioned, factor VIII dosing depends on several variables, and each case must be considered individually. Individualized pharmacokinetics may help guide treatment, particularly for serious bleeding episodes.

Alternatively, factor VIII can be administered as a continuous infusion when prolonged treatment is required (eg, in the perioperative period or for serious bleeding episodes). Infusion rates ranging from 2 to 4 units/kg/h usually are given in fixed-dose continuous infusion protocols, with the aim of maintaining a steady-state level of 60% to 100%.[22] Administration of factor concentrate via continuous infusion may reduce factor requirements by 20% to 50% because unnecessarily high peaks of factor VIII that occur with bolus injections are avoided. A gradual decrease in factor VIII clearance during the first 5 to 6 days of treatment contributes to the lower factor concentrate requirements. Daily monitoring of factor level can help determine the appropriate rate of infusion.

Administration of factor VIII concentrate via continuous infusion has been shown to be safe and effective, and it may be more convenient than bolus therapy for hospitalized patients.[23] Concerns about the stability of the formulations appear to be unwarranted, as most high-purity factor VIII concentrates have been shown to remain stable for at least 7 days after reconstitution.[23] However,

TABLE 101-5 Guidelines for Factor Replacement Therapy for Hemorrhage in Hemophilia A and B

Site of Hemorrhage	Desired Hemostatic Factor Level (% of Normal)	Comments
Joint	50%-70%, 2-3 days	Rest/immobilization/physical therapy rehabilitation following bleed; several doses may be necessary to prevent or treat target joint
Muscle	30%-50% for most sites 70%-100% for thigh, iliopsoas, or nerve compression	Risk of significant blood loss with a thigh or iliopsoas bleed; bed rest for iliopsoas or thigh bleeding
Oral mucosa	30%-50%	May try antifibrinolytic or topical thrombin prior to factor replacement for minor bleeding; higher factor levels are needed for tongue swelling or risk of airway compromise; antifibrinolytic therapy should be used following factor replacement
GI	Initially 100%, then 40%-60%	Endoscopy is highly recommended; antifibrinolytic therapy may be useful. Continue until healing occurs
Hematuria	30%-50% if no trauma 70%-100% if traumatic	If no pain or trauma, consider bed rest and fluids for 24 hours; factor should be given if hematuria persists; evaluate if hematuria persists; if trauma to abdomen or back, perform imaging and give aggressive factor replacement
CNS	Initially 100%, then 50%-100% for 10-21 days	Lumbar puncture requires prophylactic factor coverage
Trauma or surgery	Initially 100%, then 50%-100% until wound healing complete	Perioperative and postoperative management plan must be in place preoperatively; evaluation for inhibitors is crucial prior to elective surgery

aPCC, activated prothrombin complex concentrate; PCC, prothrombin complex concentrate.

exposure of factor VIII to light for 10 hours after reconstitution can decrease activity by 30%.[23] Therefore, it would be prudent to shield the container with foil wrap or an appropriate bag.

Other Pharmacologic Therapy

Treatment with desmopressin acetate often is adequate for minor bleeding episodes in patients with mild hemophilia A. A synthetic analog of the antidiuretic hormone vasopressin, desmopressin causes release of vWF and factor VIII from endogenous endothelial storage sites. It appears to be most effective in patients with higher baseline factor VIII levels (0.1-0.15 units/mL).[24] The recommended dose of desmopressin is 0.3 mcg/kg diluted in 50 mL of normal saline and infused IV over 15 to 30 minutes.[24] Patients with mild or moderate hemophilia A should undergo a desmopressin trial to determine their response to this medication. At least a twofold rise in factor VIII to a minimal level of 0.3 units/mL within 60 minutes is considered an adequate response.[1,22] Infusion of desmopressin can be repeated daily for up to 2 to 3 days. Tachyphylaxis, an attenuated response with repeated dosing, may develop after that time due to the depletion of factor stores. The factor increase after the second dose of desmopressin is about 30% lower than after the initial dose.[24] Factor concentrate therapy may be necessary if the patient requires additional treatment. Factor levels should be measured to ensure that an adequate response has been achieved. Treatment with desmopressin will not result in hemostasis in patients who have severe hemophilia and those who are only marginally responsive. Desmopressin should not be used as primary therapy for life-threatening bleeding episodes such as intracranial hemorrhage or for major surgical procedures.[1]

Desmopressin can be administered intranasally via a concentrated nasal spray.[24] It elicits a slower and less marked response, with a peak effect in 60 to 90 minutes after administration, which is somewhat longer than with IV administration.[22,24] The dosage is one spray (150 mcg) in one nostril for patients who weigh less than 50 kg and two sprays (300 mcg) (one in each nostril) for those who weigh more than 50 kg.[22] The nasal spray may serve as an alternative to the IV formulation, especially in patients with mild bleeding episodes. Few adverse effects are associated with desmopressin. The most commonly observed side effect is facial flushing.[24] Less frequently reported side effects include mild headaches, increased heart rate, and decreased blood pressure. Desmopressin has the potential to cause water retention because of its antidiuretic effects, which may lead to severe hyponatremia. This may be a particular problem in children younger than 2 years and therefore should be used with caution in this age group.[22] Fluid restriction for 24 hours after the desmopressin dose and monitoring of urine output are recommended with desmopressin administration.[22]

Antifibrinolytic therapy inhibits clot lysis and therefore is a useful adjunctive therapy for the treatment of hemophilia, primarily with mucocutaneous bleeding. Antifibrinolytic agents are particularly beneficial for treatment of oral bleeding because of a high concentration of fibrinolytic enzymes in saliva. Antifibrinolytic therapy can also be helpful as adjuvant therapy in GI bleeding, epistaxis and menorrhagia. Antifibrinolytic therapy should be used with caution in patients with urinary bleeding, due to the risk of obstruction and subsequent renal toxicity. The two currently available antifibrinolytics include aminocaproic acid and tranexamic acid. Aminocaproic acid is given at a dosage of 100 mg/kg (maximum 6 g) every 6 hours and can be administered orally or IV.[5] The dosage of tranexamic acid is 25 mg/kg (maximum 1.5 g) orally every 6 to 8 hours.[5]

Hemophilia B

Therapeutic options for hemophilia B have improved greatly over the past several years, first with the development of monoclonal antibody-purified plasma-derived products and then with the licensure of recombinant factor IX. Products currently available in the United States for treatment of hemophilia B are listed in Table 101-4.

Recombinant Factor IX

Recombinant factor IX was not available until 1998, which is 6 years after the first recombinant factor VIII product.[25] Recombinant factor IX is produced in Chinese hamster ovary cells transfected with the factor IX gene. Since blood and plasma products are not used to produce recombinant factor IX or to stabilize the final product, recombinant factor IX has an excellent viral safety profile.[5,25] Clinical trials have shown the product to be safe and efficacious in the treatment of acute bleeding episodes and in the management of bleeding associated with surgical procedures.[5,25] Although the half-life of recombinant factor IX is similar to that of the plasma-derived products, recovery is about 30% lower.[25] As a result, doses of recombinant factor IX concentrate must be higher than those of plasma-derived products to achieve equivalent plasma levels. Because individual pharmacokinetics may vary, recovery and survival studies should be performed to determine optimal treatment.[5] Recombinant factor IX is considered the treatment of choice for hemophilia B.[1]

Plasma-Derived Factor IX Products

High-purity factor IX plasma concentrates have been available in the United States since the early 1990s.[5,25] These products are derived from plasma through biochemical purification and monoclonal immunoaffinity techniques. Other viral inactivation measures, such as solvent detergent or chemical treatment, are also used. High-purity factor IX concentrates have excellent efficacy in the treatment of bleeding episodes and in the control of bleeding associated with surgical procedures.[25] Their viral safety profile has been reported to be excellent and the risk of thromboembolic complications is low.[25]

Before the high-purity products were approved for use, hemophilia B patients were treated with factor IX concentrates that also contained other vitamin K-dependent proteins (factors II, VII, and X), known as prothrombin complex concentrates (PCCs). These products contain small amounts of activated factors generated during processing, and their use has been associated with thrombotic complications, including deep-vein thrombosis, pulmonary embolism, myocardial infarction, and disseminated intravascular coagulation.[5,25] The risk of such complications is highest in patients who are receiving high or repeated doses of PCCs, in those who have hepatic disease (the liver produces antithrombotic factors and removes the activated factors from circulation), in neonates, and in patients who have experienced crush injuries or who are undergoing major surgery.[5,25] Concomitant use of PCCs and antifibrinolytics should be avoided because of the risk for thrombosis. Because of the lower purity of PCCs and their thrombogenic potential, these products are not first-line treatment for hemophilia B.

Factor IX Concentrate Replacement

Factor IX is a relatively small protein. Unlike factor VIII, it is not limited to the intravascular space; it also passes into the extravascular compartment.[25] Therefore, it has a volume of distribution that is about twice that of factor VIII. For plasma-derived factor IX concentrates, each unit of factor IX infused per kilogram of actual body weight results in about a 1% rise in the plasma level of factor IX (range, 0.67%-1.28%).[5] The following equation can be used to calculate the initial dose:

$$\text{Plasma-derived factor IX (units)} = (\text{Desired level} - \text{Baseline level}) \times (\text{Weight [in kilograms]})$$

As with the factor VIII dose calculation, the baseline level term can be omitted from the formula if it is negligible compared to the desired level. Because recovery of recombinant factor IX is lower than that of the plasma-derived products, the following adjustment is made:

Pediatric dosing:

$$\text{Recombinant factor IX (units)} = (\text{Desired level} - \text{Baseline level}) \times 1.4 \times (\text{Weight [in kilograms]})$$

Adult dosing:

$$\text{Recombinant factor IX (units)} = (\text{Desired level} - \text{Baseline level}) \times 1.2 \times (\text{Weight [in kilograms]})$$

A recovery study to determine optimal dosing is recommended for patients who receive recombinant factor IX because of the wide interpatient variability in pharmacokinetics. Because the half-life of factor IX is about 24 hours, dosing can be less frequent than with factor VIII. Table 101-5 provides general guidelines for dosing factor IX based on the site and severity of the bleeding episode.

Prophylaxis Versus On Demand Therapy

One approach to treating hemophilia patients is to administer the necessary factor only for acute bleeding episodes; this is referred to as *on demand therapy*. However, recurrent joint bleeding can damage the joint and lead to the development of severe physical disability. It is therefore advisable to prevent bleeding episodes and avoid the resultant damage. This is the rationale for the second approach to treatment known as *prophylactic factor replacement therapy*. The goal of this approach is to maintain a patient's minimum factor level at or above 0.01 units/mL (1%) with regular infusions of factor products. In developed countries, prophylaxis for patients with severe hemophilia is considered standard of care. It is also recommended by the World Health Organization and the World Federation of Hemophilia.[6] Prophylaxis is sometimes required in patients with moderate hemophilia and is rarely used in patients with mild hemophilia.

Prophylactic replacement therapy converts severe hemophilia into a milder form of the disease. The rationale for this approach is that patients with moderate hemophilia rarely experience spontaneous hemarthroses, and they have a much lower risk of chronic arthropathy. Recent pediatric clinical trials have demonstrated the efficacy of prophylaxis in pediatric patients.[26] The first pediatric randomized clinical trial comparing prophylaxis to enhanced episodic treatment in boys (age less than 30 months) with severe hemophilia demonstrated that prophylaxis prevented joint damage and decreased the frequency of joint and other hemorrhages.[27] More recently, a European randomized clinical trial of prophylaxis in pediatric patients with hemophilia A confirmed the efficacy of prophylaxis in preventing bleeds and arthropathy.[26] The efficacy of prophylaxis in adult patients with hemophilia is still unclear.

The dosing for prophylactic regimens varies considerably and no one regimen has been proven to be superior.[27] A common regimen for patients with hemophilia A is 20 to 40 units/kg of factor VIII given every other day or three times per week.[28] For hemophilia B, the usual dosage ranges between 25 and 60 units/kg of factor IX given twice weekly because of the intrinsically longer half-life of factor IX.[25] The recent introduction of longer lasting factor products has made prophylaxis a more feasible approach. Patients with hemophilia A can now be dosed with the Fc fusion product at a dose of 25 to 65 units/kg at 3 to 5 day intervals depending on their individual response.[28] Similarly, patients with hemophilia B can be dosed with the corresponding Fc fusion protein product either 50 units/kg once weekly or 100 units/kg every 10 days.[28]

Controversy exists regarding the ideal timing for the initiation of prophylaxis. Primary prophylaxis is regular replacement therapy started at a young age (usually before age 2 years), prior to the onset of joint bleeding.[27] Secondary prophylaxis begins after significant joint bleeding has already occurred.[27] In 2001, the Medical and Scientific Advisory Council of the National Hemophilia Foundation of the United States recommended primary prophylaxis beginning at age 1 to 2 years for children with severe hemophilia. Prophylaxis regimens are best administered in the morning to protect the patient during daily activities.[1]

Clinical **Controversy...**

Despite the evidence based support for prophylaxis in children, controversy still exists over its benefit in adults. Appropriate time to initiate prophylaxis in children, and appropriate dosing for prophylaxis has still yet to be clearly defined.

Prophylaxis therapy comes with its own set of challenges. In addition to the paucity of evidence regarding dosing and initiation, a prohibitive challenge is the high cost of this approach. The cost to treat a patient with hemophilia A in the United States has been estimated to be about $300,000 per year.[29] Other issues to consider are the inconvenience to families and possible difficulties with adherence. Central venous lines may be necessary for frequent administration of factor concentrates, particularly in children younger than 2 years, who are at the age targeted for initiation of primary prophylaxis regimens. Potential complications of central venous access include surgical risks, infection, and catheter-related deep-vein thrombosis. Finally, routine use of primary prophylaxis may initially overtreat some patients with severe hemophilia who do not have a severe clinical phenotype. For these reasons, the use of primary prophylaxis has not been widely adopted in the United States. Many institutions continue to use some form of secondary prophylaxis, in which prophylaxis is started after a pattern of bleeding has been established.

Treatment of Inhibitors in Hemophilia

Neutralizing antibodies to factors VIII and IX, known as *inhibitors*, develop in a subset of patients with hemophilia. (4) The development of an inhibitor is the most serious complication of factor replacement therapy and is associated with considerable morbidity and a decreased quality of life. The incidence of new factor VIII inhibitors in patients with severe factor VIII deficiency is about 30%.[2,32] Inhibitors are less common in patients with mild or moderate hemophilia occurring in about 5% to 10% of patients.[1] The risk of developing inhibitors in patients with hemophilia B is much lower, occurring in only 3% of patients.[2,5]

Most inhibitors develop in childhood, after relatively few exposure days (median 10-15 days).[30] Patients with severe hemophilia are much more likely to develop inhibitors than those with milder forms of the disease.[30] It is possible that the low levels of factor produced in patients with mild or moderate hemophilia induce immune tolerance in these individuals. In contrast, factor levels are undetectable in patients with severe hemophilia, so infused factor VIII is regarded as a foreign protein, which may provoke an antibody response. The rate of inhibitor formation varies even among patients with identical mutations, which suggests that host factors modify the risk. The development of an inhibitor is the result of a complex interaction between a patient's immune system and genetic and environmental risk factors.

An inhibitor is a polyclonal high-affinity immunoglobulin G (IgG) directed against the factor VIII or IX protein.[31] Inhibitors interfere with infused factor concentrate, rendering them ineffective. The presence of an inhibitor is suspected when a decreased clinical response to factor replacement is observed or it may be discovered incidentally on routine laboratory screening. Inhibitors are measured with the Bethesda assay, and titers are reported in Bethesda units (BUs). One BU is the amount of inhibitor needed to inactivate half of the factor VIII or factor IX in a mixture of inhibitor-containing plasma and pooled normal plasma.[5] Patients with inhibitors to factor VIII or factor IX are divided into two groups: low responders, who have low levels of inhibitors (<5 BU/mL) and generally have little or no rise in antibody titers after exposure to the factor; and high responders (>5 BU/mL), who have higher inhibitor levels and develop an increase in antibody titer after exposure (anamnestic response).[2]

Clinical **Controversy...**

The risk of inhibitor formation has been reported to be higher in recombinant products as compared with plasma-derived products. However, it is difficult to compare the cumulative incidence from different studies because of differences in patient population (eg, heterogeneity in risk factors for inhibitor formation), study methodology, frequency of inhibitor testing, and length of follow-up. The results of several reviews have been contradictory. To address this very important clinical question, a prospective international randomized clinical trial (SIPPET—Survey of Inhibitors in Plasma Product Exposed Toddlers) is currently comparing inhibitor incidence in previously untreated patients exposed to either plasma or recombinant factor products.

Therapy for patients with inhibitors involves treatment of acute bleeding episodes and treatment directed at eradicating the inhibitor. The inhibitor titer, the site and magnitude of bleeding, and the patient's past response to bypassing therapy determine the approach to the treatment of acute bleeding. For patients with a low inhibitor titer, administration of high doses of the specific factor often can control bleeding episodes. Two to three times the usual replacement dose and more frequent dosing intervals are often necessary to overcome the antibody. Factor-level monitoring and clinical assessments help to evaluate the adequacy of treatment. Additional supportive measures, such as immobilization and administration of antifibrinolytic agents, should be used, where appropriate.

In the presence of a high-titer inhibitor, it is impossible to administer enough factor VIII or factor IX to neutralize the antibody and achieve a hemostatic plasma level. Therefore, the treatment of bleeding episodes consists of agents that bypass the factor to which the antibody is directed. These bypassing agents include PCCs, activated prothrombin complex concentrates (aPCCs), and recombinant factor VIIa. PCCs contain the vitamin K-dependent factors II, VII, IX, and X. Small quantities of activated factors are present in these products. Activated PCCs contain greater quantities of the activated factors primarily factor X and prothrombin. The only available aPCC product in the United States is FEIBA® (Factor Eight Inhibitor Bypassing Agent). The recommended dosage is 50 to 100 units/kg administered every 8 to 12 hours, depending on the severity of the bleeding episode and the maximum dose should not exceed 200 units/kg/day.[28] Activated PCCs appear to be more effective than PCCs and are preferred in patients with inhibitors. As previously mentioned, there is a risk of serious thrombotic complications, including pulmonary emboli, deep-vein thrombosis, and myocardial infarction associated with use of PCCs and aPCCs.[28] Other minor side effects include dizziness, nausea, hives, flushing, and headaches. Patients with factor IX inhibitors occasionally develop severe allergic reactions in response to infusion of factor IX-containing products, so these patients should be monitored closely.[25]

5 Recombinant factor VIIa is effective for the treatment of acute bleeds in patients with hemophilia A or B who have developed inhibitors. Recombinant factor VIIa is a bypassing agent which is thought to be hemostatically active only at the site of tissue injury where the tissue factor is present. Recombinant factor VIIa is not a plasma-derived product, so both viral transmission and anamnestic responses to factor VIII or factor IX are unlikely. The initial recommended dose for bleeding episodes is 90 mcg/kg.[28] However, depending on a patient's response, higher doses up to 300 mcg/kg can be used. A drawback is the product's short half-life, which necessitates initial dosing every 2 hours. Continuous infusion of recombinant factor VIIa, which may be more convenient and cost-effective, has been reported.[33] Patients treated with bypassing agents must be monitored clinically because no laboratory test directly measures the effectiveness of treatment.

Both recombinant factor VIIa and aPCCs have been demonstrated to be effective in the treatment of bleeding for patients with inhibitors. In determining which bypassing product to use in an individual patient, the clinician must consider multiple factors. In a patient with a newly diagnosed inhibitor, it is prudent to use recombinant factor VIIa because aPCCs contain a small amount of factor VIII or IX and have been shown to increase the inhibitor titer. It is also important to consider an individual's response to specific bypassing agents because of the significant variability in response between individuals. In some patients, bleeding can be unresponsive to monotherapy and may require alternating products.[34] Due to the risk of developing thrombosis or disseminated intravascular coagulation from alternating bypassing agents, this therapy should be used with caution and only in an inpatient setting.[35]

In the past, plasma derived porcine factor VIII was an alternative therapeutic option for patients who have hemophilia A and inhibitors. It was removed from the market secondary to contamination with porcine parvovirus. The rationale for its use is that porcine factor VIII is enough like human factor VIII to participate in the coagulation cascade, yet most factor VIII inhibitors have absent or only weak neutralizing activity against nonhuman factor VIII making this an effective agent to treat an acute bleed. Unfortunately, cross-reactivity with porcine factor VIII does occur, and a high titer of antibody against porcine factor VIII can develop and hypersensitivity to porcine proteins can occur. Recently a recombinant porcine factor VIII has been approved (Obizur®), but only for treatment of acute bleeds in patients with acquired hemophilia A.[28]

The current hemostatic therapies for patients with an inhibitor have limited effectiveness leading to significant morbidity and a decreased quality of life. The ideal therapy for patients with an inhibitor is total eradication so that optimal hemostatic treatment with either factor VIII or IX is possible. At this time, the only proven method for inhibitor eradication is immune tolerance induction (ITI), which involves the regular infusion of factor VIII to induce antigen-specific tolerance. This approach is not recommended for patients with hemophilia B who have developed inhibitors due to the risk of hypersensitivity reactions and anaphylaxis associated with factor IX administration in this group.

Multiple immune tolerance registries were established to help determine patient- and treatment-related factors associated with immune tolerance outcome.[36,37] Across these registries, a patient's peak historical factor VIII inhibitor titer (<200 BU) and the inhibitor titer at the time of ITI induction (<10 BU) were associated with successful immune tolerance. The overall ITI success rate from these registries ranges from 51% to 79%;[36,37] the variability is likely related to a lack of standardization in study methodologies, treatment protocols, and eradication definitions.

The relationship between factor VIII dose and ITI success rate is not clear. A variety of different dosing regimens, ranging from 25 units/kg every other day to more than 200 units/kg every day, have been used. The International Immune Tolerance Registry demonstrated improved ITI success with high doses (200 IU/kg), while the North American and Spanish Immune Tolerance Registries showed improved success with lower dosing strategies.[37] The International Immune Tolerance Study is a multicenter randomized clinical trial that compared high-dose (200 units/kg/day) to low-dose (50 units/kg three times/wk) regimens in patients with severe hemophilia A and high titer inhibitors

(>5 BU).[7,38] This study was stopped early due to an increased risk of bleeding events in the low-dose arm. At the stopping point, the proportion of ITI success was not significantly different between the two arms, but the time to achieve ITI success was shorter in the high-dose arm. Because the study was stopped early, it lacked statistical power to demonstrate therapeutic equivalence below the 30% boundary of equivalence. It appears that a high-dose strategy achieves tolerance at a faster rate, which explains the lower bleeding rate.

Some studies report better success rates for ITI in patients receiving plasma-derived factor products containing vWF, which may be related to the role of vWF in factor VIII function, stabilization, and immunogenicity.[39,40] vWF binding to the C2 domain of factor VIII, a common site for inhibitor formation, may result in epitope masking and decreased inhibitor activity.[40] The use of vWF-containing products may also extend the plasma half-life of factor VIII during ITI, thus increasing antigen presentation and possibly contributing to its overall success.[39]

Although not commonly used in ITI protocols, immune modulation has been reported as a method to improve tolerance success. Agents, such as cyclophosphamide and intravenous immune globulin, have been used in an effort to reduce inhibitor titers and make ITI more successful.[7] Another immune modulating agent, rituximab, an anti-CD20 monoclonal antibody that inhibits B-cells and interferes with IgG production, has been used with some success. In a phase II trial of rituximab in patients with high titer inhibitors, only 3 out of 16 subjects (18.8%) had a major response (decline in the inhibitor to <5 BU without an increase in the inhibitor titer after rechallenge to factor VIII).[41] When used as a single agent in previously treated patients with inhibitors, rituximab had a modest effect, but further studies are needed to determine the activity of rituximab combined with ITI. Figure 101-1 summarizes the therapeutic options in the management of hemophilia A patients with inhibitors.

Gene Therapy in Hemophilia

Hemophilia is an excellent candidate for gene therapy because tight control of gene expression is not required. Even low levels of factor expression can reduce bleeding episodes in patients with severe hemophilia, which is similar to the rationale for prophylactic factor replacement. The goal of gene therapy would be to achieve a sustainable factor activity level of over 5%, which is sufficient to convert patients with severe disease to a much milder phenotype.[42] If a treatment strategy could produce consistent factor activity levels of around 50%, it would be considered curative.[42] Gene therapy for the treatment of hemophilia remains in the early clinical stages. Advances are most apparent in hemophilia B, which has been attributed to the smaller size (about 1.4 kb) of its complementary DNA (cDNA).[42] Recently, a landmark clinical trial reported the results of a single peripheral venous infusion of an adenovirus associated factor IX transgene vector under the control of a liver-restricted promoter in six patients with severe hemophilia B.[43] All of the study subjects demonstrated long-term (over 2 years) expression of the factor IX transgene with therapeutic levels of factor IX (plateau factor IX levels from 1% to 6%).[43,44] At this time, gene therapy for factor VIII deficiency has not progressed as far due to the considerably larger size of its cDNA (about 9 kb).[42] Potential benefits to gene therapy include patient convenience, viral safety, and decreased cost. Possible drawbacks to gene therapy include a risk of inhibitor formation, tumorigenesis related to possible integration of the viral vector, possible germ-line transmission of the viral vector, and concerns about long-term gene expression.

Pain Management in Hemophilia

Pain, both acute and chronic, can be a common occurrence in patients with hemophilia. The most likely cause of acute pain is

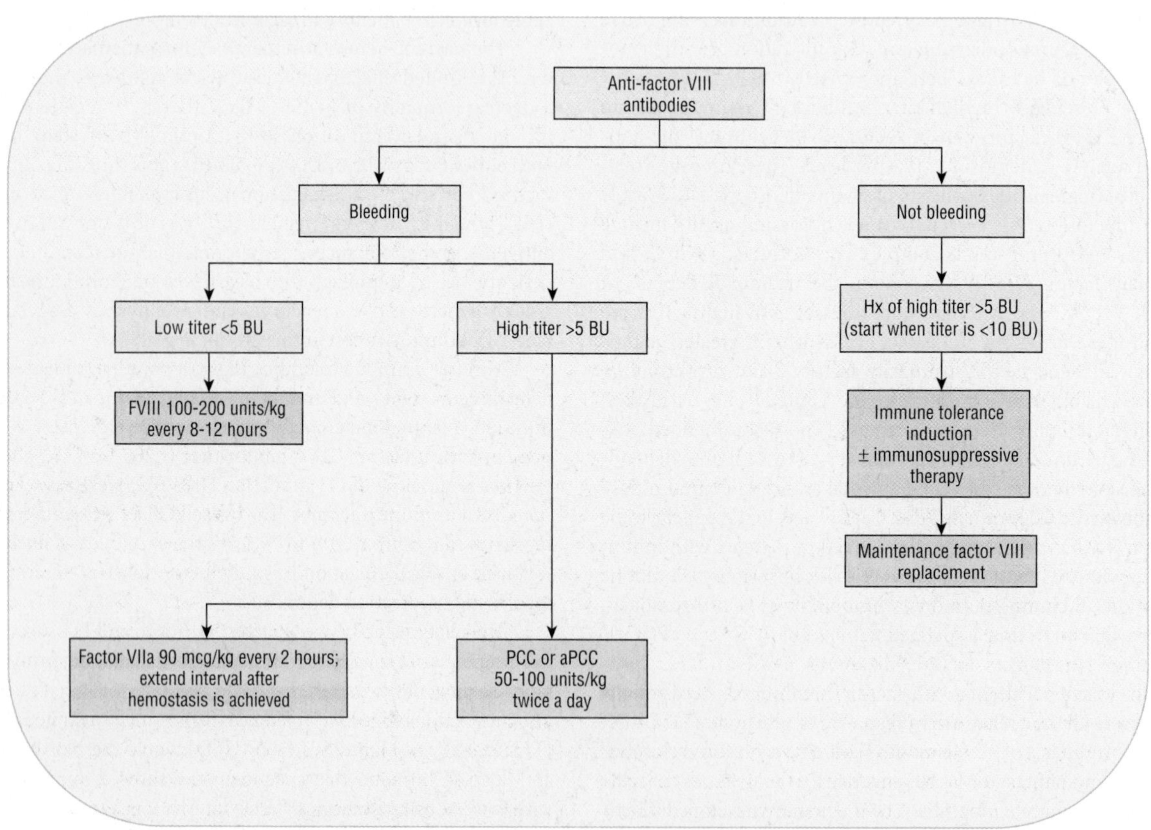

FIGURE 101-1 Treatment algorithm for the management of patients with hemophilia A and factor VIII antibodies. (aPCC, activated prothrombin complex concentrate; BU, Bethesda unit; PCC, prothrombin complex concentrate.)

bleeding, and treatment should include factor replacement to stop the bleeding, and RICE (Rest, Ice, Compression, and Elevation).[7,45] Acetaminophen can be used for mild pain, although narcotic analgesia may be required for more severe pain. Nonsteroidal anti-inflammatory drugs impair platelet function and may increase bleeding and should not be used during acute bleeding episodes. Cyclooxygenase-2 inhibitors have less antiplatelet activity and are an option for acute and chronic pain management.[1,45]

Chronic pain in patients with hemophilia is typically secondary to hemophilic arthropathy. Hemophilic arthropathy is the direct result of recurrent hemarthrosis. Persistent blood in the joint leads to inflammation, synovial hypertrophy and inflammation, cartilage destruction, and finally bony erosion. Cyclooxygenase-2 inhibitors can also be helpful in managing chronic pain. Surgical interventions may help to alleviate chronic pain. Synovectomy (removal of the hypertrophied synovium) can reduce chronic pain from recurrent bleeding. Patients with more advanced joint disease could benefit from joint replacement.

Surgery in Hemophilia

In patients with severe hemophilia, the dose of replacement factor required in the perioperative period will depend on the surgery, the inhibitor status, and the patient's previous response to factor products. Ideally, the patient's factor activity level should be maintained in the range of 50% to 100% depending on clinical status and type of procedure. Intermittent dosing or continuous infusion factor replacement may accomplish this goal.[1,33,46] Before surgery, factor concentrate is usually infused to obtain a plasma level of 1 unit/mL (100%). Replacement therapy is continued to maintain plasma levels greater than 0.5 units/mL (50%) for 5 to 7 days or longer, depending on the type of surgery and the patient's clinical response. Preoperative evaluation for elective procedures should include measurement of an inhibitor titer no longer than 2 weeks prior to procedure and assessment of the recovery and half-life of infused factor in the patient.[1] For those patients with inhibitors undergoing surgical procedures, there is evidence to support the use of both activated factor VII and aPCCs.[1,33]

Personalized Pharmacotherapy

The newest approach in hemophilia treatment is "personalized" prophylaxis.[47] Traditionally, standard prophylaxis is prescribed based on a weight-based calculation to increase a patient's trough factor level to greater than 0.01 units/mL (1%). Although this approach is successful for many patients, some may still experience breakthrough bleeding, which suggests that prophylactic dosing and timing may need to be personalized to prevent bleeding. Many factors can contribute to breakthrough bleeding including the patient's activity level, individual pharmacokinetics, the presence of a target joint, synovial hypertrophy, and the degree of hemophilic arthropathy present.[47] The prophylaxis regimen should take into account these factors and be adjusted accordingly.

Since inhibitor formation is the most significant treatment complication in hemophilia, targeted pharmacotherapy is being evaluated to decrease a patient's risk of inhibitor formation. For example, researchers are working to identify immunodominant epitopes in factor VIII that could lead to the development of new therapeutic factor VIII products for high-risk individuals.[48]

Evaluation of Therapeutic Outcomes

The main goal in the treatment of hemophilia is to control and prevent bleeding episodes and their long-term sequelae such as chronic arthropathies. Pharmacologic and nonpharmacologic interventions should be aimed at achieving this goal. Treatment response can be monitored through clinical parameters such as cessation of bleeding and resolution of symptoms. Monitoring plasma factor levels also may be helpful, particularly for severe bleeding episodes. Home therapy for administration of factor concentrates is common among patients with hemophilia because this approach can lead to earlier treatment and more independence for the patient. Diaries in which the patient documents symptoms, the dose of factor replacement, adjuvant therapies used, and treatment response can help the caregiver to evaluate the success of home therapy. Monitoring the number and type of bleeding episodes and trough plasma factor levels makes it possible to evaluate the adequacy of prophylactic regimens. Physical examination with evaluation of joint range of motion and radiographic imaging of target joints indicates the long-term success of preventing and treating arthropathies.

Clinicians should check for the development of inhibitors, especially in patients with severe disease and exposure to factor concentrates, at least yearly and with any suspicion of poor treatment response. The development of inhibitors challenges the management and control of bleeding episodes. A full understanding of the clinical situation and the titer of the inhibitor are mandatory to address all treatment options for each patient. Because no laboratory test measures the effectiveness of bypassing therapy in patients with inhibitors, close clinical monitoring for worsening or resolution of symptoms is essential for optimizing the outcome.

VON WILLEBRAND DISEASE

von Willebrand disease (vWD) is the most common congenital bleeding disorder in the United States and in the world, with a prevalence of 1% to 2%.[49,50] vWD refers to a family of disorders caused by a quantitative and/or qualitative defect of vWF, a glycoprotein that plays a role in both platelet aggregation and coagulation (Table 101-6). vWF mediates platelet adhesion to injured blood vessel sites and promotes platelet aggregation. It binds factor VIII and protects it from degradation by plasma proteases, thus prolonging its half-life. Unlike hemophilia, vWD has an autosomal inheritance pattern, resulting in an equal frequency of disease in males and females.

The gene for vWF is located on chromosome 12 and is 178 kb in length.[49,53] Transcription and translation produce a large primary product that subsequently undergoes complex modifications, resulting in vWF multimers of various sizes with molecular weights ranging from 500 to 20,000 kDa.[51,52] vWF is synthesized in endothelial cells, where it is either stored in Weibel–Palade bodies or secreted constitutively. It is also synthesized in megakaryocytes and stored in α-granules, from which it is released following platelet activation.[53,54]

von Willebrand factor is important for both primary and secondary hemostases. In response to vascular injury, it promotes platelet adhesion by interacting with the glycoprotein Ib receptor on platelets.[53] It can facilitate platelet aggregation by binding to the platelet glycoprotein IIb/IIIa receptor, although fibrinogen is the main ligand for this receptor.[55] The highest-molecular-weight vWF multimers appear to be the most important in platelet adhesion because their large surface area contains numerous binding sites for various ligands and receptors. vWF is also the carrier molecule for circulating factor VIII, protecting it from premature degradation and removal.[53,54] A deficiency of vWF reduces the half-life of

TABLE 101-6 von Willebrand Disease

von Willebrand factor (vWF)
Large multimeric glycoprotein that is necessary for normal platelet adhesion, normal bleeding time, and stabilization of factor VIII
von Willebrand factor antigen (vWF:Ag)
Antigenic determinant(s) on vWF measured by immunoassays; usually low in types 1 and 2; virtually absent in type 3
Ristocetin cofactor activity (RCo)
Functional assay of vWF activity based on platelet aggregation with ristocetin. Reduced by the same degree as vWF:Ag in types 1 and 3, but to a greater extent in type 2 disease (except 2B)

CLINICAL PRESENTATION von Willebrand Disease

Signs and Symptoms

- Clinical manifestations are variable; some patients are asymptomatic
- Mucocutaneous bleeding: epistaxis, gingival bleeding with minor manipulation, menorrhagia
- Easy bruising
- Postoperative bleeding

factor VIII and decreases plasma factor VIII levels. Therefore, vWF plays a dual role in hemostasis, affecting both platelet function and coagulation.

Classification of von Willebrand Disease

von Willebrand Disease consists of a heterogeneous group of disorders that can be classified into three major subtypes. The National Institutes of Health has developed a classification scheme that characterizes vWD according to both the quantity of the von Willebrand clotting factors and their functionality (Table 101-7). Types 1 and 3 are associated with quantitative defects in vWF; type 2 mutations refer to functional abnormalities in vWF.[50,53] It is important to determine disease subtype because it influences treatment.

Type 1 vWD is the most common type, accounting for 70% to 80% of cases.[50,56] It is characterized by a mild-to-moderate quantitative reduction in the level of vWF (although its multimeric structure is normal) and a similar reduction in the level of factor VIII. It usually is inherited in an autosomal-dominant fashion with variable penetrance and expression.[53] Bleeding symptoms often are very mild to moderate.[53] Patients with vWD can experience mucocutaneous bleeding such as nosebleeds, bruising, gastrointestinal, or menstrual bleeding. Subjects may be at risk of bleeding following surgery, traumatic injury, or childbirth.[53]

Type 2 vWD, diagnosed in 20% to 30% of affected patients, is characterized by a qualitative abnormality of vWF.[50] Bleeding manifestations may be more severe than with type 1 disease. Inheritance most often is autosomal dominant but may be recessive.[53] Type 2 vWD can be subdivided into four variants. Type 2A is the most frequent subtype and is characterized by a reduced vWF–platelet interaction and an absence of high- and intermediate-molecular-weight factor multimers. Type 2B is a less common variant characterized by an abnormal vWF that has an increased affinity for the platelet glycoprotein Ib receptor. This subtype is associated with thrombocytopenia, which is usually mild. In addition, high-molecular-weight forms of vWF are usually absent. A platelet-type pseudo-vWD has been characterized in which vWF is normal but a defect in the platelet glycoprotein Ib receptor causes an increased affinity for normal vWF.[53] As a result, platelet-type pseudo-vWD is phenotypically similar to type 2B disease but should be distinguished from it because the treatment is different. Type 2M arises from a qualitative defect in vWF that impairs its binding to platelets; it is similar to type 2A, except there is no measurable reduction in the high-molecular-weight multimers.[53] Finally, type 2N vWD (Normandy) is a rare form of the disease in which vWF has a markedly reduced affinity for factor VIII. This subtype leads to a moderate-to-severe reduction of factor VIII plasma levels with normal vWF levels.[53]

Type 3 vWD refers to a severe quantitative variant of the disease in which vWF is nearly undetectable and factor VIII levels are very low (<20 IU/dL [<0.2 IU/mL]). It is often inherited in an autosomal recessive fashion.[56] Type 3 vWD is rare and accounts for 1% to 3% of all cases.[50] The clinical phenotype is severe, reflecting major deficits in primary hemostasis and coagulation.

Acquired vWD is a rare bleeding disorder that is similar to the congenital form of the disease. It has been reported primarily in association with autoimmune disorders, such as systemic lupus erythematosus, lymphoproliferative disorders, myeloproliferative disorders, hypothyroidism, and certain neoplastic diseases such as Wilms' tumor and lymphoma. It has been reported in situations of high shear stress such as aortic stenosis.[57] Certain medications have been associated with acquired vWD, including valproic acid, griseofulvin,

TABLE 101-7 von Willebrand Disease Classification and Laboratory Values (Modified from Nichols 2009)

Condition	Description	vWF-RCo (IU/dL)[1]	vWF-Ag (IU/dL)[1]	FVIII	vWF-RCo/vWF-Ag Ratio
Definite Type 1	Partial quantitative vWF deficiency	<30	<30	↓ or Normal	>0.5-0.7
"Probable type 1"		30-50	30-50	Normal	>0.5-0.7
Type 2A	↓ vWF-dependent platelet adhesion with selective deficiency of high-MW vWF multimer	<30	<30-200	↓ or Normal	<0.5-0.7
Type 2B	↑ vWF affinity for platelet GP 1b; + ↓ platelet numbers	<30	<30-200	↓ or Normal	Usually <0.5-0.7
Type 2M	↓ vWF-dependent platelet adhesion without selective deficiency of high MW vWF multimers	<30	<30-200	↓ or Normal	<0.5-0.7
Type 2N	Markedly ↓ vWF binding affinity for FVIII	30-200	30-200	↓↓	>0.5-0.7
Type 3	Virtually complete deficiency of vWF	<3	<3	↓↓↓ (<10 IU/dL)	Not applicable
Normal		50-200	50-200	Normal	>0.5-0.7

vWF, von Willebrand factor; RCo, ristocetin cofactor.

To calculate levels of vWF-RCo and vWF-Ag in units of IU/mL multiply the corresponding value expressed in IU/dL by 0.010.

Modified from Nichols WL, Rick ME, Ortel TL. Clinical and laboratory diagnosis of von Willebrand disease: A synopsis of the 2008 NHLBI/NIH guidelines. Am J Hematol 2009;84:366-370.

hydroxyethyl starch, and ciprofloxacin.[57] Bleeding manifestations vary from mild to severe, and the condition often resolves with treatment of the underlying disease. Various mechanisms have been proposed, including autoantibodies to vWF resulting in rapid removal from the plasma, adsorption to tumor cells or activated platelets, increased proteolysis, or mechanical destruction.[57]

Diagnosis

When a patient has a lifelong history of mucocutaneous bleeding and a family history of abnormal bleeding, vWD should be suspected. For a review of clinical questions to ask the patient, refer to the National Heart, Lung, and Blood Institute guidelines (Table 101-8).[58]

Several different laboratory tests are helpful in the diagnosis of this hemostatic abnormality. Initial screening tests include determinations of PT, activated partial thromboplastin time (aPTT), and platelet count. PT is normal, while aPTT may be normal or prolonged in relation to the reduction in plasma factor VIII levels. A normal aPTT does not rule out vWD; specific laboratory assessment of the vWF is required. The platelet count usually is normal, although thrombocytopenia is common in type 2B and platelet-type pseudo-vWD. The platelet function analysis (PFA-100), or the less commonly used bleeding time, may be prolonged but can be normal in patients with milder forms of the disease.[53,59]

Specific laboratory tests for the diagnosis of vWD include measurement of vWF antigen (vWF:Ag) level, factor VIII assay, determination of vWF ristocetin cofactor (vWF:RCo) activity, and vWF multimer analysis (see Table 101-6). Unfortunately, these levels vary considerably and often indeterminate or unreliable results can lead to confusion in the diagnosis. For example, the cutoff normal values for vWF:Ag, vWF:RCo, and other specialized tests vary between laboratories. This coupled with the natural variation of plasma concentrations of vWF can make interpretation of these results complicated.[53] Plasma concentrations of vWF have been shown to increase with age, stress, cigarette smoking, exercise, pregnancy starting in the second trimester, infection, and with the use of certain medications such as corticosteroids, high-dose estrogen birth control pills, and desmopressin. Repeated test measurements may be necessary due to this physiologic variability.[53]

Electroimmunoassay, immunoradiometric assay or enzyme-linked immunosorbent assay (ELISA) can be used to quantify vWF:Ag.[53] vWF:Ag levels are known to vary with different ABO blood types. Individuals with type O blood exhibit up to a 25% decrease in vWF levels when compared to those with type A due to increased plasma protein clearance.[53] The vWF:Ag level is usually low in types 1 and 2 vWD and virtually absent in type 3 disease. Factor VIII levels are normal or mildly decreased in patients with type 1 or 2 disease and very low (<10%) in those with type 3 disease.[53] Ristocetin, an antibiotic that causes platelet aggregation in the presence of functional vWF, is used to measure vWF activity. The assay is performed by mixing platelet-free patient plasma, normal formalin-fixed platelets, and ristocetin and then quantitating the extent of platelet agglutination.[52] Ristocetin cofactor activity usually is reduced in parallel to vWF:Ag levels in types 1 and 3 disease and decreased to a greater extent than vWF:Ag in type 2 disease (except type 2B).[53] Low-dose ristocetin-induced platelet agglutination (LD-RIPA) is useful for further distinguishing type 2B disease, as a low concentration of ristocetin induces excessive aggregation in type 2B disease (see Table 101-7).[53]

von Willebrand factor, secreted as high molecular weight multimers, is cleaved in plasma to increasingly small protein fragments. The distribution of these multimer sizes can be helpful in determining the type of vWD. All multimer sizes are present in type 1 disease, whereas reduced levels of intermediate- and high-molecular-weight multimers are characteristic of type 2 disease. Type 3 patients lack all types of vWF multimers. Molecular genetic testing for vWD is now a feasible option in some instances. Genetic testing may be used to clarify diagnostic uncertainty that may remain after coagulation testing and clinical evaluation.[53]

TABLE 101-8 Questions to Ask Patients

1. Have you or a blood relative ever needed medical attention for a bleeding problem or been told you have a bleeding disorder or problem?
   - During or after surgery?
   - With dental procedures or extractions?
   - During childbirth or for heavy menses?
   - Ever had bruises with lungs?
2. Do you have or have you ever had:
   - Liver or kidney disease?
   - A blood or bone marrow disorder?
   - A high or low platelet count?
3. Do you take aspirin, NSAIDs, clopidogrel, warfarin, heparin?

If yes to any of the above questions, ask additional questions:

1. Do you have a blood relative who has a bleeding disorder, such as von Willebrand disease or hemophilia?
2. Have you ever had prolonged bleeding from trivial wounds, lasting more than 15 minutes or recurring spontaneously during the 7 days after the wound?
3. Have you ever had heavy, prolonged, or recurrent bleeding after surgical procedures, such as tonsillectomy?
4. Have you ever had bruising, with minimal or no apparent trauma, especially if you could feel a lump under the bruise?
5. Have you ever had a spontaneous nosebleed that required more than 10 minutes to stop or needed medical attention?
6. Have you ever had heavy, prolonged, or recurrent bleeding after dental extractions that required medical attention?
7. Have you ever had blood in your stool, unexplained by a specific anatomic lesion (such as an ulcer in the stomach or polyp in the colon) that required medical attention?
8. Have you ever had anemia requiring treatment or received a blood transfusion?
9. For women, have you ever had heavy menses, characterized by the presence of clots greater than an inch in diameter and/or changing a pad or tampon more than hourly or resulting in anemia or low iron level?

NSAID, non-steroidal antiinflammatory drug.

Adapted from Nichols WL, Rick ME, Otel TL, et al. Clinical and laboratory diagnosis of von Willebrand disease: a synopsis of the 2008 NHLBI/NIH guidelines. Am J Hematol 2009;84:366-370.

TREATMENT

6 The specific type of vWD and the location and severity of bleeding determine the approach to treatment. The comprehensive care of patients with vWD requires a team approach. The desired outcome is to prevent bleeding episodes and their short-term and long-term consequences so that patients with vWD can live active and productive lives. Local measures, including pressure, ice, and topical thrombin, often can control superficial bleeding. Systemic treatment is used for bleeding that cannot be controlled in this manner and for prevention of bleeding with surgery. The goal of systemic therapy is to correct platelet adhesion and coagulation defects by stimulating the release of endogenous vWF or by administering products that contain vWF and factor VIII.[60] General guidelines for treatment of vWD are shown in Fig. 101-2.

Replacement Therapy

7 The treatment of choice for patients with types 2B, 2M, and 3 vWD and for patients with type 1 or 2A vWD who are unresponsive to desmopressin (which is discussed in the next section) is replacement therapy with plasma-derived vWF-containing products.[56] Several virus-inactivated, intermediate- or high-purity plasma derived factor VIII concentrates contain sufficient amounts of functional vWF for treatment in this patient population (see Table 101-4).

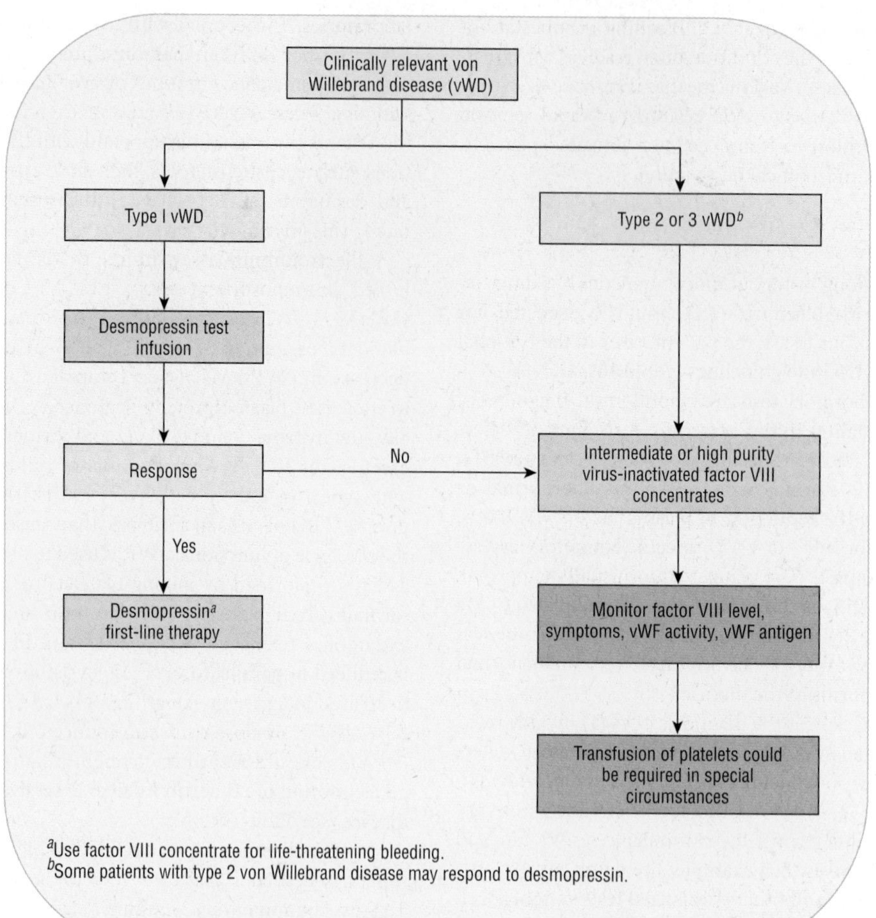

FIGURE 101-2 Guidelines for treatment of von Willebrand disease.

Ultrahigh-purity (monoclonal antibody-derived) plasma-derived products contain only negligible amounts of vWF and recombinant factor VIII products contain no vWF and are inadequate for treatment of vWD. Developing improved factor replacement products is an active area of research at this time. A recent prospective first-in-human clinical trial of a combination of recombinant vWF and recombinant factor VIII in a fixed ratio was completed. The study showed the combination product to be safe and well tolerated with only minor and transient adverse effects similar to those seen in patients receiving plasma derived products. The pharmacokinetics of the recombinant combination were also comparable to the plasma derived vWF with the added benefit of enhanced factor VIII stabilization, resulting in no additional factor VIII product required for adequate hemostasis.[62]

Cryoprecipitate contains about 80 to 100 units of vWF per unit (5 to 10 times more vWF and factor VIII than fresh-frozen plasma), and historically it was the mainstay of therapy for vWD. However, because cryoprecipitate is not virally inactivated, it should not be used as first-line treatment. General guidelines for the dosing of replacement therapy in patients with vWD unresponsive to desmopressin are provided in Table 101-9. The vWD guidelines are also available at the National Heart, Lung and Blood Institute Web site (*http://www.nhlbi.nih.gov/guidelines/vwd/index.htm*). In addition, a consensus guideline for the treatment of vWD and other bleeding disorders in women was published in 2009.[61]

Other Pharmacologic Therapy

8 Desmopressin stimulates the endothelial cell release of vWF and factor VIII. It is temporarily effective for patients with vWD who have adequate endogenous stores of functional vWF, which includes most patients with type 1 disease and some patients with type 2A disease. Conversely, desmopressin is not appropriate for patients with type 3 disease, who lack stores of vWF. Desmopressin usually is not recommended for treatment of type 2B disease because the release of additional abnormal vWF may exacerbate thrombocytopenia, but it has been reported to be beneficial in some patients with type 2B disease.[59] If desmopressin is used for treatment of type 2B disease, close monitoring is necessary.

TABLE 101-9 Replacement Therapy in von Willebrand Disease[a]

Condition	Therapy
Major surgery	Maintain factor VIII level ≥50% for 1 week
	Prolonged treatment in type 3 patients (>7 days)
Minor surgery	Maintain factor VIII level ≥50% for 1-3 days
	Maintain factor VIII level >20%-30% for an additional 4-7 days
Dental extraction	Single infusion to achieve factor VIII level >50%
	Desmopressin prior to procedure for type I
Spontaneous or posttraumatic bleeding	Usually single infusion of 20-40 units/kg

[a]The yield of factor VIII after first infusion is similar to that observed in hemophilia A (about 2% increment over baseline amount for every 1 unit/kg of factor VIII infused).

Clinical **Controversy...**

The use of desmopressin in treating acute bleeds in patients with type 2B vWD is controversial. There is some evidence that it may put patients at risk of severe thrombocytopenia.

The dose of desmopressin used for treatment of vWD is identical to that used for treatment of mild factor VIII deficiency, 0.3 mcg/kg given IV over 15 to 30 minutes.[28] Patients with vWD generally have a better response to desmopressin than those with hemophilia, with an average threefold to fivefold increase in vWF and factor VIII levels.[59] These levels remain elevated for about 6 to 8 hours. The response to desmopressin in a given patient usually is consistent, and a desmopressin trial should determine if the medication likely will be effective for the individual. Desmopressin is preferable to use of plasma-derived products for patients who have an adequate response because desmopressin does not carry a risk of viral transmission. An added benefit is the substantially lower cost of desmopressin compared to the plasma-derived products. (For a discussion of the side effects of desmopressin, see Treatment of Hemophilia A discussed earlier.)

Desmopressin can be administered every 12 to 24 hours, but the response diminishes with repeated treatment. After three to four doses, desmopressin often is no longer effective and alternative replacement therapy may be necessary if prolonged treatment is required. Laboratory monitoring, including vWF:Ag measurements, factor VIII assays, vWF:activity assessments, and clinical examinations, will determine the adequacy of treatment.[59] Intranasal administration of desmopressin, at the same dosage as that used for mild factor VIII deficiency, can be useful for treatment of mild bleeding episodes. One or two doses administered at the start of menses may be helpful in controlling menorrhagia. Oral contraceptives may also be very effective in controlling this symptom. Antifibrinolytic agents, such as aminocaproic acid and tranexamic acid, may be of special value in bleeds associated with tissues rich in plasminogen activators, such as the mouth, especially with tooth extractions.[59] These agents can also be used in the management of epistaxis, GI bleeding, and menorrhagia. However, these agents should be avoided in urinary tract bleeding because of the risk of thrombosis and obstruction.

In acquired vWD, low levels of plasma vWF are the result of accelerated removal of protein from plasma through the action of different pathogenic mechanisms. Acquired vWD may be associated with monoclonal gammopathy, lymphoproliferative or myeloproliferative syndromes, or cardiovascular disease. The treatment of the underlying lymphoproliferative disease with rituximab, a monoclonal antibody against CD20 on lymphocytes, has been reported to be relatively ineffective in the management of acquired vWD.[57] IV immune globulin remains a therapeutic option in acquired vWD, along with vWF concentrate and/or desmopressin.

Gene Therapy

Patients with the most severe bleeding phenotypes of vWD (type 3 and some severe cases of types 1 and 2) may be the most likely candidates for gene therapy, which offers the potential of a long-term, if not lifelong, correction of vWF deficiency. Studies placing vWF cDNA into a lentiviral vector are currently ongoing.[51] Preclinical trials are being conducted to test the feasibility of gene transfer in the management of vWD.

Personalized Pharmacotherapy

Current treatment of individual patients with vWD is personalized. Although the general goal of systemic therapy is to correct platelet adhesion and coagulation defects by stimulating the release of vWF or administering products that contain vWF, each patient's bleeding risk factors must be taken into consideration, and therapy tailored to the individual. The proposed regimen should take into account these risk factors and the most appropriate individualized therapy should be provided.

Evaluation of Therapeutic Outcomes

Since the main goal in the treatment of vWD is to prevent or control bleeding and the consequences of such bleeding, bleeding episodes can be monitored via clinical and laboratory parameters. Monitoring the number and types of bleeding episodes and measurement of plasma concentrations of vWF and factor VIII make it possible to evaluate the effectiveness of specific prophylactic and treatment regimens. As with hemophilia patients, assessment of patients' activities of daily living gives clinicians a better appreciation of the success of the treatment plan.

OTHER CONGENITAL FACTOR DEFICIENCIES

Rare bleeding disorders constitute 3% to 5% of all inherited coagulation factor deficiencies.[63] These rare bleeding disorders include congenital deficiencies in fibrinogen, in factors II, V, VII, X, XI, and XIII, and in combinations of factor deficiencies. Contact factor abnormalities, including deficiencies in factor XII, high-molecular-weight kininogen, and prekallikrein, prolong the aPTT but do not lead to any bleeding diathesis. Identification of these disorders is important so that inappropriate treatment is not given. The only contact factor deficiency associated with bleeding symptoms is factor XI deficiency. Also known as hemophilia C, this deficiency is particularly common in people of Ashkenazi Jewish descent.[61] Bleeding manifestations are variable. Bleeding usually does not occur spontaneously, but excessive bleeding may occur after trauma or surgery. Most other deficiencies are inherited as autosomal recessive disorders and are rare. Some patients with abnormal molecules, such as a dysfibrinogenemia, may have an increased tendency to develop thromboembolic disease. Most of these deficiencies are treated with fresh-frozen plasma. Newer specific concentrates are becoming available. For example, a factor XIII plasma-derived concentrate is available, and recombinant factor VIIa is approved for use in patients with congenital VII deficiency. Cryoprecipitate, which is rich in fibrinogen, or fibrinogen concentrates (RiaSTAP®), can be used to treat patients with fibrinogen deficiency or dysfunctional fibrinogen (dysfibrinogenemia).

COMPLICATIONS OF REPLACEMENT THERAPY

As discussed previously, transmission of bloodborne infectious diseases is always a concern when blood and blood-derived products are used. Most patients with hemophilia who received plasma-derived products were infected with hepatitis viruses and HIV during the 1980s prompting the development of viral inactivation methods for use during the manufacturing of factor concentrates.[28] All currently available plasma-derived factor concentrates come from screened donors and undergo viral inactivation procedures in an effort to reduce the risk of viral transmission. Heat treatment, which includes dry and wet heat, is one method of viral inactivation. Wet heat is applied while the concentrate is in suspension or in solution (pasteurization) and appears to be more effective than dry heat. Other methods of viral inactivation include chemical (solvent detergent) and affinity chromatography with monoclonal antibodies. Solvent detergent treatment inactivates lipid-coated viruses, such as HIV and hepatitis B and C, but it is not effective against parvovirus

B19, transfusion transmitted virus, hepatitis A, or prions.[5] Parvovirus B19 has been found in both plasma-derived and recombinant factor VIII concentrates (due to the use of albumin as a stabilizer in some recombinant products).[5,14] Parvovirus B19 may be particularly important for patients with hemophilia and HIV infection because it can cause chronic anemia in patients with immune deficiency. Prions are not inactivated by either solvent detergent treatment or by heat, so there is a risk of transmission.[7]

Other complications associated with factor administration include allergic reactions, fever, chills, urticaria, and nausea. PCCs and aPCCs also have the potential to cause thromboembolic complications, including deep-vein thrombosis, pulmonary embolism, myocardial infarction and DIC, likely related to the presence of activated factors.[28] Antifibrinolytic agents should not be given to patients receiving PCCs or aPCCs to avoid thrombotic complications.

Porcine factor VIII, used in the treatment of patients with inhibitors to factor VIII, is not known to transmit human viruses. However, allergic-type reactions (eg, fever, chills, skin rashes, nausea, and headaches) have been reported.[28] Patients who experience these reactions can be treated with steroids and/or diphenhydramine. Thrombocytopenia is another potential complication of porcine factor VIII use.[28]

CONCLUSION

Coagulation disorders, such as hemophilia and vWD, affect a small subset of the overall population, but their treatment can be costly and complicated, requiring knowledgeable healthcare professionals and an interprofessional team approach for optimal outcomes to be achieved. Exciting progress is being made in the development of new strategies for treating these types of disorders. The development of new factor products with improved pharmacokinetic properties as well as the advances in gene therapy may soon redefine the therapeutic landscape for these patients and improve their overall experience.

ABBREVIATIONS

aPCC	activated prothrombin complex concentrate
aPTT	activated partial thromboplastin time
BU	Bethesda unit
ELISA	enzyme-linked immunosorbent assay
HIV	human immunodeficiency virus
ITI	immune tolerance induction
LD-RIPA	low-dose ristocetin-induced platelet agglutination
PCC	prothrombin complex concentrate
PT	prothrombin time
RICE	Rest, Ice, Compression, and Elevation
SIPPET	Survey of Inhibitors in Plasma Product Exposed Toddlers
vWD	von Willebrand disease
vWF:Ag	von Willebrand factor antigen
vWF:RCo	vWF ristocetin cofactor

REFERENCES

1. Srivastava A, Brewer AK, Mauser-Bunschoten EP, et al. Guidelines for the management of hemophilia. *Haemophilia* 2013;19:e1-e47.
2. Valentino LA, Ismael Y, Grygotis M. Novel drugs to treat hemophilia. *Expert Opin Emerg Drugs* 2010;15(4):597-612.
3. Ay C, Thom K, Abu-Hamdeh F, et al. Determinants of factor VIII plasma levels in carriers of hemophilia A and in control women. *Haemophilia* 2010;16:111-117.
4. Weinspach S, Sieperman M, Schaper J, et al. Intracranial hemorrhage in a female leading to the diagnosis of severe hemophilia A and Turner syndrome. *Klin Padiatr* 2009;221:167-171.
5. Lee C, Berntorp E, Hoots W, eds. *Textbook of Hemophilia*, 2nd ed. Chichester, West Sussex, UK: Wiley-Blackwell, 2010.
6. http://www.factorviii-db.org.
7. Benavides S, Nahata MC, eds. *Pediatric Pharmacotherapy*. American College of Clinical Pharmacy, Lenexa, Kansas, USA: 2013.
8. http://www.factorix.org.
9. Kurachi S, Huo JS, Ameri A, et al. An age-related homeostasis mechanism is essential for spontaneous amelioration of hemophilia B Leyden. *Proc Natl Acad Sci USA* 2009;106:7921-7926.
10. Khorana AA, Streiff MB, Farge D, et al. Venous thromboembolism prophylaxis and treatment in cancer: A consensus statement of major guidelines panels and call to action. *J Clin Oncol* 2009;27:4919-4926.
11. Peyvandi F, Garagiola I, Mortarino M. Prenatal diagnosis and preimplantation genetic diagnosis: Novel technologies and state of the art of PGD in different regions of the world. *Haemophilia* 2011;17(Suppl 1):14-17.
12. Tsui NB, Kadir RA, Chan KC, et al. Noninvasive prenatal diagnosis of hemophilia by microfluidics digital PCR analysis of maternal plasma DNA. *Blood* 2011;117:3684-3691.
13. Steele M, Cochrane A, Wakefield C, et al. Hepatitis A and B immunization for individuals with inherited bleeding disorders. *Haemophilia* 2009;15:437-447.
14. Franchini M. The modern treatment of haemophilia: A narrative review. *Blood Transfus* 2012;4:1-6.
15. Berntorp E, Shapiro AD. Modern haemophilia care. *Lancet* 2012;379: 1447-1456.
16. Escobar MA. Advances in the treatment of inherited coagulation disorders. *Haemophilia* 2013;19:648-659.
17. Bensen-Kennedy D. Bringing new therapy options to the hemophilia community. *Thromb Res* 2013;131:S15-S18.
18. Lillicrap D. Improvements in factor concentrates. *Curr Opin Hematol* 2010;17:393-397.
19. Nolan B, Mahlangu J, Perry D, et al. Long-term safety and efficacy of recombinant factor VIII Fc fusion protein (rFVIIIFc) in subjects with hemophilia A. *Haemophilia* 2015;22(1):72-80.
20. Franchini M, Lippi G. Recombinant factor VIII concentrates. *Semin Thromb Hemost* 2010;36:493-497.
21. Jemel A, Siegel R, Ward E, Hao Y, Xu J, Thun MJ. Cancer statistics, 2009. *CA Cancer J Clin* 2009;59:225-249.
22. Micromedex® Healthcare Series. Greenwood Village, CO: Thomson Reuters (Healthcare). Updated November 19, 2014
23. Schulman S. Continuous infusion. *Haemophilia* 2003;9:368-375.
24. Franchini M, Zaffanello M, Lippi G. The use of desmopressin in mild hemophilia A. *Blood Coagul Fibrinolysis* 2010;21:615-619.
25. Franchini M, Frattini F, Crestani S, Bonfanti C. Haemophilia B: Current pharmacotherapy and future directions. *Expert Opin Pharmacother* 2012;13:2053-2063.
26. Gringeri A, Lundin B, von Mackensen S, Mantovani L, Mannucci PM. A randomized clinical trial of prophylaxis in children with hemophilia A (the ESPRIT Study). *J Thromb Haemost* 2011;9:700-710.
27. Blanchette VS. Prophylaxis in the haemophilia population. *Haemophilia* 2010;16(Suppl 5):181-188.
28. Lexicomp Online®, Pediatric & Neonatal Lexi-Drugs®, Hudson, Ohio: Lexi-Comp, Inc.; January 29, 2015.
29. Ponder K. Merry Christmas for patients with hemophilia B. *N Engl J Med* 2011;365:2424-2425.
30. Gouw SC, van den Berg HM. The multifactorial etiology of inhibitor development in hemophilia: Genetics and environment. *Semin Thromb Hemost* 2009;35:723-734.
31. Fulcher CA, de Graaf Mahoney S, Zimmerman TS. FVIII inhibitor IgG subclass and FVIII polypeptide specificity determined by immunoblotting. *Blood* 1987;69:1475-1480.
32. Chambost H. Assessing risk factors: Prevention of inhibitors in haemophilia. *Haemophilia* 2010;16:10-15.
33. Santagostino E, Escobar M, Ozelo M, et al. Recombinant activated factor VII in the treatment of bleeds and for the prevention of surgery-related bleeding in congenital haemophilia with inhibitors. *Blood Rev* 2015(Suppl 1);29:S9-S18.
34. Gringeri A, Fischer K, Karafoulidou A, et al. Sequential combined bypassing therapy is safe and effective in the treatment of unresponsive bleeding in adults and children with haemophilia and inhibitors. *Haemophilia* 2011;17:630-635.
35. Ingerslev J, Sorensen B. Parallel use of by-passing agents in haemophilia with inhibitors: A critical review. *Br J Haematol* 2011; 155:256-262.
36. Coppola A, Margaglione M, Santagostino E, et al. Factor VIII gene (F8) mutations as predictors of outcome in immune tolerance induction of hemophilia A patients with high-responding inhibitors. *J Thromb Haemost* 2009;7:1809-1815.

37. Dimichele D. The North American Immune Tolerance Registry: Contributions to the thirty-year experience with immune tolerance therapy. *Haemophilia* 2009;15:320-328.
38. Hay CR, DiMichele DM. The principal results of the International Immune Tolerance Study: A randomized dose comparison. *Blood* 2012;119:1335-1344.
39. Coppola A, Di Minno MN, Santagostino E. Optimizing management of immune tolerance induction in patients with severe haemophilia A and inhibitors: Towards evidence-based approaches. *Br J Hematol* 2010;150:515-528.
40. Franchini M, Lippi G. Von Wilebrand factor-containing factor VIII concentrates and inhibitors in haemophilia A. *Thromb Haemost* 2010;104:931-940.
41. Leissinger C, Kruse-Jarres R, Granger S, et al. Phase II trial of rituximab in the treatment of inhibitors in congenital hemophilia A: Results of the RICH study. *Blood (ASH Annual Meeting Abstracts)* 2011;118:27.
42. Walsh CE, Batt KM. Hemophilia clinical gene therapy: Brief review. *Transl Res* 2013;161:307-312.
43. Nathwani AC, Tuddenham EG, Rangarajan S, et al. Adenovirus-associated virus vector-mediated gene transfer in hemophilia B. *N Engl J Med* 2011;365:2357-2365.
44. High KA. The gene therapy journey for hemophilia: Are we there yet? *Hematology Am Soc Hematol Educ Program* 2012;2012:375-381.
45. Riley RR, Witkop M, Hellman E, Akins S. Assessment and management of pain in haemophilia patients. *Haemophilia* 2011;17:839-845.
46. Mensah PK, Gooding R. Surgery in patients with inherited bleeding disorders. *Anaesthesia* 2015;70(Suppl 1):112-120.
47. Collins PW. Personalized prophylaxis. *Haemophilia* 2012;18(Suppl 4): 131-135.
48. Howard TE, Yanover C, Mahlangu J, et al. Haemophilia management: Time to get personal? *Haemophilia* 2011;17:721-728.
49. Blomback M, Eikenboom J, Lane D, Denis C, Lillicrap DP. von Willebrand disease biology. *Haemophilia* 2012;18(Suppl 4):141-147.
50. Windyga J, von Depka-Prondzinski M. Efficacy and safety of a new generation von Willebrand factor/factor VIII concentrate (Wilate) in the management of perioperative haemostasis in von Willebrand disease patients undergoing surgery. *Thromb Haemost* 2011;105:1072-1079.
51. DeMeyer SF, Deckmyn H, Vanhoorelbeke K. von Willebrand factor to the rescue. *Blood* 2009;113:5049-5057.
52. Bolton-Maggs PH, Favaloro EJ, Hillarp A, Jennings I, Kohler H. Difficulties and pitfalls in the laboratory diagnosis of bleeding disorders. *Haemophilia* 2012;18(Suppl 4):66-72.
53. Ng C, Motto DG, Di Paola J. Diagnostic approach to von Willebrand disease. *Blood* 2015;125:2029-2037.
54. Kessler CM, Friedman K, Schwartz B, et al. The pharmacokinetic diversity of two von Willebrand factor (VWF)/factor VIII (FVIII) concentrates in subjects with congenital von Willebrand disease. *Thromb Haemost* 2011;106:279-288.
55. Buga-Corbu I, Arion C, Davila C, et al. Up to date concepts about von Willebrand disease and the diagnose of this hemostatic disorder. *J Med Life* 2014;7:327-334.
56. Federici AB, James P. Current management of patients with severe von Willebrand disease type 3: A 2012 update. *Acta Haematol* 2012;128:88-99.
57. Callaghan MU, Wong TE, Federici AB. Treatment of acquired von Willebrand syndrome in childhood. *Blood* 2013;122: 2019-2022.
58. Nichols WL, Rick ME, Ortel TL. Clinical and laboratory diagnosis of von Willebrand disease: A synopsis of the 2008 NHLBI/NIH guidelines. *Am J Hematol* 2009;84:366-370.
59. Laffan MA, Lester W, O'Donnell JS, et al. The diagnosis and management of von Willebrand disease: A United Kingdom Haemophilia Centre Doctors Organization guideline approved by the British Committee for Standards in Haematology. *Br J Haematol* 2014;167:453-465.
60. Peyvandi F, Klamroth R, Carcao M. Management of bleeding disorders in adults. *Haemophilia* 2012;18(Suppl 2):24-36.
61. James AH, Kouides PA, Abdul-Kadir R. Von Willebrand disease and other bleeding disorders in women: Consensus on diagnosis and management from an international expert panel. *Am J Obstet Gynecol* 2009;201:12e1-12e8.
62. Mannucci PM, Kempton C, Millar C, et al. Pharmacokinetics and safety of a novel recombinant human von Willebrand factor manufactured with a plasma-free method: A prospective trial. *Blood* 2013;122:648-657.
63. James P, Salomon O, Mikovic D, et al. Rare bleeding disorders—bleeding assessment tools, laboratory aspects and phenotype and therapy of FXI deficiency. *Haemophilia* 2014;20:71-75.

102

Sickle Cell Disease

C. Y. Jennifer Chan and Melissa Frei-Jones

KEY CONCEPTS

1. Sickle cell disease is an inherited disorder caused by a defect in the gene for β-globin, a component of hemoglobin, and is called a qualitative hemoglobinopathy. Patients can have one defective gene (sickle cell trait) or two defective genes (sickle cell disease).
2. Although sickle cell disease usually occurs in persons of African ancestry, other ethnic groups can be affected. Multiple mutation variants are responsible for differences in clinical manifestations.
3. Sickle cell disease involves multiple organ systems. Usual clinical signs and symptoms include anemia, pain, splenomegaly, and pulmonary symptoms. Sickle cell disease is identified through routine newborn screening programs available in all 50 states. Early diagnosis allows early preventive and comprehensive care.
4. Patients with sickle cell disease are at risk for infection. Prophylaxis against pneumococcal infection reduces death during childhood in children with sickle cell anemia or hemoglobin SS.
5. Hydroxyurea decreases the incidence of painful episodes, but patients treated with hydroxyurea should be carefully monitored.
6. Neurologic complications caused by vasoocclusion can lead to stroke. Screening with transcranial Doppler ultrasound to identify children at risk accompanied by chronic transfusion therapy programs can decrease the risk of overt and silent stroke in children with sickle cell disease.
7. Patients with fever greater than 38.5°C (101.3°F) should be evaluated, and appropriate antibiotics administered immediately, including coverage for encapsulated organisms, especially pneumococcal organisms.
8. Pain episodes can often be managed at home. Hospitalized patients require parenteral analgesics. Analgesic options include opioids, nonsteroidal anti-inflammatory agents, and acetaminophen. The patient characteristics and the severity of the pain should determine the choice of agent and regimen.
9. Patients with sickle cell disease should be followed regularly for healthcare maintenance issues and monitored for changes in organ function.

(1) Sickle cell syndromes, which can be divided into sickle cell trait (SCT) and sickle cell disease (SCD), are a group of hereditary conditions characterized by the presence of sickle cell hemoglobin (HbS) in red blood cells. SCT is the heterozygous inheritance of one normal β-globin gene producing HbA and one sickle gene, producing HbS (HbAS). Individuals with SCT are asymptomatic. SCD can be of homozygous or compounded heterozygous inheritance. Homozygous HbS (HbSS) has historically been referred to as sickle cell anemia (SCA) which now also includes HbSβ^0-thal due to similarities in clinical severity. The heterozygous inheritance of HbS with another qualitative or quantitative β-globin mutation results in sickle cell hemoglobin C (HbSC), sickle cell β-thalassemia (HbSβ^+-thal and HbSβ^0-thal), and some other rare phenotypes.[1,2]

Over the years, progress has been made in understanding the relationship between clinical severity and genotype, as well as the natural history of common morbidities associated with SCD. Ongoing research focuses on pharmacotherapies to treat SCD and prevent organ damage. Recent advances in the care of SCD patients have increased life expectancy. Therefore, the transition from pediatric to adult medical care has become a focus to further improve survival and quality of life.[1-7]

SCD is a chronic illness with significant psychosocial consequences for patients, caregivers and society. Frequent hospitalizations can interrupt schooling and result in employment difficulties.[8-10] Acute complications of the disease can be unpredictable, rapidly progressive, and life threatening. Later in life, chronic organ damage and cognitive or emotional impairment can develop.[1,2,7] Because of the complexity and gravity of the illness, it is essential that comprehensive care is available to all patients and that all providers involved have a good understanding of the disease and its management.[1,2,8,11]

EPIDEMIOLOGY

(2) SCD affects millions of people worldwide and is most common in people with African heritage.[1,12] The most common SCD genotype is HbSS (~60%-65%), followed by HbSC (~25%-30%), HbSβ^+-thal and HbSβ^0-thal (~5%-10%). Other variants account for less than 1% of patients.[1,2] The disease is common among those with ancestors from sub-Saharan Africa, India, Saudi Arabia, and Mediterranean countries.[2,13] In the United States, about 100,000 Americans have SCD with a prevalence of 1 in 2,500 newborns, 1 in 365 African Americans and 1 in 36,000 Hispanic births.[1,14,15] About 2 million Americans have SCT with a prevalence rate of 1 in 13 African Americans and 1 in 100 Hispanics.[15,16]

About 275,000 babies are born with SCD every year with 85% of births in Africa.[2,12] The prevalence of SCD in the region is determined by the frequencies of SCT. The distribution of SCT reflects the survival advantage in regions where malaria is endemic as the gene mutation offers partial protection against serious malarial infection. Red blood cells (RBCs) carrying the abnormal sickle hemoglobin prevent the normal growth and development of *Plasmodium falciparum* within RBCs. Individuals with SCT are more likely to survive acute malarial illness whereas individuals with SCD-HbSS often present with more severe disease. The incidence of the sickle gene in a population correlates with the historical incidence of malaria and SCT results in partial resistance to the disease.[1,2,12,17]

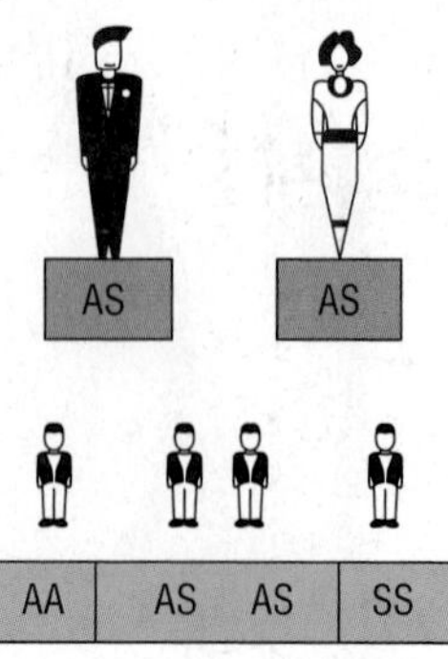

FIGURE 102-1 Sickle cell gene inheritance scheme for both parents with sickle cell trait (SCT). Possibilities with each pregnancy: 25% normal (AA); 50% SCT (AS); 25% sickle cell anemia (SS). (A, normal hemoglobin; S, sickle cell hemoglobin)

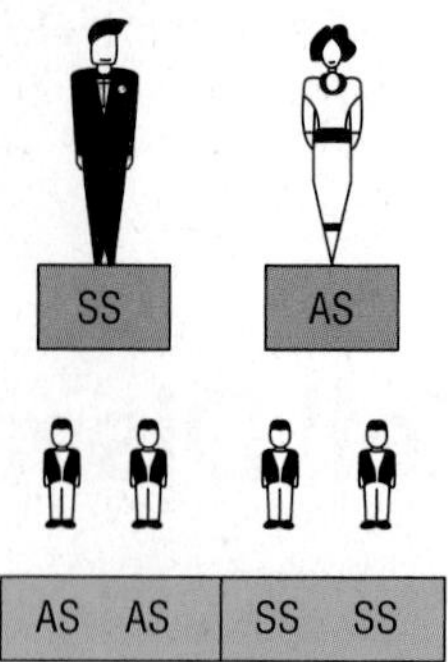

FIGURE 102-3 Sickle cell gene inheritance scheme for one parent with sickle cell trait (SCT) and one parent with sickle cell anemia (SCA). Possibilities with each pregnancy: 50% SCA (SS); 50% SCT (AS). (A, normal hemoglobin; S, sickle cell hemoglobin)

The prevalence of SCD is highest in sub-Saharan Africa. Other areas where the sickle mutation can be found include the Arabian Peninsula, the Indian subcontinent, and the Mediterranean region. Genetic analysis shows that the mutation found in Arabic patients is different from the mutation in those of African descent. SCD gene variants associated with different geographic locations may be responsible for variations in clinical manifestations.[3,5,13]

ETIOLOGY

Normal hemoglobin (hemoglobin A [HbA]) is composed of two α chains and two β chains ($\alpha_2\ \beta_2$). The biochemical defect that leads to the development of HbS involves the substitution of valine for glutamic acid as the sixth amino acid in the β-polypeptide chain. Another abnormal hemoglobin, hemoglobin C (HbC), is produced by the substitution of lysine for glutamic acid as the sixth amino acid in the β-chain. Structurally, the α chains of HbS, HbA, and HbC are identical. Therefore, it is the chemical differences in the β-chain that account for sickling and its related sequelae.[1-3,7]

Homozygous HbSS is the most common form of SCD and occurs when an individual inherits both maternal and paternal β-globin alleles that code for HbS. Figures 102-1 to 102-4 show the probability of inheritance with each pregnancy for the offspring of parents with HbA, SCT, and HbSS. If both parents are carriers, the offspring will have a 25% risk of inheriting SCD and a 50% risk of SCT (see Fig. 102-1). β-Thalassemia is a quantitative hemoglobinopathy resulting from a genetic defect in β-globin production. β-Thalassemia can be co-inherited with HbS and may vary from no β-globin production (β^0) to some β-globin production (β^+). Individuals with HbSS and HbSβ^0-thal have a more severe course than those with HbSC and HbSβ^+-thal and are now both referred to as SCA.[2,7,13]

Several haplotypes characterize the sickle gene, resulting in different clinical and hematologic courses. The three most common haplotypes in the United States are the Bantu haplotype, characterized by severe disease; the Senegal haplotype, characterized by mild disease; and the Benin haplotype, characterized by a course intermediate to that of the other two haplotypes. Although there are a number of other haplotypes seen around the world, the major types outside of the United States include Saudi Arabian and Cameroon, both with milder courses of illness.[2,3,5,7]

PATHOPHYSIOLOGY

Normal adult RBCs contain predominantly HbA (96%-98%). Other forms of hemoglobin are HbA_2 (2%-3%) and fetal hemoglobin (<1%). Normal RBCs are biconcave shape and able to deform to squeeze through capillaries.[1-3,18] Fetal hemoglobin (HbF) is present predominantly in fetal RBCs and is a tetramer of two α-globin chains and two γ-globin chains ($\alpha_2\gamma_2$). Prior to birth, HbF is the predominant hemoglobin type. At around 32 weeks gestation, a switch from the production of γ chains to β chains occurs and consequently, an increase in HbA production is seen. Increased HbF production is seen under severe erythroid stress, such as anemia, post-hematopoietic stem cell transplantation, or chemotherapy or in the hereditary condition, hereditary persistence of fetal hemoglobin (HPFH) where a mutation in the β-globin gene cluster results in continued HbF production after birth. HPFH is a benign, asymptomatic condition.[3,5,19]

In the pathogenesis of SCD, the following are responsible for the various clinical manifestations: impaired circulation, destruction of RBCs, stasis of blood flow and ongoing inflammatory responses. These changes result directly from two major disturbances involving

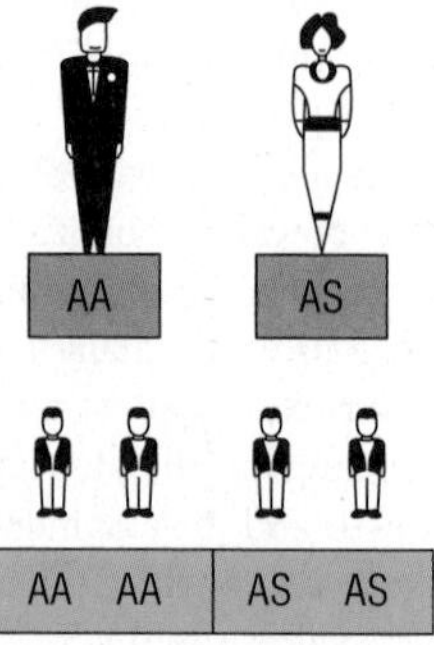

FIGURE 102-2 Sickle cell gene inheritance scheme for one parent with sickle cell trait (SCT) and one parent with no sickle cell gene. Possibilities with each pregnancy: 50% normal (AA); 50% SCT (AS). (A, normal hemoglobin; S, sickle cell hemoglobin)

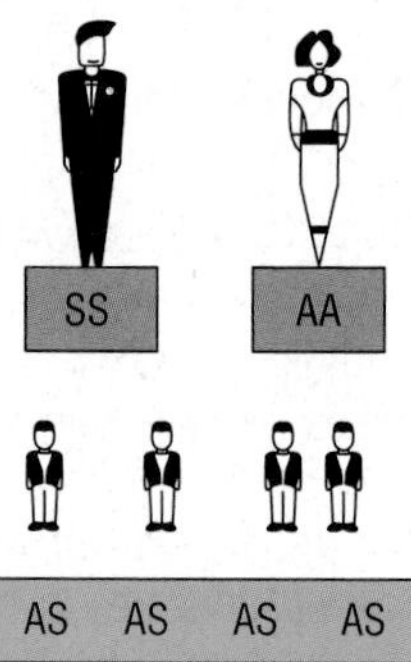

FIGURE 102-4 Sickle cell inheritance scheme for one parent without sickle cell gene and one parent with sickle cell anemia (SCA). Possibilities with each pregnancy: 100% SCT (AS). (A, normal hemoglobin; S, sickle cell hemoglobin)

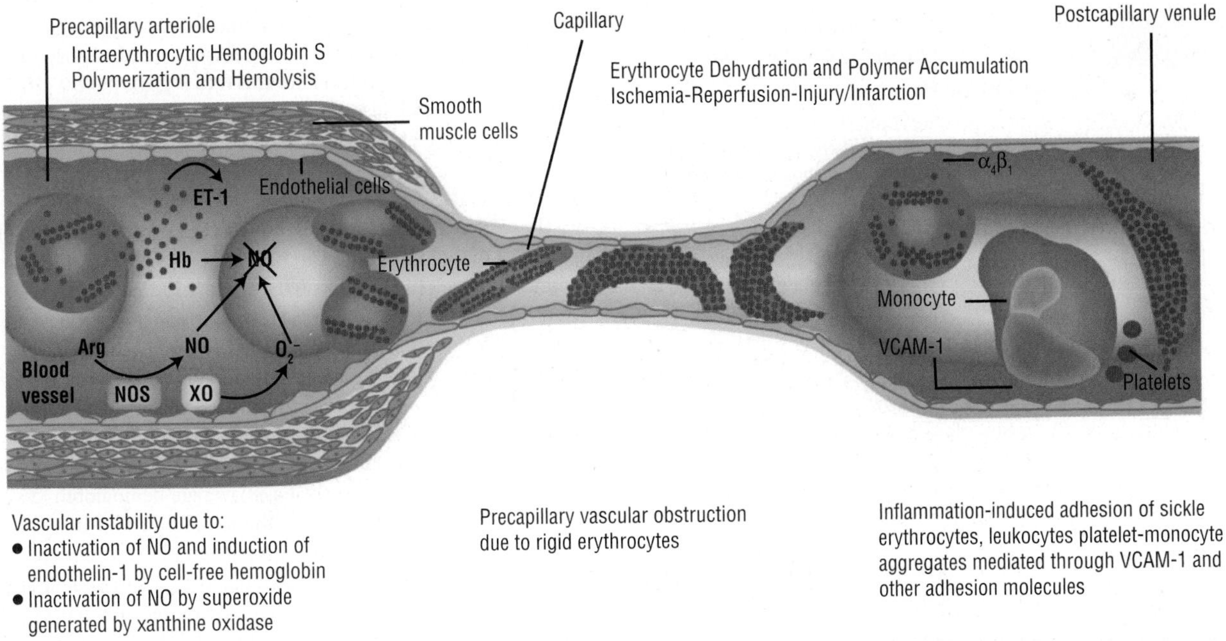

FIGURE 102-5 Pathophysiology of sickle cell disease. (Arg, arginine; ET-1, endothelin-1; Hb, hemoglobin; NO, nitric oxide; NOS, nitrous oxide synthase; VCAM-1, vascular cell adhesion molecule 1; XO, xanthine oxidase.) *(Reproduced with permission from Kato GJ, Gladwin MT. Sickle cell disease. In: Hall JB, Schmidt GA, Wood LDH. Principles of Critical Care, 3rd ed. New York: McGraw-Hill, 2005:1658.)*

RBCs: abnormal hemoglobin polymerization and membrane damage (Fig. 102-5).

The solubilities of HbS and HbA are the same under conditions of normal oxygenation. Because of increased hydrophobicity as a result of the valine substitution, solubility of deoxygenated HbS is reduced. Saturation of deoxy-HbS leads to intermolecular binding and formation of thin bundles of fibers, which initially are unstable. However, the increased binding of deoxy-HbS eventually results in cross-linked fibers and stable polymers. This process is influenced by mean corpuscular hemoglobin concentration (MCHC), temperature, intracellular pH, and the circulating amount of HbS. Polymerization allows deoxygenated hemoglobin molecules to exist as a semisolid gel that protrudes into the cell membrane, leading to distortion of RBCs (sickle shaped) and loss of deformability. The presence of sickled RBCs increases blood viscosity and encourages sludging in the capillaries and postcapillary venules. Such obstructive events lead to local tissue hypoxia, which tends to accentuate the pathologic process.[1,2,6]

When reoxygenated, polymers within the RBCs are lost and the RBCs eventually return to normal shape. This process contributes to the vasoocclusive manifestation in that HbS-containing RBCs are able to enter the microvasculature when oxygenated, but sickle when deoxygenated. The cycle of sickling and unsickling results in damage to the cell membrane, loss of membrane flexibility, and rearrangement of surface phospholipids. Membrane damage also alters ion transport, resulting in potassium and water loss, which can lead to a dehydrated state enhancing the formation of sickled forms. After continual repetitions of the process, the RBC membrane develops into rigid irreversibly sickled cells (ISC). Unlike the reversible sickled cells (RSC), which have normal morphology when oxygenated, ISCs are elongated cells and remain sickled when oxygenated. More rigid membranes of HbS-containing RBCs retard flow, particularly through the microcirculation. In addition, sickled RBCs tend to adhere to vascular endothelial cells, which further increase polymerization and obstruction.[1,2,6]

Intermolecular binding and polymer formation are reduced by HbF and to a lesser degree by HbA_2. RBCs that contain HbF sickle less readily than cells without. ISCs, not surprisingly, have a low HbF level. Increased levels of HbF, as in the case of the Saudi Arabian genotype, result in a more benign form of SCD. The amount of HbF and HbA_2 in relation to HbS influences the clinical manifestations and accounts for some of the variability in severity among SCD genotypes.[2,3,5]

Intravascular destruction of sickle cells can occur at an accelerated rate. The stresses of circulation and repetitive sickle–unsickle cycles lead to cell fragmentation. Damage to the cell membrane promotes cell recognition by macrophages. Rigid ISCs are easily trapped, resulting in short circulatory survival and chronic hemolysis. The typical sickled cell survives for about 10 to 20 days, while the life span of a normal RBC is 120 days.[7] Anemia triggers the release of immature RBCs (reticulocytes) from the bone marrow prematurely. Surface adhesion proteins that maintain the reticulocytes inside the marrow adhere to the endothelium in postcapillary venules further blocking the mature HbS-containing RBCs leading to complete occlusion of microvessels.[6,7]

In addition to sickling, other factors contribute to the clinical manifestations associated with SCD. Sickled cells also interact with leukocytes, endothelial cells, and platelets to form an occlusive clot. Hemolysis releases free hemoglobin resulting in generation of reactive oxygen species, nitric oxide (NO) depletion, and vascular inflammation. Chronic NO depletion contributes to vasoconstriction, activation of platelet, and adhesion molecules such as vascular cell adhesion molecule 1 (VCAM-1) and production of potent vasoconstrictor and endothelin 1 (ET-1).[2,20]

Obstruction of blood flow to the spleen by sickle cells can result in functional asplenia, defined as the loss of splenic function with an intact spleen. These patients can also have deficient opsonization. Impaired splenic function increases susceptibility to infection by encapsulated organisms, particularly pneumococcal bacteria. Coagulation abnormalities in SCD can be the result of continuous activation of the hemostatic system or disorganization of the membrane layer.[2,6,7,20]

CLINICAL PRESENTATION

3 SCD is usually identified on routine newborn screening programs in the United States. Since 2006, universal newborn screening for SCD is performed in all 50 states. The sensitivity and specificity

TABLE 102-1 Clinical Features of Sickle Cell Trait and Common Types of Sickle Cell Disease

Type	Clinical Features
Sickle cell trait (SCT)	Rare painless hematuria; normal Hb level; heavy exercise under extreme conditions can provoke gross hematuria and complications (normal Hb)
Sickle cell anemia (SCA- HbSS)	Pain episodes, microvascular disruption of organs (spleen, liver, bone marrow, kidney, brain, and lung), gallstones, priapism, leg ulcers; anemia (Hb 6-9 g/dL [60-90 g/L; 3.72-5.59 mmol/L])
Sickle cell hemoglobin C (HbSC)	Painless hematuria and rare aseptic necrosis of bone; pain episodes are less common and occur later in life; other complications are ocular disease and pregnancy-related problems; mild anemia (Hb 9-14 g/dL [90-140 g/L; 5.59-8.69 mmol/L])
Sickle cell β^{+}-thalassemia (HbSβ^{+}-thal)	Rare pain; milder severity than HbSS because production of some HbA; Hb 9-12 g/dL (90-120 g/L; 5.59-7.45 mmol/L) with microcytosis
Sickle cell β^{0}-thalassemia (HbSβ^{0}-thal)	No HbA production; severity similar to SCA; Hb 7-9 g/dL (70-90 g/L; 4.34-5.59 mmol/L) with microcytosis

Hb, hemoglobin; HbA, hemoglobin A.

Data from references 1, 2, 13, 14 and 22.

of screening methods such as isoelectric focusing high-performance liquid chromatography and hemoglobin electrophoresis approaches 100%. For infants with a positive screening result, a second test should be performed before 2 months of age to confirm the diagnosis. More than 98% newborns in the United States are screened for SCD to identify the disease. Despite universal screening, some infants with SCD escape identification at birth because of extreme prematurity, prior blood transfusion, or inability to contact family.[2,19,21]

SCD involves multiple organ systems, and its clinical manifestations vary greatly between genotypes (Table 102-1).[1,2,13,22] Persons with SCT are usually asymptomatic and SCT is not considered a disease. However, under certain extreme situations where hemoglobin oxygenation is altered, RBC sickling can occur. Sickling of RBCs in the renal medulla, an area with low-oxygen tension, can result in the inability to concentrate urine. Individuals with such impairment can be at risk of dehydration. Microscopic hematuria has been observed, and gross hematuria can occur after heavy exercise. Other reported complications associated with SCT are venous thromboembolism, particularly pulmonary embolism, renal medullary carcinoma and chronic kidney disease.[14,17] Individuals with SCT should be cautious when participating in exercise under extreme conditions, such as athletic or military training. The US Sudden Death in Athletes Registry reported that 0.9% of 2,462 deaths occurred in athletes with SCT. The events in those 23 athletes with SCT were sudden cardiovascular collapse followed by several minutes of gradually worsening symptoms including dyspnea, fatigue and weakness during or after vigorous physical activity.[23] Preventive strategies such as gradual conditioning, adequate rest and hydration are recommended to minimize risk of sudden death in personnel undergoing athletic or military training.[17,23]

The cardinal features of SCD are hemolytic anemia and vaso-occlusion. In individuals with HbSS, anemia usually develops from 4 to 6 months after birth. The delay is due to the presence of HbF in fetal RBCs. HbF production is gradually replaced by HbS, leading to the clinical manifestations of the disease, such as pain and swelling of the hands and feet, commonly referred to as *hand-and-foot syndrome* or *dactylitis* in infants.[1,2]

The common clinical signs and symptoms associated with HbSS include chronic anemia and pallor; fever; arthralgia; scleral icterus; abdominal pain; weakness; anorexia; fatigue; enlargement of the liver, spleen, and heart; and hematuria. Laboratory findings include low hemoglobin level around 6 to 9 g/dL (60-90 g/L; 3.72-5.59 mmol/L), elevated reticulocytes of 10% to 25%, and elevated platelet and white blood cell (WBC) counts. Mean corpuscular volume (MCV) is normal. The peripheral blood smear demonstrates sickled red cell forms.[1,2,14]

Individuals with HbSC disease present with less severe symptoms than that of HbSS and can be characterized primarily by mild anemia (hemoglobin levels of 9-14 g/dL [90-140 g/L; 5.59-8.69 mmol/L] and reticulocytes of 5%-10%), infrequent episodes of pain, persistence of splenomegaly into adult life, and excessive target cells in the peripheral blood smear. In individuals with heterozygous HbS-β-thalassemia syndrome, severity of disease depends on the thalassemia gene involved.[1,2]

Predictors for severe disease in children have not been established. Dactylitis before 1 year of age, average hemoglobin less than 7 g/dL (70 g/L; 4.34 mmol/L) in the second year of life, and leukocytosis in the absence of infection are markers of disease severity previously described but not validated in a subsequent study.[24] The Cooperative Study of Sickle Cell Disease recently reported that reticulocytosis is associated with increased risk of death and stroke in infants.[25] Early acute chest syndrome during the first 3 years of life is a predictor for recurrent episodes throughout childhood. Children with concomitant SCD and asthma have increased frequencies of acute chest syndrome and pain episodes and increased mortality.[26] Factors associated with decreased survival in adults with SCD include frequency of sickle cell pain, elevated WBC, cerebrovascular events, renal failure, proteinuria and pulmonary hypertension.[26,27] With improved survival for SCD, chronic manifestations of the disease contribute to the increased morbidity later in life.

COMPLICATIONS

Acute Complications

Fever and Infection

Functional asplenia and failure to make antibodies against encapsulated organisms contribute to the high risk of overwhelming sepsis in individuals with SCD. Penicillin prophylaxis and vaccination have significantly reduced the overall risk of *Streptococcus pneumonia* bacteremia, but nonvaccine serotypes of *Streptococcus pneumonia* has been reported.[2] Children with SCD remain at a greater risk of invasive pneumococcal infections when compared to those with other underlying diseases or healthy children.[28] This is not specific to SCD but to the presence of vascular device and is not due to asplenia. Would like to rephrase and move.[29] Other encapsulated organisms are *Haemophilus influenzae, Neisseria meningitidis,* and *Salmonella*, with the latter known to cause osteomyelitis and pneumonia in SCD. *Mycoplasma pneumoniae* and *Chlamydia pneumoniae* should be considered in older children with infiltrates on chest radiograph. Viral infections (eg, influenza and parvovirus B19) can result in severe morbidity.[1,2] In children with SCD admitted for bacteremia, coagulase-negative *Staphylococcus* was associated with central venous access;[29] and should be considered for those with central line placed for chronic transfusion. In adults, overt pneumococcal bacteremia is less common and pathogens such as *Staphylococcus aureus* and gram-negative organisms are associated with immunosuppression, indwelling catheter and bone and joint infections.[30]

All SCD patients with fever greater than 38.5°C (101.3°F) must be evaluated to determine the risk of infection or sepsis; and those with temperature 39.5°C (103.1°F) and appear ill should be hospitalized. Evaluation should include physical examination, complete blood count with reticulocyte count, blood culture, chest radiograph, urinalysis, and urine culture. Lumbar puncture may be

TABLE 102-2 Acute Sickle Cell Complications

Vasoocclusive pain episodes[a]
Clinical features: Acute painful infarction without changes in Hb; almost all patients with SCA will have episodes of acute pain. Recurrent acute pain results in bone, joint, and organ damage and chronic pain. Vasoocclusive episodes most commonly involve the bones, liver, spleen, brain, lungs, and penis. Acute long bone pains can be accompanied by signs of inflammation, making it difficult to differentiate from osteomyelitis. Abdominal involvement can resemble a surgical abdomen. Precipitating factors include infection, extreme weather conditions, dehydration, and stresses.
Signs and symptoms: Deep throbbing pain; local tenderness, erythema, and swelling can be seen. Fever and leukocytosis are common. Dactylitis usually occurs in young infants. Jaundice and increased transaminases can be present if liver is involved.
Evaluation: Frequent physical examination, CBC, reticulocyte count, and urinalysis. Based on symptomatology, the following may be needed: needle aspiration to rule out osteomyelitis, abdominal studies (radiograph, computed tomography scan, etc.), liver function tests, bilirubin, culture, and chest radiograph.
Aplastic crisis[b]
Clinical features: Acute decrease in Hb with decreased reticulocyte count (usually <1%); transient suppression of RBC production in response to bacterial or viral infection, most common being parvovirus B19.
Signs and symptoms: Headache, fatigue, dyspnea, pallor, and tachycardia; can also present with fever, upper respiratory or gastrointestinal infection symptoms.
Evaluation: CBC, reticulocyte count, radiograph, cultures (blood, urine, and throat), evaluation of viral infection (eg, parvovirus titers).
Acute splenic sequestration[c]
Clinical features: Acute exacerbation of anemia due to sequestration of large blood volume by the spleen. More commonly seen in patients with functioning spleens (eg, infants with HbSS and older children and rarely adults with HbSC disease); onset often is associated with viral or bacterial infections; recurrences are common and can be fatal.
Signs and symptoms: Sudden onset of fatigue, dyspnea, and distended abdomen; rapid decrease in Hb and Hct with elevated reticulocyte count, abdominal pain, splenomegaly, vomiting, hypotension, and shock.
Evaluation: Close monitoring of vital signs, spleen size, and oxygen saturation, CBC, reticulocyte count, and cultures.

CBC, complete blood count; Hb, hemoglobin; HbSC, sickle cell hemoglobin C; HbSS, Homozygous; Hct, hematocrit; RBC, red blood cell.

[a]*Data from references 1, 14, 37 and 38.*

[b]*Data from references 1, 2, 14, 22 and 30.*

[c]*Data from references 1, 2, 14, 22 and 39.*

needed, especially in young and toxic-appearing children. Fever in a patient with SCD should be considered a medical emergency with rapid administration of intravenous antibiotics due to risk of overwhelming sepsis.[1,22]

Children with SCD may experience a severe complication due to infection that results in impaired production of RBCs. An aplastic crisis is characterized by a decrease in the reticulocyte count and the rapid development of severe anemia (Table 102-2). The bone marrow becomes hypoplastic and is most often associated with a viral infection, particularly parvovirus B19.[1,2,14]

Neurologic

Neurologic abnormalities and cognitive deficits are well documented in patients with SCD. Vasoocclusive processes can lead to cerebrovascular occlusion that manifests as signs and symptoms of overt stroke, such as headache, paralysis, aphasia, visual disturbances, facial droop and convulsions. The risk of stroke is highest for HbSS and lowest for HbSβ^+-thal. The incidence of cerebral infarct in HbSS is 11% by age 20 years and 24% by age 45 years with a recurrence rate as high as 70% in 3 years. The highest risk occurs during the first decades, in particular ages 2 to 5. The risk is lowest before age 2 secondary to the protective effect of HbF. Ischemic strokes occur in 54% of cerebrovascular accidents with the highest risk before age 10 years and after 30 years of age; whereas hemorrhagic strokes are more common when patients are in their 20s and is associated with poor outcome.[1,2,7,31,32]

In addition to neurologic examination, evaluation of acute events include computed tomography (CT) scan and magnetic resonance imaging (MRI). Asymptomatic or silent infarcts are detected by screening MRI; and transcranial Doppler ultrasound (TCD) is important in primary stroke prevention and is used. In addition, electroencephalography (EEG) can be used if there is a history of seizure.[1,2,22]

About 10% to 30% of SCD who have HbSS with no prior history of stroke have been found to have changes on MRI of the brain consistent with infarction or ischemia. Silent cerebral infarcts can be associated with increased risk of stroke, decreased neurocognitive functions, behavioral changes and poor academic performances. Ongoing intermittent cerebral ischemia episodes have been found in asymptomatic children without concurrent illness.[33] Finally, lower intelligence, visual-motor impairments and neuropsychological dysfunctions have been reported in patients not affected by acute or silent strokes and are associated with severity of anemia.[1,2,31,33]

Acute Chest Syndrome

Acute chest syndrome (ACS) is the second most common cause of hospitalization and responsible for about 25% of deaths among individuals with SCD. ACS is defined as a new pulmonary infiltrate associated with one or more of the following: cough, dyspnea, tachypnea, chest pain, fever, wheezing, and new-onset hypoxia. As many as one-half of individuals with SCD experience at least one episode of ACS.[2,18,34]

Risk factors for ACS and recurrence include young age (peak incidence between age 2 and 4 years), lower HbF, higher leukocytes, history of asthma or bronchial hyper-responsiveness, and smoke exposure. Genotype and haplotype also influence the occurrence. Patients with HbSS and HbSβ^0-thal have higher incidence than those with HbSC and HbSβ^+-thal. The prevalence is higher with African haplotypes than that of Saudi Arabia.[1,18,26]

The primary etiology for ACS is pulmonary vascular occlusion. Infections, fat emboli released from bone marrow or direct adhesion of RBCs to the pulmonary vasculature lead to the inflammation and injury of the lung. The most common cause of ACS is infection. Viral causes are more common in children than adults. Bacteria that cause community acquired pneumonias can be the pathogens, which include *Mycoplasma pneumonia*, *Chlamydia pneumoniae*, and *Streptococcus pneumoniae*.[2,18,34]

ACS is more common in children but more severe in adults. Hypoxia is a predictor for severity and outcome. In addition to physical examinations, evaluations may include complete blood count and chest radiographs. In severe cases, CT scan, perfusion scintigraphy, transthoracic echocardiography and bronchoscopy may also be considered to exclude other etiologies. Pulmonary changes often involve the lower lobes of the lungs and may cause pleural effusions. Bilateral infiltrates or multiple lobe involvement may be an indication of poor prognosis.[2,18,26] Pulmonary manifestations must be recognized early and managed aggressively as ACS can rapidly progress to pulmonary failure and death.[26]

Priapism

Stasis and sickling of RBCs within the sinusoids of the corpora cavernosa is the primary mechanism of priapism, a sustained painful erection. In recent years, a better understanding of pathophysiology of priapism has identified other mechanisms at molecular level, such as abnormal NO signaling as result of chronic NO depletion. Stuttering priapism is repeated intermittent attacks up to several hours before remission; ischemic priapism is a persistent painful erection greater than 4 hours and should be considered as an emergency. Thirty percent to 45% of males with SCD will present with at least one episode of priapism during their lifetime and the first episodes often occur during childhood. Impotence has been reported after repeated episodes and is directly related to the duration prior to treatment.[1,35,36]

Sickle Cell Pain

Acute episodes of pain are the most common symptoms and reason for seeking treatment in SCD. Sickle cell pain may be caused by bone or muscle infarction due to vasoocclusion (see Table 102-2). Although fever, infections, dehydration, hypoxia, acidosis, and sudden temperature alterations can precipitate pain, multiple factors often contribute to its development.[2,37,38] The back, chest and extremities are the most common locations of pain but pain can occur in any location such as abdomen or head and lead to confusion with other acute complications such as stroke.[1,22]

Individuals with HbSS experience more frequent episodes of pain than those with HbSC or other variants. Risk factors associated with painful episodes include older age, iron overload, higher Hb and lower HbF.[1,2,14,38] Biomarkers for severity of pain during vasoocclusion episodes include elevated C-reactive protein and lactate dehydrogenase (LDH).[4] Dactylitis (hand-and-foot syndrome) is a subtype of sickle cell pain, occurring in infancy and early childhood and is characterized by redness and swelling of the dorsal aspects of the hands, feet, fingers, and toes. The episodes are painful but usually do not result in permanent damage.[1,2]

Splenic Sequestration

Splenic sequestration is the sudden massive enlargement of the spleen resulting from the sequestration of sickled RBCs in the splenic parenchyma (see Table 102-2). Hematocrit and hemoglobin concentrations dramatically fall, with reticulocytosis and no evidence of marrow failure or accelerated hemolysis. The trapping of the sickled RBCs by the spleen also leads to a decrease in circulating blood volume, which can result in hypotension and shock. The condition is most often seen in infants and children because their spleens are intact, and can cause sudden death in young children. Splenic enlargement may also be acutely painful due to rapid capsular expansion. Over time, repeated splenic infarctions lead to autosplenectomy and the spleen can no longer become engorged. Sequestration usually occurs between one to 4 years of age and is uncommon beyond 5 year for children with HbSS and HbSβ^0-thal because autoinfarction usually is completed by then. For HbSC and HbSβ^+-thal, autoinfarction is delayed and sequestration can occur even during adulthood.[1,2,22,39]

Chronic Complications

Pulmonary

Over 90% of children survive into adulthood, increasing the contribution of pulmonary manifestations to the morbidity and mortality of SCD. Physical exam and history should be performed to identify signs and symptoms of respiratory conditions such as asthma, restrictive lung disease and chronic obstructive pulmonary disease. Pulmonary function testing is recommended to determine the cause in symptomatic patients but not as a routine screening tool.

Pulmonary hypertension, defined as a resting mean pulmonary arterial pressure (PAP) 25 mmHg or greater by right heart catheterization, is associated with increased morbidity and mortality in SCD. Symptoms of pulmonary hypertension include shortness of breath during normal activities, fatigue, syncope, and peripheral edema. A less invasive test, tricuspid regurgitant jet velocity by Doppler echocardiography, is frequently performed initially to estimate PAP. Serum NT-pro-BNP measurement is an alternative test that can be used in patients with normal renal function when Doppler echocardiography is not an option. The American Thoracic Society recommends assessment of mortality risk using noninvasive (indirect) or invasive direct measurement to guide management of pulmonary hypertension (Table 102-3).[22,26,40,41]

The prevalence of asthma in children with SCD is similar to that of general population. Symptoms of asthma exacerbation can overlap with ACS making it difficult to differentiate the two. Asthma and wheezing in individuals with SCD have been associated with ACS and vasoocclusive pain episodes and increased mortality. Early screening for asthma and other signs of respiratory conditions has been recommended.[1,22] In general, the national asthma education and prevention program asthma management guideline should be utilized in the management of asthma in children with SCD. Inhaled corticosteroids are first line for persistent symptoms.[42]

Skeletal and Skin Diseases

Bone diseases are common in SCD and vitamin D level has been suggested to be the biomarker.[4] Osteonecrosis, particularly of the femoral or humeral heads, causes permanent damage and disability.[14,22,43,44] Low bone mineral density can occur early with a prevalence of over 70% reported in adults with SCD.[43] Osteopenia and osteoporosis associated with low bone formation has been reported in both males and females with SCD.[43,44] Children with SCD also have an increased incidence of osteomyelitis; the organism most

TABLE 102-3 Risk Stratification and Management Recommendation for Pulmonary Hypertension

	Recommendations	Strength	Evidence Quality
Increased risk for mortality[a]	Hydroxyurea	Strong	Moderate
Increased risk for mortality, unresponsive or not candidates for hydroxyurea	Chronic transfusion therapy	Weak	Low
RHC-confirmed PH, venous thromboembolism, no risk factors for hemorrhage	Indefinite anticoagulant therapy	Weak	Low
Elevated TRV alone Elevated NT-pro-BNP alone	No PAH therapy[b]	Strong	Moderate
RHC-confirmed marked elevation of pulmonary vascular resistance, normal pulmonary artery wedge pressure, presence of related symptoms	• A trial of prostacyclin agonist or endothelin receptor antagonist	Weak	Very low
	• Phosphodiesterase-5 inhibitor should not be used as first-line therapy	Moderate	Moderate

[a]Increased risk for mortality: (1) Tricuspid regurgitant jet velocity (TRV) greater than or equal to 2.5 m/s, (2) an N-terminal pro-brain natriuretic peptide (NT-pro-BNP) level greater than or equal to 16 pg/mL (ng/L; 1.9 pmol/L) or (3) right heart catheterization (RHC)-confirmed pulmonary hypertension (PH).

[b]PAH therapy: (1) prostacyclin agonist (epoprostenol, treprostinil, iloprost), (2) soluble guanylate cyclase stimulator (riociguat), (3) endothelin receptor antagonist (bosentan, macitentan, ambrisentan), (4) phosphodiesterase-5 inhibitor (sildenafil, vardenafil, tadalafil).

Data from references 40 and 41.

often responsible is *Salmonella*.[30,44] In addition to necrosis of joints, chronic leg ulcers most commonly seen in the medial and lateral malleolus (ankles) can become a difficult and painful problem for adult. Ulcers are often seen after trauma or infection and are usually slow to heal.[22]

Ocular Manifestations

Ocular problems seen in patients with SCD include transient monocular blindness, visual field defects from retinal hemorrhage, retinal detachment, vitreous hemorrhage, venous microaneurysms, and neovascularization. The incidence of proliferative sickle retinopathy and vitreous hemorrhage is up to 50%. Vasoocclusion in the eye can occur as early as 20 months of age, and clinically detectable retinal diseases usually occur during adolescence and early adulthood. Despite the less systemic manifestations, individuals with HbSC develop serious retinal complications more often and earlier than those with HbSS. Annual retinal examination is recommended for patients with SCD to prevent blindness from retinopathy and other complications.[22,45]

Hepatobiliary Diseases

Cholelithiasis is a common complication of SCD resulting from chronic hemolysis and increased bilirubin production, and leading to biliary sludge and/or stone formation. The risk of gallstones increases with age: 12% for age 2 to 4 years, 43% by age 15 to 18 years and 70% to 75% in adults. Cholecystitis, exemplified by pain in the right upper quadrant, can be confused with an acute sickle pain episode in the abdomen. Mild baseline hepatomegaly and elevation of lever function tests are found in individuals with SCD. Cirrhosis occurred in 18% of young adults with SCD. Causes for development of chronic hepatic disease include repeated occlusion in the liver, iron overload, and hepatitis.[22,46]

Cardiac Diseases

Cardiovascular complications associated with anemia, including cardiac enlargement and various murmurs, can occur in patients with SCD. Patients experience various degrees of exertional dyspnea, tachycardia, and palpitation because of the decreased oxygen-carrying capacity of the blood. Left ventricular diastolic dysfunction has been reported in 18% of adults with SCD and is associated with increased mortality, especially in patients with pulmonary hypertension. Left ventricular stiffness and left ventricular hypertrophy have been reported, and the progression is speculated to lead to diastolic dysfunction later in life. Acute myocardial infarction in adults with SCD may be under-recognized due to the high incidence of sickle cell acute chest pain.[7,47,48]

Renal Diseases

Renal dysfunction in SCD begins during infancy as evidenced by glomerular hyperfiltration. Other manifestations include inability to concentrate urine, hematuria, tubular acidosis, papillary necrosis, glomerulonephritis, microalbuminuria, and proteinuria. Enuresis, as a result of increased urine production, occurs in 42% of children ages 6 to 8 and 9% in young adults age 18 to 20. Microalbuminuria is typically the first sign of chronic kidney disease, which has been associated with increased mortality.[22,49,50]

Growth and Development

Delayed growth and sexual maturation are common in patients with SCD. Despite normal birth weight and length, growth retardation occurs between 6 months and 4 years with height, weight and bone mass index being affected. The poor growth cannot be explained by nutritional factors alone. Alternations in growth factors as well as increased metabolic rate are factors contributing to the growth failure. Pubertal delay by 1 to 2 years is common in adolescents with SCD and fertility problems have been reported in both men and women with SCD.[14,51-53]

Psychiatric

Depression and anxiety are more common in children and adults with SCD than in the general population and have a significant impact on quality of life.[54,55] Depression is associated with pain episodes in children with SCD. In addition, depression is associated with social support for parents as well as individuals with SCD.[54] DSM-IV psychiatric diagnoses in adolescents with SCD include attention-deficit-hyperactivity, oppositional defiant, conduct, major depressive and anxiety disorders.[56]

Pregnancy

Pregnancy introduces an increased risk for the mother with SCD and for the fetus. Some women experience increased pain episodes during pregnancy and the anemia of SCD can lead to intrauterine growth retardation. Preterm labor and premature delivery are common in mothers with SCD, and the risk of spontaneous abortion is increased. The incidence of cesarean delivery and pregnancy-related complications are higher when compared to mothers who do not have SCD.[22,57,58]

TREATMENT

Desired Outcomes

The goal of treatment is to reduce hospitalizations, complications, and mortality. Treatment for SCD involves the use of general measures to meet the unique demands for increased erythropoiesis. Additional interventions can be aimed at preventing or treating complications of the disease. When an acute complication occurs, the type and severity of the episode determines the appropriate therapeutic plan.

With availability of public health programs and comprehensive care, most children in developed countries survive through childhood.[2,14] The median survival rate is estimated to be 42 years for males and 48 years for females for HbSS, and 60 years for males and 68 years for females for HbSC.[12,59] With increased life expectancy, outcome evaluation for management of SCD therefore should include assessment of health-related quality of care in both adults and children.

Patients with SCD require lifelong multidisciplinary care. All patients with SCD should receive regularly scheduled comprehensive medical evaluations. Because of the complexity of the disease, a multidisciplinary team is needed to provide high quality medical care, education, counseling, and psychosocial support. Appropriate comprehensive care can have a positive impact on both longevity and quality of life. This care includes the use of evidence based treatment combining general symptomatic supportive care, preventative medical therapies and specific disease modifying therapies aimed at altering hematologic capacity and function.

Routine Health Maintenance

SCD is a complex chronic disease involving multiple organs. In addition to the preventive care recommended for the general population, individuals with SCD also need health maintenance and screenings that are focused on minimizing complications from the disease (Table 102-4).

Immunizations

Administration of routine immunizations is crucial preventive care in managing SCD. Children 6 months and older and adults with SCD should receive influenza vaccine annually. The most updated immunization and catch-up schedules are provided by the Centers for Disease Control and Prevention (http://www.cdc.gov/vaccines/schedules.)

TABLE 102-4 Health Maintenance

Invasive Pneumococcal Infection Prevention[a]

1. Oral penicillin until age 5 for children with HbSS
    a. Discontinue penicillin prophylaxis at age 5 unless have had splenectomy or invasive pneumococcal infection
2. Consider no penicillin prophylaxis for children with HbSC disease and HbS—thal unless they have had a splenectomy

Immunization[b]

1. All individuals should receive immunization according to The Advisory Committee on Immunization Practices
2. Pneumococcal Vaccine
    a. All infants should receive complete series of PCV13.
    b. All children should receive PPSV23 at age 2 years and second dose at age 5 years.
    c. Children age 6-18 years with functional or anatomic asplenia should receive 1 dose of PCV13.
    d. Adults (age ≥ 19 years) with functional or anatomic asplenia.
        i. Not previously received PCV13 or PPSV23
            1. One dose PCV13; followed by PPSV23 at least 8 weeks later
        ii. Previously received PPSV23
            1. One dose PCV13 at least 1 year after last PPSV23
        iii. For individual age 19-64 years, a second dose of PPSV23 should be 5 years after first dose and no sooner than 8 weeks after PCV13
3. Haemophilus Influenza (Hib) Vaccine
    a. Children age greater than 5 years who have not previously received Hib vaccine should receive one dose
4. Meningococcal Vaccine (indicated for persons have functional or anatomic asplenia)
    a. 4-dose primary series to be administered with Hib-MenCY-TT (2, 4, 6, and 12-15 months) or MenACWY-CRM (2, 4, 6, and 12 months)
    b. Booster dose to be administered with MenACWY-CRM or MenACWY-D
        i. Primary series completed prior to age 7: booster dose 3 years after primary series and repeat every 5 years thereafter
        ii. Primary series completed age 7 or older: booster dose 5 years after primary series and repeat every 5 years thereafter
    c. Unvaccinated children 7-23 months: 2 doses of MenACWY-CRM with second dose at least 12 weeks after the first dose AND after first birthday
    d. Unvaccinated children age 2 years or older and adults: 2 doses of MenACWY-CRM or MenACWY-D 8-12 weeks apart
        i. MenACWY-D to be given at least 4 weeks after completion of all PCV13 doses
    e. Adults previously vaccinated should receive MenACWY-CRM or MenACWY-D every 5 years
5. Influenza vaccine annually for age ≥ 6 months

Renal[c]

1. Screen for proteinuria by age 10 and annually if negative
2. Initiate ACE inhibitor for adults with microalbuminuria or proteinuria without apparent cause

Pulmonary Hypertension (PH)[d]

1. Noninvasive tests (Doppler echocardiography or alternatively, serum NT-pro-BNP measurement) can be used to assess mortality risk
2. Echocardiogram to screen for PH and associated cardiac problems by age 8 for those with frequent cardiorespiratory symptoms
3. The optimal frequency for Doppler echocardiography is unknown but every 1-3 years seems to be reasonable
4. Children with evidence of PH by echocardiogram should be further evaluated: pulmonary function test, polysomnography, oxygenation assessment and thromboembolic disease
5. Cardiac catheterization should be performed before initiation of PAH-specific therapy

Ophthalmological Evaluation[c]

1. Eye examination begins at age 10 and rescreen at 1-2 year intervals

Stroke Prevention[c]

1. Children with SCA: transcranial Doppler (TCD) annually beginning at age 2 until at least age 16
2. Chronic transfusion therapy for stroke prevention in children with elevated (>200 cm/s) TCD results

PCV13, 13-valent conjugate pneumococcal vaccine; PPSV23, 23-valent pneumococcal polysaccharide vaccine; ACE Inhibitor, angiotensin converting enzyme inhibitor; NT-pro-BNP, N-terminal pro-brain natriuretic peptide; PAH, pulmonary artery hypertension; PH, pulmonary hypertension.

[a]*Data from references 2, 22 and 24.*

[b]*Data from references 60-63.*

[c]*Data from reference 22.*

[d]*Data from references 40 and 41.*

Impaired splenic function increases susceptibility to infection by encapsulated organisms, particularly *S. pneumoniae*. Prior to the routine use of penicillin prophylaxis and the development of pneumococcal vaccines, invasive pneumococcal disease was 20- to 100-fold more common in children with SCD than in healthy children. Reduced mortality has been associated with the introduction of pneumococcal vaccines.[2,30]

Two different pneumococcal vaccines are available. The 13-valent pneumococcal conjugate vaccine (PCV13; Prevnar®) induces good antibody responses in infants and children less than 2 years of age. Immunization with the PCV13 is recommended for all children, regardless of SCD status, younger than 24 months of age. Infants should receive the first dose after 6 weeks of age. Two additional doses should be given at 2-month intervals, followed by a fourth dose at age 12 to 15 months. One dose of PCV13 should be given to children age 6 to 18 years and adults with functional or anatomic asplenia (see Table 102-4). The 23-valent pneumococcal polysaccharide vaccine (PPSV23; Pneumovax®23) is recommended for all children with functional or acquired asplenia but must be given after 2 years of age because of poor antibody response. To cover different serotypes, PPSV23 should be given starting at 2 years of age, and be administered 2 months after the last dose of the PCV13. A booster dose of PPSV23 is recommended 5 years after the first dose.[22,60,61]

The risk of meningococcal disease is also higher in SCD and vaccination is recommended for individuals with functional or acquired asplenia. Three different meningococcal vaccines are available: Meningococcal groups C and Y and *Haemophilus* b tetanus toxoid conjugate vaccine (Hib-MenCY-TT), and quadrivalent (serogroups A, C, Y, and W-135) meningococcal conjugate vaccines, MenACWY-CRM and MenACWY-D. Infants with functional asplenia should receive 4-dose series with Hib-MenCY-TT at 2, 4, 6, and 12 through 15 months or MenACWY-CRM at 2, 4, 6, and 12 months. If the first dose of Hib-MenCY-TT is given at or after 12 months of age, 2 doses should be given at least 8 weeks apart. Children over 2 years and adults with functional or acquired asplenia should receive a primary immunization series with two doses of the quadrivalent vaccine given 8 weeks apart. MenACWY-D should be given at age 2 years or older and at least 4 weeks after completion of all PCV13. A booster is recommended every 5 years for individuals with SCD.[22,62,63]

Penicillin

4 Penicillin prophylaxis until at least 5 years of age is recommended in children with SCD HbSS or HbSβ^0-thal, even if they have received PCV13 or PPSV23 immunization, as prophylaxis against invasive pneumococcal infections. An effective regimen that reduces the risk of pneumococcal infections by 84% is penicillin V potassium at a dosage of 125 mg orally twice daily until the age of 3 years, followed by 250 mg twice daily until the age of 5 years. Individuals who are allergic to penicillin can be given erythromycin 20 mg/kg per day. Penicillin prophylaxis is not routinely given in older children, based on a study demonstrating no benefit over placebo beyond the age of 5 years. However, continuation of oral pneumococcal prophylaxis should be considered on a case-by-case basis, and is recommended for anyone with a history of invasive pneumococcal infection or surgical splenectomy.[22,24]

Clinical **Controversy...**

The need for routine penicillin prophylaxis in HbSC and HbSβ^+-thal patients is controversial because these patients have less severe disease. The original trial showing decreased morbidity from invasive infection included children with HbSS or SCA. But some clinicians recommend that children with any genotype should start penicillin prophylaxis as severe and fatal pneumococcal infections can occur with HbSC and HbSβ^+-thal.

Fetal Hemoglobin Inducers

HbF reduces polymer formation of HbS due to its high-oxygen affinity. Increased HbF levels significantly correlate with decreased RBC sickling and RBC adhesion and observational studies show a relationship between HbF concentration and severity of SCD. Individuals with SCD and low HbF levels experience more frequent pain and higher mortality. HbF levels of 20% or greater reduce the risk of acute sickle cell complications. Based on these observations, HbF induction has become a treatment modality for patients with SCD.

Hydroxyurea

Hydroxyurea (HU), a chemotherapeutic agent, stimulates HbF production and increases the number of HbF-containing reticulocytes and intracellular HbF. The antineoplastic activity of HU is related to inhibition of DNA synthesis by blocking the conversion of ribonucleoside to deoxyribonucleotides. The exact mechanism of HbF production is unknown, but is postulated that the cytotoxic effect in the bone marrow stimulates stress erythropoiesis and triggers rapid erythroid regeneration and shifts erythrocyte hemoglobin production to HbF. In addition, HU increases NO levels, reduces neutrophils and monocytes, has antioxidant properties, alters the RBC membrane, increases RBC deformability by increasing intracellular water content, and decreases RBC adhesion to the endothelium.[1,22,24]

HU can decrease the frequency of acute sickle cell pain and is FDA approved for adults with SCD based on the results of the Multicenter Study of Hydroxyurea in Sickle Cell Anemia (MSH Trial), a double-blind, placebo-controlled randomized controlled trial. In that study, HU significantly reduced the frequency of painful episodes, risk of ACS, need for blood transfusions, and number of hospitalizations. The incidence of death, stroke, and hepatic sequestration in the HU and placebo groups was not significantly different during the evaluation period. However, a follow-up study showed a 40% reduction in mortality with HU over a 9-year period. The original 299 patients from the MSH study were followed for 17.5 years and the results suggest improved survival with the long-term use of HU.[2,7,64,65]

Studies in pediatric patients have demonstrated similar results to the MSH Trial with no adverse effects on growth and development. In addition, some patients treated with HU therapy had possible recovery or preservation of splenic and brain functions, including cognitive performances. The Transcranial Doppler with Transfusions Converting to Hydroxyurea study (TWiTCH) closed early after interim analysis found that HU was not inferior to chronic blood transfusions to prevent primary stroke. However, the Stroke with Transfusions Changing to Hydroxyurea (SWiTCH) trial also closed early when the interim analysis showed that HU was inferior to chronic transfusions to prevent recurrent stroke. Therefore, chronic transfusions with iron chelation remain the best therapy to prevent stroke.[2,7,24] Initiating HU early and prior to development of complications may be beneficial. The Pediatric HU Phase III Clinical Trial (BABY HUG) evaluated HU therapy in young children ages 9 to 18 months.[66] Infants were randomized between HU and a placebo; the primary endpoints were splenic and renal function. Investigators found no significant difference in the primary endpoints but did find fewer episodes of pain and dactylitis with no significant toxicities. HU reduced the risk of painful events, ACS, renal enlargement, hospitalizations, and transfusions. In addition, improved urine concentration ability as demonstrated by higher urine osmolality was reported.[66-68] In a retrospective study of children aged 3 to 18 years with SCD, significant reduction in mortality, fewer hospitalizations and emergency visits and shorter admissions were reported.[69]

The most common adverse effect of HU is bone marrow suppression, resulting in neutropenia, thrombocytopenia, anemia, and decreased reticulocyte count. These hematologic adverse effects usually recover within 2 weeks of therapy discontinuation. Other side effects include dry skin and hyperpigmentation of skin or nails.[2,67,68,70] Long-term adverse effects of HU therapy in patients with SCD are not fully known although no serious adverse effects were reported in the long term (17.5 years) follow-up study of the MSH trial.[65] Studies in children have not demonstrated delays in growth or puberty, increased risk of infections or genotoxicity.[70,71] Myelodysplasia, acute leukemia, and chronic opportunistic infection associated with T-lymphocyte abnormalities have been reported in other patient populations treated with higher doses of HU. Reproductive toxicity is also a concern. High-dose HU has been shown to be teratogenic in animals, but normal pregnancies have been reported in women with SCD who received HU during pregnancy.[53]

Although HU is only FDA approved for adults with SCD, the National Institutes of Health (NIH) has supported its use in children and adolescents (Table 102-5).[22] Clinical indications for HU include frequent painful episodes, severe symptomatic anemia, a history of ACS, or other severe vasoocclusive complications. The starting dose for adult is 15 mg/kg per day rounded to the nearest 500 mg as a single daily dose (Fig. 102-6). A lower dose of 5 to 10 mg/kg per day is used for patients with chronic disease. The Baby HUG study found that children can be safely started at 20 mg/kg. Dosage can be increased by 5 mg/kg up to a maximum of 35 mg/kg in 8 week intervals if the patient does not demonstrate significant adverse effects and blood counts are stable. HU dosage should be individualized based on response and toxicity. In general, 3 to 6 months of therapy are required before improvement is observed. Medication adherence can be an issue. Since the MCV generally increases as the level of HbF increases, monitoring MCV is an inexpensive and convenient method to monitor response and adherence.[2,22,66,72]

5 Patients receiving HU should be closely monitored for toxicity. Blood counts should be checked every 4 weeks during dose titration and every 8 weeks thereafter. Treatment should be interrupted if hematologic indices fall below the following values: absolute neutrophil count, 2,000 cells/mm^3 (2×10^9/L); platelet count,

TABLE 102-5 Recommendations on Hydroxyurea Therapy

	Recommendation	Strength	Evidence Quality
Adults with HbSS or Sβ⁰-thalassemia			
1. Three or more sickle cell associated moderate to severe pain crises per year	Treat with hydroxyurea	Strong	High
2. Sickle cell associated pain that interferes with daily activities and quality of life		Strong	Moderate
3. History of severe and/or recurrent ACS		Strong	Moderate
4. Severe symptomatic chronic anemia that interferes with daily activities or quality of life		Strong	Moderate
Infants 9 months of age and older, children, and adolescents with HbSS or Sβ⁰-thalassemia regardless clinical severity	Offer hydroxyurea	Strong	High (age 9-42 months); Moderate (>42 months)
Chronic kidney disease and taking erythropoietin	Hydroxyurea can be added	Weak	Low
HbSC or HbSβ⁺-thalassemia with recurrent sickle cell associated pain that interferes with daily activities or quality of life	Consider hydroxyurea	Moderate	Low
History of stroke and unable to implement chronic transfusion	Initiate hydroxyurea	Moderate	Low

Data from references 22 and 64.

80,000 cells/mm^3 (80 × 10^9/L); hemoglobin, 5 g/dL (50 g/L; 3.1 mmol/L); or reticulocytes, 80,000 cells/mm^3 (80 × 10^9/L) if the hemoglobin concentration is less than 9 g/dL (90 g/L; 5.59 mmol/L). Other laboratory abnormalities warranting temporary discontinuation of therapy are a 50% increase in serum creatinine and a 100% increase in transaminases. After recovery has occurred, treatment should be resumed at a dose that is 5 mg/kg per day lower than the dose associated with toxicity. If no toxicity occurs after 12 weeks with the lower dose, the dose can be increased by 2.5 to 5 mg/kg per day. If the increased dose produces hematologic toxicity, the patient should be maintained at the last tolerated dose with no further escalation except for normal growth or weight gain.[22,64,72]

Chronic Transfusion Therapy

RBC transfusions play an important role in the management of SCD. In acute illness, transfusions can be life saving and the guidelines for acute transfusion are discussed in a later section. Chronic transfusion programs can prevent serious complications of SCD. The primary indication for chronic transfusion is primary and secondary stroke prevention and amelioration of organ damage.[1,2,73] Blood transfusions can be administered as a simple transfusion, a manual exchange or an automated exchange called erythrocytapheresis. Exchange transfusion frequently requires permanent venous access and is associated with higher cost but has the advantage of increasing normal (donor) HbA, limiting volume, minimizing hyperviscosity and transfusional iron overload.[22]

6 In children with an overt stroke, chronic transfusions are used as secondary stroke prevention and reduce stroke recurrence from about 50% to about 10% over 3 years. An initial stroke in SCD can be devastating and transfusions can be given for primary stroke prevention. Prophylactic transfusions significantly reduced the incidence of first stroke over a 2-year period in children 2 to 16 years of age who were at an increased risk for stroke based on TCD. The risk of stroke was reduced from 16% in patients receiving usual care to 2% in those who received prophylactic transfusions.[1,4,73] Chronic transfusions should be considered in selected children and adults with previous stroke or children with abnormal TCD measurements.[22] Chronic transfusions have also been used in patients with severe or recurrent ACS, debilitating pain, splenic sequestration, recurrent priapism, chronic organ failure, intractable leg ulcers, severe chronic anemia with cardiac failure, and complicated pregnancies, although data supporting the efficacy of chronic transfusion in these situations are limited.[1,74]

The goal of transfusions is to achieve and maintain an HbS concentration of less than 30% of total hemoglobin in the primary and secondary prevention of neurologic complications. Transfusions are usually given every 3 to 4 weeks, but the frequency of transfusion is adjusted to maintain the desired HbS levels. The risk of recurrent stroke decreases after 2 years of transfusion therapy and, in the absence of recurrent stroke, many clinicians will liberalize the HbS goal to less than 50%.[2,14] The optimal duration of primary prophylactic transfusion therapy in children with abnormal TCD is not clear, but discontinuation of transfusions has been associated with a 50% stroke recurrence rate within 12 months and abnormal blood flow velocity on TCD in children with SCD. The results of the TWiTCH trial suggest that some patients can safely transition to HU therapy after normalization of TCD and no evidence of cerebral vasculopathy with at least a 6-month overlap in transfusions and HU therapy. For secondary stroke prevention, transfusions should be continued indefinitely.[2,14,73] A pilot study suggested that HU could be started prior to discontinuation of transfusion for secondary stroke prevention with at least a 6-month overlap with transfusions. However, the phase III trial of switching HU for transfusion in secondary stroke prevention, the SWiTCH trial, was closed early due to an increased risk of recurrent strokes in the HU arm when compared to the transfusions arm.[14,31] The NIH recommends HU for prevention of recurrent stroke only if implementation of a transfusion program is not possible.[22]

Although the benefits of transfusion therapy are clear in some clinical situations, its role in other situations such as an acute pain episode remains controversial.[22] The risks of transfusion therapy must be weighed against possible benefits. The risks associated with transfusion therapy include alloimmunization (sensitization to the blood received), hyperviscosity, viral transmission, volume overload, iron overload, and nonhemolytic transfusion reactions. The use of leukocyte-reduced RBC transfusions in chronically transfused patients can reduce the risk of nonhemolytic transfusion reactions and viral transmission.[2,14] Transfusion-related infections also remain a concern. All patients should be immunized with hepatitis A and B vaccines. Other viruses that can be transmitted through blood products are parvovirus B19, hepatitis,[74] and cytomegalovirus. The risk of contracting human immunodeficiency virus from blood transfusions, although still of concern, has decreased with routine blood screening.[2,30]

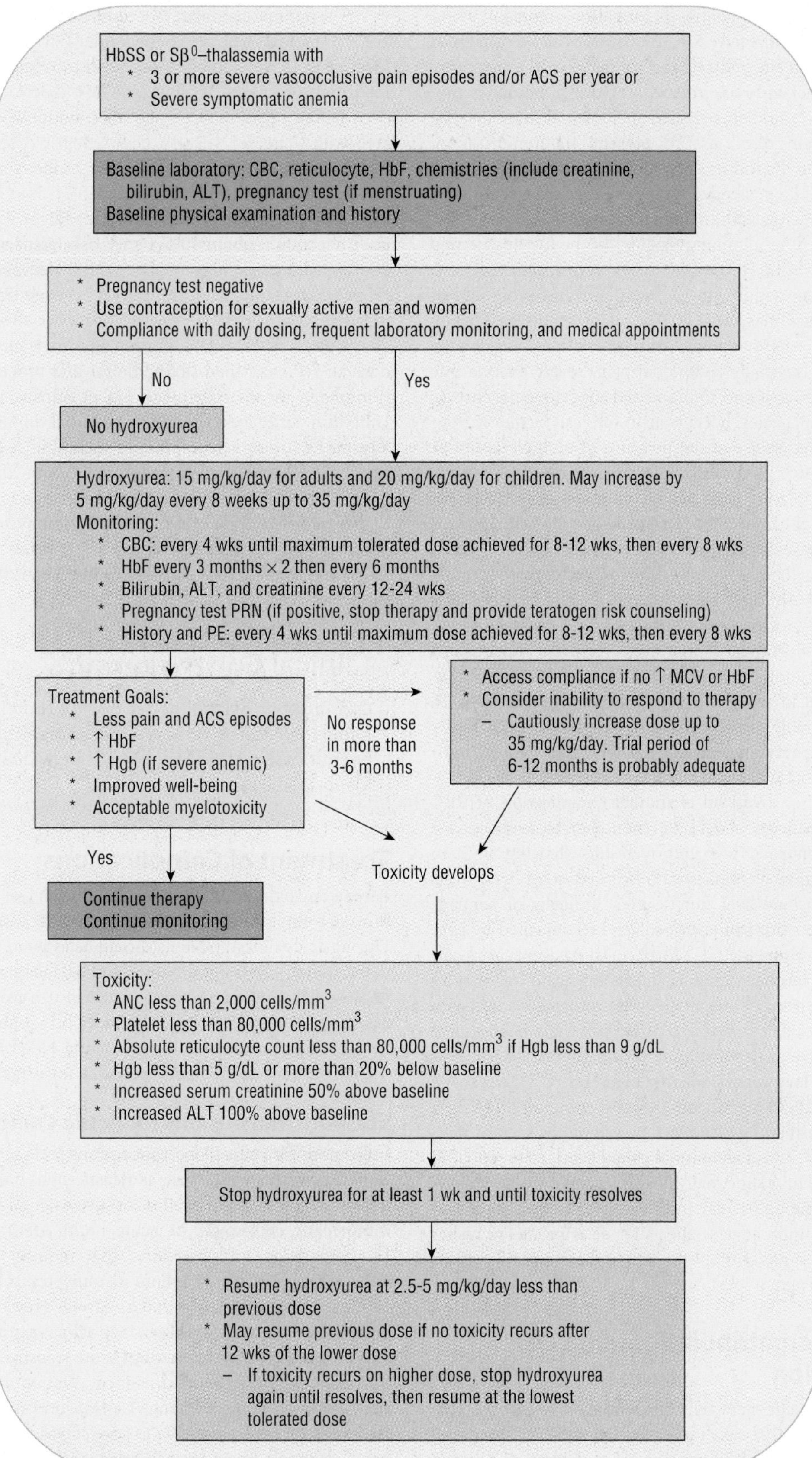

FIGURE 102-6 Hydroxyurea use in sickle cell disease. (ACS, acute chest syndrome; ALT, alanine aminotransferase; ANC, absolute neutrophil count; CBC, complete blood cell count; Hb, hemoglobin; HbF, fetal hemoglobin; HbSS, homozygous sickle cell hemoglobin; HbSSβ^0, sickle cell β^0-thalassemia; MCV, mean corpuscular volume; PE, physical examination; PRN, as needed; RBC, red blood cell) *(Data from references 1, 22 and 64.)*

Alloimmunization or alloantibody formation occurs in 19% to 37% of SCD patients who receive RBC transfusions and results from antigen differences on the red cell surface between the primarily Caucasian donor pool and recipients with SCD. Alloimmunization can make it difficult to find cross-matched blood and cause delayed hemolytic transfusion reactions. To prevent alloimmunization, patients receiving chronic transfusions should receive the best cross-matched blood including extended typing of other red cell antigens especially C, E, and Kell or full RBC phenotyping.[22,73,74]

The development of alloimmunization can be life threatening for individuals with SCD. Delayed hemolytic transfusion reactions (DHTR) usually occur within 7 to 10 days after transfusion but can occur as early as 2 days or as late as 20 days after transfusion. During a DHTR, patients develop symptoms consistent with hemolysis such as worsening pain, especially abdominal pain, severe anemia due to hemolysis of the transfused unit and reticulocytopenia, further aggravating the anemia. Subsequent transfusions can further worsen the clinical situation because of the presence of multiple antibodies making cross-matching difficult. Life-threatening events can be treated with steroids and intravenous immunoglobulin. Recombinant erythropoietin has been used in patients with reticulocytopenia.[73] Recovery, as evidenced by reticulocytosis with a gradual increase in the hemoglobin level, may occur only after further transfusions are withheld. Although some patients tolerate further transfusions after recovery, especially if the donor unit is negative for the offending alloantibody, others cannot avoid recurrent transfusions and may experience another hemolytic transfusion reaction. Rituximab has been used in two patients to prevent recurrent DHTR. It is generally preferable to prevent the development of DHTR by performing RBC phenotyping and, at a minimum, transfusing individuals with blood that is C, E, and Kell negative.[2,22,74]

Transfusional iron overload is another complication of RBC transfusions, and patients should be counseled to avoid excess dietary iron.[73,74] Abnormal liver biopsy results showing mild to moderate inflammation or fibrosis have been reported. Iron overload assessments include liver function test annually or semiannually and serum ferritin. Iron overload can be confirmed by liver biopsy or less invasively by MRI.[22,75] Three chelating agents are available. Deferoxamine has been used as a chelating agent for decades but must be administered by subcutaneous or intravenous infusion. Oral chelation agents, deferasirox and deferiprone have been shown to be equally effective as deferoxamine with demonstrated acceptable safety profile in long-term studies up to 5 years.[7,75-77] Deferasirox is given once daily (20-30 mg/kg) and the most common side effects are transient skin rash and gastrointestinal symptoms such as nausea, vomiting, diarrhea, and abdominal pain. Deferiprone has good oral bioavailability but a short half-life. The usual dose for deferiprone is 75 to 100 mg/kg per day in three divided dose. Similar to deferasirox, the common adverse effects for deferiprone are rashes and gastrointestinal symptoms but the most concerning side effects are neutropenia and agranulocytosis.[75-77]

Allogeneic Hematopoietic Stem Cell Transplantation

Allogeneic hematopoietic stem cell transplantation (HSCT) is currently the only therapy that can cure patients with SCD. The overall survival rate and disease-free survival rate for children and young adults with sibling matched donors, has been reported at 95% to 98% and 87% to 92%, respectively.[78,79] The reported incidences of acute and chronic GVHD ranged from 5% to 17% and 0% to 3%, respectively. Other complications included seizures, marrow rejection, and sepsis. Improved growth, stabilization or improvement of CNS abnormalities and recovery of splenic dysfunction were observed in posttransplant SCD patients, but gonadal failure and delayed sexual development in females requiring hormonal replacement have been reported.[80]

The optimal candidates for unrelated matched allogeneic HSCT are SCD patients who are younger than 16 years of age, have a severe form of SCD and complications such as refractory pain, stroke, or recurrent ACS. Because allogeneic HSCT performed in young children before organ damage and alloimmunization occur is associated with increased success, counseling and screening for sibling matched donors during the first year of life is now recommended. The risks associated with allogeneic HSCT must be carefully considered, as the transplant-related mortality rate is about 5% to 10%, and graft rejection is about 10%. Other risks associated with allogeneic HSCT include secondary malignancies. Neurologic events, such as intracranial hemorrhage and seizures during transplant, were seen more frequently in patients with a history of stroke.[81-83]

Unfortunately, many children who are eligible for HSCT do not have an HLA-matched sibling donor and unrelated HLA-matched transplants are associated with higher transplant-related mortality. Umbilical cord blood is another potential donor source with some advantages over marrow donors including a lower incidence of severe GVHD and a larger donor pool from which to select donors, but such advantages are offset by longer time to engraftment and a higher rate of graft rejection.[80,82] Use of nonmyeloablative allogeneic HSCT in adults and pediatric patients reported mixed donor-recipient chimerism and reversal of SCD in several clinical trials and has the advantage of less acute toxicity.[78-80]

Clinical **Controversy...**

Consideration of HSCT before disease complications develop rather than waiting for severe problems to manifest has been advocated for asymptomatic individuals with HLA-identical sibling.

Treatment of Complications

Parents and older children should be educated on the signs and symptoms of complications and conditions that require urgent evaluation. During acute illness, patients should be evaluated promptly because deterioration can occur rapidly. Fluid balance should be maintained because dehydration and fluid overload can worsen complications associated with SCD. Oxygen saturation by pulse oximetry should be maintained at least 92% or at baseline. New or increasing supplemental oxygen requirements should be investigated.

Episodic Transfusions for Acute Complications

Indications for acute blood transfusions include (1) acute exacerbation of baseline anemia, such as aplastic crisis if the anemia is severe, hepatic or splenic sequestration, or severe hemolysis; (2) ACS, stroke, intrahepatic cholestasis, or acute multisystem organ failure; and (3) preparation for procedures that require the use of general anesthesia.[22] Patients in whom chronic transfusions can be useful include primary or secondary stroke prevention, patients with complicated obstetric problems, refractory leg ulcers, or refractory and protracted painful episodes. Acute transfusion is not indicated for priapism, uncomplicated pain or asymptomatic anemia. Simple transfusion or partial exchange transfusion can be used though red cell exchange has been shown to have superior outcomes when compared to simple transfusion in overt stroke. If simple transfusion is used, volume overload leading to congestive heart failure can occur if anemia is corrected too rapidly in patients with severe anemia. In addition, increases in hemoglobin levels to greater than 10 g/dL (100 g/L; 6.21 mmol/L) can cause hyperviscosity and should be avoided.[14,22]

Infection and Fever

Patients with SCD should be evaluated as soon as possible for any fever greater than 38.5°C (101.3°F). Criteria for hospitalization include an infant younger than 1 year, history of previous bacteremia or sepsis, temperature greater than 39.5°C (103.1°F), WBC greater than 30,000 cells/mm^3 (30 × 10^9/L) or less than 5,000 cells/mm^3 (5 × 10^9/L) and/or platelets less than 100,000 cells/mm^3 (100 × 10^9/L), and evidence of other acute complications or toxic appearance. Outpatient management can be considered in older nontoxic children with reliable family caregivers. Antibiotic choice should provide adequate coverage for encapsulated organisms.[2,22,30]

7 Ceftriaxone should be used for outpatient management because it provides coverage for 24 hours. If admitted, cefotaxime can also be used. For patients with cephalosporin allergy, clindamycin can be used. Vancomycin should be considered for acutely ill children or if *Staphylococcus* is suspected. A macrolide antibiotic should be added if *Mycoplasma pneumoniae* is suspected such as in ACS. Penicillin prophylaxis should be discontinued while the patient is receiving broad-spectrum antibiotics. Acetaminophen or ibuprofen can be used for fever control. Increased fluid requirements may be present because of poor oral intake and/or increased insensible losses contributing to dehydration.[1,30]

Cerebrovascular Accidents

Patients with acute neurologic events must be hospitalized and monitored closely. Physical and neurologic examination should be performed every 2 hours. Acute treatment for children should include exchange transfusion to maintain hemoglobin at about 10 g/dL (100 g/L; 6.21 mmol/L) and HbS less than 30%, anticonvulsants for patients with a seizure history, and therapy for increased intracranial pressure if needed. Chronic transfusion therapy should be initiated for children with ischemic stroke as discussed earlier. In adults presenting with ischemic stroke related to atherosclerotic disease and not occlusion by sickled red cells, thrombolytic therapy should be considered if it is less than 3 hours since the onset of symptoms.[1,2,32]

Acute Chest Syndrome

Patients with ACS should use incentive spirometry frequently (eg, at least every 2 hours while awake) to reduce atelectasis development. In addition, proper management of pain is important. The goal is to provide relief while avoiding analgesic-induced hypoventilation. Appropriate fluid therapy is important as overhydration can cause pulmonary edema and exacerbate respiratory distress. Early use of broad-spectrum antibiotics, including a macrolide or quinolone in adults, is also recommended. Studies indicate that infection is the most common cause of ACS and can involve gram-positive, gram-negative, or atypical bacteria. Oxygen therapy is indicated for all patients who are hypoxic or in acute distress. In a patient with a history of reactive airway disease, asthma or wheezing on examination, a trial of bronchodilators is appropriate. Transfusions are indicated for severe ACS with worsening hypoxia and increased work of breathing.[1,14,18]

Steroids can decrease inflammation and endothelial cell adhesion. Glucocorticoids can decrease the duration of hospitalization and need for transfusions and other supportive care but can also increase the readmission rate for other sickle cell-related complications. Another potential therapy is the use of NO, which relaxes and dilates blood vessels. Its hematologic effects include inhibition of platelet aggregation and reduction in the polymerization tendency of HbS. Marked improvement of pulmonary status and cardiac output were reported in case reports of patients with ACS.[1,14,34]

Priapism

Stuttering priapism, episodes that last a few minutes to 2 hours, may resolve spontaneously with exercise, warm bath and oral analgesics. Prolonged episodes lasting more than 2 to 3 hours require prompt medical attention. The initial goals of treatment are to provide appropriate analgesic therapy, reduce anxiety, produce detumescence, and preserve testicular function and fertility. Treatment given within 4 to 6 hours can usually reduce erection. Aggressive hydration and adequate pain control should be initiated. Use of ice packs is not recommended. Heat (hot water bottles, hot packs, or sitz baths) can provide comfort without precipitating pain crisis. Although transfusions have been given to these patients, transfusions are not recommended for this use because they have not been shown to be efficacious and are associated with severe neurologic sequelae.[1,24]

Clinicians have used both vasoconstrictors and vasodilators in the treatment of priapism. Vasoconstrictors, such as diluted phenylephrine (10 mcg/mL) or epinephrine (1:1,000,000), are thought to work by forcing blood out of the corpus cavernosum into the venous return. In one uncontrolled open-label study, aspiration followed by intrapenile irrigation with a 1:1,000,000 solution of epinephrine was effective and well tolerated with 37 of 39 episodes experiencing resolution. Detumescence can be achieved more rapidly using penile irrigation than simple transfusion but the procedure should be performed by an urologist with experience in the treatment of priapism.[36,84]

Vasodilators, such as terbutaline and hydralazine, relax the smooth muscle of the vasculature. This relaxation allows oxygenated arterial blood to enter the corpus cavernosum, which displaces or washes out the damaged sickle cells that are stagnant in the corpus cavernosum. Terbutaline has been used to treat priapism, but it has not been formally studied in patients with SCD.[36,84] In one case report, a single oral sildenafil dose at onset of priapism aborted episodes. However, long-term studies of sildenafil have shown an increase in the frequency of pain episodes.[84,85] Surgical interventions used in severe refractory priapism have included a variety of shunt procedures. These surgical procedures have been successful in some cases, but they have a high failure rate and potential serious complications, which include impotence, skin sloughing, cellulitis, and urethral fistulas.[36,84]

Modalities to prevent priapism are limited and not well studied. Pseudoephedrine (30 or 60 mg/day given orally at bedtime) and leuprolide, a gonadotropin-releasing hormone, have been used to decrease the number of recurrent episodes of priapism. HU therapy can also be used, but the effect of HU on risk of priapism has not been formally investigated. Finally, antiandrogens (bicalutamide and finasteride) have been used in SCD for treatment of recurrent or refractory priapism without major side effects.[84] The role of chronic transfusion in preventing priapism remains unclear and transfusion is not recommended for long-term management.[22,84]

Clinical **Controversy...**

Some clinicians transfuse patients to maintain an HbS level less than 30% to prevent recurrent priapism. Duration of such regimens should be limited to 6 to 12 months. Clinical practice guidelines do not recommend chronic transfusion to prevent recurrent priapism.

Aplastic Crisis

Treatment of aplastic crisis is primarily supportive, and most patients recover spontaneously within 5 to 10 days. The only treatment may be blood transfusion if the anemia is severe or symptomatic. The reticulocyte count is used to detect the suppression of red cell production and the need for transfusion. The most common cause, parvovirus B19, is contagious and infected patients should be placed in isolation. In addition, contact with pregnant healthcare providers should be avoided because parvovirus infection during the midtrimester of pregnancy can result in hydrops fetalis and stillbirth.[1,2,30]

Splenic Sequestration

Splenic sequestration is a major cause of mortality in young children with SCD. The sequestration of RBCs in the spleen can result in a rapid drop of hemoglobin, leading to hypovolemia, shock, and death. Immediate treatment with fluid resuscitation and blood transfusions is indicated to correct hypovolemia. Broad-spectrum antibiotic therapy, which includes coverage for *S. pneumoniae* and *H. influenzae*, can also be beneficial if the patient is febrile as infection can precipitate sequestration.[14,22]

Recurrent episodes occur in about half of patients and are associated with increased mortality. Options for management of recurrence include observation and splenectomy.[22] Increased risk of invasive infection after splenectomy is a concern in very young children, but most experts agree individuals with HbSS develop splenic dysfunction as early as 6 months of age and have acquired asplenia by 5 years of age and by 10 to 12 years for those with HbSC. Splenectomy is probably indicated, even after a single sequestration crisis, if that sequestration was life threatening. Splenectomy should be considered after repetitive episodes, even if they are less serious. For children younger than 2 years of age, chronic blood transfusions are recommended by some experts to prevent sequestration and delay splenectomy until the age of 2 years, when the risk of post-splenectomy septicemia is lower and pneumococcal vaccination has been completed. Finally, splenectomy should also be considered for patients with chronic hypersplenism.[1,2,22,39]

Acute Sickle Cell Pain

Hydration and analgesia are the mainstays of treatment for vaso-occlusive (painful) episodes (Table 102-6). Patients with mild pain crisis can be treated as outpatients with rest, increased fluid intake, warm compresses, and oral analgesics. Hospitalization is necessary for moderate-to-severe pain or when oral analgesics fail to relieve pain. A pain episode may be precipitated by several risk factors including infection. In the setting of pain and fever, an infectious etiology should be evaluated, and appropriate empiric therapy should be initiated in patients. In patients with severe symptomatic anemia, transfusions may be indicated. Fluid replacement given intravenously or orally to correct or prevent hydration at 1 to 1.5 times the maintenance requirement is recommended. Close monitoring of fluid status is essential as aggressive hydration, particularly with sodium-containing fluids, can lead to volume overload, ACS, and heart failure.[1,22,24]

TABLE 102-6 Management of Acute Pain of Sickle Cell Disease

Principles

1. Treat underlying precipitating factors
2. Avoid delays in analgesia administration
   a. Initiate analgesic within 30 minutes of triage or 60 minutes of registration
3. Use pain scale to assess severity
4. Choice of initial analgesic should be based on previous pain pattern, history of response, current status, and other medical conditions
5. Schedule pain medication; avoid as-needed dosing
6. Provide rescue dose for breakthrough pain
7. If adequate pain relief can be achieved with one or two doses of morphine, consider outpatient management with a weak opioid; otherwise hospitalization is needed for parenteral analgesics
8. Frequently assess to evaluate pain severity and side effects; titrate dose as needed
9. Treating adverse effects of opioids is part of pain management
10. Consider nonpharmacologic intervention (eg, relaxation techniques, guided imagery, deep breathing)
11. Transition to oral analgesics as the patient improves; choose an oral agent based on previous history, anticipated duration, and ability to swallow tablets; if sustained-release products are used, a product with a rapid onset is also needed for breakthrough pain

Analgesic regimens

Mild-to-moderate pain: nonopioid ± weak opioid
Moderate-to-severe pain: weak opioid or low dose of a strong opioid ± nonopioid
Severe pain: strong opioid + nonopioid

Other adjunct therapy

Hydration, heating pads, relaxation, and distraction
Laxatives for constipation
Antihistamine for itching
Antiemetics for nausea or vomiting

Data from references 86-88.

The frequency and severity of acute pain episodes associated with SCD are variable. Pain should be assessed and analgesic therapy should be tailored for each patient and each individual episode. Several verbal and nonverbal pain assessment tools are available and should be used to measure the intensity of pain. Unfortunately, they have not been validated for sickle cell pain. However, pain scales validated for use in children, such as the Wong-Baker FACES scale should be used in pediatric patients with SCD pain. The healthcare provider should choose one tool appropriate for age and use it routinely to assess pain. Other useful information to guide choice of analgesics should include previous effective agents and their dosages, response to therapy and previous clinical course, and duration of pain episodes.[86-88]

8 Aggressive therapy that relieves pain and enables the patient to attain maximum functional ability should be initiated in patients with acute pain. Mild-to-moderate pain should be treated with nonsteroidal anti-inflammatory drugs (NSAIDs) or acetaminophen, unless there are contraindications to their use. Ketorolac may be useful for patients requiring intravenous therapy. Because of increased risk of gastrointestinal bleeding, it is recommended to limit the duration of therapy to 5 days or less. Ketorolac has also been associated with acute nonreversible kidney failure in a patient with SCD and should be used with caution and renal function monitored appropriately. When acetaminophen is used, it is important to monitor the total dose of acetaminophen administered in patients who may also be receiving the agent for fever or another acetaminophen-containing product for pain. If mild-to-moderate pain persists, an opioid should be added.[14,22,86,87]

Severe pain should be treated aggressively until the pain is tolerable. Commonly used opioids include morphine, hydromorphone, fentanyl, and methadone. The weak opioids, codeine, and hydrocodone, are used to manage mild-to-moderate pain usually in the outpatient setting. Meperidine has no advantages as an analgesic and many disadvantages. Meperidine toxicity is caused by accumulation of the metabolite normeperidine which can cause central nervous system side effects, ranging from dysphoria to seizures. Effective combination therapy, such as an NSAID and an opioid, can enhance analgesic efficacy while decreasing side effects.

Both prior history and current assessment should be considered in the management of acute sickle cell pain. For patients whose typical pain improves in a short time, preparations with a short duration of action are appropriate. For patients whose pain requires many days to resolve, sustained-release preparations combined with a short-acting product for breakthrough pain are more appropriate. If the patient has been on long-term opioid therapy at home, tolerance can develop. In these cases, the acute pain can be treated with an opioid of different potency or a larger dose of the same medication. Intravenous administration provides a rapid onset of action and therefore is preferred for severe pain. Intramuscular injections should be avoided. Children may actually deny pain due to fear of injections. Analgesics should be titrated to pain relief. In patients with continuous pain, the analgesic should be given as a scheduled dose or continuous infusion. Continuous infusion has the advantage of less fluctuation of blood levels between dosing intervals. As needed dosing is only indicated for breakthrough pain. Patient-controlled analgesia (PCA) is commonly prescribed for severe pain episodes. When used properly, PCA allows patients to have control over pain therapy and minimizes the lag time between perception of pain and administration of analgesics. Studies have shown PCA use reduced cumulative dosage required for pain control. The transdermal fentanyl patch has also been used successfully, but its role in sickle cell acute pain crisis is unclear because of its slow onset of onset of pain relief (12-16 hours) and fixed dosage form, which makes it difficult to titrate the dose. Other alternative pain management techniques such as physical therapy, massage, biofeedback, and relaxation therapy can be helpful as adjunct therapy.[86-88]

Suboptimal pain relief has been reported in both emergency room and hospitalized patients. The most common cause of suboptimal pain control in children and adults with SCD is the suspicion of addiction.[22] This obstacle is especially common in adolescents. In one study, 53% of emergency physicians believed that 20% of SCD patients are psychologically addicted to opioid analgesics. Another barrier to effective pain control is the difference in perception between patients, family, and healthcare providers. Patients with SCD have been reported to experience pain over 50% of days, and they develop coping strategies including flat affect. Patients who have inadequate pain control can exhibit anxiety and drug-seeking behavior for fear of pain. Tolerance to opioids may also be misinterpreted as drug addiction by healthcare providers and families. Aggressive pain control, frequent monitoring of pain during episodes, and tapering medication according to response are factors that minimize physical dependence. The use of a protocol has been shown to result in optimal management of pain control in SCD.[24,86-89]

With better understanding of NO and inflammation on vasculopathy, therapy targeting blood rheology, endothelium adhesion or inflammation have been explored as adjunct therapy. Inhaled NO has been studied as therapy to abort pain at onset of episodes. Significant reduction of pain scores in adult patients received inhaled NO in the emergency room. However, no differences in duration of episodes, hospital stay, or opioid use when given to hospitalized adult and pediatric patients were observed.[90,91] In a randomized controlled trial in children hospitalized for painful episodes, arginine, the precursor for NO, reduced total opioid use by more than 50%. Length of hospital stay was not reduced significantly but the pain scores were significantly lower at discharge when compared to placebo.[92] Systemic corticosteroids, methylprednisolone and dexamethasone have also been evaluated as an adjunct therapy for pain control. Shorter duration of analgesic therapy and duration of hospitalization were reported but increased risk of readmission was also reported.[93]

Chronic Sickle Cell Pain

As the number of adults living with SCD increases due to improved survival, the prevalence of disease morbidities including chronic pain also increases. Most of the published research has focused on the prevention of pain and the management of acute pain episodes. The mechanisms of chronic pain development in SCD are poorly understood and no systematic studies have evaluated risk factors for chronic pain development. Central sensitization and peripheral neural sensitization have been hypothesized to play a role in the development of chronic SCD pain.[37,38,94] Currently, there are no published reports of other medications such as selective serotonin reuptake inhibitors, serotonin–norepinephrine reuptake inhibitors and anticonvulsants commonly used to treat chronic pain in patients with SCD. Treatment of chronic pain in SCD requires a multidisciplinary approach and most physicians with expertise in treating SCD recommend following established guidelines for chronic pain.[95]

PERSONALIZED PHARMACOTHERAPY

The mainstay of treatment in SCD involves medical therapy both for supportive care and disease modification. Classically, pharmacotherapy is individualized by weight-based dosing. However, new research is evaluating approaches to further personalize therapy. For example, many adults with SCD have abnormal renal function due to intrarenal sickling. HU, the most important disease modifying medication, is renally excreted with urinary recovery of 40% of the administered dose in adults with SCD. A lower initial dose of 5 to 10 mg/kg per day is recommended for individuals with creatinine clearance of less than 60 mL/min (1 mL/s).[22] Pharmacokinetic differences between adult and pediatric patients were not reported in initial studies. As a result, investigators designed a prospective clinical trial, the Hydroxyurea Study of Long-Term Effects (HUSTLE, NCT00305175), to evaluate interpatient variability among children taking HU. For the first-dose pharmacokinetic studies, 51 of 87 patients showed a "fast" absorption profile with an earlier and higher maximum concentration after a single dose of 20 mg/kg. Although several parameters were associated with maximum tolerated dose (MTD) and HbF at MTD, the investigators concluded that standardized dose titration to myelosuppression remains the best option.[96]

Adults and children with SCD require the use of acute and chronic pain medications including opioids to control painful episodes. Some patients have clinically demonstrated inadequate relief to analgesic dosing with codeine. Children who failed oral therapy with codeine were found to carry a polymorphism in the *CYP2D6* gene resulting in a poor metabolizer phenotype. The CYP2D6 isoenzyme mediates the metabolism of codeine to morphine. These results have led to early discontinuation of codeine analgesics in children with SCD if no response is seen after their first dose and use of alternative oral analgesics for the treatment of pain at home. Often in treating individuals with SCD, analgesia is not obtained even with very high intravenous opioid doses. A recent review highlighted several enzymes that play a role in morphine metabolism that may be altered in patients with SCD including UGT2B7, a morphine-metabolizing enzyme; OPRM1, a mu opioid receptor or ABCB1, a transporter protein at the blood brain barrier. However, further investigation is needed and genetic testing has not been used to guide morphine dosing.[97,98]

The concept of individualized therapy in SCD is being tested with the identification of single nucleotide polymorphisms (SNPs) associated with severity of disease and HbF responses to HU therapy. Increases in HbF with HU appeared to be related to baseline levels suggesting that genomic profiles may contribute to the differences. Genome-wide association studies have identified several loci in HbF expression. BCL11A is a transcription factor that regulates hemoglobin switching and could account for the variability of HbF levels between individuals with high and low HbF. Different biomarkers have been studied in SCD to identify complications and phenotypic variability. The potential use of biomarkers and genome-based modification of phenotype in SCD may allow a personalized therapeutic approach in the future.[97]

EVALUATION OF THERAPEUTIC OUTCOMES

9 SCD is a complex disorder that requires multidisciplinary comprehensive care. All patients should receive regular medical evaluation to provide preventive care, establish baseline symptoms and laboratory values, monitor changes, and provide education appropriate for age. For infants younger than 1-year-old, medical evaluations every 2 to 4 months are recommended. Beyond 2 years of age, evaluation can be extended to every 6 to 12 months with modifications depending on severity of the illness.

Routine laboratory evaluation including complete blood cell counts and reticulocyte counts every 3 to 6 months up to 2 years of age, then every 6 to 12 months; HbF level should be screened annually until 2 years of age. Evaluation of renal, hepatobiliary, and pulmonary function should be done annually. TCD screening is recommended to start at age 2 years and performed annually for children with HbSS and HbSβ. Ophthalmologic examination to screen for retinopathy is recommended at around age 10 to 12 years for those with HbSC and 14 years for HbSS. In patients with recurrent ACS, pulmonary function tests should be done to establish baseline values and identify declines in lung function as well as an evaluation by pulmonology to screen for lower airway hyper-responsiveness.

It is essential that immunizations and prophylactic antibiotics be given. When infections do occur, appropriate antibiotic therapy should be initiated, and the patient should be monitored for laboratory and clinical improvement. The efficacy of HU can be measured as a decrease in the number, severity, and duration of sickle cell pain episodes. HbF concentrations or MCV values can also provide some indication of the patient's response to therapy. When painful episodes do occur, the effectiveness of analgesics can be measured by subjective assessments made by the patient, and healthcare practitioners. The success of poststroke blood transfusions can be measured by clinical progression or the occurrence of subsequent strokes. Finally, indicators can be used for measurements of quality of care for children with SCD.

ABBREVIATIONS

ACS	acute chest syndrome
CT	computed tomography
ET-1	endothelin 1
GVHD	graft-versus-host disease
HbA	hemoglobin A
HbAS	one normal (hemoglobin A) and one sickle cell hemoglobin (hemoglobin S) gene
HbC	hemoglobin C
HbF	fetal hemoglobin
HbS	sickle cell hemoglobin
HbSβ^+-thal	hemoglobin sickle cell β^+-thalassemia
HbSβ^0-thal	hemoglobin sickle cell β^0-thalassemia
HbSC	sickle cell hemoglobin C
HbSS	homozygous sickle cell hemoglobin (hemoglobin S)
HLA	human leukocyte antigen
HPFH	hereditary persistence of fetal hemoglobin
HSCT	hematopoietic stem cell transplantation
HU	hydroxyurea
ISC	irreversibly sickled cell
MCHC	mean corpuscular hemoglobin concentration
MCV	mean corpuscular volume
MRI	magnetic resonance imaging
MSH	Multicenter Study of Hydroxyurea in Sickle Cell Anemia
MTD	maximum tolerated dose
NIH	National Institutes of Health
NO	nitric oxide
NSAID	nonsteroidal anti-inflammatory drug
NT-pro-BNP	N-terminal pro-brain natriuretic peptide
PAH	pulmonary artery hypertension
PAP	pulmonary arterial pressure
PCA	patient-controlled analgesia
PCV7	7-valent pneumococcal conjugate vaccine
PCV13	13-valent pneumococcal conjugate vaccine
PPSV23	23-valent pneumococcal polysaccharide vaccine
RBC	red blood cell
SCA	sickle cell anemia
SCD	sickle cell disease
SCT	sickle cell trait
TCD	transcranial Doppler ultrasound
VCAM-1	vascular cell adhesion molecule 1
WBC	white blood cell

REFERENCES

1. McCavit TL. Sickle cell disease. *Pediatr Rev* 2012;33:195-204; quiz 5-6.
2. Quinn CT. Sickle cell disease in childhood: from newborn screening through transition to adult medical care. *Pediatr Clin North Am* 2013;60:1363-1381.
3. Steinberg MH, Sebastiani P. Genetic modifiers of sickle cell disease. *Am J Hematol* 2012;87:795-803.
4. Rees DC, Gibson JS. Biomarkers in sickle cell disease. *Br J Haematol* 2012;156:433-445.
5. Eridani S, Mosca A. Fetal hemoglobin reactivation and cell engineering in the treatment of sickle cell anemia. *J Blood Med* 2011;2:23-30.
6. Odievre MH, Verger E, Silva-Pinto AC, Elion J. Pathophysiological insights in sickle cell disease. *Indian J Med Res* 2011;134:532-537.
7. Kanter J, Kruse-Jarres R. Management of sickle cell disease from childhood through adulthood. *Blood Rev* 2013;27:279-287.
8. Dampier C, LeBeau P, Rhee S, et al. Health-related quality of life in adults with sickle cell disease (SCD): a report from the comprehensive sickle cell centers clinical trial consortium. *Am J Hematol* 2011;86:203-205.
9. Dale JC, Cochran CJ, Roy L, et al. Health-related quality of life in children and adolescents with sickle cell disease. *J Pediatr Health Care* 2011;25:208-215.
10. Swanson ME, Grosse SD, Kulkarni R. Disability among individuals with sickle cell disease: literature review from a public health perspective. *Am J Prev Med* 2011;41(Suppl 4):S390-S397.
11. Wang CJ, Kavanagh PL, Little AA, et al. Quality-of-care indicators for children with sickle cell disease. *Pediatrics* 2011;128:484-493.
12. Aygun B, Odame I. A global perspective on sickle cell disease. *Pediatr Blood Cancer* 2012;59:386-390.
13. Apanah S, Rizzolo D. Sickle cell disease: taking a multidisciplinary approach. *JAAPA* 2013;26:28-33.
14. Steinbert M. In the clinic: sickle cell disease. *Ann Intern Med* 2011;155:ITC3-1-15.
15. National Institutes of Health, Division of Blood Diseases and Resources, Public Health Service. Who Is at Risk for Sickle Cell Anemia? *http://www.nhlbi.nih.gov/health/health-topics/topics/sca/atrisk.html*. Last accessed, October 13, 2015.
16. Hamideh D, Alvarez O. Sickle cell disease related mortality in the United States (1999-2009). *Pediatr Blood Cancer* 2013;60: 1482-1486.
17. Key NS, Connes P, Derebail VK. Negative health implications of sickle cell trait in high income countries: from the football field to the laboratory. *Br J Haematol* 2015;170:5-14.
18. Knight-Madden J, Greenough A. Acute pulmonary complications of sickle cell disease. *Paediatr Respir Rev* 2014;15:13-16.
19. Benson JM, Therrell BL. History and current status of newborn screening for hemoglobinopathies. *Semin Perinatol* 2010;34: 134-144.
20. Pakbaz Z, Wun T. Role of the hemostatic system on sickle cell disease pathophysiology and potential therapeutics. *Hematol Oncol Clin North Am* 2014;28:355-374.
21. Therrell BL, Lloyd-Puryear MA, Eckman JR, Mann MY. Newborn screening for sickle cell diseases in the United States: a review of data spanning 2 decades. *Semin Perinatol* 2015;39:238-251.
22. National Institutes of Health, National Heart Lung and Blood Institute. Evidence-Based Management of Sickle Cell Disease: Expert Panel Report. *http://www.nhlbi.nih.gov/health-pro/guidelines/sickle-cell-disease-guidelines/*. Last accessed, October 15, 2015.
23. Maron BJ, Harris KM, Thompson PD, et al. Eligibility and disqualification recommendations for competitive athletes with cardiovascular abnormalities: task force 14: sickle cell trait: a scientific statement from the American Heart Association and American College of Cardiology. *Circulation* 2015;132:e343-e345.
24. Meier ER, Miller JL. Sickle cell disease in children. *Drugs* 2012;72: 895-906.
25. Meier ER, Wright EC, Miller JL. Reticulocytosis and anemia are associated with an increased risk of death and stroke in the newborn cohort of the Cooperative Study of Sickle Cell Disease. *Am J Hematol* 2014;89:904-906.
26. Miller AC, Gladwin MT. Pulmonary complications of sickle cell disease. *Am J Respir Crit Care Med* 2012;185:1154-1165.
27. Elmariah H, Garrett ME, De Castro LM, et al. Factors associated with survival in a contemporary adult sickle cell disease cohort. *Am J Hematol* 2014;89:530-535.
28. Payne AB, Link-Gelles R, Azonobi I, et al. Invasive pneumococcal disease among children with and without sickle cell disease in the United States, 1998 to 2009. *Pediatr Infect Dis J* 2013;32:1308-1312.

29. Ellison AM, Ota KV, McGowan KL, Smith-Whitley K. Epidemiology of bloodstream infections in children with sickle cell disease. *Pediatr Infect Dis J* 2013;32:560-563.
30. Sobota A, Sabharwal V, Fonebi G, Steinberg M. How we prevent and manage infection in sickle cell disease. *Br J Haematol* 2015;170:757-767.
31. Brousse V, Kossorotoff M, de Montalembert M. How I manage cerebral vasculopathy in children with sickle cell disease. *Br J Haematol* 2015;170:615-625.
32. Kassim AA, Galadanci NA, Pruthi S, DeBaun MR. How I treat and manage strokes in sickle cell disease. *Blood* 2015;125:3401-3410.
33. Quinn CT, McKinstry RC, Dowling MM, et al. Acute silent cerebral ischemic events in children with sickle cell anemia. *JAMA Neurol* 2013;70:58-65.
34. Howard J, Hart N, Roberts-Harewood M, et al. Guideline on the management of acute chest syndrome in sickle cell disease. *Br J Haematol* 2015;169:492-505.
35. Anele UA, Le BV, Resar LM, Burnett AL. How I treat priapism. *Blood* 2015;125:3551-3358.
36. Crane GM, Bennett NE. Priapism in sickle cell anemia: emerging mechanistic understanding and better preventative strategies. *Anemia* 2011;297364:1-6.
37. Ballas SK, Gupta K, Adams-Graves P. Sickle cell pain: a critical reappraisal. *Blood* 2012;120:3647-3656.
38. Darbari DS, Ballas SK, Clauw DJ. Thinking beyond sickling to better understand pain in sickle cell disease. *Eur J Haematol* 2014;93: 89-95.
39. Brousse V, Elie C, Benkerrou M, et al. Acute splenic sequestration crisis in sickle cell disease: cohort study of 190 paediatric patients. *Br J Haematol* 2012;156:643-648.
40. Klings ES, Machado RF, Barst RJ, et al. An official American Thoracic Society clinical practice guideline: diagnosis, risk stratification, and management of pulmonary hypertension of sickle cell disease. *Am J Respir Crit Care Med* 2014;189:727-740.
41. Abman SH, Hansmann G, Archer SL, et al. Pediatric pulmonary hypertension: guidelines from the American Heart Association and American Thoracic Society. *Circulation* 2015;132:2037-2099.
42. Gomez E, Morris CR. Asthma management in sickle cell disease. *Biomed Res Int* 2013;604140:1-12.
43. Osunkwo I. An update on the recent literature on sickle cell bone disease. *Curr Opin Endocrinol Diabetes Obes* 2013;20:539-546.
44. da Silva Jr GB, Daher Ede F, da Rocha FA. Osteoarticular involvement in sickle cell disease. *Rev Bras Hematol Hemoter* 2012;34:156-164.
45. Lim JI. Ophthalmic manifestations of sickle cell disease: update of the latest findings. *Curr Opin Ophthalmol* 2012;23:533-536.
46. Ebert EC, Nagar M, Hagspiel KD. Gastrointestinal and hepatic complications of sickle cell disease. *Clin Gastroenterol Hepatol* 2010;8:483-489.
47. Voskaridou E, Christoulas D, Terpos E. Sickle-cell disease and the heart: review of the current literature. *Br J Haematol* 2012;157:664-673.
48. Fitzhugh CD, Lauder N, Jonassaint JC, et al. Cardiopulmonary complications leading to premature deaths in adult patients with sickle cell disease. *Am J Hematol* 2010;85:36-40.
49. Nath KA, Hebbel RP. Sickle cell disease: renal manifestations and mechanisms. *Nat Rev Nephrol* 2015;11:161-171.
50. McClellan AC, Luthi JC, Lynch JR, et al. High one year mortality in adults with sickle cell disease and end-stage renal disease. *Br J Haematol* 2012;159:360-367.
51. Hyacinth HI, Adekeye OA, Yilgwan CS. Malnutrition in sickle cell anemia: implications for infection, growth, and maturation. *J Soc Behav Health Sci* 2013;7:23-34.
52. Bennett EL. Understanding growth failure in children with homozygous sickle-cell disease. *J Pediatr Oncol Nurs* 2011;28:67-74.
53. Smith-Whitley K. Reproductive issues in sickle cell disease. *Blood* 2014;124:3538-3543.
54. Sehlo MG, Kamfar HZ. Depression and quality of life in children with sickle cell disease: the effect of social support. *BMC Psychiatry* 2015;15:78-85.
55. Unal S, Toros F, Kutuk MO, Uyaniker MG. Evaluation of the psychological problems in children with sickle cell anemia and their families. *Pediatr Hematol Oncol* 2011;28:321-328.
56. Benton TD, Boyd R, Ifeagwu J, et al. Psychiatric diagnosis in adolescents with sickle cell disease: a preliminary report. *Curr Psychiatry Rep* 2011;13:111-115.
57. Parrish MR, Morrison JC. Sickle cell crisis and pregnancy. *Semin Perinatol* 2013;37:274-279.
58. Oteng-Ntim E, Meeks D, Seed PT, et al. Adverse maternal and perinatal outcomes in pregnant women with sickle cell disease: systematic review and meta-analysis. *Blood* 2015;125:3316-3325.
59. Quinn CT, Rogers ZR, McCavit TL, Buchanan GR. Improved survival of children and adolescents with sickle cell disease. *Blood* 2010;115:3447-3452.
60. Nuorti JP, Whitney CG. Prevention of pneumococcal disease among infants and children—use of 13-valent pneumococcal conjugate vaccine and 23-valent pneumococcal polysaccharide vaccine—recommendations of the Advisory Committee on Immunization Practices (ACIP). *MMWR Recomm Rep* 2010;59(RR-11):1-18.
61. Bennett N. Use of 13-valent pneumococcal conjugate vaccine and 23-valent pneumococcal polysaccharide vaccine for adults with immunocompromising conditions: recommendations of the Advisory Committee on Immunization Practices (ACIP). *MMWR Morb Mortal Wkly Rep* 2012;61:816-819.
62. Cohn AC, MacNeil JR, Clark TA, et al. Prevention and control of meningococcal disease: recommendations of the Advisory Committee on Immunization Practices (ACIP). *MMWR Morb Mortal Wkly Rep* 2013;62(RR-2):1-28.
63. MacNeil JR, Rubin L, McNamara L, et al. Use of MenACWY-CRM vaccine in children aged 2 through 23 months at increased risk for meningococcal disease: recommendations of the Advisory Committee on Immunization Practices, 2013. *MMWR Morb Mortal Wkly Rep* 2014;63:527-530.
64. Wong TE, Brandow AM, Lim W, Lottenberg R. Update on the use of hydroxyurea therapy in sickle cell disease. *Blood* 2014;124:3850-3857.
65. Steinberg MH, McCarthy WF, Castro O, et al. The risks and benefits of long-term use of hydroxyurea in sickle cell anemia: a 17.5 year follow-up. *Am J Hematol* 2010;85:403-408.
66. Wang WC, Ware RE, Miller ST, et al. Hydroxycarbamide in very young children with sickle-cell anaemia: a multicentre, randomised, controlled trial (BABY HUG). *Lancet* 2011;377:1663-1672.
67. Thornburg CD, Files BA, Luo Z, et al. Impact of hydroxyurea on clinical events in the BABY HUG trial. *Blood* 2012:120:4304-4310.
68. Alvarez O, Miller ST, Wang WC, et al. Effect of hydroxyurea treatment on renal function parameters: results from the multi-center placebo-controlled BABY HUG clinical trial for infants with sickle cell anemia. *Pediatr Blood Cancer* 2012;59:668-674.
69. Lobo CL, Pinto JF, Nascimento EM, et al. The effect of hydroxycarbamide therapy on survival of children with sickle cell disease. *Br J Haematol* 2013;161:852-860.
70. McGann PT, Flanagan JM, Howard TA, et al. Genotoxicity associated with hydroxyurea exposure in infants with sickle cell anemia: results from the BABY-HUG Phase III Clinical Trial. *Pediatr Blood Cancer* 2012;59:254-257.
71. Rana S, Houston PE, Wang WC, et al. Hydroxyurea and growth in young children with sickle cell disease. *Pediatrics* 2014;134:465-472.
72. Ware RE. Hydroxycarbamide: clinical aspects. *C R Biol* 2013;336: 177-182.
73. Chou ST. Transfusion therapy for sickle cell disease: a balancing act. *Hematology Am Soc Hematol Educ Program* 2013;2013:439-446.
74. Smith-Whitley K, Thompson AA. Indications and complications of transfusions in sickle cell disease. *Pediatr Blood Cancer* 2012;59:358-364.
75. Ware HM, Kwiatkowski JL. Evaluation and treatment of transfusional iron overload in children. *Pediatr Clin North Am* 2013;60:1393-1406.
76. Chaudhary P, Pullarkat V. Deferasirox: appraisal of safety and efficacy in long-term therapy. *J Blood Med* 2013;4:101-110.
77. Calvaruso G, Vitrano A, Di Maggio R, et al. Deferiprone versus deferoxamine in sickle cell disease: results from a 5-year long-term Italian multi-center randomized clinical trial. *Blood Cells Mol Dis* 2014;53:265-271.
78. Fitzhugh CD, Abraham AA, Tisdale JF, Hsieh MM. Hematopoietic stem cell transplantation for patients with sickle cell disease: progress and future directions. *Hematol Oncol Clin North Am* 2014;28:1171-1185.
79. Walters MC, De Castro LM, Sullivan KM, et al. Indications and results of HLA-identical sibling hematopoietic cell transplantation for sickle cell disease. *Biol Blood Marrow Trans* 2016;22:207-211.
80. Thompson LM, Ceja ME, Yang SA. Stem cell transplantation for treatment of sickle cell disease: bone marrow versus cord blood transplants. *Am J Health Syst Pharm* 2012;69:1295-1302.
81. Khoury R, Abboud MR. Stem-cell transplantation in children and adults with sickle cell disease: an update. *Expert Rev Hematol* 2011;4:343-351.
82. Al Jefri AH. Advances in allogeneic stem cell transplantation for hemoglobinopathies. *Hemoglobin* 2011;35:469-475.
83. Angelucci E, Matthes-Martin S, Baronciani D, et al. Hematopoietic stem cell transplantation in thalassemia major and sickle cell disease: indications and management recommendations from an international expert panel. *Haematologica* 2014;99:811-820.

84. Olujohungbe A, Burnett AL. How I manage priapism due to sickle cell disease. *Br J Haematol* 2013;160:754-765.
85. Lane A, Deveras R. Potential risks of chronic sildenafil use for priapism in sickle cell disease. *J Sex Med* 2011;8:3193-3195.
86. Zempsky WT. Evaluation and treatment of sickle cell pain in the emergency department: paths to a better future. *Clin Pediatr Emerg Med* 2010;11:265-273.
87. Jerrell JM, Tripathi A, Stallworth JR. Pain management in children and adolescents with sickle cell disease. *Am J Hematol* 2011;86:82-84.
88. Wright J, Ahmedzai SH. The management of painful crisis in sickle cell disease. *Curr Opin Support Palliat Care* 2010;4:97-106.
89. Krishnamurti L, Smith-Packard B, Gupta A, et al. Impact of individualized pain plan on the emergency management of children with sickle cell disease. *Pediatr Blood Cancer* 2014;61:1747-1753.
90. Head CA, Swerdlow P, McDade WA, et al. Beneficial effects of nitric oxide breathing in adult patients with sickle cell crisis. *Am J Hematol* 2010;85:800-802.
91. Gladwin MT, Kato GJ, Weiner D, et al. Nitric oxide for inhalation in the acute treatment of sickle cell pain crisis: a randomized controlled trial. *JAMA* 2011;305:893-902.
92. Morris CR, Kuypers FA, Lavrisha L, et al. A randomized, placebo-controlled trial of arginine therapy for the treatment of children with sickle cell disease hospitalized with vaso-occlusive pain episodes. *Haematologica* 2013;98:1375-1382.
93. Vandy Black L, Smith WR. Evidence-based mini-review: are systemic corticosteroids an effective treatment for acute pain in sickle cell disease? *Hematology Am Soc Hematol Educ Program* 2010;2010:416-417.
94. Brandow AM, Farley RA, Panepinto JA. Early insights into the neurobiology of pain in sickle cell disease: A systematic review of the literature. *Pediatr Blood Cancer* 2015;62:1501-1511.
95. Lanzkron S, Haywood C, Jr. The five key things you need to know to manage adult patients with sickle cell disease. *Hematology Am Soc Hematol Educ Program* 2015;2015:420-425.
96. Ware RE, Despotovic JM, Mortier NA, et al. Pharmacokinetics, pharmacodynamics, and pharmacogenetics of hydroxyurea treatment for children with sickle cell anemia. *Blood* 2011;118:4985-4991.
97. Fertrin KY, Costa FF. Genomic polymorphisms in sickle cell disease: implications for clinical diversity and treatment. *Expert Rev Hematol* 2010;3:443-458.
98. Yee MM, Josephson C, Hill CE, et al. Cytochrome P450 2D6 polymorphisms and predicted opioid metabolism in African American children with sickle cell disease. *J Pediatr Hematol Oncol* 2013;35:e301-e305.

Drug-Induced Hematologic Disorders

e103

Elisa M. Greene and Tracy M. Hagemann

KEY CONCEPTS

1. The most common drug-induced hematologic disorders include aplastic anemia, agranulocytosis, megaloblastic anemia, hemolytic anemia, and thrombocytopenia.
2. Drug-induced hematologic disorders are generally rare adverse effects associated with drug therapy.
3. The incidence of rare adverse drug reactions (ADRs) is usually established by postmarketing surveillance and reporting.
4. Rechallenging a patient with an agent suspected of inducing a blood disorder is not generally recommended.
5. Drug-induced hematologic disorders can occur by two mechanisms: direct drug or metabolite toxicity or an immune reaction.
6. The primary treatment of drug-induced hematologic disorders is removal of the drug in question and symptomatic support of the patient.

INTRODUCTION

1 Hematologic disorders have long been a potential risk of modern pharmacotherapy. Granulocytopenia (agranulocytosis) was reported in association with one of medicine's early therapeutic agents, sulfanilamide, in 1938.[1] Some agents cause predictable hematologic disease (eg, antineoplastics), but others induce idiosyncratic reactions not directly related to the drugs' pharmacology. The most common drug-induced hematologic disorders include aplastic anemia, agranulocytosis, megaloblastic anemia, hemolytic anemia, and thrombocytopenia.

2 The incidence of idiosyncratic drug-induced hematologic disorders varies depending on the condition and the associated drug. Few epidemiologic studies have evaluated the actual incidence of these adverse reactions, but these reactions appear to be rare. Women are generally more susceptible than men to the hematologic effects of drugs. The incidence varies based on geography, which suggests that genetic differences may be important determinants of susceptibility. Drug-induced thrombocytopenia is the most common drug-induced hematologic disorder, with reports suggesting that between 0.1% and 5% of patients who receive heparin develop heparin-induced thrombocytopenia (HIT).[2,3] The Berlin Case-Control Surveillance Study was conducted from 2000 to 2009 to assess the incidence and risks of drug-induced hematologic disorders and found that almost 30% of all cases of blood dyscrasias were "possibly" attributable to drug therapy.[4]

Although drug-induced hematologic disorders are less common than other types of adverse reactions, they are associated with significant morbidity and mortality. Aplastic anemia is the leading cause of death followed by thrombocytopenia, agranulocytosis, and hemolytic anemia.[5] Similar to most other adverse drug reactions (ADRs), drug-induced hematologic disorders are more common in elderly adults than in the young; the risk of death also appears to be greater with increasing age.

3 The MedWatch program supported by the Food and Drug Administration[6] is the most common avenue for postmarketing surveillance to establish the incidence of ADRs. Many facilities have similar drug-reporting programs to follow ADR trends and to determine whether an association between a drug and an ADR is causal or coincidental. These programs enable practitioners to confirm that an adverse event is the result of drug therapy rather than one of many other potential causes; general guidelines are readily available.[7,8]

4 Because drug-induced blood disorders are potentially dangerous, rechallenging a patient with a suspected agent in an attempt to confirm a diagnosis is not recommended. In vitro studies with the offending agent and cells or plasma from the patient's blood can be performed to determine causality.[9] These methods are often expensive, however, and require facilities and expertise that are not generally available. Laboratory confirmation of drug causation is not always necessary to warrant interruption or discontinuation of therapy. Therefore, it is extremely important that practitioners be able to clinically evaluate suspect drugs quickly and to interrupt therapy when necessary.

Through the use of surveillance programs, lists of drugs that may be associated with adverse events have been published. These lists include a large number of commonly used drugs. Although these lists may help clinicians identify specific drug causes of adverse events, the large number of agents implicated may make this a difficult process. The absence of a drug from such a list should not discourage the investigation and reporting of a suspected agent associated with an adverse event. It is imperative that clinicians use a rational approach to determine causality and identify the agents associated with a reaction. The clinician should focus on the issue, perform a rigorous investigation, develop appropriate criteria, use objective criteria to grade the response, and complete a quantitative summary. A complete, thorough, and detailed drug and exposure history must be obtained from the patient in order to best determine any potential for drug causation.

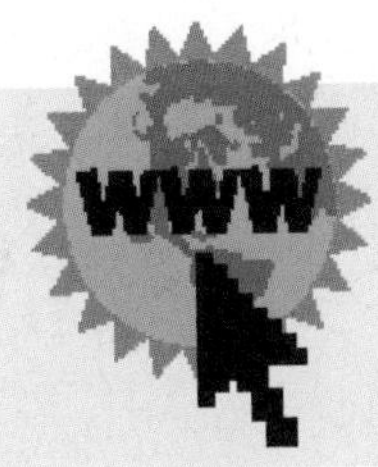

The complete chapter, learning objectives, and other resources can be found at **www.pharmacotherapyonline.com.**

Laboratory Tests to Direct Antimicrobial Pharmacotherapy

e104

Michael J. Rybak, Jeffrey R. Aeschlimann, and Kerry L. LaPlante

KEY CONCEPTS

1. Understanding the difference between normal host flora and typical pathogens will help to determine whether a patient is truly infected or merely colonized.
2. Direct examination of tissue and body fluids by Gram stain provides rapid information about the causative pathogen.
3. Isolation of the offending organism by culture or rapid diagnostic testing assists in the diagnosis of infection and allows for more definitive directed treatment.
4. Development of molecular testing systems (or rapid diagnostic testing) has improved our ability to diagnose infection and determine the antimicrobial susceptibilities for numerous pathogens, including fastidious or slow growing mycobacteria and viruses.
5. Although highly standardized, in vitro antimicrobial susceptibility testing has limitations and often cannot truly mimic the conditions found at the site of an infection. This can cause discordance between in vitro susceptibility results and in vivo response to therapy.
6. Laboratory evaluation of antimicrobial activity is an important component of the pharmacotherapeutic management of infectious diseases.
7. When used appropriately, rapid automated susceptibility test systems appear to improve therapeutic outcomes of patients with infection, especially when they are linked with other clinical information systems.
8. Laboratory tests such as the minimum inhibitory and minimum bactericidal concentration tests, time-kill tests, postantibiotic effect tests, and antimicrobial combination testing are important for the clinician to understand because they help to determine antimicrobial pharmacodynamic properties.
9. Routine monitoring of serum concentrations is currently used for a select few antimicrobials (eg, aminoglycosides and vancomycin) in an attempt to minimize toxicity and maximize efficacy.
10. Appropriate timing for the collection of serum samples when measuring antimicrobial serum concentrations is crucial to ensure that proper data are generated on the pharmacokinetics of antimicrobials.
11. Monitoring of aminoglycoside serum concentrations and the use of extended-interval doses can help to maximize the probability of therapeutic success and minimize the probability of aminoglycoside-related toxicity for certain infections.
12. Vancomycin and aminoglycoside serum concentration monitoring should be routinely done to ensure adequate serum concentrations, minimize toxicity, and avoid the potential for resistance.
13. Antimicrobial pharmacodynamics have become a crucial consideration for the selection of both empirical and pathogen-directed therapy in the current era of antimicrobial resistance.
14. Optimization of antimicrobial pharmacodynamic parameters such as the ratio of the peak serum concentration to minimum inhibitory concentration (MIC) or the time that the antibiotic serum concentration remains above the MIC and area above the curve over MIC can improve infection treatment outcomes.

Selection of an appropriate antimicrobial therapeutic regimen for a given infection requires knowledge of the infecting pathogen, host characteristics, and the drug's expected activity against the pathogen. The most fundamental aspect of therapy starts with an appropriate diagnosis. A vast array of laboratory tests including rapid diagnostic technology is available to assist in verifying the presence of infection and for monitoring the response to therapy. Although rigorous standardization of these tests is desirable, many of the tests may be difficult to interpret correctly and therefore, often they should be considered complementary to sound clinical judgment. Organism susceptibility to the administered antimicrobials is key to determining the outcome from therapy. Host characteristics, however, such as immune status, infection site location, and body organ function, play a significant role in selecting the most appropriate antimicrobial for a given individual.[1] This chapter reviews the routine laboratory tests that are used to assist in the diagnosis and treatment of infection.

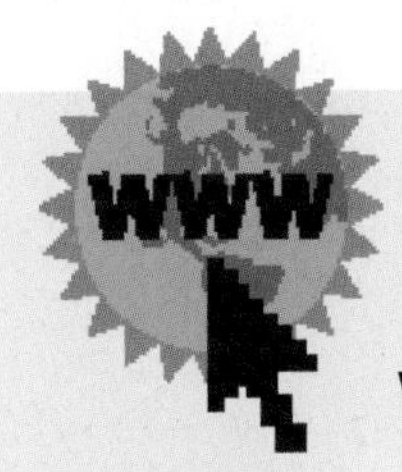

The complete chapter, learning objectives, and other resources can be found at **www.pharmacotherapyonline.com.**

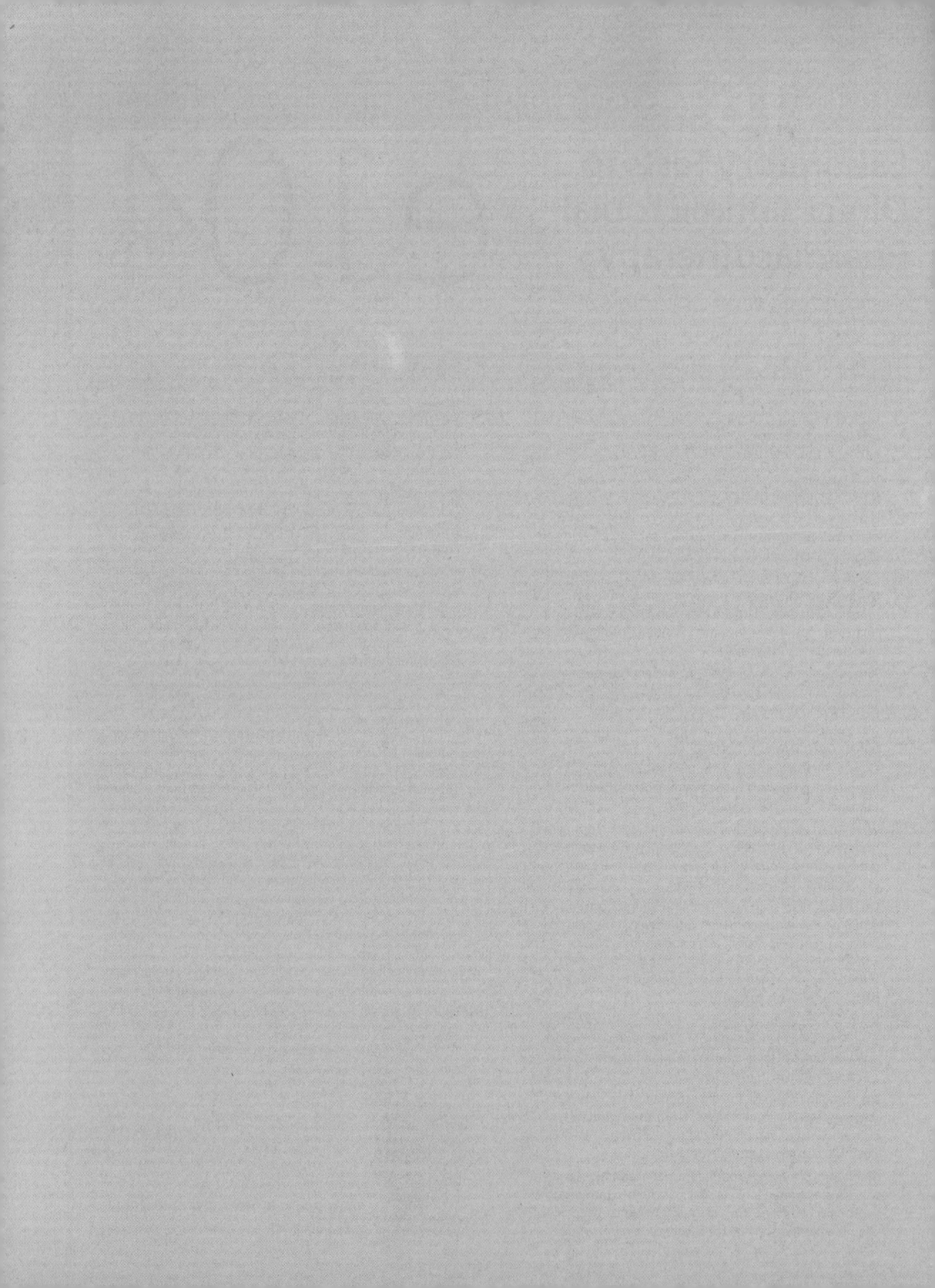

Antimicrobial Regimen Selection

105

Grace C. Lee and David S. Burgess

KEY CONCEPTS

1. Every attempt should be made to obtain specimens for culture and sensitivity testing prior to initiating antibiotics.
2. Empirical antibiotic therapy should be based on knowledge of likely pathogens for the site of infection, information from patient history (eg, recent hospitalizations, work-related exposure, travel, and pets), and local susceptibility.
3. Patients with delayed dermatologic reactions (ie, rash) to penicillin generally can receive cephalosporins. Patients with type I hypersensitivity reactions (ie, anaphylaxis) to penicillins should not receive cephalosporins. Alternatives to the cephalosporins include aztreonam, quinolones, sulfonamide antibiotics, or vancomycin based on type of coverage indicated.
4. Creatinine clearance should be estimated for every patient who is to receive antibiotics and the antibiotic dose interval adjusted accordingly. Hepatic function should be considered for drugs eliminated through the hepatobiliary system, such as clindamycin, erythromycin, and metronidazole.
5. All concomitant drugs and nutritional supplements should be reviewed when an antibiotic is added to a patient's therapy to ensure drug–drug interactions will be avoided.
6. Combination antibiotic therapy may be indicated for polymicrobial infections (eg, intra-abdominal and gynecologic infections), to produce synergistic killing (such as β-lactam plus aminoglycoside vs *Pseudomonas aeruginosa*), or to prevent the emergence of resistance.
7. All patients receiving antibiotics should be monitored for resolution of infectious signs and symptoms (eg, decreasing temperature and white blood cell count) and adverse drug events.
8. Antibiotics with the narrowest effective spectrum of activity are preferred. Antibiotic route of administration should be evaluated daily, and conversion from IV to oral therapy should be attempted as signs of infection improve for patients with functioning GI tracts (general exceptions are endocarditis and CNS infections).
9. Patients not responding to an appropriate antibiotic treatment in 2 to 3 days should be reevaluated to ensure (a) the correct diagnosis, (b) that therapeutic drug concentrations are being achieved, (c) that the patient is not immunosuppressed, (d) that the patient does not have an isolated infection (ie, abscess and foreign body), or (e) that resistance has not developed.
10. The main goals of antimicrobial stewardship programs (ASPs) are to optimize antimicrobial selection, dosing, duration, and route of administration while minimizing adverse drug events and the emergence of antimicrobial resistance.

Antimicrobials are among the most widely used classes of drugs. In the United States, expenditures for antimicrobial agents exceed $10 billion annually. Approximately 20% to 40% of hospitalized patients receive antibiotics. The use of antibiotics is the main driver in creating selective pressure for the emergence of antimicrobial resistant pathogens; nevertheless, antibiotic overuse remains common. Selecting appropriate antimicrobial agent(s) to treat an infection has proven to be a challenging task.[1,2] Although the choice of a single agent or a combination of agents should be individualized for each patient, certain general principles of therapy should guide the selection of specific drugs (Table 105-1).

The initial selection of antimicrobial therapy is nearly always empirical, which is prior to documentation and identification of the offending organism. Infectious diseases generally are acute, and a delay in antimicrobial therapy can result in serious morbidity or even mortality. Thus, empirical antimicrobial therapy selection should be based on information gathered from the patient's history and physical examination and results of Gram stains or of rapidly performed tests on specimens from the infected site. This information, combined with knowledge of the most likely offending organism(s) and an institution's local susceptibility patterns, should result in a rational selection of antibiotics to treat the patient. This chapter introduces a systematic approach to the selection of antimicrobial therapeutic regimens.

CONFIRMING THE PRESENCE OF INFECTION

An infectious disease diagnosis is determined by assessing the presence of signs and symptoms of an infection, determining the site of infection, and establishing a microbiological diagnosis, when possible.

Fever

The presence of a temperature greater than the expected 37°C (98.6°F) "normal" body temperature is considered a hallmark of infectious diseases. Body temperature is controlled by the hypothalamus. In addition, the circadian rhythm, a built-in temperature cycle, is also operational. The daily temperature rhythm can vary for each individual. In a healthy person, the internal thermostat is set between the morning low temperature and the afternoon peak as controlled by the circadian rhythm. During fever, the hypothalamus is reset at a higher temperature level.

Fever is defined as a controlled elevation of body temperature above the normal range. The average normal body temperature range taken orally is 36.7°C to 37°C (98°F-98.6°F). Body temperatures obtained rectally generally are 0.6°C (1°F) higher and axillary temperatures are 0.6°C (1°F) lower than oral temperatures, respectively. Skin temperatures are also less than the oral temperature but can vary depending on the specific measurement method.

TABLE 105-1 Systematic Approach for Selection of Antimicrobials

Confirm the presence of infection
Careful history and physical examination
Signs and symptoms
Predisposing factors
Identification of the pathogen (see Chapter e25)
Collection of infected material
Stains
Serologies
Culture and sensitivity
Selection of presumptive therapy considering every infected site
Host factors
Drug factors
Monitor therapeutic response
Clinical assessment
Laboratory tests
Assessment of therapeutic failure

Fever can be a manifestation of disease states other than infection. Collagen vascular (autoimmune) disorders and several malignancies can have fever as a manifestation. Fever of unknown or undetermined origin is a diagnostic dilemma and is reviewed extensively elsewhere.[3]

Many drugs have been identified as causes of fever. *Drug-induced fever* is defined as persistent fever in the absence of infection or other underlying condition. The fever must coincide temporally with the administration of the offending agent and disappear promptly on its withdrawal, after which the temperature remains normal. Possible mechanisms of drug-induced fever are either a hypersensitivity reaction or development of antigen–antibody complexes that result in the stimulation of macrophages and the release of interleukin 1 (IL-1). While fever is not a common drug effect (accounting for no more than 5% of all drug reactions), it should be suspected when obvious reasons for fever are not present. Almost any medication can produce fever, but β-lactam antibiotics, anticonvulsants, allopurinol, hydralazine, nitrofurantoin, sulfonamides, phenothiazines, and methyldopa appear to be responsible more often than others.

Noninfectious etiologies of fever can be referred to as "false-positives." Although these certainly can confuse the clinician, even more troublesome are false-negatives: the absence of fever in a patient with signs and symptoms consistent with an infectious disease. Careful questioning of the patient or family is vital to assess the ingestion of any medication that can mask fever (eg, aspirin, acetaminophen, nonsteroidal anti-inflammatory agents, and corticosteroids). The use of antipyretics should be discouraged during the treatment of infection unless absolutely necessary because they can mask a poor therapeutic response. Moreover, elevated body temperature, unless very high (greater than 40.5°C [greater than 105°F]), is not harmful and may be beneficial.

Signs and Symptoms

White Blood Cell Count

Most infections result in elevated white blood cell (WBC) counts (leukocytosis) because of the increased production and mobilization of granulocytes (neutrophils, basophils, and eosinophils), lymphocytes, or both to ingest and destroy invading microbes. The generally accepted range of normal values for WBC counts is between 4,000 and 10,000 cells/mm^3 (4×10^9 and 10×10^9/L). Values above or below this range hold important prognostic and diagnostic value.

Bacterial infections are associated with elevated granulocyte counts, often with immature forms (band neutrophils) seen in peripheral blood smears. Mature neutrophils are also referred to as *segmented neutrophils* or *polymorphonuclear* (PMN) *leukocytes.* The presence of immature forms (left shift) is an indication of an increased bone marrow response to the infection. With infection, peripheral WBC counts can be very high, but they are rarely higher than 30,000 to 40,000 cells/mm^3 (30×10^9/L-40×10^9/L). Because leukocytosis indicates the normal host response to infection, low leukocyte counts after the onset of infection indicate an abnormal response and generally are associated with a poor prognosis.

The most common granulocyte defect is neutropenia, a decrease in absolute numbers of circulating neutrophils. A thorough description of the consequences of neutropenia is given in Chapter e99. Lymphocytosis, even with normal or slightly elevated total WBC counts, generally is associated with tuberculosis and viral or fungal infections. Increases in monocytes can be associated with tuberculosis or lymphoma, and increases in eosinophils can be associated with allergic reactions to drugs or infections caused by metazoa. Many types of infections can be accompanied by a completely normal WBC count and differential.

Local Signs

The classic signs of pain and inflammation can manifest as swelling, erythema, tenderness, and purulent drainage. Unfortunately, these are only visible if the infection is superficial or in a bone or joint. The manifestations of inflammation in deep-seated infections (eg, meningitis, pneumonia, endocarditis, and urinary tract infection) must be ascertained by examining tissues or fluids. For example, the presence of neutrophils in spinal fluid, lung secretions (sputum), or urine is highly suggestive of a bacterial infection.

Symptoms referable to an organ system must be sought out carefully because not only do they help in establishing the presence of infection, but they also aid in narrowing the list of potential pathogens. For example, a febrile patient with complaints of flank pain and dysuria can well have pyelonephritis. In this situation, enteric Gram-negative bacilli, especially *Escherichia coli*, are the predominant pathogens. If a febrile patient has no symptoms suggestive of an organ system but only constitutional complaints, the list of possible infectious diseases is lengthy.[3] A febrile individual with cough and sputum production probably has a pulmonary infection. What is not so evident, however, is the etiologic organism in this situation, because it can be caused by bacteria, mycobacteria, viruses, *Chlamydia*, or mycoplasmas.[4] In this situation, attention to the patient's history and background disease states is important. Even more important is a careful examination of the infected material (in this case sputum) to ascertain the identity of the pathogen.

IDENTIFICATION OF THE PATHOGEN

Microbiological Studies

1 Identification and antimicrobial susceptibility of a suspected pathogen are the most important factors in determining the choice of antimicrobial therapy. Generally, infected body materials must be sampled, if at all possible or practical, before or concurrently with institution of any antimicrobial therapy for two reasons. First, a Gram stain of the material might reveal bacteria, or an acid-fast stain might detect mycobacteria or actinomycetes. Second, the premature use of antimicrobials can suppress the growth of pathogens which might result in false-negative cultures results or alterations in the cellular and chemical composition of infected fluids. This is particularly true in patients with vertebral osteomyelitis, urinary tract infections, subacute endocarditis, meningitis, and septic arthritis.[5-9]

Blood cultures usually should be performed in the acutely ill febrile patient. Blood culture collection should coincide with sharp elevations in temperature, suggesting the possibility of microorganisms or microbial antigens in the bloodstream. Ideally, blood should be obtained from peripheral sites as two sets (one set consists of an aerobic bottle and one set an anaerobic bottle) from two different sites approximately 1 hour apart. In selected infections, bacteremia is qualitatively continuous (eg, endocarditis), so cultures can be obtained at any time.[9]

In addition to the infected materials produced by the patient (eg, blood, sputum, urine, stool, and wound or sinus drainage), other less accessible fluids or tissues must be obtained if they are suspected to be the infected site (eg, spinal fluid in meningitis and joint fluid in arthritis). Abscesses and cellulitic areas also should be aspirated.

When a pathogenic microorganism is identified, the next step for the majority of clinical microbiological laboratories is antimicrobial susceptibility testing which measures the ability of a select organism to grow in the presence of an antimicrobial agent. These methods are described in detail in Chapter e25. Once a microorganism is identified and its susceptibilities are known, specific definitive antimicrobial therapy should be promptly administered.

Over the last decade, there has been an explosion in the development of rapid diagnostic methods that provide simultaneous organism identification and resistance marker detection. These methods include nonamplified probe technologies (peptide nucleic-acid-fluorescence in situ hybridization), proteomics, and nucleic acid amplification methods combined with microarray technologies. These tests can significantly reduce time to organism identification; thereby, can reduce time to effective antimicrobial therapy, overall antimicrobial use, and health outcomes among patients with infectious diseases.[10-12]

Interpreting Results

After a positive Gram stain, culture results, or both are obtained, the clinician must be cautious in determining whether the organism recovered is a true pathogen, a contaminant, or a part of the normal flora (see Chapter e25). The latter consideration is especially problematic with cultures obtained from the skin, oropharynx, nose, ears, eyes, throat, and perineum. These surfaces are heavily colonized with a wide variety of bacteria, some of which can be pathogenic in certain settings. For example, coagulase-negative staphylococci are found in cultures of all the aforementioned sites, yet are seldom regarded as pathogens unless recovered from blood, venous access catheters, or prosthetic devices.

Importantly, cultures of specimens from purportedly infected sites that are obtained by sampling from or through one of these contaminated areas might contain significant numbers of the normal flora. For urine cultures, the urinalysis should be used in combination with culture results to assess the presence of WBCs, nitrite, and leukocyte esterase to help confirm infection and rule out colonization.[13]

Particularly problematic are expectorated sputum specimens that must be evaluated carefully by determination of the presence of squamous epithelial cells and leukocytes.[4] A predominance of epithelial cells in sputum specimens reduces the likelihood that recovered bacteria are pathogenic, especially when multiple types of organisms are seen on Gram stain. In contrast, the discovery of leukocytes in large numbers with one predominant type of organism is a more reliable indicator of a valid collection. In general, however, sputum evaluation has poor sensitivity and specificity as a diagnostic test.

Gram-staining techniques, culture methods, and serologic identification, as well as susceptibility testing, are discussed in detail in Chapter e25. Emphasis must be placed on the proper collection and handling of specimens and careful assessment of Gram stain or other test results in guiding the clinician toward appropriate selection of initial antimicrobial therapy.[14]

SELECTION OF PRESUMPTIVE THERAPY

2 In many instances, empiric therapy must be instituted before microbiological results are available. To select rational antimicrobial therapy for a given clinical situation, a variety of factors must be considered. These include the severity and acuity of the disease, local epidemiology and antibiogram, patient history, host factors, factors related to the drugs used, and the necessity for using multiple agents. In addition, there are generally accepted drugs of choice for the treatment of most pathogens (see **Appendix 105-1**).

Antibiogram

Drugs of choice are compiled from a variety of sources and are intended as guidelines rather than as specific rules for antimicrobial use. These choices are influenced by local antimicrobial susceptibility data rather than information published by other institutions or national compilations. Each institution should publish an annual summary of antibiotic susceptibilities (antibiogram) for organisms cultured from patients. Antibiograms contain both the number of nonduplicate isolates for common species and the percentage susceptible to the antibiotics tested. To further guide empirical antibiotic therapy, some hospitals publish unit-specific antibiograms in unique patient care areas, such as intensive care units or burn units.

Susceptibility of bacteria can differ substantially among hospitals within a community. For example, the prevalence of hospital-acquired methicillin-resistant *Staphylococcus aureus* (HA-MRSA) in some centers is quite high, whereas in other centers the problem might be nonexistent. This particular situation will influence the selection of therapy for possible *S. aureus* infection, where the clinician must choose either a β-lactam or vancomycin. The problem of differing susceptibilities is not limited only to Gram-positive bacteria but also is evident in Gram-negative organisms, and all drug classes are affected.

Patient History

Empirical therapy is directed at organisms that are known to cause the infection in question. These organisms are discussed for different sites of infection in Chapters 83 to e103. To define the most likely infecting organisms, a careful history and physical examination must be performed. The place where the infection was acquired should be determined, for example, the home (community acquired), nursing home environment, or hospital acquired (nosocomial). Nursing home patients can be exposed to potentially more resistant organisms because they are often surrounded by ill patients who are receiving antibiotics. Important considerations when selecting empiric antimicrobial therapy include: 1) prior knowledge of colonization or infections, 2) previous antimicrobial use, 3) the site of infection and the organisms most likely pathogens, and 4) local antibiogram and resistance patterns for important pathogens. Other questions to ask infected patients regarding the history of present illness include: 1) Are any other people sick at home, especially children? 2) Are any unusual pets kept in the home? 3) Where are you employed (ie, are you exposed to contaminated meat or infectious biohazards)? and 4) Has there been any recent travel (ie, to endemic areas of fungal infections or developing countries)?

Host Factors

Several host factors should be considered when evaluating a patient for antimicrobial therapy. The most important factors are drug allergies, age, pregnancy, genetic or metabolic abnormalities, renal and hepatic function, site of infection, concomitant drug therapy, and underlying disease states.

Allergy

3 Allergy to an antimicrobial agent generally precludes its use. Careful assessment of allergy histories must be performed because many patients confuse common adverse drug effects (ie, GI disturbance) with true allergic reactions.[15-17] Among the most commonly cited antimicrobial allergies are those to penicillin, penicillin-related compounds, or both. In the absence of complete penicillin skin testing capabilities, a rule of thumb for giving cephalosporins to patients allergic to penicillin is to avoid giving them to patients who give a good history for immediate or accelerated reactions (eg, anaphylaxis, laryngospasm) and to give them under close supervision in patients with a history of delayed reactions, such as a rash.[18] If a Gram-negative infection is suspected or documented, therapy with a monobactam may be appropriate because cross-reactivity with other β-lactams is nonexistent.

Age

The patient's age is an important factor both in trying to identify the likely etiologic agent and in assessing the patient's ability to eliminate the drug(s) to be used. The best example of an age determinant of organisms is in bacterial meningitis, where the pathogens differ as the patient grows from the neonatal period through infancy and childhood into adulthood.[5,19]

For neonates, hepatic and liver functions are not well developed. Therefore, bilirubin excretion is decreased resulting in increased concentration of unconjugated bilirubin that can cause kernicterus. Neonates (especially when premature) can develop kernicterus when given sulfonamides. This results from displacement of bilirubin from serum albumin. In addition, neonates have more body water content that results in a larger volume of distribution leading to adjustments in antibiotic dosing regimens. Additional special drug considerations for pediatric patients include low frequency of adverse effects and compliance-enhancing features (eg, absorption not affected by food, once- to twice-daily dosing, and good taste).[7,20,21]

The major physiologic change in persons older than 65 years of age is a decline in the number of functioning nephrons that, in turn, results in decreased renal function.[22] This is usually manifested by an increased incidence of side effects caused by antimicrobials that are eliminated renally. For example, renal toxicity caused by aminoglycosides may be apparent much sooner during therapy in older adults than in younger patients.

Pregnancy

During pregnancy, not only is the fetus at risk for drug teratogenicity, but the pharmacokinetic disposition of certain drugs can be altered.[23] Penicillins, cephalosporins, and aminoglycosides are cleared from the peripheral circulation more rapidly during pregnancy. This is probably a result of marked increases in intravascular volume, glomerular filtration rate, and hepatic and metabolic activities. The net result is that maternal serum antimicrobial concentrations can be as much as 50% lower during this period than in the nonpregnant state. Increased dosages of certain compounds might be necessary to achieve therapeutic levels during late pregnancy.[24]

Metabolic or Genetic Variation

Inherited or acquired metabolic abnormalities will influence the therapy of infectious diseases in a variety of ways. For example, patients with impaired peripheral vascular flow may not absorb drugs given by intramuscular injection. In addition, certain metabolic states can predispose patients to enhanced drug toxicity. For instance, patients who are phenotypically slow acetylators of isoniazid are at greater risk for peripheral neuropathy.[25] Patients with severe deficiency of glucose-6-phosphate dehydrogenase can develop significant hemolysis when exposed to such drugs as sulfonamides, nitrofurantoin, nalidixic acid, antimalarials, and dapsone. Although mild deficiencies are found in African Americans, the more severe forms of the disease generally are confined to persons of eastern Mediterranean origin. Another example is the antiretroviral drug abacavir, which is associated with a severe hypersensitivity reaction, consisting of fever, rash, abdominal pain, and respiratory distress. This risk has been associated with the presence of a human leukocyte antigen allele HLA-B*5701. Routine screening for the presence of this allele before initiating treatment with abacavir is a recommendation in the current HIV treatment guidelines. Furthermore, the hepatic cytochrome P450 system is a major pathway for a large number of antimicrobials. While differential host expressions of these enzymes occur, insufficient clinical data are currently available to recommend routine screening for antimicrobial therapy.

Organ Dysfunction

4 Patients with diminished renal or hepatic function or both will accumulate certain drugs unless the dosage is adjusted. It is common for patents requiring antimicrobial therapy to have some degree of renal impairment. Because many of the commonly used antimicrobials are primarily cleared by the kidneys, it is imperative to adjust the dosing regimen or therapy.[26,27] Recommendations for dosing antibiotics in patients with liver dysfunction are not as formalized as guidelines for patients with renal dysfunction. Antibiotics that should be adjusted in severe liver disease include clindamycin, erythromycin, metronidazole, and rifampin. Significant accumulation can occur when both liver dysfunction and renal dysfunction are present for the following drugs: cefotaxime, nafcillin, piperacillin, and sulfamethoxazole.[28]

Concomitant Drugs

5 Any concomitant therapy that the patient is receiving can influence the drug selection, dose, and monitoring. For instance, administration of isoniazid to a patient who is also receiving phenytoin can result in phenytoin toxicity secondary to inhibition of phenytoin metabolism by isoniazid. Furthermore, drugs that possess similar adverse effect profiles can increase the risk for effects (ie, two drugs that cause nephrotoxicity or neutropenia). A detailed review of drug interactions is beyond the scope of this chapter, but an excellent textbook on this subject is available.[29] Lists of potentially severe drug–drug interactions are provided in Table 105-2.

Concomitant Disease States

Concomitant disease states can influence the selection of therapy. Certain diseases will predispose patients to a particular infectious disease or will alter the type of infecting organism. For example, patients with diabetes mellitus and the resulting peripheral vascular disease often develop infections of the lower extremity soft tissue. Moreover, the alterations in peripheral blood flow associated with the disease and perhaps altered immunity make such infections more difficult to treat than in nondiabetics. Patients with chronic lung disease or cystic fibrosis develop frequent pulmonary infections that can be caused by somewhat different microorganisms than are found in otherwise normal hosts.

Patients with immunosuppressive diseases, such as malignancies or acquired immunologic deficiencies, are highly predisposed to infections, and the types of causative or pathogenic organisms can be vastly different from what would be expected (see Chapter e99). For instance, patients undergoing chemotherapy for acute forms of leukemia often are profoundly granulocytopenic and are predisposed to infections caused by bacteria and fungi.[30] Patients with the acquired immunodeficiency syndrome (AIDS) often become infected with an enormous variety of organisms (see Chapter e103).

TABLE 105-2 Major Drug Interactions with Antimicrobials

Antimicrobial	Other Agent(s)	Mechanism of Action/Effect	Clinical Management
Aminoglycosides	Neuromuscular blocking agents	Additive adverse effects	Avoid
	Nephrotoxins (N) or ototoxins (O) (eg, amphotericin B [N], cisplatin [N/O], cyclosporine [N], furosemide [O], NSAIDs [N], radiocontrast [N], vancomycin [N])	Additive adverse effects	Monitor aminoglycoside SDC and renal function
Amphotericin B	Nephrotoxins (eg, aminoglycosides, cidofovir, cyclosporine, foscarnet, pentamidine)	Additive adverse effects	Monitor renal function
Azoles	See Chapter 98		
Chloramphenicol	Phenytoin, tolbutamide, ethanol	Decreased metabolism of other agents	Monitor phenytoin SDC, blood glucose
Foscarnet	Pentamidine IV	Increased risk of severe nephrotoxicity/hypocalcemia	Monitor renal function/serum calcium
Isoniazid	Carbamazepine, phenytoin	Decreased metabolism of other agents (nausea, vomiting, nystagmus, ataxia)	Monitor drug SDC
Macrolides/azalides	Digoxin	Decreased digoxin bioavailability and metabolism	Monitor digoxin SDC; avoid if possible
	Theophylline	Decreased metabolism of theophylline	Monitor theophylline SDC
Metronidazole	Ethanol (drugs containing ethanol)	Disulfiram-like reaction	Avoid
Penicillins and cephalosporins	Probenecid, aspirin	Blocked excretion of β-lactams	Use if prolonged high concentration of β-lactam desirable
Ciprofloxacin/norfloxacin	Theophylline	Decreased metabolism of theophylline	Monitor theophylline
Quinolones	Classes Ia and III antiarrhythmics	Increased Q-T interval	Avoid
	Multivalent cations (antacids, iron, sucralfate, zinc, vitamins, dairy, citric acid), didanosine	Decreased absorption of quinolone	Separate by 2 hours
Rifampin	Azoles, cyclosporine, methadone propranolol, PIs, oral contraceptives, tacrolimus, warfarin	Increased metabolism of other agent	Avoid if possible
Sulfonamides	Sulfonylureas, phenytoin, warfarin	Decreased metabolism of other agent	Monitor blood glucose, SDC, PT
Tetracyclines	Antacids, iron, calcium, sucralfate	Decreased absorption of tetracycline	Separate by 2 hours
	Digoxin	Decreased digoxin bioavailability	Monitor digoxin SDC; avoid if possible

PI, protease inhibitor; PT, prothrombin time; SDC, serum drug concentrations.

Azalides: azithromycin; azoles: fluconazole, itraconazole, ketoconazole, and voriconazole; macrolides: erythromycin and clarithromycin; protease inhibitors: amprenavir, indinavir, lopinavir/ritonavir, nelfinavir, ritonavir, and saquinavir; quinolones: ciprofloxacin, gemifloxacin, levofloxacin, and moxifloxacin.

Many factors predisposing to infection are related to disruption of the host's integumentary barriers. For example, trauma, burns, and iatrogenic wounds induced in surgery can lead to a substantial risk of infection depending on the severity and location of the injury or disruption. For a complete discussion of the various risks involved in surgical procedures, see Chapter 100.

Drug Factors

Pharmacokinetic and Pharmacodynamic Considerations

Integration of both pharmacokinetic and pharmacodynamic properties of an agent is important when choosing antimicrobial therapy to ensure efficacy and to prevent resistance.[31] Early researchers relied solely on pharmacokinetic properties such as the area under the (drug concentration) curve (AUC), maximum observed concentration (peak), and drug half-life to optimize therapy. Pharmacodynamics is the study of the relationship between drug concentration and the effects on the microorganism. There is an important relationship between both pharmacokinetic and microbiologic parameters that has resulted in measurements such as AUC:minimal inhibitory concentration (MIC) ratio, peak:MIC ratio, and time (T) the concentration is above MIC ($T >$ MIC).[32-35]

Aminoglycosides exhibit concentration-dependent bactericidal effects. An example of the integration of pharmacokinetics and microbiologic activity is the use of high-dose, once-daily aminoglycosides. For these regimens, the drug is given as a single large daily dose to maximize the peak:MIC ratio. Aminoglycosides also possess a postantibiotic effect (persistent suppression of organism growth after concentrations decrease below the MIC) that appears to contribute to the success of high-dose, once-daily administration. Fluoroquinolones exhibit concentration-dependent killing activity, but optimal killing appears to be characterized by the AUC:MIC ratio.

β-Lactams display time-dependent bactericidal effects. Killing activity is enhanced only marginally if drug concentration exceeds the MIC. Therefore, the important pharmacodynamic relationship for these antimicrobials is the duration that drug concentrations exceed the MIC ($T >$ MIC). Effective dosing regimens require serum drug concentrations to exceed the MIC for at least 40% to 50% of the dosing interval. Frequent small doses, continuous infusion, or prolonged infusion of β-lactams appears to be correlated with positive outcomes.

A detailed discussion on antimicrobial pharmacokinetics–pharmacodynamics is beyond the scope of this chapter. However, excellent sources of information on this topic are available.[31,32,35]

Tissue Penetration

The importance of tissue penetration varies with site of infection. Some of the difficulties in interpreting data include a lack of correlation with clinical outcomes and poor understanding of whether the antimicrobial agents are present in a biologically active form. An example of the former problem is the recognized efficacy of drugs with low biliary fluid concentrations in the treatment of cholecystitis, cholangitis, or both and the absence of the enhanced efficacy of drugs whose primary route of elimination is biliary excretion of active drug. An example of the latter difficulty is with penetration to deep infections, such as abscesses, where various factors such as acid pH, WBC products, and various enzymes can inactivate even high concentrations of certain drugs.

The CNS is one body site where antimicrobial penetration is relatively well defined, and correlations with clinical outcomes are established.[5,36] CSF concentrations of antimicrobial agents necessary to cure bacterial meningitis have been defined, and drugs that do not reach significant concentrations in the CSF should be either avoided or instilled directly, if feasible.

Caution must be exercised when selecting an antimicrobial agent for clinical use on the basis of tissue or fluid penetration. Body fluids where drug concentration data are clinically relevant include CSF, urine, synovial fluid, and peritoneal fluid. Apart from these areas, more attention should be paid to clinical efficacy, antimicrobial spectrum, toxicity, and cost than to comparative data on penetration into a given body site.

The proper route of administration for an antimicrobial depends on the site of infection. Parenteral therapy is warranted when patients are being treated for febrile neutropenia or deep-seated infections such as meningitis, endocarditis, and osteomyelitis. Severe pneumonia often is treated initially with IV antibiotics and switched to oral therapy as clinical improvement is evident.[4,37,38] Patients treated in the ambulatory setting for upper respiratory tract infections (eg, pharyngitis, bronchitis, sinusitis, and otitis media), lower respiratory tract infections, skin and soft-tissue infections, uncomplicated urinary tract infections, and selected sexually transmitted diseases can usually receive oral therapy.

Drug Toxicity

It is incumbent on health professionals to avoid toxic drugs whenever possible. Antibiotics associated with CNS toxicities, usually when not dose-adjusted for renal function, include penicillins, cephalosporins, quinolones, and imipenem. Hematologic toxicities generally are manifested with prolonged use of nafcillin (neutropenia), piperacillin (platelet dysfunction), cefotetan (hypoprothrombinemia), chloramphenicol (bone marrow suppression, both idiosyncratic and dose-related toxicity), and trimethoprim (megaloblastic anemia). Reversible nephrotoxicity classically is associated with aminoglycosides and vancomycin. Irreversible ototoxicity can occur with aminoglycosides. In the outpatient setting, patients must be counseled regarding photosensitivity with azithromycin, quinolones, tetracyclines, pyrazinamide, sulfamethoxazole, and trimethoprim. Lastly, all antibiotics have been implicated in causing diarrhea and colitis secondary to *Clostridium difficile* (see Chapter 91).[39] List of potential antibiotic adverse drug reactions is provided in Table 105-3.

Aside from consideration of drug toxicity, some antimicrobial use requires more intensive risk–benefit analysis. An example of this is the decision to use isoniazid prophylactically to prevent tuberculosis. Because the hepatotoxicity of isoniazid increases in frequency with age, older persons (greater than 45 years of age) who are candidates for isoniazid prophylaxis (positive skin test) must have additional risk factors for tuberculosis to balance the potential toxic effects. These include evidence of recent skin test conversion, immunosuppression, or previous gastrectomy. Older patients without additional risk factors are more likely to suffer toxicity from isoniazid than derive benefit from its use.

Combination Antimicrobial Therapy

6 In selecting a drug regimen for a given patient, consideration must be given to the necessity of using more than one drug. Inappropriate or inadequate antimicrobial therapy has been associated with increased morbidity and mortality.[40] Combinations of antimicrobials generally are used to broaden the spectrum of coverage for empirical therapy, achieve synergistic activity against the infecting organism, and prevent the emergence of resistance.

Broadening the Spectrum of Coverage

Increasing the coverage of antimicrobial therapy generally is necessary in two scenarios. First is in mixed infections where multiple organisms are likely to be present. This is the case in intra-abdominal and female pelvic infections, in which a variety of aerobic and anaerobic bacteria can produce disease.[41] Traditionally, a combination of a drug active against aerobic Gram-negative bacilli (such as an aminoglycoside) and a drug active against anaerobic bacteria (such as metronidazole or clindamycin) is selected. Newer compounds, which possess good activity against both of these types of organisms, such as the β-lactam/β-lactamase inhibitor combinations, carbapenems, or glycylcyclines, might be adequate to replace the combination and thereby reduce the cost of therapy. The second scenario is for critically ill patients with presumed health care-associated infections in which an increased spectrum of activity is desirable.[37] Health care-associated infections are frequently caused by multi-drug resistant pathogens; combination therapy is used in this setting to ensure that at least one of the antimicrobials will be active against the pathogen(s).

Synergism

The achievement of synergistic antimicrobial activity is advantageous for infections caused by enteric Gram-negative bacilli in immunosuppressed patients. Laboratory tests to identify synergy between antibiotic combinations are described in Chapter 24. Traditionally, combinations of aminoglycosides and β-lactams have been used because these drugs together generally act synergistically against a wide variety of bacteria. However, the data supporting superior efficacy of synergistic over nonsynergistic combinations are weak. At best, synergistic combinations appear to produce better results in infections caused by *Pseudomonas aeruginosa* and *Enterococcus* species.[33,42-44]

The most obvious example of the use of synergy is the treatment of enterococcal endocarditis. The causative organism is usually only inhibited by penicillins, but it is killed rapidly by the addition of streptomycin or gentamicin to a penicillin. The need for bactericidal activity in the treatment of endocarditis underscores the need for these synergistic combinations.[9,45]

Preventing Resistance

The use of antimicrobial combinations to prevent the emergence of resistance is applied widely but not often realized. The only circumstance where this has been clearly effective is in the treatment of tuberculosis. The prevalence of resistance to a first-line drug such as isoniazid or rifampin in a population of organisms may be as high as 1 in 10^6 to 10^8. Because the bacterial load in a patient with active tuberculosis often exceeds this, two drugs are given to reduce the likelihood of encountering resistance to less than 1 in 10. There is ample evidence from in vitro data and experimental bacterial infections that combinations of drugs with different mechanisms are effective in the prevention of the emergence of resistance. Data from clinical trials, however, either are conflicting or do not convincingly support this concept.[42]

Clinical **Controversy...**

Rapid initiation of appropriate antibiotic therapy is associated with improved outcomes among patients with infections. Therefore, there is a great need for reliable methods to rapidly screen patient risk factors for infections due to multi-drug resistant pathogens. However, prediction tools or criteria definitions may lack sensitivity and or specificity, and may lead to inadequate therapy or to

TABLE 105-3 Antimicrobial Adverse Drug Reactions

Antimicrobial Class	Adverse Drug Reaction	Monitoring Parameters	Comments
Penicillins	Hypersensitivity reactions and rash, drug fever, diarrhea, emesis, abdominal pain, hepatitis, interstitial nephritis, leukopenia, thrombocytopenia, Coomb's positive-hemolytic anemia, *C. difficile* colitis, electrolyte abnormalities, seizures	Monitor for hypersensitivity reactions (eg, bronchospasm, anaphylaxis, angioneurotic edema, immediate urticaria). During prolonged therapy and/or high-dose regimens, periodically monitor renal function, hepatic function, and CBC	Most serious reaction is immediate IgE-mediated anaphylaxis. Incidence is 0.05%, but 5%-10% can be fatal
Cephalosporins	Hypersensitivity reactions and rash, drug fever, diarrhea, interstitial nephritis, Coomb's positive-hemolytic anemia, leukopenia, thrombocytopenia, coagulopathy, hepatitis, *C. difficile* colitis	Monitor for hypersensitivity reactions (eg, bronchospasm, anaphylaxis, angioneurotic edema, immediate urticaria) and rash, renal function, hepatic function, and CBC	Patients with a history of IgE-mediated allergic reactions to penicillins should not receive a cephalosporin
Carbapenems	Hypersensitivity reactions and rash, headache, nausea, diarrhea, seizures, drug fever, eosinophilia, thrombocytopenia, hepatitis, *C. difficile* colitis	Monitor for hypersensitivity reactions (eg, bronchospasm, anaphylaxis, angioneurotic edema, immediate urticaria) and rash, renal function, hepatic function, and CBC	Skin test cross-sensitivity with penicillin reported to be up to 50%, but clinically significant cross-sensitivity reactions in penicillin-allergic patients reported to be as low as 1% Highest incidence of seizures with use of imipenem–cilastatin. More frequent in patients who are elderly, have history of seizure disorders and renal dysfunction
Monobactams	Rash, diarrhea, nausea, hepatitis, thrombocytopenia, *C. difficile* colitis	Monitor renal and hepatic function	May be used in patients with allergy to penicillins/cephalosporins
Aminoglycosides	Tubular necrosis and renal failure, vestibular and cochlear toxicity, neuromuscular blockade, vertigo, anemia, hypersensitivity	Monitor renal function, SDC, serum calcium, magnesium, sodium. Monitor for nausea, vomiting, nystagmus, and vertigo	Nephrotoxicity can be reversible. More frequent in patients with the following risk factors: elderly, history of renal dysfunction, concomitant administration of nephrotoxic drug (ie, cyclosporine, amphotericin B, radiocontrast, vancomycin), and duration of therapy Ototoxicities can be irreversible
Glycopeptides	Red man syndrome, phlebitis, renal dysfunction, neutropenia, leukopenia, eosinophilia, thrombocytopenia, drug fever	Monitor renal function, CBC, and SDC	Red man syndrome is associated with rapid infusion and nonspecific histamine release. May be prevented by prolonging infusions to over at least 60 minutes and pretreatment with antihistamines
Lipopeptides (daptomycin)	Hepatotoxicity, CPK elevation with or without myopathy, diarrhea, eosinophilic pneumonia, *C. difficile* colitis	Monitor LFTs, development of muscle pain/weakness, or neuropathy Obtain serum CPK levels at baseline and weekly (or more frequently in patients with prior or concomitant statin, renal dysfunction, or patients with elevations in CPK)	CPK elevation is dose-dependent. Obtain baseline and weekly CPK levels. Discontinue daptomycin if CPK exceeds 10 times normal level or if patient develops myopathy and CPK >1,000 international units/L (>16.7 μkat/L). Consider stopping statin therapy during treatment with daptomycin
Oxazolidinones	Myelosuppression (thrombocytopenia, leukopenia, and anemia), peripheral neuropathy, optic neuropathy, blindness, lactic acidosis, diarrhea, nausea, serotonin syndrome, interstitial nephritis	Monitor for signs and symptoms of serotonin syndrome particularly in patients with prior or concomitant serotonergic agents, CBC with differential. For prolonged therapy, perform visual function tests, monitor visual acuity and visual field defect	Myelosuppression is reversible and associated with treatment duration >2 weeks
Tetracyclines	GI upset, nausea, vomiting, diarrhea, hepatotoxicity, esophageal ulcerations, photosensitivity, azotemia, visual disturbances, vertigo, hyperpigmentation, deposition on teeth, hemolytic anemia, pseudotumor cerebri, pancreatitis, *C. difficile* colitis	Monitor CBC with differential, LFTs, and renal function	Doxycycline preferred in patients with renal dysfunction Vestibular symptoms more frequent in women than in men Avoid use during pregnancy and in children
Chloramphenicol	Myelosuppression, aplastic anemia, "gray baby syndrome," optic neuritis, peripheral neuropathy, digital paresthesias, GI upset, *C. difficile* colitis, hypersensitivity	Obtain baseline CBC with differential and every 2 days during therapy. Monitor SDC (particularly in children and in patients with hepatic or renal insufficiency), liver and renal function	Bone marrow suppression associated with doses >4 g/day. Serum levels >50 mcg/mL (mg/L; 155 μmol/L) are associated with increased risk for "gray baby syndrome"
Rifamycines	Discoloration of urine, tears, contact lens, sweat, hepatotoxicity, GI upset, flu-like syndrome, hypersensitivity, thrombocytopenia, leukopenia, drug fever, interstitial nephritis, thrombocytopenia	Monitor LFTs, bilirubin, renal function, CBC at baseline; continue to monitor every 2-4 weeks in patients with hepatic impairment or receiving concomitant hepatotoxic drugs	Increased potential for hepatitis with concomitant hepatotoxic drugs (ie, TB drugs)

(*continued*)

TABLE 105-3 Antimicrobial Adverse Drug Reactions (*Continued*)

Antimicrobial Class	Adverse Drug Reaction	Monitoring Parameters	Comments
Macrolides/azalide	GI intolerance, diarrhea, prolonged QTc, cholestatic hepatitis, reversible ototoxicity, torsade de pointes, rash, hypothermia, exacerbation of myasthenia gravis	Monitor LFTs and ECG in high-risk patients	
Clindamycin	Diarrhea, *C. difficile* colitis, nausea, vomiting, generalized rash, hypersensitivity	For prolonged therapy, monitor liver and renal function	
Fluoroquinolones	GI intolerance, headache, malaise, insomnia, dizziness, photosensitivity, QTc prolongation, tendon rupture, peripheral neuropathy, crystalluria, seizure, interstitial nephritis, Stevens-Johnson syndrome, allergic pneumonitis, *C. difficile* colitis	Monitor renal function, encephalopathic changes (eg, confusion, hallucinations, and tremor)	Tendon rupture more frequently seen in the elderly and kidney, heart, and lung transplant recipients, and with concurrent use of corticosteroids
Polymyxins	Nephrotoxicity, neurotoxicity (paresthesia, vertigo, ataxia, blurred vision, slurred speech), neuromuscular blockade, bronchospasm (administered via inhalation)	Obtain baseline renal function tests and regularly during therapy. Monitor for signs of neuromuscular blockade (eg, respiratory depression, apnea, muscle weakness)	Nephrotoxicity is dose-dependent
Sulfonamides and trimethoprim	GI intolerance, rash, hyperkalemia, bone marrow suppression (anemia with folate deficiency, thrombocytopenia, and leukopenia), serum sickness, hepatitis, photosensitivity, crystalluria with azotemia, urolithiasis, methemoglobinemia, Stevens-Johnson syndrome, toxic epidermal necrolysis, aseptic meningitis, pancreatitis, interstitial nephritis, Sweet syndrome, neurologic toxicity	Monitor for hypersensitivity reactions and rash, CBC, renal and hepatic function, serum potassium, serum glucose	HIV-infected patients are at increased risk for developing adverse drug reactions Methemoglobinemia due to severe G6PD deficiency
Metronidazole	GI intolerance, headache, metallic taste, dark urine, peripheral neuropathy, disulfiram reactions with alcohol, insomnia, stomatitis, aseptic meningitis, dysarthria	Monitor hepatic function, mental/neurologic status	Peripheral neuropathy is reversible and associated with prolonged treatment

CBC, complete blood count; CPK, creatine phosphokinase; LFT, liver function test; SDC, serum drug concentrations; TB, tuberculosis.

overuse of broad-spectrum antibiotic therapy. For example, there have been numerous studies evaluating the utility of the healthcare-associated pneumonia (HCAP) criteria in guiding empiric broad-spectrum therapy. Despite evidence of high sensitivity in identifying potential multi-drug resistant pathogens, other studies have demonstrated that HCAP criteria have low specificity for identifying specific organisms, such as MRSA or Pseudomonas, and may lead to overuse of antibiotics. Currently, whether the HCAP criteria appropriately guide broad-spectrum empiric therapy remains a debate.

Disadvantages of Combination Therapy

Although there are potentially beneficial effects from combining drugs, there also are potential disadvantages, including increased cost, greater risk of drug toxicity such as nephrotoxicity with aminoglycosides, amphotericin, and possibly vancomycin, and superinfection with even more resistant bacteria.[42,44,46]

The combination of two or more antibiotics can result in antagonistic effects. For example, the effect of antagonism may be evident when one drug induces β-lactamase production and another drug is β-lactamase unstable. Cefoxitin and imipenem are examples of drugs capable of inducing β-lactamases and may result in more rapid inactivation of penicillins when used together.

MONITORING THERAPEUTIC RESPONSE

7 After antimicrobial therapy has been instituted, the patient must be monitored carefully for a therapeutic response. Culture and sensitivity reports from specimens sent to the microbiology laboratory must be reviewed and the therapy changed accordingly. Use of agents with the narrowest spectrum of activity against identified pathogens is recommended. If anaerobes are suspected, even if they are not identified, anti-anaerobic therapy should be continued.

Patient monitoring should include many of the same parameters used to diagnose the infection. The WBC count and temperature should start to normalize. Physical complaints from the patient also should diminish (ie, decreased pain, shortness of breath, cough, or sputum production). Appetite should improve. However, radiologic improvement can lag behind clinical improvement.

Determinations of serum (or other fluid) levels of antimicrobials can be useful in ensuring outcome, preventing toxicity, or both. There are only a few antimicrobials that require serum concentration monitoring and then only in selected situations. These include the aminoglycosides, vancomycin, flucytosine, and chloramphenicol. Achievement of adequate aminoglycoside concentrations within the first few days of therapy of Gram-negative infection has been correlated with better therapeutic outcome.[47]

Changes in the volume of distribution can have a significant impact on the efficacy, safety, or both of therapy. An unexpectedly low volume of distribution (such as in the dehydrated patient) will result in higher, potentially toxic drug concentrations, whereas a larger-than-expected volume of distribution (such as in patients with edema or ascites) will result in low, potentially subtherapeutic concentrations. The most effective methods use measured serum concentrations of the drugs rather than estimations from renal function tests to assess true drug clearance from the body.

8 As patients improve clinically, the route of administration should be reevaluated. Streamlining therapy from parenteral to oral (switch therapy) has become an accepted practice for many infections.[5] Criteria that should be present to justify a switch to oral therapy include (a) overall clinical improvement, (b) lack of fever for 8 to 24 hours, (c) decreased WBC count, and (d) a functioning GI tract. Drugs that exhibit excellent oral bioavailability when compared with IV formulations include ciprofloxacin, clindamycin, doxycycline, levofloxacin, metronidazole, moxifloxacin, linezolid, and trimethoprim–sulfamethoxazole.

FAILURE OF ANTIMICROBIAL THERAPY

9 A variety of factors may be responsible for an apparent lack of response to therapy. Patients who fail to respond over 2 to 3 days require a thorough reevaluation. It is possible that the disease is not infectious or is nonbacterial in origin, or there is an undetected pathogen in a polymicrobial infection. Other factors include those directly related to drug selection, the host, or the pathogen. Laboratory error in identification, susceptibility testing, or both (presence of inoculum effect or resistant subpopulations) is a rare cause of antimicrobial failure.

Failures Caused by Drug Selection

Factors related directly to the drug selection include an inappropriate drug selection, dosage, or route of administration. Malabsorption of a drug product because of GI disease (such as a short-bowel syndrome) or a drug interaction (such as complexation of fluoroquinolones with multivalent cations resulting in reduced absorption) can lead to potentially subtherapeutic serum concentrations. Accelerated drug elimination is also possible. This can occur in patients with cystic fibrosis or during pregnancy, when more rapid clearance or larger volumes of distribution can result in low serum concentrations, particularly for aminoglycosides. A common cause of failure of therapy is poor penetration into the site of infection. This is especially true for sites such as the CNS, eye, and prostate gland. Drug failure also can result from drugs that are highly protein bound or that are chemically inactivated at the site of infection.

Failures Caused by Host Factors

Host defenses must be considered when evaluating a patient who is not responding to antimicrobial therapy. Patients who are immunosuppressed (eg, granulocytopenia from chemotherapy or AIDS) may respond poorly to therapy because their defenses are inadequate to eradicate the infection despite seemingly adequate drug regimens. A good example is the poor response of infection in granulocytopenic patients that is seen when their WBC counts remain low during therapy. This contrasts with a much better response when granulocyte counts increase during therapy.

Other host factors are related to the need for surgical drainage of abscesses or removal of foreign bodies, necrotic tissue, or both. If these situations are not corrected, they result in persistent infection and, occasionally, bacteremia despite adequate antimicrobial therapy.

Failures Caused by Microorganisms

There are two types of resistance, intrinsic and acquired resistance. Intrinsic resistance is when the antimicrobial agent never had activity against the bacterial species. For example, Gram-negative bacteria are naturally resistant to vancomycin because the drug cannot penetrate the outer membrane of Gram-negative bacteria. Acquired resistance is when the antimicrobial agent was originally active against the bacterial species but the genetic makeup of the bacteria has changed so the drug can no longer be effective.[48]

The strategies used by bacteria to develop acquired resistance are primarily classified into four general mechanisms of resistance: (a) alteration in the target site, (b) change in membrane permeability, (c) efflux pump, and (d) drug inactivation. Bacteria can use one or more of these mechanisms against a specific antibiotic class. Furthermore, a single mechanism of resistance can result in resistance to multiple related or unrelated classes of antibiotics.

Drug inactivation through either β-lactamases or aminoglycoside-modifying enzymes is the predominant mechanism of resistance. For example, β-lactamases can be either plasmid or chromosomally mediated. In addition, the expression of β-lactamases can be induced or constitutive. There are now multiple types and classes of β-lactamases identified, which is beyond the scope of this chapter. However, there are several outstanding papers discussing all of the different types of β-lactamases.[49-51]

The increase in resistance among bacteria is believed to be a result of continued overuse of antimicrobials in the community, as well as in hospitals, and the increasing prevalence of immunosuppressed patients receiving long-term suppressive antimicrobials for the prevention of infections. These resistance patterns are regionally variable, and susceptibility patterns in the community (or hospital) should be monitored closely to promote rational antimicrobial selection.[48]

Enterococci have been isolated with multiple resistance patterns. They may be resistant to β-lactams (by virtue of β-lactamase production, altered penicillin-binding proteins [PBPs], or both), vancomycin (via alterations in peptidoglycan synthesis), and high levels of aminoglycosides (via enzymatic degradation). Pneumococci resistant to penicillins, certain cephalosporins, and macrolides are increasingly common. These organisms generally are susceptible to vancomycin, the new fluoroquinolones, and cefotaxime or ceftriaxone. However, antimicrobial agents such as linezolid, daptomycin, telavancin, and tigecycline have been targeted at resistant Gram-positive bacteria.

Treatment of an infection caused by *Enterobacter*, *Citrobacter*, *Serratia*, or *P. aeruginosa* with a third-generation cephalosporin or aztreonam may produce an initial clinical response by eradicating all the susceptible bacteria in the population. Within a few days, however, the highly resistant subpopulations have a selective advantage and can overgrow the infection site to produce a relapse. These bacteria usually retain susceptibility to aminoglycosides, carbapenems, and fluoroquinolones but are resistant to all other β-lactams. Host defenses are extremely important in this scenario. Debilitated patients with pulmonary infections, abscesses, or osteomyelitis are at high risk for drug failure. In these situations, a combination regimen to prevent the emergence of resistance or the use of carbapenem or a fluoroquinolone may be warranted for empirical therapy.

ANTIMICROBIAL STEWARDSHIP

The importance of the selection and continuation of appropriate antimicrobial therapy in acute care hospitals are part of a wide movement that is referred to as 'antimicrobial stewardship'. Antimicrobial stewardship programs are aimed at "optimizing antimicrobial selection, dosing, route, and duration of therapy to maximize clinical cure or prevention of infection while limiting the unintended consequences, such as the emergence of resistance, adverse drug events, and cost."

Many institutions have developed an antibiotic stewardship program. The team is generally a multidisciplinary group including representation from microbiology, infection control, administration, information technology, pharmacy including infectious disease-trained clinical pharmacists, and physicians from several disciplines, including infectious disease. Components of antimicrobial stewardship activities include formulary restriction, prospective audit and feedback of antimicrobial prescriptions to clinicians, education, use of clinical order sets and guidelines, de-escalation of therapy, and intravenous to oral antimicrobial conversion.[52,53]

Antibiotic Formulary

One of the main roles of an antimicrobial stewardship team is to decide which antibiotics to include on their formularies. The decision to have a formulary remains controversial; however, restricting choices does encourage familiarity with a core of antibiotics for residents and attending physicians. Open formularies allow the empirical use of any commercially available antibiotics, with recommended guidelines for changes when culture and sensitivity results are finalized. The implementation of the guidelines and restrictions requires the cooperation of the entire medical staff. Education is vital to the success of the antibiotic formulary.

Keeping Current

Attention must be paid to the literature on antimicrobials to assist in the selection of therapy. Evidence-based practice guidelines from the Infectious Diseases Society of America can aid clinicians to direct appropriate therapy for specific infectious disease syndromes. In addition, the results from prospective, controlled, randomized clinical trials should be evaluated whenever possible when considering appropriate antimicrobial therapy. Results from prelicensing open trials offer only limited information that can be useful in this regard because patients in these trials generally are not seriously ill and are not infected with multiple resistant bacteria. Other confounding factors found in most clinical situations are excluded by virtue of the study design. Therefore, comparative data in more seriously ill patients are essential for the appropriate application of new agents.

Postmarketing trials are also important because results can demonstrate superiority of one regimen over another, in efficacy, safety, or cost-effectiveness. Appropriate antimicrobial therapy can change as new organisms are discovered, susceptibility patterns change, new drugs become available, and new clinical trial results are published. Classical thinking in the treatment of infectious diseases will continue to change and evolve to maintain antimicrobial efficacy. Optimal use of modern antimicrobials is just beginning to be defined.

ABBREVIATIONS

AIDS	acquired immunodeficiency syndrome
AST	antimicrobial susceptibility testing
AUC	area under the curve
CSF	cerebrospinal fluid
HA-MRSA	hospital-acquired methicillin-resistant *Staphylococcus aureus*
IL-1	interleukin 1
MIC	minimal inhibitory concentration
PBP	penicillin-binding protein
PMN	polymorphonuclear
WBC	white blood cell

REFERENCES

1. Boucher HW, Talbot GH, Bradley JS, et al. Bad bugs, no drugs: No ESKAPE! An update from the Infectious Diseases Society of America. *Clin Infect Dis* 2009;48:1-12.
2. Spellberg B, Guidos R, Gilbert D, et al. Infectious Diseases Society of A. The epidemic of antibiotic-resistant infections: A call to action for the medical community from the Infectious Diseases Society of America. *Clin Infect Dis* 2008;46:155-64.
3. Mackowiak PA DD. Fever of unknown origin. In: Mandell GL BJ, Dolin R, ed. Mandell, Douglas and Bennett's Principles and Practice of Infectious Diseases. New York: Churchill Livingstone; 2010: 779-190.
4. Mandell LA, Wunderink RG, Anzueto A, et al. Infectious Diseases Society of A, American Thoracic S. Infectious Diseases Society of America/American Thoracic Society consensus guidelines on the management of community-acquired pneumonia in adults. *Clin Infect Dis* 2007;44 Suppl 2:S27-72.
5. Brouwer MC, Tunkel AR, van de Beek D. Epidemiology, diagnosis, and antimicrobial treatment of acute bacterial meningitis. *Clin Microbiol Rev* 2010;23:467-92.
6. van de Beek D, Drake JM, Tunkel AR. Nosocomial bacterial meningitis. *N Engl J Med* 2010;362:146-54.
7. Liu C, Bayer A, Cosgrove SE, et al. Infectious Diseases Society of A. Clinical practice guidelines by the infectious diseases society of america for the treatment of methicillin-resistant *Staphylococcus aureus* infections in adults and children. *Clin Infect Dis* 2011;52:e18-55.
8. Berbari EF, Kanj SS, Kowalski TJ, et al. 2015 Infectious Diseases Society of America (IDSA) Clinical Practice Guidelines for the Diagnosis and Treatment of Native Vertebral Osteomyelitis in Adultsa. *Clin Infect Dis* 2015.
9. Baddour LM, Wilson WR, Bayer AS, et al. Committee on Rheumatic Fever E, Kawasaki D, Council on Cardiovascular Disease in the Y, Councils on Clinical Cardiology S, Cardiovascular S, Anesthesia, American Heart A, Infectious Diseases Society of A. Infective endocarditis: Diagnosis, antimicrobial therapy, and management of complications: A statement for healthcare professionals from the Committee on Rheumatic Fever, Endocarditis, and Kawasaki Disease, Council on Cardiovascular Disease in the Young, and the Councils on Clinical Cardiology, Stroke, and Cardiovascular Surgery and Anesthesia, American Heart Association: Endorsed by the Infectious Diseases Society of America. Circulation 2005;111:e394-434.
10. Jenkins SG, Schuetz AN. Current concepts in laboratory testing to guide antimicrobial therapy. *Mayo Clin Proc* 2012;87:290-308.
11. Goff DA, Jankowski C, Tenover FC. Using rapid diagnostic tests to optimize antimicrobial selection in antimicrobial stewardship programs. *Pharmacotherapy* 2012;32:677-87.
12. Avdic E, Carroll KC. The role of the microbiology laboratory in antimicrobial stewardship programs. *Infect Dis Clin North Am* 2014;28:215-35.
13. Gupta K, Hooton TM, Naber KG, et al. Infectious Diseases Society of A, European Society for M, Infectious D. International clinical practice guidelines for the treatment of acute uncomplicated cystitis and pyelonephritis in women: A 2010 update by the Infectious Diseases Society of America and the European Society for Microbiology and Infectious Diseases. *Clin Infect Dis* 2011;52:e103-20.
14. Croft AC WG. Specimen collection and handling for diagnosis of infectious diseases. In: McPherson RA PM, ed. McPherson: Henry's Clinical Diagnosis and Management by Laboratory Methods. Pennsylvania: Elsevier Saunders; 2011:1239-54.
15. Granowitz EV, Brown RB. Antibiotic adverse reactions and drug interactions. *Crit Care Clin* 2008;24:421-42, xi.
16. Macy E. Penicillin and beta-lactam allergy: Epidemiology and diagnosis. *Curr Allergy Asthma Rep* 2014;14:476.
17. Macy E, Contreras R. Health care use and serious infection prevalence associated with penicillin "allergy" in hospitalized patients: A cohort study. *J Allergy Clin Immunol* 2014;133:790-6.
18. Gruchalla RS, Pirmohamed M. Clinical practice. Antibiotic allergy. *N Engl J Med* 2006;354:601-9.
19. Hameed N, Tunkel AR. Treatment of drug-resistant pneumococcal meningitis. *Curr Infect Dis Rep* 2010;12:274-81.
20. Bradley JS, Byington CL, Shah SS, et al. Pediatric Infectious Diseases S, the Infectious Diseases Society of A. The management of community-acquired pneumonia in infants and children older than 3 months of age: Clinical practice guidelines by the Pediatric Infectious Diseases Society and the Infectious Diseases Society of America. *Clin Infect Dis* 2011;53:e25-76.

21. Bradley JS LS. Principles of anti-infective therapy. In: Long SS PL, Prober CG, ed. Principles and Practice of Pediatric Infectious Diseases: Elsevier Saunders; 2012:1412-518.
22. Weber S, Mawdsley E, Kaye D. Antibacterial agents in the elderly. *Infect Dis Clin North Am* 2009;23:881-98, viii.
23. Crider KS, Cleves MA, Reefhuis J, Berry RJ, Hobbs CA, Hu DJ. Antibacterial medication use during pregnancy and risk of birth defects: National Birth Defects Prevention Study. *Arch Pediatr Adolesc Med* 2009;163:978-85.
24. Briggs GG FR, Yaffe SJ. Drugs in Pregnancy and Lactation. 9 ed. Philadelphia, PA, USA: Lippincott Williams & Wilkins; 2011.
25. Roy PD, Majumder M, Roy B. Pharmacogenomics of anti-TB drugs-related hepatotoxicity. *Pharmacogenomics* 2008;9:311-21.
26. Patel N, Scheetz MH, Drusano GL, Lodise TP. Determination of antibiotic dosage adjustments in patients with renal impairment: elements for success. *J Antimicrob Chemother* 2010;65:2285-90.
27. Matzke GR, Aronoff GR, Atkinson AJ, Jr, et al. Drug dosing consideration in patients with acute and chronic kidney disease-A clinical update from Kidney Disease: Improving Global Outcomes (KDIGO). *Kidney Int* 2011;80:1122-37.
28. Verbeeck RK. Pharmacokinetics and dosage adjustment in patients with hepatic dysfunction. *Eur J Clin Pharmacol* 2008;64:1147-61.
29. Piscitelli S. RK, Pai MP. Drug Interactions in Infectious Diseases. 3 ed. New York: Springer Science; 2012.
30. Freifeld AG, Bow EJ, Sepkowitz KA, et al. Infectious Diseases Society of A. Clinical practice guideline for the use of antimicrobial agents in neutropenic patients with cancer: 2010 Update by the Infectious Diseases Society of America. *Clin Infect Dis* 2011;52:427-31.
31. Drusano GL. Pharmacokinetics and pharmacodynamics of antimicrobials. *Clin Infect Dis* 2007;45 Suppl 1:S89-95.
32. Ambrose PG, Bhavnani SM, Rubino CM, et al. Pharmacokinetics-pharmacodynamics of antimicrobial therapy: It's not just for mice anymore. *Clin Infect Dis* 2007;44:79-86.
33. DeRyke CA, Lee SY, Kuti JL, Nicolau DP. Optimising dosing strategies of antibacterials utilising pharmacodynamic principles: Impact on the development of resistance. *Drugs* 2006;66:1-14.
34. George JM, Towne TG, Rodvold KA. Prolonged infusions of beta-lactam antibiotics: Implication for antimicrobial stewardship. *Pharmacotherapy* 2012;32:707-21.
35. Nightingale CH AP, Drusano GL, Murakawa T. Antimicrobial Pharmacodynamics in Theory and Clinical Practice. 2 ed. New York: Informa Healthcare; 2007.
36. Sinner SW, Tunkel AR. Antimicrobial agents in the treatment of bacterial meningitis. *Infect Dis Clin North Am* 2004;18:581-602, ix.
37. American Thoracic S, Infectious Diseases Society of A. Guidelines for the management of adults with hospital-acquired, ventilator-associated, and healthcare-associated pneumonia. *Am J Respir Crit Care Med* 2005;171:388-416.
38. Bradley JS, Byington CL, Shah SS, et al. Pediatric Infectious Diseases S, the Infectious Diseases Society of A. Executive summary: The management of community-acquired pneumonia in infants and children older than 3 months of age: Clinical practice guidelines by the Pediatric Infectious Diseases Society and the Infectious Diseases Society of America. *Clin Infect Dis* 2011;53:617-30.
39. Cohen SH, Gerding DN, Johnson S, et al. Society for Healthcare Epidemiology of A, Infectious Diseases Society of A. Clinical practice guidelines for *Clostridium difficile* infection in adults: 2010 update by the society for healthcare epidemiology of America (SHEA) and the infectious diseases society of America (IDSA). *Infect Control Hosp Epidemiol* 2010;31:431-55.
40. Shorr AF, Micek ST, Welch EC, Doherty JA, Reichley RM, Kollef MH. Inappropriate antibiotic therapy in Gram-negative sepsis increases hospital length of stay. *Crit Care Med* 2011;39:46-51.
41. Solomkin JS, Mazuski JE, Bradley JS, et al. Diagnosis and management of complicated intra-abdominal infection in adults and children: Guidelines by the Surgical Infection Society and the Infectious Diseases Society of America. *Surg Infect (Larchmt)* 2010;11:79-109.
42. Tamma PD, Cosgrove SE, Maragakis LL. Combination therapy for treatment of infections with Gram-negative bacteria. *Clin Microbiol Rev* 2012;25:450-70.
43. Leekha S, Terrell CL, Edson RS. General principles of antimicrobial therapy. *Mayo Clin Proc* 2011;86:156-67.
44. Paul M, Leibovici L. Combination antimicrobial treatment versus monotherapy: The contribution of meta-analyses. *Infect Dis Clin North Am* 2009;23:277-93.
45. Liu C, Bayer A, Cosgrove SE, et al. Clinical practice guidelines by the infectious diseases society of america for the treatment of methicillin-resistant *Staphylococcus aureus* infections in adults and children: Executive summary. *Clin Infect Dis* 2011;52:285-92.
46. Bliziotis IA, Samonis G, Vardakas KZ, Chrysanthopoulou S, Falagas ME. Effect of aminoglycoside and beta-lactam combination therapy versus beta-lactam monotherapy on the emergence of antimicrobial resistance: A meta-analysis of randomized, controlled trials. *Clin Infect Dis* 2005;41:149-58.
47. Turnidge J. Pharmacodynamics and dosing of aminoglycosides. *Infect Dis Clin North Am* 2003;17:503-28, v.
48. Chen LF, Chopra T, Kaye KS. Pathogens resistant to antibacterial agents. *Med Clin North Am* 2011;95:647-76, vii.
49. Patel G, Bonomo RA. "Stormy waters ahead": Global emergence of carbapenemases. *Front Microbiol* 2013;4:1-17.
50. Bush K, Jacoby GA. Updated functional classification of beta-lactamases. *Antimicrob Agents Chemother* 2010;54:969-76.
51. Bush K. The ABCD's of beta-lactamase nomenclature. *J Infect Chemother* 2013;4:549-59.
52. Dellit TH, Owens RC, McGowan JE, Jr, et al. Infectious Diseases Society of A, Society for Healthcare Epidemiology of A. Infectious Diseases Society of America and the Society for Healthcare Epidemiology of America guidelines for developing an institutional program to enhance antimicrobial stewardship. *Clin Infect Dis* 2007;44:159-77.
53. Srinivasan A, Fishman N. Antimicrobial stewardship 2012: Science driving practice. *Infect Control Hosp Epidemiol* 2012;33:319-21.

Appendix 105-1

Drugs of Choice, First Choice, *Alternative(s)*

GRAM-POSITIVE COCCI

Enterococcus faecalis (generally not as resistant to antibiotics as *Enterococcus faecium*)

- Serious infection (endocarditis, meningitis, pyelonephritis with bacteremia)
  - Ampicillin (or penicillin G) + (gentamicin or streptomycin)
  - Vancomycin + (gentamicin or streptomycin), daptomycin, linezolid, tedizolid, telavancin, tigecycline[a]
- Urinary tract infection
  - Ampicillin, amoxicillin
  - *Fosfomycin* or *nitrofurantoin*

E. faecium (generally more resistant to antibiotics than *E. faecalis*)

- Recommend consultation with infectious disease specialist
  - Linezolid, quinupristin/dalfopristin, daptomycin, tigecycline[a]

Staphylococcus aureus/Staphylococcus epidermidis

- Methicillin (oxacillin)-sensitive
  - Nafcillin or oxacillin
  - *FGC,[b,c] trimethoprim–sulfamethoxazole, clindamycin, BL/BLI[d]*
- Hospital-acquired methicillin (oxacillin)–resistant
  - Vancomycin ± (gentamicin or rifampin)
  - *Ceftaroline, daptomycin, linezolid, telavancin, tigecycline,[a] trimethoprim–sulfamethoxazole, quinupristin–dalfopristin*
- Community-acquired methicillin (oxacillin)–resistant
  - Clindamycin, trimethoprim–sulfamethoxazole, doxycycline[a]
  - *Ceftaroline, dalbavancin, daptomycin, linezolid, oritivancin, tedizolid, telavancin, tigecycline,[a]* or *vancomycin*

Streptococcus (groups A, B, C, G, and *Streptococcus bovis*)

- Penicillin G or V or ampicillin
- *FGC,[b,c] erythromycin, azithromycin, clarithromycin*

Streptococcus pneumoniae

- Penicillin-sensitive (minimal inhibitory concentration [MIC] <0.1 mcg/mL [mg/L])
  - Penicillin G or V or ampicillin
  - *FGC,[b,c] doxycycline,[a] azithromycin, clarithromycin, erythromycin*
- Penicillin intermediate (MIC 0.1-1 mcg/mL [mg/L])
  - High-dose penicillin (12 million units/day for adults) or ceftriaxone[c] or cefotaxime[c]
  - *Levofloxacin,[a] moxifloxacin,[a] gemifloxacin,[a] or vancomycin*
- Penicillin-resistant (MIC ≥1.0 mcg/mL [mg/L])
  - Recommend consultation with infectious disease specialist.
    - *Vancomycin ± rifampin*
    - *Per sensitivities: ceftaroline, cefotaxime, ceftriaxone,[c] levofloxacin,[a] moxifloxacin,[a] or gemifloxacin[a]*

Streptococcus, viridans group

- Penicillin G ± gentamicin[e]
- *Cefotaxime,[c] ceftriaxone,[c] erythromycin, azithromycin, clarithromycin,* or *vancomycin ± gentamicin*

GRAM-NEGATIVE COCCI

Moraxella (Branhamella) catarrhalis

- Amoxicillin–clavulanate, ampicillin–sulbactam
- *Trimethoprim–sulfamethoxazole, erythromycin, azithromycin, clarithromycin, doxycycline,[a] SGC,[c,f] cefotaxime,[c] ceftriaxone,[c]* or *TGCPO[c,g]*

Neisseria gonorrhoeae (also give concomitant treatment for *Chlamydia trachomatis*)

- Disseminated gonococcal infection
  - Ceftriaxone[c] or cefotaxime[c]
  - *Oral follow up: cefpodoxime,[c] ciprofloxacin,[a]* or *levofloxacin[a]*
- Uncomplicated infection
  - Ceftriaxone,[c] cefotaxime,[c] or cefpodoxime[c]
  - *Ciprofloxacin[a]* or *levofloxacin[a]*

Neisseria meningitides

- Penicillin G
- *Cefotaxime[c]* or *ceftriaxone[c]*

GRAM-POSITIVE BACILLI

Clostridium perfringens

- Penicillin G ± clindamycin
- *Metronidazole,[a] clindamycin, doxycycline,[a] cefazolin,[c] carbapenem[h,i]*

Clostridium difficile

- Oral metronidazole[a]
- *Oral vancomycin* or *fidaxomicin*

GRAM-NEGATIVE BACILLI

Acinetobacter spp.

- Doripenem, imipenem, or meropenem ± aminoglycoside[j] (amikacin usually most effective)
- *Ampicillin–sulbactam, polymyxins,[i]* or *tigecycline[a]*

Bacteroides fragilis (and others)

- Metronidazole[a]
- *BL/BLI,[d] clindamycin, cefoxitin,[c] cefotetan,[c] ceftolozane-azobactam, ceftazidime-avibactam,* or *carbapenem[h,i]*

Enterobacter spp.

- Carbapenem[h] or cefepime ± aminoglycoside[j]
- *ceftolozane-tazobactam, ceftazidime-avibactam, ciprofloxacin,[a] levofloxacin,[a] piperacillin–tazobactam, ticarcillin–clavulanate*

Escherichia coli

- Meningitis
  - Cefotaxime,[c] ceftriaxone,[c] meropenem
- Systemic infection
  - Cefotaxime[c] or ceftriaxone[c]
  - *BL/BLI,[d] fluoroquinolone,[a,k] carbapenem[h,i]*
- Urinary tract infection
  - Most oral agents: check sensitivities
  - Ampicillin, amoxicillin–clavulanate, doxycycline,[a] or cephalexin[c]
  - *Aminoglycoside,[j] FGC,[b,c] nitrofurantoin, fluoroquinolone[a,k]*

Gardnerella vaginalis

- Metronidazole[a]
- *Clindamycin*

Haemophilus influenzae

- Meningitis
  - Cefotaxime[c] or ceftriaxone[c]
  - *Meropenem[i]*

- Other infections
  - BL/BLI,[d] or if β-lactamase-negative, ampicillin or amoxicillin
  - *Trimethoprim–sulfamethoxazole, cefuroxime,*[c] *azithromycin, clarithromycin,* or *fluoroquinolone*[a,k]

Klebsiella pneumoniae

- BL/BLI,[d] cefotaxime,[c] ceftriaxone,[c] cefepime[c]
- Carbapenem,[h,i] *ceftolozane-tazobactam, ceftazidime-avibactam,* fluoroquinolone[a,k]

Legionella spp.

- Azithromycin, erythromycin ± rifampin, or fluoroquinolone[a,k]
- Trimethoprim–sulfamethoxazole, clarithromycin, or doxycycline[a]

Pasteurella multocida

- Penicillin G, ampicillin, amoxicillin
- *Doxycycline,*[a] *BL/BLI,*[d] *trimethoprim–sulfamethoxazole* or *ceftriaxone*[c]

Proteus mirabilis

- Ampicillin
- *Trimethoprim–sulfamethoxazole*

Proteus (indole-positive) (including *Providencia rettgeri, Morganella morganii,* and *Proteus vulgaris*)

- Cefotaxime,[c] ceftriaxone,[c] or fluoroquinolone[a,k]
- *BL/BLI,*[d] *aztreonam,*[l] *aminoglycosides,*[j] *carbapenem,*[h,i] *ceftolozane-tazobactam, ceftazidime-avibactam*

Providencia stuartii

- Amikacin, cefotaxime,[c] ceftriaxone,[c] fluoroquinolone[a,k]
- *Trimethoprim–sulfamethoxazole, aztreonam,*[l] *carbapenem*[h,i]

Pseudomonas aeruginosa

- Urinary tract infection only
  - Aminoglycoside[j]
  - *Ciprofloxacin,*[a] *levofloxacin*[a]
- Systemic infection
  - Cefepime,[c] ceftazidime,[c] doripenem,[i] imipenem,[i] meropenem,[i] piperacillin–tazobactam, or ticarcillin–clavulanate + aminoglycoside[j]
  - *Aztreonam,*[l] *ceftolozane-tazobactam, ceftazidime-avibactam, ciprofloxacin,*[a] *levofloxacin,*[a] *polymyxin*[i]

Salmonella typhi

- Ciprofloxacin,[a] levofloxacin,[c] ceftriaxone,[c] cefotaxime[c]
- *Trimethoprim–sulfamethoxazole*

Serratia marcescens

- Ceftriaxone,[c] cefotaxime,[c] cefepime,[c] ciprofloxacin,[a] levofloxacin[a]
- *Aztreonam,*[l] *carbapenem,*[h,i] *piperacillin–tazobactam, ticarcillin–clavulanate*

Stenotrophomonas (Xanthomonas) maltophilia (generally very resistant to all antimicrobials)

- Trimethoprim–sulfamethoxazole.
- *Check sensitivities to ceftazidime,*[c] *doxycycline,*[a] *minocycline,*[a] and *ticarcillin–clavulanate*

MISCELLANEOUS MICROORGANISMS

Chlamydia pneumoniae

- Doxycycline[a]
- *Azithromycin, clarithromycin, erythromycin, or fluoroquinolone*[a,k]

C. trachomatis

- Azithromycin or doxycycline[a]
- *Levofloxacin,*[a] *erythromycin*

Mycoplasma pneumoniae

- Azithromycin, clarithromycin, erythromycin, fluoroquinolone[a,k]
- *Doxycycline*[a]

SPIROCHETES

Treponema pallidum

- Neurosyphilis
  - Penicillin G
  - *Ceftriaxone*[c]
- *Primary* or *secondary*
  - Benzathine, penicillin G
  - *Ceftriaxone*[c] or *doxycycline*[a]

Borrelia burgdorferi (choice depends on stage of disease)

- Ceftriaxone[c] or cefuroxime axetil,[c] doxycycline,[a] amoxicillin
- *High-dose penicillin, cefotaxime*[c]

[a]Not for use in pregnant patients or children.
[b]First-generation cephalosporins—IV: cefazolin; orally: cephalexin, cephradine, or cefadroxil.
[c]Some penicillin-allergic patients may react to cephalosporins.
[d]β-Lactam/β-lactamase inhibitor combination—IV: ampicillin–sulbactam, piperacillin–tazobactam, and ticarcillin–clavulanate; orally: amoxicillin–clavulanate.
[e]Gentamicin should be added if tolerance or moderately susceptible (MIC >0.1 mcg/mL [mg/L]) organisms are encountered; streptomycin is used but can be more toxic.
[f]Second-generation cephalosporins—IV: cefuroxime; orally: cefaclor, cefditoren, cefprozil, cefuroxime axetil, and loracarbef.
[g]Third-generation cephalosporins—orally: cefdinir, cefixime, cefetamet, cefpodoxime proxetil, and ceftibuten.
[h]Carbapenem: doripenem, ertapenem, imipenem/cilastatin, and meropenem.
[i]Reserve for serious infection.
[j]Aminoglycosides: gentamicin, tobramycin, and amikacin; use per sensitivities.
[k]Fluoroquinolones IV/orally: ciprofloxacin, levofloxacin, and moxifloxacin.
[l]Generally reserved for patients with hypersensitivity reactions to penicillin.

Central Nervous System Infections

106

Ramy H. Elshaboury, Aileen S. Ahiskali, Jessica S. Holt, and John C. Rotschafer

KEY CONCEPTS

1. The four most common pathogens of acute bacterial meningitis in the United States are *Streptococcus pneumoniae*, group B *Streptococcus*, *Neisseria meningitidis*, and *Haemophilus influenzae* type b, although routine vaccinations are having a dramatic effect on the incidence and distribution of these pathogens.
2. In cases of bacterial meningitis, initial findings can include (a) presenting signs and symptoms: fever, headache, nuchal rigidity (the classic triad), Brudzinski's or Kernig's sign, and altered mental status; and (b) abnormal cerebrospinal fluid (CSF) chemistries: elevated white blood cell (WBC) count (greater than 1,000 cells/mm^3[greater than 1×10^2/L]), elevated protein (greater than 50 mg/dL [greater than 500 mg/L]), and decreased glucose levels (less than 45 mg/dL [less than 2.5 mmol/L]).
3. Two main microbiologic tests that should be obtained include a gram stain and culture of the CSF. Molecular testing such as polymerase chain reaction (PCR), latex coagglutination, and enzyme immunoassay (EIA) tests can provide for the rapid identification of several causes of meningitis.
4. Three primary goals of treatment in meningitis include (a) eradication of infection, (b) amelioration of signs and symptoms, and (c) prevention of the development of neurologic sequelae, such as seizures, deafness, coma, and death.
5. When selecting antibiotics, the clinician must consider the antibiotic concentration at the site of infection as well as the spectrum of antibacterial activity. Empirical choices should be based on age, predisposing conditions, vaccination history, and comorbidities. (a) Ceftriaxone or cefotaxime and vancomycin are reasonable initial choices for empirical coverage of community-acquired meningitis in adult patients. (b) *Listeria monocytogenes* is a common pathogen in infants and elderly; therefore, ampicillin with or without gentamicin should be empirically added to antimicrobial regimens.
6. Empirical coverage with an appropriate antibiotic should be started as soon as possible when clinical suspicion of meningitis exists. If there is a delay in obtaining a lumbar puncture (even 30-60 minutes), or if the patient is to undergo neuroimaging, the first dose of an antibiotic should not be withheld.
7. Antibiotic dosages for the treatment of meningitis should be optimized to ensure adequate CNS therapeutic concentrations.
8. The duration of antibiotic treatment for meningitis has not been standardized; however, it is generally based on the causative organism and the individual case, and may range from 7 to 21 days.
9. Close contacts and relatives of the index case should be assessed for appropriate chemoprophylaxis and vaccinations, particularly for *N. meningitidis* and *H. influenzae* meningitis.
10. Steroid treatment includes dexamethasone of 0.15 mg/kg per dose given four times daily for 4 days in infants and children older than 2 months of age with proven or strongly suspected bacterial meningitis. Steroids should be started prior to the first dose of antibiotics.

Central nervous system (CNS) infections are caused by a variety of pathogens, including bacteria, viruses, fungi, and parasites. Infections are the result of hematogenous spread from a primary infection site, seeding from a parameningeal focus, reactivation from a latent site, trauma, or congenital defects within the CNS. Newer diagnostic techniques have enabled more rapid and definitive diagnoses, thus diminishing the number of unknown "aseptic meningitis" diagnoses and improving targeted therapy. Bacteria resistant to multiple antibiotics present new challenges in the management of CNS infections. This chapter presents the etiology, pathophysiology, therapy, and prophylaxis of these infections, concentrating predominantly on bacterial meningitis.

EPIDEMIOLOGY

Approximately 4,100 cases of acute community-acquired bacterial meningitis, excluding epidemics, occurred annually in the United States between 2003 and 2007, resulting in approximately 500 deaths.[1] Risk factors and mortality rates widely vary depending on the causative microorganism and age group, and as high as 20% (range 12.3%-35.3%) of survivors will experience one or more neurologic disabilities.[2] Neurologic sequelae frequently associated with bacterial meningitis include seizures, sensorineural hearing loss, and hydrocephalus. While risk for the development of neurologic sequelae depends on the infecting organism, pneumococcal meningitis is typically associated with the highest risk.[2,3] Despite the availability of antimicrobial therapy against the most common CNS pathogens, CNS infections continue to pose significant morbidity and mortality.

ETIOLOGY

1 CNS infections are caused by a variety of microorganisms. Historically, infections were primarily community-acquired; however, an increasing number of cases are now nosocomial.[4] *Haemophilus*

influenzae type b (Hib) was the most commonly identified cause of bacterial meningitis until the introduction of the Hib conjugate vaccine in 1990,[5] when *Streptococcus pneumoniae* became the most commonly identified cause.[1,6] Between 2003 and 2007 in the United States, *S. pneumoniae* accounted for 58% of all bacterial meningitis cases, followed by group B *Streptococcus* (18.1%), *Neisseria meningitidis* (13.9%), *H. influenzae* (6.7%), and *L. monocytogenes* (3.4%).[1] Other causative organisms included gram-negative organisms and *Staphylococcus* spp.[4,6]

Following the release of the pneumococcal heptavalent protein-polysaccharide conjugate vaccine (PCV7) in 2000, the rate of invasive pneumococcal disease (IPD), including pneumococcal meningitis, steadily dropped from 24.3 cases per 100,000 people in 1999 to 17.3 cases per 100,000 in 2001 and 13.5 cases per 100,000 in 2007.[7] The largest impact was in children younger than 2 years of age, where a nearly 70% decline in infection rate was reported as a result of implementation in the routine childhood vaccination schedule. This positive effect carried into the adult population with significant reduction in IPD across all age groups, despite stagnant adult vaccination coverage.[8] Further reductions in IPD in the United States and Europe were also noted following the introduction of the 13-valent pneumococcal conjugate vaccine (PCV13) in 2010 for routine childhood vaccination, and later for high-risk and older adults.[9,10] Widespread availability of childhood vaccination against Hib starting in 1980s in the United States has also resulted in a dramatic reduction of invasive infections, including meningitis, in the past 20 to 30 years. Finally, targeted meningococcal vaccination for high-risk infants, adolescents, and adults have similarly impacted the epidemiology and risk of meningococcal meningitis, and further changes are expected following the availability of meningococcal group B vaccines in the United States.[11] As a result of the rapid decline of acute community-acquired bacterial meningitis rates in children, the median age of patients increased from 30.3 years in 1998 to 41.3 years in 2007 in the United States.[1]

Both the Hib and pneumococcal vaccines are of limited availability in low-income and developing countries where cost is often prohibitive. Thus rates of invasive disease, neurologic sequelae, and case fatalities among children and adults continue to be substantially higher than western developed countries.[2]

ANATOMY AND PHYSIOLOGY OF THE CENTRAL NERVOUS SYSTEM

Meninges

The skull and vertebrae protect the CNS from blunt or penetrating trauma (Fig. 106-1). The brain is suspended in these structures by cerebrospinal fluid (CSF) and is surrounded by the meninges. The meninges are made up of three separate membranes: dura mater, arachnoid, and pia mater.[12] Dura mater, or pachymeninges, lies directly beneath and is adherent to the skull. The other two membranes are referred to collectively as leptomeninges. Pia mater lies directly over brain tissue. Arachnoid, the middle layer, lies between the dura mater and the pia mater. The subarachnoid space, located between the arachnoid and the pia mater, is the conduit for CSF. By definition, meningitis refers to inflammation of the subarachnoid space or spinal fluid, whereas encephalitis is an inflammation of the brain tissue itself. Since infectious microorganisms frequently are an underlying cause of these inflammatory processes, the terms meningitis, encephalitis, or meningoencephalitis are frequently used to denote an infectious process.

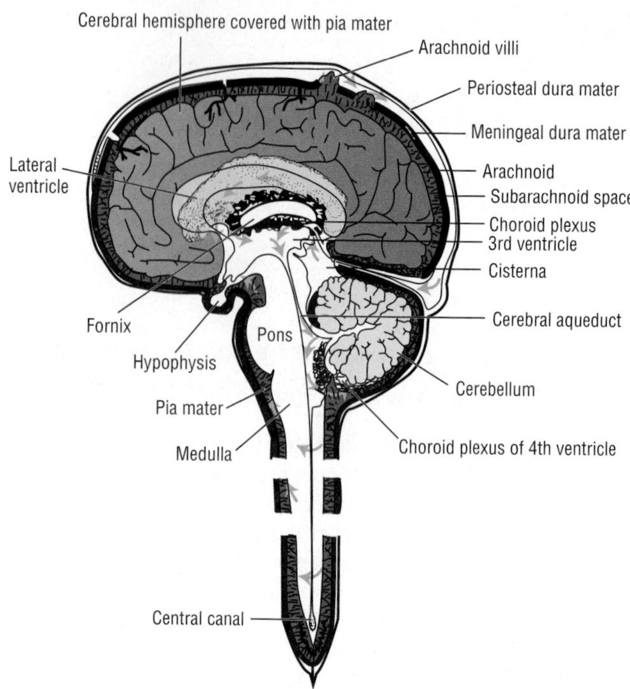

FIGURE 106-1 Diagram of the central nervous system.

Cerebrospinal Fluid

Approximately 85% of the CSF is produced within the third, fourth, and lateral ventricles by the choroid plexus (Fig. 106-1). CSF volume in the CNS is related to patient age: infants have approximately 40 to 60 mL of CSF, older children have 60 to 100 mL, while adults have 115 to 160 mL. Normally, CSF is produced at the rate of approximately 500 mL/day and flows unidirectionally downward through the spinal cord. The CSF is removed by the arachnoid villi and vertebral venous plexus located in the spinal cord and does not recommunicate with the point of production.[12]

2 The CSF normally is clear, with a protein content of less than 50 mg/dL (500 mg/L), a glucose concentration of approximately 50% to 60% of the simultaneous peripheral serum glucose concentration, and a pH of approximately 7.4. Also, it typically contains fewer than five WBCs per cubic millimeter (fewer than 5×10^6/L), all of which should be lymphocytes (Table 106-1).[13-17] As meninges become inflamed, the constituency of the CSF changes, and these abnormalities can be used diagnostically as markers of CNS infections.

TABLE 106-1 Mean Values of the Components of Normal and Abnormal Cerebrospinal Fluid[13-17]

Type	Normal	Bacterial	Viral	Fungal	Tuberculosis
WBC (cells/mm³ or 10^6/L)	<5 (<30 in newborns)	1,000-5,000	5-500	100-400	25-500
Differential[a]	Monocytes	Neutrophils	Lymphocytes	Lymphocytes	Variable
Protein (mg/dL)	<50 (<500 mg/L)	Elevated	Mild elevation	Elevated	Elevated
Glucose (mg/dL)	45-80 (2.5-4.4 mmol/L)	Low	Normal	Low	Low
CSF/blood glucose ratio	50%-60%	Decreased	Normal	Decreased	Decreased

[a]Initial cerebrospinal fluid (CSF), while blood cell (WBC) count may reveal a predominance of polymorphonuclear neutrophils (PMNs).

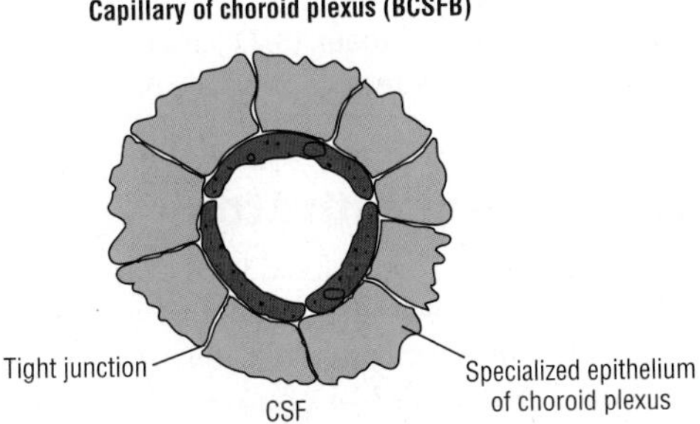

FIGURE 106-2 Schematic representation of a blood–cerebrospinal fluid barrier capillary, brain tissue capillary, and normal tissue capillary (*below*).

Blood–Brain Barrier/Blood–CSF Barrier

Natural barriers to the exchange of drugs and endogenous compounds among the blood, brain, and CSF are the blood–brain barrier (BBB) and the blood–CSF barrier (BCSFB) (Fig. 106-2). The BBB consists of tightly joined capillary endothelial cells. Drug entry into brain tissue is accomplished by direct passage through the capillary endothelial cells and further penetration of the glial cells that envelop the capillary structure.[12] Passage of drugs into the CSF is controlled by the BCSFB. This barrier is created by ependymal cells of the choroid plexus, which function as an active-transport system similar to the renal tubular epithelial cells. The inflammatory process associated with meningitis can also inhibit the active-transport system of the choroid plexus.[18]

PATHOPHYSIOLOGY OF THE CNS INFECTION

The development of bacterial meningitis occurs following bacterial invasion of the host and CNS, bacterial multiplication with subsequent inflammation of the CNS; specifically the subarachnoid and the ventricular spaces; pathophysiologic alterations owing to progressive inflammation, and the resulting neuronal damage.[14] The critical first step in the acquisition of acute bacterial meningitis is nasopharyngeal colonization of the host. Immunoglobulins (Igs), such as secretory IgA, are found in high concentrations within nasopharyngeal secretions and work to inhibit bacterial colonization. However, this mucus barrier is deteriorated by IgA proteases secreted by bacteria, which then extend pili allowing adherence to the host cell surface receptors. Bacterial pathogens tightly attach to nasopharyngeal epithelial cells and are then phagocytized into the host's bloodstream. After accessing the patient's bloodstream, bacteria must overcome the host's defense mechanisms. Commonly, CNS bacterial pathogens produce an extensive polysaccharide capsule resistant to neutrophil phagocytosis and complement opsonization. Therefore, *H. influenzae*, Escherichia *coli*, and *N. meningitidis* strains lacking polysaccharide capsules are unable to cause meningitis. Capsular polysaccharides activate the alternate complement pathway, which promotes phagocytosis and clearance of infecting pathogens. Patients unable to activate the alternative complement pathway, such as asplenic and sickle cell patients, are predisposed to bacterial infections caused by encapsulated microorganisms and therefore are at increased risk for meningitis.[14]

Although the exact site and mechanism of bacterial invasion into the CNS is unknown, studies suggest invasion into the subarachnoid space occurs by continuous exposure of the CNS to large bacterial inoculum. Bacteremia with inoculum densities of at least 10^3 colony-forming units (CFU)/mL [10^6 CFU/L] appears to be essential for subarachnoid space invasion.[19] Although several sites of bacterial invasion have been theorized, the most plausible sites are the choroid plexus and/or the cerebral microvasculature. Host defense mechanisms within the subarachnoid space are inadequate to combat bacterial pathogens; therefore, bacteria replicate freely within the CSF until either overgrowth occurs or an effective antibiotic regimen is administered that terminates the process.

The effects of meningitis, namely, inflammation within the subarachnoid space and the ensuing neurologic damage, are not necessarily a direct result of the pathogens themselves. The neurologic sequelae occur due to the activation of the host's inflammatory pathways, a process induced by the pathogen or its products. Bacterial cell lysis and subsequent death can result in the release of cell-wall components, such as lipopolysaccharide (LPS), lipid A (endotoxin), lipoteichoic acid, teichoic acid, and peptidoglycan, depending on whether the pathogen is gram-positive or gram-negative (Fig. 106-3). These cell-wall components cause capillary endothelial cells and CNS macrophages to release cytokines (interleukin-1 [IL-1] and tumor necrosis factor [TNF]) and other inflammatory mediators (IL-6, IL-8, platelet-activating factor [PAF], nitric oxide, arachidonic acid metabolites [eg, prostaglandin and prostacycline], and macrophage-derived proteins). Proteolytic products and toxic oxygen radicals are

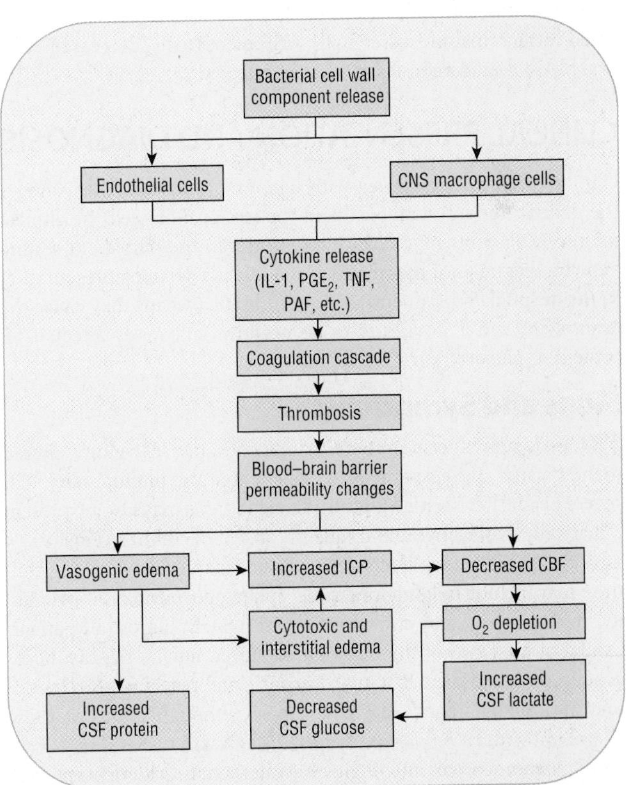

FIGURE 106-3 Hypothetical schema of pathophysiologic events that occur during bacterial meningitis. CBF, cerebral blood flow; CSF, cerebrospinal fluid; ICP, intracranial pressure; IL-1, interleukin-1; PAF, platelet-activating factor; PGE$_2$, prostaglandin E$_2$; TNF, tumor necrosis factor.

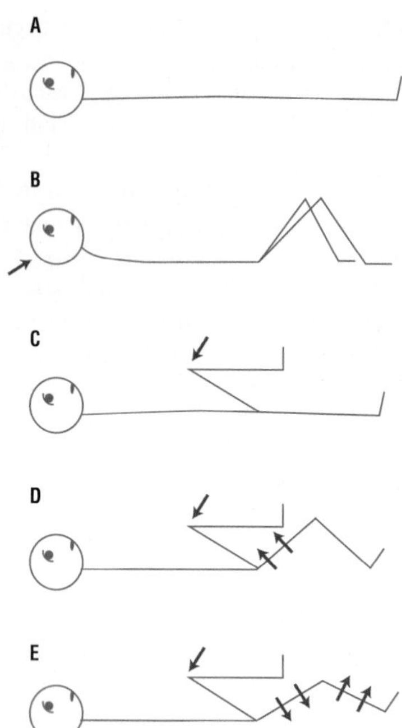

FIGURE 106-4 (A and B) Brudzinski's neck signs. (B) Hip and knee flexion occurs as a result of flexion of the neck. (C to E) Brudzinski's leg signs. (C) Patient's leg is flexed by examiner (*arrow*). (D) The contralateral leg begins to flex—identical contralateral sign (*arrows*). (E) The contralateral leg now begins to extend spontaneously, resembling a little kick (*arrows*).

released from the capillary endothelium, causing an alteration in the permeability of the BBB. PAF activates the coagulation cascade, and arachidonic acid metabolites stimulate vasodilation. These events propagate other sequential events that lead to cerebral edema, elevated intracranial pressure (ICP), CSF pleocytosis, decreased cerebral blood flow, cerebral ischemia, and death.[14,19]

CLINCAL PRESENTATION AND DIAGNOSIS

Clinical presentation varies with age, and generally, the younger the patient, the more atypical and the less pronounced the clinical picture is. Patients may receive antibiotics in the outpatient setting before a diagnosis of meningitis is made, thus delaying presentation to the hospital. Subsequently, prior antibiotic therapy may cause the gram stain and CSF culture to be negative, but rarely affects CSF protein or glucose.

Signs and Symptoms

2 Classic signs and symptoms include fever, nuchal rigidity, altered mental status (*the classic triad*), chills, vomiting, photophobia, and severe headache; Kernig's and Brudzinski's signs may also be present but are poorly sensitive and frequently absent in children (Figs. 106-4 **and** 106-5). Additionally, clinical signs and symptoms in young children may include bulging fontanelle, apneas, purpuric rash, irritability, refusal to eat, and convulsions.[20] Ultimately, almost all patients exhibit at least two of these symptoms: fever, nuchal rigidity, headache, and altered mental status.[3] Purpuric and petechial skin lesions may indicate meningococcal involvement, although lesions may also be present with *H. influenzae* meningitis and skin rashes rarely occur with pneumococcal meningitis.[5] Waterhouse–Friderichsen syndrome, a rapid eruption of multiple hemorrhagic lesions associated with a shock-like state, is associated with meningococcal meningitis. *H. influenzae* and meningococcal meningitis both can cause involvement of the joints during the illness. Finally, history of head trauma with or without skull fracture or presence of a chronically draining ear may be associated with pneumococcal involvement.

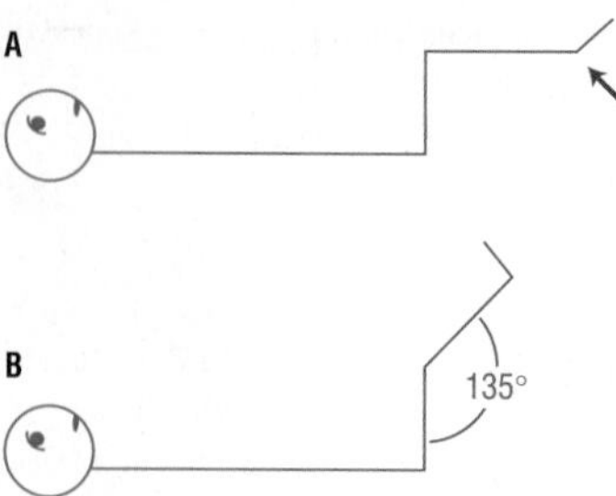

FIGURE 106-5 Kernig's sign. (A) Knees are raised to form a 90-degree angle relative to the trunk, and the examiner attempts to extend the knees. (B) Once the knee angle reaches approximately 135 degrees, contracture or extensor spasm occurs.

Bacterial Meningitis Score

Bacterial Meningitis Score is a validated clinical decision tool aimed to identify children older than 2 months with CSF pleocytosis who are at low risk of acute bacterial meningitis.[21,22] This tool incorporates clinical features such as positive CSF gram stain, presence of seizure, serum absolute neutrophil count 10,000 cells/mm^3 or more (10×10^9/L or more), CSF protein 80 mg/dL or more (800 mg/L or more), and CSF neutrophil count 1,000 cells/mm^3 or more (1×10^9/L or more). Treatment is recommended when one or more criteria are present. Certain pediatric patients are excluded including those with purpura, CSF shunt, recent neurosurgery, Lyme disease (LD), and those who received oral or intravenous antibiotics within 72 hours. This scoring tool was validated in several studies showing high accuracy in excluding acute bacterial meningitis. One meta-analysis of eight validation studies between 2002 and 2012 showed the tool to be highly accurate, with combined sensitivity of 99.3%, specificity of 62.1%, and negative predictive value of 99.7%.[22]

Laboratory Tests

Several tubes of CSF are collected via lumbar puncture for chemistry, cytology, microbiology, and hematology tests. Theoretically, the first tube has a higher likelihood of being contaminated with both blood and bacteria during the puncture, although the total volume is more important in practice than the tube cultured. CSF should not be refrigerated or stored on ice. Analysis of CSF chemistries includes measurement of glucose and total protein concentrations. An elevated CSF protein of more than or equal to 50 mg/dL (500 mg/L or more) and a CSF glucose concentration of less than 50% of the simultaneously obtained peripheral value suggest bacterial meningitis (Table 106-1).[13-17] The values for CSF glucose, protein, and WBC found with bacterial meningitis overlap significantly with those with viral, tuberculous, and fungal meningitis (Table 106-1).[13-17] Therefore, CSF WBC counts and CSF glucose and protein concentrations cannot always distinguish the different etiologies of meningitis.

Other Diagnostic Tests[13,15,23,24]

In patients presenting with new-onset seizures, signs of space-occupying lesions, or moderate to severe impairment of consciousness, cranial imaging via magnetic resonance imaging (MRI) or cranial computed tomography (CT) should precede a lumbar puncture. MRI is generally preferred, as it more clearly identifies areas of cerebral edemas. In these instances, the withdrawal of CSF fluid from a lumbar puncture reduces counterpressure that may result in compression of the brain with risk of brain herniation complicating the clinical course. Neuroimaging should not, however, delay initiation of appropriate antibiotic therapy as doing so can result in a poor outcome in this disease.[25,26] Finally, MRI is considered the preferred imaging modality for the diagnosis of encephalitis due to higher specificity and sensitivity than CT.[15]

Blood and other specimens should be cultured according to clinical judgment as meningitis frequently can arise via hematogenous dissemination or can be associated with infections at other sites. 3 Gram stain and culture of the CSF should be performed for suspected meningitis, and gram stain continues to be the most rapid and accurate method for presumptive diagnosis. When performed before antibiotic therapy is initiated, gram stain is both rapid and sensitive and can confirm the diagnosis of bacterial meningitis in 75% to 90% of cases. However, the sensitivity of the gram stain decreases to 40% from 60% in patients who received prior outpatient antibiotic therapy. Procalcitonin (PCT) has emerged as a predictive biomarker for invasive infections, including meningitis, owing to specificity to bacterial infections. Elevation of serum PCT levels was mostly studied in lower respiratory tract and blood stream infections, but some data support its association with bacterial meningitis.[27] Utility of PCT in predicting bacterial meningitis and differentiating bacterial from viral etiologies is controversial, and more studies are needed to confirm the impact of serum PCT monitoring on clinical outcomes.

Polymerase chain reaction (PCR) techniques can be used to diagnose meningitis caused by *N. meningitidis*, *S. pneumoniae*, and Hib. PCR is considered to be highly sensitive and specific, but expense and availability can be limiting. A multiplex PCR system with a meningitis panel is currently under review by the U.S. Food and Drug Administration (FDA) for approval. The panel includes tests for six bacterial, eight viral, and two yeast targets, with a turnaround time of appoximately 1 hour. Latex fixation, latex coagglutination, and enzyme immunoassay (EIA) tests provide for the rapid identification of several bacterial causes of meningitis, including *S. pneumoniae*, *N. meningitidis*, and Hib. Rapid-identification latex tests work by bringing potential capsular antigens of the pathogen causing meningitis in contact with a specific antibody, causing an antigen-antibody reaction. This capsular antigen-antibody reaction can be quickly observed visually without waiting for culture results. The sensitivity and specificity of latex fixation and coagglutination tests can vary with the manufacturer of the antibody, density of the antigen present in the CSF, and pathogen being tested. Latex agglutination is considered most useful for patients who have been previously treated with antimicrobials and whose CSF gram stain and culture remain negative.[15]

Diagnosis of tuberculosis meningitis employs acid-fast stain, culture, and PCR of the CSF. Also, PCR testing of the CSF is the preferred method for diagnosing most viral meningitis/encephalitis infections. Finally, the standard diagnostic tests for fungal meningitis include culture, direct microscopic examination of stained and unstained specimens of CSF, antigen detection of cryptococcal or histoplasmal antigens, and antibody assay of serum and/or CSF.

TABLE 106-2 Bacterial Meningitis: Most Likely Etiologies and Empirical Therapy by Age Group[13-15]

Age	Most Likely Organisms	Empirical Therapy[a]
<1 month	*S. agalactiae* Gram-negative enterics[b] *L. monocytogenes*	Ampicillin + cefotaxime *or* ampicillin + aminoglycoside
1-23 months	*S. pneumoniae* *N. meningitidis* *H. influenzae* *S. agalactiae*	Vancomycin[c] + 3rd generation cephalosporin (cefotaxime *or* ceftriaxone)
2-50 years	*N. meningitidis* *S. pneumoniae*	Vancomycin[c] + 3rd generation cephalosporin (cefotaxime *or* ceftriaxone)
>50 years	*S. pneumoniae* *N. meningitidis* Gram-negative enterics[b] *L. monocytogenes*	Vancomycin[c] + ampicillin + 3rd generation cephalosporin (cefotaxime *or* ceftriaxone)

[a]All recommendations are A-III.

[b]*E. coli*, *Klebsiella* spp, Enterobacter spp common.

[c]Vancomycin use should be based on local incidence of penicillin-resistant *S. pneumoniae* and until cefotaxime or ceftriaxone minimum inhibitory concentration results are available.

Strength of recommendation: (A) Good evidence to support a recommendation for use; should always be offered. (B) Moderate evidence to support a recommendation for use; should generally be offered.[15]

Quality of evidence: (I) Evidence from 1or more properly randomized, controlled trial. (II) Evidence from 1 or more well-designed clinical trial, without randomization; from cohort or case-controlled analytic studies (preferably from 1 or more center) or from multiple time-series. (III) Evidence from opinions of respected authorities, based on clinical experience, descriptive studies, or reports of expert committees.[15]

TREATMENT

Desired Outcome

4 Goals for the treatment of CNS infections should include eradication of infection, amelioration of signs and symptoms, prevention or reduction of morbidity and mortality, initiation of appropriate antimicrobials and supportive care, and prevention of disease through timely introduction of vaccination and chemoprophylaxis. Understanding antibiotic selection and the issues surrounding antibiotic penetration will assist in meeting the goals of treatment.

General Approach to Treatment and Nonpharmacologic and Supportive Therapy

Until a pathogen is identified, prompt empirical antibiotic coverage is often needed. 5 Based on the patient's profile (ie, allergies, age, and concurrent medical conditions), extent of antibiotic CNS penetration,[28] and spectrum of activity; appropriate recommendations can be made, and therapy should last at least 48 to 72 hours or until the diagnosis of bacterial meningitis can be ruled out (Tables 106-2 and 106-3).[13-15,28] 6 The first dose of antibiotics should not be withheld, even when lumbar puncture is delayed or neuroimaging is being performed, as changes in the CSF after antibiotic administration usually take up to 12 to 24 hours to occur. Continued therapy should be based on the assessment of clinical improvement, culture, and susceptibility testing results. Once a pathogen is identified, antibiotic therapy should be tailored to the specific pathogen (Tables 106-4 and 106-5).[13,15,24] Throughout the course of treatment, efficacy parameters such as signs and symptoms, microbiologic findings, and CSF examination should be followed to evaluate the success of meeting the desired outcomes.

Supportive care, particularly early in the course of treatment, is critically important. Administration of fluids, electrolytes, antipyretics, and analgesics are indicated for patients presenting with a possible CNS infection. Additionally, venous thromboembolism prophylaxis and ICP monitoring are often needed. Patients may require the administration of osmotic diuretics such as mannitol 25% or hypertonic 3% saline to maintain an ICP of less than 15 mm Hg (less than 2 kPa) and a cerebral perfusion pressure of 60 mm Hg or more (8 kPa or more). Other supportive care measures may include respiratory and circulatory supports, gastrointestinal (GI) care and maintaining normal body temperature. Although supportive care is important initially, appropriate antibiotic therapy (empirical or definitive) should be started as soon as possible.[25,26]

7 Several factors influence the transfer of antibiotic from capillary blood into the CNS. Notably, antibiotic penetration is increased through inflamed meninges due to damage to tight junctions between capillary endothelial cells and reduction of the activity of energy-dependent efflux pumps in the choroid plexus responsible for movement of penicillins and, to a lesser extent, fluoroquinolones and aminoglycosides (Table 106-3).[28] Antibiotics having low molecular weights are passed more easily through biologic barriers than compounds of higher molecular weight. Furthermore, only nonionized antibiotics at physiologic or pathologic pH are capable of diffusion. Highly lipid-soluble compounds penetrate more readily than water-soluble compounds. Antibiotics not extensively bound

TABLE 106-3 Penetration of Antimicrobial Agents into the CSF[a,28]

Therapeutic Levels in CSF With or Without Inflammation	
Acyclovir	Levofloxacin
Chloramphenicol	Linezolid
Ciprofloxacin	Metronidazole
Fluconazole	Moxifloxacin
Flucytosine	Pyrazinamide
Foscarnet	Rifampin
Fosfomycin	Sulfonamides
Ganciclovir	Trimethoprim
Isoniazid	Voriconazole
Therapeutic Levels in CSF With Inflammation of Meninges	
Ampicillin ± sulbactam	Imipenem
Aztreonam	Meropenem
Cefepime	Nafcillin
Cefotaxime	Ofloxacin
Ceftazidime	Penicillin G
Ceftriaxone	Piperacillin/tazobactam[b]
Cefuroxime	Pyrimethamine
Colistin	Quinupristin/dalfopristin
Daptomycin	Ticarcillin ± clavulanic acid[b]
Ethambutol	Vancomycin
Nontherapeutic Levels in CSF With or Without Inflammation	
Aminoglycosides	Cephalosporins (second generation)[d]
Amphotericin B	Doxycycline[e]
β-Lactamase inhibitors[c]	Itraconazole[f]
Cephalosporins (first generation)	

[a]Using recommended CNS dosing and compared to MIC of target pathogens.

[b]May not achieve therapeutic levels against organisms with higher MIC, as in *P. aeruginosa*. Tazobactam does not penetrate BBB.

[c]Includes clavulanic acid, sulbactam, and tazobactam.

[d]Cefuroxime is an exception.

[e]Documented effectiveness for *B. burgdorferi*.

[f]Achieves therapeutic concentrations for *Cryptococcus neoformans* therapy.

to plasma proteins provide a larger free fraction of drug capable of passing into the CSF. Passage of large, polar antibiotics into the CSF may be assisted, however, by a carrier transport system. Antibiotic dosages in the treatment of CNS infections must be optimized to ensure adequate penetration to the site of infection.

Problems of CSF penetration were traditionally overcome by direct instillation of antibiotics intrathecally, intracisternally, or intraventricularly. Advantages of direct instillation, however, must be weighed against the risks of invasive CNS procedures and adverse effects. Intrathecal administration of antibiotics is unlikely to produce therapeutic concentrations in the ventricles possibly owing to the unidirectional flow of CSF.[4] Although intraventricular administration from a therapeutic standpoint may be preferred over intrathecal administration, the former requires neurosurgical placement of a subcutaneous reservoir. Intraventricular delivery may be necessary in patients who have shunt infections that are difficult to eradicate or who cannot undergo surgical interventions.[15] Antimicrobial agents often utilized for bacterial meningitis treatment have adequate CSF penetration, which has limited the need for direct CNS instillation. The European Guidelines for meningitis treatment recommend considering the use of intrathecal or intraventricular antibiotics only in patients who fail conventional treatment.[13]

(8) Although the length of treatment for bacterial meningitis is generally based on the causative organism, there is no universally accepted standard (Table 106-4).[13,15,17] Meningitis caused by *S. pneumoniae* has been treated successfully with 10 to 14 days of antibiotic therapy, while cases caused by *N. meningitidis* or *H. influenzae* usually can be treated with a 7-day course. In contrast, a longer duration (21 days or more) has been recommended for patients with *L. monocytogenes*, gram-negative or pseudomonal meningitis. Nonetheless, antibiotic treatments for bacterial meningitis should be individualized, and some patients may require enduring courses.

Causative Organisms

Streptococcus pneumoniae (Pneumococcus or Diplococcus)

(1) *S. pneumoniae* is the leading cause of meningitis in patients 2 months of age or older, and causes over 50% of all cases of bacterial meningitis in the United States with an overall case-fatality rate of approximately 18%.[1] Despite the decline in rates of pneumococcal meningitis since the introduction of PCV7 vaccination in 2000, case-fatality rate did not significantly change from pre-PCV7 era. Approximately 50% of cases are secondary infections resulting from primary infections of parameningeal foci, such as the ear or paranasal sinuses. Pneumonia, endocarditis, CSF leak secondary to head trauma, splenectomy, alcoholism, sickle cell disease, and bone-marrow transplantation may predispose the patient to the development of pneumococcal meningitis.

Neurologic complications, such as coma, hearing impairment, and seizures, are common with pneumococcal meningitis. The prognosis of pneumococcal meningitis depends on a variety of factors, including chronic comorbidities, low Glasgow Coma Scale Score, focal neurological deficits on admission, low CSF leukocyte count, pneumonia, bacteremia, and intracranial and systemic complications.[29]

Based on resistance patterns and the fact that sufficient CSF concentrations of penicillin are difficult to achieve with standard intravenous doses, penicillin should not be used as empirical therapy if *S. pneumoniae* is a suspected pathogen. Furthermore, appropriate Clinical Laboratory Standards Institute (CLSI)-approved testing of all CSF isolates for penicillin resistance is recommended. Ceftriaxone and cefotaxime have served as alternatives to penicillin in the treatment of penicillin-resistant pneumococci. Of note, higher cephalosporins minimum inhibitory concentration (MIC) and higher cephalosporin resistance rates were shown in penicillin-resistant isolates.[30] Therapeutic approaches to cephalosporin-resistant pneumococcus include the addition of vancomycin and rifampin. However, only data from animal and experimental trials supporting the use of rifampin are available.[31] (6) Therefore, the combination of vancomycin and ceftriaxone has been suggested as empirical treatment until the results of antimicrobial susceptibility testing are available. Vancomycin should not be used alone even for highly penicillin- and cephalosporin-resistant strains.[13,15] Finally, some pneumococcal strains exhibit tolerance to vancomycin and were linked to increased meningitis mortality.[32,33]

Given the limited therapeutic options for penicillin- and cephalosporin-resistant pneumococcal meningitis, newer agents have been evaluated. Meropenem is approved by the US FDA for the treatment of bacterial meningitis in children aged 3 months and older and has shown similar clinical and microbiologic efficacies to cefotaxime or ceftriaxone. Meropenem is currently recommended as an alternative to a third-generation cephalosporin in penicillin nonsusceptible isolates. Some caution is warranted with the use of imipenem for CNS infections because of the possibility of drug-induced seizures, especially when dosing is not adjusted for declining renal function. Of note, seizures may be caused by meningitis itself or by imipenem, and the cause is often difficult to differentiate. The newer fluoroquinolones (levofloxacin and moxifloxacin) represent another therapeutic option with favorable activity against

TABLE 106-4 Antimicrobial Agents of First Choice and Alternative Choice in the Treatment of Meningitis Caused by Gram-Positive and Gram-Negative Microorganisms[13,15,17]

Organism	Antibiotics of First Choice	Alternative Antibiotics	Recommended Duration of Therapy
Gram-Positive Organisms			
Streptococcus pneumoniae[a]			10-14 days
Penicillin susceptible MIC ≤ 0.06 mcg/mL (mg/L)	Penicillin G or Ampicillin (A-III)	Cefotaxime (A-III), Ceftriaxone (A-III), Cefepime (B-II), or Meropenem (B-II)	
Penicillin resistant MIC > 0.06 mcg/mL (mg/L)	Vancomycin[b,c] + Cefotaxime or Ceftriaxone (A-III)	Moxifloxacin (B-II)	
Ceftriaxone resistant MIC > 0.5 mcg/mL (mg/L)	Vancomycin[b,c] + Cefotaxime or Ceftriaxone (A-III)	Moxifloxacin (B-II)	
Staphylococcus aureus			14-21 days
Methicillin susceptible	Nafcillin or Oxacillin (A-III)	Vancomycin (A-III) or Meropenem (B-III)	
Methicillin resistant	Vancomycin[b,c] (A-III)	TMP-SMX or Linezolid (B-III)	
Group B *Streptococcus*	Penicillin G or Ampicillin (A-III) ± Gentamicin[b,c]	Ceftriaxone or Cefotaxime (B-III)	14-21 days
S. epidermidis	Vancomycin[b,c] (A-III)	Linezolid (B-III)	14-21 days[d]
L. monocytogenes	Penicillin G or Ampicillin ± Gentamicin[b,c,e] (A-III)	Trimethoprim-sulfamethoxazole (A-III), Meropenem (B-III)	≥21 days
Gram-Negative Organisms			
Neisseria meningitis			7-10 days
Penicillin susceptible	Penicillin G or Ampicillin (A-III)	Cefotaxime or Ceftriaxone (A-III)	
Penicillin resistant	Cefotaxime or Ceftriaxone (A-III)	Meropenem or Moxifloxacin (A-III)	
Haemophilus influenzae			7-10 days
β-lactamase negative	Ampicillin (A-III)	Cefotaxime (A-III), Ceftriaxone (A-III), Cefepime (A-III) or Moxifloxacin (A-III)	
β-lactamase positive	Cefotaxime or Ceftriaxone (A-I)	Cefepime (A-I) or Moxifloxacin (A-III)	
Enterobacteriaceae[f]	Cefotaxime or Ceftriaxone (A-II)	Cefepime (A-III), Moxifloxacin (A-III), Meropenem (A-III) or Aztreonam (A-III)	21 days
Pseudomonas aeruginosa	Cefepime or Ceftazidime (A-II) ± Tobramycin[b,c] (A-III)	Ciprofloxacin (A-III), Meropenem (A-III), Piperacillin plus Tobramycin[a,b] (A-III), Colistin sulfomethate[g] (B-III), Aztreonam (A-III)	21 days

[a]European Guidelines recommend considering the addition of rifampin to vancomycin therapy.

[b]Direct CNS administration maybe considered if failed conventional treatment.

[c]Monitor serum drug levels.

[d]Based on clinical experience; no clear recommendations.

[e]European guidelines recommend adding gentamicin for the first 7 days of treatment.

[f]Includes *E. coli and Klebsiella* spp.

[g]Should be reserved for multidrug-resistant pseudomonal or *Actinetobacter* infections for which all other therapeutic options have been exhausted.

See Table 106-2 footnotes for rating scale of evidence.

multidrug-resistant pneumococci and good penetration into the CSF.[31,34]

Intravenous linezolid, daptomycin, and ceftaroline have also emerged as viable therapeutic options for treating multidrug-resistant gram-positive infections. Linezolid in combination with ceftriaxone has been used to treat a limited number of cases of pneumococcal meningitis with outcomes similar to standard treatment.[35] Daptomycin was as effective or better than ceftriaxone plus vancomycin for pneumococcal strains exhibiting penicillin and ceftriaxone resistance, respectively, in a rabbit model.[36] Additionally, daptomycin may reduce the inflammatory response caused by cell-wall components in pneumococcal meningitis compared with ceftriaxone in animal models.[37] Finally, ceftaroline achieved 14% penetration into inflamed meninges and 3% into uninflamed meninges in an experimental rabbit meningitis model.[38]

Pneumococcal vaccines help in reducing the risk of IPD. Virtually all serotypes of *S. pneumoniae* exhibiting intermediate or complete resistance to penicillin are included in the 23-serotype pneumococcal polysaccharide vaccine (PPV23). Due to low vaccination rates among people 65 years of age and older, the U.S. Centers for Disease Control and Prevention (CDC) issued stronger recommendations for the use of the PPV, calling for vaccination of the following high-risk groups: persons over the age of 65 years; persons aged 2 to 64 years who have a chronic illness, who live in high-risk environments (eg, Alaskan natives and residents of long-term care facilities), and who lack a functioning spleen (eg, sickle cell disease and splenectomy); and immunocompromised persons over the age of 2 years, including those with human immunodeficiency virus (HIV) infection.[39] Additionally, the question of whether or not college students living in dormitories, a possible high-risk environment, should be vaccinated remains debatable.

Use of the heptavalent pneumococcal conjugate vaccine (PCV7), introduced in 2000, significantly reduced the incidence of invasive pneumococcal infections, including sepsis and meningitis.[7,40] In the decade following its introduction, rate of invasive disease caused by non-PCV7 strains increased considerably, especially serotype 19A, leading to the development of a newer vaccine with expanded coverage.[7] In 2010, the FDA approved a PCV13 in replacement of PCV7, leading to a rapid and significant reduction of IPD in children younger than 5 years of age. In the first 3 years after the introduction of PCV13 in the United States, investigators estimated over 30,000 cases of IPD and 3,000 deaths were averted.[9] In 2011, the FDA

TABLE 106-5 Dosing of Antimicrobial Agents by Age Group Antimicrobial[13,15]

Agent	Infants and Children	Adults	Monitoring/Comments
Antibacterial			
Ampicillin	75 mg/kg every 6 h	2 g every 4 h	
Aztreonam	—	2 g every 6-8 h	Alternative for penicillin allergy
Cefepime	50 mg/kg every 8 h	2 g every 8 h	Consider prolonged infusion
Cefotaxime	75 mg/kg every 6-8 h	2 g every 4-6 h	Preferred in neonates
Ceftazidime	50 mg/kg every 8 h	2 g every 8 h	
Ceftriaxone	100 mg/kg daily	2 g every 12 h	Avoid in neonates
Ciprofloxacin	10 mg/kg every 8 h	400 mg every 8-12 h	Consider higher doses for *P. aeruginosa*
Colistin	5 mg/kg/day	5 mg/kg/day	Consider intraventricular doses Only for MDR organisms Monitor renal function
Gentamicin	2.5 mg/kg every 8 h	2 mg/kg every 8 h *or* 5-7 mg/kg daily	TDM is recommended Monitor renal function
Levofloxacin	—	750 mg daily	May prolong QTc
Linezolid	10 mg/kg every 8 h	600 mg every 12 h	May cause thrombocytopenia and peripheral neuropathy
Meropenem	40 mg/kg every 8 h	2 g every 8 h	Consider prolonged infusion
Moxifloxacin	—	400 mg daily	May prolong QTc
Oxacillin/Nafcillin	50 mg/kg every 6 h	2 g every 4 h	Nafcillin preferred if renal dysfunction
Penicillin G	0.05 million Units/kg every 4 h	4 million Units every 4 h	
Polymyxin B	—	1.25-1.5 mg/kg every 12 h	Only for MDR organisms No data in pediatric patients
Tobramycin	2.5 mg/kg every 8 h	2.5 mg/kg every 8 h *or* 5-7 mg/kg daily	TDM is recommended Monitor renal function
Trimethoprim-sulfmathoxazole	5 mg/kg every 6-12 h	5 mg/kg every 6-12 h	Dose based on trimethoprim
Vancomycin	15 mg/kg every 6 h	15-20 mg/kg every 8-12 h	TDM is recommended Monitor renal function
Antimycobacterials			
Isoniazid	10-15 mg/kg daily	5 mg/kg daily	Supplemental vitamin B_6 is recommended
Rifampin	10-20 mg/kg daily (max 600 mg daily)	600 mg daily	Many drug-drug interactions
Pyrazinamide	15-30 mg/kg daily	15-30 mg/kg daily	Rarely causes hepatotoxicity
Ethambutol	15-25 mg/kg daily	15-25 mg/kg daily	May cause neutropenia
Antifungals			
Amphotericin B	1 mg/kg daily	0.7-1 mg/kg daily	Monitor renal function Maintain adequate hydration
Lipid amphotericin B	5 mg/kg once daily	3-5 mg/kg daily	Monitor renal function Maintain adequate hydration
Flucytosine	25 mg/kg every 6 h	25 mg/kg every 6 h	Consider TDM to avoid bone marrow suppression
Fluconazole	6-12 mg/kg daily	800-1,200 mg daily	Monitor liver function
Itraconazole			Consider TDM Suspension form is preferred
Posaconazole	—	400 mg every 12 h	Variable absorption No data in pediatric patients
Voriconazole	7 mg/kg every 12 h	6 mg/kg every 12 h × 2 doses then 4 mg/kg every 12 h	Consider TDM Many drug-drug interactions Monitor liver function
Antivirals			
Acyclovir	10-20 mg/kg every 8 h	10-20 mg/kg every 8 h	Monitor renal function Maintain adequate hydration
Ganciclovir	—	5 mg/kg every 12 h	Monitor renal function
Foscarnet	—	60 mg/kg every 8 h *or* 90 mg/kg every 12 h	Monitor renal function Maintain adequate hydration

TDM, therapeutic drug monitoring.

approved the use of PCV13 in adults 50 years and older as it produced antibody levels that were either comparable to or higher than the levels achieved by PPV23, for the 12 common serotypes included in PCV13. The Advisory Committee on Immunization Practices (ACIP) in 2014 recommended routine use of PCV13 in series with PPV23 for all adults 65 years of age or older.[41] Although the total number of pneumococcal meningitis cases in the United States remained the same with PCV13, the proportion of PCV13 serotypes and antibiotic-resistant strains significantly decreased, mainly serotype 19A.[42] PCV13 is recommended for all healthy infants younger than 2 years of age to be immunized at 2, 4, 6, and 12 to 15 months; all adults of 65 years or older; and high-risk individuals.[39,41,43] High-risk persons include those with cochlear implants, CSF leaks, who lack a functioning spleen, and immunocompromised persons.

Neisseria meningitidis (Meningococcus)

1 *N. meningitidis* is a leading cause of bacterial meningitis among children and young adults in the United States and around the world.[1,44] Five of the thirteen serogroups of *N. meningitidis* (A, B, C, Y, and W-135) are primarily responsible for invasive meningococcal disease. Clusters of disease, defined as two or more cases of the same serogroup that are closer in time and space than expected for the population or group under observation, generally are associated with crowding as in schools, dormitories, and military barracks.[45] Other significant risk factors for meningococcal disease include complement deficiency, persons without a functioning spleen, and active smokers.[11] Serogroups B, C, and Y cause the majority of disease in the United States, while serogroup A, although associated with meningococcal outbreaks in Africa and Asia, is a rare cause of disease in the United States.[46] Routine vaccine recommendations has significantly decreased the prevalence of serogroup C meningococcal disease; however, this led to a surge in serogroup B infections, especially in infants.[47] Overall incidence of meningococcal disease in the United States has been declining since the late 1990s; however, incidence remains highest in infants aged older than 1 year with a second peak in adolescents and young adults 16 to 23 years of age. *N. meningitidis* accounted for 13.9% of all meningitis cases in the United States during 2003 to 2007, with a case-fatality rate of approximately 10%.[1]

Initially, patients are colonized and, at some point, develop bacteremia, which most likely occurs prior to hospital admission. Meningitis occurs after the bacteria seed into the meninges. After the acute phase of meningitis has resolved, there is a unique immune reaction that distinguishes meningococcal meningitis from other bacterial causes. 2 The patient develops a characteristic immunologic reaction of fever, arthritis (usually involving large joints), and pericarditis approximately 10 to 14 days after the onset of disease despite successful treatment. At this time, examination of the synovial fluid may reveal a large number of polymorphonuclear cells, elevated protein concentrations, normal glucose concentrations, and sterile cultures. The reaction may last a week or longer, and no additional antibiotic therapy is required; however, patients may benefit from nonsteroidal anti-inflammatory agents and supportive care.[5,48]

Seizures and coma are uncommon with meningococcal meningitis. Also, patients may develop deafness and transiently impaired ocular movements. Deafness unilaterally or, more commonly, bilaterally may develop early or late in the disease course. Hearing loss secondary to sensory nerve damage (sensorineural hearing) is usually permanent, whereas conductive hearing impairment, such as damage to the tympanic membrane, is often reversible. The presence of petechiae may be the primary clue that the underlying pathogen is *N. meningitidis*. Approximately 60% of adults and up to 90% of pediatric patients with meningococcal meningitis have purpuric lesions, petechiae, or both.[5] Patients may have an obvious or subclinical picture of disseminated intravascular coagulation (DIC), which may progress to infarction of the adrenal glands and renal cortex and cause widespread thrombosis and rapid death.

6 Third-generation cephalosporins (ie, cefotaxime and ceftriaxone) are the recommended empiric treatment for meningococcal meningitis (Table 106-4).[13,15,17] When final culture results are available, penicillin G or ampicillin is recommended for penicillin-susceptible isolates. Meropenem and fluoroquinolones are also suitable alternatives for the treatment of penicillin nonsusceptible meningococci.[13,15]

N. meningitidis is spread by direct person-to-person close contact, including respiratory droplets and pharyngeal secretions. Close contacts of patients contracting meningococcal meningitis are at an increased risk of developing meningitis. Close contacts include daycare center contacts, members of the household, or anyone who has been exposed to respiratory or oral secretions through activities such as coughing, sneezing, or kissing. Secondary cases of meningitis usually develop within the first week following exposure, but may take up to 60 days after contact with the index case.[11] Young children are at the greatest risk of contracting *N. meningitidis*; however, all ages are at risk, especially close contacts exposed via household, daycare, or military contact.

9 Prophylaxis of close contacts should be started only after consultation with the local health department. In general, rifampin, ceftriaxone, ciprofloxacin, or azithromycin are given for prophylaxis. A systematic review of available data suggests an increased rate of rifampin-resistant isolates.[49] Also, cases of ciprofloxacin-resistant isolates were reported in North America. Further discussion of who should receive prophylaxis is beyond the scope of this chapter; interested readers can refer to current recommendations from the CDC.[11]

Until recently, only two meningococcal vaccines were available in the United States; but as of 2015, six products became available. Two quadrivalent meningococcal conjugate vaccines are available with antigens to serogroups A, C, W-135, and Y. In 2012, a bivalent conjugate combination vaccine was licensed in the United States, and contains antigens to serogroups C and Y, and *H. influenzae* type b. Until late 2014, serogroup B meningococcal vaccines (MenBs) were unavailable in the United States. Following an outbreak of meningococcal meningitis due to serogroup B on two college campuses in 2013, two MenB vaccines were subsequently granted breakthrough therapy designations for rapid approval. In 2015, ACIP recommended routine administration for persons 10 to 25 years of age identified as being at increased risk due to serogroup B meningococcal disease outbreak or certain medical conditions (complement deficiencies and functional/anatomic asplenia). For full details of vaccination recommendation in various age groups and for those with significant risk factors, readers should refer to current recommendations from the ACIP.

Haemophilus influenzae type b

1 Historically, *H. influenzae* type b was the most common cause of community-acquired bacterial meningitis in children 6 months to 3 years of age. Since the introduction of effective vaccines, the incidence of Hib disease in the Unite States has declined dramatically.[5,50] Widespread vaccination of infants and children has effectively decreased the incidence of bacterial meningitis due to Hib in children between the ages of 1 month and 5 years, resulting in a significant decline in all cases of bacterial meningitis.[1] In children older than 3 years and adults, meningitis caused by Hib may indicate a parameningeal focus of infection, such as middle ear infection, paranasal sinus infection, or CSF leakage. Spread of the organism occurs either through direct spread from infected sinuses, draining of these areas via the veins, or bacteremia originating from the local focus of infection.[51]

6 Third-generation cephalosporins (cefotaxime and ceftriaxone) are the drugs of choice for empirical therapy for *H. influenzae* type b meningitis as they are active against β-lactamase–producing and non–β-lactamase–producing strains.[15] In addition, they are relatively free of toxicity and do not require serum concentration

monitoring. Cefepime and fluoroquinolones are suitable alternatives regardless of β-lactamase activity.

9 Prophylaxis is to protect close contacts from the index case by eliminating nasopharyngeal and oropharyngeal carriages of *H. influenzae*. Invasive disease should be reported to the local public health department and the CDC. Prophylaxis of close contacts should be started only after consultation with the local health department. Widespread vaccination has limited the need for chemoprophylaxis. Further discussion of who should receive prophylaxis is beyond the scope of this chapter; interested readers can refer to the recommendations of the American Academy of Pediatrics.

Vaccination includes a series of doses and usually is begun in children at 2 months of age. In addition to pediatric immunization, the vaccine also should be considered in patients older than 5 years of age with the following underlying conditions: sickle cell disease, asplenia, and immunocompromising diseases. As noted earlier, a bivalent conjugate combination vaccine, MenHibrix®, containing antigens to meningococcal serogroups C and Y, and *H. influenzae* type b became available in 2012. Refer to chapter in this text for further information on vaccine dosing and administration schedules.

Streptococcus agalactiae (Streptococcus Group B)

1 Streptococcus group B (GBS) is a leading cause of neonatal meningitis in the United States and around the world.[1,52,53] The causative organism, *Streptococcus agalactiae*, is a gram-positive bacterium with β-hemolytic properties that is often implicated in neonatal sepsis, pneumonia, and meningitis. GI and genitourinary colonization in pregnant women is common, up to 25%.[54] Neonates acquire this infection through vertical transmission while passing through the vaginal canal during birth.

Early-onset infections are those occurring within the first week of life, while late-onset infections occur after the first week of the child's birth. Universal prenatal screening and intrapartum antimicrobial prophylaxis of colonized pregnant women have significantly decreased rate of early onset invasive disease.[55] While rates of GBS meningitis in the United States did not change significantly during 1998 to 2008, including cases in patients less than 2 months of age, most cases during 2002 to 2007 were late-onset infections that are not affected by intrapartum prophylaxis.[1,53] Furthermore, neonatal GBS meningitis survivors carry substantial long-term morbidity and up to 11% die before the age of 3 years.[54]

6 Ampicillin and penicillin G are the recommended agents for the treatment of presumed GBS. Addition of an aminoglycoside should also be considered for confirmed GBS meningitis. GBS continues to be susceptible to ampicillin and penicillin; however, reports of isolates with increased MIC have been published.[55]

Investigations are undergoing to develop vaccines to reduce maternal colonization and prevent fetal transmission of GBS. Clinical trials have shown promising results; however, to date there are no licensed vaccines available for GBS.

Listeria monocytogenes

L. monocytogenes is a gram-positive diphtheroid-like organism. This disease primarily affects neonates, alcoholics, immunocompromised adults, and the elderly; while infections in healthy individuals are rare. *L. monocytogenes* is implicated in approximately 10% of meningitis cases in those older than 65 years of age and carries a case-fatality rate of approximately 18% in the United States.[1]

Transmission usually involves colonization of the patient's GI tract with the organisms, which then penetrate the gut lumen. Soft cheeses and raw produce are common causes of listeriosis outbreaks. Coleslaw, unpasteurized milk, ready-to-eat foods, and raw beef and poultry have also been identified as sources of this foodborne pathogen.[14] If a sufficient cell-mediated immune response (T-lymphocytes, macrophages) is not produced, bacteremia, meningitis, meningoencephalitis, or cerebritis may develop. Infection of the CNS may be diffuse or localized, possibly involving the cerebral hemispheres, thalamus, and brain stem.

Incidence of *L. monocytogenes* meningitis tends to peak in the summer and early fall. As with gram-negative meningitis, presentation may be subtle and insidious, and clinical suspicion should prompt lumbar puncture. 2 *L. monocytogenes* produces primarily a mononuclear CSF response.[56] One common laboratory error seen with *L. monocytogenes* is a tendency to misidentify the organism on gram stain as a diphtheroid, streptococcus, or a poorly staining gram-negative rod.

Treatment of *L. monocytogenes* meningitis with penicillin G or ampicillin may result in only a bacteriostatic effect and possible persistence of infection. Usually the combination of penicillin G or ampicillin with an aminoglycoside results in a bactericidal effect. 8 Patients should be treated for a minimum of 3 weeks.[15] European Guidelines for meningitis treatment recommend considering combination therapy for the first 7 to 10 days of treatment, with the remaining course of therapy completed with penicillin G or ampicillin alone.[13] Despite in-vitro activity against *L. monocytogenes*, vancomycin was associated with high failure rates. Also, third-generation cephalosporins lack in-vitro activity against *L. monocytogenes*. Trimethoprim-sulfamethoxazole and meropenem may be effective alternatives as adequate CSF penetration is achieved.[13,15]

Gram-Negative Meningitis

Gram-negative bacilli, excluding *H. influenzae*, are an uncommon but increasing cause of nosocomial meningitis in adults.[57] The most common pathogens are *E. coli* and *Pseudomonas* species in adults, while neonates are also at risk for gram-negative meningitis with *E. coli* and *Klebsiella pneumoniae* responsible for 40% to 50% of cases.[58] A 2013 study identified urinary tract infections as the most important independent factor associated with higher risk of gram-negative meningitis in adults.[57] Several additional factors predispose patients to the development of gram-negative meningitis include: congenital defects involving the CNS, accidental cranial trauma, neurosurgery, the use of antimicrobial agents with exclusive gram-positive activity preoperatively in neurosurgery, any form of communication between the skin and subarachnoid space (such as a dermal sinus), diabetes, malignancy, cirrhosis, parameningeal infection, spinal anesthesia, advanced age, immunosuppression, and hospitalization in general.[57]

Elderly debilitated patients are at an increased risk of gram-negative meningitis but typically lack the classic signs and symptoms of the disease. Nuchal rigidity may be difficult to detect secondary to cervical arthritis. Presence of a low-grade fever and changes in mental status without other obvious cause should prompt consideration of meningitis and a lumbar puncture.

Treatment of gram-negative meningitis is complex because of the variety of organisms implicated in these cases. The treatment of meningitis due to *Pseudomonas aeruginosa* remains a unique problem because antibiotics showing good antibacterial activity, such as antipseudomonal penicillins and aminoglycosides, penetrate the CSF poorly.[28] Furthermore, many isolates of *P. aeruginosa* are resistant to multiple, if not all, commonly used agents, and this trend in resistance is increasing. 6 Initially, cases of *P. aeruginosa* meningitis should be treated with an extended-spectrum β-lactam such as ceftazidime or cefepime, or alternatively aztreonam, ciprofloxacin, or meropenem.[4,15] The addition of an aminoglycoside, usually tobramycin, to one of the aforementioned agents should also be considered. Since aminoglycosides penetrate the CSF poorly, their inclusion is predominant to aid in the treatment of extracerebral infections. If multidrug-resistant *P. aeruginosa* is suspected initially, intraventricular administration of an aminoglycoside should be considered along with intravenous administration. Preservative-free forms of gentamicin and tobramycin are available and should be used for direct administration into the CSF. Since CSF flows unidirectionally with gravity, intraventricular aminoglycoside administration is more likely to produce therapeutic concentrations throughout the CSF than intrathecal administration. While intraventricular administration of aminoglycosides is considered for treatment of *P. aeruginosa* meningitis, this method produced higher mortality in a sample of infants treated for gram-negative bacillary meningitis.[59] Thus intraventricular administration of aminoglycosides to infants is not recommended routinely.

Multidrug-resistant *P. aeruginosa* and *Acinetobacter* infections are of concern to clinicians because of the limited therapeutic options available. This concern has led to the reemergence of the use of older antibiotics, such as colistin and polymyxin B. Colistin can be used, both intravenously and intrathecally, in the treatment of multidrug-resistant *P. aeruginosa* or *Acinetobacter* CNS infections.[60] Furthermore, synergistic activity with the combination of colistin and ceftazidime against multidrug-resistant *P. aeruginosa* was demonstrated in an *in vitro* model.[61] The use of colistin should be reserved for only the most severe cases. New cephalosporin-β-lactamase inhibitor combination agents (ceftolozane-tazobactam and ceftazidime-avibactam) have yet to be studied in patients with CNS infections, but may be future alternative therapies for multidrug resistant gram-negative organisms.

Other gram-negative organisms causing meningitis, excluding *P. aeruginosa* and *Acinetobacter* spp., most likely can be treated with a third- or fourth-generation cephalosporin, such as cefotaxime, ceftriaxone, ceftazidime, or cefepime. Ceftazidime, however, may not be the best choice of empirical antibiotic for situations where the offending organism is not known initially because of its lack of reliable gram-positive coverage. Cefotaxime should be used in place of ceftriaxone in the neonatal period because of the potential for the displacement of bilirubin from albumin-binding sites.

Trimethoprim-sulfamethoxazole is useful in the management of the Enterobacteriaceae family and also may be useful in the management of *L. monocytogenes*. One advantage of trimethoprim-sulfamethoxazole is that its penetration into the CSF does not depend on meningeal inflammation.[28] However, trimethoprim-sulfamethoxazole is not bactericidal which limits its routine use for the acute management of CNS infections. Fluoroquinolones exhibit good penetration into the CSF and are effective in animal models of both gram-negative and gram-positive meningitis; however, there are limited data on their efficacy in clinical practice. Ciprofloxacin is recommended as an alternative agent for the treatment of *E. coli*, other Enterobacteriaceae, and *P. aeruginosa*.[15] Cefepime, meropenem, and aztreonam represent other therapeutic options for the treatment of gram-negative bacterial meningitis.[13,15]

8 CSF cultures may remain positive for several days or more with a regimen that eventually will be curative. Therapeutic efficacy can be monitored through bacterial colony counts every 2 or 3 days, which should decrease progressively over the period of therapy. Therapy for gram-negative meningitis should be continued for a minimum of 21 days from the start of treatment with an effective agent.[13,15]

Clinical **Controversy...**

Multidrug resistant gram-negative meningitis is an ongoing concern due to the limited number of therapeutic options available. Therapy is often limited to older, and more toxic, antibiotics, such as colistin and polymyxin B. Although new agents with extended spectrum of activity have been developed, they are yet to be studied in patients with CNS infections. Two cephalosporin-β-lactamase inhibitor combination agents (ceftolozane-tazobactam and ceftazidime-avibactam) may be future alternative therapies for multidrug resistant gram-negative organisms, but currently lack data to support their use in clinical settings.

Bacillus anthracis

Bacillus anthracis is a large, endospore-forming, aerobic, gram-positive bacteria capable of producing infection via the cutaneous, pulmonary, or GI routes. Cases of meningitis have been reported following both cutaneous and inhalational infections. According to the CDC, and prior to the bioterrorism-related outbreak in 2001, only a handful of sporadic cases had occurred in the United States in the 20th century, with the last occurrence in 2011. Mortality rates due to uncomplicated cutaneous, GI and inhaled anthrax infections are estimated to be less than 2%, 40% or more, and 45%, respectively, while cases of anthrax meningitis are often fatal.[62]

The major neurologic complication of anthrax infection is fulminant, rapidly fatal hemorrhagic meningoencephalitis. The inhalational form of anthrax seems to be a potent inducer of neurologic symptoms, and death usually occurs within a week for those with neurologic complications.[62] *B. anthracis* typically is susceptible to penicillin, amoxicillin, erythromycin, doxycycline, and ciprofloxacin. The bioterrorism-related strain in 2001 was susceptible to fluoroquinolones, rifampin, tetracycline, vancomycin, imipenem, meropenem, chloramphenicol, clindamycin, and aminoglycoside; but resistant to third-generation cephalosporins and trimethoprim-sulfamethoxazole. Recommendations for the treatment of systemic anthrax with possible or confirmed meningitis call for the use of three active antibacterial agents. Empiric regimens that include high doses of intravenous fluoroquinolones (ciprofloxacin, levofloxacin, or moxifloxacin) along with a carbapenem (meropenem, doripenem, or imipenem) and a protein synthesis inhibitor (eg, linezolid or clindamycin) are recommended. Once penicillin susceptibility is confirmed, the carbapenem can be deescalated to intravenous penicillin G or Ampicillin.[62] Also, adjunctive corticosteroids should be considered for patients with suspected or confirmed anthrax meningitis. Doxycycline is not recommended for the treatment of anthrax meningitis owing to poor CNS penetration, compared to MIC of most bacterial pathogens, but can be utilized for cases of inhaled or cutaneous anthrax once CNS involvement has been ruled out.[62] Finally, in 2015 the U.S. FDA approved an intravenous anthrax immune globulin for the treatment of inhalation anthrax in adults and pediatric patients along with appropriate antibacterial treatments.

Dexamethasone as an Adjunctive Treatment for Bacterial Meningitis

In addition to antibiotics, dexamethasone is a commonly used adjunctive therapy in the treatment of meningitis. Corticosteroids inhibit the production of TNF and IL-1, both potent proinflammatory cytokines. In clinical trials that measured inflammatory mediators, lower levels of TNF, PAF, or IL-1 were detected in patients treated with dexamethasone.[63-65] A series of animal studies, however, suggest adjuvant dexamethasone may aggravate neuronal injury by increasing apoptosis, programmed cell death, in the hippocampus of infant rats with pneumococcal and in rabbits with *E. coli* meningitis.[66] A series of early clinical studies assessing the outcomes of dexamethasone therapy for the initial treatment of bacterial meningitis showed conflicting results.[67] Subsequently, a systematic review in 2004 indicated that treatment with corticosteroids reduced both mortality and neurological sequelae in adults with community-acquired bacterial meningitis.[68] However, large randomized clinical trials showed conflicting results. A fundamental problem with corticosteroid investigations to date is that the majority of patients in the trials had *H. influenzae* meningitis, which has decreased dramatically following the introduction of polysaccharide conjugate vaccines in early 1980s. Additionally, the majority of studies examining dexamethasone use for pneumococcal meningitis were conducted before widespread penicillin-resistant pneumococcus emerged or in parts of the world where penicillin resistance is minimal.

A systematic review of 25 randomized controlled trials involving 4,121 participants showed corticosteroid use in bacterial meningitis was associated with lower rates of severe hearing loss, any hearing loss, and neurological sequelae, but did not reduce overall mortality nor was associated with beneficial effects in low-income countries. Additionally, subgroup analyses showed reduced overall mortality in pneumococcal meningitis and severe hearing loss in children with *H. influenzae* meningitis.[69] While a previous meta-analysis of five randomized, double-blinded, placebo-controlled trials of dexamethasone for bacterial meningitis in patients of all ages showed that adjunctive dexamethasone did not seem to significantly reduce death or neurological disability.[70] Thus, adjunctive corticosteroid use in the management of bacterial meningitis remains controversial.

Most clinical trials on the use of adjunctive dexamethasone in bacterial meningitis have involved children. A retrospective analysis of pediatric patients with pneumococcal meningitis and one unblinded, noncontrolled trial suggested that adjunctive steroids may decrease the neurologic sequelae and mortality associated with *S. pneumoniae* meningitis.[63,71] Also, a meta-analysis in 1997 suggested benefits in *H. influenza* meningitis and, if commenced with or before antibiotics, suggested benefit for pneumococcal meningitis in childhood.[72] Finally, a large multicenter trial did not demonstrate reduction in mortality when adjunctive dexamethasone was used for children with meningococcal or pneumococcal meningitis, but potential benefit in preventing long-term hearing loss was observed.[73]

(10) Current recommendations call for the use of adjunctive dexamethasone in infants and children (6 weeks of age and older) with *H. influenza* meningitis.[15] The recommended intravenous dose is 0.15 mg/kg every 6 hours for 2 to 4 days, initiated 10 to 20 minutes prior to or concomitant with, but not after, the first dose of antibiotics. Clinical outcome is unlikely to improve if dexamethasone is given after the first dose of antimicrobial and should therefore be avoided. For infants and children 6 weeks of age and older with pneumococcal meningitis, adjunctive dexamethasone may be considered after weighing the potential benefits and possible risks.[15,74] If adjunctive dexamethasone is used, careful monitoring of signs and symptoms of GI bleeding and hyperglycemia should be employed. Moreover, the use of dexamethasone may interfere with the interpretation of clinical response to treatment, such as resolution of fever.

If pneumococcal meningitis is suspected or proven, it is recommended that adults receive dexamethasone 0.15 mg/kg (up to 10 mg) every 6 hours for 2 to 4 days with the first dose administered 10 to 20 minutes prior to first dose of antibiotics. Similar to the pediatric population, clinical outcome is unlikely to improve if dexamethasone is given after the first dose of antibiotics and should therefore be avoided.[13,15] It is often difficult to ascertain the responsible pathogen on presentation; therefore, some clinicians recommend initiating dexamethasone in all adult patients presenting with community-acquired bacterial meningitis. Dexamethasone is not routinely recommended for patients with acute community-acquired bacterial meningitis due to other bacterial etiologies.[13,15]

Routine use of dexamethasone in meningitis is not without controversy. A potential concern is adjunctive dexamethasone therapy that may reduce the penetration of antibiotics into the CSF by inhibiting or reducing meningeal inflammation. In early experimental models of meningitis, steroids decreased the CSF concentrations of ampicillin, rifampin, vancomycin, and gentamicin.[65,75] Yet, ceftriaxone and vancomycin penetration into CSF was unaffected by concurrent dexamethasone administration in pediatric patients.[76,77] Appropriate concentrations of vancomycin in CSF may be obtained even when adjunctive dexamethasone is used, but the small number of subjects studied limits the generalization of these findings.[78]

Bacterial Brain Abscess

Approximately 1,500 to 2,500 cases of brain abscess occur annually in the United States, with decreasing incidence due to contiguous spread of infection from the oropharynx, middle ear, and paranasal sinuses and increasing incidence due to contiguous spread from cranial trauma or neurosurgical procedures.[79,80] Other sources of infection include hematogenous spread from distant foci of infection, such as endocarditis or intra-abdominal infection. Mortality rates have declined significantly in the past 50 years, with 70% of survivors expected to have no to minimal neurologic sequelae.[81]

(2) The clinical presentation varies depending on the number, size, and location of the abscess(es). Headache, mental status changes, focal neurologic deficits, and fever are the most common symptoms of brain abscess, but seizures and nausea and vomiting may also be seen.[81,82] Diagnosis of brain abscess can be facilitated by CT or MRI, with preference given to MRI due to the ability to better differentiate cerebral tumor, stroke, and abscess. Lumbar puncture is not routinely recommended in patients with brain abscess, while CT-guided aspiration and biopsy can be both diagnostic and therapeutic.[81]

The etiology of brain abscess depends on the initial site of infection. Those arising from spread of infection from oropharynx, middle ear, and paranasal sinuses are commonly caused by streptococci and oral anaerobes (eg, *Actinomyces* spp., *Bacteroides* spp., *Fusobacterium* spp., *Peptostreptococcus*). Staphylococci, aerobic and gram-negative bacilli are commonly involved in postoperative abscesses or those following head trauma. *P. aeruginosa* and *Nocardia* spp. can also cause brain abscesses but are more commonly seen in immunocompromised patients.[81]

(6) Because brain abscesses are commonly polymicrobial, empiric antimicrobial therapy should include antibiotics with activity against gram-positive, gram-negative, and anaerobic organisms. For example, the regimen could include vancomycin plus a third- or fourth-generation cephalosporin plus metronidazole, depending on risk factors. A carbapenem (such as meropenem) could replace the cephalosporin and metronidazole. De-escalation of therapy should occur once a causative organism is identified. While no consensus on treatment duration for brain abscesses exists, duration of therapy should be determined for each individual patient and should include consideration of the causative pathogen, size of abscess, use of surgical treatment, and response to therapy. Because seizure is a common complication of brain abscesses, anticonvulsant therapy is recommended for at least 1 year and may be discontinued when an EEG shows no epileptic activity. (10) The benefit of dexamethasone in the treatment of brain abscess is unclear and not routinely recommended, unless signs of cerebral edema are identified.[81]

Cryptococcus neoformans

Cryptococcus spp. are encapsulated soil yeasts acquired by inhalation of spores from the environment leading to CNS infection and less commonly pulmonary disease. The two main pathogenic species are *Cryptococcus neoformans* and *C. gattii*. While cryptococcal infections mainly affect persons with underlying impaired immunity such as HIV-positive (approximately 80%-95% of cases) and HIV-negative immunosuppressed patients, infections in nonimmunosuppressed individuals have been reported in North America.[83] Globally, approximately 958,000 cases of cryptococcal meningitis occur annually, mostly in Sub-Saharan Africa, resulting in an overall 3-months case-fatality rate of over 600,000.[84]

The incubation period in acquired immunodeficiency syndrome (AIDS) patients may be very short, as opposed to a relatively normal host, in whom it may be very long. Symptoms of *C. neoformans* meningitis are insidious and may be present for varying periods, depending on the host involved, before the definitive diagnosis is made. (2) Fever and a history of headaches are the most common symptoms, although altered mentation and evidence of focal neurologic deficits may be present. Examination of the CSF usually reveals mildly elevated WBCs, primarily lymphocytes (Table 106-1). (3) Diagnosis is based on the presence of a positive CSF, blood, sputum, or urine culture for *C. neoformans*. Organisms may be seen by microscope when stained with India ink and are more likely to be seen in AIDS patients compared with other hosts. An additional rapid test helpful in diagnosis is latex agglutination, which detects the presence of cryptococcal antigens. Latex agglutination is associated with overall sensitivities and specificities of 93% to 100% and 93% to 98%, respectively.[83] A cryptococcal antigen detection test needs to be considered in any patient presenting initially with meningitis. Risk factors predictive of a poor outcome include lethargy at presentation, nonimmunosuppressed patients, high CSF cryptococcal antigen titer, low CSF WBC count, low CD4 cell count, fungemia, and elevated CSF pressure.[85-87]

Rapid sterilization of CNS through rapid fungicidal activity is the main approach of induction therapy, which ranges from 2 to 6 weeks, followed by consolidation therapy for 8 weeks.[88] Despite poor penetration into the CSF, amphotericin B has long been the drug of choice for the treatment of acute cryptococcal meningitis due to its rapid fungicidal activity.[85] A landmark clinical trial showed amphotericin B (1 mg/kg/day) combined with flucytosine (100 mg/kg/day) for 2 weeks was more effective than amphotericin alone for 4 weeks or in combination with fluconazole (400 mg twice daily) for 2 weeks in HIV-positive patients.[89] Additionally, this combination was associated with the most rapidly fungicidal activity, when compared with amphotericin alone, in combination with fluconazole or in combination with fluconazole and flucytosine.[90]

Clinical **Controversy...**

Timing of HAART initiation following acute cryptococcal meningitis in patients with HIV-AIDS remains an area of clinical controversy. Conflicting results from earlier studies prompted a recent prospective trial (COAT Trial) of adult HIV-positive patients with acute cryptococcal meningitis comparing early (1-2 weeks) and late (5 weeks) initiation of HAART following diagnosis. Late HAART initiation was associated with a significant reduction in 26-week mortality. Current HIV and cryptococcal meningitis treatment guidelines recommend a short delay (2-10 weeks) between diagnosis and HAART initiation; however, more definitive recommendations remain an area of clinical debate.

Unfortunately, in the AIDS population, flucytosine is often poorly tolerated, causing bone marrow suppression and GI distress. Careful monitoring of hematologic parameters, therapeutic drug monitoring (TDM) and dose adjustment for patients with renal insufficiency are recommended to avoid flucytosine-associated toxicities. Amphotericin B alone or in combination with high-dose fluconazole may be reasonable alternatives to standard treatment.[91,92] Lipid formulations of amphotericin B at higher doses (3-5 mg/kg/day) can be used for HIV-positive patients with or predisposed to renal dysfunction and are recommended for organ-transplant recipients.[88]

Azole therapy is the most studied alternative regimen for the treatment of *C. neoformans* meningitis in HIV-positive patients. Fluconazole and itraconazole have been studied as monotherapy with mixed results. If used alone or in combination with flucytosine, higher fluconazole doses of 800 to 2,000 mg/day are recommended due to higher success rates.[93] To note, the rate of fluconazole-resistant *C. neoformans* has been increasing in recent years.[94] Itraconazole has limited utility in induction therapy due to limited CSF levels of the active drug. Generally, itraconazole suspension is preferred due to better absorption, and TDM is recommended to ensure optimal drug levels.[88] Voriconazole in combination with amphotericin B showed similar rate of clearance of cryptococcal CFU in CSF samples compared with standard therapy.[91] Posaconazole has demonstrated clinical activity against cryptococcal and other fungal infections of the CNS in patients with refractory disease or otherwise intolerant to standard antifungal agents. Posaconazole appeared well tolerated at oral doses of 800 mg/day and may be an alternative in the treatment of fungal CNS infection due to *C. neoformans*.[95] More data are needed to determine what role the new azole antifungal agents will play in future treatment of cryptococcal meningitis. Also, widespread TDM of new azole antifungals will be needed to ensure adequate CNS therapeutic concentrations.

HIV-positive persons often require extended maintenance or suppressive therapy, minimum of 12 months, because of high relapse rates following primary therapy (induction and consolidation phases) for *C. neoformans*. A large multicenter, controlled trial compared fluconazole 200 mg/day and amphotericin B 1 mg/kg/wk in the prevention of relapse. Two percent of patients receiving fluconazole versus 18% of patients on amphotericin B relapsed. In addition, the amphotericin B group had significantly more frequent bacterial infections, bacteremia, and drug-related toxicity.[96] Fluconazole was also superior to itraconazole in the prevention of relapse.[97] Current guidelines recommend continuing maintenance therapy until immune reconstitution takes place. Guidelines for the prevention of opportunistic infections in HIV-infected persons are updated frequently and can be found at www.aidsinfo.nih.gov. Readers interested in treatment guidelines for cryptococcal meningitis in HIV-negative immunosuppressed, such as transplant recipients, and nonimmunosuppressed individuals are encouraged to review the Infectious Diseases Society of America Guidelines for the management of cryptococcal disease.[88]

Viral Encephalitis

Encephalitis is defined by the presence of an inflammatory process of the brain in association with clinical evidence of neurologic dysfunction.[24] Patients with metabolic disturbances, organ dysfunction, and noninfectious encephalitis, including postimmunization encephalitis or encephalomyelitis, can have similar clinical presentation to those with infectious encephalitis. Several infectious organisms have been identified to cause encephalitis, with viral etiologies being the most commonly diagnosed.[98,99] Additionally, meningoencephalitis is a term commonly used to describe meningeal inflammation along with encephalitis.

The epidemiology of viral encephalitis in the United States has changed dramatically since the mid-1960s because of the introduction of large-scale polio, rubella, varicella-zoster virus (VZV), and mumps immunization programs. Worldwide, mumps remains a causative agent of viral encephalitis in countries with low vaccination rates. Poliomyelitis, once a significant cause of encephalitis, is now confined to only a few less-developed countries. While a confirmed or probable pathogen is identified in less than 50% of cases, common causes of viral encephalitis and meningoencephalitis in the United States include herpes simplex virus (HSV), West Nile virus (WNV), and the enteroviruses.[98,99] Additionally, viral encephalitis is caused by a variety of other pathogens, such as arboviruses, adenoviruses, influenzae virus A and B, rotavirus, corona virus, cytomegalovirus (CMV), VZV, Epstein-Barr virus, and lymphocytic choriomeningitis. Collectively, about 20,000 encephalitis-associated hospitalizations are expected per year in the United States, with a case fatality rate of more than 5% and total health-care burden of nearly $2 billion.[56,99]

Viral encephalitis is acquired primarily by hematogenous spread or, alternatively, by neuronal spread of the causative pathogen. After entry into the host, viral replication occurs, resulting in dissemination through the reticuloendothelial system or vasculature. Infection of the capillary endothelial cells and choroid plexus may provide a conduit for CNS infections. Viruses such as polio, HSV, and VZV may also gain access to the CNS by axonal retrograde transmission from peripheral nerve endings. Once a virus gains access to the CNS, the course of infection depends on the virulence of the particular virus and the host immune response. Subsequent neuronal injury is caused by direct cell damage due to viral replication, but inflammatory and immune-mediated responses also contribute to neurological damage.[16,17]

In contrast with purulent meningitis, host response to viral encephalitis is mediated primarily through cytotoxic T-lymphocytes. Increases in concentrations of IL-1, IL-6, and interferon (INF)-α, -β and -γ may occur. While cytokine assays are available for investigational use, they are not used routinely in the clinical diagnosis of viral encephalitis.[16,17] 2 The clinical syndrome associated with viral encephalitis generally is independent of viral etiology and may vary depending on the patient's age. Common signs in adults include headache, mild fever, nuchal rigidity, malaise, drowsiness, nausea, vomiting, and photophobia. Only fever and irritability may be evident in the infant, and acute bacterial meningitis must be ruled out as a cause of fever when no other localized findings are observed in a child. Duration of symptoms generally is 1 to 2 weeks, and specific manifestations outside the meninges can also occur depending on the viral etiology.

Laboratory examination of the CSF usually reveals a pleocytosis with 100 to 1,000 WBC/mm^3 (0.1-1 × 10^9/L), which are primarily lymphocytic; however, 20% to 75% of patients with viral encephalitis may have a predominance of polymorphonuclear cells on initial examination of the CSF. On repeat lumbar puncture, 90% of patients presenting initially with a predominance of neutrophils experience a shift to a predominance of mononuclear cells. Other laboratory findings include normal to mildly elevated protein concentrations and normal or mildly reduced glucose concentrations (see Table 106-1).[16,17]

3 As mentioned earlier, pathogens responsible for viral encephalitis are often not identified. Poor laboratory recovery of viral pathogens and limited treatment options for viral encephalitis made the need for specific identification of pathogens of questionable value. Advances in diagnostic laboratory techniques and the potential for decreased costs associated with longer duration of hospitalization for patients with unconfirmed viral encephalitis have led to a reevaluation of the need for confirmatory pathogen diagnosis. When clinical signs warrant pathogen identification, appropriate laboratory diagnostic techniques, including PCR and serologic testing, should be undertaken. Molecular methods are preferred to conventional laboratory tests, such as viral cultures and brain biopsy, in the diagnosis of viral encephalitis owing to improved sensitivity and specificity, higher yield and rapid results.[23,24]

Supportive and symptomatic treatments of patients with viral encephalitis are of great importance due to limited treatment options for most viral etiologies. Such treatments may include seizure control, hemodynamic management, venous thromboembolism prevention, ICP management, and secondary bacterial infection prevention. Corticosteroid therapy is generally not recommended in most viral encephalitis cases; however, treatment should be considered for patients with cerebral edema and increased ICP.[23,24]

Although there are numerous pathogenic causes of viral encephalitis, much of the clinical presentation, diagnosis, and treatment are similar. The most commonly isolated viral etiologies are described here. Both HSV type 1 (HSV1) and HSV type 2 (HSV2) are considered the most common treatable causes of viral encephalitis. HSV1 is associated with encephalitis in adults, whereas HSV2 is associated predominantly with encephalitis in newborns.[99,100] Sexually active adults acquire HSV meningitis during or after an attack of genital or rectal HSV, whereas neonates acquire the virus during passage through the vaginal canal of mothers with active HSV infection. HSV PCR testing on CSF specimens should be performed for all patients with presumed encephalitis. Moreover, repeat testing should be considered for patients with an initial negative test after 3 to 7 days.[24] Establishing the correct diagnosis as early as possible is paramount because of high mortality rate without treatment (approaches 70%), and unlike other viral etiologies, specific and effective therapy is available. As a result, empirical therapy of suspected HSV encephalitis, while laboratory results are pending, is necessary. Delaying antiviral therapy has been consistently associated with unfavorable outcomes and increased mortality across several studies. In one retrospective study of 184 patients with HSV encephalitis, administration of intravenous acyclovir within first day of hospital admission was associated with a lower mortality rate (13% vs 31%).[26] Additionally, a clinical decision to treat may need to be made regardless of test results.

Acyclovir is the drug of choice for HSV encephalitis. In adult patients with normal renal function, acyclovir is usually administered as 10 mg/kg intravenously every 8 hours for 2 to 3 weeks.[23,24] Higher doses of acyclovir (20 mg/kg every intravenously every 8 hours) have been used in neonates and are associated with lower mortality rates.[101] HSV resistance to acyclovir has been reported with increasing incidence, particularly in immunocompromised patients with prior or chronic exposures to acyclovir, ranging from 3.5% to 10% in immunocompromised patients.[102] The alternative treatment for acyclovir-resistant HSV is foscarnet. The dose for patients with normal renal function is 40 to 60 mg/kg infused over 1 hour every 8 to 12 hours for 3 weeks, with the higher dose typically reserved for HIV-infected individuals.[23] Ensuring adequate hydration is imperative to decrease risk of acyclovir- and foscarnet-induced nephrotoxicity. In addition, patients receiving foscarnet should be monitored for seizures related to alterations in plasma electrolyte levels. Finally, a recent prospective study examined the utility of long-term antiviral treatment on overall survival with no or mild neuropsychological impairment. Adult patients who completed standard initial HSV encephalitis treatment followed by an additional 3-month course of oral valacyclovir did not show improvements in neuropsychological testing 12 months later compared to placebo.[103]

Because of the recent epidemic in the United States, a separate discussion of the WNV is warranted. Although primarily mosquitoes transmit WNV, transmissions via blood products, organ transplantation, transplacental transfer, and breast milk have been documented. Similar to other arboviruses, the incubation period for WNV ranges from 3 days to 2 weeks. Infection with WNV is asymptomatic in most adults or causes a mild flu-like syndrome characterized by fever, malaise, myalgia, and lymphadenopathy. Among 41,762 reported cases of WNV in the United States between 1999 and 2014, the overall mortality rate was approximately 4% (9% in patients with neuroinvasive disease).[104] Many patients develop a maculopapular, erythematous rash, which is more common in children than in adults and is uncommon in other forms of viral encephalitis. The other neurologic manifestations include fever, nausea, vomiting, headache, altered mental status, movement disorders, and/or a syndrome much like poliomyelitis.[105] The primary risk factor for this manifestation seems to be advanced age, but alcohol abuse, diabetes, hypertension, immunosuppression, and cardiovascular disease were also identified as potential risk factors for neuroinvasive disease and worse outcomes.[105,106] The poliomyelitis syndrome is characterized by an early prodromic phase of fevers and weakness followed by the sudden onset of flaccid paralysis. CSF examination of WNV encephalitis typically shows pleocytosis and a slightly elevated CSF protein concentration. Several diagnostic methods have been developed for WNV, including a PCR assay and enzyme-linked immunosorbent assay (ELISA) tests. However, serologic tests (ELISA) can cross-react with other flaviviruses causing a false-positive result. Moreover, serum IgM antibodies for WNV can persist for up to 1 year, leading to confusion regarding whether the infection is an acute or previous infection. Ribavirin has shown inhibitory effects on the WNV in neural tissue cultures, but this has not been studied in controlled trials. Finally, DNA vaccines were studied in animals and have shown positive results.[105] Treatment is typically supportive, including treatment for seizures and increased ICP, and in the majority of cases, the disease is self-limiting.[23,24]

CMV has emerged as a major cause of morbidity and mortality in immunocompromised patients, including HIV-infected individuals and transplant recipients on immunosuppressants. CNS infections with CMV are often difficult to treat, with higher failure rates and poor outcomes. Combination therapy with ganciclovir and foscarnet is recommended for induction treatment due to higher failure rates and lack of survival benefits when monotherapy with either agent is utilized.[23,24] In adult patients, ganciclovir 5 mg/kg every 12 hours and foscarnet 60 mg/kg every 8 hours (or 90 mg/kg every 12 hours) for 3 weeks are recommended during the induction phase, followed by maintenance phase with either agent. Other interventions that may improve survival outcomes include the initiation of highly active antiretroviral therapy (HAART) in untreated HIV-infected patients and reduction of immunosuppression intensity in transplant recipients.

HIV encephalitis is a common CNS complication associated with AIDS. Frequently, patients may complain of headache, photophobia, or stiff neck at the time of presumed seroconversion. As the disease progresses neurologic symptoms are frequently reported secondary to other opportunistic infections. Diagnosis of viral encephalitis is difficult because mental status and neurologic examinations are not sensitive enough to detect early changes. Direct evidence of HIV encephalitis can be obtained through CSF culture, p24 antigen testing, or qualitative or quantitative PCR for HIV RNA. Diagnostic workup of other potential copathogens, such as HSV, *Toxoplasma gondii*, *Mycobacterium tuberculosis*, *Aspergillus* spp, and *Cryptococcus*, should also be performed. Refer to chapter on HIV infection for a complete discussion of infectious complications in HIV-positive individuals.

Other Etiologies

Mycobacterium Tuberculosis

M. tuberculosis is the primary cause of tuberculous meningitis and remains the most life-threatening form of extrapulmonary tuberculosis. The incidence of tuberculosis, in general, has decreased to three cases per 100,000 individuals in the United States in 2013.[107]

The CDC recommends an initial regimen of four drugs for empirical treatment of *M. tuberculosis*. This regimen consists of isoniazid, rifampin, pyrazinamide, and ethambutol for the first 2 months, generally followed by isoniazid plus rifampin for the remaining duration of therapy.[108] The recommended therapy for HIV-positive individuals is the same as for immunocompetent patients, although rifabutin may be considered in place of other rifamycins in an effort to minimize drug interactions with protease inhibitors and nonnucleoside reverse-transcriptase inhibitors. Therapy in HIV-negative and HIV-positive patients should be individualized based on susceptibility patterns and guidelines from the CDC and the American Thoracic Society, which are updated frequently and available on the Internet (www.cdc.gov/nchstp/tb/pubs/mmwrhtml/maj_guide.htm). Patients with *M. tuberculosis* meningitis should be treated for 9 to 12 months or longer with multiple-drug therapy, and patients with rifampin-resistant strains may receive up to 18 to 24 months of therapy.

Treponema pallidum (Neurosyphilis)

Infection of the CNS by *Treponema pallidum* can occur at any stage of the disease although is most commonly seen in tertiary or latent syphilis many years, even decades, after the initial exposure. According to the CDC, incidence of late latent syphilis, which includes neurosyphilis, can develop in 15% of people who do not receive treatment for syphilis.[109] Patients with neurosyphilis may be asymptomatic, or present with signs and symptoms consistent with acute meningitis. Diagnosis is based on CSF findings, neurologic manifestations, and serologic evidence of exposure.[110] Aqueous penicillin G is recommended for treatment dosed either 3 to 4 million Units every 4 hours or 18 to 24 million units as a continuous infusion for a duration of 10 to 14 days.[109] If CSF pleocytosis is initially present, CSF examination should be repeated every 6 months until the cell count is normal. For further reading on the manifestations and treatment of syphilis we refer you to chapter on sexually transmitted infections in this text.

Toxoplasma gondii

Toxoplasmic encephalitis (TE) is caused by the protozoan *T. gondii*. Approximately 22.5% of the U.S. population 12 years and older have been infected with *T. gondii*. In other parts of the world, up to 95% of populations are infected. The primary routes of transmission are foodborne, animal-to-human (cats serving as the definitive host), mother-to-child (congenital), blood transfusions, and organ transplantation.[111] TE is typically caused by the reactivation of disease in immunocompromised patients, especially those with AIDS, or intrauterine infection in newborns. Clinical manifestations include extrapyramidal signs and symptoms, headache, seizures, confusion, hemiparesis, cranial nerve abnormalities, or fever.[24] In congenital toxoplasmosis, patients may also present with hydrocephalus, intracerebral calcification, microcephaly, convulsions, or chorioretinitis.[24,112] Definitive diagnosis of TE requires a clinical sample via a brain biopsy; therefore, TE is presumptively diagnosed on the basis of clinical symptoms, positive serology for antitoxoplasma IgG antibodies, and identification of space-occupying lesions on CT, MRI, or other radiologic imaging. In patients with AIDS, MRI typically shows multiple ring-enhancing lesions. *T. gondii* can also be detected by PCR in CSF; however, the sensitivity is low (50%) and the result is usually negative once treatment has started.[24,112,113] First-line treatment for TE in adults consists of pyrimethamine plus sulfadiazine plus leucovorin. Leucovorin is typically added to the treatment regimen to reduce the likelihood of hematologic toxicity associated with pyrimethamine. In patients who are unable to tolerate sulfadiazine, clindamycin may be used as an alternative. Other alternative treatment options include trimethoprim-sulfamethoxazole, atovaquone plus pyrimethamine plus leucovorin, atovaquone plus sulfadiazine, atovaquone monotherapy, or pyrimethamine plus leucovorin plus azithromycin. Treatment recommendations are the same in pediatric patients; however, several of the alternative regimens have not been studied in children.[24,112,113]

Borrelia burgdorferi

LD is caused by the spirochete *Borrelia burgdorferi* and is the most common tick-borne infection in North America and Europe.[114] Lyme neuroborreliosis (LNB) is an infectious disorder of the nervous system caused by *B. burgdorferi* and has been reported in up to 10% to 15% of patients with untreated LD. CNS involvement may include meningitis, myelitis, cerebral vasculitis, or encephalitis. Clinical manifestations include fever, headache, fatigue, photosensitivity, phonosensitivity, confusion, hemiparesis, cranial neuropathy (facial neuropathy being the most common), cerebellar ataxia, ocular flutter, apraxia, opsoclonus-myoclonus syndrome, or Parkinson-like symptoms. Poliomyelitis-like syndromes and acute stroke-like symptoms caused by cerebral vasculitis have been documented in single-case reports but are considered rare. Unlike the European LD, the North American LD is also characterized by a skin rash called erythema migrans.[114,115] Currently there is no international consensus for the diagnosis of LNB. Diagnosis is primarily based on the presence of neurological symptoms without other obvious reasons, CSF analysis (lymphocytic pleocytosis, moderately elevated protein, normal glucose), intrathecal *B. burgdorferi* antibody production, blood and CSF serologic testing (ELISA plus Western blot), and MRI demonstrating areas of inflammation.[24,114,115] PCR testing for detection of *B. burgdorferi* in CSF has a sensitivity of less than 10% to 30% and has an unknown specificity, therefore is not routinely recommended. Parenteral treatment with ceftriaxone once daily is recommended as first-line treatment of LNB. Patients with cranial neuropathy without clinical signs of meningitis may be treated with oral amoxicillin, doxycycline, or cefuroxime axetil. The European Federation of Neurological Societies (EFNS) guidelines also recommend oral doxycycline as a first-line option for patients with symptoms confined to the meninges, cranial nerves, nerve roots, or peripheral nerves based on its CSF penetration, ability to achieve CSF concentrations above the MIC, and several Class III studies showing similar short- and long-term efficacy to various parenteral regimens.[115] Alternative parenteral options to ceftriaxone include cefotaxime or penicillin G. For patients intolerant to β-lactams, doxycycline oral or intravenous is suggested.

EVALUATION OF THERAPEUTIC OUTCOMES

Signs and Symptoms

Because of the potential for rapid deterioration associated with CNS infections, signs and symptoms of fever, headache, meningismus (eg, nuchal rigidity, Brudzinski's or Kernig's sign), vital signs, and signs of cerebral dysfunction should be evaluated every 4 hours for the initial 3 days and then daily thereafter. The Glasgow Coma Scale should be used in severely ill patients. Trends in improvement and resolution rather than single evaluations in time are more important in monitoring the signs and symptoms of meningitis.

Microbiologic Findings

CSF and blood samples for gram-stain, cultures, and sensitivity testing should be taken prior to starting antibiotic therapy. If lumbar puncture is delayed, however, antibiotics should be started. Although the CSF cultures may be negative, antibiotic therapy rarely interferes with the protein and/or glucose concentrations in the CSF. Furthermore, if the laboratory is made aware of the antibiotic therapy, steps can be taken to diminish the effects of the antibiotic during the detection process. Gram stain results can be obtained immediately and can guide empirical antibiotic treatment. Identification of the organism can be made within 24 hours, and sensitivities should be available within 48 hours. Repeat cultures should be performed to help determine if sterilization is achieved. A second tube of blood should be taken to allow for latex agglutination tests of antigens to common meningeal pathogens (*H. influenzae*, *S. pneumoniae*, *N. meningitidis*, *E. coli*, and group B *Streptococcus*) if the gram stain has not been helpful.

CSF Examination

In bacterial meningitis, the CSF WBC count usually is greater than 1,000 cells/mm^3 (1,000 × 10^6/L), the CSF protein concentration is elevated, and the CSF glucose concentration (hypoglycorachia) is often low (45 mg/dL or less [2.5 mmol/L or less] or 50%-60% of a simultaneous blood glucose value). Viral encephalitis, in contrast, results in relatively normal CSF protein and glucose levels and typically does not result in greater than 90% polymorphonuclear neutrophils (PMNs) in the CSF (Table 106-1).

ABBREVIATIONS

ACIP	Advisory Committee on Immunization Practices
AIDS	acquired immunodeficiency syndrome
BBB	blood–brain barrier
BCSFB	blood–cerebrospinal fluid barrier
CBF	cerebral blood flow
CDC	US Centers for Disease Control and Prevention
CFU	colony forming unit
CLSI	Clinical and Laboratory Standards Institute
CMV	cytomegalovirus
CNS	central nervous system
CSF	cerebrospinal fluid
CT	computed tomography
DIC	disseminated intravascular coagulation
EFNS	European Federation of Neurological Societies
EIA	enzyme immunoassay
ELISA	enzyme-linked immunosorbent assay
FDA	US Food and Drug Administration
GBS	group B *Streptococcus*
GI	gastrointestinal
HAART	highly active antiretroviral therapy
Hib	*Haemophilus influenzae* type b
HIV	human immunodeficiency virus
HSV	herpes simplex virus
ICP	intracranial pressure
Ig	immunoglobulin
IPD	invasive pneumococcal disease
IL-1	interleukin-1
INF	interferon
LNB	lyme neuroborreliosis
LPS	lipopolysaccharide
MenB	serogroup B meningococcal vaccine
MIC	minimum inhibitory concentration
MRI	magnetic resonance imaging
PAF	platelet-activating factor
PCR	polymerase chain reaction
PCT	procalcitonin
PCV7	heptavalent pneumococcal conjugate vaccine
PCV13	13-valent pneumococcal conjugate vaccine
PGE2	prostaglandin E_2
PMN	polymorphonuclear neutrophil
PPV23	23-valent pneumococcal polysaccharide vaccine
TDM	therapeutic drug monitoring
TE	toxoplasmic encephalitis
TNF	tumor necrosis factor
VZV	varicella-zoster virus
WBC	white blood cell
WNV	West Nile virus

REFERENCES

1. Thigpen MC, Whitney CG, Messonnier NE, et al. Bacterial meningitis in the United States, 1998-2007. *N Engl J Med* 2011;364:2016-2025.
2. Edmond K, Clark A, Korczak VS, et al. Global and regional risk of disabling sequelae from bacterial meningitis: a systematic review and meta-analysis. *Lancet Infect Dis* 2010;10:317-328.
3. van de Beek D, de Gans J, Spanjaard L, et al. Clinical features and prognostic factors in adults with bacterial meningitis. *N Engl J Med* 2004;351:1849-1859.
4. van de Beek D, Drake JM, Tunkel AR. Nosocomial bacterial meningitis. *N Engl J Med* 2010;362:146-154.
5. Brouwer MC, Tunkel AR, van de Beek D. Epidemiology, diagnosis, and antimicrobial treatment of acute bacterial meningitis. *Clin Microbiol Rev* 2010;23:467-492.
6. Castelblanco RL, Lee M, Hasbun R. Epidemiology of bacterial meningitis in the USA from 1997 to 2010: a population-based observational study. *Lancet Infect Dis* 2014;14:813-819.
7. Pilishvili T, Lexau C, Farley MM, et al. Sustained reductions in invasive pneumococcal disease in the era of conjugate vaccine. *J Infect Dis* 2010;201:32-41.
8. Williams WW, Lu PJ, O'Halloran A, et al. Noninfluenza vaccination coverage among adults—United States, 2012. *MMWR Morb Mortal Wkly Rep* 2014;63:95-102.

9. Moore MR, Link-Gelles R, Schaffner W, et al. Effect of use of 13-valent pneumococcal conjugate vaccine in children on invasive pneumococcal disease in children and adults in the USA: analysis of multisite, population-based surveillance. *Lancet Infect Dis* 2015;15:301-309.
10. Harboe ZB, Dalby T, Weinberger DM, et al. Impact of 13-valent pneumococcal conjugate vaccination in invasive pneumococcal disease incidence and mortality. *Clin Infect Dis* 2014;59:1066-1073.
11. Cohn AC, MacNeil JR, Clark TA, et al. Prevention and control of meningococcal disease: recommendations of the Advisory Committee on Immunization Practices (ACIP). *MMWR Recomm Rep* 2013;62:1-28.
12. Bleck T, Greenlee J. Anatomic considerations in central nervous system infections. In: Mandell GL, Bennett JE, Dolin R, eds. *Principles and Practice of Infectious Diseases*, 5th ed. New York: Churchill Livingstone; 2000:950-959.
13. Chaudhuri A, Martinez-Martin P, Kennedy PG, et al. EFNS guideline on the management of community-acquired bacterial meningitis: report of an EFNS Task Force on acute bacterial meningitis in older children and adults. *Eur J Neurol* 2008;15:649-659.
14. Mace SE. Acute bacterial meningitis. *Emerg Med Clin North Am* 2008;26:281-317, viii.
15. Tunkel AR, Hartman BJ, Kaplan SL, et al. Practice guidelines for the management of bacterial meningitis. *Clin Infect Dis* 2004;39:1267-1284.
16. Wright EJ, Brew BJ, Wesselingh SL. Pathogenesis and diagnosis of viral infections of the nervous system. *Neurol Clin* 2008;26:617-633, vii.
17. Ziai WC, Lewin JJ, 3rd. Update in the diagnosis and management of central nervous system infections. *Neurol Clin* 2008;26:427-468, viii.
18. Spector R, Lorenzo AV. Inhibition of penicillin transport from the cerebrospinal fluid after intracisternal inoculation of bacteria. *J Clin Invest* 1974;54:316-325.
19. Kim KS. Emerging molecular targets in the treatment of bacterial meningitis. *Expert Opin Ther Targets* 2003;7:141-152.
20. Curtis S, Stobart K, Vandermeer B, et al. Clinical features suggestive of meningitis in children: a systematic review of prospective data. *Pediatrics* 2010;126:952-960.
21. Nigrovic LE, Kuppermann N, Malley R. Development and validation of a multivariable predictive model to distinguish bacterial from aseptic meningitis in children in the post-Haemophilus influenzae era. *Pediatrics* 2002;110:712-719.
22. Nigrovic LE, Malley R, Kuppermann N. Meta-analysis of bacterial meningitis score validation studies. *Arch Dis Child* 2012;97:799-805.
23. Steiner I, Budka H, Chaudhuri A, et al. Viral meningoencephalitis: a review of diagnostic methods and guidelines for management. *Eur J Neurol* 2010;17:999-e57.
24. Tunkel AR, Glaser CA, Bloch KC, et al. The management of encephalitis: clinical practice guidelines by the Infectious Diseases Society of America. *Clin Infect Dis* 2008;47:303-327.
25. Auburtin M, Wolff M, Charpentier J, et al. Detrimental role of delayed antibiotic administration and penicillin-nonsusceptible strains in adult intensive care unit patients with pneumococcal meningitis: the PNEUMOREA prospective multicenter study. *Crit Care Med* 2006;34:2758-2765.
26. Poissy J, Wolff M, Dewilde A, et al. Factors associated with delay to acyclovir administration in 184 patients with herpes simplex virus encephalitis. *Clin Microbiol Infect* 2009;15:560-564.
27. Vikse J, Henry BM, Roy J, et al. The role of serum procalcitonin in the diagnosis of bacterial meningitis in adults: a systematic review and meta-analysis. *Int J Infect Dis* 2015;38:68-76.
28. Nau R, Sorgel F, Eiffert H. Penetration of drugs through the blood-cerebrospinal fluid/blood-brain barrier for treatment of central nervous system infections. *Clin Microbiol Rev* 2010;23:858-883.
29. Kastenbauer S, Pfister H-W. Pneumococcal meningitis in adults: spectrum of complications and prognostic factors in a series of 87 cases. *Brain* 2003;126:1015-1025.
30. Fenoll A, Gimenez MJ, Robledo O, et al. Influence of penicillin/amoxicillin non-susceptibility on the activity of third-generation cephalosporins against Streptococcus pneumoniae. *Eur J Clin Microbiol Infect Dis* 2008;27:75-80.
31. Hameed N, Tunkel AR. Treatment of drug-resistant pneumococcal meningitis. *Curr Infect Dis Rep* 2010;12:274-281.
32. Gillis LM, White HD, Whitehurst A, Sullivan DC. Vancomycin-tolerance among clinical isolates of Streptococcus pneumoniae in Mississippi during 1999-2001. *Am J Med Sci* 2005;330:65-68.
33. Rodriguez CA, Atkinson R, Bitar W, et al. Tolerance to vancomycin in pneumococci: detection with a molecular marker and assessment of clinical impact. *J Infect Dis* 2004;190:1481-1487.
34. Rodriguez-Cerrato V, McCoig CC, Saavedra J, et al. Garenoxacin (BMS-284756) and moxifloxacin in experimental meningitis caused by vancomycin-tolerant pneumococci. *Antimicrob Agents Chemother* 2003;47:211-215.
35. Faella F, Pagliano P, Fusco U, et al. Combined treatment with ceftriaxone and linezolid of pneumococcal meningitis: a case series including penicillin-resistant strains. *Clin Microbiol Infect* 2006;12:391-394.
36. Vivas M, Force E, Garrigos C, et al. Experimental study of the efficacy of daptomycin for the treatment of cephalosporin-resistant pneumococcal meningitis. *J Antimicrob Chemother* 2014;69:3020-3026.
37. Grandgirard D, Burri M, Agyeman P, Leib SL. Adjunctive daptomycin attenuates brain damage and hearing loss more efficiently than rifampin in infant rat pneumococcal meningitis. *Antimicrob Agents Chemother* 2012;56:4289-4295.
38. Cottagnoud P, Cottagnoud M, Acosta F, Stucki A. Efficacy of ceftaroline fosamil against penicillin-sensitive and -resistant streptococcus pneumoniae in an experimental rabbit meningitis model. *Antimicrob Agents Chemother* 2013;57:4653-4655.
39. Use of 13-valent pneumococcal conjugate vaccine and 23-valent pneumococcal polysaccharide vaccine for adults with immunocompromising conditions: recommendations of the Advisory Committee on Immunization Practices (ACIP). *MMWR Morb Mortal Wkly Rep* 2012;61:816-819.
40. Isaacman DJ, Fletcher MA, Fritzell B, et al. Indirect effects associated with widespread vaccination of infants with heptavalent pneumococcal conjugate vaccine (PCV7; Prevnar). *Vaccine* 2007;25:2420-2427.
41. Tomczyk S, Bennett NM, Stoecker C, et al. Use of 13-valent pneumococcal conjugate vaccine and 23-valent pneumococcal polysaccharide vaccine among adults aged ≥65 years: recommendations of the Advisory Committee on Immunization Practices (ACIP). *MMWR Morb Mortal Wkly Rep* 2014;63:822-825.
42. Olarte L, Barson WJ, Barson RM, et al. Impact of the 13-valent pneumococcal conjugate vaccine on pneumococcal meningitis in US children. *Clin Infect Dis* 2015;61:767-775.
43. Centers for Disease Control and Prevention (CDC). Use of 13-valent pneumococcal conjugate vaccine and 23-valent pneumococcal polysaccharide vaccine among children aged 6-18 years with immunocompromising conditions: recommendations of the Advisory Committee on Immunization Practices (ACIP). *MMWR Morb Mortal Wkly Rep* 2013;62:521-524.
44. Harrison LH, Trotter CL, Ramsay ME. Global epidemiology of meningococcal disease. *Vaccine* 2009;27(suppl 2):B51-B63.
45. Harrison LH. Epidemiological profile of meningococcal disease in the United States. *Clin Infect Dis* 2010;50(suppl 2):S37-S44.
46. Wang X, Shutt KA, Vuong JT, et al. Changes in the population structure of invasive Neisseria meningitidis in the United States after quadrivalent meningococcal conjugate vaccine licensure. *J Infect Dis* 2015;211:1887-1894.
47. MacNeil JR, Bennett N, Farley MM, et al. Epidemiology of infant meningococcal disease in the United States, 2006-2012. *Pediatrics* 2015;135:e305-e311.
48. Weinstein L. Bacterial meningitis. Specific etiologic diagnosis on the basis of distinctive epidemiologic, pathogenetic, and clinical features. *Med Clin North Am* 1985;69:219-229.
49. Zalmanovici Trestioreanu A, Fraser A, Gafter-Gvili A, et al. Antibiotics for preventing meningococcal infections. *Cochrane Database Syst Rev* 2013;10:CD004785.
50. MacNeil JR, Cohn AC, Farley M, et al. Current epidemiology and trends in invasive Haemophilus influenzae disease—United States, 1989-2008. *Clin Infect Dis* 2011;53:1230-1236.
51. Tang LM, Chen ST, Wu YR. Haemophilus influenzae meningitis in adults. *Diagn Microbiol Infect Dis* 1998;32:27-32.
52. Thaver D, Zaidi AK. Burden of neonatal infections in developing countries: a review of evidence from community-based studies. *Pediatr Infect Dis J* 2009;28:S3-S9.
53. Weston EJ, Pondo T, Lewis MM, et al. The burden of invasive early-onset neonatal sepsis in the United States, 2005-2008. *Pediatr Infect Dis J* 2011;30:937-941.
54. Libster R, Edwards KM, Levent F, et al. Long-term outcomes of group B streptococcal meningitis. *Pediatrics* 2012;130:e8-e15.
55. Verani JR, McGee L, Schrag SJ. Prevention of perinatal group B streptococcal disease—revised guidelines from CDC, 2010. *MMWR Recomm Rep* 2010;59:1-36.
56. Brouwer MC, van de Beek D, Heckenberg SG, et al. Community-acquired Listeria monocytogenes meningitis in adults. *Clin Infect Dis* 2006;43:1233-1238.

57. Pomar V, Benito N, Lopez-Contreras J, et al. Spontaneous gram-negative bacillary meningitis in adult patients: characteristics and outcome. *BMC Infect Dis* 2013;13:451.
58. Zaidi AK, Thaver D, Ali SA, Khan TA. Pathogens associated with sepsis in newborns and young infants in developing countries. *Pediatr Infect Dis J* 2009;28:S10-S18.
59. McCracken GH, Jr, Mize SG, Threlkeld N. Intraventricular gentamicin therapy in gram-negative bacillary meningitis of infancy. Report of the Second Neonatal Meningitis Cooperative Study Group. *Lancet* 1980;1:787-791.
60. Kim BN, Peleg AY, Lodise TP, et al. Management of meningitis due to antibiotic-resistant Acinetobacter species. *Lancet Infect Dis* 2009;9:245-255.
61. Gunderson BW, Ibrahim KH, Hovde LB, et al. Synergistic activity of colistin and ceftazidime against multiantibiotic-resistant Pseudomonas aeruginosa in an in vitro pharmacodynamic model. *Antimicrob Agents Chemother* 2003;47:905-909.
62. Hendricks KA, Wright ME, Shadomy SV, et al. Centers for Disease Control and Prevention expert panel meetings on prevention and treatment of anthrax in adults. *Emerg Infect Dis* 2014;20.
63. Girgis NI, Farid Z, Mikhail IA, et al. Dexamethasone treatment for bacterial meningitis in children and adults. *Pediatr Infect Dis J* 1989;8:848-851.
64. Lebel MH, Freij BJ, Syrogiannopoulos GA, et al. Dexamethasone therapy for bacterial meningitis. Results of two double-blind, placebo-controlled trials. *N Engl J Med* 1988;319:964-971.
65. Schaad UB, Lips U, Gnehm HE, et al. Dexamethasone therapy for bacterial meningitis in children. Swiss Meningitis Study Group. *Lancet* 1993;342:457-461.
66. Peltola H, Leib SL. Performance of adjunctive therapy in bacterial meningitis depends on circumstances. *Pediatr Infect Dis J* 2013;32:1381-1382.
67. Bookstaver PB, Miller Quidley A. CNS infections in immunocompetent hosts. In: Murphy JE, Lee MW, eds. *Pharmacotherapy Self-Assessment Program, 2015 Book 1. Infectious Diseases.* Lenexa, KS: American College of Clinical Pharmacy; 2015:217-233.
68. van de Beek D, de Gans J, McIntyre P, Prasad K. Steroids in adults with acute bacterial meningitis: a systematic review. *Lancet Infect Dis* 2004;4:139-143.
69. Brouwer MC, McIntyre P, Prasad K, van de Beek D. Corticosteroids for acute bacterial meningitis. *Cochrane Database Syst Rev* 2013;6:CD004405.
70. van de Beek D, Farrar JJ, de Gans J, et al. Adjunctive dexamethasone in bacterial meningitis: a meta-analysis of individual patient data. *Lancet Neurol* 2010;9:254-263.
71. Kennedy WA, Hoyt MJ, McCracken GH, Jr. The role of corticosteroid therapy in children with pneumococcal meningitis. *Am J Dis Child* 1991;145:1374-1378.
72. McIntyre PB, Berkey CS, King SM, et al. Dexamethasone as adjunctive therapy in bacterial meningitis. A meta-analysis of randomized clinical trials since 1988. *JAMA* 1997;278:925-931.
73. Peltola H, Roine I, Fernandez J, et al. Adjuvant glycerol and/or dexamethasone to improve the outcomes of childhood bacterial meningitis: a prospective, randomized, double-blind, placebo-controlled trial. *Clin Infect Dis* 2007;45:1277-1286.
74. American Academy of Pediatrics. Pneumococcal infections. In: Kimberlin DW, Brady MT, Jackson MA, Long SS, eds. *Red Book®: 2015 REPORT OF THE COMMITTEE ON INFECTIOUS DISEASES.* American Academy of Pediatrics; Elk Grove Village, IL; 2015:626-638.
75. Paris MM, Hickey SM, Uscher MI, et al. Effect of dexamethasone on therapy of experimental penicillin- and cephalosporin-resistant pneumococcal meningitis. *Antimicrob Agents Chemother* 1994;38:1320-1324.
76. Gaillard JL, Abadie V, Cheron G, et al. Concentrations of ceftriaxone in cerebrospinal fluid of children with meningitis receiving dexamethasone therapy. *Antimicrob Agents Chemother* 1994;38:1209-1210.
77. Klugman KP, Friedland IR, Bradley JS. Bactericidal activity against cephalosporin-resistant Streptococcus pneumoniae in cerebrospinal fluid of children with acute bacterial meningitis. *Antimicrob Agents Chemother* 1995;39:1988-1992.
78. Ricard JD, Wolff M, Lacherade JC, et al. Levels of vancomycin in cerebrospinal fluid of adult patients receiving adjunctive corticosteroids to treat pneumococcal meningitis: a prospective multicenter observational study. *Clin Infect Dis* 2007;44:250-255.
79. Carpenter J, Stapleton S, Holliman R. Retrospective analysis of 49 cases of brain abscess and review of the literature. *Eur J Clin Microbiol Infect Dis* 2007;26:1-11.
80. Honda H, Warren DK. Central nervous system infections: meningitis and brain abscess. *Infect Dis Clin North Am* 2009;23:609-623.
81. Brouwer MC, Tunkel AR, McKhann GM, 2nd, van de Beek D. Brain abscess. *N Engl J Med* 2014;371:447-456.
82. Brouwer MC, Coutinho JM, van de Beek D. Clinical characteristics and outcome of brain abscess: systematic review and meta-analysis. *Neurology* 2014;82:806-813.
83. Sloan DJ, Parris V. Cryptococcal meningitis: epidemiology and therapeutic options. *Clin Epidemiol* 2014;6:169-182.
84. Park BJ, Wannemuehler KA, Marston BJ, et al. Estimation of the current global burden of cryptococcal meningitis among persons living with HIV/AIDS. *AIDS* 2009;23:525-530.
85. Bicanic T, Meintjes G, Wood R, et al. Fungal burden, early fungicidal activity, and outcome in cryptococcal meningitis in antiretroviral-naive or antiretroviral-experienced patients treated with amphotericin B or fluconazole. *Clin Infect Dis* 2007;45:76-80.
86. Nguyen MH, Husain S, Clancy CJ, et al. Outcomes of central nervous system cryptococcosis vary with host immune function: results from a multi-center, prospective study. *J Infect* 2010;61:419-426.
87. Vidal JE, Gerhardt J, Peixoto de Miranda EJ, et al. Role of quantitative CSF microscopy to predict culture status and outcome in HIV-associated cryptococcal meningitis in a Brazilian cohort. *Diagn Microbiol Infect Dis* 2012;73:68-73.
88. Perfect JR, Dismukes WE, Dromer F, et al. Clinical practice guidelines for the management of cryptococcal disease: 2010 update by the infectious diseases society of america. *Clin Infect Dis* 2010;50:291-322.
89. Day JN, Chau TT, Wolbers M, et al. Combination antifungal therapy for cryptococcal meningitis. *N Engl J Med* 2013;368:1291-1302.
90. Brouwer AE, Rajanuwong A, Chierakul W, et al. Combination antifungal therapies for HIV-associated cryptococcal meningitis: a randomised trial. *Lancet* 2004;363:1764-1767.
91. Loyse A, Wilson D, Meintjes G, et al. Comparison of the early fungicidal activity of high-dose fluconazole, voriconazole, and flucytosine as second-line drugs given in combination with amphotericin B for the treatment of HIV-associated cryptococcal meningitis. *Clin Infect Dis* 2012;54:121-128.
92. Pappas PG, Chetchotisakd P, Larsen RA, et al. A phase II randomized trial of amphotericin B alone or combined with fluconazole in the treatment of HIV-associated cryptococcal meningitis. *Clin Infect Dis* 2009;48:1775-1783.
93. Milefchik E, Leal MA, Haubrich R, et al. Fluconazole alone or combined with flucytosine for the treatment of AIDS-associated cryptococcal meningitis. *Med Mycol* 2008;46:393-395.
94. Pfaller MA, Diekema DJ, Gibbs DL, et al. Results from the ARTEMIS DISK Global Antifungal Surveillance Study, 1997 to 2007: 10.5-year analysis of susceptibilities of noncandidal yeast species to fluconazole and voriconazole determined by CLSI standardized disk diffusion testing. *J Clin Microbiol* 2009;47:117-123.
95. Flores VG, Tovar RM, Zaldivar PG, Martinez EA. Meningitis due to cryptococcus neoformans: treatment with posaconazole. *Curr HIV Res* 2012;10(7):620-623.
96. Powderly WG. Therapy for cryptococcal meningitis in patients with AIDS. *Clin Infect Dis* 1992;14(suppl 1):S54-S59.
97. Saag MS, Cloud GA, Graybill JR, et al. A comparison of itraconazole versus fluconazole as maintenance therapy for AIDS-associated cryptococcal meningitis. National Institute of Allergy and Infectious Diseases Mycoses Study Group. *Clin Infect Dis* 1999;28:291-296.
98. Bloch KC, Glaser CA. Encephalitis surveillance through the Emerging Infections Program, 1997-2010. *Emerg Infect Dis* 2015;21:1562-1567.
99. Vora NM, Holman RC, Mehal JM, et al. Burden of encephalitis-associated hospitalizations in the United States, 1998-2010. *Neurology* 2014;82:443-451.
100. Granerod J, Ambrose HE, Davies NW, et al. Causes of encephalitis and differences in their clinical presentations in England: a multicentre, population-based prospective study. *Lancet Infect Dis* 2010;10:835-844.
101. Whitley R. Neonatal herpes simplex virus infection. *Curr Opin Infect Dis* 2004;17:243-246.
102. Piret J, Boivin G. Resistance of herpes simplex viruses to nucleoside analogues: mechanisms, prevalence, and management. *Antimicrob Agents Chemother* 2011;55:459-472.
103. Gnann JW Jr, Skoldenberg B, Hart J, et al. Herpes simplex encephalitis: lack of clinical benefit of long-term valacyclovir therapy. *Clin Infect Dis* 2015;61:683-691.
104. ArboNET, Arboviral Diseases Branch, US Centers for Disease Control and Prevention (CDC). West Nile Virus Statistics, Surveillance, and Control. February 12, 2015. Available at: http://www.cdc.gov/westnile/resourcepages/survresources.html. (Accessed September 2015)

105. Murray KO, Walker C, Gould E. The virology, epidemiology, and clinical impact of West Nile virus: a decade of advancements in research since its introduction into the Western Hemisphere. *Epidemiol Infect* 2011;139:807-817.
106. Patel H, Sander B, Nelder MP. Long-term sequelae of West Nile virus-related illness: a systematic review. *Lancet Infect Dis* 2015;15:951-959.
107. CDC. Reported Tuberculosis in the United States, 2013. Atlanta, GA: U.S. Department of Health and Human Services, CDC, October 2014. Available at: http://www.cdc.gov/tb/statistics/reports/2013/pdf/report2013.pdf. (Accessed September 2015)
108. American Thoracic Society; CDC; Infectious Diseases Society of America. Treatment of tuberculosis. *MMWR Recomm Rep* 2003;52:1-77.
109. Workowski KA, Bolan GA. Sexually transmitted diseases treatment guidelines, 2015. *MMWR Recomm Rep* 2015;64:1-137.
110. Mitsonis CH, Kararizou E, Dimopoulos N, et al. Incidence and clinical presentation of neurosyphilis: a retrospective study of 81 cases. *Int J Neurosci* 2008;118:1251-1257.
111. Global Health—Division of Parasitic Diseases and Malaria. Centers for Disease Control and Prevention. Parasites—Toxoplasmosis (Toxoplasma infection). Atlanta, GA: U.S. Department of Health and Human Services. Available at: http://www.cdc.gov/parasites/toxoplasmosis/epi.html. (Accessed August 2015)
112. Panel on Opportunistic Infections in HIV-Exposed and HIV-Infected Children. Guidelines for the Prevention and Treatment of Opportunistic Infections in HIV-Exposed and HIV-Infected Children. Department of Health and Human Services. Available at: http://aidsinfo.nih.gov/contentfiles/lvguidelines/oi_guidelines_pediatrics.pdf. (Accessed August 2015)
113. Panel on Opportunistic Infections in HIV-Infected Adults and Adolescents. Guidelines for the prevention and treatment of opportunistic infections in HIV-infected adults and adolescents: recommendations from the Centers for Disease Control and Prevention, the National Institutes of Health, and the HIV Medicine Association of the Infectious Diseases Society of America. Available at: http://aidsinfo.nih.gov/contentfiles/lvguidelines/adult_oi.pdf. (Accessed August 2015)
114. Wormser GP, Dattwyler RJ, Shapiro ED, et al. The clinical assessment, treatment, and prevention of lyme disease, human granulocytic anaplasmosis, and babesiosis: clinical practice guidelines by the Infectious Diseases Society of America. *Clin Infect Dis* 2006;43:1089-1134.
115. Mygland A, Ljostad U, Fingerle V, et al. EFNS guidelines on the diagnosis and management of European Lyme neuroborreliosis. *Eur J Neurol* 2010;17:8-16, e1-4.

Lower Respiratory Tract Infections

107

Martha G. Blackford, Mark L. Glover, and Michael D. Reed

KEY CONCEPTS

1. Respiratory infections remain a major cause of morbidity from acute illness in the United States and likely represent the most common reasons why patients seek medical attention.
2. The majority of pulmonary infections follow colonization of the upper respiratory tract with potential pathogens, whereas microbes less commonly gain access to the lungs via the blood from an extrapulmonary source or by inhalation of infected aerosol particles. The competency of a patient's immune status is an important factor influencing the susceptibility to infection, etiologic cause, and disease severity.
3. An appropriate treatment regimen for the patient with uncomplicated lower respiratory tract infection can be established by evaluating the patient history, physical examination, chest radiograph, and properly collected sputum for culture interpreted in light of current knowledge of the most common lung pathogens and their antibiotic susceptibility patterns within the community.
4. Acute bronchitis is caused most commonly by respiratory viruses and almost always is self-limiting. Therapy targets associated symptoms, such as lethargy, malaise, or fever and may include fluids for rehydration. Routine use of antibiotics should be avoided and medication to suppress cough is rarely indicated.
5. Chronic bronchitis is caused by several interacting factors, including inhalation of noxious agents (most prominent are cigarette smoke and exposure to occupational dusts, fumes, and environmental pollution) and host factors including genetic factors and bacterial (and possibly viral) infections. The hallmark of this disease is a chronic cough, accompanied by excessive production, and expectoration of sputum with a persistent presence of microorganisms in the patient's sputum.
6. Treatment of acute exacerbations of chronic bronchitis includes attempts to mobilize and enhance sputum expectoration (chest physiotherapy, humidification of inspired air), oxygen if needed, aerosolized bronchodilators in select patients with demonstrated benefit, and possibly antibiotics.
7. Respiratory syncytial virus is the most common cause of acute bronchiolitis, an infection that mostly affects infants during their first year of life. In the well infant, bronchiolitis usually is a self-limiting viral illness.
8. The most prominent pathogen causing community-acquired pneumonia in otherwise healthy adults is *Streptococcus pneumoniae*, whereas the most common pathogens causing hospital-acquired are *Staphylococcus aureus* and gram-negative aerobic bacilli. Anaerobic bacteria are the most common etiologic agents in pneumonia that follow aspiration of gastric or oropharyngeal contents.
9. Treatment of community-acquired pneumonia may consist of humidified oxygen for hypoxemia, bronchodilators when bronchospasm is present, rehydration fluids, and chest physiotherapy for marked accumulation of retained respiratory secretions. Antibiotic regimens should be selected based on presumed causative pathogens and pulmonary distribution characteristics and should be adjusted to provide optimal, targeted therapy against pathogens identified by culture (sputum or blood).
10. Treatment of hospital-acquired pneumonia requires aggressive therapy with careful consideration of the dominance and susceptibility patterns of the pathogens present within the institution.

(1) Respiratory tract infections remain a major cause of morbidity from acute illness in the United States and most likely represent the single most common reason patients seek medical attention. This chapter focuses on bacterial and viral infections involving the lower respiratory tract, which includes the tracheobronchial tree and lung parenchyma.

(2) The respiratory tract has an elaborate system of host defenses, including humoral immunity, cellular immunity, and anatomic mechanisms.[1] When functioning properly, respiratory tract host defenses are markedly effective in protecting against pathogen invasion and removing potentially infectious agents from the lungs. For the most part, infections in the lower respiratory tract occur only when these defense mechanisms are impaired, as in cases of dysgammaglobulinemia or compromised ciliary function, such as that caused by the chronic inflammation accompanying cigarette smoking. In addition, local defenses may be overwhelmed when a particularly virulent microorganism or excessive inoculum invades lung parenchyma. The majority of pulmonary infections follow colonization of the upper respiratory tract with potential pathogens, which, after achieving sufficiently high concentrations, gain access to the lung via aspiration of oropharyngeal secretions. Less commonly, microbes enter the lung via the blood from an extrapulmonary source or by inhalation of infected aerosolized particles. The specific type of pulmonary infection caused by an invading microorganism is determined by a variety of host factors, including age, anatomic features of the airway, and specific characteristics of the infecting agent.

The most common infections involving the lower respiratory tract are bronchitis, bronchiolitis, and pneumonia. Bronchitis and bronchiolitis are inflammatory conditions of the large and small airways, respectively, of the tracheobronchial tree. The inflammatory process does not extend to the alveoli. Bronchitis frequently is classified as acute or chronic; acute bronchitis occurs in individuals of all ages, whereas chronic bronchitis primarily affects adults. Bronchiolitis is a disease of infancy.

Lower respiratory tract infections in children and adults most commonly result from either viral or bacterial invasion of lung parenchyma. The diagnosis of viral infections rests primarily on the recognition of a characteristic constellation of clinical signs and symptoms. Because treatment is largely supportive, only occasionally does the diagnosis require laboratory confirmation; this is achieved through serologic tests or identification of the organism by culture or antigen detection in respiratory secretions.[2] Laboratory techniques using polymerase chain reaction (PCR), microarrays, and multiplex ligation-dependent probe amplification, to name a few, have emerged as a means to identify specific pathogens rapidly and accurately.[3]

In contrast, because bacterial pneumonia usually necessitates expedient, effective, and specific antibiotic therapy, its management depends, in large part, on an understanding of the risk factors for acquiring pneumonia, predominant pathogens within the community, and, if necessary, isolation of the etiologic agent by culture from lung tissue or secretions.[4-6] The pharynx is colonized with many organisms that can cause pneumonia; therefore, culture of expectorated sputum can be misleading unless the specimen is examined to ensure that it has originated from the lower respiratory tract. The Gram stain provides the easiest method for distinguishing lower from upper respiratory tract secretions; moreover, through determination of the shape and color of the bacteria, the Gram stain frequently narrows the microbiologic differential diagnosis sufficiently to allow accurate initial therapy. Scanned under low-power microscopy, Gram-stained expectorated upper respiratory tract secretions contain many irregularly shaped epithelial cells with little evidence of inflammation and may not reflect the pathogen. In contrast, a lower-tract specimen from a patient with bacterial pneumonia usually contains multiple neutrophils per high-powered field and a single or predominant bacterial species. More aggressive procedures can be performed in an attempt to more accurately identify responsible pathogens including respiratory secretion samples obtained via bronchoscopy or bronchoalveolar lavage (BAL). Culture of specimens confirmed to originate from the lower tract by Gram stain or collection via BAL provides valuable diagnostic information for the majority of patients with bacterial pneumonia. In addition, pneumonia promotes the release of inflammatory mediators and acute-phase proteins, such as C-reactive protein, which is significantly elevated in serum in the presence of respiratory tract infections.[7] Unfortunately with the exception of pathogen identification by culture, elevations in C-reactive protein, changes in sputum color or peripheral white blood count, etc., are not specific for determining viral, bacterial, or fungal etiology. Newer genomic testing may add tremendously in determining the identity of responsible pathogen(s) and then selection of optimal antimicrobial therapy.

3 An appropriate treatment regimen for the patient with an uncomplicated lower respiratory tract infection usually can be established by history, physical examination, chest radiograph, and properly collected sputum cultures interpreted in light of the most common lung pathogens and their antibiotic susceptibility patterns within the community.[2,5] More sophisticated or invasive diagnostic methods (eg, computed tomography, bronchoscopy, and lung biopsy)[2] are reserved for severely ill patients who are unable to expectorate sputum or who are not responding to empirical therapy or for pulmonary infections occurring in immunocompromised patients.

BRONCHITIS

Acute Bronchitis

Epidemiology and Etiology

Acute bronchitis occurs year round, but more commonly during the winter months. Acute bronchitis is responsible for at least 10 million office and urgent care visits annually, underscoring its major financial impact on the healthcare system. Acute bronchitis is characterized by inflammation of the epithelium of the large airways resulting from infection or exposure to irritating environmental triggers (eg, air pollution and cigarette smoke). Acute (viral) infection and or smoking are the most common precipitants of attacks, which usually manifest initially as a persistent cough.

4 Respiratory viruses are the predominant infectious agents associated with acute bronchitis, accounting for 85% to 95% of occurrences. The most common infecting agents include influenza A and B, respiratory syncytial virus (RSV), and parainfluenza virus, whereas the common cold viruses (rhinovirus and coronavirus) and adenovirus are encountered less frequently. Although far less common, bacterial pathogens are involved in a minority of cases and involve pathogens often associated with community-acquired pneumonia (CAP), including *Mycoplasma pneumoniae, Streptococcus pneumonia, Haemophilus influenzae, Moraxella catarrhalis*, and less commonly *Chlamydophila pneumoniae* and *Bordetella pertussis*, the agent responsible for whooping cough. Although a primary bacterial etiology for acute bronchitis appears rare, secondary bacterial infection may be involved, particularly in patients with underlying disease(s).[8]

Pathogenesis

4 Since acute bronchitis is primarily a self-limiting illness and rarely a cause of death, few data describing the pathology are available. In general, infection of the trachea and bronchi yields inflammation-induced hyperemic and edematous mucous membranes with an increase in bronchial secretions. Destruction of respiratory epithelium can range from mild to extensive and may affect bronchial mucociliary function. In addition, the increase in desquamated epithelial cells and bronchial secretions, which can become thick and tenacious, further impairs mucociliary activity. The probability of permanent damage to the airways as a result of acute bronchitis remains unclear but appears unlikely. However, epidemiologic evaluations support the belief that recurrent acute respiratory infections may be associated with increased airway hyperreactivity and possibly the pathogenesis of asthma, chronic obstructive pulmonary disease (COPD), or possibly the asthma-COPD overlap syndrome.[9,10]

Clinical Presentation

Acute bronchitis usually begins as an upper respiratory infection with nonspecific complaints.[8,11] Cough is the hallmark of acute bronchitis and occurs early. The onset of cough may be insidious or abrupt, and the symptoms persist despite resolution of nasal or nasopharyngeal complaints; cough may persist for up to 3 or more weeks. Frequently, the cough initially is nonproductive, but then progresses, yielding mucopurulent sputum. In older children and adults, the sputum is raised and expectorated; in the young child, sputum often is swallowed and can result in gagging and vomiting. Substantial discomfort may result from the coughing. Dyspnea, cyanosis, or signs of airway obstruction are observed rarely unless the patient has underlying pulmonary disease, such as emphysema or COPD. Fever, when present, rarely exceeds 39°C (102.2°F) and appears most commonly with adenovirus, influenza virus, and *M. pneumoniae* infections. The diagnosis typically is made on the basis of a characteristic history and physical examination, and should be differentiated from asthma or bronchiolitis as these latter diseases are usually associated with wheezing, shortness of breath, and hypoxemia. Bacterial cultures of expectorated sputum are of limited use because of the inability to avoid normal nasopharyngeal flora by the sampling technique. Similarly, viral cultures are unnecessary. In the absence of important risk factors, including COPD, congestive heart failure, or immune compromise, throat/sputum cultures have no role in the routine care of patients with acute bronchitis. As newer antigen-based PCR and genetic diagnostic tests for identifying specific pathogens become more routinely available,[12] specific etiologic causes of acute bronchitis will be identified. However, for the vast majority of affected patients, an etiologic diagnosis is unnecessary and will not change the prescribing of routine supportive care for the management of these patients.

TREATMENT

Desired Outcome

In the absence of a complicating bacterial superinfection, acute bronchitis almost always is self-limiting. The goals of therapy are to provide comfort to the patient and, in the unusually severe case, to treat associated dehydration and respiratory compromise.[8]

General Approach to Treatment

4 Treatment of acute bronchitis is symptomatic and supportive in nature. Reassurance and antipyretics frequently are all that are needed. Bedrest for comfort may be instituted as desired. Patients should be encouraged to drink fluids to prevent dehydration and possibly to decrease the viscosity of respiratory secretions. Mist therapy (use of a vaporizer) may promote the thinning and loosening of respiratory secretions.

Pharmacologic Therapy

Mild analgesic–antipyretic therapy often is helpful in relieving the associated lethargy, malaise, and fever. Aspirin or acetaminophen (650 mg/dose in adults [maximum less than 4 g/day] or 10-15 mg/kg/dose in children [maximum 60 mg/kg/day]) administered every 4 to 6 hours or ibuprofen (200-800 mg/dose in adults [maximum 3.2 g/day] or 10 mg/kg/dose in children [maximum 40 mg/kg/day]) should be administered every 6 to 8 hours. Aspirin should be avoided in children less than 19 years of age with a fever-causing illness and acetaminophen or ibuprofen used as the preferred agents because of a possible, but unclear and unproven, association between aspirin use and the possible development of Reye's syndrome.[13]

Use of ibuprofen as an antipyretic has increased. The drug's antipyretic efficacy appears identical to that of aspirin or acetaminophen, although its duration of antipyretic effect may be slightly longer (eg, 3-4 hours for aspirin and acetaminophen vs more than 5-6 hours for ibuprofen). A possible association with acetaminophen use during pregnancy or childhood and the subsequent development of asthma has raised some question as to the viability of routine acetaminophen use during childhood.[14] For these reasons, ibuprofen has become a preferred analgesic and antipyretic by many pediatric practitioners. However, caution should be exercised with the use of ibuprofen in patients younger than 6 months, elderly patients, and individuals with poor renal function. Aspirin, ibuprofen, and other nonsteroidal anti-inflammatory drugs inhibit prostaglandin synthesis and may adversely influence renal function in these predisposed patient populations.

Patients may present with mild-to-moderate wheezing. In otherwise healthy patients, no meaningful benefits have been described with the routine use of oral or aerosolized β_2-receptor agonists[15] and/or oral or aerosolized corticosteroids. Corticosteroids should be avoided in patients with acute bronchitis. A Cochrane review concluded (based on benefit vs potential for adverse effects) there is no evidence to support the use of β_2-receptor agonists in either pediatric or adult patients with acute bronchitis; however, in adults with airflow obstruction, there was a trend toward improvement.[15] Some clinicians, despite no data, may initiate a brief trial (eg, ~5-7 days) of β_2-receptor agonists and even oral or inhaled corticosteroid for patients with a persistent (>14-20 days), troublesome cough. This is rarely if ever necessary in patients with uncomplicated acute bronchitis and should be avoided. Cough may persist for 3+ weeks and airway hyperresponsiveness for 5-6 weeks in as many as 50% of affected patients. In contrast, COPD patients experiencing an acute exacerbation can (will) benefit from a short course of corticosteroid. Studies do not support the use of mucolytic agents in patients with acute bronchitis.

Patients suffering from acute bronchitis frequently medicate themselves with nonprescription cough and cold remedies containing various combinations of antihistamines, sympathomimetics, and antitussives despite the lack of definitive evidence supporting their effectiveness. The tendency of these agents to dehydrate bronchial secretions could aggravate and prolong the recovery process. Although not recommended for routine use, persistent, mild cough, which may be bothersome, can be treated with dextromethorphan; more severe coughs may require intermittent codeine or other similar agents.[16] In severe cases, the cough may be persistent enough to disrupt sleep, and use of a mild sedative-hypnotic, concomitantly with a cough suppressant (eg, codeine), may be desirable. However, antitussives should be used cautiously when the cough is productive. The primary or supplemental use of expectorants is questionable because their clinical effectiveness has not been well established.

Routine use of antibiotics for treatment of acute bronchitis should be strongly discouraged due to limited benefit.[8,17] In previously healthy patients who exhibit persistent fever or respiratory symptoms for more than 5 to 7 days or for predisposed patients (eg, elderly/frail, COPD, and immune compromised), the possibility of a concurrent bacterial infection should be suspected. When possible, antibiotic therapy should be directed toward anticipated respiratory pathogen(s) (eg, *S. pneumoniae* and *H. influenza*). *M. pneumoniae*, if suspected by history or if confirmed by culture serology or PCR, can be treated with azithromycin. Alternatively and empirically, a fluoroquinolone antibiotic with activity against these suspected pathogens (eg, levofloxacin) can be used, but due to the increasing rate of pathogen resistance to current antimicrobial drugs, the use of antibiotics in patients with acute bronchitis should be reserved for only those patients not responding adequately to supportive care and deemed at risk of associated complications. During known epidemics involving the influenza A virus, amantadine or rimantadine may have been effective in minimizing associated symptoms if administered early in the course of the disease, though treatment with these drugs, the adamantanes, is no longer recommended by the Centers for Disease Control and Prevention due to increasing influenza resistance and associated adverse effects.[18] The neuraminidase inhibitors (eg, zanamivir and oseltamivir) are active against both influenza A and B viral infections and may reduce the severity and duration of the influenza episode if administered promptly during the onset of the viral infection and are the preferred treatment (see Chapter 109).[19] Unfortunately, the incidence of influenza virus resistance to available antiviral drugs is increasing,[20] necessitating reconsideration of how we administer antiviral drugs for prophylaxis and treatment. The concept of antiviral drug combinations has emerged as a successful approach to effectively treat systemic viral infections.[21]

Chronic Bronchitis

Epidemiology and Etiology

Chronic bronchitis, most often a component of COPD, is a clinical diagnosis for a nonspecific, heterogenic disease that primarily affects adults. An in-depth presentation of the spectrum and management of COPD is given in Chapter 27; this section will focus solely on chronic bronchitis. In developed countries, the prevalence of chronic bronchitis is slightly higher in men than in women and possibly more common in Whites. Depending on the definition used for chronic bronchitis, it is estimated that 3.4% to 22% of adults have chronic bronchitis and that 14% to 74% of COPD patients suffer from chronic bronchitis.[22]

5 Chronic bronchitis is defined clinically as the presence of a chronic cough productive of sputum lasting more than 3 consecutive months of the year for 2 consecutive years without an underlying etiology of bronchiectasis or tuberculosis. The disease is a result of several contributing factors; the most prominent include cigarette smoking, exposure to occupational dusts, fumes, and environmental pollution, and host factors (eg, genetic factors and bacterial [and possibly viral] infections). The contribution of each of these factors and of others (either alone or in combination) to chronic bronchitis is unknown.[23] Cigarette smoke is a well-known airway irritant and is a predominant factor in the etiology of chronic bronchitis. Although previously assumed the most common etiologic cause of chronic bronchitis, more strict prohibition of public smoking, and the resultant decrease in chronic tobacco smokers, particularly in developed countries, underscores the importance of other factors as causes of this chronic disease. Approximately 4% to 22% of patients with chronic bronchitis report never smoking.[22] Additional airway irritants including occupational dust, chemicals, or air pollution, either alone or more likely in combination, are also responsible for the pathogenesis of chronic bronchitis.[22,23] Furthermore, genome-wide association studies have begun to expand our understanding of the molecular pathways that may have clinical relevance in this very heterogeneous disease; see Chapter 27. Lastly, the influence of recurrent respiratory tract infections during childhood or young adult life on the later development of chronic bronchitis remains obscure, but recurrent respiratory infections may predispose individuals to the development of chronic bronchitis. Whether these recurrent respiratory tract infections are a result of unrecognized anatomic abnormalities of the airways or impaired pulmonary defense mechanisms is unclear.

Numerous consensus statements and published authoritative guidelines define chronic bronchitis and emphysema as the two main components of COPD/chronic obstructive lung disease.[24-26] The Global Initiative for Chronic Obstruction Lung Disease (GOLD) guidelines document does not distinguish these two diagnoses (eg, emphysema or chronic bronchitis) in the definition of COPD, but it does define COPD as a disease characterized by airflow obstruction that is not fully reversible and progressive. The GOLD guidelines (www.goldcopd.com) provide a COPD classification scoring system according to severity that can be helpful in staging patients for intensity of therapy, acute/chronic therapy, and prognosis. Unfortunately, differences in definitions between authoritative organizations may cause confusion in the assignment of patients in clinical trials and thus in assessment and application of study results to clinical care.

Pathogenesis

Chronic inhalation of an irritating noxious substance compromises the normal secretory and mucociliary function of bronchial mucosa.[27] Bronchial biopsy specimens in bronchitic patients underscore the importance of T-cell derived proinflammatory cytokines (eg, interleukins IL-4, 5, 13, and interferon gamma) in the pathogenesis and propagation of the observed inflammatory changes. In chronic bronchitis, the bronchial wall is thickened, and the number of mucus-secreting goblet cells on the surface epithelium of both larger and smaller bronchi is increased markedly. In contrast, goblet cells generally are absent from the smaller bronchi of normal individuals. In addition to the increased number of goblet cells, hypertrophy of the mucous glands and dilation of the mucous gland ducts are observed. As a result of these changes, chronic bronchitics have substantially more mucus in their peripheral airways, further impairing normal lung defenses. This increased quantity (overproduction and hypersecretion) of tenacious secretions within the bronchial tree frequently causes mucous plugging of the smaller airways. Accompanying these changes are squamous cell metaplasia of the surface epithelium, edema, and increased vascularity of the basement membrane of larger airways and variable chronic inflammatory cell infiltration. In addition, the amounts of several proteases derived from inflammatory cells are increased and due to COPD-induced defective antiproteases lead to continued destruction of connective tissue. Continued progression of this pathology can result in residual scarring of small bronchi and peribronchial fibrosis augmenting airway obstruction and weakening of bronchial walls.[22]

Clinical Presentation

5 The hallmark of chronic bronchitis is a cough that may range from a mild to a severe and incessant coughing productive of purulent sputum. Coughing may be precipitated by multiple stimuli, including simple, normal conversation. Expectoration of the largest quantity of sputum usually occurs on arising in the morning, although many patients expectorate sputum throughout the day. The expectorated sputum usually is tenacious and can vary in color from white to yellow-green. Patients with chronic bronchitis often expectorate as much as 100 mL/day more than normal. As a result, many patients complain of a frequent bad taste in their mouth and of halitosis. It is important to recognize that sputum color provides no prognostic indication of infection or cause of an infectious disease exacerbation, that is, viral versus bacterial cause. Although sputum color of more green and yellow can be a predictor of potentially pathogenic bacteria this is unreliable clinically.[28] The diagnosis of an acute exacerbation requires consideration of a number of different factors all occurring within a discrete timeframe, (eg, increased/worsening respiratory symptoms including dyspnea, sputum volume and/or clearance, cough, etc). The tracking of the number of acute exacerbations and their consequences (decline in forced expiratory volume in 1 second (FEV1), persistent/worsening of symptoms annually is extremely important for prognostication and defining ongoing treatment strategies. Each acute exacerbation of chronic bronchitis results in continual declines in lung function.

The diagnosis of chronic bronchitis is based primarily on clinical assessment and history. Any patient who reports coughing sputum on most days for at least 3 consecutive months each year for 2 consecutive years presumptively has chronic bronchitis.[22] The diagnosis of chronic bronchitis is made only when the possibilities of bronchiectasis, cardiac failure, cystic fibrosis, and lung carcinoma, amongst others, have been effectively excluded. In an attempt to be more specific in the diagnosis, some investigators have added the criteria of lost wages for 3 or more weeks. In addition, many clinicians attempt to subdivide their patients based on severity of disease to guide therapeutic interventions. Two primary classification proposals are most often used in an attempt to determine the severity of the underlying disease as well as the occurrence/impending occurrence of an acute exacerbation of chronic bronchitis; for disease severity and acute exacerbations the prognostic tools advocated by GOLD are very helpful including classification based on spirometry ("mild" postbronchodilator FEV1 greater than or equal to 80% predicted to "very severe" postbronchodilator FEV1 less than 30% predicted: see Chapter 27); the COPD assessment test (8-item measure of health status), the Clinical COPD Questionnaire (a measure of clinical control) and the Modified Medical Research Council Questionnaire to predict future mortality. The other simple classification system is that proposed by Anthonisen and colleagues in 1987[29] that is still used to categorize patients in many therapeutic clinical trials. The use of patient symptom diaries can also be

TABLE 107-1 Clinical Presentation of Chronic Bronchitis

Signs and symptoms
- Excessive sputum expectoration
- Cough
- Cyanosis (advanced disease)

Physical examination
- Chest auscultation usually reveals inspiratory and expiratory rales, rhonchi, and mild wheezing with an expiratory phase that is frequently prolonged
- Hyperresonance on percussion with obliteration of the area of cardiac dullness
- Normal vesicular breathing sounds are diminished
- Clubbing of digits (advanced disease)
- Obesity

Chest radiograph
- Increase in anteroposterior diameter of the thoracic cage (barrel chest)
- Depressed diaphragm with limited mobility

Laboratory tests
- Erythrocytosis (advanced disease), that is, increased hematocrit

Pulmonary function tests
- Decreased vital capacity
- Prolonged expiratory flow

helpful in compliant patients. The importance of accurate classification for grouping patients of similar disease involvement cannot be overemphasized with respect to assessing publications outlining treatment strategies for these patients. Although gross, these classifications attempt to capture specific phenotypes of chronic bronchitis patients. The typical clinical presentation of chronic bronchitis is listed in Table 107-1. Comparison of the trends in changes in a patient's physical activity, symptoms, and clinical/physical findings from the patient's "routine" is extremely helpful in determining the presence and severity of an acute exacerbation.

In more advanced stages of chronic bronchitis, physical findings associated with cor pulmonale, including cardiac enlargement, hepatomegaly, and edema of the lower extremities, are observed. In general, chronic bronchitics tend to maintain at least normal body weight and commonly are obese. Radiographic studies are of limited value in either the diagnosis or follow-up of a patient. The microscopic and laboratory assessments of sputum are used in the overall evaluation of patients with chronic bronchitis. Gram staining of the sputum often reveals a mixture of both gram-positive and gram-negative bacteria, reflecting normal oropharyngeal flora and chronic tracheal colonization (in order of frequency) by nontypable *H. influenzae*, *S. pneumoniae*, and *M. catarrhalis*. Table 107-2 lists the most common bacterial isolates identified from sputum culture for patients experiencing an acute exacerbation of chronic bronchitis. For patients with more severe airflow disease (eg, FEV_1 less than 40% predicted), enteric gram-negative bacilli, *Escherichia coli*, *Klebsiella* species, *Enterobacter* species, and *Pseudomonas aeruginosa* may be significant pathogens during acute exacerbations.

TABLE 107-2 Common Bacterial Pathogens Isolated from Sputum of Patients with Acute Exacerbation of Chronic Bronchitis

Pathogen	Percent of Cultures
H. influenzae[a,b]	45
M. catarrhalis[a]	30
S. pneumoniae[c]	20
E. coli, *Enterobacter* species, *Klebsiella* species, *P. aeruginosa*	5

[a]Often β-lactamase positive.
[b]Vast majority are nontypable strains.
[c]More than 25% of strains may have intermediate or high resistance to penicillin.

TREATMENT

Desired Outcome

The goals of therapy for chronic bronchitis are twofold: to reduce the severity of chronic symptoms and to ameliorate acute exacerbations and achieve prolonged exacerbation-free intervals.

General Approach to Treatment

The approach to treatment of chronic bronchitis is multifactorial.[22] First and foremost, attempts must be made to reduce the patient's exposure to known bronchial irritants (eg, smoking and workplace pollution). A complete occupational and environmental history for determination of exposure to noxious, irritating gases as well as preference toward cigarette smoking must be assessed. Often easier discussed than accomplished, honest, yet reasonable attempts should be made with the patient to reduce or eliminate the number of cigarettes smoked daily and to reduce exposure to secondhand smoke. An organized, coordinated, smoking cessation program, including counseling, possibly hypnotherapy, and the adjunctive use of nicotine substitutes (eg, nicotine gum or patch) or other pharmacotherapy (eg, bupropion and varenicline) may promote the reduction or complete withdrawal from cigarette smoking. Often just as difficult is modification of exposure to irritating substances within the home and workplace.

The importance of pulmonary rehabilitation has been realized in improving the quality of life for patients with chronic respiratory diseases.[30] Pulmonary rehabilitation is broadly defined as an interdisciplinary program individualized for patients with chronic respiratory impairment designed to optimize each patient's physical and social performance and autonomy. A personalized exercise training program including resistance and aerobic exercise are central to these programs. Pulmonary rehabilitation programs relieve dyspnea and fatigue, improve a patient's emotional function, and enhance their sense of control over their disease and life. These improvements are often moderately large and clinically relevant.[30] The challenge for the future is to determine what components of a comprehensive pulmonary rehabilitation program provide the greatest benefit.

6 Measures to provide chest physiotherapy (eg, pulmonary "toilet") can be instituted.[31] Clearly the cost-effectiveness of chest physiotherapy needs to be better described but their short-term effects have been demonstrated and may be of symptomatic value to many patients experiencing an acute exacerbation of the chronic bronchitis. During acute pulmonary exacerbations of the disease, the patient's ability to mobilize and expectorate sputum may be reduced dramatically. In these instances, attempts at postural drainage techniques, with instruction and or active participation from a respiratory therapist, may assist in promoting clearance of pulmonary secretions. In addition, humidification of inspired air may promote the hydration (liquefaction) of tenacious secretions, allowing for removal that is more productive. Use of aerosolized mucolytic aerosols, such as *N*-acetylcysteine (NAC) and DNAse, is of questionable therapeutic value, particularly considering their propensity to induce bronchospasm (NAC) and their excessive cost. NAC cleaves the disulfide bonds of mucous, decreasing its elastic property that is important for upward mobility and then expectoration. A Cochrane meta-analysis of aerosol mucolytic therapy in subjects with chronic bronchitis or COPD found that treatment with mucolytics was associated with a small reduction in acute exacerbations and did not cause any harm, improve quality of life, or slow the decline of lung function.[32] The clinical benefit may be greater for chronic bronchitics/COPD patients who have frequent or prolonged exacerbations and are unable to utilize inhaled corticosteroids or long-acting β_2-agonists.[32] Although limited data are available, chronic use of oral or aerosolized bronchodilators may be of benefit by increasing

mucociliary and cough clearance. For patients with moderate to severe COPD, combination therapy with a long-acting β_2-agonist and inhaled corticosteroid led to decreased exacerbations and rescue medication use, while it also improved quality of life, lung function, and symptom scores compared with long-acting β_2-agonist monotherapy.

Pharmacologic Therapy

Patients should be up to date with vaccinations, particularly pneumococcal and an annual influenza vaccine; however, the clinical utility of vaccination against haemophilus disease is questionable. For patients who consistently demonstrate clinical limitation in airflow, a therapeutic challenge of a short-acting β_2-agonist bronchodilator (eg, as albuterol aerosol) should be considered. Pulmonary function tests should be performed before and after β_2-agonist aerosol administration for more objective determination of a patient's propensity to benefit from supplemental aerosol therapy. Sufficient published experience supports the use of inhalation therapy with a β_2-agonist for patients with chronic bronchitis (COPD) to improve pulmonary function and exercise tolerance and to reduce the sense of breathlessness.[22] Regular use of a long-acting β-receptor agonist aerosol (eg, salmeterol and formoterol) in responsive patients are more effective and probably more convenient than short-acting β_2-receptor agonists.[33] The aerosol route for β_2-receptor agonist and/or corticosteroid administration is favored over systemic formulations for improved patient acceptance and compliance and to minimize the number and magnitude of associated adverse effects. Chronic inhalation of a long-acting β-receptor agonist (LABA) and a poorly absorbed corticosteroid combination (eg, salmeterol/fluticasone and formoterol/mometasone) has been associated with improved pulmonary function and quality of life.[34] However, chronic use of aerosolized corticosteroid is associated with increased side effects including hoarseness, sore throat, thrush, pneumonia, and osteoporosis. Nevertheless, caution should be exercised in withdrawing inhaled glucocorticoid administration in patients with severe COPD receiving triple inhalation therapy as it may lead to increased frequency of acute exacerbations and a greater decrease in lung function.

Published experience with inhaled anticholinergic drugs, including ipratropium and tiotropium, is increasing and defining an important role in the chronic management of patients with chronic bronchitis and COPD.[35] Numerous studies are now available demonstrating the clinical effectiveness of inhaled long-acting muscarinic antagonists (LAMAs) alone or more frequently when administered in combination with a LABA, in improving lung function and real benefits in symptom control and reductions in the number of acute exacerbations. Triple combination inhalation therapy (eg, LABA + LAMA + an inhaled corticosteroid) is being evaluated in patients with more severe COPD with promising findings.[36] The exact role of triple therapy remains to be defined. Although once prescribed extensively for patients with chronic bronchitis, chronic theophylline therapy is used with decreasing frequency in favor of aerosolized β_2-receptor agonists, LABA, LAMA, etc. Nevertheless, long-acting theophylline remains an effective "add on" therapy for many patients, particularly those with more severe chronic bronchitis/COPD due to the drugs beneficial effects of bronchodilation, improved ciliary function and increased beat frequency, possibly increased mucus hydration, and low cost.[22]

Phosphodiesterase 4 inhibitors (PDE-4), compared with the nonselective phosphodiesterase inhibitor theophylline, only affect phosphodiesterase in the airway smooth muscle, immune (eosinophils, monocytes, and neutrophils), and proinflammatory cells. Roflumilast is a highly specific (second generation) PDE-4 inhibitor which is most often reserved for use in patients with moderate to severe COPD. Considering that many of the published studies assessing the viability of second-generation PDE-4 inhibitors in patients with COPD involved patients with chronic cough and increased sputum production, it is inferred that these drugs would be of value in patients with chronic bronchitis as well. The GOLD guidelines suggest roflumilast reduces exacerbations in COPD patients with chronic bronchitics treated with oral glucocorticosteroids. A review of clinical trials and observational studies found that roflumilast only provides a net benefit to patients at high risk of severe exacerbations.[37] A lower 30-day readmission rate in patients hospitalized for COPD with roflumilast therapy was reported.[38] Others have found that PDE-4 inhibitors improved lung function over placebo and reduced the likelihood of exacerbations; they had little impact on a patient's symptoms or quality of life. Nevertheless, the major limitation to the use of PDE-4 inhibitors is their side effect profiles. Patients receiving roflumilast often experience nausea, vomiting, headache, decreased appetite, sleep disturbances, and an increased risk of psychiatric events.[39] The exact role of roflumilast in chronic lung disease is evolving but many guidelines suggest its greatest use is in the more severely affected patients.

Use of antimicrobials for treatment of chronic bronchitis has been controversial, but is becoming more accepted in specific circumstances. Numerous comparative evaluations, including placebo-controlled studies of antibiotic administration with acute and chronic treatment of chronic bronchitics, have suggested clinical benefit. The antibiotics selected most frequently possess variable in vitro activity against the common sputum isolates *H. influenzae*, *S. pneumoniae*, *M. catarrhalis*, and *M. pneumoniae*. Conflicting published results appear independent of the antibiotic used or the regimen compared. A wide disparity that existed in the published results from older studies, served as the basis for the enormous controversy that surrounded the use of antibiotics for the treatment of acute exacerbations of chronic bronchitis. Overall, good clinical results have been observed with the use of standard antibiotic regimens (eg, macrolides, azalides, oral cephalosporins, and the combination drug amoxicillin/clavulanate, trimethoprim/sulfamethoxazole, and tetracyclines) as well as with the use of fluoroquinolones.[40-45] The goal is to select the most effective antibiotic drug for the patient based on their history of previous exacerbations and response to drug therapy. The introduction of genome expression profiling of sputum and other biologic fluids can facilitate specific pathogen diagnosis and focused therapy.[46]

A useful paradigm for the assessment and treatment of acute exacerbations of chronic bronchitis and antibiotic decision making is shown in Fig. 107-1. Many clinicians use the so-called Anthonisen criteria to determine if antibiotic therapy is indicated.[29] With the Anthonisen criteria, if a patient exhibits two of the following three criteria during an acute exacerbation of chronic bronchitis (AECB), the patient will most likely benefit from antibiotic therapy and, thus, should receive a treatment course: (a) increase in shortness of breath; (b) increase in sputum volume; and (c) production of purulent sputum. There are greater healthcare costs for patients who are noncompliant with their antibiotic regimen for their AECB.

The increasing resistance of the common bacterial pathogens to first-line agents further complicates antibiotic selection. As many as 30% to 40% of *H. influenzae* isolates and 95% to 100% of *M. catarrhalis* isolates produce β-lactamases. Moreover, up to 40% of *S. pneumoniae* isolates demonstrate resistance to penicillin (minimum inhibitory concentration [MIC] = 0.1-2 mg/L), with approximately 20% of isolates being highly resistant (MIC greater than 2 mg/L). Concern regarding *S. pneumoniae* resistance is increasing, and resistance is now greater than or equal to 30% for macrolides. Despite these changes in bacterial susceptibility, the current recommendation is to initiate therapy with first-line antimicrobial agents in less severely affected patients (see Fig. 107-1). Trimethoprim/sulfamethoxazole has been extremely useful for patients with less-severe disease.[47] For patients with more moderate to severe disease, many clinicians will begin antibiotic therapy with the second-line

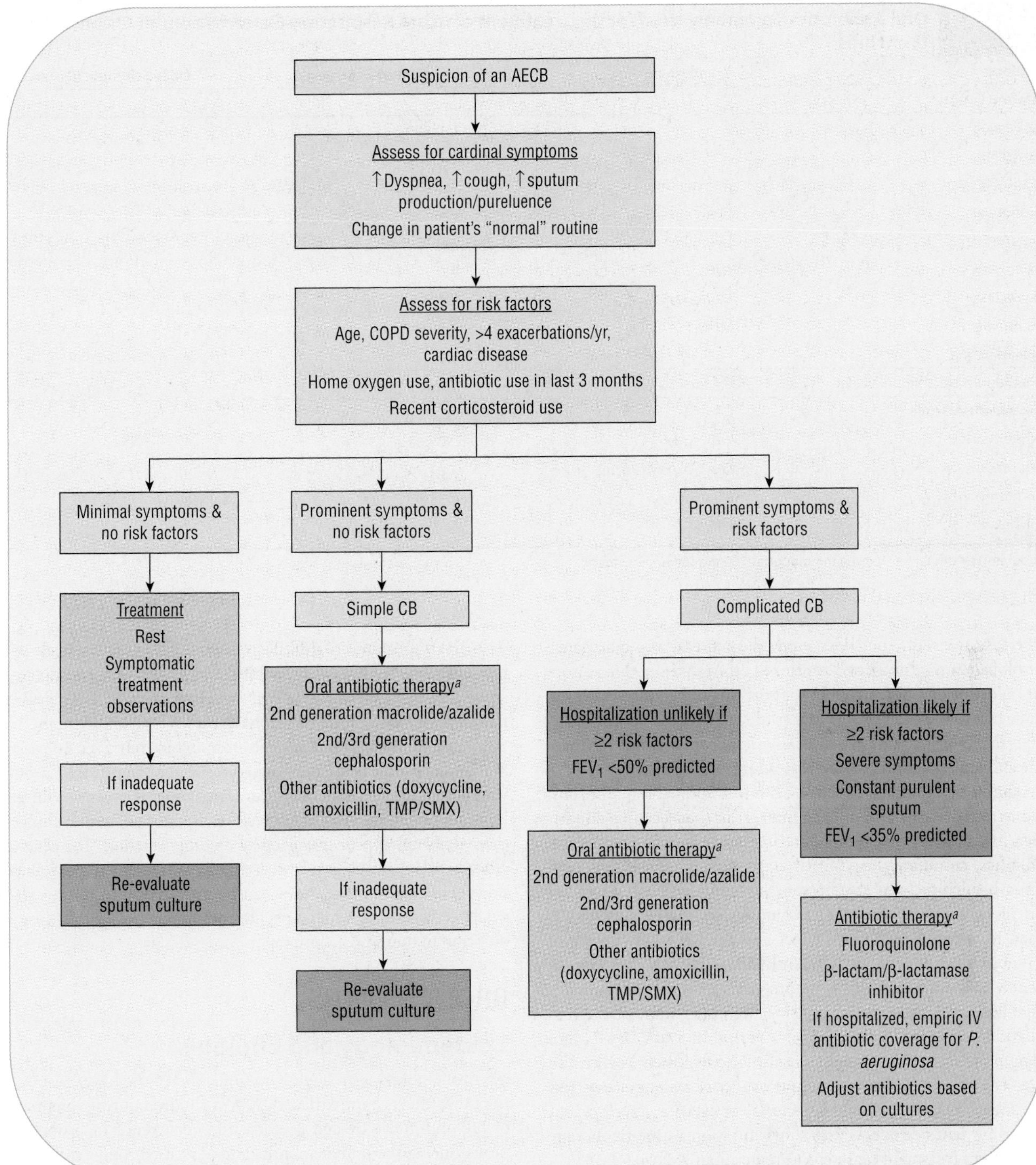

FIGURE 107-1 Clinical algorithm for the diagnosis and treatment of chronic bronchitic patients with an acute exacerbation incorporating the principles of the clinical classification system. (AECB, acute exacerbation of chronic bronchitis; COPD, chronic obstructive pulmonary disease; CB, chronic bronchitis; TMP/SMX, trimethoprim/sulfamethoxazole.) [a]See Table 107-3 for commonly used antibiotics and doses. *(Adapted from reference 110.)*

agents, amoxicillin/clavulanate, a macrolide (such as azithromycin or clarithromycin, although they are being used less frequently), and more frequently with a fluoroquinolone, such as levofloxacin and moxifloxacin (see Fig. 107-1).

Regardless of the antibiotic selected, predetermined outcome measures should be monitored closely for each patient to determine the success or failure of the therapeutic intervention. Oral antibiotics with broader antibacterial spectra (eg, amoxicillin/clavulanate and fluoroquinolones) that possess potent in vitro activity against sputum isolates are increasingly becoming first-line antibiotics as initial therapy for treatment of acute exacerbations of chronic bronchitis.

An important clinical outcome variable directing drug selection and criteria for beginning antibiotics in individual patients is the infection-free period when chronic bronchitics are off antibiotics. The length of the infection-free time period and the change in the number of physician office visits and hospital admissions with a particular antibiotic regimen are extremely important to identify, whenever possible, for each patient. The antibiotic regimen that results in the longest infection-free period defines the "regimen of choice" for specific patients for future acute exacerbations of their disease. Trials of long-term prophylactic antibiotic use may provide a slight benefit in decreasing exacerbation rates, but does not appear

TABLE 107-3 Oral Antibiotics Commonly Used for the Treatment of Acute Respiratory Exacerbations in Chronic Bronchitis

Antibiotic	Brand Name	Usual Adult Dose (mg)	Dose Schedule (Doses/Day)
Preferred Drugs			
Ampicillin	–	250-500	4-3
Amoxicillin	–	500-875	3-2
Amoxicillin/clavulanate	Augmentin®	500-875	3-2
Ciprofloxacin	Cipro®	500-750	2
Levofloxacin	Levaquin®	500-750	1
Moxifloxacin	Avelox®	400	1
Doxycycline	Monodox®	100	2
Minocycline	Minocin®	100	2
Tetracycline HCl	–	500	4
Trimethoprim/sulfamethoxazole[a]	Bactrim DS™/Septra DS®	1 DS	2
Supplemental Drugs			
Azithromycin	Zithromax®	250-500	1
Erythromycin	Ery-Tab®/Erythrocin®	500	4
Clarithromycin	Biaxin®	250-500	2
Cephalexin	Keflex®	500	4

[a]DS, double-strength tablet (160-mg trimethoprim/800-mg sulfamethoxazole).

to decrease mortality, but does markedly increase the emergence and colonization of antibiotic-resistant pathogens. For this reason, most guidelines do not currently support this indication. However, chronic macrolide/azalide use reduces the incidence of acute exacerbations in COPD patients in a clinically significant manner[48,49] (macrolide and anti-inflammatory activity addressed later).

Antibiotics that are effective against responsible pathogens, demonstrate the least risk of drug interactions, and can be administered in a manner that promotes compliance should be selected. Antibiotics, commonly used for treatment of these patients with chronic bronchitis, and their respective adult starting doses are listed in Table 107-3. Doses of antibiotics should be adjusted as needed to the desired clinical effect and the lowest incidence of acceptable side effects. A frequently used clinical strategy to enhance the duration of symptom-free periods incorporates higher-dose antibiotic regimens using the upper limit of the recommended daily antibiotic dose for a period of 5 to 7 days. More clinicians are electing to limit their antibiotic treatment regimen to 5 days as compelling data continue to support equal efficacy, less exposure potentially reducing bacterial resistance development and possibly less side effects with short-duration antibiotic therapy versus longer treatment regimens (greater than 7 days).[41,42]

With the exception of long-term macrolide/azalide administration, chronic antibiotic therapy is rarely indicated in the management of patients with chronic bronchitis. Such approaches lead to marked increase in cost and occurrence of multidrug resistant (MDR) pathogens. Conversely, long-term macrolide (erythromycin, clarithromycin, and roxithromycin) or azalide (azithromycin) administration has been associated with a clinically significant reduction in the incidence of acute exacerbations in patients with chronic bronchitis and COPD.[48-50] The benefit of these drugs is attributed to their antibacterial, anti-inflammatory, and immunomodulatory activity. These drugs reduce bacterial adherence and toxin production, inhibit biofilm function, and reduce the generation of oxygen free radicals, modulate mucin gene protein production controlling mucus hypersecretion, and improve mucociliary clearance. These drugs also decrease neutrophil chemotaxis, promote downregulation of adhesion molecule expression, and inhibit transcription factors leading to decreased production of pro-inflammatory cytokines.[50]

The importance of multifactorial cellular oxidative stress in the pathogenesis of chronic bronchitis and COPD has prompted the study of the efficacy of antioxidants and in particular, the oral administration of NAC, other mucolytic agents and antioxidants.[32,51,52] Some guidelines suggest their use for more severely affected patients. Studies with oral NAC have suggested a dose-dependent response with 600 mg once to twice daily and it may slightly decrease the exacerbation rate in COPD patients not using inhaled steroids; however, there does not appear to any effect on lung function. The exact role of antioxidant in the care of these patients remains to be defined—no specific recommendations can be provided until more data are available regarding which specific compound (as well as dose and duration of therapy) is optimal.

BRONCHIOLITIS

Epidemiology and Etiology

7 Bronchiolitis is an acute viral infection of the lower respiratory tract that affects approximately 50% of children during the first year of life and 100% by age 2 years. The occurrence of bronchiolitis peaks during the winter months and persists through early spring. Bronchiolitis remains the major reason for hospital admission during the first year of life. The incidence of bronchiolitis appears to be more common in males than in females.[53]

Respiratory syncytial virus is the most common cause of bronchiolitis, accounting for up to 75% of all cases. During epidemic periods, the incidence of RSV-induced bronchiolitis may approach 90% of cases. Other detectable viruses include parainfluenza, adenovirus, and influenza. Bacteria serve as secondary pathogens in a minority of cases.[53,54]

Clinical Presentation

The clinical presentation of bronchiolitis (Table 107-4) is often preceded by 1 to 4 days of symptoms (eg, nasal congestion, rhinorrhea, cough, and low-grade fever) indicative of an upper respiratory tract infection. Due to limited oral intake because of coughing combined with fever, vomiting, and diarrhea, infants frequently are dehydrated. The increased work of breathing and tachypnea most likely contribute to increased fluid loss. In most cases, bronchiolitis

TABLE 107-4 Clinical Presentation of Bronchiolitis

Signs and symptoms
Prodrome with irritability, restlessness, and mild fever
Cough and coryza
Vomiting, diarrhea, noisy breathing, and increased respiratory rate as symptoms progress
Labored breathing with retractions of the chest wall, nasal flaring, and grunting
Physical examination
Tachycardia and respiratory rate of 40-80/min in hospitalized infants
Wheezing and inspiratory rales
Mild conjunctivitis in one third of patients
Otitis media in 5%-10% of patients
Laboratory tests
Peripheral white blood cell count normal or slightly elevated
Abnormal arterial blood gases (hypoxemia and, rarely, hypercarbia)

is self-limiting and typically symptoms improve within 7 to 10 days with resolution within 28 days without the need for hospitalization. In patients who require hospitalization, the average length of stay is approximately 3 days.[54]

The diagnosis of bronchiolitis is based primarily on history and clinical findings. It is important for the clinician to attempt to differentiate between bronchiolitis and a host of other clinical entities affecting infants, which may produce a similar picture of dyspnea and wheezing. Asthma, congestive heart failure, anatomic airway abnormalities, cystic fibrosis, foreign bodies, and gastroesophageal reflux are the primary disease entities that may present with wheezing in children. Isolation of a viral pathogen in the respiratory secretions of a wheezing child establishes a presumptive diagnosis of infectious bronchiolitis. However, the ability to identify specific viral pathogens often is hindered by the limited availability of special virology laboratories. In addition, in the elderly and in immunocompromised patients, antigen detection lacks adequate sensitivity, and patients frequently seek medical care after the acute stage of the infection, thus compromising the ability of the available tests to diagnose RSV. However, the proliferation of commercial enzyme-linked immunosorbent assays and fluorescent antibody staining techniques of nasopharyngeal secretions has increased the ability to identify viral antigens within several hours. Identification of RSV by PCR should be available from most clinical laboratories, but its relevance to the clinical management of bronchiolitis remains obscure and therefore routine testing is not recommended.[53,54]

Multiple clinical laboratory determinations have been used to assist in the management of cases of bronchiolitis. Radiographic evaluation of the chest in children with bronchiolitis yields variable findings and rarely alters therapeutic decisions. Thus, the routine use of chest radiography is not recommend; however, in hospitalized patients who fail to demonstrate expected improvement, they may help to distinguish bronchiolitis from other entities characterized by wheezing so that appropriate treatment may be initiated. In children requiring hospitalization, abnormalities in blood gas tensions are frequent and appear to relate to disease severity. Hypoxemia is common and increases the respiratory drive, whereas hypercarbia is seen in only the most severe cases. Despite the presence of moderate degrees of hypoxemia, clinical cyanosis is unusual.[54]

TREATMENT

Desired Outcome

7 In the well infant, bronchiolitis usually is a self-limiting illness, and reassurance, antipyretics, and adequate fluid intake usually are all that are necessary while waiting for resolution of the underlying viral infection. In-hospital support is necessary for the child suffering from respiratory failure or marked dehydration; underlying cardiac and pulmonary diseases potentiate these conditions.[54]

General Approach to Treatment

7 Almost all otherwise healthy babies with bronchiolitis can be followed as outpatients. Such infants are treated for fever, provided generous amounts of oral fluids, and observed closely for evidence of respiratory deterioration.[55] In severely affected children, the mainstays of therapy for bronchiolitis are oxygen therapy and IV fluids. In a subset of patients, aerosolized bronchodilators may have a role. For selected infants, particularly those with underlying pulmonary disease, cardiac disease, or both, therapy with the antiviral agent ribavirin can be considered.[54]

Pharmacologic Therapy

7 Aerosolized β_2-adrenergic therapy appears to offer little benefit for the majority of patients and may even be detrimental.[53,56,57] However, this therapy may offer some benefit to the child with a predisposition toward bronchospasm. In addition, although clinical trials have demonstrated varied results, nebulized epinephrine seems to be more efficacious than albuterol in hospitalized patients with bronchiolitis.[53,58] For such patients, bronchodilator therapy may be offered initially, but should not be pursued in the absence of a clear-cut clinical benefit. Furthermore, given their overall ineffectiveness, neither aerosolized β_2-adrenergic nor nebulized epinephrine therapies are recommended by the American Academy of Pediatrics for the treatment of bronchiolitis.[57]

Similarly, controlled trials of corticosteroids in bronchiolitic infants have not shown therapeutic effects or significant harmful effects, though viral shedding may be prolonged.[54,57] As a result, the routine use of systemically administered corticosteroids is not recommended by the American Academy of Pediatrics and is therefore discouraged.[57] Conversely, the combined use of oral dexamethasone with nebulized epinephrine may act synergistically to reduce hospital admissions and shorten the time to discharge and the duration of symptoms; however, more trials are needed to confirm these findings.[58,59] Although placing children with bronchiolitis in mist tents has been common practice, no data have documented the effectiveness of this practice.

The American Academy of Pediatric guidelines support the use of nebulized hypertonic saline (eg, 3% saline) for the treatment of bronchiolitis in hospitalized infants and children. As such, although nebulized hypertonic saline has proven to be safe and effective for the symptomatic improvement in patients with bronchiolitis after 1 day of use, the benefit of a reduction in length of hospital stay appears to be limited to patients whose mean length of hospital stay generally exceeds 3 days. Thus, this latter benefit may be less applicable to patients in the United States where the mean length of hospital stay due to bronchiolitis is approximately 3 days.[56,57]

Ribavirin may offer benefit to a subset of infants with bronchiolitis. Ribavirin, a synthetic nucleoside, possesses in vitro antiviral properties against a variety of RNA and DNA viruses, including influenza A, influenza B, parainfluenza, and adenovirus, it is approved only in aerosolized form against RSV. Use of the aerosol drug formulation requires special equipment (small-particle aerosol generator) and specially trained personnel for administration via oxygen hood or mist tent. Special care must be taken to avoid drug particle deposition and the resulting clogging of respiratory tubing and valves in mechanical ventilators. Among hospital admissions for RSV infection, ribavirin therapy failed to decrease length of hospital stay, number of days in the intensive care unit, or number of days receiving mechanical ventilation. Consequently, the American Academy of Pediatrics does not recommend the routine use of ribavirin in children with bronchiolitis[57] and most experts recommend reserving use of ribavirin for severely ill patients.

Clinical **Controversy...**

Despite the overall lack of demonstrated benefit of aerosolized β_2-adrenergic agonist, nebulized epinephrine, and corticosteroids in clinical trials, they continue to be prescribed to some patients presenting with bronchiolitis.

For infants with underlying pulmonary or cardiovascular disease, prophylaxis against RSV may be warranted. When administered monthly during the RSV season, both RSV immune globulin and palivizumab (a monoclonal antibody for RSV) may decrease the number of RSV episodes and the need for hospitalization. Between the two, palivizumab is preferred, given its ease of administration, lack of administration-related adverse effects, and noninterference with select immunizations.[60] Despite continuing research, there is no vaccine marketed for RSV.

PNEUMONIA

Epidemiology

Pneumonia remains one of the most common causes of severe sepsis and infectious cause of death in children and adults in the United States, with a mortality rate of 30% to 40%.[5,61] Pneumonia occurs throughout the year, with the relative prevalence of disease resulting from different etiologic agents varying with the seasons. It occurs in persons of all ages, although the clinical manifestations are most severe in the very young, the elderly, and the chronically ill.

Pathogenesis

Microorganisms gain access to the lower respiratory tract by three routes. They may be inhaled as aerosolized particles, enter the lung via the bloodstream from an extrapulmonary site of infection or via aspiration of oropharyngeal contents. Aspiration is a common occurrence in both healthy and ill people during sleep and is a major mechanism by which pulmonary pathogens gain access to the lower airways and alveoli. When pulmonary defense mechanisms are functioning optimally, aspirated microorganisms are cleared from the region before infection can become established; however, aspiration of potential pathogens from the oropharynx can result in pneumonia if lung defenses are impaired. Factors that promote aspiration, such as altered sensorium and neuromuscular disease, may result in an increase in the size of the inoculum delivered to the lower respiratory tract, thereby overwhelming local defense mechanisms. Lung infections with viruses suppress the antibacterial activity of the lung by impairing alveolar macrophage function and mucociliary clearance, thus setting the stage for secondary bacterial pneumonia. Mucociliary transport is also depressed by ethanol and narcotics and by obstruction of bronchi by mucus, tumor, or extrinsic compression. All these factors can severely impair pulmonary clearance of aspirated bacteria. Any alteration of the normal lung microbiome by infection and/or disease can evolve to pneumonia requiring antimicrobial treatment.[62]

8 The most prominent pathogen causing CAP in otherwise healthy adults is *S. pneumoniae* and accounts for up to 35% (12%-68%) of all acute cases. Other common pathogens include *H. influenza* (2.5%-45%), the atypical pathogens *M. pneumoniae*, *Legionella species*, and *C. pneumoniae* (~20%), and a variety of viruses including influenza.[63,64] Healthcare-associated pneumonia was a classification that has been used to distinguish nonhospitalized patients at risk for MDR pathogens from those with CAP however this has fallen out of use.[4,6,65] The term *atypical* may be applied to pneumonia to indicate that the pneumonia may be caused by an atypical pathogen (eg, bilateral lobar pneumonia with a negative sputum Gram stain).[66]

Gram-negative aerobic bacilli, *S. aureus*, and MDR pathogens are the leading causative agents in hospital-acquired pneumonia (HAP).[6] Anaerobic bacteria are the most common etiologic agents in pneumonia that follows the aspiration of gastric or oropharyngeal contents. Ventilator-associated pneumonia (VAP) is also associated with MDR pathogens.

Pneumonia in infants and children is caused by a wider range of microorganisms, and, unlike adults, nonbacterial pathogens predominate. Most pneumonias occurring in the pediatric age group are caused by viruses, especially RSV, parainfluenza, and adenovirus.[5] *M. pneumoniae* is an important pathogen in older children. Beyond the neonatal period, *S. pneumoniae* is the major bacterial pathogen in childhood pneumonia, followed by group A *Streptococcus* and *S. aureus*. *H. influenzae* type b, once a major childhood pathogen, has become an infrequent cause of pneumonia since the introduction of active vaccination against this organism in the late 1980s.

Based on the differences in severity and outcome for patients with CAP, genetic factors likely play a role.[67,68] Multiple variations in genes affecting inflammation, cough and airway protection, pattern recognition molecules, and organ function along with environmental factors may alter a patient's response to CAP. In the future, when disease response is better associated with specific genetic polymorphisms, therapy should become better targeted.

Clinical Presentation

Bacterial pneumonia is caused most commonly by gram-positive streptococci and staphylococci and by gram-negative organisms that normally inhabit the GI tract (enterics) or soil and water (nonenterics). In addition, *Legionella*, itself a weakly staining gram-negative nonenteric organism, accounts for a small percentage of CAP and HAP, although the true incidence may be underreported.[66] Finally, *M. tuberculosis*, an acid-fast staining bacillus, still remains an important cause of pneumonia in urban centers throughout the United States even though the incidence is much lower compared to other countries.[69,70]

Even though a wide array of gram-positive and gram-negative organisms can cause pneumonia, they usually present a similar clinical appearance (Table 107-5); thus, the epidemiologic and clinical clues will render one more likely than the other. *S. pneumoniae*,

TABLE 107-5 Clinical Presentation of Pneumonia

Signs and symptoms
Abrupt onset of fever, chills, dyspnea, and productive cough
Rust-colored sputum or hemoptysis
Pleuritic chest pain
Physical examination
Tachypnea and tachycardia
Dullness to percussion
Increased tactile fremitus, whisper pectoriloquy, and egophony
Chest wall retractions and grunting respirations
Diminished breath sounds over affected area
Inspiratory crackles during lung expansion
Chest radiograph
Dense lobar or segmental infiltrate
Laboratory tests
Leukocytosis with predominance of polymorphonuclear cells
Low oxygen saturation on arterial blood gas or pulse oximetry

S. aureus, the enteric gram-negative rods, and occasionally other organisms may produce local irritation or destruction of blood vessels leading to rust-colored sputum or hemoptysis. Pleural effusions, both sterile and emphysematous, may be associated with many of these entities, as evidenced by distant breath sounds and a wide area of dulled percussion. The chest radiograph and sputum examination and culture are the most useful diagnostic tests for gram-positive and gram-negative bacterial pneumonia, especially for hospitalized patients; urine antigen testing for *L. pneumophila* and *S. pneumoniae* is recommended for patients with severe CAP.[4,71] Typically, the chest radiograph reveals a dense lobar or segmental infiltrate. However, patchy consolidation may be seen occasionally with virtually all these pathogens. Occasionally, pneumonia resulting from hematogenous spread of the organisms results in a diffuse, alveolar pattern on chest radiograph. Gram stain of the expectorated sputum demonstrates many polymorphonuclear cells per high-powered field in the presence of a predominant organism, which is reflected as heavy growth of a single species on culture. Other laboratory tests are less sensitive or specific. Blood cultures may be helpful in identifying the offending organism, but are positive in only a minority of patients. The complete blood count usually reflects a leukocytosis with a predominance of polymorphonuclear cells; in some instances, particularly with *S. pneumoniae*, elevation of the white blood cell (WBC) count may be pronounced. Normal or mildly elevated WBC counts, however, do not exclude bacterial pneumonic disease. The patient also may be hypoxic, as reflected by low oxygen saturation on arterial blood gas or pulse oximetry.

Community-Acquired Pneumonia

8 *S. pneumoniae* is the most common community-acquired bacterial pneumonia in adult and pediatric patients.[4,5,64] It is particularly prevalent and severe for patients with splenic dysfunction, diabetes mellitus, chronic cardiopulmonary or renal disease, or HIV infection. Community-acquired disease with *S. aureus* is identified most frequently in young infants, patients with cystic fibrosis, and those recovering from an antecedent respiratory viral infection. Group A *Streptococcus* is an uncommon cause of CAP, but when it does occur, it frequently follows a viral respiratory tract infection. Only occasionally is it associated with streptococcal pharyngitis. The organism is pyogenic, and the presentation can be severe. Community-acquired enteric gram-negative pneumonia is identified most frequently among patients with chronic illness, especially alcoholism and diabetes mellitus. In preschool-aged children, viral pathogens more commonly cause CAP compared with bacterial pathogens.[5]

Severity scores (eg, CRB65, CURB-65, and PSI), with varying strengths and weaknesses, assist healthcare professionals in predicting intensive care hospitalization and outcomes for patients with CAP.[4,71-73] Definitions of severe CAP may vary depending on the institution; however, patients with severe CAP are more likely to require intensive care or mechanical ventilation, or develop complications with sepsis, bacteremia, or multiorgan failure. Severe CAP may also be difficult to distinguish from HCAP or HAP; however, the pathogens, *S. pneumoniae*, *H. influenzae*, and anaerobic bacteria are not usually MDR. Patients at greater risk for severe CAP are those with underlying medical conditions or at risk for aspiration, animal exposure, or exposure to other infected patients or seasonal epidemics.[65]

Hospital-Acquired Pneumonia

After the urinary tract and the bloodstream, the lungs are the most frequent site for infections acquired in the hospital. HAP is seen most commonly in critically ill patients and is usually caused by bacteria.[6] Factors predisposing patients to the development of HAP include the severity of illness, duration of hospitalization, supine positioning, witnessed aspiration, coma, acute respiratory distress syndrome, patient transport, and prior antibiotic exposure (Table 107-6). The strongest predisposing factor, however, is mechanical ventilation (intubation). The length of stay for hospital admissions is increased by a mean of 7 to 9 days for patients who develop HAP.[6,65]

The organisms most commonly associated with HAP are *S. aureus* and enteric (eg, *K. pneumoniae* or *E. coli*) and nonenteric (eg, *P. aeruginosa*) gram-negative bacilli, organisms that colonize the pharynx of the hospitalized, critically ill patient. Patients with longer lengths of hospital admission or IV antibiotic use within the previous 90 days prior to the development of HAP are more likely to have MDR organisms.[6] The diagnosis of HAP usually is established by the presence of a new infiltrate on chest radiograph, fever, worsening respiratory status, and the appearance of thick, neutrophil-laden respiratory secretions. The diagnosis often is difficult to make in the intensively ill patient with underlying lung pathology that itself can be associated with an abnormal changing radiograph, as occurs

TABLE 107-6 Pneumonia Classifications and Risk Factors

Type of Pneumonia	Definition	Risk Factors
Community acquired (CAP)	Pneumonia developing in patients with no contact to a medical facility	• Age >65 years • Diabetes mellitus • Asplenia • Chronic cardiovascular, pulmonary, renal and/or liver disease • Smoking and/or alcohol abuse
Hospital acquired (HAP)	Pneumonia developing >48 hours after hospital admission	• Witnessed aspiration • COPD, ARDS, or coma • Administration of antacids, H_2-antagonists, or proton pump inhibitor • Supine position • Enteral nutrition, nasogastric t ube • Reintubation, tracheostomy, or patient transport • Head trauma, ICP monitoring • Age >60 years • MDR risk (eg. MRSA, MDR *Pseudomonas*) if IV antibiotic use within 90 days
Ventilator associated (VAP)	Pneumonia developing >48 hours after intubation and mechanical ventilation	• Same as hospital acquired • MDR risk with septic shock, ARDS, acute renal replacement therapy, or 5+ days of hospitalization

ARDS, adult respiratory distress syndrome; CAP, community-acquired pneumonia; COPD, chronic obstructive pulmonary disease; HAP, hospital-acquired pneumonia; ICP, intracranial pressure; MDR, multidrug resistant; MRSA, methicillin-resistant S. aureus VAP, ventilator-associated pneumonia.

with congestive heart failure or chronic lung disease. If a patient develops fever, leukocytosis, and purulent sputum, and has positive sputum/tracheal cultures, but radiographic imaging does not indicate new infiltrates, the patient may have tracheobronchitis as opposed to HAP.[6] Broad-spectrum antibiotics frequently are started empirically even in equivocal circumstances, with bronchoscopy reserved for poorly responsive patients.[6]

Ventilator-Associated Pneumonia

VAP is defined as pneumonia occurring more than 48 hours postendotracheal intubation. The risk for developing pneumonia in the hospital increases by 6 to 21 times after a patient is intubated because the natural airway defenses against the migration of upper respiratory tract organisms into the lower tract are bypassed.[6] This situation is exacerbated by the wide use of acid-reducing drugs (eg, H_2-receptor blocking agents and proton pump inhibitors) in the intensive care unit, which increases the pH of gastric secretions and may promote the proliferation of microorganisms in the upper GI tract. Subclinical microaspirations are events that occur routinely in intubated patients and result in the inoculation of bacteria-contaminated gastric contents into the lung and a higher incidence of nosocomial pneumonia.[75] Pneumonia that develops within 4 days of hospitalization is more likely to be caused by an antibiotic sensitive organism such as *S. pneumoniae*, *S. aureus*, or *Haemophilus* species, whereas infections developing later are more likely to be MDR (eg, *P. aeruginosa*, MRSA, and *Acinetobacter* species). Outbreaks of VAP may be caused occasionally by contaminated respiratory therapy equipment.

To date, there is no "gold standard" for diagnosing VAP; thus, an accurate diagnosis is challenging. Most intensivists agree that VAP should be suspected if new or persistent infiltrates are found on chest radiograph along with two or more of the following: purulent tracheal secretions, leukocytosis or leucopenia, and body temperature greater than 38.3°C (100.9°F).[75,76] Noninvasive sampling techniques are recommended over invasive techniques (eg, bronchoalveolar lavage) for obtaining samples of lower respiratory tract secretions for culture and sensitivity testing.[6]

Special Populations

Pneumonia in the HIV-Infected Patient A broad range of pathogens can cause pneumonia in HIV infection (Table 107-7) including opportunistic infections such as *P. jiroveci* and *Mycobacterium* species.[77] These patients may be afflicted with pneumonia multiple times, particularly in the advanced stages of the disease, and a given episode may be caused by more than one species. The clinical presentation of pneumonia in HIV-infected persons frequently is not helpful in distinguishing one pathogen from another. The pneumonia usually is subacute in onset and consists of fever, nonproductive cough, and dyspnea. Radiographically, most of these entities produce a multilobular or diffuse pattern. Some practitioners initially treat the HIV-infected patient with pneumonia empirically; however, given the wide array of possible pathogens, more frequently a specific microbiologic diagnosis is aggressively pursued early in the patient's course through sputum induction or bronchoalveolar lavage to allow a rational choice of an antimicrobial regimen. The diagnosis and treatment of HIV-infected patients with pulmonary disease is discussed in detail in Chapter 126.

TABLE 107-7 Pulmonary Complications of Human Immunodeficiency Virus Infection

Infections
Viruses
Cytomegalovirus
Herpes simplex virus
Varicella-zoster virus
Respiratory syncytial virus and other common respiratory pathogens (parainfluenza virus, adenovirus)
Measles virus
Bacteria
Pyogenic organisms (especially *S. pneumoniae, H. influenzae*; in late disease, *S. aureus* and gram-negative organisms)
M. tuberculosis
M. avium complex and other nontuberculous mycobacteria
Fungi
Histoplasma capsulatum
Coccidioides immitis
Cryptococcus neoformans
Candida species
Aspergillus species
Parasites
Pneumocystis carinii
Toxoplasma gondii
Cryptosporidia
Strongyloides stercoralis
Malignancies
Kaposi's sarcoma
Non-Hodgkin's lymphoma
Smooth muscle tumors
Lymphocytic interstitial pneumonitis
Nonspecific interstitial pneumonitis
Drug-induced pneumonitis

Pneumonia in the Neutropenic Host Neutropenia in the cancer patient is a common complication of aggressive chemotherapy, but occasionally results from the cancer itself. The risk of infection for the cytopenic patient is increased significantly when the absolute neutrophil count falls less than 500 cell/mm^3 (0.500×10^9/L) and the neutropenia persists for more than 7 days. For many patients, the duration of chemotherapy-induced cytopenia can be reduced by judicious application of colony-stimulating factors.[78]

The organisms that cause pneumonia in the cytopenic cancer patient include a broad range of bacteria and fungi. The most prominent among these are gram-positive bacteria (staphylococci and streptococci); others include enteric and nonenteric (particularly *P. aeruginosa*) gram-negative rods as well as the fungi (*Candida, Aspergillus*). The chest radiograph may reveal the lobar pattern typical of bacterial infection in the normal host, or it may exhibit a diffuse pattern. The pneumonia may remain invisible by chest radiograph until the neutropenia resolves. Noninfectious entities that may cause pulmonary symptoms include toxicity from radiation or chemotherapy or infiltration of the lung parenchyma by the tumor itself.

Common Pathogens

Gram-Positive Bacteria

S. aureus is a prominent cause of HAP and may result from hematogenous spread from a distant source. It is characteristically severe and accompanied by the formation of pneumatoceles (air-containing cavities within the lung). Infections caused by MDR organisms, such as MRSA and vancomycin-intermediate and vancomycin-resistant *S. aureus* are increasing among patients with HAP. IV antibiotic use within the past 90 days increases the risk for MRSA and other MDR pathogens causing HAP and VAP.6 Group B *Streptococcus*, although rare in adults, is the most common cause of bacterial pneumonia among neonates and typically causes a clinical and radiographic picture nearly indistinguishable from hyaline membrane disease.[79]

Enteric Gram-Negative Bacteria

The enteric gram-negative bacteria are leading causes of HAP because the upper respiratory tract becomes rapidly colonized with gram-negative organisms after hospitalization, particularly among critically ill patients and those receiving antibiotics.[80] *K. pneumoniae* is the most frequently encountered pathogen among the gram-negative enteric bacteria, although the relative prominence of these organisms varies among hospitals. The gram-negative bacilli are associated with high mortality, sometimes exceeding 50%; their potential to produce significant morbidity and mortality has been enhanced by the emergence of highly MDR organisms in some hospital settings.[6]

Nonenteric Gram-Negative Bacteria

The most prominent nonenteric gram-negative rods associated with pneumonia include *P. aeruginosa*, *H. influenzae*, and *M. catarrhalis*. Like the enteric gram-negative organisms, *P. aeruginosa* is a frequent cause of HAP and is particularly prominent among neutropenic and burn patients.[6] In addition, cystic fibrosis patients suffer from chronic, multilobar infections with *P. aeruginosa*, as well as other *Pseudomonas* species, and *S. maltophilia* is an emerging pathogen[81]; these infections are punctuated with acute exacerbations. Dual coverage for *P. aeruginosa* is only suggested if patients are at risk for antimicrobial resistance, if resistance is >10% towards a monotherapy agent based on antibiogram, or if resistance patterns are not known.[6] *H. influenzae* type b has been a prominent pathogen in childhood pneumonia. The incidence of all invasive disease due to this organism in the pediatric age group has dropped dramatically since the introduction of the conjugated *Haemophilus* vaccines in the late 1980s. However, two different clinical presentations of *H. influenzae* pneumonia continue to be observed in adults. The most common by far is the bronchopneumonia form, which develops most frequently for patients with underlying chronic lung disease and is believed to represent, in most patients, an exacerbation of chronic bronchitis. In the second form of *H. influenzae* pneumonia, segmental or lobar involvement predominates. The course of this illness is more acute, with sudden onset of cough, fever, and pleuritic chest pain. Finally, *M. catarrhalis*, an important cause of otitis media and sinusitis, is an increasingly important cause of lower respiratory tract infections in immunocompromised and hospitalized patients.

Anaerobic Bacteria

Anaerobic pneumonitis is most likely to occur in individuals predisposed to aspiration by impaired consciousness or dysphagia as the source for the anaerobic bacteria is generally the oral cavity/gingival crevice.[82] Bronchogenic carcinoma is an associated underlying condition. A variety of gram-positive and gram-negative anaerobic bacteria indigenous to the upper airway may cause pneumonitis when large quantities of oropharyngeal secretions are aspirated into the lower airways. The most common organisms identified are *B. melaninogenicus*, *Fusobacteria*, and anaerobic streptococci; polymicrobial infections with anaerobes and aerobes, such as *S. aureus*, *S. pneumoniae*, and gram-negative bacilli, are common.[82]

Early in the infection, clinical symptoms are similar to CAP with patients presenting with cough, low-grade fever, pulmonary infiltrates, and leukocytosis. The course of anaerobic pneumonia is typically indolent and patients are unlikely to have rigors. Other characteristic features are lung abscess, necrotizing pneumonia, and empyema. Anaerobic infections should be suspected if patients are predisposed to aspiration or have a chronic course, putrid sputum/breath, pulmonary necrosis, or empyema.[82] Chest radiographs reveal infiltrates typically located in dependent lung segments, and lung abscesses develop in 20% of patients 1 to 2 weeks into the course of the illness.

Atypical Pneumonia

Legionella species, *Mycoplasma* species, *Chlamydia* species, viruses, and fungi are recognized causes of pneumonia syndromes in all age groups. The designation *atypical pneumonia* has been used to describe pneumonia caused by many of these agents, since it is distinct from the typical bacterial pneumonia course seen most commonly in adults.[67]

Legionella pneumophila

Of the several *Legionella* species known to cause pneumonia in humans, *L. pneumophila* is by far the most important, accounting for 2% to 9% of all CAPs in North America and Europe.[66,83,84] *Legionella*, a small, gram-negative, non–spore-forming bacilli, is an aquatic organism that is transmitted by inhalation of aerosols containing the organism or by microaspiration of contaminated water. Outbreaks of illness caused by *L. pneumophila* have been linked to excavation sites and to contaminated water from air conditioners and showers. Person-to-person transmission has not been demonstrated. In addition to epidemics, *L. pneumophila* causes sporadic illness that peaks in summer and fall. Individuals who are more than 50 years of age, have chronic lung disease, smoke cigarettes, or immunocompromised are at increased risk.[66,83,84]

Infection with *L. pneumophila* is characterized by multisystem involvement and the severity of the infection can range from mild to severe rapidly progressive pneumonia.[73,83] It has a gradual onset with prominent constitutional symptoms (eg, malaise, lethargy, weakness, and anorexia) occurring early in the course of the illness. A dry, nonproductive cough is present initially and becomes productive of mucoid or purulent sputum over several days. Fevers exceeding 38.8°C (101.8°F) develop in more than half of patients (greater than 20% with fevers exceeding 40°C[104°F]) and typically are unremitting and associated with a relative bradycardia. Pleuritic chest pain and progressive dyspnea may be seen. Along with pneumonia, extrapulmonary symptoms, particularly diarrhea, nausea, vomiting, and neurologic symptoms (headache, hallucinations, seizures, and focal neurologic findings), should increase the suspicion for *L. pneumophila*; the GI symptoms may remain evident throughout the course of the illness.[83,84] Myalgias, arthralgias, and chills also occur. Substantial changes in the patient's mental status, often out of proportion to the degree of fever, are seen in approximately one fourth of patients. Chest radiographs initially reveal patchy alveolar infiltrates that may be bilateral and asymmetric. Pulmonary infiltrates may worsen even when the patient is receiving appropriate antibiotics. Progression to lobar or multilobar consolidation is frequent, as are small pleural effusions.

Laboratory findings include leukocytosis with a predominance of mature and immature granulocytes in 50% to 75% of patients. Urinalysis may reveal proteinuria, hematuria, and casts; abnormal liver function tests, increases in serum creatine phosphokinase, hyponatremia, and hypophosphatemia (typically occurring early in infection) have been reported in patients with *L. pneumophila*.[83] Because *L. pneumophila* stains poorly, routine microscopic examination of sputum is of little diagnostic value. Although it exhibits slow growth and has highly selective growth requirements, *L. pneumophila* has been isolated successfully from tissue using a specialized medium. Direct fluorescent antibody examination of respiratory tract secretions, lung tissue, or pleural fluid is the most rapid means of establishing the diagnosis. The sensitivity of this method approaches 70% for sputum and 90% for lung tissue, and diagnostic specificity is high for both. Commercially available urine antigen tests have been developed for *L. pneumophila* (primarily Lp1, the most virulent strain) that allow for detection within 2 to 3 days from the onset of symptoms. These tests are 56% to

99% sensitive and remain positive for weeks even after effective antibiotics have been started. Thus, routine testing in the United States is not recommended, but should be considered for patients not responding to outpatient therapy, those with severe pneumonia, and those with risk factors mentioned above.[83]

M. pneumoniae

The mycoplasmas are included in their own taxonomy labeled *Mollicutes*. Although their small size and filterability are similar to viruses, the structure of their ribosomal RNA indicates that they have evolved from bacteria, and, unlike any virus, they contain cytoplasm and can replicate in an extracellular environment. They are distinguished from eubacteria by their low genetic content and have a parasitic relationship with their hosts.[66] In addition, the mycoplasmas lack a cell wall and are surrounded instead by a lipid membrane. The latter characteristic explains the resistance of these pathogens to cell wall–active antibiotics.

M. pneumoniae causes human disease throughout the year, with a slightly increased incidence in fall and early winter. During the summer months when other causes of pneumonia are less common, *M. pneumoniae* is responsible for a greater proportion of cases. Both infection and disease from *M. pneumoniae* are common, with 10% to 30% of the cases of CAP in children and young adults attributed to this organism.[85] In enclosed populations, such as military recruits and college dormitory residents, it may cause more than 50% of the cases of CAP. Infection is spread by close person-to-person contact and the incubation period is 2 to 3 weeks. *M. pneumoniae* infections are unusual in children younger than 5 years old and show a peak incidence in older children and young adults. Only 3% to 10% of persons infected with *M. pneumoniae* develop pneumonia, with the majority of respiratory tract involvement manifested as pharyngitis and tracheobronchitis. Asymptomatic infection is common.

M. pneumoniae usually presents with a gradual onset of fever, headache, and malaise, with the appearance 3 to 5 days after the onset of illness of a persistent, hacking cough that initially is nonproductive. Sore throat, ear pain, and rhinorrhea often are present. Chills are seen only occasionally and pleuritic pain is uncommon. Lung findings generally are limited to rales and rhonchi; findings of consolidation are rare. Nonpulmonary manifestations of *M. pneumoniae* are extremely common and include nausea, vomiting, diarrhea, myalgias, arthralgias, polyarticular arthritis, and skin rashes (eg, mucositis and Steven's Johnson Syndrome); myocarditis, pericarditis, hemolytic anemia, meningoencephalitis, cranial neuropathies, and Guillain-Barré syndrome have also been reported.[66,86,87] Systemic symptoms generally clear in 1 to 2 weeks, whereas respiratory symptoms may persist for up to 4 weeks. Although the course of mycoplasma pneumonia usually is benign and self-limited, severe respiratory disease may develop in patients with sickle cell disease, agammaglobulinemia, COPD, and in those who have undergone a splenectomy.[66]

Radiographic and CT findings generally are more impressive than the patient's physical findings and include patchy or interstitial infiltrates, consolidations, centrilobular nodules, and bronchial wall thickening.[88] Small unilateral, transient pleural effusions are common; large effusions and empyema are rare. Radiographic abnormalities resolve slowly and 4 to 6 weeks may be required for complete resolution.

Sputum Gram stain may reveal mononuclear or polymorphonuclear leukocytes, with no predominant organism. Although *M. pneumoniae* can be cultured from respiratory secretions using specialized medium, its growth is slow as 2 to 3 weeks may be necessary for culture identification. Indirect evidence of infection by *M. pneumoniae* is the presence of elevated levels of serum cold hemagglutinins. These immunoglobulin M antibodies develop in approximately half of patients with mycoplasmal pneumonia and can be elevated in other illnesses, especially viral infections. A definitive diagnosis also can be made by demonstrating a fourfold or greater rise in serum antibodies to *M. pneumoniae*.[88] However, because this test also requires 2 to 4 weeks for results, the diagnosis of mycoplasmal pneumonia during the acute phase of the illness must be based on the characteristic history, appropriate clinical setting, and typical physical findings.

C. pneumoniae

C. pneumoniae has received the new taxonomic classification of *Chlamydophila*; however, it may still be referred to as *Chlamydia pneumoniae* in some references.[89] *C. pneumoniae*, formally designated the Taiwan acute respiratory agent after the laboratory designations for the first two isolates, is antigenically similar to *C. psittaci*. *C. pneumoniae* infection is ubiquitous worldwide; approximately 80% of the population has been infected by adulthood,[66] but only a small percentage of infections result in clinically apparent pneumonia. Conversely, approximately 5% to 15% of pneumonia is associated with this pathogen.[89] Primary infection with *Chlamydia* pneumonia typically occurs in young adults and is characterized by mild respiratory symptoms with a gradual onset (eg, incubation period about 21 days). Constitutional manifestations, particularly fever, headache, and hoarseness, are common.[66] The radiographic findings are nonspecific and usually consist of multilobular interstitial infiltrates with circumscribed lesions. Immunity is incomplete, and reinfection with *C. pneumoniae* is common, particularly among the elderly. Definitive diagnosis of *C. pneumoniae*–associated pneumonia depends on identification of the organism in sputum. Culture of this organism is difficult and commercially available antigen detection systems are insensitive.

Viral Pneumonia

Viruses are an uncommon cause of pneumonia in adults, except in the immunosuppressed.[6] When viral pneumonia does occur, the influenza virus (usually type A) is the most common cause in the adult civilian population[4]; other viruses causing adult CAP include RSV, adenoviruses, parainfluenza, and human metapneumovirus.[4] In contrast, viruses are by far the most common agents producing pneumonia in infants and young children with a prevalence of up to 80% in those less than 2 years of age, with RSV accounting for most cases. Other common viruses in children include parainfluenza, adenovirus, human metapneumovirus, bocavirus, and rhinovirus.[5,53,66]

Viral respiratory tract infections occur more commonly in the winter and typically spread rapidly from person to person through susceptible populations. Underlying cardiac or pulmonary disease predisposes one to an increased incidence and severity of viral lower respiratory tract infection, especially with influenza virus in adults and RSV in children. Radiographic findings are nonspecific, include bronchial wall thickening and perihilar, and diffuse interstitial infiltrates. Pleural effusions may be seen, especially in adenovirus and parainfluenza pneumonia.

The clinical pictures produced by respiratory viruses are sufficiently variable and overlap to such a degree that an etiologic diagnosis cannot be made confidently based on clinical grounds alone. Although virus isolation in tissue culture is still considered the gold standard, it is time consuming and technically demanding; a period of 7 or more days often is required for virus identification[3] and thus this method usually cannot be used for definitive diagnosis during the acute phase of illness. Serologic tests for virus-specific antibodies are used often in epidemiologic and surveillance studies of viral infections since the diagnostic fourfold rise in titer between acute and convalescent phase sera may require 2 to 3 weeks to develop.[3] Rapid antigen testing for the influenza virus (some tests distinguishing types A and B) and RSV is available; however, cost, high false-positive rates, and 50% to 70% sensitivity are considerations for its utility during nonpeak seasons.[3,4,6] Viral testing with molecular techniques provides increased utility for patient care with high sensitivity, rapid results, and the ability to detect new and emerging pathogens. Although not universally available in the United States, these include real-time PCR, solid and liquid microarrays, mass spectrometry, target-enriched multiplexing PCR, and multiplex ligation-dependent probe amplification, to name a few.[3]

Viruses that have emerged in recent decades and caused significant outbreaks include avian influenza H5N1, severe acute respiratory syndrome coronavirus (SARS-CoV), swine influenza H1N1, variant influenza A H3N2, and Middle Eastern respiratory syndrome coronavirus (see Chapter 109 for further discussion of these viruses).[90,91] In general, signs and symptoms of these viral infections are similar to other viral subtypes; however, there have been unique differences with several of the strains. Pneumonia, respiratory distress syndrome, lymphopenia, and clotting abnormalities tend to occur rapidly in patients infected with H5N1. The H1N1 virus affected normally healthy young adults as opposed to other flu viruses, which tend to be more severe in the young and the elderly, and resulted in serious infections requiring hospitalization and death. The SARS-CoV is an extremely contagious atypical pneumonia[92,93] causing high fever, myalgias, headache, diarrhea, and a dry nonproductive cough, however, for unclear reasons, SARS appears to be less severe for pediatric patients.

Tuberculosis

The acid-fast bacillus *M. tuberculosis* causes tuberculosis and is spread person to person by inhalation of droplets. After years of steady decline, the number of cases of pneumonia caused by *M. tuberculosis* in the United States began to increase in the middle to late 1980s. The new epidemic was a consequence of an increased incidence among prison inmates, IV drug abusers, immigrants, and, most prominently, HIV-infected patients. It is most prominent in urban neighborhoods afflicted with crowded conditions and poor access to healthcare; thus, groups prone to tuberculosis include the homeless and patients in chronic care facilities and homes for the elderly. Unlike previous eras in which tuberculosis was seen most frequently in elderly men, infection currently is identified in increasing numbers of young minority adults. Multidrug resistant strains of *M. tuberculosis* have become more common and treatment regimens for these patients should involve consultation with a specialist. (See Chapter 112 for a detailed discussion of tuberculosis pathophysiology, diagnosis, and treatment.)

TREATMENT

Desired Outcome

Eradication of the offending organism through selection of the appropriate antibiotic and subsequent complete clinical cure are the goals of therapy for all bacterial infections. Therapy should minimize associated morbidity, including one or both of the following: reversible or irreversible disease and drug-induced organ toxicity (eg, renal, lung, or hepatic dysfunction). Most cases of viral pneumonia are self-limiting, although therapy of influenza pneumonia with specific antiviral agents (oseltamivir and zanamivir) may hasten recovery. All efforts should focus on the design of the most cost-effective approach to therapy. Whenever possible, the oral (vs parenteral) route for drug administration should be selected, encouraging outpatient management rather than hospitalization. Optimal treatment of infection/lower respiratory tract infection requires a rapid and accurate diagnosis, rapid initiation of effective antimicrobial therapy, and proper antimicrobial stewardship. The sooner proper antimicrobial therapy is instituted, the better the outcome. Comprehensive principles of optimal antimicrobial therapy and infectious diseases stewardship are discussed in detail in Chapter 105.

General Approach to Treatment

9 The first priority in assessing the patient with pneumonia is to evaluate the adequacy of respiratory function and to determine the presence of signs of systemic illness, specifically dehydration or sepsis with resulting circulatory collapse. Oxygen or, in severe cases, mechanical ventilation and fluid resuscitation should be provided as necessary. Further supportive care of the patient with pneumonia includes humidified oxygen for hypoxemia, administration of bronchodilators (albuterol) when bronchospasm is present, and chest physiotherapy with postural drainage if evidence of retained secretions. Additional therapeutic adjuncts include adequate hydration (IV if necessary), optimal nutritional support, and control of fever. Appropriate sputum samples may be obtained to determine the microbiologic etiology. In more severely ill—hospitalized patients cultures of lower respiratory tract secretions obtained by protected specimen brush bronchoscopy or via BAL along with blood cultures can be helpful in identifying causative pathogens. Rehydration should be provided to replace losses that may have occurred as a result of fever, poor intake, and/or associated vomiting. Selection of an appropriate antimicrobial must be made based on the patient's probable or documented microbiology and its distribution in the respiratory tract, side effects, and cost. Respiratory tract infection diagnosis and treatment guideline reports have been published by authoritative professional organizations that focus on proper treatment regimens and should be consulted for evidence-based treatment recommendations across the spectrum of community- and/or hospital-associated pneumonias.[94]

An increasingly important challenge to effective treatment of lower respiratory tract infections is the ability of bacteria and fungi to form biofilms—colonies of organisms protected by an extracellular polymer matrix of polysaccharides and extracellular DNA. These are complex, multicellular structures that adhere to surfaces (anatomical or devices, eg, indwelling IV lines) and are responsible for the chronicity and poor microbial eradication rates of many hospital-acquired as well as chronic infections, for example, cystic fibrosis (see Chapter 29). Biofilms display specific properties and serve as a reservoir for pathogen dissemination and resultant systemic infection. The colonies of pathogens they harbor can be resistant to antimicrobial drug (eg, aminoglycosides) and immune cell penetration—biofilms may contain single or mixed microbial communities. Other drug classes like fluoroquinolones may penetrate certain biofilms well, but still do not eradicate 100% of the biofilm microorganisms. Biofilm-based microorganisms can produce a number of small, diffusible "communication" molecules—some are signaling molecules regulating cell density within the biofilm and other intracellular functions. An in depth assessment of biofilms is beyond the scope of this chapter, but a good understanding of their many characteristics and approaches to combat them are pivotal to the design of effective treatment of (lower respiratory tract) infections.[95]

Clinical **Controversy...**

Various adjunctive therapy options have been studied for their potential benefits in CAP in recent years. Drugs that have been studied include corticosteroids, prostaglandin inhibitors, statins, immunoglobulin therapy, mediator-specific immunomodulators, angiotensinogen-converting enzyme inhibitors, and oral hypoglycemic agents. Proposed mechanisms for some of the drugs have centered on protective effects (eg, vasodilation and cough reflex) and antiinflammatory effects. Due to differences in study design and patient populations, the actual benefits of these therapies in the treatment of CAP remains undetermined.[96]

Pharmacologic Therapy

Antibiotic Concentrations

Antibiotic concentrations in respiratory secretions in excess of the pathogen MIC are necessary for successful treatment of pulmonary infections.[97] The concept of a blood–bronchus barrier, analogous but dissimilar to the blood–brain barrier, has been used to describe the characteristics of drug penetration into pulmonary secretions. The ability of a drug to penetrate respiratory secretions depends on multiple physicochemical factors, including molecular size, lipid solubility, and degree of ionization at serum and biologic fluid pH and the extent of protein binding. Studies performed in animals and cystic fibrosis patients suggest that larger molecular size favors the accumulation of drugs in bronchial secretions. This finding contrasts with data on drug penetration of other physiologic compartments, such as the cerebrospinal fluid, and may be a result of the trapping of lower-molecular-weight compounds in mucin pores. Nevertheless, the rate at which a drug may accumulate in certain respiratory secretions appears to remain an important factor relative to the drug's clinical efficacy in treating pulmonary infections. The unionized form of drug and lipid solubility also appears to favor drug penetration. Of note, the pH of the infected bronchi often is more acidic than that of normal tissue and blood. These factors combined underscore the importance of considering the inhaled route of antimicrobial drugs for the treatment of patients with moderate to severe pneumonia, particularly in high-risk patient groups.[98]

Clinical **Controversy...**

Prior to the availability of newer β-lactam and fluoroquinolone antibiotics possessing consistently potent activity against multiple gram-negative pathogens, some investigators promoted the administration of antibiotics by direct endotracheal instillation. This method of drug administration attempts to provide increased topical concentrations of antibiotics that do not appear to penetrate respiratory secretions effectively while reducing the likelihood of systemic toxicity. In addition, greater local concentrations of antibiotics, particularly of the polymyxins (eg, colistin) and aminoglycosides are believed to overcome partially the substantial decrease in antibiotic bioactivity observed when these agents interact with the purulent material present in infectious foci. Despite these potential theoretical advantages, the role of antibiotic aerosols or direct endotracheal instillation in clinical practice remains controversial and guidelines do not recommend the routine use of aerosolized antibiotics.[6, 99-102] Nevertheless, positive efficacy and safety data combined with the increasing incidence of serious infections caused by MDR pathogens is fostering the continued study of antibiotic aerosols.

Limited data are available for assessing the influence of drug protein binding on the rate and amount of respiratory secretion penetration. Clearly, it is the free antibiotic fraction reaching the infected site capable of binding to the bacterial cell target that is responsible for antibacterial activity. Given that the degree of protein binding influences a drug's ability to traverse membranes, a similar relationship would be expected within the lung. However, focusing on the absolute amount of an antibiotic bound to plasma/tissue proteins without accounting for the drug's overall antibacterial potency is errant. To completely assess an antibiotic's therapeutic potential in the treatment of pneumonia or any infectious process, it is prudent to assess the antibiotic's integrated pharmacokinetic-pharmacodynamic (PK-PD) characteristics (eg, bacterial killing may be concentration dependent, time dependent, or a hybrid) that account for the drug's degree of binding to serum proteins, tissue distribution, and in vitro potency. These concepts relating to antibiotic activity and overall drug penetration of respiratory secretions underscore the importance of applying the well-defined concepts of antimicrobial PK and PD to the design of optimal antibiotic dosing regimens. A primary example of effectively applying antibiotic PK-PD–designed optimal dosing is reflected in the clinical practice of administering certain antibiotics (once daily dosing of aminoglycosides) to achieve high peak serum concentrations on the assumption that higher (and possibly more effective) biologic fluid concentrations of the drug will be achieved. The aminoglycosides are large polar molecules that diffuse poorly into tissue and respiratory secretions; however, with increasing concentrations obtained with once-daily dosing, increased target-tissue concentrations would be expected with increasing individual doses. Further, recognizing that the peak drug concentration-to-pathogen MIC ratio (Cmax:MIC) is the primary PK-PD correlate for aminoglycosides and that the target Cmax:MIC ratio for aminoglycosides is approximately 10, the single daily dose strategy is most likely to achieve the desired PK-PD target at the desired anatomic site. Similar is the case for the so-called respiratory fluoroquinolones (eg, levofloxacin, moxifloxacin, and gemifloxacin) higher individual dose therapy targeting a greater Cmax:MIC ratio or the more commonly targeted area under the concentration–time curve (AUC)-to-pathogen MIC ratio, that is, AUC:MIC, for fluoroquinolones. The target 24-hour AUC:MIC ratio for fluoroquinolones was originally greater than 35 (possible minimum of 25) for gram-positive and greater than 125 (possible minimum of 100) for gram-negative pathogens. However, with the increasing incidence of antibiotic-resistant bacteria many clinicians are targeting higher ratios of greater than 100 to 200 to suppress possibly resistant mutants of gram-negative pathogens. For greatest probability of success, the antibiotic concentrations projected in these PK-PD correlates should include the expected free (not protein-bound) antibiotic concentration. Conversely, concentration-dependent killing characteristics best correlate with successful therapy with the β-lactam/-carbapenem and macrolide classes of antimicrobials (see Chapter e104 and Chapter 105 for more in-depth discussion of antibiotic concepts).[99,103]

Sputum collection and gram-staining and culture can still be helpful in determining the causative pathogens for respiratory tract infections since it may serve as a reservoir for pathogen growth and possibly represent the PD interface for pulmonary infections. Investigators have assessed antibiotic concentrations in sputum, frequently describing sputum drug concentrations as a ratio of serum to sputum drug concentration; however, caution should be exercised in the interpretation of these data. Data describing sputum drug concentrations is often difficult to interpret because of differences in analytic techniques, method of sputum sampling, and random nature of sampling times relative to drug dose. To more accurately describe the distribution characteristics of antimicrobial agents in sputum, research studies should be designed to allow sequential repeated sputum sampling over a specified dosage interval under both first-dose and steady-state conditions. Thus, until greater sophistication is achieved in our understanding of the relationships between antibiotic concentrations in specific anatomic sites, plasma (blood)-based integrated PK-PD correlates should be used for antibiotic and dose selection.

Recognizing the many deficiencies of using sputum drug concentration correlates for prognosticating antibacterial therapy, most investigators now prefer the determination of drug concentrations in pulmonary epithelial lining fluid and alveolar macrophages.[97] Assessing drug concentrations in specific compartments may provide greater insight into drug selection and efficacy (eg, epithelial lining fluid may reflect the extracellular fluid space and thus the important site for extracellular pathogens, *S. pneumoniae*, *M. catarrhalis*, and *H. influenza*). Although characterizing antimicrobial disposition into these compartments is desirable, access to obtain these samples requires invasive procedures (eg, BAL).

Selection of Antimicrobial Agents

Treatment of bacterial pneumonia, like the treatment of most infectious diseases, initially involves the empirical use of a relatively broad-spectrum antibiotic that is effective against probable pathogens after appropriate cultures and specimens for laboratory evaluation have been obtained.[63,94] Therapy should be narrowed to cover specific pathogens after the results of cultures are known. Multiple factors that help to define the potential pathogens involved include patient age, previous and current medication history, underlying disease(s), major organ function, and present clinical status. These factors must be evaluated to select an appropriate and effective empirical antibiotic regimen as well as the most appropriate route for drug administration (oral vs parenteral). (For a more detailed discussion on the principles of antibiotic selection, see Chapter 105.)

Many antibiotics are effective in the treatment of bacterial pneumonia. Superiority of one antibiotic over another when both demonstrate similar dose-normalized in vitro activity and tissue distribution characteristics is difficult to define. Our opinions on appropriate empirical choices for the treatment of bacterial pneumonias relative to a patient's underlying disease are listed in Table 107-8 for adults and Table 107-9 for children. A complete listing of antimicrobial agents for specific pathogens is beyond the scope of this chapter and is presented in Chapter 105.

TABLE 107-8 Evidence-Based Empirical Antimicrobial Therapy for Pneumonia in Adults[a]

Clinical Setting	Usual Pathogens	Empirical Therapy
Outpatient/Community Acquired		
Previously healthy	*S. pneumoniae*, *M. pneumoniae*, *H. influenzae*, *C. pneumoniae*, *M. catarrhalis*	Macrolide/azalide,[b] or tetracycline[c]
Comorbidities (diabetes, heart/lung/liver/renal disease, and alcoholism)	Viral MDR S. pneumoniae	Oseltamivir or zanamivir if <48° from onset of symptoms Fluoroquinolone[d] or β-lactam + macrolide[b]
Elderly Regions with >25% rate of macrolide-resistant *S. pneumoniae*	*S. pneumoniae*, gram-negative bacilli	Piperacillin/tazobactam or cephalosporin[e] or carbapenem[f] Fluoroquinolone[d] or β-lactam + macrolide[b]/tetracycline
Inpatient/Community Acquired		
Non-ICU	*S. pneumoniae*, *H. influenzae*, *M. pneumoniae*, *C. pneumoniae*, *Legionella* sp.	Fluoroquinolone[d] or β-lactam + macrolide[b]/tetracycline
ICU	*S. pneumoniae*, *S. aureus*, *Legionella* sp., gram-negative bacilli, *H. influenzae*	β-Lactam + macrolide[b]/fluoroquinolone[d]
	If *P. aeruginosa* suspected	Piperacillin/tazobactam or meropenem or cefepime + fluoroquinolone[d]/AMG/azithromycin; or β-lactam + AMG + azithromycin/respiratory fluoroquinolone[d]
	If MRSA suspected	Above + vancomycin or linezolid
	Viral	Oseltamivir or zanamivir ± antibiotics for 2° infection
Hospital Acquired or Ventilator Associated		
No risk factors for MDR pathogens (single agent *Pseudomonal* coverage)	*S. pneumoniae*, *H. influenzae*, MSSA, enteric gram-negative bacilli	Piperacillin/tazobactam, cefepime, levofloxacin, imipenem or meropenem
Risk factors for MDR pathogen (dual agent *Pseudomonal* coverage)	*P. aeruginosa*, *K. pneumoniae* (ESBL), *Acinetobacter* sp.	Antipseudomonal cephalosporin[e] or antipseudomonal carbapenem or β-lactam/β-lactamase + antipseudomonal fluoroquinolone[d] or AMG[g]
	If MRSA or *Legionella* sp. suspected	Above + vancomycin or linezolid
Aspiration	*S. aereus*, enteric gram-negative bacilli Anaerobes	Penicillin or clindamycin or piperacillin/tazobactam + AMG[g] Clindamycin, β-lactam/β-lactamase, or carbapenem
Atypical Pneumonia[h]		
Legionella pneumophila		Fluoroquinolone,[d] doxycycline, or azithromycin
Mycoplasma pneumonia		Fluoroquinolone,[d] doxycycline, or azithromycin
Chlamydophila pneumonia		Fluoroquinolone,[d] doxycycline, or azithromycin
SARS		Fluoroquinolone[d] or macrolides[b]
Avian influenza		Oseltamivir
H1N1 influenza		Oseltamivir

MRSA, methicillin-resistant *Staphylococcus aureus*; AMG, aminoglycoside; SARS, severe acute respiratory syndrome; ESBL, extended-spectrum β-lactamases; MDR, multidrug resistant; MSSA, methicillin-sensitive *Staphylococcus aureus*.

[a]See the section Selection of Antimicrobial Agents.

[b]Macrolide/azalide: erythromycin, clarithromycin, and azithromycin.

[c]Tetracycline: tetracycline, HC1, and doxycycline.

[d]Fluoroquinolone: ciprofloxacin, levofloxacin, and moxifloxacin.

[e]Antipseudomonal cephalosporin: cefepime and ceftazidime.

[f]Antipseudomonal carbapenem: imipenem and meropenem.

[g]Aminoglycoside: amikacin, gentamicin, and tobramycin.

[h]For tuberculosis, see Chapter 112.

Data from references 4, 6, 66.

TABLE 107-9 Empirical Antimicrobial Therapy for Pneumonia in Pediatric Patients[a]

Clinical Setting	Usual Pathogen(s)	Empirical Therapy
Outpatient/Community Acquired		
<1 month	Group B *Streptococcus*, *H. influenzae* (nontypable), *E. coli*, *S. aureus*, *Listeria* CMV, RSV, adenovirus	Ampicillin/sulbactam, cephalosporin,[b] carbapenem[c] Ribavirin for RSV[d]
1-3 months	*C. pneumoniae*, possibly *Ureaplasma*, CMV, *Pneumocystis carinii* (afebrile pneumonia syndrome) *S. pneumoniae*, *S. aureus*	Macrolide/azalide,[e] trimethoprim–sulfamethoxazole Semisynthetic penicillin[f] or cephalosporin[g]
Preschool-aged children	Viral (rhinovirus, RSV, influenza A and B, parainfluenzae, adenovirus, human metapneumovirus, coronavirus)	Antimicrobial therapy not routinely required
Previously healthy, fully immunized infants and preschool children with suspected mild–moderate bacterial CAP	*S. pneumoniae* *M. pneumoniae*, other atypical	Amoxicillin, cephalosporin[b,g] Macrolide/azalide or fluoroquinolone
Previously healthy, fully immunized school-aged children and adolescents with mild–moderate CAP	*S. pneumoniae* *M. pneumoniae*, other atypical	Amoxicillin, cephalosporin,[b,g] or fluoroquinolone Macrolide/azalide, fluoroquinolone, or tetracycline
Moderate–severe CAP during influenza virus outbreak	Influenza A and B, other viruses	Oseltamivir or zanamivir
Inpatient/Community Acquired		
Fully immunized infants and school-aged children	*S. pneumoniae* CA-MRSA *M. pneumoniae*, *C. pneumoniae*	Ampicillin, penicillin G, cephalosporin[b] β-Lactam + vancomycin/clindamycin β-Lactam + macrolide/fluoroquinolone/ doxycycline
Not fully immunized infants and children; regions with invasive penicillin-resistant pneumococcal strains; patients with life-threatening infections	*S. pneumoniae, PCN resistant* MRSA *M. pneumoniae*, other atypical pathogens	Cephalosporin[b] Add vancomycin/clindamycin Macrolide/azalide[e] + β-lactam/doxycycline/ fluoroquinolone

CMV, cytomegalovirus; RSV, respiratory syncytial virus; CAP, community-acquired pneumonia; MRSA, methicillin resistant *Staphylococcus aureus*.

[a]See the section Selection of Antimicrobial Agents.

[b]Third-generation cephalosporin: ceftriaxone and cefotaxime. Note that cephalosporins are not active against *Listeria*.

[c]Carbapenem: imipenem–cilastatin and meropenem.

[d]See text for details regarding possible ribavirin treatment for RSV infection.

[e]Macrolide/azalide: erythromycin and clarithromycin/azithromycin.

[f]Semisynthetic penicillin: nafcillin, and oxacillin.

[g]Second-generation cephalosporin: cefuroxime and cefprozil.

Data from reference 5.

A patient's medical history of responding or not responding to one of these antibiotics in the recent past will assist greatly in the decision to continue their use. For infected patients with risk factors, regardless of whether the patient resides in the community, long-term care facility, or acute care hospital, the fluoroquinolone antibiotics represent important treatment tools based on their highly favorable PK (tissue and intracellular distribution) and PD (potency, broad spectrum) characteristics combined with ease of administration (IV, oral) and patient tolerability. Furthermore, optimal dosing directed by the projected 24-hour free fluoroquinolone AUC-to-pathogen MIC ratio (see earlier) has fostered maximal bacteriologic kill and enhanced patient safety.

Table 107-10 lists dosages for selected antibiotics used for the treatment of bacterial pneumonia. The large number of expensive drugs mandates critical evaluation for formulary selection and clinical use. Similarities of in vitro activity, resistance to bacterial-inactivating enzymes, and overall effectiveness often make rational therapeutic decisions difficult and even appear random. However, some general principles can be applied to guide rational antibiotic choice, including direct comparison of the antibiotic's likely attainment of the defined PK-PD target correlate for specific bacterial species within the infected site. An understanding and application of inherent drug characteristics appears to be of the utmost importance for the selection of an optimal therapeutic regimen. Thus, whenever possible, identification of the causative pathogen and expected/defined antibiotic susceptibility (eg, MIC) is of paramount importance to the selection/design of the optimal antibiotic regimen. Lastly, the importance of meaningful and continuous antimicrobial stewardship in combating the rate of pathogen resistance cannot be overemphasized.

Community-Acquired Pneumonia

Tables 107-8 and 107-9 provide evidence-based guidelines for the treatment of CAP in adults[4] and children,[5] respectively. The bacterial causes are relatively constant, even across geographic areas and patient populations. Unfortunately, pathogen resistance to standard antimicrobials is increasing (eg, penicillin-resistant pneumococci), which necessitates careful attention by the clinician to local and regional bacterial susceptibility patterns.[104] Thus, whenever possible, initial therapy should be based on presumed antibacterial susceptibility and consist of older, less-expensive agents, with newer and more expensive antibiotics reserved for unresponsive illness or special circumstances. Indiscriminate use of recently introduced agents increases healthcare costs and, in some instances (eg, widespread use of fluoroquinolones), induces resistance among a significant percentage of community-acquired organisms.[4] The rapidly evolving epidemiology of bacterial resistance, including the increasing emergence of penicillin-resistant *S. pneumoniae* in many areas of the United States and Europe, forces the clinician to be vigilant and knowledgeable about antibiotic sensitivity patterns in each community.

TABLE 107-10 Antibiotic Doses for Treatment of Bacterial Pneumonia

			Daily Antibiotic Dose[a]	
Antibiotic Class	**Antibiotic**	**Brand Name**	**Pediatric**	**Adult (Total Dose/Day)**
Penicillin	Ampicillin ± sulbactam	Unasyn®	150-200 mg/kg/day	6-12 g
	Amoxicillin ± clavulanate[b]	Augmentin®	45-100 mg/kg/day	0.75-1 g
	Piperacillin/tazobactam	Zosyn®	200-300 mg/kg/day	12-18 g
	Penicillin		100,000-250,000 units/kg/day	12-18 million units
Extended-spectrum cephalosporins	Ceftriaxone	Rocephin®	50-75 mg/kg/day	1-2 g
	Cefotaxime	Claforan®	150 mg/kg/day	2-12 g
	Ceftazidime	Fortaz®/Tazicef®	90-150 mg/kg/day	4-6 g
	Cefepime	Maxipime®	100-150 mg/kg/day	2-6 g
Macrolide/azalide	Clarithromycin	Biaxin®	15 mg/kg/day	0.5-1 g
	Erythromycin	Ery-Tab®	30-50 mg/kg/day	1-2 g
	Azithromycin	Zithromax®	10 mg/kg × 1 day (× 2 days if parenteral), and then 5 mg/kg days 2-5	500 mg × 1 day (× 2 days if parenteral), and then 250 mg days 2-5
Fluoroquinolones[c]	Moxifloxacin	Avelox®	–	400 mg
	Gemifloxacin	Factive®	–	320 mg
	Levofloxacin	Levaquin®	8-20 mg/kg/day	750 mg
	Ciprofloxacin	Cipro®	30 mg/kg/day	1.2 g
Tetracycline[d]	Doxycycline	Monodox®/Doxy 100™	2-5 mg/kg/day	100-200 mg
	Tetracycline HCl		25-50 mg/kg/day	1-2 g
Aminoglycosides	Gentamicin		7.5-10 mg/kg/day	7.5 mg/kg
	Tobramycin		7.5-10 mg/kg/day	7.5 mg/kg
Carbapenems	Imipenem	Primaxin®	60-100 mg/kg/day	2-4 g
	Meropenem	Merrem®	30-60 mg/kg/day	1-3 g
Other	Vancomycin		45-60 mg/kg/day	2-3 g
	Linezolid	Zyvox®	20-30 mg/kg/day	1.2 g
	Clindamycin	Cleocin®	30-40 mg/kg/day	1.8 g

[a]Doses can be increased for more severe disease and may require modification for patients with organ dysfunction.

[b]Higher-dose amoxicillin and amoxicillin/clavulanate (eg, 90 mg/kg/day) are used for penicillin-resistant *S. pneumoniae*.

[c]Fluoroquinolones have been avoided for pediatric patients because of the potential for cartilage damage; however, they have been used for MDR bacterial infection safely and effectively in infants and children (see text).

[d]Tetracyclines are rarely used in pediatric patients, particularly in those younger than 8 years because of tetracycline-induced permanent tooth discoloration.

Interestingly, the European National Institute for Health and Care Excellence pneumonia guidelines recommend point of care C reactive protein tests to assist in determining if antibiotics should be prescribed to patients with lower respiratory tract infections when pneumonia has not been diagnosed clinically.[71] Indiscriminate use of antimicrobials for treatment of pneumonia has contributed to the problem of antimicrobial resistance, underscoring the need for defining the optimal antibiotic regimen for each patient.

9 Evidence-based empirical therapy differs among outpatients, hospitalized patients, and hospitalized patients admitted to an intensive care unit (see Tables 107-8 and 107-9).[4,5] Antimicrobial therapy should be initiated for hospitalized patients with acute pneumonia within 8 hours of admission because an increase in mortality has been demonstrated when therapy was delayed beyond 8 hours of admission.

Hospital-Acquired Pneumonia

10 Antibiotic selection within the hospital environment demands greater care because of constant changes in antibiotic resistance patterns in vitro and in vivo. Ironically, some β-lactam antibiotics, which were developed to treat MDR hospital-acquired organisms, can themselves induce broad-spectrum bacterial β-lactamases and thereby lead to even greater problems with resistance.[99] These facts underscore the importance of regularly documenting the epidemiology of pathogens and infectious diseases within a specific practice or institution and tailoring empiric antibiotic therapy based on local antibiograms.[6] As a result, an antimicrobial agent for a specific infectious disease favored in one practice site may not be the most desirable selection in another site despite similarities in size and patient profile. Strict and careful control and, possibly, rotation of empirical antibiotics in the hospital environment may help to limit the emergence of resistant organisms. Newer antibiotics developed for treatment of resistant, hospital-acquired pathogens are costly; therefore, their use must be moderated to some extent in an era where capitated hospital costs and mandated budget cuts will not tolerate careless antibiotic use. Broad-spectrum antibiotics are more appropriate choices for patients with risk factors for MDR pathogens or if HAP develops after at least 5 days of hospitalization (see Table 107-8 for recommended antimicrobial therapy).[6] For most patients, a 7 day course of antibiotics is appropriate.[6]

Ventilator-Associated Pneumonia

The approach to treating VAP is similar to antibiotic selection in HAP (see Table 107-8). Patients should be carefully evaluated to determine whether they are at risk for MDR pathogens as this is essential in selecting appropriate empirical antibiotic therapy.[6] Risk factors for MDR VAP include septic shock, ARDS, acute renal replacement therapy, IV antibiotic use within the previous 90 days and/or being hospitalized at least 5 days prior to VAP.[6] It is also important to identify patients with VAP early since delays in initiating appropriate antibiotic therapy are associated with increased mortality. Current guidelines support shorter antibiotic courses (7 days versus 8-15 days) for VAP even for gram negative bacilli infections since mortality and clinical cure rates were not significantly affected with shorter courses.[6] Aerosolized antibiotic delivery has been considered for more targeted therapy; but is currently only recommended if patients are not responding to IV antibiotic therapy.[6, 106] Inhaled plus systemic aminoglycosides or colistin can be used if the identified pathogen is only sensitive to one of those antibiotics.[6]

Atypical Pneumonia

Pneumonia caused by atypical pathogens may be more difficult to treat with antibiotics than "typical" pathogens. It is debatable whether empirical treatment for hospitalized patients with CAP should include antibiotic coverage of atypical pathogens; however, for patients requiring ICU admission, combination therapy including coverage for atypical pathogens has been associated with improved mortality.[107] There does not appear to be any benefit in terms of survival or clinical efficacy to providing atypical coverage for all outpatients unless they have risk factors for a poor outcome (eg, history of CHD, lung or liver disease, immunosuppression, DM, or malignancy) (see Table 107-8 for a summary of the evidence-based guidelines on management).[107]

For *Legionella* pneumonia, azithromycin and levofloxacin are recommended although other respiratory fluoroquinolones, tetracyclines, or macrolides could be utilized but may result in more side effects.[84] Double antibiotic coverage is not recommended if one of these agents is used, even in severe pneumonia, due to limited evidence of improved efficacy.[84] *Mycoplasma* pneumonia is difficult to treat similar to the other atypical pathogens due to the organism's lack of a cell wall, limiting the use of certain antibiotics, and because it is found on epithelial cells in the respiratory tract instead of inside the cells.[66] Macrolides and tetracyclines are generally effective against *Mycoplasma*; however, macrolide-resistant strains have been emerging over the past decade.[85] *Chlamydophila* organisms are sensitive to macrolides, doxycycline, and fluoroquinolones. Symptoms, such as cough and malaise, may be present for months following antibiotic therapy.[66] The management of tuberculosis is further discussed in Chapter 112.

For viral causes of pneumonia, antivirals such as oseltamivir and occasionally amantadine can be used, depending on viral susceptibility.[91] Treatment for H5N1 and H1N1 is primarily supportive; patients with H5N1 generally require aggressive oxygen therapy and intensive monitoring, while the majority of those with H1N1 are treated as outpatients. Both viruses are resistant to amantadine; therefore, the neuraminidase inhibitors oseltamivir and zanamivir are recommended if antivirals are administered. Treatment of SARS involves primarily supportive care and procedures to prevent transmission to others. Owing to the uncertainty associated with the diagnosis of SARS, empirical therapy with broad-spectrum antibiotics should be used including fluoroquinolones or macrolides/azalides. Although evidence for its efficacy is limited, oral ribavirin also has been used to treat patients with noninfluenza respiratory viral infections.[108] High dose systemic corticosteroids are not routinely recommended in severe viral respiratory infections due the risk of avascular osteonecrosis and prolonged viral shedding.[91]

Prevention

Prevention of some cases of pneumonia is possible through the use of vaccines and medications against selected infectious agents. Polyvalent polysaccharide vaccines are available for two of the leading causes of bacterial pneumonia, *S. pneumoniae* and *H. influenzae* type b. Children should be vaccinated against *S. pneumoniae*, *H. influenzae* type b, pertussis, and influenza while caregivers for infants less than 6 months should also be vaccinated against influenza and pertussis. Immune prophylaxis for RSV is only recommended for high-risk infants during RSV season. To minimize the risk of developing VAP, healthcare providers should seek to minimize colonization of the aerodigestive tract, prevent aspiration (head raised 45 degree), and limit the length of mechanical ventilation of patients.[75] In addition, evidence-based guidelines for preventing HCAP have been published (Table 107-11) (see Chapter 109 for a full discussion of influenza postexposure prophylaxis and Chapter 125 for vaccines.)[109]

TABLE 107-11 Evidenced-Based Guidelines for Preventing Healthcare-Associated Pneumonia

Recommendation	Recommendation Grade[a]
For nebulizers, use aerosolized medications in single-dose vials. If multidose medication vials are used, follow manufacturers' instructions for handling, storing, and dispensing the medications	1B
Pneumococcal vaccination is recommended for patients at high risk for severe pneumococcal infections	1A
Unless contraindicated, administer a macrolide to any person who has had close contact with persons having pertussis	1B
In acute care settings, offer vaccine to inpatients and outpatients at high risk for complications from influenza beginning in September and throughout the influenza season	1A
Unless contraindicated, provide prophylactic treatment to all patients without influenza illness in the involved unit with amantadine, rimantadine, or oseltamivir for a minimum of 2 weeks or until approximately 1 week after the end of the outbreak	1A
Unless contraindicated, patients with influenza should receive amantadine, rimantadine, oseltamivir, or zanamivir within 48 hours of the onset of symptoms	1A

[a]Grade 1A, strongly recommended for implementation and strongly supported by well-designed experimental, clinical, or epidemiologic studies; grade 1B, strongly recommended for implementation and supported by certain clinical or epidemiologic studies and by strong theoretical rationale.

EVALUATION OF THERAPEUTIC OUTCOMES

After therapy has been instituted, appropriate clinical parameters should be monitored to ensure the efficacy and safety of the therapeutic regimen. For patients with bacterial infections of the upper or lower respiratory tract, the time to resolution of initial presenting symptoms and the lack of appearance of new associated symptomatology are important to determine. For patients with CAP or pneumonia from any source of mild to moderate clinical severity, the time to resolution of cough, decreasing sputum production, and fever as well as other constitutional symptoms of malaise, nausea, vomiting, and lethargy, should be noted. If the patient requires supplemental oxygen therapy, the amount and need should be assessed regularly. A gradual and persistent improvement in the resolution of these symptoms and therapies should be observed. Initial resolution of infection should be observed within the first 2 days of therapy and progression to complete resolution within 5 to 7 days (usually no more than 10 days).

For patients with HAP, substantial underlying diseases, or both, additional parameters can be followed, including the magnitude and character of the peripheral blood WBC count, chest radiograph, and blood gas determinations. Similar to patients with less severe disease, some resolution of symptoms should be observed within 2 days of instituting antibiotic therapy. If no resolution of symptoms is observed within 2 days of starting seemingly appropriate antibiotic therapy or if the patient's clinical status is deteriorating, the appropriateness of initial antibiotic therapy should be critically reassessed. The patient should be evaluated carefully for deterioration of underlying concurrent disease(s). Additionally, the caregiver should consider the possibility of changing the initial antibiotic therapy to expand antimicrobial coverage not included in the original regimen (eg, *Mycoplasma*, *Legionella*, and anaerobes). Furthermore, the need for antifungal therapy (eg, triazoles, echinocandins) should be considered. Some resolution of symptoms should be observed within 2 days of starting proper antibiotic therapy, with complete resolution expected within 10 to 14 days.

ABBREVIATIONS

AECB	acute exacerbation of chronic bronchitis
AUC	area under the concentration curve
BAL	bronchoalveolar lavage
CAP	community-acquired pneumonia
Cmax	maximum concentration
COPD	chronic obstructive pulmonary disease
FEV_1	forced expiratory volume in the first second of expiration
GOLD	Global Initiative for Chronic Obstructive Lung Disease
HAP	hospital-acquired pneumonia
HIV	human immunodeficiency virus
LABA	long-acting β-receptor agonist
LAMA	long-acting muscarinic antagonist
MDR	multidrug resistant
MIC	minimum inhibitory concentration
MRSA	methicillin-resistant *Staphylococcus aureus*
NAC	*N*-acetyl cysteine
PCR	polymerase chain reaction
PDE4	phosphodiesterase 4
PK-PD	pharmacokinetic–pharmacodynamic
RSV	respiratory syncytial virus
SARS	severe acute respiratory syndrome
SARS-CoV	severe acute respiratory syndrome coronavirus
VAP	ventilator-associated pneumonia
WBC	white blood cell

REFERENCES

1. Eddens T, Kolls JK. Host defenses against bacterial lower respiratory tract infection. *Curr Opin Immunol* 2012;24:424-430.
2. Jaroszewski DE, Webb BJ, Leslie KO. Diagnosis and management of lung infections. *Thorac Surg Clin* 2012;22:301-324.
3. Yan Y, Zhang S, Tang YW. Molecular assays for the detection and characterization of respiratory viruses. *Semin Respir Crit Care Med* 2011;32:512-526.
4. Mandell L, Wunderink R, Anzeuto A, et al. Infectious Diseases Society of America/American Thoracic Society consensus guidelines on the management of community-acquired pneumonia in adults. *Clin Infect Dis* 2007;44(Suppl 2):S27-S72.
5. Bradley JS, Byington Cl, Shah SS, et al. The management of community-acquired pneumonia in infants and children older than 3 months of age: Clinical practice guidelines by the Pediatric Infectious Diseases Society and the Infectious Diseases Society of America. *Clin Infect Dis* 2011;53:e25-e76.
6. Kalil AC, Metersky ML, Klompas M, et al. Management of adults with hospital-acquire and ventilator-associated pneumonia: 2016 Clinical practice guidelines by the Infections Diseases Society of America and the American Thoracic Society. *Clin Infect Dis*. Advanced Access published July 14, 2016.
7. Lippi G, Meschi T, Cervellin G. Inflammatory biomarkers for the diagnosis, monitoring and follow-up of community-acquired pneumonia: Clinical evidence and perspectives. *Eur J Intern Med* 2011;22:460-465.
8. Tackett KL, Atkins A. Evidence-based acute bronchitis therapy. *J Pharm Pract* 2012;25:586-590.
9. Nielsen M, Barnes CB, Ulrik CS. Clinical characteristics of the asthma-COPD overlap syndrome—a systematic review. *Int J Chron Obstruct Pulmon Dis* 2015;10:1443-1454.
10. Gibson PG, McDonald VM. Asthma-COPD overlap 2015: Now we are six. *Thorax* 2015;70:683-691.
11. Blush RR. Acute bronchitis: Evaluation and management. *Nurse Pract* 2013;38:14-20.
12. Gelfer G, Leggett J, Meyers J, Wang L, Gilbert DN. The clinical impact of the detection of potential etiologic pathogens of community-acquired pneumonia. *Diagn Microbiol Infect Dis* 2015;83:400-406.
13. Beutler AI, Chesnut GT, Mattingly JC, Jamieson B. FPIN's Clinical Inquiries. Aspirin use in children for fever or viral syndromes. *Am Fam Physician* 2009;80:1472.
14. Weatherall M, Ioannides S, Braithwaite I, Beasley R. The association between paracetamol use and asthma: Causation or coincidence? *Clin Exp Allergy* 2015;45:108-113.
15. Becker LA, Horn J, Villasis-Keever M, et al. Beta2-agonists for acute bronchitis. *Cochrane Database Syst Rev* 2011;Jul 6;(7):CD001726.
16. Martin MJ, Harrison TW. Causes of chronic productive cough: An approach to management. *Respir Med* 2015;109:1105-1113.
17. Smith SM, Fahey T, Smucny J, Becker LA. Antibiotics for acute bronchitis. *Cochrane Database Syst Rev* 2014;3:CD000245.
18. Fiore AE, Fry A, Shay D, et al. Antiviral agents for the treatment and chemoprophylaxis of influenza—Recommendations of the Advisory Committee on Immunization Practices (ACIP). *MMWR Recomm Rep* 2011;60:1-24.
19. Jefferson T, Jones MA, Doshi P, et al. Neuraminidase inhibitors for preventing and treating influenza in healthy adults and children. *Cochrane Database Syst Rev* 2014;4:CD008965.
20. Spanakis N, Pitiriga V, Gennimata V, Tsakris A. A review of neuraminidase inhibitor susceptibility in influenza strains. *Expert Rev Anti Infect Ther* 2014;12:1325-1336.
21. Dunning J, Baillie JK, Cao B, Hayden FG. Antiviral combinations for severe influenza. *Lancet Infect Dis* 2014;14:1259-1270.
22. Kim V, Criner GJ. Chronic bronchitis and chronic obstructive pulmonary disease. *Am J Respir Crit Care Med* 2013;187:228-237.
23. Cai Y, Schikowski T, Adam M, et al. Cross-sectional associations between air pollution and chronic bronchitis: An ESCAPE meta-analysis across five cohorts. *Thorax* 2014;69:1005-1014.
24. Celli BR, Decramer M, Wedzicha JA, et al. An Official American Thoracic Society/European Respiratory Society Statement: Research questions in chronic obstructive pulmonary disease. *Am J Respir Crit Care Med* 2015;191:e4-e27.
25. Criner GJ, Bourbeau J, Diekemper RL, et al. Prevention of acute exacerbations of COPD: American College of Chest Physicians and Canadian Thoracic Society Guideline. *Chest* 2015;147:894-942.
26. Overington JD, Huang YC, Abramson MJ, et al. Implementing clinical guidelines for chronic obstructive pulmonary disease: barriers and solutions. *J Thorac Dis* 2014;6:1586-1596.
27. Braman SS. Chronic cough due to chronic bronchitis: ACCP evidence-based clinical practice guidelines. *Chest* 2006;129(1 Suppl): 104S-115S.
28. Miravitlles M, Kruesmann F, Haverstock D, et al. Sputum colour and bacteria in chronic bronchitis exacerbations: A pooled analysis. *Eur Respir J* 2012;39:1354-1360.
29. Anthonisen N, Manfreda J, Warren CP, et al. Antibiotic therapy in exacerbations of chronic obstructive pulmonary disease. *Ann Intern Med* 1987;106:196-204.
30. McCarthy B, Casey D, Devane D, et al. Pulmonary rehabilitation for chronic obstructive pulmonary disease. *Cochrane Database Syst Rev* 2015;2:CD003793.
31. McIlwaine MP, Less Son NM, Richmond ML. Physiotherapy and cystic fibrosis: What is the evidence base? *Curr Opin Pulm Med* 2014;20:613-617.
32. Poole P, Black PN, Cates CJ. Mucolytic agents for chronic bronchitis or chronic obstructive pulmonary disease. *Cochrane Database Syst Rev* 2012;8:CD001287.
33. Santus P, Radovanovic D, Paggiaro P, et al. Why use long acting bronchodilators in chronic obstructive lung diseases? An extensive review on formoterol and salmeterol. *Eur J Intern Med* 2015;26:379-384.
34. Kew KM, Dias S, Cates CJ. Long-acting inhaled therapy (beta-agonists, anticholinergics and steroids) for COPD: A network meta-analysis. *Cochrane Database Syst Rev* 2014;3:CD010844.
35. Singh D, New combination bronchodilators for chronic obstructive pulmonary disease: Current evidence and future perspectives. *Br J Clin Pharmacol* 2015;79:695-708.
36. Cazzola M, Matera MG. Triple combinations in chronic obstructive pulmonary disease—Is three better than two? *Expert Opin Pharmacother* 2014;15:2475-2478.
37. Yu T, Fain K, Boyd CM, et al. Benefits and harms of roflumilast in moderate to severe COPD. *Thorax* 2014;69:616-622.

38. Fu AZ, Sun SX, Huang X, Amin AN. Lower 30-day readmission rates with roflumilast treatment among patients hospitalized for chronic obstructive pulmonary disease. *Int J Chron Obstruct Pulmon Dis* 2015;10:909-915.
39. Lipari M, Benipal H, Kale-Pradhan P. Roflumilast in the management of chronic obstructive pulmonary disease. *Am J Health Syst Pharm* 2013;70:2087-2095.
40. Korbila IP, Manta KG, Siempos II, Dimopoulos G, Falagas ME. Penicillins vs trimethoprim-based regimens for acute bacterial exacerbations of chronic bronchitis: Meta-analysis of randomized controlled trials. *Can Fam Physician* 2009;55:60-67.
41. Gotfried MH, Grossman RF. Short-course fluoroquinolones in acute exacerbations of chronic bronchitis. *Expert Rev Respir Med* 2010;4:661-672.
42. Nicolau DP, Sutherland C, Winget D, Baughman RP. Bronchopulmonary pharmacokinetic and pharmacodynamic profiles of levofloxacin 750 mg once daily in adults undergoing treatment for acute exacerbation of chronic bronchitis. *Pulm Pharmacol Ther* 2012;25:94-98.
43. Chuchalin A, Zakharova M, Dokic D, et al. Efficacy and safety of moxifloxacin in acute exacerbations of chronic bronchitis: A prospective, multicenter, observational study (AVANTI). *BMC Pulm Med* 2013;13:5.
44. Rohde GG, Koch A, Welte T. Randomized double blind placebo-controlled study to demonstrate that antibiotics are not needed in moderate acute exacerbations of COPD—The ABACOPD study. *BMC Pulm Med* 2015;15:5.
45. Laopaiboon MR, Panpanich R, Swa Mya K. Azithromycin for acute lower respiratory tract infections. *Cochrane Database Syst Rev* 2015;3:CD001954.
46. Euba B, Moleres J, Segura V, et al. Genome expression profiling-based identification and administration efficacy of host-directed antimicrobial drugs against respiratory infection by nontypable Haemophilus influenzae. *Antimicrob Agents Chemother* 2015;59:7581-7592.
47. Korbila I, Manta KG, Siempos II, Dimopoulos G, Falagas ME. Penicillins vs trimethoprim-based regimens for acute bacterial exacerbations of chronic bronchitis: Meta-analysis of randomized controlled trials. *Can Fam Physician* 2009;55:60-67.
48. Herath SC, Poole P. Prophylactic antibiotic therapy for chronic obstructive pulmonary disease (COPD). *Cochrane Database Syst Rev* 2013;11:CD009764.
49. Herath SC, Poole P. Prophylactic antibiotic therapy in chronic obstructive pulmonary disease. *JAMA* 2014;311:2225-2226.
50. Spagnolo P, Fabbri LM, Bush A. Long-term macrolide treatment for chronic respiratory disease. *Eur Respir J* 2013;42:239-251.
51. Tse HN, Tseng CZ. Update on the pathological processes, molecular biology, and clinical utility of N-acetylcysteine in chronic obstructive pulmonary disease. *Int J Chron Obstruct Pulmon Dis* 2014;9:825-836.
52. Fischer BM, Voynow JA, Ghio AJ. COPD: Balancing oxidants and antioxidants. *Int J Chron Obstruct Pulmon Dis* 2015;10:261-276.
53. Stempel HE, Martin ET, Kuypers J, Englund JA, Zerr DM. Multiple viral respiratory pathogens in children with bronchiolitis. *Acta Paediatr* 2009;98:123-126.
54. Teshome G, Gattu R, Brown R. Acute bronchiolitis. *Pediatr Clin North Am* 2013;60:1019-1034.
55. Schuh S. Update on management of bronchiolitis. *Curr Opin Pediatr* 2011;23:110-114.
56. Schroeder AR, Mansbach JM. Recent evidence on the management of bronchiolitis. *Curr Opin Pediatr* 2014;26:328-333.
57. Ralston SL, Lieberthal AS, Meissner HC, et al. Clinical practice guideline: The diagnosis, management, and prevention of bronchiolitis. *Pediatrics* 2014;134:e1474-e502.
58. Plint AC, Johnson DW, Patel H, et al. Epinephrine and dexamethasone in children with bronchiolitis. *N Engl J Med* 2009;360:2079-2089.
59. Hartling L, Fernandes RM, Bialy L, et al. Steroids and bronchodilators for acute bronchiolitis in the first two years of life: Systematic review and meta-analysis. *BMJ* 2011;342:d1714.
60. Perrin KM, Begue RE. Use of palivizumab in primary practice. *Pediatrics* 2012;129:55-61.
61. Nseir S, Mathieu D. Antibiotic treatment for severe community-acquired pneumonia: Beyond antimicrobial susceptibility. *Crit Care Med* 2012;40:2500-2502.
62. Segal LN, Rom WN, Weiden MD. Lung microbiome for clinicians. New discoveries about bugs in healthy and diseased lungs. *Ann Am Thorac Soc* 2014;11:108-116.
63. Musher DM, Thorner AR. Community-acquired pneumonia. *N Engl J Med* 2014;371:1619-1628.
64. Prina E, Ranzani OT, Torres A. Community-acquired pneumonia. *Lancet* 2015;386:1097-1108.
65. Anand N, Kollef M. The alphabet soup of pneumonia: CAP, HAP, HCAP, NHAP, and VAP. *Semin Respir Crit Care Med* 2009;30:3-9.
66. Marrie TJ, Costain N, La Scola B, et al. The role of atypical pathogens in community-acquired pneumonia. *Semin Respir Crit Care Med* 2012;33:244-256.
67. Waterer GW. Community-acquired pneumonia: Genomics, epigenomics, transcriptomics, proteomics, and metabolomics. *Semin Respir Crit Care Med* 2012;33:257-265.
68. Wang H, Zhang K, Qin H, et al. Genetic association between CD143 rs4340 polymorphism and pneumonia risk: A meta analysis. *Medicine (Baltimore)* 2015;94:e883.
69. Gordin FM, Masur H. Current approaches to tuberculosis in the United States. *JAMA* 2012;308:283-289.
70. Mitruka K, Oeltmann JE, Ijaz K, Haddad MB. Tuberculosis outbreak investigations in the United States, 2002-2008. *Emerg Infect Dis* 2011;17:425-431.
71. Eccles S, Pincus C, Higgins B, Woodhead M. Diagnosis and management of community and hospital acquired pneumonia in adults: Summary of NICE guidance. *BMJ* 2014;349:g6722.
72. Buising KL, Thursky KA, Black JF, et al. A prospective comparison of severity scores for identifying patients with severe community acquired pneumonia: Reconsidering what is meant by severe pneumonia. *Thorax* 2006;61:419-424.
73. Pereira JM, Paiva JA, Rello J. Assessing severity of patients with community-acquired pneumonia. *Semin Respir Crit Care Med* 2012;33:272-283.
74. Zilberberg M, Shorr A. Epidemiology of healthcare-associated pneumonia (HCAP). *Semin Respir Crit Care Med* 2009;30:10-15.
75. Hunter JD. Ventilator associated pneumonia. *BMJ* 2012;344:e3325.
76. Porzecanski I, Bowton D. Diagnosis and treatment of ventilator-associated pneumonia. *Chest* 2006;130:597-604.
77. Punpanich W, Groome M, Muhe L, Qazi SA, Madhi SA. Systematic review on the etiology and antibiotic treatment of pneumonia in human immunodeficiency virus-infected children. *Pediatr Infect Dis J* 2011;30:e192-e202.
78. Smith TJ, Khatcheressian J, Lyman GH, et al. 2006 update of recommendations for the use of white blood cell growth factors: an evidence-based clinical practice guideline. *J Clin Oncol* 2006;24:3187-3205.
79. Pettersson K. Perinatal infection with Group B streptococci. *Semin Fetal Neonatal Med* 2007;12:193-197.
80. Falcone M, Venditti M, Shindo Y, Kollef MH. Healthcare-associated pneumonia: Diagnostic criteria and distinction from community-acquired pneumonia. *Int J Infect Dis* 2011;15:e545-e550.
81. de Vrankrijker AM, Wolfs TF, van der Ent CK. Challenging and emerging pathogens in cystic fibrosis. *Paediatr Respir Rev* 2010;11:246-254.
82. Bartlett JG. Anaerobic bacterial infection of the lung. *Anaerobe* 2012;18:235-239.
83. Cunha BA, Burillo A, Bouza E. Legionnaires' disease. *Lancet* 2016; 387:376-85.
84. Phin N, Parry-Ford F, Harrison T, et al. Epidemiology and clinical management of Legionnaires' disease. *Lancet Infect Dis* 2014;14:1011-1021.
85. Morozumi MT, Takahashi T, Ubukata K. Macrolide-resistant Mycoplasma pneumoniae: Characteristics of isolates and clinical aspects of community-acquired pneumonia. *J Infect Chemother* 2010;16:78-86.
86. Narita M. Pathogenesis of extrapulmonary manifestations of Mycoplasma pneumoniae infection with special reference to pneumonia. *J Infect Chemother* 2010;16:162-169.
87. Olson D, Watkins LK, Demirjian A, et al. Outbreak of Mycoplasma pneumoniae-Associated Stevens-Johnson Syndrome. *Pediatrics* 2015;136:e386-e394.
88. Saraya T, Kurai D, Nakagaki K, et al. Novel aspects on the pathogenesis of Mycoplasma pneumoniae pneumonia and therapeutic implications. *Front Microbiol* 2014;5:410.
89. Blasi FP, Tarsia P, Aliberti S. Chlamydophila pneumoniae. *Clin Microbiol Infect* 2009;15:29-35.
90. Centers for Disease Control and Prevention (CDC). Update: Novel influenza A (H1N1) virus infections—Worldwide, May 6, 2009. *MMWR Morb Mortal Wkly Rep* 2009;58:453-458.
91. Hui DS, Zumla A. Emerging respiratory tract viral infections. *Curr Opin Pulm Med* 2015;21:284-292.

92. Sampathkumar P, Temesgen Z, Smith T, Thompson R. SARS: Epidemiology, clinical presentation, management, and infection control measures. *Mayo Clin Proc* 2003;78:882-890.
93. Coughlin MM, Prabhakar BS. Neutralizing human monoclonal antibodies to severe acute respiratory syndrome coronavirus: Target, mechanism of action, and therapeutic potential. *Rev Med Virol* 2012;22:2-17.
94. Ottosen J, Evans H. Pneumonia: Challenges in the definition, diagnosis, and management of disease. *Surg Clin North Am* 2014;94:1305-1317.
95. Lebeaux D, Ghigo JM, Beloin C. Biofilm-related infections: Bridging the gap between clinical management and fundamental aspects of recalcitrance toward antibiotics. *Microbiol Mol Biol Rev* 2014;78:510-543.
96. Wunderink RG, Mandell L. Adjunctive therapy in community-acquired pneumonia. *Semin Respir Crit Care Med* 2012;33:311-318.
97. Rodvold KA, George JM, Yoo L. Penetration of anti-infective agents into pulmonary epithelial lining fluid: Focus on antibacterial agents. *Clin Pharmacokinet* 2011;50:637-664.
98. Kollef MH, Hamilton CW, Montgomery AB. Aerosolized antibiotics: Do they add to the treatment of pneumonia? *Curr Opin Infect Dis* 2013;26:538-544.
99. Owens RJ, Shorr A. Rational dosing of antimicrobial agents: Pharmacokinetic and pharmacodynamic strategies. *Am J Health Syst Pharm* 2009;66(Suppl 4):S23-S30.
100. Safdar A, Shelburne S, Evans S, Dickey B. Inhaled therapeutics for prevention and treatment of pneumonia. *Expert Opin Drug Saf* 2009;8:435-449.
101. Palmer L. Aerosolized antibiotics in critically ill ventilated patients. *Curr Opin Crit Care* 2009;15:413-418.
102. Muscedere J, Dodek P, Keenan S, et al. Comprehensive evidence-based clinical practice guidelines for ventilator-associated pneumonia: Diagnosis and treatment. *J Crit Care* 2008;23:138-147.
103. Sharpe B. Guideline-recommended antibiotics in community-acquired pneumonia: Not perfect, but good. *Arch Intern Med* 2009;169:1462-1464.
104. Feldman C, Anderson R. Antibiotic resistance of pathogens causing community-acquired pneumonia. *Semin Respir Crit Care Med* 2012;33:232-243.
105. Pugh R, Grant C, Cooke RP, Dempsey G. Short-course versus prolonged-course antibiotic therapy for hospital-acquired pneumonia in critically ill adults. *Cochrane Database Syst Rev* 2015;8:CD007577.
106. Luyt C, Combes A, Nieszkowska A, et al. Aerosolized antibiotics to treat ventilator-associated pneumonia. *Curr Opin Infect Dis* 2009;22:154-158.
107. Gattarello S. What is new in antibiotic therapy in community-acquired pneumonia? An evidence-based approach focusing on combined therapy. *Curr Infect Dis Rep* 2015;17:501.
108. Gross AE, Bryson ML. Oral ribavirin for the treatment of noninfluenza respiratory viral infections: A systematic review. *Ann Pharmacother* 2015;49:1125-1135.
109. Tablan O, Anderson L, Besser R, et al. Guidelines for preventing health-care–associated pneumonia, 2003: Recommendations of CDC and the Healthcare Infection Control Practices Advisory Committee. *MMWR Recomm Rep* 2004;53:1-36.
110. Hayes DJ, Meyer K. Acute exacerbations of chronic bronchitis in elderly patients: Pathogenesis, diagnosis, and management. *Drugs Aging* 2007;24:555-572.

108

Upper Respiratory Tract Infections

Christopher Frei and Bradi Frei

KEY CONCEPTS

1. Many upper respiratory tract infections will resolve spontaneously without pharmacologic therapy.
2. The most common bacterial causes are *Streptococcus pneumoniae* (acute otitis media and acute rhinosinusitis) and group A β-hemolytic *Streptococcus* (acute pharyngitis).
3. Vaccination against influenza and pneumococcus may decrease the risk of acute otitis media.
4. Because upper respiratory tract infections are so common, antibiotics used to treat them serve as catalysts for the emergence and spread of antibiotic resistance, thereby making prudent antibiotic use critically important.
5. When antibiotics are prescribed, the empirical medications of choice are amoxicillin or amoxicillin-clavulanate for acute otitis media, amoxicillin-clavulanate for acute rhinosinusitis, and amoxicillin or penicillin for acute pharyngitis.
6. For acute otitis media, high-dose amoxicillin (80-90 mg/kg/day in two divided doses) is recommended.

More patients present to physicians' offices and emergency departments for upper respiratory tract infections than any other infectious disease.[1,2] Otitis media, rhinosinusitis, and pharyngitis are the three most common upper respiratory tract infections. Because they are so common, community and emergency health care workers must be familiar with the diagnosis, assessment, and management of patients with these infections. Furthermore, antibiotics used for the treatment of upper respiratory tract infections serve as catalysts for the emergence and spread of antibiotic resistance, thereby making prudent antibiotic use critically important.

ACUTE OTITIS MEDIA

The term *otitis media* comes from the Latin *oto-* for "ear," *itis* for "inflammation," and *medi-* for "middle"; otitis media, then, is an inflammation of the middle ear. There are three subtypes of otitis media: acute otitis media, otitis media with effusion, and chronic otitis media. Acute otitis media is the subtype with the greatest role for antibiotics and will be discussed in detail.

Epidemiology

Otitis media is one of the leading reasons for physicians' office visits and emergency department visits in the United States, accounting for more than 16 million clinic and emergency department visits annually.[1,2] There are more than 709 million cases of otitis media worldwide each year; half of these cases occur in children under 5 years of age.[3] Many patients with otitis media will receive a prescription, and the costs associated with managing otitis media are $2.3 billion annually in the United States.[4]

Etiology

(1) When comprehensive and sensitive microbiologic methods have been used in patients with a certain diagnosis of acute otitis media, bacteria have been found in more than 90% of cases; with standard diagnostic and microbiologic testing, bacteria have been found in approximately 70% of cases.[5]

(2) Common bacterial pathogens include *Streptococcus pneumoniae*, nontypeable *Haemophilus influenzae*, and *Moraxella catarrhalis*.[6] The microbial etiology has changed as a result of the introduction and widespread use of the pneumococcal conjugate vaccines. Specifically, the proportion of *S. pneumoniae* cases has declined, and the proportion of *H. influenzae* cases has risen.[7] Today, these two pathogens occur in approximately equal proportions.[5]

S. pneumoniae, *H. influenzae*, and *M. catarrhalis* can all possess resistance to β-lactams. *S. pneumoniae* develops resistance through alteration of penicillin-binding proteins, whereas *H. influenzae* and *M. catarrhalis* produce β-lactamases. Up to 40% of *S. pneumoniae* isolates in the United States are penicillin nonsusceptible, and up to half of these have high-level penicillin resistance.[8] Approximately 30% to 40% of *H. influenzae* and greater than 90% of *M. catarrhalis* isolates from the upper respiratory tract produce β-lactamases.[9]

Pathophysiology

Acute otitis media usually follows a viral upper respiratory tract infection that impairs the mucociliary apparatus and causes Eustachian tube dysfunction in the middle ear.[6] The middle ear is the space behind the tympanic membrane, or eardrum. A noninfected ear has a thin, clear tympanic membrane. In otitis media, this space becomes blocked with fluid, resulting in a bulging and erythematous tympanic membrane. Bacteria that colonize the nasopharynx enter the middle ear and are not cleared properly by the mucociliary system. The bacteria proliferate and cause infection. Children tend to be more susceptible to otitis media than adults because the anatomy of their Eustachian tube is shorter and more horizontal, facilitating bacterial entry into the middle ear.

Clinical Presentation

Patients or caregivers frequently characterize acute otitis media as having an acute onset of otalgia (ear pain). For parents of young children, irritability and tugging on the ear are often the first clues that a child has acute otitis media.

The American Academy of Pediatrics (AAP) guidelines have stringent diagnostic criteria to ensure accurate diagnosis. Children should be diagnosed with acute otitis media if they have middle ear effusion *and* either (1) moderate to severe bulging of the tympanic membrane *or* new onset otorrhea not due to acute otitis externa or (2) mild bulging of the tympanic membrane *and* onset of ear pain within the last 48 hours or intense erythema of the tympanic membrane. Middle ear effusion should be identified based on pneumatic otoscopy and/or tympanometry.[5]

CLINICAL PRESENTATION Acute Otitis Media

General

- Cases of acute otitis media often follow viral upper respiratory tract infections. Nonverbal children with ear pain might hold, rub, or tug their ear. Very young children might cry, be irritable, and have difficulty sleeping.

Signs and Symptoms

- Bulging of the tympanic membrane
- Otorrhea
- Otalgia (considered to be moderate or severe if pain lasts at least 48 hours)
- Fever (considered to be severe if temperature is 39°C [102.2°F] or higher)

Compiled from references 5 and 6.

The diagnoses of acute otitis media and otitis media with effusion are easily confused, and careful attention to history, signs, and symptoms is important. Otitis media with effusion is characterized by fluid in the middle ear without signs and symptoms of acute ear infection, such as pain and a bulging eardrum.[6,7]

TREATMENT

Desired Outcomes

6 Treatment goals include pain management and prudent antibiotic use. These will be discussed in detail, but, first, it is important to consider primary prevention of acute otitis media through the use of bacterial and viral vaccines.

3 Clinicians should recommend pneumococcal conjugate vaccine and annual influenza vaccine to all children according the Advisory Committee on Immunization Practices (ACIP) schedule from the United States Centers for Disease Control and Prevention.[5] A systematic review demonstrated that the seven-valent pneumococcal conjugate vaccine (PCV7) reduced the occurrence of acute otitis media episodes by 6% to 7% when the vaccine was administered during infancy.[10] Finally, because acute otitis media cases often follow influenza cases, influenza vaccination should be considered as a possible means to prevent acute otitis media.

General Approach to Treatment

The first step is to differentiate acute otitis media from otitis media with effusion or chronic otitis media, as the latter two types do not benefit substantially from antibiotic therapy. If the child has acute otitis media, then consider if the disease severity warrants antibiotic therapy. Recognize that amoxicillin is the mainstay of therapy and that penicillin resistance can be overcome, in many cases, with higher doses of amoxicillin. Address the child's pain as described below. The therapeutic strategy should be changed if complications develop or if symptoms fail to resolve within 3 days.

Nonpharmacologic Therapy

Children with acute otitis media should be assessed for pain. Those with pain should be offered treatment to reduce pain regardless of the decision to administer antibiotics.[5] This is largely because antibiotics do not reduce pain in the first 24 hours. Furthermore, some children may experience some pain up to 3 to 7 days even after antibiotics are started. Choice of pain treatment depends on possible benefits and risks to the individual patient. Acetaminophen and ibruprofen are mainstays of treatment, are effective analgesics for mild to moderate pain, and are readily available. Eardrops with a local anesthetic may offer additional, but brief, benefit over acetaminophen in patients at least 5 years of age.[5]

Pharmacologic Therapy

National clinical practice guidelines for appropriate diagnosis and management of acute otitis media were updated in 2013, by the AAP.[5] These guidelines are focused on children 6 months to 12 years of age with uncomplicated cases and without underlying conditions that may alter the natural course of the disease.

The decision to administer antibiotics depends on patient age, symptom severity, laterality, and joint decision-making with parents/caregivers. Children 6 months to 12 years of age, with moderate to severe ear pain or temperature of 39°C (102.2°F) or higher should receive antibiotics. Children 6 to 23 months of age, with nonsevere bilateral acute otitis media should also receive antibiotics. Children 6 to 23 months, with nonsevere unilateral acute otitis media, and children 24 months to 12 years of age, with nonsevere acute otitis media, may receive *initial antibiotics* or *initial observation*. Initial observation should be based on joint decision-making with parents/caregivers, and must include a plan to initiate antibiotics if the child's symptoms worsen or decline within 48 to 72 hours of symptom onset.[5] The central principle is to administer antibiotics quickly when the diagnosis is certain, but to withhold antibiotics, at least initially, when the diagnosis is uncertain.

4 Antibiotic therapy for upper respiratory diseases must be balanced with possible increases in adverse drug events and increased antibiotic pressure. Systematic reviews and randomized controlled trials suggest a moderate benefit of antibiotics for the treatment of acute otitis media, particularly in patients with severe symptoms.[7,11-14] On the other hand, rates of adverse effects, such as diarrhea and diaper rash, are more than double in children who received antibiotics for acute otitis media.[13,14]

5 If antibiotics are to be administered, then amoxicillin should be given to most children.[5] Exceptions include: children who have received amoxicillin in the last 30 days, have concurrent purulent conjunctivitis, or have a history of recurrent infection unresponsive to amoxicillin. These patients should receive amoxicillin-clavulanate instead of amoxicillin. Patients with otitis conjunctivitis syndrome are more likely to be infected with nontypeable *H. influenzae*, hence the need for a β-lactamase inhibitor.[5] Clinicians should reassess the plan if the child's symptoms worsen or decline within 48 to 72 hours of symptom onset.[5] Table 108-1 lists antibiotic recommendations for acute otitis media.

High-dose amoxicillin (80-90 mg/kg/day in two divided doses) is recommended for most patients. Amoxicillin has the best pharmacodynamic profile against drug-resistant *S. pneumoniae* of all available oral antibiotics. In addition, amoxicillin has a long record of safety, possesses a narrow spectrum of activity, is inexpensive, and is more palatable than other options. Higher middle ear fluid concentrations of amoxicillin, as a result of higher dosing, overcome most drug-resistant *S. pneumoniae*.[5] Its excellent efficacy against *S. pneumoniae* outweighs the issue of β-lactamase-producing

TABLE 108-1 Antibiotics and Doses for Acute Otitis Media

Antibiotic	Brand Name	Dose	Comments[a]
Initial Diagnosis			
Amoxicillin	Amoxil®	80-90 mg/kg/day orally divided twice daily	First-line
Amoxicillin-clavulanate	Augmentin®	90 mg/kg/day orally of amoxicillin plus 6.4 mg/kg/day orally of clavulanate, divided twice daily	First-line if certain criteria are present[b]
Cefdinir, cefuroxime, cefpodoxime	Omnicef®, Ceftin®, Vantin®	cefdinir (14 mg/kg/day orally in 1-2 doses) cefuroxime (30 mg/kg/day orally in 2 divided doses) cefpodoxime (10 mg/kg/day orally in 2 divided doses)	Second-line or nonsevere penicillin allergy
Ceftriaxone (1-3 days)	Rocephin®	50 mg/kg/day IM or IV for 3 days	Second-line or nonsevere penicillin allergy
Failure at 48-72 Hours			
Amoxicillin-clavulanate[b]	Augmentin®	90 mg/kg/day orally of amoxicillin plus 6.4 mg/kg/day orally of clavulanate, divided twice daily	First-line
Ceftriaxone (1-3 days)	Rocephin®	50 mg/kg/day IM or IV for 3 days	First-line or nonsevere penicillin allergy
Clindamycin	Cleocin®	30-40 mg/kg/day orally in 3 divided doses plus third-generation cephalosporin	Second-line or nonsevere penicillin allergy

[a]If a patient has received amoxicillin in the last 30 days, has concurrent purulent conjunctivitis, or has a history of recurrent infection unresponsive to amoxicillin.

[b]Amoxicillin-clavulanate 90:6.4 or 14:1 ratio is available in the United States; 7:1 ratio is available in Canada (use amoxicillin 45 mg/kg for one dose, amoxicillin 45 mg/kg with clavulanate 6.4 mg/kg for second dose).

IM, intramuscular; IV, intravenous; po, orally.

Data from reference 5.

H. influenzae and *M. catarrhalis*, against which amoxicillin may not be effective. This is because both *H. influenzae* and *M. catarrhalis* are more likely than *S. pneumoniae* to lead to a spontaneous resolution of the infection.

If a patient has received amoxicillin in the last 30 days, has concurrent purulent conjunctivitis, or has a history of recurrent infection unresponsive to amoxicillin, then they should receive high-dose amoxicillin-clavulanate (90 mg/kg/day of amoxicillin, with 6.4 mg/kg/day of clavulanate, in two divided doses) instead of amoxicillin. Amoxicillin-clavulanate has activity against β-lactamase-producing *H. influenzae* and *M. catarrhalis* as well as drug-resistant *S. pneumoniae*.[5] Other antibiotic choices include cefdinir, cefuroxime, cefpodoxime, and intramuscular or intravenous ceftriaxone.[5] Second-generation cephalosporins, though β-lactamase stable, are expensive, have an increased incidence of side effects, and may increase selective pressure for resistant bacteria. Furthermore, most cephalosporins do not achieve adequate middle ear fluid concentrations against drug-resistant *S. pneumoniae* for the desired duration of the dosing interval. Use of trimethoprim-sulfamethoxazole and erythromycin-sulfisoxazole is discouraged because of high rates of resistance. Intramuscular ceftriaxone is the only antibiotic, other than amoxicillin, that achieves middle ear fluid concentrations above the minimal inhibitory concentration (MIC) for greater than 40% of the dosing interval. Although single doses of ceftriaxone have been used, daily doses for 3 days are recommended to optimize clinical outcomes.[5] Ceftriaxone is more expensive than amoxicillin and the intramuscular injections are painful. Patients with a penicillin allergy can be treated with several alternative antibiotics, including a cephalosporin in cases absent severe or type 1 penicillin allergy, or clindamycin. Notably, clindamycin lacks efficacy against *H. influenzae*, whereas macrolides lack efficacy against both *H. influenzae* and *S. pneumoniae*; therefore, macrolides are not recommended. Finally, tympanocentesis can also be considered for treatment failure or persistent acute otitis media. It has a therapeutic effect of relieving pain and pressure and can be used to collect fluid to identify the causative agent.

There is ongoing debate regarding the optimal duration of therapy for acute otitis media. Traditional recommendations call for 10 days of antibiotic therapy; however, some experts have speculated that patients can be treated for as little as 5 to 7 days. Unfortunately, the data to support the shorter courses are inconclusive, with some studies demonstrating similar outcomes and others demonstrating worse outcomes with short-course therapy.[7] Short-course treatment is not recommended in children younger than 2 years of age. In children at least 6 years of age who have mild to moderate acute otitis media, a 5- to 7-day course may be used.[5]

Clinical **Controversy...**

The 2013 AAP guidelines for acute otitis media recommend an *initial observation* approach prior to administering antibiotics in selected patients.[5] This is because many cases of acute otitis media will resolve without antibiotics, and the guideline authors believe that delayed therapy might serve as a mechanism to reduce antibiotic overuse. A systematic review supports this view, maintaining that antibiotics had only a slight benefit on pain after the first day and only a modest effect on the number of children with tympanic perforations, contralateral otitis episodes, and abnormal tympanometry findings.[12] However, others believe that the modest benefit seen in these systematic reviews is because as many as half of the included patients did not have acute otitis media.[15,16] A placebo-controlled trial, with precise diagnostic criteria, *did* find that antibiotics reduced the time to resolution of middle ear effusion and normal otoscopy findings in children with otitis media.[11] This debate will continue, but there seems to be general agreement that precise diagnostics are key.[5] Unfortunately, there is also debate as to whether such diagnostic approaches are possible in the general clinical setting.[15,17]

Recurrent acute otitis media is defined as at least 3 episodes in 6 months or 4 episodes in 1 year, with 1 episode in the preceding 6 months. Recurrent episodes are of concern because children younger than 3 years of age are at high risk for hearing loss and language and learning disabilities. Clinicians should not prescribe antibiotics as prophylaxis against recurrent episodes, but they may offer tympanostomy tubes (T tubes).[5]

Personalized Pharmacotherapy

Procalcitonin increases in response to bacterial infection and declines as the infection resolves. Clinicians are starting to use procalcitonin blood levels to decide when to initiate and discontinue antibiotics in patients with acute upper respiratory infections (URIs).[18] A Cochrane systematic review of 14 trials with 4,221 participants found that procalcitonin protocols significantly reduced antibiotic consumption without negatively impacting patient survival or treatment failure.[19] The finding was driven by lower prescription rates in primary care and shorter durations of antibiotic therapy in emergency departments and intensive care units.[19] Despite the enthusiasm for this approach, there are still several aspects of procalcitonin monitoring that need to be resolved, including the timing of levels, the procalcitonin cutoff values for different clinical decision points, and the cost-effectiveness of this technology.[20]

Evaluation of Therapeutic Outcomes

Patients with acute otitis media should be reassessed after 48 to 72 hours. By this time, there should be clinical improvement in the signs and symptoms of infection, including pain, fever, and erythema/bulging of the tympanic membrane. If the patient has not responded and antibiotics were withheld initially, they should be instituted now. If the patient initially received an antibiotic, then the antibiotic should be changed (Table 108-1). Most children will become asymptomatic at 7 days.

Early reevaluation of the eardrum when signs and symptoms are improving can be misleading because effusions persist. Over a period of 1 week, changes in the eardrum normalize, and the pus becomes serous fluid. Air-fluid levels are apparent behind the eardrum, at which point the stage is now referred to as *otitis media with effusion*. This does not represent ongoing infection, nor are additional antibiotics required.[5]

Immediate reevaluation is appropriate if hearing loss results from persistent middle ear effusions following infection. Complications of otitis media are infrequent but include mastoiditis, bacteremia, meningitis, and auditory sequelae with the potential for speech and language impairment.[5]

ACUTE BACTERIAL RHINOSINUSITIS

Sinusitis is an inflammation and/or infection of the paranasal sinuses, or membrane-lined air spaces, around the nose.[21] The term *rhinosinusitis* is now preferred because sinusitis typically also involves the nasal mucosa.[21] Even though the majority of rhinosinusitis infections are viral in origin, antibiotics are frequently prescribed. It is thus important to differentiate between viral and bacterial rhinosinusitis to avoid antibiotic overuse.

Clinical practice guidelines for acute bacterial rhinosinusitis were published in 2012.[21] Several of the recommendations in these guidelines differ substantially from prior guidelines.

Epidemiology

1 Nearly 30 million cases of rhinosinusitis are diagnosed annually in the United States.[22] Acute bacterial rhinosinusitis is overdiagnosed; thus, antibiotics are overprescribed. Most rhinosinusitis infections have a viral etiology, and yet, antibiotics are frequently prescribed. Adults with rhinosinusitis miss an average of 6 workdays/y with these infections.[23] Patients with rhinosinusitis are significantly more likely to use the emergency room, spend more than $500/y on medical care, and see a medical specialist.[23]

Etiology

2 Acute bacterial rhinosinusitis is caused, most often, by the same bacteria implicated in acute otitis media: *S. pneumoniae* and *H. influenzae*. These organisms are responsible for approximately 50% to 70% of bacterial causes of acute bacterial rhinosinusitis in both adults and children.[21] *M. catarrhalis* is also sometimes implicated in adults and children (approximately 8%-16%).[21] *Streptococcus pyogenes*, *Staphylococcus aureus*, gram-negative bacilli, and anaerobes are associated less frequently with acute bacterial rhinosinusitis.[21] Issues of bacterial resistance are similar to those found with acute otitis media.

Pathophysiology

Similar to acute otitis media, acute bacterial rhinosinusitis is often preceded by a viral respiratory tract infection that causes mucosal inflammation. This can lead to obstruction of the sinus ostia—the pathways that drain the sinuses.[6] Mucosal secretions become trapped, local defenses are impaired, and bacteria from adjacent surfaces begin to proliferate. The maxillary and ethmoid sinuses are most frequently involved.[6] The pathogenesis of chronic rhinosinusitis has not been well studied. Whether it is caused by more persistent pathogens or a subtle defect in the host's immune function, some patients develop chronic symptoms after their acute infection.

Clinical Presentation

The greatest barrier to efficient use of antibiotics in acute bacterial rhinosinusitis is the lack of a simple and accurate diagnostic test. The gold standard for diagnosis is sinus puncture with recovery of bacteria in high density (10^4 colony-forming units/mL [10^7 cfu/L]

CLINICAL PRESENTATION Acute Bacterial Rhinosinusitis

General

- There are three clinical presentations that are most consistent with acute bacterial versus viral rhinosinusitis:
- Onset with *persistent* signs or symptoms compatible with acute rhinosinusitis, lasting for ≥ 10 days without any evidence of clinical improvement
- Onset with *severe* signs or symptoms of high fever (≥39°C [102.2°F]) and purulent nasal discharge or facial pain lasting for at least 3 to 4 consecutive days at the beginning of illness
- Onset with *worsening* signs or symptoms characterized by new-onset fever, headache, or increase in nasal discharge following a typical viral URI that lasted 5 to 6 days and were initially improving ("double sickening")

Signs and Symptoms

- Purulent anterior nasal discharge, purulent or discolored posterior nasal discharge, nasal congestion or obstruction, facial congestion or fullness, facial pain or pressure, fever, headache, ear pain/pressure/fullness, halitosis, dental pain, cough, and fatigue

Data from reference 21.

or greater)[21]; however, sinus puncture is invasive and costly, and can be painful, so it is not routinely done. Sinus radiography can help, but it is not routinely recommended. Because there is no simple and accurate office-based test for acute bacterial rhinosinusitis, clinicians rely on clinical findings to make the diagnosis.

TREATMENT

Desired Outcomes

The goals of treatment for acute bacterial rhinosinusitis are to reduce signs and symptoms, achieve and maintain patency of the ostia, limit antibiotic treatment to those who may benefit, eradicate the bacterial infection with appropriate antibiotic therapy, minimize the duration of illness, prevent complications, and prevent progression from acute disease to chronic disease.

General Approach to Treatment

4 The first step is to delineate viral and bacterial rhinosinusitis. This is based on disease duration, initial severity of illness, and worsening symptomatology. Viral rhinosinusitis typically improves in 7 to 10 days; therefore, a diagnosis of acute bacterial rhinosinusitis requires persistent symptoms (10 days or greater) or a worsening of symptoms after 5 to 6 days. Acute bacterial rhinosinusitis may also be suspected if the patient has severe symptoms at the beginning of his/her illness. Amoxicillin-clavulanate is now recommended as the first-line antibiotic therapy for patients with acute bacterial rhinosinusitis.[21] Adjuvant, nonantibiotic therapies have a limited role.

The next step is to decide if the patient needs to be referred to a specialist. Potential reasons for referral include mental status changes, visual disturbances, immunosuppressive illness, nosocomial infections, anatomic defects causing obstruction and possibly requiring surgery, unusually severe symptoms, multiple recurrent episodes (3-4/y), unilateral findings, significant coexisting illnesses, risk factors for unusual or resistant pathogens, and history of antibiotic failure. The specialist may perform computed tomography to assess the severity and extent of disease and identify the underlying causes.

Nonpharmacologic Therapy

Several nonprescription therapies are used in the management of *nonbacterial rhinosinusitis* for symptomatic relief. These include nasal decongestant sprays that reduce inflammation by vasoconstriction. Use should be limited to no more than 3 days to prevent the development of tolerance and/or rebound congestion. Oral decongestants may also aid in nasal/sinus patency. Irrigation of the nasal cavity with saline and steam inhalation may be used to increase mucosal moisture, and mucolytics (eg, guaifenesin) may be used to decrease the viscosity of nasal secretions.

In contrast, if a patient is suspected of having *acute bacterial rhinosinusitis*, then decongestants and antihistamines are not recommended.[21] These can dry mucosa and disturb clearance of mucosal secretions. Other therapies are recommended to be used as adjuncts to antibiotics for patients with acute bacterial rhinosinusitis. Intranasal saline irrigation with either physiologic or hypertonic saline is recommended for adults,[21] but the evidence from a Cochrane review is unimpressive.[24] Intranasal corticosteroids are now recommended for patients with a history of allergic rhinitis.[25]

Pharmacologic Therapy

Several prestigious groups have published statements and clinical practice guidelines for the management of patients with acute bacterial rhinosinusitis, including the Academy of Pediatrics, the Sinus and Allergy Health Partnership, the American Academy of Otolaryngology—Head and Neck Surgery, the Agency for Healthcare Research and Quality, and the Joint Task Force on Practice Parameters, representing the American Academy of Allergy, Asthma, and Immunology, the American College of Allergy, Asthma, and Immunology, and the Joint Council of Allergy, Asthma, and Immunology. The Infectious Diseases Society of America (IDSA) published their clinical practice guideline in 2012;[21] these guidelines are the primary source for many of the statements in this chapter.

5 Amoxicillin-clavulanate is now the first-line treatment for acute bacterial rhinosinusitis in children and adults (Tables 108-2 and 108-3).[21] In contrast, prior guidelines, including the ones published by the Canadian government in 2011,[26] list amoxicillin as the first-line treatment option due to its safety, narrow spectrum of activity, good tolerability, and favorable cost. A randomized controlled trial questioned the value of amoxicillin in nonsevere cases of acute bacterial rhinosinusitis.[27] The IDSA guidelines support the choice of amoxicillin-clavulanate based on (a) the emergence of *H. influenzae* as a more common cause of upper respiratory tract infections in children than in the past[7,28] and (b) the high prevalence of β-lactam-producing respiratory pathogens in acute bacterial rhinosinusitis (particularly *H. influenzae* and *M. catarrhalis*). Recall that approximately 30% to 40% of *H. influenzae* and greater than 90% of *M. catarrhalis* isolates from the upper respiratory tract produce β-lactamases.[9] The advantage of using amoxicillin-clavulanate, as compared with amoxicillin, is a greater spectrum of coverage. The disadvantages are increased cost, greater risk of adverse effects including diarrhea, and an added risk of hypersensitivity to the clavulanate component.[21] No other antibiotics are recommended as first-line for initial empirical therapy.

High-dose amoxicillin-clavulanate is recommended as second-line for initial empirical therapy in children and adults; doxycycline is also second-line for adults but should be avoided in children.[21] High-dose amoxicillin-clavulanate is preferred in the following situations: (a) geographic regions with high endemic rates (10% or greater) of invasive penicillin-nonsusceptible *S. pneumoniae*, (b) severe infection, (c) attendance at daycare, (d) age less than 2 or greater than 65 years, (e) recent hospitalization, (f) antibiotic use within the last month, and (g) immunocompromised persons.[21] Severe infections are those with "evidence of systemic toxicity with fever of 39°C (102.2°F) or higher, and threat of suppurative complications."[21]

Clinical **Controversy...**

The IDSA guidelines support the use of intranasal corticosteroids for patients with acute bacterial rhinosinusitis, especially those who also have a history of allergic rhinitis; however, the guidelines are silent regarding the use of oral corticosteroids.[21] A Cochrane systematic review identified four randomized controlled trials with a total of 1,008 adult participants with acute bacterial rhinosinusitis.[29] All participants received oral antibiotics and either oral corticosteroids (prednisone 24-80 mg daily or betamethasone 1 mg daily) or a control treatment (placebo in three trials, nonsteroidal antiinflammatory drugs in one trial). All four trials observed faster resolution or improvement in symptoms among the patients who received oral corticosteroids. These studies did not report any information regarding the long-term effects of oral corticosteroids, such as relapse and recurrence of acute bacterial rhinosinusitis. This systematic review supports the use of oral corticosteroids as adjuvant therapy to antibiotics for the treatment of acute bacterial rhinosinusitis.

If a child has a β-lactam allergy, he/she may receive levofloxacin monotherapy or clindamycin plus cefixime or cefpodoxime combination therapy.[21] Adults may receive doxycycline, levofloxacin, or

TABLE 108-2 Antibiotics and Doses for Acute Bacterial Rhinosinusitis in Children

Antibiotic	Brand Name	Dose	Comments
Initial Empirical Therapy			
Amoxicillin-clavulanate	Augmentin®	45 mg/kg/day orally twice daily	First-line
Amoxicillin-clavulanate	Augmentin®	90 mg/kg/day orally twice daily	Second-line
***β*-Lactam Allergy**			
Clindamycin plus cefixime or cefpodoxime	Cleocin®, Suprax®, Vantin®	Clindamycin (30-40 mg/kg/day orally three times daily) plus cefixime (8 mg/kg/day orally twice daily) or cefpodoxime (10 mg/kg/day orally twice daily)	Non-type 1 allergy
Levofloxacin	Levaquin®	10-20 mg/kg/day orally every 12-24 hours	Type 1 allergy
Risk for Antibiotic Resistance or Failed Initial Therapy			
Amoxicillin-clavulanate	Augmentin®	90 mg/kg/day orally twice daily	
Clindamycin plus cefixime or cefpodoxime	Cleocin®, Suprax®, Vantin®	Clindamycin (30-40 mg/kg/day orally three times daily) plus cefixime (8 mg/kg/day orally twice daily) or cefpodoxime (10 mg/kg/day orally twice daily)	
Levofloxacin	Levaquin®	10-20 mg/kg/day orally every 12-24 hours	
Severe Infection Requiring Hospitalization			
Ampicillin-sulbactam	Unasyn®	200-400 mg/kg/day IV every 6 hours	
Ceftriaxone	Rocephin®	50 mg/kg/day IV every 12 hours	
Cefotaxime	Claforan®	100-200 mg/kg/day IV every 6 hours	
Levofloxacin	Levaquin®	10-20 mg/kg/day IV every 12-24 hours	

Data from reference 21.

moxifloxacin monotherapy.[21] The guidelines also provide several options for patients at risk for antibiotic resistance, who failed initial therapy, or who have a severe infection requiring hospitalization (Tables 108-2 and 108-3).[21] Notably, cephalosporins are no longer recommended as monotherapy due to variable rates of resistance against *S. pneumoniae*.[21] Macrolides are no longer recommended because of high rates of *S. pneumoniae* resistance.[21] Trimethoprim-sulfamethoxazole has not been recommended for some time due to resistance among *S. pneumoniae* and *H. influenzae*.[21]

The duration of therapy for the treatment of acute bacterial rhinosinusitis is not well established. Most trials have used 10- to 14-day antibiotic courses for uncomplicated rhinosinusitis, and the guidelines support this treatment duration in children.[21] For adults, the recommended duration is only 5 to 7 days.[21]

Personalized Pharmacotherapy

There is limited evidence to suggest that people with certain genetic polymorphisms may be at greater risk for chronic rhinosinusitis[30]; however, no such link has been identified for acute bacterial rhinosinusitis. Furthermore, patient genetics are not currently used to guide selection of antibiotic therapy for this condition. It is important to consider patient weight and renal function when selecting

TABLE 108-3 Antibiotics and Doses for Acute Bacterial Rhinosinusitis in Adults

Antibiotic	Brand Name	Dose	Comments
Initial Empirical Therapy			
Amoxicillin-clavulanate	Augmentin®	500 mg/125 mg orally three times daily, or 875 mg/125 mg orally twice daily	First-line
Amoxicillin-clavulanate	Augmentin®	2,000 mg/125 mg orally twice daily	Second-line
Doxycycline		100 mg orally twice daily or 200 mg orally once daily	Second-line
***β*-Lactam Allergy**			
Doxycycline		100 mg orally twice daily or 200 mg orally once daily	
Levofloxacin	Levaquin®	500 mg orally once daily	
Moxifloxacin	Avelox®	400 mg orally once daily	
Risk for Antibiotic Resistance or Failed Initial Therapy			
Amoxicillin-clavulanate	Augmentin®	2,000 mg/125 mg orally twice daily	
Levofloxacin	Levaquin®	500 mg orally once daily	
Moxifloxacin	Avelox®	400 mg orally once daily	
Severe Infection Requiring Hospitalization			
Ampicillin-sulbactam	Unasyn®	1.5-3 g IV every 6 hours	
Levofloxacin	Levaquin®	500 mg orally once daily	
Moxifloxacin	Avelox®	400 mg orally once daily	
Ceftriaxone	Rocephin®	1-2 g IV every 12-24 hours	
Cefotaxime	Claforan®	2 g IV every 4-6 hours	

Data from reference 21.

antibiotic therapy for acute bacterial rhinosinusitis. Notice that all of the antibiotics recommended for children are dosed according to patient weight. Furthermore, most of the recommended antibiotics are excreted through the kidneys and should be adjusted for renal function as described in the package labeling.

Evaluation of Therapeutic Outcomes

If symptoms persist or worsen after 48 to 72 hours of appropriate antibiotic therapy, then the patient should be reevaluated and alternative antibiotics should be considered.[21] Patients who do not respond to first- or second-line therapies should be referred to a specialist and worked up more aggressively, potentially with direct sinus aspiration or contrast-enhanced computed tomography.[21]

ACUTE PHARYNGITIS

1 2 Pharyngitis is an acute infection of the oropharynx or nasopharynx.[31] It is responsible for 1% to 2% of all outpatient visits.[32] Although viral causes are most common, group A β-hemolytic *Streptococcus* (GABHS; also known as *S. pyogenes*), is the primary bacterial cause;[31] pharyngitis due to GABHS is commonly known as "strep throat."

Clinical practice guidelines for GABHS were published in 2012.[31] Several of the recommendations in these guidelines differ substantially from prior guidelines.

Epidemiology

Acute pharyngitis accounts for approximately 2 million emergency department and outpatient department visits/y,[2] at a cost of up to $539 million for children alone.[31] Although viral causes are most common, GABHS is the primary bacterial cause and is associated with rare but severe sequelae if not treated appropriately.[31] Suppurative and nonsuppurative complications include acute rheumatic fever, acute glomerulonephritis, reactive arthritis, peritonsillar abscess, retropharyngeal abscess, cervical lymphadenitis, mastoiditis, otitis media, rhinosinusitis, and necrotizing fasciitis.

Although all age groups are susceptible, epidemiologic data demonstrate certain groups are at higher risk. Children 5 to 15 years of age are most susceptible; parents of school-age children and those who work with children are also at increased risk. Pharyngitis in a child younger than 3 years of age is rarely caused by GABHS.[31]

Seasonal outbreaks occur, and the incidence of GABHS is highest in winter and early spring.[31] The incubation period is 2 to 5 days, and the illness often occurs in clusters.[31] Spread occurs via direct contact (usually from hands) with droplets of saliva or nasal secretions, and transmission is thus worse in institutions, schools, families, and crowded areas.[31] Untreated, patients with streptococcal pharyngitis are infectious during the acute illness and for another week thereafter. Effective antibiotic therapy reduces the infectious period to about 24 hours.

Acute rheumatic fever is rarely seen in developed countries. In the United States, acute rheumatic fever secondary to GABHS infection was a cause of concern in the 1950s and was the major reason for penicillin therapy, but the annual incidence of this disease today is extremely rare (1 case or more per 1 million population); however, some risk does remain. Outbreaks have been reported in the United States as recently as the late 1980s and early 1990s. Furthermore, acute rheumatic fever is widespread in developing countries.

Etiology

1 Viruses cause the majority of acute pharyngitis cases. Specific etiologies include rhinovirus (20%), coronavirus (5%), adenovirus (5%), herpes simplex virus (4%), influenza virus (2%), parainfluenza virus (2%), and Epstein–Barr virus (1%).[31,32]

4 A bacterial etiology is far less likely. Of all the bacterial causes, GABHS is the most common (10%-30% of persons of all ages with pharyngitis) and is the only commonly occurring form of acute pharyngitis for which antibiotic therapy is indicated.[31] In the pediatric population, GABHS causes 15% to 30% of pharyngitis cases. In adults, GABHS is responsible for 5% to 15% of all symptomatic episodes of pharyngitis.[31]

Other, less common causes of acute pharyngitis, are groups C and G *Streptococcus*, *Corynebacterium diphtheriae*, *Neisseria gonorrhoeae*, *Mycoplasma pneumoniae*, *Arcanobacterium haemolyticum*, *Yersinia enterocolitica*, and *Chlamydia pneumoniae*.[31] Treatment options for these organisms are not addressed in this chapter.

Pathophysiology

The mechanism by which GABHS causes pharyngitis is not well defined. Asymptomatic pharyngeal carriers of the organism may have an alteration in host immunity (eg, a breach in the pharyngeal mucosa) and the bacteria of the oropharynx may migrate to cause an infection. Pathogenic factors associated with the organism itself may also play a role. These include pyrogenic toxins, hemolysins, streptokinase, and proteinase.

Clinical Presentation

Sore throat is the most common symptom of pharyngitis. Accurate differentiation of GABHS from pharyngitis caused by other agents is important for treatment decisions; however, this can be difficult even for experienced clinicians. Therefore, microbiologic testing is recommended for symptomatic patients unless they have symptoms suggestive of viral etiology or are younger than 3 years of age.[31]

In previous guidelines, clinical scoring systems, such as the Centor criteria or modifications of the Centor criteria, have been advocated for clinical diagnosis in adults as a way to overcome the lack of sensitivity and specificity of clinician judgment and to avoid laboratory testing of all patients; however, guidelines from Infectious Disease Society of America and the American Heart Association suggest testing be done in all patients with signs and symptoms of streptococcal pharyngitis.[31] Only those with a positive test for GABHS require antibiotic treatment.[31,33] Laboratory tests should not be performed unless the patient has symptoms consistent with GABHS pharyngitis. This is because a positive test does not necessarily indicate disease. A positive test may simply indicate that the patient is a carrier for GABHS and is not actively infected.

Approximately 20% of children are carriers; the prevalence is lower among adults.[31] There are several options to test for GABHS. A throat swab can be sent for culture or used for the RADT. Cultures are the gold standard, but they require 24 to 48 hours for results. The RADT is more practical in that it provides results quickly, it can be performed at the bedside, and it is less expensive than culture. If RADT is positive, it does not require a follow-up throat culture.[31] If RADT yields negative test results, it is generally recommended to follow up with a throat culture to confirm the results for children and adolescents, but not necessary in adults.[31] Delaying therapy while awaiting culture results does not affect the risk of complications (although some argue that symptomatic benefit is postponed, and contagion remains), and patients must be educated as to the value of waiting, given the low false-negative rate of RADT.[33]

TREATMENT

Desired Outcomes

The goals of treatment for pharyngitis are to improve clinical signs and symptoms, minimize adverse drug reactions, prevent transmission to close contacts, and prevent acute rheumatic fever and suppurative complications, such as peritonsillar abscess, cervical lymphadenitis, and mastoiditis.[31]

General Approach to Treatment

Once the diagnosis of GABHS pharyngitis has been made, the clinician must decide appropriate supportive care, when to initiate antibiotic therapy, the appropriate antibiotic, and the duration of therapy. The selection of appropriate antibiotic therapy will involve careful consideration of cost, safety, efficacy, potential for regimen adherence, and bacterial resistance rates. Clinicians should be aware of local resistance patterns, which may differ from the national patterns.

4 Antibiotic overuse has been well documented.[31,32] Antibiotics are prescribed for 60% of patients who visit their provider with a complaint of "sore throat."[34,35] This rate is well above the incidence of GABHS pharyngitis. Antibiotic therapy should be reserved for those patients with clinical and epidemiologic features of GABHS pharyngitis, preferably with a positive laboratory test. Empirical therapy is not recommended unless there is a high index of suspicion based on clinical or epidemiologic data and laboratory results are pending. However, it is important to discontinue empirical antibiotics if laboratory results are negative.

Nonpharmacologic Therapy

Supportive care should be offered to all patients with acute pharyngitis. Little evidence is available for nonpharmacologic therapy for pharyngitis. However, pharmacologic supportive care interventions include antipyretic medications, analgesics, and nonprescription lozenges and sprays containing menthol and topical anesthetics for temporary relief of pain.[31] There are limited data for use of corticosteroids to reduce the symptoms of GABHS pharyngitis, and given the risk of adverse effects, their use is not recommended.[31] Because pain is often the primary reason for visiting a physician, emphasis on analgesics such as acetaminophen and nonsteroidal antiinflammatory drugs to aid in pain relief is strongly recommended.

Pharmacologic Therapy

The clinical practice guidelines published by the IDSA in 2012 are the primary source for many of the recommendations in this chapter.[31] Tables 108-4 and 108-5 outline dosing for acute GABHS pharyngitis and chronic carriers of GABHS.

5 For over 30 years, GABHS isolated in the United States have been susceptible to penicillin, with no reported cases of GABHS resistance to penicillin.[31] Because penicillin and amoxicillin have a narrow spectrum of activity and are readily available, safe, and inexpensive, they are considered to be the treatments of choice.[31,33] In a controlled study that demonstrated that antibiotic therapy prevents rheumatic fever following GABHS pharyngitis was done with procaine penicillin, which was later replaced with benzathine penicillin.[33] Penicillin given by other routes is assumed to be equally efficacious. The ability of other antibiotics to eradicate GABHS has led to extrapolation that these antibiotics will also prevent rheumatic fever.[33]

Amoxicillin may be preferable for children with GABHS pharyngitis because the suspension is more palatable than penicillin.[31] Gastrointestinal (GI) adverse effects and rash are more common with amoxicillin. A once-daily, extended-release formulation of amoxicillin has been approved for treatment of GABHS pharyngitis in adults and children aged 12 years and older.[31]

If patients are unable to take oral medications, intramuscular benzathine penicillin can be given, although it is painful.[31] In penicillin-allergic patients, azithromycin, clarithromycin, clindamycin, or a first-generation cephalosporin such as cephalexin can be used if the reaction is non–immunoglobulin E (IgE)-mediated.[31,33] Newer macrolides, such as azithromycin and clarithromycin, are equally effective as erythromycin and cause fewer GI adverse effects; therefore, these newer macrolides are preferred to erythromycin. GABHS resistance to macrolides is low (5%-8%) in the United States, but is higher in some other areas of the world.[31]

In previous pharyngitis guidelines, clindamycin was only an alternative to erythromycin-resistant strains; however, it is now considered an acceptable alternative for penicillin-allergic patients due to the low GABHS resistance rate of 1%.[31,33] Tonsillectomy is not recommended because a Cochrane review found that its impact on "sore throat" due to pharyngitis is unpredictable.[36]

GABHS resistance rates to tetracyclines are high. Sulfonamides and trimethoprim-sulfamethoxazole have poor eradication rates for GABHS; therefore, use of these antibiotics is no longer recommended.[31] Fluoroquinolones are not recommended due to poor activity of the older agents. The newer fluoroquinolones have activity against GABHS, but are expensive and have a broad spectrum of activity.[31,33]

CLINICAL PRESENTATION Group A Streptococcal Pharyngitis

General

- A sore throat of sudden onset that is mostly self-limited
- Fever and constitutional symptoms resolving in about 3 to 5 days
- Clinical signs and symptoms are similar for viral causes and nonstreptococcal bacterial causes

Signs and Symptoms of GABHS Pharyngitis

- Sore throat
- Pain on swallowing
- Fever
- Headache, nausea, vomiting, and abdominal pain (especially in children)
- Erythema/inflammation of the tonsils and pharynx with or without patchy exudates
- Enlarged, tender lymph nodes
- Red swollen uvula, petechiae on the soft palate, and a scarlatiniform rash

Signs Suggestive of Viral Origin for Pharyngitis

- Conjunctivitis
- Coryza
- Cough

Laboratory Tests

- Throat swab and culture
- Rapid antigen-detection test (RADT)

Data from reference 31.

TABLE 108-4 Antibiotics and Doses for Group A β-Hemolytic Streptococcal Pharyngitis

Antibiotic	Brand Name	Dose	Duration	Rating
Preferred Antibiotics				
Penicillin V	Pen-V®	Children: 250 mg twice daily or three times daily orally Adult: 250 mg four times daily or 500 mg twice daily orally	10 days	IB
Penicillin G benzathine	Bicillin L-A®	< 27 kg: 0.6 million units; 27 kg or greater: 1.2 million units intramuscularly	One dose	IB
Amoxicillin[a]	Amoxil®	50 mg/kg once daily (maximum 1,000 mg); 25 mg/kg (maximum 500 mg) twice daily	10 days	IB
Penicillin Allergy				
Cephalexin	Keflex®	20 mg/kg/dose orally twice daily (maximum 500 mg/dose)	10 days	IB
Cefadroxil	Duricef®	30 mg/kg orally once daily (maximum 1 g)	10 days	IB
Clindamycin	Cleocin®	7 mg/kg/dose orally thrice daily (maximum 300 mg/dose)	10 days	IIaB
Azithromycin[b]	Zithromax®	12 mg/kg orally once daily (maximum 500 mg) for one day, then 6mg/kg orally once daily (maximum 250 mg) for four days	5 days	IIaB
Clarithromycin[b]	Biaxin®	15 mg/kg orally per day divided in two doses (maximum 250 mg twice daily)	10 days	IIaB

These guidelines provide a systematic weighting of the strength of the recommendation (Class I, conditions for which there is evidence and/or general agreement that a given procedure or treatment is beneficial, useful, and effective; Class II, conditions for which there is conflicting evidence and/or a divergence of opinion about the usefulness/efficacy of a procedure or treatment; Class IIa, weight of evidence/opinion is in favor of usefulness/efficacy; Class IIb, usefulness/efficacy is less well established by evidence/opinion; Class III, conditions for which there is evidence and/or general agreement that a procedure/treatment is not useful/effective and in some cases may be harmful) and quality of evidence (A, data derived from multiple randomized clinical trials or meta-analyses; B, data derived from a single randomized trial or nonrandomized studies; C, only consensus opinion of experts, cases studies, or standard of care).

[a]Standard formulation, not extended release.

[b]Resistance of group A β-hemolytic *Streptococcus* (GABHS) to these agents may vary and local susceptibilities should be considered with these agents.

Data from reference 31.

The ideal time to start antibiotics has not been established. The immediate start of antibiotics does not affect the risk of developing rheumatic fever, and no evidence suggests that it reduces recurrent infection.[33] Clinical guidelines recommend withholding antibiotics unless the patient has a positive laboratory result.[31,33]

The impact of appropriate antibiotic therapy is limited to decreasing the duration of signs and symptoms. It can decrease the severity of pharyngitis symptoms and communicability of the disease after 24 hours of antibiotic therapy.[37] The duration of therapy for GABHS pharyngitis is 10 days, except for benzathine penicillin and azithromycin, to maximize bacterial eradication.[31] A Cochrane review, published in 2012, examined short course therapy and concluded that 3 to 6 days of oral antibiotics had comparable efficacy to oral penicillin for 10 days.[38] Although some clinicians have proposed shorter courses of treatment for pharyngitis, confounding factors from these studies, such as the lack of strict entry criteria or differentiation between new and failed infections, limit the widespread application of short antibiotic courses at this time.[31]

Approximately 33% of household contacts of a person with acute GABHS pharyngitis harbor GABHS in their upper respiratory tracts.[31] Routine testing and/or treating of asymptomatic household contacts of an index patient is not recommended.[31] GABHS carriers do not need antimicrobial therapy due to very low risk of spreading GABHS pharyngitis or developing suppurative or nonsuppurative complications.[31] If tested, it is not necessary to treat these asymptomatic carriers. It is difficult to ascertain the cause of symptomatic pharyngitis in carriers of GABHS if they do develop symptoms. Providers should pay close attention to the symptoms to help differentiate viral versus bacteriologic cause of pharyngitis because laboratory tests will be positive in these patients.[31]

TABLE 108-5 Antibiotics and Doses for Eradication of Group A β-Hemolytic Streptococcal Pharyngitis in Chronic Carriers

Antibiotic	Brand Name	Dose
Clindamycin	Cleocin®	20-30 mg/kg/day orally in three divided doses (maximum 300 mg/dose)
Amoxicillin-clavulanate	Augmentin®	40 mg/kg/day orally in three divided doses (maximum 2,000 mg/day of amoxicillin)
Penicillin V and rifampin	Pen-V®, Rifadin®	Penicillin V: 50 mg/kg/day orally in four doses for 10 days (maximum 2,000 mg/day); *and* rifampin: 20 mg/kg/day orally in one dose for the last 4 days of treatment (maximum 600 mg/day)
Penicillin G benzathine and rifampin	Bicillin L-A®, Rifadin®	Penicillin G benzathine: < 27 kg—0.6 million units; 27 kg or greater—1.2 million units intramuscularly; *and* rifampin: 20 mg/kg/day orally in two doses during last 4 days of treatment with penicillin (maximum 600 mg/day)

Data from reference 31.

Clinical **Controversy...**

The ISDA pharyngitis guidelines recommend a 10-day course of appropriate antibiotics to achieve maximal rates of pharyngeal eradication of GABHS.[31] However, there has been increased interest in shorter courses of treatment to help improve adherence. Three antibiotics have been approved for 5-day course of therapy for GABHS pharyngitis, but these agents are not recommended as first-line therapy. The clinical trials for shorter course of antibiotic therapy tend to have less strict entry criteria, no assessment of adherence to therapy, and do not report details of outcomes, such as treatment failure or new infection. A Cochrane Review showed comparable efficacy for 3- to 6-day courses of therapy as compared to a 10-day course of oral penicillin.[38] The feasibility of shorter course therapy becoming a first-line recommendation needs to be determined in additional studies.

When acute GABHS pharyngitis occurs in a carrier, a treatment course of appropriate antibiotics is recommended.[31,33] In the treatment of recurring episodes of culture-positive GABHS pharyngitis, there are limited data to support a particular antibiotic regimen. Several alternative antibiotics are preferred over penicillin or amoxicillin with GABHS carriers and recurrent pharyngitis. Amoxicillin-clavulanate, clindamycin, penicillin/rifampin combination, and benzathine penicillin G/rifampin combination may be considered for recurrent episodes of pharyngitis to maximize bacterial eradication in potential carriers and to counter copathogens that produce β-lactamases.[31] Table 108-5 outlines dosing for eradication of GABHS in chronic carriers and those who experience symptomatic episodes.

Patients with documented histories of rheumatic fever (including cases manifested solely by Sydenham's chorea) and those with definite evidence of rheumatic heart disease should receive continuous prophylaxis initiated as soon as the patient is diagnosed and the initial infection has been treated. The duration of secondary prophylaxis is individualized based on patient risk of recurrence of rheumatic fever and/or rheumatic heart disease. Intramuscular benzathine penicillin G every 4 weeks is the recommended regimen for secondary prevention in the United States in most circumstances.[33] Additional options for secondary prophylaxis include oral penicillin V and sulfadiazine. Medication adherence is critical for successful secondary prevention with oral antibiotics. Sulfadiazine is an effective antibiotic for the prevention of infection and is appropriate if the patient is penicillin-allergic. Sulfonamides are not appropriate for treatment of GABHS pharyngitis because they are not effective for eradication of GABHS. If individuals are allergic to penicillin and sulfadiazine, a macrolide or azalide is recommended; however, this recommendation is based on expert opinion rather than clinical trial data.[33]

Personalized Pharmacotherapy

Currently, there are no pharmacogenetic or genomic factors involved in the diagnosis or treatment of GABHS pharyngitis. Factors that should be considered when personalizing therapy for a patient include allergy status, prior antibiotic use, and adherence. Those with a history of antibiotic use for acne may be at higher risk for resistant strains of GABHS. Short-course antibiotics or penicillin G benzathine may be considered in patients with a history of nonadherence.

Evaluation of Therapeutic Outcomes

Most pharyngitis cases are self-limited; however, antibiotics hasten resolution when given early for proven cases of GABHS pharyngitis.[31] Generally, fever and other symptoms resolve within 3 to 4 days of onset without antibiotics; however, symptoms will improve 0.5 to 2.5 days earlier with antibiotic therapy.[31] Follow-up testing is generally not necessary for index cases or asymptomatic contacts;[31] however, throat cultures 2 to 7 days after completion of antibiotics are warranted for patients who remain symptomatic or when symptoms recur despite completion of treatment.[33]

ABBREVIATIONS

AAP	American Academy of Pediatrics
ACIP	Advisory Committee on Immunization Practices
CFU	colony-forming unit
GABHS	group A β-hemolytic streptococci
GI	gastrointestinal
IDSA	Infectious Diseases Society of America
IgE	immunoglobulin E
MIC	minimal inhibitory concentration
PCV7	seven-valent pneumococcal conjugate vaccine
RADT	rapid antigen-detection test
T tube	tympanostomy tube
URI	upper respiratory infection

REFERENCES

1. Hsiao CJ, Cherry DK, Beatty PC, Rechtsteiner EA. National Ambulatory Medical Care Survey: 2007 summary. *Natl Health Stat Report* 2010;27:1-32.
2. Hing E, Hall MJ, Ashman JJ, Xu J. National Hospital Ambulatory Medical Care Survey: 2007 outpatient department summary. *Natl Health Stat Report* 2010;28:1-32.
3. Monasta L, Ronfani L, Marchetti F, et al. Burden of disease caused by otitis media: systematic review and global estimates. *PLoS One* 2012;7:e36226.
4. Roemer, M. Health care expenditures for the five most common children's conditions, 2008: estimates for U.S. civilian noninstitutionalized children, ages 0-17. Statistical Brief #349. December 2011. Agency for Healthcare Research and Quality, Rockville, MD, http://meps.ahrq.gov/mepsweb/data_files/publications/st349/stat349.shtml.
5. Lieberthal AS, Carroll AE, Chonmaitree T, et al. The diagnosis and management of acute otitis media. *Pediatrics* 2013;131:e964-999.
6. Wald ER. Acute otitis media and acute bacterial sinusitis. *Clin Infect Dis* 2011;52(suppl 4):S277-S283.
7. Coker TR, Chan LS, Newberry SJ, et al. Diagnosis, microbial epidemiology, and antibiotic treatment of acute otitis media in children: a systematic review. *JAMA* 2010;304:2161-2169.
8. Jones RN, Sader HS, Moet GJ, Farrell DJ. Declining antimicrobial susceptibility of *Streptococcus pneumoniae* in the United States: report from the SENTRY Antimicrobial Surveillance Program (1998-2009). *Diagn Microbiol Infect Dis* 2010;68:334-336.
9. Harrison CJ, Woods C, Stout G, Martin B, Selvarangan R. Susceptibilities of *Haemophilus influenzae, Streptococcus pneumoniae*, including serotype 19A, and *Moraxella catarrhalis* paediatric isolates from 2005 to 2007 to commonly used antibiotics. *J Antimicrob Chemother* 2009;63:511-519.
10. Jansen AG, Hak E, Veenhoven RH, Damoiseaux RA, Schilder AG, Sanders EA. Pneumococcal conjugate vaccines for preventing otitis media. *Cochrane Database Syst Rev* 2009;2:CD001480.
11. Tapiainen T, Kujala T, Renko M, et al. Effect of antimicrobial treatment of acute otitis media on the daily disappearance of middle ear effusion: a placebo-controlled trial. *JAMA Pediatr* 2014;168:635-641.
12. Venekamp RP, Sanders SL, Glasziou PP, Del Mar CB, Rovers MM. Antibiotics for acute otitis media in children. *Cochrane Database Syst Rev* 2015;6:CD000219.
13. Tahtinen PA, Laine MK, Huovinen P, Jalava J, Ruuskanen O, Ruohola A. A placebo-controlled trial of antimicrobial treatment for acute otitis media. *N Engl J Med* 2011;364:116-126.
14. Hoberman A, Paradise JL, Rockette HE, et al. Treatment of acute otitis media in children under 2 years of age. *N Engl J Med* 2011;364:105-115.
15. Pichichero ME. Antibiotics for children with acute otitis media—reply. *JAMA* 2015;313:1575.
16. Pichichero ME. Antibiotics for acute otitis media: yes or no. *JAMA* 2015;313:294-295.
17. Del Mar C, Venekamp RP, Sanders S. Antibiotics for children with acute otitis media. *JAMA* 2015;313:1574-1575.
18. Schuetz P, Briel M, Christ-Crain M, et al. Procalcitonin to guide initiation and duration of antibiotic treatment in acute respiratory infections: an individual patient data meta-analysis. *Clin Infect Dis* 2012;55:651-662.
19. Schuetz P, Muller B, Christ-Crain M, et al. Procalcitonin to initiate or discontinue antibiotics in acute respiratory tract infections. *Cochrane Database Syst Rev* 2012;9:CD007498.
20. Schuetz P, Amin DN, Greenwald JL. Role of procalcitonin in managing adult patients with respiratory tract infections. *Chest* 2012;141:1063-1073.
21. Chow AW, Benninger MS, Brook I, et al. Infectious Diseases Society of A. IDSA clinical practice guideline for acute bacterial rhinosinusitis in children and adults. *Clin Infect Dis* 2012;54:e72-e112.
22. Schiller JS, Lucas JW, Ward BW, Peregoy JA. Summary health statistics for U.S. adults: National Health Interview Survey, 2010. *Vital Health Stat 10* 2012;252:1-207.
23. Bhattacharyya N. Contemporary assessment of the disease burden of sinusitis. *Am J Rhinol Allergy* 2009;23:392-395.
24. Kassel JC, King D, Spurling GK. Saline nasal irrigation for acute upper respiratory tract infections. *Cochrane Database Syst Rev* 2010;3:CD006821.

25. Zalmanovici A, Yaphe J. Intranasal steroids for acute sinusitis. *Cochrane Database Syst Rev* 2009;4:CD005149.
26. Desrosiers M, Evans GA, Keith PK, et al. Canadian clinical practice guidelines for acute and chronic rhinosinusitis. *J Otolaryngol Head Neck Surg* 2011;40(suppl 2):S99-S193.
27. Garbutt JM, Banister C, Spitznagel E, Piccirillo JF. Amoxicillin for acute rhinosinusitis: a randomized controlled trial. *JAMA* 2012;307:685-692.
28. Casey JR, Adlowitz DG, Pichichero ME. New patterns in the otopathogens causing acute otitis media six to eight years after introduction of pneumococcal conjugate vaccine. *Pediatr Infect Dis J* 2010;29:304-309.
29. Venekamp RP, Thompson MJ, Hayward G, et al. Systemic corticosteroids for acute sinusitis. *Cochrane Database Syst Rev* 2011;12:CD008115.
30. Mfuna-Endam L, Zhang Y, Desrosiers MY. Genetics of rhinosinusitis. *Curr Allergy Asthma Rep* 2011;11:236-246.
31. Shulman ST, Bisno AL, Clegg HW, et al. Clinical practice guideline for the diagnosis and management of group A streptococcal pharyngitis: 2012 update by the Infectious Diseases Society of America. *Clin Infect Dis* 2012;55(10):1279-1282.
32. Wessels MR. Clinical practice. Streptococcal pharyngitis. *N Engl J Med* 2011;364:648-655.
33. Gerber MA, Baltimore RS, Eaton CB, et al. Prevention of rheumatic fever and diagnosis and treatment of acute Streptococcal pharyngitis: a scientific statement from the American Heart Association Rheumatic Fever, Endocarditis, and Kawasaki Disease Committee of the Council on Cardiovascular Disease in the Young, the Interdisciplinary Council on Functional Genomics and Translational Biology, and the Interdisciplinary Council on Quality of Care and Outcomes Research: endorsed by the American Academy of Pediatrics. *Circulation* 2009;119:1541-1551.
34. Dooling KL, Shapiro DJ, Van Beneden C, Hersh AL, Hicks LA. Overprescribing and inappropriate antibiotic selection for children with pharyngitis in the United States, 1997-2010. *JAMA Pediatr* 2014;168:1073-1074.
35. Barnett ML, Linder JA. Antibiotic prescribing to adults with sore throat in the United States, 1997-2010. *JAMA Intern Med* 2014;174:138-140.
36. Burton MJ, Glasziou PP. Tonsillectomy or adeno-tonsillectomy versus non-surgical treatment for chronic/recurrent acute tonsillitis. *Cochrane Database Syst Rev* 2009;1:CD001802.
37. Regoli M, Chiappini E, Bonsignori F, Galli L, de Martino M. Update on the management of acute pharyngitis in children. *Ital J Pediatr* 2011;37:10.
38. Altamimi S, Khalil A, Khalaiwi KA, Milner RA, Pusic MV, Al Othman MA. Short-term late-generation antibiotics versus longer term penicillin for acute streptococcal pharyngitis in children. *Cochrane Database Syst Rev* 2012;8:CD004872.

109

Influenza

Jessica C. Njoku

KEY CONCEPTS

1. Influenza is a viral illness associated with high mortality and high hospitalization rates among persons older than 65 years of age. The aging of the population is contributing to an increased disease burden in the United States.
2. Seasonal influenza epidemics are the result of viral antigenic drift, which is why the influenza vaccine is changed on an yearly basis. Antigenic drift forms the foundation of the recommendation for annual influenza vaccination.
3. The acquisition of a new hemagglutinin and/or neuraminidase by the influenza virus is called *antigenic shift*, which results in a novel influenza virus that has the potential to cause a pandemic.
4. The primary route of influenza transmission is person-to-person via inhalation of respiratory droplets, and transmission can occur for as long as the infected person is shedding virus from the respiratory tract.
5. Clinical diagnosis of influenza is difficult. Classic signs and symptoms include abrupt onset of fever, muscle pain, headache, malaise, nonproductive cough, sore throat, and rhinitis. These signs and symptoms usually resolve within 1 week of presentation.
6. In the United States, the primary mechanism of influenza prevention is annual vaccination. Vaccination not only prevents influenza illness and influenza-related hospitalizations and deaths but may also decrease healthcare resource use and the overall cost to society.
7. The inactivated influenza vaccine (IIV) and the live-attenuated influenza vaccine (LAIV) are commercially available for prevention of seasonal influenza. Both vaccines contain influenza A subtypes H3N2 and H1N1, and influenza B virus, which are initially grown in hens' eggs.
8. Antiviral drugs for prophylaxis of influenza should be considered adjuncts to vaccine and are not replacements for annual vaccination.
9. The sooner antiviral drugs are started after the onset of illness, within 48 hours of symptom onset, the more effective they are.
10. Oseltamivir, zanamivir, and peramivir are neuraminidase inhibitors that have activity against both influenza A and influenza B viruses. Although the adamantanes inherently have activity against influenza A H1N1 viruses, they are no longer used clinically due to overwhelming viral resistance.

Influenza causes significant morbidity and mortality, particularly among young children and the elderly. Seasonal influenza epidemics result in 25 to 50 million influenza cases, approximately 200,000 hospitalizations, and more than 30,000 deaths each year in the United States.[1] Globally, influenza causes nearly 500,000 deaths each year. More people die of influenza than of any other vaccine-preventable illness. Significant societal consequences associated with influenza include visits to physicians' offices and emergency departments and days lost from school and/or work. The societal costs associated with influenza are more than $40 billion in the United States[1] and $16 billion in those older than or equal to 50 years alone.[2]

Vaccination is the primary mechanism of influenza prevention in the United States. The antiviral armamentarium for treatment and prophylaxis of influenza is limited, which further emphasizes the importance of prevention with vaccination and appropriate use of infection control measures during outbreaks. Research toward the development of novel antivirals and vaccines is needed for effective control of seasonal epidemics and for pandemic preparedness.

ETIOLOGY AND EPIDEMIOLOGY

Influenza infection can occur at any time during the year with the highest rates of influenza-associated illness during the winter months. The highest rate of infection occurs in children, but the highest rates of severe illness, hospitalization, and death occur among those older than age 65 years, young children (younger than 2 years old), and those who have underlying medical conditions, including pregnancy and cardiopulmonary disorders, that increase their risk of complications from influenza. (1) The seasonal influenza epidemics from 2012 to 2015 resulted in an average annual laboratory confirmed influenza-associated hospitalization rate of 48.1 per 100,000 person-years.[3] In 2012 to 2013 influenza season alone, the rate of influenza associated hospitalization was 202 (95% confidence interval, 143-260) per 100,000 person-years.[4] Influenza-associated hospitalization rates were four times higher among children aged 0 to 4 years compared with among those aged 5 to 17 years.[3] Similarly, influenza-associated hospitalization rates were 17 times higher, and 6 times higher, among persons older than or equal to 65 years compared with among those aged 18 to 49 years, and 50 to 64 years, respectively.[3] During the 2009 pandemic influenza H1N1pdm09 outbreak, an estimated 137,414 hospital discharges were attributed to influenza.[5] Influenza-related deaths is three times higher in high-risk individuals. From 1997 to 2009, influenza A/H3N2 accounted for 71% of influenza-related mortality, while influenza B was attributed with the most deaths (51%-95%).[7] Approximately 90% of seasonal influenza-related deaths occur in those older than age 65 years, with about 70% of deaths occuring among those older than or equal to 75 years.[6] In 2012 to 2013 influenza season, the rate of influenza associated death was 54.6 (95% confidence interval, 36.2-73.0) per 100,000 person-years among those age 65 years or older, compared to a rate of 1.1, less than18 years or 1.7, 18 to 64 years old.[4] Thus, the aging of the population is contributing to an increased disease burden. Deaths associated with influenza often result from secondary bacterial pneumonia, primary viral pneumonia, and/or exacerbation of underlying comorbidities.[7]

Influenza Viruses A, B, and C

Influenza virus types A, B, and C are members of the Orthomyxoviridae family and affect many species, including humans, pigs, horses, and birds. Influenza A and B viruses are the two types that cause disease in humans. Influenza A viruses are responsible for the regular, seasonal epidemics of the flu, whereas influenza B viruses are typically associated with sporadic outbreaks, particularly among residents of long-term care facilities. Influenza A viruses are further categorized into different subtypes based on changes in two surface antigens—hemagglutinin and neuraminidase (NA). Influenza B viruses are not categorized into subtypes.

Hemagglutinin allows the influenza virus to enter host cells by attaching to sialic acid receptors and is the major antigen to which antibodies are directed on exposure.[8] NA allows the release of new viral particles from host cells by catalyzing the cleavage of linkages to sialic acid.[8]

Sixteen hemagglutinin subtypes (H1-H16) and nine NA subtypes (N1-N9) of influenza A have been isolated from birds. However, the only influenza A subtypes that have circulated among humans since the 1918 pandemic (see Antigenic Drift and Antigenic Shift in the following sections) are H1 to H3 and N1 and N2.[8] The primary subtypes of influenza A that have been circulating among humans for the past three decades are H3N2 and H1N1.

Antigenic Drift and Antigenic Shift

2 Immunity to influenza virus occurs as a result of the development of antibody directed at the surface antigens, particularly hemagglutinin. However, immunity to one influenza subtype does not offer protection against other subtypes or types of influenza. Moreover, immunity to one antigenic variant of a subtype of influenza may not confer protection against other antigenic variants. Antigenic variants are created by point mutations in the surface antigens of a particular subtype, resulting in small changes in the hemagglutinin and/or NA molecules, which is called *antigenic drift*. Antigenic drift is the basis for seasonal epidemics of influenza, the reason for changes in the annual influenza vaccine, and the rationale behind the recommendation for annual vaccination.

Immunity to one subtype of influenza does not confer protection against other subtypes or types. 3 Antigenic shift occurs when the influenza virus acquires a new hemagglutinin and/or NA via genetic reassortment rather than point mutations.[4] Most likely, the genetic reassortment occurs when an animal that supports the growth of multiple subtypes of influenza, such as a pig, is concurrently infected with two subtypes of the influenza virus. Conversely, antigenic shift may occur directly from avian strains that have gained competency in the human host. Antigenic shift results in the emergence of a novel influenza virus and carries the potential of causing a pandemic. However, novelty alone is insufficient to cause an influenza pandemic; the virus must be able to replicate in humans, spread person-to-person, and affect a susceptible population.[8]

Spanish Influenza of 1918

The influenza pandemic of 1918 was the most significant infectious disease outbreak known to humans, causing approximately 40 to 50 million deaths in a year, with more than 500,000 deaths occurring in the United States.[9,10] The pandemic occurred almost concurrently in Europe, Asia, and North America.[9]

The 1918 pandemic was caused by a particularly virulent influenza A H1N1 virus, which was entirely of avian origin.[10,11] In contrast to the other pandemics of the 20th century, the 1918 pandemic resulted in an unusual mortality pattern. The mortality peaked for those younger than 4 years of age, those between the ages of 25 and 35 years, and those older than 65 years of age, which resulted in a W-shaped mortality curve, as opposed to the U- or J-shaped curve typically associated with influenza.[10,12] Over half of the deaths occurred in persons aged 20 to 40 years. The death toll associated with this pandemic culminated in an almost 10-year drop in the life expectancy of the population at the time.[10]

Asian Influenza of 1957

The Asian flu pandemic began when a new H2 subtype of influenza A surfaced in Hunan province in China in 1957.[10] The virus appeared to have formed from coinfection with an avian H2N2 virus and a human H1N1 virus in a common host, possibly a pig or a human.[11] The H2N2 virus quickly spread to Japan, South America, the United States, New Zealand, and Europe, resulting in approximately 4 million deaths worldwide, with 70,000 deaths occurring in the United States.[10] Unlike the Spanish flu of 1918, the mortality curve for the Asian flu pandemic was U- or J-shaped, with infants and elderly being most affected.[12]

Hong Kong Influenza of 1968

The H2N2 virus of the Asian flu circulated in the human population until 1968, when a new H3 subtype emerged in China and Hong Kong[12] following genetic reassortment with the H2N2 virus.[10,11] The H3N2 virus quickly spread to the United States and later to Europe. This pandemic caused more than 30,000 deaths in the United States and approximately 2 million deaths worldwide.[10,12] The lower morbidity and mortality associated with the Hong Kong flu may be explained by previous exposure of the population to the N2 subtype, and the availability of antibiotics for the management of secondary bacterial pneumonia. Similar to the Asian flu of 1957, the mortality curve for the Hong Kong flu pandemic was U- or J-shaped, primarily affecting infants and elderly.[12]

Avian Influenza

Influenza viruses are in circulation in southern China during all months of the year.[4] Given this fact and the close proximity of dense populations of people, pigs, and wild and domestic birds, this area proves ideal for the development of new influenza viruses via genetic reassortment (antigenic shift), as demonstrated by the pandemics of 1957 and 1968 and, most recently, the emergence of what is known as avian influenza.[8]

The first report of human infection with the avian H5N1 virus occurred in 1997 in Hong Kong in a 3-year-old who had a direct link with chickens and later died.[13] This was followed by 18 confirmed cases and 6 deaths.[14] The virus reemerged in 2003 as an antigenically and genetically different virus that has spread widely through wild and domestic bird populations in Asia, Africa, and Europe as well as infecting humans in 16 countries: Azerbaijan, Bangladesh, Cambodia, Canada, China, Djibouti, Egypt, Indonesia, Iraq, Lao People's Democratic Republic, Myanmar, Nigeria, Pakistan, Thailand, Turkey, and Vietnam.[12,15] From 2003 to September 10, 2015, a total of 844 cases and 449 deaths caused by H5N1 infection have been reported.[15,16] The current overall case fatality is 53%.

The novel avian influenza H7N9 virus infection was first reported in humans in March 2013, in China.[17] Since the outbreak, only one case of influenza H7N9 has been reported outside of China, and this occurred in Canada in February 2015. Avian influenza A(H7N9) is a subtype of influenza viruses that have been detected in birds in the past, but no previous infection had been documented in animals or people until recently. Other emerging avian H7 virus subtypes with documented infections in humans are H7N3 in Canada, 2004; H7N2 in New York, 2003, and H7N7 in Netherlands, 2003.[18] Majority of avian H7N9 human infection cases have been among those with recent exposure to live poultry or potentially contaminated environments, especially markets where live birds are sold.[17,18] Presently, the virus does not appear to transmit easily from person to person, and sustained human-to-human transmission has not been reported. Nevertheless, the disease is of concern because patients become severely ill. As of July 16, 2015, a total of 677 cases and 275 deaths caused by H7N9 virus infection have been reported.[16,17] The current overall case fatality is 41%.

In May 2013, the first case of novel avian influenza H6N1 human infection, was reported in Taiwan,[18] and since May 2014, four laboratory-confirmed human case of avian influenza A(H5N6) virus infection were reported to World Health Organization (WHO) from China.[16] To date no evidence of human-to-human transmission of the viruses has been documented. Other influenza A(H5) subtypes, such as influenza A(H5N2), A(H5N3), and A(H5N8), continue to be detected in birds in West Africa, Asia, Europe, and North America.[16] Although influenza A(H5N2), A(H5N3), and A(H5N8) viruses might have the potential to cause disease in humans, so far no human cases of infection have been reported.[16] Other novel avian influenza strains emerging in 1999 (H9N2), with two cases of human infections, and in 2013 (H10N8), with three cases of infections, all in China, continue to be of concern.[18]

The spread of avian influenza viruses from person to person has been reported very rarely, and has been limited, inefficient, and unsustained.[18,19] The precise mode of transmission is unknown, but most cases have occurred as a result of contact with poultry, contaminated environment, and prolonged person-to-person contact.[15-18] Cases of transmission via aerosolization have not been reported.[20] Clinical presentation includes high fever and influenza-like illness, and watery diarrhea without blood may occur up to 1 week prior to respiratory symptoms.[21] Almost all patients have clinically apparent pneumonia. Progression to death, most commonly as a consequence of respiratory failure, occurs a mean of 9 to 10 days after the onset of illness.[15-17,20] The NA inhibitors, oseltamivir, zanamivir, and peramivir, have activity against the avian influenza viruses, although higher doses may be needed. Oseltamivir resistance has been detected in several patients infected with the H5N1 virus who were treated with oseltamivir.[20] Amantadine and rimantadine are ineffective against avian influenza viruses. An inactivated monovalent[22] and an adjuvanted monovalent[23] influenza virus vaccine, against H5N1 is available for vaccination of persons 18 to 64 years of age at increased risk of exposure to the H5N1 influenza virus. The recommended dose is two 1-mL injections given intramuscularly 28 days apart (range, 21 to -35 days) if non-adjuvanted vaccine,[22] or two 0.5-mL injections given 21 days apart if adjuvanted vaccine is used.[23] The vaccines are supplied in a 5-mL multi-dose vial, with ~50 mcg thimerosal per dose in the non-adjuvanted vaccine[22], and 5 mcg thimerosal per dose in the adjuvanted vaccine[23], added as a preservative. The monovalent adjuvanted vaccine is supplied in two separate vials, a vial of H5N1 antigen and a vial of AS03 adjuvant, that must be combined before use, for the final volume per vial that provides 10 doses at 0.5 ml per dose.[23] At the present time, the vaccines are being stockpiled for use if H5N1 begins transmitting easily from person to person. Individuals at high risk, for example, those who work with poultry and H5N1 poultry outbreak responders, are encouraged to receive annual seasonal influenza vaccine to minimize the risk of coinfection with human and avian influenza A viruses.

The potential for avian viruses H5N1 and H7N9 to cause a pandemic is of concern as it could spread more quickly than pandemics of the past because of the mobility of people in today's world. International travel has increased 73% since 1990, with 763 million people crossing international borders in 2004.[21] In 2012 alone, international tourist travels worldwide was projected at 1 billion, which was a 48% increase since 2000.[24] In 2009, the US residents made over 61 million travels outside the country, which was a 5% increase since 1999.[24] A severe pandemic, like that of 1918, could cause more than 9 million hospitalizations and more than 1.9 million deaths, whereas a moderate pandemic, like those of 1957 and 1968, could result in more than 800,000 hospitalizations and more than 200,000 deaths in the United States alone.[12,24]

Swine Influenza of 2009

An outbreak of a novel influenza A H1N1 (formerly swine origin influenza virus [SOIV]) was initially detected in Mexico in March 2009 and subsequently in the United States in April 2009 in California and Texas.[25,26] The virus then spread throughout North America, Europe, Asia, and subsequently worldwide, prompting the WHO on June 11, 2009 to declare phase 6, indicating widespread human infection, for the influenza pandemic.[26] Since 1998, triple reassortant swine influenza A (H1) viruses, containing genes from swine, avian, and human lineages, have circulated among swine in the United States.[25,27]

However, the novel influenza A H1N1 virus is unique in that although much of the genome is similar to the triple reassortant swine viruses previously seen in the United States, the genes encoding for NA and matrix (M) proteins are most similar to those circulating in the Eurasian swine population. This particular genetic combination has not been seen before.[25] The virus, now formally known as influenza A(H1N1) pdm09, has since become the predominant influenza A H1N1 in circulation, effectively replacing traditional seasonal influenza A (H1N1).

Several characteristics of the novel influenza A H1N1 outbreak differ from those of a typical seasonal influenza outbreak. Symptomatology associated with the novel influenza include fever (94%), cough (92%), sore throat (66%), diarrhea (25%), and vomiting (25%).[25,26] An estimated 43 to 89 million cases of 2009 H1N1 occurred between April 2009 and April 2010 with a median 274,000 hospitalizations. Globally, 18,500 laboratory-confirmed H1N1-related deaths were reported; however, this may represent an underestimation of true disease burden.[28] The majority of the cases occurred in otherwise healthy children and young adults younger than 65 years of age including pregnant women, with the highest incidence reported among those aged 18 to 64 years.[28] Contrary to seasonal influenza where about 60% of hospitalizations and 90% of deaths occur in people older than or equal to 65 years, approximately 90% and 87% of 2009 H1N1-related hospitalizations and deaths, respectively, occurred in people younger than 65 years. However, like seasonal influenza, people with underlying health conditions had greater risk of hospitalizations and death. Among those who were deceased due to novel H1N1 infection, the median age was ~40 years and 59% of deaths (respiratory and cardiovascular) occurred in Southeast Asia and Africa.[28]

Variant Influenza A (H3N2v), 2012

H3N2v is a non-human influenza virus that normally circulates in pigs and that has infected humans.[29] In August 2011, the US Centers for Disease Control and Prevention (CDC) reported the first case of an influenza infection due to influenza A H3N2 variant virus (H3N2v).[29] Since then, 345 cases have been documented from 13 states in the United States resulting in 20 hospitalizations and 1 death.[30] Human infections with H3N2v have been limited to the United States. The H3N2v is considered a variant virus because it is different from influenza A viruses circulating among humans. Infections due to variant influenza viruses, for example, A(H1N1)v, A(H3N2)v, and A(H1N2)v of swine origin, have been documented in the past.[29] The H3N2v virus contains genes from avian, swine, and human viruses and the M gene from the 2009 H1N1 pandemic virus (A[H1N1]pdm09).[29] The virus was originally detected in pigs in 2010 but human infection was first documented in July 2011. The virus appears to spread more readily from pigs to people than other variant viruses, but has limited person-to-person transmission. The main risk factor for infection with the virus based on evaluation of available cases is exposure to pigs, mostly in fair settings.[29] Since the virus is related to human flu viruses from the 1990s, most adults have some immunity against it.[29] Hence, most cases to date have occurred in children, who have little immunity against this virus.

The symptoms and severity of H3N2v have mostly been mild and similar to those of seasonal influenza (fever, cough, sore throat, body aches, etc.), but like seasonal influenza, serious illness with H3N2v infection is possible.[29] Vaccination remains key to preventing H3N2v infection. Additionally, the CDC has encouraged people at high risk of influenza complications to stay away from swine barns at fairs.[29,30] People who are at high risk of serious complications from influenza, including H3N2v virus infection, are: children younger than 5 years, people older than or equal to 65 years, pregnant women, and people with certain chronic medical conditions (asthma, diabetes, heart disease, immunocompromised, and neurologic or neurodevelopmental conditions). The treatment of H3N2v virus infection is similar to that of seasonal influenza. NA inhibitors are the mainstay of treatment. The adamantanes should not be used due to high resistance.[29]

PATHOGENESIS

4 The route of influenza transmission is person-to-person via inhalation of respiratory droplets, which can occur when an infected person coughs or sneezes.[31] Transmission may also occur if a person touches an object contaminated with respiratory secretions and then touches his or her mucus membranes. The incubation period for influenza ranges between 1 and 7 days, with an average incubation

CLINICAL PRESENTATION Diagnosis of Influenza

General

- The clinical diagnosis of influenza can be difficult because the presentation is similar to a number of other respiratory illnesses. The sensitivity of clinical diagnosis ranges from 40% for children to 70% for adults and largely depends on the relative prevalence of influenza and other respiratory viruses circulating in a community.[34]
- The clinical course and outcome are affected by age, immunocompetence, viral characteristics, smoking, comorbidities, pregnancy, and the degree of preexisting immunity.
- Complications of influenza may include exacerbation of underlying comorbidities, primary viral pneumonia, secondary bacterial pneumonia or other respiratory illnesses (eg, sinusitis, bronchitis, otitis), encephalopathy, transverse myelitis, myositis, myocarditis, pericarditis, and Reye's syndrome.

Signs and Symptons

- 5 Classic signs and symptoms of influenza include rapid onset of fever, myalgia, headache, malaise, nonproductive cough, sore throat, and rhinitis.
- Nausea, vomiting, and otitis media are also commonly reported in children.[35]
- Signs and symptoms typically resolve in approximately 3 to 7 days, although cough and malaise may persist for more than 2 weeks.
- Primary viral pneumonia, occurring predominantly in pregnant women and in those with underlying cardiovascular disease, usually begins with fever and dry cough, which changes to a productive cough of bloody sputum. This rapidly progresses to dyspnea, hypoxemia, and cyanosis with radiologic evidence of bilateral interstitial infiltrates.[34]
- Secondary bacterial pneumonia is usually seen in individuals with underlying pulmonary disorders and presents during the early stages of defervescence from the influenza infection. These patients usually present with fever, productive cough, and radiologic evidence of consolidation.[34]

Laboratory Tests

- Complete blood count and chemistry panels should be obtained to assess the overall status of the patient.
- The gold standard for diagnosis of influenza are reverse-transcription polymerase chain reaction (RT-PCR) or viral culture, which can provide information on the specific strain and subtype. Viral culture has a high sensitivity but can take as long as a week to develop, limiting the clinical relevance of the results.
- Tests such as the antigen-based rapid influenza diagnostic tests ([RIDTs], also known as point-of-care [POC] tests), direct (DFA) or indirect (IFA) fluorescence antibody tests, and the RT-PCR assay may be used for rapid detection of virus.[36]

Other Diagnostic Tests

- Cultures of potential sites of infection should be obtained if coinfection, superinfection, or secondary infection is suspected.
- Chest radiograph should be obtained if pneumonia is suspected.

Rapid Tests

- RIDTs have allowed for prompt diagnosis and initiation of antiviral therapy and decreased inappropriate use of antibiotics. RIDTs use enzyme immunoassay (EIA) technology to provide results within 1 hour of specimen collection. Appropriate specimens for collection, in decreasing order of sensitivity, are nasopharyngeal aspirates, nasopharyngeal swabs/washes, and oropharyngeal swabs.[36] RIDTs allow for differentiation of influenza viruses A and B, with sensitivity and specificity ranging from 50% to 70% and 85% to 99%, respectively.[36,37] In general, the use of RIDTs is contraindicated in those who have had symptoms for longer than 3 days, and results may be confounded following recent immunization with live-attenuated influenza vaccine (LAIV).[36]
- DFA testing requires more technical expertise and infrastructure than RIDTs. The advantages of DFA are increased sensitivity over RIDTs and simultaneous detection of other respiratory viruses, such as respiratory syncytial virus and adenovirus.[36] DFA provides results between 1 and 4 hours after specimen collection.
- RT-PCR assay is a nucleic acid amplification test and is the most sensitive, specific, and versatile diagnostic test for influenza.[36] RT-PCR is a gold standard diagnostic test and can determine the type, subtype, and strain of influenza. Results are provided within 1 to 6 hours of specimen collection.

of 2 days.[31] Transmission can occur for as long as the infected person is shedding virus from the respiratory tract. Adults are considered infectious within 1 day before until 7 days after onset of illness. Children, especially younger children, might potentially be infectious for longer periods (more than 10 days).[29,32] Viral shedding can persist for weeks to months in severely immunocompromised people.

The pathogenesis of influenza in humans is not well understood. The severity of the infection is determined by the balance between viral replication and the host immune response.[8] Severe illness is likely a result of both a lack of ability of host defense mechanisms to inhibit viral replication and an overproduction of cytokines leading to tissue damage in the host.[33]

PREVENTION

The best means to decrease the morbidity and mortality associated with influenza is to prevent infection through vaccination.[31,32] Appropriate infection control measures, such as hand hygiene, basic respiratory etiquette (eg, cover your cough, throw tissues away), and contact avoidance, are also important in preventing the spread of influenza. Additionally, chemoprophylaxis is useful in certain situations.

Vaccination

6 The primary means of influenza prevention used in the United States is annual vaccination. Vaccination can help prevent hospitalization and death among those at high risk, decrease influenza-like illness, decrease visits to physicians' offices and emergency rooms, decrease otitis media in children, and prevent school and/or work absenteeism. Annual vaccination is recommended for all persons aged 6 months or older and caregivers (eg, parents, teachers, babysitters, nannies) of children younger than 6 months. Vaccination is also recommended for those who live with and/or care for people who are at high risk, including household contacts and healthcare workers.

The ideal time for all influenza vaccination is during October or November to allow for the development and maintenance of immunity during the peak of the influenza season.[31,32] Table 109-1 lists the vaccination coverage rates and goals for various patient populations.

7 The two vaccine types currently available for prevention of seasonal influenza are the inactivated influenza vaccine (IIV), and the LAIV. IIV is available as trivalent (IIV3) and quadrivalent (IIV4) formulations, while LAIV is a quadrivalent formulation. Both vaccines contain two influenza A subtypes (H3N2 and H1N1) and influenza B virus; the specific strains included in the vaccine each year change based on antigenic drift. The viruses used for both vaccines are initially grown in embryonated hens' eggs, which explain the precautionary measures for vaccination of persons with a severe allergic reaction to eggs.[31] Of the two vaccines produced using nonegg based technologies, recombinant trivalent vaccine [RIV3 (Flublok®)] and cell-culture quadrivalent vaccine [ccIIV4 (Flucelvax Quadrivalent®)], only Flublok® is considered egg-free. Flucelvax® contains an estimated maximum of 5x10-8 mcg/0.5 mL dose of total egg protein ovalbumin. The Advisory Committee on Immunization Practices (ACIP) has made the following recommendations regarding the vaccinations of persons with reports of egg allergy: (a) Vaccination with any age appropriate IIV or RIV3 vaccine, for persons with a history of egg allergy that involves only hives. (b) Persons with severe allergic reactions (i.e. symptoms other than hives), such as angioedema, respiratory distress, light-headedness, or recurrent emesis or required epinephrine after an egg exposure may be immunized with any licensed IIV or RIV3 that is appropriate for age and health status. Vaccine should be administered in an inpatient or outpatient medical setting (including but not necessarily limited to hospitals, clinics, health departments, and physician offices), under the supervision of a health care provider who is able to recognize and manage severe allergic conditions. (c) Severe allergic reaction to influenza vaccine is a contraindication to receiving future vaccinations. (d) Vaccine providers should consider observing all patients for 15 minutes after vaccination to decrease the risk for injury should a patient experiences syncope.[31] The CDC encourages individuals to use the Vaccine Adverse Event Reporting System to aide in collecting and analyzing adverse events following influenza vaccinations.[31]

TABLE 109-1 Influenza Vaccination Rates and Goals by Patient Population[32,42]

Patient Population	Vaccination Coverage (%)	Vaccination Coverage National Goal (2013)
Children aged 6 months-7 years	47[a]	70%
Persons aged 18 or greater	38[a]	70%
Nursing home residents	62[b]	90%
Pregnant women	27[c]	80%
Healthcare workers	56[a]	90%

[a]2010-2011 data.

[b]2005 data.

[c]2008-2009 data.

Trivalent and Quadrivalent Influenza Vaccine

7 Intramuscular IIV is FDA approved for use in people older than 6 months of age, regardless of their immune status. Of note, several commercial products are available and are approved for different age groups (Table 109-2). The intradermal IIV4, Fluzone Intradermal®, is approved by FDA for use in adults 18 to 64 years of age and is another vaccination option for people in this age group. IIV is made with killed viruses, meaning it cannot cause signs and symptoms of influenza-like illness (Table 109-3). Age and immune status can affect the efficacy of IIV as can the similarity of the vaccine to the viruses in circulation. Afluria® brand of IIV3 vaccine is contraindicated in patients with hypersensitivity to neomycin or polymyxin. Afluria® is also not recommended first line in children 6 months to 8 years, due to reports of high febrile episodes following administration.[31]

In children between 6 and 24 months of age, a 2-year randomized study of intramuscular IIV3 exhibited 89% seroconversion and efficacy of 66% in year 1 and 7% in year 2 versus culture-confirmed influenza.[38] In children between 1 and 15 years of age, the efficacy of IIV3 was 91.4% and 77.3% against culture-confirmed influenza A H1N1 and H3N2, respectively. Two doses of IIV are important for children under the age of 9 years, supporting the rationale for the recommendation of a booster dose of IIV at least 1 month after the initial dose in children between 6 months and less than 9 years of age if no previous vaccination (see Table 109-2).[31] Booster dose is also recommended for children 2 years to 8 years at least 6 weeks after the initial dose if no previous vaccination.

IIV is also effective in adult populations under and older than the age of 65 years. A double-blind, randomized controlled trial evaluating intramuscular IIV3 in healthy adults younger than the age of 65 years demonstrated an efficacy of 50% against serologically confirmed influenza during a season in which the vaccine and the circulating viruses were not well matched and an efficacy of 86% during a season in which the vaccine and the circulating viruses were well matched.[39] Vaccination of those younger than 65 years old during seasons when the virus and vaccine are well matched results in decreased work absenteeism and healthcare resource use.[38,39]

Intradermal IIV4 in adults 18 to 64 years of age provides immune response similar to the IIV3 intradermal injection for matched strains.[40] However, for both B strains intradermal IIV4, provides immune response superior to intradermal IIV3 without the corresponding B strain. Both vaccines were similar in their safety profile. In clinical trials, Fluzone® intradermal was noninferior to Fluzone® intramuscular in eliciting immune response as

TABLE 109-2 Approved Influenza Vaccines for Different Age Groups—United States, 2016-2017 Season[31,32]

Vaccine	Trade Name	Manufacturer	Dose/Presentation	Thimerosal Mercury Content (mcg Hg/0.5 mL dose)	Age Group	Number of Doses
Inactivated						
IIV3	Fluvirin	Seqirus Vaccines	0.5-mL prefilled syringe 5-mL multi-dose vial	≤1 25	≥4 years ≥4 years	1 or 2[a] 1 or 2[a]
IIV3	Afluria	Seqirus	0.5-mL prefilled syringe 5-mL multidose vial	0 24.5	≥9 years ≥9 years via needle/syringe or 18-64 years via jet injector	1 1
ccIIV4	Quadrivalent	Seqirus Vaccines	0.5-mL prefilled syringe	0	≥4 years	1
RIV3	Flublok	Protein Sciences	0.5-ml single dose vial	0	≥18 years	1
IIV3 High Dose	Fluzone HD	Sanofi Pasteur	0.5-mL prefilled syringe	0	≥65 years	1
aIIV3	Fluad	Seqirus	0.5 mL single dose prefilled syringe	0	≥65 years	1
IIV4	Quadrivalent	ID Biomedical Corporation	5-mL multidose vial	<25	≥3 years	1
IIV4	Fluarix Quadrivalent	GlaxoSmithKline	0.5-mL prefilled syringe	0	≥3 years	1
IIV4	Fluzone Quadrivalent	Sanofi Pasteur	0.25-mL prefilled syringe 0.5-mL prefilled syringe 0.5-mL single-dose vial 5-mL multi-dose vial	0 0 0 25	≥6-35 months ≥36 months ≥36 months ≥6 months	1 or 2[a] 1 or 2[a] 1 or 2[a] 1 or 2[a]
IIV4 intradermal	Fluzone Intradermal Quadrivalent	Sanofi Pasteur	0.1-mL prefilled microinjection system	0	18-64 years	1[b]
LAIV	FluMist Quadrivalent[c]	MedImmune	0.2-mL sprayer	0	2-49 years	1 or 2[d]

LAIV, live-attenuated influenza vaccine; IIV3, trivalent influenza vaccine; IIV4, quadrivalent influenza vaccine; ccIIV3, cell culture-based trivalent influenza vaccine; RIV3, recombinant trivalent influenza vaccine; aIIV3, adjuvanted inactivated influenza vaccine, trivalent, standard dose.

[a]Two doses administered at least 1 month apart are recommended for children aged 6 months to less than 9 years who are receiving influenza vaccine for the first time or received one dose in first year of vaccination during the previous influenza season.

[b]*Given intradermally.* A 0.1-mL dose contains 9 mcg of each vaccine antigen (27 mcg total).

[c]ACIP recommends that FLumist (LAIV4) not be used during the 2016-2017 season.

[d]Two doses administered 4 weeks apart are recommended for children aged 2 to less than 9 years who are receiving influenza vaccine for the first time.

measured by hemagglutination inhibition antibody geometric mean titers (GMTs).[41] The rate of seroconversion was similar between the two vaccines against influenza strains A (H1N1 and H3N2), but not for strain B. The most common adverse reactions were injection site related, which were transient (resolving in 3-7 days), and include erythema (greater than 75%), swelling (greater than 50%), induration (greater than 50%), pain (greater than 50%), and pruritus (greater than 40%). Compared with the intramuscular vaccine, Fluzone® intradermal contains 40% less antigen (Table 109-2).

Adults older than the age of 65 years benefit from influenza vaccination, including prevention of complications, decreased risk of influenza-related hospitalization, and death. However, people in this population may not generate a strong antibody response to the vaccine and may remain susceptible to infection. In patients older than the age of 60 years who do not reside in a long-term care facility, IIV efficacy was 58% against influenza illness.[42] Although the efficacy against influenza illness for those living in long-term care facilities is between 30% and 40%, the vaccine is 50% to 60% effective in preventing influenza-related hospitalization or pneumonia and 80% effective in preventing influenza-related death.[42]

TABLE 109-3 Comparison of Inactivated Influenza Vaccine (IIV) and Live-Attenuated Influenza Vaccine (LAIV)

Characteristic	IIV (IIV3/IIV4)	LAIV
Age groups approved for use	>6 months	2-49 years
Immune status requirements	Immunocompetent or immunocompromised	Immunocompetent
Viral properties	Inactivated (killed) influenza A (H3N2), A (H1N1), and B viruses	Live-attenuated influenza A (H3N2), A (H1N1), and B viruses
Route of administration	Intramuscular/Intradermal	Intranasal
Immune system response	High serum IgG antibody response	Lower IgG response and high serum IgA mucosal response

The most frequent adverse effect associated with IIV is soreness at the injection site that lasts for less than 48 hours. IIV may cause fever and malaise in those who have not previously been exposed to the viral antigens in the vaccine.[31,42] Allergic-type reactions (hives, systemic anaphylaxis) rarely occur after influenza vaccination and are likely a result of a reaction to residual egg protein in the vaccine.

The 1976 swine influenza vaccine was linked to a rise in the incidence of Guillain-Barré syndrome (GBS), and this has propagated the belief that IIV may cause GBS.[42] However, there is insufficient evidence to establish causality. Although several studies have failed to establish a relationship between influenza vaccination and increased frequency of GBS, two studies have demonstrated a small but significant increase in GBS following influenza vaccination.[43,44] Therefore, vaccination should be avoided in persons who are not at high risk for influenza complications and who have experienced GBS within 6 weeks of receiving a previous influenza vaccine.[31,42] The potential benefits of influenza vaccination in terms of prevention of severe illness, hospitalization, and mortality significantly outweigh the risks of GBS, and vaccination is recommended for all groups previously discussed.

The multidose vials and a few of the single-dose preparations of intramuscular IIV contain trace to small amounts of a preservative, thimerosal, which is a mercury-containing compound (see Table 109-2). Some individuals are concerned about thimerosal exposure, particularly among children, because of the unfounded belief that thimerosal exposure is linked to the development of autism. No scientifically persuasive evidence exists to suggest harm from thimerosal exposure from a vaccine. Conversely, accumulating evidence reports the lack of harm from such exposure.[45-47] Thus, similar to GBS, the potential benefits of influenza vaccination in terms of prevention of severe illness, hospitalization, and mortality significantly outweigh the theoretical risk associated with thimerosal exposure, and vaccination is recommended for all groups previously discussed. However, to maximize the public health benefit and placate concerned individuals, thimerosal-free vaccine is available (see Table 109-2).

Live-Attenuated Influenza Vaccine

7 LAIV is made with live, attenuated viruses and is approved for intranasal administration in healthy people between 2 and 49 years of age (see Table 109-3). Advantages of LAIV include its ease of administration, intranasal rather than intramuscular administration, and the potential induction of broad mucosal and systemic immune response.[31] The mucosal response occurs at the site of viral entry and may prevent infection before viral replication occurs. LAIV is more expensive than IIV and is approved for use in a more limited population. Originally licensed as a trivalent vaccine, in February 2012, the FDA approved FluMist® Quadrivalent vaccine for influenza prevention in people aged 2 to 49 years.[48] FluMist® Quadrivalent vaccine contains four strains of the influenza viruses, two influenza A strains and two influenza B strains. The inclusion of a second B strain in the vaccine is thought to increase the likelihood of adequate protection against circulating influenza B strains.

Studies of FluMist® trivalent, in addition to three new clinical trials with the quadrivalent vaccine in 4,000 children (2-17 years) and adults (18-49 years) in the United States, provide supporting evidence on the efficacy and safety of FluMist® Quadrivalent.[48-50] The studies show that immune responses were similar between FluMist® Quadrivalent and FluMist® trivalent. LAIV recipients aged 2 to 5 years had 52.5% and 54.4% fewer cases of influenza illness against matched and mismatched strains, respectively, as compared with IIV3 recipients.[49]

Although LAIV is FDA approved for adults younger than the age of 49 years, LAIV is effective in healthy adults between 18 and 64 years old.[50] Vaccination reduced the number of severe febrile illnesses by 18.8% and febrile upper respiratory tract illnesses by 23.6%.[50] Additionally, vaccination led to fewer days of illness, fewer days lost from work, fewer visits to healthcare providers, and decreased use of prescription antibiotics and nonprescription medications.[50]

Adverse reactions of LAIV are similar among those receiving FluMist® Quadrivalent and FluMist® trivalent. The adverse effects typically associated with LAIV administration include runny nose, congestion, sore throat, and headache. Because LAIV contains live, attenuated viruses, viral shedding may occur for several days following vaccination with LAIV, although this should not be equated with person-to-person transmission.[31] Additionally, because LAIV contains live, attenuated viruses, which carry a theoretical infection risk, LAIV should not be given to immunosuppressed patients or given by healthcare workers who are severely immunocompromised. Moreover, for the reasons discussed in IIV above, LAIV should not be administered to persons with a history of GBS or hypersensitivity to eggs. Although the quadrivalent vaccine has replaced the trivalent vaccine since 2012, for 2016-2017 influenza season vaccination, the ACIP has recommended against the use of LAIV due to low effectiveness against influenza A(H1N1)pdm09 in the United States in the past 2 influenza seasons. (Table 109-2).

Clinical **Controversy...**

LAIV is not recommended in several populations, including people older than 50 years and pregnant women, largely because the vaccine has not been studied extensively in these populations. However, many clinicians believe the use of LAIV in these populations is acceptable.

Postexposure Prophylaxis

8 Antiviral drugs available for prophylaxis of influenza should be considered adjuncts but are not replacements for annual vaccination. Historically, the adamantanes and NA inhibitors are two classes of antiviral drugs available for influenza prophylaxis and treatment. However, the adamantanes are no longer recommended for prophylaxis or treatment in the United States (because of widespread resistance among influenza viruses) until susceptibility is reestablished among influenza A virus.[51-54] Therefore, the NA inhibitors oseltamivir, zanamivir, and peramivir are the only drugs available for the treatment of influenza infection.[52] Peramivir is not approved for chemoprophylaxis, however, oseltamivir and zanamivir, are effective prophylactic agents against influenza in terms of preventing laboratory-confirmed influenza when used for seasonal prophylaxis (67% and 85% effective for zanamivir and oseltamivir, respectively) and preventing influenza illness among persons exposed to a household contact who was diagnosed with influenza (79%-81% and 68%-89% effective for zanamivir and oseltamivir, respectively).[52,53] Additionally, oseltamivir was 92% effective against influenza and also reduced associated complications when used as seasonal prophylaxis among immunized, institutionalized, elderly patients.[55] Both of these agents remain active against all influenza viruses, including influenza A H3N2v (Tables 109-4 and 109-5). Oseltamivir is FDA approved for the treatment of influenza in individuals 14 days and older, and for chemoprophylaxis in individuals 1 year and older. However, the CDC, the American Academy of Pediatrics (AAP), and the Pediatric Infectious Diseases Society (PIDS) provide an expanded recommendation for treatment in those less than 14 days, and chemoprophylaxis in those 3 months and older.[32,52,54] Table 109-6 gives dosing recommendations.

In those patients who did not receive the influenza vaccination and are receiving an antiviral drug for prevention of disease during the influenza season, the medication should optimally be taken for the entire duration of influenza activity in the community. The use of prophylaxis requires clinical judgment and depends on a variety of

TABLE 109-4 Antiviral Susceptibilities of Circulating Viruses

	Oseltamivir	Zanamivir	Peramivir	Adamantanes
Variant influenza A (H3N2), 2015	Susceptible	Susceptible	Susceptible	Resistant
Novel influenza A (H1N1)	Susceptible[a]	Susceptible	Susceptible[a]	Resistant
Seasonal A (H3N2)	Susceptible	Susceptible	Susceptible	Resistant
Influenza B	Susceptible	Susceptible	Susceptible	Resistant
Avian influenza (H5N1)	Susceptible	Susceptible	Susceptible	Variable

[a]Small number of isolates shown to be resistant to oseltamivir and peramivir.

TABLE 109-5 Interim Recommendations for the Selection of Antiviral Treatment Based on Confirmed Influenza Subtypes[32,52]

Laboratory Test	Preferred[a]	Alternative
Not performed or negative, but influenza suspected clinically[a]	Oseltamivir or zanamivir or peramivir	None
Positive variant H3N2v	Oseltamivir or zanamivir or peramivir	None
Positive novel H1N1	Oseltamivir or zanamivir or peramivir	None
Positive A (H3N2), or B	Oseltamivir or zanamivir or peramivir	None
Positive A + B	Oseltamivir or zanamivir or peramivir	None

[a]Viral surveillance data might help guide antiviral choices if oseltamivir resistance becomes more prevalent.

factors, but prophylaxis for seasonal influenza should be considered during influenza season for the following groups of patients after exposure to an infectious source:[52]

1. Persons at high risk of serious illness and/or complications who are exposed to an infectious person and cannot be vaccinated.
2. Persons at high risk of serious illness and/or complications who are vaccinated but exposed to an infectious person during the first two weeks following vaccination. The development of sufficient antibody titers after vaccination takes approximately 2 weeks.
3. Persons with severe immune deficiency or who may have an inadequate response to vaccination (eg, advanced human immunodeficiency virus [HIV] disease, persons receiving immunosuppressive medications), after exposure to an infectious person.
4. Long-term care facility residents, regardless of vaccination status, when an outbreak has occurred in the institution.

LAIV should not be administered until 48 hours after influenza antiviral therapy has stopped, and influenza antiviral drugs should not be administered for 2 weeks after the administration of LAIV because the antiviral drugs inhibit influenza virus replication.[31,48] No contraindication exists for concomitant use of IIV and influenza antiviral drugs.

Pregnant Women and Immunocompromised Hosts

Pregnant women and immunocompromised hosts are special populations at increased risk of influenza complications and are also populations in whom careful consideration must be given in regard to prevention strategies.

Pregnant women, regardless of trimester, should receive annual influenza vaccination with IIV but not with LAIV.[31,52] No studies have demonstrated an increased incidence of adverse effects in mothers or their infants related or potentially related to IIV, but no such data exist for LAIV.[31] Influenza vaccination of pregnant women reduced hospitalization of their infants by 92% during the first 6 months of life.[56] IIV is also safe for breast-feeding mothers. No data exist for LAIV and breast-feeding, but caution is warranted because of the potential for viral shedding.[31]

TABLE 109-6 Recommended Daily Dosage of Influenza Antiviral Medications for Treatment and Prophylaxis—United States[32,52,54]

Drug	Adult Treatment	Adult Prophylaxis[a]	Pediatric Treatment[b]	Pediatric Prophylaxis[c]
Oseltamivir	75-mg capsule twice daily for 5 days	75-mg capsule daily	<1 year: 3 mg/kg/dose twice daily 9-11 months[d]: 3.5 mg/kg/dose twice daily ≥1 year ≤15 kg: 30 mg twice daily 16-23 kg: 45 mg twice daily 23-40 kg: 60 mg twice daily >40 kg: 75 mg twice daily Duration: All for 5 days	3-8 months, 3 mg/kg/dose daily Not recommended if <3 months 9-11 months, 3.5 mg/kg/dose daily ≥1 year ≤15 kg: 30 mg daily 16-23 kg: 45 mg daily 23-40 kg: 60 mg daily >40 kg: 75 mg daily Duration: All for 10 days
Zanamivir	2 inhalations twice daily × 5 days	2 inhalations daily	2 inhalations twice daily × 5 days for ≥7 years old	2 inhalations daily for ≥5 years old for 10 days
Peramivir[e]	600 mg via intravenous infusion for 15-30 minutes once	None	None	None
Rimantadine[f]	200 mg/day in one to two doses × 7 days	200 mg/day in one to two doses	1-9 years old or <40 kg: 6.6 mg/kg/day divided twice daily (maximum 150 mg/day) ≥10 years old: 200 mg/day in one to two doses Treat 5-7 days	1-9 years old: 5 mg/kg daily (maximum 150 mg/day) ≥10 years old: 200 mg/day in one to two doses
Amantadine[f]	200 mg/day in one to two doses until 24-48 hours after symptom resolution	Same as treatment doses	>12 years old: same as adult 1-9 years old: 5 mg/kg/day in one to two doses; maximum 150 mg/day ≥10-12 years old: 100 mg orally twice daily	Same as treatment doses

[a]If influenza vaccine is administered, prophylaxis can generally be stopped 14 days after vaccination for noninstitutionalized persons. When prophylaxis is being administered following an exposure, prophylaxis should be continued for 10 days after the last exposure. In persons at high risk for complications from influenza for whom vaccination is contraindicated or expected to be ineffective, chemoprophylaxis should be continued for the duration that influenza viruses are circulating in the community during influenza season.

[b]Oseltamivir dosing for preterm infants—<38 weeks, 1 mg/kg/dose every 12 h; 38-40 weeks, 1.5mg/kg/dose every 12; >40 weeks, 3mg/kg/dose every 12 hours.[32]

[c]Alternate dosing by IDSA/PIDS (2011) is: 3-8 months—3 mg/kg/dose daily; 9-23 months—3.5 mg/kg/dose daily.[54]

[d]Unlabeled dosing.[54]

[e]Only approved for use in adults ≥18 years. Adjust dose if CrCl <50 mL/min (<0.83 mL/s)

[f]*Note:* Although amantadine and rimantadine have been used historically for the treatment and prophylaxis of influenza A viruses, due to high resistance, the CDC no longer recommends the use of these agents for the treatment and/or prophylaxis of influenza.

Immunocompromised hosts should receive annual influenza vaccination with IIV but not with LAIV. IIV was 100% effective against laboratory-confirmed influenza in HIV-positive patients with no significant effect on viral load or CD4 cell count.[57] However, antibody titers may not be as high as in immunocompetent individuals and are not improved with a second dose of vaccine.[58] Similarly, antibody titers may not be as high in solid-organ transplant patients as in immunocompetent persons, but, conversely, antibody titers were increased significantly after a second dose of IIV in adult liver transplant patients.[59] Although this suggests a potential benefit from a two-dose regimen, such a regimen is not currently recommended for solid-organ transplant recipients. Likewise, immune responses in patients receiving chemotherapy for either solid or hematologic tumors are lower (fourfold rise, 17%-52%) than in those who had completed chemotherapy (50%-83%) and healthy patients (67%-100%).[60] Data are currently limited in this arena for the intradermal IIV. In a study of intradermal IIV3 involving immunocompromised patients compared with healthy controls, humoral responses (GMTs and protection rates [PRs]) were significantly better among healthy controls than those among immunocompromised patients.[61] This is not surprising given an already attenuated immune system. But it was also noted that compared with the standard intramuscular IIV, GMTs and PRs were similar within all tested groups. Immune response to vaccine may be less than desired in immunocompromised patients.[31]

Large clinical trials evaluating the use of influenza antivirals for prophylaxis are lacking in immunocompromised hosts. Viral shedding occurs for prolonged periods in this population and may promote the development of antiviral resistance, which has been documented with oseltamivir in immunocompromised patients.[62-64]

TREATMENT

When prevention efforts fail or are not used, clinicians must turn to the agents available for treatment of influenza. Currently, the antiviral treatment options are limited, particularly in the face of resistance to the adamantanes and oseltamivir.

Goals of Therapy

The four primary goals of therapy of influenza are to control symptoms, prevent complications, decrease work and/or school absenteeism, and prevent the spread of infection.

General Approach to Treatment

In the era of pandemic preparedness and increasing resistance, early and definitive diagnosis of influenza is crucial. (9) The currently available antiviral drugs are most effective if started within 48 hours of the onset of illness. Moreover, the sooner the antiviral drugs are started after the onset of illness, the more effective they are. Antiviral drugs shorten the duration of illness and provide symptom control. Adjunct agents, such as acetaminophen for fever or an antihistamine for rhinitis, may be used concomitantly with the antiviral drugs.

Nonpharmacologic Therapy

Patients suffering from influenza should get adequate sleep and maintain a low level of activity. They should stay home from work and/or school in order to rest and prevent the spread of infection. Appropriate fluid intake should be maintained. Cough/throat lozenges, warm tea, or soup may help with symptom control (cough, sore throat).

Pharmacologic Therapy

The NA inhibitors, oseltamivir, zanamivir, and peramivir are the only antiviral drugs available for the treatment and prophylaxis of influenza.[52] Peramivir is the only intravenous formulation commercially available. The adamantanes (amantadine and rimantadine) are no longer recommended due to high resistance among influenza viruses. A limited discussion of adamantanes can be found in the following section, but the focus will be on oseltamivir, zanamivir, and peramivir.

Adamantanes

The adamantanes (amantadine and rimantadine) block the M2 ion channel, which is specific to influenza A viruses, and inhibit viral uncoating. Historically, the adamantanes were used for the treatment of seasonal influenza A H1N1, as they do not have activity against influenza A H3N2 or influenza B viruses. The novel influenza A H1N1 that emerged during the 2009 to 2010 influenza season, which has now replaced seasonal influenza A H1N1 as the predominant seasonal virus, was found to be discriminatorily resistant to the adamantanes. Data from the 2014 to 2015 influenza season showed that more than 99% of influenza A H3N2 and H1N1pdm09 were resistant to adamantanes.[51,52] As a result, the CDC only recommends the use of NA inhibitors for the treatment and prophylaxis of influenza A, until susceptibility of adamantanes is reestablished among influenza A viruses. Resistance to adamantanes is often conferred by a single-point mutation, and this is problematic because it results in cross-resistance to the entire class.[53]

Neuraminidase Inhibitors

(10) Oseltamivir, zanamivir, and peramivir are NA inhibitors that have activity against both influenza A and influenza B viruses.[52,53] Without NA, release of the virus from infected cells is impaired, and, thus, viral replication is decreased. When administered within 48 hours of the onset of illness, NA inhibitors may reduce the duration of illness by approximately 1 day versus placebo.[53] In a pivotal trial, oseltamivir reduced the time to return to normal health in adults by 1.9 days and the time to return to normal activity by 2.8 days.[65] These reductions have a significant effect on not only the quality of life for the patient but also the societal costs associated with influenza. (9) Of note, the benefits of treatment are highly dependent on the timing of the initiation of treatment, with the ideal initiation period being within 12 hours of illness onset.[66] However, select observational studies have reported a lower risk for severe outcomes with oral oseltamivir started 4 and 5 days after onset of illness in critically ill patients with suspected or confirmed influenza.[67,68]

Oseltamivir treatment in adults and adolescents with documented influenza illness resulted in a 26.7% reduction in overall antibiotic use, a 55% reduction in lower respiratory tract complications (bronchitis, pneumonia), and a 59% reduction in hospitalizations.[69] Zanamivir treatment in adults and adolescents with influenza-like illness resulted in a 28% reduction in antibiotic use and a 40% reduction in lower respiratory tract complications.[70] The data in these studies largely come from healthy individuals rather than those at highest risk for complications associated with influenza. The impact of appropriate treatment in high-risk populations may be even greater than that which has been documented to date.

Oseltamivir is approved for treatment in those 14 days and older, zanamivir for treatment in those older than the age of 7 years, and peramivir for those 18 years and older.[51] The recommended doses vary by agent and age (see Table 109-6). The recommended duration of treatment for both oseltamivir and zanamivir is 5 days, and one dose for one day for peramivir.

The FDA approved single dose peramivir injection (Rapivab®) for intravenous use for the treatment of acute uncomplicated influenza in people 18 years and older.[71] Peramivir is as effective as oseltamivir, without severe adverse events.[72] Therefore, peramivir is an effective option in patients who are unable to tolerate or absorb oral or enterically-administered oseltamivir due to gastric stasis, malabsorption, or gastrointestinal bleeding. Based on an observational study, the 14-day, 28-day, and 56-day survival rates of 31 patients with severe H1N1pdm09 infection treated with peramivir were 77%, 67%, and 59%, respectively.[73] Peramivir shortened duration of influenza symptoms in outpatient adults with uncomplicated influenza by about 1 day, with a corresponding reduction in median time to resumption of usual activities to about 1.5 days.[74] Studies exploring the use of peramivir beyond 1 day have not shown a benefit. A randomized trial of influenza treatment in hospitalized patients younger than 6 years, with intravenous peramivir at a dosage of 600 mg once daily (10 mg/kg once daily in children) for five days plus standard of care compared with placebo plus standard did not demonstrate a clinical benefit.[75]

Neuropsychiatric complications consisting of delirium, seizures, hallucinations, and self-injury in pediatric patients (mostly from Japan) have been reported following treatment with oseltamivir, and peramivir.[66,76] Since influenza itself can be associated with neuropsychiatric manifestations, a causal relationship between oseltamivir or peramivir and neuropsychiatric effects has not been delineated.[42] However, the labels for oseltamivir and peramivir have been updated to include neuropsychiatric events as a precaution, and their occurrence with use of these agents should not be ignored.

Influenza resistance to the NA inhibitors has been documented but cross-resistance between the NA inhibitors has not been reported.[51-53] Antiviral resistance remains relatively low. During the 2014 to 2015 influenza season, 98.4% of the tested 2009 H1N1 viruses were susceptible to oseltamivir and peramivir, and 100% of the 2009 H1N1 viruses tested were susceptible to zanamivir; 100% of influenza A (H3N2) tested were susceptible to both oseltamivir and zanamivir; and 100% of influenza B viruses tested were susceptible to both oseltamivir and zanamivir.[52,77] Antiviral susceptibility testing of circulating viruses confirmed that seasonal influenza A H3N2 and variant influenza H3N2 maintain susceptibility to oseltamivir, peramivir, and zanamivir.[30,51] The burden of surveillance rests on clinicians to identify local patterns of influenza circulation to guide antiviral therapy.

Clinical **Controversy...**

Some clinicians debate the cost–benefit of the use of diagnostic tests for influenza as well as treatment of influenza in otherwise healthy individuals who are likely to experience resolution without treatment. This controversy is compounded by the fact that the diagnostic tests and the benefits associated with treatment of influenza are highest early in the disease process and many patients present after this time period.

Special Populations

Inadequate data exist regarding the use of antiinfluenza medications in special populations, such as immunocompromised hosts. Furthermore, limited data exist regarding use of influenza antivirals during pregnancy. The adamantanes are embryotoxic and teratogenic in rats, and limited case reports of adverse fetal outcomes following amantadine use in humans have been published. Oseltamivir and zanamivir have been used but lack solid safety clinical data in pregnant women. Pregnancy should not be considered a contraindication to oseltamivir or zanamivir use. Oseltamivir is preferred for the treatment of pregnant women because of its systemic activity; however, the drug of choice for chemoprophylaxis is not yet defined. Zanamivir may be preferred because of its limited systemic absorption, but respiratory complications need to be considered, especially in women with underlying respiratory diseases. Both the adamantanes and the NA inhibitors are excreted in breast milk and should be avoided by mothers who are breast-feeding their infants. More studies are needed in these populations who are at high risk for serious disease and complications from influenza.

Clinical **Controversy...**

Some debate exists regarding the benefit of antiviral administration more than 48 hours after onset. While clinicians agree that the most benefit is achieved the earlier the medications are started, some data suggest benefit even beyond 48 hours after onset, albeit more limited.

PANDEMIC PREPAREDNESS

This chapter is not meant to provide an exhaustive review of the biology of influenza or pandemic preparedness. This topic is rapidly changing and interested readers are referred to the following websites: *www.flu.gov*, *www.who.int/influenza/human_animal_interface/en/*, and *www.cdc.gov/h1n1flu*.

A vital component of pandemic preparedness is forethought—plans must be established for how to effectively triage large numbers of ill patients, prioritize and/or ration vaccine and antivirals, and communicate with the public through mass media during a period of severe labor shortage (a result of stress and illness among healthcare workers) and supply shortfall (a result of societal and economic disruption).

EVALUATION OF THERAPEUTIC OUTCOMES

Patients should be monitored daily for resolution of signs and symptoms associated with influenza, such as fever, myalgia, headache, malaise, nonproductive cough, sore throat, and rhinitis. These signs and symptoms will typically resolve within approximately 1 week. If the patient continues to exhibit signs and symptoms of illness beyond 10 days or a worsening of symptoms after 7 days, a physician visit is warranted as this may be an indication of a secondary bacterial infection. Ideally, antiviral therapy should not be started until influenza is confirmed via the laboratory. However, therapy should be initiated within 48 hours of illness onset, emphasizing the need for rapid diagnosis. Repeat diagnostic tests to demonstrate clearance of the virus are not necessary.

ABBREVIATIONS

AAP	American Academy of Pediatrics
ACIP	Advisory Committee on Immunization Practices
CDC	US Centers for Disease Control and Prevention
DFA	direct fluorescence antibody
EIA	enzyme immunoassay
GBS	Guillain-Barré syndrome
GMTs	geometric mean titers
HIV	human immunodeficiency virus
IFA	indirect fluorescence antibody
IIV	inactivated influenza vaccine
IIV3	trivalent influenza vaccine
IIV4	quadrivalent influenza vaccine
LAIV	live-attenuated influenza vaccine
M	matrix
NA	neuraminidase
PIDS	Pediatric Infectious Diseases Society
POC	point of care
PRs	protection rates
RIDTs	Rapid Influenza Diagnostic Tests
RT-PCR	reverse-transcription polymerase chain reaction
SOIV	swine origin influenza virus
WHO	World Health Organization

REFERENCES

1. American Lung Association. Trends in Pneumonia and Influenza Morbidity and Mortality. American Lung Association. New York: Research and Scientific Affairs Epidemiology and Statistics Unit, 2010.
2. McLaughlin JM, McGinnis JJ, Tan L, et al. Estimated human and economic burden of four major adult vaccine-preventable diseases in the United States, 2013. *J Primary Prevent* 2015;36:259-273.
3. Chaves SS, Lynfield R, Lindegren ML, et al. The US influenza hospitalization surveillance network. *Emerg Infect Dis* 2015;21(9):1543-1550.
4. Reed C, Chaves SS, Daily Kirley P, et al. Estimating influenza disease burden from population-based surveillance data in the United States. *PLoS ONE* 2015;10:e0118369. Available at: *http://dx.doi.org/10.1371/journal.pone.0118369.*
5. Uscher-Pines L (RAND), Elixhauser A (AHRQ). Emergency Department Visits and Hospital Inpatient Stays for Seasonal and 2009 H1N1 Influenza, 2008-2009. HCUP Statistical Brief #147. January 2013. Agency for Healthcare Research and Quality, Rockville, MD. Available at: *http://www.hcup-us.ahrq.gov/reports/statbriefs/sb147.pdf.*
6. Matias G, Taylor R, Haguinet F, et al. Estimates of mortality attributable to influenza and RSV in the United States during 1997-2009 by influenza type or subtype, age, cause of death, and risk status. *Influenza Resp Viruses* 2014;8(5):507-515.
7. Reed C, Chaves SS, Perez A, et al. Complications among adults hospitalized with influenza: a comparison of seasonal influenza and the 2009 H1N1 pandemic. *Clin Infect Dis* 2014;59(2):166-174.
8. Nicholson KG, Wood JM, Zambon M. Influenza. *Lancet* 2003;362(9397):1733-1745.
9. Taubenberger JK, Morens DM. 1918 influenza: The mother of all pandemics. *Emerg Infect Dis* 2006;12(1):15-22.
10. Palese P. Influenza: Old and new threats. *Nat Med* 2004;10(12 Suppl): S82-S87.
11. Belshe RB. The origins of pandemic influenza—Lessons from the 1918 virus. *N Engl J Med* 2005;353(21):2209-2211.
12. Monto AS, Comanor L, Shay DK, et al. Epidemiology of pandemic influenza: Use of surveillance and modeling for pandemic preparedness. *J Infect Dis* 2006;194(Suppl 2):S92-S97.
13. Yuen KY, Chan PK, Peiris M, et al. Clinical features and rapid viral diagnosis of human disease associated with avian influenza A H5N1 virus. *Lancet* 1998;351(9101):467-471.
14. Mounts AW, Kwong H, Izurieta HS, et al. Case–control study of risk factors for avian influenza A (H5N1) disease, Hong Kong, 1997. *J Infect Dis* 1999;180(2):505-508.
15. Anonymous. Epidemic and Pandemic Alert and Response: Avian Influenza. Available at: *http://www.who.int/csr/disease/avian_influenza/en/index.html.*
16. World Health Organization. Avian Influenza Weekly Update Number 499, September 2015. Available at: *http://www.wpro.who.int/emerging_diseases/ai-weekly-499-wpro-20150911.pdf?ua=1.*
17. Anonymous. Avian influenza A(H7N9) virus. Available at: *http://www.who.int/influenza/human_animal_interface/influenza_h7n9/en/.*
18. Trombetta C, Piccirella S, Perini D, et al. Emerging influenza strains in the last two decades: A threat of a new pandemic? *Vaccines (Basel)* 2015;3(1):172-185.
19. Yang Y, Halloran ME, Sugimoto JD, et al. Detecting human-to-human transmission of avian influenza A (H5N1). *Emerg Infect Dis* 2007;13:1348-1353.
20. Beigel JH, Farrar J, Han AM, et al. Avian influenza A (H5N1) infection in humans. *N Engl J Med* 2005;353(13):1374-1385.
21. Hill DR. The burden of illness in international travelers. *N Engl J Med* 2006;354(2):115-117.
22. Avian Influenza H5N1 Vaccine. Available at: *http://www.fda.gov/downloads/BiologicsBloodVaccines/Vaccines/ApprovedProducts/UCM112836.pdf.*
23. Influenza A (H5N1) Virus Monovalent Vaccine, Adjuvanted. Available at: *http://www.fda.gov/downloads/BiologicsBloodVaccines/SafetyAvailability/VaccineSafety/UCM376464.pdf.*
24. Harvey K, Esposito DH, Han P, et al. Centers for Disease Control and Prevention (CDC). surveillance for travel-related disease--GeoSentinel Surveillance System, United States, 1997-2011. *MMWR Surveill Summ* 2013;62:1-23.
25. Dawood FS, Jain S, Finelli L, et al. Novel swine-origin influenza A (H1N1) virus investigation team. Emergence of a novel swine-origin influenza A (H1N1) virus in humans. *N Engl J Med* 2009;360:2605-2615.
26. Centers for Disease Control and Prevention. Update: Novel influenza A (H1N1) virus infections—Worldwide, May 6, 2009. *MMWR Morb Mortal Wkly Rep* 2009;58:453-458.
27. Shinde V, Bridges CB, Uyeki TM, et al. Triple-reassortant swine influenza A (H1) in humans in the United States, 2005-2009. *N Engl J Med* 2009;360(25):2616-2625.
28. Dawood FS, Iuliano AD, Reed C, et al. Estimated global mortality associated with the first 12 months of 2009 pandemic influenza A H1N1 virus circulation: A modeling study. *Lancet Infect Dis* 2012;12: 687-695.
29. Jhung MA, Epperson S, Biggerstaff M, et al. Outbreak of variant influenza A(H3N2) virus in the United States. *Clin Infect Dis* 2013;57(12):1703-1712.
30. Centers for Disease Control and Prevention. Influenza A (H3N2) Variant Virus Outbreaks. Available at *http://www.cdc.gov/flu/swineflu/h3n2v-case-count.htm.*
31. Grohskopf LA, Sokolow LZ, Broder KR, et al. Prevention and Control of Seasonal Influenza with Vaccines. *MMWR Recomm Rep* 2016; 65(No. RR-5):1 -54. DOI: http://dx.doi.org/10.15585/mmwr.rr6505a1.
32. American Academy of Pediatrics, Committee on Infectious Diseases. Policy, statement—Recommendations for prevention and control of influenza in children, 2015-2016. *Pediatrics* 2015;136(4):2015-2920.
33. Geiler J, Michaelis M, Sithisarn P, et al. Comparison of pro-inflammatory cytokine expression and cellular signal transduction in human macrophages infected with different influenza A viruses. *Med Microbiol Immunol* 2011;200(1):53-60.
34. Marzoratti L, Iannella HA, Gómez VF, et al. Recent advances in the diagnosis and treatment of influenza pneumonia. *Curr Infect Dis Rep* 2012;14(3):275-283.
35. Fraaij PL, Heikkinen T. Seasonal influenza: the burden of disease in children. *Vaccine* 2011;29(43):7524-7528.
36. Centers for Disease Control and Prevention (CDC). Guidance for clinicians on the use of rapid influenza diagnostic tests. Available at *http://www.cdc.gov/flu/pdf/professionals/diagnosis/clinician_guidance_ridt.pdf.*
37. Chartrand C, Leeflang MM, Minion J, et al. Accuracy of rapid influenza diagnostic tests: a meta-analysis. *Ann Intern Med.* 2012;156(7): 500-511.
38. Hoberman A, Greenberg DP, Paradise JL, et al. Effectiveness of inactivated influenza vaccine in preventing acute otitis media in young children: A randomized controlled trial. *JAMA* 2003;290(12):1608-1616.
39. Bridges CB, Thompson WW, Meltzer MI, et al. Effectiveness and cost–benefit of influenza vaccination of healthy working adults: A randomized controlled trial. *JAMA* 2000;284(13):1655-1663.
40. Gorse GJ, Falsey AR, Ozol-Godfrey A, et al. Safety and immunogenicity of a quadrivalent intradermal influenza vaccine in adults. *Vaccine* 2015;33(9):1151-1159.
41. Fluzone Intradermal Quadrivalent vaccine [Package insert]. Swiftwater, PA: Sanofi Pasteur; 2015.
42. Hamborsky J, Kroger A, Wolfe S, eds. Centers for Disease Control and Prevention. Influenza. In: *Epidemiology and Prevention of Vaccine-Preventable Diseases*, 13th ed. Washington D.C. Public Health Foundation, 2015. Available at *http://www.cdc.gov/vaccines/pubs/pinkbook/downloads/flu.pdf.*
43. Juurlink DN, Stukel TA, Kwong J, et al. Guillain-Barré syndrome after influenza vaccination in adults: A population-based study. *Arch Intern Med* 2006;166(20):2217-2221.
44. Lasky T, Terracciano GJ, Magder L, et al. The Guillain-Barré syndrome and the 1992-1993 and 1993-1994 influenza vaccines. *N Engl J Med* 1998;339(25):1797-1802.
45. Centers for Disease Control and Prevention (CDC). Summary of the joint statement on thimerosal in vaccines. American Academy of Family Physicians, American Academy of Pediatrics, Advisory Committee on Immunization Practices, Public Health Service. *MMWR Morb Mortal Wkly Rep* 2000;49(27):622-631.
46. Price CS, Thompson WW, Goodson B, et al. Prenatal and infant exposure to thimerosal from vaccines and immunoglobulins and risk of autism. *Pediatrics* 2010;126:656-664.
47. Institute of Medicine. Adverse Effects of Vaccines: Evidence and Causality. August 25, 2011. Available at *http://www.iom.edu/Reports/2011/Adverse-Effects-of-Vaccines-Evidence-and-Causality.aspx.*
48. FluMist Quadrivalent Vaccine [prescribing information]. Gaithersburg, MD: MedImmune, LLC, 2015.
49. Belshe RB, Ambrose CS, Yi T. Safety and efficacy of live attenuated influenza vaccine in children 2-7 years of age. Vaccine 2008;26(Suppl 4): D10-D16.
50. Nichol KL, Mendelman PM, Mallon KP, et al. Effectiveness of live, attenuated intranasal influenza virus vaccine in healthy, working adults: A randomized controlled trial. *JAMA* 1999;282(2):137-144.

51. Blanton L, Kniss K, Smith S, et al. Update: Influenza Activity—United States and Worldwide, May 24-September 5, 2015. *MMWR Morb Mortal Wkly Rep* 2015;64(36):1011-1016.
52. Centers for Diseases Control and Prevention. Influenza Antiviral Medications: Summary for Clinicians 2015-2016. Available at *http://www.cdc.gov/flu/pdf/professionals/antivirals/antiviral-summary-clinician.pdf.*
53. Fiore AE, Fry A, Shay D, et al. Centers for Disease Control and Prevention (CDC). Antiviral agents for the treatment and chemoprophylaxis of influenza—recommendations of the Advisory Committee on Immunization Practices (ACIP). *MMWR Recomm Rep* 2011;60(1):1-24.
54. Bradley JS, Byington CL, Shah SS, et al. The management of community-acquired pneumonia in infants and children older than 3 months of age: Clinical practice guidelines by the Pediatric Infectious Diseases Society and the Infectious Diseases Society of America. *Clin Infect Dis* 2011;53(7):e25-e76.
55. Peters PH Jr, Gravenstein S, Norwood P, et al. Long-term use of oseltamivir for the prophylaxis of influenza in a vaccinated frail older population. *J Am Geriatr Soc* 2001;49(8):1025-1031.
56. Benowitz I, Esposito DB, Gracey KD, et al. Influenza vaccine given to pregnant women reduces hospitalization due to influenza in their infants. *Clin Infect Dis* 2010;51(12):1355-1361.
57. Tasker SA, Treanor JJ, Paxton WB, et al. Efficacy of influenza vaccination in HIV-infected persons. A randomized, double-blind, placebo-controlled trial. *Ann Intern Med* 1999;131(6):430-433.
58. Kroon FP, van Dissel JT, de Jong JC, et al. Antibody response after influenza vaccination in HIV-infected individuals: A consecutive 3-year study. *Vaccine* 2000;18(26):3040-3049.
59. Soesman NM, Rimmelzwaan GF, Nieuwkoop NJ, et al. Efficacy of influenza vaccination in adult liver transplant recipients. *J Med Virol* 2000;61(1):85-93.
60. Shehata MA, Karim NA. Influenza vaccination in cancer patients undergoing systemic therapy. *Clin Med Insights Oncol* 2014;8:57-64.
61. Gelinck LB, van den Bemt BJ, Marijt WA, et al. Intradermal influenza vaccination in immunocompromized patients is immunogenic and feasible. Vaccine 2009;27(18):2469-2474.
62. Whitley RJ, Monto AS. Prevention and treatment of influenza in high-risk groups: Children, pregnant women, immunocompromised hosts, and nursing home residents. *J Infect Dis* 2006;194(Suppl 2):S133-S138.
63. Ison MG, Gubareva LV, Atmar RL, et al. Recovery of drug-resistant influenza virus from immunocompromised patients: A case series. *J Infect Dis* 2006;193(6):760-764.
64. Shetty AK, Ross GA, Pranikoff T, et al. Oseltamivir-resistant 2009 H1N1 influenza pneumonia during therapy in a renal transplant recipient. *Pediatr Transplant* 2012;16(5):E153-E157.
65. Treanor JJ, Hayden FG, Vrooman PS, et al. Efficacy and safety of the oral neuraminidase inhibitor oseltamivir in treating acute influenza: A randomized controlled trial. US Oral Neuraminidase Study Group. *JAMA* 2000;283(8):1016-1024.
66. Aoki FY, Macleod MD, Paggiaro P, et al. Early administration of oral oseltamivir increases the benefits of influenza treatment. *J Antimicrob Chemother* 2003;51(1):123-129.
67. Louie JK, Yang S, Acosta M, et al. Treatment with neuraminidase inhibitors for critically ill patients with influenza A (H1N1)pdm09. *Clin Infect Dis* 2012;55(9):1198-1204.
68. Siston AM, Rasmussen SA, Honein MA, et al. Pandemic 2009 influenza A(H1N1) virus illness among pregnant women in the United States. *JAMA* 2010;303(15):1517-1525.
69. Kaiser L, Wat C, Mills T, et al. Impact of oseltamivir treatment on influenza-related lower respiratory tract complications and hospitalizations. *Arch Intern Med* 2003;163(14):1667-1672.
70. Kaiser L, Keene ON, Hammond JM, et al. Impact of zanamivir on antibiotic use for respiratory events following acute influenza in adolescents and adults. *Arch Intern Med* 2000;160(21):3234-3240.
71. Peramivir (Rapivab)® [Package Insert]. Durham, NC 27703: BioCryst Pharmaceuticals, Inc. 2015
72. Ison MG, Hui DS, Clezy K, et al. A clinical trial of intravenous peramivir compared with oral oseltamivir for the treatment of seasonal influenza in hospitalized adults. *Antivir Ther* 2013;18(5):651-661.
73. Hernandez JE, Adiga R, Armstrong R, et al. Clinical experience in adults and children treated with intravenous peramivir for 2009 influenza A (H1N1) under an emergency IND program in the United States. *Clin Infect Dis* 2011;52:695.
74. Kohno S, Kida H, Mizuguchi M, et al. Efficacy and safety of intravenous peramivir for treatment of seasonal influenza virus infection. *Antimicrob Agents Chemother* 2010; 54(11):4568-4574.
75. de Jong MD, Ison MG, Monto AS, et al. Evaluation of intravenous peramivir for treatment of influenza in hospitalized patients. *Clin Infect Dis* 2014;59(12):172-185.
76. Tamiflu [prescribing information]. San Francisco, CA: Genentech USA, Inc/Roche Group, August 2012, Available at: *http:/www.rocheusa.com/products/tamiflu/pi.pdf.*
77. Centers for Disease Prevention and Control. Influenza Antiviral Drug Resistance. Available at: *http://www.cdc.gov/flu/about/qa/antiviralresistance.htm.*

110 Skin and Soft-Tissue Infections

Douglas N. Fish

KEY CONCEPTS

1. Folliculitis, furuncles (boils), and carbuncles begin around hair follicles and are caused most often by *Staphylococcus aureus*. Folliculitis and small furuncles are generally treated with warm, moist heat to promote drainage; larger furuncles and carbuncles require incision and drainage. Purulent, moderately severe infections (eg, with fever or other systemic signs of infection) have a higher suspicion for community-associated methicillin-resistant *S. aureus* (MRSA) and empiric treatment should include trimethoprim–sulfamethoxazole or a tetracycline such as doxycycline.
2. Erysipelas, a superficial skin infection with extensive lymphatic involvement, is caused by *Streptococcus pyogenes*. The treatment of choice is penicillin, administered orally or parenterally, depending on the severity of the infection.
3. Impetigo is a superficial skin infection that occurs most commonly in children. It is characterized by fluid-filled vesicles that develop rapidly into pus-filled blisters that rupture to form golden-yellow crusts. Effective therapy includes penicillinase-resistant penicillins (dicloxacillin), first-generation cephalosporins (cephalexin), and topical mupirocin or retapamulin. *S. aureus* is the primary cause of impetigo, with infections caused by MRSA emerging in recent years.
4. Lymphangitis, an infection of the subcutaneous lymphatic channels, is generally caused by *S. pyogenes*. Acute lymphangitis is characterized by the rapid development of fine, red, linear streaks extending from the initial infection site toward the regional lymph nodes, which are usually enlarged and tender. Penicillin is the drug of choice.
5. Cellulitis is an infection of the epidermis, dermis, and superficial fascia most commonly caused by *S. pyogenes* and *S. aureus*. Lesions generally are hot, painful, and erythematous, with nonelevated, poorly defined margins. Oral trimethoprim–sulfamethoxazole, doxycycline, or minocycline is used for initial treatment of suspected MRSA in patients with purulent, moderately severe cellulitis (ie, lesion with purulent drainage or exudate, or nondrainable abscess plus systemic signs of infection). Treatment of nonpurulent cellulitis generally consists of penicillin VK, a penicillinase-resistant penicillin (dicloxacillin), first-generation cephalosporin (cephalexin), or clindamycin for 5 days, with the option of adding coverage for MRSA in certain patients. More severe infections in hospitalized and/or immunocompromised patients should receive empiric therapy with parenteral agents active against streptococci (nonpurulent infections) or both streptococci and MRSA (purulent infections).
6. Necrotizing fasciitis is a rare but life-threatening infection of subcutaneous tissue that results in progressive destruction of superficial fascia and subcutaneous fat. Early and aggressive surgical debridement is an essential part of therapy for treatment of necrotizing fasciitis. Mixed infections are treated with broad-spectrum regimens that cover streptococci, gram-negative aerobes, and anaerobes. Infections caused by *S. pyogenes* or *Clostridium* species should be treated with the combination of penicillin and clindamycin.
7. Diabetic foot infections are managed with a comprehensive treatment approach that includes both proper wound care and antimicrobial therapy. Potential pathogens include staphylococci, streptococci, aerobic gram-negative bacilli, and obligate anaerobes. Antimicrobial regimens for diabetic foot infections are based on severity of the infection, expected treatment setting, and risk factors for infection with more resistant pathogens such as MRSA and *Pseudomonas aeruginosa*. Outpatient therapy with oral antimicrobials should be used whenever possible for less severe infections, while more severe infections initially require IV therapy.
8. Prevention is the single most important aspect in the management of pressure sores. After a sore develops, successful local care includes a comprehensive approach consisting of relief of pressure, proper cleaning (debridement), disinfection, and appropriate antimicrobial therapy if an infection is present. Good wound care is crucial to successful management.
9. All bite wounds (either animal or human) should be irrigated thoroughly with large volumes of sterile normal saline, and the injured area should be immobilized and elevated. Depending on the severity of the bite wound, amoxicillin–clavulanic acid or ampicillin–sulbactam is often used for treatment of animal bites because of their coverage of *Pasteurella* species, streptococci, *S. aureus*, and anaerobes typically present in the oral flora of dogs and cats.
10. Antimicrobial prophylaxis (early preemptive therapy) of animal bites is not recommended routinely; however, patients at high risk of infection (eg, immunocompromised, moderate to severe bite injuries especially to the hands and face, penetration of the periosteum or joint capsule) should be given prophylactic antimicrobial therapy for 3 to 5 days. Infected bite wounds should be treated for 7 to 14 days with oral or IV antibiotics having activity against *Eikenella corrodens*, streptococci, *S. aureus*, and β-lactamase–producing anaerobes.

Skin and soft-tissue infections (SSTIs) may involve any or all layers of the skin (epidermis, dermis, subcutaneous fat), fascia, and muscle. They may also spread far from the initial site of infection and lead to more severe complications, such as endocarditis, gram-negative sepsis, or streptococcal glomerulonephritis. Sometimes the treatment of SSTIs may necessitate both medical and surgical management. This chapter presents details of the pathogenesis and management of some of the most common infections involving the skin and soft tissues, ranging in severity from superficial to life-threatening.

EPIDEMIOLOGY

Bacterial infections of the skin can be classified as primary or secondary (Table 110-1).[1-3] Primary bacterial infections usually involve areas of previously healthy skin and are caused by a single pathogen. In contrast, secondary infections occur in areas of previously damaged skin and are frequently polymicrobic. SSTIs are also classified as complicated or uncomplicated. Complicated infections are those that involve deeper skin structures (eg, fascia, muscle layers), require significant surgical intervention, or occur in patients with compromised immune function (eg, diabetes mellitus, human immunodeficiency virus [HIV] infection).[4] Other categories that are crucial for successful treatment are the differentiation of necrotizing versus nonnecrotizing, as well as purulent versus nonpurulent, SSTIs.[4-7]

SSTIs are among the most common infections seen in community and hospital settings.[8,9] However, most infections are believed to be mild and are treated in an outpatient setting, making it difficult to accurately quantify community-acquired SSTIs. SSTIs were diagnosed in 0.8% of physician office visits between 1993 and 2005; this corresponded to approximately 82 million diagnoses of SSTI, being more common among those 70 years of age and older.[3] Emergency room visits for SSTIs have increased dramatically in recent years, attributed primarily to an increase in community-associated methicillin-resistant *Staphylococcus aureus* (CA-MRSA) cellulitis and abscesses.[10,11] A study of emergency department visit rates between 1997 and 2007 found a 3.1-fold increase (11% per year) for abscess SSTIs, with only a minimal increase in nonabscess SSTIs.[11] According to an Agency for Healthcare Research and Quality report, in 2009 SSTIs were responsible for nearly 600,000 hospitalizations and represented 2% of all admissions in males and 1.2% in females.[9] While the exact incidence of SSTIs is unknown, the frequency of infections caused by drug-resistant gram-positive cocci has been increasing.[4-7] The high incidence of healthcare-associated MRSA (HA-MRSA) has been a major concern for many years and the emergence of CA-MRSA is even more problematic.[5-7,12-18] CA-MRSA are characteristically isolated from patients lacking typical risk factors (eg, prior hospitalization, long-term care facility) and are often susceptible to non–β-lactam antibiotics such as trimethoprim–sulfamethoxazole, doxycycline, and clindamycin.[1,12,13,15,17-19] They also differ genetically from HA-MRSA with methicillin resistance carried on the type IV or type V staphylococcal chromosomal cassette *mec* (SCC*mec*) element of the *mecA* gene.[1,12,18] CA-MRSA strains often harbor genes for Panton-Valentine leukocidin (PVL), a cytotoxin responsible for leukocyte destruction and tissue necrosis. In contrast, HA-MRSA strains usually lack genes for PVL and are associated with SCC*mec* alleles I to III.[1,12,15,18] While the incidence of HA-MRSA has declined in recent years,[20] the incidence of CA-MRSA has dramatically increased; nearly half (46%) of all culture-positive SSTIs are caused by MRSA.[4-7,8,19] Clinicians should suspect CA-MRSA in geographic areas with a high prevalence of these strains, or in recurrent or persistent infections that are not responding to appropriate β-lactam therapy. In addition to the emergence of CA-MRSA, treatment choices for SSTIs have been further complicated by the increased incidence of macrolide-resistant strains of *S. aureus* and *Streptococcus pyogenes*.[15,19,21] Data from the Minnesota Department of Health found erythromycin susceptibility among CA-MRSA strains decreased from 45% to 13% during the years 2000 to 2005.[19] There is concern about the use of clindamycin for CA-MRSA infections due to the risk of inducible clindamycin resistance in *S. aureus* strains that are erythromycin-resistant, but clindamycin-susceptible.[18,19] A double-disk test (D-zone test) is recommended to identify erythromycin-resistant strains with inducible clindamycin resistance if treatment with clindamycin is desired.[6,7,12] A positive D-zone test, indicating the presence of inducible resistance conferred by the *erm* gene, suggests the possibility of the emergence of clindamycin resistance during therapy.[12]

TABLE 110-1 Bacterial Classification of Important Skin and Soft-Tissue Infections [1-3]

Primary Infections	
Erysipelas	Group A streptococci (*Streptococcus pyogenes*)
Impetigo	*Staphylococcus aureus* (including methicillin-resistant strains), group A streptococci
Lymphangitis	Group A streptococci; occasionally *S. aureus*
Cellulitis	Group A streptococci, *S. aureus* (potentially including methicillin-resistant strains); occasionally other gram-positive cocci, gram-negative bacilli, and/or anaerobes
Necrotizing fasciitis	
Type I	Anaerobes (*Bacteroides* spp., *Peptostreptococcus* spp.) and facultative bacteria (streptococci, Enterobacteriaceae)
Type II	Group A streptococci
Type III	*Clostridium perfringens*
Secondary Infections	
Diabetic foot infections	*S. aureus*, streptococci, Enterobacteriaceae, *Bacteroides* spp., *Peptostreptococcus* spp., *Pseudomonas aeruginosa*
Pressure sores	*S. aureus* including methicillin-resistant strains, streptococci, Enterobacteriaceae, *Bacteroides* spp., *Peptostreptococcus* spp., *P. aeruginosa*
Bite wounds	
Animal	*Pasteurella* spp., *S. aureus*, streptococci, *Bacteroides* spp.
Human	*Eikenella corrodens*, *S. aureus*, streptococci, *Corynebacterium* spp., *Bacteroides* spp., *Peptostreptococcus* spp.
Burn wounds	*P. aeruginosa*, Enterobacteriaceae, *S. aureus*, streptococci

ETIOLOGY

The majority of SSTIs are caused by gram-positive organisms present on the skin surface.[7,22] Gram-positive bacteria (coagulase-negative staphylococci, diphtheroids) are the predominant flora of the skin, with gram-negative organisms being relatively uncommon (Table 110-2).[1-3] *S. aureus*, as well as a variety of gram-negative

TABLE 110-2 Predominant Microorganisms of Normal Skin [1-3]

Bacteria
Gram-positive
- Coagulase-negative staphylococci
- Micrococci (*Micrococcus luteus*)
- *Corynebacterium* species (diphtheroids)
- *Propionibacterium* species

Gram-negative
- *Acinetobacter* species

Fungi
Malassezia species
Candida species

bacteria, including *Acinetobacter* species, can be found in moist intertriginous areas (eg, axilla, groin, and toe webs) of the body.[1,2,23] Approximately 30% to 35% of healthy individuals are reported to be colonized with *S. aureus* on the skin or in the anterior nares.[1,3] Colonization, whether transient or permanent, provides a nidus for infection should the integrity of the epidermis be compromised.[1,2,10]

S. aureus and *S. pyogenes* account for the majority of community-acquired SSTIs.[1,10,22] Data from large surveillance studies showed *S. aureus* to be the most common cause of SSTIs in hospitalized patients, with often 30%-40% of these being caused by MRSA.[3,8,9] Other common nosocomial pathogens included *Pseudomonas aeruginosa* (11%), enterococci (9%), and *Escherichia coli* (7%).[3,8,9]

PATHOPHYSIOLOGY

The skin serves as a barrier between humans and their environment, therefore functioning as a primary defense mechanism against infections. The skin and subcutaneous tissues normally are extremely resistant to infection but may become susceptible under certain conditions. Even when high concentrations of bacteria are applied topically or injected into the soft tissue, resulting infections are rare.[1-3,24,25] Although the human skin supports an abundant and diverse microbiome of bacteria and fungi,[1,2] several host factors act together to confer protection against skin infections. Continuous renewal of the epidermal layer results in the shedding of keratocytes, as well as skin bacteria.[2] In addition, sebaceous secretions are hydrolyzed to form free fatty acids that strongly inhibit the growth of many bacteria and fungi. A normal commensal skin microbiome itself serves a protective function by not allowing space or environmental conditions favorable to colonization with more pathogenic strains.[1,2] Conditions that may predispose a patient to the development of skin infections include (a) high concentrations of bacteria (more than 10^5 microorganisms), (b) excessive moisture of the skin, (c) inadequate blood supply, (d) availability of bacterial nutrients, and (e) damage to the corneal layer allowing for bacterial penetration.[2,3,24,25]

The best defense against SSTI is intact skin.[2,24] The majority of SSTIs result from the disruption of normal host defenses by processes such as skin puncture, abrasion, or underlying diseases (eg, diabetes).[1,2,24,26] The nature and severity of the infection depend on both the type of microorganism present and the site of inoculation.

FOLLICULITIS, FURUNCLES, AND CARBUNCLES

1 Folliculitis is inflammation of the hair follicle and is caused by physical injury, chemical irritation, or infection. Infection occurring at the base of the eyelid is referred to as a stye. While folliculitis is a superficial infection with pus present only in the epidermis,[10,22] furuncles and carbuncles occur when a follicular infection extends from around the hair shaft to involve deeper areas (subcutaneous tissue) of the skin.[26] A furuncle, commonly known as a *boil*, is a walled-off mass of purulent material arising from a hair follicle.[10] The lesions are called *carbuncles* when adjacent furuncles coalesce to form a single inflamed area.[10] This aggregate of infected hair follicles forms deep masses that generally open and drain through multiple sinus tracts.[12,26] *S. aureus* is the most common cause of folliculitis, furuncles, and carbuncles.[12,26] Inadequate chlorine levels in whirlpools, hot tubs, and swimming pools have been responsible for outbreaks of folliculitis caused by *P. aeruginosa*.[1,26] Outbreaks of furunculosis caused by *S. aureus* and CA-MRSA have been reported in settings involving close contact (eg, families, prisons), especially when skin injury was common (such as with sports).[12,26] In addition, some individuals experience repeated episodes of furunculosis.[22] A major predisposing factor in recurrent infection is the presence of *S. aureus* in the anterior nares.[15,22,26]

TREATMENT
Folliculitis, Furuncles, and Carbuncles

Desired Outcomes

The goals of treatment include relieving discomfort, preventing further spread of the infection, and preventing recurrence. Controlling recurrent furunculosis is key due to the difficulty in treating chronic furunculosis.[22] Treatments should be effective and inexpensive and have minimal adverse effects.

CLINICAL PRESENTATION

Folliculitis

- Clustering, pruritic papules localized to hair follicles.
- Generally develop in areas subject to friction and perspiration.
- Papules are generally 5 mm or less in diameter and erythematous.
- Papules evolve into pustules that generally spontaneously rupture in several days.
- Systemic signs (fever, malaise) are uncommon.

Furuncles

- Inflammatory, draining nodule involving a hair follicle.
- Generally develop in areas subject to friction and perspiration.
- Lesions are discrete, whether occurring as singular or multiple nodules.
- Lesion starts as a firm, tender, red nodule that becomes painful and fluctuant.
- Lesions often drain spontaneously.
- Lesions caused by CA-MRSA often have necrotic centers characteristic of "spider bites."
- Systemic signs are uncommon.

Carbuncles

- Formed when adjacent furuncles coalesce to form a single inflamed area.
- Form broad, swollen, erythematous, deep, and painful follicular masses.
- Commonly develop on the back of the neck and are more likely to occur in patients with diabetes.
- Commonly associated with systemic signs (fever, chills, malaise).
- Bacteremia with secondary spread to other tissues is common.

Treatment

Table 110-3 summarizes evidence-based treatment recommendations from clinical guidelines for SSTIs.[3,5,6,15,27-29] Treatment of folliculitis generally requires only local measures, such as warm moist compresses or topical therapy (eg, clindamycin, erythromycin, mupirocin, or benzoyl peroxide).[3,26] Topical agents generally are applied two to four times daily for 7 days. Small furuncles generally can be treated with moist heat, which promotes localization and drainage of pus.[3,26] Large and/or multiple furuncles and carbuncles require incision and drainage.[3,4,12,15,28] Systemic antibiotics are usually not necessary unless accompanied by fever or extensive cellulitis.[4,15] Treatment of more severe infections (eg, accompanied by systemic signs of infection) should include oral trimethoprim–sulfamethoxazole or a tetracycline (either doxycycline or minocycline) for 5 to 10 days due to a higher suspicion for MRSA (refer to Table 110-4 for adult and pediatric doses).[4,6,15,22,28] For individuals with nasal colonization, application of mupirocin ointment twice daily in the anterior nares for the first 5 days of each month decreases recurrent furunculosis by almost half.[15,22] Daily chlorhexidine washes and daily washing of personal items such as towels, bedding, and clothes may also be recommended.[15]

Evaluation of Therapeutic Outcomes

Many follicular infections resolve spontaneously without medical or surgical intervention. Lesions should be incised if they do not respond to a few days of moist heat and nonprescription topical agents. Following drainage, most lesions begin to heal within several days without antimicrobial therapy. Any patient who is unresponsive to several days of systemic antibiotic therapy or suffers recurrent infection should have a culture and sensitivity test performed to guide continued antibiotic selection.

ERYSIPELAS

2 Erysipelas is a distinct form of cellulitis involving the more superficial layers of the skin and cutaneous lymphatics.[5,12,22,30] The intense red color and burning pain associated with this skin infection led to the common name of "St. Anthony's fire." The infection is almost always caused by β-hemolytic streptococci, with the organisms gaining access via small breaks in the skin. Group A streptococci (*S. pyogenes*) are responsible for most infections.[3,15,22] Infections are more common in infants, young children, the elderly, and patients with nephrotic syndrome.[3,6] Erysipelas also commonly occurs in areas of preexisting lymphatic obstruction or edema.[3,12] Diagnosis is made on the basis of the characteristic lesion.

TREATMENT
Erysipelas

Desired Outcomes

The goal of treatment of erysipelas is rapid eradication of the infection, thereby providing relief of symptoms (pain, tenderness, fever).[30] Preventing recurrent infection is also important, as recurrence is a primary complication, occurring in approximately 20% of patients.[22,30] Treatments should be effective and inexpensive and have minimal adverse effects.

Treatment

Mild to moderate cases of erysipelas are treated with intramuscular procaine penicillin G or penicillin VK for 7 to 10 days (see Table 110-4).[3,22] Recommended doses and monitoring parameters for selected antibiotics are given in Tables 110-5 and 110-6. Penicillin-allergic patients can be treated with clindamycin. For more serious infections, the patient should be hospitalized and aqueous penicillin G administered IV.[3,22] Marked improvement usually is seen within 48 hours, and the patient often may be switched to oral penicillin to complete the course of therapy. Although one study has shown that the median time for cure, IV antibiotics, and hospital stay was reduced in patients receiving prednisolone in addition to antibiotics, further studies are needed before corticosteroids can be recommended for routine use.[3,15,31]

Evaluation of Therapeutic Outcomes

Erysipelas generally responds quickly to appropriate antimicrobial therapy. Temperature and white blood cell count should return to normal within 48 to 72 hours. Erythema, edema, and pain also should resolve gradually.

IMPETIGO

3 Impetigo is a superficial skin infection that is seen most commonly in children.[6,22,33] The infection is generally classified as bullous or nonbullous based on clinical presentation.[10,33] Impetigo is most common during hot, humid weather, which facilitates microbial colonization of the skin.[3,6,22,33] Minor trauma, such as scratches or insect bites, allows entry of organisms into the superficial layers of skin, and infection ensues.[3,22,26,33] Impetigo is highly communicable and readily spreads through close contact, especially among siblings and children in daycare centers and schools.[3,22,33]

CLINICAL PRESENTATION Erysipelas

General

- Lower extremities are the most common sites.

Symptoms

- Flu-like symptoms (fever, chills, malaise) common prior to the appearance of the lesion.
- Infected area described as painful or as a burning pain.

Signs

- Lesion is intensely erythematous and edematous, often with lymphatic streaking.
- Lesion has raised border, which is sharply demarcated from uninfected skin.
- Temperature is often mildly elevated.

Laboratory Tests

- Causative organism usually cannot be cultured from the surface skin.
- Needle aspiration or punch biopsies occasionally identify organism.
- Cultures considered for more severe cases (eg, atypical clinical findings such as fluid-filled blisters).

Other Diagnostic Tests

- A complete blood count is often performed because leukocytosis is common.
- C-reactive protein is also generally elevated.

TABLE 110-3 Evidence-Based Recommendations for Treatment of Skin and Soft-Tissue Infections[3,5,6,15,27-29]

Recommendations	Recommendation Grade[a]
Folliculitis, Furuncles, Carbuncles	
Gram stain and culture of pus from carbuncles and abscesses are recommended, but treatment without cultures is reasonable in most patients	Strong, moderate
Carbuncles, abscesses and large furuncles of mild severity should be treated with incision and drainage	Strong, high
Administration of antibiotics with activity against *Staphylococcus aureus* as an adjunct to incision and drainage should be based on presence or absence of systemic signs of infection	Strong, low
Antibiotics with activity against MRSA are recommended for patients with carbuncles or abscesses of higher severity who have failed initial antibiotic therapy, have severe systemic signs of infection, or are immunocompromised	Strong, low
Erysipelas	
Most infections are caused by *Streptococcus pyogenes*. Penicillin (oral or IV depending on clinical severity) is the drug of choice	A-I
If *S. aureus* is suspected, a penicillinase-resistant penicillin or first-generation cephalosporin should be used	A-I
Impetigo	
Gram stain and culture of pus or exudates should be obtained to help identify causative pathogens	Strong, moderate
Bullous and nonbullous impetigo should be treated with either mupirocin or retapamulin for 5 days	Strong, high
Impetigo should be treated with oral antibiotics active against S. aureus unless cultures show streptococci alone. Dicloxacillin or cephalexin is recommended for 7 days. Doxycycline, clindamycin, or sulfamethoxazole-trimethoprim should be used when MRSA is suspected or confirmed	Strong, moderate
Cellulitis	
Cultures of blood or cutaneous aspirates, biopsies or swabs are not routinely recommended	Strong, moderate
Blood cultures are recommended, and cultures of cutaneous aspirates, biopsies, or swabs should be considered, in patients receiving chemotherapy for malignancies, neutropenia, severe cell-mediated immunodeficiency, immersion injuries, or animal bites	Strong, moderate (blood) Weak, moderate (other cultures)
Typical cases of mild nonpurulent cellulitis should be treated with antibiotics active against streptococci	Strong, moderate
Systemic antibiotics are recommended for moderate nonpurulent cellulitis with systemic signs of infection. Use of antibiotics active against methicillin-susceptible *S. aureus* could be considered	Weak, low
Patients with severe nonpurulent cellulitis associated with penetrating trauma, MRSA infection in another location, MRSA nasal colonization, injection drug use, or systemic signs of infection should be treated with vancomycin or other antibiotics active against both MRSA and streptococci	Strong, moderate
Broad-spectrum antibiotic therapy with vancomycin plus either piperacillin–tazobactam, imipenem, or meropenem may be considered for empiric treatment of severe nonpurulent cellulitis in severely immunocompromised patients	Weak, moderate (need for broad-spectrum therapy) Strong, moderate (recommended broad-spectrum antibiotic regimen if used)
A treatment duration of 5 days is recommended for cellulitis, but may be extended if lack of clinical response within that time	Strong, high
Elevation of the affected area and treatment of predisposing factors are recommended for cellulitis	Strong, moderate
Systemic corticosteroids for 7 days can be considered for adjunctive treatment of cellulitis in nondiabetic patients	Weak, moderate
Patients with mild nonpurulent cellulitis who do not have systemic signs of infection, altered mental status, or hemodynamic instability should be treated as outpatients	Strong, moderate
Hospitalization is recommended for patients with moderate to severe nonpurulent cellulitis who have failed outpatient therapy, have poor adherence to therapy, are immunocompromised, or in whom there is a concern for deeper or necrotizing infection	Strong, moderate
Empiric antibiotics for outpatients with purulent cellulitis should provide activity against community-associated MRSA; coverage of β-hemolytic streptococci is likely not required. Mild–moderate infections can generally be treated with oral agents (dicloxacillin, cephalexin, clindamycin) unless resistance is high in the community	A-II
Recommended antibiotics for empiric coverage of MRSA in outpatients include orally administered trimethoprim–sulfamethoxazole, doxycycline, minocycline, clindamycin, and linezolid	A-II for all listed options
If coverage of both β-hemolytic streptococci and community-associated MRSA is desired, empiric antibiotic regimens for outpatient therapy include orally administered clindamycin alone; linezolid alone; or trimethoprim–sulfamethoxazole, doxycycline, or minocycline in combination with amoxicillin	A-II for all listed options
Hospitalized patients with complicated or purulent cellulitis should receive IV antibiotics with activity against MRSA pending culture data. Antibiotic options include vancomycin, linezolid, daptomycin, telavancin, and clindamycin	A-I for all except clindamycin; clindamycin A-III
In the treatment of *S. aureus* infections, trough serum vancomycin concentrations should always be maintained >10 mg/L (>7 μmol/L) to avoid development of resistance	B-III
Necrotizing Fasciitis	
Patients with severe nonpurulent cellulitis characterized by aggressive infection and associated with signs of systemic toxicity, necrotizing fasciitis, or gas gangrene should have prompt surgical consultation	Strong, low

(continued)

TABLE 110-3 Evidence-Based Recommendations for Treatment of Skin and Soft-Tissue Infections[3,5,6,15,27-29] (*Continued*)

Recommendations	Recommendation Grade[a]
Early and aggressive surgical debridement of all necrotic tissue is essential	A-III
Necrotizing fasciitis should be empirically treated with broad-spectrum antibiotics such as vancomycin or linezolid plus piperacillin–tazobactam or a carbapenem, or vancomycin or linezolid plus ceftriaxone and metronidazole	Strong, low
Necrotizing fasciitis caused by *S. pyogenes* should be treated with the combination of clindamycin and penicillin	Strong, low
In the treatment of necrotizing fasciitis caused by methicillin-resistant *S. aureus* infections, trough serum vancomycin concentrations of 15-20 mg/L (10-14 μmol/L) are recommended	B-II
Clostridial gas gangrene (myonecrosis) should be treated with clindamycin and penicillin	B-III
Diabetic Foot Infections	
Clinically uninfected wounds should not be treated with antibiotics	A-III
Empiric antibiotic regimens should be selected based on severity of infection and likely pathogens	A-III
Antibiotic therapy should target only aerobic gram-positive cocci in patients with mild to moderate infection who have not received antibiotics within the previous month	C-III
Broad-spectrum empiric antibiotic therapy should be initiated in most patients with severe infections, until culture and susceptibility data are available	A-III
Empiric antibiotics directed against *Pseudomonas aeruginosa* are usually unnecessary except in patients with specific risk factors for infection with this pathogen: patient has been soaking feet, patient has failed previous antibiotic therapy with nonpseudomonal agents, or clinically severe infection	A-III
Empiric antibiotics directed against MRSA should be considered in patients with specific risk factors, including: prior history of infection or colonization with MRSA, high local prevalence of MRSA (eg, ≥50% for mild infections, ≥30% for severe infection), or clinically severe infection	C-III
Oral agents with high bioavailability may be used in the treatment of most mild, and many moderate, infections	A-II
Parenteral therapy is initially preferred for all severe, and some moderate, infections. After initial response, step-down therapy to oral agents can be considered	C-III
Definitive therapy should be based on results of appropriately collected cultures and sensitivities, as well as clinical response to empiric antimicrobial agents	A-III
Appropriate wound care, in addition to appropriate antimicrobial therapy, is often necessary for healing of infected wounds	A-III
Antibiotic therapy should only be continued until resolution of signs/symptoms of infection, but not necessarily until the wound is fully healed. The duration of therapy should initially be 1-2 weeks for mild infections and 2-3 weeks for moderate to severe infection	C-III
Animal Bites	
Preemptive early antibiotics should be administered for 3-5 days in patients with any of the following: immunocompromised; asplenic; advanced liver disease; preexisting or resultant edema of the bitten area; moderate to severe bite-related injuries, especially to the hands or face; or bite injuries that have penetrated the periosteum or joint capsule	Strong, low
Amoxicillin–clavulanic acid or other antibiotics active against both aerobic and anaerobic bacteria should be used for treatment of infected animal bites	Strong, moderate
Serious infections requiring IV antimicrobial therapy can be treated with a β-lactam/β-lactamase inhibitor combination or second-generation cephalosporin with activity against anaerobes (eg, cefoxitin)	B-II
Penicillinase-resistant penicillins, first-generation cephalosporins, macrolides, and clindamycin should not be used for treatment of infected wounds because of their poor activity against *Pasteurella multocida*	D-III
Human Bites	
Antimicrobial therapy should provide coverage against *Eikenella corrodens*, *S. aureus*, and β-lactamase–producing anaerobes	B-III

[a]Cited evidence-based guidelines utilize different systems for grading the strengths of recommendation and quality of the associated evidence. Qualitative (descriptive) recommendations are from reference 16; letter- and roman numeral-based recommendations are from the other cited guidelines. Readers are advised to consult the original documents for full explanations of the grading systems and definitions used in individual guidelines.

Strength of recommendation: A, good evidence for use; B, moderate evidence for use; C, poor evidence for use, optional; D, moderate evidence to support not using; E, good evidence to support not using. *Quality of evidence*: I, evidence from ≥1 properly randomized controlled trials; II, evidence from ≥1 well-designed clinical trials without randomization, case–control analytic studies, multiple time series, or dramatic results from uncontrolled experiments; III, evidence from expert opinion, clinical experience, descriptive studies, or reports of expert committees.

Qualitative (descriptive) recommendations: *Strong, high*: strong recommendation, high-quality evidence from well-performed randomized controlled trials (RCTs) or exceptionally strong evidence from unbiased observational studies; *Strong, moderate*: strong recommendation, moderate quality evidence from RCTs with important limitations or exceptionally strong evidence from unbiased observational studies; *Strong, low*: strong recommendation, low-quality evidence for at least 1 critical outcome from observational studies, RCTs with serious flaws, or indirect evidence; *Weak, moderate*: weak recommendation, moderate quality evidence from RCTs with important limitations or exceptionally strong evidence from unbiased observational studies; *Weak, low*: weak recommendation, low-quality evidence for at least one critical outcome from observational studies, RCTs with serious flaws, or indirect evidence.

TABLE 110-4 Recommended Oral Drugs for Outpatient Treatment of Mild–Moderate Skin and Soft-Tissue Infections

Infection	Adults	Children
Folliculitis	None; warm saline compresses usually sufficient	
Furuncles and carbuncles	Trimethoprim–sulfamethoxazole[a,b] Doxycycline[a,b] Minocycline[a,b]	Trimethoprim–sulfamethoxazole[a,b] Clindamycin[a,b]
Erysipelas	Procaine penicillin G Penicillin VK Clindamycin[a] Erythromycin[a]	Penicillin VK Clindamycin[a] Erythromycin[a]
Impetigo	Mupirocin ointment[a] Retapamulin ointment[a] Dicloxacillin Cephalexin Trimethoprim–sulfamethoxazole[a,b] Clindamycin[a,b] Doxycycline[a,b]	Mupirocin ointment[a] Retapamulin ointment[a] Dicloxacillin Cephalexin Trimethoprim–sulfamethoxazole[a,b] Clindamycin[a,b]
Lymphangitis	Initial IV therapy, followed by penicillin VK Clindamycin[a]	Initial IV therapy, followed by penicillin VK Clindamycin[a]
Diabetic foot infections	Dicloxacillin Clindamycin Cephalexin Amoxicillin–clavulanate Levofloxacin ± metronidazole or clindamycin[a,c] Ciprofloxacin ± metronidazole or clindamycin[a,c] Moxifloxacin	
Bite wounds (animal or human)	Amoxicillin–clavulanate Doxycycline[a] Moxifloxacin[a] Trimethoprim–sulfamethoxazole + metronidazole or clindamycin[a] Levofloxacin or ciprofloxacin + metronidazole or clindamycin[a] Cefuroxime axetil + metronidazole or clindamycin Dicloxacillin + penicillin VK	Amoxicillin–clavulanate Trimethoprim–sulfamethoxazole + metronidazole or clindamycin[a] Cefuroxime axetil + metronidazole or clindamycin Dicloxacillin + penicillin VK

[a]May be used in patients with penicillin allergy.

[b]Recommended if CA-MRSA is suspected.

[c]Fluoroquinolone alone may be suitable for mild infections, while addition of drugs with antianaerobic activity may be recommended for more severe infections.

TABLE 110-5 Drug Dosing Table[a]

Drug	Brand Name	Initial Dose	Usual Range	Special Population Dose	Other
Oral Agents					
Amoxicillin–clavulanate	Augmentin®	875/125 mg orally two times daily	875/125 mg orally two times daily	Pediatric: 40 mg/kg (of the amoxicillin component) orally in two divided doses	
Cefaclor	Ceclor®	500 mg orally every 8 hours	500 mg orally every 8 hours	Pediatric: 20-40 mg/kg/day (not to exceed 1 g) orally in three divided doses	
Cefadroxil	Duricef®	500 mg orally every 12 hours	250-500 mg orally every 12 hours	Pediatric: 30 mg/kg orally in two divided doses	
Cefuroxime axetil	Ceftin®	500 mg orally every 12 hours	250-500 mg orally every 12 hours	Pediatric: 20-30 mg/kg orally in two divided doses	
Cephalexin	Keflex®	250-500 mg orally every 6 hours	250-500 mg orally every 6 hours	Pediatric: 25-50 mg/kg orally in four divided doses	
Ciprofloxacin	Cipro®	500 mg orally every 12 hours	500-750 mg orally every 12 hours		
Clindamycin	Cleocin®	300-600 mg orally every 6-8 hours	300-600 mg orally every 6-8 hours	Pediatric: 10-30 mg/kg/day orally in three to four divided doses[4]	May be used for oral treatment of MRSA infection
Dicloxacillin	Dynapen®	250-500 mg orally every 6 hours	250-500 mg orally every 6 hours	Pediatric: 25-50 mg/kg orally in four divided doses	
Doxycycline	Vibramycin®	100-200 mg orally every 12 hours	100-200 mg orally every 12 hours		May be used for oral treatment of MRSA infection

(continued)

TABLE 110-5 Drug Dosing Table[a] (*Continued*)

Drug	Brand Name	Initial Dose	Usual Range	Special Population Dose	Other
Erythromycin	E-Mycin® Erythrocin®	250-500 mg orally every 6 hours	250-500 mg orally every 6 hours	Pediatric: 30-50 mg/kg orally in four divided doses[a]	
Levofloxacin	Levaquin®	500-750 mg orally once daily	500-750 mg orally once daily		
Linezolid	Zyvox®	600 mg orally every 12 hours	600 mg orally every 12 hours	Pediatric: 20-30 mg/kg/day orally in two to three divided doses	For oral treatment of MRSA infection
Metronidazole	Flagyl®	250-500 mg orally every 8 hours	250-500 mg orally every 8 hours	Pediatric: 30 mg/kg orally in three to four divided doses	
Moxifloxacin	Avelox®	400 mg orally once daily	400 mg orally once daily		
Mupirocin ointment	Bactroban®	Apply to affected areas every 8 hours	Apply to affected areas every 8 hours	Pediatric: apply to affected areas every 8 hours	
Penicillin VK	Veetids® Pen-V®	250-500 mg orally every 6 hours	250-500 mg orally every 6 hours	Pediatric: 25,000-90,000 units/kg orally in four divided doses	
Retapamulin ointment	Altabax®	Apply to affected area every 12 hours	Apply to affected area every 12 hours	Pediatric: apply to affected area every 12 hours	
Tedizolid	Sivextro®	200 mg orally once daily	200 mg orally once daily		For oral treatment of MRSA infection
Trimethoprim–sulfamethoxazole	Bactrim® Septra® Cotrimoxazole®	160/800 mg orally every 12 hours	160/800 mg orally every 12 hours	Pediatric: 4-6 mg/kg (of the trimethoprim component) orally every 12 hours	Up to double the usual dose may be considered for oral treatment of MRSA infection
Parenteral Agents					
Ampicillin	Omnipen® Polycillin® Principen®	2 g IV every 6 hours	1-2 g IV every 4-6 hours	Pediatric: 200-300 mg/kg/day IV in four to six divided doses	
Aztreonam	Azactam®	1 g IV every 6 hours	1 g IV every 6 hours	Pediatric: 100-150 mg/kg/day IV in four divided doses	
Cefazolin	Ancef® Kefzol®	1 g IV every 8 hours	1 g IV every 6-8 hours	Pediatric: 75 mg/kg/day IV in three divided doses	
Cefepime	Maxipime®	2 g IV every 12 hours	1-2 g IV every 12 hours	Pediatric: 100 mg/kg/day IV in two divided doses	
Cefotaxime	Claforan®	2 g IV every 6 hours	1-2 g IV every 6 hours	150-200 mg/kg/day in three to four divided doses	
Cefoxitin	Mefoxin®	1-2 g IV every 6 hours	1-2 g IV every 6 hours	Pediatric: 30-40 mg/kg/day IV in four divided doses	
Ceftazidime	Fortaz®	2 g IV every 8 hours	1-2 g IV every 8 hours	Pediatric: 150 mg/kg/day IV in three divided doses	
Ceftaroline	Teflaro®	600 mg IV every 12 hours	600 mg IV every 12 hours		For MRSA infection
Ceftriaxone	Rocephin®	1 g IV once daily	1 g IV once daily		
Cefuroxime	Zinacef®	1.5 g IV every 8 hours	0.75-1.5 g IV every 8 hours	Pediatric: 150 mg/kg/day IV in three divided doses	
Ciprofloxacin	Cipro®	400 mg IV every 8-12 hours	400 mg IV every 8-12 hours		
Clindamycin	Cleocin®	300-600 mg IV every 6-8 hours	300-600 mg IV every 6-8 hours; 600-900 mg IV every 6-8 hours for necrotizing fasciitis	Pediatric: 30-50 mg/kg/day IV in three to four divided doses	

(*continued*)

TABLE 110-5 Drug Dosing Table[a] (*Continued*)

Drug	Brand Name	Initial Dose	Usual Range	Special Population Dose	Other
Dalbavancin	Dalvance®	1,000 mg IV once on Day 1 of therapy	500 mg IV once on Day 8 of therapy		For MRSA infection
Daptomycin	Cubicin®	4 mg/kg IV once daily	4 mg/kg IV once daily		For MRSA infection
Doripenem	Doribax®	500 mg IV every 8 hours	500 mg IV every 8 hours		
Ertapenem	Invanz®	1 g IV once daily	1 g IV once daily	Pediatric: 30 mg/kg/day IV in one to two divided doses	
Gentamicin	Garamycin®	Traditional: 2 mg/kg loading dose, followed by 1.5 mg/kg IV every 8 hours. Alternative: 5-7 mg/kg IV once daily	Traditional dosing: guided by measured serum concentrations	Pediatric: 5-7 mg/kg/day IV in three divided doses; doses guided by serum concentrations	
Imipenem–cilastatin	Primaxin®	500 mg IV every 6 hours	250-500 mg IV every 6-8 hours	Pediatric: 40-80 mg/kg/day IV in four divided doses	
Levofloxacin	Levaquin®	750 mg IV once daily	500-750 mg IV once daily		
Linezolid	Zyvox®	600 mg IV every 12 hours	600 mg IV every 12 hours	Pediatric: 20-30 mg/kg/day IV in two to three divided doses	For MRSA infection
Meropenem	Merrem®	1 g IV every 8 hours	1 g IV every 8 hours	Pediatric: 60 mg/kg/day IV in three divided doses	
Metronidazole	Flagyl®	500 mg IV every 8 hours	500 mg IV every 8 hours	Pediatric: 30-50 mg/kg/day IV in three divided doses	
Moxifloxacin	Avelox®	400 mg IV once daily	400 mg IV once daily		
Nafcillin	Nafcil®	2 g IV every 6 hours	1-2 g IV every 4-6 hour	Pediatric: 100-200 mg/kg/day IV in four to six equally divided doses	
Oritavancin	Orbactiv®	1,200 mg IV once	(no additional doses)		For MRSA infection
Penicillin G	Pfizerpen® Bicillin® Wycillin®	1-2 million units IV every 4-6 hours	1-2 million units IV every 4-6 hours	Pediatric: 100,000-200,000 units/kg/day IV in four divided doses[a]	
Piperacillin–tazobactam	Zosyn®	4.5 g IV every 6 hours	3.375-4.5 g IV every 6 hours	Pediatric: 250-350 mg/kg/day IV in three to four divided doses	
Procaine penicillin G	Bicillin C-R®	600,000 units IM every 12 hours	600,000-1.2 million units IM every 12 hours	Pediatric: 25,000-50,000 units/kg (maximum 1.2 million units) IM once daily	
Tedizolid	Sivextro®	200 mg IV once daily	200 mg IV once daily		For MRSA infection
Telavancin	Vibativ®	10 mg/kg IV once daily	10 mg/kg IV once daily		For MRSA infection
Tigecycline	Tigacil®	100 mg IV once, and then 50 mg IV every 12 hours	100 mg IV once, and then 50 mg IV every 12 hours		
Tobramycin	Nebcin®	Traditional: 2 mg/kg loading dose, followed by 1.5 mg/kg IV every 8 hours. Alternative: 5-7 mg/kg IV once daily	Traditional dosing: guided by measured serum concentrations	Pediatric: 5-7 mg/kg/day IV in three divided doses; doses guided by serum concentrations	
Vancomycin	Vancocin®	30-40 mg/kg/day IV in two divided doses	Dosing guided by serum concentrations to achieve trough of 15-20 mg/L	Pediatric: 40-60 mg/kg/day IV in three to four divided doses; doses guided by serum concentrations	For MRSA infection

IM, intramuscularly; MRSA, methicillin-resistant *S. aureus*.

[a]Dosing guidelines in patients with normal renal function.

TABLE 110-6 Drug Monitoring

Drug	Adverse Reaction	Monitoring Parameters	Comments
Aminoglycosides (tobramycin, gentamicin)	Nephrotoxicity	Serum creatinine, urine output, serum concentrations	Extended-interval ("once-daily") dosing potentially associated with less renal toxicity, similar efficacy to traditional dosing. Goal trough concentration <1 mcg/mL (mg/L; <2 μmol/L) during extended-interval dosing
Daptomycin	Myopathy	Serum creatine phosphokinase	Most creatinine phosphokinase elevations will be asymptomatic; risk of myopathy may be increased with concomitant use of HMG-coA reductase inhibitors
Imipenem–cilastatin	CNS toxicities, seizures	Serum creatinine, mental status, CNS function	Increased incidence with higher dose, failure to adjust dose/interval for reduced renal function. Increased risk compared with meropenem or doripenem
Linezolid	Myelosuppression, thrombocytopenia, optic/peripheral neuropathy, serotonin syndrome	CBC, vision changes, serum lactate, heart rate, blood pressure, temperature, myoclonus	Myelosuppression and neuropathy more common with prolonged use. Weak MAO inhibitor, serotonin syndrome possible with other serotonergic drugs such as SSRIs and SNRIs
Nafcillin	Interstitial nephritis	Serum creatinine, urine output	Reversible, requires switch to alternative β-lactam
Vancomycin	Nephrotoxicity, infusion reactions	Serum creatinine, urine output, blood pressure, heart rate, serum concentrations	Dose adjustment required for renal dysfunction. Pretreatment and slow infusion may decrease incidence of infusion reaction. Goal trough concentration 15-20 mcg/mL (mg/L; 10-14 μmol/L) for serious infections, including necrotizing fasciitis

CBC, complete blood count; MAO, monoamine oxidase; SNRI, serotonin–norepinephrine reuptake inhibitor; SSRI, selective serotonin reuptake inhibitor.

Although historically caused by *S. pyogenes*, *S. aureus* has emerged as a principle cause of impetigo (either alone or in combination with *S. pyogenes*).[22,33] The bullous form is caused by strains of *S. aureus* capable of producing exfoliative toxins.[22,33] The bullous form most frequently affects neonates,[34] and accounts for approximately 30% of all cases of impetigo.[3,33] Similar to other SSTIs, impetigo has been reported to be increasingly due to MRSA.[22,33]

TREATMENT
Impetigo

Desired Outcomes

The goals of treatment include relieving discomfort, improving the cosmetic appearance of lesions, preventing further spread of the infection, and preventing recurrence. Preventing transmission to others is also important.[22,33] Treatments should be effective and inexpensive and have minimal adverse effects.[33]

Treatment

Although impetigo may resolve spontaneously, antimicrobial treatment is indicated to relieve symptoms, prevent formation of new lesions, and prevent complications such as cellulitis. A review of interventions for impetigo by the Cochrane Collaboration found that topical mupirocin and oral antibiotics (except penicillin and erythromycin) were equally effective for the treatment of impetigo;[34] topical mupirocin ointment or retapamulin ointment for 5 days are now recommended as first-line treatment of mild cases of impetigo not involving multiple lesions or the face.[15,22,33] Penicillinase-resistant penicillins (such as dicloxacillin) are preferred for treatment because of the increased incidence of infections caused by *S. aureus*.[15,22,33] First-generation cephalosporins (eg, cephalexin) are

CLINICAL PRESENTATION Impetigo

General

- Exposed skin, especially the face, is the most common site.

Symptoms

- Pruritus is common.
- Systemic signs and symptoms of infection are minimal.
- Weakness, fever, and diarrhea occasionally seen with bullous form.

Signs

Nonbullous:

- Lesions start as small, fluid-filled vesicles.
- Vesicles rapidly develop into pustules that rupture readily.
- Purulent discharge dries to form characteristic golden yellow crusts.

Bullous:

- Lesions start as vesicles that rapidly progress into bullae containing clear yellow fluid.
- Bullae soon rupture, forming thin, light brown crusts.
- Regional lymph nodes may be enlarged.

Laboratory Tests

- Cultures should be collected.
- Crusted tops of lesions should be raised to obtain purulent material at the base for culture.
- Open, draining pustules should not be cultured as they may be colonized with skin flora.

Other Diagnostic Tests

- Complete blood count often performed as leukocytosis is common.

also commonly used.[15,22,33] Penicillin, administered as a single intramuscular dose of benzathine penicillin G or as oral penicillin VK, is effective for infections known to be caused by *S. pyogenes*. Penicillin-allergic patients, or those known to be infected with MRSA, can be treated with clindamycin, doxycycline, or trimethoprim–sulfamethoxazole. The duration of therapy is 7 days.[15] With proper treatment, healing of skin lesions generally is rapid and occurs without residual scarring. Removal of crusts by soaking in soap and warm water also may be helpful in providing symptomatic relief.[3,22,33]

Evaluation of Therapeutic Outcomes

Clinical response should be seen within 5-7 days of initiating antimicrobial therapy for impetigo. Treatment failures could be a result of noncompliance or antimicrobial resistance. A followup culture of exudates should be collected for culture and sensitivity, with treatment modified accordingly.

LYMPHANGITIS

4 Acute lymphangitis is an inflammation involving the subcutaneous lymphatic channels. Lymphangitis usually occurs secondary to puncture wounds, infected blisters, or other skin lesions. Most infections are caused by *S. pyogenes*.[35]

TREATMENT
Lymphangitis

Desired Outcomes

The goal of treatment of lymphangitis is rapid eradication of the infection, thereby providing relief of symptoms (pain, tenderness, fever). Prevention of systemic complications is also an important goal as thrombophlebitis and abscess formation are possible. Treatments should be effective and inexpensive and have minimal adverse effects.

Treatment

Penicillin is the antibiotic of choice. Because these infections are potentially serious and rapidly progressive, initial treatment should be with IV penicillin G 1 to 2 million units every 4 to 6 hours. Parenteral treatment should be continued for 48 to 72 hours, followed by oral penicillin VK for a total of 10 days.[35] Nondrug therapy includes immobilization and elevation of the affected extremity and warm-water soaks every 2 to 4 hours.[35] For penicillin-allergic patients, clindamycin may be used.

Evaluation of Therapeutic Outcomes

Lymphangitis usually responds rapidly to appropriate therapy; signs and symptoms often are decreased markedly or absent within 24 hours of starting antibiotics.

CELLULITIS

5 Cellulitis is an acute infectious process that initially affects the epidermis and dermis and may spread subsequently within the superficial fascia.[10] Cellulitis is considered a serious disease because of the propensity of the infection to spread through lymphatic tissue and to the bloodstream. *S. pyogenes* and *S. aureus* are the most frequent bacterial causes.[5,7,12,21,26] However, many bacteria have been implicated in various types of cellulitis (Table 110-1). Approximately 4 million patients were hospitalized for cellulitis between 1998 and 2006, representing 10% of all infection-related admissions.[8,9,36] The rising incidence of infections caused by methicillin-resistant *S. aureus* (MRSA) is a major concern in both the community and hospital settings.[13-18]

Injection drug users are predisposed to several infectious complications, including abscess formation and cellulitis at the site of injection.[15] These SSTIs are often polymicrobic in nature and are believed to originate from the skin and/or oropharynx, as well as from contaminated needles, syringes, and diluents.[15] *S. aureus*, including MRSA, is the most common pathogen isolated from injection drug users.[15,6,37] Anaerobic bacteria, especially oropharyngeal

CLINICAL PRESENTATION Lymphangitis

General

- Lymphadenitis (acute or chronic inflammation of the lymph nodes) may occur when microorganisms reach the lymph nodes.

Symptoms

- Systemic signs and symptoms (ie, fever, chills, malaise, and headache) often develop rapidly before any sign of infection is evident at the initial site of inoculation, or after the initial lesion has subsided.
- Systemic signs and symptoms often are more profound than would be expected based on examination of the cutaneous lesion.

Signs

- Peripheral lesion associated with proximal red linear streaks directed toward the regional lymph nodes is diagnostic of acute lymphangitis.
- Lymph nodes usually are enlarged and tender.
- Peripheral edema of the involved extremity often is present.
- Thrombophlebitis and acute lymphangitis in the lower extremities may be confused because both are associated with red linear streaking and tender areas; however, in thrombophlebitis, no portal of entry is identifiable.

Laboratory Tests

- Cultures of the affected lesions often yield negative results.
- Pathogens often identified by Gram stain of the initial lesion if done early in the course of the disease.

Other Diagnostic Tests

- Complete blood count often performed as leukocytosis is common.

CLINICAL PRESENTATION Cellulitis

General

- Usually a history of an antecedent wound from minor trauma, abrasion, ulcer, or surgery.

Symptoms

- Patients often experience fever, chills, or malaise and complain that the affected area feels hot and painful.
- Systemic findings such as hypotension, dehydration, and altered mental status are common.

Signs

- Characterized by erythema and edema of the skin.
- Lesions are nonelevated and have poorly defined margins.
- Affected areas generally are warm to touch.
- Inflammation generally is present with little or no necrosis or suppuration of soft tissue.
- Lesions may be associated with purulent drainage, exudates, and/or abscesses.
- Tender lymphadenopathy associated with lymphatic involvement is common.

Laboratory Tests

- Cultures should be collected when possible.
- Gram stain of fluid obtained by injection and aspiration of 0.5 mL of saline (using a small 22-gauge needle) into the advancing edge of the lesion may aid the microbiologic diagnosis but often yields negative results.
- Diagnosis usually is made on clinical grounds rather than by culture.

Other Diagnostic Tests

- Complete blood count often performed as leukocytosis is common.
- Blood cultures often useful because bacteremia may be present in up to 30% of cases.

anaerobes, are also found commonly, particularly in polymicrobic infections.[15] Outbreaks caused by *Clostridium* species have also been reported in injection drug users.[15]

Acute cellulitis with mixed aerobic and anaerobic pathogens may occur in diabetics, following traumatic injuries, at sites of surgical incisions to the abdomen or perineum, or where host defenses have been otherwise compromised (vascular insufficiency).[6,10,26] In older patients, cellulitis of the lower extremities also may be complicated by thrombophlebitis. Other complications of cellulitis include local abscess, osteomyelitis, and septic arthritis.[15,38]

TREATMENT
Cellulitis

Desired Outcomes

The goals of therapy of acute bacterial cellulitis are rapid eradication of the infection and prevention of further complications. Effective treatment of cellulitis includes avoidance of unnecessary antimicrobials that contribute to increased resistance, and minimizing toxicities and cost of therapy.

Drug and Nondrug Management of Cellulitis

Local care of cellulitis includes elevation and immobilization of the involved area to decrease swelling.[5,15,38] Cool sterile saline dressings may decrease pain and can be followed later with moist heat to aid in localization of the cellulitis. Surgical intervention (incision and drainage) as a mode of therapy is rarely indicated in the treatment of uncomplicated cellulitis, but may play an important role in management of more severe or complicated cases. Antimicrobial therapy is directed against the type of bacteria either documented or suspected to be present based on the clinical presentation. Particular attention must be paid to patients with risk factors for more atypical or resistant bacterial pathogens when selecting antibiotics for treatment of cellulitis. Such organisms include particularly MRSA, but also aerobic gram-negative bacteria and anaerobes.

Because staphylococcal and streptococcal cellulitis are indistinguishable clinically,[21,38] and because of concern regarding appropriate recognition and treatment of MRSA infections, guidelines from the Infectious Diseases Society of America provide detailed recommendations for empiric antibiotic therapy of cellulitis.[15,28] Antibiotic selection for treatment of cellulitis is chiefly determined by clinical findings such as appearance of the infected lesion and presence of more severe systemic illness. Cellulitis may be broadly classified as either purulent or nonpurulent for purposes of determining likely pathogens and appropriate empiric antibiotic therapy. Purulent cellulitis is defined as infection associated with purulent drainage or exudate in the absence of a simple drainable abscess; the presence of abscesses are also often associated with purulent cellulitis but by definition that is not the only clinical feature.[15,28] Incision and drainage of any abscesses and good wound care are the primary therapies for mild purulent infections when no systemic findings of infection are present. Systemic antibiotic therapy is often unnecessary in such cases.[15,28] Antibiotic therapy is recommended along with incision and drainage in patients with more complicated abscesses and/or moderately severe purulent cellulitis including the following: those with systemic signs of infection; multiple sites of infection; rapidly progressive infection in the presence of associated cellulitis; complicating factors such as extremes of age, comorbidities, or immunosuppression; abscesses in areas that are difficult to drain, such as hands, face, and genitalia; or lack of response to previous drainage alone.[15,28,38,40-43] Such patients are usually treated as outpatients using orally administered antibiotics with activity against MRSA; infection due to streptococci is less likely in this situation and specific coverage is not required.[28,44-46] Oral agents recommended for moderate purulent cellulitis include trimethoprim–sulfamethoxazole and doxycycline (Fig. 110-1).[15] Oral linezolid is also recommended in such cases but is significantly more expensive and apparently no more efficacious than other treatment options.[28] Tedizolid, a newer oxazolidinone, is also indicated for the treatment of complicated SSTI but the relative advantages or role of tedizolid compared to linezolid have not been well established.[15]

Severe purulent cellulitis is defined as purulent infections occurring in patients who have failed incision and drainage plus oral antibiotic therapy, patients with systemic signs of infection (defined

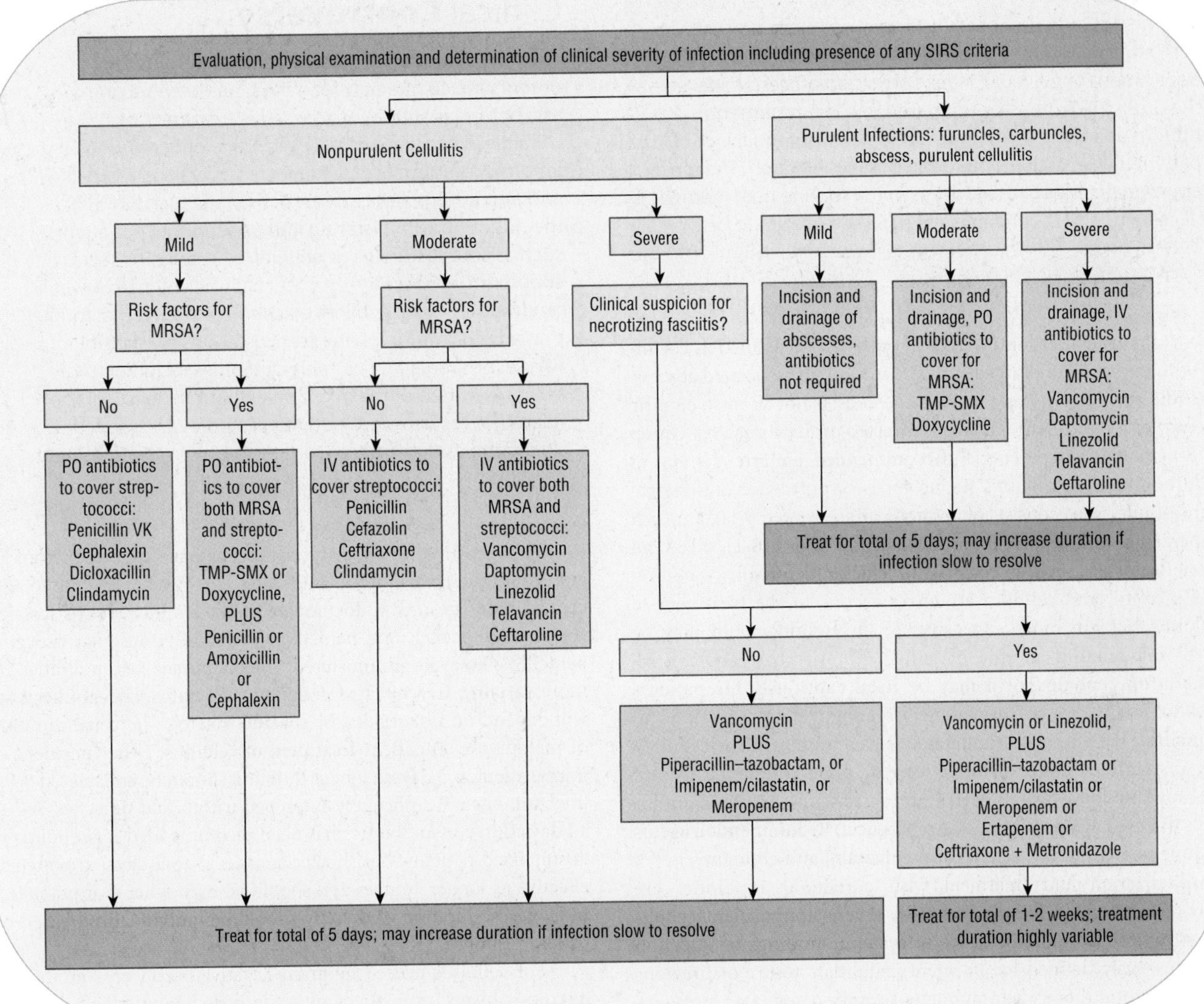

FIGURE 110-1 Recommended treatment algorithm for initial empiric management of selected purulent and nonpurulent skin and soft tissue infections. (GNR, aerobic gram-negative rods; GPC, aerobic gram-positive cocci; IV, intravenous; MRSA, methicillin-resistant *Staphylococcus aureus*; PO, oral; SIRS, systemic inflammatory response syndrome; TMP-SMX, trimethoprim–sulfamethoxazole.)

as temperature more than 38°C, heart rate more than 90 beats/minute, respiratory rate more than 24 breaths/minute, or white blood cell count more than 12,000 or less than 400 cells/μL[less than 12×10^9/L or <0.4×10^9/L]), or immunocompromised patients. Appropriate clinical specimens for culture and susceptibility testing should be collected whenever possible in such patients.[5,15,28,38] Patients with severe purulent cellulitis should be hospitalized for empiric treatment with parenteral antibiotics having activity against MRSA. Vancomycin, daptomycin, linezolid, televancin, and ceftaroline are all acceptable treatment options with comparable efficacy in adults (Fig. 110-1).[3,15,28,47] In children, vancomycin, linezolid, or clindamycin is the preferred treatment option.[15]

Linezolid, tedizolid, daptomycin, ceftaroline, and telavancin all exhibit excellent activity against resistant gram-positive pathogens.[40-43,47] However, significantly higher cost compared with vancomycin, as well as lack of demonstrated advantages in efficacy, makes them most appropriate for the treatment of complicated or refractory infections, or those documented as caused by multidrug-resistant pathogens, rather than as initial therapy. The availability of orally administered linezolid and tidezolid may provide cost-effective "step-down" options as alternatives to prolonged treatment with parenteral agents for many patients with more complicated infections and/or those patients who require initial hospitalization.[44]

Carbapenems (ie, imipenem, meropenem, ertapenem, and doripenem) and the β-lactam–β-lactamase inhibitor combination antibiotics (ampicillin–sulbactam, ticarcillin–clavulanate, and piperacillin–tazobactam) appear to be equivalent to standard therapies in adults.[3,5,15,38] However, the greater cost of these agents without increased efficacy compared with other reliable regimens, particularly given the increasing problem of MRSA, makes them less desirable for empiric therapy except in serious polymicrobic infections.[5,15,38]

Clinical **Controversy...**

The appropriate roles of dalbavancin and oritavancin, two newer drugs indicated for the treatment of complicated SSTI and with good activity against MRSA, are not well defined at this time. Dalbavancin exhibits a terminal elimination half-life of approximately 14 days and is administered as only two doses given one week apart, while oritavancin has a half-life of approximately 10 days and is administered as a single one-time dose. The ability to provide an entire course of therapy with only one or two doses is attractive in terms of convenience, negating any drug adherence concerns with oral therapy, and potentially saving hospitalization costs with administration of effective therapy in the emergency department or even outpatient physician offices. However, the drugs are expensive compared to other treatment options and there are concerns related to potential lack of patient follow-up for monitoring of their infection. The most appropriate roles of these drugs in the routine management of cellulitis and other complicated SSTIs have yet to be determined.

Nonpurulent cellulitis ("typical cellulitis") is defined as cellulitis without purulent drainage or exudate and no associated abscess. The role of MRSA in these types of infection is not clear, so empiric therapy of nonpurulent cellulitis is directed primarily against Group A β-hemolytic streptococci.[48] Recommended empiric therapy of mild nonpurulent cellulitis (ie, no focus of purulence or systemic signs of infection) consists of an orally administered β-lactam such as penicillin VK, cephalexin or dicloxacillin (Fig. 110-1).[15,28,38] Oral cephalosporins, such as cefadroxil, cefaclor, cefprozil, cefpodoxime proxetil, and cefdinir, are also effective in the treatment of cellulitis but are more expensive.[15,38] Oral clindamycin may be used in penicillin-allergic patients.[15,28,38] Alternatively, a first-generation cephalosporin may be used cautiously for patients without a history of immediate or anaphylactic reactions to penicillin. Patients with moderately severe nonpurulent cellulitis (ie, systemic evidence of infection) or poor adherence to oral therapy should be hospitalized and treated with parenteral antibiotics directed against Group A streptococci. Recommended agents include penicillin VK, ceftriaxone, cefazolin, and clindamycin.[15,48] Hospitalization and treatment with parenteral antibiotics are also recommended for patients with severe nonpurulent cellulitis as indicated by the presence of systemic findings of infection (as previously defined for purulent cellulitis), failure of previous oral antibiotic therapy, immunocompromised states, or presence of clinical signs of deeper infection such as bullae, skin sloughing, hypotension, or organ dysfunction.[15] Empiric antibiotics for severe nonpurulent cellulitis should provide a broad spectrum of activity against MRSA and streptococci, as well as gram-negative and anaerobic bacteria. Recommended regimens include vancomycin plus piperacillin–tazobactam, and vancomycin plus imipenem-cilastatin or meropenem.

Empiric treatment of MRSA should be considered for patients with either moderate or severe nonpurulent cellulitis that is associated with penetrating trauma, evidence of MRSA infection at another site or nasal colonization with MRSA, injection drug use, or in patients meeting SIRS criteria (fever, tachycardia, tachypnea, or leukocytosis or leukopenia as previously defined).[15,28] Recommended drugs for the coverage of MRSA in this setting are the same as those for purulent cellulitis. Clindamycin has reasonably good activity against β-hemolytic streptococci, but the activities of trimethoprim–sulfamethoxazole and the tetracyclines against this organism are not well defined.[28] Therefore, if empiric coverage of both MRSA and β-hemolytic streptococci is desired for patients with nonpurulent cellulitis, they should receive clindamycin alone or amoxicillin in combination with trimethoprim–sulfamethoxazole, doxycycline, or minocycline.[28] Hospitalized patients with nonpurulent cellulitis who are not initially treated for MRSA should have their antibiotic changed to an agent with activity against MRSA if there is unsatisfactory clinical response.[28] Although often used for treatment of uncomplicated outpatient cellulitis, fluoroquinolones (eg, levofloxacin, moxifloxacin) are not recommended for routine use due to their unnecessarily broad spectrum of activity, concerns for resistance, and higher cost compared with other preferred options.

Clinical **Controversy...**

The administration of systemic corticosteroids (eg, prednisone 40 mg daily for 7 days) has been recommended as a potential option for adjunctive treatment of cellulitis in nondiabetic patients. Since patients who are immunocompromised are at increased risk of severe SSTI and also potentially resistant pathogens such as MRSA, the notion of administering immunosuppressant agents such as corticosteroids to patients with cellulitis seems counterintuitive and even potentially harmful. However, a randomized, double-blind, placebo-controlled trial found that administration of oral corticosteroids plus antibiotics was associated with favorable outcomes including more rapid resolution of the infection without increased risk of relapse or recurrence.[32] Additional studies are needed to define the optimal role of corticosteroids in the treatment of cellulitis.

Patients in whom specific pathogens have been identified by culture should have empiric antibiotics narrowed according to susceptibility test results. If documented to be a mild cellulitis secondary to streptococci, oral penicillin VK or intramuscular procaine penicillin G may be administered. Since *S. aureus* susceptibilities are more variable, treatment of documented staphylococcal infections will depend on test results for specific isolates. The usual duration of therapy for outpatient treatment of cellulitis, either purulent or nonpurulent, is 5 days; a longer duration should be considered if the infection has not sufficiently improved within that time.[3,15,38] A 7 to 14 day course of antibiotics has been recommended for cellulitis in hospitalized patients, but shorter courses (5 to 7 days) are often as effective as longer courses and should be used whenever possible.[15] In all cases, duration of therapy should be individualized based on patient response.[15,28]

For cellulitis caused by gram-negative bacilli or a mixture of microorganisms, immediate antimicrobial chemotherapy, as determined by Gram stain, is essential. Surgical debridement of necrotic tissue and drainage also may be appropriate. Gram-negative cellulitis may be treated appropriately with an aminoglycoside (such as gentamicin or tobramycin), or a first- or second-generation cephalosporin (eg, cephalexin, cefaclor, or cefuroxime). Ceftriaxone, ceftazidime, and the fluoroquinolones are also effective in the treatment of cellulitis caused by both gram-negative and gram-positive bacteria.[3,5,15,38] If gram-positive aerobic bacteria are also present on Gram stain, an additional agent such as penicillin G or a penicillinase-resistant penicillin may need to be added to provide coverage against staphylococci or streptococci as appropriate.[28] Addition of an agent active against MRSA (eg, vancomycin) may need to be considered for severe, complicated infections in hospitalized patients.[3,5,15,28,38] Ceftaroline is potentially advantageous in this setting since it has activity against MRSA and streptococci as well as gram-negative aerobic bacteria.

Because some polymicrobic infections may also involve anaerobic bacteria, antibiotic therapy may need to be broadened to include agents with good activity against these organisms. Many different treatment regimens are possible depending on the bacteriology of the lesion (Fig. 110-1). Orally administered antibiotics, as monotherapy or in combination regimens, may be appropriately used in the treatment of mild to moderate infections in outpatients. Monotherapy or combination regimens of IV antibiotics may be necessary for more severe infections in hospitalized patients. Therapy should be 5 to 7 days in duration, with longer durations potentially needed in patients who do not respond to therapy in that time.[3,15,38]

Because gram-negative and mixed aerobic–anaerobic cellulitis can progress quickly to serious tissue invasion, therapeutic intervention should be immediate.[3,15,38] If treated early, a rapid response can be seen. Unfortunately, because these infections often occur in patients with compromised immune defenses, they may still progress, even with therapeutic intervention. If the infectious process is secondary to a systemic cause (eg, diabetes), the treatment course often is prolonged and may be associated with high morbidity and mortality.[3,15,38]

Infections in injection drug users generally are treated similarly to those in other types of patients.[3,15,38] It is important that blood cultures be obtained in these cases because 25% to 35% of patients may be bacteremic.[3,15] Also, patients should be assessed for the presence of abscesses; incision, drainage, and culture of these lesions are of extreme importance.[15] Initial antimicrobial therapy while awaiting culture results of abscesses should include broad coverage for gram-negative and anaerobic organisms, in addition to MRSA and streptococci.[3,15,38]

Evaluation of Therapeutic Outcomes

If treated promptly with appropriate antibiotics, the majority of patients with cellulitis are cured rapidly. Culture and sensitivity results should be evaluated carefully for both the adequacy of culture material and the presence of resistant organisms. Additional high-quality samples for culture may be needed for microbiologic analysis. Failure to respond to therapy also may be indicative of an underlying local or systemic problem or a misdiagnosis.

NECROTIZING SOFT-TISSUE INFECTIONS

Necrotizing soft-tissue infections consist of a group of extremely severe infections, associated with high morbidity and mortality, that require early and aggressive surgical debridement in addition to appropriate antibiotics and intensive supportive care.[4,7,49-52] Different terms have been used to classify necrotizing infections based on factors such as predisposing conditions, onset of symptoms, pain, skin appearance, etiologic agent, gas production, muscle involvement, and systemic toxicity.[5,26,50] However, while many types of necrotizing soft-tissue infections have been designated as unique infectious processes, they all share similar pathophysiologies, clinical features, and treatment approaches.[49-52] The major clinical entities of necrotizing infections are *necrotizing fasciitis* and *clostridial myonecrosis* (gas gangrene).[49-51]

6 Necrotizing fasciitis is a rare but severe infection of the subcutaneous tissue that may be caused by aerobic and/or anaerobic bacteria and results in progressive destruction of the superficial fascia and subcutaneous fat.[3,5,12,50,51] Type I necrotizing fasciitis is the most common and accounts for approximately 80% of necrotizing soft-tissue infections.[50,51] It generally occurs after trauma or surgery and involves a mixture of anaerobes (*Bacteroides*, *Peptostreptococcus*) and facultative bacteria (streptococci and Enterobacteriaceae) that act synergistically to cause destruction of fat and fascia.[7,50] Type I necrotizing fasciitis is also reported more commonly among injection drug users.[49-52] In type I infections, the skin may be spared, and the speed at which the infection spreads (3 to 5 days) is somewhat slower than that in type II.[26] Necrotizing fasciitis affecting the male genitalia is termed *Fournier gangrene*.[50] Type II necrotizing fasciitis is caused by virulent strains of *S. pyogenes* and is commonly referred to as *streptococcal gangrene*.[7,50] This type of infection has often been called "flesh-eating bacteria" by the lay press. Unlike previous reports of streptococcal gangrene that affected older individuals with underlying diseases, recent reports have occurred primarily in young, previously healthy adults following some type of minor trauma. It differs from type I infections in its clinical presentation. Type II infections have rapidly extending necrosis (ie, 24 to 72 hours) of subcutaneous tissues and skin, gangrene, severe local pain, and systemic toxicity.[26,49-52] They are also highly associated with an early onset of shock and organ failure and are present in approximately half the cases of streptococcal toxic shock-like syndrome.[26,49,50] Of note, MRSA is increasingly reported in type II infections, either as a single organism or in combination with streptococci.[9,50,51] Clinicians should consider MRSA in areas that are endemic for MRSA or if patients have risk factors for these organisms.

Clostridial myonecrosis (type III necrotizing fasciitis) is a necrotizing infection that involves the skeletal muscle.[9,50] Type III infections account for less than 5% of necrotizing infections.[50] Gas production and muscle necrosis are prominent features of this infection, which readily explains why this infection is commonly referred to as *gas gangrene*.[49-51] The infection advances rapidly, often over a matter of a few hours.[49-51] Most infections occur after surgery or trauma, with *Clostridium perfringens* identified as the most common etiologic agent.[50]

TREATMENT
Necrotizing Soft-Tissue Infections

Desired Outcomes

The goals of therapy of acute bacterial cellulitis are rapid eradication of the infection, prevention of further complications, and reduction in mortality. Effective treatment of necrotizing soft-tissue infections includes avoidance of unnecessary antimicrobials that contribute to increased resistance, and minimizing toxicities and cost of therapy.

Management of Necrotizing Infections

Immediate and aggressive surgical debridement of all necrotic tissues is essential in all patients with suspected or confirmed necrotizing fasciitis.[9,15,49-53] Initial surgical debridement performed greater than 14 hours after the diagnosis of necrotizing infection was independently associated with increased patient mortality, including a 34-fold increased risk of death in patients with septic shock.[53] Patients often require further surgical intervention following initial debridement to ensure that all necrotic tissue has been removed.[15,49-53] Type I necrotizing fasciitis must be empirically treated with broad-spectrum antibiotics that include coverage against streptococci, Enterobacteriaceae, and anaerobes. Piperacillin–tazobactam plus vancomycin is specifically recommended as appropriate empiric therapy of necrotizing fasciitis, although a number of antibiotic regimens are also appropriate to successfully treat necrotizing soft-tissue infections (see Fig. 110-1). These antibiotic regimens are generally similar to regimens used for polymicrobic cellulitis.[3,49-52] Antibiotic therapy can be modified after Gram stain and culture reports are available.

If a diagnosis of either type II (streptococcal) or type III (clostridial) necrotizing fasciitis is established, broad-spectrum empiric therapy should be replaced with the combination of penicillin plus clindamycin.[15,49-51] Although *S. pyogenes* remains susceptible to penicillin, the combination with clindamycin is more effective.[49,51] Several factors have been postulated to explain the greater efficacy of clindamycin, including the mechanism of action (inhibition of protein synthesis) that may cause decreased production of bacterial exotoxins.[49-52] In addition, clindamycin has immunomodulatory properties that may account for the higher efficacy.[49,51] Clindamycin is also effective against strains of MRSA.[50] Hyperbaric oxygen is potentially beneficial for clostridial myonecrosis, but its use is not currently recommended due to lack of clear evidence of improved patient outcomes.[15,49-52] Likewise, the use of intravenous immunoglobulin (IVIG) has not yet been proven beneficial in the treatment of necrotizing streptococcal infections and its use is not routinely recommended.[15]

Evaluation of Therapeutic Outcomes

Because of the high mortality associated with necrotizing infections, rapid and complete debridement of all devitalized and necrotic tissue is essential. Surgical debridement, coupled with appropriate

CLINICAL PRESENTATION Necrotizing Infections

General

- Most frequently involve the abdomen, perineum, and lower extremities.
- Predisposing factors such as diabetes mellitus, local trauma or infection, or recent surgery often present.
- Rapid diagnosis is critical due to the aggressive nature and high associated mortality (20% to 50%).

Symptoms

- Systemic symptoms generally are marked (eg, fever, chills, and leukocytosis) and may include shock and organ failure, especially in patients with type II infections.
- Pain in the affected area and systemic toxicity are characteristically more pronounced than with cellulitis.

Signs

- May be difficult to differentiate between necrotizing fasciitis and cellulitis early in infection.
- Affected area is initially hot, swollen, and erythematous without sharply demarcated margins.
- Affected area is often shiny, exquisitely tender, and painful.
- Diffuse swelling of the area is followed by the appearance of bullae filled with clear fluid.
- Rapidly progressive infection with the frequent development of a maroon or violaceous color of the skin after several days.
- Infection may rapidly evolve into a frank cutaneous gangrene, sometimes with myonecrosis.

Laboratory Tests

- Tissue samples should be obtained for histologic examination, and culture and susceptibility testing.
- Clostridial myonecrosis shows little inflammation on histologic examination.

Other Diagnostic Tests

- Surgical exploration is the best and most rapid diagnosis of necrotizing infections; computed tomography and magnetic resonance imaging may also be helpful.
- Blood samples should be collected for complete blood count and chemistry profile, as well as for bacterial culture.
- Laboratory tests that may aid in the diagnosis of necrotizing infections (LRINEC score) include C-reactive protein, white blood cell count, hemoglobin, sodium, creatinine, and glucose.

antimicrobial therapy and supportive measures for management of shock and organ failure, should stabilize the patient. Vital signs and laboratory tests should be monitored carefully for signs of resolution of the infection. Change in antimicrobial therapy or additional surgical debridement may be needed in patients who do not show signs of improvement.

DIABETIC FOOT INFECTIONS

Three major types of foot infections are seen in diabetic patients: deep abscesses, cellulitis of the dorsum, and mal perforans ulcers.[54,55] Most deep abscesses involve the central plantar space (arch) and are caused by minor penetrating trauma or by an extension of infection of a nail or web space of the toes. Infections of the dorsal area generally arise from infections in the toes that are related to routine care of the nails, nail beds, and calluses of the toes. Mal perforans ulcer is a chronic ulcer of the sole of the foot. The ulcer develops on thickened, hardened calluses over the first or fifth metatarsal. Mal perforans ulcers are associated with neuropathic changes, which are responsible for the misalignment of the weight-bearing bones of the foot.[54,55] Osteomyelitis is one of the most serious complications of diabetic foot infection (DFI) and may occur in 30% to 40% of infections.[27,54]

Epidemiology

DFI is among the most common complications of diabetes, accounting for as many as 20% of all hospitalizations in diabetic patients at an annual cost of $200 to $350 million.[27,54,56] Approximately 15% of diabetic patients experience significant soft-tissue infection during their lifetime.[56] Approximately 71,000 lower-extremity amputations, often sequelae of uncontrolled infection, are performed each year on diabetic patients; this represents up to 70% of all nontraumatic amputations in the United States.[27,54,56] Approximately 20% of diabetics will undergo additional surgery or amputation of a second limb within 12 months of the initial amputation.[27,54]

Etiology

Mild cases of DFI are often monomicrobial. However, more severe infections are typically polymicrobic; up to 60% of hospitalized patients have polymicrobial infections (Table 110-7).[27,54,55,57-62] Wide ranges in the frequency of various bacteria in DFI reflect differences in culture techniques as well as variation among different types and severity of infections. Staphylococci and streptococci are the most common pathogens, although gram-negative bacilli and/or anaerobes occur in up to 50% of cases.[27,57-62] Although *P. aeruginosa* is an important pathogen in DFI, it is usually reported to occur in <10% of wounds and is most commonly associated with more severe infections.[27,58] Obligate anaerobes are also more commonly associated with severe infections in patients with chronic foot ischemia.[27,57,58] MRSA is increasingly important in DFI and has been reported in 10% to 30% of infected wounds.[27,58,59,62-64] The presence of MRSA in DFI has been associated with increased risk of treatment failure and worse patient outcomes, but these findings have not been consistent among studies and the clinical relevance of MRSA in this setting is still unclear.[27,55,63]

Identifying causative pathogens from cultures of diabetic wounds is often difficult. The chronic nature of DFI means that these wounds are often heavily colonized by organisms not playing a role in the infection. Superficial swab cultures are not as reliable as culture specimens obtained from deep tissues via biopsy, tissue scraping (curettage), or needle aspiration of drainage or abscess fluid.[59,62] Therefore, cultures and sensitivity tests should be done with specimens obtained from a deep culture of the wound base whenever possible. Before the wound is cultured, it should be scrubbed vigorously with saline-moistened sterile gauze to remove any overlying necrotic debris and further debrided as necessary.[27,59] Bone cultures should also be performed when there is diagnostic uncertainty regarding the presence of osteomyelitis or when therapeutic decisions are dependent on knowing the exact etiology of infection.[27,59]

TABLE 110-7 Bacterial Isolates from Foot Infections in Diabetic Patients[27,54,55,57-63,65]

Organisms	Percentage of Lsolates
Aerobes	63-100
Gram-positive	24-100
Staphylococcus aureus (all)	10-80
S. aureus (MRSA)	1-37
Streptococcus spp.	3-37
Enterococcus spp.	2-25
Coagulase-negative staphylococci	6-10
Other gram-positive aerobes	0-19
Gram-negative	16-73
Proteus spp.	3-7
Enterobacter spp.	1-9
Escherichia coli	3-10
Klebsiella spp.	1-6
Pseudomonas aeruginosa	1-48
Other gram-negative bacilli	3-13
Anaerobes	1-40
Peptostreptococcus spp.	4-28
Bacteroides fragilis group	2-9
Other *Bacteroides* spp.	3-6
Clostridium spp.	0-2
Other anaerobes	7-19

Pathophysiology

Three key factors are involved in the development of diabetic foot problems: neuropathy, angiopathy and ischemia, and immunologic defects. Any of these disorders can occur in isolation; however, they frequently occur together.[56]

Neuropathic changes to the autonomic nervous system as a consequence of diabetes may affect the motor nerve supply of small intrinsic muscles of the foot, resulting in muscular imbalance, abnormal stresses on tissues and bone, and repetitive injuries.[54,56] Diminished sensory perception causes an absence of pain and unawareness of minor injuries and ulceration. The sympathetic nerve supply may be damaged, resulting in an absence of sweating that may lead to dry cracked skin and secondary infection.[27,54,56]

Atherosclerosis is more common, appears at a younger age, and progresses more rapidly in the diabetic than in the nondiabetic. Diabetics may have problems with both small vessels (microangiopathy) and large vessels (macroangiopathy) that can result in varying degrees of ischemia, ultimately leading to skin breakdown and infection.

Diabetic patients typically have normal humoral immunity, normal levels of immunoglobulins, and normal antibody responses. Patients with diabetes, however, have impaired phagocytosis and intracellular microbicidal function as compared with nondiabetics; this may be related to angiopathy and low tissue levels of oxygen.[27,54,56] These defects in cell-mediated immunity make patients with diabetes more susceptible to certain types of infection and impair the patients' ability to heal wounds adequately.[54-56]

TREATMENT
Diabetic Foot Infections

Desired Outcomes

7 The goals of therapy in the management of DFI include the following: (a) successfully treat infected wounds by using effective nondrug and antibiotic therapy; (b) prevent additional infectious complications; (c) preserve as much normal limb function as possible; (d) avoid unnecessary use of antimicrobials that contribute to increased resistance; and (e) minimize toxicities and cost while increasing patient quality of life.

MANAGEMENT

Up to 90% of infections can be treated successfully with a comprehensive treatment approach that includes both wound care and antimicrobial therapy.[27,55,59,60] After carefully assessing the extent of the lesion and obtaining necessary cultures, necrotic tissue must be thoroughly debrided, with wound drainage and amputation as required. Wounds must be kept clean and dressings changed frequently (two to three times daily). Because of the relationship

CLINICAL PRESENTATION Diabetic Foot Infections

General

- Infections are often much more extensive than they appear initially.

Symptoms

- Patients with peripheral neuropathy often do not experience pain; simple complaints of swelling or edema are common.

Signs

- Clinical signs of infection may not be present secondary to angiopathy and neuropathy.
- Lesions vary in size and clinical features (eg, erythema, edema, warmth, presence of pus, draining sinuses, pain, and tenderness).
- Foul-smelling odor suggests the presence of anaerobic organisms.
- Temperature may be mildly elevated or normal.

Laboratory Tests

- Specimens for culture and sensitivities should be collected.
- Deep-tissue samples obtained during surgical debridement are most useful for culture and susceptibility testing.
- Wounds must be cultured for both aerobic and anaerobic organisms.

Other Diagnostic Tests

- Possible presence of osteomyelitis also must be assessed via radiograph, bone scan, or both, as appropriate.

between hyperglycemia and immune system defects, glycemic control must be maximized to ensure optimal wound healing. In addition, the patient's activities should be restricted initially to bed-rest for leg elevation and control of edema, if present. Adequate pressure relief from a foot wound (ie, off-loading) is crucial to the healing process.[27,56,59] Finally, appropriate antimicrobials must be initiated.[27,55,56,59,60] However, the optimal antimicrobial therapy for DFI has yet to be defined. Empiric therapy that is totally comprehensive in its coverage of all possible pathogens does not seem to be necessary unless the infection is life- or limb-threatening, assuming that adequate wound care is also being performed.[27,55,59,60] This is particularly true regarding MRSA, *P. aeruginosa*, and anaerobes; the perceived need for empiric coverage of these organisms often leads to use of excessively broad-spectrum drug regimens. Several studies have shown good antimicrobial treatment efficacy despite the fact that the regimens did not have consistently good activity against these particular organisms.[27,59,61-63,65]

Proper selection of empiric antibiotics for DFI begins with thorough patient assessment and classification of the severity of the infection. Specific drug regimens, route of administration, and duration of therapy are all then largely dependent on the severity of infection. Although a number of classification systems are available, the most recent DFI treatment guidelines use those summarized in Table 110-8.[27,59] Wounds with no local signs of infection often do not require antibiotic therapy, and the majority of mild, uncomplicated infections can be managed successfully on an outpatient basis with highly bioavailable oral antimicrobials and good wound care (Tables 110-8 and 110-9).[37,55,61,62] Antibiotics for treatment of mild infections should be largely limited to those with activity against skin flora such as streptococci and methicillin-susceptible *S. aureus* (MSSA), except in those patients with risk factors for infection with other types of pathogens (Fig. 110-2).[27,59] Patients with specific risk factors for MRSA (Table 110-9) should empirically receive trimethoprim–sulfamethoxazole or doxycycline orally, while those who have received antibiotics within the past month should also receive empiric antibiotics that provide activity against gram-negative bacilli. Oral antimicrobials should be used cautiously in DFI complicated by osteomyelitis, extensive ulceration, areas of necrosis, or a combination of these. The use of topical antimicrobials, including medical-grade honey, has been advocated for the treatment of DFI in an attempt to minimize the cost of therapy and systemic antibiotic exposure leading to adverse effects and resistance. Although the most recent guidelines allow for consideration of topical therapy in mild infection in selected patients, use of topical agents is quite controversial and not routinely recommended.[27,55,59,66,67]

Appropriate initial therapy for patients with moderate to severe infection is also dependent on the presence of specific risk factors that increase the likelihood of infection with more resistant pathogens such as *P. aeruginosa* and MRSA (Table 110-9).[27,59] Many moderate infections can be successfully treated with orally administered antibiotics that provide activity against MSSA, streptococci, and gram-negative aerobic bacilli; coverage of obligate anaerobes may also be considered in patients with chronic or previously treated wounds (Fig. 110-3).[27,59] The addition of orally administered agents with activity against MRSA is recommended in patients with moderate or severe infection and specific risk factors for MRSA; such patients may also be considered for hospitalization and initial treatment with parenteral antibiotics in order to ensure adequate antibiotics for potentially more complex infections.[27,59] Patients with more extensive or chronically unhealed wounds, even though assessed as moderate in severity, may also be more appropriately treated initially with parenteral antibiotics in the hospital setting.[27,59]

All patients with severe DFI should be hospitalized initially and treated with broad-spectrum IV antibiotics (Table 110-9 and Fig. 110-3).[27,59] Severe infection is considered a risk factor for *P. aeruginosa*, so most patients with severe DFI will be initially started on antipseudomonal antibiotics.[27,59] Many patients will also be initially started on antibiotics that provide activity against MRSA due to risk-versus-benefit considerations, but assessment of risk factors in individual patients should still be performed in order to minimize the use of excessively broad-spectrum antibiotics when possible.

Clinical **Controversy...**

The decision whether or not to provide empiric coverage for MRSA and/or *P. aeruginosa* in the empiric treatment of diabetic foot infections remains controversial. Although proposed risk factors and treatment recommendations are provided in recent guidelines, these recommendations are somewhat broad due to lack of definitive data defining patients at high risk for infection with these pathogens. The nonspecific nature of the current recommendations may potentially lead to use of unnecessarily broad-spectrum antibiotic therapy in order to cover patients who are not actually at risk for infection with such drug-resistant pathogens. Additional studies defining specific patient risk factors are needed in order to more specifically and accurately guide empiric antibiotic management of diabetic foot infections.

TABLE 110-8 Classifications and Treatment Strategies for Diabetic Foot Infections of Varying Severity[27]

Clinical Signs/Symptoms of Infection	Infection Severity	Treatment Setting
None	Uninfected	Outpatient management; nonantibiotic wound management only
Local infection present (≥2 of the following): local swelling or induration, erythema, local tenderness or pain, local warmth, purulent discharge		
Local infection involving only skin and subcutaneous tissue, without involvement of deeper tissues or SIRS criteria present; if erythema is present, must be >0.5 and ≤2 cm around ulcer	Mild	Outpatient management; topical or oral antibiotics
Local infection with erythema >2 cm around ulcer, or involving structures deeper than skin and subcutaneous tissue (eg, abscess, osteomyelitis, septic arthritis, fasciitis); no SIRS criteria present	Moderate	Outpatient (or initial inpatient) management; oral (or initial parenteral) antibiotics
Local infection with ≥2 SIRS criteria: • Temperature >38°C or <36°C (>100.4°F or <96.8°F) • HR >90 • RR >20 • WBC >12,000 or <4,000, or >10% bands (>12 x 10^9/L or <4 x 10^9/L, or ≥0.10 bands)	Severe	Inpatient, followed by outpatient, management; initial parenteral antibiotics, followed by switch to oral when possible

TABLE 110-9 Suggested Antibiotic Regimens for Empiric Treatment of Diabetic Foot Infections[27]

Severity of Infection	Probable Pathogens	Drug(s)[a]	Duration of Therapy
Mild	*Staphylococcus aureus* (MSSA) *Streptococcus* spp. *S. aureus* (MRSA) • Patients with history of MRSA infection or colonization in past year • Prevalence of MRSA ≥50% in local geographic area • Recent hospitalization	Amoxicillin–clavulanate Cephalexin Dicloxacillin Clindamycin Levofloxacin Moxifloxacin[b]	1-2 weeks; may increase up to 4 weeks if infection slow to resolve
Moderate to severe (initially oral or IV antibiotics for moderately severe infections, IV antibiotics for severe infections)	MSSA *Streptococcus* spp. Enterobacteriaceae Obligate anaerobes	Ampicillin/Sulbactam Cefoxitin Ceftriaxone Imipenem/cilastatin Ertapenem Levofloxacin Moxifloxacin Tigecycline Levofloxacin or ciprofloxacin + clindamycin	Moderately severe infection: 1-3 weeks; severe infection: 2-4 weeks
	MRSA • Patients with history of MRSA infection or colonization in past year • Prevalence of MRSA ≥30% in local geographic area • Recent hospitalization • Infection severe enough that not empirically covering MRSA poses unacceptable risk of treatment failure	Add to one of the above regimens: • Vancomycin • Linezolid • Daptomycin	
	Pseudomonas aeruginosa • Patient has been soaking feet • Patient has previously failed therapy with nonpseudomonal antibiotic regimen • Severe infection	Piperacillin/tazobactam	
	Mixed infections potentially including all of the above	Cefepime, ceftazidime, or aztreonam + metronidazole or clindamycin + vancomycin[c] *Or* piperacillin–tazobactam or imipenem–cilastatin or meropenem[b] + vancomycin[c]	

MRSA, methicillin-resistant *S. aureus*; MSSA, methicillin-susceptible *S. aureus*.

[a]Agents not shown in any particular order of preference.

[b]Not specifically recommended in IDSA guidelines but may be appropriate treatment option.

[c]Linezolid or daptomycin may be used in place of vancomycin.

Guidelines for management of DFI include options for both monotherapy and combination regimens (Table 110-9).[27] Monotherapy, along with appropriate medical or surgical management, or both, is often effective in treating DFI, including those in which osteomyelitis is present.[27,55,60,61] Monotherapy is particularly attractive because of the potential advantages of convenience, cost, and avoidance of toxicities. Microbiologic and clinical cure rates ranging from 60% to 90% may be expected from any of these agents.[61] Selection of a specific regimen is determined by patient-specific factors including allergies, renal function, history of previous antibiotic use, and cost. In penicillin-allergic patients, metronidazole or clindamycin plus a fluoroquinolone, aztreonam, or possibly a third- or fourth-generation cephalosporin is appropriate.[27,55,60] Vancomycin also is used frequently in severe infections because of its excellent activity against gram-positive pathogens. Linezolid, daptomycin, and tigecycline are specifically recommended alternatives for the treatment of this pathogen.[27,55,59,60] Tigecycline may be particularly useful in this setting because of its activity against gram-negative aerobes and anaerobic bacteria, thus allowing it to be used as monotherapy for the treatment of mixed infections in patients where coverage of *P. aeruginosa* is not of great concern. Ceftaroline fosamil has in vitro activity that is suitable for DFI but has not been studied for this indication and its role is not yet defined. Because many patients already have some degree of diabetic nephropathy that may place them at higher risk of nephrotoxicity, strong recommendations have been made against the use of aminoglycoside antibiotics unless no alternative agents are available.[27,55] When an aminoglycoside is used, care must be taken to avoid further compromising renal function. All antibiotic regimens should be adjusted as necessary for renal dysfunction.

Duration of therapy for DFI depends on the severity of the infection, ranging from 1 to 2 weeks for mild infections up to 2 to 4 weeks or more for severe infections.[27,55] In the cases of underlying osteomyelitis, treatment should continue for 6 to 12 weeks.[27,55,60] After healing of the infection has occurred, a well-designed program for the prevention of further infections should be instituted. The use of adjunctive agents such as colony-stimulating factors, growth factors, and hyperbaric oxygen for either prevention or treatment of DFIs is controversial and not widely recommended.[27]

Evaluation of Therapeutic Outcomes

Therapy should be reevaluated carefully after 48 to 72 hours to assess favorable response. Change in therapy (or route of administration, if oral) should be considered if clinical improvement is not observed at this time. For optimal results, drug therapy should be appropriately modified according to information from deep-tissue culture and the clinical condition of the patient. Infections in diabetic patients often require extended courses of therapy because of impaired host immunity and poor wound healing.

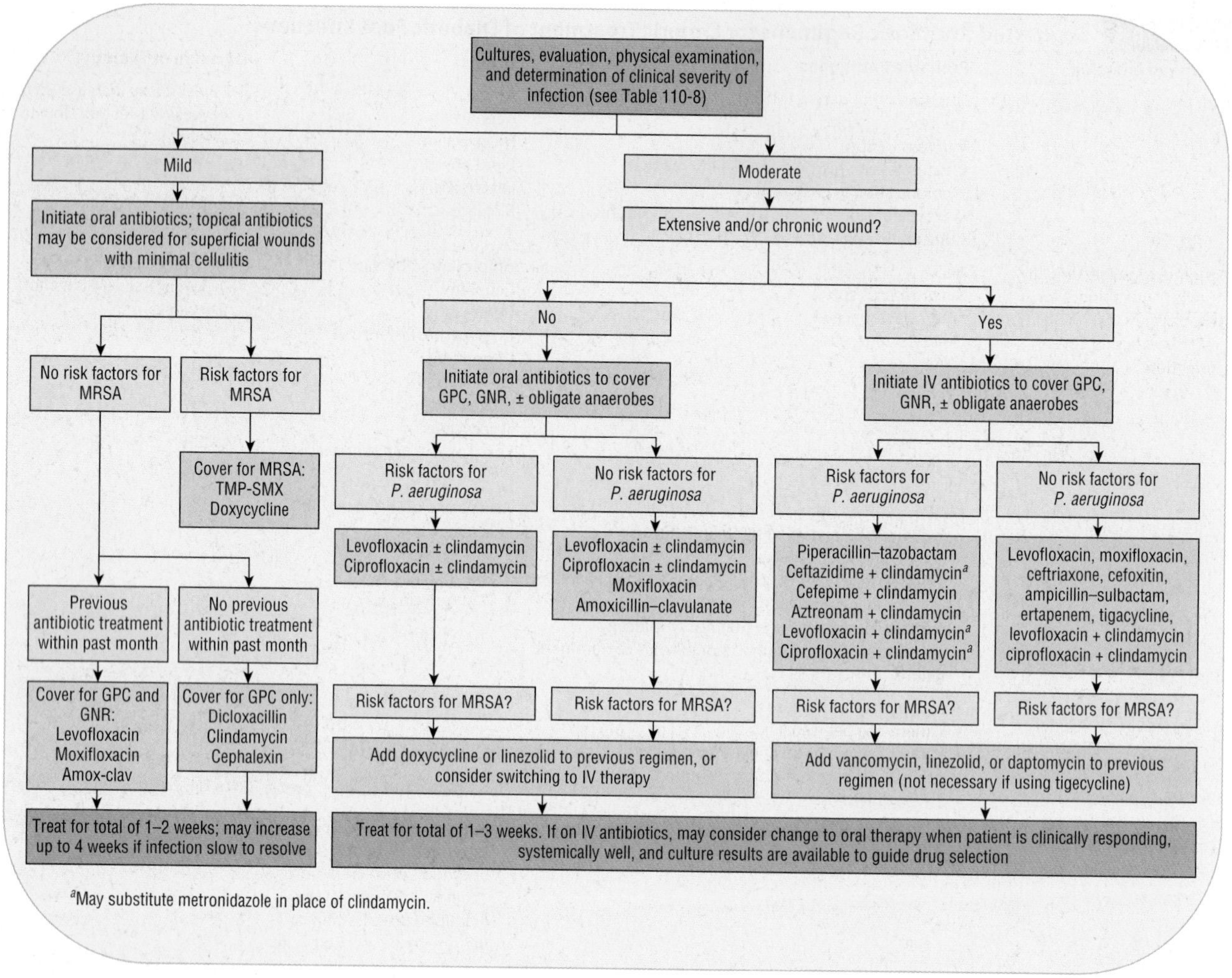

Cultures, evaluation, physical examination, and determination of clinical severity of infection (see Table 110-8)
Mild
Initiate oral antibiotics; topical antibiotics may be considered for superficial wounds with minimal cellulitis
No risk factors for MRSA
Risk factors for MRSA
Cover for MRSA: TMP-SMX Doxycycline
Previous antibiotic treatment within past month
No previous antibiotic treatment within past month
Cover for GPC and GNR: Levofloxacin Moxifloxacin Amox-clav
Cover for GPC only: Dicloxacillin Clindamycin Cephalexin
Treat for total of 1–2 weeks; may increase up to 4 weeks if infection slow to resolve
Moderate
Extensive and/or chronic wound?
No
Initiate oral antibiotics to cover GPC, GNR, ± obligate anaerobes
Risk factors for P. aeruginosa
No risk factors for P. aeruginosa
Levofloxacin ± clindamycin Ciprofloxacin ± clindamycin
Levofloxacin ± clindamycin Ciprofloxacin ± clindamycin Moxifloxacin Amoxicillin–clavulanate
Risk factors for MRSA?
Risk factors for MRSA?
Add doxycycline or linezolid to previous regimen, or consider switching to IV therapy
Yes
Initiate IV antibiotics to cover GPC, GNR, ± obligate anaerobes
Risk factors for P. aeruginosa
No risk factors for P. aeruginosa
Piperacillin–tazobactam Ceftazidime + clindamycin[a] Cefepime + clindamycin Aztreonam + clindamycin Levofloxacin + clindamycin[a] Ciprofloxacin + clindamycin[a]
Levofloxacin, moxifloxacin, ceftriaxone, cefoxitin, ampicillin–sulbactam, ertapenem, tigacycline, levofloxacin + clindamycin ciprofloxacin + clindamycin
Risk factors for MRSA?
Risk factors for MRSA?
Add vancomycin, linezolid, or daptomycin to previous regimen (not necessary if using tigecycline)
Treat for total of 1–3 weeks. If on IV antibiotics, may consider change to oral therapy when patient is clinically responding, systemically well, and culture results are available to guide drug selection
[a]May substitute metronidazole in place of clindamycin.

FIGURE 110-2 Recommended treatment algorithm for initial empiric management of mild to moderate diabetic foot infections. (GNR, aerobic gram-negative rods; GPC, aerobic gram-positive cocci; MRSA, methicillin-resistant *Staphylococcus aureus*; TMP-SMX, trimethoprim–sulfamethoxazole.)

Cultures, evaluation, physical examination, and determination of clinical severity of infection (see Table 110-8)
Severe
Initial IV therapy to cover MSSA, streptococci, GNR, Pseudomonas aeruginosa, and obligate anaerobes
No risk factors for MRSA
Piperacillin–tazobactam Imipenem–cilastatin Ceftazidime + clindamycin or metronidazole Cefepime + clindamycin or metronidazole
Risk factors for MRSA
Cover MRSA in addition to the previous organisms: Vancomycin[a] + any of the following: Piperacillin–tazobactam imipenem–cilastatin Ceftazidime + clindamycin or metronidazole Cefepime + clindamycin or metronidazole Aztreonam + clindamycin or metronidazole
Treat for total of 2–4 weeks may consider change to oral therapy when patient is clinically responding, systemically well, and culture results are available to guide drug selection
[a]May substitute linezolid or daptomycin for vancomycin.

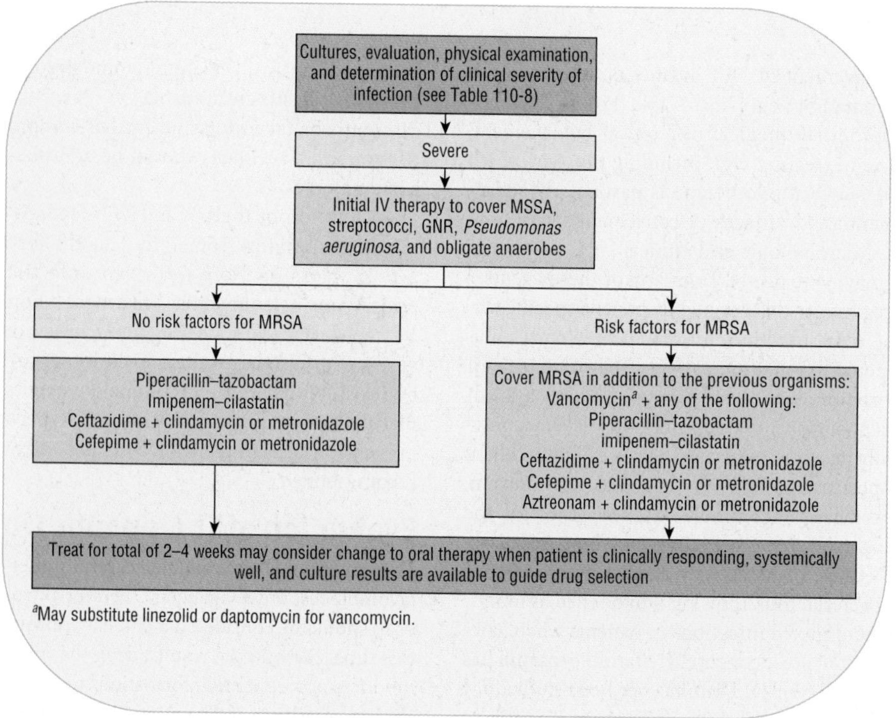

FIGURE 110-3 Recommended treatment algorithm for initial empiric management of severe diabetic foot infections. (GNR, aerobic gram-negative rods; MRSA, methicillin-resistant *Staphylococcus aureus*; MSSA, methicillin-susceptible *S. aureus*.)

PRESSURE SORES

The terms *decubitus ulcer*, *bed sore*, and *pressure sore* are used interchangeably.[68,69] The decubitus ulcer and the bed sore are types of pressure sores. The term *decubitus ulcer* is derived from the Latin word *decumbere*, meaning "lying down." Pressure sores, however, can develop regardless of a patient's position.

Numerous systems for classification of pressure sores have been described. The 2007 recommendations of the National Pressure Ulcer Advisory Panel are shown in Table 110-10 and illustrate the various stages of progression through which a pressure sore may pass.[70]

Complications of pressure sores are common and may be life-threatening. Infection is one of the most serious and most frequently encountered complications of pressure ulcers.[69] Although most pressure sore wounds are heavily colonized, the majority of these eventually heal.[71-73] When true infection is present, however, there is bacterial invasion of previously healthy tissue. Without treatment, an initial small, localized area of ulceration can rapidly progress to large ulcers within days. The visible ulcer is just a small portion of the actual wound[74]; up to 70% of the total wound is below the skin. A pressure-gradient phenomenon is created by which the wound takes on a conical nature; the smallest point is at the skin surface, and the largest portion of the defect is at the base of the ulcer (Fig. 110-4).

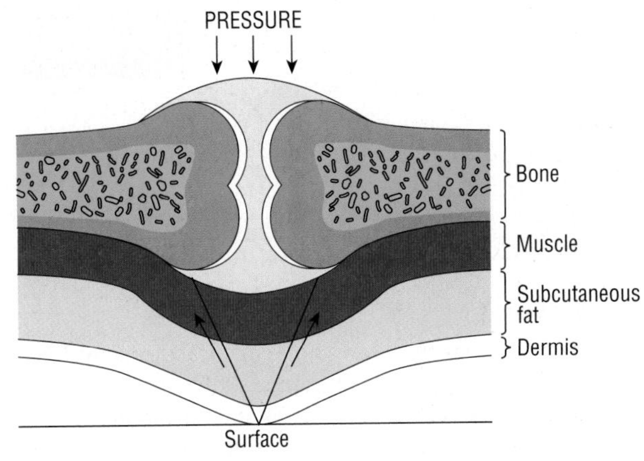

FIGURE 110-4 Distribution of forces involved with sore formation in a conical fashion.

Epidemiology

Pressure sores are most common among chronically debilitated persons, the elderly (70% involve persons greater than 70 years of age), and persons with serious spinal cord injury.[25,69,74,75] Generally, patients who are at risk for pressure sores are elderly or chronically ill young patients who are immobilized, in either bed or a wheelchair, and who may have altered mental status and/or incontinence.[69,74,75]

Etiology

Similar to DFIs, a large variety of aerobic gram-positive and gram-negative organisms, as well as anaerobes, frequently are isolated from wound cultures.[25] Most pressure sores are colonized with microorganisms, making assessment for infection a clinical challenge.[25,71] Curettage of the ulcer base after debridement provides more reliable culture information than does needle aspiration.[71-73] Biopsy specimens give the most reliable data but may not be practical to obtain. Deep-tissue cultures from different sites may give different results. Cultures collected from pressure ulcers reveal polymicrobial growth. A culture collected by swab is likely to identify surface bacteria colonizing the wound rather than to diagnose the infection.[71]

Pathophysiology

Many factors apparently predispose patients to the formation of pressure sores: paralysis, paresis, immobilization, malnutrition, anemia, infection, and advanced age. Factors thought to be most critical to their formation are pressure, shearing forces, friction, and moisture[25,76]; however, there is still debate as to the exact pathophysiology of pressure sore formation.[76]

Pressure is the essential element in the formation of pressure sores.[25,69,74,76] The areas of highest pressure are generated most often over the bony prominences.[25,68,69,71,75,76] Both the degree of pressure and the length of time that the pressure is applied are important.[69,76]

Shearing occurs when two surfaces move in opposite directions.[25,76] This situation can occur when the head of a bed is raised, causing the upper torso to slide downward, transmitting pressure to the sacrum and other areas. This effect results in occlusion or distortion of vessels, leading to compromise of the dermis. At the same time, sitting and gravity create shearing forces; the posterior sacral skin area can become fixed secondary to friction with the bed. The effects of friction and shearing forces combine, resulting in transmission of force to the deep portion of the superficial fascia and leading to further damage of soft-tissue structures.[25,71,76]

Compounding the problems of shearing and friction forces are the macerating effects of excessive moisture in the local environment, resulting from incontinence and perspiration. This factor is of critical importance because when combined with the other forces, it increases the risk of pressure sore formation fivefold.[25,72,76]

TABLE 110-10 Pressure Sore Classification

Suspected deep-tissue injury	Area of discolored intact skin or blood-filled blister due to damage of underlying soft tissue from pressure and/or shear. Area may be preceded by tissue that is painful, firm, mushy, boggy, warmer or cooler as compared with adjacent tissue
Stage 1	Pressure sore is generally reversible, is limited to the epidermis, and resembles an abrasion. Intact skin with nonblanchable redness of a localized area, usually over a bony prominence. The area may be painful, firm, soft, warmer or cooler as compared with adjacent tissue
Stage 2	A stage 2 sore also may be reversible; partial thickness loss of dermis presenting as a shallow open ulcer with a red pink wound bed. May also present as an intact or open/ruptured serum-filled blister, or as a shiny or dry shallow ulcer
Stage 3[a]	Full thickness tissue loss. Subcutaneous fat may be visible, but bone, tendon, or muscles are not exposed. May include undermining and tunneling. Depth of the ulcer varies by anatomical location; may range from shallow to extremely deep over areas of significant adiposity
Stage 4[a]	Full thickness tissue loss with exposed bone, tendon, or muscle; can extend into muscle and/or supporting structures (eg, fascia, tendon, or joint capsule) making osteomyelitis possible. Often includes undermining and tunneling; depth of the ulcer varies by anatomical location
Unstageable[a]	Full thickness tissue loss in which the base of the ulcer is covered by slough (yellow, tan, gray, green, or brown) and/or eschar (tan, brown, or black) in the wound bed. True depth, and therefore stage, cannot be determined

[a]Stage 3, stage 4, and unstageable lesions are unlikely to resolve on their own and often require surgical intervention.

Data from reference 70.

CLINICAL PRESENTATION Pressure Sores

General

- Most pressure sores are in the pelvic region and lower extremities; see Fig. 110-5.
- Most common sites: sacral and coccygeal areas, ischial tuberosities, and greater trochanter.

Symptoms

- Patients commonly have other medical problems that may mask signs and symptoms of infection.
- Pain may be present with or without infection; continuous pain may indicate infection.

Signs

- A dark red color on the surface of a pressure sore may indicate local infection.
- Surrounding erythema, swelling, and heat are commonly present with infection.
- Purulent discharge, foul odor, and systemic signs (eg, fever and leukocytosis) of infection may be present.

Laboratory Tests

- Cultures should be collected from either a biopsy or fluid obtained by needle aspiration.

Other Diagnostic Tests

- Complete blood count often performed for assessment of potential infection.
- Consider magnetic resonance imaging if suspicious of underlying osteomyelitis.

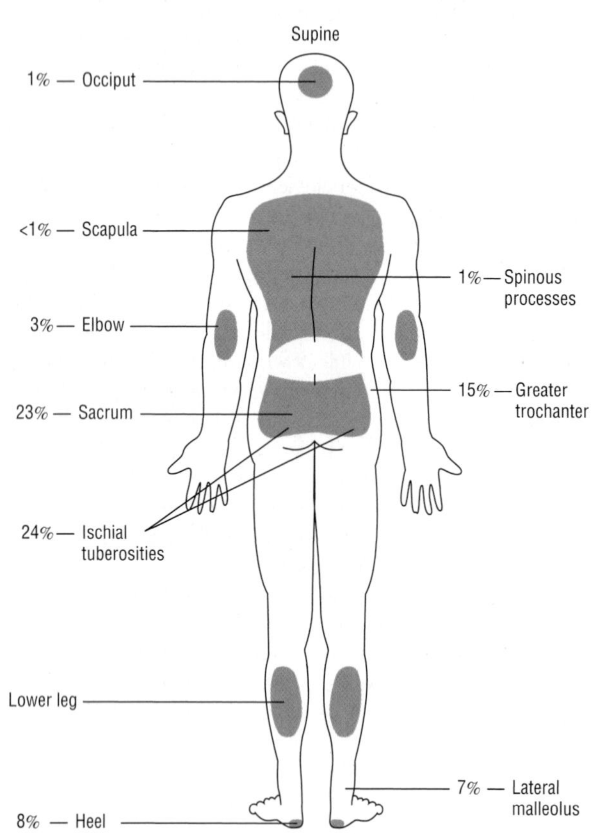

FIGURE 110-5 Supine view of areas where pressure sore formation tends to occur.

TREATMENT
Pressure Sores

Desired Outcomes

The primary goal for pressure sores is prevention. Once a pressure sore has developed, the goals of therapy are prevention of complications (ie, infections), preventing sores from growing larger, and preventing the development of sores in other locations.[74] Eradication of infection should include good wound care and topical therapies, and avoidance of broad-spectrum antimicrobials unless guided by results from appropriately collected cultures or in patients with bacteremia, sepsis, cellulitis, or osteomyelitis.

Drug and Nondrug Management

8 Prevention is the single most important aspect in the management of pressure sores. Skin surveillance and frequent repositioning (ie, pressure reduction) are key in preventing pressure sores.[69,74] Prevention is far easier and less costly than the intensive care necessary for the healing and eventual closure of pressure sores. Of primary importance, then, is the ability to identify patients who are at high risk so that preventive measures may be instituted. Relief of pressure through proper positioning, and periodic repositioning, is probably the single most important factor in preventing pressure sore formation. Relief for a period of only 5 minutes once every 2 hours is believed to give protection against pressure sore formation.[69,71-74] Repositioning seated patients every 15 to 60 minutes is also recommended.[25,74] Pressure relief devices such as mattresses or overlays filled with air, water, gel, or foam are helpful in preventing pressure sores.[77] Cushions and ankle or heel protectors should also be encouraged.[69,71] Skin care and prevention of soilage are also important, with the intent being to keep the surface relatively free of moisture. Patients with problems of incontinence should be cleaned frequently, and efforts should be made to keep the involved areas dry.[68]

The medical approach to the treatment of pressure sores depends on the stage of the disease. Medical management generally is indicated for lesions that are of moderate size and relatively shallow depth (stage 1 or 2 lesions) and are not located over a bony prominence. Depending on their location and severity, from 30% to 80% of these ulcers will heal without an operation. Surgical intervention is almost always necessary for ulcers that extend through superficial layers or into bone (stage 3, stage 4, and unstageable lesions).[70]

The goal of therapy is to clean and decontaminate the ulcer in order to permit formation of healthy granulation tissue that promotes wound healing or prepares the wound for an operative procedure. The main factors to be considered for successful topical therapy (local care) are (a) relief of pressure, (b) debridement of necrotic tissue as needed, (c) wound cleansing, (d) dressing selection, and (e) prevention, diagnosis, and treatment of infection.[25,69,71,74,75]

Relief of pressure is important once a pressure sore has developed. The same repositioning methods and pressure-reducing devices used for preventive care also apply to treatment.[25,69]

The goals of debridement and cleansing measures are removal of devitalized tissue and reduction of bacterial contamination, which can slow granulation time and impede healing.[25,69] Debridement can be accomplished by surgical, mechanical, or chemical means.[25,69] Surgical debridement rapidly removes necrotic material from the wound and is recommended for urgent situations (eg, cellulitis and sepsis).[71-73] Mechanical debridement generally involves wet-to-dry dressing changes. Saline-soaked gauze is applied to the wound; after drying, the gauze is removed and with it any adherent necrotic tissue. Other effective mechanical therapies include hydrotherapy (use of the whirlpool [Hubbard tank] to remove necrotic tissue and debris), wound irrigation, and dextranomers (beads placed in the wound to absorb exudate and bacteria).[25,69] Chemical debridement includes enzymatic and autolytic agents. Enzymatic debridement involves application of topical debriding agents to remove devitalized tissue. This method is recommended for patients who cannot tolerate surgery or are in a long-term care or home setting.[25,69] Autolytic debridement involves the use of synthetic dressings that allow devitalized tissue to self-digest via enzymes present in wound fluids. Autolytic debridement is contraindicated in the treatment of infected pressure sores.[25]

Pressure sore wounds should be cleaned with normal saline.[69] No cleansing solution or technique has demonstrated greater efficacy on healing.[77] Cleansing agents that are cytotoxic, such as povidone–iodine, iodophor, sodium hypochlorite solution, hydrogen peroxide, and acetic acid, should be avoided.[69,72,73] Many of these agents destroy granulation tissue and impair healing. Many different types of dressings are available for pressure sores.[25] Wound dressing materials should keep the wound moist, allow free exchange of air, act as a physical barrier to bacteria, and prevent physical damage.[25,69] Controlled studies of the various types of wound dressings have shown no significant differences in healing outcomes.[68] Occlusive dressings (hydrocolloid, such as DuoDERM™ or Tegaderm™) and transparent dressings (eg, 3M Tegaderm™) are not recommended for infected wounds.[25,69] If occlusive dressings are used, any infection should be controlled or the dressing frequency increased.

A 2-week trial of topical antibiotics (silver sulfadiazine or triple antibiotic) may be considered for a clean ulcer that is not healing or is producing a moderate amount of exudate despite appropriate care.[72] Systemic treatment of pressure ulcers is generally for infections associated with bacteremia, sepsis, cellulitis, or osteomyelitis.[72,73] Empiric therapy for infected pressure sores or associated infectious complications should cover MRSA, anaerobes, enterococci, and more resistant gram-negative bacteria such as *Pseudomonas* (see Table 110-5).[69] Thereafter, antibiotics should be guided by results from appropriately collected cultures.

Other nonpharmacologic approaches to shorten the healing time have included the use of hyperbaric oxygenation, hydrotherapy, high-frequency/high-intensity sound waves, and electrotherapy.[72,73,77] Electrical stimulation is the only adjunctive therapy that is proven effective.[72,73] Various comorbid conditions (diabetes mellitus, smoking, peripheral vascular disease, malnutrition) may impair wound healing. Eliminating or optimizing these factors is recommended, although studies have not demonstrated benefit.[25,69,74-76]

Evaluation of Therapeutic Outcomes

With appropriate wound care and antimicrobial therapy, infected pressure sores can heal. A reduction in erythema, warmth, pain, and other signs and symptoms should be seen in 48 to 72 hours.

ANIMAL AND HUMAN BITE WOUNDS

Approximately half the population in the United States will be bitten by either an animal or another human sometime during their lifetimes.[78,79] Animal bites (typically from dogs or cats) are common causes of injury, particularly to children, and are associated with significant risk of infection without prompt attention to appropriate management. Likewise, human bite wounds are often deceptively severe and frequently require aggressive management to reduce the risk of infectious complications. If left untreated, soft-tissue infection and osteomyelitis may occur, possibly requiring extensive debridement or amputation.

Epidemiology

Dog bites account for approximately 60% of all animal bite wounds requiring medical attention.[78] The Centers for Disease Control and Prevention reports that nearly 350,000 individuals seek emergency room attention for dog bites annually.[79] The rate of dog bite–related injuries is highest in children aged 5 to 9 years. Most dog bites are to the extremities,[78] but the majority of bites to children less than 5 years of age are to the face and neck.[79] Cat bites are the second most common cause of bite wounds in the United States, accounting for up to 20% of all animal bites.[78] Cat bites occur most commonly on the upper extremities and face, with most injuries reported in women and the elderly.[78,80] Human bites are the third most frequent type of bites requiring medical attention.

Infection rates after dog and cat bites are estimated at 20% overall. However, infection may occur in up to 30% to 80% of serious cat bites, a rate more than double those seen with dog bites.[80] Also, bite wounds to the hands become infected in 30% to 40% of cases.[78] Patients at greatest risk of acquiring animal bite–related infection have had a puncture wound (usually to the hand), have not sought medical attention within 8 hours of the injury, and are older than 50 years of age.[78,80]

Infected human bites can occur as bites from the teeth or from blows to the mouth (clenched-fist injuries). Bites by others can occur to any part of the body, but most often involve the hands. Infectious complications occur in 10% to 50% of patients with human bites.[80]

Etiology

Infections in bite wounds are caused predominantly by mouth flora from the animal or human biter, and from the victim's own skin flora (Table 110-11).[78,80-84] Most infections are polymicrobial, with a median of three to nine bacterial isolates per culture.[78,80-84] *Pasteurella* is the most frequent isolate from both dog and cat bites. *Pasteurella multocida* is part of the normal oral flora of up to 90% of cats; dog bites more commonly involve *P. canis* (approximately 26% of infections).[80,82] Tularemia (*Pasteurella tularensis*) and cat scratch disease (*Bartonella henselae*) have also been transmitted by cat bites, while rabies is associated with dog bites, particularly in developing countries.[82,83,85] Human bite wounds are notable for potential involvement of *Eikenella corrodens* in approximately 30% of infections.

Pathophysiology

The potential for infection from an animal bite is great owing to the pressure that can be exerted during the bite and the vast number of potential pathogens that make up the normal oral flora.[78,80-83] Cats' teeth are slender and extremely sharp. Their teeth easily penetrate into bones and joints, resulting in a higher incidence of septic arthritis and osteomyelitis.[78,80-83] Although a dog's teeth may not be as sharp, they can exert a pressure of 200 to 450 lb/in^2 (~1,400 to 3,100 kPa) and therefore result in a serious crush injury with much devitalized tissue.[78,80-83] In addition, the polymicrobic (aerobic and anaerobic) nature of animal bites provides a synergistic relationship, thus making an infection harder to eradicate.[81]

Human bites generally are more serious and more prone to infection than animal bites, particularly clenched-fist injuries.[81] While the force of a punch may sever a tendon or nerve or break a bone, it most often causes a breach in the capsule of the metacarpophalangeal joint, leading to direct inoculation of bacteria into the joint or bone.[81,83] When the hand is relaxed, the tendons carry bacteria into deeper spaces of the hand, resulting in more extensive infection.[81,83]

TABLE 110-11 Bacterial Isolates from Infections in Animal and Human Bite Wounds [78,80-83]

	Percentage of Isolates	
Organisms	**Dog and Cat**	**Human**
Aerobes	74-90	44
Pasteurella spp.	50-75	—
Streptococcus spp.	46-50	52-84
S. anginosus	—	52
S. mitis	22	12
S. pyogenes	12	14
S. mutans	12	2
Staphylococcus spp.	35-46	54
S. aureus	20	30
S. epidermidis	18	22
Neisseria spp.	32-35	4
Moraxella spp.	10-35	2
Corynebacterium spp.	12-28	12
Enterococcus spp.	10-12	6
Bacillus spp.	8-11	—
Eikenella corrodens	2	30
Enterobacteriaceae	6-12	8-15
Anaerobes	50-70	40-90
Fusobacterium spp.	32-33	32-34
Porphyromonas spp.	28-30	2
Bacteroides spp.	18-28	4
Prevotella spp.	19-28	22-36
Propionibacterium spp.	18-20	4
Peptostreptococcus spp.	8-16	22
Veillonella spp.	2	24
Mixed aerobic and anaerobic	50-75	40-66

TREATMENT

Desired Outcomes

The goals of therapy of bite wounds, whether caused by animals or humans, are twofold: to provide effective prophylaxis against infection, when appropriate, and to achieve rapid eradication of established infection and prevent further complications. Effective treatment of bite wounds includes avoidance of unnecessary antimicrobials that contribute to increased resistance, and minimizing toxicities and cost of therapy.

Management of Bite Wounds

9 Bite wounds should be irrigated thoroughly with a copious volume of sterile water or saline, and the wound washed vigorously with soap or povidone–iodine in order to reduce the bacterial count in the wound.[80,83] Surgical debridement and immobilization of the affected area is often required in dog and human bites associated with more extensive tissue injury. Clinical failures due to edema have occurred despite appropriate antibiotic therapy.[78] Therefore, it is important to stress to patients that the affected area should be elevated for several days or until edema has resolved. In the case of animal bites, an immunization history of the animal should be obtained. It is also important for the patient's tetanus immune status to be determined. Because transmission of viruses (HIV, herpes, hepatitis B and C) is a possibility with human bites, information about the biter is important. Although the possibility of acquiring HIV through saliva alone is believed to be unlikely, the presence of virus-containing blood in the saliva makes disease transmission possible.[86,87] Bite victims exposed to blood-tainted saliva may be offered antiretroviral chemoprophylaxis, but each case should be individually assessed based on the potential for significant exposure and potential risks and benefits of antiretroviral therapy.[86,87]

Patients with clenched-fist injuries should be seen by a specialist in hand care to evaluate for penetration into the synovium, joint capsule, and bone.[15,81] Primary closure for human bites generally is not recommended. Tetanus toxoid and antitoxin may be indicated.

10 All patients with human bite injuries should receive prophylactic antibiotic therapy ("early preemptive therapy") for 3 to 5 days due to high infection risk (Table 110-4).[83,84,87] Prophylactic antimicrobial agents should be given as soon as possible to all patients, regardless of the appearance of the wound, unless it can be documented that the wound does not involve hands, feet, or joints and penetrates no deeper than the epidermis.[15,72,83]

The role of prophylactic antimicrobial therapy for early, noninfected animal bite wounds remains controversial.[15,78,80,81,83] Recommendations from the Infectious Diseases Society of America suggest that prophylactic or early preemptive therapy seems to provide only marginal benefit for most patients in the absence of specific factors that increase the risk of infection.[15] The decision to administer prophylactic antibiotics is therefore based on an assessment of wound severity and host immune competence. Specifically, prophylaxis is more strongly recommended in patients with the following factors associated with increased risk for infection: immunocompromised; asplenic; advanced liver disease; preexisting or resultant edema of the affected area; moderate to severe bite-related injuries, especially to the hands or face; or bite injuries that have penetrated the periosteum or joint capsule.[15] A 3- to 5-day course of prophylactic antibiotics is recommended when such therapy is considered to be appropriate.[15,80,81,83]

Empiric antibiotics for the treatment of established infection of bite wounds should be directed at a variety of aerobic and anaerobic flora (Table 110-4). Amoxicillin–clavulanic acid is most commonly recommended for oral outpatient therapy due to excellent activity against all likely pathogens, including *Pasteurella* and *Eikenella*.[15,78,80,81,83] Alternative oral agents include moxifloxacin or doxycycline alone, or trimethoprim–sulfamethoxazole, levofloxacin, ciprofloxacin, or a second- or third-generation cephalosporin in combination with metronidazole or clindamycin to provide activity against oropharyngeal anaerobes. Although the combination of penicillin VK plus dicloxacillin has been recommended traditionally for the treatment of bite wounds, its use has become less common in favor of other alternatives. Failure to provide adequate initial treatment of bite wounds results in treatment failures and increased need for hospitalization for parenteral antibiotics.[15,78,80-83]

Hospitalization for minor wounds is unnecessary if surgical repair of vital structures has not been performed. Patients with clenched-fist or other serious bite injuries and severe resultant infection may be considered for IV antibiotics. Treatment options for patients requiring IV therapy include β-lactam–β-lactamase inhibitor combinations (ampicillin–sulbactam, piperacillin–tazobactam), second-generation cephalosporins with antianaerobic activity (eg, cefoxitin), and ertapenem.[15,83] The combination of doxycycline or a fluoroquinolone with metronidazole or clindamycin may be used in patients with severe β-lactam allergies. The length of antimicrobial therapy depends on the severity of the injury/infection. However, therapy should generally be continued from 7 to 14 days.[15,78,87-91]

Tetanus does not occur commonly after dog bites; however, it is possible. If the immunization history of a patient with anything other than a clean, minor wound is unknown, or if the last known vaccination was longer than 10 years ago, tetanus–diphtheria (TD) toxoids should be administered.[88,89] Both TD toxoids and tetanus immune globulin should be administered to patients who have never been immunized.[83,90]

CLINICAL PRESENTATION Bite Wounds

General

Animal bites:

- Only general wound care is required for most patients with dog bites who present early (<12 hours) after injury; infection is more likely in patients presenting late (≥12 hours) after injury.

Human bites:

- Most patients with clenched-fist injuries present for medical care after infection is already established.

Symptoms

- Patients often seek medical care for infection-related complaints (ie, pain, purulent discharge, and swelling) at the site of the injury.
- Wounds often have a purulent discharge, and decreased range of motion may be present.

Signs

- Erythema, swelling, and clear or purulent discharge at site of infected wound.

Animal bites:

- If *P. multocida* is present, a rapidly progressing cellulitis is observed within 24 to 48 hours of initial injury.
- Fever is uncommon.
- Adenopathy or lymphangitis is uncommon.

Human bites:

- Lymphadenopathy is common.
- In clenched-fist injuries, edema may limit the ability of tendons to glide in their sheaths, thereby limiting a joint's range of motion.

Laboratory Tests

- Samples for bacterial cultures (aerobic and anaerobic) should be obtained from infected wounds.
- Wounds seen <8 hours or more than 24 hours after injury that show no signs of infection may not need to be cultured.
- White blood counts should be monitored for resolution of infection if initially elevated.

Other Diagnostic Tests

- Radiographic evaluation should be performed if damage to a bone or joint is suspected.

Because the rabies virus can be transmitted via saliva, rabies may be a potential complication of a bite. When the symptoms of rabies develop after a bite, the prognosis for survival is poor. Roughly 3% of rabies cases documented in animals were in dogs (the most frequent vectors are skunks, raccoons, and bats).[85,91] In the United States, recommendations for postexposure prophylaxis after a dog bite depend on the health of the dog. If the animal is healthy and able to be observed for a 10-day period, active prophylaxis is only required if the dog develops signs of rabies.[78,80,85] If the dog is known or suspected to be rabid, postexposure procedures should be initiated; current treatment guidelines should be consulted for appropriate management recommendations.[85,91] Outside of the United States, locally applicable guidelines such as those from the World Health Organization should be consulted.[92]

Evaluation of Therapeutic Outcomes

Evaluation of treatment for either animal or human bites should follow the same general guidelines. Bite victims treated on an outpatient basis with oral antimicrobials should be followed up within 24 hours by either phone or office visit.[15] Hospitalization or change to IV therapy should be considered if the infection has progressed. For hospitalized patients with no improvement in signs and symptoms following 24 hours of appropriate therapy, surgical debridement may be needed. Physical therapy may be needed to improve complications such as residual joint stiffness and loss of function, particularly after human bites involving clenched-fist injuries.

PERSONALIZED PHARMACOTHERAPY

Desired treatment outcomes for the various types of SSTIs described in this chapter are achieved through close monitoring and frequent patient assessment, including judicious evaluation of antimicrobial therapies. SSTIs are challenging in that cultures are often not performed due to the unavailability of easily obtained culturable specimens and the low yield of common culturing techniques. Empiric antibiotic selection based on most likely pathogens is an effective strategy in less severe infections such as erysipelas, impetigo, and furuncles. However, treatment of more severe infections such as cellulitis, DFI, and necrotizing fasciitis should be individualized based on properly obtained culture specimens and documented pathogens and susceptibilities whenever possible. Aggressive antimicrobial use must be balanced against unnecessary administration of drugs that may lead to increased antimicrobial resistance, adverse effects, and cost. Proper evaluation of an individual patient's severity of infection and risk of complications allows for selection of appropriate antimicrobials for the treatment of infection and selection of appropriate treatment settings (eg, inpatient vs outpatient), both of which may allow for the most cost-effective therapy.

ABBREVIATIONS

CA-MRSA	community-associated methicillin-resistant *S. aureus*
DFI	diabetic foot infection
HA-MRSA	healthcare-associated methicillin-resistant *Staphylococcus aureus*
HIV	human immunodeficiency virus
MRSA	methicillin-resistant *Staphylococcus aureus25*
MSSA	methicillin-susceptible *Staphylococcus aureus*
PVL	Panton-Valentine leukocidin
SCC*mec*	staphylococcal chromosomal cassette *mec*
SSTI	skin and soft-tissue infection
TD	tetanus–diphtheria

REFERENCES

1. Grice EA, Segre JA. The skin microbiome. *Nat Rev Microbiol* 2011;9:244-253.
2. Sanford JA, Gallo RL. Functions of the skin microbiota in health and disease. *Sem Immunol* 2013;25:370-377.

3. Pasternak MS, Swartz MN. Cellulitis, necrotizing fasciitis, and subcutaneous tissue infections. In: Bennett JE, Dolin R, Blaser MJ, eds. *Mandell, Douglas, and Bennett's Principles and Practice of Infectious Diseases*, 8th ed. Philadelphia: Elsevier, 2015:1194-1215.
4. Rajan S. Skin and soft-tissue infections: Classifying and treating a spectrum. *Cleveland Clin J Med* 2012;79:57-66.
5. Gunderson CG. Cellulitis: Definition, etiology, and clinical features. *Am J Med* 2011;124:1113-1122.
6. Breen JO. Skin and soft tissue infections in immunocompetent patients. *Am Fam Physician* 2010;81:893-899.
7. Napolitano LM. Severe soft tissue infections. *Infect Dis Clin North Am* 2009;23:571-591.
8. Ray GT, Suaya JA, Baxter R. Incidence, microbiology, and patient characteristics of skin and soft-tissue infections in a U.S. population: a retrospective population-based study. *BMC Infect Dis* 2013;13:252-262.
9. Suaya JA, Mera RM, Cassidy A, et al. Incidence and cost of hospitalizations associated with *Staphylococcus aureus* skin and soft infections in the United States from 2001 through 2009. *BMC Infect Dis* 2014;14:296-303.
10. Dawson AL, Dellavalle RP, Elston DM. Infectious skin diseases: A review and needs assessment. *Dermatol Clin* 2012;30:141-151.
11. Qualls ML, Mooney MM, Camargo CA Jr, Zucconi T, Hooper DC, Pallin DJ. Emergency department visit rates for abscess versus other skin infections during the emergence of community-associated methicillin-resistant *Staphylococcus aureus*, 1997-2007. *Clin Infect Dis* 2012;55:103-105.
12. Stevens DL. Treatments for skin and soft-tissue and surgical site infections due to MDR gram-positive bacteria. *J Infect* 2009;59:532-539.
13. Stryjewski ME, Chambers HF. Skin and soft tissue infections caused by community-acquired methicillin-resistant *Staphylococcus aureus*. *Clin Infect Dis* 2008;46(Suppl 5):S368-S377.
14. Tenover FC, Goering RV. Methicillin-resistant *Staphylococcus aureus* strain USA300: Origin and epidemiology. *J Antimicrob Chemother* 2009;64:441-446.
15. Stevens DL, Bisno AL, Chambers HF, et al. Practice guidelines for the diagnosis and management of skin and soft-tissue infections: 2014 update by the Infectious Diseases Society of America. *Clin Infect Dis* 2014;59:e10-e52.
16. Daum RS. Skin and soft tissue infections caused by methicillin-resistant *Staphylococcus aureus*. *N Engl J Med* 2007;357:380-390.
17. Chen LF, Chastain C, Anderson DJ. Community-acquired methicillin-resistant *Staphylococcus aureus* skin and soft-tissue infections: management and prevention. *Curr Infect Dis Rep* 2011;13:442-450.
18. David MZ, Daum RS. Community-acquired methicillin-resistant *Staphylococcus aureus*: Epidemiology and clinical consequences of an emerging epidemic. *Clin Microbiol Rev* 2010;23:616-687.
19. Como-Sabetti K, Harriman KH, Buch JM, Giennen A, Boxrud DJ, Lynfield R. Community-associated methicillin-resistant *Staphylococcus aureus*: Trends in case and isolate characteristics from six years of prospective surveillance. *Public Health Rep* 2009;124:427-435.
20. Centers for Disease Control and Prevention. Active Bacterial Core Surveillance Report, Emerging Infections Program Network, Methicillin-Resistant *Staphylococcus aureus*. 2010, *http://www.cdc.gov/abcs/reports-findings/survreports/mrsa10.html*.
21. Jeng A, Beheshti M, Li J, Nathan R. The role of beta-hemolytic streptococci in causing diffuse, nonculturable cellulitis. *Medicine (Baltimore)* 2010;89:217-226.
22. Napierkowski D. Uncovering common bacterial skin infections. *Nurs Pract* 2013;38:30-37.
23. Yu Y, Cheng AS, Wang L, et al. Hot tub folliculitis or hand–foot syndrome caused by *Pseudomonas aeruginosa*. *J Am Acad Dermatol* 2007;57:596-600.
24. Reichel M, Heisig P, Kampf G. Identification of variables for aerobic bacterial density at clinically relevant skin sites. *J Hosp Infect* 2011;78:5-10.
25. Jaul E. Assessment and management of pressure ulcers in the elderly. *Drugs Aging* 2010;27:311-325.
26. Dryden MA. Complicated skin and soft tissue infection. *J Antimicrob Chemother* 2010;65(Suppl 3):iii35-iii44.
27. Lipsky BA, Berendt AR, Cornia PB, et al. 2012 Infectious Diseases Society of America clinical practice guidelines for the diagnosis and treatment of diabetic foot infections. *Clin Infect Dis* 2012;54:132-173.
28. Liu C, Bayer A, Cosgrive SE, et al. Clinical practice guidelines by the Infectious Diseases Society of America for the treatment of methicillin-resistant *Staphylococcus aureus* infections in adults and children. *Clin Infect Dis* 2011;52:1-38.
29. Rybak MJ, Lomaestro BM, Rotschafer JC, et al. Vancomycin therapeutic guidelines: A summary of consensus recommendations from the Infectious Diseases Society of America, the American Society of Health-System Pharmacists, and the Society of Infectious Diseases Pharmacists. *Am J Health Syst Pharm* 2009;66:82-98.
30. Krasagakis K, Valachis A, Maniatakis P, Kruger-Krasagakis S, Samonis G, Tosca AD. Analysis of epidemiology, clinical features and management of erysipelas. *Int J Dermatol* 2010;49:1012-1017.
31. Kilburn SA, Featherstone P, Higgins B, Brindle R. Interventions for cellulitis and erysipelas. *Cochrane Database Syst Rev* 2010;(6):CD004299.
32. Bergkvist PI, Sjobeck K. Antibiotic and prednisolone therapy of erysipelas: A randomized, double-blind, placebo-controlled study. *Scan J Infect Dis* 1997;29:377-382.
33. Bangert S, Levy M, Hebert AA. Bacterial resistance and impetigo treatment trends: A review. *Pediatr Dermatol* 2012;29:243-248.
34. Koning S, Van der Sande R, Verhagen AP, et al. Interventions for impetigo. *Cochrane Database Syst Rev* 2012;1:CD003261.
35. Pasternak MS, Swartz MN. Lymphadenitis and lymphangitis. In: Bennett JE, Dolin R, Blaser MJ, eds. *Mandell, Douglas, and Bennett's Principles and Practice of Infectious Diseases*, 8th ed. Philadelphia: Elsevier, 2015:1226-1237.
36. Seelang K, Manning ML, Saks M, Winstead Y. Skin and soft tissue infection management, outcomes, and follow-up in the emergency department of an urban academic hospital. *Adv Emerg Nurs J* 2014;36:348-359.
37. Odell CA. Community-associated methicillin-resistant *Staphylococcus aureus* (CA-MRSA) skin infections. *Curr Opin Pediatr* 2010;22:273-277.
38. Stevens DL, Eron LL. Cellulitis and soft tissue infections. *Ann Intern Med* 2009;150:ITC1–ITC11.
39. Bailey E, Kroshinsky D. Cellulitis: Diagnosis and management. *Dermatol Ther* 2011;24:229-239.
40. Gorwitz RJ, Jernigan DB, Powers JH, et al. Strategies for Clinical Management of MRSA in the Community: Summary of an Experts' Meeting Convened by the Centers for Disease Control and Prevention. 2006, *http://www.cdc.gov/ncidod/dhqp/ar_mrsa_ca.html*.
41. Tong SYC, Davis JS, Eichenberger E, Holland TL, Fowler VG Jr. *Staphylococcus aureus* infections: Epidemiology, pathophysiology, clinical manifestations, and management. *Clin Microbiol Rev* 2015;28:603-661.
42. Odell CA. Community-associated methicillin-resistant *Staphylococcus aureus* skin infections. *Curr Opin Pediatr* 2010;22:273-277.
43. Nathwani D, Morgan M, Masterton RG, et al. Guidelines for UK practice for the diagnosis and management of methicillin-resistant *Staphylococcus aureus* (MRSA) infections presenting in the community. *J Antimicrob Chemother* 2008;61:976-994.
44. McKinnon PS, Sorensen SV, Liu LZ, Itani KM. Impact of linezolid on economic outcomes and determinants of cost in a clinical trial evaluating patients with MRSA complicated skin and soft-tissue infections. *Ann Pharmacother* 2006;40:1017-1023.
45. Ruhe JJ, Menon A. Tetracyclines as an oral treatment option for patients with community onset skin and soft tissue infections caused by methicillin-resistant *Staphylococcus aureus*. *Antimicrob Agents Chemother* 2007;51:3298-3303.
46. Cenizal MJ, Skiest D, Luber S, et al. Prospective randomized trial of empiric therapy with trimethoprim–sulfamethoxazole or doxycycline for outpatient skin and soft tissue infections in an area of high prevalence of methicillin-resistant *Staphylococcus aureus*. *Antimicrob Agents Chemother* 2007;51:2628-2630.
47. Dryden MS. Novel antibiotic treatment for skin and soft tissue infection. *Curr Opin Infect Dis* 2014;27:116-124.
48. Jeng A, Beheshti M, Li J, et al. The role of beta-hemolytic streptococci in causing diffuse, nonculturable cellulitis: A prospective investigation. *Medicine (Baltimore)* 2010;89:217-226.
49. Kaafarani HMA, King DR. Necrotizing skin and soft tissue infections. *Surg Clin N Am* 2014;94:155-163.
50. Ustin JS, Malangoni MA. Necrotizing soft-tissue infections. *Crit Care Med* 2011;39:2156-2162.
51. Morgan MS. Diagnosis and management of necrotizing fasciitis: A multiparametric approach. *J Hosp Infect* 2010;75:249-257.
52. Bellapianta JM, Ljungquist K, Tobin E, et al. Necrotizing fasciitis. *J Am Acad Orthop Surg* 2009;17:174-182.
53. Boyer A, Vargas F, Coste F, et al. Influence of surgical treatment timing on mortality from necrotizing soft tissue infections requiring intensive care management. *Intensive Care Med* 2009;35:847-853.
54. Hobizal KB, Wukich DK. Diabetic foot infections: Current concept review. *Diabetic Foot Ankle* 2012;3;1-8.

55. Abbas M, Uckay I, Lipsky BA. In diabetic foot infections antibiotics are to treat infection, not to heal wounds. *Exp Opin Pharmacother* 2015;16:821-832.
56. Tecilazich F, Dinh T, Veves A. Treating diabetic ulcers. *Expert Opin Pharmacother* 2011;12:593-606.
57. Uckay I, Gariani K, Pataky Z, Lipsky BA. Diabetic foot infections: State-of-the-art. *Diabetes Obesity Metab* 2013;16:305-316.
58. Lipsky BA, Tabak YP, Johannes RS, et al. Skin and soft tissue infections in hospitalized patients with diabetes: Culture isolates and risk factors associated with mortality, length of stay and cost. *Diabetologia* 2010;53:914-923.
59. Lipsky BA, Peters EJG, Senneville E, et al. Expert opinion on the management of infections in the diabetic foot. *Diabetes Metab Res Rev* 2012;28(Suppl 1):163-178.
60. Peters EJG, Lipsky BA. Diagnosis and management of infection in the diabetic foot. *Med Clin N Am* 2013;97:911-946.
61. Crouzet J, Lavigne JP, Richard JL, et al. Diabetic foot infection: A critical review of recent randomized clinical trials on antibiotic therapy. *Int J Infect Dis* 2011;15:e601-e610.
62. Malone M, Bowling FL, Gannass A, Jude EB, Boulton AJM. Deep wound cultures correlate well with bone biopsy culture in diabetic foor osteomyelitis. *Diabetes Metab Res Rev* 2013;29:546-550.
63. Eleftheriadou I, Tentolouris N, Argiana V, et al. Methicillin-resistant *Staphylococcus aureus* in diabetic foot infections. *Drugs* 2010;70:1785-1797.
64. Zenelaj B, Bouvet C, Lipsky BA, et al. Do diabetic foot infections with methicillin-resistant *Staphylococcus aureus* differ from those with other pathogens? *Int J Lower Extrem Wounds* 2014;13:263-272.
65. Lipsky BA, Armstrong DG, Citron DM, et al. Ertapenem versus piperacillin/tazobactam for diabetic foot infections (SIDESTEP): Prospective, randomized, controlled, double-blinded, multicentre trial. *Lancet* 2005;366:1695-1703.
66. Lipsky BA, Hoey C. Topical antimicrobial therapy for treating chronic wounds. *Clin Infect Dis* 2009;49:1541-1549.
67. Chang J, Cuellar NG. The use of honey for wound care management. *Home Healthcare Nurs* 2009;27:309-316.
68. Reddy M, Gill SS, Kalkar SR, et al. Treatment of pressure ulcers. A systematic review. *JAMA* 2008;300:2647-2662.
69. Smith ME, Totten A, Hickam DH, et al. Pressure ulcer treatment strategies: A systematic comparative effectiveness review. *Ann Intern Med* 2013;159:39-50.
70. Black J, Baharestani M, Cuddigan J, et al. National Pressure Ulcer Advisory Panel's updated pressure ulcer staging system. *Dermatol Nurs* 2007;19:343-349.
71. Niederhauser A, Lukas CV, Parker V, Ayello EA, Zulkowski K, Berlowitz D. Comprehensive programs for preventing pressure ulcers: A review of the literature. *Adv Skin Wound Care* 2012;25:167-188.
72. Cushing CA, Phillips LG. Evidence-based medicine: Pressure sores. *Plast Recontruct Surg* 2013;132:1720-1732.
73. Ho CH, Bogie K. The prevention and treatment of pressure ulcers. *Phys Med Rehab Clin North Am* 2007;18:235-253.
74. Tchanque-Fossuo CN, Kuzon WM Jr. An evidence-based approach to pressure sores. *Plast Reconstr Surg* 2011;127:932-939.
75. Markova A, Mostow EN. US skin disease assessment: Ulcer and wound care. *Dermatol Clin* 2012;30:107-111.
76. Dealey C. Skin care and pressure ulcers. *Adv Skin Wound Care* 2009;22:421-428.
77. Brolmann FE, Ubbink DT, Nelson EA, Munte K, van der Horst CM, Vermeulen H. Evidence-based decisions for local and systemic wound care. *Br J Surg* 2012;99:1172-1183.
78. Oehler RL, Velez AP, Mizrachi M, et al. Bite-related and septic syndromes caused by cats and dogs. *Lancet Infect Dis* 2009;9:439-447.
79. Centers for Disease Control and Prevention. Leading causes of nonfatal injury reports, 2001-2013. Available at: *http://webappa.cdc.gov/sasweb/ncipc/nfilead2001.html.*
80. Thomas N, Brook I. Animal bite-associated infections: Microbiology and treatment. *Expert Rev Anti Infect Ther* 2011;9:215-226.
81. Aziz H, Rhee P, Pandit V, Tang A, Gries L, Joseph B. The current concepts in management of animal (dog, cat, snake, scorpion) and human bite wounds. *J Trauma Acute Care Surg* 2015;78:641-648.
82. Abrahamian FM, Goldstein EJC. Microbiology of animal bite wound infection. *Clin Microbiol Rev* 2011;24:231-246.
83. Goldstein EJC, Abrahamian FM. Bites. In: Bennett JE, Dolin R, Blaser MJ, eds. *Mandell, Douglas, and Bennett's Principles and Practice of Infectious Diseases*, 8th ed. Philadelphia: Elsevier, 2015:3510-3515.
84. Kennedy SA, Stoll LE, Lauder AS. Human and other mammalian bite injuries of the hand: Evaluation and management. *J Am Acad Ortho Surg* 2015;23:47-57.
85. Rupprecht CE, Briggs D, Brown CM, et al. Use of a reduced (4-dose) vaccine schedule for postexposure prophylaxis to prevent human rabies: Recommendations of the Advisory Committee on Immunization Practices. *MMWR Recomm Rep* 2010;59(RR02):1-9.
86. Smith DK, Grohskopf LA, Black RJ, et al. Antiretroviral postexposure prophylaxis after sexual, injection-drug use, or other nonoccupational exposure to HIV in the United States. Recommendations from the U.S. Department of Health and Human Services. *MMWR Recomm Rep* 2005;54(RR-2):1-20.
87. Harrison M. A 4-year review of human bite injuries presenting to emergency medicine and proposed evidence-based guidelines. *Injury* 2009;40:826-830.
88. Kretsinger K, Broder KR, Cortese MM, et al. Preventing tetanus, diphtheria, and pertussis among adults: Use of tetanus toxoid, reduced diphtheria toxoid and acellular pertussis vaccine. Recommendations of the Advisory Committee on Immunization Practices (ACIP). *MMWR Recomm Rep* 2006;55(RR-17):1-33.
89. Broder KR, Cortese MM, Iskander JJ, et al. Preventing tetanus, diphtheria, and pertussis among adolescents: Use of tetanus toxoid, reduced diphtheria toxoid and acellular pertussis vaccine. Recommendations of the Advisory Committee on Immunization Practices (ACIP). *MMWR Recomm Rep* 2006;55(RR-3):1–34.
90. Kroger AT, Pickering LK, Wharton M, Mawle A, Hinman AR, Orenstein WA. Immunization. In: Bennett JE, Dolin R, Blaser MJ, eds. *Mandell, Douglas, and Bennett's Principles and Practice of Infectious Diseases*, 8th ed. Philadelphia: Elsevier, 2015:3516-3553.
91. Nigg AJ, Walker PL. Overview, prevention, and treatment of rabies. *Pharmacotherapy* 2009;29:1182-1195.
92. World Health Organization. WHO guide for rabies pre and post exposure prophylaxis in humans. Updated 2013. Available at: *http://www.who.int/rabies/WHO_Guide_Rabies_Pre_Post_Exposure_Prophylaxis_Humans_2013.pdf?ua=1&ua=1.*

111

Infective Endocarditis

Angie Veverka, Brian L. Odle, and Jeffrey A. Kyle

KEY CONCEPTS

1. Infective endocarditis usually occurs in adult patients with specific risk factors (eg, IV drug abuse, heart failure, valvular disease, and healthcare exposure) and those with implanted cardiac material (eg, prosthetic heart valves).
2. Three groups of organisms cause a majority of infective endocarditis cases: streptococci, staphylococci, and enterococci.
3. The clinical presentation of infective endocarditis is highly variable and nonspecific, although a fever and murmur are usually present. Classic peripheral manifestations (eg, Osler's nodes) may or may not occur.
4. The diagnosis of infective endocarditis requires the integration of clinical, laboratory, and echocardiographic findings. The two major diagnostic criteria are bacteremia and echocardiographic changes (eg, valvular vegetation).
5. Treatment of infective endocarditis involves isolation of the infecting pathogen and determination of antimicrobial susceptibilities, followed by high-dose, parenteral, bactericidal antibiotics for an extended period.
6. Surgical replacement of the infected heart valve is an important adjunct to endocarditis treatment in certain situations (eg, patients with acute heart failure).
7. β-Lactam antibiotics, such as penicillin G (or ceftriaxone), nafcillin, and ampicillin, remain the drugs of choice for streptococcal, staphylococcal, and enterococcal endocarditis, respectively.
8. Aminoglycoside antibiotics are essential to obtain a synergistic bactericidal effect in the treatment of enterococcal endocarditis. Adjunctive aminoglycosides also may decrease the emergence of resistant organisms (eg, prosthetic valve endocarditis caused by coagulase-negative staphylococci) and hasten the pace of clinical and microbiologic response (eg, some streptococcal and staphylococcal infections).
9. Vancomycin is reserved for patients with immediate β-lactam allergies and the treatment of resistant organisms.
10. Antimicrobial prophylaxis is used to prevent infective endocarditis for patients who are at the highest risk (such as persons with prosthetic heart valves) before a bacteremia-causing procedure (eg, dental extraction).

Endocarditis is an inflammation of the endocardium, the membrane lining the chambers of the heart and covering the cusps of the heart valves.[1,2] More commonly, *endocarditis* refers to infection of the heart valves by various microorganisms. Although it typically affects native valves, it also may involve nonvalvular areas or implanted material (eg, prosthetic heart valves, cardiac defibrillators, pacemakers, and catheters). Bacteria primarily cause endocarditis, but fungi and other atypical microorganisms can lead to the disease; hence, the more encompassing term *infective endocarditis* is preferred.[1,3]

Endocarditis is often referred to as *acute* or *subacute* depending on the pace and severity of the clinical presentation. The acute, fulminating form is associated with high fevers and systemic toxicity. Virulent bacteria, such as *Staphylococcus aureus*, frequently cause this syndrome, and if untreated, death may occur within days to weeks. On the other hand, subacute infective endocarditis is more indolent, is caused by less invasive organisms, such as viridans streptococci, and usually occurs in preexisting valvular heart disease. Although infective endocarditis is often referred to as acute or subacute, it is best classified based on the etiologic organism, the anatomic site of infection, and pathogenic risk factors.[1,4,5] Infection may also occur following surgical insertion of a prosthetic heart valve, resulting in prosthetic valve endocarditis (PVE), or insertion of a cardiac implantable electronic device, resulting in cardiac device infective endocarditis (CDIE).[6,7]

EPIDEMIOLOGY AND ETIOLOGY

Infective endocarditis is an uncommon, but not rare, infection. Population-based studies have reported annual incidence rates of 2 to 15 cases per 100,000 person-years.[8,9] In the United States, the infection is listed as the primary or secondary diagnosis of 34,000 hospital discharges.[10] The mean male-to-female ratio is approximately 2:1.[11] As the population ages and as valve replacement surgery becomes more common, the mean age of patients with infective endocarditis increases. Most cases occur in individuals older than 50 years of age, and it is less common in children.[11-14] PVE and CDIE account for 20% and 6.4% of cases of infective endocarditis, respectively.[5,11,15] Those with a history of IV drug abuse (IVDA) are also at high risk. Of note, the incidence of healthcare-associated infective endocarditis is rising, especially in the elderly population.[11,12] Other conditions associated with a higher incidence of infective endocarditis include diabetes, long-term hemodialysis, and poor dental hygiene.[5,13]

(1) Most persons with infective endocarditis have risk factors, such as preexisting cardiac valvular abnormalities. Many types of structural heart disease result in turbulent blood flow that increases the risk for infective endocarditis. A predisposing risk factor, however, may be absent in up to 25% of cases. Some of the more important risk factors include:[4,5,7,11,13,16]

1. Presence of a prosthetic valve (highest risk)
2. Previous endocarditis (highest risk)
3. Healthcare-related exposure (high risk)
4. Congenital heart disease (CHD)
5. Chronic IV access
6. Diabetes mellitus

TABLE 111-1 Etiologic Organisms in Infective Endocarditis[a]

Agent	Percentage of Cases
Staphylococci	30-70
Coagulase positive	20-68
Coagulase negative	3-26
Streptococci	9-38
Viridans streptococci	10-28
Other streptococci	3-14
Enterococci	5-18
Gram-negative aerobic bacilli	1.5-13
Fungi	1-9
Miscellaneous bacteria	<5
Mixed infections	1-2
"Culture negative"	<5-17

[a]Values encompass community-acquired, healthcare-associated, native valve, and prosthetic valve infective endocarditis.

Data from references 3, 11, and 16.

7. Acquired valvular dysfunction (eg, rheumatic heart disease)
8. Cardiac implantable device
9. Chronic heart failure
10. Mitral valve prolapse with regurgitation
11. IVDA

Rheumatic heart disease was a prevalent risk factor for infective endocarditis, but the incidence of this disease continues to decline. The risk of infective endocarditis in persons with mitral valve prolapse and regurgitation is small; however, because the condition is prevalent, it is an important contributor to the overall number of infective endocarditis cases.[5,11] PVE occurs in 1% to 3% of patients undergoing valve replacement surgery in the first postoperative year.[11,17]

2 Nearly every organism causing human disease may cause infective endocarditis, but three groups of organisms result in a majority of cases: streptococci, staphylococci, and enterococci (Table 111-1).[3-5,11,16] The incidence of staphylococci, particularly *S. aureus*, continues to increase primarily due to healthcare exposure, and case series have documented that staphylococci have surpassed viridans streptococci as the leading cause of infective endocarditis.[4,11,16] In general, streptococci cause infective endocarditis in patients with community-acquired disease and underlying cardiac abnormalities, such as mitral valve prolapse or rheumatic heart disease. Staphylococci (*S. aureus* and coagulase-negative staphylococci) are the most common cause of PVE within the first year after valve surgery, and *S. aureus* is common in those with a history of IVDA. Although polymicrobial infective endocarditis is uncommon, it is encountered most often in association with IVDA.[11,16] Enterococcal endocarditis tends to follow genitourinary manipulations or obstetric procedures.[17] There are many exceptions to the preceding generalizations; thus, isolation of the causative pathogen and determination of its antimicrobial susceptibilities offer the best chance for successful therapy.

The mitral and aortic valves are affected most commonly in cases involving a single valve. Subacute endocarditis tends to involve the mitral valve, whereas acute disease often involves the aortic valve. Up to 35% of cases involve concomitant infections of both the aortic and the mitral valves. Infection of the tricuspid valve is less common, with a majority of these cases occurring in patients with a history of IVDA. It is rare for the pulmonary valve to be infected.[11,16,17]

Pathophysiology

The development of infective endocarditis via hematogenous spread, the most common route, requires the sequential occurrence of several factors. These components are complex and not fully elucidated.[2,18,19]

1. *The endothelial surface of the heart is damaged.* This injury occurs with turbulent blood flow associated with the valvular lesions previously described.
2. *Platelet and fibrin deposition occurs on the abnormal epithelial surface.* These platelet-fibrin deposits are referred to as *nonbacterial thrombotic endocarditis.*
3. *Bacteremia gives organisms access to and results in colonization of the endocardial surface.* Bacteremia is the result of trauma to a mucosal surface with a high concentration of resident bacteria such as the oral cavity and GI tract. Transient bacteremia commonly follow certain dental, GI, urologic, and gynecologic procedures. Staphylococci, viridans streptococci, and enterococci are most likely to adhere to nonbacterial thrombotic endocarditis, probably because of production of specific adherence factors such as dextran by some oral streptococci and glycocalyx for staphylococci. Gram-negative bacteria rarely adhere to heart valves and are uncommon causes of infective endocarditis.
4. *After colonization of the endothelial surface, a "vegetation" of fibrin, platelets, and bacteria forms.* The protective cover of fibrin and platelets allows unimpeded bacterial growth to concentrations as high as 10^9 to 10^{10} organisms per gram of tissue.

The pathogenesis of early PVE or CDIE differs from infective endocarditis acquired by the hematogenous route because surgery may directly inoculate prosthetic material with bacteria from the patient's skin or operating room personnel. In the case of early PVE, a recently placed nonendothelialized valve is more susceptible to bacterial colonization than are native valves. Bacteria also may colonize the new valve from contaminated bypass pumps, cannulas, and pacemakers or from a nosocomial bacteremia subsequent to an intravascular catheter.[7,16,17] The mechanism of bacterial colonization and pathogenesis in late PVE is similar to native valve endocarditis (NVE).[17]

The vegetations seen in infective endocarditis may be single or multiple and vary in size from a few millimeters to centimeters. Bacteria within the vegetation grow slowly and are protected from antibiotics and host defenses. The adverse effects of infective endocarditis and the resulting lesions can be far-reaching and include: (a) local perivalvular damage, (b) embolization of septic fragments with potential hematogenous seeding of remote sites, and (c) formation of antibody complexes.[17,19]

Formation of vegetations may destroy valvular tissue, and continued destruction can lead to acute heart failure via perforation of the valve leaflet, rupture of the chordae tendineae or papillary muscle, or, for patients with PVE, valve dehiscence. Occasionally, valvular stenosis may occur. Abscesses can develop in the valve ring or in myocardial tissue itself. Even with resolution of the process, fibrosis of tissue with some residual dysfunction is possible.

Vegetations may be friable, and fragments may be released downstream. These infected particles, termed *septic emboli*, can result in organ abscess or infarction. Septic emboli from right-sided endocarditis commonly lodge in the lungs, causing pulmonary abscesses. Emboli from left-sided vegetations commonly affect organs with high blood flow such as the kidneys, spleen, and brain.[4,17,19]

Circulating immune complexes consisting of antigen, antibody, and complement may deposit in organs, producing local inflammation, and damage (eg, glomerulonephritis in the kidneys). Other potential pathologic changes that result from immune-complex deposition or septic emboli include the development of "mycotic" aneurysms (although the aneurysm is usually bacterial in origin, not fungal), cerebral infarction, splenic infarction and abscess, and skin manifestations such as petechiae, Osler's nodes, and Janeway's lesions.[1,17,19]

CLINICAL PRESENTATION

3 The clinical presentation of infective endocarditis is highly variable and nonspecific. Fever is the most common finding and is often accompanied by other vague symptoms (Table 111-2). Fever may be relatively low grade, particularly in subacute cases. Heart murmurs are found in a majority of patients, most often preexisting, with some documented as new or changing. Infective endocarditis usually begins insidiously and worsens gradually. Patients may present with nonspecific findings such as fever, chills, weakness, dyspnea, night sweats, weight loss, or malaise. In contrast, patients with acute disease, such as those with a history of IVDA and *S. aureus* infective endocarditis, may appear with classic signs of sepsis.

Splenomegaly is a frequent finding for patients with prolonged endocarditis. Other important clinical signs especially prevalent in subacute illness may include the following peripheral manifestations ("stigmata") of endocarditis:[11,12,16,19]

1. Osler's nodes: Purplish or erythematous subcutaneous papules or nodules on the pads of the fingers and toes. These lesions are 2 to 15 mm in size and are painful and tender. These nodes are not specific for infective endocarditis and may be the result of embolism, immunologic phenomena, or both.
2. Janeway's lesions: Hemorrhagic, painless plaques on the palms of the hands or soles of the feet. These lesions are believed to be embolic in origin.
3. Splinter hemorrhages: Thin, linear hemorrhages found under the nail beds of the fingers or toes. These lesions are not specific for infective endocarditis and more commonly are the result of traumatic injuries. Distal lesions are more likely the result of trauma, whereas proximal lesions tend to be associated with infective endocarditis.
4. Petechiae: Small (usually 1-2 mm in diameter), erythematous, painless, hemorrhagic lesions. These lesions appear anywhere on the skin but more frequently on the anterior trunk, buccal mucosa and palate, and conjunctivae. Petechiae are nonblanching and resolve after a few days.
5. Clubbing of the fingers: Proliferative changes in the soft tissues about the terminal phalanges observed in long-standing endocarditis.
6. Roth's spots: Retinal infarct with central pallor and surrounding hemorrhage.
7. Emboli: Embolic phenomena occur in up to one third of cases and may result in significant complications. Left-sided endocarditis can result in renal artery emboli causing flank pain with hematuria, splenic artery emboli causing abdominal pain, and cerebral emboli, which may result in hemiplegia or alteration in mental status. Right-sided endocarditis may result in pulmonary emboli, causing pleuritic pain with hemoptysis.

TABLE 111-2 Clinical Presentation of Infective Endocarditis

General
The clinical presentation of infective endocarditis is highly variable and nonspecific
Symptoms
The patient may complain of fever, chills, weakness, dyspnea, night sweats, weight loss, and/or malaise
Signs
Fever is common, as is a heart murmur (sometimes new or changing). The patient may have embolic phenomenon, splenomegaly, or skin manifestations (eg, Osler's nodes, Janeway's lesions)
Laboratory tests
The patient's white blood cell count may be normal or only slightly elevated
Nonspecific findings include anemia (normocytic, normochromic), thrombocytopenia, an elevated erythrocyte sedimentation rate or C-reactive protein, and altered urinary analysis (proteinuria/microscopic hematuria)
The hallmark laboratory finding is continuous bacteremia; three sets of blood cultures should be collected over 24 hours
Other diagnostic tests
An electrocardiogram, chest radiograph, and echocardiogram are commonly performed. Echocardiography to determine the presence of valvular vegetations plays a key role in the diagnosis of infective endocarditis; it should be performed in all suspected cases

Patients with infective endocarditis typically have laboratory abnormalities; however, none of these changes is specific for the disease. Anemia (normocytic, normochromic), leukocytosis, and thrombocytopenia may be present. The white blood cell count is often normal or only slightly elevated, sometimes with a mild left shift. Acute bacterial endocarditis, however, may present with an elevated white blood cell count, consistent with a fulminant infection. The erythrocyte sedimentation rate (ESR) and C-reactive protein (CRP) may be elevated in approximately 60% of patients. Often the urinary analysis is abnormal, with proteinuria and microscopic hematuria occurring in approximately 25% of individuals.[11,19]

The hallmark of infective endocarditis is a continuous bacteremia caused by bacteria shedding from the vegetation into the bloodstream; 90% to 95% of patients with infective endocarditis have positive blood cultures.[1,11,17] In most cases, three sets of blood cultures, each from separate venipuncture sites, should be collected promptly, with the first and last set drawn at least 1 hour apart. This allows expedient initiation of empiric antibiotic therapy and can help guide early decisions regarding other potential interventions. "Culture-negative" endocarditis describes a patient in whom a clinical diagnosis of infective endocarditis is likely but blood cultures do not yield a pathogen. This condition is often the consequence of previous antibiotic therapy, improperly collected blood cultures, or unusual organisms.[4] When blood cultures from patients suspected of having infective endocarditis show no growth after 48 to 72 hours, cultures should be held for up to a month to detect growth of fastidious organisms.[4]

An electrocardiogram, chest radiograph, and echocardiogram are performed for patients suspected of endocarditis. The electrocardiogram rarely shows important diagnostic findings but may reveal heart block, suggesting extension of the infection. The chest radiograph may provide more diagnostic information, especially in a patient with right-sided endocarditis. Septic pulmonary emboli may occur, leading to multiple lung foci. The echocardiogram is the most important test and should be performed for all patients suspected of this infection.

Echocardiography plays an important role in the diagnosis and management of infective endocarditis.[4,5] The chosen approach, transthoracic echocardiography (TTE) or transesophageal echocardiography (TEE), depends on the clinical setting. The TEE technique is more sensitive for detecting vegetations (85%-90%) as compared with TTE (58%-75%), and TEE maintains good specificity (>90%).[1,5] In addition to helping in the diagnosis of infective endocarditis, the echocardiogram allows the physician to evaluate hemodynamic stability and the need for urgent surgical intervention; it also provides a rough estimate of the likelihood of embolism.[4,20] An initial TTE will be performed in most patients due to the rapidity (ie, fasting state unnecessary) and accessibility (ie, 24-hour service available in most institutions) of testing. This may be the only evaluation needed for children or adults in whom the clinical suspicion of infective endocarditis is relatively low.[4,21] An initial or follow-up TEE is recommended in high-risk patients such as those with many CHDs, previous endocarditis, new murmur, heart failure, or other stigmata of endocarditis.[4,20,22] For those patients with suspected PVE or CDIE, TEE should be considered mandatory. The lack of vegetation on echocardiogram does not exclude infection even if the transesophageal approach is used. In these cases, there is an evolving role for advanced imaging modalities such as 3D TEE, ^{18}F-fluorodeoxyglucose positron emission tomography, single-photon emission computed tomography, and multidetector computed tomography.[4,5,20]

DIAGNOSIS

4 The signs and symptoms of infective endocarditis are not specific, and the diagnosis is often unclear. The identification of infective endocarditis requires the integration of clinical, laboratory, and echocardiographic findings. The Duke diagnostic criteria include major and minor variables (Table 111-3).[23,24] Based on the number of major and minor criteria that are fulfilled, patients suspected of infective endocarditis are categorized into three separate groups: definite infective endocarditis, possible infective endocarditis, or infective endocarditis rejected.[24]

TABLE 111-3 Diagnosis of Infective Endocarditis According to the Modified Duke Criteria

Major Criteria
Blood culture positive for infective endocarditis
Typical microorganisms consistent with infective endocarditis from two separate blood cultures:
Viridans streptococci, *S. gallolyticus*, HACEK group, *S. aureus*; or
Community-acquired enterococci, in the absence of a primary focus; or
Microorganisms consistent with infective endocarditis from persistently positive blood cultures, defined as follows:
At least two positive cultures of blood samples drawn greater than 12 hours apart; or
All of three or a majority of four or more separate cultures of blood (with first and last sample drawn at least 1 hour apart)
Single positive blood culture for *Coxiella burnetii* or antiphase I immunoglobulin G antibody titer >1:800
Evidence of endocardial involvement
Echocardiogram positive for infective endocarditis (transesophageal echocardiography recommended for patients with prosthetic valves, rated at least "possible infective endocarditis" by clinical criteria, or complicated infective endocarditis [paravalvular abscess]; transthoracic echocardiography as first test for other patients), defined as follows:
Oscillating intracardiac mass on valve or supporting structures, in the path of regurgitant jets or on implanted material in the absence of an alternative anatomic explanation; or abscess; or
New partial dehiscence of prosthetic valve
New valvular regurgitation (worsening or changing of preexisting murmur not sufficient)
Minor Criteria
Predisposition, predisposing heart condition, or injection drug use
Fever, temperature >38°C (100.4°F)
Vascular phenomena, major arterial emboli, septic pulmonary infarcts, mycotic aneurysm, intracranial hemorrhage, conjunctival hemorrhages, and Janeway's lesions
Immunologic phenomena: glomerulonephritis, Osler's nodes, Roth's spots, and rheumatoid factor
Microbiologic evidence: positive blood culture but does not meet a major criterion as noted above or serologic evidence of active infection with organism consistent with infective endocarditis
Echocardiographic minor criteria eliminated

HACEK, *Haemophilus* species (*H. parainfluenzae, H. aphrophilus, H. paraphrophilus*), *Aggregatibacter* species, *Cardiobacterium hominis*, *Eikenella corrodens*, and *Kingella kingae*.

Note: Cases are defined clinically as *definite* if they fulfill two major criteria, one major criterion plus three minor criteria, or five minor criteria; cases are defined as *possible* if they fulfill one major and one minor criterion or three minor criteria. Cases are rejected if there is a firm alternate diagnosis explaining evidence of infective endocarditis; resolution of infective endocarditis syndrome with antibiotic therapy for <4 days; no pathologic evidence of infective endocarditis at surgery or autopsy, with antibiotic therapy for <4 days; or criteria for possible infective endocarditis are not met, as above.

Data from references 23 and 24.

The outcome for endocarditis is improved with rapid diagnosis, appropriate treatment (ie, antimicrobial therapy, surgery, or both), and prompt recognition of complications should they arise. Factors associated with increased mortality include: (a) heart failure, (b) increasing age, (c) endocarditis caused by resistant organisms, such as fungi or gram-negative bacteria, (d) left-sided endocarditis caused by *S. aureus*, (e) paravalvular complications, (f) healthcare-acquired infection, and (g) PVE.[4,5,11,16] The presence of heart failure has the greatest negative impact on the short-term prognosis.[4] For left-sided native valve infective endocarditis, mortality rates range from 15% to 45%; lower rates (4%-16%) occur with community-acquired disease that is most commonly caused by viridans streptococci. Higher rates (25%-45%) occur with healthcare-associated disease that is more commonly caused by enterococci and staphylococci.[25] Even higher rates of mortality are seen with unusually encountered organisms (eg, mortality > 80% for fungi).[4,5] The mortality rate for right-sided infective endocarditis associated with IVDA is generally low (eg, <10%).[4,25] For those who relapse after treatment for infective endocarditis, most will do so within the first 2 months after discontinuation of antimicrobials. Relapse rates for viridans streptococcus are generally low (2%), whereas relapse is more likely in those with enterococcal infection (8%-20%) and PVE (10%-15%).[17] After appropriate treatment and recovery, the risk of morbidity and mortality following infective endocarditis persists for years, although it gradually declines annually. Morbidity remains elevated because of a greater likelihood of recurrent infective endocarditis, heart failure, and embolism or, if a valve is replaced, the risk of anticoagulation, valve thrombosis, or additional valve surgery.[22]

TREATMENT

Desired Outcomes

The desired outcomes for treatment and prophylaxis of infective endocarditis are to:

1. Relieve the signs and symptoms of the disease
2. Decrease morbidity and mortality associated with the infection
3. Eradicate the causative organism with minimal drug exposure
4. Provide cost-effective antimicrobial therapy determined by the likely or identified pathogen, drug susceptibilities, hepatic and renal function, drug allergies, and anticipated drug toxicities
5. Prevent infective endocarditis from occurring or recurring in high-risk patients with appropriate prophylactic antimicrobials

General Approach to Treatment

Specific treatment recommendations from the American Heart Association (AHA) provide guidance for the management of infective endocarditis, and these were last updated in 2015.[4] Guidelines published by the European Society of Cardiology (ESC) remain consistent, for the most part, with the AHA guidelines.[5] Both now provide important recommendations for the combination of early diagnosis, early antibiotic therapy, and early surgery; but there are some subtle differences. For the first time, the ESC guidelines recommend that an "endocarditis team" is crucial for the management of infective endocarditis. The team should include cardiologists, cardiac surgeons, and specialists in infectious disease. The AHA guidelines place more emphasis on a team-based approach when assessing the timing and need for surgical intervention. The ESC guidelines also provide recommendations for specific situations, including infective endocarditis in the intensive care unit, in patients with cancer, and in patients with nonbacterial endocarditis.[5]

The AHA and ESC guidelines use an evidence-based scoring system where recommendations are given a classification as well as level of evidence. Class I recommendations are conditions for which there is evidence, general agreement, or both that a given procedure or treatment is useful and effective. Class II recommendations are conditions for which there is conflicting evidence, a divergence of opinion, or both about the usefulness/efficacy of a procedure or treatment (IIa implies that the weight of evidence/opinion is in favor of usefulness/efficacy, whereas IIb implies that usefulness/efficacy is less well established by evidence/opinion). Class III recommendations are conditions for which there is evidence, general agreement, or both that the procedure/treatment is not useful/effective and in some cases may be harmful. Level of evidence is listed as A (data derived from multiple randomized clinical trials), B (data derived from a single randomized trial or nonrandomized studies), and C (consensus opinion of experts).

5 The most important approach in the treatment of infective endocarditis is isolation of the infecting pathogen and determination of antimicrobial susceptibilities, followed by high-dose, parenteral, and bactericidal antibiotics for an extended period.[1,4,5,6,19] Identification of susceptibilities is crucial given the escalating level of antibiotic resistance to commonly encountered pathogens. Treatment usually is started in the hospital, but for select patients it is often completed in the outpatient setting so long as defervescence has occurred and follow-up blood cultures show no growth.[26] Large doses of parenteral antimicrobials usually are necessary to achieve bactericidal concentrations within vegetations. An extended duration of therapy is required, even for susceptible pathogens, because microorganisms are enclosed within valvular vegetations and fibrin deposits. These barriers impair host defenses and protect microbes from phagocytic cells. In addition, high bacterial concentrations within vegetations may result in an inoculum effect that further resists killing (see Chapter 24 for additional discussion). Many bacteria are not actively dividing, further limiting the rate of bacterial death. For most patients, a minimum of 4 to 6 weeks of therapy is required.[4,5]

Nonpharmacologic Therapy

6 Surgery is an important adjunct in the management of both NVE and PVE and is now performed in up to 50% of patients.[27] In most surgical cases, valvectomy and valve replacement are performed to remove infected tissue and to restore hemodynamic function. Indications for surgery include heart failure, persistent bacteremia, persistent vegetation, an increase in vegetation size, or recurrent emboli despite prolonged antibiotic treatment, valve dysfunction, paravalvular extension (eg, abscess), or endocarditis caused by resistant organisms (eg, fungi or gram-negative bacteria).[4-6] More controversial is the appropriate timing of surgery as well as duration of antibiotic therapy post-surgery. Additionally, studies evaluating postsurgical outcomes and associated mortality are limited such that a specific risk prediction system has not been established.[28-32] Early surgery (eg, within 48 hours) may be appropriate in patients with severe heart failure and large vegetations, whereas patients with septic shock, advanced age, or neurologic complications of infective endocarditis may have more detrimental outcomes.[28,29,33,34] The multiple factors that need to be considered in evaluating the need for and timing of surgery is why a multidisciplinary management approach (ie, "endocarditis team") is critical.[4,5,19]

Clinical **Controversy...**

The role of surgery in the management of infective endocarditis is increasing; however, the duration of antibiotic therapy post-surgery is unclear and can depend on whether prosthetic material was inserted and if resected tissue is culture positive or culture negative.

Pharmacologic Therapy

7 β-Lactam antibiotics, such as penicillin G (or ceftriaxone), nafcillin, and ampicillin, remain the drugs of choice for streptococcal, staphylococcal, and enterococcal endocarditis, respectively. Tables 111-4 to 111-7 summarize these recommendations, which are discussed in more detail in the following sections. Tables 111-8 and 111-9 list drug dosing and monitoring recommendations for adult and pediatric patients. Because these guidelines focus on common causes of endocarditis, readers are referred to other references for more in-depth discussion of unusually encountered organisms.[4,5,35-38]

8 For some pathogens, such as enterococci, the use of synergistic antimicrobial combinations (including an aminoglycoside) is essential to obtain a bactericidal effect. Combination antibiotics also may decrease the emergence of resistant organisms during treatment (eg, PVE caused by coagulase-negative staphylococci) and hasten the pace of clinical and microbiologic response (eg, some streptococcal and staphylococcal infections). Occasionally, combination treatment will result in a shorter treatment course.

Streptococcal Endocarditis

Streptococci are a common cause of infective endocarditis, with most isolates being viridans group streptococci. Viridans group streptococci refers to a large number of different species, such as *Streptococcus sanguinis, Streptococcus oralis, Streptococcus salivarius, Streptococcus mutans*, and *Gemella morbillorum*.[4] These bacteria are common inhabitants of the human mouth and gingiva, and they are especially common causes of endocarditis involving native valves.[4,16,25] During dental surgery, and even when brushing the teeth, these organisms can cause a transient bacteremia. In susceptible individuals, this may result in infective endocarditis. Streptococcal endocarditis is usually subacute, and the response to medical treatment is very good. *Streptococcus gallolyticus* (formerly known as *Streptococcus bovis*) is not a viridans group streptococcus, but it is included in this treatment group because it is penicillin sensitive and requires the same treatment. *S. gallolyticus* is a nonenterococcal group D *Streptococcus* that resides in the GI tract. Infective endocarditis caused by this organism is often associated with a GI pathology, especially colon carcinoma. Endocarditis caused by *Streptococcus pneumoniae, Streptococcus pyogenes*, and group B, C, and G streptococci are uncommon, and their treatment is not well defined.[4,5]

Antimicrobial regimens for viridans group streptococci are well studied, and in uncomplicated cases, the cure rate is expected to be more than 95%.[4,5] Viridans group streptococci are penicillin susceptible, although some are more susceptible than others. Most are highly sensitive to penicillin G and have minimal inhibitory concentrations (MICs) of less than 0.12 mcg/mL (mg/L).[4] Approximately 10% to 20% are moderately susceptible (MIC 0.12-0.5 mcg/mL [mg/L]). This different in vitro susceptibility led to recommendations that the MIC be determined for all viridans streptococci and that the results be used to guide therapy. Some streptococci are deemed tolerant to the killing effects of penicillin, where the minimal bactericidal concentration (MBC) exceeds the MIC by 32 times. A tolerant organism is inhibited but not killed by an antibiotic normally considered bactericidal.[4] Bactericidal activity is required for successful treatment of infective endocarditis; therefore, infections with a tolerant organism may relapse after treatment. Despite some animal studies of endocarditis suggesting that tolerant strains do not respond as readily to β-lactam therapy as nontolerant ones, this phenomenon is primarily a laboratory finding with little clinical significance.[4] Treatment for tolerant strains is identical to that for nontolerant organisms, and measurement of the MBC is not recommended.[4]

An assortment of regimens can be used to treat uncomplicated NVE caused by fully susceptible viridans group streptococci (see Table 111-4). Two single-drug regimens consist of high-dose

TABLE 111-4 Treatment Options for Native Valve Endocarditis by Causative Organism

Agent[a]	Duration	Strength of Recommendation	Comments
Highly Penicillin-Susceptible (MIC ≤ 0.12 mcg/mL [mg/L]) Viridans Group Streptococci and *S. Gallolyticus*			
Aqueous crystalline penicillin G sodium[b]	4 weeks	IIaB	2-week regimens are not intended for the following patients:
Ceftriaxone	4 weeks	IIaB	• Most patients >65 years of age • Children
Aqueous crystalline penicillin G sodium[b] plus gentamicin	2 weeks	IIaB	• Impairment of the eighth cranial nerve function • Renal function with a creatinine clearance <20 mL/min (<0.33 mL/s)
Ceftriaxone plus gentamicin	2 weeks	IIaB	• Known cardiac or extracardiac abscess • Infection with *Abiotrophia, Granulicatella*, or *Gemalla* species
Vancomycin	4 weeks	IIaB	Recommended only for patients unable to tolerate penicillin or ceftriaxone
Viridans Group Streptococci and *S. Gallolyticus* Relatively Resistant to Penicillin (MIC >0.12 to ≤0.5 mcg/mL [mg/L])			
Aqueous crystalline penicillin G sodium[b] plus gentamicin	4 weeks 2 weeks	IIaB	
Ceftriaxone plus gentamicin	4 weeks 2 weeks	IIbC	
Vancomycin	4 weeks	IIaB	Recommended only for patients unable to tolerate penicillin or ceftriaxone
Oxacillin-Susceptible Staphylococci[c]			
Nafcillin or oxacillin	6 weeks	1C	
Cefazolin	6 weeks	1B	For use in patients with nonanaphylactoid-type penicillin allergies; patients with an unclear history of immediate-type hypersensitivity to penicillin should be considered for skin testing
Vancomycin	6 weeks	1B	For use in patients with anaphylactoid-type hypersensitivity to penicillin and/or cephalosporins
Daptomycin	6 weeks	IIaB	For use in patients with immediate-type hypersensitivity reactions to penicillin
Oxacillin-Resistant Staphylococci			
Vancomycin	6 weeks	1C	
Daptomycin	6 weeks	IIbB	

Please refer to Table 111-6 for treatment of NVE caused by enterococci.

[a]See Tables 111-8 and 111-9 for appropriate dosing, administration, and monitoring information.

[b]May use ampicillin in the event of a penicillin shortage.

[c]Regimens indicate treatment for left-sided endocarditis or complicated right-sided endocarditis; uncomplicated right-sided endocarditis may be treated for shorter durations and is described in the text.

Data from references 4 and 20.

parenteral penicillin G or ceftriaxone for 4 weeks. If short term, 2 week therapy is desired, the guidelines suggest either high-dose parenteral penicillin G or ceftriaxone in combination with an aminoglycoside.[4] When used in select patients, this combination is as effective as 4 weeks of penicillin alone. Although streptomycin was listed in previous guidelines, gentamicin is the preferred aminoglycoside because serum drug concentrations are obtained easily, clinicians are more familiar with its use, and the few strains of streptococci resistant to the effects of streptomycin-penicillin remain susceptible to gentamicin–penicillin. Other aminoglycosides are not recommended.

The decision of which regimen to use depends on the perceived risk versus benefit. For example, a 2-week course of gentamicin in an elderly patient with renal impairment may be associated with ototoxicity, worsening renal function, or both. Furthermore, the 2-week regimen is not recommended for patients with known extracardiac infection. On the other hand, a 4-week course of penicillin alone generally entails greater expense, especially if the patient remains in the hospital. Monotherapy with once-daily ceftriaxone offers ease of administration, facilitates home healthcare treatment, and may be cost-effective.[4,5,25]

The British Society for Antimicrobial Chemotherapy guidelines suggest that all of the following conditions be present to consider a 2-week treatment regimen for penicillin-sensitive streptococcal endocarditis:[35]

1. Penicillin-sensitive viridans streptococcus or *S. gallolyticus* (penicillin MIC <0.1 mcg/mL [mg/L])
2. No cardiovascular risk factors such as heart failure, aortic insufficiency, or conduction abnormalities
3. No evidence of thromboembolic disease
4. Native valve infection
5. No vegetation of greater than 5 mm diameter on echocardiogram
6. Low risk of nephrotoxicity
7. Not at risk for *Clostridium difficile*
8. Clinical response within 7 days (the temperature should return to normal, the patient should feel well, and the patient's appetite should return to normal)

9 When a patient has a history of an immediate-type hypersensitivity to penicillin, vancomycin should be chosen for infective endocarditis caused by viridans streptococci. When vancomycin is used, the addition of gentamicin is not recommended.[4] Most patients who report a penicillin allergy have a negative penicillin skin test and consequently are at low risk of anaphylaxis.[39] The published experience with penicillin is more extensive than with alternative regimens; consequently, a thorough allergy history must be obtained before a second-line therapy is administered.

For patients with complicated infections (eg, extracardiac foci) or when the streptococcus has an MIC of 0.12 to less than or equal to 0.5 mcg/mL (mg/L), combination therapy with an aminoglycoside for the first 2 weeks and penicillin (higher dose) or ceftriaxone is recommended, followed by penicillin or ceftriaxone alone for an

TABLE 111-5 Treatment Options for Prosthetic Valve Endocarditis (PVE) by Causative Organism

Agent[a]	Duration	Strength of Recommendation	Comments
Highly Penicillin-Susceptible (MIC ≤ 0.12 mcg/mL [mg/L]) Viridans Group Streptococci and *S. Galloyticus*			
Aqueous crystalline penicillin G sodium[b] with or without gentamicin	6 weeks 2 weeks	IIaB	Combination therapy with gentamicin has not demonstrated superior cure rates compared with monotherapy with a penicillin or cephalosporin and should be avoided in patients with CrCl <30 mL/min (<0.50 mL/s)
Ceftriaxone with or without gentamicin	6 weeks 2 weeks	IIaB	
Vancomycin	6 weeks	IIaB	Recommended only for patients unable to tolerate penicillin or ceftriaxone
Relatively Resistant or Fully Resistant (MIC > 0.12 mcg/mL [mg/L]) Viridans Group Streptococci and *S. Gallolyticus*			
Aqueous crystalline penicillin G sodium[b] plus gentamicin	6 weeks	IIaB	
Ceftriaxone plus gentamicin	6 weeks	IIaB	
Vancomycin[c]	6 weeks	IIaB	Recommended only for patients unable to tolerate penicillin or ceftriaxone
Oxacillin-Susceptible Staphylococci			
Nafcillin or oxacillin plus rifampin plus gentamicin	≥6 weeks ≥6 weeks 2 weeks	1B	Cefazolin may be substituted for nafcillin or oxacillin in patients with non-immediate-type hypersensitivity
Vancomycin plus rifampin plus gentamicin	≥6 weeks ≥6 weeks 2 weeks	1B	Recommended only for patients with anaphylactoid-type hypersensitivity to penicillin and/or cephalosporins
Oxacillin-Resistant Staphylococci			
Vancomycin plus rifampin plus gentamicin	≥6 weeks ≥6 weeks 2 weeks	1B	

Please refer to Table 111-6 for treatment of PVE caused by enterococci.

[a]See Tables 111-8 and 111-9 for appropriate dosing, administration, and monitoring information.

[b]May use ampicillin in the event of a penicillin shortage.

[c]The ESC 2015 guidelines recommend gentamicin (3 mg/kg/day) be administered with vancomycin for the initial 2 weeks of therapy in patients with relatively resistant strains to penicillin.

Data from references 4, 5, and 20.

TABLE 111-6 Treatment Options for Native or Prosthetic Valve Endocarditis Caused by Enterococci

Agent[a]	Duration[b]	Strength of Recommendation	Comments
Ampicillin-, Penicillin-, and Vancomycin-Susceptible Strains			
Ampicillin plus gentamicin	4-6 weeks	IIaB	Native valve plus symptoms present for <3 months: use 4-week regimen
Aqueous crystalline penicillin G sodium plus gentamicin	4-6 weeks	IIAB	Prosthetic valve or native valve plus symptoms present for >3 months: use 6-week regimen
Ampicillin plus ceftriaxone	6 weeks	IIaB	Recommended regimen if creatinine clearance is <50 mL/min (<0.83 mL/s; at baseline or due to therapy with a gentamicin-containing regimen)
Vancomycin plus gentamicin	6 weeks	IIaB	Recommended only for patients unable to tolerate penicillin or ampicillin
Gentamicin-Resistant Strains			
If susceptible, use streptomycin in place of gentamicin in the regimens listed above as long as creatinine clearance is >50 mL/min (>0.83 mL/s), cranial nerve VIII function is intact and there is laboratory capability for rapid streptomycin serum concentrations.			
Penicillin-Resistant Strains			
Ampicillin–sulbactam plus gentamicin (β-lactamase–producing strain)	6 weeks	IIbC	
Vancomycin plus gentamicin (intrinsic penicillin resistance[c])	6 weeks	IIbC	May also use in patients with β-lactamase–producing strains who have known intolerance to ampicillin–sulbactam
***Enterococcus Faecium* Strains Resistant to Penicillin, Aminoglycosides, and Vancomycin[d]**			
Linezolid	>6 weeks	IIbC	Antimicrobial cure rates may be <50%; bacteriologic cure may only be achieved with cardiac valve replacement
Daptomycin	>6 weeks	IIbC	

[a]See Tables 111-8 and 111-9 for appropriate dosing, administration, and monitoring information.

[b]All patients with prosthetic valves should be treated for at least 6 weeks.

[c]Infectious disease consult highly recommended.

[d]Patients should be managed by a multidisciplinary team that includes specialists in cardiology, cardiovascular surgery, infectious diseases, and clinical pharmacy.

Data from reference 4.

TABLE 111-7 Treatment Options for Culture-Negative Endocarditis and Endocarditis Caused by Gram-Negative Organisms[a]

Agent[b]	Duration[c]	Strength of Recommendation	Comments
HACEK[d] Microorganisms			
Ceftriaxone	4 weeks	IIaB	Other third- or fourth-generation cephalosporins may be used as an alternative
Ampicillin or Ampicillin–sulbactam	4 weeks	IIaB	Should only use if growth is adequate for in vitro susceptibility testing; otherwise, consider organism to be resistant
Ciprofloxacin	4 weeks	IIbC	Recommended for patients with known intolerance to cephalosporins or ampicillin; other fluoroquinolones may be used as an alternative
Culture-Negative Endocarditis, Native Valve[e]			
Vancomcyin plus cefepime	4-6 weeks	IIaC	Recommended when onset is acute (days); *S. aureus*, β-hemolytic streptococci, and aerobic gram-negative bacilli should be covered
Vancomycin plus ampicillin-sulbactam	4-6 weeks	IIaC	Recommended when onset is subacute (weeks); *S. aureus*, viridans group streptococci, HACEK, and enterococci should be covered
Culture-Negative Endocarditis, Early (<1 Year) Prosthetic Valve[e]			
Vancomycin plus cefepime plus rifampin plus gentamicin	6 weeks	IIaC	Staphylococci, enterococci, and aerobic gram-negative bacilli should be covered
Culture-Negative Endocarditis, Late (>1 Year) Prosthetic Valve[e]			
Vancomycin plus ceftriaxone	6 weeks	IIaC	Staphylococci, viridans group streptococci, and enterococci should be covered
Suspected *Bartonella*, Culture-Negative			
Ceftriaxone plus gentamicin with or without doxycycline	6 weeks 2 weeks 6 weeks	IIaB	
Culture-Positive *Bartonella*			
Doxycycline plus gentamicin	6 weeks 2 weeks	IIaB	Rifampin is recommended as an alternative in patient who cannot be given gentamicin

[a]Infectious disease consult highly recommended.

[b]See Tables 111-8 and 111-9 for appropriate dosing, administration, and monitoring.

[c]All patients with prosthetic valves should be treated for 6 weeks.

[d]*Haemophilus species (H. parainfluenzae, H. aphrophilus, and H. paraphrophilus), Aggregatibacter* species, *Cardiobacterium hominis, Eikenella corrodens*, and *Kingella kingae*.

[e]Duration of therapy for culture-negative endocarditis may be variable and should be based on clinical course and recommendations from infectious diseases consult.

Haemophilus parainfluenzae, *Haemophilus aphrophilus, Actinobacillus actinomycetemcomitans, Cardiobacterium hominis, Eikenella corrodens*, and *Kingella kingae*.

Data from references 4 and 5.

additional 2 weeks (see Table 111-4).[4] Some viridans streptococci, previously referred to as nutritionally variant streptococci, have biologic characteristics that complicate diagnosis and treatment. *Abiotrophia defectiva* and *Granulicatella* species have nutritional deficiencies that hinder growth in routine culture media.[4] These organisms require special broth supplemented with pyridoxal hydrochloride or cysteine. For patients infected with nutritionally variant streptococci or when the *Streptococcus* has an MIC of more than 0.5 mcg/mL (mg/L), treatment should follow the enterococcal endocarditis treatment guidelines.[4]

The rationale for combination therapy of penicillin-susceptible viridans streptococci is that enhanced activity against these organisms usually is observed when cell-wall–active agents are combined with aminoglycosides in vitro.[40] Combined treatment results in quicker sterilization of vegetations in animal models of endocarditis and probably explains the high response rates observed for patients treated for a total of 2 weeks.[4,41] The combined treatment, however, is not superior to penicillin alone. Some authors question the need for combination therapy in relatively resistant streptococci, emphasizing that few human data suggest that patients with endocarditis caused by these organisms respond less well to penicillin alone.[40,42]

For patients with endocarditis of prosthetic valves or other prosthetic material caused by viridans group streptococci and *S. gallolyticus*, choices of treatment are similar to those without prosthetic material (eg, penicillin or ceftriaxone); however, treatment courses are extended to 6 weeks (see Table 111-5) for both the β-Lactam and the aminoglycoside. Whether extended-interval aminoglycoside dosing has a role in infective endocarditis continues to be debated. At this time, data support extended-interval dosing for the treatment of streptococcal infective endocarditis, and as compared with three-times-daily dosing this approach may have greater efficacy.[43,44] One study specifically evaluated the combination of ceftriaxone (2 g daily) with gentamicin (3 mg/kg daily) for 2 weeks compared with ceftriaxone (2 g daily) alone for 4 weeks for penicillin-sensitive streptococci. Both regimens were safe and effective with similar clinical cure rates at 3 months following treatment.[41]

Staphylococcal Endocarditis

Endocarditis caused by staphylococci has become more prevalent, mainly because of increased IVDA, more frequent use of peripheral and central venous catheters, and increased frequency of valve replacement surgery.[45,46] *S. aureus* is the most common organism causing infective endocarditis among those with IVDA and persons with venous catheters. Coagulase-negative staphylococci (usually *Staphylococcus epidermidis*) and *S. aureus* are prominent causes of PVE.

Staphylococcal endocarditis is not a homogeneous disease; appropriate management requires consideration of several questions: Is the organism methicillin resistant? Should combination therapy be used? Is the infection on a native or prosthetic valve? Does the patient have a history of IVDA? Is the infection on the left or right side of the heart? Another consideration in staphylococcal endocarditis is that some organisms may exhibit tolerance to antibiotics.

TABLE 111-8 Drug Dosing Table for Treatment of Infective Endocarditis[a]

Drug	Brand Name	Recommended Dose	Pediatric (Ped) Dose[b]	Additional Information
Ampicillin	NA	2 g IV every 4 hours	50 mg/kg every 4 hours or 75 mg/kg every 6 hours	24-hour total dose may be administered as a continuous infusion: 12 g IV every 24 hours
Ampicillin–sulbactam	Unasyn®	2 g IV every 4 hours	50 mg/kg every 4 hours or 75 mg/kg every 6 hours	
Aqueous crystalline penicillin G sodium	NA			24-hour total dose may be administered as a continuous infusion: 12-18 million units IV every 24 hours (Ped: 200,000 units/kg IV/24 hours)
• MIC <0.12 mcg/mL (mg/L) (native valve only)		3 million units IV every 4 hours or every 6 hours	50,000 units/kg IV every 6 hours	
• All other indications		4 million units IV every 4 hours or 6 million units IV every 6 hours	50,000 units/kg IV every 4 hours or 75,000 units/kg IV every 6 hours	24 million units IV every 24 hours (Ped: 300,000 units/kg IV every 24 hours)
Cefazolin	Ancef®	2 g IV every 8 hours	33 mg/kg IV every 8 hours	
Cefepime	Maxipime®	2 g IV every 8 hours	50 mg/kg IV every 8 hours	
Ceftriaxone sodium	Rocephin®	2 g IV or IM every 24 hours 2 g IV or IM every 12 hours (*E. faecalis only*)	100 mg/kg IV or IM every 24 hours	
Ciprofloxacin	Cipro®	400 mg IV every 12 hours or 500 mg po every 12 hours	20-30 mg/kg IV or po every 12 hours	Avoid use if possible in patients <18 years of age
Daptomycin	Cubicin®	≥8 mg/kg IV every 24 hours	6 mg/kg IV every 24 hours	Doses as high as 10-12 mg/kg IV every 24 hours have been used in adults with enterococcus resistant to penicillin, aminoglycosides and vancomycin; doses should be calculated using actual body weight
Doxycline	Vibramycin®	100 mg IV or po every 12 hours	1-2 mg/kg IV or po every 12 hours	
Gentamicin sulfate	NA	3 mg/kg IV or IM every 24 hours or 1 mg/kg IV or IM every 8 hours[c]	1 mg/kg IV or IM every 8 hours	Once-daily dosing is only recommended for treatment of streptococcal infections.
Linezolid	Zyvox®	600 mg IV or po every 12 hours	10 mg/kg IV every 8 hours	
Nafcillin or oxacillin	NA	2 g IV every 4 hours	50 mg/kg IV every 6 hours	
Rifampin	Rifadin®	300 mg IV or po every 8 hours	5-7 mg/kg IV or po every 8 hours	
Streptomycin	NA	7.5 mg/kg IV or IM every 12 hours		
Vancomycin	Vancocin®	15-20 mg/kg IV every 8 hours or every 12 hours	15 mg/kg IV every 6 hours	A loading dose of 25-30 mg/kg may be administered in adults; doses should be calculated using actual body weight; single doses should not exceed 2 g

[a]All doses assume normal renal function.

[b]Should not exceed adult dosage.

[c]Actual body weight should be used when the full aminoglycoside dose is administered once daily; when administered in three divided doses, use ideal body weight or adjusted body weight when actual body weight is >120% ideal body weight.

TABLE 111-9 Drug Monitoring of Select Agents

Drug	Major Adverse Drug Reactions	Monitoring Parameters	Comments
Daptomycin	Myopathy, rhabdomyolysis	Creatinine phosphokinase (CPK) at least weekly; monitor for signs and symptoms of muscle pain	More frequent monitoring may be warranted in patients with renal dysfunction or receiving concomitant therapy with HMG-CoA reductase inhibitors; discontinue if symptomatic and CPK >5 times the upper limit of normal (ULN) or if CPK ≥10 times ULN
Gentamicin	Nephrotoxicity, ototoxicity, neuromuscular blockade	When dosed three times daily: • Target peak serum concentrations of 3-4 mcg/mL (mg/L; 6.3-8.4 μmol/L) and trough serum concentrations of <1 mcg/mL (mg/L; <2.1 μmol/L)	Avoid concomitant use of other nephrotoxic agents such as diuretics, nonsteroidal antiinflammatory drugs, and radiocontrast media. Avoid rapid IV administration
Linezolid	Thrombocytopenia, optic, or peripheral neuropathy	Platelet counts at baseline and weekly, visual changes	More common with prolonged therapy (≥2 weeks for thrombocytopenia, >28 days for visual symptoms); avoid concomitant myelosuppressive agents
Rifampin	Hepatotoxicity	Baseline liver function tests, and then at least every 2-4 weeks during therapy	Avoid concomitant medications that cause hepatotoxicity; may cause red or orange discoloration of bodily secretions (urine, sweat, tears)
Vancomycin	Nephrotoxicity, red man syndrome	Target trough concentrations of 15-20 mcg/mL[a] (mg/L; 10-14 μmol/L)	Red man syndrome may be managed by prolonging the infusion time from 1 to 2 hours; administration of an antihistamine prior to loading or maintenance doses may also be considered

[a]Measuring peak serum vancomycin concentrations is no longer recommended.

Similar to streptococci, however, the concern for tolerance among staphylococci should not affect antibiotic selection.[4]

Any patient who develops staphylococcal bacteremia is at risk for endocarditis. Many investigators have attempted to develop criteria that identify the bacteremic patient likely to have infective endocarditis.[45] In the past, patients were considered to be at high risk for infective endocarditis if *S. aureus* bacteremia was community acquired versus hospital acquired; however, nosocomial *S. aureus* bacteremia is now considered as a major criterion for development of infective endocarditis.[23,24] The prevalence of infective endocarditis in patients with *S. aureus* bacteremia is approximately 25%, leading some authors to suggest that screening echocardiography be performed in all patients.[47] In hospitalized patients with *S. aureus* bacteremia and an identified focus of infection, such as a vascular catheter, the risk of concomitant infective endocarditis is low, and treatment of the bacteremia can be reduced to 2 weeks. This approach applies only if the patient does not have a prosthetic valve or additional clinical evidence for endocarditis.[48] Additionally, the following parameters predict higher risk of infective endocarditis for patients with *S. aureus* bacteremia: (a) the absence of a primary site of infection, (b) metastatic signs of infection, and (c) valvular vegetations detected by echocardiography.[24,47]

The recommended therapy for patients with left-sided, native valve infective endocarditis caused by methicillin-sensitive *S. aureus* (MSSA) is 6 weeks of nafcillin or oxacillin; a longer duration of therapy may be needed for complicated infections (ie, presence of perivalvular abscess or septic metastases). The AHA and ESC guidelines no longer recommend the addition of gentamicin because clinical benefit has not been demonstrated and there is an increase risk of toxicity (see Table 111-4). From in vitro studies, the combination of an aminoglycoside and penicillinase-resistant penicillin or vancomycin enhances the activity of these drugs for MSSA. In animal models of endocarditis, combinations of penicillin with an aminoglycoside eradicate organisms from vegetations more rapidly than penicillins alone.[5,40,49] In most human studies, the addition of an aminoglycoside to nafcillin hastens the resolution of fever and bacteremia, but it does not affect survival or relapse rates and can increase renal toxicity.[40,50,51] One small cohort study has demonstrated a decrease in recurrent bacteremia with combination therapy.[52]

If a patient has a mild, delayed allergy to penicillin, first-generation cephalosporins (such as cefazolin) are effective alternatives, but they should be avoided for patients with a history of immediate-type hypersensitivity reactions to penicillins (see Table 111-4). The potential for a true immediate-type allergy should be assessed carefully. A penicillin skin test should be conducted before giving antibiotic treatment to any patient with infective endocarditis caused by MSSA if there is a questionable penicillin allergy.[53] 9 For a patient with a positive skin test or a history of immediate hypersensitivity to penicillin, vancomycin is an option. Vancomycin, however, kills *S. aureus* slowly and is regarded as inferior to penicillinase-resistant penicillins for MSSA.[4] Alternatively, patients with immediate-type hypersensitivity reactions to penicillin can be considered for penicillin desensitization or daptomycin, a lipopeptide antibiotic approved for right sided infective endocarditis and *S. aureus* bacteremia.[4,5] Unfortunately, left-sided infective endocarditis caused by *S. aureus* continues to have a poor prognosis, with a mortality rate between 25% and 40%.[4] For reasons discussed in the following section, those with infective endocarditis associated with IVDA have a more favorable response to therapy.

During the past decade, staphylococci more commonly have become resistant to penicillinase-resistant penicillins (ie, methicillin-resistant *S. aureus* [MRSA]). 9 Although vancomycin is still the most commonly selected alternative in these cases (see Table 111-4), susceptibility reports with MIC more than 2 mcg/mL (mg/L) and reports of vancomycin-resistant *S. aureus* strains are increasing.[21] Success with daptomycin or linezolid has been demonstrated for these patients.[54-59] Based on available data, daptomycin (at a dose of 6 mg/kg/day) was approved by the FDA in 2006 for the treatment of *S. aureus* bacteremia associated with right-sided NVE and is now a recommended alternative.[21,55] Higher doses of daptomycin (8-10 mg/kg/day) have been used in clinical practice and may be preferred by some experts, although prospective, randomized clinical trials are lacking.[21,60-63] To date, linezolid has not been approved by the FDA for use in endocarditis as most available data are based on case reports, and there is concern regarding use of a bacteriostatic agent for this condition.[21,54] Furthermore, the FDA issued a warning for linezolid in 2007 following reports from one study that patients with catheter-related bacteremia treated with linezolid had an increased incidence of death due to gram-negative bacillary infections.[64] The presence or lack of a prosthetic heart valve in patients with a methicillin-resistant organism guides therapy and determines whether vancomycin should be used alone or, if a prosthetic valve is present, whether combination therapy is necessary (see Table 111-5).[4]

Clinical **Controversy...**

Use of daptomycin in clinical practice may extend beyond the FDA-indication of right-sided NVE. Selection as an alternative to vancomycin in patients with left-sided NVE (MRSA or MSSA) and in those with MSSA NVE and severe allergy to penicillins or cephalosporins may be observed (ie, in the setting of vancomycin failure or resistance). Furthermore, although the data for use of high-dose daptomycin (8-10 mg/kg/day) is limited, the favorable drug tolerability and the potential for decreased treatment-emergent resistance may compel some prescribers to opt for high-dose therapy in complicated cases.

Staphylococcus Endocarditis: IV Drug Abuser

Infective endocarditis in those with IVDA is frequently (60%-70%) caused by *S. aureus*, although other organisms may be common in certain geographic locations.[25] In this setting, the tricuspid valve is frequently infected, resulting in right-sided infective endocarditis. Most patients have no history of valve abnormalities, are usually otherwise healthy, and have a good response to medical treatment. Nonetheless, surgery may be required.

As previously mentioned, an uncomplicated, left-sided MSSA endocarditis may be treated sufficiently with 6 weeks of monotherapy with penicillinase-resistant penicillin.[4] However, the clinical response with right-sided MSSA endocarditis in the IVDA is usually excellent and may be treated effectively (clinical and microbiologic cure exceeding 85%) with a 2-week course of nafcillin, oxacillin or daptomycin.[4] Previous guidelines emphasized combination therapy with an aminoglycoside for the 2-week duration based on earlier studies.[65-67] The current recommendation for monotherapy is based on data showing that a 2-week regimen of a penicillinase-resistant penicillin alone, without the addition of an aminoglycoside, is as effective as combined therapy in MSSA tricuspid valve endocarditis.[68] Additionally, a post-hoc analysis comparing daptomycin monotherapy with combination treatment (daptomycin plus 4 days of gentamicin) showed no difference in success rates but higher rates of renal toxicity.[50] Selection of a 2-week duration of treatment may be appropriate as long as the following criteria are fulfilled:[5]

- Pathogen identified as MSSA
- Good response to treatment
- Absence of metastatic sites of infection or empyema
- Absence of cardiac and extracardiac complications

- Absence of associated prosthetic valve or left sided valve infection
- Vegetation size less than 20 mm
- Absence of severe immunosuppression (<200 CD4 cells/μL [<0.200 × 10^9/L]) with or without acquired immune deficiency syndrome (AIDS)

Short, 2-week, courses of vancomycin in IVDAs are not recommended because of limited bactericidal activity, poor penetration into vegetations, and increased drug clearance in this population. The standard 6-week regimen should therefore be used. While vancomycin and daptomycin are both options for native valve MRSA infective endocarditis in IVDAs, daptomycin would be the drug of choice in cases where the vancomycin MIC is more than 1 mcg/mL (mg/L).[5]

An intriguing therapeutic approach for staphylococcal endocarditis in those with IVDA is oral treatment. One study indicated that short-course IV treatment (primarily nafcillin; mean: 16 days) followed by oral treatment (dicloxacillin or oxacillin; mean: 26 days) might be effective for tricuspid valve MSSA endocarditis.[69] The positive results of this trial can be explained by the relatively long duration of IV antibiotics (>2 weeks). Two other studies that predominantly used oral therapy (ciprofloxacin and rifampin) demonstrated efficacy (cure rates exceeding 90%) in addicts with uncomplicated right-sided endocarditis caused by MSSA.[70,71] At this time, concerns with resistance (eg, ciprofloxacin), patient adherence, and limited published data preclude routine use of oral antibacterial regimens for the treatment of infective endocarditis in IVDAs.[4]

Staphylococcal Endocarditis: Prosthetic Valves

Prosthetic valve endocarditis accounts for 10% to 30% of all infective endocarditis cases.[5,8] Staphylococcal, fungi, and gram-negative bacilli are the main causes of early PVE, while the microbiology of late PVE mirrors that of NVE. An episode of PVE occurring within 2 months of surgery strongly suggests that the cause is staphylococci implanted during the procedure. Yet the risk of staphylococcal endocarditis remains elevated for up to 12 months after valve replacement.[72] Because this type of infective endocarditis is typically a nosocomial infection, methicillin-resistant organisms are common, and vancomycin is the cornerstone of therapy. Combination antimicrobials are recommended because of the high morbidity and mortality associated with PVE and its refractoriness to therapy.[4,5,11,21] Although the addition of rifampin to a penicillinase-resistant penicillin or vancomycin does not result in predictable bacterial synergism, rifampin may have unique activity against staphylococcal infection that involves prosthetic material, where its addition results in a higher microbiologic cure rate.[4] Combination therapy also decreases the emergence of resistance to rifampin, which frequently occurs when it is used alone. For methicillin-resistant staphylococci (both MRSA and coagulase-negative staphylococci), vancomycin is recommended with rifampin for 6 weeks or more (see Table 111-5). An aminoglycoside is added for the first 2 weeks if the organism is aminoglycoside susceptible; traditional dosing should be used as once-daily regimens have not been adequately evaluated in PVE and are not recommended.[4]

For MSSA, penicillinase-resistant penicillin is administered in place of vancomycin. PVE responds poorly to medical treatment and has a higher mortality compared with NVE. Valve dehiscence and incompetence can result in acute heart failure, and surgery is often a component of treatment.[4,33]

The use of anticoagulation is controversial in PVE. In general, those who require anticoagulation for a prosthetic valve should continue the anticoagulant cautiously during endocarditis therapy, unless a contraindication to therapy exists. It is recommended to hold all anticoagulation for at least 2 weeks for patients with *S. aureus* PVE if a recent CNS embolic event has occurred.[4]

Enterococcal Endocarditis

Enterococci are normal inhabitants of the human GI tract and, occasionally, of the anterior urethra. These organisms are usually of low virulence but can become pathogens following healthcare intervention or in predisposed patients (most commonly elderly with comorbid conditions such as diabetes or need for hemodialysis).[25] Historically, enterococci were considered group D streptococci, but they have been reclassified into the genus *Enterococcus* (*E. faecalis* and *E. faecium*). *E. faecalis* is the most common clinical isolate (approximately 97%) of the two species. Enterococci are the third leading cause of infective endocarditis, but they are more resistant to therapy than staphylococci and streptococci.[73] Enterococci are noteworthy for the following reasons: (a) no single antibiotic is bactericidal, (b) MICs to penicillin are relatively high (1-25 mcg/mL [mg/L]), (c) intrinsic resistance occurs to all cephalosporins and relative resistance occurs to aminoglycosides (eg, "low-level" aminoglycoside resistance), (d) combinations of a cell-wall–active agent such as a penicillin or vancomycin and an aminoglycoside are necessary for killing, and (e) resistance to all available drugs is increasing.[4,74-76]

Monotherapy with penicillin for infective endocarditis caused by enterococci results in relapse rates of 50% to 80%. When used alone, penicillins are only bacteriostatic against enterococci, and thus combination therapy is always recommended for susceptible strains.[4,75] The killing of enterococci by the bactericidal combination of an aminoglycoside antibiotic and a penicillin is the best clinical example of antibiotic synergy. Because the aminoglycoside cannot penetrate the bacterial cell in the absence of the penicillin, enterococci usually will appear to be resistant to aminoglycosides by routine susceptibility testing (low-level resistance). However, in the presence of an agent that disrupts the cell wall such as penicillin, the aminoglycoside can gain entry, attach to bacterial ribosomes, and cause rapid cell death. An aminoglycoside–vancomycin combination is also synergistic against enterococci and is appropriate therapy for the penicillin-allergic patient.[4,75-77]

Enterococcal endocarditis ordinarily requires 4 to 6 weeks of ampicillin or high-dose penicillin G plus an aminoglycoside for cure (see Table 111-6). Recent literature suggests that ampicillin plus ceftriaxone is as effective as ampicillin plus gentamicin and should be considered as a treatment option.[4,5] Ampicillin has greater in vitro activity than penicillin G, although there are no clinical data to document differences in efficacy. A 6-week course is recommended for patients with symptoms lasting longer than 3 months and those with PVE. Streptomycin and gentamicin have similar efficacy, but gentamicin is preferred due to the inability to obtain streptomycin serum levels in most labs.[75] Because of resistance, other aminoglycosides, such as tobramycin and amikacin, cannot be substituted routinely. In the treatment of enterococcal endocarditis, relatively low serum concentrations of aminoglycosides appear adequate for successful therapy, such as a gentamicin peak concentration of approximately 3 to 4 mcg/mL (mg/L; 6.3-8.4 μmol/L).[4,75,77] Treatment of enterococcal endocarditis does not have the high success rate seen with infective endocarditis caused by viridans streptococci, presumably because the organism is more resistant to killing.

Although some data support the use of extended-interval aminoglycoside dosing for other types of endocarditis (ie, streptococci), the data are more vague regarding this strategy in enterococcal infective endocarditis.[78] Some studies suggest that extended-interval aminoglycoside dosing and short-interval (traditional) dosing are clinically equivalent, discordant studies imply otherwise.[79-83] Newer evidence suggests that extended-interval dosing is appropriate in the setting of non-high level aminoglycoside resistant (MIC < 500 mcg/mL [mg/L]) *E. faecalis* IE and this strategy has been adopted by the new European Society of Cardiology Guidelines.[5,84,85] As such, the duration of therapy can be shortened from 4 to 6 weeks to 2 weeks. This recommendation differs from the current AHA guidelines, which continue to support traditional dosing.[4]

Resistance among enterococci to penicillins and aminoglycosides is increasing.[4] Enterococci that exhibit high-level resistance to streptomycin (MIC > 2,000 mcg/mL [mg/L]) are not synergistically killed by penicillin and streptomycin because the aminoglycoside either no longer binds to the ribosome or is inactivated by an aminoglycoside-modifying enzyme, streptomycin adenylase.[75] Because enterococci will appear resistant to aminoglycosides on routine susceptibility testing, the only way to distinguish high-level from low-level resistance is by performing special susceptibility tests using 500 to 2,000 mcg/mL (mg/L) of the aminoglycoside.[77] High-level streptomycin-resistant enterococci occur with a frequency approaching 60%, and high-level resistance to gentamicin is now found in 10% to 50% of isolates. Although most gentamicin-resistant enterococci are resistant to all aminoglycosides (including amikacin), 30% to 50% remain susceptible to streptomycin.[86] High-level gentamicin resistance is mediated by a bifunctional aminoglycoside-modifying enzyme, 6-acetyltransferase/2-phosphotransferase, and most strains also possess streptomycin adenylase. The incidence of high-level aminoglycoside resistance is increasing; however, data on appropriate therapy are sparse, and therapeutic options are few.[75,86,87]

In addition to isolates with high-level aminoglycoside resistance, β-lactamase–producing enterococci (especially *E. faecium*) have been reported. If these organisms are discovered, use of vancomycin or ampicillin–sulbactam in combination with gentamicin should be considered. Vancomycin-resistant enterococci are reported increasingly, primarily with *E. faecium*. Vancomycin resistance occurs when the bacterium replaces the normal vancomycin target with a peptidoglycan precursor that does not bind vancomycin.[76,87,88]

Treating multidrug-resistant enterococci is difficult, and data on appropriate therapy are sparse. Guidelines suggest either linezolid or daptomycin, although the latter agent has produced conflicting results.[89-95] Surgery and replacement of the infected cardiac valve may be the only cure.

HACEK Group

Fastidious gram-negative bacteria from the group of bacteria including *Haemophilus parainfluenzae, Haemophilus aphrophilus, Aggregatibacter* species, *Cardiobacterium hominis, Eikenella corrodens,* and *Kingella kingae* (HACEK group) account for 0.8% to 6% of infective endocarditis cases.[96] Frequently, these types of infective endocarditis present as subacute illnesses with large vegetations and emboli.[96,97] These oropharyngeal organisms typically are slow growing and should be considered as possible causes of "culture-negative" endocarditis.[97] With proper treatment, infectious endocarditis caused by HACEK organisms has a low mortality rate.[96] β-lactamase–producing organisms are occurring more often; hence, HACEK organisms should be considered resistant to ampicillin alone and should not be used unless in vitro susceptibility testing is adequate. Ceftriaxone, or an alternate third- or fourth-generation cephalosporin, is the preferred treatment in most cases. Ciprofloxacin may be considered as an option if an allergy to cephalosporins is present (see Table 111-7).[4,5] Treatment is usually for 4 weeks, but it should be extended to 6 weeks in PVE caused by one of these organisms.

Less Common Types of Infective Endocarditis

Atypical Microorganisms

Endocarditis caused by organisms, such as *Bartonella*; *Coxiella burnetii*; *Brucella, Candida,* and *Aspergillus* spp.; *Legionella*; and gram-negative bacilli (eg, *Pseudomonas*), is relatively uncommon. Medical therapy for infective endocarditis caused by these organisms is usually unsuccessful.[4,5] Consultation with an infectious disease expert is warranted when these microorganisms are identified.

In addition to *Pseudomonas* spp., other gram-negative bacilli that have been implicated include *Salmonella* spp., *Escherichia coli, Citrobacter* spp., *Klebsiella–Enterobacter* spp., *Serratia marcescens, Proteus* spp., and *Providencia* spp.[37] Generally, these infections have a poor prognosis, with mortality rates as high as 60% to 80%.[37] Cardiac surgery in concert with extended-course antibacterial therapy is recommended (class IIa; level of evidence: B) for most patients with gram-negative bacillary infective endocarditis. Readers are referred to the AHA guidelines for more extensive review of treatment regimens for infective endocarditis *due to Pseudomonas* spp. and unusual gram-negative bacteria.[4]

Fungi cause less than 2% of endocarditis cases; most patients with fungal endocarditis have undergone recent cardiovascular surgery, are IV drug abusers, have received prolonged treatment with indwelling central venous catheters, or are immunocompromised.[36,98] *Candida* spp. and *Aspergillus* spp. are the most commonly involved, and the mortality rate is high (>80%) for the following reasons: (a) large, bulky vegetations that often form, (b) systemic septic embolization that may occur, (c) the tendency of fungi to invade the myocardium, (d) poor penetration of vegetations by antifungals, (e) the low toxic-to-therapeutic ratio of agents such as amphotericin B, and (f) the lack of consistent fungicidal activity of available antifungal agents.[3,5,99] When fungal infective endocarditis is identified, a combined medical–surgical approach is warranted. Because these infections occur infrequently, scant clinical data are available to make solid treatment recommendations. Amphotericin B with or without flucytosine or an enchinocandin (high dose) is the recommended pharmacologic approach for *Candida* IE while voriconazole with the addition of amphotericin B or enchinocandin is suggested for those with Aspergillus IE.[5,37] Greater than 6 weeks of therapy is usually recommended; subsequent life-long suppressive therapy with an oral azole may be recommended for some.[4,5,37]

C. burnetii (Q fever) may be recovered from blood cultures, but infection is more likely to be identified via serologic tests. It is a common cause of infective endocarditis in certain areas of the world where goat, cattle, and sheep farming are widespread. The most favorable therapy for Q fever is unknown but may include doxycycline with hydroxychloroquine, trimethoprim–sulfamethoxazole, rifampin, or fluoroquinolones for at least 18 months.[100] *Brucella* are facultative intracellular gram-negative bacilli. Humans are infected by this organism after ingesting infected unpasteurized milk or undercooked meat, inhaling infectious aerosols, or contacting infected tissues. This type of infective endocarditis is more common in veterinarians and livestock handlers. Cure requires valve replacement and antimicrobial agents including doxycycline with streptomycin or gentamicin or doxycycline with trimethoprim–sulfamethoxazole or rifampin for an extended period (6 weeks to months).[101]

Culture-Negative Endocarditis

Sterile blood cultures are reported in up to 31% of patients with infective endocarditis if strict diagnostic criteria are used.[1,5] This type of infective endocarditis may occur as a result of unidentified subacute right-sided infective endocarditis, previous antibiotic therapy, slow-growing fastidious organisms, nonbacterial etiologies (eg, fungi), noninfective endocarditis, and improperly collected blood cultures. When blood cultures from patients suspected of infective endocarditis show no growth after 48 to 72 hours, cultures should be held for up to a month and special testing techniques (eg, serological analysis, polymerase chain reaction) pursued to detect fastidious or nonbacterial organisms.[4,36,97]

The AHA guidelines provide very general recommendations for culture-negative infective endocarditis (see Table 111-7) and suggest that therapy should be guided based on the individual patient's past medical history and epidemiological risks identified. Selection of treatment can be difficult, balancing the need to cover all likely organisms against potential toxic drug effects (eg, aminoglycosides). Antimicrobial selection should involve consultation with an infectious disease specialist. Irrespective of the chosen treatment, extended antimicrobial therapy is required. The empirical approaches for culture-negative infective endocarditis highlight the need for proper collection and monitoring of blood cultures and an extensive medication history.

PERSONALIZED PHARMACOTHERAPY

Infective endocarditis remains an uncommon disease, but the cost of treatment can be substantial. In the past, the long duration of hospitalization required to administer IV antimicrobials was the major expense. In select cases, abbreviated and/or outpatient, oral antimicrobial therapy may appreciably reduce the cost of care.

Shorter-course antimicrobial regimens are advocated when possible. For instance, in sensitive streptococcal endocarditis (MICs <0.12 mcg/mL [mg/L]), a 2-week regimen of high-dose parenteral penicillin G or ceftriaxone in combination with an aminoglycoside is as effective as 4 weeks of penicillin alone.[4] Uncomplicated right-sided MSSA endocarditis in the IV drug abuser may be treated with a 2-week course of nafcillin, oxacillin, or daptomycin.

The initiation of outpatient parenteral antibiotics should be considered early in the treatment of infective endocarditis, after the patient is stable clinically and responds favorably to initial antibiotics. Outpatient treatment is safe and cost-effective in select situations.[26,102,103] Patients considered for home therapy must be hemodynamically stable, compliant with therapy, have careful medical monitoring, understand the potential complications of the disease, and have immediate access to medical care. Advances in technology allow for the outpatient administration of complex antibiotic regimens that significantly reduce the cost of therapy. Simple regimens, such as single daily doses of ceftriaxone for streptococcal infective endocarditis, are particularly attractive. Although endocarditis is common in those with a history of IVDA and home healthcare would substantially reduce the cost of treatment, many clinicians are uncomfortable with outpatient IV therapy because central venous access is required. Sudden cardiac decompensation in an outpatient setting is also of concern.[4]

EVALUATION OF THERAPEUTIC OUTCOMES

The evaluation of patients treated for infective endocarditis includes assessment of disease signs and symptoms, blood cultures, microbiologic tests, inflammatory markers, serum drug concentrations, and other tests that evaluate organ function.

Signs and Symptoms

Fever usually subsides within 1 week of initiating therapy.[17] Persistence of fever may indicate ineffective antimicrobial therapy, emboli, right-sided endocarditis, intravascular catheter infections, or drug reactions. For some patients, low-grade fever may persist even with appropriate antimicrobial therapy. With defervescence, the patient should begin to feel better, and other symptoms, such as lethargy or weakness, should subside. Echocardiography should be performed when antibiotic therapy has been completed to determine new baseline cardiac function (ie, ventricular size and function). A TTE is usually sufficient.

Blood Cultures

After initiation of appropriate therapy, blood cultures should be negative within a few days, although microbiologic response to vancomycin may be slower. If bacteria continue to be isolated from blood beyond the first few days of therapy, it may indicate that the antimicrobials are inactive against the pathogen or that the doses are not producing adequate concentrations at the site of infection. If this is the case, therapeutic adjustments should be made and blood cultures should be rechecked until negative. During the remainder of therapy, frequent blood cultures are not necessary but should be obtained if fever recurs.[4]

Microbiologic Tests

For all isolates from blood cultures, MICs should be determined; MBCs are no longer recommended.[4] The agent currently being used should be tested, as well as alternatives that may be required if intolerance, allergy, or resistance occurs. Occasionally, it is useful to determine whether synergy exists for antimicrobial combinations, although synergistic regimens usually can be predicted from the literature. Chapter 24 summarizes the methods for in vitro determinations of synergy.

Inflammatory Markers

Inflammatory markers are commonly used in infectious disease processes for diagnosing, monitoring of clinical outcomes, as well as assisting clinicians with evaluating the efficacy of antibiotic therapy. Currently only one inflammatory marker, rheumatoid factor (RF), is part of the modified Duke criteria for diagnosis. Other inflammatory markers, such as ESR, CRP, and procalcitonin (PCT), have all been investigated for evaluating the outcomes of patients with in endocarditis.[104] High PCT levels (eg, >0.5 ng/mL [mcg/L]) indicate the need for surgical intervention and correlate with poor outcomes (ie, death or serious infectious complications).[105,106] While these markers may be beneficial in assessing clinical outcomes, further evidence is needed to establish routine use for infective endocarditis.

Serum Drug Concentrations

Of the agents used commonly for infective endocarditis, measurement of serum drug concentrations is routinely available for aminoglycosides (except streptomycin) and vancomycin. Few data, however, support attaining any specific serum concentrations for patients with infective endocarditis. In general, serum concentrations of the antimicrobial should exceed the MIC of the organisms.

When aminoglycosides are administered for infective endocarditis caused by gram-positive cocci with a traditional three-times-daily regimen, peak serum concentrations are recommended to be on the low side of the traditional ranges (3-4 mcg/mL [mg/L; 6.3-8.4 μmol/L] for gentamicin). If extended-interval dosing is used, which is only recommended in streptococcal infective endocarditis, the most appropriate method of monitoring has not been determined. When vancomycin is administered, the primary goal is to ensure adequate trough concentrations, in this case 15 to 20 mcg/mL (mg/L; 10-14 μmol/L), are achieved.[107]

PREVENTION

10 Antimicrobial prophylaxis is used as an attempt to prevent infective endocarditis for patients who are at the highest risk.[6,5,18] The use of antimicrobials for this purpose requires consideration of (a) cardiac conditions associated with endocarditis, (b) procedures causing bacteremia, (c) organisms likely to cause endocarditis, and

(d) pharmacokinetics, spectrum, cost, adverse effects, and ease of administration of available antimicrobial agents. The objective of prophylaxis is to diminish the likelihood of infective endocarditis in high-risk individuals from procedures that result in bacteremia. Although there are no prospective, controlled human trials demonstrating that prophylaxis in high-risk individuals protects against the development of endocarditis during bacteremia-inducing procedures, animal studies suggest possible benefit.[18] However, other studies have questioned the benefit of antibiotic prophylaxis prior to invasive procedures.[108] Furthermore, many causes of infective endocarditis appear not to be secondary to an invasive procedure. Bacteremia as a consequence of daily activities may, in fact, be the major culprit, and the value of antibiotic prophylaxis before bacteremia-causing procedures has been questioned.[109] The literature lacks adequate evidence to prove the effectiveness or ineffectiveness of antibiotic prophylaxis, and the common practice of using antimicrobial therapy in this setting remains controversial.[110] The mechanism of a beneficial effect in humans is unclear, but antibiotics may decrease the number of bacteria at the surgical site, kill bacteria after they are introduced into the blood, and prevent adhesion of bacteria to the valve.

Clinical **Controversy...**

The common practice of administering antibiotics to high-risk individuals before a bacteremia-causing procedure is controversial. Despite limited data supporting this approach and the fact that 100% compliance with AHA preventative guidelines would have only a modest benefit, the use of single-dose antibiotics for the prevention of endocarditis remains a standard of care.

Regardless of the controversy about whether prophylactic antibiotics should be used, infective endocarditis prophylaxis is recommended in select situations, specifically dental procedures, in those with underlying high-risk cardiac conditions. The AHA released updated guidelines that better define who should and should not receive infective endocarditis prophylaxis.[18] The appropriateness of the new guidelines, however, has been called into question due to epidemiological studies showing an increase in the overall incidence of IE, especially due to *Streptococcus*.[8]

Key points of this report are that (a) only a small number of cases of infective endocarditis might be prevented with antibiotic prophylaxis for dental procedures, even if 100% effective; (b) infective endocarditis prophylaxis for dental procedures should be recommended only for patients with underlying cardiac conditions associated with the highest risk; (c) for those with high-risk underlying cardiac conditions, prophylaxis is recommended for all dental procedures involving manipulation of gingival tissue or the periapical region of teeth or perforation of the oral mucosa; (d) prophylaxis is not recommended based solely on an increased lifetime risk of acquisition of infective endocarditis; and (e) administration of antibiotics solely to prevent endocarditis is not recommended for patients who undergo a genitourinary or GI tract procedure.

To determine whether a patient should receive prophylactic antibiotics, one needs to assess the patient's risk and whether he or she is undergoing a procedure resulting in bacteremia. When antibiotic prophylaxis is appropriate, a single 2 g dose of amoxicillin is recommended for adult patients at risk, given 30 to 60 minutes before undergoing procedures associated with bacteremia. Because the duration of antimicrobial prophylaxis appears to be relatively short, guidelines do not advocate a second oral dose of amoxicillin, which was recommended previously. Alternative prophylaxis regimens for patients allergic to penicillins or those unable to take oral medications are also provided. A summary of guideline recommendations is available in Table 111-10. Consultation of the full AHA guideline is suggested for more detailed information.[18]

TABLE 111-10 Prophylaxis of Infective Endocarditis

Highest Risk Cardiac Conditions	Presence of a prosthetic heart valve Prior diagnosis of infective endocarditis Cardiac transplantation with subsequent valvulopathy Congenital heart disease (CHD)[a]	
Types of procedures	Any that require perforation of the oral mucosa or manipulation of the periapical region of the teeth of gingival tissue	
Antimicrobial Options	**Adult Doses[b]**	**Pediatric Doses[b] (mg/kg)**
Oral amoxicillin	2 g	50
IM or IV ampicillin[c]	2 g	50
IM or IV cefazolin or ceftriaxone[c,d,e]	1 g	50
Oral cephalexin[d,e,f]	2 g	50
Oral clindamycin[e]	600 mg	20
Oral azithromycin or clarithromycin[e]	500 mg	15
IV or IM clindamycin[c,e]	600 mg	20

[a]Includes only the following: unrepaired cyanotic CHD, prophlyaxis within the first 6 months of implanting prosthetic material to repair a congenital heart defect, and repaired CHD with residual defects at or adjacent to prosthetic material.

[b]All one-time doses administered 30-60 minutes prior to initiation of the procedure.

[c]For patients unable to tolerate oral medication.

[d]Should be avoided in patients with immediate-type hypersensitivity reaction to penicillin or ampicillin (eg, anaphylaxis, urticaria, or angioedema).

[e]Option for patients with nonimmediate hypersensitivity reaction to penicillin or ampicillin.

[f]May substitute with an alternative first- or second-generation cephalosporin at an equivalent dose.

Data from reference 18.

ABBREVIATIONS

AHA	American Heart Association
CDIE	cardiac device infective endocarditis
CHD	congenital heart disease
CRP	C-reactive protein
ESC	European Society of Cardiology
ESR	erythrocyte sedimentation rate
HACEK	the group of bacteria including *Haemophilus parainfluenzae, Haemophilus aphrophilus, Aggregatibacter* species, *Cardiobacterium hominis, Eikenella corrodens*, and *Kingella kingae*
IE	infective endocarditis
IVDA	IV drug abuse
MBC	minimal bactericidal concentration
MIC	minimal inhibitory concentration
MRSA	methicillin-resistant *Staphylococcus aureus*
MSSA	methicillin-sensitive *Staphylococcus aureus*
NVE	native valve endocarditis
PCT	procalcitonin
PVE	prosthetic valve endocarditis
RF	rheumatoid factor
SBT	serum bactericidal titer
TEE	transesophageal echocardiography
TTE	transthoracic echocardiography

REFERENCES

1. Thuny F, Grisoli D, Cautela J, et al. Infective endocarditis: Prevention, diagnosis, and management. *Can J Cardiol* 2014;30:1046-1057.
2. Sandoe JAT, Watkin RW, Elliott TSJ. Infective endocarditis in the adult patient. *Medicine* 2013;41:689-692.
3. Fernandez Guerrero ML, Alvarez B, Manzarbeitia F, Renedo G. Infective endocarditis at autopsy: A review of pathologic manifestations and clinical correlates. *Medicine* 2012;91:152-164.
4. Baddour LM, Wilson WR, Bayer AS, et al. Infective endocarditis in adults: Diagnosis, antimicrobial therapy, and management of complications: A scientific statement for healthcare professionals from the American Heart Association: Endorsed by the Infectious Diseases Society of America. Circulation 2015;132:DOI: 10.1161/CIR.0000000000000296 First published online: 15 September 2015.
5. Habib G, Lancellotti P, Antunes MJ, et al. 2015 ESC guidelines for the management of infective endocarditis: The Task Force for the Mangement of Infective Endocarditis of the European Society of Cardiology. *Eur Heart J* 2015; DOI: http://dx.doi.org/10.1093/eurheartj/ehv319 First published online: 29 August 2015.
6. Nishimura RA, Otto CM, Bonow RO, et al. 2014 AHA/ACC guideline for the management of patients with valvular heart disease: A report of the American College of Cardiology/American Heart Association Task Force on Practice Guidelines. *Circulation* 2014;129:e521-e643.
7. Baddour LM, Epstein AE, Erickson CC, et al. On behalf of the American Heart Association Rheumatic Fever, Endocarditis, and Kawasaki Disease Committee of the Council on Cardiovascular Disease in the Young; Council on Cardiovascular Surgery and Anesthesia; Council on Cardiovascular Nursing; Council on Clinical Cardiology; and the Interdisciplinary Council on Quality of Care and Outcomes Research. Update on cardiovascular implantable electronic device infections and their management: A scientific statement from the American Heart Association. *Circulation* 2010;121:458-477.
8. Pant S, Patel NJ, Deshmukh A, et al. Trends in infective endocarditis incidence, microbiology, and valve replacement in the United States from 2000 to 2011. *J Am Coll Cardiol* 2015;65:2070-2076.
9. Bin Abdulhak AA, Baddour LM, Erwin PJ, et al. Global and regional burden of infective endocarditis, 1990-2010. *Glob Heart* 2014;9:131-143.
10. Mozaffarian D, Benjamin EJ, Go AS, et al. On behalf of the American Heart Association Statistics Committee and Stroke Statistics Subcommittee. Heart disease and stroke statistics—2015 update: A report from the American Heart Association. *Circulation* 2015;131:e29-e322.
11. Murdoch DR, Corey GR, Hoen B, et al. Clinical presentation, etiology, and outcome of infective endocarditis in the 21st century: The International Collaboration on Endocarditis-Prospective Cohort Study. *Arch Intern Med* 2009;169:463-473.
12. Durante-Mangoni E, Bradley S, Selton-Suty C, et al. Current features of infective endocarditis in elderly patients: Results of the International Collaboration on Endocarditis Prospective Cohort Study. *Arch Intern Med* 2008;168:2095-2103.
13. Chirouze C, Hoen B, Duval X. Infective endocarditis epidemiology and consequences of prophylaxis guidelines modifications: The dialectical evolution. *Curr Infect Dis Rep* 2014;16:440-448.
14. Elder RW, Baltimore RS. The changing epidemiology of pediatric endocarditis. *Infect Dis Clin N Am* 2015;29:513-524.
15. Athan E, Chu VH, Tattevin P, et al. Clinical characteristics and outcome of infective endocarditis involving implantable cardiac devices. *JAMA* 2012;307:1727-1735.
16. Benito N, Miro JM, de Lazzari E, et al. Health care-associated native valve endocarditis: Importance of non-nosocomial acquisition. *Ann Intern Med* 2009;150:586-594.
17. Hill EE, Herijgers P, Herregods MC, Peetermans WE. Evolving trends in infective endocarditis. *Clin Microbiol Infect* 2006;12:5-12.
18. Wilson W, Taubert KA, Gewitz M, et al. Prevention of infective endocarditis: Guidelines from the American Heart Association: A guideline from the American Heart Association Rheumatic Fever, Endocarditis, and Kawasaki Disease Committee, Council on Cardiovascular Disease in the Young, and the Council on Clinical Cardiology, Council on Cardiovascular Surgery and Anesthesia, and the Quality of Care and Outcomes Research Interdisciplinary Working Group. *Circulation* 2007;116:1736-1754.
19. Klein M, Wang A. Infective Endocarditis. *J Intensive Care Med* 2014; DOI: 10.1177/0885066614554906 First published online: 15 Oct 2014.
20. Bruun NE, Habib G, Thuny F, Sogaard P. Cardiac imaging in infectious endocarditis. *Eur Heart J* 2014;35:624-632.
21. Liu C, Bayer A, Cosgrove SE, et al. Clinical practice guidelines by the Infectious Diseases Society of America for the treatment of methicillin-resistant *Staphylococcus aureus* infections in adults and children. *Clin Infect Dis* 2011;52(3):e18-55.
22. Thuny F, Grisoli D, Collart F, et al. Management of infective endocarditis: Challenges and perspectives. *Lancet* 2012;379:965-975.
23. Durack DT, Lukes AS, Bright DK. New criteria for diagnosis of infective endocarditis: Utilization of specific echocardiographic findings. Duke Endocarditis Service. *Am J Med* 1994;96:200-209.
24. Li JS, Sexton DJ, Mick N, et al. Proposed modifications to the Duke criteria for the diagnosis of infective endocarditis. *Clin Infect Dis* 2000;30:633-638.
25. Qui Y, Moreillon P. Infective endocarditis. *Nat Rev Cardiol* 2011;8: 322-336.
26. Tice AD, Rehm SJ, Dalovisio JR, et al. Practical guidelines for outpatient parenteral antimicrobial therapy. *Clin Infect Dis* 2004;38: 1651-1672.
27. Duval X, Delahaye F, Alla F, et al. Temporal trends in infective endocarditis in the context of prophylaxis guideline modifications. *J Am Coll Cardiol* 2012;59:1968-1976.
28. Gelsomino S, Maessen JG, van der Veen F, et al. Emergency surgery for native mitral valve endocarditis: The impact of septic and cardiogenic shock. *Ann Thorac Surg* 2012;93:1469-1476.
29. Ramirez-Duque N, Garcia-Cabrera E, Ivanova-Georgieva R, et al. Surgical treatment for infective endocarditis in elderly patients. *J Infect* 2011;63:131-138.
30. Manne MB, Shrestha NK, Lytle BW, et al. Outcomes after surgical treatment of native and prosthetic valve infective endocarditis. *Ann Thorac Surg* 2012;93:489-494.
31. Kiefer T, Park L, Tribouilloy C, et al. Association between valvular surgery and mortality among patients with infective endocarditis complicated by heart failure. *JAMA* 2011;306:2239-2247.
32. De Feo M, Cotrufo M, Carozza A, et al. The need for a specific risk prediction system in native valve infective endocarditis surgery. *Sci World J* 2012;2012:307571. doi:10.1100/2102/307571.
33. Byrne JG, Rezai K, Sanchez JA, et al. Surgical management of endocarditis: The Society of Thoracic Surgeons clinical practice guideline. *Ann Thorac Surg* 2011;91:2012-2019.
34. Kang DH, Kim YJ, Kim SH, et al. Early surgery versus conventional treatment for infective endocarditis. *N Engl J Med* 2012;366:2466-2473.
35. Gould FK, Denning D, Elliot T, et al. Guidelines for the antibiotic treatment of endocarditis in adults: Report of the Working Party of the British Society for Antimicrobial Chemotherapy. *J Antimicrob Chemother* 2012;67(2):269-289.
36. Tattevin P, Revest M, Lefort A, Michelet C, Lortholary O. Fungal endocarditis: Current challenges. *Int J Antimicrob Agents* 2014;44:290-294.
37. Morpeth S, Murdoch D, Cabell CH, et al. Non-HACEK gram-negative bacillus endocarditis. *Ann Intern Med* 2007;147:829-835.
38. Pappas PG, Kauffman CA, Andes D, et al. Clinical practice guidelines for the management of candidiasis: 2009 update by the Infectious Diseases Society of America. *Clin Infect Dis* 2009;48:503-535.
39. Gruchalla RS, Pirmohamed M. Clinical practice. Antibiotic allergy. *N Engl J Med* 2006;354:601-609.
40. Falagas ME, Matthaiou DK, Bliziotis IA. The role of aminoglycosides in combination with a beta-lactam for the treatment of bacterial endocarditis: A meta-analysis of comparative trials. *J Antimicrob Chemother* 2006;57:639-647.
41. Sexton DJ, Tenenbaum MJ, Wilson WR, et al. Ceftriaxone once daily for four weeks compared with ceftriaxone plus gentamicin once daily for two weeks for treatment of endocarditis due to penicillin-susceptible streptococci. Endocarditis Treatment Consortium Group. *Clin Infect Dis* 1998;27:1470-1474.
42. Paul M, Leibovici L. Combination antimicrobial treatment versus monotherapy: The contribution of meta-analyses. *Infect Dis Clin North Am* 2009;23:277-293.
43. Francioli P, Ruch W, Stamboulian D. Treatment of streptococcal endocarditis with a single daily dose of ceftriaxone and netilmicin for 14 days: A prospective multicenter study. *Clin Infect Dis* 1995;21: 1406-1410.
44. Gavalda J, Pahissa A, Almirante B, et al. Effect of gentamicin dosing interval on therapy of viridans streptococcal experimental endocarditis with gentamicin plus penicillin. *Antimicrob Agents Chemother* 1995;39:2098-2103.
45. Fernandez Guerrero ML, Gonzalez Lopez JJ, Goyenechea A, et al. Endocarditis caused by *Staphylococcus aureus*: A reappraisal of the epidemiologic, clinical, and pathologic manifestations with analysis of factors determining outcome. *Medicine (Baltimore)* 2009;88:1-22.

46. Ferderspiel J, Stearns SC, Peppercorn AF, et al. Increasing US rates of endocarditis with *Staphylococcus aureus*: 1999-2008. *Arch Intern Med* 2012;172:363-365.
47. Rasmussen RV, Host U, Arpi M, et al. Prevalence of infective endocarditis in patients with *Staphylococcus aureus* bacteremia: The value of screening with echocardiography. *Eur J Echocardiogr* 2011;12:414-420.
48. Mermel LA, Allon M, Bouza E, et al. Clinical practice guidelines for the diagnosis and management of intravascular catheter-related infection: 2009 update by the Infectious Diseases Society of America. *Clin Infect Dis* 2009;49:1-45.
49. Graham JC, Gould FK. Role of aminoglycosides in the treatment of bacterial endocarditis. *J Antimicrob Chemother* 2002;49:437-444.
50. Cosgrove SE, Vigliani GA, Fowler VG Jr, et al. Initial low-dose gentamicin for *Staphylococcus aureus* bacteremia and endocarditis is nephrotoxic. *Clin Infect Dis* 2009;48:713-721.
51. Korzeniowski O, Sande MA. Combination antimicrobial therapy for *Staphylococcus aureus* endocarditis in patients addicted to parenteral drugs and in nonaddicts: A prospective study. *Ann Intern Med* 1982;97:496-503.
52. Lemonovich TL, Haynes K, Lautenbach E, et al. Combination therapy with an aminoglycoside for *Staphylococcus aureus* endocarditis and/or persistent bacteremia is associated with a decreased rate of recurrent bacteremia: A cohort study. *Infection* 2011;39:549-554.
53. Dodek P, Phillips P. Questionable history of immediate-type hypersensitivity to penicillin in staphylococcal endocarditis: Treatment based on skin-test results versus empirical alternative treatment—A decision analysis. *Clin Infect Dis* 1999;29:1251-1256.
54. Falagas ME, Manta KG, Ntziora F, Vardakas KZ. Linezolid for the treatment of patients with endocarditis: A systematic review of the published evidence. *J Antimicrob Chemother* 2006;58:273-280.
55. Fowler VG Jr, Boucher HW, Corey GR, et al. Daptomycin versus standard therapy for bacteremia and endocarditis caused by *Staphylococcus aureus*. *N Engl J Med* 2006;355:653-665.
56. Moore CL, Osaki-Kiyan P, Haque N, et al. Daptomycin versus vancomycin for bloodstream infections due to methicillin-resistant *Staphylococcus aureus* with a high vancomycin minimum inhibitory concentration: A case control study. *Clin Infect Dis* 2012;54:51-58.
57. Levine DP, Lamp KC. Daptomycin in the treatment of patients with infective endocarditis: Experience from a registry. *Am J Med* 2007;120(10 Suppl 1):S28-S33.
58. Rehm SJ, Boucher H, Levine D, et al. Daptomycin versus vancomycin plus gentamicin for treatment of bacteraemia and endocarditis due to *Staphylococcus aureus*: Subset analysis of patients infected with methicillin-resistant isolates. *J Antimicrob Chemother* 2008;62:1413-1421.
59. Segreti JA, Crank CW, Finney MS. Daptomycin for the treatment of gram-positive bacteremia and infective endocarditis: A retrospective case series of 31 patients. *Pharmacotherapy* 2006;26:347-352.
60. Wu G, Abraham T, Rapp J, et al. Daptomycin: Evaluation of a high-dose treatment strategy. *Int J Antimicrob Agents* 2011;38:192-196.
61. Dutante-Mangoni E, Casillo R, Bernardo M, et al. High-dose daptomycin for cardiac electronic device-related infective endocarditis. *Clin Infect Dis* 2012;54:347-354.
62. Kullar R, Davis SL, Levine DP, et al. High-dose daptomycin for treatment of complicated gram-positive infections: A large, multicenter, retrospective study. *Pharmacotherapy* 2011;31:527-536.
63. Carugati M, Bayer AS, Miro JM, et al. High-dose daptomycin therapy for left-sided infective endocarditis: A prospective study from the International Collaboration on Endocarditis. *Antimicrob Agents Chemother* 2013;57:6213-6222.
64. Information for Healthcare Professionals: Linezolid (Marketed as Zyvox). 2012, http://www.fda.gov/Drugs/DrugSafety/PostmarketDrugSafetyInformationforPatientsandProviders/DrugSafetyInformationforHeathcareProfessionals/ucm085249.htm.
65. Chambers HF, Miller RT, Newman MD. Right-sided *Staphylococcus aureus* endocarditis in intravenous drug abusers: Two-week combination therapy. *Ann Intern Med* 1988;109:619-624.
66. DiNubile MJ. Short-course antibiotic therapy for right-sided endocarditis caused by *Staphylococcus aureus* in injection drug users. *Ann Intern Med* 1994;121:873-876.
67. Yung D, Kottachchi D, Neupane B, et al. Antimicrobials for right-sided endocarditis in intravenous drug users: A systematic review. *J Antimicrob Chemother* 2007;60:921-928.
68. Ribera E, Gomez-Jimenez J, Cortes E, et al. Effectiveness of cloxacillin with and without gentamicin in short-term therapy for right-sided *Staphylococcus aureus* endocarditis. A randomized, controlled trial. *Ann Intern Med* 1996;125:969-974.
69. Parker RH, Fossieck BE Jr. Intravenous followed by oral antimicrobial therapy for staphylococcal endocarditis. *Ann Intern Med* 1980;93:832-834.
70. Dworkin RJ, Lee BL, Sande MA, et al. Treatment of right-sided *Staphylococcus aureus* endocarditis in intravenous drug users with ciprofloxacin and rifampicin. *Lancet* 1989;2:1071-1073.
71. Heldman AW, Hartert TV, Ray SC, et al. Oral antibiotic treatment of right-sided staphylococcal endocarditis in injection drug users: Prospective randomized comparison with parenteral therapy. *Am J Med* 1996;101:68-76.
72. Lopez J, Revilla A, Vilacosta I, et al. Definition, clinical profile, microbiological spectrum, and prognostic factors of early-onset prosthetic valve endocarditis. *Eur Heart J* 2007;28:760-765.
73. Chirouze C, Athan E, Alla F, et al. Enterococcal endocarditis in the beginning of the 21st century: Analysis from the International Collaboration on Endocarditis-Prospective Cohort Study. *Clin Microbiol Infect* 2013;19(12):1140-1147.
74. Reyes K, Zervos M. Endocarditis caused by resistant enterococcus: An overview. *Curr Infect Dis Rep* 2013;15:320-328.
75. Pericás JM, Zboromyrska Y, Cervera C, et al. Enterococcal endocarditis revisited. *Future Microbiol* 2015;10:1215-1240.
76. O'Driscoll T, Christopher CW. Vancomycin-resistant enterococcal infections: Epidemiology, clinical manifestations, and optimal management. *Infect Drug Resist* 2015;8:217-230.
77. Arias CA, Contreras GA, Murray BE. Management of multidrug-resistant enterococcal infections. *Clin Microbiol Infect* 2010;16(6):555-562.
78. Tam VH, Preston SL, Briceland LL. Once-daily aminoglycosides in the treatment of gram-positive endocarditis. *Ann Pharmacother* 1999;33:600-606.
79. Gavalda J, Cardona PJ, Almirante B, et al. Treatment of experimental endocarditis due to *Enterococcus faecalis* using once-daily dosing regimen of gentamicin plus simulated profiles of ampicillin in human serum. *Antimicrob Agents Chemother* 1996;40:173-178.
80. Houlihan HH, Stokes DP, Rybak MJ. Pharmacodynamics of vancomycin and ampicillin alone and in combination with gentamicin once daily or thrice daily against *Enterococcus faecalis* in an in vitro infection model. *J Antimicrob Chemother* 2000;46:79-86.
81. Schwank S, Blaser J. Once-versus thrice-daily netilmicin combined with amoxicillin, penicillin, or vancomycin against *Enterococcus faecalis* in a pharmacodynamic in vitro model. *Antimicrob Agents Chemother* 1996;40:2258-2261.
82. Fantin B, Carbon C. Importance of the aminoglycoside dosing regimen in the penicillin–netilmicin combination for treatment of *Enterococcus faecalis*-induced experimental endocarditis. *Antimicrob Agents Chemother* 1990;34:2387-2391.
83. Marangos MN, Nicolau DP, Quintiliani R, et al. Influence of gentamicin dosing interval on the efficacy of penicillin-containing regimens in experimental *Enterococcus faecalis* endocarditis. *J Antimicrob Chemother* 1997;39:519-522.
84. Olaison L, Schadewitz K. Enterococcal endocarditis in Sweden, 1995–1999: Can shorter therapy with aminoglycosides be used? *Clin Infect Dis* 2002;34:159-166.
85. Miro JM, Pericas JM, del Rio A. A new era for treating Enterococcus faecalis endocarditis: Ampicillin plus short-course gentamicin or ampicillin plus ceftriaxone: That is the question! *Circulation* 2013;127:1763-1766.
86. Fernandez Guerrero ML, Goyenechea A, Verdejo C, et al. Enterococcal endocarditis on native and prosthetic valves: A review of clinical and prognostic factors with emphasis on hospital-acquired infections as a major determinant of outcome. *Medicine (Baltimore)* 2007;86:363-377.
87. Sood S, Malhotra M, Das BK, et al. Enterococcal infections & antimicrobial resistance. *Indian J Med Res* 2008;128:111-121.
88. Fair RJ, Tor Y. Antibiotics and bacterial resistance in the 21st Century. *Perspect Medicin Chem* 2014;6:25-64.
89. Forrest GN, Arnold RS, Gammie JS, et al. Single center experience of a vancomycin resistant enterococcal endocarditis cohort. *J Infect* 2011;63:420-428.
90. Sierra-Hoffman M, Iznaola O, Goodwin M, et al. Combination therapy with ampicillin and daptomycin for treatment of Enterococcus faecalis endocarditis. *Antimicrob Agents Chemother* 2012;56(11):6064.
91. Kullar R, Davis SL, Levine DP, et al. High-dose daptomycin for treatment of complicated gram-positive infections: A large, multi-center, retrospective study. *Pharmacotherapy* 2011;31(6):527-536.
92. Sakoulas G, Bayer AS, Pogliano J, et al. Ampicillin enhances daptomycin- and cationic host defense peptide-mediated killing of ampicillin- and vancomycin-resistant Enterococcus faecium. *Antimicrob Agents Chemother* 2011;56(2):838-844.

93. Hidron AI, Edwards JR, Patel J, et al. NHSN annual update: Antimicrobial-resistant pathogens associated with healthcare-associated infections: Annual summary of data reported to the National Healthcare Safety Network at the Centers for Disease Control and Prevention, 2006–2007. *Infect Control Hosp Epidemiol* 2008;29(11):996-1011.
94. Kelesidis T, Humphries R, Uslan DZ, et al. Daptomycin nonsusceptible enterococci: An emerging challenge for clinicians. *Clin Infect Dis* 2011;52(2):228-234.
95. Enoch DA, Phillimore N, Karas JA, et al. Relapse of enterococcal prosthetic valve endocarditis with aortic root abscess following treatment with daptomycin in a patient not fit for surgery. *J Med Microbiol* 2010;59(Pt 4):482-485.
96. Chambers ST, Murdoch D, Morris A, et al. HACEK infective endocarditis: Characteristics and outcomes from a large, multi-national cohort. *PLoS ONE* 2013;8(5):e63181.
97. Katsouli A, Massa MG. Current issues in the diagnosis and management of blood culture-negative infective and non-infective endocarditis. *Ann Thorac Surg* 2013;95:1467-1474.
98. Bor DH, Woolhandler S, Nardin R, Brusch J, Himmelstein DU. Infective endocarditis in the U.S., 1998–2009: A nationwide study *PLoS ONE* 2013;8:e60033.
99. Pierrotti LC, Baddour LM. Fungal endocarditis, 1995–2000. *Chest* 2002;122:302-310.
100. Kersh GJ. Antimicrobial therapies for Q fever. *Expert Rev Anti Infect Ther* 2013;11:1207-1214.
101. Solera J. Update on brucellosis: Therapeutic challenges. *Int J Antimicrob Agents* 2010;36(Suppl 1):S18-S20.
102. Rehm S, Campion M, Katz DE, et al. Community-based outpatient parenteral antimicrobial therapy (CoPAT) for *Staphylococcus aureus* bacteraemia with or without infective endocarditis: Analysis of the randomized trial comparing daptomycin with standard therapy. *J Antimicrob Chemother* 2009;63:1034-1042.
103. Htin AK, Friedman ND, Hughes A, et al. Outpatient parenteral antimicrobial therapy is safe and effective treatment of infective endocarditis: A retrospective cohort study. *Intern Med J* 2013;43(6): 700-705.
104. Rybak M, Lomaestro B, Rotschafer JC, et al. Therapeutic monitoring of vancomycin in adult patients: A consensus review of the American Society of Health-System Pharmacists, the Infectious Diseases Society of America, and the Society of Infectious Diseases Pharmacists. *Am J Health Syst Pharm* 2009;66:82-98.
105. Watkins RR, Lemonovich TL. Role of inflammatory markers in the diagnosis and management of infective endocarditis. *Infect Dis Clin Pract* 2010;18:87-90.
106. Kocaxeybek B, Kucukoglu S, Oner YA. Procalcitonin and C-reactive protein in infective endocarditis: correlation with etiology and prognosis. *Chemotherapy* 2003;49:76-84.
107. Cornelissen CG, Frechen DA, Schreuner K, et al. Inflammatory parameters and prediction of prognosis in infective endocarditis. *BMC Infect Dis* 2013;13:272-278.
108. Duval X, Alla F, Hoen B, et al. Estimated risk of endocarditis in adults with predisposing cardiac conditions undergoing dental provedures with or without antibiotic prophylaxis. *Clin Infect Dis* 2006;42(12): e102-e107.
109. Mougeot FK, Saunders SE, Brennan MT, Lockhart PB. Associations between bacteremia from oral sources and distant-site infections: Tooth brushing versus single tooth extraction. *Oral Surg Oral Med Oral Pathol Oral Radiol* 2015;119(4):430-435.
110. Glenny AM, Oliver R, Roberts GJ, Hooper L, Worthington HV. Antibiotics for the prophylaxis of bacterial endocarditis in dentistry. *Cochrane Database Syst Rev* 2013;10:CD003813.

112

Tuberculosis

Rocsanna Namdar, Michael Lauzardo, and Charles A. Peloquin

KEY CONCEPTS

1. Tuberculosis (TB) is the most prevalent communicable infectious disease on earth; and it remains out of control in many developing nations. These nations require medical and financial assistance from developed nations in order to control the spread of TB globally.
2. In the United States, TB disproportionately affects the foreign born and other ethnic minorities, reflecting immigration patterns and greater ongoing transmission in these communities. Additional TB surveillance and preventive treatments are required within these communities.
3. TB is the leading cause of death in human immunodeficiency virus (HIV) infection worldwide. Coinfection with HIV and TB accelerates the progression of both diseases, thus requiring rapid diagnosis and treatment of both diseases.
4. Mycobacteria are slow-growing organisms; in the laboratory, they require special stains, special growth media, and long periods of incubation to isolate and identify.
5. TB can produce atypical signs and symptoms in infants, the elderly, and immunocompromised hosts, and it can progress rapidly in these patients.
6. Latent TB infection (LTBI) can lead to reactivation disease years after the primary infection occurred.
7. The patient suspected of having active TB disease must be isolated until the diagnosis is confirmed and the patient is no longer contagious. Often, isolation takes place in specialized "negative-pressure" hospital rooms to prevent the spread of TB.
8. Isoniazid and rifampin are the two most important drugs in the treatment of TB. Organisms resistant to both these drugs (multidrug-resistant TB [MDR-TB]) are much more difficult to treat.
9. Directly observed treatment (DOT) should be used whenever possible to reduce treatment failures and the selection of drug-resistant isolates.
10. To avoid the development of resistance, never add a single drug to a failing TB treatment regimen.

(1) Tuberculosis (TB) remains a leading infectious killer globally. TB is caused by *Mycobacterium tuberculosis*, which can produce either a silent, latent infection or a progressive, active disease.[1] Left untreated or improperly treated, TB causes progressive tissue destruction and, eventually, death. Because of renewed public health efforts, TB rates in the United States continue to decline. In contrast, TB remains out of control in many developing countries and—one third of the world's population currently is infected.[1] Given increasing drug resistance, it is critical that a major effort be made to control TB before the most potent drugs are no longer effective.

TB rates generally have risen with increasing urbanization and overcrowding because it is easier for an airborne disease to spread when people are living in closer proximity to each other. Hence, TB became a significant pathogen in Europe during the Middle Ages and peaked during the Industrial Revolution, when it caused significant mortality in Europe and in the United States.[1] This dire threat led to the rise of public health departments and to procedures such as the isolation of infected patients. Thus, TB was directly responsible for many of the healthcare practices that are used today. Unfortunately, in developing nations, some of these practices are not widely available, and TB continues to rage unabated.

EPIDEMIOLOGY

Globally, approximately 2 billion people are infected by *M. tuberculosis*, and roughly 1.5 million people die from active TB each year despite the fact that it is curable.[1] In the United States, an estimated 9 million people are latently infected with *M. tuberculosis*, meaning that they are not currently sick but that they could fall ill with TB at any time.[2] In 2014, 9,412 new TB cases were reported in the United States, which is 2.2% lower than in 2013.[2] The annual incidence of TB in the United States declined by approximately 5% per year from 1953 to 1983.[2] In 1984, this decline slowed, and then the incidence of TB rose from 1988 reaching its peak in 1992 (Fig. 112-1). Since 1993, more effective infection control practices and treatment protocols have reduced TB rates significantly as mentioned above. Despite this good news, the eradication of TB from the United States remains difficult. One reason is that TB among immigrants to the United States from high incidence countries remains a problem.[1,2]

Risk Factors for Infection

The following section will discuss the risk factors for infection including location, race, ethnicity, and human immunodeficiency virus (HIV) coinfection. Risk factors and likelihood of progression from infection to disease will also be discussed.

Location and Place of Birth

California, Florida, New York, and Texas accounted for 51% of the TB cases reported nationally in 2014.[2] Within these states, TB is most prevalent in large urban areas and among those born outside the United States in high TB incidence countries.[2]

In 2014, the TB rate among foreign-born persons was 13.4 times that of US-born persons.[2] The percentage of foreign-born TB patients in the United States has increased annually, reaching 66.5% in 2014.[2] with a total of 6,181 TB cases reported among foreign-born persons. In 2014, 55.3% of foreign-born persons with TB originated from five countries: Mexico, the Philippines, Vietnam, India, and China.[2] Therefore, healthcare workers must consider TB when caring for patients from these countries who experience symptoms such as cough, fever, and weight loss. Furthermore, in 2013, foreign-born persons accounted for 90.6% of the multidrug-resistant (MDR) TB cases.

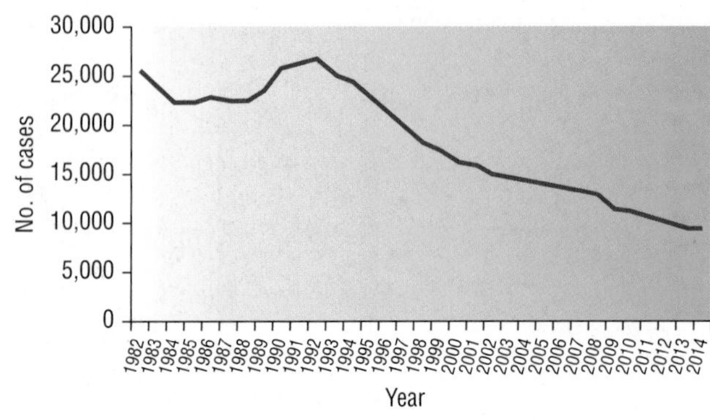

FIGURE 112-1 Reported cases of tuberculosis, United States, 1982-2011. *Updated as of June 5, 2015. *(Reproduced from Centers for Disease Control and Prevention. Reported Tuberculosis in the United States, 2014. Atlanta, GA: US Department of Health and Human Services, CDC, 2014, Available at: http://www.cdc.gov/tb/.)*

Close contacts of pulmonary TB patients such as family members, coworkers, or coresidents in places such as prisons, shelters, or nursing homes are the most likely to become infected. The more prolonged the contact, the greater is the risk, with infection rates as high as 30%.[2,3] TB patients frequently have limited access to healthcare, live in crowded conditions, or are homeless.[2,3] Many patients have histories of alcohol abuse or illicit drug use, and are coinfected with hepatitis B or HIV. These concurrent social and health problems make treating some TB patients particularly difficult.

Race, Ethnicity, Age

2 In the United States, TB disproportionately affects the foreign born and other ethnic minorities. In 2014, Asians had the largest percentage of total TB cases; however, the incidence rate among Asians decreased from 18.6 per 100,000 in 2013 to 17.9 in 2014.[2,4] TB rates among Hispanics remained relatively constant whereas rates decreased among blacks, whites, and Asians. In the American Indian/Alaska Native, Native Hawaiian or other Pacific Islander TB rates increased from 3.8 in 2013 to 4.3 in 2014.[2,4] Despite declines in the rates of TB among foreign and US-born individuals, the TB rate among foreign-born individuals was 13 times higher than among US-born individuals.[2,4] Among US-born group, non-Hispanic blacks were the ethnic group with the greatest number of TB cases and the largest disparity compared with US-born whites.[2,4]

TB is most common during adulthood primarily in the 25- to 44-year-age group and the 45- to 64-year-age group. In 2013, the case rates of TB declined from the previous years in all age groups except among children aged 14 years or younger, which remained the same from the previous year.[2]

Coinfection with Human Immunodeficiency Virus

3 In patients who have latent TB infection, HIV is the most important risk factor for progressing to active TB, especially among people between ages 25 and 44 years.[2,4,5] TB and HIV to act synergistically within patients and across populations, making each disease worse than it might otherwise be. In 2014, 6.3% of incident cases of TB in the United States were coinfected with HIV.[2,5] These numbers are estimates because laws and regulations in some states prohibit sharing HIV status of TB patients with the TB program. HIV coinfection may not increase the risk of acquiring *M. tuberculosis* infection, but it does increase the likelihood of progression to active disease.[1,5] There is evidence for higher mortality rates in HIV coinfected with MDR and extensively drug-resistant (XDR) TB.[5]

Risk Factors for Disease

Close contacts of pulmonary TB patients such as family members, coworkers, or coresidents in places such as prisons, shelters, or nursing homes are the most likely to become infected. The more prolonged the contact, the greater is the risk, with infection rates as high as 30%.[2-4] TB patients frequently have limited access to healthcare, live in crowded conditions, or are homeless.[2-4] Many patients have histories of alcohol abuse or illicit drug use, and are coinfected with hepatitis B or HIV. These concurrent social and health problems make treating some TB patients particularly difficult.

Once infected with *M. tuberculosis*, a person's lifetime risk of active TB is approximately 10%.[2-4] The greatest risk for active disease occurs during the first 2 years after infection. Children younger than 2 years and adults older than 65 years have two to five times greater risk for active disease compared with other age groups. Patients with underlying immune suppression (eg, renal failure, cancer, and immunosuppressive drug treatment) have 4 to 16 times greater risk than other patients.[2] Finally, HIV-infected patients with *M. tuberculosis* infection are 100 times more likely to develop active TB than normal hosts.[2-4] HIV-infected patients have an annual risk of active TB of approximately 10%, rather than a lifetime risk at that rate.[5] Therefore, all patients with HIV infection should be screened for tuberculous infection, and those known to be infected with *M. tuberculosis* should be tested for HIV infection.

ETIOLOGY

M. tuberculosis is a slender bacillus with a waxy outer layer.[2,6] It is 1 to 4 μm in length, and under the microscope, it is either straight or slightly curved in shape.[6] It does not stain well with Gram stain, so the Ziehl-Neelsen stain or the fluorochrome stain must be used instead.[6] After Ziehl-Neelsen staining with carbol-fuchsin, mycobacteria retain the red color despite acid–alcohol washes. Hence, they are called *acid-fast bacilli* (AFB).[6] On culture, *M. tuberculosis* grows slowly, doubling about every 20 hours. This is slow compared with gram-positive and gram-negative bacteria, which double about every 30 minutes.

Culture and Susceptibility Testing

All clinical specimens suspected of containing mycobacteria should be cultured. Culture is required for species identification and for drug susceptibility testing.

4 Direct susceptibility testing involves inoculating specialized media with organisms taken directly from a concentrated, smear-positive specimen.[1,6] This approach produces susceptibility results in 2 to 3 weeks. Indirect susceptibility testing involves inoculating the test media with organisms obtained from a pure culture of the organisms, which can take several more weeks. The most common agar method, known as the *proportion method*, uses the ratio of colony counts on drug-containing agar to that on drug-free agar.[1,6] In the United States, the critical proportion for resistance is 1%. That means that if a drug-containing plate shows 1% or more of the growth seen on a drug-free plate, some of the organisms from the specimen were resistant to that drug. Therefore, it is likely that many of the organisms in the patient also are resistant to that drug, and in general it should not be used to treat that patient.

The proportion method's limitations include many weeks to obtain results, drug degradation during the incubation, and a qualitative result (susceptible or resistant). The newer mycobacterial growth indicator tube (Becton Dickson, Sparks, MD) systems use liquid media and detect live mycobacteria in as few as 9 to 14 days.[6,7]

Rapid-identification tests are now available, but cost and care of equipment, remain an issue in many parts of the world. Nucleic acid amplifications tests use DNA probes to identify the presence of complementary ribosomal ribonucleic acid (rRNA) for several mycobacterial species.[6,7] DNA fingerprinting using restriction-fragment-length polymorphism analysis has been used to identify clusters of cases.[1,7,8] Amplification of the genetic material can be achieved through polymerase chain reaction (PCR), the amplified *M. tuberculosis* direct (MTD) test, and strand-displacement amplification.[7] Thin-layer chromatography, high-performance liquid chromatography for mycolic acid identification, and gas chromatography for short-chain fatty acids (methyl esters) have been used to speciate mycobacterial isolates.[6-9] The Enhanced Amplified *Mycobacterium Tuberculosis* Direct Test (E-MTD) has been approved for use by the US Food and Drug Administration in AFB smear-positive and smear-negative specimen in patients with fewer than 7 days of antimycobacterial therapy and the Gene X-pert MTB/RIF assay in patients with fewer than 3 days of treatment. The Amplicor *Mycobacterium Tuberculosis* Test has been approved for smear-positive samples.[9-12]

The Hain test, a line-probe assay that diagnoses resistance to isoniazid and rifampin by detecting several gene mutations responsible for drug resistance, has also entered into limited clinical use in the United States. The Gene X-pert MTB/RIF test simultaneously identifies *M. tuberculosis* and rapidly determines if resistance to rifampin is present.[9,13] The test has excellent performance in both smear-positive and -negative patients, and high accuracy for determination of rifampicin resistance.[11] Colorimetric redox indicator and nitrate reduction assays for rapid detection of rifampicin and isoniazid resistance are both inexpensive and have rapid turnaround times of 1 week. Microscopic observation drug susceptibility assay is simple test using sputum samples to detect characteristic patterns of growth of *M. tuberculosis* and resistance patterns. Time to diagnosis is 7 days and drug susceptibilities are available at the time of diagnosis.[11] Most patients with microscopic observation drug susceptibility assays are diagnosed within 2 weeks and it is similarly efficient irrespective of bacterial burden.[12]

Other tests are designed to detect common genetic changes associated with drug resistance, such as changes in the *katG* gene associated with isoniazid resistance and the *rpoB* gene associated with rifampin resistance.[5,8,13] Probe assays do not eliminate the need for conventional culture and susceptibility testing; conventional drug susceptibility testing is needed to diagnose XDR TB. The decision to use nucleic acid amplification tests should be individualized.

Transmission

M. tuberculosis is transmitted from person to person by coughing or other activities that cause the organism to be aerosolized.[2,3] These particles, called *droplet nuclei*, contain one to three bacilli and are small enough (1-5 mm) to reach the alveolar surface. This produces "droplet nuclei" that are dispersed in the air. Each droplet nuclei contains one to three organisms. Approximately 30% of individuals who experience prolonged contact with an infectious TB patient will become infected.

A person with cavitary, pulmonary TB and a cough is considered very infectious and may infect greater than 30% of contacts until that person is treated effectively, although this percentage and the absolute number can vary significantly. A person with the uncommon laryngeal form of TB can spread organisms even when talking, so the transmission rates can be even higher.

PATHOPHYSIOLOGY

The following section will discuss the pathophysiology of primary infection, reactivation disease, and the influence of HIV on the pathogenesis of *M. tuberculosis* infections.

Immune Response

T-lymphocyte responses are essential to controlling *M. tuberculosis* infections.[2,3,14,15] In the mouse model, two different T-cell responses—the T-helper type 1 (TH_1) response and the T-helper type 2 (TH_2) response—have been described. The TH_1 response is the preferred response to TB, and the TH_2 response, including the potentially subversive influence of interleukin (IL) 4, is undesirable.[2,14,15] Some workers have argued that this dichotomy is clearer in the mouse model, and in many humans, the T-cell response may be classified as TH_0 (elements of both TH_1 and TH_2).[14] In either case, T lymphocytes activate macrophages that, in turn, engulf and kill mycobacteria. T lymphocytes also destroy immature macrophages that harbor *M. tuberculosis* but are unable to kill the invaders.[14,15] CD4+ cells are the primary T cells involved, with contributions by $\gamma\ \delta$ T cells and CD8+ T cells.[14] CD4+ T cells produce interferon-γ (INF-γ) and other cytokines, including IL-2 and IL-10, that coordinate the immune response to TB.[14] Because CD4+ cells are depleted in HIV-infected patients, these patients are unable to mount an adequate defense to TB.[14,15]

Although B-cell responses and antibody production can be demonstrated in TB-infected mammals, these humoral responses do not appear to contribute much to the control of TB within the host.[3,14] Tumor necrosis factor-α (TNF-α) and INF-γ are important cytokines involved in coordinating the host's cell-mediated response. Rheumatoid arthritis patients treated with TNF-α inhibitors (such as infliximab) have high rates of reactivation TB.[16] Therefore, patients known to be deficient in the activity of TNF-α or INF-γ should be screened for TB infection and offered appropriate treatment.

M. tuberculosis has several ways of evading or resisting the host immune response.[14,15] In particular, *M. tuberculosis* can inhibit the fusion of lysosomes to phagosomes inside macrophages. This prevents the destructive enzymes found in the lysosomes from getting to the bacilli captured in the phagosomes. This inhibition of destructive mechanisms allows time for *M. tuberculosis* to escape into the cytoplasm. Virulent *M. tuberculosis* is able to multiply in the macrophage cytoplasm, thus perpetuating their spread. Finally, lipoarabinomannan (LAM), the principal structural polysaccharide of the mycobacterial cell wall, inhibits the host immune response.[14,15] LAM induces immunosuppressive cytokines, thus blocking macrophage activation; additionally, LAM scavenges O_2, thus preventing attack by superoxide anions, hydrogen peroxide, singlet oxygen, and hydroxyl radicals.[14,15] These survival mechanisms make *M. tuberculosis* a particularly difficult organism to control. Any defects in the host immune system make it likely that *M. tuberculosis* will not be controlled and that active disease will ensue.

Primary Infection

Primary infection usually results from inhaling airborne particles that contain *M. tuberculosis*.[3,15] The progression to clinical disease depends on three factors: (a) the number of *M. tuberculosis* organisms inhaled (infecting dose), (b) the virulence of these organisms, and (c) the host's cell-mediated immune response.[3,15,17] At the alveolar surface, the bacilli that were delivered by the droplet nuclei are ingested by pulmonary macrophages. If these macrophages inhibit or kill the bacilli, infection is aborted.[15] If the macrophages cannot do this, the organisms continue to multiply. The macrophages eventually rupture, releasing many bacilli, and these mycobacteria are then phagocytized by other macrophages. This cycle continues over several weeks until the host is able to mount a more coordinated response.[15] During this early phase of infection, *M. tuberculosis* multiplies logarithmically.[15]

Some of the intracellular organisms are transported by the macrophages to regional lymph nodes in the hilar, mediastinal, and retroperitoneal areas. The cycle of phagocytosis and cell rupture continues. During lymph node involvement, the mycobacteria may be held in check. More frequently, *M. tuberculosis* spreads throughout the body through the bloodstream.[3,15] When this intravascular dissemination occurs, *M. tuberculosis* can infect any tissue or organ in the body. Most commonly, *M. tuberculosis* infects the posterior apical region of the lungs. This may be so because of the high oxygen content, and it may be because of a less vigorous immune response in this area.

After about 3 weeks of infection, T lymphocytes are presented with *M. tuberculosis* antigens. These T cells become activated and begin to secrete INF-γ and the other cytokines noted earlier.

The processes described in the Immune Response section above then begin to occur. First, T lymphocytes stimulate macrophages to become bactericidal.[15] Large numbers of activated microbicidal macrophages surround the solid caseous (cheese-like) tuberculous foci (the necrotic area of infection).[15] This process of creating activated microbicidal macrophages is known as *cell-mediated immunity* (CMI).[15]

At the same time that CMI occurs, delayed-type hypersensitivity (DTH) also develops through the activation and multiplication of T lymphocytes. DTH refers to the cytotoxic immune process that kills nonactivated immature macrophages that are permitting intracellular bacillary replication.[15] These immature macrophages are killed when the T lymphocytes initiate Fas-mediated apoptosis (programmed cell death).[15] The bacilli released from the immature macrophages then are killed by the activated macrophages.[15]

By this time (more than 3 weeks), in most recently infected individuals, macrophages have begun to form granulomas to contain the organisms. In a typical tuberculous granuloma, activated macrophages accumulate around a caseous lesion and prevent its further extension.[15] At this point, the infection is largely under control, and bacillary replication falls off dramatically. Depending on the inflammatory response, tissue necrosis and calcification of the infection site plus the regional lymph nodes may occur.

Over 1 to 3 months, activated lymphocytes reach an adequate number, and tissue hypersensitivity results. In practical terms, this is the reason why tests to diagnose latent TB infection, purified protein derivative (PPD) skin test, and the INF-γ release assays, take between 2 and 12 weeks to become positive. Any remaining mycobacteria are believed to reside primarily within granulomas or within macrophages that have avoided detection and lysis, although some residual bacilli have been found in various types of cells.[3,14]

Approximately 90% of infected patients have no further clinical manifestations. Most patients only show a positive skin test (70%), whereas some also have radiographic evidence of stable granulomas. This radiodense area on chest radiograph is called a *Ghon's complex*. Approximately 5% of patients (usually children, the elderly, and the immunocompromised) experience "progressive primary" disease that occurs before skin test conversion, which presents as a progressive pneumonia, usually in the lower lobes.[18] Disease frequently spreads, leading to meningitis and other severe forms of TB.[18] Because of this risk of severe disease, very young, elderly, and immunocompromised patients, including those with HIV, should be evaluated and treated for latent or active TB.

Reactivation Disease

6 Roughly 10% of infected patients develop reactivation disease at some point in their lives. Nearly half of these cases occur within 2 years of infection.[3,15] In the United States, most cases of TB are believed to result from reactivation. Reinfection is uncommon in the United States because of the low rate of exposure and because previously sensitized individuals possess some degree of immunity to reinfection.[3,15] Exceptions include patients coinfected with HIV who live in areas of higher exposure to *M. tuberculosis*.

The apices of the lungs are the most common sites for reactivation (85% of cases).[3] For reasons that are not entirely known (waning cellular immunity, loss of specific T-cell clones, blocking antibody), organisms within granulomas emerge and begin multiplying extracellularly.[15] The inflammatory response produces caseating granulomas, which eventually will liquefy and spread locally, leading to the formation of a hole (cavity) in the lungs.

The immune response contributes to the severity of the lung damage, and DTH allows for intracellular mycobacterial multiplication.[14,15] In addition, there is "innocent bystander" killing of host cells and locally thrombosed blood vessels.[15] The killing of mycobacteria, macrophages, and neutrophils that have entered the battle releases cytokines and lysozymes into the infectious foci. This toxic mixture can be too much for the surrounding alveoli and airway cells, causing regional necrosis and structural collapse.[3,15] These unstable foci liquefy, spreading the infection to neighboring areas of the lung, creating a cavity. Some of this necrotic material is coughed out, producing droplet nuclei. Bacterial counts in the cavities can be as high as 10^8 per milliliter (or 10^{11}/L) of cavitary fluid. Partial healing may result from fibrosis, but these lesions remain unstable and may continue to expand.[3,15] If left untreated, pulmonary TB continues to destroy the lungs, resulting in hypoxia, respiratory acidosis, and eventually death.

Extrapulmonary and Miliary Tuberculosis

Caseating granulomas at extrapulmonary sites can undergo liquefaction, releasing tubercle bacilli and causing symptomatic disease.[3] Extrapulmonary TB without concurrent pulmonary disease is uncommon in normal hosts but more common in HIV-infected patients. Because of these unusual presentations, the diagnosis of TB is difficult and often delayed in immunocompromised hosts.[3] Lymphatic and pleural diseases are the most common forms of extrapulmonary TB, followed by bone, joint, genitourinary, meningeal, and other forms.[3] Occasionally, a massive inoculum of organisms enters the bloodstream, causing a widely disseminated form of the disease known as *miliary TB*. It is named for the millet seed appearance of the small granulomas seen on chest radiographs, and it can be rapidly fatal.[14] Miliary TB is a medical emergency requiring immediate treatment.

Influence of Human Immunodeficiency Virus Infection on Pathogenesis

3 HIV infection is the strongest single risk factor for progressing to active TB.[3,14] As CD4+ lymphocytes multiply in response to the mycobacterial infection, HIV multiplies within these cells and selectively destroys them. In turn, the TB-fighting lymphocytes are depleted.[14] This vicious cycle puts HIV-infected patients at 100 times the risk of active TB compared with HIV-negative people.[19,20] In addition, the combination of HIV infection and certain social behaviors increases the risk of newly acquired TB. In select areas of the United States during the resurgence of TB during the early 1990s, up to 50% of new TB cases were the result of recent infection, particularly among HIV-infected individuals.[1,19,20]

As mycobacteria spread throughout the body, HIV replication accelerates in lymphocytes and macrophages. This leads to progression of HIV disease.[14,19,20] HIV-infected patients who are infected with TB deteriorate more rapidly unless they receive antimycobacterial chemotherapy.[19,20] Most clinicians now recommend integrated antiretroviral therapy (ART) beginning TB treatment first, and then beginning HIV treatment within 2 to 12 weeks.[21-23] However, the timing needs to be individualized based on degree of immunosuppression from HIV and the patient's tolerance of the treatment regimen. Immune reconstitution inflammatory syndrome or a paradoxical worsening of TB can occur, especially in patients with more severe immunosuppression; this appears to result from a reinvigorated inflammatory response to TB.[21-23] HIV-positive patients, should be screened for tuberculous infection or disease soon after they are shown to be HIV-positive.[21,22]

CLINICAL PRESENTATION

The classical presentation of TB is weight loss, fatigue, a productive cough, fever, and night sweats. The onset of TB may be gradual, and the diagnosis may not be considered until a chest radiograph is performed. Unfortunately, many patients do not seek medical attention until more dramatic symptoms, such as hemoptysis, occur. At this point, patients typically have large cavitary lesions in the lungs. These cavities are loaded with *M. tuberculosis*. Expectoration or

CLINICAL PRESENTATION Tuberculosis

Signs and Symptoms

- Patients typically present with cough weight loss, fatigue, fever, and night sweats.[3,14,15]
- Frank hemoptysis usually occurs late in the course of disease but may present earlier.

Physical Examination

- Dullness to chest percussion, rales, and increased vocal fremitus are observed frequently on auscultation but a normal lung examination is very common compared to the degree of radiological lung involvement.
- Patient is usually thin with evidence or recent weight loss.

Laboratory Tests

- Moderate elevations in the white blood cell (WBC) count with a lymphocyte predominance.
- High platelet count (thrombocytosis) and mild to moderate anemia are common.

Diagnostic Considerations

- Positive-sputum smear
- Fiber-optic bronchoscopy (if sputum tests are inconclusive and suspicion is high)

Chest Radiograph

- Patchy or nodular infiltrates in the apical areas of the upper lobes or the superior segment of the lower lobes.[3,14,15]
- Cavitation that may show air–fluid levels as the infection progresses.

swallowing of infected sputum may spread the disease to other areas of the body.[1,3,17] Physical examination is nonspecific but suggestive of progressive pulmonary disease.

Human Immunodeficiency Virus

5 Patients coinfected with HIV may have atypical presentations.[1,3,17] As their CD4+ counts decline, HIV-positive patients are less likely to have positive skin tests, cavitary lesions, or fever. Pulmonary radiographic findings may be minimal or absent. HIV-positive patients have a higher incidence of extrapulmonary TB and are more likely to present with progressive primary disease. Because their symptoms are not specific to TB, a thorough workup for TB is essential.[3,14,15]

Extrapulmonary

Extrapulmonary TB typically presents as a slowly progressive decline in organ function.[3,17] Patients may have low-grade fever and other constitutional symptoms. Patients with genitourinary TB may present with sterile pyuria and hematuria. Lymphadenitis often involves the cervical and supraclavicular nodes and may appear as a neck mass with spontaneous drainage. Tuberculous arthritis and osteomyelitis occur most commonly in the elderly and usually affect the lower spine and weight-bearing joints. TB of the spine is known as *Pott's disease*.[3] Abnormal behavior, headaches, or convulsions suggest tuberculous meningitis. Involvement of the peritoneum, pericardium, larynx, and adrenal glands also occurs.[3,17]

The Elderly

5 TB in the elderly is easily confused with other respiratory diseases. Many clinical findings are muted or absent altogether. Compared with younger patients, TB in the elderly is far less likely to present with positive skin tests, fevers, night sweats, sputum production, or hemoptysis.[2,19,24] Weight loss may occur but is nonspecific. In contrast, mental status changes are twice as common in the elderly, and mortality is six times higher.[3,17] TB is a preventable cause of death in the elderly that should not be overlooked.

Children

5 TB in children, especially those younger than 12 years, may present as a typical bacterial pneumonia and is called *progressive primary TB*.[17,18] Clinical disease often begins 1 to 2 months after exposure and precedes skin-test positivity. Unlike adults, pulmonary TB in children often involves the lower and middle lobes.[17,18] Dissemination to the lymph nodes, GI and genitourinary tracts, bone marrow, and meninges is common. Because of delays in recruitment of cellular immunity, cavitary disease is infrequent, and the number of organisms present typically is smaller than in an adult. Because cavitary lesions are uncommon, children do not spread TB readily. However, TB can be rapidly fatal in a child, and it requires prompt chemotherapy.

DIAGNOSIS

The following section focuses on diagnostic testing for infection with *M. tuberculosis*. If active disease is suspected based on clinical presentation, additional diagnostic tests are also reviewed to confirm active disease.

Diagnostic Testing

The key to stopping the spread of TB is early identification of infected individuals.[3,17] Table 112-1 lists the populations most likely to benefit from testing (column 1 patients are at highest risk for TB, followed by those in column 2). Members of these high-risk groups should be tested for TB infection and educated about the disease.

The Mantoux test is a quantitative TB skin test that uses tuberculin PPD. The standard 5-tuberculin-unit PPD dose is placed intracutaneously on the volar aspect of the forearm with a 26- or 27-gauge needle.[3,17,24] This injection should produce a small, raised, blanched wheal. An experienced professional should read the test in 48 to 72 hours. The area of induration (the "bump") is the important end point, not the area of redness. Table 113-1 lists the criteria for interpretation.[3,17,24] The Centers for Disease Control and Prevention (CDC) does not recommend the routine use of anergy panels.[24-26] Aplisol and Tubersol 5-tuberculin-unit products are available commercially and are similar in sensitivity, specificity, and reactivity. It is important, however, to use one product and notify appropriate users when switching between products.[27,28]

The "booster effect" occurs for patients who do not respond to an initial skin test but show a positive reaction if retested about a

TABLE 112-1 Criteria for Tuberculin Positivity by Risk Group

Reaction 5 mm of Induration	Reaction ≥10 mm of Induration	Reaction ≥15 mm of Induration
HIV-positive persons	Recent immigrants (ie, within the last 5 years) from high-prevalence countries	Persons with no risk factors for TB
Recent contacts of TB case patients	Injection-drug users	
Fibrotic changes on chest radiograph consistent with prior TB	Residents and employees[a] of the following high-risk congregate settings: prisons and jails, nursing homes and other long-term care facilities for the elderly, hospitals and other healthcare facilities, residential facilities for patients with AIDS, homeless shelters	
Patients with organ transplants and other immunosuppressed patients (receiving the equivalent of ≥15 mg/day of prednisone for 1 month or more)[b]	Mycobacteriology laboratory personnel Persons with the following clinical conditions that place them at high risk: silicosis, diabetes mellitus, chronic renal failure, some hematologic disorders (eg, leukemias and lymphomas), other specific malignancies (eg, carcinoma of the head or neck and lung), weight loss of ≥10% of ideal body weight, gastrectomy, jejunoileal bypass Children younger than 4 years or infants, children, and adolescents exposed to adults at high risk	

AIDS, acquired immunodeficiency syndrome; HIV, human immunodeficiency virus; TB, tuberculosis.

[a]For persons who are otherwise at low risk and who are tested at the start of employment, a reaction of ≥15 mm induration is considered positive.

[b]Risk of TB for patients treated with corticosteroids increases with higher dose and longer duration.

Adapted from Screening for tuberculosis and tuberculosis infection in high-risk populations: Recommendations of the Advisory Council for the Elimination of Tuberculosis. MMWR Recomm Rep *1995;44(RR-11):19-34.*

week later or longer.[17,26] Patients with past *M. tuberculosis* infection and some patients with past immunization with bacillus Calmette-Guérin (BCG) vaccine or past infection with other mycobacteria may "boost" with a second skin test. Individuals who require periodic skin testing, such as healthcare workers, should receive a two-stage test initially.[17,26,29] Once they are shown to be skin-test negative, any positive skin test later shows recent infection, and this requires an evaluation to consider treatment.

The PPD skin test is an imperfect diagnostic tool. Up to 20% of patients with active TB are falsely skin-test negative, presumably because they may be immunocompromised.[14,26] False-positive results are more common in low-risk patients and those recently vaccinated with BCG. Despite BCG vaccination, one should not ignore a positive PPD result especially if the induration is more than 15 mm.[24] These patients require careful evaluation for active disease, and they may be offered preventive treatment because many come from areas where TB infection is common.

Interferon-γ release assays (IGRA) measure the release of INF-γ in blood in response to the TB antigens.[30] They may provide quick and specific results for identifying *M. tuberculosis*. IGRAs do not trigger a booster effect and are more specific for testing *M. tuberculosis* than the PPD. The QuantiFERON-TB Gold test (QFT-G) is an enzyme-linked immunosorbent assay (ELISA) and the T-SPOT.TB, is an enzyme-linked immunospot assay[30,31] Both tests can be used for diagnosing latent TB infection (LTBI) and TB disease caused by *M. tuberculosis*. However, these are tests desgined to diagnose LTBI and are not to be used to confirm or reject a diagnosis of active TB disease. For active TB, the IGRAs provide supporting evidence for the diagnosis but need to be interpreted in light of other evidence of active TB disease such as epidemiological risk factors and other studies. The antigenic proteins are absent from BCG vaccine strains and from most non-TB mycobacteria. Therefore, QFT-G does not trigger a booster effect and is more specific for testing of *M. tuberculosis* than the PPD. Although these tests can provide results to diagnose both latent infection and disease, they cannot differentiate between the two. Results are available within 24 hours, instead of the 2 to 3 days required for the traditional PPD skin test; and the patient does not have to return to the clinic as required by the PPD skin test. The CDC has approved the use of these tests in all circumstances in which the PPD is currently used. IGRAs may be preferred for testing in patients that are suspected not to return for follow up PPD reads or in patients who have received the BCG vaccine. The sensitivity for young children (younger than 5 years) and in immunocompromised patients has not clearly established.[30–34] The American Academy of Pediatrics recommends IGRAs in place of PPD skin test in immunocompetent children aged 5 years or older who have received BCG vaccination to confirm TB infection.[32] However, an increasing number of experts are using the IGRAs in children 2 years or older.

IGRAs perform similarly to the PPD in detecting TB in HIV-infected patients with LTBI. Both PPD and IGRA have suboptimal sensitivity for active TB especially in the severely immunocompromised.[30,35]

Culture and Staining

When active TB is suspected, attempts should be made to isolate *M. tuberculosis* from the site of infection.[3,17,26] Sputum collected in the morning usually has the highest yield.[3,17] Daily sputum collection over 3 consecutive days is recommended. Microscopic examination is the most rapid and inexpensive TB diagnostic tool. After staining, microscopic examination ("smear") detects about 8,000 to 10,000 organisms per milliliter (8×10^6/L to 10×10^6/L) of specimen, so a patient can be "smear-negative" but still grow *M. tuberculosis* on culture. Microscopic examination also cannot determine which of the more than 100 mycobacterial species is present or whether the organisms in the original samples were alive or dead.[1,6]

For patients unable to expectorate, sputum induction with aerosolized hypertonic saline may produce a diagnostic sample. Bronchoscopy, in older children, or aspiration of gastric fluid via a nasogastric tube, in children (5 years or younger), may be attempted for select patients.[17] For patients with suspected extrapulmonary TB, samples of draining fluid, biopsies of the infected site, or both may be attempted. Blood cultures are positive occasionally, especially in acquired immunodeficiency syndrome (AIDS) patients.[17,36]

TREATMENT

Drugs used in the treatment of active disease are divided into first-line and second-line agents. First-line agents should be the preferred options unless susceptibility results dictate otherwise. Treatment in special populations is also addressed.

Desired Outcome

The desired outcomes during the treatment of TB are:

1. Rapid identification of a new TB case.
2. Initiation of specific anti-TB treatment.
3. Eradicating *M. tuberculosis* infection.
4. Achievement of a noninfectious state in the patient, thus ending isolation.
5. Preventing the development of resistance.
6. Adherence to the treatment regimen by the patient.
7. Cure of the patient as quickly as possible (generally at least 6 months of treatment).

It is also important that patients with active disease are isolated to prevent spread of the disease and that appropriate samples for smears and cultures are collected. Secondary goals are identification of the index case that infected the patient, identification of all persons infected by both the index case and the new case of TB ("contact investigation"), and completion of appropriate treatments for those individuals.

General Approaches

Drug treatment is the cornerstone of TB management.[3,37] Monotherapy can be used only for infected patients who do not have active TB (latent infection, as shown by a positive skin test or positive IGRA). Once active disease is present, a minimum of two drugs, and generally three or four drugs, must be used simultaneously.[37] The duration of treatment depends on the condition of the host, extent of disease, presence of drug resistance, and tolerance of medications. The shortest duration of treatment generally is 6 months, and 18 to 24 months of treatment may be necessary for cases of MDR-TB.[37] Because the duration of treatment is so long and because many patients feel better after a few weeks of treatment, careful follow-up is required. Directly observed therapy (DOT) by a healthcare worker is a cost-effective way to ensure completion of treatment and is considered the standard of care.[37-39]

Principles for Treating Latent Infection and for Treating Disease

Asymptomatic patients with tuberculous infection have a bacillary load of about 10^3 organisms, compared with 10^{11} organisms in a patient with cavitary pulmonary TB.[3,7] As the number of organisms increases, the likelihood of naturally occurring drug-resistant mutants also increases. Naturally occurring resistant mutants are found at rates of 1 in 10^6 to 1 in 10^8 organisms for the anti-TB drugs.[3,7,37] When treating asymptomatic latent infection with isoniazid monotherapy, the risk of selecting out isoniazid-resistant organisms is low. The isoniazid mutation rate is about 1 in 10^6, but only about 10^3 organisms are present in the body. In contrast, the risk of selecting out isoniazid-resistant organisms is unacceptably high for patients with cavitary TB. One can prevent selection of these resistant mutants by adding more drugs because the rates for resistance mutations to multiple drugs are additive functions of the individual rates. For example, only 1 in 10^{13} organisms would be naturally resistant to both isoniazid (1 in 10^6) and rifampin (1 in 10^7).[3,7,37] It is unlikely that such rare organisms are present in a previously untreated patient.

Combination chemotherapy is required for treating active TB disease. The patient should receive at least two drugs to which the isolate is susceptible, and, generally, four drugs are given at the outset of treatment. Rifampin and isoniazid are the best drugs for preventing drug resistance, followed by ethambutol, streptomycin, and pyrazinamide.[3,7,37,40]

Three subpopulations of mycobacteria are proposed to exist within the body, and each appears to respond to certain drugs.[7,37] Most numerous are the extracellular, rapidly dividing bacteria, often found within cavities (about 10^7 to 10^9 organisms). These are killed most readily by isoniazid, followed by rifampin, streptomycin, and the other drugs. A second group resides within caseating granulomas (possibly 10^5 to 10^7 organisms). These organisms appear to be in a semidormant state, with occasional bursts of metabolic activity. Pyrazinamide, through its conversion within *M. tuberculosis* to pyrazinoic acid, appears most active against these organisms. Rifampin and isoniazid also may be active against this subpopulation. The third subset is the intracellular mycobacteria present within macrophages (10^4 to 10^6). Rifampin, isoniazid, and the quinolones appear to be most active against intracellular *M. tuberculosis*. While this appears to explain what happens during the treatment of TB, there is no practical way to quantitate these populations within a given patient.

Nonpharmacologic Therapy

7 Nonpharmacologic interventions aim to (a) prevent the spread of TB, (b) find where TB has already spread using contact investigation, and (c) replenish the weakened (consumptive) patient to a state of normal weight and well-being. The first two items are performed by public health departments. Clinicians involved in the treatment of TB should verify that the local health department has been notified of all new cases of TB.

Workers in hospitals and other institutions must prevent the spread of TB within their facilities.[7,24,27] All such workers should learn and follow each institution's infection control guidelines. This includes using personal protective equipment, including properly fitted respirators, and closing doors to "negative-pressure" rooms. These hospital isolation rooms draw air in from surrounding areas rather than blowing air (and *M. tuberculosis*) into these surrounding areas. The air from the isolation room may be treated with ultraviolet lights and then vented safely outside. However, these isolation rooms work properly only if the door is closed.

Debilitated TB patients may require therapy for other medical problems, including substance abuse and HIV infection, and some may need nutritional support. Therefore, clinicians involved in substance abuse rehabilitation and nutritional support services should be familiar with the needs of TB patients. Surgery may be needed to remove destroyed lung tissue, space-occupying infected lesions (*tuberculomas*), and certain extrapulmonary lesions.[37] BCG is the only clinically relevant vaccine for TB in use today. Although it is one of the most commonly administered vaccines in history, it is of limited value, and cannot prevent infection by *M. tuberculosis*. BCG (discussed further) may prevent extreme forms of TB in infants.[37,41]

Pharmacologic Therapy

Treating Latent Infection

Isoniazid is the preferred drug for treating LTBI.[24,37] Generally, isoniazid alone is given for 9 months. The treatment of LTBI reduces a person's lifetime risk of active TB from approximately 10% to approximately 1%. Because TB is spread easily through the air, each case prevented also prevents a second wave of cases that each prevented case would have produced. The treatment of LTBI has is called *prophylaxis*. Table 112-2 lists the LTBI treatment options.

Because young children, the elderly, and HIV-positive patients are at greater risk of active disease once infected with *M. tuberculosis*, they require careful evaluation. Once active TB is ruled out, they should receive treatment for latent infection.[24,37]

The keys to successful treatment of LTBI are (a) infection by an isoniazid-susceptible isolate, (b) adherence to the regimen, and (c) no exogenous reinfection.[24] Isoniazid adult doses are usually 300 mg daily (5-10 mg/kg of body weight)[37] (see Table 112-2). Lower doses are less effective.[24,42,43] Isoniazid should be given on an empty stomach, and antacids should be avoided within 2 hours

TABLE 112-2 Recommended Drug Regimens for Treatment of LTBI in Adults

Drug	Interval and Duration	Comments	Rating[a] (Evidence)[b] HIV–	HIV+
Isoniazid	Daily for 9 months[b,c]	In HIV-infected patients, isoniazid may be administered concurrently with NRTIs, protease inhibitors, or NNRTIs	A (II)	A (II)
	Twice weekly for 9 months[b,c]	DOT must be used with twice-weekly dosing	B (II)	B (II)
Isoniazid	Daily for 6 months[c]	Not indicated for HIV-infected persons, those with fibrotic lesions on chest radiographs, or children	B (I)	C (I)
	Twice weekly for 6 months[c]	DOT must be used with twice-weekly dosing	B (II)	C (I)
Rifampin	Daily for 4 months	For persons who are contacts of patients with isoniazid-resistant, rifampin-susceptible TB who cannot tolerate pyrazinamide	B (II)	B (III)
Isoniazid and rifapentine	Once weekly for 3 months	DOT must be used with once-weekly dosing. Not recommended for the following: children <2 years old, HIV/AIDS patients taking antiretroviral treatment, isoniazid- or rifampin-resistant strains, pregnant women or women expecting to become pregnant within the 12-week regimen	B (II)	B (II)

AIDS, acquired immunodeficiency syndrome; DOT, directly observed therapy; HIV, human immunodeficiency virus; LTBI, latent tuberculosis infection; NNRTIs, non-nucleoside reverse transcriptase inhibitors; NRTIs, nucleoside reverse transcriptase inhibitors.

[a]Strength of recommendation: A, preferred; B, acceptable alternative; C, offer when A and B cannot be given.

[b]Quality of evidence: I, randomized clinical trial data; II, data from clinical trials that are not randomized or were conducted in other populations; III, expert opinion.

[c]Recommended regimen for children younger than 18 years of age.

Adapted from Targeted tuberculin testing and treatment of latent tuberculosis infection. American Thoracic Society. MMWR Recomm Rep 2000;49(RR-6):31.

of dosing. Rifampin 600 mg daily for 4 months can be used when isoniazid resistance is suspected or when the patient cannot tolerate isoniazid.[24,37] There is a growing body of evidence that 4 months of rifampin may be a safer and more cost-effective alternative to 9 months of isoniazid. Four months of rifampin was significantly cheaper per patient completing treatment because of better completion and fewer adverse events.[44] The combination of pyrazinamide plus rifampin is no longer recommended because of higher than expected rates of hepatotoxicity. Rifabutin 300 mg daily might be substituted for rifampin for patients at high risk of drug interactions. When resistance to isoniazid and rifampin is suspected in the isolate causing infection, there are no randomized controlled trials to prove what regimen should be used to treat LTBI among contacts.[24,37] However, a course of 12-month regimen of a fluoroquinolone was effective in reducing the incidence of progression to active TB disease for MDR-TB contacts.[45] Regimens that *might* be effective include ethambutol plus levofloxacin, but data regarding efficacy are lacking.

In 2011, a randomized controlled trial compared 12 weeks of once-weekly isoniazid and rifapentine by DOT with daily self-administered isoniazid for 9 months.[46] This study, with over 8,000 participants, showed that the 12 weeks of weekly isoniazid and rifapentine given by DOT was not inferior in efficacy to 9 months of self-administered isoniazid, had a significantly higher completion rate (82% vs 69%), and was associated with fewer grade 3 or 4 adverse reactions (1.6% vs 3%).[46] Hypersensitivity reactions were more common with the isoniazid/rifapentine regimen and close clinical follow-up should be undertaken while experience is gained with this new regimen for LTBI therapy. The CDC now recommends the 12-week isoniazid/rifapentine regimen as an equal alternative to 9 months of daily isoniazid for treating LTBI in otherwise healthy patients aged older than or 12 years who have a predictive factor for greater likelihood of TB developing, which included recent exposure to contagious TB, conversion from negative to positive on an indirect test for infection (ie, IGRA or tuberculin skin test), and radiographic findings of healed pulmonary TB.[47] HIV-infected patients who are otherwise healthy and are not taking antiretroviral medications are also included in this category. However, precautions should be taken as HIV-infected patients are more likely to have extrapulmonary TB or pulmonary TB with normal findings on chest radiograph. For recent skin-test converters of all ages, the risk of active TB outweighs the risk for drug toxicity.[24,37] Pregnant women, alcoholics, and patients with poor diets who are treated with isoniazid should receive pyridoxine (vitamin B_6) 10 to 50 mg daily to reduce the incidence of central nervous system (CNS) effects or peripheral neuropathies. All patients who receive treatment of LTBI should be monitored monthly for adverse drug reactions and for possible progression to active TB.

Treating Active Disease

8 The CDC, American Thoracic Society (ATS), and the Infectious Diseases Society of America have published an algorithm for the treatment of TB (Fig. 112-2). The treatment of active TB requires the use of multiple drugs. There are two primary anti-TB drugs, isoniazid and rifampin, with the rest of the drugs having specific roles.[37,40] Isoniazid and rifampin should be used together whenever possible. Typically, *M. tuberculosis* is either very susceptible or very resistant to a given drug. Theoretically, minimal inhibitory concentration (MIC) results could be used to guide dosing in the treatment of moderately resistant *M. tuberculosis*, but this remains to be studied prospectively.[37,42]

Drug susceptibility testing should be done on the initial isolate for all patients with active TB. These data should guide the selection of drugs over the course of treatment.[12,37] However, some patients are unable to provide a suitable specimen for laboratory testing. If susceptibility data are not available for a given patient, the drug susceptibility data for the suspected source case or regional susceptibility data should be used.[12,37]

Drug resistance should be expected for patients presenting for the retreatment of TB. These patients require retesting of drug susceptibility using freshly collected specimens. It is imperative to learn what drugs the patient received and for how long the patient received them.[12,37] A treatment history, often called a "*drug-o-gram*," shows the start and stop dates of all antimycobacterial drugs on a horizontal bar graph.[37] A drug-o-gram should be constructed for all retreatment patients.

9 The standard TB treatment regimen is isoniazid, rifampin, pyrazinamide, and ethambutol for 2 months, followed by isoniazid and rifampin for 4 months, a total of 6 months of treatment.[37] If susceptibility to isoniazid, rifampin, and pyrazinamide is shown,

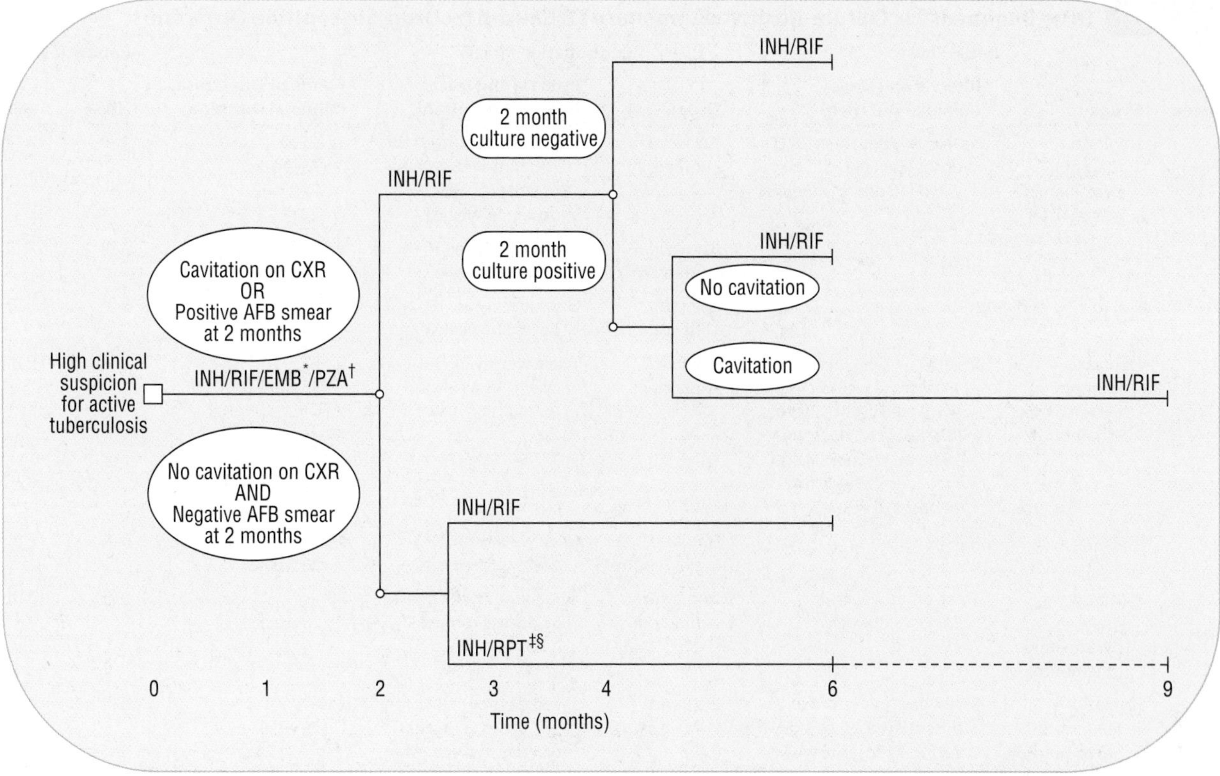

FIGURE 112-2 Treatment algorithm for tuberculosis (TB). Note: Patients in whom TB is proved or strongly suspected should have treatment initiated with isoniazid, rifampin, pyrazinamide, and ethambutol for the initial 2 months. A repeat smear and culture should be performed when 2 months of treatment has been completed. If cavities were seen on the initial chest radiograph or the acid-fast smear is positive at completion of 2 months of treatment, the continuation phase of treatment should consist of isoniazid and rifampin daily or twice weekly for 4 months to complete a total of 6 months of treatment. If cavitation was present on the initial chest radiograph and the culture at the time of completion of 2 months of therapy is positive, the continuation phase should be lengthened to 7 months (total of 9 months of treatment). If the patient has HIV infection and the CD^+ cell count is <100/μL (<100 × 10^6/L), the continuation phase should consist of daily or three-times-weekly isoniazid and rifampin. In HIV-uninfected patients having no cavitation on chest radiograph and negative acid-fast smears at completion of 2 months of treatment, the continuation phase may consist of either once-weekly isoniazid and rifapentine, or daily or twice-weekly isoniazid and rifampin, to complete a total of 6 months (bottom). Patients receiving isoniazid and rifapentine, and whose 2-month cultures are positive, should have treatment extended by an additional 3 months (total of 9 months). (CXR, chest radiograph; EMB, ethambutol; INH, isoniazid; PZA, pyrazinamide; RIF, rifampin; RPT, rifapentine.) [a]EMB may be discontinued when results of drug susceptibility testing indicate no drug resistance. [b]PZA may be discontinued after it has been taken for 2 months (56 doses). [c]RPT should not be used in HIV-infected patients with tuberculosis or in patients with extrapulmonary tuberculosis. [d]Therapy should be extended to 9 months if the 2-month culture is positive. *(Reproduced from American Thoracic Society, Centers for Disease Control and Prevention, Infectious Diseases Society of America. Treatment of tuberculosis. MMWR Recomm Rep 2003;52(RR-11):1-7.)*

ethambutol can be stopped at any time. Without pyrazinamide, a total of 9 months of isoniazid and rifampin treatment is required. Table 112-3 shows the recommended treatment regimens. When intermittent therapy is used, DOT is essential. Doses missed during an intermittent TB regimen decrease its efficacy and increase the relapse rate. Note that Table 112-3 shows recommendations that differ for HIV-negative and HIV-positive patients. HIV-positive patients should not receive highly intermittent regimens. In general, regimens given daily five times each week or three times weekly can be used for HIV-positive patients. Less frequent dosing is associated with higher failure and relapse rates and the selection of rifampin-resistant organisms.[37]

When a patient's sputum smears convert to a negative, the risk of the patient infecting others is greatly reduced, but it is not zero.[15,17,37] Such patients can be removed from respiratory isolation, but they must be careful not to cough on others and should meet with others only in well-ventilated places. Smear-negative patients still may be culture positive, so they still can transmit TB to others.

Clinical **Controversy...**

Effective therapy exists for the treatment of patients latently infected with drug susceptible TB; however, the data are limited for the latent treatment of drug-resistant strains of *M. tuberculosis.* Data for treatments of MDR-TB exposure are even more limited and treatment is often based on the resistance profile. Two or three drugs are used for 6 to 12 months while the patient is monitored in hopes that active disease does not develop. Randomized controlled trials are still needed to determine the best approach to treating those with exposure to MDR-TB.[48]

Patients who are slow to respond clinically, those who remain culture-positive at 2 months of treatment, those with cavitary lesions on chest radiograph, and perhaps HIV-positive patients should be treated for a total of 9 months and for at least 6 months from the time that they convert to smear and culture negativity.[37] Some authors

TABLE 112-3 Drug Regimens for Culture-Positive Pulmonary TB Caused by Drug-Susceptible Organisms

	Initial Phase		Continuation Phase			Rating[a] (Evidence)[b]	
Regimen	Drugs	Interval and Dose[c] (Minimal Duration)	Drugs	Interval and Doses[c,d] (Minimal Duration)	Range of Total Doses (Minimal Duration)	HIV–	HIV+
1	Isoniazid, rifampin, pyrazinamide, ethambutol	Seven days per week for 56 doses (8 weeks) or 5 days/wk for 40 doses (8 weeks)[e]	Isoniazid/rifampin	Seven days per week for 126 doses (18 weeks) or 5 days/wk for 90 doses (18 weeks)[e]	182-130 (26 weeks)	A (I)	A (II)
			Isoniazid/rifampin	Twice weekly for 36 doses (18 weeks)	92-76 (26 weeks)	A (I)	A (II)[f]
			Isoniazid/rifapentine[g]	Once weekly for 18 doses (18 weeks)	74-58 (26 weeks)	B (I)	E (I)
2	Isoniazid, rifampin, pyrazinamide, ethambutol	Seven days per week for 14 doses (2 weeks), then twice weekly for 12 doses (6 weeks) or 5 days/wk for 10 doses (2 weeks),[e] and then twice weekly for 12 doses (6 weeks)	Isoniazid/rifampin	Twice weekly for 36 doses (18 weeks)	62-58 (26 weeks)	A (II)	B (II)[f]
			Isoniazid/rifapentine[g]	Once weekly for 18 doses (18 weeks)	44-40 (26 weeks)	B (I)	E (I)
3	Isoniazid, rifampin, pyrazinamide, ethambutol	Three times weekly for 24 doses (8 weeks)	Isoniazid/rifampin	Three times weekly for 54 doses (18 weeks)	78 (26 weeks)	B (I)	B (II)
4	Isoniazid, rifampin, ethambutol	Seven days per week for 56 doses (8 weeks) or 5 days/wk for 40 doses (8 weeks)[e]	Isoniazid/rifampin	Seven days per week for 217 doses (31 weeks) or 5 days/wk for 155 doses (31 weeks)[e]	273-195 (39 weeks)	C (I)	C (II)
			Isoniazid/rifampin	Twice weekly for 62 doses (31 weeks)	118-102 (39 weeks)	C (I)	C (II)

[a]Ratings: A, preferred; B, acceptable alternative; C, offer when A and B cannot be given.

[b]Evidence ratings: I, randomized clinical trial; II, data from clinical trials that were not randomized or were conducted in other populations; III, expert opinion.

[c]When directly observed therapy is used, drugs may be given 5 days/wk, and the necessary number of doses adjusted accordingly. Although there are no studies that compare five with seven daily doses, extensive experience indicates this would be an effective practice.

[d]Patients with cavitation on initial chest radiograph and positive cultures at completion of 2 months of therapy should receive a 7-month (31-week; either 217 doses [daily] or 62 doses [twice weekly]) continuation phase.

[e]Five-day-a-week administration is always given by directly observed therapy. Rating for 5-day-per-week regimens is A (III).

[f]Not recommended for HIV-infected patients with CD4+ cell counts <100 cells/μL (<100 × 10^6/L).

[g]Should be used only in HIV-negative patients who have negative sputum smears at the time of completion of 2 months of therapy and who do not have cavitation on initial chest radiograph (see text). For patients started on this regimen and found to have a positive culture from the 2-month specimen, treatment should be extended an extra 3 months.

Adapted from American Thoracic Society, Centers for Disease Control and Prevention, Infectious Diseases Society of America. Treatment of tuberculosis. MMWR Recomm Rep *2003;52(RR-11):1–77.*

recommend therapeutic drug monitoring (TDM) the use of serum drug concentrations to optimize therapy for such patients.[40,42,49] When isoniazid and rifampin cannot be used, treatment durations become 2 years or more regardless of immune status.[37,40]

Adjustments to the regimen should be made once the susceptibility data are available.[37] If the organism is drug-resistant, careful consideration of the remaining therapeutic options must be made. Two or more drugs with in vitro activity against the patient's isolate and that the patient has not received previously should be added to the regimen, as needed.[37,40,48] 10 There is no standard regimen for MDR-TB.[37,48] Each patient's exposure history, treatment history (including toxicity and adherence issues), and current susceptibility data must be considered simultaneously. *It is critical to avoid monotherapy, and it is critical to never add a single drug to a failing regimen.*[37,40] Adding one drug at a time leads to the sequential selection of drug resistance until there are no drugs left. TB specialists should be consulted regarding cases of MDR-TB. It may take several months for a patient with MDR-TB to become culture-negative because the drugs used lack the potency of isoniazid and rifampin.[37,40] Consequently, prolonged respiratory isolation may be required.

Drug resistance should be considered in the following situations:

1. Patients who have received prior therapy for TB.
2. Patients from areas with a high prevalence of resistance (South Africa, Dominican Republic, Peru, Southeast Asia, the Baltic countries, and the former Soviet states).
3. Patients who are homeless, institutionalized, IV drug abusers, or infected with HIV.
4. Patients who still have AFB-positive sputum smears after 1 to 2 months of therapy.
5. Patients who still have positive cultures after 2 to 4 months of therapy.
6. Patients who fail treatment or relapse after treatment.
7. Patients known to be exposed to MDR-TB cases.

Empirical therapy with four or more drugs may be needed for acutely ill patients.[37] These regimens may be altered when the susceptibility pattern becomes known. If the index case is known, then the same effective regimen should be employed for the new case. Again, MDR-TB cases should be referred to specialists. A new term in use, *XDR-TB*, refers to "extensively drug-resistant TB." Such organisms are resistant to at least isoniazid, rifampin, a fluoroquinolone, and one second-line injectable drug (amikacin, capreomycin, or kanamycin).[48-50]

Special Populations

Tuberculous Meningitis and Extrapulmonary Disease

Patients with CNS TB usually are treated for longer periods (9-12 months instead of 6 months).[37] In general, isoniazid, pyrazinamide, ethionamide, and cycloserine penetrate the cerebrospinal fluid readily, but rifampin, ethambutol, and streptomycin have variable CNS penetration.[43] Of the quinolones, levofloxacin may be preferred based on current data. Extrapulmonary TB of the soft tissues can be treated with conventional regimens.[37] TB of the bone typically is treated for 9 months, occasionally with surgical debridement.[37]

Children TB in children may be treated with regimens similar to those used in adults, although some physicians still prefer to extend treatment to 9 months.[17,18,37] Pediatric doses of isoniazid and rifampin on a milligram-per-kilogram basis are higher than those used in adults (Table 112-4).[37]

Pregnancy Women with TB should be cautioned against becoming pregnant because the disease poses a risk to the fetus and to the mother. If already pregnant, the usual treatment is isoniazid, rifampin, and ethambutol for 9 months.[51] Isoniazid and ethambutol are relatively safe for use in pregnant women.[37,43,51] B vitamins are particularly important during pregnancy and should be provided to women being treated for TB. Rifampin is associated rarely with birth defects, including limb reduction and CNS lesions.[43] In general, rifampin is used in pregnant women with TB. Pyrazinamide has not been studied in large numbers of pregnant women, but anecdotal data suggest that it may be safe.[37]

Streptomycin use during pregnancy may lead to hearing loss in the newborn, including complete deafness. Streptomycin and the other aminoglycosides must be reserved for critical situations where alternatives do not exist.[37] Although the polypeptide capreomycin has not been studied, it probably carries the same risks.

Ethionamide may cause premature delivery and congenital deformities when used during pregnancy.[37,43] Down syndrome also has been reported with ethionamide, so it cannot be recommended in this setting. *p*-Aminosalicylic acid has been used safely in pregnancy, but specific data are lacking.[37,43] Cycloserine is known to cross the placenta, but the effects on the developing fetus are not known. Therefore, cycloserine generally cannot be recommended during pregnancy.[43]

Ciprofloxacin, levofloxacin, moxifloxacin, and the other quinolones are associated with permanent damage to cartilage in the weight-bearing joints of immature animals, especially dogs and rabbits.[37,43] Although these drugs do not frequently cause joint problems in humans, other anti-TB agents should be used during pregnancy.

Pregnant women with LTBI are not at the same level of risk compared with those with active disease. Therapy with isoniazid for LTBI may be delayed until after pregnancy. However in the case of recent infection documented by a skin-test conversion or a newly positive IGRA and in immunosuppressed women who are found to have LTBI while pregnant, treatment for LTBI is started during the second trimester of pregnancy.[37,43,51] Although most anti-TB drugs are excreted in breast milk, the amount of drug received by the infant through nursing is insufficient to cause toxicity. Quinolones should be avoided in nursing mothers, if possible.

HIV Infection For drug susceptible strains of tuberculosis, patients with AIDS and other immunocompromised hosts may be managed with chemotherapeutic regimens similar to those used in immunocompetent individuals, although treatment is often extended to 9 months (see Table 112-3).[37] The precise duration to recommend remains a matter of debate. Highly intermittent regimens (twice or once weekly) are not recommended for HIV-positive TB patients. Rifamycin based treatments are most effective; however, agents should be selected based on susceptibility and HIV drug interactions. Prognosis has been particularly poor for HIV-infected patients infected with MDR-TB, so all efforts should be made to reduce the time between clinical presentation, diagnosis of TB, and start of appropriate treatment. Recommendations for management of HIV and TB published by the World Health Organization and others have provided guidance on monitoring of treatment, side effects, and drug interactions of HIV and TB, MDR, XDR-TB.[5,50,52,53] Differentiation must be made between infection with *M. tuberculosis* and nontuberculous mycobacteria, such as *Mycobacterium avium* complex (MAC), because the drugs used are different. While awaiting laboratory results, the patient can be treated empirically for TB if there is any doubt about the causative organism. Some patients with AIDS malabsorb their oral medications; this is discussed in Therapeutic Drug Monitoring below.[40,42,49]

Renal Failure For nearly all patients, isoniazid and rifampin do not require dose modification in renal failure. They are eliminated primarily by the liver.[40,43,54] In the unlikely event that peripheral neuropathies develop, the frequency of isoniazid dosing may be reduced. Pyrazinamide and ethambutol typically require a reduction in dosing frequency from daily to three times weekly (Table 112-5).[37,54]

Renally cleared TB drugs include the aminoglycosides (amikacin, kanamycin, and streptomycin), capreomycin, ethambutol, cycloserine, and levofloxacin.[37,43,55] Dosing intervals need to be extended for these drugs (Table 112-5). Ciprofloxacin and moxifloxacin are approximately 50% cleared by the kidneys but may not require a change in dose from once daily, as used for TB. The metabolites of isoniazid, pyrazinamide, and *p*-aminosalicylic acid are cleared primarily by the kidneys. The role of these metabolites in causing toxicity is unknown, so their accumulation in renal failure may carry some risk.

Ethionamide and its sulfoxide metabolite are hepatically cleared, so dosing is unchanged.[37,55] *p*-Aminosalicylic acid is converted largely to metabolites prior to renal elimination; these metabolites may accumulate in renal failure.[55] For patients on hemodialysis, the usual 12-hour dosing interval for *p*-aminosalicylic acid granules seems to be safe. Dialysis will remove the metabolites. Serum concentration monitoring must be performed for cycloserine to avoid dose-related toxicities in renal failure patients.[40,42,55]

Hepatic Failure Anti-TB drugs that rely on hepatic clearance for most of their elimination include isoniazid, rifampin, pyrazinamide, ethionamide, and *p*-aminosalicylic acid.[43] Ciprofloxacin and moxifloxacin are approximately 50% cleared by the liver. Elevations of serum transaminase concentrations generally are not correlated with the residual capacity of the liver to metabolize drugs, so these markers cannot be used as guides for drug dosing. Furthermore, isoniazid, rifampin, pyrazinamide, and, to a lesser degree, ethionamide, *p*-aminosalicylic acid, and, rarely, ethambutol may cause hepatotoxicity.[37,40,43] For some patients with drug-susceptible TB, a "liver-sparing" regimen of streptomycin, levofloxacin, and ethambutol may be used, at least temporarily.[37,40,43] Because this regimen requires 18 or more months of treatment to be successful, patients usually are switched to isoniazid- and rifampin-containing regimens as soon as they are able.

Morbid Obesity Data are not available for dosing the TB drugs for patients with morbid obesity.[43] Relatively hydrophilic drugs (isoniazid, pyrazinamide, the aminoglycosides, capreomycin, ethambutol,

TABLE 112-4 Doses[a] of Antituberculosis Drugs for Adults and Children[b,c]

Drug	Preparation	Adults/ Children	Typical Doses: Daily	1× Per Week	2× Per Week	3× Per Week
First-Line Drugs						
Isoniazid	Tablets (50, 100, 300 mg); elixir (50 mg/5 mL); aqueous solution (100 mg/mL) for IV or intramuscular injection	Adults[c]	5 mg/kg	15 mg/kg	15 mg/kg	15 mg/kg
		Children[c]	10-15 mg/kg	—	20-30 mg/kg	—
Rifampin	Capsule (150, 300 mg); powder may be suspended for oral administration; aqueous solution for IV injection	Adults[d,c]	10 mg/kg	—	10 mg/kg	10 mg/kg
		Children[c]	10-20 mg/kg	—	10-20 mg/kg	—
Rifabutin	Capsule (150 mg)	Adult[d,c]	5 mg/kg	—	5 mg/kg	5 mg/kg
		Children	Appropriate dosing for children is unknown	Appropriate dosing for children is unknown	Appropriate dosing for children is unknown	Appropriate dosing for children is unknown
Rifapentine	Tablet (150 mg, film coated)	Adults[c]	—	10 mg/kg (continuation phase) (600 mg usual adult dose)	—	—
		Children	The drug is not approved for use in children	The drug is not approved for use in children	The drug is not approved for use in children	The drug is not approved for use in children
Pyrazinamide	Tablet (500 mg, scored)	Adults[c]	40-55 kg: 1,000 mg	—	40-55 kg: 2,000 mg	40-55 kg: 1,500 mg
			56-75 kg: 1,500 mg	—	56-75 kg: 3,000 mg	56-75 kg: 2,500 mg
			76-90 kg: 2,000 mg	—	76-90 kg: 4,000 mg	76-90 kg: 3,000 mg
		Children[c]	15-30 mg/kg	—	50 mg/kg	—
Ethambutol	Tablet (100, 400 mg)	Adults[c]	40-55 kg: 800 mg	—	40-55 kg: 2,000 mg	40-55 kg: 1,200 mg
			56-75 kg: 1,200 mg	—	56-75 kg: 2,800 mg	56-75 kg: 2,000 mg
			76-90 kg: 1,600 mg	—	76–90 kg: 4,000 mg	76-90 kg: 2,400 mg
		Children[d,c]	15-20 mg/kg daily	—	50 mg/kg	—
Second-Line Drugs						
Cycloserine	Capsule (250 mg)	Adults[c]	10-15 mg/kg/day, usually 500-750 mg/day in two doses[e]	No data	No data	No data
		Children[c]	10-15 mg/kg/day	—	—	—
Ethionamide	Tablet (250 mg)	Adults[f,c]	15-20 mg/kg/day, usually 500-750 mg/day in a single daily dose or two divided doses[f]	No data	No data	No data
		Children[c]	15-20 mg/kg/day	No data	No data	No data
Streptomycin	Aqueous solution (1-g vials) for IV or intramuscular administration	Adults[c]	15 mg/kg/day[g]	[g]	[g]	[g]
		Children[c]	20-40 mg/kg/day	—	20 mg/kg	—
Amikacin/ kanamycin	Aqueous solution (500-mg and 1-g vials) for IV or intramuscular administration	Adults[c]	15 mg/kg/day[g]	[g]	[g]	[g]
		Children[c]	15-30 mg/kg/day IV or intramuscular as a single daily dose	—	15-30 mg/kg	—
Capreomycin	Aqueous solution (1-g vials) for IV or intramuscular administration	Adults[c]	15 mg/kg/day[g]	[g]	15-30 mg/kg	[g]
		Children[c]	15-30 mg/kg/day as a single daily dose	—		—
p-Aminosalicylic acid (PAS)	Granules (4-g packets) can be mixed with food; tablets (500 mg) are still available in some countries, but not in the United States; a solution for IV administration is available in Europe	Adults[c]	8-12 g/day in two or three doses	No data	No data	No data
		Children[c]	200-300 mg/kg/day in two to four divided doses	No data	No data	No data

(continued)

The AHA guidelines provide very general recommendations for culture-negative infective endocarditis (see Table 111-7) and suggest that therapy should be guided based on the individual patient's past medical history and epidemiological risks identified. Selection of treatment can be difficult, balancing the need to cover all likely organisms against potential toxic drug effects (eg, aminoglycosides). Antimicrobial selection should involve consultation with an infectious disease specialist. Irrespective of the chosen treatment, extended antimicrobial therapy is required. The empirical approaches for culture-negative infective endocarditis highlight the need for proper collection and monitoring of blood cultures and an extensive medication history.

PERSONALIZED PHARMACOTHERAPY

Infective endocarditis remains an uncommon disease, but the cost of treatment can be substantial. In the past, the long duration of hospitalization required to administer IV antimicrobials was the major expense. In select cases, abbreviated and/or outpatient, oral antimicrobial therapy may appreciably reduce the cost of care.

Shorter-course antimicrobial regimens are advocated when possible. For instance, in sensitive streptococcal endocarditis (MICs <0.12 mcg/mL [mg/L]), a 2-week regimen of high-dose parenteral penicillin G or ceftriaxone in combination with an aminoglycoside is as effective as 4 weeks of penicillin alone.[4] Uncomplicated right-sided MSSA endocarditis in the IV drug abuser may be treated with a 2-week course of nafcillin, oxacillin, or daptomycin.

The initiation of outpatient parenteral antibiotics should be considered early in the treatment of infective endocarditis, after the patient is stable clinically and responds favorably to initial antibiotics. Outpatient treatment is safe and cost-effective in select situations.[26,102,103] Patients considered for home therapy must be hemodynamically stable, compliant with therapy, have careful medical monitoring, understand the potential complications of the disease, and have immediate access to medical care. Advances in technology allow for the outpatient administration of complex antibiotic regimens that significantly reduce the cost of therapy. Simple regimens, such as single daily doses of ceftriaxone for streptococcal infective endocarditis, are particularly attractive. Although endocarditis is common in those with a history of IVDA and home healthcare would substantially reduce the cost of treatment, many clinicians are uncomfortable with outpatient IV therapy because central venous access is required. Sudden cardiac decompensation in an outpatient setting is also of concern.[4]

EVALUATION OF THERAPEUTIC OUTCOMES

The evaluation of patients treated for infective endocarditis includes assessment of disease signs and symptoms, blood cultures, microbiologic tests, inflammatory markers, serum drug concentrations, and other tests that evaluate organ function.

Signs and Symptoms

Fever usually subsides within 1 week of initiating therapy.[17] Persistence of fever may indicate ineffective antimicrobial therapy, emboli, right-sided endocarditis, intravascular catheter infections, or drug reactions. For some patients, low-grade fever may persist even with appropriate antimicrobial therapy. With defervescence, the patient should begin to feel better, and other symptoms, such as lethargy or weakness, should subside. Echocardiography should be performed when antibiotic therapy has been completed to determine new baseline cardiac function (ie, ventricular size and function). A TTE is usually sufficient.

Blood Cultures

After initiation of appropriate therapy, blood cultures should be negative within a few days, although microbiologic response to vancomycin may be slower. If bacteria continue to be isolated from blood beyond the first few days of therapy, it may indicate that the antimicrobials are inactive against the pathogen or that the doses are not producing adequate concentrations at the site of infection. If this is the case, therapeutic adjustments should be made and blood cultures should be rechecked until negative. During the remainder of therapy, frequent blood cultures are not necessary but should be obtained if fever recurs.[4]

Microbiologic Tests

For all isolates from blood cultures, MICs should be determined; MBCs are no longer recommended.[4] The agent currently being used should be tested, as well as alternatives that may be required if intolerance, allergy, or resistance occurs. Occasionally, it is useful to determine whether synergy exists for antimicrobial combinations, although synergistic regimens usually can be predicted from the literature. Chapter 24 summarizes the methods for in vitro determinations of synergy.

Inflammatory Markers

Inflammatory markers are commonly used in infectious disease processes for diagnosing, monitoring of clinical outcomes, as well as assisting clinicians with evaluating the efficacy of antibiotic therapy. Currently only one inflammatory marker, rheumatoid factor (RF), is part of the modified Duke criteria for diagnosis. Other inflammatory markers, such as ESR, CRP, and procalcitonin (PCT), have all been investigated for evaluating the outcomes of patients with in endocarditis.[104] High PCT levels (eg, >0.5 ng/mL [mcg/L]) indicate the need for surgical intervention and correlate with poor outcomes (ie, death or serious infectious complications).[105,106] While these markers may be beneficial in assessing clinical outcomes, further evidence is needed to establish routine use for infective endocarditis.

Serum Drug Concentrations

Of the agents used commonly for infective endocarditis, measurement of serum drug concentrations is routinely available for aminoglycosides (except streptomycin) and vancomycin. Few data, however, support attaining any specific serum concentrations for patients with infective endocarditis. In general, serum concentrations of the antimicrobial should exceed the MIC of the organisms.

When aminoglycosides are administered for infective endocarditis caused by gram-positive cocci with a traditional three-times-daily regimen, peak serum concentrations are recommended to be on the low side of the traditional ranges (3-4 mcg/mL [mg/L; 6.3-8.4 μmol/L] for gentamicin). If extended-interval dosing is used, which is only recommended in streptococcal infective endocarditis, the most appropriate method of monitoring has not been determined. When vancomycin is administered, the primary goal is to ensure adequate trough concentrations, in this case 15 to 20 mcg/mL (mg/L; 10-14 μmol/L), are achieved.[107]

PREVENTION

10 Antimicrobial prophylaxis is used as an attempt to prevent infective endocarditis for patients who are at the highest risk.[6,5,18] The use of antimicrobials for this purpose requires consideration of (a) cardiac conditions associated with endocarditis, (b) procedures causing bacteremia, (c) organisms likely to cause endocarditis, and

Approximately 50% of whites and blacks and 80% to 90% of Asians and Native Alaskans are rapid acetylators. Slow acetylators have isoniazid half-lives of 3 to 4 hours and may be at an increased risk of neurotoxicity. The association of acetylator status and risk of hepatotoxicity, however, appears to be weak.[58] Poor absorption and rapid clearance of isoniazid for patients receiving highly intermittent therapy are associated with poor clinical outcomes.[59,60]

Transient elevations of the serum transaminases occur in 12% to 15% of patients receiving isoniazid and usually occur within the first 8 to 12 weeks of therapy.[37] Overt hepatotoxicity, however, occurs in only 1% of cases. Risk factors for hepatotoxicity include patient age, preexisting liver disease, excessive alcohol intake, pregnancy, co-administration of other medications that are potentially hepatotoxic, and the postpartum state. Isoniazid also may result in neurotoxicity, most frequently presenting as peripheral neuropathy or, in overdose, as seizures and coma. Patients with pyridoxine deficiency, such as pregnant women, alcoholics, children, and the malnourished, are at increased risk. Isoniazid may inhibit the metabolism of phenytoin, carbamazepine, primidone, and warfarin.[40] Patients who are being treated with these agents should be monitored closely, and appropriate dose adjustments should be made when necessary.

Rifampin The introduction of rifampin into routine use during the 1970s allowed for true short-course treatment of TB (6-9 months).[37] Without rifampin, treatment is generally 18 months or longer. Drug resistance to rifampin is an ominous prognostic factor because it is frequently associated with isoniazid resistance and leaves the patient with few good therapeutic options. Clinicians

TABLE 112-5 Dosing Recommendations for Adult Patients with Reduced Renal Function and for Adult Patients Receiving Hemodialysis

Drug	Change in Frequency?	Recommended Dose and Frequency for Patients with Creatinine Clearance <30 mL/min (<0.50 mL/s) or for Patients Receiving Hemodialysis[a,b,c,d]
Isoniazid	No change	300 mg once daily, or 900 mg three times per week
Rifampin	No change	600 mg once daily, or 600 mg three times per week
Pyrazinamide	Yes	25-35 mg/kg per dose three times per week (not daily)
Ethambutol	Yes	15-25 mg/kg per dose three times per week (not daily)
Levofloxacin	Yes	750-1,000 mg per dose three times per week (not daily)
Cycloserine	Yes	250 mg once daily, or 500 mg/dose three times per week[e]
Ethionamide	No change	250-500 mg/dose daily
p-Aminosalicylic acid	No change	4 g/dose, twice daily
Streptomycin	Yes	12-15 mg/kg per dose two or three times per week (not daily)
Capreomycin	Yes	12-15 mg/kg per dose two or three times per week (not daily)
Kanamycin	Yes	12-15 mg/kg per dose two or three times per week (not daily)
Amikacin	Yes	12-15 mg/kg per dose two or three times per week (not daily)

[a]Standard doses are given unless there is intolerance.

[b]The medications should be given after hemodialysis on the day of hemodialysis.

[c]Monitoring of serum drug concentrations should be considered to ensure adequate drug absorption, without excessive accumulation, and to assist in avoiding toxicity.

[d]Data currently are not available for patients receiving peritoneal dialysis. Until data become available, begin with doses recommended for patients receiving hemodialysis and verify adequacy of dosing, using serum concentration monitoring.

[e]The appropriateness of 250-mg daily doses has not been established. There should be careful monitoring for evidence of neurotoxicity.

Adapted from American Thoracic Society, Centers for Disease Control and Prevention, Infectious Diseases Society of America. Treatment of tuberculosis. MMWR Recomm Rep 2003;52(RR-11):1–77.

Mycobacterium bovis and *M. kansasii*.[61] It also is active against a broad array of other bacteria. Alteration of the target site on RNA polymerase, primarily through changes in the *rpoB* gene, leads to most forms of rifampin resistance.[37,61]

Rifampin usually is given orally, but it also can be given as a 30-minute IV infusion.[61] Oral doses are best given on an empty stomach.[62] Patients with AIDS, diabetes, and other GI problems appear to have difficulty absorbing rifampin after oral doses, and this has been associated with therapeutic failures in some cases.[40,42,60,63] Rifampin is metabolized to 25-desacetyl rifampin, which retains some of rifampin's activity; most of rifampin and its metabolite are cleared in the bile. Rifampin generally is given at 600 mg daily or intermittently, although this dose does not take full advantage of rifampin's concentration-dependent killing.[40,42] Higher doses should be tested in humans within the context of clinical trials.

...tions in hepatic enzymes have been attributed to rifampin ... with overt hepatotoxicity occurring in ... ffects of rifampin include ... been

doses 900 mg or more twice weekly. These reactions may take the form of a flu-like syndrome with development of fever, chills, headache, arthralgias, and, rarely, hypotension and shock.[37] Alternatively, hemolytic anemia or acute renal failure may occur, requiring permanent discontinuation.

Rifampin's potent induction of hepatic enzymes, especially cytochrome P450 3A4, may enhance the elimination of many other drugs, most notably the protease inhibitors used to treat HIV (Table 112-6). HIV-positive patients may benefit from the use of rifabutin instead of rifampin.[25,37,52,64] Furthermore, women who use oral contraceptives must use another form of contraception during therapy because increased clearance of the hormones may lead to unexpected pregnancies. Patient records should be reviewed for potential drug interactions before dispensing rifampin. Rifampin may turn urine and other secretions orange-red and may permanently stain some types of contact lenses.

Other Rifamycins Rifabutin is used for disseminated *M. avium* infection in AIDS patients and is quite active against *M. tuberculosis*. Most rifampin-resistant organisms are resistant to rifabutin. Because rifabutin is a less potent enzyme inducer than rifampin, it may be used for patients who are receiving protease inhibitors.[37,52,64,65] For HIV-positive patients, the ATS/CDC recommends regimens with three or more doses of the TB drugs per week (see Table 112-3). Rifapentine is a long-acting rifamycin that can be used once weekly in the continuation phase of treatment (after the first 2 months) in carefully selected HIV-negative patients. It is approximately as potent an enzyme inducer as rifampin, so similar drug interactions are likely.[37,52,64,65]

Pyrazinamide Adding pyrazinamide to the first 2 months of treatment with isoniazid and rifampin shortens the duration to 6 months for most patients.[37] Pyrazinamide may be bacteriostatic or bactericidal depending on the concentration and the susceptibility of the organism. It is usually well absorbed and displays a fairly long half-life.[66,67] The most common toxicities of pyrazinamide are GI distress, arthralgias, and elevations in the serum uric acid concentrations.[37] Most patients do not experience true gout. Hepatotoxicity is the major limiting adverse effect and is dose-related when pyrazinamide is given daily.

A fixed-combination product (Rifater, Aventis) of rifampin 120 mg, isoniazid 50 mg, and pyrazinamide 300 mg is designed to prevent drug resistance by keeping the self-medicating patient from using only one drug at a time. If the patient is receiving DOT, there is no particular advantage to this product. The typical dose of Rifater will be five to six tablets daily. When pyrazinamide is discontinued after 2 months of treatment, the combination product Rifamate (isoniazid 150 mg and rifampin 300 mg) can be substituted.

Ethambutol Ethambutol replaced *p*-aminosalicylic acid as a first-line agent in the 1960s because it was better tolerated by patients.[37] It is used as a fourth drug for TB while awaiting susceptibility data.[37] If the organism is susceptible to isoniazid, rifampin, and pyrazinamide, ethambutol can be stopped. Ethambutol is active against most mycobacteria, by inhibiting synthesis of metabolites and impairing cell metabolism, and is generally bacteriostatic.

Ethambutol should not be given with antacids.[68] For patients with renal failure, the ethambutol dose should be reduced to three times per week.[54,69] Retrobulbar neuritis is the major adverse effect. Patients may complain of a change in visual acuity, the inability to see the color green, or both. They should be monitored monthly while on the drug using Snellen wall charts for visual acuity and Ishihara red-green color discrimination cards.[31,37]

Second-Line Antituberculosis Drugs

Streptomycin Streptomycin is one of three aminoglycoside ...tibiotics (along with amikacin and kanamycin) that are active

) pharmacokinetics, spectrum, cost, adverse effects, and ease of ministration of available antimicrobial agents. The objective of phylaxis is to diminish the likelihood of infective endocarditis igh-risk individuals from procedures that result in bacteremia. ough there are no prospective, controlled human trials demon- ng that prophylaxis in high-risk individuals protects against evelopment of endocarditis during bacteremia-inducing pro- s, animal studies suggest possible benefit.[18] However, other have questioned the benefit of antibiotic prophylaxis prior sive procedures.[108] Furthermore, many causes of infective ditis appear not to be secondary to an invasive procedure. ia as a consequence of daily activities may, in fact, be the prit, and the value of antibiotic prophylaxis before bacteremia- rocedures has been questioned.[109] The literature lacks ade- ence to prove the effectiveness or ineffectiveness of anti- hylaxis, and the common practice of using antimicrobial his setting remains controversial.[110] The mechanism of a fect in humans is unclear, but antibiotics may decrease of bacteria at the surgical site, kill bacteria after they d into the blood, and prevent adhesion of bacteria to

Controversy...

practice of administering antibiotics to high- before a bacteremia-causing procedure is espite limited data supporting this approach t 100% compliance with AHA preventative d have only a modest benefit, the use of iotics for the prevention of endocarditis d of care.

controversy about whether prophylactic anti- infective endocarditis prophylaxis is recom- ons, specifically dental procedures, in those sk cardiac conditions. The AHA released better define who should and should not litis prophylaxis.[18] The appropriateness of ver, has been called into question due to wing an increase in the overall incidence tococcus.[8]

rt are that (a) only a small number of is might be prevented with antibiotic ocedures, even if 100% effective; hylaxis for dental procedures should tients with underlying cardiac con- ghest risk; (c) for those with high- ions, prophylaxis is recommended ng manipulation of gingival tissue eth or perforation of the oral ecommended based solely on an on of infective endocarditis; and olely to prevent endocarditis is undergo a genitourinary or GI

t should receive prophylactic tient's risk and whether he or g in bacteremia. When antibi- 2 g dose of amoxicillin is rec- ven 30 to 60 minutes before h bacteremia. Because the pears to be relatively short, dose of amoxicillin, which prophylaxis regimens for

TABLE 111-10 Prophylaxis of Infective Endocarditis

Highest Risk Cardiac Conditions	Presence of a prosthetic heart valve Prior diagnosis of infective endocarditis Cardiac transplantation with subsequent valvulopathy Congenital heart disease (CHD)[a]	
Types of procedures	Any that require perforation of the oral mucosa or manipulation of the periapical region of the teeth of gingival tissue	
Antimicrobial Options	**Adult Doses[b]**	**Pediatric Doses[b] (mg/kg)**
Oral amoxicillin	2 g	50
IM or IV ampicillin[c]	2 g	50
IM or IV cefazolin or ceftriaxone[c,d,e]	1 g	50
Oral cephalexin[d,e,f]	2 g	50
Oral clindamycin[e]	600 mg	20
Oral azithromycin or clarithromycin[e]	500 mg	15
IV or IM clindamycin[c,e]	600 mg	20

[a]Includes only the following: unrepaired cyanotic CHD, prophylaxis within the first 6 months of implanting prosthetic material to repair a congenital heart defect, and repaired CHD with residual defects at or adjacent to prosthetic material.

[b]All one-time doses administered 30-60 minutes prior to initiation of the procedure.

[c]For patients unable to tolerate oral medication.

[d]Should be avoided in patients with immediate-type hypersensitivity reaction to penicillin or ampicillin (eg, anaphylaxis, urticaria, or angioedema).

[e]Option for patients with nonimmediate hypersensitivity reaction to penicillin or ampicillin.

[f]May substitute with an alternative first- or second-generation cephalosporin at an equivalent dose.

Data from reference 18.

patients allergic to penicillins or those unable to take oral medications are also provided. A summary of guideline recommendations is available in Table 111-10. Consultation of the full AHA guideline is suggested for more detailed information.[18]

ABBREVIATIONS

AHA	American Heart Association
CDIE	cardiac device infective endocarditis
CHD	congenital heart disease
CRP	C-reactive protein
ESC	European Society of Cardiology
ESR	erythrocyte sedimentation rate
HACEK	the group of bacteria including *Haemophilus parainfluenzae, Haemophilus aphrophilus, Aggregatibacter* species, *Cardiobacterium hominis, Eikenella corrodens*, and *Kingella kingae*
IE	infective endocarditis
IVDA	IV drug abuse
MBC	minimal bactericidal concentration
MIC	minimal inhibitory concentration
MRSA	methicillin-resistant *Staphylococcus aureus*
MSSA	methicillin-sensitive *Staphylococcus aureus*
NVE	native valve endocarditis
PCT	procalcitonin
PVE	prosthetic valve endocarditis
RF	rheumatoid factor
SBT	serum bactericidal titer
TEE	transesophageal echocardiography
TTE	transthoracic echocardiography

TABLE 112-6 Recommended Regimens for the Concomitant Treatment of TB and HIV Infection in Adults

Combined Regimen for Treatment of HIV and TB	PK Effect of the Rifamycin	Tolerability/Toxicity	Antiviral Activity When Used with Rifamycin	Recommendations (Comments)
Efavirenz-based antiretroviral therapy[a] with rifampin-based TB treatment	Well-characterized, modest decrease in concentrations in some patients	Low rates of discontinuation	Excellent	Preferred (efavirenz should not be used during the first trimester of pregnancy)
PI-based antiretroviral therapy[a] with rifabutin-based TB treatment	Little effect of rifabutin on PI concentrations, but marked increases in rifabutin concentrations	Low rates of discontinuation (if rifabutin is appropriately dose-reduced)	Favorable, although published clinical experience is not extensive	Preferred for patients unable to take efavirenz[b] (caution to ensure patients who discontinue PI not to continue to receive reduced rifabutin dose)
Nevirapine-based antiretroviral therapy with rifampin-based TB treatment	Moderate decrease in concentrations	Concern about hepatotoxicity when used with isoniazid, rifampin, and pyrazinamide	Suboptimal when nevirapine is initiated using once-daily dosing largely favorable when nevirapine is given twice daily throughout co-treatment	Alternative for patients who cannot take efavirenz, though efavirenz is preferred (nevirapine should not be initiated among women with CD4>250 [>200 × 10^6/L] or men with CD4>400 cells/μL[>400 ×10^6/L])
Raltegravir-based antiretroviral therapy with rifampin-based TB treatment	Significant decrease in concentrations with standard dosing	Limited experience	Limited published clinical experience	Alternative at higher doses for patients who cannot take efavirenz and who have baseline viral load <100,000 copes/mL (<100 × 10^6/L)
Zidovudine/lamivudine/abacavir/tenofovir with rifampin-based TB treatment	50% decrease in zidovudine, possible effect on abacavir not evaluated	Anemia	No published clinical experience, but this regimen is less effective than efavirenz or atazanavir basd regimens in person not taking rifampin	Alternative for patients who cannot take efavirenz or nevirapine and if rifabutin not available
Zidovudine/lamivudine/tenofovir with rifampin-based TB treatment	50% decrease in zidovudine, no other effects predicted	Anemia	Favorable, but not evaluated in a randomized trial	Alternative for patients who cannot take efavirenz and abacavir and if rifabutin not available
Zidovudine/lamivudine/abacavir with rifampin-based TB treatment	50% decrease in zidovudine, possible effect on abacavir not evaluated	Anemia	Early favorable experience, but this combination is less effective than efavirenz or nevirapine based regimens in persons not taking rifampin	Alternative for patients who cannot take efavirenz and tenofovir and if rifabutin not available
Superboosted[c] lopinavir-based antiretroviral therapy or double dose lopinavir/ritonavir based therapy with rifampin-based TB treatment	Moderate decrease in concentrations	Hepatitis	Early favorable experience of super-boosting among young children and double dose among adults already on antiretroviral drugs at the time of rifampin initiation	Alternative if rifabutin not available; double dose an option among adults already taking lopinavir based antiretroviral therapy and virologically suppressed at the time of tuberculosis treatment initiation; super boosting has not been adequately tested in adults ut may be effective

ART, antiretroviral therapy; HIV, human immunodeficiency virus; TB, tuberculosis.

[a]With two nucleoside analogues.

[b]Includes patients with NNRTI-resistant HIV, those unable to tolerate efavirenz, and women during the first one to two trimesters of pregnancy.

[c]Super boosting of lopinavir is achieved by giving lopinavir 400 mg together with 400 mg ritonavir twie daily. Doble dose lopinavir/ritonavir is lopinavir 800 mg plus ritonavir 200 mg twice daily.

Adapted from Centers for Disease Control and Prevention. Managing Drug Interactions in the Treatment of HIV Related Tuberculosis. 2013.

against mycobacteria. It is quite active against MAC and several other mycobacteria, enterococci, *Brucella*, *Yersinia*, and various other bacteria. Although labeled only for intramuscular dosing, streptomycin can be given safely as IV infusions (100 mL of 5% dextrose in water or normal saline) over 30 minutes, similar to the other aminoglycosides.[70] Streptomycin, like other aminoglycosides, is renally cleared by glomerular filtration and must be given less often to patients with renal dysfunction.[37,40]

Streptomycin occasionally causes nephrotoxicity, although it tends to be mild and reversible. It also is capable of causing ototoxicity (vestibular and cochlear), which may become permanent with continued use.[37] Older patients and those receiving long durations of treatment are most likely to experience hearing loss, whereas vestibular toxicity is highly unpredictable.

Resistance to amikacin and kanamycin is frequently linked but independent of resistance to streptomycin and independent of resistance to capreomycin. Therefore, susceptibility tests should guide the selection of these injectable drugs.

***p*-Aminosalicylic Acid** In the United States, only the enteric-coated, sustained-release granule form (Paser) is available.[71-73] GI disturbances are the most common adverse effects from *p*-aminosalicylic acid. Diarrhea is usually self-limited, with symptoms improving after the first 1 to 2 weeks of therapy. Occasionally, a few doses of an opioid will resolve the problem. It also is important to tell the patient that the empty granules will appear in the stool. Although FDA-approved for three daily doses, pharmacokinetic data support twice-daily dosing.[72]

Various types of malabsorption, including steatorrhea, were reported with previous dosage forms of *p*-aminosalicylic acid. Hypersensitivity and, rarely, severe hepatitis may occur. *p*-Aminosalicylic acid is known to produce goiter, with or without myxedema, which seems to occur more frequently with concomitant ethionamide therapy.

Cycloserine Cycloserine is only used to treat MDR-TB. It is well absorbed orally and is best taken on an empty stomach.[74] It is cleared primarily through the kidneys by glomerular filtration and requires dosage reduction in renal failure. Cycloserine can produce dose-related CNS toxicity, including lethargy, confusion, or unusual behavior. Seizures, although reported, are exceedingly rare in US patients.[37] Therapy is improved by maintaining 2-hour postdose serum concentrations between 20 and 35 mcg/mL (mg/L; 200 and 349 μmol/L).[40,42] Most patients reach a dose of 750 mg daily, divided unevenly into two doses. This can be achieved by starting with 250 mg daily for 2 days, followed by 250 mg increments over 2-day intervals. This dose of cycloserine can be maintained if the patient complains of only occasional mild CNS effects, such as difficulty concentrating. Serum concentrations can be checked 1 to 2 weeks into therapy. The addition of pyridoxine 50 mg daily may improve patient tolerance of cycloserine.

Ethionamide Ethionamide shares structural features with two other antimycobacterial agents, isoniazid and, more distantly, thiacetazone, a drug not used in the United States. Prothionamide, the *n*-propyl derivative of ethionamide, is used in Europe. Ethionamide is only active against organisms of the genus *Mycobacterium*, and it should be considered primarily bacteriostatic because it is difficult to achieve serum concentrations that would be bactericidal.[37,40,42]

GI toxicity is the dose-limiting adverse effect. The drug should be introduced gradually in 250 mg increments, as described earlier for cycloserine. Rarely will a patient tolerate more than 1,000 mg daily in divided oral doses. Ethionamide may be administered with a light snack or prior to bedtime to minimize GI intolerance. Food does not affect absorption significantly.[75] Little ethionamide is recovered in the urine, so doses remain the same in renal failure. Ethionamide may cause goiter with or without hypothyroidism (especially when given with *p*-aminosalicylic acid), gynecomastia, alopecia, impotence, menorrhagia, photodermatitis, and acne. The management of diabetes also may be more difficult for patients receiving ethionamide. Because of these problems, ethionamide only is used when necessary.

Clofazimine Clofazimine is a drug with good activity against *Mycobacterium leprae* and some activity against *M. tuberculosis* and *M. avium*. It is used in doses of 100 mg daily in advanced cases of MDR-TB or MAC, especially when therapeutic options are limited.[37,40] The drug has a terminal elimination half-life that is weeks long. GI distress and skin discoloration are the most important adverse reactions. Although uncommon, severe GI pain may occur because of deposition of clofazimine crystals within the intestines; this may require surgical correction.

Thiacetazone This is a weak agent used rarely in parts of the developing world because of its low cost. Skin reactions, including rash and Stevens-Johnson syndrome, may occur. Thiacetazone must be discontinued permanently as soon as a rash appears. Similar to trimethoprim–sulfamethoxazole, the incidence of skin reactions is much higher for AIDS patients.[76]

Quinolones Levofloxacin, moxifloxacin, and gatifloxacin (outside of the United States), are sometimes used to treat MDR-TB because of their excellent activity against *M. tuberculosis*. Several studies have suggested a potential role for moxifloxacin as a possible replacement for certain first-line agents.[40,77-79] Moxifloxacin has been compared with isoniazid and ethambutol during the first 8 weeks of therapy for pulmonary TB. It did not demonstrate a significant increase in 8-week culture negativity when compared with isoniazid. However, shorter time to culture conversion was seen when compared with ethambutol.[78] Quinolones are useful because most are available in oral and IV dosage forms, so they can be used in critically ill patients. However, resistance of MTB to the fluoroquinolones is a major concern. Resistance is attributed to mutations in the *gyrA* and *gyrB* genes and can develop in a relatively short period of time.[80]

Macrolides/Azalides The macrolide clarithromycin and azalide azithromycin represent substantial advances in the treatment of MAC but demonstrate limited activity against *M. tuberculosis* and are not used frequently for TB.[37,40]

New Drugs and Delivery Systems Several promising compounds are currently under development for the treatment of MTB.

Bedaquiline is a diarylquinoline, approved for use by the FDA, which works through targeting the ATP synthase pump, and does not demonstrate cross-resistance with existing TB drugs. The WHO and CDC have issued recommendations stating that bedaquiline may be used at a dose of 400 mg daily for 2 weeks and then 200 mg three times a week for 22 weeks of treatment in adults with pulmonary MDR-TB when an effective treatment regimen cannot otherwise be provided.[81] Bedaquiline may be used on a case-by-case basis in children, HIV-infected persons, pregnant women, and extrapulmonary TB. Patients treated with bedaquiline should be closely monitored every week for potential side effects and an electrocardiogram (QT monitoring) should be performed at baseline and at weeks 2, 12, and 24.[81] The QT monitoring is required due to a black box warning issued by the FDA as a result of increased rates of death due to QT prolongation in patients receiving bedaquiline.

Delamanid, PA-824 and TBA-354 are all nitroimidazole derivatives which are chemically related to metronidazole and work through inhibiting mycolic acid synthesis. All of these agents have potent in vitro and in vivo activity with very low MICs against *M. tuberculosis*.[82-84] Delamanid has centralized marketing authorization by the European Medicines Agency for use in the European Union.[81,83,85] PA-824 is undergoing phase two studies and TBA-354 has shown benefit in preclinical trials. Combinations of PA-824 with other anti-TB drugs are also being investigated. AZD-5847 is another potentially new drug currently being investigated in Phase 2a trials.[86] Linezolid has also been used in some patients with MDR-TB.[87] Long-term use of linezolid requires careful monitoring of hematologic indices for potential anemia and thrombocytopenia. It may be possible to reduce the incidences of these toxicities by giving linezolid 600 mg daily or 300 mg twice daily for the slow-growing *M. tuberculosis* rather than the usual 600 mg twice-daily dose used for gram-positive organisms. Liposomes have been investigated as delivery systems for various agents against mycobacteria, including isoniazid, rifampin, and the aminoglycosides. By changing the pharmacokinetic profile of such agents, their use in the treatment of mycobacterial infections could be enhanced greatly. Currently, no such product is licensed for use against TB.

Corticosteroids Adjunctive therapy with corticosteroids may be of benefit for some patients with tuberculous meningitis or pericarditis to relieve inflammation and pressure.[37] They should be avoided in most other circumstances because they detract from the immune response to TB.

Bacille Calmette-Guérin Vaccine The BCG vaccine is an attenuated, hybridized strain of *M. bovis*. It was developed in 1921 and is used as a prophylactic vaccine against TB. Administration of BCG vaccine is compulsory in many developing countries and is officially recommended in many others. Vaccination with BCG produces a subclinical infection resulting in sensitization of T lymphocytes and cross-immunity to *M. tuberculosis*, as well as cutaneous hypersensitivity and, in many cases, a positive tuberculin skin test.

The efficacy of several different BCG preparations ranged from negative 56% (some patients did worse with the vaccine) to positive 80%.[37] Trials within the United States and Puerto Rico have shown efficacy rates of 6% to 29%. The primary benefit of BCG vaccination appears to be the prevention of severe forms of TB in children. Data from the BCG trials show that the incidence of tuberculous meningitis and miliary TB is 52% to 100% lower and that the incidence of pulmonary TB is 2% to 80% lower in vaccinated children younger than 15 years than it was in unvaccinated controls.

Unfortunately, BCG does not appear to be reliable in preventing disease by *M. tuberculosis* in other segments of the population. Side effects occur in 1% to 10% of vaccinated persons and usually include severe or prolonged ulceration at the vaccination site, lymphadenitis, and lupus vulgaris. Pregnant women and patients with impaired immune systems, including those with HIV infection, should avoid vaccination. The World Health Organization had recommended, however, that in populations where the risk of TB is high, HIV-infected infants who are asymptomatic should receive BCG vaccine at birth or as soon as possible thereafter. Because BCG infection has occurred in AIDS patients given the vaccine, individuals with symptomatic HIV infection should not be vaccinated.[37]

In the United States, BCG vaccination is recommended only for uninfected children who are at unavoidable risk of exposure to TB and for whom other methods of prevention and control have failed or are not feasible.[37] Its use is very limited.

PERSONALIZED PHARMACOTHERAPY

Desired treatment outcomes for tuberculosis infections require aggressive treatment and rapid identification and both latent and active disease states. Treatment must be individualized based antimicrobial susceptibilities. Appropriate treatment selection is critical to avoid resistance. TDM may be necessary in certain populations. Extended durations of therapy are required for treatment of Mycobacterial diseases so health care professionals should develop a plan to monitor efficacy, adherence, adverse drug reactions, and interactions to TB therapy through regular assessments and monitoring. Directly observed therapy may be required to assure compliance. Patients coinfected with HIV will require special attention because of their immunocompromised state and increased risk of drug interactions.

Therapeutic Drug Monitoring

TDM, or applied pharmacokinetics, generally should be used if patients are failing appropriate treatment (no clinical improvement after 2-4 weeks or smear positive after 4-6 weeks).[40,42,88,89] Patients with AIDS, diabetes, obesity, cystic fibrosis, various GI disorders, or MDR-TB may be tested prospectively, before problems arise, to ensure adequate treatment. Blood samples collected at 2 and 6 hours after a dose have been used with some success, although they may not be the optimal sampling times for all the drugs. Finally, TDM of the TB and HIV drugs is perhaps the most logical way to untangle the complex drug interactions that take place.[90,91]

Clinical **Controversy...**

Some TB centers employ TDM for many of their patients at the outset of treatment in order to identify drug-delivery problems early. Other centers wait to see how the patient responds and perform TDM only if problems arise. An argument can be made for either approach. The latter can save money in the short-term, but delays in effective treatment can affect the patient's outcome adversely.

EVALUATION OF THERAPEUTIC OUTCOMES

Monitoring of the Pharmaceutical Care Plan

The most serious problem with TB therapy is patient nonadherence to the prescribed regimens.[92] Unfortunately, there is no reliable way to identify such patients a priori. Noncompliance rates of up to 89% have been reported with TB therapy.[92] It is critical to the control of TB that such adherence rates be improved dramatically. The most effective way to achieve this end is with DOT.[37] Despite criticisms that it will cost more money, it is far cheaper in the long run to prevent the further spread of disease with DOT than to track down and treat additional cases of TB continuously.

The homeless and other underprivileged individuals are assumed to constitute the group of patients considered "unreliable," and DOT should be reserved for them; it is also assumed that "responsible" patients cared for by private physicians may be treated with daily, unsupervised therapy. A study conducted in Baltimore, however, compared outcomes (sputum culture conversion to negative at 3 months) for patients with pulmonary TB who were treated by private physicians with outcomes for patients treated via DOT in a city-run clinic. Surprisingly, 3-month culture conversion occurred in only 40% of the private-care patients, compared with 90% in the city clinic-care patients.[3] Clearly, expansion of the use of DOT to nearly all patients with TB may be of benefit.

Patients who are AFB-smear positive should have sputum samples sent for AFB stains every 1 to 2 weeks until two consecutive smears are negative. This provides early evidence of a response to treatment.[37] Once on maintenance therapy, sputum cultures can be performed monthly until two consecutive cultures are negative, which generally occurs over 2 to 3 months. If sputum cultures continue to be positive after 2 months, drug susceptibility testing should be repeated, and serum concentrations of the drugs should be checked.

Serum chemistries, including blood urea nitrogen, creatinine, aspartate transaminase, and alanine transaminase, and a complete blood count with platelets should be performed at baseline and periodically thereafter, depending on the presence of other factors that may increase the likelihood of toxicity (eg, advanced age, alcohol abuse, pregnancy)[37] (Table 112-7). Hepatotoxicity should be suspected for patients whose serum transaminases exceed five times the upper limit of normal or whose total bilirubin concentration exceeds 3 mg/dL (51.3 μmol/L) and for patients with symptoms such as nausea, vomiting, or jaundice. At this point, the offending agent(s) should be discontinued. Sequential reintroduction of the drugs with frequent testing of liver enzymes is often successful in identifying the offending agent; other agents may be continued.

TABLE 112-7 Antituberculosis Drug Monitoring Table

Drug	Adverse Effects	Monitoring
Isoniazid	Asymptomatic elevation of aminotransferases, clinical hepatitis, fatal hepatitis, peripheral neurotoxicity, CNS effects, lupus-like syndrome, hypersensitivity, monoamine poisoning, diarrhea	LFT monthly in patients who have preexisting liver disease or who develop abnormal liver function that does not require discontinuation of drug; dosage adjustments may be necessary in patients receiving anticonvulsants or warfarin
Rifampin	Cutaneous reactions, GI reactions (nausea, anorexia, abdominal pain), flu-like syndrome, hepatotoxicity, severe immunologic reactions, orange discoloration of bodily fluids (sputum, urine, sweat, tears), drug interactions due to induction of hepatic microsomal enzymes	Liver enzymes and interacting drugs as needed (eg, warfarin)
Rifabutin	Hematologic toxicity, uveitis, GI symptoms, polyarthralgias, hepatotoxicity, pseudojaundice (skin discoloration with normal bilirubin), rash, flu-like syndrome, orange discoloration of bodily fluids (sputum, urine, sweat, tears)	Drug interactions are less problematic than rifampin
Rifapentine	Similar to those associated with rifampin	Drug interactions are being investigated and are likely similar to rifampin
Pyrazinamide	Hepatotoxicity, GI symptoms (nausea, vomiting), nongouty polyarthralgia, asymptomatic hyperuricemia, acute gouty arthritis, transient morbilliform rash, dermatitis	Serum uric acid can serve as a surrogate marker for adherence; LFTs in patients with underlying liver disease
Ethambutol	Retrobulbar neuritis, peripheral neuritis, cutaneous reactions	Baseline visual acuity testing and testing of color discrimination; monthly testing of visual acuity and color discrimination in patients taking >15–20 mg/kg, having renal insufficiency, or receiving the drug for >2 months
Streptomycin	Ototoxicity, neurotoxicity, nephrotoxicity	Baseline audiogram, vestibular testing, Romberg's testing, and SCr Monthly assessments of renal function and auditory or vestibular symptoms
Amikacin/kanamycin	Ototoxicity, nephrotoxicity	Baseline audiogram, vestibular testing, Romberg's testing, and SCr; monthly assessments of renal function and auditory or vestibular symptoms
Capreomycin	Nephrotoxicity, ototoxicity	Baseline audiogram, vestibular testing, Romberg's testing, and SCr Monthly assessments of renal function and auditory or vestibular symptoms Baseline and monthly serum K^+ and Mg^{2+}
p-Aminosalicylic acid	Hepatotoxicity, GI distress, malabsorption syndrome, hypothyroidism, coagulopathy	Baseline LFTs and TSH TSH every 3 months
Moxifloxacin	GI disturbance, neurologic effects, cutaneous reactions	No specific monitoring recommended

CNS, central nervous system; GI, gastrointestinal; LFT, liver function test; SCr, serum creatinine; TSH, thyroid-stimulating hormone.

Adapted from American Thoracic Society, Centers for Disease Control and Prevention, Infectious Diseases Society of America. Treatment of tuberculosis. MMWR Recomm Rep *2003;52(RR-11):1-77.*

Alternative agents should be selected as needed. Audiometric testing should be performed at baseline and monthly for patients who must receive aminoglycosides for more than 1 to 2 months. Vision testing (Snellen visual acuity charts and Ishihara color discrimination plates) should be performed on all patients who receive ethambutol. All patients diagnosed with TB should be tested for HIV infection.

ABBREVIATIONS

AFB	acid-fast bacillus
ATS	American Thoracic Society
BCG	bacillus Calmette-Guérin
CDC	Centers for Disease Control and Prevention
CMI	cell-mediated immunity
DOT	directly observed treatment
DTH	delayed-type hypersensitivity
ELISA	enzyme-linked immunosorbent assay
HIV	human immunodeficiency virus
IGRA	interferon-γ release assay
IL	interleukin
INF	interferon
LAM	lipoarabinomannan
LTBI	latent tuberculosis infection
MAC	*Mycobacterium avium* complex
MDR	multidrug resistant
MIC	minimal inhibitory concentration
MTD	*M. tuberculosis* direct
PCR	polymerase chain reaction
PPD	purified protein derivative
QFT-G	QuantiFERON-TB Gold test
rRNA	ribosomal ribonucleic acid
SDA	strand-displacement amplification
TB	tuberculosis
TDM	therapeutic drug monitoring
TH_1	T-helper type 1
TH_2	T-helper type 2
TNF	tumor necrosis factor
WBC	white blood cell
XDR	extensively drug-resistant

REFERENCES

1. WHO. Report on the Global Tuberculosis Epidemic. Geneva: World Health Organization, 2014.
2. Centers for Disease Control and Prevention. Reported Tuberculosis in the United States, 2014. Atlanta, GA: US Department of Health and Human Services, CDC, 2014, Available at: http://www.cdc.gov/tb/statistics/reports/2014/default.htm. Accessed December 2015.
3. Fitzgerald DW, Sterling TR. *Mycobacterium tuberculosis.* In: Mandell GL, Bennett JE, Dolin R, eds. *Principles and Practice of*

Infectious Diseases, 5th ed. New York, NY: Churchill-Livingstone, 2010:3129-3164.

4. Scott C, Kirking HL, Jeffries C, et al. Tuberculosis trends. *MMWR* 2015; 64(10): 265-269.
5. WHO. Global HIV/AIDS reponse. Epidemic update and health sector progress towards universal access. Geneva: World Health Organization, 2011.
6. Magee JG. *Mycobacterium tuberculosis* . In: Ollar RA., Connell ND, eds. *Molecular Mycobacteriology: Techniques and Clinical.* New York, NY: Marcel Dekker Inc., 1999.
7. Issa R, Mohd Hassan NA, Abdul H, et al. Detection and discrimination of *Mycobacterium tuberculosis* complex. *Diagn Microbiol Infect Dis* 2012;72:62-67.
8. McNabb SJN, Braden CR, Navin TR. DNA fingerprinting of *Mycobacterium tuberculosis*, lessons learned an implication for the future. *Emerg Infect Dis* 2002;8:1314-1319.
9. Boehme CC, Nabeta P, Hillemann D, Nicol MP, et al. Rapid molecular detection of tuberculosis and rifampin resistance. *N Engl J Med* 2010;363(11):1005.
10. Availability of an assay for detecting *Mycobacterium tuberculosis*, including rifampin-resistant strains, and considerations for its use - United States, 2013. Centers for Disease Control and Prevention. *MMWR Morb Mortal Wkly Rep* 2013;62:821-827.
11. Helb D, Jones M, Boehme C, et al. Rapid detection of *Mycobacterium tuberculosis* and rifampin resistance by use of on-demand, near patient technology. *J Clin Microbiol* 2010; 48:229-237.
12. Wallis RS. Biomarkers and diagnostics for tuberculosis: Progress, needs, and translation into practice. *Lancet* 2010;375:1845-1938.
13. Somoskovi A, Parsons LM, Salfinger M. The molecular basis of resistance to isoniazid, rifampin, and pyrazinamide in *Mycobacterium tuberculosis. Respir Res* 2001;2:164-168.
14. Daniel TM, Boom WH, Ellner JJ. Immunology of tuberculosis. In: Reichman LB, Hershfield ES, eds. *Tuberculosis: A Comprehensive International Approach*, 2nd ed. New York, NY: Marcel Dekker, 2000:157-185.
15. Piessens WF, Nardell EA. Pathogenesis of tuberculosis. In: Reichman LB, Hershfield ES, eds. *Tuberculosis: A Comprehensive International Approach*, 2nd ed. New York, NY: Marcel Dekker, 2000:241-260.
16. Long, R, Gardam, M. Tumour necrosis factor-α inhibitors and the reactivation of latent tuberculosis infection. *Can Med Assoc J* 2003;168:1153-1156.
17. American Thoracic Society/Centers for Disease Control and Prevention. Diagnostic standards and classification of tuberculosis in adults and children. *Am J Respir Crit Care Med* 2000;161:1376-1395.
18. Cruz AT, Stark JR. Clinical manifestations of tuberculosis in children. *Paediatr Respir Rev* 2007;8:107-117.
19. Kwan CK, Ernst JD. HIV and tuberculosis: A deadly human syndemic. *Clin Microbiol Rev* 2011;24:351-376.
20. Swaminathan S, Padmapriyadarsini C, Narendran G. HIV-associated tuberculosis: Clinical update. *Clin Infect Dis* 2010;50:1377.
21. Panel on Opportunistic Infections in HIV-Infected Adults and Adolescents. Guidelines for the prevention and treatment of opportunistic infections in HIV-infected adults and adolescents: Recommendations from the Centers for Disease Control and Prevention, the National Institutes of Health, and the HIV Medicine Association of the Infectious Diseases Society of America. Available at: http://aidsinfo.nih.gov/contentfiles/lvguidelines/adult_oi.pdf. Accessed September 1, 2015.
22. Naidoo K, Yende-Zuma N, Padayatch N, et al. The immune reconstitution inflammatory syndrome after antiretroviral therapy initiation in patients with tuberculosis: Findings from the SAPiT trial. *Ann Intern Med* 2012;157:313.
23. Uthman OA, Okwundu C, Gbenga K, et al. Optimal timing of antiretroviral therapy initiation for HIV-infected adults with newly diagnosed pulmonary tuberculosis: A systematic review and meta-analysis. *Ann Intern Med* 2015;163:32-39.
24. American Thoracic Society/Centers for Disease Control and Prevention. Targeted tuberculin skin testing and treatment of latent tuberculosis infection. *Am J Respir Crit Care Med* 2000;161:S221-S247.
25. Akolo C, Adetifa I, Sheppard S, Volmink J. Treatment of latent tuberculosis infection in HIV infected persons. *Cochrane Database Syst Rev* 2010;(1):CD000171.
26. Anergy skin testing and preventive therapy for HIV-infected persons: Revised recommendations. Centers for Disease Control and Prevention. *MMWR Recomm Rep* 1997;46:1-0.
27. Jensen PA, Lambert LA, Iademarco MF, Ridzon R; Centers for Disease Control and Prevention. Guidelines for preventing the transmission of *Mycobacterium tuberculosis* in health care settings. *MMWR Recomm Rep* 2005;54(RR-17):1-141.
28. Villarino ME, Burman WJ, Wang Y et al. Comparable specificity of two commercial tuberculin reagents in persons at low risk for tuberculosis infection. *JAMA* 1999;281:169-171.
29. Menzies D. Interpretation of repeated tuberculin tests. Boosting, conversion, and reversion. *Am J Respir Crit Care Med* 1999;159:15.
30. Mazurek GH, Jereb J, Varnon A, et al. Updated guidelines for interferon gamma release assay to detect *Mycobacterium tuberculosis* infection, United States. *MMWR Recomm Rep* 2010;59(RR-5):1-25.
31. Barnes PF. Weighing gold or counting spots. *Am J Respir Crit Care Med* 2006;174:731-735.
32. Starke JR, Committee on Infectious Diseases. Interferon-γ release assays for diagnosis of tuberculosis infection and disease in children. *Pediatrics* 2014;134:e1763.
33. Bergamini BM, Losi M, Vaienti F, et al. Performance of commercial blood tests for the diagnosis of latent tuberculosis infection in children and adolescents. *Pediatrics* 2009;123:e419-e424.
34. Lighter J, Rigaud M, Eduardo R, Peng CH, et al. Latent tuberculosis diagnosis in children by using the quantiferon-TB gold in tube test. *Pediatrics* 2009;123:30-37.
35. Richeldi L, Losi M, D'Amico R, et al. Performance of tests for latent tuberculosis in different groups of immunocompromised patients. *Chest* 2009;136:198-204.
36. Perry S, Catanzaro A. Use of clinical risk assessments in evaluation of nucleic acid amplification tests for HIV/tuberculosis. *Int J Tuberc Lung Dis* 2000;4:S34.
37. American Thoracic Society/Centers for Disease Control/Infectious Disease Society of America. Treatment of tuberculosis. *Am J Respir Crit Care Med* 2003;167:603-662.
38. Fujiwara PI, Larkin C, Frieden TR. Directly observed therapy in New York City. *Clin Chest Med* 1997;18:135-148.
39. Cruz AT, Starke JR. Increasing adherence for latent tuberculosis infection therapy with health department-administered therapy. *Pediatr Infect Dis J* 2012;31:193.
40. Peloquin CA. Pharmacological issues in the treatment of tuberculosis. *Ann NY Acad Sci* 2001;953:157-164.
41. Fourie PB, Ellner JJ, Johnson JL. Whither *Mycobacterium vaccae*—Encore. *Lancet* 2002;360:1032-1033.
42. Alsultan A, Peloquin CA. Therapeutic drug monitoring in the treatment of tuberculosis: An update. *Drugs* 2014;74:839-854.
43. Peloquin CA. Antituberculosis drugs: Pharmacokinetics. In: Heifets LB, ed. *Drug Susceptibility in the Chemotherapy of Mycobacterial Infections.* Boca Raton, FL: CRC Press, 1991:59-88.
44. Aspler A, Long R, Trajman A, et al. Impact of treatment completion, intolerance and adverse events on health system costs in a randomized trial of 4 months of rifampin or 9 months isoniazid for latent TB. *Thorax* 2010;65:582-587.
45. Bamrah S., Brostrom R. Dorina F. et al. Treatment for LTBI in contacts of MDR-TB patients, Federated States of Micronesia, 2009-2012. *Int J Tuberc Lung Dis* 2014;18(8):912-918.
46. Sterling TR, Villarino ME, Borisov AS, et al. Three months of once-weekly rifapentine and isoniazid for *M. tuberculosis* infection. *N Engl J Med* 2011;365:2155-2166.
47. Centers for Disease Control and Prevention. Recommendations for use of isoniazid–rifapentine regimen with direct observation to treat *Mycobacterium tuberculosis* infection. *MMWR Morb Mortal Wkly Rep* 2011;60:1650-1653.
48. Zumla A, Abubaker I, Raviglione M, et al. Drug resistant tuberculosis - current dilemmas, unanswered questions, challenges, and priority needs. *J Infect Dis* 2012;205:S228-S240.
49. Heysell SK, Moore JL, Keller SJ, Houpt ER. Therapeutic drug monitoring for slow response to tuberculosis in a state control program. *Emerg Infect Dis* 2010;16:1546-1553.
50. Lawn SD, Wilkinson R. Extensively drug resistant tuberculosis. *BMJ* 2006;333:559-560.
51. Mnyani CN, McIntyre JA. Tuberculosis in pregnancy. *Br J Obstet Gynecol* 2011;118:226-231.
52. WHO. Tuberculosis care with TB-HIV co-management: Integrated management of adolescent and adult illness. Geneva: World Health Organization, 2007.
53. Centers for Disease Control and Prevention. Managing drug interactions in the treatment of HIV-related tuberculosis. 2013. Available at: http://www.cdc.gov/tb/TB_HIV_Drugs/default.htm. Accessed September 1, 2015.
54. Malone RS, Fish DN, Spiegel DM, et al. The effect of hemodialysis on isoniazid, rifampin, pyrazinamide, and ethambutol. *Am J Respir Crit Care Med* 1999;159:1580-1584.
55. Malone RS, Fish DN, Spiegel DM, et al. The effect of hemodialysis on cycloserine, ethionamide, *para*-aminosalicylate, and clofazimine. *Chest* 1999;116:984-990.

56. Crabbe SJ. Drug InfoSearch—Intravenous isoniazid. *P&T* 1990;15: 1483-1484.
57. Peloquin CA, Namdar R, Dodge AA, Nix DE. Pharmacokinetics of isoniazid under fasting conditions, with food, and with antacids. *Int J Tuberc Lung Dis* 1999;3:70-710.
58. Berning SE, Peloquin CA. Antimycobacterial agents: Isoniazid. In: Yu VL, Merigan TC, Barriere S, White NJ, eds. *Antimicrobial Chemotherapy and Vaccines*. Baltimore: Williams & Wilkins, 2010:654-663.
59. Weiner M, Burman W, Vernon A, et al. Low isoniazid concentration associated with outcome of tuberculosis treatment with once-weekly isoniazid and rifapentine. *Am J Respir Crit Care Med* 2003;167:1341-1347.
60. Weiner M, Benator D, Burman W, et al. Association between acquired rifamycin resistance and the pharmacokinetics of rifabutin and isoniazid among patients with HIV and tuberculosis. *Clin Infect Dis* 2005;40:1481-1491.
61. Morris AB, Kanyok TP, Scott J, et al. Rifamycins. In: Yu VL, Merigan TC, Barriere S, White NJ, eds. *Antimicrobial Chemotherapy and Vaccines*. Baltimore: Williams & Wilkins, 1998:901-963.
62. Peloquin CA, Namdar R, Singleton MD, Nix DE. Pharmacokinetics of rifampin under fasting conditions, with food, and with antacids. *Chest* 1999;115:12-18.
63. Barroso EC, Pinheiro VG, Facanha MC, et al. Serum concentrations of rifampin, isoniazid, and intestinal absorption, permeability in patients with multidrug resistant tuberculosis. *Am J Trop Med Hyg* 2009;81:322-329.
64. Mofenson LM, Brady MT, Danner SP, et al. Guidelines for the prevention and treatment of opportunistic infections among HIV-exposed and HIV-infected children: Recommendations from the CDC, the National Institutes of Health, the HIV Medicine Association of Infectious Diseases Society of America, the Pediatric Infectious Disease Society and the American Academy of Pediatrics. *MMWR Recomm Rep* 2009;58:1-166.
65. Burman WJ, Gallicano K, Peloquin CA. Comparative pharmacokinetics and pharmacodynamics of the rifamycin antibiotics. *Clin Pharmacokinet* 2001;40:327-341.
66. Peloquin CA, Jaresko GS, Yong CL, et al. Population pharmacokinetic modeling of isoniazid, rifampin, and pyrazinamide. *Antimicrob Agents Chemother* 1997;41:2670-2679.
67. Peloquin CA, Bulpitt AE, Jaresko GS, et al. Pharmacokinetics of pyrazinamide under fasting conditions, with food, and with antacids. *Pharmacotherapy* 1998;18:1205-1211.
68. Peloquin CA, Bulpitt AE, Jaresko GS, et al. Pharmacokinetics of ethambutol under fasting conditions, with food, and with antacids. *Antimicrob Agents Chemother* 1999;43:568-572.
69. Summers KK, Hardin TC. Treatment of tuberculosis in hemodialysis patients. *J Infect Dis Pharmacother* 1996;2:37-55.
70. Peloquin CA, Berning SE. Comment: Intravenous streptomycin. *Ann Pharmacother* 1993;27:1546-1547.
71. Peloquin CA, Henshaw TL, Huitt GA, et al. Pharmacokinetic evaluation of *p*-aminosalicylic acid granules. *Pharmacotherapy* 1994;14:40-46 (Correction. *Pharmacotherapy* 1994;14:2).
72. Peloquin CA, Berning SE, Huitt GA, et al. Once-daily and twice-daily dosing of *p*-aminosalicylic acid (PAS) granules. *Am J Respir Crit Care Med* 1999;159:932-934.
73. Peloquin CA, Zhu M, Adam RD, et al. Pharmacokinetics of *p*-aminosalicylate under fasting conditions, with orange juice, food, and antacids. *Ann Pharmacother* 2001;35:1332-1338.
74. Zhu M, Nix DE, Adam RD, et al. Pharmacokinetics of cycloserine under fasting conditions, with orange juice, food, and antacids. *Pharmacotherapy* 2001;21:891-897.
75. Zhu M, Namdar R, Stambaugh JJ, et al. Population pharmacokinetics of ethionamide in patients with tuberculosis. *Tuberculosis* 2002;82: 91-96.
76. Elliott AM, Foster SD. Thiacetazone: Time to call a halt? *Tuber Lung Dis* 1996;77:27-29.
77. Burman WJ, Goldberg S, Johnson JL, et al. Moxifloxacin versus ethambutol in the first 2 months of treatment for pulmonary tuberculosis. *Am J Respir Crit Care Med* 2006;174:331-338.
78. Conde MB, Efron A, Loredo C, et al. Moxifloxacin versus ethambutol in the initial treatment of tuberculosis: A double blind, randomized, controlled phase II trial. *Lancet* 2009;373:1183-1189.
79. Dorman SE, Johnson JL, Goldberg S, et al. Substitution of moxifloxacin for isoniazid during intensive phase treatment of pulmonary tuberculosis. *Am J Respir Crit Care Med* 2009;180:273-280.
80. Devasia RA, Blackman A, Gebretsadik T, et al. Fluoroquinolone resistance in *Mycobacterium tuberculosis*: The effect of duration and timing of fluoroquinolone exposure. *Am J Respir Crit Care Med* 2009;180:365-370.
81. Mase S, Chorba T, Lobue P, Castro K. Provisional CDC guidelines for the use and safety monitoring of bedaquiline fumarate for the treatment of multidrug resistant tuberculosis. *MMWR* 2013;62:1-9.
82. Diacon AH, Pym A, Grobusch M, et al. The diarylquinoline TMC207 for multidrug resistant tuberculosis. *N Engl J Med* 2009;360:2397-2405.
83. Diacon AH, Dawson R, Hanekom M, et al. Early bactericidal activity of delamanid (OPC-67683) in smear-positive pulmonary tuberculosis patients. *Int J Tuberc Lung Dis* 2011;15:949-954.
84. Hu Y, Coates AR, Mitchison DA. Comparison of the sterilizing activities of the nitroimidazopyran PA-824 and moxifloxacin against persisting *Mycobacterium tuberculosis*. *Int J Tuberc Lung Dis* 2008;12:69-73.
85. Gler MT, Skripconoka V, Sanchez-Garavito E, et al. Delamanid for multidrug resistant pulmonary tuberculosis. *N Engl J Med* 2012;366:2151-2160.
86. Zhenkum MA. Global tuberculosis drug development pipeline: The need and the reality. *Lancet* 2010;375:2011-2109.
87. Forun J, Martin-Davila P, Navas E, et al. Linezolid for the treatment of multidrug resistant tuberculosis. *J Antimicrob Chemother* 2005;56:180-185.
88. Chaulk CP, Friedman M, Dunning R. Modeling the epidemiology and economics of directly observed therapy in Baltimore. *Int J Tuberc Lung Dis* 2000;4:201-207.
89. Tappero JW, Bradford WZ, Agerton TB, et al. Serum concentrations of antimycobacterial drugs in patients with pulmonary tuberculosis in Botswana. *Clin Infect Dis* 2005;41:461-469.
90. Perlman DC, Segal Y, Rosenkranz S, et al. The clinical pharmacokinetics of rifampin and ethambutol in HIV-infected persons with tuberculosis. *Clin Infect Dis* 2005;41:1638-1647.
91. Peloquin CA. Agents for tuberculosis. In: Piscitelli SC, Rodvold KA, eds. *Drug Interactions in Infectious Diseases*. Totowa, NJ: Humana Press, 2001:109-120.
92. Brudney K, Dobkin J. Resurgent tuberculosis in New York City: Human immunodeficiency virus, homelessness, and the decline of tuberculosis control programs. *Am Rev Respir Dis* 1991;144:745-749.

Gastrointestinal Infections and Enterotoxigenic Poisonings

113

Andrew Roecker, Brittany Bates, and Steven Martin

KEY CONCEPTS

1. Infectious diarrhea is a disease that causes significant morbidity and mortality worldwide. Its etiology includes various bacteria, viruses, and protozoans, with viral causes being most predominant globally.
2. Two types of infectious diarrhea include watery or enterotoxigenic diarrhea and dysentery or bloody diarrhea. Common pathogens responsible for watery diarrhea are viruses and enterotoxigenic *Escherichia coli*. Common pathogens responsible for dysentery diarrhea are *Shigella* spp., *Campylobacter jejuni*, nontyphoid *Salmonella*, and enterohemorrhagic *E. coli*.
3. Fluid and electrolyte replacement is the cornerstone of therapy for diarrheal illnesses. Oral rehydration therapy is preferred in most cases of mild and moderate diarrhea.
4. The use of antibacterial therapy for infectious diarrhea is not commonly indicated due to the mild and self-limited nature of the infection, or viral etiology. Antibiotic therapy is recommended in cases of severe diarrhea, moderate-to-severe cases of traveler's diarrhea, most cases of febrile dysenteric diarrhea, and culture-proven bacterial diarrhea in high-risk patients.
5. Loperamide and diphenoxylate/atropine may offer symptomatic relief in patients with moderate watery diarrhea; however, use of antimotility agents should be avoided in patients with watery and dysentery diarrhea.
6. Diarrheal illness can be largely prevented by procedures to prevent contaminated food or water supplies and with appropriate personal hygiene.
7. Oral vancomycin is recommended in patients with severe *Clostridium difficile* infection (CDI). Metronidazole is the drug of choice for mild to moderate disease and fidaxomicin may offer an advantage in patients at high risk for disease recurrence.
8. Common traveler's diarrheal pathogens include enterotoxigenic *E. coli*, *Shigella* spp., *Campylobacter* spp., *Salmonella* spp., and viruses.
9. Patient education on prevention strategies and appropriate self-treatment of traveler's diarrhea is preferred, and prophylaxis with antibacterials is not recommended.
10. Pathogens commonly responsible for food poisoning include *Staphylococcus* spp., *Salmonella* spp., *Shigella* spp., and *Clostridium* spp.

Gastrointestinal (GI) infections and enterotoxigenic poisonings encompass a wide variety of medical conditions characterized by inflammation of the GI tract. Inflammation-induced vomiting and diarrhea are responsible for much of the morbidity and mortality of these conditions. Diarrhea is defined as a decrease in consistency of bowel movements (ie, unformed stool) and an increase in frequency of stools to three or more per day.[1,2] Acute disease is commonly associated with diarrhea lasting 14 days or less in duration while persistent diarrhea lasts more than 14 days.

This chapter focuses on infectious etiologies of acute GI infections and enterotoxigenic poisonings. A wide variety of viral, bacterial, and parasitic pathogens are responsible for these infections. Chapter e115 discusses the common protozoans that cause gastroenteritis. This chapter will focus on pathogenesis and management of common viral and bacterial etiologies. Because the clinical consequences of dysenteric diarrhea can be more severe compared with cases of watery diarrhea, the chapter is organized accordingly. Epidemiology, clinical presentation, diagnosis, treatment, and prevention strategies are discussed for all GI infections generally, and further elaborated in subsequent sections for specific diseases such as *Clostridium difficile*–associated diarrhea, traveler's diarrhea, and foodborne illnesses.

EPIDEMIOLOGY

Dehydration resulting from acute infectious diarrhea is the second leading cause of mortality in children younger than 5 years, killing 760,000 annually.[2] Globally, 1.7 billion cases of infectious diarrhea occur yearly and cause over 2 million deaths.[2] The incidence of diarrhea for all children younger than age 5 years is estimated to be 2.9 episodes per child per year. The incidence of diarrhea is higher in younger children, with 4.5 episodes per child per year among children aged 6 to 11 months, compared with 2.3 episodes per child per year for children aged 24 to 59 months.[3] Younger children also have a higher risk of death from acute dehydrating diarrhea, and diarrheal disease is still the leading global cause of malnutrition in children younger than 5 years.[2] Although the incidence of childhood diarrhea has been declining, diarrhea remains a major health problem in children, especially in those younger than 1 year.

In the United States, 179 million episodes of acute gastroenteritis occur each year, resulting in more than 600,000 hospitalizations and more than 5,000 deaths.[4,5] The highest mortality risk from infectious diarrhea in the United States occurs in the elderly, which contrasts to the developing world where the risk of death is highest among young children.[4] A study of the McDonnell-Douglas Health Information System database revealed that 25% of all hospitalizations and 85% of all mortality associated with diarrhea involved the elderly (age 60 years and older).[4] In addition to children and the elderly, other groups at risk for GI infections include travelers and campers, patients in chronic care facilities, military personnel stationed abroad, and immunocompromised patients.

ETIOLOGY

1 The etiology of GI infections and enterotoxigenic poisonings includes a wide variety of viruses, bacteria, and parasites, although the specific incidence of each is difficult to quantify. Etiologic agents

TABLE 113-1 Acute Infectious Diarrhea Clinical Syndromes: Watery versus Dysentery

	Watery	Dysentery
Percentage of patients	90-95	5-10
Stools		
Appearance	Watery	Bloody
Volume	Increased: ++/+++	Increased: +/++
Number per day	<10	>10
Reducing substances	0 to +++	0
pH	5-7.5	6-7.5
Occult blood	Negative	Positive
Fecal polymorphonuclear cells	Absent or few	Many
Mechanisms	Toxins Reduced absorption	Toxins Mucosal invasion
Complications		
Dehydration	Could be severe	Mild
Others	Acidosis, shock, electrolyte imbalance	Tenesmus, rectal prolapse, seizures
Etiology	*Vibrio cholerae*	*Shigella* spp.
	Enterotoxigenic *Escherichia coli* (ETEC)	*Salmonella* spp.
	Rotaviruses	*Campylobacter* spp.
	Noroviruses	*Yersinia* spp.
		Enterohemorrhagic *E. coli* (EHEC)
		Clostridium difficile

are rarely identified due to the infrequent collection of stool samples, or inability of many laboratories to detect the full range of pathogenic organisms. In this chapter, discussions of pathogens responsible for enterotoxigenic diarrhea focus on viral pathogens (rotavirus and norovirus), enterotoxigenic *Escherichia coli* (ETEC), and cholera. Common pathogens associated with dysenteric diarrhea discussed will be *Shigella* spp., *Salmonella* spp., *Campylobacter* spp., enterohemorrhagic *E. coli* (EHEC), *Yersinia enterocolitica*, and *Clostridium difficile*. Characteristics of watery and dysenteric diarrhea and common pathogens responsible for them are outlined in Table 113-1.

Viruses are now recognized as the leading global cause of infectious diarrhea. Noroviruses, previously known as Norwalk-like viruses, account for greater than 90% of viral gastroenteritis among all age groups, and 50% of outbreaks worldwide. In the United States, noroviruses have been estimated to cause 21 million cases of acute gastroenteritis annually including more than 70,000 hospitalizations and nearly 800 deaths.[5,6] Outbreaks occur throughout the year and have been documented in families, healthcare systems, cruise ships, and college dormitories.

In infants and children, rotavirus, a double-stranded, wheel-shaped, RNA virus, is the most common cause of infectious diarrhea globally, and 1 million people die annually from the infection.[7] In the United States, approximately 3.5 million cases of diarrhea, 500,000 physician visits, 50,000 hospitalizations, and 20 deaths occur each year in children younger than 5 years.[7] Rotavirus is a ubiquitous contagion, infecting the vast majority of children younger than 5 years. After the initial infection, 40% of children are protected against subsequent rotavirus infection, 75% are protected against subsequent gastroenteritis, and up to 88% are protected against severe gastroenteritis. Other viral etiologies include astrovirus, enteric adenovirus, pestivirus, coronavirus, and enterovirus. These viruses are increasingly identified as causative etiologies of diarrhea. Characteristics of viral pathogens causing gastroenteritis are outlined in Table 113-2.

2 In the United States, bacterial causes of acute gastroenteritis account for more than 5.2 million cases of diarrhea annually, including 46,000 hospitalizations and 1,500 deaths.[4] However, there appears to be substantial underreporting of disease, and the cause is identified in less than 3% of cases. Common pathogens responsible for watery diarrhea in the United States are norovirus and ETEC, while those most commonly associated with dysentery diarrhea are *Campylobacter* spp., EHEC, *Salmonella* spp., and *Shigella* spp. Other organisms that are responsible for dysentery include *Aeromonas* spp., noncholera *Vibrio*, and *Y. enterocolitica*. Characteristics of acute bacterial pathogens causing gastroenteritis are summarized in Table 113-3.

Cholera has been rare in the United States because of advanced water and sanitation systems; although slight increases in its incidence have occurred in recent years without clear causes.[8] It is endemic on the Indian subcontinent and sub-Saharan Africa. *Vibrio cholerae* is a gram-negative bacillus sharing similar characteristics with the family Enterobacteriaceae. Cholera is caused by toxigenic *V. cholerae* serogroups O1 or O139. Infections due to *V. cholerae* result in severe and voluminous diarrhea that can quickly result in dehydration. Approximately half of those persons infected with *V. cholerae* O1 are symptomatic, whereas only 1% to 5% of those infected with *V. cholerae* O139 manifest symptoms.[9]

E. coli is a gram-negative bacillus commonly found in the human GI tract, and *E. coli*-associated diarrhea may be differentiated into several distinct categories based on pathogenic features of diarrheal disease: enteroaggregative *E. coli* (EAEC), EHEC, enteroinvasive *E. coli* (EIEC), enteropathogenic *E. coli* (EPEC), and ETEC. ETEC occurs most commonly, and accounts for about half of all

TABLE 113-2 Characteristics of Agents Responsible for Acute Viral Gastroenteritis

Virus	Peak Age of Onset	Time of Year	Duration	Mode of Transmission	Common Symptoms
Rotavirus	6 months to 2 years	October to April	3-7 days	Fecal–oral, water, food	Nausea, vomiting, diarrhea, fever, abdominal pain, lactose intolerance
Norovirus	All age groups	Peak in winter	2-3 days	Fecal–oral, food, water, environment	Nausea, vomiting, diarrhea, abdominal cramps, myalgia
Astrovirus	<7 years	Winter	1-4 days	Fecal–oral, water, shellfish	Diarrhea, headache, malaise, nausea
Enteric adenovirus	<2 years	Year-round	7-9 days	Fecal–oral	Diarrhea, respiratory symptoms, vomiting, fever
Pestivirus	<2 years	NR	3 days	NR	Mild
Coronavirus-like particles	<2 years	Fall and early winter	7 days	NR	Respiratory disease
Enterovirus	NR	NR	NR	NR	Mild diarrhea, secondary organ damage

NR, not reported.

TABLE 113-3 Characteristics of Acute Bacterial Gastroenteritis

Bacteria	Incubation Period	Duration	Mode of Transmission	Common Symptoms
Watery Diarrhea				
Vibrio cholerae	2-3 days	1-3 days	Contaminated food or water with human feces usually in areas of inadequate treatment of sewage and drinking water	Profuse watery diarrhea, vomiting, and leg cramps Death can occur within hours without treatment
Enteroaggregative *E. coli*	NR	NR	Contaminated food or water with animal or human feces	Chronic, watery, mucoid, secretory diarrhea with low-grade fever in immunocompromised persons (HIV infections)
Enteroinvasive *E. coli*	10-18 hours	NR	Contaminated food or water with animal or human feces	Watery diarrhea in young children in the developing world
Enteropathogenic *E. coli*	9-12 hours	NR	Contaminated food or water with animal or human feces	Acute onset of profuse watery diarrhea, vomiting, and low-grade fever in young children (<2 years of age) in the developing world
Enterotoxigenic *E. coli*	1-3 days	3-4 days	Contaminated food or water with animal or human feces	Watery diarrhea and abdominal cramping
Dysentery Diarrhea				
Campylobacter jejuni	2-5 days	5-7 days	Contaminated food (particularly poultry), water, or contact with infected animals	Diarrhea (often bloody), cramping, abdominal pain, and fever
Enterohemorrhagic *E. coli*	3-4 days	5-7 days	Contaminated food (particularly cattle) or water with animal or human feces	Severe stomach cramps, diarrhea (often bloody), and vomiting Approximately 5-10% develop hemolytic uremic syndrome
Nontyphoid *Salmonella*	12-36 hours	1-5 days	Contaminated food, water, or contact with infected animals	Diarrhea (sometimes bloody), fever, and abdominal cramps
Shigella	1-3 days	1-7 days	Fecal–oral Contaminated food or water with infected human feces	Watery or bloody diarrhea (8-10 stools/day), severe abdominal pain, fever, and malaise
Yersinia	4-7 days	1-3 weeks	Contaminated food or water	Fever, abdominal pain, and diarrhea (often bloody)

NR, not reported.

cases of *E. coli* diarrhea. There are an estimated 79,000 cases of ETEC in the United States each year.[4] ETEC is also the most common cause of traveler's diarrhea and a common cause of food- and water-associated outbreaks. Infections with EIEC and EPEC are primarily a disease of children in developing countries.[10] EAEC strains are implicated in persistent diarrhea (≥14 days) in human immunodeficiency virus (HIV)-infected patients.[11] EHEC, also known as Shiga toxin–producing *E. coli* (STEC), causes watery diarrhea that becomes bloody in 1 to 5 days in 80% of patients.[10]

EHEC is believed to be the major etiologic factor responsible for the development of hemorrhagic colitis and hemolytic uremic syndrome (HUS). The annual disease burden of STEC in the United States is more than 20,000 infections and as many as 250 deaths; however, the failure of many clinical laboratories to screen for this organism greatly complicates any estimates.[12] In the United States, STEC causes 50% to 60% of all EHEC infections, but in the southern hemisphere, including Argentina, Australia, Chile, and South Africa, non-STEC serotypes are often more prevalent. Non-STEC strains generally produce a lower frequency of dysentery than STEC-positive strains (62% vs 85%).

The *Campylobacter* spp., are flagellated, curved, gram-negative rods. Although there are 14 different species, *Campylobacter jejuni* is the species responsible for more than 99% of *Campylobacter*-associated gastroenteritis. Approximately 2.4 million persons are affected each year in the United States, involving almost 1% of the entire population.[4]

Salmonella enterica is a gram-negative bacilli belonging to the family Enterobacteriaceae. The most prevalent *S enterica* serotypes are Typhi and Paratyphi, which cause enteric fever. Gastroenteritis is caused by *S enterica* serotypes Typhimurium or Enteritidis. In the United States, the largest burden of *Salmonella* infection is due to nontyphoidal serotypes, causing approximately 1.4 million cases of salmonellosis, 16,000 hospitalizations, and 600 deaths, occurring annually.[13]

Approximately 165 million cases of shigellosis occur worldwide with 450,000 cases from the United States annually.[14] *Shigella* spp., are gram-negative bacilli belonging to the family Enterobacteriaceae. Four species most often associated with disease are *Shigella dysenteriae* type 1, *Shigella flexneri*, *Shigella boydii*, and *Shigella sonnei*.[14] *Shigella sonnei* and *S. flexneri* are the most common causes of gastroenteritis in the United States. The other two *Shigella* spp., are more commonly acquired during travel to developing countries. Poor sanitation or personal hygiene, inadequate water supply, malnutrition, and increased population density are associated with an increased risk of *Shigella* gastroenteritis epidemics.

Yersinia spp., are non–lactose-fermenting gram-negative coccobacilli that are widely distributed in nature. The genus *Yersinia* includes six species known to cause disease in humans. *Yersinia enterocolitica* and, to a lesser extent, *Y. pseudotuberculosis* are most likely associated with intestinal infection, but overall both are a relatively infrequent cause of diarrhea and abdominal pain. More than 50 serotypes of *Y. enterocolitica* exist; of these, serotypes 0:3, 0:8, and 0:9 are associated most frequently with enterocolitis.[15] Children are most likely to experience illness with *Y. enterocolitica* infection.

PATHOPHYSIOLOGY

Acute gastroenteritis and its resulting diarrhea are caused by altered movement of ions and water resulting in increased colonic secretion. Under normal conditions, the GI tract has tremendous capacity to absorb fluid and electrolytes, allowing only 100 to 200 mL of fluid to be excreted in the stool daily.[16] The classic enteric pathogen that causes secretary diarrhea is *V. cholerae*, but ETEC and rotavirus also cause watery diarrhea and are much more predominant etiologies in the United States.

V. cholerae is an enteric pathogen that causes classical secretory diarrhea due to changes in ion secretion and absorption. Among the toxins produced by *V. cholerae*, the most important is cholera toxin.[9] Cholera toxin consists of two subunits, A and B. The B subunits are responsible for delivery of the A subunit into the cell. The A subunit stimulates adenylate cyclase, which increases intracellular cyclic adenosine monophosphate (cAMP) and results in protein kinase A-mediated activation of cystic fibrosis transmembrane conductance regulator. This leads to increased chloride secretion and decreased sodium absorption producing the severe watery diarrhea characteristic of the disease.[17] The toxin likely acts along the entire intestinal tract, but most fluid loss occurs in the duodenum. The net effect of the cholera toxin is isotonic fluid secretion early in the intestinal tract that exceeds the absorptive capacity of the latter intestinal tract.

ETEC also causes watery diarrhea characterized by severe intestinal water secretion by producing plasmid-mediated enterotoxins: heat-labile toxin and heat-stable toxin. The heat-labile toxin has two subunits (A and B) that have similar antigenic properties and action on the gut mucosa as cholera toxin. Heat-labile toxins increase chloride secretion via activation of cAMP. The net effect is luminal accumulation of electrolytes that draws water into the intestine, and production of a cholera-like secretory diarrhea.[18] Heat-stable toxin is thought to be non-antigenic and produces watery diarrhea by acting on the small intestine.

Rotavirus induces changes in transepithelial fluid balance, and causes malabsorption as a consequence of destruction of the epithelial lining of intestine, and vascular damage and ischemia in villi. Once rotavirus infects small intestinal villus cells, viroplasms are formed and its toxin, nonstructural protein 4, is released. The viral enterotoxin increases intracellular calcium, and the increase in calcium disrupts microvillus cytoskeleton, as well as barrier function. Changes to the villi include shortening of villus height, crypt hyperplasia, and mononuclear cell infiltration of the lamina propria.[19]

Inflammatory diarrhea is caused by two groups of organisms—enterotoxin-producing, noninvasive bacteria (eg, EAEC, EHEC) or invasive organisms (eg, *Campylobacter* spp., *Salmonella* spp., *Shigella* spp.). The enterotoxin-producing organisms adhere to the mucosa, activate cytokines, and stimulate the intestinal mucosa to release inflammatory mediators. Invasive organisms, which can also produce enterotoxin, invade the intestinal mucosa to induce an acute inflammatory reaction, involving the activation of local and systemic cytokines and inflammatory mediators.

Ingestion of as few as 10 to 200 viable organisms of the *Shigella* spp., causes disease in healthy adults.[14] *Shigella* multiply and spread within the submucosa of the small bowel, but they rarely extend beyond the mucosa. Inflammatory diarrhea is caused by the pathogens invading the epithelial barrier through M cells where they encounter and eliminate macrophages. The destruction of macrophages after emergence from M cells causes an initial release of interleukin (IL)-1β. This initial inflammatory process is exacerbated by free bacteria binding to toll-like receptor that causes the production of IL-6 and IL-8. Both IL-1β and IL-8 attract polymorphonucleocytes.[20] Release of polymorphonucleocytes activates chloride secretion and subsequent diarrhea. Degranulation and release of toxic substances by neutrophils cause ulceration of the epithelium, distortion of the crypts, death to intestinal epithelium, sloughing of mucosal cells, bloody mucoid exudate into the gut lumen, and submucosal accumulation of inflammatory cells with microabscess formation.[21] Microabscesses eventually may coalesce, forming larger abscesses. *Shigella* will frequently affect the entire colon. In addition to the virulence characteristics of invasiveness, *S. dysenteriae* type 1 and, to a lesser degree, *S. flexneri* and *S. sonnei* produce a cytotoxin or Shiga toxin, which can lead to HUS.[10]

The pathogenicity of EHEC is related to the production of Shiga-like toxins, so named because of their resemblance to the Shiga toxin of *S. dysenteriae*.[16] The cytotoxic effect of Shiga-like toxins disrupts the mucosal integrity of the large intestine, causing diarrhea. In addition, the toxin is able to pass through the intestinal epithelium to reach the endothelial cells lining small blood vessels that supply the gut, kidney, and other viscera, causing the myriad metabolic events that could eventually lead to HUS.

CLINICAL PRESENTATION

Gastroenteritis is an illness characterized by diarrhea, which may be accompanied by nausea, vomiting, fever, and abdominal pain. For effective diagnosis and management, it is important to distinguish noninflammatory diarrhea that produces watery diarrhea from inflammatory diarrhea or dysentery. Most enteric pathogens produce acute diarrhea and pathogens associated with dysentery will often result in grossly bloody stools and mucus. Systemic symptoms of gastroenteritis, such as fever, are often associated with dysentery of infectious origin. Symptoms of enteric pathogens that cause watery and dysentery diarrhea are listed in Table 113-1.

A physical examination and careful history that includes information about symptoms and symptom duration, the number of individuals affected, and recent history of travel, diet, and medications are important factors in making a diagnosis. Infections with norovirus or ETEC will often result in mild, self-limiting disease, whereas cholera will commonly produce severe dehydrating diarrhea. Infections with enteric pathogens such as *Campylobacter* spp., EHEC, *Salmonella* spp., *Shigella* spp., and *Y. enterocolitica* can result in severe symptomatology due to dysentery. The utilization of serum C-reactive protein (CRP) in young adult patients with infectious diarrhea may be able to help differentiate between noninflammatory and inflammatory causes.[22] Assessing CRP could assist with diagnosis, prognosis, and treatment selection. The clinical presentation of acute viral and bacterial gastroenteritis is summarized in Tables 113-2 and 113-3, respectively.

3 Stool culture is an important tool in making an organism-specific diagnosis and determining susceptibility to antimicrobial agents. Due to the low yield, stool cultures are not recommended in most mild to moderate watery diarrhea. Instead, indications for stool cultures include dysenteric diarrhea, persistent diarrhea in immunocompromised patients (ie, persons aged 65 years and older with comorbid diseases, neutropenia, or HIV infection), and diarrhea where an outbreak is suggested.[1] An appropriately-obtained stool culture identifies the presence of *Campylobacter*, *Salmonella*, and *Shigella* spp. The yield of stool cultures for other pathogens is increased if the test is ordered specifically based on history and physical examination. For dysenteric diarrhea, the laboratory should be instructed to evaluate for EHEC including STEC (*E. coli* O157:H7). In hospitalized patients who develop diarrhea 3 days after hospitalization or in those with recent exposure to antimicrobials or chemotherapy, stool specimen should be sent for *C. difficile* toxins A and B. In addition to stool cultures, microscopic examination for fecal polymorphonuclear cells, or a simple immunoassay for the neutrophil marker lactoferrin, can further provide evidence of an inflammatory process and increase the yield of cultures in patients presenting with dysenteric diarrhea.[1]

Complications

Complications associated with acute diarrhea most likely result from dehydration so treatment focuses primarily on rehydration therapy, regardless the etiology. Dysenteric diarrhea is more likely to have severe complications, especially in children younger than 5 years and in elderly. Bacteremia is the most common complication of gastroenteritis and can be seen after infections with nontyphoid *Salmonella*, *C. jejuni* or *C. fetus*, and *Y. enterocolitica*.[12] Nontyphoid *Salmonella* is most common in children younger than 5 years, elderly, and patients with hemoglobinopathy, malaria, or immunosuppression. Bacteremia due to *Campylobacter* spp., has been reported in patients with HIV infection, malignancy, transplantation, and hypogammaglobulinemia. *Y. enterocolitica* bacteremia has been rarely reported, but has an increased prevalence in patients with diabetes mellitus, severe anemia, hemochromatosis, iron overload (frequent transfusion), cirrhosis, malignancy, and in the elderly.[23] Persistent bacteremia with these pathogens will commonly result in prolonged intermittent fever with chills. Potentially complicating the diagnosis, stool cultures frequently are negative and leukocyte counts are often within the normal range. Vascular complications such as seeding of atherosclerotic plaques or aneurysms in arterial vessels occur in 10% to 25% of adults with bacteremia. Localized infections involving bone, cysts, heart, kidney, liver, lungs, pericardium, and spleen develop in 5% to 10% of patients with bacteremia.

A severe complication in patients infected with EHEC is HUS. HUS is defined by the triad of acute renal failure, thrombocytopenia, and microangiopathic hemolytic anemia and is more commonly observed in children younger than 5 years and in the elderly.[24] Approximately 2% to 7% of cases infected with STEC strains are complicated by development of HUS, which increases mortality associated with this infection. *S. dysenteriae* type 1 can also cause HUS, although more rarely than observed with EHEC.[14]

Shigella infection may also lead to complications such as generalized seizures, sepsis, toxic megacolon, perforated colon, arthritis, and protein-losing enteropathy. Mortality is rare, but it may be more likely with *S. dysenteriae* type I. Less than 3% of persons who are infected with *S. flexneri* will later develop Reiter syndrome, characterized by pains in the joints, irritation of the eyes, and painful urination. This can lead to chronic arthritis.[25]

Infection with *C. jejuni* has been associated with Guillain-Barré syndrome (GBS), but the relationship is not well understood.[26] The risk of developing GBS after *C. jejuni* infection appears to be low (approximately 1 case of GBS per 1,000 *C. jejuni* infections). The weakness associated with GBS usually starts in the legs, with difficulty in walking, and may progress to a complete paralysis of all extremities that lasts several weeks and usually requires intensive care.

Approximately 10% to 30% of adult patients develop a reactive arthritis 1 to 2 weeks after recovery from gastroenteritis secondary to *S. flexneri*, *Salmonella* spp., *C. jejuni*, and *Y. enterocolitica*. This arthritis, involving the knees, ankles, toes, fingers, and wrists, usually resolves in 1 to 4 months but may persist in approximately 10% of patients.[26] This complication is more common in persons with the HLA-B27 antigen.

A general complication that could occur long after an infectious gastroenteritis, especially with dysentery and toxin-mediated dysentery, is postinfectious irritable bowel syndrome (IBS). This is classified as IBS symptoms for at least 3 months following an episode of gastroenteritis or traveler's diarrhea showing recurrent abdominal pain or discomfort.[27] Albeit rare, some long-term complications associated with these infections strengthen the need for appropriate diagnosis and treatment.

TREATMENT

Mortality associated with infectious diarrhea has declined substantially in the past 2 decades, especially among children younger than 1 year. Preventative measures including improved sanitation, breastfeeding and weaning practices, and increased use of oral rehydration therapy (ORT) for affected individuals, are responsible for the decrease in case-fatality rates.

General Approach to Treatment

The cornerstone of management for all GI infections and enterotoxigenic poisonings is to prevent dehydration by correcting fluid and electrolyte imbalances. In mild, self-limiting acute gastroenteritis, a diet of oral fluids and easily digestible foods is recommended. In patients with severe dehydrating watery diarrhea and dysenteric diarrhea, IV rehydration therapy, antibiotics, and/or antimotility treatments are needed.

Rehydration Therapy

Initial assessment of fluid loss is essential for successful rehydration therapy and should include acute weight loss, as it is the most reliable means of determining the extent of water loss. However, if accurate baseline weight is not available, clinical signs are helpful in determining approximate deficits (Table 113-4). Physical assessment generally is more reliable in young children and infants than in adults.

3 Fluid replacement is the cornerstone of therapy for dehydration due to diarrhea regardless of etiology. For the treatment of mild to moderate dehydration, ORT is superior to administration of IV fluids. Oral replacement therapy reverses dehydration in nearly all patients with mild to moderate diarrhea with 94% to 97% efficacy.[1] It offers advantages of being inexpensive, noninvasive, and not requiring inpatient administration. Moreover, thirst drives use of ORT and provides a safeguard against overhydration. Replacement of ongoing losses as well as continuation of normal feeding should also be addressed.

The necessary components of oral rehydration solutions (ORS) include carbohydrates (typically glucose), sodium, potassium, chloride, and water. Using both salt and glucose in the ORS takes advantage of glucose-coupled sodium transport in the small bowel and enhances sodium and subsequently water transport across intestinal walls. In 2002, the World Health Organization/United Nations Children's Fund (WHO/UNICEF) endorsed a reduced osmolarity solution (osmolarity ≤250 mOsm/L) as the use of these solutions reduced stool volume, shortened duration of diarrhea, and decreased need for unscheduled IV therapy when compared with previously used ORS more than or equal to 310 mOsm/L.[28] The newer formulation of ORS less than or equal to 250 mOsm/L was, however, more likely to cause hyponatremia (blood sodium levels <130 mmol/L).[29] If commercial ORS are unavailable, one can be roughly duplicated by mixing ½ teaspoon of salt with 6 teaspoons of sugar in 1 L of water.[30]

In restoring fluid and electrolyte balance in cholera infections, polymer-based ORS may be more efficacious than glucose-based ORS. Polymer-based ORS contains rice, wheat, sorghum, or maize. This polymer-based ORS releases glucose more slowly after digestion, and when absorbed in the small bowel, enhances the reabsorption of water and electrolyte secreted into the bowel lumen during diarrhea. In a meta-analysis of 34 trials, polymer-based ORS has been shown to reduce the duration of diarrhea in adults with cholera when compared with glucose-based ORS more than or equal to 310 and less than or equal to 270 mOsm/L.[31]

Guidelines for rehydration therapy based on the degree of dehydration and replacement of ongoing losses are outlined in Table 113-4. ORS should be given in small and frequent volumes (5 mL every 2 to 3 minutes in a teaspoon or oral syringe). Nasogastric administration of ORS is an alternative method of administration in a child with persistent vomiting. For breast-fed infants, nursing should be continued. The composition of commercial ORS and commonly consumed beverages is listed in Table 113-5. Clear fluids, such as soft drinks, sweetened fruit drinks, chicken broth, and sports drinks, should be avoided in the treatment of dehydration. These hyperosmolar solutions may cause an osmotic diarrhea.

In the treatment of severe dehydration, the primary goal of therapy is rapid restoration of fluid losses, correction of metabolic acidosis, and replacement of potassium deficiency. Severely dehydrated patients should be resuscitated initially with IV lactated Ringer solution or normal saline to restore hemodynamic stability.

TABLE 113-4 Clinical Assessment of Degree of Dehydration in Children Based on Percentage of Body Weight Loss[a]

Variable	Minimal or No Dehydration (<3% Loss of Body Weight)	Mild to Moderate (3%-9% Loss of Body Weight)	Severe (≥10% Loss of Body Weight)
Blood pressure	Normal	Normal	Normal to reduced
Quality of pulses	Normal	Normal or slightly decreased	Weak, thready, or not palpable
Heart rate	Normal	Normal to increased	Increased (bradycardia in severe cases)
Breathing	Normal	Normal to fast	Deep
Mental status	Normal	Normal to listless	Apathetic, lethargic, or comatose
Eyes	Normal	Sunken orbits/decreased tears	Deeply sunken orbits/absent tears
Mouth and tongue	Moist	Dry	Parched
Thirst	Normal	Eager to drink	Drinks poorly; too lethargic to drink
Skin fold	Normal	Recoil in <2 seconds	Recoil in >2 seconds
Extremities	Warm, normal capillary refill	Cool, prolonged capillary refill	Cold, mottled, cyanotic, prolonged capillary refill
Urine output	Normal to decreased	Decreased	Minimal
Hydration therapy	None	ORS 50-100 mL/kg over 3-4 hours	Lactated Ringer's solution or normal saline 20 mL/kg over 15-30 minutes IV until mental status or perfusion improves Followed by 5% dextrose/0.45% sodium chloride IV at higher maintenance rates or ORS 100 mL/kg over 4 hours.
Replacement of ongoing losses	For each diarrheal stool or emesis <10 kg body weight: 60-120 mL ORS >10 kg body weight: 120-240 mL ORS	Same as minimal dehydration	If unable to tolerate ORS, administer through nasogastric tube or administer 5% dextrose/0.45% sodium chloride with 20 mEq/L (20 mmol/L) potassium chloride IV

ORS, oral rehydration solution.

[a]Percentages vary among authors for each dehydration category; hemodynamic and perfusion status is most important; when unsure of category, therapy for more severe category is recommended.

Lactated Ringer solution is preferred initially over normal saline because normal saline does not assist in correcting a metabolic acidosis. As GI and renal perfusion should be addressed aggressively, rapid IV administration is preferred over prolonged administration regimens for restoring extracellular fluids and electrolytes.[32] After rehydration, maintenance fluid is given based on accurate recording of intake and output volumes. ORT should be instituted as soon as it can be tolerated.

Early refeeding with age-appropriate unrestricted diet is recommended in children. A meta-analysis of 12 trials showed that early refeeding during or immediately following the start of rehydration did not increase the risk of complications such as unscheduled IV fluids, vomiting, or development of persistent diarrhea compared with late refeeding that ranged from 20 to 48 hours after start of rehydration.[32] Initially, easily digested foods such as bananas, applesauce, and cereal should be introduced and foods high in fiber, sodium, and sugar should be avoided. One caveat would be that lactase deficiency may be exacerbated among known lactase-deficient patients and may persist up to 10 days.

Antimicrobial Therapy

4 The indiscriminate use of antimicrobial therapy produces increases in antimicrobial resistance, side effects of antimicrobial agents, and the threat of superinfections owing to eradication of normal flora. Increasing fluoroquinolone resistance in *Campylobacter* and multidrug resistance in *Salmonella* spp. worldwide reinforces the importance of judicious use of antibiotics and prudent infection control measures.[33,34] Antibiotic therapy is recommended in severe cases of diarrhea, moderate-to-severe cases of traveler's diarrhea, most cases of febrile dysenteric diarrhea, and culture-proven bacterial diarrhea. Antimicrobial therapy is not recommended in EHEC diarrhea as it may increase HUS risk.

Antibiotic therapy is recommended in severe cases of cholera and ETEC diarrhea. In cases of cholera, antibiotics shorten the

TABLE 113-5 Comparison of Common Solutions Used in Oral Rehydration and Maintenance

Product	Na (mEq/L)[b]	K (mEq/L)[b]	Base (mEq/L)	Carbohydrate (mmol/L)	Osmolarity (mOsm/L)
WHO/UNICEF (2002)	75	20	30	75	245
Pedialyte	45	20	30	140	250
Infalyte	50	25	30	70	200
Oralyte	60	20	0	90	260
Rehydralyte	75	20	30	140	250
Cola[a]	2	0	13	700	750
Apple juice[a]	5	32	0	690	730s
Chicken broth[a]	250	8	0	0	500
Sports beverage[a]	20	3	3	255	330

[a]These solutions should be avoided in dehydration.

[b]Concentration of monovalent ions expressed in mEq/L is numerically equivalent to mmol/L concentration.

duration of diarrhea, decrease fluid loss, and shorten the duration of the carrier state.[9] It is important to consider local susceptibility patterns in the selection of the antimicrobial regimen. In areas of high fluoroquinolone resistance, azithromycin has been effective in patients with cholera. In patients with ETEC diarrhea, empiric antibiotics reduce severity and duration of diarrhea. A short course of therapy with fluoroquinolones is the most commonly recommended therapy due to increased resistance among other drug classes.[35] Rifaximin has been effective for ETEC for travel in Mexico.[36] Further discussions of antibiotic prophylaxis and treatment can be found in the section on traveler's diarrhea. Table 113-6 summarizes antibiotic recommendations. Further details regarding treatment of *C. difficile*–associated diarrhea, traveler's diarrhea, and foodborne illnesses are discussed in respective sections.

Antibiotic therapy is indicated in at-risk and febrile patients with dysenteric diarrhea. In shigellosis, antibiotics shorten the period of fecal shedding and attenuate the clinical illness. Antibiotic therapy is reserved for the elderly, those who are immunocompromised, children in daycare centers, malnourished children, and healthcare workers. In the United States, *Shigella* spp., remain susceptible to fluoroquinolones. Fluoroquinolone resistance among *Shigella* spp., is of increasing concern in developing countries, and azithromycin may be a better choice in patients with a recent history of travel to a developing region.[14] Similar antibiotic regimens can be used for high-risk patients who develop *Yersinia* bacteremia (ie, infants younger than 3 months and patients with cirrhosis or iron overload) or in patients with bone and joint infections.[37] With Campylobacteriosis, antibiotics are not useful unless started within 4 days of the start of the illness because they do not shorten the duration or severity of diarrhea and only shorten the duration of bacterial excretion. Antibiotics are warranted in patients with high fevers, severe bloody diarrhea, prolonged illnesses (more than 1 week), pregnancy, and immunocompromised states, including HIV infection. Fluoroquinolone resistance among *Campylobacter* spp., has increased, and is now 10% to 13% in the United States and 41% to 88% in Europe and Asia. Resistance may be the result of the use of fluoroquinolone antibiotics in poultry and other animal feed, and the frequent use of these agents internationally in treating enteric infections. Macrolides such as erythromycin and azithromycin are recommended especially in patients with a recent history of travel to Asia.[35]

Nontyphoid *Salmonella* infection leads to bacteremia in approximately 8% of otherwise healthy adults. However, patients with increased risk of bacteremia should be treated with antibiotics if appropriate diagnosis is made. High-risk patients include neonates or infants younger than 1 year, persons older than 50 years, and patients with primary or secondary immunodeficiency such as acquired immunodeficiency syndrome (AIDS) or chemotherapy-induced inflammatory bowel disease, sickle cell disease, vascular abnormalities (prostatic heart valve or abdominal aneurysm), or prosthetic joints.[14] If cultures are positive for Salmonellosis and antibacterial therapy is warranted, susceptibility testing should be done for appropriate targeted therapy due to concern of resistance.

Outcomes of some bacterial diarrheal illnesses may be worsened by the use of antibacterials, therefore precluding their use. In patients infected with EHEC, use of a fluoroquinolone or

TABLE 113-6 Recommendations for Antibiotic Therapy

Pathogen	Children	Adults
Watery Diarrhea		
Enterotoxigenic *Escherichia coli*	Azithromycin 10 mg/kg/day given orally once daily × 3 days; ceftriaxone 50 mg/kg/day given IV once daily × 3 days	Ciprofloxacin 750 mg orally once daily × 1-3 days. Alternatives: rifaximin 200 mg orally three times daily × 3 days; azithromycin 1,000 mg orally × 1 day *or* 500 mg orally daily × 3 days
Vibrio cholerae O1	Erythromycin 30 mg/kg/day divided every 8 hours orally × 3 days; azithromycin 10 mg/kg/day given orally once daily × 3 days	Doxycycline 300 mg orally × 1 day Alternatives: tetracycline 500 mg orally four times daily × 3 days; erythromycin 250 mg orally every 8 hours × 3 days; azithromycin 500 mg orally once daily × 3 days
Dysenteric Diarrhea		
Campylobacter species[a]	Azithromycin 10 mg/kg/day given orally once daily × 3-5 days; erythromycin 30 mg/kg/day divided into two to four doses orally × 3-5 days	Azithromycin 500 mg orally once daily × 3 days; erythromycin 500 mg orally every 6 hours × 3 days
Salmonella Nontyphoidal[a]	Ceftriaxone 100 mg/kg/day divided IV every 12 hours × 7-10 days; azithromycin 20 mg/kg/day orally once daily × 7 days	Ciprofloxacin 750 mg orally once daily × 7-10 days; levofloxacin 500 mg orally once daily × 7-10 days Alternatives: azithromycin 500 mg orally once daily × 7 days For immunocompromised patients, duration should be increased to 14 days for both fluoroquinolones and azithromycin
Shigella species[a]	Azithromycin 10 mg/kg/day given orally once daily × 3 days; ceftriaxone 50 mg/kg/day given IV once daily × 3 days	Ciprofloxacin 750 mg orally once daily × 3 days; levofloxacin 500 mg orally once daily × 3 days Alternatives: azithromycin 500 mg orally once daily × 3 days
Yersinia species[a]	Treat as shigellosis	Treat as shigellosis
***Clostridium difficile*-Associated Diarrhea**		
Clostridium difficile	Metronidazole 7.5 mg/kg (maximum: 500 mg) orally or IV every 8 hours × 10-14 days; vancomycin 10 mg/kg (maximum: 125 mg) orally every 6 hours × 10-14 days	Mild to moderate disease: metronidazole 500 mg orally or IV every 8 hours daily × 10-14 days Severe disease: vancomycin 125 mg orally every 6 hours × 10-14 days Alternatives: fidaxomicin 200 mg orally every 12 hours × 10-14 days
Traveler's Diarrhea		
Prophylaxis[a]		Norfloxacin 400 mg or ciprofloxacin 750 mg orally daily; rifaximin 200 mg one to three times daily up to 2 weeks
Treatment		Ciprofloxacin 750 mg orally × 1 day or 500 mg orally every 12 hours × 3 days; levofloxacin 1,000 mg orally × 1 day or 500 mg orally daily × 3 days; rifaximin 200 mg three times daily × 3 days; azithromycin 1,000 mg orally × 1 day or 500 mg orally daily × 3 days

[a]For high-risk patients only. See the preceding text for the high-risk patients in each infection.

trimethoprim–sulfamethoxazole may increase the risk of HUS by increasing the production of Shiga-like toxin.[37] Empiric antimicrobial therapy should be withheld when clinical suspicion is high due to the high local prevalence EHEC, patient clinical presentation suggestive of EHEC infection, or a known foodborne outbreak of dysentery with an incubation period of longer than 2 days. Antibiotics should not be given to infants or children due to a higher incidence of HUS in this population. Treatment of EHEC infection is primarily limited to supportive care, which may include fluid replacement therapy, hemodialysis, hemofiltration, transfusion red blood cells and/or platelets, and other interventions as indicated clinically. Severe disease may lead to chronic kidney failure and potential need of renal transplantation.

Antimotility Agents

5 Antimotility drugs such as diphenoxylate/atropine and loperamide offer symptomatic relief in patients with watery diarrhea by reducing the number of stools. However, in both enterotoxigenic and dysenteric diarrhea, slowing of fecal transit time with these agents is thought to result in extended toxin-associated damage, worsening symptomatology and leads to complications. Therefore, antimotility drugs should be avoided if possible and are not recommended in patients with toxin-mediated dysenteric diarrhea (ie, EHEC, pseudomembranous colitis, shigellosis). However, some evidence suggests that in adults with dysenteric diarrhea these agents do not appear to be harmful if given concomitantly with antibacterial therapy.[37]

Clinical **Controversy...**

Diphenoxylate/atropine and loperamide slow gastric motility and can prolong exposure to enterotoxins in watery and toxin-mediated dysentery diarrheas. Caution is warranted with use of these agents in infectious diarrhea and further, these agents should not be administered to patients with dysenteric symptomatology.

Probiotics

Probiotics are preparations of microorganisms and most commercial products have been derived from food sources, particularly cultured milk products (ie, lactobacilli and bifidobacteria). When used in the treatment or prophylaxis of infectious diarrhea and antibiotic-associated diarrhea, efficacy is variable. Most individual studies have not shown significant benefit from the use of probiotics and meta-analyses have shown conflicting results, with one demonstrating efficacy when trials were assessed in aggregate[38] and another demonstrating no benefit.[39] No serious adverse effects have been reported in otherwise healthy persons, however, there are data suggesting a rare but increased incidence of fungemia or bacterial sepsis with probiotic use. With these potential adverse events and limited efficacy data, probiotics should not be recommended for prophylaxis or treatment of initial antibiotic-associated diarrhea.

Oral Zinc Supplementation

Zinc deficiency is largely due to inadequate dietary intake and is common in many developing countries where morbidity and mortality associated with acute diarrhea in children remains high. In children older than 6 months who demonstrate moderate signs of malnutrition, zinc supplementation may shorten the duration of diarrhea by approximately 27 hours (95% CI −14.62 to −39.34).[40] Therefore, oral zinc supplementation of 20 mg/day for 1 to 2 weeks may have an additional benefit over ORS alone in reducing childhood mortality in developing countries. Common side effects include metallic taste and vomiting. At high doses, zinc supplementation may cause epigastric pain, lethargy, and fatigue.

PREVENTION OF GASTROINTESTINAL INFECTIONS

6 Public health measures of improved water supply and sanitation facilities and the quality control of commercial products are important for the control of the majority of GI infections. In addition, following simple rules of personal hygiene and safe food preparation can prevent many diarrheal diseases. Hand washing with soap and running water is instrumental in preventing the spread of illness and should be emphasized for caregivers and persons with diarrheal illnesses. Safe food handling and preparation practices can significantly decrease the incidence of certain enteric infections.

Reporting suspected outbreaks and cases of notifiable illness to local health authorities is vital to investigation of threats of enteric infection arising from increasingly global and industrialized food supplies. The reporting of specific infectious diseases to the appropriate public health authorities is the cornerstone of public health surveillance, outbreak detection, and prevention and control efforts.

Vaccines are used to boost specific immune processes directed against the bacteria themselves or against adherence appendages, cytotoxins, or enterotoxins. Unfortunately, there are only a few vaccines available for prevention of gastroenteritis. Vaccines for typhoid fever are the parenteral Vi capsular polysaccharide vaccine (ViCPS) and the oral live-attenuated Ty21a vaccine.[41] Efficacy rates for both vaccines range from 50% to 80%. The ViCPS is indicated for children who are 2 years or older a booster dose is administered 2 years later. The Ty21a vaccine is indicated for children 6 years or older; one capsule should be swallowed whole every other day for a total of four doses at least 1 week before the potential exposure. A booster should be taken every 5 years if continued protection is needed.

In the United States, routine rotavirus vaccination is recommended for all infants beginning at age 2 months. There are two vaccines, RotaTeq (RV5) and Rotarix (RV1), available for reducing rotaviral gastroenteritis.[42] The RV5 vaccine is a live, oral vaccine that offers 74% efficacy against gastroenteritis of any severity and 98% efficacy against severe disease. This vaccine also decreased office visits by 86%, emergency department visits by 94%, and hospitalizations by 96%. The RV1 vaccine is a live-attenuated human rotavirus vaccine. This vaccine has clinical efficacy of 79% against gastroenteritis of any severity and 96% efficacy against severe rotavirus disease. Rotarix reduced hospitalizations by 100% and medically attended visits by 92% in the first rotavirus season, and reduced hospitalizations by 96% through two seasons.[42] The RV5 vaccine is administered orally in a three-dose series at ages 2, 4, and 6 months while the RV1 vaccine is administered orally in a two-dose series at ages 2 and 4 months. The first dose may be given between 6 weeks and 14 weeks and 6 days of age and all doses should be given before 8 months of age. The vaccines are contraindicated in infants with severe allergic reactions to vaccine components, diagnosed with severe combined immunodeficiency, and with history of intussusception.[43]

Although not available in the United States, two oral vaccines against diarrheal pathogens are available in other countries. Dukoral consists of killed *V. cholerae* O1 organisms and the cholera B subunit, and is licensed in over 60 countries. Shanchol consists of killed whole cells from a mix of pathogenic strains of *V. cholerae* (O1 and O139) and is licensed in India.[9] Both vaccines are given in two doses (three doses of Dukoral are required for children aged 2-5 years) and administered about 7 to 14 days apart (up to 42 days apart for Dukoral). Dukoral must be administered with a buffer that requires 75 to 150 mL of clean water while Shanchol does not require the buffer. Both vaccines demonstrated protective efficacy of 47% to 87% after two doses but almost none after a single dose. Protection is achieved in approximately 1 week following the last dose and persists for approximately 2 years. The common side effects of the vaccines were considered mild and included abdominal pain, headache, fever, and nausea. The WHO does not require vaccination for international travel to or from endemic areas because vaccines require two doses and provide incomplete protection for a relatively short period of time.

There are vaccines in development for common enteric pathogens including ETEC and *Shigella* spp., with the potential for combining them in a single vaccine. These are still in preliminary and animal-based studies, but could significantly affect global public health if they come to fruition for human administration, especially in the infants and children.[44]

EVALUATION OF THERAPEUTIC OUTCOMES

Appropriate follow-up care of patients with acute diarrhea is based on successful restoration of fluid losses. The clinical signs and symptoms that lead to the diagnosis also can assess adequate rehydration, and should be monitored frequently. With ORT preferred, routine laboratory testing often is unnecessary. Electrolytes should be measured in those receiving IV fluids, when oral replacement fails, or when signs of hypernatremia or hypokalemia are present. Follow-up stool samples to ensure complete evacuation of the infecting pathogen may be necessary only in patients who are at high risk to initiate or contribute to a community outbreak. All patients should be monitored for complications associated with the infecting pathogen, resolution of the diarrhea, and adverse reactions to the pharmacologic agents used. Prompt discharge of hospitalized patients is recommended when rehydration is achieved, IV fluids have not been required, oral intake equals or exceeds losses, or adequate education and medical follow-up are ensured. For most patients, discharge can occur in 16 to 24 hours.

CLOSTRIDIUM DIFFICILE

Epidemiology

C. difficile is the most commonly recognized cause of infectious diarrhea in healthcare settings with high rates of disease in long-term care facilities and in the elderly. CDI is associated with use of broad-spectrum antimicrobials and accounts for approximately 20% to 30% of all cases of antibiotic-associated diarrhea.[45] The antibiotics most commonly associated with CDI include clindamycin, ampicillin, cephalosporins, and fluoroquinolones. Other agents that have been implicated, albeit at a lower incidence rate, include aminoglycosides, macrolides, trimethoprim-sulfamethoxazole, vancomycin, and metronidazole. CDI often occurs during or shortly after completion of antimicrobial therapy, however, disease onset can be delayed for 2 or more months.[46] Those at high risk for CDI include the elderly or debilitated, patients undergoing surgery or nasogastric intubation, those with cancer, and those receiving antibiotics, proton pump inhibitors (PPIs), or frequent laxatives. A meta-analysis of 23 studies (~300,000 patients) suggests that PPIs increase the incidence of CDI by 65%.[47,48]

Clinical **Controversy...**

Decreasing gastric acid has been suggested as the mechanism by which PPIs may allow for *C. difficile* toxins to proliferate. This relationship has been observed in both chronic PPI users, as well as inpatients on PPIs for stress ulcer prophylaxis. PPIs have been successful in reducing ICU-related upper GI hemorrhage; however, PPI use has been identified as an independent risk factor for CDI.

Attributable mortality from CDI has been steadily increasing over the past 2 decades and has been reported as high as 38%, with many studies demonstrating a mortality rate of 15% or greater.[49] Increased mortality is thought to be due to the emergence of a hypervirulent strain, North American pulsed-field type [NAP-1], which carries a gene mutation producing higher concentrations of toxin, and responsible for more serious disease.[50] The NAP-1 strain has been associated with fluoroquinolone use, and may be refractory to standard antibiotic therapy.

Pathogenesis

C. difficile is a gram-positive spore-forming anaerobic bacillus and causes a toxin-mediated disease. Once antibiotics disrupt normal colonic flora and colonization of *C. difficile* occurs, two toxins (A and B) are released to mediate diarrhea and colitis. Toxin production is essential for disease manifestation. Toxin A is the major pathogenic factor and has been characterized as an enterotoxin that causes intestinal fluid secretion, mucosal injury, and inflammation through actin disaggregation, intracellular calcium release, and damage to neurons. Toxin B is a nonenterotoxic cytotoxin that causes depolymerization of filamentous actin and mediates more potent damage to human colonic mucosa than toxin A. Initially, raised white and yellowish plaques form in the colon, and the surrounding mucosa may be inflamed. With progression of disease, pseudomembranous plaques become enlarged and scatted over the colorectal mucosa.[46]

Clinical Presentation

Clinical diagnosis is based on the onset of diarrhea, defined as 3 unformed stools in 24 hours, during or after antimicrobial use, and often associated with abdominal discomfort, fever, and polymorphonuclear leukocytosis. The spectrum of disease ranges from mild diarrhea to life-threatening toxic megacolon and pseudomembranous entercolitis.[45,46] In colitis without pseudomembrane formation, patients present with malaise, abdominal pain, nausea, anorexia, watery diarrhea, low-grade fever, and leukocytosis. Fulminant disease is characterized by severe abdominal pain, perfuse diarrhea, high fever, marked leukocytosis, and classic pseudomembrane formation evident with sigmoidoscopic examination.

CDI should be suspected in patients experiencing diarrhea with a recent history of antibiotic use (within the previous 3 months) or in those whose diarrhea began 72 hours after hospitalization. Diagnosis can be established by detection of toxin A or B in the stool, stool culture for *C. difficile*, or endoscopy. The most common methods of laboratory diagnosis includes cytotoxin assay, enzyme-linked immunosorbent assay (ELISA), and molecular methods such as polymerase chain reaction (PCR) testing. The cytotoxin assay was the traditional gold standard, however, today its use is limited due to its long time to test completion (1-3 days) and high cost. ELISA tests are easy to perform and provide rapid results within hours, but have a low sensitivity leading to the possibility of false-negative results. PCR is quickly becoming the test of choice in the United States due to its high sensitivity and specificity coupled with a quick turnaround time of less than 2 hours.[50] Endoscopy should be reserved for situations where rapid diagnosis is needed, ileus is present, stool is not available, or other colonic diseases are in the differential diagnosis. Many hospitalized patients may be colonized with *C. difficile*, so a careful history should be taken and routine screening is not recommended.[45]

TREATMENT

Supportive care of CDI includes fluid and electrolyte replacement therapy, in addition to discontinuation of the offending antimicrobial if possible. Antibiotic therapy is based on disease severity and may

TABLE 113-7 *Clostridium difficile* Infection Severity and Treatment[45,51]

Severity	Markers of Disease Severity	Recommended Treatment
Mild to moderate	WBC ≤15,000 cells/mm³ (15 × 10⁹/L) SCr <1.5 × premorbid level	Metronidazole 500 mg orally every 8 hours for 10-14 days
Severe	WBC >15,000 cells/mm³ (15 × 10⁹/L) SCr >1.5 × premorbid level Temperature >38.3°C Albumin <2.5 g/dL (25 g/L) Age ≥60 Pseudomembranes present ICU admission	Vancomycin 125 mg orally every 6 hours for 10-14 days
Severe, complicated	Hypotension or shock Ileus and/or megacolon Organ failure Coagulopathy	Metronidazole 500 mg IV every 8 hours *PLUS* vancomycin 500 mg every 6 hours via NG or orally (if ileus present use rectally)

NG, nasogastric; SCr, serum creatinine; WBC, white blood cell.

vary for first episode or recurrent infection.[45,51] Table 113-7 outlines CDI disease severity and treatment regimens for initial episodes.

7 Once determination of disease severity has been made, treatment should be initiated with an antibiotic effective against *C. difficile*. In the United States, metronidazole, vancomycin, and fidaxomicin are the most commonly prescribed agents.[52] Treatment courses are typically 10 to 14 days and repeat stool testing is not recommended as a test of cure.[44] Metronidazole is the drug of choice for mild to moderate CDI because its oral formation is less expensive than vancomycin or fidaxomicin, and there are concerns for vancomycin resistant-enterococci with oral vancomycin use.[51] In patients with severe disease, contraindication or intolerance to metronidazole, and inadequate response to metronidazole, oral vancomycin or fidaxomicin is recommended. Vancomycin must be administered orally because IV vancomycin does not achieve adequate gut lumen concentrations for effective bacterial elimination. Due to cost, many institutions choose to use the injectable form of vancomycin to prepare an oral formulation. Fidaxomicin is a macrocyclic antibiotic (200 mg administered orally twice daily) that has minimal bioavailability, and is bacteriostatic against *C. difficile*. Fidaxomicin was approved by the FDA after the current Infectious Diseases Society of America (IDSA)/Society for Healthcare Epidemiology of America (SHEA) guidelines were published; thus its place in therapy remains unclear. When vancomycin has been compared to fidaxomicin, the rate of initial cure was not significantly different between treatment groups; however, fidaxomicin demonstrated a significant improvement in recurrence.[53]

In patients with severe or complicated CDI, practice guidelines suggest combination therapy with IV metronidazole and vancomycin. The route of vancomycin administration is patient-dependent; oral is preferred, but if ileus is present, rectal administration via retention enema is suggested. This recommendation for combination therapy was based on expert opinion and has been supported by a small retrospective study of 88 patients, but further studies are suggested to define optimal regimens and dosing.[54]

Recurrence of CDI occurs in approximately 25% of cases within 30 days and the risk doubles after two or more recurrences.[55] Risk factors for recurrent CDI include a history of recurrence, emergency hospital admission, previous GI hospital admission, recent (within 4-12 weeks) hospitalization, increasing age, use of additional antimicrobials, and an inadequate protective immune response to *C. difficile* toxins.[56] Management of the first relapse is identical to a primary episode because relapse is rarely due to resistance to the initial agent of treatment. Instead, relapse occurs because treatment fails to eradicate the spore forms of the pathogen, or treatment leads to opportunistic infection. Fidaxomicin inhibits *C. difficile* spore production. Clinical trials have demonstrated fewer episodes of recurrence with fidaxomicin treatment compared to vancomycin.[54,57]

The optimal management of patients with multiple relapses is not clear. A prolonged tapered and pulse-dosing of oral vancomycin has been suggested for second episodes of relapse.[58] Other regimens that have shown efficacy include stepped therapy with vancomycin followed by rifaximin.[59] Alternative treatments effective against CDI include intravenous immunoglobulin (IVIG) and fecal microbiota transplantation (FMT). Individuals with low concentration of circulating IgG antitoxin are susceptible to more severe disease and frequent relapses. IVIG has been investigated in patients with intractable, recurrent CDI, and while case reports suggest promising results, high cost may preclude its use.[60] Initial methods of FMT involved preparing a small amount of fresh feces from a healthy donor suspended in saline, filtering the suspension and administering through a nasogastric tube or by retention enema. Data from case series show that FMT is efficacious; however, many practitioners are reluctant to offer this therapy to patients. Administering frozen, prepared capsules of FMT from healthy volunteers is safe and effective in treating CDI, resulting in a 90% resolution rate.[61] The FDA states that FMT should only be used in patients with recurrent CDI who have signed consents and if donor stool has been tested for transmittable diseases.

Agents in clinical trials for treatment or prevention of CDI include new antibiotics, monoclonal antibodies, and *C. difficile* toxoid vaccines.[55] Rifampin, bacitracin, and fusidic acid have lost favor in the treatment of CDI. Concerns with these regimens include drug interactions, development of resistance, and a potential increase in mortality with rifampin observed in several studies.[52] Anion exchange resins such as cholestyramine and colestipol have been used to treat CDI; however, they bind vancomycin and are no longer recommended. Drugs that inhibit peristalsis, such as diphenoxylate/atropine and loperamide, are contraindicated in CDI.[46] Slowing of fecal transit time is thought to result in extended toxin-associated damage.

Prevention of CDI involves both preventing the acquisition of the infection and stopping transmission of *C. difficile* and its spores to other patients. CDI has become the focus of antimicrobial stewardship efforts aimed at eliminating unnecessary antibiotics and reducing durations of therapy. The use of probiotics to prevent CDI has been studied in adults and children. While some studies and meta-analyses have shown no benefit, some evidence supports probiotic safety and efficacy in preventing CDI.[55] Hand washing and contact precautions are imperative measures in preventing the spread of the organism. Alcohol-based hand gels are ineffective against *C. difficile* spores; use of soap and water is recommended to prevent disease transmission. Proper environmental disinfecting measures in healthcare settings include use of chloride-containing cleaning agents or other sporicidial agents.[45]

TRAVELER'S DIARRHEA

Traveler's diarrhea describes the clinical syndrome manifested by malaise, anorexia, and abdominal cramps followed by the sudden onset of diarrhea that incapacitates many travelers. It interferes with planned activities or work in 30% of those affected. In particular, an increased risk lies with North Americans and Northern Europeans traveling to Latin America, southern Europe, Africa, and Asia. The highest risk is observed with patients with immunocompromised conditions, achlorhydria, inflammatory bowel disease, and people with chronic debilitating medical conditions. Overall, 20% to 50% of people traveling to high-risk areas will develop the illness.[35]

8 The onset of symptoms usually occurs during the first week of travel but can occur anytime during the visit or after returning home.

Traveler's diarrhea is caused by contaminated food or water. The most common pathogens are bacterial and include ETEC (20%-72%), *Shigella* spp., (3%-25%), *Campylobacter* spp., (3%-17%), and *Salmonella* spp., (3%-7%).[8] Viral causes could occur in up to 30% of cases. Parasitic etiologies are rare during short-term travels, accounting for less than 5% of cases of traveler's diarrhea. Enterotoxigenic *E. coli* is predominantly pathogenic in Latin America, Africa, and South Asia. The invasive enteric pathogens (*Campylobacter* spp., *Salmonella* spp., and *Shigella* spp.) are more important causes of traveler's diarrhea in Asia.

The severity of the syndrome is determined by the number of stools per day and the presence of cramping, nausea, and vomiting. Mild diarrhea is defined as 1 to 3 loose stools per day that are associated with abdominal cramps lasting less than 14 days. Moderate diarrhea indicates more than 4 loose stools daily associated with dehydration, and severe diarrhea is defined as the presence of blood in stools or a fever. Traveler's diarrhea is rarely life-threatening and in most cases, symptoms resolve in several days without treatment. Travelers to high-risk areas should pack a kit that includes a thermometer, loperamide, antibiotics (3-day course) (see "Treatment" section below), ORS salts, and a water purification method.[35]

Prevention

9 Patient education in avoiding high-risk food and beverages should be the best method for minimizing the risk. High-risk foods and beverages include raw or undercooked meat and seafood, moist foods served at room temperature, fruits that cannot be peeled, vegetables, milk from a questionable source, hot sauces on the table, tap water, unsealed bottled water, iced drinks, and food from street vendors. Although education is readily available, a meta-analysis concluded that the incidence of diarrhea was similar in travelers who followed advice and those who engaged in riskier eating habits.[62] Rationales for this include that cooking foods does not always kill pathogens and food should not be considered safe unless it is cooked until steaming hot. Nonetheless, advisement of avoidance measures regarding safe foods, beverages, and eating establishments is recommended to heighten awareness.

Bismuth subsalicylate 524 mg (2 tablets or 2 tablespoonfuls) orally four times daily for up to 3 weeks is a commonly recommended prophylactic regimen.[35] Bismuth subsalicylate may inhibit enterotoxin activity and prevent diarrhea. Persons taking this regimen should be informed of adverse events, including temporary black discoloration of tongue and stools, and, rarely, tinnitus.

Although the efficacy of prophylactic antibiotics has been documented, their use is not recommended for most travelers due to the potential side effects of antibiotics (eg, photosensitivity), predisposition to other infections such as CDI or vaginal candidiasis, the increased risk of selection of drug-resistant organisms, cost, lack of data on the safety and efficacy of antibiotics given for more than 2 or 3 weeks, and availability of rapidly effective antibiotics for treatment. Prophylactic antibiotics are recommended only in high-risk individuals or in situations in which short-term illness could ruin the purpose of the trip, such as a military mission. A fluoroquinolone is the drug of choice when traveling to most areas of the world.[35] Due to fluoroquinolone resistance among *Campylobacter* spp., azithromycin can be considered when traveling to South and Southeast Asia.

Rifaximin is a nonabsorbed oral rifamycin that has activity against enteric pathogens and may have a role in the prevention of traveler's diarrhea in select populations. A randomized, double-blind trial of rifaximin 200 mg once, twice, or three times daily with meals for 2 weeks resulted in equal protection of 72% for each of the three dosing regimens compared with placebo.[36] Since rifaximin is effective against traveler's diarrhea due to noninvasive strains of *E. coli*, this agent should be reserved for travel regions where *E. coli* predominates, such as Latin America and Africa. Rifaximin has a tolerability and safety profile comparable to that of placebo. The concern with the class rifamycin is the emergence of resistance when used as monotherapy.

TREATMENT

The goals of treatment are to avoid dehydration, reduce the severity and duration of symptoms, and prevent interruption of planned activities. Fluid and electrolyte replacement should be initiated at the onset of diarrhea. ORT is generally not required in otherwise healthy individuals; flavored mineral water offers a good source of sodium and glucose. In infants and young children, elderly, and those with chronic debilitating medical conditions, ORT is recommended. For symptom relief, loperamide is preferred because of its quicker onset and longer duration of relief relative to bismuth. Standard dosing of loperamide is 4 mg orally initially and then 2 mg with each subsequent loose stool to a maximum of 16 mg/day in patients without bloody diarrhea and fever. Loperamide should be discontinued if symptoms persist for more than 48 hours. Other symptomatic therapy in mild diarrhea includes bismuth subsalicylate 524 mg every 30 minutes for up to eight doses.[35] As previously discussed, there is insufficient evidence to warrant the recommendation of probiotics.

Since behavioral modification has limited efficacy and chemoprophylaxis is not recommended in most travelers, the current recommendation relies on self-treatment. A single dose of antibiotic and up to 3 days of treatment will improve the condition within 24 to 36 hours, shortening the duration of diarrhea by 1 to 2 days.[35] A single dose of fluoroquinolone is recommended initially and if diarrhea is improved within 12 to 24 hours, antibiotics should be discontinued. Otherwise, it can be continued for up to 3 days. A fluoroquinolone is recommended when traveling to most areas of the world. Where fluoroquinolone-resistant *Campylobacter* is common, such as in South and Southeast Asia, azithromycin should be used.[35] Azithromycin can also be used in pregnant women and children younger than age 16 years. Empiric treatment of young children should be instituted with caution.

Rifaximin was as effective as a 3-day course of ciprofloxacin in shortening the duration of diarrhea in noninvasive traveler's diarrhea. However, rifaximin was not as effective in patients with fever and bloody diarrhea and in those with invasive pathogens. Therefore, a 3-day course of rifaximin has been approved for the treatment of traveler's diarrhea caused by noninvasive strains of *E. coli* in people 12 years or older and can be considered when traveling to areas where *E. coli*–associated traveler's diarrhea is common, such as Mexico and Jamaica.[35]

For rapid improvement in symptoms, antibiotic therapy with adjunctive treatment with loperamide has shown benefit.[63] All clinical trials concluded that the combination therapy was safe, and the worsening of the disease with the use of antimotility treatment has not been encountered.

Clinical **Controversy...**

Prevention strategies are the most important measure for traveler's diarrhea. Although rifaximin is indicated for some traveler's diarrhea associated with ETEC, its cost and availability versus fluoroquinolones and macrolides may make it a nonpreferred choice.

FOOD POISONING

10 Foodborne illnesses result from the ingestion of food containing pathogenic microorganisms that cause GI infections or preformed toxins that were produced by microorganisms that cause enterotoxigenic poisonings. In the United States, foodborne diseases cause approximately 76 million illnesses, 325,000 hospitalizations, and 5,200 deaths each year.[4] Foodborne transmission may account

for up to 80% of acute gastroenteritis. However, the incidence and outbreaks of foodborne illness has declined in recent years.[64] Common enteric pathogens responsible for foodborne diseases have been discussed in the previous sections (*Campylobacter* spp., *E. coli*, norovirus, nontyphoidal *Salmonella*, *Shigella*). Common foodborne pathogens that cause enterotoxigenic poisonings include *Bacillus cereus*, *Clostridium botulinum*, *Clostridium perfringens*, and *Staphylococcus aureus*. Characteristics of pathogens responsible for foodborne illnesses are summarized in Table 113-8.

Because foodborne disease can appear as sporadic cases or outbreaks, the diagnosis should be suspected whenever two or more people present with acute GI or neurologic manifestations after sharing a meal within the previous 72 hours. Important clues about etiologic agents can be gathered from demographic information (age, gender, etc.), the clinical syndrome, incubation period, and medical history, type of foods consumed, seasonality, and geographic location of the outbreak.

Enterotoxigenic poisonings result from ingestion of food contaminated by preformed toxins. Therefore, symptoms are rapid in onset, but most cases of food poisoning are of short duration with recovery occurring within 1 to 2 days. *B. cereus* causes two different types of clinical syndromes. The first one is characterized by a short incubation period and vomiting. The second syndrome has a longer incubation period and is characterized by diarrhea. Foodborne *C. perfringens* infection may present as two distinct syndromes. Type A organisms are seen in Western Hemisphere nations and result in a 24-hour illness characterized by watery diarrhea and epigastric pain. Type C organisms can be found in undercooked pork and occur in underdeveloped tropical regions. They can produce a toxin-related syndrome called *enteritis necroticans*, which is a coagulative transmural necrosis of the intestinal wall.[65] This syndrome can result in intestinal perforation leading to sepsis and mortality in approximately 40% of victims.

Foodborne botulism results from the ingestion of food contaminated with preformed toxins or toxin-producing spores from *C. botulinum*. *C. botulinum* poisoning is rare; only 110 cases are reported per year in the United States.[65] Botulism is almost always associated with improper preparation or storage of food. Seven distinct toxins (A to G) have been described. The toxins prevent the release of acetylcholine at the peripheral cholinergic nerve terminal. Toxin activity has prompted the use of minute locally injected doses to treat select spastic disorders, such as blepharospasm, hemifacial spasm, and certain dystonias. Foodborne botulism is suspected when patients present with acute GI symptoms concurrently or just prior to the onset of a symmetric descending paralysis without sensory or central nervous system involvement. Diagnosis is made by culturing *C. botulinum* from the stool. The clinical presentation may resemble GBS associated with *C. jejuni* infection. The difference lies in the onset of neurologic symptoms, which typically occur 1 to 3 weeks after the onset of *C. jejuni* infection, and the condition usually is manifested by an ascending paralysis in *C. jejuni*–associated GBS.

Treatment consists primarily of respiratory support and use of botulinum antitoxin.[66] If evaluation is performed within several hours of ingestion, gastric lavage or induction of vomiting is suggested.

TABLE 113-8 Food Poisonings

Organism	Principal Foods	Peak Incidence (United States)	Time to Symptoms	Duration	Common Symptoms
Enterotoxigenic Poisonings					
Bacillus cereus	Fried rice, dairy products, spices, bean sprouts, vegetables	None	1-6 hours 6-24 hours	1 day 1 day	Nausea, vomiting Diarrhea
Clostridium botulinum	Home-canned fruits, vegetables, meats, honey	None	18-36 hours		Double vision, blurred vision, drooping eyelids, slurred speech, difficulty swallowing, dry mouth, and muscle weakness
Clostridium perfringens (type A)	Meats, poultry, gravies, dried or precooked foods	Fall, winter, spring	8-12 hours	1 day	Abdominal cramps, diarrhea
Staphylococcus aureus	Salad, pastries, ham, sandwiches, puddings, unpasteurized milk, cheese products	Summer	1-6 hours	1 day	Nausea, vomiting, abdominal cramps, diarrhea
GI Infections					
Campylobacter spp.	Poultry, dairy products, clams, water	Spring, summer	2-5 days	7 days	Diarrhea (may be bloody), cramping, abdominal pain, fever
Enteropathogenic *E. coli*	Water	None	1-3 days	5-7 days	Severe diarrhea, vomiting, dehydration
Enterotoxigenic *E. coli*	Water, ice, food	None	1-3 days	3-4 days	Profuse watery diarrhea, abdominal cramping
Salmonella spp.	Beef, poultry, water, eggs, dairy products	Summer	12-72 hours	4-7 days	Diarrhea (sometimes bloody), fever, abdominal cramps
Shigella spp.	Salad, water	Summer	1-2 days	5-7 days	Diarrhea (often bloody), fever, abdominal cramps
Vibrio cholerae	Water	None	2 hours to 5 days	2-3 days	Profuse watery diarrhea, vomiting, leg cramps
Vibrio parahemolyticus	Shellfish (oysters)	Spring, summer, fall	24 hours	3 days	Watery diarrhea, abdominal cramping, nausea, vomiting, fever, chills
Yersinia enterocolitica	Dairy products, raw or undercooked pork products	None	4-7 days	1-3 weeks	Fever, abdominal pain, diarrhea (often bloody)

Cathartics and enemas also can be used to remove residual toxin from the bowel, but they are contraindicated in cases of ileus. Botulinum antitoxin is a concentrated preparation of equine globulins obtained from horses immunized with toxins A, B, and E. Because trivalent antitoxin is equine in origin, patients should be tested for hypersensitivity before receiving the product intravenously. Newer and more effective methods of treatment and prevention are under development, including a botulinum toxin vaccine consisting of nontoxic botulinum fragments. Prevention always should be stressed. Botulinum toxins are heat labile and readily destroyed by 10 minutes of boiling. All home-canned foods should be processed according to directions and boiled, not just warmed, prior to consumption.

In foodborne illnesses, the cornerstone of therapy remains supportive care. ORT is preferred in replenishing and maintaining fluid and electrolyte balance, and IV fluid therapy should be reserved for those who are severely ill and cannot tolerate oral therapy. Antiemetics and antimotility agents offer symptomatic relief, but the latter should not be given in patients who present with high fever, bloody diarrhea, or fecal leukocytes. Antimicrobial therapy is not effective in the management of *S. aureus*, *C. perfringens*, or *B. cereus* food poisonings. In developed countries, many of the foodborne illnesses can be prevented with proper food selection, preparation, and storage. However, in developing countries, sanitation and clean water supply are larger concerns.

ABBREVIATIONS

AIDS	acquired immunodeficiency syndrome
cAMP	cyclic adenosine monophosphate
CDI	*Clostridium difficile* infection
CRP	C-reactive protein
EAEC	enteroaggregative *Escherichia coli*
EHEC	enterohemorrhagic *Escherichia coli*
EIEC	enteroinvasive *Escherichia coli*
EPEC	enteropathogenic *Escherichia coli*
ETEC	enterotoxigenic *Escherichia coli*
FDA	Food and Drug Administration
FMT	fecal microbiota transplant
GBS	Guillain-Barré syndrome
HIV	human immunodeficiency virus
HUS	hemolytic uremic syndrome
IDSA	Infectious Diseases Society of America
IBS	irritable bowel syndrome
IL	interleukin
IVIG	intravenous immune globulin
NAP-1	North American pulsed-field type 1
ORS	oral rehydration solution
ORT	oral rehydration therapy
PKA	protein kinase A
PPI	proton pump inhibitor
SHEA	Society for Healthcare Epidemiology of America
STEC	Shiga toxin–producing *Escherichia coli*
UNICEF	United Nations Children's Fund
ViCPS	Vi capsular polysaccharide vaccine
WHO	World Health Organization

REFERENCES

1. Guerrant RL, Van Gilder T, Steiner TS, et al. Practice guidelines for the management of infectious diarrhea. *Clin Infect Dis* 2001;32(3):331-351.
2. World Health Organization: Diarrheoal disease: Available at: http://www.who.int/mediacentre/factsheets/fs330/en/. Accessed: 9/30/2015.
3. Fischer Walker CL, Perin J, Aryee MJ, Boschi-Pinto C, Black RE. Diarrhea incidence in low- and middle-income countries in 1990 and 2010: A systematic review. *BMC Public Health* 2012;12:220.
4. Jones TF, McMillian MB, Scallan E, et al. A population-based estimate of the substantial burden of diarrhoeal disease in the United States; FoodNet, 1996-2003. *Epidemiol Infect* 2007;135(2):293-301.
5. Scallan E, Griffin PM, Angulo FJ, Tauxe RV, Hoekstra RM. Foodborne illness acquired in the United States—Unspecified agents. *Emerg Infect Dis* 2011;17(1):16-22.
6. Scallan E, Hoekstra RM, Angulo FJ, et al. Foodborne illness acquired in the United States—Major pathogens. *Emerg Infect Dis* 2011;17(1):7-15.
7. Charles MD, Holman RC, Curns AT, Parashar UD, Glass RI, Bresee JS. Hospitalizations associated with rotavirus gastroenteritis in the United States, 1993-2002. *Pediatr Infect Dis J* 2006;25(6):489-493.
8. Crim SM, Griffen PM, Tauxe R, et al. Preliminary incidence and trends of infection with pathogens transmitted commonly through food—Foodborne Diseases Active Surveillance Network, 10 U.S. Sites, 2006-2014. *MMWR* 2015; 64(18):495-499.
9. Sack DA, Sack RB, Nair GB, Siddique AK. Cholera. *Lancet* 2004; 363(9404):223-233.
10. Holtz LR, Neill MA, Tarr PI. Acute bloody diarrhea: A medical emergency for patients of all ages. *Gastroenterology* 2009;136(6): 1887-1898.
11. Flores J, Okhuysen PC. Enteroaggregative *Escherichia coli* infection. *Curr Opin Gastroenterol* 2009;25(1):8-11.
12. Pfeiffer ML, DuPont HL, Ochoa TJ. The patient presenting with acute dysentery—A systematic review. *J Infect* 2012;64(4):374-386.
13. Voetsch AC, Van Gilder TJ, Angulo FJ, et al. FoodNet estimate of the burden of illness caused by nontyphoidal *Salmonella* infections in the United States. *Clin Infect Dis* 2004;38(Suppl 3):S127-S134.
14. Niyogi SK. Shigellosis. *J Microbiol* 2005;43(2):133-143.
15. Sabina Y, Rahman A, Ray RC, Montet D. *Yersinia enterocolitica*: Mode of transmission, molecular insights of virulence, and pathogenesis of infection. *J Pathog* 2011;2011:429069.
16. Hodges K, Gill R. Infectious diarrhea: Cellular and molecular mechanisms. *Gut Microbes* 2010;1(1):4-21.
17. Li C, Dandridge KS, Di A, et al. Lysophosphatidic acid inhibits cholera toxin-induced secretory diarrhea through CFTR-dependent protein interactions. *J Exp Med* 2005;202(7):975-986.
18. Lucas ML. Enterocyte chloride and water secretion into the small intestine after enterotoxin challenge: Unifying hypothesis or intellectual dead end? *J Physiol Biochem* 2008;64(1):69-88.
19. Greenberg HB, Estes MK. Rotaviruses: From pathogenesis to vaccination. *Gastroenterology* 2009;136(6):1939-1951.
20. Rallabhandi P, Awomoyi A, Thomas KE, et al. Differential activation of human TLR4 by *Escherichia coli* and *Shigella flexneri* 2a lipopolysaccharide: Combined effects of lipid A acylation state and TLR4 polymorphisms on signaling. *J Immunol* 2008;180(2):1139-1147.
21. Fernandez MI, Sansonetti PJ. *Shigella* interaction with intestinal epithelial cells determines the innate immune response in shigellosis. *Int J Med Microbiol* 2003;293(1):55-67.
22. Kim DH, Kang SH, Jeong WS, et al. Serum C-reactive protein (CRP) levels in young adults can be used to discriminate between inflammatory and non-inflammatory diarrhea. *Dig Dis Sci* 2013;58:504-508.
23. Haverly RM, Harrison CR, Dougherty TH. *Yersinia enterocolitica* bacteremia associated with red blood cell transfusion. *Arch Pathol Lab Med* 1996;120(5):499-500.
24. Panos GZ, Betsi GI, Falagas ME. Systematic review: Are antibiotics detrimental or beneficial for the treatment of patients with *Escherichia coli* O157:H7 infection? *Aliment Pharmacol Ther* 2006;24(5):731-742.
25. Garg AX, Pope JE, Thiessen-Philbrook H, Clark WF, Ouimet J. Arthritis risk after acute bacterial gastroenteritis. *Rheumatology (Oxford)* 2008;47(2):200-204.
26. Allos BM. *Campylobacter jejuni* infections: Update on emerging issues and trends. *Clin Infect Dis* 2001;32(8):1201-1206.
27. Connor BA, Riddle MS. Post-infectious sequelae of traveler's diarrhea. *J Travel Med* 2013;20(5):303-312.
28. Hahn S, Kim S, Garner P. Reduced osmolarity oral rehydration solution for treating dehydration caused by acute diarrhoea in children. *Cochrane Database Syst Rev* 2002;(1):CD002847.
29. Musekiwa A, Volmink J. Oral rehydration salt solution for treating cholera: ≤ 270 mOsm/L solutions vs ≥ 310 mOsm/L solutions. *Cochrane Database Syst Rev* 2011;(12):CD003754.
30. Barr W and Smith A. Acute diarrhea. *Am Fam Physician* 2014;89(3): 180-189.
31. Gregorio GV, Gonzales ML, Dans LF, Martinez EG. Polymer-based oral rehydration solution for treating acute watery diarrhoea. *Cochrane Database Syst Rev* 2009;(2):CD006519.
32. Gregorio GV, Dans LF, Silvestre MA. Early versus delayed refeeding for children with acute diarrhoea. *Cochrane Database Syst Rev* 2011;(7): CD007296.

33. Payot S, Bolla JM, Corcoran D, Fanning S, Megraud F, Zhang Q. Mechanisms of fluoroquinolone and macrolide resistance in *Campylobacter* spp. *Microbes Infect* 2006;8(7):1967-1971.
34. Parry CM, Threlfall EJ. Antimicrobial resistance in typhoidal and nontyphoidal salmonellae. *Curr Opin Infect Dis* 2008;21(5):531-538.
35. Hill DR, Ericsson CD, Pearson RD, et al. The practice of travel medicine: Guidelines by the Infectious Diseases Society of America. *Clin Infect Dis* 2006;43(12):1499-1539.
36. DuPont HL, Jiang ZD, Okhuysen PC, et al. A randomized, double-blind, placebo-controlled trial of rifaximin to prevent travelers' diarrhea. *Ann Intern Med* 2005;142(10):805-812.
37. DuPont HL. Clinical practice. Bacterial diarrhea. *N Engl J Med* 2009; 361(16):1560-1569.
38. Hempel S, Newberry SJ, Maher AR, et al. Probiotics for the prevention and treatment of antibiotic-associated diarrhea: a systemic review and meta-analysis. *JAMA* 2012;307(18):1959-1969.
39. Allen SJ, Wareham K, Wang D, et al. Lactobacilli and bifidobacteria in the prevention of antibiotic-associated diarrhoea and *Clostridium difficile* diarrhoea in older patients (PLACIDE): a randomised, double-blind, placebo-controlled, multicentre trial. *Lancet* 2013;382(9900):1249-1257.
40. Lazzerini M, Ronfani L. Oral zinc for treating diarrhoea in children. *Cochrane Database Syst Rev* 2012;6:CD005436.
41. Steinberg EB, Bishop R, Haber P, et al. Typhoid fever in travelers: Who should be targeted for prevention? *Clin Infect Dis* 2004;39(2): 186-191.
42. Cortese MM, Parashar UD. Prevention of rotavirus gastroenteritis among infants and children: Recommendations of the Advisory Committee on Immunization Practices (ACIP). *MMWR Recomm Rep* 2009;58(RR-2):1-25.
43. Centers for Disease Control and Prevention. Addition of history of intussusception as a contraindication for rotavirus vaccination. *MMWR* 2011;60(41):1427.
44. Walker RI. An assessment of enterotoxigenic *Escherichia coli* and *Shigella* vaccine candidates for infants and children. *Vaccine* 2015;33:954-65.
45. Cohen SH, Gerding DN, Johnson S, et al. Clinical Practice Guidelines for *Clostridium difficile* Infection in Adults: 2010 Update by the Society for Healthcare Epidemiology of America (SHEA) and the Infectious Diseases Society of America (IDSA). *Infect Control Hosp Epidemiol* 2010;31(5):431-455.
46. Leffler DA, Lamont JT. Treatment of *Clostridium difficile*-associated disease. *Gastroenterology* 2009;136(6):1899-1912.
47. Janarthanan S, Ditah I, Adler DG, Ehrinpreis MN. *Clostridium difficile*-associated diarrhea and proton pump inhibitor therapy: A meta-analysis. *Am J Gastroenterol* 2012;107(7):1001-1010.
48. Buendgens L, Bruensing J, Matthes M, Duckers H, et al. Administration of proton pump inhibitors in critically ill medical patients is associated with increased risk of developing *Clostridium difficile*-associated diarrhea. *J Crit Care* 2014;29(4):696.e11-696.e15.
49. Mitchell BG, Gardner A. Mortality and *Clostridium difficile* infection: A review. *Antimicrob Resist Infect Control* 2012;1(1):20.
50. Kachrimanidou M, Malisiovas N. *Clostridium difficile* infection: A comprehensive review. *Crit Review Mircobiol* 2011;37(3):178-187.
51. Zar FA, Bakkanagari SR, Moorthi KM, Davis MB. A comparison of vancomycin and metronidazole for the treatment of *Clostridium difficile*-associated diarrhea, stratified by disease severity. *Clin Infect Dis* 2007;45(3):302-307.
52. Dimitri DM, Butler M, MacDonald R, et al. Comparative effectiveness of *Clostridium difficile* treatments. *Ann Intern Med* 2011;155 (12): 839-847.
53. Louie TJ, Miller MA, Mullane KM, et al. Fidaxomicin versus vancomycin for *Clostridium difficile* infection. *N Engl J Med* 2011; 364(5):422-431.
54. Rokas EE, Johnson JW, Beardsley JR, Ohl CA, Luther VP, Willaimson JC. The addition of intravenous metronidazole to oral vancomycin is associated with improved mortality in critically ill patients with *Clostridium difficile* infection. *Clin Infect Dis* 2015;61(6):934-941.
55. Goldberg EJ, Bhalodia S, Jacob S, et al. *Clostridium difficile* infection: A brief update on emerging therapies. *Am J Health-Syst Pharm* 2015;72: 1007-1012.
56. Eyre DW, Walker AS, Wyllie D, et al. Predictors of first recurrence of *Clostridium difficile* infection: Implications for initial management. *Clin Infect Dis* Aug 2012;55 Suppl 2:S77-87.
57. Babakhani F, Bouillaut L, Gomez A, Sears P, Nguyen L, Sonenshein AL. Fidaxomicin inhibits spore production in *Clostridium difficile*. *Clin Infect Dis* 2012;55(Suppl 2):S162-169.
58. Kelly C. A 76-year-old man with recurrent *Clostridium difficile*-associated diarrhea. *JAMA* 2009;301(9):954-962.
59. Johnson S, Galang M, et al. Interruption of recurrent *Clostridium difficile*-associated diarrhea episodes by serial therapy with vanocmycin and rifaximin. *Clin Infect Dis* 2007;44:846-848.
60. Shah N, Shaaban H, Spira R, Slim J, Boghossian J. Intravenous immunoglobulin in the treatment of severe *Clostridium difficile* colitis. *J Glob Infect Dis* 2014;6(2):82-85.
61. Youngster I, Russell GH, Pindar C, Ziv-Baran T, Sauk J, Hohmann EL. Oral, capsulized, frozen fecal microbiota transplantation for relapsing *Clostridium difficile* infection. *JAMA* 2014;312(17):1772-1778.
62. Shlim D. Looking for evidence that personal hygiene precautions prevent traveler's diarrhea. *Clin Infect Dis* 2005;41(Suppl 8): S531-S535.
63. Riddle MS, Arnold S, Tribble DR. Effect of adjunctive loperamide in combination with antibiotics on treatment outcomes in traveler's diarrhea: A systematic review and meta-analysis. *Clin Infect Dis* 2008; 47(8):1007-1014.
64. Imanishi M, Manikonda K, Murthy BP, Gould LH. Factors contributing to decline in foodborne disease outbreak reports, United States. *Emerg Infect Dis* 2014;20(9):1551-1553.
65. Sobel J, Tucker N, Sulka A, McLaughlin J, Maslanka S. Foodborne botulism in the United States, 1990-2000. *Emerg Infect Dis* 2004;10(9): 1606-1611.
66. Sobel J. Botulism. *Clin Infect Dis* 2005;41(8):1167-1173.

114 Intra-Abdominal Infections

Alan E. Gross, Keith M. Olsen and Joseph T. DiPiro

KEY CONCEPTS

1. Most intra-abdominal infections are "secondary" infections that are polymicrobial and are caused by a defect in the gastrointestinal (GI) tract that must be treated by surgical drainage, resection, and/or repair.
2. Primary peritonitis is generally caused by a single organism (*Staphylococcus aureus* in patients undergoing chronic ambulatory peritoneal dialysis [CAPD] or *Escherichia coli* in patients with cirrhosis).
3. Secondary intra-abdominal infections are usually caused by a mixture of bacteria, including enteric Gram-negative bacilli and anaerobes, which enhance the pathogenic potential of the bacteria.
4. For peritonitis, early and aggressive IV fluid resuscitation and electrolyte replacement therapy are essential. A common cause of early death is hypovolemic shock caused by inadequate intravascular volume and tissue perfusion.
5. Treatment is generally initiated on a "presumptive" or empirical basis and should be based on the likely pathogen(s) and local resistance patterns.
6. Antimicrobial regimens for secondary intra-abdominal infections should include coverage for enteric Gram-negative bacilli and anaerobes. Antimicrobials that may be used for the treatment of secondary intra-abdominal infections depending on severity of illness and microbiology data include (a) third-generation cephalosporin (ceftriaxone) with metronidazole, (b) piperacillin–tazobactam, (c) a carbapenem (imipenem, meropenem, doripenem, and ertapenem), and (d) quinolone (levofloxacin or ciprofloxacin) plus metronidazole or moxifloxacin alone.
7. Treatment of patients with peritoneal dialysis-associated peritonitis should include an antistaphylococcal antimicrobial such as a first-generation cephalosporin (cefazolin) or vancomycin (intraperitoneal administration is preferred).
8. The duration of antimicrobial treatment should be for 4 days after source control for most secondary intra-abdominal infections.
9. Patients treated for intra-abdominal infections should be assessed for the occurrence of drug-related adverse effects, particularly hypersensitivity reactions (β-lactam antimicrobials), diarrhea (most agents), fungal infections (most agents), and nephrotoxicity (aminoglycosides).

Intra-abdominal infections are those contained within the peritoneal cavity or retroperitoneal space. The peritoneal cavity extends from the undersurface of the diaphragm to the floor of the pelvis and contains the stomach, small bowel, large bowel, liver, gallbladder, and spleen. The duodenum, pancreas, kidneys, adrenal glands, great vessels (aorta and vena cava), and most mesenteric vascular structures reside in the retroperitoneum. Intra-abdominal infections may be generalized or localized, complicated or uncomplicated, and community or healthcare-associated. Uncomplicated intra-abdominal infections are confined within visceral structures, such as the liver, gallbladder, spleen, pancreas, kidney, or female reproductive organs while complicated intra-abdominal infections involve anatomical disruption, extend beyond a single organ, and yield peritonitis and/or abscess. *Peritonitis* is defined as the acute inflammatory response of the peritoneal lining to microorganisms, chemicals, irradiation, or foreign-body injury. This chapter deals only with peritonitis of infectious origin.

An *abscess* is a purulent collection of fluid separated from surrounding tissue by a wall consisting of inflammatory cells and adjacent organs. It usually contains necrotic debris, bacteria, and inflammatory cells. These processes differ considerably in presentation and approach to treatment.

EPIDEMIOLOGY

Peritonitis may be classified as primary, secondary, or tertiary.[1-5] Primary peritonitis, also called *spontaneous bacterial peritonitis*, is an infection of the peritoneal cavity without an evident source in the abdomen.[6] Bacteria may be transported from the bloodstream to the peritoneal cavity, where the inflammatory process begins. In secondary peritonitis, a focal disease process is evident within the abdomen. Secondary peritonitis may involve perforation of the gastrointestinal (GI) tract (possibly because of ulceration, ischemia, or obstruction), postoperative peritonitis, or posttraumatic peritonitis (blunt or penetrating trauma). Tertiary peritonitis occurs in critically ill patients and is infection that persists or recurs at least 48 hours after apparently adequate management of primary or secondary peritonitis.[7,8]

1 Primary peritonitis occurs in both children and adults, although the incidence and mortality rates in both populations have been declining.[4] Primary peritonitis develops in up to 10% to 30% of patients with alcoholic cirrhosis.[4-6,9,10] Patients undergoing chronic ambulatory peritoneal dialysis (CAPD) average one episode of peritonitis every 20 to 33 months.[11,12] Epidemiologic data for secondary and tertiary intra-abdominal infections are less understood. Secondary peritonitis may be caused by perforation of a peptic ulcer; traumatic perforation of the stomach, small or large bowel, uterus, or urinary bladder; appendicitis; pancreatitis; diverticulitis; bowel infarction; inflammatory bowel disease; cholecystitis; operative contamination of the peritoneum; or diseases of the female genital tract, such as septic abortion, postoperative uterine infection, endometritis, and salpingitis. Appendicitis is one of the most common causes of intra-abdominal infection. In 2010, 305,000 appendectomies were performed in the United States for suspected appendicitis.[13] Most healthcare-associated intra-abdominal infections occur as complications following intra-abdominal surgeries.

ETIOLOGY

Primary peritonitis in adults occurs most commonly in association with alcoholic cirrhosis, especially in its end stage, or with ascites caused by postnecrotic cirrhosis, chronic active hepatitis, acute viral hepatitis, congestive heart failure, malignancy, systemic lupus erythematosus, or nephritic syndrome. It may also result from the use of a peritoneal catheter for dialysis or CNS ventriculoperitoneal shunting for hydrocephalus. Rarely, primary peritonitis occurs without apparent underlying disease.

Table 114-1 summarizes many of the potential causes of bacterial peritonitis. Causes include inflammatory processes of the GI tract or abdominal organs, bowel obstruction, vascular occlusions that may lead to gangrene of the intestines, and neoplasia that may cause intestinal perforation or obstruction. Other possible causes include those resulting from traumatic injuries, postoperative infections, or solid organ transplant in the abdomen.

Abscesses are the result of chronic inflammation and may occur without preceding generalized peritonitis. They may be located within one of the spaces of the peritoneal cavity or within one of the visceral organs, and may range from a few milliliters to a liter or more in volume. These collections often have a fibrinous capsule and may take from a few weeks to years to form.

The causes of intra-abdominal abscess overlap those of peritonitis and, in fact, may occur sequentially or simultaneously. Appendicitis is the most frequent cause of abscess. Other potential causes of intra-abdominal abscess include pancreatitis, diverticulitis, lesions of the biliary tract, genitourinary tract infections, perforation in the abdomen, trauma, and leaking intestinal anastomoses. In addition, pelvic inflammatory disease in women may lead to tuboovarian abscess. For some diseases, such as appendicitis and diverticulitis, abscesses occur more frequently than generalized peritonitis.

Microflora of the Gastrointestinal Tract and Female Genital Tract

A full appreciation of intra-abdominal infection requires an understanding of the normal microflora within the GI tract. There are striking differences in bacterial species and concentrations of flora within the various segments of the GI tract (Table 114-2), and this bacterial environment usually determines the severity of infectious processes in the abdomen. Generally, the low gastric pH eradicates bacteria that enter the stomach. With achlorhydria, bacterial counts may rise to 10^5 to 10^7 organisms/mL (10^8 to 10^{10}/L). The normally low bacterial count may also increase by 1,000-or 10,000-fold with gastric outlet obstruction, hemorrhage, gastric cancer, and in patients receiving histamine 2 (H2)-receptor antagonists, proton pump inhibitors, or antacids.[14,15] A two to threefold increase in Spontaneous bacterial peritonitis has been demonstrated with the use of proton pump inhibitors.

The biliary tract (gallbladder and bile ducts) is sterile in most healthy individuals, but in people older than 70 years, those with acute cholecystitis, jaundice, or common bile duct stones, it is likely to be colonized by aerobic Gram-negative bacilli (particularly *Escherichia coli* and *Klebsiella* spp.) and enterococci.[16,17] Patients with biliary tract bacterial colonization are at greater risk of intra-abdominal infection.

In the distal ileum, bacterial counts of aerobes and anaerobes are quite high. In the colon, there may be 500 to 600 different types of bacteria in stool, with concentrations often reaching 10^{11} organisms/mL (10^{14}/L) and anaerobic bacteria outnumbering aerobic bacteria by more than 1,000 to 1.[2,18] In fact, up to 50% of the dry mass of stool is *Bacteroides* spp. Fortunately, most colonic bacteria are not pathogens because they cannot survive in environments outside the colon. Perforation of the colon results in the release of large numbers of anaerobic and aerobic bacteria into the peritoneum.

The colonic flora are generally consistent unless broad-spectrum antimicrobials have been used. Depending on the type of antibiotic and spectrum, the duration of use, route of administration, and the pharmacokinetic and pharmacodynamic properties, antibiotics can cause shifts in the normal GI microflora including causing increased drug resistance.[19]

The lower female genital tract is generally colonized by a large number of aerobic and anaerobic bacteria. Anaerobes may number 10^9 organisms/mL (10^{12}/L) and often include lactobacilli, eubacteria, clostridia, anaerobic streptococci, and, less frequently, *Bacteroides fragilis*. Aerobic bacteria most often are streptococci and *Staphylococcus epidermidis*, and these may number 10^8 organisms/mL (10^{11}/L).

TABLE 114-2 Usual Microflora of the GI Tract

Site	Commonly Found Bacteria	Approximate Concentration (No. Organisms/mL [×10³/L]) Aerobes	Anaerobes
Stomach[a]	*Streptococcus, Lactobacillus*	10-100	Rare
Biliary tract	Normally sterile (*Escherichia coli, Klebsiella*, or enterococci in some patients)	0	0
Proximal small bowel	*Streptococcus* (including enterococci), *E. coli, Klebsiella, Lactobacillus*, diphtheroids	100	Few
Distal ileum	*E. coli, Klebsiella, Enterobacter*, enterococci, *Bacteroides fragilis, Clostridium*, peptostreptococci	10^4-10^6	10^5-10^7
Colon	*Bacteroides* spp., peptostreptococci, *Clostridium, E. coli, Klebsiella*, enterococci, *Enterobacter*, *Candida*, and many others	10^5-10^8	10^9-10^{11}

GI, gastrointestinal.

[a]With achlorhydria, acid suppressive therapy, gastric cancer, or gastric outlet obstruction, bacterial counts may rise to 10^5/mL (10^8/L).

TABLE 114-1 Causes of Bacterial Peritonitis

Primary (spontaneous) bacterial peritonitis
- Peritoneal dialysis
- Cirrhosis with ascites
- Nephrotic syndrome

Secondary bacterial peritonitis
- Miscellaneous causes
  - Diverticulitis
  - Appendicitis
  - Inflammatory bowel diseases
  - Salpingitis
  - Biliary tract infections
  - Necrotizing pancreatitis
  - Neoplasms
  - Intestinal obstruction
  - Perforation
- Mechanical GI problems
  - Any cause of small bowel obstruction (adhesions, hernia)
- Vascular causes
  - Mesenteric arterial or venous occlusion (atrial fibrillation)
  - Mesenteric ischemia without occlusion
- Trauma
  - Blunt abdominal trauma with rupture of intestine
  - Penetrating abdominal trauma
- Iatrogenic intestinal perforation (endoscopy)
- Intraoperative events
  - Solid organ transplant in the abdomen
- Peritoneal contamination during abdominal operation
- Leakage from GI anastomosis

GI, gastrointestinal.

PATHOPHYSIOLOGY

Intra-abdominal infection results from bacterial entry into the peritoneal or retroperitoneal spaces or from bacterial collections within intra-abdominal organs. In primary peritonitis, bacteria may enter the abdomen via the bloodstream or the lymphatic system by transmigration through the bowel wall, through an indwelling peritoneal dialysis catheter, or via the fallopian tubes in females. Hematogenous bacterial spread (through the bloodstream) occurs more frequently with tuberculosis peritonitis or peritonitis associated with cirrhotic ascites. When peritonitis results from peritoneal dialysis, skin surface flora are introduced via the peritoneal catheter. In secondary peritonitis, bacteria most often enter the peritoneum or retroperitoneum as a result of perforation of the GI or female genital tracts caused by diseases or traumatic injuries. In addition, peritonitis or abscess may result from contamination of the peritoneum during a surgical procedure or following anastomotic leak.

The physiologic characteristics of the peritoneal cavity determine the nature of the response to infection or inflammation within it.[1,4] The peritoneum is lined by a highly permeable serous membrane with a surface area approximately that of skin. The peritoneal cavity is lubricated with less than 100 mL of sterile, clear yellow fluid, normally with fewer than 250 cells/mm^3 (0.25×10^9/L), a specific gravity below 1.016, and protein content below 3 g/dL (30 g/L). These conditions change drastically with peritoneal infection or inflammation, as described below.

After bacteria are introduced into the peritoneal cavity, there is an immediate response to contain the insult. Humoral and cellular defenses respond first; then the omentum adheres to the affected area. A limited bacterial inoculum is handled rapidly by defense mechanisms, including complement activation and a leukocyte response. Under certain conditions, the bacterial insult is not contained, and bacteria disseminate throughout the peritoneal cavity, resulting in peritonitis. This is more likely to occur in the presence of a foreign body, hematoma, dead tissue, a large bacterial inoculum, continuing bacterial contamination, and contamination involving a mixture of synergistic organisms. Protein–calorie malnutrition, antecedent steroid therapy, and diabetes mellitus may also contribute to the formation of an intra-abdominal abscess.

When bacteria become dispersed throughout the peritoneum, the inflammatory process involves most of the peritoneal lining. There is an outpouring into the peritoneum of fluid containing leukocytes, fibrin, and other proteins that form exudates on the inflamed peritoneal surfaces and begin to form adhesions between peritoneal structures. This process, combined with a paralysis of the intestines (ileus), may result in confinement of the contamination to one or more locations within the peritoneum. Fluid also begins to collect in the bowel lumen and wall, and distension may result.

The fluid and protein shift into the abdomen (called *third-spacing*) may be so dramatic that circulating blood volume is decreased, which may cause decreased cardiac output and hypovolemic shock. Accompanying fever, vomiting, or diarrhea may worsen the fluid imbalance. A reflex sympathetic response, manifested by sweating, tachycardia, and vasoconstriction, may be evident. With an inflamed peritoneum, bacteria and endotoxins are absorbed easily into the bloodstream (translocation), and this may result in septic shock.[1,4,5] Other foreign substances present in the peritoneal cavity potentiate peritonitis. These adjuvants, notably feces, dead tissues, barium, mucus, bile, and blood, have detrimental effects on host defense mechanisms, particularly on bacterial phagocytosis.

Many of the manifestations of intra-abdominal infections, particularly peritonitis, result from cytokine activity. Inflammatory cytokines, such as tumor necrosis factor-α (TNF-α), interleukin (IL) 1, IL-6, IL-8, and interferon γ (INF-γ), are produced by macrophages and neutrophils in response to bacteria and bacterial products or in response to tissue injury resulting from the surgical incision.[1,4] These cytokines produce wide-ranging effects on the vascular endothelium of organs, particularly the liver, lungs, kidneys, and heart. With uncontrolled activation of these mediators, sepsis may result (see Chapter 119 Sepsis and Septic Shock).[20-22]

Peritonitis may result in death because of the effects on major organ systems. Fluid shifts, cytokines and endotoxin may result in hypovolemia, hypoperfusion, and shock. Hypoalbuminemia may result from protein loss into the peritoneum exacerbating intravascular volume loss. Pulmonary function may be compromised by the inflamed peritoneum, producing splinting (muscle rigidity caused by pain) that inhibits adequate diaphragmatic movement leading to atelectasis and pneumonia. Increased lung vascular permeability and resulting shunting of blood may induce onset of the respiratory distress syndrome and associated hypoxemia and hypercarbia. With fluid loss and hypotension, renal and hepatic perfusion may be compromised, and acute renal and hepatic failure are potential threats.

If peritoneal contamination is localized but bacterial elimination is incomplete, an abscess results. This collection of necrotic tissue, bacteria, and white blood cells may be at single or multiple sites and may be within one of the spaces of the peritoneal cavity or in one of the visceral organs. The location of the abscess is often related to the site of primary disease. For example, abscesses resulting from appendicitis tend to appear in the right lower quadrant or the pelvis; those resulting from diverticulitis tend to appear in the left lower quadrant or pelvis.

An abscess begins by the combined action of inflammatory cells (such as neutrophils), bacteria, fibrin, and other inflammatory mediators. Bacteria may release heparinases that cause local thrombosis and tissue necrosis or fibrinolysins, collagenases, or other enzymes that allow extension of the process into surrounding tissues. Neutrophils gathered in the abscess cavity die in 3 to 5 days, releasing lysosomal enzymes that liquefy the core of the abscess. A mature abscess may have a fibrinous capsule that isolates bacteria and the liquid core from antimicrobials and immunologic defenses.

Within the abscess, the oxygen tension is low and anaerobic bacteria thrive; thus, the size of the abscess may increase because it is hypertonic, resulting in an additional influx of fluid. Hypertonicity promotes the formation of bacterial L forms, which are resistant to antimicrobial agents that disrupt cell walls. Abscess formation may continue and mature for long periods of time and may not be readily evident to either patient or physician. In some instances, the abscess may resolve spontaneously, and, infrequently, it may erode into adjacent organs or rupture and cause diffuse peritonitis. If the abscess erodes through the skin, it may result in an enterocutaneous fistula, connecting bowel to skin, or in a draining sinus tract.

The overall outcome from an intra-abdominal infection depends on key factors: inoculum size, virulence of the contaminating organisms, the presence of adjuvants within the peritoneal cavity that facilitate infection, the adequacy of host defenses, source control, and the adequacy of initial treatment.[9,23,24]

Microbiology of Intra-Abdominal Infection

2 Primary bacterial peritonitis is often caused by a single organism. In children, the pathogen is usually group A *Streptococcus*, *E. coli*, *Streptococcus pneumoniae*, or *Bacteroides* species.[4,25-28] When peritonitis occurs in association with cirrhotic ascites, *E. coli* is isolated most frequently. Other potential pathogens are: *Haemophilus influenzae*, *Klebsiella* spp., *Pseudomonas* spp., anaerobes, and *S. pneumoniae*.[29] Occasionally, primary peritonitis may be caused by *Mycobacterium tuberculosis*. Peritonitis in patients undergoing peritoneal dialysis is caused most often by common skin organisms, such as coagulase-negative staphylococci, *Staphylococcus aureus*, streptococci, and enterococci. Gram-negative bacteria associated with peritoneal dialysis infections include *E. coli*, *Klebsiella* spp., and *Pseudomonas* spp.[6] The mortality rate from primary peritonitis caused by Gram-negative bacteria is much greater than that from Gram-positive bacteria.[4,5]

TABLE 114-3 Pathogens Isolated from Patients with Intra-Abdominal Infection

	Secondary Peritonitis[3,33] (%)	Community-Acquired Infection[33] (%)	Nosocomial Infection[33] (%)
Gram-Negative Bacteria			
Escherichia coli	32-61	29	22.5
Enterobacter	8-26	5.2	8.0
Klebsiella	6-26	2.8	4.5
Proteus	4-23	1.7	2.4
Pseudomonas	5-13	5	13
Gram-Positive Bacteria			
Enterococcus	18-24	10.6	18
Streptococcus	6-55	13.7	10
Staphylococcus	6-16	3.1	4.8
Anaerobic Bacteria			
Bacteroides	25-80	13.7	10.3
Clostridium	5-18	3.5	3.4
Fungi	2-5	3	4

3 Because of the diverse bacteria present in the GI tract, secondary intra-abdominal infections are often polymicrobial.[2] The mean number of different bacterial species isolated from infected intra-abdominal sites ranged from 2.9 to 3.7, including an average of 1.3 to 1.6 aerobes and 1.7 to 2.1 anaerobes.[29,30] With proper anaerobic specimen collection, anaerobic organisms are isolated in most patients. In one report of patients with gangrenous and perforated appendicitis, an average of 10.2 different organisms was isolated from each patient, including 2.7 aerobes and 7.5 anaerobes.[31] Purely aerobic or anaerobic infections are uncommon, as are infections caused by fungi. Table 114-3 gives the frequencies with which specific bacteria were isolated from patients with peritonitis and other intra-abdominal infections.[3,32] Nosocomial infections tend to have a more diverse array of pathogens, are more likely to involve *Pseudomonas* spp., and have a higher likelihood of multidrug-resistance compared with isolates from community-acquired infections.[33]

Visceral organ abscesses differ in character from the typical intra-abdominal abscess. Hepatic abscesses may be polymicrobial (involving *E. coli*, *Klebsiella* spp., and anaerobes) or occasionally may be caused by amoeba.[18] Pancreatic abscesses are often polymicrobial, involving enteric bacteria that ascend through the biliary system. Splenic abscesses usually result from hematogenous dissemination of bacteria, such as *E. coli*, *S. aureus*, *Proteus mirabilis*, *Enterococcus* spp., and *Klebsiella pneumoniae*, as well as anaerobes.[18] Pelvic inflammatory disease is associated initially with *Neisseria gonorrhoeae* or *Chlamydia trachomatis.* However, tuboovarian abscesses are usually polymicrobial, having a mix of Gram-positive and Gram-negative aerobes and anaerobes.

Bacterial Synergism

The size of the bacterial inoculum and the number and types of bacterial species present in intra-abdominal infections influence patient outcome. The combination of aerobic and anaerobic organisms appears to greatly increase the severity of infection. In animal studies, combinations of aerobic and anaerobic bacteria were much more lethal than infections caused by aerobes or anaerobes alone.

Facultative bacteria may provide an environment conducive to the growth of anaerobic bacteria.[2] Although many bacteria isolated in mixed infections are nonpathogenic by themselves, their presence may be essential for the pathogenicity of the bacterial mixture.[9] The role of facultative bacteria in mixed infections can include (a) promotion of an appropriate environment for anaerobic bacterial growth through oxygen consumption, (b) production of nutrients necessary for anaerobes, and (c) production of extracellular enzymes that promote tissue invasion by anaerobes.

Rat models of intra-abdominal infection demonstrate that uncontrolled infection with an implanted mix of aerobes and anaerobes leads to a two-stage (biphasic) infectious process. There is an early peritonitis phase with a high mortality rate and isolation of *E. coli* from blood and a late abscess formation phase in all survivors with isolation of anaerobes such as *B. fragilis* and *Fusobacterium varium*. These experiments and others support the concept that aerobic enteric organisms and anaerobes are pathogens in intra-abdominal infection. Aerobic bacteria, particularly *E. coli*, appear responsible for the early mortality from peritonitis, whereas anaerobic bacteria are major pathogens in abscesses, with *B. fragilis* predominating.[34]

Enterococcus can be isolated from many intra-abdominal infections in humans, but its role as a pathogen is not clear. Enterococcal infection occurs more commonly in postoperative peritonitis, in the presence of specific risk factors indicating failure of the host's defenses (immunocompromised patients), or with the use of broad-spectrum antibiotics.[35,36]

CLINICAL PRESENTATION

Intra-abdominal infections have a wide spectrum of clinical features often depending on the specific disease process, the location and magnitude of bacterial contamination, and concurrent host factors. Peritonitis is usually recognized easily, but intra-abdominal abscess may often continue for considerable periods of time, either going unrecognized or being attributed to an unrelated disease process. Patients with primary and secondary peritonitis present quite differently (Table 114-4).[1,4,5]

Primary peritonitis can develop over a period of days to weeks and is usually a more indolent process than secondary peritonitis. The first sign of peritonitis may be a cloudy dialysate in patients undergoing peritoneal dialysis or worsening encephalopathy in a cirrhotic patient.

The patient with generalized bacterial peritonitis presents most often in acute distress. The patient lies still, usually on his or her back, possibly with the hips slightly flexed. Any movement of the patient, including rocking the bed or breathing, worsens the generalized abdominal pain.

If peritonitis continues untreated, the patient may experience hypovolemic shock from third-space fluid loss into the peritoneum, bowel wall, and lumen. This may be accompanied by sepsis because the inflamed peritoneum absorbs bacteria and toxins into mesenteric blood vessels and lymph nodes, initiating production of inflammatory cytokines. Hypovolemic shock is the major factor contributing to mortality in the early stage of peritonitis.

Intra-abdominal abscess may pose a difficult diagnostic challenge because the symptoms are neither specific nor dramatic. The patient may complain of abdominal pain or discomfort, but these symptoms are not reliable. Fever is usually present; often it is low grade, but it may be high, with a spiking pattern. The patient may have a paralytic ileus and abdominal distension. The abdominal examination is unreliable; tenderness and pain may be present, and a mass may be palpated.

Peritonitis may result from an abscess that ruptures, spreading bacteria and toxins throughout the peritoneum. In other patients, the entry of bacterial toxins into the systemic circulation from the abscess may lead to sepsis and progressive multisystem organ failure (eg, renal, hepatic, pulmonary, or cardiovascular).

Laboratory studies are not generally helpful in the diagnosis of intra-abdominal abscess, although most patients will have leukocytosis. Some patients may have positive blood cultures, whereas

TABLE 114-4 Clinical Presentation of Peritonitis

Primary Peritonitis

General
The patient may not be in acute distress, particularly with peritoneal dialysis

Signs and symptoms
The patient may complain of loss of appetite, bloating, nausea, vomiting (sometimes with diarrhea), and abdominal tenderness
Temperature may be only mildly elevated or not elevated in patients undergoing peritoneal dialysis
Bowel sounds are hypoactive
The cirrhotic patient may have worsening encephalopathy
Cloudy dialysate fluid with peritoneal dialysis

Laboratory tests
The patient's WBC count may be only mildly elevated
Ascitic fluid usually contains greater than 250 leukocytes/mm^3 (0.25×10^9/L), and bacteria may be evident on Gram stain of a centrifuged specimen
In 60%-80% of patients with cirrhotic ascites, the Gram stain is negative

Other diagnostic tests
Culture of peritoneal dialysate or ascitic fluid should be positive, particularly if collected prior to initiation of antibiotics
Procalcitonin in conjunction with clinical findings is a sensitive test for bacterial peritonitis[37]

Secondary Peritonitis

Signs and symptoms
Generalized abdominal pain
Tachypnea
Tachycardia
Nausea and vomiting
Temperature is normal initially then increases to 37.8-38.9°C (100-102°F) within the first few hours and may continue to rise for the next several hours
Hypotension, hypoperfusion, and shock if volume is not restored
Decreased urine output due to vascular volume depletion

Physical examination
Voluntary abdominal guarding changing to involuntary guarding and a "board-like abdomen"
Abdominal tenderness and distension
Faint bowel sounds that cease over time

Laboratory tests
Leukocytosis (15,000-20,000 WBC/mm^3 [15×10^9 to 20×10^9/L]), with neutrophils predominating and an elevated percentage of immature neutrophils (bands)
Elevated hematocrit and blood urea nitrogen because of dehydration
Patient progresses from early alkalosis because of hyperventilation and vomiting to metabolic acidosis

Other diagnostic tests
Abdominal radiographs may be useful because free air in the abdomen (indicating intestinal perforation) or distension of the small or large bowel is often evident

WBC, white blood cell.

others, particularly diabetics, may have hyperglycemia. The finding of *Bacteroides* or any two enteric bacteria in the bloodstream is often indicative of an intra-abdominal infectious process.

Radiographic methods are used to make the diagnosis of an intra-abdominal abscess. Plain radiographs may show air–fluid levels or a shift of normal intra-abdominal contents by the abscess mass. GI contrast studies may also demonstrate this displacement of abdominal structures. Both of these modalities provide indirect evidence of abscess presence but are not generally helpful in precisely locating the abscess.

Ultrasound is a frequent first diagnostic method used when an intra-abdominal abscess is suspected. The procedure may be done at the bedside, which is particularly helpful when the patient is in the intensive care unit.

Computed tomographic (CT) scanning is the preferred modality used to evaluate the abdomen for the presence of an abscess and is the imaging study of greatest value. If not contraindicated, an oral radiocontrast agent should be given to allow differentiation of the abscess from the bowel. IV radiocontrast material will be taken up preferentially in the wall of the abscess, creating a unique radiographic appearance, so-called rim enhancement. Magnetic resonance imaging offers no significant advantage when compared with CT scanning.

Intra-abdominal infection caused by disease processes at specific sites often produces characteristic manifestations that are helpful in diagnosis. For example, a patient with diverticulitis may exhibit stabbing left-lower-quadrant abdominal pain and constipation. Fever and leukocytosis are frequently present, and a tender mass is sometimes palpable. With appendicitis, the findings may be inconsistent, but many patients have a sudden onset of periumbilical or epigastric pain that is usually colicky and later shifts to the right lower quadrant. The location of pain may vary because the appendix can be in many locations (eg, retrocecal or pelvic) in the abdomen. A mass may be palpable on abdominal, pelvic, or rectal examination. The patient's temperature is generally mildly elevated early and then increases. If perforation and peritonitis occur, findings would include diffuse abdominal pain, rigidity, and sustained fever. More often, however, appendiceal perforation results in a local abscess.

TREATMENT

Desired Outcome

The primary goals of treatment are correction of the intra-abdominal disease processes or injuries that have caused infection and the drainage of purulent collections (abscesses). A secondary objective is to achieve a resolution of infection without major organ system complications (pulmonary, hepatic, cardiovascular, or renal failure) or adverse drug effects. Ideally, the patient should be discharged from the hospital after treatment with full function for self-care and routine daily activities.

General Approach to Treatment

The treatment of intra-abdominal infection most often requires hospitalization and the coordinated use of three major modalities: (a) prompt drainage of the infected site, (b) hemodynamic resuscitation and support of vital organ functions, and (c) early administration of appropriate antimicrobial therapy to treat infection not eradicated by surgery.[2]

Antimicrobials are an important adjunct to drainage procedures in the treatment of secondary intra-abdominal infections; however, the use of antimicrobial agents without surgical intervention is usually inadequate. For most cases of primary peritonitis, drainage procedures may not be required, and antimicrobial agents become the mainstay of therapy.

4 In the early phase of serious intra-abdominal infections, attention should be given to the maintenance of organ system functions. With generalized peritonitis, large volumes of IV fluids are required to restore vascular volume, to improve cardiovascular function, and to maintain adequate tissue perfusion and oxygenation. Adequate urine output should be maintained to ensure adequate resuscitation and proper renal function. Respiratory function can be assisted by a variety of methods, including oxygen therapy, pulmonary physiotherapy, and ventilatory support in severely ill patients. Often the critically ill patient with intra-abdominal infection will require intensive care management, particularly if there is cardiovascular or respiratory instability. In addition, isolation procedures may be required if the infectious process poses a threat to other hospitalized patients.

An additional important component of therapy is nutrition. Intra-abdominal infections often directly involve the GI tract or disrupt its function (paralytic ileus). The return of GI motility may take days, weeks, and, occasionally, months. In the interim, enteral or parenteral nutrition as indicated facilitates improved immune function and wound healing to ensure recovery.

Nonpharmacologic Treatment

Drainage Procedures

Primary peritonitis is treated with antimicrobials and rarely requires drainage. Secondary peritonitis requires surgical correction of the underlying pathology. The drainage of the purulent material is the critical component of management of an intra-abdominal abscess. Without adequate drainage of the abscess, antimicrobial therapy and fluid resuscitation can be expected to fail.

Secondary peritonitis is treated surgically; this is often called *source control*, which refers to all the physical measures undertaken to eradicate the focus of infection.[2,5] At the time of laparotomy (surgical opening and exploration of the abdomen), attempts are made to correct the cause of the peritonitis. This may include patching a perforated ulcer with omentum, removal of a segment of perforated colon, or excision of a portion of gangrenous small intestine. In addition, the surgeon may elect to leave the abdomen open after the laparotomy, plan a re-laparotomy at a later time regardless of the patient's condition, or, perform re-laparotomy if the patient develops reinfection.[5] The goal of all these procedures is to repair or remove the inflamed or gangrenous viscus and to prevent further bacterial contamination. The presence of active inflammation increases the difficulty of the surgical procedure, which results in a higher morbidity and mortality rate than if the same procedures were performed in an elective setting without inflammation.

The presence of active inflammation may make it technically impossible to perform the definitive surgical procedure. In this situation, attempts are made to provide drainage of the infected or gangrenous structures. If an intra-abdominal abscess, separate from any intra-abdominal organ, is discovered during an exploratory laparotomy, it may be debrided, excised, or drained. If the intra-abdominal abscess involves an abdominal structure, then a resection of part or of the entire organ may be required. An example of this situation is an abscess associated with diverticular disease of the colon. Management may include drainage of the abscess and resection of the involved part of the colon. All foreign material, necrotic tissue, feces, blood, or pus should be removed from the operative field, and the peritoneum should be copiously irrigated with 0.9% sodium chloride to decrease the concentrations of bacteria or other noxious substances.

After an abscess is located, it must be drained. This may be performed surgically or with percutaneous, image-guided techniques.[5,38] Typically, image-guided techniques employ ultrasonography or CT scanning. The management of an intra-abdominal abscess with percutaneous catheter drainage may be sufficient to resolve the infection. Some patients may require a subsequent procedure to treat the underlying GI conditions; however, a significant advantage is obtained by first draining the abscess percutaneously. This allows the surgical procedure to be performed on a patient who is no longer suffering the systemic manifestations of uncontrolled infection. Drainage techniques may be performed using endoscopy or laparoscopy. These minimal-access techniques may offer advantages when compared with traditional surgery but will probably be used less often than radiologically assisted percutaneous drainage techniques.

The most valuable microbiologic information may be obtained at the time of percutaneous or operative abscess drainage. If pus or fluid is found that is believed to be infected, it is best to aspirate 2 to 3 mL into a syringe, remove any air, and tightly cap the syringe. The specimen should be taken promptly to the microbiology laboratory, where a Gram stain should be performed immediately and cultures prepared for identification of aerobic and anaerobic bacteria. If no fluid is available for collection, culture swab devices may be applied to the infected area; however, anaerobic organisms often are not isolated from swabs.

Fluid Therapy

4 Patients should be evaluated for signs of hypovolemia, hypoperfusion, and shock. Aggressive fluid repletion and management are required for successful treatment of intra-abdominal infections. The Surviving Sepsis Campaign: International Guidelines for Management of Severe Sepsis and Septic Shock recommend treatment goals during the first 6 hours or resuscitation: (a) central venous pressure (CVP) 8 to 12 mm Hg, (b) mean arterial pressure (MAP) more than or equal to 65 mm Hg, and (c) maintain urine output more than or equal to 0.5 mL/kg/h.[39,40] If the patient is mechanically ventilated a target CVP 12 to 15 mm Hg should be achieved.[39] Fluid therapy is instituted for the purposes of achieving or maintaining proper intravascular volume to ensure adequate cardiac output, tissue perfusion, and correction of acidosis. Loss of fluid through vomiting, diarrhea, or nasogastric suction contributes to dehydration. Intravascular volume can be assessed by blood pressure and heart rate but more accurately by measurement of CVP or urinary output. When a contracted vascular volume is accompanied by hemorrhage, the initial hematocrit may be normal, but if there is no associated hemorrhage, the hematocrit is usually elevated as an indication of hemoconcentration. Urine output should be monitored continuously in severely ill patients by use of a urinary bladder catheter, quantitated hourly, and should equal or exceed 0.5 mL/kg of body weight per hour.

In patients with peritonitis, hypovolemia is often accompanied by metabolic acidosis. IV fluids should consist of a bolus of crystalloids or colloids with additional fluids targeting predefined therapeutic goals.[39,40] In the initial hour of treatment, large volumes of solution may be required to restore intravascular volume. Thereafter, fluids may be required at a rate of 1 L/h or higher. Once targeted therapeutic goals are reached, maintenance fluids should be instituted with 0.9% sodium chloride and potassium chloride (20 mEq/L [mmol/L]) or 5% dextrose and 0.45% sodium chloride with potassium chloride (20 mEq/L [mmol/L]). The administration rate should be based on estimated daily fluid loss through urine and nasogastric suction, including 0.5 to 1 L for insensible fluid loss. Potassium would not be included routinely if the patient is hyperkalemic or has renal insufficiency. If appropriate fluid management fails to restore target goals of perfusion, vasopressor therapy should be initiated.[39] A more thorough discussion of fluid and vasopressor therapy are presented elsewhere in this text (23, 24, and 119).

In patients with significant blood loss, blood transfusion may be indicated. This is generally in the form of packed red blood cells. The criteria for blood transfusion are controversial, but a hematocrit of 25% is generally accepted. In the individual patient, the decision is often determined by the overall clinical status and the ability of the patient to compensate for the reduction in oxygen-carrying capacity associated with an acute anemia. Additional blood component therapy with fresh-frozen plasma or platelets is also based on the needs of the individual patient. Aggressive fluid therapy must often be continued in the postoperative period because fluid will continue to sequester in the peritoneal cavity, bowel wall, and lumen.

Pharmacologic Treatment

Antimicrobial Therapy

The goals of antimicrobial therapy are (a) to control any bacteremia and prevent the establishment of metastatic foci of infection, (b) to reduce suppurative complications (eg, abscess formation) after bacterial contamination, and (c) to prevent local spread of existing

TABLE 114-5 Likely Intra-Abdominal Pathogens

Type of Infection	Aerobes	Anaerobes
Primary (Spontaneous) Bacterial Peritonitis		
Children	Group A *Streptococcus*, *E. coli*, pneumococci	—
Cirrhosis	*E. coli*, *Klebsiella*, pneumococci (many others)	—
Peritoneal dialysis	*Staphylococcus*, *Streptococcus*, *E. coli*, *Klebsiella*, *Pseudomonas*	—
Secondary Bacterial Peritonitis		
Gastroduodenal	*Streptococcus*, *E. coli*	—
Biliary tract	*E. coli*, *Klebsiella*, enterococci	*Clostridium* or *Bacteroides* (infrequent)
Small or large bowel	*E. coli*, *Klebsiella*, *Proteus*	*B. fragilis* and other *Bacteroides*, *Clostridium*
Appendicitis	*E. coli*, *Pseudomonas*	*Bacteroides*
Abscesses	*E. coli*, *Klebsiella*, *Streptococcus*, enterococci	*B. fragilis* and other *Bacteroides*, *Clostridium*, anaerobic cocci
Liver	*E. coli*, *Klebsiella*, *Streptococcus*, enterococci, *Staphylococcus*, amoeba	*Bacteroides* (infrequent)
Spleen	*Staphylococcus*, *Streptococcus*, *E. coli*, *Salmonella*	

infection. After suppuration has occurred, a cure by antibiotic therapy alone is very difficult to achieve; antimicrobials may serve to improve the results obtained with surgery.

5 An empirical antimicrobial regimen should be started as soon as the presence of intra-abdominal infection is suspected. Therapy must be initiated based on the likely pathogens, potential resistance, and severity of patient illness. Increased resistance among Gram-negative pathogens to fluoroquinolones and ampicillin–sulbactam emphasize the importance of using local susceptibility data to guide empiric therapy and tailoring the antibiotic regimen based on susceptibility results. Predominant pathogens, as discussed in the preceding section, vary depending on the site of intra-abdominal infection and the underlying disease process. Table 114-5 lists the likely pathogens against which antimicrobial agents should be directed.

Antimicrobial Experience Many studies have been conducted evaluating or comparing the effectiveness of antimicrobials for the treatment of intra-abdominal infections. Substantial differences in patient outcomes from treatment with a variety of agents have not generally been demonstrated.[41]

Important findings from over 20 years of clinical trials regarding selection of antimicrobials for intra-abdominal infections are the following:

1. Antimicrobial regimens used for secondary infections should cover a broad spectrum of aerobic and anaerobic bacteria from the GI tract. Empiric treatment should be guided by the local epidemiology of resistant pathogens, patient-specific risk factors for resistant pathogens, and patient severity of illness.
2. Single-agent regimens (such as cephalosporins with anaerobic activity, extended-spectrum penicillins with β-lactamase inhibitors, and carbapenems) are as effective but have the benefit of being less nephrotoxic compared to combinations of aminoglycosides with antianaerobic agents. This is also true for antimicrobial treatment of acute bacterial contamination from penetrating abdominal trauma.[42,43]
3. Resistance is prevalent among *B. fragilis* to clindamycin and cefotetan and Enterobacteriaceae to ampicillin–sulbactam and quinolones and therefore these agents should not be routinely used empirically for complicated intra-abdominal infections.[44,45]
4. If the causative pathogens are susceptible and the patient has clinically responded, antimicrobial treatment can be completed orally with amoxicillin–clavulanate, metronidazole with either ciprofloxacin or levofloxacin, or moxifloxacin.[46]
5. Four days of antimicrobial treatment is sufficient for most intra-abdominal infections with adequate source control.[47,48]

Intra-abdominal infections present in many different ways and with a wide spectrum of severity. The regimen employed and duration of treatment depends on the specific clinical circumstances (ie, the nature of the underlying disease process, severity of illness, and risk of resistant pathogens).

Recommendations 6 For most intra-abdominal infections, the antimicrobial regimen should be effective against both aerobic and anaerobic bacteria.[48,49] When initial antimicrobial therapy is inactive, morbidity and mortality rates are higher than when initially active therapy is used.[48] Generally, agents with activity against enteric Gram-negative bacilli such as *E. coli* and *Klebsiella* spp., and anaerobes including *B. fragilis* should be administered. If most of the organisms can be eliminated through drainage or antimicrobials, the synergistic effect may be removed, and the patient's defenses may be able to resolve the remaining infection.

Table 114-6 presents the recommended agents for treatment of community-acquired complicated intra-abdominal infections from the Infectious Diseases Society of America and the Surgical

TABLE 114-6 Recommended Agents for the Treatment of Community-Acquired Complicated Intra-Abdominal Infections in Adults

Agents Recommended for Mild-to-Moderate Infections	Agents Recommended for High Risk or High Severity Infections
Single Agent	
Cefoxitin[a]	Piperacillin–tazobactam
Moxifloxacin[b] Ertapenem[c]	Imipenem–cilastatin,[c] meropenem,[c] doripenem[c]
Combination Regimens	
Cefazolin,[a] cefuroxime,[a] ceftriaxone, cefotaxime each in combination with metronidazole	Cefepime or ceftazidime each in combination with metronidazole
Ciprofloxacin[b] or levofloxacin[b] each in combination with metronidazole	Ciprofloxacin[b] or levofloxacin[b] each in combination with metronidazole

[a]Empiric first- and second-generation cephalosporin use should be avoided unless local antibiograms show >80% to 90% susceptibility of *E. coli* to these agents.

[b]Use of quinolones may be associated with treatment failure due to increasing resistance of enteric pathogens including *E. coli*. Empiric quinolone use should be avoided unless local antibiograms show >80% to 90% susceptibility of *E. coli* to quinolones.

[c]Carbapenems should be reserved for settings where there is a high risk of resistance to other agents.

Data from reference 48.

Infection Society.[48] These recommendations were formulated using an evidence-based approach. Table 114-7 lists additional evidence-based recommendations for the treatment of complicated intra-abdominal infections. Most community-acquired infections are of mild-to-moderate severity whereas healthcare-associated infections tend to be more severe, more difficult to treat, and more commonly due to resistant pathogens. Table 114-8 presents guidelines for treatment and alternative regimens for specific situations. These are general guidelines; there are many factors that cannot be incorporated into such a table including local resistance patterns to commonly used agents such as quinolones.

Most patients with severe intra-abdominal infection, sepsis of intra-abdominal source, or healthcare-associated infection should be placed on piperacillin–tazobactam, cefepime with metronidazole, or a carbapenem with *Pseudomonas* activity such as imipenem, doripenem, or meropenem. In patients with IgE-mediated allergic reactions to β-lactams (hives/urticaria, bronchospasm, angioedema, or anaphylaxis), combination therapy with aztreonam, vancomycin and metronidazole may be used. The benefits of systemic empiric antifungal (with fluconazole or an echinocandin antifungal) have not been established for intra-abdominal infection and should not be routinely used.[50]

Aminoglycoside-based treatment regimens are not routinely recommended due to their narrow therapeutic index (nephrotoxicity, ototoxicity) relative to the recommended agents such as β-lactams. Aminoglycosides are reserved primarily for infections due to presumed or proven multidrug-resistant pathogen(s) or perhaps in patients with IgE-mediated allergic reactions to alternative agents.[41,48]

The initial dosage for aminoglycosides should be determined based on the patient's weight and renal function. Traditionally, gentamicin and tobramycin were administered multiple times daily with specific peak (6-10 mcg/mL) [mg/L; 13-21 μmol/L]) and trough (less than 1-2 mcg/mL) [mg/L; less than 2-4 μmol/L]) concentration targets. Because aminoglycosides have concentration-dependent killing and have a relatively long postantibiotic effect for aerobic Gram-negative bacilli, extended-interval dosing of aminoglycosides is possible. For most patients and indications, extended-interval aminoglycoside dosing (ie, 5-7 mg/kg once daily for tobramycin or gentamicin, 15-20 mg/kg once daily for amikacin) has replaced traditional dosing given equivalent efficacy and decreased nephrotoxicity.[51-53]

Antimicrobial resistance continues to rise worldwide.[54-56] These problematic multidrug-resistant bacteria include enteric pathogens producing extended-spectrum β-lactamases (ESBL) which have been increasingly isolated from intra-abdominal cultures.[44] For patients with ESBL-producing pathogens, carbapenems are typically the drugs of choice. With the increased use of carbapenems, pathogens continue to evolve with the development of β-lactamases that hydrolyze carbapenems (e.g., *Klebsiella pneumoniae* carbapenemase [KPC]), multidrug-resistant *Pseudomonas* spp., and carbapenem-resistant *Acinetobacter* spp. Especially in patients with healthcare-associated intra-abdominal infections, these multidrug-resistant pathogens have forced clinicians to use more toxic and potentially less effective agents such as the polymyxins, tigecycline, and aminoglycosides. For example, the product labeling for tigecycline now carries a Black Box Warning as it has been associated with an increased risk of mortality relative to comparator agents based on pooled data collected from randomized controlled trials including patients with intra-abdominal infections, skin and skin structure infections, and ventilator-associated pneumonia.[57-59] The limited safe and effective therapeutic options for resistant organisms highlights the need, from an individual patient and public health standpoint, for pharmacists and other clinicians to ensure that antimicrobials are selected appropriately, at the optimal dose, and for the correct duration.[60,61]

Clinical **Controversy...**

Ceftolozane/tazobactam and ceftazidime/avibactam were FDA-approved in 2014 and 2015, respectively, for the treatment of complicated intra-abdominal infections in combination with metronidazole.[62,63] These agents are useful as they may be active against multidrug-resistant pathogens including *Pseudomonas* spp., ESBL-producing *Enterobacteriaceae* and KPC-producing *Enterobacteriaceae* (ceftazidime/avibactam only). However, clinical effectiveness and safety data are limited, especially with ceftazidime/avibactam, which was approved prior to completion of Phase III studies. Ceftolozane/tazobactam may not be as effective as meropenem and metronidazole in the treatment of complicated intra-abdominal infections.[64-66] Despite this, these agents are highly valuable in terms of their activity against multidrug-resistant pathogens and as such, their use should be reserved for patients with a suspected or confirmed infection due to a pathogen resistant to all other β-lactams, including carbapenems.

With intra-abdominal contamination from the upper GI tract (perforation of a peptic ulcer or biliary tract disease), anaerobes such as *B. fragilis* are uncommon pathogens, and therefore other empiric agents such as ampicillin, penicillin, or first-generation cephalosporins are reasonable. Anaerobic coverage is also not necessary for primary peritonitis associated with cirrhosis and third-generation cephalosporins, such as cefotaxime or ceftriaxone, remain the treatments of choice.[67]

Coverage of *Enterococcus* in mild-to-moderate community-acquired intra-abdominal infections is not recommended.[48] The failure of host defenses may be a critical factor in the pathogenicity of enterococci. In patients with severe community-acquired intra-abdominal infection or patients with healthcare-associated infection, it is recommended to include coverage of *Enterococcus faecalis* in the initial regimen.[48] Ampicillin remains the drug of choice for this indication because it is most active in vitro against *E faecalis.* Vancomycin is active against most enterococci; however, rates of vancomycin-resistant enterococci are increasing, particularly in select patient populations (eg, liver transplantation, immunocompromised patients).[68] Agents including linezolid or daptomycin are commonly used for vancomycin-resistant *Enterococcus* infections. Table 114-7 lists additional evidence-based recommendations for *Enterococcus* spp. coverage.

7 Intraperitoneal administration of antibiotics is preferred over IV therapy in the treatment of peritonitis that occurs in patients undergoing CAPD.[69] The International Society of Peritoneal Dialysis guidelines for the diagnosis and pharmacotherapy of peritoneal dialysis-associated infections provide dosing recommendations for intermittent and continuous therapy based on the modality of dialysis (continuous or intermittent) and the extent of the patient's residual renal function.[70]

Antimicrobial agents effective against both Gram-positive (including *S. aureus*) and Gram-negative organisms should be used for initial intraperitoneal empiric therapy for peritonitis in peritoneal dialysis patients. The most important factors to take into consideration for initial antimicrobial selection are the dialysis center's and the patient's history of infecting organisms and their sensitivities. For empiric intraperitoneal therapy in patients on continuous peritoneal dialysis, cefazolin (loading dose [LD] 500 mg/L; maintenance dose [MD] 125 mg/L) or vancomycin (LD 1,000 mg/L; MD 25 mg/L) in cases of high prevalence of methicillin-resistant *S. aureus* (MRSA) or β-lactam allergy may be used for Gram-positive coverage. A meta-analysis based on a limited

TABLE 114-7 Evidence-Based Recommendations for Treatment of Complicated Intra-abdominal Infections

	Grade of Recommendation[a]
Elements of Appropriate Intervention	
An appropriate source control procedure to drain infected foci, control ongoing peritoneal contamination by diversion or resection, and restore anatomic and physiological function to the extent feasible is recommended for nearly all patients with intra-abdominal infection	B-2
Community-Acquired Infections of Mild-to-Moderate Severity in Adults	
Antibiotics used for empiric treatment of community-acquired intra-abdominal infections should be active against enteric Gram-negative aerobic and facultative bacilli and enteric Gram-positive streptococci	A-1
For patients with mild-to-moderate community-acquired infections regimens with substantial anti-pseudomonal activity are not required (Table 114-6)	A-1
Empiric coverage of *Enterococcus* is not necessary in patients with mild-to-moderate severity community-acquired intra-abdominal infection	A-1
The use of agents listed as appropriate for higher-severity community-acquired infection and healthcare-associated infection is not recommended for patients with mild-to-moderate community-acquired infection, because such regimens may carry a greater risk of toxicity and facilitate acquisition of more resistant organisms	B-2
High-Risk or High-Severity Community-Acquired Infections in Adults[b]	
The empiric use of antimicrobial regimens with broad-spectrum activity against Gram-negative organisms including *Pseudomonas* spp., such as meropenem, imipenem–cilastatin, doripenem, piperacillin–tazobactam, ciprofloxacin or levofloxacin in combination with metronidazole, or ceftazidime or cefepime in combination with metronidazole, is recommended for patients with high-severity community-acquired intra-abdominal infection (Table 114-6)	A-1
Aztreonam plus metronidazole is an alternative, but addition of an agent effective against Gram-positive cocci is recommended	B-3
Healthcare-Associated Infections in Adults	
Empiric antibiotic therapy for healthcare-associated intra-abdominal infection should be driven by local microbiologic results	A-2
To achieve empiric coverage of likely pathogens, multidrug regimens that include agents with expanded spectra of activity against Gram-negative aerobic and facultative bacilli may be needed. These agents include meropenem, imipenem–cilastatin, doripenem, piperacillin–tazobactam, or ceftazidime or cefepime in combination with metronidazole. Aminoglycosides or colistin may be required	B-3
Antimicrobial Agents Not Recommended	
Ampicillin–sulbactam is not recommended for use because of high rates of resistance to this agent among community-acquired *E. coli*	B-2
Quinolone-resistant *E. coli* have become common in some communities, and quinolones should not be used unless hospital surveys indicate 90% susceptibility of *E. coli* to quinolones	A-2
Cefotetan and clindamycin are not recommended for use because of increasing prevalence of resistance to these agents among *Bacteroides fragilis*	B-2
Because of the availability of less toxic agents demonstrated to be at least equally effective, aminoglycosides are not recommended for routine use in adults with community-acquired intra-abdominal infection	B-2
Oral Completion Therapy	
For adults recovering from intra-abdominal infection, completion of the antimicrobial course with oral forms of moxifloxacin, ciprofloxacin plus metronidazole, levofloxacin plus metronidazole, an oral cephalosporin with metronidazole, or amoxicillin–clavulanic acid is acceptable in patients able to tolerate an oral diet and in patients in whom susceptibility studies do not demonstrate resistance	B-2
Duration of Therapy	
Antimicrobial therapy of established infection should be limited to 4 days, unless it is difficult to achieve adequate source control. Longer durations of therapy have not been associated with improved outcome[c]	A-1
For acute stomach and proximal jejunum perforations, in the absence of acid-reducing therapy or malignancy and when source control is achieved within 24 hours, prophylactic anti-infective therapy directed at aerobic Gram-positive cocci for 24 hours is adequate	B-2
Bowel injuries attributable to penetrating, blunt, or iatrogenic trauma that are repaired within 12 hours and any other intraoperative contamination of the operative field by enteric contents should be treated with antibiotics for ≤24 hours	A-1
Acute appendicitis without evidence of perforation, abscess, or local peritonitis requires only prophylactic administration of narrow spectrum regimens active against aerobic and facultative and obligate anaerobes; treatment should be discontinued within 24 hours	A-1
The administration of prophylactic antibiotics to patients with severe necrotizing pancreatitis prior to the diagnosis of infection is not recommended	A-1
Anaerobic Coverage	
Coverage for obligate anaerobic bacilli should be provided for distal small bowel, appendiceal, and colon-derived infection and for more proximal GI perforations in the presence of obstruction or paralytic ileus	A-1
Antifungal Therapy	
Antifungal therapy for patients with severe community-acquired or healthcare-associated infection is recommended if *Candida* is grown from intra-abdominal cultures	B-2
Anti-MRSA Therapy	
Empiric antimicrobial coverage directed against MRSA should be provided to patients with healthcare-associated intra-abdominal infection who are known to be colonized with the organism or who are at risk of having an infection due to this organism because of prior treatment failure and significant antibiotic exposure	B-2
Vancomycin is recommended for treatment of suspected or proven intra-abdominal infection due to MRSA	A-3

(continued)

TABLE 114-7 Evidence-Based Recommendations for Treatment of Complicated Intra-abdominal Infections (*Continued*)

	Grade of Recommendation[a]
Antienterococcal Therapy	
Antimicrobial therapy for enterococci should be given when enterococci are recovered from patients with healthcare-associated infection	B-III
Empiric antienterococcal therapy is recommended for patients with high-risk community-acquired infections and healthcare-associated intra-abdominal infections, particularly those with postoperative infection, those who have previously received cephalosporins or other antimicrobial agents selecting for *Enterococcus* species, immunocompromised patients, and those with valvular heart disease or prosthetic intravascular materials	B-II
Initial empiric antienterococcal therapy should be directed against *Enterococcus faecalis*. Antibiotics that can potentially be used against this organism, on the basis of susceptibility testing of the individual isolate, include ampicillin, piperacillin/tazobactam, and vancomycin	B-III
Empiric therapy directed against vancomycin-resistant *Enterococcus faecium* is not recommended unless the patient is at very high risk for an infection due to this organism, such as a liver transplant recipient with an intra-abdominal infection originating in the hepatobiliary tree or a patient known to be colonized with vancomycin-resistant *E. faecium*	B-III

MRSA, methicillin-resistant *Staphylococcus aureus.*

[a]Strength of recommendations: A, B, C = good, moderate, and poor evidence to support recommendation, respectively. Quality of evidence: 1 = Evidence from ≥1 properly randomized, controlled trial. 2 = Evidence from ≥1 well-designed clinical trial without randomization, from cohort or case-controlled analytic studies; from multiple time series, or from dramatic results from uncontrolled experiments. 3 = Evidence from opinions of respected authorities, based on clinical experience, descriptive studies, or reports of expert communities.

[b]Criteria for high risk or high severity community-acquired infection: APACHE II score ≥15, delay in initial intervention >24 hours), advanced age, comorbidity and degree of organ dysfunction, low albumin level, poor nutritional status, degree of peritoneal involvement or diffuse peritonitis, inability to achieve adequate debridement or control of drainage, and presence of malignancy.

[c]After IDSA/SIS guideline publication a randomized controlled trial was published and demonstrated that 4 days of therapy after source control is adequate[47]

Data from reference 48.

number of studies found that glycopeptide-containing regimens (vancomycin or teicoplanin) were more likely to achieve complete cure compared to first generation cephalosporins.[69] However the study contributing most of the weight in this meta-analysis used a lower than recommended cefazolin dose.[71] One of these Gram-positive agents should be combined with a Gram-negative agent such as ceftazidime (LD 500 mg/L; MD 125 mg/L) or cefepime (LD 500 mg/L; MD 125 mg/L) or an aminoglycoside (gentamicin or tobramycin LD 8 mg/L; MD 4 mg/L). Another option is monotherapy with cefepime or imipenem–cilastatin (LD 250 mg/L; MD 50 mg/L). Antimicrobial doses should empirically be increased by 25% in patients with residual renal function (more than 100 mL/day urine output).[70] Antimicrobial therapy should be continued for at least 1 week after the dialysate fluid is clear and for a total of at least 14 days. The reader is referred to these guidelines for additional information.[70]

After acute bacterial contamination, such as with abdominal trauma where GI contents spill into the peritoneum, antibiotics should be administered. If the patient is seen soon after injury (within 2 hours) and surgical measures are instituted promptly, antianaerobic cephalosporins (such as cefoxitin), a third-generation cephalosporin (such as ceftriaxone) with metronidazole, or piperacillin/tazobactam are effective in preventing most infectious complications. Antimicrobials should be administered as soon as possible after injury.

For appendicitis, the antimicrobial regimen used should depend on the appearance of the appendix at the time of operation, which may be normal, inflamed, gangrenous, or perforated. Because the condition of the appendix is unknown preoperatively, it is advisable to begin antimicrobial agents before the appendectomy is performed. Reasonable regimens would be antianaerobic cephalosporins or, if the patient is seriously ill, piperacillin–tazobactam or an anti-pseudomonal carbapenem. If, at operation, the appendix is normal or inflamed, postoperative antimicrobials are not required. If the appendix is gangrenous or perforated, a treatment course of 4 days with the agents listed in Table 114-6 is appropriate.

(8) Acute intra-abdominal contamination, such as after a traumatic injury, may be treated with a very short antimicrobial course (24 hours).[72] For established infections (ie, peritonitis or intra-abdominal abscess), an antimicrobial course limited to 4 days is appropriate.[47] This allows eradication of bacteria remaining in the peritoneum after a surgical procedure that may enter the peritoneum through healing suture lines. Under certain conditions, therapy for longer than 4 days would be justified (eg, when a focus of infection in the abdomen is still present). For some abscesses, such as pyogenic liver abscess, antimicrobials may be required for a month or longer.

Clinical **Controversy...**

The Infectious Diseases Society of America/Surgical Infection Society guidelines for complicated intra-abdominal infections recommend 4 to 7 days of antimicrobial therapy after attainment of source control.[48] Despite this, therapy has historically continued for longer durations, likely due to an initial lack of high quality data supporting this recommendation.[73] A subsequent randomized controlled trial of 518 patients with intra-abdominal infection and adequate source control compared the clinical outcomes of 4 days of antimicrobial therapy after the index source control procedure versus 2 days of therapy after normalization of leukocytosis, temperature, and diet (median 8 days of therapy).[47] This study found no difference in the rate of surgical site infections, recurrent intra-abdominal infections, or mortality between treatment groups; this suggests 4 days of therapy after source control is likely adequate. Although the study was stopped after enrolling approximately 50% of the patients initially planned, the proportion of patients meeting primary or secondary outcomes were similar in the total cohort as well as in multiple patient subgroups defined a priori. Because the study only assessed patients with source control, the optimal duration of antimicrobial therapy in patients with uncontrolled sources of intra-abdominal infection remains unknown. In these cases, should antimicrobial therapy be continued until the source is controlled? Or, if source control is not possible in the near term and the patient is clinically stable with minimal signs of systemic inflammatory response, can antimicrobial therapy be safely withheld and the patient closely monitored so as to limit long durations of antimicrobial therapy and associated adverse effects?

TABLE 114-8 Guidelines for Empiric Antimicrobial Agents for Intra-Abdominal Infections[48,70]

	Primary Agents	Alternatives
Primary (Spontaneous) Bacterial Peritonitis		
Cirrhosis	Ceftriaxone, cefotaxime	1. Piperacillin–tazobactam, carbapenems 2. Aztreonam combined with an agent active against *Streptococcus* spp. (eg, vancomycin) or quinolones with significant *Streptococcus* spp. activity (levofloxacin, moxifloxacin)
Peritoneal dialysis	Initial empiric regimens should be active against both Gram-positive (including *S. aureus*) and Gram-negative pathogens: Gram-positive agent (first-generation cephalosporin or vancomycin) plus a Gram-negative agent (third-generation cephalosporin or aminoglycoside)	1. Cefepime or carbapenems may be used alone 2. Aztreonam or an aminoglycoside may be used in place of ceftazidime or cefepime as long as combined with a Gram-positive agent 3. Quinolones may be used in place of Gram-negative agents if local susceptibilities allow
	1. *Staphylococcus* spp.: oxacillin/nafcillin or first-generation cephalosporin	1. Vancomycin should be used if concern for methicillin-resistant *Staphylococcus* spp. 2. Add rifampin for 5-7 days with vancomycin for methicillin-resistant *S. aureus*
	2. *Streptococcus* or *Enterococcus*: ampicillin	1. An aminoglycoside may be added for *Enterococcus* spp. 2. Linezolid or daptomycin should ideally be used to treat vancomycin-resistant *Enterococcus* spp. not susceptible to ampicillin
	3. Aerobic Gram-negative bacilli: ceftazidime or cefepime	1. The regimen should be based on in vitro sensitivity tests
	4. *Pseudomonas aeruginosa*: two agents with differing mechanisms of action, such as an oral quinolone plus ceftazidime, cefepime, tobramycin, or piperacillin	
Secondary Bacterial Peritonitis		
Perforated peptic ulcer	First-generation cephalosporins	1. Ceftriaxone, cefotaxime, or antianaerobic cephalosporins[a]
Other	Third- or fourth-generation cephalosporin with metronidazole, piperacillin–tazobactam or carbapenem	1. Ciprofloxacin[b] or levofloxacin[b] each with metronidazole or *moxifloxacin*[b] alone 2. Aztreonam with vancomycin and metronidazole 3. Antianaerobic cephalosporins[a]
Abscess		
General	Third- or fourth-generation cephalosporin with metronidazole, or piperacillin–tazobactam	1. Imipenem–cilastatin, meropenem, doripenem, or ertapenem 2. Ciprofloxacin[b] or levofloxacin[b] each with metronidazole or moxifloxacin alone
Liver	As above	Use metronidazole if amoebic liver abscess is suspected
Spleen	Ceftriaxone or cefotaxime	Moxifloxacin[b] or levofloxacin[b]
Other Intra-abdominal Infections		
Appendicitis	Same management as for community-acquired complicated intra-abdominal infections as listed in Table 114-6[39]	
Community-acquired acute cholecystitis	Ceftriaxone or cefotaxime	Severe infection, piperacillin/tazobactam, antipseudomonal carbapenem, aztreonam with metronidazole
Cholangitis	Ceftriaxone or cefotaxime each with or without metronidazole	Vancomycin with aztreonam with or without metronidazole
Acute contamination from abdominal trauma	Antianaerobic cephalosporins[a] or metronidazole with either ceftriaxone or cefotaxime	1. Piperacillin/tazobactam or a carbapenem 2. Ciprofloxacin[b] or levofloxacin[b] each with metronidazole or moxifloxacin alone

[a]Cefoxitin or ceftizoxime; these agents should be avoided empirically unless local antibiograms show >80% to 90% susceptibility of *E. coli* to these agents.

[b]Use of quinolones may be associated with treatment failure due to increasing resistance of enteric pathogens including *E. coli*. Empiric quinolone use should be avoided unless local antibiograms show >80% to 90% susceptibility of *E. coli* to quinolones.

Intraperitoneal irrigation of antimicrobial agents for treatment of intra-abdominal infection has been studied, often with conflicting results.[74] Intraoperative antimicrobial irrigation does not improve patient outcomes in comparison with copious intraoperative irrigation with normal saline. Possibly the most important aspect of peritoneal irrigation is the dilutional effect on bacteria and adjuvants that promotes infection (intestinal contents and hemoglobin). Most systemically administered antimicrobials easily cross the peritoneal membrane so that peritoneal fluid concentrations are similar to serum. Confined areas, such as an abscess, can be expected to attain much lower antimicrobial concentrations.

EVALUATION OF THERAPEUTIC OUTCOMES

Whichever antimicrobial regimen is chosen, the patient should be reassessed continually to determine the success or failure of therapies. The clinician should recognize that there are many reasons for poor patient outcomes with intra-abdominal infections; improper antimicrobial administration is only one. The patient may be immunocompromised, which decreases the likelihood of successful outcome with any regimen. There may be surgical reasons for poor patient outcome. Failure to identify all intra-abdominal foci of infection or leaks from a GI anastomosis may cause continued infection. Finally, antimicrobial resistance may contribute to treatment failure as isolates from intra-abdominal infections are increasingly drug resistant.[75]

The outcome from intra-abdominal infection is not determined solely by what transpires in the abdomen. Unsatisfactory outcomes in patients with intra-abdominal infections may result from complications that arise in other organ systems, including renal or respiratory failure. Furthermore, pneumonia is a complication that is commonly associated with mortality after intra-abdominal infection.[76] A high APACHE (Acute Physiology and Chronic Health Evaluation) II score, low serum albumin concentration, and high New York Heart Association cardiac function status were independently associated with increased mortality from intra-abdominal infection.[77]

9 Once antimicrobials are initiated and the other important therapies described earlier are used, most patients should show improvement within 2 to 3 days. Usually, temperature will return to near normal, vital signs should stabilize, and the patient should not appear in distress, with the exception of recognized discomfort and pain from incisions, drains, and the nasogastric tube. At 24 to 48 hours, aerobic bacterial culture results should return. If a suspected pathogen is not sensitive to the antimicrobial agents being given, the regimen should be changed if the patient has not shown sufficient improvement. If the isolated pathogen is susceptible to a narrower spectrum agent, therapy should be deescalated.

With anaerobic culturing techniques and the slow growth of these organisms, anaerobes are often not identified until 4 to 7 days after culture. A report indicating that anaerobes were not isolated should not be the sole justification for discontinuing antianaerobic drugs because anaerobic bacteria that were present in the infectious process may not have been transported properly to the microbiology laboratory, or other problems may have led to cell death in vitro.

Reasons for antimicrobial failure may not always be apparent. Even when antimicrobial susceptibility tests indicate that an organism is susceptible in vitro to the antimicrobial agent, therapeutic failures may occur. Possibly there is poor penetration of the antimicrobial agent into the focus of infection, or bacterial resistance may develop after initiation of antimicrobial therapy. In addition, it is possible that an antimicrobial regimen may encourage the development of infection by organisms not susceptible to the regimen being used. Superinfection in patients being treated for intra-abdominal infection can be caused by *Candida*; however, enterococci or opportunistic Gram-negative bacilli such as *Pseudomonas* may be involved.

Treatment regimens for intra-abdominal infection can be judged as successful if the patient recovers from the infection without recurrent peritonitis or intra-abdominal abscess and without the need for additional antimicrobials. A regimen can be considered unsuccessful if a significant adverse drug reaction occurs, reoperation or percutaneous drainage is necessary, or patient improvement is delayed beyond 1 or 2 weeks. The costs of treatment can be significantly reduced if parenteral antimicrobials can be switched to oral agents for completion of therapy.[78]

ABBREVIATIONS

APACHE	acute physiology and chronic health evaluation
CAPD	chronic ambulatory peritoneal dialysis
CT	computed tomography
CVP	central venous pressure
ESBL	extended-spectrum β-lactamase
IL	interleukin
INF	interferon
KPC	*Klebsiella pneumoniae* carbapenemase
LD	loading dose
MAP	mean arterial pressure
MD	maintenance dose
MRSA	methicillin-resistant *Staphylococcus aureus*
TNF	tumor necrosis factor

REFERENCES

1. Shirah GR, O'Neill PJ. Intra-abdominal infections. *Surg Clin North Am* 2014;94:1319-1333.
2. Marshall JC. Intra-abdominal infections. *Microbes Infect* 2004;6:1015-1025.
3. Marshall JC, Innes M. Intensive care unit management of intra-abdominal infection. *Crit Care Med* 2003;31:2228-2237.
4. Levison ME, Bush LM. Peritonitis and intraperitoneal abscesses. In: Bennett JE, Dolin R, Blaser MJ, eds. *Mandell, Douglas, and Bennett's Principles and Practice of Infectious Diseases,* 8th ed. Philadelphia: Saunders, 2015:935-959 [chapter 76].
5. Sartelli M, Viale P, Koike K et al. WSES consensus conference: Guidelines for the first-line management of intra-abdominal infections. *World J Emerg Surg* 2011;6:1-29.
6. Wiest R, Krag A, Gerbes A. Spontaneous bacterial peritonitis: Recent guidelines and beyond. *Gut* 2012;61:297-310.
7. Ginès P, Angeli P, Lenz K, et al. EASL clinical practice guidelines on the management of ascites, spontaneous bacterial peritonitis, and hepatorenal syndrome in cirrhosis. *J Hepatol* 2010;53:397-417.
8. Jalan R, Fernandez J, Wiest R, et al. Bacterial infections in cirrhosis: A position statement based on the EASL Special Conference 2013. *J Hepatol* 2014;60:1310-1324.
9. Dever JB, Sheikh MY. Spontaneous bacterial peritonitis—Diagnosis, treatment, and prevention. *Aliment Pharmacol Ther* 2015;41:1116-1131.
10. Schmidt ML, Barritt AS, Orman ES, Hayashi PH. Decreasing mortality in patients hospitalized with cirrhosis in the United States from 2002 through 2010. *Gastroenterology* 2015;148;967-977.
11. Mujais S. Microbiology and outcomes of peritonitis in North America. *Kidney Int* 2006;70:555-562.
12. Piraino B, Bernardini J. Catheter-related peritonitis. *Perit Dial Int* 2013;33:592-595.
13. National Hospital Discharge Survey 2010. U.S. Department of Health and Human Services Centers for Disease Control and Prevention. National Center for Health Statistics. Available at: http://www.cdc.gov/nchs/nhds.htm. Accessed 18 August, 2016.
14. Deshpande A, Pasupuleti V, Thota P, et al. Acid-suppressive therapy is associated with spontaneous bacterial peritonitis in cirrhotic patients: A meta-analysis. *J Gastroenterol Hepatol* 2013;28:235-242.
15. Ratelle M, Perreault S, Villeneuve JP, Tremblay L. Association between proton pump inhibitor use and spontaneous bacterial peritonitis in cirrhotic patients with ascites. *Can J Gastroenterol Hepatol* 2014;28:330-334.
16. Toloza EM, Wilson SE. Cholecystitis and cholangitis. In: Fry DE, ed. *Surgical Infections.* Boston: Little, Brown, 1995:254-263.
17. Sartelli M, Catena F, Di Saverio S, et al. The challenge of antimicrobial resistance in managing intra-abdominal infections. *Surg Infect (Larchmt)* 2015;16:213-220.
18. Brook I. Microbiology and management of abdominal infections. *Dig Dis Sci* 2008;53:2585-2591.
19. Jernberg C, Lofmark S, Edlund C, Jansson JK. Long-term impacts of antibiotic exposure on the human intestinal microbiota. *Microbiology* 2010;156:3216-3223.
20. Riche FC, Cholley BP, Panis YH, et al. Inflammatory cytokine response in patients with septic shock secondary to generalized peritonitis. *Crit Care Med* 2000;28:433-437.
21. Solomkin JS, Mazuski J. Intra-abdominal sepsis: Newer interventional and antimicrobial therapies. *Infect Dis Clin North Am* 2009;23:593-608.
22. Schietroma M, Piccione F, Carlei F, Sista F, Cecilia EM, Amicucci G. Peritonitis from perforated peptic ulcer and immune response. *J Invest Surg* 2013;26:294-304.
23. Malangoni MA. Contributions to the management of intra-abdominal infection. *Am J Surg* 2005;190:255-259.
24. Herzog T, Chromic, Uhl W. Treatment of complicated intra-abdominal infections in the era of multidrug resistant bacteria. *Eur J Med Res* 2010;15:525-532.
25. Thompson AE, Marshall JC, Opal SM. Intra-abdominal infections in infants and children: Descriptions and definitions. *Pediatr Crit Care Med* 2005;6:S30-S35.
26. Rice-Townsend SE, Lawrence Moss R, Rangel SJ. Peritonitis. In: Long SS, Pickering LK, Prober CG, eds. *Principles and Practice of Pediatric Infectious Diseases,* 4th ed. Elsevier Churchill Livingstone; 2012.
27. Guillet-Caruba C, Cheikhelard A, Guillet M, et al. Bacteriologic epidemiology and empirical treatment of pediatric complicated appendicitis. *Diagn Microbiol Infect Dis* 2011;69:376-381.
28. Lee SL, Islam S, Cassidy LD, et al. Antibiotics and appendicitis in the pediatric population: An American Pediatric Surgical Association Outcomes and Clinical Trials Committee systematic review. *J Pediatr Surg* 2010;45:2181-2185.
29. Johnson DH, Cuhna BA. Infections in cirrhosis. *Infect Dis Clin North Am* 2001;15:363-371.
30. Brook I, Frazier EH. Aerobic and anaerobic microbiology of retroperitoneal abscesses. *Clin Infect Dis* 1998;26:938-941.
31. Bennion RS, Baron EJ, Thompson JE, et al. The bacteriology of gangrenous and perforated appendicitis—Revisited. *Ann Surg* 1990;211:165-171.

32. Sawyer RG, Rosenlof LK, Adams RB, et al. Peritonitis into the 1990s: Changing pathogens and changing strategies in the critically ill. *Am Surg* 1992;58:82-87.
33. Montravers P, Lepape A, Dubreuil L, et al. Clinical and microbiological profiles of community-acquired and nosocomial infections: Results of the French prospective, observational EBIIA study. *J Antimicrob Chemother* 2009;63:785-794.
34. Onderdonk AB, Bartlett JG, Louie T, et al. Microbial synergy in experimental intra-abdominal abscess. *Infect Immun* 1997;13:22-26.
35. Donskey CJ, Chowdhry TK, Hecker MT, et al. Effect of antibiotic therapy on the density of vancomycin-resistant enterococci in the stool of colonized patients. *Ann Surg* 2000;343:1925-1932.
36. Sitges-Serra A, Lopez MJ, Girvent M, et al. Postoperative enterococcal infection after treatment of complicated intra-abdominal sepsis. *Br J Surg* 2002;89:361-367.
37. Yang SK, Xiao L, Zhang H, et al. Significance of serum procalcitonin as biomarker for detection of bacterial peritonitis: A systematic review and meta-analysis. *BMC Infect Dis* 2014;14:452.
38. Jaffe TA, Nelson RC, Delong DM, Paulson EK. Practice patterns in percutaneous image-guided intra-abdominal abscess drainage: Survey of academic and private practice centers. *Radiology* 2004;233:750-756.
39. Dellinger RP, Levy MM, Rhodes A, et al. Surviving Sepsis Campaign: International guidelines for management of severe sepsis and septic shock: 2012. *Crit Care Med* 2013; 41:580-637.
40. Rivers E, Nguyen B, Havstad S, et al. Early goal-directed therapy in the treatment of severe sepsis and septic shock. *N Engl J Med* 2001;345:1368-1377.
41. Wong PF, Gilliam AD, Kumar S, et al. Antibiotic regimens for secondary peritonitis of gastrointestinal origin in adults. *Cochrane Database Syst Rev* 2007;2:CD004539.
42. Hooker KD, DiPiro JT, Wynn JJ. Aminoglycoside combinations versus single β-lactams for penetrating abdominal trauma: A meta-analysis. *J Trauma* 1991;31:1155-1160.
43. Solomkin JS, Dellinger EP, Christou NV, et al. Results of a multicenter trial comparing imipenem/cilastatin to tobramycin/clindamycin for intra-abdominal infections. *Ann Surg* 1990;212:581-591.
44. Hoban DJ, Bouchillon SK, Hawser SP, Badal RE, Labombardi VJ, DiPersio J. Susceptibility of gram-negative pathogens isolated from patients with complicated intra-abdominal infections in the United States, 2007–2008: Results of the Study for Monitoring Antimicrobial Resistance Trends (SMART). *Antimicrob Agents Chemother* 2010;54:3031-3034.
45. Snydman DR, Jacobus NV, McDermott LA, et al. Lessons learned from the anaerobe survey: Historical perspective and review of the most recent data (2005–2007). *Clin Infect Dis* 2010;50(Suppl 1): S26-S33.
46. Hawser SP, Bouchillon SK, Hoban DJ, Badal RE. In vitro susceptibilities of aerobic and facultative anaerobic Gram-negative bacilli from patients with intra-abdominal infections worldwide from 2005–2007: Results from the SMART study. *Int J Antimicrob Agents* 2009;34:585-588.
47. Sawyer RG, Claridge JA, Nathens AB, et al. Trial of short-course antimicrobial therapy for intra-abdominal infection. *N Engl J Med* 2015;372:1996-2005.
48. Solomkin JS, Mazuski JE, Bradley JS, et al. Diagnosis and management of complicated intra-abdominal infection in adults and children: Guidelines by the Surgical Infection Society and the Infectious Diseases society of America. *Clin Inf Dis* 2010;50:133-164.
49. Gauzit R, Pean Y, Mistretta F, Lalaude O. Epidemiology, management, and prognosis of secondary non-postoperative peritonitis: A French prospective observational multicenter study. *Surg Infect* 2009;10:119-127.
50. Knitsch W, Vincent J-L, Utzolino S, et al. A randomized, placebo-controlled trial of preemptive antifungal therapy for the prevention of invasive candidiasis following gastrointestinal surgery for intra-abdominal infections. *Clin Infect Dis* 2015;61:1671-1678.
51. Nicolau DP, Freeman CD, Belliveau PP, Nightingale CH, Ross JW, Quintiliani R. Experience with a once-daily aminoglycoside program administered to 2184 adult patients. *Antimicrob Agents Chemother* 1995;39:650-655.
52. Rybak MJ, Abate BJ, Kang SL, Ruffing MJ, Lerner SA, Drusano GL. Prospective evaluation of the effect of an aminoglycoside dosing regimen on rates of observed nephrotoxicity and ototoxicity. *Antimicrob Agents Chemother* 1999;43:1549-1555.
53. Olsen KM, Rudis MA, Rebuck JA, Gelmont D, Mehdian R, Nelson C, Rupp ME. Effect of single daily dose vs. multiple daily dosing of tobramycin on alanine aminopeptidase and *N*-acetyl-β-D-glucosaminidase excretion. *Crit Care Med* 2004;32:1678-1682.
54. Boucher HW, Talbot GH, Bradley JS, et al. Bad bugs, no drugs: No ESKAPE! An update from the Infectious Diseases Society of America. *Clin Infect Dis* 2009;48:1-12.
55. Centers for Disease Control and Prevention. Antibiotic resistance threats in the United States, 2013. Available at: http://www.cdc.gov/drugresistance/threat-report-2013/. Accessed January 4, 2015.
56. World Health Organization. Antimicrobial resistance: Global report on surveillance. Geneva: Switzerland; 2014.
57. Tasina E, Haidich AB, Kokkali S, Arvanitidou M. Efficacy and safety of tigecycline for the treatment of infectious diseases: A meta-analysis. *Lancet Infect Dis.* 2011 Nov;11(11):834-844.
58. Prasad P, Sun J, Danner R, Natanson C. Excess deaths associated with tigecycline after approval based on non-inferiority trials. *Clin Infect Dis* 2012;54:1699-1709.
59. US Food and Drug Administration. FDA Drug Safety Communication: Increased risk of death with Tygacil (tigecycline) and approved new Boxed Warning. US Food and Drug Administration. Sept. 27, 2013. Available at: http://www.fda.gov/Drugs/DrugSafety/ucm369580.htm. Accessed November 27, 2015.
60. Barlam TF, Cosgrove SE, Abbo LM, et al. Implementing an antimicrobial stewardship program: Guidelines by the Infectious Diseases Society of America and the Society for Healthcare Epidemiology of America. *Clin Infect Dis* 2016;62(10):e51-e77.
61. Wilde AM, Gross AE. A new practitioner's guide to antimicrobial stewardship. *Am J Health Syst Pharm* 2013;70:2180-2183.
62. Ceftolozane/tazobactam Package Insert. Cubist. Lexington, MA. May 2015.
63. Ceftazidime/avibactam Package Insert. Forest Pharmaceuticals. Cincinnati, OH. September 2015.
64. Solomkin J, Hershberger E, Miller B, et al. Ceftolozane/tazobactam plus metronidazole for complicated intra-abdominal infections in an era of multidrug resistance: Results from a randomized, double-blind, phase 3 trial (ASPECT-cIAI). *Clin Infect Dis* 2015;60:1465-1471.
65. Spellberg B, Brass, EP. Noninferiority doesn't mean not inferior. *Clin Infect Dis* 2016;62(4):525-6.
66. Solomkin JS, Hershberger E, Eckmann C. Response to Spellberg and Brass. *Clin Infect Dis* 2016;62(4):526.
67. Runyon BA. Management of adult patients with ascites due to cirrhosis: Update 2012. Available at: http://www.aasld.org/publications/practice-guidelines-0. Accessed January 5, 2016.
68. Deshpande LM, Fritsche TR, Moet GJ, Biedenbach DJ, Jones RN. Antimicrobial resistance and molecular epidemiology of vancomycin-resistant enterococci from North America and Europe: A report from the SENTRY antimicrobial surveillance program. *Diagn Microbiol Infect Dis* 2007;58:163-170.
69. Ballinger AE, Palmer SC, Wiggins KJ, et al. Treatment for peritoneal dialysis-associated peritonitis. *Cochrane Database Syst Rev* 2014;(4): CD005284.
70. Li PK, Szeto CC, Piraino B, et al. International Society for Peritoneal Dialysis Peritoneal dialysis-related infections recommendations: 2010 update. *Perit Dial Int* 2010;30:393-423.
71. Flanigan MJ, Lim VS. Initial treatment of dialysis associated peritonitis: A controlled trial of vancomycin versus cefazolin. *Perit Dial Int* 1991;11:31-37.
72. Bozorgzadeh A, Pizzi WF, Barie PS, et al. The duration of antibiotic administration in predicting abdominal trauma. *Am J Surg* 1999;172:125-135.
73. Riccio LM, Popovsky KA, Hranjec T, et al. Association of excessive duration of antibiotic therapy for intra-abdominal infection with subsequent extra-abdominal infection and death: A study of 2,552 consecutive infections. *Surg Infect (Larchmt)* 2014;15:417-424.
74. Schein M, Gecelter G, Freinkel W, et al. Peritoneal lavage in abdominal sepsis: A controlled clinical study. *Arch Surg* 1990;125:1132-1135.
75. Baquero F, Hsueh P, Paterson DL, et al. In vitro susceptibilities of aerobic and facultatively anaerobic gram-negative bacilli isolated from patients with intra-abdominal infections worldwide: 2005 results from study for monitoring antimicrobial resistance trends. *Surg Infect* 2009;10:99-104.
76. Merlino JI, Yowler CJ, Malangoni MA. Nosocomial infections adversely affect the outcomes of patients with serious intra-abdominal infections. *Surg Infect (Larchmt)* 2004;5:21-27.
77. Christou NV, Barie PS, Dellinger EP, et al. Surgical infection society intra-abdominal infection study. *Arch Surg* 1993;128:193-199.
78. Paladino JA, Gilliland-Johnson KK, Adelman MH, Coohn SM. Pharmacoeconomics of ciprofloxacin plus metronidazole vs. piperacillin–tazobactam for complicated intra-abdominal infections. *Surg Infect* 2008;9:325.

Parasitic Diseases

Jason M. Cota and JV Anandan

e115

KEY CONCEPTS

1. Nitazoxanide and tinidazole are Food and Drug Administration (FDA)-approved for giardiasis treatment. While the FDA has not approved metronidazole for this indication, it has been widely accepted as the mainstay of giardiasis therapy for the past 50 years.
2. Human immunodeficiency virus (HIV)-infected patients with cryptosporidiosis must receive antiretroviral therapy as the mainstay of therapy in addition to antiparasitic therapy.
3. Serologic detection assays are required to diagnose *Entamoeba histolytica* infection because stool sample analysis is insensitive and does not distinguish between *E. histolytica* and the nonpathogenic *E. dispar* or *E. moshkovskii.*
4. Metronidazole and tinidazole are tissue-acting agents against amoeba; whereas, paromomycin, iodoquinol, and diloxanide furoate are luminal amebicides.
5. The drugs that have been used to treat *Trypanosoma cruzi* infections include benznidazole and nifurtimox, but are not currently approved by the FDA. Both are available from the Centers for Disease Control and Prevention (CDC) under an Investigational New Drug program.
6. Chloroquine has been the recommended drug for malaria chemoprophylaxis, but clinicians have increasingly prescribed alternative antimalarial drugs such as atovaquone-proguanil, doxycycline, primaquine, and mefloquine because these regimens retain effectiveness in areas where chloroquine-resistant *Plasmodium falciparum* exposure is likely.
7. Administration of corticosteroids or other immunosuppressive drugs to an infected individual can result in hyperinfections and disseminated strongyloidiasis.
8. Antihelminthic therapy destroys parasites and may cause increased inflammation and worsening of neurocysticercosis symptoms.
9. For head lice, the American Academy of Pediatrics recommends either nonprescription 1% permethrin or pyrethrins plus piperonyl butoxide topical preparations as agents of choice unless local resistance to these agents is documented.
10. A single application of 5% permethrin results in cure rates in more than 90% of subjects with scabies at 14 and 28 days, but a second dose should be applied 1 week later because its ovicidal efficacy remains unclear.

Parasitic diseases remain a significant global health problem causing approximately one million deaths per year and affecting more than 1.7 billion people worldwide.[1-5] In the United States, immunocompromised patients, ethnic/racial minorities, immigrants, those with recent travel to developing regions, individuals living in poor sanitary conditions, and people who lack access to basic health care services appear to be at highest risk for developing parasitic disease.[6] However, people in every income and social strata can become infected. In fact, the Centers for Disease Control and Prevention (CDC) has referred to five diseases as neglected parasitic infections and has prioritized these for increased public health action.[7] They include Chagas disease, cysticercosis, toxocariasis, toxoplasmosis, and trichomoniasis.[8]

This chapter discusses the major parasitic diseases including protozoan disease (giardiasis, cryptosporidiosis, Chagas disease, amebiasis, and malaria), helminthic infections (strongyloidiasis, cysticercosis, and toxocariasis), and ectoparasitic infestations (lice and scabies).

HOST–PARASITE RELATIONSHIP

Symbiosis is the association of two species for the purpose of obtaining food for either one or the other. *Parasitism* is a symbiotic relationship in which one species, the host, is injured through the activities of the other. Through evolution, parasites have made specific morphologic adaptations. Adaptation to the host has taken a number of forms: loss of locomotor organelles in the protozoan *Sporozoa*; partial and complete lack of digestive systems in the trematodes and cestodes, respectively; elaboration of proteolytic enzymes to penetrate the host intestinal mucosa by *Entamoeba histolytica*; the cercariae of the blood fluke that penetrate the skin of the host by elaborate enzymes; and, finally, the ability to infect an intermediate host to increase reproductive capacity, as seen among the cestodes and trematodes.[9]

Parasites normally inflict some degree of injury to the host, the extent of which depends on such factors as parasite load, nutritional status, and immunologic competence of the host. *E. coli* is considered commensal because it subsists on the bacterial flora of the gut and does not cause any harm to the host. Unlike *E. coli*, *Fasciolopsis buski*, the giant intestinal fluke, can produce severe local damage to the intestinal wall. *Ascaris*, the roundworm, can perforate the bowel wall, cause intestinal obstruction, and invade the appendix and bile duct. Malarial parasites destroy red blood cells by multiplying inside them. *Diphyllobothrium latum*, or the broad fish tapeworm, removes vitamin B_{12} from the gastrointestinal (GI) tract, resulting in megaloblastic anemia.[9]

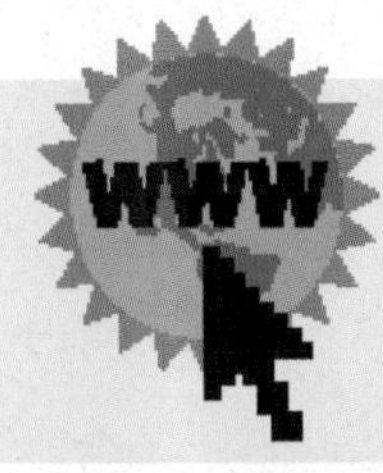

The complete chapter, learning objectives, and other resources can be found at **www.pharmacotherapyonline.com.**

Urinary Tract Infections and Prostatitis

116

Elizabeth A. Coyle and Randall A. Prince

KEY CONCEPTS

1. Urinary tract infections (UTIs) can be classified as uncomplicated and complicated. *Uncomplicated* refers to an infection in an otherwise healthy, premenopausal female who lacks structural or functional abnormalities of the urinary tract. Most often complicated infections are associated with a predisposing lesion of the urinary tract; however, the term may be used to refer to all other infections, except for those in the otherwise healthy, premenopausal adult female.
2. Recurrent UTIs are considered either reinfections or relapses. Reinfection usually happens more than 2 weeks after the last UTI and is treated as a new uncomplicated UTI. Relapse usually happens within 2 weeks of the original infection, and is a relapse of the original infection either because of unsuccessful treatment of the original infection, a resistant organism, or anatomical abnormalities.
3. Majority (75%-90%) of uncomplicated UTIs are caused by *Escherichia coli* and the remainder are caused primarily by *Staphylococcus saprophyticus*, *Proteus* spp., and *Klebsiella* spp. Complicated infections may be associated with other gram-negative organisms and *Enterococcus faecalis*.
4. Symptoms of lower UTIs include dysuria, urgency, frequency, nocturia, and suprapubic heaviness, whereas upper UTIs involve more systemic symptoms such as fever, nausea, vomiting, and flank pain.
5. Significant bacteriuria traditionally has been defined as bacterial counts of greater than 10^5 organisms (colony-forming unit [CFU])/mL (10^8 CFU/L) of a midstream clean catch urine. However, this is too general and significant bacteriuria in patients with symptoms of a UTI may be defined as greater than 10^2 organisms (CFU)/mL (10^5 CFU/L).
6. The goals of treatment of UTIs are to eradicate the invading organism(s), prevent or treat systemic consequences of infections, prevent the recurrence of infection, and prevent antimicrobial resistance.
7. Uncomplicated UTIs can be managed most effectively with short-course therapy (3 days) with either trimethoprim–sulfamethoxazole, one dose of fosfomycin, or 5 days of nitrofurantoin. Fluoroquinolones should be reserved for suspected pyelonephritis or complicated infections.
8. In choosing appropriate antibiotic therapy, practitioners need to be cognizant of antibiotic resistance patterns, particularly to *E. coli*. Trimethoprim–sulfamethoxazole has diminished activity against *E. coli* in some areas of the country, with reported resistance in some areas greater than 20%.
9. Acute bacterial prostatitis can be managed with many agents that have activity against the causative organism. Chronic prostatitis requires prolonged therapy with an agent that penetrates the prostatic tissue and secretions. Therapy with fluoroquinolone or trimethoprim–sulfamethoxazole is preferred for up to 6 weeks.

Infections of the urinary tract represent a wide variety of syndromes, including urethritis, cystitis, prostatitis, and pyelonephritis. Urinary tract infections (UTIs) are the most commonly occurring bacterial infections and one of the most common reasons for antibiotic exposure, especially in females of childbearing age.[1-3] Approximately 60% of females will develop a UTI during their lifetime with about one-fourth having a recurrence within a year.[2] Infections in men occur much less frequently until the age of 65 years at which point the incidence rates in men and women are similar.

A UTI is defined as the presence of microorganisms in the urinary tract that cannot be accounted for by contamination. The organisms present have the potential to invade the tissues of the urinary tract and adjacent structures. Infection may be limited to the growth of bacteria in the urine, which frequently may not produce symptoms. A UTI can present as several syndromes associated with an inflammatory response to microbial invasion and can range from asymptomatic bacteriuria (ASB) to pyelonephritis with bacteremia or sepsis.

UTIs are classified by lower and upper UTIs. Typically, they have been described by anatomic site of involvement. Lower tract infections correspond to cystitis (bladder), and pyelonephritis (an infection involving the kidneys) represents upper tract infection.

1 Also, UTIs are designated as uncomplicated or complicated. Uncomplicated infections occur in individuals who lack structural or functional abnormalities of the urinary tract that interfere with the normal flow of urine or voiding mechanism. These infections occur in premenopausal females of childbearing age (15-45 years) who are otherwise normal, healthy individuals. Infections in males generally are not classified as uncomplicated because these infections are rare and most often represent a structural or neurologic abnormality.

Complicated UTIs are usually the result of a predisposing lesion of the urinary tract, such as a congenital abnormality or distortion of the urinary tract, a stone, indwelling catheter, prostatic hypertrophy, obstruction, or neurologic deficit that interferes with the normal flow of urine and urinary tract defenses. Complicated infections occur in both genders and frequently involve the upper and lower urinary tract.

2 Recurrent UTIs in healthy nonpregnant women—two or more UTIs occurring within 6 months or three or more UTIs within 1 year—are a common problem. They are characterized by multiple symptomatic infections with asymptomatic periods occurring between each episode and may be either reinfections or relapses. Reinfections are caused by a different organism than originally isolated and account for the majority of recurrent UTIs. Relapses are

TABLE 116-1 Diagnostic Criteria for Significant Bacteriuria

$\geq 10^2$ CFU coliforms/mL ($\geq 10^5$ CFU/L) or $\geq 10^5$ CFU noncoliforms/mL ($\geq 10^8$ CFU/L) in a symptomatic female
$\geq 10^4$ CFU bacteria/mL ($\geq 10^7$ CFU/L) in a symptomatic male
$\geq 10^5$ CFU bacteria/mL ($\geq 10^8$ CFU/L) in asymptomatic individuals on two consecutive specimens
Any growth of bacteria on suprapubic catheterization in a symptomatic patient
$\geq 10^{2-5}$ CFU bacteria/mL ($\geq 10^{5-8}$ CFU/L) in a catheterized patient

CFU, colony-forming unit.

the development of repeated infections with the same initial organism and usually indicate a persistent infectious source.[2]

ASB is a common finding, particularly among those 65 years of age and older when there is significant bacteriuria (more than 10^5 bacteria/mL [more than 10^8/L] of urine) in the absence of symptoms. Symptomatic abacteriuria or acute urethral syndrome consists of symptoms of frequency and dysuria in the absence of significant bacteriuria. This syndrome is commonly associated with *Chlamydia* infections.

Significant abacteriuria is a term used to distinguish the presence of microorganisms that represent true infection versus contamination of the urine as it passes through the distal urethra prior to collection. Historically, bacterial counts equal to or greater than 100,000 organisms/mL (10^8/L) of urine in a "clean-catch" specimen were judged to indicate true infection.[4-6] Counts less than 100,000 organisms/mL (10^8/L) of urine, however, may represent true infection in certain situations. For example, with concurrent antibacterial drug administration, rapid urine flow, low urinary pH, or upper tract obstruction.[6] Table 116-1 lists the clinical definitions of significant bacteriuria, which are dependent on the clinical setting and the method of specimen collection.[6] These criteria allow for more appropriate specificity and sensitivity in documenting infection under differing clinical circumstances.

EPIDEMIOLOGY

The prevalence of UTIs varies with age and gender. In newborns and infants up to 6 months of age, the prevalence of abacteriuria is approximately 1% and is more common in boys. Most of these infections are associated with structural or functional abnormalities of the urinary tract and also have been correlated with noncircumcision.[7] Between the ages of 1 and 6 years, UTIs occur more frequently in females. The prevalence of abacteriuria in females and males of this age group is 3% to 7% and 1% to 2%, respectively.[7,8] Infections occurring in preschool boys usually are associated with congenital abnormalities of the urinary tract. These infections are difficult to recognize because of the age of the patient, but they often are symptomatic. In addition, the majority of renal damage associated with UTI develops at this age.[7,8]

Through grade school and before puberty, the prevalence of UTI is approximately 1%, with 5% of females reported to have significant bacteriuria prior to leaving high school. This percentage increases dramatically to 1% to 4% after puberty in nonpregnant females primarily as a result of sexual activity. Approximately one in five women will suffer a symptomatic UTI at some point in their lives. Many women have recurrent infections with a significant proportion of these women having a history of childhood infections. In contrast, the prevalence of bacteriuria in adult men is very low (less than 0.1%).[9]

In the elderly, the ratio of bacteriuria in women and men is dramatically altered and is approximately equal in persons older than 65 years.[10] The overall incidence of UTI increases substantially in this population with the majority of infections being asymptomatic. The rate of infection increases further for elderly persons who are residing in nursing homes, particularly those who are hospitalized frequently. The increase is probably the result of factors such as obstruction from prostatic hypertrophy in males, poor bladder emptying as a result of prolapse in females, fecal incontinence in demented patients, and neuromuscular disease including strokes and increased urinary instrumentation (catheterization).

ETIOLOGY

3 The bacteria causing UTIs usually originate from bowel flora of the host. Although virtually every organism is associated with UTIs, certain organisms predominate as a result of specific virulence factors. The most common cause of uncomplicated UTIs is *Escherichia coli*, which accounts for 80% to 90% of community-acquired infections. Additional causative organisms in uncomplicated infections include *Staphylococcus saprophyticus*, *Klebsiella pneumoniae*, *Proteus* spp., *Pseudomonas aeruginosa*, and *Enterococcus* spp.[11] Because *S. epidermidis* is frequently isolated from the urinary tract, it should be considered initially a contaminant. Repeat cultures should be performed to help confirm the organism as a real pathogen.

Organisms isolated from individuals with complicated infections are more varied and generally are more resistant than those found in uncomplicated infections. *E. coli* is a frequently isolated pathogen, but it accounts for less than 50% of infections. Other frequently isolated organisms include *Proteus* spp., *K. pneumoniae*, *Enterobacter* spp., *P. aeruginosa*, staphylococci, and enterococci. Enterococci represent the second most frequently isolated organisms in hospitalized patients.[11-13] In part, this finding may be related to the extensive use of third-generation cephalosporin antibiotics, which are not active against the enterococci. Vancomycin-resistant *E. faecalis* and *E. faecium* (vancomycin-resistant enterococci) have become more widespread, especially in patients with long-term hospitalizations or underlying malignancies. Vancomycin-resistant enterococci are major therapeutic and infection control issues because these organisms are susceptible to few antimicrobials.[12,13]

S. aureus infections may arise from the urinary tract, but they are more commonly a result of bacteremia producing metastatic abscesses in the kidney. *Candida* spp. are common causes of UTI in the critically ill and chronically catheterized patient.

Most UTIs are caused by a single organism; however, in patients with stones, indwelling urinary catheters, or chronic renal abscesses, multiple organisms may be isolated. Depending on the clinical situation, the recovery of multiple organisms may represent contamination and a repeat evaluation should be done.

PATHOPHYSIOLOGY

Route of Infection

Organisms typically gain entry into the urinary tract via three routes: the ascending, hematogenous (descending), and lymphatic pathways. The female urethra usually is colonized by bacteria believed to originate from the fecal flora. The short length of the female urethra and its proximity to the perirectal area make colonization of the urethra likely. Other factors that promote urethral colonization include the use of spermicides and diaphragms as methods of contraception.[2,3] Although there is evidence in females that bladder infections follow colonization of the urethra, the mode of ascent of the microorganisms is incompletely understood. Massage of the female urethra and sexual intercourse allow bacteria to reach the bladder.[14] Once bacteria have reached the bladder, the organisms quickly multiply and can ascend the ureters to the kidneys. This sequence of events is more likely to occur if vesicoureteral reflux (reflux of urine into the ureters and kidneys while voiding) is present. UTIs are more common in females than in males because the anatomic differences in location and length of the urethra tend to support the ascending route of infections as the primary acquisition route.

Infection of the kidney by hematogenous spread of microorganisms usually occurs as the result of dissemination of organisms from a distant primary infection in the body. Infections via the descending route are uncommon and involve a relatively small number of invasive pathogens. Bacteremia caused by *S. aureus* may produce renal abscesses. Additional organisms include *Candida* spp., *Mycobacterium tuberculosis*, *Salmonella* spp., and enterococci. Of particular interest, it is difficult to produce experimental pyelonephritis by IV administration of common gram-negative organisms such as *E. coli* and *P. aeruginosa*. Overall, less than 5% of documented UTIs result from hematogenous spread of microorganisms.

There appears to be little evidence supporting a significant role for renal lymphatics in the pathogenesis of UTIs. There are lymphatic communications between the bowel and kidney, as well as between the bladder and kidney. There is no evidence, however, that microorganisms are transferred to the kidney via this route.

After bacteria reach the urinary tract, three factors determine the development of infection: the size of the inoculum, the virulence of the microorganism, and the competency of the natural host defense mechanisms. Most UTIs reflect a failure in host defense mechanisms.

Host Defense Mechanisms

The normal urinary tract generally is resistant to invasion by bacteria and is efficient in rapidly eliminating microorganisms that reach the bladder. The urine under normal circumstances is capable of inhibiting and killing microorganisms. The factors thought to be responsible include a low pH, extremes in osmolality, high urea concentration, and high organic acid concentration. Bacterial growth is further inhibited in males by the addition of prostatic secretions.[14,15]

The introduction of bacteria into the bladder stimulates micturition with increased diuresis and efficient emptying of the bladder. These factors are critical in preventing the initiation and maintenance of bladder infections. Patients who are unable to void urine completely are at greater risk of developing UTIs and frequently have recurrent infections. Also, patients with even small residual amounts of urine in their bladder respond less favorably to treatment than patients who are able to empty their bladders completely.[16]

An important virulence factor of bacteria is their ability to adhere to urinary epithelial cells resulting in colonization of the urinary tract, bladder infections, and pyelonephritis. Various factors that act as anti-adherence mechanisms are present in the bladder preventing bacterial colonization and infection. The epithelial cells of the bladder are coated with a urinary mucus or slime called *glycosaminoglycan*. This thin layer of surface mucopolysaccharide is hydrophilic and strongly negatively charged. When bound to the uroepithelium, it attracts water molecules and forms a layer between the bladder and urine. The anti-adherence characteristics of the glycosaminoglycan layer are nonspecific and when the layer is removed by dilute acid solutions, rapid bacterial adherence results.[17]

In addition, the Tamm–Horsfall protein is a glycoprotein produced by the ascending limb of Henle and distal tubule that is secreted into the urine and contains mannose residues. These mannose residues bind *E. coli* that contain small surface-projecting organellae on their surfaces called *pili* or *fimbriae*. Type 1 fimbriae are mannose-sensitive and this interaction prevents the bacteria from binding to similar receptors present on the mucosal surface of the bladder. Other factors that possibly prevent adherence of bacteria include immunoglobulins (Ig) G and A. Investigators have documented both systemic and local kidney Ig synthesis in upper tract infections. The role of Igs in preventing bladder infection is less clear. Patients with reduced urinary levels of secretory IgA are, however, at increased risk of infections of the urinary tract.

After bacteria have invaded the bladder mucosa, an inflammatory response is stimulated with the mobilization of polymorphonuclear leukocytes (PMNs) and resulting phagocytosis. PMNs are primarily responsible for limiting the tissue invasion and controlling the spread of infection in the bladder and kidney. They do not play a role in preventing bladder colonization or infections and actually contribute to renal tissue damage.

Other host factors that may play a role in the prevention of UTIs are the presence of *Lactobacillus* in the vaginal flora and circulating estrogen levels. In premenopausal women, circulating estrogen supports the vaginal tract growth of lactobacilli, which produce lactic acid to help maintain a low vaginal pH, thereby preventing *E. coli* vaginal colonization.[18] Topical estrogens are used for the prevention of UTI in postmenopausal women who have more than three recurrent UTI episodes per year and are not on oral estrogens.[19]

Bacterial Virulence Factors

Pathogenic organisms have differing degrees of pathogenicity (virulence), which play a role in the development and severity of infection. Bacteria that adhere to the epithelium of the urinary tract are associated with colonization and infection. The mechanism of adhesion of gram-negative bacteria, particularly *E. coli*, is related to bacterial fimbriae that are rigid, hair-like appendages of the cell wall.[9] These fimbriae adhere to specific glycolipid components on epithelial cells. The most common type of fimbriae is type 1, which binds to mannose residues present in glycoproteins. Glycosaminoglycan and Tamm–Horsfall protein are rich in mannose residues that readily trap those organisms that contain type 1 fimbriae, which are then washed out of the bladder.[20] Other fimbriae are mannose resistant and are associated more frequently with pyelonephritis, such as P fimbriae, which bind avidly to specific glycolipid receptors on uroepithelial cells. These bacteria are resistant to washout or removal by glycosaminoglycan and are able to multiply and invade tissue, especially the kidney. In addition, PMNs, as well as secretory IgA antibodies, contain receptors for type 1 fimbriae, which facilitate phagocytosis, but are lacking receptors for P fimbriae.

Other virulence factors include the production of hemolysin and aerobactin.[21] Hemolysin is a cytotoxic protein produced by bacteria that lyses a wide range of cells, including erythrocytes, PMNs, and monocytes. *E. coli* and other gram-negative bacteria require iron for aerobic metabolism and multiplication. Aerobactin facilitates the binding and uptake of iron by *E. coli*; however, the significance of this property in the pathogenesis of UTIs remains unknown.[22]

PREDISPOSING FACTORS TO INFECTION

The normal urinary tract typically is resistant to infection and colonization by pathogenic bacteria. In patients with underlying structural abnormalities of the urinary tract, the typical host defenses previously discussed usually are lacking or compromised. There are several known abnormalities of the urinary tract system that interfere with its natural defense mechanisms, the most important of which is obstruction. Obstruction can inhibit the normal flow of urine disrupting the natural flushing and voiding effect in removing bacteria from the bladder and resulting in incomplete emptying. Common conditions that result in residual urine volumes include prostatic hypertrophy, urethral strictures, calculi, tumors, bladder diverticula, and drugs such as anticholinergic agents. Additional causes of incomplete bladder emptying include neurologic malfunctions associated with stroke, diabetes, spinal cord injuries, tabes dorsalis, and other neuropathies. Vesicoureteral reflux represents a condition in which urine is forced up the ureters to the kidneys. Urinary reflux is associated not only with an increased incidence of UTIs and pyelonephritis, but also with renal damage.[8,16] Reflux may

CLINICAL PRESENTATION Urinary Tract Infections in Adults

Signs and Symptoms

- Lower UTI: Dysuria, urgency, frequency, nocturia, and suprapubic heaviness
- Gross hematuria
- Upper UTI: Flank pain, fever, nausea, vomiting, and malaise

Physical Examination

- Upper UTI: Costovertebral tenderness

Laboratory Tests

- Bacteriuria
- Pyuria (WBC count more than 10/mm^3 [more than 10 × 10^6/L])
- Nitrite-positive urine (with nitrite reducers)
- Leukocyte esterase-positive urine
- Antibody-coated bacteria (upper UTI)

be the result of a congenital abnormality or, more commonly, bladder overdistension from obstruction.

Other risk factors include urinary catheterization, mechanical instrumentation, pregnancy, and the use of spermicides and diaphragms.

CLINICAL PRESENTATION

4 The presenting signs and symptoms of UTIs in adults are recognized easily. Women frequently will report gross hematuria. Systemic symptoms, including fever, typically are absent in this setting. Unfortunately, large numbers of patients with significant bacteriuria are asymptomatic. These patients may be normal, healthy patients, elderly patients, children, pregnant patients, and patients with indwelling catheters. It is important to note that attempts at differentiating upper tract from lower tract infections on the basis of symptoms alone are not reliable.

Elderly patients frequently do not experience specific urinary symptoms, but they will present with altered mental status, change in eating habits, or gastrointestinal (GI) symptoms. In addition, patients with indwelling catheters or neurologic disorders commonly will not have lower tract symptoms. Instead, they may present with flank pain and fever. Many of the aforementioned patients, however, frequently will develop upper tract infections with bacteremia and no or minimal urinary tract symptoms.

Symptoms alone are unreliable for the diagnosis of bacterial UTIs. The key to the diagnosis of UTI is the ability to demonstrate significant numbers of microorganisms in an appropriate urine specimen to distinguish contamination from infection. The type and extent of laboratory examination required depends on the clinical situation.

Urine Collection

Examination of the urine is the cornerstone of laboratory evaluation for UTIs. There are three acceptable methods of urine collection. The first is the *midstream clean-catch method.* After cleaning the urethral opening area in both men and women, 20 to 30 mL of urine is voided and discarded. The next part of the urine flow is collected and should be processed immediately (refrigerated as soon as possible). Specimens that are allowed to sit at room temperature for several hours may result in falsely elevated bacterial counts. The midstream clean-catch is the preferred method for the routine collection of urine for culture. When a routine urine specimen cannot be collected or contamination occurs, alternative collection techniques must be used.

The two acceptable alternative methods include catheterization and suprapubic bladder aspiration. Catheterization may be necessary for patients who are uncooperative or who are unable to void urine. If catheterization is performed carefully with aseptic technique, the method yields reliable results. Note, however, that introduction of bacteria into the bladder may result and the procedure is associated with infection in 1% to 2% of patients. Suprapubic bladder aspiration involves inserting a needle directly into the bladder and aspirating the urine. This procedure bypasses the contaminating organisms present in the urethra and any bacteria found using this technique generally are considered to represent significant bacteriuria.[23-26] Suprapubic aspiration is a safe and painless procedure that is most useful in newborns, infants, paraplegics, seriously ill patients, and others in whom infection is suspected and routine procedures have provided confusing or equivocal results.

Bacterial Count

5 The diagnosis of UTI is based on the isolation of significant numbers of bacteria from a urine specimen. Microscopic examination of a urine sample is an easy-to-perform and reliable method for the presumptive diagnosis of bacteriuria. The examination may be performed by preparing a Gram stain of unspun or centrifuged urine. The presence of at least one organism per oil-immersion field in a properly collected uncentrifuged specimen correlates well with more than 100,000 CFU/mL (10^5 CFU/mL or 10^8 CFU/L) of urine. For detecting smaller numbers of organisms, a centrifuged specimen is more sensitive. Such examinations detect more than 10^5 bacteria (CFU)/mL (10^8 CFU/L) with a sensitivity of greater than 90% and a specificity of greater than 70%.[23,24] A quantitative count of greater than or equal to 10^5 CFU/mL (10^8 CFU/L) is considered indicative of a UTI; however, up to 50% of women will present with clinical symptoms of a UTI with lower counts (10^3 CFU/mL) [10^6 CFU/L].[4]

Pyuria, Hematuria, and Proteinuria

Microscopic examination of the urine for leukocytes is used to determine the presence of pyuria. The presence of pyuria in a symptomatic patient correlates with significant bacteriuria.[25] Pyuria is defined as a white blood cell (WBC) count of greater than 10 WBC/mm^3 (10×10^6/L) of urine. A count of 5 to 10 WBC/mm^3 (5×10^6 to 10×10^6/L) is accepted as the upper limit of normal. It should be emphasized that pyuria is nonspecific and signifies only the presence of inflammation and not necessarily infection. Thus patients with pyuria may or may not have infection. Sterile pyuria has long been associated with urinary tuberculosis, as well as chlamydial and fungal urinary infections.

Hematuria, microscopic or gross, is frequently present in patients with UTI, but is nonspecific. Hematuria may indicate the presence of other disorders, such as renal calculi, tumors, or glomerulonephritis. Proteinuria is found commonly in the presence of infection.

Chemistry

Several biochemical tests have been developed for screening urine for the presence of bacteria. A common dipstick test detects the presence of nitrite in the urine, which is formed by bacteria that reduce nitrate normally present in the urine. False-positive tests are uncommon. False-negative tests are more common and frequently are caused by the presence of gram-positive organisms or *P. aeruginosa* that do not reduce nitrate.[26] Other causes of false tests include low urinary pH, frequent voiding, and dilute urine.

The leukocyte esterase dipstick test is a rapid screening test for detecting the presence of pyuria. Leukocytes esterase is found in primary neutrophil granules and indicates the presence of WBCs. The leukocyte esterase test is a sensitive and highly specific test for detecting more than 10 WBC/mm^3 (10×10^6/L) of urine. When the leukocyte esterase test is used with the nitrite test, the reported positive predictive value and specificity is 79% and 82%, respectively, for the detection of bacteriuria.[27,28] These tests can be useful in the outpatient evaluation of uncomplicated UTIs. However, urine culture is still the "gold standard" test in determining the presence of UTIs.

Culture

The most reliable method of diagnosing UTI is by quantitative urine culture. Urine in the bladder is normally sterile making it statistically possible to differentiate contamination of the urine from infection by quantifying the number of bacteria present in a urine sample. This criterion is based on a properly collected midstream clean-catch urine specimen. Patients with infection usually have greater than 10^5 bacteria/mL (10^8/L) of urine. It should be emphasized that as many as one-third of women with symptomatic infection have less than 10^5 bacteria/mL (10^8/L). Also, a significant portion of patients with UTIs, either symptomatic or asymptomatic, have less than 10^5 bacteria/mL (10^8/L) of urine.

Several laboratory methods are used to quantify bacteria present in the urine. The most accurate method is the pour-plate technique. This method is unsuitable for a high-volume laboratory because it is expensive and time-consuming. The streak-plate method is an alternative that involves using a calibrated-loop technique to streak a fixed amount of urine on an agar plate. This method is used most commonly in diagnostic laboratories because it is simple to perform and less costly.

After identification and quantification are complete, the next step is to determine the susceptibility of the organism. There are several methods by which bacterial susceptibility testing may be performed. Knowledge of bacterial susceptibility and achievable urine concentration of the antibiotics puts the clinician in a better position to select an appropriate agent for treatment.

Infection Site

Several methods have been evaluated to determine the location of infection within the urinary system and differentiate upper tract from lower tract involvement. The most direct method is a ureteral catheterization procedure as described by Stamey and colleagues.[29] The method involves the passage of a catheter into the bladder and then into each ureter, where quantitative cultures are obtained. History and physical examination were of little value in predicting the site of infection. Although this method provides direct quantitative evidence for UTI, it is invasive, technically difficult, and expensive. The Fairley bladder washout technique is a modification of the Stamey procedure that involves Foley catheterization only.[30] After the catheter is passed into the bladder, bladder samples are obtained and the bladder is washed out with culture samples taken at 10, 20, and 30 minutes. The procedure shows that up to 50% of patients have renal involvement, regardless of signs and symptoms. Other investigators found 10% to 20% of tests to be equivocal.[30]

Noninvasive methods of localization may be more acceptable for routine use; however, they have limited clinical value. Patients with pyelonephritis can have abnormalities in urinary concentrating ability. The use of concentrating ability for localization of UTIs, however, is associated with high false-positive and false-negative responses and is not useful clinically.[26] The antibody-coated bacteria test is an immunofluorescent method that detects bacteria coated with Ig in freshly voided urine indicating upper UTI. The sensitivity and specificity of this test to localize the site of infection are reported to average 88% and 76%, respectively.[31] Because of the high incidence of false-positive and false-negative results, antibody-coated bacteria testing is not used routinely in the management of UTIs.

Virtually all patients with uncomplicated lower tract infections can be cured with a short course of antibiotic therapy and this assumption sometimes can be used to distinguish between patients with lower and upper tract infections. Patients who do not respond or who relapse may do so because of upper tract involvement. It is rarely necessary to localize the site of infection to direct the clinical management of such patients.

TREATMENT

Desired Outcomes

6 The goals of UTI treatments are (a) to eradicate the invading organism(s), (b) to prevent or to treat systemic consequences of infection, (c) to prevent the recurrence of infection, and (d) to decrease the potential for collateral damage with too broad of antimicrobial therapy.

Management

The management of a patient with a UTI includes initial evaluation, selection of an antibacterial agent, and duration of therapy and follow-up evaluation. The initial selection of an antimicrobial agent for the treatment of UTI is based primarily on the severity of the presenting signs and symptoms, the site of infection and whether the infection is determined to be uncomplicated or complicated. Other considerations include antibiotic susceptibility, side-effect potential, cost, current antimicrobial exposure, and the comparative inconvenience of different therapies.[1]

Various pharmacologic factors may affect the action of antibacterial agents. Certainly, the ability of the agent to achieve appropriate concentrations in the urine is of utmost importance. Factors that affect the rate and extent of excretion through the kidney include the patient's glomerular filtration rate and whether or not the agent is actively secreted. Filtration depends on the molecular size and degree of protein binding of the agent. Agents such as sulfonamides, tetracyclines, and aminoglycosides enter the urine via filtration. As the glomerular filtration rate is reduced, the amount of drug that enters the urine is reduced. Most β-lactam agents and quinolones are filtered and are actively secreted into the urine. For this reason, most of these agents achieve high urinary concentrations despite unfavorable protein-binding characteristics or the presence of renal dysfunction.

The ability to eradicate bacteria from the urine is related directly to the sensitivity of the microorganism and the achievable concentrations of the antimicrobial agent in the urine. Unfortunately, most susceptibility testing is directed at achievable concentrations in the blood. There is a poor correlation between achievable blood concentrations of antimicrobial agents and the eradication of bacteria from the urine.[32] In the treatment of lower tract infections, plasma concentrations of antibacterial agents may not be important, but achieving appropriate plasma concentrations appears critical in patients with bacteremia and renal abscesses.

Nonspecific therapies have been advocated in the treatment and prevention of UTIs. Fluid hydration has been used to produce rapid dilution of bacteria and removal of infected urine by increased voiding. A critical factor appears to be the amount of residual volume remaining after voiding. As little as 10 mL of residual urine can alter the eradication of infection significantly.[16] Paradoxically, increased diuresis also may promote susceptibility to infection by diluting the normal antibacterial properties of the urine. Often in clinical practice the concentrations of antimicrobial agents in the urine are so high that dilution has little effect on efficacy.

The antibacterial activity of the urine is related to the low pH, which is the result of high concentrations of various organic acids. Large volumes of cranberry juice increase the antibacterial activity of the urine and prevent the development of UTIs.[3,33,34] Apparently, the fructose and other unknown substances (condensed tannins, proanthocyanidin) in cranberry juice may act to interfere with adherence mechanisms of some pathogens, thereby preventing infection or reinfection. Acidification of the urine by cranberry juice does not appear to play a significant role. The use of other agents (ascorbic acid) to acidify the urine to hinder bacterial growth does not achieve significant acidification. Consequently, attempts to acidify urine with systemic agents are not recommended. *Lactobacillus* probiotics also may aid in the prevention of female UTIs by decreasing the vaginal pH, thereby decreasing *E. coli* colonization.[19,34,35] In postmenopausal women, estrogen replacement may be of help in the prevention of recurrent UTIs. After 1 month of topical estrogen replacement, decreases in vaginal *Lactobacillus*, as well as decreases in vaginal pH and *E. coli* colonization, have been found.[18,34]

Clinical **Controversy...**

The use of cranberry juice or lactobacilli in the prevention of UTIs has long been discussed. *Lactobacillus* potentially helps keep the vaginal pH in the normal range (pH 4-4.5), regulating genitourinary bacteria therefore aiding in the prevention of UTIs.[33] Possible clinical benefits with cranberry juice in sexually active adult women with recurrent UTI by decreasing the adherence of bacteria to the bladder epithelial cells. However, adhesion research and clinical trials show no significant effectiveness with cranberry juice.[33,36] Unfortunately, the consistency of study results has varied, as have the types of cranberry products tested, leading to overall inconclusive evidence.[33,34,37,38] More reliable and thorough studies on the overall effectiveness of cranberry juice or lactobacilli need to be performed before a uniform opinion on the role of these agents in UTIs can be stated.

Urinary analgesics such as phenazopyridine hydrochloride are used frequently by many clinicians.[3] If the pain or dysuria present in a UTI is a consequence of infection, then urinary analgesics have little clinical role because most patients' symptoms respond quite rapidly to appropriate antibacterial therapy. Also, urinary analgesics may mask signs and symptoms of UTIs not responding to antimicrobial therapy.[35,39,40]

Clinical **Controversy...**

Phenazopyridine hydrochloride is an over-the-counter urinary anesthetic/analgesic that can be used for symptom relief in UTIs. Common brand names are Pyridium®, Azo-Standard®, and Uristat®. It is used frequently by patients as self-medication to alleviate the dysuria associated with UTIs. The use of phenazopyridine in the treatment of UTIs is controversial. It has no antimicrobial properties and has a number of adverse effects such as red-orange discoloration of body fluids, rash, anaphylaxis, and rare effects such as hemolytic anemia, methemoglobinemia, and acute renal failure. In addition, its use can mask the symptoms of an untreated or inappropriately treated UTI. Unfortunately, there are not any guidelines for its role in the treatment of UTIs; however, experts agree that if phenazopyridine is used, only use the recommended dose (maximum 200 mg three times a day) and it should be limited to 1 to 2 days for symptomatic relief of the dysuria with UTIs.[35,39] In addition, it should be used with the combination of appropriate antibiotic therapy.

Pharmacologic Therapy

Ideally, the antimicrobial agent chosen should be well tolerated, well absorbed, achieve high urinary concentrations, and have a spectrum of activity limited to the known or suspected pathogen(s). Table 116-2 lists the most common agents used in the treatment of UTIs along with comments concerning their general use. Table 116-3 presents an overview of various therapeutic options for outpatient therapy of UTI. Table 116-4 describes empirical treatment regimens for selected clinical situations.

8 The therapeutic management of UTIs is best accomplished by first categorizing the type of infection: acute uncomplicated cystitis, symptomatic abacteriuria, ASB, complicated UTIs, recurrent infections, or prostatitis. In choosing the appropriate antibiotic therapy, it is important to be aware of the increasing resistance of *E. coli* and other pathogens to many frequently prescribed antimicrobials.[41] Resistance to *E. coli* is as high as 37% for amoxicillin and ampicillin.[1,42] Overall, most *E. coli* remain susceptible to trimethoprim–sulfamethoxazole, although resistance is continuing to increase and has been reported as high as 27%.[43] Although resistance to the fluoroquinolones remains low, these agents are being used more frequently and the incidence of fluoroquinolone-resistant *E. coli* is increasingly being reported and is of great concern.[42-48] Current or recent antibiotic exposure is the most significant risk factor associated with *E. coli* resistance and with the extensive use of the fluoroquinolones and trimethoprim–sulfamethoxazole for various infections, including UTIs, resistance will continue to increase.[42-47] In addition, broad-spectrum antimicrobials such as fluoroquinolones and broad-spectrum cephalosporins have a high impact on GI flora, increasing the risk of collateral damage (term used to refer to ecological adverse effects of antibiotic therapy) or the selection of resistant *E. coli* pathogens.[42-45,48,49] In light of rising resistance and in order to decrease the overuse of broad-spectrum antimicrobials, agents such as nitrofurantoin and fosfomycin are now considered first-line treatments along with trimethoprim–sulfamethoxazole in acute uncomplicated cystitis. Both nitrofurantoin and fosfomycin have little effects on the gut flora and *E. coli* susceptibility still remains high.[33,49-53] Antibiotic therapy should be determined based on the geographic resistance patterns, as well as the patient's recent history of antibiotic exposure.

Acute Uncomplicated Cystitis

Acute uncomplicated cystitis is the most common form of UTI. These infections typically occur in women of childbearing age and often are related to sexual activity. Although the presence of dysuria, frequency, urgency, and suprapubic discomfort frequently is associated with lower tract infection, a significant number of patients have upper tract involvement as well.[3] Because these infections are predominantly caused by *E. coli*, antimicrobial therapy initially should be directed against this organism. Other common causes include *S. saprophyticus* and occasionally *K. pneumoniae* and *Proteus mirabilis*. Because the causative organisms and their susceptibility generally are known, many clinicians advocate a cost-effective approach to management. This approach includes a urinalysis and initiation of empirical therapy without a urine culture (Fig. 116-1).[1]

TABLE 116-2 Commonly Used Antimicrobial Agents in the Treatment of UTIs

Drug	Adverse Drug Reactions	Monitoring Parameters	Comments
Oral Therapy			
Trimethoprim–sulfamethoxazole	Rash, Stevens–Johnson Syndrome, renal failure, photosensitivity, hematologic (neutropenia, anemia, etc.)	Serum creatinine, BUN, electrolytes, signs of rash, and CBC	This combination is highly effective against most aerobic enteric bacteria except *P. aeruginosa*. High urinary tract tissue concentrations and urine concentrations are achieved, which may be important in complicated infection treatment. Also effective as prophylaxis for recurrent infections
Nitrofurantoin	GI intolerance, neuropathies, and pulmonary reactions	Baseline serum creatinine and BUN	This agent is effective as both a therapeutic and prophylactic agent in patients with recurrent UTIs. Main advantage is the lack of resistance even after long courses of therapy
Fosfomycin trometamol	Diarrhea, headache, and angioedema	No routine tests recommended	Single-dose therapy for uncomplicated infections, low levels of resistance, use with caution in patients with hepatic dysfunction
Fluoroquinolones Ciprofloxacin Levofloxacin	Hypersensitivity, photosensitivity, GI symptoms, dizziness, confusion, and tendonitis (black box warning)	CBC, baseline serum creatinine, and BUN	The fluoroquinolones have a greater spectrum of activity, including *P. aeruginosa*. These agents are effective for pyelonephritis and prostatitis. Avoid in pregnancy and children. Moxifloxacin should not be used owing to inadequate urinary concentrations
Penicillins Amoxicillin–clavulanate	Hypersensitivity (rash, anaphylaxis), diarrhea, superinfections, and seizures	CBC, signs of rash, or hypersensitivity	Due to increasing *E. coli* resistance, amoxicillin–clavulanate is the preferred penicillin for uncomplicated cystitis
Cephalosporins Cefaclor Cefpodoxime-proxetil	Hypersensitivity (rash, anaphylaxis), diarrhea, superinfections, and seizures	CBC, signs of rash, or hypersensitivity	There are no major advantages of these agents over other agents in the treatment of UTIs, and they are more expensive. These agents are not active against enterococci
Parenteral Therapy			
Aminoglycosides Gentamicin Tobramycin Amikacin	Ototoxicity, nephrotoxicity	Serum creatinine and BUN, serum drug concentrations, and individual pharmacokinetic monitoring	These agents are renally excreted and achieve good concentrations in the urine. Amikacin generally is reserved for multidrug-resistant bacteria
Penicillins Ampicillin–sulbactam Piperacillin–tazobactam	Hypersensitivity (rash, anaphylaxis), diarrhea, superinfections, and seizures	CBC, signs of rash, or hypersensitivity	These agents generally are equally effective for susceptible bacteria. The extended-spectrum penicillins are more active against *P. aeruginosa* and enterococci and often are preferred over cephalosporins. They are very useful in renally impaired patients or when an aminoglycoside is to be avoided
Cephalosporins Ceftriaxone Ceftazidime Cefepime	Hypersensitivity (rash, anaphylaxis), diarrhea, superinfections, and seizures	CBC, signs of rash, or hypersensitivity	Second- and third-generation cephalosporins have a broad spectrum of activity against gram-negative bacteria, but are not active against enterococci and have limited activity against *P. aeruginosa*. Ceftazidime and cefepime are active against *P. aeruginosa*. They are useful for nosocomial infections and urosepsis due to susceptible pathogens
Carbapenems/monobactams Imipenem–cilistatin Meropenem Doripenem Ertapenem Aztreonam	Hypersensitivity (rash, anaphylaxis), diarrhea, superinfections, and seizures	CBC, signs of rash, or hypersensitivity	Carbapenems have a broad spectrum of activity, including gram-positive, gram-negative, and anaerobic bacteria. Imipenem, meropenem, and doripenem are active against *P. aeruginosa* and enterococci, but ertapenem is not. Aztreonam is a monobactam that is only active against gram-negative bacteria, including some strains of *P. aeruginosa*. Generally useful for nosocomial infections when aminoglycosides are to be avoided and in penicillin-sensitive patients
Fluoroquinolones Ciprofloxacin Levofloxacin	Hypersensitivity, photosensitivity, GI symptoms, dizziness, confusion, and tendonitis (black box warning)	CBC, baseline serum creatinine, and BUN	These agents have broad-spectrum activity against both gram-negative and gram-positive bacteria. They provide urine and high-tissue concentrations and are actively secreted in reduced renal function

BUN, blood urea nitrogen; CBC, complete blood count; GI, gastrointestinal; UTIs, urinary tract infections.

TABLE 116-3 Overview of Outpatient Antimicrobial Therapy for Lower Tract Infections in Adults

Indications	Antibiotic	Dose	Interval	Duration
Lower tract infections				
Uncomplicated	Trimethoprim–sulfamethoxazole	1 DS tablet	Twice a day	3 days
	Nitrofurantoin monohydrate	100 mg	Twice a day	5 days
	Fosfomycin trometamol	3 g	Single dose	1 day
	Ciprofloxacin	250 mg	Twice a day	3 days
	Levofloxacin	250 mg	Once a day	3 days
	Amoxicillin–clavulanate	500 mg	Every 8 hours	5-7 days
	Pivmecillinam	400 mg	Twice a day	3 days
Complicated	Trimethoprim–sulfamethoxazole	1 DS tablet	Twice a day	7-10 days
	Ciprofloxacin	250-500 mg	Twice a day	7-10 days
	Levofloxacin	250 mg	Once a day	10 days
		750 mg	Once a day	5 days
	Amoxicillin–clavulanate	500 mg	Every 8 hours	7-10 days
Recurrent infections	Nitrofurantoin	50 mg	Once a day	6 months
	Trimethoprim–sulfamethoxazole	1/2 SS tablet	Once a day	6 months
Acute pyelonephritis	Trimethoprim–sulfamethoxazole	1 DS tablet	Twice a day	14 days
	Ciprofloxacin	500 mg	Twice a day	14 days
		1,000 mg ER	Once a day	7 days
	Levofloxacin	250 mg	Once a day	10 days
		750 mg	Once a day	5 days
	Amoxicillin–clavulanate	500 mg	Every 8 hours	14 days

DS, double strength; SS, single strength.

Dosing intervals for normal renal function.

TABLE 116-4 Evidence-Based Empirical Treatment of UTIs and Prostatitis

Diagnosis	Pathogens	Treatment Recommendation	Comments
Acute uncomplicated cystitis	*Escherichia coli*, *Staphylococcus saprophyticus*	1. Nitrofurantoin × 5 days (A,I)[a] 2. Trimethoprim–sulfamethoxazole × 3 days (A,I)[a] 3. Fosfomycin trometamol × 1 dose (A,I)[a] 4. Fluoroquinolone × 3 days (A,I)[a] 5. β-Lactams × 3-7 days (B,I)[a] 6. Pivmecillinam × 3-7 days (A,I)	Short-course therapy more effective than single dose Reserve fluoroquinolones as alternatives to development of resistance (A-III)[a] β-Lactams as a group are not as effective in acute cystitis then trimethoprim–sulfamethoxazole or the fluoroquinolones, do not use amoxicillin or ampicillin[a] Pivmecillinam not available in United States
Pregnancy	As above	1. Amoxicillin–clavulanate × 7 days 2. Cephalosporin × 7 days 3. Trimethoprim–sulfamethoxazole × 7 days	Avoid trimethoprim–sulfamethoxazole during the third trimester
Acute pyelonephritis			
Uncomplicated	*E. coli*	1. Quinolone × 7 days (A,I)[a] 2. Trimethoprim–sulfamethoxazole (if susceptible) × 14 days (A,I)[a]	Can be managed as outpatient
	Gram-positive bacteria	1. Amoxicillin or amoxicillin–clavulanic acid × 14 days	
Complicated	*E. coli* *P. mirabilis* *K. pneumoniae* *P. aeruginosa* *Enterococcus faecalis*	1. Quinolone × 14 days 2. Extended-spectrum penicillin plus aminoglycoside	Severity of illness will determine duration of IV therapy; culture results should direct therapy Oral therapy may complete 14 days of therapy
Prostatitis	*E. coli* *K. pneumoniae* *Proteus* spp. *P. aeruginosa*	1. Trimethoprim–sulfamethoxazole × 4-6 weeks 2. Quinolone × 4-6 weeks	Acute prostatitis may require IV therapy initially Chronic prostatitis may require longer treatment periods or surgery

UTI, urinary tract infection.

[a]Strength of recommendations: A, good evidence for; B, moderate evidence for; C, poor evidence for and against; D, moderate against; E, good evidence against. Quality of evidence: I, at least one proper randomized, controlled study; II, one well-designed clinical trial; III, evidence from opinions, clinical experience, and expert committees.

Data from reference 1.

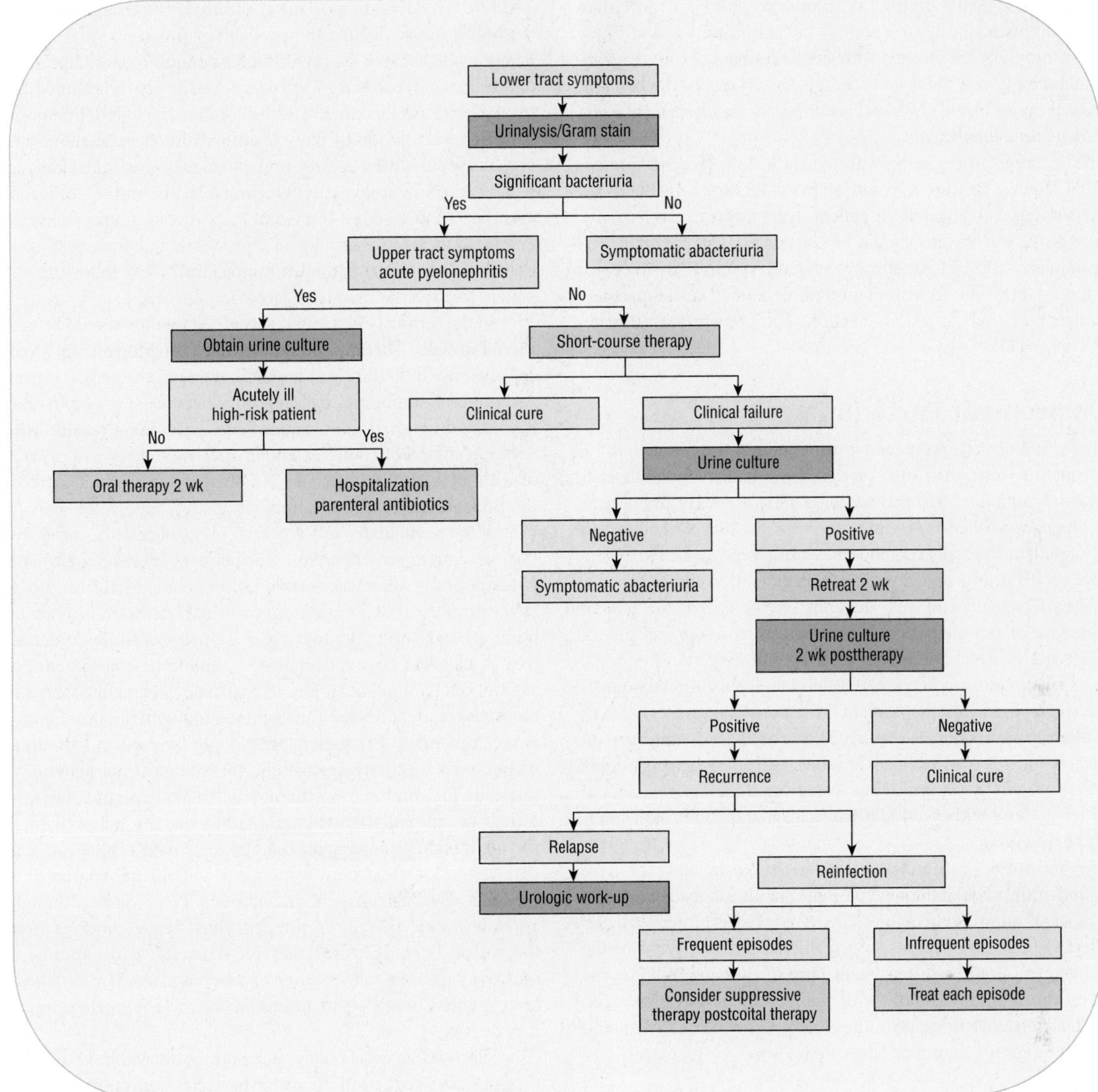

FIGURE 116-1 Management of urinary tract infections in females.

Therefore, the susceptibility patterns of the geographic area drive the choice of empiric therapy.

The goal of treatment for uncomplicated cystitis is to eradicate the causative organism and to reduce the incidence of recurrence caused by relapse or reinfection. The ability to reduce the chance of recurrence depends on the agent's efficacy in eradicating the uropathogenic bacteria from the vaginal and GI reservoir. In the past, conventional therapy consisted of an effective oral antibiotic administered for 7 to 14 days. However, acute cystitis is a superficial mucosal infection that can be eradicated with much shorter courses of therapy (3 days). Advantages of short-course therapy include increased adherence, fewer side effects, decreased cost, and less potential for the development of resistance.

7 Three-day courses of trimethoprim–sulfamethoxazole or a fluoroquinolone (eg, ciprofloxacin or levofloxacin, not moxifloxacin) are superior to single-dose therapies.[52,54-56] Although the fluoroquinolones have shown excellent efficacy in acute cystitis, the newest guidelines recommend reserving these agents for patients with suspected or possible pyelonephritis due to the collateral damage risk. Instead, a 3-day course of trimethoprim--sulfamethoxazole, a 5-day course of nitrofurantoin, or a one-time dose of fosfomycin should be considered as first-line therapy[1,50,51,55,57] In areas where there is more than 20% resistance of *E. coli* to trimethoprim–sulfamethoxazole, nitrofurantoin or fosfomycin should be used. Amoxicillin or ampicillin should not be used due to the high incidence of resistant *E. coli*. Instead, if a β-lactam must be used, amoxicillin/-clavulanate, cefdinir, cefaclor, or cefpodoxime proxetil for 3 to 7 days are the preferred choices. For most adult females, short-course therapy is the treatment of choice for uncomplicated lower UTIs. Short-course therapy is inappropriate for patients who have had previous infections caused by resistant bacteria, for male patients, and for patients with complicated UTIs. If symptoms recur or do not respond to therapy, a urine culture should be obtained and conventional therapy with a suitable agent instituted.[1]

Symptomatic Abacteriuria

Symptomatic abacteriuria or acute urethral syndrome represents a clinical syndrome in which females present with dysuria and pyuria, but the urine culture reveals less than 10^5 bacteria/mL

(10^8/L) of urine. Acute urethral syndrome accounts for more than half the complaints of dysuria seen in the community today. These women most likely are infected with small numbers of coliform bacteria, including *E. coli*, *Staphylococcus* spp., or *Chlamydia trachomatis*. Additional causes include *Neisseria gonorrhoeae*, *Gardnerella vaginalis*, and *Ureaplasma urealyticum*.

Most patients presenting with pyuria will, in fact, have infection that requires treatment. If antimicrobial therapy is ineffective, a culture should be obtained. If the patient reports recent sexual activity, therapy for *C. trachomatis* should be considered. Chlamydial treatment should consist of 1 g azithromycin or doxycycline 100 mg twice daily for 7 days. Often, concomitant treatment of all sexual partners is required to cure chlamydial infections and prevent reacquisition (see Chapter 117).

Asymptomatic Bacteriuria

ASB is the finding of two consecutive urine cultures with more than 10^5 organisms/mL (more than 10^8/L) of the same organism in the absence of urinary symptoms. Most patients with ASB are elderly and female. Also, pregnant women frequently present with ASB. Although this group of patients typically responds to treatment, relapse and reinfection are very common and chronic ASB is difficult to eradicate.

The management of ASB depends on the age of the patient and whether or not the patient is pregnant. In children, because of a greater risk of developing renal scarring and long-standing renal damage, treatment should consist of the same conventional courses of therapy as used for symptomatic infection. The greatest risk of renal damage occurs during the first 5 years of life.[58] In nonpregnant females, therapy is controversial; however, treatment has little effect on the natural course of infections. Two groups characterize ASB in the elderly: those with persistent bacteriuria and those with intermittent bacteriuria.

Several studies in hospitalized elderly subjects, however, have not found antimicrobial therapy to be efficacious for abacteruria.[59-62] A number of questions remain unanswered. For example: What is the effect of eradication of bacteriuria on life expectancy? What are the cost-effectiveness and risk-to-benefit ratio of therapy? What is the effect on morbidity? Certainly with the information available and the high adverse reaction rate in the elderly, vigorous treatment and screening programs cannot be advocated.

Complicated Urinary Tract Infections

Acute Pyelonephritis

The presentation of high-grade fever (more than 38.3°C [more than 100.9°F]) and severe flank pain should be treated as acute pyelonephritis and warrants aggressive management. Severely ill patients with pyelonephritis should be hospitalized and IV antimicrobials administered initially (see Table 116-4). However, milder cases may be managed with orally administered antibiotics in an outpatient setting. Signs and symptoms of nausea, vomiting, and dehydration may require hospitalization.

At the time of presentation, a Gram stain of the urine should be performed along with a urinalysis, culture, and sensitivity tests. The Gram stain should indicate the morphology of the infecting organism(s) and help direct the selection of an appropriate antibiotic. However, the precise identity and susceptibility of the infecting organism(s) will be unknown initially, warranting empirical therapy. The goals of treatment include the achievement of therapeutic concentrations of an antimicrobial agent in the bloodstream and urinary tract to which the invading organism is susceptible and sufficient therapy to eradicate residual infection in the tissues of the urinary tract.

In the mildly to moderately symptomatic patient in whom oral therapy is considered, an effective agent should be administered for 7 to 14 days, depending on the agent used.[1,63-68] Oral antibiotics that are highly active against the probable pathogens and that are sufficiently bioavailable are preferred. Fluoroquinolones (ciprofloxacin or levofloxacin) orally for 7 to 10 days are the first-line choice in mild to moderate pyelonephritis. Other options include trimethoprim–sulfamethoxazole for 14 days. If amoxicillin/clavulanate or an oral cephalosporin is used, it is recommended to give an initial long-acting parenteral antimicrobial such as ceftriaxone first and continue the oral agent for 10 to 14 days. If a Gram stain reveals gram-positive cocci, *Enterococcus faecalis* should be considered and treatment directed against this potential pathogen (ampicillin). Close follow-up of outpatient treatment is mandatory to ensure success.

In the seriously ill patient, parenteral therapy should be administered initially. Therapy should provide a broad spectrum of coverage and should be directed toward bacteremia or sepsis, if present. A number of antibiotic regimens have been used as empirical therapy, including an IV fluoroquinolone, an aminoglycoside with or without ampicillin, and extended-spectrum cephalosporins with or without an aminoglycoside.[1,69] Other options include aztreonam, the β-lactamase inhibitor combinations (eg, ampicillin–sulbactam, ticarcillin–clavulanate, and piperacillin–tazobactam), carbapenems (eg, imipenem, meropenem, doripenem, or ertapenem), or IV trimethoprim–sulfamethoxazole.[70] If the patient has been hospitalized within the past 6 months, has a urinary catheter, or is a nursing home resident, the possibility of *P. aeruginosa* and enterococci, as well as multiple resistant organisms, should be considered. In this setting, ceftazidime, ticarcillin–clavulanate, piperacillin, aztreonam, meropenem, or imipenem in combination with an aminoglycoside is recommended. Ertapenem should not be used in this situation owing to its inactivity against enterococci and *P. aeruginosa*.[67] The rationale for combination therapy is that in experimental animals 3 days of aminoglycoside combination therapy followed by non-aminoglycoside single-agent therapy for 7 days resulted in a 100% cure rate.[63,68] If the patient responds to initial combination therapy, the aminoglycoside may be discontinued after 3 days. Although the aminoglycoside therapy is stopped, renal tissue concentrations of the aminoglycoside will persist for days. Based on antimicrobial sensitivity data, the patient then can be maintained or switched to a less expensive single agent and ultimately, an appropriate oral agent may be used.

Effective therapy should stabilize the patient within 12 to 24 hours. A significant reduction in urine bacterial concentrations should occur in 48 hours. If bacteriologic response has not occurred, an alternative agent should be considered based on susceptibility testing. If the patient fails to respond clinically within 3 to 4 days or has persistently positive blood or urine cultures, further investigation is needed to exclude bacterial resistance, possible obstruction, papillary necrosis, intrarenal or perinephric abscess, or some other disease process. Usually by the third day of therapy, the patient is afebrile and significantly less symptomatic. In general, after the patient has been afebrile for 24 hours, parenteral therapy may be discontinued and oral therapy instituted to complete a 2-week course. Follow-up urine cultures should be obtained 2 weeks after completion of therapy to ensure a satisfactory response and detect possible relapse.

Urinary Tract Infections in Males

The management of UTIs in males is distinctly different and often more difficult than in females. Infections in male patients are considered to be complicated because endogenous bacteria in the presence of functional and/or structural abnormalities that disrupt the normal defense mechanisms of the urinary tract cause them. The incidence of infections in males younger than 60 years is much less than the incidence in females. During the adult years, the occurrence of infection can be related directly to some manipulation of the urinary tract. The most common causes are instrumentation of the urinary tract, catheterization, and renal and urinary stones.

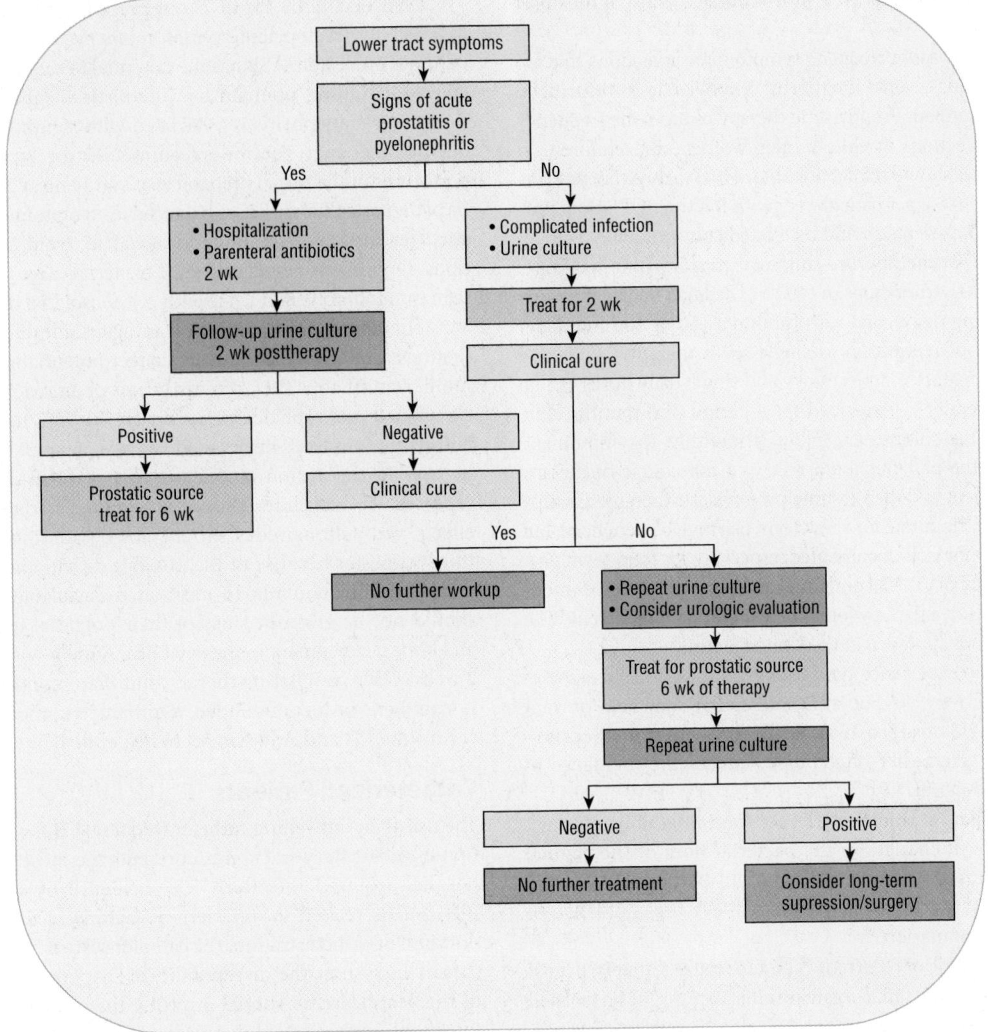

FIGURE 116-2 Management of urinary tract infections in males.

Uncomplicated infections are rare, but they may occur in young males as a result of homosexual activity, noncircumcision, and having sex with partners who are colonized with uropathogenic bacteria. As the patient ages, the most common cause of infection is related to bladder outlet obstruction because of prostatic hypertrophy. In addition, the prostate gland may become infected and provide a nidus for recurrent infection in males.

The conventional view is that therapy in males requires prolonged treatment (Fig. 116-2). A urine culture should be obtained before treatment because the cause of infection in men is not as predictable as in women. Single-dose or short-course therapy is not recommended in males. Considerably fewer data are available comparing various antimicrobial agents in males as compared with females. If gram-negative bacteria are presumed, trimethoprim–sulfamethoxazole or the quinolone antimicrobials should be considered because these agents achieve high renal tissue, urine, and prostatic concentrations.[71]

Initial therapy should be for 10 to 14 days. Factors associated with treatment success are isolation of a single organism, the absence of significant obstruction or anatomic abnormalities, a normally functioning urinary tract, and the absence of prostatic involvement. Parenteral therapy may be required in certain situations, such as in severely ill patients, in the presence of acute prostatitis or epididymitis and in patients who cannot tolerate oral medications. A comparison of 2-week versus 6-week therapy in males with recurrent infections who were given trimethoprim–sulfamethoxazole had cure rates of 29% and 62%, respectively.[72] Other investigators advocate longer treatment periods in males, as well.[73] Follow-up cultures at 4 to 6 weeks after treatment are important in males to ensure bacteriologic cure. Many patients require longer periods of treatment and possible alterations in antibiotics, depending on culture and sensitivity results and clinical response.

Recurrent Infections

Recurrent episodes of UTI account for a significant portion of all UTIs. Of the patients suffering from recurrent infections, 80% can be considered reinfections, that is, the recurrence of infection by an organism different from the organism isolated from the preceding infection. These patients most commonly are female and recurrence develops in approximately 20% of females with cystitis. Reinfections can be divided into two groups: those with less than three episodes per year and those who develop more frequent infections. Treatment strategies are continuing to develop, as well as, an understanding of the role of the microbiome.[74,75] An excellent overview of the various treatment modalities for recurrent UTI in women has been published.[76]

Management strategies depend on predisposing factors, number of episodes per year, and the patient's preference. Factors commonly associated with recurrent infections include sexual intercourse and diaphragm or spermicide use for birth control. Therapeutic options include self-administered therapy, postcoital therapy, and continuous low-dose prophylaxis. In patients with infrequent infections (less than three infections per year), each episode may be treated as a separately occurring infection. Short-course therapy is appropriate in this setting. Many women have been treated successfully with self-administered short-course therapy at the onset of symptoms.[40,77]

In patients with more frequent symptomatic infections and no apparent precipitating event, long-term prophylactic antimicrobial therapy may be instituted. Prophylactic therapy reduces the frequency of symptomatic infections in elderly men, women, and children. In women, most studies show a reinfection rate of two to three per patient-year reduced to 0.1 to 0.2 per patient-year with treatment.[77] Before prophylaxis is initiated, patients should be treated conventionally with an appropriate agent. Trimethoprim–sulfamethoxazole (one-half of a single-strength tablet), trimethoprim (100 mg daily), a fluoroquinolone (levofloxacin 500 mg daily), and nitrofurantoin (50 or 100 mg daily) all reduce the rate of reinfection as single-agent therapy.[77] Full-dose therapy with these agents is unnecessary and single daily doses can be used. Therapy generally is prescribed for a period of 6 months, during which time urine cultures are followed monthly. If symptomatic episodes develop, the patient should receive a full course of therapy with an effective agent and then resume prophylactic therapy. Therapy with methenamine hippurate for short term use may be beneficial, but its overall utility is not well documented, especially for long-term prophylaxis.[78] The utility of OM-89 oral immunotherapy has been demonstrated to be an effective therapy for some women with recurrent UTI; however, its use is not approved in the United States.[79]

In women who experience symptomatic reinfections in association with sexual activity, voiding after intercourse may help prevent infection. Also, single-dose prophylactic therapy with trimethoprim–sulfamethoxazole taken after intercourse reduces the incidence of recurrent infection significantly.[77]

In postmenopausal women with recurrent infections, the lack of estrogen results in changes in the bacterial flora of the vagina, resulting in increased colonization with uropathogenic *E. coli*. Topically administered estrogen cream reduces the incidence of infections in this population.[18,19]

The remaining 20% of recurrent UTIs are relapses, that is, persistence of infection with the same organism after therapy for an isolated UTI. The recurrence of symptomatic or ASB after therapy usually indicates that the patient has renal involvement, a structural abnormality of the urinary tract or chronic bacterial prostatitis. In the absence of structural abnormalities, relapse often is related to renal infection and requires a long duration of treatment. Women who relapse after short-course therapy should receive a 2-week course of therapy. In patients who relapse after 2 weeks of therapy, therapy should be continued for another 2 to 4 weeks. If relapse occurs after 6 weeks of therapy, urologic evaluation should be performed and any obstructive lesion should be corrected. If this is not possible, therapy for 6 months or longer may be considered. Asymptomatic adults who have no evidence of urinary obstruction should not receive long-term therapy.

In males, relapse usually indicates bacterial prostatitis, the most common cause of persistent bacteriuria. Although many agents have been used for long-term therapy of relapses, trimethoprim–sulfamethoxazole and the fluoroquinolones appear to be highly effective.

Special Conditions

Urinary Tract Infections in Pregnancy

During pregnancy, significant physiologic changes occur to the entire urinary tract that dramatically alter the prevalence of UTIs and pyelonephritis. Severe dilation of the renal pelvis and ureters, decreased ureteral peristalsis, and reduced bladder tone occur during pregnancy.[80] These changes result in urinary stasis and reduced defenses against reflux of bacteria to the kidneys. In addition, increased urine content of amino acids, vitamins, and nutrients encourages bacterial growth. All of these factors increase the incidence of bacteriuria resulting in symptomatic infections, especially during the third trimester.

ASB occurs in 4% to 7% of pregnant patients. Of these, 20% to 40% will develop acute symptomatic pyelonephritis during pregnancy. If untreated, ASB has the potential to cause significant adverse effects, including prematurity, low birth weight, and stillbirth.[81,82] Because pyelonephritis is associated with significant adverse events during pregnancy, routine screening tests for bacteriuria should be performed at the initial prenatal visit and again at 28 weeks gestation. In patients with significant bacteriuria, symptomatic or asymptomatic, treatment is recommended so as to avoid possible complications. Organisms associated with bacteriuria are the same as those seen in uncomplicated UTIs with *E. coli* isolated most frequently.

Therapy should consist of an agent administered for 7 days that has a relatively low adverse effect potential and is safe for the mother and baby. The administration of amoxicillin, amoxicillin–clavulanate, or cephalexin is effective in 70% to 80% of patients. Nitrofurantoin has been used in pregnancy; however, it must be used with caution as occurrences of birth defects have been reported. Tetracyclines should be avoided because of teratogenic effects and sulfonamides should not be administered during the third trimester because of the possible development of kernicterus and hyperbilirubinemia. In addition, the available fluoroquinolones should not be given because of their potential to inhibit cartilage and bone development in the newborn. A follow-up urine culture 1 to 2 weeks after completing therapy and then monthly until gestation is complete is recommended. Optimal treatment for preventing recurrent UTI and ASB has yet to be defined.[83]

Catheterized Patients

The use of an indwelling catheter frequently is associated with infection of the urinary tract and represents the most common cause of hospital-acquired infection. The incidence of catheter-associated infection is related to a variety of factors, including method and duration of catheterization, the catheter system (open or closed), the care of the system, the susceptibility of the patient, and the technique of the healthcare personnel inserting the catheter. Catheter-related infections are reasonably preventable infections and are now considered one of the hospital-acquired complications chosen by the Centers for Medicare and Medicaid Services in which hospitals will no longer receive reimbursement for treatment.[84,85]

Bacteria may enter the bladder in a number of ways. During the catheterization, bacteria may be introduced directly into the bladder from the urethra. Once the catheter is in place, bacteria may pass up the lumen of the catheter via the movement of air bubbles, by motility of the bacteria, or by capillary action. In addition, bacteria may reach the bladder from around the exudative sheath that surrounds the catheter in the urethra. Cleaning the periurethral area thoroughly and applying an antiseptic (povidone-iodine) can minimize infection occurring during insertion of the catheter. The use of closed drainage systems has reduced significantly the ability of bacteria to pass up the lumen of the catheter and cause infection. Presently, a bacterium passing around the catheter sheath in the urethra is probably the most important pathway for infection. Avoiding manipulation of the catheter and trauma to the urethra and urethral meatus can minimize this path of acquisition.

Patients with indwelling catheters acquire UTIs at a rate of 5% per day.[84-86] The closed systems are capable of preventing bacteriuria in most patients for up to 10 days with appropriate care. After 30 days of catheterization, however, there is a 78% to 95% incidence of bacteriuria, despite use of a closed system.[85,87] Unfortunately, UTI symptoms in catheterized patient are not clearly defined. Fever, peripheral leukocytosis, and urinary signs and symptoms may be of little predictive value.[84,85] When bacteriuria occurs in the asymptomatic, short-term catheterized patient (less than 30 days), the use of systemic antibiotics should be withheld and the catheter removed as soon as possible. If the patient becomes symptomatic, the catheter should be removed and treatment as described for complicated infections started.

The optimal duration of therapy is unknown. In the long-term catheterized patient (more than 30 days), bacteriuria is inevitable.[84,85] The administration of systemic antibiotics active against the infecting organism will sterilize the urine; however, reinfection occurs rapidly in more than 50% of patients. In addition, resistant organisms recolonize the urine. Symptomatic patients must be treated because they are at risk of developing pyelonephritis and bacteremia. Bacteria adhere to the catheter and produce a biofilm consisting of bacterial glycocalyces, Tamm–Horsfall protein, as well as apatite and struvite salts, that act to protect the bacteria from antibiotics.[86] Biofilm mechanisms and their treatment continue to be examined and more fully understood.[88] Recatheterization with a new sterile unit should be performed in those symptomatic patients, if the existing catheter has been in place for more than 2 weeks.

Various methods have been proposed to prevent the development of bacteriuria and infection in the patient with an indwelling catheter (see Table 116-4). The success of these methods depends on the type of catheter and the length of time it is in place. The use of constant bladder irrigation with antiseptic or antibacterial solutions reduces the incidence of infection in those with open drainage systems, but this approach has no advantage in those with closed systems. The use of prophylactic systemic antibiotics in patients with short-term catheterization reduces the incidence of infection over the first 4 to 7 days.[85,87] In long-term catheterized patients, however, antibiotics only postpone the development of bacteriuria and lead to the emergence of resistant organisms. Therefore, antibiotic prophylaxis should not be utilized in short-term or long-term catheterized patients.

PROSTATITIS

Bacterial prostatitis is an inflammation of the prostate gland and surrounding tissue as a result of infection. It is classified as either acute or chronic. By definition, pathogenic bacteria and significant inflammatory cells must be present in prostatic secretions and urine to make the diagnosis of bacterial prostatitis. Prostatitis occurs rarely in young males, but it is commonly associated with recurrent infections in persons older than 30 years. As many as 50% of all males develop some form of prostatitis at some period in their life.[89-91] The acute form typically is an acute infectious disease characterized by a sudden onset of fever, tenderness, and urinary and constitutional symptoms. Chronic prostatitis presents with few symptoms related to the prostate but rather symptoms of urinating difficulty, low back pain, perineal pressure, or a combination of these. It represents a recurring infection with the same organism that results from incomplete eradication of bacteria from the prostate gland.

Pathogenesis and Etiology

The exact mechanism of bacterial infection of the prostate is not well understood. The possible routes of infection are the same as those for UTIs. Reflux of infected urine into the prostate gland is thought to play an important role in causing infection. Intraprostatic reflux of urine occurs commonly and results in direct inoculation of infected urine into the prostate.[89-91] In addition, intraprostatic reflux of sterile urine can result in a chemical prostatitis and may be the cause of nonbacterial prostatitis. Sexual intercourse may contribute to infection of the prostate gland because prostatic secretions from men with chronic prostatitis and vaginal cultures from their sexual partners grow identical organisms. Other known causes of bacterial prostatitis include indwelling urethral and condom catheterization, urethral instrumentation, and transurethral prostatectomy in patients with infected urine.

Physiologic factors are believed to contribute to the development of prostatitis. Functional abnormalities found in bacterial prostatitis include altered prostate secretory functions. Prostatic fluid obtained from normal males contains prostatic antibacterial factor. This heat-stable, low-molecular-weight cation is a zinc-complexed polypeptide that is bactericidal to most urinary tract pathogens.[92] The antibacterial activity of prostatic antibacterial factor is related directly to the zinc content of prostatic fluid. Prostate fluid zinc levels and prostatic antibacterial factor activity also appear diminished in patients with prostatitis, as well as in the elderly.[92] Whether these changes are a cause or effect of prostatitis remains to be determined.

The pH of prostatic secretions in patients with prostatitis is altered.[93] Normal prostatic secretions have a pH in the range of 6.6 to 7.6. With increasing age, the pH tends to become more alkaline. In patients with inflammation of the prostate, prostatic secretions may have an alkaline pH in the range of 7 to 9. These changes suggest a generalized secretory dysfunction of the prostate that not only can affect the pathogenesis of prostatitis but also can influence the mode of therapy.

Gram-negative enteric organisms are the most frequent pathogens in acute bacterial prostatitis.[89-91] *E. coli* is the predominant organism, occurring in 75% of cases. Other gram-negative organisms frequently isolated include *K. pneumoniae*, *P. mirabilis*, and less frequently, *P. aeruginosa*, *Enterobacter* spp., and *Serratia* spp. Infrequently, cases of gonococcal and staphylococcal prostatitis occur.

E. coli most commonly causes chronic bacterial prostatitis with other gram-negative organisms isolated less frequently. The importance of gram-positive organisms in chronic bacterial prostatitis remains controversial. *S. epidermidis*, *S. aureus*, and diphtheroids have been isolated in some studies.

Clinical Presentation

Acute bacterial prostatitis presents as other acute infections. Massage of the prostate will express a purulent discharge that will readily grow the pathogenic organism. Prostatic massage is contraindicated in acute bacterial prostatitis, however, because of the risk of inducing bacteremia and the associated local pain. The diagnosis of acute bacterial prostatitis can be made from the patient's clinical presentation

CLINICAL PRESENTATION Bacterial Prostatitis

Signs and Symptoms

- Acute bacterial prostatitis: High fever, chills, malaise, myalgia, localized pain (perineal, rectal, sacrococcygeal), frequency, urgency, dysuria, nocturia, and retention
- Chronic bacterial prostatitis: Voiding difficulties (frequency, urgency, dysuria), low back pain, and perineal and suprapubic discomfort

Physical Examination

- Acute bacterial prostatitis: Swollen, tender, tense, or indurated gland
- Chronic bacterial prostatitis: Boggy, indurated (enlarged) prostate in most patients

Laboratory Tests

- Bacteriuria
- Bacteria in EPSs

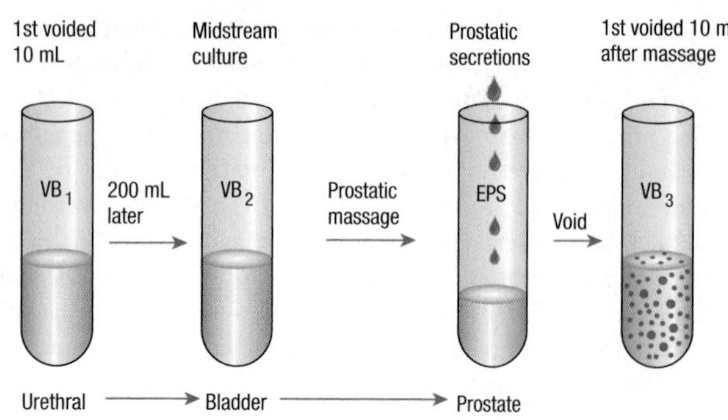

FIGURE 116-3 Segmented cultures of the lower tract in men. (EPS, expressed prostatic secretions; VB_1, voiding bladder 1; VB_2, voiding bladder 2; VB_3, voiding bladder 3.)

and the presence of significant bacteriuria. As with other UTIs, the infecting organism can be isolated from a midstream specimen.

In contrast, chronic bacterial prostatitis is more difficult to diagnose and treat. Chronic bacterial prostatitis typically is characterized by recurrent UTIs with the same pathogen and is the most common cause of recurrent UTI in males. The patient's clinical presentation can vary widely. Many adults, however, are asymptomatic.

Because physical examination of the prostate is often normal, urinary tract localization studies are critical to the diagnosis of chronic bacterial prostatitis. The method of quantitative localization culture, as described by Meares and Stamey,[15,94] remains the diagnostic standard (Fig. 116-3). The method compares the bacterial growth in sequential urine and prostatic fluid cultures obtained during micturition. The first 10 mL of voided urine is collected (voiding bladder 1, or VB_1) and constitutes urethral urine. After approximately 200 mL of urine has been voided, a 10-mL midstream sample is collected (VB_2). This specimen represents bladder urine. After the patient voids, the prostate is massaged and expressed prostatic secretions (EPS) are collected. After prostatic massage, the patient voids again and 10 mL of urine is collected (VB_3).

The diagnosis of bacterial prostatitis is made when the number of bacteria in EPS is 10 times that of the urethral sample (VB_1) and midstream sample (VB_2). If no EPS is available, the urine sample following massage (VB_3) should contain a bacterial count 10-fold greater than that of VB_1 or VB_2. If significant bacteriuria is present, ampicillin, cephalexin, or nitrofurantoin should be given for 2 to 3 days to sterilize the urine prior to performing the localization study.

TREATMENT

9 In general, the goals in the management of bacterial prostatitis are the same as those for UTIs. Acute bacterial prostatitis responds well to appropriate antimicrobial therapy that is directed at the most commonly isolated organisms. Prostatic penetration of antimicrobials occurs because the acute inflammatory reaction alters the cellular membrane barrier between the bloodstream and the prostate. Most patients can be managed with oral antimicrobial agents, such as trimethoprim–sulfamethoxazole and the fluoroquinolones (eg, ciprofloxacin, levofloxacin) (see Table 116-4). Other effective agents in this setting include cephalosporins and β-lactam–β-lactamase combinations. Although IV therapy is rarely necessary for total treatment, IV to oral sequential therapy with trimethoprim–sulfamethoxazole or the fluoroquinolones is appropriate. The conversion to an oral antibiotic can be considered after the patient is afebrile for 48 hours or after 3 to 5 days of IV therapy. The total course of antibiotic therapy should be 4 weeks in order to reduce the risk of development of chronic prostatitis, although in some cases 2 weeks may be sufficient. Therapy may be prolonged with chronic prostatitis (6-12 weeks). Long-term suppressive therapy also may be initiated for recurrent infections, such as three times weekly ciprofloxacin, trimethoprim–sulfamethoxazole regular-strength tablet daily, or nitrofurantoin 100 mg daily.[94]

Chronic bacterial prostatitis often presents a more vexing situation because cures are obtained rarely. Despite high serum concentrations of antibacterial drugs in excess of the minimal inhibitory concentrations of the infecting organisms, bacteria persist in prostatic fluid. Most likely the failure to eradicate sensitive bacteria is caused by the inability of antibiotics to reach sufficient concentrations in the prostatic fluid and cross the prostatic epithelium.

Several factors that determine antibiotic diffusion into prostatic secretions were delineated from the canine model. Lipid solubility is a major determinant in the ability of drugs to diffuse from plasma across epithelial membranes. The degree of ionization in plasma also affects the diffusion of drugs. Only unionized molecules can cross the lipid barrier of prostatic cells, and the drug's pK_a (negative logarithm of acid ionization constant) directly determines the fraction of unchanged drug.

The pH gradient across the membrane has an influence on tissue penetration, as well. A pH gradient of at least one pH unit between separate compartments allows for ion trapping. As the unionized drug crosses the epithelial barrier into prostatic fluid, it becomes ionized allowing less drug to diffuse back across the lipid barrier. In early studies with the canine model, the prostatic pH was reported to be acidic (6.4).[93] In humans, however, the pH of prostatic secretions from an inflamed prostate is actually basic (8.1-8.3).[93]

The choice of antibiotics in chronic bacterial prostatitis should include agents that are capable of reaching therapeutic concentrations in the prostatic fluid and which possess the spectrum of activity to be effective. Agents that achieve therapeutic prostatic concentrations include trimethoprim and the fluoroquinolones. Sulfamethoxazole penetrates poorly and probably contributes very little to trimethoprim activity when used in combination. The fluoroquinolones appear to provide the best therapeutic options in the management of chronic bacterial prostatitis. Therapy should be continued for 4 to 6 weeks initially. Longer treatment periods may be necessary in some cases. If therapy fails with these regimens, chronic suppressive therapy may be used or surgery considered.

PERSONALIZED PHARMACOTHERAPY

Patient-centered pharmacotherapy and management of UTIs require knowledge of the pathogenesis and causative organisms associated with the various clinical syndromes described in this chapter.[22] Individualizing the antimicrobial therapy will depend on many factors, first and foremost being the susceptibility of the offending pathogen. As was discussed in the chapter, *E. coli* resistance is continuing to increase, therefore, it is imperative for the healthcare professional to be familiar with the resistance trends in their geographical area when prescribing therapy. In addition, the prevention of increasing resistance and collateral damage should be considered when selecting antimicrobial therapy.[1] Other factors to consider in selecting therapy would be a patient's allergies and recent antimicrobial exposure. Lastly, cost may factor into compliance enhancing the effectiveness of therapy. The costs include both direct and indirect costs associated with treatment.

Direct costs are those associated with diagnosis, treatment, and follow-up. The cost of pharmaceuticals varies according to the agents used and the duration of therapy. Trimethoprim–sulfamethoxazole and amoxicillin–clavulanate are rather inexpensive. However, when considering rates of resistance leading to therapeutic failure, overall costs increase dramatically. The fluoroquinolones also are highly effective agents, but generally are more expensive and a rise in their utilization is now being associated with increasing resistance.[69,95]

In general, the outcome and total cost depend on whether therapy is empirical or definitive (based on a culture diagnosis for acute infection) and if the individual patient is adherent with the regimen. As a healthcare professional, working with and/or within the healthcare team is necessary to select appropriate therapies and maximize the possibility of positive therapeutic outcomes.

ABBREVIATIONS

ASB	asymptomatic bacteriuria
CFU	colony-forming unit
EPS	expressed prostatic secretions
GI	gastrointestinal
PMN	polymorphonuclear leukocyte
UTI	urinary tract infection
WBC	white blood cell

REFERENCES

1. Gupta K, Hooton TM, Naber KG, et al. International clinical practice guidelines for the treatment of acute uncomplicated cystitis and pyelonephritis in women: A 2010 update by the infectious diseases society of america and the european society for microbiology and infectious diseases. *Clin Infect Dis* 2011;52(5):e103-e120.
2. Naber KG, Cho YH, Matsumoto T and Schaeffer AJ. Immunoactive prophylaxis of recurrent urinary tract infections: A meta-analysis. *Int J Antimicrob Agents* 2009;33(2):111-119.
3. Kallen AJ, Welch HG and Sirovich BE. Current antibiotic therapy for isolated urinary tract infections in women. *Arch Intern Med* 2006;166(6):635-639.
4. Nicolle LE. Uncomplicated urinary tract infection in adults including uncomplicated pyelonephritis. *Urol Clin North Am* 2008;35(1):1-12, v.
5. Little P, Turner S, Rumsby K, et al. Developing clinical rules to predict urinary tract infection in primary care settings: Sensitivity and specificity of near patient tests (dipsticks) and clinical scores. *Br J Gen Pract* 2006;56(529):606-612.
6. Platt R. Quantitative definition of bacteriuria. *Am J Med* 1983;75(1b):44-52.
7. Alper BS and Curry SH. Urinary tract infection in children. *Am Fam Physician* 2005;72(12):2483-2488.
8. Habib S. Highlights for management of a child with a urinary tract infection. *Int J Pediatr* 2012;2012:943653.
9. Sobel J and Kaye D. *Urinary Tract Infections*. 7th ed. Philadelphia: Churchill Livingstone/Elsevier; 2010.
10. Shortliffe LM and McCue JD. Urinary tract infection at the age extremes: Pediatrics and geriatrics. *Am J Med* 2002;113(Suppl 1A):55s-66s.
11. Nicolle L, Anderson PA, Conly J, et al. Uncomplicated urinary tract infection in women. Current practice and the effect of antibiotic resistance on empiric treatment. *Can Fam Physician* 2006;52:612-618.
12. Shigemura K, Arakawa S, Tanaka K and Fujisawa M. Clinical investigation of isolated bacteria from urinary tracts of hospitalized patients and their susceptibilities to antibiotics. *J Infect Chemother* 2009;15(1):18-22.
13. Heintz BH, Halilovic J and Christensen CL. Vancomycin-resistant enterococcal urinary tract infections. *Pharmacotherapy* 2010;30(11):1136-1149.
14. Stamatiou C, Bovis C, Panagopoulos P, et al. Sex-induced cystitis—patient burden and other epidemiological features. *Clin Exp Obstet Gynecol* 2005;32(3):180-182.
15. Stamey TA, Fair WR, Timothy MM and Chung HK. Antibacterial nature of prostatic fluid. *Nature* 1968;218(5140):444-447.
16. Shand DG, Nimmon CC, O'Grady F and Cattell WR. Relation between residual urine volume and response to treatment of urinary infection. *Lancet* 1970;760(1):1305-1306.
17. Parsons CL, Shrom SH, Hanno PM and Mulholland SG. Bladder surface mucin. Examination of possible mechanisms for its antibacterial effect. *Invest Urol* 1978;16(3):196-200.
18. Raz R and Stamm WE. A controlled trial of intravaginal estriol in postmenopausal women with recurrent urinary tract infections. *N Engl J Med* 1993;329(11):753-756.
19. Stamm WE. Estrogens and urinary-tract infection. *J Infect Dis* 2007;195(5):623-624.
20. Orskov I, Ferencz A and Orskov F. Tamm-horsfall protein or uromucoid is the normal urinary slime that traps type 1 fimbriated escherichia coli. *Lancet* 1980;1(8173):887.
21. Measley RE Jr and Levison ME. Host defense mechanisms in the pathogenesis of urinary tract infection. *Med Clin North Am* 1991;75(2):275-286.
22. Flores-Mireles AL, Walker JN, Caparon M and Hultgren SJ. Urinary tract infections: Epidemiology, mechanisms of infection and treatment options. *Nat Rev Microbiol* 2015;13(5):269-284.
23. Jenkins RD, Fenn JP and Matsen JM. Review of urine microscopy for bacteriuria. *JAMA* 1986;255(24):3397-3403.
24. Pezzlo M. Detection of urinary tract infections by rapid methods. *Clin Microbiol Rev* 1988;1(3):268-280.
25. Stamm WE. Measurement of pyuria and its relation to bacteriuria. *Am J Med* 1983;75(1b):53-58.
26. Pappas PG. Laboratory in the diagnosis and management of urinary tract infections. *Med Clin North Am* 1991;75(2):313-325.
27. St John A, Boyd JC, Lowes AJ and Price CP. The use of urinary dipstick tests to exclude urinary tract infection: A systematic review of the literature. *Am J Clin Pathol* 2006;126(3):428-436.
28. Nys S, van Merode T, Bartelds AI and Stobberingh EE. Urinary tract infections in general practice patients: Diagnostic tests versus bacteriological culture. *J Antimicrob Chemother* 2006;57(5):955-958.
29. Stamey TA, Govan DE and Palmer JM. The localization and treatment of urinary tract infections: The role of bactericidal urine levels as opposed to serum levels. *Medicine (Baltimore)* 1965;44:1-36.
30. Fairley KF, Bond AG, Brown RB and Habersberger P. Simple test to determine the site of urinary-tract infection. *Lancet* 1967;2(7513):427-428.
31. Thomas VL and Forland M. Antibody-coated bacteria in urinary tract infections. *Kidney Int* 1982;21(1):1-7.
32. Stamey TA, Fair WR, Timothy MM, et al. Serum versus urinary antimicrobial concentrations in cure of urinary-tract infections. *N Engl J Med* 1974;291(22):1159-1163.
33. Barbosa-Cesnik C, Brown MB, Buxton M, et al. Cranberry juice fails to prevent recurrent urinary tract infection: Results from a randomized placebo-controlled trial. *Clin Infect Dis* 2011;52(1):23-30.
34. Barrons R and Tassone D. Use of lactobacillus probiotics for bacterial genitourinary infections in women: A review. *Clin Ther* 2008;30(3):453-468.
35. Zelenitsky SA and Zhanel GG. Phenazopyridine in urinary tract infections. *Ann Pharmacother* 1996;30(7-8):866-868.
36. Stapleton AE, Dziura J, Hooton TM, et al. Recurrent urinary tract infection and urinary escherichia coli in women ingesting cranberry juice daily: A randomized controlled trial. *Mayo Clin Proc* 2012;87(2):143-150.
37. Jepson RG, Williams G and Craig JC. Cranberries for preventing urinary tract infections. *Cochrane Database Syst Rev* 2012;10:CD001321.
38. Stapleton AE. Cranberry-containing products are associated with a protective effect against urinary tract infections. *Evid Based Med* 2013;18(3):110-111.
39. Gaines KK. Phenazopyridine hydrochloride: The use and abuse of an old standby for UTI. *Urol Nurs* 2004;24(3):207-209.
40. Masson P, Matheson S, Webster AC and Craig JC. Meta-analyses in prevention and treatment of urinary tract infections. *Infect Dis Clin North Am* 2009;23(2):355-385.
41. Chen YH, Ko WC and Hsueh PR. Emerging resistance problems and future perspectives in pharmacotherapy for complicated urinary tract infections. *Expert Opin Pharmacother* 2013;14(5):587-596.
42. Olson RP, Harrell LJ and Kaye KS. Antibiotic resistance in urinary isolates of escherichia coli from college women with urinary tract infections. *Antimicrob Agents Chemother* 2009;53(3):1285-1286.
43. Colgan R, Johnson JR, Kuskowski M and Gupta K. Risk factors for trimethoprim-sulfamethoxazole resistance in patients with acute uncomplicated cystitis. *Antimicrob Agents Chemother* 2008;52(3):846-851.
44. Bergman M, Nyberg ST, Huovinen P, et al. Association between antimicrobial consumption and resistance in escherichia coli. *Antimicrob Agents Chemother* 2009;53(3):912-917.
45. Talan DA, Krishnadasan A, Abrahamian FM, et al. Prevalence and risk factor analysis of trimethoprim-sulfamethoxazole- and fluoroquinolone-resistant escherichia coli infection among emergency department patients with pyelonephritis. *Clin Infect Dis* 2008;47(9):1150-1158.
46. Paterson DL. "Collateral damage" from cephalosporin or quinolone antibiotic therapy. *Clin Infect Dis* 2004;38(Suppl 4):S341-S345.

47. Karlowsky JA, Hoban DJ, Decorby MR, et al. Fluoroquinolone-resistant urinary isolates of escherichia coli from outpatients are frequently multidrug resistant: Results from the north american urinary tract infection collaborative alliance-quinolone resistance study. *Antimicrob Agents Chemother* 2006;50(6):2251-2254.
48. Johnson L, Sabel A, Burman WJ, et al. Emergence of fluoroquinolone resistance in outpatient urinary escherichia coli isolates. *Am J Med* 2008;121(10):876-884.
49. Wagenlehner FM, Weidner W and Naber KG. An update on uncomplicated urinary tract infections in women. *Curr Opin Urol* 2009;19(4):368-374.
50. Kashanian J, Hakimian P, Blute M Jr, et al. Nitrofurantoin: The return of an old friend in the wake of growing resistance. *BJU Int* 2008;102(11):1634-1637.
51. Knottnerus BJ, Nys S, Ter Riet G, et al. Fosfomycin tromethamine as second agent for the treatment of acute, uncomplicated urinary tract infections in adult female patients in the netherlands? *J Antimicrob Chemother* 2008;62(2):356-359.
52. Tice AD. Short-course therapy of acute cystitis: A brief review of therapeutic strategies. *J Antimicrob Chemother* 1999;43(Suppl A):85-93.
53. Stein GE. Comparison of single-dose fosfomycin and a 7-day course of nitrofurantoin in female patients with uncomplicated urinary tract infection. *Clin Ther* 1999;21(11):1864-1872.
54. Cox CE, Marbury TC, Pittman WG, et al. A randomized, double-blind, multicenter comparison of gatifloxacin versus ciprofloxacin in the treatment of complicated urinary tract infection and pyelonephritis. *Clin Ther* 2002;24(2):223-236.
55. Iravani A, Klimberg I, Briefer C, et al. A trial comparing low-dose, short-course ciprofloxacin and standard 7 day therapy with co-trimoxazole or nitrofurantoin in the treatment of uncomplicated urinary tract infection. *J Antimicrob Chemother* 1999;43(Suppl A): 67-75.
56. Stass H and Kubitza D. Pharmacokinetics and elimination of moxifloxacin after oral and intravenous administration in man. *J Antimicrob Chemother* 1999;43(Suppl B):83-90.
57. Gupta K, Hooton TM, Roberts PL and Stamm WE. Short-course nitrofurantoin for the treatment of acute uncomplicated cystitis in women. *Arch Intern Med* 2007;167(20):2207-2212.
58. Chang SL and Shortliffe LD. Pediatric urinary tract infections. *Pediatr Clin North Am* 2006;53(3):379-400.
59. Nicolle LE, Bradley S, Colgan R, et al. Infectious diseases society of america guidelines for the diagnosis and treatment of asymptomatic bacteriuria in adults. *Clin Infect Dis* 2005;40(5):643-654.
60. Screening for asymptomatic bacteriuria in adults: U.S. Preventive services task force reaffirmation recommendation statement. *Ann Intern Med* 2008;149(1):43-47.
61. Juthani-Mehta M, Quagliarello V, Perrelli E, et al. Clinical features to identify urinary tract infection in nursing home residents: A cohort study. *J Am Geriatr Soc* 2009;57(6):963-970.
62. Nicolle LE, Bjornson J, Harding GK and MacDonell JA. Bacteriuria in elderly institutionalized men. *N Engl J Med* 1983;309(23):1420-1425.
63. Neal DE Jr. Complicated urinary tract infections. *Urol Clin North Am* 2008;35(1):13-22.
64. Talan DA, Stamm WE, Hooton TM, et al. Comparison of ciprofloxacin (7 days) and trimethoprim-sulfamethoxazole (14 days) for acute uncomplicated pyelonephritis pyelonephritis in women: A randomized trial. *JAMA* 2000;283(12):1583-1590.
65. van Nieuwkoop C, van't Wout JW, Assendelft WJ, et al. Treatment duration of febrile urinary tract infection (futirst trial): A randomized placebo-controlled multicenter trial comparing short (7 days) antibiotic treatment with conventional treatment (14 days). *BMC Infect Dis* 2009;Aug 19;9:131.
66. Katchman EA, Milo G, Paul M, et al. Three-day vs longer duration of antibiotic treatment for cystitis in women: Systematic review and meta-analysis. *Am J Med* 2005;118(11):1196-1207.
67. Peterson J, Kaul S, Khashab M, et al. A double-blind, randomized comparison of levofloxacin 750 mg once-daily for five days with ciprofloxacin 400/500 mg twice-daily for 10 days for the treatment of complicated urinary tract infections and acute pyelonephritis. *Urology* 2008;71(1):17-22.
68. Brown P, Ki M and Foxman B. Acute pyelonephritis among adults: Cost of illness and considerations for the economic evaluation of therapy. *Pharmacoeconomics* 2005;23(11):1123-1142.
69. Curran M, Simpson D and Perry C. Ertapenem: A review of its use in the management of bacterial infections. *Drugs* 2003;63(17):1855-1878.
70. Wagenlehner FM, Wagenlehner C, Redman R, et al. Urinary bactericidal activity of doripenem versus that of levofloxacin in patients with complicated urinary tract infections or pyelonephritis. *Antimicrob Agents Chemother* 2009;53(4):1567-1573.
71. Naber KG. Management of bacterial prostatitis: What's new? *BJU Int* 2008;101(Suppl 3):7-10.
72. Gleckman R, Crowley M and Natsios GA. Therapy of recurrent invasive urinary-tract infections of men. *N Engl J Med* 1979;301(16):878-880.
73. Lipsky BA. Urinary tract infections in men. Epidemiology, pathophysiology, diagnosis, and treatment. *Ann Intern Med* 1989;110(2):138-150.
74. Whiteside SA, Razvi H, Dave S, et al. The microbiome of the urinary tract--a role beyond infection. *Nat Rev Urol* 2015;12(2):81-90.
75. O'Brien VP, Hannan TJ, Schaeffer AJ and Hultgren SJ. Are you experienced? Understanding bladder innate immunity in the context of recurrent urinary tract infection. *Curr Opin Infect Dis* 2015;28(1):97-105.
76. Geerlings SE, Beerepoot MA and Prins JM. Prevention of recurrent urinary tract infections in women: Antimicrobial and nonantimicrobial strategies. *Infect Dis Clin North Am* 2014;28(1):135-147.
77. Lichtenberger P and Hooton TM. Antimicrobial prophylaxis in women with recurrent urinary tract infections. *Int J Antimicrob Agents* 2011; Dec;38 Suppl:36-41.
78. Lee BS, Bhuta T, Simpson JM and Craig JC. Methenamine hippurate for preventing urinary tract infections. *Cochrane Database Syst Rev* 2012;Oct 17;10.
79. Renard J, Ballarini S, Mascarenhas T, et al. Recurrent lower urinary tract infections have a detrimental effect on patient quality of life: A prospective, observational study. *Infect Dis Ther.* 2015 Mar; 4(1): 125–135.
80. Macejko AM and Schaeffer AJ. Asymptomatic bacteriuria and symptomatic urinary tract infections during pregnancy. *Urol Clin North Am* 2007;34(1):35-42.
81. Christensen B. Which antibiotics are appropriate for treating bacteriuria in pregnancy? *J Antimicrob Chemother* 2000;46 (Suppl 1):29-34.
82. McDermott S, Daguise V, Mann H, et al. Perinatal risk for mortality and mental retardation associated with maternal urinary-tract infections. *J Fam Pract* 2001;50(5):433-437.
83. Schneeberger C, Geerlings SE, Middleton P and Crowther CA. Interventions for preventing recurrent urinary tract infection during pregnancy. *Cochrane Database Syst Rev.* 2012 Nov 14;11.
84. Saint S, Meddings JA, Calfee D, et al. Catheter-associated urinary tract infection and the medicare rule changes. *Ann Intern Med* 2009;150(12):877-884.
85. Hooton TM, Bradley SF, Cardenas DD, et al. Diagnosis, prevention, and treatment of catheter-associated urinary tract infection in adults: 2009 international clinical practice guidelines from the infectious diseases society of america. *Clin Infect Dis* 2010;50(5):625-663.
86. Ohkawa M, Sugata T, Sawaki M, et al. Bacterial and crystal adherence to the surfaces of indwelling urethral catheters. *J Urol* 1990;143(4):717-721.
87. Johnson JR, Kuskowski MA and Wilt TJ. Systematic review: Antimicrobial urinary catheters to prevent catheter-associated urinary tract infection in hospitalized patients. *Ann Intern Med* 2006;144(2):116-126.
88. Kostakioti M, Hadjifrangiskou M and Hultgren SJ. Bacterial biofilms: Development, dispersal, and therapeutic strategies in the dawn of the postantibiotic era. *Cold Spring Harb Perspect Med* 2013;3(4):a010306.
89. Murphy AB, Macejko A, Taylor A and Nadler RB. Chronic prostatitis: Management strategies. *Drugs* 2009;69(1):71-84.
90. Sharp VJ, Takacs EB and Powell CR. Prostatitis: Diagnosis and treatment. *Am Fam Physician* 2010;82(4):397-406.
91. Lipsky BA, Byren I and Hoey CT. Treatment of bacterial prostatitis. *Clin Infect Dis* 2010;50(12):1641-1652.
92. Fair WR, Couch J and Wehner N. Prostatic antibacterial factor. Identity and significance. *Urology* 1976;7(2):169-177.
93. Pfau A, Perlberg S and Shapira A. The pH of the prostatic fluid in health and disease: Implications of treatment in chronic bacterial prostatitis. *J Urol* 1978;119(3):384-387.
94. Wagenlehner FM and Naber KG. Current challenges in the treatment of complicated urinary tract infections and prostatitis. *Clin Microbiol Infect* 2006;12(Suppl 3):67-80.
95. Alam MF, Cohen D, Butler C, et al. The additional costs of antibiotics and re-consultations for antibiotic-resistant escherichia coli urinary tract infections managed in general practice. *Int J Antimicrob Agents* 2009;33(3):255-257.

Sexually Transmitted Diseases 117

Leroy C. Knodel, Bryson Duhon, and Jacqueline Argamany

The editors are deeply appreciative for the excellent contributions of Dr Leroy Knodel over all 10 editions of this book. This chapter was in preparation at the time of Dr Knodel's death. We thank Dr. Bryson Duhon for his timely work to complete the chapter.

KEY CONCEPTS

1. All recommended treatment regimens for gonorrhea include antibiotic therapy directed against *Chlamydia* species because of the high prevalence of coexisting infections, unless chlamydia has been ruled out.
2. Parenteral penicillin is the treatment of choice for all syphilis infections. For patients who are penicillin-allergic, few well-studied alternative agents are available, and most are oral medications that require 2 to 4 weeks of therapy to be effective. Patient compliance and thus efficacy are a concern when alternative regimens must be used.
3. Chlamydia genital tract infections represent the most frequently reported communicable disease in the United States. In females, these infections are frequently asymptomatic or minimally symptomatic and, if left untreated, are associated with the development of pelvic inflammatory disease and attendant complications such as ectopic pregnancy and infertility. As a result, all sexually active females younger than 25 years and sexually active women with multiple sexual partners should be screened annually for this infection.
4. Oral acyclovir, famciclovir, and valacyclovir are effective in reducing viral shedding, duration of symptoms, and time to healing of first-episode genital herpes infections, with maximal benefits seen when therapy is initiated at the earliest stages of infection. The benefit of these agents for recurrent infections has not been demonstrated. Patient-initiated, episodic antiviral therapy started within one day of lesion onset or during the prodrome preceding an outbreak offers an alternative to continuous suppressive therapy of recurrent infection in some individuals.
5. Metronidazole and tinidazole are the only agents currently approved in the United States to treat trichomoniasis. Although a single 2-g dose of either agent is widely used for compliance and other reasons, single-dose therapy should be avoided for treating recurrent infections.

The spectrum of sexually transmitted diseases (STDs) has broadened from the classic venereal diseases—gonorrhea, syphilis, chancroid, lymphogranuloma venereum, and granuloma inguinale—to include a variety of pathogens known to be spread by sexual contact (Table 117-1). Because of the large number of infected individuals, the diversity of clinical manifestations, the changing drug-susceptibility patterns of some pathogens, and the high frequency of multiple STDs occurring simultaneously in infected individuals, the diagnosis and management of patients with STDs are much more complex today than they were even a decade ago.[1-4] Approximately 20 million new infections occur annually in the United States, with a total prevalence of 110 million infections resulting in a total medical cost of $116 billion to the US healthcare system.[5,6]

Although the annual number of new infections is roughly equal between genders, the complications of STDs generally are more frequent and severe in women.[5] In particular, serious effects on maternal and infant health during pregnancy are well documented.[1,4] Damage to reproductive organs, increased risk of cancer, complications associated with pregnancy, and transmission of disease to the fetus or newborn are associated with several STDs. As a result of the physiologic, psychosocial, and economic consequences of STDs, and because of the increasing prevalence of some viral STDs, such as human immunodeficiency virus (HIV) and genital herpes, for which curative therapy is not available, there is continuing research into STDs and the primary prevention of these diseases.[2-4,7]

With the exception of HIV infection, which is reviewed in detail in Chapter 126, the most frequently occurring STDs in the United States are discussed in this chapter. For other less common STDs, only recommended treatment regimens are presented. The most current information on the epidemiology, diagnosis, and treatment of STDs provided by the US Centers for Disease Control and Prevention (CDC) can be obtained at the CDC Web site (www.cdc.gov).

Numerous interrelated factors contribute to the epidemic nature of STDs. Sociocultural, demographic, and economic factors, together with patterns of sexual behavior, host susceptibility to infection, changing properties of the causative pathogens, disease transmission by asymptomatic individuals, and environmental factors, are important determinants of the frequency and distribution of STDs in the United States and worldwide.

Age is one of the most important demographic determinants of STD incidence. Approximately half of all new STD cases each year occur in persons in their teens and twenties, the peak years of sexual activity. With increasing age, the incidence of most STDs decreases exponentially. In sexually active teenagers, STD rates are highest in the youngest, suggesting that physiologic differences may contribute to increased susceptibility.[2-4,7]

Age-specific rates of STDs are historically higher in men than in women; however, reported rates may not represent true gender differences but rather may reflect greater ease of detection in men. In recent years, the ratio of male-to-female cases for most STDs has

TABLE 117-1 Sexually Transmitted Diseases

Disease	Associated Pathogens
Bacterial	
Gonorrhea	*Neisseria gonorrhoeae*
Syphilis	*Treponema pallidum*
Chancroid	*Haemophilus ducreyi*
Granuloma inguinale	*Calymmatobacterium granulomatis*
Enteric disease	*Salmonella* spp., *Shigella* spp., *Campylobacter* fetus
Campylobacter infection	*Campylobacter jejuni*
Bacterial vaginosis	*Gardnerella vaginalis, Mycoplasma hominis, Bacteroides* spp., *Mobiluncus* spp.
Group B streptococcal infections	Group B *Streptococcus*
Chlamydial	
Nongonococcal urethritis	*Chlamydia trachomatis*
Lymphogranuloma venereum	*C. trachomatis*, type L
Viral	
Acquired immunodeficiency syndrome	Human immunodeficiency virus
Herpes genitalis	Herpes simplex virus, types I and II
Viral hepatitis	Hepatitis A, B, C, and D viruses
Condylomata acuminata	Human papillomavirus
Molluscum contagiosum	Poxvirus
Cytomegalovirus infection	Cytomegalovirus
Mycoplasmal	
Nongonococcal urethritis	*Mycoplasma genitalium*
Protozoal	
Trichomoniasis	*Trichomonas vaginalis*
Amebiasis	*Entamoeba histolytica*
Giardiasis	*Giardia lamblia*
Fungal	
Vaginal candidiasis	*Candida albicans*
Parasitic	
Scabies	*Sarcoptes scabiei*
Pediculosis pubis	*Phthirus pubis*
Enterobiasis	*Enterobius vermicularis*

declined, and in some cases reversed, possibly reflecting improvements in the diagnosis of STDs in asymptomatic women or changes in female sexual behavior following the availability of improved methods of contraception. Although some racial disparity exists for rates of STD infection, it is possible that this is a reflection of socioeconomic differences.[1-5,7]

The single greatest risk factor for contracting STDs is the number of sexual partners. As the number of sexual partners increases, the risk of being exposed to someone infected with an STD increases. Sexual preference also plays a major role in the transmission of STDs. For all major STDs, rates are disproportionately greater in men who have sex with men (MSM) than in heterosexuals. In addition, a number of less common STDs, including several caused by enteric protozoans and bacterial pathogens, occur primarily in MSM. The major risk factors for MSM appear to be related to the greater number of sexual partners and the practice of unprotected anal–genital, oral–genital, and oral–anal intercourse. In addition, prostitution and illicit drug use are associated with a higher incidence of most STDs.[1-4,7]

Some of the most serious sequelae of STDs are associated with congenital or perinatal infections. Most neonatal infections are acquired at birth, after infant passage through an infected cervix or vagina. Neonatal *Chlamydia trachomatis, Neisseria gonorrhoeae*, and herpes simplex virus (HSV) infections are associated with this type of spread. For pregnant women with syphilis, infection is usually transmitted transplacentally, producing a congenital infection. Depending on the organism, neonatal infections can manifest in a variety of ways, produce significant morbidity, and in some cases result in infant death.[1-4]

Other than complete abstinence, the most effective way to prevent STD transmission is by maintaining a mutually monogamous sexual relationship between uninfected partners. Short of this, use of barrier contraceptive methods, such as the male and female condoms, diaphragm, cervical cap, vaginal sponges, and vaginal spermicides alone or in combination, provides varying degrees of protection from a number of STDs. When used correctly and consistently, male latex condoms with or without spermicide are more effective than natural skin condoms in protecting against STD transmission, including HIV, gonorrhea, chlamydia, trichomoniasis, HSV, and human papillomavirus (HPV). When lubrication is desired with latex condoms, water-based products, such as K-Y jelly, are recommended because oil-based agents (eg, petroleum jelly) can weaken latex condoms and reduce their effectiveness. For latex-allergic individuals, other synthetic condoms (eg, polyurethane) appear to possess efficacy against STD transmission similar to latex condoms. The female condom is a lubricated polyurethane sheath with a diaphragm-like ring on each end that can be used as a protective device for women with male sexual partners who do not desire to use a condom. Limited data suggest that the female condom blocks penetration of viruses, including HIV; for nonviral STDs, the female condom provides STD protection similar to the male condom.[1,3,7,8] At one time, use of nonoxynol-9, a vaginal spermicide with cytolytic activity, was advocated to reduce the transmissibility of several STDs. This was based in large part on in vitro and animal data. However, nonoxynol-9 does not reduce the risk of transmission of common STDs and actually can increase the risk of HIV transmission. Frequent use of nonoxynol-9 damages vaginal, cervical, and rectal epithelium, leading to increased transmissibility of HIV and possibly other STDs. Diaphragms may protect against cervical gonorrheal, chlamydial, and trichomonal infections.[1,7-10]

The varied spectrum of clinical syndromes produced by common STDs is determined not only by the etiologic pathogen(s) but also by differences in male and female anatomy and reproductive physiology. For a number of STDs, the signs and symptoms overlap sufficiently to prevent accurate diagnosis without microbiologic confirmation. Frequently, symptoms are minimal or absent despite the presence of infection. Table 117-2 lists common clinical syndromes associated with STDs.[1-4]

GONORRHEA

Epidemiology and Etiology

The gram-negative diplococcus *N. gonorrhoeae* is the causative organism of gonorrhea. Although the rate of reported cases in the United States has remained relatively stable over the past decade, 333,000 new cases were reported in 2013, representing an 8.2% increase from 2009.[11] Due to the increasing incidence of resistance to available antibiotics, there is concern that this number may continue to increase in the future.[1,12] Of concern also are the substantial number of infections that remain undiagnosed and unreported.[1,12] Humans are the only known natural host of this intracellular parasite. Because of its rapid incubation period and the large number of infected individuals with asymptomatic disease, gonorrhea is difficult to control.[1,13-18]

Although the risk of a female acquiring a cervical infection after a single episode of vaginal intercourse with an infected male

TABLE 117-2 Selected Syndromes Associated with Common Sexually Transmitted Pathogens

Syndrome	Commonly Implicated Pathogens	Common Clinical Manifestations[a]
Urethritis	*Chlamydia trachomatis*, herpes simplex virus, *Neisseria gonorrhoeae*, *Trichomonas vaginalis*, *Ureaplasma Mycoplasma genitalium*	Urethral discharge, dysuria
Epididymitis	*C. trachomatis*, *N. gonorrhoeae*	Scrotal pain, inguinal pain, flank pain, urethral discharge
Cervicitis/ vulvovaginitis	*C. trachomatis*, *Gardnerella vaginalis*, herpes simplex virus, human papillomavirus, *N. gonorrhoeae*, *T. vaginalis*	Abnormal vaginal discharge, vulvar itching/irritation, dysuria, dyspareunia
Genital ulcers (painful)	*Haemophilus ducreyi*, herpes simplex virus	Usually multiple vesicular/pustular (herpes) or papular/pustular (*H. ducreyi*) lesions that can coalesce; painful, tender lymphadenopathy[b]
Genital ulcers (painless)	*Treponema pallidum*	Usually single papular lesion
Genital/anal warts	Human papillomavirus	Multiple lesions ranging in size from small papular warts to large exophytic condylomas
Pharyngitis	*C. trachomatis* (?), herpes simplex virus, *N. gonorrhoeae*	Symptoms of acute pharyngitis, cervical lymphadenopathy, fever[c]
Proctitis	*C. trachomatis*, herpes simplex virus, *N. gonorrhoeae*, *T. pallidum*	Constipation, anorectal discomfort, tenesmus, mucopurulent rectal discharge
Salpingitis	*C. trachomatis*, *N. gonorrhoeae*	Lower abdominal pain, purulent cervical or vaginal discharge, adnexal swelling, fever[d]

[a]For some syndromes, clinical manifestations can be minimal or absent.

[b]Recurrent herpes infection can manifest as a single lesion.

[c]Most cases of pharyngeal gonococcal infection are asymptomatic.

[d]Salpingitis increases the risk of subsequent ectopic pregnancy and infertility.

partner is high and increases with multiple exposures, the risk of transmission from an infected female to an uninfected male is not as great following a single act of coitus. No data are available on the risk of transmission after other types of sexual contact.[13-17]

Pathophysiology

On contact with a mucosal surface lined by columnar, cuboidal, or noncornified squamous epithelial cells, the gonococci attach to cell membranes by means of surface pili and are then pinocytosed. The virulence of the organism is mediated primarily by the presence of pili and other outer membrane proteins. After mucosal damage is established, polymorphonuclear (PMN) leukocytes invade the tissue, submucosal abscesses form, and purulent exudates are secreted.[13-18]

Clinical Presentation

Individuals infected with gonorrhea can be symptomatic or asymptomatic, have complicated or uncomplicated infections, and have infections involving several anatomic sites. Interestingly, most of the symptomatic patients who are not treated become asymptomatic within 6 months, with only a few becoming asymptomatic carriers of the disease.[13-16] Up to 50% of women experience nonspecific symptoms, including mucopurulent vaginal discharge and vaginal bleeding, especially following sexual intercourse. In comparison, 90% of males experience symptoms within 2 to 6 days following exposure, most commonly mucopurulent penile discharge and dysuria.[19] The most common clinical features of gonococcal infections are presented in Table 117-3.

Complications associated with untreated gonorrhea appear more pronounced in women, likely a result of a high percentage who experience signs and symptoms that are nonspecific and minimally symptomatic. As a result, many women do not seek treatment until after the development of serious complications, such as pelvic inflammatory disease (PID). Approximately 15% of women with gonorrhea develop PID. Left untreated, PID can be an indirect cause of infertility and ectopic pregnancies. In 0.5% to 3% of patients with gonorrhea, the gonococci invade the bloodstream and produce disseminated disease. Disseminated gonococcal infection (DGI) is three times more common in women than in men. The usual clinical manifestations of DGI are tender necrotic skin

TABLE 117-3 Presentation of Gonorrhea Infections

	Males	Females
General	Incubation period 1-14 days	Incubation period 1-14 days
	Symptom onset in 2-8 days	Symptom onset in 10 days
Site of infection	Most common: urethra	Most common: endocervical canal
	Others: rectum (usually caused by rectal intercourse in MSM), oropharynx, eye	Others: urethra, rectum (usually caused by perineal contamination), oropharynx, eye
Symptoms	Commonly symptomatic, may be asymptomatic	Can be asymptomatic or minimally symptomatic
	Urethral infection: dysuria and urinary frequency	Endocervical infection: usually asymptomatic or mildly symptomatic
	Anorectal infection: asymptomatic to severe rectal pain	Urethral infection: dysuria, urinary frequency
	Pharyngeal infection: asymptomatic to mild pharyngitis	Anorectal and pharyngeal infection; symptoms same as for men
Signs	Purulent urethral or rectal discharge can be scant to profuse Anorectal: pruritus, mucopurulent discharge, bleeding	Abnormal vaginal discharge or uterine bleeding; purulent urethral or rectal discharge can be scant to profuse
Complications	Rare (epididymitis, prostatitis, inguinal lymphadenopathy, urethral stricture)	Pelvic inflammatory disease and associated complications (ie, ectopic pregnancy, infertility)
	Disseminated gonorrhea	Disseminated gonorrhea (three times more common than in men)

MSM, men who have sex with men.

lesions, tenosynovitis, and monoarticular arthritis.[1,13-17] Additionally, HIV infection is more easily transmitted in patients coinfected with gonorrhea.

Diagnosis

Diagnosis of gonococcal infections can be made by gram-stained smears, culture, or methods based on the detection of cellular components of the gonococcus (eg, enzymes, antigens, DNA, or lipopolysaccharide [LPS]) in clinical specimens. Various stains have been used to identify gonococci microscopically, with the Gram stain the most widely used in clinical practice. Gram-stained smears are positive for gonococci when gram-negative diplococci of typical kidney bean morphology are identified within PMN leukocytes.[1,13-17] In urethral smears from men with symptomatic urethritis, the smear is highly sensitive and specific, and is considered diagnostic for infection. However, due to lower sensitivity, gram-stained smears are not recommended in the diagnosis of endocervical, rectal, cutaneous, and asymptomatic male urethral infections. Because of the presence of nonpathogenic *Neisseria* in the pharynx, the Gram stain is not useful in the diagnosis of pharyngeal infection.[1,13,15-17]

Although culture is highly sensitive and specific, limitations including prolonged turnaround times and difficulty maintaining viable samples preclude widespread usage. Additionally, culture requires invasive specimen collection for processing (endocervical or urethral swab). As a result, direct culture is primarily utilized in cases of suspected or documented treatment failures, as a test of cure following use of an alternative treatment regimen, or for detection of rectal, oropharyngeal, and conjunctival gonococcal infections.[1]

With the exception of Gram stain for symptomatic gonococcal urethritis, alternative methods of diagnosis, including enzyme immunoassay (EIA), DNA probe techniques, and nucleic acid amplification techniques (NAATs) offer increased sensitivity and/or specificity over traditional diagnostic methods.[13,16,17,20] Additionally, many of these tests can provide a more rapid means of diagnosis than culture. Of particular clinical importance is the high sensitivity of NAATs for detecting *N. gonorrhoeae* using noninvasive specimens (eg, self-collected urine specimens, vaginal swabs). NAAT is recommended by the CDC for detection of gonorrhea in FDA-cleared specimen types specific to each NAAT manufacturer.[1] This technology is also being used to concurrently test for *C. trachomatis* using a single specimen. However, a major drawback of NAATs is their inability to provide resistance data on isolated gonococcal strains. In cases of documented treatment failure, antimicrobial susceptibility testing is recommended, as previously mentioned.[1,12,17,18,20]

TREATMENT

1 In 2010, the CDC issued an update to their recommended treatment regimens for gonorrhea. This update eliminated oral cephalosporins from the recommended treatment regimens for gonorrhea, leaving single-dose intramuscular ceftriaxone as the only recommended agent for treating gonorrhea[18] (Table 117-4). The ceftriaxone-based regimens are the only regimens that have well-documented efficacy in the treatment of urethral, cervical, rectal, and pharyngeal infections, curing 99.2% of uncomplicated cases and 98.9% of pharyngeal cases.[12] A 400 mg oral dose of cefixime may be substituted if ceftriaxone is unavailable, however, a test of cure is often recommended two weeks later due to reduced bactericidal levels and efficacy (97.5% in uncomplicated cases and 92.3% in pharyngeal gonorrhea) compared to ceftriaxone. Additionally, only ceftriaxone is effective in treating pharyngeal gonorrhea and eradicating both gonorrhea and incubating syphilis in a patient coinfected with both organisms. The latter is particularly beneficial in areas with a high rate of syphilis.[1,13,15-18]

Coexisting chlamydial infection, which is documented in up to 50% of women and 20% of men with gonorrhea, constitutes the major cause of postgonococcal urethritis, cervicitis, and salpingitis in patients treated for gonorrhea for whom concurrent chlamydial infection has not been ruled out.[1,17] As a result, concomitant treatment with azithromycin or doxycycline is recommended in all patients treated for gonorrhea. Azithromycin 1,000 mg given orally as a one-time dose is currently preferred to doxycyline due to advantages of single-dose therapy and increased resistance of gonococcal resistance to tetracycline. Doxycycline 100 mg orally twice a day may be used in cases of azithromycin allergy.[1] While azithromycin (2 g) as a single dose appears highly effective in eradicating both gonorrhea and chlamydia, it is not recommended as a preferred alternative to ceftriaxone because of concerns regarding the development of resistance. Alternative therapies can be used for in cephalosporin-allergic individuals. Single-dose regimens consisting of oral gemifloxacin or intramuscular gentamicin in combination with azithromycin were associated with high cure rates (99.5% and 100%, respectively), however, high rates gastrointestinal side effects may limit their applicability [1,17,21,22,23] Pregnant women infected with *N. gonorrhoeae* should be treated with ceftriaxone. For presumed or diagnosed concurrent *C. trachomatis* infection, azithromycin is the preferred treatment.[1,13,14]

Ceftriaxone is the recommended therapy for DGI, gonococcal meningitis, endocarditis, and any type of gonococcal infection in children. In cases of DGI, patients should be hospitalized and treated with ceftriaxone or one of the alternative parenteral cephalosporin antibiotics (see Table 117-4). Although marked improvement is usually noted within 48 hours of initiating therapy, treatment should be continued for at least 7 days, with longer durations necessary for serious infections, such as meningitis and endocarditis[1,16,17] Gonococcal ophthalmia is highly contagious in adults and neonates and requires ceftriaxone therapy. Single-dose therapy is adequate for gonococcal conjunctivitis, although some physicians recommend continuing therapy until cultures are negative at 48 to 72 hours. Topical antibiotics are not sufficiently effective when used alone for ocular infections and are not necessary with appropriate systemic therapy. Infants with any evidence of ocular infection should be evaluated for signs of DGI.[1,13,16,17,24]

Clinical **Controversy...**

The American College of Obstetricians and Gynecologists (ACOG) supports expedited partner therapy, or the treatment of sexual partners of those infected with gonorrhea and chlamydial without first examining these partners, in order to reduce reinfection rates. This is particularly useful in cases when the patient's partner is unwilling to seek medical care. However, many legal and social barriers exist which prevent widespread acceptance of this philosophy.

Treatment of gonorrhea during pregnancy is essential to prevent ophthalmia neonatorum. Gonococcal infection in newborns results primarily from passage through an infected birth canal, but it also can be transmitted in utero. Conjunctival involvement usually develops within 7 days of delivery and is characterized by intense, bilateral conjunctival inflammation with chemosis. If not treated promptly, corneal ulceration and blindness can develop. Because the law in most states requires neonatal prophylaxis with topical ocular antimicrobials, gonococcal ophthalmia neonatorum is rare in the United States. The CDC recommends that erythromycin (0.5%) ophthalmic ointment be instilled in each conjunctival sac immediately postpartum.[1,13-17,24]

TABLE 117-4 Treatment of Gonorrhea

Type of Infection	Recommended Regimens[a]	Alternative Regimens[a]
Uncomplicated infections of the cervix, urethra, and rectum in adults	Ceftriaxone 250 mg IM once *plus* Azithromycin 1 g orally once	Cefixime 400 mg orally once *plus* Azithromycin 1 g orally once, or doxycycline 100 mg PO twice daily for 7 days[b,c] or Gemifloxacin 320 mg orally once or gentamicin 240 mg IM[e] *plus* Azithromycin 2 g orally once
Uncomplicated infections of the pharynx	Ceftriaxone 250 mg IM once *plus* Azithromycin 1 g orally once	Consult with infectious disease expert
Disseminated gonococcal infection in adults (>45 kg)	Ceftriaxone 1-2 g IM or IV every 12-24 hour[e] *plus* Azithromycin 1 g orally once	Cefotaxime 1 g IV every 8 hours[e] or ceftizoxime 1 g IV every 8 hours[e] *plus* Azithromycin 1 g orally once
Uncomplicated infections of the cervix, urethra, pharynx, and rectum in children (<45 kg)	Ceftriaxone 25-50 mg/kg IV or IM once (not to exceed 125 mg)	
Disseminated gonococcal infection in children (<45 kg)	Ceftriaxone 50 mg/kg IV or IM once daily (not to exceed 1 g)	
Gonococcal conjunctivitis in adults	Ceftriaxone 1 g IM once[f]	
Ophthalmia neonatorum	Ceftriaxone 25-50 mg/kg IV or IM once (not to exceed 125 mg)	
Disseminated gonococcal infection in neonates	Ceftriaxone 25-50 mg/kg/day IV or IM once daily or cefotaxime 25 mg/kg IV or IM twice daily for 7 days, or 10-14 days if meningitis is suspected[h]	
Infants born to mothers with gonococcal infection (prophylaxis)	Erythromycin (0.5%) ophthalmic ointment in a single application[g] Ceftriaxone 25-50 mg/kg IM or IV once (not to exceed 125 mg)	

CDC, Centers for Disease Control and Prevention; *C. trachomatis, Chlamydia trachomatis*; NAAT, Nucleic Acid Amplification Test; *N. gonorrhoeae, Neisseria gonorrhoeae*.

[a]Recommendations are those of the CDC.

[b]Tetracyclines are contraindicated during pregnancy. Pregnant women should be treated with recommended cephalosporin-based combination therapy. In severe cephalosporin allergy, consulation with an infectious diseases expert is recommended.

[c]Patients who are treatment failures with alternative regimens should be treated with ceftriaxone 250 mg IM once plus azithromycin 1 g PO once in consultation with an infectious disease expert.

[d]For patients with severe cephalosporin allergy.

[e]Parenteral treatment duration should be determined in consultation with an infectious diseases expert. Parenteral therapy for meningitis should be continued for at least 10-14 days and at least 4 weeks in endocarditis.

[f]A single lavage of the infected eye with normal saline should be considered; empiric therapy for *C. trachomatis* is recommended.

[g]Efficacy in preventing chlamydial ophthalmia is unclear.

[h]Caution should be taken when administering ceftriaxone to hyperbilirubinemic neonates.

Recent sex partners (within 60 days of preceding onset of symptoms or diagnosis) should be referred to for evaluation and treatment. Sex partners should abstain from unprotected sexual intercourse for 7 days after both have completed treatment and symptoms have resolved.[1]

Evaluation of Therapeutic Outcomes

In the past, persistence of gonorrhea symptoms a short time following treatment with a recommended regimen against gonorrhea usually indicated reinfection rather than treatment failure and, as such, reflected the need for improved patient education and sex partner referral. However, with antimicrobial resistance increasingly being reported in recent years, reinfection can no longer be assumed as the cause. As a result, the CDC recommends that all apparent treatment failures be assessed using culture and sensitivity testing. Persistence of symptoms also can be due to other infectious causes, such as *C. trachomatis*.[1,13-18] While the CDC does not recommend a test-of-cure of patients treated with a recommended regimen, it is recommend that any patient treated for gonorrhea be retested 3 months after treatment, and if not possible, whenever the patient next presents for medical care in the following 12 months. Patients who require retreatment should be tested for cure 7-14 days following the second regiment.[1]

SYPHILIS

Epidemiology and Etiology

Although nearly eradicated in 2000, cases of syphilis more than doubled in the United States from 2005 to 2013, with an annual total of primary and secondary syphilis diagnoses of around 16,000. Of these newly diagnosed cases, 91% were reported in men, the majority of whom were reported as MSM.[25] In addition to being highly contagious, syphilis is of major concern because, if left untreated, it can progress to a chronic systemic disease that can be fatal or seriously disabling.[26-35] Syphilis usually is acquired by sexual contact with infected mucous membranes or cutaneous lesions, although on rare occasions it can be acquired by nonsexual personal contact, accidental inoculation, or blood transfusion. The causative organism of syphilis is *Treponema pallidum*, a spirochete. The risk of acquiring syphilis from an infected individual after a single sexual encounter is approximately 50% to 60%. After sexual contact, the organism penetrates the intact mucous membrane or a break in the cornified epithelium, and spirochetemia occurs.[27,30,31-35]

There is strong evidence of an association between syphilis and HIV infection. Syphilis, similar to other sexually transmitted genital ulcer diseases, can increase the risk of acquiring HIV in exposed individuals. In addition, immunologic defects in HIV-infected individuals can produce an atypical serologic response to syphilis. In particular, the possibility of delayed seroreactivity, markedly elevated serologic titers, and increased false-positive results could complicate the diagnosis, as well as assessment of treatment efficacy, in HIV-positive individuals infected with syphilis. Furthermore, anecdotal evidence suggests that compromised immune function can result in an accelerated progression of syphilis, particularly to neurosyphilis, requiring more aggressive antibiotic therapy in comparison with an immunocompetent host. As a result of this association, the CDC recommends that all patients diagnosed with syphilis be tested for HIV infection.[1,26,28-30,32,33]

Clinical Presentation

The clinical presentation of syphilis is varied with progression through multiple stages possible in untreated or inadequately treated patients (Table 117-5).

Primary Syphilis

The primary stage, characterized by the appearance of a chancre on cutaneous or mucocutaneous tissue exposed to the organism, is highly infectious. Even without treatment, chancres persist only for 1 to 8 weeks before healing spontaneously. Because syphilitic chancres can be confused with other infectious etiologies, appropriate diagnostic testing is important.[26-30,32,34]

TABLE 117-5 Presentation of Syphilis Infections

General	
Primary	Incubation period 10-90 days (mean, 21 days)
Secondary	Develops 2-8 weeks after initial infection in untreated or inadequately treated individuals
Latent	Develops 4-10 weeks after secondary stage in untreated or inadequately treated individuals
Tertiary	Develops in approximately 30% of untreated or inadequately treated individuals 10-30 years after initial infection
Site of Infection	
Primary	External genitalia, perianal region, mouth, and throat
Secondary	Multisystem involvement secondary to hematogenous and lymphatic spread
Latent tertiary	Potentially multisystem involvement (dormant)
	CNS, heart, eyes, bones, and joints
Signs and Symptoms	
Primary	Single, painless, indurated lesion (chancre) that erodes, ulcerates, and eventually heals (typical); regional lymphadenopathy is common; multiple, painful, purulent lesions possible but uncommon
Secondary	Pruritic or nonpruritic rash, mucocutaneous lesions, flulike symptoms, lymphadenopathy
Latent	Asymptomatic
Tertiary	Cardiovascular syphilis (aortitis or aortic insufficiency), neurosyphilis (meningitis, general paresis, dementia, tabes dorsalis, eighth cranial nerve deafness, blindness), gummatous lesions involving any organ or tissue

CNS, central nervous system.

Secondary Syphilis

The secondary stage of syphilis is characterized by a variety of mucocutaneous eruptions resulting from widespread hematogenous and lymphatic spread of *T. pallidum*. Skin lesions can be either generalized or localized to a small portion of the body and, with the exception of follicular lesions, are nonpruritic. Generalized lymphadenopathy also is seen in the majority of patients, as are nonspecific symptoms such as mild and transitory malaise, fever, pharyngitis, headache, anorexia, and arthralgia. If untreated, secondary syphilis disappears in 4 to 10 weeks; however, lesions can recur at any time within 4 years.[26-34]

Latent Syphilis

By definition, persons with a positive serologic test for syphilis but with no other evidence of disease have latent syphilis. Latent syphilis is further divided into early and late latency. During early latency, the patient is considered potentially infectious because of the 25% risk of spontaneous mucocutaneous relapse. The CDC defines early latency as 1 year from the onset of infection, although other investigators propose a longer interval, such as 2 to 4 years. With the exception of pregnancy in which the mother can pass the disease to the fetus, late latency is considered noninfectious, although the patient remains a host.[1,26-34]

Most untreated patients with late latent syphilis have no further sequelae; however, approximately 25% to 30% progress either to neurosyphilis or to late syphilis with clinical manifestations other than neurosyphilis. Treatment of all patients with latent syphilis is essential because there is no way to predict which patients will have progression of their disease.[26-34]

Tertiary Syphilis and Neurosyphilis

If left untreated, syphilis can slowly produce an inflammatory reaction in virtually any organ in the body. Manifestations of this disease progression were referred to previously as *tertiary syphilis*. These clinical manifestations now are differentiated into two subgroups based on the presence or absence of central nervous system (CNS) involvement: neurosyphilis or tertiary syphilis (ie, gumma and cardiovascular syphilis).[1,26-34]

Currently, the term *neurosyphilis* encompasses any patient with cerebrospinal fluid (CSF) abnormalities consistent with CNS infection. Approximately 40% of patients with primary or secondary syphilis exhibit such abnormalities, although most remain asymptomatic. Persistence of CSF abnormalities into late latency is associated with a greater risk of progression to symptomatic neurosyphilis. Although data are conflicting, some investigators suggest that HIV-infected patients are at greater risk of developing symptomatic neurosyphilis than patients with intact immune systems.[1,26-34]

Rarely seen, the most common manifestations of disease progression from late latency are benign gumma formation and cardiovascular syphilis. The gumma, a nonspecific granulomatous lesion, is the classic lesion of late syphilis and develops in 50% of patients with disease progression. These chronic, destructive lesions characteristically infiltrate the skin, bone, soft tissue, and liver but can be found in any organ or tissue. Gummas of critical organs, such as the heart or brain, can be fatal.[1,26-30,33]

Congenital Syphilis

In pregnant women with syphilis, *T. pallidum* can cross the placenta at any time during pregnancy. The risk of fetal infection is greatest in pregnant women with primary and secondary syphilis and declines in pregnant women with late disease. Transmission of syphilis during pregnancy occurs primarily transplacentally and can result in fetal death, prematurity, or congenital syphilis. Symptoms can be seen during the first months of life (early congenital syphilis) or later in childhood or adolescence (late congenital syphilis). Manifestations of early congenital syphilis resemble those of secondary syphilis, whereas those of late congenital syphilis correspond to the tertiary stage in adults.[26,28-30]

Diagnosis

Because *T. pallidum* is difficult to culture in vitro, diagnosis is based primarily on microscopic examination of serous material from a suspected syphilitic lesion or on results from serologic testing. In primary syphilis, diagnosis is established by the presence of *T. pallidum* on dark-field microscopic examination of material from cutaneous lesions and enlarged lymph nodes in patients with secondary syphilis. In incubating syphilis, confirmation frequently is by dark-field microscopic examination because serologic tests can be unreactive early in the disease. Another method of direct microscopic examination, the direct fluorescent-antibody (test) for *T. pallidum* (DFA-TP), which uses monoclonal or polyclonal antibodies specific for *T. pallidum*, has greater specificity and sensitivity than dark-field examination, and does not require the immediate examination of fresh specimens.[30-35]

Serologic tests are the mainstay in the diagnosis of syphilis and traditionally are categorized as nontreponemal or treponemal. Common nontreponemal tests include the Venereal Disease Research Laboratory (VDRL) slide test, rapid plasma reagin (RPR) card test, unheated serum reagin (USR) test, and the toluidine red unheated serum test (TRUST). Nontreponemal tests, which are inexpensive and easily performed, rely on the detection of treponemal antibodies directed against an alcoholic solution of cardiolipin, lecithin, and cholesterol contained in these tests. A positive nontreponemal test can indicate the presence of any stage of syphilis or congenital syphilis, although incubating syphilis and very early primary syphilis produce a negative reaction; however, because they are nonspecific tests, false-positive reactions occur, making them inappropriate to confirm the diagnosis alone. Transiently false-positive results can be seen in patients with acute febrile illnesses, after immunizations, and during pregnancy. Chronic false-positive results are commonly associated with heroin addiction, aging, chronic infections, autoimmune diseases, and malignant disease. In some cases, false-positive reactions are familial and are related to abnormal serum globulin levels. As such, patients with a positive nontreponemal test should always receive a treponemal test for diagnosis confirmation.[1,29-35]

Nontreponemal tests are used primarily as screening tests; however, because *T. pallidum* antibody titers also can be quantitated by testing serial dilutions of the patient's serum for reactivity, they are useful in following the progression of the disease, recovery after therapy, and possible reinfection. Because antibody titers vary to some extent between tests, it is important that sequential serologic testing be performed using the same method each time. In patients treated successfully for primary and secondary syphilis, nontreponemal tests usually decline over time and may return to seronegativity. If these tests are going to return to negative in patients with early latent syphilis, they will do so within the first 4 years after adequate therapy; patients with disease of longer duration usually remain seropositive for life. In addition to their use in serologic testing, nontreponemal tests often are used on CSF to diagnose neurosyphilis.[29-35]

In some patients with secondary syphilis, a prozone phenomenon occurs that produces a negative VDRL test despite the presence of high reaginic antibody titers. This is corrected by diluting the patient's serum prior to testing.[32,33] For HIV-positive individuals with syphilis, the reactivity of nontreponemal tests can vary depending on the stage of the HIV infection. In the early stages, reaginic titers higher than in non–HIV-infected patients have been seen, resulting in the prozone phenomenon. During the later stages of HIV infection, however, when immune function deteriorates to a greater extent, serologic responses can be reduced or delayed. As a result, the diagnosis of syphilis in HIV-infected individuals can be more difficult.[1,30-35]

Use of only one serologic test for diagnosis of syphilis is insufficient as false-positives can occur in those without syphilis and false-negatives in those with primary syphilis. In diagnosing all stages of syphilis, treponemal tests are more sensitive than nontreponemal tests. Because these tests are technically more demanding and are more expensive, they have been used as confirmatory rather than as screening tests. However, patients with a positive treponemal test should have a nontreponemal test with titer reflexively drawn in order to guide management decisions and to monitor response to therapy. If the nontreponemal test is negative, a different treponemal test should be used to confirm the initial positive result. If a second treponemal test is positive, previously untreated patients should be offered treatment. Those with a previous history of treatment require no further management unless sexual history indicates likelihood of re-exposure, in which case a repeat nontreponemal test is recommended in 2 to 4 weeks.[1]

For many years, the fluorescent treponemal antibody absorption (FTA-ABS) test was the most frequently used treponemal test. The FTA-ABS test uses the *T. pallidum* antigen to detect specific antibodies to treponemal organisms. However, the FTA-ABS test has largely been replaced by card assays such as the *T. pallidum* hemagglutination assay (TPHA), the microhemagglutination assay for antibodies to *T. pallidum* (MHA-TP), and the *T. pallidum* particle agglutination assay (TPPA) which can be automated and are less expensive to perform. Despite adequate antibiotic therapy for any stage of syphilis, the antibody tests usually remain reactive for life and therefore are not useful in assessing serologic response to therapy, relapse, or reinfection, hence the need for a reflex nontreponemal test.[1,30-35]

Several EIAs for *T. pallidum* have become available and are gaining wide use as confirmatory tests. Polymerase chain reaction (PCR)-based tests also are being investigated, particularly in situations in which serologic testing has poor sensitivity and specificity (eg, congenital syphilis, early primary syphilis, and neurosyphilis). Additionally, multiplex PCR tests that can identify the presence of *T. pallidum*, herpes simplex virus type 1 (HSV-1) and herpes simplex virus type 2 (HSV-2), and *Haemophilus ducreyi* from genital ulcer specimens are under study. The CDC recommends that all patients diagnosed with syphilis be tested for HIV infection.[1,28-30,35]

TREATMENT

Table 117-6 presents the CDC's treatment recommendations.[1] Parenteral penicillin G is the treatment of choice for all stages of syphilis. Because *T. pallidum* multiplies slowly, single doses of short- or intermediate-acting penicillins do not provide the prolonged, low-level exposure to penicillin required for eradication of the treponeme. As a result, benzathine penicillin G is the only penicillin effective for single-dose therapy.[1,28-34]

The recommended treatment for syphilis of less than 1 year's duration is benzathine penicillin G 2.4 million units as a single dose. Although the relapse rate for this regimen is less than 3%, some investigators advocate that 2.4 million units be administered once a week for two consecutive weeks. In patients with late latent syphilis and normal CSF examination, benzathine penicillin G is administered weekly for three successive doses. Although not specifically recommended by the CDC, this three-dose regimen is used by some experts to treat HIV-infected patients with syphilis of less than 1 year's duration based on data suggesting a greater risk of treatment failure with single-dose therapy.[1,30-34]

Patients with abnormal CSF findings should be treated as having neurosyphilis. Preferred regimens for neurosyphilis provide treatment over 10 to 14 days with 18 to 24 million units per day of parenteral penicillin G administered as 3 to 4 million units every 4 hours

TABLE 117-6 Drug Therapy and Follow-up of Syphilis

Stage/Type of Syphilis	Recommended Regimens[a,b]	Follow-up Serology
Primary, secondary, or early latent syphilis (<1 year's duration)	Adults: Benzathine penicillin G 2.4 million units IM in a single dose Children: Benzathine penicillin G 50,000 units/kg IM in a single dose, up to 2.4 million units	Quantitative nontreponemal tests at 6 and 12 months for primary and secondary syphilis; at 6, 12, and 24 months for early latent syphilis[c]
Late latent syphilis (>1 year's duration) or latent syphilis of unknown duration or tertiary syphilis or retreatment	Adults: Benzathine penicillin G 2.4 million units IM once a week for 3 successive weeks (7.2 million units total) Children: Benzathine penicillin G 50,000 units/kg IM once a week for 3 successive weeks, up to 7.2 million units total	Quantitative nontreponemal tests at 6, 12, and 24 months[d,e]
Neurosyphilis	Aqueous crystalline penicillin G 18-24 million units IV (3-4 million units every 4 hours or by continuous infusion) for 10-14 days[f] *or* Aqueous procaine penicillin G 2.4 million units IM daily plus probenecid 500 mg orally four times daily, both for 10-14 days[f]	CSF examination every 6 months until the cell count is normal; if it has not decreased at 6 months or is not normal by 2 years, retreatment should be considered
Congenital syphilis (infants with proven or highly probable disease)	Aqueous crystalline penicillin G 50,000 units/kg/dose IV every 12 hours during the first 7 days of life and every 8 hours thereafter for a total of 10 days *or* Procaine penicillin G 50,000 units/kg IM daily for 10 days	Serologic follow-up only recommended if antimicrobials other than penicillin are used
Penicillin-Allergic Patients[g]		
Primary, secondary, or early latent syphilis	Doxycycline 100 mg orally two times daily for 14 days[g,h] *or* Tetracycline 500 mg orally four times daily for 14 days[h] *or* Ceftriaxone 1-2 g IM or IV daily for 10-14 days	Same as for non–penicillin-allergic patients
Late latent syphilis (>1 year's duration) or syphilis of unknown duration	Doxycycline 100 mg orally twice a day for 28 days[h,i] *or* Tetracycline 500 mg orally four times daily for 28 days[h,i]	Same as for non–penicillin-allergic patients

CDC, Centers for Disease Control and Prevention; CSF, cerebrospinal fluid; HIV, human immunodeficiency virus.

[a]Recommendations are those of the CDC.

[b]The CDC recommends that all patients diagnosed with syphilis be tested for HIV infection.

[c]More frequent follow-up (ie, 3, 6, 9, 12, and 24 months) recommended for HIV-infected patients.

[d]More frequent follow-up (ie, 6, 12, 18, and 24 months) recommended for HIV-infected patients.

[e]No specific recommendations exist for tertiary syphilis because of the lack of available data.

[f]Some experts administer benzathine penicillin G 2.4 million units IM once per week for up to 3 weeks after completion of the neurosyphilis regimens to provide a total duration of therapy comparable to that used for late syphilis in the absence of neurosyphilis.

[g]For nonpregnant patients; pregnant patients should be treated with penicillin after desensitization.

[h]Pregnant patients allergic to penicillin should be desensitized and treated with penicillin.

[i]Limited data suggest that ceftriaxone may be effective, although the optimal dosage and treatment duration are unclear.

or by continuous infusion. Benzathine penicillin G alone in standard weekly doses and procaine penicillin G in doses under 2.4 million units do not consistently provide treponemicidal levels in the CSF and have resulted in treatment failures. Because *T. pallidum* resistance to penicillin has not emerged, the primary need for alternative drugs in treating syphilis is for penicillin-allergic patients.[1,30-34]

2 Alternative regimens recommended for penicillin-allergic patients are doxycycline 100 mg orally twice daily or tetracycline 500 mg orally four times daily for 2 to 4 weeks depending on the duration of syphilis infection. These regimens should be used only in cases of documented penicillin allergy, and given concerns regarding patient compliance with these regimens, follow-up serologic testing is of particular importance.[1,30-34]

Other antibiotics used successfully in treating syphilis include various beta lactam antibiotics; however, none offers significant advantages over benzathine penicillin G. Even though ceftriaxone is considered effective in eradicating incubating syphilis when given as a single 125-mg dose, higher doses and more frequent administration (eg, 1-2 g daily for 10-14 days) appear necessary for more advanced syphilis, and treatment failures are reported in HIV-infected patients. Although azithromycin 2 g as a single dose produces good results in patients with early syphilis, treatment failures and resistance to azithromycin are reported.[1,27,30-34]

Clinical **Controversy...**

One clinical trial recently reported positive results on the use of high dose amoxicillin (3 g) plus probenecid for treatment of patients coinfected with HIV and syphilis. This method might prove particularly useful in countries where benzathine penicillin is not available or for treatment of patients who are unlikely to follow-up for weekly injections.

For pregnant patients, penicillin is the treatment of choice at the dosage recommended for that particular stage of syphilis. To ensure treatment success and prevent transmission to the fetus, some experts advocate an additional IM dose of benzathine penicillin G 2.4 million units 1 week after completion of the recommended regimen. In women allergic to penicillin, safe and effective alternatives are not available; therefore, skin testing should be performed to confirm a penicillin allergy. It is recommended that women with positive skin tests undergo penicillin desensitization and receive the appropriate treatment regimen for their stage of disease.[1,28-30]

Most patients treated for primary and secondary syphilis experience the Jarisch-Herxheimer reaction after treatment. This benign, self-limiting reaction is characterized by flulike symptoms, such as transient headache, fever, chills, malaise, arthralgia, myalgia, tachypnea, peripheral vasodilation, and aggravation of syphilitic lesions. The exact mechanism of the reaction is unknown, although proposed etiologies, including immunologic mechanisms and release of endotoxin or other toxic treponemal products, are not substantiated. The Jarisch-Herxheimer reaction is independent of the drug and dose used and should not be confused with penicillin allergy. It usually begins within 2 to 4 hours of initiating therapy, peaks at 8 hours, and is complete within 12 to 24 hours. Most reactions can be managed symptomatically with analgesics, antipyretics, and rest. Steroids and antihistamines have been administered prior to initiation of syphilitic therapy but are of limited value.[1,28-30]

Evaluation of Therapeutic Outcomes

Table 117-6 lists the CDC recommendations for serologic follow-up of patients treated for syphilis.[1] Quantitative nontreponemal tests should be performed at 6 and 12 months in all patients treated for primary and secondary syphilis and at 6, 12, and 24 months for early and late latent disease. Patients indicated for retreatment should receive three weekly treatments of IM 2.4 million units of benzathine penicillin G, unless neurosyphilis is present. The CDC recommends more frequent monitoring of HIV-infected individuals (ie, 3, 6, 9, 12, and 24 months after therapy). In general, the time to reach seronegativity is proportional to the duration of the disease. Table 117-6 also includes specific testing recommendations for other stages of syphilis. Despite adequate therapy, some patients can remain seropositive based on nontreponemal test results. In these cases, stabilization of low antibody titers is indicative of adequate therapy. For women treated during pregnancy, monthly quantitative nontreponemal tests are recommended in those at high risk of reinfection.[28-30]

CHLAMYDIA TRACHOMATIS

Epidemiology and Etiology

Based on CDC data for 2013, over 1.4 million cases of chlamydia infection were reported, making it the second most frequently reported infectious disease in the United States behind HPV.[1,5] Because of the silent nature of many infections, the presumptive treatment of many cases, and the underreporting of many cases, it is estimated that more than double this number of cases actually occur annually. Chlamydial infections also are the primary causes of nongonococcal urethritis (NGU), accounting for as much as 50% of such infections.[1,36-40]

Pathophysiology

C. trachomatis is an obligate intracellular parasite that shares properties of both viruses and bacteria. Like viruses, chlamydiae require cellular material from host cells for replication; however, unlike viruses, chlamydiae maintain their cellular identity throughout development. Although *C. trachomatis* lacks a cell-wall peptidoglycan, its major outer membrane is similar to gram-negative bacteria. At least 18 serovars (subspecies) of *C. trachomatis* exist, of which only the lymphogranuloma venereum strains produce potentially invasive infections. The remaining serovars are involved primarily with superficial infection of epithelial cells.[36-40]

The risk of transmissibility of chlamydia after exposure is unknown but is believed to be less than that following exposure to *N. gonorrhoeae*. Coinfection with chlamydia occurs in a substantial number of individuals with gonorrhea and all individuals diagnosed with *N. gonorrhoeae* should be assumed also to have *C. trachomatis* present, if chlamydial infection has not been ruled out.[1] Of major concern is that chlamydial infections are associated with a significantly increased risk of acquiring HIV infection. In addition to genital infections, ocular infections in adults owing to autoinoculation and infants owing to vaginal delivery through an infected birth canal are reported. Pharyngeal and rectal infections can develop secondary to orogenital or receptive anal intercourse, respectively, with an infected individual.[1,36-43]

Clinical Presentation

In comparison with gonorrhea, chlamydial genital tract infections are more frequently asymptomatic, and when present, symptoms tend to be less noticeable. Urethral discharge usually is less profuse and more mucoid or watery than the urethral discharge associated with gonorrhea.[37-40] Table 117-7 summarizes the usual clinical presentation of chlamydial infections.

Similar to gonorrhea, chlamydia can be transmitted to an infant during contact with infected cervicovaginal secretions. Nearly two-thirds of infants acquire chlamydial infection after endocervical exposure, with the primary morbidity associated with seeding of the infant's eyes, nasopharynx, rectum, or vagina. In exposed infants, neonatal conjunctivitis develops in as many as 50%, and pneumonia develops in up to 16%. Inclusion conjunctivitis in newborns is usually self-limited, but it can result in scarring and micropannus of the cornea. Interstitial pneumonitis occurring secondary to carriage in the nasopharynx typically is mild, but it can be severe and require hospitalization.[1,37-40,42]

Diagnosis

(3) Because of the high rate of asymptomatic disease and the high prevalence of chlamydial infection in sexually active females 25 years of age or younger and sexually active women with new sex partners or multiple sex partners, the CDC recommends routine annual screening in these individuals. Laboratory confirmation of chlamydial infection is important because of the relative lack of specificity of symptoms when present.[1]

Cell culture is the reference standard against which all other diagnostic tests are measured. Because chlamydiae are obligate

TABLE 117-7 Presentation of *Chlamydia* Infections

	Males	Females
General	Incubation period: 35 days Symptom onset: 7-21 days	Incubation period: 7-35 days Usual symptom onset: 7-21 days
Site of infection	Most common: urethra Others: rectum (receptive anal intercourse), oropharynx, eye	Most common: endocervical canal Others: urethra, rectum (usually caused by perineal contamination), oropharynx, eye
Symptoms	More than 50% of urethral and rectal infections are asymptomatic Urethral infection: mild dysuria, discharge Pharyngeal infection: asymptomatic to mild pharyngitis	More than 66% of cervical infections are asymptomatic Urethral infection: usually subclinical; dysuria and frequency uncommon Rectal and pharyngeal infection: symptoms same as for men
Signs	Scant to profuse, mucoid to purulent urethral or rectal discharge Rectal infection: pain, discharge, bleeding	Abnormal vaginal discharge or uterine bleeding, purulent urethral or rectal discharge can be scant to profuse
Complications	Epididymitis, Reiter's syndrome (rare)	Pelvic inflammatory disease and associated complications (ie, ectopic pregnancy, infertility) Reiter's syndrome (rare)

intracellular parasites, specimens for culture must be obtained from endocervical (women) or urethral (men) epithelial cell scrapings rather than from urine or urethral discharges. Although tissue culture techniques have close to 100% specificity, the sensitivity is reported to be as low as 70% in part because of problems of improper specimen collection, transport, or processing. Because of the technical demands, expense, and length of time until results are available (3-7 days), culture is not used widely for diagnostic purposes today. However, culture remains the diagnostic standard in medicolegal cases such as sexual assault and child abuse because of its high specificity and ability to detect only viable organisms.[37-40,43-46]

Tests that detect chlamydial antigens and nucleic acid provide more rapid results, are technically less demanding to perform, are less costly, and in some situations have greater sensitivity than culture. Commonly used nonculture tests for detection of *C. trachomatis* are the enzyme immunosorbent assay (EIA), DNA hybridization probe, and NAATs.[38,40,43,45]

Although still widely used both as rapid office tests and as laboratory-based tests, EIA methods for diagnosis of *C. trachomatis* are no longer recommended because of their poor sensitivity in comparison to NAATs. NAATs, which can detect small amounts of chlamydial DNA, are highly sensitive and specific for detecting infection in urogenital and anal specimens, as well as in urine. Use of self-collected vaginal or anal specimens or first-void urine samples offers greater patient acceptability, particularly when used to screen asymptomatic individuals. A further advantage of tests that can screen urine for the presence of infection is that up to 30% of women are reported to have urethral infection only, which would be missed using a test on endocervical samples. Because of their ability to detect as little as a single gene copy in a specimen, nucleic acid residues that persist following successful antibiotic therapy of a chlamydial infection can result in a false-positive test for several weeks following eradication of the organism.[39,40]

TREATMENT

A number of antimicrobials, including tetracyclines, macrolides, azithromycin, and some fluoroquinolones, display good in vitro and in vivo activity against *C. trachomatis*. In most clinical trials, cure rates exceeding 90% are reported for these agents. All these antimicrobials also appear to have good efficacy against *Ureaplasma urealyticum*, the second most common cause of NGU.[37-40]

Azithromycin 1 g orally as a single dose and doxycycline 100 mg orally twice daily for 7 days are the regimens of choice for the treatment of uncomplicated chlamydial infections[1] (Table 117-8). Because of its prolonged serum and tissue half-life, azithromycin is the only single-dose therapy that is effective in treating *C. trachomatis*. Delayed-release doxycycline (Doryx) given as 200 mg orally once daily for 7 days may be considered as an alternative regimen for the treatment of urogenital *C. trachomatis* infection. In a double-blind, randomized, controlled trial it was as effective as generic doxycycline and was associated with a lower frequency of gastrointestinal side effects, but this regimen is more costly.[47] Of the fluoroquinolones, ofloxacin and levofloxacin are included in the CDC recommendations, but neither appears to offer an advantage over other first-line nor alternative therapies. Although ciprofloxacin and some other fluoroquinolones have activity against *C. trachomatis* and *U. urealyticum*, high dosages have not consistently eradicated chlamydial infections.[1,37-43]

For pregnant women with chlamydial urogenital infections, treatment can reduce the risk of pregnancy complications and transmission to the newborn significantly. Because the use of tetracyclines and fluoroquinolones is contraindicated during pregnancy, azithromycin is the recommended drug treatment (see Table 117-8).

TABLE 117-8 Treatment of *Chlamydial* Infections

Infection	Recommended Regimens[a]	Alternative Regimen
Uncomplicated urethral, endocervical, or rectal infection in adults	Azithromycin 1 g orally once, or doxycycline 100 mg orally twice daily for 7 days	Erythromycin base 500 mg orally four times daily for 7 days, or erythromycin ethylsuccinate 800 mg orally four times daily for 7 days, or levofloxacin 500 mg orally once daily for 7 days, or ofloxacin 300 mg orally twice daily for 7 days
Urogenital infections during pregnancy	Azithromycin 1 g orally as a single dose or amoxicillin 500 mg orally three times daily for 7 days	Amoxicillin 500 mg orally three times daily for 7 days, or erythromycin base 500 mg orally four times daily for 7 days, or erythromycin base 250 mg orally four times daily for 14 days, or erythromycin ethylsuccinate 800 mg orally four times daily for 7 days, or erythromycin ethylsuccinate 400 mg orally four times daily for 14 days
Conjunctivitis of the newborn or pneumonia in infants	Erythromycin base or ethylsuccinate 50 mg/kg/day orally in four divided doses for 14 days[b,c]	Azithromycin suspension 20 mg/kg/day orally once daily for 3 days[c]

CDC, Centers for Disease Control and Prevention; IHPS, infantile hypertrophic pyloric stenosis.

[a]Recommendations are those of the CDC.

[b]Topical therapy alone is inadequate for ophthalmia neonatorum and is unnecessary when systemic therapy is administered. Effectiveness of erythromycin treatment is approximately 80%; therefore, a second course of therapy may be required.

[c]An association between oral erythromycin and azithromycin and IHPS has been reported in infants aged <6 weeks. Infants treated with either of these antimicrobials should be followed for signs and symptoms of IHPS.

When compliance with a multiday regimen is a concern, azithromycin is the preferred treatment in women, regardless of pregnancy status. Additionally, adherence can be maximized by providing onsite, directly observed single-dose therapy with azithromycin. It is recommended that test-of-cure be obtained for pregnant patients treated for chlamydial infections to ensure eradication of the infection. Persons treated for chlamydia should abstain from sexual intercourse for 7 days after single-dose therapy or until completion of a 7-day regimen and resolution of symptoms if present.[1,40-43,48,49]

C. trachomatis transmission during perinatal exposure can result in infections of the eye, oropharynx, lungs, urogenital tract, and rectum of the neonate or infant. Despite its efficacy in preventing gonococcal ophthalmia, topical erythromycin ointment (0.5%) appears less effective in preventing chlamydial ophthalmia. Additionally, topical therapy has no effect on nasal carriage or colonization of other parts of the infant's body, so the potential for other infections, including pneumonia, remains. Because of the high percentage of treatment failures, topical therapy is not recommended to treat ophthalmia caused by *C. trachomatis*. Instead, an oral erythromycin regimen is recommended.[1,37-40]

Evaluation of Therapeutic Outcomes

Treatment of chlamydial infections with the recommended regimens is highly effective; therefore, posttreatment laboratory testing is not recommended routinely unless symptoms persist or there are other specific concerns (eg, pregnancy). Posttreatment tests should not be performed for at least 3 weeks following completion of therapy.[1] When posttreatment tests are positive, they usually represent noncompliance, failure to treat sexual partners, or laboratory error rather than inadequate therapy or resistance to therapy. Infants with pneumonitis should receive follow-up testing because erythromycin is only 80% effective, and a second course of therapy can be necessary.[1,37-40]

GENITAL HERPES

Epidemiology and Etiology

Genital herpes infections represent the most common cause of genital ulceration seen in the United States. More than 50 million Americans have genital herpes, and this number is increasing by at least 500,000 each year.[1,50-55] Because of its morbidity, recurrent nature, and potential for complications, as well as its ability to be transmitted asymptomatically, genital herpes is of major public health importance.[52-61] Of note, the CDC does not recommend screening for HSV in the general population.[1] Similar to syphilis and other STDs, the presence of genital herpes lesions is associated with an increased risk of acquiring HIV following exposure.[1,50-56]

Pathophysiology

Herpes comes from the Greek word meaning "to creep" and is used to describe two distinct but antigenically related serotypes of HSV. HSV-1 is associated most commonly with oropharyngeal disease, and HSV-2 is associated most closely with genital disease; however, each virus is capable of causing clinically indistinguishable infections in both anatomic areas.[50-52,55]

Humans are the sole known reservoir for HSV. Infection is transmitted via inoculation of virus from infected secretions onto mucosal surfaces (eg, urethra, oropharynx, cervix, and conjunctivae) or through abraded skin. Evidence that the virus survives for a limited time on environmental surfaces suggests the possibility of fomitic transfer as a nonvenereal route of transmission.[50-52,55]

The cycle of HSV infection occurs in five stages: primary mucocutaneous infection, infection of the ganglia, establishment of latency, reactivation, and recurrent infection. After viral inoculation, HSV infection is associated with cytoplasmic granulation, ballooning degeneration of cells, and production of mononucleated giant cells. Initially, the cellular response is predominantly PMN, followed by a lymphocytic response. Replication occurs with viral spread to contiguous cells and peripheral sensory nerves. Latency then is established in sensory or autonomic nerve root ganglia. Latency appears to be lifelong, interrupted only by reactivation of the viral infection. It is unclear what factors are important in maintaining latency, but immune responses and emotional and physical stresses appear important in reactivating latent virus.[50-52,55]

Clinical Presentation

The signs and symptoms of genital herpes infection are influenced by many factors, including previous exposure to HSV, viral type, and host factors such as age and site of infection. Because a high percentage of initial and recurrent infections are asymptomatic, and because viral shedding can occur in the absence of apparent lesions or symptoms, identification and education of individuals with genital herpes are essential in controlling its transmission.[50-59] A summary of the clinical presentation of genital herpes is provided in Table 117-9.

TABLE 117-9 Presentation of Genital Herpes Infections

General	Incubation period 2-14 days (mean, 4 days) Can be caused by either HSV-1 or HSV-2
Classification of infection	
First-episode primary	Initial genital infection in individuals lacking antibody to either HSV-1 or HSV-2
First-episode nonprimary	Initial genital infection in individuals with clinical or serologic evidence of prior HSV (usually HSV-1) infection
Recurrent	Appearance of genital lesions at some time following healing of first-episode infection
Signs and symptoms	
First-episode infections	Most primary infections are asymptomatic or minimally symptomatic Multiple painful pustular or ulcerative lesions on external genitalia developing over a period of 7-10 days; lesions heal in 2-4 weeks (mean, 21 days) Flulike symptoms (eg, fever, headache, malaise) during first few days after appearance of lesions Others—local itching, pain, or discomfort; vaginal or urethral discharge, tender inguinal adenopathy, paresthesias, urinary retention Severity of symptoms greater in females than in males Symptoms are less severe (eg, fewer lesions, more rapid lesion healing, fewer or milder systemic symptoms) with nonprimary infections Symptoms more severe and prolonged in the immunocompromised On average viral shedding lasts approximately 11-12 days for primary infections and 7 days for nonprimary infections
Recurrent	Prodrome seen in approximately 50% of patients prior to appearance of recurrent lesions; mild burning, itching, or tingling are typical prodromal symptoms Compared to primary infections, recurrent infections associated with (1) fewer lesions that are more localized, (2) shorter duration of active infection (lesions heal within 7 days), and (3) milder symptoms Severity of symptoms greater in females than in males Symptoms more severe and prolonged in the immunocompromised On average viral shedding lasts approximately 4 days Asymptomatic viral shedding is more frequent during the first year after infection with HSV
Therapeutic implications of HSV-1 versus HSV-2 genital infection	Primary infections caused by HSV-1 and HSV-2 virtually indistinguishable Recurrent infections and subclinical viral shedding are less frequent with HSV-1 Recurrent infections with HSV-2 tend to be more severe
Complications	Secondary infection of lesions; extragenital infection because of autoinoculation; disseminated infection (primarily in immunocompromised patients); meningitis or encephalitis; neonatal transmission

HSV-1, herpes simplex virus type 1; HSV-2, herpes simplex virus type 2.

Complications

Complications from genital herpes infections result from both genital spread and autoinoculation of the virus and occur most commonly with primary first episodes. Lesions at extragenital sites, such as the eye, rectum, pharynx, and fingers, are not uncommon. CNS involvement is seen occasionally and can take several forms, including an aseptic meningitis, transverse myelitis, or sacral radiculopathy syndrome.[50-59]

A major concern is the effect of genital herpes on neonates exposed during pregnancy. Neonatal herpes is associated with a high mortality and significant morbidity. It is transmitted to the newborn primarily through exposure to HSV in the birth canal but, in rare cases, also is transmitted transplacentally. The risk of transmission during birth appears much greater for first-episode primary infections than for recurrent infections. Neonatal herpes infection has a case-fatality rate of approximately 50%, with a large proportion of surviving infants experiencing significant morbidity, including permanent neurologic damage.[50,51,55]

Diagnosis

Confirmation of a genital herpes infection can be made only with laboratory testing. Tissue culture is the most specific (100%) and sensitive method (80%-90%) of confirming the diagnosis of first-episode genital herpes; however, culture is relatively insensitive in detecting HSV in ulcers in the latter stages of healing and in recurrent infections, as a result, in part, of reduced viral load. Viral culture is expensive and time-consuming, and improper collection or transport of specimens can result in false-negative results. In most situations, HSV isolation on tissue culture takes 48 to 96 hours. Following isolation, it is recommended that typing of the virus be performed because of prognostic implications. HSV-1 is associated with a lower rate of asymptomatic and symptomatic recurrence, while HSV-2 is characterized by more frequent recurrences and subclinical shedding. In instances in which rapid detection is necessary, such as an impending birth, other detection methods can be more useful. Amplified culture techniques that combine cell culture for 24 hours and subsequent staining for HSV antigen have sensitivities and specificities only slightly less than those of culture.[50-55,60-62]

Several serologic tests capable of distinguishing HSV-1 and HSV-2 antibodies are available. These tests detect antibodies to type-specific HSV-1 and HSV-2 proteins gG-1 and gG-2, respectively. Although antibody formation begins immediately following a primary herpes infection, complete seroconversion (ie, complete antibody development) can take several months. Until the full expression of all antigenic determinants of HSV-1 and HSV-2 occurs, these tests are not useful in differentiating HSV-1 and HSV-2 infection. Older antibody detection tests, some of which are still marketed, are unable to distinguish between HSV-1 and HSV-2 owing to the considerable cross-reactivity between the two serotypes. Given the high prevalence of HSV-1 antibody in the adult population, accurate interpretation of positive results is not possible.[50-55,60-62]

PCR assays that detect HSV DNA and differentiate HSV-1 and HSV-2 infections are more sensitive than culture and are considered the diagnostic test of choice for suspected CNS infections (ie, HSV encephalitis and HSV meningitis). PCR assays are highly sensitive in detecting asymptomatic viral shedding.[50-55,60-62]

Although the diagnosis of genital herpes can be confirmed only by laboratory tests, less stringent diagnostic criteria (eg, characteristic physical findings or clinical history) frequently are used in clinical practice. A presumptive diagnosis of genital herpes commonly is made based on the presence of dark-field-negative, vesicular, or ulcerative genital lesions. A history of similar lesions or recent sexual contact with an individual with similar lesions also is useful in making the diagnosis. Other STDs, including chancroid, lymphogranuloma venereum, and granuloma inguinale, and causes such as trauma, allergic reactions, and bacterial or fungal infections are considered in the differential diagnosis.[50-55,60-62]

TREATMENT

The most achievable goals in the management of genital herpes are to relieve symptoms and to shorten the clinical course, to prevent complications and recurrences, and to decrease disease transmission. Although research has focused primarily on the treatment of active infection and suppression of recurrences, increasing emphasis is being placed on various approaches, including immunotherapy that might provide protection from disease transmission or possibly eliminate established latency.[54-55]

Palliative and supportive measures are the cornerstone of therapy for patients with genital herpes. Pain and discomfort usually respond to warm saline baths or the use of analgesics, antipyretics, or antipruritics; good genital hygiene can prevent the development of bacterial superinfection.

4 Specific chemotherapeutic approaches to treating genital herpes include antiviral compounds, topical surfactants, photodynamic dyes, immune modulators, vaccines, and interferons. Few of these have undergone extensive evaluation, however, and only the antiviral agents have demonstrated any consistent clinical efficacy. The most recent CDC recommendations for the treatment of genital herpes include the antiviral agents acyclovir, valacyclovir, and famciclovir (Table 117-10).[1] The overall efficacy of these agents in treating genital HSV infection appears comparable, although patient compliance can be improved with regimens requiring less frequent dosing.[1,50,51]

First-Episode Infections

Oral formulations of acyclovir, famciclovir, and valacyclovir have demonstrated efficacy in reducing viral shedding, duration of symptoms, and time to healing of first-episode genital herpes infections, with maximal benefits seen when therapy is initiated at the earliest stages of infection. Table 117-10 lists the recommended acyclovir, famciclovir, and valacyclovir oral regimens for first-episode infections. The CDC recommends that all patients with first episodes of genital herpes receive systemic antiviral therapy to prevent severe or prolonged symptoms associated with newly acquired genital herpes. Additionally, topical antiviral therapy offers minimal clinical benefit and is not recommended.[1] In immunocompromised patients or those with severe symptoms or complications necessitating hospitalization, parenteral acyclovir can be beneficial; however, the IV regimen has been associated with renal, GI, bone marrow, and CNS toxicity, particularly in patients with renal dysfunction receiving high doses. No antiviral regimen is known to prevent latency or alter the subsequent frequency and severity of recurrences in humans.[1,50-55,58,59,63-66]

Recurrent Infections

There are two approaches to management of recurrent episodes: episodic or chronic suppressive therapy. Episodic therapy is initiated early during the course of the recurrence, preferably within 6 to 12 hours of the onset of prodromal symptoms but no more than 24 hours after the appearance of lesions. Patients should be instructed to initiate treatment immediately when symptoms begin. In most patients, appreciable effects on symptomatology are not seen. Patients with prolonged episodes of recurrent infection or severe symptomatology are most likely to benefit from episodic therapy. Table 117-10 lists the recommended acyclovir, famciclovir, and valacyclovir suppressive regimens. One concern with episodic therapy is that some patients continue to shed virus despite the

TABLE 117-10 Treatment of Genital Herpes

Type of Infection	Recommended Regimens[a,b]	Alternative Regimen
First clinical episode of genital herpes[c]	Acyclovir 400 mg orally three times daily for 7-10 days,[d] *or* Acyclovir 200 mg orally five times daily for 7-10 days,[d] *or* Famciclovir 250 mg orally three times daily for 7-10 days,[d] *or* Valacyclovir 1 g orally twice daily for 7-10 days[d]	Acyclovir 5-10 mg/kg IV every 8 hours for 2-7 days or until clinical improvement occurs, followed by oral therapy to complete at least 10 days of total therapy[e]
Recurrent infection		
Episodic therapy	Acyclovir 400 mg orally three times daily for 5 days,[f] *or* Acyclovir 800 mg orally twice daily for 5 days,[f] *or* Acyclovir 800 mg orally three times daily for 2 days,[f] *or* Famciclovir 125 mg orally twice daily for 5 days,[f] *or* Famciclovir 1 g orally twice daily for 1 day,[f] *or* Famciclovir 500 mg orally once, followed by 250 mg orally twice daily for 2 days,[f] *or* Valacyclovir 500 mg orally twice daily for 3 days,[f] *or* Valacyclovir 1 g orally once daily for 5 days[f]	
Suppressive therapy	Acyclovir 400 mg orally twice daily, *or* Famciclovir 250 mg orally twice daily[h], *or* Valacyclovir 500 mg or 1,000 mg orally once daily[i]	

CDC, Centers for Disease Control and Prevention; HIV, human immunodeficiency virus; IV, intravenous.

[a]Recommendations are those of the CDC.

[b]HIV-infected patients can require more aggressive therapy.

[c]Primary or nonprimary first episode.

[d]Treatment duration can be extended if healing is incomplete after 10 days.

[e]Only for patients with severe symptoms or complications that necessitate hospitalization. HSV encephalitis requires 21 days of IV therapy.

[f]Requires initiation of therapy within 24 hours of lesion onset or during the prodrome that precedes some outbreaks.

[g]Consider discontinuation of treatment after one year to assess frequency of recurrence.

[h]Famcicolvir appears less effective for suppression of viral shedding.

[i]Valacyclovir 500 mg appears less effective than other valacyclovir and acyclovir regimens in patients with 10 or more recurrences per year.

absence of lesions or presence of prodromal symptoms. Because of the relative mildness and brevity of recurrent infections, parenteral administration of acyclovir usually is not justifiable.[1,50-55,58,59,63-66]

Suppressive therapy with recommended antivirals reduces the frequency and severity of recurrences in 70% to 80% of patients experiencing frequent recurrences. Furthermore, many patients with frequent recurrences experience an improved quality of life with suppressive therapy as compared to episodic therapy.[1,67] Asymptomatic viral shedding is markedly reduced in patients receiving suppressive therapy; however, the extent to which this decreases disease transmission to sexual partners remains to be determined. Despite antiviral suppressive therapy, low-level virus shedding still occurs. However, this virus shedding may be less than that seen in patients treated episodically for recurrences, and thus may be associated with a lower risk of disease transmission. Although antiviral therapy with acyclovir, famciclovir, or valacyclovir appears equally effective for episodic treatment, famciclovir appears somewhat less effective for suppression of viral shedding.[1,68] Because the frequency of recurrences tends to diminish over time, periodic "drug holidays" are advocated to assess changes in the underlying recurrence rate and determine if continued suppressive therapy is warranted.[1,50-55,58,59,63-66]

Resistant HSV isolates have been identified in some patients experiencing breakthrough recurrences while taking acyclovir. Strains resistant to acyclovir are also resistant to valacycylovir, and most are also resistant to famciclovir. Although there is concern about the development of resistant strains with suppressive therapy, clinical trials have found no evidence of cumulative toxicity or significant resistance in patients treated continuously with the recommended antivirals.[50-55]

Selected Populations

Immunocompromised patients are at greatest risk for severe and recurrent HSV infections. Acyclovir, valacyclovir, and famciclovir have been used to prevent reactivation of infection in patients seropositive for HSV who undergo transplantation procedures or induction chemotherapy for acute leukemia. Immunocompromised individuals, such as patients with acquired immunodeficiency syndrome (AIDS), who fail treatment or prophylaxis with recommended antiviral doses frequently demonstrate improved response with higher doses. If resistance is suspected or confirmed with recommended first-line antivirals, foscarnet is usually effective. However, its use is associated with a greater risk of serious adverse effects. Intravenous cidofovir or topical imiquimod may be effective alternatives to forscarnet. Lesional application of an extemporaneous compounded cidofovir (1%) gel or trifluridine ophthalmic solution appears to offer some benefits also.[1,50-55]

The safety of acyclovir, famciclovir, and valacyclovir during pregnancy is not established, although considerable experience with acyclovir in pregnant patients has produced no evidence of teratogenic effects. Because of the high maternal and infant morbidity associated with first-episode primary genital infections or severe recurrent infections at or near term, many clinicians advocate the use of systemic acyclovir as the standard of care in such cases; however, the effectiveness of such therapy is unknown. The use of acyclovir to suppress recurrent episodes near term is more controversial primarily because of the lack of data demonstrating significant benefits in this situation.[1,50-55,69-72]

With the increasing prevalence of genital herpes worldwide, the potential exists for widespread use and misuse of acyclovir, valacyclovir, and famciclovir, resulting in development of resistant HSV isolates. In vitro resistance to these three agents usually is mediated by alterations in viral thymidine kinase; most resistant isolates are either thymidine kinase-deficient or have altered thymidine kinase. The incidence and clinical implications of HSV resistance require further study particularly with respect to immunocompromised hosts, in whom resistance can develop with greater frequency and be of greater clinical importance. Importantly, a study in hematopoietic stem-cell transplant recipients found that persons receiving daily suppressive antiviral therapy were less likely to develop acyclovir-resistance as compared with those receiving episodic therapy.[73] Unlike acyclovir, valacyclovir, and famciclovir, foscarnet does not require the presence of thymidine kinase to be effective.[50-55]

Numerous agents for the prophylaxis and treatment of genital herpes infections are being studied. Neither topical nor systemic interferons have demonstrated consistent beneficial effects in genital HSV infections; however, a reduction in pain and time of healing of lesions has been reported with an interferon preparation incorporated into a gel containing nonoxynol-9. Other treatments under investigation include cidofovir and immune modulators such as topical imiquimod and resiquimod.[50-55] Agents that can eliminate ganglionic latency and prevent recurrent HSV infections are not expected to be available in the near future. Development of vaccines capable of protecting against HSV infection has proved challenging given the relative lack of protection offered by humoral and cell-mediated immunity in preventing naturally occurring recurrent infections. Safety concerns with live attenuated virus vaccines resulted in research focused primarily on recombinant protein vaccines that have exhibited relatively poor immunogenicity. Use of heterologous vaccines (bacillus Calmette–Guérin and influenza vaccines) to stimulate the immune system in patients with recurrent genital herpes has proved of no significant benefit.[50-55,74]

Evaluation of Therapeutic Outcomes

Available antiviral compounds are of greatest benefit in patients experiencing first-episode primary infections, immunocompromised patients, and patients with frequent or severe recurrent infections. Antivirals, however, are palliative and not curative, and patients receiving these agents should be monitored closely for adverse drug effects. CDC guidelines suggest that discontinuation of suppressive therapy after 1 year should be considered to assess for possible changes in the patient's intrinsic pattern of recurrence. In many patients, decreases in recurrence rates and the severity of symptoms occur over time. However, some clinicians prefer to continue suppressive therapy indefinitely because it significantly reduces asymptomatic viral shedding, a potential benefit in reducing the risk of disease transmission to uninfected sexual partners.[1,50-55]

TRICHOMONIASIS

Epidemiology and Etiology

Trichomonas vaginalis, a flagellated, motile protozoan is responsible for 3 to 5 million cases of trichomoniasis annually in the United States. Humans are host to two other *Trichomonas* species, *T. tenax* and *T. hominis*, but *T. vaginalis* is the only species thought to be pathogenic. Although infection by nonsexual contact is reported, it is rare. Contamination of inanimate objects and spread of infection via communal bathing or contact with infected bath or toilet articles is possible because *T. vaginalis* can survive for up to 45 minutes on moist surfaces. Neonatal infections also represent another possible nonvenereal route of disease transmission.[75-79]

Coinfection with other STDs is not unusual in patients diagnosed with trichomoniasis. Women infected with *T. vaginalis* are three times more likely to have gonorrhea than those who do not have trichomoniasis; approximately 20% of men with gonococcal urethritis also have trichomoniasis.[65-69] In patients treated appropriately for genital *C. trachomatis* or *U. urealyticum* infection, persistent urethritis can result from coexisting trichomonal infection. Although not well documented, the inflammatory response produced by trichomoniasis may increase the risk of acquiring HIV by two- to threefold.[1,75-81]

Pathophysiology

Trichomonads typically can be isolated from the vagina, urethra, and paraurethral ducts and glands in the majority of infected women. Infrequently, they are recovered from the endocervix. Extragenital sites are epidemiologically important because infection can persist and result in reinfection of the vagina if local therapy alone is used. This may account for the higher relapse rates reported for local versus systemic therapy. After attachment to the vaginal or urethral mucosa, trichomonads usually elicit an inflammatory response that manifests as a discharge containing large numbers of PMN leukocytes.[75-80,82-85]

Clinical Presentation

Trichomonal infections are reported more commonly in women than in men. In part this might be because of the smaller number of organisms found in the male urethra making detection more difficult, greater disease transmission rates from males to females, and the nature of male infections, which have a high spontaneous cure rate even in the absence of treatment.[76,77,80,82,82,86] The typical clinical presentation of trichomoniasis in males and females is presented in Table 117-11.

Diagnosis

T. vaginalis produces nonspecific symptoms also consistent with bacterial vaginosis; as a result, laboratory diagnosis is required. Because *T. vaginalis* requires a pH range of 4.9 to 7.5 for survival, a vaginal discharge pH of greater than 5 usually indicates the presence of either *T. vaginalis* or *Gardnerella vaginalis*, a common cause of bacterial vaginosis. The simplest and most reliable means of diagnosis is a wet-mount examination of the vaginal discharge.[77,80,82,83,86] Trichomoniasis is confirmed if characteristic pear-shaped, flagellating

TABLE 117-11 Presentation of Trichomonas Infections

	Males	Females
General	Incubation period 3-28 days Organism can be detectable within 48 hours after exposure to infected partner	Incubation period 3-28 days
Site of infection	Most common: urethra Others: rectum (usually caused by rectal intercourse in MSM), oropharynx, eye	Most common: endocervical canal Others: urethra, rectum (usually caused by perineal contamination), oropharynx, eye
Symptoms	Can be asymptomatic (more common in males than females) or minimally symptomatic Urethral discharge (clear to mucopurulent) Dysuria, pruritus	Can be asymptomatic or minimally symptomatic Scant to copious, typically malodorous vaginal discharge (50%-75%) and pruritus (worse during menses) Dysuria, dyspareunia
Signs	Urethral discharge	Vaginal discharge Vaginal pH 4.5-6 Inflammation/erythema of vulva, vagina, and/or cervix Urethritis
Complications	Epididymitis and chronic prostatitis (uncommon) Male infertility (decreased sperm motility and viability)	Pelvic inflammatory disease and associated complications (ie, ectopic pregnancy, infertility) Premature labor, premature rupture of membranes, and low–birth-weight infants (risk of neonatal infections is low) Cervical neoplasia

MSM, men who have sex with men.

organisms are observed. The wet mount is only 51% to 65% sensitive in detecting the presence of trichomonads, with lower sensitivities reported in men and in women with low-grade, subacute, or chronic infections.[78-80,83,85,87]

Although the presence of trichomonads may be reported on a Papanicolaou smear (Pap), the sensitivity of this cytologic technique is less than for wet mount and also is associated with a high number of false-positive and false-negative results. Stained smears of cervical specimens have been used in diagnosis, but they are less sensitive and more time-consuming than the wet mount and therefore are not recommended. Culture techniques for trichomonads are highly specific up to 100% and more sensitive, 75% to 96% than the wet mount, but they are not useful in rapid diagnosis because up to 48 hours or longer is necessary for growth. Cultures can be necessary, however, to confirm the diagnosis in the absence of a positive wet mount or to determine antimicrobial susceptibility in intractable cases.[1,75-80,82,83,85,86,88]

Newer diagnostic tests such as monoclonal antibody or DNA probe techniques, as well as PCR tests that can detect small amounts of trichomonal DNA, have been developed. These office-based tests are highly sensitive and specific for detecting infection in both vaginal specimens and urine. The CDC now recommends the use of these highly sensitive and specific tests for detecting *T. vaginalis*.[1,75-79]

In males, demonstration of trichomonads in urethral specimens or urine sediment by wet mount is difficult, and diagnosis depends largely on culture. Specimens from males should be taken prior to first voiding because the small number of trichomonads in males may be reduced by micturition.[75-80,82]

TABLE 117-12 Treatment of Trichomoniasis

Type	Recommended Regimen[a]	Alternative Regimen
Symptomatic and asymptomatic infections	Metronidazole 2 g orally in a single dose or Tinidazole 2 g orally in a single dose[b]	Metronidazole 500 mg orally two times daily for 7 days[c,d]
Persistent or recurrent infections	Metronidazole 500 mg orally two times daily for 7 days[c]	Metronidazole 2 g orally for 7 days[e] or Tinidazole 2 g orally for 7 days[e]
Treatment in pregnancy	Metronidazole 2 g orally in a single dose[e]	

CDC, Centers for Disease Control and Prevention; HIV, human immunodeficiency virus.

[a]Recommendations are those of the CDC.

[b]Randomized controlled trials comparing single 2 g doses of metronidazole and tinidazole suggest that tinidazole is equivalent to, or superior to, metronidazole in achieving parasitologic cure and resolution of symptoms.

[c]Metronidazole labeling approved by the FDA does not include this regimen. Dosage regimens for treatment of trichomoniasis included in the product labeling are the single 2 g dose; 250 mg three times daily for 7 days; and 375 mg twice daily for 7 days. The 250 mg and 375 mg dosage regimens are currently not included in the CDC recommendations.

[d]Recommended treatment regimen for women with HIV coinfection.

[e]For treatment failures with metronidazole 2 g as a single dose and metronidazole 500 mg orally two times daily for 7 days.

[f]Symptomatic pregnant women can be treated with this regimen at any stage of pregnancy.

TREATMENT

Recommended and alternative treatment regimens for *T. vaginalis* include either metronidazole or tinidazole, both of which produce high cure rates in these infections. In only a few cases have *T. vaginalis* isolates been resistant to standard metronidazole or tinidazole doses. In these instances, longer courses of therapy or doses higher than those recommended routinely as initial therapy usually produce a cure.[1,75-79,83,86,89]

Table 117-12 provides treatment recommendations for trichomonas infections.[1] The standard therapy for trichomoniasis is either metronidazole or tinidazole 2 g orally as a single dose; cure rates are comparable with the recommended alternative regimen of metronidazole 500 mg twice daily for 7 days. When sexual partners are treated simultaneously, cure rates greater than 95% are reported. If sexual partners are not treated concurrently, cure rates are somewhat lower. In limited clinical testing, single metronidazole doses of less than 1.5 g are associated with high failure rates.[1,75-79,83,86,89]

Advantages of single-dose therapy over the multidose alternative regimen include better patient compliance, lower total dose, lower cost, and shorter exposure of the patient's GI and urogenital anaerobic bacterial flora to the drug. As a result of the latter, the likelihood of developing pseudomembranous colitis or symptomatic candidal vulvovaginitis is decreased.[75-79,83] Because high doses of metronidazole have mutagenic effects in bacteria and oncogenic effects in mice, a reduced time of exposure in humans can be beneficial. There is no conclusive evidence for either of these effects in humans after short-term therapy with recommended doses. GI complaints (eg, anorexia, nausea, vomiting, and diarrhea) are more common with the single 2-g dose of either metronidazole or tinidazole, occurring in 5% to 10% of treated patients. Some patients also complain of a bitter metallic taste in the mouth with metronidazole. Patients intolerant of the single 2-g dose because of GI adverse effects usually tolerate the alternative metronidazole multidose regimen.[75-79,83,86,89]

5 To achieve maximal cure rates and prevent relapse with either metronidazole or tinidazole as a single 2-g dose, simultaneous treatment of infected sexual partners is necessary. Tinidazole is at least equivalent, or potentially superior, to metronidazole in achieving microbiologic and clinical cure.[90] In women treated with the alternative 7-day course, however, relapse rates are not appreciably different regardless of whether or not sexual partners are treated. It is speculated that in men, spontaneous resolution of trichomonal infection or a reduction in the number of trichomonads below the inoculum necessary to transmit disease may occur during the 7 days of a female's therapy. The 7-day metronidazole treatment regimen is also recommended in women coinfected with HIV and may be more effective than a single 2-g dose in these patients.[91] In patients who fail to respond to an initial course of metronidazole therapy, a second course of therapy with metronidazole 500 mg twice daily for 7 days or a single 2-g dose of tinidazole is recommended. Patients refractory to a second course of treatment usually respond to a regimen using higher 2 g daily for 7 days of either agent. Good response rates also are reported for tinidazole 2 to 3 g orally plus intravaginal tinidazole for 14 days.[1,70,75-79,82,89,92] Topical vaginal therapy alone is associated with low cure rates because infections involving the urethra or periurethral glands are unaffected and can serve as the source of reinfection.[77] Use of IV metronidazole can be warranted for rare cases of intolerance to oral medication or infections resistant to high-dose oral metronidazole. Sexual partners of all patients who require retreatment also should be treated or retreated because the majority of apparent treatment failures appear to be caused by reinfection or noncompliance.[75-79]

Concerns regarding the use of metronidazole in women who are pregnant or breast-feeding have been raised. Because metronidazole is secreted in breast milk, it is recommended that breast-feeding be interrupted for 12 to 24 hours after maternal ingestion of a single 2-g dose. Metronidazole (pregnancy category B) and tinidazole (pregnancy category C) are contraindicated during the first trimester of pregnancy based on FDA-approved labeling. Although some experts recommend avoiding use of either agent throughout pregnancy, others advocate the use of metronidazole during any stage of pregnancy because of the potential adverse pregnancy outcomes associated with trichomoniasis. The CDC now recommends that all symptomatic pregnant women, regardless of pregnancy stage, be tested and considered for treatment with metronidazole 2 g orally in a single dose.[1,75-79]

Several other nitroimidazole antibiotics related to metronidazole and tinidazole (eg, nimorazole, ornidazole, and carnidazole) are being investigated worldwide for the treatment of trichomoniasis. Unfortunately, none of these agents differs significantly from metronidazole or tinidazole in terms of efficacy (ie, cross-resistance is high) or toxicity against metronidazole-susceptible strains of *T. vaginalis*.[75-79]

EVALUATION OF THERAPEUTIC OUTCOMES

Follow-up was previously considered unnecessary in patients who become asymptomatic after treatment with recommended therapy; however, retesting is now recommended for all sexually active women within 3 months following initial treatment due to the high rates or reinfection. When patients remain symptomatic, it is important to determine if reinfection has occurred. In these cases, a repeat course of therapy, as well as identification and treatment or retreatment of infected sexual partners, is recommended. In situations in which reinfection can be excluded, a relative resistance to metronidazole or tinidazole should be assumed, and an alternative regimen should be prescribed. Culture and sensitivity are warranted for infections unresponsive to alternative regimens.

HUMAN PAPILLOMAVIRUS AND OTHER SEXUALLY TRANSMITTED DISEASES

Several STDs other than those just discussed occur with varying frequency in the United States and throughout the world. Although an in-depth discussion of these diseases is beyond the scope of this chapter, Table 117-13 lists recommended treatment regimens.[1] Of notable importance among these other STDs, however, is genital HPV infection, the most common viral STD in the United States. More than 100 HPV types have been characterized by genomic makeup, with approximately 30 types associated with genital tract lesions.[94-96] Of these, types 6 and 11 are associated most commonly with the

TABLE 117-13 Treatment Regimens for Miscellaneous Sexually Transmitted Diseases

Infection	Recommended Regimen[a]	Alternative Regimen
Chancroid (*Haemophilus ducreyi*)	Azithromycin 1 g orally in a single dose, *or* Ceftriaxone 250 mg IM in a single dose, *or* Ciprofloxacin 500 mg orally twice daily for 3 days,[b] *or* Erythromycin base 500 mg orally four times daily for 7 days	
Lymphogranuloma venereum	Doxycycline 100 mg orally twice daily for 21 days[c]	Erythromycin base 500 mg orally four times daily for 21 days[d]
HPV infection		
External genital/perianal warts	*Provider-Administered Therapies:* Cryotherapy (eg, liquid nitrogen or cryoprobe); repeat weekly as necessary, *or* Podophyllin resin 10%-25% in compound tincture of benzoin applied to lesions; repeat weekly as necessary,[e,f] *or* TCA 80%-90% *or* BCA 80%-90% applied to warts; repeat weekly as necessary, *or* Surgical removal (tangential scissor excision, tangential shave excision, curettage, or electrosurgery) *Patient-Applied Therapies:* Podofilox 0.5% solution or gel applied twice daily for 3 days, followed by 4 days of no therapy; cycle is repeated as necessary for up to four cycles,[f] *or* Imiquimod 3.75% or 5% cream applied at bedtime three times weekly for up to 16 weeks,[f] *or* Sinecatechins 15% ointment applied three times daily for up to 16 weeks	Intralesional interferon *or* Photodynamic therapy *or* Topical cidofovir
Vaginal and anal warts	Cryotherapy with liquid nitrogen, or TCA or BCA 80%-90% as for external HPV warts; repeat weekly as necessary[g] Surgical removal (not for vaginal or urethral meatus warts)	
Urethral meatus warts	Cryotherapy with liquid nitrogen, or podophyllin resin 10%-25% in compound tincture of benzoin applied at weekly intervals[f,h]	
Prevention	Gardasil® (HPV quadrivalent [types 6, 11, 16, and 18]) recombinant vaccine 0.5 mL IM on day 1; a second and third dose are administered 2 and 6 months following the first dose[i,j,k] Cervarix® (HPV bivalent [types 16 and 18]) recombinant vaccine 0.5 mL IM on day 1; a second and third dose are administered 1 and 6 months following the first dose[i,l] Gardasil9®(HPV 9-valent [types 6, 11, 16, 18, 31, 33, 45, 52, 58]) recombinant vaccine 0.5 mL IM on day 1; a second and third dose are administered 1 and 6 months following the first dose[i]	

BCA, bichloracetic acid; HPV, human papillomavirus; TCA, trichloroacetic acid.

[a]Recommendations are those of the Centers for Disease Control and Prevention (CDC).

[b]Ciprofloxacin is contraindicated for pregnant and lactating women and for persons aged <18 years.

[c]Azithromycin 1 g PO once weekly for 3 weeks can be effective.

[d]Pregnant patients should be treated with erythromycin.

[e]Some experts recommended washing podophyllin off after 1-4 hours to minimize local irritation.

[f]Safety during pregnancy is not established.

[g]Surgical removal of anal warts is also a recommended treatment.

[h]Some specialists recommend the use of podofilox and imiquimod for treating distal meatal warts.

[i]CDC recommendations: vaccination is recommended in girls 11-12 years of age, and in females aged 13-26 years who either were not previously vaccinated, or who did not complete the vaccination series.

[j]FDA approved labeling for Gardasil®: indicated in girls and women 9 through 26 years of age for the prevention of cervical, vulvar, vaginal, and anal cancer caused by HPV types 16 and 18, genital warts (condyloma acuminata) caused by HPV types 6 and 11, and precancerous or dysplastic lesions caused by HPV types 6, 11, 16, and 18.

[k]Vaccination is recommended in males aged 9-26 years to prevent genital warts and anal cancer.

[l]FDA approved labeling for Cervarix®: indicated in females 9 through 25 years of age for the prevention of cervical cancer, cervical intraepithelial neoplasia grade 2 or worse, adenocarcinoma in situ, and cervical intraepithelial neoplasia grade 1 caused by HPV types 16 and 18.

development of low-grade dysplasia manifested as exophytic genital warts. In most individuals, genital infection with HPV is subclinical, and patients with visible acuminate warts represent less than 1% of all infected individuals. When present, genital warts can be large and multifocal, producing variable degrees of discomfort. Based on HPV DNA detection methods, most warts will regress spontaneously within 1 to 2 years of their initial appearance. However, reinfection is common in young, sexually active populations.[1,93,94]

Infection with several HPV types, particularly HPV-16 and HPV-18, is considered the major risk factor for the development of cervical neoplasia, the second most common cancer in women worldwide. Although epidemiologic, virologic, and clinical data strongly support this association, HPV infection alone is insufficient to cause cervical cancer development because only a small percentage of infected women develop the disease. It appears that the interplay of host immune defenses, genetic factors, and infection with HPV types containing a more aggressive variant all contribute to the risk of developing cervical neoplasia.[93,94]

The Pap smear is the most frequently used and cost-effective diagnostic test for detecting clinical and subclinical (ie, no visible signs of condylomata) HPV in women. However, Pap smears are neither specific for HPV nor useful in detecting latent infections. Frequently, visual inspection of genital surfaces under magnification can assist in making the diagnosis. Various tests for detecting HPV DNA, RNA, or capsid protein also are available, and unlike the Pap smear do not require subjective interpretation of the results. The HPV-specific tests are only approved in women with abnormal Pap smears or women older than 30 years. However, use of HPV DNA testing as a routine screening test in lieu of Pap smears is expected in the near future. In women identified to have high-risk HPV infections by these tests, follow-up cytology would be performed.[93,94]

No consensus exists on the best approach to treating patients with genital HPV infection, particularly because most cases appear to be transient with spontaneous regression of lesions. A number of treatments are recommended (see Table 117-13), but none is clearly superior to the others. Treatment generally is directed toward patients with manifestations of genital warts, with the goal of removing or destroying these lesions and grossly infected surrounding tissue. Because such treatment neither stops viral expression in surrounding tissue nor eliminates viral latency, recurrence of lesions is not uncommon.[93,94]

Clinical **Controversy...**

Recent research has indicated that HPV (particularly HPV-16) may be implicated in the development of intractable childhood epilepsy. As such, women of child-bearing age should be educated regarding the fetal risk associated with the HPV infection in order to improve vaccination rates.

Three HPV vaccines are marketed in the United States. Cervarix, a bivalent vaccine for HPV-16 and 18, Gardasil, a quadrivalent vaccine for HPV-6, 11, 16, and 18, and Gardasil 9, a 9-valent vaccine for HPV-6, 11, 16, 18, 31, 33, 45, 52, and 58. All vaccines are indicated for preventing cervical precancers and cervical cancer in females 9 to 26 years of age. In addition, Gardasil and Gardasil 9 are indicated in unvaccinated males 9 to 21 years of age. Specific populations (MSM, immunocompromised) are recommended to receive the vaccination up to the age of 26.[1] Clinically important differences in the magnitude and duration of the immune response, as well as prevention of HPV infections and cervical cancer remain to be determined.[95-97]

ABBREVIATIONS

AIDS	acquired immunodeficiency syndrome
CDC	Centers for Disease Control and Prevention
CSF	cerebrospinal fluid
DFA-TP	direct fluorescent-antibody (test) for *T. pallidum*
DGI	disseminated gonococcal infection
EIA	enzyme immunoassay
FTA-ABS	fluorescent treponemal antibody absorption
HIV	human immunodeficiency virus
HPV	human papillomavirus
HSV	herpes simplex virus
HSV-1	herpes simplex virus type 1
LPS	lipopolysaccharide
MHA-TP	microhemagglutination assay for antibodies to *T. pallidum*
MSM	men who have sex with men
NAATs	nucleic acid amplification tests
NGU	nongonococcal urethritis
Pap	Papanicolaou smear
PCR	polymerase chain reaction
PID	pelvic inflammatory disease
PMN	polymorphonuclear
RPR	rapid plasma reagin
STD	sexually transmitted disease
TPHA	*T. pallidum* hemagglutination assay
TPPA	*T. pallidum* particle agglutination assay
TRUST	toluidine red unheated serum test
USR	unheated serum reagin
VDRL	Venereal Disease Research Laboratory

REFERENCES

1. Workowski KA, Bolan GA. Sexually transmitted diseases treatment guidelines, 2015. *MMWR Recomm Rep* 2015;64:1-135.
2. Marrazzo JM, Holmes KK. Sexually transmitted diseases: Overview and clinical approach. In: Longo DL, Fauci AS, Kasper DL, Hauser SL, Jameson JL, Loscalzo J, eds. *Harrison's Principles of Internal Medicine,* 18th ed. [electronic version]; New York, NY: McGraw-Hill, 2012. Available at: http://www.accessmedicine.com.libproxy.uthscsa.edu/content.aspx?aID=9119937.
3. Aral SO, Holmes KK. The epidemiology of STIs and their social and behavioral determinants: Industrialized and developing countries. In: Holmes KK, Sparling PF, Stamm WE, et al., eds. *Sexually Transmitted Diseases,* 4th ed. New York, NY: McGraw-Hill, 2008:53-92.
4. Sulak PJ. Sexually transmitted diseases. *Semin Reprod Med* 2003;21:399-413.
5. Satterwhite CL, Torrone E, Meites E, et al. Sexually transmitted infections among U.S. women and men: Prevalence and incidence estimates, 2008. *Sex Transm Dis* 2013;40(3):187-193.
6. Owusu-Edusei K, Chesson HW, Gift TL, et al. The estimated direct medical cost of selected sexually transmitted infections in the United States, 2008. *Sex Transm Dis* 2013;40(3):197-201.
7. Cohen MS. Approach to the patient with a sexually transmitted disease. In: Goldman L, Schafer AI, eds. *Goldman's Cecil Medicine,* 24th ed. [electronic version]; 2011. Available at: http://www.mdconsult.com.libproxy.uthscsa.edu/books/page.do?eid=4-u1.0-B978-1-4377-1604-7.00293-1&isbn=978-1-4377-1604-7&uniqId=368839637-2#4-u1.0-B978-1-4377-1604-7..00293-1–c00293.
8. Steiner MJ, Warner L, Stone KM, Cates W Jr. Condoms and other barrier methods for prevention of STD/HIV infection and pregnancy. In: Holmes KK, Sparling PF, Stamm WE, et al., eds. *Sexually Transmitted Diseases,* 4th ed. New York, NY: McGraw-Hill, 2008:1821-1829.
9. Obiero J, Mwethera PG, Wiysonge CS. Topical microbicides for prevention of sexually transmitted infections. *Cochrane Database Syst Rev* 2012;6:CD007961.
10. Food and Drug Administration, HHS. Over-the-counter vaginal contraceptive and spermicide drug products containing nonoxynol 9; required labeling. Final rule. *Fed Regist* 2007;72:71769-71785.

11. Sexually Transmitted Disease Surveillance 2013. Available at: http://www.cdc.gov/std/stats13/surv2013-print.pdf. Accessed September 27, 2015.
12. Centers for Disease Control and Prevention. Sexually Transmitted Disease Surveillance, 2010. Atlanta, GA: U.S. Department of Health and Human Services, 2011.
13. Ram S, Rice PA. Gonococcal infections. In: Longo DL, Fauci AS, Kasper DL, Hauser SL, Jameson JL, Loscalzo J, eds. *Harrison's Principles of Internal Medicine,* 18th ed. [electronic version]. 2012. Available at: http://www.accessmedicine.com.libproxy.uthscsa.edu/content.aspx?aID=9121197.
14. Marrazzo JM, Handsfield HH, Sparling PF. *Neisseria gonorrhoeae.* In: Mandell GL, Bennett JE, Dolin R, eds. *Mandell, Douglas, and Bennett's Principles and Practice of Infectious Diseases,* 7th ed. [electronic version]; MD Consult, 2010. Available at: http://www.mdconsult.com.libproxy.uthscsa.edu/book/player/book.do?method=display&type=aboutPage&decorator=header&eid=4-u1.0-B978-0-443-06839-3.X0001-X-TOP&isbn=978-0-443-06839-3&uniq=177288689.
15. Newman LM, Moran JS, Workowski KA. Update on the management of gonorrhea in adults in the United States. *Clin Infect Dis* 2007;44:S84-S101.
16. Marrazzo JM, Hofmann J. Infections due to *Neisseria.* In: Nabel EG (editor in chief), Federman DD (founding editor). *ACP Medicine* [electronic version]; 2009. Available at: http://online.statref.com.libproxy.uthscsa.edu/Document/Document.aspx?docAddress=SaoWxNG8S1byvtPckclkVw%3d%3d&offset=7&SessionId=11469E6MHHSOSKLN.
17. Centers for Disease Control and Prevention. Cephalosporin-resistant *Neisseria gonorrhoeae* public health response plan. Atlanta, GA: U.S. Department of Health and Human Services, 2012. Available at: http://www.cdc.gov/std/treatment/Ceph-R-ResponsePlanJuly30-2012.pdf.
18. Centers for Disease Control and Prevention. Update to CDC's sexually transmitted diseases treatment guidelines, 2010: Oral cephalosporins no longer a recommended treatment for gonococcal infections. *MMWR Morb Mortal Wkly Rep* 2012;61(31):590-594. Available at: http://www.cdc.gov/mmwr/preview/mmwrhtml/mm6131a3.htm?s_cid=mm6131a3_w.
19. McCormack WM, Stumacher RJ, Johnson K, et al. Clinical spectrum of gonococcal infection in women. *Lancet* 1977;1:1182-1185.
20. Gaydos CA. Nucleic acid amplification tests for gonorrhea and chlamydia: Practice and applications. *Infect Dis Clin North Am* 2005;19:367-386.
21. Lyss SB, Kamb ML, Peterman TA, et al. *Chlamydia trachomatis* among patients infected with and treated for *Neisseria gonorrhoeae* in sexually transmitted disease clinics in the United States. *Ann Intern Med* 2003;139:178-185.
22. Ison CA. Antimicrobial resistance in sexually transmitted infections in the developed world: Implications for rational treatment. *Curr Opin Infect Dis* 2012;25:73-78.
23. Kirkcaldy RD, Weinstock HS, Moore PC, et al. The efficacy and safety of gentamicin plus azithromycin and gemifloxacin plus azithromycin as treatment of uncomplicated gonorrhea. *Clin Infect Dis* 2014;59:1083-1091.
24. Woods CR. Gonococcal infections in neonates and young children. *Semin Pediatr Infect Dis* 2005;16:258-270.
25. Patton ME, Su JR, Nelson R, Weinstock H. Primary and Secondary Syphilis – United States, 2005–2013. *MMWR Morb Mort Wkly Rep* 2013;63(18):402-406.
26. LaFond RE, Lukehart SA. Biological basis for syphilis. *Clin Microbiol Rev* 2006;19:29-49.
27. Carlson JA, Dabiri G, Cribier B, Sell S. The immunopathobiology of syphilis: The manifestations and course of syphilis are determined by the level of delayed-type hypersensitivity. *Am J Dermatopathol* 2011;33:433-460.
28. Lukehart SA. Syphilis. In: Longo DL, Fauci AS, Kasper DL, Hauser SL, Jameson JL, Loscalzo J, eds. *Harrison's Principles of Internal Medicine,* 18th ed. [electronic version]; 2012. Available at: http://www.accessmedicine.com.libproxy.uthscsa.edu/content.aspx?aid=9102029.
29. Augenbraun M. Syphilis. In: Klausner JD, Hook EW III, eds. *Current Diagnosis & Treatment of Sexually Transmitted Diseases* [electronic version]; AccessMedicine, 2007. Available at: http://www.accessmedicine.com.libproxy.uthscsa.edu/content.aspx?aID=3025480.
30. Sparling PF, Swartz MN, Musher DM, Healy BP. Clinical manifestations of syphilis. In: Holmes KK, Sparling PF, Stamm WE, et al., eds. *Sexually Transmitted Diseases,* 4th ed. New York, NY: McGraw-Hill, 2008:661-688.
31. Lee V, Kinghorn G. Syphilis: An update. *Clin Med* 2008;8:330-333.
32. Goh BT. Syphilis in adults. *Sex Transm Infect* 2005;81:448-452.
33. Kent ME, Romanelli F. Reexamining syphilis: An update on epidemiology, clinical manifestations, and management. *Ann Pharmacother* 2008;42:226-236.
34. Eccleston K, Collins L, Higgins SP. Primary syphilis. *Int J STD AIDS* 2008;19:145-151.
35. Sena AC, White BL, Sparling PF. Novel *Treponema pallidum* serologic tests: A paradigm shift in syphilis screening for the 21st century. *Clin Infect Dis* 2010;51:700-708.
36. Hafner L, Beagley K, Timms P. *Chlamydia trachomatis* infection: Host immune responses and potential vaccines. *Mucosal Immunol* 2008;1:116-130.
37. Stamm WE, Batteiger BE. *Chlamydia trachomatis* (trachoma, perinatal infections, lymphogranuloma venereum, and other genital infections). In: Mandell GL, Bennett JE, Dolin R, eds. *Mandell, Douglas, and Bennett's Principles and Practice of Infectious Diseases,* 7th ed [electronic version]; MD Consult, 2010. Available at: http://www.mdconsult.com.libproxy.uthscsa.edu/book/player/book.do?method=display&type=aboutPage&decorator=header&eid=4-u1.0-B978-0-443-06839-3.X0001-X-TOP&isbn=978-0-443-06839-3&uniq=177288689.
38. Gaydos CA, Quinn TC. Chlamydial infections. In: Longo DL, Fauci AS, Kasper DL, Hauser SL, Jameson JL, Loscalzo J, eds. *Harrison's Principles of Internal Medicine,* 18th ed. [electronic version]; 2012. Available at: http://www.accessmedicine.com.libproxy.uthscsa.edu/content.aspx?aid=9102676.
39. Stamm WE. *Chlamydia trachomatis* infections of the adult. In: Holmes KK, Sparling PF, Stamm WE, et al., eds. *Sexually Transmitted Diseases,* 4th ed. New York, NY: McGraw-Hill, 2008:575-593.
40. Geisler WM, Stamm WE. Genital chlamydial infections. In: Klausner JD, Hook EW III, eds. *Current Diagnosis & Treatment of Sexually Transmitted Diseases* [electronic version]; AccessMedicine, 2007. Available at: http://www.accessmedicine.com.libproxy.uthscsa.edu/content.aspx?aID=3025480.
41. Mylonas I. Female genital *Chlamydia trachomatis* infection: Where are we heading? *Arch Gynecol Obstet* 2012;285:1271-1285.
42. Zar HJ. Neonatal chlamydial infections: Prevention and treatment. *Paediatr Drugs* 2005;7:103-110.
43. Paavonen J. *Chlamydia trachomatis* infections of the female genital tract: State of the art. *Ann Med* 2012;44:18-28.
44. Kalwij S, Macintosh M, Baraitser P. Screening and treatment of *Chlamydia trachomatis* infections. *BMJ* 2010;340:912-917.
45. Bebear C, de Barbeyrac B. Genital *Chlamydia trachomatis* infections. *Clin Microbiol Infect* 2009;5:4-10.
46. Hammerschlag MR, Kohlhoff SA. Treatment of chlamydial infections. *Expert Opin Pharmacother* 2012;13:545-552.
47. Geisler WM, Koltun WD, Abdelsayed N, et al. Safety and efficacy of WC2031 versus vibramycin for the treatment of uncomplicated urogenital *Chlamydia trachomatis* infection: A randomized, double-blind, double-dummy, active-controlled, multicenter trial. *Clin Infect Dis* 2012;55:82-88.
48. Geisler WM. Diagnosis and management of uncomplicated *Chlamydia trachomatis* infections in adolescents and adults: Summary of evidence reviewed for the 2010 Centers for Disease Control and Prevention Sexually Transmitted Diseases Treatment Guidelines. *Clin Infect Dis* 2011;53(Suppl 3):S92-S98.
49. Anonymous. Drugs for sexually transmitted infections. *Treat Guidel Med Lett* 2010;8:53-50. [Erratum appears in Treat Guidel Med Lett 2010;8:82]
50. Leone P. Genital Herpes. In: Klausner JD, Hook EW III, eds. *Current Diagnosis & Treatment of Sexually Transmitted Diseases* [electronic version]; AccessMedicine, 2007. Available at: http://www.accessmedicine.com.libproxy.uthscsa.edu/content.aspx?aID=3025480.
51. Schiffer, JT, Corey L. Herpes simplex virus. In: Mandell GL, Bennett JE, Dolin R, eds. *Mandell, Douglas, and Bennett's Principles and Practice of Infectious Diseases,* 7th ed. [electronic version]; MD Consult, 2010. Available at: http://www.mdconsult.com.libproxy.uthscsa.edu/book/player/book.do?method=display&type=aboutPage&decorator=header&eid=4-u1.0-B978-0-443-06839-3.X0001-X-TOP&isbn=978-0-443-06839-3&uniq=177288689.
52. Gupta R, Warren T, Wald A. Genital herpes. *Lancet* 2007;370:2127-2137.
53. Kimberlin DW, Rouse DJ. Genital herpes. *N Engl J Med* 2004;350:1970-1977.
54. Corey L, Wald A. Genital herpes. In: Holmes KK, Sparling PF, Stamm WE, et al., eds. *Sexually Transmitted Diseases,* 4th ed. New York, NY: McGraw-Hill, 2008:399-437.
55. Corey L. Herpes simplex viruses. In: Fauci AS, Kasper DL, Longo DL, et al., eds. *Harrison's Principles of Internal Medicine,* 17th ed.

[electronic version]; 2008. Available at: http://online.statref.com.libproxy.uthscsa.edu/Document/Document.aspx?docAddress=41ATb9F8ccLkXnJpdO9gbw%3d%3d&offset=71&SessionId=11465DDAHROTSXMQ.

56. Dwyer DE, Cunningham AL. Herpes simplex and varicella-zoster virus infections. *Med J Aust* 2002;177:267-273.
57. Chayavichitslip P, Buckwalter JV, Krakowski AC, Friedlander SF. Herpes simplex. *Pediatr Rev* 2009;30:119-130.
58. Simmons A. Clinical manifestations and treatment considerations of herpes simplex virus infection. *J Infect Dis* 2002;186(Suppl 1):S71-S77.
59. Beauman JG. Genital herpes: A review. *Am Fam Physician* 2005;72:1527-1534.
60. Wald A, Ashley-Morrow R. Serological testing for herpes simplex virus (HSV)-1 and HSV-2 infection. *Clin Infect Dis* 2002;35(Suppl 2):S173-S182.
61. Wald A. Testing for genital herpes: How, who, and why. *Curr Clin Top Infect Dis* 2002;22:166-180.
62. Scoular A. Using the evidence base on genital herpes: Optimising the use of diagnostic tests and information provision. *Sex Transm Infect* 2002;78:160-165.
63. Cernik C, Gallina K, Brodell RT. The treatment of herpes simplex infections: An evidence-based review. *Arch Intern Med* 2008;168:1137-1144.
64. Martinez V, Caumes E, Chosidow O. Treatment to prevent recurrent genital herpes. *Curr Opin Infect Dis* 2008;21:42-48.
65. Mell HK. Management of oral and genital herpes in the emergency department. *Emerg Med Clin North Am* 2008;26:457-473.
66. Patel R, Stanberry L, Whitley RJ. Review of recent HSV recurrent-infection treatment studies. *Herpes* 2007;14:23-26.
67. Bartlett BL, Tyring SK, Fife K, et al. Famciclovir treatment options for patients with frequent outbreaks of recurrent genital herpes: The RELIEF trial. *J Clin Virol* 2008;43:190-195.
68. Wald A, Selke S, Warren T, et al. Comparative efficacy of famciclovir and valacyclovir for suppression of recurrent genital herpes and viral shedding. *Sex Transm Dis* 2006;33:529-533.
69. Hill J, Roberts S. Herpes simplex virus in pregnancy: New concepts in prevention and management. *Clin Perinatol* 2005;32:657-670.
70. Mills J, Mindel A. Genital herpes simplex infections: Some therapeutic dilemmas. *Sex Transm Dis* 2003;30:232-233.
71. Jones CA. Vertical transmission of genital herpes: Prevention and treatment options. *Drugs* 2009;69:421-434.
72. Hollier LM, Wendell GD. Third trimester antiviral prophylaxis for preventing maternal genital herpes simplex virus (HSV) recurrences and neonatal infection. *Cochrane Database Syst Rev* 2008;1:CD004946.
73. Erard V, Wald A, Corey L, et al. Use of long-term suppressive acyclovir after hematopoietic stem-cell transplantation: Impact on herpes dimplex virus (HSV) disease and drug-resistant HSV disease. *J Infect Dis* 2007;196:266-270.
74. Stanberry LR. Clinical trials of prophylactic and therapeutic herpes simplex virus vaccines. *Herpes* 2004;11(Suppl 3):161A-169A.
75. Weller PF. Protozoal intestinal infections and trichomoniasis. In: Fauci AS, Kasper DL, Longo DL, et al., eds. *Harrison's Principles of Internal Medicine,* 17th ed. [electronic version]; 2008. Available at: http://online.statref.com.libproxy.uthscsa.edu/Document/Document.aspx?docAddress=41ATb9F8ccLkXnJpdO9gbw%3d%3d&offset=71&SessionId=11465DDAHROTSXMQ.
76. Soper D. Trichomoniasis: Under control or undercontrolled? *Am J Obstet Gynecol* 2004;190:281-290.
77. Hobbs MM, Sena AC, Swygard H, Schwebke JR. *Trichomonas vaginalis* and trichomoniasis. In: Holmes KK, Sparling PF, Stamm WE, et al., eds. *Sexually Transmitted Diseases,* 4th ed. New York, NY: McGraw-Hill, 2008:771-793.
78. Schwebke J. Trichomoniasis. In: Klausner JD, Hook EW III, eds. *Current Diagnosis & Treatment of Sexually Transmitted Diseases* [electronic version]; AccessMedicine, 2007. Available at: http://www.accessmedicine.com.libproxy.uthscsa.edu/content.aspx?aID=3025480.
79. Schwebke JR. *Trichomonas vaginalis.* In: Mandell GL, Bennett JE, Dolin R, eds. *Mandell, Douglas, and Bennett's Principles and Practice of Infectious Diseases,* 7th ed. [electronic version]; MD Consult, 2010. Available at: http://www.mdconsult.com.libproxy.uthscsa.edu/book/player/book.do?method=display&type=aboutPage&decorator=header&eid=4-u1.0-B978-0-443-06839-3.X0001-X-TOP&isbn=978-0-443-06839-3&uniq=177288689.
80. Schwebke JR, Burgess D. Trichomoniasis. *Clin Microbiol Rev* 2004;17:794-803.
81. McClelland RS, Sangare L, Hassan WM, et al. Infection with *Trichomonas vaginalis* increases the risk of HIV-1 acquisition. *J Infect Dis* 2007;195:698-702.
82. Wendel KA, Workowski KA. Trichomoniasis: Challenges to appropriate management. *Clin Infect Dis* 2007;44(Suppl 3):S123-S129.
83. Say PJ, Jacyntho C. Difficult-to-manage vaginitis. *Clin Obstet Gynecol* 2005;48:753-768.
84. Faro S. *Vaginitis: Differential Diagnosis and Management.* Boca Raton, FL: Parthenon Publishing, 2004:67-92.
85. Eckert LO. Acute vulvovaginitis. *N Engl J Med* 2006;355:1244-1252.
86. Sobel JD. What's new in bacterial vaginosis and trichomoniasis. *Infect Dis Clin North Am* 2005;19:387-406.
87. Nye MB, Schwebke JR, Body BA. Comparison of APTIMA Trichomonas vaginalis transcription-mediated amplification to wet mount microscopy, culture, and polymerase chain reaction for diagnosis of trichomoniasis in men and women. *Am J Obstet Gynecol* 2009;200:e181-e187.
88. Forna F, Gülmezoglu AM. Interventions for treating trichomoniasis in women. *Cochrane Database Syst Rev* 2003;2:CD000218.
89. Cudmore SL, Delgaty KL, Hayward-McClelland SF, et al. Treatment of infections caused by metronidazole-resistant *Trichomonas vaginalis. Clin Microbiol Rev* 2004;17:783-793.
90. Forna F, Gulmezoglu AM. Interventions for treating trichomoniasis in women. *Cochrane Database Syst Rev* 2003;2:CD000218.
91. Kissinger P, Mena L, Levison J, et al. A randomized treatment trial: Single versus 7-day dose of metronidazole for the treatment of *Trichomonas vaginalis* among HIV-infected women. *J Aquir Immune Defic Syndr* 2010;55:565-571.
92. Huh WK. Human papillomavirus infection: A concise review of natural history. *Obstet Gynecol* 2009;114:139-143.
93. Winer RL, Koutsky LA. Genital human papillomavirus infection. In: Holmes KK, Sparling PF, Stamm WE, et al., eds. *Sexually Transmitted Diseases,* 4th ed. New York, NY: McGraw-Hill, 2008:489-508.
94. Hutchinson DJ, Klein KC. Human papillomavirus disease and vaccines. *Am J Health Syst Pharm* 2008;65:2105-2112.
95. Hershey JH, Velez LF. Public health issues related to HPV vaccination. *J Public Health Manag Pract* 2009;15:384-392.
96. Hager WD. Human papilloma virus infection and prevention in the adolescent population. *J Pediatr Adolesc Gynecol* 2009;22:197-204.
97. Medeiros LR, Rosa DD, da Rosa MI, et al. Efficacy of human papillomavirus vaccines: A systematic quantitative review. *Int J Gynecol Cancer* 2009;19:1166-1176.

Bone and Joint Infections

118

Marcella N. Honkonen, Ziad Shehab, and Edward P. Armstrong

KEY CONCEPTS

1. The most common cause of osteomyelitis (particularly that acquired by hematogenous spread) and infectious arthritis is *Staphylococcus aureus*.
2. Culture and susceptibility information are essential as a guide for antimicrobial treatment of osteomyelitis and infectious arthritis.
3. Joint aspiration and examination of synovial fluid are extremely important to evaluate the possibility of infectious arthritis.
4. The most important treatment modality of acute osteomyelitis is the administration of appropriate antibiotics in adequate doses for a sufficient length of time.
5. Antibiotics generally are given in high doses so that adequate antimicrobial concentrations are reached within the infected bone and joints.
6. Oral antimicrobial therapies can be used for osteomyelitis to follow a parenteral regimen in children who have a good clinical response to IV antibiotics and in adults without diabetes mellitus or peripheral vascular disease when the organism is susceptible to the oral antimicrobial, a suitable oral agent is available, and adherence is ensured.
7. The standard duration of antimicrobial treatment for acute osteomyelitis is 4 to 6 weeks.
8. The three most important therapeutic approaches to the management of infectious arthritis are appropriate antibiotics, joint drainage, and joint rest.
9. Monitoring of antibiotic therapy is important and typically involves noting clinical signs of inflammation, periodic white blood cell (WBC) counts, C-reactive protein, and erythrocyte sedimentation rate (ESR) determinations.

Bone and joint infections are comprised of two disease processes known, respectively, as *osteomyelitis* and *septic* or *infectious arthritis*. They are unique and separate infectious entities with different signs and symptoms and infecting organisms. Despite advances in therapy, these infections continue to cause significant morbidity from residual damage and chronic or recurring infections. Emphasis on initiating antibiotic therapy as soon as possible is important in reducing long-term complications.

EPIDEMIOLOGY

Osteomyelitis

1 Osteomyelitis generally is an uncommon disease. One classic publication reported that 247 patients had osteomyelitis in a prominent American teaching hospital during a 4-year period.[1] Acute osteomyelitis has an estimated annual incidence of 0.4 per 1,000 children. In adults, osteomyelitis caused by contiguous spread, including postoperative, direct puncture, and that associated with adjacent soft tissue infections, comprises 47% of infections. *Hematogenous osteomyelitis* comprises 19% of infections, and osteomyelitis occurring in patients with significant peripheral vascular disease comprises 34% of infections.

The bacteriology of *hematogeous osteomyelitis* is unique in that one pathogen, *Staphylococcus aureus*, is responsible for more than 80% of these infections, with group A Streptococci and *Streptococcus pneumoniae* accounting for a few cases. *Kingellakingae*, an organism that is part of the oral flora is emerging as a pathogen in children less than 3 years of age. *Haemophilus influenzae* type b which used to be an important pathogen has been almost completely eliminated with the use of the conjugate vaccine and is now a rare pathogen in bone and joint infections.[2] Pneumococcal disease will likely decrease in prevalence as invasive pneumococcal disease is prevented by the use of the conjugate pneumococcal vaccine in infants. *Osteomyelitis* in neonates can result from infections with group B streptococcus, *Escherichia coli*, and most commonly *S. aureus*.

Vertebral osteomyelitis has several unique features and occurs most commonly in adults 50 to 60 years of age typically presenting with recalcitrant back pain unresponsive to usual symptomatic therapies, elevated inflammatory markers and who may or may not be having fever.[3] The lumbar and thoracic regions are the locations of most infections. Hematogenous infections are most likely to develop in the vascular areas near the subchondral plate region of the vertebral body. These infections are typically monomicrobial and are caused principally by Staphylococci that cause approximately 60% of these infections; however, Gram-negative organisms now play a significant role.[3-5] These Gram-negative organisms are most commonly Enterobacteriaceae species, particularly *E. coli* and *Klebsiella pneumoniae*, and most likely originate within the urinary tract or intra-abdominal cavity.[5]*Mycobacterium tuberculosis* and *Coccidioidesimmitis/posadasii* also are known to cause infections in the spine. Skin and respiratory tract infections are other sources of infection known to lead to vertebral infections. While infections of the spine can involve the vertebrae in 1% to 2% of older children with osteomyelitis, they more commonly involve the disk space of the lumbar vertebrae in children less than 5 years of age.

Contiguous-spread disease has several important differences compared with *hematogeous osteomyelitis*. Although *S. aureus* is still the most common organism isolated, polymicrobial infections, including with Gram-negative bacilli, occur frequently. *Pseudomonas aeruginosa*, streptococcus, *E. coli*, *Staphylococcus epidermidis*, and anaerobes can be isolated.

When anaerobes are grown from cultures, they usually are found in association with other organisms, including aerobic bacteria. Predisposing factors in patients who have anaerobic osteomyelitis include vascular disease, bites, contiguous infections, peripheral neuropathy, hematogenous spread, and trauma. Osteochondritis resulting from puncture injuries to the foot is associated with Gram-negative infection often times caused by *P. aeruginosa*. *S. aureus* is also a significant pathogen in these patients. The anaerobic infections in association with diabetes mellitus almost always involve the foot and are mixed. *Bacteroides fragilis* and *Bacteroides melaninogenicus* comprise the majority of anaerobic isolates.

Infectious Arthritis

Infectious or septic arthritis is an inflammatory reaction within the joint space. Septic arthritis is one of the most common causes of new cases of arthritis. The incidence of proven or likely septic arthritis is 4 to 10 cases per 100,000 patient-years.[6] The incidence of septic arthritis increases to 70 cases per 100,000 patient-years among patients that have rheumatoid arthritis.[7]

Neonates may have infectious arthritis because of a broad range of organisms, with *S. aureus*, group B Streptococcus, and Gram-negative organisms being most common. *S. aureus* and *Streptococcus pyogenes* are the most common pathogens in children younger than 5 years of age. *Hemophilus influenzae* type b (Hib) which used to be the most common pathogen in these children has essentially been eliminated by immunization with the conjugate Hib vaccine. Pneumococcal arthritis is also decreasing in incidence as a result of conjugate pneumococcal vaccine administration to infants. If the child has not been fully vaccinated or is immunocompromised, *H. influenzae* type b may be a cause.

Some organisms, such as *Neisseria gonorrhoeae*, are especially likely to infect a joint during bacteremia. Gonococcal arthritis is a common manifestation of disseminated gonococcal infection occurring in 42% to 85% of such patients.[8] Gonococcal arthritis is now uncommon in North America and Europe although it remains an important concern in developing countries.

Within the adult population, *S. aureus* is responsible for 37% to 65% of nongonococcal bacterial arthritis.[8] Streptococcal infections are the second most common followed by Gram-negative organisms. Among the latter, *E. coli* is the most common; however, *P. aeruginosa* is the most frequent organism in intravenous drug abusers.

Although rare, osteomyelitis and infectious arthritis can be caused by fungi and in the case of arthritis by viruses such as varicella-zoster, rubella or parvovirus.[9] Arthritis is rarely caused by Salmonella, Corynebacteria, Brucella, *Neisseria meningitidis*, *Mycoplasma pneumoniae* or *Ureaplasmaurealyticum*. Penetrating injury of the joint can result in an infection due to Pasteurella in dog bites, Capnocytophaga in human bites and Pantoea when the injury is induced by a thorn.

ETIOLOGY

Osteomyelitis

The most common method of classifying osteomyelitis is based on the mode of acquisition of the bone infection. Disease that results from spread through the bloodstream is termed *hematogeous osteomyelitis*, while that reaching the bone from an adjoining soft tissue infection is termed *contiguous osteomyelitis*. Patients with peripheral vascular disease are at risk for the development of contiguous osteomyelitis, and they present unique management features. Osteomyelitis that results from direct inoculation, such as from trauma, puncture wounds, or surgery, generally is also classified as inoculation osteomyelitis.

Osteomyelitis also can be classified based on the duration of the disease. Acute osteomyelitis describes infections of recent onset, usually several days to 1 week, whereas chronic infections are those of a longer duration. Some authors describe chronic infections as those with symptoms for more than 1 month before therapy, whereas other authors define chronic infections as relapse of an initial infection. *Hematogeous osteomyelitis* almost always involves one bone whereas contiguous osteomyelitis can present in multiple bones, especially when vascular insufficiency is an underlying risk factor.

Infectious Arthritis

Infectious arthritis can occur from many different types of microorganisms. Most infecting organisms produce an infection in a single joint, termed *monoarticular infection*; however, infections also can involve two or more joints. As with osteomyelitis, joint infections also can be classified according to the mechanisms by which the infecting organism reaches the joint. Infectious arthritis can result by spread from an adjacent bone infection, direct contamination of the joint space, or hematogenous dissemination. Hematogenous spread of the disease comprises the majority of infections; spread from osteomyelitis and direct inoculation is much less frequent. Septic arthritis is most prevalent in children and the elderly. Approximately, one-third of people with septic arthritis are children younger than 2 years of age.[8]

Unlike children, adults often have significant systemic diseases that predispose them to infectious arthritis, such as diabetes mellitus, immunosuppressive states (eg, cancer or liver disease), or preexisting arthritis. Risk factors associated with adult infectious arthritis (more than one factor may be present) are systemic corticosteroid use, preexisting arthritis, arthrocentesis, distant infection, diabetes mellitus, trauma, and other diseases. Intravenous drug abusers and individuals with intravascular infections such as endocarditis also are prone to develop septic arthritis.

PATHOPHYSIOLOGY

Osteomyelitis

Hematogenous Osteomyelitis

Hematogeous osteomyelitis is typically a disease of the growing bone and most cases occur in patients younger than 16 years of age. Less commonly, these infections occur in adults. Table 118-1 summarizes the primary characteristics of osteomyelitis.

Unique features of the anatomy and vascular supply of long bones appear to predispose them to become infected.[2] The hematogenous infections begin within the metaphyses (Fig. 118-1) as the

TABLE 118-1 Types of Osteomyelitis, Age Distribution, Common Sites, and Risk Factors

Type of Osteomyelitis	Typical Age (years)	Site(s) Involved	Risk Factors
Hematogenous	<1	Long bones and joints	Prematurity, umbilical or other central venous catheter or venous cut-down, respiratory distress syndrome, and perinatal asphyxia
	1-20	Long bones (femur, tibia, and humerus)	Infection (pharyngitis, cellulitis, and respiratory infections), trauma, and sickle cell disease
	Older than 50	Vertebrae	Diabetes mellitus, blunt trauma to spine, and urinary tract infection
Contiguous	Older than 50	Femur, tibia, and mandible	Hip fractures and open fractures
Puncture	<18	Foot	Puncture injury to foot
Vascular insufficiency	Older than 50	Feet and toes	Diabetes mellitus, peripheral vascular disease, and pressure sores

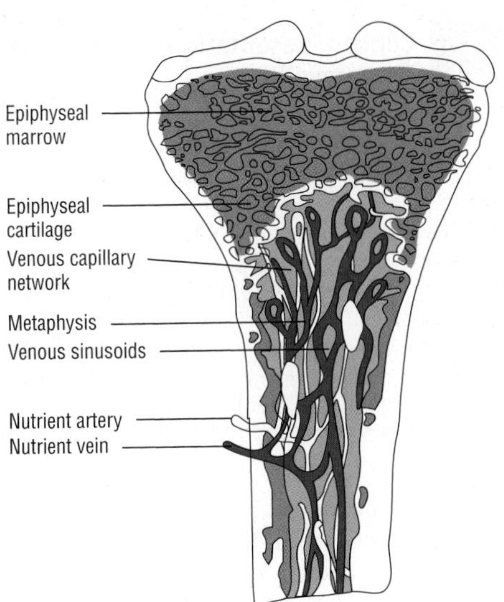

FIGURE 118-1 Cross-section of normal bone.

nutrient arteries of the long bones divide within the medullary canal of the bone into small arterioles. These end in hairpin turns near the growth plate and flow into veins, of much wider diameter, that drain the medullary cavity.[1] The infection is initiated within the bend of the arterioles where there is considerable slowing of blood flow in the hairpin capillary loops. This sludging of blood flow allows bacteria present within the bloodstream to settle and initiate an inflammatory response. They have access to the bone by gaps in the endothelium and the absence of a basement membrane. In addition to these structural features, phagocytosis is less active within the metaphysis. After the bacteria settle in the bone, avascular necrosis can occur from occlusion of the nutrient vessels and release of bacterial enzymes. Once the infection is initiated, exudate begins to form within the bone marrow and the fluid accumulates under increased pressure. The age of the patient largely determines the next stage in the pathophysiology.

Neonatal infections commonly involve multiple bones. The vascular supply of long bones in neonates has unique anatomic characteristics that affect their clinical presentation. Bridging blood vessels go across the epiphyseal plate from the metaphysis into the epiphysis thus enabling an infection that started within the metaphyseal area to spread easily to involve the epiphyses and then break into the joint. Therefore, in infants, not only can the infection spread under the periosteum or break through the periosteum and the shaft as in older children, but the infection also can spread directly through the bridging blood vessels to involve the joint.

In children older than 12 to 18 months, *hematogeous osteomyelitis* typically involves a single bone and has a predilection for involvement of the long bones, such as the femur, tibia, humerus, and fibula. The infection that started in the metaphysis of a long bone is prevented from spreading into the epiphysis and the adjacent joint space because of the epiphyseal growth plate which acts as a physical barrier; however, the exudate often dissects from the medulla through the soft cortex to the subperiosteal space as the periosteum in these children is loosely attached to the underlying cortex. The periosteum is thick and not easily ruptured thus containing the pus in the subperiosteal space, sometimes forming a subperiosteal abscess. If there is significant damage to the periosteum, the pus can decompress into a soft tissue abscess. The cortex obtains most of its blood supply from the periosteum and a subperiosteal abscess can impair the blood flow to the outer portion of the cortical bone resulting in a devitalized piece of dead bone termed a *sequestrum*. The elevated periosteum remains viable because its blood supply, derived from the overlying muscle, is unaffected. The raised periosteum will continue to produce bone; however, this new bone is now separated from the cortex because the periosteum has been raised from the infection. This new bone that is deposited under the periosteum is termed *involucrum*. In addition to these anatomic and functional features, there is some evidence that trauma is associated with developing an infection in specific bones. Children who develop *hematogeous osteomyelitis* may report some type of trauma before the onset of their symptoms and animal data indicate that traumatized bone is more likely to become infected than normal bone.

In adults, the periosteum is tightly bound to the cortex which is thick. These anatomic features generally cause the infections to remain intramedullary. As expected, subperiosteal abscess formation is less common in this population. The infection can spread to subperiosteal structures through the Haversian and Volkmann canals.

Osteomyelitis of the vertebrae is also acquired hematogenously and occurs most frequently in patients older than 50 years of age.[10,11] Vertebral disease in young children usually involve the disk space and the two vertebral facets adjoining it because of the nature of the vascular supply of the vertebrae at that age. This entity is known as diskitis. Vertebral osteomyelitis involving the body of the vertebra can be seen in children older than 8 years of age.

Chronic osteomyelitis is more likely to occur if large segments of bone become avascular and necrotic. This results in a piece of devitalized bone to which antimicrobial delivery is impaired. As a result, this infection is prone to exacerbations and may lead to weakening of that bone or to the formation of draining sinuses to the skin.

Direct Inoculation Osteomyelitis

This category of osteomyelitis includes infections caused by direct entrance of organisms from a source outside the body. Penetrating wounds (eg, trauma), open fractures, and various invasive orthopedic procedures can result in direct inoculation of organisms into the bone. More than 80% of cases of postoperative osteomyelitis are known to occur following open reduction of fractures. Specifically, these infections occur most commonly after internal fixation of a hip fracture or femoral or tibial shaft fracture. Inoculation osteomyelitis can also occur as a result of penetrating foreign bodies most commonly nail puncture injuries to the foot.

Contiguous Spread Osteomyelitis

Osteomyelitis secondary to spread from an adjacent soft tissue infection is called contiguous osteomyelitis. It can result from pressure ulcers or from adjacent soft tissue infections and most often involves the distal extremities. Less commonly, infections can spread from infected teeth to involve the mandible or occurs secondary to sinus infections by spreading through the mucosal lining of the sinuses into the vascular system surrounding the bone.

In contrast to *hematogeous osteomyelitis*, which occurs most commonly in children, contiguous-spread osteomyelitis occurs most commonly in patients older than age 50, most likely because of predisposing factors, such as hip fractures or vascular disease, are more common in this age group.

Patients with osteomyelitis in association with severe vascular insufficiency are extremely difficult to manage.[12] As anticipated, most of these patients have diabetes mellitus or severe atherosclerosis, and they develop their infections by contiguous spread. Generally, these patients are between the ages of 50 and 70 years. Frequently, patients with vascular disease develop osteomyelitis in their toes and fingers, and there is usually an adjacent area of infection, such as cellulitis or dermal ulcers. Importantly, infections in these patients are almost always polymicrobial and often include staphylococcus and streptococcus or the combination of staphylococcus, streptococcus, and Enterobacteriaceae. Enterococci and anaerobic organisms also can be involved.

TABLE 118-2 Characteristics of Acute Infectious Arthritis

Feature	Finding
Peak incidence	Children younger than 16 years Adults older than 50 years
Clinical findings	Fever of 38-40°C (100.4-104°F) in children; painful swollen joint in the absence of trauma Physical examination: Effusion, restriction of joint motion, tenderness, redness, and warmth of joint
Most commonly affected joints	Knee, hip, ankle, elbow, wrist, and shoulder
Laboratory findings	
Erythrocyte sedimentation rate	Elevated in 90% of cases
White blood cell count	Elevated in 30%-60% of cases
Left shift	Seen in two thirds of patients
Blood culture	Positive in 40% of cases
Needle aspiration of joint	Gram-stain diagnostic in 30%-50% of cases. Synovial fluid cultures are positive in 60%-80% of cases. Synovial fluid differential reveals 90% polymorphonuclear leukocytes. Synovial fluid glucose decreased relative to serum glucose. Lactic acid levels elevated in nongonococcal infectious arthritis, but not in gonococcal infectious arthritis

Infectious Arthritis

Infectious arthritis usually is acquired by hematogenous spread. The synovial tissue is highly vascular and does not have a basement membrane, so organisms in the blood can easily reach the synovial fluid. Table 118-2 summarizes the characteristics of acute infectious arthritis.

Preexisting abnormal joint architecture, joint trauma, and surgery are risk factors because chronic inflammation or trauma makes the joint more susceptible to infection. Individuals with rheumatoid arthritis can be prone to bacterial infection because of an inherent phagocytic defect, as well as concomitant corticosteroid therapy.

Organisms can gain access to the joint from a deep-penetrating wound injury, intra-articular steroid injections, arthroscopy, prosthetic joint surgery, and spread to the joint from a contiguous focus of osteomyelitis. After bacteria gain access to the joint, the organisms begin to multiply and produce a purulent exudate within the joint. If this joint effusion is present beyond 7 days, chronic, and sometimes irreversible, damage can occur to the bone and joint as a result of proteolytic enzymes and pressure necrosis. Purulent effusions can promote cartilage destruction by increasing leukocyte enzyme activity. In conjunction with the development of the effusion, almost all patients will develop a hot, swollen, painful joint.

CLINICAL PRESENTATION

Osteomyelitis

The clinical presentation of acute *hematogeous osteomyelitis* is summarized in Table 118-3. Although neonatal *hematogeous osteomyelitis* can spread rapidly to involve the joint, often there are few associated systemic symptoms.[13] A joint effusion is present in 60% to 70% of neonatal infections. Decreased limb motion or edema over the affected area may be the only signs from which to suspect the diagnosis. While it is sometimes acute in onset, the disease is often insidious in children.

Vertebral osteomyelitis produces nonspecific symptoms, such as constant back pain, fever or night sweats, and weight loss.[14] The pain typically is present at rest and increases in severity with movement. Serious neurologic complications can occur if the infection extends and compresses the spinal cord.

The presentation of osteomyelitis after surgery or trauma depends on the precipitating cause. If the infection follows surgery

TABLE 118-3 Clinical Presentation of Hematogenous Osteomyelitis

Signs and symptoms
Significant tenderness of the affected area, pain, swelling, fever, chills, decreased motion, and malaise

Laboratory tests
Elevated erythrocyte sedimentation rate, C-reactive protein, and white blood cell count
50% of patients will have positive blood cultures

Diagnostic studies
Bone changes observed on radiographs 10-14 days after the onset of infection. Magnetic resonance imaging and technetium scans positive as early as 1 day after the onset of infection

or bone trauma, the symptoms usually are noted within 1 month. The most frequent symptom is pain in the area of infection. Less commonly, patients also can develop a fever and elevated WBC count.

With contiguous-spread osteomyelitis there is often an area of localized tenderness, warmth, edema, and erythema over the infected site. Patients with significant vascular insufficiency usually have local symptoms, such as pain, swelling, and redness. Less commonly, they also can have fever and elevated WBC count.

Infectious Arthritis

Patients with nongonococcal bacterial arthritis almost always present with a fever, and 50% of patients have an elevated WBC count (see Table 118-2). The average initial synovial WBC count is $10 \times 10^3/mm^3$ ($10 \times 10^9/L$) or greater in nongonococcal bacterial disease. Nongonococcal bacterial arthritis is almost always monoarticular. The knee is the most commonly involved joint, but infections also can occur in the shoulder, wrist, hip, ankle, interphalangeal joints, and elbow joints. Usually, the initial focus of infection that acted as the portal of entry can be identified. Common routes for bacterial entrance include infections of the respiratory tract, skin, and urinary tract or previous bacteremia; often no specific source can be identified. Blood cultures are important in these patients because they can be positive in 50% of patients.

The most frequent initial sign of disseminated gonococcal infections is the triad of dermatitis, tenosynovitis (inflammation and swelling of a tendon) and migratory polyarthralgia or polyarthritis. Women are more prone to develop disseminated gonococcal infections than men by a ratio of 4:1. The second and third trimesters of pregnancy and the time of menses appear to be the times of greatest risk for developing gonococcal bacteremia, hypothesized to be associated with mucosal vascularity. Common joints involved include the knee, wrist, elbow, and ankle. Presentation varies slightly depending on whether or not the woman is pregnant. In non-pregnant women, duration of symptoms are longer, presence of joint effusion is more likely, and white blood cells are more often present within the synovial fluid.[15]

Another type of infectious arthritis occurs following prosthetic joint surgery. The most common symptom is pain. Local signs of inflammation and fever are common in acute infections while chronic infections present in a more subtle fashion, typically with pain alone and often loosening of the prosthesis. With these infections, the C-reactive protein usually is elevated, although a leukocytosis often is absent. Infections that result from postoperative contamination usually become apparent within 1 year of surgery.

Radiologic and Laboratory Tests

Osteomyelitis

2 The evaluation of a patient who may have osteomyelitis has several unusual aspects. Radiographs of the involved area should be obtained to rule out other processes such as a fracture; bone changes

characteristic of osteomyelitis appear late and are not typically seen until at least 10 to 14 days after the onset of the infection as more than 50% of the bone matrix must be decalcified before the lesions can be detected radiologically. Magnetic resonance imaging (MRI) is the most sensitive and commonly used diagnostic imaging modality and offers the advantage of better anatomic definition, especially of abscesses or joint effusions. Radionuclide bone scanning (technetium/gallium) computed tomographic scanning or positive emission tomography scanning is useful in identifying the focus of osteomyelitis in patients unable to have an MRI.[16]

Despite the seriousness of osteomyelitis, often there are few laboratory abnormalities. The erythrocyte sedimentation rate (ESR), C-reactive protein, and WBC count may be the only laboratory abnormalities. The degree of abnormality of these laboratory findings does not correlate with the disease outcome; however, these inflammatory markers are useful for monitoring therapy. C-reactive protein is generally the more sensitive marker of response to therapy and often increases and decreases before the ESR.

When a clinical assessment of osteomyelitis is suspected, it is important to establish a bacteriologic diagnosis by culture of the infected bone and blood. Accurate culture information is especially important as a guide for treatment of osteomyelitis in this era of increasing antimicrobial resistance. Bone aspiration or bone biopsy are valuable in determining an accurate bacteriologic diagnosis. In addition, they help determine whether or not there is an abscess present. If an abscess is identified, it must be drained and the pus cultured, and a Gram stain performed. Aspirates of subperiosteal pus or metaphyseal fluid yield a pathogen in 70% of cases. Cultures should be done for both aerobic and anaerobic bacteria. A Gram stain of the aspirate can be useful in initiating appropriate empirical antibiotic therapy.

If a specimen is obtained from a previously undrained or unopened wound abscess, the pathogen usually can be identified. In chronic osteomyelitis, however, identification can be more difficult. Open wounds and draining sinuses frequently are contaminated with other organisms and thus provide inaccurate culture information.[17] They cannot be relied on to reflect the pathogen unless consecutive deep sinus tract cultures reveal the same pathogens.[18] Cultures of loculated pus aspirates in the area of orthopedic devices removed from infected bone can be trusted, however, to identify the infecting organism. The preferable time to obtain culture material in a patient with a chronic draining sinus is at the time of open surgical debridement.

In addition to performing cultures from the involved bone, it also is important to obtain cultures from any site believed to be the primary source of a bacteremia. Blood cultures should be obtained. Approximately 50% of patients with *hematogeous osteomyelitis* will have positive blood cultures and may obviate the need for bone aspiration in these patients.

Infectious Arthritis

3 Radiographs of infected joints often reveal distension of the joint capsule with soft tissue swelling in the adjacent space. Magnetic resonance imaging can be helpful in identifying an infected joint, especially the shoulder and hip. In patients who have developed an infected prosthetic joint, loosening of the prosthesis can be seen radiographically.

When evaluating the possibility of a patient having infectious arthritis, immediate joint aspiration with analysis of the synovial fluid is extremely important. The presence of purulent fluid usually indicates the presence of a septic joint. The synovial fluid WBC count is usually 50×10^3-200×10^3/mm^3 (50×10^9-200×10^9/L) when an infection is present. As with osteomyelitis, most patients will have an elevated C-reactive protein concentration and ESR. However, serum WBC, ESR, and C-reactive protein may not be useful acutely in septic arthritis.[19]Approximately half the patients with an infected joint have a low synovial glucose level, usually less than 40 mg/dL (2.2 mmol/L). Gram stains of joint fluid demonstrate bacteria in 50% of patients with septic arthritis; however, such stains are positive in only 25% of patients with gonococcal arthritis. Synovial fluid cultures usually are positive in patients with nongonococcal infections. Both blood and joint fluid should be cultured aerobically and anaerobically in a patient suspected of having an infected joint. Blood cultures are positive in one-half of patients with nongonococcal infections but in only 20% of those with gonococcal infections. Pharyngeal, rectal, cervical, or urethral smears and cultures, as well as cultures of cutaneous lesions, should be performed if a disseminated gonococcal infection is considered. Nucleic acid based assays should also be used for the diagnosis of genital gonococcal infection.

TREATMENT

Desired Outcome(s)

Osteomyelitis

The goals of treatment are resolution of the infection and prevention of long-term sequelae. The ultimate outcome of osteomyelitis depends on the acute or chronic nature of the disease and how rapidly appropriate therapy including surgical drainage where appropriate is initiated. Patients with acute osteomyelitis have the best prognosis. Cure rates exceeding 80% can be expected for patients with acute osteomyelitis who have surgery when indicated and receive appropriate antibiotics for 4 to 6 weeks. When the growth plate is involved in children, discrepancies in the growth of bones or angular bone deformities can result.

In contrast, patients with chronic osteomyelitis have a much poorer prognosis. Dead bone and other necrotic material from the infection act as a bacterial reservoir and make the infection very difficult to eliminate. Adequate surgical debridement to remove all the dead bone and necrotic material, combined with prolonged administration of antibiotics, provides the best chance to obtain a cure.[20] The inability to remove all the dead bone can allow residual infection and require suppressive antibiotics to control the infection.

Infectious Arthritis

While many patients who develop infectious arthritis recover with no long-term sequelae, 50% are left with decreased joint function or mobility. Gonococcal arthritis usually resolves rapidly with antibiotics and has fewer sequelae. Individuals at greatest risk for long-term sequelae are those who have symptoms present for more than 7 days before starting therapy and those with infections occurring within the hip joint and infections caused by Gram-negative organisms. Common long-term residual effects following infectious arthritis are limited joint motion and persistent pain.

During the initial phase of the infection, weight bearing, such as walking on the joint should be avoided. Passive range-of-motion exercises should be initiated when the pain begins to subside to maintain joint mobility. Approximately one-third of patients with bacterial arthritis have a poor joint outcome, such as severe functional deterioration. Poor joint outcomes are associated with older patients, those with preexisting joint disease, and patients with an infected joint containing synthetic material.

General Approach to Treatment

Osteomyelitis

4 Following completion of the steps needed to determine the infecting organism, the most important treatment modality of acute osteomyelitis is the administration of appropriate antibiotics in adequate doses for a sufficient length of time. It is important to stress that early antibiotic therapy can mitigate the need for surgery, subsequent sepsis, chronic infection, disruption of longitudinal bone growth and angular deformity of the bone.[21] A delay in treatment can allow bone

TABLE 118-4 Empiric Treatment of Osteomyelitis

Patient Subtype	Likely Infecting Organism	Antibiotic[a]	Recommendation Grades[b]
Newborn	*Staphylococcus aureus*, group B *Streptococci, Escherichia coli*	Nafcillin or oxacillin 50-150 mg/kg/day IV plus cefotaxime 100-200 mg/kg/day IV	B-3
Children 5 years of age or younger	1. If vaccinated for *Haemophilus influenzae* type b: *S. aureus* or Streptococci 2. If not vaccinated against *H. influenzae* type b	1. Nafcillin or oxacillin 150-200 mg/kg/day IV orcefazolin 100 mg/kg/day IV 2. Cefuroxime 150 mg/kg/day IV	B-3 B-3
Children older than 5 years of age	*S. aureus*	Nafcillin or oxacillin 150-200 mg/kg/day IV or cefazolin 100 mg/kg/day IV	A-3
Adults	*S. aureus*	Nafcillin or oxacillin 2 g IV every 4 hours or cefazolin 2 g IV every 8 hours	A-3
IV drug abusers	*Pseudomonas*	Ciprofloxacin 750 mg orally twice daily or ceftazidime or cefepime 2 g IV every 8 hours	B-3
Postoperative or posttrauma patients	Gram-positive and Gram-negative organisms	Nafcillin or oxacillin 2 g IV every 4 hours plus ceftazidime or cefepime 2 g IV every 8 hours or ticarcillin–clavulanate 3.1 g IV every 4 hours	B-3
Patients with vascular insufficiency	Gram-positive and Gram-negative organisms	Nafcillin or oxacillin 2 g IV every 4 hours or cefazolin 2 g IV every 8 hours plus ceftazidime or cefepime 2 g IV every 8 hours	B-3
	If anaerobes suspected	Cefotetan 2 g IV every 12 hours or clindamycin 900 mg IV every 8 hours plus ceftazidime or cefepime 2 g IV every 8 hours	C-3

IV, intravenous.

[a]Dosage should be adjusted for some agents in patients with renal and/or hepatic dysfunction.

[b]Strength of recommendations: A, B, C = good, moderate, and poor evidence to support recommendation, respectively. Quality of evidence: 1 = Evidence from more than one properly randomized, controlled studies or multiple time series; or dramatic results from uncontrolled experiments. 2 = Evidence from more than one well-designed clinical trial with randomization, from cohort or case-controlled analytic studies. 3 = Evidence from opinions of respected authorities, based on clinical experience, descriptive studies, or reports of expert communities.

necrosis to occur and make eradication of the infection much more difficult. In these patients with chronic osteomyelitis, exacerbations of the infection can result if all necrotic tissue is not removed surgically and all microorganisms eliminated. Chronic suppressive antimicrobial therapy and adjunctive treatment with hyperbaric oxygen or antibiotic-impregnated implants during surgery also has been used.

If a patient with *hematogeous osteomyelitis* does not respond by having a decrease in fever, local swelling, redness, and pain following the initiation of adequate antibiotic therapy, the patient should undergo surgical debridement of the infected area. It is important to emphasize the priority of starting antibiotics immediately after the cultures have been obtained.

Infectious Arthritis

Patients with infectious arthritis are typically admitted to the hospital to obtain synovial fluid and blood cultures and initiate antimicrobial therapy. Attempt to decrease bacterial burden in the joint space is obtained by performing either open or arthroscopic debridement. Empiric antibiotics are started as soon as culture specimens are collected. As with osteomyelitis, it is important to stress early initiation of antibiotic therapy to avoid complications such as avascular necrosis, limb-length discrepancy, and pathologic fractures.[22]

In patients with prosthetic joint devices, it is imperative that orthopedic surgeons work alongside infectious disease practitioners to determine the best course of action.[23] The gold standard treatment method includes resection of the implant, placement of temporary antibiotic-impregnated cement spacer, and delayed component re-implantation. Although it may be decided to retain the implant in certain cases for which patients will receive irrigation and debridement in addition to antibiotic therapy, or antibiotic therapy alone in patients unable to tolerate surgical procedures.[24]

Pharmacologic Therapy

Osteomyelitis

Antibiotic Selection A critical component in the management of osteomyelitis is the selection of appropriate antibiotics. Empiric therapy must be selected on the basis of the most likely infecting organism while the results of culture and susceptibility data are pending. Once culture and susceptibility results are obtained the antimicrobial therapy should be tailored. Table 118-4 summarizes empiric therapy recommendations.

With staphylococcus being the most common bacteria in osteomyelitis, resistance patterns must be considered when deciding on an empiric agent. For communities showing low evidence of resistant strains of *S. aureus*, nafcillin is the drug of choice.[25]Although cefazolin or cephalexin are often chosen to treat susceptible strains due to ease of dosing compared to nafcillin. Clindamycin can be used in less severe cases.[25,26] If 10% or more of the surrounding community *S. aureus* isolates are methicillin resistant, then an agent active against MRSA should be selected. Vancomycin is the drug of choice in this case.[25,26] If the patient is severely ill, then both vancomycin and nafcillin should be used for empiric treatment, as nafcillin is superior for the treatment of methicillin susceptible *S. aureus*.[25]

In the setting of vertebral osteomyelitis, empiric therapy should be initiated in conjunction with culture if the patient is hemodynamically unstable, septic or experiencing neurologic compromise; otherwise, it is recommended empiric therapy be held 1 to 2 weeks while awaiting culture results.[3]

Antibiotic Bone Concentration

5 Antibiotics used in the management of acute osteomyelitis generally are given in high doses (adjusted for weight, renal function, hepatic function, or both) so that adequate antimicrobial concentrations are reached within the infected bone and joint.[27] Table 118-5 summarizes antibiotics doses that have been successful in the treatment of osteomyelitis.

Oral Antibiotic Therapy

6 Criteria for the use of oral outpatient antibiotic therapy for osteomyelitis includes all of the following:

- Confirmed osteomyelitis
- Initial clinical response to parenteral antibiotics
- Suitable oral agent available
- Adherence ensured

TABLE 118-5 Antimicrobial Agents for the Treatment of Osteomyelitis

Antimicrobial	Dose[a]	Comments
Amoxicillin	Adult: 500-875 mg orally every 8 hours[21]	
Amoxicillin/Clavulanate	Adult: 875/125 mg orally every 8 hours[21]	
Ampicillin	Adult: 2 g IV every 4 hours[21] Children: 150-200 mg/kg/day in 4 equal doses (max 8-12 g daily)[29] VO:12 g IV every 24 hours, continuous, or in 6 divided doses[3]	May add IV aminoglycoside for treatment of *Enterococcus* spp[21] VO:For enterococcus, add 4-6 weeks of aminoglycoside therapy in patients with infective endocarditis[3]
Ampicillin/Sulbactam	Adult: 1.5-3 g IV every 6 hours[21]	
Anti-staphylococcal (cloxacillin, flucloxacillin, dicloxacillin, nafcillin, oxacillin)	Adult: Nafcillin or oxacillin 1-2 g IV every 4-6 hours[21,28] Children: ≤200 mg/kg/day in 4 equal doses (max dose 8-12 g daily)[29] VO: Nafcillin or oxacillin 1.5-2 g IV every 4-6 hours or continuous infusion[3]	VO: 6 week duration[3]
Aztreonam	VO: 2g IV every 8 hours[3]	VO: 6 week duration. Double coverage for *P. aeruginosa* may be considered. Use only for severe penicillin allergy and quinolone-resistant strains[3]
Cefepime	Adult: 2 g IV every 24 hours[21,28] VO: 2 g IV every 8-12 hours[3]	Add IV ciprofloxacin for treatment of *P. aeruginosa*[28] VO: 6 week duration. Double coverage for *P. aeruginosa* may be considered. For Enterobacteriaceae, 2 g IV every 12 hours[3]
Cefotetan	Adult: 2 g IV every 12 hours[28]	
Ceftazidime	Adult: 2 g IV every 8-12 hours[21] VO: 2 g IV every 8 hours[3]	VO: 6 week duration. Double coverage for *P. aeruginosa* may be considered[3]
Ceftriaxone	Adult:1-2 g IV every 24 hours[21,28] VO: 2 g IV every 24 hours[3]	VO: 6 week duration. For *Salmonella*, 6-8 week duration[3]
Chloramphenicol	Children: 75 mg/kg/day in 3 equal doses (max dose 2-4 g daily)[29]	To be used if safer agents are not available or affordable[29]
Ciprofloxacin	Adult: 400 IV every 8-12 hours[21,28] or 500-750 mg PO every 12 hours[21,23] VO: 500-750 mg orally every 12 hours, or 400 mg IV every 8 hours[3]	VO: 6 week duration. Double coverage for *P. aeruginosa* may be considered. For *Salmonella*, 6-8 week duration[3]
Clindamycin	Adult: 600 mg IV every 6 hours[21,28] or 300-600 mg orally every 6 hours[21,23] Children: ≥40 mg/kg/day in 4 equal doses (max dose 3 g daily)[29] VO: 600-900 mg IV every 8 hours, or 300-450 mg orally twice daily[3]	VO: 6 week duration, not recommended for MRSA. Recommended as second line for sensitive staphylococcal infection[3]
Daptomycin	Adult: 4-6 mg/kg IV every 24 hours[21] VO: 6-8 mg/kg IV every 24 hours[3]	VO: 6 week duration. For enterococcus, 6 mg/kg IV every 24 hours plus 4-6 weeks of aminoglycoside therapy in patients with infective endocarditis[3]
Doripenem	VO: 500 mg IV every 8 hours[3]	VO: 6 week duration. Double coverage for *P. aeruginosa* may be considered[3]
Doxycycline	Adult: 100 mg orally twice daily[23]	VO: Can be used in addition to rifampin for brucellar infection
Ertapenem	VO: 1 g IV every 24 hours[3]	VO: 6 week duration[3]
First Generation Cephalosporin (Cefazolin, Cephalexin)	Adult: Cefazolin 1-1.5 g IV every 6 hours[28] or 1-2 g IV every 6-8 hours[21] Cephalexin 500 mg orally every 6 hours[21] Children: ≥150 mg/kg/day in 4 equal doses (max dose 2-4 g daily)[29] VO: Cefazolin 1-2 g IV every 8 hours[3]	VO: 6 week duration[3]
Fusidic acid	Adult: 500 mg orally three times daily[23]	
Imipenem/cilastatin	Adult: 1 g IV every 8 hours[28]	Add IV aminoglycoside for treatment of *P. aeruginosa*[28]
Levofloxacin	Adult: 500-750 mg IV once daily[21,28] or 750 mg PO once daily[23] or 500 mg orally twice daily[23] VO: 500-750 mg orally once daily[3]	Add IV rifampin for treatment of MRSA[28] VO: Add rifampin 600 mg orally daily for all staphylococcus strains, duration 6 weeks of combination therapy[3]
Linezolid	Adult: 600 mg IV or orally every 12 hours[21,23,28] Children: 30 mg/kg/day in 3 equal doses (max dose 1.2 g for no more than 28 days)[29] VO: 600 mg IV or orally every 12 hours[3]	VO: 6 week duration. For enterococcus, add 4-6 weeks of aminoglycoside therapy in patients with infective endocarditis[3]
Meropenem	Adult: 1 g IV every 8 hours[21] VO: 1 g IV every 8 hours[3]	VO: 6 week duration. Double coverage for *P. aeruginosa* may be considered[3]

(continued)

TABLE 118-5 Antimicrobial Agents for the Treatment of Osteomyelitis (*Continued*)

Antimicrobial	Dose	Comments
Metronidazole	Adult: 500 mg IV every 6-8 hours[21,28] or 500 mg orally three to four times a day[23] VO: 500 mg orally three to four times daily[3]	VO:F *Bacteroides* species and other susceptible anaerobes[3]
Minocycline	Adult: 200 mg orally initially, then 100 mg daily[28] or 100 mg PO twice daily[23]	
Moxifloxacin	Adult: 400 mg orally once daily[23] VO: 400 mg orally once daily[3]	VO: For Enterobacteriaceae and other susceptible aerobic Gram-negative organisms. Not recommended for staphylococcal infection[3]
Penicillin G	Adult: 2-4 million units IV every 4 hours[28] or 10-20 million units IV continuous every 24 hours[21] VO:20-24 million units IV every 24 hours, continuously, or in 6 divided doses[3]	VO: For enterococcus, add 4-6 weeks of aminoglycoside therapy in patients with infective endocarditis[3]
Piperacillin/Tazobactam	Adult: 3.375 g IV every 6 hours[28]	Add IV ciprofloxacin for treatment of *P. aeruginosa*[28]
Rifampin	Adult: 600 mg IV every 12 hours[28] or 600-900 mg orally every 24 hours[21,23] or 300-450 mg orally twice daily[23]	Only to be used in combination with another antimicrobial
Ticarcillin/Clavulanate	Adult: 3.1 g IV every 4 hours[28]	
Trimethoprim-Sulfamethoxazole	Adult: 1 double-strength tablet orally every 12 hours[28] or 1 double-strength tablet orally three times a day[23] VO: 1-2 double-strength tablets orally twice daily[3]	VO: Second line agent for Enterobacteriaceae and other susceptible aerobic Gram-negative organisms. May need to monitor sulfamethoxazole levels[3]
Vancomycin	Adult: 1 g IV every 12 hours[28] or 15 mg/kg IV every 12 hours[21] Children: ≤40 mg/kg/day in 4 equal doses[29] VO: 15-20 mg/kg IV every 12 hours[3]	Adjust based on patient and pharmacokinetic parameters. Target trough of 15-20 mcg per milliliter[29] VO: Consider loading dose for MRSA and enterococcus, 6 week duration. For enterococcus, add 4-6 weeks of aminoglycoside therapy in patients with infective endocarditis. For enterococcus, use only if patient is penicillin allergic or bacteria is penicillin resistant[3]

IV, intravenous;MRSA, methicillin susceptible *staphylococcus aureus*;VO, vertebral osteomyelitis.

[a]Dosage should be adjusted for some agents in patients with renal and/or hepatic dysfunction.

Suitable candidates are children with good clinical response to intravenous therapy and adults without diabetes mellitus or peripheral vascular disease.

The use of oral antibiotics is well studied in children.[30] Typically, injectable antibiotics are used initially and then switched to oral antibiotics when there was a decrease in the signs of inflammation and the ESR or when the patient was afebrile for 3 days. If pus was obtained on the initial needle aspirate, or if a reduction in fever, local swelling, and tenderness did not occur despite adequate rest, immobilization, and intensive antibiotic therapy, the patients underwent surgical drainage. The patients enrolled in oral antibiotic trials generally had disease of recent onset, identification of a specific infecting organism, enforced adherence, and surgery as indicated. In patients who meet these criteria, oral antibiotics appear to offer a great advantage in the treatment of osteomyelitis. Patients not meeting these criteria may have a higher risk of developing chronic osteomyelitis if oral therapy is inappropriate or not strictly adhered to. When oral antibiotics are used, the total duration of oral and injectable therapy is usually at least 4 weeks. Limited retrospective data in adults indicated that parenteral therapy for less than 4 weeks followed by oral therapy may be effective.[31]

Duration of Antibiotic Therapy

7 Following debridement, bone takes 3 to 4 weeks to revascularize thus the basis of treatment duration.[32] The specific duration of antibiotic therapy needed in the management of osteomyelitis is usually 4 to 6 weeks.[33] Failure rates approaching 20% have been observed in children treated with parenteral antibiotics for 3 weeks or less. One analysis in children with *hematogeous osteomyelitis* recommended 20 days of antibiotic therapy after initial parenteral therapy as long as the C-reactive protein level normalized within 7 to 10 days.[34] Although these data were largely evaluated in children, this duration of therapy recommendation is also used in adults. Treatment failures may be due to the presence of infected necrotic bone or infected hardware (wires, plates, screws, and rods) that could not be removed.[35]Improvement in the patient's clinical signs and symptoms and normalization of the C-reactive protein level or ESR are important parameters to assess therapy.[36] If signs or symptoms are still present at 6 weeks, therapy should be extended. In some cases of chronic osteomyelitis, lifelong suppressive therapy might be the most appropriate option.[37]

Duration of antibiotic administration for vertebral osteomyelitis may vary depending on the infecting organism. With Gram-negative bacteria a longer duration (greater than or equal to 8 weeks) is associated with less rates of recurrence compared to shorter durations (4-6 weeks).[5] One study compared 6 weeks versus 12 weeks duration in patients with pyogenic vertebral osteomyelitis and found the shorter duration to be non-inferior.[38] However, many factors remained left for questioning and it is uncertain whether or not it is safe to use a shorter duration for patients with extensive bone destruction or abscesses.[38,39] The IDSA guidelines recommend a minimum of 6 weeks of parenteral therapy or highly bioavailable oral therapy.[3]

Clinical **Controversy...**

Vertebral osteomyelitis—The exact duration of antimicrobial therapy for a patient with vertebral osteomyelitis is unknown. Many factors play a role in determining the severity of the infection and risk of recurrence. Longer courses might be needed in patients with Gram negative infections or infections complicated by abscesses.

Special Populations

Osteomyelitis in the intravenous drug user has unique features.[40] More than 50% of such infections involve the vertebral column and less than 20% of infections are located in either the sternoarticular or pelvic girdle. Infections are much less frequent within the extremities. They also have an unusual spectrum of organisms with Gram-negative organisms being responsible for 88% of infections. *P.aeruginosa*, either singly or in combination with other organisms, is cultured in 78% of all such infections. *Klebsiella, Enterobacter*, and *Serratia* species also can be found but less commonly. In addition, staphylococcal and streptococcal organisms are sometimes cultured.

Patients with sickle cell anemia and related hemoglobinopathies also represent a unique population in that two-thirds of bone infections in these patients are caused by *Salmonella* species, while the rest are usually caused by staphylococci and other Gram negative organisms.[41] Bowel infarctions from the sickle cell disease can facilitate the entry of salmonellae from the colon into the bloodstream with resultant hematogenous spread to the bone. Osteomyelitis in patients with sickle cell disease may occur in any bone, but it most commonly involves the medullary cavity of long or tubular bones. Because of the difficulty in separating bone pain during a sickle cell crisis from that of an infection, osteomyelitis can be relatively advanced in these patients by the time the diagnosis is made.

Infectious Arthritis

Antibiotic Selection

8 The three most important therapeutic maneuvers in the management of infectious arthritis are appropriate antibiotics, joint drainage, and joint rest. Smears of the synovial fluid can be useful to select appropriate antibiotic therapy initially.[8] If bacteria are not observed on the Gram stain in a patient who has a purulent joint effusion, antibiotics still should be initiated because of the low sensitivity of the Gram stain. A delay in initiating antibiotics significantly increases the likelihood for long-term complications. The specific antibiotic selected depends on the most likely infecting organism. When staphylococcal infection is suspected, rifampin is often added to the anti-staphylococcal or anti-MRSA agent, especially in the setting of prosthetic hardware.[42]

Antibiotic Joint Space Concentration

The antibiotics selected usually are administered parenterally to achieve sufficient concentrations within the synovial fluid, and thus intra-articular antibiotic injections are unnecessary.

In prosthetic joint infections, antimicrobial cement spacers are often used to aide in delivery of the antimicrobial to the site of infection. The most common antimicrobials used include vancomycin and aminoglycosides, tobramycin and gentamicin.[43,44]However, the doses of each agent are widely variable and it is uncertain whether the placement of antimicrobial cement spacers adds outcome benefit to systemic therapy.[43] The thought of antimicrobial cement spacer providing local exposure of the antimicrobial agent without systemic consequences has been questioned.[45] Ameta-analysis reported the incidence of acute kidney injury in patients receiving treatment with antimicrobial cement spacers at 4.8%, incidence range varied from 2% to 17% based on the definition of acute kidney injury used.[43]

Clinical **Controversy...**

Antimicrobial cement spacers—The use of antimicrobial cement spacers is routine for patients with prosthetic joint infections. The antimicrobial agents used locally may place the patient at risk for systemic adverse reactions with little benefit added to systemic therapy. In addition, the exact dose of the antimicrobials used is unknown.

Similar to osteomyelitis, once the infection is confirmed if initial response to parenteral therapy is achieved, the culture susceptibilities have resulted, and adherence is ensured, then selected oral antibiotics can be used for the treatment of infectious arthritis. Shorter durations of antimicrobial therapy are needed to treat infectious arthritis compared to osteomyelitis. A randomized trial compared 10 days versus 30 days of antimicrobial therapy and found no difference between the groups.[34] The treatment duration may be extended to 20 days if the adjacent bone is affected.[46]

Home Antibiotic Therapy

Because the management of bone and joint infections frequently requires prolonged parenteral antibiotics, newer antibiotic regimens have been used. Administration of antibiotics in the home environment and the use of antibiotics with extended elimination half-lives are commonly used. Although acute osteomyelitis is one of the more common infectious diseases that can be treated with home intravenous antibiotics, not all patients are acceptable candidates for home administration. Patients must be screened to include only those who are receiving a stable treatment program, those who are interested and are motivated in participating, and those who have good venous access, as well as those who have support from family members or neighbors and have home facilities for storage and refrigeration. Patients with adequate vascular access may be able to use a peripheral intravenous catheter; however, a central intravenous catheter may be required if venous access difficulties occur. Certain exclusion criteria also must be considered. Complications of other preexisting diseases, such as diabetic retinopathy, intention tremor, disabling inflammation or degenerative joint disease, coagulopathies, or various neurologic disorders can prevent individuals from receiving home antibiotics. A history of alcoholism or of intravenous drug abuse also is important exclusion criteria. Patients who are fluent in only a foreign language and patients who are illiterate or hard of hearing may have to be excluded if a qualified guardian is unavailable. In addition to meeting these initial screening criteria, patients must successfully complete a thorough training program before hospital discharge. Aseptic technique, proper catheter care, and correct administration techniques must be documented. Once a patient is receiving therapy in the home environment, continued monitoring of their antimicrobial therapy and drug levels when indicated is important. It is vital to ensure compliance with the antimicrobial regimen. Catheter-related complications are common in patients receiving prolonged courses of parenteral antibiotics.

In addition, the specific antibiotic regimen characteristics must be considered when evaluating a patient for home antibiotics. Some important features are microbiologic culture and susceptibility data, the number of required daily antimicrobial doses, antibiotic stability data, and requirements for unique monitoring for the specific antimicrobial regimen, such as serum creatinine and drug level monitoring with aminoglycosides or vancomycin. Although an organism can be susceptible to several antimicrobial agents, one antibiotic can provide practical benefits over other agents.

PERSONALIZED PHARMACOTHERAPY

Individualized therapy is important in the treatment of osteomyelitis and infectious arthritis. Patient quality of life can be significantly diminished if long-term sequelae develop, such as impaired joint motion or draining sinus tracts, or if amputation is required. Patient demographics, infection characteristics (eg, infecting organism and its susceptibility patterns), treatment cost, and quality-of-life issues all play a major role in evaluating individualized treatment alternatives (oral therapy or home antibiotic treatment) rather than requiring patients to remain hospitalized to receive 4 to 6 weeks of parenteral antibiotics. In addition, adverse events commonly occur with prolonged outpatient parenteral antibiotic therapy. One study in 45 children noted that 85.7% of patients receiving vancomycin had adverse drug events and 42.9% of patients required the drug be discontinued.[47] This analysis also noted that cefazolin had the lowest rate of adverse drug events in this population. Monitoring is important to ensure that personalized therapy is effective to both cure the infection as well as minimize the risk for complications.

EVALUATION OF THERAPEUTIC OUTCOMES

Monitoring of the Pharmaceutical Care Plan

9 Patients with bone and joint infections must be monitored closely. Table 118-6 summarizes a pharmaceutical care monitoring protocol. An assessment of a therapy's success or failure is based on the patient's clinical findings and laboratory values. The clinical signs of inflammation, such as swelling, tenderness, pain, redness, and fever, should resolve with appropriate therapy. Initially, the clinical signs are assessed daily until improvement and then periodically thereafter. Elevations in WBC count also should decline gradually. The ESR usually is determined weekly. Elevations in the C-reactive protein or ESR may not return to normal until after several weeks of therapy. The WBC count usually is obtained once or twice per week until it returns to the normal range. If by the end of the 4- to 6-week antibiotic course the clinical findings of osteomyelitis are no longer present and the C-reactive protein and ESR are within normal limits, the patient can be considered a clinical cure. Patients can relapse, however, after initially appearing to be cured. No relapse for 1 year generally is considered a complete cure.

If a patient fails to resolve the clinical signs and symptoms of inflammation after appropriate empirical antibiotics, suspicion for an abscess should be raised and imaging by MRI and surgical debridement may be needed. In addition, the patient might have a resistant or an atypical infecting organism that may require a modification of the antibiotic therapy. It is especially important to identify the infecting organism and its susceptibility pattern. Follow-up cultures at subsequent debridements can be useful to assess the antibiotic therapy.

TABLE 118-6 Monitoring Protocol

Parameter	Frequency	Notes
Culture and susceptibility	At initiation of treatment	
White blood cell count	One time per week until within normal range	
C-reactive protein or erythrocyte sedimentation rate	Weekly	May not decrease to normal range until several weeks of therapy
Clinical signs of inflammation (redness, pain, swelling, tenderness, and fever)	Daily during initiation of therapy	
Adherence of outpatient therapy	Reinforce before starting oral therapy and with each healthcare visit	Adherence is critical if treatment is to be successful
Complete blood count	Weekly	Certain antimicrobial agents may cause blood dyscrasias when used for long term therapy (eg, linezolid, trimethoprim/sulfamethoxazole)

Despite apparently adequate surgery and antibiotics, some patients can fail therapy and have recurrent relapses in their infection.[39] This scenario is more common in those with chronic osteomyelitis. These patients can require long-term oral suppressive antimicrobial therapy to keep the infection under control.

ABBREVIATIONS

ESR	erythrocyte sedimentation rate
MRSA	methicillin-resistant *Staphylococcus aureus*
WBC	white blood cell
PO	orally
VO	vertebral osteomyelitis

REFERENCES

1. Waldvogel FA, Medoff G, Swartz MN. Osteomyelitis: A review of clinical features, therapeutic considerations and unusual aspects. *N Engl J Med* 1970;282:198-206, 260-266, 316-322.
2. Harik NS, Smeltzer MS. Management of acute hematogenous osteomyelitis in children. *Expert Anti Infect Ther* 2010;8:175-181.
3. Berbari EF, Kanj S, Kowalski TJ, et al. 2015 Infectious Disease Society of America (IDSA) Clinical Practice Guidelines for the diagnosis and treatment of native vertebral osteomyelitis in adults. *Clin Infect Dis* 2015;61:859-63.
4. Dartnell J, Ramachandran M, Katchburian M. Haematogenous acute and subacute paediatric osteomyelitis. *J Bone Joint Surg Br* 2012;94:584-595.
5. Park K, Cho OH, Jung M, et al. Clinical characteristics and outcomes of hematogenous vertebral osteomyelitis caused by Gram-negative bacteria. *J Infect* 2014;69:42-50.
6. Mathews CJ, Weston VC, Jones A, Field M, Coakley G. Bacterial septic arthritis in adults. *Lancet* 2010;375:846-855.
7. Garcia-De La Torre I, Nava-Zavala A. Gonococcal and nongonococcal arthritis. *Rheum Dis Clin North Am* 2009;35:63-73.
8. Garcia-Arias M, Balsa A, Mola EM. Septic arthritis. *Best Pract Res Clin Rheumatol* 2011;25:407-421.
9. Horowitz DL, Katzap E, Horowitz S, Barilla-LaBarca ML. Approach to septic arthritis. *Am Fam Physician* 2011;84:653-660.
10. Zimmerli W. Vertebral osteomyelitis. *N Engl J Med* 2010;362:1022-1029.
11. Pigrau C, Rodriguez-Pardo D, Fernandez-Hidalgo N, et al. Health care associated hematogenous pyogenic vertebral osteomyelitis: A severe and potentially preventable infectious disease. *Medicine* 2015;94(3):e365.
12. Howell WR, Goulston C. Osteomyelitis: an update for hospitalists. *Hosp Pract (Minneap)* 2011;39:153-160.
13. Copley LAB. Pediatric musculoskeletal infection: trends and antibiotic recommendations. *J Am Acad Orthop Surg* 2009;17:618-626.
14. Conrad DA. Acute hematogenous osteomyelitis. *Pediatr Rev* 2010;31:464-471.
15. Bleich AT, Sheffield JS, Wendel GD, Sigman A, Cunningham FG. Disseminated gonococcal infection in women. *Obstet Gynecol* 2012;119(3);597-602.
16. Jaramillo D. Infection: musculoskeletal. *Pediatr Radiol* 2011;41(Suppl 1): S127-S134.
17. Elamurugan TP, Jagdish S, Kate V, Parija SC. Role of bone biopsy specimen culture in the management of diabetic foot osteomyelitis. *Int J Surg* 2011;9:214-216.
18. Bernard L, Uckay I, Vuagnat A, et al. Two consecutive deep sinus tract cultures predict the pathogen of osteomyelitis. *Int J Infect Dis* 2010;14:e390-e393.
19. Carpenter CR, Schuur JD, Everett WW, Pines JM. Evidence-based diagnostics: adult septic arthritis. *Acad Emerg Med* 2011;18:781-786.
20. Garcia-Lechuz J, Bouza E. Treatment recommendations and strategies for the management of bone and joint infections. *Expert Opin Pharmacother* 2009;10:35-55.
21. Rao N, Ziran BH, Lipsky BA. Treating osteomyelitis: antibiotics and surgery. *Plast Reconstr Surg* 2011;127(Suppl 1):S177-S187.
22. Dodwell ER. Osteomyelitis and septic arthritis in children: current concepts. *Curr Opin Pediat* 2013;25:58-63.
23. Sendi P, Zimmerli W. Antimicrobial treatment concepts for orthopaedic device-related infection. *Clin Microbial Infect* 2012;18:1176-1184.
24. Parvizi J, Adeli B, Zmistowski BS, Restrepo C, Greenwald AS. Management of periprosthetic joint infection: The current knowledge. *J Bone Joint Surg Am* 2012;94:e104(1-9).

25. Kaplan SL. Recent lessons for the management of bone and joint infections. *J Infect* 2014;68:S51-S56.
26. Pendleton A, Kocher MS. Methicillin-resistant *Staphylococcus aureus* bone and joint infections in children. *J Am Acad Orthop Surg* 2015;23:29-37.
27. Pea F. Penetration of antibacterials into bone. What do we really need to know for optimal prophylaxis and treatment of bone and joint infections. *Clin Pharmacokinet* 2009;48:125-127.
28. Hatzenbuehler J, Pulling TJ. Diagnosis and Management of Osteomyelitis. *Am Fam Physician* 2011;84(9):1027-1033.
29. Peltola H, Paakkonen M. Acute Osteomyelitis in children. *N Engl J Med* 2014;370:352-360.
30. Zaoutis T, Localio AR, Leckerman K, et al. Prolonged intravenous therapy versus early transition to oral antimicrobial therapy for acute osteomyelitis in children. *Pediatrics* 2009;123:636-642.
31. Daver NG, Shelburne SA, Atmar RL, et al. Oral step-down therapy is comparable to intravenous therapy for *Staphylococcus aureus* osteomyelitis. *J Infect* 2007;54:539-544.
32. White CN, Rolston KV. Osteomyelitis: Drug bioavailability and bone penetration are key. *J Am Acad Physician Assist* 2012;25(7);21-27.
33. Howard-Jones AR, Isaacs D. Systematic review of systemic antibiotic treatment for children with chronic and sub-acute pyogenic osteomyelitis. *J Paediatr Child Health* 2010;46:736-741.
34. Peltola H, Paakkonen M, Kallio P, Kallio MJT. Prospective, randomized trial of 10 days versus 30 days of antimicrobial treatment, including a short-term course of parenteral therapy, for childhood septic arthritis. *Clin Infect Dis* 2009;48:1201-1210.
35. Haidar R, Boghossian AD, Atiyeh B. Duration of post-surgical antibiotics in chronic osteomyelitis: Empiric or evidence-based? *Int J Infect Dis* 2010;14:e752-e758.
36. Paakkonen M, Peltola H. Simplifying the treatment of acute bacterial bone and joint infections in children. *Expert Rev Anti Infect Ther* 2011;9:1125-1131.
37. Thompson S, Townsend R. Pharmacological agents for soft tissue and bone infected with MRSA: Which agent and for how long? *Injury. Int J Care Injured* 2011;42:S5, S7-S10.
38. Bernard L, Dinh A, Ghout I, et al. Antibiotic treatment for 6 weeks versus 12 weeks in patients with pyogenic vertebral osteomyelitis: An open-label, non-inferitority, randomized, controlled trial. *Lancet* 2015;385:875-882.
39. Lora-Tamayo J, Murillo O. Shorter treatments for vertebral osteomyelitis. *Lancet* 2015;385:836-837.
40. Chihara S, Segreti J. Osteomyelitis. *Dis Mon* 2010;56:6-31.
41. Marti-Carvajal AJ, Agreda-Perez LH, Cortes-Jofre M. Antibiotics for treating osteomyelitis in people with sickle cell disease. *Cochrane Database of Systematic Reviews* 2009;2:CD007175.
42. Coiffier G, Alber JD, Arvieux C, Guggenbuhl P. Optimizing combination rifampin therapy for staphylococcal osteoarticular infections. *Joint Bone Spine* 2013;80:11-17.
43. Larikov D, Demian H, Rubin D, et al. Choice and doses of anti-bacterial agents for cement spacers in treatment of prosthetic joint infections: review of published studies. *Clin Infect Dis* 2012;55(11): 1474-1480.
44. Luu A, Syed F, Raman G, et al. Two-stage arthroplasty for prosthetic joint infection: A systematic review of acute kidney injury, systemic toxicity and infection control. *J Arthroplasty* 2013;28:1490-1498.e1.
45. Noto MJ. Detectable serum tobramycin levels in patients with renal dysfunction and recent placement of antibiotic-impregnated cement knee or hip spacers. *Clin Infect Dis* 2014;58(12):1783-1784.
46. Peltola H, Paakkonen M, Kallio P, Kallio MJ. Short- versus long-term antimicrobial treatment for acute hematogenous osteomyelitis of childhood: Prospective, randomized trial on 131 culture-positive cases. *Pediatr Infect Dis J* 2010;29:1123-1128.
47. Faden D, Faden HS. The high rate of adverse drug events in children receiving prolonged outpatient parenteral antibiotic therapy for osteomyelitis. *Pediatr Infect Dis J* 2009;28:539-541.

119

Sepsis and Septic Shock

S. Lena Kang-Birken

KEY CONCEPTS

1. Gram-negative organisms are isolated in 50% to 62% of patients with severe sepsis or septic shock, followed by gram-positive bacteria in 37% to 47%, anaerobic organisms in 5%, and fungi in 8% to 19%.
2. Candidemia is a major cause of morbidity and mortality. *Candida albicans* remains the most common pathogen (45.6%); however, non–*albicans Candida* species collectively is more frequently isolated (54.4%).
3. Sepsis presents a complex pathophysiology, characterized by the activation of multiple overlapping and interacting cascades leading to systemic inflammation, a procoagulant state, and decreased fibrinolysis.
4. Mortality rates with sepsis are higher for older patients with preexisting disease, intensive care unit (ICU) care, and multiple organ failure.
5. Prompt initiation of one or more parenteral antibiotics within 1 hour of recognition of septic shock and severe sepsis without septic shock is required and the regimen should be assessed daily for potential de-escalation.
6. A significant volume of fluid leaks from the vasculature occurs with sepsis, and initial fluid resuscitation with large volumes of fluid is required. Crystalloid solutions are generally recommended for fluid resuscitation because of the absence of any clear benefit with colloids solutions in addition to the lower cost of crystalloids.
7. Norepinephrine is the preferred vasopressor to correct hypotension in septic shock, and epinephrine should be considered the first alternative to patients intolerant to norepinephrine.
8. Implementation of protocolized, quantitative resuscitation bundle within 6 hours of recognition of sepsis-induced hypoperfusion has been shown to decrease the mortality rates as well as the ICU length of stay.
9. A blood glucose level less than 180 mg/dL (10 mmol/L) is recommended for the majority of critically ill patients to reduce morbidity and mortality without the detrimental effects associated with hypoglycemia.
10. IV hydrocortisone is recommended for adult patients with septic shock whose blood pressure is unresponsive to fluids and vasopressors.

Sepsis and severe sepsis continue to pose major healthcare burden. The Nationwide Inpatient Sample years 2003 to 2009 reported hospitalizations with sepsis claims including septicemia sepsis, severe sepsis, and septic shock increased from 359 per 100,000 US residents to 535 per 100,000, a 49% increase.[1] Despite aggressive medical care and advances, overall in-hospital deaths remains at 15% to 40%, with over one-third of patients discharged to a long-term care facility.[2] Given the public health and financial burden, there is a vital need for clinicians to comprehend the pathophysiology and the optimal management approaches for acutely ill patients with severe sepsis or septic shock.

DEFINITIONS

Periods of bacteremia, systemic inflammatory response syndrome (SIRS), sepsis, severe sepsis, septic shock, or multiple-organ dysfunction syndrome (MODS) often overlap, and they signify an important continuum of progressive physiologic decline (Fig. 119-1). *Severe sepsis* refers to patients with an acute organ dysfunction, such as acute renal failure or respiratory failure. Sepsis-induced hypotension is defined as a systolic blood pressure less than 90 mm Hg or mean arterial pressure (MAP) less than 70 mm Hg (<9.3 kPa) (Table 119-1).[3] *Septic shock* refers to sepsis patients with sepsis-induced hypotension that is refractory to adequate fluid resuscitation, thus requiring vasopressor administration. Sepsis-induced tissue hypoperfusion is defined as infection-induced hypotension, elevated lactate, or oliguria.[3,4]

INFECTION SITES AND PATHOGENS

Predisposing factors of septic shock include age, nonwhite ethnic origin in North Americans, comorbid diseases especially chronic obstructive pulmonary disease, malignancy, immunodeficiency or immunocompromised state, chronic organ failure, alcohol dependence, and genetic factors.[1,5,6] Male gender has been associated with higher incidence of sepsis and severe sepsis in the past. However, the difference between the genders appears to be diminishing.[1,2]

The primary sites of microbiologically documented infections that lead to sepsis are the respiratory tract (39%-50%), intra-abdominal space (8%-16%), and urinary tract (5%-37%).[1,2,7-9]

Gram-Positive Bacterial Sepsis

1 In international studies, gram-negative organisms were isolated in 50% to 62% of patients with severe sepsis or septic shock, gram-positive bacteria in 37% to 47%, anaerobic organisms in 5%, and fungi in 8% to 19%.[7,9] The most common gram-positive organisms are *Staphylococcus aureus, Streptococcus pneumoniae*, coagulase-negative staphylococci, and *Enterococcus* species.[8-11] *S. aureus* bacteremia is associated with an overall mortality rate ranging between 10% and 30%.[12] Factors related to a higher mortality include older age, shock, preexisting renal failure, and the presence of a rapidly fatal underlying disease. *Staphylococcus epidermidis* is most often related to infected intravascular devices, artificial heart valves and stents, and the use of IV and intra-arterial catheters. Enterococci are isolated most commonly isolated from blood cultures following a prolonged hospitalization and treatment with broad-spectrum cephalosporins.

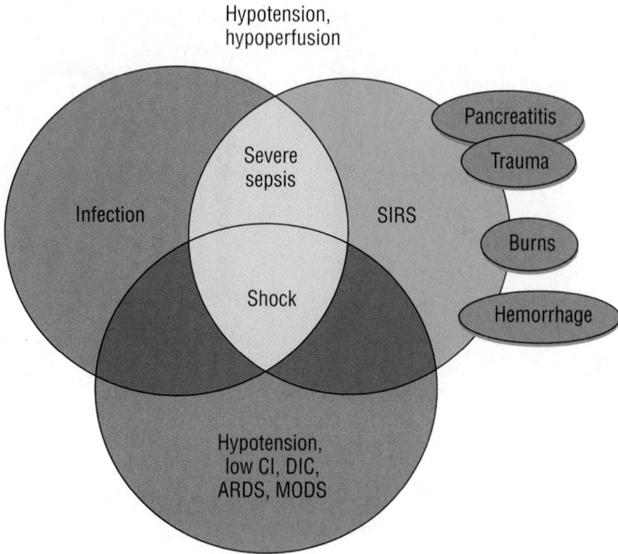

FIGURE 119-1 Relationship of infection, systemic inflammatory response syndrome (SIRS), sepsis, severe sepsis, and septic shock. (ARDS, acute respiratory distress syndrome; CI, cardiac index; DIC, disseminated intravascular coagulation; MODS, multiple-organ dysfunction syndrome.)

TABLE 119-1 Definitions Related to Sepsis

Condition	Definition
Bacteremia (fungemia)	Presence of viable bacteria (fungi) in the bloodstream
Infection	Inflammatory response to invasion of normally sterile host tissue by the microorganisms
SIRS	Systemic inflammatory response to a variety of clinical insults, which can be infectious or noninfectious. The response is manifested by two or more of the following conditions: temperature >38°C (>100.4°F) or <36°C (<96.8°F); HR >90 beats/min; RR >20 breaths/min or $PaCO_2$<32 mm Hg (<4.3 kPa); WBC >12,000 cells/mm^3 (>12 × 10^9/L), <4,000 cells/mm^3 (<4 × 10^9/L), or >10% (>0.10) immature (band) forms
Sepsis	SIRS secondary to suspected or documented infection Additional criteria include general variables (altered mental status, positive fluid balance of >20 mL/kg over 24 hours, hyperglycemia >120 mg/dL [>6.7 mmol/L]); inflammatory variables (plasma C-reactive protein/procalcitonin >2 SD above normal value); hemodynamic variables (arterial hypotension <90mm Hg (<12.0 kPa) or MAP <70 mm Hg (<9.3 kPa), elevated mixed venous oxygen saturation of >70% (>0.70); CI >3.5 L/min (>0.058 L/s); organ-dysfunction variables (arterial hypoxemia; acute oliguria of <0.5ml/kg/hr or 45 ml/hr for at least 2 hr, creatinine increase >0.5 mg/dL (>0.44 μmol/L), coagulation abnormalities, paralytic ileus, platelets <100,000 /mm^3 (<100 × 10^9/L), bilirubin >4 mg/dL (>68 μmol/L); tissue-perfusion variable (hyperlactatemia >1 mmol/L, decreased capillary refill)
Severe sepsis	Sepsis associated with one or more organ dysfunctions, hypoperfusion, or hypotension. Hypoperfusion and perfusion abnormalities may include but not limited to arterial hypoxemia (PaO_2/FiO_2<300) lactic acidosis, oliguria, increase in creatinine, coagulation abnormalities (INR>1.5), and elevated bilirubin
Septic shock	Sepsis with persistent hypotension despite fluid resuscitation (intravenous fluid of 30 mL/kg) or hyperlactatemia >1 mmol/L

CI, cardiac index; HR, heart rate; INR, international normalized ratio; RR, respiratory rate; SD, standard deviation; SIRS, systemic inflammatory response syndrome; T, temperature; WBC, white blood cell (count).

Adapted from Levy MM, Fink MP, Marshall JC, et al. 2001 SCCM/ESICM/ACCP/ATS/SIS International Sepsis Definitions Conference. Crit Care Med 2003;31:1250-1256.

Gram-Negative Bacterial Sepsis

Escherichia coli (8%-30%), *Klebsiella* species (8%-23%), and *Pseudomonas aeruginosa* (7%-18%) are the most commonly isolated gram-negative microorganisms in sepsis.[8-11,13,14] Other common gram-negative pathogens include *Serratia* species, *Enterobacter* species, and *Proteus* species. *P. aeruginosa* and *Acinetobacter* species are more likely to be associated with prior antibiotic exposure.[13]

A greater proportion of patients with gram-negative bacteremia develop sepsis, and also more likely to produce septic shock in comparison to gram-positive organisms, 50% versus 25%, respectively.[8,9,11] Specifically, *P. aeruginosa* sepsis has been associated with a higher mortality rate.[9,13] Mortality increased significantly with increasing severity of sepsis (3.5% for sepsis, 9.9% in severe sepsis, and 28,6% in septic shock).[14] Furthermore, severity of any underlying conditions is another major factor associated with the outcome of gram-negative sepsis. Patients with rapidly fatal conditions, such as acute leukemia, aplastic anemia, cirrhosis, and human immunodeficiency virus (HIV) have a significantly worse prognosis than those patients with nonfatal underlying conditions such as diabetes mellitus and chronic renal insufficiency.[2]

Anaerobic and Miscellaneous Bacterial Sepsis

Anaerobic bacteria such as *Bacteroides fragilis* and *Clostridium* species are usually considered low-risk organisms for the development of sepsis. If present, anaerobes are often found together with other pathogenic bacteria that are commonly found in sepsis. Polymicrobial infections accounted for 5% to 39% of sepsis.[1,9-11,13] Mortality rates associated with polymicrobial infections are similar to sepsis caused by a single organism. Although some clinicians believe the particular combination of organisms present in polymicrobial sepsis can provide clues to the source of infection, no clear source for the infection can be identified in up to 25% of cases.

Fungal Sepsis

3 Candidemia is among the most common fungal etiologic agents of bloodstream infections. Although *Candida albicans* was the most commonly isolated fungus from blood cultures (45.6%), collectively, non-*albicans Candida* species were more frequently isolated (54.4%).[10-11,15-17] Non-*albicans Candida* species include *C. glabrata* (26%), *C. parapsilosis* (15.7%), *C. tropicalis* (8.1%), and *C. krusei* (2.5%). Other fungi identified as causes of sepsis are *Cryptococcus*, *Coccidioides*, *Fusarium*, and *Aspergillus*.[10] Traditionally, risk factors for fungal infection include abdominal surgery, poorly controlled diabetes mellitus, prolonged granulocytopenia, broad-spectrum antibiotic treatment, corticosteroid treatment, prolonged hospitalization, central venous catheter, total parenteral nutrition, hematologic malignancy, and chronic indwelling bladder (Foley) catheter. A large retrospective analysis also reported patients with candidemia and severe sepsis and septic shock were more likely to have been admitted from nursing homes or transferred from outside hospitals.[17] Recent exposure to azoles is an important risk factor for infection with fluconazole-resistant *Candida* spp.[18] There is a close correlation between antibacterial drug exposure and bloodstream infection with *C. glabrata* and fluconazole-resistant *Candida* isolates.[18]

A multicenter analysis of patients with septic shock due to candidemia between 2009 and 2011 reported overall 30-day mortality rate of 54%. A higher in-hospital mortality was reported (61%) among patients with healthcare-associated candidemia.[16] The highest mortality rate of 52.9% was observed in patients with *C. krusei* candidemia; *C. parapsilosis* candidemia was associated with the lowest 12-week mortality rate (23.7%).

PATHOPHYSIOLOGY

Sepsis is the result of complex interactions among the invading pathogen, the host immune system, and the inflammatory responses. The inflammatory response leads to damage to host tissue, and the anti-inflammatory response causes leukocytes to activate. Once the balance to control the local inflammatory process and to eradicate the invading pathogens is lost, systemic inflammatory response occurs, converting the infection to sepsis, severe sepsis, or septic shock.

Cellular Components for Initiating the Inflammatory Process

The pathophysiologic focus of gram-negative sepsis has been on the lipopolysaccharide component of the gram-negative bacterial cell wall. Commonly referred to as endotoxin, this substance is unique to the outer membrane of the gram-negative cell wall and is generally released with bacterial lysis. Lipid A, the innermost region of the lipopolysaccharide, is highly immunoreactive and is considered responsible for most of the toxic effects. Although lipid A can affect tissues directly, its predominant effect is to activate macrophages and trigger inflammatory cascades critical in the progression to sepsis and septic shock.[19] Endotoxin forms a complex with an endogenous protein called a lipopolysaccharide-binding protein, which then engages the CD14 receptor on the surface of a macrophage. Subsequently, cytokine mediators are activated and released by the macrophages.

In gram-positive sepsis, the exotoxin peptidoglycan on the cell wall surface appears to exhibit proinflammatory activity. Although it competes with lipid A for similar binding sites on CD14, the potency of peptidoglycan is less than that of endotoxin.[19] However, an important feature of gram-positive bacteria such as *S. aureus* and *Streptococcus pyogenes* is the production of potent exotoxins, some of which have been associated with septic shock.

Pro- and Anti-inflammatory Mediators

A complex interaction between proinflammatory and anti-inflammatory mediators plays a major role in the pathogenesis of sepsis. In general, proinflammatory reactions are directed at eliminating invading pathogens and the anti-inflammatory reactions are important for limiting local and systemic tissue injury. The key proinflammatory mediators are tumor necrosis factor-α (TNF-α), interleukin-1 (IL-1), and interleukin-6 (IL-6), which are released by activated macrophages.[19-21] Other mediators that may be important for the pathogenesis of sepsis are interleukin-8 (IL-8), platelet-activating factor (PAF), leukotrienes, and thromboxane A_2.

The TNF-α levels in plasma can be increased in patients with a variety of diseases and in many healthy people. However, there is a correlation of plasma TNF-α levels with the severity of sepsis. It is highly elevated early in the inflammatory response in most patients with sepsis.[20,21] The TNF-α release leads to activation of other cytokines (IL-1 and IL-6) associated with cellular damage. In addition, TNF-α stimulates the release of cyclooxygenase-derived arachidonic acid metabolites (thromboxane A_2 and prostaglandins) that contribute to vascular endothelial damage. Higher levels of IL-6 and IL-8 have been reported in patients with septic shock than those with SIRS.

The significant anti-inflammatory mediators include interleukin-1 receptor antagonist (IL-1RA), IL-4, and IL-10.[19,20,22] These anti-inflammatory cytokines inhibit the production of the proinflammatory cytokines and down regulate some inflammatory cells. Levels of IL-10 and IL-1RA are higher in septic shock than in sepsis, and higher levels are found among nonsurviving patients than in survivors.[20-22]

The activation and secretion of pro- and anti-inflammatory mediators in septic shock occur as a simultaneous immune response as early as the first 24 hours of diagnosis, but the balance between pro- and anti-inflammatory mechanisms determines the degree of inflammation, ranging from local antibacterial activity to systemic tissue toxicity, organ failure, or death.[20,21]

Cascade of Sepsis

3 The cascade leading to development of sepsis is complex and multifactorial, involving causative pathogen (virulence and organism load) and host characteristics (comorbidities and immunosuppression) triggering various mediators and cell lines. Endothelial cells produce a variety of cytokines that mediate a primary mechanism of injury in sepsis. When injured, endothelial cells allow circulating cells such as granulocytes and plasma constituents to enter inflamed tissues, which can result in organ damage.

The microcirculation is affected by sepsis-induced inflammation. The arterioles become less responsive to either vasoconstrictors or vasodilators. The capillaries are less perfused even at the early phases of septic shock, and there is neutrophil infiltration and protein leakage into the venules.[23]

The inflammatory process in sepsis is also directly linked to the coagulation system. Proinflammatory mechanisms that promote sepsis are also procoagulant and antifibrinolytic, whereas fibrinolytic mechanisms can be anti-inflammatory.[24] A key endogenous substance involved in inflammation of sepsis is activated protein C, which enhances fibrinolysis and inhibits inflammation. Levels of protein C are reduced in patients with sepsis.[24]

COMPLICATIONS

Septic shock is the most ominous complication associated with sepsis. Of the patients who presented to the emergency department with sepsis 3.6% progressed to septic shock within 4 hours, and 8.4% progressed to septic shock between 4 and 48 hours.[25] The predictors for progression to septic shock included female gender, non-persistent hypotension, band neutrophils of at least 10% in blood, lactate of at least 4.0 mmol/L, and past medical of coronary artery disease.[25] Septic shock may lead to several complications including disseminated intravascular coagulation (DIC), acute respiratory distress syndrome (ARDS), and multiple organ failure. The organs that failed most frequently in patients with severe sepsis were kidneys (49%), lungs (48%), and heart (42%).[2] The less frequent complications are hematologic failure (18%), metabolic failure (17%), neurologic failure (11%), and hepatic failure (5%).[2] Mortality occurs in approximately half of the patients with septic shock.

Disseminated Intravascular Coagulation

DIC is the inappropriate activation of the clotting cascade that causes formation of microthrombi, resulting in consumption of coagulation factors, organ dysfunction, and bleeding. Sepsis remains the most common cause of DIC, and the incidence of DIC increases as the severity of sepsis increases. In sepsis alone, the incidence was 16% in comparison to 38% in septic shock.[26,27] DIC occurs in up to 50% of patients with gram-negative sepsis, but it is also common in patients with gram-positive sepsis.

DIC begins with the activation and production of the proinflammatory cytokines, such as TNF, IL-1, and IL-6, which appear to be the principal mediators, along with endotoxin. The combination of excessive fibrin formation, compromised fibrin removal from a depressed fibrinolytic system, and endothelial injury result in microvascular thrombosis and DIC.[27]

Complications of DIC vary and depend on the target organ affected and the severity of the coagulopathy. DIC can produce acute renal failure, hemorrhagic necrosis of the gastrointestinal (GI) mucosa, liver failure, acute pancreatitis, ARDS, and pulmonary failure. Furthermore, as the procoagulant state appears to be the key in the pathogenesis of MODS, coagulation dysfunction and MODS often coexist in sepsis.

Acute Respiratory Distress Syndrome

Pulmonary dysfunction, the most common organ dysfunction in sepsis, usually precedes other organs, and it can even initiate the development of SIRS with resultant MODS. Activated neutrophils and platelets adhere to the pulmonary capillary endothelium, initiating multiple inflammatory cascades with a release of a variety of toxic substances. There is diffuse pulmonary endothelial cell injury, increased capillary permeability, and alveolar epithelial cell injury. Consequently, interstitial pulmonary edema occurs that gradually progresses to alveolar flooding and collapse. The end result is loss of functional alveolar volume, impaired pulmonary compliance, and profound hypoxemia.

Coagulation is locally upregulated in the injured lung, whereas fibrinolytic activity is depressed. These abnormalities occur concurrently and favor alveolar fibrin deposition, leading to local inflammation, macrophage migration, and increased vascular permeability. Anticoagulant interventions that block the extrinsic coagulation pathway can protect against the development of pulmonary fibrin deposition as well as lung dysfunction and acute inflammation.[27] Overall, fibrin deposition in the injured lung and abnormalities of coagulation and fibrinolysis are integral to the pathogenesis of ARDS.

Hemodynamic Effects

The hallmark of the hemodynamic effect of sepsis is the hyperdynamic state characterized by high cardiac output and an abnormally low systemic vascular resistance (SVR).[23,28] TNF-α and endotoxin directly depress cardiovascular function. Endotoxin depresses left ventricular (LV) function independent of changes in LV volume or vascular resistance. Myocardial dysfunction is common in severe sepsis and septic shock, affecting 64% of patients, and involves LV in more than half of the patients.[28]

Persistent hypotension raises concern for the balance of oxygen delivery (DO_2) to the tissues and oxygen consumption (VO_2) by the tissues. Sepsis results in a distributive shock characterized by inappropriately increased blood flow to particular tissues at the expense of other tissues, which is independent of specific tissue oxygen needs. This perfusion defect is accentuated by an increased precapillary atrioventricular shunt. If perfusion decreases, oxygen extraction increases, and the arteriovenous oxygen gradient widens. Cellular DO_2 is decreased, but VO_2 remains unaffected. When increased oxygen demand occurs without increased blood flow, the increased VO_2 is compensated by increased oxygen extraction. If perfusion decreases sufficiently in the face of high metabolic demands, then the reserve DO_2 can be exceeded, and tissue ischemia results. Significant tissue ischemia leads to organ dysfunction and failure. Therefore, systemic DO_2 relative to VO_2 should be optimized by increasing oxygen delivery or decreasing oxygen consumption in a hypermetabolic patient.

Acute Renal Failure

Early acute kidney injury occurs in 42% to 64% of adult patients with sepsis and septic shock.[29] Without normal urine output, fluid overload in extravascular space including the lungs develops, leading to impairment of pulmonary gas exchange and severe hypoxemia. Consequently, compromised oxygen delivery exacerbates peripheral ischemia and organ damage. Adequate renal perfusion and a trial of loop diuretics should be initiated promptly in oliguric or anuric patients with MODS along with dialysis to facilitate volume and electrolytes.

CLINICAL PRESENTATION

The clinical features of sepsis vary significantly depending on multiple factors including the patient's underlying health status, site and severity of infection, and time course of sepsis before therapy. Table 119-2 lists some of the common clinical features of sepsis. The initial clinical presentation can be referred to as signs and symptoms of early sepsis, defined as the first 6 hours. They are typically fever, chills, and change in mental status. Hypothermia can occur with a systemic infection, and this is often associated with a poor prognosis.[30] In patients with sepsis caused by gram-negative bacilli, hyperventilation can occur even before fever and chills, and it can lead to respiratory alkalosis as the earliest metabolic change.

Progression of uncontrolled sepsis leads to clinical evidence of organ system dysfunction as represented by the signs and symptoms attributed to late sepsis. With the exception of rapidly progressing cases as in meningococcemia, *P aeruginosa*, or *Aeromonas* infection, the onset of shock is somewhat delayed and usually follows a period of several hours of hemodynamic instability. Oliguria often follows hypotension. Increased glycolysis with impaired clearance of the resulting lactate by the liver and kidneys and tissue hypoxia because of hypoperfusion result in elevated lactate levels, contributing to metabolic acidosis. Altered glucose metabolism, including impaired gluconeogenesis and excessive insulin release, is evidenced by either hyperglycemia or hypoglycemia.

PROGNOSIS

4 As the patient progresses from SIRS to sepsis, severe sepsis, or septic shock, mortality increases in a stepwise fashion. Mortality rates are higher for patients with advanced age, preexisting disease, including chronic obstructive pulmonary disease, neoplasm, and HIV disease, intensive care unit (ICU) care, more failed organs, positive blood cultures, and *Pseudomonas* species infection.[1,2,12] The highest mortality was seen in patients with intra-abdominal infection secondary to ischemic bowel (75%) whereas the source associated with the lowest hospital mortality was obstructive uropathy-associated urinary tract infection (26%).[7] Mortality from severe sepsis and MODS is most closely related to the number of dysfunctioning organs. As the number of failing organs increased from two to five, mortality increased from 29% to 65% (Fig. 119-2).[2] Duration of organ dysfunction can also affect the overall mortality rate.

TABLE 119-2 Signs and Symptoms Associated with Sepsis

Early Sepsis	Late Sepsis
Fever or hypothermia	Lactic acidosis
Rigors, chills	Oliguria
Tachycardia	Leukopenia
Tachypnea	DIC
Nausea, vomiting	Myocardial depression
Hyperglycemia	Pulmonary edema
Myalgia	Hypotension (shock)
Lethargy, malaise	Hypoglycemia
Proteinuria	Azotemia
Hypoxia	Thrombocytopenia
Leukocytosis	ARDS
Hyperbilirubinemia	GI hemorrhage
Delirium	Coma

ARDS, acute respiratory distress syndrome; DIC, disseminated intravascular coagulation.

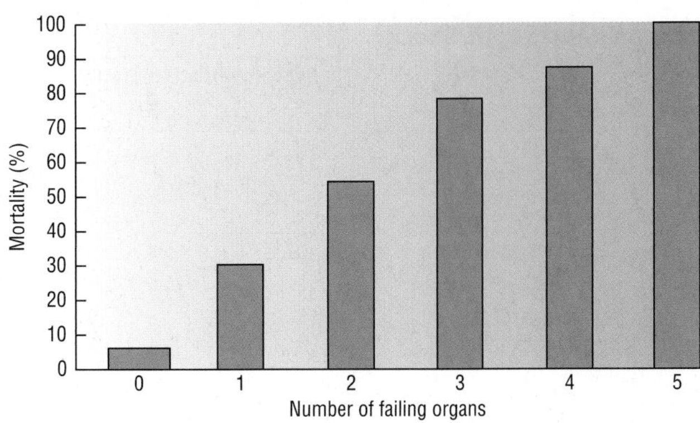

FIGURE 119-2 Mortality related to the number of failing organs.

An elevated lactate concentration of more than 4 mmol/L in the presence of SIRS significantly increases ICU admission rates, and persistent elevations in lactate for more than 24 hours are associated with an increased mortality rate. Furthermore, 28-day mortality rate was the highest (44.8%) among patients with septic shock and hyperlactatemia more than 2.5 mmol/L, followed by hyperlactatemia without vasopressor need (35.3%), and no hyperlactemia with vasopressor need (27.7%). Hyperlactemia increased the risk of 28-day mortality independent of vasopressor need (odds ratio 3.0, 95% confidence interval 2.1-4.1 for lactate of >4 mmol/L).[31]

Diagnosis and Identification of Pathogen

The presence of clinical features suggesting sepsis should prompt further evaluation of the patient. In addition to obtaining a careful history of any underlying conditions and recent travel, injury, animal exposure, infection, or use of antibiotics, a complete physical examination should be performed to determine the source of the infection.

A collection of specimens should be sent for culture prior to initiating any antimicrobial therapy. Minimally two sets of blood cultures (both aerobic and anaerobic bottles) should be collected without temporal separation between the sets.[3,32] With suspected catheter-related infection, a pair of blood cultures should be drawn through every lumen of each vascular access device.[32] In severe community-acquired pneumonia, blood cultures and respiratory secretions must be obtained. Urinary antigen detection of *Legionella* sero group 1 is recommended during outbreaks. To document a soft tissue infection, a Gram stain and bacterial culture of any obvious wound exudates should be performed. A needle aspiration of a closed infection such as cellulitis or abscess may be needed for stain and bacterial culture. In abdominal infections, fluid collections identified by imaging studies should be aspirated for Gram stains and aerobic and anaerobic cultures. Development of accurate and rapid identification tests has demonstrated positive impact on prescribing appropriate therapy in bloodstream infections such as methicillin-resistant *Staphylococcus aureus* (MRSA) and *Candida* spp.[3,33,34] The surviving sepsis guidelines recommend the use of 1,3 β-D-glucan assay in case of invasive candidiasis.[3]

A lumbar puncture is indicated with mental alteration, severe headache, or a seizure, assuming that there are no focal cranial lesions identified by computed tomography (CT) scan. Further tests may be indicated to assess any systemic organ dysfunction caused by severe sepsis. The laboratory tests should include hemoglobin, white blood cell (WBC) count with differential, platelet count, complete chemistry profile, coagulation parameters, serum lactate, and arterial blood gases. The potential role of biomarkers such as procalcitonin (PCT) levels or C-reactive protein for diagnosis of infection in patients with severe sepsis remain undefined as there is no definitive way to discriminate the acute inflammatory pattern of sepsis from other generalized inflammation.[3]

TREATMENT

In 2012, a "surviving sepsis" campaign guideline for management of severe sepsis and septic shock updated the earlier publication of an international effort to increase awareness and improve outcome in severe sepsis.[3,35] The primary goals of therapy for patients with sepsis are (a) timely diagnosis and identification of the pathogen, (b) rapid elimination of the source of infection medically and/or surgically, (c) early initiation of aggressive antimicrobial therapy, (d) interruption of pathogenic sequence leading to septic shock, and (e) avoidance of organ failure. Supportive care such as stress ulcer prophylaxis and nutritional support is important to prevent complications during the stay in the ICU. Table 119-3 describes the summary of the surviving sepsis campaign treatment recommendations.

Elimination of the Source of Infection

After the source of infection is identified, prompt efforts to eradicate that source should be made.[3] With an infected intravascular catheter, the catheter should be removed and cultured. Urinary tract catheters should be removed if association with sepsis is suspected. Suspicion of soft tissue (cellulitis or wound infection) or bone involvement should lead to aggressive debridement of the affected area. Evidence of an abscess or sepsis associated with any intraabdominal pathology should prompt surgical intervention.

Antimicrobial Therapy

5 The Surviving Sepsis Campaign guidelines recommended starting IV administration of one or more antibiotics within 1 hour of recognition of septic shock and severe sepsis without septic shock.[3] Early administration (within 1 hour vs 6 hours of diagnosis) of broad-spectrum antibiotics was independently associated with lower hospital mortality in patients with severe sepsis and septic shock, regardless of the number of organ failure.[36,37] Delays in the initiation of effective antimicrobial therapy especially after the onset of hypotension were significant predictors of mortality.[38] In addition to the timing of the empiric antibiotic, administration of appropriate antibiotic, especially for multidrug-resistant bacteria has a great impact in reducing mortality.[14,39,40] Inappropriate initial antimicrobial therapy occurred in about 20% of patients with septic shock, and was associated with a fivefold reduction in survival in comparison to those who received appropriate therapy (52.0% vs 10.3%, respectively).[11] Therefore, early administration of appropriate antimicrobial therapy is critical in the treatment of severe sepsis and septic shock.

Pharmacokinetics of Antimicrobial Agents in Critically Ill Patients

Pathophysiologic changes in sepsis can affect drug distribution, and adjusted dosing regimens are required in critically ill patients with sepsis.[41] Initially, high creatinine clearance can be seen in patients with normal serum creatinine because of increased renal preload. Volume of distribution can increase because of fluid accumulation from leaky capillaries and/or altered protein binding. Consequently, some antimicrobial agents, especially for hydrophilic antimicrobials including aminoglycosides, β-lactams, carbapenems, and vancomycin can result in lower peak serum concentrations with usual doses.[42] However, as sepsis progresses, organ perfusion decreases because of significant myocardial depression and leads to multiple organ dysfunction. Consequently, clearance of antimicrobial agents is decreased, prolonging the elimination half-life and accumulation of metabolites. Hence, in addition to selecting the most appropriate antimicrobial agents, a clinician must ensure effective antibiotic usage, such as proper dosing, interval of administration, optimal

TABLE 119-3 Evidence-Based Treatment Recommendations for Sepsis and Septic Shock

Recommendations	Recommendation Grades[a]
Initial Resuscitation (First 6 Hours)	
Quantitative resuscitation of patients with sepsis-induced tissue hypoperfusion, CVP 8-12 mm Hg (1.1-1.6 kPa), MAP ≥65 mm Hg (≥8.6 kPa), urine output > 0.5 mL/kg/hr, $SCVO_2$ ≥70% (≥0.70)	1C
Antibiotic Therapy	
IV broad-spectrum antibiotic within 1 hour of diagnosis of septic shock and severe sepsis against likely bacterial/fungal pathogens	1B
Reassess antibiotic therapy daily with microbiology and clinical data to narrow coverage (de-escalation)	1B
Combination empirical therapy for neutropenic patients with severe sepsis and patients with difficult-to-treat, multidrug-resistant bacterial pathogens such as *Acinetobacter* and *Pseudomonas* spp. for no more than 3-5 days and then de-escalate	2B
Fluid Therapy	
Crystalloids as the initial fluid of choice	1B
Minimum of 30 mL/kg of crystalloids for initial fluid challenge, but more rapid and greater amount may be needed	1C
Albumin when patients require substantial amounts of crystalloids	2C
Vasopressors	
Initiate vasopressor therapy to maintain MAP ≥65 mm Hg (≥8.6 kPa)	1C
Norepinephrine as the first choice vasopressor	1B
Epinephrine when an additional agent is needed to maintain adequate blood pressure	2B
Dopamine as an alternative vasopressor to norepinephrine in selective patients with low risk of tachyarrhythmia and bradycardia	2C
Inotropic Therapy	
Use dobutamine up to 20 mcg/kg/min or added to vasopressor when cardiac output remains low or ongoing signs of hypoperfusion despite adequate MAP	1C
Glucose Control	
Use insulin dosing protocol in ICU patients when 2 consecutive blood glucose levels are >180 mg/dL (>10 mmol/L), targeting an upper blood glucose <180 mg/dL (≤10 mmol/L)	1A
Steroids	
IV hydrocortisone 200 mg per day for septic shock only when hypotension remains poorly responsive to adequate fluid resuscitation and vasopressors	2C
Hydrocortisone should be tapered when vasopressors are no longer required	2D
Deep Vein Thrombosis Prophylaxis	
Use daily low-molecular-weight heparin and intermittent pneumatic compression device whenever possible	1B
If creatinine clearance is <30 mL/min (<0.5 mL/s), use unfractionated heparin or dalteparin	1A, 1A
If heparin is contraindicated, use mechanical prophylactic treatment	2C
Stress Ulcer Prophylaxis	
Stress ulcer prophylaxis should be given to patients who have bleeding risk factors	1B
Proton pump inhibitors are preferred over H2 receptor blockers	2C

CVP, central venous pressure; MAP, mean arterial pressure.

[a]Grades of Recommendation, Assessment, Development, and Evaluation (GRADE) system: a structured system for rating quality of evidence and grading strength of recommendation in clinical practice. Quality of evidence: high (grade A), moderate (grade B), low (grade C), or very low (grade D). Strength of recommendation: strong (grade 1) or weak (grade 2).

Adapted from Dellinger RP, Levy MM, Rhodes A, et al. Surviving sepsis campaign: International guidelines for management of severe sepsis and septic shock: 2012. Crit Care Med 2013;41:580-637.

duration of treatment, monitoring of drug levels when appropriate, and avoidance of unwanted drug interactions. The lack of adherence to these requirements can lead to suboptimal or excessive tissue concentrations that can promote antibiotic resistance, toxicity, and inadequate efficacy despite appropriate antibiotic selection.

Selection of Antimicrobial Agents

The selection of an empiric regimen should be based on the suspected site of infection, the most likely pathogens, acquisition of the organism from the community or hospital, the patient's immune status, recent exposure to antibiotics within past 3 months, and the antibiotic susceptibility and resistance profile for the institution. All patients should be treated initially with parenteral antibiotics for optimal drug concentrations within the first hour of recognition of severe sepsis after appropriate cultures have been taken.[3] Empiric therapy for an immunocompromised patient should be broad enough to cover likely pathogens and penetrate adequately into the presumed infection site. Once the pathogen and its susceptibility pattern are known, the antimicrobial regimen should be modified accordingly.

Table 119-4 lists antimicrobial regimens that can be used empirically based on the possible source of infection. In the non-neutropenic patient with a urinary tract infection, ceftriaxone or a fluoroquinolone is generally recommended. When there is increased risk of *P. aeruginosa* in sepsis or hospital-acquired infections, an antipseudomonal antibiotic, such as ceftazidime is recommended.[43]

S. pneumoniae is the most common cause of community-acquired pneumonia, and it accounts for approximately 60% of all deaths. The steady prevalence of penicillin-resistant *S pneumoniae* requires empiric use of newer "respiratory" fluoroquinolones. Levofloxacin or moxifloxacin can be used as monotherapy, as they

TABLE 119-4 Empiric Antimicrobial Regimens in Sepsis

Infection (Site or Type)	Antimicrobial Regimen: Community-Acquired	Antimicrobial Regimen: Hospital-Acquired
Urinary tract	Ceftriaxone or ciprofloxacin/levofloxacin	Ciprofloxacin/levofloxacin or ceftriaxone or ceftazidime
Respiratory tract	Levofloxacin[a]/moxifloxacin or ceftriaxone + clarithromycin/azithromycin	Piperacillin/tazobactam or ceftazidime or cefipime + levofloxacin/ciprofloxacin or aminoglycoside carbapenem[b]
Intraabdominal	Ertapenem or ciprofloxacin/levofloxacin + metronidazole	Piperacillin/tazobactam or carbapenem[b]
Skin/soft tissue	Vancomycin or linezolid or daptomycin	Vancomycin + piperacillin/tazobactam
Catheter-related		Vancomycin
Unknown		Piperacillin/tazobactam or ceftazidime/ cefipime or imipenem/meropenem } ± vancomycin

[a]750 mg orally once daily.

[b]Imipenem, meropenem, and doripenem.

offer excellent coverage against penicillin-resistant pneumococci and aerobic gram-negative bacteria, as well as atypical pathogens, including *Legionella pneumophila, Mycoplasma pneumoniae*, and *Chlamydophila pneumoniae*.[44] Addition of a macrolide to a β-lactam empirical therapy improves outcome in severe pneumonia, and clarithromycin and azithromycin are effective against atypical pathogens and better tolerated than erythromycin.[45]

In nosocomial pneumonia, enteric gram-negative bacteria such as *Enterobacter* and *Klebsiella* species and *P. aeruginosa* are the major pathogens in addition to *S. aureus*. If *P. aeruginosa* infection is suspected, β-lactam antipseudomonal agents (ceftazidime or cefepime), antipseudomonal fluoroquinolone (ciprofloxacin or levofloxacin), or an aminoglycoside should be included in the regimen.[3,46] When *S. aureus* is likely to be methicillin-resistant, linezolid may be preferred to vancomycin because of the poor penetration of vancomycin into the lungs, as well as the worldwide emergence of glycopeptide intermediately resistant *S. aureus*.[47] Televancin, a bactericidal, lipoglycopeptide was evaluated in treatment of hospital-acquired pneumonia due to gram-positive organisms against vancomycin in two randomized trials.[48] MRSA was the most commonly isolated microorganism from both respiratory specimens and blood. Televancin was noninferior to vancomycin in terms of clinical responses. However, vancomycin dosing and the subsequent serum trough levels were slightly lower than the current practice. Further use in clinical settings will define its role.

Abdominal infections are frequent causes of sepsis and septic shock in the ICU and are associated with adverse outcomes. ICU mortality was higher in patients with abdominal infections than in those with other infections (29.4% vs 24.2%, $p < 0.001$).[49] Microbiological cultures were positive in 67%, and polymicrobial infections were present in 40.1% of the patients. *E. coli* was isolated most frequently, followed by *Pseudomonas* spp. and *Klebsiella* spp. among gram-negative isolates. *Enterococcus* was the most common gram-positive isolate.[49] Because of widespread resistance of *E. coli* to ampicillin/sulbactam, it is no longer recommended.[50] Emerging fluoroquinolone-resistant *E. coli* and the local prevalence of extended-spectrum β-lactamase-producing strains of *Klebsiella* species and *E. coli* should be considered in choosing empiric therapy. *Bacteroides fragilis*, the major pathogen, has shown uniform susceptibility to metronidazole, carbapenems, and β-lactam/β-lactamase inhibitors.[51] High resistance rates were observed for clindamycin and moxifloxacin (as high as 60% for clindamycin and >80% for moxifloxacin), with relatively stable low resistance (5.4%) for tigecycline.

In addition to surgical intervention, broad-spectrum antibiotics, such as a β–lactam/β-lactamase inhibitor combination agent (piperacillin/tazobactam) is appropriate in treating intraabdominal infections.[50] Carbapenems such as imipenem, meropenem, and doripenem are indicated in the treatment of resistant pathogens, including Enterobacteriaceae and *P. aeruginosa* in critically ill patients.[50]

Skin and soft tissue infections (SSTIs) range from cellulitis to rapidly progressive necrotizing fasciitis, which may be associated with septic shock and toxic shock syndrome. Staphylococci and streptococci long have been the leading causes of SSTIs, but severe SSTIs can be caused also by indigenous aerobes and anaerobes such as *Clostridium* species.[52] Early initiation of appropriate empiric broad-spectrum antimicrobial therapy is essential and should include coverage against MRSA due to the high prevalence of community-associated MRSA strains.[47,52] Vancomycin, daptomycin, and linezolid have comparable clinical efficacy and safety data for complicated skin and skin-structure infections caused by MRSA.[47,53] Daptomycin resulted in a 70% success rate for septic patients bacteremic with MRSA, vancomycin-resistant *Enterococcus* (VRE) *faecium* or coagulase-negative staphylococci.[54]

Combination therapy does not appear to be more effective than monotherapy in reducing organ failure or mortality in low risk patients.[10,55] However, multidrug resistance in sepsis due to gram-negative bacteremia was strongly associated with the receipt of inappropriate empiric therapy and a three-fold increase in the risk of hospital mortality.[40] As such, the greatest benefit of combination therapy appeared to be in patients with *Pseudomonas* or multidrug-resistant gram-negative bacteremia and in neutropenic patients with severe sepsis or septic shock.[3,55-57]

Empiric combination therapy should not be administered for longer than 3 to 5 days.[3] The antimicrobial regimen should be reassessed daily based on the microbiological and clinical data. This creates a potential de-escalation opportunity as part of good antibiotic stewardship to narrow down the spectrum when possible to prevent drug toxicities and the development of nosocomial super infections with *Candida* species, *Clostridium difficile*, or VRE.[3,58] Furthermore, improved patient care outcomes have been demonstrated with such de-escalation of antibiotic therapy.[59] De-escalation of antimicrobial therapy in patients admitted to the ICU with severe sepsis or septic shock had a protective factor.[60] The hospital mortality rate was 27.4% in patients in whom therapy was de-escalated, 32.6% in the category of "no change", and 42.9% in the escalation group.[60]

Antifungal Therapy

Patients with candidemia are generally acutely sicker based on higher APACHE II scores, have presence of septic shock, and mechanical ventilation, and the mortality is significantly higher in comparison to patients with bacteremia (47% vs 28%, respectively).[17]

Septic shock caused by *C. albicans* demonstrated 24.6% survival with initial appropriate therapy but only 4.6% survival without (ninefold decrease).[11] Of the patients with candidemia, delayed appropriate antifungal treatment, especially in presence of septic shock and failure to achieve timely source control were independently associated with a greater risk of hospital mortality.[15,61,62] Hence, accurate and rapid identification of candida is critical in prompt initiation of appropriate therapy.[3,34]

Treatment of invasive candidiasis involves echinocandins, triazoles, or a formulation of amphotericin B. The choice depends on the clinical status of the patient, the fungal species and its susceptibility, relative drug toxicity, presence of organ dysfunction that would affect drug clearance, and the patient's prior exposure to antifungal agents.

Empirical fluconazole therapy for suspected nosocomial bloodstream infections can be appropriate for hospitalized patients at high risk for fungal infections, including those receiving total parenteral nutrition, with bowel perforation, *Candida* colonization, malignancy, emergency surgery, or with persistent or new signs and symptoms of infections despite receiving broad-spectrum antibacterial therapy.[63,64] However, recent exposure to antibiotics and fluconazole have been associated with fluconazole-resistant *Candida* species.[18,65] A global survey evaluating Candida bloodstream infections reported a low overall fluconazole resistance (5% of ICU isolates and 4.4% of non-ICU isolates).[66] *C. glabrata* was the only species to exhibit resistance to both azoles and echinocandins. Of 1,669 bloodstream infection isolates of *C. glabrata* reported resistance to fluconazole was 9.7%, of which 8% to 9.3% were resistant to enchinocandins.[67]

Echinocandins are potent against all *Candida* species, including *C. glabrata, C. krusei*, and *Candida lusitaniae*, as well as *Aspergillus* species. IV caspofungin was equally effective but better tolerated than amphotericin B deoxycholate for invasive candidiasis.[68] In an international, randomized, double-blind trial, micafungin 100-mg was noninferior to caspofungin for the treatment of candidemia and other forms of invasive candidiasis (76.4% vs 72.3%).[69] All three echinocandins appear to be comparable in terms of efficacy, pharmacology, and adverse effects, and the guidelines do not make a distinction or a preferred agent.[64,70]

In general, suspected systemic mycotic infection leading to sepsis in nonneutropenic patients should be treated empirically with parenteral fluconazole or an enchinocandin.[64] However, an echinocandin is preferred for a patient with recent azole exposure or if the patient is clinically unstable because of its greater activity against fluconazole-resistant *Candida* species and non-*albicans* species, including *C. glabrata* and *C. krusei*.[64] In neutropenic patients, an echinocandin, or voriconazole is recommended. Azoles should be avoided for empiric therapy in patients who have received an azole for prophylaxis.[64]

Antiviral Therapy

Early antiviral treatment of suspected or confirmed influenza is recommended among persons with severe influenza or at higher risk for influenza complications. A neuramidase inhibitor such as oseltamivir or zanamivir is generally effective but susceptibility among the seasonal influenza virus should be considered.[3] While cytomegalovirus in the bloodstream has been associated with poor prognosis, the role of cytomegalovirus and other herpesviruses in septic patients in mildly immunocompromised state remains unclear.

Duration of Therapy

The average duration of antimicrobial therapy in a patient with sepsis is 7 to 10 days, and fungal infections can require 10 to 14 days.[3,46,64] However, the duration can be longer in patients with a slow clinical response, undrainable focus of infection, bacteremia with *S. aureus*, or neutropenia. In a neutropenic patient, therapy is usually continued until the patient is no longer neutropenic and has been afebrile for at least 72 hours. After the patient is hemodynamically stable, afebrile for 48 to 72 hours, has a normalizing WBC count, and is able to take oral medications, then a "step-down" from parenteral to oral antibiotics can be considered for the remaining duration of therapy.

PCT is a biomarker that increases in response to endotoxins and inflammatory cytokines that are released during systemic bacterial infections. Hence, PCT has been studied as a marker to initiate and discontinue antibiotics in patients with severe sepsis or septic shock and surgical intensive care patients.[71] However, aside from the shortened length of antibiotic therapy, the survival benefit has not been clearly defined.

Clinical **Controversy...**

The biomarkers such as PCT rise early in severe sepsis by pneumonia and bloodstream infections, and a growing body of evidence supports the use of PCT to differentiate bacterial from viral diagnoses, to help risk stratify patients, and to guide antibiotic therapy decisions in terms of initiating and optimizing duration of therapy.[71,72]

A meta-analysis of randomized controlled clinical trials or cohort studies investigating PCT guided therapy in ICU patients with severe sepsis and septic shock found no significant difference in both hospital mortality and 28-day mortality between PCT-guided therapy and standard treatment groups.[73] Duration of antimicrobial therapy was significantly reduced in favor of PCT group. However, the length of stay in the ICU and in hospital did not differ between groups. The Procalcitonin and Survival Study Group in Demark found no significant difference in ICU mortality between the PCT arm and the standard of care arm with a strategy of escalation of broad-spectrum antimicrobials and intensified diagnostics based on daily PCT measurements.[74] PCT-guided antimicrobial escalation leads to increased use of broad-spectrum antimicrobials, organ-related harm, and prolonged admission to the ICU. Further trials are needed to determine the safety and efficacy of antibiotic sparing PCT strategies in critically ill patients.

Hemodynamic Support

A high cardiac output and a low SVR characterize septic shock. Patients can have hypotension as a result of low SVR and abnormal distribution of blood flow in the microcirculation, resulting in compromised tissue perfusion. Because approximately half of patients with septic shock die of multiple organ system failure, they should be monitored carefully, and aggressive hemodynamic support should be initiated. The Surviving Sepsis Guidelines recommend a MAP of at least 65 mm Hg (8.6 kPa) in patients with septic shock.[3] A large, controlled trial randomized patients to either a high (MAP of 80-85 mm Hg [10.6-11.3 kPa]) or low (MAP of 65-70 mm Hg [8.6-9.3 kPa]) target and found no significant difference in mortality at 28 days.[75] Among patients with chronic hypertension, those in the high-target group had less renal dysfunction and need for renal-replacement therapy. However, the high-target group had an increased risk of new atrial fibrillation in comparison to the low-target group. Hence, the question of an ideal MAP for septic shock still remains unanswered.

Hemodynamic support can be divided into three main categories: fluid therapy, vasopressor therapy, and inotropic therapy.

Fluid Therapy

6 Septic patients have enormous fluid requirements as a result of peripheral vasodilation and capillary leakage. In approximately 50% of septic patients who initially present with hypotension, fluids alone

will reverse hypotension and restore hemodynamic stability. Rapid fluid resuscitation improves the 28-day survival rate in patients with sepsis-induced hypoperfusion.[3] The goal of fluid therapy is to maximize cardiac output by increasing the LV preload, which will ultimately restore tissue perfusion. Fluid administration should be titrated to clinical end points such as heart rate, urine output, blood pressure, and mental status. Increased serum lactate, a by-product of cellular anaerobic metabolism, should normalize as tissue perfusion improves.

Isotonic crystalloids, such as 0.9% sodium chloride (normal saline) and lactated Ringer solution, are commonly used for fluid resuscitation. A patient in septic shock may require up to 10 L of crystalloid solution during the first 24-hour period. These solutions distribute into the extracellular compartment, and approximately 25% of the infused volume of crystalloid remains in the intravascular space, whereas the balance distributes to extravascular spaces. Although this could impair diffusion of oxygen to tissues, clinical impact is unproven.

The most commonly used colloids are 5% albumin, a naturally occurring plasma protein, and 6% hetastarch, a synthetic colloid formulation. These solutions offer more rapid restoration of intravascular volume because they produce greater intravascular volume expansion per quantity of volume infused. Colloids produce less peripheral edema than crystalloid, but there is no significant clinical impact. However, synthetic colloids cause dose-related acute kidney injury and increased bleeding.[3,76] The use of colloid solutions and blood products can be particularly important if there is significant blood loss associated with sepsis or if the patient had severe preexisting anemia.

There was no difference in 28-day mortality in critically ill patients given saline or albumin in the Saline versus Albumin Fluid Evaluation (SAFE) trial.[77] There was no significant difference in the mortality rate at 28 days for patients admitted to ICU with severe sepsis or septic shock given 20% albumin or crystalloid solution (31.8% vs 32.0%) and at 90 days (41.1% vs 43.6%).[78]

Crystalloid solutions are generally recommended for fluid resuscitation because of the absence of any clear benefit with colloids solutions in addition to the lower cost of crystalloids. For initial fluid challenge, a minimum of 30 mL/kg of normal saline is recommended. More rapid administration and greater amounts of fluid may be needed in some patients. The fluid administration should be continued as long as there is hemodynamic improvement either based on changes in pulse pressure, stroke volume, arterial pressure, and heart rate.[3]

Patients receiving fluid challenges require close monitoring of volume status to avoid pulmonary and systemic edema. Aggressive volume expansion can cause an increase in pulmonary capillary pressure, leading to an increase in lung water and associated hypoxemia. In a retrospective cohort of 405 patients with severe sepsis and septic shock, fluid overload was seen in 67% at day 1, and 48% had persistent fluid overload, exhibiting pulmonary vascular congestion and/or pleural effusions and requiring medical interventions including thoracentesis and diuretics.[79] Fluid overload was also associated with increased hospital mortality (odds ratio, 1.92; confidence interval, 1.16-3.22).

Vasopressor and Inotropic Therapy

When fluid resuscitation alone provides inadequate arterial pressure and organ perfusion, vasopressors and inotropic agents should be initiated. Inotropic agents such as dopamine and dobutamine have been effective in improving cardiac output by increasing cardiac contractility. Vasopressors such as norepinephrine should be considered when a systolic blood pressure is less than 90 mm Hg (12.0 kPa) or MAP is less than 65 mm Hg (<8.6 kPa) after adequate LV preload and inotrope therapy. Although inotropes and vasopressors are effective in life-threatening hypotension and in improving cardiac index (CI), there are significant complications such as tachycardia and myocardial ischemia and infarction as a result of the change in myocardial oxygen consumption in patients with coexisting coronary disease. Thus, a catecholamine infusion should be titrated gradually to restore MAP without impairing stroke volume.

Fluids and vasoactive agents have a strong influence on mortality. Mortality was lowest when vasoactive agents were started within 1 to 6 hours after onset of septic shock, with more than 1 L of fluid in the initial hour.[80]

7 Agents commonly considered for vasopressor or inotropic support include dopamine, dobutamine, norepinephrine, phenylephrine, and epinephrine (Table 119-5). Norepinephrine should generally be considered to be the first-choice vasopressor in septic shock after failure to restore adequate blood pressure and organ perfusion with appropriate fluid resuscitation.[3] Norepinephrine is a potent α-adrenergic agent with less pronounced β-adrenergic activity. It increases MAP and SVR because of its vasoconstrictive effects on peripheral vascular beds. Doses of 0.01 to 3 mcg/kg/min can reliably increase blood pressure with little changes in heart rate or CI. Despite the earlier concern of decreased renal blood flow associated with norepinephrine, data in humans and animals demonstrate a norepinephrine-induced renal blood flow as well as urine and cardiac output.[81] Norepinephrine is a more potent agent than dopamine in refractory septic shock. Norepinephrine resulted in greater increases in arterial blood pressure in comparison to patients with septic shock who were treated with dopamine (93% with norepinephrine vs 31% with dopamine).[81] In a meta-analysis evaluation the randomized trials comparing norepinephrine and dopamine, dopamine was associated with a higher risk of death and more frequently associated with arrythmias.[82]

Dopamine is a natural precursor of norepinephrine and epinephrine, and it exhibits dose-dependent pharmacologic effects. It is an α- and β-adrenergic agent with dopaminergic activity. Doses greater than 5 mcg/kg/min increase MAP and cardiac output, primarily because of the increase in heart rate and cardiac contractility through stimulation of β-adrenergic receptors. At higher doses, α-adrenergic effects predominate, resulting in arterial vasoconstriction. Because of combined vasopressor and inotropic effects, dopamine is more useful in patients with hypotension and compromised systolic function. However, it is also more arrhythmogenic and can cause more tachycardia.[3,81,82] It should be used with caution in patients who have underlying heart disease. Norepinephrine was more frequently used in 61,122 patients admitted with septic shock in US hospitals as initial vasopressor (77.6%) over dopamine, and

TABLE 119-5 Receptor Activity of Cardiovascular Agents Commonly Used in Septic Shock

Agent	α_1	α_2	β_1	β_2	Dopaminergic
Dopamine	++/+++	?	++++	++	++++
Dobutamine	+	+	++++	++	0
Norepinephrine	+++	+++	+++	+/++	0
Phenylephrine	++/+++	+	?	0	0
Epinephrine	++++	++++	++++	+++	0

α_1, α_1-adrenergic receptor; α_2, α_2-adrenergic receptor; β_1, β_1-adrenergic receptor; β_2, β_2-adrenergic receptor; 0, no activity; ++++, maximal activity; ?, unknown activity.

patients who received dopamine experienced greater hospital mortality (25% norepinephrine vs 23.7% dopamine).[83]

Epinephrine is a nonspecific α- and β-adrenergic agonist. Ranging from 0.1 to 0.5 mcg/kg/min, cardiac output is increased at lower doses, and vasoconstriction occurs predominantly at higher doses. Despite human and animal studies suggesting epinephrine impairing blood flow to the splanchnic system and increasing lactate level, clinical data demonstrating worse clinical outcomes as in mortality is lacking. The 2012 guidelines recommend epinephrine as the first alternative to patients intolerant to norepinephrine.[3]

Phenylephrine, a selective α-1-agonist, has rapid onset, short duration, and primary vascular effects, and it is least likely to produce tachycardia. Limited data suggest it can increase blood pressure modestly in fluid-resuscitated patients. Phenylephrine may decrease the stroke volume. Hence, it is only recommended when norepinephrine is associated with serious arrhythmias, cardiac output is known to be high, or as a salvage therapy when all other vasopressors have failed to achieve target MAP.[3,81]

During hypotension, endogenous vasopressin levels should increase and maintain arterial blood pressure, as vasopressin is a direct vasoconstrictor without inotropic or chronotropic effects. However, there is a vasopressin deficiency in septic shock most likely caused by inadequate production. Low doses of vasopressin produce a significant increase in MAP in septic shock, and it may be beneficial to add vasopressin in severe sepsis and septic shock that is refractory to other vasopressors.[77] Although vasopressin 0.03 units/min can be used to increase MAP or reduce norepinephrine requirements, this has not been shown to improve mortality rates.[3,84]

Dobutamine is a β-adrenergic inotropic agent that many clinicians consider to be the preferred drug for improvement of cardiac output and oxygen delivery, particularly in early sepsis before significant peripheral vasodilation has occurred. Doses of 2 to 20 mcg/kg/min increase the CI, ranging from 20% to 66%. However, heart rate often increases significantly.[81] Dobutamine should be considered in severely septic patients with low CI but adequate filling pressures and blood pressure.[3] A vasopressor such as norepinephrine and dobutamine can be used in combination to maintain both MAP and cardiac output.

In summary, for the septic patients with clinical signs of shock and significant hypotension unresponsive to aggressive fluid therapy, norepinephrine is the preferred agent for increasing MAP. In comparison to dopamine, it is less arrhythmogenic and studies have shown benefits in mortality. Epinephrine is an alternative to norepinephrine for refractory hypotension. Dopamine and epinephrine are more likely to induce or exacerbate tachycardia than norepinephrine. Phenylephrine is only recommended as a salvage therapy only if tachycardia or arrhythmia makes norepinephrine and epinephrine intolerable. In a septic patient with low CI after adequate fluid therapy and adequate MAP, dobutamine is the first-line agent for its strong inotropic effect, increasing cardiac output with minimal effect on SVR.

Initial Resuscitation

8 Initial resuscitation of patients in severe sepsis or sepsis-induced tissue hypoperfusion should begin within 6 hours of recognition of the syndrome. A randomized, controlled trial evaluated the timing of the goal-directed therapy involving adjustments of cardiac preload, afterload, and contractility to balance oxygen delivery with demand prior to admission to the ICU.[85] The goals during the first 6 hours included central venous pressure (CVP) of 8 to 12 mm Hg (1.1-1.6 kPa), MAP more than or equal to 65 mm Hg (≥8.6 kPa), urine output more than or equal to 0.5 mL/kg/h, and a central venous or mixed venous oxygen saturation ($Scvo_2$) more than or equal to 70% (≥0.70). During the first 6 hours of resuscitation, this early goal-directed therapy (EGDT) group had a central venous catheter placed and received more fluid than with traditional therapy (5 vs 3.5 L), dobutamine therapy to a maximum of 20 mcg/kg/min, and red blood cell transfusions. The 28-day mortality rate was 30% in the EGDT group, in comparison to 46.5% in the traditional therapy group consisting of fluid resuscitation, followed by vasopressor therapy if required. Increased oxygen delivery from the red blood cell transfusions to achieve a hematocrit of ≥30% (≥0.30) in the EGDT group appeared to be the primary difference between the two groups. However, a decade later, new data challenges the effect of EGDT on patient outcomes.[86-89]

Clinical **Controversy...**

The benefit of EGDT is controversial. EGDT emerged over a decade ago, as a novel approach for reducing mortality due to sepsis.[85] The impressive 15.9% absolute reduction in 28-day mortality rate is the result of invasive monitoring to guide resuscitation with aggressive IV fluids, vasopressors, red cell transfusions, and inotropes. Three large multicenter, randomized trials of 4,183 patients were conducted to validate the effect of EGDT on morbidity and mortality. The Protocolized Care for Early Septic Shock (ProCESS) trial was conducted in the United States at 31 academic hospitals. The patients with septic shock were randomly assigned to one of the three treatment groups: EGDT with continuous monitoring of CVP and Scvo2, protocolized standard therapy without continuous monitoring, and usual care. The EGDT group was most likely to receive vasopressors, inotropes, and red cell transfusions. However, there was no significant change in 60-day mortality (21.0% EGDT vs 18.9% usual care).[87] The Australasian Resuscitation in Sepsis Evaluation (ARISE) trial in Australia and New Zealand enrolled patients from 51 urban and rural hospitals who were diagnosed with septic shock.[88] No significant difference in 90-day mortality (18.6% EGDT vs 18.8% usual care) was noted. The Protocolised Management of Sepsis (ProMISe) trial in England showed similar findings as the ProCESS and ARISE.89. There was no significant difference in the 90-day mortality (29.5% EGDT vs 29.2% usual care), but the patients in the EGDT group had higher organ failure at 6 hours and longer stays in the ICU. Furthermore a meta-analysis of 11 published randomized clinical trials of EGDT did not show improved survival for patients in the EGDT group but rather had an increase admission to ICU from the emergency room for an invasive monitoring.[90]

The 2012 Surviving Sepsis Campaign recommends implementation of hospital-based performance improvement efforts such as a core set ("bundle") as they have been associated with improved patient outcomes. A 7.5-year study assessing the level of compliance with the 2004 Surviving Sepsis Campaign performance bundle and its effect on mortality in the United States, South America, and Europe reported lower mortality in high resuscitation compliance (29.0%) versus low compliance sites (38.6%).[91] In addition, hospital mortality rates dropped 0.7% per site for every three months of participation and the hospital and ICU length of stay decreased 4% for every 10% increase in site compliance. The 2012 guidelines have created the resuscitation bundle based on the time from of 3 hours and 6 hours with the recommended targets from the guidelines (Table 119-6).

Adjunctive Therapies

ARDS and hypoxia are common in septic patients, even in those without pulmonary infection. Oxygen therapy is indicated to

TABLE 119-6 Initial Resuscitation Bundle for Sepsis and Septic Shock

Within 3 hours
• Measure lactate level • Obtain blood cultures x 2 prior to antibiotic administration • Initiate empiric broad spectrum antibiotics • Fluid resuscitation with crystalloid for hypotension or lactate >4mmol/L
Within 6 hours
• Vasopressors if not responsive to initial fluid resuscitation to maintain MAP >65 mm Hg (≥8.6 kPa) • Measure for target CVP of ≥8 mm Hg (≥1.1 kPa), $SCVO_2$ of ≥70% (≥0.70) and normalization of lactate

CVP, central venous pressure; MAP, mean arterial pressure; $SCVO_2$, saturation of central venous oxygen.

Adapted from Dellinger RP, Levy MM, Rhodes A, et al. Surviving sepsis campaign: International guidelines for management of severe sepsis and septic shock: 2012. Crit Care Med 2013;41:580-637.

maintain oxygen saturation greater than 90% (0.90), and with progressive pulmonary insufficiency, the patient may require assisted ventilation.

9 Hyperglycemia and insulin resistance are frequently associated with sepsis regardless of the presence of diabetes prior to sepsis, and more severe hyperglycemia is associated with higher morbidity and mortality.[3] However, intensive insulin therapy is no longer the standard of care in critically ill patients. Patients receiving intensive insulin therapy (target serum glucose of 81-108 mg/dL [4.5-6 mmol/L]) had a higher incidence of severe hypoglycemia and increased mortality at 90 days compared with patients receiving conventional insulin therapy (target ≤180 mg/dL [≤10.0 mmol/L]).[92] Further analysis of patients with moderate (41-70 mg/dL [2.3-3.9 mmol/L]) and severe hypoglycemia (≤40 mg/dL [≤2.2 mmol/L]) reported death rate of 23.5% with moderate hypoglycemia and 35.4% with severe hypoglycemia.[93] Severe hypoglycemia in the absence of insulin therapy was also associated with a higher risk of death. The 2012 guidelines recommend blood glucose levels more than 180 mg/dL (>10 mmol/L) to initiate an insulin protocol with an upper target blood glucose level than 180 mg/dL (10 mmol/L) for the majority of critically ill patients to improve the outcome while reducing the risk of hypoglycemia.[3]

10 Cortisol levels vary widely in patients with septic shock, and some studies have suggested increased mortality associated with both low and high serum cortisol levels. Corticosteroids have been studied as adjunct therapy in patients with severe sepsis and septic shock to decrease the duration of shock and to decrease mortality.

A significant reduction in 28-day all–cause mortality and hospital mortality was reported in patients unresponsive to vasopressor therapy and receiving prolonged courses (>5 days) of low-dose corticosteroid therapy (<300 mg hydrocorortisone or equivalent/day) compared to placebo (38% vs 44%; relative risk 0.84).[94] There was no benefit for those patients without adrenal insufficiency. However, the large multicenter trial, the Corticosteroid Therapy of Septic Shock (CORTICUS) found no survival benefit among patients who received prolonged courses of hydrocortisone, but reported a trend in shock reversal for patients who received hydrocortisone.[95] The use of adrenocorticotropic hormone (ACTH) stimulation test to identify those patients who have a relative adrenal insufficiency did not predict the faster resolution of shock. The differences between the studies appear to arise from the study design of considering the response of septic shock patients to fluid and vasopressor therapy prior to hydrocortisone therapy. The CORTICUS study included patients with septic shock regardless of their responsiveness to vasopressor therapy. The guidelines recommend using IV hydrocortisone only if hemodynamic stability is not achieved after adequate fluid resuscitation and vasopressor therapy, regardless of the state of adrenal insufficiency, negating the ACTH stimulation test.[3] The guidelines also suggest using continuous infusion of hydrocortisone rather than repetitive bolus injections to avoid increased hyperglycemia and hypernatremia. Data on optimal duration of hydrocortisone therapy and the comparative clinical trials comparing whether steroid should be abruptly discontinued or tapered are sparse. Patients should be tapered from steroid therapy when vasopressors are no longer required.[3]

Deep vein thrombosis prophylaxis with daily subcutaneous low-molecular weight heparin should be initiated in all patients admitted to the ICU with severe sepsis and septic shock.[3] There was no significant difference in asymptomatic venous thromboembolism (VTE) between the low-molecular heparin group versus unfractionated heparin twice daily group but the proportion of patients with pulmonary embolism on CT scan was much lower in the low-molecular weight heparin group.[3] In patients with creatinine clearance of less than 30 mL/min (0.5 mL/s), dalteparin did not accumulate while data on the low-molecular weight heparin products is lacking. Dalteparin or unfractionated heparin is recommended for critically ill patients with acute renal injury.[3]

The systemic inflammatory events of sepsis may further predispose septic patients to VTE. A combination of pharmacologic therapy and intermittent pneumatic compression devices is recommended whenever possible. If heparin use is contraindicated, mechanical prophylactic treatment should be considered.[3] The incidence of venous thromboembolism (VTE) was 37.2% in patients admitted to the ICU with severe sepsis and septic shock despite thromboprophylaxis and resulted in increased ICU length of stay (18.2 vs 13.4 days).[96]

Stress ulcer prophylaxis should be initiated in all patients with severe sepsis and septic shock.[3] Proton pump inhibitors and H_2 receptor antagonists are equivalent in their ability to increase gastric pH. However, proton pump inhibitors may be more effective in GI bleeding protection over H_2 receptor antagonists.

PERSONALIZED PHARMACOTHERAPY

Patients presenting with severe sepsis and septic shock are critically ill and their management in an intensive care setting can be overwhelming. While it is critical to manage the complications involving multiple organ systems to ultimately sustain life during the initial hours, initial resuscitation of sepsis-induced tissue hypoperfusion and infection source identification are imperative as severe sepsis and subsequent multiorgan dysfunction arise from an uncontrolled infection and septic shock. Clinical presentation of each patient should be considered carefully and should prompt further evaluation of any underlying conditions, recent travel, injury, animal exposure, infection or use of antibiotics along with a complete physical examination to determine the possible source of infection. Based on the individual patients' findings and the most likely source of infection, the empiric regimen may be completely different from one patient to another. A patient presenting with sepsis secondary to a community-acquired pneumonia may receive ceftriaxone and azithromycin where another patient presenting with secondary peritonitis as a consequence of perforation of the GI tract may require a broad-spectrum regimen such as ertapenem or piperacillin/tazobactam.[44,45,50] Catheter-related sepsis may require a removal of the line as well as initiating vancomycin. There is abundant evidence in the literature demonstrating a correlation between the prompt and appropriate antibiotics and the overall survival rate.[36,37] Severe sepsis and complications such as shock, ARDS, and DIC result from an acute infection. As such, prompt identification of the source of infection in an individual patient and customizing the empiric antibiotic regimen while maintain hemodynamic stability may be the key to controlling the multiorgan dysfunctions and overall mortality rate.

ABBREVIATIONS

ACTH	adrenocorticotropic hormone
ARDS	acute respiratory distress syndrome
CI	cardiac index
CORTICUS	Corticosteroid Therapy of Septic Shock (trial)
CT	computed tomography
CVP	central venous pressure
DIC	disseminated intravascular coagulation
DO_2	oxygen delivery to tissues
EGDT	Early goal-directed therapy
GI	gastrointestinal
HIV	human immunodeficiency virus
ICU	intensive care unit
IL	interleukin
IL-1RA	interleukin-1 receptor antagonist
LV	left ventricular
MAP	mean arterial pressure
MODS	multiple-organ dysfunction syndrome
MRSA	methicillin-resistant *Staphylococcus aureus*
PAF	platelet activating factor
PCT	procalcitonin
$Scvo_2$	central venous oxygen saturation
SIRS	systemic inflammatory response syndrome
SSTIs	skin and soft tissue infections
SVR	systemic vascular resistance
TNF	tumor necrosis factor
VO_2	oxygen consumption
VRE	vancomycin-resistant enterococci
VTE	venous thromboembolism
WBC	white blood cell

REFERENCES

1. Walkey AJ, Lagu T, Lindenauer PK. Trends in sepsis and infection sources in the United States. A population-based study. *Ann Am Thorac Soc* 2015;12:216-220.
2. Kumar G, Kaumar N, Taneja A, et al. Nationwide trends of severe sepsis in the 21st century (2000-2007). *Chest* 2011;140:1223-1231.
3. Dellinger RP, Levy MM, Rhodes A, et al. Surviving sepsis campaign: International guidelines for management of severe sepsis and septic shock: 2012. *Crit Care Med* 2013;41:580-637.
4. Levy MM, Fink MP, Marshall JC, et al. 2001 SCCM/ESICM/ACCP/ATS/SIS International Sepsis Definitions Conference. *Crit Care Med* 2003;31:1250-1256.
5. Tiruvoipati R, Ong K, Gangopadhyay H, et al. Hypothermia predicts mortality in critically ill elderly patients with sepsis. *MCB Geriatr* 2010;10:70-78.
6. Netea MG, van der Meer JWM. Immunodeficiency and genetic defects of pattern-recognition receptors. *N Engl J Med* 2011;364: 60-70.
7. Leligdowicz A, Dodek PM, Norena M, et al. Association between source of infection and hospital mortality in patients who have septic shock. *Am J Respi Crit Care Med* 2014;189:1204-1212.
8. Zahar JR, Timsit JF, Garrouste-Orgeas M, et al. Outcomes in severe sepsis and patients with septic shock: Pathogen species and infection sites are not associated with mortality. *Crit Care Med* 2011;39:1886-1895.
9. Vincent JL, Rello J, Marshall J, et al. International study of the prevalence and outcomes of infection in intensive care units. *JAMA* 2009;302:2323-2329.
10. Brunkhorst FM, Oppert M, Marx G, et al. Effect of empirical treatment with moxifloxacin and meropenem vs meropenem on sepsis-related organ dysfunction in patients with severe sepsis. *JAMA* 2012;307:2390-2399.
11. Kumar A, Ellis P, Arabi Y, et al. Initiation of inappropriate antimicrobial therapy results in a fivefold reduction of survival in human septic shock. *Chest* 2009;136:1237-1248.
12. van Hal SJ, Jensen SO, Vaska VL, et al. Predictors of mortality in *Staphylococcus aureus* bacteremia. *Clin Microbiol Rev* 2012;25: 362-386.
13. Johnson MT, Reichley R, Hoppe-Bauer J, et al. Impact of previous antibiotic therapy on outcome of gram-negative severe sepsis. *Crit Care Med* 2011;39:1859-1865.
14. Burnham JP, Lane MA, Kollef MH. Impact of sepsis classification and multidrug-resistance status on outcome among patients treated with appropriate therapy. *Crit Care Med* 2015;43:1580-1586.
15. Bassetti M, Righi E, Ansaldi F, et al. A multicenter study of septic shock due to candidemia: outcomes and predictors of mortality. *Intensiv Care Med* 2014;40:839-845.
16. Diekema D, Arbefeville S, Boyken L, et al. The changing epidemiology of healthcare-associated candidemia over three decades. *Diagn Microb Infect Dis* 2012;73:45-48.
17. Guillamet CV, Vazquez R, Micek ST, et al. Development and validation of a clinical prediction rule for candidemia in hospitalized patients with severe sepsis and septic shock. *J Crit Care* 2015;30:715-720.
18. Ben-Ami R, Olshtain-Pops K, Krieger M, et al. Antibiotic exposure as a risk factor for fluconazole-resistant *Candida* bloodstream infection. *Antimicrob Agents Chemother* 2012;56:2518-2523.
19. Tamayo E, Fernandez A, Almansa R, et al. Pro- and anti-inflammatory responses are regulated simultaneously from the first moments of septic shock. *Eur Cytokine Network* 2011;22:82-87.
20. Andaluz-Ojeda D, Bobillo E, Iglesias V, et al. A combined score of pro- and anti-inflammatory interleukins improves mortality prediction in severe sepsis. *Cytokine* 2012;57:332-336.
21. De Pablo R, Monserrat J, Reyes E, et al. Mortality in patients with septic shock correlates with anti-inflammatory but not proinflammatory immunomodulatory molecules. *J Intensive Care Med* 2011;26:125-132.
22. Carlyn C, Andersen N, Baltch A, et al. Analysis of septic biomarker patterns: prognostic value in predicting septic state. *Diagn Microb Infect Dis* 2015;83:312-318.
23. Kanoore Edul VS, Enrico C, Laviolle B, et al. Quantitative assessment of the microcirculation in healthy volunteers and in patients with septic shock. *Crit Care Med* 2012;40:1443-1448.
24. Fourrier F. Severe sepsis, coagulation, and fibrinolysis: Dead end or one way? *Crit Care Med* 2012;40:2704-2708.
25. Capp R, Horton CL, Takhar SS, et al. Predictors of patients who presnt to the emergency department with sepsis and progress to septic shock between 4 and 48 hours of emergency department arrival. *Crit Care Med* 2015;43:983-988.
26. Semeraro N, Ammollo CT, Semeraro F, et al. Sepsis-associated disseminated intravascular coagulation and thromboembolic disease. *Mediter J Hematol Infect Dis* 2010;2:e2010024.
27. Levi M, van der Poll T. Inflammation and coagulation. *Crit Care Med* 2010;38:S26-S34.
28. Pulido JN, Afessa B, Masaki M, et al. Clinical spectrum, frequency, and significance of myocardial dysfunction in severe sepsis and septic shock. *Mayo Clin Proc* 2010;87:620-628.
29. Bagshaw SM, Lapinsky S, Dial S, et al. Acute kidney injury in septic shock: Clinical outcomes and impact of duration of hypotension prior to initiation of antimicrobial therapy. *Intensive Care Med* 2009;35:871-881.
30. Cunha BA. With sepsis: If fever is good, then hypothermia is bad! *Crit Care Med* 2012;40:2926-2927.
31. Thomas-Rueddel D, Poidinger B, Weiss M, et al. Hyperlactatemia is an independent predictor of mortality and denotes distinct subtypes of severe sepsis and septic shock. *J Crit Care* 2015;30:439.e1-439.e6.
32. Coelho FR, Martins JO. Diagnostic methods in sepsis: The need of speed. *Rev Assoc Med Bras* 2012;58:498-504.
33. Davies J, Gordon CL, Tong SY, et al. Impact of results of a rapid *Staphylococcus aureus* diagnostic test on prescribing of antibiotics for patients with clustered gram-positive cocci in blood cultures. *J Clin Microbiol* 2012;50:2056-2058.
34. Aittakorpi A, Kuusela P, Koukila-Kahkola P, et al. Accurate and rapid identification of *Candida* spp. frequently associated with fungemia by using PCR and the microarray-based Prove-it sepsis assay. *J Clin Microbiol* 2012:50:3635-3640.
35. Dellinger RP, Levy MM, Cartlet JM, et al. Surviving sepsis campaign: International guidelines for management of severe sepsis and septic shock: 2008. *Crit Care Med* 2008;36:296-327.
36. Ferrer R, Martin-Loeches I, Phillips G, et al. Empiric antibiotic treatment reduces mortality in severe sepsis and septic shock from the first hour: results from a guideline-based performance improvement program. *Crit Care Med* 2014;42:1749-1755.
37. Gaieski DF, Mikkelsen ME, Band RA, et al. Impact of time to antibiotics on survival in patients with severe sepsis or septic shock

in whom early goal-directed therapy was initiated in the emergency department. *Crit Care Med* 2010;38:1045-1053.

38. Kumar A, Roberts D, Wood KE, et al. Duration of hypotension before initiation of effective antimicrobial therapy is the critical determinant of survival in human septic shock. *Crit Care Med* 2006;34:1589-1596.
39. Vazquez-Guillamet C, Scolari M, Zilberberg MD, et al. Using the number needed to treat as assess appropriate antimicrobial therapy as a determinant of outcome in severe sepsis and septic shock. *Crit Care Med* 2014;42:2342-2349.
40. Zilbergerg MD, Shorr AF, Micek ST, et al. Multi-drug resistance, inappropriate initial antibiotic therapy and mortality in Gram-negative severe sepsis and septic shock: A retrospective cohort study. *Crit Care* 2014;18:596-608.
41. Pea F. Plasma pharmacokinetics of antimicrobial agents in critically ill patients. *Curr Clin Pharmacol* 2013;8:5-12.
42. Baptista JP, Sousa E, Martins PJ, et al. Augmented renal clearance in septic patients and implications for vancomycin optimisation. *Int J Antimicrob Agents* 2012;39:420-423.
43. Hooton TM, Bradley SF, Cardenas DD, et al. Diagnosis, prevention, and treatment of catheter-associated urinary tract infection in adults: 2009 International clinical practice guidelines from the Infectious Diseases Society of America. *Clin Infect Dis* 2010;50:625-663.
44. Mandell LA, Wunderinnk RG, Anzueto A, et al. Infectious Disease Society of America/American Thoracic Society consensus guidelines on management of community-acquired pneumonia in adults. *Clin Infect Dis* 2007;44:S27-S72.
45. Pereira JM, Paiva JA, Rello J. Severe sepsis in community-acquired pneumonia—Early recognition and treatment. *Eur J Intern Med* 2012;23:412-419.
46. American Thoracic Society Documents. Guidelines for the management of adults with hospital-acquired, ventilator-associated, and healthcare-associated pneumonia. *Am J Respir Crit Care Med* 2005;171:388-416.
47. Liu C, Bayer A, Cosgrove SE, et al. Clinical practice guidelines by the Infectious Diseases Society of America for the treatment of methicillin-resistant *Staphylococcus aureus* infections in adults and children. *Clin Infect Dis* 2011;52:1-38.
48. Rubinstein E, Lalani T, Corey GR. Televancin versus vancomycin for hospital-acquired pneumonia due to Gram-positive pathogens. *Clin Infect Dis* 2011;52:31-40.
49. De Waele J, Lipman J, Sakr Y, et al. Abdominal infections in the intensive care unit: characteristics, treatment and determinants of outcome. *BMC Infect Dis* 2014;14:420-437.
50. Solomkin JS, Mazuski JE, Bradley JS, et al. Diagnosis and management of complicated intra-abdominal infection in adults and children: Guidelines by the Surgical Infection Society and the Infectious Diseases Society of America. *Clin Infect Dis* 2010;50: 133-164.
51. Snydman DR, Jacobus NV, McDermott LA, et al. Update on resistance of *Bacteroides fragilis* group and related species with special attention to carbapenems 2006–2009. *Anaerobe* 2011;17: 147-151.
52. Lipsky BA, Moran GJ, Napolitano LM, et al. A prospective, multicenter, observational study of complicated skin and soft tissue infections in hospitalized patients: Clinical characteristics, medical treatment, and outcomes. *BMC Infect Dis* 2012;12:227.
53. Stevens DL, Bisno AL, Chambers HF, et al. Practice guidelines for the diagnosis and management of skin and soft tissue infections: 2014 update by the Infectious Diseases Society of America. *Clin Infect Dis* 2014;59:147-159.
54. Brown JE, Fominaya C, Christensen KJ, et al. Daptomycin experience in critical care patients: Results from a registry. *Ann Pharmacother* 2012;46:495-502.
55. Tamma PD, Cosgrove SE, Maragakis LL. Combination therapy for treatment of infections with gram-negative bacteria. *Clin Microbiol Rev* 2012;25:450-470.
56. Vasquez-Grande G, Kumar A. Optimizing antimicrobial therapy of sepsis and septic shock: focus on antibiotic combination therapy. *Semin Respir Crit Care Med* 2015;36:154-166.
57. Qureshi ZA, Paterson DL, Potoski BA, et al. Treatment outcome of bacteremia due to KPC-producing *Klebsiella pneumoniae*: Superiority of combination antimicrobial regimens. *Antimicrob Agents Chemother* 2012;56:2108-2113.
58. Dellit TH, Owens RC, McGowan JE Jr, et al. Infectious Disease Society of America and the Society for Healthcare Epidemiology of America guidelines for developing an institutional program to enhance antimicrobial stewardship. *Clin Infect Dis* 2007;44:159-177.
59. Heenen S, Jacobs F, Vincent JL. Antibiotic strategies in severe nosocomial sepsis: Why do we not de-escalate more often? *Crit Care Med* 2012;40:1404-1409.
60. Garnacho-Montero J, Gutierrez-Pizarraya A, Escoresc-Ortega A, et al. De-escalation of empirical therapy is associated with lower mortality in patients with severe sepsis and septic shock. *Intensive Care Med* 2014;40:32-40.
61. Grim SA, Berger K, Teng C, et al. Timing of susceptibility-based antifungal drug administration in patients with *Candida* bloodstream infection: Correlation with outcomes. *J Antimicrob Chemother* 2012;67:707-714.
62. Kollef M, Micek S, Hampton N, et al. Septic shock attributed to *Candida* infection: Importance of empiric therapy and source control. *Clin Infect Dis* 2012;54:1739-1746.
63. Azoulay E, Dupont H, Tabah A, et al. Systemic antifungal therapy in critically ill patients without invasive fungal infection. *Crit Care Med* 2012;40:813-822.
64. Pappas PG, Kauffman CA, Andes D, et al. Clinical practice guidelines for management of candidiasis: 2009 update by the Infectious Diseases Society of America. *Clin Infect Dis* 2009;48:503-535.
65. Shah DN, Yau R, Lasco TM, et al. Impact of prior inappropriate fluconazole dosing on isolation of fluconazole-nonsusceptible *Candida* species in hospitalized patients with candidemia. *Antimicrob Agents Chemother* 2012;56:3239-3243.
66. Pfaller MA, Messer SA, Moet GJ, et al. Candida bloodstream infections: Comparison of species distribution and resistance to echinocandin and azole antifungal agents in Intensive Care Unit (ICU) and non-ICU settings in the SENTRY Antimicrobial Surveillance Program (2008–2009). *Int J Antimicrob Agents* 2011;38: 65-69.
67. Pfaller MA, Castanheira M, Lockhart SR, et al. Frequency of decreased susceptibility and resistance to echinocandins among fluconazole-resistant bloodstream isolates of *Candida glabrata*. *J Clin Microbiol* 2012;50:1199-1203.
68. Mora-Duarte J, Betts R, Rotstein R, et al. Comparison of caspofungin and amphotericin B for invasive candidiasis. *N Engl J Med* 2002;347: 2020-2029.
69. Pappas PG, Rotstein CMF, Betts RF, et al. Micafungin versus caspofungin for treatment of candidemia and other forms of invasive candidiasis. *Clin Infect Dis* 2007;45:883-893.
70. Reboli AC, Rotstein C, Pappas PG, et al. Anidulafungin versus fluconazole for invasive candidiasis. *N Engl J Med* 2007;356: 2472-2482.
71. Schroeder S, Hochreiter M, Koehler T, et al. Procalcitonin-guided algorithm reduces length of antibiotic treatment in surgical intensive care patients with severe sepsis: Results of a prospective randomized study. *Langenbecks Arch Surg* 2009;394:221-226.
72. Layios N, Lambermont B, Canivet JL, et al. Procalcitonin usefulness for the initiation of antibiotic treatment in intensive care unit patients. *Crit Care Med* 2012;40:2304-2309.
73. Prkno A, Wacker C, Brunkhorst F, et al. Procalcitonin-guided therapy in intensive care unit patients with severe sepsis and septic shock – a systematic review and meta-analysis. *Crit Care* 2013;17:R291-R302.
74. Jensen JU, Hein L, Lundgren B, et al. Procalcitonin-guided interventions against infections to increase early appropriate antibiotics and improve survival in the intensive care unit: A randomized trial. *Crit Care Med* 2011;39:2048-2058.
75. Asfar P, Meziani F, Hamel FJ, et al. High versus low blood-pressure target in patients with septic shock. *N Engl J Med* 2014;370: 1583-1594.
76. Bayer O, Reinhart K, Kohl M, et al. Effects of fluid resuscitation with synthetic colloids or crystalloids alone on shock reversal, fluid balance, and patient outcomes in patients with severe sepsis: A prospective sequential analysis. *Crit Care Med* 2012;40:2543-2551.
77. Finfer S, Bellomo R, Boyce N, et al. A comparison of albumin and saline for fluid resuscitation in the intensive care unit. *N Engl J Med* 2004;350:2247-2256.
78. Caironi P, Tognoni G, Masson S, et al. Albumin replacement in patients with severe sepsis or septic shock. *N Engl J Med* 2014;370: 1412-1422.
79. Kelm DJ, Perrin JT, Cartin-Ceba R, et al. Fluid overload in patients with severe sepsis and septic shock treated with early goal-directed therapy is associated with increased acute need for fluid-related medical interventions and hospital death. *Shock* 2015;43:68-73.
80. Waechter J, Kumar A, Lapinsky SE, et al. Interaction between fluids and vasoactive agents on mortality in septic shock: a multicenter, observational study. *Crit Care Med* 2014;42:2158-2168.

81. Hollenberg SM. Inotrope and vasopressor therapy of septic shock. *Crit Care Nurs Clin North Am* 2011;23:127-148.
82. Backer DD, Aldecoa C, Njimi H, et al. Dopamine versus norepinephrine in the treatment of septic shock: A meta-analysis. *Crit Care Med* 2012;40:725-730.
83. Fawzy A, Evans SR, Walkey AJ. Practice patterns and outcomes associated with choice of initial vasopressor therapy for septic shock. *Crit Care Med* 2015;43:2141-2146.
84. Russell JA, Walley KR, Singer J, et al. VASST Investigators: Vasopressin versus norepinephrine infusion in patients with septic shock. *N Engl J Med* 2008;358:877-887.
85. Rivers E, Nguyen B, Havstad S, et al. Early goal–directed therapy in the treatment of severe sepsis and septic shock. *N Engl J Med* 2001;345:1368-1377.
86. Rivers EP, Katranji M, Jaehne KA, et al. Early interventions in severe sepsis and septic shock: A review of the evidence one decade later. *Minerva Anesthesiol* 2012;78:712-724.
87. The ProCESS Investigators A randomized trial of protocol-based care for early septic shock. *N Engl J Med* 2014;370:1683-1693.
88. The ARISE Investigators and the ANZICS Clinical Trials Group. Goal-directed resuscitation for patients with early septic shock. *N Engl J Med* 2014;371:1496-1506.
89. Mouncey PR, Osborn TM, Power GS, et al. Trial of early, goal-directed resuscitation for septic shock. *N Engl J Med* 2015;372: 1301-1311.
90. Angus DC, Barnato AE, Bell D, et al. A systematic review and meta-analysis of early goal-directed therapy for septic shock: the ARISE, ProCESS and ProMISe Investigators. *Intensive Care Med* 2015;41:1549-1560.
91. Levy MM, Thodes A, Phillips GS, et al. Surviving sepsis campaign: association between performance metrics and outcomes in a 7.5-year study. *Crit Care Med* 2015;43:3-12.
92. The NICE-SUGAR Investigators. Intensive versus conventional glucose control in critically ill patients. *N Engl J Med* 2009;360: 1283-1297.
93. The NICE-SUGAR Investigators. Hypoglycemia and risk of death in critically ill patients. *N Engl J Med* 2012;367:1108-1118.
94. Annane D, Bellissant E, Bollaert PE, et al. Corticosteroids in the treatment of severe sepsis and septic shock in adults: A systematic review. *JAMA* 2009;301:2362-2375.
95. Sprung CL, Annane D, Keh D, et al. Hydrocortisone therapy for patients with septic shock. *N Engl J Med* 2008;358:111-124.
96. Kaplan D, Casper C, Elliott G, et al. VTE incidence and risk factors in patients with severe sepsis and septic shock. *Chest* 2015;148:1224-1230.

Superficial Fungal Infections

120

Thomas E. R. Brown and Linda D. Dresser

KEY CONCEPTS

1. Vulvovaginal candidiasis (VVC) is a fungal infection of the vagina that can be classified as uncomplicated or complicated. This classification is useful in determining appropriate pharmacotherapy.
2. *Candida albicans* is the major pathogen responsible for VVC. The number of cases of non-*C. albicans* species appears to be increasing.
3. Signs and symptoms of VVC are not pathognomonic, and reliable diagnosis must be made with laboratory tests including vaginal pH, saline microscopy, and 10% potassium hydroxide (KOH) microscopy.
4. *C. albicans* is the predominant species causing all forms of mucosal candidiasis. Important host and exogenous risk factors have been identified that predispose an individual to the development of mucosal candidiasis. In oropharyngeal and esophageal candidiasis, the key risk factor is impaired host immune system.
5. Topical antimycotic agents such as nystatin or clotrimazole are the first choice for treating oropharyngeal candidiasis (OPC). Systemic therapy can be used in patients who are not responding to an adequate trial of topical treatment or are unable to tolerate topical agents and in those at high risk for systemic candidiasis. Fluconazole and itraconazole remain first line antimycotic agents.
6. For esophageal candidiasis, topical agents are not of proven benefit; fluconazole or itraconazole solution is the first choice.
7. Optimal antiretroviral therapy is important for the prevention of recurrent and refractory candidiasis in patients with human immunodeficiency virus (HIV) infection.
8. Primary or secondary prophylaxis of fungal infection is not recommended routinely for HIV-infected patients; use of secondary prophylaxis should be individualized for each patient.
9. Topical antimycotic agents are first-line treatment for fungal skin infections. Oral therapy is preferred for the treatment of extensive or severe infection and those with tinea capitis or onychomycosis.
10. New topical antifungal agents efinaconazole and tavaborole are recommended for mild-moderate toenail fungal infections.

Superficial mycoses are among the most common infections in the world and the second most common vaginal infections in North America. Mucocutaneous candidiasis can occur in three forms—oropharyngeal, esophageal, and vulvovaginal disease—with oropharyngeal and vulvovaginal disease being the most common. Over the past 15 to 20 years, the occurrence rates of some fungal infections have increased dramatically. The prevalence of fungal skin infections varies throughout different parts of the world, from the most common causes of skin infections in the tropics to relatively rare disorders in the United States. This chapter reviews the pharmacotherapy of vulvovaginal candidiasis (VVC), oropharyngeal and esophageal candidiasis, and common dermatophyte infections.

VULVOVAGINAL CANDIDIASIS

1 Vulvovaginal candidiasis refers to infections in individuals with or without symptoms who have positive vaginal cultures for *Candida* species. Depending on episodic frequency, VVC can be classified as either sporadic or recurrent.[1] This classification is essential to understand the pathophysiology, as well as the pharmacotherapy, of VVC. Furthermore, VVC may be defined as uncomplicated, which refers to sporadic infections that are susceptible to all forms of antifungal therapy regardless of the duration of treatment, or complicated, in which consideration of factors affecting the host, microorganism, and pharmacotherapy all have an essential role in successful treatment.[1] Complicated VVC includes recurrent VVC, severe disease, non-*Candida albicans* candidiasis, and host factors, including diabetes mellitus, immunosuppression, and pregnancy.[1]

Epidemiology

There is minimal information on the incidence and prevalence of VVC. Healthcare workers are not required to report cases of VVC; therefore, estimates are derived from self-reported histories. Epidemiologic data are limited because VVC usually is diagnosed without microscopy and/or cultures, and antifungal nonprescription preparations are available for self-treatment.[1] By 25 years of age, approximately 50% of college women will have had at least one episode of VVC.[1] It is rare before menarche and increases dramatically at about 20 years of age, with the peak incidence between age 30 and 40 years. It is associated with the initial act of sexual intercourse. As many as 75% of women experience one bout of symptomatic VVC in their lifetime. Between 40% and 50% of women who experience one episode of VVC experience a second episode, and 5% experience recurrent VVC.[2,3] Black women appear to be at higher risk than white women of developing VVC (62.8% vs 55%, respectively).[4] The incidence after menopause remains unknown. However, one study of 149 healthy postmenopausal women with vulvar conditions reported significantly more women taking hormone replacement therapy (HRT) were prone to developing VVC than those who were not taking HRT (culture-positive, clinical VVC in 49% on HRT versus 1% on those not on HRT).[5]

Costs from VVC can be direct (medical visits and self-treatment) and indirect (nonmedical expenses, eg, time losses from work, costs of travel, and time required in obtaining treatment). There are an estimated 6 million visits to healthcare providers each year, resulting in more than $1 billion spent annually on these medical visits and self-treatment.[6] These costs could reach $3.1 billion by 2014.[7]

Pathophysiology

2 *C. albicans* is the major pathogen responsible for VVC, accounting for 80% to 92% of symptomatic episodes. The remainder are caused by non-*C. albicans* species, with *Candida glabrata* dominating.[8] The number of cases of non-*C. albicans* candidiasis appears to be increasing, possibly related to the use of nonprescription vaginal antifungal preparations and short-course therapy and/or the increased use of long-term maintenance therapy in preventing recurrent infections.[1]

Candida species can act as commensal members of the vaginal flora. Asymptomatic colonization with *Candida* species has been found in 10% to 20% of women of reproductive age.[8,9] *Candida* organisms are dimorphic; blastospores are responsible for colonization (transmission and spread), whereas germinated *Candida* forms are associated with tissue invasion and symptomatic infections.[10] To colonize the vagina, *Candida* species must be able to attach to the mucosa. The attachment process is complex. Not only are candidal surface structures important for attachment, but appropriate receptors for attachment must be present in the epithelial tissue. Not all women have the same range of receptors, which may explain variation in colonization.[9] Changes in the host's vaginal environment or response are necessary to induce a symptomatic infection. Unfortunately, in most cases of symptomatic VVC, no precipitating factor can be identified.[10]

Risk Factors

Several factors predispose a woman to VVC. VVC is not considered to be a sexually transmitted disease, although sexual factors can be important. There is a dramatic increase in the frequency of VVC when women become sexually active. In addition, oral-genital contact can increase the risk.[1] However, current guidelines do not recommend the treatment of asymptomatic partners.[8] Contraceptive agents, including the diaphragm with spermicide, the contraceptive sponge, and the intrauterine device, increase the risk of VVC. An in vitro study demonstrated that four different isolates of *Candida* species were capable of adhering to the contraceptive vaginal ring.[11] Oral contraceptive users demonstrated increased risk of candidiasis; however, these reports were with the higher-dose oral contraceptive pills, and the risk may not be as great with the lower-estrogen-dose oral contraceptives.[12]

Antibiotic use can increase the risk of VVC, but it is significant in only a small number of women. The mechanism by which antibiotics can increase the risk of VVC is unknown; colonization, however, is a prerequisite.[1] A small pilot study showed that 3 days of antibiotics increased the prevalence of asymptomatic vaginal colonization of *Candida* and the incidence of symptomatic VVC.[13] Diet (excess refined carbohydrates), douching, and tight-fitting clothing often are listed as important risk factors; however, no association has been established between these factors and increased risk of VVC.[1]

Clinical Presentation

3 These signs and symptoms of VVC (Table 120-1) are not pathognomonic, and a reliable diagnosis cannot be made without laboratory tests.[1,8] Self-diagnosis has a sensitivity of 35%, a specificity of 89%, and a positive predictive value of 62%.[4] More than 50% of women who had self-diagnosed VVC did not have yeast as the causative agent.[14] This limits the value of self-diagnosis and the success of self-treatment. The American College of Obstetricians and Gynecologists (ACOG) recommends that whenever possible women requesting treatment for VVC should be examined and evaluated. They only recommend self-diagnosis in compliant women with multiple confirmed prior cases of VVC who report the same symptoms. They further recommend that if these individuals fail to improve on a short course of therapy, they be evaluated for a further diagnosis.[15] Therefore, in most instances the diagnosis should be based on both clinical presentation and investigations, including vaginal pH, saline microscopy, and 10% potassium hydroxide (KOH) microscopy. The vaginal pH remains normal in VVC, and microscopic investigations should detect blastospores or pseudohyphae. *Candida* cultures usually are not required in the diagnosis of uncomplicated VVC; however, they are recommended when an individual presents with classic signs and symptoms of VVC, has a normal vaginal pH, but microscopy is inconclusive or recurrence is suspected.[8]

TABLE 120-1 Clinical Presentation of Vulvovaginal Candidiasis

General	Often involves both the vulva and the vagina
Symptoms	Intense vulvar itching, soreness, irritation, burning on urination, and dyspareunia
Signs	Erythema, fissuring, curdy "cheese"-like discharge, satellite lesions, edema
Laboratory tests	Vaginal pH—normal, saline and 10% KOH microscopy—blastospores or pseudohyphae
Other diagnostic tests	*Candida* cultures not recommended unless classic signs and symptoms with normal vaginal pH and microscopy are inconclusive or recurrence is suspected

KOH, potassium hydroxide.

TREATMENT

Goals of Therapy

The goal of therapy is complete resolution of symptoms in patients who have symptomatic VVC. A test of the cure is not necessary if symptoms resolve.[8] Antimycotic agents used in the treatment of VVC do not meet the definition of being fungicidal agents because of their slower killing rate. At the end of therapy, the number of viable organisms drops below the detectable range. However, by 6 weeks after a course of therapy, 25% to 40% of women will have positive yeast cultures and remain asymptomatic.[1] Asymptomatic colonization with *Candida* species does not require therapy.

General Approaches to Treatment

The approach to therapy is to remove or improve any predisposing factors if they can be identified. A pharmacologic antimycotic agent should have limited local and systemic side effects, a high cure rate, and easy administration. Additionally, it would be advantageous to use a therapy that is able to resolve symptoms within 24 hours, that has broad antimycotic activity (to cover increasing rates on non-*C. albicans* species), that prevents recurrence, and that can be used over a shortened period of time, such as 1 to 3 days. Many topical azoles medications (such clotrimazole, miconazole, etc.) are available without a prescription, and although this may increase public access to these medications, there is concern that having them available without a prescription may lead to inappropriate use. Patient actors who visited 60 pharmacies found that vaginal antimycotics were more likely to be supplied to appropriate individuals as more information was exchanged, if interactions involved a pharmacist, and if questions regarding specific symptoms were used.[16]

Patients should be advised to avoid harsh soaps and perfumes that can cause or worsen vulvar irritation. The genital area must be kept clean and dry by avoiding constrictive clothing and frequent or prolonged exposure to hot tub use.[3] Douching is not recommended for either prevention or treatment.[14] Cool baths can soothe the skin.[3] The oral use of lactobacillus remains unclear. The addition of oral lactobacillus to single dose oral fluconazole VVC treatment augmented the cure rate compared to the use of fluconazole alone.[17] A mixture of oral consumption of bee-honey and yogurt showed some efficacy with mycotic cure rates of 76.9% compared to cure rates with antifungal agents of 91.5%.[18] Daily ingestion of 240 mL yogurt containing *Lactobacillus acidophilus* decreased colonization and symptomatic infections of VVC in women with recurrent infections.[19] However, a subsequent study showed that the addition of oral lactobacillus to itraconazole therapy in the treatment of recurrent VVC did not confer any additional benefit. Treatment using classic homeopathy was less effective than the use of itraconazole in recurrent VVC.[20] The use of probiotic remains controversial. A Cochrane Collaborative protocol has been developed to determine the role of probiotics in the treatment of VVC in nonpregnant women.[21]

Treatment of VVC will be considered to have positive outcomes if the symptoms of VVC are resolved within 24 to 48 hours and no adverse medication events are experienced. Self-assessment of symptom relief is appropriate for most cases of VVC. If symptoms remain unresolved or recur, then further testing and treatment can be required.

Pharmacologic Treatments

Uncomplicated Vulvovaginal Candidiasis

Cure rates for uncomplicated VVC are between 80% and 95% with topical or oral azoles and between 70% and 90% with nystatin preparations. Table 120-2 lists available topical and oral preparations for the treatment of uncomplicated VVC. There are many topical nonprescription preparations for the treatment of VVC. No significant differences in in vitro activity or clinical efficacy exist between the topical azole agents.[1,3,8,15] The selection of a topical azole antimycotic agent should be based primarily on an individual patient's preference as to product formulation. Some topical products can cause vaginal burning, stinging, or irritation; conversely, the vehicle used in topical creams or gels can provide initial symptomatic relief.[1] Of note, most topical preparations can decrease the efficacy of latex condoms and diaphragms.

TABLE 120-2 Treatment for Uncomplicated Vulvovaginal Candidiasis

Active Ingredient	Preparation	Regimen
Nonprescription/Topical Vaginal Products		
Butoconazole	2% cream	One applicator × 3 days
Clotrimazole	1% cream 100 mg tablet 2% cream	One applicator × 7-14 days One 100 mg tablet × 7 days One applicator × 3 day
Miconazole[a]	100 mg suppository 200 mg suppository 1,200 mg ovule	One 100 mg suppository × 7 days One 200 mg suppository × 3 days One ovule × 1 day
Ticonazole	6.5% cream	One applicator × 1 day
Prescription/Topical		
Nystatin Butoconazole	100,000 unit tablet 2% cream	One tablet × 14 days One applicator x 1 day
Terconazole	0.4% cream	One applicator × 7 days
	0.8% cream 80 mg suppository	One applicator × 3 days One suppository × 3 days
Oral Products		
Fluconazole	150 mg	One tablet × 1 day

[a]The FDA warns of the possible increase in the anticoagulant effects of warfarin with concomitant use.

Oral azoles (such as fluconazole or itraconazole) have been used in the treatment of VVC. Patients may prefer oral therapy because of its convenience.[22] A Cochrane review of 19 trials analyzing 22 oral versus topical antifungal comparisons concluded that there were no differences between the routes of administration in short-term mycologic cure rates. There was a significant difference between long-term cure rates in favor of long-term follow up; however, the authors stated that the clinical significance of this finding is uncertain.[1,23]

In the treatment of uncomplicated VVC, the duration of therapy is not critical. Cure rates with different lengths of treatment have not demonstrated that one duration of therapy is significantly better.[22-24] Shorter-duration therapies (eg, clotrimazole 1-day therapy) consist of higher concentrations of azoles that maintain the local therapeutic effect for up to 72 hours and allow for resolution of signs and symptoms.[25] A review of 14 trials that examined 1-day treatments showed less than 7% difference in short-term cure rates or improvement between any two treatments in any two studies and no significant differences in short- or long-term clinical cure rates among 1-day regimens.[24] Table 120-2 lists the therapeutic options recommended by the Centers for Disease Control and Prevention for the treatment of uncomplicated VVC.[26]

Clinical Controversy...

Although there are a few clinical trials evaluating the use of lactobacillus formulations. The use of probiotics alone or in combination with an anti-mycotic agent remains unclear.

Complicated Vulvovaginal Candidiasis

Complicated VVC occurs in patients who are immunocompromised or have uncontrolled diabetes mellitus.[1] These individuals need a more aggressive treatment plan.[15] Current recommendations are to lengthen therapy to 10 to 14 days regardless of the route of administration.[15] Therapeutic options include those listed in Table 120-2; however, regimens should be continued for 10 to 14 days. A study of oral fluconazole therapy in women with complicated VVC demonstrated that cure rates increased from 67% with single-dose therapy to 80% when the 150 mg dose of fluconazole was repeated 72 hours after the initial dose.[27]

VVC during pregnancy can be considered complicated because consideration of host factors such as hormonal changes that can affect normal flora are essential in selecting therapeutic regimens. Topical agents are considered to be safe throughout pregnancy. A systematic review of 10 trials demonstrated that imidazole topical agents (such as fluconazole) were more effective than nystatin. Two of the trials showed that treatment for 7 days was more effective than treatments of 4 days or less.[28] Oral agents are contraindicated in pregnancy because of the concern for fetal complications. A prospective assessment of pregnancy outcomes in 226 women exposed to fluconazole in the first trimester did not indicate increased risk of congenital abnormalities or other adverse outcomes.[29] A Danish registry based cohort found that oral fluconazole may increase the risk of tetratology of Fallot.[30] The ACOG recommends avoiding oral therapy, and recommends a topical imidazole therapy for 7 days.[14]

Recurrent Vulvovaginal Candidiasis

Recurrent vulvovaginal candidiasis (RVVC) is defined as having more than four episodes of VVC within a 12-month period.[1,7] The prevalence of RVVC is higher than once thought, as high as 7% to 8%.[31] A proper diagnosis should be obtained to rule out other infections or nonmycotic contact dermatitis. RVVC is best treated in two stages: an initial intensive stage followed by prolonged antifungal therapy to achieve mycologic remission. Ninety percent of women randomly receiving 150 mg fluconazole daily for 10 days followed by 6 months of either fluconazole 150 mg weekly or placebo were symptom free for the 6 months following initial treatment (during the weekly fluconazole therapy), and there were 50% fewer symptomatic episodes in the 6 months following weekly suppressive therapy.[32] The Infectious Diseases Society of America recommends 10 to 14 days of induction therapy with a topical or oral azole, followed by 150 mg of fluconazole once weekly for 6 months for recurring *Candida* VVC.[33] Future directions in pharmacotherapy include the development of anti-Candida vaccines. Clinical investigations have begun to determine the effectiveness of these vaccines in preventing RVVC.[34]

ANTIFUNGAL-RESISTANT VULVOVAGINAL CANDIDIASIS

Resistance to azole antimycotics should be considered in individuals who have persistently positive yeast cultures and fail to respond to therapy despite adherence to prescribed regimens.[1] These infections can be treated with boric acid or 5-flucytosine.[35,36] Boric acid is administered as a 600 mg intravaginal capsule daily for 14 days of induction therapy, followed by a maintenance regimen of one capsule intravaginally twice weekly. Boric acid should not be administered orally, as it is toxic. 5-Flucytosine cream is administered vaginally, 1,000 mg inserted nightly for 7 days. The prevalence of *C. glabrata* with VVC is higher in those with diabetes, 68% had isolates for *C. glabrata* compared with 28.8% for *C. albicans*. Those with *C. glabrata* had significantly higher mycological cure rates with 600 mg of boric acid suppositories for 14 days compared with a single dose of fluconazole 150 mg.[37]

OROPHARYNGEAL AND ESOPHAGEAL CANDIDIASIS

Oropharyngeal candidiasis (OPC), or *thrush*, is a common and localized infection of the oral mucosa caused by the yeast *Candida*. *C. albicans*, a common oral commensal organism, is the most frequent infecting species. OPC is also referred to as *candidiasis* (or the more correct but less commonly used term *candidosis*). The infection may extend into the esophagus, causing esophageal candidiasis.

Epidemiology and Etiology

Candida is a commensal fungus found in the oral cavity in up to 65% of healthy individuals with higher prevalence in healthy children and young adults.[38,39] *Candida* carriage increases under immunocompromised conditions and also among hospitalized patients.[39] Even in the era of highly active antiretroviral therapy (HAART) up to 80% of human immunodeficiency virus (HIV)-infected persons may demonstrate oral yeast colonization.[40] The organism is capable of transition to a pathogen causing symptomatic mucosal infections in association with predisposing host factors.[39] *C. albicans* is the predominant colonizing *Candida* species (70%-80%), but any of the non-*C. albicans* species such as *C. glabrata* and *C. tropicalis* which may account for 5% to 8%, respectively, can be colonizers.[40] Colonization rates are influenced by the severity and nature of the underlying medical illness and the duration of hospitalization, as well as age (highest in infants younger than 18 months of age and in adults older than 60 years of age). A variety of host and exogenous factors (Table 120-3) can lead to the transformation of asymptomatic colonization to symptomatic disease, such as oropharyngeal and esophageal candidiasis. *C. albicans* is the most common species causing all forms of mucosal candidiasis in humans. Less frequently, non-*C. albicans* species can be pathogenic and cause disease. These include *C. glabrata*, *Candida tropicalis*, *Candida krusei*, and *Candida parapsilosis*.[41,42] *Candida krusei*, although relatively uncommon, generally is recovered from mucosal surfaces of neutropenic patients with hematologic malignancies.[42] Another species, *Candida dubliniensis*, has been identified in both HIV-infected and noninfected patients, and may cause ~15% of infections previously ascribed to *C. albicans*.[42] In patients with cancer, non-*C. albicans* species account for almost half of all *Candida* infections.

OPC is the most common opportunistic infection in patients with HIV disease, and it may be the first clinical manifestation of the HIV infection in the majority of untreated patients. OPC occurs in 50% to 90% of HIV-infected patients at some point during the progressive course of the disease to acquired immunodeficiency syndrome (AIDS),[38,41,42] although significant reductions in the incidence have been observed after the introduction of HAART. The absolute CD4 T-cell count is the primary risk factor for development of OPC with the greatest risk at CD4 T-cell levels less than 200 cells/mm^3 (less than 0.2×10^9/L). Also, the HIV viral load is a predictor of OPC development; OPC is thought to increase with HIV viral loads greater than 10,000 copies/mL (greater than 10×10^6/L). This finding correlates with the observation that initiation of antiretroviral therapy and subsequent increase in CD4 T-cell counts does not fully account for the decrease in OPC incidence.[41] Regardless of the CD4 T-cell count, or HIV viral load OPC is predictive for the development of AIDS-related illnesses if left untreated.[38,42]

In non-HIV diseases, such as cancer, the incidence of OPC varies depending on the type of malignant neoplastic disease, level of immune suppression, and type and duration of treatment, but it is less common than in HIV-infected patients. OPC was initially reported in ~25% of patients with solid tumors and up to 60% in those with hematologic malignancies or bone marrow transplant recipients.[43] Rates of OPC have decreased significantly in these patients because of widespread use of antifungal prophylaxis. Incidence in other patient populations predisposed to OPC such as the hospitalized patient administered broad-spectrum antibiotics or denture and other oral appliance users is not well quantified, however, do represent at-risk individuals where the clinical pharmacist has an important patient-care role.[39,43]

OPC can predispose patients to develop more invasive disease, including esophageal candidiasis.[43] The esophagus is the second most common site of GI candidiasis. The prevalence of esophageal candidiasis has increased mainly because of the number of individuals with AIDS, as well as the increased numbers of other severely immunocompromised patients, especially those with hematologic malignancies.[42] Esophageal candidiasis is the first opportunistic infection in 3% to 10% of HIV-infected patients and is the second most common AIDS-defining disease after *Pneumocystis jiroveci* pneumonia.[42] The mean incidence of esophageal candidiasis among HIV-infected patients is less than OPC and ranges from 15% to 20%.[42] The risk of esophageal candidiasis is increased in HIV-infected patients when the CD4 T-cell count has dropped below 100 to 200 cells/mm^3 (0.1×10^9 to 0.2×10^9/L), as well as in those with OPC.[43,44] However, the absence of OPC does not necessarily exclude the possibility of esophageal disease. Like OPC, the presence of esophageal candidiasis can help predict HIV disease progression and prognosis.[43] The incidence of esophageal candidiasis in non-HIV-infected immunocompromised patients is not well established. *C. albicans* is the most common cause of esophageal candidiasis, accounting for ~80% of cases, with the rest being caused by non-*C. albicans* species.[41]

The introduction of HAART appears to have resulted in a significant decline in the incidence of OPC and esophageal candidiasis.[41,42,45] In addition, the widespread use of the azole agents for treatment and prophylaxis has led to a decline in the prevalence of mucosal candidiasis while leading to the emergence of refractory infections that are more challenging to treat.

TABLE 120-3 Risk Factors for the Development of Oropharyngeal and/or Esophageal Candidiasis

Local Factors	Potential Mechanisms
Use of steroids and antibiotics	Suppression of cellular immunity and inhibition of phagocytosis by steroids, including chronic use of inhaled and topical steroids
	Alteration of endogenous oral flora by broad-spectrum antibiotics, especially when used with steroids, creates a milieu for proliferation of *Candida* species because of reduced environmental and nutritional competition
Dentures	Enhanced adherence of *Candida* species to the acrylic material of dentures, reduced saliva flow under surfaces of denture fittings, improperly fitted dentures, and poor oral hygiene provide a milieu conducive to the survival of microorganisms
Xerostomia caused by drugs (eg, tricyclic antidepressants and phenothiazine), chemotherapy, radiotherapy to the head/neck, and various diseases (eg, Sjögren's syndrome, HIV, and cancer of the head/neck), as well as bone marrow transplant recipients	Reduced dilutional and cleansing effect caused by low secretion rate and low pH in saliva: Saliva and mucosa secretions have defense factors, such as lactoferrin, sialoperoxidase, isozyme, histidine-rich polypeptide, secretory IgA antibodies, specific anti-*Candida* antibodies that help prevent adhesion and overgrowth of *Candida* species
Smoking	
Disruption of oral mucosa caused by chemotherapy and radiotherapy, ulcers, endotracheal intubation trauma, and burns	Oral mucositis induced by radiation and breaks in the physical barrier of the oral epithelium, which is protective against invasion by microorganisms; altered rate of mucosa regeneration by cancer chemotherapy, which increases vulnerability to infection
Systemic Factors	**Potential Mechanisms**
Drugs (eg, cytotoxic agents, corticosteroids, and immunosuppressants after organ transplant), omeprazole, and environmental chemicals (eg, benzene and pesticides)	Reduced immunity because of drug-induced neutropenia or cell-mediated immunity; potent inhibition of gastric acid by PPIs can facilitate the growth of *Candida* species; PPIs also can inhibit the cytotoxic effect of lymphocytes and reduce salivary secretion
Neonates or the elderly	Immature immune system of neonates who usually acquire infection during birth to a mother with vaginal candidiasis or from exposure to infected bottle nipples or to skin of adult caregiver
	Elderly—unclear if this is the direct effect of age per se or contribution from dentures or underlying comorbidity
HIV infection/AIDS	Depletion of CD4 T lymphocytes especially below 200-300 cells/mm^3 (0.2×10^9-0.3×10^9/L); anti-*Candida* protective mechanism of T lymphocytes at a mucosal level is unclear but can be caused by altered cytokines, especially interferon-γ, that inhibit transformation of *Candida* blastoconidia to the more invasive hyphal phase
Diabetes	Higher than normal numbers of *C. albicans* cultured from saliva of diabetic patients; can be related to the elevated glucose levels and reduced chemotactic factor in saliva, altered neutrophil function, and reduced saliva volume and flow
Malignancies (eg, leukemia and head/neck cancer)	Use of intensive radiotherapy and chemotherapy can disrupt oral mucosa and cause xerostomia; prolonged use of broad-spectrum antibiotics in neutropenic patients can alter the normal oral flora; because of the prolonged neutropenia, the principal immune defect, seen especially in leukemic patients, the initial oropharyngeal candidiasis can become systemic or invasive
Nutritional deficiencies (eg, iron, folate, and vitamins B1, B2, B6, B12, and C)	Can be related to dietary restriction or GI absorption problems; deficiencies can serve to enhance the pathogenic potential of the *Candida* inhabitants, alter host defense mechanisms, or change epithelial barrier integrity

AIDS, acquired immunodeficiency syndrome; GI, gastrointestinal; HIV, human immunodeficiency virus; IgA, immunoglobulin A; PPI, proton pump inhibitor.

Pathophysiology

The pathogenesis of OPC is most clearly elucidated in the setting of HIV infection. There appear to be several levels of immune defense against the development of OPC in HIV-infected persons, and they involve both systemic and local immunity. The primary line of host defense against *C. albicans* is cell-mediated immunity (CMI) at the mucosal surfaces, which is mediated by CD4 T cells.[38] The efficacy of the CD4 T cells is reduced when the number of cells drops below a protective threshold, and protection against infection becomes dependent on secondary or local immune mechanisms.[38,41] When the number of CD4 T cells drops too low, recruitment of these cells to the oral cavity is impaired. The CD4 T-cell count is the hallmark predictor for development of OPC. However, HIV viral load may have a stronger association with OPC than CD4 cell number.[41,46] The possibility that HIV plays a strong role in susceptibility to infection is supported clinically by the observation that OPC is more common in HIV-infected persons than in those with similar immunosuppression, such as lymphoma and bone marrow transplant. When the primary line of defense fails, the secondary host defenses become crucial. These include the CD8 T cells, salivary cytokines, and other innate immune cells, such as the neutrophils, macrophages, and epithelial cells (with anti-*Candida* activity). Deficiencies or dysfunction in any of these can result in increased susceptibility to OPC. The problem with the CD8 T cells is caused more by a dysfunction of the microenvironment, specifically, reduction in the E-cadherin adhesion molecule that promotes migration of the cells through mucosal tissues.[42] The role of humoral immunity by antibodies as a protective mechanism is unclear and controversial. The changeover of the role of *Candida* species from commensal to pathogenic in the human host usually occurs when breakdown in these host defenses occurs. The pathogenesis of OPC is still not completely understood. It is important to develop a better understanding of the pathogenesis and role of host defenses, including the mechanism of CD8 T-cell activity, reduced adhesion molecules, and whether other cofactors, such as HIV viral load, HAART, and injection drug use, play a role. Immunotherapeutic modalities can then be developed to eliminate the susceptibility factors and significantly reduce OPC in the at-risk populations.

TABLE 120-4 Clinical Classification of Oropharyngeal Candidiasis

Types	Population at Risk	Clinical Signs and Appearance
Pseudomembranous (thrush)	Neonates, patients with HIV or cancer, the debilitated elderly, patients on broad-spectrum antibiotics or steroid inhalers, patients with dry mouth from various causes, and smokers	Classic "cottage cheese" appearance, yellowish white, soft plaques (or milk curds) overlying areas of erythema on the buccal mucosa, tongue, gums, and throat; plaques are easily removed by vigorous rubbing but can leave red or bleeding sites when removed; lesions on the tongue dorsum give it a bald, depapillated appearance
Erythematous (atrophic)	Patients with HIV, patients on broad-spectrum antibiotics or steroid inhalers	Sensitive and painful erythematous mucosa with few, if any, white plaques; lesions are generally on the dorsal surface of the tongue or the hard palate, occasionally on the soft palate, but any part of the mucosa can be involved; appear as flat red patches on the palate or atrophic patches on the tongue dorsum with loss of papillae. Can be acute or chronic
Hyperplastic (candidal leukoplakia)	Smokers; uncommon in patients with HIV	Thick white and adherent keratotic plaques commonly seen on the buccal mucosa and lateral border of the tongue; can also be seen on the lips and the bottom of the mouth; plaques cannot be easily scraped off or only partially removed; this condition is distinct from oral hairy leukoplakia, and it can progress to severe dysplasia or malignancy
Angular cheilitis	Patients with HIV, denture wearers	Painful red, ulcerative, cracking, or fissuring lesion at one or both comers of the mouth because of an inflammatory reaction; usually lesions are small and rather punctate, but occasionally they can extend in a linear fashion from the angles onto the facial skin
Denture stomatitis (chronic atrophic)	Denture wearers who tend to be elderly and have poor oral hygiene	Red, flat lesions on the mucosa beneath the denture and extend right up to the denture border; more commonly located beneath a maxillary denture, although they can be encountered beneath a mandibular denture
Central papillary atrophy (median rhomboid glossitis)	Uncommon (<1% prevalence), men more commonly infected than women (3:1)	Rhomboid-shaped hypertrophic or atrophic plaque in the mid-doral tongue. Lesions may not resolve completely

HIV, human immunodeficiency virus.

Significant differences exist in the virulence among *Candida* species in mucosal candidiasis. One virulence factor is the ability of the organism to adapt and survive in response to changes in the host environment.[41] The genes required for virulence are regulated in response to the environmental signals indigenous to the host environment (eg, temperature, pH, osmotic pressure, iron and calcium ion concentrations, oxygenation, and carbon and nitrogen availability). The ability of *C. albicans* to undergo reversible morphologic transition between the budding pseudohyphal and the more invasive hyphal growth forms is also a determinant of virulence, and genes are recognized to play a role.[38] Other virulence factors are the adhesive ability of *C. albicans* to epithelial cells and proteins and its ability to invade host cells by means of phospholipase and proteinase enzymes. This may be one of the factors leading to OPC in non-HIV-infected individuals. Other components of the pathogenesis in the absence of HIV that have been postulated are the ability of the *Candida* species to adhere to buccal epithelial cells. A close correlation between adhesion of *Candida* species and their ability to cause infection has been demonstrated in animal model studies.[47] This is hypothesized to be a key element in the development of OPC in patients with altered microflora, including those receiving broad-spectrum antimicrobial therapy.

Risk Factors

4 Several host and exogenous factors contribute to the ability of *Candida* species to cause infection (see Table 120-3). Local and systemic factors, as well as characteristics of the organism itself, can increase the susceptibility of an individual to *Candida* infections.[38] Endocrine disorders besides diabetes mellitus, such as hypothyroidism, hypoparathyroidism, and hypoadrenalism, also can predispose patients to *Candida* species overgrowth. Patients with primary immune deficiencies such as lymphocytic abnormalities, phagocytic dysfunction, immunoglobulin A (IgA) deficiency, viral-induced immune paralysis, and severe congenital immunodeficiencies are also at risk for OPC as well as disseminated candidiasis. Oral mucosal disease, such as lichen planus, can be preexistent causes of candidiasis. Smoking may be a predisposing risk factor. In many cases, multiple concurrent predisposing factors to candidiasis can exist, for example, xerostomia with mucositis and a break in the epithelial surface or immunosuppression, such as might occur in a leukemic patient receiving radiation and chemotherapy. The severity and extent of *Candida* infections increase with the number and severity of predisposing risk factors.[39]

Clinical Presentation and Diagnosis

OPC can manifest in several major forms (Table 120-4).[38,39] The clinical signs and symptoms of OPC and the locations of the lesions can be quite diverse (Table 120-5). A presumptive diagnosis of OPC usually is made by the characteristic appearance on the oral mucosa, with resolution of signs and symptoms after antifungal therapy. Pseudomembranous candidiasis, commonly known as *oral thrush*, is the classic and most common form seen in immunosuppressed and immunocompetent hosts. Erythematous and hyperplastic candidiasis and angular cheilitis occur less commonly in the HIV-infected population. Dysphagia, odynophagia, and retrosternal chest pain are common complaints of esophageal candidiasis, which is usually, but not always, accompanied by the presence of OPC. Clinical symptomatology, along with a therapeutic trial of antifungal, can provide a reliable presumptive diagnosis of esophageal candidiasis. If antifungal therapy does not lead to resolution, more invasive tests such as upper GI endoscopy can be undertaken.

TREATMENT

Desired Outcomes

The primary desired outcome in the management of OPC is a clinical cure, that is, elimination of clinical signs and symptoms. Even when the patient is relatively asymptomatic, it is important to treat the initial episode of OPC to avoid progression to more extensive disease. In the most severe cases, the patient's quality of life can be impaired; this can result in decreased fluid and nutritional intake.

TABLE 120-5 Clinical Presentation of Oropharyngeal and Esophageal Candidiasis

Oropharyngeal Candidiasis	Esophageal Candidiasis
General	**General**
The clinical features can be quite diverse (see Table 98-4)	This usually occurs as an extension of OPC; however, the esophagus can be the only site involved; the distal two-thirds, rather than the proximal one-third, is the most common site
Symptoms	**Symptoms**
Symptoms are diverse and range from none to a sore, painful mouth, burning tongue, metallic taste, and dysphagia and odynophagia with involvement of the hypopharynx	Typically, the symptoms are dysphagia, odynophagia, and retrosternal chest pain but can be asymptomatic in some patients; although rare, epigastric pain can be the dominant symptom
Signs	**Signs**
Signs are variable and can include diffuse erythema and white patches on the surfaces of the buccal mucosa, throat, tongue, or gums; constitutional signs are absent	Constitutional signs, including fever, occasionally occur; physical findings can range from a few to numerous white or beige plaques of variable size Plaques can be hyperemic or edematous, with ulceration in more severe cases Most advanced cases can occur with increased mucosal friability and narrowing of lumen Uncommon complications include perforation and aortic–esophageal fistula formation
Laboratory tests	**Laboratory tests**
Scraping of an active lesion for microscopic examination can help confirm the diagnosis (presence of pseudohyphae and budding yeast) but is usually not necessary Cultures are not necessary because isolation of *Candida* species does not distinguish between colonization and true infection; cultures can be taken in patients responding poorly to therapy to determine the infecting species and to predict likely drug resistance	The best test is upper GI endoscopy (more useful than barium swallow); helps exclude other causes of esophagitis (eg, viral, aphthous ulcers); diagnosis is confirmed by the histologic presence of *Candida* species in biopsy lesions taken during endoscopy Cultures to look for drug-resistant *Candida* species are warranted in patients who require endoscopy

GI, gastrointestinal; OPC, oropharyngeal candidiasis.

Lack of appropriate treatment of OPC can lead to more extensive oral disease, especially in patients who are immunocompromised. The most serious complication of untreated OPC is extension of the infection to esophageal candidiasis. Because esophageal candidiasis is more debilitating, the patient's quality of life is more affected. It is important to initiate appropriate antifungal therapy for both OPC and esophageal candidiasis. Preventing or minimizing the number of future recurrences of both types of candidiasis is an equally important outcome. The approach depends largely on the underlying predisposing conditions. Mycologic cure is not a necessary treatment outcome because it may not be feasible or realistic, given that *Candida* species exist commonly as part of the normal mouth flora.

Minimizing toxicities and drug–drug interactions of systemic antifungal agents, as well as maximizing adherence by ensuring that the patient understands the importance of therapy and the directions to take the medication appropriately, are important secondary outcomes of therapy.

General Approach to Treatment

The management of OPC should be individualized for each patient, taking into consideration the underlying immune status, other concurrent mucosal and medical diseases, concomitant medications, and exogenous infectious sources. In HIV-infected patients with inadequately controlled disease, antifungal treatment produces only a transient clinical response, and the relapse rates are higher than in other patient populations. These patients usually require frequent courses of antifungal treatment. Therefore, in patients with HIV disease, treatment with effective HAART is paramount because this would provide the best prophylaxis against recolonization and recurrence of symptoms.[39,41,48]

Whenever feasible, it is desirable to minimize all predisposing factors, such as administration of corticosteroids, chemotherapeutic agents, and antimicrobials, as well as institute proper oral hygiene and resolve concurrent conditions, such as denture stomatitis. Selection of an appropriate antifungal agent for treatment of candidiasis requires consideration of several factors, including the patient's drug adherence, adequate saliva for dissolution of solid topical medications, risk of caries from sucrose- or dextrose-containing preparations, potential drug interactions, coexisting medical conditions (eg, liver disease), location and severity of the infection, and the need for long-term maintenance therapy. Another factor that could affect drug selection is overuse of fluconazole, leading to the emergence of fluconazole-resistant species of *C. albicans*, and in some cases to all azoles, and other intrinsically more resistant species, such as *C. krusei*, *C. glabrata*, and *C. tropicalis*.

5 Topical antimycotic therapies should be the first choice for milder forms of infections.[48] The efficacy of antimycotic agents for OPC varies in different patient populations. Until the polyene antimycotic agents became available in the 1950s, gentian violet, an aniline dye, was used to treat OPC. Problems with gentian violet include fungal resistance, skin irritation, and especially the unaesthetic staining of the oral mucosa. In resource limited areas gentian violet remains a therapeutic option. A 0.00165% gentian violet solution does not stain the oral mucosa and has potent antifungal activity.[49] Topical agents, such as nystatin and clotrimazole, have been the standard of treatment for uncomplicated OPC and generally are effective for treatment in otherwise healthy adults and infants with no underlying immunodeficiencies. Topical agents are available in an assortment of formulations, including oral rinses (suspension), troches, powder, vaginal tablets, creams and most recently as a mucoadhesive tablet[43,48,50] (Table 120-6).

Topical agents require frequent applications because of the short contact time with the oral mucosa; the ideal contact time is 20 to 30 minutes. Sufficient saliva is needed to dissolve clotrimazole troches, and this can be problematic for patients with xerostomia. Also, the rough surface of the tablet can become irritating to the oral soft tissue. Troches also contain dextrose, which has cariogenic potential. Nystatin suspension might be a better choice for patients with xerostomia, but it is difficult to maintain adequate contact time with the oral mucosa. Some patients complain of the unpleasant taste of nystatin, which can cause nausea and vomiting; this is especially problematic in cancer patients experiencing chemotherapy-induced nausea. The high sucrose content of nystatin suspension is

TABLE 120-6 Therapeutic Options for Mucosal Candidiasis

Initial Episodes of OPC:[a] Treat for 7-14 Days	Common/Significant Side Effects
Clotrimazole 10 mg troche: hold 1 troche in mouth for 15-20 minutes for slow dissolution 5 times daily (B-2)	Altered taste, mild nausea, vomiting
Nystatin 100,000 units/mL suspension: 5 mL swish and swallow 4 times daily (B-2)	Mild nausea, vomiting, diarrhea
Miconazole 50 mg mucoadhesive buccal tablets 50 mg daily (A-1)	Diarrhea, headache, nausea, dysgeusia, upper abdominal pain, and vomiting
Fluconazole 100 mg tablets:[b] 100-200 mg daily (A-1)	GI upset, hepatitis not common
Itraconazole 10 mg/mL solution:[c] 200 mg daily (A-2)	GI upset, not common: hepatotoxicity, CHF, pulmonary edema with long-term usee
Posaconazole 40 mg/mL suspension: 400 mg daily with a full meal (A-2)	GI upset, fever, headache, increased hepatic transaminases not common
Fluconazole-Refractory OPC: Treat for ≥14 Days	
Itraconazole 10 mg/mL solution: 200 mg daily (A-3)	See above
Voriconazole 200 mg tablets: 200 mg twice daily (>40 kg), taken on empty stomach (A-3)	GI upset, rash, reversible visual disturbance (altered light perception, photopsia, chromatopsia, photophobia), increased hepatic transaminases, hallucinations, or confusion
Posaconazole 40 mg/mL suspension: 400 mg twice daily × 3 days, then 400 mg daily × 28 days (A-2)	See above
Amphotericin B 100 mg/mL suspension:[d] 1-5 mL swish and swallow 4 times daily (B-2)	Oral: nausea, vomiting, diarrhea with higher dose
Amphotericin B deoxycholate 50 mg injection: 0.3-0.7 mg/kg/day IV daily (B-2)	IV: fever, chills, sweats, nephrotoxicity, electrolyte disturbances, bone marrow suppression
Caspofungin 50 mg IV daily (B-2)	Fever, headache, infusion-related reactions (<5%) (eg, rash, facial swelling, pruritus, vasodilation), hypokalemia, increased hepatic transaminases, anemia, neutropenia
Micafungin 150 mg IV daily (B-2)	Similar to caspofungin
Anidulafungin 200 mg IV daily (B-2)	Similar to caspofungin
Esophageal Candidiasis:[a] Treat for 14-21 Days	
Fluconazole 100 mg tablets: 200-400 mg (3-6 mg/kg) daily (A-1)	See above
Echinocandin: see above (B-2)	See above
Amphotericin B deoxycholate 50 mg injection: 0.3-0.7 mg/kg/day IV daily (B-2)	See above
Posaconazole 40 mg/mL suspension: 400 mg twice daily (A-3)	See above
Itraconazole 10 mg/mL solution:[c] 200 mg daily (A-3)	See above
Voriconazole 200 mg tablets: 200 mg twice daily (>40 kg) (A-3)	See above
Voriconazole and echinocandins (A-1): generally reserved for refractory cases	See above
Fluconazole-Refractory EC: Treat for 21-28 Days	
Itraconazole 10 mg/mL solution: 200 mg daily (A-2)	See above
Posaconazole 40 mg/mL suspension: 400 mg twice daily (A-3)	See above
Voriconazole 200 mg tablets: 200 mg twice daily (>40 kg), taken on empty stomach (A-3)	See above
Caspofungin 50 mg IV daily (B-2)	See above
Micafungin 150 mg IV daily (B-2)	Similar to caspofungin
Anidulafungin 100 mg IV on day 1, then 50 mg IV daily (B-2)	Similar to caspofungin
Amphotericin B deoxycholate: 0.3-0.7 mg/kg/day IV, or lipid-based amphotericin 3-5 mg/kg/day IV (B-2)	See above

CHF, congestive heart failure; GI, gastrointestinal; OPC, oropharyngeal candidiasis.

[a]Initial episodes of OPC can be adequately treated first with topical agents before resorting to systemic therapy (B-2), but systemic therapy is required for effective treatment of esophageal candidiasis. (A-2) Suppressive therapy is recommended for patients with frequent or severe recurrences (A-1).

[b]Fluconazole is more effective than ketoconazole (A-1).

[c]Solution is more effective than capsule (A-1); solution is better taken on an empty stomach.

[d]Suspension is not marketed; can be prepared extemporaneously by pharmacy.[50]

[e]See discussion under onychomycosis.

Recommendation grades:

Strength of recommendation: **A**—Both strong evidence for efficacy and substantial clinical benefit to support recommendation for use. *Should always be offered.* **B**—Moderate evidence for efficacy but only limited clinical benefit, to support recommendation for use. *Should generally be* offered. **C**—Evidence for efficacy is insufficient to support recommendation for or against use; or evidence for efficacy might not outweigh adverse consequences or cost of the treatment under consideration. *Optional.* **D**—Moderate evidence for lack of efficacy or adverse outcome supports a recommendation against use. *Should generally not be offered.*

Quality of evidence: **1**—Evidence from at least one properly designed randomized, controlled trial. **2**—Evidence from at least one well-designed trial without randomization, from cohort or case-controlled analytic studies (preferably from more than one center), or from multiple time-series studies, or dramatic results from uncontrolled experiments. **3**—Evidence from opinions of respected authorities based on clinical experience, descriptive studies, or reports of expert committees. (UR) Evidence currently unrated.

cariogenic in dentate patients, and it should be used with caution in diabetic patients.[39,43] Miconazole 50 mg mucoadhesive tablets are the first buccal adherent miconazole product approved for the local treatment of OPC in adults and adolescents older than age 16 years.[51] This product offers the advantage of a once-daily formulation that is tasteless, odorless, and sugar free.[50] Topical creams, such as clotrimazole, ketoconazole, miconazole, and nystatin (usually mixed with a steroid), are more appropriate for application three times daily to the corners of the mouth in treating angular cheilitis, the inflammation, drying, and cracking of the corners of the mouth.[48]

Systemic therapy is necessary in patients with OPC that is refractory to topical treatment, those who cannot tolerate topical agents, moderate-to-severe disease, and those at high risk for disseminated systemic or invasive candidiasis. Effective treatment of esophageal candidiasis generally requires the use of systemic antifungal agents. However, these agents have the disadvantage of producing more side effects (see Table 120-6) and drug–drug interactions (see Chapter e99). Fluconazole is inexpensive and generally well tolerated, and its absorption is unaffected by food or gastric acidity. Ketoconazole requires gastric acidity for absorption, which can be problematic in AIDS patients with achlorhydria; hence, it is best given with an acidic beverage. Ketoconazole is not recommended today with the availability of more effective triazoles. Itraconazole capsules also have the same absorption problem and are no longer recommended. In contrast, itraconazole solution has enhanced absorption and is best taken in a fasting state; in addition, the solution provides the benefit of both topical effects to the oral mucosa and systemic effects and is beneficial to patients with mucositis or swallowing problems. Whenever possible, it is generally beneficial to limit the use of systemic azole agents to prevent unnecessary drug exposure and to minimize the potential for occurrence of drug-resistant candidiasis, particularly from fluconazole resistance.

When patients become unresponsive to topical agents or fluconazole and itraconazole, alternative agents are available.[43,44,48,52,53] These include amphotericin B and newer triazoles such as voriconazole and posaconazole and echinocandins (caspofungin, micafungin, and anidulafungin) (see discussion below). Although posaconazole is now available in three formulations; the original suspension as well as oral tablets and an intravenous product, only the suspension has an FDA indication for the treatment of OPC.[54]

Clinical **Controversy...**

The optimal strategy for the management of recurrent oral mucosal candidiasis is unclear. Primary and secondary prophylaxis is not routinely recommended in HIV infected patients. The decision to use secondary prophylaxis should be made on an individual case basis.

Oropharyngeal Candidiasis: Human Immunodeficiency Virus-Infected Patients

It is appropriate to start therapy with topical agents for initial or recurrent episodes of OPC, provided that clinical symptoms are not severe and that there is minimal risk of esophageal involvement.[42,48] Clinical responses with the resolution of signs and symptoms generally occur within 5 to 7 days of initiating treatment. Clotrimazole appears to be the most effective topical agent and demonstrates comparable clinical response rates with both fluconazole and itraconazole.[42,48] However, topical therapy is associated with more frequent relapses than with fluconazole.[44,48] This may be of limited clinical significance in patients receiving effective HAART because of their decreased susceptibility to opportunistic infection. In practice, nystatin suspension is still used frequently in initial episodes of OPC, although it is the least effective agent and is associated with frequent treatment failures and early relapses, especially in patients with advanced HIV disease or neutropenia.[39,43] Miconazole mucoadhesive tablets (MMT) 50 mg once daily was noninferior to clotrimazole troches 10 mg five times daily for the treatment of OPC in HIV infected patients (61% vs 65%, respectively for intention to treat cure rate), (68% vs 74%, respectively per protocol) populations at the test of cure visit. Safety and tolerability was also similar between treatment groups.[51]

Systemic oral azoles should be reserved for use in the more severe episodes of OPC unresponsive to topical agents or in patients with concurrent esophageal involvement.[43,48] In clinical practice, fluconazole usually is the systemic azole agent of choice because of its proven efficacy, favorable absorption, safety, and drug-interaction profiles, and it is relatively inexpensive. Fluconazole is superior to ketoconazole and itraconazole capsules.[42,48] A fluconazole regimen of 100 to 200 mg/day for 7 to 14 days is recommended.[48] A single dose of fluconazole 750 mg orally is as effective as fluconazole 150 mg orally for 14 days, which warrants further evaluation, given the potential advantages of adherence and cost-effectiveness.[52] Itraconazole oral solution with an improved absorption profile compared with the capsule formulation is as effective as fluconazole, with comparable clinical and mycologic response and relapse rates.[43,48] However, it carries a higher risk of drug interactions because it is a potent inhibitor of the cytochrome P450 (CYP) enzymes, and it is associated with more nausea than fluconazole. Posaconazole is an extended-spectrum triazole with potent in vitro activity against both *C. albicans* and non-*C. albicans* species. It is equivalent to fluconazole in terms of efficacy, safety, and tolerability.[53] Posaconazole has joined itraconazole solution and voriconazole as the azole alternatives to fluconazole in the management of moderate-to-severe OPC.[47] Other agents that are effective are amphotericin B and the echinocandins (caspofungin, micafungin, and anidulafungin). They are better reserved for refractory OPC, however, because of their greater toxicity. They are also more expensive and are less convenient to use.

Oropharyngeal Candidiasis: Non-Human Immunodeficiency Virus-Infected Patients

This patient population includes patients with hematologic malignancy (eg, leukemias) or blood and bone marrow transplantation (BMT) with a long duration of neutropenia and chronic graft-versus-host disease, patients with solid tumors, patients with solid-organ transplants who are receiving immunosuppressive therapy, and patients with diabetes mellitus, as well as patients on prolonged courses of antibiotics or corticosteroids and the debilitated elderly. Factors to consider in deciding whether to use topical or systemic antifungal therapy include the severity and extent of mucosal involvement (oropharyngeal vs esophageal), predisposing risk factors, and risk for dissemination. Patients who develop neutropenia (eg, leukemic and BMT patients) are usually at high risk for disseminated and invasive fungal disease, and treatment of oral candidiasis is more aggressive. Patients with cell-mediated immune deficits but normal or near-normal granulocyte function and number (eg, solid tumors, solid-organ transplants, or diabetic patients) are at low risk for dissemination of infection.

Specific antifungal therapy can be unnecessary for asymptomatic patients at relatively low risk for disseminated candidiasis, such as those who are not granulocytopenic or who are expected to have a short duration of granulocytopenia.[43] Many of these infections will clear spontaneously after recovery of the granulocytes or discontinuation of antibiotic and/or immunosuppressive therapy. However, antifungal therapy usually is required for patients who have persistent infection or significant symptoms, usually pain, or who are granulocytopenic with a relatively high risk of fungal dissemination. Topical agents can be given a first therapeutic trial depending on the severity of infection and the degree of immunosuppression.

Although both nystatin and clotrimazole can be effective in treating OPC, nystatin suspension does not effectively reduce the incidence of either oropharyngeal or systemic *Candida* infections in immunocompromised patients receiving chemotherapy or radiation; its use often is associated with treatment failures and early relapses.[48] Clotrimazole appears to be more effective in reducing colonization and treating acute episodes in cancer patients who are immunocompromised. MMTs were superior to miconazole oral gel in achieving a complete response in patients with head and neck cancer.[55] MMT has not been studied against clotrimazole in this patient population specifically but is approved for use in adults with OPC.

Systemic azole agents are used for treating OPC in patients who have failed or who are unable to take topical therapy.[43,48,53] The preceding discussion on the relative efficacy of fluconazole, itraconazole, and ketoconazole in HIV-infected patients can be extrapolated to the non-HIV-infected population. Oral fluconazole 100 to 200 mg daily is used more commonly because of more extensive experience with its use, and it is more effective and has a more favorable absorption and side-effect profile compared with other available azoles.[48] If the oral route is not feasible for reasons such as severe chemotherapy-induced mucositis, fluconazole can be administered IV. In patients unresponsive to azoles, IV amphotericin B in relatively low doses of 0.1 to 0.3 mg/kg/day can be tried.[48] Because of the higher risk for dissemination in patients who are severely neutropenic (less than 0.1×10^9 neutrophils/L) or clinically unstable (hypotensive or febrile), some clinicians prefer to initiate therapy with IV amphotericin B at 0.6 mg/kg/day, with therapy continued until the neutropenia has resolved or an echinocandin.[48] The echinocandins caspofungin, micafungin, and anidulafungin have all been found to be effective for treatment of OPC, thus offering another option, with fewer adverse effects in the patient with refractory disease.[48]

Topical therapy with clotrimazole or nystatin for 7 days is usually adequate for treating mucocutaneous candidiasis in most solid-organ transplant patients.[43] Use of topical therapy will reduce the number of systemic drugs that these patients receive and hence minimize the risk of drug–drug interactions. Failure to respond to topical agents warrants the use of fluconazole. Low-dose amphotericin B solution as "swish and swallow" (100 mg/mL, 1 mL four times daily) for 7 to 10 days is reserved for the unusual cases of treatment failure.

Patients who develop OPC because of prolonged antibiotic use or aerosolized corticosteroids use can be managed successfully by discontinuation of the offending agent, and the infection usually will resolve. If there is a strong desire to treat because of discomfort or need to hasten symptom resolution or an inability to stop the offending agent, therapy with a topical agent, either miconazole MT, clotrimazole or nystatin, is effective in most cases. The advantage of systemic azoles is the convenience of less frequent dosing. Symptoms usually improve in 3 or 4 days. Infants should be given smaller amounts more frequently (eg, nystatin 100,000 units every 2-3 hours) to ensure better contact time. For denture-related OPC, or candidal stomatitis, effective therapy requires treatment of both the mouth and the dentures to avoid relapse. The dentures must be brushed vigorously and disinfected every night by soaking in antiseptic solution, such as chlorhexidine gluconate 0.25% or a product such as Polident or Efferdent.[43,48] Topical antifungal therapy of the oral cavity is required. Consistent proper oral hygiene and care of the dentures can help prevent relapse.

Esophageal Candidiasis: Human Immunodeficiency Virus-Infected Patients

6 Treatment of esophageal candidiasis has not been as well studied as OPC. Because of the significant morbidity of esophageal candidiasis and the absence of evidence supporting the efficacy of topical antifungals, treatment requires systemic antifungal agents.[3] Fluconazole is superior to ketoconazole and itraconazole capsules with respect to endoscopic cure and clinical response and usually produces a more rapid onset of action and resolution of symptoms. Fluconazole is as effective as itraconazole solution, with reported response rates of greater than 80% to 90%.[39,43] However, itraconazole solution causes more nausea and drug interactions because of inhibition of the CYP enzymes. Amphotericin B, voriconazole, posaconazole, and the echinocandins are also effective in esophageal candidiasis, but they are generally reserved for patients with advanced or inadequately controlled HIV disease where the candidiasis tends to recur or becomes refractory to azole therapy.[56-59]

Esophageal Candidiasis: Non-Human Immunodeficiency Virus-Infected Patients

As in the case of HIV-infected patients, treatment of esophageal candidiasis requires systemic therapy. Patients can be started on fluconazole 200 to 400 mg/day for 14 to 21 days.[48] Higher fluconazole doses (up to 400 mg/day) have been suggested for patients with severe symptoms or those who are neutropenic.[60] Other agents currently recommended if fluconazole is not an option are an echinocandin or amphotericin B at 0.3 to 0.7 mg/kg. Itraconazole solution, posaconazole, and voriconazole are effective alternatives that may be considered for those not responding adequately to fluconazole. An echinocandin or IV amphotericin B may be selected over fluconazole for initial therapy in neutropenic patients who present with severe symptoms or who are at high risk for dissemination of *Candida* species, such as those receiving other aggressive immunosuppressive therapy (eg, corticosteroids, total-body irradiation, or antithymocyte globulin) and who have documented evidence of esophageal candidiasis or who have failed an initial empirical trial of oral nonabsorbable agents or systemic azoles.[48] Therapy should be continued at least until the neutropenia resolves. For patients whose symptoms have resolved and who are afebrile and clinically stable, therapy should be discontinued, and the patients should be monitored closely for infection recurrence. In high-risk patients, particularly those with persistent fever and neutropenia, the potential presence of clinically occult, diffuse GI or disseminated candidiasis should be considered. The echinocandins and newer azole agents (voriconazole and posaconazole) offer less toxic alternatives or oral agents and are preferred in patients who are intolerant of amphotericin B deoxycholate or who have preexisting renal impairment.[43,60,61] There are limited data on the clinical efficacy of anidulafungin compared with fluconazole, 95% versus 89% cure rates, respectively, in the non-HIV-infected patients.[60]

Antifungal-Refractory Oral Mucosal Candidiasis

Treatment failure is generally defined as persistence of signs and symptoms of OPC or esophageal candidiasis after an appropriate trial of antifungal therapy.[42] Treatment of refractory oral mucosal candidiasis is frequently unsatisfactory, and clinical response is usually short-lived, with rapid and periodic recurrences. The key risk factors for occurrence of refractory candidiasis are advanced stage of AIDS with low CD4 cell counts (less than 50 cells/mm^3 [less than 0.05×10^9/L]) and repeated or prolonged courses of various systemic antifungal agents, in particular systemic azoles.[43,48] Frequent or prolonged use of fluconazole can be associated with fluconazole-refractory candidiasis because of selection of more resistant non-*C. albicans* species. An important initial management strategy is to assess and optimize the antiretroviral therapy of the patient with refractory OPC to help improve the immune function. With the widespread use of HAART, fluconazole-refractory OPC is now less commonly encountered. It is also important to identify and rectify potentially correctable causes of clinical failures of mucosal candidiasis, such as poor drug adherence, adequate dosing, reduced drug absorption associated with hypochlorhydria, and drug–drug interactions.

There have been few controlled studies that assess the effectiveness of antifungal agents. Doubling of the fluconazole dosage to 400 or 800 mg/day can be effective in some patients with infection caused by *Candida* species of intermediate resistance, although the response may be only transient.[44] Fluconazole oral suspension can be beneficial in some patients because of increased salivary concentrations obtained when the suspension is taken with the swish and swallow technique.[48] Patients with fluconazole-refractory mucosal candidiasis can be treated with itraconazole oral suspension because it can be effective in 64% to 80% of patients; however, the benefit is short-lived if chronic suppressive therapy is not maintained.[42,48] Posaconazole suspension has been reported to be successful in ~74% of patients with refractory oral or esophageal candidiasis; voriconazole may also be efficacious in these patients. Amphotericin B oral suspension is another alternative for azole-refractory patients.[44,48] It has broad-spectrum activity against many fungal species and low likelihood of *Candida* species resistance. There are limited data and experience on its use in immunosuppressed patients, and results from small studies have yielded mixed results.[62] Amphotericin B suspension is no longer available commercially in the United States, but it can be prepared extemporaneously by the pharmacy.[62]

Clinical **Controversy...**

There are several alternatives to fluconazole refractory candidiasis, no drug of choice has been definitively identified, selection will depend on disease severity, route of administration effect on cytochrome P450 enzymes and side effect profile.

Until recently, IV amphotericin B deoxycholate has been the alternative for patients with endoscopically proven disease who have failed fluconazole or itraconazole therapy. Patients with severe disease unresponsive to other agents require IV amphotericin B 0.3 to 0.7 mg/kg/day for 7 to 10 days to achieve clinical response; higher dose or longer treatment duration can be needed in more severe disease.[44,48] After response, suppressive therapy with amphotericin B is required to increase disease-free intervals. Patients who fail to respond to amphotericin B and require greater than 1 mg/kg/day might be candidates for liposomal amphotericin B preparations because of renal and/or bone marrow toxicities, although at a markedly higher cost. Flucytosine usually is not used as monotherapy because of rapid development of resistance but can be used in combination with an azole or amphotericin B.[44] Less toxic agents that are also effective are voriconazole and the echinocandins.[60,61] Voriconazole, a triazole antifungal available in both oral and IV preparations, appears to be as effective as fluconazole for esophageal candidiasis, and it has shown success in treatment of fluconazole-refractory disease.[59] However, voriconazole has more side effects and multiple pharmacokinetic drug interactions compared to fluconazole.[59] Caspofungin, micafungin, and anidulafungin are approved for this indication. All three echinocandins have similar efficacy and tolerability profile as fluconazole, although caspofungin and anidulafungin have higher relapse rates compared with fluconazole.[48,61] Because the echinocandins require IV administration and are expensive, they are primarily used in patients who are refractory to the triazoles or have serious triazole-related adverse effects. As a class, the echinocandins have a favorable adverse effect profile. They are less toxic than amphotericin B (see Table 120-6) and have less impact on the CYP enzymes than either itraconazole or voriconazole. Immunomodulation with adjunctive granulocyte-macrophage colony-stimulating factor and interferon have been used for refractory oral candidiasis in very limited numbers of patients.[48]

Antifungal Prophylaxis

7 Ensuring that the HIV-infected patient is receiving appropriate antiretroviral therapy to enhance the immune system is perhaps the most important measure in preventing future episodes of mucosal candidiasis (oropharyngeal, esophageal, and vulvovaginal).[48] Initial success of treatment often is followed by symptomatic recurrences, especially in patients with advanced or poorly controlled HIV disease. Long-term suppressive therapy with fluconazole is effective in preventing recurrences or new infections of OPC in HIV disease and in patients with cancer.[48] However, the indications for antifungal prophylaxis and the best long-term management strategy still have not been well established. Fluconazole does not provide complete protection, and breakthrough infections can occur.[44] The reduced risk of recurrence of OPC also has not been demonstrated to improve survival. In addition, chronic exposure to azole therapy is a concern in that it might lead to the development of refractory disease or emergence of azole resistance.[48] However, in a randomized trial of continuous versus episodic fluconazole therapy, continuous therapy did not result in a higher rate of refractory OPC or esophageal disease.[63] HIV specialists do not recommend primary or secondary prophylaxis for OPC.[44] The rationale includes effectiveness of therapy for acute episodes of OPC, low incidence of serious invasive fungal disease, low mortality associated with mucosal candidiasis, potential for drug interactions, potential for emergence of drug resistance, and the prohibitive long-term cost of prophylaxis.

8 The decision to use secondary prophylaxis should be individualized for each patient. Secondary prophylaxis can be considered in patients with multiple recurrent episodes of symptomatic OPC or when the disease is sufficiently severe and affecting the quality of life.[44] Patients with a history of one or more episodes of documented esophageal candidiasis and a CD4 T-cell count still less than 200 cells/mm^3 (less than 0.2×10^9/L) despite being on HAART are candidates for secondary prophylaxis. Oral fluconazole 100 mg daily is the usual regimen recommended for OPC and esophageal candidiasis,[44,48] although 200 mg three times weekly also appears to be effective.[63] Once-weekly oral fluconazole (200 mg) is also effective for preventing OPC recurrences in those with less-advanced AIDS.[44] Itraconazole solution 200 mg daily orally is an alternative as suppressive therapy for OPC.[48]

Patients with malignant neoplastic diseases who are receiving irradiation, cytotoxic, and/or immunosuppressive therapy are at high risk for fungal infections in addition to bacterial and viral infections. Prophylaxis of *Candida* infection is controversial, and the results of studies have been conflicting and difficult to evaluate. In the hematopoietic stem cell transplant (HSCT) population, fluconazole prophylaxis is recommended prior to engraftment. Cross-resistance to other azoles may occur among *Candida* species; this should be a treatment consideration in a patient who develops a breakthrough fungal infection. Micafungin is an alternative to fluconazole prophylaxis of candidiasis.[64] The value of antifungal prophylaxis in these patients needs to be considered in the broader context of not only reducing colonization and the risk of superficial candidiasis but also, more importantly, reducing the risk for invasive candidiasis and improving survival. Management of these infections in this patient population is discussed further in Chapter 100.

Evaluation of Therapeutic Outcomes

Efficacy end points for oropharyngeal and esophageal candidiasis include rapid relief of symptoms and prevention of complications without early relapse after completion of the course of therapy.[44,48] Sterilization of the oral cavity is not a feasible end point because mycologic eradication is rarely achievable, especially in HIV-positive patients. Symptomatic relief of presenting signs and symptoms (see Table 120-5) generally occurs within 48 to 72 hours of starting therapy, with complete resolution by 7 to 10 days. Patients should be

TABLE 120-7 Patient Counseling Tips for Managing Oropharyngeal Candidiasis

1. Clean the oral cavity prior to administering the topical antifungal agent. Daily fluoride rinses can help reduce the risk of caries when using an agent containing sucrose or dextrose.
2. Use the topical antifungal agent after meals, as saliva flow and mouth movements can reduce the contact time.
3. Troches should be slowly dissolved in the mouth, not chewed or swallowed whole, over 15-20 minutes, and the saliva swallowed.
4. Suspension should be swished around the mouth in the oral cavity to cover all areas for as long as possible, ideally at least 1 minute, then gargled and swallowed.
5. Remove dentures while medication is being applied to the oral tissues.
6. Use a suspension or buccal mucoadhesive tablet instead of a troche if xerostomia is present; if a troche is preferred, the patient should rinse or drink water prior to dosing. For xerostomia, suggest nonpharmacologic measures for symptomatic relief (eg, ice chips, sugarless gum or hard candy, citrus beverages).
7. Dentures should be removed and disinfected overnight using an antiseptic solution (eg, chlorhexidine 0.12%-0.2%). Disinfect oral tissues in addition to dental prosthesis.
8. Complete treatment course even though symptomatic improvement can occur in 48-72 hours.
9. Maintain good oral hygiene. Brush teeth daily (twice daily) and floss, rinse mouth, or brush teeth after eating sweets.
10. Stop smoking; avoid alcohol.

Data from reference 52.

advised about the time course and told to return for reassessment when signs and symptoms recur. It is usually unnecessary for the patient to be reassessed soon after finishing the treatment course. However, HIV patients should be questioned and examined for the occurrence of mucosal candidiasis as part of their regular follow-up. The frequency of monitoring can be more often in neutropenic patients because of concern for dissemination of candidiasis. During the period of neutropenia, temperature should be monitored daily, as well as signs of dissemination.

Efficacy of the antifungal agent is partly influenced by patient adherence to the medication regimen. Patients must be counseled on proper administration and dosing, in particular for topical agents (Table 120-7).[60] Safety end points include monitoring for occurrence of the relevant drug side effects and drug interactions (see Table 120-6). Mild GI intolerance can occur with topical therapy, but serious adverse effects are rare. It is still prudent to monitor for hypersensitivity reactions, especially rash and pruritus that might occur with any medication. GI intolerance is more associated with the oral azoles. Hepatotoxicity can occur when azole therapy is prolonged beyond 7 to 10 days or high doses are used. Periodic monitoring of liver enzymes (alanine transaminase and aspartate amino-transferase) should be considered, especially if prolonged therapy (longer than 21 days) is anticipated. Patients who are receiving IV amphotericin B require daily monitoring by a pharmacist.

MYCOTIC INFECTIONS OF THE SKIN, HAIR, AND NAILS

Superficial cutaneous mycoses affect up to 20% to 25% of the global population.[65] The usual pathogens are the dermatophytes classified by genera: *Trichophyton*, *Epidermophyton*, and *Microsporum*. Less frequently infection is caused by nondermatophyte fungi (eg, *Malassezia furfur*) and Candida species. Dermatophytes have the ability to penetrate keratinous structures of the body and therefore infections are limited to hair, nails and skin. These infections affect both male and female genders and all races. Reservoirs of mycotic infections include humans, animals, and soil.[65,66] Individuals can develop an infection if they come in contact with a reservoir in addition to having a conducive environment for mycotic growth (ie, moist conditions).[67] Risk factors for the development of an infection include prolonged exposure to sweat or soaking in water, maceration, intertriginous folds, sharing personal belongings such as combs, close living quarters (dormitories, barracks).[66,67]

Mycotic infections of the skin have a classic appearance that consists of a central clearing surrounded by an advancing red, scaly, elevated border, also referred to as an "active" border.[67,68] The central clearing of the lesion may distinguish dermatophytoses from other skin eruptions such as psoriasis or lichen planus which have a more uniform inflammatory presentation.[68] Infections of the nail can appear chalky and dull yellow or white and become brittle and crumbly.

Diagnosis usually is based on patient history, as well as the physical examination.[69] Diagnostic tests include direct microscopic examination of a specimen after the addition of KOH or fungal cultures. The KOH test is quick, inexpensive, and easy to perform, whereas cultures are more expensive and take longer to obtain results. Diagnostic tests are recommended when systemic therapy is likely to be prescribed.[69]

9 A general approach to treatment of superficial mycotic infections includes keeping the infected area dry and clean and limiting exposure to the infected reservoir. Topical agents generally are considered to be first-line therapy for infections of the skin. Oral therapy is preferred when the infection is extensive or severe or when treating tinea capitis or onychomycosis. Table 120-8 lists specific treatments for each mycotic infection. Superficial mycotic infections are categorized by the pattern and site of infection.[66] The most commonly occurring infections in North America are detailed in the following sections.

Tinea Pedis

Tinea pedis is the most common dermatophytoses (affecting ~70% of adults). It is better known as "athlete's foot" and occurs in hot weather, with exposure to surface reservoirs (locker room floors), and with use of occlusive footwear.[67] Tinea pedis has three common presentations. The most common is the interdigital form which is characterized by fissuring, maceration and scaling of the spaces between the toes (most frequently the fourth and fifth toes). Patients often complain of itching and burning. The "moccasin-like" distribution presentation is usually caused by *Trichophyton* rubrum. In this form the plantar surface becomes chronically scaly and thickened with accompanying erythema of the soles, heels, and sides of the foot. The third presentation, vesiculobulous tinea pedis, is characterized by the formation of vesicles, pustules and occasionally bullae typically on the soles of the foot. Contact dermatitis, pustular psoriasis and eczema would be in the differential diagnosis. Disruption of skin integrity with tinea pedis is a risk factor for streptococcal cellulitis as a complication.[68] Treatment with topical therapy for 2 to 4 weeks often is adequate for mild infections; however, severe infections or involvement of the nails require oral therapy[67] (see Table 120-8). A new 2% gel formulation of naftifine has been approved by the FDA for the treatment of interdigital tinea pedis. In clinical trials of naftifine 2% gel for tinea pedis (interdigital and moccasin-type) found that there was continued improvement even after the therapy was completed with clinical and mycological cure rates increasing from 5.4% and 39.1%, respectively at the 2 weeks end of treatment time point to 21.5% and 62% at week 6.[70] This finding suggests a depot effect of naftifine gel which is supported by the results of studies demonstrating the epidermal level of naftifine at application site remains relatively constant over several weeks post-treatment.[71] Naftifine is not approved for moccasin-type tinea pedis but is the only agent formally studied for this indication in a randomized double-blind vehicle controlled trial. Naftifine 2% gel resulted in a complete cure rate at week 6 of 19.6% compared to 0.7% for vehicle treated patients. Treatment effectiveness at week 6 was 51% for the naftifine versus 6% for the vehicle group.[70] Luliconazole 1% cream once daily for 2 weeks was approved for the topical management of interdigital tinea pedis, tinea cruris and tinea corporis in patients 18 years or older. Similar to naftifine, luliconazole 1% cream

TABLE 120-8 Treatment of Mycoses of the Skin, Hair, and Nails

	Topical[a,b]	Oral[c]
Tinea pedis	Butenafine, daily Sertaconazole, twice daily Luliconazole daily Naftifine cream daily, gel daily	Fluconazole 150 mg 1 per week × 1-4 weeks
Tinea manuum	Ciclopirox, twice daily	Ketoconazole 200 mg daily × 4 weeks
Tinea cruris	Clotrimazole, twice daily Luliconazole, daily Naftifine cream daily,	Itraconazole 200-400 mg/day × 1 week
Tinea corporis	Econazole, daily Haloprogin, twice daily Ketoconazole cream, daily Luliconazole daily Miconazole, twice daily Naftifine cream, daily; Oxiconazole, twice daily Sulconazole, twice daily Terbinafine, twice daily Tolnaftate, twice daily Triacetin cream, solution, 3 times daily Undecylenic acid, various preparations: apply as directed	Terbinafine 250 mg/day × 2 weeks Fluconazole 150 mg once weekly × 4 weeks
Tinea capitis	Shampoo only in conjunction with oral therapy or for treatment of asymptomatic carriers	Terbinafine 250 mg/day × 4-8 weeks Fluconazole 150 mg/week × 4 weeks
Tinea barbae	Ketoconazole twice weekly × 4 weeks Selenium sulfide daily × 2 weeks	Ketoconazole 200 mg daily × 4 weeks Itraconazole 100-200 mg/day × 4-6 weeks Griseofulvin 500 mg/day × 4-6 weeks
Pityriasis versicolor	Clotrimazole, twice daily Econazole, daily Haloprogin, twice daily Ketoconazole, daily Miconazole, twice daily Oxiconazole cream only, twice daily Sulconazole, twice daily Tolnaftate, three times daily	Ketoconazole Fluconazole Itraconazole 200 mg daily × 3-7 days
Onychomycosis	Ciclopirox 8% nail lacquer: apply solution at night for up to 48 weeks (fingernails and toenails) Efinaconazole 10% topical solution daily for 48 weeks (toenails) Tavaborole 5% topical solution daily for 48 weeks (toenails)	Terbinafine 250 mg/day × 6 weeks (fingernail), 12 weeks (toenail) Itraconazole 200 mg twice daily × 1 week/month for 2 months (fingernail); 200 mg daily × 12 weeks (toenail) Fluconazole 50 mg daily or 300 mg once weekly for ≥6 months (fingernail) or 12 months (toenail)

[a]Other products are available, including combination products.

[b]Length of therapy depends on mycotic sensitivity and severity of infection.

[c]Only capsule formulation studied; give with food for increased absorption.

applied once daily for interdigital tinea pedis resulted in continued improvement even after therapy was completed.[72] Recurrence of infection occurs in up to 70% of individuals especially if there is concomitant onychomycosis. Prolonged treatment with either topical or systemic therapy may be required.[65,66] Other nonpharmacologic measures such as disinfecting footwear, avoidance of walking barefoot in public places, controlling hyperhidrosis, wearing absorbent socks and nonocclusive shoes should be advised.[67]

Tinea Manuum

Tinea manuum is a superficial fungal infection of one or infrequently both hands, and can involve the feet (tinea pedis). The infection presents with dry and hyperkeratotic palmar surface of the hand. The fingernails, when involved, may present with vesicles and scaling. Contact dermatitis, eczema, psoriasis and callus formation should be in the differential diagnosis.[68] Treatment of this infection is similar to tinea pedis (see Table 120-8). Emollients that contain lactic acid also can be useful.[65] Relapse or recurrence is frequent especially if tinea pedis or onychomycosis is present.[68]

Tinea Cruris

Tinea cruris is an infection of the proximal thighs and buttocks.[68] It is referred to as "jock itch" and is more common in males. Tinea cruris and tinea pedis often occur concurrently. High humidity and warm temperatures along with wet or tight-fitting clothes contribute to the development of tinea cruris. The scrotum and penis often are spared from infection. The lesions are red, scaling with raised borders. Pustules or vesicles and maceration are usually found along the active border. Itching and burning are the most common patient complaint. The differential diagnosis would include candida infection, erythrasma, mechanical intertrigo, psoriasis, and seborrheic dermatitis.[68] Treatment with topical therapy is recommended and should continue for 1 to 2 weeks after symptom resolution. Severe infections can require oral therapy (see Table 120-8). Relief of pruritus and burning can be facilitated by the use of short-term (2 or 3 days) topical steroids (2.5% hydrocortisone).[67] The feet of the patient should also be examined as a source of infection. Non-pharmacological measures such as keeping the area dry or avoiding prolonged exposure to moisture are important patient counselling points.[68]

Tinea Corporis

Tinea corporis, also known as ringworm, is an infection of the glabrous skin of the trunk, extremities, or face.[68] Lesions of tinea corporis may be singular or multiple and appear as round, scaly lesions with central clearing and a raised border with sharp margination.

The border may exhibit pustules. The degree of pruritis is variable. The differential diagnosis includes nummular eczema, contact dermatitis, psoriasis, pityriasis rosea, tinea versicolor, granuloma annulare and Lyme disease.[68] Prior use of topical corticosteroid preparations may alter the appearance such that the central clearing and raised borders are no longer apparent impacting diagnosis. Diagnosis should be confirmed with KOH examination of skin scrapings of the edge of the lesion. Therapy is similar to that for tinea pedis, tinea manuum, and tinea cruris (see Table 120-8). If the infection is very widespread systemic antifungal therapy may be necessary.[68]

Tinea Capitis

Tinea capitis is a mycotic infection involving the scalp, hair follicles, and adjacent skin that primarily affects children.[68,73] Approximately, 90% to 95% of tinea capitis cases are due to *Trichophyton tonsurans*. Inanimate objects such as hats, brushes, or pillowcases are often the source of transmission particularly in the setting of poor hygiene. Viable organisms can be recovered from shed hairs for up to a year.[68] The lesions are characterized by irregular, frequently well-demarcated areas of alopecia with scaling. The alopecia is a result of infected hairs breaking off a few millimeters from the scalp; sometimes called "black dot alopecia." A "kerion" is a sterile, inflammatory scalp mass, often accompanied with cervical and occipital lymphadenopathy, due to a cell-mediated immune response to the infecting pathogen and is another manifestation of tinea capitis. The differential diagnosis will be influenced by the appearance of the lesions. For lesions that are predominantly scaly in inflamed consider seborrheic dermatitis, atopic dermatitis or psoriasis. If alopecia is the primary presenting feature rule out alopecia areata, traction alopecia and trichotillomania (obsessive hair pulling). The diagnosis of tinea capitis can be made in children based on the presence of at least 3 clinical features: scalp scaling, scalp pruritis, occipital adenopathy and diffuse patchy or discrete alopecia.[74] However, given the broad differential diagnoses and the need for prolonged treatment required diagnosis should be confirmed with microscopic examination or fungal culture. Treatment should consist of oral therapy, as well as the cleaning of combs and brushes, which can be contaminated (see Table 120-8). Topical therapy will not penetrate into hair follicles. Daily shampooing is recommended for removal of scales. An antifungal shampoo (eg, selenium sulfide 1%, ketoconazole 2%) in addition to oral therapy is recommended to eliminate the shedding of viable spores.[75] Some children and adults can be asymptomatic carriers, thereby facilitating spread of the infection. Family members who culture positive for *T. tonsurans* should be treated with an antifungal shampoo (eg, ketoconazole, selenium sulfide, or povidone-iodine).[68]

Tinea Barbae

Tinea barbae affects the hairs and follicles of beards and mustaches of adult men and hirsute women.[68] Tinea barbae will present with scaling, follicular pustules and erythema. The differential diagnosis included bacterial folliculitis, contact dermatitis, perioral dermatitis, pseudofolliculitis barbae and herpes simplex. One clue to the diagnosis of tinea barbae is that hair removal with shaving is painless. Treatment is similar to that for tinea capitis (see Table 120-8). Removal of the beard or mustache is recommended.[67]

Pityriasis Versicolor

Hyper- and hypopigmented scaly patches characterize pityriasis versicolor, which is also known as *tinea versicolor*. It is caused by yeasts of the *Malassezia* genus which with the exception of *Malassezia pachydermatis*, are all lipophilic. The seborrheic areas (scalp, face, back and front of the trunk) of the human body are always colonized by one or more *Malassezia* spp., such as *M. globosa*, *M. sympodialis*, *M. sloffiae*, and *M. restricta* are the most common colonizers; *M. globosa* and *M. furfur* are most frequent clinical infection isolates. This is not considered a contagious infection given the source is normal flora. It is more common in adults and in areas with tropical ambient temperatures. The lesions are found on the trunk, face and extremities.[64] Lesions are described as well-demarcated and scaling thin plaques with various degrees of pigmentation. Most patients are asymptomatic or may complain of mild pruritis. Many are concerned about the cosmetic appearance and possible contagion.[76] Topical treatment usually is adequate unless there is extensive involvement, recurrent infections, or failure of topical therapy. Ketoconazole 2% shampoo was significantly more effective than selenium sulfide 2.5% shampoo (89% vs 35% cure rate).[77] Oral imidazole antifungal agents (ketoconazole, itraconazole, or fluconazole) are safe and effective options for oral therapy of extensive pityriasis versicolor. Recurrence of infection after cessation of treatment may be as high as 60% in the first year and 80% the second year. Suppressive maintenance therapy either orally or topically may be used in these cases although data is lacking to definitively identify the most optimal drug, dose or route.[76]

Onychomycosis (Tinea Unguium)

Onychomycosis is a fungal infection of the nail apparatus and is the most common single cause of nail dystrophy, affecting up to 8% of the general population and accounting for up to 50% of all nail problems.[78] Onychomycosis more commonly affects the toenails (2%-14% of adults), ~4 to 19 times more frequently than fingernails, with prevalence increasing with age.[78] This can be because of the slower growth of toenails (three times slower than fingernails), making it easier for fungi to establish infection. Onychomycosis has a significant impact on quality of life, both functional and psychosocial. In addition, the affected nails can disrupt the integrity of the surrounding skin, potentially increasing the risk of secondary bacterial infections.[78,79]

Onychomycosis is due to infection by dermatophytes (tinea unguium), yeasts and nondermatophyte fungi.[80] Dermatophytes are the most frequent causes of onychomycosis (~90% in toenail and ~50% in fingernail infections).[77] The dermatophytes responsible for causing >90% of cases of onychomycosis are *Trichophyton rubrum* (71%) and *Trichophyton mentagrophytes* (20%).[73] Less common fungi causing onychomycosis are the nondermatophytic molds (2.3%-11%) and yeasts (5.6%). *C. albicans* is the most commonly isolated yeast and typically affects fingernails rather than toenails.[77,81] Risk factors for dermatophytic onychomycosis are increasing age (especially older than 40 years), family history and genetic factors, immunodeficiency (eg, HIV, renal transplant, immunosuppressive therapy, and defective polymorphonuclear chemotaxis), diabetes mellitus, psoriasis, peripheral vascular disease, smoking, prevalence of tinea pedis, frequent nail trauma, and sporting activities such as swimming.[81,82] These risk factors also appear to apply to recurrence of onychomycosis. Mold onychomycosis does not seem to be associated with systemic or local predisposing factors, but there is a risk of systemic dissemination in immunosuppressed patients.[77] *Candida* onychomycosis seems to always occur in immunosuppressed patients.[81]

Onychomycosis can present in in a variety of clinical forms. The five major clinical patterns are i) lateral distal subungual onychomycosis (DLSO), ii) white superficial onychomycosis (WSO), iii) proximal subungual onychomycosis (PSO), iv) endonyx onychomycosis, and v) total dystrophic onychomycoisis (TDO).[78,79] In DSO, the most common type, the nail plate, the nail bed, and, in advanced cases, the matrix are all affected, and *T. rubrum* is the most common etiologic cause. The worst case of onychomycosis is progression of the infection to total dystrophic onychomycosis, characterized by almost complete destruction of the nail plate. WSO is usually caused by *T. mentagrophytes*, where the infection is localized to the surface of the nail plate. In PSO, the fungi

TABLE 120-9 Differential Diagnosis of Fungal Nail Infections

Diagnosis	Features Consistent with Diagnosis
Psoriasis	Nail pitting, rash elsewhere on body, family history of psoriasis
Lichen planus	Nail atrophy, scarring at proximal aspect of the nail
Periungual squamous cell carcinoma	Single nail affected, pain, warty nail fold change, or ooze from the edge of nail
Yellow nail syndrome	Multiple nails turn yellow, grow slowly, increased longitudinal and transverse curvature, intermittent pain and shedding, associated with chronic sinusitis, bronchiectasis, lymphedema
Trauma	Single nail affected, homogeneous alteration of nail color and altered shape of nail

Data from Reference 24.

TABLE 120-10 Factors That May Impact Treatment Decisions and Outcomes

- Type and severity of onychomycosis
- Causative organism—dermatophyte vs molds or yeast
- Infection of the finger vs toenail
- Extent of disease—involvement of matrix, one or two lateral edges, number of nails
- Thickness of nail plate
- Other sites of mycotic infection (palms, soles, toe webs)
- Other nail alterations affecting outcome (onycholysis, paronychia, dermatophytoma, etc.)
- Other nail diseases and symptoms
- Age and underlying medical conditions (diabetes, poor perfusion, immunocompromised)
- Drug interactions and adverse effects
- Cost of therapy

Data from references 67, 76, 78, and 79.

(usually *T. rubrum*) invade the nail through the proximal nail fold and spread to the nail plate and matrix. Although PSO is relatively uncommon in the general population, it occurs most frequently in severely immunocompromised patients and is often considered a marker for AIDS.[82,83] In endonyx onychomycosis the fungus directly invades the nail plate keratin instead of the nail plate margin.[78] Because of the multifactorial etiology of onychomycosis, it is important to differentiate onychomycosis from other causes of nail dystrophies (eg, psoriasis, lichen planus, chronic trauma, eczema, yellow nail syndrome, lamellar onychoschizia, periungual squamous cell carcinoma, malignant melanoma, and myxoid cyst) so that the patient receives appropriate therapy and is not subjected to prolonged treatment with unnecessary drugs.[79] Besides clinical history and physical examination, proper diagnosis of onychomycosis can include the combination of direct microscopy of scrapings from the appropriate nail area to look for fungal hyphae and fungal cultures, and, if necessary, histologic examination.[78,79,81] Table 120-9 provides a differential diagnosis for fungal nail diseases.[84]

TREATMENT

General Approach

Onychomycosis merits proper assessment and treatment consideration because it is a debilitating disease and can exert a negative impact on quality of life (eg, cosmetic and psychosocial effects, pain, discomfort, and decreased ambulation).[78,79] It is reasonable to not treat persons with minimal toenail involvement and no associated symptoms.[84] Although definitive data are lacking regarding the risk of progression of untreated disease, it can lead to complications such as cellulitis or reduced mobility, which can further compromise peripheral circulation in those with diabetes or peripheral vascular disease; additionally, infected nails can serve as a source of transmission of fungi to other areas of the body, as well as to other people, such as close household contacts, or in communal bathing places.[78,85] Treatment decisions should be made on an individual basis. The primary end point of treatment is eradication of the organism, with secondary end points being clinical cure and improvement. Assessment of clinical success (cure or improvement) requires follow-up for several months after the end of treatment because of the slow growth rate of nails, especially toenails (1 mm/mo).[78] Successful eradication of the fungus does not always result in normalization of the nails because they can have been dystrophic prior to infection. This can cause patient dissatisfaction, especially if this is not explained before starting treatment.[79] There are several factors that must be taken into account on a patient-by-patient basis to ensure appropriate treatment decisions (Table 120-10). The impact of patient adherence on the success of treatment cannot be overemphasized. Patients need to be educated about their disease, expectations of treatment, and prevention of recurrence, and various strategies have been suggested to improve treatment success.[79]

In general, onychomycosis of the toenail is more difficult to treat than fingernails, requires longer treatment duration, and is associated with a higher recurrence. The treatment options for onychomycosis include oral and topical therapies, mechanical or chemical nail avulsion, or a combination of these. Mechanical or chemical nail avulsion is used primarily as adjunct to oral therapy in patients with total dystrophic onychomycosis, in whom there is severe onycholysis and extensive nail thickening or longitudinal spikes. This is to enhance penetration of the antifungal agent to the entire nail plate and unit.[78,79,85]

Topical Therapy

Diffusion of topically applied drugs is impeded by the hard keratin and compact structure of the dorsal nail plate. The hydrophilic nature of the nail plate also inhibits absorption of most lipophilic molecules.[78]

(10) Conventional topical antifungal products are available as creams, ointments, powders, and solutions. Because these formulations do not penetrate through the nail plate to the nail bed, they are most appropriately used when the nail plate has been removed.[80,85] Even then cure rates are still low and variable and are influenced by patient adherence.[80,81] Efinaconazole is a new triazole antifungal formulated as a topical solution with a novel applicator and tavaborole, a novel boron-based molecule that is the latest development in the management of onychomycosis.[85,86]

The most often recommended topical therapies for onychomycosis include amorolfine, ciclopirox, and the newer agents efinaconazole and tavaborole.[85] Amorolfine 5% and ciclopirox 8% solution (Penlac), are available as nail lacquers, the latter being the only one approved in the United States for the treatment of mild-to-moderate onychomycosis caused by *T. rubrum* without lunula involvement.[79,85] The volatile vehicle, used to deliver the drug, evaporates and leaves an occlusive film with a high drug concentration on the nail surface.[78,85] Ciclopirox, a hydroxypyridine, has a broad spectrum of antifungal activity (dermatophytes, *Candida* species, and some molds) and requires treatment for 1 year. Although ciclopirox was significantly better than vehicle alone, the mycologic cure rate was only 32% with ciclopirox versus 10% for vehicle alone after 48 weeks of treatment; the overall treatment cure (mycologic cure with 0%-10% involvement of the target nail) was 9% versus 0.9% for drug and vehicle, respectively.[85] Concomitant nail debridement accompanied treatment in most ciclopriox studies. Higher mycologic cure rates of 45% to 65% have been reported in open-label trials involving 6 to 12 months of treatment.[86] Amorolfine appears to produce higher mycologic and treatment cure rates than ciclopirox but is not approved for use in the United States or Canada.[80,85] Efinaconazole is a triazole antifungal approved as a 10% topical solution for the treatment of DLSO. Efinaconazole was evaluated in two phase III randomized controlled trials enrolling adult patients with mild to moderate DLSO of the great toenail. Patients were treated with once daily administration for 48 weeks without concomitant nail debridement. At 4 weeks post-treatment there was significantly greater mycological cure rates in the eficonazole group (55.2%) versus the vehicle controls (16.8%).[86]

Tavaborole 5% solution is a novel boron-based antifungal agent approved for the treatment of toenail onychomycosis involving 20% to 60% of the nail without spikes and lunula involvement. Tavaborole 5% solution applied to the affected great toenail once daily for 48 weeks was compared to vehicle in two phase III trials. Complete cure was achieved in 6.5% of tavaborole treated patients versus 0.5% vehicle controls in trial 1 and 9.1% versus 1.5% respectively in trial 2. Mycologic cure rates were significantly higher with tavaborole compared to vehicle control at 31.1% and 35.9% versus 7.2% and 12.2% in trials 1 and 2, respectively.[87] Unfortunately no studies comparing any of the approved agents head to head have been conducted. Most experts consider topical therapy a feasible option when the infection is superficial involving the nail plate without matrix involvement, such as WSO, involves a partial area of the nail plate not exceeding 50% (owing to difficulty of applying treatment to the margin of the nail), is limited to a few (three or four) nails, is in the very early stages of DSO when infection is still confined to the distal edge of the nail, or when systemic therapy is contraindicated.[78,79] Combining topical therapy with debridement of the affected nail (thus diminishing the amount of nail requiring treatment) may increase the likelihood of successful treatment, although there is no strong supporting evidence and this practice has not been a consistent component of clinical trials.[84,85,86] Topical therapy is not associated with systemic adverse effects or drug interactions. Any adverse effect will be localized to the application site, such as mild erythema in the adjacent skin area.

Clinical **Controversy...**

Treatment of onychomycosis is associated with a high failure rate of 20% to 50%. There appears to be a sound pharmacologic rationale behind the use of topical therapy and concomitant nail debridement to improve overall efficacy. However, this approach had not been consistently employed in clinical trials making it unclear if nail debridement should be routinely performed nor is it possible to compare outcomes between studies that have included debridement to those that have not.

Systemic Therapy

Oral antifungal therapy is considered to be more effective than topical for treating onychomycosis. Terbinafine and itraconazole (capsule), the current first-line agents for treatment, have yielded higher efficacy rates using shorter treatment periods (generally 3 months or shorter) for toenail and fingernail onychomycosis compared with the traditional agents, such as griseofulvin and ketoconazole, which are rarely used nowadays. Terbinafine, an allylamine, exerts fungicidal activity and demonstrates the greatest in vitro activity against dermatophytes compared with the other oral antifungals; it has good activity against nondermatophyte molds and only marginal activity against *Candida* species.[78,85] Like other azoles, itraconazole is fungistatic, has a broad antifungal spectrum, and is very active against dermatophytes, nondermatophytes, and *Candida* species.[78] Both agents have lipophilic and keratinophilic properties, which explains their excellent penetration (appearing in the nail plate within days of treatment initiation) and accumulation in the nails, achieving concentrations far exceeding the minimal inhibitory concentration (MIC) of most dermatophytes. Nail terbinafine concentrations are detected within 1 week of starting therapy, whereas itraconazole can be detected 1 (fingernails) to 2 weeks (toenails) after starting therapy.[81] Both drugs are slowly eliminated from the nail, with effective drug concentrations persisting in nails for 30 to 36 weeks after completion of treatment with terbinafine and for 27 weeks with itraconazole.[83] The persistence of drug in the nails explains in part the long-term protection against relapses after the end of treatment and also permits use of intermittent (pulse) dosing.

The treatment of toenail onychomycosis requires a 12-week course, whereas a 6-week course is adequate for fingernail onychomycosis with either drug.[83,85] In general, cure rates of 80% to 90% for fingernail infection and 70% to 80% for toenail infection can be expected.[79] Terbinafine is approved for daily dosing (see Table 120-8).[79,83] Various terbinafine pulse regimens have been evaluated;[78] in some trials, pulse dosing was less effective than continuous dosing, and it did not provide clear safety advantages.[81] Pulse terbinafine had similar efficacy to continuous therapy had better outcomes compared with pulse itraconazole treatment.[88] Itraconazole pulse therapy is the preferred method over continuous dosing for fingernail infections, and it is licensed as twice-daily dosing for a 1-week cycle per month for 2 consecutive months (ie, two pulses), or as daily therapy for 6 weeks (see Table 120-8).[83] Although itraconazole pulse therapy is not approved by the U.S. Food and Drug Administration (FDA), three or four pulses are effective for toenail infections; otherwise, half the dose is taken daily for 3 months (see Table 120-8).[83] In addition to lower drug cost, the potential advantages of itraconazole pulse therapy compared with continuous therapy are a lower risk of adverse drug effects and improved patient adherence.

Terbinafine is generally considered by most experts as the first-line agent for onychomycosis; itraconazole is the alternative. It is more effective than itraconazole by continuous or pulse dosing.[78,79] Mycologic cure rates for terbinafine range from 77% to 100% depending on the study.[81,89,90] In a cumulative meta-analysis of randomized, controlled trials, mycologic cure rates for terbinafine, itraconazole pulse, itraconazole continuous, fluconazole, and griseofulvin were 76%, 63%, 59%, 60%, and 48%, respectively.[91] An earlier meta-analysis and systematic review also reported that continuous terbinafine was the most effective therapy for toenail onychomycosis.[91-93] In addition, terbinafine was reported to achieve high cure rates in high-risk immunosuppressed patients, such as diabetics and organ transplant recipients, comparable to the immunocompetent population, with no significant adverse effects or drug interactions. It also appears to be effective in HIV patients and nondermatophyte infections.[78,94] A pharmacoeconomic analysis of oral and topical (ciclopirox) therapies showed that from a managed-care perspective, terbinafine was the most cost-effective therapy in terms of highest success rate, lowest relapse rate, and highest number of disease-free days for both fingernail and toenail infections.[95] The cost per cure with the use of oral terbinafine (based on cure rates from clinical trials) ranged from $2,439 to $7,944, depending on disease severity.[96] Compared with the amount of money a patient would consider reasonable to spend on treatment, the current charges for a course of systemic therapy are considerably higher.[96,97]

Both terbinafine and itraconazole generally are well tolerated. The more common adverse effects reported with terbinafine are GI (eg, diarrhea, dyspepsia, nausea, and abdominal pain), dermatologic (eg, rash, urticaria, and pruritus), and headache; less common adverse effects are taste disturbances, fatigue, inability to concentrate, and asymptomatic liver enzyme abnormalities.[81,85] Terbinafine can cause transient decrease in absolute lymphocyte counts; hence, monitoring of complete blood counts can be useful, especially in immunocompromised patients.[98] Although uncommon, severe adverse effects have been reported with terbinafine, including erythema multiforme, Stevens-Johnson's syndrome, toxic epidermal necrolysis, pancytopenia, lupus erythematosus, psoriasis, hair loss, and hepatotoxicity. Although the incidence of severe hepatotoxicity is considered rare, the FDA issued a public health advisory in 2001 regarding the association of terbinafine tablets with 16 possible cases of liver failure, including 2 liver transplants and 11 deaths.[99] Terbinafine thus is not recommended for patients with chronic or active liver disease, although hepatotoxicity can occur in patients with no preexisting liver disease or serious underlying medical condition. Prior to initiating terbinafine treatment, it is recommended to obtain appropriate nail specimens for laboratory testing to confirm the diagnosis of onychomycosis. Liver function parameters (serum transaminases) should be assessed at baseline and periodically during treatment with terbinafine.[98,99]

The common adverse effects of itraconazole are similar to those of terbinafine, such as GI disturbance, dermatologic disorders, and headache; less common adverse effects include dizziness, fatigue, fever, decreased libido, and asymptomatic liver enzyme abnormalities (1%-5% with continuous dosing and ~2% with pulse dosing).[83,100] Although still considered rare, 24 serious cases of liver failure, including transplantation and death, have been reported with the use of itraconazole, resulting in an FDA public health advisory warning.[99] Some of these patients did not have preexisting liver disease or serious underlying medical conditions, and some developed within the first week of treatment. Itraconazole should be avoided in patients with elevated liver enzymes or active liver disease or in those who have experienced other drug-induced liver toxicity. Liver function parameters (serum transaminases) should be assessed prior to and periodically during treatment. However, some experts have suggested that frequent monitoring is not as necessary if pulse therapy is used because symptomatic hepatotoxicity has not been reported with pulse therapy.[100] In addition, there is an FDA warning on the risk of developing congestive heart failure (CHF) associated with the use of itraconazole, possibly related to its potential negative inotropic effect.[78,89] Therefore, itraconazole should not be used in patients with evidence of ventricular dysfunction, such as CHF. Symptomatic assessment for the development of CHF also should be included as part of therapy monitoring. Before a patient is subjected to several months of itraconazole treatment, it is important to confirm the diagnosis of onychomycosis.

In contrast to the azoles, terbinafine does not inhibit the CYP 3A4 isoenzymes, but it is a potent inhibitor of the CYP2D6 isoenzymes, which are responsible for metabolism of tricyclic antidepressants and other psychotropic drugs.[78,83,98] The most significant drug interactions with terbinafine are decreased clearance of 33% by cimetidine and increased clearance of 100% by rifampin. Other drug interactions of variable clinical significance are tricyclic antidepressants, cyclosporine, caffeine, theophylline, and terfenadine. Itraconazole and its major metabolite can inhibit the CYP3A4 isoenzymes and result in numerous clinically significant drug interactions where coadministration with several drugs are contraindicated (eg, alprazolam, midazolam, triazolam, pimozide, lovastatin, simvastatin, cisapride, and terfenadine).[78,83,98]

Fluconazole is also active against dermatophytes, *Candida* species, and some nondermatophytes;[78,83] however, it does not have current FDA-approved indication for treatment of onychomycosis. The overall mycologic cure rate of fluconazole is 48%, which is lowest compared with all other oral agents.[91] The most effective dose and treatment duration have not been clearly established, with a variety of dosing regimens used, ranging from 50 mg daily to 300 mg once weekly for 6 to 12 months (see Table 120-8).[87,98] The advantages of fluconazole include a relatively good safety profile and fewer drug interactions compared with itraconazole.[83,98]

These three oral antifungal agents have superseded the use of griseofulvin and ketoconazole as treatments of choice for onychomycosis.[78,79] Griseofulvin has a narrow antifungal spectrum, low clinical efficacy, especially for toenail infections, high relapse rates, and the need for prolonged treatment duration (up to 12-18 months for toenails). Use of ketoconazole is also associated with high relapse rates, and the prolonged treatment duration carries an increased risk of hepatotoxicity.

Treatment Response and Recurrence

Treatment failures and recurrence rates of infection following initial cure are high, ranging from 20% to 50%.[78,79,84] Recurrence could be either a relapse (original infection not completely cured) or reinfection (new infection after achieving a cure of the original). Factors associated with poor response to systemic therapy include a compromised immune system (AIDS), reduced blood flow (diabetes, peripheral vascular disease, vasculitis, connective tissue disease, and CHF), coexisting nail disease (psoriasis), nail factors (slow growth, thick nails, and severe disease), drug-resistant organisms because of extensive prior drug exposure, and reduced bioavailability (absorption problems, poor compliance, and drug interactions).[83,84] To improve treatment outcomes and reduce recurrence, patients should be counseled on the importance of proper foot hygiene, for example, wearing breathable footwear and 100% cotton socks with frequent changes, keeping the nails short and clean, keeping the feet dry, protecting the feet in shared bathing areas, treating tinea pedis, and controlling other predisposing medical conditions.[84]

The use of combination therapy (topical–oral) has been suggested to provide antifungal synergy, broader antifungal spectrum, increased cure rates, suppression of resistant mutants and enhancement of tolerability and safety.[78] Combination therapy could shorten treatment duration of therapy, as this approach provides complementary mechanisms of attack.[78] Ciclopirox, amorolfine and topical imidazoles have all been studied in combination with systemic antifungal agents (eg, tioconazole 28% with griseofulvin 1 g for 1 year; amorolfine 5% with pulsed itraconazole; amorolfine 5% with oral terbiafine) and reported favorable results. Conversely, a study of combination amorolfine 5% or ciclopriox 8% nail lacquer with pulsed oral terbinafine did not offer any advantage over pulsed oral terbinafine monotherapy.[101] To date, no specific combination has been approved or endorsed for use.

Clinical **Controversy...**

The optimal dosing regimen of terbinafine therapy in onychomycosis remains unclear. Either continuous, or pulse therapy can be used, Selection should be based on cost and adherence to therapy.

ABBREVIATIONS

ACOG	American College of Obstetricians and Gynecologists
AIDS	acquired immunodeficiency syndrome
BMT	bone marrow transplantation
CHF	congestive heart failure
CMI	cell-mediated immunity
CYP	cytochrome P450
DSO	distal subungual onychomycosis
FDA	Food and Drug Administration
GI	gastrointestinal
HAART	highly active antiretroviral therapy
HIV	human immunodeficiency virus
HRT	hormone replacement therapy
HSCT	hematopoietic stem cell transplant

IgA	immunoglobulin A
KOH	potassium hydroxide
MMT	miconazole mucoadhesive tablet
OPC	oropharyngeal candidiasis
PSO	proximal subungual onychomycosis
RVVC	recurrent vulvovaginal candidiasis
VVC	vulvovaginal candidiasis
WSO	white superficial onychomycosis

REFERENCES

1. Sobel JD, Faro S, Force R, et al. Vulvovaginal candidiasis: Epidemiologic, diagnostic and therapeutic considerations. *Am J Obstet Gynecol* 1998; 178:203-211.
2. Center for Disease Control and Prevention. *Vaginal Discharge-STD Treatment Guidelines*. 2006, *www.cdc.gov/std/treatment/2006/vaginaldischarge.htm.*
3. Haefner HK. Current evaluation and management of vulvovaginitis. *Clin Obstet Gynecol* 1999;42:184-195.
4. Foxman B, Barlow R, D'arcy H, et al. *Candida* vaginitis self-reported incidence and associated costs. *Sex Transm Dis* 2000;27:230-235.
5. Fischer G, Bradford J. Vulvovaginal candidiasis in postmenopausal women: The role of hormone replacement therapy. *J Low Genit Tract Dis* 2011;15:263-237.
6. Lipsky MS, Waters T, Sharp LK. Impact of vaginal antifungal products on utilization of health care services: Evidence from physician visits. *J Am Board Fam Pract* 2000;13:178-182.
7. Foxman B, Barlow R, D'Arcy H, Gillespie B, Sobel JD. Candida vaginitis: Self-reported incidence and associated costs. *Sexual Trans Dis* 2000;27:230-235.
8. Clinical Effectiveness Group. National guideline for the management of vulvovaginal candidiasis. *Sex Transm Infect* 1999;75(suppl 1): S19-S20.
9. Larsen B. Vaginal flora in health and disease. *Clin Obstet Gynecol* 1993; 36:107-121.
10. Sobel JD. Clinical vulvovaginitis. *Clin Obstet Gynecol* 1993;36:153-165.
11. Camacho DP, Consolaro ME, Patussi EV, Donatti L, Gasparetto A, Svidzinski TL. Vaginal yeast adherence to the combined contraceptive vaginal ring (CCVR). *Contraception* 2007;76:439-443.
12. Barbone F, Austin H, Louv WC, Alexander WJ. A follow-up study of the methods of contraception, sexual activity, and rates of trichomoniasis, candidiasis, and bacterial vaginosis. *Am J Obstet Gynecol* 1990;163:510-514.
13. Xu J, Schwartz K, Bartoces M, Monsur J, Severson RK, Sobel JD. Effect of antibiotics on vulvovaginal candidiasis: A MetroNet study. *J Am Board Fam Med* 2008;21:261-268.
14. Ferris DG, Dekle C, Litaker MS. Women's use of over-the-counter antifungal pharmaceutical products for gynecologic symptoms. *J Fam Pract* 1996;42:595-600.
15. ACOG practice bulletin: Clinical management guidelines for obstetrician-gynecologists. *Obstet Gynecol* 2006;107: 1195-1206.
16. Watson MC, Bond CM, Grimshaw J, Johnston M. Factors predicting the guideline compliant supply (or non-supply) of non-prescription medicines in the community pharmacy setting. *Qual Saf Health Care* 2006;15:53-57.
17. Martinez RC, Franceschini Sa, Patta MC, et al. Improved treatment of vulvaovaginal candidiasis with fluconazole plus probiotic *Lactobacillus rhamnosus* GR-1 and *Lactobacillus reuteri* RC-14. *Lett Appl Microbiol* 2009;48:269-274.
18. Abdelmonem AW, Rasheed SM, Mohamed AS. Bee-honey and yogurt: A novel mixture for treating patients with vulvovaginal candidiasis during pregnancy. *Arch Gynecol Obstet* 2012;8: Epub ahead of print.
19. Hilton E, Isenberg HD, Alperstein P, et al. Ingestion of yogurt containing *Lactobacillus acidophilus* as prophylaxis for candidal vaginitis. *Ann Intern Med* 1992;116:353-357.
20. Witt A, Kaufmann U, Bitschnau M, et al. Monthly itraconazole versus classic homeopathy for the treatment of recurrent vulvovaginal candidiasis: A randomized trial. *Br J Obstet Gynecol* 2009;116:1499-1505.
21. Cooke G, Watson C, Smith J, Pirotta M, van Driel ML. Treatment for recurrent vulvovaginal candidiasis (thrush) (Protocol). *Cochrane Database Syst Rev* 2011(5).
22. Tooley PJ. Patient and doctor preferences in the treatment of vaginal candidiasis. *The Practitioner* 1985;229:655-662.
23. Nurbhai M, Grimshaw J, Watson M, Bond CM, Mollison JA, Ludbrook A. Oral versus intravaginal imidazole and triazole antifungal treatment of uncomplicated vulvovaginal candidiasis (thrush). *Cochrane Database Syst Rev* 2007;4:CD002845, doi:10.1002/14651858.CD002845.pub2.
24. Edelman DA, Grant S. One-day therapy for vaginal candidiasis: A review. *J Reprod Med* 1999;44:543-547.
25. Mendling W, Plempel M. Vaginal secretion levels after 6 days, 3 days and 1 day of treatment with 100-, 200-, 500-mg vaginal tablets of clotrimazole and their therapeutic efficacy. *Chemotherapy* 1982;28(suppl 1):43-47.
26. Centers for Disease Control and Prevention. Sexually transmitted diseases treatment guidelines. *MMWR* 2010;59(RR-12):61-63.
27. Sobel JD, Kapernick PS, Zervos M, et al. Treatment of complicated candida vaginitis: Comparison of single and sequential doses of fluconazole. *Am J Obstet Gynecol* 2001;185:363-369.
28. Young G, Jewell D. Topical treatment for vaginal candidiasis (thrush) in pregnancy. *Cochrane Database Syst Rev* 2001;4:CD000225, doi:10.1002/14651858.CD000225.
29. Mastroiacovo P, Mazzone T, Botto L, et al. Prospective assessment of pregnancy outcomes after first-trimester exposure to fluconazole. *Am J Obstet Gynecol* 1996;175:1645-1650.
30. Molgaard-Nielsen D, Pasternak B, Hviid A. Use of oral fluconazole during pregnancy and the risk of birth defects. *N Engl J Med* 2013; 369:830-839.
31. Foxman B, Muraglia R, Dietz JP, Sobel JD, Wagner J. Prevalence of recurrent vulvovaginal candidiasis in 5 European countries and the United States: Results from an internet panel survey. *J Low Genit Tract Dis* 2013:17:340-345.
31. Sobel JD, Wiesenfeld HC, Martens M, et al. Maintenance fluconazole therapy for recurrent vulvovaginal candidiasis. *N Engl J Med* 2004; 351:363-369.
33. Pappas PG, Kauffman CA, Andes DA, et al. Clinical practice guidelines for the management of candidiasis: 2009 update by the infectious diseases society of America. *Clin Infect Dis* 2009;48:503-535.
34. Cassone A. Vulvovaginal candid albicans infections: Pathogenesis, immunity and vaccine prospects. *BJOG* 2015;122:785-794.
35. Sobel JD, Chiam W, Nagappan V, Leaman D. Treatment of vaginitis caused by *Candida glabrata*: Use of topical boric acid and flucytosine. *Am J Obstet Gynecol* 2003;189:1297-1300.
36. Sobel JD, Chaim W. Treatment of *Torulopsis glabrata* vaginitis: Retrospective review of boric acid therapy. *Clin Infect Dis* 1996; 22:336-340.
37. Ray D, Goswami R, Banerjee U, et al. Prevalence of *Candida glabrata* and its response to boric acid vaginal suppositories in comparison with oral fluconazole in patients with diabetes and vulvovaginal candidiasis. *Diabetes Care* 2007;30:312-317.
38. Leigh JE, Shetty K, Fidel Jr PL. Oral opportunistic infections in HIV-positive individuals: Review and role of mucosal immunity. *AIDS Patient Care STDS* 2004;18:443-456.
39. Farah CS, Lynch N, McCullough MJ. Oral fungal infections: An update for the general practitioner. *Aust Dent J* 2010;55(1 suppl):48-54.
40. Muzyka BC, Epifanio RN. Update on oral fungal infections. *Dent Clin N Am* 2013;57:561-581
41. Thompson III GR, Patel PK, Kirkpatrick WR, et al. Oropharyngeal candidiasis in the era of antiretroviral therapy. *Oral Surg Oral Med Oral Pathol Oral Radiol Endod* 2010;109:488-495.
42. Delgado ACD, de Jesus PR, Aoki FH, et al. Clinical and microbiological assessment of patients with long-term diagnosis of human immunodeficiency virus infection and *Candida* oral colonization. *Clin Microbiol Infect* 2009;15:364-371.
43. Laudenbach JM, Epstein JB. Treatment strategies for oropharyngeal candidiasis. *Expert Opin Pharmaocother* 2009;10(9):1413-1421.
44. Benson CA, Kaplan JE, Masur H, et al. Treating opportunistic infections among HIV-infected adults and adolescents: Recommendations from CDC, the National Institutes of Health, and the HIV Medicine Association/Infectious Diseases Society of America. *Clin Infect Dis* 2004;40:S131-S235.
45. Patuwo C, Young K, Lin M,, et al. The changing role of HIV-associated oral candidiasis in the era of HAART. *CDA J* 2015;43:87-92.
46. Mercante DE, Leigh JE, Lilly EA, et al. Assessment of the association between HIV viral load and CD4 cell count on the occurrence of oropharyngeal candidiasis in HIV-infected patients. *J Acquir Immune Defic Syndr* 2006;42:578-583.
47. Soysa NS, Samaranayake LP, Ellepola ANB. Antimicrobials as a contributory factor in oral candidosis: A brief overview. *Oral Dis* 2008;14:138-143.
48. Pappas PG, Kauffman CA, Andes D, et al. Guidelines for management of candidiasis: 2009 update by the Infectious Diseases Society of America. *Clin Infect Dis* 2009;48:503-535.

49. Jurevic RJ, Traboulsi RS, Mukherjee PK, et al. Identification of gentian violet concentration that does not stain oral mucosa, possesses anti-candidal activity and is well tolerated. *Eur J Clin Microbiol Infect Dis* 2011;30(5):629-633.
50. Lalla RV, Bensadoun RJ. Miconazole mucoadhesive tablet for oropharyngeal candidiasis. *Expert Rev Anti Infect Ther* 2011;9(1):13.
51. Vazquez JA, Patton LL, Epstein JB,, et al. Randomized, comparative, double-blind, double-dummy, multicenter trial of miconazole buccal tablet and clotrimazole troches for the treatment of oropharyngeal candidiasis: Study of Miconazole Lauriad® Efficacy and Safety (SMiLES). *HIV Clin Trials* 2010;11(4):186-196.
52. Hamza OJM, Matee MIN, Bruggemann RJM, et al. Single-dose fluconazole versus standard 2-week therapy for oropharyngeal candidiasis in HIV-infected patients: A randomized, double-blind, double-dummy trial. *Clin Infect Dis* 2008;47:1270-1276.
53. Vasquez JA, Skiest DJ, Nieto L, et al. A multicenter randomized trial evaluating posaconazole versus fluconazole for the treatment of oropharyngeal candidiasis in subjects with HIV/AIDS. *Clin Infect Dis* 2006;42:1179-1186.
54. *Posaconazole Product Monograph*, revised July, 2015, Merck. http://www.merck.com/product/usa/pi_circulars/n/noxafil/noxafil_pi.pdf; accessed October, 2015.
55. Bensadoun RJ, Daoud J, El Gueddari B,, et al. Comparison of the efficacy and safety of miconazole 50 mg mucoadhesive buccal tablets with miconazole 500 mg gel in the treatment of oropharyngeal candidiasis: A prospective, randomized, single-blind, multicenter, comparative, phase III trial in patients treated with radiotherapy for head and neck cancer. *Cancer* 2008;112(1):204-211.
56. Villanueva A, Arathoon EG, Gotuzzo E, et al. A randomized double-blind study of caspofungin versus amphotericin for the treatment of candidal esophagitis. *Clin Infect Dis* 2001;33:1529-1535.
57. Arathoon EG, Gotuzzo E, Noriega LM, et al. Randomized, double-blind, multicenter study of caspofungin versus amphotericin B for treatment of oropharyngeal and esophageal candidiasis. *Antimicrob Agents Chemother* 2002;46:451-457.
58. Villanueva A, Gotuzzo E, Arathoon EG, et al. A randomized, double-blind study of caspofungin versus fluconazole for the treatment of esophageal candidiasis. *Am J Med* 2002;113:294-299.
59. Deresinski SC, Stevens DA. Caspofungin. *Clin Infect Dis* 2003;36:1445-1457.
60. Akpan A, Morgan R. Oral candidiasis. *Postgrad Med J* 2002;78:455-459.
61. Morris MI, Villmann. Echinocandins in the management of invasive fungal infections, part 1. *Am J Health Syst Pharm* 2006;63:1693-1703.
62. Grim SA, Smith KM, Romanelli F, Ofotokun I. Treatment of azole-resistant oropharyngeal candidiasis with topical amphotericin B. *Ann Pharmacother* 2002;36:1383-1386.
63. Goldman M, Cloud GA, Wade KD, et al. A randomized study of the use of fluconazole in continuous versus episodic therapy in patients with advanced HIV infection and a history of oropharyngeal candidiasis: AIDS clinical trials group study 323/mycoses study group 40. *Clin Infect Dis* 2005;41:1473-1480.
64. Marr KA, Bow E, Chiller T, et al. Fungal infection prevention after hematopoietic cell transplantation. *Bone Marrow Transplant* 2009;44:483-487.
65. Routt ER, ON SCJ, Zeichner JA, et al. What is new in fungal pharmacotherapeutics? *J Drugs Dermatol* 2015:13(4):391-395.
66. Mendez-Tovar LJ. Pathogenesis of dermatophytosis and tinea versicolor. *Clin Dermatol* 2010;28:185-189.
67. Goldstein AO, Smith KM, Ives TJ, Goldstein B. Mycotic infections. Effective management of conditions involving the skin, hair, and nails. *Geriatrics* 2000;55:40-52.
68. Hainer BL. Dematophyte infections. *Am Fam Physician* 2003;67:101-108.
69. Drake LA, Dinehart SM, Farmer ER, et al. Guidelines of care for superficial mycotic infections of the skin: Tinea capitis and tinea barbae. *J Am Acad Dermatol* 1996;34:290-294.
70. Stein Gold LF, Parish LC, Vlahovic T,, el al. Efficacy and safety of naftitine HCL gel 2% in the treatment of interdigital and moccasin type tinea pedis: Pooled results from two multicenter, randomized, double-blind, vehicle-controlled trials. *J Drugs Dermatol* 2013;12(8):911-918.
71. Plaum S, Verma A, Fleischer A,, et al. Detection and relevance of naftifine hydrochloride in the stratum corneum up to four weeks following the last application of naftifine cream and gel 2%. *J Drugs Dermatol* 2013;12(9):1004-1008.
72. Jarratt M, Jones T, Kempers S, et al. Luliconazole for the treatment of interdigital tinea pedis: A double blind, vehicle controlled study. *Cutis* 2013:91:203-210.
73. Higgins EM, Fuller LC, Smith CH. Guidelines for the management of tinea capitis. *Br J Dermatol* 2000;143:53-58.
74. Hubbard TW. The predictive value of symptoms in diagnosing childhood tinea capitis. *Arch Pediatr Adolesc Med* 1999;153:1130-1153.
75. Meadows-Oliver M. Tinea capitis: Diagnostic criteria and treatment options. *Pediatric Nursing* 2009;35(1):53-57.
76. Hu SW. Pityriasis versicolor. *Arch Dermatol* 2010;46(10):1132-1140.
77. Ansarun H, Ghaffarpour G. Comparison of effectiveness between ketoconazole 2% and selenium sulfide 2% shampoos in the treatment of tinea versicolor. *Iranian J Derm* 2005;8:21-25.
78. Ameen M, Lear JT, Madan V et al. British Association of Dermatologists' guidelines for the management of onychomycosis 2014. *Br J Dermatol* 2014;171:937-958.
79. Eisman S, Sincalir R. Fungal nail infection: Diagnosis and management. *BMJ*. 2014;348:g1800 doi:10.1136/bmj.g1800 (published 24, March2104).
80. Welsh O, Vera-Cabrera L, Welsh E. Onychomycosis. *Clin Dermatol* 2010;28:151-159.
81. Baran R, Kaoukhov A. Topical antifungal drugs for the treatment of onychomycosis: An overview of current strategies for monotherapy and combination therapy. *J Eur Acad Dermatol Venereol* 2005;19:21-29.
82. Tosti A, Hay R, Arenas-Guzman R. Patients at risk of onychomycosis—Risk factor identification and active prevention. *J Eur Acad Dermatol Venereol* 2005;19(suppl 1):13-16.
83. Iorizzo M, Piraccini BM, Rech G, Tosti A. Treatment of onychomycosis with oral antifungal agents. *Expert Opin Drug Deliv* 2005;2:435-440.
84. de Berker D. Fungal nail disease. *N Engl J Med* 2009;360:2108-2116.
85. Gupta AK, Daigle D, Foley KA. Topical therapy for toenail onychomycosis: An evidence-based review. *Am J Clin Dermatol* 2014; 15:489-502.
86. Elewski BE, Rich P, Pollak R, et al. Efinaconazole 10% solution in the treatment of toenail onychomycosis: Two phase III multicenter, randomized, double-blind studies. *J Am Acad Dermatol* 2013;68(4):600-608.
87. Elewski BE, Aly R, Baldwin SL, et al. Efficacy and safety of tavaborole topical solution, 5%, a novel boron-based antifungal agent, for the treatment of toenail onychomycosis: Results from 2 randomized phase-III studies. *J Am Acad Dermatol* July 2015: http://dx.doi.org/10.1016/j.jaad.2015.04.010.
88. Gupta AK, Lynch LE, Kogan N, et al. The use of intermittent terbinafine for the treatment of dermatophyte toenail onychomycosis. *J Eur Acad Dermatol Venereol* 2009;23:256-262.
89. Sigurgeirsson B, Elewski EE, Rich PA, et al. Intermittent versus continuous terbinafine in the treatment of toenail onychomycosis: A randomized, double-blind, comparison. *J Dermatol Treat* 2006;17:38-44.
90. Warshaw EM, Fett DD, Bloomfield HE, et al. Pulse versus continuous terbinafine for onychomycosis: A randomized, double-blind, controlled trial. *J Am Acad Dermatol* 2005;53:578-584.
91. Gupta AK, Ryder JE, Johnson AM. Cumulative meta-analysis of systemic antifungal agents for the treatment of onychomycosis. *Br J Dermatol* 2004;150:537-544.
92. Haugh M, Helou S, Boissel JP, Cribier BJ. Terbinafine in fungal infections of the nails: A meta-analysis of randomized clinical trials. *Br J Dermatol* 2002;147:118-121.
93. Crawford F, Young P, Godfrey C, et al. Oral treatments for toenail onychomycosis: A systematic review. *Arch Dermatol* 2002;138:811-816.
94. Cribier BJ, Bakshi R. Terbinafine in the treatment of onychomycosis: A review of its efficacy in high-risk populations and in patients with nondermatophyte infections. *Br J Dermatol* 2004;150:414-420.
95. Casciano J, Amaya K, Doyle J, et al. Economic analysis of oral and topical therapies for onychomycosis of the toenails and fingernails. *Manag Care* 2003;12:47-54.
96. Schram SE, Warshaw EM. Costs of pulse versus continuous terbinafine for onychomycosis. *J Am Acad Dermatol* 2007;56:525-527.
97. Cham PM, Chen SC, Grill JP, et al. Reliability of self-reported willingness-to-pay and annual income in patients treated for toenail onychomycosis. *Br J Dermatol* 2007;156:922-928.
98. Gupta AK, Ryder JE, Skinner AR. Treatment of onychomycosis: Pros and cons of antifungal agents. *J Cutan Med Surg* 2004;8:25-30.
99. *Food and Drug Administration*. FDA issues health advisory regarding the safety of Sporanox products and Lamisil tablets to treat finger nail infections. 2001, *www.fda.gov/cder/drug/advisory/sporanox-lamisil/advisory.htm*.
100. Gupta AK, Chwetzoff, Del Rosso J, Baran R. Hepatic safety of itraconazole. *J Cutan Med Surg* 2002;6:210-213.
101. Avner S, Nir N, Henri T. Combination of oral terbinafine and topical ciclopirox compared to oral terbinafine for the treatment of onychomycosis. *J Dermatol Treat* 2005;16:327-330.

121

Invasive Fungal Infections

Peggy L. Carver

KEY CONCEPTS

1. Systemic mycoses can be caused by pathogenic fungi and include histoplasmosis, coccidioidomycosis, cryptococcosis, blastomycosis, paracoccidioidomycosis, and sporotrichosis, or infections by opportunistic fungi such as *Candida albicans*, *Aspergillus* species, *Trichosporon*, *Candida glabrata*, *Fusarium*, *Alternaria*, and *Mucor*.
2. The diagnosis of fungal infection generally is accomplished by careful evaluation of clinical symptoms, results of serologic tests, and histopathologic examination and culture of clinical specimens. Rapid, accurate diagnostic laboratory tests are currently under development.
3. Histoplasmosis is caused by *Histoplasma capsulatum* and is endemic in parts of the central United States along the Ohio and Mississippi River valleys. Although most patients experience asymptomatic infection, some can experience chronic, disseminated disease.
4. Asymptomatic patients with histoplasmosis are not treated, although patients who do not have acquired immune deficiency syndrome (AIDS) patients with evident disease are treated with either oral ketoconazole or IV amphotericin B; AIDS patients are treated with amphotericin B and then receive lifelong suppression.
5. Blastomycosis is caused by *Blastomyces dermatitidis*. In the immunocompetent host, acute pulmonary blastomycosis can be mild and self-limited and may not require treatment. However, consideration should be given to treating all infected individuals to prevent extrapulmonary dissemination. All persons with moderate to severe pneumonia, disseminated infection, or those who are immunocompromised require antifungal therapy.
6. Coccidioidomycosis is caused by *Coccidioides immitis* and is endemic in some parts of the southwestern United States. It can cause nonspecific symptoms, acute pneumonia, or chronic pulmonary or disseminated disease. Primary pulmonary disease (unless severe) frequently is not treated, whereas extrapulmonary disease is treated with amphotericin B, and meningitis is treated with fluconazole.
7. Cryptococcosis is caused by *Cryptococcus neoformans*, which occurs primarily in immunocompromised patients, and *Cryptococcus gattii*, which occurs primarily in nonimmunocompromised patients. Patients with acute meningitis are treated with amphotericin B with flucytosine. Patients infected with human immunodeficiency virus (HIV) often require long-term suppressive therapy with fluconazole or itraconazole.
8. A variety of *Candida* species (including *C. albicans*, *C. glabrata*, *Candida tropicalis*, *Candida parapsilosis*, and *Candida krusei*) can cause diseases such as mucocutaneous, oral, esophageal, vaginal, and hematogenous candidiasis, as well as candiduria. Candidemia can be treated with a variety of antifungal agents; the optimal choice depends on previous patient exposure to antifungal agents, potential drug interactions and toxicities of each agent, and local epidemiology of intensive care unit (ICU) or hematology–oncology centers.
9. Aspergillosis can be caused by a variety of *Aspergillus* species that can cause superficial infections, pneumonia, allergic bronchopulmonary aspergillosis (BPA), or invasive infection. Voriconazole has emerged as the drug of choice of most clinicians for primary therapy of most patients with invasive aspergillosis (IA). Combination therapy, while widely used, lacks clinical trial data to support its use.

1 Advances in medical technology including organ and bone marrow transplantation, cytotoxic chemotherapy, the widespread use of indwelling IV catheters, and the increased use of potent broad-spectrum antimicrobial agents all have contributed to the dramatic increase in the incidence of fungal infections worldwide.[1-3] Problems remain in the diagnosis, prevention, and treatment of fungal infections.[1,4-6] The Infectious Diseases Society of America (IDSA) publishes guidelines regarding the prophylaxis and treatment of many commonly encountered fungal infections.[7-12]

MYCOLOGY

Fungi are eukaryotic organisms with a defined nucleus enclosed by a nuclear membrane; a cytoplasmic membrane containing lipids, glycoproteins, and sterols, mitochondria, golgi apparatus, and ribosomes bound to endoplasmic reticulum; and a cytoskeleton with microtubules, microfilaments, and intermediate filaments. Fungi have rigid cell walls composed of chitin, cellulose, or both that stain with Gomori methenamine silver or periodic acid–Schiff reagent. Most fungi, except *Candida* species, are too weakly Gram-positive to be seen well on Gram stain. *Cryptococcus neoformans* has a polysaccharide capsule surrounding the cell wall.[1]

Morphologically, pathogenic fungi can be grouped as either filamentous molds or unicellular yeasts (Fig. 121-1). *Molds* grow as multicellular branching, threadlike filaments (hyphae) that are either septate (divided by transverse walls) or coenocytic (multinucleate without cross walls). Yeasts are oval or spherically shaped unicellular forms that generally produce pasty or mucoid colonies on agar medium similar to those observed with bacterial cultures. Yeasts have rigid cell walls and reproduce by budding, a process in which daughter cells arise from pinching off a portion of the parent cell.

Many pathogenic fungi, termed *dimorphic fungi*, exist as either a yeast or a mold, depending on pathogen, site of growth (in the host or in the laboratory setting), and temperature. Usually yeasts are the parasitic form that invades human or animal host tissue,

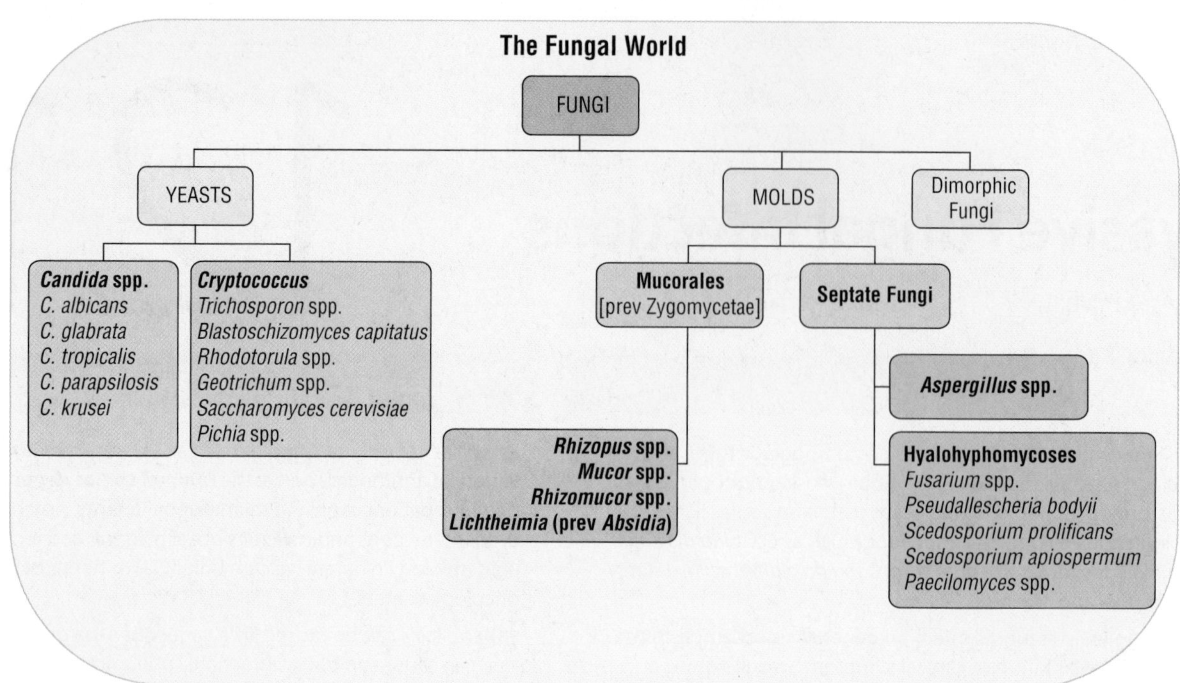

FIGURE 121-1 Morphologically, pathogenic fungi can be grouped as either filamentous molds or unicellular yeasts. *Molds* grow as multicellular branching, thread-like filaments (hyphae) that are either septate (divided by transverse walls) or coenocytic (multinucleate without cross walls).

whereas molds are the free-living form found in the environment. For example, *Histoplasma capsulatum* exists as a yeast in humans and as a mold in the laboratory.[1]

Clinical Versus Microbial Resistance

Host factors contribute greatly to clinical outcome. A patient may respond clinically to treatment with an antifungal agent despite resistance to that agent in vitro because the patient's own immune system may eradicate the infection, or the agent may reach the site of infection in high concentrations.[13] Thus, in vitro susceptibility does *not* necessarily equate with in vivo clinical success, and in vitro resistance might *not* always correlate with treatment failure.

It is important to distinguish between clinical resistance and microbial resistance. *Clinical resistance* refers to failure of an antifungal agent in the treatment of a fungal infection that arises from factors other than microbial resistance, such as failure of the antifungal agent to reach the site of infection or inability of a patient's immune system to eradicate a fungus whose growth is retarded by an antifungal agent.[13,14]

Microbial resistance can refer to *primary* or *secondary* resistance, as determined by in vitro susceptibility testing using standardized methodology. *Primary* or *intrinsic resistance* refers to resistance recorded prior to drug exposure in vitro or in vivo. *Secondary* or *acquired resistance* develops on exposure to an antifungal agent and can be either reversible, owing to transient adaptation, or acquired as a result of one or more genetic alterations. It is possible for a patient to respond clinically to treatment with an antifungal agent, despite resistance to that agent in vitro, because the patient's own immune system may eradicate the infection, or the agent reaches the site of infection in high concentrations.[6]

Susceptibility Testing of Antifungal Agents

Most laboratories do not routinely perform susceptibility tests on fungal isolates, but standardized methods for performing these tests are being developed and are now available for testing selected yeasts. As the prevalence of nosocomial and community-acquired fungal infections become more prominent, the need for in vitro susceptibility testing increases. Susceptibility testing occasionally is indicated, for example, in a patient with prolonged fungemia with a presumed susceptible isolate, and is most helpful in dealing with infections caused by non-*albicans* species of *Candida*.[5-7]

Clinical breakpoints (CBPs) are antimicrobial concentrations (MICs) obtained from susceptibility testing, which are used to define isolates as susceptible, intermediate, or resistant. No CBPs have been established for posaconazole or amphotericin B versus *Candida*, or for antifungal agents and filamentous fungi such as *Aspergillus*.[6] CBPs can be used to differentiate strains for which there is a high likelihood of treatment success (organisms which are clinically susceptible, or (S), from those for which treatment is more likely to fail (clinically resistant [R]). (Tables 121-1 and 121-2). A clinically intermediate (I) or susceptible dose-dependent (SDD) category can be assigned to pathogens for which the level of antimicrobial agent activity is associated with uncertain therapeutic effect, implying that infections due to the isolate may be appropriately treated in body sites where the drugs are physically concentrated or when a high dosage of drug can be used. Although CBPs are designed to guide therapy, they do not distinguish between fungal isolates with or without resistance mechanisms, nor do they always allow for early detection of resistant isolates. Table 121-3 shows the currently approved Interpretive CBPs for *Candida* species.

Resistance to Antifungal Agents

Understanding mechanisms of resistance is an important process in the optimization of antifungal therapy. The most exhaustive and definitive accounts of antifungal resistance have been described in *Candida* species, in particular *Candida albicans* and, to a lesser extent, *Candida glabrata*, *Candida tropicalis*, and *Candida krusei*, as well as in a few *C. neoformans* isolates.[13,14] *C. glabrata* isolates are increasingly resistant to both azole and echinocandin antifungal agents.

There are four different mechanisms that result in azole resistance: (a) mutations or upregulation of *ERG11* (an enzyme involved in the ergosterol biosynthesis pathway), (b) expression of multidrug efflux transport pumps that decrease antifungal drug accumulation

TABLE 121-1 General Patterns of Susceptibility and Interpretive Breakpoints of *Candida* Species[a]

	Patterns of Susceptibility								
	Azoles					*Echinocandins*			*Amphotericin*
***Candida* Species**	**Fluconazole**	**Itraconazole**	**Voriconazole**	**Posaconazole**	**Isavuconazole**	**Caspofungin**	**Micafungin**	**Anidulafungin**	**Amphotericin B**
C. albicans	+++ S	+++ S	+++ S	S	S	+++	+++	+++	+++
C. tropicalis	+++ S	+++ S	+++ S	+++ S	S	+++ S	+++ S	+++ S	+++ S
C. parapsilosis	S	S	S	S	S	S[d]	S[d]	S[d]	S
C. glabrata	++ S-DD to R[b]	++ S-DD to R[c]	++	S	S	S	S	S	S-I[e]
C. krusei	R	S-DD to R[c]	S	S	S	S	S	S	S-I[e]
C. lusitaniae	S	S	S	S	S	S	S	S	S to R[f]

For antifungal drugs and pathogens for which susceptibility breakpoints have been established (fluconazole, itraconazole, voriconazole): S, susceptible; S-DD, susceptible-dose dependent (see the text); I, intermediate; R, resistant; NA, not applicable (has not been established for this antifungal against this pathogen).

[a]Except for amphotericin B, interpretations are based on the use of a broth sensitivity test.

[b]Approximately 15% of C. glabrata isolates are resistant to fluconazole.

[c]Approximately 46% of C. glabrata isolates and 31% of C. krusei isolates are resistant to itraconazole.

[d]Most isolates of C. parapsilosis have reduced susceptibility to echinocandins.

[e]A significant proportion of C. glabrata and C. krusei isolates has reduced susceptibility to amphotericin B.

[f]Although frank resistance to amphotericin B is not observed in all isolates, it is well described for isolates of C. lusitaniae

within the fungal cell, (c) alteration of the structure or concentration of antifungal drug target proteins, and (d) alteration of membrane sterol proteins (Fig. 121-2). Although detailed analysis of each of the elucidated mechanism of resistance is beyond the scope this chapter, interested readers are referred to several recent publications which have comprehensively summarized this topic.[13,14]

The most commonly reported mechanisms of azole resistance among *C. albicans* isolates include reduced permeability of the fungal cell membrane to azoles, modification or overproduction of the target fungal enzymes (cytochrome P450, CYP) resulting in decreased binding of the azole to the target site, alterations in sterol synthesis, and activation of efflux pumps capable of actively pumping azoles from the target pathogen.

Fluconazole resistance is observed most frequently in *C. glabrata*, which may appear S-DD, or resistant, and in *C. krusei*, for which fluconazole resistance is universal.

Azole resistance among *Aspergillus* spp. (specifically *A. fumigatus*) is predominantly mediated by specific point mutations in TR/L98H in the CYP51A gene promoter region, causing amino acid changes and tandem repeats, and often results in cross-resistance with azole antifungals.

With the increase in echinocandin use, there has been an increase in the number of reports of echinocandin-resistant isolates from patients failing therapy. Echinocandin exposure and previous episodes of *C. glabrata* are predictors of FKS gene mutations in *Candida*.[15-17]

TABLE 121-2 General Patterns of In Vitro Susceptibility of Non-*Candida* Fungal Pathogens[a]

	Patterns of Susceptibility								
	Azoles					*Echinocandins*			*Amphotericin B*
Pathogen	**Fluconazole**	**Itraconazole**	**Voriconazole**	**Posaconazole**	**Isavuconazole**	**Caspofungin**	**Micafungin**	**Anidulafungin**	**Amphotericin B**
Aspergillus	No	Yes	Yes	Yes	Yes	Yes	Yes	Yes	Yes
A. fumigatus	No	Yes	Yes	Yes		Yes	Yes	Yes	Yes
A. flavus	No	Yes	Yes			Yes			No
A. terreus									
Fusarium	No	No	Yes (but breakthrough infections are seen)	Conflicting data (species dependent)	Variable	No	No	No	Yes but occasional resistance
Scedosporium	No	No	Yes	Yes (apiospermum)	Variable	No	No	No	No
Zygomycetes[b]	No	No	No	Yes	Yes	No	No	No	Yes
Trichosporon	No	No	Yes	Yes	Yes	No	No	No	No
Cryptococcus	Yes	Yes	Yes	Yes	Yes	No	No	No	
Histoplasma	Yes	Yes	Yes	Yes	Yes	No[c]	No[c]	No[c]	Yes
Coccidioides	Yes	Yes	Yes	Yes	Yes	No[c]	No[c]	No[c]	Yes

[a]No = has minimal or no in vitro activity versus the pathogen; Yes = possesses adequate in vitro activity versus the pathogen.

[b]Includes *Rhizopus*, *Mucor*, and *Absidia* species.

[c]While the echinocandins display activity against the mycelial forms of endemic fungi such as *Histoplasma* spp., *Blastomyces* spp., and *Coccidioides* spp., they display significantly higher MIC values against the yeast forms of these organisms, and should not be used to treat these infections.

Data from references 6, 75, and 100.

TABLE 121-3 Clinical Breakpoints for Anole Antifungal Agents

	Interpretive Clinical Breakpoints[5,6]		
	Susceptible	**Susceptible-Dose Dependent**	**Resistant**
Fluconazole	***C. albicans, C. tropicalis,* and *C. parapsilosis***		
	≤2	4	≥8
	C. glabrata		
	—	≤32	≥64
	Susceptible	**Intermediate**	**Resistant**
Voriconazole	***C. albicans, C. tropicalis,* and *parapsilosis***		
	≤0.125	0.25-0.5	≥1
	C. krusei		
	≤0.5	1	≥2
Caspofungin Micafungin Anidulafungin	***C. albicans, C. tropicalis,* and *C. krusei***		
	≤0.25	0.5	≥1
	C. parapsilosis		
	≤2	4	≥8
Caspofungin Anidulafungin	***C. glabrata***		
	≤0.12	0.25	≥0.5
Micafungin	≤0.06	0.12	≥0.25
Posaconazole		Interpretive criteria have not been established	
Amphotericin B		Interpretive criteria have not been established	

Data from references 5 and 6.

Although, to date, the rate of amphotericin B resistance remains low, the exact incidence remains difficult to quantify and the response to antifungal agents difficult to characterize. As such, no consensus for therapy has been formulated at this time, although clinicians should keep in mind that *C. glabrata*, *Candida guilliermondii*, *C. krusei*, and *Candida lusitaniae* may have a higher propensity to developing resistance than other species.

Acquired resistance of *Aspergillus* species during long-term azole exposure to azoles, while still relatively uncommon, is emerging, and varies widely between geographic centers. Acquisition of primary-resistant isolates is also increasing, due to the agricultural use of azoles.[18,19] Cross-resistance of azole-resistant strains of *Aspergillus* to amphotericin B has not been described.

PATHOGENESIS AND EPIDEMIOLOGY

Systemic mycoses caused by primary or pathogenic fungi include histoplasmosis, coccidioidomycosis, cryptococcosis, blastomycosis, paracoccidioidomycosis, and sporotrichosis. Primary pathogens can cause disease in both healthy and immunocompromised individuals, although disease generally is more severe or disseminated in the immunocompromised host. In contrast, mycoses caused by opportunistic fungi such as *C. albicans*, *Aspergillus* species, *Trichosporon*, *Torulopsis (Candida) glabrata*, *Fusarium*, *Alternaria*, and *Mucor* generally are found only in the immunocompromised host.[1]

Most fungal infections are acquired as a result of accidental inhalation of airborne conidia. For example, *H. capsulatum* is found in soil contaminated by bat, chicken, or starling excreta, and *C. neoformans* is associated with pigeon droppings. Although some fungi, including *C. albicans*, *C. neoformans*, and *Aspergillus* species, are ubiquitous pathogens with worldwide distribution, other fungi have regional distributions associated with specific geographic environments.[1]

IFIs are a major cause of morbidity and mortality in the immunocompromised patient.[20,21] In patients with hematologic malignancies and following hematopoietic stem cell transplantation (HSCT), there has been a shift in the most commonly encountered IFIs from *Candida* spp. to *Aspergillus* spp. *Candida* species (primarily *C. albicans*) are the fourth most commonly isolated bloodstream isolate and account for 78% of all nosocomial fungal infections.

Nosocomially acquired fungal infections can arise from either exogenous or endogenous flora. Endogenous flora can include normal commensal organisms of the skin, GI, genitourinary, or respiratory tract. *C. albicans* is found as a normal commensal of the GI tract in 20% to 30% of humans. A complex interplay of host and pathogen factors influences the acquisition and development of fungal infections. Intact skin or mucosal surfaces serve as primary barriers to infection. Alterations in the balance of normal flora caused by the use of antibiotics or alterations in nutritional status can allow the proliferation of fungi such as *Candida*, increasing the likelihood of systemic invasion and infection.[1]

Patients with decreased neutrophil counts or decreased neutrophil function are at higher risk of infections, particularly infections

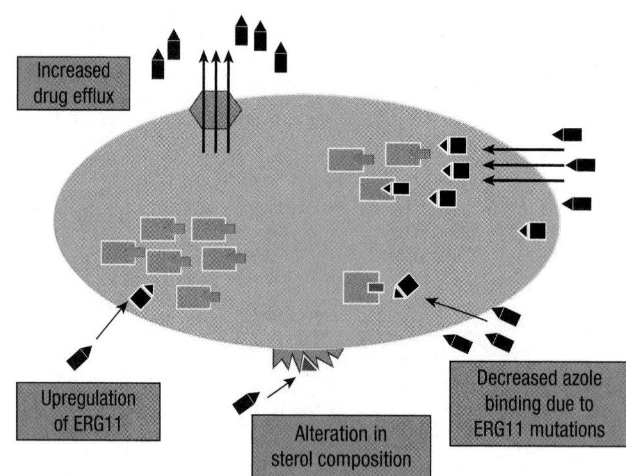

FIGURE 121-2 Mechanisms of azole resistance. Four different mechanisms result in azole resistance: (a) mutations or upregulation of *ERG11*, the target enzyme of azoles, (b) expression of multidrug efflux transport pumps that decrease antifungal drug accumulation within the fungal cell, (c) alteration of the structure or concentration of antifungal drug target proteins, and (d) alteration of membrane sterol proteins.

caused by *Candida* and *Aspergillus* species. Fungal cells sometimes can persist within macrophages without being killed, perhaps because of resistance to the effects of lysosomal enzymes.[1]

Risk Factors for Fungal Infections

Increasing use of aggressive and intensive cancer chemotherapeutic regimens, immunosuppressive therapy for autoimmune disorders, and transplantation have led to an increase in the number of susceptible hosts, contributing to the changing epidemiology of fungal infections. Infection epidemiology can drastically vary depending on patients' underlying concomitant conditions, comorbidities, confounding risk factors and geographical area.

A clinical indicator for a patient's immunologic status is the quantitation of absolute neutrophil count (ANC). Neutropenia, defined as an ANC less than equal to 500/mm^3 (less than equal to 0.5×10^9/L), dramatically escalates the risk of acquiring and opportunistic infection. However, recent studies have demonstrated that the shift in fungemic pathogens occur in both neutropenic and nonneutropenic patients.

There is an increased prevalence of fungemia in the general in-patient setting and in critically-ill, neutropenic, and transplant patients.[22-26] Major risk factors for *Candida* blood stream infections (BSIs) in ICU patients include the use of central venous catheters (CVCs), receipt of multiple antibiotics or parenteral nutrition (PN), extensive surgery and burns, renal failure and hemodialysis, mechanical ventilation, and prior fungal colonization.[27]

Diagnosis and Rapid Diagnostic Tests

2 Traditionally, the diagnosis of invasive fungal infections (IFIs) is accomplished by careful evaluation of clinical symptoms, results of serologic tests, and histopathologic examination and culture of clinical specimens. While traditional direct microscopy, culture and histological techniques constitute the 'gold standard' for diagnosis, obtaining biopsies from sterile body sites for these studies is a highly invasive approach that may not be possible in severely ill patients. Also, histopathology lacks sensitivity and selectivity, as several filamentous fungi may exhibit undistinguishable morphologies. Further, the finding of a positive culture from a sterile site may indicate transient colonization and not true infection, especially for opportunistic fungi. Fungi may require special laboratory conditions, with additional time (up to 4 days) required in order to obtain species identification and the results of susceptibility testing. Some species, such as *C. glabrata*, tend to grow more slowly; initial identification of yeast from blood averages 100 hours (~4 days) in most institutions.[28] Several rapid, accurate diagnostic laboratory tests, including matrix-assisted laser desorption ionization time-of-flight mass spectrometry (MALDI-TOF), peptide nucleic acid (PNA) in situ hybridization (PNA-FISH), PCR, galactomannan, and T2 magnetic resonance assays, have been developed which have the potential to enhance sensitivity and speed of diagnosis of IFIs.[29,30]

New laboratory methods that allow for early differentiation of IFIs due to *Aspergillus* species versus zygomycetes and other moulds would be helpful in allowing clinicians in the earlier initiation of appropriate antifungal therapy. These underscore the need for rapid diagnosis and identification of clinically significant isolates to species level, and the need for susceptibility testing.[31]

TREATMENT
Invasive Mycoses

Strategies for the prevention or treatment of invasive mycoses can be classified broadly as prophylaxis, early empirical therapy, empirical therapy, and secondary prophylaxis or suppression.[1] In patients undergoing cytotoxic chemotherapy, antifungal therapy is directed primarily at the prevention or treatment of infections caused by *Candida* and *Aspergillus* species. Prophylactic therapy with topical, oral, or IV antifungal agents is administered prior to and throughout periods of granulocytopenia (absolute neutrophil count less than 1,000 cells/L [less than 1×10^9/L]). The potential benefits of prophylactic therapy must be weighed against the potential risks inherent in each regimen, including safety, efficacy, cost, the prevalence of infection, and the potential consequences (eg, resistance) of widespread use.

Early empirical therapy is the administration of systemic antifungal agents at the onset of fever and neutropenia. Empirical therapy with systemic antifungal agents is administered to granulocytopenic patients with persistent or recurrent fever despite the administration of appropriate antimicrobial therapy.

Secondary prophylaxis (or suppressive therapy) is the administration of systemic antifungal agents (generally prior to and throughout the period of granulocytopenia) to prevent relapse of a documented invasive fungal infection that was treated during a previous episode of granulocytopenia.

Although these treatment classifications also have been applied to the treatment of fungal infections in acquired immunodeficiency syndrome (AIDS), patients with AIDS rarely acquire systemic infections caused by *Candida* or *Aspergillus* species, unless they become granulocytopenic because of disease or drugs.

HISTOPLASMOSIS

In humans, histoplasmosis is caused by inhalation of dust-borne microconidia of the dimorphic fungus *H. capsulatum*. Although there exist two dimorphic varieties of *H. capsulatum*, the small-celled (2-5 microns) form (var. *capsulatum*) occurs globally, whereas the large-celled (8-15 microns) form (var. *duboisii*) is confined to the African continent and Madagascar. In tissues stained by conventional techniques, *H. capsulatum* appears as an oval or round, narrow-pore, budding, unencapsulated yeast.[32]

Epidemiology

3 Although histoplasmosis is found worldwide, certain areas of North and Central America are recognized as endemic areas. In the United States, most disease is localized along the Ohio and Mississippi River valleys, where more than 90% of residents may be affected. Precise reasons for this endemic distribution pattern are unknown but are thought to include moderate climate, humidity, and soil characteristics. *H. capsulatum* is found in nitrogen-enriched soils, particularly those heavily contaminated by avian or bat guano, which accelerates sporulation. Blackbird or pigeon roosts, chicken coops, and sites frequented by bats, such as caves, attics, or old buildings, serve as "microfoci" of infections; once contaminated, soils yield *Histoplasma* for many years. Although birds are not infected because of their high body temperature, bats (mammals) may be infected and can pass yeast forms in their feces, allowing the spread of *H. capsulatum* to new habitats. Air currents carry the spores for great distances, exposing individuals who were unaware of contact with the contaminated site.[32]

Pathophysiology

At ambient temperatures, *H. capsulatum* grows as a mold. The mycelial phase consists of septate branching hyphae with terminal micro- and macroconidia that range in size from 2 to 14 microns in diameter. When soil is disturbed, these conidia become aerosolized and reach the bronchioles or alveoli.[32]

Animal studies demonstrate that within 2 to 3 days after reaching lung tissue, the conidia germinate, releasing yeast forms that begin multiplying by binary fission. During the next 9 to 15 days, organisms are ingested but not destroyed by large numbers of macrophages that are recruited to the infected site, resulting in small infiltrates. Infected macrophages migrate to the mediastinal lymph nodes and other sites within the mononuclear phagocyte system, particularly the spleen and liver. At this time, the onset of specific T-cell immunity in the nonimmune host activates the macrophages, rendering them capable of fungicidal activity. Tissue granulomas form, many of which develop central caseation and necrosis over the next 2 to 4 months. Over a period of several years, these foci become encapsulated and calcified, often with viable yeast trapped within the necrotic tissue.[32]

Cellular immunity, as measured by histoplasmin skin-test reactivity, wanes in the absence of occasional reexposure. Although exposure to heavy inocula can overcome these immune mechanisms, resulting in severe disease, reinfection occurs frequently in endemic areas. In the immune individual, the reactions of acquired immunity begin 24 to 48 hours after the appearance of yeast forms, resulting in milder forms of illness and little proliferation of organisms. Although viable organisms can be found within granulomas years after initial infection, the organisms appear to have little ability to proliferate within the fibrous capsules, except in immunocompromised patients.[32]

Clinical Presentation

The outcome of infection with *H. capsulatum* depends on a complex interplay of host, pathogen, and environmental factors.[10,32] Host factors include the degree of immunosuppression and the presence of immunity (from prior infection). Environmental factors include inoculum size, exposure within an enclosed area, and duration of exposure. Hematogenous dissemination from the lungs to other tissues probably occurs in all infected individuals during the first 2 weeks of infection before specific immunity has developed but is nonprogressive in most cases, which leads to the development of calcified granulomas of the liver and/or spleen. Progressive pulmonary infection is common in patients with underlying centrilobular emphysema.

Acute and chronic manifestations of histoplasmosis appear to result from unusual inflammatory or fibrotic responses to the pathogen, including pericarditis and rheumatologic syndromes during the first year after exposure, with chronic mediastinal inflammation or fibrosis, broncholithiasis, and enlarging parenchymal granulomas later in the course of disease.

Acute Pulmonary Histoplasmosis

In the vast majority of patients, low-inoculum exposure to *H. capsulatum* results in mild or asymptomatic pulmonary histoplasmosis. The course of disease generally is benign, and symptoms usually abate within a few weeks of onset. Patients exposed to a higher inoculum during an acute primary infection or reinfection can experience an acute, self-limited illness with flu-like pulmonary symptoms, including fever, chills, headache, myalgia, and a nonproductive cough. Patients with diffuse pulmonary histoplasmosis can have diffuse radiographic involvement, become hypoxic, and require ventilatory support. A low percentage of patients present with arthritis, erythema nodosum, pericarditis, or mediastinal granuloma.

Chronic Pulmonary Histoplasmosis

Chronic pulmonary histoplasmosis generally presents as an opportunistic infection imposed on a preexisting structural abnormality, such as lesions resulting from emphysema. Patients demonstrate chronic pulmonary symptoms and apical lung lesions that progress with inflammation, calcified granulomas, and fibrosis. Patients with early, noncavitary disease often recover without treatment. Progression of disease over a period of years, seen in 25% to 30% of patients, is associated with cavitation, bronchopleural fistulas, extension to the other lung, pulmonary insufficiency, and often death.

Disseminated Histoplasmosis

In patients exposed to a large inoculum and in immunocompromised hosts, successful containment of the organism within macrophages may not occur, resulting in a progressive illness characterized by yeast-filled phagocytic cells and an inability to produce granulomas. This disease, termed *disseminated histoplasmosis*, is characterized by persistent parasitization of macrophages. The clinical severity of the diverse forms of disseminated histoplasmosis (Table 121-4) generally parallels the degree of macrophage parasitization observed.

Acute (infantile) disseminated histoplasmosis is characterized by massive involvement of the mononuclear phagocyte system by yeast-engorged macrophages. Classically, this severe type of infection is seen in infants and young children and (rarely) in adults with Hodgkin's disease or other lymphoproliferative disorders. In infants or children, acute disseminated histoplasmosis is characterized by unrelenting fever, anemia, leukopenia or thrombocytopenia, enlargement of the liver, spleen, and visceral lymph nodes, and GI symptoms, particularly nausea, vomiting, and diarrhea. The chest roentgenogram often demonstrates remnants of the initiating acute pulmonary lesion. Untreated disease is uniformly fatal in 1 to 2 months. A less severe "subacute" form of the disease, which occurs in both infants and immunocompetent adults, is characterized by focal destructive lesions in various organs, weight loss, weakness, fever, and malaise. Untreated disease generally is fatal in approximately 10 months.

Most adults with disseminated histoplasmosis demonstrate a mild, chronic form of the disease. Untreated patients often are ill for 10 to 20 years, demonstrating long asymptomatic periods interrupted by relapses of clinical illness characterized primarily by weight loss, weakness, and fatigue. Chronic disseminated histoplasmosis can be seen in patients with lymphoreticular neoplasms (Hodgkin's disease) and patients undergoing immunosuppressant chemotherapy for organ transplantation or for rheumatic diseases. Although CNS involvement occurs in 10% to 20% of patients with severe underlying immunosuppressive conditions, focal organ involvement is uncommon. The disease is characterized by the development of focal granulomatous lesions, often with bone marrow involvement resulting in thrombocytopenia, anemia, and leukemia. Fever, hepatosplenomegaly, and GI ulceration are common.

Histoplasmosis in HIV-Infected Patients

Adult patients with AIDS demonstrate an acute form of disseminated disease that resembles the syndrome seen in infants and children. Progressive disseminated histoplasmosis (PDH), which is defined as a clinical illness that does not improve after at least 3 weeks of observation and that is associated with physical or radiographic findings and/or laboratory evidence of involvement of extrapulmonary tissues, can occur as the direct result of initial infection or because of the reactivation of dormant foci. In endemic areas, 50% of AIDS patients demonstrate PDH as the first manifestation of their disease. PDH is characterized by fever (75% of patients), weight loss, chills, night sweats, enlargement of the spleen, liver, or lymph nodes, and anemia. Pulmonary symptoms occur in only one third of patients and do not always correlate with the presence of infiltrates on chest roentgenogram. A clinical syndrome resembling septicemia is seen in approximately 25% to 50% of patients.[10]

Diagnosis

The diagnosis of histoplasmosis is made on the basis of histopathology, cultures, antigen detection, and serologic tests for *Histoplasma*-specific antibodies. Detection of single, ovoid cells 2 to 5 microns in diameter with narrow-based budding by direct examination or by histologic study of blood smears or tissues should raise strong suspicion of infection with *H. capsulatum* because colonization does not occur as with

TABLE 121-4 Clinical Manifestations and Therapy of Histoplasmosis

Type of Disease and Common Clinical Manifestations	Approximate Frequency (%)[a]	Therapy/Comments
Nonimmunosuppressed Host		
Acute pulmonary histoplasmosis		
Asymptomatic or mild to moderate disease	50-99	*Asymptomatic, mild, or symptoms <4 weeks:* No therapy generally required. Itraconazole (200 mg three times daily for 3 days and then 200 mg once or twice daily for 6-12 weeks) is recommended for patients who continue to have symptoms for 11 months *Symptoms >4 weeks:* Itraconazole 200 mg once daily × 6-12 weeks[b]
Self-limited disease	1-50	*Self-limited disease:* Amphotericin B[c] 0.3-0.5 mg/kg/day × 2-4 weeks (total dose 500 mg) or ketoconazole 400 mg orally daily × 3-6 months can be beneficial in patients with severe hypoxia following inhalation of large inocula; antifungal therapy generally not useful for arthritis or pericarditis; NSAIDs or corticosteroids can be useful in some cases
Mediastinal granulomas	1-50	Most lesions resolve spontaneously; surgery or antifungal therapy with amphotericin B 40-50 mg/day × 2-3 weeks or itraconazole 400 mg/day orally × 6-12 months can be beneficial in some severe cases; mild to moderate disease can be treated with itraconazole for 6-12 months
Moderately severe to severe diffuse pulmonary disease		Lipid amphotericin B 3-5 mg/kg/day followed by itraconazole 200 mg twice daily for 3 days then twice daily for a total of 12 weeks of therapy; alternatively, in patients at low risk for nephrotoxicity, amphotericin B deoxycholate 0.7-1 mg/kg/day can be utilized; methylprednisolone (0.5-1 mg/kg daily IV) during the first 1-2 weeks of antifungal therapy is recommended for patients who develop respiratory complications, including hypoxemia or significant respiratory distress
Inflammatory/fibrotic disease	0.02	*Fibrosing mediastinitis:* The benefit of antifungal therapy (itraconazole 200 mg twice daily × 3 months) is controversial but should be considered, especially in patients with elevated ESR or CF titers ≤1:32; surgery can be of benefit if disease is detected early; late disease cannot respond to therapy *Sarcoid-like:* NSAIDs or corticosteroids[d] can be of benefit for some patients *Pericarditis:* Severe disease: corticosteroids 1 mg/kg/day or pericardial drainage procedure
Chronic cavitary pulmonary histoplasmosis	0.05	Antifungal therapy generally recommended for all patients to halt further lung destruction and reduce mortality *Mild–moderate disease:* Itraconazole 200 mg three times daily for 3 days and then one or two times daily for at least 1 year; some clinicians recommend therapy for 18-24 months due to the high rate of relapse; itraconazole plasma concentrations should be obtained after the patient has been receiving this agent for at least 2 weeks *Severe disease:* Amphotericin B 0.7 mg/kg/day for a minimum total dose of 25-35 mg/kg is effective in 59%-100% of cases and should be used in patients who require hospitalization or are unable to take itraconazole because of drug interactions, allergies, failure to absorb drug, or failure to improve clinically after a minimum of 12 weeks of itraconazole therapy
Histoplasma endocarditis		Amphotericin B (lipid formulations may be preferred, due to their lower rate of renal toxicity) plus a valve replacement is recommended; if the valve cannot be replaced, lifelong suppression with itraconazole is recommended
CNS histoplasmosis		Amphotericin B should be used as initial therapy (lipid formulations at 5 mg/kg/day, for a total dosage of 175 mg/kg may be preferred, due to their lower rate of renal toxicity) for 4-6 weeks, followed by an oral azole (fluconazole or itraconazole 200 mg two or three times daily) for at least a year; some patients may require lifelong therapy; response to therapy should be monitored by repeat lumbar punctures to assess *Histoplasma* antigen levels, WBC, and CF antibody titers; blood levels of itraconazole should be obtained to ensure adequate drug exposure
Immunosuppressed Host		
Disseminated histoplasmosis	0.02-0.05	*Disseminated histoplasmosis:* Untreated mortality 83%-93%; relapse 5%-23% in non-AIDS patients; therapy is recommended for all patients
Acute (Infantile)		*Nonimmunosuppressed patients:* Ketoconazole 400 mg/day orally × 6-12 months or amphotericin B 35 mg/kg IV
Subacute		*Immunosuppressed patients (non-AIDS) or endocarditis or CNS disease:* Amphotericin B >35 mg/kg × 3 months followed by fluconazole or itraconazole 200 mg orally twice daily × 12 months
Progressive histoplasmosis (immunocompetent patients and immunosuppressed patients without AIDS)		*Moderately severe to severe:* Liposomal amphotericin B (3 mg/kg daily), amphotericin B lipid complex (ABLC, 5 mg/kg daily), or deoxycholate amphotericin B (0.7-1 mg/kg daily) for 1-2 weeks, followed by itraconazole (200 mg twice daily for at least 12 months) *Mild to moderate:* Itraconazole (200 mg twice daily for at least 12 months)
Progressive disease of AIDS	25-50[e]	Amphotericin B 15-30 mg/kg (1-2 g over 4-10 weeks)[f] or itraconazole 200 mg three times daily for 3 days then twice daily for 12 weeks, followed by lifelong suppressive therapy with itraconazole 200-400 mg orally daily; although patients receiving secondary prophylaxis (chronic maintenance therapy) might be at low risk for recurrence of systemic mycosis when their $CD4^+$ T-lymphocyte counts increase to >100 cells/μL (>0.1 × 10^9/L) in response to HAART, the number of patients who have been evaluated is insufficient to warrant a recommendation to discontinue prophylaxis

AIDS, acquired immunodeficiency syndrome; CF, complement fixation; ESR, erythrocyte sedimentation rate; HAART, highly active antiretroviral therapy; NSAIDs, nonsteroidal antiinflammatory drugs; PO, orally.

[a]As a percentage of all patients presenting with histoplasmosis.

[b]Itraconazole plasma concentrations should be measured during the second week of therapy to ensure that detectable concentrations have been achieved. If the concentration is below 1 mcg/mL (mg/L; 1.4 μmol/L), the dose may be insufficient or drug interactions can be impairing absorption or accelerating metabolism, requiring a change in dosage. If plasma concentrations are greater than 10 mcg/mL (mg/L; 14 μmol/L), the dosage can be reduced.

[c]Deoxycholate amphotericin B.

[d]Effectiveness of corticosteroids is controversial.

[e]As a percentage of AIDS patients presenting with histoplasmosis as the initial manifestation of their disease.

[f]Liposomal amphotericin B (AmBisome) may be more appropriate for disseminated disease.

Data from references 10 and 32.

Aspergillus or *Candida* infection. In patients with acute self-limited histoplasmosis, extensive testing to verify the diagnosis may not be necessary.[32,33]

In most patients, serologic evidence (complement fixation test or immunodiffusion testing) remains the primary method in the diagnosis of histoplasmosis. Detection of *Histoplasma* antigen by enzyme immunoassay (EIA) in the urine, blood, or bronchoalveolar lavage fluid of infected patients provides rapid diagnostic information and is particularly useful in patients who are severely ill. The highest sensitivity is obtained by testing both urine and serum.[34] *Histoplasma* EIA has also been used to monitor the course of therapy and to detect relapses in patients with AIDS, and the clearance of antigen from serum and urine correlates with clinical efficacy during maintenance therapy.[35]

TREATMENT

Non-HIV-Infected Patient

4 Table 121-4 summarizes the recommended therapy for the treatment of histoplasmosis. In general, asymptomatic or mildly ill patients and patients with sarcoid-like disease do not benefit from antifungal therapy. In the vast majority of patients, low-inoculum exposure to *H. capsulatum* results in *mild* or *asymptomatic* pulmonary histoplasmosis. The course of disease generally is benign, and symptoms usually abate within a few weeks of onset. Therapy can be helpful in symptomatic patients whose conditions have not improved during the first month of infection. Fever persisting more than 3 weeks can indicate that the patient is developing progressive disseminated disease, which can be aborted by antifungal therapy. Whether antifungal therapy hastens recovery or prevents complications is unknown because it has never been studied in prospective trials.

Fluconazole remains a second-line agent for the treatment of histoplasmosis. Clinical data regarding the use of newer azoles such as voriconazole and posaconazole are limited. While both have activity against *Histoplasma*, posaconazole appears to be more active than itraconazole in the immune compromised and nonimmune compromised mouse model of infection, while voriconazole has not been tested in animal models. Both agents have been used successfully in a few patients. Of note, the echinocandins have no activity against *Histoplasma*.

Patients with mild, self-limited disease, chronic disseminated disease, or chronic pulmonary histoplasmosis who have no underlying immunosuppression usually can be treated with either oral itraconazole or IV amphotericin B. The goals of therapy are resolution of clinical abnormalities, prevention of relapse, and eradication of infection whenever possible, although chronic suppression of infection can be adequate in immunosuppressed patients, including those with HIV disease.[10]

HIV-Infected Patient

In AIDS patients, intensive 12-week primary antifungal therapy (induction and consolidation therapy) is followed by lifelong suppressive (maintenance) therapy with itraconazole. Amphotericin B dosages of 50 mg/day (up to 1 mg/kg per day) should be administered IV to a cumulative dose of 15 to 35 mg/kg (1-2 g) in patients who require hospitalization. Amphotericin B can be replaced with itraconazole 200 mg orally twice daily when the patient no longer requires hospitalization or IV therapy to complete a 12-week total course of induction therapy. In patients who do not require hospitalization, itraconazole therapy for 12 weeks can be used.

Fluconazole 800 mg/day orally as induction, followed by 400 mg/day, was effective in 88% of patients, but relapses occurred in approximately one third of patients, and in vitro resistance developed in approximately 50% of patients who relapsed.

In regions experiencing high rates of histoplasmosis (greater than 5 cases/100 patient-years), itraconazole 200 mg/day is recommended as prophylactic therapy in HIV-infected patients. Fluconazole is not an acceptable alternative because of its inferior activity against *H. capsulatum* and its lower efficacy for the treatment of histoplasmosis.[10]

Although patients receiving secondary prophylaxis (chronic maintenance therapy) might be at low risk for recurrence of systemic mycosis when their CD4$^+$ T lymphocyte counts increase to greater than 100 cells/μL (greater than 0.1×10^9/L) in response to highly active antiretroviral therapy (HAART), the number of patients who have been evaluated is insufficient to warrant a recommendation to discontinue prophylaxis.

Evaluation of Therapeutic Outcomes

Response to therapy should be measured by resolution of radiologic, serologic, and microbiologic parameters and by improvement in signs and symptoms of infection. Although investigators are limited by the lack of standardized criteria to quantify the extent of infection, degree of immunosuppression, or treatment response, response rates (based on resolution or improvement in presenting signs and symptoms) of greater than 80% have been reported in case series in AIDS patients receiving varied dosages of amphotericin B. Rapid responses are reported, with the resolution of symptoms in 25% and 75% of patients by days 3 and 7 of therapy, respectively.

After the initial course of therapy for histoplasmosis is complete, lifelong suppressive therapy with oral azoles or amphotericin B (1-1.5 mg/kg weekly or biweekly) is recommended because of the frequent recurrence of infection. Relapse rates in AIDS patients not receiving maintenance therapy range from 50% to 90%.[10]

Antigen testing can be useful for monitoring therapy since concentrations decrease with therapy and increase with relapse.

BLASTOMYCOSIS

North American blastomycosis is a systemic fungal infection caused by *Blastomyces dermatitidis*, a dimorphic fungus that infects primarily the lungs. Patients, however, can present with a variety of pulmonary and extrapulmonary clinical manifestations. Pulmonary disease can be acute or chronic and can mimic infection with tuberculosis, pyogenic bacteria, other fungi, or malignancy. Blastomycosis can disseminate to virtually every other body organ, and approximately 40% of patients with blastomycosis present with skin, bone and joint, or genitourinary tract involvement without any evidence of pulmonary disease.[8,36]

Pulmonary infection probably occurs by inhalation of conidia, which convert to the yeast form in the lung. A vigorous inflammatory response ensues, with neutrophilic recruitment to the lungs followed by the development of cell-mediated immunity and the formation of noncaseating granulomas.

Epidemiology

Blastomycosis was renamed *North American blastomycosis* in 1942, when Conant and Howell named a similar fungus endemic to South America, *Blastomyces braziliensis*, and the disease it caused *South American blastomycosis*. Although the disease is now recognized to be endemic to the southeastern and south central states of the United States (especially those bordering on the Mississippi and Ohio River basins) and the midwestern states and Canadian provinces bordering the Great Lakes, numerous cases of North American blastomycosis have been diagnosed in Africa, northern parts of South America, India, and Europe. Endemic areas have been defined primarily by analysis of sporadic cases and epidemics or clusters of disease because the lack of a dependable skin or laboratory test makes wide-scale epidemiologic testing to determine the incidence of infection unfeasible at present.[8,36] Although initial review of sporadic cases suggested that males with outdoor occupations that exposed them to soil were at greatest risk for blastomycosis, there is no sex, age, or occupational predilection for blastomycosis.[8,36]

Although *B. dermatitidis* generally is considered to be a soil inhabitant, attempts to isolate the organism in nature frequently have been unsuccessful. *B. dermatitidis* has been isolated from soil containing decayed vegetation, decomposed wood, and pigeon manure, frequently in association with warm, moist soil of wooded areas that is rich in organic debris.[8,36]

Pathophysiology and Clinical Presentation

Colonization does not occur with *Blastomyces*[8,36] *Acute pulmonary blastomycosis* generally is an asymptomatic or self-limited disease characterized by fever, shaking chills, and productive, purulent cough, with or without hemoptysis, in immunocompetent individuals. The clinical presentation can be difficult to differentiate from other respiratory infections, including bacterial pneumonia, on the basis of clinical symptoms alone.

Sporadic (nonepidemic) pulmonary blastomycosis can present as a more chronic or subacute disease, with low-grade fever, night sweats, weight loss, and productive cough that resembles tuberculosis rather than bacterial pneumonia. *Chronic pulmonary blastomycosis* is characterized by fever, malaise, weight loss, night sweats, chest pain, and productive cough. Patients often are thought to have tuberculosis and frequently have evidence of disseminated disease that can appear 1 to 3 years after the primary pneumonia has resolved. Reactivation of disease can occur in the lungs or as the focus of new infection in other organs.

In approximately 40% of patients, dissemination is not accompanied by reactivation of pulmonary disease. The most common sites for disseminated disease include the skin and bony skeleton, although less commonly the prostate, oropharyngeal mucosa, and abdominal viscera are involved. CNS disease, while exceedingly uncommon, is associated with the highest mortality rate.

Laboratory and Diagnostic Tests

The simplest and most successful method of diagnosing blastomycosis is by direct microscopic visualization of the large, multinucleated yeast with single, broad-based buds in sputum or other respiratory specimens following digestion of cells and debris with 10% potassium hydroxide.[8,36] Histopathologic examination of tissue biopsies and culture of secretions also should be used to identify *B. dermatitidis*, although it can require up to 30 days to isolate and identify a small inoculum.

No reliable skin test exists to determine the incidence and prevalence of disease in endemic populations, and reliable serologic diagnosis of blastomycosis has long been hampered by the lack of specific and standardized reagents. Serologic response does not always correlate with clinical improvement, although some investigators have noted that a decline in the number of precipitins or CF titers can offer evidence of a favorable prognosis in patients with established disease.

Acute pulmonary blastomycosis generally is an asymptomatic or self-limited disease characterized by fever, shaking chills, and productive, purulent cough, with or without hemoptysis, in immunocompetent individuals. The clinical presentation can be difficult to differentiate from other respiratory infections, including bacterial pneumonia, on the basis of clinical symptoms alone. Sporadic (nonepidemic) cases of pulmonary blastomycosis can present as a more chronic or subacute disease with low-grade fever, night sweats, weight loss, and productive cough that resembles tuberculosis rather than bacterial pneumonia.

TREATMENT

Non-HIV-Infected Patient

5 In the immunocompetent host, acute pulmonary blastomycosis can be mild and self-limited and may not require treatment. However, consideration should be given to treating all infected individuals to prevent extrapulmonary dissemination. All individuals with moderate to severe pneumonia, disseminated infection, or those who are immunocompromised require antifungal therapy.

In patients with mild to moderate pulmonary blastomycosis, itraconazole is effective; however, in patients with moderately severe to severe pulmonary disease, the clinical presentation of the patient, the immune competence of the patient, and the toxicity of the antifungal agents are the main determinants of the choice of antifungal therapy. All immunocompromised patients and patients with progressive pulmonary disease or with extrapulmonary disease should be treated (Table 121-5). In the case of disease limited to the lungs, cure might have occurred without treatment before the diagnosis is made. Regardless of whether or not the patient receives treatment, however, he or she must be followed carefully for many years for evidence of reactivation or progressive disease.[8,36]

Some authors recommend azole therapy for the treatment of self-limited pulmonary disease, with the hope of preventing late extrapulmonary disease; however, data supporting the efficacy of these regimens are lacking.[8,36] Itraconazole 200 to 400 mg/day demonstrated 90% efficacy as a first-line agent in the treatment of nonlife-threatening non-CNS blastomycosis, and for compliant patients who completed at least 2 months of therapy, a success rate of 95% was noted. No therapeutic advantage was noted with the higher (400 mg) dosage as compared with patients treated with 200 mg.

All patients with disseminated blastomycosis, as well as those with extrapulmonary disease, require therapy. Due to its adverse effects, variable oral absorption, and lack of CNS penetration, ketoconazole is now reserved as an alternative therapy for mild to moderate pulmonary and non-CNS disease. However, older studies demonstrate that ketoconazole 400 mg/day orally for 6 months cures more than 80% of patients with chronic pulmonary and nonmeningeal disseminated blastomycosis. Amphotericin B is more efficacious but more toxic and therefore is reserved for noncompliant patients and patients with overwhelming or life-threatening disease, CNS infection, and treatment failures.[8,36] Lipid preparations of amphotericin B have largely replaced conventional amphotericin B for treatment of blastomycosis, despite their higher cost, due to their decreased renal toxicity. Surgery has only a limited role in the treatment of blastomycosis.

HIV-Infected Patient

For unclear reasons, blastomycosis is an uncommon opportunistic disease among immunocompromised individuals, including AIDS patients; however, blastomycosis can occur as a late (CD4 lymphocytes less than 200 cells/mm^3 [less than 0.2×10^9/L]) and frequently fatal complication of HIV infection. In this population, overwhelming disseminated disease with frequent involvement of the CNS is common.[8,36] Following induction therapy with amphotericin B (total cumulative dose of 1 g), HIV-infected patients should receive chronic suppressive therapy with an oral azole antifungal.[8,36]

COCCIDIOIDOMYCOSIS

Epidemiology

Coccidioidomycosis is caused by infection with *Coccidioides immitis*, a dimorphic fungus found in the southwestern and western United States,

TABLE 121-5 Therapy of Blastomycosis

Type of Disease	Preferred Treatment
Pulmonary[a]	
Moderately severe to severe disease	Lipid formulation of amphotericin B 3-5 mg/kg IV daily or amphotericin B[b] 0.7-1 mg/kg IV daily (total dose 1.5-2.5 g) × 1-2 weeks or until improvement is noted, followed by itraconazole[c,d] 200 mg orally three times daily for 3 days, then 200 mg twice daily, × total of 6-12 months
Mild to moderate disease	Itraconazole[c,d] 200 mg orally three times daily for 3 days, then 200 mg twice daily, for a total of 6 months[c]
CNS disease	*Induction:* Lipid formulation of amphotericin B 5 mg/kg IV daily × 4-6 weeks, followed by an oral azole as consolidation therapy *Consolidation:* Fluconazole[d] 800 mg orally daily, or itraconazole[d] 200 mg two or three times orally daily, or voriconazole[d] 200-400 mg orally twice daily, for ≥12 months and until resolution of CSF abnormalities
Disseminated or Extrapulmonary Disease	
Moderately severe to severe disease	Lipid formulation of amphotericin B 3-5 mg/kg IV daily or amphotericin B[b] 0.7-1 mg/kg IV daily × 1-2 weeks or until improvement is noted, followed by itraconazole[c,d] 200 mg orally three times daily for 3 days, then 200 mg twice daily × 6-12 months. Treat osteoarticular disease with 12 months of antifungal therapy Most clinicians prefer to step-down to itraconazole[d] therapy once the patient's condition improves
Mild to moderate	Itraconazole[c,d] 200 mg orally three times daily for 3 days, then 200 mg once or twice daily × ≥12 months. Treat osteoarticular disease with 12 months of antifungal therapy
Immunocompromised Host (Including Patients with AIDS, Transplants, or Receiving Chronic Glucocorticoid Therapy)	
Acute disease	Lipid formulation of amphotericin B 3-5 mg/kg IV daily or amphotericin B[b] 0.7-1 mg/kg IV daily × 1-2 weeks or until improvement is noted, then give suppressive therapy for a total of at least 12 months of therapy
Suppressive therapy	Itraconazole[c,d] 200 mg orally three times daily for 3 days, then 200 mg twice daily for a total of at least 12 months of therapy; lifelong suppressive therapy with oral itraconazole[d] 200 mg daily may be required for immunosuppressed patients in whom immunosuppression cannot be reversed, and in patients who experience relapse despite appropriate therapy

AIDS, acquired immunodeficiency syndrome.

[a]In the immunocompetent host, acute pulmonary blastomycosis can be mild and self-limited and may not require treatment.

[b]Desoxycholate amphotericin B.

[c]Serum levels of itraconazole should be determined after the patient has received itraconazole for ≥2 weeks, to ensure adequate drug exposure.

[d]Azoles should not be used during pregnancy.

Data from reference 8.

as well as in parts of Mexico and South America. In North America, the endemic regions encompass the semiarid areas of the southwestern United States from California to Texas known as the Lower Sonoran Zone, where there is scant annual rainfall, hot summers, and sandy, alkaline soil. *C. immitis* grows in the soil as a mold, and mycelia proliferate during the rainy season. During the dry season, resistant arthroconidia form and become airborne when the soil is disturbed.

Although generally considered to be a regional disease, coccidioidomycosis has increased in importance in recent years because of the increased tourism and population in endemic areas, the increased use of immunosuppressive therapy in transplantation and oncology, and the AIDS epidemic. Although there is no racial, hormonal, or immunologic predisposition for acquiring primary disease, these factors affect the risk of subsequent dissemination of disease (Table 121-6).[37]

TABLE 121-6 Factors for Severe, Disseminated Infection with Coccidioidomycosis

Race (Filipinos > African Americans > Native Americans > Hispanics > Asians)
Pregnancy (especially when infection is acquired or reactivated in the second or third trimester)
Compromised cellular immune system, including
- AIDS patients
- Patients receiving
- Corticosteroids
- Immunosuppressive agents
- Chemotherapy

Male gender
Neonates
Patients with B or AB blood types

AIDS, acquired immune deficiency syndrome.

Data from reference 37.

Pathophysiology

When individuals come in contact with contaminated soil during ranching, dust storms, or proximity to construction sites or archaeologic excavations, arthroconidia are inhaled into the respiratory tree, where they transform into spherules, which reproduce by cleavage of the cytoplasm to produce endospores. The endospores are released when the spherules reach maturity. Similar to histoplasmosis, an acute inflammatory response in the tissue leads to infiltration of mononuclear cells, ultimately resulting in granuloma formation.[37]

Clinical Presentation of Coccidioidomycosis

Coccidioidomycosis encompasses a spectrum of illnesses ranging from primary uncomplicated respiratory tract infection that resolves spontaneously to progressive pulmonary or disseminated infection.[37] Initial or primary infection with *C. immitis* almost always involves the lungs. Although approximately one third of the population in endemic areas is infected, the average incidence of symptomatic disease is only approximately 0.43%.

Signs and Symptoms

Primary Coccidioidomycosis ("*Valley Fever*"): Approximately 60% of infected patients have an asymptomatic, self-limited infection without clinical or radiological manifestations. The remaining 40% of patients exhibit nonspecific symptoms that are often indistinguishable from ordinary upper respiratory infections, including fever, cough, headache, sore throat, myalgias, and fatigue that occur 1 to 3 weeks after exposure to the pathogen. More commonly, a diffuse, mild erythroderma or maculopapular rash is observed. Patients can have pleuritic chest pain and peripheral eosinophilia.

A fine, diffuse rash can appear during the first few days of the illness. Primary pneumonia can be the first manifestation of disease, characterized by a productive cough that can be blood-streaked, as well as single or multiple soft or dense homogeneous hilar or basal infiltrates on chest roentgenogram. *Chronic, persistent pneumonia or persistent pulmonary coccidioidomycosis* (primary disease lasting more than 6 weeks) is complicated by hemoptysis, pulmonary scarring, and the formation of cavities or bronchopleural fistulas.

Necrosis of pulmonary tissue with drainage and cavity formation occurs commonly. Most parenchymal cavities close spontaneously or form dense nodular scar tissue that can become superinfected with bacteria or spherules of *C. immitis*. These patients often have persistent cough, fevers, and weight loss.

Disseminated disease occurs in less than 1% of infected patients. The most common sites for dissemination are the skin, lymph nodes, bone, and meninges, although the spleen, liver, kidney, and adrenal gland also can be involved. Occasionally, miliary coccidioidomycosis occurs, with rapid, widespread dissemination, often in concert with positive blood cultures for *C. immitis*. Patients with AIDS frequently present with miliary disease. Coccidioidomycosis in AIDS patients appears to be caused by reactivation of disease in most patients. Dissemination also is more likely if infection occurs during pregnancy, especially during the third trimester or in the immediate postpartum period.[37]

CNS infection occurs in approximately 16% of patients with disseminated coccidioidomycosis. Patients can present with meningeal disease without previous symptoms of primary pulmonary infection, although disease usually occurs within 6 months of the primary infection. The signs and symptoms are often subtle and nonspecific, including headache, weakness, changes in mental status (lethargy and confusion), neck stiffness, low-grade fever, weight loss, and occasionally, hydrocephalus. Space-occupying lesions are rare, and the main areas of involvement are the basilar meninges.

Diagnosis

The diagnoses of coccidioidomycosis generally utilizes identification or recovery of *Coccidioides* spp. from clinical specimens and detection of specific anticoccidioidal antibodies in serum or other body fluids.

TREATMENT

General Guidelines

6 Therapy for coccidioidomycosis is difficult, and the results are unpredictable. Guidelines[11] are available for treatment of this disease; however, optimal treatment for many forms of this disease still generates debate. The efficacy of antifungal therapy for coccidioidomycosis often is less certain than that for other fungal etiologies, such as blastomycosis, histoplasmosis, or cryptococcus, even when in vitro susceptibilities and the sites of infections are similar. The refractoriness of coccidioidomycosis can relate to the ability of *C. immitis* spherules to release hundreds of endospores, maximally challenging host defenses.[37] Fortunately, only approximately 5% of infected patients require therapy.

Goals of Therapy

Desired outcomes of treatment are resolution of signs and symptoms of infection, reduction of serum concentrations of anticoccidioidal antibodies, and return of function of involved organs. It would also be desirable to prevent relapse of illness on discontinuation of therapy, although current therapy is often unable to achieve this goal.

Specific Agents Used for the Treatment of Coccidioidomycosis

Azole antifungals, primarily fluconazole and itraconazole, have replaced amphotericin B as initial therapy for most chronic pulmonary or disseminated infections. Amphotericin B is now usually reserved for patients with respiratory failure because of infection with *Coccidioides* species, those with rapidly progressive coccidioidal infections, or women during pregnancy. Therapy often ranges from many months to years in duration, and in some patients, lifelong suppressive therapy is needed to prevent relapses. Specific antifungals (and their usual dosages) for the treatment of coccidioidomycosis include IV amphotericin B (0.5-1.5 mg/kg per day), ketoconazole (400 mg/day orally), IV or oral fluconazole (usually 400-800 mg/day, although dosages as high as 1,200 mg/day have been used without complications), and itraconazole (200-300 mg orally twice daily or three times daily, as either capsules or solution).[37] If itraconazole is used, measurement of serum concentrations can be helpful to ascertain whether oral bioavailability is adequate.

Amphotericin B generally is preferred as initial therapy in patients with rapidly progressive disease, whereas azoles generally are preferred in patients with subacute or chronic presentations. The lipid formulations of amphotericin B have not been studied extensively in coccidioidal infection but can offer a means of giving more drugs with less toxicity. Fluconazole probably is the most frequently used medicine given its tolerability, although high relapse rates have been reported in some studies. Relapse rates with itraconazole therapy can be lower than those with fluconazole.[37]

The usefulness of newly available antifungal agents of possible benefit for the treatment of refractory coccidioidal infections has not been adequately assessed and they are not yet FDA approved for use in this population. Case reports have suggested that voriconazole can be effective in selected patients. Caspofungin has been effective in treating experimental murine coccidioidomycosis, but in vitro susceptibility of isolates varies widely, and there is only one report regarding its value. Posaconazole was shown to be an effective treatment in a small clinical trial and in patients with refractory infections. Its efficacy relative to other triazole antifungals is unknown.

Clinical **Controversy...**

Although there is continued disagreement among experts in endemic areas whether antifungal therapy in patients with uncomplicated early coccidioidal infection might shorten the course of illness or reduce the development of more serious complications, prospective randomized trials addressing this question are lacking. The excellent tolerability of oral azoles has lowered the threshold for deciding to treat primary infection, and clinicians should treat patients with significantly debilitating illness, those with extensive pulmonary disease, and with who are frail due to advanced age, concurrent diabetes or comorbidities.[11]

Combination therapy with members of different classes of antifungal agents has not been evaluated in patients, and there is a hypothetical risk of antagonism. However, some clinicians feel that outcome in severe cases is improved when amphotericin B is combined with an azole antifungal. If the patient improves, the dosage of amphotericin B can be slowly decreased while the dosage of azole is maintained.[37]

Primary Respiratory Infection

Although most patients with symptomatic primary pulmonary disease recover without therapy, management should include followup visits for 1 to 2 years to document resolution of disease or to identify as early as possible evidence of pulmonary or extrapulmonary complications.

Patients with a large inoculum, severe infection, or concurrent risk factors (eg, HIV infection, organ transplant, pregnancy, or high doses of corticosteroids) probably should be treated, particularly those with high CF titers, in whom incipient or occult dissemination is likely. Because some racial or ethnic populations have a higher risk of dissemination, some clinicians advocate their inclusion in the high-risk group. Common indicators used to judge the severity of infection include weight loss (greater than 10%), intense night sweats persisting more than 3 weeks, infiltrates involving more than one half of one lung or portions of both lungs, prominent or persistent hilar adenopathy, CF antibody titers of greater than 1:16, failure to develop dermal sensitivity to coccidial antigens, inability to work, or symptoms that persist for more than 2 months.[37]

Commonly prescribed therapies include currently available oral azole antifungals at their recommended doses for courses of therapy ranging from 3 to 6 months.[37] In patients with diffuse pneumonia with bilateral reticulonodular or miliary infiltrates, therapy usually is initiated with amphotericin B; several weeks of therapy generally are required to produce clear evidence of improvement. Consolidation therapy with oral azoles can be considered at that time. The total duration of therapy should be at least 1 year, and in patients with underlying immunodeficiency, oral azole therapy should be continued as secondary prophylaxis.

Infections of the Pulmonary Cavity

Many pulmonary infections that are caused by *C. immitis* are benign in their course and do not require intervention. In the absence of controlled clinical trials, evidence of the benefit of antifungal therapy is lacking, and asymptomatic infections generally are left untreated. Symptomatic patients can benefit from oral azole therapy, although recurrence of symptoms can be seen in some patients once therapy is discontinued. Surgical resection of localized cavities provides resolution of the problem in patients in whom the risks of surgery are not too high.[37]

Extrapulmonary (Disseminated) Disease

Nonmeningeal Disease

Almost all patients with disease located outside the lungs should receive antifungal therapy; therapy usually is initiated with 400 mg/day of an oral azole. Amphotericin B is an alternative therapy and can be necessary in patients with worsening lesions or with disease in particularly critical locations such as the vertebral column. Approximately 50% to 75% of patients treated with amphotericin B for nonmeningeal disease achieve a sustained remission, and therapy usually is curative in patients with infections localized strictly to skin and soft tissues without extensive abscess formation or tissue damage. The efficacy of local injection into joints or the peritoneum, as well as intraarticular or intradermal administration, remains poorly studied. Amphotericin B appears to be most efficacious when cell-mediated immunity is intact (as evidenced by a positive coccidioidin or spherulin skin test or low CF antibody titer). Controlled trials that document these clinical impressions are lacking, however.[37]

Meningeal Disease

Fluconazole has become the drug of choice for the treatment of coccidioidal meningitis. A minimum dose of 400 mg/day orally leads to a clinical response in most patients and obviates the need for intrathecal amphotericin B. Some clinicians will initiate therapy with 800 or 1,000 mg/day, and itraconazole dosages of 400 to 600 mg/day are comparably effective. It is also clear, however, that fluconazole only leads to remission rather than cure of the infections; thus suppressive therapy must be continued for life. Ketoconazole cannot be recommended routinely for the treatment of coccidioidal meningitis because of its poor CNS penetration following oral administration. Patients who do not respond to fluconazole or itraconazole therapy are candidates for intrathecal amphotericin B therapy with or without continuation of azole therapy. The intrathecal dose of amphotericin B ranges from 0.01 to 1.5 mg given at intervals ranging from daily to weekly. Therapy is initiated with a low dosage and is titrated upward as patient tolerance develops.[37]

CRYPTOCOCCOSIS

Epidemiology

Cryptococcosis is a noncontagious, systemic mycotic infection caused by the ubiquitous encapsulated soil yeast *Cryptococcus*, which is found in soil, particularly in pigeon droppings, although disease occurs throughout the world, even in areas where pigeons are absent. Infections caused by *C. neoformans* var. *grubii* (serotype A) are seen worldwide among immunocompromised hosts, followed by *C. neoformans* var. *neoformans* (serotype D). On the other hand, *Cryptococcus gattii* (serotypes B and C) is geographically more restricted and in contrast to *C. neoformans*, rarely infects immunosuppressed patients, is not associated with HIV infection, and the infections are more difficult to treat. *C. gattii* is not associated with birds; its main reservoir was thought to be limited to certain species of eucalyptus tree. Until recently, it was most common in tropical and subtropical areas, such as Australia, South America, Southeast Asia, and central Africa, with the highest incidence in Papua New Guinea and Northern Australia, although infections occur in nontropical areas such as North America and Europe. *C. gattii* emerged on Vancouver Island, British Columbia, Canada, in 1999, and subsequently spread to the Vancouver lower mainland, Washington state, and Oregon.[38]

Infection is acquired by inhalation of the organism. The incidence of cryptococcosis has risen dramatically in recent years, reflecting the increased numbers of immunocompromised patients, including those with malignancies, diabetes mellitus, chronic renal failure, and organ transplants and those receiving immunosuppressive agents. In most developed countries, widespread use of HAART has significantly decreased the incidence of cryptococcosis; however, the incidence and mortality of this infection are still extremely high in areas with limited access to HAART and a high incidence of HIV.[39]

Disease can remain localized in the lungs or can disseminate to other tissues, particularly the CNS, although the skin also can be affected. Hematogenous spread generally occurs in the immunocompromised host, although it also has been seen in individuals with intact immune systems.

Clinical Presentation of Cryptococcosis

Primary cryptococcosis in humans almost always occurs in the lungs, although the pulmonary focus usually produces a subclinical infection.[38,39] Symptomatic infections usually are manifested by cough, rales, and shortness of breath that generally resolve spontaneously. Cryptococcus can present as part of an immune reconstitution inflammatory syndrome (IRIS), a paradoxical worsening of preexisting infectious processes following the initiation of HAART in HIV-infected individuals. In non-AIDS patients, the symptoms of cryptococcal meningitis are nonspecific. Headache, fever, nausea, vomiting, mental status changes, and neck stiffness generally are observed. Less common symptoms include visual disturbances (photophobia and blurred vision), papilledema, seizures, and aphasia. In AIDS patients, fever and headache are common, but meningismus and photophobia are much less common than in non-AIDS patients. Approximately 10% to 12% of AIDS patients have asymptomatic disease, similar to the rate observed in non-AIDS patients.[39,40] Intracerebral mass lesions (cryptococcomas) are more common in *C. gattii* than in *C. neoformans*, presumably due to their different host immune responses.[38]

Laboratory Tests

With cryptococcal meningitis, the CSF opening pressure generally is elevated. There is a CSF pleocytosis (usually lymphocytes), leukocytosis, a decreased glucose concentration, and an elevated CSF protein concentration. There is also a positive cryptococcal antigen (detected by LA). The test is rapid, specific, and extremely sensitive, but false-negative results can occur. False-positive tests can result from cross-reactivity with rheumatoid factor and *Trichosporon beigelii*. *C. neoformans* can be detected in approximately 60% of patients by India ink smear of CSF, and it can be cultured in more than 96% of patients. Occasionally, large volumes of CSF are required to confirm the diagnosis.

The CSF parameters in patients with AIDS are similar to those seen in non-AIDS patients, with the exception of a decreased inflammatory response to the pathogen, resulting in a strikingly low number of leukocytes in CSF and extraordinarily high cryptococcal antigen titers.

TREATMENT

The choice of treatment for disease caused by *C. neoformans* depends on both the anatomic sites of involvement and the host's immune status, and thus, treatment recommendations are divided into three specific risk groups: (a) HIV-infected individuals, (b) transplant recipients, and (c) non–HIV-infected and nontransplant hosts (Table 121-7).[9] The management of cryptococcosis includes systemic antifungal therapy, control of elevated intracranial pressure (ICP), and supportive care. When possible, immune defects should be addressed. Although no randomized clinical trials have been performed to address this, outcomes of treatment for CNS cryptococcosis (without mass lesions or hydrocephalus) appear to be similar for disease due to either *C. neoformans* or *C. gattii*.[38]

Nonimmunocompromised Patients

7 Prior to the introduction of amphotericin B, cryptococcal meningitis was an almost uniformly fatal disease; approximately 86% of patients died within 1 year. The use of large (1-1.5 mg/kg) daily doses of amphotericin B resulted in cure rates of approximately 64%. When amphotericin B is combined with flucytosine, a smaller dose of amphotericin B can be employed because of the in vitro and in vivo synergy between the two antifungal agents. Resistance develops to flucytosine in up to 30% of patients treated with flucytosine alone, limiting its usefulness as monotherapy.[41] Combination therapy with amphotericin B and flucytosine will sterilize the CSF within 2 weeks of treatment in 60% to 90% of patients, and most immunocompetent patients will be treated successfully with 6 weeks of combination therapy.[39] However, because of the need for prolonged IV therapy and the potential for renal and hematologic toxicity with this regimen, alternative regimens utilizing lipid formulations of amphotericin B and the use of shorter (2 weeks) courses of amphotericin B followed by consolidation therapy with fluconazole for 8 weeks, then maintenance therapy with a lower dosage of fluconazole for 6 to 12 months has been advocated.[9,40,42]

For asymptomatic, immunocompetent hosts with isolated mild to moderate pulmonary disease and no evidence of CNS disease, careful observation can be warranted; in the case of symptomatic infection, fluconazole for 6 to 12 months is warranted. In individuals with non-CNS cryptococcemia, a positive serum cryptococcal antigen titer (greater than 1:8), cutaneous infection, a positive urine culture, or prostatic disease, the clinician must decide whether to follow the regimen for isolated pulmonary disease or the more aggressive regimen for patients with CNS (disseminated) disease.[9]

Pilot studies evaluating combination therapy with fluconazole plus flucytosine as initial therapy yielded unsatisfactory results, and this approach is discouraged even in "low-risk" patients. Ketoconazole has been used successfully in the treatment of cutaneous cryptococcosis, but it is not useful in the treatment of CNS disease, probably because of its poor penetration into the CNS.[9]

Despite low CSF concentrations of amphotericin B (2%-3% of those observed in plasma), the use of intrathecal amphotericin B is not recommended for the treatment of cryptococcal meningitis except in very ill patients or in patients with recurrent or progressive disease despite aggressive therapy with IV amphotericin B. The dosage of amphotericin B employed is usually 0.5 mg administered through the lumbar, cisternal, or intraventricular (through an Ommaya reservoir) route two or three times weekly. Side effects of intrathecal amphotericin B include arachnoiditis and paresthesias. Intrathecal amphotericin B therapy should be administered in combination with IV amphotericin B.[42]

The recommended management of raised ICP in cryptococcal meningitis (without hydrocephalus, a mass lesion, or a shift on computed tomography [CT] scan) has been repeated CSF removal by spinal tap. Those who do not respond and have ongoing raised ICP should have ophthalmologic monitoring for possible vision loss, and should be considered for ventriculoperitoneal shunt surgery. Neither corticosteroids (in the absence of IRIS) nor acetazolamide is recommended for management of raised ICP. Symptomatic, medically refractory mass lesions that may be compressing vital structures should be considered for surgical therapy.[38]

Immunocompromised Patients

Immunocompromised hosts with isolated severe pulmonary and extrapulmonary disease (including cryptococcemia) without CNS disease should be treated similarly to nonimmunocompromised patients with CNS disease. Immunocompromised patients with CNS infection require more prolonged therapy; treatment regimens are based on those used in the HIV-infected population and follow induction therapy with amphotericin B and consolidation therapy with 6 to 12 months of suppressive therapy with fluconazole.[9]

Organ Transplant Recipients

Cryptococcosis has been documented in an average of 2.8% of solid-organ transplant recipients. The median time to disease onset is 21 months after transplantation; 68.5% of the cases occur greater than 1 year after transplantation.

Induction therapy for solid organ transplant recipients with cryptococcal meningoencephalitis consists of liposomal amphotericin B or amphotericin B lipid complex (ABLC) plus flucytosine for at least 2 weeks. Fluconazole maintenance therapy should be continued for at least 6 to 12 months. Immunosuppressive management should include sequential or stepwise reduction of immunosuppressants, with consideration of lowering the corticosteroid dose first.[43] Amphotericin B should be used with caution in transplant recipients and is not recommended as first-line therapy in this patient population due to the risk of nephrotoxicity in this population that frequently has reduced renal function. If used, the tolerated dosage of amphotericin B is uncertain, but 0.7 mg/kg daily is suggested with frequent renal function monitoring. Regardless of the agent utilized, all antifungal dosages need to be carefully monitored.[43]

HIV-Infected Patients

Primary antifungal prophylaxis for cryptococcosis is not routinely recommended in HIV-infected patients in the United States and Europe. However, in areas with limited HAART availability, high levels of antiretroviral drug resistance, and a high burden of disease, clinicians may wish to consider the use of either prophylactic therapy or a preemptive strategy with serum cryptococcal antigen testing for asymptomatic antigenemia.[9]

Early studies confirmed the benefit of early high-dose amphotericin B use, the usefulness of flucytosine added to amphotericin B for induction therapy, and the slight superiority of fluconazole over itraconazole for consolidation therapy.

Amphotericin B combined with flucytosine during the two-week induction phase of therapyis the initial treatment of choice. In patients who cannot tolerate flucytosine, amphotericin B alone is an acceptable alternative. After the initially successful 2-week induction period, consolidation therapy with fluconazole can be administered for 8 weeks or until CSF cultures are negative. In patients in whom fluconazole cannot be given, itraconazole is an acceptable, albeit less effective, alternative. Combination therapy with fluconazole plus flucytosine is effective; however, it is recommended as an alternative

TABLE 121-7 Therapy of Cryptococcosis[a,b]

Type of Disease and Common Clinical Manifestations	Therapy/Comments
Nonimmunocompromised Patients (Non–HIV-Infected, Nontransplant)	
Meningoencephalitis *without* neurological complications, in patients in whom CSF yeast cultures are negative after 2 weeks of therapy	*Induction:* Amphotericin B[c] IV 0.7-1 mg/kg/day *plus* flucytosine 100 mg/kg/day orally in four divided doses × ≥4 weeks A lipid formulation of amphotericin B may be substituted for amphotericin B in the second 2 weeks
Follow all regimens with suppressive therapy	*Consolidation:* Fluconazole 400-800 mg orally daily × 8 weeks *Maintenance:* Fluconazole 200 mg orally daily × 6-12 months
Meningoencephalitis *with* neurological complications	*Induction:* Same as for patients without neurologic complications, but consider extending the induction therapy for a total of 6 weeks. A lipid formulation of amphotericin B may be given for the last 4 weeks of the prolonged induction period *Consolidation:* Fluconazole 400 mg orally daily × 8 weeks
Mild-to-moderate pulmonary disease (Nonmeningeal disease)	Fluconazole 400 mg orally daily × 6-12 months
Severe pulmonary cryptococcosis	*Same as CNS disease × 12 months*
Cryptococcemia (nonmeningeal, nonpulmonary disease)	*Same as CNS disease × 12 months*
Immunocompromised Patients	
Severe pulmonary cryptococcosis	*Same as CNS disease × 12 months*
HIV-infected Patients	
Primary therapy; induction and consolidation[g]	*Preferred regimen*: *Induction:* Amphotericin B[d] IV 0.7-1 mg/kg IV daily *plus* flucytosine 100 mg/kg/day orally in four divided doses for ≥2 weeks
Follow all regimens with suppressive therapy	*Consolidation:* Fluconazole 400 mg [6 mg/kg] orally daily × ≥8 weeks Liposomal amphotericin B 3-4 mg/kg IV daily, or amphotericin B lipid complex (ABLC) 5 mg/kg IV daily, for ≥2 weeks can be substituted for amphotericin B[d] in patients with or at risk for renal dysfunction *Alternative regimens, in order of preference:* Amphotericin B[d] IV 0.7-1 mg/kg IV daily × 4-6 weeks *or* liposomal amphotericin B 3-4 mg/kg IV daily[f] × 4-6 weeks *or* ABLC 5 mg/kg IV daily × 4-6 weeks *or* Amphotericin B[d] IV 0.7 mg/kg IV daily, *plus* fluconazole 800 mg (12 mg/kg) orally daily × 2 weeks, followed by fluconazole 800 mg (12 mg/kg) orally daily × ≥8weeks *or* Fluconazole ≥800 mg (1,200 mg/day is preferred) orally daily *plus* flucytosine 100 mg/kg/day orally in four divided doses × 6 weeks *or* Fluconazole 800-1,200 mg/day orally daily × 10-12 weeks (a dosage ≥1,200 mg/day is preferred when fluconazole is used alone)[e] *or* Itraconazole 200 mg orally twice daily × 10-12 weeks (use of itraconazole, which produces minimal concentrations of active drug in the CSF is discouraged)[i]
Suppressive/maintenance therapy[h]	Preferred: Fluconazole 200 mg orally daily × ≥1 year *or* Itraconazole[i] 200 mg orally twice daily × ≥1 year *or* Amphotericin B[j] IV 1 mg/kg weekly × ≥1 year
Organ Transplant Recipients	
Mild-moderate non-CNS disease or mild-to-moderate symptoms without diffuse pulmonary infiltrates	Fluconazole 400 mg (6 mg/kg) orally daily × 6-12 months
CNS disease, moderately severe or severe CNS disease or disseminated disease without CNS disease, or severe pulmonary disease without evidence of extrapulmonary or disseminated disease	*Induction:* Liposomal amphotericin B 3-4 mg/kg IV daily,[f] or ABLC 5 mg/kg IV daily *plus* flucytosine 100 mg/kg/day orally in four divided doses × ≥2 weeks If induction therapy does not include flucytosine, consider a lipid formulation of amphotericin B for ≥4-6 weeks of induction therapy. Consider the use of a lipid formulation of amphotericin B lipid formulation (6 mg/kg IV daily) in patients with a high-fungal burden disease or relapse of disease *Consolidation:* Fluconazole 400-800 mg (6-12 mg/kg) per day orally for 8 weeks *Maintenance:* Fluconazole 200-400 mg per day orally for 6-12 months

HIV, human immunodeficiency virus; IT, intrathecal.

[a]When more than one therapy is listed, they are listed in order of preference.

[b]See the text for definitions of induction, consolidation, suppressive/maintenance therapy, and prophylactic therapy.

[c]Deoxycholate amphotericin B.

[d]In patients with significant renal disease, lipid formulations of amphotericin B can be substituted for deoxycholate amphotericin B during the induction.

[e]Or until cerebrospinal fluid (CSF) cultures are negative.

[f]Liposomal amphotericin B has been given safely up to 6 mg/kg daily; could be considered in treatment failure or in patients with a high fungal burden.

[g]Initiate HAART therapy 2-10 weeks after commencement of initial antifungal treatment.

[h]Consider discontinuing suppressive therapy during HAART in patients with a CD4 cell count ≥100 cells/μL (≥0.1 × 10^9/L) and an undetectable or very low HIV RNA level sustained for ≥3months (with a minimum of 12 months of antifungal therapy). Consider reinstitution of maintenance therapy if the CD4 cell count decreases to <100 cells/μL (<0.1 × 10^9/L).

[i]Drug level monitoring is strongly advised.

[j]Use is discouraged except in azole intolerant patients, since it is less effective than azole therapy, and is associated with a risk of IV catheter-related infections.

Data from reference 9.

to the preceding therapies because of its potential for toxicity. Lipid formulations of amphotericin B are effective, but the optimal dosage is unknown.[9]

In HIV-infected patients, mortality is highly associated with elevated ICP (CSF opening pressure greater than 250 mm H_2O [greater than 2.5 kPa]). At the initiation of antifungal therapy, lumbar drainage should remove enough CSF to reduce the opening pressure by 50%. Patients initially should undergo daily lumbar punctures to maintain CSF opening pressure in the normal range. When the CSF pressure is normal for several days, the procedure can be suspended. Adjunctive steroid treatment is not recommended because therapy has resulted in mixed results and its impact on outcome is unclear. Similarly, neither mannitol nor acetazolamide therapy provides any clear benefit in the management of elevated ICP.[9]

Suppressive (Maintenance) Therapy for Cryptococcal Meningitis in the HIV-Infected Patient

Relapse of *C. neoformans* meningitis occurs in approximately 50% of AIDS patients after completion of primary therapy. Persistence of asymptomatic urinary *C. neoformans* has been documented in a high percentage of AIDS patients despite seemingly adequate courses of therapy for primary meningeal disease. The prostate appears to act as a sequestered reservoir of infection in these patients, resulting in systemic relapse.

Patients appear to be at low risk for recurrence of cryptococcosis when they have successfully completed a course of initial therapy for cryptococcosis, remain asymptomatic with regard to signs and symptoms of cryptococcosis, have received antifungal therapy for greater than 3 of the previous 6 months, have a serum cryptococcal antigen titer less than 1:512, or have a sustained increase (eg, greater than 6 months) in their $CD4^+$ T-lymphocyte counts to greater than 100 to 200 cells/μL (greater than 0.1×10^9-0.2×10^9/L) and an HIV viral load of less than 50 copies/mL (50×10^3/L).[9,40,42]

After the completion of induction/consolidation phases of therapy, long-term chronic suppression with fluconazole (200 mg orally daily) should be continued for a minimum of one year. Maintenance therapy can be discontinued after one year in patients who have successfully completed primary therapy, are free of symptoms and signs of active cryptococcosis, and have been receiving HAART with a sustained CD4 cell count greater than 100 cells/mL (greater than 0.100×10^6/L) and an undetectable viral load.[9]

Evaluation of Therapeutic Outcomes

Once the CNS is involved, the usual course is weeks to months of progressive deterioration, with 80% of untreated patients dying within the first year. The prognosis of cryptococcal meningitis depends largely on the underlying predisposing factors of the host. Although cryptococcal antigen is positive in 90% of patients with cryptococcal meningitis, fewer than one half of the patients with cryptococcal meningitis develop antibody to capsular polysaccharide. Those who produce antibody have a slightly improved prognosis. In contrast, the presence of headache is a favorable symptom, presumably because it leads to an earlier diagnosis. A favorable outcome is also associated with a normal mental status on diagnosis and a CSF white blood cell (WBC) count of less than 20 cells/mm³ (20×10^6/L). A poor outcome is predicted, however, by the presence of one or more underlying diseases (including hematopoietic disorders and AIDS), corticosteroid or immunosuppressive therapy, pretreatment serum cryptococcal antigen titers of 1:32, and posttherapy serum antigen titers of 1:8. In non-AIDS patients, the cryptococcal antigen titer can be followed during therapy to assess response to antifungal therapy. In AIDS patients, decreasing titers are not necessarily predictive of success, and titers rarely become negative at the completion of therapy.

CANDIDA INFECTIONS

Candida species are yeasts that exist primarily as small (4-6 microns), unicellular, thin-walled, ovoid cells that reproduce by budding. On agar medium, they form smooth, white, creamy colonies resembling staphylococci. Although there are more than 150 species of *Candida*, eight species—*C. albicans, C. tropicalis, Candida parapsilosis, C. krusei, Candida stellatoidea, C. guilliermondii, C. lusitaniae,* and *C. glabrata*—are regarded as clinically important pathogens in human disease.[17] Yeast forms, hyphae, and pseudohyphae can be found in clinical specimens.

Pathophysiology

8 *C. albicans* is a normal commensal of the skin, female genital tract, and entire GI tract of humans. Therefore, the mere presence of hyphae or pseudohyphae in a clinical specimen is insufficient for the diagnosis of invasive disease. The majority of infections with *C. albicans* are acquired endogenously, although human-to-human transmission also can occur. Although the term *fungemia* refers to the presence of fungi in the blood, the most commonly isolated organism is *C. albicans*. Candidiasis can cause mucocutaneous or systemic infection, including endocarditis, peritonitis, arthritis, and infection of the CNS. (Mucocutaneous infections caused by *Candida* are discussed in further detail in Chapter 98.)

Adherence of *C. albicans* is important in the pathogenesis of oral candidiasis and subsequent colonization of the GI tract. Because evidence suggests that the GI tract is often the portal of entry for *Candida* in disseminated disease, factors that alter the adherence of *Candida* are crucial in the development of local and systemic infection. *C. tropicalis* adheres to intravascular catheters at a higher rate than *C. albicans*, a factor that may help to account for the increased incidence of systemic infections caused by this pathogen.

CANDIDEMIA AND ACUTE HEMATOGENOUSLY DISSEMINATED CANDIDIASIS

Epidemiology

Candidemia has increased substantially in the past 2 decades, and the fourth most common bloodstream infection (BSI) in US hospitals.[44] It is associated with high mortality, increased length of hospital stay, and significant economic burden.[44-54] Although patients with neutropenia are at high risk for IFIs, the use of antifungal prophylaxis and prompt initiation of antifungal therapy in persistently febrile patients with neutropenia who do not respond to antibioticshas resulted in a reduction in the frequency of *Candida* BSIs in this population.[7] In fact, most BSIs due to *Candida* species now occur in nonneutropenic patients who have been hospitalized in ICUs, especially adult ICUs and neonatal ICUs.

The most commonly encountered clinical species of *Candida* include *C. albicans, C. glabrata, C. tropicalis, C. parapsilosis, C. lusitaniae, C. krusei, and C. guilliermondii.* While *C. albicans* is still the most common species of *Candida* causing candidemia, its relative frequency is decreasing, while the frequency of the other, non-*albicans* species, including *C. glabrata, C. tropicalis, C. krusei,* and *C. parapsilosis*, have increased.[44,52,55-57] The change in species is of concern clinically, as certain pathogens, such as *C. krusei* and *C. glabrata*, are intrinsically more resistant to commonly used triazole drugs.[58,59] Although risk factors for the development of *Candida* BSIs in ICU patients can be identified, factors that lead to the acquisition of specific species are still unclear.[27]

Patients' characteristics influence the distribution of *Candida* species: *C. glabrata* infections are more common in the elderly,

C. krusei in immunocompromised patients, while *C. parapsilosis* is most common in children and neonates. *C. lusitaniae* infections are a cause of breakthrough fungemia in cancer patients; *C. parapsilosis* has emerged as the second most common pathogen, following *C. albicans*, in neonatal ICU patients, where it is often associated with central lines and PN, and fungemias in patients outside the United States, in particular in South America. Fungemia caused by *C. glabrata* is observed more commonly in adults older than 65 years of age.[32]

Pathophysiology

Candida generally is acquired via the GI tract, although organisms also can enter the bloodstream via indwelling IV catheters. Immunosuppressed patients, including those with lymphoreticular or hematologic malignancies, diabetes, and immunodeficiency diseases and those receiving immunosuppressive therapy with high-dose corticosteroids, immunosuppressants, antineoplastic agents, or broad-spectrum antimicrobial agents, are at high risk for IFIs (Table 121-8). Major risk factors include the use of CVCs, total PN, receipt of multiple antibiotics, extensive surgery and burns, renal failure and hemodialysis, mechanical ventilation, and prior fungal colonization. Patients who have undergone surgery (particularly surgery of the GI tract) are increasingly susceptible to disseminated candidal infections.[20,46]

TABLE 121-8 Risk Factors for Invasive Candidiasis

Colonization
Corrected colonization index (CCI) ≥0.4[a]
Colonization index (CI) ≥0.8[a]
Candida spp. cultured from sites other than blood
Candiduria
Antibiotic use
Number of antibiotics prior to infection (per additional antibiotics)
Use of two or more antibiotics
Use of broad-spectrum antibiotics in previous 10 days
Surgery
Surgery on ICU admission
Gastro-abdominal surgery
Abdominal drainage
Elective surgery
Cardiopulmonary bypass time >120 minutes
Hickman catheter
Foreign devices
Central venous catheter
Triple lumen catheter in patients who have undergone surgery
Bladder catheter
Renal failure and dialysis
Prior hemodialysis
Hemofiltration procedures
Increased serum creatinine[b]
New-onset hemodialysis within 3 days of admission to ICU
Acute renal failure
Underlying disease/baseline characteristics
Total PN
Diabetes mellitus
Apache II (per point)
Signs of severe sepsis
Diarrhea at any time
Mechanical ventilation ≥10 days
Hospital-acquired bacterial infection
Bacterial peritonitis by ICU day 11
GI disease
ICU length of stay
Transferred from other hospital
Use of corticosteroids
Profound neutropenia (ANC < 100/mm³ [<0.100 ×10⁹/L])

[a]CI = the ratio of number of nonblood distinct body sites (dbs) heavily colonized with identical strains to the total number of dbs; CCI = the product of the CI and the ratio of the number of dbs showing heavy growth (≥10⁵ CFU/mL [≥10⁸ CFU/L]) to the total of dbs growing *Candida* spp.

[b]Serum creatinine >1.2 mg/dL (>106 μmol/L) in females, >1.6 mg/dL (>141 μmol/L) in males.

Data from reference 27.

Clinical Presentation of Hematogenous Candidiasis

Dissemination of *C. albicans* can result in infection in single or multiple organs, particularly the kidney, brain, myocardium, skin, eye, bone, and joints.[60] In most patients, multiple micro- and macroabscesses are formed. Infection of the liver and spleen is becoming recognized as a particularly common and difficult-to-treat site of infection that characteristically occurs in patients undergoing chemotherapy for acute leukemia or lymphoma.

Laboratory Tests

The interpretation of positive surveillance cultures of the skin, mouth, sputum, feces, or urine is hampered by their occurrence as commensal pathogens and in distinguishing colonization from invasive disease. A rapid presumptive identification of *C. albicans* can be made by incubation of *Candida* in serum; formation of a germ tube (the beginning of hyphae, which arise as perpendicular extensions from the yeast cell, with no constriction at their point of origin) within 1 to 2 hours offers a positive identification of *C. albicans*. Unfortunately, *C. dubliniensis* also can produce a germ tube, and a negative germ tube test does not rule out the possibility of *C. albicans*, but further biochemical tests must be performed to differentiate between other non-*albicans* species.

The PNA fluorescence in situ hybridization (FISH) method uses fluorescein-labeled PNA probes that target *C. albicans* 26S rRNA for the identification of *C. albicans*. The test has excellent sensitivity (99%-100%) and specificity (100%) in the direct identification of *C. albicans* from blood cultures.[61]

Matrix-assisted laser desorption/ionization time-of-flight intact cell mass spectrometry (MALDI-TOF-ICMS) and T2 Magnetic Resonance Assays, are promising tools for the rapid detection and identification of pathogenic *Candida* species.[29,30,61]

TREATMENT

The list of risk factors for invasive candidiasis in critically ill patients is extensive, and trying to decipher which patients may benefit from antifungal prophylaxis or empirical therapy based on risk factors in an ICU is exceedingly difficult. In addition, the number of risk factors present in ICU patients changes over time, and the majority of ICU patients will have more than one risk factor. Clinically useful, practical predictive algorithms and "scoring systems" to identify high-risk patients early during their ICU admission have not proved successful thus far. To maximize its clinical utility as a decision-making tool, the ideal algorithm would identify high-risk populations (ones with a rate of invasive candidiasis of 10%-15%), providing clinicians with a means of administering prophylaxis to a minimal number of patients, while preventing the maximal number of invasive candidiasis cases.[27]

Hematogenous Candidiasis

There is a high rate of mortality in nonneutropenic patients with fungal blood cultures. Delays in the initiation of antifungal therapy significantly increase mortality.[62,63] Treatment of candidiasis should be guided by knowledge of the infecting species, the clinical status of the patient, and when available, the antifungal susceptibility of the infecting isolate. Therapy should be continued for 2 weeks after documented clearance of blood cultures, with resolution of all signs and symptoms of infection. All patients should undergo dilated fundiscopic exam within the 1st week of therapy. Susceptibility testing of the infecting isolate is a useful adjunct to species identification during selection of a therapeutic approach, since it can be used to identify isolates that are unlikely to respond to fluconazole or amphotericin B.[7] However, this is not currently available at many institutions.

Clinical **Controversy...**

Role of Catheter Removal

Although it is common practice in today's standard of care to place indwelling catheters in patients for the administration of medications and parenteral nutrition (TPN), catheter-related infections are a common complication. These foreign bodies (especially triple lumen catheters) double as entry ports for normal skin flora or other nosocomial pathogens, and they provide a readily available site for the binding of pathogens via microbiotic biofilms. Their subsequent role as a source of BSIs is facilitated by frequent use, TPN, and the potential for contamination of catheters by medical staff who are colonized with *Candida* species.

Most consensus recommendations urge removal of all existing tunneled CVCs and implantable devices, particularly in patients with fungemia caused by *C. parapsilosis*, which is very frequently associated with catheters, as it has been associated with reduced mortality in adults, and a shorter duration of candidemia.[7] Arguments against the removal of all catheters in patients with candidemia include the prominent role of the gut as a source for disseminated candidiasis, the significant cost and potential for complications, and the problems that can be encountered in patients with difficult vascular access.[7,64,65] However, in an individual patient it is often difficult to determine the relative contribution of gut versus catheter as the primary source of fungemia.[66-69] The evidence for this recommendation is weakest in cancer patients with severe neutropenia and mucositis (eg, acute leukemia, stem cell transplant), in whom candidemia is almost always primarily of gut origin, and removal of CVCs is least likely to have an impact on mortality.[66-69]

Nonimmunocompromised Patient

Prophylaxis

In ICUs, the use of fluconazole for prophylaxis or empirical therapy has increased exponentially in the past decade. However, studies that demonstrated benefit in the prevention of invasive candidal BSIs did so either by using highly selective criteria or by studying patients in an unusually high-risk ICU setting, and the role of antifungal prophylaxis in the surgical ICU remains extremely controversial. For a study to demonstrate efficacy in clinical trials, the baseline rate of invasive candidiasis must be greater than 10%, and that prophylaxis must result in greater than fourfold reduction of disease.[7] Although ICU-specific, a greater than 10% rate of invasive candidiasis is generally found only in the setting of high-risk transplant patients (eg, patients undergoing liver transplantation), or in patients with one or more of the following risk factors by day 3 of their ICU stay: new-onset dialysis, receipt of broad-spectrum antibiotics, the presence of diabetes, and in patients receiving PN.[70,71] Prophylactic antifungals are indicated in patients with recurrent intestinal perforations and/or anastomotic leak as these patients are at extremely high risk for invasive candidiasis (35%) and the use of empiric fluconazole has been shown to significantly decrease the incidence of infection to 4%.[27]

"Empirical" Therapy (Also Known as Preemptive Therapy)

The term "preemptive" antifungal therapy is often used to describe early antifungal therapy given to high-risk patients with persistent signs and symptoms and clinical, laboratory, or radiologic surrogate markers of infection but without mycological evidence of infection, or those heavily colonized with *Candida*. Few data are available for assessing the role of antifungals as empirical therapy for *suspected* fungemia in patients who do not yet exhibit a positive blood culture, or for isolates other than *C. albicans*. The empiric use of fluconazole did not significantly decrease the incidence of invasive candidiasis; thus, its use is not recommended at this time.[72]

Initial Antifungal Therapy in Non-neutropenic Patients with Documented Candidemia, in Whom the Species is Not Yet Identified and Results of Antifungal Susceptibility Testing are Not Known

Several large randomized studies in non-neutropenic patients have demonstrated that azoles (fluconazole or voriconazole), echinocandins, and deoxycholate amphotericin B (d-AmB) are similarly effective for the therapy of documented candidemia; however, fewer adverse effects are observed with azole therapy.[45] Similarly, echinocandins are at least as effective as amphotericin B or fluconazole in (primarily non-neutropenic) adult patients with candidemia with fewer drug-related adverse events. Although the use of combination therapy (high-dose fluconazole plus amphotericin B) was demonstrated to be superior to treatment with fluconazole alone, it was associated with a higher rate of nephrotoxicity, and the routine use of combination therapy in this patient population is not yet recommended.[7]

For empiric therapy in non-neutropenic adults, IDSA guidelines (Table 121-9) recommend use of an echinocandin or fluconazole as initial therapy. Echinocandins are recommended for patients with moderately severe to severe illness, and patients with recent azole exposure. Patients may be transitioned to fluconazole if their *Candida* isolates are known/likely to be susceptible to fluconazole (eg, *C. albicans*, *C. parapsilosis*) in patients who are clinically stable. Fluconazole may be used initially in patients who are less critically ill, with no recent azole exposure, who are not at high risk for *C. glabrata* or with central nervous system or endocardial disease.[7,45]

Among the lipid-associated formulations of amphotericin B, only liposomal amphotericin B (AmBisome) and ABLC (Abelcet) have been approved for use in proven cases of candidiasis; however, patients with invasive candidiasis also have been treated successfully with amphotericin B colloid dispersion (ABCD, Amphotec or Amphocil). The lipid-associated formulations are less toxic but as effective as amphotericin B deoxycholate.

Antifungal Therapy for Specific *Candida* Species

C. krusei infections should be treated with large doses of amphotericin B (greater than equal to 1 mg/kg per day) or with caspofungin. *C. tropicalis*, and *C. parapsilosis* can be treated with either amphotericin B at or fluconazole.[7] Amphotericin B resistance remains relatively rare despite more than 45 years of clinical use, although it has been reported in *C. lusitaniae* (now *Clavispora lusitaniae*) and *C. guilliermondii*. *Candida rugosa* often is considered to be "polyene tolerant," and these isolates are believed to be selected owing to the wide use of amphotericin B.

Immunocompromised Patients

In immunocompromised patients, the optimal agent, dose, and duration of therapy are unclear, and patients must be monitored carefully with serial blood cultures and careful physical examinations,

TABLE 121-9 Antifungal Therapy of Invasive Candidiasis[7,34]

Type of Disease and Common Clinical Manifestations	Therapy/Comments
Prophylaxis of Candidemia	
Nonneutropenic patients[a]	Not recommended except for severely ill/high-risk patients in whom fluconazole IV/PO 400 mg daily should be used (see the text)
Neutropenic patients[a]	The optimal duration of therapy is unclear but at a minimum should include the period at risk for neutropenia: Fluconazole IV/PO 400 mg daily *or* itraconazole solution 2.5 mg/kg every 12 hours orally *or* micafungin 50 mg (1 mg/kg in patients under 50 kg) IV daily
Solid-organ transplantation, liver transplantation	*Patients with two or more key risk factors[b]:* Amphotericin B IV 10-20 mg daily *or* liposomal amphotericin B (AmBisome) 1 mg/kg/day *or* fluconazole 400 mg orally daily
Empirical (Preemptive) Antifungal Therapy	
Suspected disseminated candidiasis in febrile nonneutropenic patients	None recommended; data are lacking defining subsets of patients who are appropriate for therapy (see the text)
Initial Antifungal Therapy (Documented Candidemia with Unknown Candida Species)	
Febrile neutropenic patients with prolonged fever despite 4-6 days of empirical antibacterial therapy	*Treatment duration:* Until resolution of neutropenia An echinocandin[d] is a reasonable alternative; voriconazole can be used in selected situations (see the text)
Less critically ill patients with no recent azole exposure	An echinocandin[d] or fluconazole (loading dose of 800 mg [12 mg/kg], then 400 mg [6 mg/kg] daily)
Additional mold coverage is desired	Voriconazole
Antifungal Therapy of Documented Candidemia and Acute Hematogenously Disseminated Candidiasis, Unknown Species	
Nonimmunocompromised host[c]	*Treatment duration:* 2 weeks after the last positive blood culture and resolution of signs and symptoms of infection *Remove existing central venous catheters when feasible plus fluconazole (loading dose of 800 mg [12 mg/kg], then 400 mg [6 mg/kg] daily) or an echinocandin[d]*
Patients with recent azole exposure, moderately severe or severe illness, or who are at high risk of infection due to *C. glabrata* or *C. krusei*	An echinocandin[d] Transition from an echinocandin to fluconazole is recommended for patients who are clinically stable and have isolates (eg, *C. albicans*) likely to be susceptible to fluconazole
Patients who are less critically ill and who have had no recent azole exposure	Fluconazole
Antifungal Therapy of Specific Pathogens	
C. albicans, C. tropicalis, and *C. parapsilosis*	Fluconazole IV/PO 6 mg/kg/day *or* an echinocandin[d] or amphotericin B IV 0.7 mg/kg/day *plus* fluconazole IV/orally 800 mg/day; amphotericin B deoxycholate 0.5-1 mg/kg daily or a lipid formulation of amphotericin B (3-5 mg/kg daily) are alternatives in patients who are intolerant to other antifungals; transition from amphotericin B deoxycholate or a lipid formulation of amphotericin B to fluconazole is recommended in patients who are clinically stable and whose isolates are likely to be susceptible to fluconazole (eg, *C. albicans*); voriconazole (400 mg [6 mg/kg] twice daily × two doses then 200 mg [3 mg/kg] twice daily thereafter) is efficacious, but offers little advantage over fluconazole; it may be utilized as step-down oral therapy for selected cases of candidiasis due to *C. krusei* or voriconazole-susceptible *C. glabrata* *Patients intolerant or refractory to other therapy[e]:* Amphotericin B lipid complex IV 5 mg/kg/day Liposomal amphotericin B IV 3-5 mg/kg/day Amphotericin B colloid dispersion IV 2-6 mg/kg/day
C. krusei	Amphotericin B IV ≤1 mg/kg/day *or* an echinocandin[d]
C. lusitaniae	Fluconazole IV/orally 6 mg/kg/day
C. glabrata	An echinocandin[d] (transition to fluconazole or voriconazole therapy is not recommended without confirmation of isolate susceptibility)
Neutropenic host[f]	*Treatment duration:* Until resolution of neutropenia *Remove existing central venous catheters when feasible, plus:* Amphotericin B IV 0.7-1 mg/kg/day (total dosages 0.5-1 g) *or patients failing therapy with traditional amphotericin B:* Lipid formulation of amphotericin B IV 3-5 mg/kg/day
Chronic disseminated candidiasis (hepatosplenic candidiasis)	*Treatment duration:* Until calcification or resolution of lesions *Stable patients:* Fluconazole IV/orally 6 mg/kg/day *Acutely ill or refractory patients:* Amphotericin B IV 0.6-0.7 mg/kg/day
Urinary candidiasis	*Asymptomatic disease:* Generally no therapy is required *Symptomatic or high-risk patients[g]:* Removal of urinary tract instruments, stents, and Foley catheters, +7-14 days therapy with fluconazole 200 mg orally daily *or* amphotericin B IV 0.3-1 mg/kg/day

PO, orally.

[a]Patients at significant risk for invasive candidiasis include those receiving standard chemotherapy for acute myelogenous leukemia, allogeneic bone marrow transplants, or high-risk autologous bone marrow transplants. However, among these populations, chemotherapy or bone marrow transplant protocols do not all produce equivalent risk, and local experience should be used to determine the relevance of prophylaxis.

[b]Risk factors include retransplantation, creatinine of more than 2 mg/dL (177 μmol/L), choledochojejunostomy, intraoperative use of 40 units or more of blood products, and fungal colonization detected within the first 3 days after transplantation.

[c]Therapy is generally the same for acquired immunodeficiency syndrome (AIDS)/non-AIDS patients except where indicated and should continued for 2 weeks after the last positive blood culture and resolution of signs and symptoms of infection. All patients should receive an ophthalmologic examination. Amphotericin B can be switched to fluconazole (IV or oral) for the completion of therapy. Susceptibility testing of the infecting isolate is a useful adjunct to species identification during selection of a therapeutic approach because it can be used to identify isolates that are unlikely to respond to fluconazole or amphotericin B. However, this is not currently available at most institutions.

[d]Echinocandin = caspofungin 70 mg loading dose, then 50 mg IV daily maintenance dose, or micafungin 100 mg daily, or anidulafungin 200 mg loading dose, then 100 mg daily maintenance dose.

[e]Often defined as failure of ≥500 mg amphotericin B, initial renal insufficiency (creatinine ≥2.5 mg/dL [≥221 μmol/L] or creatinine clearance <25 mL/min [< 0.42 mL/s]), a significant increase in creatinine (to 2.5 mg/dL [221 μmol/L] for adults or 1.5 mg/dL [133 μmol/L] for children), or severe acute administration-related toxicity.

[f]Patients who are neutropenic at the time of developing candidemia should receive a recombinant cytokine (granulocyte colony-stimulating factor or granulocyte–monocyte colony-stimulating factor) that accelerates recovery from neutropenia.

[g]Patients at high risk for dissemination include neutropenic patients, low-birth-weight infants, patients with renal allografts, and patients who will undergo urologic manipulation.

Data from reference 7.

TABLE 121-10 Comparative Trials for Initial Antifungal Therapy in the Febrile Neutropenic Host

Year Published	Study Drugs	Study Design	Results and Comments
1982	Placebo versus amphotericin B	Randomized	Favored amphotericin B
1989	Placebo versus amphotericin B	Randomized	Favored amphotericin B
1996	Fluconazole versus amphotericin B	Randomized	Defervescence: equivalence; safety analysis favored fluconazole
1998	Fluconazole versus amphotericin B	Randomized	Composite: equivalence; secondary analysis favored fluconazole
2000	Fluconazole versus amphotericin B	Randomized	Composite: equivalence; safety analysis favored fluconazole
1999	Liposomal amphotericin B versus amphotericin B	Randomized, double blind	Composite: equivalence; secondary analysis favors liposomal amphotericin B
2000	Liposomal amphotericin B versus amphotericin B lipid complex	Randomized, double blind	Liposomal amphotericin B had superior safety versus amphotericin B lipid complex and a similar therapeutic success rate
2001	Itraconazole versus amphotericin B	Randomized, open label	Composite: equivalence; secondary analysis favors itraconazole
2002	Voriconazole versus liposomal amphotericin B	Randomized, open label	Composite: equivalence; secondary analysis variable (voriconazole failed to meet criteria for noninferiority); fewer breakthrough infections with voriconazole
2004	Caspofungin versus liposomal amphotericin B	Randomized, double blind	Composite: equivalence; secondary analysis favored caspofungin for treatment of baseline infections
2005	Liposomal amphotericin B loading regimen (10 mg/kg/day × 14 day) vs standard dosing (3 mg/kg/day)	Randomized, prospective, double blind	Loading regimen did not demonstrate any benefit in overall response or survival and was associated with higher rates of nephrotoxicity and hypokalemia

Data from reference 74.

particularly of the retina. Patients who are neutropenic at the time of developing candidemia should receive a recombinant cytokine (granulocyte colony-stimulating factor or granulocyte-monocyte colony-stimulating factor) that accelerates recovery from neutropenia.[7]

Prophylaxis

Recognition of the role of the GI tract in invasive *Candida* infections has led to efforts to decrease infections by prophylactic administration of topical or systemically absorbed antifungal agents in immunocompromised patients. The use of systemically absorbable agents such as azole antifungal agents appears to decrease the risk of IFIs.[7]

Several antifungal agents, including fluconazole (400 mg/day), posaconazole (200 mg three times daily), micafungin or caspofungin (50 mg daily) administered from the start of the conditioning regimen until day 75, can reduce the frequency of invasive *Candida* infections and decrease mortality in patients undergoing allogeneic bone marrow transplantation.[7,21,73]

Similarly, in less risk-selected patients with hematologic malignancies who are undergoing remission-induction chemotherapy, fluconazole, posaconazole, or caspofungin, during induction chemotherapy for the duration of neutropenia, are effective in preventing systemic infection and death caused by *Candida* species.[7]

For solid-organ transplant recipients, fluconazole or liposomal amphotericin B is recommended as postoperative antifungal prophylaxis for liver, pancreas, and small bowel transplant recipients at high risk of candidiasis.[7,20]

Widespread use of prophylactic fluconazole in all ICU patients is not warranted and may lead to an increase in resistance and adverse events. If utilized, prophylactic fluconazole should target high-risk patients with a presumed risk of invasive candidiasis of 10% to 15%.[7,27]

Empirical Therapy for Febrile Neutropenic Patients

Many clinicians advocate early institution of empirical IV amphotericin B in patients with neutropenia and persistent (greater than 5-7 days) fever.[21] However, the potential toxicities (particularly nephrotoxicity) of this agent preclude its routine use in all patients. Suggested criteria for the empirical use of amphotericin B include: (a) fever of 5 to 7 days' duration that is unresponsive to antibacterial agents, (b) neutropenia of more than 7 days' duration, (c) no other obvious cause for fever, (d) progressive debilitation, (e) chronic adrenal corticosteroid therapy, and (f) indwelling intravascular catheters. In patients who fail therapy with amphotericin B, lipid formulations of amphotericin B can be used. Lipid formulations of amphotericin B can be used as alternatives to amphotericin B deoxycholate for empirical therapy. Although they do not appear to be substantially more effective, there is less drug-related toxicity (Table 121-10).[74]

Itraconazole and fluconazole have demonstrated efficacy equivalent to that of d-AmB in patients with hematologic malignancy (not treated with allogeneic HSCT). However, as fluconazole is not active against filamentous fungi, its use in patients at high risk for these pathogens should be avoided. If itraconazole is used, the IV formulation should be used because the bioavailability of the oral formulations (including the solution) is unreliable; however, it is no longer available. Voriconazole and caspofungin were compared with liposomal amphotericin B in large randomized, multicenter trials of empirical antifungal therapy in febrile neutropenic patients. Voriconazole did not fulfill the protocol-defined criteria for noninferiority; however, it was superior in reducing documented breakthrough infections, infusion-related toxicity, and nephrotoxicity. Patients who received voriconazole had more frequent episodes of transient visual disturbances and hallucinations. Caspofungin demonstrated equivalent efficacy but was superior in the successful treatment of baseline IFIs.[74,75]

Specific Therapy

Amphotericin B, the azoles, and the echinocandins have roles in the treatment of hematogenous candidiasis, and the choice of therapy is guided by weighing the greater activity of amphotericin B for some non-*albicans* species (eg, *C. krusei*) against the lower toxicity and ease of administration of fluconazole and the echinocandins.[7]

Most clinicians recommend amphotericin B in total dosages of 0.5 to 1 g administered over approximately 1 to 2 weeks in patients with *Candida* endophthalmitis and in all neutropenic patients with candidemia. Longer courses of therapy can be needed in some patients.[17] Fluconazole and amphotericin B appear similarly effective for the treatment of *C. albicans* BSIs in the neutropenic patient; controlled data, however, are lacking. In patients with uncomplicated *C. albicans* fungemia who have not received systemic prophylaxis with antifungal azoles, therapy with fluconazole 400 to 800 mg/day IV can be considered. However, in patients who have undergone allogeneic HSCT, the role of fluconazole is becoming more limited because of its widespread use for antifungal prophylaxis. In this setting, particularly if the patient has been treated previously with an azole antifungal agent, the possibility of microbiologic resistance must be considered. Infections with fluconazole-resistant *Candida* species, including *C. glabrata*, *C. krusei*, and fluconazole-resistant *C. albicans*, or with *Aspergillus* species are more likely.

Clinical **Controversy...**

Treatment of Candidemia in Non-Neutropenic Adults Once the *Candida* Species Is Identified

Expert opinion is divided regarding the optimal therapy of infections caused by *C. glabrata*.[76,77] Since *C. glabrata* often demonstrate reduced susceptibility to fluconazole, treatment with echinocandins, or amphotericin B at a dosage of 0.7 mg/kg/day is often recommended as initial therapy although there are successful treatment outcomes reported in response to fluconazole therapy of 6 to 12 mg/kg/day, and may be suitable in less critically ill patients.[76,77] The severity of illness and choice of antifungal predict response in patients with *C. glabrata* fungemia, and the choice of antifungal (fluconazole or an echinocandin) does not influence mortality. Failure is associated with admission to an intensive care unit. When fluconazole is dosed appropriately, (Table 121-9) *C. glabrata* fluconazole susceptibility breakpoints are predictive of clinical and microbiological response. Echinocandin therapy is independently associated with treatment success, but not survival, in invasive candidiasis due to *C. glabrata*.[77]

Amphotericin B, at a dosage of 1 mg/kg/day, is recommended for the management of systemic *C. krusei* infections. *C. tropicalis* and *C. parapsilosis* may be treated with either amphotericin B at 0.6 mg/kg/day or fluconazole at 6 mg/kg/day. Candidemia due to *C. parapsilosis* has increased in frequency among pediatric populations and appears to be associated with a lower mortality rate than other species of *Candida*. Since many, but not all isolates of *C. lusitaniae* are resistant to amphotericin B, fluconazole at 6 mg/kg/day is the preferred agent for treatment of this species.

In patients with *C. parapsilosis* candidemia, guidelines[7] recommend the use of fluconazole, since MICs of echinocandins tend to be higher for *C. parapsilosis*. However, a meta-analysis of 5 randomized, blinded, comparative trials for treatment of candidemia or invasive candidiasis concluded that the overall treatment success of echinocandins versus other agents was similar: 76.5% versus 73%.[78,79] In patients with *Candida glabrata* candidemia, guidelines recommend the use of an echinocandin.[7] Treatment should be continued for 2 weeks, in the absence of metastatic complications of disease. It is important to note when counting days of therapy that the days of treatment 'begin' on the first day of documented clearance of *Candida* species from bloodstream, with the use of an effective antifungal agent to which the species is susceptible.

Updated IDSA and European guidelines have recently been published.[7,31,80] In the European Guidelines, important recommendations include the recommendation for daily blood cultures until negative, and that patients can be switched to oral therapy after 10 days of IV therapy. They also recommend the use of amphotericin or echinocandins preferentially if catheters cannot be removed.[31,80,81]

CANDIDURIA

Within the urinary tract, most common lesions are either *Candida* cystitis or hematogenously disseminated renal abscesses. *Candida* cystitis often follows catheterization or therapy with broad-spectrum antimicrobial agents. The diagnosis of *Candida* cystitis can be problematic because of the frequent presence of *Candida* pseudohyphae and yeast cells in urine specimens secondary to urethral colonization. The usefulness of urine colony counts or antibody coating techniques is questionable. The recovery of 10,000 organisms or visualization of both yeast and pseudohyphae from fresh midstream urine or from bladder urine obtained by single catheterization (not indwelling) is suggestive of genitourinary candidiasis. In most patients, the infection is asymptomatic and clears spontaneously without specific antifungal therapy.

Initial therapy of candidal cystitis should focus on removal of urinary catheters whenever possible. Changing the catheter will eliminate candiduria in only 20% of patients, whereas discontinuation will eradicate *Candida* in 40% of patients. Asymptomatic candiduria rarely requires therapy. Therapy should be used in symptomatic patients and in neutropenic patients, as well as in patients with renal allografts and those who will undergo urologic manipulation, because of the risk of dissemination.[82,83]

Fluconazole 200 mg/day for 14 days hastens the time to a negative urine culture as compared with placebo treatment, but 2 weeks after the end of therapy, the frequency of a negative urine culture remains the same with both treatments.[83] Short courses of therapy are not recommended; treatment should include removal of catheters and stents whenever possible plus 7 to 14 days of therapy. Bladder irrigation with amphotericin B (50 mg in 500 mL sterile water instilled twice daily into the bladder via a three-way catheter) is only transiently effective. Minimal quantities (less than 3%) of amphotericin B are absorbed systemically from the bladder.[83,84]

ASPERGILLOSIS

Saprophytic molds belonging to the *Aspergillus* spp. can be found around the world, of which, *Aspergillus fumigatus* is the most commonly observed pathogen, followed by *Aspergillus flavus*. Guidelines for the prophylaxis and empiric treatment of IA in neutropenic hosts can be referred to for more comprehensive details.[85]

IA is the second most common IFI, with increasing incidence over the last 20 years along with the advances in the treatment of hematological malignancies. The infection most commonly affects immunocompromised patients and patients with acute myeloid leukemia (AML) and those who undergo allogeneic HSCT who have prolonged durations (more than 10 days) of neutropenia are at highest risk. In the highest risk group, IA rates can reach 25%. The frequency of IA and infections caused by other molds has increased over the past 2 decades. Despite heightened awareness of the profiles of patients at risk, for *Aspergillus* infections, and despite the advent of liposomal formulations of amphotericin B, IA continues to be associated with extremely high mortality rates.[12,86] The crude mortality approaches 80% to 90% in patients with AIDS and bone marrow transplant patients. Major target sites for primary invasive disease include the lungs and sinuses; frequently, secondary infections involve the central nervous system. The appropriate duration of treatment is based on the extent of the infection, response to therapy, and host factors.[12]

Epidemiology

Aspergillus is a ubiquitous mold that grows well on a variety of substrates, including soil, water, decaying vegetation, moldy hay or straw, and organic debris. Although more than 300 species of *Aspergillus* have been characterized, three species are most commonly pathogenic: *A. fumigatus*, *A. flavus*, and *Aspergillus niger*. The varying degrees of pathogenicity of each species depend on their relative geographic prevalence, conidial size and shape, thermotolerance, and production of mycotoxins. For example, transport of *A. fumigatus* conidia into the lungs is facilitated by their smaller diameter in comparison with *A. flavus* and *A. niger*.

9 The term *aspergillosis* may be broadly defined as a spectrum of diseases attributed to allergy, colonization, or tissue invasion caused by members of the fungal genus *Aspergillus*. A single satisfactory classification system for these disease entities is difficult because different populations of patients can develop the same type of infection. For example, osteomyelitis can result from local trauma or hematogenous dissemination in an immunocompromised host. Colonization in normal hosts can lead to allergic diseases ranging from asthma to allergic BPA or, rarely, invasive disease.[87]

Pathophysiology

Aspergillosis generally is acquired by inhalation of airborne conidia that are small enough (2.5-3 microns) to reach alveoli or the paranasal sinuses. Each conidiophore releases 10^4 conidia that remain suspended for long periods and are viable for months in dry locations. Although some authors advocate monitoring of hospital air for *Aspergillus* conidia, guidelines for interpreting results do not exist. The use of high-efficiency particulate air (HEPA) filters in operating rooms and laminar flow rooms and removal of immunocompromised patients from hospital renovation sites can be helpful in preventing infection in this population.

Superficial or locally invasive infections of the ear, skin, or appendages often can be managed with topical antifungal therapy. Skin infections in patients with burn wounds, although uncommon, can progress to deep-tissue invasion despite the use of topical or parenteral antifungal agents. Risk factors for deep infection include extensive thermal injuries, malnutrition, cirrhosis, and previous infection with *Pseudomonas aeruginosa*.[88-90]

Allergic manifestations of *Aspergillus* range in severity from mild asthma to allergic BPA. BPA, which is almost always caused by *A. fumigatus*, is characterized by severe asthma with wheezing, fever, malaise, weight loss, chest pain, and a cough productive of blood-streaked sputum. Following recurrent episodes of severe asthma, the disease usually progresses to fibrosis and bronchiectasis with granuloma formation. When *Aspergillus* conidia become trapped in the viscous mucus of asthmatic patients, BPA develops. The fungus grows, releasing toxins and antigens. The resulting host sensitization results in a variety of immune reactions. Early in the course of disease, an immunoglobulin E (IgE)-mediated (type I) immune reaction results in bronchospasm, eosinophilia, and immediate skin reactivity. The ensuing fibrosis and pulmonary infiltrates appear to be mediated by circulating or precipitating antibody complexes of IgG antibody, followed by granuloma formation and mononuclear infiltration because of a type IV delayed hypersensitivity reaction. Therapy is aimed at minimizing the quantity of antigenic material released in the tracheobronchial tree. Management of acute asthma attacks minimizes trapping of *Aspergillus* by bronchial secretions, and administration of parenteral corticosteroids clears lung infiltrates.[88-90] Antifungal therapy generally is not indicated in the management of allergic manifestations of aspergillosis, although some patients have demonstrated a decrease in their corticosteroid dose following therapy with itraconazole.[91]

Aspergilloma

In the nonimmunocompromised host, *Aspergillus* infections of the sinuses most commonly occur as saprophytic colonization (aspergillomas or "fungus balls") of previously abnormal sinus tissue. An aspergilloma is composed of intertwined *Aspergillus* hyphae matted together with fibrin, mucus, and cellular debris. Infection usually is localized in the maxillary sinus and rarely is associated with local invasion of adjacent bone or brain tissue. Sinus aspergillosis also can present as allergic sinusitis with nasal drainage of brownish mucous plugs. Therapy with corticosteroids and surgery generally is successful. In the immunocompromised host, subacute, chronic, or fulminant invasive disease can be seen, and a combination of antifungal and surgical therapy generally is required.[85]

Pulmonary aspergillomas are fungus balls arising in preexisting cavities because of tuberculosis, histoplasmosis, lung tumors, or radiation fibrosis, although occasionally no previous pulmonary disease is present. The diagnosis of aspergilloma generally is made on the basis of chest radiographs, on which aspergillomas appear as a solid rounded mass, sometimes mobile, of water density within a spherical or ovoid cavity and separated from the wall of the cavity by an airspace of variable size and shape. Patients generally experience chest pain, dyspnea, and sputum production. Hemoptysis is observed in 50% to 80% of patients, probably because of ulceration of the epithelial lining of the cavity with formation of granulation tissue, and hemoptysis is the cause of death in up to 26% of patients with aspergilloma. A poor prognosis is associated with increasing size or number of aspergillomas, immunosuppression (including corticosteroids), increasing *Aspergillus*-specific titers, underlying sarcoidosis, and HIV infection. Although *Aspergillus* can be cultured in only 50% to 60% of patients, precipitating antibodies are positive in virtually 100% of patients.

Invasive disease occurs rarely, and therapy therefore is controversial. There are no controlled clinical trials with which to guide therapy, and recommendations for treatment have been generated from uncontrolled trials and case reports.[85] Concern regarding the risk of severe hemorrhage has led some clinicians to use aggressive surgical excision of aspergillomas or pulmonary resection in patients with hemoptysis. Complications, including bronchopulmonary fistulas, hemorrhage, empyema, and persistent airspace problems, have led to the recommendation that surgical intervention be reserved for patients with severe (greater than 500 mL/24 h) hemoptysis, however. Bronchial artery embolization has been used to occlude the vessel that supplies the bleeding site in patients experiencing hemoptysis. Unfortunately, bronchial artery embolization generally is unsuccessful or only temporarily effective. Collateral circulation eventually develops, supplying blood flow to the affected area, and hemoptysis often recurs; consequently, reembolization is often unsuccessful. Bronchial artery embolization should be used as a temporizing procedure in a patient with life-threatening disease who might respond to more definitive therapy if hemoptysis is stabilized. Mild to moderate hemoptysis should be managed conservatively. Although IV amphotericin B generally is not useful in eradicating aspergillomas, inhaled or intracavitary instillation of amphotericin B has been employed successfully in a limited number of patients. Itraconazole has been efficacious in uncontrolled studies; however, the dose and duration of therapy have not been standardized. Hemoptysis generally ceases when the aspergilloma is eradicated.[85]

Invasive Aspergillosis

IA remains a disease of very high mortality: for example, in HSCT recipients with a diagnosis of invasive aspergillosis, the 3-month post HSCT mortality rate is 53.8% for autologous transplant recipients but approaches 90% for allogeneic HSCT recipients. However, the overall 1-year survival rate is only about 20% for autologous and allogeneic HSCT recipients with proven or probable invasive mold infections.[92-94]

Although exposure to *Aspergillus* conidia is nearly universal, impaired host defenses are required for the development of invasive disease. Phagocytes (neutrophils, monocytes, and macrophages) rather than antibodies or lymphocytes constitute the primary host defense system against invasive disease with aspergillosis. Macrophages prevent germination of conidia and also eradicate conidia, providing the first line of defense against invasive disease. Administration of corticosteroids appears to impair the killing of conidia by macrophages and to impair mobilization of neutrophils. Neutrophils halt hyphal growth and dissemination and kill mycelia, constituting a second line of defense. Prolonged neutropenia appears to be the most important predisposing factor to the development of IA, accounting for the high frequency of disease in patients with acute leukemia.[87]

Invasive disease with *Aspergillus* can arise de novo or from any of the allergic or colonizing forms of aspergillosis. Predisposing factors to the development of IA include glucocorticoid therapy, particularly following chronic administration or with higher dosages (30-200 mg/day of prednisone), cytotoxic agents, and recent or concurrent therapy with broad-spectrum antimicrobial agents. Patients with chronic hepatitis, alcoholism, diabetes mellitus, chronic granulomatous disease, leukopenia (less than 1,000 cells/mm^3 [less than 1×10^9/L]), leukemia (particularly acute lymphocytic or myelogenous leukemia), lymphoma, and acute rejection of an organ transplant are also at a higher risk of invasive disease. Although rare, IA has been reported in apparently normal hosts.[87] Aspergillosis is an uncommon fungal infection in patients with AIDS. AIDS patients may be at less risk for aspergillosis than other fungal infections because the primary cellular defect in AIDS patients is in the T-lymphocytes, whereas neutrophils and macrophages constitute the primary lines of defense to infection with aspergillosis.

Clinical Presentation

The lung is the most common site of invasive disease.[87] In the immunocompromised host, aspergillosis is characterized by vascular invasion leading to thrombosis, infarction, necrosis of tissue, and dissemination to other tissues and organs in the body. If bone marrow function returns, cavitation of the pulmonary lesion generally occurs, and the spread of infection can be halted. The progressive nature of the disease and its refractoriness to therapy are, in part, caused by the organism's rapid growth and its tendency to invade blood vessels.

Signs and Symptoms

Patients with IPA generally have blunted or non-specific signs and symptoms of infection due to impaired inflammatory responses.[95] Patients often present with classic signs and symptoms of acute pulmonary embolus: pleuritic chest pain, fever, hemoptysis, and friction rubs. The CNS, liver, spleen, heart, GI tract, pericardium, and other body sites are involved in a substantial minority of cases. In neutropenic patients with *Aspergillus* pneumonia, hyphae invade the walls of bronchi and surrounding parenchyma, resulting in an acute necrotizing, pyogenic pneumonitis. As a result, patients often present with classic signs and symptoms of acute pulmonary embolus: pleuritic chest pain, fever, hemoptysis, and friction rubs.

Diagnosis

The diagnosis of aspergillosis is complicated by the presence of *Aspergillus* as a normal commensal in the human GI tract and respiratory secretions, and establishment of a definitive diagnosis of disease is difficult. Demonstration of *Aspergillus* by repeated culture and microscopic examination of tissue provides the most firm diagnosis. A definitive diagnosis of invasive pulmonary aspergillosis (IPA) can be made by obtaining a biopsy of lung tissue; however, thrombocytopenia often limits clinicians' ability to perform this procedure. The appearance of *Aspergillus* in tissues varies with increasing host resistance from the normal vegetative hyphae found with necrotic tissue and exudate in the alveoli of immunocompromised hosts to the compact, tangled filaments (*granules*) observed in fungal balls. Identification of *Aspergillus* generally is based on the appearance of 2- to 4-micron-wide septate hyphae that are dichotomously branched at 45° angles. Sporulation is observed rarely in tissue. Although growth on Sabouraud dextrose or brain-heart infusion agar can be used for primary culture, bronchoscopy or bronchoalveolar lavage cultures are positive in only 40% of histopathologically identified specimens. Blood, CSF, and bone marrow cultures are rarely positive for *Aspergillus*.

Currently, the diagnosis is determined with the use of high resolution CT, in which IPA will manifest early on as "halo sign" (an area of low attenuation surrounding a nodular lung lesion, caused by edema or bleeding surrounding an ischemic area). In late IA nodular lesions, diffuse pulmonary infiltrates, consolidation, or ground glass opacities can be observed, and CT scans may demonstrate the crescent sign (an air crescent near the periphery of a lung nodule caused by contraction of infarcted tissue), while chest radiographs can demonstrate wedge-shaped, pleural-based infiltrates or cavities.[95] These signs are not specific to IPA, however, as bacteria and other fungal infections may produce similar findings. CT abnormalities are best documented in neutropenic marrow transplant recipients and commonly precede plain chest radiograph abnormalities.

Diagnostic Tests

New laboratory methods that allow for early differentiation of IFIs due to *Aspergillus* species versus zygomycetes and other moulds would be helpful in allowing clinicians in the earlier initiation of appropriate antifungal therapy. Although PCR-based testing is being performed in some centers, and appears promising, no FDA-approved method is commercially available.

The galactomannan test is an enzyme-linked immunosorbent assay (ELISA) (Platelia *Aspergillus* EIA test; Bio-Rad Laboratories) that detects galactomannan, an antigen released from *Aspergillus* hyphae upon invasion of host tissue. The clinical utility of this assay has been assessed in the clinical setting by sampling serum, BAL fluid, cerebrospinal fluid (CSF), and pleural fluid; however, the currently approved test is performed on serum. Additionally, while FDA-approved for use in the diagnosis of IA in HSCT recipients and in patients with leukemia; its usefulness in solid-organ transplant and pediatric populations needs to be established. In most patients, circulating antigen can be detected at a mean of 8 days before diagnosis by other means. The test has a sensitivity ranging from 30% to 100% and a specificity of approximately 85%; however, the sensitivity of the assay is decreased in patients receiving mold-active drugs on the day of sampling.[95] False positives can occur, particularly in patients receiving cyclophosphamide, piperacillin–tazobactam and amoxicillin–clavulanate, those with bifidobacteria infections, and in neonates.[96,97] And there are differences in the cutoff values for a positive result in the United States versus Europe. False negatives can occur during the concomitant use of antifungals, presumably because the level of galactomannan is related to the fungal burden.[95] In addition, it is important to note that the utility of galactomannan testing in the setting of prophylaxis has not been defined.[94]

1,3-*β*-D-glucan is a component of fungal cell walls that can be detected colorimetrically in clinical samples, including blood and bronchoalveolar lavage specimens, using a chromogenic variant of the limulus amoebocyte lysate assay. However, the current FDA-approved test (Fungitell; Associates of Cape Cod) is performed only on serum. The 1,3-*β*-D-glucan test can be used to detect most fungi, including *Fusarium*, *Trichosporon*, *Saccharomyces*, and *Acremonium*, which are less common but very important fungal pathogens, with a sensitivity of 55% to 100% and a specificity of 52% to 100%. However, the test does not detect the zygomycetes or cryptococci, and it can produce false positives in patients undergoing hemodialysis with cellulose membranes, and in other cases for unclear reasons.[95] Although a positive test result for the presence of (1,3)-*β*-D-glucan [BG] does not identify the infecting fungus, the practical application of this test includes its use as a screening assay (presumptive marker) for invasive fungal infection to allow the earlier initiation of antifungal therapy. Other tests are necessary for the confirmation and identification of the fungal pathogen.

TREATMENT

Invasive Aspergillosis

Therapy for IA is far from optimal at this time in part because of the difficulties in establishing a diagnosis and in part because of a lack of truly effective antifungal agents. Administration of amphotericin B appears to decrease mortality from more than 90% to approximately 45%. These data, however, are difficult to interpret because many patients were diagnosed postmortem, or amphotericin B therapy was not administered until the patient had very advanced disease. Mortality from pulmonary aspergillosis in bone marrow transplant recipients exceeds 94% regardless of therapy.[87] Although early diagnosis and administration of antifungal therapy can result in higher response rates, correction of underlying immune deficits (in particular, return of neutrophil counts) is of paramount importance in eradication of infection.[87]

Until the diagnosis of aspergillosis can be determined more rapidly and definitively, empirical therapy must be instituted when invasive disease is suspected. In patients at highest risk for invasive disease (acute leukemia and bone marrow transplant recipients), the most important predisposing factors include prolonged severe neutropenia (less than 100 cell/μL [less than 0.1×10^9/L] for more than 1 week), graft rejection, chronic administration of corticosteroids, and tissue damage from preexisting infection.[87]

Non-HIV-Infected Patient

Prophylaxis

As noted above in the discussion of prophylaxis for *Candida* infections in immunocompromised hosts, prophylaxis with azoles or echinocandins can reduce the incidence of aspergillosis in select high-risk populations.

Specific Therapy

Even though older azole antifungal agents (miconazole and ketoconazole) possess poor in vitro activity against *Aspergillus* species, newer triazoles demonstrate improved activity both in vitro and in animal models of infection. Antifungal agents with in vitro activity against *Aspergillus* species include amphotericin B, the echinocandins, and the azoles itraconazole, voriconazole, posaconazole, and isavuconazole. Historically, high dosages (1-1.5 mg/kg/day) of d-AmB were utilized for the treatment of suspected or proven invasive aspergillosis. Lipid formulations of amphotericin B are overall less nephrotoxic and at least as effective as amphotericin B, and that they can be effective when amphotericin Bis not.[98] They are indicated when preexisting or arising nephrotoxicity or concomitant nephrotoxic agents preclude high-dose amphotericin B therapy or when treatment with amphotericin Bappears to fail. Use of the highest approved dosages of the lipid formulations for treatment of suspected or documented infections is strongly advocated. However, randomized data from clinical trials are limited for most agents. Thus, while open-label trials support the potential of posaconazole and the echinocandins for treatment of invasive aspergillosis in immunocompromised patients, current guidelines from the US and other countries, consider voriconazole as the agent of choice for the primary treatment of aspergillus.

Voriconazole has emerged as the drug of choice of most clinicians for primary therapy of most patients with IA, based on a pivotal study in which a randomized comparison of voriconazole and d-AmB followed by other licensed antifungal agents for primary therapy for invasive aspergillosis demonstrated superior antifungal efficacy and improved survival at week 12 in the voriconazole arm.[99]

Isavuconazole was recently approved for the primary treatment of aspergillosis, based upon the results of a double blind, randomized, multi-national trial in subjects with proven or probable invasive fungal disease caused by *Aspergillus* spp. or other filamentous fungi. Isavuconazole was well tolerated, with fewer drug-related adverse effects than voriconazole.[100,101]

In patients who are unable to tolerate voriconazole, amphotericin B can be used. Because *Aspergillus* is only moderately susceptible to amphotericin B, full doses (1-1.5 mg/kg/day) are generally recommended, with response measured by defervescence and radiographic clearing. To treat microfoci, therapy should be continued after resolution of clinical and radiographic abnormalities until cultures (if they can be obtained) are negative, and reversible underlying predispositions have abated.

Clinical response rather than any arbitrary total dose should guide duration of therapy. The optimal dosage or duration of treatment of invasive disease is unknown and dependent on the extent of disease, the response to therapy, and the patient's underlying disease(s) and immune status. Response to therapy is largely related to the extent of aspergillosis at the time of diagnosis, and host factors, such as resolution of neutropenia and the return of neutrophil function, lessening immunosuppression, and the return of graft function from a bone marrow or organ transplant.

Lipid formulations of amphotericin B can be indicated in patients with impaired renal function, and in those patients who develop nephrotoxicity while receiving d-AmB. The lipid-based formulations may be preferred as initial therapy in patients with marginal renal function or in patients receiving other nephrotoxic drugs. Although these preparations appear less toxic than standard preparations, only limited data regarding their relative efficacy for IA are available at this time, as the studies with the lipid preparations have been open-label or with historical conventional amphotericin B controls.[70,74]

Although caspofungin (and other echinocandins) have in vitro activity against *Aspergillus* species, echinocandins are unable to completely kill or inhibit *Aspergillus* species. Caspofungin is approved by the FDA for use as salvage therapy in patients who are refractory to or intolerant of other therapies such as conventional amphotericin B, lipid formulations of amphotericin B, and/or itraconazole.[18,75] However, for primary therapy of aspergillosis, response rates are lower with caspofungin than those obtained with voriconazole and amphotericin B.[102]

The role of azoles in the management of azole-resistant aspergillosis remains unclear. In patients infected with azole-resistant strains of *Aspergillus*, limited data suggests that combination therapy with liposomal amphotericin B or a combination of voriconazole or posaconazole with an echinocandin may be effective.

Clinical **Controversy...**

The Role of Combination Antifungal Therapy for the Treatment of Invasive Aspergillosis

The outcome of invasive aspergillosis (IA) continues to be associated with significant attributable mortality, especially in patients with hematological malignancies and in HSCT recipients. Based on extensive experience in the management of bacterial, and more recently, retroviral infections, the use of combination agents for synergistic or additive effects is now common practice, particularly for the treatment of IA. However, while the advantages of combination therapy include the possibility of more rapid, synergistic killing, disadvantages include the possibility of antagonism, as well as increased cost and the increased risk of drug interactions and adverse effects.

A 'proof of principle' study demonstrated that combination antifungal therapy could provide superior outcomes versus single agent therapy in the treatment of candidemia. High-dose fluconazole, alone or in combination with amphotericin B, in non-immunocompromised patients with candidemia demonstrated no antagonism and a trend toward improved success and more rapid clearance of *Candida* from the bloodstream. However, renal toxicity (from amphotericin B) was higher in the combination therapy arm.[103] Whether these adverse effects would be similar, if lipid formulations were used instead of the deoxycholate formulation of amphotericin B, is not known.

In a recent large study, combination therapy with voriconazole plus anidulafungin, versus voriconazole alone in the subgroup of patients with invasive aspergillosis demonstrated only a trend toward increased 6 week survival.[104] Thus, there are as yet no firm recommendations regarding the use of such combinations in humans.[104,105]

Secondary Prophylaxis

The use of prophylactic antifungal therapy to prevent primary infection or reactivation of aspergillosis during subsequent courses of chemotherapy is controversial.[12] Studies assessing the utility of IV administration of amphotericin B in low doses (0.1 mg/kg per day) as prophylactic therapy or with higher dosages (0.5-0.6 mg/kg per day) as empirical therapy for IFIs in patients with granulocytopenia have not included sufficient numbers of patients to enable detection of differences in the number of *Aspergillus* infections.

In granulocytopenic patients who recover from an episode of IA, the risk of relapse of aspergillosis during subsequent courses of chemotherapy is greater than 50%. Secondary prophylaxis of aspergillosis with empirical administration of high-dose amphotericin B decreases the risk of relapse. Amphotericin B 1 mg/kg per day is started 24 to 48 hours prior to the start of chemotherapy and continued throughout the period of granulocytopenia.

TREATMENT OPTIONS FOR EMERGING PATHOGENS

The increased frequency of fungal pathogens that were once rare is gaining attention from the medical community. Mucormycosis, previously known zygomycosis, is a term describing infections caused by fungi belonging to the order Mucorales. Permissive environmental conditions, selective antifungal pressure, and increased numbers of immunosuppressed patients have led to increased numbers of infections caused by the Mucorales, which include *Rhizomucor* spp., *Absidia* spp. (now *Lichtheimia* spp.), *Rhizopus* spp., *Mucor* spp., and *Cunninghamella* spp. Prompt initiation of antifungal therapy is crucial, as treatment delays are associated with increased mortality.[106]

Of currently available systemic antifungals, only amphotericin B (including the lipid formulations) and posaconazole exhibit good in vitro activity against the Mucorales. Isavuconazole displays variable in vitro activity against the Mucorales, with wide MIC ranges. Prompt initiation of antifungal therapy is crucial, as treatment delays are associated with increased mortality.[106]

Mucor Infections

European guidelines recommend surgical debridement, in addition to therapy with a liposomal or lipid-complex formulation of amphotericin B at a dosage of greater than equal to 5 mg/kg/day. Isavuconazole was approved for the primary treatment of invasive mold infections, and as salvage therapy of patients who were intolerant of or failing prior antifungal therapy.[100,101] The approval was based upon the results of an open-label, noncomparative trial of patients with IFIs caused by rare molds, including members of the order Mucorales and patients with invasive aspergillosis and renal impairment.[101,107]

Fusarium and *Scedosporium*

Unfortunately, the early presentation of *Fusarium* and *Scedosporium* infections often mimics that of aspergillosis. On histopathology, *Scedosporium* species resembles *Aspergillus* species with dichotomously branching, septate hyphae and has a tendency for invasion of vascular structures.[106] These pathogens often demonstrate intrinsic resistance to amphotericin B and are associated with high mortality rates. Interpretive CBPs for antifungal MICs and *Scedosporium* spp. are not available, and the optimal choice and duration of therapy is unknown.[108] Voriconazole is FDA approved for the treatment of serious fungal infections caused by *S. apiospermum* and *Fusarium* species, including *Fusarium solani*, in patients intolerant of or refractory to other therapy.[58]

ANTIFUNGAL THERAPY

Pharmacists must have working knowledge of mechanism of action, spectrum of activity, dosing, and adverse effects of azole antifungals in order to provide appropriate recommendations for therapy. Dosing adjustments are needed for many antifungal agents in the setting of renal or hepatic dysfunction. A summary of the most common adverse effects of systemic antifungal agents are summarized in Fig. 121-3 and described in the text below.[58]

The antifungal armamentarium for the treatment of IFIs includes: (a) inhibitors of the fungal cell membrane such as polyenes (eg, amphotericin B) and azole antifungals, (b) inhibitors of DNA (5-flucytosine), and (c) inhibitors of cell wall biosynthesis (echinocandins).[58]

Antifungal therapy generally includes one or more antifungal agents, depending on the severity of infection and the patients' immune status. Rarely are the agents used in combination. Often therapy is initiated with an IV agent such as amphotericin B, and therapy is changed to an oral (azole) regimen as the patient's clinical status improves and oral therapy is tolerated.

Amphotericin B

Amphotericin B remains the therapy of choice for many systemic fungal infections despite a lack of controlled clinical trials documenting the optimal dosage, duration of therapy, or relative efficacy of this agent in comparison with newer azole antifungal agents. During pregnancy, amphotericin B remains the treatment of choice for most fungal infections because azole antifungals are teratogenic.[84,109] The side effects of amphotericin B generally are categorized as acute (infusion-related) or long term. Amphotericin B commonly causes renal functional impairment, including decreased glomerular filtration rate, hypokalemia, hypomagnesemia, metabolic acidosis due to distal (or type 1) renal tubular acidosis (RTA), and polyuria due to nephrogenic diabetes insipidus. The nephrotoxicity associated with amphotericin B is usually reversible with discontinuation of therapy. However, recurrent renal dysfunction can occur if treatment is reinstituted. The risk of amphotericin B nephrotoxicity is increased by higher daily doses and concurrent therapy with other nephrotoxins, such as an aminoglycoside or cyclosporine. The incidence and severity of nephrotoxicity can be minimized by administering amphotericin B in lipid-based formulations; liposomal amphotericin B may be less nephrotoxic than the ABLC.[58,110]

Adverse Effects of Systemic Antifungal Agents

Adverse Effect	AmB	Flucon	Itra	Vori	Posa	Echino
Nephrotoxicity	✓	✗	✗ (possible with IV)	✗ (possible with IV)	✗	✗
Abdominal Discomfort	✗	✓	✓	✓	✓	✗
↑ Hepatic transaminases	✓	✓	✓	✓	✓	✓
Rash, photosensitivity	✗	✓	✓	✓ (vori-malignancy)	✓	✓
Infusion-related Reactions/ Histamine Release	✓	✗	✗	✗	✗	✓
CNS & Visual Disturbances	✗	✗	✗	✓	✗	✗
Cardiomyopathy (itra), ↑ QT (azoles), ?echinos	✗	✓	✓	✓	✓	?

FIGURE 121-3 Adverse Effects of Systemic Antifungal Agents.

Lipid Formulations of Amphotericin B

The use of d-AmB frequently is associated with the development of induced nephrotoxicity. In an attempt to decrease the incidence of nephrotoxicity, three lipid formulations of amphotericin B have been developed and approved for use in humans: ABLC (Abelcet; Enzon Pharmaceuticals), ABCD (Amphotec; Intermune Pharmaceuticals), and liposomal amphotericin B (AmBisome; Gilead Pharmaceuticals). In these preparations, amphotericin B is incorporated into the phospholipid bilayer membrane rather than in the enclosed aqueous phase.

The various lipid formulations of amphotericin B exhibit markedly different pharmacokinetics; however, whether these differences result in different outcomes in the treatment of specific types of infections (eg, CNS infections) is unclear. Although larger doses of these preparations are required to achieve similar pharmacologic effects as the deoxycholate form of amphotericin B, the toxicity appears to be much lower. Although the FDA-approved dosages of these agents are 5 mg/kg per day (ABLC), 3 to 6 mg/kg per day (ABCD), and 3 to 5 mg/kg per day (liposomal amphotericin B), the agents appear generally equipotent. The optimal dose of these compounds for serious *Candida* infections is unknown; however, dosages of 3 to 5 mg/kg per day appear reasonable.[7]

Lipid formulations of amphotericin B are indicated for patients intolerant of, refractory to, or at high risk of being intolerant to conventional antifungal therapy.[7,110] Intolerance generally is defined as initial renal insufficiency (creatinine greater than 2.5 mg/dL [greater than 221 μmol/L] or creatinine clearance less than 25 mL/min [less than 0.42 mL/s]), a significant increase in creatinine (to 2.5 mg/dL [221 μmol/L] for adults or 1.5 mg/dL [133 μmol/L] for children), or severe acute administration-related toxicity, whereas refractory infections are defined as therapeutic failure of more than 500 mg amphotericin B.

Clinical **Controversy...**

Owing to the higher cost and paucity of randomized trials showing the efficacy of lipid-associated formulations of amphotericin B against proven invasive candidiasis, many clinicians limit their first-line use for the treatment of these infections to individuals who are intolerant to, at high risk of intolerance to, or refractory to amphotericin B deoxycholate. However, the data demonstrating up to a 6.6-fold increase in mortality in patients with amphotericin B-induced nephrotoxicity have convinced other clinicians that high-risk patients (eg, residence in an ICU care or intermediate care unit at the time of initiation of amphotericin B therapy) warrant first-line therapy with these agents.[7,110]

Flucytosine

Flucytosine (also known as 5-flucytosine) is a fluorinated pyrimidine analog that is highly water-soluble. Patients with creatinine clearances of less than 40 mL/min (0.67 mL/s) should receive careful dosage adjustments. Peak serum concentrations (2 hours after an oral dose) should be monitored in all patients (particularly those with a creatinine clearance of less than 10 mL/min [0.17 mL/s]) to maintain peak serum concentrations of more than 100 mg/L (775 μmol/L).[41]

Flucytosine generally is associated with few side effects in patients with normal renal, GI, and hematologic function, although rash, GI discomfort, diarrhea (5%-10%), and reversible elevations in hepatic enzymes are observed occasionally. In patients with renal dysfunction or concomitant amphotericin B therapy, leukopenia, thrombocytopenia, and (rarely) enterocolitis can occur. Although studies have suggested that little or no conversion of flucytosine to fluorouracil occurs in vitro, serum concentrations of greater than 1,000 ng/mL (1 mg/L; ~7.7 μmol/L) (therapeutic for the treatment of malignancies) have been documented in some patients. Investigators have theorized that flucytosine may be secreted into the GI tract, deaminated by intestinal bacteria, and reabsorbed as 5-fluorouracil.[41]

Flucytosine is used in combination with amphotericin B or fluconazole in the treatment of cryptococcosis or (less commonly) candidiasis. The rapid development of resistance to flucytosine, however, precludes its use as single-agent therapy. Mechanisms for drug resistance can include loss of deaminase and decreased permeability to the drug.[41]

Echinocandins

The echinocandins (caspofungin, micafungin, and anidulafungin) are a new class of antifungal agents that act as concentration-dependent, noncompetitive inhibitors of BG synthase, an essential component of the cell wall of susceptible filamentous fungi that is absent in mammalian cells.[75,111]

All echinocandins display linear pharmacokinetics following administration of IV dosages, and are degraded primarily by the liver (also in the adrenals and spleen) by hydrolysis and *N*-acetylation. Following initial distribution, echinocandins are taken up by red blood cells (micafungin) and the liver (caspofungin and micafungin) where they undergo slow degradation to mainly inactive metabolites, although two uncommon metabolites of micafungin possess antifungal activity. Degradation products are excreted slowly over many days, primarily through the bile. Among the echinocandins, anidulafungin is unique in being eliminated almost exclusively by slow chemical degradation rather than undergoing hepatic metabolism.[75]

Echinocandins are available only as parenteral formulations, are not dialyzable, and do not require dosage adjustment in patients with renal insufficiency. They have minimal CSF penetration, largely because of their high protein binding and large molecular weights, although the clinical relevance of these findings can be disputed, given that several other antifungal agents (amphotericin B and itraconazole) are effective for the treatment of fungal meningitis despite low CSF concentrations.

Adverse effects of echinocandins include histamine release resulting in rash, facial swelling, and itchiness. Limited experience suggests that caspofungin and micafungin are safe to use in pediatric patients; the safety and effectiveness of anidulafungin in pediatric patients has not been established. At the time of FDA approval, there were concerns regarding the safety of caspofungin when combined with cyclosporine. However, three retrospective analyses of the use of caspofungin and cyclosporine in patients do not support a risk of clinically relevant hepatotoxicity.[75,111]

Azole Antifungal Agents

Adverse effects of azoles include GI disturbances (primarily nausea, vomiting, epigastric pain, and diarrhea), which appear to be more common in patients receiving ketoconazole and the solution formulation of itraconazole. Although cyclodextrin is not absorbed following oral administration, use of the IV formulations of itraconazole and voriconazole is limited to 2 weeks because of concerns for potential nephrotoxicity secondary to accumulation of the cyclodextrin vehicle, although recent studies suggest that this is of less concern than previously thought.[112] Fluconazole is well tolerated; intestinal complaints are the most frequently reported, followed by headaches and rash.[113] Unlike ketoconazole, fluconazole does not inhibit testicular or adrenal steroidogenesis in healthy volunteers or hospitalized patients. Reversible alopecia occurs not infrequently and usually appears after several months of treatment with higher doses of fluconazole.[114] Azoles are potentially teratogenic and should be avoided in pregnant women.[58,109]

Azole antifungals have been implicated in idiosyncratic drug induced liver injury with the incidence and pattern of injury varying between specific agents.[114-116] The exact mechanism of toxicity has not been elucidated and there is varying level of evidence with regards to the effect of dose on the development of the toxicity. It is recommended that baseline liver function tests (LFTs) be obtained for patients being started on therapy with these agents and periodically monitored. In general, hepatotoxicity can occur at any time after initiation of the antifungal with most cases occurring in the first month of therapy. The liver injury is usually reversible with discontinuation of the offending agent. Several reports support that substitution of the offending azole antifungal with a different azole antifungal can occur without impacting resolution of the toxicity.

Itraconazole

Itraconazole is triazole antifungal with a broad spectrum of antifungal activity. Despite its marked structural similarity to ketoconazole, itraconazole differs in several important respects. Itraconazole appears to have greater specificity against fungal versus mammalian CYP, resulting in greater potency and a decrease in CYP-mediated side effects. In addition, itraconazole possesses excellent in vitro activity against *Aspergillus* and *Sporothrix* species.[58,114]

Like ketoconazole, the capsule formulation of itraconazole depends on the availability of low gastric pH for dissolution and absorption. Administration with food appears to enhance significantly the bioavailability of itraconazole capsules, whereas it decreases the bioavailability of the oral solution. Because itraconazole exhibits pH-dependent dissolution and absorption, absorption of the capsule formulation is impaired in patients receiving antacids or H_2-receptor antagonists and in patients with achlorhydria.[112] Plasma concentrations of itraconazole following a single oral dose (capsules) in HIV-infected patients are approximately 50% lower than concentrations observed in healthy volunteers. The capsule formulation of itraconazole exhibits unpredictable oral bioavailability, particularly in subjects with hypochlorhydria and in patients with enteropathy caused by mucositis or graft versus host disease GVHD of the gut. An oral suspension formulation of itraconazole is available; that uses cyclodextrin as a solubilizing vehicle to increase the solubility of the drug. The oral bioavailability of the solution is unaffected by alterations in gastric pH or in patients with enteropathy.[58,112,114]

Fluconazole

Fluconazole is a triazole antifungal agent with markedly different pharmacologic features than other marketed azole antifungals. The small molecular weight, low protein binding, and increased water solubility of fluconazole result in rapid, essentially complete absorption of drug following oral administration. Because fluconazole is excreted primarily (greater than 80%) as unchanged drug in the urine, dosage adjustments are necessary in patients with renal dysfunction.[58]

Voriconazole

The hepatic biotransformation of voriconazole is fairly complex and involves CYP2C19, CYP3A4, and CYP2C9, with most metabolism mediated through CYP2C19. Two of the CYPs involved in voriconazole metabolism (CYP2C19 and CYP2C9) exhibit genetic polymorphism; variability in the CYP2C19 genotype accounts for approximately 30% of the overall between subject variability in voriconazole pharmacokinetics. About 3% to 5% of white and African human populations are poor metabolizers, while 15% to 20% of Asian populations are poor metabolizers. Drug levels can be as much as fourfold greater in poor metabolizers than in individuals who are homozygous extensive metabolizers. Coadministration of voriconazole with drugs that are potent CYP450 enzyme inducers can significantly reduce voriconazole levels. Voriconazole drug interactions are dose-dependent, as they exhibit unpredictable nonlinear pharmacokinetics; thus, drug interactions are more difficult to predict and manage.[117]

The most common side effect of voriconazole is a reversible disturbance of vision (photopsia), which occurs in approximately 30% of patients but rarely leads to discontinuation of the drug. Symptoms tend to occur during the first week of therapy and decrease or disappear despite continued therapy.

Patients experience altered color discrimination, blurred vision, the appearance of bright spots and wavy lines, and photophobia. Patients should be cautioned that driving can be hazardous because of the risk of visual disturbances. The visual effects are associated with changes in electroretinogram tracings, which revert to normal when treatment with the drug is stopped; no permanent damage to the retina has been demonstrated.[58,118-120]

Clinical Controversy...

Controversy has arisen about whether single-drug therapy or combination therapy (eg, voriconazole plus an echinocandin or voriconazole plus a lipid formulation of amphotericin B) is optimum therapy. At present, the highest interest concerns combination therapy in the treatment of aspergillosis, given the continued high mortality of these infections.[83] However, in vitro and animal data have produced conflicting results. Several retrospective studies have suggested an improvement in mortality with combination therapy with two or three antifungal agents; however, prospective, controlled human studies are lacking. Thus, there are as yet no firm recommendations regarding the use of such combinations in humans.[12]

Posaconazole

Posaconazole has a broad spectrum of antifungal activity, including *Aspergillus* and *Candida* species and zygomycetes. In vitro studies demonstrate that posaconazole is an inhibitor but not a substrate of hepatic (but not total) CYP3A4, and both a substrate and an inhibitor of P-glycoprotein (Pgp), suggesting that it may exhibit a drug interaction profile similar to other azoles. In addition, posaconazole undergoes glucuronidation by uridine diphosphate (UDP)-glucuronosyltransferase enzymes.[117]

Posaconazole was initially developed as an oral suspension for the prevention of IFIs in immunocompromised patients, including hematologic malignancy patients with prolonged neutropenia from chemotherapy as well as HSCT patients with GVHD.[121] However, to ensure adequate absorption, the suspension formulation had to be administered 2 to 3 times daily, with a high fat meal or a nutritional supplement. Most patients with GVHD, and many with chemotherapy-associated nausea or vomiting, mucositis or diarrhea, were unable to comply with the requirement for a fatty meal, resulting in decreased plasma concentrations of posaconazole and an increased risk of breakthrough fungal infection.[121-124] More recently, the development of IV and delayed-release tablet formulations of posaconazole have circumvented these absorption issues. In addition, the tablet formulation allows once daily oral administration of posaconazole following administration of a twice daily loading dose on the first day of therapy.[125]

Isavuconazole

Isavuconazole, is available both orally and IV, has a broad spectrum of activity against a number of clinically important yeasts and molds, including *Candida* spp., *Aspergillus* spp., *C. neoformans*, *Trichosporon* spp., and variable activity against the Mucorales. The most commonly reported adverse events, which are mild and limited in nature, include nausea, diarrhea and elevated liver function tests. Its drug interaction potential appears similar to other azole antifungals, but less than those observed with voriconazole. The potential advantage of this agent over other currently available broad-spectrum azole antifungals is as a clinically useful alternative to voriconazole for the treatment of invasive aspergillosis, due to its lack of genetically determined variability in plasma levels, and more favorable and predictable drug interaction profile. Preliminary studies suggest that it may also prove useful for the treatment of invasive mold infections; however, these indications await the results of clinical trials.[100,101]

Drug Interactions with Antifungal Agents

Drug interactions with azole antifungals generally can be placed into three broad categories: (a) decreases in azole bioavailability because of chelation or secondary to increases in gastric pH, (b) interactions with other CYP-metabolized drugs, and (c) interactions caused by inhibition of Pgp. Drug interactions in the latter two categories can result in increases or decreases in the azole antifungal, in the interacting drug, or in both drugs.[117]

The interaction of azole antifungal agents with other CYP-metabolized drugs is well recognized. The azoles appear to be metabolized almost entirely via the CYP3A4 subfamily. As expected, they interact with other drugs metabolized partly or wholly through this enzyme pathway. In addition, fluconazole and voriconazole use the CYP2C19 pathway. Numerous clinically significant interactions have been documented with azole antifungals and a variety of other drugs. In most cases, the azole interferes with the metabolism of the other CYP-metabolized drug.[117]

Relative to ketoconazole and itraconazole, fluconazole appears to be intermediate in its ability to inhibit human cytochromes P450. The magnitude of fluconazole-induced inhibition of cyclosporine metabolism appears, however, to depend on the dosage of fluconazole.[117]

Predictably, drugs such as rifampin, rifabutin, isoniazid, phenytoin, and carbamazepine, which are known to induce the activity of cytochromes P450, result in increased metabolism of the azole antifungals and can result in therapeutic failures. Increased dosages of azole antifungals can be required in patients receiving these combinations of drugs.[117]

Itraconazole is an inhibitor of intestinal Pgp. Significant increases in digoxin (a Pgp substrate) have been observed in patients receiving both agents concurrently. Interactions with other substrates of Pgp would be expected to occur.[117]

Echinocandins are not inducers of CYP enzymes, nor do they interact with Pgp, and are considered poor substrates of CYP3A4. Nevertheless, drug interactions are noted with caspofungin and cyclosporine and tacrolimus; the mechanism for these interactions is not yet known. Rifampin both inhibits (acutely) and induces (after chronic administration) caspofungin metabolism, and a dosage increase is recommended in patients receiving other enzyme inducers, such as efavirenz, nevirapine, phenytoin, dexamethasone, and carbamazepine. Although micafungin does not significantly affect the clearance (or area under the plasma-concentration vs time curve [AUC]) of tacrolimus, it increases the AUCs of sirolimus and nifedipine and decreases the clearance of cyclosporine.[75,126]

Therapeutic Drug Monitoring (TDM) of Antifungal Agents

The available, good-quality, prospectively obtained data in the prophylactic or therapeutic setting are insufficient to justify the routine use of therapeutic drug monitoring. In addition, logistics, cost, and incorporation of therapeutic drug monitoring have yet to be worked out in modern prophylactic algorithms. However, under certain circumstances, serum or plasma concentration monitoring is warranted. Given the tremendous interpatient and intrapatient variability in voriconazole metabolism, TDM is warranted in most patients, Also, given the poor oral bioavailability of itraconazole capsules, and posaconazole solution, monitoring is recommended, particularly in patients with GVHD of the gut, mucositis, or diarrhea, or poor oral intake or those receiving concomitant therapy with proton-pump inhibitors.[127-131] Although the use of posaconazole tablets may result in a decreased need for TDM, recent data suggest that patients with a higher weight and those experiencing diarrhea are more likely to have lower levels.[65] Additional settings

TABLE 121-11 Plasma Concentration Monitoring of Antifungal Agents[127-132]

	Serum Concentration Monitoring Necessary?	Target Concentration Range	Timing of Sample
Echinocandins	No	NA	NA
Amphotericin B (including lipids)	No	NA	NA
Fluconazole	No	NA	NA
Itraconazole	Yes, to ensure absorption and efficacy	*Efficacy:* Prophylaxis: >0.5 mcg/mL (mg/L; >0.7 μmol/L) Treatment: >1 mcg/mL (mg/L; >1.4 μmol/L) *Toxicity:* <5 mcg/mL (mg/L; <7 μmol/L)	Trough 7 days after initiation of therapy
Voriconazole	Probably yes—in all patients treated for IFI, altered liver function, potential drug–drug interactions, lack of response *Low* concentrations are associated with poor outcome; *high* concentrations are associated with adverse effects Variable metabolism due to nonlinear PK and genetic variability in CYP2C19 → unpredictable dose–exposure relationship	*Efficacy:* Prophylaxis: trough >0.5-2 mcg/mL (mg/L; >1.4-5.7 μmol/L) Treatment: trough >1-2 mcg/mL (mg/L; >2.9-5.7 μmol/L) Concentrations >2.05 mcg/mL (mg/L; >5.7 μmol/L) are associated with improved outcome; 2-5.5 mcg/mL (mg/L; 5.7-15.7 μmol/L) is probably the best target *Toxicity:* concentrations >5.5 mcg/mL (mg/L; >15.7 μmol/L) are associated with ↑ risk of visual and hepatic adverse events	Trough after 5-7 days therapy if no loading dose administered; 48 hours after administration of loading dose in critically ill patient (time to steady state is unpredictable due to nonlinear metabolism)
Posaconazole	Maybe Outcomes (but not adverse events) correlate with higher plasma concentrations in prophylaxis and possibly treatment	*Efficacy:* Prophylaxis: >0.7 mcg/mL (mg/L; >1 μmol/L) Treatment: Not well studied; concentrations >1.25 mcg/mL (mg/L;1.78 μmol/L) needed ? *Toxicity:* Correlation with toxicity poorly defined	Random level at SS (>7 days therapy). The long $t_{1/2}$ ensures little fluctuation in peaks and troughs at SS
Flucytosine	Yes—High concentrations are associated with toxicity	*Toxicity:* "Peak" <80-100 mcg/mL (mg/L; <620-775 μmol/L) *Efficacy:* Trough >30 mcg/mL (mg/L; >232 μmol/L)	2 hours postdose "peak", 3-5 days after initiation of therapy

NA, not applicable.

include patients susceptible to flucytosine toxicity, to document adequate oral absorption of poorly bioavailable azoles in cases of suspected treatment failure or concern about compliance or absorption, solubility and finally, when drug interactions that might reduce or accelerate the metabolism of azoles is suspected.[127,132] Recommendations regarding plasma concentration monitoring of antifungals are summarized in Table 121-11.

ABBREVIATIONS

AIDS	acquired immunodeficiency syndrome
ABCD	amphotericin B colloid dispersion
ABLC	amphotericin B lipid complex
AUC	area under the plasma-concentration versus time curve
BG	(1,3)-β-D-glucan
BPA	bronchopulmonary aspergillosis
BSI	bloodstream infection
CBP	clinical breakpoint
CT	computed tomography
CVC	central venous catheter
CSF	cerebrospinal fluid
CYP	cytochrome P450
d-AmB	deoxycholate amphotericin B
ELISA	enzyme-linked immunosorbent assay
FISH	fluorescence in situ hybridization
GVHD	graft-versus-host disease
HEPA	high-efficiency particulate air
HAART	highly active antiretroviral therapy
HSCT	hematopoietic stem cell transplantation
ICP	intracranial pressure
ICUs	intensive care units
IDSA	Infectious Diseases Society of America
IPA	invasive pulmonary aspergillosis
IRIS	immune reconstitution inflammatory syndrome
MALDI-TOF-ICMS	matrix-assisted laser desorption ionization time-of-flight mass spectrometry
PDH	progressive disseminated histoplasmosis
PN	parenteral nutrition
PNA	peptide nucleic acid
SDD	susceptible dose-dependent
TDM	therapeutic plasma drug concentration monitoring
WBC	white blood cell

REFERENCES

1. Bennett JE. Introduction to mycoses. In: Bennett JED, Raphael; Blaser, Martin J. ed. *Mandell, Douglas, and Bennett's Principles and Practice of Infectious Diseases*. Philadelphia, PA: Elsevier/Saunders, 2015:2874-78.
2. Pfaller MA, Jones RN, Messer SA, Edmond MB, Wenzel RP. National Surveillance of Nosocomial Blood Stream Infection due to *Candida albicans*: Frequency of Occurrence and Antifungal Susceptibility in the SCOPE Program. *Diagnostic Microbiology and Infectious Disease* 1998;1:327-332.
3. Pfaller MA, Jones RN, Doern GV, et al. International Surveillance of Blood Stream Infections due to *Candida* species in the European SENTRY Program: Species Distribution and Antifungal Susceptibility Including the Investigational Triazole and Echinocandin Agents. SENTRY Participant Group (Europe). *Diagnostic Microbiology and Infectious Disease* 1999;1:19-25.
4. Pfaller MA, Diekema DJ. Progress in Antifungal Susceptibility Testing of *Candida* spp. by use of Clinical and Laboratory Standards Institute broth Microdilution Methods, 2010 to 2012. *Journal of Clinical Microbiology* 2012;9:2846-2856.
5. Pfaller MA, Andes D, Diekema DJ, Espinel-Ingroff A, Sheehan D, Testing CSfAS. Wild-type MIC distributions, epidemiological cutoff values and species-specific clinical breakpoints for fluconazole and Candida: Time for harmonization of CLSI and EUCAST broth microdilution methods. *Drug Resistance Updates: Reviews and Commentaries in Antimicrobial and Anticancer Chemotherapy* 2010;6:180-195.

6. Eschenauer GA, Carver PL. The evolving role of antifungal susceptibility testing. *Pharmacotherapy* 2013;5:465-475.
7. Pappas PG, Kauffman CA, Andes D, et al. Clinical practice guidelines for the management of candidiasis: update by the Infectious Diseases Society of America. *Clinical Infectious Diseases: An Official Publication of the Infectious Diseases Society of America* 2016;4:e1-e50.
8. Chapman SW, Dismukes WE, Proia LA, et al. Clinical practice guidelines for the management of blastomycosis: 2008 update by the Infectious Diseases Society of America. *Clinical Infectious Diseases: An Official Publication of the Infectious Diseases Society of America* 2008;12:1801-1812.
9. Perfect JR, Dismukes WE, Dromer F, et al. Clinical practice guidelines for the management of cryptococcal disease: 2010 update by the infectious diseases society of america. *Clinical Infectious Diseases: An Official Publication of the Infectious Diseases Society of America* 2010;3:291-322.
10. Wheat LJ, Freifeld AG, Kleiman MB, et al. Clinical practice guidelines for the management of patients with histoplasmosis: 2007 update by the Infectious Diseases Society of America. *Clinical Infectious Diseases: An Official Publication of the Infectious Diseases Society of America* 2007;7:807-825.
11. Galgiani JN, Ampel NM, Blair JE, et al. 2016 Infectious Diseases Society of America (IDSA) Clinical Practice Guideline for the Treatment of Coccidioidomycosis. Clinical infectious diseases : an official publication of the Infectious Diseases Society of America 2016.
12. Walsh TJ, Anaissie EJ, Denning DW, et al. Treatment of aspergillosis: Clinical practice guidelines of the Infectious Diseases Society of America. *Clinical Infectious Diseases: An Official Publication of the Infectious Diseases Society of America* 2016;4:e1-e60.
13. Cowen LE, Sanglard D, Howard SJ, Rogers PD, Perlin DS. *Mechanisms of Antifungal Drug Resistance*. Cold Spring Harbor perspectives in medicine 2015;7:a019752.
14. Perlin DS. Echinocandin resistance, susceptibility testing and prophylaxis: Implications for patient management. *Drugs* 2014;14: 1573-1585.
15. Alexander BD, Johnson MD, Pfeiffer CD, et al. Increasing echinocandin resistance in Candida glabrata: Clinical failure correlates with presence of FKS mutations and elevated minimum inhibitory concentrations. *Clinical Infectious Diseases: An Official Publication of the Infectious Diseases Society of America* 2013;12:1724-1732.
16. Shields RK, Nguyen MH, Press EG, et al. The presence of an FKS mutation rather than MIC is an independent risk factor for failure of echinocandin therapy among patients with invasive candidiasis due to Candida glabrata. *Antimicrobial Agents and Chemotherapy* 2012;9:4862-4869.
17. Beyda ND, John J, Kilic A, Alam MJ, Lasco TM, Garey KW. FKS mutant *Candida glabrata*: Risk factors and outcomes in patients with candidemia. *Clinical Infectious Diseases: An Official Publication of the Infectious Diseases Society of America* 2014;6:819-825.
18. Aigner M, Lass-Florl C. Treatment of drug-resistant Aspergillus infection. *Expert Opinion on Pharmacotherapy* 2015;1-4.
19. Vermeulen E, Lagrou K, Verweij PE. Azole resistance in *Aspergillus fumigatus*: A growing public health concern. *Current Opinion in Infectious Diseases* 2013;6:493-500.
20. Eschenauer GA, Lam SW, Carver PL. Antifungal prophylaxis in liver transplant recipients. *Liver Transplantation: Official Publication of the American Association for the Study of Liver Diseases and the International Liver Transplantation Society* 2009;8:842-858.
21. McCoy D, Depestel DD, Carver PL. Primary antifungal prophylaxis in adult hematopoietic stem cell transplant recipients: Current therapeutic concepts. *Pharmacotherapy* 2009;11:1306-1325.
22. Rabin AS, Givertz MM, Couper GS, et al. Risk factors for invasive fungal disease in heart transplant recipients. *The Journal of Heart and Lung Transplantation: The Official Publication of the International Society for Heart Transplantation* 2015;2:227-232.
23. Barchiesi F, Mazzocato S, Mazzanti S, et al. Invasive aspergillosis in liver transplant recipients: Epidemiology, clinical characteristics, treatment, and outcomes in 116 cases. *Liver Transplantation: Official Publication of the American Association for the Study of Liver Diseases and the International Liver Transplantation Society* 2015;2:204-212.
24. Quindos G. Epidemiology of candidaemia and invasive candidiasis: A changing face. *Revista Iberoamericana de Micologia* 2014;1:42-48.
25. Paramythiotou E, Frantzeskaki F, Flevari A, Armaganidis A, Dimopoulos G. Invasive fungal infections in the ICU: How to approach, how to treat. *Molecules* 2014;1:1085-1119.
26. Colombo AL, Guimaraes T, Sukienik T, et al. Prognostic factors and historical trends in the epidemiology of candidemia in critically ill patients: An analysis of five multicenter studies sequentially conducted over a 9-year period. *Intensive Care Medicine* 2014;10:1489-1498.
27. Lam SW, Eschenauer GA, Carver PL. Evolving role of early antifungals in the adult intensive care unit. *Critical Care Medicine* 2009;5:1580-1593.
28. Fernandez J, Erstad BL, Petty W, Nix DE. Time to positive culture and identification for Candida blood stream infections. *Diagnostic Microbiology and Infectious Disease* 2009;4:402-407.
29. Teles F, Seixas J. The future of novel diagnostics in medical mycology. *Journal of Medical Microbiology* 2015;(Pt 4):315-22.
30. Halliday CL, Kidd SE, Sorrell TC, Chen SC. Molecular diagnostic methods for invasive fungal disease: The horizon draws nearer? *Pathology* 2015;3:257-269.
31. Schelenz S, Barnes RA, Barton RC, et al. British Society for Medical Mycology best practice recommendations for the diagnosis of serious fungal diseases. *The Lancet Infectious Diseases* 2015;4:461-474.
32. Deepe GS. Chapter 265. *Histoplasma capsulatum* (Histoplasmosis). In: Bennett JED, Raphael; Ir, Martin J. ed. *Mandell, Douglas, and Bennett's Principles and Practice of Infectious Diseases*. Philadelphia, PA: Elsevier/Saunders, 2015:2949-2962.
33. Riddell JT, Kauffman CA, Smith JA, et al. *Histoplasma capsulatum* Endocarditis: Multicenter case series with review of current diagnostic techniques and treatment. *Medicine* 2014;5:186-193.
34. Hage CA, Ribes JA, Wengenack NL, et al. A multicenter evaluation of tests for diagnosis of histoplasmosis. *Clinical Infectious Diseases: An Official Publication of the Infectious Diseases Society of America* 2011;5:448-454.
35. Hage CA, Kirsch EJ, Stump TE, et al. Histoplasma antigen clearance during treatment of histoplasmosis in patients with AIDS determined by a quantitative antigen enzyme immunoassay. *Clinical and Vaccine Immunology: CVI* 2011;4:661-666.
36. Bradsher RW. Chapter 266, Blastomycosis. In: Bennett JED, Raphael; Blaser, Martin J. ed. *Mandell, Douglas, and Bennett's Principles and Practice of Infectious Diseases*. Philadelphia, PA: Elsevier/Saunders, 2015:2963-2973.
37. Galgiani JN. Chapter 267. Coccidioidomycosis (Coccidioides Species). In: Bennett JED, Raphael; Blaser, Martin J. ed. *Mandell, Douglas, and Bennett's Principles and Practice of Infectious Diseases*. Philadelphia, PA: Elsevier/Saunders, 2015:2974-2984.
38. Hoang LMN, Philips P, Galanis E. *Cryptococcus gattii*: A review of the epidemiology, clinical presentation, diagnosis, and management of this endemic yeast in the Pacific Northwest. *Clinical Microbiology Newsletter* 2011;24:187-195.
39. Bennett JE, Dismukes WE, Duma RJ, et al. A comparison of amphotericin B alone and combined with flucytosine in the treatment of cryptoccal meningitis. The New England *Journal of Medicine* 1979;3: 126-131.
40. Saag MS, Powderly WG, Cloud GA, et al. Comparison of amphotericin B with fluconazole in the treatment of acute AIDS-associated cryptococcal meningitis. The NIAID Mycoses Study Group and the AIDS Clinical Trials Group. *The New England Journal of Medicine* 1992;2:83-89.
41. Francis P, Walsh TJ. Evolving role of flucytosine in immunocompromised patients: New insights into safety, pharmacokinetics, and antifungal therapy. *Clinical Infectious Diseases: An Official Publication of the Infectious Diseases Society of America* 1992;6:1003-1018.
42. van der Horst CM, Saag MS, Cloud GA, et al. Treatment of cryptococcal meningitis associated with the acquired immunodeficiency syndrome. National Institute of Allergy and Infectious Diseases Mycoses Study Group and AIDS Clinical Trials Group. *The New England Journal of Medicine* 1997;1:15-21.
43. Perfect JR. Chapter 264. Cryptococcosis (*Cryptococcus neoformans* and *Cryptococcus gattii*) In: Bennett JED, Raphael; Blaser, Martin J. ed. *Mandell, Douglas, and Bennett's Principles and Practice of Infectious Diseases*. Philadelphia, PA: Elsevier/Saunders, 2015:2934-2948.
44. Wisplinghoff H, Bischoff T, Tallent SM, Seifert H, Wenzel RP, Edmond MB. Nosocomial bloodstream infections in US hospitals: Analysis of 24,179 cases from a prospective nationwide surveillance study. *Clinical Infectious Diseases: An Official Publication of the Infectious Diseases Society of America* 2004;3:309-317.
45. Eschenauer GA, Nguyen MH, Clancy CJ. Is fluconazole or an echinocandin the agent of choice for candidemia. *The Annals of Pharmacotherapy* 2015;9:1068-1074.
46. Wey SB, Mori M, Pfaller MA, Woolson RF, Wenzel RP. Hospital-acquired candidemia: The attributable mortality and excess length of stay. *Archives of Internal Medicine* 1988;12:2642-2645.
47. Wey SB, Mori M, Pfaller MA, Woolson RF, Wenzel RP. Risk factors for hospital-acquired candidemia. A matched case-control study. *Archives of Internal Medicine* 1989;10:2349-2353.

48. Diekema DJ, Messer SA, Brueggemann AB, et al. Epidemiology of candidemia: 3-year results from the emerging infections and the epidemiology of Iowa organisms study. *Journal of Clinical Microbiology* 2002;4:1298-1302.
49. Pfaller MA, Messer SA, Hollis RJ, et al. Trends in species distribution and susceptibility to fluconazole among blood stream isolates of *Candida* species in the United States. *Diagnostic Microbiology and Infectious Disease* 1999;4:217-222.
50. Wisplinghoff H, Ebbers J, Geurtz L, et al. Nosocomial bloodstream infections due to Candida spp. in the USA: Species distribution, clinical features and antifungal susceptibilities. *International Journal of Antimicrobial Agents* 2014;1:78-81.
51. Edmond MB, Wallace SE, McClish DK, Pfaller MA, Jones RN, Wenzel RP. Nosocomial bloodstream infections in United States hospitals: a three-year analysis. *Clinical Infectious Diseases: An Official Publication of the Infectious Diseases Society of America* 1999;2:239-244.
52. Trick WE, Fridkin SK, Edwards JR, Hajjeh RA, Gaynes RP. Secular trend of hospital-acquired candidemia among intensive care unit patients in the United States during 1989-1999. *Clinical Infectious Diseases: An Official Publication of the Infectious Diseases Society of America* 2002;5:627-630.
53. Nguyen MH, Peacock JE Jr, Morris AJ, et al. The changing face of candidemia: emergence of non-Candida albicans species and antifungal resistance. *The American Journal of Medicine* 1996;6:617-623.
54. Morgan J, Meltzer MI, Plikaytis BD, et al. Excess mortality, hospital stay, and cost due to candidemia: A case-control study using data from population-based candidemia surveillance. *Infection Control and Hospital Epidemiology: The official Journal of the Society of Hospital Epidemiologists of America* 2005;6:540-547.
55. Horn DL, Neofytos D, Anaissie EJ, et al. Epidemiology and outcomes of candidemia in 2019 patients: Data from the prospective antifungal therapy alliance registry. *Clinical Infectious Diseases: An Official Publication of the Infectious Diseases Society of America* 2009;12:1695-1703.
56. Pfaller MA, Diekema DJ. Epidemiology of invasive candidiasis: A persistent public health problem. *Clinical Microbiology Reviews* 2007;1:133-163.
57. Pfaller MA, Castanheira M, Messer SA, Moet GJ, Jones RN. Variation in *Candida* spp. distribution and antifungal resistance rates among bloodstream infection isolates by patient age: report from the SENTRY Antimicrobial Surveillance Program (2008-2009). *Diagnostic Microbiology and Infectious Disease* 2010;3:278-283.
58. Lewis RE. Current concepts in antifungal pharmacology. *Mayo Clinic Proceedings Mayo Clinic* 2011;8:805-817.
59. Maubon D, Garnaud C, Calandra T, Sanglard D, Cornet M. Resistance of *Candida* spp. to antifungal drugs in the ICU: Where are we now? *Intensive Care Medicine* 2014;9:1241-1255.
60. Edwards JE. Chapter 258. *Candida* species. In: Bennett JED, Raphael; Blaser, Martin J. ed. *Mandell, Douglas, and Bennett's Principles and Practice of Infectious Diseases*. Philadelphia, PA: Elsevier/Saunders, 2015:2879-2894.
61. Kothari A, Morgan M, Haake DA. Emerging technologies for rapid identification of bloodstream pathogens. *Clinical Infectious Diseases: An Official Publication of the Infectious Diseases Society of America* 2014;2:272-278.
62. Garey KW, Rege M, Pai MP, et al. Time to initiation of fluconazole therapy impacts mortality in patients with candidemia: a multi-institutional study. *Clinical Infectious Diseases: An Official Publication of the Infectious Diseases Society of America* 2006;1:25-31.
63. Morrell M, Fraser VJ, Kollef MH. Delaying the empiric treatment of candida bloodstream infection until positive blood culture results are obtained: A potential risk factor for hospital mortality. *Antimicrobial Agents and Chemotherapy* 2005;9:3640-3645.
64. Nucci M, Anaissie E. Should vascular catheters be removed from all patients with candidemia? An evidence-based review. *Clinical Infectious Diseases: An Official Publication of the Infectious Diseases Society of America* 2002;5:591-599.
65. Nucci M, Anaissie E. Revisiting the source of candidemia: Skin or gut? *Clinical Infectious Diseases: An Official Publication of the Infectious Diseases Society of America* 2001;12:1959-1967.
66. Rex JH, Bennett JE, Sugar AM, et al. Intravascular catheter exchange and duration of candidemia. NIAID Mycoses Study Group and the Candidemia Study Group. *Clinical Infectious Diseases: An Official Publication of the Infectious Diseases Society of America* 1995;4:994-996.
67. Cheng S, Clancy CJ, Hartman DJ, Hao B, Nguyen MH. *Candida glabrata* intra-abdominal candidiasis is characterized by persistence within the peritoneal cavity and abscesses. *Infection and Immunity* 2014;7:3015-3022.
68. Clancy CJ, Nguyen MH. Finding the "missing 50%" of invasive candidiasis: How nonculture diagnostics will improve understanding of disease spectrum and transform patient care. *Clinical Infectious Diseases: An Official Publication of the Infectious Diseases Society of America* 2013;9:1284-1292.
69. Bassetti M, Marchetti M, Chakrabarti A, et al. A research agenda on the management of intra-abdominal candidiasis: Results from a consensus of multinational experts. *Intensive Care Medicine* 2013;12:2092-2106.
70. Eggimann P, Francioli P, Bille J, et al. Fluconazole prophylaxis prevents intra-abdominal candidiasis in high-risk surgical patients. *Critical Care Medicine* 1999;6:1066-1072.
71. Rocco TR, Reinert SE, Simms HH. Effects of fluconazole administration in critically ill patients: Analysis of bacterial and fungal resistance. *Archives of Surgery* 2000;2:160-165.
72. Winston DJ, Hathorn JW, Schuster MG, Schiller GJ, Territo MC. A multicenter, randomized trial of fluconazole versus amphotericin B for empiric antifungal therapy of febrile neutropenic patients with cancer. *The American Journal of Medicine* 2000;4:282-289.
73. Ullmann AJ, Lipton JH, Vesole DH, et al. Posaconazole or fluconazole for prophylaxis in severe graft-versus-host disease. *The New England Journal of Medicine* 2007;4:335-347.
74. Segal BH, Almyroudis NG, Battiwalla M, et al. Prevention and early treatment of invasive fungal infection in patients with cancer and neutropenia and in stem cell transplant recipients in the era of newer broad-spectrum antifungal agents and diagnostic adjuncts. *Clinical Infectious Diseases: An Official Publication of the Infectious Diseases Society of America* 2007;3:402-409.
75. Eschenauer G, Depestel DD, Carver PL. Comparison of echinocandin antifungals. *Therapeutics and Clinical Risk Management* 2007;1:71-97.
76. Eschenauer GA, Carver PL, Lin SW, et al. Fluconazole versus an echinocandin for *Candida glabrata fungaemia*: A retrospective cohort study. *The Journal of Antimicrobial Chemotherapy* 2013;4: 922-926.
77. Andes DR, Safdar N, Baddley JW, et al. Impact of treatment strategy on outcomes in patients with candidemia and other forms of invasive candidiasis: A patient-level quantitative review of randomized trials. *Clinical Infectious Diseases: An Official Publication of the Infectious Diseases Society of America* 2012;8:1110-1122.
78. Kale-Pradhan PB, Wilhelm SM, Johnson LB. Clinical relevance of in vitro resistance of echinocandins: A focus on *Candida parapsilosis*. Current Fungal Infection Reports 2012;2:107-112.
79. Kale-Pradhan PB, Morgan G, Wilhelm SM, Johnson LB. Comparative efficacy of echinocandins and nonechinocandins for the treatment of *Candida parapsilosis* infections: A meta-analysis. Pharmacotherapy 2010;12:1207-13.
80. Cornely OA, Bassetti M, Calandra T, et al. ESCMID* guideline for the diagnosis and management of Candida diseases 2012: Non-neutropenic adult patients. *Clinical Microbiology and Infection: The Official Publication of the European Society of Clinical Microbiology and Infectious Diseases* 2012;19-37.
81. Tagliaferri E, Menichetti F. Treatment of invasive candidiasis: Between guidelines and daily clinical practice. *Expert Review of Anti-Infective Therapy* 6:685-689.
82. Kauffman CA, Vazquez JA, Sobel JD, et al. Prospective multicenter surveillance study of funguria in hospitalized patients. The National Institute for Allergy and Infectious Diseases (NIAID) Mycoses Study Group. *Clinical Infectious Diseases: An Official Publication of the Infectious Diseases Society of America* 2000;1:14-18.
83. Sobel JD, Kauffman CA, McKinsey D, et al. Candiduria: A randomized, double-blind study of treatment with fluconazole and placebo. The National Institute of Allergy and Infectious Diseases (NIAID) Mycoses Study Group. *Clinical Infectious Diseases: An Official Publication of the Infectious Diseases Society of America* 2000;1:19-24.
84. Gallis HA, Drew RH, Pickard WW. Amphotericin B: 30 years of clinical experience. *Reviews of Infectious Diseases* 1990;2:308-329.
85. Bohme A, Ruhnke M, Buchheidt D, et al. Treatment of fungal infections in hematology and oncology—guidelines of the Infectious Diseases Working Party (AGIHO) of the German Society of Hematology and Oncology (DGHO). Annals of hematology 2003;S133-40.
86. Martin-Pena A, Aguilar-Guisado M, Espigado I, Cisneros JM. Antifungal combination therapy for invasive aspergillosis. *Clinical*

Infectious Diseases: An Official Publication of the Infectious Diseases Society of America 2014;10:1437-1445.

87. Patterson TF. Chapter 259. *Aspergillus* species. In: Bennett JED, Raphael; Blaser, Martin J. ed. *Mandell, Douglas, and Bennett's Principles and Practice of Infectious Diseases*. Philadelphia, PA: Elsevier/Saunders, 2015:2895-2908.
88. Blyth CC, Gilroy NM, Guy SD, et al. Consensus guidelines for the treatment of invasive mould infections in haematological malignancy and haemopoietic stem cell transplantation, 2014. *Internal Medicine Journal* 2014;12b:1333-1349.
89. Fleming S, Yannakou CK, Haeusler GM, et al. Consensus guidelines for antifungal prophylaxis in haematological malignancy and haemopoietic stem cell transplantation, 2014. *Internal Medicine Journal* 2014;12b:1283-1297.
90. Sugui JA, Kwon-Chung KJ, Juvvadi PR, Latge JP, Steinbach WJ. *Aspergillus fumigatus and Related Species*. Cold Spring Harbor Perspectives in Medicine 2015;2:a019786.
91. Stevens DA, Schwartz HJ, Lee JY, et al. A randomized trial of itraconazole in allergic bronchopulmonary aspergillosis. *The New England Journal of Medicine* 2000;11:756-762.
92. Mavor AL, Thewes S, Hube B. Systemic fungal infections caused by Candida species: Epidemiology, infection process and virulence attributes. *Current Drug Targets* 2005;8:863-874.
93. Garcia-Vidal C, Upton A, Kirby KA, Marr KA. Epidemiology of invasive mold infections in allogeneic stem cell transplant recipients: biological risk factors for infection according to time after transplantation. *Clinical Infectious Diseases: An Official Publication of the Infectious Diseases Society of America* 2008;8:1041-1050.
94. Nam HS, Jeon K, Um SW, et al. Clinical characteristics and treatment outcomes of chronic necrotizing pulmonary aspergillosis: A review of 43 cases. *International Journal of Infectious Diseases: IJID: Official Publication of the International Society for Infectious Diseases* 2010;6:e479-482.
95. Reichenberger F, Habicht JM, Gratwohl A, Tamm M. Diagnosis and treatment of invasive pulmonary aspergillosis in neutropenic patients. *The European Respiratory Journal: Official journal of the European Society for Clinical Respiratory Physiology* 2002;4:743-755.
96. Gerlinger MP, Rousselot P, Rigaudeau S, et al. False positive galactomannan Platelia due to piperacillin-tazobactam. *Medecine et Maladies Infectieuses* 2012;1:10-14.
97. Alhambra A, Cuetara MS, Ortiz MC, et al. False positive galactomannan results in adult hematological patients treated with piperacillin-tazobactam. *Revista Iberoamericana de Micologia* 2007;2:106-112.
98. Walsh TJ, Hiemenz JW, Seibel NL, et al. Amphotericin B lipid complex for invasive fungal infections: Analysis of safety and efficacy in 556 cases. *Clinical Infectious Diseases: An Official Publication of the Infectious Diseases Society of America* 1998;6:1383-1396.
99. Herbrecht R, Denning DW, Patterson TF, et al. Voriconazole versus amphotericin B for primary therapy of invasive aspergillosis. *The New England Journal of Medicine* 2002;6:408-415.
100. Pettit NN, Carver PL. Isavuconazole: A new option for the management of invasive fungal infections. *The Annals of Pharmacotherapy* 2015;7:825-42.
101. Miceli MH, Kauffman CA. Isavuconazole: A new broad-spectrum triazole antifungal agent. *Clinical Infectious Diseases: An Official Publication of the Infectious Diseases Society of America* 2015;10:1558-65.
102. Viscoli C, Herbrecht R, Akan H, et al. An EORTC Phase II study of caspofungin as first-line therapy of invasive aspergillosis in haematological patients. *The Journal of Antimicrobial Chemotherapy* 2009;6:1274-1281.
103. Rex JH, Pappas PG, Karchmer AW, et al. A randomized and blinded multicenter trial of high-dose fluconazole plus placebo versus fluconazole plus amphotericin B as therapy for candidemia and its consequences in nonneutropenic subjects. *Clinical Infectious Diseases: An Official Publication of the Infectious Diseases Society of America* 2003;10:1221-1228.
104. Marr KA, Schlamm HT, Herbrecht R, et al. Combination antifungal therapy for invasive aspergillosis: A randomized trial. *Annals of Internal Medicine* 2015;2:81-89.
105. Martín-Peña A, Aguilar-Guisado M, Espigado I, Cisneros JM. Antifungal combination therapy for invasive aspergillosis. *Clinical Infectious Diseases* 2014;10:1437-1445.
106. Kontoyiannis DPL, Russell E. Chapter 260. Agents of mucormycosis and entomophthoramycosis. In: Bennett JED, Raphael; Blaser, Martin J. ed. *Mandell, Douglas, and Bennett's Principles and Practice of Infectious Diseases*. Philadelphia, PA: Elsevier/Saunders, 2015:2909-2919.
107. van Burik JA, Hare RS, Solomon HF, Corrado ML, Kontoyiannis DP. Posaconazole is effective as salvage therapy in zygomycosis: a retrospective summary of 91 cases. *Clinical Infectious Diseases: An Official Publication of the Infectious Diseases Society of America* 2006;7:e61-65.
108. Tortorano AM, Richardson M, Roilides E, et al. ESCMID and ECMM joint guidelines on diagnosis and management of hyalohyphomycosis: Fusarium spp., Scedosporium spp. and others. *Clinical Microbiology and Infection: The Official Publication of the European Society of Clinical Microbiology and Infectious Diseases* 2014;27-46.
109. King CT, Rogers PD, Cleary JD, Chapman SW. Antifungal therapy during pregnancy. *Clinical Infectious Diseases: An Official Publication of the Infectious Diseases Society of America* 1998;5:1151-1160.
110. Ostrosky-Zeichner L, Marr KA, Rex JH, Cohen SH. Amphotericin B: Time for a new "gold standard". *Clinical Infectious Diseases: An Official Publication of the Infectious Diseases Society of America* 2003;3:415-425.
111. Kauffman CA, Carver PL. Update on echinocandin antifungals. *Seminars in Respiratory and Critical Care Medicine* 2008;2:211-219.
112. Stevens DA. Itraconazole in cyclodextrin solution. *Pharmacotherapy* 1999;5:603-611.
113. Shear NH. Alopecia associated with fluconazole therapy. *Annals of Internal Medicine* 1996;2:53-54.
114. Kauffman CA, Carver PL. Use of azoles for systemic antifungal therapy. *Advances in Pharmacology* 1997;143-189.
115. Song JC, Deresinski S. Hepatotoxicity of antifungal agents. *Current Opinion in Investigational Drugs* 2005;2:170-177.
116. Leise MD, Poterucha JJ, Talwalkar JA. Drug-induced liver injury. *Mayo Clinic Proceedings Mayo Clinic* 2014;1:95-106.
117. Saad AH, DePestel DD, Carver PL. Factors influencing the magnitude and clinical significance of drug interactions between azole antifungals and select immunosuppressants. *Pharmacotherapy* 2006;12:1730-1744.
118. Zrenner E, Tomaszewski K, Hamlin J, Layton G, Wood N. Effects of multiple doses of voriconazole on the vision of healthy volunteers: a double-blind, placebo-controlled study. *Ophthalmic Research* 2014;1:43-52.
119. Kinoshita J, Iwata N, Ohba M, Kimotsuki T, Yasuda M. Mechanism of voriconazole-induced transient visual disturbance: Reversible dysfunction of retinal ON-bipolar cells in monkeys. *Investigative Ophthalmology & Visual Science* 2011;8:5058-5063.
120. Gao H, Pennesi M, Shah K, et al. Safety of intravitreal voriconazole: Electroretinographic and histopathologic studies. *Transactions of the American Ophthalmological Society* 2003;183-189; discussion 89.
121. Frampton JE, Scott LJ. Posaconazole: A review of its use in the prophylaxis of invasive fungal infections. *Drugs* 2008;7:993-1016.
122. Dolton MJ, Ray JE, Chen SC, Ng K, Pont L, McLachlan AJ. Multicenter study of posaconazole therapeutic drug monitoring: Exposure-response relationship and factors affecting concentration. *Antimicrobial Agents and Chemotherapy* 2012;11: 5503-5510.
123. Dolton MJ, Ray JE, Marriott D, McLachlan AJ. Posaconazole exposure-response relationship: Evaluating the utility of therapeutic drug monitoring. *Antimicrobial Agents and Chemotherapy* 2012;6: 2806-2813.
124. Kersemaekers WM, Dogterom P, Xu J, et al. Effect of a high-fat meal on the pharmacokinetics of 300-milligram posaconazole in a solid oral tablet formulation. *Antimicrobial Agents and Chemotherapy* 2015;6:3385-3389.
125. McKeage K. Posaconazole: A review of the gastro-resistant tablet and intravenous solution in invasive fungal infections. *Drugs* 2015;4: 397-406.
126. Carver PL. Micafungin. *The Annals of Pharmacotherapy* 2004;10: 1707-1721.
127. Laverdiere M, Bow EJ, Rotstein C, et al. Therapeutic drug monitoring for triazoles: A needs assessment review and recommendations from a Canadian perspective. *The Canadian Journal of Infectious Diseases & Medical Microbiology = Journal Canadien des Maladies Infectieuses et de la Microbiologie Medicale/AMMI Canada* 2014;6:327-343.
128. Ashbee HR, Barnes RA, Johnson EM, Richardson MD, Gorton R, Hope WW. Therapeutic drug monitoring (TDM) of antifungal agents: guidelines from the British Society for Medical Mycology. *Journal of Antimicrobial Chemotherapy* 2014;5:1162-1176.
129. Seyedmousavi S, Mouton JW, Verweij PE, Bruggemann RJ. Therapeutic drug monitoring of voriconazole and posaconazole

for invasive aspergillosis. *Expert Review of Anti-Infective Therapy* 2013;9:931-941.

130. Heinz WJ, Einsele H, Helle-Beyersdorf A, et al. Posaconazole concentrations after allogeneic hematopoietic stem cell transplantation. *Transplant Infectious Disease: An Official Journal of the Transplantation Society* 2013;5:449-56.

131. Gross BN, Ihorst G, Jung M, Wasch R, Engelhardt M. Posaconazole therapeutic drug monitoring in the real-life setting: A single-center experience and review of the literature. *Pharmacotherapy* 2013;10:1117-25.

132. Hussaini T, Ruping MJ, Farowski F, Vehreschild JJ, Cornely OA. Therapeutic drug monitoring of voriconazole and posaconazole. *Pharmacotherapy* 2011;2:214-225.

Infections in Immunocompromised Patients

122

Scott W. Mueller and Douglas N. Fish

KEY CONCEPTS

1. An *immunocompromised host* is a patient with defects in host defenses that predispose to infection. Risk factors include neutropenia, immune system defects (from disease or immunosuppressive drug therapy), compromise of natural host defenses, environmental contamination, and changes in normal flora of the host.

2. Immunocompromised patients are at high risk for a variety of bacterial, fungal, viral, and protozoal infections. Bacterial infections caused by gram-positive cocci (staphylococci and streptococci) occur most frequently, followed by gram-negative bacterial infections caused by Enterobacteriaceae and *Pseudomonas aeruginosa*. Fungal infections caused by *Candida* and *Aspergillus*, as well as certain viral infections (herpes simplex virus [HSV], cytomegalovirus [CMV]), are also important causes of morbidity and mortality.

3. Risk of infection in neutropenic patients is associated with both the severity and duration of neutropenia. Patients with severe neutropenia (absolute neutrophil count less than 500 cells/mm^3 [less than 0.5×10^9/L]) for greater than 7 to 10 days are considered to be at high risk of infection.

4. Fever (single oral temperature of greater than or equal to 38.3°C [greater than or equal to 101°F], or a temperature of greater than or equal to 38°C [greater than or equal to 100.4°F] for greater than or equal to 1 hour) is the most important clinical finding in neutropenic patients and is usually the stimulus for further diagnostic workup and initiation of antimicrobial treatment. Infection should be considered as the cause of fever until proven otherwise. Usual signs and symptoms of infection may be altered or absent in neutropenic patients. Appropriate empiric broad-spectrum antimicrobial therapy must be rapidly instituted to prevent excessive morbidity and mortality.

5. Empiric antimicrobial regimens for neutropenic infections should take into account patients' individual risk factors, as well as institutional infection and susceptibility patterns. The significant morbidity and mortality associated with gram-negative infections require that initial empiric regimens for treatment of febrile neutropenia have good activity against *P. aeruginosa* and Enterobacteriaceae. Parenteral regimens most commonly recommended for initial inpatient treatment include monotherapy with an antipseudomonal *β*-lactam, or a combination regimen consisting of an antipseudomonal *β*-lactam, plus an aminoglycoside. Low-risk patients may be successfully treated with oral antibiotics (ciprofloxacin plus amoxicillin-clavulanate), with the treatment setting determined by the patient's clinical status.

6. Neutropenic patients who remain febrile after 3 to 5 days of initial antimicrobial therapy should be reevaluated to determine whether treatment modifications are necessary. Common regimen modifications include addition of vancomycin (if not already administered) and antifungal therapy (amphotericin B, an echinocandin, or fluconazole). Therapy should be directed at causative organisms, if identified, but broad-spectrum regimens should be maintained during neutropenia.

7. The optimal duration of therapy for febrile neutropenia is controversial. The decision to discontinue antimicrobials is based on resolution of neutropenia, defervescence, culture results, and clinical stability of the patient.

8. Prophylactic antimicrobials are administered to cancer patients expected to experience prolonged neutropenia, as well as to hematopoietic stem cell and solid-organ transplant recipients. Prophylactic regimens may include antibacterial, antifungal, antiviral, or antiprotozoal agents, or a combination of these, selected according to risk of infection with specific pathogens. Optimal prophylactic regimens should take into account individual patient risk for infection and institutional infection and susceptibility patterns.

9. Patients undergoing hematopoietic stem cell transplantation are at an extremely high risk of infection because of prolonged neutropenia following intensive chemotherapy with or without irradiation, while solid-organ transplant recipients are at high risk because of prolonged administration of immunosuppressive drugs. Fungal (*Aspergillus*) and viral (CMV) infections are particularly troublesome in these populations, and prophylactic regimens directed against these pathogens are commonly used. When documented, these infections must be treated aggressively in order to optimize patient outcomes. Nevertheless, mortality rates are often high despite appropriate and aggressive antimicrobial therapy.

10. Immunocompromised patients must be continuously assessed for evidence of infection and response to antimicrobial therapy. Because a large number of antimicrobials may potentially be used, the occurrence of drug-related adverse effects must also be carefully assessed. Efforts should be directed at designing cost-effective treatment strategies that promote optimal patient outcomes.

An immunocompromised host is a patient with intrinsic or acquired defects in host immune defenses that predispose to infection. Advances in modern medicine have created more immunocompromised hosts than ever before. Historically, many of these patients died of their underlying diseases. Dramatic improvements in survival have been achieved by more aggressive therapy of underlying diseases and improved supportive care. However, because such aggressive therapy often renders patients profoundly immunosuppressed for long periods, opportunistic infections remain important causes of morbidity and mortality. This chapter focuses on risk factors for infection, common pathogens and infection sites, and prevention and management of suspected or documented infections in cancer patients (including hematopoietic stem cell transplantation [HSCT] patients) and solid-organ transplant (SOT) recipients. Chapter e103 discusses infectious complications associated with human immunodeficiency virus (HIV) infection.

RISK FACTORS FOR INFECTION/ EPIDEMIOLOGY

Many factors influence the degree of immunosuppression and also influence the epidemiology of the associated infections.

Neutropenia

1 2 3 Neutropenia is defined as an abnormally reduced number of neutrophils circulating in peripheral blood. Although exact definitions of neutropenia can vary, an absolute neutrophil count (ANC) of less than 1,000 cells/mm^3 (1.0×10^9/L) indicates a reduction sufficient to predispose patients to infection.[1] ANC is the sum of the absolute numbers of both mature neutrophils (polymorphonuclear cells [PMNs], also called *polys* or *segs*) and immature neutrophils (*bands*). The absolute number of PMNs and bands is determined by dividing the total percentage of these cells (obtained from the white blood cell [WBC] differential) by 100 and then multiplying the quotient obtained by the total number of WBCs.

The degree or severity of neutropenia, rate of neutrophil decline, and duration of neutropenia are important risk factors for infection.[1-4] All neutropenic patients are considered to be at risk for infection, but those with ANC less than 500 cells/mm^3 (0.5×10^9/L) are at greater risk than those with ANCs of 500 to 1,000 cells/mm^3 (0.5×10^9 to 1.0×10^9/L). Most treatment guidelines use ANC less than 500 cells/mm^3 (0.5×10^9/L) as the critical value in making therapeutic decisions regarding the management of suspected or documented infections.[1-4] Risk of infection and death are greatest among patients with less than 100 neutrophils/mm^3 (0.1×10^9/L) ("profound neutropenia").[1-3,5] In patients with chemotherapy-induced neutropenia, the risk of infection is also increased according to both the rapidity of ANC decline and duration of neutropenia. Patients with severe neutropenia of more than 7 to 10 days' duration are considered to be at especially high risk for serious infections.[1-3,6] The duration of chemotherapy-induced neutropenia varies considerably among subsets of cancer patients according to the specific chemotherapeutic agents used and the intensity of treatment. Patients undergoing HSCT may have no detectable granulocytes in peripheral blood for up to 3 to 4 weeks and are at particular risk for severe infections with a variety of pathogens.[5]

Bacteria and fungi commonly cause infections in neutropenic patients. Gram-positive cocci (*Staphylococcus aureus, Staphylococcus epidermidis,* and other coagulase-negative staphylococci, streptococci, and enterococci) have emerged as the most common cause of acute bacterial infections among neutropenic patients. Gram-negative bacilli (*Escherichia coli, Klebsiella pneumoniae, Pseudomonas aeruginosa*) traditionally were the most common causes of bacterial infection and remain frequent pathogens.[4,6-9] Although now not as common as gram-positive bacteria, the incidence of gram-negative infections may again be increasing and account for nearly half of bacterial infections.[2,6-9] Gram-negative infections are associated with significant morbidity and mortality, in large part due to increasing antibiotic resistance.[7-9] Patients who are neutropenic for extended periods and who receive broad-spectrum antibiotics are at high risk for fungal infections, usually due to *Candida* or *Aspergillus* spp.[1-3,6,10,11] Viral infections, although not as common as bacterial and fungal infections, also may cause severe infection in neutropenic patients.[1,2,5,6] Successful treatment of infections in neutropenic patients depends on resolution of neutropenia.[1,2]

Although not readily quantifiable, abnormalities may exist in granulocyte function as well as in cell numbers. Defects in phagocyte function may be caused by underlying disease (eg, leukemia) or its treatment (eg, corticosteroids, antineoplastic agents including monoclonal antibodies, and radiation).[2,6]

Immune System Defects

In addition to neutropenia, defects in T-lymphocyte and macrophage function (cell-mediated immunity), B-cell function (humoral immunity), or both predispose patients to infection. Cellular immune dysfunction is the result of underlying disease or immunosuppressive drug therapy; these defects result in a reduced ability of the host to defend against intracellular pathogens. Patients with malignancies and transplant patients receiving a wide variety of immunosuppressive drugs, such as cyclosporine, tacrolimus, sirolimus, mycophenolate, corticosteroids, azathioprine, and antineoplastic agents, are at risk for a variety of bacterial, fungal, viral, and protozoal infections (Table 122-1). Although some of these pathogens are associated with asymptomatic or mild disease in normal hosts, they may cause disseminated, life-threatening infections in immunocompromised hosts.

Underlying disease also frequently causes defects in humoral immune function. Patients with multiple myeloma and chronic lymphocytic leukemia have progressive hypogammaglobulinemia that results in defective humoral immunity. Splenectomy performed as a part of the staging process for Hodgkin's disease places patients at risk for infectious complications. Disease states with humoral immune dysfunction predispose the patient to serious, life-threatening infection with encapsulated organisms such as *Streptococcus pneumoniae, Haemophilus influenzae,* and *Neisseria meningitidis.*

Destruction of Protective Barriers

Loss of protective barriers is a major factor predisposing immunocompromised patients to infection. Damage to skin and mucous membranes by surgery, venipuncture, IV and urinary catheters, radiation, and chemotherapy disrupts natural host defense systems, leaving patients at high risk for infection. Chemotherapy-induced mucositis may erode mucous membranes of the oropharynx and GI tract and establish a portal for subsequent infection by bacteria, HSV, and *Candida.*[1,2,5] Medical and surgical procedures, such as transplant surgery, indwelling IV catheter placement, bone marrow aspiration, biopsies, and endoscopy, further damage the integument and predispose patients to infection. Infections resulting from disruption of protective barriers usually are a result of skin flora, such as *S. aureus, S. epidermidis,* and various streptococci.[1,2,6]

Environmental Contamination/Alteration of Microbial Flora

Infections in immunocompromised patients are caused by organisms either colonizing the host or acquired from the environment. Microorganisms may be transferred easily from patient to patient on the hands of hospital personnel unless strict infection control guidelines are followed. Contaminated equipment, such as nebulizers or ventilators, and contaminated water supplies have been responsible for outbreaks of *P. aeruginosa* and *Legionella pneumophila* infections, respectively. Foods, such as fruits and green leafy vegetables, which often are colonized with gram-negative bacteria and fungi, are sources of microbial contamination in immunocompromised hosts.[1,5]

Most infections in cancer patients are caused by organisms colonizing body sites, such as the skin, oropharynx, and GI tract and are therefore caused by the patient's own endogenous flora.[1,2,5,6] The GI tract is a common site from which infections in immunocompromised hosts originate. Periodontitis, pharyngitis, esophagitis, colitis,

TABLE 122-1 Risk Factors and Common Pathogens in Immunocompromised Patients

Risk Factor	Patient Conditions	Common Pathogens
Neutropenia	Acute leukemia Chemotherapy	Bacteria: *Staphylococcus aureus, Staphylococcus epidermidis, Escherichia coli, Klebsiella pneumoniae, Pseudomonas aeruginosa*, streptococci, enterococci Fungi: *Candida, Aspergillus*, Mucorales (*Mucor*) Viruses: Herpes simplex
Impaired cell-mediated immunity	Lymphoma Immunosuppressive therapy (steroids, cyclosporine, chemotherapy)	Bacteria: *Listeria, Nocardia, Legionella*, Mycobacteria Fungi: *Cryptococcus neoformans, Candida, Aspergillus, Histoplasma capsulatum* Viruses: Cytomegalovirus, varicella-zoster, herpes simplex Protozo: *Pneumocystis jiroveci*
Impaired humoral immunity	Multiple myeloma Chronic lymphocytic leukemia Splenectomy Immunosuppressive therapy (steroids, chemotherapy)	Bacteria: *S. pneumoniae, H. influenzae, N. meningitidis*
Loss of protective skin barriers	Venipuncture, bone marrow aspiration, urinary catheterization, vascular access devices, radiation, biopsies	Bacteria: *S. aureus, S. epidermidis, Bacillus* spp., *Corynebacterium jeikeium* Fungi: *Candida*
Mucous membranes	Respiratory support equipment, endoscopy, chemotherapy, radiation	Bacteria: *S. aureus, S. epidermidis*, streptococci, Enterobacteriaceae, *P. aeruginosa, Bacteroides* spp. Fungi: *Candida* Viruses: Herpes simplex
Surgery	Solid-organ transplantation	Bacteria: *S. aureus, S. epidermidis*, Enterobacteriaceae, *P. aeruginosa, Bacteroides* spp. Fungi: *Candida* Viruses: Herpes simplex
Alteration of normal microbial flora	Antimicrobial therapy Chemotherapy Hospital environment	Bacteria: Enterobacteriaceae, *P. aeruginosa, Legionella, S. aureus, S. epidermidis* Fungi: *Candida, Aspergillus*
Blood products, donor organs	Bone marrow transplantation Solid-organ transplantation	Fungi: *Candida* Viruses: Cytomegalovirus, Epstein–Barr virus, hepatitis B, hepatitis C Protozo: *Toxoplasma gondii*

perirectal cellulitis, and bacteremias are caused predominantly by normal flora of the gut; bloodstream infections are thought to arise from microbial translocation across injured GI mucosa.[1,5,6] Normal flora may be significantly disrupted and altered; oropharyngeal flora rapidly change to primarily gram-negative bacilli in hospitalized patients. Many cancer patients may already be colonized with gram-negative bacilli on admission as a result of frequent prior hospitalizations and clinic visits. In hospitalized cancer patients, however, many infections are caused by colonizing organisms acquired after admission.[1]

Although hospitalization and severity of illness are important risk factors for colonization by gram-negative bacilli, administration of broad-spectrum antimicrobial agents has the greatest impact on flora of immunocompromised hosts. Use of these agents disrupts GI tract flora and predisposes patients to infection with more virulent pathogens. Antineoplastic drugs (eg, cyclophosphamide, doxorubicin, and fluorouracil) and acid-suppressive therapy (eg, H_2-receptor antagonists, proton-pump inhibitors, and antacids) also may result in changes in GI flora and possibly predispose patients to infection.[1,2]

Numerous factors, such as underlying disease, immunosuppressive drug therapy, and antimicrobial administration, determine the immunocompromised host's risk of developing infection. Several risk factors are present concomitantly in many patients (see Table 122-1).

ETIOLOGY OF INFECTIONS IN NEUTROPENIC CANCER PATIENTS

2 Infection remains a significant cause of morbidity and mortality in neutropenic cancer patients. More than 50% of febrile neutropenic patients have an established or occult infection.[1,2] Patients with profound neutropenia are at greatest risk for systemic infection, with at least 20% of these individuals developing bacteremia.[1,2] Areas of impaired or damaged host defenses, such as the oropharynx, lungs, skin, sinuses, and GI tract, are common sites of infection. These local infections may progress to cause systemic infection and bacteremia.[2] Febrile episodes in neutropenic cancer patients can be attributed to microbiologically documented infection in approximately 30% to 40% of cases, about half of which are due to bacteremia. Further, infections can be documented clinically (but not microbiologically) in another 30% to 40% of patients, with the remaining 20% to 40% of patients manifesting infection only by fever.[2,4,6]

Table 122-1 lists organisms commonly infecting immunocompromised patients. Approximately 45% to 70% of bacteremic episodes in cancer patients are the result of gram-positive organisms compared with less than 30% of episodes documented during the 1970s and 1980s.[1,4,6-8] This shift is attributed to the frequent use of indwelling central and peripheral IV catheters, frequent use of broad-spectrum antibiotics with excellent gram-negative activity but relatively poor gram-positive coverage, higher rates of mucositis caused by aggressive cancer treatments, and prophylaxis with trimethoprim–sulfamethoxazole or quinolones.[1,4,6-8,12] Staphylococci (especially *S. epidermidis*) account for most infections, but *Bacillus* spp. and *Corynebacterium jeikeium* are also important pathogens.[1,2,6] Rates of infection due to methicillin-resistant *S. aureus* (MRSA) have increased in the hospital and community setting.[2,5,13] Viridans streptococci, which may be resistant to β-lactams, also have emerged as important pathogens, particularly in patients with chemotherapy-induced mucositis of the oropharynx.[2,4,5,12] Enterococci, including vancomycin-resistant strains, also may be problematic in many institutions.[2,5,12] Bacteremia caused by vancomycin-resistant enterococci (VRE) in neutropenic patients is associated with a mortality rate up to 30%.[4,14]

Gram-positive infections do not always cause immediately life-threatening infections and are associated with somewhat lower mortality rates (approximately 5%-10%) compared with gram-negative infections.[1,2,7] However, increasing rates of antibiotic resistance have made treatment of gram-positive infections in immunocompromised patients more challenging.[2,6,7] MRSA infections are associated with increased morbidity, mortality, and hospital costs compared with susceptible organisms.[15,16] Methicillin resistance among coagulase-negative staphylococci, which may cause 40% to 80% of infections in certain populations, is common (70%-90% of isolates).[1,2,5-7] Organisms that are resistant to vancomycin are increasing in importance.[1,2,4,7,14] Thus, prevention and timely diagnosis and treatment of gram-positive infections are clearly of great importance in the management of neutropenic cancer patients.

Gram-negative infections remain important causes of morbidity and mortality (approximately 20%-30%) in immunocompromised cancer patients.[7] However, the relative frequency of infection owing to specific pathogens has been shifting among gram-negative infections. *E. coli* and *Klebsiella* remain the most common isolates at many centers.[2,6] Strains of Enterobacteriaceae producing plasmid-mediated extended-spectrum β-lactamases that hydrolyze extended-spectrum cephalosporins, and carbapenemases that hydrolyze carbapenems have emerged and are cause for concern.[1,2,6,7,12] The global spread of carbapenem-resistant Enterobacteriaceae (CRE) is especially concerning. The frequency of infections resulting from other gram-negative organisms, such as *Enterobacter*, *Serratia*, and *Citrobacter*, has been increasing.[1,2] Infections with these particular organisms may be difficult to treat because of the ease of β-lactamase induction and the more frequent development of resistance to multiple antibiotics.[1,2,6,12]

P. aeruginosa has long been an important pathogen in cancer patients. *P. aeruginosa* infection rates are decreasing in patients with solid tumors but not in patients with hematologic malignancies.[4,6,7] Infections caused by *P. aeruginosa* are associated with significant morbidity and mortality in neutropenic patients, with mortality rates of 31% to 75% reported.[1,3,7] The frequency of infection caused by difficult-to-treat organisms such as *Stenotrophomonas maltophilia* appear to be increasing at many centers, probably because of selective pressures of broad-spectrum antimicrobial use.[6,8] As with gram-positive organisms, antibiotic resistance among gram-negative organisms has continued to increase at alarming rates and has made appropriate antibiotic selection for treatment of febrile neutropenia more difficult.[1,13] Although the GI tract is a common site of bacterial infection, severe infections caused by anaerobic organisms are relatively infrequent. Anaerobes are found most frequently in mixed infections, such as perirectal cellulitis and mucositis-associated oropharyngeal infections.[2,6]

In addition to bacterial infections, neutropenic cancer patients are at risk for invasive fungal infections. Patients with extended periods of profound neutropenia who have been receiving broad-spectrum antibiotics, corticosteroids, or both are at the highest risk for invasive fungal infection. Up to one third of febrile neutropenic patients who do not respond to 1 week of broad-spectrum antibiotic therapy will have a systemic fungal infection.[1,2,8] Large autopsy studies have documented a change over time in invasive fungal infections. Whereas from 1989 to 2003 over 30% of autopsies of patients with hematologic malignancies found deep fungal infection (75% of which were undiagnosed prior to death), this number decreased to 19% from 2004 to 2008 (49% of which were undiagnosed prior to death). These improvements may be due to improved awareness, diagnostic techniques and treatments. One single center estimated the average prevalence of invasive fungal infections was 30% in those autopsied over the 20 year period. Causative pathogens were usually either *Aspergillus* spp., *Candida* spp., or Mucorales fungi (such as *Mucor* spp.).[17]

Candida albicans is a common fungal pathogen in neutropenic cancer patients, especially those with solid tumors.[1,2,4,11,17,18] However, non-*albicans* species of *Candida* including *Candida glabrata*, *Candida tropicalis*, *C. parapsilosis*, and *C. krusei* are being isolated with increasing frequency and are more common than *C. albicans* infections in some studies.[11,18] Increased infections caused by pathogens such as *Trichosporon* spp., *Fusarium* spp., and *Curvularia* spp. have also been reported.[10,11,17] The shift toward more frequent infection with non-*albicans Candida* is important because of significantly decreased rates of susceptibility among many of these strains.[19] Because *Candida* spp. are normal flora, alteration of body host defenses is an important risk factor for the development of these infections. Oral thrush is the most common clinical manifestation of fungal infection. Mucous membranes damaged from chemotherapy and radiation serve as areas of *Candida* surface colonization and subsequent entry into the bloodstream; disease then may disseminate throughout the body. Organs such as the liver, spleen, kidney, and lungs are commonly involved in disseminated disease.[1,2,17] Hepatosplenic candidiasis is a particularly important infection in patients with hematologic malignancies.[6,17,24] Diagnosis of *Candida* infections is difficult and often requires invasive tissue sampling.[6] In patients with invasive candidiasis, overall attributable mortality is as high as 35% to 50%.[4,11,18]

Invasive infections caused by *Aspergillus* spp. are a serious complication of neutropenia. Mortality rates have historically approached 80% in patients with prolonged neutropenia and/or patients undergoing allogeneic HSCT; however, mortality is now reported as low as 35%.[4,10] These infections are particularly prevalent and more common in patients with hematologic malignancies and in patients undergoing HSCT.[4,10,11,17,20] Infections resulting from *Aspergillus* species (including *A. fumigatus*, *A. terreus*, *A. flavus*, and *A. niger*) usually are acquired via inhalation of airborne spores. After colonizing the lungs, *Aspergillus* invades the lung parenchyma and pulmonary vessels, resulting in hemorrhage, pulmonary infarcts, and a high mortality rate. Invasive pulmonary disease is the dominant manifestation of infection in patients with neutropenia. However, *Aspergillus* also may cause other infections, including sinusitis, cutaneous infection, and disseminated disease involving multiple organs, including the CNS.[17,20] Prolonged neutropenia is the primary risk factor for invasive pulmonary aspergillosis in patients with acute leukemia; use of corticosteroids also may predispose patients to disease.[20] Invasive aspergillosis should be suspected in neutropenic cancer patients colonized with *Aspergillus* (in sputum and/or nasal cultures) who remain persistently febrile despite at least 1 week of broad-spectrum antibiotic therapy.[1,2,20] Increased infections caused by other yeasts (such as *Trichosporon*) and molds (such as Mucorales, *Fusarium*, and *Curvularia*) have also been reported.[10,11,17]

Chemotherapy-induced mucous membrane damage may predispose neutropenic cancer patients to reactivation of HSV, manifesting as gingivostomatitis or recurrent genital infections. Untreated oropharyngeal HSV infections may spread to involve the esophagus and often coexist with *Candida* infections. Clinical disease resulting from HSV occurs most often in patients with serologic evidence (eg, serum antibodies to HSV) of prior infection. Both HSV-seropositive HSCT patients and HSV-seropositive leukemics receiving intensive chemotherapy are at high risk for recurrent HSV disease during periods of immunosuppression.[2,4,5]

Pneumocystis jiroveci and *Toxoplasma gondii* are the most common parasitic pathogens found in immunocompromised cancer patients. Patients with hematologic malignancies and those receiving high-dose corticosteroids as part of chemotherapy regimens are at the greatest risk of infection.[2,4,5] Routine use of trimethoprim–sulfamethoxazole prophylaxis has reduced substantially the incidence of these infections.[1,2,5]

Because the majority of infecting organisms in cancer patients are from the host's own flora, some centers have used routine surveillance cultures in an attempt to prospectively identify causes of fever and suspected infection. In a typical surveillance culture program, cultures of the nose, mouth, axillae, and perirectal area are performed twice weekly, and culture results are correlated with the clinical status of the patient. Because these cultures are costly and have low diagnostic yield, the utility of surveillance culture programs is believed to be limited.[1,2] However, surveillance cultures are useful as research tools and in patients with prolonged profound neutropenia and in institutions that have high rates of antimicrobial resistance or have problems with virulent pathogens such as *P. aeruginosa* or *Aspergillus* spp. Surveillance cultures should be limited to the anterior nares for detecting colonization with MRSA, *Aspergillus*, and penicillin-resistant pneumococci and to the rectum for detecting VRE, *P. aeruginosa*, and multiple-antibiotic-resistant gram-negative rods (such as CRE).[1,2]

Knowledge of infection rates and local susceptibility patterns is essential for guiding optimal management of febrile neutropenia. These parameters must be monitored closely because the spectrum of infectious complications is related to multiple factors, including cancer chemotherapy regimens and antimicrobial therapy used for treatment and prophylaxis.

CLINICAL PRESENTATION

(4) The most important clinical finding in the neutropenic cancer patient is fever. Because of the potential for significant morbidity and mortality associated with infection in these patients, fever should be considered to be the result of infection until proved otherwise.[1-3,6] At the appearance of fever, the patient should be evaluated carefully for other signs and symptoms of infection.

TREATMENT

Management of patients with febrile neutropenia, including both treatment and prophylaxis of infectious complications, can be extremely challenging. Although published guidelines are available, the most optimal clinical management of these patients remains unclear in many aspects.

Febrile Episodes in Neutropenic Cancer Patients

DESIRED OUTCOMES 121-1

(4) (5) The goals of therapy in neutropenic cancer patients with fever are the following: (a) protect the neutropenic patient from early death caused by undiagnosed infection; (b) prevent breakthrough bacterial, fungal, viral, and protozoal infections during periods of neutropenia; (c) effectively treat established infections; (d) reduce morbidity and allow for administration of optimal antineoplastic therapy; (e) avoid unnecessary use of antimicrobials that contribute to increased resistance; and (f) minimize toxicities and cost of antimicrobial therapy while increasing patient quality of life. Empirical broad-spectrum antibiotic therapy is effective at reducing early mortality.[7]

Approach to Treatment

General guidelines for management of febrile episodes and documented infections in neutropenic patients are shown in Figs. 122-1 and 122-2.[1] Although many controversies remain regarding optimal

CLINICAL PRESENTATION Febrile Neutropenia[1-6]

General

- Due to high risk for serious infections, frequent (at least daily) careful clinical assessments must be performed to search for possible evidence of infection
- Physical assessment should include examination of all common sites of infection, including mouth/pharynx, nose and sinuses, respiratory tract, GI tract, urinary tract, skin, soft tissues, perineum, and intravascular catheter insertion sites

Symptoms

- Usual signs and symptoms of infection may be absent or altered in neutropenic patients owing to low numbers of leukocytes and an inability to mount an inflammatory response (eg, no infiltrate on chest x-ray film, urinary tract infection without pyuria)
- Pain may be present at the infection site(s)

Signs

- Fever in this setting is defined as a single oral temperature ≥38.3°C (≥101°F) in the absence of other causes or temperature ≥38°C (≥100.4°F) for 1 hour or more. Other causes of fever unrelated to infection in this patient population include reactions to blood products, chemotherapeutic agents (and other drugs, including biologics), cell lysis, and underlying malignancy
- Usual signs of infection may be absent or altered; patients with bacteremia commonly exhibit no signs of infection other than fever

Laboratory Tests

- Neutropenia (ANC ≤1,000 cells/mm^3 [≤1.0 × 10^9/L])
- Blood cultures (two or more sets, including vascular access devices) for bacteria and fungi; cultures of other suspected infection sites (infection can be documented microbiologically in only about 30% of cases, about half of which are due to bacteremia)
- Other cultures should be obtained as indicated clinically according to the presence of signs or symptoms
- Recent surveillance cultures (nasal, rectal) should be reviewed, if available
- Complete blood count and blood chemistries should be obtained frequently to monitor neutropenia, plan supportive care, guide drug dosing, and assess patient's overall status

Other Diagnostic Tests

- Chest x-ray film
- Aspiration, biopsy of skin lesions
- Other diagnostic tests as indicated clinically on the basis of physical examination and other assessments

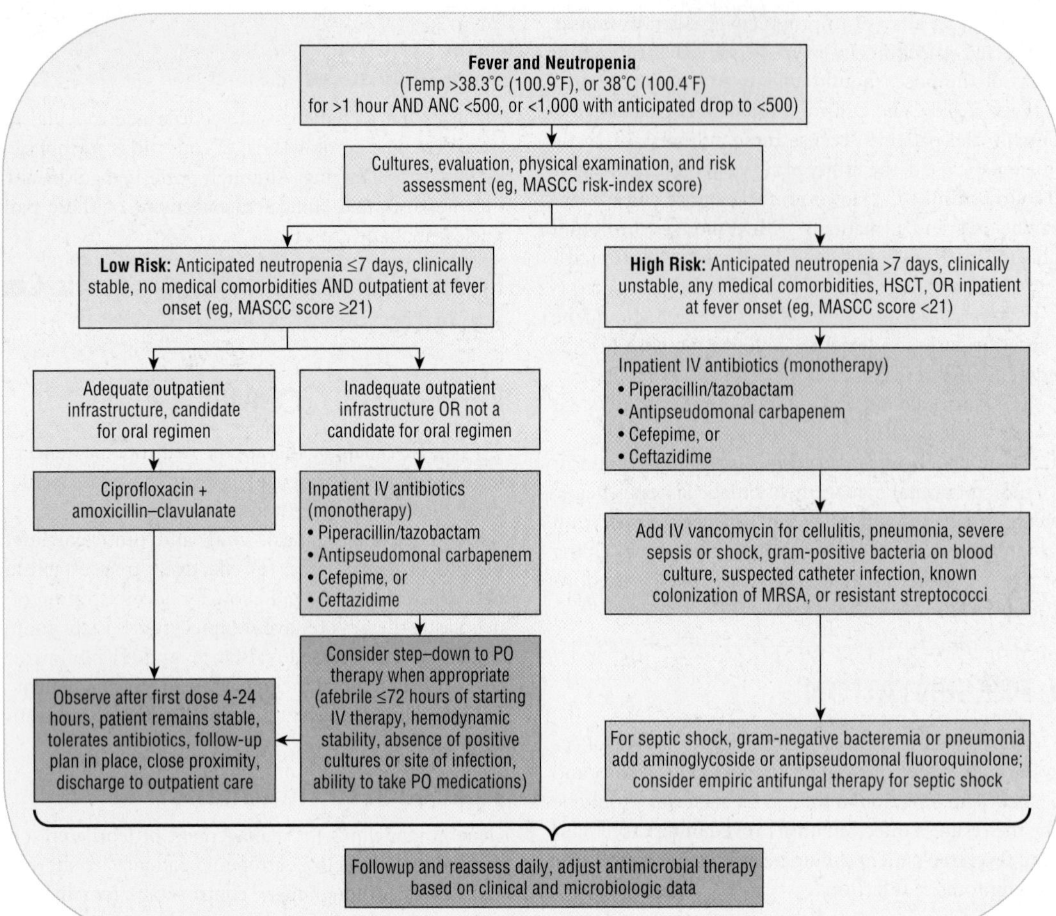

FIGURE 122-1 Initial management of febrile episodes in neutropenic patients. (ANC, absolute neutrophil count; HSCT, hematopoietic stem cell transplantation; MASCC, Multinational Association for Supportive Care in Cancer; PO, oral.)

management of these patients, updated evidence-based guidelines from the Infectious Diseases Society of America (IDSA) for the management of febrile neutropenia were published in 2010.[1] Similarly, the National Comprehensive Cancer Network (NCCN) published updated clinical practice guidelines for the prevention and treatment of cancer-related infections in 2015.[2] Selected specific recommendations are discussed in the following sections of this chapter, and their associated evidence-based rankings are summarized in Table 122-2.

Fever in the neutropenic cancer patient is considered to be caused by infection until proved otherwise. High-dose broad-spectrum bactericidal, usually parenteral, empirical antibiotic therapy should be initiated at the onset of fever or at the first signs or symptoms of infection. Withholding antibiotic therapy until an organism is isolated results in unacceptably high mortality rates. Undiagnosed infection in immunocompromised patients can rapidly disseminate and result in death if left untreated or if treated improperly. Failure to initiate appropriate antibiotic therapy for *P. aeruginosa* bacteremia at the onset of fever in neutropenic cancer patients resulted in mortality rates of 15% and 70% within 12 and 48 hours, respectively.[1,2] Empirical antibiotic therapy is 70% to 90% effective at reducing early morbidity and mortality.[1,2,7] Therapy must be appropriate and initiated promptly. Antimicrobial therapy must also be initiated promptly in afebrile cancer patients with clinical signs and symptoms of infection.

When designing optimal empirical antibiotic regimens, clinicians must consider infection patterns and antimicrobial susceptibility trends in their respective institutions. Patient factors such as risk for infection, drug allergies, concomitant nephrotoxins, and previous antimicrobial exposure (including prophylaxis) must be considered.[1,2,4] Assessment of the patient's risk of infection will help determine the appropriate route and setting for antibiotic administration (Fig. 122-1). Neutropenic patients with fever can be divided into low- and high-risk groups for complications of severe infection. Risk stratification drives both type and setting of antimicrobial therapy. The Multinational Association for Supportive Care in Cancer (MASCC) risk-index score is recommended by many clinical guidelines to assess a patient's risk of complications.[1,2] Most experts agree that, in general, low-risk patients have an anticipated duration of neutropenia less than or equal to 7 days, are clinically stable, and have no or few comorbidities and no bacterial focus or systemic signs of infection other than fever. In contrast, high-risk patients are those with an anticipated duration of neutropenia greater than 7 days or profound neutropenia, are clinically unstable or have comorbid medical problems (eg, focal or systemic signs of infection, GI symptoms, nausea, vomiting, diarrhea, hypoxemia, and chronic lung disease), or have a high-risk cancer (eg, acute leukemia) and/or have undergone high intensity chemotherapy. High-risk patients (MASCC less than 21) should be hospitalized for parenteral antibiotics whereas low-risk patients may be candidates for oral or outpatient antibiotics. Even with such classifications, careful selection of low-risk patients for oral outpatient management is important (discussed in "Oral Antibiotic Therapy for Management of Febrile Neutropenia" section below).[1,2,21]

The optimal antibiotic regimen for empirical therapy in febrile neutropenic cancer patients remains controversial, but it is clear that no single regimen can be recommended for all patients. Because of their frequency and relative pathogenicity, *P. aeruginosa* and other gram-negative bacilli and staphylococci remain the primary targets

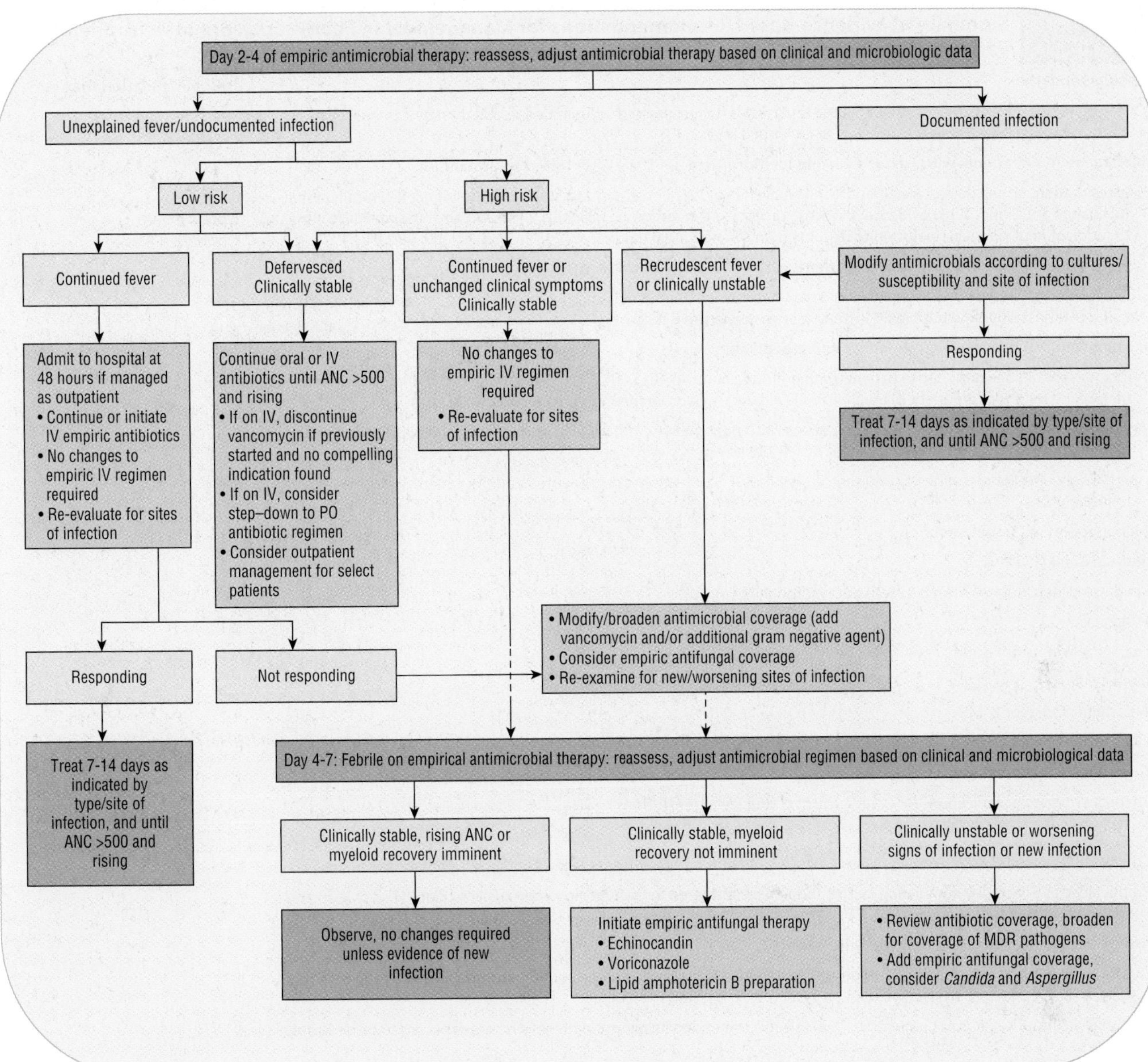

FIGURE 122-2 Subsequent management of febrile episodes in neutropenic patients who have already received empirical antimicrobial therapy for 2-4 days. (ANC, absolute neutrophil count; MDR, multidrug-resistant; PO, oral.)

TABLE 122-2 Summary of Evidence-Based Recommendations for Management of Febrile Episodes in Neutropenic Patients

Recommendations	Recommendation Grades[a]
Oral antibiotics are feasible for treatment of carefully selected patients at low risk for complications	A-1
Monotherapy with appropriate antibiotics is as effective as combination regimens for initial empirical treatment of febrile neutropenic episodes	A-1
Patients at high risk for serious life-threatening infections must be initially treated with IV antibiotics. Patients at low risk can be treated with either IV or oral drugs (see text for risk stratification criteria)	A-2
Patients who become afebrile within 2-4 days of beginning initial empirical antibiotic therapy and in whom specific organisms have been identified should be treated for ≥7 days (until cultures are negative and patient has clinically recovered). Low-risk patients in whom no organism is identified can be switched to oral antibiotics if desired, whereas patients originally classified as high risk should continue on IV antibiotics	B-2
Management of Patients with Persistent Fever During First 2-4 Days of Treatment	
In patients initially receiving monotherapy or a two-drug regimen *not* including vancomycin, addition of vancomycin can be considered if any criteria for use of vancomycin are present (see the text for specific criteria)	B-3
In patients *already* receiving vancomycin as part of the initial empirical regimen, withdrawal of vancomycin should be considered after 2 days in the absence of a documented pathogen requiring continued therapy	A-2

(Continued)

TABLE 122-2 Summary of Evidence-Based Recommendations for Management of Febrile Episodes in Neutropenic Patients (*Continued*)

Recommendations	Recommendation Grades[a]
Other initial antibiotics can be continued if the disease has not progressed, or switched to oral therapy if the patient was classified as low risk even in the presence of continued fever	A-1
Management of Patients with Fever Persisting for More Than 2-4 Days After Initial Treatment	
Reassess patient after 2 days of treatment. If still febrile by day 4, then: (a) continue the same antibiotics if clinically stable; (b) change antibiotics if any evidence of disease progression or antibiotic toxicities; or (c) add an antifungal drug if the duration of neutropenia is expected to be more than 5-7 additional days	Option a: A-1 Option b: A-3 Option c: A-3
Continuation of Antibiotics in Afebrile Patients with no Identified Infection	
Antibiotic therapy can be discontinued after 3 days of treatment if patient is afebrile for ≥48 hours and absolute neutrophil count (ANC) is ≥500 cells/mm^3 (≥0.5 × 10^9/L) for two consecutive days	A-2
If patient remains neutropenic, continue IV or oral antibiotics	A-2
Antibiotics should be continued in patients with profound neutropenia (ANC <100 cells/mm^3 [<0.1 × 10^9/L]), mucous membrane lesions of mouth or GI tract, unstable vital signs, or other identified risk factors	A-2
Antibiotics can be stopped after 2 weeks in patients with prolonged neutropenia of unclear continued duration, no identified site of infection, and who can be closely observed	C-3
Alternatively, antibiotics can be discontinued after 4 days if no infection is documented and the patient shows no response to therapy	C-3
Management of Fungal Infections	
Suspected candidiasis:	
Lipid-associated amphotericin B (LAMB) or caspofungin[b]	A-1
Voriconazole	B-1
Fluconazole or itraconazole	B-1
Candidemia:	
An echinocandin[b] or LAMB	A-2
Fluconazole or voriconazole	B-3
Granulocyte Transfusions	
There are no specific indications for routine use of granulocyte transfusions	C-2
Colony-Stimulating Factors	
Colony-stimulating factors are not indicated for routine treatment of neutropenia in either febrile or afebrile patients	B-2
Prophylactic use of colony-stimulating factors should be considered for patients in whom the anticipated risk of fever and neutropenia is ≥20%	A-2
Antimicrobial Prophylaxis in Neutropenic Patients	
Fluoroquinolone prophylaxis should be considered for high-risk patients with profound neutropenia (ANC <100 cells/mm^3 [<0.1 × 10^9/L]) expected to last 7-10 days	B-1
Antibacterial prophylaxis is not required in routinely recommended in low-risk patients who are expected to be neutropenic <7 days	A-3
Prophylaxis with trimethoprim–sulfamethoxazole should be administered to all patients at risk for *Pneumocystis jiroveci* pneumonia, regardless of whether they are neutropenic	A-1
Prophylaxis with fluconazole, posaconazole, voriconazole, or caspofungin[b] is recommended in high-risk patients, starting with induction chemotherapy and continued for duration of neutropenia; itraconazole is an effective alternative agent	A-1 for all agents except voriconazole and caspofungin[b] (both B-2)
In HSCT, prophylaxis with fluconazole, micafungin[b], posaconazole, itraconazole, voriconazole, or LAMB is recommended during the period of risk of neutropenia	A-1 for fluconazole and micafungin[b], all others B-2
In HSCT patients with graft-versus-host disease, or neutropenic patients with hematologic malignancies, prophylaxis with posaconazole is recommended for prevention of invasive fungal infections	A-1
HSV-seropositive patients undergoing HSCT or leukemia induction therapy should receive acyclovir prophylaxis during neutropenia, and for at least 30 days after HSCT	A-1 for prophylaxis, A-2 for duration
In HSCT, prophylaxis with acyclovir should be administered during neutropenia and for at least 1 year afterward to prevent VZV infection or reactivation	A-2

[a]Strength of recommendations: A, B, C = good, moderate, and poor evidence to support recommendation for use, respectively; D = moderate evidence to support a recommendation against use.

[b]Expert opinion indicates all echinocandins are likely interchangeable and equally effective.

Quality of evidence: 1 = evidence from ≥1 properly randomized, controlled trial; 2 = evidence from ≥1 well-designed clinical trial without randomization, from cohort or case–control analytic studies, from multiple time series, or from dramatic results from uncontrolled experiments; 3 = evidence from opinions of respected authorities, based on clinical experience, descriptive studies, or reports of expert committees.

Data from references 1, 2, 5, 18, and 20.

of empirical antimicrobial therapy.[1,2] Although *P. aeruginosa* may be documented in fewer than 5% of bloodstream infections in the population of hospitalized patients, adequate antipseudomonal antibiotic coverage still must be included in empirical regimens because of the significant morbidity and mortality associated with this pathogen.[1,4,13] All empirical regimens must be carefully monitored and appropriately revised on the basis of documented infections, susceptibilities of bacterial isolates, development of more defined clinical signs and symptoms of infection, or a combination of these factors.

TABLE 122-3 Comparative Advantages and Disadvantages of Various Antibiotic Regimens for Empiric Therapy of Febrile Neutropenic Cancer Patients

Regimen	Potential Advantages	Potential Disadvantages
β-Lactam monotherapy (ceftazidime, cefepime, piperacillin–tazobactam, imipenem–cilastatin, or meropenem)	Efficacy comparable to combination regimens; decreased drug toxicities; ease of administration; possibly less expensive	Possibly less efficacy in profound neutropenia or prolonged neutropenia; limited gram-positive activity; no potential for additive/synergistic effects; increased selection of resistant organisms; increased colonization and superinfection rates
Antipseudomonal β-lactam plus aminoglycoside (eg, gentamicin or tobramycin + cefepime, ceftazidime, or piperacillin–tazobactam)	Traditional regimen, broad-spectrum coverage; optimal therapy of *Pseudomonas aeruginosa*; rapidly bactericidal; synergistic activity; decreased bacterial resistance; reduction of superinfections	Limited gram-positive activity; potential for nephrotoxicity; need for therapeutic monitoring of aminoglycoside concentrations
Antipseudomonal β-lactam plus fluoroquinolone (ciprofloxacin or higher-dose levofloxacin + ceftazidime, cefepime, or piperacillin–tazobactam)	Efficacy similar to other regimens when used in combination therapy; no cross-resistance with β-lactams; possibility for oral administration; may be useful in patients with renal impairment in whom aminoglycosides are undesirable	Marginal gram-positive activity; fluoroquinolones not recommended as monotherapy; resistance may develop rapidly
Empirical regimens containing vancomycin (added to antipseudomonal β-lactam ± aminoglycoside or fluoroquinolone)	Early effective therapy of gram-positive infections	No demonstrated benefit of vancomycin empirical therapy versus addition of vancomycin if needed later; increased risk of selection for vancomycin-resistant enterococci; risk of toxicities; excessive cost; need for therapeutic monitoring of vancomycin concentrations
Oral antibiotic regimens (eg, ciprofloxacin or levofloxacin + amoxicillin–clavulanate or clindamycin)	Efficacy comparable with parenteral therapy in low-risk patients; less expensive; reduced exposure of patients to nosocomial pathogens	Least studied treatment approach; less potent than parenteral antibiotics; requires compliant patient with 24-hour access to medical care should clinical instability develop

Data from references 1-3, 7, 22, and 26.

Although there are some differences among them, consensus guidelines generally recognize three different types of empirical parenteral antibiotic regimens: (a) monotherapy with an antipseudomonal β-lactam such as a cephalosporin (cefepime or ceftazidime), a carbapenem (imipenem–cilastatin or meropenem), or piperacillin–tazobactam; (b) two-drug combination therapy with an antipseudomonal β-lactam plus either an aminoglycoside or an antipseudomonal fluoroquinolone (ciprofloxacin or levofloxacin); and (c) monotherapy or two-drug combination therapy as above, plus the addition of vancomycin (Fig. 122-1).[1,2] Each of these regimens has advantages and disadvantages, which are summarized in Table 122-3. There is no overwhelming evidence that any one of these regimens is superior to the others. The overall response to empirical antibiotic regimens in febrile neutropenic cancer patients is approximately 70% to 90% regardless of whether a pathogen is isolated or which antimicrobial regimen is used.[1,2,4,7] Additionally, other alternative regimens may also appropriate based on specific patient characteristics or susceptibilities of suspected pathogens.

β-Lactam Monotherapy

Monotherapy with an antipseudomonal β-lactam is recommended by IDSA 2010 and NCCN 2015 guidelines as initial parenteral therapy for management of febrile neutropenia without suspected or proven resistant organisms or complications (eg, pneumonia, hypotension, vascular access infection, etc.).[1,2] Several β-lactam antibiotics in current use have been evaluated as monotherapy for management of febrile episodes in neutropenic cancer patients, including antipseudomonal cephalosporins (ceftazidime and cefepime), piperacillin–tazobactam, and antipseudomonal carbapenems (imipenem–cilastatin and meropenem).[1,2] Three different meta-analyses assessing as many as 46 clinical trials involving more than 7,600 patients found no significant differences overall between monotherapy and combination therapy (β-lactam/aminoglycoside) in rates of survival, treatment response, and bacterial/fungal superinfections.[2] One study also found a higher rate of adverse effects in aminoglycoside-containing combination regimens.[22] In addition, one analysis found that cefepime monotherapy was associated with a significantly higher risk of mortality compared with the other β-lactams evaluated.[1,2,23] A follow-up analysis conducted by the FDA using additional studies and patient-level data failed to confirm an increased risk of mortality with cefepime, concluding that it is as efficacious as other β-lactams.[1,23,24] Significantly lower response rates for ceftazidime (but not cefepime) monotherapy have been reported in another review of the clinical literature.[1,2] However, until the results of these studies can be validated, ceftazidime is still among the monotherapy regimens routinely recommended as appropriate initial therapy of febrile neutropenic patients, although with a lower strength of evidence in 2015 NCCN guidelines.[1,2,23,24] Institutional susceptibility patterns and patient characteristics should drive drug selection.

Doripenem, ceftazidime-avibactam, and ceftolozane-tazobactam have appropriate overall spectrum of antibacterial activity with good activity against *P. aeruginosa* and other gram-negative organisms as well as many gram-positive pathogens. Neither the 2015 NCCN nor the 2010 IDSA consensus guidelines specifically recommend these agents as appropriate for monotherapy due to a lack of supportive clinical evidence at the time the guidelines were written.[1,2] They are, however, considered by some clinicians to be reasonable treatment options depending on patient- and institution-specific factors related to risk of infection with MDR pathogens.

Use of monotherapy has several potential advantages and disadvantages (see Table 122-3). Perhaps the most common concerns are those regarding the selection of resistant strains of organisms, such as *P. aeruginosa*, *Enterobacter* spp., and *Serratia* spp., through extended-spectrum β-lactamases and type 1 β-lactamases, especially with ceftazidime.[1,2,7,12] Activity against gram-positive organisms such as coagulase-negative staphylococci, MRSA, enterococci (including VRE), penicillin-resistant *S. pneumoniae*, and some strains of viridans streptococci is poor with some single β-lactams, but cefepime and antipseudomonal carbapenems have good activity against viridans streptococci and pneumococci.[1,2] Although ceftazidime has been studied widely and used for treatment of febrile neutropenia, newer agents may be more effective owing to ceftazidime's susceptibility to β-lactamase induction and lower activity against gram-positive organisms.[1,2,7,12,23] Ertapenem, a carbapenem, and tigecycline, a glycylcycline antibiotic, have excellent activity against many gram-negative organisms but should not be used in the empirical treatment of febrile neutropenia due to their weaker activity against *P. aeruginosa*. For the same reason ceftaroline, a cephalosporin active against MRSA, is not an acceptable option for empiric monotherapy in most patients.

As with all empirical antibiotic regimens, patients receiving monotherapy should be monitored closely for treatment failure, secondary infections, and development of resistance. Use of monotherapy may not be appropriate in institutions with high rates of gram-positive infections or infections caused by relatively resistant gram-negative pathogens such as *P. aeruginosa* and *Enterobacter*. The carbapenems are less susceptible to inducible β-lactamases and often may be used effectively in these institutions. Overall, similar efficacy has been observed with monotherapy with antipseudomonal β-lactams compared to aminoglycoside combination therapy for treatment of *P. aeruginosa* infections.[1,2,22]

Aminoglycoside Plus Antipseudomonal β-Lactam

Regimens consisting of an aminoglycoside plus an antipseudomonal β-lactam traditionally have been the most commonly used for empirical treatment of febrile neutropenia, although many such regimens may lack adequate gram-positive activity (see Table 122-3).[1,2] This relative lack of activity remains a concern because of the increasing frequency of gram-positive infections. The choice of aminoglycoside and β-lactam for inclusion in empirical regimens should be based on institutional epidemiology and antimicrobial susceptibility patterns. Similar efficacy is observed with an antipseudomonal β-lactam in combination with an aminoglycoside.[1,2,22]

Combinations of broad-spectrum β-lactams and aminoglycosides may provide synergistic activity against bacteria commonly infecting neutropenic patients. The exact role of synergy in the outcome of febrile neutropenic patients treated with empirical antibiotic therapy is somewhat controversial, particularly in light of the efficacy of single-drug regimens and nephrotoxicity associated with aminoglycosides.[22] Nevertheless, combinations of antibiotics appear to be beneficial in patients with persistent profound neutropenia.

Aminoglycoside toxicity may be a concern in patients receiving these regimens who are already receiving other nephrotoxic drugs, such as cisplatin and cyclosporine. Administration of aminoglycosides in large single daily doses (once-daily dosing) may be as effective, less costly, and no more toxic than conventional dosing methods. Although once-daily aminoglycoside dosing regimens appear to be safe and effective in these patients, standard dosing regimens are recommended for infections where data are not sufficient to recommend once-daily dosing (eg, endocarditis).[1,2]

Fluoroquinolones as a Component of Empirical Regimens

Because the fluoroquinolone antibiotics have broad-spectrum activity (particularly against gram-negative pathogens), rapid bactericidal activity, and favorable pharmacokinetic and toxicity profiles, these agents have been investigated as empirical therapy for febrile neutropenic patients. Ciprofloxacin is the preferred agent for use in this clinical setting because of its relatively better activity against *P. aeruginosa* and more extensive evidence-based support for its use.[1,2] Response rates to quinolone-containing combination regimens are comparable to those obtained with the other regimens described previously.[1,2,4] Ciprofloxacin is not recommended for monotherapy, however, because of its relatively poor activity against gram-positive pathogens, particularly streptococci, and variable response rates in clinical studies.[1,2] Fluoroquinolones should also not be used as empirical therapy in patients who have received quinolones as infection prophylaxis because of the risk of drug resistance.[1,2] Rates of fluoroquinolone resistance are increasing, and streptococcal treatment failures are a concern.[12,13] Although fluoroquinolones are not generally considered first-line empirical therapy, they may be useful as one component of combination regimens in patients with allergies or other contraindications to first-line agents.[1,2]

Empirical Regimens Containing Vancomycin

The inclusion of vancomycin in initial empirical therapy of febrile neutropenic cancer patients is not currently recommended by IDSA 2010 or NCCN 2015 guidelines unless the patient has specific risk factors; however, this remains an ongoing debate. This controversy continues because of the increasing incidence of gram-positive infections in this population, particularly MRSA. One approach is to include vancomycin in the initial empirical antibiotic regimen, thereby providing early effective treatment of possible gram-positive infections. Inclusion of vancomycin in initial empirical regimens may be more appropriate today because of higher rates of MRSA infections as well as aggressive chemotherapy regimens causing significant mucosal damage that increases the risk for streptococcal infections. Decreased mortality from penicillin-resistant viridans streptococcal infections has been observed when vancomycin was included in initial therapy.[1,5,25] A second approach is to withhold vancomycin from initial empirical regimens, later adding the drug if gram-positive organisms are isolated from cultures or if there is clinical deterioration. Support for both these approaches can be found in the medical literature.[1,2,25,26] Prospective studies and multiple meta-analyses have failed to document increased response rates or decreased mortality with the routine addition of vancomycin to initial empirical regimens, provided that vancomycin can be added later as needed.[1,2,25,26] In addition to increased costs of therapy, vancomycin was also associated with increased adverse effects, including nephrotoxicity.[2] Finally, concerns remain regarding selection of resistant gram-positive bacteria such as VRE with excessive vancomycin use.[1,2]

Vancomycin is currently recommended for inclusion in initial empirical regimens only in patients at high risk for gram-positive infection, particularly due to MRSA and coagulase-negative staphylococci (including patients with evidence of infection of central venous catheters and other indwelling lines), high risk for viridans streptococcal infection due to severe mucositis, or pneumonitis or soft tissue infection in hospitals with high rates of MRSA infections.[1,2,7,25] Rates of β-lactam resistance among viridans streptococci range up to 25%.[1,2] Empirical vancomycin use may be justified in institutions using empirical or prophylactic antibiotic regimens without good activity against streptococci (eg, ciprofloxacin) and in patients known to be colonized with MRSA or β-lactam–resistant pneumococci. In patients with preliminary culture results indicating gram-positive infection, empirical vancomycin is appropriate while the susceptibility results are pending. Lastly, empirical use of vancomycin may be recommended in patients with hypotension or other evidence of cardiovascular impairment or sepsis without an identified pathogen.[1,2] If empirical vancomycin therapy is initiated and no evidence of gram-positive infection is found after 48 to 72 hours, the drug should be discontinued.[1,2] Continuing vancomycin when not warranted results in higher costs, more toxicities, and greater risk of development of VRE.[1,2]

Other antimicrobial agents, such as quinupristin–dalfopristin, linezolid, daptomycin, telavancin, and ceftaroline, should be reserved for documented infections caused by multiresistant gram-positive pathogens that are not susceptible to, or are unresponsive to, vancomycin. The role of these drugs in the routine treatment of fever in neutropenic patients is undetermined, and linezolid is associated with risk of myelosuppression.[1,2]

Oral Antibiotic Therapy for Management of Febrile Neutropenia

An individual patient's risk for complications of severe infection determines appropriate antibiotic therapy and the proper setting for administration (see Table 122-3).[1,4,5] Risk stratification is based on several parameters (eg, MASCC score as mentioned above) as well as response to empirical antimicrobial therapy if IV therapy is initially given.[1] Because of the excellent spectrum of activity and favorable pharmacokinetics of currently available oral antibiotics, particularly the fluoroquinolones, oral antibiotics have an important role in the management of selected patients. In patients at low risk for severe or complicated bacterial infection, empirical therapy with broad-spectrum oral antibiotic agents achieves similar patient outcomes as parenteral antibiotics, with response rates of 77% to 95%.[1,2,4,21] This has made possible the treatment of febrile neutropenia in low-risk patients in the outpatient setting. Patients judged to be low risk with reliable follow-up may be appropriate candidates for oral antibiotic therapy administered on an outpatient basis.[1,2,4,21] Ciprofloxacin in combination with amoxicillin–clavulanate (or clindamycin for penicillin-allergic patients) for enhanced gram-positive coverage has been most commonly studied for outpatient therapy in low-risk patients and is recommended by IDSA and NCCN guidelines.[1,2] In general, monotherapy with ciprofloxacin should be avoided due to relatively poor gram-positive activity. Levofloxacin has been used as monotherapy for outpatient treatment of low-risk patients, due to enhanced gram-positive activity; however, this regimen has not been well studied and is not formally recommended by IDSA or NCCN guidelines. If used, only the higher-dose levofloxacin 750 mg regimen should be administered in order to provide adequate activity against organisms such as *P. aeruginosa*.[1,2] Moxifloxacin has been endorsed as an option by NCCN guidelines, however, the lack of *P. aeruginosa* activity warrants special consideration.[2] Careful patient selection obviously is required for such management strategies. Important criteria include patient and provider comfort, a history of medication compliance, good caregiver support, a follow-up plan, and close proximity, prompt access and transportation to appropriate medical care around the clock in the event of failure to respond to outpatient antibiotic therapy. If a patient qualifies for oral therapy based on social and clinical status, the first dose of oral regimen should be given and the patient observed for 4 to 24 hours to ensure tolerance and the patient remains clinically stable. Benefits of oral therapy on an outpatient basis include increased convenience and quality of life for patients and caregivers and reduced exposure to multidrug-resistant institutional pathogens.[1,2] Outpatient therapy of low-risk patients now is common practice in most institutions.

In patients at low risk for severe bacterial infection who were initiated on IV antibiotics, oral antibiotics may play a role in step-down therapy. Carefully selected neutropenic patients may be safely switched from broad-spectrum parenteral therapy to oral antibiotic regimens (eg, ciprofloxacin plus amoxicillin–clavulanate) with response rates comparable to patients remaining on IV therapy.[1,21] Patient selection criteria generally include defervescence within 72 hours of initiation of parenteral therapy, hemodynamic stability, absence of positive cultures or a discernible site of infection, and ability to take oral medications. Many of these patients are able to complete their course of therapy at home.[1,2,21] Changing parenteral antimicrobials to oral regimens in carefully selected patients is now relatively common practice and allows for less expensive hospitalizations and earlier patient discharges.

Antimicrobial Therapy After Initiation of Empirical Therapy

6 After initiation of empirical antimicrobial therapy (Table 122-4), judicious assessment of febrile neutropenic cancer patients is mandatory to evaluate response, clinical status, laboratory data, and potential need for therapy adjustments. After 2 to 4 days of empirical antimicrobial therapy, the clinical status and culture results of febrile neutropenic patients should be reevaluated to determine whether therapeutic modifications are necessary (Fig. 122-2). Modifications of antimicrobial therapy should be based on clinical and laboratory data; antibiotic therapy should be optimized based on culture results. However, during periods of neutropenia, patients generally should continue to receive broad-spectrum therapy because of risk of secondary infections or breakthrough bacteremias when antimicrobial coverage is too narrow.[1,2] The treatment duration for a documented infection should be appropriate for the particular organism and site, and should continue for at least the duration of neutropenia (until ANC greater than or equal to 500 cells/mm^3 [greater than or equal to 0.5×10^9/L]) or longer if clinically necessary.

In patients who become afebrile after 2 to 4 days of therapy with no infection identified, it is generally optimal to continue antibiotic therapy until neutropenia has resolved (ANC greater than or equal to 500 cells/mm^3 [greater than or equal to 0.5×10^9/L]). Some clinicians switch therapy to an oral regimen (eg, ciprofloxacin plus amoxicillin–clavulanate) after 2 days of IV therapy in low-risk patients who become afebrile and have no evidence of infection. In high-risk patients, parenteral antibiotic regimens should be continued until resolution of neutropenia.[1,2] However, in afebrile patients with prolonged neutropenia but no signs or symptoms of infection, consideration can be given to discontinuing antibiotic therapy or switching to fluoroquinolone prophylaxis (discussed in "Prophylaxis of Infections in Neutropenic Cancer Patients" below), provided that patients can be observed carefully and have ready access to medical care.

The optimal management of patients who remain febrile in the absence of microbiologic or clinical documentation of infection remains highly controversial. Persistently febrile patients should be evaluated carefully, but modifications generally are not made to initial antimicrobial regimens within the first 2 to 4 days of therapy unless there is evidence of clinical deterioration (see Fig. 122-1).[1,2,4] It is important to note that the persistence of fever does not necessarily mean failure of a given antimicrobial regimen; up to 25% of neutropenic patients have fever due to noninfectious causes.[6] This is particularly true if patients are otherwise clinically stable. Fever after 2 or more days of antibiotic therapy can be due to a number of causes, including nonbacterial infection, resistant bacterial infection or infection slow to respond to therapy, emergence of a secondary infection, inadequate drug concentrations, drug fever, fever at an avascular site (eg, catheter infection or abscess), or noninfectious causes such as tumor or administration of blood products.[1,2,4] Patients with documented infection who are receiving appropriate antimicrobial therapy (based on in vitro susceptibility tests) often remain febrile until resolution of neutropenia occurs. Therefore, the same antibiotic regimen can be continued in patients who remain febrile despite 2 to 4 days of antibiotic therapy but are otherwise clinically stable, especially if neutropenia is expected to resolve within 1 week. However, antibiotic regimens may require modification in patients experiencing toxicities (Table 122-5) as well as in patients with evidence of progressive disease, clinical instability, or documentation of an organism not covered by the initial regimen.[1,2,4] If not already part of the regimen, vancomycin should be considered as warranted by clinical and laboratory findings. However, if vancomycin was included in the initial empirical regimen and the patient is still febrile after 2 to 3 days of therapy without isolating a gram-positive pathogen, discontinuation of vancomycin should be considered to reduce the risk of toxicities or resistance.[1,2]

TABLE 122-4 Drug Dosing Table[a]

Drug	Brand Name	Initial Dose	Usual Range	Special Population Dose	Other
Antibacterial Agents					
Amoxicillin–clavulanate	Augmentin®	875 mg orally two times daily	875 mg orally two times daily		In combination with ciprofloxacin for outpatient treatment
Ceftazidime	Fortaz®	2 g IV every 8 hours	1-2 g IV every 8 hours		
Ceftazidime-avibactam	Avycaz®	2.5 g IV every 8 hours	2.5 g IV every 8 hours		Not studied in febrile neutropenia, but spectrum is appropriate if high rates of MDR gram-negative bacteria (esp. CRE)
Cefepime	Maxipime®	2 g IV every 12 hours	1-2 g IV every 12 hours		
Ceftaroline	Teflaro®	600 mg IV every 12 hours	600 mg IV every 12 hours		Activity against methicillin-resistant *S. aureus*
Ceftolozane-tazobactam	Zerbaxa®	1.5 g IV every 8 hours	1.5 g IV every 8 hours		Not studied in febrile neutropenia, but spectrum is appropriate if high rates of MDR gram-negative bacteria
Piperacillin–tazobactam	Zosyn®	4.5 g IV every 6 hours	3.375-4.5 g IV every 6 hours		
Imipenem–cilastatin	Primaxin®	500 mg IV every 6 hours	250-500 mg IV every 6 hours		
Meropenem	Merrem®	1 g IV every 8 hours	1 g IV every 8 hours		
Doripenem	Doribax®	500 mg IV every 8 hours	500 mg IV every 8 hours		
Tobramycin	Nebcin®	Traditional: 2 mg/kg loading dose, followed by 1.5 mg/kg IV every 8 hours. Alternative: 5-7 mg/kg IV once daily	Traditional dosing: Guided by measured serum concentrations		
Gentamicin	Garamycin®	Traditional: 2 mg/kg loading dose, followed by 1.5 mg/kg IV every 8 hours. Alternative: 5-7 mg/kg IV once daily	Traditional dosing: Guided by measured serum concentrations		
Amikacin	Amikin®	Traditional: 7.5 mg/kg IV every 12 hours. Alternative: 15-20 mg/kg IV once daily	Traditional dosing: Guided by measured serum concentrations		
Ciprofloxacin	Cipro®	400 mg IV every 8 hours	400 mg IV every 8-12 hours	Outpatient treatment: 750 mg PO every 12 hours	May be given orally in low-risk patients in combination with amoxicillin-clavulanate
Levofloxacin	Levaquin®	750 mg IV once daily	500-750 mg IV once daily	Outpatient treatment: 750 mg PO once daily	May be given orally in low-risk patients
Moxifloxacin	Avelox®	400 mg IV/PO once daily	400 mg IV/PO once daily	Outpatient treatment: 400 mg PO once daily	For select outpatient use, lacks *P. aeruginosa* activity
Vancomycin	Vancocin®	30–40 mg/kg/day IV in two divided doses	Dosing guided by serum concentrations to achieve trough of 15-20 mg/L		For methicillin-resistant *S. aureus* infection
Nafcillin	Nafcil®	2 g IV every 6 hours	1-2 g IV every 4-6 hours		For methicillin-susceptible *S. aureus* infection
Daptomycin	Cubicin®	Skin/soft tissue infections: 4 mg/kg IV once daily; bacteremia: 6 mg/kg IV once daily	Skin/soft tissue infections: 4 mg/kg IV once daily; bacteremia: 6 mg/kg IV once daily		For infection (esp. bacteremia) due to methicillin-resistant *S. aureus*, vancomycin-resistant enterococci

(continued)

TABLE 122-4 Drug Dosing Table[a] (*Continued*)

Drug	Brand Name	Initial Dose	Usual Range	Special Population Dose	Other
Linezolid	Zyvox®	600 mg IV or orally every 12 hours	600 mg IV or orally every 12 hours		For infection due to vancomycin-resistant enterococci
Ampicillin	Omnipen®, Polycillin®, Principen®	2 g IV every 4 hours	1-2 g IV every 4-6 hours		In combination with gentamicin for *Listeria* infection
Erythromycin	E-mycin®, Erythrocin®	1 g IV every 6 hours	1-2 g IV every 4-6 hours		For *Legionella* infection
Antifungal Agents					
Clotrimazole	Mycelex Troche®	10 mg orally five times daily	10 mg orally five times daily		Administered as oral troche; dissolve in mouth
Nystatin	Nystatin Oral®	100,000 units orally every 6 hours	100,000 units orally every 4-6 hours		Administered as suspension; swish and swallow
Fluconazole	Diflucan®	800 mg IV or orally once, then 400 mg IV or orally once daily	100-800 mg IV or orally once daily	Prophylaxis of *Candida* infection: 400 mg IV or orally once daily	
Itraconazole	Sporanox®	200 mg orally twice daily	200-400 mg/day orally divided twice daily	Prophylaxis of *Candida* infection: 200 mg orally twice daily	Therapeutic drug monitoring recommended
Voriconazole	Vfend®	6 mg/kg IV every 12 hours for two doses, then 4 mg/kg IV every 12 hours	4 mg/kg IV or 200 mg orally every 12 hours	Prophylaxis in high-risk patients: 200 mg orally twice daily	Therapeutic drug monitoring recommended
Posaconazole	Noxafil®	Suspension: 800 mg orally per day in two to four divided doses Oral DR or IV: 300 mg every 12 hours × 2 doses, then 300 mg daily	Suspension: 400 mg orally two times daily Oral DR or IV: 300 mg every 12 hours × 2 doses then 300 mg daily	Prophylaxis in high-risk patients: 200 mg orally three times daily	DR formulation has improved bioavailability, administered with food. Suspension: administer with full meal or enteral nutritional supplements Therapeutic drug monitoring recommended
Isavuconazonium	Cresemba®	372 mg IV/PO every 8 hours × 6 doses, then 372 mg daily	372 mg IV/PO every 8 hours × 6 doses, then 372 mg daily		Limited clinical experience
Lipid-associated amphotericin B (LAMB)	AmBisome®, Abelcet®	3-5 mg/kg IV once daily	3-5 mg/kg IV once daily	Prophylaxis in high-risk patients: 1 mg/kg IV once daily	
5-Flucytosine	Ancobon®	25 mg/kg/day orally four times daily	25 mg/kg/day orally four times daily		In combination with LAMB for cryptococcal meningitis. Therapeutic drug monitoring recommended
Caspofungin	Cancidas®	70 mg IV once, then 50 mg IV once daily	50 mg IV once daily		
Micafungin	Mycamine®	100 mg IV once daily	100 mg IV once daily	Prophylaxis in high-risk patients: 50 mg IV once daily	
Anidulafungin	Eraxis®	200 mg IV once, then 100 mg IV once daily	100 mg IV once daily		
Antiviral Agents					
Acyclovir	Zovirax®	5 mg/kg IV every 8 hours, or 800 mg orally five times daily	5-10 mg/kg IV every 8 hours, or 800 mg orally two to five times daily	Prophylaxis of HSV or VZV: 800-1,600 mg orally twice daily; CMV prophylaxis in allogeneic HSCT: 800 mg orally four times daily; HSV or VZV encephalitis: 10mg/kg IV every 8 hours	

(*continued*)

TABLE 122-4 Drug Dosing Table[a] (*Continued*)

Drug	Brand Name	Initial Dose	Usual Range	Special Population Dose	Other
Valacyclovir	Valtrex®	1 g orally three times daily	1 g orally three times daily	Prophylaxis of HSV or VZV: 500 mg orally two or three times daily; CMV prophylaxis in allogeneic HSCT: 2 g orally four times daily	
Ganciclovir	Cytovene®	CMV treatment or preemptive therapy: 5 mg/kg IV daily for 2 weeks	CMV treatment or preemptive therapy: After first 2 weeks, 5-6 mg/kg IV daily 5 days/wk	CMV prophylaxis: 5-6 mg/kg IV daily 5 days/wk	
Valganciclovir	Valcyte®	CMV preemptive therapy: 900 mg orally twice daily for 2 weeks	CMV preemptive therapy: After first 2 weeks, 900 mg orally daily	CMV prophylaxis: 900 mg orally daily	
Foscarnet	Foscavir®	CMV treatment: 90 mg/kg IV every 12 hours for 2 weeks; CMV preemptive therapy: 60 mg/kg IV every 12 hours for 2 weeks	CMV treatment: after first 2 weeks, 120 mg/kg IV daily; CMV preemptive therapy: after first 2 weeks, 90 mg/kg IV daily 5 days/wk	CMV prophylaxis: 60 mg/kg IV two or three times daily for 7 days, then 90-120 mg/kg IV daily	
CMV hyperimmune globulin	Cytogam®	400 mg/kg IV every other day for three to five doses	400 mg/kg IV every other day for three to five doses		Consider as adjunct to ganciclovir or foscarnet for treatment of CMV pneumonia; IVIG considered equally effective
Antiprotozoal/Antiparasitic Agents					
Trimethoprim–sulfamethoxazole	Bactrim®, Cotrimoxazole®	15-20 mg/kg/day IV divided every 6 hours[b]	15-20 mg/kg/day IV divided every 6 hours[b]	Prophylaxis of *P. jiroveci*: 160 mg/800 mg orally daily or three times per week	
Atovaquone	Mepron®	750 mg orally every 12 hours	750 mg orally every 12 hours		
Pentamidine	Pentam®	4 mg/kg IV once daily	4 mg/kg IV once daily		
Clindamycin	Cleocin®	450-600 mg orally every 6 hours	450-600 mg orally every 6 hours		In combination with primaquine for *P. jiroveci*, or with pyrimethamine for toxoplasmosis
Primaquine	Aralen® Primaquine®	15 mg orally once daily	15 mg orally once daily		In combination with clindamycin for *P. jiroveci*
Dapsone	Dapsone®	100 mg orally once daily	100 mg orally once daily		In combination with trimethoprim for *P. jiroveci*
Trimethoprim	Triprim®	15-20 mg/kg/day orally divided every 6 hours	15-20 mg/kg/day orally divided every 6 hours		In combination with dapsone for *P. jiroveci*
Pyrimethamine	Daraprim®	50 mg orally once daily[c]	50-100 mg orally once daily[c]		In combination with sulfadiazine for toxoplasmosis
Sulfadiazine	Sulfadiazine®	1 g orally every 6 hours	1 g orally every 4-6 hours		In combination with pyrimethamine for toxoplasmosis
Thiabendazole	Mintezol®	25 mg/kg orally every 12 hours	25 mg/kg orally every 12 hours (maximum 3 g/day)		For *Strongyloides* and other intestinal worm infections

CMV, cytomegalovirus; CRE, carbapenem-resistant Enterobacteriaceae; DR, delayed-release; HSV, herpes simplex virus; MDR, multidrug-resistant; VZV, varicella zoster virus.

[a]Dosing guidelines in patients with normal renal and hepatic function.

[b]Based on the trimethoprim component of the combination.

[c]Folinic acid (5-10 mg/day) often recommended in conjunction with pyrimethamine-containing regimens for prevention of bone marrow toxicity.

TABLE 122-5 Drug Monitoring of Selected Antimicrobials for Febrile Neutropenia, HSCT, and SOT

Drug	Adverse Reaction	Monitoring Parameters	Comments
Antibaterial Agents			
Aminoglycosides (Tobramycin, Gentamicin, Amikacin)	Nephrotoxicity	Serum creatinine, urine output, serum concentrations	Extended-interval ("once daily") dosing potentially associated with less renal toxicity, similar efficacy to traditional dosing. Goal trough concentration <1 mcg/mL (mg/L; or <2 µmol/L) during extended-interval dosing
Imipenem–cilastatin	CNS toxicities, seizures	Serum creatinine, mental status, CNS function	Increased incidence with higher dose, failure to adjust dose/interval for reduced renal function. Increased risk compared to meropenem or doripenem
Linezolid	Myelosuppression, thrombocytopenia, optic/peripheral neuropathy, serotonin syndrome	CBC, vision changes, serum lactate, heart rate, blood pressure, temperature, myoclonus	Myelosuppression and neuropathy more common with prolonged use. Short course unlikely to affect marrow recovery in HSCT. Weak MAO inhibitor, serotonin syndrome possible with other serotonergic drugs such as SSRIs and SNRIs
Nafcillin	Interstitial nephritis	Serum creatinine, urine output	Reversible, requires switch to alternative β-lactam
Vancomycin	Nephrotoxicity, infusion reactions	Serum creatinine, urine output, blood pressure, heart rate, serum concentrations	Dose adjustment required for renal dysfunction. Pretreatment and slow infusion may decrease incidence of infusion reaction. Goal trough concentration 15-20 mcg/mL (mg/L; 10-14 µmol/L) for serious infections
Antifungal Agents			
Amphotericin B (lipid-associated)	Nephrotoxicity, hepatotoxicity, electrolyte disturbances, infusion reactions	Serum creatinine, electrolytes, LFTs, blood pressure, heart rate	Liposomal preparations associated with less renal toxicity, similar efficacy to standard preparation. Electrolyte disturbances occur before creatinine alterations. Pretreatment and slow infusion may decrease incidence of infusion reaction
5-Flucytosine	Myelosuppression, GI toxicities	CBC, GI symptoms, serum creatinine, 5-flucytosine serum concentrations	Dose adjustment required for renal dysfunction. Goal serum concentrations are peak <100 mcg/mL (<775 µmol/L) and trough 20-40 mcg/mL (155-310 µmol/L)
Posaconazole	Hepatotoxicity, rash; interactions with CYP450 3A4	LFTs, skin, posaconazole serum concentrations	Poor absorption with suspension, goals of >1 mcg/mL (>1.4 µmol/L) for treatment and >0.7 mcg/mL (>1 µmol/L) for prophylaxis. Parenteral formulation contains SBECD, not recommended for patients with CrCL<50 mL/min (<0.83 mL/s). Multiple interactions with drugs metabolized by CYP 3A4, including immunosuppressants; close monitoring needed.
Voriconazole	Mental status changes, headache, hallucinations, visual disturbances, hepatotoxicity, QTc prolongation; interactions with CYP450 2C9, 2C19, and 3A4	Mental status, visual function, LFTs, ECG, voriconazole serum concentrations	Mental status/visual changes associated with elevated troughs >5.5 mcg/mL (>16 µmol/L); goal trough 1-5.5 mcg/mL (3-16 µmol/L) for treatment and prophylaxis, target trough of >2 mcg/ml (>6 µmol/L) in disease with poor prognosis. Parenteral formulation contains SBECD, not recommended for patients with CrCL<50 mL/min (<0.83 mL/s). Multiple interactions with drugs metabolized by CYP enzymes, including immunosuppressants; close monitoring needed
Antiviral Agents			
Foscarnet	Nephrotoxicity, hypocalcemia	Serum creatinine, electrolytes	IV hydration prior to administration. Dose adjustment required for renal dysfunction
Ganciclovir, valganciclovir	Myelosuppression, thrombocytopenia	CBC, serum creatinine	Dose adjustment required for renal dysfunction
Antiprotozoal/Antiparasitic Agents			
Dapsone	Hemolytic anemia, hypersensitivity (fever, jaundice, eosinophilia), peripheral neuropathy	CBC, bilirubin, LFTs, muscle strength, G6PD testing before use	Higher incidence of hemolytic anemia in G6PD-deficient patients
Pentamidine (IV)	Nephrotoxicity, leukopenia, hypotension, QTc prolongation, pancreatitis, hypo/hyperglycemia	Serum creatinine, serum blood glucose, blood urea nitrogen, CBC, blood pressure, heart rate; ECG	Adequate hydration recommended
Primaquine	Hemolytic anemia	CBC, bilirubin, G6PD testing before use	Avoid use in G6PD-deficient patients (hemolytic anemia)
Pyrimethamine	Bone marrow suppression	CBC	Folinic acid 5-10 mg/day often used for prevention of bone marrow toxicity
Trimethoprim–sulfamethoxazole	Myelosuppression, hyperkalemia, rash	Serum creatinine, electrolytes, CBC, skin	Dose adjustment required for renal dysfunction

CBC, complete blood count; ECG, electrocardiogram; G6PD, glucose-6-phosphate dehydrogenase; HSCT; hematopoietic stem cell transplantation; LFT, liver function test; MAO, monoamine oxidase; PFT, pulmonary function test; QTc, corrected Q-T interval; SBECD, sulfobutylether-β-cyclodextrin; SOT, solid-organ transplantation; SSNRI, selective serotonin–norepinephrine reuptake inhibitor; SSRI, selective serotonin reuptake inhibitor.

Therapeutic drug monitoring recommendations from reference 33.

Initiation of Antifungal Therapy

Neutropenic patients who remain febrile despite more than 4 to 7 days of broad-spectrum antibiotic therapy are candidates for antifungal therapy. A high percentage of febrile patients who die during prolonged neutropenia have evidence of invasive fungal infection on autopsy, even though many had no evidence of fungal disease before death.[17] Persistence of fever or development of a new fever during broad-spectrum antibiotic therapy may indicate the presence of a fungal infection, most commonly due to *Candida* or *Aspergillus* spp.[10,11,17] Blood cultures are positive in fewer than 50% of neutropenic patients with invasive fungal infections.[10,17] Sensitivity and specificity of fungal galactomannan assay may vary and should only be used when *Aspergillus* is suspected. Rapid, sensitive diagnostic tests for fungi such as serum β-D-glucan or fungal DNA assay are not yet in common usage, and waiting for isolation of fungal organisms is associated with high morbidity and mortality. The empirical addition of antifungal therapy is thus justified in this clinical setting.[1,2] Therefore, empirical antifungal therapy should be initiated after 4 to 7 days of broad-spectrum antibiotic therapy in persistently febrile patients if the duration of neutropenia is expected to be greater than 1 week. Administered doses must be adequate to treat undiagnosed fungal infection and prevent fungal superinfection in high-risk febrile neutropenic patients.[1,2,18]

Evidence-based recommendations from published guidelines for management of suspected or documented fungal infections in neutropenic patients are summarized in Table 122-2.[18,20] Empirical coverage for both *Candida* spp. and *Aspergillus* should be considered because these organisms are responsible for more than 90% of fungal infections in neutropenic cancer patients.[5,10,11,17] *Aspergillus* is particularly common in patients with hematologic malignancies and in patients with hematologic malignancies undergoing HSCT; therefore, amphotericin B traditionally has been preferred for these patients.[1,2,27] In the setting of febrile neutropenia, lipid-associated amphotericin B (LAMB) products are similar in efficacy to conventional amphotericin B while causing fewer toxicities. LAMB products are thus almost exclusively recommended over conventional amphotericin B despite the significantly higher cost without clear improvement in efficacy.[1,2,18,20,27] Although the use of higher doses of LAMB has been advocated in an effort to improve efficacy, lower doses (3 mg/kg) of liposomal amphotericin B may be as efficacious as higher doses (10 mg/kg) with lower cost and fewer toxicities.[2]

The azole compounds are also used in the management of febrile neutropenia.[1,2,18,20] Despite the increased cost and toxicities of LAMB, concerns regarding the emergence of *Candida* strains with decreased azole susceptibility and unclear efficacy advantages relative to other agents have prevented these agents from replacing amphotericin B as the gold standard in persistently febrile neutropenic patients.[20,27] Fluconazole has good efficacy against *C. albicans* but lacks activity against molds such as *Aspergillus*. The use of fluconazole as an alternative to amphotericin B for empirical antifungal therapy is thus perhaps most appropriate in hospitals in which infections due to *Aspergillus* or non-*albicans* strains of *Candida* are not common.[1,2,27] If fluconazole is used as antifungal prophylaxis in cancer patients, it should not be included in empirical antifungal regimens. Voriconazole is effective in the treatment of documented invasive fungal infections and is recommended as a reliable option for febrile neutropenia. Despite failing to meet noninferiority criteria when compared against LAMB for empiric therapy in febrile neutropenic patients, voriconazole is a preferred agent for invasive aspergillosis (especially pulmonary) due to improved survival and less toxicity when compared to amphotericin B.[1,2,20,27-31] Itraconazole has similar efficacy as amphotericin B, with fewer toxicities. However, current lack of a parenteral dosage form, sometimes erratic oral absorption, numerous potential drug–drug interactions, and availability of many other antifungal options limit the use of itraconazole for empiric therapy.[29,30] Posaconazole has extended activity against some Mucorales and rare molds in addition to *Candida* and *Aspergillus*, but is only approved for prophylaxis of fungal infections in neutropenic patients. The improved bioavailability of the delayed-release tablets and availability of a parenteral dosage form make posaconazole an attractive option, however, clinical data remain limited.[2] Isavuconazonium, the prodrug of isavuconazole, is approved for the treatment of invasive aspergillosis and mucormycosis with overall activity generally comparable to voriconazole and posaconazole. Although not addressed by recent clinical guidelines, isavuconazonium showed mortality and treatment success similar to voriconazole in a largely neutropenic patient population with hematologic malignancies and suspected invasive fungal infections including a subgroup of proven or probable aspergillosis.[32] Therapeutic drug monitoring has been recommended for some azole antifungals given potential for interpatient variability, therapeutic failure associated with subtherapeutic concentrations, and toxicities associated with supratherapeutic concentrations (Table 122-5).[2,33]

The echinocandin antifungals (caspofungin, micafungin, and anidulafungin) are attractive agents for treatment of febrile neutropenia because of their broad spectrum of antifungal activity and favorable adverse effect profiles. Caspofungin is as effective as, and also generally better tolerated than, liposomal amphotericin B for empirical treatment of neutropenic patients with persistent fever.[1,2,30] Therefore, caspofungin is considered an appropriate alternative to LAMB and voriconazole.[1,2,18,20,27,30] Micafungin and anidulafungin have not been as well studied specifically in this capacity; however, most experts consider them likely as effective.[1,2,18,20]

Clinical **Controversy...**

The optimal choice of antifungal agents for treatment of invasive fungal infections in immunocompromised patients (neutropenic patients as well as those undergoing HSCT and SOT) is currently not well defined. Newer agents such as posaconazole and isavuconazonium (isazuconazole) have excellent, broad-spectrum *in vitro* activity against many yeasts and fungi. These agents are also available in both oral and intravenous dosage forms with good bioavailability of the oral products, and their adverse effect and toxicity profiles are favorable compared to other available agents. However, their labeled indications are relatively narrow and clinical data in the treatment of invasive disease caused by *Aspergillus*, *Mucor*, and other difficult pathogens are still relatively limited compared to agents such as voriconazole and LAMB which have been much more extensively used over longer periods of time. Although attractive for more routine clinical use, the optimal role of newer agents remains to be defined.

Initiation of Antiviral Therapy

Febrile neutropenic patients with vesicular or ulcerative skin or mucosal lesions should be evaluated carefully for infection due to HSV or varicella-zoster virus (VZV). Mucosal lesions from viral infections provide a portal of entry for bacteria and fungi during periods of immunosuppression. If viral infection is presumed or documented, neutropenic patients should receive aggressive antiviral therapy to aid healing of primary lesions and prevent disseminated disease. Acyclovir traditionally has been used in this population. However, the newer antivirals valacyclovir and famciclovir have better oral absorption and more convenient dosing schedules. Routine use of antiviral agents in the management of patients without mucosal lesions or other evidence of viral infection generally is not recommended.[1,2] Treatment recommendations for viral infections are given in Table 122-6.

TABLE 122-6 Infectious Complications During Neutropenia, and After Hematopoietic Stem Cell and Solid-Organ Transplantation: Syndromes of Disease and Treatment Guidelines

Pathogen	Syndromes of Disease	Recommended Treatment
Bacterial		
Gram-negative aerobic bacilli (Enterobacteriaceae, *Pseudomonas aeruginosa*, *Haemophilus influenzae*)	Blood, urinary tract, pulmonary, abdomen	*Empiric:* Ceftazidime + aminoglycoside,[a,b] cefepime + aminoglycoside[a,b]; piperacillin–tazobactam; imipenem–cilastatin ± aminoglycoside[a,b] *Definitive:* According to culture and sensitivity results
Gram-positive cocci (*Staphylococcus aureus*, *Staphylococcus epidermidis*, *Streptococcus pneumoniae*, *Enterococcus faecalis*)	Skin, blood, urinary tract, pulmonary, abdomen	*Empiric:* Nafcillin; vancomycin *Definitive:* According to culture and sensitivity results
Legionella spp.	Pulmonary	Erythromycin; ciprofloxacin; levofloxacin
Listeria monocytogenes	CNS	Ampicillin with gentamicin[a]; trimethoprim–sulfamethoxazole
Nocardia spp.	Skin, pulmonary, CNS	Sulfadiazine; trimethoprim–sulfamethoxazole
Fungal		
Candida spp.[c]	Blood, urinary tract, mucous membranes, skin, disseminated disease	Clotrimazole; nystatin; fluconazole; itraconazole; amphotericin B ± 5-flucytosine; lipid-associated amphotericin B (LAMB); caspofungin; micafungin; anidulafungin
Aspergillus spp.[d]	Skin, pulmonary, CNS	Voriconazole; LAMB; caspofungin; micafungin; posaconazole; itraconazole
Cryptococcus neoformans	Skin, pulmonary, CNS	LAMB + 5-flucytosine; fluconazole
Mucorales (*Mucor*)	Rhinocerebral disease	LAMB; posaconazole
Viral		
Herpes simplex virus	Skin, CNS, mucous membranes, pulmonary	Acyclovir; foscarnet
Human herpesvirus-6	CNS, hepatic, bone marrow	Ganciclovir; foscarnet
Cytomegalovirus	Pulmonary, blood, urinary tract, GI tract	Ganciclovir; foscarnet; immunoglobulin
Varicella-zoster virus	Skin, disseminated disease	Acyclovir; foscarnet
Epstein–Barr virus	Lymphoproliferative disease	Rituximab
Papovaviruses (BK, JC)	Skin, CNS	No effective treatment
Protozoal/Parasitic		
Pneumocystis jiroveci	Pulmonary	Trimethoprim–sulfamethoxazole; atovaquone; pentamidine; dapsone + trimethoprim; clindamycin + primaquine
Toxoplasma gondii	CNS	Pyrimethamine + sulfadiazine; pyrimethamine + clindamycin
Strongyloides stercoralis	Pulmonary, CNS	Thiabendazole

[a]Choice of specific agent determined according to institutional susceptibilities to individual drugs.

[b]For penicillin-allergic adults, use aztreonam or ciprofloxacin + an aminoglycoside.

[c]Refer to the Clinical Practice Guidelines of the Infectious Diseases Society of America (*reference 18*) for selection and dosing of antifungal agents for specific infections.

[d]Refer to the Clinical Practice Guidelines by the Infectious Diseases Society of America (*reference 20*) for selection and dosing of antifungal agents for specific infections.

Duration of Antimicrobial Therapy

7 The optimal duration of antimicrobial therapy in the neutropenic cancer patient remains controversial. Decisions regarding discontinuation of empirical antimicrobial therapy often are more difficult and complex than those regarding initiation of therapy (see Fig. 122-1). One point on which experts agree, however, is that the most important determinant of the total duration of antibiotic therapy is the patient's ANC.[1,2] If ANC is greater than or equal to 500 cells/mm^3 (greater than or equal to 0.5×10^9/L) for two consecutive days, if the patient is afebrile and clinically stable for 48 hours or more, and if no pathogen has been isolated, then antibiotics can be discontinued. Some clinicians advocate that patients with ANC less than 500 cells/mm^3 (0.5×10^9/L) be maintained on antibiotic therapy until resolution of neutropenia, even if they are afebrile. However, prolonged antibiotic use has been associated with superinfections resulting from resistant bacteria and fungi and increases the risk of antibiotic-related toxicities.[1,2] If low-risk patients are stable clinically with negative cultures but the ANC still is less than 500 cells/mm^3 (0.5×10^9/L) antibiotics may be discontinued after a total of 5 to 7 afebrile days. However, patients with profound neutropenia (ANC greater than 100 cells/mm^3 [greater than 0.1×10^9/L]), mucosal lesions, or unstable vital signs or other risk factors should continue to receive antibiotics until ANC has increased greater than or equal to 500 cells/mm^3 (greater than or equal to 0.5×10^9/L) and the patient is stable clinically.[1,2]

Patients who are persistently neutropenic and febrile, but who are stable clinically with no active site of infection, often can be successfully discontinued from antimicrobials after at least 2 weeks of therapy. However, these patients must be monitored carefully because reinstitution of antibiotics may be necessary.[1,2] An alternative approach is to place these patients on antimicrobial prophylaxis (discussed in "Prophylaxis of Infections in Neutropenic Cancer Patients" below). Patients with documented infections should receive antimicrobial therapy until the infecting organism is eradicated and signs and symptoms of infection have resolved (at least 10-14 days of therapy).

Consensus guidelines provide useful information regarding the management of febrile episodes in cancer patients with neutropenia.[1,2] However, therapy (including initial empirical regimens, modifications, and duration of treatment) must be individualized based on individual patient parameters and response to therapy.

Colony-Stimulating Factors

Because resolution of neutropenia is arguably the most important determinant of patient outcome from both febrile episodes and documented infections, numerous studies have evaluated hematopoietic colony-stimulating factors (CSFs) (sargramostim [granulocyte-macrophage colony-stimulating factor] and filgrastim [granulocyte colony-stimulating factor]) as adjunct therapy to antimicrobial treatment of febrile neutropenic cancer patients. A meta-analysis found that use of CSFs is associated with reduced total duration and severity of chemotherapy-related neutropenia, reduced duration of antibiotic use, fewer hospitalizations, and decreased hospital length of stay.[34] However, this meta-analysis failed to demonstrate a benefit of CSFs in relation to important outcomes such as decreased overall mortality or infection-related mortality.[34] Evidence-based guidelines from the IDSA, American Society of Clinical Oncology (ASCO), and the NCCN recommend that CSFs should not be routinely initiated in patients with uncomplicated fever and neutropenia.[1,2,35,36] However, CSFs should be considered in patients who are at high risk for infection-associated complications, or who have factors that are predictive of poor clinical outcomes.[2,35,36] These factors are summarized in Table 122-7. Patients with prolonged neutropenia and documented severe infections who are not responding to appropriate antimicrobial therapy may also benefit from treatment with CSFs.[35,36] Clinical judgment must be exercised in determining which patients may benefit from judicious use of these expensive agents.

Direct transfusion of neutrophils has also been studied for treatment of febrile neutropenia or documented infections.[3,37] Routine use of neutrophil transfusions is not generally supported by data demonstrating improved clinical outcomes. However, use may be considered in patients with profound prolonged neutropenia with severe documented infections and in whom causative organisms have not been eradicated with appropriate antimicrobial therapy in combination with CSFs.[2] At present, the use of neutrophil transfusions is not recommended for routine management of febrile neutropenic patients.[2]

TABLE 122-7 Recommendations for Use of Colony-Stimulating Factors in the Management of Neutropenic Cancer Patients and Those Undergoing Hematopoietic Stem Cell Transplantation

A Primary prophylaxis of febrile neutropenia

1. Colony-stimulating factors (CSFs) (filgrastim, pegfilgrastim, or sargramostim) may be considered in patients who have a high risk of febrile neutropenia (>20% incidence) based on myelotoxicity of the planned chemotherapy regimen
2. When risk of febrile neutropenia is 10%-20%, CSFs may be considered in the presence of certain patient and clinical factors predisposing to increased complications from prolonged neutropenia, including: patient age >65 years; poor performance status; extensive prior treatment including large radiation ports; administration of combined chemoradiotherapy; cytopenias due to bone marrow involvement by tumor; poor nutritional status; presence of open wounds or active infections; previous surgery; poor renal function; liver dysfunction, particularly when evidenced by increased bilirubin; and lack of antibiotic prophylaxis

B Secondary prophylaxis of febrile neutropenia

1. CSFs (filgrastim, pegfilgrastim, or sargramostim) recommended for patients who experienced neutropenic complications from prior cycles of chemotherapy, and in which a reduced dose may compromise disease-free or overall survival or treatment outcome

C Therapeutic use in febrile neutropenia

1. CSFs should not be routinely used for patients with neutropenia who are afebrile
2. CSFs (filgrastim or sargramostim only) may be considered in patients with febrile neutropenia who are at high risk for infection-associated complications, or who have prognostic factors that are predictive of poor clinical outcomes, including: profound neutropenia (absolute neutrophil count <100 cells/mm^3 [<0.1 × 10^9/L]); expected prolonged period of neutropenia (>10 days); patient age >65 years; uncontrolled primary disease; sepsis syndrome, or severe infection manifest by hypotension and multiorgan dysfunction; pneumonia; invasive fungal infection; other clinically documented infection; hospitalized at the time of the development of fever; or severe complications during previous episode of febrile neutropenia

D Reduction in duration of neutropenia in HSCT

1. CSFs are recommended to mobilize peripheral-blood progenitor cells (PBPC) prior to chemotherapy and to reduce the duration of neutropenia after autologous PBPC transplantation

Data from references 2, 35, and 36.

Prophylaxis of Infections in Neutropenic Cancer Patients

8 Owing to the potential morbidity and mortality of infections in neutropenic cancer patients, environmental modifications and prophylactic antimicrobial regimens have been implemented to prevent these complications. The overall goal of antimicrobial prophylaxis in cancer patients is to decrease the number and severity of systemic infections during prolonged periods of neutropenia. As with febrile neutropenia, patient risk factors for development of infection and complications should be assessed prior to initiation of prophylaxis (Table 122-8).

General Measures

Because approximately 50% of pathogens infecting neutropenic cancer patients are acquired in the hospital, reducing acquisition of infectious organisms from the environment is a basic component in controlling nosocomial infections.[1,2,5] Neutropenic patients should be placed in reverse isolation (isolation to protect patients from contracting infections after exposure to others) with standard barrier precautions, and strict adherence to infection control guidelines by hospital personnel.[1,2,5] Plants and fresh or dried flowers are usually prohibited as part of standard neutropenic precautions in order to minimize risk of exposure to pathogenic bacteria. Proper meticulous handwashing by hospital personnel is a simple yet very effective infection control measure. Most neutropenic patients do not require specific room ventilation; however, HSCT recipients should be placed in a private positive-pressure room with greater than 12 air exchanges per hour and HEPA filtration.[1,2,5]

Bacterial Infections

Combinations of oral nonabsorbable antibiotics, such as gentamicin, nystatin, vancomycin, polymyxin B, and colistin, have been widely studied as a means of reducing colonization of the GI tract with virulent pathogens. Although selective intestinal decontamination with oral nonabsorbable antibiotics successfully reduces infections, these regimens are not routinely recommended for prophylaxis because of problems that include unpalatability, cost, frequent adverse effects (eg, nausea, vomiting, and diarrhea), and development of resistance.[1-5]

Prophylaxis with orally administered, systemically available antibiotics such as trimethoprim–sulfamethoxazole and fluoroquinolones is effective at reducing gram-negative infections.[1,2] Although trimethoprim–sulfamethoxazole is effective as prophylaxis against *P. jiroveci*, its lack of activity against *P. aeruginosa* is worrisome when used as prophylaxis against bacterial infection, particularly

TABLE 122-8 Risk-Based Prophylactic Strategies for Patients with Neutropenia

Risk Group	Patient Characteristics	Prophylactic Strategies
High risk	*Neutropenia:* Severe (absolute neutrophil count <100/mm^3 [<0.1 × 10^9/L]) and/or prolonged (≥10 days) *Malignancy/treatment:* Hematologic malignancy (acute leukemia), allogeneic HSCT, GVHD with high dose steroids, or use of alemtuzumab	Consider bacterial prophylaxis with fluoroquinolone for duration of neutropenia. Give fungal prophylaxis with product and duration based on patient-specific factors. Consider viral prophylaxis with product and duration based on patient-specific factors
Moderate risk	*Neutropenia:* Moderate duration (7-10 days) *Malignancy/treatment:* Autologous HSCT, multiple myeloma, lymphoma, chronic lymphocytic leukemia, purine analog therapy	Consider bacterial prophylaxis with fluoroquinolone for duration of neutropenia. Consider fungal prophylaxis with product and duration based on patient-specific factors. Give/consider viral prophylaxis with product and duration based on patient-specific factors
Low risk	*Neutropenia:* Short duration (≤7 days) *Malignancy/treatment:* Solid tumor treated with conventional chemotherapy	Antibacterial and antifungal prophylaxis not indicated. Viral prophylaxis considered during neutropenia if patient has prior HSV episode

GVHD, graft versus host disease; HSCT, hematopoietic stem cell transplant; HSV, herpes simplex virus.

Data from references 1, 2, 5, 21, 38, and 39.

in institutions where pseudomonal infections are frequent.[1] Other concerns with trimethoprim–sulfamethoxazole prophylaxis include selection of resistant organisms, predisposition to development of oral fungal infections, and delay in bone marrow recovery resulting in prolonged neutropenic episodes.[1,2,5]

Fluoroquinolones are more effective than placebo in preventing all-cause mortality, infection-related mortality, febrile episodes and gram-negative infections in neutropenic cancer patients.[1,2,5,38] However, there are several potential limitations to their use. In particular, ciprofloxacin may lack adequate gram-positive activity and may not be the preferred fluoroquinolone for this reason. Although fluoroquinolone prophylaxis has been associated with the development of resistant gram-negative organisms, these findings have not been consistent in various studies.[1,2,8,38] Also the risk of colonization or infection with strains resistant to the prophylactic agent is lower with fluoroquinolones than with trimethoprim–sulfamethoxazole.[38] However, patients experiencing breakthrough infection during fluoroquinolone prophylaxis should not be subsequently placed on a fluoroquinolone-containing empirical antibiotic regimen.[1,2]

Clinical **Controversy...**

A primary concern with the use of fluoroquinolones for prophylaxis of infections in neutropenic cancer patients is the development of antimicrobial resistance and subsequent infection with fluoroquinolone-resistant bacteria. A meta-analysis which included 56 clinical trials found that fluoroquinolone prophylaxis was associated with an increase in colonization with quinolone-resistant bacteria but that this increase was not statistically significant compared with placebo (Relative Risk [RR] 1.68; 95% Confidence Interval [CI], 0.71-4.00). This same study also found no difference in the incidence of infections caused by quinolone-resistant bacteria (RR 1.04; 95% CI, 0.73-1.50).[2] Although this and other studies have not documented increased fluoroquinolone resistance in association with prophylaxis, other potentially unfavorable outcomes such as increased risk of *Clostridium difficile* infection should also be considered in weighing the potential benefits of fluoroquinolone prophylaxis.[1,2,8,38]

Although the benefits of prophylaxis with fluoroquinolones outweigh the potential risks in neutropenic patients with intermediate to high risk for infection (Table 122-8), antibacterial prophylaxis in general remains somewhat controversial due to continued concerns regarding the potential for development of resistant bacteria, high cost, and lack of impact on patient survival.[1,2,8] Therefore, antibacterial prophylaxis is not recommended routinely for all neutropenic patients. Prophylaxis with ciprofloxacin or levofloxacin generally is indicated for intermediate- to high-risk patients expected to be profoundly neutropenic for more than 1 week, such as HSCT patients.[1,2,5] High dose levofloxacin may be preferred by some clinicians due to enhanced gram-positive activity, but many other clinicians consider them similar in efficacy. If fluoroquinolone prophylaxis is used, strategic monitoring of gram-negative resistance to the drugs should be employed. Neutrophil recovery eliminates the need for continued prophylaxis, and recovery may be facilitated by use of CSFs.[35] CSFs have also been formally recommended by ASCO and NCCN for primary prevention of febrile neutropenia in high-risk patients (see Table 122-7).[1,2]

Fungal Infections

Because neutropenic patients are at risk for mucocutaneous and invasive fungal infections that are difficult to diagnose and treat in this population, antifungal prophylaxis can be considered in intermediate- to high-risk patients at institutions where fungal infections in cancer patients occur frequently.[1,2] The goal of antifungal prophylaxis is to prevent development of invasive fungal infections during periods of risk, thereby reducing morbidity and mortality. A meta-analysis of antifungal prophylaxis in 38 trials involving more than 7,000 cancer patients reported a decrease in the use of parenteral antifungal therapy, superficial and invasive systemic fungal infections, and fungal infection-related mortality rate.[39] Antifungal prophylaxis in these studies resulted in decreased mortality in patients with prolonged neutropenia and HSCT.

Although the choice of antifungal prophylaxis agents remains controversial, fluconazole prophylaxis has been particularly well studied and reduces the incidence of both superficial and systemic fungal infections; it also significantly decreases mortality from fungal infections in patients with leukemia and HSCT recipients.[2,39] However, use of fluconazole prophylaxis has contributed to the emergence of infections caused by *C. krusei* and *C. glabrata*, pathogens that frequently are resistant to fluconazole and other azole-type antifungal agents.[2,19] When compared to prophylaxis with mold-active agents, patients on fluconazole have higher rate of aspergillosis and invasive fungal-related mortality but lower rate of adverse events leading to discontinuation.[40] Therefore, antifungal prophylaxis with oral fluconazole, itraconazole, voriconazole, posaconazole, an echinocandin, or LAMB is recommended for prophylaxis in select patients starting at the time of induction chemotherapy.[2] The choice of a specific agent should be determined by the types of fungal isolates at individual institutions and the chemotherapeutic regimen.[1,2,18] Patients in whom prophylaxis should be considered include those at intermediate to high infection risk as shown in

Table 122-8. After initiation, antifungal prophylaxis should be continued until resolution of neutropenia or the need for institution of antifungal therapy for suspected/documented infection.[2,18]

Itraconazole, low to moderate doses of amphotericin B, intranasal and aerosolized amphotericin B, LAMB products, voriconazole, posaconazole and the echinocandins have all been investigated for *Aspergillus* prophylaxis in neutropenic patients.[2,5,20,40] Posaconazole was more effective than either fluconazole or itraconazole in the prevention of *Aspergillus* and other invasive fungal infections in patients with hematologic malignancies and prolonged neutropenia.[2,20]

Other Infections

Use of trimethoprim–sulfamethoxazole in cancer patients at risk for *P. jiroveci* pneumonia has substantially reduced the incidence of this protozoal infection.[1,2] Antiviral prophylaxis with acyclovir, valacyclovir, or famciclovir is used in most centers to reduce the risk of HSV reactivation in patients with acute leukemia undergoing intensive chemotherapy. Varicella vaccine provides good protection (90%) in leukemic children and may be useful in seronegative adults, although the vaccine has been less well studied in this population.

When considering use of antimicrobial (antibacterial, antifungal, antiprotozoal, and antiviral) prophylaxis in neutropenic patients with cancer, the risks and benefits of prophylaxis must be weighed against issues with development of resistance, toxicities, and other concerns.

Evaluation of Therapeutic Outcomes

10 Close monitoring of febrile neutropenic patients, including both clinical and laboratory parameters, is essential for early detection and treatment of infectious complications. Three general therapeutic outcomes have been defined in the setting of febrile neutropenia: (a) success (survival during the febrile episode until resolution of neutropenia by judicious selection of empirical antimicrobial therapy), (b) success with modification (same as [a] but with additions/modifications to empirical therapy), and (c) failure (death during febrile neutropenia).[13] Because many of the drugs that can be used in this setting (eg, aminoglycosides and amphotericin B) have significant toxicity potential, careful attention must be paid to prevention and management of drug-related adverse effects. Evaluations of the parameters given in the Clinical Presentation are appropriate to help monitor and guide therapy. In addition, the NCCN guidelines for febrile neutropenia provide comprehensive recommendations on clinical/laboratory monitoring parameters, including schedules.[2] The reader is referred to individual chapters within this book for more detailed discussions of monitoring parameters related to specific types of infections (eg, pneumonia and urinary tract infections).

INFECTIONS IN PATIENTS UNDERGOING HSCT

1 Infection remains a major barrier to successful HSCT.[1,2,5,41] Recipients of HSCT are at enhanced risk for infection because of prolonged periods of neutropenia. In addition, patients receiving allogeneic or matched unrelated donor transplants receive prolonged immunosuppressive drug therapy for prevention and treatment of graft-versus-host disease (GVHD). Intensive pretransplant conditioning regimens (high-dose chemotherapy and total-body irradiation), as well as GVHD itself, often disrupt protective barriers, such as mucous membranes, skin, and the GI tract, placing patients at further risk of infection. Although infectious complications are still associated with considerable morbidity and mortality, studies have documented significant reduction in mortality after HSCT in association with reductions in disease caused by bacterial, fungal, and viral infections.[41]

Etiology and Clinical Presentation of Infections

2 10 The timing with which specific types of infections typically occur following HSCT is shown in Fig. 122-3, but the relative incidence and importance of specific pathogens vary greatly according to the specific type of HSCT performed. Patients receiving allogeneic transplants are at greatest risk for infection after HSCT and are predisposed to earlier and more severe infections with opportunistic pathogens such as *Aspergillus*. The presence of GVHD also has an impact on the incidence and timing of various infections, including invasive fungal infections.

After administration of intensive conditioning regimens to eliminate malignant cells and prevent rejection of donor cells, patients may remain profoundly neutropenic for 3 to 4 weeks. During this preengraftment period, patients are at risk for the same types of infectious complications that occur in other granulocytopenic cancer patients (eg, bacterial and fungal infections) and should be managed accordingly (see Table 122-1). Table 122-6 lists regimens for treatment of specific infections.

HSCT recipients remain at high risk for infection after bone marrow engraftment has occurred.[2,5,41] Significant defects in neutrophil function and cell-mediated and humoral immunity, persisting for several months after transplantation, predispose patients to infectious complications. Acute and chronic GVHD also result in prolonged periods of immunosuppression and increased infection rates.

Patients undergoing HSCT are at significant risk for serious bacterial infections.[2,5,41,42] The risk of bacterial infection is particularly increased in patients undergoing allogeneic transplantation and those with GVHD. Gram-negative bacteremia occur in approximately 20% of patients, and mortality rates may reach 25%.[42]

Fungal infections, especially those caused by *Candida* and *Aspergillus* spp., are serious and often result in fatal complications. Fungi remain a serious cause of infection, particularly in allogeneic HSCT recipients, for up to 1 to 2 years following transplantation and may occur in as many as 20% of patients.[5,41,43] Significant mortality is associated with invasive aspergillosis and mucormycosis infections.[5,10,41-43]

HSCT recipients are also at risk for serious viral infections, particularly HSV and cytomegalovirus (CMV). HSV infections may include gingivostomatitis, esophagitis, genital lesions, and, rarely, pneumonia during the first month after transplant.[2,5,6,44,45] Clinical disease is more common in patients with serologic evidence of prior exposure and latent HSV infection pretransplant. Therefore, reactivation of latent disease during periods of immunosuppression is the most common etiology of HSV infection. Without prophylaxis, as many as 80% of HSV-seropositive patients experience mucocutaneous disease after intensive chemotherapy compared with less than 25% of seronegative patients.[2,6,44,45] HSV infections often coexist with *Candida* infection and mucositis secondary to chemotherapy, radiation, or both.[2,44,45] Painful swallowing associated with these conditions often makes it difficult for patients to take oral medications and maintain adequate nutritional intake. Because of the considerable morbidity associated with HSV reactivation after transplantation, the HSV serologic status of patients should be determined prior to transplant.

HSCT recipients are at high risk for CMV infections during the early postengraftment period. Infections range in severity from asymptomatic infection with viral shedding (urine, throat, and lungs), to life-threatening disseminated disease and interstitial pneumonia.[2,44,45]

As with HSV, patients seropositive for CMV before transplantation are at high risk for reactivation of infection during periods of immunosuppression; up to 70% of seropositive patients develop reactivation after transplantation compared with only 3%

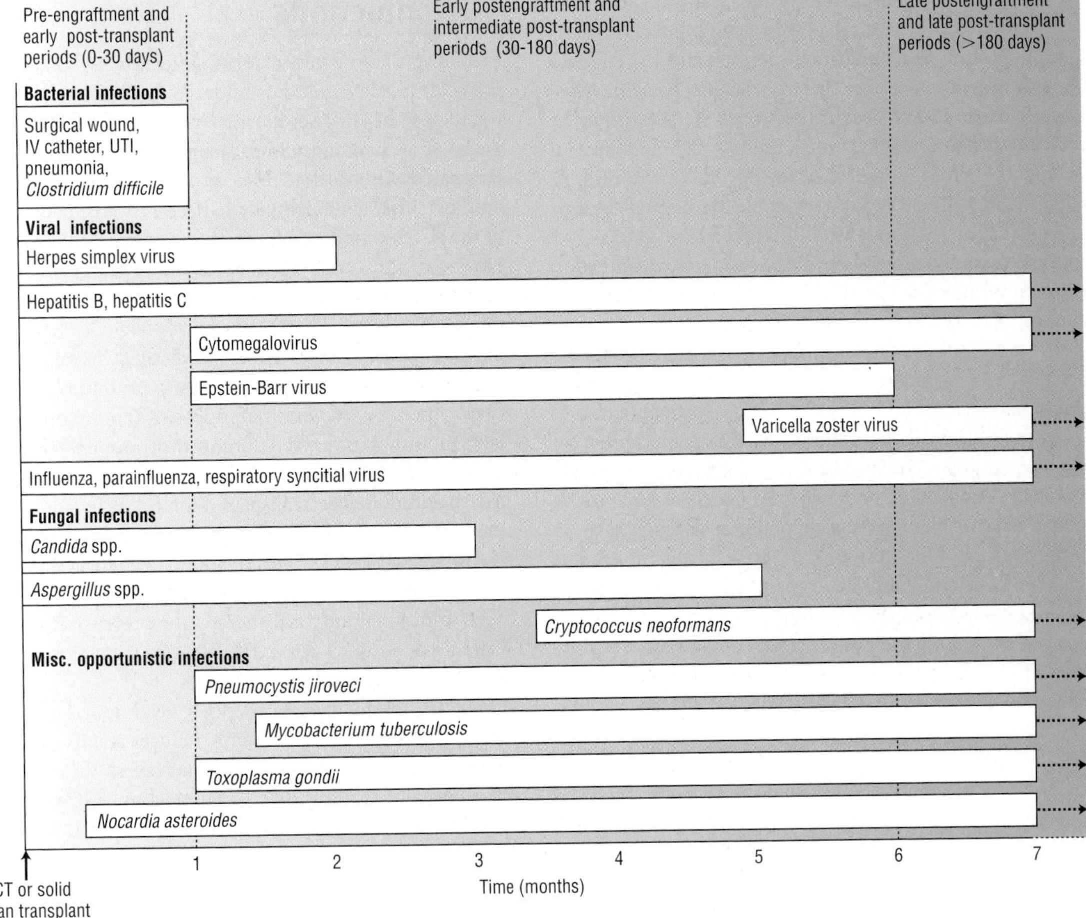

FIGURE 122-3 Timetable for the occurrence of infections in hematopoietic stem cell transplantation (HSCT) and solid-organ transplant patients. (UTI, urinary tract infection.)

of seronegative patients.[2,41,44,45] Other risk factors for CMV infection in HSCT patients include advanced age, human lymphocyte antigen mismatch, total-body irradiation, multiagent conditioning regimens, and presence of GVHD.[2,5,44,45] Patients without evidence of latent CMV infection (CMV-seronegative) before transplantation may develop primary CMV infection after receiving bone marrow or blood products from CMV-seropositive donors. Although the typical onset of both primary and recurrent CMV infection is 1 to 2 months after transplantation, late-onset infections may occur more than 100 days after transplantation.[2,5,41,44,45] Patients receiving allogeneic transplants are at highest risk for CMV reactivation, with progression to clinical disease in approximately 10% to 30% of patients.[44,45]

The most serious clinical manifestation of CMV disease and a leading cause of infectious death in HSCT recipients is interstitial pneumonia, which is associated with an 85% mortality rate if left untreated.[44,45] This clinical syndrome manifests as fever, dyspnea, hypoxia, nonproductive cough, and diffuse pulmonary infiltrates. As many as 40% of allogeneic HSCT patients will develop interstitial pneumonia; a significant proportion are viral in etiology.[44,45] Interstitial pneumonia also may result from other infectious (*P. jiroveci*, VZV) and noninfectious causes (pulmonary damage by radiation and chemotherapy).[2,44,45]

During the late postengraftment period (beginning approximately 180 days after transplantation), infections remain a major problem in patients suffering from chronic GVHD. Infections common during the late postengraftment period include those caused by encapsulated bacteria, such as *S. pneumoniae* and *H. influenza*, fungi, and viruses, including CMV and VZV.[2,5] Patients not undergoing allogeneic transplantation or suffering from chronic GVHD generally have few infections in this period.

Up to 50% of all patients surviving up to 10 months after transplantation develop an infection caused by VZV.[44,45] Infection with VZV is most common in allogeneic HSCT recipients with acute or chronic GVHD.[44,45] Both primary (varicella) or recurrent disease (herpes zoster) usually present as skin lesions, most of which remain contained to local areas; however, 30% to 45% of these infections may disseminate to other cutaneous areas or body organs, causing mortality as high as 50%.[44,45]

TREATMENT

Desired Outcomes

The goals of therapy in managing HSCT recipients from the neutropenic period through the late postengraftment period are: (a) protect the patient from early death caused by undiagnosed infection; (b) employ effective prophylactic therapy to prevent common bacterial, fungal, viral, and protozoal/parasitic infections; (c) effectively and aggressively treat established infections; (d) avoid unnecessary use of antimicrobials that contribute to increased resistance; and (e) minimize toxicities and cost while increasing patient quality of life.

Prophylaxis and Management of Infections in Recipients of HSCT

8 9 The overall goal of prophylaxis and treatment of infection in HSCT patients is prevention of infectious morbidity and mortality.

Specific goals of antimicrobial drug use in HSCT patients include (a) prevention of bacterial, fungal, viral, and protozoal infections during preengraftment and postengraftment periods and (b) effective treatment of established infections. These goals must be achieved at the lowest possible toxicity and cost. Prophylactic therapy should be aimed specifically at pathogens known to cause a high incidence of infection within the HSCT population, the specific institution, or both. In addition, prophylactic therapy should be limited to regimens proved to be effective through well-designed clinical trials.

Appropriate immunizations should be a primary consideration in the prevention of infections in HSCT recipients. Immunizations against common bacterial and viral pathogens are timed to avoid periods of severe immunosuppression following HSCT when the protective response to vaccination potentially would be decreased.[2,5] Recommendations for immunization of HSCT patients include three doses each of diphtheria–pertussis–tetanus (or diphtheria–tetanus), inactivated polio, conjugated *H. influenzae* type b, conjugated 13-valent pneumococcal, and two doses each of hepatitis A and B, and one dose of meningococcal conjugate vaccines 6 to 12 months post-transplant. One dose of the 23-valent pneumococcal vaccine should follow after 12 months. The influenza vaccine should be resumed at least 4 to 6 months after transplantation, and continued annually for life. Family members, close contacts, and healthcare providers of HSCT patients also should be vaccinated annually against influenza. Finally, the measles–mumps–rubella vaccine should be administered no sooner than 24 months after HSCT if the patient is considered to be immunocompetent. The varicella vaccine may be considered on a case by case basis owing to the live-attenuated nature of the product and the risk of VZV infection, but if administered should occur no sooner than 24 months after transplant. The injectable inactivated influenza vaccine is preferred both before and after HSCT due to severe underlying illnesses pretransplant and contraindication of the live-attenuated intranasal product posttransplant.[1,2,5]

Bacterial Infections

Prophylaxis of infections in HSCT patients is similar in many ways to that used in other neutropenic patients. Oral antibacterial prophylaxis is used commonly; considerations are the same as those discussed previously in the "Prophylaxis of Infections in Neutropenic Cancer Patients" section. Although rates of bacteremia and other bacterial infections are decreased after HSCT, overall mortality rates have not been consistently reduced.[1,2,5,44] Therefore, routine use of prophylactic antibiotics in HSCT is still controversial but should be considered in patients at moderate to high risk of infection (Table 122-8). Fluoroquinolones are the most frequently used agents, with levofloxacin preferred over ciprofloxacin due to enhanced gram-positive activity.[1,2,5,44] These regimens usually are started either within 72 hours of beginning the chemotherapy conditioning regimens or on the day of hematopoietic stem cell infusion and continued throughout the neutropenic period. Patients who become febrile while receiving prophylaxis should be managed according to general guidelines for febrile neutropenic patients.

Antibiotic prophylaxis against bacterial infection is also recommended in the late postengraftment period (greater than 100 days after transplantation) in certain high-risk patients, specifically allogeneic transplant recipients with chronic GVHD.[2,6] Antibiotics should be targeted against encapsulated bacteria, particularly *S. pneumonia*, and should be selected based on local susceptibility patterns for these organisms; penicillin is preferred in areas with low rates of penicillin-resistant pneumococci.[2] Patients receiving trimethoprim–sulfamethoxazole for prophylaxis of other opportunistic infections may be protected adequately and do not necessarily require an additional antibiotic.[2,5] Prophylaxis should be continued as long as the chronic GVHD is being actively treated.

Viral Infections

Prophylaxis of recurrent HSV infection is recommended for all HSV-seropositive patients undergoing HSCT.[1,2,5,44,45] Approximately 0% to 10% of HSV-seropositive patients receiving acyclovir experienced viral shedding, clinical symptoms of viral reactivation, or both compared with 60% to 80% of patients receiving placebo.[5,44,45] IV acyclovir therapy eventually is necessary in many patients because of the development of severe mucositis from conditioning regimens. However, oral acyclovir, valacyclovir, or famciclovir is effective and considerably less expensive in patients who can take oral medications. Valacyclovir has replaced acyclovir as first-line therapy in many institutions.[2,5,44] The antiviral agent usually is started at the time of the conditioning regimen and continued until bone marrow engraftment or resolution of mucositis (approximately 30 days after HSCT), although longer durations of prophylaxis may be considered in allogeneic HSCT recipients with GVHD or frequent HSV reactivations before transplantation.[2,5,44,45] In addition to preventing recurrence of HSV disease, acyclovir prophylaxis may reduce the incidence of CMV reactivation.[2,5] Patients receiving ganciclovir or foscarnet for prophylaxis or treatment of CMV infection do not need additional antiviral therapy for prevention of HSV or VZV.[2] Patients developing active HSV or VZV infection should be treated with high-dose acyclovir.[2,44,45]

Oral acyclovir or valacyclovir given for up to 12 months after transplantation also significantly reduces reactivation of VZV infections and prevents the occurrence of severe VZV disease.[1,2] Patients receiving either allogeneic or autologous HSCT may therefore be considered for long-term (up to 1 year after transplantation) prophylaxis against VZV.[2] Patients who received HSCT within the previous 24 months, or those more than 24 months after HSCT who have chronic GVHD or are undergoing immunosuppressive therapy, should receive varicella-zoster immunoglobulin 625 units intramuscularly within 48 to 96 hours after close contact with persons with chickenpox or shingles for prevention of VZV-related disease.[5]

Acyclovir-resistant HSV has been reported occasionally in HSCT patients receiving acyclovir prophylaxis. Foscarnet is a drug of choice for treatment of documented infection with acyclovir-resistant HSV and should be reserved for this use.[2,5,44,45]

Prevention of CMV disease is a well-accepted indication for prophylaxis in HSCT patients because of the high associated infectious morbidity and mortality. If possible, CMV-seronegative patients should receive donor cells and supportive blood products from seronegative donors only; however, CMV-seropositive patients are not at significant additional risk by receiving blood or donor cells from seropositive donors.[44,45] Although acyclovir has relatively poor in vitro activity against CMV, a decrease in CMV infection and an improvement in overall survival were reported in HSV- and CMV-seropositive allogeneic HSCT recipients receiving IV acyclovir.[2,5,45]

Ganciclovir has been well studied for prophylaxis because of its superior activity against CMV compared with acyclovir.[2,5] Oral valganciclovir has also been well studied in the setting of HSCT.[2,5] Valganciclovir has excellent pharmacokinetics and produces serum levels of ganciclovir which are at least similar to those achieved after IV administration. Valganciclovir is routinely used in many centers based on the favorable pharmacokinetic properties and convenience of oral dosing in certain patients.[2,5] Although administration of prophylactic ganciclovir to CMV-seropositive patients may significantly decrease the occurrence of CMV disease, there is no clear survival benefit, and ganciclovir-related bone marrow suppression frequently was problematic. Therefore, ganciclovir prophylaxis is somewhat controversial and is not universally recommended for routine use, and a preemptive approach is reasonable.[2,5,44] It may, however, be considered for allogeneic HSCT recipients for the first 100 days after transplantation.[2,5,44]

Perhaps a more appropriate role for ganciclovir and valganciclovir is preemptive therapy, in which ganciclovir is administered at first isolation of CMV from the blood or bronchoalveolar lavage fluid. Detection of CMV can be accomplished by use of either a monoclonal antibody-based test for viral antigens or by detection of viral DNA through polymerase chain reaction (PCR)-based tests. Preemptive therapy significantly reduced the occurrence of CMV disease (including CMV pneumonia) and improved survival significantly up to 180 days after transplantation.[2,44] Because CMV viremia and bronchoalveolar lavage cultures are highly predictive of subsequent CMV disease, preemptive ganciclovir or valganciclovir therapy should be considered for autologous HSCT recipients within the first 100 days after transplantation or in allogeneic HSCT recipients at any time after transplantation.[2,5,44] The doses of ganciclovir or valganciclovir for preemptive therapy are the same as those used for prophylaxis. Foscarnet can also be used for either prophylaxis or preemptive therapy of CMV disease in patients intolerant of ganciclovir.

CSFs are beneficial in this setting (Table 122-6), providing benefits similar to those noted in neutropenic patients with acquired immunodeficiency syndrome receiving ganciclovir therapy for CMV retinitis. Prophylaxis of CMV disease with either IV immunoglobulin (IVIG) or cytomegalovirus hyperimmune globulin (CMVIG) produced variable and inconclusive results, and their use is not currently recommended.[46,47]

Ganciclovir or valganciclovir are the drugs of choice for treatment of active CMV infection in HSCT patients (see Table 122-5). Foscarnet also may be of benefit for treatment or prevention of infections in HSCT patients and may be used as an alternative to ganciclovir/valganciclovir because of its relative lack of bone marrow toxicity. Foscarnet-related nephrotoxicity may be problematic, however, especially in the post-transplant period when patients may be receiving other nephrotoxic agents. Cidofovir has not been well studied in HSCT patients and is also associated with nephrotoxicity, but this agent may also be considered for preemptive therapy or treatment of active disease.[2]

Numerous single-agent treatments such as interferon and ganciclovir have been used unsuccessfully as treatment for CMV pneumonitis. However, the combination of high-dose IVIG and ganciclovir may decrease the mortality of the syndrome from 85% to 30% to 50%.[44,46,48] Ganciclovir plus hyperimmune CMVIG also is considered effective for treatment of CMV disease, although this regimen has not been studied as extensively in the HSCT population in a controlled fashion. However, CMVIG was not more effective than IVIG, therefore ganciclovir plus IVIG is considered as the treatment regimen of choice for severe or life-threatening CMV disease based on benefit-versus-risk considerations more than definitive clinical data.[2] The potential for ganciclovir-associated bone marrow suppression prior to marrow engraftment and in patients who are just recovering from granulocytopenia remains a concern, especially in patients with unstable renal function.

Fungal Infections

Prophylaxis with antifungal agents is efficacious and generally recommended for prevention of mucocutaneous and disseminated fungal infections in high-risk HSCT patients (Tables 122-2 and 122-8).[2,5,18,40,49-51] Patients specifically recommended for prophylaxis include all allogeneic recipients and autologous transplant recipients who are expected to have prolonged neutropenia, have received intensive conditioning regimens associated with extensive mucositis, or have recently received fludarabine.[2,5,18,49,50] Fluconazole is the most commonly used agent; it is started on the day of transplantation and continued until resolution of neutropenia or, in allogeneic HSCT, for at least 75 days after transplantation.[2,5,18,44,50] The variable activity of fluconazole against non-*albicans* species of *Candida* may be problematic in this population, as is lack of activity against *Aspergillus*.[2,19,50] Prophylaxis with fluconazole (as well as itraconazole), although effectively reducing colonization and infection with yeasts, has not consistently been demonstrated to reduce overall mortality or invasive infections such as aspergillosis in HSCT recipients.[2,40,49-51] Micafungin was more efficacious than fluconazole in the prevention of early-onset *Candida* infections in patients with neutropenia prior to engraftment, and also showed a trend to fewer episodes of invasive aspergillosis.[2] Posaconazole was also more effective than fluconazole in the late prevention of invasive *Aspergillus* and other fungal infections in HSCT patients with GVHD. In a meta-analysis, prophylaxis with agents active against *Aspergillus* were also associated with a 33% reduction in mortality related to invasive fungal infections compared to fluconazole.[40] Fluconazole, itraconazole, voriconazole, posaconazole, echinocandins, and LAMB products are all recommended for prophylaxis of fungal infections in HSCT. Posaconazole is the preferred agent in high-risk HSCT patients with GVHD (Table 122-2).[2,20,49-51]

Protozoal Infections

Pulmonary infection with *P. jiroveci* is a relatively infrequent complication of HSCT. However, mortality rates in this population are approximately 60% and are especially high in patients with GVHD.[2,5] Prophylactic trimethoprim–sulfamethoxazole is recommended for a period of 3 to 6 months after autologous HSCT, and for at least 6 months and while receiving immunosuppressive therapy after allogeneic HSCT. Toxoplasmosis is not a common infection in HSCT patients but is associated with mortality rates of approximately 70%.[52] Toxoplasmosis should also be prevented by trimethoprim–sulfamethoxazole prophylaxis.[2,5]

Use of Colony-Stimulating Factors

Filgrastim, pegfilgrastim, and sargramostim have been studied in HSCT patients in an effort to speed bone marrow recovery, reduce the period of neutropenia, and decrease infectious complications. CSFs appear effective as well as safe following autologous transplantation, although increased rates of GVHD and mortality have been reported with use of CSFs following allogeneic transplantation.[35] The use of CSFs is now routinely recommended to mobilize blood progenitor cells and reduce the period of neutropenia in autologous transplants (Table 122-6).[2,35,36]

Evaluation of Therapeutic Outcomes

10 Close monitoring of HSCT patients, including clinical and laboratory data, is essential for early detection and treatment of infectious complications. In addition, because many of the drugs commonly used in this setting (eg, ganciclovir, amphotericin B, and trimethoprim–sulfamethoxazole) have significant toxicity potential in HSCT patients, careful attention must be paid to prevention and management of drug-related adverse effects. Monitoring parameters related to specific types of infections (eg, pneumonia and urinary tract infections) should be applied as appropriate. The reader is referred to other chapters within this book for more specific information.

INFECTIONS IN SOLID-ORGAN TRANSPLANT RECIPIENTS

Solid-organ transplantation (SOT) has become an established mode of treatment for end-stage diseases of the heart, lungs, kidney, liver, pancreas, and small bowel. Patient and allograft survival rates have greatly improved due to improvements in immunosuppressive drug therapy, candidate selection, and transplant surgery techniques as well as more experience in the management of complications (including infection) in these patients. Despite advances in diagnostic techniques and antimicrobial therapy, infectious complications remain important causes of morbidity and mortality after SOT.

Risk Factors

1 Many risk factors for infection are present in SOT patients (see Table 122-1). The most important risk factor in this population is immunosuppressive drug therapy for prevention and treatment of allograft rejection. Risk of infection depends on specific immunosuppressive drug regimens as well as the intensity (numbers and doses of drugs) and duration of immunosuppression. Most opportunistic infections in transplant patients occur during the first 6 months after transplantation, when the intensity and total cumulative doses of immunosuppressive therapy are very high.[53,54]

Immunosuppressive drugs, often in escalated doses, are used to treat episodes of graft rejection and include immunoglobulins directed against T cells (eg, antithymocyte globulin), murine monoclonal antibodies (muromonab), antibodies against interleukin 2 receptors (daclizumab and basiliximab), T-cell–depleting antibodies (alemtuzumab), and high-dose corticosteroids. Rejection episodes often occur during the period 2 to 4 months post-transplant when the overall cumulative dose or net state of immunosuppression is highest.[53,55] Therefore, patients already at risk for infection are placed at even higher risk if additional immunosuppressive therapy is needed to treat one or more episodes of graft rejection. Immunosuppressive drug therapy must be evaluated carefully when infections occur because, in many cases, immunosuppression may have to be reduced to allow patients to survive the infectious episode, at the expense of increased risk of graft rejection. Risk of increased infectious complications from immunosuppressive therapy used to treat rejection episodes is determined, at least in part, by the specific therapy used.[53-55]

Etiology

2 As with cancer patients, microorganisms infecting SOT patients are present before transplantation or are acquired from exogenous sources. All transplant recipients are at risk for mucocutaneous candidiasis from species colonizing body sites. Invasive fungal infection is less common following kidney and pancreas transplantation (5%-15%) but may occur in 30% to 60% of heart, lung, liver, and small bowel transplant recipients. Rates are highest following lung, liver, and small bowel transplantation and are associated with mortality rates up to 60% to 80%.[53,56-60] Approximately 50% to 90% of all systemic fungal infections in transplant recipients are caused by *Candida* spp.[53,56,57] Abdominal surgery, especially the more complex procedures required for liver and small bowel transplantation, predispose patients to serious fungal disease, most likely as a consequence of entering an area already colonized with *Candida* spp.[56] Lung and heart transplant recipients are particularly at risk for invasive aspergillosis; these infections may occur in up to 15% of patients and in lung transplant recipients may be more common than infections caused by *Candida* spp.[56-59] Liver and lung transplant recipients are at high risk for serious gram-negative bacterial infections as a result of the technically difficult surgical procedures.[53] Although opportunistic viral, fungal, and protozoal infections may occur commonly, bacterial infections remain the most frequent infectious complications after transplantation in all allograft recipients.

Organisms present as latent tissue infections may reactivate and cause clinical disease with administration of immunosuppressive drug therapy. Disease resulting from infection reactivation has been noted with viruses (HSV, human herpesvirus-6, CMV, VZV, Epstein–Barr virus [EBV]), protozoa (*T. gondii*, *P. jiroveci*), and mycobacteria (*Mycobacterium tuberculosis*).[61,62] Serologic or immunologic tests are performed prior to transplantation to assess the risk for reactivation infection and identify other subclinical infections (eg, hepatitis B virus [HBV], hepatitis C virus [HCV], *Legionella*). Many patients with reactivated infection have no clinical symptoms; often the only evidence of active infection is a rise in antibody titer from the pretransplant baseline, positive culture, or histologic evidence. Reactivation of latent infection may result in severe life-threatening disease in immunosuppressed hosts.[62]

Exogenous sources of infection in transplant patients include environmental contamination and transmission of microorganisms via transplanted organs and blood products. Environmental sources of infection are similar to those noted in other immunocompromised hosts, such as cancer patients. Airborne pathogens, especially fungi such as *Aspergillus* and *Cryptococcus neoformans*, may cause infections in transplant patients; this is thought to be a direct cause of increased *Aspergillus* infections among lung transplant patients.[53,56] Transplant patients are at high risk for nosocomial infections (MRSA, *P. aeruginosa*, *Acinetobacter*). Optimal prevention and management of nosocomial infections in transplant patients require knowledge of the current epidemiology of infections and susceptibility patterns in the institution.

Infections transmitted via donor organs or blood products are major causes of morbidity and mortality in transplant patients and may include HSV, *T. gondii*, HBV, and HCV. The most important infections transmitted from the donor, however, are caused by CMV. These infections may cause serious disease, and predispose patients to other opportunistic infections, and contribute to acute and chronic allograft dysfunction or rejection, post-transplant lymphoproliferative disorders (particularly associated with EBV), and cardiac complications and atherosclerosis in heart transplant recipients.[53,63] In contrast to reactivation disease, transplant patients contracting primary CMV disease are at increased risk for serious life-threatening infections.[53,64-66] The most important source of primary CMV infection in transplant patients is the donor organ. Efforts are made to avoid transplanting organs from CMV-seropositive donors into CMV-seronegative recipients because of the potentially severe consequences. With the relative scarcity of suitable organs and the rapidity with which transplant decisions often must be made, however, this is not always possible. The consequences of transplanting an organ from a CMV-seropositive donor into an already CMV-seropositive recipient are less clear. CMV reinfection (as well as reactivation) syndromes may occur in these patients.[53,54,66] In addition to transmission from donor organs, primary CMV disease may be transmitted from seropositive blood products, although this is a much less common mode of transmission.

Organs from donors seropositive for *T. gondii* or HSV generally are not withheld from seronegative patients. Organs from known HIV-infected donors, however, are not used for transplantation. Asymptomatic HIV-seropositive individuals with $CD4^+$ lymphocyte count greater than 100 cells/mm^3 (0.1×10^9/L) and no active opportunistic infection or malignancy may be considered for SOT (as well as HSCT) without prohibitively high risk for acceleration of HIV disease.[66] The impact of protease inhibitors and highly active antiretroviral therapy on long-term outcome of HIV-infected patients following transplantation is not precisely known but is believed to have improved the overall feasibility of transplanting these individuals.[66]

Timing of Infections After Transplantation

As with HSCT, the overall time course for infections can be divided into three general periods after transplantation (see Fig. 122-3). Although risk of infection with specific pathogens varies with the type of transplant, the time course of infections is similar in all transplant recipients. During the early post-transplant period (within the first month after transplantation), patients are at risk for infections already present and brought forward from the pretransplant period (eg, HBV); postoperative infections, such as surgical wound and catheter infections; infection resulting from colonized donor organs (pneumonia following lung transplant); and reactivation of HSV.[53,54,62] In the intermediate post-transplant period (2-6 months after transplant), risk is highest for viral infections, including CMV,

EBV, HBV, and HCV. The combination of these "immunomodulating" viruses plus sustained immunosuppressive therapy leads to a high risk for opportunistic infections with pathogens such as *P. jiroveci*, *Aspergillus*, and *Nocardia asteroides*.[53,54,56,62] In the late post-transplant period (greater than 6 months after transplant), patients are at risk for persistent infections (particularly viral) from earlier post-transplant periods, reactivation of VZV and *C. neoformans*, and routine infections affecting the general population.[53] In addition, patients who required additional immunosuppression therapy for acute or chronic rejection are at continued high risk for opportunistic infections (*Aspergillus* and *P. jiroveci*).[53,54,56] Although Fig. 122-3 illustrates infection patterns common to all solid-organ transplants, the relative incidence and importance of a particular pathogen vary according to the type of transplant.

Types of Infections and Clinical Presentation

10 Transplant patients are at risk for infections occurring at a variety of sites, including skin, surgical wound, urinary tract, lungs, blood, abdomen, and CNS. However, most infections occur at or near the site of the transplanted organ. For example, heart transplant and heart and lung transplant recipients most often are infected within the lungs or thoracic cavity. Urinary tract infections remain an important cause of morbidity in renal transplant patients, especially in the early post-transplant period. Administration of prophylactic antibiotics (eg, trimethoprim–sulfamethoxazole) to these patients has reduced the incidence and severity of urinary tract infections.[53,54] Serious bacterial and fungal infections originating from the abdomen and GI tract are most common after liver transplantation and are related to variables such as length of surgery and surgical procedures performed. Risk of bacteremia, usually originating from the gut, is highest in liver transplant patients. Renal transplant recipients are at the lowest risk for infections and infectious deaths, whereas patients receiving heart, lung, and liver transplants are at the highest risk for infection-related morbidity and mortality.[53,54,56]

In contrast to febrile neutropenic patients, the threshold for initiating empirical antimicrobial therapy is higher in febrile transplant patients. Appropriate therapy for the large numbers of pathogens that may cause infections in transplant patients varies greatly from organism to organism (Table 122-5). Therefore, careful attempts at definitive diagnosis of suspected infections must be made. If comprehensive workup reveals no source of infection, careful observation of the febrile transplant patient (rather than empirical therapy) is common practice. Surveillance cultures may be useful during the first 3 months for detecting CMV and HSV infections.[53,56,64,65,67,68] Management and monitoring of documented infections are similar to that in other types of patients.

TREATMENT

Desired Outcomes

The goals of therapy in managing SOT recipients are similar to those in HSCT and include: (a) protect the patient from early death caused by undiagnosed infection, from the surgical procedure through the

CLINICAL PRESENTATION Infections in Solid-Organ Transplant Patients

General

- Because transplant patients are at high risk for serious infections, frequent (at least daily), careful clinical assessments must be performed to search for evidence of infection
- Clinical presentation of infection is variable and depends on the type and site of infection, type of transplant, time after transplantation, immune status of the host, and dose and duration of immunosuppressive therapy
- Primary viral disease usually is more symptomatic and severe than disease caused by reactivation
- Physical assessment should include examination of all common sites of infection, including mouth/pharynx, nose and sinuses, respiratory tract, GI tract, urinary tract, skin, soft tissues, perineum, and intravascular catheter insertion sites

Symptoms

- Usual signs and symptoms of infection may be absent or altered in patients receiving intensive immunosuppressive regimens owing to an inability to mount a typical inflammatory response (eg, no infiltrate on chest x-ray film, urinary tract infection without pyuria)
- Pain may be present at infection site(s)

Signs

- Fever is the single most important clinical sign indicating the presence of infection. Other causes of fever unrelated to infection in this patient population include reactions to blood products, drugs, embolic events, and ischemic injury
- Usual signs of infection may be absent or altered
- Signs of allograft dysfunction may be related to infection. Distinguishing fever caused by allograft rejection from that caused by infection often is difficult and frequently requires allograft biopsy

Laboratory Tests

- Blood cultures (at least two sets, including vascular access devices) for bacteria and fungi; cultures of other suspected or potential infection sites (urine, lungs, surgical wounds, and soft tissue infections)
- Other cultures should be obtained as clinically indicated according to the presence of signs or symptoms
- Complete blood count and chemistries should be obtained frequently to monitor allograft function, plan supportive care, guide drug dosing, and assess patient's overall status
- Surveillance cultures for CMV and HSV may be useful during first 3 months after transplantation for early detection of infection

Other Diagnostic Tests

Chest x-ray film

- Aspiration, biopsy of skin lesions
- Other diagnostic tests as indicated clinically on the basis of physical examination and other assessments

late postengraftment period; (b) prevent common bacterial, fungal, viral, and protozoal/parasitic infections; (c) effectively and aggressively treat established infections; (d) avoid unnecessary use of antimicrobials; and (e) minimize toxicities and cost while increasing patient quality of life and avoiding harm to the engrafted organ(s).

Prevention of Infection in Solid-Organ Transplantation

8 The goals of antimicrobial drug use in solid-organ transplant recipients are (a) prevention of infectious complications in the immediate postoperative period, (b) prevention of late infectious complications associated with prolonged periods of immunosuppression, and (c) effective treatment of established infections in order to prevent graft dysfunction and rejection and decrease patient morbidity and mortality. All of these goals must be achieved at the lowest possible toxicity and cost.

Prevention of infection in the transplant patient can be accomplished in a number of ways. First, risk of environmental contamination should be minimized.[69] Patients should be protected from institutional infectious outbreaks. Transplant patients should receive the pneumococcal vaccine once and the influenza vaccine yearly; however, their immunologic responses to these vaccines may be suboptimal due to immunosuppressive therapy.[53] Timing of reinstitution of regular vaccinations in relation to transplantation is less clear, but is probably similar to that previously discussed for HSCT recipients.[70]

Because the most important source of primary CMV infection is an infected donor organ, CMV-seronegative patients should not receive organs or blood products from seropositive donors if possible. A number of pharmacologic strategies have been studied in an attempt to prevent CMV infection. Prophylaxis with IV ganciclovir or oral valganciclovir is effective in reducing the incidence of both primary and reactivated CMV infection in SOT.[48,53,54,63-66] Ganciclovir prophylaxis also may significantly reduce reactivation of CMV infection in seropositive patients receiving antithymocyte globulin or muromonab for treatment of acute rejection.[54,65,66] High-dose oral acyclovir effectively reduces the incidence of CMV infection and disease following renal transplantation. However, acyclovir is less efficacious in high-risk renal transplant patients (donor positive, recipient negative for CMV serum antibodies) and other nonrenal transplant types.[53,54,63-66,71] Preemptive ganciclovir or valganciclovir (initiated after actual isolation of CMV from blood, urine, bronchoalveolar lavage fluid, or other site) is more effective than acyclovir in preventing CMV disease in liver transplant recipients. Preemptive ganciclovir effectively prevents CMV disease in other types of solid-organ transplants as well.[64,65,68] Ganciclovir-related bone marrow suppression is not as problematic in solid-organ transplant recipients as in HSCT patients; most studies report that the drug is reasonably well tolerated.[48,53,64,65,68,71]

Whether prophylaxis or preemptive therapy is the best approach to preventing CMV disease in SOT is controversial.[48,53,60,64-66,68,72-74] Prophylaxis is effective and easy to administer without the need for careful discrimination among suitable patients. However, universal prophylaxis results in unnecessary exposure of low-risk individuals to adverse effects of drugs, and there are concerns that prolonged exposure may increase the risk of viral resistance to drugs.[64,65,71-73] Preemptive therapy is effective and results in exposure of fewer patients to drugs. Prophylactic therapy is recommended primarily in patients at highest risk of disease (ie, seronegative patients receiving organs from seropositive donors), whereas other lower-risk patients are often recommended to receive only preemptive therapy.[53,64,65,68,71-74] However, the risk of CMV infection and disease in lung transplant recipients is so high and is associated with such severe consequences (ie, chronic graft dysfunction, decreased survival) that prophylaxis is routinely recommended for all lung transplant recipients.[62,68,72-74] The duration of prophylactic therapy in SOT recipients is typically 100 days (typically using valganciclovir), although the duration may be extended to 6 months in high-risk kidney transplant recipients and to 12 months in high-risk lung and heart transplant patients.[62,68,72-75]

Clinical **Controversy...**

Sirolimus and everolimus are classified as mTOR (mammalian target of rapamycin) inhibitors and are often used, either alone or in combination with calcineurin inhibitors (CNI), in immunosuppressive regimens in SOT recipients. Experimental and clinical data suggest that mTOR inhibitors exert a marked anti-CMV effect through reduction in viral replication and/or potent immunomodulating properties.[76] In a meta-analysis, patients receiving immunosuppressant regimens containing mTOR inhibitors (with or without CNI) displayed a nearly three-fold reduced incidence of CMV infections compared to patients receiving CNI alone; it has even been suggested that routine prophylaxis of CMV infection may be eliminated in patients receiving mTOR inhibitors.[76] The potential for mTOR inhibitors to reduce the need for CMV prophylaxis in favor of preemptive treatment of CMV infection is the subject of extreme clinical interest, but will remain controversial until prospective clinical trials can be conducted.

Although use of prophylactic acyclovir in HSV-seropositive patients undergoing HSCT is well accepted, prophylaxis in solid-organ transplant recipients remains controversial. Reactivation disease caused by HSV occurs in approximately 25% of HSV-seropositive patients who are not receiving prophylaxis.[53] Oral or genital mucocutaneous disease is the most common presentation, but HSV pneumonitis also is seen occasionally and is associated with a mortality rate of approximately 75%.[53] Acyclovir is therefore used at some centers because of the high incidence of clinical HSV infection after transplantation. Acyclovir for prophylaxis of HSV infection may be considered in patients following a preemptive strategy for management of CMV infection, but would not be necessary in patients receiving ganciclovir or valganciclovir for CMV prophylaxis.

Prophylactic antimicrobial agents are also of benefit to SOT patients in certain other clinical situations. Antibiotic prophylaxis, with agents such as cefazolin started perioperatively and continued for less than 24 hours, is considered to reduce wound infection rates effectively following renal transplantation.[53,54,68] Although the benefits of perioperative prophylaxis have not been well demonstrated in other types of transplantation procedures, surgical prophylaxis usually is considered mandatory for liver, heart, lung, or small bowel transplant patients because of the high risk of perioperative bacterial infections.[53,68] Pulmonary infections are particularly common in lung and heart-lung transplant recipients. They often are caused by bacteria colonizing the airways of the diseased organs prior to transplantation. Therefore, perioperative antibiotics for lung and heart and lung procedures often are selected based on pretransplant sputum cultures and/or known colonizations.[53,68] In addition, posttransplant antibiotic prophylaxis is effective in decreasing the number of bacterial infections in renal transplant patients. Prophylactic trimethoprim–sulfamethoxazole traditionally has been used because it is inexpensive and well tolerated; other antibiotics, such as the fluoroquinolones, also have been evaluated.[53] Administration of oral low-dose trimethoprim–sulfamethoxazole (one double-strength tablet, either daily or 3 times/week) for 6 to 12 months for prevention of *P. jiroveci* infection following heart and lung transplantation is common, although the efficacy and optimal duration are somewhat controversial.[53,74] Selective bowel decontamination with nonabsorbable antibiotics in combination with a low-bacterial diet (no fresh fruits and vegetables) effectively reduces oropharyngeal and GI colonization with gram-negative aerobes and *Candida* in liver transplant patients. However, selective bowel contamination is less efficacious when administered for a period of less than 1 week prior to transplantation.[68,77] Because liver transplantation usually is performed without advance notice as organs become emergently available, the practice of selective bowel decontamination remains controversial and is not recommended routinely.[53,68]

Because immunosuppressed transplant recipients are at risk for mucocutaneous fungal infections, prophylactic oral or topical antifungal agents may be indicated in these patients. Liver, pancreas, and small bowel transplant recipients are clearly at high risk for invasive fungal infections and should receive prophylaxis with fluconazole.[18,53,56,73] Antifungal prophylaxis has also been suggested for lung and heart–lung transplant recipients due to the high incidence of invasive fungal infections in these patients (up to 25% of patients, with mortality rates up to 82%).[78] Prophylaxis with inhaled LAMB, itraconazole, voriconazole, and echinocandins have all been reported; however, data from well-designed trials supporting either the general recommendation for prophylaxis or choice of specific agent are largely lacking and center-to-center variability is great.[18,56,60,73] Oral voriconazole or inhaled LAMB for a period of 3 to 6 months post-transplant are most often recommended for prophylaxis of invasive fungal infection in lung and heart lung transplant recipients.[78] Concentrations of immunosuppressant drugs should be monitored closely in transplant patients receiving azole-type antifungal agents (fluconazole, itraconazole, and voriconazole).

Transplant patients, especially heart and heart and lung recipients, without serologic evidence of prior exposure to *T. gondii* who receive organs from seropositive donors are at high risk for toxoplasmosis.[53,60,68] Many of these patients will be receiving trimethoprim–sulfamethoxazole for prophylaxis of *P. jiroveci* infection; this agent will also provide effective prophylaxis against *T. gondii* as well as *N. asteroides*. Although prophylaxis is not given routinely at all centers, this therapy for a period of up to 12 months may be justified in high-risk patients because of the delays in diagnosis and serious infections associated with toxoplasmosis.[53,60,68,75]

PERSONALIZED PHARMACOTHERAPY

Desired treatment outcomes in febrile neutropenia and in HSCT and SOT recipients are achieved through close monitoring and frequent patient assessment, including judicious evaluation of antimicrobial therapies based on suspected or documented infections. Treatment of known infections must be individualized based on documented pathogens and antimicrobial susceptibilities; effective treatment may require durations of therapy well beyond recovery of ANC in febrile neutropenic patients. High intensity of immunosuppression regimens in HSCT and SOT, as well as the presence of GVHD in HSCT, also dictate aggressive antimicrobial use with potentially long durations of therapy. However, such aggressive antimicrobial use must be balanced against unnecessary administration of drugs, which may lead to increased antimicrobial resistance, adverse effects, and cost. Proper evaluation of an individual patient's risk of complications during febrile neutropenia or after transplantation allows for determination of proper prophylaxis regimens, selection of appropriate antimicrobials for treatment of infection, and selection of appropriate treatment settings (eg, inpatient versus outpatient), all of which may allow for the most cost-effective therapy and contribute to an increased quality of life for the patient.

ABBREVIATIONS

ANC	absolute neutrophil count
ASCO	American Society of Clinical Oncology
CMV	cytomegalovirus
CMVIG	cytomegalovirus hyperimmune globulin
CRE	carbapenem-resistant Enterobacteriaceae
CSF	colony-stimulating factor
EBV	Epstein-Barr virus
GVHD	graft-versus-host disease
HBV	hepatitis B virus
HCV	hepatitis C virus
HIV	human immunodeficiency virus
HSCT	hematopoietic stem cell transplantation
HSV	herpes simplex virus
IDSA	Infectious Diseases Society of America
IVIG	intravenous immunoglobulin
LAMB	lipid-associated amphotericin B
MASCC	Multinational Association for Supportive Care in Cancer
MRSA	methicillin-resistant *Staphylococcus aureus*
NCCN	National Comprehensive Cancer Network
PCR	polymerase chain reaction
PMN	polymorphonuclear leukocyte
SOT	solid-organ transplantation
VRE	vancomycin-resistant enterococci
VZV	varicella-zoster virus
WBC	white blood cell

REFERENCES

1. Freifeld AG, Bow EJ, Sepiowitz KA, et al. Clinical practice guideline for the use of antimicrobial agents in neutropenic patients with cancer: 2010 update by the infectious disease society of America. *Clin Infect Dis* 2011;52(4):e56-e93.
2. National Comprehensive Cancer Network. Prevention and treatment of cancer-related infections. Clinical Practice Guidelines in Oncology (NCCN Guidelines®), v.2.2015. September 20, 2015. *http://www.nccn.org/professionals/physician_gls/pdf/infections.pdf.*
3. Bodey GP. Fever and neutropenia: the early years. *J Antimicrob Chemother* 2009;63(S1):i3-i13. doi:10.1093/jac/dkp074.
4. Ellis M. Febrile neutropenia. Evolving strategies. *Ann NY Acad Sci* 2008;1138:329-350.
5. Tomblyn M, Chiller T, Einsele H, et al. Guidelines for preventing infectious complications among hematopoietic cell transplantation recipient: A global perspective. *Biol Blood Marrow Transplant* 2009;15:1143-1238.
6. Nesher L, Rolston KVI. The current spectrum of infection in cancer patients with chemotherapy related neutropenia. *Infection* 2014;42:5-13.
7. Klastersky J, Awada A, Paesmans MM, Aoun M. Febrile neutropenia: A critical review of the initial management. *Crit Rev Oncol Hematol* 2011;78:185-194.
8. Trecarichi E, Tumbarello M. Antimicrobial-resistant gram-negative bacteria in febrile neutropenic patients with cancer: current epidemiology and clinical impact. *Curr Opin Infect Dis* 2014;27:200-210.
9. Feld R. Bloodstream infections in cancer patients with febrile neutropenia. *Int J Antimicrob Agents* 2008;32(Suppl):S30-S33.
10. Neofytos D, Horn D, Anaissie E, et al. Epidemiology and outcome of invasive fungal infection in adult hematopoietic stem cell transplant recipients: analysis of multicenter prospective antifungal therapy (PATH) alliance registry. *Clin Infect Dis* 2009;48(3):265-273 doi:10.1086/595846.
11. Azie N, Neofytos D, Pfaller M, et al. The PATH (prospective antifungal therapy) alliance® registry and invasive fungal infections: update 2012. *Diagn Microbiol Infect Dis* 2012;73(4):293-300. doi:10.1016/j.diagmicrobio.2012.06.012.
12. Bow EJ. Fluoroquinolones, antimicrobial resistance and neutropenic cancer patients. *Curr Opin Infect Dis* 2011;24:545-553.
13. Hidron A, Edwards JR, Patel J, et al. Antimicrobial-resistant pathogens associated with healthcare-associated infections: Annual summary of data reported to the National Healthcare Safety Network at the Centers for Disease Control and Prevention, 2006-2007. *Infect Control Hosp Epidemiol* 2008;29(11):996-1011.
14. Cho SY, Lee DG, Choi SM, et al. Impact of vancomycin resistance on mortality in neutropenic patients with enterococcal blood stream infection: a retrospective study. *BMC Infect Dis* 2013;13:504. doi:10.1186/1471-2334-13-504.

15. Hanberger H, Walther S, Leone M, et al. Increased mortality associated with methicillin-resistant Staphylococcus aureus (MRSA) infection in the intensive care unit: results from the EPIC II study. *Int J Antimicrob Agents* 2011;38(4):331-335.
16. Nelson RE, Jones M, Lie CF, et al. The impact of healthcare-associated methicillin-resistant Staphylococcus aureus infections on post-discharge healthcare costs and utilization. *Infect Control Hosp Epidemiol* 2015:36(5):534-542.
17. Lewis RE, Cahyame-Zuniga L, Leventakos K, et al. Epidemiology and site of involvement of invasive fungal infections in patients with haematological malignancies: a 20-year autopsy study. *Mycoses* 2013;56:638-645.
18. Pappas PG, Kauffman CA, Andes D, et al. Clinical practice guidelines for the management of candidiasis: 2009 update by the Infectious Diseases Society of America. *Clin Infect Dis* 2009;48:503-535.
19. Ruan S-Y, Chu C-C, Hsueh P-R. In vitro susceptibilities of invasive isolates of Candida species: Rapid increase in rates of fluconazole susceptible-dose dependent Candida glabrata isolates. *Antimicrob Agents Chemother* 2008;52:2919-2922.
20. Walsh TJ, Anaissie EJ, Denning DW, et al. Treatment of aspergillosis: Clinical practice guidelines of the Infectious Diseases Society of America. *Clin Infect Dis* 2008;46:327-360.
21. Carstensen M, Sorensen JB. Outpatient management of febrile neutropenia: Time to revise the present treatment strategy. *J Support Oncol* 2008;6:199-208.
22. Paul M, Dickstein Y, Schlesinger A, et al. Beta-lactam versus beta-lactam-aminoglycoside combination therapy in cancer patients with neutropenia *Cochrane Database Syst Rev* 2013;6:CD003038.
23. Paul M, Yahav D, Bivas A, Fraser A, Leibovici L. Anti-pseudomonal beta-lactams for the initial, empirical, treatment of febrile neutropenia: Comparison of beta-lactams. *Cochrane Database Syst Rev* 2010;10(11):CD005197.
24. U.S. Food and Drug Administration. Information for Healthcare Professionals: Cefepime (marketed as Maxipime), 2009. Retrieved September 26, 2012, from *http://www.fda.gov/Drugs/DrugSafety/PostmarketDrugSafetyInformationforPatientsandProviders/DrugSafetyInformationforHeathcareProfessionals/ucm167254.htm.*
25. Gea-Banacloche J. Evidence-based approach to treatment of febrile neutropenia in hematologic malignancies. *Hematology Am Soc Hematol Educ Program* 2013;2013:414-422.
26. Paul M, Dickstein Y, Borok S, Vidal L. Empirical antibiotics targeting gram-positive bacteria for the treatment of febrile neutropenic patients with cancer. *Cochrane Database Syst Rev* 2014;1:CD003914.
27. Goldberg E, Gafter-Gvili A, Robenshtok E, et al. Empirical antifungal therapy for patients with neutropenia and persistent fever: Systematic review and meta-analysis. *Eur J Cancer* 2008;44:2192-2203.
28. Moen MD, Lyseng-Williamson KA, Scott LJ. Liposomal amphotericin B: A review of its use as empirical therapy in febrile neutropenia and in the treatment of invasive fungal infections. *Drugs* 2009;69:361-392.
29. Lass-FlÖrl C. Triazole antifungal agents in invasive fungal infections: A comparative review. *Drugs* 2011;71(18):2405-2419.
30. Rogers TR, Frost S. Newer antifungal agents for invasive fungal infections in patients with haematological malignancy. *Br J Haematol* 2009;144:629-641.
31. Blyth CC, Gilroy NM, Guy SD, et al. Consensus guidelines for the treatment of invasive mould infections in haematological malignancy and haemopoietic stem cell transplantation, 2014. *Intern Med J* 2014;44(12b):1333-1349.
32. McCormack PL. Isavuconazonium: first global approval. *Drugs* 2015;75:817-822.
33. Ashbee HR, Barnes RA, Johnson EM, et al. Therapeutic drug monitoring (TDM) of antifungal agents: guidelines from the British Society for Medical Mycology. *J Antimicrob Chemother* 2014;69:1162-1176.
34. Mhaskar R, Clark OA, Lyman G, et al. Colony-stimulating factors for chemotherapy-induced febrile neutropenia. *Cochrane Database Syst Rev* 2014;10:CD003039.
35. Smith TJ, Bohlke K, Lyman GH, et al. Recommendations for the use of WBC growth factors: American Society of Clinical Oncology clinical practice guideline update. *J Clin Oncol* 2015;33:3199-3212.
36. National Comprehensive Cancer Network. Myeloid growth factors. National Comprehensive Cancer Network. Clinical Practice Guidelines in Oncology (NCCN Guidelines®), v.1.2015; September 26, 2015. *http://www.nccn.org/professionals/physician_gls/pdf/myeloid_growth.pdf.*
37. Seidel MG, Peters C, Wacker A, et al. Randomized phase III study of granulocyte transfusions in neutropenic patients. *Bone Marrrow Transplant* 2008;42:679-684.
38. Gafter-Gvili A, Fraser A, Paul M, et al. Antibiotic prophylaxis for bacterial infections in afebrile neutropenic patients following chemotherapy. *Cochrane Database Syst Rev* 2014;1:CD004386.
39. Bow EJ, Laverdiere M, Lussier N, et al. Antifungal prophylaxis for severely neutropenic chemotherapy recipients: A meta-analysis of randomized-controlled clinical trials. *Cancer* 2002;94:3230-3246.
40. Ethier MC, Science M, Beyene J, Briel M, Lehrnbecher T, Sung L. Mould-active compared with fluconazole prophylaxis to prevent invasive fungal diseases in cancer patient receiving chemotherapy or haematopoietic stem-cell transplantation: a systematic review and meta-analysis of randomized controlled trials. *Br J Cancer* 2012;106:1626-1637.
41. Gooley TA, Chien JW, Pergam SA, et al. Reduced mortality after allogeneic hematopoietic-cell transplantation. *N Engl J Med* 2010;363:2091-2101.
42. Mikulska M, Del Bono V, Raiola AM, et al. Blood stream infections in allogeneic hematopoietic stem cell transplant recipients: Reemergence of gram-negative rod and increasing antibiotic resistance. *Biol Blood Marrow Transplant* 2009;15:47-53.
43. Camps IR. Risk factors for invasive fungal infections in haematopoietic stem cell transplantation. *Int J Antimicrob Agents* 2008;32(Suppl 2):S119-S123.
44. Angarone M, Ison MG. Prevention and early treatment of opportunistic viral infections in patients with leukemia and allogeneic stem cell transplantation recipients. *J Natl Compr Canc Netw* 2008;6:191-201.
45. Lin R, Liu Q. Diagnosis and treatment of viral diseases in recipients of allogeneic hematopoietic stem cell transplantation. *J Hematol Oncol* 2013;6:94. doi:10.1186/1756-8722-6-94.
46. Ichihara H, Nakamae H, Hirose A, et al. Immunoglobulin prophylaxis against cytomegalovirus infection in patients at high risk of infection following allogeneic hematopoietic cell transplantation. *Transplant Proc* 2011;43:3927-3932.
47. Raanani P, Gafter-Gvili A, Paul M, et al. Immunoglobulin prophylaxis in hematopoietic stem cell transplantation: Systematic review and meta-analysis. *J Clin Oncol* 2008;27:770-781.
48. Crumpacker CS. Cytomegalovirus. In: Bennett JE, Dolin R, Blaser MJ, eds. Mandell, Douglas, and Bennett's Principles and Practice of Infectious Diseases, 8th ed. Philadelphia: Elsevier, 2015:1738-1753.
49. Ziakas PD, Kourbeti IS, Voulgarelis MV, Mylonakis E. Effectiveness of systemic antifungal prophylaxis in patients with neutropenia after chemotherapy: A meta-analysis of randomized controlled trials. *Clin Ther* 2010;32:2316-2336.
50. Michallet M, Ito JI. Approaches to the management of invasive fungal infections in hematological malignancy and hematopoietic cell transplantation. *J Clin Oncol* 2009;27:3398-3409.
51. Nucci M, Anaissie E. Fungal infections in hematopoietic stem cell transplantation and solid-organ transplantation—Focus on aspergillosis. *Clin Chest Med* 2009;30:295-306.
52. Cavattoni I, Ayuk F, Zander AR, et al. Diagnosis of *Toxoplasma gondii* infection after allogeneic stem cell transplant can be difficult and requires intensive scrutiny. *Leuk Lymphoma* 2010;51:1530-1535.
53. Fishman JA, Issa NC. Infection in organ transplantation: Risk factors and evolving patters of infection. *Infect Dis Clin N Am* 2010;24: 273-283.
54. Grim SA, Clark NM. Management of infectious complications in solid-organ transplant recipients. *Clin Pharmacol Ther* 2011;90:333-342.
55. Issa NC, Fishman JA. Infectious complications of antilymphocyte therapies in solid organ transplantation. *Clin Infect Dis* 2009;48:772-786.
56. Person AK, Kontoyiannis DP, Alexander BD. Fungal infections in transplant and oncology patients. *Infect Dis Clin N Am* 2010;24:439-459.
57. San Juan R, Aguado JM, Lumbreras C, et al. Incidence, clinical characteristics and risk factors of late infection in solid organ transplant recipients: Data from the RESITRA study group. *Am J Transplant* 2007;7:964-971.
58. Neofytos D, Treadway S, Ostrander D, et al. Epidemiology, outcomes, and mortality predictors of invasive mold infections among transplant recipients: a 10-year, single-center experience. *Transpl Infect Dis* 2013;15:233-242.
59. Neofytos D, Fishman JA, Horn D, et al. Epidemiology and outcome of invasive fungal infections in solid organ transplant recipients. *Transpl Infect Dis* 2012;12:220-229.
60. Kotton CN. Zoonoses in solid-organ and hematopoietic stem cell transplant recipients. *Clin Infect Dis* 2007;44:857-866.
61. Weikert BC, Blumberg EA. Viral infection after renal transplantation: Surveillance and management. *Clin J Am Soc Nephrol* 2008;3: S76-S86.

62. Razonable RR. Management strategies for cytomegalovirus infection and disease in solid organ transplant recipients. *Infect Dis Clin N Am* 2013;27:317-342.
63. Jancel T, Penzak SR. Antiviral therapy in patients with hematologic malignancies, transplantation, and aplastic anemia. *Semin Hematol* 2009;46:230-247.
64. Zhang L-F, Wang Y-T, Tian J-H, et al. Preemptive versus prophylactic protocol to prevent cytomegalovirus infection after renal transplantation: A meta-analysis and systematic review of randomized controlled trials. *Transpl Infect Dis* 2011;13:622-632.
65. Torres-Madriz G, Boucher HW. Immunocompromised hosts: Perspectives in the treatment and prophylaxis of cytomegalovirus disease in solid-organ transplant recipients. *Clin Infect Dis* 2008;47:702-711.
66. Grossi PA. Update in HIV infection in organ transplantation. *Curr Opin Organ Transplant* 2012;17:586-593.
67. Kotton CN. CMV: prevention, diagnosis, and therapy. *Am J Transplant* 2013;13:24-40.
68. Lee B, Michaels MG. Prophylactic antimicrobials in solid organ transplant. *Curr Opin Crit Care* 2014;20:420-425.
69. Razonable RR. Management of viral infections in solid organ transplant recipients. *Exp Rev Antiinfect Ther* 2011;9:685-700.
70. Pittet LF, Posfay-Barbe KM. Immunization in transplantation: review of the recent literature. *Curr Opin Organ transplant* 2013;18:543-548.
71. Hantz S, Garnier-Geoffroy F, Mazeron M-C, et al. Drug-resistant cytomegalovirus in transplant recipients: A French cohort study. *J Antimicrob Chemother* 2010;65:2628-2640.
72. Subramanian AK. Antimicrobial prophylaxis regimens following transplantation. *Curr Opin Infect Dis* 2011;24:344-349.
73. Patel N, Snyder LD, Finlen Copeland CA, Palmer SM. Is prevention the best treatment? CMV after lung transplantation. *Am J Transplant* 2012;12:539-544.
74. Sims KD, Blumberg EA. Common infections in the lung transplant recipient. *Clin Chest Med* 2011;32:327-341.
75. Kittleson MM, Kobashigawa JA. Long-term care of the heart transplant patient. *Curr Opin Organ Transplant* 2014;19:515-524.
76. Andrassy J, Hoffmann VS, Rentsch M, et al. Is cytomegalovirus prophylaxis dispensable in patients receiving an mTOR inhibitor-based immunosuppression? A systematic review and meta-analysis. *Transplantation* 2012;94:1208-1217.
77. Kim SI. Bacterial infection after liver transplantation. *World J Gastroenterol* 2014;20:6211-6220.
78. Schaenman JM. Is universal antifungal prophylaxis mandatory in lung transplant patients? *Curr Opin Infect Dis* 2013;26:317-325.

Antimicrobial Prophylaxis in Surgery

123

Salmaan Kanji

KEY CONCEPTS

1. Prophylactic antibiotic therapy differs from presumptive and therapeutic antibiotic therapy in that the latter two involve treatment regimens for presumed or documented infections, whereas the goal of prophylactic therapy is to prevent infections in high-risk patients or procedures.
2. The risk of a surgical site infection (SSI) is determined from both the type of surgery and the patient-specific risk factors; however, most commonly used classification systems account for only procedure-related risk factors.
3. The timing of antimicrobial prophylaxis is of paramount importance. Antibiotics should be administered within 1 hour before surgery to ensure adequate drug levels at the surgical site prior to the initial incision.
4. Antimicrobial agents with short half-lives (eg, cefazolin) may require intraoperative redosing during procedures last more than 3 hours or 2.5 half-lives of the antimicrobial used.
5. The type of surgery, intrinsic patient risk factors, most commonly identified pathogenic organisms, institutional antimicrobial resistance patterns, and cost must be considered when choosing an antimicrobial agent for prophylaxis.
6. Single-dose prophylaxis is appropriate for many types of surgery. First-generation cephalosporins (eg, cefazolin) are the mainstay for prophylaxis in most surgical procedures because of their spectrum of activity, safety, and cost.
7. Vancomycin as a prophylactic agent should be limited to patients with a documented history of life-threatening *β*-lactam hypersensitivity or those in whom the incidence of infections with organisms resistant to cefazolin (eg, methicillin-resistant *Staphylococcus aureus*) is documented or high enough to justify use.

According to the National Center for Health Statistics and the National Hospital Discharge Survey, nearly 57 million outpatient and 51 million in patient surgical procedures are performed annually in the United States.[1,2] Infection is the most common complication of surgery.[3] Surgical site infections (SSIs) occur in ~3% to 6% of patients and prolong hospitalization by an average of 7 days at a direct annual cost of $5 billion to $10 billion.[4,5] SSIs are the third (14%-16%) most frequent cause of nosocomial infections among hospitalized patients and the primary (40%) cause of nosocomial infection in surgical patients.[4] Prophylactic administration of antibiotics decreases the risk of infection after many surgical procedures and represents an important component of care for this population.

Antibiotics administered prior to the contamination of previously sterile tissues or fluids are called prophylactic antibiotics. The goal of prophylaxis is to prevent an infection from developing. Although eradication of distal (preexisting, unrelated to surgery) infections lowers the risk for subsequent postoperative infections, it does not per se constitute a prophylactic regimen. In fact, surgical prophylaxis should be prescribed concurrently under these circumstances because of important antimicrobial spectrum- and timing-related concerns. Both SSIs and hospital-acquired infections not directly related to the surgical site (eg, urinary tract infections and pneumonia) are termed *nosocomial.* Prevention of hospital-acquired infections is a major goal of antibiotic prophylaxis.

1 Presumptive antibiotic therapy is administered when an infection is suspected but not yet proven. Clinical scenarios where presumptive therapy is used commonly include acute cholecystitis, open compound fractures, and acute appendicitis of less than 24 hours' duration. In these situations, if signs of perforation, contamination or infection are absent during surgery, then routine prophylactic treatment rather than presumptive therapy is warranted. An operative finding of a gangrenous gallbladder or a perforated appendix, however, is suggestive of an established infectious process, and a therapeutic antibiotic regimen is required.[4]

According to the Centers for Disease Control and Prevention's (CDC) National Nosocomial Infections Surveillance System (NNIS),[4] SSIs can be categorized as either incisional (eg, cellulitis of the incision site) or organ/space (eg, meningitis; Fig. 123-1). Incisional SSIs are subcategorized into superficial (involving only the skin or subcutaneous tissue) and deep (fascial and muscle layers) infections. Organ/space SSIs can involve any anatomic area other than the incision site. For example, a patient who develops bacterial peritonitis after bowel surgery has an organ/space SSI. By definition, SSIs must occur within 30 days of surgery. If a prosthetic implant is involved, a deep incisional or organ/space SSI can be reported up to 1 year from the date of surgery. Although microbiologic testing of surgical drainage material or sites may help to guide care, the specificity of a negative culture is poor and generally does not rule out an SSI.[4]

RISK FACTORS FOR SURGICAL SITE INFECTIONS

2 SSI incidence depends on both procedure- and patient-related factors. The risk for SSIs has been stratified by surgical procedure in a classification system developed by the National Research Council (NRC; Table 123-1).[6] The NRC classification system proposes that the risk of an SSI depends on the microbiology of the surgical site, the presence of a preexisting infection, the likelihood of contaminating previously sterile tissue during surgery, and the events during

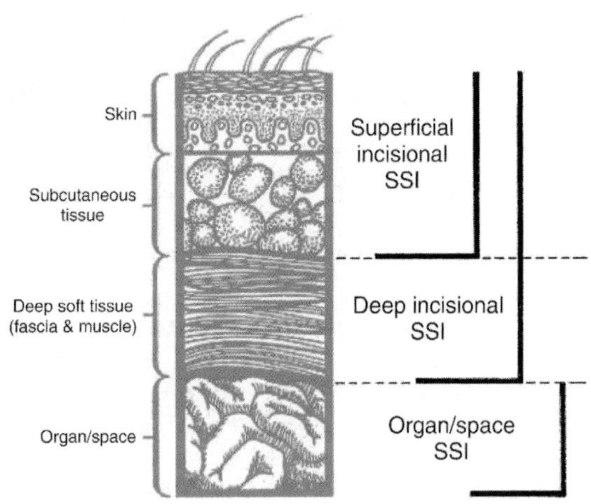

FIGURE 123-1 Cross section of abdominal wall depicting Centers for Disease Control and Prevention classifications of surgical site infections (SSI). *(Reprinted from Alexander JW, Solomkin JS, Edwards MJ. Updated recommendations for control of surgical site infections. Ann Surg 2011;253:1082-1093. Copyright © 2011 with permission from Elsevier.)*

and after surgery.[6,7] A patient's NRC procedure classification is the primary determinant of whether antibiotic prophylaxis is warranted. However, because a patient's NRC wound classification is influenced by surgical findings (eg, gangrenous gallbladder) and perioperative events (eg, major technique breaks), categorization generally occurs intraoperatively.[8]

Inherent Patient Risk

The NRC classification system does not account for the influence of underlying patient risk factors for SSI development, instead categorizing the risks for SSIs simply based on a specific surgical procedure. Disease states and conditions known to increase SSI risk are listed in Table 123-2. Preexisting distal infections increase SSI rates and should be resolved prior to surgery whenever possible. Diabetic patients have an increased risk for SSIs, especially those with uncontrolled perioperative blood sugars. Preoperative smoking is an independent risk factor for SSI because of the deleterious effects of nicotine on wound healing. Preoperative immunosuppression, including corticosteroid use, may increase infection risk. Patients coinfected with human immunodeficiency virus (HIV) and hepatitis C are at approximately double the risk of SSI as the general population.[9] Malnutrition is a well-described risk factor for postoperative complications, including SSI, impaired wound and colonic anastomosis healing, and prolonged hospital stay. Although enteral feeding during the perioperative period can reduce bacterial translocation by maintaining the integrity of the intestinal mucosa, nutritional supplementation does not decrease the incidence of infection.[10]

Colonization of the nares with *S. aureus* is a well-described SSI risk factor.[4] A large multicenter study involving more than 38,000 patients undergoing more than 42,000 cardiac and orthopedic procedures showed that pre-operative screening for carriers of *S. aureus* followed by intranasal mupirocin administration and chlorhexidine bathing for five days before surgery significantly reduced *S. aureus* SSI from 0.36% to 0.2%.[11] Although the absolute risk difference is small, this represents a 44% relative risk reduction. The potential impact on patient outcomes and health resource utilization is large given the number of surgeries performed annually. However, the logistics and cost of pre-screening and treatment of colonized patients represents a challenge. Other factors shown to increase the risk of SSI are age, length of preoperative hospital stay, and obesity.[4]

TABLE 123-2 Patient and Operation Characteristics That May Influence the Risk of Surgical Site Infection

Patient	Operation
Age	Duration of surgical scrub
Nutritional status	Preoperative skin preparation
Diabetes	Preoperative shaving
Smoking	Duration of operation
Obesity	Antimicrobial prophylaxis
Coexisting infections at distal body sites	Operating room ventilation
Colonization with resistant microorganisms	Sterilization of instruments
Altered immune response	Implantation of prosthetic materials
Length of preoperative stay	Surgical drains Surgical technique

Reprinted from Alexander JW, Solomkin JS, Edwards MJ. Updated recommendations for control of surgical site infections. Ann Surg 2011;253:1082-1093. Copyright © 2011 with permission from Elsevier.

Identifying SSI Risk

Two large epidemiologic studies have objectively quantified SSI risk based on specific patient- and procedure-related factors. The Study

TABLE 123-1 National Research Council Wound Classification, Risk of Surgical Site Infection, and Indication for Antibiotics

	SSI Rate (%)			
Classification	Preoperative Antibiotics	No Preoperative Antibiotics	Criteria	Antibiotics
Clean	5.1	0.8	No acute inflammation or transection of GI, oropharyngeal, genitourinary, biliary, or respiratory tracts; elective case, no technique break	Not indicated unless high-risk procedure[a]
Clean–contaminated	10.1	1.3	Controlled opening of aforementioned tracts with minimal spillage/minor technique break; clean procedures performed emergently or with major technique breaks	Prophylactic antibiotics indicated
Contaminated	21.9	10.2	Acute, nonpurulent inflammation present; major spillage/technique break during clean–contaminated procedure	Prophylactic antibiotics indicated
Dirty	N/A	N/A	Obvious preexisting infection present (abscess, pus, or necrotic tissue present)	Therapeutic antibiotics required

N/A, not applicable; SSI, surgical site infection.

[a]High-risk procedures include implantation of prosthetic materials and other procedures where surgical site infection is associated with high morbidity (see the text).

Data from references 5 and 11.

TABLE 123-3 Surgical Site Infection Incidence (%) Stratified by NRC Wound Classification and SENIC Risk Factors[a]

Number of SENIC Risk Factors	Clean	Clean–Contaminated	Contaminated	Dirty
0	1.1	0.6	N/A	N/A
1	3.9	2.8	4.5	6.7
2	8.4	8.4	8.3	10.9
3	15.8	17.7	11.0	18.8
4	N/A	N/A	23.9	27.4

N/A, not applicable; NRC, National Research Council; SENIC, Study on the Efficacy of Nosocomial Infection Control.

[a]Study on the Efficacy of Nosocomial Infection Control (SENIC) risk factors include abdominal operation, operations lasting >2 hours, contaminated or dirty procedures by National Research Council (NRC) classification, and more than three underlying medical diagnoses.

Used with permission from Wilson AP, Hodgson B, Liu M, et al. Reduction in wound infection rates by wound surveillance with postdischarge follow-up and feedback. Br J Surg 2006;93:630-638. Copyright © 2006 Wiley & Sons.

on the Efficacy of Nosocomial Infection Control (SENIC) analyzed more than 100,000 surgery cases to identify and validate risk factors for SSI.[12] Abdominal operations, operations lasting longer than 2 hours, contaminated or "dirty" procedures (as per NRC classification), and more than three underlying medical diagnoses each was associated with an increased incidence of SSI. When NRC classification was stratified by number of SENIC risk factors present, SSI incidence varied by as much as a factor of 15 within the same NRC operative category (Table 123-3).[13]

In a subsequent analysis of more than 84,000 surgical cases, the NNIS attempted to simplify and refine the SENIC system by quantifying intrinsic patient risk using the American Society of Anesthesiologists' (ASA) preoperative assessment score (Table 123-4).[14,15] An ASA score greater than or equal to 3 was a strong predictor for the development of an SSI. Other factors associated with increased SSI incidence are contaminated or "dirty" operations (NRC criteria) and surgical procedures lasting longer than average. As in the SENIC study, the SSI rate was linked to the number of risk factors present and varied considerably within NRC class. The NNIS basic SSI risk index is composed of the following criteria: ASA score = 3, 4, or 5; wound class; and duration of surgery. Overall, for 34 of the 44 NNIS procedure categories, SSI rates increased proportionally with the number of risk factors present.[16] The SSI rate was generally lower when the procedure was done laparoscopically.

Although evidence-based recommendations for antimicrobial prophylaxis during surgery are best established using the results of randomized clinical trials, many studies have small sample sizes and do not stratify patients according to overall SSI risk. Future studies, particularly those involving clean procedures, should be stratified by SSI risk so that the subset of high-risk patients who might benefit the most from prophylaxis is clearly established.

TABLE 123-4 American Society of Anesthesiologists' Physical Status Classification

Class	Description
1	Normal healthy patient
2	Mild systemic disease
3	Severe systemic disease that is not incapacitating
4	Incapacitating systemic disease that is a constant threat to life
5	Not expected to survive 24 hours with or without operation

Data from reference 15.

BACTERIOLOGY

The most important consideration when choosing antibiotic prophylaxis is the bacteriology of the surgical site. Organisms involved in an SSI are acquired by one of two ways: endogenously (from the patient's own normal flora) or exogenously (from contamination during the surgical procedure). Based on the type and anatomic location of the procedure and the NRC classification (see Table 123-1), resident flora can be predicted and appropriate antibiotic choices made. According to NNIS data, *S. aureus*, coagulase-negative staphylococci, enterococci, *Escherichia coli*, and *Pseudomonas aeruginosa* are the pathogens most commonly isolated (Table 123-5).[14] With the widespread use of broad-spectrum antibiotics, however, *Candida* species and methicillin-resistant *Staphylococcus aureus* (MRSA) are becoming more prevalent.[14]

Factors affecting the ability of an organism to induce an SSI depend on organism count, organism virulence, and host immunocompetency. Organisms in the commensal flora generally are not pathogenic. These organisms often serve the host as a form of protection against invasive organisms that otherwise would colonize the surgical site. Opportunistic organisms usually are kept in check by normal flora and rarely are problematic unless they are present in large numbers. The loss of normal flora through the use of broad-spectrum antibiotics can destabilize homeostasis, allowing pathogenic bacteria to proliferate and infection to occur.[5]

Normal flora translocated to a normally sterile tissue site or fluid during a surgical procedure can become pathogenic. For example, *S. aureus* or *Staphylococcus epidermidis* may be translocated from the surface of the skin to deeper tissues or *E. coli* from the colon to the peritoneal cavity, bloodstream, or urinary tract. Studies in animals and healthy volunteers have shown bacterial virulence to be an important determinant in the development of secondary infections.[17,18] Whereas more than one million *S. aureus* per square centimeter or gram of tissue are required to produce infection in animals, less than 100,000 *Streptococcus pyogenes* per square centimeter or gram of tissue are required at the same site.[18,19]

Impaired host defense reduces the number of bacteria required to establish an infection. A breach of normal host defenses through surgical intervention (eg, insertion of a prosthetic device) may enable organisms to cause infection. In addition, the loss of specific immune factors, such as complement activation, tissue-derived inhibitors (eg, proinflammatory cytokines), cell-mediated response

TABLE 123-5 Major Pathogens in Surgical Wound Infections

Pathogen	Percent of Infections[a]
Staphylococcus aureus	20
Coagulase-negative staphylococci	14
Enterococci	12
Escherichia coli	8
Pseudomonas aeruginosa	8
Enterobacter species	7
Proteus mirabilis	3
Klebsiella pneumoniae	3
Other *Streptococcus* species	3
Candida albicans	3
Group D streptococci	2
Other gram-positive aerobes	2
Bacteroides fragilis	2

[a]Data reported by the National Nosocomial Infections Surveillance System from January 1992 through June 2004.

Data from reference 5.

(eg, T-cell function), and granulocytic or phagocytic function (eg, neutrophils or macrophages) can greatly increase the risk for SSI development.[20] Vascular occlusive states related to the surgical procedure or those occurring from hypovolemic shock can greatly affect blood flow to the surgical site, thus diminishing host defense mechanisms against microbial invasion. Traumatized tissue, hematomas, and the presence of foreign material also lead to more infections. When a foreign body is introduced during a surgical procedure, fewer than 100 bacterial colony-forming units are required to cause an SSI.[21] Studies examining *S. aureus*-contaminated wound infections on the skin of healthy volunteers demonstrate a 10,000-fold reduction in the number of organisms required to establish a wound infection if sutures are not present.[17]

ANTIMICROBIAL RESISTANCE

Colonization of the host with antibiotic-resistant hospital flora prior to or during surgery may lead to an SSI that is unresponsive to routine antibiotic therapy. The most common cause of nosocomially acquired multiresistant organisms is transmission from hospital personnel.[22] Patients treated with broad-spectrum antibiotic therapy are at increased risk for colonization with hospital flora.

With cephalosporins established as first-line agents for prophylaxis, organisms resistant to cephalosporins represent the majority of pathogens causing SSIs. MRSA and coagulase-negative staphylococci have emerged as the most common pathogens in patients who develop SSIs despite prophylaxis with cephalosporins particularly in cardiothoracic, vascular, orthopedic, and neurologic surgery. Methicillin resistance not only limits the treatment/-prophylaxis options available, but it also is associated with increased mortality, longer hospital lengths of stay, and increased costs.[23,24] Although the use of vancomycin for prophylaxis may be appropriate for some operations performed in hospitals with a high rate of infection due to MRSA, there is little guidance on what constitutes a "high rate" of MRSA infection and whether providing prophylaxis with vancomycin alone will result in fewer SSIs.[25] A more effective strategy would be to screen elective surgical candidates for MRSA colonization preoperatively. MRSA colonization is predictive of MRSA SSI and thus effective prophylaxis with vancomycin is then reserved for carriers only. Some single center studies evaluating the decolonization of MRSA carriers preoperatively (ie, with intranasal mupirocin, chlorhexidine showers) yield mixed results and may not be cost-effective.[26,27]

Although cefazolin remains a mainstay in cardiovascular SSI prophylaxis, its failure has been reported in cases involving methicillin-sensitive *Staphylococcus aureus* (MSSA). In a comparison trial between cefamandole and cefazolin, significantly more failures were attributed to cefazolin, even though the primary pathogen was MSSA.[28] However, a similar trial comparing cefazolin and cefuroxime did not show any difference in SSI incidence between the two regimens.[28] The β-lactamase expressed by some MSSA may be capable of hydrolyzing cefazolin more readily than cefuroxime or cefamandole. Although this trend is disturbing, the overall incidence of cefazolin failure remains low, and cefazolin remains the drug of choice for SSI prophylaxis in cardiovascular surgery.[28]

The increase in frequency of fungal infections in surgical patients has drawn concern. In hospitalized patients, the incidence of nosocomial *Candida* infections nearly doubled from 1992 to 2004.[14,29] Overzealous use of broad-spectrum antibiotics is the most likely cause for this increase. A study of patients undergoing cardiovascular surgery identified female sex, length of stay in the ICU, and duration of central venous catheterization as risk factors for postoperative *Candida* infections.[30] Although presurgical *Candida* colonization is associated with a higher risk of fungal SSIs, routine preoperative use of prophylactic antifungal agents is not being advocated at this time.[29,31]

SCHEDULING ANTIBIOTIC ADMINISTRATION

3 4 The following principles must be considered when providing antimicrobial surgical prophylaxis: (a) the agents should be delivered to the surgical site prior to the initial incision, and (b) bactericidal antibiotic concentrations should be maintained at the surgical site throughout the surgical procedure. Although animal and human models have demonstrated the efficacy of a single dose of an antibiotic administered just prior to bacterial contamination, long operations often require intraoperative doses of antibiotics to maintain adequate concentrations at the surgical site for the duration of surgery.[32] Antibiotic administration should be completed within 60 minutes prior to the initial incision, preferably at the time of anesthetic induction. Since the administration duration varies between antimicrobials, this needs to be considered when determining when to start the infusion. Administration of antibiotics too early may result in concentrations below the MIC toward the end of the operation, and administration too late leaves the patient unprotected at the time of initial incision. In a study examining the timing of antibiotic administration to 2,847 patients receiving prophylaxis, Classen et al.[32] evaluated patients who received prophylaxis early (2-24 hours before surgery), preoperative prophylaxis (0-2 hours prior to surgery), perioperative prophylaxis (up to 3 hours after first incision), and postoperative prophylaxis (greater than 3 hours after the first incision). The risk of infection was lowest (0.6%) for patients who received preoperative prophylaxis, moderate (1.4%) for those who received perioperative antibiotics, and greatest for those who received postoperative antibiotics (3.3%) or preoperative antibiotics too early (3.8%). The risk for an SSI increases dramatically with each hour from the time of initial incision to the time when antibiotics are eventually administered. For these reasons, prophylactic antibiotics should not be prescribed to be given "on call to the operating room (OR)," which can occur two or more hours prior to the initial incision, nor should concurrent therapeutic antibiotics be relied on to provide adequate protection. In both situations, the chance for improperly timed doses is high. Although the landmark study by Classen et al.[32] confirmed that antimicrobial prophylaxis should be administered within 2 hours prior to the initial incision, administration immediately prior to the incision may not allow enough time for the drug to distribute throughout the tissues involved in the surgery.

In a large prospective observational study of 3,836 visceral, trauma, and vascular surgeries where antimicrobial prophylaxis with cefuroxime and metronidazole was employed, the incidence of SSIs was analyzed according to the timing of antimicrobial administration. When antimicrobial prophylaxis was administered within 30 minutes or between 1 and 2 hours before the initial incision, the risk of SSI was greater when compared to antimicrobial prophylaxis administered 30 to 59 minutes prior to the initial incision. The authors conclude that the optimal window for antimicrobial (cefuroxime and metronidazole) is between 30 and 59 minutes prior to the initial incision.[33] This effect may be a function of the pharmacodynamics and pharmacokinetics of the antimicrobial chosen for the prophylactic regimen. A larger study of 4,472 patients undergoing cardiac, orthopedic, and gynecologic surgery with a variety of antimicrobial prophylactic regimens also evaluated the temporal relationship between SSI occurrence and the timing of antibiotics. After excluding patients who received drugs with prolonged infusion times (ie, fluoroquinolones and vancomycin), there was a nonsignificant trend toward fewer SSIs in patients who received their prophylactic regimen within the 30 minutes prior to incision as compared with those who received the regimen 31 to 60 minutes prior to incision (odds ratio, OR: 1.74; 95% confidence interval: 0.98-3.04).[34]

Despite the importance of appropriately timed prophylactic antibiotic therapy, many patients receive antibiotics outside of the optimal time window in relation to surgery. Potential barriers include antibiotics ordered after the patient has arrived in the OR, delayed antibiotic preparation or delivery, and use of antibiotics that require long infusion times. One retrospective study assessed the timing of prophylactic antibiotics in more than 32,000 patients and found that 91.9% of patients received an antibiotic dose within 60 minutes of the initial surgical incision.[35]

Although most studies comparing single versus multiple doses of prophylactic antibiotics have failed to show a benefit of multidose regimens, the duration of operations in these studies may not be as long as that frequently observed in clinical practice. Proponents of administering a second antibiotic dose during lengthy operations suggest that the risk for SSI is just as great at the end of surgery (during wound closing) as it is during the initial incision. One study of patients undergoing cleancontaminated operations suggests that procedures longer than 3 hours require a second intraoperative dose of cefazolin or substitution of cefazolin with a longer-acting antimicrobial agent.[5] A second study of patients undergoing elective colorectal surgery suggests that low serum antimicrobial concentrations at the time of surgical closure is the strongest predictor of postoperative SSI.[36] Studies of patients undergoing cardiac surgery also have demonstrated a higher infection rate among patients with undetectable antibiotic serum concentrations at the conclusion of the procedure.[37] Ideally antibiotic prophylaxis should be repeated when surgeries last longer than two half-lives of chosen antibiotic (ie, four hours for cefazolin) or if intraoperative blood loss exceeds 1.5 L.[38]

One strategy to ensure appropriate redosing of prophylactic antibiotics during long operations is use of a visual or auditory reminder system. One hospital reported its experience with such a system, finding that an automated reminder improved compliance and reduced SSIs. However, even with the reminder system, intraoperative redosing was done in only 68% of eligible patients.[39] Another strategy currently being evaluated is the role of continuous infusions of cefazolin, which one pilot study has found to be a feasible way to ensure adequate serum concentrations of antibiotic during prolonged surgeries.[40] Further trials are required before such an intervention can be recommended.

ANTIMICROBIAL CHOICE

5 The choice of prophylactic antibiotic depends on the type of surgical procedure, the most frequent pathogens seen with this procedure, safety and efficacy profiles of the antimicrobial agent, current literature evidence supporting its use, and cost. Although most SSIs involve the patient's normal flora, antimicrobial selection also must take into account the susceptibility patterns of nosocomial pathogens within each institution. Typically, gram-positive coverage should be included in the choice of surgical prophylaxis because organisms such as *S. aureus* and *S. epidermidis* are encountered commonly as skin flora. The decision to broaden antibiotic prophylaxis to agents with gram-negative and anaerobic spectra of activity depends on both the surgical site (eg, upper respiratory, GI, or genitourinary tract) and whether the operation will transect a hollow viscous or mucous membrane that may contain resident flora.[4]

Although antimicrobial prophylaxis can be administered through a variety of routes (eg, oral, topical, or intramuscular), the parenteral route is favored because of the reliability by which adequate tissue concentrations may be acheived.[41] Cephalosporins are the most commonly prescribed agents for surgical prophylaxis because of their broad antimicrobial spectrum, favorable pharmacokinetic profile, low incidence of adverse side effects, and low cost. First-generation cephalosporins, such as cefazolin, are the preferred choice for surgical prophylaxis, particularly for clean surgical procedures.[4,5,8] In cases where broader gram-negative and anaerobic coverage is desired, antianaerobic cephalosporins, such as cefoxitin and cefotetan, are appropriate choices. Although third-generation cephalosporins (eg, ceftriaxone) have been advocated for prophylaxis because of their increased gram-negative coverage and prolonged half-lives, their inferior gram-positive and anaerobic activity and high cost have discouraged the widespread use of these agents.[4,5,8]

Allergic reactions are the most common side effects associated with cephalosporin use. Reactions can range from minor skin manifestations at the site of infusion to rash, pruritus, and rarely anaphylaxis (less than 0.02%). The structural similarity between penicillins and cephalosporins (each contains a β-lactam ring) has led to considerable confusion about the cross-allergenicity between these two classes of drugs. Twenty percent of the general population is labeled "penicillin allergic," yet of these patients, only 10% to 20% have positive results of a penicillin skin test.[42] The rate of cross-reactivity with cephalosporins is ~2%, but as only 20% of all "penicillin-allergic" patients truly are penicillin allergic, the true incidence of cross-reactivity likely is less than 1%. Routine penicillin skin testing is not cost-effective.[42] The administration of cephalosporins is both safe and cost-effective for many patients who are labeled "penicillin allergic," and they can be used by patients who have not experienced an immediate or type I penicillin allergy.

Vancomycin can be considered for prophylactic therapy in surgical procedures involving implantation of a prosthetic device in which the rate of MRSA is high.[24,43] If the risk of MRSA is low, and a β-lactam hypersensitivity exists, clindamycin can be used for many procedures instead of cefazolin to limit vancomycin use. Infusion-related side effects, such as thrombophlebitis and hypotension, particularly with vancomycin, usually can be controlled by adequate dilution and slower administration rates.[44]

Pseudomembranous colitis secondary to cephalosporins is uncommon and generally easily treated with a short course of oral metronidazole. Although infrequent, bleeding abnormalities related to cephalosporin use have been reported.[45] The primary hematologic effect appears to be inhibition of vitamin K-dependent clotting factors that results in prolongation of the prothrombin time. The mechanism for this effect, most commonly seen with cefotetan, is related to the methylthiotetrazole side chain of the β-lactam molecule. Patients at greatest risk for this hypoprothrombinemic effect have received a prolonged course of these agents and have underlying risk factors for vitamin K deficiency, such as malnutrition.[46]

Because inappropriate prophylactic antibiotic use not only can induce antibiotic resistance but also can negatively affect an institution's antibiotic budget, initiatives to curtail inappropriate antibiotic use have become the focus of many drug use evaluation efforts. Potential sources of inappropriate antibiotic prophylaxis include the use of broad-spectrum antimicrobials when a narrow-spectrum agent is warranted, extending prophylaxis for durations beyond that recommended in published guidelines, and using expensive antibiotics when equivalent, less expensive agents are available. The most effective tools for ensuring appropriate prophylactic antibiotic prescribing are knowledge of the institutional postoperative infection rate for each type of surgical procedure and familiarity with the bacterial epidemiology patterns for each surgical population. Individualized institutional guidelines that take into account the best literature evidence, institution-based antibiotic susceptibility data, and surgeon preference are important tools for rationalizing antibiotic prophylaxis use.[47]

RECOMMENDATIONS FOR SPECIFIC TYPES OF SURGERY

Guidelines for surgical prophylaxis usually are structured according to the tissues affected during an operation. Although many different surgical procedures may be performed at any one anatomic site, this method of categorization still is optimal because the factors related to the success of a prophylactic regimen, such as the endogenous flora that are expected and the pharmacokinetics, pharmacodynamics, and spectrum of selected antimicrobials, generally are constant for a particular surgical site (see the discussion above). The choice of antimicrobial prophylaxis is always best evaluated using the results of properly conducted clinical trials. In the absence of studies specific to the procedure in question, extrapolation from data on regimens for different procedures in the same anatomic site in question usually can be made. Subsequent modifications to each prophylactic regimen should be based on intraoperative findings or events.

6 A comprehensive review of the surgical prophylaxis literature is beyond the scope of this chapter, but important factors are reviewed here for each type/site of surgery. Specific recommendations are summarized in Table 123-6. The reader is referred to published guidelines and review articles.[3-5,8,41,48,49]

Gastrointestinal Surgery

GI surgery can be categorized according to surgical site and infectious risk. Gastroduodenal surgery and hepatobiliary surgery generally are considered to be clean or clean–contaminated surgeries, with SSI rates generally less than 5%. Colorectal surgery, including appendectomies, is considered contaminated because of the large quantities and polymicrobial nature of bacterial flora within the colon. SSI rates for these types of surgeries generally range from 15% to 30%. Emergent abdominal surgery involving bowel perforation or peritonitis is considered a dirty surgical procedure, associated with a greater than 30% risk of SSI, and should be treated with therapeutic rather than prophylactic antibiotics.[4]

Gastroduodenal Surgery

Insignificant numbers of bacteria usually are found in the stomach and duodenum because of their acidity. The rate of SSIs in gastroduodenal surgery generally is low, so procedures in this region can be classified as clean. The risk for an SSI in this population increases with any condition that can lead to bacterial overgrowth, such as obstruction, hemorrhage, or malignancy, or increasing the pH of gastroduodenal secretions with concomitant acid suppression therapy. Antimicrobial prophylaxis is of clinical benefit only in this high-risk population. In most cases, a single dose of IV cefazolin will provide adequate prophylaxis.[50] For patients with a β-lactam allergy, oral ciprofloxacin is as efficacious as parenteral cefuroxime as prophylactic therapy for gastroduodenal surgery.[50] Antimicrobial prophylaxis is indicated in esophageal surgery only in the presence of obstruction. Postoperative therapeutic antibiotics may be indicated if perforation is detected during surgery, depending on whether an established infection is present.

Use of antibiotic prophylaxis for percutaneous endoscopic gastrostomy placement is also warranted. Postoperative peristomal infection can occur in up to 30% of patients and a systematic review of 12 trials involving 1,271 patients found a significant reduction in peristomal infections with antimicrobial prophylaxis (OR 0.36, 95% CI 0.26-0.50).[51] A single dose of cefazolin given 30 minutes preoperatively is preferred over longer regimens.

There are no well-designed clinical trials of antimicrobial prophylaxis in bariatric surgery. However, given that obesity is a consistently identified risk factor for SSIs, guidelines do promote antimicrobial prophylaxis with cefazolin but at higher doses.[8]

Hepatobiliary Surgery

Although bile normally is sterile, and the SSI rate after biliary surgery is low, antibiotic prophylaxis is of benefit in this population. Bile contamination (bactobilia) can increase the frequency of SSIs and is present in many patients (eg, those with acute cholecystitis or biliary obstruction and those of advanced age).[48] In general, however, the correlation between bactobilia in surgical specimens and the subsequent pathogens implicated in an SSI is poor. The most frequently encountered organisms are *E. coli*, *Klebsiella* species, and enterococci. *Pseudomonas* is an uncommon finding in the absence of cholangitis. Most of the SSI literature on biliary tract surgery pertains to cholecystectomy while more recent trials pertain to laparoscopic procedures which have eclipsed the traditional open cholecystectomy because of a reduction in recovery time and hospital stay. The evidence in open cholecystectomy strongly supports the use of antimicrobial prophylaxis while the evidence for laparoscopic procedures is less impressive.[8] Trials comparing first-, second-, and third-generation cephalosporins have not demonstrated benefit over single-dose cefazolin prophylaxis even in high-risk patients (eg, age greater than 60 years, previous biliary surgery, acute cholecystitis, jaundice, obesity, diabetes, and common bile duct stones).[52] Ciprofloxacin and levofloxacin are effective alternatives for β-lactam-allergic patients undergoing open cholecystectomy.[53,54] In fact, orally levofloxacin appears to provide similar intraoperative gallbladder tissue concentrations.[54] For patients undergoing elective laparoscopic cholecystectomy, antibiotic prophylaxis is not of benefit and is not recommended.[55,56] Detection of an active infection during surgery (eg, gangrenous gallbladder and suppurative cholangitis) is an indication for a course of postoperative therapeutic antibiotics. The risk for SSIs in cirrhotic patients undergoing transjugular intrahepatic portosystemic shunt surgery may be reduced with a single prophylactic dose of ceftriaxone,[57] but not with single doses of shorter-acting cephalosporins.[58]

Appendectomy

Acute appendicitis can be broadly categorized as complicated (evidence of perforation, gangrene, peritonitis or abscess formation) or uncomplicated. Complicated appendicitis should be treated as an active intra-abdominal infection. While appendectomy for uncomplicated appendicitis is more common it has been associated with SSI rates of 9% to 30% in the absence of antimicrobial prophylaxis. Randomized controlled trials do suggest that pre-operative antimicrobials are effective at reducing this risk and should be administered in all cases.[59] Numerous antibiotic regimens, all with activity against gram-positive and gram-negative aerobes and anaerobic pathogens, are effective in reducing SSI incidence.[48] A cephalosporin with antianaerobic activity, such as cefoxitin or cefotetan, is recommended as first-line therapy; however, a comparative trial of cefoxitin and cefotetan suggests that cefotetan may be superior, possibly because of its longer duration of action.[60] Alternatively, cefazolin in combination with metronidazole is also effective. In patients with β-lactam allergy, metronidazole in combination with gentamicin is an effective regimen. Broad-spectrum antibiotics covering nosocomial pathogens (eg, *Pseudomonas*) do not further reduce SSI risk and instead may increase the cost of therapy and promote bacterial resistance.[61] Although single-dose therapy with cefotetan is adequate, prophylaxis with cefoxitin may require intraoperative redosing if the procedure extends beyond 3 hours.

Colorectal Surgery

In the absence of adequate prophylactic therapy, the risk for SSI after colorectal surgery is high because of the significant bacterial counts in fecal material present in the colon (frequently greater than 10^9 per gram). Anaerobes and gram-negative aerobes predominate, but gram-positive aerobes also may play an important role. Reducing this bacterial load with a thorough bowel preparation regimen (4 L of polyethylene glycol solution or 90 mL of sodium phosphate solution administered orally the day before surgery) is controversial; however, 99% of surgeons in a survey routinely use mechanical preparation.[62] Risk factors for SSIs include age over 60 years, hypoalbuminemia, poor preoperative bowel preparation, corticosteroid therapy, malignancy, and operations lasting longer than 3.5 hours.[8]

TABLE 123-6 Most Likely Pathogens and Specific Recommendations for Surgical Prophylaxis

Type of Operation	Likely Pathogens	Recommended Prophylaxis Regimen[a]	Comments	Grade of Recommendation[b]
GI Surgery				
Gastroduodenal	Enteric gram-negative bacilli, gram-positive cocci, oral anaerobes	Cefazolin 1 g × 1	High-risk patients only (obstruction, hemorrhage, malignancy, acid suppression therapy, morbid obesity)	IA
Cholecystectomy	Enteric gram-negative bacilli, anaerobes	Cefazolin 1 g × 1 for high-risk patients Laparoscopic: none	High-risk patients only (open biliary tract procedures, acute cholecystitis, common duct stones, previous biliary surgery, jaundice, age >60 years, obesity, diabetes mellitus)	IA
Transjugular intrahepatic portosystemic shunt (TIPS)	Enteric gram-negative bacilli, anaerobes	Ceftriaxone 1 g × 1	Longer-acting cephalosporins preferred	IA
Appendectomy	Enteric gram-negative bacilli, anaerobes	Cefoxitin or cefotetan 1 g × 1 or cefazolin 1 g plus metronidazole 1 g × 1	Second intraoperative dose of cefoxitin may be required if procedure lasts longer than 3 hours	IA
Colorectal	Enteric gram-negative bacilli, anaerobes	Orally: neomycin 1 g + erythromycin base 1 g at 1, 2, and 11 PM 1 day preoperatively plus mechanical bowel preparation IV: cefoxitin or cefotetan 1 g × 1	Role of mechanical bowel preparation is controversial. It is widely used despite evidence suggesting it may have no effect on SSI or other clinical outcomes	IA
GI endoscopy	Variable, depending on procedure, but typically enteric gram-negative bacilli, gram-positive cocci, oral anaerobes	Orally: amoxicillin 2 g × 1 IV: ampicillin 2 g × 1 or cefazolin 1 g × 1	Recommended only for high-risk patients undergoing high-risk procedures (see the text)	IA
Urologic Surgery				
Prostate resection, shock-wave lithotripsy, ureteroscopy	*Escherichia coli*	Ciprofloxacin 500 mg orally or Trimethoprim–sulfamethoxazole 1 DS tablet	All patients with positive preoperative urine cultures should receive a course of antibiotic treatment	IA–IB
Removal of external urinary catheters, cystography, urodynamic studies, simple cystourethroscopy	*E. coli*	Ciprofloxacin 500 mg orally or Trimethoprim–sulfamethoxazole 1 DS tablet	Should be considered only in patients with risk factors (see the text)	IB
Gynecological Surgery				
Cesarean section	Enteric gram-negative bacilli, anaerobes, group B streptococci, enterococci	Cefazolin 2 g × 1	Most guidelines recommend administration before incision. Administration after cord clamping may be as effective based on conflicting studies.	IA
Hysterectomy	Enteric gram-negative bacilli, anaerobes, group B streptococci, enterococci	Vaginal: cefazolin 1 g × 1 Abdominal: cefotetan 1 g × 1 or cefazolin 1 g × 1	Metronidazole 1 g IV × 1 is recommended alternative for penicillin allergy	IA
Head and Neck Surgery				
Maxillofacial surgery	*Staphylococcus aureus*, streptococci oral anaerobes	Cefazolin 2 g or clindamycin 600 mg	Repeat intraoperative dose for operations longer than 4 hours	IA
Head and neck cancer resection	*S. aureus*, streptococci oral anaerobes	Clindamycin 600 mg at induction and every 8 hours × 2 more doses	Add gentamicin for clean–contaminated procedures	IA

(continued)

TABLE 123-6 Most Likely Pathogens and Specific Recommendations for Surgical Prophylaxis (*Continued*)

Type of Operation	Likely Pathogens	Recommended Prophylaxis Regimen[a]	Comments	Grade of Recommendation[b]
Cardiothoracic Surgery				
Cardiac surgery	*S. aureus*, *S. epidermidis*, *Corynebacterium*	Cefazolin 1 g every 8 hours × 48 hours Intranasal mupirocin twice daily for 5 days preoperatively for patients colonized with *S. aureus*	Patients >80 kg (>176 lb) should receive 2 g of cefazolin instead; in areas with high prevalence of *S. aureus* resistance, vancomycin should be considered	IA
Thoracic surgery	*S. aureus*, *S. epidermidis*, *Corynebacterium*, enteric gram-negative bacilli	Cefuroxime 750 mg IV every 8 hours × 48 hours	First-generation cephalosporins are deemed inadequate, and shorter durations of prophylaxis have not been adequately studied	IA
Vascular Surgery				
Abdominal aorta and lower extremity vascular surgery	*S. aureus*, *S. epidermidis*, enteric gram-negative bacilli	Cefazolin 1 g at induction and every 8 hours × 2 more doses	Although complications from infections may be infrequent, graft infections are associated with significant morbidity	IB
Orthopedic Surgery				
Joint replacement	*S. aureus*, *S. epidermidis*	Cefazolin 1 g × 1 preoperatively, then every 8 hours × 2 more doses Intranasal mupirocin twice daily for 5 days preoperatively for patients colonized with *S. aureus*	Vancomycin reserved for penicillin-allergic patients or where institutional prevalence of methicillin-resistant *S. aureus* warrants use	IA
Hip fracture repair	*S. aureus*, *S. epidermidis*	Cefazolin 1 g × 1 preoperatively, then every 8 hours for 48 hours	Compound fractures are treated as if infection is presumed	IA
Open/compound fractures	*S. aureus*, *S. epidermidis*, gram-negativebacilli, polymicrobial	Cefazolin 1 g × 1 preoperatively, then every 8 hours for a course of presumed infection	Gram-negative coverage (ie, gentamicin) often indicated for severe open fractures	IA
Neurosurgery				
CSF shunt procedures	*S. aureus*, *S. epidermidis*	Cefazolin 1 g every 8 h ours × 3 doses or ceftriaxone 2 g × 1	No agents have been shown to be better than cefazolin in randomized comparative trials	IA
Spinal surgery	*S. aureus*, *S. epidermidis*	Cefazolin 1 g × 1	Limited number of clinical trials comparing different treatment regimens	IB
CSF shunt procedures	*S. aureus*, *S. epidermidis*	Cefazolin 1 g every 8 h ours × 3 doses or ceftriaxone 2 g × 1	No agents have been shown to be better than cefazolin in randomized comparative trials	IA
Craniotomy	*S. aureus*, *S. epidermidis*	Cefazolin 1 g × 1 or cefotaxime 1 g × 1	Vancomycin 1 g IV × 1 can be substituted for patients with penicillin allergy	IA

CSF, cerebrospinal fluid; DS, double strength.

[a]One-time doses are optimally infused at induction of anesthesia except as noted. Repeat doses may be required for long procedures. See the text for references.

[b]Strength of recommendations:

Category IA: Strongly recommended and supported by well-designed experimental, clinical, or epidemiologic studies.

Category IB: Strongly recommended and supported by some experimental, clinical, or epidemiologic studies and strong theoretical rationale.

Category II: Suggested and supported by suggestive clinical or epidemiologic studies or theoretical rationale.

Antimicrobial prophylaxis reduced mortality from 11.2% to 4.5% in a pooled analysis of trials comparing antimicrobial prophylaxis with no prophylaxis for colon surgery.[63] Effective antibiotic prophylaxis consisting of an oral and IV regimen reduces even further the risk for an SSI. A Cochrane review comparing oral, IV and combination regimens found that while each one was more effective at reducing SSI than placebo, combination therapy (oral and IV) was superior to oral regimens alone (OR 0.52 [0.35, 0.76]) and IV regimens alone (OR 0.55 [0.43, 0.71]).[64]

Several oral regimens designed to reduce bacterial counts in the colon have been studied.[48] The combination of 1 g neomycin and 1 g erythromycin base given orally 19, 18, and 9 hours preoperatively is the regimen most commonly used in the United States.[65] Neomycin is poorly absorbed, but provides intraluminal concentrations that are high enough to effectively kill most gram-negative aerobes. Oral erythromycin is only partially absorbed but still produces concentrations in the colon that are sufficient to suppress common anaerobes. If surgery is postponed, the antibiotics must be readministered to maintain efficacy. Optimally, the bowel preparation regimen (if used) should be completed prior to starting the oral antibiotic regimen. This is of particular concern because most procedures now are performed electively on a "same-day surgery" basis. In this case, the bowel preparation regimen is self-administered by the patient at home on the day prior to hospital admission, and compliance cannot be monitored carefully.

Single dose cephalosporins are the most used and studied preoperative IV antimicrobial. Cefoxitin or cefotetan is used most commonly, but other second- and some third-generation cephalosporins also are effective.[66] The role of metronidazole in combination with cephalosporin therapy is unclear. Only retrospective evidence suggests that the addition of metronidazole to a cephalosporin or extended-spectrum penicillin provides additional benefit.[67] Until this finding is confirmed in prospective studies, metronidazole should be reserved for combination therapy with cephalosporins with poor anaerobic coverage (eg, cefazolin). At this time, the evidence recommending the addition of metronidazole to cephalosporins with anaerobic activity (eg, cefotaxime, cefoxitin, and ceftriaxone) is insufficient.[68] For β-lactam-allergic patients, perioperative doses of gentamicin and metronidazole have been used. Combination therapy (ie, oral and IV therapy) is controversial. Postoperative antibiotics generally are unnecessary in the absence of any untoward events or findings during surgery. IV antibiotics are required for colostomy reversal and rectal resection because enterally administered antibiotics will not reach the distal segment that is to be reanastomosed or resected.[69]

Clinical **Controversy...**

A randomized trial of 380 patients undergoing elective colorectal surgery suggests that SSIs are not reduced by preoperative mechanical bowel preparation.[70] This finding was confirmed in two meta-analyses showing that mechanical bowel preparation does not reduce the risk of anastomotic leakage or other complications, including postoperative infection.[71,72] Despite this new evidence, mechanical bowel preparations continue to be a standard of practice prior to elective bowel surgery.

Gastrointestinal Endoscopy

Despite the large number of endoscopic procedures performed each year, the rate of postprocedural infection is relatively low. The highest bacteremia rates have been reported in patients undergoing esophageal dilation for stricture or sclerotherapy for management of esophageal varices. Although postprocedural bacteremia can occur in as many as 22% of patients, the bacteremia usually is transient (less than 30 minutes) and rarely results in clinically significant infection. Therefore, antimicrobial prophylaxis is routinely recommended only for high-risk patients (eg, patients with prosthetic heart valves, a history of endocarditis, systemic-pulmonary shunt, synthetic vascular graft less than 1 year old, complex cyanotic congenital heart disease, obstructed bile duct, or liver cirrhosis, as well as immunocompromised patients) undergoing high-risk procedures (eg, stricture dilation, variceal sclerotherapy, and endoscopic retrograde cholangiopancreatography, ERCP).[73] Single-dose preprocedural regimens similar to those for endocarditis prophylaxis are most common (amoxicillin for patients who can tolerate oral premedication or either IV ampicillin or cefazolin). A meta-analysis of antimicrobial prophylaxis for endoscopic placement of percutaneous feeding tubes also suggests that a single preoperative dose of antibiotics reduces the risk of postoperative infection compared with no antibiotic (6.4% vs 24%).[74] Consensus guidelines have adopted this recommendation and suggest a single dose of cefazolin within 30 minutes prior to the procedure.[73]

Urologic Surgery

Preoperative bacteriuria is the most important risk factor for development of an SSI after urologic surgery. All patients should have a preoperative urinalysis and should receive therapeutic antibiotics if bacteriuria is detected. Patients undergoing clean urologic procedures with sterile urine preoperatively are at low risk for developing an SSI and antimicrobial prophylaxis is not recommended.[8] Antibiotic prophylaxis is recommended for all patients undergoing transurethral resection of the prostate or bladders tumors, shock-wave lithotripsy, percutaneous renal surgery, or ureteroscopy.[75] The exact incidence of SSIs in this population is obscured by the frequent use of postoperative urinary catheters and the subsequent risk of bacteriuria. *E. coli* is the most frequently encountered organism. Routine use of broad-spectrum antibiotics, such as third-generation cephalosporins and fluoroquinolones, does not decrease SSI rates more than cefazolin, but the ability to administer fluoroquinolones orally rather than IV makes antimicrobial prophylaxis with ciprofloxacin easier and less expensive.[76] First- or second-generation cephalosporins are considered the antimicrobial agents of choice for patients undergoing open or laparoscopic procedures involving entry into the urinary tract and any urologic surgical procedures involving the intestine, rectum, vagina, or implanted prosthesis.[75] The evidence supporting antimicrobial prophylaxis for the removal of external urinary catheters, cystography, urodynamic studies, simple cystourethroscopy, and open or laparoscopic urologic procedures that do not involve entry into the urinary tract is not as evident. Only patients considered to have risk factors (patients of advanced age; those with anatomic anomalies, poor nutritional history, externalized catheters, colonized endogenous/exogenous material, or distant coexistent infection; smokers; immunocompromised patients; and those who are hospitalized for a prolonged stay) should receive antimicrobial prophylaxis.[75]

Obstetric and Gynecologic Surgeries

Cesarean Section

Cesarean section is the most frequently performed surgical procedure in the United States.[8] Prophylactic antibiotics are given to prevent endometritis, the most commonly occurring SSI. In the past, antibiotics were recommended for only high-risk patients, including those with premature membrane rupture or those not receiving prenatal care. Several large trials, as well as a meta-analysis of 81 trials, have shown benefit in administering prophylactic antibiotics to all women undergoing emergent or elective cesarean section regardless of their underlying risk factors.[77] Cefazolin remains the drug of choice despite the wide spectrum of potential pathogens, and a single 2 g dose appears to be superior to single or multiple 1 g doses.[78] Providing a broader spectrum of coverage with cefoxitin (for anaerobes) or piperacillin (for *Pseudomonas* or enterococci) does not further reduce postoperative infection rates. For patients with a β-lactam allergy, preoperative metronidazole is an acceptable alternative.[77]

Clinical **Controversy...**

During a cesarean section, unlike other surgical procedures, the most appropriate timing of antibiotic administration is controversial. Traditionally, antimicrobials were administered after the initial incision and when the umbilical cord was clamped in an attempt to minimize infant drug exposure, which theoretically could mask the signs of infection and induce antimicrobial resistance. Published guidelines recommend administering prophylactic antibiotics pre-incision but recent trials and meta-analyses show conflicting results.[78-80]

Hysterectomy

The most important factor affecting the incidence of SSI after hysterectomy is the type of procedure performed. Vaginal hysterectomies are associated with a high rate of postoperative infection when performed without the benefit of prophylactic antibiotics because of the polymicrobial flora normally present at the operative site.[81] As with cesarean sections, cefazolin is the drug of choice for vaginal hysterectomies despite the wide spectrum of possible pathogens.[81] The American College of Obstetricians and Gynecologists (ACOG) recommends a single dose of either cefazolin or cefoxitin.[82] For patients with a β-lactam allergy, a single preoperative dose of either metronidazole or doxycycline also is effective.[82]

Prophylactic antibiotics are recommended for abdominal hysterectomy despite the lack of bacterial contamination from the vaginal flora. Both cefazolin and antianaerobic cephalosporins (eg, cefoxitin and cefotetan) have been studied extensively. Single-dose cefotetan is superior to single-dose cefazolin,[83] and the investigators suggest that cefotetan should be the drug of choice for abdominal hysterectomies. However, other investigators suggest that either agent is appropriate, provided 24 hours of antimicrobial coverage is not exceeded.[8] The ACOG guidelines suggest that first-, second-, or third-generation cephalosporins can be used for prophylaxis.[82] Metronidazole plus an aminoglycoside or fluoroquinolone is also effective and can be used if patients are allergic to β-lactam antibiotics. Antibiotic prophylaxis may not be required in laparoscopic gynecologic surgery or tubal microsurgery.[84] As with other surgical procedures, perioperative events and findings may require the use of therapeutic antibiotics after surgery.

Head and Neck Surgery

The use of prophylactic antibiotics during head and neck surgery depends on the procedure type. Clean procedures (per NRC definition), such as thyroidectomy, lymph node excision and simple tooth extraction, are associated with a low incidence of SSI. Antimicrobial prophylaxis is not recommended for these procedures. Head and neck surgeries involving an incision through a mucosal layer are associated with a higher risk for SSI but antimicrobial prophylaxis is not always associated with a reduction in SSI (ie, adenoidectomy, tonsillectomy and septoplasty).[8] The normal flora of the mouth is polymicrobial; both anaerobes and gram-positive aerobes predominate. Although typical doses of cefazolin usually are ineffective for anaerobic infections, a 2 g dose produces concentrations high enough to inhibit these organisms. A pharmacokinetic study suggested that a single dose of clindamycin is adequate for prophylaxis in maxillofacial surgery unless the procedure lasts longer than 4 hours, when a second dose should be administered intraoperatively.[85] The greatest evidence for antimicrobial prophylaxis is in head and neck cancer resection surgeries. For most head and neck cancer resection surgeries, including free-flap reconstruction, 24 hours of clindamycin is appropriate, and no additional benefit of extending therapy beyond 24 hours is seen. A combination of clindamycin and gentamicin to cover aerobic, anaerobic, and gram-negative bacteria in clean-contaminated oncologic surgery is recommended.[86] Topical therapy with clindamycin, amoxicillin–clavulanate, and ticarcillin–clavulanate has been described in small trials, but the exact role of topical antibiotics is not defined.[87] Antimicrobial prophylaxis is not indicated for endoscopic sinus surgery without nasal packing.[41]

Cardiothoracic Surgery

Although cardiac surgery generally is considered a clean procedure, antibiotic prophylaxis lowers SSI incidence.[48] The substantial morbidity related to an SSI in this population, coupled with the routine implementation of prosthetic devices, further justifies the routine use of prophylaxis.[88] Patients who develop SSIs after coronary artery bypass graft surgery have a mortality rate of 22% at 1 year compared with 0.6% for those who do not develop an SSI.[89] Risk factors for developing an SSI after cardiac surgery include obesity, renal insufficiency, connective tissue disease, reexploration for bleeding, and poorly timed administration of antibiotics.[88] Skin flora pathogens predominate; gram-negative organisms are rare.

Cefazolin has been studied extensively and is considered the drug of choice. Although several studies and a meta-analysis advocate the use of second-generation cephalosporins (eg, cefuroxime) rather than cefazolin, various methodologic flaws in these studies have limited the extrapolation of these results to practice. Cefazolin was as effective as cefuroxime in a large randomized trial of 702 patients undergoing open heart surgery and thus remains the standard of care.[90] Both patient weight and timing of cefazolin administration relative to surgery must be considered when developing a dosing strategy. Patients weighing greater than 80 kg (greater than 176 lb) should receive 2 g cefazolin rather than 1 g. Doses should be administered no earlier than 60 minutes before the first incision and no later than the beginning of induction.[86] Extending therapy beyond 48 hours does not further reduce SSI rates. Single-dose cefazolin therapy may be sufficient but is not recommended by the Society of Thoracic Surgeons at this time pending further study.[91]

7 Routine vancomycin administration may be justified in hospitals having a high incidence of MRSA or when sternal wounds are to be explored surgically for possible mediastinitis. However, a large comparative trial enrolling almost 900 patients in a single center with a high prevalence of MRSA infections found that both cefazolin and vancomycin had similar efficacy in preventing SSI in patients undergoing cardiac surgery that required sternotomy.[92] Mediastinitis constitutes a failure of a prior prophylactic regimen. Continued postoperative vancomycin should be guided by culture and sensitivity data.[42] Subsequent antibiotic therapy is guided by intraoperative findings.

Since *S. aureus* is routinely identified as the most common pathogen in SSIs after cardiac surgery, several studies have investigated alternative methods for preoperative eradication including nasal mupirocin administration (ie, twice daily for 5 days pre-operatively) and chlorhexidine body wash (ie, daily pre-operatively for up to 5 days). A bundled approach (ie, more than one intervention implemented together) in addition to pre-operative antimicrobials appears to further reduce the risk of postoperative SSI in both cardiac and orthopedic surgeries.[11,93]

Pulmonary resection is associated with significant SSI risk, and prophylactic antibiotics have an established role in preventing postoperative infectious morbidity. Pleuropulmonary infections are much more common than wound infections, and pathogenic organisms likely migrate from the oral cavity or pharynx.[94] First-generation cephalosporins are inadequate; 48 hours of cefuroxime is preferred. A regimen of ampicillin–sulbactam is superior to first-generation cephalosporins, but further studies are required before this agent can be recommended as first-line prophylactic therapy.[95]

Vascular Surgery

Vascular surgery, like cardiac surgery, generally is considered clean by NRC criteria. Although vascular graft infections occur infrequently (3%-5%), the associated morbidity and mortality are extensive because treatment often requires surgical graft removal along with therapeutic antibiotic therapy.[96] Prophylactic antibiotics are of benefit, particularly for procedures involving the abdominal aorta, lower extremities or the implantation of prosthetic devices. Cefazolin is regarded as the drug of choice.[97] Twenty-four hours of prophylaxis with cefazolin is adequate; longer courses may lead to bacterial resistance.[98] For patients with β-lactam allergy, 24 hours of oral ciprofloxacin was effective.[96]

Orthopedic Surgery

Most orthopedic surgery is clean by definition; thus, prophylactic antibiotics generally are indicated only when prosthetic materials (eg, pins, plates, and artificial joints) are implanted.[21] A late-occurring infectious complication in this surgical population can result in substantial morbidity and may lead to prosthesis failure and subsequent removal. Staphylococci species are the most frequently encountered pathogens; gram-negative aerobes are infrequent. The use of cefazolin is supported by substantial evidence in the literature and therefore is the prophylactic agent of choice. Vancomycin, although effective, is not recommended for routine use unless a patient has a documented history of a serious allergy to β-lactams, or the propensity for MRSA infections at a particular institution necessitates its use. The current recommended duration of prophylaxis for joint replacement and hip fracture surgery is 24 hours.[8] Antibiotic-impregnated cement and beads have been used to lower SSI rates, but conclusive data regarding their efficacy are lacking.[21]

Duration of prophylaxis for the surgical repair of long bone fractures depends on the nature of the fracture. Multiple doses of prophylactic antibiotics offer no advantage over a single preoperative dose for repair of closed bone fractures and is more cost effective.[99,100] Patients suffering open (compound) fractures are particularly susceptible to infection because bacterial contamination almost always has occurred already. Under these circumstances, the use of antibiotics is presumptive. In this setting, cefazolin often is combined with an aminoglycoside, but controlled trials are lacking.[101] A clinical trial comparing clindamycin and cloxacillin suggests that clindamycin is superior and may be appropriate as monotherapy for Gustilo type I and II open fractures but not for type III fractures, for which added gram-negative activity is recommended.[102] Duration of antibiotic therapy is highly variable and depends on surgical findings during debridement, results of intraoperative cultures, and clinical status. A prospective trial comparing short (less than 24 hours) and long (greater than 24 hours) courses of antimicrobial prophylaxis for severe trauma suggests that longer courses of antibiotics do not offer additional benefit and may be associated with the development of resistant infections.[103] However, established joint infections and osteomyelitis require an extended course of therapeutic antibiotics.

As in cardiac surgery, there is evidence to support the use of preoperative intranasal mupirocin and chlorhexidine body wash for patients colonized with *S. aureus*. For elective procedures patients would be instructed to administer these at home in the days prior to the surgery. This bundled approach appears to further reduce the risk of postoperative SSI in addition to preoperative antimicrobials.[11,93]

Neurosurgery

The rates of SSI after clean neurosurgical operations (ie, craniotomy, spinal procedures) are low, however, the morbidity and mortality of central nervous system SSI, should they occur, are high. Pre-operative antibiotics are effective at reducing SSI rates and are recommended even in clean procedures.[104,105] While many antimicrobials have been studied, a single dose of cefazolin is what is recommended.[8]

Procedures involving cerebrospinal fluid (CSF) shunt placement should be considered separately because this procedure involves placement of a foreign body and is associated with higher infection rates. A study of 780 patients undergoing neurosurgical procedures that included shunt surgery reported that single doses of cefotaxime and trimethoprim–sulfamethoxazole were equally effective in preventing SSIs.[106] Most studies of procedures involving a shunt have been small in size and do not consistently show lower infection rates with antibiotic prophylaxis, although the results of a systematic review and meta-analysis suggest that a significant improvement in the incidence of shunt infection with 24 hours of systemic antibiotics (ie, cefazolin) and the use of antibiotic-impregnated catheters independently.[107]

SSIs associated with spinal surgery are rare but devastating when they occur. The use of antimicrobial prophylaxis in this setting is warranted and recommended by a meta-analysis.[108] Large randomized, controlled trials are lacking, but cefazolin is the antibiotic recommended most commonly. Cephalosporin penetration into the vertebral disk has been questioned. Some small studies suggest that the addition of gentamicin, which has better penetration, might be warranted; however, there is a paucity of clinical trials comparing these two regimens.[109]

NONPHARMACOLOGIC INTERVENTIONS

Strategies other than antimicrobial and aseptic technique for reducing postoperative infections have been investigated in different types of surgeries. The most commonly cited and practiced interventions include intraoperative maintenance of normothermia, provision of supplemental oxygen in the perioperative period, and aggressive perioperative glucose control.

Clinical **Controversy...**

Although interventions to maintain normothermia intraoperatively, provide supplemental oxygen in the perioperative period, and aggressively control perioperative glucose show a significant reduction in SSI, they cannot be generalized to all types of surgeries. However, given the simplicity and low cost of these interventions, many clinicians consider applying these measures outside of the studied population(s). At this time, pending further research, these interventions can be recommended for routine use only in the type of patient or surgery for which they were studied.

Core body temperature can fall by 1 to 1.5°C intraoperatively in patients under general anesthesia. Intraoperative hypothermia has been associated with impaired immune function, decreased blood flow to the surgical site, decreased tissue oxygen tension, and an increased risk of SSI. Efforts to maintain intraoperative normothermia should be exercised and may include the use of warming blankets and IV fluid warmers to maintain core body temperature between 36 and 38°C. One prospective trial of 200 patients undergoing colorectal surgery found that maintenance of normothermia reduced postoperative infection rates along with other morbidity parameters, including length of stay.[110]

Clinical **Controversy...**

Several studies have investigated the role of specialized enteral formulas fortified with a variety of immunomodulating micronutrients thought to enhance the immune response and gut function after trauma or surgery. Although many clinicians are exploring the role of supplements such as glutamine, arginine, omega fatty acids, and nucleotides, no study to date has shown a significant reduction in postoperative infection rates using these formulations.

Low oxygen tension in the tissues that make up the surgical site increases the risk of bacterial colonization and subsequent SSI by decreasing the efficiency of neutrophil activity. Administration of high concentrations of oxygen (80% via ventilator or 12 L/min via a nonrebreather mask) reduced postoperative infection rates significantly in a multicenter randomized trial of 500 patients undergoing colorectal surgery.[111]

Diabetes and poor glucose control are well-known risk factors for SSI. The increased risk of infection is thought to be due to both macrovascular (vasculopathy and venoocclusive disease) and microvascular (subtle immunologic deficiencies, including neutrophil dysfunction and reduced complement and antibody activity) complications. Aggressive control of perioperative blood glucose level decreases the incidence of SSI in diabetics undergoing cardiac surgery and is being evaluated in other types of surgery and in nondiabetic patients.[112] Perioperative blood glucose levels should be checked in all patients and conventional glucose targets (blood glucose less than 10 mmol/L [180 mg/dL]) should be encouraged. Hypoglycemia is similarly associated with poor outcomes and thus blood glucose levels less than 4.1 mmol/L (74 mg/dL) should be avoided.[8]

PERSONALIZED PHARMACOTHERAPY

Prophylactic antibiotics are only effective when therapeutic concentrations in the surgical field are maintained for the entire duration of the surgery. While consideration of drug half-life in the context of the duration of surgery has been discussed earlier in this chapter, other patient-related factors may influence the effectiveness of antibiotic prophylaxis and warrant consideration when choosing a prophylactic regimen (Table 123-7).

TABLE 123-7 Strategies for Implementing an Institutional Program to Ensure Appropriate Use of Antimicrobial Prophylaxis in Surgery

1. **Educate**
   Develop an educational program that enforces the importance and rationale of timely antimicrobial prophylaxis
   Make this educational program available to all healthcare practitioners involved in the patient's care
2. **Standardize the ordering process**
   Establish a protocol (eg, a preprinted order sheet) that standardizes antibiotic choice according to current published evidence, formulary availability, institutional resistance patterns, and cost
3. **Standardize the delivery and administration process**
   Use system that ensures antibiotics are prepared and delivered to the holding area in a timely fashion
   Standardize the administration time to <1 hour preoperatively
   Designate responsibility and accountability for antibiotic administration
   Provide visible reminders to prescribe/administer prophylactic antibiotics (eg, checklists)
   Develop a system to remind surgeons/nurses to readminister antibiotics intraoperatively during long procedures
4. **Provide feedback**
   Follow up with regular reports of compliance and infection rates

Obese patients require larger doses of prophylactic antibiotics to maintain therapeutic drug levels when compared to nonobese patients. Patients with a body mass index greater than 40 are more likely to have subtherapeutic concentrations at the end of surgery with cefazolin 1 g preoperatively (and intraoperative for surgeries greater than 3 hours) and thus should receive 2 g doses.[113,114] Underlying disease states that may affect antibiotic metabolism and/or elimination should be considered when developing a prophylactic regimen. For example, patients with thermal burn and spinal cord injuries eliminate certain classes of antibiotics, primarily the aminoglycosides and β-lactams, at unusually high rates compared with controls and will need more frequent intraoperative dosing. Conversely, individuals with renal failure may need less frequent dosing of renally cleared antibiotics. For example, while intraoperative dosing for cefazolin should be every 3 to 4 hours in patients with normal renal function, this interval should be extended to 8 hours for patients with creatinine clearances of less than 50 mL/min (0.83 mL/s). Individuals who are aggressively fluid resuscitated pre- or intraoperatively or those undergoing cardiac bypass may have altered antibiotic disposition related to increased volume of distribution and reduced total body clearance and may need larger doses (ie, 2 g cefazolin).

EVALUATION OF THERAPEUTIC OUTCOMES

When evaluating the outcome of surgical antibiotic prophylaxis, it is important to differentiate any potential SSI from other postoperative infection or complication. Although fever and leukocytosis are common in the immediate postoperative period, they typically resolve with prompt ambulation, timely removal of invasive devices, prevention and/or resolution of atelectasis through optimal respiratory care, and effective analgesia. It is important to remember that the emergence of distal infections, such as pneumonia, does not constitute a failure of surgical prophylaxis. Prophylaxis should be as short as possible because prolonged prophylactic regimens may contribute to the selection of resistant organisms and may make any infection more difficult to treat.

Surgical site appearance is the most important determinant of the presence of an infection. Drainage of pus from the incision accompanied by redness, warmth, and pain or tenderness is highly suggestive of an SSI. By definition, any surgical site that requires incision and drainage by the surgeon is considered infected regardless of appearance. Failure to heal and wound dehiscence also are seen with SSIs, although the surgical technique and nutritional status may be important contributing factors.

The presentation of signs and symptoms consistent with an SSI in relation to previous surgery is an important consideration when evaluating therapeutic outcomes after surgical prophylaxis. Many SSIs will not be evident during acute hospitalization. In fact, SSIs may not become evident until up to 30 days later or, in the case of prosthesis implantation, up to 1 year later. Thus, the true incidence of SSI can be determined only by completing comprehensive postdischarge surveillance. All studies investigating the efficacy of surgical prophylaxis must include adequate postdischarge follow-up to be able to thoroughly assess the success of any prophylactic regimen.

ABBREVIATIONS

ACOG	American College of Obstetricians and Gynecologists
ASA	American Society of Anesthesiologists
CDC	Centers for Disease Control and Prevention
CSF	cerebrospinal fluid
MRSA	methicillin-resistant *Staphylococcus aureus*
MSSA	methicillin-sensitive *Staphylococcus aureus*

NNIS National Nosocomial Infections Surveillance System
NRC National Research Council
SENIC Study on the Efficacy of Nosocomial Infection Control
SSI surgical site infection

REFERENCES

1. Hollingsworth JM, Krein SL, Ye Z, et al. Opening of ambulatory surgery centers and procedure use in elderly patients: Data from Florida. *Arch Surg* 2011;146:187-193.
2. National Hospital Discharge Survey. ftp://ftp.cdc.gov/pub/Health_Statistics/NCHS/Datset_Documentation/NHDS/NHDS_2010_Documentation.pdf Last accessed Oct. 19, 2015.
3. Alexander JW, Solomkin JS, Edwards MJ. Updated recommendations for control of surgical site infections. *Ann Surg* 2011;253:1082-1093.
4. Mangram AJ, Horan TC, Pearson ML, et al. Guideline for prevention of surgical site infection, 1999. Centers for Disease Control and Prevention (CDC) Hospital Infection Control Practices Advisory Committee. *Am J Infect Control* 1999;27:97-132.
5. Hendrick TL, Anastacio MM, Sawyer RG. Prevention of surgical site infection. *Expert Rev Anti Infect Ther* 2006;4:223-233.
6. National Academy of Sciences, National Research Council. Postoperative wound infections: The influence of ultraviolet irradiation of the operating room and of various other factors. *Ann Surg* 1964;160:32-135.
7. Cruse PJE, Foord R. A five-year prospective study of 23,649 surgical wounds. *Arch Surg* 1973;107:206-210.
8. Bratzler DW, Dellinger EP, Olsen KM, et al. Clinical practice guidelines for antimicrobial prophylaxis in surgery. *Am J Health Syst Pharm* 2013;70:195-283.
9. Drapeau CMJ, Pan A, Bellacosa C, et al. Surgical site infections in HIV-infected patients: Results from an Italian prospective multicenter observational study. *Infection* 2009;37:455-460.
10. Dionigi R, Rovera F, Dionigi G, et al. Risk factors in surgery. *J Chemother* 2001;13:6-11.
11. Schweizer ML, Chiang HY, Septimus E, et al. Association of a bundled intervention with surgical site infections among patients undergoing cardiac, hip or knee surgery. *JAMA* 2015;313:2162-2171.
12. Haley RW, Culver DH, Morgan WM, et al. Identifying patients at high risk of surgical wound infection: A simple multivariate index of patient susceptibility and wound contamination. *Am J Epidemiol* 1985;127:206-215.
13. Wilson AP, Hodgson B, Liu M, et al. Reduction in wound infection rates by wound surveillance with postdischarge follow-up and feedback. *Br J Surg* 2006;93:630-638.
14. National Nosocomial Infections Surveillance (NNIS) System Report, data summary from January 1992 through June 2004 issued October 2004. *Am J Infect Control* 2004;32:470-485.
15. Owens WD, Felts JA, Spitznagel EL. ASA physical status classifications: A study of consistency of ratings. *Anesthesiology* 1978;49:239-243.
16. Gaynes RP, Culver DH, Horan TC, et al. Surgical site infection (SSI) rates in the United States, 1992-1998: The National Nosocomial Infections Surveillance System basic SSI risk index. *Clin Infect Dis* 2001;33(Suppl 2):S69-S77.
17. Elek SD, Conen PE. The virulence of *Staphylococcus pyogenes* for man: A study of the problems of wound infection. *Br J Exp Pathol* 1958;38:573-586.
18. Burke JF. Identification of the sources of staphylococci contaminating the surgical wound during operation. *Ann Surg* 1963;158:898-904.
19. Kaiser AB, Kernodle DS, Parker RA. Low-inoculum model of surgical wound infection. *J Infect Dis* 1992;166:393-399.
20. Esposito S. Immune system and surgical site infection. *J Chemother* 2001;13:12-16.
21. De Lalla F. Antibiotic prophylaxis in orthopedic prosthetic surgery. *J Chemother* 2001;13:48-53.
22. Halwani M, Solaymani-Dodaran M, Grundman H, et al. Cross transmission of nosocomial pathogens in an adult intensive care unit: Incidence and risk factors. *J Hosp Infect* 2006;63:39-46.
23. Crawford T, Rodvold KA, Solomkin JS. Vancomycin for surgical prophylaxis? *Clin Infect Dis* 2012;54:1474-1479.
24. Weigelt JA, Lipsky BA, Tabak YP, et al. Surgical site infection: Causative pathogens and associated outcomes. *Am J Infect Control* 2010;38:112-120.
25. Chambers D, Worthy G, Myers L, et al. Glycopeptide vs. non-glycopeptide antibiotics for prophylaxis of surgical site infections: A systematic review. *Surg Infect (Larchmt)* 2010;11:455-462.
26. Ramirez MC, Marchessault M, Govednik-Horny C, et al. The impact of MRSA colonization on surgical site infection following major gastrointestinal surgery. *J Gastrointest Surg* 2013;17:144-152.
27. Kim DH, Spencer M, Davidson SM, et al. Institutional prescreening for detection and eradication of methicillin-resistant *Staphylococcus aureus* in patients undergoing elective orthopaedic surgery. *J Bone Joint Surg Am* 2010;92:1820-1826.
28. Lowy FD, Waldhausen JA, Miller M, et al. Report of the National Heart, Lung and Blood Institute–National Institute of Allergy and Infectious Diseases working group on antimicrobial strategies and cardiothoracic surgery. *Am Heart J* 2004;147:575-581.
29. Munoz P, Burrillo A, Bouza E. Criteria used when initiating antifungal therapy against *Candida* spp. in the intensive care unit. *Int J Antimicrob Agents* 2000;15:83-90.
30. Lipsett PA. Surgical critical care: Fungal infections in surgical patients. *Crit Care Med* 2006;34:S25-S24.
31. McKinnon PS, Goff DA, Kern JW, et al. Temporal assessment of *Candida* risk factors in the surgical intensive care unit. *Arch Surg* 2001;136:1401-1408.
32. Classen DC, Evans RS, Pestotnik SL, et al. The timing of prophylactic administration of antibiotics and the risk of surgical wound infection. *N Engl J Med* 1992;326:281-286.
33. Weber WP, Marti WR, Zwahlen M, et al. The timing of surgical antimicrobial prophylaxis. *Ann Surg* 2008;247:918-926.
34. Steinberg JP, Braun BI, Hellinger WC, et al. Timing of antimicrobial prophylaxis and the risk of surgical site infections: Results from the trial to reduce antimicrobial prophylaxis errors. *Ann Surg* 2009;250:10-16.
35. Hawn MT, Richman JS, Vicks CC, et al. Timing of surgical antibiotic prophylaxis and the risk of surgical site infection. *JAMA Surg* 2013;148:649-657.
36. Zelenitzky SA, Ariano RE, Harding GKM, et al. Antibiotic pharmacodynamics in surgical prophylaxis: An association between intraoperative antibiotic concentrations and efficacy. *Antimicrob Agents Chemother* 2002;46:3026-3030.
37. Goldman DA, Hopkins CC, Karchmer AW. Cephalothin prophylaxis in cardiac valve surgery: A prospective, double-blind comparison of two-day and six-day regimen. *J Thorac Cardiovasc Surg* 1977;73:470-479.
38. Cataife G, Weinberg DA, Wong HH, et al. The effect of Surgical Care Improvement Project (SCIP) compliance on surgical site infection (SSI). *Med Care* 2014;52(Suppl 1):S66-S73.
39. Zanetti G, Flanagan HL Jr, Cohn LH, et al. Improvement of intraoperative antibiotic prophylaxis in prolonged cardiac surgery by automated alerts in the operating room. *Infect Control Hosp Epidemiol* 2003;24:7-9.
40. Waltrip T, Lewis R, Young V, et al. A pilot study to determine the feasibility of continuous cefazolin infusion. *Surg Infect* 2002;3:5-9.
41. Weed HG. Antimicrobial prophylaxis in the surgical patient. *Med Clin North Am* 2003;27:59-75.
42. Salkind AR, Cuddy PG, Foxworth JW. The rational clinical examination: Is this patient allergic to penicillin? An evidence-based analysis of the likelihood of penicillin allergy. *JAMA* 2001;285:2498-2505.
43. Gemmel CG, Edwards DI, Fraise AP, et al. Guidelines for the prophylaxis and treatment of methicillin *Staphylococcus aureus* (MRSA) infections in the UK. *J Antimicrob Chemother* 2006;57:589-608.
44. Hadaway L, Chamallas SN. Vancomycin: New perspectives on an old drug. *J Infus Nurs* 2003;26:278-284.
45. Wong RS, Cheng G, Chang NP, et al. Use of cefoperazone still needs a caution for bleeding from induced vitamin K deficiency. *Am J Hematol* 2006;81:76.
46. Williams KJ, Bax RP, Brown H, Machin SJ. Antibiotic treatment and associated prolonged prothrombin time. *J Clin Pathol* 1991;44:738-741.
47. Frighetto L, Marra CA, Stiver HG, et al. Economic impact of standardized orders for antimicrobial prophylaxis program. *Ann Pharmacother* 2000;34:154-160.
48. Bratzler DW, Houck PM. Antimicrobial prophylaxis for surgery: An advisory statement from the National Surgical Infection Prevention Project. *Clin Infect Dis* 2004;38:1706-1715.
49. Anderson DJ. Surgical site infections. *Infect Dis Clin North Am* 2011;25:135-153.
50. McArdle CS, Morran CG, Anderson JR, et al. Oral ciprofloxacin as prophylaxis in gastroduodenal surgery. *J Hosp Infect* 1995;30:211-216.
51. Lipp A, Lusardi G. Systemic antimicrobial prophylaxis for percutaneous endoscopic gastrostomy. *Cochrane Database Syst Rev* 2013;11:CD005571.

52. Jewesson PJ, Stiver G, Wai A, et al. Double-blind comparison of cefazolin and ceftizoxime for prophylaxis against infections following elective biliary tract surgery. *Antimicrob Agents Chemother* 1996;40:70-74.
53. Agrawal CS, Sehgal R, Singh RK, Gupta AK. Antibiotic prophylaxis in elective cholecystectomy: A randomized, double-blinded study comparing ciprofloxacin and cefuroxime. *Ind J Physiol Pharmacol* 1999;43:501-504.
54. Swoboda S, Oberdorfer K, Klee F, et al. Tissue and serum concentrations of levofloxacin 500 mg administered intravenously or orally for antibiotic prophylaxis in biliary surgery. *J Antimicrob Chemother* 2003;51:459-462.
55. Zhou H, Shang J, Wang Q, et al. Meta-analysis: Antibiotic prophylaxis in elective laparascopic cholecystectomy. *Aliment Pharmacol Ther* 2009;29:1086-1095.
56. Choudhary A, Bechtold ML, Puli SR, et al. Role of prophylactic antibiotics in laparoscopic cholecystectomy: A meta-analysis. *J Gastrointest Surg* 2008;12:1847-1853.
57. Gulberg V, Deibert P, Ochs A, et al. Prevention of infectious complications after transjugular intrahepatic portosystemic shunt in cirrhotic patients with a single dose of ceftriaxone. *Hepatogastroenterology* 1999;46:1126-1130.
58. Deibert P, Schwartz S, Olschewski M, et al. Risk factors and prevention of early infection after implantation or revision of transjugular intrahepatic portosystemic shunts: Results of a randomized study. *Dig Dis Sci* 1998;43:1708-1713.
59. Andersen BR, Kallehave FL, Andersen HK. Antibiotics versus placebo for prevention of postoperative infection after appendicectomy. *Cochrane Database Syst Rev* 2005;3:CD001439.
60. Liberman MA, Greason KL, Frame S, Ragland JJ. Single-dose cefotetan or cefoxitin versus multiple-dose cefoxitin as prophylaxis in patients undergoing appendectomy for acute nonperforated appendicitis. *J Am Coll Surg* 1995;180:77-80.
61. Colliza S, Rossi S. Antibiotic prophylaxis and treatment of surgical abdominal sepsis. *J Chemother* 2001;13:193-201.
62. Zmora O, Wexner SD, Hajjar L, et al. Trend in preparation for colorectal surgery: Survey of the members of the American Society of Colon and Rectal Surgeons. *Am Surg* 2003;69:150-154.
63. Baum ML, Anish DS, Chalmers TC, et al. A survey of clinical trials of antibiotic prophylaxis in colon surgery: Evidence against further use of no-treatment controls. *N Engl J Med* 1981;305:795-799.
64. Nelson RL, Gladman E, Barbateskovic M. Antimicrobial prophylaxis for colorectal surgery. *Cochrane Database Syst* Rev 2014;5:CD001181.
65. Solla JA, Rothenberger DA. Preoperative bowel preparation: A survey of colon and rectal surgeons. *Dis Colon Rectum* 1990;33:154-159.
66. Fujita S, Saito N, Yamada T, et al. Randomized, multicenter trial of antibiotic prophylaxis in elective colorectal surgery: Single dose vs 3 doses of a second-generation cephalosporin without metronidazole and oral antibiotics. *Arch Surg* 2007;142:657-661.
67. Mittelkotter U. Antimicrobial prophylaxis for abdominal surgery: Is there a need for metronidazole? *J Chemother* 2001;13:27-34.
68. Kobayashi M, Mohri Y, Tonouchi H, et al. Randomized clinical trial comparing intravenous antimicrobial prophylaxis alone with oral and intravenous antimicrobial prophylaxis for the prevention of a surgical site infection in colorectal cancer surgery. *Surg Today* 2007;37:383-388.
69. Ghorra SG, Rzeczycki TP, Natarajan R, Pricolo VE. Colostomy closure: Impact of preoperative risk factors on morbidity. *Am Surg* 1999;65:266-269.
70. Zmora O, Mahajna A, Bar-Zakai B, et al. Colon and rectal surgery without mechanical bowel preparation: A randomized, prospective trial. *Ann Surg* 2003;237:363-367.
71. Cao F, Li J, Li F. Mechanical bowel preparation for elective colorectal surgery: Updated systematic review and meta-analysis. *Int J Colorectal Dis* 2012;27:803-810.
72. Dahabreh IJ, Steele DW, Shah N, Trikalinos TA. Oral Mechanical Bowel Preparation for Colo-rectal Surgery. Comparative Effectiveness Review No. 128. AHRQ Publication No. 14-EHC018-EF. Rockville, MD: Agency for Healthcare Research and Quality; April 2014. www.effectivehealthcare.ahrq.gov/reports/final.cfm Accessed Oct. 19, 2015.
73. ASGE Standards of Practice Committee. Antibiotic prophylaxis for GI endoscopy. *Gastrointest Endosc* 2015;81:81-89.
74. Sharma VK, Howden CW. Meta-analysis of randomized, controlled trials of antibiotic prophylaxis before percutaneous endoscopic gastrostomy. *Am J Gastroenterol* 2001;96:1951-1952.
75. Wolf Jr JS, Bennett CJ, Dmochowski RR, Hollenbeck BK, Pearles MS, Schaeffer AJ. Best practice policy statement on urologic surgery antimicrobial prophylaxis. *J Urol* 2008;179:1379-1390.
76. Christiano AP, Hollowell CM, Kim H, et al. Double-blind, randomized comparison of single-dose ciprofloxacin versus intravenous cefazolin in patients undergoing outpatient endourologic surgery. *Urology* 2000;55:182-185.
77. Smaill F, Hofmeyr GJ. Antibiotic prophylaxis for cesarean section. *Cochrane Database Syst Rev* 2002;2:CD000933.
78. Rouzi AA, Khalifa F, Ba'aqeel H, et al. The routine use of cefazolin in cesarean section. *Int J Gynaecol Obstet* 2000;69:107-112.
79. Heesen M, Klohr S, Rossaint R, et al. Concerning the timing of antibiotic administration in women undergoing caesarean section: A systematic review and meta-analysis. *BMJ Open* 2013;3:e002028.
80. Mackeen AD, Packard RE, Ota E, Berghella V, Baxter JK. Timing of intravenous prophylactic antibiotics for preventing postpartum infectious morbidity in women undergoing cesarean delivery. *Cochrane Database Syst Rev* 2014;12:CD009516.
81. Guaschino S, De Santo D, De Seta F. New perspectives in antibiotic prophylaxis for obstetric and gynaecological surgery. *J Hosp Infect* 2002;50(Suppl A):S13-S16.
82. American College of Obstetricians and Gynecologists. Antibiotic prophylaxis for gynecologic procedures. *Obstet Gynecol* 2009;113:1180-1189.
83. Hemsell DL, Johnson ER, Hemsell PG, et al. Cefazolin is inferior to cefotetan as single dose prophylaxis for women undergoing elective total abdominal hysterectomy. *Clin Infect Dis* 1995;20:677-684.
84. Sturlese E, Retto G, Pulia A, et al. Benefits of antibiotic prophylaxis in laparoscopic gynaecological surgery. *Clin Exp Obstet Gynecol* 1999;26:217-218.
85. Meuller SC, Henkel KO, Neumann J, et al. Perioperative antibiotic prophylaxis in maxillofacial surgery: Penetration of clindamycin into various tissues. *J Craniomaxillofac Surg* 1999;27:172-176.
86. Simo R, French G. The use of prophylactic antibiotics in head and neck oncological surgery. *Curr Opin Otolaryngol Head Neck Surg* 2006;14:55-61.
87. Grandis JR, Vickers RM, Rihs JD, et al. Efficacy of topical amoxicillin plus clavulanate–ticarcillin plus clavulanate and clindamycin in contaminated head and neck surgery: Effect of antibiotic spectra and duration of therapy. *J Infect Dis* 1994;170:729-732.
88. Roy MC. Surgical-site infections after coronary artery bypass graft surgery: Discriminating site-specific risk factors to improve prevention efforts. *Infect Control Hosp Epidemiol* 1998;19:229-233.
89. Hollenbeak CS, Murphy DM, Koenig S, et al. The clinical and economic impact of deep chest surgical site infections following coronary artery bypass graft surgery. *Chest* 2000;118:397-402.
90. Curtis JJ, Boley TM, Walls JT, et al. Randomized, prospective comparison of first- and second-generation cephalosporins as infection prophylaxis for cardiac surgery. *Am J Surg* 1993;166:734-737.
91. Edwards FH, Egleman RM, Houck P, et al. The society of thoracic surgeons practice guidelines series: Antibiotic prophylaxis in cardiac surgery, part 1: Duration. *Ann Thorac Surg* 2006;81:397-404.
92. Finkelstein R, Rabino G, Masiah T, et al. Vancomycin versus cefazolin prophylaxis for cardiac surgery in the setting of a high prevalence of methicillin-resistant staphylococcal infections. *J Thorac Cardiovasc Surg* 2002;123:326-332.
93. Schweizer ML, Perencevich E, McDaniel J, et al. Effectiveness of a bundled intervention of decolonization and prophylaxis to decrease Gram positive surgical site infections after cardiac or orthopedic surgery: Systematic review and meta-analysis. *BMJ* 2013;346:f2743.
94. Sok M, Dragas AZ, Erzen J, et al. Sources of pathogens causing pleuropulmonary infections after lung cancer resection. *Eur J Cardiothorac Surg* 2002;22:23-27.
95. Boldt J, Piper S, Uphus D, et al. Preoperative microbiologic screening and antibiotic prophylaxis in pulmonary resection operations. *Ann Thorac Surg* 1999;68:208-211.
96. Pratesi C, Russo D, Dorigo W, et al. Antibiotic prophylaxis in clean surgery: Vascular surgery. *J Chemother* 2001;13:123-128.
97. Douglas A, Udy AA, Wallis S, et al. Plasma and tissue pharmacokinetics of cefazolin in patients undergoing elective and semielective abdominal aortic aneurysm open repair surgery. *Antimicrob Agents Chemother* 2011;55:5238-5242.
98. Terpstra S, Noorkhoek GT, Voesten HG, et al. Rapid emergence of resistant coagulase-negative staphylococci on the skin after antibiotic prophylaxis. *J Hosp Infect* 1999;43:195-202.
99. Slobogean GP, Kennedy SA, Davidson D, et al. Single- versus multiple-dose antibiotic prophylaxis in the surgical treatment of closed fractures: A meta-analysis. *J Orthop Trauma* 2008;22:264-269.
100. Slobogean PG, O'Brien PJ, Brauer CA. Single-dose versus multiple-dose antibiotic prophylaxis for the surgical treatment of closed fractures: A cost-effective analysis. *Acta Orthop* 2010;81:256-262.

101. Gillespie WJ, Walenkamp G. Antibiotic prophylaxis for surgery for proximal femoral and other closed long bone fractures. *Cochrane Database Syst Rev* 2001;1:CD000244.
102. Vasenius J, Tulikoura I, Vainionpaa S, Rokkanen P. Clindamycin versus cloxacillin in the treatment of 240 open fractures: A randomized, prospective study. *Ann Chir Gynaecol* 1998;87:224-228.
103. Velmahos GC, Toutouzas KG, Sarkisyan G, et al. Severe trauma is not an excuse for prolonged antibiotic prophylaxis. *Arch Surg* 2002;137:537-541.
104. Barker FG II. Efficacy of prophylactic antibiotics against meningitis after craniotomy: A meta-analysis. *Neurosurgery* 2007;60:887-894.
105. Watters WC 3rd, Baisden J, Bono CM, et al. Antibiotic prophylaxis in spine surgery:an evidence-based clinical guideline for the sue of prophylactic antibiotics in spine surgery. *Spine J* 2009;9:142-146.
106. Whitby M, Johnson BC, Atkinson RL, et al. The comparative efficacy of intravenous cefotaxime and trimethoprim/sulfamethoxazole in preventing infection after neurosurgery: A prospective, randomized study. Brisbane Neurosurgical Infection Group. *Br J Neurosurg* 2000;14:13-18.
107. Ratilal B, Costa J, Sampaio C. Antibiotic prophylaxis for surgical introduction of intracranial ventricular shunts: A systematic review. *J Neurosurg Pediatr* 2008;1:48-56.
108. Barker FG. Efficacy of prophylactic antibiotic therapy in spinal surgery: A meta-analysis. *Neurosurgery* 2002;51:391-400.
109. Riley LH 3rd. Prophylactic antibiotics for spine surgery: Description of a regimen and its rationale. *J South Orthop Assoc* 1998;7:212-217.
110. Kurz A, Sessler DI, Lenhardt R. Perioperative normothermia to reduce the incidence of surgical-wound infection and shorten hospitalization. Study of Wound Infection and Temperature Group. *N Engl J Med* 1996;334:1209-1215.
111. Greif R, Akca O, Horn EP, et al. Supplemental perioperative oxygen to reduce the incidence of surgical-wound infection. Outcomes Research Group. *N Engl J Med* 2000;342:161-167.
112. Kao LS, Meeks D, Moyer VA, Lally KP. Peri-operative glycaemic control regimens for preventing surgical site infections in adults. *Cochrane Database Syst Rev* 2009;3:CD006806.
113. Edmiston CE, Krepel C, Kelly H, et al. Perioperative antibiotic prophylaxis in the gastric bypass patient: Do we achieve therapeutic levels? *Surgery* 2004;136:738-747.
114. Ho VP, Nicolau DP, Dakin GF, et al. Cefazolin dosing for surgical prophylaxis in morbidly obese patients. *Surg Infect (Larchmt)* 2012;13:33-37.

e124

Travel Health

Douglas Slain and Scott Kincaid

KEY CONCEPTS

1. Travelers should consult practitioners with travel health expertise when going to tropical or developing countries.
2. For the pretravel consultation recommendations, travelers should be given written material to reinforce and supplement verbal instructions.
3. The pretravel screening appointment should include a discussion of items that should be contained in a travel medical kit.
4. Pregnant travelers should consult obstetric and travel medicine experts prior to traveling to developing countries.
5. Immunocompromised patients may need longer periods of pretravel preparatory time to allow for adequate immunization, given their sometimes blunted antibody responses to vaccines.
6. Travelers to sub-Saharan Africa, Southern Asia, Central and South America, and the Caribbean experience higher rates of infection than those traveling to other parts of the world.
7. Although prophylactic antibiotic use may reduce the risk of traveler's diarrhea, such use is generally not recommended, primarily because of the risk of developing drug resistance or *Clostridium difficile* infection.
8. Prevention strategies are essential for limiting vector-borne infections during travel.
9. The mainstay of therapy in all altitude-related illnesses is descent to a lower altitude (typically at least a 300-meter reduction in altitude).
10. Patients who have previously been diagnosed with depression should continue their prescribed medications and minimize alcohol consumption while traveling.

Global (international) travel has increased dramatically over the past 20 years. A sizable proportion of this increased travel can be explained by individuals traveling from developed countries to developing countries.[1] Reasons for travel to developing countries are variable, but include work-related travel, leisure travel, medical tourism, adventure travel, medical mission or outreach, and study abroad programs.

Travel to distant lands has always been associated with risks to mental and physical health. Twenty-two percent to 64% of travelers experience health problems while traveling.[2] Travel to developing and/or tropical countries can be associated with even higher risks to traveler health than travel to developed or temperate countries. Many health problems arising during travel are self-limiting or not bothersome enough for travelers to seek medical care. However, approximately10% of travelers seek help from physicians either during or soon after traveling.[3] In addition to infectious and noninfectious health problems, global travelers face potential dangers from vehicle and pedestrian traffic accidents, drowning, animal attacks, and assaults. This chapter focuses on health risks and diseases that affect global travelers, with primary emphasis on travel from developed countries to developing or tropical countries. Some travel-related information is included in other chapters, and readers will be referred accordingly.

PRETRAVEL PREPARATION

Travelers should review information about their destinations and itinerary and consider potential self-care options for health issues that may arise during travel. Pretravel preparation often involves the assistance of healthcare providers, which is typically more important for patients with chronic health conditions and those traveling internationally, especially to the developing world. Travelers from North American and Europe heading to developing countries seek pretravel health advice 35% to 50% of the time.[4] Of these, only about 10% to 20% of travelers consult travel medicine experts or travel clinics. Informed primary care providers without extensive travel health expertise can provide adequate advice to travelers en route to low-risk destinations, but (1) travelers should consult practitioners with travel health expertise when going to tropical or developing countries.[4]

Travel clinics and travel health experts are often underutilized.[4] Global travelers may not seek specialty travel advice because health insurance may not cover expenses associated with pretravel care.[5] In addition, immigrants living in developed countries, going back to their home countries to visit friends and relatives (VFR) often believe they are immune to local diseases and do not feel the need to seek advice.[6] Unfortunately, VFR travelers often display some of the highest rates of travel health problems.[4,6] U.S. residents traveling on global VFR trips make up about 33% of all travelers.[7] Other global travelers may not seek travel expert advice for travel to resorts in nearby countries. For example, Caribbean travel was associated with a higher proportion of travelers who did not seek pretravel advice among ill-returning travelers than travelers to other regions.[8] Even travelers staying at all-inclusive Caribbean resorts are subject to travel health issues.

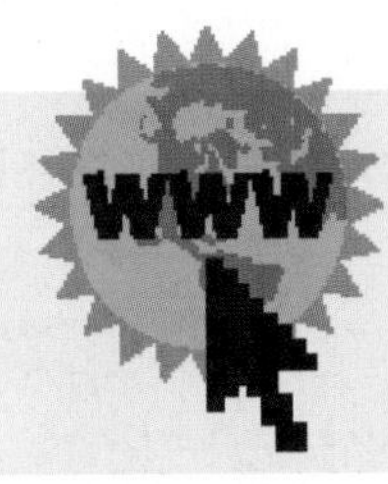

The complete chapter, learning objectives, and other resources can be found at **www.pharmacotherapyonline.com.**

Vaccines and Immunoglobulins

125

Mary S. Hayney

KEY CONCEPTS

1. Live vaccines may confer life-long immunity but cannot be administered to immunosuppressed patients.
2. Inactivated and subunit vaccines and toxoids often require multiple doses to protect from infection, and generally booster doses are needed following the primary series.
3. Children less than 2 years of age are unable to mount T-cell–independent immune responses that are elicited by polysaccharide vaccines.
4. Severely immunocompromised individuals should not receive live vaccines, and their responses to inactivated, polysaccharide, toxoid, and recombinant vaccines may be poor.
5. The childhood and adult immunization schedules are updated frequently and published annually. These documents can be used to develop an immunization plan.
6. Immunoglobulin (Ig) provides short term, rapid postexposure protection from measles, hepatitis A, varicella, and other infections.
7. Ig adverse effects are often secondary to infusion rate. Slowing the IV infusion rate ameliorate chills, nausea, and fever that may develop during administration.
8. Rh_0(D) Ig prevents Rh-negative mothers from mounting an immune response against hemolytic disease of the newborn. Hemolytic disease of the newborn results when Rh-negative mothers are sensitized to the Rh(D) antigen on the red blood cells of their fetuses.

Immunization is defined as rendering a person protected from an infectious agent. Immunity to an infectious agent can be acquired by exposure to the disease, by transfer of antibodies from mother to fetus, through administration of immunoglobulin (Ig), and from vaccination. Immunization is the process of introducing an antigen into the body to induce protection against the infectious agent without causing disease. An *antigen* is a substance that induces an immune response. An *antibody* produced by the humoral arm of the immune system usually is the response that is measured as evidence of successful vaccination. However, cellular immune responses, which are more difficult to measure, are also an important aspect of vaccine responses.

This chapter introduces the clinical use of vaccines and immunoglobulins. Agents with a limited use, such as agents for bioterrorism or travel, are beyond the scope of this chapter.

PRODUCTS USED TO IMMUNIZE

Vaccines induce active immunity—that is, immunity generated by a natural immunologic response to an antigen. Vaccines can be live attenuated or inactivated. Inactivated vaccines may consist of whole or a particle of the pathogen that induces a protective immune response. Bacterial vaccines generally are inactivated specific bacterial antigens or conjugates. Live-attenuated vaccines induce an immunologic response more consistent with that occurring with natural infection. (1) Because the organisms in live-attenuated vaccines undergo limited replication in the vaccinated individual after administration, they may confer lifelong immunity with one dose (as does a natural infection). (2) Multiple doses of inactivated vaccines usually are needed to induce long-lasting, effective immunity. Additional doses at varying time intervals (booster doses) often are required to maintain immunity. Booster doses of such vaccines elicit memory responses from the B cells that produce immunoglobulin G (IgG). The immune system already has developed an array of antibodies to the antigen. Upon restimulation with a booster dose, the B cells, which produce the most specific antibodies against the antigen, are activated. Restimulation allows the most active antibodies against the antigen to be selected and maintained in the "immunologic memory." Thus, the booster dose results in a rapid, intense antibody response that is long lasting. Inactivated vaccines can also differ in immunity potential, depending on their composition. For example, polysaccharide vaccines tend to be poorly immunogenic in infants, whereas protein–polysaccharide conjugated vaccines of the same antigen tend to be highly immunogenic (eg, pneumococcal polysaccharide vaccine vs pneumococcal conjugated vaccine). (3) T-cell–independent immune response is made to polysaccharide antigens that stimulate B cells directly.[1] There is no maturation or booster response with a T-cell–independent immune response, and children younger than 2 years cannot make this type of response. Protein–polysaccharide conjugate vaccines stimulate T cells and promote interactions between T cells and B cells when producing the protective immune responses consisting of immunologic memory and high-affinity IgG.

Toxoids are inactivated bacterial toxins that generally are combined with aluminum salts to enhance their antigenicity by prolonging antigen absorption and exposure. These adjuvants also increase local tissue irritation when injected. Toxoids stimulate the production of antibodies against the bacterial toxins rather than the infecting bacterial pathogens.

Immunoglobulins are sterile solutions containing antibody derived from human (Ig) sources. Igs are derived from donor pools of blood plasma and are processed using cold ethanol fractionation in order to inactivate known potential pathogens. These products are indicated for induction of passive immunity (temporary immunity to infection as a result of administration of antibodies not produced by the host; see Other Immunoglobulins below).

In addition to the active component in a vaccine, other active and inert ingredients are often present. Suspending agents, such as water, saline, or complex fluids containing proteins (eg, albumin), are used as the vehicle for the vaccines. Preservatives, stabilizers, and antibiotics may be added to help maintain the integrity of the product. Immunized individuals may respond with allergic reactions not to the agent itself but to the other components of the pharmaceutical preparation. Different manufacturers of the vaccines have different active and inert ingredients or different quantities of these ingredients in their products.

Certain vaccines manufactured by various companies are considered interchangeable. Hepatitis A, hepatitis B, and *Haemophilus influenzae* type b (Hib) conjugate vaccines from different manufacturers used for the primary series of three doses are considered interchangeable. It is preferable to use diphtheria, tetanus toxoids, and acellular pertussis (DTaP) vaccine from the same manufacturer to complete the entire primary series. However, immunization should not be delayed if the particular type of vaccine administered for the initial doses cannot be ascertained easily.[1]

FACTORS AFFECTING RESPONSE TO IMMUNIZATION

Various factors are known to affect response to vaccines. Viability of the antigen is an important factor (live attenuated vs. inactivated), as discussed previously. Total dose also is important because there seems to exist a threshold dose above which no further increase in antibody titer is seen. The interval between immunization doses, number of doses given, or both may change immune response to an agent. Among hepatitis B vaccine nonresponders, a significant proportion of individuals mount a vaccine response when given additional doses of vaccine.[2] In contrast, additional doses of influenza vaccine are minimally effective in individuals with chronic illness.[3] Generally, intervals longer than those recommended between vaccine doses do not reduce immune response.[1]

The route and site of administration of the immunobiologic are important. This is best illustrated by the hepatitis B vaccine, which elicits a satisfactory antibody response when given in the deltoid muscle but not a consistent response when administered in the gluteal area. Injections should be administered at a site with little likelihood of site damage. Vaccines containing adjuvants should be given into a muscle mass because they can cause irritation when given subcutaneously or intradermally.[1]

Host factors influence vaccine response. Immunocompromise, increasing age, underlying disease, and genetic background have been associated with poor response rates.[1,4–6]

VACCINE ADMINISTRATION

Subcutaneous injections should be administered into the thigh of infants and in the upper arm area over the triceps of older children and adults. A $^5/_8$-inch, 25-gauge needle (0.508 mm × 1.6 cm) should be used, taking care not to administer the dose intradermally or intramuscularly (IM). For IM injection, the anterolateral aspect of the upper thigh (infants and toddlers) or the deltoid muscle of the upper arm (children and adults) should be used. When giving an IM injection to an adult weighing less than 60 kg, a $^5/_8$-inch or 1-inch needle (1.6 cm or 2.5 cm) can be used. If a $^5/_8$-inch needle (1.6 cm) is used, the skin over the injection site must be stretched tight, and the needle must enter the skin at a 90° to assure that the needle reaches the muscle. A 1-inch needle (2.5 cm) should be used for adults who weigh 60 to 70 kg. Immunizers can choose either a 1-inch or $1^1/_2$-inch needle (2.5 cm or 3.8 cm) for women who weigh 70 to 90 kg and for men who weigh 70 to 118 kg. For women weighing more than 90 kg and men who weigh more than 118 kg, a $1^1/_2$-inch needle (3.8 cm) must be used.[1] The buttock should not be used because of the potential for inadequate immunologic response and the potential risk of injury to the sciatic nerve. When the buttock must be used (as for large doses of Ig), only the upper outer quadrant should be used with the needle inserted anteriorly. An influenza vaccine for intradermal administration over the deltoid is supplied in an injection device that reliably delivers the vaccine to the intradermal space.[3]

The rotavirus vaccines are administered orally. The tube of vaccine should be squeezed inside the infant's mouth toward the inner cheek until the dosing tube is empty. If the infant regurgitates or spits out the vaccine, readministration is not recommended.[8]

Live-attenuated influenza vaccine is administered intranasally.[3] A specially designed sprayer is inserted just inside the nostril, and the dose is sprayed by rapidly depressing the plunger of the sprayer. The clip is removed from the plunger so that the second half of the dose can be administered into the other nostril. The vaccinated individual should breathe normally. The dose does not need to be repeated if the individual sneezes during or shortly after administration.

Questions often arise concerning the simultaneous administration of vaccines. In general, inactivated and live-attenuated vaccines can be administered simultaneously at separate sites. If two or more inactivated vaccines cannot be administered simultaneously, they can be administered without regard to spacing between doses. Inactivated and live vaccines can be administered simultaneously or, if they cannot be administered simultaneously, at any interval between doses, except for cholera (killed) and yellow fever (live) vaccines, which should be given at least 3 weeks apart. If live vaccines are not administered simultaneously, their administration should be separated by at least 4 weeks. Live viral vaccines may interfere with purified protein derivative response; thus, tuberculin testing should be postponed for 4 to 6 weeks after administration of live-virus vaccine.[1]

Simultaneous administration of Ig and live-attenuated vaccines may interfere with host antibody response. A dose relationship exists between administration of Ig and inhibition of immune response to a vaccine (Table 125-1). Whole blood and other blood products containing antibodies may interfere with the response to the measles, mumps, and rubella (MMR) and varicella vaccines. In any individual, if vaccination with MMR or varicella is followed by emergency Ig administration, the vaccine can be repeated or seroconversion to viral antigens can be confirmed after sufficient time has elapsed (see Table 125-1). Ig does not interfere with the response to oral vaccines, zoster vaccine, or yellow fever vaccine.[1]

Inactivated vaccines and Igs may be administered simultaneously. However, different sites are recommended for killed vaccine and Ig administration.

VACCINE STORAGE

Appropriate storage is critical to maintaining the integrity of vaccines because improperly stored vaccines can fail to protect the individuals to whom they are administered. Refrigerator temperature is defined as between 2°C and 8°C (36°F to 46°F) and freezer temperature as −50°C (−58°F) to −15°C (5°F). Inactivated vaccines are stored refrigerated. Varicella and zoster vaccines must be stored frozen. MMR vaccine can be stored in either the freezer or refrigerator. Live-attenuated influenza vaccine is stored in the refrigerator. Specific storage conditions for individual vaccines can be found in the package insert.

IMMUNIZATION OF SPECIAL POPULATIONS

Groups of individuals may have precautions to vaccines. Many precautions are temporary, and vaccines can be administered later.

Infants

The age of the recipient is an important determining factor in vaccine response. In the first few months of life, passively transferred maternal antibodies acquired during the third trimester of gestation protect an infant. However, the maternal antibodies also inhibit

TABLE 125-1 Recommended Intervals Between Administration of Immunoglobulin and Measles- or Varicella-Containing Vaccine[1]

Product/Indication	Dose, Including mg Immunoglobulin G(IgG)/kg Body Weight	Recommended Interval Before Measles or Varicella-Containing[a] Vaccine Administration
RSV monoclonal antibody (Synagis®)[b]	15 mg/kg intramuscularly (IM)	None
TIG	250 units (10 mg IgG/kg) IM	3 months
HAIG		
Contact prophylaxis	0.02 mL/kg (3.3 mg IgG/kg) IM	3 months
International travel	0.06 mL/kg (10 mg IgG/kg) IM	3 months
HBIG	0.06 mL/kg (10 mg IgG/kg) IM	3 months
RIG	20 IU/kg (22 mg IgG/kg) IM	4 months
Measles prophylaxis IG		
Standard (ie, nonimmunocompromised) contact	0.25 mL/kg (40 mg IgG/kg) IM	5 months
Immunocompromised contact	0.5 mL/kg (80 mg IgG/kg) IM	6 months
Blood transfusion		
RBCs, washed	10 mL/kg negligible IgG/kg IV	None
RBCs, adenine-saline added	10 mL/kg (10 mg IgG/kg) IV	3 months
Packed RBCs (Hct 65%) [0.650][c]	10 mL/kg (60 mg IgG/kg) IV	6 months
Whole blood (Hct 35%–50%)[0.35–0.50][c]	10 mL/kg (80–100 mg IgG/kg) IV	6 months
Plasma/platelet products	10 mL/kg (160 mg IgG/kg) IV	7 months
Cytomegalovirus IV immunoglobulin (IGIV)	150 mg/kg maximum	6 months
IVIG		
Replacement therapy for immune deficiencies[d]	300-400 mg/kg IV[c]	8 months
Immune thrombocytopenic purpura	400 mg/kg IV	8 months
Immune thrombocytopenic purpura	1 g/kg IV	10 months
Postexposure varicella prophylaxis[e]	400 mg/kg IV	8 months
Kawasaki's disease	2 g/kg IV	11 months

HAIG, Hepatitis A IG; HBIG, Hepatitis B IG; RBCs, Red blood cells; RIG, Rabies IG; TIG, Tetanus IG.

[1]This table is not intended for determining the correct indications and dosages for using antibody-containing products. Unvaccinated persons might not be fully protected against measles during the entire recommended interval, and additional doses of Ig or measles vaccine might be indicated after measles exposure. Concentrations of measles antibody in an Ig preparation can vary by manufacturer's lot. Rates of antibody clearance after receipt of an Ig preparation also might vary. Recommended intervals are extrapolated from an estimated half-life of 30 days for passively acquired antibody and an observed interference with the immune response to measles vaccine for 5 months after a dose of 80 mg IgG/kg.

[a]Varicella-containing vaccine, as used here, does not include zoster vaccine. Zoster vaccine may be given without regard to antibody-containing blood products.

[b]Contains antibody only to respiratory syncytial virus (RSV).

[c]Assumes a serum IgG concentration of 16 mg/mL (g/L).

[d]Measles and varicella vaccinations are recommended for children with asymptomatic or mildly symptomatic human immunodefi ciency virus (HIV) infection but are contraindicated for persons with severe immunosuppression from HIV or any other immunosuppressive disorder.

[e]The investigational product VariZIG, similar to licensed VZIG, is a purified human Ig preparation made from plasma containing high levels of anti-varicella antibodies (immunoglobulin class G [IgG]). The interval between VariZIG and varicella vaccine is 5 months.

the immune response to live vaccines because the circulating antibodies neutralize the vaccine before the infant has the opportunity to mount an immune response. For this reason, measles, mumps, rubella, and varicella vaccines are not administered until maternal antibodies have waned, generally by infant age 12 months.

Premature infants should be vaccinated at the same chronologic age using the same schedule and precautions for full-term infants. The full recommended doses of vaccines should be used, regardless of age or birth weight. Breastfed infants should be vaccinated according to standard pediatric schedules.

Pregnant Women and Postpartum Immunization

The benefit of most vaccines outweighs the risk for administration to pregnant females. As with most drugs, a lack of information regarding risks to the fetus exists rather than any actual known risk. No adverse birth outcome has ever been attributed to vaccine exposure.[1] For example, no cases of congenital rubella syndrome from inadvertent administration of rubella vaccine to a pregnant woman have ever been reported. Universal influenza immunization is recommended for women who will be or are pregnant during influenza season. Pregnant women should receive Tdap during the late second trimester or third trimester of pregnancy.[4] Although live vaccines generally are avoided because of the theoretical risk of transmission of the vaccine organism to the fetus, inactivated vaccines may be administered to pregnant women when the benefits outweigh the risks.[1] Hepatitis B, hepatitis A, meningococcal, and inactivated polio vaccines should be administered to pregnant females if they are otherwise indicated. Insufficient evidence is available for pneumococcal vaccines, and the human papillomavirus (HPV) series should be deferred during pregnancy.[5]

Administration of live vaccines, such as rubella or varicella, are deferred until pregnancy is completed and are routinely recommended for new mothers who do not have evidence of immunity prior to hospital discharge. These live vaccines can be administered without regard to administration of $Rh_0(D)$ Ig in the postpartum period. Additionally, Tdap is recommended for all new mothers who have not received a Tdap before because household contacts are frequently implicated as the source of pertussis infection in a young infant.[4]

Immunocompromised Hosts

4 Immununization of individuals with chronic disease, such as immunocompromise, diabetes or connective tissue disease, alcoholism, or those with cancer or HIV disease, must be individualized based on the disease state and its treatment. In general, severely immunocompromised individuals should not receive live vaccines. Administration of other vaccines may be indicated, but responses may be lower than those mounted by healthy individuals, but may still confer protection.[6]

Patients with chronic pulmonary, renal, hepatic, or metabolic disease who are not receiving immunosuppressants can receive both live-attenuated and killed vaccines and toxoids to induce active immunity. These patients often need higher doses of vaccines or more frequent dosing to induce immunity. Generally, immunization should be considered early in the course of the disease in an attempt to induce immunity at a point when the disease is less severe.[2]

Patients with active malignant disease can receive killed vaccines or toxoids but should not be given live vaccines. The MMR vaccine is not contraindicated for close contacts, however. Live-virus vaccines can be administered to persons with leukemia who have not received chemotherapy for at least 3 months. Vaccines should be timed so that they do not coincide with the start of chemotherapy or radiation therapy.[6] Zoster vaccine should be administered at least 2 weeks prior to the start of immunosuppressing therapy.[7] Annual influenza vaccine should be administered 2 weeks prior to chemotherapy or between cycles.[6] If vaccines cannot be given at least 2 weeks before the start of these therapies, immunization should be postponed until 3 months after the therapy has been completed. Passive immunization with Ig can be used in place of active immunization regardless of the history of immunization.

Glucocorticoids may cause suppressed responses to vaccines. For the purposes of immunization, the immunosuppressing dose of corticosteroids is prednisone 20 mg or more daily or 2 mg/kg daily, or an equivalent dose of another steroid, for at least 2 weeks. Patients receiving long-term, alternate-day steroid therapy with short-acting agents, administration of maintenance physiologic doses of steroids (eg, 5 to 10 mg/day of prednisone) topical, aerosol, intraarticular, bursal, or tendon steroid injections require no special consideration for immunization. If patients have been receiving high-dose corticosteroids or have had a course lasting longer than 2 weeks, then at least 1 month should pass before immunization with live-virus vaccines.[1]

Patients with HIV infection require special consideration. Responses to live and inactivated vaccines generally are suboptimal and decrease as the disease progresses because HIV produces defects in cell-mediated immunity and humoral immunity. The routinely recommended vaccines should be administered to children. MMR should be administered to anyone older than 12 months of age without evidence of immunity and are not severely immunocompromised (CD4% greater than 15% and CD4 count greater than 200 lymphocytes/mm^3 [greater than equals to 0.2×10^9/L] for at least 6 months).[8] Two doses of varicella vaccine separated by 3 months are recommended for those with no evidence of immunosuppression. Adults should receive routinely recommended vaccines. Zoster vaccine may be administered to individuals with HIV infection who do not have clinical manifestations of AIDS and have CD4 counts greater than 200/mm^3 (greater than 0.200×10^9/L).[7]

Solid Organ Transplant Patients

Organ transplantation has become routine treatment of end-stage organ disease of many causes. Solid-organ transplant patients remain on immunosuppressive regimens for the rest of their lives. These immunosuppressive regimens result in a higher risk of infection and decrease the protection conferred by immunization.[9]

Whenever possible, transplant patients should be immunized prior to transplantation. Live vaccines generally are not given after transplantation. Posttransplantation diphtheria, tetanus, pneumococcal, and influenza vaccine responses are unpredictable. Decreased immune response has been documented following hepatitis B vaccine.

Hematopoietic Stem Cell Transplant Patients

Reimmunization of patients with hematopoietic stem cell transplantation is necessary because antibody concentrations wane rapidly. Annual influenza immunization may begin as soon as 6 months after successful engraftment. Reimmunization with inactivated vaccines should begin approximately 6 months after hematopoietic stem cell transplantation. Hematopoietic stem cell transplant recipients are at increased risk for fulminant infection with encapsulated bacteria, so 13-valent pneumococcal vaccine (PCV13), the 23-valent pneumococcal polysaccharide vaccine (PPSV23), meningococcal vaccines, and Hib vaccines are recommended. MMR vaccine (MMR) can be administered at 24 months. Varicella vaccine is not routinely recommended but can be considered on a case-by-case basis. Immunization of household contacts and healthcare workers also is necessary.[1,6]

CONTRAINDICATIONS AND PRECAUTIONS

There are few contraindications to the use of vaccines except those outlined earlier. The contraindications include a history of anaphylactic reactions to the vaccine or a component of the vaccine. Unexplained encephalopathy occurring within 7 days of a dose of pertussis vaccine is a contraindication to future doses of pertussis vaccines. Immunosuppression and pregnancy are temporary contraindications to live vaccines. An interval of time must elapse based on the dose of Ig before a live vaccine can be administered (see Table 125-1). Precautions for DTaP administration include hypotonic hyporesponsive episode, fever of 40.5°C (104.9°F) or greater, crying lasting more than 3 hours within 48 hours of a previous dose, and seizures with or without fever within 3 days after a dose. A personal or family history of seizures is a precaution for receiving the combination MMR–varicella (MMRV) vaccine. Immunizers should use MMR and varicella vaccines separately.[1] Generally, mild-to-moderate local reactions, mild acute illnesses, concurrent antibiotic use, prematurity, family history of adverse events, diarrhea, and lactation or breastfeeding are not contraindications to immunization.

OBTAINING AN IMMUNIZATION HISTORY

An immunization history should be obtained from every patient, regardless of the reason for the healthcare visit. Ideally, any history provided by the patient from memory should be verified by reviewing the patient's personal written immunization record or a database that contains the complete immunization history. State-based or other public health jurisdiction-based immunization information systems, also called immunization registries, have been developed to improve immunization coverage by allowing healthcare providers access to records at any contact with the healthcare system. Registries are aimed primarily at facilitation of childhood immunization records.[10] If an official written record is not available, patient characteristics (eg, military service, travel history, and occupation) may provide clues to the immunization history. Serologic testing for immunity against certain diseases can provide specific information but is used routinely for only a few selected diseases (eg, measles, rubella, hepatitis A and B, and varicella) and selected circumstances (eg, employment in a healthcare facility). If a written record does not exist, one should be generated at the time of initiation of immunization. Patients without a written record should be considered susceptible, and an immunization program started and completed unless a serious adverse reaction occurs. As a general rule, the risks associated with overimmunization are minimal relative to the risks associated with contracting vaccine-preventable diseases.[1]

Every healthcare visit, regardless of its purpose, should be viewed as an opportunity to review a patient's immunization status and to administer needed vaccines. Immunization is perhaps the most cost-effective health intervention available. Each visit should include assessment of individuals' vaccine needs, administration of indicated vaccines, and documentation of immunization histories. The outcome measurement of what percentage of patients in a particular practice site is completely immunized is extremely important because the benefits of optimal vaccine use extend beyond the individual patient to the public as a whole.

NATIONAL VACCINE INJURY COMPENSATION PROGRAM

The National Childhood Vaccine Injury Act of 1986 was passed by the US Congress in response to reports of vaccine side effects and liability concerns of vaccine manufacturers and healthcare providers. With vaccine safety being questioned and manufacturers ceasing the development and marketing of vaccines, the National Vaccine Injury Compensation Program was implemented to offer a no-fault alternative means to compensate individuals for injury following vaccination. The program offers liability protection to manufacturers and an efficient means of recovering damages for individuals potentially injured by vaccines. The types of vaccine-related injuries that are considered for compensation are outlined in the Health Resources and Services Administration's Vaccine Injury Table (http://www.hrsa.gov/vaccinecompensation/vaccinetable.html). Healthcare providers must report all events requiring medical attention within 30 days of vaccination to the Vaccine Adverse Event Reporting System (VAERS), which serves as a central depot for vaccine-related adverse effects. Only a temporal association between the adverse event and vaccine administration is required. No adverse event rates can be determined because only the number of adverse events reported is known; the number of vaccines administered is not known. This database can be used to survey for changes in the frequencies of adverse events, to evaluate risk factors for adverse events, and to find rare adverse events.[11] VAERS report forms can be obtained by calling 1-800-822-7967, or reports can be made online at https://vaers.hhs.gov/esub/index.

USE OF VACCINES

The Advisory Committee on Immunization Practices (ACIP) makes recommendations for use of vaccines for the United States. Other professional organizations, for example, the American Academy of Pediatrics, the American Academy of Family Physicians, or the American College of Obstetrics and Gynecology, publish guidelines. Usually, these guidelines are the same as those issued by the ACIP or the groups try to reconcile their recommendations.

5 The appendices show the recommended schedules for routine immunization of children and adults. The latest vaccine schedules can be found at http://www.cdc.gov/vaccines/schedules/hcp/index.html. All states require children to be fully immunized prior to entering elementary school; however, optimal protection is achieved by immunizing at the recommended ages, which requires special attention to children younger than 2 years. Adults and adolescents also require vaccination and often are unaware of this need. An early adolescent preventive health visit is recommended. This visit is an opportunity to catch up on missed immunizations and to administer meningococcal conjugate, Tdap, and HPV vaccines. All individuals older than 6 months of age should receive an annual seasonal influenza vaccine. Adults should receive routine tetanus–diphtheria (Td) or Tdap boosters and be immune to measles, mumps, rubella, and varicella by either immunization or history of infection. Older adults need zoster vaccine after age 60 years, and pneumococcal vaccines after age 65 years. Certain individuals with conditions or lifestyles that put them at high risk for vaccine-preventable diseases also should be immunized as described in the following text and outlined in the immunization schedules in the appendices.

Clinical **Controversy**

Some parents and clinicians consider an alternative schedule for the immunization of young children. The advantages of the alternative schedule are that fewer injections and fewer vaccines are administered in any single visit and the child is immunized using more visits. Disadvantages to the use of an alternative immunization schedule are that childhood vaccines are subject to concomitant use studies to investigate immunogenicity and safety when administered at the same time. Second, delaying vaccines leaves the child susceptible to vaccine-preventable diseases until the vaccine is administered. Finally, studies show that an infant is no more stressed by one injection than multiple injections in a single visit as measured by cortisol production.[12]

VACCINES

Diphtheria Toxoid Adsorbed

Diphtheria is an acute illness caused by the toxin released by a *Corynebacterium diphtheriae* infection. The toxin inhibits cellular protein synthesis, and membranes form on mucosal surfaces. Systemic toxemia can result in myocarditis, neuritis, and thrombocytopenia. Membrane formation can cause respiratory obstruction, and significant toxin absorption can lead to severe illness and death.

Diphtheria toxoid adsorbed is a sterile suspension of modified toxins of *C. diphtheriae* that induces immunity against the exotoxin of this organism. Two strengths of diphtheria toxoid are available in the United States: pediatric strength (D) and adult strength (d), which contains less antigen. The widespread use of diphtheria toxoid essentially has eliminated diphtheria from the United States.

Primary immunization with diphtheria toxoid (D) is indicated for children older than 6 weeks. The toxoid is given in combination with tetanus toxoid and acellular pertussis vaccine (as DTaP or in combination with additional childhood vaccines that have been licensed to decrease the number of injections required to complete the childhood immunization recommendations) at age 2, 4, and 6 months. Additional doses are given at age 15 to 18 months and again at age 4 to 6 years.[13] Booster doses should be given every 10 years.

For unimmunized adults, a complete three-dose series of diphtheria toxoid should be administered, with the first two doses given at least 4 weeks apart and the third dose given 6 to 12 months after the second. One of the vaccine doses in this series should be Tdap. The combined Td preparation is used for adults because it contains less diphtheria toxoid than the pediatric dose and is associated with fewer reactions to the diphtheria component. All adults should receive booster doses of Td every 10 years.[14] Adverse effects of diphtheria toxoid include mild-to-moderate tenderness, erythema, and induration at the injection site. Systemic reactions occur very rarely.

Haemophilus Influenzae Type B Vaccines

Before 1995, Hib was responsible for thousands of cases of serious illnesses (eg, meningitis, epiglottitis, pneumonia, sepsis, and septic arthritis). The incidence of Hib disease has declined more than 99% since the introduction of the conjugate vaccines based on the organism's capsular substance, polyribosylribitol phosphate (PRP).[15]

The Hib vaccines are conjugate products consisting of either a polysaccharide or an oligosaccharide of PRP covalently linked to a protein carrier. The protein carrier is important because it provides for T-lymphocyte–dependent immunologic response, whereas earlier Hib vaccines that consisted of only unconjugated PRP elicited a response that was T-cell independent. T-cell involvement in the response provides for (a) a greater antibody response regardless of the age of the patient receiving the vaccine, (b) immunologic response at an earlier age (including infants), and (c) a booster effect on subsequent exposure to the Hib capsule, whether through revaccination or natural exposure. The protein carrier is not considered a vaccine and should not be substituted for immunization against tetanus, diphtheria, or *Neisseria meningitidis*.

Hib conjugate vaccines are indicated for routine use in all infants and children younger than 5 years. Multiple products in various combinations are available for use in infants and children of different ages. The primary series of Hib vaccination consists of a 0.5-mL IM dose at ages 2, 4, and 6 months. If Hib PRP-OMP (outer membrane protein of *Neisseria meningitides* as the protein conjugate) is being used, the primary series consists of doses given at ages 2 and 4 months. The series should not be initiated in an infant younger than 6 weeks. Although use of one product for the entire primary series is desirable, adequate protection is achieved even when different products are used during the initial series. Following the primary series, a booster dose is recommended at age 12 to 15 months. Any of the Hib conjugate vaccines are suitable for the booster dose regardless of which conjugate was used for the primary series of doses.[15]

Schedules are more complex for infants who do not begin Hib immunization at the recommended age or who have fallen behind in the immunization schedule. For infants 7 to 11 months of age who have not been vaccinated, three doses of Hib vaccine should be given: two doses spaced 4 weeks apart and then a booster dose at age 12 to 15 months (but at least 8 weeks since the second dose). For unvaccinated children ages 12 to 14 months, two doses should be given, with an interval of 2 months between doses. In a child older than 15 months, a single dose of any of the vaccine preparations is indicated.[15]

Vaccines for Hib are recommended for routine use only for children up to age 59 months; beyond this age, the incidence of invasive Hib disease is very low. Patients with certain underlying conditions (eg, HIV infection, IgG_2 subclass deficiency, sickle cell disease, splenectomy, and hematopoietic stem cell transplants and those receiving chemotherapy for malignancies) are at higher than normal risk for Hib infection, and use of at least one dose of vaccine in these patients should be considered.[13-15]

Adverse reactions to the Hib vaccine are uncommon. Erythema and induration at the injection site occur in approximately 5% to 30% of children and resolve within 12 to 24 hours. Fever, diarrhea, and vomiting are reported occasionally.[15]

Hepatitis Vaccines

Information on vaccination for viral hepatitis is given in Chapter 40.

Human Papillomavirus Vaccine

HPV infections are the most common sexually transmitted infections, with the highest prevalence of infection in sexually active young adults. Although more than 120 different HPV types have been identified, at least 40 different types of HPV infect the anogenital tract. These 40 different viruses are grouped into low-risk and high-risk types. Low-risk types can cause genital warts and mild abnormalities on Papanicolaou (Pap) tests. Ninety percent of all cases of genital warts and the majority of respiratory papillomatosis are caused by types 6 and 11. As many as 18 types are considered high risk as they have the ability to penetrate the nucleus of an epithelial cell to transform it to a precancerous cell. They cause abnormal Pap test results and may lead to cancer of the cervix, vulva, vagina, anus, or penis. Types 16 and 18 cause about 70% of all cervical cancers. Another 10% of HPV-related cancers are caused by types 31, 33, 45, 52, and 58. Men who have sex with men (MSM) are at a higher risk for infection with HPV, genital warts, and anal cancer.[16] The incidence of cancers associated with HPV is higher among MSM, and the rate of anal cancer among MSM continues to rise.[16,17] High-risk HPV infections are necessary but not sufficient for the development of cervical cancer and for the majority of other anogenital and oral squamous cell cancers.

A nine valent HPV vaccine against types 6 and 11 and 16, 18, 31, 33, 45, 52, and 58 is licensed for the prevention of HPV. ACIP recommends HPV vaccine for the prevention of HPV-related disease in females aged 9 to 26 years. The nine valent vaccine can be used for males aged 9 to 26 years. This vaccine is administered as a three-dose series using a schedule of 0, 1 to 2, and 6 months.[18] The vaccines are recommended for adolescents aged 11 to 12 years and for all females aged 13 to 26 years. Males should be immunized routinely up to age 21 years. Males who have sex with males and the immunocompromised should be immunized through age 26 years. Males aged 22 to 26 years may receive the series.[18]

The vaccine is well tolerated, with injection-site reactions and systemic reactions (eg, headache and fatigue) occurring as commonly in immunized individuals as in the groups receiving placebo. Although syncope is possible with any immunization, the target population of adolescents and young adults has a higher incidence of syncope, including with administration of the HPV vaccine.[19]

The effective vaccine is an important advance, but the need for a Pap test for cervical cancer screening remains. Surveillance for the duration of protection conferred by the vaccine series is ongoing; the need for future booster doses is not yet known.

Influenza Virus Vaccine

Information on vaccination for influenza is given in Chapter e88.

Measles Vaccine

Measles (rubeola) is a highly contagious viral illness characterized by rash and high fever. Complications of measles infections include severe diarrhea, otitis media, pneumonia, and encephalitis. Measles results in one to two deaths per 1,000 cases, with a much higher death rate in developing countries. With widespread vaccination, measles is on the verge of elimination from the Western Hemisphere.

The measles vaccine is a live-attenuated viral vaccine that produces a subclinical, noncommunicable infection. Approximately 95% of vaccine recipients mount a protective immune response after a single dose, and most individuals are protected for life.[25] Most persons who do not respond to the first dose of measles vaccine will respond after receiving a second dose, and this forms the basis for the two-dose vaccine strategy that was implemented in the United States in 1989.

The measles vaccine is administered subcutaneously as a 0.5-mL dose in the arm (or in the thigh if the patient is younger than 15 months). The vaccine is administered routinely for primary immunization to persons 12 to 15 months of age. Two combinations of measles containing vaccines are available—measles–mumps–rubella (MMR) or measles–mumps–rubella–varicella (MMRV). The measles vaccine is not administered earlier than 12 months (except in certain outbreak circumstances or for travel) because persisting maternal antibody that was acquired transplacentally late in gestation can neutralize the vaccine virus before the vaccinated person can mount an immune response. A second dose of measles-containing vaccine is recommended when children are 4 to 6 years old.[8] The second dose of vaccine results in seroconversion in 95% of individuals who were first-dose nonresponders.

Measles-containing vaccine should not be given to pregnant women or immunosuppressed patients. An exception is HIV-infected patients, who are at very high risk for severe complications if they develop measles. Adults with HIV infection who have no evidence of measles immunity should be immunized as long as they are not severely immunocompromised (CD4 greater than 200 lymphocytes/mm^3 [greater than equals to 0.2×10^9/L] for at least 6 months). The second dose should be given 1 month later.[8] Children with HIV who are not severely immunocompromised can be immunized according to the childhood immunization schedule at 12 months and 4 to 6 years of age.[8,13]

Recent administration of Ig interferes with measles vaccine response, so the recommended interval between the Ig and vaccine is determined by the dose of Ig (see Table 125-1).[1] Live vaccines not administered during the same visit must be delayed for at least 30 days following measles or MMR vaccine. Live measles vaccine may suppress a positive tuberculin skin test for up to 6 weeks postadministration.[1]

Measles vaccine is indicated in all persons born after 1956 or in those who lack documentation of wild virus infection by either history or antibody titers. Two doses of a measles-containing vaccine separated by at least one month are required for children, college students, and healthcare workers who were born in 1957 or later.[13,14]

The measles vaccine has an excellent safety record. The most common side effect following vaccination is fever, which occurs in 5% to 15% of vaccinees. Transient generalized rash may occur in approximately 5% of vaccine recipients. These reactions generally appear 5 to 12 days postvaccination and last 2 to 5 days. Other adverse effects, such as headache, cough, sore throat, eye pain, malaise, and transient thrombocytopenia, occur less frequently.[8]

Meningococcal Vaccines

N. meningitidis is a leading cause of meningitis and sepsis in children and young adults in the United States. Five serotypes, A, B, C, W-135, and Y, cause almost all infections in humans. The infection is transmitted by respiratory droplets from infected individuals and asymptomatic carriers. Symptoms include severe headache, sensitivity to light, stiff neck, nausea and vomiting, and high fever. Mortality occurs in 24 to 48 hours following onset of symptoms in 10% to 13% of infected individuals.[33] Immunization is recommended for high-risk populations, such as those exposed to the infection, those in the midst of uncontrolled outbreaks, travelers to areas with epidemic or hyperendemic meningococcal disease, and individuals who have terminal complement component deficiencies or asplenia.

MenACYW Conjugate and Polysaccharide Vaccines

Two meningococcal conjugate vaccines combining the same serotypes are licensed for use in individuals aged 9 months to 55 years old (Menactra®, Sanofi-Pasteur) or 2 to 55 years old (Menveo®, Novartis). A quadrivalent vaccine containing capsular polysaccharides for serotypes A, C, Y, and W-135 (Menimmune®, Sanofi-Pasteur) has been available since the early 1970s.

The meningococcal conjugate vaccine is recommended for adolescents at ages 11 to 12 years with a second dose at age 16 years. Reimmunization at 5-year intervals is recommended for individuals who are at high risk.[34] The polysaccharide vaccine should be reserved for those older than 55 years of age who require immunization.

Injection-site reactions are the most common adverse effects following administration of either the meningococcal conjugate or polysaccharide vaccine.

MenB vaccines

Meningococcal serogroup B (MenB) vaccines use other antigens from the bacterial capsule, specifically factor H binding protein, Neisseria adhesin A, and neisserial neparin binding antigen. Two MenB vaccines have been licensed for the prevention of invasive disease caused by *N. meningitidis* serogroup B for individuals aged 10 to 25 years. The ACIP recommends either of the two MenB vaccines, Trumenba® and Bexsero®, for individuals at high risk for invasive meningococcal disease.[20] Additionally, MenB vaccine use is acceptable for adolescents and young adults. Trumenba® requires two or three dose series administered at 0 and 6 months or 0, 2, and 6 month intervals. Bexsero® requires two doses with at least one month between doses. Both vaccines were licensed based upon antibody response studies.[20] The most common adverse events after MenB vaccines are pain at the injection site, fatigue, headache, myalgia, and chills.

Mumps Vaccine

Mumps is a viral illness that classically causes bilateral parotitis 16 to 18 days after exposure. Fever, headache, malaise, myalgia, and anorexia may precede the parotitis. Serious complications are rare but more common in adults.

The mumps vaccine is a lyophilized live-attenuated vaccine. The vaccine is available in combinations with measles, rubella (as MMR), and varicella (MMRV) vaccines.

The vaccine is administered as a 0.5-mL subcutaneous injection in the upper arm. Dosing recommendations coincide with those for measles vaccine, with the first dose administered at age 12 to 15 months and the second dose prior to the child's entry into elementary school. Two doses of mumps-containing vaccine are recommended for school-aged children, international travelers, students in post-high school educational institutions, and healthcare workers born after 1956.[8] A single dose of vaccine is acceptable documentation of immunity to mumps for other adults considered at lower risk of mumps infection, including adults born after 1956 and those with an uncertain history of wild virus infection. Mumps vaccine should not be given to pregnant women or immunosuppressed patients.[1]

Serious adverse reactions to the vaccine are reported rarely. Fever, parotitis, rash, and lymphadenopathy occur rarely. Local reactions, including soreness, burning, and stinging, may occur at the injection site.[8]

Pertussis Vaccine

Pertussis is caused by a bacterial infection with *Bordetella pertussis*. The infection starts with signs and symptoms of an acute respiratory infection, called the catarrhal stage. The coughing spells manifest about a week later. Typically, young children will have the characteristic whoop as they struggle to inhale while coughing. Adolescents and adults are more likely to have prolonged periods of coughing. Pertussis can affect any age group, but young infants are at much higher risk for pneumonia, seizures, brain damage, and death. Their rate of hospitalization is much higher than for other age groups. The individual is contagious during the catarrhal stage and the first two weeks of the cough.[4,21]

Acellular pertussis vaccines contain components of the *B. pertussis* organism. All acellular vaccines contain pertussis toxin, and some contain one or more additional bacterial components (eg, filamentous hemagglutinin, pertactin [a 69-kDa outer membrane protein], and fimbriae types 2 and 3). Acellular pertussis vaccine is recommended for all doses of the pertussis schedule at 2, 4, 6, and 15 to 18 months of age. A fifth dose of pertussis vaccine is given to children 4 to 6 years of age.[13] Pertussis vaccine is administered in combination with diphtheria and tetanus (DTaP). Administration of an acellular pertussis-containing vaccine is also recommended for adolescents once between ages 11 and 18 years. In addition, they should receive a pertussis-containing vaccine with their next dose of Td toxoids.[13,21] Special attention is warranted for the immunization of individuals who have close contact with young infants. Tdap should be administered to women in their late second or third trimester of pregnancy. Tdap should also be administered to all close contacts, including household contacts and out of home care providers.[4]

Local administration site reactions are relatively common. Systemic reactions, such as moderate fever, occur in 3% to 5% of vaccinees. Very rarely, high fever, febrile seizures, persistent crying spells, and hypotonic hyporesponsive episodes occur following vaccination. Encephalopathy without known cause within 7 days of a pertussis vaccine are contraindications to future doses of this vaccine.[1]

Pneumococcal Vaccines

Streptococcus pneumoniae is a common pathogen with a range of manifestations, including asymptomatic upper respiratory tract colonization, sinusitis, acute otitis media, pharyngitis, pneumonia, meningitis, and bacteremia. Rates of invasive infections are highest in children younger than 2 years and in the elderly.[35,36] Invasive pneumococcal infections cause approximately 40,000 deaths annually. Most of the deaths occur in the elderly or in those with underlying medical conditions. Approximately half the deaths could be preventable by vaccine. Two pneumococcal vaccine preparations, PCV13 and 23-valent pneumococcal polysaccharide vaccine (PPV23) are available. The vaccines have different indications and are not interchangeable.

Pneumococcal Polysaccharide Vaccine

Pneumococcal polysaccharide vaccine (Pneumovax 23) is a mixture of highly purified capsular polysaccharides from 23 of the most prevalent or invasive types of *S. pneumoniae* seen in the United States. Serotypes included are 1, 2, 3, 4, 5, 6B, 7F, 8, 9N, 9V, 10A, 11A, 12F, 14, 15B, 17F, 18C, 19A, 19F, 20, 22F, 23F, and 33F. These 23 types represent 85% to 90% of all blood isolates and 85% of pneumococcal isolates from other generally sterile sites seen in the United States. The vaccine is administered IM or subcutaneously as a single 0.5-mL dose.

PPSV23 is recommended for the following individuals:[22]

1. Persons 65 years and older (if an individual received vaccine more than 5 years earlier and was younger than 65 years at the time of administration, revaccination should be given).
2. Persons aged 2 to 64 years with a chronic illness (congestive heart failure, cardiomyopathy, chronic pulmonary disease, diabetes, alcoholism, and liver disease).
3. Persons aged 2 to 64 years with functional or anatomic asplenia (when splenectomy is planned, PPSV23 should be given at least 2 weeks before surgery; a single revaccination is recommended at 5 years in subjects older than 10 years and at 3 years in subjects younger than 10 years).
4. Persons aged 19 to 64 years who smoke cigarettes or have asthma.
5. Persons with cochlear implants.

PPSV23 is recommended for immunocompromised persons 2 years and older with (a) HIV infection, (b) leukemia, (c) lymphoma, (d) Hodgkin disease, (e) multiple myeloma, (f) generalized malignancy, (g) chronic renal failure or nephrotic syndrome, (h) patients receiving immunosuppressive therapy including corticosteroids, and (i) organ and bone marrow transplant recipients. A single revaccination should be given if 5 years or more have passed since the first dose in subjects older than 10 years. In subjects 10 years of age and younger, revaccination should be given 3 years after the previous dose.

PPSV23 induces type-specific antibodies (T-cell-independent mechanisms) with a twofold rise within 2 to 3 weeks in 80% of young healthy adults. No correlation of antibody levels and protection has been determined. Antibody levels to these strains remain elevated for at least 5 years. In certain individuals, these levels decline within 10 years. Children may be protected for only 3 to 5 years. Elderly individuals and patients with chronic disease may have lower antibody levels produced with the vaccine. Children younger than 2 years do not respond adequately to the vaccine.

A number of other groups, including immunocompromised patients (eg, leukemia, lymphoma, and multiple myeloma), dialysis patients, and patients with acquired immune deficiency syndrome, have reduced antibody production with the vaccine. Asymptomatic HIV-infected patients respond sufficiently to the vaccine. Patients with Hodgkin disease respond to the vaccine better before splenectomy, chemotherapy, or radiation therapy.

PPSV23 vaccine efficacy has been debated in the literature. Study results generally point to a reduction in invasive pneumococcal disease in the general population and in the elderly. In immunosuppressed populations, the reduction in invasive disease is estimated at 50% to 80% with immunization.[37] Adults hospitalized with community-acquired pneumonia are significantly less likely to die if they have been immunized. In addition, immunized patients were less likely to have respiratory failure and had hospitalization stays that were shorter by 2 days.[38]

PPSV23 safety is well documented. Local reactions occur frequently within the first 48 hours and generally are mild. Local erythema and induration (30%), local discomfort (40%), and local swelling (3%) are the side effects observed most commonly. Revaccination has been associated with self-limited injection-site reactions more commonly than after the first dose. Severe systemic reactions occur rarely and consist of weakness, myalgia, headache, photophobia, chills, and fever.

Pneumococcal Conjugate Vaccine

Invasive pneumococcal disease occurs even more frequently in children younger than 2 years than in those older than 65 years. The infection ranges goes from nasopharyngeal carriage to bacteremia and meningitis. Because of the lack of immune responsiveness in children younger than 2 years when exposed to polysaccharide vaccines, a conjugate vaccine was developed to protect young children from certain strains of *S. pneumoniae*. However, the 13-valent vaccine is also licensed for individuals aged 50 years and older. The 13 valent vaccine (Prevnar-13) contains the conjugated capsular polysaccharides of serotypes 1, 3, 4, 5, 6A, 6B, 7F, 9V, 14, 18C, 19A, 19F, and 23F. In clinical use, the vaccine is associated with a dramatic decline in invasive disease not only in immunized young children but also in individuals in all age groups.[23]

Immunization of Children PCV13 is administered as a 0.5-mL IM injection at 2, 4, and 6 months of age and between 12 and 15 months of age. A single dose of PCV13 should be administered to children aged 6 to 18 years with sickle cell disease or splenic dysfunction, HIV infection, immunocompromising conditions, cochlear implant, or cerebral spinal fluid leak should be immunized. PPSV23 can be used in conjunction with PCV13. PPSV23 should be administered after age 2 years and at least 2 months after the last dose of PCV13.[24,25]

Immunization of Adults The PCV13 offers some additional protection over PPSV23 alone in adult high-risk populations protection is at least as good as PPSV23. PCV13 is safe in these populations. Based on this information, the ACIP recommended PCV13 for adults with immunocompromising conditions and for those 65 years of age and older.[26,27] (Table 125-2). PCV13 should be administered prior to PPSV23 in adults who have not been immunized previously. PCV13 should be administered with at least a year interval

TABLE 125-2 ACIP Recommendations for Use of PCV13 and PPSV23[40]

Vaccine naïve adults
- PCV13 first with PPSV23 administered at least 8 weeks later
- Second dose of PPSV23 at 5-year interval and PPSV23 at age 65 years and at least 5 years after last dose

PPSV23-immunized adults
- PCV13 at least 1 year after last dose of PPSV23
- Second dose of PPSV23 at 5 year interval and PPSV23 at age 65 years and at least 5 years after last dose

Indications for PCV13 for adults 19 years and older
- Functional or anatomic asplenia
- Immunocompromising conditions
  - Congenital or acquired immunodeficiencies
  - HIV infection
  - Chronic renal failure or nephrotic syndrome
  - Leukemias, lymphomas, Hodgkin's lymphoma
  - Generalized malignancy
  - Diseases requiring treatment with immunosuppressive drugs, including long-term systemic corticosteroids or radiation therapy
  - Solid organ transplantation
  - Multiple myeloma
- Cerebral spinal fluid leaks or cochlear implants

PCV13, 13-valent pneumococcal conjugate vaccine. PPSV23, 23-valent pneumococcal polysaccharide vaccine.

in those adults for whom it has been recommended and have already received one or more doses of PPSV23.

Poliovirus Vaccines

Poliomyelitis is a contagious viral infection that usually causes asymptomatic infection; however, in its serious form it causes acute flaccid paralysis. Poliovirus is spread via the fecal–oral route. The virus replicates in the upper respiratory tract, GI tract, and local lymphatics. The vast majority of polio infections are subclinical and asymptomatic. Polio has been eliminated from the United States since 1979, and the last case in Western Hemisphere was reported in 1991. Global eradication efforts are entering the final stages, and the eradication of polio should be accomplished in the next few years.

An inactivated trivalent vaccine developed by Jonas Salk was licensed for use in 1955. In 1987, an enhanced-potency inactivated polio vaccine (IPV) was introduced and has replaced the original inactivated vaccine. A live-attenuated oral polio vaccine (OPV) was developed by Albert Sabin in 1962. OPV was the primary immunizing agent for poliovirus infection. Widespread OPV use is responsible for the elimination of wild-type polio in most of the world. However, with no poliovirus circulation in the United States for years, IPV is the recommended vaccine for the primary series and booster dose for children.[28] OPV will continue to be used in areas of the world that have circulating poliovirus. The CDC maintains a stockpile of OPV to be used only in case of an outbreak.

The IPV series is administered routinely to children at ages 2, 4, and 6 to 18 months, and 4 to 6 years.[13] Primary poliomyelitis immunization is recommended for all children up to age 18 years. Primary immunization of adults over age 18 years is not recommended routinely because a high level of immunity already exists in this age group, and the risk of exposure in developed countries is exceedingly small. However, unimmunized adults who are at increased risk for exposure because of travel, residence, or occupation should receive IPV series. Incompletely immunized adults or children should complete the series of IPV regardless of the interval since initiation of primary immunization. Adults do not need a booster dose routinely unless they are at increased risk of exposure (travel), in which case a single dose of IPV can be given.[29]

No serious side effects are attributable to IPV. Pregnant women should be given IPV only if there is a clear need, such as women who will be traveling or living in an area with endemic or epidemic poliovirus.

Rabies Vaccine and Immunoglobulin

Rabies is a virtually universally fatal infection in humans. Although all mammals are susceptible to rabies, carnivorous mammals are reservoirs of the virus and responsible for persistence of the virus in nature. In the United States, most human cases of rabies are from exposure to rabid bats, but raccoons, foxes, skunks, and coyotes are also associated with possible exposure. Worldwide, canines are the primary vectors. Transmission of rabies can occur via percutaneous, permucosal, or airborne exposure to the rabies virus. Circumstances favoring such transmission include animal bites and attacks and contamination of scratches, cuts, abrasions, and mucous membranes with saliva or other infectious material (brain tissue). Unprovoked attacks and daytime attacks by nocturnal animals are considered highly suspect. A few cases of person-to-person transmission have been reported.

Symptoms of rabies are nonspecific during the prodomal stage—fever, headache, malaise, irritability, nausea, and vomiting. The acute neurologic phase is characterized by hyperexcitability, hyperactivity, hallucinations, salivation, a fear of water, and air. A minority of patients present with limp paralysis. Patients die within 5 days of presentation with these neurologic symptoms.

Human diploid cell vaccine, and purified chick embryo cell rabies vaccine are killed vaccines used for preexposure and postexposure rabies virus prophylaxis. Preexposure indications for rabies vaccine include persons whose vocation or avocation place them at high risk for rabies exposure, such as veterinarians, animal handlers, laboratory workers in rabies research or diagnostic laboratories, cavers, wildlife officers where animal rabies is common, and anyone who handles bats. Travelers who will be in a country or area of a country where there is a constant threat of rabies, whose stay is likely to extend beyond 1 month, and who may not have readily available medical services (eg, Peace Corps workers and missionaries) should be considered for preexposure prophylaxis. Rabies immunization of immunocompromised individuals should be postponed until the immunosuppression has resolved, or activities should be modified to minimize the potential exposure to rabies. If the vaccine is used in immunocompromised persons, antibody titers should be checked postimmunization. Pregnancy is not a contraindication if the risk of rabies is great. Both vaccine preparations can be administered for preexposure prophylaxis as a three-dose series of 1 mL IM on days 0 and 7 and once between days 21 and 28.[30] Individuals with ongoing risk of exposure—either continuous risk (eg, research laboratory staff or those involved in rabies biologics production) or individuals with frequent exposures (eg, those involved with rabies diagnosis, spelunkers, veterinarians, animal control workers, and wildlife workers in rabies-enzootic areas)—should undergo serologic testing every 6 months and 2 years, respectively, to monitor rabies antibody concentrations. A booster dose is recommended if the complete virus neutralization is less than 1:5 serum dilution by the rapid fluorescent focus inhibition test.

Preexposure prophylaxis does not eliminate the need for postexposure therapy. Persons previously immunized with rabies vaccine or those who previously received postexposure prophylaxis should receive two 1-mL IM doses of rabies vaccine on postexposure days 0 and 3.[31] Rabies Ig should not be given to this group.

Postexposure prophylaxis should be given after percutaneous or permucosal exposure to saliva or other infectious material from a high-risk source. Each case must be considered individually. Consideration needs to be given to the geographic area, species of animal, circumstances of the incident, and type of exposure. Local or state health departments should be contacted for assistance. Thorough cleansing of the wound with soap and water followed by irrigation with a virucidal agent such as povidone–iodine solution is an extremely important part of the management of rabies-prone wounds. Individuals who have not been immunized previously should receive the recommended regimen of rabies Ig (see Rabies Immunoglobulin below) and four doses of rabies vaccine 1 mL IM on days 0, 3, 7, and 14 after exposure. However, a fifth dose in a series should be considered if the exposed individual is immunocompromised. Vaccine response for these immunocompromised individuals should be checked.[31] Rabies vaccine must be administered in the deltoid muscle in adults and in the anterolateral thigh in children. The gluteal region should not be used.[1,31]

Adverse reactions to rabies biologicals are less common and less serious with the currently available vaccines compared with previously used preparations. Local or mild systemic symptoms can typically be managed with anti-inflammatory medications or antihistamines. Systemic allergic reactions ranging from hives to anaphylaxis occur in a very small number of subjects. Given the lack of alternative therapy and the fact that rabies infection is almost always fatal, persons exposed to rabies who do have adverse reactions should continue the vaccine series in a setting with medical support services.[30]

Human rabies Ig is used in conjunction with rabies vaccine as part of postexposure rabies management for previously unvaccinated individuals. The product is derived from plasma obtained from donors who have been hyperimmunized with rabies vaccine and have high titers of circulating antibody.

In persons who previously have not been immunized against rabies, rabies Ig is given simultaneously with rabies vaccine to provide optimal coverage in the interval before immune response to the vaccine occurs. The efficacy of this regimen has been clearly demonstrated as it provides virtually complete protection from rabies when administered with the vaccine series promptly following exposure.[31] Rabies Ig does not interfere with vaccine-induced antibody formation. Its use is not recommended beyond 8 days after initiation of the vaccine series nor in persons previously immunized to rabies.

Human rabies Ig is administered in a dose of 20 international units/kg (0.133 mL/kg). If anatomically feasible, the entire dose should be infiltrated around the wound(s). Any remaining volume should be administered IM at a site distant from the rabies vaccination site. This product should never be administered by the IV route. Because other antibodies in the rabies Ig may interfere with the response to live-virus vaccines (MMR and varicella), it is recommended that these immunizations be delayed for 3 months.[1]

Side effects are rare but may include local soreness at the wound or IM injection site and mild temperature elevations. Caution is advised when administering the product to persons with known systemic allergies to Ig or thimerosal. Pregnancy is not a contraindication to its use.

Rubella Vaccine

Rubella (German measles) is characterized by an erythematous rash, lymphadenopathy, arthralgia, and low-grade fever. The most important consequence of rubella infection occurs during pregnancy, particularly during the first trimester. Congenital rubella syndrome is associated with auditory, ophthalmic, cardiac, and neurologic defects. Rubella infection during pregnancy can also result in miscarriage or stillbirth. The primary goal of rubella immunization is to prevent congenital rubella syndrome. Rubella is no longer endemic in the United States, but high immunization rates are necessary to prevent rubella outbreaks from imported cases.[8]

Rubella vaccine contains lyophilized live-attenuated rubella virus grown in human diploid cell culture. The vaccine is available in combinations with measles and mumps (as MMR), or varicella (MMRV) vaccines.

Rubella vaccine induces antibodies that are protective against wild-virus infection. The duration of immunity has not been established. A second dose is recommended, however, at the same time measles vaccine is administered (as a second dose of MMR). The vaccine is indicated for children older than 1 year of age. Individuals born before 1957 are assumed to be immune to rubella except for females who could become pregnant. Therefore, all females of childbearing potential should have documentation of receiving at least one dose of a rubella-containing vaccine or laboratory evidence of immunity.[8] The vaccine should not be given to immunosuppressed individuals, although MMR vaccine should be administered to individuals with HIV infection without evidence of immunity (see Measles).[8] The vaccine should not be given to individuals who have experienced anaphylactic reactions to neomycin.

Adverse effects of the rubella virus vaccine tend to increase with the age of the recipient. Mild symptoms are similar to wild-virus infection and include lymphadenopathy, rash, urticaria, fever, malaise, sore throat, headache, myalgias, and paresthesias of the extremities. These symptoms occur 7 to 12 days after vaccination and last 1 to 5 days. Joint symptoms occur more often in susceptible postpubertal females. Arthralgia occurs in 25% of vaccinees, and 10% have arthritis-like symptoms. These symptoms usually begin 1 to 3 weeks after vaccination, persist for 1 day to 3 weeks, and rarely recur.[8] The vaccine may cause suppression of tuberculin skin tests for up to 6 weeks after vaccination.

The rubella vaccine has never been associated with congenital rubella syndrome, but its use during pregnancy is contraindicated. However, routine pregnancy testing prior to vaccination is not recommended. Females should be counseled not to become pregnant for 4 weeks following vaccination.[8] Termination of pregnancy is not indicated in women who are accidentally given the vaccine or who become pregnant during the month after vaccination.

Tetanus Toxoid Adsorbed and Tetanus Immunoglobulin

Tetanus is a severe acute illness caused by the exotoxin of *Clostridium tetani*. Tetanus is the only vaccine-preventable disease that is not contagious as it is acquired from the environment. Tetanus toxin interferes with neurotransmitters that promote muscle relaxation, leading to continuous muscle spasms that are characteristic of tetanus. Death can be due to the tetanus toxin itself or secondary to a complication such as aspiration pneumonia, dysregulation of the autonomic nervous system, or pulmonary embolism.

Tetanus toxoid adsorbed (adsorbed onto aluminum hydroxide, phosphate, or potassium sulfate to increase antigenicity) is a sterile suspension of the toxoid derived from *C. tetani*. A series of three 0.5-mL doses of tetanus toxoid elicits protection in virtually all individuals. Primary vaccination provides protection for at least 10 years.[21] Additional doses of tetanus toxoid (combined with diphtheria toxoid, ie, Td) are recommended as part of wound management if a patient has not received a dose of tetanus toxoid within the preceding 5 years. For minor or clean wounds, no dose is given. Table 125-3 summarizes these recommendations. Tetanus Ig should be given to

TABLE 125-3 Tetanus Prophylaxis[20]

Vaccination History	Clean, Minor		All Other	
	Td[a]	TIG	Td[a]	TIG
Unknown or fewer than three doses	Yes	No	Yes	Yes
Three or more doses	No[a,b]	No	No[a,c]	No

[a]A single dose of Tdap should be used for the next dose of tetanus-diphtheria toxoid for individuals aged >10 years.

[b]Yes, if more than 10 years since last dose.

[c]Yes, if more than 5 years since last dose.

individuals who have received fewer than three doses of tetanus toxoid and have more serious wounds. It can be administered with tetanus toxoid, provided that separate syringes and separate injection sites are used.

In children, primary immunization against tetanus usually is offered in conjunction with diphtheria and pertussis vaccination (using DTaP or a combination vaccine that includes other antigens used to decrease the number of injections to complete the childhood immunization schedule). A 0.5-mL dose is recommended at age 2, 4, 6, and 15 to 18 months.[13] In children 7 years and older and in adults who have not been immunized previously, a series of three 0.5-mL doses of a tetanus toxoid-containing vaccine is administered IM initially. The first two doses are given 1 to 2 months apart, and the third dose is recommended at 6 to 12 months after the second dose. Boosters are recommended every 10 years, and unless there is contraindication to diphtheria toxoid, Td should be used. Tetanus toxoid can be given simultaneously with other killed and live vaccines, and, if indicated, it can be given to immunosuppressed patients.[21]

Adverse reactions to tetanus toxoid include mild-to-moderate local reactions at the injection site, such as warmth, erythema, and induration. Occasionally, a nodule at the injection site develops and remains for a few weeks. This type of reaction is indicative of high preexisting antibody concentrations, and additional doses of toxoid should not be given any sooner than 10 years. Local reactions do not limit the use of the toxoid for further dosing.[21]

Tetanus Ig is a sterile, concentrated, nonpyrogenic solution of Igs prepared from hyperimmunized humans. It is used to provide passive immunity to tetanus after the occurrence of traumatic wounds in nonimmunized or suboptimally immunized persons (see Table 125-3).[32] A dose of 250 to 500 units IM should be administered. When administered with tetanus toxoid, separate sites for administration should be used. Tetanus Ig also is used for treatment of tetanus. In this setting, a single dose of 3,000 to 6,000 units IM is administered.

Adverse effects of tetanus Ig include pain, tenderness, erythema, and muscle stiffness at the injection site, which may persist for several hours. Systemic reactions occur rarely. IV administration has been associated with severe adverse reactions and is not recommended.

Varicella and Zoster Vaccines

Varicella is a highly contagious disease caused by varicella-zoster virus. The clinical illness is characterized by the appearance of successive waves of pruritic vesicles that rapidly crust over. Malaise and fever are common and last for 2 to 3 days. The virus remains dormant in the dorsal ganglia and reactivates as herpes zoster, also known as *shingles*. Although the exact stimulus for reactivation is unknown, a decrease in varicella-specific cell-mediated immunity associated with age or immunosuppression appears to be necessary but not sufficient for reactivation.

Varicella Vaccine

Live-attenuated varicella vaccine contains the Oka/Merck strain of varicella virus, which was attenuated by propagation through several different cell culture lines. Varicella vaccine is a lyophilized product that must be kept frozen and protected from light. Once reconstituted, it must be administered subcutaneously within 30 minutes. Each 0.5-mL dose contains a minimum of 1,350 plaque-forming units of virus as well as 12.5 mg of hydrolyzed gelatin and trace amounts of neomycin, fetal bovine serum, and residual components from cell culture.[33]

The varicella vaccine is safe and immunogenic in healthy children and adults. In clinical studies, varicella vaccine has been 70% to more than 95% effective in preventing chickenpox. Vaccinated individuals who develop chickenpox typically experience milder disease, often with low or no fever and fewer skin lesions, many of which do not vesiculate.[33]

The varicella vaccine is recommended for all children at 12 to 18 months of age, with a second dose prior to entering school between ages 4 and 6 years.[13] A second dose is also recommended for individuals older than this age if they have not already had chickenpox. Varicella vaccine can be used for postexposure prophylaxis. The vaccine is effective in the prevention or modification of varicella infection when given within 3 days and possibly 5 days of exposure. Because the varicella vaccine is a live vaccine, it is contraindicated in pregnant women and in immunocompromised individuals. An exception is children with asymptomatic or mildly symptomatic HIV infection, who should receive two doses of varicella vaccine 3 months apart. In addition, children with humoral immune deficiencies may be immunized. Varicella vaccination is contraindicated in individuals with a history of anaphylactic reaction to any component of the vaccine. Persons who have received blood, plasma, or Ig products in the recent past should not receive varicella vaccine because of concern that passively acquired antibody will interfere with response to the vaccine. The recommended time interval between antibody-containing products and varicella vaccine depends on the dose of Ig (see Table 125-1).[1] Although no adverse events associated with salicylate use after vaccination have been reported, salicylates should be avoided for 6 weeks after vaccination because of the association of salicylate use and Reye syndrome following varicella infection.[33]

The varicella vaccine has an excellent safety record. Pain, local swelling, and erythema at the injection site occur in up to 32% of patients and fever in 10% to 15%. A varicella-like rash occurs in approximately 4% of vaccinees, accompanied by few, if any, systemic symptoms. The rash may be localized at the injection site or generalized. Lesions usually are few in number (2 to 10) and often papular rather than vesicular. Transmission of vaccine virus to susceptible close contacts has occurred but is rare and believed to occur only when the vaccinee develops a rash. Because the risk of vaccine virus transmission is very low and primary infection can be very severe, vaccination of household contacts of immunocompromised patients is recommended to prevent introduction of varicella into the household.[33]

Zoster Vaccine

After the primary infection with varicella-zoster virus manifested as chicken pox, the virus remains latent in the dorsal ganglia. Herpes zoster, more commonly known as *shingles*, occurs upon reactivation of varicella-zoster virus replication. Herpes zoster can occur at any age, but the incidence dramatically increases with increasing age. The rate of disease increases sharply after age 50 years. The disease rate in individuals older than 80 years of age is 15 cases per 1,000 person-years.[34] Patients with HIV, cancer, or other conditions associated with immunosuppression are at increased risk for disease.[35] The development of the disease is associated with declining cellular immunity to varicella-zoster virus.

The clinical presentation of herpes zoster usually is a vesicular eruption limited to one dermatome. The most common complication is postherpetic neuralgia, which is pain that persists after the skin lesions have healed. Postherpetic neuralgia can persist for weeks to years. The risk of postherpetic neuralgia increases dramatically with age. Virtually no risk of developing postherpetic neuralgia with herpes zoster exists prior to age 50 years, but the risk increases to 50% to 75% after ages 60 and 75 years, respectively. The pain can be so severe as to limit activities of daily living and quality of life.[7]

The zoster vaccine contains 19,000 plaque-forming units of Oka/Merck strain live varicella-zoster virus. Although the same strain of vaccine virus is contained in the childhood varicella vaccines, the doses of vaccine virus are dramatically different, and the vaccines are *not* interchangeable. Zoster vaccine reduces the burden of disease by 60%. The burden of disease is a composite measure considering incidence, severity, and duration of herpes zoster. The incidence of zoster is cut in half and the development of postherpetic

TABLE 125-4 Zoster Vaccine Use in Special Populations[7]

- Immunize patients with a history of shingles
- Screening patients for a history of chickenpox is not necessary. Assume anyone born before 1980 is immune to varicella[47]
- Zoster vaccine may be administered to individuals on inhaled, topical or intraarticular steroids or low dose oral steroids
- Zoster vaccine may be administered to individuals treated with low-dose methotrexate (less than 0.4 mg/kg/wk) or mercaptopurine (less than 1.5 mg/kg/day). These therapies are often used for autoimmune diseases
- The vaccine may be administered to individuals anticipating immunosuppressive therapy. The minimum duration between immunization and initiation of immunosuppressive therapy is 14 days, and some clinicians recommend 1 month
- Stop antiviral therapy at least 24 hours before immunization and restart it at least 14 days after immunization
- Zoster vaccine can be administered without regard to blood product or immunoglobulin administration
- Do not administer zoster vaccine to
  - Individuals with AIDS or clinical manifestations of HIV, such as a $CD4^+$ count less than 200 per mm^3
  - Patients on high doses of steroids (prednisone or its equivalent of 20 mg daily or more for more than 2 weeks)
- Risks and benefits of administering zoster vaccine to individuals on immune modulators, such as tumor necrosis factor agents, must be determined on a case-by-case basis. Immunize prior to initiating therapy if possible

neuralgia can be decreased by 67%.[36] The duration of protection from the vaccine is about 8 years for prevention of zoster and about 10 years for decrease in burden of disease which includes incidence, severity, and complications of zoster.[37]

The zoster vaccine is licensed for individuals 50 years of age and older. However, the ACIP recommends the zoster vaccine for routine use in individuals aged 60 years and older. This live vaccine should not be used in immunocompromised individuals, including those on high-dose corticosteroids or with HIV (CD4 cell count less than $200/mm^3$) [less than $0.200 \times 10^9/L$] or malignancies.[7] Immunization of some special populations can be done (see Table 125-4).

Varicella-Zoster Immunoglobulin

Varicella-zoster Ig is used after exposure to varicella for passive immunization of susceptible immunodeficient patients or other susceptible individuals at particularly high risk for complications of varicella infection. Postexposure prophylaxis with varicella-zoster Ig is indicated for the following susceptible individuals: (a) immunocompromised patients without evidence of immunity, (b) neonates whose mothers develop varicella within 5 days before or 2 days after delivery, (c) hospitalized premature infants (more than 28 weeks of gestation) whose mothers have no evidence of immunity (d) hospitalized preterm infants (less than 28 weeks' gestation or weight less than 1,000 g), and (e) susceptible pregnant women.[38] If varicella is prevented, vaccination should be offered at a later date. Exposure to varicella is defined as direct indoor contact for more than 1 hour with an infectious person. A negative history of clinical disease is not a reliable indicator of varicella susceptibility. Most people with a negative clinical history will have detectable antibody on laboratory testing. Caution is warranted when interpreting a low-positive result in an immunosuppressed patient who has received blood products or Ig because the circulating antibody may be acquired passively.

For maximum effectiveness, varicella-zoster Ig must be given as soon as possible and not more than 10 days following exposure.[38] Because this agent may only attenuate infection, patients who receive varicella-zoster Ig still may have a period of communicability, and varicella-zoster Ig may prolong the incubation period to 28 days. Antiviral therapy can be initiated if signs and symptoms of varicella infection become apparent.

Administration of varicella-zoster Ig is by the IM route at doses of 125 plaque-forming units per 10 kg of body weight up to 625 units (five vials) for patients weighing more than 40 kg. The dose for newborn infants is 125 units.[38]

OTHER IMMUNOBIOLOGICS

Immunoglobulin

Ig is available as both an intramuscular immunoglobulin (IMIG) and an IV immunoglobulin (IVIG) preparation. The IMIG preparation, or the Cohn fraction II, is prepared from pooled plasma of several thousand donors by cold ethanol fractionation. It typically contains greater than 95% IgG and trace amounts of IgM, IgA, and other plasma proteins. Because Ig is harvested from a large donor pool, it contains a wide spectrum of IgG antibodies to the pathogens prevalent in the area from which the donors were obtained. In the fractionation process, high-molecular-weight IgG aggregates are formed, which can activate complement in the absence of antigen and precipitate anaphylactoid reactions. For this reason, IMIG is unsuitable for IV administration. IMIG typically contains 15% to 18% protein and not less than 90% IgG. A number of IVIG preparations are available commercially in the United States. Generally, these preparations contain greater than 90% IgG monomers and trace to small amounts of IgA. These products are available as lyophilized powders or solutions.

When administered either IV or IM, Ig distributes in approximately 5% of the body weight of the recipient. The plasma half-life of Ig ranges from 18 to 32 days. This range of half-life probably is attributable to the variation in the half-life of IgG subclasses. Peak serum concentrations occur immediately with IVIG but within 2 days with IMIG. After the initial period of equilibration, circulating IgG levels are superimposable between IV and IM equivalent dosages. No dosage adjustment is necessary in patients with renal insufficiency, hepatic insufficiency, or both, dialysis patients, or geriatric patients.

6 Ig is indicated in a wide variety of circumstances to provide passive immunity to individuals. The indications for IMIG differ from those for IVIG. IMIG is indicated for providing passive immunity in patients with hepatitis A infections in those less than 1 year and older than 39 years, hepatitis B exposures (however, hepatitis B Ig is significantly more effective), measles, varicella, and primary immunodeficiency diseases. Although IMIG is indicated for the treatment of primary immunodeficiency, IVIG is better tolerated and is more effective. IMIG is not indicated for prevention of rubella, mumps, or poliomyelitis. Table 125-5 lists the suggested dosages of IMIG for prevention or attenuation of various infectious diseases.

There are many licensed indications, as well as off-label uses, for IVIG.[39] The therapeutic dose of IVIG is set empirically at

TABLE 125-5 Indications and Dosage of Intramuscular Immunoglobulin in Infectious Diseases

Primary immunodeficiency states	1.2 mL/kg IM then 0.6 mL/kg every 2-4 weeks
Hepatitis A exposure	0.02 mL/kg IM within 2 weeks if <1 year or >39 years of age
Hepatitis A prophylaxis	0.02 mL/kg IM for exposure <3 months' duration
	0.06 mL/kg IM for exposure up to 5 months' duration
Hepatitis B exposure	0.06 mL/kg (HBIG preferred in known exposures)
Measles exposure	0.25 mL/kg (maximum dose 15 mL) as soon as possible
	0.5 mL/kg (maximum dose 15 mL) as soon as possible for immunocompromised individuals

2 g/kg, often given as five daily doses of 400 mg/kg each.[40] Mechanisms of IVIG action for treatment of these conditions have been hypothesized.[41]

1. *Primary Immunodeficiency States.*[42] In primary immunodeficiency states, monthly doses of between 100 and 800 mg/kg are administered; the average dose is 200 to 400 mg/kg. The immunodeficiency states for which IVIG is indicated include both antibody deficiencies and combined immune deficiencies. Significant reactions can occur in patients with low intrinsic levels of IgA given IVIG with greater amounts of IgA. An IVIG product with very low amounts of IgA should be used for these patients.
2. *Immune Thrombocytopenia.*[43] For the treatment of hemorrhage associated with immune thrombocytopenia (ITP), doses of 1 g/kg daily for 2 to 3 days plus high-dose methylprednisolone are indicated. Adults tend to respond less well to IVIG than do children. IVIG is acceptable for treatment of both chronic and acute ITP, and IVIG has been used for ITP associated with pregnancy without adverse effects on the fetus. Corticosteroids remain the drugs of choice for adult ITP. In thrombotic thrombocytopenia purpura, IVIG is reported to be effective in patients who do not respond to plasmapheresis. Other platelet disorders in which IVIG may be useful include neonatal immune thrombocytopenia, perinatal autoimmune thrombocytopenia, drug-induced thrombocytopenia, thrombocytopenia secondary to infection, and transfusion-refractory thrombocytopenia; however, the data supporting these uses are minimal.
3. *Chronic Lymphocytic Leukemia.* IVIG is used as a prophylactic measure in patients with chronic lymphocytic leukemia who have had a serious bacterial infection. Doses of 400 mg/kg every 3 to 4 weeks are used.
4. *Kawasaki Disease.*[44] This disease, which generally occurs in children, carries the hallmark of development of coronary artery abnormalities. Generally, the American Academy of Pediatrics recommends that if the strict criteria for Kawasaki disease are met, an IVIG dose of 400 mg/kg/day for 4 consecutive days be used or, preferably, 2 g/kg as a single dose. The dose should be administered within 10 days of disease onset. Aspirin therapy also should be initiated.
5. *Pediatric HIV infection.*[45] IVIG prevents serious bacterial infections in children with HIV infection. However, in the era of highly active anti-retroviral therapy, its use has waned.
6. *Allogeneic bone marrow transplantation.*[41]
7. *Chronic inflammatory demyelinating polyneuropathy.*[46] This disabling neuropathy often responds to corticosteroids, IVIG, or plasmapheresis.
8. *Multifocal motor neuropathy*[47] IVIG is considered first line therapy.
9. *Kidney transplantation involving a recipient with high antibody concentrations or an ABO-incompatible donor.*[48] Some transplant recipients have antibody concentrations that present an immunological barrier to transplantation. Desensitization can be accomplished using IVIG.

Many other proposed uses of IVIG have been identified. It is important to note that these uses are off-label but may be generally accepted in the medical community for routine treatment.[39,41]

7 Adverse effects of Ig vary with the route of administration. Following IMIG, pain, tenderness, and muscle stiffness persisting for hours or days are common. Repeat courses may cause sensitization with resulting allergic reactions. Chills, fever, nausea, and vomiting often are related to the rate of the infusion.[49] Infusion should be given at a rate of 0.01 to 0.02 mL/kg/min for 30 minutes. If no reactions occur, then the rate can be increased to 0.02 to 0.04 mL/kg/min. If reactions do occur, the infusion should be stopped for 30 minutes and restarted at a lower rate. Although recommendations for infusion rate vary slightly depending on the preparation, the guidelines presented can be followed for the various IV preparations.

Most adverse reactions are mild and transient. Arthralgia, myalgia, fever, pruritus, nausea, vomiting, chest tightness, palpitations, diaphoresis, dizziness, pallor, and respiratory distress have been reported. Rarely, aseptic meningitis has occurred from a few hours to 2 days after high-dose infusion. The syndrome resolves within days without sequelae. Acute renal failure has been reported, primarily in individuals with underlying renal dysfunction, diabetes, sepsis, volume depletion, or other nephrotoxic drugs or in patients older than 65 years. To minimize the risk, ensure adequate hydration prior to infusion and choose an IVIG product that does not contain high sucrose concentrations for individuals at high risk.[49]

Ig products are derived from human blood. Precautions such as donor screening and fractionation procedures and solvent–detergent treatment during the manufacturing process render the IVIG products free of HIV and hepatitis B and C viruses. Although no manufacturing process can guarantee no viral contamination, the potential infection risk from Ig preparations is very small.

Rh_o(D) Immunoglobulin

Second only to the ABO blood group system, Rhesus antigen D [Rh_o(D)] is an important antigen in human blood. The Rh_o(D) locus encodes this antigen, but this locus is absent in approximately 15% of the population. 8 Individuals lacking the Rh_o(D) locus are Rh_o(D) negative and have the potential to mount an antibody response to erythrocytes with the Rh_o(D) present. Rh_o(D) incompatibility during pregnancy can lead to sensitization of the mother. The maternal antibodies developed following normal fetal leakage of erythrocytes to the mother can cause hemolytic disease of the newborn during subsequent pregnancies.

Rh_o(D) Ig is a sterile solution of Igs prepared from human sera with high titers of Rh_o(D) antibody. Rh_o(D) Ig suppresses the antibody response and formation of anti-Rh_o(D) in Rh_o(D)-negative women exposed to Rh_o(D)-positive blood. Administration of Rh_o(D) Ig prevents hemolytic disease of the newborn in subsequent pregnancies with a Rh_o(D)-positive fetus. When administered within 72 hours of delivery of a full-term infant, Rh_o(D) Ig reduces active antibody formation from 1% to about 0.2%.[50] The reduction in antibody formation is lower when Rh_o(D) Ig is given beyond 72 hours postpartum. Smaller doses of Rh_o(D) Ig are used after abortion, miscarriage, amniocentesis, or abdominal trauma. In addition, Rh_o(D) Ig is used in the case of a premenopausal woman who is Rh_o(D) negative and has inadvertently received Rh_o(D)-positive blood or blood products.[50]

The dosage of Rh_o(D) Ig varies with the indication. A standard dose of 300 mcg is given within 72 hours of a term delivery. Occasionally, when the fetus is known to be Rh_o(D) positive, a 300-mcg dose is given at 28 weeks' gestation and within 72 hours after delivery. For postpregnancy termination occurring up to 13 weeks' gestation, one microdose (50 mcg) vial is given within 72 hours. For pregnancy termination after 13 weeks, one standard dose (300 mcg) is given within 72 hours. In other circumstances, such as in abdominal trauma, amniocentesis, or transfusion accidents, the dosage (number of standard dose vials) is based on the estimated packed red blood cell volume of fetal/maternal hemorrhage divided by 15. Rh_o(D) Ig is administered IM only.

When considering use of Rh_o(D) Ig use, the mother's Rh_o(D) antigen status must be known with certainty. Rh_o(D) Ig should not be given to individuals positive for this antigen or to those with

TABLE 125-6 Web Resources for Vaccine Information

Recommended Internet Sites for Vaccine Information	
http://www.cdc.gov/vaccines/	Vaccines & Immunizations Centers for Disease Control and Prevention
www.immunize.org	Immunization Action Coalition
www.nfid.org/	National Foundation for Infectious Diseases
www.cdc.gov/mmwr/	Morbidity and Mortality Weekly Report
http://iom.nationalacademies.org/	Institute of Medicine of the National Academies
http://www.hrsa.gov/vaccinecompensation/	Vaccine Injury Compensation Program
http://www.chop.edu/service/vaccine-education-center/	Vaccine Education Center Children's Hospital of Philadelphia
http://vaers.hhs.gov/index	Vaccine Adverse Event Reporting System
Recommended Electronic Newsletters	
www.immunize.org/express	The Immunization Action Coalition's newsletter
www.cdc.gov/mmwr/	Morbidity and Mortality Weekly Report

anti-Rh_o(D) antibodies. Occasionally, a large fetal bleed of Rh_o(D)-positive blood may make cross-matching of the mother difficult. In these cases, Rh_o(D) Ig should be given only if previous tests have shown that the mother is Rh_o(D) negative with no anti-Rh_o(D) antibody.

Adverse reactions to Rh_o(D) Ig include injection-site tenderness and fever. Rh_o(D) does not interfere with response to rubella vaccine. Rubella-seronegative women should be immunized at hospital discharge even if they received Rh_o(D) Ig postpartum.

VACCINE INFORMATION RESOURCES

The field of vaccinology is developing even more rapidly, with numerous changes in recommendations for vaccine use made each year. Keeping up to date with the current recommendations can be a challenge. The childhood, adolescent, and adult immunization schedules are updated frequently and published annually. Recommendations for the use of influenza vaccine are issued annually. Healthcare providers involved in primary care and immunization delivery must keep themselves abreast of these changes in a systematic way. Reading electronic newsletters and browsing reliable Websites are efficient methods for obtaining information (Table 125-6). Although several excellent, reliable, and timely Websites exist, hundreds of sites with misleading and incorrect information also exist. Many of these sites are targeted at parents.

Although the medical community has moved past the controversy, the public still has questions regarding the possible connection between vaccine exposure and autism. The only study to demonstrate a link between vaccines and autism was a series of case reports published in 1998 that has since been withdrawn, and its lead author has been accused of fraud.[51] None of ten studies that have been conducted have found a connection between vaccine exposure and the development of autism.[52] The Vaccine Education Center at the Children's Hospital of Philadelphia has several documents for parents who have questions about vaccine safety. *http://www.chop.edu/centers-programs/vaccine-education-center/vaccine-safety/are-vaccines-safe#.VhHMbyta0rI* The CDC is another source of information for parents. *http://www.cdc.gov/vaccines/vac-gen/safety/*.

PERSONALIZED PHARMACOTHERAPY

Immunization programs are an important part of public health for all people. Therefore, immunization schedules are used across the population with little consideration of individual variability. Recommendations for some vaccines are based on risks, occupation, life-style, or age.

However, pharmacogenomics can be used to predict which individuals may be likely to have a vigorous or poor response to a vaccine. Some apparently healthy individuals fail to mount an immune response to a particular vaccine.[53] The consequence of these research findings are not yet ready to be used in clinical care of patients. As the field matures, these polymorphisms may be considered for vaccine design, immunization scheduling or vaccine safety.

Vaccines are the only class of medications to which nearly every patient is exposed. Knowledge of these agents is critical to providing pharmaceutical care. Dramatic progress in public health has been made through the appropriate use of immunization. Additional improvements in quality of life and mortality can be made through continued increases in vaccination coverage with careful attention to this aspect of care by all healthcare providers.

ABBREVIATIONS

ACIP	Advisory Committee on Immunization Practices
CDC	US Centers for Disease Control and Prevention
DTaP	diphtheria, tetanus toxoids, and acellular pertussis
HBIG	Hepatitis B immune globulin
Hib	*Haemophilus influenzae* type b
HPV	human papillomavirus
Ig	immunoglobulin
IMIG	intramuscular immunoglobulin
IPV	inactivated polio vaccine
ITP	idiopathic (immune) thrombocytopenic purpura
IVIG	IV immunoglobulin
MenB	Meningococcal serogroup B
MMR	measles–mumps–rubella vaccine
MMRV	measles–mumps–rubella-varicella vaccine
MSM	men who have sex with men
OPV	oral polio vaccine
PCV	pneumococcal conjugate vaccine
PPSV23	23-valent pneumococcal polysaccharide vaccine
PRP	polyribosylribitol phosphate
Td	tetanus–diphtheria
Tdap	tetanus–diphtheria–acellular pertussis
TIG	Tetanus immune globulin
VAERS	Vaccine Adverse Event Reporting System

REFERENCES

1. Centers for Disease Control and Prevention. General recommendations on immunization. Recommendations of the Advisory Committee on Immunization Practices (ACIP). *MMWR Morb Mortal Wkly Rep* 2011;60:1-64.
2. Centers for Disease Control and Prevention. A comprehensive immunization strategy to eliminate transmission of hepatitis B virus infection in the United States. Recommendations of the Advisory Committee on Immunization Practices (ACIP) Part II: Immunization of adults. *MMWR Morb Mortal Wkly Rep* 2006;55:1-33.
3. Centers for Disease Control and Prevention. Prevention and control of influenza with vaccines: Recommendations of the Advisory Committee on Immunization Practices, United States, 2015-16 influenza season. *MMWR Morb Mortal Wkly Rep* 2015;64:818-825.
4. Centers for Disease Control and Prevention. Updated recommendations for use of tetanus toxoid, reduced diphtheria toxoid and acellular pertussis (Tdap) vaccine in pregnant women and persons who have or anticipate having close contact with an infant aged <12 months—Advisory Committee on Immunization Practices (ACIP), 2011. *MMWR Morb Mortal Wkly Rep* 2011;60:1424-1426.
5. Centers for Disease Control and Prevention. Guidelines for vaccinating pregnant women http://www.cdc.gov/vaccines/pubs/preg-guide.htm Accessed March 2014.
6. Rubin LG, Levin MJ, Ljungman P, et al. 2013 IDSA clinical practice guideline for vaccination of the immunocompromised host. *Clin Infect Dis* 2013;58:309-318.
7. Centers for Disease Control and Prevention. Prevention of herpes zoster. Recommendations of the Advisory Committee on Immunization Practices (ACIP). *MMWR Morb Mortal Wkly Rep* 2008;57:1-30.
8. Centers for Disease Control and Prevention. Prevention of measles, rubella, congenital rubella syndrome, and mumps, 2013. Summary recommendations of the Advisory Committee on Immunization Practices (ACIP). *MMWR Morb Mortal Wkly Rep* 2013;62:1-33.
9. Danziger-Isakov L, Kumar D, the A. S. T. Infectious Diseases Community of Practice. Vaccination in solid organ transplantation. *Am J Transplant* 2013;13:311-317.
10. Centers for Disease Control and Prevention. Progress in Immunization Information Systems—United States, 2012. *MMWR Morb Mortal Wkly Rep* 2013;62:1005-1008.
11. Lopalco PL, DeStefano F. The complementary roles of Phase 3 trials and post-licensure surveillance in the evaluation of new vaccines. *Vaccine* 2015;33:1541-1548.
12. Hanson D, Hall W, Mills LL, et al. Comparison of distress and pain in infants randomized to groups receiving standard versus multiple immunizations. *Infant Behav Dev* 2010;33:289-296.
13. Centers for Disease Control and Prevention. Recommended immunization schedules for persons aged 0 through 18 years—United States, 2015. 2015:1-6.
14. Centers for Disease Control and Prevention. Recommended adult immunization schedule—United States, 2015. 2015:1-5.
15. Centers for Disease Control and Prevention. Prevention and control of *Haemophilus influenzae* type b disease. Recommendations of the Advisory Committee on Immunization Practices (ACIP). *MMWR Morb Mortal Wkly Rep* 2015;63:1-14.
16. Centers for Disease Control and Prevention. Recommendations on the use of quadrivalent human papillomavirus vaccine in males--Advisory Committee on Immunization Practices (ACIP), 2011. *MMWR Morb Mortal Wkly Rep* 2011;60:1705-1708.
17. Palefsky JM, Giuliano AR, Goldstone S, et al. HPV vaccine against anal HPV infection and anal intraepithelial neoplasia. *N Engl J Med* 2011;365:1576-85.
18. Centers for Disease Control and Prevention. Use of 9-valent human papillomavirus (HPV) vaccine: Updated HPV vaccination recommendations of the the Advisory Committee on Immunization Practices (ACIP). *MMWR Morb Mortal Wkly Rep* 2015;64:300-4.
19. Angelo M-G, Zima J, Tavares Da Silva F, et al. Post-licensure safety surveillance for human papillomavirus-16/18-AS04-adjuvanted vaccine: More than 4 years of experience. *Pharmacoepidemiol Drug Safety* 2014;23:456-465.
20. Centers for Disease Control and Prevention. Use of serogroup B meningococcal vaccines in persons aged ≥10 years at increased risk for serogroup B meningococcal disease: Recommendation of the Advisory Committee on Immunization Practices, 2015. *MMWR Morb Mortal Wkly Rep* 2015;62:608-612.
21. Centers for Disease Control and Prevention. Updated recommendations for use of tetanus toxoid, reduced diphtheria toxoid and acellular pertussis (Tdap) vaccine from the Advisory Committee on Immunization Practices, 2010. *MMWR Morb Mortal Wkly Rep* 2011;60:13-15.
22. Centers for Disease Control and Prevention. Updated recommendations for the prevention of invasive pneumococcal disease among adults using the 23-valent pneumococcal polysaccharide vaccine (PPSV23). *MMWR Morb Mortal Wkly Rep* 2010;59:1102-1106.
23. Pingali SC, Warren JL, Mead AM, et al. Association between local pediatric vaccination rates and patterns of pneumococcal disease in adults. *J Infect Dis* 2015.
24. Centers for Disease Control and Prevention. Prevention of pneumococcal disease among infants and children-Use of 13-valent pneumococcal conjugate vaccine and 23-valent pneumococcal polysaccharide vaccine. Recommendations of the Advisory Committee on Immunization Practices (ACIP). *MMWR Morb Mortal Wkly Rep* 2010;59:1-18.
25. Centers for Disease Control and Prevention. Use of 13-valent pneumococcal conjugate vaccine and 23-valent pneumococcal polysaccharide vaccine among children aged 6-18 years with immunocompromising conditions: Recommendations of the Advisory Committee on Immunization Practices (ACIP). *MMWR Morb Mortal Wkly Rep* 2013;62:521-524.
26. Centers for Disease Control and Prevention. Updated recommendations for prevention of invasive pneumococcal disease among adults using the 23-valent pneumococcal polysaccharide vaccine (PPSV23). *MMWR Morb Mortal Wkly Rep* 2010;59:1102-1106.
27. Centers for Disease Control and Prevention. Use of 13-valent pneumococcal conjugate vaccine and 23-valent pneumococcal polysaccharide vaccine among adults aged ≥65 years: Recommendations of the Advisory Committee on Immunization Practices (ACIP). *MMWR Morb Mortal Wkly Rep* 2014;63:822-825.
28. Centers for Disease Control and Prevention. Updated recommendations of the Advisory Committee on Immunization Practices (ACIP) regarding routine poliovirus vaccination. *MMWR Morb Mortal Wkly Rep* 2009;58:829-830.
29. Centers for Disease Control and Prevention. Poliomyelitis prevention in the United States: Updated recommendations of the Advisory Committee on Immunization Practices (ACIP). *MMWR Morb Mortal Wkly Rep* 2000;49:1-22.
30. Centers for Disease Control and Prevention. Human rabies prevention—United States, 2008. Recommendations of the Advisory Committee on Immunization Practices. *MMWR Morb Mortal Wkly Rep* 2008;57:1-28.
31. Centers for Disease Control and Prevention. Use of a reduced (4-dose) vaccine schedule for postexposure prophylaxis to prevent human rabies. Recommendations of the Advisory Committee on Immunization Practices. *MMWR Morb Mortal Wkly Rep* 2010;59:1-9.
32. Centers for Disease Control and Prevention. Preventing tetanus, diphtheria, and pertussis among adults: Use of tetanus toxoid, reduced diphtheria toxoid and acellular pertussis vaccines. Recommendations fo the Advisory Committee on Immunization Practices (ACIP) and Recommendation of ACIP, supported by the Healthcare Infection Control Practices Advisory Committee (HIPAC), for the Use of Tdap Among Health-Care Personnel. *MMWR Morb Mortal Wkly Rep* 2006;55:1-37.
33. Centers for Disease Control and Prevention. Prevention of varicella. Recommendations of the Advisory Committee on Immunization Practices (ACIP). *MMWR Morb Mortal Wkly Rep* 2007;56:1-39.
34. McLaughlin J, McGinnis J, Tan L, et al. Estimated human and economic burden of four major adult vaccine-preventable diseases in the United States, 2013. *J Primary Prevent* 2015;36:259-273.
35. Zhang J, Xie F, Delzell E, et al. Association between vaccination for herpes zoster and risk of herpes zoster infection among older patients with selected immune-mediated diseases. *JAMA* 2012;308:43-49.
36. Centers for Disease Control and Prevention. Update on recommendations for the use of herpes zoster vaccine. *MMWR Morb Mortal Wkly Rep* 2014;63:729-731.
37. Morrison VA, Johnson GR, Schmader KE, et al. Long-term persistence of zoster vaccine efficacy. *Clin Infect Dis* 2015;60:900-909.
38. Centers for Disease Control and Prevention. Updated recommendations for use of VariZIG—United States, 2013. *MMWR Morb Mortal Wkly Rep* 2013;62.

39. Robert P, Hotchko M. Polyvalent immune globulin usage by indication in the United States, 2012: A quantitative analysis of the use of polyvalent immune globulin (intravenous and subcutaneous) by medical indication in the United States in 2012. *Transfusion* 2015;55:S6-S12.
40. Stiehm ER, Orange JS, Ballow M, et al. Therapeutic use of immunoglobulins. *Advances in Pediatrics* 2010;57:185-218.
41. Gelfand EW. Intravenous immune globulin in autoimmune and inflammatory diseases. *N Engl J Med* 2012;367:2015-2025.
42. Berger M. Choices in IgG replacement therapy for primary immune deficiency diseases: Subcutaneous IgG vs intravenous IgG and selecting an optimal dose. *Curr Opin Allergy Clin Immunol* 2011;11:532-538.
43. Thota S, Kistangari G, Daw H, Spiro T. Immune thrombocytopenia in adults: An update. *Cleve Clin J Med* 2012;79:641-650.
44. Greco A, De Virgilio A, Rizzo MI, et al. Kawasaki disease: An evolving paradigm. *Autoimmun Rev* 2015;14:703-709.
45. Wong PH, White KM. Impact of immunoglobulin therapy in pediatric disease: A review of immune mechanisms. *Clin Rev Allergy Immunol* 2015; Ahead of print.
46. Nobile-Orazio E, Gallia F. Update on the tretament of chronic inflammatory demyelinating polyradiculoneuropathy. *Curr Opin Neurol* 2015;28:480-485.
47. Živković S. Intravenous immunoglobulin in the treatment of neurologic disorders. *Acta Neurol Scand* 2015:n/a-n/a.
48. Songsaroj P, Kahwaji J, Vo A, Jordan SC. Modern approaches to incompatible kidney transplantation. *World J Nephrol* 2015;4:354-362.
49. Späth PJ, Granata G, La Marra F, et al. On the dark side of therapies with immunoglobulin concentrates: The adverse events. *Front Immunol* 2015;6:11.
50. Crowther C, Middleton P, McBain R. Anti-D administration in pregnancy for preventing Rhesus alloimmunisation (Review). *Cochrane Database Syst Rev* 2013:1-27.
51. Hawkes N. College investigates whether Wakefield was guilty of scientific fraud. *BMJ* 2011;342.
52. Centers for Disease Control and Prevention. Vaccines and autism: A summary of CDC conducted or sponsored studies. 2013:1-3.
53. Thomas C, Moridani M. Interindividual variations in the efficacy and toxicity of vaccines. *Toxicology* 2010;278:204-210.

Human Immunodeficiency Virus Infection

126

Peter L. Anderson, Thomas N. Kakuda, and Courtney V. Fletcher

KEY CONCEPTS

1. Infection with human immunodeficiency virus (HIV) occurs through three primary routes: sexual, parenteral, and perinatal. Sexual intercourse, primarily receptive anal and vaginal intercourse, is the most common method for transmission.
2. HIV infects cells expressing cluster of differentiation 4 (CD4) receptors, such as T-helper lymphocytes, monocytes, macrophages, dendritic cells, and brain microglia. Infection occurs via an interaction between glycoprotein 160 (gp160) on HIV with CD4 (primary interaction) and chemokine coreceptors (secondary interactions) present on the surfaces of these cells.
3. The hallmark of untreated HIV infection is profound CD4 T-lymphocyte depletion and severe immunosuppression that puts patients at significant risk for infectious diseases caused by opportunistic pathogens. Opportunistic infections (OIs) in settings without access to antiretroviral drugs are the chief cause of morbidity and mortality associated with HIV infection.
4. The current goal of combination antiretroviral therapy (ART) is to achieve maximal and durable suppression of HIV replication, taken to be a level of HIV-RNA in plasma (viral load) less than the lower limit of quantitation. Another equally important outcome is an increase in CD4 lymphocytes because this closely correlates with the risk for developing OIs.
5. General principles for the management of OIs include preventing or reversing immunosuppression with ART, preventing exposure to pathogens, vaccination, prospective immunologic monitoring, primary chemoprophylaxis, treatment of acute episodes, secondary chemoprophylaxis, and discontinuation of such prophylaxes following ART and subsequent immune recovery.
6. Clinical use of antiretroviral agents is complicated by drug–drug interactions. Some interactions are beneficial and used purposely; others may be harmful, leading to dangerously elevated or inadequate drug concentrations. For these reasons, clinicians involved in the pharmacotherapy of HIV infection must exercise constant vigilance and maintain a current knowledge of drug interactions.
7. Recommendations for the initial treatment of HIV advocate a minimum of three active antiretroviral agents from at least two drug classes. The typical regimen consists of two nucleoside/nucleotide analogs with either a protease inhibitor (PI; pharmacokinetically enhanced by coadministration with a CYP3A inhibitor) or an integrase strand transfer inhibitor (InSTI).
8. Inadequate suppression of viral replication allows HIV to select for antiretroviral-resistant HIV variants, a major factor limiting the ability of antiretroviral drugs to inhibit virus replication. Recommendations for treating drug-resistant HIV include choosing at least two drugs (preferably three) to which the patient's virus is susceptible. Susceptibility can be assessed using either genotypic or phenotypic resistance testing.
9. The reduction of viral load with ART lowers the risk of transmission to others. Additionally, prophylaxis with antiretroviral agents in at-risk persons lowers HIV acquisition risk.
10. The longer life span conferred by ART has given rise to other medical issues. A wide spectrum of complications associated with older age have become common, some of which overlap with adverse effects from antiretroviral drugs. Medical management of these contemporary HIV complications is constantly evolving.

Acquired immunodeficiency syndrome (AIDS) was first recognized in a cohort of young, previously healthy homosexual men with new-onset profound immunologic deficits, *Pneumocystis carinii* (now *P. jirovecii*) pneumonia (PCP), and/or Kaposi's sarcoma. A retrovirus, human immunodeficiency virus type 1 (HIV-1), is the major cause of AIDS. A second retrovirus, HIV-2, also is recognized to cause AIDS, although it is less virulent, transmissible, and prevalent than HIV-1. These retroviruses are transmitted primarily by sexual contact and by contact with infected blood or blood products. Several risk behaviors for the acquisition of HIV infection have been identified in the United States, most notably the practice of anorectal intercourse and the sharing of blood-contaminated needles by injection-drug users. In many resource-limited countries, the majority of HIV transmission occurs via heterosexual intercourse and from childbearing women to their offspring. Initially, the medical management of HIV consisted of repeated treatments for opportunistic infections (OIs) and eventual palliative care. In the mid-1990s, a new era in the pharmacotherapy for HIV, known as *combination antiretroviral therapy* (ART), was born. ART consists of combinations of antiretroviral agents with different mechanisms of action that potently and durably suppress HIV replication, delay the onset of AIDS, reverse HIV-associated immunologic deficits, reduce HIV transmissions, and significantly prolong survival. Despite the effectiveness of ART, established HIV infection cannot be cured due in part to the integration of the HIV genome into host cells, creating a latent reservoir. Modern antiretroviral drugs and ART regimens have improved upon tolerability and efficacy. Nevertheless, therapeutic challenges remain in the ART era and include the need for continuous adherence to medication and care, drug–drug interactions, drug-resistant HIV, acute and long-term drug toxicities, and other complications associated with a prolonged life span. Despite progress in the treatment access for this disease, large numbers of

HIV-infected persons remain outside of care, nationally and globally. Significant efforts to develop an HIV vaccine have not been fruitful, but prophylactic use of antiretroviral drugs effectively prevents HIV infection in persons exposed to the virus.

EPIDEMIOLOGY

The epidemiologic characteristics of HIV infection differ according to geographic region and depend upon the mode of transmission, governmental prevention efforts and resources, and cultural factors.[1,2]

1 Infection with HIV occurs through three primary modes: sexual, parenteral, and perinatal. Sexual intercourse, primarily anal and vaginal intercourse, is the most common method for transmission. The probability of HIV transmission depends upon the type of sexual exposure. The highest risk appears to be from receptive anorectal intercourse at about 1.4 transmissions per 100 sexual acts.[3] Transmission risk is lower for receptive vaginal intercourse, and insertive sex acts have lower risk than receptive acts. Condom use reduces risk of transmission by approximately 80%.[3] Other factors that affect the probability of infection include the stage of HIV disease and viral load in the index partner. For example, transmission is significantly higher when the index partner has early or late HIV compared with asymptomatic HIV, as these disease stages are associated with higher viral loads.[3] Individuals with genital ulcers or sexually transmitted diseases are at greater risk for contracting HIV. HIV incidence and prevalence are lower in cultures that advocate male circumcision, which is estimated to reduce risk of male acquisition of HIV approximately 50%.[3] Casual contact with patients with AIDS or HIV infection is not a significant risk factor for HIV transmission.

Prevention of sexual transmission has focused primarily on education that encourages safer sex practices such as use of condoms and reduction of high-risk behavior (eg, intercourse or promiscuity with partners of unknown HIV status).[4] A powerful tool for HIV prevention is combination ART for the infected individual, as this dramatically lowers viral replication and infectiousness, significantly reducing the risk of transmission to others.[3,5] Another effective prevention tool is chemoprophylaxis with antiretroviral drugs, as this significantly reduces HIV acquisition risk among uninfected individuals.[6-8] A combined approach has been advocated for optimal prevention.[4] Prevention strategies under investigation include HIV vaccines and topical vaginal/rectal microbicides.[9,10]

Parenteral transmission of HIV broadly encompasses infections due to infected blood exposure from needle sticks, IV injection with used needles, receipt of blood products, and organ transplants. Use of contaminated needles or other injection-related paraphernalia by drug abusers has been the main cause of parenteral transmissions. The risk of HIV transmission from sharing needles is approximately 0.67 per 100 episodes.[3,11] Prevention strategies include stopping drug abuse, obtaining needles from credible sources (eg, pharmacies), never reusing any paraphernalia, using sterile procedures in all injecting activities, and safely disposing of used paraphernalia.[4]

Before widespread screening, HIV was readily transmitted in blood products.[11] However, blood and tissue products in the healthcare system are now rigorously screened for HIV. The estimated risk for receiving tainted blood or blood products in the United States is well below 1:1,000,000 and that for receiving a tainted tissue transplant is 1:55,000.[12,13] Healthcare workers have a small but definite occupational risk of contracting HIV through accidental exposure. Most cases of occupationally acquired HIV have been the result of a percutaneous needle stick injury, which carries an estimated 0.3% risk of transmitting HIV.[3,14] Mucocutaneous exposures (eg, tainted blood splash in eyes, mouth, nose) carries a transmission risk of approximately 0.09%.[14] Significant risk factors for seroconversion with a needle stick include deep injury, injury with a device visibly contaminated with blood, and advanced HIV disease in the index patient (high viral load). The risk of transmission from an HIV-infected healthcare worker to a patient is extremely remote. Comprehensive medical guidelines, including antiretroviral drug prophylaxis, have been developed to minimize the hazard of HIV transmission for healthcare workers and for persons exposed by rape or other means.[11,14]

Perinatal infection, or vertical transmission, is the most common cause of pediatric HIV infection. Most infections occur during or near to the time of birth, although a fraction can occur in utero.[2] The risk of mother-to-child transmission is approximately 25% in the absence of ART. Factors that increase the likelihood of vertical transmission include prolonged rupture of membranes, chorioamnionitis, genital infection during pregnancy, preterm delivery, vaginal delivery, birth weight less than 2.5 kg, illicit drug use and cigarette smoking during pregnancy, and high maternal viral load.[15] Breast-feeding also can transmit HIV. The estimated frequency of breast milk transmission is approximately 5% to 10% in the first 6 months and 15% to 20% through 18 to 24 months.[16] High levels of virus in breast milk and in the mother are associated with higher risk of transmission. Formula feeding prevents breast milk transmission of HIV but may not improve mortality from other causes early in life in resource limited settings.[16] In the United States, HIV-infected mothers are recommended not to breast-feed.[17] A separate and comprehensive set of medical guidelines including antiretroviral drug prophylaxis have been developed to minimize the hazard of mother-to-child HIV transmission.[17]

Persons with HIV infection are broadly categorized as those living with HIV and those with an AIDS diagnosis (stage 3). An AIDS diagnosis is made when the presence of HIV is laboratory-confirmed and the cluster of differentiation 4 (CD4; T-helper cell) count drops below 200 cells/mm^3 (200×10^6/L) for those older than or equal to 6 years of age, or after an AIDS indicator condition is diagnosed.[18] Further distinctions regarding the stage of HIV and AIDS (stage 3) are given in the Revised Centers for Disease Control and Prevention (CDC) surveillance case definition (Table 126-1).[18] In the United States, the CDC estimates HIV epidemiology using models that rely on surveillance data from state and local health departments.[19] Using these models, the CDC estimates that about 1.2 million individuals are currently living with HIV (all stages) in the United States and that approximately 659,000 have died from complications of HIV infection.[19,20] Importantly, approximately 15% of persons with HIV are unaware of their infection and only approximately 45% of those who are aware of their infection are retained in care. Therefore, a majority of HIV-infected persons (~60%) are not receiving ART regularly, which significantly contributes to the ongoing transmission of HIV infection in the United States, totaling approximately 50,000 new infections per annum.[20,21]

The epidemic in the United States initially was established in men who have sex with men (MSM), and this population continues to be prominently affected by HIV, accounting for approximately 65% of new cases.[20] Heterosexual transmissions accounted for approximately 25% of new cases and approximately 75% of these are women. Injection drug use make up about 10% of new cases. For women, the main risk factor for transmission is heterosexual intercourse (~84% of cases) and injection-drug use (~16% of cases). For men the main risks are MSM (~78%), heterosexual sex (~10%), and injection-drug use (~10%).[20] African Americans and Hispanics are disproportionately affected by HIV infection. Of new infections in recent years, 44% were African American and 21% were Hispanic although these populations only make up 12% and 17% of the US population respectively. A relatively large proportion of these populations are not well linked to appropriate prevention, care, and treatment services, which represents a significant public health challenge.[19]

TABLE 126-1 Surveillance Case Definition for HIV Infection Stage Based on CD4+ T-lymphocyte Counts, United States, 2014

	Age on date of CD4+ T-lymphocyte test					
	<1 year		1-5 years		≥6 years	
Stage	Cells/μL (×10⁶/L)	%	Cells/μL (×10⁶/L)	%	Cells/μL (×10⁶/L)	%
1	≥1,500	≥34	≥1,000	≥30	≥500	≥26
2	750-1,499	26-33	500-999	22-29	200-499	14-25
3 (AIDS)	<750	<26	<500	<22	<200	<14

AIDS Indicator Conditions

Bacterial infections, multiple or recurrent (specific to children <6 years)	
Candidiasis of bronchi, trachea, or lungs	Lymphoma, Burkitt
Candidiasis, esophageal	Lymphoma, immunoblastic
Cervical cancer, invasive (specific to adults, adolescents, children >6 years)	Lymphoma, primary, or brain
Coccidioidomycosis, disseminated or extrapulmonary	*Mycobacterium avium* complex or *Mycobacterium kansasii*, disseminated or extrapulmonary
Cryptococcosis, extrapulmonary	*Mycobacterium tuberculosis*, any site (pulmonary or extrapulmonary)
Cryptosporidiosis, chronic intestinal (duration >1 month)	*Mycobacterium*, other species or unidentified species, disseminated or extrapulmonary
Cytomegalovirus disease (other than liver, spleen, or nodes), onset at age > 1 month	*Pneumocystis jirovecii* pneumonia (PCP)
Cytomegalovirus retinitis (with loss of vision)	Pneumonia, recurrent (specific to adults, adolescents, children >6 years)
Encephalopathy, HIV-related	Progressive multifocal leukoencephalopathy
Herpes simplex: chronic ulcer(s) (duration >1 month); or bronchitis, pneumonitis, or esophagitis, onset at age > 1 month	*Salmonella* septicemia, recurrent Toxoplasmosis of brain, onset at age >1 month Wasting syndrome due to HIV
Histoplasmosis, disseminated or extrapulmonary Isosporiasis, chronic intestinal (duration >1 month) Kaposi's sarcoma	

Data from reference 18.

The number of individuals living with HIV/AIDS globally has risen to approximately 35 million persons.[1,2] Recent increases are due to a longer lifespan due to wider implementation of ART worldwide. This has reduced the death rate and new infection rate in recent years. For example, the peak number of new infections was 3.3 million per year in 2002 and this has declined to 2.3 million in 2012. New infections in children (mostly due to mother to child transmission) have declined by 38% between 2009 and 2012, and overall deaths have declined by approximately 30% since 2005. Nevertheless, approximately 1.6 million people succumbed to HIV/AIDS in 2012 and HIV/AIDS is still a major contributor to the global burden of disease.[22] The highest concentration of HIV/AIDS cases in the world is in sub-Saharan Africa, where approximately 25 million people are infected. However, new infections have declined there by approximately 38% since 2000 (albeit with regional differences).[1] Heterosexual transmission is the most common mode of transmission in sub-Saharan Africa and worldwide (~80% of cases). Women in sub-Saharan Africa and resource-limited countries are at disproportionately high risk for acquiring HIV because of biological and cultural factors that foster HIV transmission, such as limited ability to refuse sex.[23] Other important epidemiologic features of the HIV epidemic include growing incidence among injection drug users in North Africa and the Middle East, as well as some regions of Eastern Europe and Central Asia (eg, Russia and Ukraine).[1]

ETIOLOGY

HIV is an enveloped single-stranded RNA virus and a member of the Lentivirinae (*lenti*, meaning "slow") subfamily of retroviruses. Lentiviruses are characterized by their indolent infectious cycle. There are two related but distinct types of HIV: HIV-1 and HIV-2. HIV-2, found mostly in western Africa, consists of seven phylogenetic lineages designated as subtypes (clades) A through G. Four groups of HIV-1 are recognized: M (main or major), N (non-M, non-O), and O (outlier) and P (pending the identification of further cases).[2] The nine subtypes of HIV-1 group M are identified as A through D, F through H, and J and K. Mixtures of subtypes are referred to as *circulating recombinant forms.* Group M, subtype B, is primarily responsible for the epidemic in North America and western Europe.[24]

The accumulated evidence suggests that HIV in humans was the result of a cross-species transmission (zoonosis) from primates infected with simian immunodeficiency virus (SIV).[24] Phylogenetic and geographic relationships suggest that HIV-2 arose from SIV that infects sooty mangabeys and HIV-1 group M and N arose from SIVcpz, a virus that infects chimpanzees (*Pan troglodytes troglodytes*). Groups O and P may have arisen from a SIV variant that infects wild gorillas. Cultural practices, such as preparation and eating of bush meat or keeping animals as pets, may have allowed the virus to cross from primates to humans. The earliest known human infection with HIV has been traced to central Africa in 1959, but cross-species transmissions probably date back to the early 1900s.[24] Modern transportation, promiscuity, and drug abuse have caused the rapid spread of the virus within the United States and throughout the world. This chapter focuses on HIV-1 group M, which is the predominant strain likely to be encountered in the western world.

PATHOGENESIS

2 Understanding the life cycle of HIV (Fig. 126-1) is necessary because the current strategies used for treatment of HIV target points in this cycle. Once HIV enters the human body, the outer glycoprotein (gp160) on its surface, which is composed of two subunits (gp120 and gp41), has affinity for CD4 receptors, proteins present on the surface of T-helper lymphocytes, monocytes, macrophages, dendritic cells, and brain microglia. The gp120 subunit is responsible for CD4 binding. Once initial binding occurs, the intimate association of HIV with the cell is enhanced by further binding to chemokine coreceptors. The two major chemokine receptors used

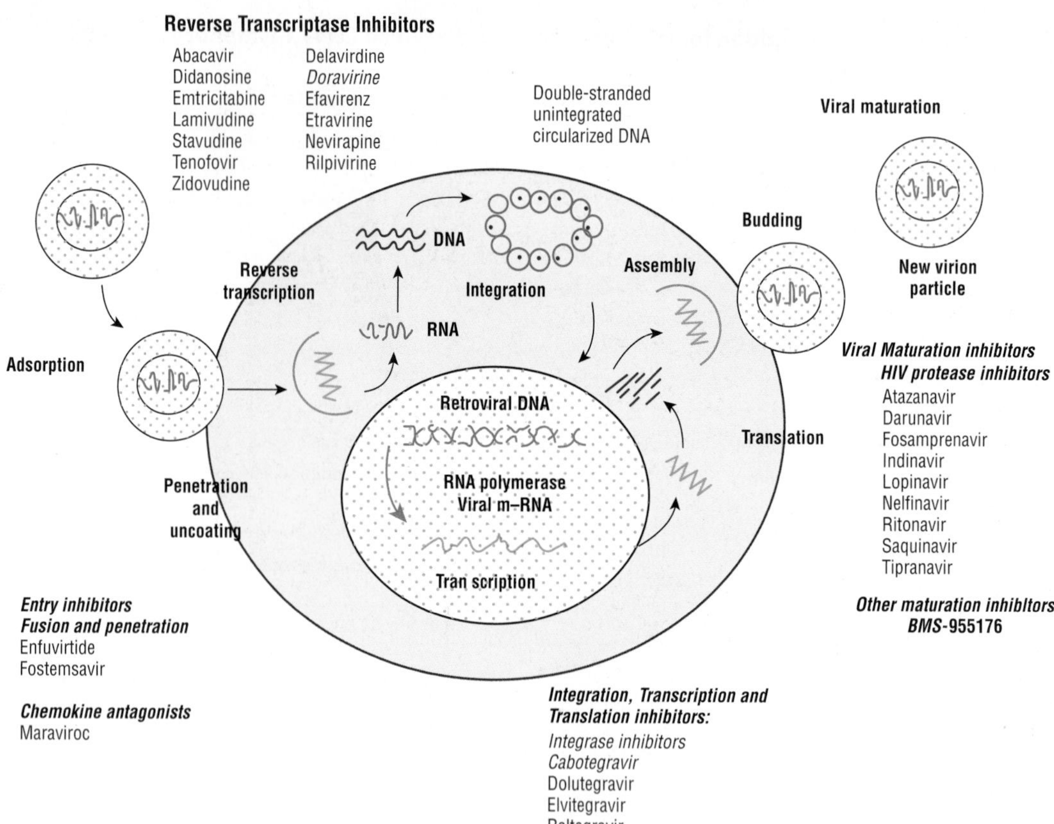

FIGURE 126-1 Life cycle of human immunodeficiency virus with potential targets where replication may be interrupted. Italicized compounds were in development at the time of this writing. *(Reprinted with permission, Courtney V. Fletcher, 2015.)*

by HIV are Chemokine (C–C motif) receptor 5 (CCR5) and chemokine (C-X-C motif) receptor 4 (CXCR4). HIV isolates may contain a mixture of viruses that target one or the other of these coreceptors, and some viral strains may be dual-tropic (ie, can use both coreceptors). The HIV strain that preferentially uses CCR5, R5 viruses, is macrophage-tropic and typically implicated in most cases of sexually transmitted HIV.[25] Individuals with a common 32-base-pair deletion in the CCR5 gene are protected from progression of HIV disease, and those who are homozygous for the 32-base-pair deletion have a degree of resistance to acquisition of HIV-1.[26] The HIV strain that targets CXCR4, designated X4 virus, is T-cell–tropic and often is predominant in the later stage of disease. CD4 and coreceptor attachment of HIV to the cell promotes membrane fusion, which is mediated by gp41, and finally internalization of the viral genetic material and enzymes necessary for replication.

After internalization, the viral protein shell surrounding the nucleic acid (capsid) is uncoated in preparation for replication.[27] The genetic material of HIV is positive-sense single-stranded RNA; the virus must transcribe this RNA into DNA (transcription normally occurs from DNA to RNA; HIV works backward, hence the name *retrovirus*). To do so, HIV is equipped with the unique enzyme RNA-dependent DNA polymerase (reverse transcriptase). HIV reverse transcriptase first synthesizes a complementary strand of DNA using the viral RNA as a template. The RNA portion of this DNA–RNA hybrid is then partially removed by ribonuclease H (RNase H), allowing HIV reverse transcriptase to complete the synthesis of a double-stranded DNA molecule. The fidelity of HIV reverse transcriptase is poor, and many mistakes are made during the process. These errors in the final DNA product contribute to the rapid mutation of the virus, which enables the virus to evade the immune response (thus complicating vaccine development), and promotes the evolution of drug resistance during partially suppressive therapy. Following reverse transcription, the final double-stranded DNA product migrates into the nucleus and is integrated into the host cell chromosome by integrase, another enzyme unique to HIV.

The integration of HIV into the host chromosome is critically important. Most notably, HIV can establish a persistent, latent infection, particularly in long-lived cells of the immune system such as memory T lymphocytes. The virus is effectively hidden in these cells, and this characteristic has greatly complicated efforts to cure HIV infection.[28] It also necessitates continuous ART therapy because virus reemerges from this reservoir if therapy is suspended.

After integration, HIV preferentially replicates in activated cells. Activation by antigens, cytokines, or other factors stimulates the cell to produce nuclear factor kappa B (NF-κB), an enhancer-binding protein. NF-κB normally regulates the expression of T-lymphocyte genes involved in growth but also can inadvertently activate replication of HIV.[29] HIV encodes six regulatory and accessory proteins: Tat, Nef, Rev, Vpu, Vif, and Vpr, which enhance replication and inhibit innate immunity. For example, the Tat protein is a potent amplifier of HIV gene expression; it binds to a specific RNA sequence of HIV that initiates and stabilizes transcription elongation.[29] Vif is a viral protein that binds human ABOBEC 3G, a cytidine deaminase that disrupts the virus' genetic code by converting viral RNA cytosine to uracil thereby providing innate cellular immunity.[30] Vpu inhibits tetherin, a human cellular membrane protein that prevents release of virus particles after budding from infected cells. Assembly of new viral particles occurs in a stepwise manner beginning with the coalescence of HIV proteins beneath the host cell lipid bilayer. The nucleocapsid subsequently is formed with viral single-stranded RNA and other components packaged inside. Once packaged, the virion then buds through the plasma membrane, acquiring the characteristics of the host lipid bilayer. After the virus buds, the maturation process begins. Within the virion, protease, another enzyme unique to HIV, cleaves a large precursor polypeptide (gag-pol) into functional proteins that are necessary to produce a complete and infectious virus. Without this enzyme, the virion is immature and unable to infect other cells.

The natural history of HIV infection exhibits three general phases: acute, chronic, and terminal (AIDS). Initial rounds of HIV replication during acute infection take place largely in the mucosal CD4+ CCR5+ T cell pools in the gut resulting in a massive CD4 T-cell depletion in these tissues.[31] Cells are destroyed by various mechanisms, including cell lysis from newly budding virions, cytotoxic T-lymphocyte–induced cell killing, and induction of apoptosis. Following this destruction of the mucosal CD4 T cell pool, which lasts for 2 to 3 weeks, a state of heightened immune activation ensues during the chronic infection phase, which can last for several years. The activated state is characterized by high levels of activation markers on circulating T cells (eg HLA-DR and CD38) and proinflammatory cytokines, and may result from HIV antigen as well as translocation of microbial antigens from the T-cell depleted gut mucosa. Heightened activation enables further HIV replication and ultimately leads to continued depletion of CD4+ CCR5+ T cells. HIV-1 exhibits a very high turnover rate during this chronic phase, with an estimated 10 billion new viruses produced each day.[32] More than 99% of these viruses are produced in newly infected activated cells. Nevertheless, for much of the chronic phase, the immune system is able to operate well enough to prevent overt OIs that herald AIDS. But eventually, the depletion of CD4 cells and the continuous cellular activation leads to a final collapse of the immune system, or AIDS. HIV may use CXCR4 coreceptor during this last phase of infection and these viruses infect a broader range of CD4 cells (naïve and central-memory) speeding the disease progression. It is this unrelenting destruction of CD4 cells that causes the profoundly compromised immune system and AIDS.

DIAGNOSIS AND CLINICAL PRESENTATION

Detection of HIV and Surrogate Markers of Disease Progression

HIV is diagnosed through a multi-step process.[33] The presence of HIV infection is screened with an enzyme-linked immunosorbent assay (ELISA), which detects antibodies against HIV-1. Although ELISA has been the mainstay of HIV screening for decades, the technology has been evolving to detect infection earlier in the time course of the disease.[34] Older ELISA tests detected IgG (2nd generation tests) but more modern tests detect IgG and IgM (3rd generation tests) and may further include detection of p24 antigen, an early marker of infection (4th generation tests). These technological advances enable earlier detection of HIV by as much as 15 to 20 days compared with older 2nd generation tests. ELISA tests are generally highly sensitive (less than 99%) and highly specific (greater than 99%), but rare false-positive results can occur particularly in those with autoimmune disorders.[33] False-negative results also occur and may be attributed to the "window-period" before adequate production of antibodies or antigen. This "window period" between HIV acquisition and detection of HIV with 4th and 3rd generation tests is approximately two and three weeks, respectively.[33] Positive screening tests are confirmed with another enzyme immunoassay to specify if the antibodies are to HIV-1 versus HIV-2. (Although HIV-2 is rare in the US, this step ensures proper diagnosis and treatment). If this follow up assay is indeterminant or negative, an HIV nucleic acid test is performed for definitive diagnosis. HIV-RNA is the earliest indicator of infection, detectable ~10 days from acquisition and about one week before 4th generation tests.[34] Several point-of-care screening kits are available for serum, plasma, whole blood, or oral fluids. While oral fluid tests are convenient, they are not as sensitive as blood assays, which may result in false negatives early in infections; this is a particular disadvantage in the setting of HIV testing prior to initiating or continuing preexposure prophylaxis (PrEP).[34]

HIV testing is recommended when HIV infection is suspected because of symptoms and/or high-risk behavior.[35,36] Additionally, the CDC now recommends routine HIV screening in all healthcare settings in persons 13 to 64 years, a policy called "opt-out" testing.[37] A focus of the recommendations is to screen persons at high risk of HIV infection (eg, MSM) at least annually and to screen pregnant women while they are in care. The policy states that consent for medical care will imply consent for HIV testing; however, the person must be informed of the test and can opt out of taking it. Because states may have different HIV consent laws, the local requirements for HIV testing should be consulted. The rationale for the opt-out strategy is to diagnose those who unknowingly carry HIV so as to initiate ART early leading to improved prognosis and reduced forward transmissions.

Once diagnosed, HIV disease is monitored primarily by two surrogate biomarkers, viral load and CD4 cell count.[38] The viral load test quantifies the degree of viremia by measuring the number of copies of viral RNA (HIV RNA) in the plasma. Methods for determining HIV RNA include reverse-transcription polymerase chain reaction (RT-PCR), branched-chain DNA, transcription-mediated amplification, and nucleic acid sequence-based assay. RT-PCR is used more widely than the other techniques.[34] Irrespective of the method used, viral load is reported as the number of viral RNA copies per milliliter of plasma. Each assay has its own lower limit of quantitation, and results can vary from one assay method to the other; therefore, it is recommended that the same assay method be used consistently for each patient. Reductions in viral load often are reported in base 10 logarithm. For example, if a patient presents initially with a viral load of 100,000 copies/mL (10^5 copies/mL or 10^8 copies/L) and subsequently has a viral load of 10,000 copies/mL (10^4 copies/mL or 10^7 copies/L), the decrease is 1 $\log_{10}$. Given that HIV RNA varies within a patient, a perceptible clinical response is generally considered when the decline in viral load is more than 0.5 $\log_{10}$.[38] Viral load is a major prognostic factor for disease progression, CD4 count decline, and death.[38,39] It is also the predominant way to assess the effectiveness of treatment.

Because HIV attacks and leads to the destruction of cells bearing the CD4 receptor, the number of CD4 lymphocytes (T-helper cells) in the blood is a critical surrogate marker of disease progression and immune system status.[38] The normal adult CD4 lymphocyte count ranges from 500 to 1,600 cells/mm^3 (500×10^6-$1{,}600 \times 10^6$/L), or 40% to 70% of total lymphocytes. CD4 counts in children are age dependent, with younger children having higher CD4 counts (see Table 126-1). The hallmark of HIV disease is depletion of CD4 cells and the associated development of OIs and malignancies especially at lower CD4 cell counts.

Clinical Presentation

3 Clinical presentation of primary HIV infection varies, but most patients (50%-90%) have an acute retroviral syndrome or mononucleosis-like illness, presumably due to the host immune response to the virus (ie, "cytokine storm") (Table 126-2).[40] Although many of these symptoms are nonspecific, the presence of aseptic meningitis, oral or genital ulcers, rash, and leukopenia should raise suspicion of acute HIV infection in the setting of a potential exposure. Symptoms often last 2 weeks, and hospitalization may be required for a small fraction of patients. Primary infection is associated with a high viral load (more than 10^6 copies/mL [more than 10^9/L]) and a precipitous drop in CD4 cells. After several weeks an immune response is mounted, the amount of HIV RNA in plasma falls substantially, CD4 cells rebound slightly, and symptoms resolve gradually. However, as described above, this clinically latent period is not virologically latent because HIV replication is continuous (~10 billion viruses per day) and immune system

TABLE 126-2 Clinical Presentation of Primary Human Immunodeficiency Virus Infection in Adults

Signs and Symptoms
Most common: Fever, headache, sore throat, fatigue, GI upset (diarrhea, nausea, vomiting) weight loss, myalgia, morbilliform or maculopapular rash usually involving the trunk, lymphadenopathy, night sweats
Less common: Aseptic meningitis, oral ulcers, leukopenia
Other
High viral load (may exceed 1,000,000 copies per milliliter or 10^9/L)
Persistent decrease in CD4 lymphocytes

Data from reference 40.

destruction is ongoing. A steady decrease in CD4 cells (approximately 50 cells/μL [50×10^6/L] per year) is the most measurable aspect of this immune system deterioration during the asymptomatic phase. Plasma viral load, on the other hand, will appear to have stabilized at a particular level or "set point." The set point correlates strongly with the CD4 cell decline and time to AIDS and morbidity. For example, prior to ART, the Multicenter AIDS Cohort Study measured viral load in 1,604 HIV-positive men and followed them for as long as 11 years. The CD4 cell count decline was approximately twice as fast in those with HIV-RNA above 30,000 copies/mL ($30,000 \times 10^3$/L) compared with those with HIV-RNA less than or equal to 500 copies/mL (less than or equal to 500×10^3/L) and mortality rates (within 6 years) were 69.5% versus 0.9%, respectively.[39] Thus, a higher viral set point is associated with faster disease progression and poorer prognosis. Not all individuals infected with HIV progress to AIDS—these so-called "long-term nonprogressors" may be infected with a defective virus (eg, nef-deficient HIV) or may have an intrinsic ability to resist infection (eg, CCR5 mutation).

Most children born with HIV are asymptomatic. On physical examination, children often present with nonspecific signs, such as lymphadenopathy, hepatomegaly, splenomegaly, failure to thrive, weight loss or unexplained low birth weight (in prenatally exposed infants), and fever of unknown origin.[41] Laboratory findings include anemia, hypergammaglobulinemia (primarily immunoglobulin [Ig]A and IgM), altered mononuclear cell function, and altered T-cell subset ratios. Of note, the normal range for CD4 cell counts in young children is much different from the range in adults (Table 126-1). Children have different susceptibility and/or exposures to OIs compared with adults. Bacterial infections, including *Streptococcus pneumoniae*, *Salmonella* spp., and *Mycobacterium tuberculosis*, may be more prevalent in children with AIDS than in adults with the disease. Kaposi's sarcoma is rare in children. Children with HIV infection may develop lymphocytic interstitial pneumonitis without evidence of *P. jirovecii* or other pathogens on lung biopsy. Some children (~25%) will progress to AIDS rapidly within the first year of life. A presentation of serious OIs such as *P. jirovecii* pneumonia, encephalopathy, failure to thrive, and a precipitous drop in CD4 cells are common in these infants. General management of the HIV-infected child involves principles similar to those used for the adult: ART, treatment and prophylaxis of OIs, and supportive care.[42,43]

TREATMENT

Desired Outcomes

4 The central goals of ART are to decrease morbidity and mortality, improve quality of life, restore and preserve immune function, and prevent further transmission.[38] The most important and effective way to achieve these goals is maximal and durable suppression of HIV replication, which is interpreted as plasma HIV RNA less than the lower limit of quantitation (ie, undetectable; usually less than 50 copies/mL [less than 50×10^3/L]). Such a profound reduction in HIV RNA is associated with reduced transmissions and long-term response to therapy (ie, durability), as well as increases in CD4 lymphocytes that closely correlates with a reduced risk for developing OIs. While undetectable HIV RNA almost always corresponds with a rise in CD4 lymphocytes, some patients respond virologically or immunologically without the other.

General Approach to Treatment

5 Combinations of three active antiretroviral agents from two pharmacologic classes profoundly inhibit HIV replication to undetectable plasma levels, prevent and reverse immune deficiency, and substantially decrease morbidity and mortality—constituting the ART era.[44] Principles that serve as a guide for the clinical use of antiretroviral agents are still relevant today[45]:

1. Ongoing HIV replication leads to immune system damage and progression to AIDS. HIV infection is always harmful, and true long-term survival free of clinically significant immune dysfunction is unusual.
2. Plasma HIV RNA levels indicate the magnitude of HIV replication and its associated rate of CD4 cell destruction, whereas CD4 cell counts indicate the extent of HIV-induced immune damage already suffered.
3. Use of potent combination ART to suppress HIV replication to below the levels of detection of sensitive plasma HIV RNA assays limits the potential for selection of antiretroviral-resistant HIV variants, the major factor limiting the ability of antiretroviral drugs to inhibit virus replication and delay disease progression. Therefore, maximum achievable suppression of HIV replication should be the goal of therapy.
4. The most effective means for accomplishing durable suppression of HIV replication is simultaneous initiation of combinations of effective anti-HIV drugs with which the patient has not been treated previously and that are not cross-resistant with antiretroviral agents with which the patient has been treated previously.
5. Each of the antiretroviral drugs used in combination therapy regimens always should be used according to optimal schedules and dosages.
6. The available effective antiretroviral drugs are limited in number and mechanism of action, and cross-resistance between specific drugs has been documented. Therefore, any change in ART increases future therapeutic constraints.
7. Women should receive optimal ART regardless of pregnancy status.
8. The same principles of ART apply to both HIV-infected children and adults, although treatment of HIV-infected children involves unique pharmacologic, virologic, and immunologic considerations.
9. Persons with acute primary HIV infections should be treated with combination ART to suppress virus replication to levels below the limit of detection of sensitive plasma HIV RNA assays.

The extent to which these principles will continue to stand the test of time is unknown; new information on the pathogenesis and treatment of HIV accrues constantly. As of December 2015, 29 antiretroviral compounds have been approved by the FDA; two (amprenavir and zalcitabine) have since been removed from the market. Table 126-3 presents the state of the art for treatment of HIV-infected individuals as of December 2015.[38] Treatment is recommended for all HIV-infected persons regardless of CD4 lymphocyte

TABLE 126-3 Treatment of Human Immunodeficiency Virus Infection: Antiretroviral Regimens Recommended in Antiretroviral-Naïve Persons

	Preferred Regimens	Selected Limitations
HIV PI-based	Darunavir + ritonavir + tenofovir disoproxil fumarate + emtricitabine (AI)	Rash (darunavir has sulfonamide moiety); GI; food requirement; CYP3A4 drug interactions
InSTI-based	Raltegravir + tenofovir disoproxil fumarate + emtricitabine (AI)	Twice daily (not once daily); interactions with polyvalent antacids; creatine kinase increases
	Elvitegravir + cobicistat + tenofovir disoproxil fumarate + emtricitabine (co-formulated) (AI)	Only if CLcr ≥70 mL/min (≥1.17 mL/s); food requirement; interactions with polyvalent antacids; CYP3A4 drug interactions; cobicistat inhibits creatinine secretion increasing Scr - distinguish vs renal dysfunction
	Elvitegravir + cobicistat + tenofovir alafenamide fumarate + emtricitabine (co-formulated) (AI)	Only if CLcr ≥30 mL/min (≥0.5 mL/s); same as above
	Dolutegravir + abacavir + lamivudine (co-formulated) (AI)	Only if HLA-B5701 negative; interactions with polyvalent antacids; dolutegravir inhibits creatinine secretion increasing Scr - distinguish vs renal dysfunction
	Dolutegravir + tenofovir disoproxil fumarate + emtricitabine (AI)	Same as above without HLA-B5701 negative requirement
Selected alternative Regimens (Some Potential Disadvantages vs Preferred Regimens)		
NNRTI-based	Efavirenz + tenofovir disoproxil fumarate + emtricitabine (co-formulated) (BI)	CNS side effects with efavirenz; CYP450 drug interactions; empty stomach dosing; teratogenic in non human primates - avoid in women planning to conceive
	Rilpivirine + tenofovir disoproxil fumarate + emtricitabine (co-formulated) (BI)	Not recommended when HIV-RNA >100,000 copies/mL (>100,000 × 10^3/L) or CD4 <200 cells/μL (<200 × 10^6/L); no proton-pump inhibitors (rilpivirine); food requirement; antacid interactions
HIV PI-based	Atazanavir + ritonavir (or cobicistat) + tenofovir disoproxil fumarate + emtricitabine (BI)	GI; food requirement; CYP3A4 drug interactions; hyperbilirubinemia leading to drug discontinuation especially in those with Gilbert's; only for CLcr ≥ 70 mL/min (≥1.17 mL/s) as cobicistat inhibits creatinine secretion increasing Scr - distinguish vs renal dysfunction
	Darunavir + ritonavir (or cobicistat) + abacavir + lamivudine (BII for ritonavir and BIII for cobicistat)	Only if HLA-B5701 negative; see issues above
	Darunavir + cobicistat + tenofovir disoproxil fumarate + emtricitabine (BII)	Only for CLcr ≥70 mL/min (≥1.17 mL/s) as cobicistat inhibits creatinine secretion increasing Scr - distinguish vs renal dysfunction; see issues above
Selected Regimens or Components that should not be used at any time		
Regimen or component		**Comment**
Any all NRTI regimen (AIBII)		Inferior virologic efficacy
Didanosine + tenofovir (AII)		Inferior virologic efficacy, CD4 declines
Didanosine + Stavudine (AII)		Toxicity including subcutaneous fat loss, peripheral neuropathy, and lactic acidosis
2 NNRTI combinations (AI)		Higher adverse events, drug interactins
Emtricitabine + lamivudine or zidovudine + stavudine (AIIAIII)		Analogs of same nucleobase, No additive benefit (or antagonistic)
Unboosted PIs (ie, darunavir, saquinavir, tipranavir) (AII)		Inadequate bioavailability
Etravirine + selected boosted PIs (AII)		Possible induction of PI metabolism, doses not established
Nevirapine in ARV naïve with higher CD4 counts (>250 for women, >400 for men) (BI)		High incidence of symptomatic hepatotoxicity

Evidence-based rating definition.

Rating strength of recommendation:

A: Strong recommendation.

B: Moderate recommendation.

C: Optional recommendation.

Rating Quality of Evidence Supporting the Recommendation:

I: Evidence from at least one correctly randomized, controlled trial with clinical outcomes and/or validated laboratory endpoints.

II: Evidence from at least one well-designed clinical trial without randomization or observational cohorts with long-term clinical outcomes.

III: Expert opinion.

Lamivudine and emtricitabine are considered interchangeable.

Data from reference 38.

count, as long as the patient is ready to adhere to therapy. Urgent indications for therapy include pregnancy, history of AIDS-defining illness, rapidly declining CD4 counts, HIV-associated nephropathy, or HIV/hepatitis B virus coinfection.

The optimal time to initiate therapy in chronic HIV infection has been a matter of debate for decades. The main arguments for postponing therapy were the concern for cumulative drug toxicity and trepidation for drug resistance and loss of therapeutic options. These concerns were well-founded when older drugs such as lopinavir/ritonavir, stavudine, zidovudine, indinavir, and efavirenz were the mainstay of therapy. Today, the availability of newer medications with different mechanisms of action (eg, InSTI and attachment inhibitors) and significantly improved adverse event profiles helps mitigate these issues.

An additional issue, until recently, was the lack of high-quality evidence of clinical benefits for initiating therapy at higher versus lower CD4 counts (eg, 500 cells/μL [500 × 10^6/L] vs 350 cells/μL [350 × 10^6/L]). This issue was addressed in 2015 with results from two large randomized controlled trials.[46,47] The START trial randomized 4,685 patients with CD4 counts above 500 cells/μL (500 × 10^6/L) to either immediate ART or to delayed ART until the CD4 count reached 350 cells/μL (350 × 10^6/L). Immediate ART resulted in significantly fewer serious AIDS events (HR 0.28, 95% CI 0.15-0.50), and non-AIDS events (HR 0.61, 0.38-0.97) as compared with delaying ART. The TEMPRANO study was conducted in the Ivory Coast where HIV and tuberculosis (TB) co-infection is endemic. The trial randomized 2,056 patients with less than or equal to 800 CD4 cells/μL (less than or equal to 800 × 10^6/L) to immediate ART, immediate ART with isoniazid TB prophylaxis, delayed ART (based upon WHO guidelines), or delayed ART with isoniazid TB prophylaxis. Again, immediate ART resulted in fewer deaths or severe HIV-related illnesses as compared with deferred ART (HR among patients with a baseline CD4 greater than or equal to 500 cells/μL [greater than or equal to 500 × 10^6/L], 0.56; 95% CI, 0.33-0.94). In addition to these important studies, immediate ART is also known to prevent ongoing HIV transmissions by as much as 96% compared with delayed ART.[5] Taken together, these studies provide high-quality evidence that untreated HIV is harmful even at high CD4 counts and immediate ART confers individual- and population-level benefit compared with delayed ART. Major policy-makers now recommend immediate ART regardless of CD4 count, including the WHO and US Department of Health and Human Services.[38,48] An excellent source for information on updated treatment guidelines *www.AIDSinfo.NIH.gov*. Additional guidelines and electronic resources for HIV clinicians are provided in reference 36.[36] Healthcare professionals involved in the care of HIV-infected persons are urged to consult the most current literature on the principles and strategies for ART therapy.

Pharmacologic Therapy

Several methods of therapeutic intervention have been evaluated against HIV including systemic antiretroviral drugs (the focus of this chapter) for direct inhibition of chronic viral replication or prevention of HIV acquisition; vaccination; immunomodulators to help stimulate and restore the immune system; and topical antiretroviral drugs or virucides (chemicals that destroy intact viruses) to prevent HIV infection. The latter three approaches are investigational at this time. Several approaches for an HIV vaccine are in development, including whole killed virus, subunit and peptide vaccination, recombinant live vector, and naked DNA delivery. Historically, vaccine progress has been slow. Genetic variability in HIV and a nascent understanding of the role of the immune system in suppressing viral replication are significant barriers to the development of an effective HIV vaccine with long-lasting and protective immunity. In the past few years, a randomized placebo-controlled trial demonstrated a modest 30% reduction in HIV transmission in a modified-intention to treat analysis of ALVAC-HIV plus AIDSVAX vaccine in 16,402 volunteers.[49] Efforts are now underway to understand the correlates of protection from this study to inform the vaccine field going forward.[50] Immunomodulators, such as aldesleukin (interleukin-2), provide mild benefits in terms of increased CD4 cells; however, aldesleukin is also associated with significant toxicities and no apparent clinical benefit.[51] Thus, the future is uncertain for immunomodulatory approaches. Topical virucidal or antiretroviral drug formulations for use vaginally or rectally to prevent sexual transmission of HIV are in various phases of development.[9] For example, vaginal application of tenofovir 1% gel before and after intercourse reduced HIV acquisition by 39% in women.[52] However, daily tenofovir 1% gel administered vaginally did not reduce HIV acquisition, an outcome that was driven by poor adherence.[53] Microbicide research is now focusing on long-acting formulations (eg, rings and intra-uterine devices) to mitigate adherence challenges.

Antiretroviral Agents Systemic delivery of antiretroviral agents for direct inhibition of viral replication has been the most clinically successful strategy for both treatment and prophylaxis. Four general classes of drugs are used today: entry inhibitors, reverse transcriptase inhibitors, InSTIs, and HIV PIs (Table 126-4).[38] As a rule, newer agents exhibit significant advantages over first generation drugs in terms of pharmacokinetics, tolerability, safety, and efficacy. This section will highlight specific advantages of newer agents over first generation drugs and will focus the discussion on newer agents used most often today. Updated drug information is available in the Department of Health and Human Services Guidelines including common adverse events and dosing recommendations for hepatic and renal insufficiency for all antiretroviral drugs.[38]

Reverse transcriptase inhibitors consist of two classes: those that are chemical derivatives of purine- and pyrimidine-based nucleosides and nucleotides (nucleoside/nucleotide reverse transcriptase inhibitors [NRTIs]) and those that are not (nonnucleoside reverse transcriptase inhibitors [NNRTIs]). NRTIs include the thymidine analogs stavudine (d4T) and zidovudine (AZT or ZDV); the deoxycytidine analogs emtricitabine (FTC) and lamivudine (3TC); the deoxyguanosine analog abacavir sulfate (ABC); and the deoxyadenosine analogs of which didanosine (ddI) is an inosine derivative and tenofovir is a deoxyadenosine-monophosphate nucleotide analog (a nucleotide is a nucleoside with one or more phosphates). **Note that drug abbreviations are provided here and below for reference, but their use is discouraged because they may lead to prescribing or administration errors.** Tenofovir comes in two prodrug formulations, tenofovir disoproxil fumarate (TDF) and tenofovir alafenamide (TAF). Tenofovir disoproxil fumarate is an ester pro drug that releases tenofovir upon first pass metabolism, producing relatively high systemic concentrations of tenofovir, which confers some risk (usually mild) of proximal tubulopathy and bone de-mineralization. On the other hand, for tenofovir alafenamide, more of the intact pro-drug reaches the systemic circulation and the pro-drug releases tenofovir within lymphoid cells via cathepsin A or hepatic cells via carboxylesterase 1. This strategy results in higher intracellular concentrations, but lower systemic tenofovir concentrations and less change in markers of proximal tubulopathy and bone de-mineralization.[54]

As a class, the NRTIs require phosphorylation to the 5′-triphosphate moiety to become pharmacologically active. Intracellular phosphorylation occurs by cytoplasmic or mitochondrial kinases and phosphotransferases (not viral kinases). The 5′-triphosphate moiety acts in two ways: (a) it competes with endogenous deoxyribonucleotides for the catalytic site of reverse transcriptase, and (b) it prematurely terminates DNA elongation, if taken up and incorporated, as it lacks the requisite 3′-hydroxyl for sugar-phosphate linking. NRTIs are active against both HIV-1 and HIV-2.[38] Emtricitabine, lamivudine, and tenofovir are also active against hepatitis B virus, and a combination of these agents should be used when possible in HIV–hepatitis B coinfected patients.

Although NRTI triphosphates (or diphosphate for tenofovir) are specific for HIV reverse transcriptase, their adverse effects may be caused in part by inhibition of mitochondrial DNA or RNA synthesis.[55] It is largely this problem that differentiates the first-generation drugs (didanosine, stavudine, and zidovudine) from the agents used most often at this time (tenofovir disoproxil fumarate, tenofovir alafenamide, emtricitabine, lamivudine, abacavir).[38,56] The mitochondrial toxicities include peripheral neuropathy, pancreatitis, lipoatrophy (subcutaneous fat loss), myopathy, anemia, and rarely life-threatening lactic acidosis with fatty liver. The newer agents exhibit less potential to cause these toxicities, but they still have their own adverse event profiles to be considered (see Table 126-4).[38]

The newer NRTI are eliminated by the kidney and dose adjustments are required for renal insufficiency, whereas abacavir is metabolized in the liver and it should not be used in advanced hepatic impairment. Resistance has been reported for all NRTIs, including cross-resistance within the class as multiple and/or specific mutations in the viral genome accrue.[57]

TABLE 126-4 Selected Pharmacologic Characteristics of Selected Antiretroviral Compounds

Drug	*F* (%)	$t_{1/2}$ (h)[a]	Adult Dose[b] (doses/day)	Plasma C_{max}/C_{min} (μM)	Distinguishing Adverse Effect(s)
Integrase Inhibitors (InSTI)					
Dolutegravir	?	14	50 mg (1)	8.3/2.5	Insomnia, headache, rash (can be severe)
Elvitegravir (coformulated with cobicistat)	?	13	150 mg (1)	3.8/1	Diarrhea, nausea
Raltegravir	?	9	400 mg (2)	1.74/0.22	Rash (can be severe), creatine phosphokinase increases
Nucleoside (Nucleotide) Reverse Transcriptase Inhibitors (NtRTIs)					
Abacavir	83	1.5/20	300 mg (2)	5.2/0.03	Hypersensitivity (HLA-B5701 test to predict)
			or		
			600 mg (1)	7.4[c]	
Didanosine	42	1.4/24	200 mg (2)	2.8/0.03	Peripheral neuropathy, pancreatitis
			or		
			400 mg (1)	5.6[c]	
Emtricitabine	93	10/39	200 mg (1)	7.3/0.04	Rarely pigmentation on soles and palms in nonwhites
Lamivudine	86	5/22	150 mg (2)	6.3/1.6	Headache
			or		
			300 mg (1)	10.5/0.5	
Stavudine	86	1.4/7	40 mg (2)	2.4/0.04	Lipoatrophy, peripheral neuropathy
Tenofovir alafenamide	?	35/150 (tenofovir component)	10 mg (1) (when combined with cobicistat)	0.07/0.03	Increased lipids
Tenofovir disoproxil fumarate	25	17/150 (tenofovir component)	300 mg (1)	1.04/0.4	Renal dysfunction (proximal tubulopathy), bone de-mineralization
Zidovudine	85	2/7	200 mg (3)	0.2	Anemia, neutropenia, myopathy
			or		
			300 mg (2)	3[c]	
Nonnucleoside Reverse Transcriptase Inhibitors (NNRTIs)					
Delavirdine	85	5.8	400 mg (3)	35/14	Rash, elevated liver function tests
			or		
			600 mg (2)		
Efavirenz	43	48	600 mg (1)	12.9/5.6	CNS disturbances and potential teratogenicity
Etravirine	?	41	200 mg (2)	1.69/0.86	Rash, nausea
Nevirapine	93	25	200 mg (2)[d]	22/14	Potentially serious rash and hepatotoxicity
Rilpivirine	?	50	25 mg (1)	0.7/0.3	Possibly depression

(*continued*)

TABLE 126-4 Selected Pharmacologic Characteristics of Selected Antiretroviral Compounds (*Continued*)

Drug	F (%)	$t_{1/2}$ (h)[a]	Adult Dose[b] (doses/day)	Plasma C_{max}/C_{min} (μM)	Distinguishing Adverse Effect(s)
Protease Inhibitors (PIs)					
Fosamprenavir[e]		8	1,400 mg (1)[e,f]	14.3/2.9	Rash
Atazanavir	68	7	400 mg (1)	3.3/0.23	Unconjugated hyperbilirubinemia
			or		
			300 mg (1)[f]	6.2/0.9	
Darunavir	82	15	800 mg (1)[f]	11.9/6.5	Hepatitis, rash
			or		
			600 mg (2)[f]		
Indinavir	60	1.5	800 mg (3)	13/0.25	Nephrolithiasis
			or		
			400-800 mg (2)[f]		
Lopinavir[g]	?	5.5	800 mg (1)	13.6/7.5	Hyperlipidemia/GI intolerance
			or		
			400 mg (2)		
Nelfinavir	?	2.6	750 mg (3)	5.3/1.76	Diarrhea
			or		
			1,250 mg (2)	7/1.2	
Ritonavir	60	3-5	600 mg (2)[d]	16/5	GI intolerance
			or		
			"Boosting doses"		
Saquinavir	4	3	1,000 mg (2)[f]	3.9/0.55	QT prolongation
Tipranavir	?	6	500 mg (2)[f]	77.6/35.6	Hepatotoxicity, intracranial hemorrhage
Entry Inhibitors—Fusion Inhibitor					
Enfuvirtide	84	3.8	90 mg (2)	1.1/0.73	Injection-site reactions
Coreceptor Inhibitor					
Maraviroc	33	15	300 mg (2)	1.2/0.066	Hepatitis, allergic reaction

C_{max}, maximum plasma concentration; C_{min}, minimum plasma concentration; *F*, bioavailability; $t_{1/2}$, elimination half-life.

[a]NtRTIs: Plasma NtRTI $t_{1/2}$/intracellular (peripheral blood mononuclear cells) NtRTI-triphosphate $t_{1/2}$; plasma $t_{1/2}$ only for other classes.

[b]Dose adjustment may be required for weight, renal or hepatic disease, and drug interactions.

[c]C_{min} concentration typically below the limit of quantification.

[d]Initial dose escalation recommended to minimize side effects.

[e]Fosamprenavir is a tablet phosphate prodrug of amprenavir. Amprenavir is no longer available.

[f]Must be boosted with low doses of ritonavir (100-200 mg).

[g]Available as coformulation 4:1 lopinavir to ritonavir.

Data from reference 38.

NNRTIs are a chemically heterogeneous group of agents that bind noncompetitively to reverse transcriptase adjacent to the catalytic site, forcing a conformation change to the enzyme. Unlike NRTIs, NNRTIs do not require intracellular activation, do not compete against endogenous deoxyribonucleotides, and do not have intrinsic antiviral activity against HIV-2. Available NNRTIs include delavirdine (DLV), efavirenz (EFV), etravirine (ETR), nevirapine (NVP), and rilpivirine (RPV).[38] As a class, the NNRTIs are generally associated with rash and elevated liver function tests, including life-threatening cases rarely, particularly for nevirapine.[55] The use of first-generation NNRTI (delavirdine, nevirapine, efavirenz) are on the decline largely because of efficacy (delavirdine) or tolerability and/or safety concerns (nevirapine, efavirenz). NNRTIs tend to have long plasma half-lives (except delavirdine) and they are mainly cleared by liver and/or gut-mediated metabolism through the cytochrome P450 (CYP) enzyme system. Caution should be used for those with advanced hepatic insufficiency (nevirapine should not be used in moderate or advanced hepatic insufficiency). NNRTI can be perpetrators of drug–drug interactions, most often associated with induction of CYP metabolism. The NNRTIs are unique in that a single mutation is needed to confer high-level cross-resistance for the class (except etravirine), which has been termed a *low-genetic barrier* to resistance.[58]

The HIV PIs include atazanavir (ATV), darunavir (DRV), fosamprenavir (FPV), indinavir (IDV), lopinavir (LPV), nelfinavir (NFV), ritonavir (RTV), saquinavir (SQV), and tipranavir (TPV). HIV PIs competitively inhibit the cleavage of the gag-pol polyprotein, which is a crucial step in the viral maturation process, thereby resulting in the production of immature, noninfectious virions. HIV PIs have activity against HIV-1 and HIV-2 (particularly darunavir, lopinavir, and saquinavir).[38] HIV PIs are generally associated with GI distress and metabolic changes, such as increased lipids, insulin insensitivity, and changes in body fat distribution. Some of these issues can be traced to formulation problems due to limited aqueous solubility, requiring high levels of excipients and large pill burdens. The first generation HIV PIs (eg, indinavir, nelfinavir, saquinavir, lopinavir) exhibited poor solubility leading to erratic absorption (eg, nelfinavir, saquinavir), crystallization of drug in urine (eg, indinavir), gastrointestinal distress (eg, nelfinavir, lopinavir), and hyperlipidemia (eg, lopinavir). Generally, the newer HIV PIs (eg, darunavir, atazanavir) improve upon (but do not eliminate) these issues. HIV PIs are cleared by liver- and gut-mediated metabolism (mainly CYP3A), and dose adjustments may be required in hepatic insufficiency (tipranavir/ritonavir should not be used in moderate to severe hepatic insufficiency). HIV PIs are almost always used with low doses of ritonavir or cobicistat, that is, CYP3A inhibitors, to increase the plasma concentrations of the HIV PI of interest. CYP3A-mediated drug interactions with concomitant medications are important considerations for PIs. Resistance to the HIV PIs generally requires the buildup of multiple mutations, termed a *high-genetic barrier*. Multiple mutations can lead to cross-resistance.[57]

There are currently two types of entry inhibitors: fusion inhibitors and CCR5 antagonists. Enfuvirtide (ENF) is the only fusion inhibitor available at this time. Enfuvirtide is a synthetic 36-amino-acid peptide that binds gp41, which inhibits envelope fusion of HIV-1 with the target cell, but does not have activity against HIV-2. Because of the peptide nature of enfuvirtide, oral delivery is impossible, and subcutaneous injection is the preferred route of administration. Injection-site reactions (pain, erythema, nodules) are the most common adverse effect, nearing 100% incidence. Enfuvirtide is cleared via protein catabolism and amino acid recycling, and it appears to have a low genetic barrier to resistance.[57] Maraviroc is a CCR5 antagonist with activity against HIV-1 and HIV-2. Unlike the other available antiretrovirals that interact with a viral target, CCR5 antagonists block a human receptor. The long-term consequences of blocking CCR5 are unknown but may include increased susceptibility to disease by flaviviruses (eg, West Nile virus and tickborne encephalitis virus).[59] One advantage of targeting a human receptor is that resistance to CCR5 antagonists may be more difficult to develop. Because CCR5 antagonists are only effective against R5 virus and not X4 virus, a viral tropism assay must be performed prior to using a CCR5 antagonist. Maraviroc is a CYP3A and P-glycoprotein substrate and is therefore susceptible to drug–drug interactions and caution should be used in those with advanced hepatic insufficiency. Maraviroc has been associated with rash and hepatotoxicity. Resistance mutations have been identified for enfuvirtide, which has a low-genetic barrier to resistance, but assays for maraviroc resistance have not been developed other than the R5 versus X4 tropism test.[38,57]

Among the newer classes of antiretroviral drugs are the InSTI including, raltegravir (RAL), dolutegravir (DTG), and elvitegravir (EVG). InSTI bind to HIV integrase while it is in a specific complex with viral DNA and inhibit the strand transfer that incorporates the proviral DNA into the chromosomal DNA. InSTI are active against HIV-1 and HIV-2. Raltegravir and dolutegravir are primarily glucuronidated by UGT1A1 and are not susceptible to CYP-mediated drug interactions, although other kinds of interactions may be important (Table 126-3). Elvitegravir is extensively metabolized by CYP3A and is co-formulated with cobicistat, a potent CYP3A inhibitor, to optimize drug exposure and enable once daily dosing. InSTI are relatively well-tolerated with adverse events that include rash, nausea, and headache. InSTI should be used with caution in advanced hepatic insufficiency. Multiple mutations have been identified conferring resistance to InSTI including cross-resistance as mutations accrue. Dolutegravir appears to have a higher genetic barrier to resistance compared with elvitegravir and raltegravir.[60]

Novel antiviral agents in the classes listed above and novel agents in new drug classes that exploit other steps in the HIV life cycle (see Fig. 126-1) are in development, with a focus on long-lasting activity (eg, nanosuspensions) and/or high activity against drug-resistant virus. In particular, nanosuspensions of a novel InSTI, cabotegravir and rilpivirine are in clinical-phase development as intermittent injections (eg, quarterly) for treatment and prophylaxis.[61,62]

The anti-herpes and anti-hepatitis B antivirals acyclovir, foscarnet, entecavir, and adefovir exhibit modest anti-HIV activity. If these antivirals are used in HIV-infected patients, it should be with suppressive ART therapy.

Drug Interactions 6 Medical use of antiretroviral agents is complicated by clinically significant drug–drug interactions that can occur with many of these agents.[38,63] Some interactions are beneficial and used purposely (eg, ritonavir and cobicistat as pharmacokinetic enhancers); others may be harmful, leading to dangerously elevated or inadequate drug concentrations. Clinicians involved in the pharmacotherapy of HIV must understand the mechanistic basis for these interactions and maintain a current knowledge of drug interactions for these reasons.

Many clinically significant antiretroviral-associated drug interactions involve CYP3A-mediated first-pass metabolism and clearance. The HIV PIs, except nelfinavir, the NNRTIs delavirdine, etravirine, and rilpivirine, the CCR5 antagonist maraviroc, and the InSTI elvitegravir are metabolized by CYP3A. In general, efavirenz, etravirine and nevirapine are inducers of CYP3A, whereas delavirdine and the PIs inhibit CYP3A. Ritonavir is a potent mechanism-based inhibitor of CYP3A-mediated metabolism and is now used exclusively at lower doses as a pharmacokinetic enhancer of other HIV PIs. Similarly, cobicistat, which is an analog of ritonavir without antiretroviral activity, is also a potent mechanism-based inhibitor of CYP3A activity and is used in a similar fashion. Darunavir, lopinavir, saquinavir, and tipranavir must be taken with ritonavir or cobicistat to achieve optimal plasma concentrations. Atazanavir, fosamprenavir, and indinavir are also primarily used with ritonavir or cobicistat for the same reason. Nelfinavir is not effectively boosted by ritonavir given its CYP2C19-mediated metabolism. Many potential concomitant drugs on the market are also metabolized by CYP3A and therefore susceptible to clinically relevant drug interactions with HIV PIs, NNRTIs, and cobicistat. Agents with narrow therapeutic indices and/or that exhibit major changes in pharmacokinetics with CYP3A inhibition are most important in this regard. Examples include, but are not limited to, simvastatin, lovastatin, corticosteroids (including inhaled and intranasal), ergot derivatives, oral hormonal contraceptives, some antiarrhythmics, and some anti-cancer agents.

The drug interaction potential of antimycobacterium agents, specifically the rifamycins, are particularly relevant given the high potential for such infections in HIV-infected patients.[63] Rifampin, a potent inducer of CYP3A metabolism and conjugation enzymes, is contraindicated with use of most HIV PIs, etravirine, rilpivirine, and maraviroc because concentrations are reduced substantially even with ritonavir enhancement. Raltegravir or dolutegravir dose should be doubled in the presence of rifampin; efavirenz is an alternative agent. Ritonavir enhancement generally allows coadministration of HIV PIs with rifabutin.[38] In such cases, the rifabutin dose will require adjustment given its CYP3A-mediated clearance. The herbal product St. John's wort (*Hypericum perforatum*) is a potent inducer of metabolism and is contraindicated with PIs, NNRTIs, and maraviroc.[38] It must be stressed that the pharmacology of CYP3A interactions may be complicated by simultaneous induction/inhibition of drug transporter-mediated (eg, P-glycoprotein) clearance and/or other phase I (eg, CYP 2B6 for RTV) or phase II enzymes.

Some antiretroviral drugs require acidic environments for optimal absorption leading to interactions with antacids, particularly proton-pump inhibitors (eg, atazanavir, rilpivirine). On the other hand, some antiretroviral agents chelate polyvalent cations in antacids, reducing absorption following concomitant dosing (eg, raltegravir, dolutegravir, elvitegravir); dosing can be temporally separated for these cases. Other potential mechanisms for drug interactions include inhibition of renal tubule secretion (eg, TFV and OAT inhibitors), and antagonistic phosphorylation for NRTI of the same nucleobase (eg, lamivudine and emtricitiabine). This list of drug interactions and mechanisms for drug interactions is not complete. Clinicians who treat HIV must stay abreast of antiretroviral drug interaction data.

Websites are available that catalog and regularly update HIV drug-interaction information (*http://www.hiv-druginteractions.org/*), and the Department of Health and Human Services guidelines for antiretroviral use provide, and regularly update, excellent summaries of known clinically relevant drug interactions.[38]

Landmarks in the Evolution of Antiretroviral Therapy (7)

ART has undergone major changes over the past decades. Illustrating these changes is important for a thorough understanding of current treatment strategies. The fundamental landmarks in the use of antiretroviral agents are as follows:

1. An early study demonstrated that zidovudine monotherapy confers a survival benefit in persons who have AIDS.[64]
2. Combination regimens of two NRTIs (eg, zidovudine and didanosine or zalcitabine) were superior to zidovudine monotherapy in immunologic and virologic parameters, particularly in patients with no previous ART, and conferred a superior survival benefit.[65] This established that NRTI monotherapy was inferior to dual NRTI therapy.
3. Dual NRTI therapy was inferior to triple therapy consisting of 2 NRTIs and the HIV PI indinavir.[66] Use of triple therapy with combinations of two NRTIs with NNRTIs or HIV PIs was associated with a durable response as well as significantly reduced incidence of OIs and improved survival, thus establishing the current paradigm of ART.[67]
4. Evolution of triple-therapy regimens utilizing boosted HIV PIs, co-formulations, new drug classes, and better tolerated agents showed improvements in convenience, tolerability, safety, and virologic efficacy, all helping usher in the current era of ART.[68, 69]

(7) Taken together, the pivotal studies described above established that HIV should not be treated with single or dual NRTIs. Recommendations for initial treatment of HIV infection advocate a minimum of three active antiretroviral agents: tenofovir disoproxil fumarate plus emtricitabine with either a ritonavir-enhanced PI (darunavir) or the InSTIs, elvitegravir/cobicistat, dolutegravir, or raltegravir. Additionally, tenofovir alafenamide/emtricitabine plus elvitegravir/cobicistat or abacavir/lamivudine plus dolutegravir are other first-line options (abacavir can only be used in patients who are HLA-B5701 negative). Multiple alternative regimens are also safe and effective, but have one or two disadvantages compared with the preferred regimens such as weaker virologic responses with high viral loads, lower tolerability, or greater risk of long-term toxicities such as subcutaneous fat loss. Preferred antiretroviral regimens are listed in Table 126-3. Recommended first line ART regimens constantly evolve (as described above) and clinical controversies emerge as data and clinical experience accrue and new strategies come under consideration.

Clinical **Controversy...**

"Induction-maintenance" therapy is a strategy whereby ART is initiated with three active drugs (conventional ART), but one or two drugs are stopped once undetectable HIV-RNA has been established (ie, maintenance therapy with mono- or dual-drugs). The hope is to reduce cost and long-term drug toxicities, especially related with older NRTIs. This led to maintenance strategies that were NRTI-sparing. Early maintenance regimens led to some elevation in risk for breakthrough viremia, which lowered enthusiasm for this approach. However, new more potent drugs have revived interest. A current example includes a maintenance dual-drug therapy with cabotegravir (investigational InSTI) and rilpivirine (NNRTI), which are under study as intermittent nanosuspension injections.

Adherence The simplest definition of adherence is the patient's follow through on taking medication as directed. As with any chronic therapy, variable adherence to ART is common, and it significantly impacts virologic response. Factors associated with poor adherence include major psychiatric illnesses, active substance abuse, unstable social circumstances, adverse events, and poor adherence with clinic visits.[38] Most, but not all, modern ART regimens consist of co-formulations and long half-life drugs allowing for once-daily dosing (sometimes without food restrictions), which facilitates adherence compared with multiple dose units, multiple doses per day, and food restrictions with dosing. Average adherence rates range from 60% to 80% for both HIV PI and NNRTI-based regimens including 30% of subjects who miss less than 7 consecutive days of dosing.[70, 71] The odds of persistent or breakthrough viremia are several-fold higher in patients with adherence below 60% to 80%, and the risk mounts with longer dosing "holidays."[72] As clinicians, it is critical to establish a relationship of trust with the patient and to communicate to the patient the importance of proper medication taking. Education should be aimed at understanding the disease process, monitoring, and goals of therapy. An individual's "readiness" to take medications should be clearly established before treatment is initiated.[38] Help from caregivers, friends, and/or family members should be leveraged by the patient because social and psychological support are among the most important factors that influence adherence in this patient population.

Efficacy Based on clinical trial data, approximately 90% of patients will achieve undetectable viral loads with modern ART regimens.[68,69] The preferred NRTI combination, tenofovir disoproxil fumarate plus emtricitabine, has demonstrated virologic and safety/tolerability advantages compared with zidovudine/lamivudine and abacavir/lamivudine (when combined with atazanavir/ritonavir or efavirenz).[73,74] Its main drawback is renal tubulopathy risk for tenofovir disoproxil fumarate, especially in those with preexisting renal dysfunction. When combined with dolutegravir, abacavir-lamivudine exhibited superior efficacy rates regardless of baseline viral load compared with efavirenz- tenofovir disoproxil fumarate-emtricitabine.[69] This finding was mainly due to fewer discontinuations arising from adverse events for the abacavir-lamivudine-dolutegravir regimen (most in the other arm were associated with efavirenz). Tenofovir alafenamide was compared with tenofovir disoproxil fumarate both given with emtricitabine- elvitegravir- cobicistat.[68] Similar efficacy was observed but changes in creatinine clearance and bone demineralization was more favorable for tenofovir alafenamide compared with tenofovir disoproxil fumarate. Together, these studies established recommendations for tenofovir disoproxil fumarate -emtricitabine, tenofovir alafenamide -emtricitabine, abacavir-lamivudine as initial NRTI therapy. Note, if abacavir is to be used in any regimen, a test for the presence of human leukocyte antigen (HLA)-B*5701 must be done as its presence has been strongly correlated with the development of abacavir hypersensitivity. Should this test be positive, an abacavir allergy should be added to the patient's chart and abacavir should not be used in the patient, as the hypersensitivity reaction can be life-threatening.

The third active agent of ART regimens has also evolved based on large, randomized, controlled trials. Efavirenz maintained a long history as the recommended third active agent until recently, when comparative trials demonstrated poorer tolerability and more therapy discontinuations for efavirenz versus InSTI.[69,75,76] CNS perturbations such as somnolence, vivid dreams, and depressive symptoms are troublesome issues for efavirenz. Similarly, atazanavir-ritonavir was a recommended third active agent until it showed higher rates of treatment discontinuations compared with raltegravir and darunavir-ritonavir.[77] Atazanavir inhibits the bilirubin conjugating enzyme resulting in asymptomatic hyperbilirubinemia, but in those with Gilbert's disease, the hyperbilirubinemia can be more pronounced leading to drug discontinuation.[78] Together, these studies support recommendations for darunavir-ritonavir and InSTIs as third active agents for preferred initial ART regimens. Many agents are available for inclusion in alternative regimens, including efavirenz and atazanavir-ritonavir, among others. Recommended preferred and alternative regimens are continuously updated as new studies are performed and longer-term follow-up data accrue. Patients with sustained undetectable HIV-RNA taking out-of-date drug regimens may be candidates to simplify to one of the preferred regimens or a more desirable alternative regimen based on past treatment history and other variables. Simplified regimens should continue to include three active drugs.

Resistance 8 Regimen failure is commonly associated with antiretroviral resistance, and testing for such resistance is a useful clinical tool.[57,58] The two types of resistance tests available are phenotype and genotype. A phenotype test determines the concentration of antiretroviral agent necessary to inhibit 50% (IC_{50}) replication of the patient's viral isolate (inhibitory concentration of 50% [IC_{50}]) in a recombinant in vitro viral assay. Results usually are expressed as a fold change in susceptibility (IC_{50}) compared with a wild-type laboratory strain virus. Generally, the fold-change in IC_{50} increases as HIV accumulates additional mutations that confer resistance to a particular drug. However, a single mutation may confer a very high fold-change in IC_{50} for some drugs (eg, lamivudine, emtricitabine, efavirenz, nevirapine) rendering them ineffective after a single mutation. Although small-to-moderate increases in the fold change suggests reduced susceptibility to that antiretroviral agent, resistance may not be absolute, and partial susceptibility may remain. Theoretically, drug concentrations may be increased to overcome reduced susceptibility. The strengths of phenotypic testing is to provide resistance information for complex mutation patterns, but it is also associated with higher cost, limited number of commercial providers, and slower turnaround time for results. Genotyping assesses genetic mutations and associated codon changes in gp41, reverse transcriptase, integrase, or protease in the patient's virus and compares it with the wild-type sequence. Certain mutations are known to confer resistance to specific drugs. An updated list of drug resistance mutations can be found at (http://www.iasusa.org/resistance_mutations). Mutations are listed by the wild-type amino acid followed by the position in the protein or enzyme and end with the mutation found in the patient's virus. For example, a common mutation caused by lamivudine and emtricitabine is the M184V mutation: a substitution of valine (V) for methionine (M) at the 184 position of reverse transcriptase. Mutations can confer varying degrees of antiretroviral drug resistance and in some cases, weighting algorithms have been developed to predict the relative impact of mutation combinations on antiretroviral activity. Algorithms have also been developed to predict a phenotype from a genotype test (ie, virtual phenotype). Not all mutations, however, are only detrimental—for example, while M184V confers significant resistance to lamivudine and emtricitabine, it is also associated with a less fit virus. Interpretation of genotype resistance tests is complex; therefore, the reader is encouraged to obtain expert advice and consult the most recent guidelines on HIV resistance testing.

Treatment of Special Populations

Pregnancy Several considerations are relevant to the treatment of pregnant women, including the health of the mother, prevention of HIV transmission to the fetus, potential for teratogenicity, and drug dosing issues based on pharmacokinetic changes during pregnancy. Treatment recommendations should be consulted to address the specific requirements for HIV-infected pregnant women and the prevention of vertical transmission.[17] Generally, pregnant women should be treated as would nonpregnant women, with the goal of maximally suppressing HIV-RNA. Efavirenz should be avoided when possible in women planning to become pregnant or who are not using effective contraception as efavirenz has been associated with neural tube defects in the first trimester, in some but not all studies.[79] Zidovudine is recommended intrapartum depending on the mother's viral load (more than 1,000 copies/mL [more than $1,000 \times 10^3$/L] or unknown), based on early studies demonstrating clear prophylactic effectiveness as well as extensive familiarity with the side effect profile.[17] Infants born to HIV infected mothers should also receive zidovudine (± several doses of nevirapine) prophylaxis for 4 to 6 weeks after birth. HIV transmission rates to their infants have been reduced to less than 0.5% for women who are treated with ART and when zidovudine prophylaxis is used. Breastfeeding is not recommended in the USA, but in resource-limited settings where lack of clean water makes breastfeeding a more favorable option, infants receive six weeks of once-daily nevirapine for prophylaxis.[17]

Chemoprophylaxis

9 In addition to fetal and infant chemoprophylaxis, protection of healthcare workers from accidental exposure to HIV and in cases of rape or high-risk postcoital and postinjection drug-use episodes are important concerns. The CDC has issued guidelines governing antiretroviral postexposure prophylaxis (PEP) of occupational and other high-risk HIV exposures that should be consulted for updates as the knowledge in this field evolves.[11,14] The principles of the guidelines are to assess the exposure risk and treat as soon as possible after high-risk exposures to prevent HIV infection. Assessing the exposure risk requires knowledge of the HIV-infection status of the source individual, which can be difficult to ascertain. The HIV status of the source should be determined as soon as possible with a rapid HIV test, whenever feasible. However, providers may have to rely on reasonable suspicion when this is not possible, so provider expertise is essential. PEP should not be delayed while waiting on the HIV status of the source, if reasonable suspicion is present. PEP should be considered an urgent medical situation. Both guidelines recommend conventional ART regimens (eg, tenofovir disoproxil fumarate -emtricitabine-rategravir), initiated as soon as possible, ideally within 1 to 2 hours of exposure. Animal studies show reduced PEP efficacy when initiated 72 hours or more after the exposure.[14] The optimal duration of treatment is unknown, but at least 4 weeks of therapy is advocated. Expert consultation is needed when exposure to drug-resistant virus is suspected or confirmed, but this should not delay initial initiation of PEP.

Preexposure prophylaxis (PrEP) involves daily tenofovir disoproxil fumarate–emtricitabine in HIV-negative persons at high risk of HIV acquisition to prevent infection should an HIV-exposure occur.[80] PrEP is effective in MSM, sero-discordant couples, at-risk heterosexual men and women, including those who inject drugs. The key considerations for PrEP are to assess HIV risk for the individual (ie, risk should be elevated) and to document a negative HIV test prior to initiating PrEP, including negative symptoms of acute HIV infection. Reports of drug resistance from PrEP failures were mostly among individuals who initiated PrEP during acute HIV infection, in the window period before the rapid HIV test could detect infection.[81] HIV-testing should be repeated at least every 3 months and renal function should be assessed every 6 months while on PrEP.[80] Promotion of adherence is critical for PrEP effectiveness. The most up-to-date PrEP guidelines should be consulted, as new PrEP strategies are currently under evaluation.

EVALUATION OF THERAPEUTIC OUTCOMES

Two laboratory tests are used to evaluate response to ART: the plasma HIV RNA and the CD4 count.[38] These tests should be performed at baseline, along with a medical history and physical, urinalysis, hematology, chemistries, serologies for coinfections, and patient education about HIV infection. A HIV resistance test is recommended upon initiation of care. After therapy is initiated, patients are generally monitored at 3-month intervals until HIV-RNA reaches undetectable levels. An assessment at 2 to 8 weeks is warranted to document early response. Monitoring may be increased to every 6 months in stabilized patients. The two main indications for a change in therapy are significant toxicity and treatment failure. Should a single agent be responsible for an intolerable side effect, that agent often can be singly changed out of the regimen, for example, the patient who experiences intolerable CNS disturbances during initiation of efavirenz can switch to a boosted PI or inSTI without changing the dual NRTI backbone. Maintaining virologic suppression is an important goal for switching therapy due to adverse events. Caution must be exercised when drugs in the regimen have overlapping toxicities, which makes changing a single agent problematic. Serious and life-threatening toxicities warrant cessation of the whole regimen before deciding upon a subsequent therapy.

As a general guide, the inability to achieve and maintain less than 200 copies/mL (200×10^3/L) of HIV-RNA represents treatment failure and should prompt consideration for changing therapy. This includes the inability to achieve less than 200 copies/mL (200×10^3/L) by 24 weeks of therapy initiation (repeat testing is suggested to confirm), or, after HIV RNA suppression, repeated detection of greater than 200 copies/mL (200×10^3/L) of HIV-RNA.

Therapeutic Failure

8 The most important measure of therapeutic failure is suboptimal suppression of viral replication. Many reasons may underlie suboptimal suppression of viral replication such as pre-ART disease factors (eg, high viral load or preexisting drug resistance), nonadherence to medication, development of new drug resistance, intolerance to one or more medications, adverse drug–drug or drug–food interactions, or pharmacokinetic–pharmacodynamic variability.[38] In cases of suboptimal suppression of viral replication, these potential causes should be investigated and addressed, if possible. As a general rule, drug resistance develops for regimens that do not maximally suppress HIV replication. Drug resistance testing is recommended while the patient is undergoing the failing regimen or within 4 weeks after stopping the regimen as long as the HIV RNA count is greater than 500 copies/mL (500×10^3/L), which is the threshold for resistance assays (~500-1,000 copies/mL [~500×10^3-1000×10^3/L]). Virus may revert to wild-type if more than 4 to 6 weeks has elapsed between regimen discontinuation and the resistance test. Most clinicians use the genotype assay because it is less expensive and results typically are available sooner compared with the phenotype assay. Resistance results usually require expert interpretation. Treating patients with drug-resistant HIV utilizes the same general treatment approaches described for initial therapy above. Patients should be treated with at least two (preferably three) fully active antiretroviral drugs based on medication history, resistance tests, and new mechanistic drug classes (eg, maraviroc and InSTIs). The goal of therapy is to suppress HIV-RNA to undetectable levels. In cases when undetectable HIV-RNA cannot be attained, maintenance on the regimen is preferred over drug discontinuation so as to prevent rapid immunological and clinical decline.

Several antiretroviral drugs are well-suited for drug-resistant HIV. For example, the HIV PI, tipranavir-ritonavir and the NNRTI, etravirine have demonstrated activity in persons with multidrug-resistant HIV in controlled clinical trials.[82,83] The drugs in the newer classes (ie, inSTI, CCR5 antagonist, and enfuvirtide) are also active against NRTI-, NNRTI-, and PI-resistant viruses in highly treatment experienced patients in controlled trials.[84,85]

Prior to the availability of new drugs and drug classes, other strategies were studied to help manage therapeutic failure including drug holidays, structured or strategic treatment interruptions, and structured intermittent therapy. The overall premise of these strategies was similar: stop all antiretrovirals to spare the patient from drug toxicities and to allow the virus to revert to wild-type. Reinitiation of therapy was intended to reestablish control of viral replication, as wild-type virus would be expected to predominate, although it was known that resistant virus was archived in long-lived cells, so viral suppression was short-lived. A landmark clinical trial showed that patients randomized to episodic therapy (drug-sparing) guided by the CD4 experienced significantly increased risk of opportunistic disease or death from any cause, including non-AIDS causes.[86,87] This and other studies have established that viral replication is damaging to the immune system and end organs and drug-sparing approaches are not advocated.

Clinical **Controversy...**

There is a strong theoretical rationale for therapeutic drug monitoring in the treatment experienced patient, but this approach is controversial. Drug susceptibility is founded on the premise that increasing drug concentration corresponds with stronger inhibition of replication up to a maximal effectiveness. This principle holds for drug-resistant variants, except higher drug concentrations are needed for the same levels of inhibition. Therefore, drug concentration monitoring could guide dose adjustments needed to attain the higher target drug concentrations required for optimal viral inhibition.Therapeutic drug monitoring is suggested as a consideration for patients with multidrug-resistant HIV as well as in other select clinical situations. However, limitations to therapeutic drug monitoring include the lack of established target concentrations, unsuitable dose formulations for minor adjustments, intrapatient pharmacokinetic variability, lack of randomized clinical trials proving benefit or cost effectiveness, and few analytical laboratories and experts available for interpretation.

COMPLICATIONS OF HIV INFECTION AND AIDS

3 In the pre-ART era, the major therapeutic focus was prevention and treatment of OIs associated with uncontrolled HIV replication and the steady decline in CD4 cells.[44] Uncontrolled HIV is an insidious disease; persons often present with OIs, a consequence of the weakened immune system rather than HIV per se. Most OIs are caused by organisms that are common in the environment and often represent the reactivation of quiescent, hidden infections common in the population. The probability of developing specific OIs is closely related to CD4 count thresholds (Fig. 126-2). These CD4 thresholds serve as a basis for initiating primary OI chemoprevention.

5 In the ART era, the main principle in the management of OIs is treating HIV infection to enable CD4 cell recovery and maintenance above safe levels.[63] Additional important principles regarding management of OIs are as follows:

1. Prevent exposure to opportunistic pathogens
2. Vaccinate to prevent first-episode disease (consult HIV-specific guidelines)
3. Use primary chemoprophylaxis at certain CD4 thresholds to prevent first-episode disease
4. Treat emergent OI
5. Use secondary chemoprophylaxis to prevent disease recurrence
6. Discontinue prophylaxes with sustained ART-associated immune recovery

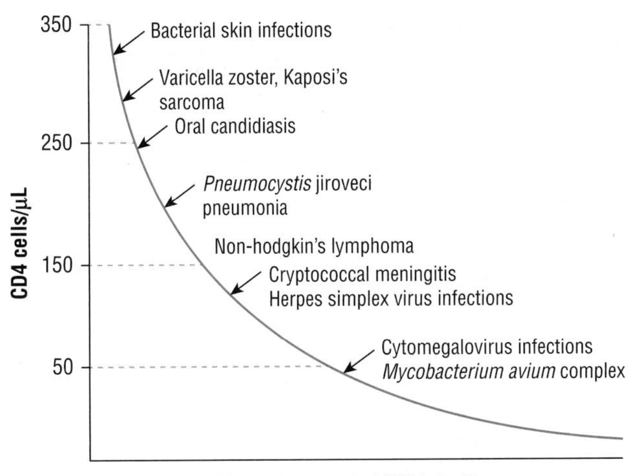

FIGURE 126-2 Natural history of opportunistic infections associated with human immunodeficiency virus infection. CD4 counts expressed as cells/µL can be converted to SI units by multiplying by 10^6/L. *(Reprinted with permission, © Courtney V. Fletcher, 2009.)*

Several considerations are required for the patient who presents with an OI and is simultaneously diagnosed with HIV and who thus needs both OI and ART treatment. Immediate initiation of ART is indicated for OIs that respond to CD4 recovery, such as cryptosporidiosis, progressive multifocal leukoencephalopathy, and mild-to-moderate Kaposi's sarcoma. Rapid initiation of ART (within days to weeks) is also indicated in the setting of other OIs such as tuberculosis, *Mycobacterium avium* complex (MAC), and PCP, but several potential issues need consideration. First, drug–drug interactions and the complexity of adhering to concomitant ART and OI regimens can be daunting. Careful review of potential interactions and adherence support should be provided. Second, clinicians must be cognizant of potentially overlapping drug toxicities (eg, rash) that creates problems when attempting to stop the perceived culprit drug. Third, an immune reconstitution syndrome (IRIS) has been associated with initiation of ART in the presence of underlying OIs. IRIS is generally characterized by fever and worsening of OI manifestations in the first few weeks to months after initiating ART.[88] Risk factors for IRIS are a low CD4 count (eg, less than 50 cells/µL [less than 50 × 10^6/L]) and a high antigenic burden. An ART-associated rapid-onset immune reconstitution against the smoldering OI infection, and resulting proinflammatory cytokine cascade, is thought to be the mechanism of IRIS. The most serious IRIS reactions involve neurological OIs such as cryptococcal meningitis, where IRIS can lead to increased morbidity and mortality. For cryptococcal meningitis, it may be prudent to delay ART until completion of the induction or induction/consolidation phase of antifungal therapy (up to 10 weeks).[63] Generally, treatment of IRIS is supportive and may include corticosteroids and/or NSAIDs, depending on the OI. Expert consultation should be used in the management of ART initiation in patients with advanced HIV infection and OIs, and the most up-to-date guidelines should be consulted.[63]

The epidemiology of specific OIs can depend upon geographical region. For instance, TB is particularly endemic on the Africa continent and is considered a major OI in that region, but the incidence of this OI is relatively uncommon in the USA.[89] Major OIs in the USA include PCP, toxoplasmosis, MAC, cytomegalovirus retinitis, and cryptococcal meningitis. All have decreased substantially in incidence with the advent of ART.[44,63,67] Furthermore, primary and secondary chemoprophylaxis for specific OIs have contributed to the same decreases.[44] Nevertheless, opportunistic diseases continue to be complications of HIV disease and occur at low CD4 lymphocyte counts in patients who are unaware of their HIV infection, or who have not responded to ART therapy or OI prophylaxis because of adherence issues or inadequate engagement with the healthcare system.[63]

Selected OIs and example recommended first-line regimens for OI treatment are given in Table 126-5, and example recommended therapies for primary OI prophylaxis are given in Table 126-6.[63] These recommendations are representative and not as extensive as in the published guidelines, which include multiple additional treatment considerations and alternatives, as well as coverage of less common OIs. The following brief discussion of PCP provides a more in depth overview of the epidemiology, diagnosis, clinical manifestations, and results of treatment and serves as an illustration for the principles discussed above.

Pneumocystis jirovecii Pneumonia

5 *Pneumocystis jirovecii* (*carinii*) pneumonia (PCP) has been and continues to be the most common life-threatening OI in patients with AIDS.[90] *P. jirovecii* was formerly named *P. carinii*; the name change was made to distinguish the organism that infects humans (*P. jirovecii*) from the strain that infects rodents (*P. carinii*). Nevertheless, the acronym PCP is still used today. Early in the AIDS epidemic 80% of patients experienced PCP at some point during their lifetime.[91] Although the incidence of PCP has fallen markedly since the advent of ART and effective prophylaxis for PCP, it still occurs in persons unaware of their HIV infection, and breakthrough PCP can occur in those with variable adherence to ART and/or prophylaxis.

P. jirovecii is a fungus that has protozoan characteristics as well.[90,91] Exposure to *P. jirovecii* is widespread; two thirds of the population have developed serum antibodies by age 2 to 4 years. The organism appears to reside without consequence in humans unless the host becomes immunologically impaired.[92] Disease associated with immunosuppression probably occurs from both new acquisition and reactivation. Ninety percent of PCP cases in AIDS patients occurred in those with CD4 counts less than 200 cells/mm^3 (200 × 10^6/L).[63] Other risk factors include oral thrush, recurrent bacterial pneumonia, unintentional weight loss, and high plasma HIV RNA. Past episodes of PCP increase risk for future episodes, which provides the basis for secondary chemoprophylaxis, as described below.

The presentation of PCP in AIDS often is insidious.[90] Characteristic symptoms include fever and dyspnea. Clinical signs are tachypnea with or without rales or rhonchi and a nonproductive or mildly productive cough occurring over a period of weeks, although more fulminant presentations can occur. Chest radiographs may show florid or subtle interstitial and bilateral infiltrates but occasionally are normal. Arterial blood gases may show minimal hypoxia (PaO_2 80 to 95 mm Hg [10.6-12.6 kPa]) but in more advanced disease may be markedly abnormal. The diagnosis of PCP usually is made by identification of the organism in induced sputum or in specimens obtained from bronchoalveolar lavage. Less commonly, transbronchial or open lung biopsy is used to locate the organism. Diagnostic PCR tests of bronchoavelor lavage is an emerging approach.[63]

Untreated PCP has a mortality rate of nearly 100%. Several potential treatments are available for PCP, but the treatment of choice is trimethoprim–sulfamethoxazole (also called cotrimoxazole), which is associated with a response rate of 60% to 100%.[63] Parenteral pentamidine is equally efficacious but significantly more toxic. Trimethoprim–sulfamethoxazole is also the regimen of choice for primary and secondary prophylaxis of PCP in patients with and without HIV.[63,90]

When used for treatment of PCP, the dose of trimethoprim–sulfamethoxazole is 15 to 20 mg/kg/day (based on the trimethoprim component) as three to four divided doses. Treatment duration typically is 21 days but also must be based on clinical response. Trimethoprim–sulfamethoxazole usually is initiated by the IV route, although oral therapy may suffice in mildly ill and reliable outpatients

TABLE 126-5 Selected Therapies for Common Opportunistic Pathogens in HIV-Infected Individuals

Clinical Disease	Preferred Initial Therapies for Acute Infection in Adults (Strength of Recommendation in Parentheses)	Common Drug- or Dose-Limiting Adverse Reactions
Fungi		
Candidiasis, oral	Fluconazole 100 mg orally for 7-14 days (AI)	Elevated liver function tests, hepatotoxicity, nausea, and vomiting
	or	
	Nystatin 500,000 units oral swish (~5 mL) four times daily for 7-14 days (BII)	Taste, patient acceptance
Candidiasis, esophageal	Fluconazole 100-400 mg orally or IV daily for 14-21 days (AI)	Same as above
	or	
	Itraconazole 200 mg/day orally for 14-21 days (AI)	Elevated liver function tests, hepatotoxicity, nausea, and vomiting
Pneumocystis jirovecii pneumonia	Trimethoprim–sulfamethoxazole IV or orally 15-20 mg/kg/day as trimethoprim component in three to four divided doses for 21 days[a] (AI) moderate or severe therapy should be started IV	Skin rash, fever, leucopenia Thrombocytopenia
	or	
	Pentamidine IV 4 mg/kg/day for 21 days[a] (AI)	Azotemia, hypoglycemia, hyperglycemia, arrhythmias
	Mild episodes	
	Atovaquone suspension 750 mg (5 mL) orally twice daily with meals for 21 days[a] (BI)	Rash, elevated liver enzymes, diarrhea
Cryptococcal meningitis	Liposomal amphotericin B 3-4 mg/kg/day IV for a minimum of 2 weeks with flucytosine 100 mg/kg/day orally in four divided doses (AI) *followed by*	Nephrotoxicity, hypokalemia, anemia, fever, chills Bone marrow suppression
	Fluconazole 400 mg/day, orally for 8 weeks or until CSF cultures are negative (AI)[a]	Same as above
Histoplasmosis	Liposomal amphotericin B 3 mg/kg/day IV for 2 weeks (AI) *followed by*	Same as above
	Itraconazole 200 mg orally thrice daily for 3 days then twice daily, for 12 months (AII)[a]	
Coccidioidomycosis	Liposomal amphotericin B 4-6 mg/kg/day IV until clinical improvement (usually after 500-1,000 mg) then switch to azole (AIII)[a]	Same as above
	or	
	Fluconazole 400-800 mg once daily (meningeal disease) (AII)[a]	Same as above
Protozoa		
Toxoplasmic encephalitis	Pyrimethamine 200 mg orally once, then 50-75 mg/day	Bone marrow suppression
	plus	
	Sulfadiazine 1-1.5 g orally four times daily	Rash, drug fever
	and	
	Leucovorin 10-25 mg orally daily for 6 weeks (AI)[a]	
Isosporiasis	Trimethoprim and sulfamethoxazole: 160 mg trimethoprim and 800 mg sulfamethoxazole orally or IV four times daily for 10 days (AII)[a]	Same as above
Bacteria		
Mycobacterium avium complex	Clarithromycin 500 mg orally twice daily, *plus* ethambutol 15 mg/kg/day orally (AI) for at least 12 months	GI intolerance, optic neuritis, peripheral neuritis, elevated liver tests
Salmonella enterocolitis or bacteremia	Ciprofloxacin 500-750 mg orally (or 400 mg IV) twice daily for 14 days (longer duration for bacteremia or advanced HIV) (AIII)	GI intolerance, headache, dizziness
Campylobacter enterocolitis (mild to moderate)	Ciprofloxacin 500-750 mg orally (or 400 mg IV) twice daily for 7-10 days (or longer with bacteremia) (BIII)	Same as above
Shigella enterocolitis	Ciprofloxacin 500-750 mg orally (or 400 mg IV) twice daily for 7-10 days (or 14 days for bacteremia) (AIII)	Same as above
Viruses		
Mucocutaneous herpes simplex	Acyclovir 5 mg/kg IV every 8 hours until lesions regress, then acyclovir 400 mg orally three times daily until complete healing (famciclovir or valacyclovir is alternative) (AIII)	GI intolerance, crystalluria
Primary varicella-zoster	Acyclovir 10-15 mg/kg every 8 hours IV for 7-10 days (severe cases), then switch to oral valacyclovir 1 g three times daily after defervescence (famciclovir or acyclovir is alternative) (AIII)	Obstructive nephropathy, CNS symptoms
Cytomegalovirus (retinitis)	Intravitreal ganciclovir (2 mg) one to four doses over 7-10 days (for sight threatening lesions) *plus* valganciclovir 900 mg twice daily for 14-21 days then once daily until immune recovery from ART (AIII)[a]	Neutropenia, thrombocytopenia
Cytomegalovirus esophagitis or colitis	Ganciclovir 5 mg/kg IV every 12 hours for 21-42 days may switch to valganciclovir 900 mg orally every 12 hours when oral therapy can be tolerated (BI)	Same as above

ART, antiretroviral therapy; CSF, cerebrospinal fluid; HIV, human immunodeficiency virus.

[a]Maintenance therapy is recommended.

See Table 126-3 for levels of evidence-based recommendations.

Data from reference 63.

TABLE 126-6 Therapies for Prophylaxis of Select First-Episode Opportunistic Diseases in Adults and Adolescents

Pathogen	Indication	First Choice (Strength of Recommendation in Parentheses)
I. Standard of care		
Pneumocystis jirovecii	CD4+ count <200/mm³ (<200 × 10⁶/L) *or* oropharyngeal candidiasis	Trimethoprim–sulfamethoxazole, one double-strength tablet orally once daily (AI) or one single-strength tablet orally once daily (AI)
Histoplasma capsulatum	CD4+ count <150/mm³, (<150 × 10⁶/L) endemic geographic area and high risk for exposures	Intraconazole 200 mg orally once daily (BI)
Mycobacterium tuberculosis		
Isoniazid-sensitive	(Active TB should be ruled out): + test for latent TB infection with no prior TB treatment history (AI) *or* – test for latent TB infection, but close contact with case of active tuberculosis (AII)	Isoniazid 300 mg orally plus pyridoxine, 25 mg orally once daily for 9 months (AII) *or* Isoniazid 900 mg orally twice weekly by directly observed therapy (BII) plus pyridoxine 25 mg orally daily for 9 months (BII)
For exposure to drug-resistant TB	Consult public health authorities	
Toxoplasma gondii	Immunoglobulin G antibody to *Toxoplasma* and CD4+ count <100/mm³ (<100 × 10⁶/L)	Trimethoprim–sulfamethoxazole one double-strength tablet orally once daily (AII)
Mycobacterium avium complex	CD4+ count <50/mm³ (<50 × 10⁶/L)	Azithromycin 1,200 mg orally once weekly (AI) or 600 mg orally twice weekly (BIII) or clarithromycin 500 mg orally twice daily (AI)
Varicella zoster virus (VZV)	Preexposure: CD4 ≥200/mm³ (≥200 × 10⁶/L), no history of varicella vaccination or infection, or, if available, negative antibody to VZV Postexposure: Significant exposure to chicken pox or shingles for patients who have no history of vaccination or either condition or, if available, negative antibody to VZV	Varicella vaccination; two doses, 3 months apart (CIII) Varicella-zoster immune globulin, 125 IU per 10 kg (maximum of 625 IU) IM, as soon as possible and within 10 days after exposure (AIII)
Streptococcus pneumoniae	Any individual regardless of CD4 count	13-valent polysaccharide vaccine, 0.5 mL intramuscularly once (AI) followed by 23-valent polysaccharide vaccine 0.5 mL 8 weeks later (CIII) Re-vaccinate with 23-valent polysaccharide vaccine every 5 years
Hepatitis B virus	All susceptible patients	HBV vaccine IM (Engerix-B 20 mcg/mL or Recombivax HB 10 mcg/mL), 0, 1, and 6 months (AII) Anti-HBs should be obtained 1 month after the vaccine series completion (BIII)
Influenza virus	All patients (annually, before influenza season)	Inactivated trivalent influenza virus vaccine (annual): 0.5 mL intramuscularly (AIII) (live-attenuated vaccine is contraindicated in all HIV-infected patients)
Hepatitis A virus	All susceptible (anti-hepatitis A virus–negative) patients at increased risk for hepatitis A infection (eg, chronic liver disease, injection drug users, men who have sex with men)	Hepatitis A vaccine: two doses (AII) antibody response should be assessed 1 month after vaccination; with revaccination as needed when CD4 >200 cells/μL (>200 × 10⁶/L)(BIII)
Human papillomavirus (HPV) infection	13-26 year old males and females	HPV quadrivalent vaccine months 0, 1-2, and 6 (BIII)

See Table 126-3 for levels of evidence-based recommendations.

Data from reference 63.

or for completion of a course of therapy after a response has been achieved with IV administration.[63,90] Patients with moderate-to-severe PCP (eg, PaO_2 more than 70 mm Hg [more than 9.3 kPa]) should be treated with corticosteroids as soon as possible after starting PCP therapy and certainly within 72 hours, in order to blunt the deterioration seen just after initiation of PCP therapy. Alternative regimens include pentamidine for moderate-to-severe disease and dapsone with trimethoprim, primaquine with clindamycin, and atovaquone for mild-to-moderate PCP.[63] Early initiation of ART (within 2 weeks) is recommended keeping in mind the potential issues described earlier.

Adverse reactions to trimethoprim–sulfamethoxazole and pentamidine are common, occurring in 20% to 85% of patients in this setting.[63] The more common adverse reactions seen with trimethoprim–sulfamethoxazole are rash (rarely including Stevens–Johnson syndrome), fever, leukopenia, elevated serum transaminase levels, and thrombocytopenia. The incidence of these adverse reactions is higher in HIV-infected individuals than in those not infected with HIV. Mild rashes should be watched closely for progression to more severe reactions but are not an absolute contraindication to continuing therapy.[63] This highlights the need for thoughtful consideration of ART components because of overlapping toxicities with some antiretrovirals such as NNRTI, which also are associated with rash and hypersensitivity, including life-threatening cases. For pentamidine, side effects are pronounced and include hypotension, tachycardia, nausea, vomiting, severe hypoglycemia or hyperglycemia, pancreatitis, irreversible diabetes mellitus, elevated serum transaminase levels, nephrotoxicity, leukopenia, and cardiac arrhythmias. Some of these reactions appear to be related to the infusion rate (eg, hypotension and tachycardia) and can be minimized by infusing pentamidine over 1 hour or more.[91] Dosage modification or pharmacokinetic monitoring can reduce the toxicity of both pentamidine and trimethoprim–sulfamethoxazole. Dose reduction of pentamidine from 4 to 3 mg/kg/day appears to be successful in minimizing further rises in serum creatinine levels.[91] As mentioned earlier, early addition of adjunctive corticosteroid therapy to anti-PCP regimens decreases the risk of respiratory failure and improves survival.[63] The adverse effects associated with corticosteroid use for this scenario are minimal, primarily an increased incidence of herpetic lesions, although some concerns exist about the potential for reactivation of tuberculosis or cytomegalovirus and/or long-term effects on bones.[91,93]

Prevention of PCP is clearly a preferable treatment strategy. Primary prophylaxis is recommended for any HIV-infected person who has a CD4 lymphocyte count less than 200 cells/mm^3 (200 × 10^6/L) (or CD4 percentage of total lymphocytes less than14%) or a history of oropharyngeal candidiasis.[63,90] Secondary PCP prophylaxis is recommended for all HIV-infected individuals who have had a previous episode of PCP.

Trimethoprim–sulfamethoxazole is the most effective and least expensive agent and is the preferred therapy for both primary and secondary prophylaxis of PCP in adults and adolescents.[63,90] It also confers cross-protection against toxoplasmosis and many bacterial infections. The recommended dose in adults and adolescents is one double-strength tablet daily, although other regimens, such as one double-strength tablet thrice weekly or one single-strength tablet daily and gradual dose escalation using liquid trimethoprim–sulfamethoxazole, have been used in an attempt to reduce the incidence of adverse reactions and improve compliance. Alternative prophylactic regimens are available if trimethoprim–sulfamethoxazole cannot be tolerated.[63]

In the ART era, the profound reduction in HIV replication and restoration in CD4 cell count to levels rarely associated with the development of OIs provides a basis for the discontinuation of primary and secondary prophylaxis.[63] For PCP, primary prophylaxis should be discontinued in patients receiving and responding to ART who have a CD4 cell count greater than 200 cells/mm^3 (200 × 10^6/L) sustained for at least 3 months, but should be reinstated if the CD4 count drops to less than 200 cells/mm^3 (200 × 10^6/L). The same criteria apply for both discontinuation and reinitiation of secondary prophylaxis of PCP. However, continued secondary prophylaxis should be considered when the original PCP episode occurred at a CD4 count greater than 200 cells/mm^3 (200 × 10^6/L).[63]

Comprehensive recommendations are available for management of PCP and other OIs in the context of HIV infection including prophylaxis, treatment, and removal of prophylaxis with the control of HIV infection.[63] Readers are advised that data continue to emerge on new OI therapies, the safety of stopping primary and secondary prophylaxis, as well as criteria for when to restart secondary prophylaxes. The most current guidelines always should be consulted. Similar OI guidelines have been developed and are updated regularly that are specific to children.[43]

Complications in the ART Era

10 As with any medication, adverse reactions occur with antiretroviral agents that can range from minor intolerances to life-threatening events. Example side effects for each antiretroviral agent are listed in Table 126-4. A comprehensive discussion of all the adverse effects during ART is beyond the scope of this chapter, but can be found in various other sources.[38,55,56] The purpose of this section is to highlight certain medical issues that have emerged in the modern ART era as HIV-infected patients live longer and are exposed to antiretroviral drugs for many years.

Given the life-prolonging effects of ART, as many as half of the HIV-infected population is over 50 years old in resource rich countries.[94] Along with older age come higher rates of well-known chronic and acute illnesses such as osteoporosis and osteopenia, renal and hepatic insufficiency, metabolic syndrome, neurocognitive decline, atherosclerotic disease, frailty, and non-AIDS malignancies. Many of these illnesses occur at higher than expected rates in older HIV-infected patients in the ART era.[95] The cause(s) of these higher rates is the focus of intense study. Initially, adverse events from antiretroviral medications were thought to contribute significantly to these conditions but evidence now suggests that ongoing inflammation and viral persistence play a critical role.[87] Therefore, a theme that emerges in this section is that ART generally protects against non-AIDS events and it is universally recommended to manage these emerging complications.

Non-AIDS malignancies are now a leading cause of mortality in the ART era.[96] While contemporary ART has reduced the incidence of HIV-related cancers such as Kaposi's sarcoma and non-Hodgkin's lymphoma, other non-AIDS-related malignancies impact HIV-infected individuals at significantly elevated rates such as Hodgkin's lymphoma and anal, lung, skin, and hepato-carcinoma.[97] Part of this risk may be attributed to elevated exposures to, or susceptibilities to human papillomavirus (oral and anal cancer), smoking (lung carcinoma), and chronic hepatitis B and/or C coinfection (liver cancer), which are modifiable risk factors. For example, primary care guidelines advocate HPV vaccination for younger HIV infected individuals, as well as increased screening for anal cancer in those with existing genital or anal warts.[36] Concern has been raised that antiretroviral drugs may contribute directly to these increased cancer rates, as some agents have been associated with cancers in retrospective studies, or were associated with cancer in laboratory animals.[98,99] However, there are similar elevated cancer rates in organ transplant recipients with medication-induced immunosuppression, suggesting it is the impairment to the immune system and/or inflammation associated with HIV-infection that is driving much of these higher cancer rates.[100] While the approach to treatment of non-AIDS-related malignancies in HIV-infected patients is similar to that in non-HIV-infected patients, treatment is complicated by drug–drug interactions that may exist between the antiretrovirals and the oncolytics.[101]

Cardiovascular disease has also emerged as a major concern for HIV infected patients. Patients with HIV infection exhibit an approximately 1.5-fold higher risk of cardiovascular disease compared with matched HIV-negative individuals.[94] This increased risk is similar in magnitude to other well-established risk factors such as hypertension and hyperlipidemia. Elevated systemic inflammation and its impact on endothelial structure and function and the clotting cascade is thought to underlie much of this risk, as elevations in circulating IL-6 and D-dimer correlate with clinical outcomes.[102] Antiretroviral drugs may contribute to risk, given the well-known relationships between PIs, efavirenz, and the thymidine analog NRTIs and dyslipidemia (increased triglycerides and low-density lipoproteins [LDL] and decreased high-density lipoproteins [HDL]), abnormal glucose homeostasis (insulin resistance and impaired glucose tolerance), body fat abnormalities (lipoatrophy of the face and extremities and central lipoaccumulation), and lactic acidosis with hepatosteatosis (all the NRTIs).[103] Many agents within these drug classes are less associated with these complications including atazanavir and darunavir for the PIs, nevirapine and rilpivirine for NNRTIs, and lamivudine, emtricitabine, tenofovir, and abacavir for the NRTIs.[103,104] The same appears to be true for InSTI and maraviroc.[104] Retrospective studies have found an association between myocardial infarction and abacavir and didanosine use, but other studies have not, so this association is controversial.[105,106] This controversy highlights the difficulty in using observational and retrospective data to attribute risk to these emerging medical conditions.

Metabolic abnormalities such as hyperlipidemia and hyperglycemia should be treated according to national guidelines for those conditions with the caveat to intensively screen for potential drug–drug interactions.[36] For instance, there is a long history of using β-hydroxy-β-methylglutaryl-coenzyme A (HMG-CoA) reductase inhibitor (statin) therapy for HIV or ART-associated hyperlipidemia. Examples of serious drug–drug interactions include the PIs and lovastatin and simvastatin where plasma area under the concentration–time curve of these statins can be increased more than 10-fold, potentially increasing the risk for rhabdomyolysis.[38] Generally, fluvastatin, pitavistatin, and pravastatin are recommended as alternatives. Atorvastatin or rosuvastatin should be used with caution including initiation with low doses with careful monitoring. There is growing interest for using statins for their anti-inflammatory effects in HIV infected individuals, given the strong relationships between inflammation and cardiovascular disease in this population.[107]

A relevant problem for HIV infected individuals with years of ART experience is body fat abnormalities, as older ART was associated with changes in body fat distribution.[108] The thymidine analogs, particularly stavudine, were associated with lipoatrophy of the subcutaneous fat in the extremities and face, and these agents and older PIs were associated with hypertrophy of the deep abdominal fat depot. Collectively these fat abnormalities were termed HIV lipodystrophy. Newer agents such as abacavir, tenofovir, emtricitabine, darunavir, and InSTI appear to be less associated with lipodystrophy compared with older agents such as stavudine, zidovudine, and indinavir. In patients still taking older ART regimens, this provides a basis for switching therapy to newer regimens, which may result in small gains in subcutaneous fat in those with existing lipoatrophy. Small controlled studies have demonstrated modest but inconsistent gains in subcutaneous fat with thiazolidinedione therapy. Central fat accumulation is difficult to treat. Lifestyle changes, such as reducing calorie intake and increasing aerobic exercise, should be the first-line approach. Metformin reduces central fat accumulation, but lean body mass and subcutaneous fat may exhibit unwanted declines. Tesamorelin, a growth hormone releasing analog was approved to safely reduce central adiposity, although a drawback is that visceral fat returns within months of discontinuation.[108] Unfortunately, both lipoatrophy and fat accumulation eventually may lead to reconstructive surgery strategies in severe or refractory cases. The best management of body fat changes is prevention through initiation of preferred regimens less likely to cause such changes (see current recommendations for initial therapy).[38]

Functional declines of end organs such as kidney, liver and brain (cognition) are another important problem for older HIV infected patients. Like above, these declines appear to be related with HIV infection itself, and some improvement may be seen with therapy, particularly for neurocognitive function.[109,110] However, certain drugs may also exacerbate these issues.[111] The NNRTI efavirenz, for instance, is commonly associated with central nervous system perturbations including somnolence, attention deficits and psychiatric issues. These effects exacerbate neurocognitive impairment, although this is controversial and difficult to disentangle from the effects of HIV.[112] The most important defense against HIV associated neurocognitive decline is durable suppression of viral replication.[111]

HIV also causes a nephropathy (termed HIVAN), most commonly a glomerulopathy that can lead to end stage renal disease in the absence of ART.[113] The incidence of this condition has declined by approximately 60% in the ART era, demonstrating that ART is the most important intervention against HIVAN. African-Americans are more likely to experience HIVAN compared with those of European ancestry. Some antiretroviral drugs impact renal health and these may exacerbate the effects of HIV. For example, atazanavir and lopinavir may crystallize in urine leading to obstruction, whereas tenofovir may injure the proximal tubule leading to fanconi syndrome in rare cases.[114] The newer tenofovir alafenamide pro-drug appears to be less likely to cause proximal tubulopathy—via lower plasma exposures of tenofovir—compared with tenofovir disoproxil.[54] Renal function should be monitored routinely in all HIV-infected patients including consideration for more frequent monitoring for patients receiving the drugs mentioned above.[38]

HIV infected patients experience co-infection with hepatitis B (HBV) and hepatitis C virus (HCV) relatively commonly, and this can influence hepatic declines in this population.[115] For example, up to 30% of HIV-infected patients in the United States have HIV–HCV (approximately 300,000 individuals) including as many as 90% of injection–drug users and 90% of hemophiliacs. HIV worsens the prognosis of HCV by reducing the chance of HCV clearance and accelerating HCV progression. With chronic HCV infection, progression to fibrosis, cirrhosis, and liver failure is several-fold faster in HIV–HCV patients versus HCV-monoinfected patients. ART reduces progression to hepatic decompensation and, among HIV–HCV coinfected population on ART, progression is faster in those who do not fully suppress HIV replication.[115,116] For these reasons, ART is recommended for HIV–HCV coinfected patients and HCV therapy should be offered according to HCV guidelines.[117] The most important consideration for co-treatment is potential drug–drug interactions between ART and HCV therapies. Again, the most recent information should be consulted in reviewing potential interaction.[38,117]

The same general principles extend to HIV-HBV coinfected patients, who comprise approximately 10% of the HIV infected population. [118] However, two unique considerations are relevant for HIV-HBV coinfection. First, the ART regimen should include tenofovir plus either lamivudine or emtricitabine given the HBV activity of these agents. Second, hepatic flares and decompensation has been reported when tenofovir-based therapy was interrupted or discontinued. If discontinuation is necessary, close monitoring of hepatic function is indicated.

PERSONALIZED PHARMACOTHERAPY

Whether the patient will ultimately mount a durable response to ART depends upon adherence, convenience/tolerability, and pharmacologic effectiveness. As discussed throughout this chapter, a great number of considerations go into choosing the optimal ART for a given patient. These factors include: pre-ART disease characteristics (eg, resistance testing, viral load and CD4 count), ART characteristics (eg, co-formulations, food requirements, drug–drug interactions, etc), co-morbid conditions (eg, preexisting renal dysfunction), potential for pregnancy (eg, efavirenz may be excluded), HLA-B5701 and/or tropism testing (if abacavir or maraviroc are being considered), and co infections (eg, TB infection). Thus, the clinician's knowledge of HIV pathophysiology and pharmacologic principles of ART will help determine therapeutic success.

ACKNOWLEDGMENT

This work was supported by Grants U01 AI106499, UM1 AI06701, R01AI093319, and R01 AI124965 from the National Institute of Allergy and Infectious Disease.

DISCLOSURES

Thomas Kakuda is an employee of Alios Biopharma, a Johnson & Johnson company and a stock holder of Johnson & Johnson.

ABBREVIATIONS

AIDS	acquired immunodeficiency syndrome
ART	antiretroviral therapy
CCR5	chemokine (C–C motif) receptor 5
CD	cluster of differentiation
CDC	Centers for Disease Control and Prevention
CXCR4	Chemokine (C-X-C motif) Receptor 4
CYP	cytochrome P450

DHHS	Department of Health and Human Services
ELISA	enzyme-linked immunosorbent assay
FDA	Food and Drug Administration
gp	glycoprotein
HCV	hepatitis C virus
HDL	high density lipoprotein
HIV	human immunodeficiency virus
HLA	human leukocyte antigen
IC_{50}	concentration of antiretroviral agent necessary to inhibit 50% of viral replication
Ig	immunoglobulin
InSTI	integrase strand transfer inhibitor
IRIS	immune reconstitution syndrome
LDL	low-density lipoprotein
LTR	long-terminal repeat
MAC	*Mycobacterium avium* complex
MSM	men who have sex with men
NNRTI	nonnucleoside reverse transcriptase inhibitor
NRTI	nucleoside/nucleotide reverse transcriptase inhibitor
OI	opportunistic infection
PCP	*Pneumocystis jirovecii* (*carinii*) pneumonia
PCR	polymerase chain reaction
PI	protease inhibitor
PEP	postexposure prophylaxis
PrEP	preexposure prophylaxis
RT-PCR	reverse-transcription polymerase chain reaction
SIV	simian immunodeficiency virus
TB	tuberculosis
TDF	tenofovir disoproxil fumarate
WHO	World Health Organization

REFERENCES

1. Fettig J, Swaminathan M, Murrill CS, et al. Global epidemiology of HIV. *Infect Dis Clin North Am* 2014;28(3):323-337.
2. Maartens G, Celum C, Lewin SR. HIV infection: epidemiology, pathogenesis, treatment, and prevention. *Lancet* 2014;384(9939):258-271.
3. Patel P, Borkowf CB, Brooks JT, et al. Estimating per-act HIV transmission risk: a systematic review. *AIDS* 2014;28(10):1509-1519.
4. Centers for Disease Control, Health Resources and Services Administration, National Institutes of Health, American Academy of HIV Medicine, Association of Nurses in AIDS Care, International Association of Providers of AIDS Care, National Minority AIDS Council, and Urban Coalition for HIV/AIDS Prevention Services. Recommendations for HIV prevention with adults and adolescents with HIV in the United States 2014. Available http://stacks.cdc.gov/view/cdc/26063. Accessed Dec. 17, 2015.
5. Cohen MS, Chen YQ, McCauley M, et al. Prevention of HIV-1 infection with early antiretroviral therapy. *N Engl J Med* 2011;365(6):493-505.
6. Baeten JM, Donnell D, Ndase P, et al. Antiretroviral prophylaxis for HIV prevention in heterosexual men and women. *N Engl J Med* 2012;367(5):399-410.
7. Chasela CS, Hudgens MG, Jamieson DJ, et al. Maternal or infant antiretroviral drugs to reduce HIV-1 transmission. *N Engl J Med* 2010;362(24):2271-2281.
8. Grant RM, Lama JR, Anderson PL, et al. Preexposure chemoprophylaxis for HIV prevention in men who have sex with men. *N Engl J Med* 2010;363(27):2587-2599.
9. Friend DR, Kiser PF. Assessment of topical microbicides to prevent HIV-1 transmission: Concepts, testing, lessons learned. *Antiviral Research* 2013;99(3):391-400.
10. Esparza J. A brief history of the global effort to develop a preventive HIV vaccine. *Vaccine* 2013;31(35):3502-3518.
11. Smith DK, Grohskopf LA, Black RJ, et al. Antiretroviral postexposure prophylaxis after sexual, injection-drug use, or other nonoccupational exposure to HIV in the United States: recommendations from the U.S. Department of Health and Human Services. *MMWR Recomm Rep* 2005;54(RR-2):1-20.
12. Zou S, Dodd RY, Stramer SL, et al. Probability of viremia with HBV, HCV, HIV, and HTLV among tissue donors in the United States. *N Engl J Med* 2004;351(8):751-759.
13. Zou S, Stramer SL, Dodd RY. Donor testing and risk: Current prevalence, incidence, and residual risk of transfusion-transmissible agents in US allogeneic donations. *Transfusion Medicine Reviews* 2012;26(2):119-128.
14. Kuhar DT, Henderson DK, Struble KA, et al. Updated US Public Health Service Guidelines for the management of occupational exposures to human immunodeficiency virus and recommendations for postexposure prophylaxis. *Infection Control and Hospital Epidemiology* 2013;34(9):875-892.
15. Magder LS, Mofenson L, Paul ME, et al. Risk factors for in utero and intrapartum transmission of HIV. *J Acquir Immune Defic Syndr* 2005;38(1):87-95.
16. World Health Organization. HIV Transmission through Breastfeeding. 2007. Available at: http://apps.who.int/iris/bitstream/10665/43879/1/9789241596596_eng.pdf. Accessed Dec. 17, 2015.
17. Panel on Treatment of HIV-Infected Pregnant Women and Prevention of Perinatal Transmission. Recommendations for Use of Antiretroviral Drugs in Pregnant HIV-1-Infected Women for Maternal Health and Interventions to Reduce Perinatal HIV Transmission in the United States. Available at: http://aidsinfo.nih.gov/contentfiles/lvguidelines/PerinatalGL.pdf. Accessed 12/17/2015.
18. Revised surveillance case definition for HIV infection--United States, 2014. MMWR Recomm Rep. 2014; 63(RR-03):1-10.
19. Centers for Disease Control and Prevention. Monitoring selected national HIV prevention and care objectives by using HIV surveillance data—United States and 6 dependent areas—2012. HIV Surveillance Supplemental Report. 2014;19(3).
20. Centers for Disease Control and Prevention. HIV/AIDS Basic Statistics. 2015; Available at: http://www.cdc.gov/hiv/statistics/basics.html. Accessed 12-17-2015.
21. Skarbinski J, Rosenberg E, Paz-Bailey G, et al. Human immunodeficiency virus transmission at each step of the care continuum in the United States. *JAMA Intern Med* 2015;175(4):588-596.
22. Ortblad KF, Lozano R, Murray CJ. The burden of HIV: insights from the flobal burden of disease study 2010. *AIDS* 2013;27(13):2003-2017.
23. UNAIDS. How AIDS Changed Everything. 2015. Available at: http://www.unaids.org/sites/default/files/media_asset/MDG6Report_en.pdf. Accessed 12-17-2015.
24. Sharp PM, Hahn BH. Origins of HIV and the AIDS Pandemic. Cold Spring Harbor perspectives in medicine. 2011;1(1).
25. Shaw GM, Hunter E. HIV transmission. Cold Spring Harbor perspectives in medicine. 2012;2(11).
26. Huang Y, Paxton WA, Wolinsky SM, et al. The role of a mutant CCR5 allele in HIV-1 transmission and disease progression. *Nat Med* 1996;2(11):1240-1243.
27. Tang H, Kuhen KL, Wong-Staal F. Lentivirus replication and regulation. *Annu Rev Genet* 1999;33:133-170.
28. Smiley ST, Singh A, Read SW, et al. Progress toward curing HIV infections with hematopoietic stem cell transplantation. *Clin Infect Dis* 2015;60(2):292-297.
29. Chan JK, Greene WC. Dynamic roles for NF-κB in HTLV-I and HIV-1 retroviral pathogenesis. *Immunological Reviews* 2012;246(1):286-310.
30. Cullen BR. Role and mechanism of action of the APOBEC3 family of antiretroviral resistance factors. J Virol. 2006;80(3):1067-1076.
31. Siewe B, Landay A. Key concepts in the early immunology of HIV-1 infection. *Current Infectious Disease Reports* 2012;14(1):102-109.
32. Ho DD, Neumann AU, Perelson AS, et al. Rapid turnover of plasma virions and CD4 lymphocytes in HIV-1 infection. *Nature* 1995;373(6510):123-126.
33. Centers for Disease Control and Prevention. Laboratory testing for the diagnosis of HIV infection: Updated recommendations. 2014. Available at: http://www.cdc.gov/hiv/pdf/hivtestingalgorithmrecommendation-final.pdf. Accessed at 12-17-2015.
34. Branson BM. HIV testing updates and challenges: when regulatory caution and public health imperatives collide. *Curr HIV/AIDS Rep* 2015;12(1):117-1126.
35. Aberg JA, Kaplan JE, Libman H, et al. Primary care guidelines for the management of persons infected with human immunodeficiency virus: 2009 update by the HIV medicine Association of the Infectious Diseases Society of America. *Clin Infect Dis* 2009;49(5):651-681.
36. Aberg JA, Gallant JE, Ghanem KG, et al. Executive summary: Primary care guidelines for the management of persons infected with

HIV: 2013 Update by the HIV Medicine Association of the Infectious Diseases Society of America. *Clin Infect Dis* 2014;58(1):1-10.

37. Branson BM, Handsfield HH, Lampe MA, et al. Revised recommendations for HIV testing of adults, adolescents, and pregnant women in health-care settings. *MMWR Recomm Rep.* 2006;55(RR-14):1-17; quiz CE1-4.
38. Panel on antiretroviral Guidelines for Adults and Adolescents. Guidelines for the use of antiretroviral agents in HIV-1-infected adults and adolescents. Department of Health and Human Services. Available at: http://www.aidsinfo.nih.gov/ContentFiles/AdultandAdolescentGL.pdf. Accessed 12/17/2015.
39. Mellors JW, Munoz A, Giorgi JV, et al. Plasma viral load and CD4+ lymphocytes as prognostic markers of HIV-1 infection. *Annals of Internal Medicine* 1997;126(12):946-954.
40. Richey LE, Halperin J. Acute human immunodeficiency virus infection. *American Journal of Medical Sciences* 2013;345(2):136-142.
41. Khoury M, Kovacs A. Pediatric HIV infection. *Clin Obstet Gynecol* 2001;44(2):243-275.
42. Panel on Antiretroviral Therapy and Medical Management of HIV-Infected Children. Guidelines for the Use of Antiretroviral Agents in Pediatric HIV Infection. Available at: http://aidsinfo.nih.gov/contentfiles/lvguidelines/pediatricguidelines.pdf. Accessed 12/17/2015.
43. Panel on Opportunistic Infections in HIV-Exposed and HIV-Infected Children. Guidelines for the Prevention and Treatment of Opportunistic Infections in HIV-Exposed and HIV-Infected Children. Department of Health and Human Services. Available at: http://aidsinfo.nih.gov/contentfiles/lvguidelines/OI_guidelines_pediatrics.pdf. Accessed 12/17/2015.
44. Walensky RP, Paltiel AD, Losina E, et al. The survival benefits of AIDS treatment in the United States. *J Infect Dis.* 2006;194(1):11-19.
45. NIH Panel to Define Principles of Therapy of HIV Infection. Report of the NIH panel to define principles of therapy of HIV infection. 1997.
46. Initiation of antiretroviral therapy in early asymptomatic HIV infection. *N Engl J Med* 2015;373(9):795-807.
47. A trial of early antiretrovirals and isoniazid preventive therapy in Africa. *N Engl J Med* 2015;373(9):808-822.
48. World Health Organization. Guideline on when to start antiretroviral therapy and pre-exposure prophylaxis for HIV. 2015. Available at: http://www.who.int/hiv/pub/guidelines/earlyrelease-arv/en/. Accessed 12/17/2015.
49. Rerks-Ngarm S, Pitisuttithum P, Nitayaphan S, et al. Vaccination with ALVAC and AIDSVAX to prevent HIV-1 infection in Thailand. *N Engl J Med* 2009.
50. Kim JH, Excler J-L, Michael NL. Lessons from the RV144 Thai Phase III HIV-1 vaccine trial and the search for correlates of protection. *Annual Review of Medicine.* 2015;66(1):423-37.
51. Abrams D, Levy Y, Losso MH, et al. Interleukin-2 therapy in patients with HIV infection. *N Engl J Med* 2009;361(16):1548-1559.
52. Abdool Karim Q, Abdool Karim SS, Frohlich JA, et al. Effectiveness and safety of tenofovir gel, an antiretroviral microbicide, for the prevention of HIV infection in women. *Science* 2010;329(5996):1168-1174.
53. Marrazzo JM, Ramjee G, Richardson BA, et al. Tenofovir-based preexposure prophylaxis for HIV infection among African women. *N Engl J Med.* 2015;372(6):509-518.
54. Mills A, Crofoot GJ, McDonald C, et al. Tenofovir alafenamide versus tenofovir disoproxil fumarate in the first protease inhibitor–based single-tablet regimen for initial HIV-1 therapy: A randomized phase 2 study. *J Acquir Immune Defic Syndr* 2015;69(4):439-445.
55. Calmy A, Hirschel B, Cooper DA, et al. A new era of antiretroviral drug toxicity. *Antivir Ther* 2009;14(2):165-1679.
56. Fernandez-Montero JV, Eugenia E, Barreiro P, et al. Antiretroviral drug-related toxicities–clinical spectrum, prevention, and management. *Expert Opin Drug Saf* 2013;12(5):697-707.
57. Hirsch MS, Gunthard HF, Schapiro JM, et al. Antiretroviral drug resistance testing in adult HIV-1 infection: 2008 recommendations of an International AIDS Society-USA panel. *Clin Infect Dis* 2008;47(2):266-285.
58. Vandamme AM, Camacho RJ, Ceccherini-Silberstein F, et al. European recommendations for the clinical use of HIV drug resistance testing: 2011 update. *AIDS Rev* 2011;13(2):77-108.
59. Telenti A. Safety concerns about CCR5 as an antiviral target. *Curr Opin HIV AIDS* 2009;4(2):131-135.
60. Park TE, Mohamed A, Kalabalik J, et al. Review of integrase strand transfer inhibitors for the treatment of human immunodeficiency virus infection. *Expert Review of Anti-infective Therapy.* 2015;13(10):1195-212.
61. Arts EJ, Hazuda DJ. HIV-1 antiretroviral drug therapy. *Cold Spring Harbor Perspectives in Medicine* 2012;2(4).
62. Spreen WR, Margolis DA, Pottage JC, Jr. Long-acting injectable antiretrovirals for HIV treatment and prevention. *Curr Opin HIV AIDS.* 2013;8(6):565-71.
63. Panel on Opportunistic Infections in HIV-Infected Adults and Adolescents. Guidelines for the prevention and treatment of opportunistic infections in HIV-infected adults and adolescents: recommendations from the Centers for Disease Control and Prevention, the National Institutes of Health, and the HIV Medicine Association of the Infectious Diseases Society of America. Available at http://aidsinfo.nih.gov/contentfiles/lvguidelines/adult_oi.pdf. Accessed 12/17/2015.
64. Fischl MA, Richman DD, Grieco MH, et al. The efficacy of azidothymidine (AZT) in the treatment of patients with AIDS and AIDS-related complex. *N Engl J Med* 1987;317:185-191.
65. Hammer SM, Katzenstein DA, Hughes MD, et al. A trial comparing nucleoside monotherapy with combination therapy in HIV-infected adults with CD4 cell counts from 200 to 500 per cubic millimeter. *N Engl J Med* 1996;335:1081-1090.
66. Hammer S, Squires K, Hughes M, et al. A controlled trial of two nucleoside analogues plus indinavir in persons with human immunodeficiency virus infection and CD4 cell counts of 200 per cubic millimeter or less. AIDS Clinical Trials Group 320 Study Team. *N Engl J Med* 1997;337:725-733.
67. Palella FJ Jr, Delaney KM, Moorman AC, et al. Declining morbidity and mortality among patients with advanced human immunodeficiency virus infection. HIV Outpatient Study Investigators. *N Engl J Med* 1998;338(13):853-860.
68. Sax PE, Wohl D, Yin MT, et al. Tenofovir alafenamide versus tenofovir disoproxil fumarate, coformulated with elvitegravir, cobicistat, and emtricitabine, for initial treatment of HIV-1 infection: two randomised, double-blind, phase 3, non-inferiority trials. *Lancet* 2015;385(9987):2606-2615.
69. Walmsley SL, Antela A, Clumeck N, et al. Dolutegravir plus abacavir-lamivudine for the treatment of HIV-1 infection. *N Engl J Med* 2013;369(19):1807-1818.
70. Genberg BL, Wilson IB, Bangsberg D, et al. Patterns of ART adherence and impact on HIV RNA among patients from the MACH14 study. AIDS. 2012.
71. Parienti J-J, Das-Douglas M, Massari V, et al. Not all missed doses are the same: Sustained NNRTI treatment interruptions predict HIV rebound at low-to-moderate adherence levels. *PLoS ONE* 2008;3(7):e2783.
72. Haberer JE, Musinguzi N, Boum Y, 2nd, et al. Duration of antiretroviral therapy adherence interruption is associated with risk of virologic rebound as determined by real-time adherence monitoring in rural Uganda. *J Acquir Immune Defic Syndr* 2015;70(4):386-392.
73. Gallant JE, DeJesus E, Arribas JR, et al. Tenofovir DF, emtricitabine, and efavirenz vs. zidovudine, lamivudine, and efavirenz for HIV. *N Engl J Med* 2006;354(3):251-260.
74. Sax PE, Tierney C, Collier AC, et al. Abacavir/Lamivudine versus tenofovir DF/emtricitabine as part of combination regimens for initial treatment of HIV: Final results. *Journal of Infectious Diseases* 2011;204(8):1191-1201.
75. Wohl DA, Cohen C, Gallant JE, et al. A randomized, double-blind comparison of single-tablet regimen elvitegravir/cobicistat/emtricitabine/tenofovir DF versus single-tablet regimen efavirenz/emtricitabine/tenofovir DF for initial treatment of HIV-1 infection: Analysis of week 144 results. *J Acquir Immune Defic Syndr* 2014;65(3):e118-e120.
76. Rockstroh JK, DeJesus E, Lennox JL, et al. Durable efficacy and safety of raltegravir versus efavirenz when combined with tenofovir/emtricitabine in treatment-naive HIV-1-infected patients: final 5-year results from STARTMRK. *J Acquir Immune Defic Syndr* 2013;63(1):77-85.
77. Lennox JL, Landovitz RJ, Ribaudo HJ, et al. Efficacy and tolerability of 3 nonnucleoside reverse transcriptase inhibitor-sparing antiretroviral regimens for treatment-naive volunteers infected with HIV-1: a randomized, controlled equivalence trial. *Ann Intern Med* 2014;161(7):461-471.
78. Gammal RS, Court MH, Haidar CE, et al. Clinical Pharmacogenetics Implementation Consortium (CPIC) Guideline for UGT1A1 and Atazanavir Prescribing. *Clin Pharmacol Ther* 2015.
79. Ford N, Mofenson L, Shubber Z, et al. Safety of efavirenz in the first trimester of pregnancy: an updated systematic review and meta-analysis. *AIDS* 2014;28Suppl 2:S123-S131.

80. Smith DK, Koenig LJ, Martin M, et al. Preexposure prophylaxis for the prevention of HIV infection – 2014: a clinical practice guideline. Available at http://stacks.cdc.gov/view/cdc/23109. Accessed Dec. 17, 2015.
81. Grant RM, Liegler T. Weighing the risk of drug resistance with the benefits of HIV preexposure prophylaxis. *J Infect Dis* 2015;211(8):1202-1204.
82. Berhan A, Berhan Y. Virologic response to tipranavir-ritonavir or darunavir-ritonavir based regimens in antiretroviral therapy experienced HIV-1 patients: a meta-analysis and meta-regression of randomized controlled clinical trials. *PLoS ONE* 2013;8(4):e60814.
83. Katlama C, Clotet B, Mills A, et al. Efficacy and safety of etravirine at week 96 in treatment-experienced HIV type-1-infected patients in the DUET-1 and DUET-2 trials. *Antivir Ther*. 2010;15(7):1045-1052.
84. Cahn P, Pozniak AL, Mingrone H, et al. Dolutegravir versus raltegravir in antiretroviral-experienced, integrase-inhibitor-naive adults with HIV: week 48 results from the randomised, double-blind, non-inferiority SAILING study. *Lancet* 2013;382(9893):700-708.
85. Gulick RM, Lalezari J, Goodrich J, et al. Maraviroc for previously treated patients with R5 HIV-1 infection. *N Engl J Med* 2008;359(14):1429-1441.
86. El-Sadr WM, Lundgren J, Neaton JD, et al. CD4+ count-guided interruption of antiretroviral treatment. *N Engl J Med.* 2006 ;355(22):2283-2296.
87. Phillips AN, Neaton J, Lundgren JD. The role of HIV in serious diseases other than AIDS. *AIDS* 2008;22(18):2409-2418.
88. Walker NF, Scriven J, Meintjes G, et al. Immune reconstitution inflammatory syndrome in HIV-infected patients. *HIV AIDS (Auckl)* 2015;7:49-64.
89. Bruchfeld J, Correia-Neves M, Källenius G. Tuberculosis and HIV coinfection. *Cold Spring Harbor Perspectives in Medicine*. 2015;5(7).
90. Krajicek BJ, Thomas CF Jr, Limper AH. Pneumocystis pneumonia: current concepts in pathogenesis, diagnosis, and treatment. *Clin Chest Med* 2009;30(2):265-278, vi.
91. Santamauro J, Stover D. Pneumocystis carinii pneumonia. *Med Clin North Am* 1997;81:299-318.
92. Kovacs JA, Masur H. Evolving health effects of Pneumocystis: one hundred years of progress in diagnosis and treatment. *JAMA* 2009;301(24):2578-2585.
93. Morse CG, Kovacs JA. Metabolic and skeletal complications of HIV infection: the price of success. *JAMA*. 2006;296(7):844-854.
94. Martin-Iguacel R, Llibre JM, Friis-Moller N. Risk of cardiovascular disease in an aging HIV population: Where are we now? *Curr HIV/AIDS Rep* 2015;12(4):375-387.
95. Hunt PW. HIV and aging: emerging research issues. *Curr Opin HIV AIDS*. 2014;9(4):302-308.
96. Smith CJ, Ryom L, Weber R, et al. Trends in underlying causes of death in people with HIV from 1999 to 2011 (D:A:D): a multicohort collaboration. *Lancet*. 2014;384(9939):241-248.
97. Brickman C, Palefsky J. Cancer in the HIV-infected host: Epidemiology and pathogenesis in the antiretroviral era. *Current HIV/AIDS Reports* 2015;12(4):388-396.
98. Wogan GN. Does perinatal antiretroviral therapy create an iatrogenic cancer risk? *Environ Mol Mutagen* 2007;48(3-4):210-214.
99. Bruyand M, Ryom L, Shepherd L, et al. Cancer risk and use of protease inhibitor or nonnucleoside reverse transcriptase inhibitor-based combination antiretroviral therapy: the D: A: D study. *J Acquir Immune Defic Syndr* 2015;68(5):568-577.
100. Grulich AE, van Leeuwen MT, Falster MO, et al. Incidence of cancers in people with HIV/AIDS compared with immunosuppressed transplant recipients: a meta-analysis. *Lancet* 2007;370(9581):59-67.
101. Mounier N, Katlama C, Costagliola D, et al. Drug interactions between antineoplastic and antiretroviral therapies: Implications and management for clinical practice. *Critical Reviews in Oncology/Hematology* 2009;72(1):10-20.
102. Deeks SG, Tracy R, Douek DC. Systemic effects of inflammation on health during chronic HIV infection. *Immunity* 2013;39(4):633-645.
103. Kotler DP. HIV and antiretroviral therapy: lipid abnormalities and associated cardiovascular risk in HIV-infected patients. *J Acquir Immune Defic Syndr* 2008;49Suppl 2:S79-S85.
104. da Cunha J, Maselli LM, Stern AC, et al. Impact of antiretroviral therapy on lipid metabolism of human immunodeficiency virus-infected patients: Old and new drugs. *World Journal of Virology* 2015;4(2):56-77.
105. Ding X, Andraca-Carrera E, Cooper C, et al. No association of abacavir use with myocardial infarction: Findings of an FDA meta-analysis. *J Acquir Immune Defic Syndr* 2012.
106. Marcus JL, Neugebauer RS, Leyden WA, et al. Use of abacavir and risk of cardiovascular disease among HIV-infected individuals. *J Acquir Immune Defic Syndr* 2015.
107. Mitka M. Exploring statins to decrease hiv-related heart disease risk. *JAMA*. 2015;314(7):657-659.
108. Stanley TL, Grinspoon SK. Body composition and metabolic changes in HIV-infected patients. *Journal of Infectious Diseases* 2012; 205(suppl 3):S383-S390.
109. Peluso MJ, Spudich S. Treatment of HIV in the CNS: effects of antiretroviral therapy and the promise of non-antiretroviral therapeutics. *Curr HIV/AIDS Rep* 2014;11(3):353-362.
110. Kalayjian RC, Franceschini N, Gupta SK, et al. Suppression of HIV-1 replication by antiretroviral therapy improves renal function in persons with low CD4 cell counts and chronic kidney disease. *AIDS* 2008;22(4):481-487.
111. Zayyad Z, Spudich S. Neuropathogenesis of HIV: From initial neuroinvasion to HIV-associated neurocognitive disorder (HAND). *Current HIV/AIDS Reports* 2015;12(1):16-24.
112. Apostolova N, Funes HA, Blas-Garcia A, et al. Efavirenz and the CNS: what we already know and questions that need to be answered. *J Antimicrob Chemother* 2015;70(10):2693-2708.
113. Rosenberg AZ, Naicker S, Winkler CA, et al. HIV-associated nephropathies: epidemiology, pathology, mechanisms and treatment. *Nature Reviews Nephrology* 2015;11(3):150-160.
114. Bagnis CI, Stellbrink HJ. Protease inhibitors and renal function in patients with HIV infection: a systematic review. *Infect Dis Ther* 2015.
115. Lo Re V, Kallan MJ, Tate JP, et al. Hepatic decompensation in antiretroviral-treated patients co-infected with HIV and hepatitis C virus compared with hepatitis C virus–monoinfected patients A cohort study. *Ann Intern Med* 2014;160(6):369-379.
116. Anderson JP, Tchetgen Tchetgen EJ, Lo Re V, 3rd, et al. Antiretroviral therapy reduces the rate of hepatic decompensation among HIV- and hepatitis C virus-coinfected veterans. *Clin Infect Dis*. 2014;58(5):719-727.
117. AASLD and IDSA. HCV Guidance: Recommendations for testing, managing, and treating hepatitis C. Available at: http://www.hcvguidelines.org/. Accessed Dec. 17, 2015.
118. Soriano V, Labarga P, de Mendoza C, et al. Emerging challenges in managing hepatitis B in HIV patients. *Curr HIV/AIDS Rep* 2015;12(3):344-352.

Cancer Treatment and Chemotherapy

127

Stacy S. Shord and Lisa M. Cordes

KEY CONCEPTS

1. Carcinogenesis is a multistep process that includes initiation, promotion, conversion, and progression.
2. Cancer cells demonstrate unique traits that distinguish them from normal cells. Cancer cells can stimulate their own growth, resist inhibitory signals, avoid programmed cell death, grow new blood vessels (angiogenesis), invade local tissues, and spread to distant sites (ie, metastases).
3. Screening programs are designed to detect cancers in asymptomatic people who are at risk of a specific cancer.
4. Diagnosis and staging informs the treatment goals and helps select the most appropriate anticancer therapy. The treatment goal may be cure, control, or palliation. The therapy typically includes a combination of surgery, radiation therapy, and systemic anticancer agents. Systemic anticancer agents include chemotherapy, targeted drugs, and biologic therapies.
5. Chemotherapy inhibits cancer growth by killing rapidly proliferating cells. These agents can be identified as either cell-cycle phase-specific, targeting one specific phase of the cell cycle, or cell-cycle phase-nonspecific, targeting all proliferating cells regardless of their place in the cell cycle. Cell-cycle phase-specific chemotherapy is generally given more frequently or as a continuous infusion and cell-cycle phase-nonspecific chemotherapy is usually given as a single dose.
6. Targeted drugs are small molecular weight drugs that inhibit kinases or enzymes responsible for the activation of various proteins that form intracellular signaling cascades. These drugs treat a cancer by correcting a dysregulated signaling pathway.
7. Biologic therapies include cytokines, vaccines, growth factors, and monoclonal antibodies (mAb) with most biologic therapies classified as a mAb. mAb recognize an antigen that is expressed preferentially on cancer cells or target growth factors responsible for cancer growth. These antibodies induce cell death by a variety of mechanisms that involve the host immune system. These antibodies can also be used to deliver drugs, radioisotopes, or toxins to the antigen-expressing cells.
8. Various factors can affect the response and toxicities a patient may experience with anticancer therapy. When determining the optimal therapy, the clinician should carefully consider patient-specific factors, tumor-specific factors, and treatment goals.
9. Myelosuppression is a common acute dose-limiting toxicity for chemotherapy agents. Dose-limiting toxicities are not commonly identified for targeted drugs and biologic therapies. The common toxicities associated with these latter systemic therapies are typically related to the interference with an intracellular signaling pathway and may occur several months after starting therapy.

INTRODUCTION

Cancer is a group of more than 100 different diseases that are characterized by uncontrolled cellular growth, local tissue invasion, and distant metastases. It is the second leading cause of death in Americans. Nearly 1.7 million cases of cancer are projected for 2016 with an estimated 600,000 lives claimed in the United States.[1] Figure 127-1 shows the estimated incidence of common cancers and cancer-related deaths. The most common cancers are prostate, breast, and lung cancer. The most common cause of cancer-related deaths in the United States is lung cancer, which accounts for about 160,000 deaths each year. These cancers are discussed in further detail in the subsequent chapters.

Health professionals treating patients with cancer should have a thorough understanding of the pharmacokinetic, pharmacodynamic, and pharmacogenomic properties of all available anticancer drugs, in addition to the reported safety and efficacy of each drug in each cancer population. Health professionals should be able to critically evaluate, summarize, and communicate the essential information to other health professionals, patients, and caregivers. This chapter defines the etiology, pathology, diagnosis, staging, screening, and treatment; provides general information on how to safely administer systemic anticancer drugs; and presents an overview of common supportive care measures for patients with cancer undergoing anticancer treatment.

ETIOLOGY OF CANCER

Normal healthy cells are strictly regulated, with stimulatory and inhibitory signals in a delicate balance. For normal cells to become cancer cells, it is believed that a physical, chemical or biological agent must damage the cell and cause a genetic or epigenetic alteration that is subsequently propagated during cell division. Cancer cells eventually acquire multiple alterations and these alterations lead to unlimited growth, invasion, and metastases.

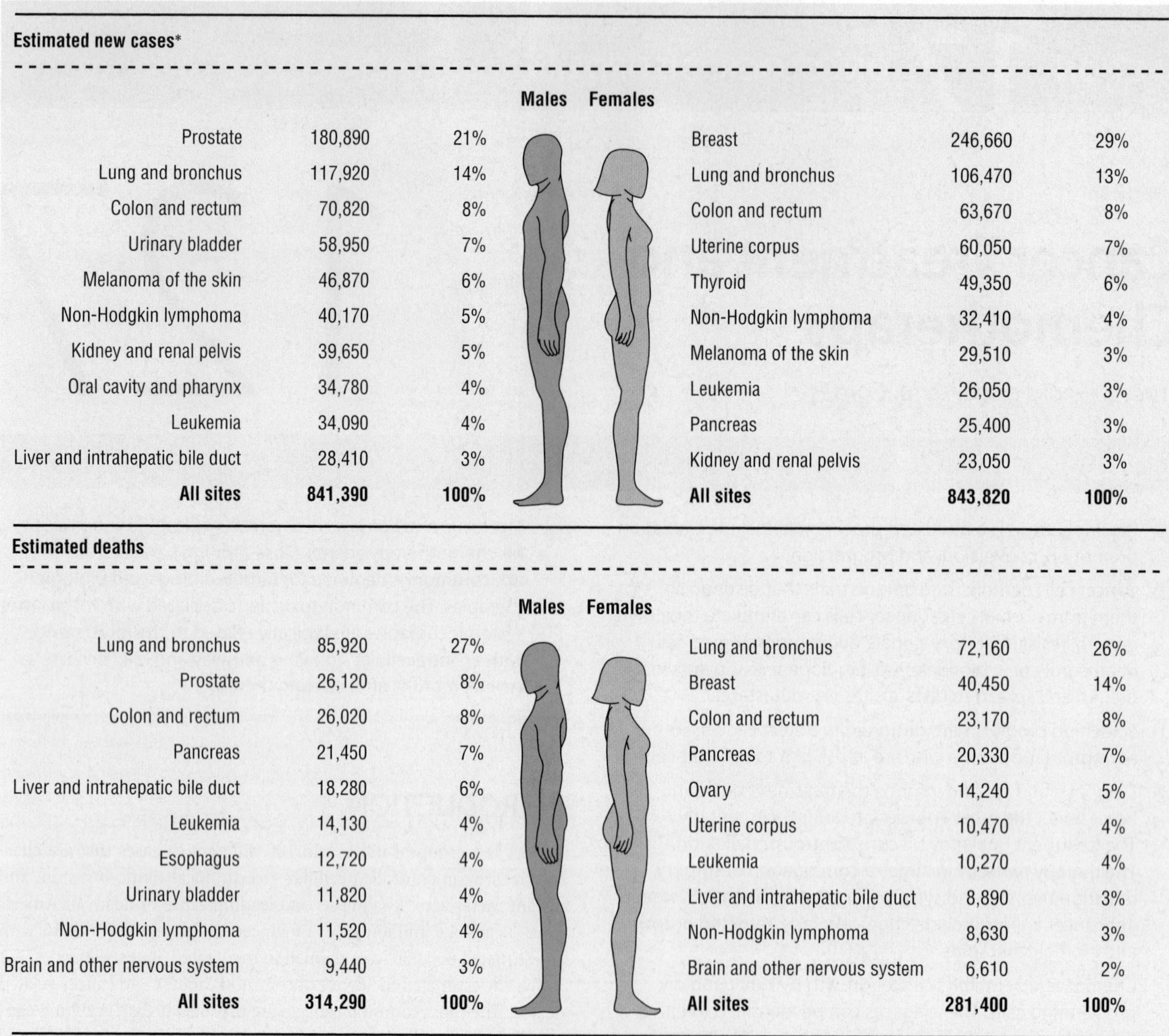

Estimated new cases*

Males			Females		
Prostate	180,890	21%	Breast	246,660	29%
Lung and bronchus	117,920	14%	Lung and bronchus	106,470	13%
Colon and rectum	70,820	8%	Colon and rectum	63,670	8%
Urinary bladder	58,950	7%	Uterine corpus	60,050	7%
Melanoma of the skin	46,870	6%	Thyroid	49,350	6%
Non-Hodgkin lymphoma	40,170	5%	Non-Hodgkin lymphoma	32,410	4%
Kidney and renal pelvis	39,650	5%	Melanoma of the skin	29,510	3%
Oral cavity and pharynx	34,780	4%	Leukemia	26,050	3%
Leukemia	34,090	4%	Pancreas	25,400	3%
Liver and intrahepatic bile duct	28,410	3%	Kidney and renal pelvis	23,050	3%
All sites	**841,390**	**100%**	**All sites**	**843,820**	**100%**

Estimated deaths

Males			Females		
Lung and bronchus	85,920	27%	Lung and bronchus	72,160	26%
Prostate	26,120	8%	Breast	40,450	14%
Colon and rectum	26,020	8%	Colon and rectum	23,170	8%
Pancreas	21,450	7%	Pancreas	20,330	7%
Liver and intrahepatic bile duct	18,280	6%	Ovary	14,240	5%
Leukemia	14,130	4%	Uterine corpus	10,470	4%
Esophagus	12,720	4%	Leukemia	10,270	4%
Urinary bladder	11,820	4%	Liver and intrahepatic bile duct	8,890	3%
Non-Hodgkin lymphoma	11,520	4%	Non-Hodgkin lymphoma	8,630	3%
Brain and other nervous system	9,440	3%	Brain and other nervous system	6,610	2%
All sites	**314,290**	**100%**	**All sites**	**281,400**	**100%**

FIGURE 127-1 Estimated 2016 cancer incidences (top) and deaths (bottom) in the United States for males and females. *Estimates are rounded to the nearest 10 and exclude basal cell and squamous cell skin cancers and in situ carcinoma except urinary bladder. *(Reproduced with permission from Siegel R, Naishadham D, Jemal A. Cancer statistics, 2016. CA Cancer J Clin 2016;66:7-30.)*

Carcinogenesis

1 The mechanisms by which cancers occur are incompletely understood. A cancer is thought to develop from a cell in which the normal mechanisms that control cell growth and proliferation are altered. Current evidence supports the concept of carcinogenesis as a multistage process that is genetically regulated.[2,3] The first step in this process is *initiation*, which requires exposure of normal cells to carcinogens. These carcinogens produce genetic alterations that, if not repaired, results in irreversible cellular changes. The changed cell may subsequently have an altered response to their environment that provides a selective growth advantage and permits the development of a clonal population of cancer cells. During the second step, known as *promotion*, carcinogens or other factors alter the environment to favor growth of the altered cell population compared to normal cells. Promotion could be affected by chemoprevention strategies (strategies to lower cancer risk), including changes in lifestyle and diet. At some point, the altered cell becomes cancerous (*conversion* or *transformation*). Depending on the cancer, 5 to 20 years may elapse between the initiation and the development of a clinically detectable cancer. The final stage, called *progression*, involves further genetic alterations that lead to increased cell proliferation. The critical elements of this phase include invasion into local tissues and the development of metastases.

Substances that may act as carcinogens include a myriad of chemical, physical, and biologic agents.[2] Chemical exposures may occur by occupational and environmental means or by lifestyle habits. Some chemicals associated with cancer include aniline dye, asbestos, and benzene. Aniline dye is a known cause of bladder cancer; benzene is a known cause of leukemia and asbestos is a known cause of mesothelioma. Some drugs and hormones used for therapeutic purposes are also classified as carcinogens (Table 127-1). Physical agents that act as carcinogens include ionizing radiation and ultraviolet light; radiation induces mutations by forming free radicals that damage deoxyribonucleic acid (DNA) and other cellular components. Biologic agents that are associated with certain cancers, include natural compounds (ie, viruses) or pollutants. The Epstein-Barr virus (EBV) may be an important factor in the initiation of Burkitt lymphoma. Likewise, infection with human papilloma virus (HPV) is a cause of cervical and head and neck cancers. Hereditary factors, age, and gender may also contribute to the development of cancer.

TABLE 127-1 Selected Drugs and Hormones Known to Cause Cancer in Humans

Drug or Hormone	Type of Cancer
Alkylating agents (eg, chlorambucil, mechlorethamine, melphalan, and nitrosoureas)	Leukemia
Anabolic steroids	Liver
Analgesics containing phenacetin	Renal, urinary bladder
Anthracyclines (eg, doxorubicin)	Leukemia
Antiestrogens (tamoxifen)	Endometrium
Coal tars (topical)	Skin
Nonsteroidal estrogens (diethylstilbestrol)	Vagina or cervix, endometrium, breast, testes
Steroidal estrogens (estrogen replacement therapy, oral contraceptives)	Endometrium, breast, liver
Epipodophyllotoxins (etoposide, teniposide)	Leukemia
Immunosuppressive drugs (cyclosporine, azathioprine)	Lymphoma, skin
Oxazaphosphorines (cyclophosphamide, ifosfamide)	Urinary bladder, leukemia

Data from Compagni A, Christofori G. Recent advances in research on multistage tumorigenesis. Br J Cancer 2000;83:1 -5 and Stricker TP, Kumar V. Neoplasia. In: Kumar V, Abbas AK, Aster JC, Fausto N, eds. Robbins and Cotran Pathologic Basis of Disease, 8th ed. Philadelphia, PA: Saunders, 2010:259-330.

Genetic Alterations

Clinical **Controversy...**

Can an anticancer drug be selected for an individual patient based on an observed genetic alteration regardless of the underlying disease? For example, a kinase inhibitor has shown to improve survival in a specific cancer. Will this drug prove effective in an individual patient with the same genetic alteration but different underlying cancer?

In recent years, there has been marked progress in our understanding of the genetic changes that lead to the development of cancer.[2,3] Two types of genes play an important role in the development of cancer: oncogenes and tumor suppressor genes. Figure 127-2 illustrates the acquired capabilities of cancer cells that differ from normal cellular function.[4]

Oncogenes

Oncogenes develop from normal genes, called proto-oncogenes. Proto-oncogenes are present in all cells and are essential regulators of normal cellular functions. Genetic alterations of the proto-oncogene through point mutation, chromosomal rearrangement, or gene amplification can activate the oncogene. Carcinogens may cause these genetic alterations or these alterations may be inherited (germ-line mutations). After activation, the oncogene produces either excessive amounts of the normal gene product or an abnormal gene product. The result is dysregulation of normal cell growth and proliferation, which imparts a distinct growth advantage to the cell and increases the probability of transformation. For example, the erythroblastic leukemia viral oncogene (ErbB) family members are oncogenes that mediate cell proliferation and differentiation through activation of intracellular signaling pathways. As an oncogene, the ErbB gene product is typically mutated, overexpressed, or amplified, resulting in excessive cellular proliferation, invasion, and metastasis and increased cell survival in several cancers. Table 127-2 lists examples of oncogenes by their cellular function.

Tumor Suppressor Genes

Tumor suppressor genes regulate and inhibit inappropriate cellular growth and proliferation.[3] Genetic alterations result in loss of control over normal cell growth. Retinoblastoma (Rb1) and TP53 are examples of tumor suppressor genes. Mutation of TP53 is one of the most common genetic alterations associated with cancer. The normal gene product of TP53 is responsible for negative regulation of the cell cycle (ie, a series of cellular events that lead to the division and duplication of a cell), allowing the cell cycle to halt for repairs, corrections, and responses to other external signals. Inactivation of TP53 following a genetic alteration removes this checkpoint, allowing genetic alterations to accumulate within a cell. Mutation of TP53

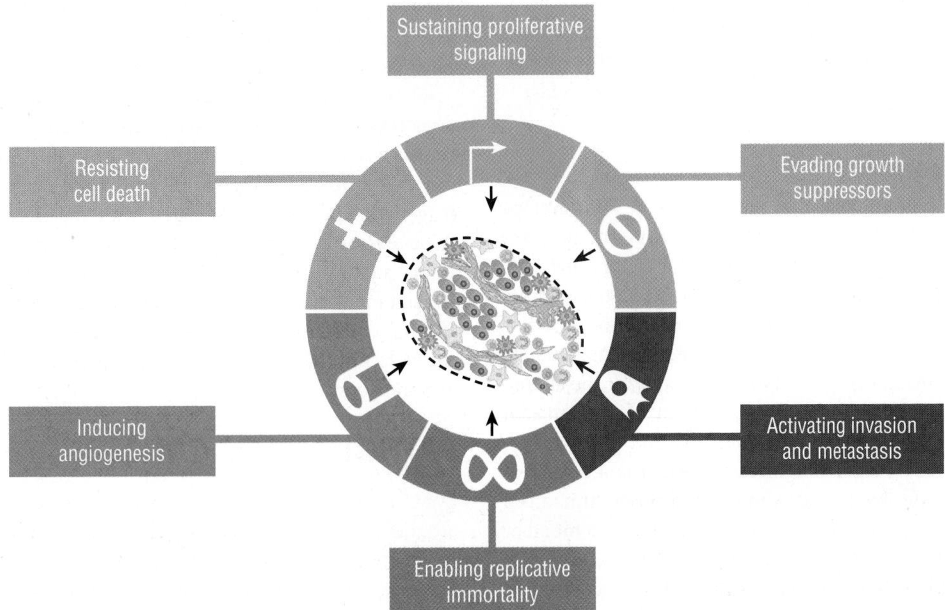

FIGURE 127-2 Functional capabilities acquired by cancer cells, including angiogenesis, self-proliferation, insensitivity to antigrowth signals and limitless growth potential, metastasis, and antiapoptotic effects. It is thought that most, if not all, cancer cells acquire these functions through a variety of mechanisms, including activation of oncogenes and mutations in tumor suppressor genes. *(Reprinted from Cell, Vol 144(5), Hanahan D, Weinberg RA, The Hallmarks of Cancer: The Next Generation, Copyright © 2011, with permission from Elsevier.)*

TABLE 127-2 Examples of Oncogenes and Tumor Suppressor Genes

Gene	Associated Human Cancer
Oncogenes	
ALK	Lung cancer, lymphomas, neuroblastoma, and ovarian cancer
BCR-ABL	Acute lymphoblastic leukemia, chronic myeloid leukemia
BCL-2	B-cell lymphomas
BRAF	Colon cancer, lung cancer, melanoma, ovarian cancer, thyroid cancer
ERBB1	Colon cancer, glioblastoma multiforme, lung cancer
ERBB2	Breast cancer, gastric cancer, lung cancer
KIT (CD117)	Acute leukemia, gastrointestinal stromal tumor, and gastrointestinal stromal tumor
MYC	Acute myeloid leukemia, breast cancer, lung cancer, pancreatic cancer, retinoblastoma, T-cell lymphomas
PI3KCA	Lung cancer, ovarian cancer
RAS (NRAS, HRAS, KRAS)	Colon cancer, melanoma, ovarian cancer, thyroid cancer
RET	Lung cancer, thyroid cancer
Tumor Suppressor Genes	
APC	Colon cancer, thymus cancers
BRCA1, BRCA2	Breast cancer, ovarian cancers
MSH2, MLH1, PMS1, PMS2, MSH6	Colon cancer
NF1, NF2	Leukemias, melanoma
TP53	Multiple cancers
PTEN	Lung cancer, ovarian cancer
RB1	Bladder cancer, retinoblastoma, sarcoma
VHL	Renal cell cancer

Data collated from My Cancer Genome found at http://www.mycancergenome.org/.

is linked to a variety of cancers. For example, a germline mutation in which an individual has only one functional copy of TP53 is associated with Li-Fraumeni syndrome, a syndrome characterized by multiple cancers by early adulthood. Another important function of TP53 may be modulation of cytotoxic drug effects; loss of TP53 is associated with anticancer drug resistance.

DNA Repair Genes

Another important type of gene that plays a role in the development of cancer is the DNA repair genes. Their normal function is to repair DNA that is damaged by environmental factors or errors in DNA that occur during replication.[3] If not corrected, these errors can result in alterations that activate oncogenes or inactivate tumor suppressor genes. Subsequently, more genetic alteration saccumulate within a cell and the risk for transformation increases for the altered cell population. Specifically, DNA repair genes can affect mismatch repair, single-strand break repair, and double-strand break repair. For example, poly ADP ribose polymerase (PARP) is a family of proteins that are responsible for DNA repair and programmed cell death by affecting multiple repair mechanisms.[5] PARP1 is a member of the PARP family that plays a role in repairing single-strand DNA breaks. Deficiencies in DNA repair genes have been discovered in breast, colon, and ovarian cancers.

Accumulation of Genetic Alterations

It has become evident that a single genetic alteration is probably insufficient to initiate cancer.[2,3] Most cancers acquire multiple somatic genetic alterations; some alterations may make no contribution to the development of the cancer (eg, passenger mutations), while other alterations likely support the ongoing survival of the cancer (eg, driver mutations). Scientists postulate that combinations of alterations are required for carcinogenesis and that each alteration is inherited by the next generation of cells. Thus, several detectable genetic alterations may be present in a cancer. Whereas early alterations are found in both premalignant lesions and established cancers, later alterations are found only in an established cancer. This theory of sequential genetic alteration resulting in cancer has been demonstrated in colon cancer. In colon cancer, the initial genetic alteration is believed to be loss of the adenomatous polyposis coli (APC) gene, which results in formation of a small benign polyp (ie, abnormal tissue growth in a mucus membrane). An oncogenic mutation of ras genes is often the next step, leading to enlargement of the polyp. Loss of function of DNA mismatch repair enzymes may occur at many points during the transformation. Loss of TP53 and another gene, believed to be the deleted in colorectal cancer (DCC) gene, completes the transformation. Loss of TP53 may be a late event in the development and progression of colon cancer, as well as other cancers.

Identification of genes and proteins involved in carcinogenesis has several important clinical implications. For example, the identification of the involvement of a gene product in the development of a cancer may lead to the development of new screening tools or anticancer drugs. As another example, specific genetic alterations may also aid in diagnosing specific cancers or identifying the most appropriate anticancer therapy. Many genetic markers have become important prognostic or predictive markers. For example, ErbB2 (also known as, human epidermal growth factor receptor 2 [HER2]) overexpression or amplification predicts response to trastuzumab in breast and gastric cancer and predicts overall survival in women with breast cancer.

Epigenetic Alterations

Epigenetics refers to changes in gene expression that occur without altering the DNA sequence.[6] The two most common mechanisms of epigenetic regulation include methylation and histone modification. DNA methylation commonly occurs at CpG dinucleotides (or islands) and is catalyzed by DNA methyltransferases (DNMTs). Histones are basic proteins associated with DNA in the nucleosome. These proteins may be modified by acetylation, methylation, or phosphorylation on their N-terminal tail. These modifications play a role in transcriptional regulation. For example, histone deacetylases (HDAC) repress transcription and histone acetylases activate transcription. Epigenetic changes may be involved in the development of cancer by either priming the cell or making it susceptible to genetic alterations associated with the development of cancer. As an example, hypermethylation at CpG dinucleotides found near tumor suppressor genes can switch these genes off and promote the development of cancer. Anticancer drugs, identified as inhibitors of DNMT or HDAC, target these modifications. Figure 127-3 shows the effects of these inhibitors on methylation, chromatin formation, and transcription.

PATHOLOGY OF CANCER

2 Cancer cells demonstrate several characteristics that differentiate them from normal cells. These traits include unlimited growth in which the cell cycle is no longer strictly regulated. Genetic alterations permit activation of multiple oncogenes and suppression of various tumor suppressor genes, releasing the cancer cells from the strict regulation observed with healthy cells. The cancer cells subsequently undergo multiple cell divisions, allowing the tumor size to increase exponentially. Cancer cells also resist programmed cell death by inhibiting apoptosis and senescence. Lastly, cancer cells

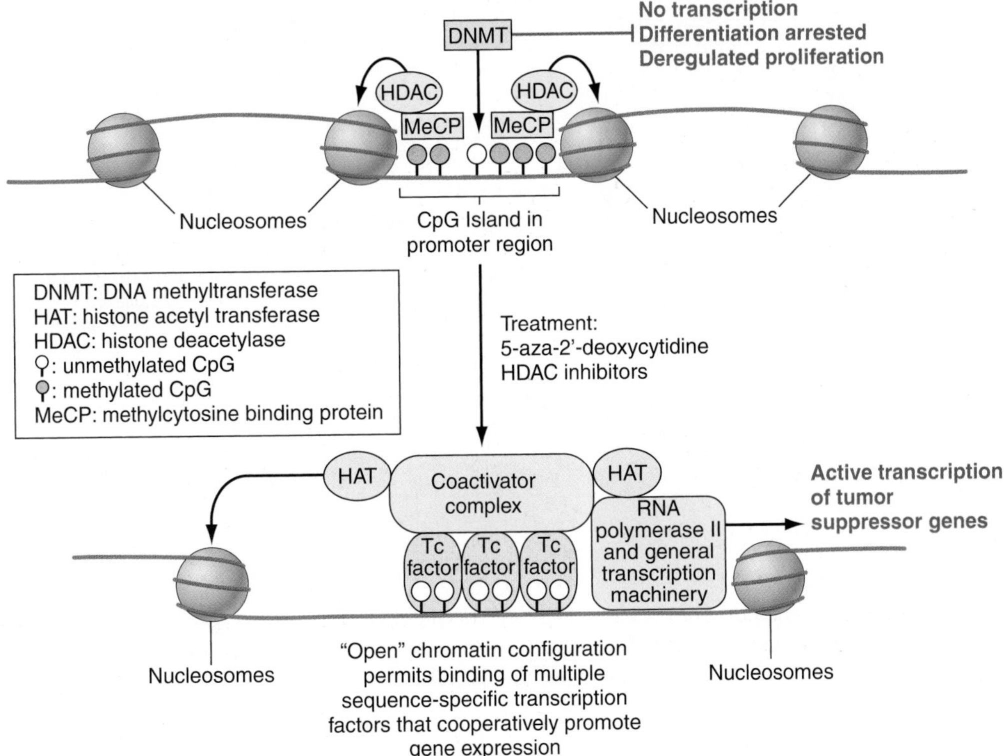

FIGURE 127-3 Epigenetic regulation of gene expression in cancer cells. CpG islands within the promoter and enhancer regions of the gene are methylated, resulting in the complexes with HDAC activity. Chromatin is in a condensed conformation that inhibits transcription (upper figure). Inhibitors of DNMT with inhibitors of HDAC confer a chromatin structure that allows transcription (lower figure). *(Reproduced with permisson from Longo DL. Cancer Cell Biology and Angiogenesis. In: Longo DL, Fauci AS, Kasper DL, et al. eds. Harrison's Principles of Internal Medicine, 18th ed. New York, NY: McGraw-Hill, 2012.)*

grow new blood vessels, invade new local tissue, and spread to distant sites.

Cell Cycle

The cell cycle incorporates a series of events by which normal and cancer cells divide and make new cells. This process is strictly regulated in healthy cells. Oncogenes and tumor suppressor genes provide the stimulatory and inhibitory signals that regulate the cell cycle. These signals converge on a molecular system in the nucleus known as the cell-cycle clock. The function of the clock in healthy cells is to integrate the signal input and to determine if the cell cycle should proceed. The clock is composed of a series of interacting proteins, the most important of which are cyclins and cyclin-dependent kinases (CDKs). Cyclins and CDK promote entry into the cell cycle and are overexpressed in several cancers. CDK inhibitors have been identified as important negative regulators of the cell cycle.

The cell cycle proceeds from one cell division to the next. The cycle involves five phases: DNA replication (S phase), cell division (M phase), two resting phases (G_1 and G_2), and a nondividing state (G_0 phase). In the first resting phase G_1, the cell grows in size and decides to commit to the cell cycle or remain in a resting state. If the cell is normal, the cell will move into the S phase to synthesize its DNA. Next, the cell enters the second resting phase G_2, in which the cell prepares to divide. In the M phase, the cell enters mitosis and yields two daughter cells. If the cell is not healthy the cell can stop dividing and initiate apoptosis. Figure 127-4 depicts the cell cycle and the phases of activity for some chemotherapy agents.

Four checkpoints exist within the cell cycle, one in each phase of the cell cycle, and these checkpoints serve as quality control checkpoints. The cell will not proceed to the next phase unless all requirements for the current phase are met. Complexes of cyclin and CDK regulate these checkpoints. These complexes lead to the activation of other proteins that are responsible for the specific events of each phase of the cell cycle. The first checkpoint is called the restriction site. Rb complexed to a transcription factor called E2F controls the restriction site. The presence of this complex prevents cell cycle progression. A cell can proceed beyond the G_1 restriction site and continue into the S phase, when cyclin–CDK complexes phosphorylate Rb and target it for degradation. A cell may alternatively withdraw into the G_0 phase in the presence of anti-mitogenic or the absence of mitogenic factors.

Defense Systems

When the normal regulatory mechanisms for cell growth fail, backup defense systems may be activated. The secondary defenses include apoptosis (programmed cell death or suicide) and cellular senescence (aging). Apoptosis is a normal mechanism of cell death required for tissue homeostasis. This process is regulated by oncogenes and tumor suppressor genes and is also a mechanism of cell death after exposure to cytotoxins. Overexpression of oncogenes responsible for apoptosis may produce an "immortal" cell, which has increased potential for malignancy. For example, the B-cell lymphoma 2 (BCL-2) is normally located on chromosome 18, but it may be translocated to chromosome 14 in proximity to the immunoglobulin heavy chain gene. This translocation leads to overexpression of BCL-2 in lymphoid malignancies, which decreases apoptosis and confers a survival advantage. As another example, loss of TP53 disrupts normal apoptotic pathways, imparting a survival advantage. Apoptosis may also play an important role as a mechanism of inherent resistance to some chemotherapy agents.

Cellular senescence is another important defense mechanism.[3] Laboratory studies demonstrate that after a cell population has undergone a preset number of doublings, growth stops, and cells die. This is known as senescence, a process that is regulated by telomeres.

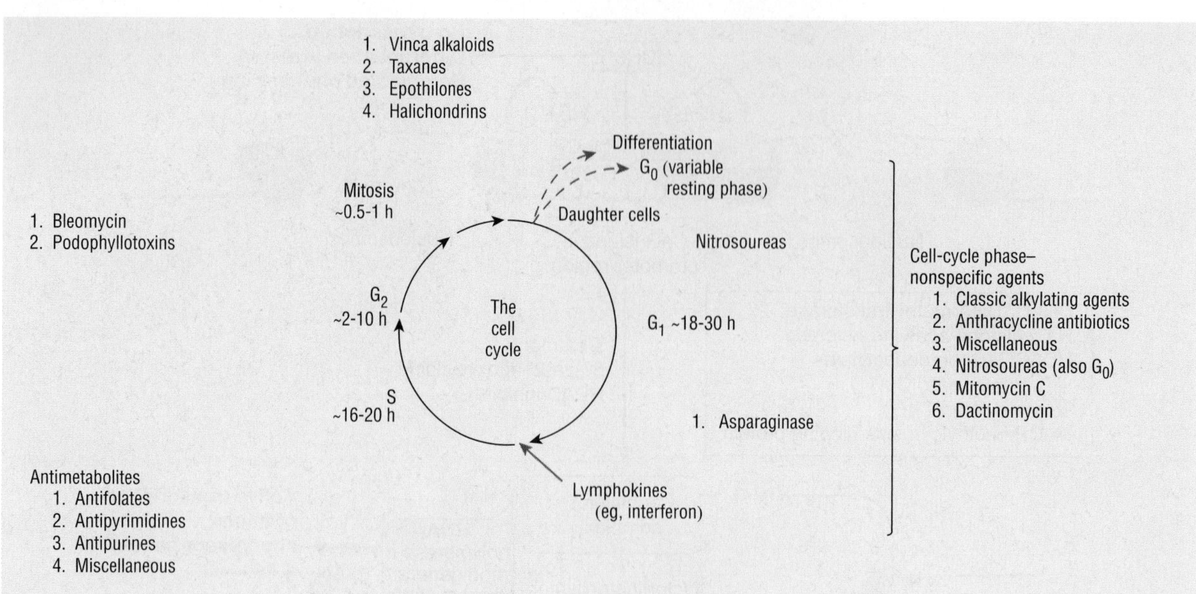

FIGURE 127-4 Cell-cycle activity for chemotherapy. Cell-cycle phase-specific chemotherapy are most active during a particular phase. Cell-cycle phase-nonspecific chemotherapy may have activity in more than one phase. In many cases, it is likely that chemotherapy cytotoxicity involves multiple intracellular sites of action and may not be linked to specific cell-cycle events.

Telomeres are the DNA segments or caps at the ends of chromosomes. They are responsible for protecting the end of the DNA from damage. With each replication, the length of the telomeres is shortened. After the telomeres are shortened to a critical length, senescence is triggered. In this way, telomeres tally and limit the number of cell doublings. In cancer cells, the function of telomeres is overcome by overexpression of an enzyme known as telomerase. Telomerase replaces the portion of the telomeres that is lost with each cell division, thereby avoiding senescence and permitting an infinite number of cell doublings.

Cancer Growth

The study of cancer growth forms the foundation for many of the basic principles of modern chemotherapy. The growth of most cancers is illustrated by the Gompertzian growth curve (Figure 127-5).[3] Gompertz was an insurance actuary who described the relationship between age and expected death. This mathematical model also approximates cancer cell proliferation. In the early stages, cancer growth is exponential, which means that the cancer takes a constant amount of time to double its size. During this early phase, most cancer cells are actively dividing. This population of cells is called the growth fraction. The doubling time, or time required for the cancer to double in size, is very short. Because systemic anticancer drugs typically have a greater effect on rapidly dividing cells, cancers are most sensitive to their effects when the cancer is small and the growth fraction is high. As the cancer grows, the doubling time is slowed. The growth fraction decreases, probably owing to the cancer outgrowing its blood and nutrient supply or the inability of blood and nutrients to diffuse throughout the mass. Wide variability exists in measured doubling times for different cancers. The doubling time of most solid tumors is about 2 to 3 months, but some cancers have doubling times of only days (eg, aggressive non-Hodgkin lymphoma [NHL]).[3]

Tumor burden impacts diagnosis and treatment (Fig. 127-5). Regarding diagnosis, it takes about 10^9 cancer cells (1 g mass, 1 centimeter in diameter) for a cancer to be clinically detectable by palpation or radiography. A cancer of this size has likely undergone about 30 doublings in cell number. It only takes 10 additional doublings for this 1 g mass to reach 1 kg in size. A cancer possessing 10^{12} cells (1 kg mass) is considered lethal. Thus, a cancer is clinically undetectable for most of its life span. Tumor burden also impacts treatment. The cell kill hypothesis states that a certain percentage of cells will be killed with each treatment course. For example, if a cancer consists of 1,000 cells and the first treatment kills 90% of the cells, then 10% or 100 cells remain. The second treatment kills another 90% of cells, and again only 10% or 10 cells remain. According to this hypothesis, the tumor burden will never reach zero. Cancers consisting of less than 10^4 cells are believed to be small enough for elimination by host factors, including immunologic mechanisms. The limitations of this theory are that it assumes all cancers are equally responsive to treatment and that resistance to anticancer drugs and the development of metastases do not occur.[3]

Invasion and Metastasis

As the cancer grows, cancer cells break away or shed from the primary site to invade surrounding tissue and metastasize to distant sites.[2,7] Metastatic disease is associated with a poorer prognosis and shortened survival compared to earlier disease. The cancer cells invade adjacent tissue or metastasize to distant sites by hematogenous or lymphatic spread but, not all of the shed cells result in a metastatic lesion. The shed cells must first find an environment suitable for growth.[7] The onset and time course for the development of metastasis depends largely on the individual cancer, as illustrated by the diverse patterns of metastasis observed for different cancers. Breast cancer, for example, tends to metastasize very early. As another example, prostate cancer commonly metastasizes to bone and colon cancer commonly metastasizes to the liver. Other less common modes of disease spread include dissemination via cerebrospinal fluid and transabdominal spread within the peritoneal cavity.

For a cancer cell to break away from the primary tumor site, the shed cell and surrounding host tissue must first secrete substances that stimulate angiogenesis.[8] The shed cells must then detach from the primary tumor by expressing proteins that degrade the extracellular matrix, such as matrix metalloproteases, and invade surrounding blood and lymph vessels. The cells must then attach to the vascular endothelium. The cells may proliferate within the lumen of the vessel, but most commonly extravasate into the surrounding tissue. The local microenvironment may provide growth factors that can serve as fertilizer to potentiate the development of a metastatic site. At every step, the potential metastatic cell must fight the host immune system. Finally, the metastasis must again initiate angiogenesis to ensure continued growth and proliferation.

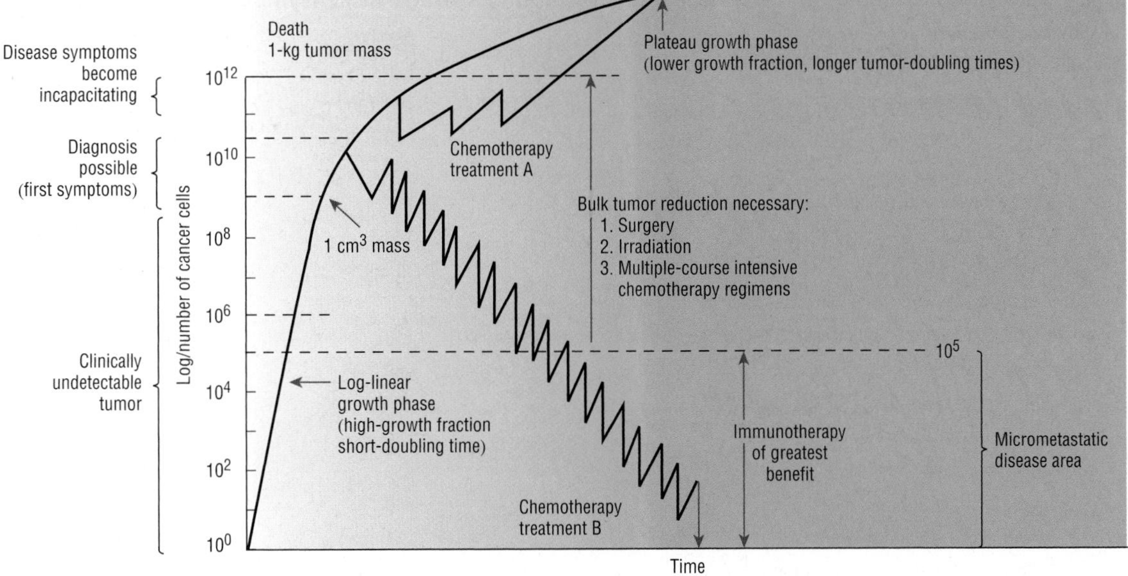

FIGURE 127-5 Gompertzian kinetics tumor-growth curve: relationship to symptoms, diagnosis, and various treatment regimens. *(Reproduced with permission from Buick RN. Cellular basis of chemotherapy. In: Dorr RT, Von Hoff DD, eds. Cancer Chemotherapy Handbook, 2nd ed. New York: Appleton & Lange/McGraw-Hill, 1994:3-14.)*

Angiogenesis is the development of new blood vessels.[9] This process becomes unregulated in several cancers and supports growth, invasion, and metastasis. Angiogenesis is regulated by pro- and anti-angiogenic growth factors, which are released in response to hypoxia and other stresses to the cell. Pro-angiogenic growth factors include vascular endothelial growth factor (VEGF), fibroblast growth factor, platelet-derived growth factor (PDGF) and tumor necrosis factor-alpha (TNF-α). Anti-angiogenic growth factors include interleukin-12 (IL-12), interferon (IFN), and tissue inhibitors of metalloproteinases. The best studied pro-angiogenic factor is VEGF, whose elevated levels have been associated with a poor prognosis and an increased risk of metastases in many cancers, including breast cancer, non-small cell lung cancer (NSCLC), ovarian cancer, and colon cancer. Similar to other growth factors, VEGF binds to specific receptors located on the extracellular domain: VEGFR1, 2, and 3. VEGFR1 and VEGFR2 are expressed primarily in endothelial cells and in some cancer cells and mediate the biologic effects of VEGF. Each of the receptors induces a different signal transduction pathway. These pathways eventually result in the generation of proteases that are necessary for the breakdown of the extracellular matrix. Inhibiting the development of new blood vessels with biologic therapies and targeted drugs can limit or prevent tumor growth.

DIAGNOSIS OF CANCER

Tumors may be either benign or malignant. Benign tumors are noncancerous growths that are often encapsulated, localized, and indolent. Benign tumors are named for the cell or tissue of origin followed by the suffix-oma. The tumor cells resemble the cells from which they developed. These masses seldom metastasize and rarely recur after being removed. In contrast to benign tumors, malignant tumors or cancers invade and destroy the surrounding tissue. The cancer cells are genetically unstable and loss of normal cell architecture results in cells that are atypical of their tissue or cell of origin. These cells lose the ability to perform their usual functions. This loss of structure and function is called anaplasia. Cancers tend to metastasize and consequently, recurrences are common after removal or destruction of the primary tumor. Cancers arising from epithelial cells are called carcinomas and those arising from muscle or connective tissue are called sarcomas. Table 127-3 lists common nomenclature by tissue type.[3]

Screening

3 Because cancers are most curable before they metastasize, early detection and treatment have obvious potential benefits. Cancer

TABLE 127-3 Tumor Classification by Tissue Type

Tissue of Origin	Benign	Malignant
Epithelium		
Surface epithelium	Papilloma	Carcinoma (squamous, epidermoid)
Glandular tissue	Adenoma	Adenocarcinoma
Connective tissue		
Fibrous tissue	Fibroma	Fibrosarcoma
Bone	Osteoma	Osteosarcoma
Smooth muscle	Leiomyoma	Leiomyosarcoma
Striated muscle	Rhabdomyoma	Rhabdomyosarcoma
Fat	Lipoma	Liposarcoma
Lymphoid tissue and hematopoietic cells		
Bone marrow elements		
Lymphoid tissue		Hodgkin and non-Hodgkin lymphoma
Plasma cell		Multiple myeloma
Neural tissue		
Glial tissue	"Benign" gliomas	Glioblastoma multiforme, astrocytoma
Nerve sheath	Neurofibroma	Neurofibrosarcoma
Melanocytes	Pigmented nevus	Melanoma
Mixed tumors		
Gonadal tissue	Teratoma	Teratocarcinoma

Adapted from Stricker TP, Kumar V. Neoplasia. In: Kumar V, Abbas AK, Aster JC, Fausto N, eds. Robbins and Cotran Pathologic Basis of Disease, 8th ed. Philadelphia, PA: Saunders, 2010:259-330. Copyright © 2010, with permission from Elsevier.

TABLE 127-4 Screening Guidelines for Early Detection of Cancer in Average-Risk, Asymptomatic Individuals

Cancer	Test or Procedure	Age (y)	Frequency
Breast[a]	Breast self-examination	≥20	Monthly[b]
	Clinical breast examination	20-39	Every 3 years
		≥40	Every year
	Mammography	≥40	Every year
Cervical[c]	Pap test (conventional or liquid based)	21-29	Every 3 years
		30-65	Every 3 years
	Pap test and HPV DNA test	30-65	Every 5 years
Colorectal	One of the following examination schedules should be followed:		
	Guaic-based fecal occult blood test (FOBT) or fecal immunochemical test (FIT)[d]	≥50	Every year
	Stool DNA test	≥50	Every 3 years
	Flexible sigmoidoscopy	≥50	Every 5 years alone or with FOBT or FIT
	Double contrast barium enema	≥50	Every 5 years
	Colonoscopy	≥50	Every 10 years
	Computed tomography colonography	≥50	Every 5 years
Endometrial	Information on risks and symptoms	Menopause	Once
Lung	Low-dose helical computed tomography	55-74 years	Annually[e]
Prostate	Digital rectal examination and prostate-specific antigen (PSA) blood test	≥50 (average-risk) or ≥45 (high-risk)	Not specified[f]

[a]Annual screening mammography and magnetic resonance imaging (MRI) starting at age 30 years is recommended for women with a known BRCA mutation, women who are untested but have a first-degree relative with a BRCA mutation or other high risk genetic syndrome with known penetrance, or women with an approximately 20% to 25% or greater lifetime risk of breast cancer based on specialized breast cancer risk estimation models capable of pedigree analysis of first degree and second-degree relatives on both the maternal and paternal sides.

[b]Beginning in their early 20s, women should be told about the benefits and limitations of breast self-examination (BSE). The importance of prompt reporting of any new breast symptoms to a healthcare professional should be emphasized. It is acceptable for women to choose not to do BSE or to do BSE irregularly or irregularly.

[c]Women age 65 years and older who have had three or more normal Pap test results and no abnormal Pap tests within the last 10 years and women who have undergone a total hysterectomy may choose to stop cervical cancer screening. Women at any age should NOT be screened annually by any screening method.

[d]Testing at home with adherence to manufacturer's recommendation for collection techniques and number of samples is recommended. FOBT with the single stool sample collected on the clinician's fingertip during a digital rectal examination in the health care setting and guaiac-based toilet bowl FOBT tests also are not recommended.

[e]Clinicians with access to high-volume, high-quality lung cancer screening and treatment centers should initiate a discussion about annual lung cancer screening with apparently healthy patients who have at least a 30 pack-year smoking history and who currently smoke or have quit within the past 15 years. A process of informed and shared decision making with a clinician related to the potential benefits, limitations, and harms associated with screening should occur before any decision is made to initiate annual lung cancer screening. Smoking-cessation counseling remains a high priority for clinical attention in discussions with current smokers.

[f]Menwho have at least a 10-year life expectancy should have an opportunity to make an informed decision with their healthcare provider about whether to be screened for prostate cancer, after receiving information about the potential benefits, risks, and uncertainties associated with prostate cancer screening. Prostate cancer screening should not occur without an informed decision-making process.

Adapted from Smith RA, Manassaram-Baptiste D, Brooks D, et al.. Cancer screening in the United States, 2015: A review of current American Cancer Society guidelines and issues in cancer screening. CA Cancer J Clin 2015;65(1):30-54.

screening programs are designed to detect cancers in individuals who have not yet developed symptoms, but they are only available for a few cancers, such as colon, prostate, breast, and cervical cancers. Available screening tools include the Papanicolaou (Pap) smear test for cervical cancer and mammography for breast cancer. Limitations of the available screening tests include false-negative test results (related to the sensitivity of the test), false-positive test results (related to the specificity), and overdiagnosis (true positives not likely to become clinically significant). For example, most abnormal test results identified by a screening mammography are false-positive, although the specificity of a mammogram exceeds 90%. For most cancers, lack of effective screening methods and inaccessible anatomic sites limit the availability of screening methods. Public education on the early warning signs of common cancers is therefore extremely important for facilitating early detection. The American Cancer Society publishes yearly guidelines for routine screening examinations (Table 127-4).[10]

Diagnosis

4 The presenting signs and symptoms vary widely and depend on the type of cancer. The presentation in adults may include any of the seven warning signs listed in Table 127-5, as well as headaches, weight loss, chronic pain, fatigue, or anorexia.[11] The warning signs of cancer in pediatrics are different and reflect the cancers more common in this population (Table 127-6).[12] The definitive diagnosis of cancer relies on the procurement of a tissue sample and pathologic assessment of this sample. This sample can be obtained by numerous methods, including an excisional, core, or needle aspiration biopsy. A tissue diagnosis is essential, because many benign tumors can masquerade as cancers and most tumors are not cancer. The diagnosis may include evaluation for genetic alterations commonly found in some tumors, such as hormone receptor status in breast cancer or epidermal growth factor receptor (EGFR) status in NSCLC.

TABLE 127-5 Cancer's Seven Warning Signs

Change in bowel or bladder habits
A sore that does not heal
Unusual bleeding or discharge
Thickening or lump in the breast or elsewhere
Indigestion or difficulty in swallowing
Obvious change in wart or mole
Nagging cough or hoarseness
If YOU have a warning signal, see your doctor!

Adapted from American Cancer Society Study Communicating Cancer Information Through Mass Distribution Leaflets–an American Cancer Society Study. CA Cancer J Clin 1967;17:291-293.

TABLE 127-6 Cancer's Warning Signs in Children

Continued, unexplained weight loss
Headaches with vomiting in the morning
Increased swelling or persistent pain in bones or joints
Lump or mass in abdomen, neck, or elsewhere
Development of a whitish appearance in the pupil of the eye
Recurrent fevers not caused by infections
Excessive bruising or bleeding
Noticeable paleness or prolonged tiredness

Staging

Following a pathologic diagnosis, cancers should be staged to determine the extent of disease (ie, tumor location and size) before starting treatment. Staging provides information on prognosis and guides treatment selection. A staging workup may involve physical examination, biopsy, imaging tests (ie, computed tomography scans, magnetic resonance imaging, and positron emission tomography scans), and laboratory tests. The laboratory tests may include tumors markers, antigens or other substances produced by the cancer but, tumor markers are often nonspecific and may be elevated in many different cancers or in patients with nonmalignant diseases. As a result, tumor markers are generally more useful for monitoring response and detecting recurrence than as diagnostic tools. For example, human chorionic gonadotropin (hCG) and alpha-fetoprotein (AFP) in testicular cancer or prostate-specific antigen (PSA) in prostate cancer are useful markers to monitor response or recurrence.[3] After starting treatment, the staging workup is usually repeated to evaluate the effectiveness of the treatment.

The most common staging system for solid tumors is the TNM system that describes the tumor (T), nodes (N) and metastases (M). A numerical value is assigned to each letter to indicate the size or extent of disease. The T describes the size of the primary tumor and spread to adjacent tissues, the N specifies the size, location and number of regional lymph nodes affected by the cancer, and the M describes the presence or absence of metastases. Each letter is followed by an Arabic number that uniquely describes that tumor, node or metastases. After the individual T, N, and M are determined; their values are combined to provide an overall stage that is identified using Roman numerals ranging from stage I to stage IV. For example, stage $T_3 N_1 M_0$, which describes a moderate- to large-sized primary mass with regional lymph node involvement and no distant metastases, is typically a stage III cancer. This simplified staging system allows health professionals to easily identify the extent of disease. For example, stage I usually indicates localized cancer, stages II and III typically indicate local and regional disease, and stage IV typically indicates distant metastases. The criteria for classifying disease extent are quite specific for each different cancer.[12] Alternative staging systems that are used in clinical practice for leukemias and lymphomas as discussed in subsequent chapters.

TREATMENT MODALITIES

Three modalities are used to treat cancer: surgery, radiation, and systemic anticancer agents. These modalities may be used alone, but are typically given sequentially or concurrently to treat a specific cancer. The timing of the different modalities relative to one another is typically based on the outcomes of a clinical trial.

Surgery is the oldest treatment modality and it plays a major role in diagnosis and treatment. It may be curative if the primary cancer has not metastasized. Surgery remains the treatment of choice for most early stage cancers, such as breast and colon cancers. Surgery typically involves removal of the primary tumor and adjacent lymph nodes. This modality may also be used to remove isolated metastases and relieve symptoms associated with metastatic disease. For example, hepatic metastases may be removed for patients with colon cancer.

Radiation therapy can be used alone for localized cancer or for cancer that may encompass a single radiation field. It was first used to treat cancer in the late 1800s and remains a mainstay of treatment for some cancers. Radiation therapy may also be used to alleviate symptoms associated with vena cava syndrome, bone metastases, spinal cord compression, and brain tumors. This modality typically damages normal tissue surrounding the cancer, but the normal tissue typically repairs itself more readily than the cancer cells. Several different types of radiation therapy are available including external beam radiation therapy, stereotactic radiation, brachytherapy, and radioisotopes. Both early and late toxicities associated with radiation therapy are dependent on the organs within the radiation field. For example, mucositis is commonly observed in patients with head and neck cancer. Secondary cancers are a devastating late toxicity that can occur following radiation therapy.

Systemic anticancer agents include chemotherapy, targeted drugs, and biologic therapies. The specific agents will be discussed later in this chapter. In general, systemic anticancer agents have been developed to destroy cancer cells while minimizing effects to healthy cells.

Combined Modality Treatment

As stated earlier in the chapter, a cancer may be treated with multiple modalities. For example, systemic anticancer agents are often administered to patients with local disease (ie, early stage) following surgery or radiation therapy, because most patients with local disease have undetectable metastatic disease (ie, micrometastases) at diagnosis. Localized anticancer treatment alone would likely fail to completely eliminate the cancer. *Adjuvant* therapy is systemic therapy administered to eradicate micrometastatic disease after surgery or radiation. The goal of adjuvant therapy is to reduce recurrence rates and prolong long-term survival. Thus, adjuvant therapy is given to patients with potentially curable cancers who have no clinically detectable disease after surgery or radiation. Because adjuvant therapy is given at a time when the cancer is undetectable (ie, no measurable disease), its effectiveness is evaluated by recurrence rates and survival. The value of adjuvant therapy has been established for the treatment of colorectal and breast cancers. As another example, systemic therapy called *neoadjuvant* or preoperative therapy may be given to patients before surgery or radiation therapy to reduce tumor burden and destroy micrometastases. Neoadjuvant therapy has been given to women with breast cancer to reduce the size of the primary tumor and allow for a less invasive surgical procedure.

The management of hematologic malignancies typically involves the use of systemic anticancer therapies and radiation therapy. Since these cancers are systemic diseases that cannot be effectively treated with localized modalities. Systemic therapy that is administered to eradicate the cancer cells is called *induction* therapy. When a complete remission (the disappearance of all signs of the cancer) is documented, postremission, or *consolidation* therapy is administered. These therapies are designed to eradicate any remaining disease, similar to adjuvant therapy for solid tumors, and can include systemic therapy, a hematopoietic stem cell transplant, or radiation therapy. *Maintenance* therapy is sometimes administered after consolidation therapy. This therapy is given to prevent the cancer from recurring and may include combination chemotherapy. Not all treatment phases are employed for a hematological malignancy.

Goals of Treatment

The goals of treatment depend on the cancer stage and patient factors, such as comorbidities. When an anticancer agent is administered to patients with local or regional disease, the treatment (ie, adjuvant therapy) is often administered to cure the patient and may be labeled as *curative* therapy. When the cancer has metastasized to distant sites, a cure is usually not possible. Anticancer therapy may be administered to patients with metastatic disease to slow the progression of cancer (ie, control) and prolong survival by months to years. If anticancer therapy is given to patients with the goal of reducing symptoms, the treatment is often called *palliative* therapy.

SYSTEMIC ANTICANCER AGENTS

Chemotherapy

5 Chemotherapy was first administered in 1941 when Goodman and Gilman gave nitrogen mustard to patients with lymphoma. These agents typically target DNA. As discussed later in the chapter, a chemotherapy agent is typically given as part of a combination regimen, in which multiple anticancer agents with different mechanisms of action and toxicities are given together. Most chemotherapy agents target rapidly proliferating cells (both normal and cancer cells) and these agents might act at one or more phases of the cell cycle. A chemotherapy agent that demonstrates major activity in a particular phase of the cell cycle is known as a cell-cycle phase-specific agent. For example, antimetabolites exert their effect during the S phase. Cell-cycle phase-specific agents may be less active in other phases of the cell cycle. A cell-cycle phase-nonspecific agent has significant activity in multiple phases. Alkylating agents, such as nitrogen mustards, are examples of cell-cycle phase-nonspecific agents. Despite this classification, it is believed that most chemotherapy agents provide cytotoxic effects following interactions with other intracellular activities, not just specific cell-cycle events. Knowledge of cell-cycle specificity has been used to optimize treatment schedules. For example, a cell-cycle phase-specific chemotherapy agent is typically administered as a continuous infusion or in multiple repeated fractions to maximize the number of cancer cells in the sensitive cell cycle phase. Thus, a cell-cycle phase-specific chemotherapy agent is also termed schedule dependent. In contrast, cell-cycle phase-nonspecific chemotherapy is active in many phases and consequently these agents are not schedule dependent. The activity of these chemotherapy agents depends on the dose, so these chemotherapies are termed dose-dependent. Chemotherapy agents are typically given in a defined repeating schedule called a cycle. The cycle length typically depends on the toxicities associated with the chemotherapy agent, such that sufficient time elapses between doses to allow a patient to adequately recover from a serious adverse event (eg, neutropenia). The number of cycles depends, in part, on the treatment goals. The number of cycles is typically defined by prior clinical trials for early stage disease, while the number of cycles is typically defined by individualized treatment response and tolerability for locally advanced or metastatic disease.

Targeted Drugs and Biologic Therapies

Biologic therapies and targeted drugs interfere with cancer cell proliferation in a different manner compared with chemotherapy. These agents stop cancer progression by blocking aberrant intracellular signaling pathways that govern cell responses, movement, and division. Some of these agents can cause cancer cell death by inducing apoptosis or stimulating the immune system to destroy the cancer cells.

The first targeted drug was developed in the late 1980s. Targeted drugs are small molecular weight drugs (less than 1,000 daltons) that have been specifically designed to interact with extracellular receptors or interfere with intracellular signaling pathways. These drugs are typically given orally once or twice daily until disease progression or unacceptable toxicity. Since resistance commonly develops with targeted drugs, some targeted drugs are administered with other anticancer agents.

Biologic therapies include growth factors, cytokines, enzymes, vaccines, and monoclonal antibodies (mAb). These agents treat cancer by boosting the host immune system and causing the patient's own body to eradicate the cancer. The most common biologic anticancer therapy is a mAb. The first mAb and cytokine for the treatment of cancer were approved in the 1990s. Similar to targeted drugs, most biologic therapies are administered with other anticancer drugs. Both mAbs and targeted drugs have been developed to interfere with intracellular signaling. Whereas mAbs target the extracellular receptors or their natural ligands and prevent ligand binding to the receptor, targeted drugs typically inhibit intracellular kinases. The net effect of both strategies is to interfere with intracellular signal transduction and decrease cell proliferation (Figure 127-6). Some common receptors and pathways affected by available targeted drugs and mAbs include ErbB2 family, mitogen-activated protein kinase (MAPK) pathway and phosphatidylinositide 3-kinase (PI3K) pathway.

ErbB Family

The ErbB family of receptors contains four known members: ErbB1 (EGFR), ErbB2 (HER2), ErbB3, and ErbB4. EGFR and HER2 are overexpressed in several cancers, including breast, lung, gastric, and colon cancers. The roles of the other receptors in cancer growth and proliferation are still under investigation. Members of this family are inactive by themselves and must form a dimer (a molecule composed of two subunits) either with a member of the same family (homodimer) or with a member of a different ErbB family (heterodimer). Dimerization of the receptor leads to kinase phosphorylation and subsequent activation of downstream pathways required to activate signal transduction and cell growth.

Intracellular Signaling Pathways

Well-described intracellular signaling pathways include PI3K, JAK-STAT (Janus kinase–signal transducers and activators of transcription), and MAPK. When these pathways are activated, they promote cell proliferation and survival. These pathways consist of a chain of proteins that ultimately communicate a signal to the DNA found in the nucleus from a cell surface receptor. A protein within a signaling pathway communicates by adding a phosphate group to its neighboring protein; the phosphate groups act as an "on" or "off" switch for the pathway. In cancer, a mutated protein permits the pathway to remain in the "on" or "off" position. The downstream effectors of these pathways also initiate cell cycle progression by promoting the expression of cyclins and repressing the expression of CDK inhibitors.

The MAPK signaling pathway regulates many fundamental cellular processes, including cell differentiation, proliferation, and senescence. These pathways relay the intracellular signals through a series of ras, raf, MEK (mitogen-activated protein kinase-extracellular signal-regulated kinase), and ERK (extracellular signaling receptor kinase) proteins that subsequently phosphorylate and regulate nuclear and cytoplasmic structures. Some of these proteins are commonly altered in pancreatic, melanoma, colorectal, hepatocellular, and other solid tumors.[13]

The PI3K signaling pathway also regulates cell proliferation, growth, survival, and mobility. PI3K becomes activated in response to growth hormones, and it ultimately activates protein kinase B (AKT), a serine–threonine kinase that serves as a master switch for the cell cycle progression. Fully activated AKT translocates to the nucleus, where it can inhibit pro-apoptotic signals and activate anti-apoptotic substrates. It can also phosphorylate mammalian target of rapamycin (mTOR). After being activated, mTOR stimulates protein synthesis by phosphorylating translation regulators. mTOR also contributes to protein degradation and angiogenesis.[14] Phosphatase and tensin homolog (PTEN) is a tumor suppressor gene that blocks intracellular signaling through this pathway and is frequently inactivated in several solid tumors.[15]

The JAK-STAT signaling pathway helps regulate the immune system. This pathway contains three main components: extracellular receptors, JAKs, and STAT. The pathway is initiated when

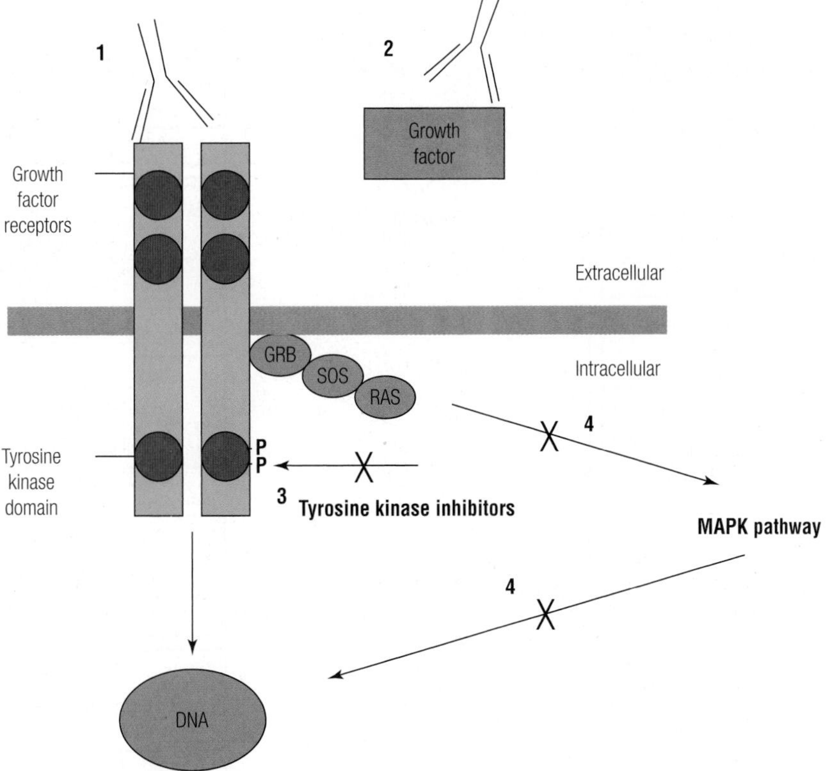

FIGURE 127-6 Common elements of intracellular signaling pathways and targeted strategies that inhibit these pathways, such as (1) mAb against the growth factor receptor, (2) mAb against a growth factor, (3) targeted drugs that inhibit intracellular kinases and prevent subsequent activation of downstream signals, and (4) targeting downstream signals. All targeted drugs have the same goal of decreasing cell proliferation and increasing cancer cell death. (MAPK, mitogen-activated protein kinase.)

cytokines or growth factors bind to the receptor, activate JAK, and subsequently recruit STAT. The STAT proteins then translocate to the nucleus and modify gene expression. Altered JAK signaling has been associated with JAK mutations in patients with myelofibrosis.[16]

Combination Therapy

Although a single anticancer agent may be administered to a cancer patient, the more common approach to systemic therapy is to administer multiple agents. Initially, this approach was based on the Goldie-Coldman hypothesis, which addresses the issue of cancer cell heterogeneity and the inevitable development of drug resistance. The individual agents selected for combination therapy should have different mechanisms of action and adverse event profiles. For example, myelosuppressive agents are typically combined with non-myelosuppressive agents to minimize myelosuppression and other sequela. The individual agents should each have significant activity against the cancer and the combination therapy should have known clinical benefit in the cancer to be treated. Combination regimens that include multiple chemotherapy agents with or without a targeted drug or biologic therapy have been used to successfully manage many cancers for decades. More recently, two targeted drugs have been given together for the treatment of melanoma. Predictive markers, such as HER2 and BRAF, may be used to identify which patients may benefit from combination therapy.

CHEMOTHERAPY

Since all chemotherapy agents interfere with the cellular synthesis of DNA, ribonucleic acid (RNA), and proteins, chemotherapy agents are commonly categorized by their mechanism of action. For example, akylators exert their effects on DNA and protein synthesis by binding to DNA and preventing the unwinding of the DNA molecule. As another example, antimetabolites resemble nucleotide bases or inhibit enzymes involved in the synthesis of DNA and proteins. Figure 127-7 shows the sites of action of common categories of anticancer agents.

The following sections discuss the biochemical classification system and the individual agents within each classification. The clinical uses, mechanisms of action, common toxicities, and practical patient management for most available chemotherapy agents are detailed below. Table 127-7 summarizes dose modifications of individual chemotherapy agents.

Antimetabolites

Antimetabolites are similar to the nucleotides that make up DNA and RNA. The body mistakes these chemotherapy agents for the naturally occurring nucleotide bases and metabolizes these agents as the natural nucleotides. These chemotherapy agents ultimately disrupt replication and cell division by interfering with the production of nucleic acids, DNA, and RNA. Unfortunately, these compounds are not selective for cancer cells and rapidly dividing normal cells may be affected by an antimetabolite. The most common toxicities associated with the antimetabolites are secondary to their effect on rapidly dividing normal cells, such as cells of the bone marrow and gastrointestinal tract. The three major classes of antimetabolites include pyrimidine analogs, purine analogs, and folate antagonists.

Pyrimidine Analogs

Cytarabine Cytarabine is a cytidine analogue commonly used to treat acute myeloid leukemia (AML), acute lymphoblastic leukemia (ALL), and NHL. It is phosphorylated to its active phosphates within cancer cells and inhibits DNA polymerase, an enzyme responsible for strand elongation. It is also incorporated directly into DNA, where it inhibits the replication of DNA and acts as a chain terminator to

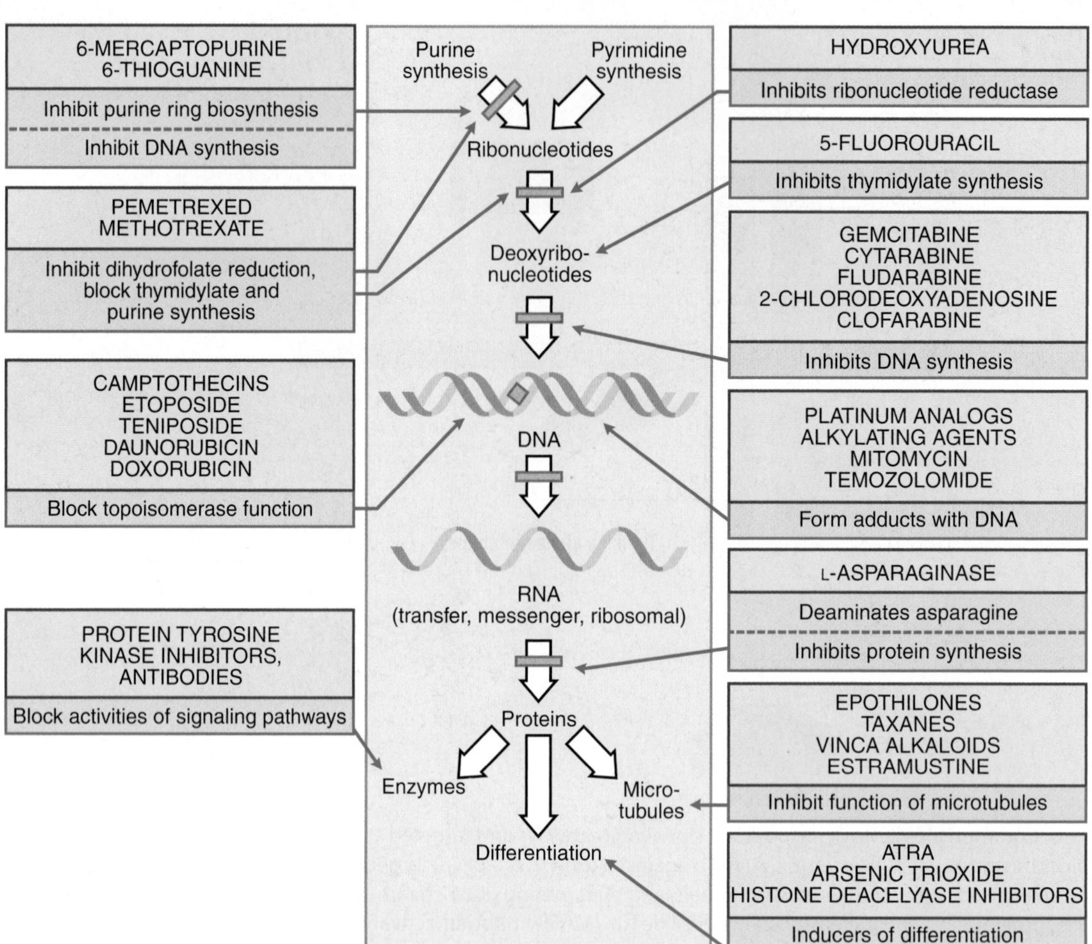

FIGURE 127-7 Mechanisms of action of commonly used anticancer agents. (ATRA, all-trans-retinoic acid) *(Reproduced with permission from Chabner BA. General Principles of Chemotherapy. In: Brunton LL, Chabner BA, Knollman BC (eds). Goodman & Gilman's The Pharmacologic Basis of Therapeutics, 12th ed. New York: McGraw-Hill, 2010.)*

TABLE 127-7 Monitoring of Anticancer Drugs[a]

Agent	Major Adverse Effects	Monitoring Parameters	Comments
Antimetabolites			
Capecitabine	Diarrhea; hand-foot syndrome (palmar–plantar erythema); mild nausea and vomiting	Stool count; hands and feet for early signs of skin breakdown	Adjust dose for renal impairment Oral prodrug of FU Warfarin results in increased anticoagulant effects; may require phenytoin dose reduction
Cladribine	Myelosuppression; fever (onset by day 6, persisting for about 3 days); immunosuppressive; severe opportunistic infections occur	CBC; signs of infection	Risk of opportunistic infections necessitate prophylactic antibiotics for PJP and other infections
Clofarabine	Myelosuppression; elevated liver enzymes; nausea and vomiting; TLS	CBC; liver function; uric acid	
Cytarabine and liposomal cytarabine for intrathecal use	Myelosuppression; nausea and vomiting; diarrhea; mucositis; TLS; flu-like syndrome; rash HDAC toxicities: worsening of above and cerebellar toxicity; conjunctivitis	CBC; signs of infection; renal function; neurologic examinations (signs of confusion)	HDAC infusions should be administered over 2-3 hours to decrease risk of CNS toxicity; use eye drops during treatment and for 48 hours after treatment to prevent conjunctivitis with HDAC Increased HDAC neurotoxicity with impaired renal function
Fludarabine	Myelosuppression, including decreased T cells; diarrhea; rare CNS toxicity: somnolence, peripheral neuropathy, hearing and visual changes, altered mental status, seizures; pulmonary toxicity; TLS	CBC; signs of infection; renal function; neurologic examinations	Adjust dose for renal impairment Risk of opportunistic infections necessitate prophylactic antibiotics for PJP and HSV
Fluorouracil	Mucositis; diarrhea; hand-foot syndrome; myelosuppression; nausea and vomiting; hyperpigmentation; photosensitivity; ocular toxicity; myocardial ischemic symptoms	CBC; stool count; hands and feet for early signs of skin breakdown	Deficiency of DPD correlates with increased toxicity Drug interaction with warfarin: increased anticoagulant effect

(continued)

TABLE 127-7 Monitoring of Anticancer Drugs[a] (*Continued*)

Agent	Major Adverse Effects	Monitoring Parameters	Comments
Gemcitabine	Myelosuppression; flu-like syndrome; rash; elevations in liver transaminases; nausea and vomiting	CBC; liver function	Rash may respond to topical steroids; fevers may respond to acetaminophen
6-Mercaptopurine	Myelosuppression; dry skin; rash; photosensitivity; hepatotoxicity; jaundice and hyperbilirubinemia; nausea and vomiting	CBC; liver function	Allopurinol increases the toxicity of 6-MP by interfering with metabolism 6-MP reduces anticoagulant effects of warfarin
Methotrexate	Myelosuppression; mucositis; renal failure at high doses; nausea and vomiting; CNS toxicity (more severe with IT administration); hepatotoxicity	CBC; liver function; renal function; urine pH and methotrexate drug levels with high-dose therapy	Adjust dose or avoid use with renal impairment; avoid drugs that decrease renal excretion of methotrexate (eg, NSAIDs, PPIs, sulfas and penicillins) Distributes readily into third-space fluids (ascites, pleural effusions), prolonging exposure and increasing toxicity; may be contraindication for use Monitor methotrexate levels with high-dose administration; these must include leucovorin rescue to prevent excessive myelosuppression; sodium bicarbonate also given for high-dose therapy to prevent nephrotoxicity (maintain urine pH >7) Use preservative-free preparations for IT and high-dose administration
Pemetrexed	Myelosuppression; stomatitis; pharyngitis; rash; desquamation	CBC; renal function; skin examinations	Avoid with renal impairment Avoid NSAIDs during administration Supplement with folic acid (400 mcg daily starting 1 week before first dose; continued days after last dose) and vitamin B_{12} (1,000 mcg IM during week before first dose and even cycles thereafter) to decrease myelosuppression Premedicate with dexamethasone (day before, the day of, and day after) to decrease incidence of rash
Trifluridineand tipiracil	Anemia, neutropenia, asthenia/fatigue, nausea, thrombocytopenia, decreased appetite, diarrhea, vomiting, abdominal pain, and pyrexia	CBC; renal function	Consider dose modifications for moderate renal impairment
Microtubule-Targeting Drugs			
Cabazitaxel	Myelosuppression; infection; hypersensitivity reactions; diarrhea; asthenia; renal failure; nausea and vomiting	CBC; signs of infection; stool count; renal function; signs of hypersensitivity reactions; liver function	Avoid with hepatic impairment Premedicate with H_1 and H_2 antagonist plus dexamethasone to decrease risk of hypersensitivity
Docetaxel	Myelosuppression; fluid retention and edema; pleural effusions; ascites; alopecia; rash; peripheral neuropathy; hypersensitivity reactions	CBC; fluid status; liver function	Contraindicated with hepatic impairment (hyperbilirubinemia, elevated transaminases, or elevated alkaline phosphatase) Premedicate with dexamethasone 8 mg orally twice daily for 3 days (starting 1 day before docetaxel) to lower risk of fluid retention
Paclitaxel and nab-paclitaxel	Myelosuppression; infection; hypersensitivity reactions; peripheral neuropathy; myalgias or arthralgias; mucositis; cardiac arrhythmias; alopecia	CBC; signs of infection; signs of hypersensitivity reactions; liver function	Avoid or adjust dose with hepatic impairment Premedicate with dexamethasone, diphenhydramine, and ranitidine 30 minutes before paclitaxel; nab-paclitaxel associated with decreased hypersensitivity reactions and does not require premedication Neurotoxicity may require discontinuation Products are not interchangeable
Vinblastine and vinorelbine	Myelosuppression; mucositis; neurotoxicity; less common than with vincristine; myalgias; SIADH (rarely); vesicant	CBC; liver function	Adjust dose with elevated bilirubin Treat extravasation injury with warm soaks and injection of hyaluronidase
Vincristine	Peripheral neuropathy (highest of vinca alkaloids); motor, sensory, autonomic, and cranial nerves may be affected (paresthesias, ileus, urinary retention, facial palsies) and can be irreversible; SIADH; vesicant	Signs of neurotoxicity (tingling in extremities; constipation, CNS toxicity); liver function	Adjust dose with elevated bilirubin Treat constipation aggressively to prevent ileus Doses are commonly capped at 2 mg to minimize neurotoxicity LETHAL if administered IT Treat extravasation similar to vinblastine

(continued)

TABLE 127-7 Monitoring of Anticancer Drugs[a] (Continued)

Agent	Major Adverse Effects	Monitoring Parameters	Comments
Eribulin	Myelosuppression; peripheral neuropathy; asthenia; alopecia; nausea; constipation	CBC; liver function; renal function; potassium and magnesium levels	Dose reduce for Child-Pugh class A or B hepatic impairment and moderate renal impairment May cause QT prolongation in patients with electrolyte or congenital abnormalities (avoid other drugs that may prolong QT interval)
Ixabepilone	Myelosuppression; peripheral neuropathy; hypersensitivity reactions; asthenia; arthralgias; alopecia	CBC; signs of infection; signs of hypersensitivity reactions; liver function	Avoid or adjust dose with hepatic impairment CYP3A4 substrate, levels may be effected by inducers or inhibitors, avoid use or dose adjustment to ixabepilone may be necessary Premedicate with H_1 and H_2 antagonist
Topoisomerase Inhibitors			
Irinotecan	Diarrhea: acute (within 1 hour of completion; related to cholinergic effects) and delayed (>12 hours after administration; usually after the second or third dose); nausea and vomiting; myelosuppression (neutropenia); alopecia; fatigue; increased liver enzymes; pulmonary toxicity: diffuse infiltrates, fever, dyspnea	CBC; GI symptoms (bowel movements); fluid and electrolytes	Acute diarrhea is best treated or prevented with atropine; delayed diarrhea is managed with antimotility agents Adjust dose (or discontinue) with elevated total bilirubin or UGT1A1 deficiency
Topotecan	Myelosuppression (neutropenia and thrombocytopenia); mucositis; reversible increased liver enzymes	CBC; liver function; renal function	Adjust dose for renal impairment
Daunorubicin and liposomal daunorubicin	Myelosuppression (dose related); mucositis; nausea and vomiting; alopecia; vesicant: severe extravasation injury; cardiac toxicities: acute—not related to cumulative dose; arrhythmias, pericarditis; chronic—cumulative injury to myocardium (total dose >550 mg/m^2)	CBC; LVEF; liver function	Adjust dose for elevated bilirubin LVEF should be >50% to administer safely Liposomal form: decreased risk of cardiac and vesicant toxicity
Doxorubicin and liposomal doxorubicin	Similar to daunorubicin; cardiac toxicity associated with cumulative doses >450-550 mg/m^2; radiation recall reactions	CBC; LVEF; liver function	Adjust dose for elevated bilirubin LVEF should be >50% to administer safely May discolor urine (red-orange) Liposomal form: decreased risk of cardiac and vesicant toxicities
Epirubicin	Similar to daunorubicin; cardiac toxicity associated with cumulative doses >900 mg/m^2	CBC; LVEF; liver function	Adjust dose for elevated bilirubin LVEF should be >50% to administer safely
Etoposide	Myelosuppression; nausea and vomiting: may be worse with oral and high-dose regimens; alopecia; mucositis; hypotension: infusion rate–related; hypersensitivity reactions	CBC; blood pressure	Adjust dose for renal impairment Requires large volumes of fluid for IV administration because of limited solubility (maximum concentration, 0.4 mg/mL) Available orally in liquid-filled gelatin capsules; ~50% bioavailability, but absorption is variable and greater at lower oral doses
Idarubicin	Similar to daunorubicin Total cumulative dose not well established; >150 mg/m^2 reported to be associated with decreased LVEF	CBC; LVEF; liver function	Adjust dose for elevated bilirubin LVEF should be >50% to administer safely
Mitoxantrone	Myelosuppression; nausea and vomiting; mucositis; alopecia; less cardiotoxic than the anthracyclines	CBC; LVEF; liver function	Not a vesicant (may cause vein irritation but not associated with severe tissue injury such as anthracyclines) May discolor urine blue-green
Alkylating Agents			
Bendamustine	Myelosuppression; infection; dermatologic reactions, including Stevens-Johnson syndrome; TLS; infusion reactions	CBC; signs of infection; signs of dermatologic toxicity; uric acid	Not studied in renal impairment Allopurinol may increase risk for Stevens-Johnson's syndrome
Busulfan	Myelosuppression; skin hyperpigmentation; pulmonary fibrosis; gynecomastia; adrenal insufficiency High (HSCT) dose toxicities: seizures; hepatic venoocclusive disease; severe nausea and vomiting	CBC; pulmonary status; liver function; signs of edema (weight gain, fluid status)	Bone marrow recovery may be delayed (3-6 weeks); pulmonary fibrosis associated with >3 years exposure, prior chest radiation Seizure prophylaxis with HSCT doses Pharmacokinetic monitoring is required with IV busulfan IV and oral preparations are not interchangeable; put tablets in gelatin capsules for easier administration with high-dose administration

(continued)

TABLE 127-7 Monitoring of Anticancer Drugs[a] (*Continued*)

Agent	Major Adverse Effects	Monitoring Parameters	Comments
Carboplatin	Myelosuppression (thrombocytopenia); nausea and vomiting (acute and delayed); risk of hypersensitivity reactions at higher cumulative doses (frequently results in cross-hypersensitivity to cisplatin)	CBC; renal function	Calvert formula used to dose carboplatin Lower incidence of nephrotoxicity, neurotoxicity, and nausea and vomiting than cisplatin
Chlorambucil	Myelosuppression; increased liver enzymes; skin rash; menstrual irregularities; pulmonary toxicity; risk of secondary malignancies; causes infertility and sterility; teratogenic	CBC; liver function; pulmonary function	Administer on an empty stomach; food decreases absorption May be dosed in low daily-dosing regimens or in higher dose, "pulse," or intermittent dosing schedules administered biweekly or monthly; pulse dosing may require patients to take several tablets (eg, 10-20 tablets) per dose
Cisplatin	Nephrotoxicity; potassium and magnesium wasting; severe nausea and vomiting (acute or delayed onset); peripheral neuropathy that is cumulative and dose related; ototoxicity; anemia seen with chronic dosing	Renal function; potassium and magnesium levels; GI symptoms (nausea and vomiting)	Adjust dose or avoid with renal impairment Hydration required (1-2 L of 0.9% sodium chloride) minimum before and after administration; ensure good urine output >100 mL/h); potassium chloride and magnesium sulfate in IV fluid to replace losses; dose reduce or consider carboplatin with impaired renal function Aggressive antiemetics required pretreatment and for 3-5 days after to prevent delayed nausea and vomiting Amifostine chemoprotective agent may reduce cisplatin renal toxicity Doses should not exceed 100 mg/m^2 (maximum single dose and per-cycle dose)
Cyclophosphamide	Hemorrhagic cystitis; nausea and vomiting (acute and delayed); myelosuppression; alopecia; SIADH: typically with high doses (>2 g/m^2); risk of secondary malignancies causes infertility and sterility	CBC; renal function; urinalysis	Adjust dose for renal impairment Hydration needed to prevent hemorrhagic cystitis (oral or IV ~3 L/day × 72 h); mesna may be required with high-dose regimens (see ifosfamide) Instruct patients to take oral tablets Administer in the morning to allow for elimination of toxic metabolite; absorbed through skin: avoid spills Drug interactions: CYP450 inducers (eg, barbiturates) may increase formation of toxic metabolites; CYP450 inhibitors (eg, cimetidine) may increase myelosuppression
Ifosfamide	Hemorrhagic cystitis; nephrotoxicity; myelosuppression; CNS effects: somnolence, confusion, disorientation, cerebellar symptoms that are dose-related; nausea and vomiting (acute and delayed); alopecia	CBC; daily urinalysis for blood; renal function	Adjust dose for renal impairment 3-4 L/day fluid for hydration; potassium, magnesium, and phosphate may be required to replace losses Mesna is always given (typically 60%-100% of ifosfamide dose), may be delivered in same IV bag CNS toxicity and nausea and vomiting may be more severe with rapid infusion; case reports suggest methylene blue may be effective treatment for CNS toxicity
Mechlorethamine	Myelosuppression; severe nausea and vomiting; vesicant; secondary malignancies; sterility and infertility	CBC; GI symptoms (nausea and vomiting)	Antidote for extravasation is sodium thiosulfate
Nitrosoureas (carmustine and lomustine)	Myelosuppression; severe nausea and vomiting; cumulative nephrotoxicity; pulmonary fibrosis; facial flushing during infusion	CBC; renal function; pulmonary function	Bone marrow recovery may require 6-8 weeks Carmustine is a vein irritatant, and facial flushing may be related to alcohol vehicle; also available in wafer form for implantation into brain tumor cavities after resection Lomustine is administered orally
Oxaliplatin	Peripheral neuropathy >50% patients: acute form: <14 days, rapid onset, reversible, exacerbated by cold; chronic form: onset >14 days and may be permanent; pharyngolaryngeal dysesthesias; nausea and vomiting; anaphylaxis risk	CBC; renal function; acute and chronic neuropathies	Adjust dose for renal impairment 1 g of magnesium and calcium before and after may be used to prevent neuropathies Avoid exposure to cold
Procarbazine	Myelosuppression; diarrhea; neurotoxicity; neuropathy; flu-like syndrome; infertility and sterility; secondary malignancies	CBC	Administer as a single daily dose on an empty stomach MAOIs that interact with tyramine-rich foods and may precipitate hypertensive crisis; drug interactions: TCAs and SSRIs, sympathomimetics; disulfiram-like reaction with alcohol

(continued)

TABLE 127-7 Monitoring of Anticancer Drugs[a] (Continued)

Agent	Major Adverse Effects	Monitoring Parameters	Comments
Thiotepa	Myelosuppression; nausea and vomiting; mucositis; pruritus and dermatitis	CBC; dermatologic toxicities	Most commonly used in HSCT preparative regimens
Trabectedin	Myelosuppression; rhabdomyolysis; hepatotoxicity; nausea and vomiting; diarrhea or constipation; cardiomyopathy	CBC; creatine phosphokinase; liver function	Extravasation may lead to tissue necrosis
Triazenes (dacarbazine and temozolamide)	Myelosuppression; severe nausea and vomiting; increased liver enzymes; flu-like syndrome (may last for several days after dacarbazine administration); facial flushing; photosensitivity	CBC; liver function	Dispense in a lightproof bags Temozolamide crosses the blood–brain barrier; may cause lymphosuppression when given with radiation therapy; requires PJP prophylaxis
Miscellaneous Agents			
Arsenic trioxide	Differentiation syndrome (pulmonary infiltrates, respiratory distress, fever, and hypotension); QT prolongation; electrolyte abnormalities (hypokalemia or hyperkalemia and hypomagnesemia); hyperglycemia; rash; lightheadedness; fatigue; musculoskeletal pain	ECG and serum electrolytes (calcium, magnesium, potassium) before each course; renal function	Differentiation syndrome must be treated promptly with corticosteroids Do not give if QTc >500 msec Replace electrolytes before therapy
Bleomycin	Anaphylaxis and hypersensitivity reactions; fever and flu-like symptoms; mucositis; pulmonary fibrosis	Obtain PFTs before use and if signs of pulmonary toxicity develop; monitor for anaphylactic reactions	Adjust dose for renal impairment Test dose (1 unit) is recommended but controversial; premedicate for subsequent doses with acetaminophen Pulmonary toxicity associated with cumulative dose >400 units and preexisting pulmonary disease
Hydroxyurea	Myelosuppression; rash; skin hyperpigmentation; TLS; secondary leukemias	CBC; uric acid	Dose may need to be adjusted with renal impairment (use with caution) Used to decrease white blood cell counts rapidly to prevent adverse effects of leukocytosis
Mitomycin C	Myelosuppression (delayed and prolonged); mucositis; nausea and vomiting; vesicant; pulmonary fibrosis; hemolytic anemia and uremic syndrome	CBC; renal function; pulmonary function	Apply ice or cold packs to site for extravasation
Omacetaxine	Myelosuppression (Thrombocytopenia, increased risk of hemorrhage; anemia and neutropenia); diarrhea; nausea; fatigue; asthenia; injection site reaction; pyrexia; infection; lymphopenia; hyperglycemia	CBC; blood glucose	Active in T315I-resistant CML
Retinoids			
Bexarotene	Peripheral edema; insomnia; headache; fever; increased triglycerides and cholesterol; hypothyroidism; leukopenia and anemia; dry skin; increased liver enzymes; pancreatitis; photosensitivity	CBC; liver function; cholesterol and triglyceride levels; thyroid function	Avoid gemfibrozil to treat elevated triglycerides Limit vitamin A supplements May cause hypoglycemia in patients receiving insulin, sulfonylureas, or metformin Teratogenic; contraindicated in pregnancy; female patients should be educated about proper contraceptive measures
Tretinoin (ATRA)	Headache; differentiation syndrome; "ATRA syndrome" consisting of pulmonary symptoms, fever, hypotension, and pleural effusions; dry skin and mucous membranes; mucositis; increases in liver enzymes and bilirubin	CBC; liver function; signs of differentiation syndrome	Differentiation syndrome must be treated promptly with corticosteroids Teratogenic; contraindicated in pregnancy; female patients should be educated about proper contraceptive measures
ALK Inhibitors			
Alectinib	Fatigue; bradycardia; hepatotoxicty; anemia; constipation; edema; myalgia; visual disturbances	CBC; liver function; heart rate; creatine phosphokinase	Administer with food
Ceritinib	Gastrointestinal toxicity; increases in liver enzymes; fatigue; visual disturbances; QT prolongation; bradycardia; hyperglycemia	CBC; renal function; liver function, blood glucose; pancreatic enzymes; cardiac monitoring; electrolytes	Administer on an empty stomach
Crizotinib	Nausea and vomiting; diarrhea; constipation; fatigue; increases in liver enzymes; visual disorders; edema; ILD; QT prolongation; bradycardia	CBC; renal function; liver function; HR and BP; cardiac monitoring; electrolytes; pulmonary symptoms	Visual disorders (visual impairment, blurred vision, and photopsia) occur in approximately half of patients

(continued)

TABLE 127-7 Monitoring of Anticancer Drugs[a] (*Continued*)

Agent	Major Adverse Effects	Monitoring Parameters	Comments
BCR-ABL Inhibitors			
Bosutinib	Nausea and vomiting; edema; pleural effusions and ascites; myelosuppression; CHF; arthralgias; rash; diarrhea; increased liver enzymes; hypophosphatemia	CBC; liver function; electrolytes; Philadelphia chromosome levels; signs of edema	Adjust dose for hepatic impairment Avoid antacids and PPIs Maintenance dose based on CBC
Dasatinib	Nausea and vomiting; edema; pleural effusions and ascites; myelosuppression; CHF; arthralgias; fatigue; rash; diarrhea; increased liver enzymes; QT prolongation; hypophosphatemia and hypocalcemia	CBC; liver function; electrolytes; signs of edema; Philadelphia chromosome levels	Avoid antacids, H_2 antagonists and PPIs Maintenance dose based on CBC
Imatinib	Nausea and vomiting; edema; pleural effusions and ascites; myelosuppression; CHF; arthralgias; rash; diarrhea; increased liver enzymes; hypophosphatemia	CBC; liver function; electrolytes; Philadelphia chromosome levels; signs of edema	Dose adjustments should be considered with severe liver and moderate renal impairment May increase warfarin effects Maintenance dose based on CBC Take with meals and a full glass of water
Nilotinib	Nausea and vomiting; edema; myelosuppression; increased lipase; hyperglycemia; arthralgias; rash; diarrhea; increased liver enzymes; QT prolongation	CBC; liver function; serum lipase; serum glucose; electrolytes; Philadelphia chromosome levels	Adjust dose for hepatic impairment Take on an empty stomach CYP3A4 substrate, avoid inhibitors Maintenance dose based on CBC
Ponatinib	Myelosuppression; hypertension; rash; abdominal pain; fatigue; headache; dry skin; constipation; arthralgia; nausea; pyrexia; thromboembolic events; hepatotoxicity; congestive heart failure; pancreatitis; hemorrhage (secondary to thrombocytopenia); fluid retention	Cardiac monitoring (CHF, arrhythmias); BP; pancreatic enzymes; fluid retention; CBC; liver function	May need to decrease or hold therapy if hepatotoxicity develops Avoid antacids and drugs that decrease gastric pH
BRAF Inhibitors			
Dabrafenib	Papilloma; arthralgia; alopecia; fatigue; headache; HFSR; pyrexia	CBC; serum glucose; electrolytes; renal function; dermatologic evaluations	Take on an empty stomach
Vemurafenib	Papilloma; arthralgia; alopecia; fatigue; headache; photosensitivity reaction; hypersensitivity reactions; QT prolongation	Liver function; electrolytes; cardiac monitoring; dermatologic evaluations	Radiation sensitization/recall
BTK Inhibitor			
Ibrutinib	Diarrhea; fatigue; musculoskeletal pain; nausea; rash; atrial fibrillation; hemorrhage; tumor lysis syndrome; bone marrow suppression	CBC; renal function; hepatic function; uric acid levels; electrolytes; cardiac monitoring	Reduce dose with hepatic impairment
CDK Inhibitor			
Palbociclib	Thromboembolic events; infection; bone marrow suppression; gastrointestinal toxicity	CBC; infection	Administer with food
DNA Methyltransferase Inhibitors			
Azacitidine and decitabine	Myelosuppression and infection; constitutional symptoms; musculoskeletal symptoms (arthralgias); cough; dyspnea	CBC; infection	
EGFR Inhibitors			
Afatinib	Rash; diarrhea; ILD; keratitis	Liver function; renal function; dermatologic evaluations; electrolytes; LVEF in patients with cardiac risk factors; pulmonary symptoms	Administer on an empty stomach
Erlotinib	Rash; diarrhea; ILD, hepatic and renal failure reported	Liver function; renal function; electrolytes; pulmonary symptoms; dermatologic evaluations	Dose reductions or delays may be required for rash, but supportive care should be attempted first Major interaction with warfarin, leading to increased bleeding risk H_2 antagonists, PPIs, and antacids may decrease drug levels Administer on an empty stomach as food increases absorption and possibly toxicity
Gefitinib	Similar to erlotinib	Liver function; renal function; electrolytes; pulmonary symptoms; dermatologic evaluations	Similar precautions and drug interactions as with erlotinib

(continued)

TABLE 127-7 Monitoring of Anticancer Drugs[a] (*Continued*)

Agent	Major Adverse Effects	Monitoring Parameters	Comments
Lapatinib	Diarrhea; rash; nausea; vomiting; fatigue; decreases in LVEF; hepatotoxicity; QT prolongation; ILD	Liver function; cardiac monitoring (LVEF, QT, MUGA); electrolytes; pulmonary symptoms	Adjust dose for severe hepatic impairment Administer on empty stomach Avoid strong CYP3A4 inhibitors, (if unavoidable, consider dose reduction); avoid strong CYP3A4 inducers (if unavoidable, consider gradual dose increases)
Osimertinib	Gastrointestinal toxicity; dermotologic toxicity; ILD/pneumonitis; pneumonia; pulmonary embolism; cardiomyopathy; QT prolongation	Cardiac monitoring (LVEF, QT); pulmonary symptoms; dermatologic evaluations	Avoid strong CYP3A4 inhibitors and inducers
Hedgehog Inhibitors			
Sonidegib	Fatigue; alopecia; amenorrhea; musculoskeletal toxicity; teratogenic effects	Pregnancy status; creatine phosphokinase; renal function; liver function	Boxed waring for severe birth defects and embryo-fetal death; advise females to use contraception during treatment and for 20 months after the last dose; advise males to use condoms during treatment and for at least 8 months after the last dose; do not donate blood during treatment and for 20 months after the last dose; do not donate sperm during treatment and for 8 months after the last dose Avoid strong and moderate CYP3A modulators; moderate CYP3A inhibitors may be used for short-term
Vismodegib	Muscle spasms; alopecia; dysgeusia; fatigue; nausea; vomiting; diarrhea; decreased appetite; constipation; arthralgias; teratogenic effects	Pregnancy status	Boxed warning for severe birth defects and embryo-fetal death; patients should not donate blood or blood products while receiving vismodegib and for at least 7 months after the last dose; verify pregnancy status within 7 days prior to treatment initiation; do not donate sperm during treatment and for 3 months after the last dose
Histone Deacetylase Inhibitors			
Belinostat	Pyrexia; nausea; fatigue; anemia; hepatotoxicity; infection; tumor lysis syndrome	Liver function; renal function; CBC; electrolytes, uric acid levels	
Panobinostat	Cardiotoxicity; nausea; vomiting; diarrhea; hemorrhage; infection; hepatotoxicity	Cardiac monitoring; electrolytes, CBC; liver function; pregnancy status	Boxed warnings for cardiovascular events and gastrointestional events
Romidepsin	Neutropenia; lymphopenia; thrombocytopenia; infection; nausea; fatigue; vomiting; anorexia; anemia; ECG T-wave changes	CBC; cardiac monitoring (ECG); electrolytes	Monitor INR if patient on warfarin
Vorinostat	Diarrhea; fatigue; nausea; thrombocytopenia; anorexia; dysgeusia; thromboembolic events; hyperglycemia	CBC; electrolytes; serum glucose; renal function	Avoid or adjust dose for hepatic impairment Increase in INR with concomitant warfarin Severe thrombocytopenia and GI bleeding have been reported with concomitant use with vorinostat and other HDAC inhibitors (eg, valproic acid)
JAK Inhibitor			
Ruxolitinib	Thrombocytopenia; anemia; bruising; dizziness; headache; infections; cardiovascular abnormalities	CBC; renal function; liver function; cardiac monitoring	Consider adjust dose for renal and hepatic impairment
MEK Inhibitor			
Trametinib	Diarrhea; lymphedema; hemorrhage; venous thromboembolism; febrile reactions; cardiomyopathy; dermatologic toxicity; hyperglycemia; hypertension; ophthalmic events	CBC; liver function; LVEF; ophthalmologic evaluation; dermatologic evaluation; BP	Capsules are stored refrigerated Administer on an empty stomach
Cobimetinib	Dermatologic toxicity; nausea and vomiting; pyrexia; hemorrhage; new primary malignancies; cardiomyopathy; ophthalmic events; hepatotoxicity; rhabdomyolysis	CBC; liver function; signs of bleeding; dermatologic evaluation; ophthalmologic evaluation; LVEF; creatine phosphokinase; electrolytes	Avoid coadministration with strong or moderate CYP3A inducers or inhibitors

(continued)

TABLE 127-7 Monitoring of Anticancer Drugs[a] (*Continued*)

Agent	Major Adverse Effects	Monitoring Parameters	Comments
mTOR Inhibitors			
Everolimus	Rash; asthenia; stomatitis; nausea; edema; anorexia; anemia; pneumonitis; hyperglycemia; hyperlipidemia; hypertriglyceridemia; hypophosphatemia; elevated liver enzymes; elevated Scr; lymphopenia; thrombocytopenia; leukopenia; infection	Blood glucose; cholesterol and triglyceride levels; CBC, renal function; liver function; electrolytes; pulmonary symptoms	Adjust dose for hepatic impairment Initiation or increase in cholesterol or diabetic medications often needed CYP3A4 and Pgp substrate, may require dose adjustment based on concurrent medication
Temsirolimus	Similar to everolimus with addition of infusion-related reactions	Similar to everolimus; infusion reactions	Adjust dose for hepatic impairment Requires diphenhydramine premedication
Multikinase Inhibitors			
Axitinib	Diarrhea; rash; HFSR; bleeding; thrombotic events; hypertension; hepatotoxicity; hypothyroidism; proteinuria; GI perforation; fatigue; rare reports of progressive multifocal leukoencephalopathy	CBC; liver function; BP; thyroid function; urine protein; neurologic evaluation; dermatologic evaluation	Adjust dose for hepatic impairment Substrate of CYP3A4, may require dose adjustment based on concurrent medication administered
Cabozantinib	Diarrhea; stomatitis; HFSR; decreased weight; decreased appetite; nausea; fatigue; oral pain; hair color changes; dysgeusia; hypertension; abdominal pain; constipation; increased liver enzymes; proteinuria; lymphopenia; neutropenia; thrombocytopenia; hypocalcemia; hypophosphatemia; GI perforations and fistulas and hemorrhage have been reported	Signs and symptoms of bleeding; BP; urine protein; CBC; liver function; thyroid function; electrolytes, dermatologic evaluation	Administer on an empty stomach CYP3A4 substrate, monitor for drug interactions
Lenvatinib	Hypertension; fatigue; diarrhea; proteinuria; stomatitis; HFSR; hypothyroidism; hepatotoxicity; thromboembolic events; renal toxicity; hypocalcemia	Liver function; renal function; thyroid function; BP; electrolytes	Adjust dose for in severe hepatic and renal impairment
Pazopanib	Diarrhea; hypertension; hair/skin hypopigmentation; nausea; anorexia; vomiting; decreased weight; fatigue; musculoskeletal pain; dysguesia; dyspnea; hypothyroidism; proteinuria; fatal hepatotoxicity; thromboembolic events	Liver function; cardiac monitoring (ECG); BP; thyroid function; urine protein; dermatologic evaluation	Adjust dose for hepatic impairment Take on empty stomach Reduce dose when administered with strong CYP3A4 inhibitors; avoid CYP3A4 inducers; concomitant use with simvastatin increases liver enzymes
Regorafenib	Asthenia; fatigue; decreased appetite; HFSR; diarrhea; mucositis; weight loss; infection; hypertension; dysphonia; hepatotoxicity; hemorrhage	Liver function; BP; dermatologic evaluation	Administer with food, low-fat breakfast that contains <30% fat Monitor INR closely if on concomitant warfarin because of an increased risk of hemorrhage with regorafenib
Sorafenib	Diarrhea; rash; HFSR; fatigue; hypertension; prolonged QT interval; cardiac events (including MI); drug-induced hepatitis	BP; liver function; cardiac monitoring; electrolytes; dermatologic evaluation	Administer on an empty stomach May increase the anticoagulation effects of warfarin
Sunitinib	Diarrhea; rash; bleeding; CHF and cardiac effects; QT prolongation; fatigue; hypertension; hepatotoxicity; thyroid dysfunction	CBC; liver function; BP; thyroid function; cardiac monitoring (CHF, ECG); electrolytes	CYP3A4 substrate, may require dose adjustment based on concurrent medication administered
Vandetanib	Diarrhea; rash; acne; nausea; hypertension; headache; fatigue; upper respiratory tract infections; decreased appetite; abdominal pain; prolonged QT interval, torsades de pointes, and sudden death; ILD; hemorrhage; increased liver enzymes	Liver function; electrolytes; cardiac monitoring (QT); BP; pulmonary symptoms; dermatologic evaluation	REMS program for QT prolongation/sudden death Adjust dose for renal impairment Avoid other medications that prolong the QT interval Advise patients to wear sunscreen and protective clothing when exposed to sun
PARP Inhibitor			
Olaparib	Fatigue; musculoskeletal pain; dermatitis; nausea/vomiting; upper respiratory infections; anemia; pneumonitis; secondary malignancies (MDS/AML)	CBC; pulmonary symptoms	
PI3K Inhibitor			
Idelalisib	Gastrointestional disorders; pneumonitis; neutropenia; fever; rash; elevated liver enzymes; dermatologic toxicity	Liver function; CBC; dermatologic evaluation; pulmonary symptoms	Boxed warnings for hepatotoxicity, diarrhea, colitis, pneumonitis, intestinal perforation

(*continued*)

TABLE 127-7 Monitoring of Anticancer Drugs[a] (*Continued*)

Agent	Major Adverse Effects	Monitoring Parameters	Comments
Proteasome Inhibitors			
Bortezomib	Fatigue or malaise; nausea; diarrhea; anorexia; constipation; vomiting; myelosuppression, especially thrombocytopenia; hyponatremia; hypokalemia; peripheral neuropathy, cumulative and dose-related; fever	CBC; thyroid function; symptoms of neuropathy; electrolytes	Adjust dose for hepatic impairment Administer IV or subcutaneous (subcutaneous administration has been shown to decrease neuropathies) Increased risk of severe neuropathy with preexisting neuropathy Co-administration with strong CYP3A4 inhibitors can increase bortezomib concentrations
Carfilzomib	Fatigue; anemia; thrombocytopenia; nausea; diarrhea; dyspnea; pyrexia; infusion-related reactions; rare reports of cardiac arrest, CHF, and MI	Symptoms of dyspnea; CBC; liver function; cardiac monitoring; infusion reactions	Premedicate with dexamethasone before all cycle 1 doses, during the first cycle of dose escalation, and if infusion reaction symptoms develop
Ixazomib	Gastrointestinal toxicity; thrombocytopenia; perhipheral neuropathy; edema; back pain; cutaneous reactions	CBC; liver function; dermatologic evaluation	Administer on an empty stomach Reduce starting dose for hepatic or renal impairment Avoid use with strong CYP3A4 inducers
Miscellaneous Small Molecule Inhibitors			
Lanreotide	Abdominal pain; musculoskeletal pain; vomiting; headache; injection site reaction; hypertension; hypo- and/or hyperglycemia; gallstones; hypothyroidism (mild)	HR and BP; blood glucose; thyroid function; gall bladder ultrasonography	
Thalidomide, lenalidomide, and pomalidomide	Thalidomide: somnolence; constipation; dizziness or orthostatic; hypotension; rash; peripheral neuropathies; thromboembolic events Lenalidomide: fatigue; peripheral neuropathy; neutropenia and thrombocytopenia; thromboembolic events	CBC; signs of thrombosis; signs of peripheral neuropathies; pregnancy status	REMS program for fetal toxicity For lenalidomide, adjust dose for renal impairment Prophylactic anticoagulation may be required
Monoclonal Antibodies that Target CD20			
Ibritumomab tiuxetan	Must consider toxicities of rituximab; delayed hematologic toxicity; infusion-related reactions; asthenia; nausea; chills; fever; tumor pain	Infusion-related reactions; CBC	Radiopharmaceutical; prepared and administered only by personnel trained in radiopharmaceuticals; patients must be trained in precautions to decrease radiation exposure
Obinutuzumab	Infusion reactions; myelosuppression; nausea; diarrhea; Progressive Multifocal Leukoencaphalopathy; HBV reactivation	CBC; hepatitis B screening at baseline; renal function; electrolytes; infusion reaction; fluid status	Antimicrobial, antiviral, and antifungal prophylaxis in select patients Antihyperuricemic prophylaxis and hydration if risk for tumor lysis syndrome HBV reactivation Premedicate with acetaminophen, an antihistamine, and a glucocorticoid
Ofatumumab	Neutropenia; pneumonia; pyrexia; cough; diarrhea; anemia; fatigue; dyspnea; rash; nausea; bronchitis; upper respiratory infection	Infusion-related reactions; CBC; hepatitis B screening at baseline	Premedicate with acetaminophen, antihistamine, and corticosteroid For dose 1 initiate infusion at a rate of 3.6 mg/h, dose 2 initiate rate at 24 mg/h, and for doses 3-12 initiate infusion at a rate of 50 mg/h; in the absence of infusional toxicity, the rate of infusion may be increased every 30 minutes
Rituximab	Hypersensitivity reactions and infusion-related reactions; TLS (especially with large tumor burden); myelosuppression and infection; rare reports of progressive multifocal leukoencephalopathy; severe skin reactions; myalgias; tachycardia	Infusion-related reactions; CBC; neurologic examination; hepatitis B screening at baseline; electrolytes, HR, BP	Patients at high risk of hepatitis B should be screened for before therapy Infusion-related reactions may be severe; increase rate of infusion gradually and premedicate with acetaminophen and diphenhydramine; use meperidine IV as needed for rigors
Tositumomab	Myelosuppression (especially thrombocytopenia and neutropenia) that is severe and prolonged; abdominal pain; diarrhea; infusion reactions; anaphylaxis may occur; hypothyroidism; asthenia; myalgias; cough; rash	Infusion-related reactions; CBC; thyroid function	Similar radiation safety procedures as ibritumomab Premedicate with acetaminophen and antihistamine Thyroprotective regimen required

(*continued*)

TABLE 127-7 Monitoring of Anticancer Drugs[a] (Continued)

Agent	Major Adverse Effects	Monitoring Parameters	Comments
Monoclonal Antibodies that Target Cell Surface Receptors			
Alemtuzumab	Myelosuppression and immunosuppression; autoimmune conditions; infection; infusion-related reactions; nausea and vomiting; fever; hypotension; rash; headache; fatigue; secondary malignancies	CBC; infusion-related reactions; CMV; CD4+ counts; HR; BP; autoimmune symptoms; symptoms of infection	Restricted distribution through REMS program to mitigate risks of autoimmune conditions, infusion reactions, and secondary malignancies Patients should be started on antiviral and PJP prophylaxis during and 6 months posttreatment
Blinatumomab	Infusion reactions; cytokine release syndrome; neurologic toxicities; infections; fever; headache; peripheral edema; rash; tumor lysis syndrome; hepatotoxicity; bone marrow suppression	CBC; liver function; neurological examination; uric acid levels; electrolytes	Boxed warnings for cytokine release syndrome and neurological toxicities Premedicate with dexamethasone prior to the first dose of each cycle, prior to a step dose or when restarting therapy after an interruption >4 hours Administered as a continuous intravenous infusion over 28 days
Brentuximab vedotin	Neutropenia; peripheral neuropathy; fatigue; nausea or vomiting; anemia; diarrhea; rash; thrombocytopenia; infusion-related reactions; TLS; rare reports of progressive multifocal leukoencephalopathy	CBC; symptoms of neuropathy; infusion-related reactions; uric acid levels, electrolytes	
Daratumumab	Infusion-related reactions; pyrexia; fatigue; upper respiratory tract infection; nausea; myelosuppression	CBC; actue or delayed infusion-related reactions	Type and screen patients prior to starting treatment as daratumumab may interfere with crossmatching and red blood cell antibody screening
Dinutuximab	Infections; infusion reactions; hyookalemia; hypotension; capillary leak syndrome; hypotension; neurological ocular toxicity; pain; bone marrow suppression; hemolytic uremic syndrome	CBC; electrolytes; renal function; BP; infusion reaction	Boxed warnings for infusion reactions and severe peripheral neuropathy Premedicate with analgesics (such as morphine), an antihistamine, acetaminophen, and intravenous hydration
Monoclonal Antibodies that Target Growth Factor Receptors and Their Ligands			
Ado-Trastuzumab Ematansine	Cardiac toxicity; thrombocytopenia; hemorrhage; hepatotoxicity; infusion reactions; peripheral neuropathy; ILD	CBC; liver function; pregnancy status; cardiac monitoring (LVEF); pulmonary symptoms	Boxed warnings for cardiotoxicity, hepatotoxicity, and embryo-fetal death Ado-Trastuzumab Ematansine and Trastuzumab are NOT interchangeable
Bevacizumab	GI bleeding or perforation, sometimes with intraabdominal abscess formation; impaired wound healing; hypertension; proteinuria; thrombotic events; rare severe pulmonary hemorrhage; rare reports of progressive multifocal leukoencephalopathy	BP; urine protein; neurologic examination; signs of GI perforation; symptoms of thromboembolism	Boxed warnings for gastrointestinal perforation, wound dehiscence, and hemorrhage
Cetuximab, Necitumumab, and Panitumumab	Rash; paronychial cracking in fingers or toes; asthenia; abdominal pain; nausea; constipation; diarrhea; infusion and hypersensitivity reactions; electrolyte wasting; cardiopulmonary arrest	Electrolytes; infusion reactions; dermatologic evaluation	Dose reductions or delays may be required for rash but supportive care should be attempted first Decreased risk of infusion-related reactions to panitumumab and does not appear to be cross reactive; therefore, a patient can receive panitumumab if they react to cetuximab
Pertuzumab	Diarrhea; nausea; alopecia; rash; neutropenia; fatigue; peripheral neuropathy; embryo and fetal toxicity; left ventricular dysfunction; infusion-related reactions	LVEF; infusion reactions; pregnancy status	Given with trastuzumab
Ramucirumab	GI bleeding or perforation; impaired wound healing; hypertension; proteinuria; thyroid dysfunction; thromboembolic events; hemorrhage	BP; urine protein; thyroid function, liver function	Boxed warnings for gastrointestinal perforation, wound dehiscence, and hemorrhage
Trastuzumab	Cardiac toxicity: congestive cardiomyopathy, usually reversible with medical management; infusion-related reactions	Infusion-related reactions; cardiac monitoring (LVEF)	Do not administer with anthracyclines because of increased cardiotoxicity
Immunomodulatory Monoclonal Antibodies			
Denosumab	Arthralgia; headache; nausea; hypocalcemia; osteonecrosis of the jaw	Dental evaluations; electrolytes	A dental examination prior to initiation of therapy
Elotuzumab	Fatigue; pyrexia; diarrhea or constipation; respiratory infections; peripherial neuropathy; hepatotoxicity; infusion-related reactions; second primary malignancies	Liver function; infusion-related reactions; infections	May interfere with the assay used to monitor M-protein which can impact the determination of complete response

(continued)

TABLE 127-7 Monitoring of Anticancer Drugs[a] (*Continued*)

Agent	Major Adverse Effects	Monitoring Parameters	Comments
Ipilimumab	Fatigue; diarrhea; pruritus; rash; immune-mediated reactions (enterocolitis, dermatitis, neuropathy, endocrinopathy, hepatitis)	Thyroid function; electrolytes; liver function; renal function; dermatologic evaluations; gastrointestinal symptoms	Treat severe immune-mediated reactions with corticosteroids
Nivolumab and Pembrolizumab	Fatigue; immune-mediated toxicities (pneumonitis, colitis, hepatitis, nephritis, thyroid dysfunction)	Liver function; renal function, thyroid function; GI symptoms	Treat severe immune-mediated reactions with corticosteroids
Siltuximab	Pruritis, weight gain, hyperuricemia, infection; gastrointestinal perforation	CBC; uric acid levels; cytokine release reactions	Do not administer live vaccines while being treated with siltuximab HIV-positive and HHV-8-positive patients excluded from the clinical trials
Cytokines			
Interferon-alfa	Flu-like symptoms; fatigue; serious or fatal neuropsychiatric (eg, depression, suicide), autoimmune, ischemic, and infectious complications; pulmonary symptoms; thyroid disorders; hyperglycemia	Neurological evaluation; infection; pulmonary and cardiac monitoring; blood glucose; thyroid function	Fatigue and Flu-like symptoms tend to decrease with duration of therapy Exists in a pegylated form that has a prolonged half-life
Interleukin-2	Flu-like syndrome: fevers, chills, malaise; vascular or capillary leak syndrome: hypotension, pulmonary and peripheral edema; GI: nausea and vomiting, diarrhea; nephrotoxicity; myelosuppression (thrombocytopenia and leukopenia); bacterial infections; CNS: somnolence, confusion; arrhythmias; rash; itching	Intense monitoring required; electrolytes; liver function; renal function; CBC; thallium stress test; pulmonary function tests; cardiac monitoring during IL-2 administration, BP, HR	Vasopressor support and fluid resuscitation may be necessary during treatment because of hypotension Pulmonary edema can be managed with cautious use of diuretics; short courses of albumin may also be beneficial Itching may respond to treatment with antihistamines; emollient skin creams or occlusive agents are effective for dry, peeling skin Avoid corticosteroids because they may counteract the antitumor effects of IL-2 Patients on beta-blockers will need to be tapered off before initiation of aldesleukin
Enzymes			
L-asparaginase	Hypersensitivity reactions (fever, hypotension, rash, dyspnea in 25%), much lower risk with polyethylene glycol form and asparaginase *E. chrysanthemi;* pancreatitis; decreased synthesis of proteins, clotting factors; CNS: lethargy	Pancreatic enzymes; liver function; coagulation parameters (fibrinogen, PT, PTT); hypersensitivity reactions; blood glucose; CBC	Skin test before administration of *E. coli*–derived asparaginase; anaphylaxis precautions Pegaspargase complexes with polyethylene glycol to decrease immunogenicity and prolong duration of action Asparaginase *E. chrysanthemi* was developed for patients who have developed hypersensitivity to *E. coli*–derived asparaginase
Fusion Proteins			
Denileukin diftitox	Pyrexia; nausea; fatigue; rigors; vomiting; diarrhea; headache; peripheral edema; cough; dyspnea; pruritus; infusion reactions; capillary leak syndrome; loss of visual acuity	Infusion reactions; fluid status; BP; serum albumin; ophthalmologic evaluation	Serum albumin should be ≥3 g/dL (30 g/L) before initiating therapy Premedicate with an antihistamine and acetaminophen
Ziv-aflibercept	Neutropenia; diarrhea; proteinuria; increases in liver enzymes; stomatitis; fatigue; thrombocytopenia; hypertension; weight decreased; decreased appetite; epistaxis; abdominal pain; dysphonia; serum creatinine increased; headache; hemorrhage; GI perforation; compromised wound healing; arterial thromboembolic events; fistula formation	BP; urine protein; signs and symptoms of hemorrhage; CBC; liver function; renal function	Should be held at least 4 weeks before elective surgery and restarted at least 4 weeks after major surgery and until the surgical wound is fully healed
Vaccines			
Sipuleucel-T	Infusion reactions; chills; fatigue; back pain; nausea; joint ache; headache; thromboembolic events have occurred	Infusion reaction	Physicians and patients must be registered Premedicate with an antihistamine and acetaminophen
Talimogene laherparepvec	Fatigue; chills; pyrexia; nausea; influenza-like illness; injection site pain; cellulitis; risk of herpetic infection	Herpetic infections; injection-site complications; immune-mediated events	Administered directly into the cutaneous, subcutaneous and/or nodal lesion(s) Precautions for accidental exposure of healthcare works and close contacts

ATRA, all-*trans*-retinoic acid; BP, blood pressure; CBC, complete blood count; CHF, congestive heart failure; CML, chronic myeloid leukemia; CMV, cytomegalovirus; CNS, central nervous system; CrCL, creatinine clearance; CYP, cytochrome P450 isoenzyme; DPD, dihydropyrimidine dehydrogenase; DVT, deep vein thrombosis; ECG, electrocardiogram; GI, gastrointestinal; G6PD, glucose-6-phosphate dehydrogenase; HDAC, high-dose cytarabine; HSV, herpes simplex virus; H_1 and H_2, histamine 1 and 2; HDAC, histone deacetylase; HSCT, hematopoietic stem cell transplantation; ILD, interstitial lung disease; INR, international normalized ration; IT, intrathecal; IM, intramuscular; LVEF, left ventricular ejection fraction; MAOI, monoamine oxidase inhibitor; MI, myocardial infarction; mTOR, mammalian target of rapamycin; MUGA, multigated acquisition scan; NSAID, nonsteroidal antiinflammatory drug; PE, pulmonary embolism; PFT, pulmonary function tests; Pgp, P-glycoprotein; PJP, *Pneumocystis jiroveci* pneumonia; PPI, proton pump inhibitor; PT, prothrombin time; PTT, partial thromboplastin time; SC, subcutaneous; Scr, serum creatinine; SIADH, syndrome of inappropriate secretion of antidiuretic hormone; SSRI, selective serotonin reuptake inhibitor; TCA, tricyclic antidepressant; TLS, tumor lysis syndrome; TSH, thyroid-stimulating hormone; UGT1A1, Uridine 5′-diphospho-glucuronosyltransferase (UDP-glucuronosyltransferase).

[a]Only approximate guidelines can be given. Consult current references before dispensing as not all dose adjustments and monitoring parameters are provided in the table.

Data from Chabner BA, Longo DL, ed. Cancer Chemotherapy and Biotherapy: Principles and Practice, 5th ed. Philadelphia: Lippincott Williams & Wilkins, 2010 and prescribing information package inserts.

prevent DNA elongation. Deaminase enzymes, particularly cytidine deaminase, degrades cytarabine.[17]

Cytarabine may be given intravenously or intrathecally. Intrathecal administration allows for cytotoxic concentrations of cytarabine to be maintained in the central nervous system (CNS) for several hours after administration of traditional cytarabine formulations and for more than 2 weeks after administration of a depot formulation. It may be given to patients with leukemia.

The dose-limiting toxicities are leukopenia and thrombocytopenia. Other common toxicities include nausea, vomiting, mucositis, and diarrhea. Following administration of high-dose cytarabine (greater than 1 g/m^2 per dose), cerebellar syndrome may occur presenting with dysarthria, nystagmus, and ataxia. The risk of cerebellar syndrome is strongly correlated with advanced age and renal dysfunction. Renal dysfunction permits accumulation of high levels of the triphosphate, which is believed to be neurotoxic. Hepatic dysfunction, high cumulative doses, and bolus dosing may also increase the risk of neurotoxicity.[17] Conjunctivitis or keratitis is another common toxicity associated with high-dose cytarabine. Prophylactic steroid or saline eye drops should be administered with high-dose cytarabine to minimize irritation as discussed later in this chapter. Allopurinol may be given with high-dose cytarabine to minimize the risk of tumor lysis syndrome, a group of metabolic complications that occur following the breakdown of dying cancer cells.

Fluoropyrimidines Fluorouracil (FU or 5-FU) is a fluorinated uracil analog that was originally synthesized in the late 1950s. It acts as a false pyrimidine and undergoes sequential phosphorylation to a mono-, di-, and triphosphate similar to natural nucleotide bases. In the presence of folates, the monophosphate binds tightly to and interferes with the function of thymidylate synthase. The triphosphate metabolite is incorporated into RNA as a false base and interferes with its function. The interference with both thymidine formation and RNA function both contribute to its cytotoxic effects. FU is commonly used to treat gastrointestinal tract and head and neck cancers.

The dosage and administration influences both the mechanism of action and toxicity profile.[17] With continuous-infusion regimens, thymidylate synthesis inhibition plays a greater role and dose-limiting toxicities are hand-foot syndrome and diarrhea. Comparatively, the incorporation into RNA plays a greater role with intermittent bolus schedules. The dose-limiting toxicity commonly associated with a bolus administration is myelosuppression.

Several pharmacologic strategies have been attempted to increase its cytotoxicity against cancer cells and decrease its toxicity to normal cells. The most common strategy combines FU with the reduced folate leucovorin. Folates increase the reduced folate pool, stabilize the monophosphate–thymidylate synthase complex and prolong the inhibition of thymidylate synthase. Clinical trials suggest that combining reduced folates with FU provides greater anticancer activity and improves tolerability.[17]

Dihydropyrimidine dehydrogenase (DPD) is a pyrimidine catabolic enzyme that is responsible for about 80% of the catabolism of FU. Reduced expression of this enzyme has been associated with drug accumulation and serious adverse events.[18] DPD deficiency is an autosomal recessive genetic disorder, with genetic variation in the DYPD gene associated with reduced enzyme activity. DPD deficiency occurs in up to 5% of the overall population. FU is contraindicated in patients with known DPD deficiency.

Capecitabine is an oral pyrimidine uracil analog used to treat breast and colon cancers. Because capecitabine is enzymatically converted to FU, it shares the same mechanisms of action. Capecitabine is typically taken twice daily with food for the first 14 days of a 21-day treatment cycle. Because chronic twice-daily oral dosing produces sustained FU levels similar to those observed with continuous infusions, hand-foot syndrome and diarrhea are the dose-limiting toxicities.

Uridine triacetate is approved for the emergency treatment of adult and pediatric patients following a FU or capecitabine overdose regardless of the presence of symptoms, or who exhibit early-onset, severe or life-threatening toxicity affecting the cardiac or central nervous system and/or early-onset, unusually severe adverse reactions within 96 hours following the FU or capecitabine administration. It is not recommended for the nonemergent treatment of adverse reactions. The safety and efficacy has not been established when more than 96 hours has elapsed following the end of FU or capecitabine administration. Few adverse events have been reported, but the most common adverse reactions are vomiting, nausea and diarrhea.

Gemcitabine Gemcitabine is a fluorine-substituted deoxycytidine analog that is related structurally to cytarabine and is used to treat pancreatic, nonsmall cell lung, breast, and bladder cancers. Its activation and mechanism of action are similar to those of cytarabine. Gemcitabine is incorporated into DNA, where it inhibits DNA polymerase activity. It also inhibits ribonucleotide reductase, which is the enzyme required to convert ribonucleotides into the deoxyribonucleotides that are needed for both DNA synthesis and repair. Compared with cytarabine, gemcitabine achieves intracellular concentrations about 20 times higher, secondary to increased penetration of cell membranes and greater affinity for the activating enzyme deoxycytidine kinase. Gemcitabine that is incorporated into DNA has a prolonged intracellular half-life. Its stereoconfiguration causes another normal base pair to be added next to the fraudulent gemcitabine base pair in the DNA strand. This "masked chain termination" protects the gemcitabine from excision and elimination. Flu-like symptoms are commonly associated with gemcitabine. These symptoms may last several days and may be treated with acetaminophen.

Trifluridine and Tipiracil Trifluridine and tipiracil are combined in a molar ration of 1:0.5 in one tablet that is approved for the treatment of metastatic colorectal cancer. Trifluridine is a thymidine-based nucleoside analogue and tipiracil is a thymidine phosphorylase inhibitor. Following uptake into cancer cells, trifluridine is incorporated into DNA, interferes with DNA synthesis and inhibits cell proliferation. Inclusion of tipiracil increases trifluridine exposure by inhibiting its metabolism by thymidine phosphorylase. The dose-limiting toxicity is myelosuppression; patients older than 65 years of age may be at greater risk for grade 3 or higher myelosuppression. Other common toxicities include asthenia/fatigue, nausea, decreased appetite, diarrhea, vomiting, abdominal pain, and pyrexia.

Purine Analogs

Cladribine and Pentostatin Cladribine and pentostatin are purine nucleoside analogs with slightly different mechanisms of action. Both agents are used to treat hairy cell leukemia. Cladribine is resistant to inactivation by adenosine deaminase and is triphosphorylated to an active form that is incorporated into DNA that inhibits DNA synthesis and early chain termination. Its anticancer activity is unusual for an antimetabolite in that it affects both actively dividing and resting cancer cells. Pentostatin is a potent inhibitor of adenosine deaminase. Adenosine deaminase is an enzyme critical in purine base metabolism and is found in high concentrations in lymphatic tissue. Both agents have immunosuppressive effects that place patients at risk for serious opportunistic infections and require the administration of prophylactic antibiotics.

Fludarabine Fludarabine is an adenine analogue used to treat chronic lymphocytic leukemia (CLL) and indolent NHL. Similar to cytarabine, fludarabine interferes with DNA polymerase, causing chain termination. Fludarabine also incorporates into RNA, resulting in inhibition of transcription. Fludarabine is immunosuppressive; it has been associated with the development of opportunistic infections, secondary to its effect on T-cells and subsequent decrease in CD4 counts. Prophylactic antibiotics and antiviral medications are recommended and should continue until CD4 counts normalize.[17]

Mercaptopurine and Thioguanine 6-Mercaptopurine (6-MP) and its analog thioguanine are oral antimetabolites used for the treatment of ALL. These antimetabolites are rapidly converted to ribonucleotides that inhibit purine biosynthesis or undergo purine interconversion reactions needed to supply purine precursors for synthesis of nucleic acids. Clinical cross-resistance is generally observed.[17] Both antimetabolites are metabolized by thiopurine methyltransferase (TPMT) and hypoxanthine phosphoribosyl transferase to produce multiple metabolites that contribute to the observed anticancer activity, hepatotoxicity, and myelosuppression. Certain genetic alterations within the TPMT gene can lead to a reduction of loss of TPMT enzyme activity. Therefore, patients who are homozygous or heterozygous for a genetic alteration that affects TPMT enzyme activity may lead to an accumulation of toxic metabolites and an increased risk of severe myelosuppression. The Clinical Pharmacogenetics Implementation Consortium (CPIC) provides primary dosing recommendations for patients with altered TPMT gene.

6-MP depends on xanthine oxidase for an initial oxidation step. Its metabolism is markedly decreased by coadministration of the xanthine oxidase inhibitor allopurinol, which may lead to the development of serious adverse events. If allopurinol is given concurrently with 6-MP to minimize tumor lysis syndrome, the dose of 6-MP must be reduced.[17]

6-MP is now available as tablets or suspension for oral administration to facilitate dosing in pediatrics.

Folate Antagonists

Methotrexate Methotrexate is commonly used to treat ALL and some lymphomas. It inhibits dihydrofolate reductase (DHFR), which results in the depletion of intracellular pools of reduced folates (tetrahydrofolates) essential for thymidylate and purine synthesis. Folates are essential cofactors for DNA and RNA synthesis and thus, lack of either thymidine or purines prevents DNA or RNA synthesis.

Chemotherapy regimens may contain low-, intermediate- or high-dose methotrexate and may incorporate methotrexate given orally, intravenously or intrathecally. High-dose methotrexate defined as doses greater than 500 mg/m^2 given intravenously as prophylaxis or treatment of CNS disease can cause severe myelosuppression and gastrointestinal toxicity. The development of these toxicities is related to both the maximal concentrations and the time that concentrations remain above 0.02 mg/L (50 nmol/L). These effects may be neutralized by supplying reduced folates exogenously, such as leucovorin (folinic acid), which bypasses the metabolic block induced by DHFR inhibitors.[19] Leucovorin should be administered until levels fall below the threshold and various dosing algorithms are available to guide leucovorin dosing based on methotrexate level. As an alternative to leucovorin, levoleucovorin may be given with high-dose methotrexate. Vigorous hydration with sodium biocarbonate to alkalinize the urine should be given to decrease the risk of renal failure. Patients with third space fluids may require prolonged leucovorin rescue, since these fluids influence methotrexate volume of distribution and elimination half-life.

Glucarpidase has been approved for the treatment of toxic plasma methotrexate concentrations in patients with delayed methotrexate clearance because of impaired renal function. It is important to note that methotrexate concentrations within 48 hours after glucarpidase administration can only be reliably measured by chromatographic methods. Immunoassays can overestimate methotrexate concentration because of interference from metabolites.

Methotrexate is highly protein bound and drugs, such as sulfonamides, salicylates, phenytoin, and tetracyclines, may displace methotrexate from albumin. Increased toxicity may be observed. Nonsteroidal anti-inflammatory drugs (NSAIDs) and vitamin C may also affect methotrexate disposition and prolong methotrexate elimination half-life. Although the exact mechanism is uncertain, proton pump inhibitors are thought to inhibit methotrexate elimination and thereby potentially increase methotrexate toxicity.

Pemetrexed Pemetrexed is a multi-targeted antifolate that is used to treat nonsquamous NSCLC and mesothelioma. It inhibits at least three biosynthetic pathways in thymidine and purine synthesis. In addition to inhibiting DHFR, it also inhibits thymidine synthase and glycinamide ribonucleotide formyltransferase, decreasing the risk of the development of drug resistance. Severe hematologic toxicity and deaths associated with neutropenic sepsis have been reported in clinical trials. Elevated baseline cystathionine or homocysteine concentrations correlated with this unexpected toxicity. Routine supplementation of folic acid and vitamin B_{12} lowers levels of these substances and lowers the risk of mortality related to neutropenic sepsis. The approved labeling of pemetrexed requires administration of folic acid and vitamin B_{12} prior to initiating pemetrexed and throughout the duration of treatment. Oral or intravenous dexamethasone should be given with pemetrexed to minimize the risk of rash.

Pralatrexate Pralatrexate is an antifolate drug approved for patients with relapsed or refractory peripheral T-cell leukemias. It competitively inhibits DHFR and polyglutamylation by the enzyme folylpolyglutamyl synthetase. This inhibition results in the depletion of thymidine and other synthesis of biological molecules that depends on single carbon transfer.[20] The most common adverse events resulting in dose reductions are pyrexia, mucositis, febrile neutropenia, sepsis, and thrombocytopenia.

Microtubule-Targeting Drugs

Microtubules are an integral part of the cytoskeleton and help maintain the shape of a cell. These structures are also involved in chromosome separation during mitosis and form the mitotic spindle responsible for separating chromosomes during cell replication. Several chemotherapy agents affect microtubule function, including epipodophyllotoxins, taxanes, vinca alkaloids, epitholones, and macrolides.

Eribulin

Eribulin is a fully synthetic antimicrotubule analogue of the macrolide halichondrin B. Eribulin inhibits tubulin polymerization by inhibiting microtubule growth, but it does not shorten or promote depolymerization of microtubules.[21] Additionally, eribulin only binds to the β-tubulin subunit and has demonstrated the ability to overcome taxane resistance conferred by β-tubulin mutations.[21] The most common toxicities are similar to other microtubule inhibitors, but eribulin demonstrates a decreased incidence of neuropathy compared with vincristine and taxanes. Eribulin is approved for the treatment of metastatic breast cancer and unresectable or metastatic liposarcoma.

Estramustine

Estramustine is approved for the treatment of metastatic prostate cancer. It structurally combines the alkylating agent nor-nitrogen mustard with estradiol. It was designed with the intent that the estradiol portion of the molecule would facilitate uptake of the alkylating agent into hormone-sensitive prostate cancer cells. Despite the inclusion of an alkylator, estramustine does not function as an alkylating agent. The estradiol is released after its administration and it is responsible for most of the toxicity associated with estramustine; the estradiol is not believed to contribute to its anticancer activity. In the mid-1980s, estramustine was redefined as an antimicrotubule agent. It binds covalently to microtubule-associated proteins that are part of the structural support for microtubules. The binding causes the separation of microtubule-associated proteins from the microtubules, inhibiting microtubule assembly and eventually causing their disassembly. Observed toxicities include gastrointestinal disorders, edema, gynecomastia, thromboembolic events, and cardiovascular events.

Ixabepilone

Ixabepilone is a synthetic epothilone approved for the treatment of metastatic breast cancer. Its binding to microtubules appears distinct from other microtubule inhibitors, such as the taxanes. Dose-limiting toxicities are leukopenia and neuropathy, consistent with other microtubule inhibitors. Other toxicities include anemia, thrombocytopenia, diarrhea, myalgia and alopecia. Premedication with antihistamines must be administered; a corticosteroid may be co-administered with the antihistamines if a patient experiences a hypersensitivity reaction to a previous dose.

Taxanes

Paclitaxel and docetaxel are taxane plant alkaloids with antimitotic activity used to treat many different solid tumors.[22] Paclitaxel and docetaxel both act by binding to tubulin, but they do not interfere with tubulin assembly. Instead, the taxanes promote microtubule assembly and interfere with microtubule disassembly. They induce tubulin polymerization, resulting in formation of inappropriately stable, nonfunctional microtubules. The stability of the microtubules damages cells by disrupting the dynamics of microtubule-dependent structures required for mitosis and other cellular functions. Taxanes also have some nonmitotic actions that can promote cancer cell death, such as inhibition of angiogenesis.

Resistance to the antitumor effects of the taxanes is attributable to alterations in tubulin or tubulin binding sites or to P-glycoprotein (Pgp)-mediated multidrug resistance. Although paclitaxel and docetaxel have very similar mechanisms of action, cross-resistance between the two chemotherapy agents is incomplete.[22]

Myelosuppression is common with both taxanes, but other toxicities differ. While fluid retention is seen with docetaxel, neurotoxicity and hypersensitivity reactions are seen with paclitaxel.[22] Both require premedications with corticosteroids; paclitaxel also requires premedication with antihistamines to decrease the likelihood of hypersensitivity reactions.

Two paclitaxel drug products are available. The original drug product contains Cremephor and ethanol. The subsequent drug product contains paclitaxel bound to albumin (nab-paclitaxel); this drug product does not contain the Cremophor excipient that is believed to contribute to the hypersensitivity reactions and exacerbate myelosuppression with the original drug product. In clinical trials, nab-paclitaxel has shown comparable activity to the original drug product with a lower incidence of hypersensitivity reactions. Peripheral neuropathy remains a common adverse event with nab-paclitaxel. Nab-paclitaxel is approved for the treatment of metastatic breast, NSCLC and pancreatic cancer. Of note, the dose differs from the original paclitaxel drug product.

Cabazitaxel is a semisynthetic derivative of docetaxel that has demonstrated anticancer activity in hormone refractory prostate cancer that has progressed following treatment with docetaxel-based chemotherapy despite having the same mechanism of action. This is partially because of its lack of affinity for Pgp that allows cabazitaxel to remain inside the cancer cells. Toxicities and premedications are similar to docetaxel.[23]

Vinca Alkaloids

Vincristine, vinblastine, and vinorelbine are natural alkaloids derived from the periwinkle (vinca) plant. These agents act as mitotic inhibitors or spindle poisons. Although these alkaloids have a very similar structure, they have different activities and patterns of toxicity. These agents are used to treat different cancers. For example, vinblastine may be used to treat testicular cancer and Hodgkin lymphoma, vincristine may be used to treat NHL and Hodgkin lymphoma, and vinorelbine may be used to treat NSCLC and breast cancer. Vinorelbine and vinblastine are associated with dose-limiting myelosuppression, while vincristine is associated with dose-limiting neurotoxicity, including constipation and paralytic ileus. All vinca alkaloids are vesicants upon extravasation; the application of local heat allows dispersal or dilution of the alkaloid to minimize the tissue damage.

Vinca alkaloids should never be administered intrathecally. Accidental overdose is associated with a very high mortality rate. It is recommended to avoid administration of intravenous and intrathecal chemotherapy on the same day to avoid accidental intrathecal administration of these alkaloids.

Vinca alkaloids bind to tubulin and disrupt the normal balance between polymerization and depolymerization of microtubules, which inhibits assembly of microtubules and disrupts microtubule dynamics. This interferes with formation of the mitotic spindle and causes cells to accumulate in mitosis. These agents also disturb a variety of microtubule-related processes in cells and induce apoptosis. Resistance to the vinca alkaloids develops primarily from Pgp-mediated multidrug resistance, which decreases drug accumulation and retention within cancer cells.[22]

Topoisomerase Inhibitors

Topoisomerases (I and II) are essential enzymes involved in maintaining DNA topologic structure during replication. During replication, these enzymes cleave DNA strands and form intermediates with the strands, producing a gap through which DNA strands can pass, and then reseal the strand breaks. Topoisomerase I produces single-strand breaks and topoisomerase II produces double-strand breaks.[24] Several important anticancer agents interact with topoisomerase enzymes: anthracyclines, camptothecins, and podophyllotoxins.

Anthracyclines

The anthracyclines include doxorubin, daunorubicin (daunomycin), idarubicin, and epirubicin. These agents share a common, four-membered anthracene ring complex with an attached aglycone or sugar portion. The ring complex is a chromophore and accounts for the intense colors of these derivatives.[24] Anthracyclines are classified as antitumor antibiotics, but they have multiple mechanisms of action, including intercalation into DNA and inhibition of topoisomerase II.[24] The production of free radicals following their metabolism may also contribute to their anticancer activity. These agents are used to treat many cancers, including leukemias, lymphomas, and multiple other cancers.

Although the dose-limiting toxicity is myelosuppression, development of cardiomyopathy is a significant concern with these agents. All patients should have a baseline study to evaluate left ventricular ejection fraction. Since the probability of congestive heart failure increases with the cumulative dose, a maximum cumulative dose has been identified for each anthracycline. The relatively low level of defensive enzymes found in cardiac muscle that scavenge against oxygen free radicals may account for the relative risk of cardiomyopathy compared to other organs. Oxygen free-radical formation likely contributes to extravasation injury associated with these agents, as well. Other common toxicities include nausea, vomiting and alopecia. Doxorubicin also causes a discoloration of the urine. Resistance to anthracyclines is usually secondary to Pgp-mediated multidrug resistance, but altered topoisomerase II activity may also contribute to the development of resistance.

Mitoxantrone is a closely related chemotherapy agent identified as an anthracendione. It was synthesized in an attempt to develop a chemotherapy agent with comparable antitumor activity to doxorubicin but with an improved safety profile. Similar to the anthracyclines, mitoxantrone is an intercalating topoisomerase II inhibitor, but its potential for free-radical formation is much less than that of the anthracyclines. This decreased tendency for free-radical formation may explain the reduced risks of cardiac toxicity and ulceration after extravasation. Mitoxantrone may be used with other anticancer agents to treat leukemias and lymphomas. Common toxicities include nausea, vomiting, alopecia and discolored urine.

Camptothecins

Topotecan and irinotecan, through its active metabolite SN-38, inhibit topoisomerase I enzyme activity. Topoisomerase I enzymes stabilize DNA single-strand breaks and inhibit strand resealing.[24] Topotecan is available for oral and intravenous administration and it is used to treat ovarian cancer and small cell lung cancer. Irinotecan is used for the treatment of colorectal cancer. Irinotecan's active metabolite SN-38 undergoes metabolism by the polymorphic enzyme uridine diphosphate glucosyltransferase. Although variant tandem repeats in the promoter of this gene have been associated with a higher risk of diarrhea and neutropenia, genotyping has not been widely adopted in clinical practice.

Liposomal irinotecan is approved for the treatment of patients with metastatic adenocarcinoma of the pancreas whose disease has progressed following gemcitabine-based therapy with FU and leucovorin. The common toxicities associated with irinotecan have been observed with liposomal irinotecan, including gastrointestinal toxicity and myelosuppression. The recommended dose is lower for patients homozygous for the UGT1A1*28 allele.

Etoposide and Teniposide

Etoposide and teniposide are semisynthetic podophyllotoxin derivatives that bind to tubulin and interfere with microtubule formation. Etoposide and teniposide also damage cancer cells by causing strand breakage through inhibition of topoisomerase II.[24] Resistance may be caused by differences in topoisomerase II levels, increased cell ability to repair strand breaks, or increased levels of Pgp. Etoposide and teniposide are usually clinically cross-resistant. They are cell-cycle phase-specific and arrest cells in the S or early G_2 phase. As a result, activity is much greater when they are administered in divided doses over several days rather than in large single doses. Etoposide may be used to treat testicular cancer and small cell lung cancer and teniposide is used to treat pediatric ALL. Both agents are associated with dose-limiting myelosuppression, as well as nausea, vomiting and alopecia.

Alkylating Agents

The alkylating agents are among the oldest and most useful classes of chemotherapy agents. Their clinical use evolved from the observation of myelosuppression and lymph node shrinkage in soldiers exposed to sulfur mustard gas warfare during World War I. In an effort to develop similar agents that might be useful in treating lymphomas, less reactive derivatives were synthesized. Their anticancer activity was confirmed by clinical trials in the mid-1940s.

All alkylating agents work by covalently bonding to highly reactive alkyl groups or substituted alkyl groups with nucleophilic groups of proteins and nucleic acids. Some agents react directly with biologic molecules, but others form an intermediate compound that reacts with these molecules. The most common binding site for alkylating agents is the seven-nitrogen group of the DNA base guanine. These covalent interactions result in cross-linking between two DNA strands or between two bases in the same strand of DNA and prevent the separation of DNA strands that needs to occur during replication. Reactions between DNA and RNA and between drug and proteins may also occur. Alkylating agents are cell-cycle phase-nonspecific, but their greatest effect is seen in rapidly dividing cells.

As a class, alkylators are cytotoxic, mutagenic, teratogenic, carcinogenic, and myelosuppressive. Resistance to these chemotherapies can occur from increased DNA repair capabilities, decreased entry into or accelerated exit from cells, increased inactivation inside cells, or lack of cellular mechanisms to result in cell death after DNA damage. They are inactivated by hydrolysis, making spontaneous degradation an important component of their elimination.[25]

Nitrogen Mustards

Bendamustine Bendamustine is an alkylating agent with a benzimidazole ring that demonstrates only partial cross-resistance in vitro with other alkylating agents.[26] It is used primarily to treat lymphoid malignancies, such as CLL and NHL. Bendamustine is incompatible with polycarbonate or acrylonitrile-butadiene-styrene found in syringes and adapters and has been shown to minimize the integrity of syringes and adapters. Typical adverse events associated with alkylating agents have been observed with bendamustine, but it appears to cause less alopecia.

Cyclophosphamide and Ifosfamide Cyclophosphamide and ifosfamide are nitrogen mustard derivatives and are widely used in the treatment of solid tumors and hematologic malignancies. These mustards are closely related in structure, clinical use, and toxicity. Neither agent is active in its parent form and must be activated by cytochrome P450 enzymes. One of the active metabolites of cyclophosphamide is phosphoramide mustard and of ifosfamide is ifosfamide mustard. The cytochrome P450-mediated metabolites 4-hydroxycyclophosphamide and 4-hydroxyifosfamide are also cytotoxic compounds. Acrolein, a metabolite of both cyclophosphamide and ifosfamide, has little anticancer activity, but is responsible for the hemorrhagic cystitis associated with ifosfamide and high-dose cyclophosphamide. Encephalopathy after ifosfamide can occur within 48 to 72 hours after the infusion and is reversible once the infusion is stopped. Methylene blue has been administered to manage neuropathy, but no clinical trials are available to support its routine use. The increased production of dechloroethylated metabolites after administration of ifosfamide compared with cyclophosphamide may explain the increased risk of CNS toxicity associated with ifosfamide.

Nitrosoureas

Carmustine and Lomustine Carmustine (BCNU) and lomustine (CCNU) are characterized by their lipophilicity and their ability to cross the blood–brain barrier; both agents are used to treat brain cancers. Carmustine is also used to treat multiple myeloma and lymphoma and in preparation for a bone marrow transplant. It is available as an intravenous preparation and as a drug-impregnated biodegradable wafer for direct application to residual tumor tissue after surgical resection of brain tumors. Both agents cause dose-limiting myelosuppression, but the nadir is typically delayed to 4 to 6 weeks after administration. The nitrosoureas decompose to reactive alkylating metabolites and to isocyanate compounds that have several effects on reproducing cells.[25]

Nonclassic Alkylating Agents

Several other chemotherapy agents appear to act as alkylators, although their structures do not include the classic alkylating groups. These agents are capable of binding covalently to cellular components and include procarbazine, dacarbazine, temozolomide, and platinum analogues.[25]

Dacarbazine and Temozolomide Dacarbazine and temozolomide undergo demethylation to the same active intermediate (monomethyl triazeno-imidazole-carboxamide [MTIC]) that interrupts DNA replication by causing methylation of guanine. Unlike dacarbazine, temozolomide does not require the liver for activation and is chemically degraded to MTIC at physiologic pH. Both agents inhibit DNA, RNA, and protein synthesis.[25]

Important pharmacokinetic differences exist between these two agents. Dacarbazine is poorly absorbed and must be administered by intravenous infusion. Temozolomide is rapidly absorbed after oral administration; it demonstrates nearly 100% bioavailability when given under fasted conditions. Dacarbazine penetrates the CNS poorly, but temozolomide readily crosses the blood–brain barrier, achieving therapeutically active concentrations in cerebrospinal fluid and brain tumor tissues.[25] Temozolomide is approved for the treatment of glioblastoma multiforme and dacarbazine was commonly used to treat melanoma. Common adverse events include nausea and vomiting, alopecia, and myelosuppression.

Platinum Analogs The platinum derivatives—cisplatin, carboplatin, and oxaliplatin—are chemotherapy agents with remarkable usefulness in cancer treatment. Recognition of cisplatin's cytotoxic activity was the result of a serendipitous observation that bacterial growth in culture was altered when an electric current was delivered to the media through platinum electrodes. The growth change was noted to be similar to that produced by alkylating agents and radiation. It was found that a platinum–chloride complex, now known as cisplatin, generated by the current was responsible for the changes. Carboplatin is a structural analog of cisplatin in which the chloride groups of the parent compound are replaced by a carboxycyclobutane moiety. It shares a similar spectrum of clinical activity with cisplatin and cross-resistance is common. Oxaliplatin is an organoplatinum compound in which the platinum is complexed with an oxalate ligand as the leaving group and to diaminocyclohexane. Its spectrum of activity differs substantially from the other platinum compounds and includes notable activity against colorectal cancers.[25]

The cytotoxicity of the platinum derivatives depends on platinum binding to DNA and the formation of intrastrand cross-links or adducts between neighboring guanines. These intrastrand links cause a major bending of the DNA. These agents may cause cellular damage by distorting the normal DNA conformation and preventing bases that are normally paired from lining up with each other. Interstrand cross-links also occur.[25]

The aquated species differ among these platinum compounds, but all of these species contribute to the anticancer activity. The cytotoxic form of cisplatin is the aquated species in which hydroxyl groups or water molecules replace the two chloride groups. This reaction occurs readily in low concentrations of chloride, such as the concentrations present within cells, and produces a positively charged compound that can react with DNA. The aquated species is responsible for both the efficacy and toxicity of cisplatin. Carboplatin also undergoes aquation but at a slower rate. Oxaliplatin becomes active when the oxalate ligand is displaced in physiologic solutions.[25]

Resistance to the therapeutic effects of platinum compounds may occur through several mechanisms. The ability to repair platinum-induced DNA damage may be increased or the compounds may be inactivated by increased levels of intracellular glutathione, metallothioneins, or other thiol-containing proteins. Altered uptake into cells may also affect sensitivity to platinum compounds.[25]

The dose-limiting toxicities differ substantially among these compounds. Cisplatin can cause serious nephrotoxicity, ototoxicity, peripheral neuropathy, emesis, and anemia, but its significant anticancer activity in many tumors makes it a valuable agent despite these toxicities. Most of these toxicities can be prevented or managed with aggressive supportive care measures. Intravenous hydration, mannitol and diuretics have been used to minimize the risk of nephrotoxicity, but it appears intravenous hydration alone is adequate to minimize the risk of nephrotoxicity. In contrast, carboplatin administration is limited by hematologic toxicity. Patients with compromised renal function require dose reductions to limit myelosuppressive toxicity.[25] The most widely used dosage schema, the Calvert formula, uses a target area-under-the-curve and renal function parameters to estimate the carboplatin dose. Carboplatin's potential to cause renal damage, peripheral neuropathy, ototoxicity, and nausea and vomiting is much less than that of comparable cisplatin doses.[25] Oxaliplatin is not nephrotoxic or ototoxic, but it can cause peripheral neuropathies and unique cold-induced neuropathies. Intravenous calcium and magnesium were commonly used to minimize the risk of neuropathy, but these measures do not appear to decrease the risk of acute neurotoxicity or cumulative sensory neurotoxicity based on the results of a controlled trial.[27] All of the platinum derivatives have potential to cause hypersensitivity reactions, including anaphylaxis, after a threshold exposure is reached. De-sensitization protocols may be successful in re-establishing tolerance to these agents.

Trabectedin Trabectedin is an alkylating drug that binds guanine residues in the minor groove of DNA. Subsequently, adducts form and cause a bending of the DNA helix towards the major groove. It is approved for the treatment of patients with unresectable or metastatic liposarcoma or leiomyosarcoma who have received a prior anthracycline-containing regimen. Possible risks associated with trabectedin include neutropenic sepsis, rhabdomyolysis, cardiomyopathy, hepatotoxicity, anaphylaxis, and extravasation leading to tissue necrosis.

Endocrine Therapies

Endocrine therapies are perhaps the earliest successful approach to target the growth processes of cancer cells. Endocrine manipulation is an option for management of cancers in which its growth is under gonadal hormonal control, such as breast, prostate, and endometrial cancers. These cancers may regress if the feeding hormone is eliminated or antagonized. Major organ system toxicity is uncommon from endocrine therapies. Specific anticancer agents such as the selective estrogen receptor modulators (SERM) and aromatase inhibitors (AI) have increased the utility of endocrine therapies in the treatment of cancer.[28,29] These therapies are discussed in detail in Chapters 128 and 131.

Corticosteroids

Corticosteroids are also useful anticancer agents because of their lymphotoxic effects. These drugs are primarily used to treat hematologic malignancies and together with chemotherapy or targeted therapy for hormone-refractory prostate cancer. In addition to their cytotoxic effects, corticosteroids have many other applications as part of supportive care measures and in the management of oncologic emergencies. Short-term corticosteroid regimens are generally well tolerated.

Miscellaneous Agents

Arsenic Trioxide

Arsenic is an organic element and a well-known poison that is an effective treatment for acute promyelocytic leukemia (APL).[30] As an anticancer agent, arsenic trioxide acts as a differentiating agent, inducing the growth progression of cancer cells into mature, more normal cells. It also induces apoptosis. This anticancer agent is discussed in more detail in Chapter 134.

Bleomycin

Bleomycin is an antitumor antibiotic used with other anticancer agents to treat Hodgkin lymphoma and testicular cancer and for pleurodesis to prevent recurrence of a pleural effusion. It is a mixture of peptides from fungal Streptomyces species. Its strength is expressed in units of drug activity and one unit is roughly equal to 1 mg of polypeptide protein. The predominant peptide is bleomycin A2, which makes up about 70% of the commercial drug product.

Its cytotoxicity is secondary to DNA strand breakage, which it produces via free-radical formation. Cytotoxicity depends on binding of the bleomycin–iron complex to DNA. The bleomycin–iron complex then reduces molecular oxygen to free oxygen radicals that cause primarily single-strand breaks in DNA. Bleomycin has greatest effect on cells in the G2 and M phases of the cell cycle.

Bleomycin is inactivated within cells by the enzyme aminohydrolase. This enzyme is widely distributed, but is present in only low concentrations in the skin and the lungs, explaining the predominant toxicities of bleomycin to those sites. Baseline pulmonary function tests and monitoring for pulmonary toxicity are necessary. The presence of hydrolase enzymes in cancer cells is the primary mechanism of resistance to bleomycin. Cells can also become resistant by repairing the DNA breaks produced by bleomycin.

Hydroxyurea

Hydroxyurea is a unique drug that inhibits ribonucleotide reductase. Cells accumulate in the S phase, because DNA synthesis is inhibited and only abnormally short DNA strands are produced.[30] This anticancer agent was used to treat chronic myeloid leukemia (CML) because of its ability to cause a rapid decline in white blood cells.

Mitomycin C

Mitomycin C is a natural product that is sometimes classified as an antitumor antibiotic.[25] It has similarities to nitrogen mustards and may function as an alkylating agent, although its toxicity pattern differs from conventional alkylating agents. It is used to treat bladder cancer. Mitomycin C may be given intravenously or as an instillation directly into the bladder. Mitomycin C causes delayed myelosuppression, so treatment is typically given every six weeks.

Omacetaxine mepesuccinate

Omacetaxine mepesuccinate is a natural ester of the alkaloid cephalotaxine. It inhibits protein translation and thus prevents the initial elongation step of protein synthesis. It is given subcutaneously for treatment of patients with CML who have failed two or more approved targeted drugs for this disease. Additionally, synergy with these approved targeted drugs has been demonstrated in a few clinical studies and additional combination trials are ongoing.[31] The most common serious adverse reactions are myelosuppression, hemorrhage and hyperglycemia.

Radium-223

Radium-223 is for the treatment of patients with castration-resistant prostate cancer, who have symptomatic bone metastases and no known visceral metastatic disease. It is an alpha-particle emitting radiotherapy that mimics calcium and forms complexes with hydroxyapatite at areas of increased bone turnover, such as bone metastases. Radium-223 shows minimal myelosuppression with gastrointestinal adverse reactions the most common toxicities observed following its administration.

Retinoids

Three retinoids are available to treat patients with cancer. Tretinoin (all-trans-retinoic acid), a naturally occurring derivative of vitamin A (retinol), is used to treat APL. Other retinoids indicated for the treatment of cancers include alitretinoin (9-cis-retinoic acid) gel for topical management of Kaposi's sarcoma lesions and bexarotene gel or capsules for treatment of cutaneous T-cell lymphoma.

Retinoids are classified as morphogens, small molecules released from one type of cell that can affect the growth and differentiation of neighboring cells. Their normal roles in the human body are to induce differentiation of some cells, stop the differentiation of others, and both suppress and induce apoptosis in different cell types. Their diverse actions come from the diversity of their receptors. The two classes of retinoid receptors are retinoid X receptors (RXR) and retinoic acid receptors (RAR). RXR are versatile; they bind to RAR and to other nuclear receptors, such as thyroid hormone receptors. After being activated, the receptors act as transcription factors that in turn regulate the expression of genes that control cellular growth and differentiation.

Tretinoin binds primarily to the RAR-α receptors. Alitretinoin is considered a pan-agonist, which means that it binds to all known retinoid receptors, producing diverse regulatory effects. Bexarotene is synthetic and is classed as a rexinoid. It is the first RXR-selective retinoid agonist. The exact mechanism of action of alitretinoin and bexarotene as anticancer agents is unknown.

The common adverse events differ for these three agents. Tretinoin may be associated with retinoic acid syndrome. This syndrome manifests with dyspnea, fever, weight gain, or peripheral edema following cytokine release from the differentiating promyelocytes. Corticosteroids should be administered to manage this syndrome. Aliretinoin is associated with pain, itching and rash and bexarotene is associated with skin reactions, thyroid disorders, hypercholesterolemia and hyperlipidemia.

TARGETED DRUGS

6 Targeted drugs are a class of small molecule drugs (molecular weight less than 1,000 daltons) that are typically identified as kinases inhibitors. Kinases are enzymatic proteins that constitute the intracellular signaling pathways, such as the JAK-STAT and MAPK/ERK pathways described earlier. Following ligand binding to an extracellular receptor, these kinases transmit signals to the cell interior that stimulates activation of the pathway. The targeted drugs turn off or inhibit these pathways by inhibiting the adenosine triphosphate (ATP) binding domain of the kinases.[32] Most of the approved kinase inhibitors are promiscuous, such that they inhibit more than one kinase. The binding to multiple kinases typically leads to off-target effects or toxicities; some toxicities are attributed to specific kinase families. For example, the VEGF family is associated with hypertension, poor wound healing and proteinuria. Although most inhibitors are given orally continuously for months to years, their anticancer activity is typically limited by the development of resistance. Some targeted drugs require identification of the target within the cancer with a companion diagnostic test before initiation of therapy.

Anaplastic Lymphoma Kinase (ALK) Inhibitors

Crizotinib

Crizotinib binds to the ATP intracellular domain of activated ALK, thereby inhibiting phosphorylation and subsequent downstream signaling. ALK rearrangements were first identified in large cell lymphomas and later in NSCLC. In NSCLC, the most common rearrangement involves inversion of chromosome 2p that is primarily fused to the echinoderm microtubule-like protein 4 (EML4), which forms the ALK-EML4 oncogene fusion protein. This rearrangement leads to the activation of downstream signaling pathways and inhibition of apoptosis.[33] ALK-EML4 has a higher prevalence in younger patients, Asians, never or light smokers and adenocarcinoma. Crizotinib also inhibits other kinases, such as ROS1, RON, and MET. Crizotinib is approved for the treatment of patients with locally advanced or metastatic NSCLC that is ALK-positive as detected by an FDA (Food and Drug Administration)-approved test.

The most common toxicities reported in patients taking crizotinib include nausea, vomiting, diarrhea, constipation, fatigue, and elevated transaminases. Visual disorders occur in about half of patients and usually occur within the first weeks of therapy. Edema is also commonly seen and is most likely attributed to the inhibition of MET. Crizotinib has been associated with interstitial lung disease/pneumonitis, hepatotoxicity, QT interval prolongation, and bradycardia.

Many patients with ALK- positive NSCLC initially respond to crizotinib, but most patients will develop resistance. Possible reasons for resistance include the development of brain metastases or development of genetic alterations in ALK.

Alectinib and Ceritinib

Alectinib and ceritinib are second-generation ALK inhibitors that are approved for the treatment of patients with metastatic ALK-positive NSCLC resistant or intolerant to crizotinib. Similar to crizotinib, alectinib and ceritinib inhibit autophosphorylation of ALK and subsequent downstream signaling. In addition to ALK, ceritinib also inhibits insulin-like growth factor 1 receptor (IGF-1R) although to a lesser extent.[34]

Toxicities that are seen with both alectinib and ceritinib include fatigue, bradycardia, and hepatotoxicity. Additional adverse effects seen in patients taking alectinib include anemia, constipation, edema, and myalgia. Patients taking ceritinib should be monitored for QT interval prolongation, gastrointestinal toxicity, pancreatitis, and hyperglycemia. Visual disturbances have been reported with alectinib and ceritinib although to a much lesser extent when compared to crizotinib. Whereas crizotinib may be taken without regard to food, alectinib should be taken with food and ceritinib should be taken on an empty stomach.

Breakpoint Cluster Region-Abelson (BCR-ABL) Inhibitors

Imatinib

Imatinib is a selective inhibitor of the tyrosine kinase activity of BCR-ABL fusion gene, the product of the Philadelphia chromosome. The Philadelphia chromosome is the hallmark finding of CML and it is a translocation of genetic material between chromosomes 9 and 22. Imatinib binds to the kinase-binding site of the BCR-ABL gene, competitively blocking access to ATP. This prevents tyrosine-kinase phosphorylation of the gene and downstream activation of cellular proliferation. An additional effect of imatinib is its ability to inhibit stem-cell factor receptor (KIT) and platelet-derived growth factor receptor (PDGFR).

Imatinib is a standard treatment option for newly diagnosed Philadelphia chromosome–positive (Ph^+) CML and for gastrointestinal stromal tumors (GIST). A major advantage of imatinib is that it can eliminate the Philadelphia chromosome, resulting in cytogenetic responses (ie, elimination of the genetic defect). Imatinib and other BCR-ABL inhibitors are further discussed in Chapter 135. Imatinib is also approved for the treatment of Ph^+ALL and other rare diseases.

Potential serious adverse events observed with imatinib include fluid retention and rash. Severe fluid retention (ie, pleural effusion, pericardial effusion, and ascites) occurs in fewer than 10% of patients taking imatinib, but patients should be monitored regularly for early signs and symptoms of fluid retention and instructed to call their health professionals when symptoms first develop. A rash may require early intervention, because Stevens-Johnson syndrome has been reported with imatinib and may require permanent discontinuation.

Dasatinib, Nilotinib, and Bosutinib

These targeted drugs are next-generation kinase inhibitors that share the same binding site on the BCR-ABL kinase ATP-binding domain with imatinib.[35,36] These inhibitors maintain clinical activity in patients with CML with some mutations in the BCR-ABL binding site that confer imatinib resistance, but none of these inhibitors are active against the genetic alteration identified as T351I. Nilotinib and dasatinib are approved for the treatment of CML and Ph^+ALL. Bosutinib is approved for the treatment of patients resistant or intolerant to the other inhibitors. Both bosutinib and dasatinib also inhibit a family of kinases called sarcoma (Src) kinases that are believed to mediate cellular differentiation, proliferation, and survival; Src kinases have been implicated in modulating multiple oncogenic signal transduction pathways.[36]

These inhibitors have a toxicity profile similar to that of imatinib with myelosuppression, nausea, vomiting, headache, and fluid retention being commonly reported. Bosutinib does not inhibit the KIT or PDGFR, which may account for its reported decrease in myelosuppression.[36]

Ponatinib

As mentioned earlier, the T351I mutation, often referred to as the gatekeeper mutation, confers resistance to the above BCR-ABL inhibitors. Ponatinib was developed with a computational chemistry-based approach to inhibit this mutated conformation of BCR-ABL and provide an effective treatment for this traditionally resistant tumor.[37] Ponatinib is also approved for the treatment of Ph^+ALL that is resistant or intolerant to prior therapy. The more common toxicities reported are similar to other BCL-ABL inhibitors, such as hypertension, rash, headache, constipation, fever, and nausea. Arterial thrombosis and hepatotoxicity have also been observed.

BRAF Inhibitors

BRAF is mutated in a variety of solid tumors with most mutations occurring at codon 600. This codon is in the activation loop of BRAF and increases downstream activity at MEK then ERK, which results in proliferation and survival of cancer cells. BRAF mutations occur in up to 50% of melanomas. The most common mutations are the V600E mutation, which replaces valine with glutamic acid at codon 600 and is seen in about 80% of BRAF mutated melanomas and the V600K mutation, which replaces valine with lysine at this codon and occurs in about 8% of BRAF mutated melanomas. Dabrafenib and vemurafenib inhibit BRAF V600E thereby blocking the MAPK pathway in BRAF-mutated cells. Both inhibitors are approved for the treatment of unresectable or metastatic melanoma with the BRAF V600E mutation as detected by an FDA-approved test. Common toxicities seen with dabrafenib and vemurafenib include papilloma, arthralgia, alopecia, fatigue, and headache. Hand-foot skin reaction (HFSR) and pyrexia are commonly seen with dabrafenib, whereas photosensitivity reactions, hypersensitivity reactions, and QT prolongation are more commonly reported with vemurafenib. Patients should be monitored for the development of new cutaneous malignancies and noncutaneous squamous cell carcinoma that have been associated with dabrafenib and vemurafenib-induced paradoxical activation of the MAPK pathway.[39]

Bruton's Tyrosine Kinase (BTK) Inhibitor

BTK is involved in the B-cell receptor (BCR) signaling pathway that leads to B-cell proliferation and differentiation upon its activation. In B-cell malignancies, the BCR signaling pathway is thought to promote disease progression although the exact mechanism of BCR stimulation has not been determined. Ibrutinib forms an irreversible covalent bond with a cysteine residue of BTK resulting in the inhibition of malignant B-cell proliferation and survival.[40] Ibrutinib is approved for the treatment of the following B-cell malignancies: Waldenstrom's macroglobulinemia; mantle cell lymphoma (MCL), and CLL. Patients should be monitored for hemorrhage, infections, cytopenias, atrial fibrillation, and tumor lysis syndrome. Additional common toxicities include diarrhea, fatigue, musculoskeletal pain, nausea, and rash.

CDK Inhibitor

As discussed earlier in this chapter, CDK play an important role in the cell cycle progression. Specifically, CDK 4/6 and cyclin D1 regulate transition from the G1 phase to the S phase by phosphorylating the retinoblastoma protein (pRb). Palbociclib reversibly inhibits CDK 4/6, which results in the blockade of pRb hyperphosphorylation and ultimately G1 arrest.[41] In breast cancer, it has been demonstrated that cyclin D1 expression and subsequent pRb phosphorylation can be maintained despite estrogen receptor (ER) antagonism. Therefore, inhibiting CDK 4/6 with palbociclib may overcome acquired resistance to hormonal therapy observed in ER-positive breast cancer.[42]

Palbociclib is approved for use with letrozole for the initial treatment of postmenopausal women with ER-positive, HER2-negative advanced breast cancer. Patients receiving palbociclib should be monitored for hematologic toxicities, infections, and pulmonary embolisms.

DNA Methyltransferase Inhibitors

Azacitidine and decitabine are approved for the treatment of patients with myelodysplastic syndrome (MDS), a disorder of hematopoietic cell maturation that can progress to AML. These inhibitors are nucleoside analogs that demonstrate dose-dependent effects. At lower doses, these analogs exert their effects by directly incorporating into DNA and inhibiting DNMT, which leads to cellular differentiation and apoptosis.[6] At higher doses, these agents might cause the formation of covalent adducts between DNMT and active drug being incorporated into DNA, particularly in cells actively dividing. Hypomethylation also appears to normalize the function of genes that control cell differentiation and proliferation, promoting normal cell maturation.[43]

These inhibitors have demonstrated efficacy in slowing the progression of MDS to AML, reducing transfusion requirements, and allowing for the improvement of normal hematopoiesis over time. The primary toxicity is myelosuppression, particularly during early phases of treatment as the malignant clone driving the MDS is cleared from the bone marrow and normal hematopoiesis is slowly restored. As a result, infections occur frequently.

EGFR Inhibitors

Erlotinib

Erlotinib is an oral first generation selective EGFR kinase inhibitor. By competing with ATP for its binding site on the EGFR kinase cytosolic domain, it blocks intracellular downstream signaling and ultimately interferes with the proliferation and growth of cancer cells. Erlotinib is approved for the first-line treatment of patients with metastatic NSCLC whose tumors have EGFR exon 19 deletions or exon 21 (L858R) substitution mutations as detected by an FDA-approved test. In addition, erlotinib is approved for the treatment of locally advanced or metastatic NSCLC as a second-line agent or as maintenance treatment for patients with NSCLC whose disease has not progressed after first-line therapy with a platinum-based regimen. Although erlotinib appears effective in patients with or without EGFR-activating mutations, it appears to be more effective in patients with these mutations.[44] Erlotinib is also approved for use in pancreatic cancer with gemcitabine.

The most common adverse events that occur with erlotinib result from the abundance of EGFR in skin and mucosa and include acneiform rash and diarrhea.[45] Some studies suggest that the development of a rash may be predictive of a response to therapy and correlates with clinical benefit.[46] Interstitial lung disease is a rare adverse event reported in patients taking erlotinib.

Afatinib

Unlike erlotinib which reversibly binds to EGFR, afatinib irreversibly blocks all kinases of the ErbB family by covalently binding to the intracellular kinase domain, which subsequently inhibits tumor growth.[47] Afatinib shares the same indication as erlotinib for patients with NSCLC and exon 19 deletions or exon 21 substitution. The safety and efficacy of afatinib have not been established in patients whose tumors have other EGFR mutations. Toxicities are similar to those seen with erlotinib, although one study reported an increased incidence of rash and diarrhea with afatinib.[47]

Gefitinib

Gefitinib similarly blocks the promotion of the development of lung cancer cells with specific EGFR mutations (exon 19 deletions and exon 21 substitution). This inhibitor was initially approved in 2003, but it was subsequently withdrawn in 2005 when the confirmatory clinical trial failed to demonstrate an improvement in survival. In 2015, gefitinib was approved for the first-line treatment of metastatic NSCLC whose tumors harbor specific types of EGFR gene mutations, as detected by an FDA-approved test. The second approval was based on a clinical trial that demonstrated an improvement in response in this population, which was supported by a retrospective analysis of another trial.[48] Gefitinib has similar adverse events compared to other EGFR inhibitors, including diarrhea and skin reactions.

Lapatinib

Lapatinib is a 4-anilinoquinazoline kinase inhibitor that inhibits the intracellular kinase domains of both EGFR (ErbB1) and HER2 (ErbB2). It has demonstrated clinical activity with capecitabine in patients with breast cancer whose tumors overexpress HER2 and who have previously received therapy with trastuzumab, an anthracycline, and a taxane. Lapatinib is also approved for use with letrozole in postmenopausal women for the treatment of hormone receptor-positive metastatic breast cancer that overexpresses HER2. Common adverse events include an increased incidence of diarrhea, hepatotoxicity, rash, and QT interval prolongation. Two specific mutations observed in the HLA-DQA and HLA-DRB genes have been associated with an increased risk of hepatotoxicity.[49,50]

Osimertinib

Osimertinib is approved for the treatment of patients with metastatic EGFR T790M mutation-positive NSCLC, as detected by an FDA-approved test, who have progressed on or after EGFR tyrosine kinase inhibitor. This mutation, referred to as the EGFR gatekeeper mutation, occurs in about 50% of patients who develop acquired resistance to first-line therapy with erlotinib or gefitinib.[37] Gastrointestinal and dermatologic toxicities are commonly reported with osimertinib. Serious adverse events include interstitial lung disease/pneumonitis, pneumonia, and pulmonary embolism.

Hedgehog Inhibitors

Sonidegib and vismodegib are oral inhibitors of the Hedgehog signaling pathway that is abnormally activated in basal cell carcinoma and medulloblastoma. Through binding to smoothened (SMO) receptor, sonidegib and vismodegib prevent downstream signaling and activation of the Hedgehog pathway leading to the inhibition of tumor growth.[51] Vismodegib is approved for metastatic or locally advanced basal cell carcinoma, while sonidegib is approved only for locally advanced disease.

The Hedgehog pathway is essential for early embryogenesis. Therefore, both sonidegib and vismodegib have been shown to be embryotoxic, fetotoxic, and teratogenic in animals. The approved labeling for both drugs contains specific recommendations regarding contraception for women of child bearing potential and for men with a pregnant partner or a female partner of child bearing potential, as well as limitations regarding blood and sperm donation during treatment and for several months following the last dose. Vismodegib is generally well tolerated and toxicities include muscle spasm, alopecia, dysgeusia, fatigue, and nausea. Sonidegib is associated with an increased risk of serious musculoskeletal toxicities and the probability of developing this adverse event appears to rise with increasing sonidegib exposure. Grades 3 and 4 serum lipase and creatine kinase elevations occurred in at least 5% of patients given the approved dose of 200 mg daily. Sonidegib uniquely has a very long elimination half-life of 28 days compared to vismodegib and other small molecular targeted drugs.

HDAC Inhibitors

Belinostat

The mechanism of HDAC inhibitors was discussed earlier in the chapter. Belinostat is an HDAC inhibitor that is approved for the treatment of relapsed or refractory peripheral T-cell lymphoma. Ongoing trials are evaluating the administration of belinostat with other anticancer agents. The most common toxicities seen with belinostat include pyrexia, nausea, fatigue, and anemia.

Panobinostat

Panobinostat is an HDAC inhibitor that has been shown to improve progression-free survival with bortezomib and dexamethasone in patients with multiple myeloma who have received at least two prior regimens, including bortezomib and an immunomodulatory agent.[52] Since severe cardiac toxicities have been reported with panobinostat, an electrocardiograph (ECG) and electrolytes should be monitored at baseline and during treatment. Nausea, vomiting, and severe diarrhea are often seen with panobinostat.

Romidepsin and Vorinostat

Similar to belinostat and panobinostat, romidepsin and vorinostat inhibit HDAC. Romidepsin is approved for the treatment of patients with cutaneous or peripheral T-cell lymphoma who have received at least one prior therapy and vorinostat is approved for the treatment of cutaneous T-cell lymphoma who have received at least two prior therapies. Patients receiving romidepsin should be monitored for myelosuppression, ECG changes, and infections. Reactivation of DNA viruses, including EBV and hepatitis B virus (HBV), have been reported with romidepsin.[53] Serious adverse events reported with vorinostat include venous thromboembolism, dose-related thrombocytopenia, and anemia.

JAK Inhibitor

Ruxolitinib is an oral inhibitor of JAK1 and JAK2 of the JAK-STAT signaling pathway; these kinases are involved in the regulation of blood and immunologic functioning. In myelofibrosis and polycythemia vera, JAK1 and JAK2 activity is dysregulated. Ruxolitinib has been shown to modulate the affected JAK1 and JAK2 activity resulting in clinical responses and symptomatic improvement.[54] Approved indications for ruxolitinib include the treatment of intermediate or high-risk myelofibrosis and the treatment of polycythemia vera in patients who have had an inadequate response to or are intolerant of hydroxyurea. The most common toxicities include thrombocytopenia, anemia, bruising, dizziness, and headache.

MEK Inhibitors

Reported resistance mechanisms of the BRAF inhibitors dabrafenib and vemurafenib include reactivation of the MAPK pathway. The combination of BRAF and MEK inhibition has demonstrated delayed resistance and decreased incidence of secondary cancers.[42] Trametinib is approved as a single agent and with dabrafenib for the treatment of unresectable or metastatic melanoma with BRAF V600E or V600K mutations as detected by an FDA-approved test. Common toxicities reported with trametinib include rash, diarrhea, and lymphedema. Serious toxicities reported with the combination dabrafenib and trametinib include hemorrhage, venous thromboembolism, and febrile reactions.

Unlike trametinib, cobimetinib is not approved as a single agent; it is only approved for the treatment of unresectable or metastatic melanoma with BRAF V600E or V600K mutations with vemurafenib. Common toxicities include diarrhea, nausea, vomiting, photosensitivity reaction, and pyrexia. Serious risks with the use of cobimetinib are new primary malignancies, hemorrhage, cardiomyopathy, severe dermatologic reactions, serous retinopathy and retinal vein occlusion, hepatotoxicity, and rhabdomyolysis.

mTOR Inhibitors

Temsirolimus

Temsirolimus and its primary active metabolite, sirolimus, bind to the intracellular protein 12-kilodalton FK506 binding protein (FKBP-12) and this protein–drug complex inhibits mTOR by blocking its kinase activity.[55] mTOR inhibition suppresses the production of proteins that regulate progression through the cell cycle resulting in G1 phase arrest. Temsirolimus is approved for the treatment of advanced renal cell carcinoma.

The most common adverse reactions with temsirolimus are rash, asthenia, mucositis, nausea, edema, and anorexia. Infusion reactions may occur and pre-treatment with an antihistamine is recommended. Lab abnormalities are common with temsirolimus including hyperglycemia and hyperlipidemia. Rare but potentially serious adverse events include interstitial lung disease, immunosuppression, and renal failure.

Everolimus

Similar to temsirolimus, everolimus is an mTOR inhibitor that reduces protein synthesis and cell proliferation by binding to FKBP-12. Everolimus has the following indications: treatment of advanced renal cell carcinoma after treatment failure with sunitinib or sorafenib; hormone receptor-positive, HER2-negative breast cancer with exemestane after letrozole or anastrozole failure in postmenopausal women; subependymal giant cell astrocytoma with tubular sclerosis complex (TSC); renal angiomyolipoma with TSC; and unresectable or metastatic pancreatic neuroendocrine tumors. Dosage forms for everolimus include traditional oral tablets and tablets for oral suspension, but it is important to note that the tablets for oral suspension do not have the same FDA approved indications. Stomatitis is one of the most common toxicities with everolimus while other adverse reactions are similar to those of temsirolimus.

Multikinase Inhibitors

Axitinib, Pazopanib, Sorafenib and Sunitinib

Several kinase inhibitors inhibit multiple kinases, such as axitinib, pazopanib, sorafenib and sunitinib. Sunitinib and sorafenib inhibit multiple growth factor receptors (VEGFR2 and PDGFR), cell surface proteins (KIT), and cytokine receptors (FLT3) and thus, disrupt multiple aberrant intracellular signaling pathways. In addition, sorafenib inhibits Raf, which is part of the MAPK signaling pathway.[56] Sunitinib is approved for GIST, pancreatic neuroendocrine tumors and advanced renal cell carcinoma and sorafenib is approved for unresectable hepatocellular carcinoma, advanced renal cell carcinoma, and locally recurrent or metastatic, progressive, differentiated thyroid carcinoma refractory to radioactive iodine treatment.

Pazopanib and axitinib are second-generation inhibitors. Pazopanib inhibits all VEGFR kinases with additional activity against KIT and PDGFR. Axitinib has enhanced potency and selectivity to all VEGFR kinases with minor activity against PDGFR and KIT.[57] Pazopanib is approved for the treatment of advanced renal cell carcinoma and axitinib is approved for the same indication after failure of one prior systemic therapy. Pazopanib has an additional indication for patients with advanced soft tissue sarcoma who have received prior chemotherapy.

Gastrointestinal toxicities such as diarrhea are common with these drugs, as are rash, fatigue, and hypertension. Patients should also be monitored for the development of thyroid dysfunction and hepatotoxicity.

Cabozantinib

Cabozantinib is a small molecule inhibitor of numerous receptor kinases, most importantly RET (rearranged during transfection), VEGFR2, and MET membrane receptor.[58] MET is required for several important processes during embryogenesis (eg, angiogenesis) and leads to abnormal growth and proliferation of several tumors. Medullary thyroid cancers express mutated RET as well as VEGFR2 and MET. Cabozantinib is approved for the treatment of metastatic medullary thyroid cancers. Toxicities reported in clinical trials included diarrhea, HFSR, lymphopenia, hypocalcemia, hypertension, transaminitis, and stomatitis.

Lenvatinib

Lenvatinib primarily inhibits VEGFR1, -2, and -3, but it can also inhibit other kinases including fibroblast growth factor receptor (FGFR) and PDGFR-alpha, KIT, and RET. Lenvatinib is approved for the treatment of locally recurrent or metastatic, progressive, radioactive iodine-refractory differentiated thyroid cancer. Common toxicities seen with lenvatinib include hypertension, fatigue, diarrhea, proteinuria, stomatitis, and HFSR.

Regorafenib

Regorafenib is multikinase inhibitor that blocks the activity of several protein kinases, including those involved in the regulation of tumor angiogenesis (VEGFR1, -2, and -3), oncogenes and downstream targets (KIT, RET, RAF1, and BRAF), as well as PDGFR and FGFR.[59] Because many of these targets are important in colon cancer and GIST, regorafenib is approved for the treatment of metastatic colorectal cancer and for advanced or metastatic GIST in patients who have previously received imatinib and sunitinib. Serious adverse events reported with regorafenib include hepatotoxicity, hemorrhage, gastrointestinal perforation, and reversible posterior leukoencephalopathy syndrome. Regorafenib should be stopped prior to surgery as wound-healing complications may occur. Common adverse reactions with regorafenib include asthenia, hypertension, mucositis, gastrointestinal toxicities, and HFSR. Regorafenib should be given with a low-fat evening meal, as the toxicities anecdotally appear minimized when given at night.

Vandetanib

Vandetanib is a small molecule inhibitor of RET, VEGFR2 and -3, and EGFR.[60] Most medullary thyroid tumors express mutated RET and vandetanib has demonstrated activity in this tumor. It is approved for the treatment of metastatic medullary thyroid cancer. Toxicities observed with vandetanib include diarrhea, hypertension, and rash. Vandetanib can prolong the QT interval and cases of Torsades de pointes and sudden death have been reported. Because of this risk, vandetanib is only available through a risk evaluation and mitigation strategy (REMS) program where prescribers and pharmacies must be certified through the program to prescribe and dispense vandetanib.

PARP Inhibitor

PARP is essential for the repair of single-stranded DNA breaks through the base-excision-repair pathway. Tumors with breast cancer gene 1 (BRCA1) or BRCA2 mutations are highly sensitive to the blockade of single-strand DNA breaks (through PARP inhibition), because they exhibit a compromised ability to repair double-strand DNA breaks. This concept is known as *synthetic lethality* and occurs when there is a lethal synergy between two nonlethal events. Olaparib inhibits PARP and induces synthetic lethality in BRCA1 and BRCA2 deficient tumor cells.[61,62] Olaparib is indicated for the treatment of deleterious or suspected deleterious germline BRCA mutated advanced ovarian cancer who have been treated with three or more prior lines of chemotherapy.

Patients receiving olaparib should be monitored for hematological toxicity as MDS/AML has been reported with olaparib. Common toxicities include fatigue, musculoskeletal pain, dermatitis, nausea and vomiting, upper respiratory infections, and anemia.

PI3K Inhibitor

Malignant B-cell proliferation and survival depend on PI3K signaling. The p110δ isoform is highly expressed in malignant lymphoid B-cells and plays a direct role in activation of the PI3K pathway. Through the selective inhibition of p110*δ*, idelalisib induces apoptosis.[63] Idelalisib is approved for the treatment of relapsed CLL with rituximab. Other indications include relapsed follicular B-cell NHL and small lymphocytic lymphoma in patients who have received at least two prior systemic therapies.

Boxed warnings for idelalisib include hepatotoxicity, severe diarrhea or colitis, pneumonitis, and intestinal perforation. Common adverse reactions include neutropenia, fever, rash, and elevated liver enzymes.

Proteasome Inhibitors

The proteasome is an enzyme complex that is responsible for degrading proteins that control the cell cycle. Some of the proteins degraded by proteasomes regulate critical functions for cancer growth, such as regulation of the cell cycle, transcription factors, apoptosis, angiogenesis, and cell adhesion.[64]

Bortezomib

Bortezomib has specific affinity for the catalytic portion of the 26S proteasome. It is a specific inhibitor of this proteasome, which results in accumulation of IκB, an inhibitor of the major transcription factor nuclear factor κB (NF-κB). NF-κB induces transcription of genes that block cell death pathways and promote cell proliferation. Its activity depends on its release from its inhibitory partner protein, IκB, in the cytoplasm and its move to the nucleus. When IκB fails to degrade, through the actions of bortezomib, NF-κB remains in the cytoplasm, preventing it from transcribing the genes that promote cancer growth. Bortezomib is approved for the treatment of multiple myeloma and MCL.[64]

The most commonly reported toxicities with bortezomib include fatigue, nausea, diarrhea, thrombocytopenia, and fever. Peripheral neuropathy may develop or worsen with the use of bortezomib. Subcutaneous administration of bortezomib has been associated with a lower incidence of peripheral neuropathy when compared with intravenous administration. Caution should be used when treating patients with existing heart disease as cardiac failure has been reported. Patients should also be monitored for hypotension and acute respiratory syndrome. At least 72 hours should elapse between consecutive doses of bortezomib to minimize cumulative toxicity by permitting the restoration of proteasome function between doses.

Carfilzomib

Carfilzomib is a second-generation proteasome inhibitor approved for relapsed or refractory multiple myeloma. Whereas bortezomib exhibits reversible inhibition of multiple proteasome targets, the inhibition with carfilzomib is irreversible. As a result, carfilzomib produces more sustained inhibition of the proteasome. Carfilzomib is a more potent and selective inhibitor of the chymotrypsin-like activity of the proteasome and immunoproteasome and has been demonstrated to overcome bortezomib resistance in cell lines.[65]

Ixazomib

Ixazomib is an oral proteasome inhibitor approved with lenalidomide and dexamethasone for the treatment of patients with multiple myeloma who have received at least one prior therapy. Common adverse reactions are gastrointestinal toxicity, thrombocytopenia, peripheral neuropathy, peripheral edema, and back pain. Ixazomib has a unique administration schedule for an oral agent (given on days 1, 8, and 15 of a 28-day cycle) and should be taken on an empty stomach.

Miscellaneous

Thalidomide, Lenalidomide, and Pomalidomide

Thalidomide, the infamous drug that caused severe limb deformities when used by pregnant women as a nonprescription sedative in the 1960s, is approved for treatment of leprosy and multiple myeloma. Thalidomide is a glutamic acid derivative and is broadly classified as an immunomodulatory drug. Lenalidomide and pomalidomide are analogs of thalidomide with similar therapeutic activity but different adverse event profiles. Lenalidomide is approved for the treatment of multiple myeloma, transfusion-dependent anemia caused by MDS with a specific mutation and MCL whose disease has relapsed or progressed after two prior therapies, including bortezomib. Pomalidomide has been approved for the treatment of multiple myeloma with disease progression after at least two prior therapies including lenalidomide and a proteasome inhibitor.

These drugs have many potential mechanisms of action, but the most important is thought to be angiogenesis inhibition, an action also linked to their teratogenic effects. Other possible mechanisms include direct inhibition of cancer cells, free radical oxidative damage to DNA, interference with adhesion of cancer cells, inhibition of TNF-α production, or alteration of cytokine secretion that affects the growth of cancer cells.

The most common toxicities for thalidomide include somnolence, constipation, dizziness, orthostatic hypotension, rash, and peripheral neuropathies. In contrast, lenalidomide is associated with much less somnolence and neuropathies compared with thalidomide. Neutropenia, thrombocytopenia, and thrombotic events are prevalent with thalidomide, lenalidomide and pomalidomide. To avoid embryo-fetal exposure and to inform health professionals and patients of the teratogenic potential, these drugs are only available under a REMS program.

Lanreotide

As an octapeptide analog of somatostatin, the mechanism of lanreotide is believed to be similar to that of natural somatostatin through the inhibition of neuroendocrine functions. Somatostatin analogues are commonly used to treat hypersecretion syndromes associated with neuroendocrine tumors, but only recently have been proven to have an antitumor effect associated with prolonged progression-free survival. Lanreotide is approved for the treatment of unresectable, well or moderately differentiated, locally advanced or metastatic gastroenteropancreatic neuroendocrine tumors. Common toxicities include abdominal pain, musculoskeletal pain, vomiting, headache, injection site reaction, and hypertension. Patients should be monitored for hypoglycemia, hyperglycemia and gallstones.

Clinical **Controversy...**

Numerous targeted agents and biologic therapies have been recently approved and although this is a very exciting time for the world of oncology, many of these new agents come at a high financial cost to the patient. What is an acceptable cost of a small increase in survival and who should make that determination? "Financial toxicity" of anticancer agents is an important conversation oncology health professionals should have with their patients and caregivers.

BIOLOGIC THERAPIES

7 Biologic therapies include cytokines, mAbs, growth factors, and vaccines. The mAb are the most common biologic therapy available to treat patients with cancer.

Monoclonal Antibodies

The mAbs are designed to target pathways critical for the survival and growth of cancer cells and improve outcomes while minimizing toxicities. The mAb can bind to either the extracellular receptor or to its natural ligand and prevent the activation of the downstream intracellular signaling. Several antibodies are available to treat both solid tumors and hematologic malignancies.

The mAbs consist of immunoglobulin sequences that are known to recognize a specific antigen or protein on the surface of cells. There are five classes of immunoglobulins, but IgG is the most commonly used therapeutically. Similar to endogenous antibodies, the Fab portion is composed of heavy and light chains that are responsible for binding to antigens and the constant region determines the effector function of the antibody. The mAb may be naked (unconjugated) or conjugated to toxin (immunotoxin), chemotherapy agent (antibody drug conjugate), or radioactive particle (radioimmunoconjugate).

Standardized nomenclature exists for naming mAbs. The suffix -mab is used for all antibodies and it is always preceded by the identification of the animal source of the product. The letters o, u, xi, and zu before the -mab suffix indicate murine, human, chimeric, and humanized, respectively. The general disease state the antibody is treating precedes the source and is identified using a code. Most approved antibodies used to treat cancer have the code -tu(m) that designates it for use against miscellaneous tumors. If the product is conjugated, a separate word is added to identify the toxin, chemotherapy, or radioactive particle. For example, the antibody-drug conjugate of trastuzumab and mertansine is named ado-trastuzumab ematansine.

The first mAb used in humans were murine, but most of the antibodies used today are humanized or human. These agents differ in the amount of foreign component. Hypersensitivity and infusion-related reactions, with or without the development of antiproduct antibodies (APA), are generally greatest with murine antibodies and least with humanized antibodies. The severity of these reactions can range from mild (eg, fever, chills, nausea, and rash) to severe, life-threatening anaphylaxis with cardiopulmonary collapse. Patients with a hypersensitivity or infusion-related reaction may also experience chest or back pain during the infusion. Patients with circulating cancer cells in the bloodstream are at highest risk for more severe reactions. Patients must be monitored closely during infusion. The reactions tend to be more severe with the initial infusion, and subside with subsequent treatments. Some mAbs require premedication, including antihistamines, acetaminophen, or steroids, to minimize hypersensitivity reactions. Recommended infusion rates may be lower for the initial dose, with incremental increases as tolerated by the patient. For patients experiencing signs or symptoms of infusion-related reactions, the infusion should be interrupted and prompt treatment with antihistamines, corticosteroids, and other supportive measures should be initiated. Other adverse events are typically determined by the selectivity of the target antigen. mAbs against antigens found on normal and cancer cells will have increased toxicity compared with tumor-specific antigens found only on tumor tissues.

Unconjugated mAbs that target antigens on the cell surface of cancer cells may induce death of cancer cells by several mechanisms. These mAbs could directly mediate cell killing through complement-dependent cytotoxicity (CDC), antibody-dependent cell-mediated cytotoxicity (ADCC), or inhibiting intracellular signaling. CDC occurs when the Fc portion of the antibody activates the complement system, leading to tumor cell lysis and ADCC occurs when effector cells that contain Fc receptors bind to the Fc portion of the antibody and either lyses or phagocytizes the antibody-containing cell. Natural killer cells, monocytes, and macrophages are all capable of mediating ADCC. Finally, antibody binding may result in the transmission of signals that induce apoptosis, or programmed cell death in the targeted cell.

Immunoconjugates deliver a payload, typically a chemotherapy agent, toxin, or radioactive particle to a cell targeted by the antibody. After the antibody binds the target antigen, the payload is internalized by the target cell and kills cancer cells through traditional mechanisms of action. In addition to killing the target cell, radioimmunoconjugates are capable of killing antigen-negative cancer cells sometimes termed the bystander effect. Theoretically, immunoconjugates conjugates deliver therapy to specific sites of disease while limiting systemic exposure to the chemotherapy, radiation, or toxin. The mAb might also contribute to the observed anticancer effects.

Monoclonal Antibodies that Target B-lymphocyte Antigens

Rituximab

Rituximab is a chimeric antibody directed against the cluster of differentiation (CD)20 antigen found on the surface of normal and cancerous B-cells. The Fab domain of rituximab binds to the CD20 antigen on B lymphocytes and the Fc domain recruits immune effector functions to mediate B-cell lysis. Possible explanations for its anticancer effect include CDC and ADCC of malignant B-cells and possibly a direct apoptotic effect.

Rituximab is approved for the treatment of low-grade or follicular, CD20-positive, B-cell NHL in multiple settings. It is also approved for the treatment of CD20-positive CLL with standard chemotherapy. Rituximab is also indicated for the treatment of a variety of immune-mediated diseases, including rheumatoid arthritis, granulomatosis with polyangiitis, and microscopic polyangiitis.

Most of the infusion-related reactions associated with rituximab occur during the first infusion and are components of an infusion-related complex secondary to the amount of circulating B-cells. After the first infusion, the incidence and the severity of these reactions decrease dramatically. Premedication and additional supportive care medications may be required depending on indication. The most common events with the infusion-related complex are transient fever, chills, nausea, asthenia, and headache. Additionally, rituximab may cause HBV reactivation and should not be administered in patients with severe, active infections.

Ofatumumab

Ofatumumab is a type I human mAb that also targets the CD20 antigen. Its mechanism of action is similar to that of rituximab, but ofatumumab targets a different epitope than rituximab, has greater affinity for the antigen, and dissociates from the epitope slower than rituximab.[66] Specifically, ofatumumab binds to two regions of the CD20 antigen, the small extracellular loop and the N-terminal region of the large extracellular loop. This allows it to demonstrate anticancer activity in patients who have progressed on rituximab in a variety of B-cell cancers.[66]

Ofatumumab is approved as a single agent for refractory, recurrent or progressive CLL and with other anticancer agents for treatment-naive CLL. Adverse reactions are similar to rituximab with fewer infusion-related reactions and a higher rate of infectious complications.

Obinutuzumab

Obinutuzumab is a type II humanized anti-CD20 mAb approved with chlorambucil. When compared with the type I anti-CD20 antibodies such as rituximab, type II agents exhibit a different elbow hinge angle and therefore bind CD20 in a different orientation. Furthermore, the Fc portion of obinutuzumab has been glycoengineered to reduce fucosylation resulting in improved receptor affinity and enhanced ADCC potency.[67,68]

Adverse events associated with obinutuzumab include infusion reactions, myelosuppression, nausea, and diarrhea. HBV reactivation and Progressive Multifocal Leukoencephalopathy (PML) have been reported with obinutuzumab use.

Ibritumomab Tiuxetan

Ibritumomab tiuxetan is a radioimmunoconjugate that consists of the murine anti-CD20 antibody ibritumomab and a linker chelator tiuxetan that allows the attachment of indium-111 (used for imaging and dosimetry) or yttrium-90 (active radiotherapy). Yttrium-90-ibritumomab is the therapeutic radiation isotope and selectively delivers radiation to B-cells that express the CD20 antigen.

The radiation-induced cytotoxicity delivered by yttrium -90-ibritumomab not only affects the cancer cells it binds but also other cells that are within the path length of the radioisotope's emissions (ie, bystander effect). Consequently, yttrium-90-ibritumomab can induce cell death in CD20-positive and -negative cancer cells and eradicates a large number of cancer cells. Ibritumomab tiuxetan also induces ADCC, CDC, and apoptosis. Ibritumomab tiuxetan is indicated to be given with rituximab for the treatment of relapsed or refractory, low-grade or follicular B-cell NHL and for previously untreated follicular NHL who achieved a response to first-line chemotherapy. The therapeutic regimen consists of two steps. Rituximab is administered on day 1, and about one week later (day 7, 8, or 9), an additional dose of rituximab is administered followed by yttrium-90-ibritumomab within 4 hours after completion of the rituximab infusion.

Adverse reactions include severe infusion-related reactions. Myelosuppression is common with ibritumomab tiuxetan as a consequence of the radioisotope. Ibritumomab tiuxetan results in prolonged thrombocytopenia and neutropenia and dose modifications are necessary based on baseline neutrophil and platelet blood counts. The median durations of thrombocytopenia and neutropenia were 24 days and 22 days, respectively. Monitoring and management of cytopenias, along with their complications is necessary for up to 3 months after completing treatment.

Tositumomab

Tositumomab is a murine anti-CD20 radioimmunoconjugate similar to ibritumomab tiuxetan. One important difference is that tositumomab is combined with the radioisotope I-131, which has therapeutic and safety implications. The mechanisms of cell death are similar to ibritumomab as is the indication for refractory NHL. The tositumomab regimen consists of four components in two steps: a dosimetric step to assess the radiation dose and a therapeutic step.

Most adverse events are similar to ibritumomab tituxetan, including infusion-related reactions and myelosuppression. Complete blood counts should be obtained weekly for 10 weeks to 12 weeks to assess recovery of normal blood counts. To prevent iodine uptake by the thyroid gland and subsequent delivery of ionizing radiation to the thyroid gland, thyroid protective agents (eg, saturated solution of potassium iodide) should be given before starting the tositumomab dosing regimen and continued for 14 days after the therapeutic dose.

Monoclonal Antibodies that Target Other Cell Surface Receptors

Alemtuzumab

Alemtuzumab is a recombinant humanized mAb that is directed against CD52. CD52 is expressed on the surface of B and T lymphocytes, natural killer cells, monocytes, and macrophages.[69] Its anticancer activity comes from binding to the CD52 antigen present on leukemic lymphocytes and inducing cell lysis and death. Alemtuzumab is indicated as a single agent for the treatment of B-cell CLL.

Alemtuzumab is associated with severe infusion-related reactions, hematologic toxicity, and opportunistic infections.[69] Hematologic toxicity consisting of severe prolonged neutropenia and thrombocytopenia occurs in most patients. Health professionals should monitor complete blood counts prior to each dose to determine the need for dose modification. Because CD52 is expressed on lymphocytes, alemtuzumab can induce profound lymphopenia including a decrease in CD4 and CD8 counts. Patients should receive prophylaxis for *Pneumocystis jiroveci* pneumonia and herpes virus, which should be continued for a minimum of 2 months after completing alemtuzumab therapy or until recovery of CD4 counts. Alemtuzumab is only available through a restricted distribution program and has a REMS program to mitigate the risks of autoimmune conditions, infusion reactions, and malignancies associated with the use of alemtuzumab.

Blinatumomab

Blinatumomab is a bispecific T-cell engaging antibody against a B-lymphocyte-specific molecule CD19. Through the formation of a synapse between CD19 on malignant B-cells and CD3 on T-cell receptors, blinatumomab potentiates T-cell induced cytotoxic cell killing. Blinatumomab is indicated for the treatment of Philadelphia chromosome-negative relapsed or refractory B-cell precursor ALL.[70]

Due to its short half-life (~2 hours) and mechanism of action, blinatumomab is administered as a continuous intravenous infusion over 28 days. In addition to possible decreased efficacy, early trials that utilized shorter infusion durations also reported a higher rate of neurologic toxicities and cytokine-release syndrome.[70] Patients receiving blinatumomab are usually hospitalized for the first 9 days of cycle 1 and the first 2 days of cycle 2 to monitor for infusion reactions. Patients receiving blinatumomab should be monitored for infusion reactions, cytokine release syndrome, neurological toxicities, and infections. Common toxicities include fever, headache, peripheral edema, and rash.

Brentuximab Vedotin

Brentuximab vedotin is an antibody–drug conjugate that targets the CD30 antigen found on cancer cells. Upon binding to the CD30 antigen, brentuximab vedotin is internalized by endocytosis, and the dipeptide bond that links the naked mAb to the chemotherapy monomethylauristatin E (MMAE) is cleaved.[71] MMAE then binds to microtubules and acts as an inhibitor of microtubule polymerization. It may also induce apoptosis by inhibiting NF-κB. Brentuximab vedotin is indicated for Hodgkin lymphoma after failure of autologous hematopoietic stem cell transplant and relapsed anaplastic large cell lymphoma. Infusion reactions, peripheral neuropathy, and neutropenia are common toxicities seen with brentuximab vedotin administration; these toxicities are common with other microtubule inhibitors.

Daratumumab

Daratumumab is a mAb that inhibits the growth of CD38 expressing tumor cells by inducing apoptosis directly through Fc mediated cross linking and immune-mediated tumor cell lysis through CDC, ADCC, and antibody dependent cellular phagocytosis. Myeloid derived suppressor cells and a subset of regulatory T cells express CD38. It is approved for the treatment of patients with multiple myeloma who have received at least three prior lines of therapy.

The most frequently reported adverse reactions were infusion reactions, fatigue, nausea, back pain, pyrexia, cough, upper respiratory tract infection, and myelosuppression. Pre-medications (corticosteroid, antipyretic, and an antihistamine) and post-infusion medications (corticosteroid) are recommended to prevent acute and delayed infusion reactions. Since daratumumab interferes with blood bank crossmatching, specifically with Indirect Antiglobulin Tests, it is recommended that a type and screen be performed prior to treatment initiation. If a blood transfusion is necessary, inform the blood bank that the patient has received daratumumab.

Dinutuximab

Glycolipid GD2 is expressed primarily on the cell surface of neuroblastoma cells and on normal tissues including neurons and peripheral sensory nerve fibers.[72,73] The function of the GD2 carbohydrate antigen is not completely understood, but is thought to play a role in the attachment of tumor cells to extracellular matrix proteins.[72] Dinutuximab is a chimeric mAb that binds GD2 inducing cell lysis through ADCC and CDC. This activity is thought to be enhanced when dinutuximab is given with granulocyte-macrophage colony-stimulating factor (GM-CSF) and IL-2.[73] Dinutuximab is approved to be given with GM-CSF, IL-2, and 13-cis-retinoic acid for the treatment of pediatric patients with high-risk neuroblastoma who achieve at least a partial response to prior first-line multiagent, multimodality therapy. Serious toxicities associated with dinutuximab include infections, infusion reactions, hypokalemia, hypotension, and capillary leak syndrome.

Monoclonal Antibodies That Target Growth Factor Receptors and Their Ligands

EGFR Inhibitors

Cetuximab is a chimeric mAb that binds specifically to the extracellular domain of EGFR on both normal and cancer cells and competitively inhibits the binding of epidermal growth factor and other ligands, such as transforming growth factor-α. Binding of cetuximab to the EGFR inhibits cell growth, induces apoptosis, and inhibits VEGF production. Cetuximab may be given as a single agent or with other anticancer agents to treat metastatic KRAS wild-type colorectal cancer and squamous cell head and neck cancer. Acneiform rash and skin reactions occur in most patients receiving cetuximab, as observed with the targeted drugs that inhibit EGFR.[46] Multiple follicular or pustular lesions generally appear within the first 2 weeks of therapy and usually resolve after cessation of treatment. Resolution can be slow, continuing beyond 28 days in nearly half of cases. In patients who develop a severe rash, dose modifications may be necessary. Interestingly, a trend for improved responses with increasing severity of skin reactions has been reported and requires further research to assess the clinical importance of these reactions.[46]

Panitumumab is a mAb that also binds to the cell surface EGFR. It is an IgG2 antibody and the first human mAb approved to treat cancer. Panitumumab is currently approved to treat KRAS wild-type metastatic colon cancer with chemotherapy for first-line treatment or as a single agent following disease progression after prior treatment. Adverse reactions are similar to cetuximab, although severe reactions appear to be less common because panitumumab does not have a murine component.

Both antibodies appear to be more effective in patients with tumors that are RAS wild type, than patients with tumors that are RAS mutation positive. Therefore, patients with metastatic colorectal cancer should not receive anti-EGFR antibody therapy if a RAS mutation is detected.[74] Genetic testing of colorectal cancers is discussed in further detail in Chapter 130.

Necitumumab is a next-generation mAb that binds to the human EGFR and blocks the binding of EGFR to its ligands. It is approved for first-line treatment of patients with metastatic *squamous* NSCLC with gemcitabine and cisplatin. Serious and clinically significant adverse events include cardiopulmonary arrest, hypomagnesemia, thromboembolic events, dermatologic toxicities, and infusion reactions. Since increased toxicity and mortality was observed when necitumumab was given with pemetrexed and cisplatin for the treatment of nonsquamous NSCLC, patients with metastatic nonsquamous NSCLC should not receive necitumumab.

HER2 Inhibitors

Trastuzumab Trastuzumab is a humanized mAb that selectively binds to HER2. HER2 is overexpressed in about 33% of breast cancers, in about 22% of gastroesophageal junction and gastric cancers, and to varying degrees in other malignancies.[75] Trastuzumab inhibits cell cycle progression by decreasing cells entering the S phase of the cell cycle, which leads to downregulation of HER2 receptors on cancer cells and decreased cell proliferation.[74] Trastuzumab also leads to ADCC and CDC and directly induces apoptosis in cells overexpressing HER2. In addition, synergy between trastuzumab and chemotherapy has been demonstrated, resulting in trastuzumab often being used in combination regimens. Trastuzumab is approved for the treatment of HER2-positive early stage and metastatic breast cancer and metastatic gastric or gastroesophageal junction adenocarcinoma. The tumor should overexpress HER2 as measured by diagnostic tests that can quantify gene amplification or protein expression.

The most serious adverse reactions caused by trastuzumab include cardiomyopathy, infusion-related reactions, hypersensitivity reactions, and increased myelosuppression. An evaluation of cardiac function should be performed before administration and extreme caution should be exercised in patients with preexisting cardiac dysfunction and in those who have received prior anthracyclines. In patients who develop a clinically significant decrease in left ventricular function (defined as greater than 16% decrease in ejection fraction from pretreatment levels or an ejection fraction below normal limits and greater than 10% decrease from baseline), discontinuation of therapy should be considered. Similar to most mAbs, the symptoms associated with a hypersensitivity reaction are most common with the initial infusions and occur infrequently thereafter. Myelosuppression is infrequent with trastuzumab alone, but the incidence of neutropenia and febrile neutropenia is higher when trastuzumab is given with myelosuppressive chemotherapy.

Ado-Trastuzumab Ematansine Ado-trastuzumab ematansine is indicated for the treatment of HER2-positive, metastatic breast cancer previously treated with trastuzumab and a taxane. Ado-trastuzumab ematansine is an antibody–drug conjugate that consists of the humanized anti-HER2 monoclonal antibody trastuzumab covalently linked to the microtubule inhibitory drug DM1 (derivative of maytansine 1).[76] Ematansine refers to the linker-payload complex. It is important to note that ado-trastuzumab ematansine and trastuzumab are not interchangeable and should not be substituted for one another. The adverse events associated with ado-trastuzumab ematansine include adverse events reported with trastuzumab and microtubule inhibitors.

Pertuzumab Pertuzumab is a humanized mAb that targets the HER2 receptor. It is synergistic with trastuzumab and is effective in tumors that have developed resistance to trastuzumab. Pertuzumab binds to extracellular domain II of HER2, a site distinct from trastuzumab, and inhibits ligand-dependent HER2–HER3 dimerization, which subsequently decreases tumor proliferation and resistance pathways.[77] Dual targeting of the HER2 receptor allows for increased efficacy against variant forms of the HER2 receptor, including truncated HER2 receptors. Similar to trastuzumab, it appears to induce ADCC in cancer cells. Pertuzumab is approved to treat HER2 overexpressed locally advanced, inflammatory or early stage breast cancer in the neoadjuvant setting or for the treatment of refractory metastatic breast cancer.

VEGF Inhibitors

Bevacizumab Bevacizumab is a humanized mAb directed against circulating VEGF. It binds to all biologically active circulating isoforms of VEGF and prevents the activation and promotion of angiogenesis. Bevacizumab is approved to treat metastatic colorectal cancer and as first-line treatment of advanced nonsquamous NSCLC. Additional indications include the following: metastatic renal cell carcinoma to be given with interferon alfa; progressive glioblastoma as a single agent; persistent, recurrent, or metastatic cervical cancer with paclitaxel and cisplatin or paclitaxel and topotecan; and for platinum-resistant recurrent ovarian, fallopian tube or primary peritoneal cancer with chemotherapy.

Several serious adverse events have been associated with bevacizumab, including hypertension, bleeding, and thrombotic events. Hypertension is more common in patients with a history of hypertension and responds to oral antihypertensive medications. Although the most common bleeding episodes are transient epistaxis, fatal CNS, and gastrointestinal hemorrhages have been reported. The product labeling includes a box warning regarding the risk of gastrointestinal perforation, wound dehiscence, and hemorrhage. Bevacizumab is not recommended for use within 28 days of major surgery and patients should be instructed to report abdominal pain (an initial sign of gastrointestinal hemorrhage) to their health professionals immediately. Paradoxically, bevacizumab also has been associated with thrombotic events, including deep vein thrombosis, pulmonary embolism, and myocardial infarction, especially in elderly patients with a history of cardiac events. Another potentially serious adverse event associated with bevacizumab is proteinuria/nephrotic syndrome, and patients should be monitored for the development or worsening of proteinuria with serial urine dipsticks. Patients with a 2+ or greater urine dipstick should undergo further assessment.

Ramucirumab Ramucirumab is a human mAb that binds to VEGFR2 resulting in the inhibition of ligand-induced proliferation. Whereas bevacizumab binds the circulating ligand (ie, VEGF), ramucirumab inhibits angiogenesis through the specific blockade of VEGFR2.[78] Ramucirumab is approved for the treatment of advanced gastric or gastroesophageal junction adenocarcinoma as a single agent or with paclitaxel. Other indications include treatment of metastatic NSCLC with docetaxel after progression with platinum-based chemotherapy and for the treatment of metastatic colorectal cancer in the second-line setting. When administered as a single agent, the most common toxicities associated with ramucirumab are hypertension and diarrhea. Boxed warnings for ramucirumab are the same as for bevacizumab. Patients should also be monitored for thromboembolic events, hypertension, proteinuria, and thyroid dysfunction.

Immunomodulatory Monoclonal Antibodies

Denosumab

Denosumab is a human mAb with affinity for the receptor activator of nuclear factor kappa-B ligand (RANKL). Giant cell tumors of bone are benign osteolytic tumors whose osteoclast-like giant cells express the receptor activator of nuclear factor kappa-B (RANK) receptor. Activation of RANK contributes to osteolysis and tumor growth.[79] Denosumab binds to RANKL thereby preventing the activation of RANK on osteoclast-like giant cells. It is approved for the treatment of adults and skeletally mature adolescents with giant cell tumor of bone that is not amenable to surgery. The most common toxicities include arthralgia, headache, nausea, and hypocalcemia. A dental examination should be performed prior to initiation of therapy and patients should be monitored for symptoms of osteonecrosis of the jaw.

Ipilimumab

Ipilimumab is a human mAb that blocks cytotoxic T-lymphocyte antigen 4 (CTLA-4) and is approved for the treatment of metastatic melanoma and adjuvant treatment of cutaneous melanoma with pathologic involvement of regional lymph nodes. CTLA-4 acts as a negative regulator of T-cell function, decreasing the ability of the immune system to mount an antitumor response. By binding to CTLA-4, ipilimumab allows for enhanced T-cell stimulation, proliferation, and antitumor activity.[80] Ipilimumab can take longer than chemotherapy to demonstrate a response because its mechanism depends on harnessing the immune system. Based on its enhanced immune response, several severe and fatal immune-mediated adverse reactions have been observed, including enterocolitis, hepatitis, dermatitis, neuropathy, and endocrinopathy.

Nivolumab

The programmed death-1 (PD-1) receptor is expressed by activated T cells and serves as an immunologic checkpoint. The PD-1 ligand (PD-L1) is expressed on numerous human tumors including melanoma and lung. Through the interaction of PD-L1 with PD-1, T-cell activity is limited and the tumor evades immunosurveillance. It has been suggested that PD-L1 expression is associated with increased tumor aggressiveness. Nivolumab, a fully human IgG4 mAb, binds to and blocks PD-1 from interacting with its receptor resulting in the restoration of T-cell activity.[81]

Nivolumab is approved for the treatment of metastatic NSCLC with progression on or after platinum-based chemotherapy, unresectable or metastatic melanoma, and metastatic renal cell carcinoma. Nivolumab is also approved with ipilimumab for the treatment of patients with BRAF V600 wild-type, unresectable or metastatic melanoma. Patients receiving nivolumab must be monitored for immune-mediated toxicities including pneumonitis, colitis, hepatitis, nephritis, and thyroid dysfunction. Depending on the severity of the reaction, corticosteroids should be administered.

Elotuzumab

Elotuzumab is an IgG mAb directed against Signaling Lymphocytic Activation Molecule Family 7 (SLAMF7). It is approved with lenalidomide and dexamethasone for the treatment of patients with previously treated multiple myeloma. The most common adverse reactions reported include fatigue, diarrhea, constipation, pyrexia, peripheral neuropathy, decreased appetite, cough, and respiratory infections. Patients should also be monitored for infusion reactions, infections, second primary malignancies, and hepatotoxicity. Of note, elotuzumab can be detected in the serum protein electrophoresis and immunofixation assays of M-protein, which may interfere with the ability to assess complete response.

Pembrolizumab

Pembrolizumab is a highly selective humanized IgG4 mAb. Similar to nivolumab, pembrolizumab binds to the PD-1 receptor thereby reversing T-cell suppression. Pembrolizumab is approved for the treatment of unresectable or metastatic melanoma. Given its similar mechanism of action, toxicities reported with pembrolizumab are similar to those reported with nivolumab.

Siltuximab

Siltuximab is an anti-IL-6 chimeric mAb approved for the treatment of multicentric Castleman Disease (MCD) who are human immunodeficiency virus (HIV)-negative and human herpes virus-8 (HHV-8)-negative. MCD is a rare lymphoproliferative disorder and although it is not considered a form of cancer, many patients with this disease develop lymphomas and it is therefore often treated with chemotherapy. Hyperplastic lymph nodes of patients with MCD produce IL-6, a cytokine that induces B-cell differentiation, and it is thought that dysregulated IL-6 plays a critical role in the manifestation of the disease. Siltuximab is an antibody to endogenous IL-6 and is not thought to bind to viral IL-6. Therefore, HIV-positive and HHV-8-positive patients were excluded from the clinical trials. The most common toxicities associated with siltuximab include pruritus, increased weight, and hyperuricemia. Patients should also be monitored for infections and siltuximab should be held in patients who develop a severe infection.

Cytokines

Interferons

Recombinant interferon-alfa is approved for hairy cell leukemia, melanoma, Kaposi's sarcoma, and CML. A pegylated interferon-alpha identified as peginterferon-alfa has been approved for adjuvant treatment of metastatic melanoma. The mechanisms by which IFNs exert their anticancer effects is unknown, but IFNs exert their effect by binding to specific membrane receptors and initiating various intracellular signaling pathways.[82] The most frequent toxicities are flu-like symptoms and elevated transaminases. Potentially serious toxicities include neuropsychiatric, autoimmune, ischemic, and infectious disorders.

Interleukin-2 (Aldesleukin)

Interleukin-2 (IL-2) is a cytokine produced by recombinant DNA technology that promotes B- and T-cell proliferation and differentiation and initiates a cytokine cascade with multiple interacting immunologic effects. The IL-2 receptor is expressed in increased amounts on activated T-cells and mediates most of the effects of aldesleukin. Anticancer activity depends on proliferation of cytotoxic immune cells that can recognize and destroy cancer cells without damaging normal cells. Some of these cytotoxic cells are natural killer cells, lymphokine-activated killer cells, and tumor-infiltrating lymphocytes.[83] Aldesleukin is approved for the treatment of metastatic renal cell carcinoma and melanoma.

Aldesleukin is a toxic therapy that requires vigorous supportive care under the supervision of experienced healthcare professionals. The most common dose-limiting toxicities are hypotension, fluid retention, and renal dysfunction. Aldesleukin decreases peripheral vascular resistance, producing peripheral vasodilation, tachycardia, and hypotension. A characteristic vascular or capillary leak syndrome produces fluid retention, which in turn can cause respiratory compromise. These toxicities require administration of vasopressors in most patients, judicious use of fluid support and diuretics, and supplemental oxygen. Patients with underlying cardiovascular or renal abnormalities are more susceptible to these toxicities, making careful patient selection important.[83] Most patients treated with aldesleukin experience thrombocytopenia, anemia, eosinophilia, reversible cholestasis, and skin erythema with burning and pruritus, and some have neuropsychiatric changes, hypothyroidism, and bacterial infections.[83] In general, the toxicities from aldesleukin reverse quickly after therapy is stopped and can be managed or prevented by careful prospective monitoring and supportive care.

Enzymes

L-Asparaginase is unique among anticancer agents in its unusual mechanism of action, patterns of toxicity, and source. It is an enzyme produced by Escherichia coli or Erwinia chrysanthemi. L-Asparagine is a nonessential amino acid that can be synthesized by most mammalian cells except cells with certain lymphoid malignancies, which have no or limited synthetase levels required for L-asparagine formation. L-Asparagine is degraded by the enzyme L-asparaginase, which depletes existing supplies and inhibits protein synthesis. Increased L-asparagine synthetase activity within cancer cells causes resistance to L-asparaginase treatment. L-Asparaginase is a component of combination chemotherapy regimen used for the treatment of ALL and multiple products are available.

Fusion Proteins

Denileukin Diftitox

Denileukin diftitox is a recombinant fusion protein that combines the active sections of both IL-2 and diphtheria toxin. Unconjugated diphtheria toxin is much too toxic to administer to humans. As the payload of the fusion protein, however, its cytotoxic effects are directed toward cells that express the high-affinity form of the IL-2 receptor, such as cancer cells of some patients with cutaneous T-cell lymphoma. When denileukin diftitox interacts with IL-2 receptors, the toxin inhibits protein synthesis in the cancer cells and causes cell death. It is approved for the treatment of cutaneous T-cell lymphomas.

Although denileukin diftitox is directed therapy, its targeting of cells that express high-affinity IL-2 receptors is not specific because these receptors are expressed on cells other than cancer cells. Denileukin diftitox produces acute hypersensitivity reactions, flu-like symptoms, diarrhea, visual impairment, and vascular leak syndrome. It differs from the vascular leak syndrome produced by high-dose aldesleukin in that it occurs in fewer patients, is delayed in onset, is usually self-limited, and does not consistently recur on retreatment.[83] Patients with an albumin concentration less than 3 g/dL (30 g/L) are at increased risk for vascular leak syndrome and use in these patients is not recommended.

Ziv-Aflibercept

Ziv-aflibercept is a soluble recombinant fusion protein that was designed to block multiple signals that stimulate the angiogenic process. It was developed by fusing sections of the VEGFR1 and VEGFR2 immunoglobulin domains to the Fc portion of human IgG1. Ziv-aflibercept blocks VEGFA, VEGFB, and phosphatidylinositol-glycan biosynthese class F by "trapping" the ligands before they get to the native transmembrane receptors and thus decreasing proangiogenic signaling and tumor growth. It is approved with chemotherapy for resistant or progressive metastatic colorectal cancer and has toxicities similar to other anti-VEGF therapies.

Vaccines

Sipuleucel-T

Sipuleucel-T is the first therapeutic vaccine approved by the FDA and has paved the way for numerous vaccines currently being investigated. Sipuleucel-T is classified as an autologous cellular immunotherapy that is indicated for the treatment of asymptomatic or minimally symptomatic metastatic castrate-resistant prostate cancer. Through leukapheresis, a patient's dendritic cells are collected and isolated then cultured ex vivo. The fusion protein (PAP-GM-CSF) is composed of prostate acid phosphatase (PAP) and GM-CSF. PAP is selectively expressed on prostatic tissues and GM-CSF is included to enhance the immune response. Antigen-presenting cells take up this antigen and are then re-infused into the donor patient to stimulate a T-cell response.[84]

Treatment with sipuleucel-T consists of three infusions separated by approximately 2 weeks. Due to the leukapheresis, ex vivo cell manipulation, and re-infusion, treatment with sipuleucel-T can be logistically challenging. Premedication consisting of acetaminophen and an antihistamine should be given prior to each infusion to decrease the chance of an infusion reaction. Common toxicities include chills, fatigue, back pain, nausea, joint ache, and headache.

Talimogene Laherparepvec

Talimogene laherparepvec (T-VEC) is an oncolytic viral therapy based on a modified herpes simplex virus (HSV) type 1. T-VEC is modified through the deletion of two HSV genes, ICP34.5 and ICP47, and is designed to lyse tumor cells and promote antitumor immunity. It is indicated for the local treatment of unresectable cutaneous, subcutaneous, and nodal lesions in patients with melanoma recurrent after initial surgery. T-VEC is injected directly into the cutaneous, subcutaneous or nodal lesion. The most common toxicities are fatigue, chills, pyrexia, nausea, influenza-like illness, and injection site pain. Pyrexia, chills, and influenza-like illness can occur any time during treatment, but were more frequent during the first 3 months of treatment. Cellulitis is the most commonly reported serious adverse event.

RESPONSE CRITERIA

The response to anticancer agents and other treatment modalities could be described as a cure, complete response (CR), partial response (PR), stable disease, or progression. A cure implies that the patient is entirely free of disease and has the same life expectancy as a cancer-free individual. Because of our inability to detect small numbers of cancer cells, we can never be absolutely certain that an individual patient is cured. Cancers that are curable with treatment are characterized by a stable plateau in the survival curve where the risk of relapse is very low. For most curable cancers, the survival curve has plateaued by about 5 years. Therefore, patients with a curable cancer who are alive 5 years from the time of diagnosis without disease recurrence are often considered "cured", but patients with some malignancies, such as breast cancer and melanoma, are still at significant risk for relapse after 5 years.

Response Evaluation Criteria for Solid Tumors

In an attempt to simplify and unify response definitions in clinical practice, clinical trials, and published reports, the response evaluation criteria in solid tumors (RECIST) criteria were developed in 2000 and revised in 2009 (RECIST 1.1).[85] At baseline, overall tumor burden and measurable disease is assessed. Target lesions are identified and measured at baseline and are later re-evaluated to determine objective tumor response. Nontarget lesions are also assessed. A CR means disappearance of all target lesions and any pathological lymph nodes must be reduced in short axis to less than 10 mm. A PR is defined as a 30% or greater decrease in the sum of diameters of target lesions from baseline. Overall objective response rates for a given treatment are calculated by adding the CR and PR rates. Progressive disease is defined as a 20% or greater increase in the sum of diameters of target lesions when compared to the smallest sum since treatment initiation. The development of one or more new lesions while receiving treatment is also considered progressive disease. A patient whose tumor size neither grows nor shrinks by the above criteria is termed to have stable disease.[85] Some patients may experience subjective improvement in cancer-related symptoms without a defined response. Although clinically important, this does not indicate an objective response. Although RECIST 1.1 is the most widely accepted criteria for the assessment of tumor response in solid tumors, it does not come without shortcomings. The modified RECIST (mRECIST) assessment may be more accurate for the evaluation of tumor burden in some cancers.[86]

Furthermore, the emergence of immunotherapy in oncology has led to the need for revised response criteria that accounts for the mechanism of immunotherapeutic agents. RECIST neglects to take into account the pseudo-progression effect ("flare") that can be seen with these agents which may result in declaring progressive disease too early. The immune-related response criteria (irRC) and immune-related RECIST (irRECIST) have been proposed to overcome the challenges of RECIST 1.1 with immunotherapy.[87,88]

The response definitions described above are applicable to solid tumors, but leukemias and multiple myeloma are not characterized by discrete, measurable masses. Responses in these cancers are measured by elimination of abnormal cells (eg, return to normal hematology parameters and normal bone marrow in leukemia), return of tumor markers to normal levels (eg, normal serum protein electrophoresis in multiple myeloma), or improved function of affected organs (eg, improved renal function after obstructive uropathy). Cytogenetic markers and molecular techniques have an increasingly important role in determining whether all cancer has been truly eliminated. For example, in CML, the Philadelphia chromosome can be detected by polymerase chain reaction techniques even when no leukemia is evident in the bone marrow or bloodstream. Patients without evidence of the Philadelphia chromosome are classified as having a complete cytogenetic response. Measuring cytogenetic responses is increasingly common in patients with known cytogenetic abnormalities, and the absence of complete cytogenetic responses may predict disease relapse.

Factors Affecting Treatment Response

8 Factors affecting response include tumor burden, cancer cell heterogeneity, drug resistance, dose intensity, and patient-specific factors. The significance of tumor burden was discussed earlier in the Principles of Tumor Growth section. Tumors consist of a heterogeneous population of cells. Because of the genetic instability of cancer cells compared with normal cells, genetic alterations commonly occur during cell division. Large tumors have therefore undergone many cell divisions and express multiple genetic alterations, resulting in genetically varied populations.[3] In 1979, Goldie and Coldman proposed that these cytogenetic changes were not completely random and were highly associated with the development of the ability of tumors to develop drug resistance. The probability of developing resistant cell populations increases as tumor size increases. It is believed that a small percentage of resistant cancer cells may survive initial therapy. Resistant populations later proliferate and eventually become the dominant population, which could explain the common pattern of an initial response to therapy followed by progressive tumor regrowth despite continuing the same treatment.

Drug resistance may be either acquired or inherited. Mechanisms of drug resistance include altered drug transport systems, metabolism, and target enzymes; inability to repair drug-induced damage; and insensitivity to drug-induced apoptosis.[3] For example, multidrug resistance has been observed with natural chemotherapies (eg, anthracyclines, vinca alkaloids, epipodophyllotoxins, and taxanes), and it occurs when some cancer cells are exposed to increasing concentrations of a specific chemotherapy. Surprisingly, these same cells also become resistant to other structurally unrelated chemotherapies and are therefore considered multidrug resistant. The resistant cancer cells overexpress the drug transporter Pgp, which enhances the export of these chemotherapies. Other potential mechanisms of drug resistance include inactivation of chemotherapy by glutathione metabolism, upregulation of drug targets, alternative intracellular signaling pathways, and decreased apoptosis. The last mechanism can be mediated by overexpression of BCL-2 or loss of TP53, as discussed earlier in the chapter.

The relationship between dose and response has been extensively explored for chemotherapy agents,[1] because dose is believed to be a critical factor in determining response for many cancers. Dose intensity is defined as the dose delivered to the patient over a specified period of time. The three main variables that determine delivered dose intensity are the dose per course, the interval between doses, and the total cumulative dose. Dose density refers to shortening of the usual interval between doses (eg, every 2 weeks instead of every 3 weeks) and is designed to maximize the effects of therapy on tumor growth kinetics. This strategy has been most extensively studied in breast cancer, with positive results from adjuvant therapy given to patients with high-risk node-positive disease. The delivery of optimal dose intensity is often compromised by the toxicities of the anticancer agent. Treatment cycles are commonly delayed because of inadequate recovery from toxicity, especially myelosuppression. Subsequent doses of the anticancer agents are often reduced to prevent or reduce the severity of these toxicities. The impact on patient outcome has been proven in studies showing reduced rates of response and survival in individuals receiving less-than-optimal doses. Understanding the pathophysiology of toxicities has led to the development of more effective agents to prevent and manage these toxicities. The development of chemoprotective agents has facilitated application of dose-intensity principles. For example, colony-stimulating factors minimize neutropenia and permit delivery of dose-intensive or dose-dense regimens that are myelosuppressive. The issue of dose intensity is particularly important in the setting of high-dose chemotherapy with autologous hematopoietic stem cell support. Although lethal myelosuppression is avoided by administering hematopoietic stem cells, other severe end-organ toxicities emerge as doses of the anticancer agents are increased.

Patient-specific factors create unpredictable variability in response to anticancer therapy. For example, interindividual variations in absorption, distribution, or elimination could lead to sub- or supratherapeutic levels of anticancer agents and their metabolites. The genetic alterations that resulted in the cancer can also affect response. For example, breast cancers that overexpress HER2 are often sensitive to anthracycline-based regimens. As a result, both efficacy and tolerability can be affected. Health professionals in oncology may modify doses based on variations in body size, blood counts, and organ function. Prospective dose modifications based on these parameters are still very important to optimize the effectiveness of therapy and minimize toxicity. But more specific tools are becoming available as we learn how to identify and apply differences in the genetic makeup of the patient and cancer to their anticancer therapy. Pharmacogenomics is the study of the role of inheritance in individual variation in drug response. In oncology, several clinically relevant genetic polymorphisms or variations have been identified that can affect pharmacokinetics and pharmacodynamics. Examples include polymorphisms in genes responsible for the activity of the enzymes DPD (responsible for FU metabolism), TPMT (responsible for thiopurine metabolism), and UGT1A1 (responsible for irinotecan metabolism). Patients with deficiencies in these enzymes can experience significant, and possibly life-threatening, toxicity. Identifying these genetic variants could permit individualization of regimens containing these agents to avoid toxicity. Monitoring concentrations of anticancer agents could also improve the therapeutic index. For example, pharmacokinetic and pharmacodynamic modeling is associated with improved responses and decreased toxicity in children with ALL.

The presence of other disease states (eg, comorbidities) may also affect response to treatment by limiting treatment options. The overall functional status of a patient may be assessed using performance status scales, such as the Karnofsky Performance Status (KPS) and Eastern Cooperative Oncology Group (ECOG) scales. These scales can be used to predict patient tolerance of anticancer therapy and to assess the effects of therapy on the patient's level of activity and quality of life. For many cancers, performance status at diagnosis is the most important prognostic indicator.

Today's oncology health professionals have a wealth of information to consider when designing a personalized treatment approach. Patient-specific factors (eg, performance status, comorbidities, organ function, and pharmacogenomics), tumor-specific factors (eg, pathology, stage, and molecular profile), and treatment goals (eg, palliation and cure) are all considered when determining the best treatment option. Treatment cost can also be an important consideration.

ADMINISTRATION

Dosing and Administration

Health professionals should monitor all clinical and laboratory values that are affected by a specific anticancer agent at baseline and periodically during treatment. For example, a complete blood count should be evaluated weekly while receiving myelosuppressive chemotherapy. In general, a neutrophil count of 3,000 cells/mm^3 (3×10^9/L) or above or an absolute neutrophil count (ANC) of 1,500 cells/mm^3 (1.5×10^9/L) or above and a platelet count of 100,000 cells/mm^3 (100×10^9/L) or above are usually required before administering myelosuppressive agents. In addition, a chemistry panel is drawn to assess organ function, especially for agents eliminated or metabolized via those routes. Table 127-7 lists agents that require dosing adjustments and require specific laboratory tests before administration; failure to follow these recommendations may result in overdosing and excessive toxicity.

Anticancer agents might be dosed based on body size (such as body weight or body surface area [BSA]) or as a fixed dose. Chemotherapy is generally dosed based on BSA. BSA is commonly used as an estimate of cardiac output and subsequent distribution to the liver and kidneys, the primary determinants of drug elimination. The most common methods used to determine BSA are the Mosteller and DuBois formulas. Body-sized dosing is also commonly used for mAbs, but the effect of body size on interpatient variability should be explored to determine the optimal dosing approach. In contrast, most oral targeted agents are based on a fixed-dose approach based on the available tablet or capsule strengths.

Other dosing methods are being used to improve tolerability and anticancer activity. For example, carboplatin is dosed based on the patient's estimated glomerular filtration rate (GFR). This method is known as the Calvert formula and has been demonstrated to achieve adequate levels of carboplatin while minimizing excessive toxicity. The dose might also be based on drug levels (eg, methotrexate) and health professionals should be proficient in these calculations before dosing and administering any chemotherapy agent. A healthcare provider should complete diagnostic tests recommended before administering some anticancer agents, such as tamoxifen, trastuzumab, vemurafenib, and crizotinib, which are only prescribed to patients whose tumor expresses a specific protein or gene. Additionally, health professionals need to be aware of the diagnostic tests associated with the drug approval and how to interpret the findings from the various tests. For example, some tests may identify if a tumor is mutation positive or negative, whereas other tests may identify the specific genetic alteration identified in the tumor.

Safety and Handling

All anticancer agents regardless of the route of administration should be handled with care to avoid inadvertent exposure of health professionals and caregivers. Consequently, all healthcare facilities should have written procedures for safely handling these agents and all personnel should be oriented to these procedures. Additionally, health professionals should provide information about safe handling and disposal to patients and their families when a patient is prescribed an oral anticancer agent. Safe handling includes avoiding skin contact and inhalation, but patient-centered guidelines regarding safe handling of oral anticancer agents have not been developed.[89]

The United States Pharmacopeia Chapter 797 regulates the preparation of extemporaneously compounded sterile preparations and should be used by providers that prepare intravenous chemotherapy. Chapter 800 is currently in draft form and should be available in the near future. The most common avenue of exposure is via inhalation or skin absorption. Individuals preparing intravenous chemotherapy should work in an International Organization for Standardization (ISO) Class 5 biologic safety cabinet and wear appropriate personal protective equipment including a gown, face mask, eye protection, hair covers, shoe covers, and double sterile chemo-type gloves. Closed-system vial-transfer devices should be used when possible. Negative-pressure techniques should be used in drug preparation to minimize aerosolization. Health professionals administering chemotherapy should take similar precautions to avoid exposure. Double chemotherapy-tested gloves, protective gowns, and protective eyewear (if there is potential for splashing) should be worn whenever handling or administering hazardous drugs. Kits for cleaning up chemotherapy spills should be located in all areas where chemotherapy is handled. Cytotoxic waste should be disposed of properly, and patients should be informed of proper methods for disposing of potentially contaminated body excreta and cytotoxic waste.

SUPPORTIVE CARE

9 The treatment of cancer is complicated by the risk of multiple serious adverse events, many of which may be life-threatening. Adverse events (or toxicities) are commonly graded on a scale from no toxicity (grade 0) to death (grade 5) with the Common Terminology Criteria for Adverse Events (CTCAE) developed by the National Cancer Institute (NCI). Specific toxicities observed with individual anticancer agents were listed earlier in the chapter. Toxicities such as myelosuppression, mucositis, nausea and vomiting, and alopecia are commonly observed with chemotherapy because these agents target rapidly dividing normal and cancer cells. Other toxicities associated with chemotherapy are infertility and carcinogenesis. The adverse event profile with biologic therapies and targeted agents typically differ from chemotherapy. The events observed with these anticancer agents depend on the altered intracellular signaling. For example, rash has been observed with agents that inhibit EGFR intracellular signaling and hemorrhage and thrombosis have been observed with agents that affect the VEGFR intracellular signaling pathway. Nutritional support and pain management are also important supportive care issues for all patients with cancer. The management of chemotherapy-induced nausea and vomiting and the basic principles of nutritional support and pain management are discussed in detail in other chapters. The basic principles for the management of some common toxicities or adverse events are described below.

Hematologic

Myelosuppression is the most common dose-limiting toxicity observed with chemotherapy, but myelosuppression may be seen with kinase inhibitors (eg, sunitinib). The risk of myelosuppression increases when chemotherapy is administered concurrently with radiation to the chest or pelvic region. The effects of myelosuppression are usually not observed immediately after administration because the currently circulating blood cells must first be consumed. For example, neutropenia is typically observed before thrombocytopenia, because white blood cells have a short life span of 6 to 12 hours compared to platelets with a life span of 5 to 10 days. Anemia typically occurs a few months after the first dose, since erythrocytes have a relatively long life span of 120 days. The lowest blood cell count (or nadir) typically occurs 10 to 14 days after chemotherapy administration, with a recovery in cell counts by 3 to 4 weeks after administration; however, the nadir commonly occurs later following administration of nitrosoureas, mitomycin C, and radiolabeled antibodies (about 4-6 weeks). Subsequent doses should be delayed until the minimum suggested blood counts are achieved to minimize additional toxicity and morbidity. Patients with leukemia or receiving a hematopoietic stem cell transplant may have a more rapid nadir of about 5 to 7 days.

A dose reduction should be considered if a patient develops severe myelosuppression such as anemia necessitating a transfusion or neutropenia with a fever. A dose reduction may be considered empirically before the first dose if the patient has a low baseline neutrophil or platelet count, has diminished bone marrow reserve, has impaired drug elimination, or is to receive a combination of several myelosuppressive agents; these patients may be at an increased risk of developing severe myelosuppression. A decreased bone marrow reserve has been observed in patients who have received multiple prior courses of myelosuppressive chemotherapy or extensive radiation therapy.

A dose reduction should be carefully balanced with the treatment goals, since reduced dose can compromise anticancer activity in some tumors (eg, breast cancer and lymphoma).[1] In patients who are responding well to treatment, some myelosuppression is accepted by most health professionals if it is not compromising the patient's quality of life and the cancer is responding to therapy. In these patients, empiric use of hematopoietic growth factors provides an alternative to dose reduction.

Anemia

Although usually not life threatening, anemia is the most common hematologic complication of chemotherapy.[90] The incidence of anemia depends on several factors, including the type and duration of therapy and the type and stage of the underlying malignancy. For example, carboplatin is more commonly associated with anemia than other chemotherapy agents. Multiple conditions can cause anemia, including gastrointestinal blood loss, nutrient deficiency (eg, iron and folate), chemotherapy and radiation therapy, bone marrow invasion, hemolysis, renal dysfunction, and anemia of chronic disease. Of all the signs and symptoms of anemia, fatigue is most common in patients with cancer. In fact, fatigue is the most commonly reported symptom overall in patients undergoing anticancer therapy. Of note, other common causes of fatigue include insomnia, depression, unrelieved pain, and the underlying malignancy.

The underlying cause of the anemia should be identified before treatment for anemia is started. Red blood cell transfusions are the mainstay of treatment, but erythropoiesis-stimulating agents (epoetin alfa and darbepoetin alfa) may be considered for patients with underlying kidney disease and for patients receiving palliative treatment. Serious adverse events related to erythropoiesis-stimulating agents include thrombosis and myocardial infarction. These events have generally occurred when the target hemoglobin of 12 g/dL (120 g/L; 7.45 mmol/L) is exceeded or the hemoglobin rises too quickly.[90] Various studies have demonstrated an increased risk of mortality with the use of erythropoiesis-stimulating agents in patients with cancer. For these reasons, epoetin alfa and darbepoetin alfa must be prescribed and used under a REMS program. Other rare and generally mild toxicities include pain at injection site, rash, flu-like symptoms, seizures, and hypertension. The presence of functional iron deficiency should be determined before administering these products. If the functional iron deficiency is identified, intravenous iron should be considered, as oral iron is poorly tolerated and absorbed in patients with cancer. Clinical practice guidelines for the treatment of cancer- and chemotherapy-related anemia are available.[90]

Neutropenia

Neutropenia in patients with cancer is associated with an increased risk of infection. The probability of developing an infection increases when ANC falls below 500 cells/mm^3 (0.5×10^9/L) or when the duration of neutropenia is prolonged.[91] Other risk factors for infection include alteration in the integrity of physical defense barriers and the functional integrity of the leukocytes. Neutrophil function can be affected by the underlying cancer, anticancer agent, or radiation therapy.

In the neutropenic patient, it can be difficult to identify an infection, as the usual signs and symptoms of infection, such as pus, abscesses, and infiltrates on chest radiography, are often absent. Subsequently, health professionals must rely on fever as an indicator of infection in these patients. Definitive culture results may take days and a septic neutropenic cancer patient can die within hours if not treated. Therefore, empiric antibiotics are promptly initiated based on reliable coverage of the most likely organisms, antibiotic sensitivities at the institution, the patient's signs and symptoms (if present), and possible adverse events.[91] The most common source of infection in these patients is self-infection with body flora, which includes both gram-positive and gram-negative bacteria. Specific treatment of infections in immunocompromised hosts is discussed in Chapter 122.

Colony-stimulating factors (CSF) may minimize the severity of neutropenia and subsequently, reduce the risk of infection.[91] These factors are naturally occurring proteins that are essential for the normal growth and maturation of blood cell components (Figure 127-8). For example, filgrastim specifically stimulates the production of neutrophilic granulocytes and sargramostim promotes the proliferation of granulocytes (neutrophils and eosinophils), monocytes and macrophages.[92] Although sargramostim stimulates megakaryocytes, no consistent effect on platelet production has been observed in clinical trials. Both factors initially enhance demargination and mobilization of mature cells from the marrow and then provide constant stimulation of stem cell progenitors. Pegfilgrastim is a peglyated filgrastim that has a substantially longer half-life compared to filgrastim. Whereas multiple daily doses of filgrastim are typically needed to increase neutrophil count, only a single dose of pegfilgrastim is needed to similarly increase neutrophil counts. Filgrastim-sndz (a biosimilar to filgrastim) and tbo-filgrastim have recently been approved for use with myelosuppressive chemotherapy.

These growth factors may be used as primary or secondary prophylaxis of neutropenia. Primary prophylaxis refers to the use of these factors to prevent neutropenia with the first cycle of chemotherapy. The National Comprehensive Cancer Network (NCCN) recommends this strategy for patients who are receiving a chemotherapy regimen with a 20% or higher risk of febrile neutropenia.[93] These guidelines also recommend primary prophylaxis for patients with risk factors receiving a chemotherapy regimen with a 10% to 20% risk of febrile neutropenia. Patient risk factors include age 65 years or older, previous chemotherapy or radiation, pre-existing conditions, poor performance status, poor organ function, and HIV-positive patients. Secondary prophylaxis refers to the use of growth factors to prevent recurrent neutropenia in patients who had experienced neutropenia with the prior cycle of chemotherapy. It is recommended that secondary prophylaxis be reserved for patients with chemosensitive cancers when a dose reduction may affect survival.

The role of these factors in the treatment of established neutropenia is less well defined. Some guidelines suggest that the administration of these factors may be considered in select patients with

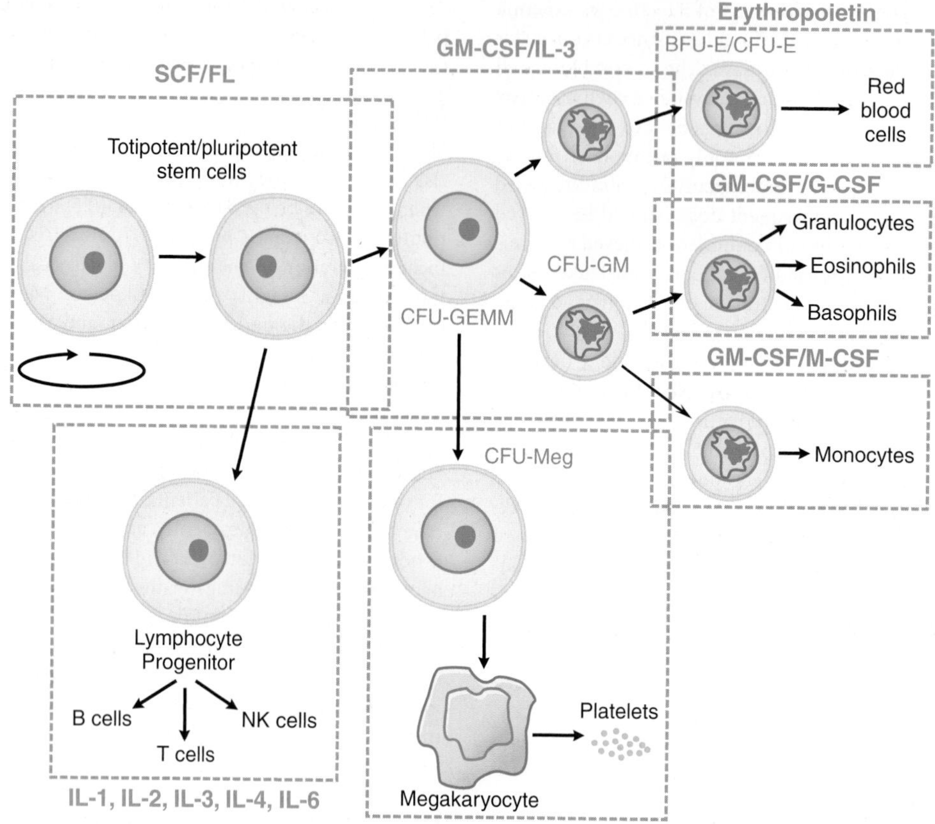

FIGURE 127-8 Sites of action of hematopoietic growth factors in the differentiation and maturation of marrow cell lines. A self-sustaining pool of marrow stem cells differentiates under the influence of specific hematopoietic growth factors to form a variety of hematopoietic and lymphopoietic cells. Stem cell factor (SCF), FTL-3 ligand (FL), interleukin-3 (IL-3), and granulocyte-macrophage colony-stimulating factor (GM-CSF), together with cell–cell interactions in the bone marrow, stimulate stem cells to form a series of burst-forming units (BFU) and colony-forming units (CFUs): CFU-GEMM, CFU-GM, CFU-Meg, BFU-E, and CFU-E (GEMM, granulocyte, erythrocyte, monocyte, and megakaryocytes; GM, granulocyte and macrophage; Meg, megakaryocyte; E, erythrocyte). After considerable proliferation, further differentiation is stimulated by synergistic interactions with growth factors for each of the major cell lines—granulocyte colony-stimulating factor (G-CSF), monocyte/macrophage-stimulating factor (M-CSF), thrombopoietin, and erythropoietin. Each of these factors also influences the proliferation; maturation; and, in some cases, the function of the derivative cell line. (NK, natural killer.) *(Reproduced with permission from Kaushansky K, Kipps TJ. Hematopoietic agents: Growth factors, minerals and vitamins. In: Brunton LL, Chabner BA, Knollman BC (eds). Goodman & Gilman's The Pharmacologic Basis of Therapeutics, 12th ed. New York: McGraw-Hill, 2010.)*

established neutropenia. High-risk patients with fever and neutropenia may include those with neutropenia for more than 10 days, ANC less than 100 cells/mm^3 (0.1×10^9/L), age greater than 65 years, and infectious complications (pneumonia, sepsis, or invasive fungal infections) as well as those who are hospitalized at the time of the development of neutropenic fever.[91]

Both filgrastim and sargramostim have also proven effective in accelerating hematopoietic engraftment and in treating graft failure after hematopoietic stem cell transplantation. Other uses for the factors include peripheral blood stem cell mobilization and congenital or idiopathic neutropenia. Growth factors should not be used in patients receiving concomitant chemotherapy and radiotherapy, especially if the radiation involves the mediastinum. These patients appear to experience more significant thrombocytopenia.

At currently recommended doses, these factors are well tolerated. Toxicities are more commonly seen with sargramostim and may be related to its ability to enhance binding of neutrophils to endothelial cells or to activation of monocytes or macrophages, which may stimulate the release of cytokines such as IL-1 and TNF-α.[92] The most common adverse event with these factors is bone pain. Other toxicities include constitutional symptoms, such as low-grade fever, myalgia, arthralgia, lethargy, and mild headache. At higher sargramostim doses, pleural and pericardial effusions, capillary leak syndrome, and thrombus formation may occur. Both factors may produce mild erythema at subcutaneous injection sites, as well as a generalized maculopapular rash. The toxicities observed with pegfilgrastim are similar to those of filgrastim.

The dosing and administration of these factors for the prophylaxis of chemotherapy-induced neutropenia is as follows: a single dose of pegfilgrastim 6 mg or daily doses of filgrastim 5 mcg/kg or sargramostim 250 mcg/m^2 until the ANC reaches a pre-specified target following the nadir. Alternative doses are used in other settings, such as mobilization. These factors should be started between 24 and 72 hours after chemotherapy. Filgrastim and sargramostim can be stopped the day before chemotherapy, but pegfilgrastim should be administered at least 14 days before the next dose of chemotherapy due to its extended half-life. Both sargramostim and filgrastim may be given intravenously, but subcutaneous administration is preferred. Because of the high cost of these agents, doses are commonly rounded to the nearest product vial size to minimize waste.

Thrombocytopenia

Thrombocytopenia increases the risk for significant bleeding. To date, platelet transfusions remain the mainstay of management. At most centers, platelet transfusions are reserved for patients with a platelet count of less than 10,000 cells/mm^3 (10×10^9/L) unless the patient is actively bleeding, must undergo a surgical procedure, or has documented infections or fever. For patients with nonmyeloid malignancies who experience significant thrombocytopenia with chemotherapy, oprelvekin (IL-11) may be considered as secondary prophylaxis in subsequent cycles.[95] When used after chemotherapy that is associated with a high risk of thrombocytopenia, oprelvekin decreased the need for platelet transfusions, as well as the number of platelets required for transfusion. Unfortunately, oprelvekin is associated with some significant toxicities, mostly related to fluid retention (eg, edema, dilutional anemia, dyspnea, and pleural effusions). Cardiac toxicity, especially tachycardia, and atrial fibrillation and flutter also have been observed. Prophylactic oprelvekin is significantly more expensive than platelet transfusions. Considering the modest clinical benefit, the toxicities, and the high cost, oprelvekin use should be reserved for patients who are at high risk for severe thrombocytopenia from chemotherapy when dose reduction is expected to compromise disease response.

Gastrointestinal

Nausea and vomiting are common toxicities observed with chemotherapy agents and some targeted drugs. Medications to minimize the risk of nausea and vomiting are typically given before administration of the anticancer drug. The medications selected depend on the underlying risk of nausea and vomiting associated with the anticancer drug. Medications should also be given for patients to take as needed if nausea or vomiting occurs at home after administration is complete. The underlying pathophysiology and available antiemetic regimens are discussed further in Chapter 35.

The gastrointestinal mucosa is a common site of toxicity associated with anticancer therapy. The subsequent inflammation (mucositis) can lead to painful ulcerations, local infection, and an inability to eat, drink, or swallow. Disruption of the gastrointestinal mucosal barrier may also provide an avenue for systemic microbial invasion. Anticancer agents most commonly associated with mucositis include FU, doxorubicin, methotrexate, multikinase inhibitors, and mTOR inhibitors. Currently, the most effective means of preventing mucositis is through good oral hygiene. Patients who are at high risk for this toxicity (those with poor dentition, high-dose chemotherapy, or radiation therapy involving the oropharynx) should be evaluated by a dentist before starting therapy and should be instructed to rinse their mouths frequently with baking soda and salt water or plain saline rinses during therapy. Clinical practice guidelines for the prevention and treatment of anticancer therapy-induced mucositis are available.

A better understanding of the pathophysiology of mucositis has resulted in identification of promising new agents that may minimize the risk of developing mucositis. The keratinocyte growth factor palifermin is approved for use in patients receiving myelotoxic therapy before hematopoietic stem cell transplantation. Palifermin is administered at a dose of 60 mcg/kg/day intravenously for 3 consecutive days immediately before the initiation of conditioning therapy and then again for 3 days after hematopoietic stem cell transplantation. The effect of palifermin on solid tumor growth is unknown, and its use in nonhematologic cancers is not recommended.

After mucositis has developed, treatment is mainly supportive, including use of topical or systemic analgesics and oral hygiene. Numerous formulations of "magic mouthwash" are commercially available or compounded and often include viscous lidocaine, diphenhydramine, and Maalox. These mouthwashes are commonly used in clinical practice, but data is currently lacking to support their use. Severe cases of mucositis may lead to dehydration and require intravenous hydration and opioid analgesics. Local infections caused by Candida species and HSV are common in these patients. Suspicious lesions should be cultured and appropriate antifungal or antiviral treatment should then be initiated. Antifungal therapy may be delivered topically for mild infections (thrush) with clotrimazole troches or nystatin oral suspension. For more severe oral or esophageal fungal infections, systemic treatment with oral or intravenous antifungals is indicated.

Mucosal damage can occur at any point along the entire length of the gastrointestinal tract. In the lower portion of the gastrointestinal tract, this damage is usually manifested as diarrhea (mild to life threatening) and abdominal pain. Intravenous fluids and electrolyte supplementation should be initiated promptly in severe cases. After infectious causes have been ruled out, diarrhea can safely be treated with agents such as diphenoxylate/atropine or loperamide. The somatostatin analog octreotide has also been used successfully to treat severe cases of chemotherapy-induced diarrhea; guidelines are available to assist health professionals in treating chemotherapy-induced diarrhea. It is important to note that patients receiving immunotherapy may experience diarrhea that is immune-mediated and corticosteroids should be administered in severe cases.

Dermatologic

Chemotherapy-induced cutaneous reactions are generally reversible and self-limiting upon dose reductions or delays. Common reactions include localized rash, photosensitivity, skin hyper- or hypopigmentation, nail changes, and HFSR or hand-foot syndrome.

Alopecia

Many patients find alopecia to be one of the most distressing toxicities associated with anticancer therapy. Alopecia from chemotherapy is usually temporary and the degree of hair loss varies widely. Hair loss is not limited to the scalp; any area of the body may be affected. Patients receiving a taxane as part of their chemotherapy regimen are especially prone to total body alopecia. Hair loss usually begins 1 to 2 weeks after chemotherapy and regrowth may begin before completing treatment. Cryotherapy (local application of ice) and scalp tourniquets have both been investigated as methods of preventing alopecia. Both techniques produce vasoconstriction, resulting in decreased exposure of hair follicles to the chemotherapy. These techniques are not uniformly effective and are contraindicated in patients with cancer whose cancer can metastasize to the scalp, such as leukemia and lymphoma.

In addition to alopecia, other hair changes may occur that may be distressing to patients. Notably, some kinase inhibitors (such as pazopanib) have been associated with hair depigmentation. This loss of pigmentation (white color) is thought to be the result of the inhibition of KIT signaling which decreases melatonin synthesis.

Extravasation

Vesicants are agents that may cause severe tissue damage if they escape from the vasculature.[94] These agents include the anthracyclines, the vinca alkaloids, the taxanes, and others. The anthracyclines are the most notorious agents and the most extensively investigated. The tissue damage may result in prolonged pain, tissue sloughing, infection, and loss of mobility. Prompt initiation of the appropriate interventions is important to minimize morbidity. Unfortunately, most information on extravasation management is anecdotal and few controlled clinical trials have been conducted to determine optimal intervention strategies. Consequently, prevention is the focus of extravasation management. The most important method of prevention is good administration technique, but extravasations may occur despite optimal administration.[94] The vein selected for administration should be on the distal portion of the arm. The large veins of the forearm are desirable because if a drug does extravasate, there is adequate soft tissue coverage to protect crucial structures such as nerves and tendons and joint function is not put at risk. The healthcare provider administering the vesicant should verify needle stability and adequate blood return regularly throughout the administration. A central venous catheter is highly recommended for the intravenous infusion of vesicants of longer duration. For extravasation of anthracyclines, antitumor antibiotics, and alkylating agents, apply ice packs to the affected area. Only a few antidotes to vesicant agents are used clinically. Topical dimethyl sulfoxide (DMSO) or intravenous dexrazoxane are recommended as antidotes for anthracycline extravasation. Topical DMSO may also be given for mitomycin C extravasation. Dry, warm compresses and hyaluronidase are recommended for the extravasation of vinca alkaloids and taxanes. Clinical practice guidelines for the management of extravasation are available.[96]

HFSR and Hand-Foot Syndrome

Although the terms HFSR and hand-foot syndrome are commonly interchanged, it is important to note that these adverse reactions are distinct in both cause and presentation. HFSR is associated with multikinase inhibitors and characteristically localizes to areas of pressure or friction on the hands and feet. Hand-foot syndrome, also known as palmar-plantar erythrodysesthesia, is associated with chemotherapy including FU, capecitabine, and liposomal doxorubicin. Hand-foot syndrome typically presents with diffuse edema and redness on the palms and soles of the feet. Both HFSR and hand–foot syndrome can be uncomfortable and interfere with daily activities. Topical moisturizers may aid in prevention. Urea cream, topical steroids, and pain medication (such as gabapentin or NSAID) may be beneficial for treatment.

Rash

Rash has been observed with some targeted drugs. For example, rash is one of the most common toxicities associated with therapy that inhibits EGFR signaling pathways. Some studies suggest that the rash may be a surrogate marker of response to these agents. Therefore, extensive patient counseling is required to prevent drug discontinuation. Patients should also be instructed to prophylactically apply sunscreen and avoid alcohol-containing skin products. Rash occurs in up to two-thirds of patients taking EGFR inhibitors, most commonly in the first month of treatment with the typical site of presentation being the face and upper torso. Anecdotal reports indicate that emollients help if patients present with dry skin, topical and systemic antibiotics may help if the rash becomes infected, and steroids may help prevent itching and inflammation.

Endocrine

Blood Glucose Dysregulation

Both hyper- and hypoglycemia have been reported with numerous targeted drugs. Hyperglycemia is most commonly associated with mTOR inhibitors. Fasting blood glucose and hemoglobin A1C should be monitored closely especially in diabetic patients. Standard guidelines should be used to adjust anti-diabetic medications as necessary. Hypoglycemia has been commonly reported with multikinase inhibitors and bexarotene. Fasting blood glucose should be closely monitored and doses of anti-diabetic medications reduced as required.

Hypothyroidism

Hypothyroidism is a common adverse event that is seen with multikinase inhibitors. Thyroid stimulating hormone (TSH) and free T4 should be measured at baseline and periodically throughout treatment. Most symptoms are mild and can be reversed with thyroid supplementation. Bexarotene has also been associated with hypothyroidism. It rapidly suppresses TSH levels and affects thyroid hormone metabolism. Free T4 levels should be monitored closely and supplementation is usually required.

Miscellaneous

Numerous other toxicities are seen with both targeted drugs and chemotherapy agents and many of these are discussed in other chapters. A few common toxicities including hypertension and ocular toxicities are discussed here.

Hypertension

Many anticancer agents, especially those that inhibit the VEGF signaling pathway, are associated with hypertension. Although the exact mechanism has yet to be established, it is thought that VEGF inhibition leads to a decrease in nitric oxide and prostacyclin production, resulting in an increase in vascular resistance and blood pressure.[97] Prior to treatment initiation, blood pressure should be well-controlled according to standard guidelines. If hypertension develops, antihypertensive therapy should be initiated or adjusted. Anticancer treatment should be held with persistent or severe hypertension.

Ocular

A broad spectrum of ocular toxicities is seen with both targeted and chemotherapy agents. Common ocular toxicities seen with a variety of anticancer agents include blurred vision, photophobia, conjunctivitis, cataracts, abnormal lacrimation, dry eye, keratitis, optic neuropathy, and retinopathy.

The ALK inhibitor, crizotinib, has been associated with common complaints of visual disturbances including blurred vision, photophobia, and vitreous floaters, among others. Although common, the ocular effects associated with crizotinib are usually self-limiting and have a minimal impact on daily activities.

It is well documented that high-dose cytarabine can cause reversible corneal toxicity. This ocular toxicity is thought to be due to the high concentration of cytarabine in tears. Ophthalmic corticosteroids or saline are recommended to prevent this toxicity. Other ocular toxicities that are associated with anticancer agents include the following: cataracts with anastrozole and tamoxifen; uveitis and retinal vein occlusion with vemurafenib; and cortical blindness with vincristine.

Thrombosis

Patients with cancer have a relatively high risk of developing a venous thromboembolism. The factors that may affect a patient's risk of developing a thromboembolism include the specific cancer (ie, lung cancer, pancreatic cancer, gastric cancer), tumor burden, anticancer treatment (ie, antiangiogenic agents and endocrine therapies) and surgical interventions. Other risk factors might include familial thrombophilia, previous venous thromboembolism, immobilization, age and indwelling catheters. Thromboembolism increases morbidity and mortality, with thromboembolic events a leading cause of death in patients with cancer.

Routine primary prophylaxis is not recommended for most patients, but it should be considered for patients undergoing major surgery or for immobilized hospitalized patients. Unfractionated heparin or a low molecular weight heparin is recommended for patients undergoing major surgery. As an example, enoxaparin or dalteparin may be administered subcutaneously daily for up to one month post-surgery. Unfractionated or low molecular weight heparin or fondaparinux is recommended for immobilized patients with cancer (ie, hospitalization). As discussed earlier in the chapter, thromboprophylaxis is recommended with thalidomide and its analogues.

For patients who develop a venous thromboembolism, treatment goals include preventing a pulmonary embolus, recurrent venous thromboembolism and long-term complications. The American College for Chest Physicians recommend treatment with a low molecular weight heparin.[99] For patients with severe renal impairment, anti-Xa activity monitoring or unfractionated heparin is recommended and dose modifications may be necessary. Treatment with oral vitamin K antagonists, such as warfarin, or other oral anticoagulants are not currently recommended as first-line treatment. The optimal duration of antithrombotic therapy for the prevention of recurrence has not been specifically studied and is often determined based on patient-specific factors including the underlying disease and anticancer treatment. Treatment duration may be a minimum of 3 to 6 months or indefinite.

Survivorship

Advances in the treatment of some cancers, such as Hodgkin lymphoma and testicular cancer, have produced long-term survivors and the opportunity to examine the late consequences of chemotherapy. Survivors should be assessed for long-term psychosocial and physical effects and survivorship guidelines are available for health professionals through the NCCN.[99] Infertility and secondary cancers have emerged as important late effects.

Infertility

The gonadal toxicities of chemotherapy have not received much attention in the past because they are not life threatening. High rates of fertility deficits and sexual dysfunction have been noted for both men and women. In men, chemotherapy can produce severe oligospermia or azoospermia, as well as infertility. Serum testosterone levels are rarely altered. The recovery of spermatogenesis after completing therapy is unpredictable. Men receiving combination chemotherapy appear to sustain more long-lasting toxicities on fertility than do men receiving single-agent chemotherapy. Age, total dose, duration of therapy, and the chemotherapy mechanism are other important variables. In women, toxic effects on the ovaries result clinically in amenorrhea, vaginal epithelial atrophy, and menopausal symptoms. These effects are related to dose and age. Younger patients are more resistant to the effects on the ovaries. As with men, the recovery of fertility is unpredictable, but women younger than 25 years of age appear to have the best outcomes. The effects of the alkylating agents on fertility have been extensively studied. These agents exert profound and consistently detrimental effects on reproductive function. The impact of this drug-induced amenorrhea on patient survival has been less clear with some trials demonstrating a benefit to patients who achieve chemotherapy-induced amenorrhea. Trial results have been mixed, however, and conclusive statements cannot be made at this time. Less is known about commonly used agents such as doxorubicin, taxanes, and platinum compounds. The risk of infertility should be discussed with all patients before they receive anticancer agents, and they should be informed about options for fertility preservation.

Secondary Malignancies

Secondary cancers induced by chemotherapy and radiation are serious long-term complications.[100] Some targeted drugs may also be associated with development of secondary cancers. Although many solid tumors have been reported as chemotherapy-induced malignancies, AML and MDS are the most common secondary cancers and have been reported after successful treatment of Hodgkin lymphoma and NHL, acute leukemias, multiple myeloma, breast cancer, and advanced ovarian cancer. For curable cancers, the relatively small risk for occurrence of secondary malignancies is far outweighed by the benefits of survival in large numbers of patients. The issue of secondary malignancies is of particular concern in patients receiving adjuvant chemotherapy. As with the late complication of infertility, the anticancer agents primarily associated with secondary cancers are the alkylating agents. Etoposide, teniposide, radioimmunoconjugates, and the anthracyclines also are linked to secondary leukemias. Solid tumors as secondary malignancies occur more commonly after treatment with radiation than with chemotherapy.

ABBREVIATIONS

6-MP	6-mercaptopurine
ADCC	antibody-dependent cell-mediated cytotoxicity
AFP	alpha-fetoprotein
AI	aromatase inhibitor
ALL	acute lymphoblastic leukemia
ALK	anaplastic lymphoma kinase
AML	acute myeloid leukemia
ANC	absolute neutrophil count
APA	antiproduct antibodies
APC	adenomatous polyposis coli
APL	acute promyelocytic leukemia
ATP	adenosine triphosphate
BCNU	carmustine
BCL-2	B-cell lymphoma 2
BCR	B-cell receptor
BCR-ABL	breakpoint cluster region-Abelson
BSA	body surface area
BTK	Bruton's tyrosine kinase
CCNU	lomustine
CD	cluster of differentiation
CDC	complement-dependent cytotoxicity
CDK	cyclin-dependent kinase
CLL	chronic lymphocytic leukemia
CML	chronic myeloid leukemia
CNS	central nervous system
CPIC	Clinical Pharmacogenetics Implementation Consortium
CR	complete response
CSF	colony-stimulating factor
CTCAE	Common Terminology Criteria for Adverse Events
CTLA-4	cytotoxic T-lymphocyte antigen 4
DCC	deleted in colorectal cancer
DHFR	dihydrofolate reductase
DM1	derivative of maytansine 1
DMSO	dimethyl sulfoxide
DNA	deoxyribonucleic acid
DNMT	DNA methyltransferase
DPD	dihydropyrimidine dehydrogenase
EBV	Epstein-Barr virus
ECG	electrocardiograph
ECOG	Eastern cooperative oncology group
EGFR	epidermal growth factor receptor
EML4	echinoderm microtubule-like protein 4
ER	estrogen receptor
ErbB	erythroblastic leukemia viral oncogene
ERK	extracellular signal-regulated kinase
FDA	Food and Drug Administration
FGFR	fibroblast growth factor receptor
FKBP-12	12-kDa FK506-binding protein
FU	fluorouracil
GFR	glomerular filtration rate
GIST	gastrointestinal stromal tumor

GM-CSF	granulocyte-macrophage colony stimulating factor
HBV	hepatitis B virus
hCG	human chorionic gonadotropin
HDAC	histone deacetylase
HER2	human epidermal growth factor receptor 2
HFSR	hand-foot skin reaction
HHV	human herpes virus
HIV	human immunodeficiency virus
HPV	human papilloma virus
HSV	herpes simplex virus
IL	interleukin
IFN	interferon
IGF-1R	insulin-like growth factor 1 receptor
irRC	immune-related response criteria
irRECIST	immune-related RECIST
ISO	International Organization for Standardization
JAK	Janus kinase
JAK-STAT	Janus kinase–signal transducers and activators of transcription
mAb	monoclonal antibody
MAPK	mitogen-activated protein kinase
MCD	multicentric Castleman's Disease
MCL	mantle cell lymphoma
MDS	myelodysplastic syndrome
MEK	mitogen-activated protein kinase- extracellular signal-regulated kinase
MMAE	monomethylauristatin E
mRECIST	modified RECIST
MTIC	monomethyl triazeno-imidazole-carboxamide
mTOR	mammalian target of rapamycin
NCCN	National Comprehensive Cancer Network
NCI	National Cancer Institute
NSAID	nonsteroidal anti-inflammatory drug
NSCLC	nonsmall cell lung cancer
NF-κB	nuclear factor-κB
NHL	non-Hodgkin lymphoma
Pap	Papanicolaou
PAP	prostate acid phosphatase
PARP	poly ADP ribose polymerase
PD-1	programmed death-1
PD-L1	programmed death ligand-1
PDGF	platelet-derived growth factor
PDGFR	platelet-derived growth factor receptor
Pgp	p-glycoprotein
Ph^+	Philadelphia chromosome-positive
PI3K	phosphatidylinositide 3-kinases
PML	progressive multifocal leukoencephalopathy
PR	partial response
pRb	retinoblastoma protein
PSA	prostate-specific antigen
PTEN	phosphatase and tensin homolog
RANK	receptor activator of nuclear factor kappa-B
RANKL	receptor activator of nuclear factor kappa-B ligand
RAR	retinoic acid receptor
Rb	retinoblastoma
RECIST	response evaluation criteria in solid tumors
REMS	risk evaluation and mitigation strategy
RET	rearranged during transfection
RNA	ribonucleic acid
RXR	retinoid X receptor
SERM	selective estrogen receptor modulator
SMO	smoothened
STAT	signal transducers and activators of transcription
T-VEC	talimogene laherparepvec
TNF-α	tumor necrosis factor-alpha
TPMT	thiopurine methyltransferase
TSC	tubular sclerosis complex
TSH	thyroid stimulating hormone
VEGF	vascular endothelial growth factor
VEGFR	vascular endothelial growth factor receptor

REFERENCES

1. Siegel R, Naishadham D, Jemal A. Cancer statistics, 2016. *CA Cancer J Clin* 2016;66:7-30.
2. Weston A, Harris CC. Chemical carcinogenesis. In: Waun KH, Bast RC, Hait WN, et al., eds. *Cancer Medicine*, 8th ed. Shelton, CT: People's Medical Publishing House-USA, 2010:225-236.
3. Stricker TP, Kumar V. Neoplasia. In: Kumar V, Abbas AK, Aster JC, Fausto N, eds. *Robbins and Cotran Pathologic Basis of Disease*, 8th ed. Philadelphia, PA: Saunders, 2010:259-330.
4. Hanahan D, Weinberg RA. Hallmarks of cancer: The next generation. *Cell* 2011;144:646-674.
5. Davar D, Beumer JH, Hamieh L, Tawbi H. Role of PARP inhibitors in cancer biology and therapy. *Curr Med Chem* 2012;19:3907-3921.
6. Duarte JD. Epigenetics primer: Why the clinician should care about epigenetics. *Pharmacotherapy* 2013;33:1362-1368.
7. Minn AJ, Massave J. Invasion and metastases. In: DeVita VT, Hellman S, Rosenberg SA, eds. *Cancer: Principles and Practice of Oncology*, 9th ed. Philadelphia, PA: Lippincott Williams & Wilkins, 2011.
8. Heymach JV, Sledge GW, Jain RK. Tumor angiogenesis. In: Waun KH, Bast RC, Hait WN, et al., eds. *Cancer Medicine*, 8th ed. Shelton, CT: People's Medical Publishing House-USA, 2010:149-169.
9. Curran MP, McKeage K. Bortezomib: A review of its use in patients with multiple myeloma. *Drugs* 2009;69:859-888.
10. Smith RA, Cokkinides V, Brawley OW. Cancer screening in the United States, 2012: A review of current American Cancer Society guidelines and issues in cancer screening. *CA Cancer J Clin* 2012;62:129-142.
11. American Cancer Society. *Warning Signs of Cancer*. Atlanta, GA: American Cancer Society, 2007.
12. Edge SB, Byrd DR, Compton CC, Fritz AG, Greene FL, Trotti A, eds. *AJCC Cancer Staging Manual*, 7th ed. New York: Springer-Verlag, 2010.
13. Santarpia L, Lippman SM, El-Naggar AK. Targeting the MAPK-RAS-RAF signaling pathway in cancer therapy. *Expert Opin Ther Targets* 2012;16:103-119.
14. Kapoor A, Figlin RA. Targeted inhibition of mammalian target of rapamycin for the treatment of advanced renal cell carcinoma. *Cancer* 2009;115:3618-3630.
15. Georgescu M-M. PTEN tumor suppressor network in PI3K-Akt pathway control. *Genes Cancer* 2010;1:1170-1177.
16. Murray PJ. The JAK-STAT signaling pathway: Input and output integration. *J Immunol* 2007;178:2623-2629.
17. Pizzorno G, Sharma S, Cheng Y-C. Pyrimidines and purine antimetabolites. In: Waun KH, Bast RC, Hait WN, et al., eds. *Cancer Medicine*, 8th ed. Shelton, CT: People's Medical Publishing House-USA, 2010:621-632.
18. Amstutz U, Froehlich TK, Largiadèr CR. Dihydropyrimidine dehydrogenase gene as a major predictor of severe 5-fluorouracil toxicity. *Pharmacogenomics* 2011;12:1321-1336.

19. Cole PD, Kamen BA, Bertino JR. Folate antagonists. In: Waun KH, Bast RC, Hait WN, et al., eds. *Cancer Medicine*, 8th ed. Shelton, CT: People's Medical Publishing House-USA, 2010:611-620.
20. Hui J, Przespo E, Elefante A. Pralatrexate: A novel synthetic antifolate for relapsed or refractory peripheral T-cell lymphoma and other potential uses. *J Oncol Pharm Pract* 2012;18:275-283.
21. Jain S, Vahdat LT. Eribulin mesylate. *Clin Cancer Res* 2011;17:6615-6622.
22. Rowinsky E. Microtubule-targeting natural products. In: Waun KH, Bast RC, Hait WN, et al., eds. *Cancer Medicine*, 8th ed. Shelton, CT: People's Medical Publishing House-USA, 2010:655-678.
23. Mita AC, Figlin R, Mita MM. Cabazitaxel: More than a new taxane for metastatic cas-trateresistant prostate cancer? *Clin Cancer Res* 2012;18:6574-6579.
24. Rubin EH, Hait WN. Drugs that target DNA topoisomerase. In: Waun KH, Bast RC, Hait WN, et al., eds. *Cancer Medicine*, 8th ed. Shelton, CT: People's Medical Publishing House-USA, 2010:645-654.
25. Colvin M. Alkylating agents and platinum antitumor compounds. In: Waun KH, Bast RC, Hait WN, et al., eds. *Cancer Medicine*, 8th ed. Shelton, CT: People's Medical Publishing House-USA, 2010:633-644.
26. Cheson BD, Rummel MJ. Bendamustine: Rebirth of an old drug. *J Clin Oncol* 2009;27:1492-1501.
27. Loprinzi CL, Qin R, Dakhil SR, et al. Phase III randomized, placebo-controlled, double-blind study of intravenous calcium and magnesium to prevent oxaliplatin-induced sensory neurotoxicity. *J Clin Oncol* 2014;32:997-1005.
28. Buzdar AU, Dawood S, Harvey HA, Jordan VC. Antiestrogens, progestins and aromatase inhibitors. In: Waun KH, Bast RC, Hait WN, et al., eds. *Cancer Medicine*, 8th ed. Shelton, CT: People's Medical Publishing House-USA, 2010:737-749.
29. Denmeade SR. Androgen deprivation strategies in the treatment of advanced prostate cancer. In: Waun KH, Bast RC, Hait WN, et al., eds. *Cancer Medicine*, 8th ed. Shelton, CT: People's Medical Publishing House-USA, 2010:750-758.
30. Powell BL, Moser B, Stock W, et al. Arsenic trioxide improves event-free and overall survival for adults with acute promyelocytic leukemia: North American Leukemia Inter-group Study C9710. *Blood* 2010;116:3751-3757.
31. Wetzler M, Segal D. Omacetaxine as an anticancer therapeutic: What is old is new again. *Curr Pharm Res* 2011;17:59-64.
32. Busse D, Yakes FM, Lenferink AE, Arteaga CL. Tyrosine kinase inhibitors: Rationale, mechanisms of action, and implications for drug resistance. *Semin Oncol* 2001;28(Suppl 16):47-55.
33. Camidge DR, Bang YJ, Kwak EL, et al. Activity and safety of crizotinib in patients with ALK-positive non-small-cell lung cancer: Updated results from a phase 1 study. *Lancet Oncol* 2012;13:1011-1019.
34. Shaw AT, Kim D, Mehra R, et al. Ceritinib in ALK-rearranged non-small-cell lung cancer. *N Engl J Med* 2014;370:1189-1197.
35. McFarland KL, Wetzstein GA. Chronic myeloid leukemia therapy: Focus of second-generation tyrosine-kinase inhibitors. *Cancer Control* 2009;16:132-140.
36. Keller-V Amsberg G, Brummendorf TH. Novel aspects of therapy with the dual Src and Abl kinase inhibitor bosutinib in chronic myeloid leukemia. *Expert Rev Anticancer Ther* 2012;12:1121-1127.
37. Gibbons DL, Pricl S, Kantarjian H, Cortes J, Quintas-Cardama A. The rise and fall of gatekeeper mutations? The BCR-ABL1 T315I paradigm. *Cancer* 2012;118:293-299.
38. Bollag G, Tsai J, Zhang J, et al. Vemurafenib: The first drug approved for BRAF-mutant cancer. *Nat Rev Drug Discov* 2012;11: 873-886.
39. Long GV, Stroyakovskiy D, Gogas H, et al. Combined BRAF and MEK inhibition versus BRAF inhibition alone in melanoma. *N Engl J Med* 2014;371:1877-1888.
40. Burger JA, Buggy JJ. Bruton tyrosine kinase inhibitor ibrutinib (PCI-32765). *Leuk Lymphoma* 2013;54:2385-2391.
41. Finn RS, Crown JP, Lang I, et al. The cyclin-dependent kinase 4/6 inhibitor palbociclib in combination with letrozole versus letrozole alone as first-line treatment of oestrogen receptor-positive, HER2 negative, advanced breast cancer (PALOMA-1/TRIO-18): A randomised phase 2 study. *Lancet Oncol* 2015;16:25-35.
42. Cadoo KA, Gucalp A, Traina TA. Palbociclib: An evidence-based review of its potential in the treatment of breast cancer. *Breast Cancer: Targets and Therapy* 2014;6:123-133.
43. Fandy TE. Development of DNA methyltransferase inhibitors for the treatment of neo-plastidiseases. *Curr Med Chem* 2009;16:2075-2085.
44. Cersosimo RJ. Gefitinib: A new antineoplastic for advanced non-small-cell lung cancer [see comment]. *Am J Health Syst Pharm* 2004;61:889-898.
45. Pallis AG, Syrigos KN. Epidermal growth factor receptor tyrosine kinase inhibitors in the treatment of NSCLC. *Lung Cancer* 2013;80:120-130.
46. Li T, Perez-Soler R, Saltz L. Skin toxicities associated with epidermal growth factor inhibitors. *Target Oncol* 2009;4:107-119.
47. Köhler J, Schuler M. Afatinib, erlotinib, and gefitinib in the first-line therapy of EGFR mutation-positive lung adenocarcinoma: A review. *Onkologie* 2013;36:510-518.
48. Iressa (gefintinib) tablets for oral use. http://www.accessdata.fda.gov/drugsatfda_docs/label/2015/206995s000lbl.pdf. Accessed 7 September 2015.
49. Spraggs CF, Budde LR, Briley LP, et al. HLA-DQA1*02:01 is a major risk factor for lapatinib-induced hepatotoxicity in women with advanced breast cancer. *J Clin Oncol* 2011;29:667-673.
50. Schaid DJ, Spraggs CF, McDonnell SK, et al. Prospective validation of HLA-DRB1*07:01 allele carriage as a predictive risk factor for lapatinib-induced liver injury. *J Clin Oncol* 2014;32:2296-2303.
51. Rudin CM. Vismodegib. *Clin Cancer Res* 2012;18:3218-3222.
52. San-Miguel JF, Hungria V, Yoon S, et al. Panobinostat plus bortezomib and dexamethasone versus placebo plus bortezomib and dexamethasone in patients with relapsed or relapsed and refractory multiple myeloma: A multicenter, randomised, double-blind phase 3 trial. *Lancet Oncol* 2014;15:1195-1206.
53. Ritchie D, Piekarz R, Blombery P, et al. Reactivation of DNA viruses in association with histone deacetylase inhibitor therapy: A case series report. *Haematologica* 2009;94:1618-1622.
54. Verstovsek S, Kantarjian H, Mesa R, et al. Safety and efficacy of INCB018424, a JAK1 and JAK2 inhibitor, in myelofibrosis. *N Engl J Med* 2010;363:1117-1127.
55. Klümpen H, Beijnen JH, Gurney H, Schellens J. Inhibitors of mTOR. *The Oncologist* 2010;15:1262-1269.
56. Rini BI, Campbell SC, Escdier B. Renal cell carcinoma. *Lancet* 2009;373:1119-1132.
57. Ward JE, Stadler WM. Pazopanib in renal cell carcinoma. *Clin Cancer Res* 2010;16:5923-5927.
58. Yakes FM, Chen J, Tan J, et al. Cabozantinib (XL184), a novel MET and VEGFR2 inhibitor, simultaneously suppresses metastasis, angiogenesis, and tumor growth. *Mol Cancer Ther* 2011;10:2298-2308.
59. Wilhelm SM, Dumas J, Adnane L, et al. Regorafenib (BAY 73-4506): A new oral multikinase inhibitor of angiogenic, stromal and oncogenic receptor tyrosine kinases with potent preclinical antitumor activity. *Int J Cancer* 2011;129:245-255.
60. Chau NG, Haddad RI. Vandetanib for the treatment of medullary thyroid cancer. *Clin Cancer Res* 2013;19:524-529.
61. Ledermann J, Harter P, Gourley C, et al. Olaparib maintenance therapy in platinum-sensitive relapsed ovarian cancer. *N Engl J Med* 2012;366:1382-1392.
62. Audeh MW, Carmichael J, Penson RT, et al. Oral poly (ADP-ribose) polymerase inhibitor olaparib in patients with BRCA1 or BRCA2 mutations and recurrent ovarian cancer: A proof-of-concept trial. *Lancet* 2010;376:245-251.
63. Lannutti BJ, Meadows SA, Herman S, et al. CAL-101, a P110δ selective phosphatidylinositol-3-kinase inhibitor for the treatment of b-cell malignancies, inhibits PI3K signaling and cellular viability. *Blood* 2011;117:591-594.
64. Curran MP, McKeage K. Bortezomib: A review of its use in patients with multiple myeloma. *Drugs* 2009;69:859-888.
65. Ruschak AM, Slassi M, Kay LE, Schimmer AD. Novel proteasome inhibitors to overcome bortezomib resistance. *J Natl Cancer Inst* 2011;103:1-11.
66. Cheson BD. Ofatumumab, a novel anti-CD20 monoclonal antibody for the treatment of B-cell malignancies. *J Clin Oncol* 2010;28:3525-3530.
67. Mössner E, Brünker P, Moser S, et al. Increasing the efficacy of CD20 antibody therapy through the engineering of a new type II anti-CD20 antibody with enhanced direct and immune effector cell-mediated b-cell cytotoxicity. *Blood* 2010;115:4393-4402.
68. Sehn LH, Assouline SE, Stewart DA, et al. A phase 1 study of obinutuzumab induction followed by 2 years of maintenance in patients with relapsed CD20-positive b-cell malignancies. *Blood* 2012;119:5118-5125.
69. Gribben JG, Hallek M. Rediscovering alemtuzumab: Current and emerging therapeutic roles. *Br J Haematol* 2009;144:818-831.
70. Portell CA, Wenzell CM, Advani AS. Clinical and pharmacologic aspects of blinatumomab in the treatment of b-cell acute lymphoblastic leukemia. *Clin Pharmacol* 2013;5(suppl 1):5-11.

71. Katz J, Janik JE, Younes A. Brentuximab vedotin (SGN-35). *Clin Cancer Res* 2011;17:6428-6436.
72. Navid F, Santana VM, Barfield RC. Anti-GD2 antibody therapy for GD2-expressing tumors. *Curr Cancer Drug Targets* 2010;10:200-209.
73. Yu AL, Gilman AL, Ozkaynak MF, et al. Anti-GD2 antibody with GM-CSF, interleukin-2, and isotretinoin for neuroblastoma. *N Engl J Med* 2010;363:1324-1334.
74. Allegra CJ, Jessup JM, Somerfield MR, et al. American Society of Clinical Oncology pro-visional clinical opinion: Testing for KRAS gene mutations in patients with metastatic colorectal carcinoma to predict response to anti-epidermal growth factor receptor monoclonal antibody therapy. *J Clin Oncol* 2009;27:2091-2096.
75. Okines AF, Cunningham D. Trastuzumab in gastric cancer. *Eur J Cancer* 2010;46:1949-1959.
76. Verma S, Miles D, Gianni L, et al. Trastuzumab emtansine for HER2-positive advanced breast cancer. *N Engl J Med* 2012;367:1783-1791.
77. Capelan M, Pugliano L, De Azambuja E, et al. Pertuzumab: New hope for patients with HER2-positive breast cancer. *Ann Oncol* 2013;24:273-282.
78. Clarke JM, Hurwitz HI. Targeted inhibition of VEGF receptor 2: An update on ramucirumab. *Expert Opin Biol Ther* 2013;13:1187-1196.
79. Branstetter DG, Nelson SD, Manivel JC, et al. Denosumab induces tumor reduction and bone formation in patients with giant-cell tumor of bone. *Clin Cancer Res* 2012;18:4415-4424.
80. Mellman I, Coukos G, Dranoff G. Cancer immunotherapy comes of age. *Nature* 2011;480:480-489.
81. Wang C, Thudium KB, Han M, et al. In vitro characterization of the anti-PD-1 antibody nivolumab, BMS-936558, and in vivo toxicology in non-human primates. *Cancer Immunol Res* 2014;2:846-856.
82. Borden EC. Interferons. In: Waun KH, Bast RC, Hait WN, et al., eds. *Cancer Medicine*, 8th ed. Shelton, CT: People's Medical Publishing House-USA, 2010:679-685.
83. Ekmekcioglu S, Grimm EA, Kurzrock R. Cytokines and hematopoietic growth factors. In: Waun KH, Bast RC, Hait WN, et al., eds. *Cancer Medicine*, 8th ed. Shelton, CT: People's Medical Publishing House-USA, 2010:686-709.
84. Di Lorenzo G, Buonerba C, Kantoff PW. Immunotherapy for the treatment of prostate cancer. *Nat Rev Clin Oncol* 2011;8:551-561.
85. Eisenhauer EA, Therasse P, Bogaerts J, et al. New response evaluation criteria in solid tumours: Revised RECIST guidelines (version 1.1). *Eur J Cancer* 2009;45:228-247.
86. Lencioni R, Llovet JM. Modified RECIST (mRECIST) assessment for hepatocellular carcinoma. *Semin Liver Dis* 2010;30:52-60.
87. Wolchok JD, Hoos A, O'Day S, et al. Guidelines for the evaluation of immune therapy activity in solid tumors: Immune-related response criteria. *Clin Cancer Res* 2009;15:7412-7420.
88. Bohnsack O, Hoos A, Ludajic K. Adaptation of the immune related response criteria: irRECIST. Abstract presented at: ESMO 2014 Congress; 2014 Sept 26-30; Madrid, Spain.
89. Goodin S, Griffith N, Chen B, et al. Safe Handling of oral chemotherapeutic agents in clinical practice: Recommendations from an international pharmacy panel. *J Oncol Pract* 2011;7:7-12.
90. The NCCN Cancer- and Chemotherapy-Induced Anemia Clinical Practice Guidelines in Oncology (version 1.2016). National Comprehensive Cancer Network, Inc. 2016, http://www.nccn.org/professionals/physician_gls/pdf/anemia.pdf.
91. Freifeld AG, Bow EJ, Sepkowitz KA, et al. Clinical practice guideline for the use of an-timicrobial agents in neutropenic patients with cancer: 2010 Update by the Infectious Diseases Society of America. *Clin Infect Dis* 2011;52:427-431.
92. Metcalf D. The colony-stimulating factors and cancer. *Nat Rev Cancer* 2010;10:425-434.
93. The NCCN Myeloid Growth Factor Clinical Practice Guidelines in Oncology (version 1.2015). National Comprehensive Cancer Network, Inc. 2015, http://www.nccn.org/professionals/physician_gls/pdf/myeloid_growth.pdf.
94. McCurdy MT, Shanholtz CB. Oncologic emergencies. *Crit Care Med* 2012;40:2212-2222.
95. Vadhan-Raj S. Management of chemotherapy-induced thrombocytopenia: Current status of thrombopoietic agents. *Semin Hematol* 2009;46(Suppl 2):S26-S32.
96. Pérez Fidalgo JA, García Fabregat L, Cervantes A, et al. Management of chemotherapy extravasation: ESMO-EONS clinical practice guidelines. *Ann Oncol* 2012;23(suppl 7):167-173.
97. Bhargava P. VEGF kinase inhibitors: How do they cause hypertension? *Am J Physiol Regul Integr Comp Physiol* 2009;297:R1-R5.
98. Kearon C1, Akl EA, Comerota AJ, et al. American College of Chest Physicians. Antithrombotic therapy for VTE disease: Antithrombotic Therapy and Prevention of Thrombosis, 9th ed: American College of Chest Physicians Evidence-Based Clinical Practice Guidelines. *Chest* 2012;141(2 Suppl):e419S-494S.
99. The NCCN Survivorship Clinical Practice Guidelines in Oncology (version 1.2015). National Comprehensive Cancer Network, Inc. 2015, http://www.nccn.org/professionals/physician_gls/pdf/survivorship.pdf.
100. Travis LB, Bhatia S, Allan JM, Oeffinger KC, Ng A. Second primary cancers. In: DeVita VT, Hellman S, Rosenberg SA, eds. *Cancer Principles and Practice of Oncology*, 9th ed. Philadelphia, PA: Lippincott Williams & Wilkins, 2011.

128

Breast Cancer

Chad M. Barnett, Bonnie Lin Boster, and Laura Boehnke Michaud

KEY CONCEPTS

1. Breast cancer is usually diagnosed in the early stages when it is a highly curable malignancy.
2. Although controversial, regular screening mammography in women younger than 50 years of age is beneficial, and many national and international studies demonstrate a reduction in the breast cancer mortality rate from annual or biennial screening mammography in women ages 50 to 74 years.
3. Local therapy of early-stage breast cancer consists of modified radical mastectomy or lumpectomy plus external-beam radiation therapy. The surgical approach to the ipsilateral axilla may consist of a lymph node mapping procedure with sentinel lymph node biopsy or a full level I/II axillary lymph node dissection.
4. Adjuvant endocrine therapy reduces the rates of relapse and death in patients with hormone receptor–positive early breast cancer. Adjuvant chemotherapy reduces the rates of relapse and death in all patients with early-stage breast cancer.
5. The choice of the most appropriate chemotherapy, endocrine therapy, and anti-*HER2* therapy regimen is complex and rapidly changing as results from ongoing randomized clinical trials are reported.
6. Neoadjuvant chemotherapy and biotherapy are appropriate for selected patients with early breast cancer and most patients with locally advanced breast cancer and inflammatory breast cancer followed by local therapy and further adjuvant systemic therapy as indicated.
7. Whereas the goal of adjuvant and neoadjuvant chemotherapy is curative, the goal of chemotherapy in the metastatic setting is palliative.
8. Anti-*HER2* therapies and other biologic or targeted agents (eg, everolimus, palbociclib) in combination with chemotherapy or endocrine therapy have significantly improved outcomes for selected patients with metastatic breast cancer (MBC).
9. Initial therapy of metastatic breast cancer in most women with hormone receptor–positive tumors should include endocrine therapy.
10. About 60% of women with metastatic breast cancer will respond to chemotherapy regimens; anthracycline- and taxane-containing regimens are the most active.

INTRODUCTION

Breast cancer is the most common site of cancer and is second only to lung cancer as a cause of cancer death in American women. It was estimated that 249,260 new cases of breast cancer will be diagnosed and that 40,890 people will die of breast cancer in 2016.[1] In addition to invasive breast cancers, it was estimated that 61,000 cases of non-invasive, or in situ, cancer will be diagnosed among women in the United States in 2016.[1]

Female breast cancer incidence rates have increased for all women combined since 1980, although the rate of increase slowed in the 1990s and has decreased starting in 2000 after peaking in 1999. The decrease in breast cancer incidence of about 7% from 2002 to 2003 is thought to be related to decreased use of menopausal hormone therapy, also known as hormone replacement therapy (HRT), in postmenopausal women.[2] Incidence rates were stable from 2007 to 2011. The incidence of DCIS also increased rapidly between the early and late 1980s and continues to increase. The increase in DCIS is largely attributed to an increased use of screening mammography because most cases of DCIS manifest solely as clustered microcalcifications seen on mammography.[2]

Female breast cancer incidence rates vary considerably across racial and ethnic groups. The average annual age-adjusted incidence rate from 2008 to 2012 was 128.1 cases per 100,000 among whites, 124.3 cases among African Americans, 91.9 cases in Hispanics, 91.9 cases in American Indians and Alaska Natives, and 88.3 cases among Asian Americans and Pacific Islanders.[1] Reasons for the higher incidence rates in whites than in other racial and ethnic groups may include differences in reproductive and lifestyle factors and access to and use of screening.

(1) For all racial and ethnic groups, most breast cancers are diagnosed at an early stage when tumors are small and localized. However, a higher proportion of disease is diagnosed at more advanced stages in African American and other minority women than in white women. The death rate is also higher among African American women than white women despite the lower incidence. From 2008 to 2012, the breast cancer death rate was highest in African Americans (31.0 cases per 100,000 women) followed by whites (21.9), American Indians and Alaska Natives (15.0), Hispanics (14.5), and Asian Americans and Pacific Islanders (11.4).[1] The cause of this disparity between white and African American women is widely debated and multifactorial, with possible explanations including access to care, socioeconomic status, cultural differences, higher stage at diagnosis, and more aggressive biologic features. Despite these differences, overall mortality rates from breast cancer in the United States have declined since 1990. These declines have been attributed to improvements in early detection and in treatment.[1] Figure 128-1 shows the temporal trends in incidence and mortality by race.

The median age at diagnosis for breast cancer is 61 years of age.[3] Although lung cancer is the leading cause of cancer deaths for women regardless of age, breast cancer is the leading cause of cancer deaths for females between the ages of 20 and 59 years.[1]

EPIDEMIOLOGY AND ETIOLOGY

The two variables most strongly associated with the occurrence of breast cancer are gender and age. Although one commonly thinks of breast cancer as a disease confined to women, about 2,600 cases

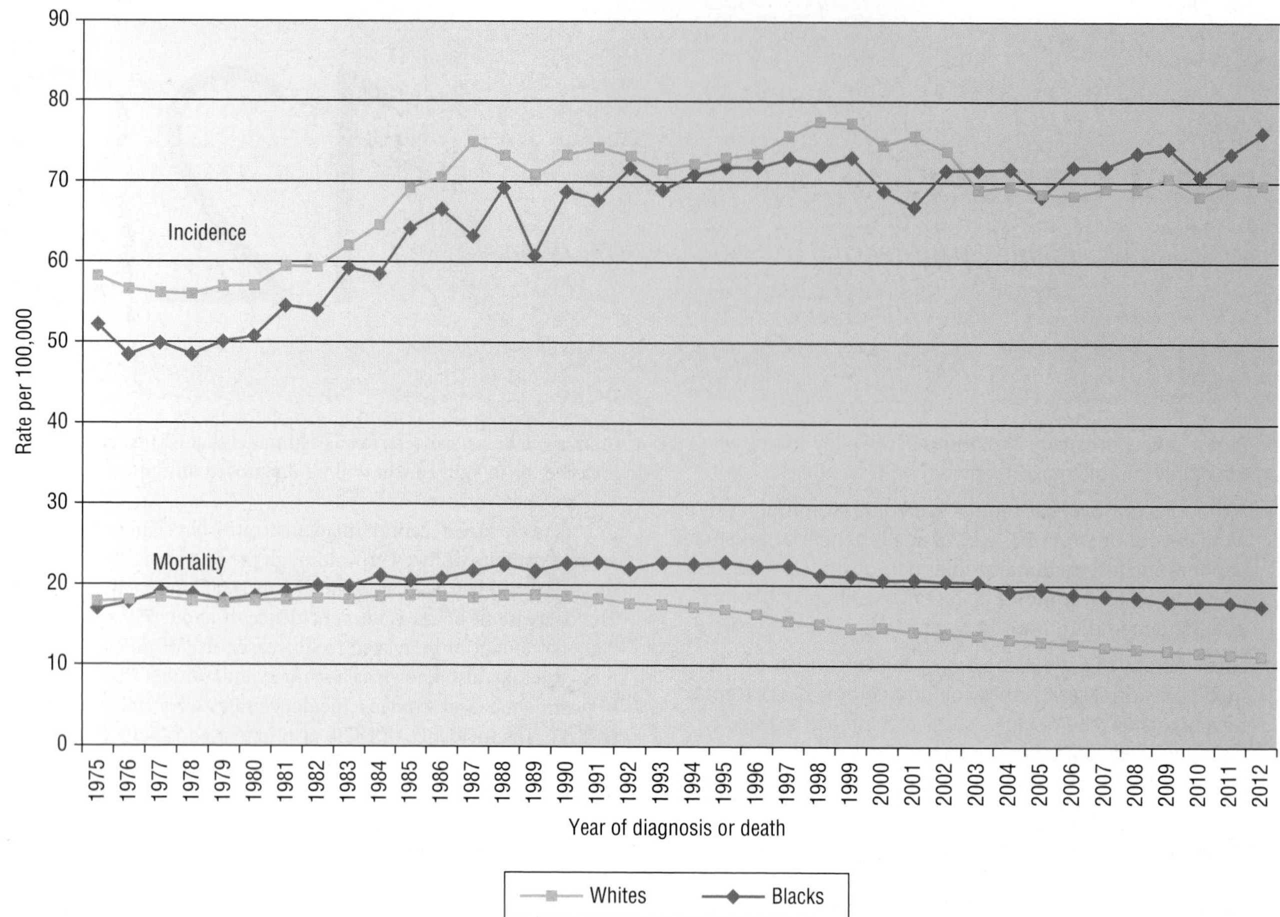

FIGURE 128-1 Breast cancer incidence and mortality rates by race, 1975 to 2009. *(Data from Howlader N, Noone AM, Krapcho M, et al. SEER Cancer Statistics Review, 1975-2012, National Cancer Institute. Bethesda, MD,* http://seer.cancer.gov/csr/1975_2012/, *based on November 2014 SEER data submission, posted to the SEER web site, April 2015.)*

of male breast cancer were estimated to be diagnosed in the United States in 2016.[1] Male gender had been considered a poor prognostic factor in some investigations, but it is now believed that higher mortality rates in men are attributable to more advanced disease at the time of diagnosis. When stage and other known prognostic factors are controlled for, the clinical outcome for men with breast cancer is comparable to that of women.[4] Treatment of breast cancer in men is similar to treatment of breast cancer in women.

The incidence of breast cancer increases with advancing age. A frequently quoted breast cancer statistic is that one in eight women will develop breast cancer during her lifetime. It should be emphasized that this is a cumulative lifetime risk of developing the disease from birth to death. The one-in-eight women figure is often misinterpreted by women who assume that it translates into one in eight women being diagnosed with breast cancer each year. A more useful method of presenting the risk data is based on age intervals.[5] Table 128-1 shows that the risk of a woman developing breast cancer before the age of 50 years is about one in 53, and more than half the risk occurs after age 60 years.

An understanding of the relationship between age and the incidence of breast cancer is particularly relevant when one discusses "risk factors" or factors other than age that increase a woman's probability of developing breast cancer. The RR of developing breast cancer for an individual woman in a defined risk group is usually multiplied by the probability of a woman developing breast cancer during her lifetime, and this figure is taken as the cumulative lifetime risk of that individual developing breast cancer. However, the risk of developing breast cancer depends on age. Therefore, a more meaningful way to counsel patients regarding their risk of developing breast cancer based on the presence of a known risk factor incorporates an age-specific incidence rate, not cumulative lifetime risk. For example, if a 40-year-old woman with a strong family history of breast cancer has a RR ratio of 2.0, her risk of developing breast cancer by the age of 50 years is only 4.6% (2 × 2.3), not 24.6% (2 × 12.3) (Table 128-1). It is also important to note that recognized risk factors are not additive in a simple mathematical sense. Finally, most women with breast cancer have no identifiable major risk factor, indicating that the search for the etiology of this disease is largely incomplete.

TABLE 128-1 Risk of Developing Breast Cancer, Women, All Races, 2009-2011

Age Interval	Probability (%) of Developing Invasive Breast Cancer During the Interval
Birth-49 y	1.9 or 1 in 53
50-59 y	2.3 or 1 in 44
60-69 y	3.5 or 1 in 29
70 y and older	6.7 or 1 in 15
From birth to death	12.3 or 1 in 8

Data from reference 2.

A number of calculators are available to estimate a patient's risk of developing breast cancer. The National Cancer Institute (NCI) has an online version of the Breast Cancer Risk Assessment Tool (*www.cancer.gov/bcrisktool/Default.aspx*). This tool is based on a statistical model known as the Gail model, derived from data from the Breast Cancer Detection and Demonstration Project, a mammography screening project conducted in the 1970s. The Breast Cancer Risk Assessment Tool was designed for healthcare professionals to project a woman's individualized risk for invasive breast cancer over a 5-year period and over her lifetime. This model has been shown to provide accurate estimates in white women, but it has not been validated for other racial and ethnic groups and other subgroups, including those with genetic risk factors. Other risk assessment models also exist, each taking into account different risk factors. Gail and colleagues have developed a similar model for assessing the risk of developing breast cancer in African American women.[6] These empiric models may not be as useful for women with a history suggestive of hereditary breast cancer. Thus, no one model is appropriate for every patient.

Endocrine Factors

A number of endocrine factors have been linked to the incidence of breast cancer.[7,8] Many of these relate to the total duration of menstrual life. Early menarche, generally defined as menstruation beginning before age 12 years, increases the cumulative lifetime risk of breast cancer development. Similarly, a late age of natural menopause (age 55 years or later) increases the risk of breast cancer development, although to a lesser degree than early menarche.[7] Conversely, bilateral oophorectomy before age 40 years reduces the risk of developing breast cancer.

Nulliparity and a late age at first birth (greater than or equal to 30 years) are reported to increase the lifetime risk of developing breast cancer. It is suggested that the period between the onset of menses and the age of first pregnancy provides a "window of initiation" for the development of breast cancer. This is a time when an unbalanced hormonal environment reacts with the abundant and highly responsive breast tissue. Investigators postulate that international differences in age of menarche, age at menopause, and childbearing may account for a substantial part of the international differences in the incidence of breast cancer.

Many studies have evaluated the relationship between exogenous hormones and the development of breast cancer. Postmenopausal HRT has been the subject of several epidemiologic studies and meta-analyses, with conflicting results. The NCI–funded Women's Health Initiative (WHI) is a series of clinical trials designed to investigate the risks and benefits of treatment strategies that could affect women's health issues, such as breast cancer. The estrogen plus progestin trial randomized more than 16,000 postmenopausal women to take conjugated equine estrogen combined with medroxyprogesterone or a placebo.[9] This study reported an increased risk of breast cancer (38 vs 30 cases per 10,000 person-years; RR ratio = 1.26; 95%; CI, 1.00–1.59) in women taking combined estrogen and progestin for an average of 5.2 years compared with those receiving placebo. Analysis of the NCI's Surveillance, Epidemiology, and End Results (SEER) registries showed that the age-adjusted incidence rate of breast cancer in women in the United States in 2003 fell by 6.7% compared with 2002.[10] This decrease in breast cancer incidence seems to be temporally associated with the first report of the WHI study and subsequent decrease in estrogen and progestin HRT use among postmenopausal women. Additional follow-up of patients in this trial confirms a decrease in breast cancer incidence after cessation of estrogen and progestin.[11] In the estrogen alone trial, more than 10,000 women who had a hysterectomy and therefore did not require progestin therapy because of a decreased risk of endometrial carcinoma were randomized to estrogen alone or placebo.[12] The risk of breast cancer was not increased in women who received estrogen alone compared with those who received placebo. With additional follow-up, the incidence of breast cancer in women in this study was actually lower in patients who received estrogen compared with those who received placebo.[13] However, the authors concluded that estrogen alone may not reduce the incidence of breast cancer in patients at increased risk and therefore should not be used specifically for breast cancer risk reduction. Unresolved issues remain as to whether lower doses or short-term use of estrogen or estrogen–progestin for menopausal symptoms can be safe and effective. A longer duration of HRT and concurrent use of progestins appear to contribute to breast cancer risk. In addition, the impact of HRT use on breast cancer risk also varies according to race, body mass index (BMI), and breast density.[14] The use of postmenopausal HRT in women with a history of breast cancer is generally contraindicated. Women who are considering HRT should carefully consider the risks versus benefits (see Chapter 82).

Epidemiologic studies of oral contraceptives do not show a consistent relationship between use of birth control pills and breast cancer risk. Results are conflicting, and assessment of the studies should consider the particular oral contraceptive products involved, daily and cumulative doses of the hormones administered, and latency period for development of breast cancer. A meta-analysis of 13 prospective cohort studies conducted between the years of 1989 and 2010 reported a nonsignificant increase in breast cancer incidence for patients who used oral contraceptives compared with those who had never used oral contraceptives.[15] Newer formulations of oral contraceptives contain lower hormone concentrations, and the authors of this meta-analysis were not able to differentiate breast cancer risk based on the formulations of oral contraceptives. It is also important to note that oral contraceptives are known to reduce the risk of ovarian and endometrial cancers. Most experts believe that the safety and benefits of low-dose oral contraceptives currently outweigh the potential risks.

Genetic Factors

Both personal and family histories influence a woman's risk of developing breast cancer. A personal history of breast cancer is associated with an increased risk of developing contralateral breast cancer. Cancers of the uterus and ovary are also associated with an increased risk of developing breast cancer. A number of cancer family syndromes include breast cancer in association with other types of cancers.

Many women have "lumpy breasts" or have a clinical diagnosis of fibrocystic breast disease or benign breast disease. Nonproliferative lesions, such as cysts or simple fibroadenomas, do not increase the risk of breast cancer. Proliferative lesions without atypia, such as intraductal papillomatosis, are associated with a mildly elevated breast cancer risk of about 1.5 to 2.0 times that of the general population. Atypical hyperplasias are classified as either ductal or lobular units, and these lesions may increase a woman's risk for breast cancer to about 4.0 times that of the general population.[16]

Dense breast tissue reduces the sensitivity of mammography in detecting breast cancer and is associated with an increased risk of breast cancer. The risk of breast cancer in women with dense breasts (defined by mammography) has been estimated to be between four to five times that of women of the same age with little density.[17] Many variables, including age, BMI, menopausal status, HRT, parity, and the ratio of fibroglandular to fatty tissue, can influence mammographic breast density. This ratio can be expressed as the percentage dense area and the absolute dense area, both of which are risk factors for breast cancer.[17] Genetic factors may also play a role in this finding because mammographic breast density has been shown to have high heritability and is also strongly associated with a positive family history of breast cancer.

The percentage of all breast cancers in the U.S. population that can be attributed to family history is about 10%. Empirical estimates of the risks associated with particular patterns of family history of breast cancer indicate the following:[18]

1. Having any first-degree relative with breast cancer increases a woman's risk of breast cancer about 1.5- to 3-fold. Risk increases with increasing numbers of affected first-degree relatives.
2. The risk is affected by both a woman's own age and the age of the relative when diagnosed. A higher risk is seen when a woman and her relative at diagnosis are younger than 50 years.
3. The risk associated with having any second-degree relative with breast cancer is complex and depends on other family history patterns. However, the risk is generally lower than that of first-degree relatives.
4. Affected family members on both the maternal and the paternal sides are important to consider in evaluation of risk.

Although women with a family history of breast cancer are at increased risk for the disease, the diagnosis of breast cancer is still uncommon in young women even with a positive family history.

Germ-line mutations in either *BRCA1* or *BRCA2* are associated with an increased risk for breast and ovarian cancer. These genes function as tumor suppressor genes, maintaining genomic integrity and DNA repair. Compared with an average woman's 13% lifetime risk of developing breast cancer, the probability of developing breast or ovarian cancer by the age of 70 years in women with a *BRCA1* or *BRCA2* mutation is estimated to be 57% and 49% for breast cancer and 40% and 18% for ovarian cancer, respectively.[19]

The probability of being a *BRCA* gene mutation carrier is related to ethnicity and family history. Jewish people of Eastern European decent (Ashkenazi Jews) have an unusually high (2.1%) carrier rate of germ-line mutations in *BRCA1* and *BRCA2* compared with the rest of the U.S. population. Conversely, it is estimated that clinically significant *BRCA* mutations occur at a frequency of about one in 300 to 500 persons in the general, non-Jewish U.S. population.[20] Testing for *BRCA1* and *BRCA2* mutations is now widely available, but testing is generally recommended only when there is personal or family history suggestive of hereditary cancer, when the test results can be adequately interpreted, and when results will assist with diagnosis and management. The decision to test an individual for a genetic mutation related to breast cancer risk is complex, and several organizations have published recommendations on genetic susceptibility testing for individuals who meet the criteria for increased risk.[20,21,22]

Although most genetic causes of breast cancer are attributed to *BRCA1* and *BRCA2,* other genes that have been identified as being associated with hereditary breast cancer include *TP53, CHEK2, PALB2, PTEN, ATM,* and others.[23]

Environmental and Lifestyle Factors

Breast cancer incidence rates vary considerably among countries, which suggests that environmental and lifestyle factors play an important role in the etiology. Compelling evidence is derived from studies of Asian women who migrated to the United States. Although the incidence of breast cancer in Asian women is quite low, the incidence of breast cancer in Asian women who were born in the United States or who migrated from Asia to the United States gradually increases over the individual's lifetime to equal that of the white population in the same geographic area.[24]

Diet is an important and modifiable environmental risk factor. Possible relationships between fat intake and steroid hormone metabolism have led to an emphasis on dietary fat as a possible etiologic agent for breast cancer. Epidemiologic data show a positive correlation between higher dietary fat intake and breast cancer risk, which is stronger in postmenopausal than in premenopausal women. In a meta-analysis of 31 case-control and 14 cohort studies on dietary fat and breast cancer, Boyd et al. reported a small but significant RR ratio of 1.13 (95% CI, 1.03-1.25) when comparing the highest and lowest fat intake categories.[25] To confirm this association prospectively, the hypothesis that low dietary fat intake reduces breast cancer risk was further tested in the WHI Randomized Controlled Dietary Modification Trial.[26] More than 48,000 postmenopausal women were randomized to a dietary intervention that consisted of reducing total fat intake to 20% of energy and consuming at least five servings of fruits and vegetables daily and six servings of grains daily versus a comparison group without any dietary interventions. Over an 8-year mean follow-up period, the incidence of invasive breast cancer was not significantly different between the two groups (annualized incidence rate, 0.42% vs 0.45%; HR, 0.91; 95% CI, 0.83-1.01). Although there is still much to be learned about the effects of diet on the risk of developing breast cancer, a low-fat diet seems to be a reasonable approach to potentially reduce the risk of breast cancer.

An additional dietary factor to be explored in the breast cancer population includes food-derived heterocyclic amines, which are known carcinogens found commonly in cooked red meat or processed meat. Studies of red or processed meat ingestion and breast cancer incidence are inconsistent, and no association was reported in one meta-analysis.[27]

Many studies have also examined the association between breast cancer and intake of dietary fiber and micronutrients, including β-carotene, and vitamins A, C, and E. The relationship between vitamins and breast cancer is unclear. No consistent benefit of fruits or vegetable consumption and the risk of breast cancer has been demonstrated.[27]

Another dietary factor that deserves mention is the possible effect of phytoestrogens on breast cancer risk. Phytoestrogens are natural plant estrogens found in soybean products, seeds, berries, and nuts. The two most studied classes of dietary phytoestrogens are isoflavones and lignans; isoflavones are richer in Asian diets, and lignans are the main source of phytoestrogens in the Western diet.[28,29] Because these compounds exhibit weak estrogenic properties, some experts believe that they may function as relative antiestrogens by displacing natural estradiol. However, studies have also reported a potential stimulatory effect on breast tissue. A meta-analysis of observational studies that evaluated phytoestrogen use and the risk of breast cancer suggests that any potential associated risk reduction is modest and may be limited to postmenopausal patients.[28] Nonetheless, the effect of phytoestrogens on breast cancer is very controversial, and further research is needed.

Both body weight and height are associated with the incidence of breast cancer. Most studies of premenopausal women show either no relationship with body weight or slightly declining breast cancer risks with increasing body weight. Most studies in postmenopausal women show increasing breast cancer risks with increasing body weight. Accordingly, a meta-analysis by Renehan et al. found that an increase in BMI was associated with an increase in the risk of breast cancer for postmenopausal women (RR, 1.12; 95% CI, 1.08-1.16; $P<0.0001$) but had the opposite effect in premenopausal women (RR, 0.92; 95% CI, 0.88-0.97; $P<0.001$).[30] An increase in circulating estrogen is postulated to be the most likely explanation for these results. Although height is not a modifiable risk factor, weight and body composition are modifiable and should be studied further. Maintaining a healthy weight and body composition appear to be beneficial and promote many different health benefits but requires further study in association with the incidence of breast cancer.

Many studies report an inverse association between physical activity and breast cancer risk.[31] A review of 7 cohort and 14 case-control studies suggests that the association is stronger for postmenopausal breast cancer than for premenopausal breast cancer. Exercise may provide modest protection against breast cancer, but the relationship is complex. Possible explanations include the effects of physical activity on menstrual characteristics (in premenopausal women), body size, weight, and serum hormone levels. Estrogen-related pathways or other metabolic hormones such as insulin and insulin-like growth factors may influence this relationship. Making healthy choices appears to be the best health advice for women.

Many epidemiologic studies have evaluated the relationship between alcohol and breast cancer. Studies indicate both a modest positive association between alcohol and breast cancer and a dose–response relationship.[32] The risk increases with consumption of alcohol in general regardless of the beverage type or woman's menopausal status. Although the exact mechanism is unknown, the most plausible biologic hypothesis relates to increased levels of estrogen or other reproductive steroid hormones caused by impaired liver function. Although a causal relationship between alcohol consumption and breast cancer has not been proven in a prospective trial, the weight of the available evidence suggests that a relationship (direct or indirect) may exist. Because alcohol consumption is a modifiable risk factor, use in moderation appears to be a sensible approach.

Radiation to the breast tissue is associated with an increased risk of breast cancer, particularly with exposure at a young age (less than 20 years), again suggesting that a "window of initiation" for breast cancer occurs at a relatively early age. Much of the knowledge about radiation-related breast cancer comes from epidemiologic studies of patients exposed to diagnostic or therapeutic radiation and of Japanese survivors of the atomic bombs.[33] Women treated with chest irradiation for Hodgkin lymphoma in childhood or adolescence and survivors of other childhood cancers (in which radiation is used as a mainstay of therapy) are among the populations at greater risk for secondary breast cancers. The risk increases linearly with radiation dose. Exposure to diagnostic x-rays, including annual screening mammography, does not impart a sufficient dose of radiation for clinical concern in the general population. However, the risk of breast cancer after radiation exposure even in low levels in those with genetic risk factors is unclear and is an ongoing area of research.

Tobacco smoke exposure has not been associated with an increased risk of breast cancer in the past. In recent years, some studies have found that heavy smoking in certain groups is linked to a higher risk, such as in women who started smoking before having their first child.[34] The 2014 US Surgeon General's report on smoking concluded that there is "suggestive but not sufficient" evidence that smoking increases the risk of breast cancer.[35]

In conclusion, numerous studies have been performed to investigate potential causative factors in the etiology of breast cancer. Several endocrine, genetic, environmental, and lifestyle factors are associated with the development of breast cancer to varying degrees. Some factors are modifiable, but others are not. Additionally, the impact of individual risk factors may vary depending on other confounding variables such as age, family history, estrogen use, and menopausal status. Although epidemiologic studies provide a large body of the current evidence, they have their limitations, and results are varied. Meta-analyses summarize numerous study results, but heterogeneity of studies may limit the applicability of the evidence. Additional prospective, randomized controlled trials are needed to confirm the importance of factors that are associated with the risk of developing breast cancer.

PREVENTION AND EARLY DETECTION

Current efforts at breast cancer prevention are directed toward the identification and removal of risk factors often referred to as risk reduction strategies. Unfortunately, a number of risk factors associated with development of breast cancer, such as family history of breast cancer or personal history of breast or other gynecologic malignancies, cannot be modified. Isolation and cloning of breast cancer susceptibility genes now allow screening of women with histories suggestive of "breast cancer families" and identification of appropriate candidates for prophylactic bilateral mastectomies or bilateral salpingo-oophorectomy. These surgeries are considered for women who are at very high risk for the development of breast or ovarian cancer, particularly if the women's breasts are difficult to evaluate by both physical examination and mammography and if the women have persistent disabling fears that they will be diagnosed with cancer. Guidelines for the incorporation of surgical risk reduction strategies are largely based on genetics and other known risk factors for the development of breast (or ovarian) cancer.

In the last 20 years, there has been increasing interest in pharmacologic risk reduction for breast cancer. The drugs with the most clinical information as risk reduction agents for breast cancer are the selective estrogen receptor modulators (SERMs), tamoxifen and raloxifene. Tamoxifen is useful as an adjunct after treatment of primary breast cancer (see Adjuvant Endocrine Therapy section for details). In randomized trials of tamoxifen as an adjuvant treatment for breast cancer, women who received tamoxifen were also found to have a reduced incidence of contralateral primary breast carcinomas.[36] In a large, randomized, placebo-controlled study, the National Surgical Adjuvant Breast and Bowel Project (NSABP) demonstrated significant reductions in risk of invasive and noninvasive breast cancers with 5 years of tamoxifen therapy (20 mg/day) in women at high risk for developing the disease.[37] Although this study (also known as P-1) is controversial, other studies from around the world also have been reported that investigated the role of tamoxifen as a risk reduction strategy. A meta-analysis of these trials indicates a consistent benefit with tamoxifen in reducing the incidence of ER-positive breast cancers (48% reduction; 95% CI, 36%-58%; $P<0.0001$).[38] Tamoxifen has been repeatedly shown to be a relatively safe drug with an acceptable toxicity profile when used to treat patients with breast cancer. However, its estrogenic effects on the uterus and the coagulation system increase the risk of serious adverse effects that may be critical for patients taking this agent as a risk reduction strategy. Toxicities associated with tamoxifen are described in the Adjuvant Endocrine Therapy section. Any decision to use tamoxifen for risk reduction should be made after a thorough discussion of the woman's risk of breast cancer, the potential benefits of tamoxifen, and the potential serious adverse events associated with tamoxifen.

A second trial has been reported that compared tamoxifen with raloxifene in high-risk postmenopausal women. The STAR (or P2) trial was published in 2006 and demonstrated a similar rate of invasive breast cancers with the two drugs.[39] However, the rates of noninvasive breast cancer were numerically higher in the raloxifene arm of the trial, although this difference did not reach statistical significance. In 2010, an updated analysis was published, reporting that raloxifene retained 76% of tamoxifen's effectiveness in preventing invasive breast cancer.[40] Rates of endometrial cancer and deep-vein thrombosis (DVT) were more frequent in the tamoxifen arm, but overall quality of life was similar between the two agents.[39] Based on these results, the Food and Drug Administration (FDA) approved raloxifene for breast cancer risk reduction in women at high risk of the disease.

After the STAR update, there has since been an update reviewing SERMs in the prevention of breast cancer. In this meta-analysis, all SERMs reduced the incidence of invasive ER-positive breast cancer not only during treatment but also for at least 5 years after completing therapy.[41] As with all preventive interventions, the risks and benefits need to be carefully considered for each woman.

A similar reduction in the incidence of contralateral primary breast cancers was demonstrated in the adjuvant clinical trials with the aromatase inhibitors (AIs), leading to the premise that AIs may also play a role in risk reduction of breast cancer.[42] Goss et al. published the first results of a randomized, placebo-controlled, phase III trial comparing exemestane with placebo for 5 years in high-risk postmenopausal women.[43] Eligibility criteria were similar to the P-1 and STAR trials, and this report represented a median follow-up period of only 35 months. Nonetheless, significant reductions were seen in the rates of invasive breast cancers with exemestane (HR, 0.35; 95% CI, 0.18-0.70; P=0.002). A second randomized, placebo-controlled, phase III trial by Cuzick et al. compared the AI anastrozole to placebo for 5 years in high-risk postmenopausal women.[44] After a median follow up of 5 years, the anastrozole arm showed significant reductions in the rates of invasive breast cancers (HR, 0.50; 95% CI, 0.32-0.76; P=0.001). In both the Goss et al. and Cuzick et al. studies, adverse events were tolerable. Based on this data, AIs appear to be a reasonable option for breast cancer risk reduction. In this setting, AIs were not compared to SERMs although both classes of agents are options. The National Comprehensive Cancer Network (NCCN) has established guidelines for risk reduction strategies, including mastectomy, oophorectomy, and pharmacologic agents.[45] These guidelines are based on risk assessment tools such as the Gail, BRCAPRO, or Claus models as well as other established risk factors. Much of the guideline depends on a woman's preferences for intervention. The American Society of Clinical Oncology (ASCO) also has published recommendations guiding the use of pharmacologic agents for breast cancer risk reduction.[46] These guidelines are similar to the NCCN guidelines in that they recommend the use of tamoxifen, raloxifene, or exemestane for postmenopausal women at high risk (as defined by the Gail or other models) and tamoxifen for premenopausal women at high risk based on the woman's wishes. Although neither exemestane nor anastrozole is FDA approved for breast cancer risk reduction, ASCO and NCCN included AIs as acceptable options for use in postmenopausal women.[45,46]

The rationale for early detection of breast cancer is based on the relationship between stage of breast cancer at diagnosis and the probability for cure. If all breast cancer cases could be detected at a very early stage of the disease (ie, small primary tumor and negative lymph nodes), then more patients theoretically could be cured of their disease. Screening guidelines for early detection of breast cancer in women at average risk have been developed by several organizations, including but not limited to the American Cancer Society (ACS), the United States Preventive Services Task Force (USPSTF), and the NCCN (See Table 128-2).[47,48,49] The ACS guidelines are most commonly cited. However, it is important to note that the expert panels developing these guidelines often differ in their approach and analysis of the available data, as is evident in the controversies that currently exist.

The ACS currently recommends that all women be informed of the benefits and limitations of breast cancer screening.[47] In the 2015 guidelines, ACS did not recommend breast self-examinations (BSEs) but noted that they did not change from their 2003 guidelines which states that beginning at age 20 years women should be told about the benefits and limitations of BSE.[47,50] Several studies have investigated the benefits of BSE. These trials were primarily conducted before the routine use of mammographic screening and demonstrated an inferential benefit in diagnosis of earlier stages of breast cancer. The Shanghai trial appeared to indicate no benefit, but there was a higher rate of biopsies in women who were taught BSE than in women who were not taught BSE.[51] The investigators from this trial caution that

TABLE 128-2 Breast Cancer Screening Guidelines

Risk Category	ACS[1]	USPTF[2]	NCCN[3]
Average Risk			
BSE	Age ≥20 y: optional (discuss benefits and limitations)	Not recommended	Age ≥25 y: breast awareness
CBE	Evidence does not support	Insufficient evidence	Age ≥25-39 y: every 1-3 y Age ≥40 y: annually
Mammography	Age 40-44 y: opportunity annually Age 45-54 y: annually Age ≥55 y: biennially or opportunity annually (as long as in good health and at least 10 years life expectancy)	Age 40-50 y: individualized decision Age 50-74 y: biennial Age >75 y: insufficient evidence	Age ≥40 y: annually
High Risk[a,b]			
BSE	NA	NA	All ages: breast awareness
CBE	NA	NA	All ages: every 6-12 months
Mammography	Age ≥30 y: annually with MRI	NA	Prior RT or strong family history or genetic predisposition, age ≥25 y: annually (+ CBE) All other categories: annually (+ CBE)
Breast MRI	Age ≥30 y: annually with mammogram	NA	Annually with mammogram + CBE for (a) prior RT, age ≥25 y; (b) lifetime risk >20%; (c) strong family history or genetic predisposition, age ≥25 y; (d) history of LCIS

ACS, American Cancer Society; BSE, breast self-examination; CBE, clinical breast examination by a healthcare professional; LCIS, lobular carcinoma in situ; MRI, magnetic resonance imaging; NA, not addressed; NCCN, National Comprehensive Cancer Network; RT, thoracic radiation therapy; USPTF, United States Preventive Task Force.

[a]High risk is defined by the ACS as women with (a) a known *BRCA1/2* gene mutation; (b) untested woman with first-degree relative with a known *BRCA1/2* gene mutation; (c) lifetime risk of breast cancer of 20%-25% or greater using a risk assessment tool based largely on family history; (d) radiation therapy to the chest between the ages of 10 and 30 years; (e) LiFraumeni syndrome, Cowden syndrome, or Bannayan-Riley-Ruvalcaba syndrome or have first-degree relatives with one of these syndromes.

[b]High risk is defined by the NCCN as women with (a) prior thoracic radiation therapy before age 30 years, (b) 5-year risk of ≥1.7% of invasive breast cancer in women ≥35 years old, lifetime risk of >20% as defined by models that are largely based on family history, (d) strong family history or genetic predisposition, (e) LCIS, (f) prior history of breast cancer.

1. Oeffinger KC, Fontham ET, Etzioni R, et al. Breast Cancer Screening for Women at Average Risk: 2015 Guideline Update From the American Cancer Society. *JAMA* 2015;314:1599-1614.

2. U.S. Preventive Services Task Force. Screening for breast cancer: U.S. Preventive Services Task Force recommendation statement. *Ann Intern Med* 2009;151:716-726.

3. NCCN Clinical Practice Guidelines in Oncology (NCCN Guidelines®) for *Breast Cancer Screening and Diagnosis Guidelines* V.1.2015 © National Comprehensive Cancer Network, Inc 2015. All rights reserved. Last accessed, September 1, 2015.

this was a study of BSE instruction and not BSE performance. Compliance and competency with the BSE were neither guaranteed nor evaluated in this trial. Because of the lack of direct evidence to support or refute a benefit with BSE and the apparent associated increase in biopsy rates, the ACS has taken the position that it is optional.[47] Other organizations have taken a similar approach to their recommendations regarding BSE or simply state that there are insufficient evidence to recommend this practice.[48,49]

Recommendations for breast examination by a healthcare professional (clinical breast examination [CBE]) vary among the screening guidelines most often cited. The rate of breast cancer detection using CBE alone is low, with even lower rates in younger women.[52] Randomized clinical trials have reported inconsistent results and often evaluated CBE in conjunction with mammograms. The ACS does not recommend CBE for women of average risk.[47] The USPSTF concluded that there is insufficient evidence to assess the benefits and risks of CBE beyond screening mammography in women older than the age of 40 years.[48]

2 The most controversial screening recommendation for breast cancer is related to annual mammography. It is clear that screening mammography decreases mortality from breast cancer. The controversies surround the balance of benefits and harms associated with a less than perfect screening test in women at average risk of developing breast cancer but of differing ages. Multiple clinical trials have been completed over the years, and multiple meta-analyses of these trials have been conducted as well. Most of the trials included women 50 to 74 years of age, and the interval between testing ranged from 12 to 33 months. The most recent meta-analysis of these data estimated an number needed to invite (NNI) for screening as 1,339 for women aged 50 to 59 years.[53] Some trials also included women aged 40 to 49 years, albeit significantly fewer women in this age group were included in the meta-analyses. The estimated NNI for women aged 39 to 49 years was reported as 1,904. The largest benefit was found in women ages 60 to 69 years with an estimated NNI of 377. None of the trials included women 75 years of age or older; therefore, there are no data to support or refute the benefit of screening mammography in this population.[53]

Incorporation of this new information into national guidelines differs with each organization. The ACS recommends annual screening mammography for women ages 45 to 54 years, biennial screening mammography for women greater than or equal to 55 years and older (as long as they are in good health and have at least a 10 year life expectancy), and the opportunity for annual screening mammography for women 40 to 44 years. Women greater than or equal to 55 years and older should have the opportunity to continue with annual screening rather than changing over to biennial screening.[47] This recommendation allows for individualized decisions to be made based on the overall health of the woman but does not limit access to younger or older women who may benefit from screening. The USPSTF took a different approach, stating that "the decision to start regular, biennial screening mammography before the age of 50 years should be an individualized one and take patient context into account, including the patient's values regarding specific benefits and harms."[48] For women 50 to 74 years of age, the USPSTF recommends biennial screening mammography. This interval recommendation was based on assumptions of risks and benefits based on the available studies. Although the upper limit for screening varies among guidelines, most experts agree that mammograms in women older than the age of 74 are not supported by the current body of evidence, but some women may benefit if they are otherwise in good health and have a life expectancy of 10 years or more. There are also many other debates within this controversial area, and readers are referred to these references for further details.[47,48,49,53]

Other radiologic methods of breast imaging are also being investigated (eg, digital mammography, ultrasonography, and magnetic resonance imaging [MRI]), and minimal data exist to support these methods in some high-risk populations. Recommendations for women with a high risk of breast cancer are not fully established, and definitions of "high risk" vary among different guidelines. See Table 128-2 for appropriate patients for breast screening MRI as an adjunct to mammography according to the ACS.[54,55] The NCCN also has adopted consensus guidelines for women at high risk of breast cancer, incorporating breast MRI with other established screening tools for women as young as 25 years old.[22]

It should also be noted that there are risks associated with any screening procedure, and they should be discussed with all patients so they are able to make an informed decision regarding these procedures. The risks involved with screening mammograms include false-negative results, false-positive results, overdiagnosis (true positives that will not become clinically significant), and radiation risk. The rate of false-negative results with the current technology is about 20%, which explains why CBE is an important adjunct to screening for many women. Although the specificity of mammography is quite high (90%), most abnormal examinations are false-positive results, leading to additional biopsies and psychological distress. The issue of overdiagnosis refers primarily to the growth in

CLINICAL PRESENTATION

General

- The patient may not have any symptoms because breast cancer may be detected in asymptomatic patients through routine screening mammography.

Local Signs and Symptoms

- A painless, palpable lump is most common.
- Less common: pain; nipple discharge, retraction, or dimpling; skin edema, redness, or warmth.
- Palpable local–regional lymph nodes may also be present.

Signs and Symptoms of Systemic Metastases

- Depends on the site of metastases, but may include bone pain, difficulty breathing, abdominal pain or enlargement, jaundice, or mental status changes.

Laboratory Tests

- Tumor markers such as cancer antigen (CA 27.29) or carcinoembryonic antigen (CEA) may be elevated.
- Alkaline phosphatase or liver function test results may be elevated in patients with metastatic disease.

Other Diagnostic Tests

- Mammography (with or without ultrasonography, breast MRI, or both).
- Biopsy for pathology review and determination of tumor ER or PR status and human epidermal growth factor receptor-2 (*HER2*) status.
- Systemic staging tests may include chest radiography, chest computed tomography (CT), bone scan, abdominal CT or ultrasonography, or MRI.

detection of DCIS from screening mammography. (See Noninvasive Carcinoma section for a detailed discussion of DCIS.) The biologic significance of these tumors is unknown because only some of them would become invasive if left in place. So the question remains: Are we treating women who do not require treatment? Experts in the field continue to debate this issue. Radiation exposure also has been discussed in the context of screening mammography, but the small doses of radiation exposure with mammograms (2-4 mGy [0.2-0.4 Rad] per standard two-view examination) appears to be overshadowed by other benefits in terms of reduction in mortality as a consequence of early cancer detection.[48]

Significant advances in the safety and efficacy of screening mammography have occurred during the last 2 decades. These advances have enabled superior visualization of breast and breast tissue with a lower dose of radiation being delivered. Despite these advances, about 10% of all palpable masses are not detected by mammography. This is most commonly observed in premenopausal women and may be directly related to the increased density of breast tissue in this estrogen-rich environment. In addition, differences exist between breast imaging quality and interpretation, and it is best to have imaging conducted at the same facility over time if possible.

CLINICAL PRESENTATION

A painless lump is the initial sign of breast cancer in most women. The typical malignant mass is solitary, unilateral, solid, hard, irregular, and nonmobile. In small numbers of cases, stabbing or aching pain is the first symptom. Less commonly, nipple discharge, retraction, or dimpling may herald the onset of the disease. In more advanced cases, prominent skin edema, redness, warmth, and induration of the underlying tissue may be observed.

The breast is a complex organ composed of skin, subcutaneous tissue, fatty tissue, and branching ductal and glandular structures (Fig. 128-2). Various diseases that affect these structures can produce a palpable mass. In addition, the physiologic changes associated with the menstrual cycle can cause normal breast changes. Common causes of breast masses in young women are fibroadenoma, fibrocystic disease, carcinoma, and fat necrosis.

Many women detect some breast abnormality themselves, but in the United States, it is increasingly common for breast cancer to be detected during routine screening mammography in asymptomatic women. It is widely accepted that the smaller the mass, the higher the likelihood of cure. Thus, the routine use of screening mammography

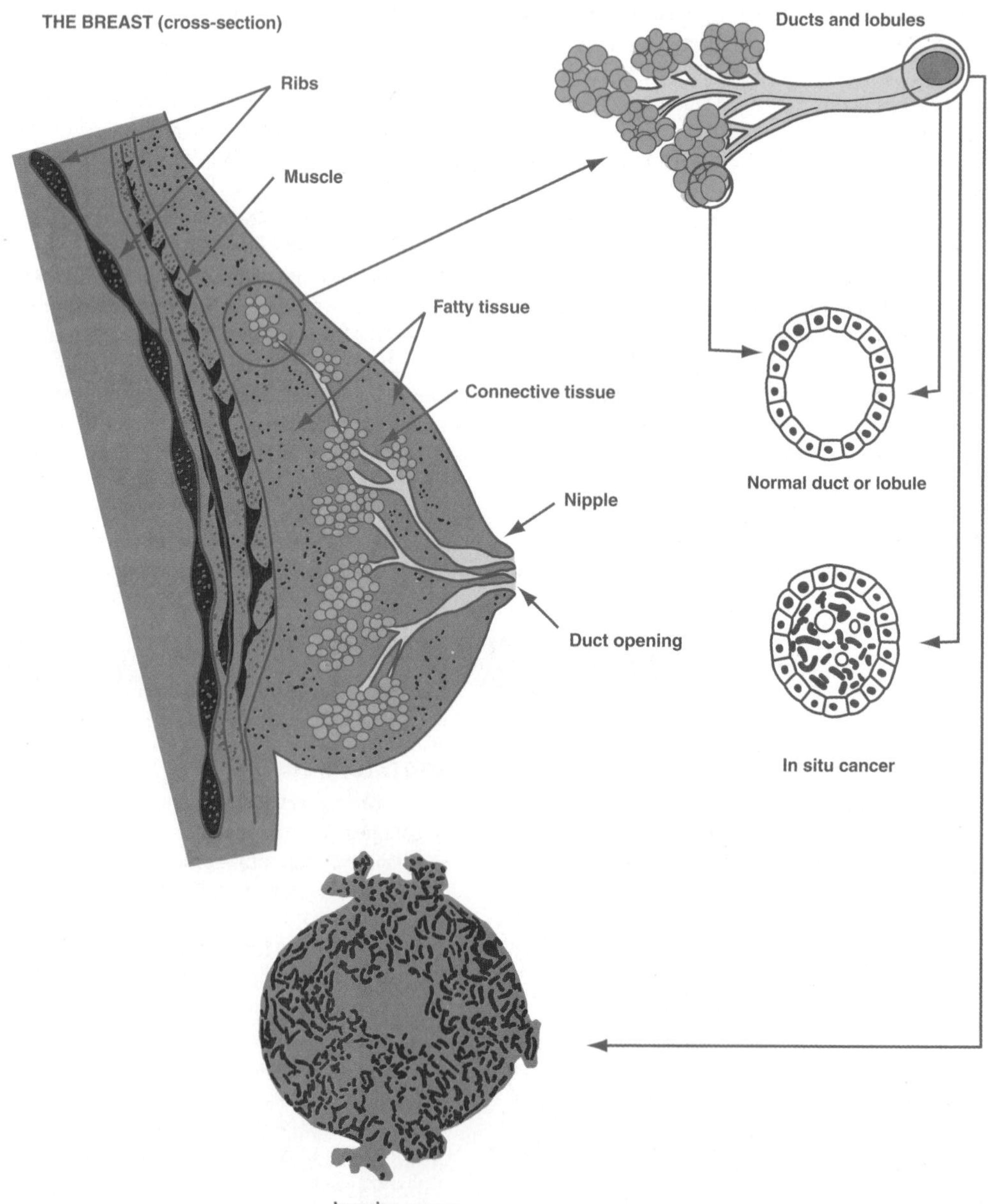

FIGURE 128-2 Breast anatomy.

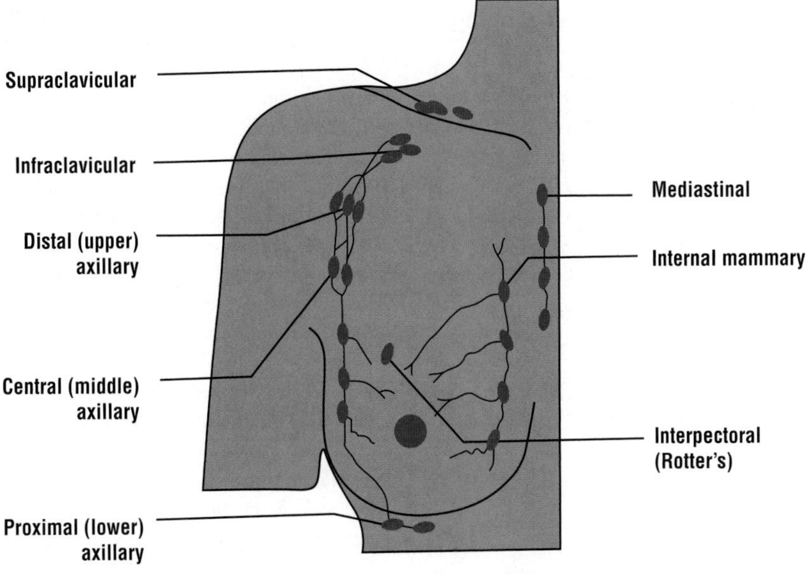

FIGURE 128-3 Lymph node anatomy.

has contributed to the recent decline in mortality rate. However, this decreasing mortality rate is also related to improved systemic therapy.

Breast cancer that is confined to a localized breast lesion is often referred to as *early*, *primary*, *localized*, or *curable*. Breast cancer that has spread to local–regional lymph nodes is still considered early stage (Fig. 128-3). Unfortunately, breast cancer cells often spread by contiguity, through lymph channels, and through the blood to distant sites. This often occurs early in breast cancer growth, and deposits of tumor cells form in distant sites that are undetected with current diagnostic methods and equipment (micrometastases). When breast cancer cells can be detected clinically or radiologically in sites distant from the breast, the disease is referred to as *advanced* or *metastatic* breast cancer (MBC). Tissues most commonly involved with distant metastases are lymph nodes (other than local–regional lymph nodes), skin, bone, liver, lungs, and brain. Symptoms of bone pain, difficulty breathing, abdominal enlargement, jaundice, and mental status changes may herald the clinical presentation of MBC. A small percentage of women have signs and symptoms of distant metastases when they first seek treatment. In virtually all of them, a neglected breast mass has been present for several months to years. In addition, 10% to 50% of all patients who initially are treated for localized disease eventually develop signs and symptoms of MBC.[56]

DIAGNOSIS

The initial workup for a woman presenting with a breast mass or symptoms suggestive of breast cancer should include a careful history, physical examination of the breast, three-dimensional mammography, and possibly other breast imaging techniques such as ultrasonography or MRI. Most breast cancers can be visualized on a mammogram as a mass, a cluster of calcifications, or a combination of these findings. Specific mammographic features associated with the highest risk of malignancy include masses with spiculated margins or an irregular shape and calcifications with a linear or segmental distribution.[57] One major factor that affects the ability of mammography to detect cancer includes breast density (the fat-to-glandular tissue ratio of the breast), which may be affected by age, menopausal status, and HRT use. Ultrasonography, MRI, and digital mammography are alternate breast imaging methods that are being investigated for women with dense breasts or other specific subsets of patients with breast cancer (eg, MRI in patients with inflammatory breast cancer [IBC]).[49] The technical quality of the examination and the expertise of the radiologist are also important factors.

Breast biopsy is indicated for a mammographic abnormality that suggests malignancy or for a palpable mass on physical examination. Three techniques are available: fine-needle aspiration, core-needle biopsy, and excisional biopsy.[58] Excisional biopsy completely removes the abnormal tissue. Needle biopsies are performed percutaneously and include both core-needle biopsy (which removes a core of tissue) and fine-needle aspiration (which removes cells from the suspicious site). Core-needle biopsy is the preferred biopsy method for mammographically detected, nonpalpable abnormalities.[49] Core-needle biopsy offers a more definitive histologic diagnosis, avoids inadequate samples, and can distinguish invasive from in situ breast cancer (which fine needle biopsy cannot). After confirmation of malignancy via core-needle biopsy, subsequent surgical procedures are performed (either before or after systemic therapy) to assure complete removal of the abnormal tissue.

STAGING AND PROGNOSIS

Breast cancer stage is defined on the basis of the primary tumor extent and size (T_{1-4}), presence and extent of lymph node involvement (N_{1-3}), and presence or absence of distant metastases (M_{0-1}) (Table 128-3 and Fig. 128-4). Although many possible combinations of T and N are possible within a given stage, simplistically, stage 0 represents carcinoma in situ (T_{is}) or disease that has not invaded the basement membrane of the breast tissue. Stage I represents a small primary invasive tumor without lymph node involvement or with micrometastatic nodal involvement, and stage II disease usually involves regional lymph nodes. Stages I and II are often referred to as *early breast cancer*. It is in these early stages that the disease is highly curable (99% 5-year survival in patients with disease confined to the breast, node negative).[2] Stage III, also referred to as *locally advanced disease*, usually represents a large tumor with extensive nodal involvement in which either node or tumor is fixed to the chest wall. Stage IV disease is characterized by the presence of metastases to organs distant from the primary tumor and is often referred to as *advanced or metastatic disease* as described earlier (26% 5-year survival rate in patients with distant metastases).[3] Most breast cancer today presents in early stages where the prognosis is favorable (93% of newly diagnosed patients have disease confined to the breast or local lymph nodes).[3]

Staging for breast cancer is separated into two groups, clinical and pathologic. Clinical staging is assigned before surgery and is based on physical examination (assessment of tumor size and presence of axillary lymph nodes), imaging (mammography, ultrasonography, and so on), and pathologic examination of tissues (eg, biopsy results).

TABLE 128-3 Tumor, Node, Metastasis Stage Grouping for Breast Cancer

Stage Grouping			
0	T_{is}	N_0	M_0
IA	T_1[a]	N_0	M_0
IB	T_0	N_1mi	M_0
	T_1[a]	N_1mi	M_0
IIA	T_0	N_1[b]	M_0
	T_1[a]T	N_1[b]	M_0
	T_2	N_0	M_0
IIB	T_2	N_1	M_0
	T_3	N_0	M_0
IIIA	T_0	N_2	M_0
	T_1[a]	N_2	M_0
	T_2	N_2	M_0
	T_3	N_1	M_0
	T_3	N_2	M_0
IIIB	T_4	N_0	M_0
	T_4	N_1	M_0
	T_4	N_2	M_0
IIIC	Any T	N_3	M_0
IV	Any T	Any N	M_1

TNM, tumor, node, metastasis.

[a]T_1 includes T_1mi.

[b]T_0 and T_1 tumors with nodal micrometastasis only are excluded from stage IIa and are classified as stage IB.

Used with the permission of the American Joint Committee on Cancer (AJCC), Chicago. The original source for this material is the AJCC Cancer Staging Manual, 7th ed. (2010) published by Springer Science and Business Media LLC, www.springer.com.

Pathologic staging occurs after surgery and uses information from clinical staging but adds data from surgical exploration and resection, such as tumor size at surgery and the involvement of micro- or macro-invasive tumor in the lymph nodes or other metastatic sites. Because of the advent of sentinel lymph node biopsy (SLNB), the assessment of lymph node status has become more complex (see the Treatment of Early Breast Cancer section). The American Joint Committee for Cancer (AJCC) publishes staging criteria for cancers, and the breast cancer criteria were most recently updated in January 2010.[59] This staging system is widely accepted and used in all breast cancer patients to determine prognosis and assist with treatment decisions. It is also used to report and track breast cancer diagnoses in tumor registries and databases.

PATHOLOGY

The pathologic evaluation of breast tissue serves to establish the histologic diagnosis and to confirm the presence or absence of other factors believed to influence prognosis.

Invasive Carcinoma

Invasive breast cancers are a histologically heterogeneous group of lesions. Most breast cancers are adenocarcinomas and are classified on the basis of their microscopic appearance as ductal or lobular, corresponding to the ducts and lobules of the normal breast (Fig. 128-2). The various histologic types of breast cancer have different prognoses, but it is unknown whether their response to therapy differs because patients in therapeutic trials are not typically stratified according to histologic type. The five most common types of invasive breast cancer are briefly described.[60]

Invasive or *infiltrating ductal carcinoma* is the most common histology, accounting for about 75% of all invasive breast cancers. These tumors commonly spread to the axillary lymph nodes, and their prognosis is poorer than for some other histologic types. *Invasive or infiltrating lobular carcinoma* accounts for 5% to 10% of breast tumors. Both clinical and radiologic findings for these tumors may be quite subtle. The typical presentation is an area of ill-defined thickening in the breast in contrast to a prominent lump characteristic of infiltrating ductal carcinoma. *Infiltrating lobular carcinoma* can also be more difficult to detect by mammography. Overall, *infiltrating lobular carcinoma* and *infiltrating ductal carcinoma* have similar likelihoods of axillary node involvement and disease recurrence and death, yet the sites of metastases may differ. Whereas *infiltrating ductal carcinoma* more frequently metastasizes to the bone or to the liver, lung, or brain, *infiltrating lobular carcinoma* tends to metastasize to the leptomeninges, peritoneal surfaces, retroperitoneum, gastrointestinal tract, reproductive organs, and other unusual sites.

The three most common special types of invasive cancer are *medullary*, *mucinous*, and *tubular*. The prognosis may be more favorable with these unusual histologies. *Medullary carcinoma* accounts for fewer than 7% of all breast carcinomas, *mucinous (or colloid) carcinoma* constitutes about 3%, *and tubular carcinoma* accounts for about 2% of all breast cancers. Histologies rarely reported include adenocystic carcinoma, carcinosarcomas, metaplastic, cribriform, and papillary carcinoma.

Special situations seen clinically and histologically include Paget's disease of the breast, phyllodes tumors, and IBC. Paget's disease of the breast occurs in 1% to 4% of all patients with breast cancer and is characterized by neoplastic cells in the nipple areolar complex. The patient presents clinically with eczematous changes in the nipple with itching, burning, oozing, bleeding, or some combination of these. In most cases, the nipple changes are associated with an underlying carcinoma in the breast that is usually palpable.

Phyllodes tumors of the breast (also known as cystosarcoma phyllodes) are rare tumors with subtypes that range from benign to malignant. These tumors often enlarge rapidly, are painless, and can appear as fibroadenomas.[61]

IBC is characterized clinically by prominent skin edema, redness and warmth, and induration of the underlying tissue. Biopsies of the involved skin reveal cancer cells in the dermal lymphatics. IBC typically has a very rapid onset and is often mistaken for an infectious cellulitis or mastitis. Although it may look somewhat similar to a neglected mass, its presentation with rapid onset and progression of local symptoms distinguishes it from other cases of locally advanced breast cancer. The prognosis of patients with IBC is poor even if the disease is apparently localized.[62]

Noninvasive Carcinoma

As with invasive carcinoma, the noninvasive lesions may be divided broadly into ductal and lobular categories. Evidence supports that the development of malignancy is a multistep process and that invasive breast cancer has a preinvasive, in situ phase. During the carcinoma in situ phase, normal epithelial cells undergo genetic alterations that result in malignant transformation. Transformed epithelial cells proliferate and pile up within lobules or ducts but lack the required genetic alterations that enable the cells to penetrate the basement membrane. Therefore, carcinoma in situ is diagnosed when malignant transformation of cells has occurred but the basement membrane is intact.

The widespread use of screening mammography with subsequent biopsy and greater recognition of noninvasive breast carcinoma by pathologists has resulted in a significant increase in the diagnosis of in situ breast cancer over the past decade. An estimated 61,000 new cases of female noninvasive (in situ) breast cancer is expected to be diagnosed in 2016.[1] The natural history of these disorders is not well described, and thus the debate continues regarding carcinoma in situ: Is carcinoma in situ preinvasive cancer or simply a marker of unstable epithelium that represents an increased risk for

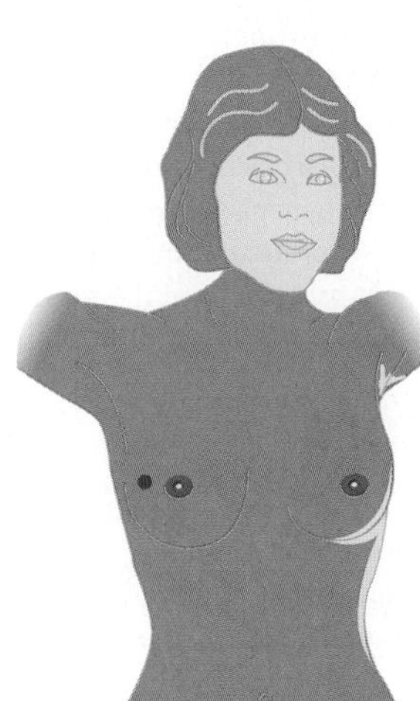

Tumor (T)

T_x Primary tumor cannot be assessed
T_0 No evidence of tumor
T_{is} Carcinoma in situ
T_1 ≤2 cm
    T_1 mic ≤0.1 cm
    T_{1a} >0.1-0.5 cm
    T_{1b} >0.5-1 cm
    T_{1c} >1-2 cm
T_2 >2-5 cm
T_3 >5 cm
T_4 Any size; with direct extension to chest wall or skin
T_{4a} Extension to chest wall (not including pectoralis muscle)
T_{4b} Edema (including peau d'orange) or ulceration of skin or satellite skin nodules
T_{4c} Both T_{4a} and T_{4b}
T_{4d} Inflammatory carcinoma

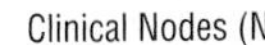

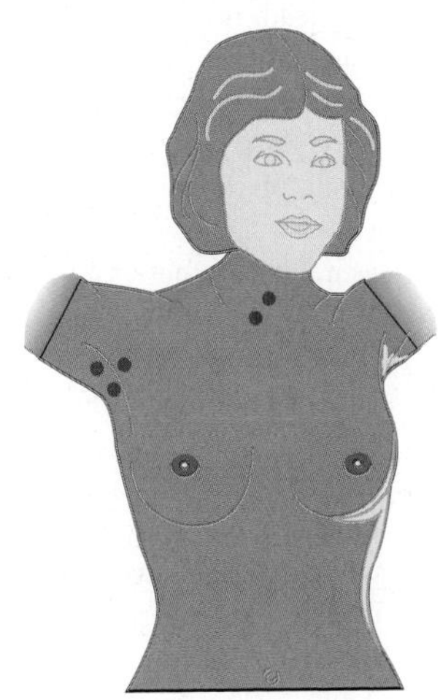

Clinical Nodes (N)

N_x Regional lymph nodes cannot be assessed (eg, previously removed)
N_0 No regional lymph node metastasis
N_1 Metastasis in movable ipsilateral axillary lymph node(s)
N_2 Metastases in ipsilateral axillary lymph nodes fixed or matted or in clinically detected ipsilateral internal mammary nodes in the absence of clinically evident axillary lymph node metastasis
    N_{2a} Metastasis in ipsilateral axillary lymph nodes fixed to one another (matted) or to other structures
    N_{2b} Metastasis only in clinically detected ipsilateral internal mammary nodes and in the absence of clinically evident axillary lymph node metastasis
N_3 Metastasis in ipsilateral infraclavicular lymph node(s) or in clinically detected ipsilateral internal mammary node(s) and in the presence of clinically evident axillary lymph node metastasis or metastasis in ipsilateral supraclavicular lymph node(s) with or without axillary or internal mammary lymph node involvement
    N_{3a} Metastasis in ipsilateral infraclavicular lymph node(s) and axillary lymph node(s)
    N_{3b} Metastasis in ipsilateral internal mammary lymph node(s) and axillary lymph node(s)
    N_{3c} Metastasis in ipsilateral supraclavicular lymph node(s)

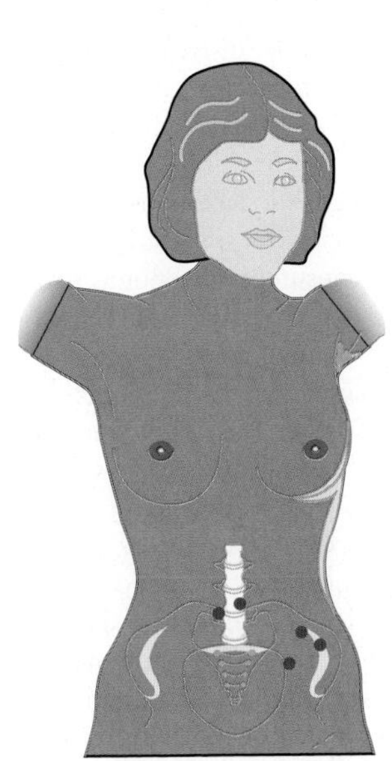

Pathologic Nodes (pN)*

pN0 No regional lymph node metastasis histologically
pN1mi Micrometastasis (>0.2 mm but none >2.0 mm)
pN1 Metastasis in one to three axillary lymph nodes and/or internal mammary nodes with microscopic disease detected by sentinel lymph node dissection but not clinically detected
pN2 Metastasis in four to nine axillary lymph nodes or in clinically detected internal mammary lymph nodes in the absence of axillary lymph node metastasis
pN3 Metastasis in 10 or more axillary lymph nodes, in infraclavicular lymph nodes, or in clinically detected ipsilateral internal mammary lymph nodes in the presence of one or more positive axillary lymph nodes; in more than three axillary lymph nodes with clinically negative microscopic metastasis in internal mammary lymph nodes; or in ipsilateral supraclavicular lymph nodes

*Based on axillary lymph node dissection with or without sentinel lymph node dissection

Metastasis (M)

M_x Distant metastasis cannot be assessed
M_0 No distant metastases
M_1 Distant metastasis

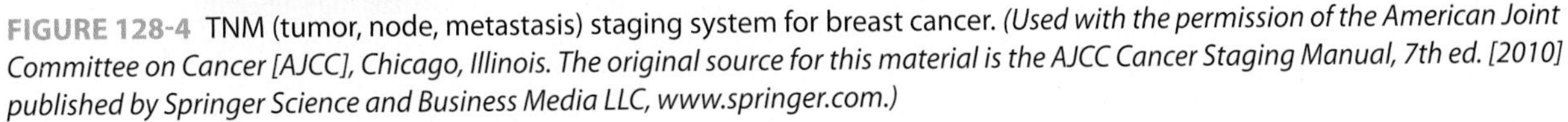

FIGURE 128-4 TNM (tumor, node, metastasis) staging system for breast cancer. *(Used with the permission of the American Joint Committee on Cancer [AJCC], Chicago, Illinois. The original source for this material is the AJCC Cancer Staging Manual, 7th ed. [2010] published by Springer Science and Business Media LLC, www.springer.com.)*

the development of subsequent aggressive cancer?[63,64] Answering this question may change the way noninvasive breast cancers are treated.

Ductal carcinoma in situ (DCIS) is more frequently diagnosed than lobular carcinoma in situ (LCIS). Most cases of DCIS today are found by biopsies performed for clustered microcalcifications seen on screening mammography, a hallmark of this disorder.

The ultimate goal of treatment for noninvasive carcinomas is to prevent the development of invasive disease. If left untreated, it is estimated that 14% to 50% of DCIS lesions will progress to invasive breast cancer.[63] Therefore, up to 50% of these tumors do not progress to invasive disease, but identifying this group of patients is not yet feasible, and all diagnoses should be treated. Locoregional treatment of DCIS depends on its location, size, and pathology.[61] Treatment options include (a) local excision alone with negative margins, (b) local excision (with negative margins) followed by breast irradiation, and (c) traditional total mastectomy with or without reconstruction. Whole-breast irradiation is recommended after excision to significantly decrease the risk of local recurrence, although there is no evidence that survival differs between the previously mentioned options.[61] Excision with negative margins alone without radiation may be considered in patients with small and low-grade DCIS. Mastectomy had been the standard treatment of DCIS for several decades, but long-term survival appears to be equivalent with mastectomy versus local excision and irradiation, and the latter option allows for breast conservation. If more than one area of the breast is involved with DCIS, a mastectomy is the preferred option. Axillary lymph node dissection (ALND) is generally not indicated, although SLNB (see the Early Breast Cancer section) may be considered in selected patients.[61] Cytotoxic chemotherapy has no role in the treatment of patients with pure DCIS. It is important to determine hormone receptor status on the cancer cells. Tamoxifen treatment for 5 years may be considered in some women with hormone receptor–positive DCIS. The NSABP B-24 trial, which randomized women with DCIS to lumpectomy with radiation plus either tamoxifen or placebo, showed a benefit with tamoxifen in reducing ipsilateral breast cancer recurrence (32% reduction; P=0.025).[65] Further subgroup analyses of this trial showed a benefit for patients with ER-positive DCIS.[66] The NSABP B-35 trial evaluated the role of the AI anastrozole compared to tamoxifen each given for 5 years in the treatment of postmenopausal hormone receptor–positive DCIS in patients who had lumpectomy with radiation therapy. Significant improvement in 10 year point estimates for the breast cancer-free interval was seen with anastrozole (89.1% for tamoxifen and 96.3% for anastrozole, HR, 0.73; P=0.02). Further subgroup analyses of this trial showed the benefit to be primarily in women less than 60 years of age.[67] These decisions are often difficult to discuss with patients because these treatments have toxicities that are worrisome. Nonetheless, an open and honest conversation regarding the risks and benefits is warranted.

LCIS is a microscopic diagnosis. In these cases, there is generally no palpable mass, and no specific clinical abnormality is noted. Unlike DCIS, LCIS does not generally demonstrate calcifications on mammography and in fact is usually undetectable by mammography. Consequently, the diagnosis of LCIS is usually an incidental finding in biopsy specimens obtained because of symptoms or mammography findings consistent with benign lesions. It is unclear whether LCIS is a precursor lesion to invasive carcinoma or serves as a marker of risk for invasive carcinoma developing somewhere in the breast. The risk for developing invasive carcinoma is about 0.5% to 1% per year, and both invasive ductal carcinoma and invasive lobular carcinoma can occur. In about 50% to 70% of patients, there are multiple foci of LCIS in the ipsilateral breast, and the contralateral breast is also affected. Thus, the risk for the development of breast cancer is equally high in either breast, which makes the management of LCIS very controversial.[64] Some experts favor a program of observation, with semiannual physical examination and annual mammography.[61] In selected patients with high-risk genetic mutations or strong family history and in women who are particularly anxious about the development of cancer, bilateral mastectomies with or without reconstruction may be considered.[45] Radiation and systemic chemotherapy have no role in the management of LCIS. The use of chemoprevention with tamoxifen in premenopausal women or tamoxifen, raloxifene, or exemestane in postmenopausal women may also be considered for risk reduction in these patients.[45] See the Prevention and Early Detection section for details.

PROGNOSTIC FACTORS

The natural history of breast cancer varies among patients, with some having extremely aggressive disease that progresses rapidly and others following a more indolent course. The ability to predict prognosis is extremely important in designing treatment recommendations to maximize quantity and quality of life. A number of pathologic prognostic and predictive factors have been identified. Prognostic factors are characteristics or measurements available at diagnosis or time of surgery that in the absence of adjuvant systemic therapy are associated with recurrence rate, death rate, or other clinical outcomes. Predictive factors are measurements available at diagnosis that are associated with response to a specific therapy. Prognostic and predictive factors fall into three general categories: (a) patient characteristics that are independent of the disease such as age; (b) cancer characteristics such as tumor size or histologic type; and (c) other biomarkers that are measurable parameters in tissues, cells, or fluids, such as hormone receptor status. Ideally, the use of prognostic and predictive factors can limit a specific treatment to patients who are most likely to derive benefit, thus sparing unwanted toxicities in those who are unlikely to benefit.

Age at diagnosis and ethnicity are patient characteristics that may affect prognosis. Some younger patients, particularly those younger than 35 years of age, have more aggressive forms of breast cancer and a worse prognosis. Younger patients are more likely to present with poor prognostic features, such as affected lymph nodes, large tumor size, and tumors negative for hormone receptors. Race and ethnicity may also play a role in breast cancer prognosis. African American women have decreased survival periods compared with white women. The cause of this racial disparity is widely debated, with possible explanations including access to care, socioeconomic status, cultural differences, higher stage at diagnosis, and more aggressive biologic features.

Potentially modifiable prognostic factors include alcohol use, dietary factors, weight, and exercise. The association between breast cancer prognosis and alcohol consumption is not as strong as with alcohol and breast cancer risk. A review of seven observational studies showed that postdiagnosis alcohol consumption was not associated with breast cancer outcomes.[68] Two randomized controlled studies examined the effects of diet on the risk of breast cancer with conflicting results, primarily focusing on lowering dietary fat.[69,70] One study found an improvement in disease-free survival (DFS) with incorporation of a low-fat diet (less than 15% dietary fat per day vs no intervention),[70] but another study found no difference in recurrence rates between two dietary intervention approaches (both incorporating a low-fat, high-fiber approach).[69] Although these studies asked different questions and had many confounding variables that potentially affected the results, most clinicians recommend that breast cancer survivors eat a low-fat, high-fiber diet and maintain a healthy weight. Obesity at the time of a breast cancer diagnosis has been shown to increase the risk of breast cancer–specific and overall mortality compared with nonobese breast cancer patients, although the impact of weight loss in this population is unclear.[68] Observational studies have reported that exercise in women after a diagnosis of breast cancer may also decrease the likelihood of breast cancer recurrence and breast cancer–related death.[68] Based on these

TABLE 128-4 Five-Year Survival Rates (%) According to Tumor Size and Axillary Lymph Node Status

	Tumor Size		
Lymph Node Status	**<2 cm**	**2-5 cm**	**>5 cm**
Negative	96	89	82
1-3 positive	87	80	73
≥4 positive	66	59	46

Data from Dillon DA, Guidi AJ, Schnitt SJ. Pathology of invasive breast cancer. In: Harris JR, Lippman ME, Morrow M, Osborne CK, eds. Diseases of the Breast, 4th ed. Philadelphia, PA: Lippincott Williams & Wilkins, 2010:374-407.

data, agencies such as the ACS have recognized that physical activity, weight control, and diet are potentially modifiable risk factors for reducing the risk of recurrent breast cancer and other comorbidities (eg, heart disease, diabetes).[71]

Disease characteristics that have been shown to provide important prognostic information include lymph node status, tumor size, histologic subtype, nuclear or histologic grade, lymphatic and vascular invasion (LVI), and proliferation indices.

Tumor size and the presence and number of involved lymph nodes are established primary factors in assessing the risk for breast cancer recurrence and subsequent metastatic disease. Table 128-4 shows 5-year survival rates according to size of the primary tumor and axillary node involvement. The major factor that influences the likelihood of recurrence is the presence of positive lymph nodes. However, regardless of lymph node status, the size of the primary tumor remains an independent prognostic factor for disease recurrence.

The number of affected lymph nodes is directly related to the risk of disease recurrence. The revised staging system for breast cancer recognizes the absolute number of positive nodes as a prognostic factor: N_1 represents one to three positive nodes, N_2 represents four to nine positive nodes, and N_3 represents 10 or more positive nodes in its pathologic staging system.[59] The relationship between tumor size and lymph node status is complex and not a simple grouping (see discussion below).

Certain histologic subtypes and clinical presentation of breast cancer have prognostic importance. As mentioned earlier, because women with pure *tubular* or *mucinous* tumors have more favorable outcomes than those with *invasive ductal carcinomas*, treatment recommendations may differ.[61] IBC, although a clinical designation and not a distinct histologic subtype, is associated with a poor prognosis.[62]

Nuclear grade and tumor (histologic) differentiation are known independent prognostic indicators. Several histologic grading systems have been developed, most of which grade tumors with a score from 1 to 3: grade 1, well differentiated; grade 2, moderately differentiated; and grade 3, poorly differentiated. Higher grade tumors are associated with higher rates of distant metastasis and poorer survival. This factor aids in making treatment decisions, particularly for patients with small tumors and negative lymph nodes.

Lymphatic and vascular invasion (LVI), defined as evidence of tumor emboli in lymphatic or vascular spaces, is a poor prognostic factor likely representing ability of the cancer to spread via hematogenous routes. However, the utility of this as a prognostic factor is largely unknown and is not currently included in either staging or treatment guidelines.[59,61]

The rate of tumor cell proliferation also is associated with risk of breast cancer recurrence. Rate of cell proliferation can be evaluated with various techniques, including (1) mitotic index, which counts the number of mitotic bodies; (2) thymidine-labeling index or S-phase fraction with DNA flow cytometry, which determines the percentage of tumor cells actively dividing; or (3) the use of monoclonal antibodies (MoABs) to antigens present on proliferating cells, such as Ki-67. In a meta-analysis of 85 studies and nearly 33,000 patients, proliferation markers (including Ki-67, mitotic index, proliferating cell nuclear antigen, and thymidine or bromodeoxyuridine labeling index) were associated with significantly shorter disease-free and OS periods.[72] These proliferation indices are additional factors that may be useful in decision making and may predict for responsiveness to chemotherapy, although this is still controversial.

Hormone receptors are not strong prognostic markers but are used clinically to predict response to endocrine therapy. Hormone receptors are nuclear transcription factors that, upon ligand binding, activate a variety of signal transduction pathways that result in cell growth and proliferation. Determination of both ER and PR status is an established procedure that is important in the management of breast cancer. Immunohistochemistry is used to determine the level (ie, quantity) of hormone receptors, which is important for predictive ability. Other methods of determining ER and PR status, such as mRNA expression, are under investigation but have not been validated as predictive markers. Hormone receptors are most valuable in predicting response to endocrine therapy. About 60% to 70% of patients with ER-positive and PR-positive tumors will respond to hormonal manipulation. More recently, the importance of PR has come under question because response to tamoxifen has been shown to be related to ER status independent of PR status.[36] Guidelines for testing of ER and PR status are available and recommend standards for what tumors to test and methodologic guidelines for pathologists.[73] The majority of patients with primary or MBC have hormone receptor–positive tumors. Hormone receptor positivity, more common in postmenopausal women, is associated with a higher response to endocrine therapy and a longer DFS.

The *HER2/neu* gene is located on chromosome 17q21 and encodes a 185-kilodaton transmembrane tyrosine kinase growth factor receptor. The *HER2* protein is normally expressed at low levels in the epithelial cells of normal breast tissue. *HER2* is a member of the HER growth factor receptor family, and its overexpression is associated with transmission of growth signals that control aspects of normal cell growth and division. *HER2* overexpression occurs in about 20% to 30% of breast cancers and is associated with increased tumor aggressiveness, increased rates of recurrence, and increased mortality rates. In some studies, *HER2* gene amplification and protein overexpression, measured by fluorescence in situ hybridization (FISH) and immunohistochemistry (IHC), respectively, correlates with factors associated with a poor prognosis. *HER2*-positive status clearly predicts response to anti-*HER2* therapy. Tumors that are either IHC 3+ or FISH positive for gene amplification are considered to be positive for *HER2*.[74] For equivocal results of IHC (2+) or FISH, confirmatory testing with the alternate test is recommended. *HER2* gene amplification or protein overexpression has traditionally been considered a poor prognostic factor. However, more recent data suggest that patients with *HER2*-positive MBC treated with trastuzumab, a MoAB directed against the extracellular domain of the *HER2* receptor, have improved survival rates compared with patients with *HER2*-negative MBC or patients with *HER2*-positive MBC who do not receive trastuzumab.[75] These results demonstrate the powerful impact trastuzumab therapy has made on improving patient outcomes.

Although there is a growing understanding of the prognostic significance of individual factors, it is not clear how each factor contributes to the overall prognosis for an individual patient. Computer-aided models, including Adjuvant! (*www.adjuvantonline.com*), are available that combine patient- and tumor-related variables to estimate overall prognosis for individual patients with early stage breast cancer (ESBC) and aid in decisions regarding adjuvant systemic therapy.[76] (See Systemic Adjuvant Therapy later).

Genetic profiling is also being used to provide prognostic and predictive information on clinical outcomes of breast cancer.[77] Commercially available multiparameter gene expression assays include

Oncotype DX, MammaPrint and Prosigna. Further details on these assays are available in the Systemic Adjuvant Therapy section later.

Novel molecular markers that have shown prognostic and predictive significance include urokinase-type plasminogen activator and its inhibitor, plasminogen activator inhibitor type 1, cyclin E, and the presence of tumor cells in bone marrow or circulating blood.[78] Prospective validation studies will determine whether these tests can be used to assist decision making in individual patients.

In summary, lymph node status and tumor size are two significant prognostic factors that assist clinicians in estimating prognosis and making treatment recommendations for most breast cancer patients (see Systemic Adjuvant Therapy later). Although the risk of recurrence is clearly high in patients with large primary tumors or lymph node–positive disease, many patients with small primary tumors and lymph node–negative disease will still develop metastases, yet our ability to accurately identify these individual patients is limited. Evaluation of additional prognostic factors can help identify which patients will have a good outcome with local therapy alone and which patients with aggressive features who would benefit from more aggressive, multimodality treatment. Despite these markers, a large proportion of patients will likely be treated unnecessarily with systemic adjuvant therapy, and better prognostic and predictive tools are needed to better select patients to undergo these toxic and costly treatments and procedures.

TREATMENT

Early Breast Cancer (Stage I and II)

Desired Outcomes

The desired therapeutic outcome of adjuvant therapy of breast cancer differs significantly from that of metastatic disease. Adjuvant therapy—chemotherapy, biologic therapy, and hormonal therapy—is administered with curative intent. The rationale for adjuvant therapy is that breast cancer, even when diagnosed in early stages when clinical evidence of distant spread is not apparent, is a systemic disease that spreads early to distant sites. Adjuvant therapy is intended to eradicate micrometastases and thus cure the patient of breast cancer. A predetermined number of cycles of adjuvant therapy or years of biologic or hormonal therapy (or both) are administered. The goals of neoadjuvant therapy are to eradicate micrometastatic disease, determine prognosis, and potentially conserve the breast tissue for a better cosmetic result. Adjuvant and neoadjuvant chemotherapy is often associated with significant toxicity. Clinicians and patients must weigh the short- and long-term risks of chemotherapy, biological therapy, and endocrine therapy with the benefits of lowering the risk of breast cancer recurrence.

Locoregional Therapy

3 Most patients presenting with breast cancer today have an in situ tumor, a small invasive tumor with negative lymph nodes (stage I), or a small invasive tumor with axillary lymph node involvement (stage II). Surgery alone can cure most, if not all, patients with in situ cancers; 70% to 80% of patients with stage I; and about half of all patients with stage II cancers. The choice of surgical procedures has changed drastically over the past 50 years. This is partly a result of changes in our understanding of the biology of breast cancer and is partly a result of a series of well-conducted clinical trials performed over this time period.

Over the years, many trials have investigated reducing the amount of surgery required to maintain acceptable cosmetic results and rates of local and distant recurrence and mortality. Breast-conserving therapy (BCT) includes removal of part of the breast, surgical evaluation of the axillary lymph node basin, and radiation therapy to the breast. The amount of breast tissue removed as a part of BCT varies from just removing the cancerous "lump" (a lumpectomy) with a small margin of adjacent normal-appearing tissue to removing the "lump" with a wider excision of adjacent normal-appearing tissue (a wide local excision) to removing the entire quadrant of the breast that includes the cancerous "lump" (a quadrantectomy). All of these techniques are referred to as a *segmental or partial mastectomy*. A meta-analysis of 18 clinical trials in almost 10,000 women found no difference in OS for patients who received BCT compared with mastectomy.[79] However, this and other meta-analyses have suggested the potential for a small increase in the risk of locoregional recurrence with BCT.[79,80]

Most patients diagnosed today with breast cancer can be treated with BCT. Several factors should be considered in selecting patients for BCT, including any additional risk the remaining breast tissue poses despite the local effects of radiation therapy. The NCCN recommends that women who carry a known *BRCA1* or *BRCA2* mutation undergo mastectomy and consider additional risk reduction strategies (eg, bilateral mastectomies).[61] Bilateral total mastectomy and oophorectomy reduce the risk of breast cancer occurrence in patients with *BRCA1* or *BRCA2* mutations, but both breast and ovarian cancers have been reported in patients who have had prophylactic removal of these organs. Multiple sites of cancer within the breast and the inability to attain negative pathologic margins on the excised breast specimen are predictive for an increased risk of recurrence with BCT and are indications for mastectomy. Some preexisting collagen vascular diseases (eg, scleroderma, systemic lupus erythematosus) are relative contraindications for the use of BCT because of an increased risk of radiation-related adverse effects. Although local recurrence after BCT has not been consistently associated with an increased mortality rate, it is distressing to the patient and requires surgical removal of the breast. In addition, reconstructive therapy is often not feasible in a breast that has previously received irradiation. Another major consideration in selecting patients for BCT is the expected cosmetic result. For some patients, preservation of a limited amount of breast tissue may not justify the inconvenience of radiation therapy. Another approach to therapy for these patients is primary (neoadjuvant) systemic therapy to potentially shrink the tumor and minimize surgery (see Systemic Adjuvant Therapy and Locally Advanced Breast Cancer sections for further details). Aside from the probability of local recurrence and the ability to achieve a satisfactory cosmetic result, consideration must be given to the availability of an external-beam radiation facility and the patient's willingness to comply with the prescribed course of radiotherapy. A meta-analysis of 10,801 patients in 17 randomized controlled trials of radiotherapy compared to no radiotherapy after breast conserving surgery demonstrated a reduction in the 10-year risk of first recurrence by 15.7% and the 15-year risk of breast cancer death by 3.8% favoring radiation.[81] In most instances, external-beam radiation therapy used in conjunction with BCT involves 3 to 5 weeks of radiation therapy directed to the entire breast tissue (typically a total of 40-50 Gy administered in 15-25 daily doses Mondays through Fridays with an optional boost of radiation to the tumor bed) to eradicate residual disease. Local tumor control is similar with shorter courses of radiation compared to longer courses, and toxicities such as breast shrinkage, telangiectasias and breast edema is less common with shorter regimens. The preferred radiation course by the NCCN is 40 to 42.5 Gy in 15 to 16 fractions.[61] Complications associated with radiation therapy to the breast are generally minor and include reddening and erythema of the breast tissue and subsequent shrinkage of the total breast mass beyond that predicted on the basis of breast tissue removal.

Clinical trials are investigating the use of accelerated partial breast irradiation, intraoperative radiotherapy, or no radiation after segmental mastectomy for certain patient populations with a very low risk of recurrence.[82] Until the results of these studies are available, the standard approach to BCT includes whole-breast radiation therapy for the majority of patients.

Postmastectomy radiation therapy to the chest wall and regional lymph nodes (if indicated) may also be required in certain situations when tumors are large or the number of positive axillary lymph nodes is high (see the Locally Advanced Breast Cancer section). However, these criteria are also widely debated and are the subject of several meta-analyses. Despite the controversy, it is clear that some women may benefit from local radiation therapy even after removal of the entire breast (ie, total mastectomy). The NCCN Guidelines state that women with four or more positive axillary lymph nodes should undergo postmastectomy radiation therapy. Patients with one to three positive ipsilateral axillary lymph nodes should strongly consider postmastectomy radiation, although conflicting data exist in this patient population. Patients with (a) positive surgical margins, (b) a tumor larger than 5 cm, or (c) tumors less than 5 cm with close margins (less than 1 mm of normal adjacent tissue) should consider postmastectomy chest wall radiation therapy. Finally, patients with surgical margins of at least 1 mm, tumor size of 5 cm or less, and negative axillary lymph nodes do not require postmastectomy chest wall radiation therapy. The optimal sequence of radiation therapy and chemotherapy is somewhat controversial. Concurrent administration of chemotherapy and radiation therapy is usually avoided because of an increase in local adverse effects. Most clinicians administer systemic chemotherapy immediately after surgery (if chemotherapy was not administered before surgery) given the hypothetical presence of systemic micrometastases that cannot be eradicated by local radiation therapy. Radiation therapy is then administered after chemotherapy, leaving hormone therapy (which is given for many years) for the end (see the Adjuvant Biologic Therapy section for a discussion of sequencing trastuzumab).

Accurate assessment of the spread of breast cancer cells to the axillary lymph nodes is critical for prognosis and the determination of the utility of both local and systemic treatments. ALND with histopathologic study of the full axillary specimen, including level I and II lymph nodes, was the gold standard for detecting axillary nodal involvement and determining the number of lymph nodes containing tumor. The number of positive axillary lymph nodes remains the most powerful predictor of breast cancer recurrence and survival, but other benefits may include a therapeutic effect of removing the lymph nodes and obtaining information to guide treatment selection. However, axillary dissection is associated with significant morbidity, including lymphedema (10%-20%), arm pain or numbness (30%), and reduction in quality of life (35%).[83] Recent studies indicate that about 60% of patients with ESBC present with lymph node–negative disease, which indicates that many women would derive no therapeutic benefit but would be exposed to the complications from the procedure.

For these reasons, a procedure involving lymphatic mapping and SLNB is recommended for patients with clinically negative lymph nodes, and guidelines regarding recommendations for this procedure are available.[84] The sentinel lymph node(s) is the first lymph node(s) that receives lymph drainage from the primary tumor. Injection of a vital blue dye, a radiocolloid, or both around the primary breast tumor identifies the sentinel lymph node(s) in most patients, and the status of this lymph node(s) may predict the status of the remaining nodes in the nodal basin. Patients with lymph nodes that are suspicious for cancer involvement either by physical examination or imaging should have a biopsy performed to exclude lymph node involvement. SLNB has become the standard of care for patients with clinically negative axillary lymph nodes.[61] Historically, patients with positive sentinel nodes should proceed to a level I and II ALND, although this has recently been called into question. Data from a single randomized trial suggest that ALND after SLNB in women with clinically node negative tumors smaller than 5 cm, fewer than three involved sentinel lymph nodes, and undergoing BCT with subsequent breast irradiation resulted in higher morbidity, no improvement in local recurrence, and no difference in DFS or OS with SLNB alone.[85] Therefore, the ASCO guidelines currently recommend that clinicians should not recommend ALND for women with ESBC with one or two positive sentinel lymph nodes who will receive BCT followed by radiation.[84] Women undergoing mastectomy with positive sentinel lymph nodes should be offered ALND.

In studies that incorporated completion axillary dissections for comparison, the SLNB procedure accurately predicted the status of the remaining axillary nodes in more than 90% of patients.[83] Greater surgeon experience improves the sensitivity of the procedure. Women with large tumors (greater than 5 cm) or locally advanced disease, IBC, or DCIS when BCT is planned should not receive SLNB.[84] Patients with multifocal or multicentric breast tumors, DCIS when mastectomy is planned, prior neoadjuvant (preoperative) chemotherapy, or prior surgery involving the breast or axilla may be offered SLNB.[84] Patients who are pregnant or lactating are not considered candidates for this procedure because of concerns regarding the effects of the blue dye or the radiocolloid on the fetus. The decision of whether to use the sentinel lymph node procedure or a full axillary dissection is complex, and readers are referred to an excellent review for further information.[83]

The early trials investigating less extensive surgical approaches to breast cancer are widely credited with the finding that BCT is an appropriate primary therapy for most women with stages I and II disease and is preferable because it arguably provides survival rates equivalent to those of modified radical mastectomy. These historical trials provided valuable information regarding the natural history of the disease and identified pathologic prognostic factors associated with early cancer spread. The preponderance of information available regarding selection of women most likely to benefit from systemic adjuvant therapy was derived from pathologic evaluation of tissues archived from these early trials. It is hoped that further investigation into less extensive local therapy (now focused on the surgical approach to the axilla and radiation therapy) will continue to provide valuable information for the future.

Systemic Adjuvant Therapy

4 *Systemic adjuvant therapy* is defined as the administration of systemic therapy after definitive local therapy (surgery, radiation, or a combination of these) when there is no evidence of metastatic disease but a high likelihood of disease recurrence. By the time breast cancers become clinically detectable, they have likely been present for a number of years and have had ample opportunity to establish distant micrometastases. Micrometastatic disease can travel from the primary breast tumor and spread to distant organs through several different routes (eg, hematogenous spread through blood vessels, lymphangitic spread through lymph channels, local extension to surrounding structures). Because local therapies such as breast surgery and irradiation do not address distant micrometastases, systemic therapy may be required to target these tumor cells that have escaped the local area of the breast. The likelihood of micrometastatic disease presence is used to attempt to identify patients with a high risk of recurrence who would require systemic adjuvant therapy. Many collaborative research groups have conducted stepwise series of studies designed to identify appropriate candidates for systemic adjuvant therapy and the optimal regimens and duration of therapy. Several hundred randomized clinical trials evaluating various systemic adjuvant modalities have been reported. Most published results confirm that administration of chemotherapy, endocrine therapy, targeted therapy, or some combination of these agents, results in improved DFS or OS for all treated patients or more commonly for patients in specific prognostic subgroups (eg, nodal involvement, menopausal status, hormone receptor status, or *HER2* status). The huge amounts of data generated by these trials have resulted in a great deal of controversy, with different conclusions being reached by various experts.

5 Interpretation of results of systemic adjuvant therapy is difficult because of differences in the patient populations studied, the variation in natural history of breast cancer, the absence of information regarding pathologic prognostic factors in many studies, and differences in treatment approach and methods of analysis. Several groups around the world have conducted meta-analyses of similar breast cancer trials in hopes of gaining more insight regarding adjuvant systemic therapy than a single study can provide. One such effort, organized by the EBCTCG, is based on a worldwide collaboration involving multiple randomized trials and is continually updated with results from new clinical trials. The EBCTCG's overview analyses are updated periodically as new data become available. The most recent updates reflect the long-term effects on breast cancer recurrence and survival for adjuvant endocrine therapy and chemotherapy.[36,56,86] Many important questions regarding the optimal way to administer adjuvant chemotherapy and endocrine therapy and the magnitude of benefit as measured by DFS or OS in clinically relevant subsets of patients have been answered by these overview analyses. Simply stated, the results of these analyses support the use of adjuvant endocrine therapy in all patients with positive hormone receptor status regardless of age, menopausal status, involvement of axillary lymph nodes, or tumor size.[36] The results of these overview analyses also support the use of adjuvant chemotherapy in most women with lymph node metastases or with primary breast cancers larger than 1 cm in diameter (both node negative and node positive).[56] It is important to note that data from clinical trials incorporating anti-*HER2* therapy into adjuvant regimens are not included in these analyses because sufficient long-term follow-up has not been reached. Results from these more recent clinical trials are discussed later.

Table 128-5 uses data from the overview analyses to show the absolute benefits of adjuvant chemotherapy in terms of age and nodal status. In the highest risk group, node-positive women younger than 50 years of age, only 44.8% were alive and disease free at 5 years with no polychemotherapy compared with 59.4% with polychemotherapy, which translates into an absolute DFS benefit of 14.6%. However, in the node-negative group, patients younger than 50 years old in whom DFS with no polychemotherapy was highest (ie, 72.6%), the addition of polychemotherapy produced an absolute benefit of only 9.9%. It should be pointed out that all of these differences in DFS are clearly statistically significant and form the basis for national and international guidelines that recommend offering cytotoxic chemotherapy to most women with ESBC.[61,87,88] However, the absolute survival benefit in node-positive women 50 to 69 years old is quite small (3%), and depending on other disease characteristics and comorbid conditions, patients may elect not to pursue treatment. Although a 3% absolute reduction in death attributable to polychemotherapy may appear small, many patients with breast cancer may accept severe toxicity from treatment to achieve as little as a 1% to 5% absolute improvement in survival.

TABLE 128-5 Absolute Benefits of Adjuvant Chemotherapy by Age and Nodal Status

	With Polychemotherapy (%)	With No Polychemotherapy (%)	Absolute Benefit (%)
Disease-Free Survival			
Age <50 years			
Node negative	82.5	72.6	9.9
Node positive	59.4	44.8	14.6
Age 50-69 years			
Node negative	85.7	80.4	5.3
Node positive	63.3	57.4	5.9
Survival[a]			
Age <50 years	67.6	57.6	10
Age 50-69 years	52.6	49.6	3

[a]Younger women, 35% node positive; older women, 70% node positive.

Data from reference 86.

Several international and national groups have developed guidelines for treatment of ESBC based on specific patient and disease characteristics and the results of the overview analyses. The three most commonly referenced guidelines are the St. Gallen International Expert Consensus Conference, European Society of Medical Oncology (ESMO), and the NCCN guidelines.[61,87,88] The St. Gallen guidelines are updated every 2 years by an international group of researchers that meets in St. Gallen, Switzerland to review available evidence and create consensus recommendations for selection of adjuvant systemic therapies in specific patient populations outside of the framework of clinical trials. The NCCN and ESMO have also developed practice guidelines for the treatment of breast cancer that are updated annually or more often based on the available evidence. Recommendations from the NCCN for patients with tumors 1 cm or larger or positive lymph nodes are summarized in Fig. 128-5. For patients with tumors smaller than 1 cm, micrometastatic lymph node involvement, or negative lymph nodes, treatment is highly individualized and based on multiple patient- and tumor-related factors, including hormone receptor status, *HER2* status, comorbidities, and patient preferences. Specific treatment recommendations are complex, and readers are referred to the guidelines for further details.

6 The use of preoperative systemic therapy is the standard of care for patients with locally advanced breast cancer and represents an important treatment option for patients with ESBC. This approach to therapy, referred to as *neoadjuvant* or *primary systemic therapy*, usually consists of chemotherapy but in special circumstances may also include endocrine therapy (eg, in inoperable patients with significant comorbidities or in patients with high sensitivity to endocrine therapy). Advantages of preoperative systemic therapy include (a) a decrease in the size of the tumor to minimize surgery, (b) determination of the response to chemotherapy or hormone therapy in vivo (an important prognostic indicator), and (c) other theoretical advantages (eg, delivery of chemotherapy through an intact vascular system). In a pivotal study conducted by the NSABP (Trial B18), preoperative chemotherapy was compared with traditional chemotherapy given after surgery (the same chemotherapy and the same number of cycles).[89,90] Although no difference was found in DFS or OS, rates of BCT were higher in the group receiving preoperative chemotherapy (67.8% vs 59.8%).[90] This study also identified a small subset of patients (13%) who had a pathologic complete response (pCR) (no tumor left at surgery) after chemotherapy. These patients went on to have a significantly longer DFS compared with patients who did not achieve a pCR ($P<0.0001$).[90] Importantly, even after 16 years of follow-up, patients who achieved a pCR continued to have superior DFS and OS compared with patients who did not achieve a pCR.[91] Although this approach to therapy was historically reserved for patients with inoperable tumors (locally advanced), the use of preoperative systemic therapy in patients with ESBC is increasing in popularity because of the ability to assess the response to therapy in vivo as well as the potential to decrease the size of the tumor, allowing for less radical surgery and better cosmetic results.

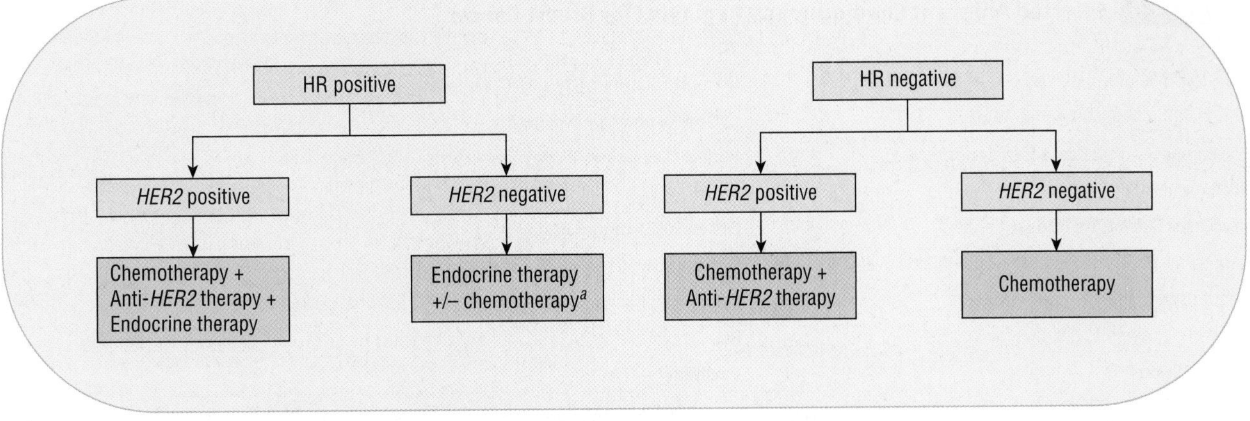

FIGURE 128-5 Treatment of patients with breast cancers larger than 1 cm or with positive lymph nodes. Refer to the text for definitions of HR and *HER2* positivity. Refer to the text for management of patients with tumors smaller than 1 cm, micrometastatic lymph node involvement, or negative lymph nodes. [a]Oncotype DX may identify patients who derive little benefit from chemotherapy (lymph node–negative patients only) (see Systemic Adjuvant Therapy section for details). (HR, hormone receptor; *HER2*, human epidermal growth factor receptor-2.)

Intensive research efforts are directed toward identifying characteristics of the primary tumor (eg, pathologic or molecular prognostic factors) that may predict for a higher or lower likelihood of distant metastases and death in node-negative patients. Although many prognostic factors are being investigated, no single factor or combination of factors sufficiently identifies those at risk of metastases or is sufficiently standardized to be reproducibly applicable to all patients. Several multiparameter gene expression assays are commercially available as decision-support tools for adjuvant chemotherapy.[77] Oncotype DX® is one of these tests that screens for expression of 21 genes using RT-PCR and results in a recurrence score that can be used to determine the risk of distant recurrence or death from breast cancer in women with ER-positive, node-negative, invasive breast cancer. A low recurrence score (less than 18) indicates a low risk of recurrence with endocrine therapy alone indicating that perhaps adjuvant chemotherapy could be avoided. A high recurrence score (greater than or equal to 31) indicates a high risk of recurrence despite endocrine therapy, suggesting a need for adjuvant chemotherapy followed by endocrine therapy. The utility of chemotherapy in patients with an intermediate score (18-30) is unclear, and is the subject of the prospective TAILORx clinical trial. Retrospective data have suggested that Oncotype DX testing may also be beneficial in selecting patients with positive lymph nodes that may derive little benefit from chemotherapy, and an ongoing clinical trial is underway to further elucidate the role of Oncotype DX in patients with one to three positive lymph nodes after surgery. Other multiparameter gene expression assays include MammaPrint and Prosigna. MammaPrint screens the tumor for 70 genes using microarray technology in breast cancer patients with ESBC, regardless of hormone receptor status. The assay reports the predicted rates of recurrence as high or low. The Microarray In Node-negative Disease may Avoid ChemoTherapy (MINDACT) trial, ongoing in Europe, will compare the predictive capabilities of MammaPrint against the standard prognostic factors to assess which patients with node-negative, ER-positive breast cancer will benefit from adjuvant chemotherapy. PAM50 (Prosigna) is a commercially available multigene test that screens the tumor for 50 genes (plus 5 control genes) to predict distant relapse-free survival and likelihood of recurrence at 10 years in postmenopausal women with ER-positive breast cancer treated with endocrine therapy regardless of nodal status.[77] Prospective data with PAM50 in this patient population is eagerly awaited. Although many clinicians use these tools for individual patients, we await further information to guide the appropriate use of these novel pharmacogenomic tools.

A clinical tool that has been widely adopted for clinical use is an Internet-based tool called Adjuvant! (*www.adjuvantonline.com*), which helps clinicians and patients make informed decisions regarding adjuvant therapy for breast, colon, and lung cancers. The tool allows healthcare professionals to estimate the risks of negative outcomes (eg, cancer recurrence, death), and the potential benefits of therapy (eg, reductions in risks of recurrence and death). This is a validated, evidence-based tool that incorporates multiple prognostic and predictive factors into a mathematical model in which each factor is weighted based on established evidence from clinical trials and is placed in the background of the SEER database for patients living in the United States.[76] By entering the patient's age, comorbidities, ER status, tumor grade, tumor size, and nodal status, the clinician can use the tool to estimate the breast cancer mortality and recurrence risk at 10 years and determine the impact of chemotherapy, hormone therapy, or both on these risks. The results are then projected in a graphic format that is easy to understand and explain to patients, although this tool should not be used directly by patients because of the importance of accurate data entry, selection of different treatment options, and appropriate interpretation of results. Some of the limitations of Adjuvant! include the limited information regarding outcome in patients with tumors that are smaller than 1 cm and no axillary lymph node involvement; it does not incorporate proliferation markers or *HER2* status of the primary tumor; and it does not consider potential adverse effects of therapy for individual patients. Estimates of outcome with the Adjuvant! program may also vary in specific subgroups of patients, such as women who are diagnosed with breast cancer at a younger age.

The most common cytotoxic drugs that have been used alone and in combination as adjuvant therapy for breast cancer include doxorubicin, epirubicin, cyclophosphamide, methotrexate, fluorouracil, carboplatin, paclitaxel, and docetaxel. Table 128-6 lists some of the most common combination chemotherapy regimens used in the adjuvant setting.

The basic principle of adjuvant therapy for any cancer type is that the regimen with the highest response rate in advanced disease should be the optimal regimen for use in the adjuvant setting. However, results from individual clinical trials investigating specific regimens in the adjuvant setting are required to identify the benefits and risks in a specific patient population. Early administration of

TABLE 128-6 Selected Adjuvant Chemotherapy Regimens for Breast Cancer

AC[b]	TC[a,c]
Doxorubicin 60 mg/m² IV, day 1	Docetaxel 75 mg/m² IV, day 1
Cyclophosphamide 600 mg/m² IV, day 1	Cyclophosphamide 600 mg/m² IV, day 1
Repeat cycles every 21 days for 4 cycles	Repeat cycles every 21 days for 4 cycles
FAC[d,m]	**TAC[a,e]**
Fluorouracil 500 mg/m² IV, days 1 and 4	Docetaxel 75 mg/m² IV, day 1
Doxorubicin 50 mg/m² IV continuous infusion over 72 hours	Doxorubicin 50 mg/m² IV bolus, day 1
Cyclophosphamide 500 mg/m² IV, day 1	Cyclophosphamide 500 mg/m² IV, day 1 (doxorubicin should be given first)
Repeat cycles every 21-28 days for 6 cycles	Repeat cycles every 21 days for 6 cycles (must be given with growth factor support)
AC → Paclitaxel[a,f]	**Paclitaxel → FAC[g,m]**
Doxorubicin 60 mg/m² IV, day 1	Paclitaxel 80 mg/m² per week IV over 1 hour every week for 12 weeks
Cyclophosphamide 600 mg/m² IV, day 1	Followed by:
Repeat cycles every 21 days for 4 cycles	Fluorouracil 500 mg/m² IV, days 1 and 4
Followed by:	Doxorubicin 50 mg/m² IV continuous infusion over 72 hours
Paclitaxel 80 mg/m² IV weekly	Cyclophosphamide 500 mg/m² IV, day 1
Repeat cycles every 7 days for 12 cycles	Repeat cycles every 21-28 days for 4 cycles[g]
FEC[h]	**CEF[i]**
Fluorouracil 500 mg/m² IV, day 1	Cyclophosphamide 75 mg/m² per day orally on days 1-14
Epirubicin 100 mg/m² IV bolus, day 1	Epirubicin 60 mg/m² IV, days 1 and 8
Cyclophosphamide 500 mg/m² IV, day 1	Fluorouracil 600 mg/m² IV, days 1 and 8
Repeat cycle every 21 days for 6 cycles	Repeat cycles every 21 days for 6 cycles (requires prophylactic antibiotics or growth factor support)
CMF[j,k]	**Dose-Dense AC → Paclitaxel[a,l,n]**
Cyclophosphamide 100 mg/m² per day orally, days 1-14	Doxorubicin 60 mg/m² IV bolus, day 1
Methotrexate 40 mg/m² IV, days 1 and 8	Cyclophosphamide 600 mg/m² IV, day 1
Fluorouracil 600 mg/m² IV, days 1 and 8	Repeat cycles every 14 days for 4 cycles (must be given with growth factor support)
Repeat cycles every 28 days for 6 cycles	Followed by:
Or	Paclitaxel 175 mg/m² IV over 3 hours
Cyclophosphamide 600 mg/m² IV, day 1	Repeat cycles every 14 days for 4 cycles (must be given with growth factor support)
Methotrexate 40 mg/m² IV, day 1	
Fluorouracil 600 mg/m² IV, days 1 and 8	
Repeat cycles every 21 days for 6 cycles	

AC, Adriamycin (doxorubicin), Cytoxan (cyclophosphamide); CAF, Cytoxan (cyclophosphamide), Adriamycin (doxorubicin), 5-fluorouracil; CEF, cyclophosphamide, epirubicin, 5-fluorouracil; CMF, cyclophosphamide, methotrexate, 5-flourouracil; FAC, 5-fluorouracil, Adriamycin (doxorubicin), cyclophosphamide; FEC, 5-fluorouracil, epirubicin, cyclophosphamide; TAC, Taxotere (docetaxel), Adriamycin (doxorubicin), cyclophosphamide; TC, Taxotere (docetaxel), cyclophosphamide.

[a]Designated as a preferred regimen in the NCCN Breast Cancer Guidelines.

[b]From Fisher B, Brown AM, Dimitrov NV, et al. Two months of doxorubicin-cyclophosphamide with and without interval reinduction therapy compared with 6 months of cyclophosphamide, methotrexate, and fluorouracil in positive-node breast cancer patients with tamoxifen-nonresponsive tumors: results from the National Surgical Adjuvant Breast and Bowel Project B-15. *J Clin Oncol* 1990;8:1483.

[c]From Jones SE, Savin MA, Holmes FA, et al. Phase III trial comparing doxorubicin plus cyclophosphamide with docetaxel plus cyclophosphamide as adjuvant therapy for operable breast cancer. *J Clin Oncol* 2006;24:5381.

[d]From Buzdar AU, Hortobagyi GN, Singletary SE, et al. In: Salmon S, ed. *Adjuvant Therapy of Cancer*, VIII. Philadelphia, PA: Lippincott-Raven, 1997:93-100.

[e]From Martin M, Dienkowski T, Mackey J, et al. Adjuvant docetaxel for node-positive breast cancer. *N Engl J Med* 2005;352:2302.

[f]From Sparano JA, Wang M, Martino S, et al. Weekly paclitaxel in the adjuvant treatment of breast cancer. *N Engl J Med* 2008;358:1663-1671.

[g]From Green MC, Buzdar AU, Smith T, et al. Weekly paclitaxel improves pathologic complete remission in operable breast cancer when compared with paclitaxel once every 3 weeks. *J Clin Oncol* 2005;23:5983.

[h]From French Adjuvant Study Group. Benefit of a high-dose epirubicin regimen in adjuvant chemotherapy for node-positive breast cancer patients with poor prognostic factors: 5-year follow-up results of French Adjuvant Study Group 05 randomized trial. *J Clin Oncol* 2001;19:602.

[i]From Levine MN, Bramwell VH, Pritchard KI, et al. Randomized trial of intensive cyclophosphamide, epirubicin, and fluorouracil chemotherapy compared with cyclophosphamide, methotrexate, and fluorouracil in premenopausal women with node-positive breast cancer. National Cancer Institute of Canada Clinical Trials Group. *J Clin Oncol* 1998;16:2651.

[j]From Bonadonna G, Brusamolino E, Valagussa P, et al. Combination chemotherapy as an adjuvant treatment in operable breast cancer. *N Engl J Med* 1976;294:405.

[k]From Fisher B, Redmond C, Dimitrov NV, et al. A randomized clinical trial evaluating sequential methotrexate and fluorouracil in the treatment of patients with node-negative breast cancer who have estrogen-receptor-negative tumors. *N Engl J Med* 1989;320:473.

[l]From Citron ML, Berry DA, Cirrincione C, et al. Randomized trial of dose-dense versus conventionally scheduled and sequential versus concurrent combination chemotherapy as postoperative adjuvant treatment of node-positive primary breast cancer: first report of Intergroup Trial C9741/Cancer and Leukemia Group B Trial 9741. *J Clin Oncol* 2003;21:1431-1439.

[m]FAC may also be given with bolus doxorubicin administration, and the fluorouracil dose is then given on days 1 and 8.

[n]Another way to give these agents in a dose-dense manner is A → P → C as sequential single agents, in the same doses indicated above, every 14 days for 4 cycles each with growth factor support.

effective combination chemotherapy at a time when the tumor burden is low should increase the likelihood of cure and minimize the emergence of drug-resistant tumor cell clones. Historically, combination chemotherapy regimens (polychemotherapy) have been more effective than single-agent chemotherapy. Anthracyclines (doxorubicin and epirubicin) and more recently taxanes (paclitaxel and docetaxel) have become the cornerstones of modern chemotherapy for the adjuvant treatment of breast cancer. The overview analysis of adjuvant chemotherapy (discussed previously) analyzed the use of CMF- or anthracycline-based chemotherapy regimens (polychemotherapy) compared with no chemotherapy. Patients who received polychemotherapy had a 23% ± 2% reduction in annual odds of recurrence and a 14% ± 2% reduction in annual odds of death compared with patients who did not receive chemotherapy, establishing adjuvant chemotherapy as a powerful option for reducing breast cancer recurrence. The authors also analyzed results from 20 trials that directly compared an anthracycline-containing regimen with a CMF-type regimen and demonstrated a significant advantage with the anthracycline regimens.[56] In that meta-analysis, anthracycline-containing regimens were modestly superior in reducing recurrence and death compared with regimens without anthracyclines. A 7% ± 3% reduction in annual odds of recurrence and a 9% ± 3% reduction in annual odds of death were reported in the 2012 update with the anthracycline-containing regimens. It should be noted that regimens with higher cumulative doses of anthracycline (at least 240 mg/m^2 of doxorubicin and at least 360 mg/m^2 of epirubicin) were associated with improvements in the RR of recurrence (11% ± 4%) and OS (16% ± 4%) compared with standard CMF regimens. The 2012 update of the meta-analysis also reported data from an additional 33 clinical trials and discovered that incorporation of a taxane reduced the risk of distant recurrence (13% ± 3%), any recurrence (14% ± 2%), and overall mortality (11% ± 3%) compared with a nontaxane regimen.[56] These trials included both sequential and concurrent taxane therapy (paclitaxel or docetaxel) in conjunction with anthracyclines (with or without cyclophosphamide, fluorouracil, or methotrexate). Proportional reductions in recurrence and breast cancer mortality were largely independent of age, nodal status, tumor size, tumor differentiation, or ER status. Most of these trials enrolled node-positive patients only, but some high-risk node-negative patients were also included. There is no apparent biologic reason why patients with node-negative disease should respond differently to the taxanes than those with node-positive disease. However, the absolute benefits for this population may not be large enough to require that all patients with node-negative disease receive an anthracycline- and taxane-based chemotherapy regimen. Because the addition of a taxane may predispose patients to peripheral neuropathy, myelosuppression, and alopecia, adverse events should also be considered. Taxane-containing, non-anthracycline regimens were not included in the meta-analysis but may be appropriate for some patients with a low risk of disease recurrence based on the results from a single randomized clinical trial.[76] However, this subject remains widely debated, and no single adjuvant chemotherapy regimen is preferred.

Cytotoxic chemotherapy is a particularly important treatment modality for patients with tumors that do not express ER or PR and do not overexpress *HER2* (so called triple negative breast cancer [TNBC]).[92] Patients with TNBC treated with anthracycline- and taxane-based chemotherapy have significantly decreased survival compared with patients with other breast cancer subtypes. Ironically, this subgroup of patients is more likely to respond to neoadjuvant chemotherapy. Therefore, patients with TNBC who achieve a pCR have an excellent long-term survival, but those who have residual disease at the time of surgery have a worse prognosis than non-TNBC patients. The optimal type and duration of chemotherapy for patients with TNBC is unknown. More recently, the addition of carboplatin to a neoadjuvant anthracycline- and taxane-based chemotherapy regimen resulted in a higher pCR rate compared to chemotherapy without carboplatin, but at the cost of increased toxicity.[92] Identification of meaningful molecular targets for this aggressive breast cancer subtype is much needed and research is ongoing. Molecular targets of interest include EGFR, mammalian target of rapamycin (mTOR), and poly-ADP ribose polymerase (PARP).

Although the optimal duration of adjuvant chemotherapy administration is unknown, it appears to be on the order of 12 to 24 weeks and depends on the regimen being used. Optimally, chemotherapy should be initiated within 12 weeks of surgical removal of the primary tumor.[93] "Dose intensity" and "dose density" appear to be critical factors in achieving optimal outcomes in adjuvant breast cancer therapy. *Dose intensity* is defined as the amount of drug administered per unit of time and is typically reported in milligrams per square meter of body surface area per week (mg/m^2/wk). Increasing dose, decreasing time between doses, or both can increase dose intensity. *Dose density* is one way of achieving dose intensity but not by increasing the amount of drug given, as occurs with dose escalation, but instead by decreasing the time between treatment cycles. The importance of dose intensity first received wide attention in 1981 when the Milan group reported in a retrospective analysis of their original CMF adjuvant study that only patients who received at least 85% of their planned CMF dose benefited significantly from adjuvant therapy, and those receiving less than 65% of the planned dose had the same DFS and OS as the group of control patients treated with surgery alone.[94] Therefore, dose reductions for standard treatment regimens should be avoided unless necessitated by severe toxicity. But increasing doses beyond those contained in standard treatment regimens does not appear to be beneficial and may be harmful.

Several studies investigating the impact of *dose density* have now been reported. Interest in this approach to adjuvant therapy was stimulated when the Cancer and Leukemia Group B (CALGB) reported results from their trial 9741, which tested not only dose density but also the question of using sequential versus combination chemotherapy regimens. Using a 2 × 2 factorial design, investigators randomized node-positive breast cancer patients after surgery to compare sequential versus concurrent chemotherapy and standard dose versus dose density.[95] The arms of the study were group 1, sequential doxorubicin (A) for 4 cycles followed by paclitaxel (P) for 4 cycles followed by cyclophosphamide (C) for 4 cycles, with all cycles given every 3 weeks; group 2, sequential A for 4 cycles followed by P for 4 cycles followed by C for cycles with all cycles given every 2 weeks with filgrastim; group 3, concurrent AC for 4 cycles followed by P for 4 cycles with all cycles given every 3 weeks; and group 4, concurrent AC for 4 cycles followed by P for 4 cycles with all cycles given every 2 weeks with filgrastim. After a median follow-up period of 36 months, the patients receiving chemotherapy every 2 weeks had a significantly prolonged DFS (at 3 years: 85% vs 81%; RR, 0.74; P=0.01) and OS (92% vs 90%; RR, 0.69; P=0.013) compared with chemotherapy every 3 weeks.[95] The use of sequential versus concurrent chemotherapy did not show a benefit for one over the other in terms of DFS or OS, but sequential therapy did appear to be less toxic. Patients in the concurrent every 2 week group (group 4) had significantly more regimen-related toxicity, including a very high rate of red blood cell transfusions for anemia (13% of cycles).[95] Red blood cell transfusions are rarely required with most other standard adjuvant chemotherapy regimens used for breast cancer.

Dose intensity appears to be important for some drugs but not for others. Many studies with anthracyclines (without taxanes) appear to indicate no benefit from a dose-dense approach to drug administration. These data seem to contradict the CALGB 9741 data. However, data with the taxanes, especially paclitaxel, appear to support a dose-dense (not intense) approach, with weekly therapy producing optimal outcomes.[96] Data with paclitaxel given weekly versus every 3 weeks indicate that this drug is more effective when given weekly in the adjuvant, neoadjuvant, and metastatic settings.[96,97,98]

Thus, some speculate that the different paclitaxel schedule is the primary reason for the success with this approach to therapy. A direct comparison between taxane dosing intervals was evaluated in the North American Breast Cancer Intergroup Trial E1199, which randomized patients to receive doxorubicin and cyclophosphamide for 4 cycles every 3 weeks followed by either weekly or every 3 week paclitaxel or docetaxel.[96]

Although this study does not directly address the question of dose density because of the lower doses given in the weekly arms, it appears to support the pharmacologic advantage of a taxane given more frequently as the essential factor driving the beneficial outcomes seen with "dose density" in the CALGB 9741 trial. Although no differences in DFS or OS were observed between the weekly or every 3 week schedule or the different taxanes in the E1199 trial, a subgroup analysis indicated that the weekly paclitaxel arm resulted in improved DFS (HR, 0.84; 95% CI, 0.73-0.96; P=0.011), but not OS (HR, 0.87; 95% CI, 0.75-1.02; P=0.09) compared with paclitaxel administered every 3 weeks. Docetaxel, when administered every 3 weeks, resulted in improved DFS (HR, 0.79; 95% CI, 0.68-0.90; P= 0.001), but not OS (HR, 0.86; 95% CI, 0.73-1.00; P=0.54) compared with paclitaxel administered every 3 weeks. DFS and OS with weekly docetaxel were not significantly different from paclitaxel administered every 3 weeks. Interestingly, a subgroup analysis of patients with TNBC demonstrated a significant benefit in DFS and OS from weekly paclitaxel compared to paclitaxel administered every 3 weeks. This benefit was not seen in patients who received every 3 week docetaxel or weekly docetaxel.[96] This remains an active area of investigation. Although other trials have attempted to investigate dose-dense regimens, they also have other variables that were altered that could potentially impact the outcomes. A meta-analysis by Bonilla et al. evaluated four trials of chemotherapy given in a dose-dense fashion compared with conventional administration.[99] In these studies, patients who received dose-dense chemotherapy had statistically improved DFS and OS compared with patients who received conventionally administered chemotherapy. Unfortunately, none of the trials, with the exception of the CALGB 9741 study, adequately evaluated the true impact of dose density. This remains an area of continued research.

The short-term toxic effects of chemotherapy used in the adjuvant setting are generally well tolerated. Although a number of investigators have demonstrated a reduction in quality of life, most patients are able to maintain a reasonable level of function and emotional and social well-being during treatment.[100] Supportive therapy of patients receiving systemic adjuvant chemotherapy has improved over the past decades. Increased attention to the impact of symptoms on quality of life may account for some of this improvement. In addition, more effective antiemetics have become available to assist in managing chemotherapy-induced nausea and vomiting, and myeloid growth factors are often helpful in preventing febrile neutropenia, particularly in elderly patients and patients receiving dose-dense chemotherapy regimens. Standard anti-nausea medications for anthracycline-based chemotherapy include serotonin receptor antagonists, dexamethasone, and neurokinin-1 antagonists.[101] The use of myeloid growth factors to support some adjuvant chemotherapy regimens may be required (eg, with dose-dense regimens), but these are not routinely used for all adjuvant chemotherapy regimens. Because erythropoiesis-stimulating agents have potential effects on cancer cells and the cellular environment that may negatively impact the antitumor effects of chemotherapy or enhance adverse effects related to the chemotherapy, they should be avoided in patients receiving chemotherapy with a curative intent.[102]

Many other side effects are common with the chemotherapy regimens used for the treatment of ESBC, and patients should be appropriately counseled regarding the likelihood of alopecia, weight gain, and fatigue. Patients who are menstruating often experience a cessation of menses that may not return; cessation of menses may be accompanied by signs and symptoms of menopause. DVT has been reported in women receiving combination chemotherapy regimens.[103] Leukemia and other hematologic disorders have long been associated with the alkylating agents (eg, cyclophosphamide) and the topoisomerase II inhibitors (eg, doxorubicin and epirubicin). Several studies have estimated a 0% to 1.5% cumulative incidence of leukemia or myelodysplasia after adjuvant chemotherapy with median follow-up period of 3 to 11 years.[104] To date, the dose-dense regimens have not been associated with an excess rate of leukemias, but the follow-up period for these trials is relatively short.

Cardiomyopathy induced by doxorubicin occurs in fewer than 1% of women whose total dose of doxorubicin is less than 320 mg/m^2.[105] This risk may be further decreased by use of continuous infusion or weekly doxorubicin. It should be noted that epirubicin in the adjuvant setting is usually given at a dose of 100 to 120 mg/m^2.[61] At this dose, epirubicin has an equal chance of causing cardiomyopathy as standard doxorubicin doses when both agents are given as bolus or short infusions. Taxanes are often associated with hypersensitivity reactions, peripheral neuropathy, or myalgias and arthralgias for a few days after the infusion.

It is important to note that the magnitude of survival benefit for adjuvant chemotherapy in stages I and II breast cancer is modest, with an absolute reduction in mortality rate of only 5% at 10 years for patients with negative axillary lymph nodes and 10% for patients with positive axillary lymph nodes. In addition, it is currently not possible to accurately predict who will attain this survival benefit. The advent of genetic prognostic tools, such as Oncotype DX, can help to identify patients who may derive little or no benefit from chemotherapy. However, these tests are only appropriate in specific subsets of patients. Many patients with breast cancer may accept toxicity from treatment to achieve as little as a 1% to 5% absolute improvement in survival. Thus, in the absence of the ability to predict who will benefit, it is likely that most patients with stage I and stage II breast cancer would choose adjuvant chemotherapy.

The optimal chemotherapy regimen for use in the adjuvant setting has yet to be identified, and the choice of chemotherapy regimen for a specific patient is complex. Many adjuvant chemotherapy regimens are available, and most of these regimens have not been directly compared in randomized clinical trials. In some cases, the choice of chemotherapy regimen may be geographic, particularly if a regimen has been developed and studied by a particular institution. Based on data from clinical trials and the previously mentioned pooled analysis, the concomitant or sequential addition of a taxane to an anthracycline-based chemotherapy regimen has become the standard of care for women with node-positive breast cancer. Data from meta-analyses and randomized trials specifically in patients with high-risk node negative disease support the use of anthracycline- and taxane-based chemotherapy regimens in this patient population.[56,76] Results from a single trial that evaluated a taxane-containing (non-anthracycline) regimen are available, and this regimen may be an appropriate treatment in a subset of patients at low risk of disease recurrence. NCCN recommendations are purposefully vague, and they do not differentiate between patients with node-positive or negative breast cancer. The NCCN has designated preferred chemotherapy regimens, as listed in Table 128-6, although detailed information is not provided regarding the rationale behind these designations.

Adjuvant Biologic Therapy As biologic agents continue to demonstrate significant activity against MBC, they are subsequently tested in the adjuvant or neoadjuvant setting. Trastuzumab is a MoAB targeted against the *HER2*-receptor protein. It has demonstrated significant survival benefits when administered with chemotherapy in women with metastatic, *HER2*-positive breast cancer. Several published trials support the use of trastuzumab in combination with or sequentially after adjuvant chemotherapy for patients with early stage, *HER2*-positive breast cancer (Table 128-7).[106]

TABLE 128-7 Selected Regimens for *HER2*-Positive Early-Stage Breast Cancer

Regimen	Drugs	Doses	Frequency	Cycles
Adjuvant				
AC ⇒ PH ⇒ H[a]	Doxorubicin	60 mg/m² IV	Every 21 days	4
	Cyclophosphamide	600 mg/m² IV	Every 21 days	4
	followed by			
	Paclitaxel	175 mg/m² IV over 3 hours	Every 21 days	4
	or			
	Paclitaxel	80 mg/m² IV over 1 hours	Every 7 days	12 weeks
	with Trastuzumab	4 mg/kg IV → 2 mg/kg IV	Every 7 days	12 weeks
	followed by			
	Trastuzumab	2 mg/kg IV or 6 mg/kg IV	Every 7 days or every 21 days	Complete 1 year
TCH[b]	Docetaxel	75 mg/m² IV	Every 21 days	6
	Carboplatin	AUC 6 IV	Every 21 days	6
	Trastuzumab	4 mg/kg IV → 2 mg/kg IV	Every 7 days	18 weeks
	followed by			
	Trastuzumab	6 mg/kg IV	Every 21 days	Complete 1 year
Chemo ⇒ H[c]	Chemotherapy	See reference for details		At least 4
	followed by			
	Trastuzumab	8 mg/kg IV→ 6 mg/kg IV	Every 21 days	1 year
AC ⇒ TH[b]	Doxorubicin	60 mg/m² IV	Every 21 days	4
	Cyclophosphamide	600 mg/m² IV	Every 21 days	4
	followed by			
	Docetaxel	100 mg/m² IV	Every 21 days	4
	Trastuzumab	4 mg/kg IV → 2 mg/kg IV	Every 7 days	12 weeks
	followed by			
	Trastuzumab	6 mg/kg IV	Every 21 days	Complete 1 year
TCHP[d]	Docetaxel	75 mg/m² IV	Every 21 days	6
	Carboplatin	AUC 6 IV	Every 21 days	6
	Trastuzumab	8 mg/kg IV → 6 mg/kg IV	Every 21 days	6
	Pertuzumab	840 mg IV → 420 mg IV	Every 21 days	6
	followed by			
	Trastuzumab	6 mg/kg IV	Every 21 days	Complete 1 year
THP ⇒ FEC[e]	Neoadjuvant Docetaxel[f]	75 mg/m² IV	Every 21 days	4
	Trastuzumab	8 mg/kg IV → 6 mg/kg IV	Every 21 days	4
	Pertuzumab	840 mg IV → 420 mg IV	Every 21 days	4
	followed by adjuvant			
	5-Fluorouracil	600 mg/m² IV	Every 21 days	3
	Epirubicin	90 mg/m² IV	Every 21 days	3
	Cyclophosphamide	600 mg/m² IV	Every 21 days	3

AC, Adriamycin (doxorubicin), Cytoxan (cyclophosphamide); FEC, fluorouracil, epirubicin, cyclophosphamide; H, Herceptin (trastuzumab); PH, paclitaxel, Herceptin (trastuzumab); TCH, Taxotere (docetaxel), carboplatin, Herceptin (trastuzumab); TCHP, Taxotere (docetaxel), carboplatin, Herceptin (trastuzumab), pertuzumab; TH, Taxotere (docetaxel), Herceptin (trastuzumab); THP, Taxotere (docetaxel), Herceptin (trastuzumab), pertuzumab.

[a]From Romond EH, Perez EA, Bryant J, et al. Trastuzumab plus adjuvant chemotherapy for operable *HER2*-positive breast cancer. *N Engl J Med* 2005;353:1673-1684.

[b]From Slamon D, Eiermann W, Robert N, et al. Adjuvant trastuzumab in *HER2*-positive breast cancer. *N Engl J Med* 2011;365:1273-1283.

[c]From Smith I, Procter M, Gelber RD, et al. 2-year follow-up of trastuzumab after adjuvant chemotherapy in *HER2*-positive breast cancer: a randomised controlled trial. *Lancet* 2007;369:29-36.

[d]From Schneeweiss A, Chia S, Hickish T, et al. Pertuzumab plus trastuzumab in combination with standard neoadjuvant anthracycline-containing and anthracycline-free chemotherapy regimens in patients with *HER2*-positive early breast cancer: a randomized phase II cardiac safety study (TRYPHAENA). *Ann Oncol* 2013;24:2278-84.

[e]From Gianni L, Pienkowski T, Im YH, et al. Efficacy and safety of neoadjuvant pertuzumab and trastuzumab in women with locally advanced, inflammatory, or early *HER2*-positive breast cancer (NeoSphere): a randomised multicentre, open-label, phase 2 trial. *The Lancet Oncology* 2012;13:25-32.

[f]Some guidelines allow the substitution of paclitaxel for docetaxel.

Results from these trials report up to a 50% reduction in the risk of recurrence with the addition of trastuzumab to an adjuvant chemotherapy regimen. A meta-analysis of the six available clinical trials investigating the addition of trastuzumab to chemotherapy involving almost 14,000 women revealed superior DFS (OR, 0.69; 95% CI, 0.59-0.80; $P<0.001$) and OS (OR, 0.78; 95% CI, 0.69-0.88; $P<0.001$) in patients with *HER2*-positive breast cancer who received trastuzumab with chemotherapy compared with those that received chemotherapy alone.[107] This difference in DFS translated into a 31% overall lower RR for disease progression or death from any cause for patients who received trastuzumab. Although the benefit of adding trastuzumab to these regimens is obvious, the type of chemotherapy, sequence of administration, and duration of trastuzumab differed among the trials, making the optimal trastuzumab-based regimen less obvious.

Most of the regimens investigated in these adjuvant trials included an anthracycline and a taxane given concurrently with trastuzumab or sequentially before trastuzumab. From the available evidence, it appears that administration of a taxane with trastuzumab may be more effective than trastuzumab administered after chemotherapy. In the previously mentioned meta-analysis, sequential and concomitant use of trastuzumab with chemotherapy both prolonged DFS compared with chemotherapy alone; whereas concomitant trastuzumab also improved OS, sequential trastuzumab did not.[107] The adjuvant use of trastuzumab without an anthracycline has been reported in one trial (Breast Cancer International Research Group 006) and appears to provide similar benefit with diminished cardiac adverse effects as compared with traditional anthracycline-containing adjuvant trastuzumab regimens.[108] The duration of trastuzumab therapy in these adjuvant trials ranges from 9 to 104 weeks in the published studies. The optimal duration of trastuzumab therapy is unknown, although the most current data support the use of trastuzumab for a total of 52 weeks. The most commonly used trastuzumab-based adjuvant chemotherapy regimens are listed in Table 128-7.

The incidence of adverse cardiac effects associated with the addition of trastuzumab appears to increase when an anthracycline is included in the regimen before administration of trastuzumab. The incidence of symptomatic heart failure with adjuvant trastuzumab ranges from 0.5% to 4% in highly selected patients who participated in the clinical trials.[108,109] The higher risk of cardiac complications may be acceptable in many patients given the significant reductions in breast cancer recurrence and death rates. Sequential administration of trastuzumab after chemotherapy (as in the HERA trial) appears to produce a lower incidence of cardiac toxicity (symptomatic congestive heart failure = 2% with trastuzumab). Also, the use of a non–anthracycline-based regimen in the BCIRG 006 trial (Table 128-7) was associated with a low incidence (0.4%) of symptomatic heart failure compared with other regimens.[108] However, cross-trial comparisons are challenging because the definition of cardiac events in each trial was different. Therefore, application of these results to individual patients is fraught with difficulties, and many different regimens may be appropriate for a given patient. Concurrent administration of trastuzumab with an anthracycline is very controversial because of potentially higher rates of cardiac dysfunction (see the Anti-*HER2* Agents of MBC section). Similar to many MoABs, trastuzumab is associated with infusion-related reactions such as fever, chills, and rigors temporally associated with trastuzumab infusions.[110] Postmarketing surveillance data have identified "pulmonary toxicity" and "anaphylaxis" as rare but potentially life-threatening reactions associated with trastuzumab. Chemotherapy-related adverse effects, including neutropenia, infection, and diarrhea, are slightly more frequent with the addition of concurrent trastuzumab therapy, but these toxicities are easily managed and do not preclude the use of trastuzumab in patients with ESBC.

All of these adjuvant trials continued trastuzumab administration during adjuvant radiation therapy and endocrine therapy. The administration of trastuzumab during radiation therapy was evaluated in patients that participated in the N9831 clinical trial. Patients that received concurrent radiation therapy with adjuvant trastuzumab did not experience a significant increase in cardiac events or acute radiation-related adverse events with the exception of transient leukopenia.[111] Therefore, if radiation therapy is clinically indicated, trastuzumab is typically administered concomitantly with radiation.

Many questions remain regarding the optimal use of trastuzumab in the adjuvant or neoadjuvant therapy of ESBC. The use of trastuzumab with chemotherapy in the adjuvant or neoadjuvant setting is now considered to be the standard of care for patients with node-positive and high-risk node-negative *HER2*-positive breast cancer.[61] Controversy exists regarding the use of anti-*HER2* therapy in patients with small, *HER2*-positive, node-negative tumors. Several retrospective analyses of patients with *HER2*-positive tumors smaller than 1 cm who did not receive trastuzumab appear to indicate a poor prognosis, suggesting that these patients may also benefit from trastuzumab-based adjuvant chemotherapy.[112] A single arm, nonrandomized clinical trial demonstrated an excellent 3-year disease-free survival (98.7%) in patients who received weekly paclitaxel and trastuzumab for 12 weeks, followed by trastuzumab every 3 weeks for a total of one year in patients with lymph-node negative, *HER2*-positive, breast cancers smaller than 3 cm.[113] The MoAB pertuzumab has become an important treatment option for patients with *HER2*-positive breast cancer in the neoadjuvant setting.[114] Two clinical trials have shown high rates of pCR at the time of surgery following chemotherapy in combination with trastuzumab and pertuzumab. Patients included in these trials were required to have tumors larger than 2 cm or positive lymph nodes. See Table 128-7 for details regarding the most commonly used regimens. A large clinical trial with pertuzumab in combination with trastuzumab and chemotherapy in the adjuvant setting for *HER2*-positive breast cancer is ongoing and results are eagerly awaited.

Clinical **Controversy...**

Trastuzumab clearly has improved the outcomes for women with lymph node–positive and high-risk lymph node–negative early-stage, *HER2*-positive breast cancer. However, patients with small (less than 1 cm) tumors with negative lymph nodes were not included in prospective clinical trials with trastuzumab. Retrospective data suggest that patients with small *HER2*-positive tumors who did not receive trastuzumab-based chemotherapy have a poor prognosis. A single arm, nonrandomized clinical trial with weekly paclitaxel and trastuzumab for 12 weeks, followed by trastuzumab every 3 weeks for a total of one year has been conducted in this patient population. Questions remain regarding optimal use of trastuzumab in this patient population, and each patient must weigh the risks versus benefits for his or her individual circumstance.

Adjuvant Endocrine Therapy Endocrine therapies that have been studied in the treatment of primary or early-stage breast cancer include tamoxifen, toremifene, oophorectomy, ovarian irradiation, luteinizing hormone–releasing hormone (LHRH) agonists, and AIs. The choice of agent(s) depends on menopausal status and is based on a multitude of clinical trials completed in this setting that establish different roles for different therapies.

Tamoxifen was traditionally the gold standard adjuvant endocrine therapy and has been used in the adjuvant setting for more than 3 decades. Tamoxifen is antiestrogenic in breast cancer cells, but it appears to have estrogenic properties in other tissues and organs.[115,116] More recent studies show that tamoxifen and other similar drugs have many estrogenic and antiestrogenic effects that depend on the tissue and the gene in question, and they are more appropriately called SERMs. Women receiving adjuvant tamoxifen therapy have reduced risk of recurrence and mortality compared with women not receiving adjuvant tamoxifen therapy.[36] In the United States, tamoxifen is generally considered the adjuvant endocrine therapy of choice for premenopausal women, although newer data also support the use of LHRH agonists or oophorectomy in combination with AIs in this group of women.

If chemotherapy and radiation therapy are not required, adjuvant endocrine therapy is generally initiated shortly after surgery or as soon as pathology results are known. When adjuvant chemotherapy is also required, endocrine therapy should be administered after chemotherapy is completed. This recommendation is based on evidence from a phase III trial suggesting tamoxifen administered concurrently with chemotherapy may antagonize the beneficial effect of chemotherapy.[117] In the phase III clinical trial, administration of sequential tamoxifen resulted in a marginally superior DFS compared with concurrent use of tamoxifen with chemotherapy (HR, 0.84; 95% CI, 0.70-1.01; P=0.061).[117] Some clinicians also advocate the initiation of endocrine therapy after completion of radiation therapy, but this subject is very controversial, and few trials have addressed the issue of concurrent versus sequential endocrine therapy and radiation therapy.

Historically, the duration of tamoxifen therapy in the adjuvant setting has been 5 years. However, the results of two recent studies have suggested that a longer duration of tamoxifen may be more effective. In the ATLAS trial, patients with ER-positive breast cancer who had 10 years of tamoxifen had improved DFS and OS compared with those with 5 years of treatment.[118] In the aTTom trial, patients with ER-positive breast cancer who received 10 years of tamoxifen had improved DFS, but not breast cancer mortality, compared with those who received 5 years of treatment.[119] Previous randomized trials comparing 5 years of tamoxifen treatment with longer than 5 years of tamoxifen treatment have shown opposite results and, in fact, were stopped early because of these detrimental outcomes.[120] Patients in the ATLAS and aTTom trials who received 10 years of tamoxifen had increased toxicities, including an increased risk of developing endometrial cancer (ATLAS and aTTom trials) and pulmonary embolism (ATLAS trial only) compared with those receiving tamoxifen for 5 years.[118,119] With this new information, administration of tamoxifen for 10 years can be considered in women with a higher risk of breast cancer recurrence, although the clinician must weigh the risk of toxicity associated with prolonged therapy.

Clinical **Controversy...**

For premenopausal women with early-stage or locally advanced hormone-receptor-positive breast cancer, tamoxifen administered for 5 years has historically been the gold standard. However, two recent clinical trials have suggested a decreased risk of breast cancer recurrence in premenopausal women with ovarian suppression and AI compared to tamoxifen and ovarian suppression for 5 years. Confounding factors include the use of ovarian suppression with tamoxifen in these trials and newer data with tamoxifen given for 10 years. Providers should discuss the risks and benefits of endocrine therapy options individually in each premenopausal patient.

The most reliable information regarding the side effects of tamoxifen comes from the NSABP Breast Cancer Prevention Trial (P-1).[37] This trial randomized 13,388 women 35 years of age or older who were at increased risk for breast cancer to placebo (n = 6,707) or to 20 mg/day of tamoxifen (n = 6,681) for 5 years. Although the primary finding of this study is that tamoxifen reduces the risk of invasive breast cancer by 49%, this study also provides an excellent opportunity to determine the risk of side effects associated with tamoxifen. Information was prospectively collected with regard to the occurrence of hot flashes, vaginal discharge, irregular menses, fluid retention, nausea, skin changes, diarrhea, and weight gain or loss. The self-administered depression scale and a global quality-of-life and a sexual function scale were administered at each follow-up visit. The only symptomatic differences noted between the placebo and tamoxifen group were related to hot flashes and vaginal discharge, both of which occurred more often in the tamoxifen group. No important differences between the two groups were observed in the various self-reporting instruments. Tamoxifen did not increase the risk of ischemic heart disease but did reduce the risk of hip radius and spine fractures. Of note, the rates of stroke, pulmonary embolism, and DVT were elevated in the tamoxifen group (stroke: RR, 1.59; pulmonary embolism: RR, 3.01; and DVT: RR, 1.60), particularly in women age 50 years or older. The rate of endometrial cancer was increased in the tamoxifen group (RR, 2.53), and this increased risk occurred predominantly in women age 50 years or older. The increased risk of endometrial carcinoma is similar in magnitude to that associated with postmenopausal estrogen replacement therapy and is likely a consequence of an estrogenic effect of tamoxifen on the endometrium. Some experts argue that this risk is acceptable because the endometrial cancer induced by tamoxifen is low stage, low grade, and easily treated with surgery or other means and does not pose a life-threatening risk to women. Tamoxifen was also associated with an increased risk of uterine sarcomas (a more aggressive form of endometrial cancer), but this risk appears to be lower than the more common endometrial cancers identified in the NSABP P-1 study. Routine endometrial biopsy is not currently recommended for women receiving tamoxifen therapy. However, women receiving tamoxifen therapy should be counseled to have regular gynecologic examinations and immediately report unusual vaginal bleeding to their primary clinicians for further evaluation.[121]

In premenopausal women, the use of LHRH agonists (ovarian suppression) or ovarian ablation provides benefit in the adjuvant setting. In the EBCTCG overview analysis published in 2005, the overall benefit of ovarian ablation or suppression was significant compared with no treatment (reduction in annual odds of recurrence = 25% ± 12% in women younger than 40 years old and 29% ± 6% in women 40-49 years old).[122] Many of the ongoing trials with the LHRH agonists were not yet included in this analysis, and most of the clinical trials analyzed included patients with hormone receptor–positive, –negative, and unknown tumor status. In an update of this analysis, study inclusion was restricted to patients treated with ovarian suppression with LHRH agonists (not ovarian oblation or oophorectomy) and patients with tumors known to be hormone receptor positive.[123] The addition of a LHRH agonist reduced the rates of recurrence by 25%, deaths after recurrence by 28%, and all deaths by 27% in women younger than 40 years; no significant reductions in recurrence or death were noted in patients older than 40 years. Also, a similar benefit was observed with goserelin as compared with CMF chemotherapy in hormone-sensitive premenopausal breast cancer patients but not in patients with hormone receptor–negative tumors.[123] It is not clear whether the benefit of chemotherapy in this population is a result of the actual effects of chemotherapy or a result of the endocrine effects of chemotherapy-induced amenorrhea. Consequently, some studies have investigated the benefits of adding ovarian ablation or suppression to chemotherapy either with or without tamoxifen. Results from these studies clearly indicate a benefit from ceasing menses regardless of whether this is caused by chemotherapy or ovarian ablation or suppression.[123] It is not clear whether the addition of an LHRH agonist to tamoxifen is advantageous in women with hormone receptor–positive tumors who continue to menstruate after chemotherapy. The optimal duration of adjuvant LHRH agonist use is unknown, with trials ranging from 18 months to 5 years of treatment. Two recently published clinical trials evaluated the benefit of combining an LHRH agonist with tamoxifen or with an AI in premenopausal women. In the TEXT trial, premenopausal patients with hormone receptor–positive early-stage breast cancer were randomized to receive 5 years of tamoxifen or exemestane, both concomitantly with triptorelin for ovarian suppression. In the SOFT trial, premenopausal patients with hormone receptor–positive early-stage breast cancer were randomized to receive 5 years of tamoxifen alone, tamoxifen with triptorelin or exemestane with triptorelin. Combined results of the tamoxifen/triptorelin arms and exemestane/triptorelin arms from the SOFT and TEXT studies demonstrated prolonged 5-year DFS with exemestane compared to tamoxifen (91% vs 87%, $P<0.001$).[124] Results from the tamoxifen only arm of the SOFT trial were not reported in this analysis. Subsequently, results from the SOFT trial were published. In this trial, the estimated 5-year DFS rate did not significantly differ with tamoxifen alone compared to tamoxifen with ovarian suppression (HR 0.78; 95% CI 0.66-1.04).[125] Not unexpectedly, patients who received tamoxifen with ovarian suppression more frequently experienced menopausal symptoms such as hot flushes, sweating, and vaginal dryness compared to patients who received tamoxifen alone. Based on this data, the combination of ovarian suppression and an AI could be considered in premenopausal women with hormone receptor-positive ESBC.

In postmenopausal women, incorporation of AIs is the standard of care in the adjuvant setting. Four different approaches to therapy have been undertaken with these agents: (a) direct comparison with tamoxifen for adjuvant endocrine therapy; (b) sequential use after 5 years of adjuvant tamoxifen therapy; (c) sequential use after 2 to 3 years of adjuvant tamoxifen; and (d) 2 years of treatment with an AI followed by 3 years of adjuvant tamoxifen. In an analysis of two trials that compared 5 years of adjuvant tamoxifen to 5 years of an AI (n = 9885), the risk of recurrence at 10 years was significantly reduced in women who received an AI compared to tamoxifen (RR 0.80; 95% CI 0.73-0.88).[86] In a separate analysis of trials investigating a switch to an AI, 12,799 patients who had completed 2 to 3 years of adjuvant tamoxifen therapy were randomized to continue tamoxifen or crossover to an AI for the remainder of 5 years.[86] The results of this analysis show a decreased risk of recurrence at 7 years after randomization in patients who switched to an AI compared with those who continued with tamoxifen alone (RR 0.90; 95% CI 0.81-0.99). The Breast International Group (BIG) 1-98 trial, which compared letrozole with tamoxifen, also included two separate arms that investigated the value of switching from tamoxifen to an AI or vice versa. With 71 months of follow-up period, the sequential arms did not improve estimated 5-year DFS compared with letrozole alone in either comparison.[61] Clinical trials are also investigating longer durations of AI use to assess the benefits and harms of continued estrogen deprivation, the results of which are greatly anticipated.

Most national and international guidelines currently recommend incorporation of an AI into the adjuvant endocrine therapy regimen for all postmenopausal, hormone-sensitive breast cancers.[61] The current NCCN guidelines for breast cancer management state that any of the following are acceptable endocrine therapy regimens for these women: (a) an AI for 5 years (or longer based on expert opinion); (b) tamoxifen for 2 to 3 years followed by an AI for a total of 5 years of endocrine therapy; or (c) tamoxifen for 5 years followed by an AI for another 5 years (total of 10 years of endocrine therapy).[61] The NCCN panel believes that the three available AIs (anastrozole, letrozole, and exemestane) have similar antitumor efficacy and toxicity profiles, and many other clinicians agree. Therefore, the optimal endocrine therapy regimen in the adjuvant setting has yet to be determined, and incorporation of biologic therapies into these regimens is also being examined. Results from ongoing trials are eagerly awaited to more clearly define a treatment strategy for women facing this clinical dilemma.

Aromatase inhibitors (AIs) are generally well tolerated. Adverse effects include bone loss or osteoporosis, hot flashes, myalgias or arthralgias, vaginal dryness or atrophy, mild headaches, and diarrhea. Although concerns surrounding loss of bone density and an increased risk of osteoporosis are evident in these adjuvant trials, the overall impact on quality of life and long-term survival are still being evaluated. Bone modifying agents are coadministered with the AI in many patients in the metastatic setting and may also be beneficial in the adjuvant setting. Other adverse events that are worrisome include questionable effects on the cardiovascular system (eg, hypercholesterolemia), cognitive functioning, and joint health. Longer follow-up from these trials will continue to provide valuable information to guide treatment decisions and management of adverse effects.

In summary, tamoxifen has been used in the adjuvant setting for nearly 30 years and has a very well-defined safety and efficacy profile in this setting. The roles of other agents such as AIs in postmenopausal women and LHRH agonists in premenopausal women have changed the landscape of adjuvant endocrine therapy, and incorporation of other biologic therapies may further impact outcomes.

The pharmacologic disposition of tamoxifen in humans is very complex and has only recently been elucidated (Fig. 128-6). Tamoxifen is now considered to be a prodrug. Although the parent compound has significant clinical activity, tamoxifen is metabolized through multiple enzymes, including CYP3A4, CYP2C19, CYP2D6, and others, to metabolites that appear to be more active than the parent compound.[126] The active metabolites 4-hydroxytamoxifen (4OH-TAM) and 4-hydroxy-*N*-desmethyltamoxifen (endoxifen) have nearly a 100-fold higher affinity for the ER compared with tamoxifen. Endoxifen is present in the serum at a 6 to 12-fold higher

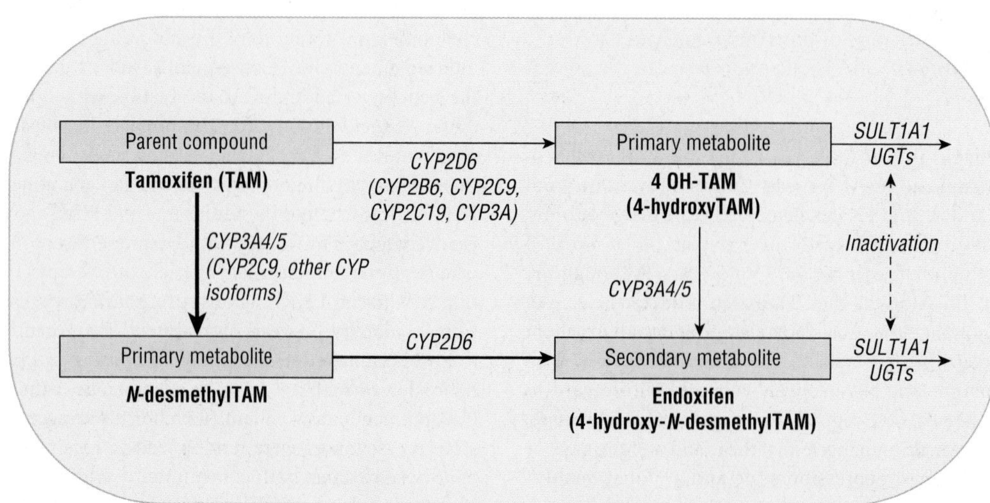

FIGURE 128-6 Tamoxifen metabolism. Widths of the arrows approximate allocation of parent compound to various metabolites.

concentrations compared with 4OH-TAM; hence, endoxifen is thought to be the most important metabolite for the clinical activity of tamoxifen. The formation of endoxifen is highly dependent on the enzymatic activity of CYP2D6. However, multiple other pathways may also be important for determining activity, including deactivation pathways (eg, SULT-1-A1, UGT). Polymorphisms in CYP2D6 can lead to increased or decreased formation of endoxifen and may be related to improved or diminished clinical outcomes, respectively. Although clinical data suggest that certain polymorphisms in CYP2D6 may result in poorer DFS or relapse-free survival in patients receiving tamoxifen, other studies show either no relationship or the opposite effect between clinical outcomes and CYP2D6 polymorphisms. Multiple commercially available assays for CYP2D6 are available, but widespread testing for patients receiving tamoxifen is not currently recommended based on available evidence.[61,87] Excellent reviews on this subject are available.[126] Potent inhibitors of CYP2D6, such as paroxetine and fluoxetine, may decrease levels of endoxifen in patients receiving tamoxifen.[126] The clinical outcomes related to such drug–drug interactions in an individual patient are largely unknown and may depend on their underlying CYP2D6 genetic status (eg, poor metabolizer, extensive metabolizer). In one population-based cohort study, concomitant use of tamoxifen and paroxetine (but not other antidepressants) resulted in increased risk of breast cancer death.[127] Even though high-quality data on strong CYP2D6 inhibitors and breast cancer outcomes in patients receiving tamoxifen are limited, common sense would dictate avoiding known strong inhibitors of CYP2D6, if possible, in patients receiving tamoxifen.

Locally Advanced Breast Cancer (Stage III)

6 *Locally advanced breast cancer* generally refers to breast carcinomas with significant primary tumor and nodal disease but in which distant metastases cannot be documented. A wide variety of clinical scenarios can be seen within this group of patients, including neglected tumors that have spread locally, to IBCs that are a unique clinical entity. IBC is associated with similar clinical findings compared with neglected, locally advanced breast tumors (eg, erythema representing skin involvement). The distinction between the two diagnoses lies in the rapidity of onset of symptoms. Many locally advanced breast cancers are diagnosed in patients who have had symptoms for months to years and have neglected to seek medical attention. Although these women have a poor prognosis because of the delay in diagnosis, they are not classified as IBC. The hallmark of IBCs is the rapid onset of symptoms within weeks to months, including erythema of the skin with or without a detectable underlying breast mass. These patients are often inappropriately treated for cellulitis with antibiotics for several weeks to months. Because of the aggressive nature of this disease, a delay in diagnosis can be fatal for some of these women.

The natural history of locally advanced breast cancer shows that even when local–regional control is accomplished, systemic relapse and death from breast cancer eventually occur in most patients if systemic therapy is not used.[128] That observation led to interest in the use of neoadjuvant or primary chemotherapy in locally advanced breast cancer, which renders inoperable tumors resectable and can increase rates of BCT. Other potential benefits related to early initiation of systemic therapy include delivery of drugs through an intact vasculature, in vivo assessment of response to therapy, and the opportunity to study the biologic effects of the systemic treatment. For patients with inoperable breast cancer, including IBC, the initial approach to therapy should be chemotherapy with the goal of achieving resectability. The NCCN guidelines addressing the management of locally advanced disease recommend primary chemotherapy with an anthracycline- and taxane-containing regimen.[61]

After neoadjuvant chemotherapy, most tumors respond with more than a 50% decrease in tumor size; about 70% of patients experience a reduction in their stage of disease. The chemotherapy regimens used in this setting are similar to those used in the adjuvant setting, but generally include an anthracycline and incorporate a taxane in some manner. For patients with *HER2*-positive tumors, the incorporation of trastuzumab and pertuzumab with chemotherapy is appropriate.[114] Neoadjuvant endocrine therapy may be an option for patients who have unresectable hormone receptor–positive tumors who are unable to receive chemotherapy (eg, multiple comorbid conditions).[129] However, this approach to therapy is not common.

Local therapy usually follows chemotherapy, and the extent of surgery is determined by response to chemotherapy, the wishes of the patient, and the cosmetic results likely to be achieved. However, many patients may be able to have BCT if an acceptable response to chemotherapy is accomplished. Adjuvant radiation therapy should be administered to all locally advanced breast cancer patients to minimize local recurrences regardless of the type of surgery used for that individual patient (eg, mastectomy or segmental mastectomy). Inoperable tumors that are unresponsive to systemic chemotherapy may require radiation therapy for local management and may not be eligible for surgical resection after radiation. These patients are not commonly encountered but have a very poor prognosis. For most patients with locally advanced breast cancer, cure is still the primary goal of therapy and can be achieved in a large number of patients when all treatment modalities are used.

Metastatic Breast Cancer (Stage IV)

7 Treatment of MBC with cytotoxic, biologic, or endocrine therapy often results in regression of disease and improvements in quality of life. The choice of therapy for metastatic disease is based on the presence or absence of certain tumor or patient characteristics and extent of disease involvement. The most important factors predicting response to therapy are the presence of *HER2*, estrogen, and progesterone receptors in the primary tumor tissue. Tumors over-expressing *HER2* receptor protein are more likely to benefit from *HER2*-targeted therapy. Tumors expressing high levels of ER, PR, or both are more likely to respond to endocrine therapy. For TNBC, investigators and clinicians are diligently searching for biologic targets that may be predictive of response to a number of agents (eg, BRCA1 mutations with the platinum agents). The extent of metastases is also an important factor to consider. Endocrine therapy is the treatment of choice for patients with hormone receptor–positive tumors who exhibit mild to no symptoms of disease, regardless of *HER2* status. For cases where hormone receptors and *HER2* receptors are over-expressed, an endocrine agent in combination with a *HER2*-targeting agent (eg, trastuzumab or lapatinib), should be considered. Data with biologic, targeted therapies (eg, everolimus, palbociclib) which appear to target endocrine resistance, have changed the approach in patients with *HER2*-negative, HR-positive MBC, favoring combination endocrine/biologic therapy as first- or second-line therapy compared to single agent endocrine therapy for some patients. Patients with symptomatic visceral or central nervous system (CNS) involvement generally have more rapidly growing cancers that require up-front chemotherapy, either alone or with *HER2*-targeted therapy. In this clinical setting, for tumors that over-express *HER2*, regimens that combine *HER2*-targeted therapy with chemotherapy are preferred.[130]

Patients who respond to initial endocrine therapy alone often respond to a second (or even third) hormonal manipulation. But the response rate is lower, and the duration of response is shorter with second (and third) hormonal manipulations. Patients who respond initially to an endocrine/biologic combination are generally treated with a second combination with varying results. Little information is known about subsequent response to therapy after biologic combinations in this setting and this is the subject of much research. Patients typically are sequentially treated with endocrine therapy (alone or with a biologic agent) until their tumors cease to respond or the patient ceases to benefit from endocrine therapy, at which time cytotoxic chemotherapy can be administered. Subsequent response to chemotherapy after endocrine/biologic therapy combinations is also currently unknown, but is frequently recommended for patients who can tolerate chemotherapy. Concurrent administration of more than one endocrine therapy or combining chemotherapy plus endocrine therapy is generally avoided in the setting of MBC because of increased toxicity and no substantial improvement in OS. Women with hormone receptor–negative tumors; with rapidly progressive or symptomatic lung, liver, or bone marrow involvement (a visceral crisis); and with progressive disease while on initial endocrine therapy (with or without a biologic agent) are usually treated with cytotoxic chemotherapy.[61]

All breast cancer patients with metastases to the bone should be considered for treatment with a bone-modifying agent (eg, pamidronate, zoledronic acid, or denosumab) because these agents have been shown to decrease the rates of skeletal-related events, such as fractures, spinal cord compression, and pain, and the need for radiation to the bones or surgery.[131] These agents do not act as anticancer agents and should be coadministered with other therapies targeting the cancer cells specifically.

Desired Outcomes

After advancing beyond local–regional disease, breast cancer is currently incurable. However, some patients live for many years with metastatic disease, making this a chronic disease requiring long-term management strategies that incorporate improvements or maintenance of quality of life. Palliation is the desired therapeutic outcome in the treatment of MBC. Optimizing benefits and minimizing toxicity are general therapeutic goals of any therapy administered in this setting. Therefore, sequential single-agent chemotherapy is often chosen over combination regimens, but individual circumstances may call for more rapid responses in which combination therapy may be indicated. Endocrine therapy is generally less toxic than chemotherapy and may be a more appropriate option for patients with hormone receptor–positive breast cancer with or without a biologic, targeted therapy. Tumor response to a particular treatment regimen may be measured by changes in laboratory tests, diagnostic imaging, and physical signs and symptoms. If a patient is tolerating therapy well, clear evidence of disease progression on imaging or physical examination is required to warrant changing therapy. Unless the patient clearly cannot tolerate the regimen or the cancer is clearly progressing at a rate that will quickly cause symptoms (or is causing symptoms already), there is not a sound reason to change therapy. Optimizing quality of life is an important therapeutic end point in the treatment of patients with MBC and eventually requires discontinuation of active cancer therapy and a shift to supportive care with hospice services. Balancing between quantity and quality of life is a frequent battle waged by many oncology clinicians in close collaboration with their patients, and difficult decisions are faced during this time.

Biologic or Targeted Therapy

Therapies that focus on molecular targets through novel mechanisms are often referred to as biologic or targeted therapy. These agents, while using the biologic knowledge gained from decades of research, are designed to specifically target cancer cells while generally sparing normal tissues. For breast cancer, several agents are available that focus on a myriad of targets that are differentially expressed in breast cancer cells and play a critical role in their proliferation and survival.

8 ***HER2*-Targeted Agents** *HER2*, in selected breast cancers, is a very important protein for maintenance of breast cancer cell proliferation and survival. Currently, four anti-*HER2* agents are available in the United States, trastuzumab, lapatinib, pertuzumab and ado-trastuzumab emtansine.

As mentioned previously, trastuzumab is a MoAB targeted against the *HER2*-receptor protein. Pertuzumab is also a MoAB but binds to a different epitope on *HER2* and prevents protein dimerization and subsequent cell signaling. Ado-trastuzumab emtansine (also called T-DM1) is a MoAB-drug conjugate with a trastuzumab backbone linked to a potent tubulin inhibitor, emtansine (DM1). Lapatinib is a small-molecule TKI targeted against the *HER2* protein and the *HER1* (EGFR) protein, leading to dual signaling blockade.

Evidence supporting the use of *HER2*-targeted therapy is found in two systematic reviews: 1) ASCO clinical practice guideline for systemic therapy for patients with advanced *HER2*-positive breast cancer published in 2014 and 2) systematic review by Cancer Care Ontario (CCO) published in 2011.[130] These systematic reviews found evidence of progression-free (PFS), time-to-progression (TTP) and overall response rate benefits with the addition of trastuzumab to chemotherapy. Additionally, the combination of trastuzumab and chemotherapy increased OS, an endpoint that had historically been stagnant for this disease. The addition of trastuzumab to endocrine therapy in the CCO review was found to increase PFS and TTP, but not OS. Based on this information, the ASCO guidelines clearly recommend the use of first-line *HER2*-directed therapy with chemotherapy for patients with *HER2*-positive MBC. Combination endocrine therapy plus *HER2*-directed therapy (either trastuzumab or lapatinib) is appropriate as first-line therapy in selected cases where the tolerability of chemotherapy may be problematic or after a patient has achieved maximal response with a chemotherapy-*HER2* therapy approach. First-line endocrine therapy alone may be considered in selected cases where disease burden is low, there is a presence of comorbidities and/or there has been a long disease-free interval.[130]

First-line therapy with a pertuzumab-trastuzumab-taxane combination is now the standard for *HER2*-overexpressing MBC. Two regimens predominate in this setting. The use of docetaxel administered every 3 weeks in combination with trastuzumab and pertuzumab (both administered every 3 weeks) has the most evidence to support its use in this setting. Substitution of docetaxel with weekly paclitaxel may be utilized if tolerability with docetaxel is problematic.[130]

Second-line *HER2*-targeted therapy for MBC that has progressed during or after first-line *HER2*-targeted therapy should include ado-trastuzumab emtansine (T-DM1). Use of this agent is largely based on a single, randomized phase III trial comparing the antibody-drug conjugate (T-DM1) to lapatinib plus capecitabine, which was previously the standard of care after progression on a trastuzumab-containing regimen. Patients on this trial had received zero to 3 prior regimens for metastatic disease. T-DM1 was associated with increased OS and PFS and fewer adverse events overall. In this trial, there were a small number of patients who had no prior therapy for metastatic disease, but the numbers were considered insufficient to draw any sound conclusions in this subset of patients. Several ongoing clinical trials are underway to explore the use of T-DM1 compared with trastuzumab-chemotherapy combination regimens and pertuzumab-trastuzumab combinations as first-line therapy and these results are eagerly awaited.[130]

Subsequent therapy (third-line) for *HER2*-positive, MBC is somewhat controversial. If a patient has not yet received pertuzumab and/or T-DM1, then these agents can be used as stated earlier. If a patient has been treated with pertuzumab and T-DM1, then use of another *HER2*-targeted regimen may be considered. This could include lapatinib plus capecitabine, a chemotherapy-trastuzumab combination, or trastuzumab plus lapatinib. For patients with tumors that are ER/PR positive, the option of endocrine therapy, alone or with trastuzumab or lapatinib, is also available. See Table 128-8 for details on *HER2*-targeted regimens.[130]

Brain metastases are very common in patients with *HER2*-positive MBC with over 50% of patients experiencing brain metastases over their lifetime. This statistic is somewhat misleading in that the rate of brain as a site of first recurrence in patients with

TABLE 128-8 Selected Regimens for *HER2*-Positive Metastatic Breast Cancer

Selected Chemotherapy/Biologic Regimens	
Docetaxel + Trastuzumab + Pertuzumab Docetaxel 75 mg/m² IV day 1 Trastuzumab 8 mg/kg IV day 1 followed by 6 mg/kg IV Pertuzumab 840 mg IV day 1 followed by 420 mg IV Repeat cycle every 21 days	**Ado-Trastuzumab Emtansine (T-DM1)** Ado-Trastuzumab Emtansine 3.6 mg/kg IV day 1 Repeat cycle every 21 days
Paclitaxel + Trastuzumab + Pertuzumab	**Trastuzumab + chemotherapy**
Paclitaxel 80 mg/m² IV days 1, 8, 15 Trastuzumab 8 mg/kg IV day 1 followed by 6 mg/kg IV Pertuzumab 840 mg IV day 1 followed by 420 mg IV Repeat cycle every 21 days	Trastuzumab 8 mg/kg IV day 1 followed by 6 mg/kg IV day 1 Repeat cycle every 21 days (for Q 21 day chemotherapy) **OR** Trastuzumab 4 mg/kg IV day 1 followed by 2 mg/kg IV day 1 Repeat cycle weekly (for weekly chemotherapy) Chemotherapy may include any one of the following: Paclitaxel, docetaxel, protein-bound paclitaxel, capecitabine, vinorelbine, gemcitabine
Selected Endocrine Therapy/Biologic Therapy Regimens	
Trastuzumab + Lapatinib Lapatinib 1,000 mg orally daily continuously Trastuzumab 8 mg/kg IV day 1 followed by 6 mg/kg IV day 1 Repeat cycle every 21 days **OR** Trastuzumab 4 mg/kg IV day 1 followed by 2 mg/kg IV day 1 Repeat cycle weekly	Trastuzumab + Anastrozole Anastrozole 1 mg orally daily continuously Trastuzumab 8 mg/kg IV day 1 followed by 6 mg/kg IV day 1 Repeat cycle every 21 days **OR** Trastuzumab 4 mg/kg IV day 1 followed by 2 mg/kg IV day 1 Repeat cycle weekly
Lapatinib + Capecitabine Lapatinib 1,250 mg orally daily continuously Capecitabine 1,000 mg/m² twice daily × 14 days Repeat cycle every 21 days	Lapatinib + Letrozole Lapatinib 1,500 mg orally daily continuously Letrozole 2.5 mg orally daily continuously

1. NCCN Clinical Practice Guidelines in Oncology (NCCN Guidelines®) for *Breast Cancer* V.3.2015 © National Comprehensive Cancer Network, Inc 2015. Last accessed, September 1, 2015.

2. Giordano SH, Temin S, Kirshner JJ, et al. Systemic therapy for patients with advanced human epidermal growth factor receptor 2-positive breast cancer: American Society of Clinical Oncology clinical practice guideline. *J Clin Oncol* 2014;32:2078-2099.

3. Herceptin (trastuzumab) product information. 2015 April 2015 [cited 2015 12/2/15]; Product information. Available from: http://www.gene.com/download/pdf/herceptin_prescribing.pdf.

4. Tykerb (lapatinib) product information. 2015 March 2015 [cited 2015 December 2]; Tykerb prescribing information]. Available from: http://www.pharma.us.novartis.com/product/pi/pdf/tykerb.pdf.

Data from references 1-4.

ESBC is still very low (1%-3%), negating the need for routine screening for brain metastases. However, a very low threshold for diagnostic testing exists if any neurologic signs or symptoms occur. Local therapy including surgery, whole-brain radiation, stereotactic radiosurgery or some combination of these approaches are considered as initial therapy. Systemic therapy will continue if the remainder of metastatic sites are stable. If extracranial metastases are progressing, changing the *HER2*-targeted therapy according to guidelines is appropriate.[132]

Clinical **Controversy...**

This phenomenon is thought to be due to the overall success of *HER2*-targeted therapy at extracranial sites and the presence of the blood-brain-barrier (BBB) which prevents *HER2*-targeted MoAB from accessing these tissues, creating a sanctuary site for breast cancer cells to flourish. There is some evidence that responses in the brain may be possible even with the large, *HER2*-targeted antibodies due to disruptions in the BBB from disease or prior local therapy (surgery or radiation). While there are anecdotal reports of responses in the brain, the likelihood is low that the patient's disease will respond in the brain. There is some evidence that the small molecule TKI, lapatinib, maybe effective in this scenario, but overall local therapies tend to offer the best approach in conjunction with systemic therapy. If local therapy fails to control disease in the brain, best supportive or palliative care may be prudent, depending on the status of their extracranial sites of disease and their overall performance status.[132]

Adverse effects of the *HER2*-targeted therapies have been identified and are primarily related to the heart. Therefore, all therapies in this class, regardless of their exact mechanism of receptor blockade, have some degree of cardiotoxicity that should be acknowledged and monitored for. The type of cardiotoxicity differs depending on the agent in question. Trastuzumab and likely pertuzumab are associated with myocardial damage leading to heart failure clinically similar to anthracycline-associated cardiomyopathy. The incidence of heart failure is approximately 5% with single-agent trastuzumab and the risk is unacceptably high when trastuzumab is given concurrently with an anthracycline.[133] Fortunately, heart failure seen with trastuzumab is somewhat reversible with pharmacologic management, and some patients have continued therapy with trastuzumab after their left ventricular ejection fraction has returned to normal with medical management. Close monitoring for clinical signs and symptoms of heart failure as well as routine echocardiography is recommended in order to intervene with appropriate cardiac treatments. The incidence of cardiotoxicity with pertuzumab administered in combination with trastuzumab is largely unknown. One early study with pertuzumab was stopped early because of cardiotoxicity that surpassed 50% at the time of study discontinuation. Subsequent studies have not demonstrated an increased rate of cardiotoxicity beyond that seen with trastuzumab alone.[114] This discrepancy is likely to be better characterized as further clinical evidence and experience is gained with this agent. Nonetheless, careful clinical monitoring is required. Cardiotoxicity with T-DM1 is largely similar to that seen with trastuzumab.

Because of concerns regarding the role of *HER2* in normal cardiac functioning, lapatinib may also increase the risk for cardiac dysfunction. However, in a review of more than 3,689 patients who received lapatinib in phase I to III trials, cardiotoxicity occurred in only 1.6% of patients.[134] Although these data are reassuring, it does not rule out the possibility of expanded toxicity when this agent is used in patients not included in the clinical trials such as those with underlying cardiac risks. Rare QT prolongation has also been reported with lapatinib, but the exact clinical significance of this effect is widely debated. Drug interactions that increase systemic exposure to lapatinib may predispose patients to this rare complication.

Adverse events associated with MoABs are seen with trastuzumab, pertuzumab and T-DM1 and include infusion-related reactions (primarily fever and chills). These occur in about 40% of patients receiving trastuzumab during the initial infusion and generally go unrecognized by patients. Other infusion-related reactions with trastuzumab include mild nausea, pain at tumor sites, rigors, headaches, dizziness, hypotension, rash, and asthenia, which are much less common.[133] A rare but more severe reaction consisting of severe hypersensitivity or pulmonary reactions has been reported in postmarketing surveillance with trastuzumab. It is important to educate patients regarding the pulmonary reactions because these may occur up to 24 hours after the infusion and can be fatal if not promptly treated. Trastuzumab may increase the incidence of infection, diarrhea, and other adverse events slightly when given with chemotherapy, but most of these increases are not clinically significant for an individual patient. The adverse effects of pertuzumab appear to be similar, with increases in febrile neutropenia and grade 3 diarrhea evident in the phase III trial with docetaxel.[114] As clinicians gain more experience with this agent outside the context of clinical trials, the true incidence and severity of these adverse events will become more evident.

Other adverse events associated with lapatinib include primarily rash and diarrhea. These adverse effects appear to be more significant when combined with chemotherapy (eg, capecitabine, paclitaxel) but are generally manageable with aggressive antidiarrheal therapy or dose reductions. Other rare effects have been reported (QT prolongation, hepatotoxicity, and interstitial lung disease), and patients should be counseled regarding these effects. Drug–drug and drug–food interactions are particularly important with lapatinib because of its metabolism through CYP 3A4 and other pharmacokinetic and pharmacodynamic issues.[135] Many of the adverse effects listed previously may be exacerbated by drug or food interactions, and careful review of patients' medication lists and education regarding these issues are extremely important.

It should be noted that only 15% to 20% of patients with MBC overexpress *HER2*. To date, there is no benefit associated with the administration of trastuzumab to patients with *HER2*-negative tumors (IHC score of 0-1+, or FISH negative) and a very questionable benefit associated with administration of trastuzumab to women with tumors that are 2+ for *HER2* by IHC staining alone. Further analyses investigating what other predictive markers may be clinically useful are currently ongoing.[136]

Other Targeted Agents As previously mentioned, treatments for MBC rarely eliminate all cancer cells, and cures are seldom seen after the cancer has spread beyond the local area of the breast and axilla. Acquired drug resistance develops in nearly all patients. Alterations in cell signaling, cell cycle control, and apoptotic signaling are among the common mechanisms of resistance with chemotherapy, endocrine therapy, and anti-*HER2* therapy. The PI3K/protein kinase-B (also called Akt) pathway includes many different proteins, one of the most important being the mTOR tyrosine kinase. mTOR is an important mediator for cell proliferation and regulation of apoptosis, angiogenesis, and cellular metabolism. Use of mTOR inhibitors to treat MBC has resulted in conflicting results. Temsirolimus, an intravenous mTOR inhibitor, was administered with letrozole as first-line therapy for MBC in a large randomized phase III trial, resulting in no improvement in PFS.[137] Everolimus, an oral mTOR inhibitor, was administered with exemestane as second-line therapy for MBC after an AI and produced significant improvements in PFS.[138] In combination with tamoxifen, everolimus demonstrated superior clinical benefit rate and TTP in a small, randomized phase II trial.[139]

Targeting mTOR also appears to be important for *HER2*-positive MBC patients progressing on trastuzumab. Limited data have explored the use of everolimus with trastuzumab–taxane combinations that appear to be promising, but added toxicities and cost are important factors to consider when adding an mTOR inhibitor to a patient's regimen.[139] The most common adverse events experienced in the everolimus–exemestane trial were mucositis, fatigue or asthenia, cough, pyrexia, and hyperglycemia.[138] As more patients receive this combination outside the context of a clinical trial, adverse effects related to metabolic effects (hypercholesterolemia, hypertriglyceridemia, hyperglycemia) and pneumonitis may become more prevalent because these are evident in patients receiving everolimus for other cancer types (eg, renal cell carcinoma).

Cell cycle regulators play an important role in drug resistance and a great deal of investigation has occurred to elucidate specific pathways at work in breast cancers. Cyclin-dependent kinases (CDK), in coordination with their regulatory cyclin partners, form CDK-cyclin heterodimer complexes that control cell cycling. CDK-4 and -6 are critical components of this process. In some breast cancer cell lines, these complexes are responsible for phosphorylating the retinoblastoma tumor suppressor gene product (RB), thus inactivating the suppression of cell division and allowing unregulated progression through the cell cycle. Palbociclib, a potent, selective inhibitor of CDK-4 and -6, effectively prevents phosphorylation of RB, leaving it in an active state that is able to appropriately regulate cell division. This action reverses some acquired resistance to tamoxifen and AIs and appears to be synergistic with trastuzumab in *HER2*-amplified cell lines. While this is encouraging and hopeful, combining these agents with DNA-damaging techniques (eg, chemotherapy, radiation) is very complex and sequencing and timing are very important.[140] To date, palbociclib has shown improved PFS in combination with letrozole (as first-line therapy) and fulvestrant (as second-line therapy). Further explanation of palbociclib's role in therapy can be found below in the Endocrine Therapy section. Preclinical data with other palbociclib combinations is promising, but remains investigational until further information on optimal timing and sequencing with specific agents is elucidated.

Targeting tumor blood vessels is another strategy to fight breast cancer and potentially reverse drug resistance. One of the most important growth factors that regulates the development of new blood vessels (angiogenesis) is VEGF. Bevacizumab is a MoAB targeted against VEGF and is FDA approved for use with chemotherapy for the management of a variety of malignancies. Bevacizumab has also been tested in clinical trials with capecitabine and paclitaxel in patients with MBC. Conflicting results have been reported with the use of bevacizumab in combination with chemotherapy in patients with MBC, and in 2012, the FDA withdrew the approval for bevacizumab in combination with paclitaxel for management of newly diagnosed MBC. Nonetheless, NCCN guidelines for management of breast cancer continue to list bevacizumab–paclitaxel as one option for the management of *HER2*-negative MBC. Continuing controversy exists regarding this agent in the management of MBC.[141,142] Many other biologic or targeted agents are being investigated and may change the overall management of breast cancer for both early and metastatic disease.

Endocrine Therapy

9 The pharmacologic goal of endocrine therapy for breast cancer is to either (a) decrease circulating levels of estrogen or (b) prevent the effects of estrogen at the breast cancer cell by blocking the hormone receptors or downregulating the presence of these receptors. Achievement of the first goal depends on the menopausal status of

the patient, but achievement of the second goal is independent of menopausal status. Many endocrine therapies are available to target either pathway, and combinations of drugs with differing mechanisms of action have also been investigated. Unfortunately, most combinations of endocrine therapy with a second endocrine therapy have not demonstrated significant benefits over single-agent hormone therapy but have increased toxicity. Therefore, combinations of endocrine agents for MBC are generally not recommended outside the context of a clinical trial. With the approval of lapatinib, everolimus and palbociclib for MBC, we now have combination endocrine regimens that are quite effective, although they introduce an increased risk of adverse events that require supportive management strategies and may limit the utility of these combinations in some patients. These combinations address de novo or acquired resistance with endocrine therapy and have demonstrated efficacy over single agents in specific patient populations. Sequential use of single endocrine agents is common in the metastatic setting when a patient is progressing on one agent after experiencing an initial response. Responsive patients are often treated with a series of endocrine agents, usually over several years, before chemotherapy is considered. In conjunction with biologic therapies, such sequential approaches are currently untested, but are being investigated and make logical sense given the indolent nature of these hormone-sensitive metastases.

Data with lapatinib, everolimus, and palbociclib put these regimens squarely in the forefront in the battle against this disease. For patients with *HER2*-positive metastases, lapatinib or trastuzumab has been administered with letrozole or anastrozole, respectively, with substantial benefits seen compared to endocrine therapy alone. Newly diagnosed patients with *HER2*-negative, HR-positive MBC should be considered for treatment with palbociclib and letrozole therapy. In this patient population, the palbociclib/letrozole regimen provided nearly double the duration of PFS compared to letrozole alone in one small, randomized phase 2 trial which was the basis for the FDA-approval of palbociclib (PALOMA-1).[143] Subsequent publication of interim results of the PALOMA-3 trial indicates a benefit is also seen with the addition of palbociclib to fulvestrant in patients who had relapsed or progressed during previous endocrine therapy (second-line therapy).[144] Limitations with these combinations include small numbers of patients, limited follow-up, and a toxicity profile that is not typical of endocrine therapy regimens. Myelosuppression, mainly neutropenia, is the dose-limiting toxicity seen with palbociclib and occurs in 50% to 80% of patients. Interestingly, the consequences of this appear to be minimal at least in the short-term data currently available. Rates of neutropenic fever are very low (less than 1%) and other infections have included only mild upper respiratory infections. Pulmonary embolism was seen in 1% to 4% of patients and other common side effects include mild fatigue and nausea. Other, confirmatory trials with palbociclib plus letrozole or exemestane are currently underway.[140]

As mentioned earlier, everolimus is now approved for use with exemestane as second-line therapy in HR-positive, *HER2*-negative MBC in patients who have progressed on a non-steroidal AI (eg, anastrozole, letrozole). Adverse events associated with this combination are more prominent than that seen with palbociclib and include metabolic syndrome, mucositis, fatigue and pneumonitis to name a few. The use of this combination after palbociclib/letrozole has not yet been reported, but concerns regarding changes in resistance patterns exist and future trials addressing sequencing these regimens are needed to determine the optimal order of administration.

Outside of these regimens that include novel targeted agents, there is little evidence that the survival benefit from one endocrine therapy is clearly superior to that achieved with other therapies in women with MBC. Prior to the availability of biologic agents, randomized controlled trials demonstrated similar OS in patients with MBC comparing antiestrogens, AIs, progestins, estrogens, and androgens as well as surgical procedures, including oophorectomy, adrenalectomy, and hypophysectomy. Consequently, the choice of a particular endocrine therapy is based primarily on the mechanism of action, toxicity, and patient preference (Tables 128-9 and 128-10). Based on these criteria, tamoxifen is the preferred initial agent when metastases are present in a premenopausal woman except when the patient's cancer recurs at the same time or within 1 year of adjuvant tamoxifen therapy. In these cases, other agents are generally used. For postmenopausal women, the AIs are generally used first followed by other endocrine therapies upon progression.[61,145]

In postmenopausal and castrated women, the main source of estrogen is derived from the peripheral conversion of androstenedione, produced by the adrenal gland, into estrone and estradiol. This conversion requires the enzyme aromatase. Aromatase also catalyzes the conversion of androgens to estrogens in the ovary in premenopausal women and in extraglandular tissue, including the breast and breast cancer cells, in postmenopausal women. Therefore, AIs effectively reduce the levels of estrogens in circulation and in the target organ. Third-generation AIs available in the United States include anastrozole, letrozole, and exemestane. A major advantage of these specific compounds is their preferable toxicity profile, which consists mainly of bone loss and/or osteoporosis, mild nausea, hot flashes, arthralgias and/or myalgias, and mild fatigue. Anastrozole and letrozole are nonsteroidal compounds that exhibit reversible, competitive inhibition of aromatase. These are triazole compounds and have no intrinsic hormonal activity. Exemestane is a steroidal compound that binds irreversibly to aromatase, forming a covalent bond. Although this mechanism may have theoretical advantages to the reversible binding seen with the nonsteroidal agents, there is no clinical evidence that this drug is superior to other agents in this class. Exemestane does possess some androgenic properties at doses that are much higher than those used clinically and may have unique toxicities in some patients.[145]

Third-generation AIs have been compared with several other endocrine therapies since their approval. Although results are somewhat mixed, there appears to be at least equivalent activity seen with all three of the AIs compared with tamoxifen as first-line therapy and megestrol acetate as second-line therapy after progression on tamoxifen in postmenopausal women with positive or unknown hormone receptor status.[145] Compared with tamoxifen, there appears to be a lower incidence of thromboembolic events and vaginal bleeding in patients who received selective AIs. As second-line therapy after tamoxifen, more nausea, vomiting, and hot flashes are seen with the AIs and more weight gain, fluid retention, and thromboembolism with megestrol acetate. Although generally considered therapeutically equivalent, the use of a steroidal AI (exemestane) after a patient progresses on a nonsteroidal inhibitor (anastrozole or letrozole) may provide some benefit and is a common practice based on limited data. The opposite sequence also has shown some benefit; thus, patients may receive two AIs (first-line and second-line) sequentially, especially patients who progress while on adjuvant tamoxifen therapy.[61]

The AIs should only be used in postmenopausal women. Based on the available evidence, pre- or premenopausal women, whose ovaries are functioning, are inappropriate candidates for these therapies. Use of the AIs in addition to ovarian ablation (eg, oophorectomy or LHRH agonists) is appropriate and acceptable after progression on tamoxifen. Interestingly, the use of AIs in men with advanced breast cancer is controversial due to concerns that the pituitary feedback loop may be activated, increasing the levels of follicle-stimulating hormone, LH, and possibly testosterone. Therefore, although objective responses are seen with single-agent AI therapy in men with breast cancer, consensus has yet to be reached regarding the clinical utility of these agents in men, and some clinicians are investigating the combination of an LHRH agonist with an AI in this population.[146]

TABLE 128-9 Therapies Used for HR-Positive Metastatic Breast Cancer

Drug	Brand Name	Initial Dose	Usual Range	Special Population Dose	Comments
Aromatase Inhibitors: Nonsteroidal					
Anastrozole	Arimidex, generic	1 mg orally daily			
Letrozole	Femara, generic	2.5 mg orally daily		Caution in severe liver impairment[a]	
Aromatase Inhibitor: Steroidal					
Exemestane	Aromasin, generic	25 mg orally daily			Take after meals
Antiestrogens: SERMs					
Tamoxifen	Nolvadex, generic	20 mg orally daily		See text regarding *CYP2D6*	See text regarding *CYP2D6*
Toremifene	Fareston	60 mg orally daily			
Antiestrogen: SERD					
Fulvestrant	Faslodex	500 mg IM every 28 days (after loading days 1, 15, 29)	250-500 mg (see text for details)	Moderate liver impairment[a] administer 250 mg IM every 28 days (after loading days 1, 15, 29)	
LHRH Agonists					
Goserelin	Zoladex	3.6 mg SC every 28 days		Premenopausal women only	
Leuprolide	Lupron (IM), generic	3.75 mg IM every 28 days	Other formulations and doses are not used for breast cancer	Premenopausal women only	Not FDA approved for breast cancer; other formulations are administered differently
Triptorelin	Trelstar	3.75 mg IM every 28 days		Premenopausal women only	Not FDA-approved for breast cancer
Progestins					
Megestrol acetate	Megace, generic	40 mg orally 4 times a day	80 mg twice daily also appropriate		Absorption maybe increased when taken with food
Medroxyprogesterone	DepoProvera, generic	400 mg IM every week	400-1,000 mg IM every week	May need to decrease dose in severe liver impairment[a]	
Androgens					
Fluoxymesterone	Androxy, generic	10 mg orally twice a day	10-20/day in divided doses	Avoid in severe renal or liver impairment[a]	
Estrogens					
Ethinyl estradiol	Multiple generics	1 mg orally 3 times a day	Lower doses not effective	Avoid in jaundice or "marked" liver disease	Take with food
Conjugated estrogens	Premarin	2.5 mg orally 3 times a day	Lower doses not effective	Avoid in jaundice or "marked" liver disease	Take with food
Biologic/Targeted Therapies					
Everolimus (+ Exemestane)	Afinitor	10 mg orally daily	2.5-10 mg daily	Adjust dose in mild, moderate and severe liver impairment; also monitor for myelosuppression, hyperglycemia, dyslipidemia, renal dysfunction. May need to adjust dose with concomitant CYP3A4 inhibitors/inducers	Do not split tablets
Palbociclib (+ Letrozole or Fulvestrant)	Ibrance	125 mg orally daily × 21 days, followed by 7 days off, repeated every 28 days	75-125 mg daily	Adjust dose for myelosuppression. Avoid concomitant strong inhibitors of *CYP3A4* and moderate/severe inducers of *CYP3A4*	Do not split tablets

IM, intramuscular; LHRH, luteinizing hormone-releasing hormone; SC, subcutaneous; SERD, selective estrogen receptor downregulator SERM, selective estrogen receptor modulator.

[a]Severe liver impairment: Child-Pugh class C; moderate liver impairment: Child-Pugh class B; minor liver impairment: Child-Pugh class A.

TABLE 128-10 Drug Monitoring for Endocrine Therapies

Drug	Adverse Drug Reaction	Monitoring Parameters	Comments
Aromatase inhibitors	Hot flashes Arthralgias or myalgias Osteoporosis Hypercholesterolemia	Patient assessment BMD Lipid panel	Interval of monitoring controversial
Antiestrogens: SERMs[a]	Hot flashes Endometrial hyperplasia or cancer Venous thromboembolism Osteopenia (premenopausal women only)	Patient assessment Annual gynecologic assessment Consider BMD for premenopausal women	Routine transvaginal ultrasonography and endometrial biopsies are not recommended in the absence of symptoms
Antiestrogens: SERDs[a]	Hot flashes Injection-site reactions	Patient assessment	
LHRH agonists	Hot flashes Injection-site reactions Osteoporosis	Patient assessment BMD	
Progestins[a]	Weight gain Vaginal bleeding or spotting Nausea Venous thromboembolism	Patient assessment Periodic weights	
Androgens[a]	Hirsutism Acne Masculinization Increased hemoglobin Nausea Venous thromboembolism	Patient assessment Complete blood counts	
Estrogens[a]	Nausea or vomiting Venous and arterial thromboembolism Fluid retention Breast tenderness Endometrial hyperplasia or cancer	Patient assessment Annual gynecologic assessment	Routine transvaginal ultrasonography and endometrial biopsies are not recommended in the absence of symptoms

BMD, bone mineral density; LHRH, luteinizing hormone-releasing hormone; SERD, selective estrogen receptor downregulator; SERM, selective estrogen receptor modulator.

[a]Liver function tests obtained periodically to screen for changes in hepatic elimination, hepatotoxicity, and the presence of hepatic metastases.

Conducting clinical trials in this patient population is fraught with limitations, making evidence-based decisions very difficult.

Antiestrogens bind to ERs, which inhibit receptor-mediated gene transcription and therefore block the effect of estrogen on the end target. This class of agents is subdivided into two pharmacologic categories, SERMs and pure antiestrogens. SERMs include tamoxifen and toremifene (and raloxifene for breast cancer risk reduction in high-risk women) and demonstrate tissue-specific activity, both estrogenic and antiestrogenic, as described previously. The agonistic activity is thought to be responsible for many of the adverse reactions seen with these agents, including the increased risk of endometrial cancer, and has led to the development of pure ER antagonists that lack estrogen agonist activity. Pure antiestrogens are also referred to as selective estrogen receptor downregulators (SERDs). These molecules bind to ER, inhibit estrogen binding, and degrade the drug–ER complex, thus decreasing the amount of ER expressed. Fulvestrant is currently the only pure antiestrogen commercially available in the United States.

Tamoxifen is generally considered to be the antiestrogen of choice in premenopausal women with MBC who have hormone receptor–positive tumors. The toxicities of tamoxifen are described in the Adjuvant Endocrine Therapy section earlier. The only additional toxicity that may be observed in the setting of MBC (specifically bone metastases) is a tumor flare or hypercalcemia, which occurs in about 5% of patients after the initiation of any SERM therapy and is not an indication to discontinue the drug. It is generally accepted that this reaction is associated with response to endocrine therapy, but patients who do not experience such a reaction may still respond. This reaction is seen less frequently with the concurrent use of bisphosphonates as a result of their inhibition of osteoclasts, subsequently preventing the release of calcium from the bone.

Toremifene is another commercially available SERM for the treatment of breast cancer. It exhibits similar efficacy and tolerability compared with tamoxifen in the metastatic setting. Cross-resistance to toremifene has been demonstrated in patients with tamoxifen-refractory disease.[147] Thus, at the current time, toremifene appears to be an alternative to tamoxifen in postmenopausal patients with positive or unknown hormone receptor status with MBC. Details regarding its metabolism are becoming available, but a lack of robust clinical data to suggest it as an alternative to tamoxifen in settings where there are concerns regarding drug interactions leaves its role in therapy unclear at this time. Raloxifene, another SERM, was originally approved for prevention of osteoporosis in postmenopausal women. Available data with raloxifene as a treatment for breast cancer show very low response rates and no significant clinical benefit. Consequently, use of this agent for breast cancer treatment should be discouraged. The use of raloxifene for breast cancer risk reduction in high-risk postmenopausal women has been reported (see Prevention and Early Detection).

Fulvestrant is approved for the second-line therapy of postmenopausal MBC patients with hormone receptor–positive tumors. Biologically, fulvestrant should produce similar outcomes in premenopausal women, but no data exist to confirm the safety or efficacy in premenopausal women in the presence of active ovarian function. In conjunction with ovarian suppression or ablation, fulvestrant is an appropriate therapy in young women. It is unique in that it is given as an intramuscular injection and the dosing of fulvestrant has been controversial. Many comparative studies used what is now thought to be an insufficient dose; therefore, its place in therapy is not clearly defined.

Studies have compared fulvestrant with anastrozole, exemestane, and tamoxifen in the treatment of postmenopausal women with MBC with varying results. Initially, comparative trials with fulvestrant and an AI (anastrozole or exemestane) demonstrated similar efficacy and safety when given after patients progressed on tamoxifen therapy.[145] When compared directly with tamoxifen as first-line therapy, fulvestrant appeared to be less effective than tamoxifen. Subsequent data confirm that the appropriate dose of fulvestrant for MBC should be 500 mg intramuscularly administered every 2 weeks for 3 doses (days 1, 15, and 29) followed by administration every 28 days. This loading approach to dosing facilitates reaching steady-state plasma levels more rapidly, allowing for a response to be seen within a clinically relevant time frame. A randomized, phase II study comparing this fulvestrant dosing strategy with anastrozole in postmenopausal women with hormone receptor–positive MBC demonstrated superior TTP and OS with fulvestrant with similar objective responses seen with subsequent hormone therapy administered to both groups.[148] Although the power of this phase II study is limited, it is encouraging to better understand how dosing may impact response with this novel endocrine agent. To accomplish this dosing, two intramuscular injections of 5 mL each are administered simultaneously. Although cumbersome and slightly more uncomfortable, patients appear to tolerate this higher dose relatively well, exhibiting similar toxicity profiles regardless of the dose administered.

Combining therapy with anastrozole and fulvestrant has been investigated in three randomized phase III trials with conflicting results. Although the combination does appear to be well tolerated, the overall benefits (if any) appear to be modest, and sequential single agents are most commonly administered in the palliative setting of metastatic disease. Adverse events related to fulvestrant include injection-site reactions, hot flashes, asthenia, and headaches.[61]

Another goal of endocrine therapy in premenopausal women is to reduce estrogen production with surgery, radiation, or medication. Ovarian ablation (surgically or chemically) is still commonly used in some parts of the United States and is considered by many specialists to be the endocrine therapy of choice in premenopausal women. The mortality rate with surgical oophorectomy is low, usually less than 3% in appropriately selected patients. While radiotherapeutic ablation of the ovaries is effective, this approach is typically not used in the United States. Chemical castration with LHRH analogs is increasingly used instead of oophorectomy in premenopausal women. Because effects with the LHRH analogs are reversible, use of these agents may also be used to determine how a patient will tolerate estrogen deprivation. If the patient tolerates this therapy, then an oophorectomy may be proposed as a permanent therapeutic intervention.

Medical castration with LHRH analogs induces responses in about one third of unselected premenopausal MBC cases. This is accomplished through downregulation of LHRH receptors in the pituitary, decreasing levels of LH, which subsequently lead to a decrease in circulating estrogen to castrated levels. Thus, the effect of LHRH analogs on circulating estrogen levels in premenopausal breast cancer simulates an oophorectomy. The three agents available and used in the United States are leuprolide, goserelin, and triptorelin, but only goserelin is FDA-approved for the treatment of MBC. These agents are administered as an injection every 4 weeks (all products have extended formulations, lasting 3 months to 1 year, but they are not recommended for the treatment of breast cancer) and are associated with minimal side effects, including amenorrhea, bone loss or osteoporosis, hot flashes, and occasional nausea (Table 128-10). LHRH analogs may also produce a flare response because of an initial surge in luteinizing hormone (LH) and estrogen production lasting 2 to 4 weeks. This flare response is similar to that seen with tamoxifen, and patients with high-volume, bulky disease should be monitored for increasing pain and hypercalcemia during the initiation period. Combining LHRH analogs with tamoxifen or an AI has been investigated with varying results. In order to safely administer AIs to premenopausal women, the ovarian function must be suppressed or ablated. The question remains as to whether the combination of an LHRH analog and an AI is superior to tamoxifen alone. Both approaches to therapy are appropriate to consider. Combining an LHRH analog with tamoxifen remains controversial, although some data in ESBC indicate a benefit may exist. This also would be an appropriate consideration in a young, premenopausal woman.[61]

Other endocrine therapies that have data to support their use in MBC include the progestins (such as megestrol acetate and medroxyprogesterone acetate), high-dose estrogens (such as ethinyl estradiol) and high-dose androgens (fluoxymesterone). Typically, these agents are less well tolerated than more contemporary agents discussed previously. The most common side effect of megestrol acetate is weight gain, occurring in 20% to 50% of patients. Other side effects associated with progestins include vaginal bleeding in 5% to 10% of patients, either while taking the progestational agent or when it is discontinued, and less than a 10% incidence of hot flashes. Thromboembolic complications are also associated with these agents.[149] About one-third of patients placed on high-dose estrogens will discontinue them because of side effects, the most important of which are thromboembolic events, vomiting, and fluid retention. Less common side effects include areolar hyperpigmentation, breast tenderness and engorgement, vaginal discharge, incontinence, hot flashes, and phlebitis. All of the effective androgens cause masculinizing effects, including hirsutism and acne, in more than 50% of patients. The mechanism by which these agents exert a therapeutic effect in breast cancer is unknown. However, these agents may inhibit aromatase, among other pharmacologic effects that antagonize estrogen.

Cytotoxic Therapy

10 The vast majority of MBC are devoid of *HER2*-overexpression and represent one of the most prevalent cancer problems facing the developing world. Investigators continue to look for acceptable targets and innovative approaches to treating this group of cancers. For hormone receptor-positive MBC, endocrine therapy should be considered first-line as stated previously. Hormone-receptor-positive tumors that fail to respond to initial endocrine therapy or become refractory to endocrine therapy, require chemotherapy. Patients with triple negative tumors require chemotherapy as initial therapy of metastases. Overall, this group of patients represents a minority population, but has a relatively poor prognosis. Therefore, cytotoxic chemotherapy is eventually required in most patients with MBC and this is an area of much needed innovation.[92]

Combination chemotherapy results in an objective response in approximately 50% to 60% of unselected, chemotherapy-naive patients. The clinical use of biomarkers and genetic panels as a means to make clinical cancer treatment decisions is relative new. In MBC the large body of evidence superseding these types of data remains informative. In the absence of a clear predictive marker, the choice of chemotherapy is chosen based on overall efficacy, but also on the prevalence of toxicity, performance status and presence of comorbidities in the patient, pace of disease (eg, indolent vs visceral crisis), and patient preferences in terms of schedules, dosing route (eg, oral versus intravenous), and frequency (eg, weekly vs every 3 weeks) of the chemotherapy. Therefore, an optimal first-line or later-line chemotherapy choice varies between patients.

While response rates are high with combination chemotherapy, sequential use of single-agent therapies utilized in succession is also an effective strategy that may be preferred due to decreased rates of adverse events. In the palliative setting, when efficacy is similar, the least toxic approach is preferred. In clinical practice, patients who require a rapid response (eg, those with symptomatic bulky metastases or a visceral crisis) may benefit from combination chemotherapy despite the added toxicity. This decision is complex and should be made on an individual patient basis.

Most patients experience partial responses to chemotherapy, but complete disappearance of disease occurs in fewer than 10% of patients treated. The median duration of response is highly variable, ranging from 5 to 18 months. Some patients with small volume metastatic disease will have an excellent response to an initial course of chemotherapy and may live 5 to 10 years or longer without evidence of disease. The median OS for patients after commonly used chemotherapy combinations ranges between 14 and 33 months. The median time to response ranges from 2 to 3 months in most studies, but this period depends on the site of measurable disease and can range from 3 weeks (skin and lymph node metastases) to 18 weeks (bone metastases). After a chemotherapy regimen has been initiated, it is usually continued until there is unequivocal evidence of progressive disease or intolerable side effects. Table 128-11 lists some selected chemotherapy agents used in the metastatic setting.[150]

Factors associated with an increased likelihood of response to chemotherapy include a good performance status, a limited number (one to two) of disease sites (or involved organ systems), and a prolonged previous response to chemotherapy or hormonal therapy (ie, long disease-free interval). Patients who have progressive disease during chemotherapy have a lower likelihood of response to a subsequent chemotherapy. However, this is not necessarily true for patients who are given chemotherapy after a treatment-free interval of substantial duration (eg, more than 1 year). Treatments may be repeated if some time has passed between therapies, but this is rarely done because of the large number of agents now available to treat breast cancer. Hormone receptor–positive tumors that are resistant to endocrine therapy are as likely to respond to chemotherapy as patients who receive upfront chemotherapy. Age, menopausal status, and receptor status do not appear to be directly associated with response to chemotherapy. However, there continues to be much debate surrounding the potential association between hormone receptor status and response to chemotherapy (eg, ER status and anthracyclines). Most clinical decisions regarding chemotherapy are not currently influenced by hormone-receptor status. Molecular tumor subtypes (eg, luminal A, luminal B, etc.) have not been extremely helpful in selecting an optimal chemotherapy regimen. TNBC is an aggressive phenotype associated with a poor prognosis. These cancers have variable responses to chemotherapy, although many of them have high chemosensitivity. Unfortunately, TNBCs have a high chance of brain metastases and shorter survival after a first metastatic event compared with other subtypes. TNBC is strongly associated with germline mutations in the BRCA-1 gene and this potentially leads to increased sensitivity to platinum agents due to lack of intact DNA repair mechanisms. Clinical implications of this mutation are being tested now, but many clinicians may add a platinum agent to the chemotherapy regimen in some patients with a BRCA-1 germline mutation.[92]

A number of chemotherapeutic agents have demonstrated activity in the treatment of breast cancer, including doxorubicin (conventional and liposomal), epirubicin, paclitaxel (conventional and protein bound), docetaxel, capecitabine, fluorouracil, cyclophosphamide, methotrexate, vinblastine, vinorelbine, gemcitabine, ixabepilone, eribulin, carboplatin, cisplatin, mitoxantrone, mitomycin C, thiotepa, and melphalan. The most active classes of chemotherapy in MBC are the anthracyclines and the taxanes, producing response rates as high as 50% to 60% in patients who have not received prior chemotherapy for metastatic disease.[150] Doxorubicin (conventional and liposomal) and epirubicin have demonstrated significant efficacy in the metastatic setting and are generally considered therapeutically equivalent when dosed appropriately. Administration of these agents is limited by their cumulative cardiotoxicity. Paclitaxel, docetaxel, and protein-bound paclitaxel are also FDA-approved for the treatment of MBC and are generally considered therapeutically equivalent, yet lack complete cross-resistance. Taxane administration is limited by cumulative peripheral neuropathy. Most patients will likely receive each of these agents at some point in the course of their MBC.

An increasing number of patients diagnosed with MBC have been exposed to adjuvant chemotherapy consisting of an anthracycline and a taxane. If metastases are found within 6 to 12 months of completing treatment with these agents, many clinicians will choose treatment from a different chemotherapy class. If it has been longer since their adjuvant therapy, then retreating with the same agents may be considered. However, given the cardiotoxicity associated with the anthracyclines, the use of these agents in the metastatic setting has been generally avoided until the availability of liposomal anthracyclines. Pegylated liposomal doxorubicin is associated with less cardiotoxicity and similar efficacy compared with conventional doxorubicin and is a viable option for women who recur more than 1 year after their adjuvant anthracycline regimen.[150]

Weekly administration of paclitaxel and protein-bound paclitaxel results in higher response rates, TTP, and survival in addition to a more favorable side effect profile compared with administration every 3 weeks.[150] The most useful weekly dose of conventional paclitaxel in the metastatic setting appears to be 80 mg/m^2/wk with no breaks in therapy. With this approach, the toxicity profile of paclitaxel changes with less myelosuppression and delayed onset of peripheral neuropathy but slightly more fluid retention and skin and nail changes. Although the incidence of hypersensitivity reactions is also slightly less at these lower doses (requiring fewer premedications), it remains at about 3% despite incorporation of all available preventive measures. There is currently debate regarding the most appropriate weekly dose of protein-bound paclitaxel in the metastatic setting. Doses of 100 to 150 mg/m^2/wk administered on days 1, 8, and 15 of a 28-day cycle have been investigated, demonstrating some evidence of a dose–response relationship. In the metastatic palliative setting, a lower dose is generally chosen, minimizing toxicity while not significantly compromising efficacy. Docetaxel is most appropriately dosed on an every-3-week schedule for MBC. Weekly dosing did not produce improvements in disease response and was associated with significantly more toxicities than the every-3-week dosing strategy.

After patients have been treated with an anthracycline and a taxane, single-agent capecitabine, vinorelbine, or gemcitabine have resulted in response rates of 20% to 25%.[150] Of these agents, only capecitabine is FDA approved as a single agent for MBC. Gemcitabine is only FDA-approved in combination with paclitaxel for MBC. However, all of these are included in most national and international guidelines as appropriate therapy for MBC. Decisions regarding which agent to choose are based on patient characteristics, expected toxicities, and previous exposure to chemotherapy.

Other antimicrotubule agents have also been approved for the management of MBC, demonstrating significant benefits in patients who have had prior exposure to multiple other chemotherapy agents. Ixabepilone is an epothilone compound with a similar but distinct mechanism of action from the taxanes, binding to β-microtubulin in a unique manner but ultimately leading to microtubule stabilization and cell death in a similar manner compared with the taxanes. It is approved for use in combination with capecitabine and as a single agent for the management of MBC. Eribulin is another antimicrotubule agent with a unique mechanism of action. The first synthetic analogue of halochondrin B, eribulin effectively inhibits polymerization of tubulin into microtubules and suppresses the microtubule growth phase similar to the vinca alkaloids. The mechanism of eribulin's antitumor efficacy differs from the vinca alkaloids in that eribulin does not appear to have any effect on the microtubule shortening phase. These subtle differences are thought to be important for eribulin's efficacy in patients who have been exposed to multiple therapies, including other antimicrotubule agents. It is approved for use as a single agent for the management of MBC patients who

TABLE 128-11 Selected Chemotherapy Regimens for *HER2*-Negative Metastatic Breast Cancer

Single-Agent Chemotherapy	
Paclitaxel[a,b] Paclitaxel 175 mg/m² IV over 3 hours Repeat cycles every 21 days *or* Paclitaxel 80 mg/m²/wk IV over 1 hour Repeat dose every 7 days	**Vinorelbine**[c] Vinorelbine 30 mg/m² IV, days 1 and 8 Repeat cycles every 21 days *or* Vinorelbine 25-30 mg/m²/wk IV Repeat cycles every 7 days (adjust dose based on absolute neutrophil count; see product information)
Docetaxel[d,e] Docetaxel 60-100 mg/m² IV over 1 hour Repeat cycles every 21 days *or* Docetaxel 30-35 mg/m²/wk IV over 30 minutes Repeat dose every 7 days	**Gemcitabine**[f] Gemcitabine 600-1,000 mg/m²/wk IV, days 1, 8, and 15 Repeat cycles every 28 days (may need to hold day 15 dose based on blood counts)q
	Ixabepilone[i] Ixabepilone 40 mg/m² IV over 3 hours Repeat cycles every 21 days
Protein-Bound Paclitaxel[g,h] Protein-bound Paclitaxel 260 mg/m² IV over 30 minutes Repeat cycles every 21 days *or* Protein-bound paclitaxel 100-150 mg/m² IV over 30 minutes on days 1, 8, and 15 Repeat cycle every 28 days	
	Eribulin[k] Eribulin 1.4 mg/m²/dose IV over 2-5 minutes on days 1 and 8 Repeat dose every 21 days
	Liposomal Doxorubicin[l] Liposomal doxorubicin 30-50 mg/m² IV over variable duration Repeat cycles every 28 days
Capecitabine[j] Capecitabine 2,000-2,500 mg/m² per day orally, divided twice daily for 14 days Repeat cycles every 21 days	
Combination Chemotherapy Regimens	
Gemcitabine + Carboplatin[m] Gemcitabine 1,000 mg/m² IV, days 1 & 8 Carboplatin AUC 2 IV, day 1 & 8 Repeat cycles every 21 days	**Paclitaxel + Gemcitabine**[n] Paclitaxel 175 mg/m² IV over 3 hours, day 1 Gemcitabine 1,250 mg/m² IV days 1 and 8 Repeat cycles every 21 days
Ixabepilone + Capecitabine[i] Ixabepilone 40 mg/m² IV over 3 hours, day 1 Capecitabine 1,750-2,000 mg/m²/day orally divided twice daily for 14 days Repeat cycles every 21 days	**Paclitaxel + Bevacizumab**[o] Paclitaxel 90 mg/m² IV over 1 hour, days 1, 8, and 15 Bevacizumab 10 mg/kg IV over 30-90 minutes, days 1 and 15 Repeat cycles every 28 days

[a]From Taxol (paclitaxel) product information. Princeton, NJ: Bristol-Myers Squibb, July 2007.

[b]From Perez EA, Vogelci, Irwin DH, et al. Multicenter phase II trial of weekly paclitaxel in women with metastatic breast cancer. *Clin Oncol* 2001;19:4216.

[c]From Zelek L, Bartheir S, Riofrio M, et al. Weekly vinorelbine is an effective palliative regimen after failure with anthracyclines and taxanes in metastatic breast carcinoma. *Cancer* 2001;92:2267.

[d]From Taxotere (docetaxel) product information. *Bridgewater*, NJ: Sanofi-Aventis, 2008.

[e]From Hainsworth JD, Burris HA 3rd, Erlaud JB, et al. Phase I trial of docetaxel administered by weekly infusion in patients with advanced refractory cancer. *J Clin Oncol* 1998;16:2164.

[f]From Carmichael J, Possinger K, Philip P, et al. Advanced breast cancer: a phase II trial with gemcitabine. *J Clin Oncol* 1995;13:2731.

[g]From Abraxane (paclitaxel protein-bound particles for injectable suspension) product information. *Bridgewater*, NJ: Abraxis Bioscience, September 2009.

[h]From Gradishar WJ, Krasnojon D, Cheporov S, et al. Significantly longer progression-free survival with nab-paclitaxel compared with docetaxel as first-line therapy for metastatic breast cancer. *J Clin Oncol* 2009;27:3611-3619.

[i]From Boehnke Michaud L. The optimal therapeutic use of ixabepilone in patients with locally advanced or metastatic breast cancer. *J Oncol Pharm Pract* 2009;15(2):95-106.

[j]From Gralow, JR. Optimizing the treatment of metastatic breast cancer. *Breast Cancer Res Treat* 2005;89(Suppl 1):S9-S15.

[k]From Halaven (eribulin) product information. *Woodcliff Lake*, NJ: Eisai Inc., February 2012.

[l]From O'Brien ME, Wigler N, Inbar M, et al. Reduced cardiotoxicity and comparable efficacy in a phase III trial of pegylated liposomal doxorubicin HCl (CAELYX/Doxil) versus conventional doxorubicin for first-line treatment of metastatic breast cancer. *Ann Oncol* 2004;15(3):440-449.

[m]From O'Shaughnessy J, Schwartzberg LS, Danso MA, et al. A randomized phase III study of iniparib (BSI-201) in combination with gemcitabine/carboplatin (G/C) in metastatic triple-negative breast cancer (TNBC). [abstract]. *J Clin Oncol* 2011;29(Suppl 15):Abstract 1007.

[n]From Gemzar (gemcitabine) product information. *Indianapolis*, IN: Eli Lilly and Co, May 2007.

[o]From Miller K, Wang M, Gralow J, et al. Paclitaxel plus bevacizumab versus paclitaxel alone for metastatic breast cancer. *N Engl J Med* 2007;357(26):2666-2676.

have received at least two prior chemotherapies for their metastatic disease.[150]

Both of these agents are associated with similar toxicities compared with the taxanes and vinca alkaloids, respectively (eg, myelosuppression, neuropathy, myalgias or arthralgias, alopecia, and skin and nail changes with ixabepilone and myelosuppression and neuropathy with eribulin). Hypersensitivity is occasionally seen with ixabepilone because it is also solubilized in Cremophor-EL, the likely causative agent in paclitaxel-associated hypersensitivity. However, eribulin has not been associated with hypersensitivity reactions and is not formulated in a complex solvent system that may predispose patients to allergic-type reactions. Neuropathy may become problematic in patients who have received numerous sequential neurotoxic chemotherapy agents; therefore, careful monitoring of the impact on quality of life is imperative because these therapies are administered in a palliative setting. Ongoing clinical trials are investigating these agents in other combinations and in earlier stages of the disease, and these results are eagerly awaited.[150]

Radiation Therapy

Radiation is an important modality in the treatment of symptomatic metastatic disease. The most common indication for treatment with radiation therapy is painful bone metastases or other localized sites of disease refractory to systemic therapy. Radiation therapy provides significant pain relief to about 90% of patients who are treated for painful bone metastases. Radiation is also an important modality in the palliative treatment of metastatic brain lesions and spinal cord lesions, which respond poorly to systemic therapy, as well as eye or orbit lesions and other sites where significant accumulation of tumor cells occurs. Skin and lymph node metastases confined to the chest wall area may also be treated with radiation therapy for palliation (eg, open wounds or painful lesions). Chemotherapy may also be added to radiation for sensitization purposes.

PERSONALIZED PHARMACOTHERAPY

Personalized pharmacotherapy is a very broad term that includes many old and new scientific approaches to predict which patients should be treated, how they should be treated, and their likelihood of response or toxicity to treatment. These approaches may be focused on the tumor(s) itself or on patient or host factors. Breast cancer clinicians have been using these approaches to therapeutic decisions for decades and continue to search for novel characteristics to further individualize the choice of therapies.

Most scientific studies in breast cancer focus on tumor-specific markers either individually or as a panel of markers. Since the mid-1970s, clinicians have been using biomarkers to individualize therapy for patients with breast cancer. Initially, the tumor's ER or PR status was used to determine whether endocrine therapy (starting with tamoxifen) would benefit patients with MBC. Although these data have been widely available for many years, ER and PR testing in all breast cancers worldwide has been a relatively new phenomenon. Other biomarkers have been developed over the decades, with *HER2* being the most widely accepted alternate marker for breast cancer. *HER2* was initially studied as a prognostic biomarker in an attempt to ascertain an individual patient's risk of breast cancer recurrence and chemotherapy sensitivity or resistance. Although these applications of *HER2* testing remain controversial, the use of *HER2* testing to establish the likelihood of response or benefit to anti-*HER2* therapies is well established and required for all breast tumors at diagnosis. (See the Adjuvant Systemic Therapy section.)

It is clear from these individual biomarker studies that breast cancers are very heterogeneous, and interaction among markers is also important. Incorporation of multiple markers into biomathematical formulas that predict the likelihood of recurrence of cancer have been developed and are used across the United States to assist clinicians and patients in making informed decisions regarding adjuvant systemic therapy (eg, Adjuvant! Online). These predictive formulas are useful but do not incorporate several markers that have since been validated individually (eg, *HER2*, Ki-67, LVI). Genetic panels such as Oncotype DX, Mammaprint, and PAM50 were developed to screen for and quantify multiple genetic markers in tumor cells and are used as prognostic biomarkers to determine the risk of recurrence in early-stage breast cancer patients. The exact role these genetic panels will play in treatment decisions in the future is uncertain, but scientists and clinicians have embraced the technology, and the copious amounts of data collected from these analyses are being analyzed and incorporated into clinical trials and new standards every day.

Although these are all examples of tools that are used to individualize or personalize pharmacotherapy, very few markers are currently used clinically to represent host or patient differences. One promising area of research is in pharmacogenomics related to drug pharmacokinetics or pharmacodynamics. Results from studies with tamoxifen and CYP2D6 genotyping have been mixed, which is probably related to the complex metabolism of tamoxifen and large number of other prognostic factors (see the Adjuvant Endocrine Therapy section). Throughout this chapter are examples of characteristics that are used to individualize therapy. As more research is done in this field, the amount of tools available to clinicians to assist with treatment decisions will expand greatly.

EVALUATION OF THERAPEUTIC OUTCOMES

The desired therapeutic outcome of adjuvant therapy of breast cancer differs significantly from that of metastatic disease. Adjuvant therapy—chemotherapy, biologic therapy, and hormonal therapy—is administered with curative intent. The rationale for adjuvant therapy is that breast cancer, even when diagnosed in early stages when clinical evidence of distant spread is not apparent, is a systemic disease that spreads early to distant sites. Adjuvant therapy is intended to eradicate micrometastases and thus cure the patient of breast cancer. Therefore, the overall goal of adjuvant therapy is to cure the disease, which is something that cannot be fully evaluated for years after initial diagnosis and treatment. In addition, because disease cannot be detected at the time adjuvant therapy is started, assessment of disease response is not possible. Instead, a predetermined number of cycles of adjuvant therapy or years of biologic or hormonal therapy are administered. Adjuvant chemotherapy is often associated with significant toxicity. Maintaining dose intensity has been demonstrated to be important in the cure of disease, and therefore optimizing supportive care measures such as antiemetics and growth factors is highly recommended. The concept of dose density, using growth factors to maintain blood counts while decreasing the interval between chemotherapy administrations, is very controversial in the management of early-stage breast cancer. Multiple studies investigating this approach to adjuvant chemotherapy have been conducted with conflicting results and many more trials continue to be analyzed in hopes of determining the long-term outcomes related to this approach to therapy. The goals of therapy with neoadjuvant chemotherapy are slightly different. These goals focus on earlier end points of tumor response so as to minimize surgery, determine prognosis, and potentially conserve the breast tissue for a better cosmetic result. The other outcomes discussed with adjuvant therapy also apply to this scenario in terms of improving survival and decreasing recurrences compared with no systemic therapy.

Palliation is the therapeutic outcome in treatment of MBC. Optimizing benefits and minimizing toxicity are general therapeutic goals of any therapy administered in this setting. Therefore, sequential single agents are often chosen over combination regimens, but individual circumstances may call for more rapid responses in which combination therapy may be indicated. Tumor response to a particular treatment regimen may be measured by changes in laboratory tests, diagnostic imaging, or physical signs or symptoms. Periodic testing is clinically useful in some circumstances, but careful interpretation of results is required. If a patient is tolerating therapy well, clear evidence of disease progression on imaging or physical examination is required to warrant changing therapy. Unless the patient clearly cannot tolerate the regimen or the cancer is clearly progressing at a rate that will quickly cause symptoms (or is causing symptoms already), there is not a sound reason to change therapy. Optimizing quality of life is an important therapeutic end point in the treatment of patients with MBC. A number of valid and reliable tools are available for objective assessment of quality of life in patients with breast cancer.

ABBREVIATIONS

ACS	American Cancer Society
AI	aromatase inhibitor
AJCC	American Joint Committee for Cancer
ALND	axillary lymph node dissection
ASCO	American Society of Clinical Oncology
BCT	breast-conserving therapy
BIG	Breast International Group
BMI	body mass index
BSE	breast self-examination
CALGB	Cancer and Leukemia Group B
CBE	clinical breast examination
CDK	cyclin-dependent kinases
CI	confidence interval
CMF	cyclophosphamide, methotrexate, fluorouracil (regimen)
CNS	central nervous system
CYP	cytochrome P450 enzyme
DCIS	ductal carcinoma in situ
DFS	disease-free survival
DVT	deep-vein thrombosis
EBCTCG	Early Breast Cancer Trialists' Collaborative Group
EGFR	epidermal growth factor receptor; also known as HER1
ER	estrogen receptor
ESBC	early stage breast cancer
ESMO	European Society of Medical Oncology
FDA	Food and Drug Administration
FISH	fluorescence in situ hybridization
HER2	human epidermal growth factor receptor-2
HR	hazard ratio
HRT	hormone replacement therapy
IBC	inflammatory breast cancer
IHC	immunohistochemistry
LCIS	lobular carcinoma in situ
LH	luteinizing hormone
LHRH	luteinizing hormone–releasing hormone
LVI	lymphatic and vascular invasion
MBC	metastatic breast cancer
MINDACT	Microarray In Node-negative Disease may Avoid ChemoTherapy
MoAB	Monoclonal antibody
MRI	magnetic resonance imaging
mTOR	mammalian target of rapamycin
NCCN	National Comprehensive Cancer Network
NCI	National Cancer Institute
NNI	number needed to invite for screening to extend one woman's life
NSABP	National Surgical Adjuvant Breast and Bowel Project
OR	odds ratio
OS	overall survival
PARP	poly-ADP ribose polymerase
pCR	pathologic complete response
PFS	progression-free survival
PI3K	phosphatidylinositol 3-kinase
PR	progesterone receptor
RR	relative risk
SEER	Surveillance, Epidemiology, and End Results
SERD	selective estrogen receptor downregulator
SERM	selective estrogen receptor modulators
SLNB	sentinel lymph node biopsy
STAR	Study of Tamoxifen and Raloxifene
TTP	Time to progression
TKI	tyrosine kinase inhibitor
TNBC	triple negative breast cancer
USPSTF	United States Preventive Services Task Force
VEGF	vascular endothelial growth factor
WHI	Women's Health Initiative

REFERENCES

1. Siegel R, Miller K and Jemal A. Cancer statistics, 2016. *CA Cancer J Clin* 2016;66:7-30.
2. American Cancer Society. Cancer Facts & Figures 2015. Atlanta: *American Cancer Society*; 2015.
3. Howlader N, Noone AM, Krapcho M, et al., eds. SEER Cancer Statistics Review, 1975-2012, National Cancer Institute. Bethesda, MD, http://seer.cancer.gov/csr/1975_2012/, based on November 2014 SEER data submission, posted to the SEER web site, April 2015.
4. Korde LA, Zujewski JA, Kamin L, et al. Multidisciplinary meeting on male breast cancer: summary and research recommendations. *J Clin Oncol* 2010;28:2114-2122.
5. Fay MP, Pfeiffer R, Cronin KA, et al. Age-conditional probabilities of developing cancer. *Stat Med* 2003;22:1837-1848.
6. Gail MH, Costantino JP, Pee D, et al. Projecting individualized absolute invasive breast cancer risk in African American women. *J Natl Cancer Inst* 2007;99:1782-1792.
7. Collaborative Group on Hormonal Factors in Breast Cancer. Menarche, menopause, and breast cancer risk: individual participant meta-analysis, including 118 964 women with breast cancer from 117 epidemiological studies. *Lancet Oncol* 2012;13:1141-1151.
8. Clemons M and Goss P. Estrogen and the risk of breast cancer. *N Engl J Med* 2001;344:276-285.
9. Rossouw JE, Anderson GL, Prentice RL, et al. Risks and benefits of estrogen plus progestin in healthy postmenopausal women: principal results from the Women's Health Initiative randomized controlled trial. *JAMA* 2002;288:321-333.
10. Ravdin PM, Cronin KA, Howlader N, et al. The decrease in breast-cancer incidence in 2003 in the United States. *N Engl J Med* 2007;356:1670-1674.
11. Chlebowski RT, Kuller LH, Prentice RL, et al. Breast cancer after use of estrogen plus progestin in postmenopausal women. *N Engl J Med* 2009;360:573-587.
12. Anderson GL, Limacher M, Assaf AR, et al. Effects of conjugated equine estrogen in postmenopausal women with hysterectomy:

the Women's Health Initiative randomized controlled trial. *JAMA* 2004;291:1701-1712.

13. Anderson GL, Chlebowski RT, Aragaki AK, et al. Conjugated equine oestrogen and breast cancer incidence and mortality in postmenopausal women with hysterectomy: extended follow-up of the Women's Health Initiative randomised placebo-controlled trial. *Lancet Oncol* 2012;13:476-486.
14. Hou N, Hong S, Wang W, et al. Hormone replacement therapy and breast cancer: heterogeneous risks by race, weight, and breast density. *J Natl Cancer Inst* 2013;105:1365-1372.
15. Zhu H, Lei X, Feng J, Wang Y. Oral contraceptive use and risk of breast cancer: a meta-analysis of prospective cohort studies. *Eur J Contracept Reprod Health Care* 2012;17:402-414.
16. Hartmann LC, Degnim AC, Santen RJ, et al. Atypical hyperplasia of the breast—risk assessment and management options. *N Engl J Med* 2015;372:78-89.
17. Pettersson A, Graff RE, Ursin G, et al. Mammographic density phenotypes and risk of breast cancer: a meta-analysis. *J Natl Cancer Inst* 2014;106:dju078. doi:10.1093/jnci/dju078.
18. Collaborative Group on Hormonal Factors in Breast Cancer. Familial breast cancer: collaborative reanalysis of individual data from 52 epidemiological studies including 58,209 women with breast cancer and 101,986 women without the disease. *Lancet* 2001;358:1389-1399.
19. Chen S and Parmigiani G. Meta-analysis of BRCA1 and BRCA2 penetrance. *J Clin Oncol* 2007;25:1329-1333.
20. Moyer VA. Risk assessment, genetic counseling, and genetic testing for BRCA-related cancer in women: U.S. Preventive Services Task Force recommendation statement. *Ann Intern Med* 2014;160:271-281.
21. Robson ME, Bradbury AR, Arun B, et al. American Society of Clinical Oncology Policy Statement Update: Genetic and Genomic Testing for Cancer Susceptibility. *J Clin Oncol* 2015;33:3660-3667.
22. NCCN Clinical Practice Guidelines in Oncology (NCCN Guidelines®) for Genetic/Familial High-Risk Assessment: *Breast and Ovarian* V.2.2015© National Comprehensive Cancer Network, Inc 2015. All rights reserved. Last accessed, September 1, 2015.
23. Lerner-Ellis J, Khalouei S, Sopik V, Narod SA. Genetic risk assessment and prevention: the role of genetic testing panels in breast cancer. *Expert Rev Anticancer Ther* 2015;15:1315-1326.
24. Velie EM, Nechuta S, Osuch JR. Lifetime reproductive and anthropometric risk factors for breast cancer in postmenopausal women. *Breast Dis* 2005;24:17-35.
25. Boyd NF, Stone J, Vogt RN, et al. Dietary fat and breast cancer risk revisited: a meta-analysis of the published literature. *Br J Cancer* 2003;89:1672-1685.
26. Prentice RL, Caan B, Chlebowski RT, et al. Low-fat dietary pattern and risk of invasive breast cancer: the Women's Health Initiative Randomized Controlled Dietary Modification Trial. *JAMA* 2006;295:629-642.
27. Thomson CA. Diet and breast cancer: understanding risks and benefits. *Nutr Clin Pract* 2012;27:636-650.
28. Velentzis LS, Cantwell MM, Cardwell C, et al. Lignans and breast cancer risk in pre- and post-menopausal women: meta-analyses of observational studies. *Br J Cancer* 2009;100:1492-1498.
29. Velentzis LS, Woodside JV, Cantwell MM, et al. Do phytoestrogens reduce the risk of breast cancer and breast cancer recurrence? What clinicians need to know. *Eur J Cancer* 2008;44:1799-1806.
30. Renehan AG, Tyson M, Egger M, et al. Body-mass index and incidence of cancer: a systematic review and meta-analysis of prospective observational studies. *Lancet* 2008;371:569-578.
31. Goncalves AK, Dantas Florencio GL, Maisonnette de Atayde Silva MJ, et al. Effects of physical activity on breast cancer prevention: a systematic review. *J Phys Act Health* 2014;11:445-454.
32. McDonald JA, Goyal A, Terry MB. Alcohol Intake and Breast Cancer Risk: Weighing the Overall Evidence. *Curr Breast Cancer Rep* 2013;5:208-221.
33. Ronckers CM, Erdmann CA, Land CE. Radiation and breast cancer: a review of current evidence. *Breast Cancer Res* 2005;7:21-32.
34. Glantz SA, Johnson KC. The surgeon general report on smoking and health 50 years later: breast cancer and the cost of increasing caution. *Cancer Epidemiol Biomarkers Prev* 2014;23:37-46.
35. U.S. Department of Health and Human Services. The Health Consequences of Smoking: 50 Years of Progress. A Report of the Surgeon General. Atlanta: U.S. Department of Health and Human Services, Centers for Disease Control and Prevention, National Center for Chronic Disease Prevention and Health Promotion, Office on Smoking and Health, 2014.
36. Early Breast Cancer Trialists' Collaborative Group (EBCTCG), Davies C, Godwin J, Gray R, et al. Relevance of breast cancer hormone receptors and other factors to the efficacy of adjuvant tamoxifen: patient-level meta-analysis of randomised trials. *Lancet* 2011;378:771-784.
37. Fisher B, Costatino JP, Wickerham DL, et al. Tamoxifen for prevention of breast cancer: report of the National Surgical Adjuvant Breast and Bowel Project P-1 Study. *J Natl Cancer Inst* 1998;90:1371-1388.
38. Cuzick J, Powles T, Veronesi U, et al. Overview of the main outcomes in breast-cancer prevention trials. *Lancet* 2003;361:296-300.
39. Vogel VG, Costatino JP, Wickerhan DL, et al. Effects of tamoxifen vs raloxifene on the risk of developing invasive breast cancer and other disease outcomes: the NSABP Study of Tamoxifen and Raloxifene (STAR) P-2 trial. *JAMA* 2006;295:2727-2741.
40. Vogel VG, Costatino JP, Wickerham DL, et al. Update of the National Surgical Adjuvant Breast and Bowel Project Study of Tamoxifen and Raloxifene (STAR) P-2 Trial: Preventing breast cancer. *Cancer Prev Res (Phila)* 2010;3:696-706.
41. Cuzick J, Sestak I, Bonanni B, et al. Selective oestrogen receptor modulators in prevention of breast cancer: an updated meta-analysis of individual participant data. *Lancet* 2013;381:1827-1834.
42. Litton JK, Arun BK, Brown PH, and Hortobagyi GN. Aromatase inhibitors and breast cancer prevention. *Expert Opin Pharmacother* 2012;13:325-331.
43. Goss PE, et al. Exemestane for breast-cancer prevention in postmenopausal women. *N Engl J Med* 2011;364:2381-2391.
44. Cuzick J, Ingle JN, Ales-Martinez JE, et al. Anastrozole for prevention of breast cancer in high-risk postmenopausal women (IBIS-II): an international, double-blind, randomised placebo-controlled trial. *Lancet* 2014;383:1041-1048.
45. NCCN Clinical Practice Guidelines in Oncology (NCCN Guidelines®) for *Breast Cancer Risk Reduction* V.2.2015 © National Comprehensive Cancer Network, Inc 2015. All rights reserved. Last accessed, September 1, 2015.
46. Visvanathan K, Hurley P, Bantug E, et al. Use of pharmacologic interventions for breast cancer risk reduction: American Society of Clinical Oncology clinical practice guideline. *J Clin Oncol* 2013;31:2942-2962.
47. Oeffinger KC, Fontham ET, Etzioni R, et al. Breast Cancer Screening for Women at Average Risk: 2015 Guideline Update From the American Cancer Society. *JAMA* 2015;314:1599-1614.
48. U.S. Preventive Services Task Force. Screening for breast cancer: U.S. Preventive Services Task Force recommendation statement. *Ann Intern Med* 2009;151:716-726.
49. NCCN Clinical Practice Guidelines in Oncology (NCCN Guidelines®) for *Breast Cancer Screening and Diagnosis Guidelines* V.1.2015 © National Comprehensive Cancer Network, Inc 2015. All rights reserved. Last accessed, September 1, 2015.
50. Smith RA, Saslow D, Sawyer KA. et al. American Cancer Society guidelines for breast cancer screening: update 2003. *CA Cancer J Clin* 2003;53:141-169.
51. Thomas DB, Gao DL, Self SG, et al. Randomized trial of breast self-examination in Shanghai: methodology and preliminary results. *J Natl Cancer Inst* 1997;89:355-365.
52. Chiarelli AM, Majpruz V, Brown P, et al. The contribution of clinical breast examination to the accuracy of breast screening. *J Natl Cancer Inst* 2009;101:1236-1243.
53. Nelson HD, Tyne K, Naik A, et al. Screening for breast cancer: an update for the U.S. Preventive Services Task Force. *Ann Intern Med* 2009;151:727-737.
54. Smith RA, Manassaram-Baptiste D, Brooks D, et al. Cancer screening in the United States, 2015: a review of current American cancer society guidelines and current issues in cancer screening. *CA Cancer J Clin* 2015;65:30-54.
55. Saslow D, Boetes C, Burke W, et al. American Cancer Society guidelines for breast screening with MRI as an adjunct to mammography. *CA Cancer J Clin* 2007;57:75-89.
56. Early Breast Cancer Trialists' Collaborative Group (EBCTCG), Peto R, Davies C, Godwin J, et al. Comparisons between different polychemotherapy regimens for early breast cancer: meta-analyses of long-term outcome among 100,000 women in 123 randomised trials. *Lancet* 2012;379:432-444.
57. Helvie MA. Imaging Analysis: Mammography. In: Harris, JR, et al., eds. *Diseases of the Breast*. Philadelphia: Lippincott Williams & Wilkins; 2001:116-130.
58. Bleicher RJ. Management of the palpable breast mass. In: Harris JR, Lippman ME, Osborne CK, Morrow M, eds. *Diseases of the Breast*. 4th ed. Philadelphia: Lippincott Williams & Wilkins; 2010:32-41.
59. Edge S, Byrd DR, Compton CC, Fritz AG, Green FL, and Trotti, A, eds. *AJCC Cancer Staging Manual*. 7th ed. New York: Springer; 2010.

60. Dillon DA, Guidi AJ and Schnitt SJ. Pathology of Invasive Breast Cancer. In: Harris JR, Lippman ME, Osborne CK, Morrow M, eds. *Diseases of the Breast*. 4th ed. Philadelphia: Lippincott Williams & Wilkins;2010:374-407.
61. NCCN Clinical Practice Guidelines in Oncology (NCCN Guidelines®) for *Breast Cancer* V.3.2015 © National Comprehensive Cancer Network, Inc 2015. Last accessed, September 1, 2015.
62. Dawood S, Merajver SD, Viens P, et al. International expert panel on inflammatory breast cancer: consensus statement for standardized diagnosis and treatment. *Ann Oncol* 2011;22:515-523.
63. Kuerer HM, Albarracin CT, Yang WT, et al. Ductal carcinoma in situ: state of the science and roadmap to advance the field. *J Clin Oncol* 2009;27:279-288.
64. Venkitaraman R. Lobular neoplasia of the breast. *Breast J* 2010;16: 519-528.
65. Wapnir IL, Dignam JJ, Fisher B, et al. Long-term outcomes of invasive ipsilateral breast tumor recurrences after lumpectomy in NSABP B-17 and B-24 randomized clinical trials for DCIS. *J Natl Cancer Inst* 2011;103:478-488.
66. Allred DC, Anderson SJ, Paik S, et al. Adjuvant tamoxifen reduces subsequent breast cancer in women with estrogen receptor-positive ductal carcinoma in situ: a study based on NSABP protocol B-24. *J Clin Oncol* 2012;30:1268-1273.
67. Margolese RG, Cecchini RS, Julian TB, et al. Anastrozole versus tamoxifen in postmenopausal patients with ductal carcinoma in situ undergoing lumpectomy plus radiotherapy (NSABP B-35): a randomized, double-blind, phase 3 clinical trial. *Lancet* 2016; in press.
68. Ligibel J. Lifestyle factors in cancer survivorship. *J Clin Oncol* 2012;30:3697-3704.
69. Pierce JP, Natarajan L, Caan BJ, et al. Influence of a diet very high in vegetables, fruit, and fiber and low in fat on prognosis following treatment for breast cancer: the Women's Healthy Eating and Living (WHEL) randomized trial. *JAMA* 2007;298:289-298.
70. Chlebowski RT, Blackburn GT, Thomson CA, et al. Dietary fat reduction and breast cancer outcome: interim efficacy results from the Women's Intervention Nutrition Study. *J Natl Cancer Inst* 2006;98:1767-1776.
71. Demark-Wahnefried W, Rogers LQ, Alfano CM, et al. Practical clinical interventions for diet, physical activity, and weight control in cancer survivors. *CA Cancer J Clin* 2015;65:167-189.
72. Stuart-Harris R, Caldas C, Pinder SE, Pharoah P. Proliferation markers and survival in early breast cancer: a systematic review and meta-analysis of 85 studies in 32,825 patients. *Breast* 2008;17:323-334.
73. Hammond ME, Hayes DJ, Dowsett M, et al. American Society of Clinical Oncology/College Of American Pathologists guideline recommendations for immunohistochemical testing of estrogen and progesterone receptors in breast cancer. *J Clin Oncol* 2010;28:2784-2795.
74. Wolff AC, Hammond ME, Hicks DG, et al. Recommendations for human epidermal growth factor receptor 2 testing in breast cancer: American Society of Clinical Oncology/College of American Pathologists clinical practice guideline update. *J Clin Oncol* 2013;31:3997-4013.
75. Dawood S, Broglio K, Duzdar AU, et al. Prognosis of women with metastatic breast cancer by HER2 status and trastuzumab treatment: an institutional-based review. *J Clin Oncol* 2010;28:92-98.
76. Anampa J, Makower D, Sparano JA. Progress in adjuvant chemotherapy for breast cancer: an overview. *BMC Med* 2015;13:195.
77. Adaniel C, Jhaveri K, Heguy A, Esteva FJ. Genome-Based Risk Prediction for Early Stage Breast Cancer. *Oncologist* 2014;19:1019-1027.
78. Harris L, Fritsche H, Mennel R, et al. American Society of Clinical Oncology 2007 update of recommendations for the use of tumor markers in breast cancer. *J Clin Oncol* 2007;25:5287-5312.
79. Yang SH, Yang KH, Li YP, et al. Breast conservation therapy for stage I or stage II breast cancer: a meta-analysis of randomized controlled trials. *Ann Oncol* 2008;19:1039-1044.
80. Jatoi I and Proschan MA. Randomized trials of breast-conserving therapy versus mastectomy for primary breast cancer: a pooled analysis of updated results. *Am J Clin Oncol* 2005;28:289-294.
81. Early Breast Cancer Trialists' Collaborative Group (EBCTCG), Darby S, McGale P, Correa C, et al. Effect of radiotherapy after breast-conserving surgery on 10-year recurrence and 15-year breast cancer death: meta-analysis of individual patient data for 10,801 women in 17 randomised trials. *Lancet* 2011;378:1707-1716.
82. Fisher CM, Rabinovitch R. Frontiers in radiotherapy for early-stage invasive breast cancer. *J Clin Oncol* 2014;32:2894-2901.
83. Rao R, Euhus D, Mayo HG, Balch C. Axillary node interventions in breast cancer: a systematic review. *JAMA* 2013;310:1385-1394.
84. Lyman GH, Temin S, Edge SB, et al. Sentinel lymph node biopsy for patients with early-stage breast cancer: American Society of Clinical Oncology clinical practice guideline update. *J Clin Oncol* 2014;32:1365-1383.
85. Giuliano AE, Hunt KK, Ballman KV, et al. Axillary dissection vs no axillary dissection in women with invasive breast cancer and sentinel node metastasis: a randomized clinical trial. *JAMA* 2011;305:569-575.
86. Early Breast Cancer Trialists' Collaborative Group (EBCTCG), Dowsett M, Forbes JF, Bradley R, et al. Aromatase inhibitors versus tamoxifen in early breast cancer: patient-level meta-analysis of the randomised trials. *Lancet* 2015;386:1341-1352.
87. Coates AS, Winer EP, Goldhirsch A, et al. Tailoring therapies-improving the management of early breast cancer: St Gallen International Expert Consensus on the Primary Therapy of Early Breast Cancer 2015. *Ann Oncol* 2015;26:1533-1546.
88. Senkus E, Kyriakides S, Ohno S, et al. Primary breast cancer: ESMO Clinical Practice Guidelines for diagnosis, treatment and follow-updagger. *Ann Oncol* 2015;26 Suppl 5: v8-v30.
89. Fisher B, Brown A, Mamounas E, et al. Effect of preoperative chemotherapy on local-regional disease in women with operable breast cancer: findings from National Surgical Adjuvant Breast and Bowel Project B-18. *J Clin Oncol* 1997;15:2483-2493.
90. Fisher B, Bryant J, Wolmark N, et al. Effect of preoperative chemotherapy on the outcome of women with operable breast cancer. *J Clin Oncol* 1998;16:2672-2685.
91. Rastogi P, Anderson SJ, Bear HD, et al. Preoperative chemotherapy: updates of National Surgical Adjuvant Breast and Bowel Project Protocols B-18 and B-27. *J Clin Oncol* 2008;26:778-785.
92. Kumar P, Aggarwal R. An overview of triple-negative breast cancer. *Arch Gynecol Obstet* 2016;293:247-269.
93. Lohrisch C, Paltiel C, Gelmon K, et al. Impact on survival of time from definitive surgery to initiation of adjuvant chemotherapy for early-stage breast cancer. *J Clin Oncol* 2006;24:4888-4894.
94. Bonadonna G, Valagussa P, Moliterni A, Zambetti M, Brambilla C. Adjuvant cyclophosphamide, methotrexate, and fluorouracil in node-positive breast cancer: the results of 20 years of follow-up. *N Engl J Med* 1995;332:901-906.
95. Citron ML, Berry DA, Cirrincione C, et al. Randomized trial of dose-dense versus conventionally scheduled and sequential versus concurrent combination chemotherapy as postoperative adjuvant treatment of node-positive primary breast cancer: first report of Intergroup Trial C9741/Cancer and Leukemia Group B Trial 9741. *J Clin Oncol* 2003;21:1431-1439.
96. Sparano JA, Zhao F, Martino S, et al. Long-Term Follow-Up of the E1199 Phase III Trial Evaluating the Role of Taxane and Schedule in Operable Breast Cancer. *J Clin Oncol* 2015;33:2353-2360.
97. Seidman AD, Berry D, Cirrincione C, et al. Randomized phase III trial of weekly compared with every-3-weeks paclitaxel for metastatic breast cancer, with trastuzumab for all HER-2 overexpressors and random assignment to trastuzumab or not in HER-2 nonoverexpressors: final results of Cancer and Leukemia Group B protocol 9840. *J Clin Oncol* 2008;26:1642-1649.
98. Green MC, Buzdar AU, Smith T, et al. Weekly paclitaxel improves pathologic complete remission in operable breast cancer when compared with paclitaxel once every 3 weeks. *J Clin Oncol* 2005;23:5983-5992.
99. Bonilla L, Ben-Aharon I, Vidal L, et al. Dose-dense chemotherapy in nonmetastatic breast cancer: a systematic review and meta-analysis of randomized controlled trials. *J Natl Cancer Inst* 2010;102:1845-1854.
100. Moore HC. Impact on quality of life of adjuvant therapy for breast cancer. *Curr Oncol Rep* 2007;9:42-46.
101. Hesketh PJ, Bohlke K, Lyman GH, et al. Antiemetics: American Society of Clinical Oncology Focused Guideline Update. *J Clin Oncol* 2016;34:381-386.
102. Rizzo JD, Brouwers M, Hurley P, et al. American Society of Clinical Oncology/American Society of Hematology clinical practice guideline update on the use of epoetin and darbepoetin in adult patients with cancer. *J Clin Oncol* 2010;28:4996-5010.
103. Levine MN, Gent M, Hirsh J, et al. The thrombogenic effect of anticancer drug therapy in women with stage II breast cancer. *N Engl J Med* 1988;318:404-407.
104. Matesich SM, Shapiro CL. Second cancers after breast cancer treatment. *Semin Oncol* 2003;30:740-748.
105. Henderson IC, Sloss LJ, Jaffe N, Blum RH, Frei III E. Serial studies of cardiac function in patients receiving adriamycin. *Cancer Treat Rep* 1978;62:923-929.

106. Costa RB, Kurra G, Greenberg L, Geyer CE. Efficacy and cardiac safety of adjuvant trastuzumab-based chemotherapy regimens for HER2-positive early breast cancer. *Ann Oncol* 2010;21:2153-2160.
107. Yin W, Jiang Y, Shen Z, Shao Z, Lu J. Trastuzumab in the adjuvant treatment of HER2-positive early breast cancer patients: a meta-analysis of published randomized controlled trials. *PLoS One* 2011;6:e21030.
108. Slamon D, Eiermann W, Robert N, et al. Adjuvant trastuzumab in HER2-positive breast cancer. *N Engl J Med* 2011;365:1273-1283.
109. Telli ML, Witteles RM. Trastuzumab-related cardiac dysfunction. *J Natl Compr Canc Netw* 2011;9:243-249.
110. Thompson LM, Eckmann K, Boster BL, et al. Incidence, risk factors, and management of infusion-related reactions in breast cancer patients receiving trastuzumab. *Oncologist* 2014;19:228-234.
111. Halyard MY, Pisansky TM, Dueck AC, et al. Radiotherapy and adjuvant trastuzumab in operable breast cancer: tolerability and adverse event data from the NCCTG Phase III Trial N9831. *J Clin Oncol* 2009;27:2638-2644.
112. Reeder-Hayes KE, Carey LA. How low should we go? The search for balance in management of small human epidermal growth factor receptor 2-positive breast cancers. *J Clin Oncol* 2014;32:2122-2124.
113. Tolaney SM, Barry WT, Dang CT, et al. Adjuvant paclitaxel and trastuzumab for node-negative, HER2-positive breast cancer. *N Engl J Med* 2015;372:134-141.
114. Jhaveri K, Esteva FJ. Pertuzumab in the treatment of HER2+ breast cancer. *J Natl Compr Canc Netw* 2014;12:591-598.
115. Love RR, Wiebe DA, Newcomb PA, et al. Effects of tamoxifen on cardiovascular risk factors in postmenopausal women. *Ann Intern Med* 1991;115:860-864.
116. Love RR, Mazess RB, Barden HS, et al. Effects of tamoxifen on bone mineral density in postmenopausal women with breast cancer. *N Engl J Med* 1992;326:852-856.
117. Albain KS, Barlow WE, Reynolds W, et al. Adjuvant chemotherapy and timing of tamoxifen in postmenopausal patients with endocrine-responsive, node-positive breast cancer: a phase 3, open-label, randomised controlled trial. *Lancet* 2009;374:2055-2063.
118. Davies C, Pan H, Godwin J, et al. Long-term effects of continuing adjuvant tamoxifen to 10 years versus stopping at 5 years after diagnosis of oestrogen receptor-positive breast cancer: ATLAS, a randomised trial. *Lancet* 2013;381:805-816.
119. Gray RG, Rea D, Handley K, et al. aTTom: Long-term effects of continuing adjuvant tamoxifen to 10 years versus stopping at 5 years in 6,953 women with early breast cancer. *J Clin Oncol* 2013;(suppl):31:abstract 05.
120. Fisher B, Dignam J, Bryant J, Wolmark N. Five versus more than five years of tamoxifen for lymph node-negative breast cancer: updated findings from the National Surgical Adjuvant Breast and Bowel Project B-14 randomized trial. *J Natl Cancer Inst* 2001;93:684-690.
121. Khatcheressian JL, Hurley B, Bantug E, et al. Breast cancer follow-up and management after primary treatment: American Society of Clinical Oncology clinical practice guideline update. *J Clin Oncol* 2013;31:961-965.
122. Early Breast Cancer Trialists' Collaborative Group (EBCTCG). Effects of chemotherapy and hormonal therapy for early breast cancer on recurrence and 15-year survival: an overview of the randomised trials. *Lancet* 2005;365:1687-1717.
123. LHRH-agonists in Early Breast Cancer Overview group, Cuzick J, Ambroisine L, Davidson N, et al. Use of luteinising-hormone-releasing hormone agonists as adjuvant treatment in premenopausal patients with hormone-receptor-positive breast cancer: a meta-analysis of individual patient data from randomised adjuvant trials. *Lancet* 2007;369:1711-1723.
124. Pagani O, Regan MM, Walley Ba, et al. Adjuvant exemestane with ovarian suppression in premenopausal breast cancer. *N Engl J Med* 2014;371:107-118.
125. Francis PA, Regan MM, Fleming GF, et al. Adjuvant ovarian suppression in premenopausal breast cancer. *N Engl J Med* 2015;372:436-446.
126. Hertz DL, McLeod HL and Irvin, WJ Jr. Tamoxifen and CYP2D6: a contradiction of data. *Oncologist* 2012;17:620-630.
127. Kelly CM, Juurlink DN, Gomes T, et al. Selective serotonin reuptake inhibitors and breast cancer mortality in women receiving tamoxifen: a population based cohort study. *BMJ* 2010;340:c693.
128. Tryfonidis K, Senkus E, Cardoso MJ and Cardoso F. Management of locally advanced breast cancer-perspectives and future directions. *Nat Rev Clin Oncol* 2015;12:147-162.
129. Charehbili A, Fontein DB, Korep JR, et al. Neoadjuvant hormonal therapy for endocrine sensitive breast cancer: a systematic review. *Cancer Treat Rev* 2014;40:86-92.
130. Giordano SH, Temin S, Kirshner JJ, et al. Systemic therapy for patients with advanced human epidermal growth factor receptor 2-positive breast cancer: American Society of Clinical Oncology clinical practice guideline. *J Clin Oncol* 2014;32:2078-2099.
131. Van Poznak CH, Temin S, Yee GC, et al. American Society of Clinical Oncology executive summary of the clinical practice guideline update on the role of bone-modifying agents in metastatic breast cancer. *J Clin Oncol* 2011;29:1221-1227.
132. Ramakrishna N, Temin S, Chandarlapaty S, et al. Recommendations on disease management for patients with advanced human epidermal growth factor receptor 2-positive breast cancer and brain metastases: American Society of Clinical Oncology clinical practice guideline. *J Clin Oncol* 2014;32:2100-2108.
133. Herceptin (trastuzumab) product information. [PDF] 2015 April 2015 [cited 2015 12/2/15]; Product information]. Available from: http://www.gene.com/download/pdf/herceptin_prescribing.pdf.
134. Perez EA, Koehler M, Byrne J, et al. Cardiac safety of lapatinib: pooled analysis of 3689 patients enrolled in clinical trials. *Mayo Clin Proc* 2008;83:679-686.
135. Tykerb (lapatinib) product information. [PDG] 2015 March 2015 [cited 2015 December 2]; Tykerb prescribing information]. Available from: http://www.pharma.us.novartis.com/product/pi/pdf/tykerb.pdf.
136. Ross JS, Slodkowska EA, Symmans WF, et al. The HER-2 receptor and breast cancer: ten years of targeted anti-HER-2 therapy and personalized medicine. *Oncologist* 2009;14:320-368.
137. Wolff AC, Lazar AA, Bondarenko I, et al. Randomized phase III placebo-controlled trial of letrozole plus oral temsirolimus as first-line endocrine therapy in postmenopausal women with locally advanced or metastatic breast cancer. *J Clin Oncol* 2013;31:195-202.
138. Baselga J, Campone M, Piccart M, et al. Everolimus in postmenopausal hormone-receptor-positive advanced breast cancer. *N Engl J Med* 2012;366:520-529.
139. Keck S, Glencer AC, Rugo HS. Everolimus and its role in hormone-resistant and trastuzumab-resistant metastatic breast cancer. *Future Oncol* 2012; 8:1383-1396.
140. Cadoo KA, Gucalp A, Traina TA. Palbociclib: an evidence-based review of its potential in the treatment of breast cancer. *Breast Cancer (Dove Med Press)* 2014;6:123-133.
141. Cortes J, Calvo, E, Gonzalez-Martin A, et al. Progress against solid tumors in danger: the metastatic breast cancer example. *J Clin Oncol* 2012;30:3444-3447.
142. Lyman GH, Burstein HJ, Buzdar AU, D'Agostino R, Ellis PA. Making genuine progress against metastatic breast cancer. *J Clin Oncol* 2012;30:3448-3451.
143. Finn RS, Crown JP, Lang I, et al. The cyclin-dependent kinase 4/6 inhibitor palbociclib in combination with letrozole versus letrozole alone as first-line treatment of oestrogen receptor-positive, HER2-negative, advanced breast cancer (PALOMA-1/TRIO-18): a randomised phase 2 study. *Lancet Oncol* 2015;16:25-35.
144. Turner NC, Huang Bartlett C, Cristofanilli M. Palbociclib in Hormone-Receptor-Positive Advanced Breast Cancer. *N Engl J Med* 2015;373:1672-1673.
145. Sainsbury R. The development of endocrine therapy for women with breast cancer. *Cancer Treat Rev* 2013;39:507-517.
146. Doyen J, Italiano A, Largillier R, et al. Aromatase inhibition in male breast cancer patients: biological and clinical implications. *Ann Oncol* 2010;21:1243-1245.
147. Stenbygaard LE, Herrstedt J, Thomsen JF, et al. Toremifene and tamoxifen in advanced breast cancer--a double-blind cross-over trial. *Breast Cancer Res Treat* 1993;25:57-63.
148. Robertson JF, Lindemann JP, Llombart-Cussac A, et al. Fulvestrant 500 mg versus anastrozole 1 mg for the first-line treatment of advanced breast cancer: follow-up analysis from the randomized 'FIRST' study. *Breast Cancer Res Treat* 2012;136:503-511.
149. Cardoso F, Bischoff J, Brain E, et al. A review of the treatment of endocrine responsive metastatic breast cancer in postmenopausal women. *Cancer Treat Rev* 2013;39:457-465.
150. Partridge AH, Rumble RB, Carey LA, et al. Chemotherapy and targeted therapy for women with human epidermal growth factor receptor 2-negative (or unknown) advanced breast cancer: American Society of Clinical Oncology Clinical Practice Guideline. *J Clin Oncol* 2014;32:3307-3329.

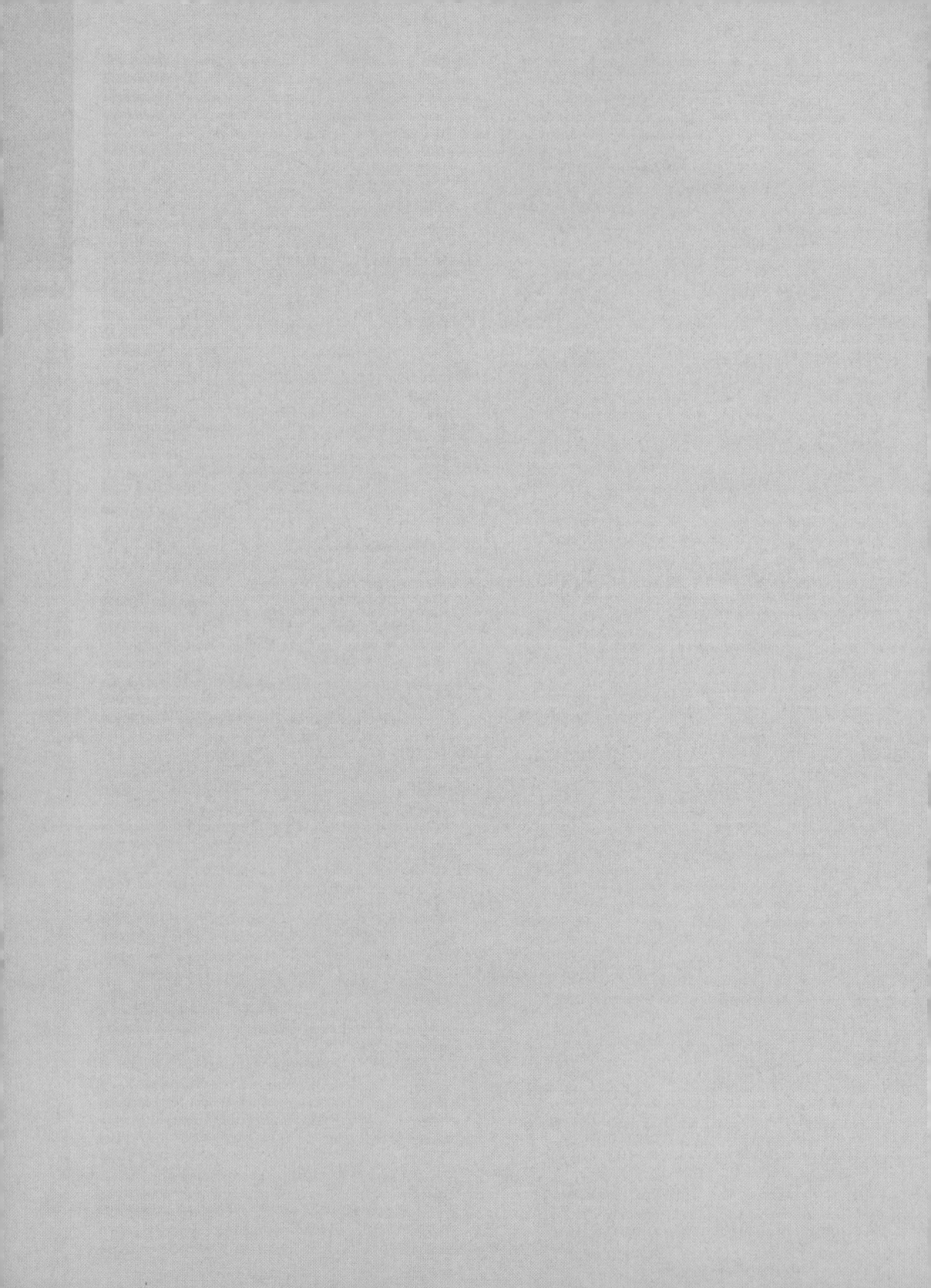

129

Lung Cancer

Val R. Adams and Sarah Scarpace Peters

KEY CONCEPTS

1. Lung cancer is the leading cause of cancer deaths in both men and women in the United States. The overall 5-year survival rate for all types of lung cancer is about 15%.
2. Cigarette smoking is responsible for most lung cancers. Smoking cessation should be encouraged, particularly in those receiving curative treatment (ie, Stages I to IIIA non-small cell lung cancer [NSCLC] and limited-stage small cell lung cancer [SCLC]).
3. NSCLC is the most commonly diagnosed type of lung cancer (about 80%). NSCLC typically has a slower growth rate and doubling time than SCLC.
4. Annual screening with low-dose computed tomography imaging (LDCT) is currently recommended to identify lung cancer in high-risk individuals. However, several studies are evaluating the optimal frequency and duration, as well as the impact of false-positive tests.
5. Treatment decisions are guided by the stage of disease (which is characterized by tumor size and spread), histology (squamous or non-squamous), and molecular features (epidermal growth factor receptor [EGFR] mutations or anaplastic lymphoma kinase [ALK] positivity) of the tumor. Patient-specific factors (ie, performance status, comorbid conditions, etc.) must also be considered when developing a treatment plan.
6. The treatment goals in lung cancer are cure (early stage disease), prolongation of survival, and maintenance or improvement of quality of life through alleviation of symptoms.
7. Early stage lung cancer has the highest cure rates when surgical resection of the tumor is used with or without chemotherapy for NSCLC and chemoradiotherapy for SCLC.
8. Advanced-stage lung cancer is primarily treated with systemic therapy. Doublet platinum-based chemotherapy regimens are superior in response to single-agent regimens and should be used when the patient can tolerate the associated toxicity. Platinum-containing doublets are first-line treatment in most cases of NSCLC and SCLC.
9. Targeted therapies for advanced-stage NSCLC are preferred over platinum-based doublets as first-line therapy in those patients whose tumors express certain genetic mutations such as EGFR exon 19 deletions or exon 21 (L858R) substitution mutations or ALK-positive.
10. Immunotherapy with anti-programmed-death receptor-1 (PD1) monoclonal antibody is currently approved for the second-line treatment of NSCLC and is a novel therapeutic class of treatment available for these patients.
11. Optimal patient care needs to include prevention and treatment of adverse events from drug therapy. Adverse events may cause delays in treatment administration, increase morbidity, and contribute to treatment failure.

Lung cancer is a major cause of morbidity and mortality. It has reached epidemic proportions in many industrialized countries and is the most frequently fatal malignancy in the world. It is estimated that 224,390 new cases of lung cancer were diagnosed in the United States in 2016.[1]

Despite major advances in the understanding and management of lung cancer, the overall 5-year survival rate for all types of lung cancer remains a dismal 18%.[1] In the United States, lung cancer accounts for about 13% of all newly diagnosed cancer in adults.[1] (1) It remains the leading cause of cancer death in both adult men and women, with about 158,080 deaths in 2016.[1] The incidence and death rate caused by lung cancer are declining, which has been attributed to decreased tobacco use over the last 50 years. In comparison to whites, the incidence and mortality of lung cancer is greater in African American men and slightly lower in African American women.[1]

The incidence of lung cancer increases with age, with about 58% of deaths occurring between 60 and 79 years.[1] Early lung cancer screening studies failed to demonstrate a survival advantage, but in November 2010, the largest trial of its kind, the National Lung Screening Trial, demonstrated a 20% reduction in the relative risk of death from lung cancer in moderate-to-high risk individuals (95% confidence interval [CI], 6.8 to 26.7; $P=0.004$). Among subjects enrolled in lung cancer screening trials, the rate of malignancy in the pulmonary nodule detected on low-dose computed tomography (LDCT) scan is low, and surgical procedures are not without risk. Consequently, patients who receive scans as part of lung cancer screening or for another purpose should have other criteria or tests done before considering a biopsy to evaluate for malignant pathology.[2]

Patients with lung cancer may undergo surgery, chemotherapy, radiation, or multimodality therapy, depending on the histologic type of the tumor, presence of genetic mutations, its size and location, and the presence of metastases at diagnosis.[3,4] Two leading oncology groups representing leading clinicians in the United States have published clinical practice guidelines for the treatment of lung cancer. The National Comprehensive Cancer Network (NCCN) has developed consensus-based guidelines that provide recommendations regarding the screening, staging, and treatment of both non-small cell lung cancer (NSCLC) and small cell lung cancer (SCLC).[3,4] The American Society of Clinical Oncology (ASCO) published evidence-based guidelines that were updated in 2015.[5] ASCO also endorsed the guidelines of other organizations related to the treatment of SCLC,[6] the use of radiotherapy for locally advanced NSCLC,[7] and the use of molecular testing for NSCLC.[8]

ETIOLOGY

Lung carcinomas arise from normal bronchial epithelial cells that have acquired multiple genetic lesions and are capable of expressing a variety of phenotypes.[9] Significant advances have been made recently in understanding the molecular genetic changes involved in lung cancer pathogenesis.[9] A large variety of molecular lesions result in abrogation of key cellular regulatory and growth control pathways. Activation of a proto-oncogene, inhibition or mutation of tumor suppressor genes, and production of autocrine (self-stimulatory) growth factors contribute to cellular proliferation and malignant transformation.[9] Many of these molecular alterations are common to both SCLC and NSCLC, but certain mutations are found more frequently in specific subtypes of lung cancer and offer more targeted interventions to prevent or treat lung cancer. In autocrine loop abnormalities, SCLC frequently overexpresses C-KIT (a protein tyrosine kinase receptor that is specific for stem cell factor [CD117]), while NSCLC frequently overexpresses epidermal growth factor receptor (EGFR). EGFR inhibitors, such as erlotinib, gefitinib, afatinib, and osimertinib, are used clinically to treat NSCLC and theoretically offer a potential method of lung cancer chemoprevention.[9-11] Crizotinib, ceritinib, and alectinib, drugs that target the EML4-ALK gene rearrangement protein, demonstrates the importance of this pathway in a subset of adenocarcinoma lung cancer patients.[12]

2 Smoking is a major cause of lung cancer, with about 80% of lung cancer deaths in the United States directly attributed to tobacco use. Tobacco smoke contains many substances, including tumor promoters, carcinogens, and cocarcinogens.[13] The association between environmental tobacco smoke (ETS; also referred to as passive smoking) and lung cancer risk in nonsmokers is not as clear. Most studies have consistently found that spouses of smokers have higher rates of lung cancer than spouses of nonsmokers (about 25% higher risk). In addition, workplace exposure to environmental smoke increases the risk of lung cancer by about 17%. It is currently estimated that ETS contributes to about 3,000 lung cancers annually. Although many of these studies have methodologic flaws, the data consistently show dose-risk relationship, with no safe level of exposure.[13] Smoking cessation is associated with a gradual decrease in the risk, but more than 5 years is necessary before an appreciable decline in risk occurs and the risk never returns to that of a nonsmoker.[13] Because of the public health implications, the United States has several, mainly state-led, tobacco control efforts, including anti-smoking campaigns, increased tobacco taxes, and smoke-free areas in many public areas. Although the prevalence of cigarette smoking has slowly decreased, it remains at about 19% in 2010 and 2011.[13]

Although most cases of lung cancer are attributable to cigarette smoking, less than 20% of smokers develop lung cancer, which suggests that other risk factors are relevant. An increased risk of lung cancer has been associated with exposure to other environmental respiratory carcinogens (eg, asbestos, benzene, and arsenic). Genetic risk factors are also important, with an increased risk of lung cancer observed in those with first-degree relatives diagnosed with the disease. Lung cancer risk is associated with polymorphisms that affect the expression and/or function of enzymes regulating metabolism of tobacco carcinogens, DNA repair, or inflammation. Patients with a history of chronic obstructive airway disease and adults with asthma are at an increased risk for lung cancer.[9,10] Further studies to better identify which patients are at highest risk of developing lung cancer will be key for new lung cancer screening trials and in chemoprevention trials.

HISTOLOGIC CLASSIFICATION

Before treatment begins, it is critical that an experienced lung cancer pathologist reviews the pathologic material because of the different treatment regimens for NSCLC and SCLC.

TABLE 129-1 Histologic Classification of Non-Small Cell Lung Carcinomas

1. Squamous cell carcinoma
   - Papillary
   - Clear cell
   - Small cell (probably should be discontinued)
   - Basaloid
2. Adenocarcinoma
   - Minimally invasive adenocarcinoma (MIA)
   - Invasive adenocarcinoma
   - Lepidic predominant (previously classified as bronchioalveolar carcinoma [BAC])
   - Acinar predominant
   - Papillary predominant
   - Micropapillary predominant
   - Solid predominant with mucin
   - Variants of invasive adenocarcinoma
   - Invasive mucinous adenocarcinoma (previously classified as BAC)
   - Colloid
   - Fetal (low and high grade)
   - Enteric
3. Large cell carcinoma
   - Variants
   - Large cell neuroendocrine carcinoma
   - Combined large cell neuroendocrine carcinoma
   - Basaloid carcinoma
   - Lymphoepithelioma-like carcinoma
   - Clear cell carcinoma
   - Large cell carcinoma with rhabdoid phenotype
4. Adenosquamous carcinoma
5. Sarcomatoid carcinomas
   - Pleomorphic carcinoma
   - Spindle cell carcinoma
   - Giant cell carcinoma
   - Carcinosarcoma
   - Pulmonary blastoma
   - Other
6. Carcinoid tumor
   - Typical carcinoid (TC)
   - Atypical carcinoid (AC)
7. Carcinomas of salivary gland type
   - Mucoepidermoid carcinoma
   - Adenoid cystic carcinoma
   - Epimyoepithelial carcinoma

Adapted from 2004 WHO classification and the 2011 IASCL/ATS/ERS classification as described in reference 16.

3 NSCLC is diagnosed in most (80%) lung cancer patients. NSCLC typically has a slower growth rate and doubling time than SCLC. The histologic classification of NSCLC is well defined and widely accepted (Table 129-1).[14] In the most recent classification, the histologic types, subtypes, and identifiable variants convey information about tumors' natural behavior and in some cases influence therapeutic decisions.[14,15]

Four major cell types of carcinomas (squamous cell, adenocarcinoma, large cell, and small cell) account for more than 90% of all lung tumors. Early studies with localized disease demonstrated that radiation could cure small cell histology, while surgery did not. Studies with the other histologic types demonstrated better outcomes with surgery than with radiation, which provided the basis for the general classification of SCLC and NSCLC. Historically, systemic treatment for NSCLC histologies was the same and resulted in a similar overall prognosis, which again supported a general classification of SCLC and NSCLC. Translation of histology and genetics in NSCLC has led to personalized medicine. Trials have clearly shown that optimal therapeutic selection requires knowledge of the histology and genetic mutational status.[8,9] For metastatic NSCLC, there are four pathways: (1) squamous cell histology, (2) non-squamous histology with an EGFR mutation (EGFR+), (3) non-squamous histology with and ALK-EML4 rearrangement (ALK+), and (4) non-squamous histology with wild type EGFR and ALK.

Squamous cell carcinoma was once the most common histology, but it now represents less than 30% of all lung cancers. Squamous cell carcinomas have a much higher incidence in smokers and among males and appear to have a strong dose-response relationship to tobacco exposure. Most of these tumors occur centrally, but the incidence of peripheral presentation is increasing. Studies describing the natural history of lung cancer in the era of screening with LDCT scans have revealed a relatively constant tumor volume doubling time (104-122 days), while the other histologies indicate that smaller tumors found with a CT scan are more indolent (eg, doubling times three to four times longer with CT-discovered tumors).[2] Squamous cell tumors are slower to metastasize, but they eventually spread to the hilar and mediastinal lymph nodes, liver, adrenal glands, kidneys, bone, and GI tract. Since it is rare that tumors of squamous histology harbor an EGFR or ALK-EML4 mutation, patients are not routinely tested for genetic mutations unless the patient is a nonsmoker or there are concerns about the adequacy of the sample.[4,9,10] Adenocarcinoma accounts for about one-half of lung cancers and is increasing in frequency. It is the most common histology in nonsmoking lung cancer patients. The natural history of adenocarcinoma in the lung shows that small tumors discovered with CT screening are relatively slow growing and the tumor doubling time increases as they get larger; volume doubling time of tumors discovered with CT screening is about 576 days, while those found with routine care double every 169 days.[2] This information is most important when considering screening programs and the potential for lead time bias. Patients with adenocarcinoma can present with a single nodule, multifocal nodules, or rapidly progressing, bilateral, diffuse processes. This histology is likely to metastasize from a relatively small tumor (often before the diagnosis of the primary tumor) and spread widely to distant sites, including the contralateral lung, liver, bone, adrenal glands, kidneys, and CNS. As a result, adenocarcinoma has a worse prognosis than squamous cell carcinoma, but the prognosis is similar when controlled for stage.[4,10]

Table 129-1 shows several sub-classifications and variants of adenocarcinoma. These tumors should undergo genetic testing for EGFR mutations and EML4-ALK rearrangements, which can influence prognosis and guide therapy for advanced tumors.

Large cell carcinomas are undifferentiated epithelial tumors, which tend to be large and bulky tumors arising in the periphery of the lung, have a propensity to metastasize in a pattern quite similar to adenocarcinomas, and are associated with a similar poor prognosis.[4,10] They also should be tested for EGFR and ELM4-ALK genetic aberrations, which provide prognostic information and guide therapy. SCLCs account for about 15% of all lung tumors. They are distinguished by their appearance as small neoplastic cells with round to oval nuclei. These tumors occur in both the major bronchi and the periphery of the lung. SCLC is a very aggressive and rapidly growing tumor, with about 60% to 70% of patients initially presenting with disseminated disease outside of the hemithorax. These tumors commonly express neuroendocrine differentiation, which may account for some of the paraneoplastic syndromes frequently associated with this disease. SCLC secretes gastrin-releasing peptide that acts as an autocrine growth factor. Secretion of other peptide hormones, cytogenetic abnormalities, and amplification and increased expression of oncogenes are also common. This disease has a propensity to metastasize to the lymph nodes, opposite lung, liver, adrenal glands and other endocrine organs, bone, bone marrow, and CNS.[3,11] They do not contain EGFR or EML4-ALK mutations and consequently are not tested for those. Current research is attempting to identify targetable genetic mutations for these tumors. Lung tumors can exhibit more than one histologic cell type (eg, adenosquamous) and mixed histology tumors should also undergo genetic testing for EGFR and EML4-ALK alterations.[8,9] Patients can also occasionally have multiple lung nodules arising in different lobes or the contralateral lung. They can be the same or different histology. This is referred to as synchronous tumors, and the nodules may be of similar or different cell types. If one tumor is pure squamous histology, then genetic testing can be omitted. Synchronous tumors worsen the patient's overall prognosis.[4]

CLINICAL PRESENTATION

At the time of diagnosis, 16% of lung cancers are localized, 22% have regional spread, and 57% have distant metastases (the remaining were not staged).[1] Location and extent of the tumor determine

CLINICAL PRESENTATION Lung Cancer

Local Signs and Symptoms Associated with Primary Tumor or Regional Spread within the Thorax

- Cough
- Hemoptysis
- Dyspnea
- Rust-streaked or purulent sputum
- Chest, shoulder, or arm pain
- Wheeze and stridor
- Superior vena cava obstruction
- Pleural effusion or pneumonitis
- Dysphagia (secondary to esophageal compression)
- Hoarseness (secondary to laryngeal nerve paralysis)
- Horner's syndrome
- Phrenic nerve paralysis
- Pericardial effusion/tamponade
- Tracheal obstruction

Extrapulmonary Signs and Symptoms Associated with Metastatic Involvement

- Bone pain and/or pathologic fractures
- Liver dysfunction
- Neurologic deficits
- Spinal cord compression

Paraneoplastic Syndromes

- Weight loss
- Cushing's syndrome
- Hypercalcemia (most commonly in squamous cell lung cancer)
- Syndrome of inappropriate secretion of antidiuretic hormone (most commonly in SCLC)
- Pulmonary hypertrophic osteoarthropathy
- Clubbing
- Anemia
- Eaton-Lambert's myasthenic syndrome
- Hypercoagulable state

the presenting signs and symptoms. A lesion in the central portion of the bronchial tree is more likely to cause symptoms at an earlier stage as compared with a lesion in the periphery of the lung, which may remain asymptomatic until the lesion is large or has spread to other areas. The most common initial signs and symptoms include cough, dyspnea, and chest pain or discomfort, with or without hemoptysis.[10] Unfortunately, many patients with lung cancer also have chronic pulmonary and/or cardiovascular diseases (usually related to smoking), and such symptoms may go unnoticed or be attributed to the concomitant disease. Many patients also exhibit systemic symptoms of malignancy such as anorexia, weight loss, and fatigue. Disseminated disease can cause extrapulmonary signs and symptoms such as neurologic deficits resulting from CNS metastases, bone pain or pathological fractures secondary to bone metastases, or liver dysfunction resulting from tumor involvement in the liver.[10]

Paraneoplastic syndromes are signs and symptoms that occur at sites away from the primary tumor or its metastases and are not associated with direct tumor involvement. They may be caused by the production of biologically active substances (eg, peptide hormones) or antibodies, or by other undefined mechanisms. Paraneoplastic syndromes occur more frequently with lung cancer than with any other tumor, and more frequently with SCLC than with NSCLC. These syndromes may be the first signs of a tumor and may prompt the search for an underlying malignancy.[11]

SCREENING AND PREVENTION

4 Most lung cancer patients are diagnosed with advanced disease, which is a key factor in the poor prognosis associated with this disease. Surgery and radiation are the most effective treatment modalities in NSCLC and SCLC, respectively, which generally limit curative intent to patients diagnosed at an early clinical stage.[3,4,6,7] Therefore, it is important to diagnose lung cancer earlier, which implies a potential improvement with screening. Several screening techniques, including chest x-ray, CT, and positron emission tomography (PET), scanning have been investigated to detect lung cancer at an earlier stage. The mortality results from screening with a chest x-ray have been negative, but positive results for LDCT scans to screen for lung cancer have been reported. A recent systematic review of the potential benefit and harm from LDCT screening was reported with accompanying recommendations.[17] The largest and only positive study was known as the National Lung Cancer Screening trial that enrolled more than 54,000 high-risk smokers. The study reported a decrease in overall (7% vs 7.5%) and lung cancer-specific (1.3% vs 1.7%) mortality with LDCT versus control, respectively. The resulting recommendation is to offer annual LDCT screening to individuals aged 55 to 74 years with a 30-pack-year history who are still smoking or have quit for less than 15 years. These recommendations come with a few caveats, including the fact that the most important step is for current smokers to quit. The optimal frequency and duration of screening is unknown and the harm from screening, including frequent false-positive findings, is unknown.[17] Consequently, patients interested in screening should be enrolled in a clinical trial so answers to these important questions can be answered.

The term *chemoprevention* refers to the use of prophylactic medications to prevent the development of cancer. Many studies of potential chemopreventive agents, including nonsteroidal anti-inflammatory drugs (NSAIDs), retinoids, inhaled glucocorticoids, vitamin E, selenium, and green tea extracts, have been conducted, but none have been successful.[18] Large randomized clinical trials have evaluated β-carotene as a lung cancer chemopreventive agent in high-risk patients (older smokers). Rather than prevent lung cancer, the trials clearly show that older people who smoke have a higher risk of developing and dying of lung cancer if they take a β-carotene supplement. Nonsmokers do not appear to have an altered risk of lung cancer with β-carotene consumption.[18] The impact of selenium and/or vitamin E supplementation was evaluated in older men as part of a large prostate cancer prevention study (Selenium and Vitamin E Cancer Prevention Trial [SELECT]). Unfortunately, no benefit was seen with selenium or vitamin E supplementation on lung cancer incidence or mortality.[18]

Because the net benefit of screening is still being defined and chemoprevention trials have not proven to provide a survival benefit, the current recommendation is to avoid smoking and maintain a healthy diet with high amounts of fruits and vegetables.[19]

DIAGNOSIS

A patient suspected of having lung cancer should undergo a diagnostic evaluation. Diagnosis of lung cancer requires both visualization of the cancerous lesion and tissue sampling for pathologic assessment. All patients must have a thorough history and physical examination with emphasis on detecting signs and symptoms of the primary tumor, regional spread of the tumor, distant metastases, and paraneoplastic syndromes. The patient's performance status should be assessed to determine whether or not a patient may be able to tolerate surgery or chemotherapy.[3,4,10,11]

Visualization of the suspected tumor provides the clinician with the information necessary to choose the most appropriate sampling technique. Chest radiographs, endobronchial ultrasound, CT scans, and PET scans are among the most valuable diagnostic tests.[10,11] Chest radiography is the primary method of lung cancer detection and may also be used to measure tumor size, establish gross lymph node enlargement, and detect other tumor-related findings, such as pleural effusion, lobar collapse, and metastatic bone involvement of ribs, spine, and shoulders. In addition, CT scans may be helpful in the evaluation of parenchymal lung abnormalities, detection of masses only suspected on the chest radiography, and assessment of mediastinal and hilar lymph nodes. PET scans are more accurate than CT scans to distinguish malignant from benign lesions, detect mediastinal lymph node metastases, and identify metastatic spread. Most recently, the use of integrated CT-PET technology has been reported to improve the diagnostic accuracy in the staging of NSCLC over either CT or PET technology alone.[10]

Once the tumor has been located, pathologic examination of tumor tissue is necessary to establish the diagnosis of lung cancer. Tissue is typically obtained through the least invasive method likely to result in an adequate sample; methods include sputum cytology, tumor biopsy by bronchoscopy, mediastinoscopy, percutaneous needle biopsy, or open-lung biopsy. The tissue sample not only confirms malignancy but is also necessary to determine the histology (ie, squamous cell, adenocarcinoma, large cell, or small cell) and to provide adequate tissue for molecular analysis. Once the diagnosis is established, additional radiologic tests may be required to evaluate lymph nodes and potential metastatic sites for accurate staging. Surgical candidates will have additional sampling of their mediastinal nodes to determine those with Stage IIIB (N_3) disease (Table 129-2).[3,4,10,11]

STAGING

5 Once the diagnosis of lung cancer is confirmed, the extent of disease must be determined to estimate prognosis and guide therapy. For NSCLC, tumor growth and spread are staged with the American Joint Committee on Cancer (AJCC) tumor, node, and metastasis (TNM) staging system. SCLC is typically staged with the Veterans Administration Lung Cancer Study Group method.[14,21]

TABLE 129-2 Tumor (T), Node (N), Metastasis (M) Staging for Non-Small Cell Lung Cancer

Primary Tumor		Description
T_1		Tumor ≤3 cm in diameter, surrounded by lung or visceral pleura, without invasion more proximal than lobar bronchus
	T_{1a}	Tumor ≤2 cm in diameter
	T_{1b}	Tumor >2 cm but ≤3 cm in diameter
T_2		Tumor >3 cm but ≤7 cm, or tumor with any of the following features: –Involves main bronchus, ≥2 cm distal to carina –Invades visceral pleura –Associated with atelectasis or obstructive pneumonitis that extends to the hilar region but does not involve the entire lung
	T_{2a}	Tumor >3 cm but ≤5 cm
	T_{2b}	Tumor >5 cm but ≤7 cm
T_3		Tumor >7 cm or any of the following: –Directly invades any of the following: chest wall, diaphragm, phrenic nerve, mediastinal pleura, parietal pericardium, main bronchus <2 cm from carina (without involvement of carina) –Atelectasis or obstructive pneumonitis of the entire lung –Separate tumor nodules in the same lobe
T_4		Tumor of any size that invades the mediastinum, heart, great vessels, trachea, recurrent laryngeal nerve, esophagus, vertebral body, carina, or with separate tumor nodules in a different ipsilateral lobe
Regional Lymph Nodes (N)		
N_0		No regional lymph node metastases
N_1		Metastasis in ipsilateral peribronchial and/or ipsilateral hilar lymph nodes and intrapulmonary nodes, including involvement by direct extension
N_2		Metastasis in ipsilateral mediastinal and/or subcarinal lymph node(s)
N_3		Metastasis in contralateral mediastinal, contralateral hilar, ipsilateral or contralateral scalene, or supraclavicular lymph node(s)
Distant Metastasis (M)		
M_0		No distant metastasis
M_1		Distant metastasis
	M_{1a}	Separate tumor nodule(s) in a contralateral lobe; tumor with pleural nodules or malignant pleural or pericardial effusion
	M_{1b}	Distant metastasis

Stage	T	N	M	5-Year Survival (%)
IA	T_{1a}-T_{1b}	N_0	M_0	73
IB	T_{2a}	N_0	M_0	58
IIA	T_{1a}, T_{1b}, T_{2a}	N_1	M_0	46
	T_{2b}	N_0	M_0	
IIB	T_{2b}	N_1	M_0	36
	T_3	N_0	M_0	
IIIA	T_{1a}, T_{1b}, T_{2a}, T_{2b}	N_2	M_0	
	T_3	N_1, N_2	M_0	24
	T_4	N_0, N_1	M_0	
IIIB	T_4	N_2	M_0	9
	Any T	N_3	M_0	
IV	Any T	Any N	M_{1a} or M_{1b}	13

Data from references 4 and 20.

Non-Small Cell Lung Cancer

Clinical staging of NSCLC with the TNM system evaluates the size of the tumor, extent of nodal involvement, and presence of metastatic sites. The TNM criteria were last updated in January 2010.[14] The combination of these three evaluations determines the stage. Clinical stages and associated survival rates are described in Table 129-2. For comparison of various therapeutic modalities, a simpler stage grouping system is used in which Stage I refers to tumors confined to the lung without lymphatic spread, Stage II refers to large tumors with ipsilateral peribronchial or hilar lymph node involvement, Stage III includes other lymph node and regional involvement, and Stage IV includes tumor with distant metastases. Local disease is associated with the highest cure and survival rates, while those with advanced disease have a 5-year survival rate of less than 10%.

Small Cell Lung Cancer

The most commonly used system of staging SCLC was developed originally by the Veterans Administration Lung Cancer Study Group.[21] This system categorizes SCLC into two stages: limited and extensive disease. When evidence of the tumor is confined to a single hemithorax and can be encompassed by a single radiation port, the disease is considered limited. Any progression beyond this point is extensive disease. About 60% to 70% of patients initially present with extensive-stage disease. The initial pretreatment evaluation of an SCLC patient should include a medical history, a clinical examination, and laboratory survey, as well as a CT scan of the chest, abdomen, and head. Typically the approach is to identify tumor spread that would demonstrate extensive stage, at which time the workup can stop. For patients without extrathoracic disease identified by these tests, a bone scan and bone marrow biopsy should be performed to confirm limited-stage disease.[3,11]

TREATMENT

Desired Outcomes

6 The desired outcomes of lung cancer treatment depend on tumor histology, stage of disease, and patient characteristics such as age, history, and performance status.[4] These aspects must be assessed before appropriate treatment can be recommended. In the development of a patient care plan, the ultimate goals of therapy should be considered. In patients with early stage disease who can tolerate aggressive treatment, a definitive cure is the desired outcome of treatment. With advanced stage disease, the desired outcomes of treating lung cancer patients who can tolerate aggressive therapy include prolongation of survival. Regardless of treatment based on survival, all therapies should ultimately improve quality of life through alleviation of symptoms. Patients should carefully consider whether to receive aggressive treatment that may prolong survival by a few months but includes a high potential for toxicity that could significantly decrease quality of life. Treatment decisions must include both the healthcare team and an informed and well-counseled patient.

Non-Small Cell Lung Cancer

If left untreated, patients with advanced NSCLC will die within 3 to 5 months and those with early stage disease treated with routine care will die within 10 to 11 months.[10] Surgery, radiation therapy, and systemic therapy with cytotoxic chemotherapy or targeted therapies are all used in the management of NSCLC patients. The applications of these treatment modalities are determined by stage and other patient-specific factors (eg, age and performance status).[4,10] Table 129-3 lists commonly used chemotherapy regimens including doses and schedules.[4,10]

Local Disease (Stage I-II)

7 Local disease is associated with a favorable prognosis, and the goal of therapy is cure. Surgery is the mainstay of treatment and may be used alone or in some situations with radiation and/or chemotherapy. Patients who have comorbid conditions preventing them from being surgical candidates can be treated with radiation in place of surgery with curative intent, although the cure rates are lower. Stage IA and IB tumors are treated with surgery alone; when complete resection is achieved, adjuvant therapy is not routinely recommended.[4,7] If surgical margins are positive, re-resection is recommended. Alternatively, patients may receive radiotherapy with or without chemotherapy. Although controversial, patients with IB tumors and high-risk features (poorly differentiated tumors, vascular invasion, wedge resection, minimal margins, tumors more than 4 cm, or visceral pleural involvement) may also receive adjuvant chemotherapy.[4,7] Postoperative radiation therapy with older techniques may be detrimental and is not recommended.[4,7]

Stage IIA and IIB disease is primarily treated with surgery, which should be followed by adjuvant chemotherapy. The adjuvant treatment regimen of choice is not clear, but the positive clinical trials used platinum-based regimens, with arguably the best clinical trial data coming from cisplatin–vinorelbine (Table 129-4).[15] The absolute benefit in terms of 5-year overall survival in large randomized trials ranges from no benefit to 15%, with a recent systematic review reporting an absolute difference of 4%. The analysis suggested little effect of the chemotherapy regimen.[15] Although genetics and histology influence systemic treatment and outcomes in advanced disease, this approach has not been tested in large randomized adjuvant therapy trials.

Adjuvant radiation should be avoided in patients who have complete resection and clean margins because it has not demonstrated to be beneficial and can be detrimental. In those with resected lung cancer and N_2 nodal disease, radiation is recommended followed by adjuvant chemotherapy. Radiation, or more commonly chemoradiotherapy, is the treatment of choice for Stage II patients who are medically inoperable. Concurrent rather than sequential administration of chemotherapy and radiation therapy is preferred. Platinum-based chemotherapy is usually given when concurrent chemoradiotherapy is given; recommended regimens include cisplatin with either etoposide or pemetrexed (only for non-squamous histology) or carboplatin with either paclitaxel or pemetrexed (only for non-squamous histology).[4] Neoadjuvant chemotherapy can be used in patients with early stage disease. The trials and meta-analysis include Stages I-III and is discussed in Stage III.

Locally Advanced Disease (Stage III)

7 Patients with more advanced local disease have large tumors, multiple tumors, and/or nodal involvement—particularly mediastinal nodal involvement (N_2). Collectively this group of patients is heterogeneous and few large clinical trials are available to guide treatment. Consequently, treatment is best planned by a multimodality team where individual features and patient input are considered. Optimal outcomes are achieved with multimodality therapy that typically includes systemic chemotherapy. Patients with operable disease should be considered for surgery preceded or followed by systemic chemotherapy. Adjuvant chemotherapy after surgery in selected patients improves overall survival (see Table 129-4).[4,15] The primary adjuvant trials included patients with Stage IIIA disease as well as early stage disease; 5-year survival in these studies improved by about 5%. Chemotherapy administration prior to surgery (ie, neoadjuvant) should also be considered. It will treat micrometastatic disease (if present) prior to surgery and reduce tumor size, making surgery easier and better tolerated. However, it is possible that the tumor will grow and become inoperable during therapy. Two meta-analyses have reported that neoadjuvant chemotherapy improves 5-year survival by about 5% compared with surgery alone.[36,37] The analysis did not analyze what stage is most likely to benefit, what regimen is best, or how it would compare to surgery followed by adjuvant therapy. It is discussed here because the potential benefit of reducing the tumor size to make the surgery easier and, in some cases, feasible is most attractive for patients with larger tumors. Although a randomized trial comparing neoadjuvant and adjuvant therapy has not been reported, it appears that both approaches are roughly equivalent and better than surgery alone.

Radiation may be given in place of surgery as the local treatment modality combined with chemotherapy. Although a large definitive trial has not been performed, this research question has been evaluated in small randomized trials. The largest trial randomized 333 Stage IIIA (N_2) patients who responded to three cycles of induction chemotherapy to radiation or surgery. No significant difference in median overall survival (17.5 vs 16.3 months for radiation and surgery, respectively) or overall 5-year survival was observed.[38] This study suggests that surgery could be avoided by administering chemoradiotherapy, but it does not improve survival. Based on the knowledge that dual-modality therapy was better than a single modality, researchers tested trimodal therapy in small studies. The results of the only phase III randomized trial (SAKK-16/00) compared neoadjuvant chemotherapy followed by surgery with sequential neoadjuvant chemoradiotherapy followed by surgery.[39] The event-free survival, overall survival, and local failure did not differ between groups. It is currently recommended that patients with resectable Stage IIIA NSCLC be treated with chemotherapy followed by surgery or radiation, depending on individual patient and tumor features.[4,7]

TABLE 129-3 Common Chemotherapy Regimens Used to Treat Advanced Stage Lung Cancer

Place in Therapy	Small Cell Lung Cancer		Non-Squamous EGFR and ALK WT		Squamous Cell		EGFR Mutation Positive		ALK Rearrangement Positive	
	Regimen	Dosage Schedule	Regimen	Drugs, Doses, Frequency	Regimen	Drugs, Doses, Frequency	Regimen	Drugs, Doses, Frequency	Regimen	Drugs, Doses, Frequency
First Line	Etoposide/cisplatin (EP)[4,11]	Cisplatin 80 mg/m² IV on day 1 Etoposide 100 mg/m² IV on days 1-3; repeat cycle every 3 weeks[83,92] or Cisplatin 60 mg/m² IV on day 1 Etoposide 120 mg/m² IV on days 1-3; repeat cycle every 3 weeks	Carboplatin/ paclitaxel/ bevacizumab[3,5,10]	Carboplatin AUC 6 IV mg/mL/min on day 1 Paclitaxel 200 mg/m² IV on day 1 Bevacizumab 15 mg/kg IV on day 1 Repeat cycle every 3 weeks × 6 cycles—continue bevacizumab until progression	Gemcitabine/ cisplatin (GC)[3,5,10]	Gemcitabine 1,000 mg/m² IV on days 1, 8, and 15 Cisplatin 100 mg/m² IV on day 1 repeat cycle every 28 days	Erlotinib[3,5,10]	Erlotinib 150 mg (one 150 mg capsule) po daily on an empty stomach	Crizotinib[3,5,12]	Crizotinib 250 mg (one 250 mg capsule) po bid without regard to meals
	Cisplatin/irinotecan (IP)[4,11]	Cisplatin 60 mg/m² IV on day 1 Irinotecan 60 mg/m² IV on days 1, 8, and 15; repeat cycle every 4 weeks Or Cisplatin 30 mg/m² IV on day 1 Irinotecan 65 mg/m² IV on days 1 and 8; repeat cycle every 3 weeks	Carboplatin/ pemetrexed[3,5,10,26]	Carboplatin AUC 5 mg/mL/min IV on day 1 Pemetrexed 500 mg/m² IV on day 1 Repeat cycle every 3 weeks	Gemcitabine/ cisplatin/ Necitumumab[3,10]	Gemcitabine 1,250 mg/m² IV on days 1 and 8 Cisplatin 75 mg/m² IV on day 1 Necitumumab 800 mg IV on day 1 and 8 Repeat cycle every 21 days	Afatinib[3,5,10]	Afatinib 40 mg (one 40 mg tablet) po daily on an empty stomach		
Second Line	Topotecan[4,11]	Topotecan 1.5 mg/m²/ day IV days 1-5 Repeat every 21 days	Docetaxel/ Ramucirumab[3]	Docetaxel 75 mg/m² IV day 1 Ramucirumab 10 mg/ kg IV day 1 Repeat every 21 days	Docetaxel/ Ramucirumab[3]	Docetaxel 75 mg/m² IV day 1 Ramucirumab 10 mg/kg IV day 1 Repeat every 21 days	Osimertinib[3]	Osimertinib 80 mg (one 80 mg tablet) po daily without regard to meals	Ceritinib[3,12]	Ceritinib 750 mg (five 150 mg capsules) po daily on an empty stomach
			Nivolumab[3]	Nivolumab 3 mg/kg IV day 1 Repeat every 2 weeks	Nivolumab[3]	Nivolumab 3 mg/kg IV day 1 Repeat every 2 weeks			Alectinib[12]	Alectinib 600 mg (four 150 mg capsules) po twice daily with food
			Pembrolizumab[3]	Pembrolizumab 2 mg/ kg IV day 1 Repeat every 3 weeks	Pembrolizumab[3]	Pembrolizumab 2 mg/kg IV day 1 Repeat every 3 weeks				

Table 129-4 Common Chemotherapy Regimens used in the Adjuvant Treatment of Non-Small Cell Lung Cancer

Regimen[4]	Drugs and Doses	Frequency and Number of Cycles
Cisplatin/ etoposide	Cisplatin 100 mg/m² IV day 1 Etoposide 100 mg/m² IV daily on days 1, 2, and 3	Every 28 days for 4 cycles
Cisplatin/ vinorelbine	Cisplatin 50 mg/m² IV days 1 and 8 Vinorelbine 25 mg/m² IV days 1, 8, 15, and 22	Every 28 days for 4 cycles
	Cisplatin 100 mg/m² IV day 1 Vinorelbine 30 mg/m² IV days 1, 8, 15, and 22	Every 28 days for 4 cycles
Carboplatin/ paclitaxel	Carboplatin AUC 6 IV day 1 Paclitaxel 200 mg/m² IV day 1	Every 21 days for 4 cycles
Cisplatin/ pemetrexed	Cisplatin 75 mg/m² IV day 1 Pemetrexed 500 mg/m² IV day 1	Every 21 days for 4 cycles (for non-squamous histology only)

Patients with Stage IIIA disease who are not surgical candidates or have a tumor that cannot reasonably be resected and nearly all Stage IIIB patients are usually treated with both an active platinum-containing regimen and concurrent radiotherapy. Patients with tumors that cannot fit safely in a radiation port may receive induction chemotherapy followed by chemoradiotherapy. Responding patients may then become surgical candidates. Patients who are not surgical candidates should continue treatment with concurrent chemotherapy and radiation. Patients who are not candidates for radiation are treated like Stage IV disease as discussed further.[4,5,7]

Clinical **Controversy...**

Multimodality therapy improves outcomes for patients with Stage III disease, but the sequence and use of surgery or radiation remains to be defined.

Advanced-Stage Disease (Stage IIIB and IV)

8 About two-thirds of NSCLC patients present with advanced disease (unresectable Stage IIIB or IV) at the time of diagnosis.[1,4,10] These advanced tumors are generally not surgically resectable. A few patients with single metastatic sites may undergo surgical resection of both the primary tumor and the metastatic site.[4,5] For patients who have a tumor that will fit in a tolerable radiation port, chemoradiotherapy should be considered, but systemic therapy is the primary treatment modality for most of these patients.

The intent of first-line therapy is to palliate symptoms, improve quality of life, and increase the duration of survival. The benefits of cytotoxic chemotherapy—as measured by overall survival and quality of life—were not clearly established until the 1990s. The Non-Small Cell Lung Cancer Collaborative Group reported in 1995 the pivotal results of a large meta-analysis of 52 clinical trials of chemotherapy in the management of NSCLC with follow-up of an additional 16 trials in 2010.[40] The results of this updated meta-analysis showed that chemotherapy, either alone or combined with surgery or radiotherapy, improves median survival for patients with advanced-stage NSCLC by 2 to 4 months and increases the 1-year absolute survival rate from 10% to 20%; this rate did not change between the years 1995-2010.[40] Since chemotherapy became the standard treatment, new agents and targeted therapies have extended these modest gains in survival, while in some cases decreasing toxicity profiles. Current guidelines and experts agree that most patients with advanced-stage disease should receive at least one antitumor regimen.[4,5]

Patient selection for treatment of advanced-stage NSCLC depends on patient-specific factors that include age, performance status, and comorbid conditions. The patient's current performance status (Eastern Cooperative Oncology Group [ECOG] performance status of 0 to 2) appears to be the most consistent predictor of a better response and improved survival after chemotherapy. All patients with a good performance status without significant comorbidities, including elderly patients, should receive first-line therapy. Patients with an ECOG performance status 2 or significant comorbidities should be considered for less intensive therapy (eg, single-agent chemotherapy). Patients with poor ECOG performance status (more than or equal to 3) do not respond well to chemotherapy. Patients with an unfavorable prognosis (poor performance status or significant concomitant diseases) should receive best supportive care and palliative radiation when necessary.[4,5]

Historically a platinum doublet has been used as first-line therapy regardless of histology and in the absence of tumor genetic markers. In many cases these regimens are still appropriate (see Table 129-3). However, translating tumor genetics to practice has led to personalized medicine for advanced NSCLC. Instead of treating all patients the same, clinicians now categorize patients in one of four groups: (1) squamous histology, (2) EGFR mutated, (3) ALK positive (EML4-ALK rearrangement), or (4) non-squamous with wild type EGFR and ALK. 9 The four groups have been defined by varied response to drug therapy and/or toxicity to therapy. Select treatments for each group are outlined in Table 129-3.

Squamous Cell Histology First-line therapy for advanced-stage squamous cell lung cancer has not changed much since the mid-1990s. The standard of care continues to be a platinum doublet, with arguably the best doublet being either carboplatin plus paclitaxel[57] or cisplatin and gemcitabine.[41] Necitumumab, in combination with cisplatin and gemcitabine, was recently approved for first-line treatment of advanced squamous cell histology patients. The international trial randomized 1,093 patients to receive cisplatin and gemcitabine with or without necitumumab. The necitumumab arm had a similar response rate (31% vs 29%), median progression-free survival (5.7 vs 5.5 months), but longer median survival (11.5 vs 9.9 months, P=0.01).[23] At this point it is too early to see if this incremental improvement is enough to change the standard of care. Although platinum-based combination regimens remain the preferred treatment, nonplatinum-based combinations are acceptable and recommended in patients with a contraindication to a platinum agent. Nonplatinum doublets (eg, gemcitabine plus paclitaxel or docetaxel) have been evaluated in the setting of first-line therapy of advanced NSCLC. The results of a meta-analysis comparing platinum-based regimens with either the same regimen without the platinum or the platinum replaced by another agent demonstrated that platinum provides a modest benefit.[42,43] One meta-analysis evaluated 17 trials with a total of 4,792 patients and found a small but significant 1-year survival benefit with a platinum-based combination regimen compared with nonplatinum combination regimens (relative risk = 1.08, 95% CI 1.01-1.16).[43] A number of trials and meta-analyses have been performed to determine if carboplatin and cisplatin are equally effective or if one is more effective in NSCLC.[44-47] Individual clinical trials have produced equivocal data and meta-analyses report conflicting results.[44,46,47] One meta-analysis of doublet regimens reported that cisplatin was slightly superior when combined with a "newer" agent; cisplatin improved survival by 11% (P=0.039).[45] Clinical trials comparing the two agents have also demonstrated a different toxicity profile. Cisplatin is associated with more GI (severe nausea and vomiting) and renal toxicity than carboplatin. However, carboplatin is associated with more hematologic toxicity (thrombocytopenia) than cisplatin.[46] Although neither is clearly superior to the other, many clinicians have historically used carboplatin because of its more tolerable renal and GI toxicity, but over the past few years the trend has reversed toward increased use of cisplatin, which could be attributed to improved antiemetics (ie, the combination of a neurokinin-1 receptor antagonist, 5-HT3 receptor antagonist, and a corticosteroid). The lack of progress for first-line treatment represents the slow translation of targeted therapies to be safe and effective in this histology.

The duration of first-line therapy has also been studied. The optimal number of cycles remains controversial.[48] Response rates and quality of life were not improved with administration of six as compared with three cycles of mitomycin, cisplatin, and vinblastine.[49] For those receiving paclitaxel–carboplatin, administration of chemotherapy until disease progression had no clinically significant benefit in survival, response rate, or quality of life, but increased toxicity as compared with administration of four cycles.[50] Many large randomized trials have used six cycles as a standard. Current guidelines recommend four to six cycles of first-line platinum-based doublet chemotherapy for advanced squamous cell lung cancer that is stable or responding to chemotherapy.[4] The one exception to this recommendation is when necitumumab is added to cisplatin plus gemcitabine, where the chemotherapy stops after six cycles, but the necitumumab continues until progression (continuation maintenance).[23]

Significant advances with targeted therapy have been made for second-line treatment. After failure of first-line therapy, second-line monotherapy with docetaxel has been the standard. Pemetrexed, erlotinib, and afatinib can be used as second-line treatment. Pemetrexed appears to lack efficacy in squamous histology and is not recommended in this histology group.[4,41] Erlotinib and afatinib (EGFR tyrosine kinase inhibitors) provide most of their benefit to patients with an EGFR mutation (rarely seen in squamous histology) and therefore are not often used.[16,51] Afatinib and erlotinib have been compared in a large randomized trial for second-line treatment of squamous cell NSCLC. The progression-free and overall survival favored the afatinib arm (2.6 vs 1.9 months, P=0.01; and 7.9 vs 6.8 months, P=0.0077, respectively) making it the EGFR tyrosine kinase inhibitor of choice for this situation.[52] The efficacy of docetaxel has recently been improved with the addition of ramucirumab, a monoclonal antibody against VEGFR2. A large randomized trial comparing docetaxel with or without ramucirumab reported an increase in progression-free survival and overall survival (4.5 vs 3 months, P<0.0001, and 10.5 vs 9.1 months, P=0.023) favoring the ramucirumab arm.[29] This trial included all NSCLC histologies and about 26% of tumors were squamous histology. Response by histology was not compared, but ramucirumab appeared to be active in all histologies. In patients with squamous cell histology, median overall survival was 9.5 months in the ramucirumab-docetaxel arm compared to 8.2 months in the docetaxel alone arm. More importantly, no safety concerns (serious and fatal bleeding) like those seem with bevacizumab and chemotherapy in squamous histology were reported.[29]

10 Perhaps the most exciting new breakthrough has been the immune checkpoint inhibitors, nivolumab and pembrolizumab (PD1 inhibitors). Nivolumab was approved as second-line therapy for advanced stage squamous histology based on a phase III trial that randomized patients to receive nivolumab or docetaxel.[33] Nivolumab increased progression-free and overall survival (3.5 vs 2.8 months, P<0.001, and 9.2 vs 6.0 months, P<0.001).[33] This data has generated significant interest because historically immune responses can be durable; in this study the 1-year survival was 42%, which is remarkable for second-line therapy.[33] Pembrolizumab was approved as second-line therapy for all NSCLC histologies. The KEYNOTE-001 study compared three different pembrolizumab arms and was designed to identify and validate tumor PD-L1 expression to identify responders.[53] The primary endpoint of the study verified that patients who have a tumor where 50% of the cells express PD-L1 are most likely to benefit (PD-L1+). The progression-free survival was 3.7 months, overall survival was 12 months, and response rate was 19% for the entire population. The outcomes for PD-L1+ patients were significantly better; progression-free survival was 6.3 months, overall survival not reached (lower boundary of the CI was 13.7 months), and response rate was 45%.[53] These numbers were impressive enough for the FDA to approve the drug and the assay to determine PD-L1 positivity. More recently, a large trial randomized 1,034 patients to pembrolizumab 2 mg/kg, pembrolizumab 10 mg/kg, or docetaxel 75 mg/m^2 as second-line therapy for NSCLC. The median progression-free survival did not differ between arms, but overall survival with pembrolizumab (both arms) was superior to docetaxel (overall survival 10.4, 12.7, and 8.5 months for pembrolizumab 2 mg/kg, 10 mg/kg, and docetaxel arms, respectively). The overall survival difference was even greater in the patients with PD-L1+ tumors. The subgroup analysis showed that pembrolizumab was better in PD-L1 negative tumors patients as compared to docetaxel. Therefore, the value of knowing PD-L1 status is likely more important for prognosis than drug selection.[35] Due to the lack of comparative trials between PD1 inhibitors, the best second-line option is yet to be defined.[4]

Third-line therapy and beyond can be considered for patients who desire treatment and have a good performance status. The best agent(s) has not been determined in clinical trials. Therapeutic decisions are based on patient specific factors including prior therapies and potential contraindications to specific agents. Most commonly the treatment selection should be monotherapy with an agent known to have activity in clinical trials.[4]

Non-Squamous Histology Patients with advanced non-squamous histology have new treatment options based on tumor genetic findings. This group needs to be considered as three separate subgroups: (1) EGFR mutation positive, (2) ALK+, and (3) non-squamous with wild type EGFR and ALK. Determining which treatment path (subgroup) to put them in begins at the time of diagnosis where tumor tissue samples should undergo genetic testing. More specifically, tumor tissue needs to be tested for mutations in the kinase domain of EGFR, exon 19 and mutation of exon 21 (del746-750 and L858R), as well as for the EML4-ALK rearrangement. Tumors that harbor one of these genetic mutations (positive findings) will have a different treatment pathway.[4]

Patients who have a tumor that harbors a *mutation in the EGFR receptor* should receive first-line EGFR tyrosine kinase inhibitor: afatinib, erlotinib, or gefitinib.[5] In prospective randomized trials, EGFR inhibitors are superior to traditional chemotherapy regimens. They result in progression-free survival times of about 11 months, which is about 4 to 5 months longer than chemotherapy.[5,27] All three agents have been approved by the FDA for first-line treatment in EGFR mutation positive patients. There are no randomized head-to-head comparisons of these agents in this group of patients so the most effective agent is unclear. A recent meta-analysis comparing the three agents to chemotherapy for progression-free survival and overall survival by the two most common mutation types (exon 19 deletion and exon 21 L858R mutation) and subgroup comparisons by EGFR inhibitor type (reversible binding versus irreversible binding) was published.[54] The analysis found that all agents were associated with a significantly longer progression-free survival in exon 19 deletion (hazard ratio [HR] 0.27, 95% CI: 0.20-0.36) and L858R (HR 0.44, 95% CI: 0.33-0.58). Interestingly, the subgroup analysis suggests that the irreversible inhibitor (afatinib) is less effective in L858R mutated tumors than the reversible inhibitors (erlotinib and gefitnib). The overall survival analysis found that patients with an exon 19 deletion had improved survival (HR 0.72, 95% CI: 0.60-0.88). The analysis was not able to account for cross over from chemotherapy to an EGFR tyrosine kinase inhibitor, which was common.[54] Although this study did not identify which type of agent was best, it clearly supports the guidelines that recommend patients with an activating EGFR mutation should receive first-line EGFR tyrosine kinase inhibitor therapy instead of chemotherapy. They also show that prognosis with exon 19 deletion is better than exon 21 L858R mutation.[54]

After failing first-line EGFR tyrosine kinase inhibitor treatment, patients may be treated with a second-line EGFR tyrosine kinase inhibitor. If erlotinib or gefitinib (reversible EGFR binding inhibitors) was given as first-line therapy, then afatinib can be used as second-line treatment. A placebo controlled randomized trial showed that afatinib generated a 7% response (all partial responses) and improved progression-free survival (3.3 vs 1.1 months, $P<0.0001$).[55] This lack of cross resistance can be attributable to the activity of afatinib in tumors that harbor an EGFR T790M mutation. This acquired mutation occurs in about half of patients treated with erlotinib and gefitinib, and impairs binding of the drug to the receptor.[56] Osimertinib, an irreversible EGFR binding TKI, was designed to bind to this mutation and recently received accelerated FDA approval for patients with a T790M mutation. The approval was based on overall response in two single arm trials where 57% and 61% of patients responded to treatment. Although complete responses were rare, the median duration of response was reported to be 12.5 months.[30] Ongoing studies will determine the true benefit of this agent and its ultimate role in therapy. Based on the current data, osimertinib is an attractive second-line therapy for patients with a T790M mutation.

Second-line chemotherapy after failing a first-line EGFR tyrosine kinase inhibitor has been the standard and is still reasonable given the lack of trials comparing second-line regimens. For those who start chemotherapy, it is not clear whether patients should start with a platinum doublet or a single agent. For patients who can tolerate aggressive treatment, most will start treatment with a platinum doublet in the same path as non-squamous advanced disease without an EGFR mutation or ALK rearrangement.[4,5]

Third-line treatment is a likely option for those patients who still have a good performance status, desire for treatment, and can tolerate chemotherapy. For patients who have received two EGFR tyrosine kinase inhibitors, they could then be treated with a platinum doublet with or without bevacizumab, similar to non-squamous patients with wild type EGFR and ALK. For patients who received second-line chemotherapy, they would also follow the treatment path for non-squamous histology second-line therapy.[4,5]

The NCCN guidelines recommend that patients whose tumors have *an ALK rearrangement* should be treated with first-line crizotinib, an ALK tyrosine kinase inhibitor.[4] A phase III trial comparing first-line crizotinib to chemotherapy in patients with ALK+ disease found crizotinib to be superior. The median progression-free survival was 10.9 months versus 7 months ($P<0.001$) favoring crizotinib. The response rate was also higher in the crizotinib group, 74% versus 45% ($P<0.001$) and the median duration of response was longer, 11.3 versus 5.3 months. Overall survival was not different at the time of analysis, which is likely due to the relatively low number of deaths and high rate of cross over from chemotherapy to crizotinib.[25]

Second-line therapy with another ALK tyrosine kinase inhibitor appears to be a viable option after failing first-line crizotinib. Ceritinib was approved based on a non-comparative trial that reported a 56% response rate in crizotinib treated patients.[31] The median progression-free survival in the NSCLC population was 7 months. Based on these findings the FDA approved ceritinib as second-line therapy for this patient population. Alectinib is another recently approved option. It was approved based on two non-comparative trials that enrolled patients who had failed first-line crizotinib. The response rate was 38% to 48% and the duration of response from 7.2 to 11.2+ months depending upon the analysis. The attractive outcome with this study occurred in patients with brain metastases; the CNS response rate was 61%, which includes an 18% complete response rate. It is unclear at this point how ceritinib and alectinib compare, but patients with brain metastases have a proven option with alectinib.[34] Second-line chemotherapy is another reasonable option given the lack of comparative data between ceritinib or alectinib and chemotherapy. Similar to the EGFR mutated process, most patients would then begin the non-squamous wild type EGFR and ALK pathway with doublet chemotherapy and continue future treatment options along that pathway.[4]

Third-line therapy and beyond for those who have failed crizotinib and ceritinib or alectinib is reasonable and would involve chemotherapy. Although we do not have any data evaluating this process, most patients would start treatment with a platinum doublet similar to the EGFR and ALK wild type pathway.[4]

Most NSCLC patients have advanced-stage disease whose tumor is *non-squamous histology and does not have an EGFR or ALK aberration*. First-line treatment options for this subgroup of patients consist of four to six cycles of a platinum doublet and with some regimens the addition of bevacizumab. Patients who have benefit will continue with maintenance therapy. Historically, platinum-based doublets consisting of cisplatin or carboplatin combined with a "newer agent" paclitaxel (nab paclitaxel), docetaxel, gemcitabine, pemetrexed, or vinorelbine are considered the standard and equally effective in this population.[4,5] Based on an intergroup study comparing four regimens, carboplatin and paclitaxel had slightly less toxicity and was considered by ECOG to be the standard of care.[57] When evaluating the addition of a targeted agent, ECOG performed a prospective randomized trial comparing carboplatin and paclitaxel for six cycles with or without bevacizumab 15 mg/kg every 3 weeks.[22] The bevacizumab was continued until progression or unacceptable toxicity. As a result of bleeding complications seen in the phase II trial, patients with squamous cell carcinoma or brain metastases were excluded. The addition of bevacizumab led to longer progression-free survival from 4.5 to 6.2 months ($P<0.001$), median overall survival from 10.3 to 12.3 months ($P=0.003$), and 1-year survival from 44% to 51%.[22] NCCN guidelines recommend the addition of bevacizumab to chemotherapy for patients with advanced NSCLC of non-squamous cell histology, no history of recent significant hemoptysis, no CNS metastasis, and not receiving therapeutic anticoagulation.[4] Interestingly, a study that randomized patients to cisplatin and gemcitabine with or without bevacizumab did not find any survival benefit with the addition of bevacizumab.[58] This trial indicates that bevacizumab may not be equally synergistic with all chemotherapy regimens and the best evidence supports its use in combination with carboplatin and paclitaxel for lung cancer.

Another attractive option, particularly for patients with a contraindication to bevacizumab is cisplatin and pemetrexed. A phase III trial comparing six cycles of cisplatin and either gemcitabine or pemetrexed included all NSCLC patients, but was analyzed for this treatment subgroup. The overall survival with cisplatin and pemetrexed was noninferior to cisplatin and gemcitabine in all patients and in those with non-squamous histology. The cisplatin and pemetrexed had less neutropenia, anemia, and thrombocytopenia but more nausea than cisplatin and gemcitabine.[41] This study supports the concept that pemetrexed has limited activity in squamous cell histology, but is as good as other new agents when combined with a platinum agent and perhaps better in non-squamous histologies. Table 129-3 lists selected regimens for non-squamous NSCLC.

Therapy beyond four to six cycles is typically a single agent and is described as maintenance therapy.[4] Several studies demonstrate that continuation or switch maintenance therapy improves survival of NSCLC patients with non-squamous histology.[5] Continuation maintenance therapy is continuing at least one of the agents used in a combination for four to six cycles until progression. Alternatively, switch maintenance therapy is starting a new agent in responding patients after four to six cycles. Pemetrexed, bevacizumab, and erlotinib are the agents that have a proven survival benefit as monotherapy maintenance (switch or continuation), although the combination of pemetrexed and bevacizumab has also been shown to be a benefit.[5] Two large trials have evaluated pemetrexed as maintenance therapy.[59,60] In the largest phase III trial, 663 patients who responded to platinum-doublet therapy were randomized to pemetrexed maintenance (switch maintenance) or no further therapy until relapse. The results show that pemetrexed maintenance therapy prolonged median overall survival (13.4 vs 10.6 months, P=0.012). Interestingly, the benefit was only seen in patients with non-squamous histology, and the best results occurred in patients with adenocarcinoma (median survival 16.8 vs 11.5 months, HR 0.73, 95% CI 0.56-0.96). This histologic-specific benefit of pemetrexed is consistent in both the first (in combination with cisplatin)- and second (as a single agent)-line settings.[59] A second large study enrolled 939 non-squamous histology patients and treated them with four cycles of cisplatin and pemetrexed. The 539 patients who showed benefit from treatment (responders and stable disease) were randomized to continuation maintenance with pemetrexed or placebo. Continuation maintenance with pemetrexed resulted in a longer median overall survival (13.9 vs 11 months) and 1-year survival (58% vs 45%).[60] These two studies clearly established maintenance therapy as standard therapy, but for patients who start a doublet with bevacizumab, it is unclear if both bevacizumab and pemetrexed should be used as continuation maintenance. Initial results from the Alimta/Avastin versus Avastin Alone (AVAPERL) study show that bevacizumab and pemetrexed are superior to bevacizumab alone based on progression-free survival.[61] However, a larger study that compared carboplatin, paclitaxel, and bevacizumab with bevacizumab continued maintenance to carboplatin, pemetrexed, and bevacizumab with bevacizumab and pemetrexed continuation maintenance found no difference in overall survival.[26] Ongoing studies will address the effectiveness of maintenance therapy in specific situations.

Another recently reported randomized phase III trial shows that maintenance therapy with erlotinib prolongs disease-free survival versus placebo (Sequential Tarceva in Unresectable NSCLC [SATURN] study).[63] A total of 1,949 patients received four cycles of a platinum doublet; the 889 patients without progressive disease were then randomized to erlotinib or placebo. Erlotinib maintenance prolonged survival by 1 month (11 vs 12 months), which included all patients (11% with EGFR mutation and 89% EGFR wild type). Erlotinib maintenance appeared to be most effective in patients with adenocarcinoma histology and in those with an EGFR mutation. Although this study is compelling, pemetrexed is more commonly used because those with an EGFR mutation should receive first-line EGFR tyrosine kinase inhibitor therapy and continue it until progression.[4,5]

Studies evaluating gemcitabine[64] and docetaxel[65] maintenance therapy have been reported with some positive data. Both studies demonstrate that maintenance therapy improved progression-free survival, with a nonsignificant trend for improved overall survival. These agents should be considered in patients with a contraindication to pemetrexed and erlotinib.

Clinical **Controversy...**

The benefit of maintenance pemetrexed and bevacizumab for patients with non-squamous cell Stage IV NSCLC is proven. However, the benefit of bevacizumab and pemetrexed versus pemetrexed alone as maintenance is unknown. Additional clinical trial results to clarify optimal maintenance therapy for patients with non-squamous Stage IV NSCLC are needed.

Monotherapy with nivolumab, pembrolizumab, docetaxel, pemetrexed, or erlotinib are options for second-line therapy in patients with a good performance status who progress during or after first-line chemotherapy.[4,5] Docetaxel was the first to receive FDA approval for the treatment of advanced NSCLC after failure of a platinum-based chemotherapy regimen. The initial docetaxel dose of 100 mg/m^2 IV over 1 hour every 21 days was decreased to 75 mg/m^2 after an interim analysis showed a greater risk of severe neutropenia with the higher dose. Docetaxel, at the 75 mg/m^2 dose, was superior to best supportive care in terms of time-to-disease progression (10.6 vs 6.7 weeks, P=0.001), median survival (7.5 vs 4.6 months; P=0.047), and 1-year survival (37% vs 11%; P=0.003).[66] Both doses had a statistically significant improvement in 1-year survival when compared with a control regimen of vinorelbine or ifosfamide (32%, 21%, and 19%, respectively).[67] The efficacy of docetaxel has recently been improved with the addition of ramucirumab. A large randomized trial comparing docetaxel with or without ramucirumab found an increase in progression-free survival and overall survival (4.5 vs 3 months, P<0.0001, and 10.5 vs 9.1 months, P=0.023) favoring the ramucirumab arm.[29] This trial included all NSCLC histologies and about 73% had non-squamous histology. Overall survival in the non-squamous histology patients was 11.1 months with ramucirumab versus 9.7 months with docetaxel alone.[29]

The second chemotherapy agent approved as second-line treatment is pemetrexed. The approval was based on results of a phase III trial that randomized 571 patients to receive either pemetrexed 500 mg/m^2 with folate and cyanocobalamin supplementation or docetaxel 75 mg/m^2. No significant differences in overall response rate, stable disease, or median survival between the pemetrexed and docetaxel arms were observed. Docetaxel had significantly more hematologic toxicities as compared with pemetrexed, leading to more hospitalizations and use of hematopoietic growth factors and erythropoiesis-stimulating agents. Patients receiving docetaxel had a significantly higher incidence of alopecia, while patients receiving pemetrexed had a significantly higher elevation of alanine aminotransferase.[68] Pemetrexed appears to be a preferred option based on this study, but it is not appropriate as second-line therapy when it is used as maintenance therapy.

Erlotinib, a relatively nontoxic agent that targets the EGFR, was approved in November 2004 as a single agent for patients with advanced NSCLC whose disease progressed after at least one prior chemotherapy regimen. Its approval was based on an international, multicenter, randomized, double-blind phase III trial (BR.21) in 731 patients with locally advanced or metastatic NSCLC who had failed at least one prior chemotherapy regimen.[69] Patients were randomized to receive either erlotinib 150 mg or placebo orally once daily. Patients in the erlotinib group had a significantly higher objective response rate (9% vs 1%, P<0.001) and longer median progression-free and overall survival (9.9 vs 7.9 weeks, P<0.001 and 6.7 vs 4.7 months, HR 0.73, P<0.001, respectively) than those in the placebo group. Patients in the erlotinib group also had significantly improved symptom control, specifically time-to-deterioration of cough, dyspnea, and pain.[69] Although these benefits are relatively modest, some individual patients show a profound response. Analysis of predictive biomarkers led to EGFR mutational testing and to the recommendation that patients who have EGFR mutation-positive tumors should receive first-line erlotinib, afatinib, or gefitinib.[4,5,24]

As described above in the section on squamous cell histologies, the PD-1 inhibitors nivolumab and pembrolizumab are options in the second-line setting. Although currently only pembrolizumab is FDA-approved for all histologies and nivolumab is only FDA-approved for squamous cell histology, data from the CHECKMATE-057 study suggests that nivolumab is also active in non-squamous histologies and improves overall survival compared to docetaxel.[32] More recently, a large trial comparing second-line pembrolizumab to docetaxel found overall survival to be better with pembrolizumab regardless of PD-L1 expression, although the survival advantage was most impressive in patients with PD-L1 positive tumors.[35] The comparative trials indicate that pemetrexed and docetaxel are equally effective,[68] and docetaxel plus ramucirumab are superior to docetaxel alone.[29] Similarly nivolumab and pembrolizumab are superior to docetaxel alone.[32] All five monotherapies and ramucirumab-docetaxel are acceptable regimens, but the NCCN guidelines list nivolumab or pembrolizumab as preferred.[4] Their recommendation is likely attributed to the impressive durability of response.

Third-line therapy and beyond is reasonable for patients who have a good performance status and can tolerate another agent. Typically monotherapy with an active agent would be used in this setting. Erlotinib was tested in all histologies in the second- or third-line setting and is an appropriate option.[69] For patients who received an immune check point inhibitor (nivolumab or pembrolizumab), docetaxel would be an option with or without ramucirumab. For those who received second-line docetaxel with or without ramucirumab, an immune checkpoint inhibitor would be an option. For patients who want treatment beyond third-line, a single agent with activity could be used.[4,5]

In summary, patients with advanced-stage NSCLC should have their tumor tested for histology and those with a non-squamous histology should be tested for an EGFR mutation or ALK rearrangement. Based on these findings there are four distinct groups that have different treatment pathways and prognosis. The good news is that better understanding of tumor biology has resulted in better drugs and drug selection, which will hopefully improve prognosis for most patients.

Elderly and Poor-Performance Status Patients Single-agent chemotherapy is an alternative in elderly patients or those with an ECOG performance status of 2.[69] First-line, single-agent chemotherapy has objective response rates of 5% to 25% with no significant effect on overall survival. Complete responses are rare and responses that do occur are of brief duration (ie, 2-4 months).[70,71] Among the most active cytotoxic chemotherapy agents in NSCLC are cisplatin, carboplatin, docetaxel, paclitaxel, etoposide, gemcitabine, ifosfamide, irinotecan, topotecan, mitomycin, vinblastine, vinorelbine, and pemetrexed.[4] Erlotinib, afatinib, and crizotinib are also active as a single agent and should be considered in patients with a mutation-positive tumor.

Historically, patients with an ECOG performance status 2 were excluded from NSCLC trials because of excessive toxicity with minimal benefit from combination cytotoxic therapy. A recent randomized phase III trial comparing single-agent weekly docetaxel with docetaxel and gemcitabine in elderly or poor performance status (35% of patients) had disappointing results.[72] No survival differences were observed between the two treatment arms in the 122 poor-performance status patients (3.8 vs 2.9 months, respectively) and the median survival is short compared with patients with good performance status.[72] Another randomized phase III trial compared single-agent gemcitabine with gemcitabine/carboplatin in patients with ECOP performance status 2.[80] The median overall survival was not different between gemcitabine and gemcitabine/carboplatin (5.1 vs 6.7 months, respectively). The authors concluded that single-agent therapy is still the standard in this setting.[72] The updated ASCO guidelines state that available data support the use of single-agent and combination chemotherapy, but are relatively weak and incorporate elderly and poor performance status patients. They emphasize the need to individualize this decision.[5] A recent meta-analysis shows that patients with performance status 2 benefit from treatment.[73] The NCCN guidelines list both single agents and combinations for patients with a performance status of 2, and best supportive care for patient with a performance status of 3 or 4 unless they have an EGFR mutation or ALK rearrangement where they can receive a tyrosine kinase inhibitor.[4]

Personalized Pharmacotherapy

The translation of basic science to the clinic has resulted in personalized pharmacotherapy plans. Treatment decisions are influenced by tumor biology as described above, but must also consider patient characteristics (eg, comorbidities and performance status). Treatment guidelines generally apply to patients who are fit and desire aggressive therapy. Patient-specific factors that can alter these recommendations include age and comorbid conditions that serve as a relative or absolute contraindication to aggressive platinum-based doublet therapy and even some targeted therapies such that the risk of toxicity outweighs the benefit.[5] For example, elderly patients or those with an ECOG performance status of 2 have a modest benefit to aggressive platinum-doublet therapy; patients with an ECOG performance status of 3 have little to no benefit and a high risk of toxicity. Other considerations include renal dysfunction and the use of a platinum agent, and history of hemoptysis and the use of bevacizumab. Although these examples appear to provide clear guidance, risk is often a continuum and it is sometimes not clear how to treat individual patients (eg, a fully functioning 50-year-old with angina and a serum creatinine of 1.7 mg/dL (150 μmol/L) and Stage IIIB squamous cell lung cancer).

Evaluation of Therapeutic Outcomes

For patients who have undergone surgical resection with or without chemotherapy, radiation, or both, a physical examination and chest radiography are recommended every 3 to 4 months for the first 2 years, then every 6 months for 3 years, and then annually. In addition, a low-dose spiral chest CT scan is recommended annually to monitor for evidence of local recurrence. Suspicious symptoms or physical findings (eg, bone pain, visual abnormalities, headache, or elevated liver function tests) should prompt an evaluation to rule out distant metastases.[4,5]

Tumor response to chemotherapy is generally evaluated at the end of the second or third cycle and at the end of every second cycle thereafter. Patients with stable disease, with objective response, or with measurable decrease in tumor size (complete or partial response) should continue until four to six cycles have been administered. Patients with non-squamous histology tumors who respond (ie, nonprogressive disease) should be considered for maintenance therapy with pemetrexed. Following initial therapy for NSCLC, patients must be monitored for evidence of disease progression.[4,5] Second-line therapy and beyond is traditionally given until progression. The immune checkpoint inhibitors can display a different response pattern than traditional chemotherapy or targeted therapy. It can take some time for the immune system to become activated and then the tumor will initially be infiltrated with cytotoxic lymphocytes that radiographically can appear as progression prior to a response.[74] Although the registry trials continue to assess response based on RECIST criteria, an immune response criterion has been proposed where essentially progression needs to be documented on two consecutive assessments at least 4 weeks apart.[75] The median time-to-response for immune checkpoint inhibitors is 10 to 12 weeks.

Small Cell Lung Cancer

Small cell lung cancer is a rapidly dividing malignancy that spreads early in the disease course. Consequently, most patients present with extensive-stage disease (about 60%-70% of new cases). When patients with SCLC are not treated, the disease quickly becomes fatal. Fortunately, SCLCs are very responsive to chemotherapy and radiation. Chemotherapy with or without radiotherapy is the treatment of choice for most patients. Even after a complete response to therapy, the cancer usually recurs within 6 to 8 months, and survival time following recurrence is typically short (about 4 months). With treatment, median survival rates for patients with limited and extensive disease are 14 to 20 and 9 to 11 months, respectively. Treatment planning starts with stage of disease (ie, limited vs extensive stage), but must also take into account other factors, including performance status (treatment usually restricted to performance status 0 or 1), patient age, comorbid conditions (eg, renal failure), and patient desire to receive treatment.[3,6]

Limited Disease

7 When a single SCLC mass is found, local therapy with radiation or surgery is considered, although the use of surgery in SCLC is limited to solitary nodules, without evidence of metastasis to lymph nodes. One of the factors differentiating SCLC and NSCLC is the fact that radiation is favored for treatment of local disease over surgery. Radiation is always combined with chemotherapy in limited-stage SCLC, and the regimen of choice is etoposide and cisplatin (the EP regimen). Carboplatin may be substituted for cisplatin to reduce nausea and vomiting, nephrotoxicity, or neurotoxicity,[76] although increased myelosuppression in the form of thrombocytopenia may result. In European countries, a three-drug combination containing an anthracycline has been the mainstay of therapy, but mounting clinical evidence shows that these regimens are inferior to EP plus concurrent radiation and have more toxicity.[77] Consequently, the guidelines recommend that the EP regimen be used with concurrent radiotherapy.[3,6] Because patients with SCLC commonly have a recurrence in the CNS, trials have been performed to evaluate the benefit of prophylactic cranial irradiation (PCI). A pivotal study showed that PCI reduces the incidence of brain metastasis and increases 3-year survival from 15% to 21%.[78,79] Therefore, patients who achieve a complete response with treatment should be offered PCI.

Extensive Disease

8 Platinum regimens are also the treatment of choice in extensive disease, and many studies have failed to show superiority to the EP regimen as first-line treatment. A combination of irinotecan and cisplatin in one Japanese study demonstrated an increased median survival time by about 3 months over the EP regimen. This regimen showed a lower incidence of severe neutropenia but exhibited higher rates of moderate-to-high grade diarrhea in an Asian population.[80] However, irinotecan and cisplatin failed to improve survival as compared with EP in a study conducted in the United States.[81] Therefore, EP remains the regimen of choice for treating extensive-stage SCLC in the United States, with irinotecan and cisplatin reserved as an acceptable alternative. Concurrent radiotherapy is not used routinely in extensive disease. However, a recent study that randomized extensive-stage patients responding to chemotherapy to observation or PCI reported that PCI decreased the 1-year risk of brain metastasis (14.6% vs 40.4%), and prolonged survival (13.3% vs 27.1% at 1 year).[82] A more recent Japanese study reported that PCI reduced the risk of brain metastases, but did not improve overall survival. The results of these studies led to guideline revisions recommending PCI for patients with limited disease responding to chemotherapy.[3,6]

Recurrent Disease

Small cell lung cancer patients who relapse or progress after first-line chemotherapy have a median survival of 4 to 5 months. Unfortunately, when disease recurs, it is usually less sensitive to chemotherapy. The decision of whether or not to use second-line chemotherapy is often based on the length of time between completion of the induction chemotherapy regimen and relapse. If this interval is less than 3 months, the patient has refractory SCLC and is unlikely to respond to second-line therapy; hence, they should receive best supportive care or be enrolled in a clinical trial. For those with greater than a 3-month time interval between first-line chemotherapy and relapse, the expected response rate to treatment is about 25%, and second-line therapy should be considered.[3,6] Topotecan (IV and oral) is the only FDA-approved second-line therapy for SCLC. The pivotal trial leading to the approval randomized patients to IV topotecan or to cyclophosphamide, doxorubicin, and vincristine (CAV) regimen.[83] The response rates, time-to-disease progression, and overall survival were not different between groups. Interestingly, the proportion of patients experiencing symptom improvement was higher in the topotecan arm. The hematologic toxicity was similar between arms, but there was slightly more neutropenia in the CAV arm and more anemia and thrombocytopenia in the topotecan arm. Nonhematologic toxicity appears to be higher in the CAV arm; 11% of patients required a dose reduction compared with 1% in the topotecan arm.[83] Oral topotecan appears to be equally effective and similar in terms of dosing, toxicity, and effectiveness as IV topotecan.[28] Based on these studies, topotecan should be considered as the second-line treatment of choice, but because of its modest efficacy other agents warrant consideration. Agents that are recommended in national guidelines include single-agent topotecan (oral or IV), irinotecan, gemcitabine, paclitaxel, docetaxel, oral etoposide, temozolomide, and vinorelbine; CAV regimen; and participation in a clinical trial.[3,6]

Personalized Pharmacotherapy

Personalized pharmacotherapy based on tumor biology has not become a standard for SCLC. However, there is significant interest to identify targeted drug therapy that will improve the outcomes of all or subpopulations of patients with SCLC. Genotyping studies to identify targetable mutations are currently being employed. If a drug inhibiting a specific pathway proves to be beneficial, then optimal treatment may be individualized based on the tumor biology. Until then, we will continue to choose treatment primarily based on stage, comorbid conditions, and performance status. Similar to NSCLC, patients without comorbid conditions and good performance status will typically receive a platinum doublet (cisplatin and etoposide), but elderly patients, those with significant comorbid conditions, or those with an ECOG performance status of 2 may receive less aggressive treatment (a single agent), and those with extensive-stage disease who are bedridden will not be given cytotoxic therapy because of a lack of benefit.

Evaluation of Therapeutic Outcomes

The effectiveness of first-line therapy is evaluated after two to three cycles of treatment. At this point, therapy is continued for four to six cycles of therapy in patients with a complete or partial response or stable disease, and discontinued or changed to a non–cross-resistant regimen in patients demonstrating evidence of progressive disease. In the case of SCLC, those with response benefit from the addition of PCI following initial therapy. After recovery from first-line therapy, follow-up visits should occur every 3 months for years 1, 2, and 3, then every 4 to 6 months for years 4 and 5, and then annually for patients with either a partial or complete response.[3,6]

Complications and Supportive Care

Patients with lung cancer frequently have numerous concurrent medical problems. Such problems may be related to invasion of the primary tumor and its metastases, paraneoplastic syndromes (see Clinical Presentation earlier), chemotherapy and radiotherapy toxicity, or concomitant disease states (eg, cardiac disease, renal dysfunction, chronic obstructive pulmonary disease, asthma, or diabetes). Depression is also common and sometimes persistent in patients with SCLC and NSCLC and should be treated. Identification, diagnosis, and treatment of the patient as a whole may improve the patient's overall quality of life and tolerance to cancer treatments.

11 The chemotherapy regimens used in the management of lung cancer are intensive and are associated with a wide variety of toxic effects. Nausea and vomiting may be severe. Cisplatin-containing regimens require the use of aggressive acute and delayed antiemetic regimens containing a serotonin antagonist, dexamethasone, and neurokinin-1 receptor antagonist.[84] Patients experiencing protracted nausea and vomiting may require IV hydration and nutritional support. Myelosuppression is often the dose-limiting toxicity associated with chemotherapy. Granulocytopenia places patients at a high risk for serious infections. Other toxic effects associated with

these chemotherapy regimens include mucositis, anemia, nephrotoxicity, peripheral neuropathies, and ototoxicity.

About 30% to 65% of advanced-stage NSCLC patients will develop bone metastases, which may lead to significant bone pain, pathologic fractures, spinal cord compression, and hypercalcemia.[85] Zoledronic acid, an IV administered bisphosphonate, has been shown to reduce skeletal-related events in patients with bone metastases at a dose of 4 mg over 15 minutes infused every 3 weeks. Although the data do not show a significant reduction in skeletal-related events, time-to-first event is significantly increased (230 vs 163 days, P=0.023), thereby making zoledronic acid a viable therapy for patients with bone metastases. Denosumab has been compared to zoledronic acid in solid tumor patients including lung cancer and found to be noninferior in preventing or delaying first on-study skeletal-related event.[86] A subgroup exploratory analysis of lung cancer patients suggests that denosumab may prolong survival by just over a month.[87] Since they are equally effective for the primary endpoint, the potential benefit in survival might be considered when selecting therapy.

Patients receiving radiation therapy may experience complications including severe esophagitis, fatigue, radiation pneumonitis, and cardiac toxicity. These toxicities are usually more common and severe when radiation is combined with chemotherapy. The patient's baseline performance status and the degree of pulmonary dysfunction (eg, chronic obstructive pulmonary disease from years of tobacco use) must be considered in decisions concerning radiation dosage and fractionation.[88]

Patients who receive an immune checkpoint inhibitor can develop immune-related adverse events. Most commonly they include the GI tract where they present as diarrhea, the skin where they present as a rash, and pneumonitis where patients present with dyspnea. Holding therapy and intervening with steroids can blunt the progression of these toxicities. The other key point is that responses to immune checkpoint inhibitors can be delayed in onset.[88] A new response criterion has been developed for immunotherapies, which differs from RECIST criteria by requiring documentation of significant tumor grown on two occasions at least 4 weeks apart to be defined as progression. However, the registry trials for pembrolizumab and nivolumab both used the traditional RECIST criteria, indicating that the immune response criteria will not become the standard.

It is readily apparent that many lung cancer patients receive complex pharmacologic regimens that may include chemotherapeutic agents, immune checkpoint inhibitors, antiemetics, antibiotics, analgesics, anticoagulants, bronchodilators, corticosteroids, anticonvulsants, and cardiovascular agents. Such regimens necessitate intensive therapeutic monitoring in order to avoid drug-related and radiotherapy-related toxic effects and to optimize therapeutic outcomes for individual patients.

ABBREVIATIONS

AJCC	American Joint Committee on Cancer
ALK	anaplastic lymphoma kinase
ASCO	American Society of Clinical Oncology
BAC	bronchioalveolar carcinoma
CAV	cyclophosphamide, doxorubicin, and vincristine
CI	confidence interval
CT	computed tomography
ECOG	Eastern Cooperative Oncology Group
EGFR	epidermal growth factor receptor
EP	etoposide and cisplatin
ETS	environmental tobacco smoke
HR	hazard ratio
LDCT	low-dose computed tomography
MIA	Minimally invasive adenocarcinoma
NCCN	National Comprehensive Cancer Network
NSAIDs	nonsteroidal antiinflammatory drugs
NSCLC	non-small cell lung cancer
PD-1	programmed death receptor-1
PCI	prophylactic cranial irradiation
PET	positron emission tomography
SATURN	Sequential Tarceva in Unresectable NSCLC
SCLC	small cell lung cancer
SELECT	Selenium and Vitamin E Cancer Prevention Trial
TNM	tumor, node, and metastasis

REFERENCES

1. Siegel RL, Miller KD, Jemal A. Cancer statistics, 2015. *CA Cancer J Clin* 2015;65:5-29.
2. Couraud S, Cortot AB, Greillier L, et al. From randomized trials to the clinic: Is it time to implement individual lung-cancer screening in clinical practice? A multidisciplinary statement from French experts on behalf of the french intergroup (IFCT) and the groupe d'Oncologie de langue francaise (GOLF). *Ann Oncol* 2012.
3. National Comprehensive Cancer Network. NCCN Small Cell Lung Cancer Clinical Practice Guidelines in Oncology, v1.2016. Available at: http://www.nccn.org. (Accessed January 1, 2016.)
4. National Comprehensive Cancer Network. NCCN Non-Small Cell Lung Cancer Clinical Practice Guidelines in Oncology, v4.2016. Available at: http://www.nccn.org. (Accessed January 1, 2016.)
5. Masters GA, Temin S, Azzoli CG, et al. Systemic therapy for stage IV non-small-cell lung cancer: American Society of Clinical Oncology Clinical Practice Guideline Update. *J Clin Oncol* 2015;33:3488-3515.
6. Rudin CM, Ismaila N, Hann CL, et al. Treatment of small-cell lung cancer: American Society of Clinical Oncology Endorsement of the American College of Chest Physicians Guideline. *J Clin Oncol* 2015;33:4106-1411.
7. Bezjak A, Temin S, Franklin G, et al. Definitive and adjuvant radiotherapy in locally advanced non-small-cell lung cancer: American Society of Clinical Oncology Clinical Practice Guideline Endorsement of the American Society for Radiation Oncology Evidence-Based Clinical Practice Guideline. *J Clin Oncol* 2015;33: 2100-2105.
8. Leighl NB, Rekhtman N, Biermann WA, et al. Molecular testing for selection of patients with lung cancer for epidermal growth factor receptor and anaplastic lymphoma kinase tyrosine kinase inhibitors: American Society of Clinical Oncology endorsement of the College of American Pathologists/International Association for the study of lung cancer/association for molecular pathology guideline. *J Clin Oncol* 2014;32:3673-3679.
9. Horn L, de Lima Araujo LH, Nana-Sinkam P, et al. Molecular biology of lung cancer. In: DeVita VT, Lawrence TS, Rosenberg SA, eds. *DeVita, Helma, and Rosenberg's Cancer: Principles and Practice of Oncology*, 10th ed. Philadelphia: Wolters Kluwer; 2014:482-494.
10. Detterbeck FC, Decker RH, Tanoue L, Lilenbaum RC. Non-small cell lung cancer. In: DeVita VT, Lawrence TS, Rosenberg SA, eds. *DeVita, Helma, and Rosenberg's Cancer: Principles and Practice of Oncology*, 10th ed. Philadelphia: Wolters Kluwer; 2014:495-535.
11. Pietanza MC, Krug LM, Wu AJ, et al. Small cell and neuroendocrine tumors of the lung. In: DeVita VT, Lawrence TS, Rosenberg SA, eds. *DeVita, Helma, and Rosenberg's Cancer: Principles and Practice of Oncology*, 10th ed. Philadelphia: Wolters Kluwer; 2014:536-559.
12. Awad MM, Shaw AT. ALK inhibitors in non-small cell lung cancer: Crizotinib and beyond. *Clin Adv Hematol Oncol* 2014;12:429-439.
13. U.S. Department of Health and Human Services. The Health Consequences of Smoking: 50 Years of Progress. A Report of the Surgeon General. Atlanta, GA: U.S. Department of Health and Human Services, Centers for Disease Control and Prevention, National Center for Chronic Disease Prevention and Health Promotion, Office on Smoking and Health, 2014.
14. Edge SB, Byrd DR, Compton CC, et al. *AJCC Cancer Staging Manual*, 7th ed. New York City: Springer; 2010.
15. Burdett S, Pignon JP, Tierney J, et al. Adjuvant chemotherapy for resected early-stage non-small cell lung cancer. *Cochrane Database Syst Rev* 2015;3:CD011430.
16. Travis WD. Pathology of lung cancer. *Clin Chest Med* 2011;32: 669-692.
17. Bach PB, Mirkin JN, Oliver TK, et al. Benefits and harms of CT screening for lung cancer: A systematic review. *JAMA* 2012;307:2418-2429.

18. Keith RL, Miller YE. Lung cancer chemoprevention: Current status and future prospects. *Nat Rev Clin Oncol* 2013;10:334-343.
19. Kushi LH, Doyle C, McCullough M, et al. American Cancer Society guidelines on nutrition and physical activity for cancer prevention: Reducing the risk of cancer with healthy food choices and physical activity. *CA Cancer J Clin* 2012;62:30-67.
20. Kligerman S, Digumarthy S. Staging of non-small cell lung cancer using integrated PET/CT. *AJR Am J Roentgenol* 2009;193:1203-1211.
21. Micke P, Faldum A, Metz T, et al. Staging small cell lung cancer: Veterans Administration lung study group versus international association for the study of lung cancer-what limits limited disease? *Lung Cancer* 2002;37:271-276.
22. Sandler A, Gray R, Perry MC, et al. Paclitaxel-carboplatin alone or with bevacizumab for non-small-cell lung cancer. *N Engl J Med* 2006;355:2542-2550.
23. Thatcher N, Hirsch FR, Luft AV, et al. Necitumumab plus gemcitabine and cisplatin versus gemcitabine and cisplatin alone as first-line therapy in patients with stage IV squamous non-small-cell lung cancer (SQUIRE): An open-label, randomised, controlled phase 3 trial. *Lancet Oncol* 2015;16:763-774.
24. Rosell R, Carcereny E, Gervais R, et al. Erlotinib versus standard chemotherapy as first-line treatment for European patients with advanced EGFR mutation-positive non-small-cell lung cancer (EURTAC): A multicentre, open-label, randomised phase 3 trial. *Lancet Oncol* 2012;13:239-246.
25. Solomon BJ, Mok T, Kim DW, et al. First-line crizotinib versus chemotherapy in ALK-positive lung cancer. *N Engl J Med* 2014;371: 2167-2177.
26. Zinner RG, Obasaju CK, Spigel DR, et al. PRONOUNCE: Randomized, open-label, phase III study of first-line pemetrexed + carboplatin followed by maintenance pemetrexed versus paclitaxel + carboplatin + bevacizumab followed by maintenance bevacizumab in patients ith advanced nonsquamous non-small-cell lung cancer. *J Thorac Oncol* 2015;10:134-142.
27. Sequist LV, Yang JC, Yamamoto N, et al. Phase III study of afatinib or cisplatin plus pemetrexed in patients with metastatic lung adenocarcinoma with EGFR mutations. *J Clin Oncol* 2013;31: 3327-3334.
28. Eckardt JR, von Pawel J, Pujol JL, et al. Phase III study of oral compared with intravenous topotecan as second-line therapy in small-cell lung cancer. *J Clin Oncol* 2007;25:2086-2092.
29. Garon EB, Ciuleanu TE, Arrieta O, et al. Ramucirumab plus docetaxel versus placebo plus docetaxel for second-line treatment of stage IV non-small-cell lung cancer after disease progression on platinum-based therapy (REVEL): A multicentre, double-blind, randomised phase 3 trial. *Lancet* 2014;384:665-673.
30. AstraZeneca. Tagrisso prescribing information. 2015.
31. Shaw AT, Kim DW, Mehra R, et al. Ceritinib in ALK-rearranged non-small-cell lung cancer. *N Engl J Med* 2014;370:1189-1197.
32. Borghaei H, Paz-Ares L, Horn L, et al. Nivolumab versus docetaxel in advanced nonsquamous non-small-cell lung cancer. *N Engl J Med* 2015;373:1627-1639.
33. Brahmer J, Reckamp KL, Baas P, et al. Nivolumab versus Docetaxel in Advanced Squamous-Cell Non-Small-Cell Lung Cancer. *N Engl J Med* 2015;373:123-135.
34. Genentech. Alecensa Prescribing Information. 2015.
35. Herbst RS, Baas P, Kim DW, et al. Pembrolizumab versus docetaxel for previously treated, PD-L1-positive, advanced non-small-cell lung cancer (KEYNOTE-010): A randomised controlled trial. *Lancet* 2016;387(10027):1540-1550.
36. Felip E, Rosell R, Maestre JA, et al. Preoperative chemotherapy plus surgery versus surgery plus adjuvant chemotherapy versus surgery alone in early-stage non-small-cell lung cancer. *J Clin Oncol* 2010;28:3138-3145.
37. Westeel V, Quoix E, Puyraveau M, et al. A randomised trial comparing preoperative to perioperative chemotherapy in early-stage non-small-cell lung cancer (IFCT 0002 trial). *Eur J Cancer* 2013;49:2654-2664.
38. van Meerbeeck JP, Kramer GWPM, Van Schil PEY, et al. Randomized controlled trial of resection versus radiotherapy after induction chemotherapy in stage IIIA-N2 non–small-cell lung cancer. *J Natl Cancer Inst* 2007;99:442-450.
39. Pless M, Stupp R, Ris HB, et al. Induction chemoradiation in stage IIIA/N2 non-small-cell lung cancer: A phase 3 randomised trial. *Lancet* 2015;386:1049-1056.
40. Non-Small Cell Lung Cancer Collaborative Group. Chemotherapy and supportive care versus supportive care alone for advanced non-small cell lung cancer. *Cochrane Database Syst Rev* 2010;(5): CD007309. doi: 10.1002/14651858.CD007309.pub2.
41. Scagliotti G, Brodowicz T, Shepherd FA, et al. Treatment-by-histology interaction analyses in three phase III trials show superiority of pemetrexed in nonsquamous non-small cell lung cancer. *J Thorac Oncol* 2011;6:64-70.
42. D'Addario G, Pintilie M, Leighl NB, et al. Platinum-based versus non-platinum-based chemotherapy in advanced non-small-cell lung cancer: A meta-analysis of the published literature. *J Clin Oncol* 2005;23:2926-2936.
43. Rajeswaran A, Trojan A, Burnand B, Giannelli M. Efficacy and side effects of cisplatin- and carboplatin-based doublet chemotherapeutic regimens versus non-platinum-based doublet chemotherapeutic regimens as first line treatment of metastatic non-small cell lung carcinoma: A systematic review of randomized controlled trials. *Lung Cancer* 2008;59:1-11.
44. Ardizzoni A, Boni L, Tiseo M, et al. Cisplatin- versus carboplatin-based chemotherapy in first-line treatment of advanced non-small-cell lung cancer: An individual patient data meta-analysis. *J Natl Cancer Inst* 2007;99:847-857.
45. Hotta K, Matsuo K, Ueoka H, et al. Meta-analysis of randomized clinical trials comparing Cisplatin to Carboplatin in patients with advanced non-small-cell lung cancer. *J Clin Oncol* 2004;22:3852-3859.
46. Jiang J, Liang X, Zhou X, et al. A meta-analysis of randomized controlled trials comparing carboplatin-based to cisplatin-based chemotherapy in advanced non-small cell lung cancer. *Lung Cancer* 2007;57:348-358.
47. Rossi A, Di Maio M, Chiodini P, et al. Carboplatin- or cisplatin-based chemotherapy in first-line treatment of small-cell lung cancer: The COCIS meta-analysis of individual patient data. *J Clin Oncol* 2012;30:1692-1698.
48. Soon YY, Stockler MR, Askie LM, Boyer MJ. Duration of chemotherapy for advanced non-small-cell lung cancer: A systematic review and meta-analysis of randomized trials. *J Clin Oncol* 2009;27:3277-3283.
49. Smith IE, O'Brien ME, Talbot DC, et al. Duration of chemotherapy in advanced non-small-cell lung cancer: A randomized trial of three versus six courses of mitomycin, vinblastine, and cisplatin. *J Clin Oncol* 2001;19:1336-1343.
50. Socinski MA, Schell MJ, Peterman A, et al. Phase III trial comparing a defined duration of therapy versus continuous therapy followed by second-line therapy in advanced-stage IIIB/IV non-small-cell lung cancer. *J Clin Oncol* 2002;20:1335-1343.
51. Vilmar AC, Sorensen JB. Customising chemotherapy in advanced nonsmall cell lung cancer: Daily practice and perspectives. *Eur Respir Rev* 2011;20:45-52.
52. Soria JC, Felip E, Cobo M, et al. Afatinib versus erlotinib as second-line treatment of patients with advanced squamous cell carcinoma of the lung (LUX-Lung 8): An open-label randomised controlled phase 3 trial. *Lancet Oncol* 2015;16:897-907.
53. Garon EB, Rizvi NA, Hui R, et al. Pembrolizumab for the treatment of non-small-cell lung cancer. *N Engl J Med* 2015;372:2018-2028.
54. Kuan FC, Kuo LT, Chen MC, et al. Overall survival benefits of first-line EGFR tyrosine kinase inhibitors in EGFR-mutated non-small-cell lung cancers: A systematic review and meta-analysis. *Br J Cancer* 2015;113:1519-1528.
55. Miller VA, Hirsh V, Cadranel J, et al. Afatinib versus placebo for patients with advanced, metastatic non-small-cell lung cancer after failure of erlotinib, gefitinib, or both, and one or two lines of chemotherapy (LUX-Lung 1): A phase 2b/3 randomised trial. *Lancet Oncol* 2012;13:528-538.
56. Ma C, Wei S, Song Y. T790M and acquired resistance of EGFR TKI: A literature review of clinical reports. *J Thorac Dis* 2011;3:10-18.
57. Schiller JH, Harrington D, Belani CP, et al. Comparison of four chemotherapy regimens for advanced non-small-cell lung cancer. *N Engl J Med* 2002;346:92-98.
58. Reck M, von Pawel J, Zatloukal P, et al. Phase III trial of cisplatin plus gemcitabine with either placebo or bevacizumab as first-line therapy for nonsquamous non-small-cell lung cancer: AVAiL. *J Clin Oncol* 2009;27:1227-1234.
59. Ciuleanu T, Brodowicz T, Zielinski C, et al. Maintenance pemetrexed plus best supportive care versus placebo plus best supportive care for non-small-cell lung cancer: A randomised, double-blind, phase 3 study. *Lancet* 2009;374:1432-1440.
60. Paz-Ares L, de Marinis F, Dediu M, et al. Maintenance therapy with pemetrexed plus best supportive care versus placebo plus best supportive care after induction therapy with pemetrexed plus cisplatin for advanced non-squamous non-small-cell lung cancer (PARAMOUNT): A double-blind, phase 3, randomised controlled trial. *Lancet Oncol* 2012;13:247-255.
61. Gray JE, Infante JR, Brail LH, et al. A first-in-human phase I dose-escalation, pharmacokinetic, and pharmacodynamic evaluation

of intravenous LY2090314, a glycogen synthase kinase 3 inhibitor, administered in combination with pemetrexed and carboplatin. *Invest New Drugs* 2015;33:1187-1196.

62. Branden E, Hillerdal G, Kolbeck K, Koyi H. Pemetrexed and gemcitabine versus carboplatin and gemcitabine in non-small cell lung cancer: A randomized noninferiority phase II study in one center. *Oncologist* 2015;20:365.
63. Cappuzzo F, Ciuleanu T, Stelmakh L, et al. Erlotinib as maintenance treatment in advanced non-small-cell lung cancer: A multicentre, randomised, placebo-controlled phase 3 study. *Lancet Oncol* 2010;11:521-529.
64. Perol M, Chouaid C, Perol D, et al. Randomized, phase III study of gemcitabine or erlotinib maintenance therapy versus observation, with predefined second-line treatment, after cisplatin-gemcitabine induction chemotherapy in advanced non-small-cell lung cancer. *J Clin Oncol* 2012;30:3516-3524.
65. Fidias PM, Dakhil SR, Lyss AP, et al. Phase III study of immediate compared with delayed docetaxel after front-line therapy with gemcitabine plus carboplatin in advanced non-small-cell lung cancer. *J Clin Oncol* 2009;27:591-598.
66. Shepherd FA, Dancey J, Ramlau R, et al. Prospective randomized trial of docetaxel versus best supportive care in patients with non-small-cell lung cancer previously treated with platinum-based chemotherapy. *J Clin Oncol* 2000;18:2095-2103.
67. Fossella FV, DeVore R, Kerr RN, et al. Randomized phase III trial of docetaxel versus vinorelbine or ifosfamide in patients with advanced non-small-cell lung cancer previously treated with platinum-containing chemotherapy regimens. The TAX 320 Non-Small Cell Lung Cancer Study Group. *J Clin Oncol* 2000;18:2354-2362.
68. Hanna N, Shepherd FA, Fossella FV, et al. Randomized phase III trial of pemetrexed versus docetaxel in patients with non-small-cell lung cancer previously treated with chemotherapy. *J Clin Oncol* 2004;22:1589-1597.
69. Shepherd FA, Rodrigues Pereira J, Ciuleanu T, et al. Erlotinib in previously treated non-small-cell lung cancer. *N Engl J Med* 2005;353:123-132.
70. Lilenbaum RC, Herndon JE, 2nd, List MA, et al. Single-agent versus combination chemotherapy in advanced non-small-cell lung cancer: the cancer and leukemia group B (study 9730). *J Clin Oncol* 2005;23:190-196.
71. Ramalingam SS, Dahlberg SE, Langer CJ, et al. Outcomes for elderly, advanced-stage non small-cell lung cancer patients treated with bevacizumab in combination with carboplatin and paclitaxel: Analysis of Eastern Cooperative Oncology Group Trial 4599. *J Clin Oncol* 2008;26:60-65.
72. Hainsworth JD, Spigel DR, Farley C, et al. Weekly docetaxel versus docetaxel/gemcitabine in the treatment of elderly or poor performance status patients with advanced nonsmall cell lung cancer: A randomized phase 3 trial of the Minnie Pearl Cancer Research Network. *Cancer* 2007;110:2027-2034.
73. Goffin J, Lacchetti C, Ellis PM, et al. First-line systemic chemotherapy in the treatment of advanced non-small cell lung cancer: A systematic review. *J Thorac Oncol* 2010;5:260-274.
74. Ferraldeschi R, Thatcher N, Lorigan P. Pemetrexed in small-cell lung cancer: Background and review of the ongoing GALES pivotal trial. *Expert Rev Anticancer Ther* 2007;7:635-640.
75. Smit EF, Burgers SA, Biesma B, et al. Randomized phase II and pharmacogenetic study of pemetrexed compared with pemetrexed plus carboplatin in pretreated patients with advanced non-small-cell lung cancer. *J Clin Oncol* 2009;27:2038-2045.
76. Kosmidis PA, Samantas E, Fountzilas G, et al. Cisplatin/etoposide versus carboplatin/etoposide chemotherapy and irradiation in small cell lung cancer: A randomized phase III study. Hellenic Cooperative Oncology Group for Lung Cancer Trials. *Semin Oncol* 1994;21:23-30.
77. Sundstrom S, Bremnes RM, Kaasa S, et al. Cisplatin and etoposide regimen is superior to cyclophosphamide, epirubicin, and vincristine regimen in small-cell lung cancer: Results from a randomized phase III trial with 5 years' follow-up. *J Clin Oncol* 2002;20:4665-4672.
78. Auperin A, Arriagada R, Pignon JP, et al. Prophylactic cranial irradiation for patients with small-cell lung cancer in complete remission. Prophylactic Cranial Irradiation Overview Collaborative Group. *N Engl J Med* 1999;341:476-484.
79. Christodoulou C, Skarlos DV. Treatment of small cell lung cancer. *Semin Respir Crit Care Med* 2005;26:333-341.
80. Noda K, Nishiwaki Y, Kawahara M, et al. Irinotecan plus cisplatin compared with etoposide plus cisplatin for extensive small-cell lung cancer. *N Engl J Med* 2002;346:85-91.
81. Hanna N, Bunn PA, Jr., Langer C, et al. Randomized phase III trial comparing irinotecan/cisplatin with etoposide/cisplatin in patients with previously untreated extensive-stage disease small-cell lung cancer. *J Clin Oncol* 2006;24:2038-2043.
82. Slotman BJ, Mauer ME, Bottomley A, et al. Prophylactic cranial irradiation in extensive disease small-cell lung cancer: Short-term health-related quality of life and patient reported symptoms: Results of an international phase III randomized controlled trial by the EORTC Radiation Oncology and Lung Cancer Groups. *J Clin Oncol* 2009;27:78-84.
83. von Pawel J, Schiller JH, Shepherd FA, et al. Topotecan versus cyclophosphamide, doxorubicin, and vincristine for the treatment of recurrent small-cell lung cancer. *J Clin Oncol* 1999;17:658-667.
84. Socinski MA, Weissman C, Hart LL, et al. Randomized phase II trial of pemetrexed combined with either cisplatin or carboplatin in untreated extensive-stage small-cell lung cancer. *J Clin Oncol* 2006;24:4840-4847.
85. Rosen LS, Gordon D, Tchekmedyian S, et al. Zoledronic acid versus placebo in the treatment of skeletal metastases in patients with lung cancer and other solid tumors: A phase III, double-blind, randomized trial—the Zoledronic Acid Lung Cancer and Other Solid Tumors Study Group. *J Clin Oncol* 2003;21:3150-3157.
86. Machiels JP, Licitra LF, Haddad RI, et al. Rationale and design of LUX-Head & Neck 1: A randomised, Phase III trial of afatinib versus methotrexate in patients with recurrent and/or metastatic head and neck squamous cell carcinoma who progressed after platinum-based therapy. *BMC Cancer* 2014;14:473.
87. Scagliotti GV, Kortsik C, Dark GG, et al. Pemetrexed combined with oxaliplatin or carboplatin as first-line treatment in advanced non-small cell lung cancer: A multicenter, randomized, phase II trial. *Clin Cancer Res* 2005;11:690-696.
88. Dolan DE, Gupta S. PD-1 pathway inhibitors: Changing the landscape of cancer immunotherapy. *Cancer Control* 2014;21:231-237.

130

Colorectal Cancer

Lisa M. Holle, Jessica M. Clement, and Lisa E. Davis

KEY CONCEPTS

1. Advancing age, inherited and acquired genetic susceptibilities, lifestyle factors, inflammatory bowel disease, type 2 diabetes mellitus, and environmental factors are associated with colorectal cancer risk.
2. Regular use of aspirin and other nonsteroidal anti-inflammatory drugs, calcium intake, and higher blood vitamin D levels may reduce risk of colorectal cancer, but they are not currently recommended for routine cancer prevention.
3. Effective colorectal cancer detection programs incorporate routine screening starting at age 50 years for average-risk individuals. Colorectal adenomas can progress to cancer and should be removed.
4. The histologic stage of colorectal cancer upon diagnosis—determined by depth of bowel invasion, lymph node involvement, and presence of metastases—is the most important prognostic factor for disease recurrence and survival.
5. The treatment goal for stages I, II, and III colon cancer is cure; surgery should be offered to all eligible patients for this purpose. Six months of fluoropyrimidine-based adjuvant systemic therapy reduces the risk of cancer recurrence and overall mortality in patients with stage III and select populations with stage II colon cancer. An oxaliplatin-containing regimen further reduces risk as compared with fluoropyrimidine alone.
6. Combined modality neoadjuvant therapy consists of fluoropyrimidine-based chemosensitized radiation therapy and surgery for patients with stage II or III cancer of the rectum and is considered standard of care to decrease risk of local and distant disease recurrence.
7. Preoperative chemotherapy may reduce tumor size and convert unresectable disease to resectable disease in selected patients with metastatic colorectal cancer. This strategy offers the potential for prolonging overall survival and cure for metastatic disease.
8. Chemotherapy is palliative for metastatic disease. A fluoropyrimidine with oxaliplatin or irinotecan improves survival compared to fluoropyrimidine monotherapy and should be offered to patients who are candidates for aggressive treatment. The ability for patients to receive all active cytotoxic agents (eg, fluoropyrimidine, oxaliplatin, and irinotecan) during the course of their disease improves their overall survival.
9. Bevacizumab plus fluoropyrimidine-based chemotherapy as initial therapy for metastatic disease is considered standard of care and provides a survival benefit as compared with combination chemotherapy alone.
10. The addition of an epidermal growth factor receptor (EGFR) inhibitor (cetuximab or panitumumab) to initial treatment for *RAS* wild-type advanced or metastatic disease may improve tumor response rates and survival. Individuals who have disease progression after initial therapy not containing an EGFR inhibitor may benefit from cetuximab or panitumumab, either alone as a single agent or combined with other drugs. However, patients with *RAS* gene mutations should not receive cetuximab or panitumumab as these tumor mutations predict lack of treatment response.

Colorectal cancer involves the colon, rectum, and anal canal. It is one of the three most common cancers in adult men and women in the United States.[1] In 2016, an estimated 134,490 new cases will be diagnosed, of which 95,270 will involve the colon and 39,220 the rectum. An additional 8,080 new cases of cancer involve the anus, anal canal, or anorectum. For both adult men and women, colorectal cancer is the third leading cause of cancer-related deaths in the United States. An estimated 49,190 deaths will occur during 2016.

Mortality and incidence rates associated with colorectal cancer in the United States have decreased steadily over the past two decades. Incidence rates vary worldwide, with the highest incidence rates in economically developed countries.[2] Colorectal cancer mortality rates have been decreasing likely due to increased screening and/or improved treatments; however, mortality rates continue to increase in less developed countries in eastern Europe and South America.[2]

Multiple factors are associated with the development of colorectal cancer, including inherited susceptibility, environmental and lifestyle factors, and certain disease states. Overall, about 40% of affected individuals undergo a surgical procedure alone intended for cure. An additional 37% of individuals can potentially be cured with surgery followed by adjuvant radiation therapy (XRT), chemotherapy, or both. Curability is influenced primarily by the depth of tumor penetration, involvement of lymph nodes, and presence of metastatic disease. Five-year survival rates are about 90% for persons with early stages of colon and rectal cancer.[3] After the tumor has spread regionally to adjacent lymph nodes or tissues, 5-year survival rates drop to about 70% for both colon and rectal cancer. Five-year survival for individuals with metastatic disease is about 13%.

Treatment modalities for colorectal cancer include surgery, XRT, chemotherapy, and targeted molecular therapies (eg, angiogenesis inhibitors and epidermal growth factor receptor inhibitors). Surgery is the important and definitive procedure associated with cure. XRT can improve curability following surgical resection in rectal cancer and may reduce symptoms and complications associated with advanced disease. Chemotherapy is used in the adjuvant setting to increase cure rates and in treatment for advanced stages of disease to prolong survival. Selected patients with metastatic disease who receive aggressive preoperative chemotherapy and targeted therapies experience higher resection rates and can be potentially cured. Much progress has been made in the treatment of advanced disease, the ability to identify candidates for potentially curative surgical procedures, and the availability of active drug regimens that improve patients' survival.

EPIDEMIOLOGY

Colorectal cancer is the third most common malignancy worldwide in men and second most common malignancy in women, accounting for more than 1.4 million new cases annually.[2] The variation in colorectal cancer occurrence worldwide is at least 20-fold.[2] The highest incidence rates are found in Australia and New Zealand, Europe, North America, and South Korea. The lowest incidence rates are seen in less-developed areas such as Africa and South Central Asia. Most recently, incidence rates have rapidly increased in newer economically developed countries where rates were historically low, such as in eastern Europe and in Japan, Kuwait, and Israel.[2] The increases in these countries is thought to be associated with an increased prevalence of risk factors associated with westernization, such as unhealthy diet, obesity, and smoking.

The incidence of invasive colon cancer is greatest among males, who have an age-adjusted incidence rate of 37.4 per 100,000, as compared with females for whom the rate is 29.9 per 100,000.[3] Invasive cancer of the rectum occurs less frequently; the incidence rate is 16.5 and 10.3 per 100,000 for males and females, respectively. Differences in colorectal cancer incidence exist among ethnic groups in the United States, where incidence is highest among African Americans followed by, American Indian/Alaska Native, Whites, Hispanic/Latino, and Asian American/Pacific Islander.[2] Cultural and genetic factors as well as disparities in access to healthcare services, may influence risk among population groups.

The overall incidence of colon and rectal cancers in the United States continues to decline, with an annual percent decrease of more than 4.3% from 2007 to 2011 in adults over the age of 50 years and 1.8% per year in adults younger than 50 years.[1] Cancer incidence rates have declined in every major ethnic group since 1975, although less among American Indian/Alaska Natives. Most recent rapid declines in incidence rates are attributed to screening and polyp removal.[1] Figure 130-1 displays trends for incidence and mortality rates among White and African American males and females in the United States.[4]

Cancer of the colon and rectum accounts for about 8% of all cancer deaths in the United States.[1] The median age for death from cancer of the colon or rectum is 74 years.[4] It is estimated that 49,190 individuals will die of colorectal cancer in the United States in 2016, which represents a continued decline in overall combined mortality for both colon and rectal cancer.[1] Overall mortality rates are highest among African American males and females, although a steep rate of decline began in the late 1990s.[3] Colorectal cancer death rates are decreasing among all ethnic groups, but mortality rates are not statistically lower in American Indian/Alaska Natives.[3] Factors contributing to the overall decline in colorectal cancer mortality include decreasing incidence rates, screening programs with early polyp removal, and more effective and better tolerated treatments. Differences among different world geographic regions, and in population groups in the United States, may also reflect variations in underlying tumor biology, stage at diagnosis, access to screening programs, and availability of effective treatments.[2]

ETIOLOGY AND RISK FACTORS

Numerous studies suggest that the development of colorectal cancer is related to both uncontrollable and modifiable risk factors. Age, family history, clinical and genetic susceptibilities cannot be controlled by individuals. However, lifestyle factors, dietary, and environmental factors that affect the bowel may influence an individual's risk of developing colorectal cancer.

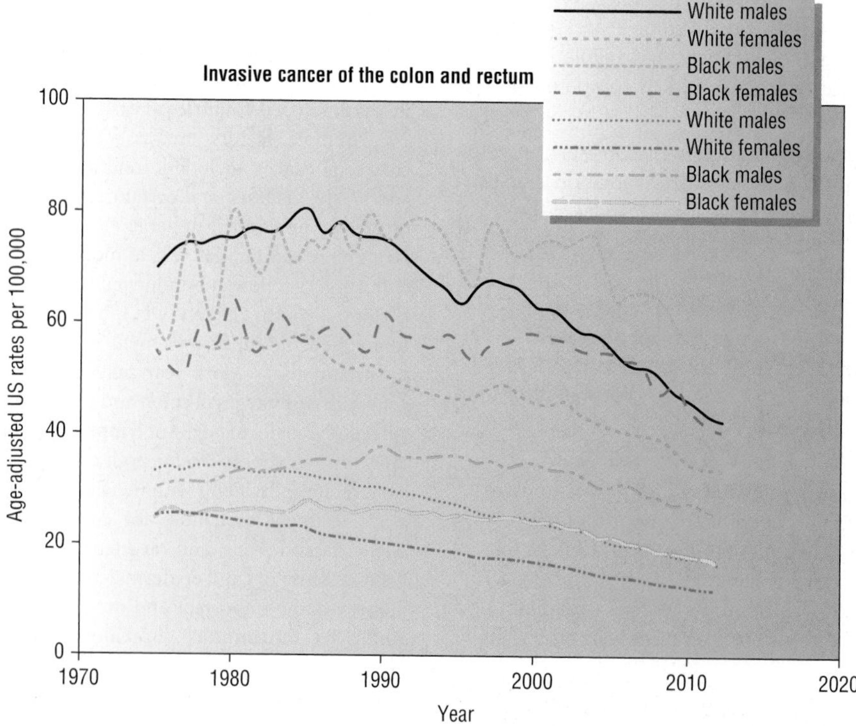

FIGURE 130–1 National Cancer Institute, Surveillance Epidemiology, and End Results (SEER) incidence and mortality rates for invasive colon and rectum cancer, 1975-2012. SEER 9 areas and US Mortality Files (National Center for Health Statistics, CDC). Rates are age adjusted to the 2000 US standard population (19 age groups—Census P25-1130). *(From reference 4.)*

Personal Medical History

Age

1 An individual's risk of developing cancer of the colon or rectum increases with advancing age, rising progressively after age 50.[3] The median age at colon cancer diagnosis is 69 years in men and 73 years in women and 63 years in men and 65 years in women for rectal cancer.[3] Although about 10% of patients are less than 50 years of age at the time of diagnosis, the incidence of colorectal cancer is increasing in this age group, in contrast to overall rates of decline among adults age 50 years and older. The reasons for this pattern are unclear, but may reflect increasing trends in obesity and detrimental dietary factors among younger people.[3]

Adenomatous Polyps or Colorectal Cancer

A prior history of high-risk adenomatous polyps, particularly multiple adenomas or size 10 mm or more, is associated with increased risk of colorectal cancer.[5] Individuals with a prior diagnosis of colon or rectal cancer have a greater risk of developing a new malignancy at another area in their colon or rectum as compared to individuals without a prior history of colorectal cancer.

Inflammatory Bowel Disease

1 Individuals with chronic inflammatory bowel disease, such as ulcerative colitis or Crohn's disease, have about a two-fold greater risk of developing colorectal cancer than the average individual.[3,6] This risk increases with the extent and duration of disease, a familial history of colorectal cancer, coexistent primary sclerosing cholangitis, and the degree of inflammation. The risk is even greater for young individuals and increases for all affected individuals with increasing extent of bowel involvement and disease duration. Recent data suggest that the overall incidence is staying steady or diminishing in Western countries. The cumulative risk of colorectal cancer is low early in life, but increases over time. The reported incidence ranges from 2% to 3% at 10 years after diagnosis to 5% to 8% at 20 years and 8% to 18% at 30 years.[6] Recent evidence suggests that the risk may be lower in these patients in more recent years because of improved screening and disease management.[3] Chronic underlying inflammation, oxidative stress, genetic instability, and release of various cytokines, including nuclear factor-kappa B and tumor necrosis factor-alpha, and intestinal microbiota appear to promote tumorigenesis.[6] The progressive dysplastic changes that bowel mucosa undergo are similar to those observed in adenomatous polyps. Overall, persons diagnosed with either disease constitute about 1% to 2% of all new cases of colorectal cancer each year.

Type 2 Diabetes Mellitus

1 Type 2 diabetes mellitus, independent of body mass size and physical activity level, is associated with increased colorectal cancer risk, although glycosylated hemoglobin (HbA_{1c}) alone as an indicator of hyperglycemia and association with colorectal cancer is inconsistent.[7] Metabolic syndrome is associated with an elevated risk of colorectal cancer. In a meta-analysis of 24 studies, diabetes was associated with a 37% increase in risk of colorectal cancer and increased risk of colorectal cancer mortality.[8] Features associated with type 2 diabetes, such as hyperinsulinemia and elevated levels of free insulin-like growth factor-1 (IGF-1), promote tumor cell proliferation.[7,9] Individuals diagnosed with colorectal cancer and type 2 diabetes have a higher risk of all-cause mortality compared to individuals without diabetes.[9] Risk of death from cardiovascular disease was higher among patients receiving insulin whereas colorectal cancer related mortality was lower with insulin use. Individuals with type 2 diabetes mellitus treated for colorectal cancer also have decreased disease-free survival (DFS) and overall survival (OS) and experience a higher incidence of treatment-related diarrhea and risk of death.

Family History and Inherited Genetic Risk

Colorectal Cancer or Adenomatous Polyps

1 Three specific patterns of colon cancer occurrence are generally observed: sporadic, familial, and recognized hereditary syndromes. Although most cases of colon cancer are sporadic in nature, about 30% of patients who develop colorectal cancer will have a family history of colorectal cancer.[10] In these families, the frequency of colorectal cancer is too high to be considered sporadic, but the pattern is not consistent with an inherited syndrome. First-degree relatives of patients diagnosed with colorectal cancer have an increased risk of the disease (2 times the risk), which is higher if the relative was diagnosed at age 45 or younger (3-6 times higher). Similarly, parents and siblings of relatives diagnosed with adenomatous polyps are at increased risk for developing colorectal cancer. The reasons for these associations are not established, but may be related to a combination of inherited genes and environmental factors.

Hereditary Syndromes

1 Colorectal cancer is a consequence of several well-defined genetic syndromes.[10] The two most common forms of hereditary colon cancer are familial adenomatous polyposis (FAP) and Lynch syndrome, historically known as *hereditary nonpolyposis colorectal cancer* (HNPCC). Both forms result from a specific germline mutation. FAP is a rare autosomal dominant trait caused by inactivating mutations of the adenomatous polyposis coli (*APC*) gene and accounts for about 1% of all colorectal cancers. The disease is manifested by hundreds to thousands of tiny sessile adenomatous polyps that carpet the colon and rectum, typically arising during adolescence. The polyps continue to proliferate throughout the colon, with eventual transformation to malignancy and have a propensity for occurring in the proximal colon. The risk of developing colorectal cancer for individuals with untreated FAP is virtually 100%; most will develop colorectal cancer by the fourth and fifth decades of life. Several variants of FAP exist and are associated with different extracolonic manifestations.

Lynch syndrome is an autosomal dominant inherited syndrome and is the most common hereditary predisposition for colorectal cancer.[10] Patients with Lynch syndrome are predisposed to many types of cancer (eg, endometrial, stomach, and ovarian), but the risk of colorectal cancer is the highest.[3] Germline mutations in one of the DNA mismatch-repair (MMR) genes, most commonly *MLH1*, *MSH2*, *MSH6*, or *PMS2*, are responsible for Lynch syndrome, which accounts for 2% to 4% of overall colorectal cancer cases.[10] A fifth germline cause of Lynch syndrome has been recently described, whereby a deletion occurs in the epithelial cell adhesion gene, but this cause is rare. The estimated lifetime risk of developing colorectal cancer is about 50% and 80% for carriers of germline MMR mutations. Multiple generations within a family are affected, and colorectal cancer develops early in life, with a mean age at time of diagnosis of about 45 years of age.[3] If Lynch syndrome is suspected in a patient diagnosed with colorectal cancer, typically due to early age at diagnosis or family cancer history, the tumor is examined for evidence of deficient MMR to distinguish between sporadic or germline genetic mutations. Criteria for diagnosis of Lynch syndrome have been established, and it is important to identify carriers of these MMR mutations so that they can be counseled and followed appropriately.[10]

Enzyme Polymorphisms

1 Increasing evidence suggests that genetic polymorphisms in drug-metabolizing enzymes, such as *N*-acetyltransferases (NAT1 and NAT2), cytochrome P450 (CYP) isoenzymes, glutathione-*S*-transferase enzymes, methylenetetrahydrofolate reductase (MTHFR), and hemochromatosis gene mutations, may confer genetic susceptibility to colorectal cancer.[11] Individuals with certain variations in

NAT1, NAT2, CYP1A2, CYP1A1, and CYP2E1 enzyme genotypes may be particularly susceptible to carcinogenic effects of a high dietary intake of meat, tobacco smoke, or other environmental factors.

Lifestyle Factors

Nonsteroidal Antiinflammatory Drug and Aspirin Use

2 Several lifestyle factors are known to affect colorectal cancer risk (Table 130-1). Observational studies have reported that regular (at least 2 doses per week) nonsteroidal antiinflammatory drug (NSAID) and aspirin use is associated with a reduced risk of colorectal cancer. In an average-risk individual, regular aspirin use is associated with a 20% to 40% reduction in the risk of colorectal adenoma and colorectal cancer.[12] In patients with prior adenomas or diagnosis of colorectal cancer, regular daily aspirin use reduces colorectal adenoma recurrence, and colorectal cancer incidence and mortality.[7,13,14]

Benefit has also been seen with NSAID and cyclooxygenase-2 inhibitor (COX-2) use. NSAID use over a 10- to 15-year period is associated with protection against adenomas and colorectal cancer, with a 30% to 45% reduction in the risk of colorectal cancer.[12] The protective effects of these agents appear to be related to their inhibition of COX-2 and free radical formation. COX-2 overexpression is seen in precancerous and cancerous lesions in the colon and is associated with decreased colon cancer cell apoptosis and increased production of angiogenesis-promoting factors.[13,14] Up to 50% of colorectal adenomas and 85% of sporadic colon carcinomas have elevated levels of COX-2, and COX-2 overexpression in colorectal cancer is associated with a worse survival. COX-2 appears to play a role in polyp formation, and COX-2 inhibition suppresses polyp growth, restores apoptosis, and decreases expression of proangiogenic factors. Inhibition of COX-2 also downregulates the phosphatidylinositol 3-kinase (PI3K) signaling pathway, which plays an important role in carcinogenesis and cancer cell resistance to apoptosis.[15]

TABLE 130-1 Lifestyle Factors Associated with Colorectal Cancer Risk

Factor	Comments
Elevated Risk	
Sedentary lifestyle	Inverse relationship between physical activity and colon cancer risk; colon cancer risk 40% lower for physically active individuals compared to less active individuals
Overweight and obesity	Elevated BMI, waist circumference, and waist-to-hip ratio directly associated with increased cancer risk
Alcohol intake	Risk of colorectal cancer 23% higher with 2-4 alcohol drinks/day compared to <1 drink/day; risk association strongest for males
Cigarette smoking	Prolonged cigarette smoking increases risk of large adenomas and carcinoma; higher colorectal cancer mortality in current smokers; risk may be higher for rectal cancer than for colon cancer and persists after smoking cessation for up to 25 years
Western diet	High caloric, saturated fat diet, processed meat and red meat (especially fried and barbecued) consumption increases cancer risk; influence of low dietary fiber intake not established
Reduced Risk	
Aspirin and nonaspirin NSAID use	Regular aspirin or NSAID use associated with 20% to 45% reduction in adenoma recurrence and colorectal cancer risk. Benefit in risk reduction requires at least 5-10 years of use
Postmenopausal hormone use	Exogenous hormone intake decreases risk of adenomas, colon, and rectal cancer by about 35%
Calcium and vitamin D intake	Vitamin D 400 international units and calcium intake of 1,000 mg/day (adults <50 years) or 1,200 mg/day (adults >50 years) may help reduce colorectal cancer risk but data remains unclear

BMI, body mass index; NSAID, nonsteroidal antiinflammatory drug.

Postmenopausal Hormone-Replacement Therapy

Exogenous postmenopausal oral hormone-replacement therapy is associated with a significant reduction in colorectal cancer risk.[16] Risk reduction is seen in postmenopausal women receiving both estrogen only and combined estrogen and progestin therapy, and persists for about 10 years after therapy is discontinued.

Several mechanisms for a protective effect of estrogens on the bowel have been identified.[7] Age-related declines in estrogen levels are associated with estrogen receptor hypermethylation, which is associated with reduced expression of the estrogen receptor gene and dysregulated colonic mucosal cell growth. Estrogen may also interact with bile acids, or alter levels of insulin and IGF-1, an important mitogen that influences cell-cycle progression in certain cells. However, because postmenopausal hormone replacement therapy increases breast cancer risk and harmful cardiovascular effects, its use is not recommended to prevent colorectal cancer.

Obesity and Physical Inactivity

1 Physical inactivity and elevated body mass index (BMI), independent of level of physical activity, are associated with an elevated risk of colon adenoma, colon cancer, and rectal cancer.[7,17-19] Individuals with a higher level of activity throughout life have the lowest risk, which may be up to 50% lower than that of physically inactive individuals. Possible hypotheses are that physical activity stimulates bowel peristalsis, resulting in decreased bowel transit time; or that exercise-induced alterations in body glucose, insulin resistance, hyperinsulinemia, and possibly other hormones reduce tumor cell growth.[18]

In most studies, a 5-unit increase above a healthy BMI was associated with increased risk of colorectal cancer in men, but the relationship is weaker and less consistent for women, possibly because of interactions with age or hormone replacement therapy.[18,19] Differences in body composition and distribution of fat weight among men and women could contribute to this discrepancy.[7,16] Several mechanisms have been proposed to explain the association between body size and colorectal cancer risk, including insulin resistance, chronic inflammation, and alterations in growth factors or steroid hormones.[7]

Alcohol and Tobacco Use

1 Alcohol consumption increases the risk of colorectal cancer, but stronger associations have been observed for men than for women, possibly because alcohol consumption is generally greater in men than in women.[7] Lifetime and baseline alcohol consumption increase risk of cancer of the colon and rectum, and an alcohol intake of about 2 to 4 alcoholic beverages per day have a 23% higher risk of colorectal cancer than those who consume less than 1 each day.[3] Proposed mechanisms include impaired folate metabolism, abnormal DNA methylation, suppressed tumor immune surveillance, and other procarcinogenic effects related to alcohol intake.[7]

Cigarette smoking is associated with an increased risk of colorectal cancer (about 18% higher) and mortality, with a stronger association for cancer of the rectum than for cancer of the colon than in nonsmokers.[20,21] The risk of colorectal cancer development persists after smoking cessation for as many as 25 years.[21] Early tobacco use may also influence risk of cancer recurrence and mortality among colon cancer survivors, possibly due to an increase in genetic alterations that influence tumor behavior.[22]

Dietary Intake and Nutrients

1 Epidemiologic studies of worldwide incidence of colorectal cancer suggest that economic development and dietary habits strongly influence its development. However, findings based on epidemiologic data are subject to potential biases and inconsistencies in how dietary factors are categorized and measured, and numerous studies have been able to clearly establish only a few specific dietary habits as independent risk factors for colorectal cancer development.

Fiber, Fruit, and Vegetables

1 Worldwide, high-fiber dietary patterns have been associated with a low incidence of colorectal cancer.[7,23,24] Dietary fiber is composed of both water-soluble and insoluble remnants of plant cells that are not processed by normal human digestive enzymes. Foods that are high in fiber include vegetables, fruits, grains, and cereals. Dietary fiber is postulated to reduce colonic mucosal cell exposure to carcinogens through the dilution or reduced absorption of carcinogens in the bowel, reduced fecal pH, reduced bowel transit time, alterations in bile acid metabolism, or increased production of short-chain fatty acids.[7] At present, the role of dietary fiber with regard to amount, source, and type and colorectal cancer risk requires further study.

Red Meat, Processed Meat, and Fat

1 Studies suggest that dietary fat intake may be associated with colorectal cancer risk.[7,23] This may have resulted from the use of dietary evaluations that focused on the quantity, origin, or type (saturated, monounsaturated, and polyunsaturated) of fat rather than on the source of dietary fat ingested. Dietary fat may promote cancer development as a result of its effect on fecal bile acid concentrations. Dietary fat ingestion stimulates the release of bile acids that are converted by colonic flora to secondary bile acids, which are associated with bowel mucosal irritation and cell proliferation responses and may promote tumor growth.[23]

The association between red, but not white, meat consumption and colorectal cancer is strongest, which may be related to the heterocyclic amines and polycyclic aromatic hydrocarbons formed during the cooking process, or the presence of specific fatty acids in red meat, such as arachidonic acid.[7,23] Processed meat products containing certain preservatives may increase exogenous exposure to carcinogenic *N*-nitroso compounds.[23] Although red and processed meat and high saturated fat intake has been associated with increased risk of colorectal cancer, the exact nature and magnitude of these risks have not been determined.

Calcium and Vitamin D

2 Inverse associations between dietary calcium, vitamin D intake, and serum 25-hydroxyvitamin D_3 levels, and colorectal cancer risk have been reported in several observational studies.[7,23,25] Calcium may exert antiproliferative effects by binding to bile and fatty acids in the small intestine, thereby reducing colonic epithelial cell exposure to mutagens.[12] In addition, calcium induces differentiating, proapoptotic, and direct growth-restraining activities on both normal and tumor cells in the gastrointestinal tract. Vitamin D also has antiproliferative and differentiation and proapoptotic effects in addition to immune response modulation on colonic epithelial cells and on a variety of tumor cells.[7,12,25] Most of its actions are mediated through a high-affinity nuclear vitamin D receptor, and the expression of this receptor is altered during different phases of colon cancer development.[12] Thus, cellular responsiveness to vitamin D and associated cancer risk is unlikely limited to dietary intake alone. Vitamin D and calcium appear to interact synergistically to protect against adenoma recurrence and colorectal cancer, but large, long-term controlled trials have yet to confirm that supplementation with calcium and vitamin D reduce colorectal cancer risk.[12]

Folate and Other Micronutrients

Folate intake has been linked to colorectal cancer risk through epidemiologic and experimental studies in cell lines, animals, and humans.[7,26] However, the underlying basis for this is complex, particularly because alcohol use, smoking, genetic variants of the *MTHFR* gene, and other factors can interfere with folate metabolism.[7,26] Cellular folates act to accept and donate methyl groups in cellular processes that influence DNA synthesis and methylation of DNA, RNA, and proteins.[26] Variations in DNA methylation of gene promoter regions influence gene expression and DNA stability. Inappropriate hypermethylation leads to inactivation of tumor suppressor gene function and hypomethylation can result in oncogene activation.[26]

The relationship between the timing of folate exposure to the development of neoplastic foci may influence what appears to be a bimodal impact of folate on tumorigenesis.[7,26] Moderate folate supplementation, if initiated prior to the establishment of neoplastic foci, may be protective, whereas excessive or increased intake might enhance growth of established early neoplastic lesions.[7,26] Thus, an adequate dietary folate intake may be enough to lower the risk of colorectal cancer, and exceeding normal intake may not be beneficial.

Epidemiologic and animal model data suggest that deficiencies in other dietary micronutrients, including vitamin B_6, selenium, vitamin C, vitamin E, and carotenoids, may increase colorectal cancer risk, but there is no convincing evidence that the incidence of colorectal cancer is greater in patients with low serum levels than in patients with adequate levels.[7,27]

PATHOPHYSIOLOGY

Anatomy and Bowel Function

The large intestine consists of the cecum; the ascending, transverse, descending, and sigmoid colon; and the rectum (Fig. 130-2). In adults, it extends about 1.5 m and has a diameter ranging from 8 cm in the cecum to 2 cm in the sigmoid colon. The function of the large intestine is to receive 500 to 2,000 mL of ileal contents per day. Absorption of fluid and solutes occurs in the right colon or the segments proximal to the middle of the transverse colon, with movement and storage of fecal material in the left colon and distal segments of the colon. Mucus secretion from goblet cells into the intestinal lumen lubricates the mucosal surface and facilitates movement of the dehydrated feces. It also serves to protect the luminal wall from bacteria and colonic irritants such as bile acids.

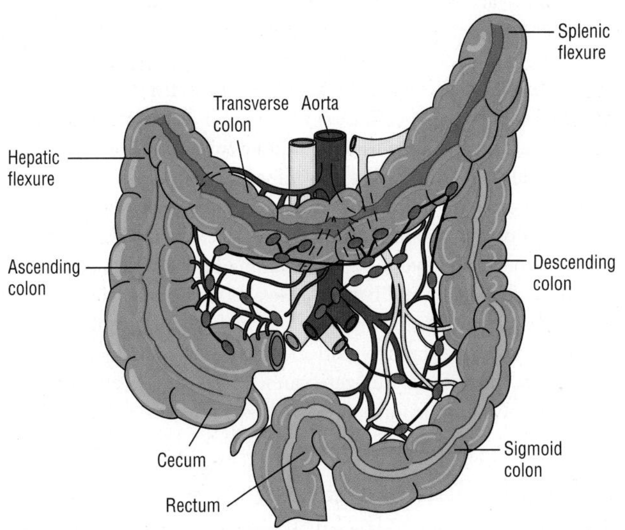

FIGURE 130-2 Colon and rectum anatomy.

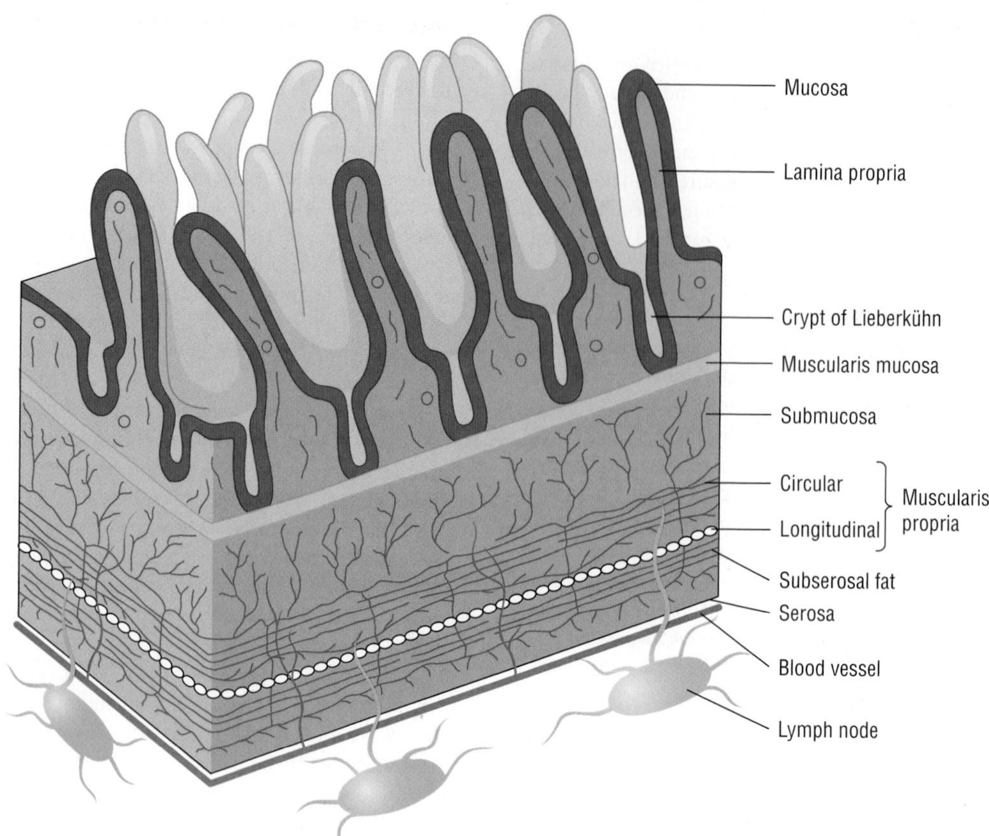

FIGURE 130-3 Cross-section of bowel wall.

Four major tissue layers, from the lumen outward, form the large intestine: the mucosa, submucosa, muscularis propria, and serosa (Fig. 130-3). Embedded in the submucosa and muscularis propria is a rich lymphatic capillary system. Lymphatic channels do not extend into the mucosa. The muscularis propria consists of circular smooth muscle and outer longitudinal smooth muscle bands. Contraction of these muscle groups moves colonic material toward the anal canal. The outermost layer of the colon, the serosa, secretes a fluid that allows the colon to slide easily over nearby structures within the peritoneum. The serosa covers only the anterior and lateral aspects of the upper third of the rectum. The lower third lies completely extraperitoneal and is surrounded by fibrofatty tissue as well as adjacent organs and structures.

The surface epithelium of the colonic mucosa undergoes continual renewal, and complete replacement of epithelial cells occurs every 4 to 8 days. Cell replication normally takes place within the lower third of the crypts, the tubular glands located within the intestinal mucosa. The cells then mature and differentiate to either goblet or absorptive cells as they migrate toward the bowel lumen. The total number of epithelial cells remains relatively constant as the number of cells migrating from the crypts is balanced by the rate of exfoliation of cells from the mucosal surface. This 2-phase process is critical to the malignant transformation of the epithelial cells. The number of dysplastic and hyperplastic aberrant crypt foci increases with increasing age; as the mass of abnormal cells accumulates at the top of the crypt and starts to protrude into the stream of fecal matter, their contact with fecal mutagens can lead to further cell mutations and eventual adenoma formation.

Colorectal Tumorigenesis

The development of a colorectal neoplasm is a multistep process involving several genetic and phenotypic alterations of normal bowel epithelium structure and function, leading to dysregulated cell growth, proliferation, and tumor development. Because most colorectal cancers develop sporadically, with no inherited or familial disposition, efforts have been directed toward identifying these alterations and learning whether detection of such changes may lead to improved cancer detection or treatment outcomes.

Features of colorectal tumorigenesis include genomic instability, activation of oncogene pathways, mutational inactivation or silencing of tumor-suppressor genes, DNA mismatch repairs, and activation of growth factor pathways.[11] A genetic model has been proposed for colorectal tumorigenesis that describes a process of transformation from adenoma to carcinoma (Fig. 130-4).[28-31] The adenoma to carcinoma sequence of tumor development reflects an accumulation of mutations within colonic epithelium that confers a selective growth advantage to the affected cells. Key elements of this process include hyperproliferation of epithelial cells to form a small benign neoplasm or adenoma in conjunction with acquisition of various genetic mutations.[29] These mutations occur early and frequently in sporadic cases of both adenomas and colorectal cancer. Somatic mutations must occur in multiple genes to produce the malignant transformation. Table 130-2 lists important genetic mutations that are associated with colorectal cancers.[11,30]

Genomic Instability

Genomic instability plays an integral role in normal colonic or rectal mucosal transformation to carcinoma.[11] Three molecular pathways that lead to genomic instability are the microsatellite instability (MSI), CpG island methylator phenotype (CIMP), and chromosomal instability (CIN) pathways. The most common type is CIN, which leads to alterations in chromosomal structure and copy number. Important consequences of CIN include imbalanced chromosome number (aneuploidy), chromosomal gene amplifications, and loss of a wild-type allele of a tumor-suppressor gene, also referred to

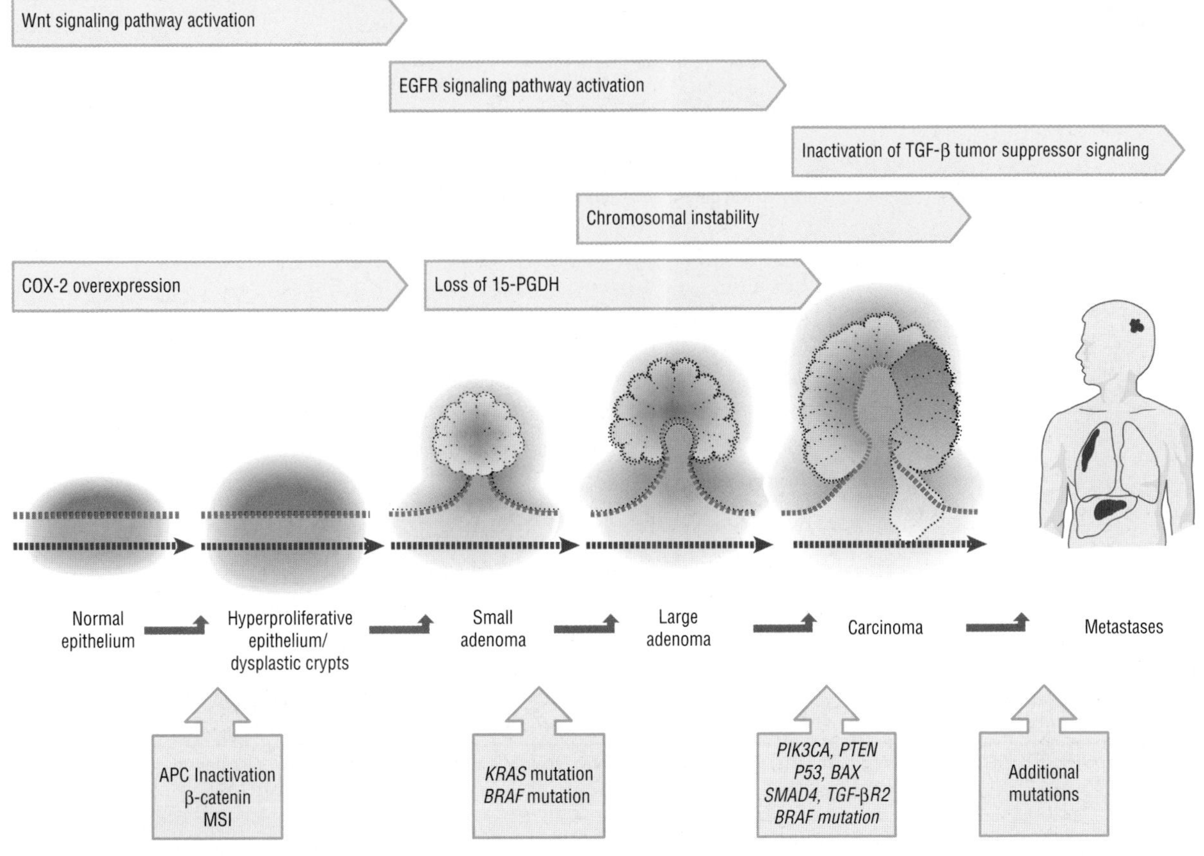

FIGURE 130-4 Genetic changes associated with the adenoma–carcinoma sequence in colorectal cancer. The accumulation of genetic changes in the pathogenesis of colorectal cancer includes microsatellite instability (MSI) initiated by aberrant DNA methylation or mismatch repair (MMR) gene mutation with subsequent disruption in transforming growth factor-β receptor type II (TGF-β2R) and BAX signaling; mutation in the adenomatous polyposis coli (*APC*) gene or abnormalities in β-catenin leading to inappropriate activation of the Wnt signaling pathway; mutational activation of cyclooxygenase-2 (COX-2) and impaired prostaglandin degradation from loss of 15-prostaglandin dehydrogenase (15-PGDH); *KRAS*, *PIK3CA*, or *BRAF* oncogene activation; increased epidermal growth factor receptor (EGFR) signaling; and deletions or mutations of tumor suppressor genes *SMAD4*, *PTEN*, *P53*. Chromosomal instability (CIN) is a common feature of sporadic disease, but causative factors are not defined. The sequence of molecular events may differ between somatic and inherited genetic alterations. *(Data from references 28-31.)*

as loss of heterozygosity (LOH). More than 50% of sporadic colorectal cancers exhibit CIN and involve tumor suppressor genes *APC* and *P53*, loss of 18q allele, and aneuploid DNA content.

Microsatellites are series of repeat nucleotide sequences that are spread out across the entire genome.[11] Microsatellite replication errors within tumor DNA occur frequently, and mutations of the MMR genes that recognize and regulate DNA MMR errors contribute to MSI and colorectal tumorigenesis. Germline mutation of MMR genes is an important characteristic of Lynch syndrome, but somatic mutations are also present in about 15% of sporadic colorectal cancers.

Alterations in gene expression or function in the absence of DNA sequence alterations are referred to as epigenetic changes, and these are usually due to methylation of DNA gene promotor regions or histone modifications.[11] CIMP is characterized by hypermethylation of a panel of multiple genes that are associated with gene silencing and subsequent loss of tumor suppressor gene function.[31] About 15% of sporadic colorectal cancers arise as a consequence of CIMP.

Oncogene and Tumor Suppressor Gene Alterations

Mutation or loss of the *APC* tumor suppressor gene is a key factor involved in tumor formation through activation of the Wnt signaling pathway, a mediator of cell-cycle progression, cell proliferation, differentiation, and apoptosis.[11] The *APC* gene encodes for APC protein that binds to and degrades cytoplasmic β-catenin, a downstream component of the Wnt signaling pathway. In the absence of functional APC, β-catenin accumulates in the cytoplasm, then enters the nucleus and activates transcription of various genes, leading to constitutive activation of the Wnt signaling pathway. Inactivation of the *APC* gene is the single gene defect responsible for FAP, and is frequently an initiating event in sporadic colorectal cancer.[11]

Mutational inactivation of *P53* represents a frequent and second key step in colorectal tumorigenesis, occurring in about 50% to 75% of colorectal cancers.[11] Normal *P53* gene expression is important for G_1 cell-cycle arrest to facilitate DNA repair during replication and to induce apoptosis. A third step in tumor progression is the mutational inactivation of the transforming growth factor-β (TGF-β) signaling pathway, which facilitates adenoma transition to high-grade dysplasia or carcinoma and also inactivates *SMAD4*. In normal epithelium, TGF-β has an antiproliferative role and induces growth arrest and apoptosis. Alterations in *SMAD4* or TGF-β receptors lead to a loss of the normal growth inhibitory response to TGF-β.

Several oncogene-activating mutations play an important role in promoting colorectal cancer.[11] Mutations in members of the *RAS* gene family—*KRAS*, *HRAS*, and *NRAS*—in addition to *BRAF*, activate the mitogen-activated protein kinase (MAPK) signaling pathway, which stimulates cell proliferation and other activities that promote carcinogenesis. Mutations of *PIK3CA*, which encodes the catalytic subunit of a PI3K survival pathway, increase

TABLE 130-2 Genetic Mutations Associated with Colorectal Cancer

Type of Mutation	Disease	Genes	Comments
Germline	Familial adenomatous polyposis (FAP)	*APC*	Multiple adenomas and carcinomas in colon and rectum
	MYH-associated polyposis	*MYH*	Autosomal recessive syndrome; wide spectrum of degree of polyposis; frequent *KRAS* mutations
	Lynch syndrome	DNA MMR genes: *MSH2, MLH1, MSH6, PMS2*	Colorectal cancer in absence of extensive polyposis; predisposition for endometrial, ovarian, gastric, hepatobiliary, urothelial, pancreatic, brain, and skin cancers
Somatic	Sporadic colorectal cancer	Oncogenes:	
		KRAS	Mutations found in about 40% of cancers
		NRAS	Mutations found in <5% of cancers
		BRAF	*BRAF* V600E mutation found in 5%-10% of cancers
		PIK3CA	Mutations found in 15%-25% of cancers
		EGFR	Gene amplification in 5%-15% of cancers
		Tumor suppressor genes:	
		P53	Loss or mutation in 60%-70% of cancers
		SMAD4	Mutations in 10%-15% of cancers
		APC	Inactivated in 70%-80% of sporadic cancers
		TGF-βR2	Inactivating mutations present in 10%-15% of cancers; mutations in more than 90% of cancers with MSI
		PTEN	Frequency of inactivating mutations about 10% but loss of PTEN protein expression evident in 15%-20% of cancers

APC, adenomatous polyposis coli; EGFR, epidermal growth factor receptor; MMR, mismatch repair; MSI, microsatellite instability; TGF-βR2, transforming growth factor-β receptor type II.

Data from references 11 and 30.

production of phosphatidylinositol-3,4,5-triphosphate, which influences cell growth, proliferation, and survival. Mutation or loss of *PTEN*, a tumor suppressor gene that antagonizes PI3K signaling, produces similar effects. Multiple additional genetic alterations contribute to carcinoma formation and metastases by altering cellular growth, metabolism, migration, and invasive capabilities, and angiogenesis.[31]

Growth Factor Signaling Pathways

Aberrant signaling of growth factor pathways plays an important role in colorectal tumorigenesis. Activation of prostaglandin signaling is an early step in the adenoma to carcinoma transformation process and is induced by upregulated expression of COX-2 and inflammation.[29] COX-2 mediates the synthesis of prostaglandin E_2, which stimulates cancer growth.[29] Furthermore, 80% of colorectal cancers have loss of 15-prostaglandin dehydrogenase (15-PGDH), the rate-limiting enzyme responsible for prostaglandin degradation. Gene amplification of the epidermal growth factor receptor (*EGFR*) gene that encodes for a transmembrane glycoprotein involved in signaling pathways which affect cell growth, differentiation, proliferation, and angiogenesis, is present in 5% to 15% of all colorectal cancers.[30] EGFR activation enables downstream signaling of the MAPK, PI3K, and Akt pathways that influence colorectal tumorigenesis. EGFR is overexpressed in up to 75% of colorectal cancers and high tumor EGFR overexpression is associated with worse prognosis.[32] These mechanisms are relevant because of the availability of pharmacologic agents that can influence these signaling pathways and affect cell growth.

Histology

Adenocarcinomas account for about 85% of tumors of the large intestine and 10% to 15% are classified mucinous adenocarcinoma.[33] The other histologic types, such as signet-ring adenocarcinoma, squamous cell carcinoma, and neuroendocrine carcinomas, are rare. Adenocarcinomas are assigned one of three tumor grade designations based on the degree of cellular differentiation, the degree to which the tumor resembles the structure, and function of its cell of origin. The most differentiated adenocarcinomas are low-grade tumors, whereas high-grade tumors are the most undifferentiated, and have frequently lost the characteristics of mature normal cells. Poorly differentiated tumors are associated with a worse prognosis than those that are relatively better differentiated.

Mucinous adenocarcinomas possess the same basic structure as adenocarcinomas but differ in that they secrete an abundant quantity of extracellular mucus. They tend to be frequent in patients with MMR mutations.[33] Signet-ring adenocarcinomas also have a characteristic appearance but are uncommon. Signet-ring histology occurs more frequently in individuals younger than 50 years of age, patients with ulcerative colitis, and tends to present at a more advanced stage of disease at diagnosis. Both mucinous and signet-ring adenocarcinoma histologies confer a poor prognosis. Patients with neuroendocrine tumors and squamous cell carcinoma often present with distant metastases and have a poor prognosis as well.

PREVENTION AND SCREENING

Cancer prevention efforts can be considered as either primary or secondary. Primary prevention strategies aim to prevent the development of colorectal cancer in a population at risk. Secondary prevention approaches are undertaken to prevent malignancy in a population that has already manifested an initial disease process. Several promising primary and secondary prevention strategies are currently undergoing study (Table 130-3).[7,24,34-40]

Diet

1 Although early studies suggest that a substantial increase in daily dietary fiber or decrease in dietary fat intake might significantly reduce colorectal cancer risk, results from prospective, controlled trials show no protective effects of fiber intake on colorectal adenoma or carcinoma risk. However, a recent meta-analysis suggests

TABLE 130-3 Prevention Strategies Under Evaluation for Colorectal Cancer

Prevention Strategy	Proposed Mechanism of Protective Effect
Aspirin, NSAIDs, and COX-2 selective inhibitors	Inhibit COX-2; downregulate PI3K signaling pathway; induce apoptosis
Calcium	Direct binding to bile and fatty acids; inhibits epithelial cell proliferation
Curcumin	Antiinflammatory and antioxidant effects; induces p53-independent apoptosis; inhibits NF-κB and PI3K/Akt/mTOR signaling pathways
Difluoromethylornithine (Eflornithine)	Inhibits cellular proliferation through alterations in polyamine metabolism via inhibition of ornithine decarboxylase
Epigallocatechin gallate (EGCG)	Major polyphenolic constituent of green tea. Strong antioxidant; inhibits lipoxygenase and COX activity; inhibits cell proliferation and angiogenesis via inhibition of cell signaling proteins and proangiogenic signaling pathways
High-fiber diet supplementation	Decreases fecal bile acids; decreases bowel transit time; direct binding to fecal mutagens; dilution of fecal material
Genistein	Flavonoid phytoestrogen; modulates cell-cycle progression, induces apoptosis; possesses antioxidant and antiinflammatory activities
HMG-CoA reductase inhibitors	Induce intestinal cell apoptosis and inhibit cell proliferation; suppress angiogenesis; synergistic COX-2 inhibition with NSAIDs
Metformin	Targets IGF pathway to influence cell growth, proliferation, and differentiation. Activation of AMPK inhibits insulin and protein synthesis, and suppresses NF-κB activity
NO-NSAIDs	Nitrous-oxide release mimics effects of prostaglandins on gastrointestinal epithelium; suppress formation of aberrant colonic crypt foci
Omega (ω)-3 polyunsaturated fatty acids (ω-3 PUFAs)	Inhibit COX-2 expression; COX-2 independent mechanisms
Probiotic bacteria	Alter intestinal microflora; inactivate carcinogens; improve host immune response; regulate cell proliferation by altering cell signaling pathways, apoptosis, and cell differentiation
Resveratrol	Antiinflammatory and antioxidant effects; induces apoptosis; influences genes that inhibit cell-cycle progression, cell proliferation, metastasis, and angiogenesis
Quercetin	Flavonoid antioxidant constituent in fruit, vegetables, tea, and wine; induces apoptosis

AMPK, AMP-activated protein kinase; COX, cyclooxygenase; EGFR, epidermal growth factor receptor; HMG-CoA, β-hydroxy-β-methylglutaryl-coenzyme A; IGF, insulin-like growth factor; MAPK, mitogen-activated protein kinase; mTOR, mammalian target of rapamycin; NF-κB, nuclear factor -kappa B; NO-NSAIDs, nitrous oxide donating nonsteroidal antiinflammatory drugs; NSAIDs, nonsteroidal antiinflammatory drugs; PI3K; phosphatidylinositol 3-kinase.

Data from references 7, 24, and 34-40.

a 10% reduction in colorectal cancer risk with 10 gram daily intake of total dietary and cereal fiber and up to a 20% risk reduction with 3 servings of whole grains daily.[23,24] There is insufficient evidence to support the use of fiber supplementation as a colorectal cancer prevention strategy at this time.

Chemoprevention

2 The most widely studied agents for the chemoprevention of colorectal cancer are aspirin, nonaspirin NSAIDs, and COX-2 selective inhibitors, but only aspirin is recommended for chemoprevention in some patients.[7,13,24,37,38] The effectiveness of these agents has been studied in high-risk individuals and within the general population.

In individuals with FAP, celecoxib, NSAIDs, and aspirin have been studied to delay development of adenomatous polyps and to reduce polyp recurrence following colectomy with a retained rectum, but they are not viewed as alternatives to surgery.[34] In randomized, controlled trials, celecoxib 400 milligrams (mg) orally twice daily as an adjunct to usual care significantly reduced the mean size and number of colorectal polyps after 6 to 9 months of treatment. However, FDA approval for celecoxib was withdrawn because of lack of data showing long-term benefit. Sulindac has been shown to induce adenoma regression, but does not appear to delay or prevent malignancy. The benefits of these agents are transient, because patients experience an increase in size and number of polyps within a few months after discontinuing treatment. Sulindac is not recommended as chemoprevention for individuals with FAP. These agents may be useful to reduce adenoma recurrence following surgery, but additional data with long-term use are needed.

Nonaspirin NSAIDs and COX-2 inhibitors were associated with reduced risk of sporadic and recurrent colorectal adenomas in cohort and case-control studies, and COX-2 inhibitors were also effective in controlled trials.[7] Celecoxib was associated with a 34% relative risk reduction in adenoma recurrence and 55% risk reduction in the incidence of advanced adenomas.[34] Optimal dosing, agents, and duration of treatment remain to be determined, and potential cardiovascular events in addition to risk of gastric ulceration and bleeding with these agents are of concern. Although NSAIDs may be appropriate for selected individuals at high risk for colorectal cancer but low risk for cardiovascular disorders, the United States Preventive Services Task Force (USPTF) has concluded that potential harms associated with NSAID use (other than aspirin) outweigh benefits for prevention of colorectal cancer in the general population.[38] However, USPTF guidelines recommend daily low-dose aspirin for at least 10 years in adults ages 50 to 59 years who have a life expectancy of at least 10 years and are not at risk for bleeding for primary to prevent both cardiovascular disease and colorectal cancer. Adults ages 60 to 69 years may also receive low-dose-daily aspirin for at least 10 years if the benefits outweigh the risks.

Clinical **Controversy...**

Emerging data support the use of aspirin as colorectal cancer chemoprevention for patients with Lynch syndrome and regular long-term aspirin use modestly reduces colorectal cancer risk in individuals without Lynch syndrome. However, because of the small risk of serious bleeding associated with even low doses, aspirin should only be used as chemoprevention in those adults ages 50-69 for a minimum of 10 years if benefits outweigh the risks.

The use of aspirin as both a primary and a secondary chemopreventive agent remains controversial. Aspirin reduces of risk of sporadic and recurrent adenomas by about 17% and advanced adenomas by 28%.[34,39] Higher aspirin doses reduced the incidence of colorectal cancer over a 23-year follow-up period by 26% among the general population, but lower doses (75-300 mg) of daily aspirin for 5 years was also associated with a risk reduction in colorectal cancer incidence and in 20-year mortality from colorectal cancer by 34%.[34,37,39] Individuals with Lynch syndrome who received aspirin 600 mg daily for at least 2 years experienced a 59% reduction in colorectal cancer risk that became evident 5 years after the aspirin was first started and had been discontinued.[39] Although the optimal aspirin dose and treatment durations are unknown, increasing evidence supports a chemoprotective effect of aspirin in select high-risk individuals and in the general population. The extent of risk reduction appears to be inversely related to duration of therapy and the chemopreventive effects of aspirin may be delayed by 5 to 10 years. However, the balance of risks and benefits with long-term aspirin use is currently unclear, and aspirin is only recommended for chemoprevention in some patients. *PIK3CA* mutations, which are present in up to 20% of colorectal cancers, and polymorphisms in genes that regulate proinflammatory processes may serve as biomarkers to identify patients who may benefit from prophylactic or adjuvant aspirin therapy.[41]

Randomized controlled trials of calcium, vitamin D, and folate supplementation as chemoprevention have also been conducted, but findings do not support their use at this time.[7,34] Individuals at high risk of colorectal cancer may experience a moderate reduction in risk of recurrent colorectal adenomas with 5 years of calcium supplementation.[20] However, individuals with adequate vitamin D levels and no known increased risk of colorectal cancer do not appear to benefit from calcium or vitamin D supplementation.[42] In two trials, folate supplementation was associated with a nonsignificant increase in adenoma recurrence. Based on these results, the use of folate supplementation to reduce colorectal cancer risk is not recommended at this time.[8] Additional intervention trials of various micronutrients, epigenetic modulators, and other chemopreventive agents have been completed or are ongoing.[7,13,24,25,34-36,40]

Surgical Resection

Surgical resection remains an option to prevent colon cancer in individuals at extremely high risk for its development.[43] Despite the effects of NSAIDs and COX-2 selective inhibitors on adenoma development and recurrence in individuals with FAP, their effects are incomplete and surgical resection is necessary for cancer prevention for these high-risk individuals. Individuals with FAP who are found to have polyposis on lower endoscopy screening examinations should undergo total proctocolectomy and ileal pouch–anal anastomosis or subtotal colectomy with an ileorectal anastomosis, typically starting around age 20 years. Because of the high incidence of metachronous (ie, consecutive development) cancers (45%) in patients with Lynch syndrome, prophylactic subtotal colectomy with an ileorectal anastomosis is recommended for individuals who are not candidates for routine close follow-up. Colonoscopic polypectomy, removal of polyps detected during screening colonoscopy, is considered the standard of care for all individuals to prevent the progression of premalignant adenomatous polyps to adenocarcinomas.

Screening

3 Colorectal cancer screening decreases mortality by detecting cancers at an early, curable stage, and by detecting and removing adenomatous polyps. Multiple screening recommendations for early detection of colorectal cancer have been established; differences exist in specific screening guidelines published by various organizations.[5,44-49] Structural tests detect colorectal polyps and cancer whereas fecal-based tests detect early cancer. This section reviews available screening techniques for colon and rectal cancer.

Colonoscopy

3 Colonoscopy facilitates examination of the entire large bowel to the cecum in most patients, and allows for simultaneous removal of premalignant lesions. Although no randomized trials show that colonoscopy decreases colorectal cancer mortality, observational studies show a 56% to 77% decrease in the incidence in colorectal cancer with colonoscopy and polyp removal and about a 50% reduction in colorectal mortality.[49] Colonoscopy allows for greater visualization of the colon, but it involves sedation, complete bowel preparation, and is associated with greater risk and inconvenience to patients. However, it is the preferred screening method based on its superior ability to detect and remove lesions in the proximal as well as distal colon and colonoscopy is therefore considered the gold standard for colorectal screening.[49] Four large-scale, randomized, prospective trials are evaluating colonoscopy versus no screening or fecal immunochemistry test (FIT).

Flexible Sigmoidoscopy

3 Flexible sigmoidoscopy (FSIG) uses a 60-cm flexible sigmoidoscope to examine the lower half of the bowel to the splenic flexure for most patients, and is thus capable of detecting 50% to 60% of cancers.[49] Randomized trials show that FSIG decreases colorectal cancer incidence and mortality by 31% and 38%, respectively. The combination of FSIG and a fecal-based test appears to improve sensitivity for lesions that will be missed by sigmoidoscopy alone, but the true benefit of this approach to general practice has not been established.[45] FSIG offers the advantage of not requiring sedation or extensive bowel preparation, but the entire colon cannot be examined with FSIG and suspicious lesions must be evaluated by colonoscopy.

Computed Tomography Colonography

3 Computed tomography colonography, also referred to as *virtual colonoscopy*, is an imaging procedure that creates 2- or 3-dimensional images of the colon by combining multiple helical computed tomography (CT) scans. Initial tests show high sensitivity and specificity for detecting adenomas at least 6 mm in size and sedation is not required. However, the procedure requires complete bowel preparation, is associated with radiation exposure, and many individuals will still be referred for colonoscopy to remove detected lesions. Individuals who refuse to undergo invasive colonoscopy or FSIG may find this screening method more acceptable.

Double-Contrast Barium Enema

3 A double-contrast barium enema (DCBE) involves coating the interior bowel with barium and distending it with air to produce an image of the entire colon in most examinations, and the retained barium outlines small polyps and mucosal lesions.[45] This approach is the least expensive method of examining the entire colon, but is considered inferior to colonoscopy for detecting polyps and colorectal cancer. In addition, DCBE requires bowel preparation cleaning, is associated with radiation exposure, and a supplemental colonoscopy is required if suspicious lesions are identified. However, DCBE is considered an alternative for individuals who do not wish to undergo or are not suitable for colonoscopy.

Fecal Occult Blood Tests

3 Fecal occult blood tests (FOBTs) are used to detect occult blood in the stool that may be associated with bleeding adenomas or cancer. Results from randomized, controlled trials of annual

TABLE 130-4 Patient Counseling Points Prior to Guaiac-Based Stool Tests

To Avoid False Positives	To Avoid False Negatives
Dietary restrictions • Avoid red meat (beef, lamb, liver) and raw vegetables with peroxidase activity (turnips, broccoli, cauliflower, and radishes) for 3 days prior to testing[a]	• Avoid vitamin C in excess of 250 mg supplements and from citrus juices and fruit for 3 days prior to testing • Avoid testing dehydrated samples (rehydrating of samples is not recommended)
Medical restrictions • Avoid rectal enemas, rectal medications, and digital rectal examinations for 3 days prior to testing • Avoid aspirin and nonsteroidal antiinflammatory drugs for up to 7 days prior to testing • Avoid testing if blood from hemorrhoids is evident in stool • Delay testing until 3 days after menstrual bleeding has ended	
Procedure for guaiac-based stool testing	
Patient uses an applicator stick to apply stool to 2 test cards on 3 separate occasions, usually from different bowel movements on consecutive days (total of 6 test cards or samples). After the sample dries, the card is mailed or returned to the healthcare professional.	

[a]Test instructions for several products no longer contain dietary vegetable or fruit restrictions.

Data from reference 45.

FOBT screening show a reduction in colorectal cancer mortality by 33%.[45,49] Unlike structural tests, FOBTs are noninvasive and do not require bowel preparation. Two main methods are available to detect occult blood in the feces: guaiac-based FOBT (gFOBT) and FITs, also known as immunochemical fecal occult blood test (iFOBT). Several gFOBTs are available that detect peroxidase activity of heme when hemoglobin comes in contact with a guaiac-impregnated paper. When a solution containing hydrogen peroxide is poured over the paper, a blue color appears if the test is positive. The testing process is complex and requires specific patient counseling to avoid inaccurate results (Table 130-4).[45]

Clinical guidelines have been developed for performing and interpreting results of gFOBT.[45] Several limitations associated with gFOBT screening are of concern. Many early-stage tumors do not bleed, and therefore the false-negative rates can be high and are variable depending on the gFOBT product used. In addition, the test results may not be valid because the test is often poorly performed both in the home and in physician office settings.[45,46] However, these concerns are addressed by testing three successive stool samples. False-positive results can prove to be very expensive and inconvenient for a patient because of the follow-up tests required to confirm a positive result. Annual screening, preferably using a high-sensitivity gFOBT (eg, Hemoccult SENSA), is an acceptable option for individuals at average risk for colorectal cancer. It should be noted that FOBT conducted in conjunction with a digital rectal exam during an office visit is not considered adequate colorectal screening.

FITs (iFOBTs) were developed to reduce false-positive and false-negative test results associated with the gFOBT. FIT uses antibodies to detect the globin protein portion of human hemoglobin. Globin is degraded by enzymes in the upper gastrointestinal tract; therefore, FIT is more specific for lower gastrointestinal bleeding. Also, immunochemical tests do not produce false-negative results in the presence of vitamin C or meat/vegetables containing peroxidase activity.[45] Moreover, testing involves a single stool sample collection annually. Comparative studies report that FIT is more accurate than gFOBT for detecting cancer and advanced adenomas, although colonoscopy identifies more adenomas.[49]

Stool DNA Screening Tests

Molecular screening strategies analyze stool samples for presence of potential markers of malignancy in cells that are shed from premalignant polyps or adenocarcinomas in the bowel.[45,49] Adenoma and carcinomas can contain certain DNA mutations and markers of MSI that can be detected using a multiple marker panel for stool DNA (sDNA) testing. One FDA-approved sDNA test is currently commercially available, but the appropriate screening interval is not clear.[49] Therefore, it is not routinely recommended as a screening option by all screening guidelines.

Screening Summary

3 Table 130-5 outlines current US screening guidelines for early detection of colorectal cancer with the goal of cancer prevention.[44-49] Men and women who are at average risk for colorectal cancer (their only risk factor is age greater than or equal to 50 years) should begin regular screening starting at age 50 years with a colonoscopy every 10 years, or annually using a sensitive gFOBT or FIT, or undergo FSIG every 5 years, alone or in conjunction with annual FOBT. Several screening methods are available, and because each method is associated with different benefits and potential harms, patient preferences and available resources should be considered for individual patients.[45] More rigorous (usually starting at an earlier age) screening recommendations are given for moderate- to high-risk individuals and colonoscopy is generally preferred for initial screening and surveillance following polyp removal in this population.[5,45,46,49] Most organizations recommend discontinuing screening and surveillance in populations when risk may outweigh benefit.[5] The United States Preventive Services Task Force (USPSTF) and NCCN recommend routine colorectal cancer screening for individuals age 50 to 75 years with different consideration given to adults 76 to 85 years and recommends against screening for adults older than 85 years.[5,49] The American College of Physicians recommends against screening adults older than age 75 years or with a life expectancy of less than 10 years.[44]

DIAGNOSIS

Signs and Symptoms

The signs and symptoms associated with colorectal cancer can be extremely varied and nonspecific. Patients with early-stage colorectal cancer are often asymptomatic, and lesions are usually found as a result of screening studies. Any change in bowel habits (eg, constipation, diarrhea, or alteration in size or shape of stool), abdominal pain, or distension may all be warning signs of a malignant process. Obstructive symptoms and changes in bowel habits frequently develop with tumors located in the transverse and descending colon. Rectal cancer may be associated with tenesmus, though bleeding is the most common symptom of rectal cancer. Bleeding may be acute or chronic and can appear as bright red blood mixed with stool or melena. Iron-deficiency anemia, presenting as weakness and fatigue, can develop as a result of chronic occult blood loss.

TABLE 130-5 Guidelines for Colorectal Cancer Screening in the United States for Individuals at Average Risk, 50 Years of Age and Older

ACS	ACG	USPSTF	ACS-USMSTF-ACR	ACP	NCCN
gFOBT[a,e]	Colonoscopy[d]	gFOBT[a,e]	gFOBT[a,e]	gFOBT[a,e]	Colonoscopy[d]
Or	*Or*	*Or*	*Or*	*Or*	*Or*
FIT[a,e]	FIT[a]	gFOBT[a,e] + FSIG[c]	FIT[a]	FIT[a]	gFOBT[a,e]
Or	*Or*	*Or*	*Or*	*Or*	*Or*
sDNA[f]	FSIG[c–d]	Colonoscopy[d]	sDNA[e]	FSIG[c]	FIT[a]
Or	*Or*	*Or*	*Or*	*Or*	*Or*
FSIG[c]	CTC[c]	FIT[a]	FSIG[c]	Colonoscopy[d]	gFOBT[a,e] + FSIG[c]
Or	*Or*		*Or*	*Or*	*Or*
gFOBT[a,e] + FSIG[c]	gFOBT[a,e]		Colonoscopy[d]	sDNA[f]	FIT[a] + FSIG[c]
Or	*Or*		*Or*	*Or*	
FIT[a,e] + FSIG[c]	sDNA[b]		DCBE[c]	DCBE[c]	
Or			*Or*	*Or*	
DCBE[c]			CTC[c]	CTC[c]	
Or					
Colonoscopy[d]					
Or					
CTC[c]					

ACG, American College of Gastroenterology; ACP, American College of Physicians; ACR, American College of Radiology; ACS, American Cancer Society; CTC, CT colonography; DCBE, double-contrast barium enema; FIT, fecal immunochemical test; FSIG, flexible sigmoidoscopy; gFOBT, guaiac-based fecal occult blood test; NCCN, National Comprehensive Cancer Network; USMSTF, US Multi-Society Task Force on Colorectal Cancer; USPSTF, US.

Preventive Services Task Force.

[a]Annually.

[b]Every 3 years.

[c]Every 5 years.

[d]Every 10 years.

[e]If more than 50% sensitivity for colorectal cancer.

[f]Interval uncertain.

Data from references 44-49.

About 20% of patients with colorectal cancer present with metastatic disease.[1] Metastatic spread occurs as a result of direct tumor invasion of the peritoneum or by lymphatic or hematogenous spread. The venous drainage of the colon and rectum influences the pattern of metastases most commonly seen. The most common site of metastasis is the liver followed by the lungs and then bones, specifically the sacrum, coccyx, pelvis, and lumbar vertebrae. Liver metastases are present in 25% of patients at presentation, with another 25% to 30% of patients developing liver metastases in the following 2 to 3 years.[50]

Workup

When a patient is suspected of having colorectal carcinoma, a complete history and physical examination should be performed. The patient history should include a past medical history and family history, especially noting the presence of inflammatory bowel disease, colorectal cancer, polyps, and familial clustering of cancers to assess risk for an inherited colorectal cancer syndrome as well as a full medication history, including prescription, over-the-counter and complementary alternative therapies. A complete physical examination includes careful abdominal examination for the presence of masses or ascites, a rectal examination, and an assessment for possible hepatomegaly and lymphadenopathy. A breast and pelvic examination is recommended in all women.

An evaluation of the entire large bowel requires a total colonoscopy and allows for tissue collection for a histologic evaluation to provide a preliminary diagnosis following the procedure. Patients with invasive cancer of the colon or rectum require a complete staging workup with laboratory testing and imaging of the abdomen, pelvis, and chest. Baseline laboratory tests should be obtained and include a complete blood cell count, platelet count, international normalized ratio, prothrombin time, activated partial thromboplastin time, liver chemistries, renal function tests, and carcinoembryonic antigen (CEA) level. Abnormal liver chemistry test results may suggest liver involvement with tumor. However, patients with metastatic disease to the liver may have normal liver chemistries. Iron studies (eg, serum ferritin, serum iron, and total iron-binding capacity) may be useful to identify iron deficiency in patients with anemia.

CEA belongs to a group of cell-surface glycoproteins termed *oncofetal proteins*, which are expressed during embryonic development and reexpressed on the cell surfaces of many carcinomas, particularly those originating from the gastrointestinal tract. CEA concentrations can be measured in the blood and can, therefore, potentially serve as a marker for colorectal cancer. Elevated CEA levels are more frequent in patients with metastatic disease, but not all colorectal cancers produce CEA. It is important to recognize, however, that several concomitant disease states are associated with an elevated CEA: liver diseases, gastritis, peptic ulcer disease, diverticulitis, chronic obstructive pulmonary disease, chronic or acute inflammatory conditions, and diabetes.[51] Most commercially available assays list a value of less than 5 ng/mL (mcg/L) as the upper limit of normal. Although CEA measurement is too insensitive and nonspecific to be used as a screening test for early-stage colorectal cancer, it is the surrogate marker of choice for monitoring colorectal cancer response to treatment, particularly if the pretreatment concentration is elevated.[51] The CEA test may have preoperative prognostic implications because it has been shown to correlate with the size and degree of differentiation of the carcinoma. Elevated preoperative CEA levels

CLINICAL PRESENTATION

General

- Patient symptoms are usually nonspecific and can vary drastically among patients.
- Most patients are asymptomatic.

Symptoms

- Change in bowel habits (generally an increase in frequency) or rectal bleeding.
- Constipation, depending on the location of the tumor.
- Nausea, vomiting, and abdominal discomfort.
- Fatigue may be present if anemia is severe.

Signs

- Blood in the stool is the most common sign in symptomatic patients.
- Hepatomegaly and jaundice in advanced disease.
- Leg edema as a consequence of lymph node involvement, thrombophlebitis, fistula formation, weight loss, and pain in the lower back or radiating down the legs may be indicative of widespread disease.

Laboratory Tests

- Positive guaiac stool test and anemia (iron deficiency) from blood loss.
- Elevated carcinoembryonic antigen (more likely in patients with higher stages at presentation).
- Elevated liver enzymes may be present with metastatic disease.

correlate with a poor survival and may predict likelihood of recurrence, regardless of tumor stage at diagnosis. However, it should not be used as an indication for adjuvant therapy. After a potentially curative resection, CEA levels should return to normal within 4 to 6 weeks. Persistently elevated CEA levels may indicate residual disease, while elevations after normalization may indicate relapsed disease.

Radiographic imaging studies are used to evaluate the extent of disease involvement for initial staging and subsequently to monitor disease response to therapy. Contrast dye-enhanced CT scans of the chest, abdomen, and pelvis are performed to evaluate for pulmonary, hepatic, and retroperitoneal involvement as well as occult abdominal and pelvic disease. In certain cases, such as patients with contrast dye allergies, magnetic resonance imaging (MRI) of the abdomen and pelvis may be performed. A glucose analog [^{18}F]-fluorodeoxyglucose-positron emission tomography (PET) scan may also be performed as the primary imaging modality or to confirm metastatic disease if findings from CT or MRI scans are not conclusive. PET imaging may provide functional information to assist in discriminating between benign and malignant disease by detecting tumor-related metabolic alterations in affected tissues. PET scans are commonly used for the detection of recurrent colorectal cancer in patients with rising CEA levels and inconclusive findings on standard imaging studies. A PET scan is often performed in conjunction with a CT scan for anatomical localization of a lesion(s). For initial rectal cancer staging, assessment of the extent of tumor spread into the surrounding mesorectum and depth of invasion within the bowel wall may be performed using MRI or endorectal ultrasound.

Because of the increased likelihood of HNPCC in patients diagnosed with colorectal cancer younger than the age of 50 years, MMR protein testing on the cancer specimen is recommended.[49] The level of MMR protein expression can be determined by immunohistochemistry, which is decreased with MMR gene mutations. Gene sequencing can also be performed to detect MSI. If immunohistochemical analysis of the tumor reveals absence of MLHI protein expression, *BRAF* gene mutation testing is recommended to distinguish between somatic and germline *MLH1* gene mutation.[49] Individuals with abnormal MMR protein expression or MSI should be referred for genetic counseling as additional testing and cancer susceptibility risk assessment may be appropriate for themselves and family members.

STAGING

4 The purpose of staging examinations is to determine the extent of disease, which allows the oncologist to develop treatment plans and estimate overall prognosis. The same TNM classification system is used for both cancers of the colon and rectum since the categories reflect similar survival outcomes.[52,53] This classification assesses three aspects of cancer growth: T (tumor penetration), N (lymph node involvement), and M (presence or absence of metastases) into account. The TNM classification also allows for various subdivisions within each of the three categories, which is then used for determining the disease stage. Table 130-6 summarizes the staging definitions used in the TNM system and corresponding 5-year survival rates.[52-54] Figure 130-5 shows the various stages of cancer based on cancer penetration through the bowel wall and extension to regional lymph nodes. Of note, an individual patient's stage is determined at the time of the initial diagnosis and does not change with progression of disease or recurrence. For example, if a patient is diagnosed with stage II colon cancer and later recurs with metastases to the liver, that patient is stage II now with metastatic disease to the liver, not stage IV.

PROGNOSIS

4 The stage of colorectal cancer upon diagnosis is the most important independent prognostic factor for survival and disease recurrence. Five-year relative survival is about 90% for individuals who present with a localized tumor stage at diagnosis as compared with about 13% for individuals with metastatic disease at diagnosis.[1]

Clinical factors present at the time of diagnosis that are associated with a poor prognosis and decreased survival include bowel obstruction or perforation, high preoperative CEA level, distant metastases, and location of the primary tumor in the rectum or rectosigmoid area.[55] Along with resection of the primary tumor, a minimum of 12 lymph nodes must be examined to accurately determine regional lymph node involvement and predict lymph node-negative disease.[55] The pathologic assessment also includes determination of TNM stage, tumor type, and histologic grade, presence of venous, and lymphatic invasion, and whether the resected margins are free of tumor.[56] Consideration of these factors plays an

TABLE 130-6 Colon Cancer by TNM Classification and Associated 5-Year Relative Survival

Stage	T	N	M	Survival (%)
0	T_{is}	N_0	M_0	95.6
I	T_1	N_0	M_0	97.4
	T_2	N_0	M_0	96.8
IIA	T_3	N_0	M_0	87.5
IIB	T_{4a}	N_0	M_0	79.6
IIC	T_{4b}	N_0	M_0	58.4
IIIA	T_1-T_2	N_1/N_{1c}	M_0	71.1
	T_1	N_{2a}	M_0	68.5
IIIB	T_3-T_{4a}	N_1/N_{1c}	M_0	60.6-68.7
	T_2-T_3	N_{2a}	M_0	53.4-81.7
	T_1-T_2	N_{2b}	M_0	62.4
IIIC	T_{4a}	N_{2a}	M_0	40.9
	T_3-T_{4a}	N_{2b}	M_0	21.8-37.3
	T_{4b}	N_1-N_2	M_0	15.7
IVA	Any T	Any N	M_{1a}	11.5
IVB	Any T	Any N	M_{1b}	

Primary Tumor (T)

T_{is}, Carcinoma in situ: intraepithelial or invasion of lamina propia.[a]

T_1, Tumor invades submucosa.

T_2, Tumor invades muscularis propria.

T_3, Tumor invades through the muscularis propria into pericolorectal tissues.

T_{4a}, Tumor penetrates to the surface of the visceral peritoneum.[b]

T_{4b}, Tumor directly invades or is adherent to other organs or structures.[b,c]

Lymph Nodes (N)

N_0, no regional lymph node metastasis

N_1, metastasis in 1-3 lymph nodes

N_{1a}, metastasis in 1 lymph node

N_{1b}, metastasis in 2-3 lymph nodes

N_{1c}, tissue tumor deposits without lymph node metastasis

N_2, metastasis in more than 4 lymph nodes

N_{2a}, metastasis in 4-6 lymph nodes

N_{2b}, metastasis in more than 7 lymph nodes

Distant Metastasis (M)

M_0, no distant metastasis

M_{1a}, metastasis confined to one site or organ

M_{1b}, metastasis in peritoneum or more than 1 site or organ

[a]T_{is} includes cancer cells confined within the glandular basement membrane (intraepithelial) or mucosal lamina propria (intramucosal) with no extension through the muscularis mucosae into the submucosa.

[b]Direct invasion in T_4 includes invasion of other organs or other segments of the colorectum as a result of direct extension through the serosa, as confirmed on microscopic examination (eg, invasion of the sigmoid colon by a carcinoma of the cecum) or, for cancers in a retroperitoneal or subperitoneal location, direct invasion of other organs or structures by virtue of extension beyond the muscularis propria (ie, respectively, a tumor on the posterior wall of the descending colon invading the left kidney or lateral abdominal wall; or a mid or distal rectal cancer with invasion of prostate, seminal vesicles, cervix, or vagina).

[c]Tumor that is adherent to other organs or structures, grossly, is classified cT_{4b}. However, if no tumor is present in the adhesion, microscopically, the classification should be pT_{1-4a} depending on the anatomical depth of wall invasion. The V and L classifications should be used to identify the presence or absence of vascular or lymphatic invasion whereas the PN site-specific factor should be used for perineural invasion.

Data from references 52-54.

important role in determining optimal strategies for treatment and appropriate follow-up.

Additional morphologic tumor features that have negative prognostic value with regard to clinical outcome include infiltrative tumor border configuration, evidence of perineural invasion, extranodal tumor deposits, and presence of tumor budding, characterized by clusters of cells that possess properties of malignant stem cells and are associated with increased risk of local and distant spread.[56] A high density of tumor-infiltrating lymphocytes in the tissue specimen is associated with a favorable outcome.[55,56]

Certain molecular markers, particularly MSI, 18q/*DCC* mutation or LOH, *BRAF* V600E mutation, and *RAS* mutations, are also associated with colorectal cancer prognosis, although the pathologic stage of disease remains the primary prognostic assessment.[57]

Colorectal cancers with allelic LOH on chromosome 18q or absent DCC protein are associated with a worse prognosis within stages II and III disease, but data are insufficient to warrant use of this test in practice at this time.[56,57] MSI can be determined through DNA sequencing or by immunohistochemistry staining for protein products of the MMR genes. Colorectal cancers that demonstrate high MSI (MSI-H) appear to be associated with a more favorable outcome and appear to predict the benefit of adjuvant fluoropyrimidines for early-stage disease.[55-57] Tumor DNA *BRAF* and *RAS* mutation status appear to be linked to OS but are not used to determine prognosis.

Although multiple prognostic biomarkers for colorectal cancer have been identified, single molecular tests other than MSI are not used routinely in clinical practice. However, several multigene

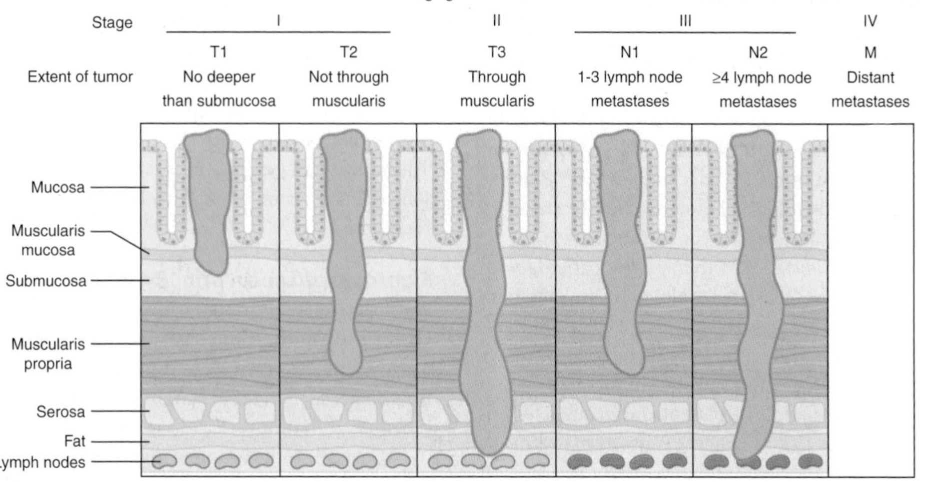

FIGURE 130-5 TNM staging for colorectal cancer. *(From Longo DL, Fauci AS, Kasper DL, Hauser SL, Jameson JL, Loscalzo J: Harrison's Principles of Internal Medicine, 18th ed. http://www.accessmedicine.com. Copyright © The McGraw-Hill Companies, Inc. All right reserved.)*

assays have been developed that provide prognostic information to assist in identifying individuals at high risk for cancer recurrence from early-stage disease.[57,58] The Onco*type* DX colon cancer assay is commercially available and has been validated in several trials as a prognostic test for stage II and III colon cancer.[57-59] Gene expression profiles classify risk of recurrence of low, intermediate, or high, and these scores are prognostic for recurrence, DFS, and OS. The Colo-Print gene expression assay characterizes risk of recurrence as low or high, and is undergoing further validation in clinical trials.[58] The ability for these and other gene signature assays in development to predict which patients may benefit from adjuvant chemotherapy has not been well established.

TREATMENT
Colorectal Cancer

Desired Outcomes

Treatment goals for cancer of the colon or rectum are based on the stage of disease at presentation. Stages I, II, and III disease are considered potentially curable and the goal of management is to eradicate potential micrometastases after surgical resection. Based on the numbers and site(s) of metastases, about 20% to 30% of patients with metastatic colorectal cancer may be cured, if their metastases are considered resectable.[58] Most patients with stage IV disease are not curable, and treatments for metastatic disease are considered palliative to reduce symptoms, avoid disease-related complications, and prolong survival. However, special attention should be given to those with oligo-lesions in the liver or lung since potential cure is still possible for some of these patients.

General Approach to Treatment

Performance status, concomitant disease states, lifestyle factors, patient preferences, and patient age (although advanced age is not an absolute contraindication for aggressive therapies) must be considered in the treatment planning process. Special or emergent conditions, such as bowel obstruction or perforation, severe pain, anemia, or other symptomatic problems, need to be addressed acutely, after which time a more long-term disease-specific plan can be developed. The treatment approaches for cancer of the colon or rectum reflect two primary treatment goals: curative therapy for localized disease and palliative therapy for metastatic cancer.

For patients for whom treatment intent is curative, surgical resection of the primary tumor is the most important component of therapy. Depending on the extent of disease and whether the tumor originated in the colon or rectum, further adjuvant chemotherapy or chemotherapy plus XRT (chemoradiation) may be appropriate. For selected patients with resectable metastases, surgical resection may be an option. However, for most patients with metastases, systemic chemotherapy is the mainstay of treatment; XRT may also be useful for disease palliation of localized symptoms. Patients with metastatic disease who are asymptomatic may benefit from initiation of therapy, and continuous treatment should be considered.

Operable Disease

Surgery

5 Individuals with operable—stages I, II, and III—cancer of the colon or rectum should undergo complete surgical resection of the primary tumor mass with regional lymphadenectomy as a curative approach for their disease.[60] The surgical approach for colon cancer generally involves complete resection of the tumor with at least a 5 cm margin of tumor-free bowel and a regional lymphadenectomy.

The preferred surgical procedure for rectal cancer is a total excision of the mesorectum, the surrounding tissue containing perirectal fat and draining lymph nodes.[60,61] If the distal margin clear of tumor is at least 1 cm, sphincter-preserving surgery may be possible for patients with cancers in the middle and lower portion of the rectum. Individuals who are not candidates for sphincter-sparing resections or have extensive local spread of tumor will require an abdominoperineal resection. This involves removal of the distal sigmoid, rectosigmoid, rectum, and anus with the establishment of a permanent sigmoid colostomy.

Colectomies for colon cancer can be performed as open procedures or laparoscopically. Laparoscopic colectomy has become an accepted procedure for colon and rectal cancer.[60] This technique appears to produce similar results to conventional surgery, with the benefits of a smaller surgical incision, shorter hospital stay, shorter duration of ileus, and reduced pain. Complications associated with colorectal surgery include infection, anastomotic leakage, obstruction, adhesion formation, sexual dysfunction, and malabsorption syndromes, depending on the site and extent of resection. Complications affecting bowel function associated with surgery for rectal cancer increase as the level of anastomosis approaches the anus.

Adjuvant Therapy for Colon Cancer

Adjuvant therapy in colorectal cancer is administered to selected individuals after complete tumor resection in an attempt to eliminate residual micrometastatic disease, thereby decreasing tumor recurrence and improving survival rates. Patients should start adjuvant therapy as soon as they are medically stable following surgery because each 4-week delay results in a 14% decrease in OS.[58] Because more than 90% of patients with stage I colon cancer are cured by surgical resection alone, adjuvant therapy is not indicated.[58,60]

Adjuvant chemotherapy is standard therapy for patients with stage III colon cancer. The presence of lymph node involvement with tumor places patients with stage III colon cancer at high risk for recurrence, and the risk of death within 5 years of surgical resection alone is as high as 70%, depending on the number of lymph nodes involved.[60] In this population of patients, adjuvant chemotherapy significantly decreases risk of cancer recurrence and death and is standard of care. Adjuvant chemotherapy should be initiated as soon as the patient is medically stable, as delays in chemotherapy have been associated with a decrease in OS.

The role of adjuvant chemotherapy for all patients without lymph node involvement (stage II) colon cancer is controversial because early studies that showed improvements in survival included patients with both stage II and III colon cancer. However, the QUASAR trial, which included patients with mostly stage II disease, showed a significant improvement in OS with adjuvant fluorouracil and leucovorin as compared to observation alone.[60]

Patients with stage II disease who are at higher risk for relapse include those with inadequate lymph node sampling, perforation of the bowel at presentation, poorly differentiated tumors, perineural invasion, and T_4 lesions (stage IIB/IIC), and many practitioners offer this therapy to selected patients, with a detailed discussion with patients regarding the potential benefits versus treatment-related toxicities.[58] Individuals with MSI-H tumors have a better prognosis compared to those with MSI-L and may not benefit or even be harmed from adjuvant fluoropyrimidine chemotherapy. In addition, subgroup analysis from the QUASAR trial indicated that individuals greater than 70 years of age did not appear to benefit from adjuvant chemotherapy.[60] Optimal dosing, administration schedule, and duration of therapy have yet to be determined, but most practitioners use the same treatment approach as that used for patients with stage III colon cancer.

Adjuvant Radiation Therapy Adjuvant XRT has a limited role in colon cancer because most recurrences are extrapelvic and occur in the abdomen. A subset of patients with recurrent disease or with T_4 tumors that have penetrated fixed structures may benefit from adjuvant fluorouracil-based chemoradiation, with consideration of intraoperative radiation.[58] Selected candidates may also be considered for preoperative fluoropyrimidine-based chemoradiation to improve resectability. Adverse effects associated with XRT in colorectal cancer can be acute or chronic. Acute effects primarily include hematologic depression, dysuria, diarrhea, abdominal cramping, and proctitis. Chronic symptoms that sometimes persist for months following discontinuation of XRT include persistent diarrhea, proctitis or enteritis, small bowel obstruction, perineal tenderness, sexual dysfunction, and impaired wound healing.

Adjuvant Systemic Chemotherapy 5 Standard adjuvant chemotherapy regimens include a fluoropyrimidine (fluorouracil [with leucovorin] or capecitabine) as a single agent and in combination with oxaliplatin.[62-69] The addition of leucovorin increases the binding affinity of the active fluorouracil metabolite to thymidylate synthase (TS), thus enhancing its cytotoxic activity. Combinations of fluorouracil plus leucovorin have been studied extensively in the adjuvant setting, based on the observation that fluorouracil plus leucovorin substantially improves response rates as compared with fluorouracil alone for metastatic disease.[58,60] Leucovorin administration prior to fluorouracil is the most effective approach to enable intracellular-reduced folates to accumulate prior to fluorouracil administration. When leucovorin is unavailable, levoleucovorin, the active isomer of racemic leucovorin, can be substituted as an alternative. The recommended levoleucovorin dose is 50% of the leucovorin dose.[70] The addition of oxaliplatin is superior to fluoropyrimidines alone in stage III colon cancer, but this benefit hasn't been observed in stage II colon cancer.[58]

Fluorouracil/Leucovorin Regimens Schedules of fluorouracil and leucovorin administration vary among the different regimens. Historically in the United States, the Roswell Park regimen and the Mayo Clinic regimen were once commonly used, while in Europe, treatments such as the de Gramont regimen favored a continuous IV schedule of fluorouracil (Table 130-7).[62-69]

Clinical studies comparing the efficacy of bolus and continuous infusion schedules generally favor continuous infusion of fluorouracil, which is probably related to its short plasma half-life and S-phase specificity for optimal TS inhibition. Continuous IV infusions also permit increased fluorouracil dose intensity, which may account for the higher response rates observed with prolonged infusions of fluorouracil. In most common combination regimens, fluorouracil is administered by both IV bolus injection and continuous IV infusion. This method of administration is now the most common method of administration in the United States and has replaced the Roswell Park and Mayo Clinic regimens.

Clinically significant differences in toxicity occur based on the dose, route, and schedule of fluorouracil administration. Leukopenia is the primary dose-limiting toxicity of IV bolus fluorouracil, although diarrhea, stomatitis, and nausea and vomiting can also occur.[71] The incidence and severity of stomatitis can be significantly reduced with the use of oral cryotherapy. In this approach, the patient is instructed to chew and hold ice chips in the mouth during the period between 5 minutes prior to and 30 minutes following the bolus injection of fluorouracil. The protective effects of this procedure are probably related to the local vasoconstriction caused by the ice chips, which temporarily reduces blood flow to the oral mucosa, thereby reducing drug exposure to the oral mucosa.

Although continuous IV infusion fluorouracil is generally well tolerated, dose-limiting toxicities can be substantial. A distinct toxicity, palmar–plantar erythrodysesthesia ("hand–foot syndrome" or PPE), and stomatitis occur most frequently with this route of administration.[71] Hand–foot syndrome occurs in 24% to 40% of patients receiving extended continuous IV infusions and is characterized by painful swelling and erythroderma of the soles of the feet, palms of the hands, and distal fingers. The skin toxicity is fully reversible on interruption of therapy or dose reduction and is not life threatening, but it can be significant and acutely disabling. The incidence of stomatitis, diarrhea, and hematologic toxicity is not substantial at standard doses, but it increases with increasing fluorouracil doses. No significant difference is noted in the incidence of mucositis, diarrhea, nausea and vomiting, or alopecia between continuous and bolus IV fluorouracil administration.[71]

An additional determinant of fluorouracil toxicity, regardless of the method of administration, is related to its catabolism and pharmacogenomic factors. Dihydropyrimidine dehydrogenase (DPD) is the main enzyme responsible for the catabolism of fluorouracil to inactive metabolites. A rare pharmacogenetic disorder characterized by complete or near-complete deficiency of this enzyme has been identified in patients with cancer. Patients with this enzyme deficiency develop severe toxicity, including death, after fluorouracil administration. Molecular studies have identified a relationship between allelic variants in the *DPYD* gene (the gene that encodes DPD) and a deficiency in DPD activity.[57]

TABLE 130-7 Chemotherapy Regimens for the Adjuvant Treatment of Colorectal Cancer

Regimen	Agents	Comments
The Historical Standard		
FOLFOX4[62]	Oxaliplatin 85 mg/m² IV day 1 Leucovorin 200 mg/m² per day IV over 2 hours days 1 and 2 Fluorouracil 400 mg/m² IV bolus, after leucovorin, then 600 mg/m² CIV over 22 hours days 1 and 2 Repeat every 2 weeks	Improved OS and DFS as compared with infusional fluorouracil-leucovorin–based regimens
The Current Standard		
mFOLFOX6[63]	Oxaliplatin 85 mg/m² IV on day 1 Leucovorin 400 mg/m² IV on day 1 Fluorouracil 400 mg/m² IV bolus, after leucovorin on day 1, then 1,200 mg/m²/day × 2 days CIV (total 2,400 mg/m² over 46-48 hours) Repeat every 2 weeks	Easier administration and better tolerated as compared to FOLFOX4; common toxicities: sensory neuropathy, neutropenia. A preferred regimen for adjuvant colon and rectal therapy
Alternative Regimens		
Capecitabine[64]	Capecitabine 1,250 mg/m² PO twice daily on days 1 through 14 Each cycle lasts 14 days and is repeated every 3 weeks × 24 weeks	Equivalent DFS as compared with the Mayo Clinic regimen with improved tolerability; hand-foot syndrome common, useful for patients without vascular access or have difficulties with travel to infusion center
CapOx[65]	Oxaliplatin 130 mg/m² IV day 1 Capecitabine 850-1,000 mg/m² twice daily orally days 1 through 14 Each cycle lasts 3 weeks × 24 weeks	Improved DFS in patients with stage III colon cancer compared to capecitabine alone; common dose-limiting toxicities: neuropathies and hand–foot syndrome. A preferred regimen for adjuvant rectal therapy.
de Gramont regimen[66]	Leucovorin 200 mg/m² per day IV over 2 hours, days 1 and 2 Fluorouracil 400 mg/m² per day IV bolus, followed by 600 mg/m² CIV over 22 hours, days 1 and 2 for 2 consecutive days after leucovorin Repeat every 2 weeks	Improved safety as compared with the Mayo Clinic regimen; hand–foot syndrome common
FLOX[67]	Oxaliplatin 85 mg/m² IV administered on weeks 1, 3, and 5 Fluorouracil 500 mg/m² IV bolus weekly × 6 Leucovorin 500 mg/m² IV weekly × 6 Each cycle lasts 8 weeks and is repeated for 3 cycles	Improved DFS as compared with bolus fluorouracil-leucovorin–based regimens. Increased toxicity (diarrhea and neuropathies) compared to FOLFOX4
Mayo Clinic regimen[68]	Leucovorin 20 mg/m² per day IV, days 1 to 5 Fluorouracil 425 mg/m² per day IV, days 1 to 5 after leucovorin Repeat every 4 to 5 weeks	Leukopenia common dose-limiting toxicity, diarrhea, and stomatitis common
Roswell Park Regimen[69]	Leucovorin 500 mg/m² IV day 1 over 2 hours Fluorouracil 500 mg/m² IV day 1 after leucovorin Repeat weekly for 6 of 8 weeks × 4 cycles	Leukopenia common dose-limiting toxicity, diarrhea, and stomatitis common
Simplified Biweekly[63]	Leucovorin 400 mg/m² per day IV Fluorouracil 400 mg IV bolus, after leucovorin, then 1,200 mg/m²/day days 1 and 2 (total 2,400 mg/m² over 46-48 hours) for 2 consecutive days Repeat every 2 weeks	Hand–foot syndrome common

CIV, continuous intravenous infusion; DFS, disease-free survival; OS, overall survival; PO, by mouth.

In summary, fluorouracil and leucovorin can be administered in a variety of treatment schedules, but none has proven superior with regard to overall patient survival and these regimens tend to be used in patients unable to tolerate an oxaliplatin-containing regimen. Table 130-7 lists examples of some of these regimens. A weekly or bimonthly schedule of leucovorin plus fluorouracil (either bolus or continuous infusion) may be more convenient for the patient in terms of fewer scheduled clinic appointments, less interference with work schedules, and ease of dose adjustments based on toxicity.

Fluorouracil Plus Oxaliplatin Regimens 5 Current National Comprehensive Cancer Network (NCCN) guidelines recommend a FOLFOX (fluorouracil/leucovorin and oxaliplatin) regimen as the preferred treatment for patients with stage III colon cancer who can tolerate combination therapy.[58] These recommendations are based on results from the Multicenter International Study of Oxaliplatin/5-Fluorouracil/Leucovorin in the Adjuvant Treatment of Colon Cancer (MOSAIC) trial, where the addition of oxaliplatin resulted in a 20% risk reduction in disease recurrence and increased 5-year DFS (73% vs 67%) as compared with fluorouracil plus leucovorin alone. With a median follow-up of 82 months, the addition of oxaliplatin resulted in a statistically significant absolute 6-year OS difference of 2.5%.[63] Oxaliplatin was associated with increased risk of paresthesia, neutropenia, and gastrointestinal toxicity (nausea, vomiting, and diarrhea) that were manageable with supportive care. This initial trial was performed with FOLFOX4 dosing schedule, more recent studies have further modified the to improve tolerability and the most current standard is mFOLFOX6 regimen.[58]

Further supporting the role of oxaliplatin in the adjuvant setting are the results of the National Surgical Adjuvant Breast and Bowel Project C-07 trial, which compared bolus fluorouracil and leucovorin, with or without oxaliplatin.[67] A significant risk reduction in disease recurrence by 20% was seen with oxaliplatin added to the fluorouracil backbone. As expected, neurotoxicity was increased with oxaliplatin. This method of administration, called the FLOX regimen (fluorouracil, leucovorin, and oxaliplatin), is associated with increased diarrhea and neuropathies as compared with the aforementioned regimen used in the MOSAIC trial. Though listed as an option according to current NCCN guidelines, its use is limited by its toxicity.[58]

Oxaliplatin has minimal renal toxicity, myelosuppression, and nausea and vomiting when compared with other platinum-based drugs. Oxaliplatin is associated with both acute and persistent neuropathies.[72] The acute neuropathies occur within 1 to 2 days of dosing and resolve within 2 weeks. The neuropathies usually occur peripherally, but may also occur in the jaw and tongue. A rare acute syndrome of pharyngolaryngeal dysesthesia (1%-2% of patients) is characterized by subjective sensations of difficulty in swallowing and shortness of breath. Overall, acute neuropathies occur in about 90% of patients, and are precipitated or exacerbated by exposure to cold temperatures or cold objects. Thus, patients should be instructed to avoid cold drinks and use of ice, and to cover skin before exposure to cold or cold objects. Several prophylactic and treatment strategies have been studied with varying degrees of success. Persistent neuropathy is typically a cumulative adverse effect, occurring after 8 to 10 cycles. The neuropathy is characterized by paresthesia, dysesthesia, and hypoesthesia, but may also include deficits in proprioception that can interfere with daily activities (eg, writing, buttoning, swallowing, and difficulty walking as a result of impaired proprioception). Persistent neuropathy occurs in about one-half of patients receiving oxaliplatin but usually resolves with dosage reductions or cessation of oxaliplatin therapy.[58,72] Prophylaxis with calcium and magnesium infusions has not been proven effective. A "stop-and-go" approach where oxaliplatin is temporarily discontinued after 3 months of therapy (or sooner with significant neuropathic symptoms) with the other drugs continued, reduces neurotoxicity without compromising OS and has been advocated.[58] Oxaliplatin can be reinitiated at disease progression in those patients that experience near complete resolution of neurotoxicity. Anticonvulsant and antidepressant agents are potentially useful to treat symptoms.

Capecitabine Regimens (5) Capecitabine has been evaluated in adjuvant studies as a replacement for fluorouracil in an attempt to improve the safety and ease of administration of the chemotherapy regimen. Capecitabine is converted to fluorouracil through a three-step activation process, the final step being activation by thymidine phosphorylase, which is present in greatest concentrations at the tumor site. These activation steps lead to about a threefold increase in tumor fluorouracil levels. The use of CapOx (capecitabine plus oxaliplatin) has been demonstrated to prolong 3-year DFS (71% vs 67%) as compared to bolus fluorouracil alone in patients with stage III disease, but no difference in OS was observed. The toxicities differed for the two regimens, with increased risks of neuropathies and hand–foot syndrome with CapOx and increased risk of neutropenia/neutropenic fever with fluorouracil.[65] Capecitabine is FDA approved as a single agent in the adjuvant setting and has been shown to be noninferior to bolus fluorouracil and leucovorin in patients with stage III colon cancer.[64] Both regimens were given for 6 months. DFS between the groups was found to be equivalent. Secondary end points of relapse-free survival (hazard ratio [HR] 0.86; $P=0.04$) and safety were improved with capecitabine. In particular, the incidence of diarrhea, stomatitis, and neutropenia was decreased with capecitabine, but the incidence of hand–foot syndrome was increased with capecitabine. Doses may need to be reduced in patients who experience side effects. Patients with renal dysfunction can accumulate drug and often require dose modification. This regimen is recommended when patients are considered unable to tolerate combination therapy.[58]

Selection of an Adjuvant Regimen Selecting a specific regimen from those listed in Table 130-7 requires an assessment of several patient-specific factors, including the performance status of the patient, comorbid conditions that may exist, and patient preferences for treatment based on lifestyle factors that are important to the patient. If a clinical trial is not an option, most patients with a good performance status will receive mFOLFOX6. Single-agent capecitabine may be the preferred option for patients with preexisting neuropathies, such as diabetic patients, or those patients wishing not to receive IV chemotherapy for any other reason. Fluorouracil and leucovorin has limited use at this time but is an acceptable option for patients who cannot receive oxaliplatin and are unable to tolerate or take oral capecitabine. For example, patients who develop severe hand–foot syndrome may tolerate bolus fluorouracil/leucovorin because this toxicity is minimal with this administration method.

Patient age should also be considered when selecting an appropriate regimen. Subset analysis of the MOSAIC and NSABP-C07 trials have demonstrated no OS benefit from adding oxaliplatin to patients older than the age of 70 years and these patients may be appropriate for fluoropyrimidine-based therapy.[60,67]

Clinical **Controversy...**

Current guidelines discourage the use of age as a sole determining factor in choosing an adjuvant chemotherapy regimen. However, subset analysis of large clinical trials has shown that patients older than the age of 70 years may not benefit from adjuvant oxaliplatin and may need to be treated differently.

Adjuvant and Neoadjuvant Therapy for Rectal Cancer

(6) Rectal cancer involves those tumors found below the peritoneal reflection in the most distal 15 cm of the large bowel, and as such is distinct from colon cancer in that it has a propensity for both local and distant recurrence. The higher incidence of local failure and overall poorer prognosis associated with rectal cancer is a result of anatomic limitations in excising adequate radial margins around the rectal tumor. Most patients with stage II or stage III rectal cancer should receive combined-modality therapy consisting of XRT and fluoropyrimidine-based chemotherapy perioperatively.[60,73]

Neoadjuvant Therapy (6) Neoadjuvant (preoperative) chemoradiation is considered standard of care for most patients with stage II or II rectal cancer because of significant reduction in local recurrence, fewer toxicities, and improved sphincter-preserving surgeries as compared to postoperative chemoradiation.[61,73] However, some patients are unable to tolerate a typical 5- to 6-week chemoradiation regimen and may be more appropriate candidates for a short course of preoperative radiation therapy alone.[73] Chemotherapy combined with XRT typically involves continuous infusion fluorouracil, oral capecitabine, or bolus fluorouracil and leucovorin; the addition of oxaliplatin to either fluoropyrimidine was associated with increased toxicities without clear improvements in complete remission rates or survival benefit.[60,73] Although oxaliplatin and other agents continue to be evaluated in this setting, the addition of oxaliplatin, irinotecan or biologic agents (eg, cetuximab, panitumumab, and bevacizumab) is currently not recommended.[73]

Adjuvant Therapy (6) Current NCCN guidelines for rectal cancer indicate that preoperative fluoropyrimidine-based chemotherapy plus XRT is the preferred initial treatment for resectable stage IIA (T_3 N_0), stage III (any T, N_{1-2}, or T_4/locally unresectable lesions).[73] This should be followed additional adjuvant chemotherapy after surgery to total 6 months of chemotherapy (combined total from preoperative and postoperative regimens). Postoperative treatment regimens include a fluoropyrimidine-based chemotherapy. FOLFOX or CapeOx are preferred regimens, but FLOX, fluorouracil, and leucovorin, and capecitabine can be used as well. Combined chemoradiation is preferred for patients that do not receive preoperative radiation therapy.[60,61,73]

Metastatic Disease: Initial Therapy

Multiple efficacious treatment options for metastatic colorectal cancer are available. Patients are generally classified as having resectable, potentially resectable, or unresectable metastatic disease. Surgery and XRT are used to manage isolated sites of tumor. Chemotherapy is for disseminated disease and the primary treatment modality for unresectable metastatic colorectal cancer. Patients with resectable or potentially resectable metastases are candidates for multimodality therapy.[74] Tumor *RAS* (*KRAS* exon 2 and nonexon 2 and *NRAS*) and *BRAF* genotyping for mutation status is recommended for patients at the time when metastatic disease is diagnosed to identify appropriate treatment options.[58,73] Testing can also be performed on archived tissue samples obtained when the cancer was initially diagnosed.

Resectable or Potentially Resectable Metastatic Colorectal Cancer

Surgery 7 Up to 25% of patients will present with hepatic metastases at the time of diagnosis, and 60% of patients with colorectal cancer will develop hepatic metastases sometime during the course of their disease.[75] The lung is the second most common site of cancer recurrence. Resection of colorectal cancer metastases (metastasectomy) can achieve 5-year OS rates between 20% and 70%, whereas 5-year OS in patients with unresectable metastatic disease is uncommon.[58] Therefore, a primary goal is surgical resection of metastases with curative intent in those individuals for whom complete surgical resection is realistically possible. Patients with no significant general medical risk factors, fewer than four hepatic lesions, CEA levels less than 200 ng/mL (mcg/L), small tumor size, lack of extrahepatic tumor, and adequate surgical margins have the best opportunity for an improved long-term outcome.[75] The primary site of tumor should also be completely resected. Complete surgical resection of discrete metastases in extrahepatic sites, such as the lung, peritoneum, abdomen, and brain, has been less studied but appears to benefit patients with small numbers of metastases who are appropriate candidates for surgery. Adjuvant systemic chemotherapy is recommended to reduce the risk of recurrence following resection.[58]

Neoadjuvant (Conversional) and Adjuvant Chemotherapy 7 Patients that present with metastatic disease isolated to the liver or lung and who undergo resection of all metastatic and primary lesions have an increased probability of survival compared with those whose metastatic lesions remain unresected.[74] Therefore, strategies to increase the success rate of these resections (or convert unresectable lesions to resectable) is the primary goal in these patients. Neoadjuvant chemotherapy, also referred to as conversional chemotherapy, is the primary method to increase complete resection rates in both patients with resectable or potentially resectable liver or lung lesions. In some cases, individuals with metastatic disease initially deemed unresectable may achieve significant tumor regression following neoadjuvant chemotherapy to then be considered for surgery.[58]

The optimal sequencing of chemotherapy for patients with initially resectable metastatic disease is controversial, as treatment options include surgery followed by chemotherapy or perioperative (pre- and postoperative) chemotherapy with surgery.[58,73] Because of the high risk of recurrence following resection of metastases, postoperative chemotherapy is always recommended. Administration of both pre- and postoperative chemotherapy is common practice, but hepatotoxicity associated with preoperative chemotherapy should be considered. Steatohepatitis occurs in 4% to 28% of patients who receive irinotecan-containing regimens and vascular sinusoidal obstructive liver injury develops in 10% to 61% of patients receiving oxaliplatin.[76] Therefore, surgery is performed as soon as possible after the disease becomes resectable. Preoperative chemotherapy is limited to a 2- to 3-month time period, and patients undergo close monitoring.

Regimens are the same for neoadjuvant and adjuvant therapy. The choice of agents depends on patient-specific factors but may include regimens such as FOLFOX, FOLFIRI, FOLFOXIRI (infusional fluorouracil and leucovorin, oxaliplatin, and irinotecan), CapOx, and FOLFOX alternating with FOLFIRI. Biologic agents have been added to the aforementioned regimens.[77] If patients receive bevacizumab, surgery should not occur within 6 weeks of the last dose of therapy, and bevacizumab should not be restarted until 6 to 8 weeks after surgery due to the risk of bleeding or wound healing complications. EGFR inhibitors are to be considered only in patients that have tumors with wild-type *RAS*. Postoperative chemotherapy should be administered to patients to complete a total of 6 months of chemotherapy (pre- and postoperative).[58]

Patients with unresectable lesions are eligible for the same chemotherapy regimens (see Table 130-7). However, because the primary goal is surgical resection whenever possible, patients should be evaluated for possible resection after every 2 months of therapy. If resection occurs, adjuvant chemotherapy should be administered to complete a total of 6 months of chemotherapy.

Hepatic-Directed Therapies 7 Individuals with liver-only or liver-predominant metastatic disease may be considered for hepatic-directed therapy in addition to or as an alternative to surgical resection. Hepatic artery infusion (HAI) involves the placement of a permanent access catheter to the hepatic artery through which chemotherapy can be infused directly into the liver.[58] This approach offers the advantage of delivering high drug concentrations to tumors locally, thereby limiting systemic toxicities. Floxuridine with dexamethasone and fluorouracil with or without leucovorin are most commonly used agents. HAI is associated with potential biliary toxicity and the technical expertise required warrants use in selected patients by experienced practitioners.[58] Another option is hepatic transarterial chemoembolization, which delivers high concentrations of cytotoxic agents directly to the tumor and results in the embolization or devascularization of the liver, blocking perfusion of the tumor and eliminating its blood supply. This procedure involves the instillation of a mixture that incorporates chemotherapeutic agents, radioactive contrast dye, and/or an embolic agent directly into the hepatic artery. Agents most commonly used include doxorubicin, mitomycin, and cisplatin, which are usually dissolved in about 10 to 15 mL of a radiographic contrast dye. Addition of an embolic agent to the mixture results in either a temporary or permanent occlusion of the hepatic artery. Alternatively, drug-eluding beads of doxorubicin or irinotecan mixed with an embolic agent have been used. Local tumor response rates with these strategies are high and most patients will experience partial or complete relief of symptoms. Toxicities include postembolization syndrome characterized by nausea, fatigue, and transient elevations in hepatic enzymes and bilirubin, gastrointestinal ulcerations, and biliary toxicity. Although various hepatic-directed therapies offer potential disease palliation in select patients with unresectable, yet limited hepatic metastases, no conclusive survival advantage has been demonstrated. XRT can also be used to sites of hepatic tumor using external beam radiation therapy or percutaneous arterial injection of micron-sized embolic particles loaded with a radioisotope (radioembolization). Other less common methods include tumor ablation procedures using radiofrequency ablation or microwave energy to generate heat that destroys localized tumor cells. Cryoablation can also be used, which includes placement of a cryoprobe into the tumor, either percutaneously or intraoperatively, and then lowering the probe temperature to −20°C to −40°C and rewarming it in cycles, resulting in formation of an ice ball that causes tumor destruction. These strategies may be useful for patients who have very small hepatic lesions and are unable to undergo liver resection surgery, but they are less successful than surgical interventions.[58]

Unresectable Metastatic Colorectal Cancer

Unless the primary tumor is causing an obstruction, surgery in patients with established unresectable disease is rarely indicated. XRT may be useful to control localized symptoms in patients with metastatic colorectal cancer. Systemic chemotherapy palliates symptoms and improves survival in patients with unresectable disease. Common treatment regimens include combinations of cytotoxic and biologic agents.

Chemotherapy 7 Accepted initial chemotherapy regimens for metastatic colorectal cancer consist of oxaliplatin-containing regimens (FOLFOX, CapOx), irinotecan-containing regimens (FOLFIRI), oxaliplatin plus irinotecan plus fluorouracil plus leucovorin (FOLFOXIRI), infusional fluorouracil plus leucovorin alone, and capecitabine alone.[58] Current guidelines recommend the addition of bevacizumab to FOLFOX, CapOx, FOLFIRI, infusional fluorouracil plus leucovorin, and capecitabine alone, or an EGFR inhibitor added to FOLFOX or FOLFIRI or administered alone, if *RAS* wild type.[58] The goals of therapy, history of prior chemotherapy, tumor *RAS* mutation status, and risk of drug-related toxicities should be considered when an appropriate management strategy is defined for each individual. Treatment regimens are the same for metastatic cancer of the colon and rectum. Table 130-8 lists common initial chemotherapeutic regimens for metastatic disease.[78-87]

Currently, most metastatic colorectal cancers are incurable, and treatment goals are to control cancer growth, reduce patient symptoms, improve quality of life, and extend survival. The benefit of palliative chemotherapy for metastatic colorectal cancer as compared to observation or supportive care alone with regard to these treatment goals has been established. Results from multiple randomized trials and meta-analyses demonstrate that chemotherapy prolongs life and improves quality of life of patients with metastatic colorectal cancer.[60,88]

Most first-line chemotherapy regimens used for metastatic colorectal cancer incorporate a fluoropyrimidine. Irinotecan or oxaliplatin added to a fluoropyrimidine-based regimen significantly improves response rates, progression-free survival (PFS), and median survival.[60] Targeted antiangiogenesis agent bevacizumab further improve response rates and survival when combined with chemotherapy as compared to chemotherapy alone. Patients considered appropriate for initial intensive chemotherapy typically receive an oxaliplatin or irinotecan-containing regimen with infusional fluorouracil plus leucovorin and bevacizumab. Capecitabine can be substituted for fluorouracil and leucovorin. Patients that are not considered appropriate candidates for initial intensive therapy may be considered for fluoropyrimidine monotherapy, a fluoropyrimidine regimen combined with bevacizumab, or EGFR inhibitor monotherapy, as appropriate.[58] Patients may receive multiple

TABLE 130-8 Initial Chemotherapeutic Regimens for Metastatic Colorectal Cancer

Regimen	Agents	Major-Dose Limiting Toxicities	Comments
Patients Appropriate for Intensive Therapy with *RAS* Mutations			
mFOLFOX4+/– bevacizumab[78]	Oxaliplatin 85 mg/m^2 IV day 1 Leucovorin 400 mg/m^2 IV day 1 Fluorouracil 400 mg/m^2 IV bolus, after leucovorin day 1, then 1,200 mg/m^2/day × 2 days CIV (total 2,400 mg/m^2 over 46-48 hours) Repeat every 2 weeks +/– Bevacizumab 5 mg/kg IV day 1 before mFOLFOX6 Repeat cycle every 2 weeks	mFOLFOX4: Sensory neuropathy, neutropenia Bevacizumab: hypertension, thrombosis, proteinuria	Easier administration as compared with original FOLFOX
CapeOX +/– bevacizumab[78]	Oxaliplatin 130 mg/m^2 IV day 1 Capecitabine 850 to 1,000 mg/m^2 orally twice a day, days 1 to 14 Repeat cycle every 3 weeks +/– Bevacizumab 7.5 mg/kg IV day 1 Repeat cycle every 3 weeks	CapeOX: Diarrhea, hand–foot syndrome, neuropathies Bevacizumab: hypertension, thrombosis, proteinuria	Reduced capecitabine dose better tolerated; patient must be able to be adherent and report side effects a timely fashion
FOLFIRI+/– bevacizumab[79]	Irinotecan 180 mg/m^2 IV day 1 Leucovorin 400 mg/m^2 IV day 1 Fluorouracil 400 mg/m^2 IV bolus, after leucovorin day 1, then 1,200 mg/m^2/day × 2 days CIV (total 2,400 mg/m^2 over 46-48 hours) +/– Bevacizumab 5 mg/kg IV day prior to FOLFIRI Repeat cycle every 2 weeks	FOLFIRI: Diarrhea, mucositis, neutropenia Bevacizumab: hypertension, thrombosis, proteinuria	May be preferred in patients who have preexisting neuropathy or those in which neuropathy may be debilitating to their line of work (eg, musician)
Fluorouracil/leucovorin +/– bevacizumab[80,81]	See Table 107-X for fluorouracil/leucovorin regimen options +/– Bevacizumab 5 mg/kg IV day prior to fluorouracil and leucovorin Repeat cycle every 2 weeks	Fluorouracil/Leucovorin: diarrhea, hand–foot syndrome, mucositis, neutropenia Bevacizumab: hypertension, thrombosis, proteinuria	Infusional fluorouracil/leucovorin regimen preferred to bolus fluorouracil regimen. Infusional regimens tend to have more hand–foot syndrome and stomatitis and bolus regimens more neutropenia; weekly or bimonthly schedule of leucovorin plus fluorouracil (either bolus or continuous infusion) may be more convenient for the patient in terms of fewer scheduled clinic appointments, less interference with work schedules, and ease of dose adjustments based on toxicity

(continued)

TABLE 130-8 Initial Chemotherapeutic Regimens for Metastatic Colorectal Cancer (*Continued*)

Regimen	Agents	Major-Dose Limiting Toxicities	Comments
Capecitabine +/– bevacizumab[82]	Capecitabine 850-1,250 mg/m² orally twice a day, days 1 to 14 +/– Bevacizumab 7.5 mg/kg IV day 1 Repeat cycle every 3 weeks	Capecitabine: Hand–foot syndrome, diarrhea, hyperbilirubinemia Bevacizumab: hypertension, thrombosis, proteinuria	May be preferred in those without a port or limited venous access; patient must be able to be adherent and report side effects a timely fashion
FOLFOXIRI +/– bevacizumab[83]	Irinotecan 165 mg/m² IV day 1 prior to oxaliplatin Oxaliplatin 85 mg/m² IV prior to leucovorin day 1 Leucovorin 400 mg/m² IV day 1 prior to fluorouracil Fluorouracil 1,600 mg/m²/day × 2 days CIV (total 3,200 mg/m² over 48 hours) Repeat cycle every 2 weeks +/– Bevacizumab 5 mg/kg IV day 1 before FOLFOXIRI Repeat cycle every 2 weeks	FOLFOXFIRI: Neutropenia, diarrhea, stomatitis, peripheral neurotoxicity, thrombocytopenia Bevacizumab: hypertension, thrombosis, proteinuria	More neutropenia and peripheral neurotoxicity compared to FOLFIRI; often used in medically fit individuals with diffuse aggressive disease to palliate symptoms and as potential conversion therapy
Patients Appropriate for Intensive Therapy with *RAS* Wild Type			
mFOLFOX4 + cetuximab or panitumumab[83,84]	mFOLFOX4 regimen + Cetuximab (400 mg/m² IV loading dose, then cetuximab 250 mg/m² IV weekly thereafter OR cetuximab 500 mg/m² IV every 2 weeks) IV before mFOLFOX 4 OR Panitumumab 6 mg/kg IV day 1 before mFOLFOX6 Repeat cycle every 2 weeks	mFOLFOX4: Sensory neuropathy, neutropenia Cetuximab: Papulopustular and follicular rash, asthenia, constipation, diarrhea, allergic reactions, hypomagnesemia Panitumumab: rash, diarrhea, hypomagnesemia	Only *RAS* wild-type tumor
FOLFIRI + cetuximab or panitumumab[83]	FOLFIRI + Cetuximab (400 mg/m² IV loading dose, then cetuximab 250 mg/m² IV weekly thereafter OR cetuximab 500 mg/m² IV every 2 weeks) IV before FOLFIRI OR Panitumumab 6 mg/kg IV day 1 before FOLFIRI Repeat cycle every 2 weeks	FOLFIRI: Diarrhea, mucositis, neutropenia Cetuximab: papulopustular and follicular rash, asthenia, constipation, diarrhea, allergic reactions, hypomagnesemia Panitumumab: Rash, diarrhea, hypomagnesemia	Only *RAS* wild-type tumor; preferred for patients with pre existing neuropathy or those in which neuropathy may be debilitating to their line of work (eg, musician)
Patients NOT Appropriate for Intensive Therapy with *RAS* Mutations			
Infusional fluorouracil + leucovorin +/– bevacizumab[85]	Fluorouracil 400 mg/m² IV bolus, after leucovorin on day 1, then 1,200 mg/m²/day × 2 days CIV (total 2,400 mg/m² over 46-48 hours) Repeat cycle every 2 weeks +/– Bevacizumab 5 mg/kg IV day 1 prior to fluorouracil and leucovorin Repeat cycle every 2 weeks	Infusional fluorouracil/leucovorin: neutropenia, diarrhea Bevacizumab: hypertension, bleeding, proteinuria	Infusional fluorouracil/leucovorin regimen preferred to bolus fluorouracil regimen
Patients NOT Appropriate for Intensive Therapy with *RAS* Wild Type			
Cetuximab[83,86]	Cetuximab 400 mg/m² IV loading dose, then cetuximab 250 mg/m² IV weekly thereafter Or Cetuximab 500 mg/m² IV every 2 weeks	Papulopustular and follicular rash, asthenia, constipation, diarrhea, allergic reactions, hypomagnesemia	Only *RAS* wild-type tumor
Panitumumab[87]	6 mg/kg IV over 60 minutes every 2 weeks	Rash, hypomagnesemia, rare allergic reactions	Only *RAS* wild-type tumor

different regimens, and the sequence of drugs used appears less important than exposure to all active agents during the course of cancer treatments.[60] Table 130-9 summarizes comparative outcome data from potentially useful chemotherapeutic treatments for metastatic colorectal cancer.[78,83,84,87,89-102] Please refer back to the *Adjuvant Systemic Chemotherapy Section* for more information on the toxicities of the regimens that are used in both the adjuvant and metastatic settings.

Fluorouracil-Based Regimens 8 Fluorouracil can be administered as a bolus, a continuous infusion, or combination of the two in the metastatic setting. Continuous IV infusion fluorouracil regimens increase the duration of drug exposure during the S-phase of the cell cycle, increase cytotoxicity, and are better tolerated than bolus administration. When combined with irinotecan or oxaliplatin, infusional fluorouracil is recommended because of improved efficacy.[58]

Fluorouracil and Leucovorin Plus Irinotecan 8 Unlike in the adjuvant setting, irinotecan added to fluorouracil plus leucovorin as initial therapy for metastatic disease improves tumor response rates, time-to-progression, and OS (see Table 130-9).[91] The most common adverse effects of irinotecan in these regimens are diarrhea, neutropenia, nausea and vomiting, dehydration, asthenia, abdominal pain,

TABLE 130-9 Comparative Outcomes from Selected Trials in Metastatic Colorectal Cancer

Trial	Number	Outcome Measures	Results
First-Line			
FOLFOX vs IROX vs IFL Goldberg[89]	795	Primary: TTP; secondary: OS, ORR, time to treatment discontinuation	Median TTP: IFL vs FOLFOX 6.9 vs 8.7 months (*P*=0.0014). Median survival 15.0 months with IFL vs 19.5 months with FOLFOX (*P*=0.001). ORR with FOLFOX (45%) higher compared to IFL (31%; *P*=0.002) and IROX (35%, *P*=0.03). TTP and OS with IROX (6.5 and 17.4 months) no different from FOLFOX.
Infusional FU/LV ± Oxaliplatin de Gramont[90]	420	Primary: PFS; secondary: ORR, OS, tolerability, QOL	Median PFS: 9.0 vs 6.2 months (*P*=0.0003); ORR: 50.7 vs 22.3% (*P*=0.0001), oxaliplatin plus infusional FU/LV vs infusional FU/LV alone; no difference in OS (16.2 vs 14.7 months) or QOL between oxaliplatin plus infusional FU/LV vs infusional FU/LV alone.
Infusional FU/LV ± Irinotecan Douillard[91]	387	Primary: ORR; secondary: TTP, response duration, TTF, OS, QOL	Significantly higher ORR with infusional IFL vs infusional FU/LV alone (35% vs 22%; *P*<0.005) by ITT; TTP longer with IFL (6.7 vs 4.4 months; *P*<0.001) and OS longer with IFL vs infusional FU/LV alone (17.4 vs 14.1 months; *P*=0.031).
Capecitabine vs FU/LV Twelves[92]	1,207	Primary: ORR; secondary: TTP, OS, response duration	Tumor response to capecitabine greater than with FU/LV (25.7 vs 16.7%; *P*<0.0002), but no difference in median TTP (4.6 vs 4.7 months) or median survival (392 vs 391 days).
Irinotecan-based regimen ± Bevacizumab Fuchs[93]	547	Primary: PFS; secondary ORR, OS, toxicity	PFS increased with FOLFIRI compared with IFL (7.6 vs 5.9 months, *P*=0.004); addition of bevacizumab improved OS (28 months for FOLFIRI + bevacizumab vs 19.2 months for IFL + bevacizumab; *P*=0.037). Capelri equivalent to IFL and not included in final analysis and not recommended.
FOLFIRI vs FOLFOX6 Tournigand[94]	226	Test the best sequence of FOLFIRI vs FOLFOX6; primary: second PFS; secondary: PFS, OS, ORR, safety	Median survival 21.5 months with FOLFIRI then FOLFOX6 vs 20.6 months with FOLFOX6 then FOLFIRI; median PFS also no different (14.2 vs 10.9 months), or ORR or median PFS with first treatment: FOLFOX6 54% and 8.0 months, vs 56% and 8.5 months with FOLFIRI.
FOLFIRI vs FOLFOXIRI Masi[83]	244	Primary: ORR; secondary: PFS, OS, rate of surgical resection, QOL	FOLFOXIRI increased median PFS (9.8 months) vs FOLFIRI (6.8 months; *P*<0.001) and median OS (23.4 vs 16.7 months; *P*=0.26). Absolute 5-year survival benefit improved by 7% with FOLFOXIRI.
FOLFOXIRI + Bevacizumab vs FOLFIRI + Bevacizumab Falcone[83]	508	Primary: PFS; secondary: OS, efficacy in *BRAF* and *RAS* molecular subgroups, ORR	FOLFOXIRI plus bevacizumab improved median OS (29.8 months) compared to FOLFIRI plus bevacizumab (25.8 months; *P*=0.03). Median OS was longer (37.1 months) in the *RAS* and *BRAF* wild-type subgroup than in the *RAS*-mutation- (25.6 months) or *BRAF*-mutation- (13.4 months) positive subgroups. There was no difference in treatment effect across molecular subgroups.
CapOx or FOLFOX or FU/LV ± Bevacizumab Hochster[78]	360	Primary: toxicity; secondary ORR, TTP, OS	Grade 3/4 toxicity not increased with bevacizumab. TTP, ORR, and OS all greater when bevacizumab added to CapOx, FOLFOX, or bolus fluorouracil/leucovorin. Median survival with bevacizumab-containing regimens was 24.4 months vs 18.4 months without bevacizumab (not a randomized trial).
XELOX or FOLFOX ± Bevacizumab Saltz[83]	1,401	Primary: PFS; secondary ORR, OS	PFS increased from 8 to 9.4 months with bevacizumab added to oxaliplatin-containing regimens (XELOX or FOLFOX); *P*=0.0023. ORR and OS not different between groups.
FOLFOX ± Cetuximab Bokemeyer[95]	337	Primary: ORR; secondary PFS, OS, toxicity	ORR and PFS increased in patients with wild-type *KRAS* treated with FOLFOX + cetuximab compared with FOLFOX alone; *KRAS* mutant patients had no benefit with cetuximab (ORR 33 vs 49%, *P*=0.106 in cetuximab + FOLFOX and FOLFOX treated patients, respectively).
FOLFIRI ± Cetuximab Van Cutsem[96]	1,198	Primary: PFS; secondary OS, toxiocity	Of the 676 KRAS WT patients, median PFS was 9.9 months vs 8.4 months with FOLFIRI plus cetuximab vs FOLFIRI alone (HR = 0.696; *P*=0.0012). OS was also significantly increased with cetuximab (23.5 months vs 20.0 months, HR = 0.797; *P*=0.0093).
Oxaliplatin-based regimen ± Cetuximab Maughan[83]	1,630	Primary: OS in *KRAS* wild-type tumors; secondary, PFS, RR	Oxaliplatin-based chemotherapy + cetuximab had no effect on OS vs the control group of chemotherapy alone (17.9 months vs 17.0 months, *P*=0.67). Additionally, no difference was seen in PFS (*P*=0.60).
mFOLFOX6 + Panitumumab vs mFOLFOX6 + Bevacizumab Schwartzberg LS 2014[83]	285	Primary: PFS; secondary: OS, safety, treatment effects in extended *RAS* analysis	Subjects were previously untreated with wild-type KRAS (codons 12 and 13). PFS was similar for both treatment groups; median OS was 34.2 months in the panitumumab treatment arm and 24.3 months with bevacizumab (HR = 0.89; *P*=0.009). A trend for longer PFS and OS favored panitumumab treatment in the wild-type extended RAS subgroup.
FOLFOX4 ± Panitumumab Douillard[84]	1,183	Primary: PFS	656 patients had *KRAS* wild-type tumors. Panitumumab + FOLFOX4 improved PFS compared with FOLFOX4 (10.0 vs 8.6 months, respectively; HR = 0.80; *P*=0.01). The median OS for individuals with wild-type *KRAS* tumor receiving panitumumab + FOLFOX4 was 23.9 months vs 19.7 months with FOLFOX4 alone (HR 0.88; *P*=0.17).
Second-Line			
Irinotecan vs Infusional Fluorouracil Rougier[97]	267	Primary: OS; secondary: PFS, ORR, symptom-free survival, adverse effects, QOL	Irinotecan improved median PFS (4.2 vs 2.9 months; *P*=0.030) compared with infusion fluorouracil and 1-year survival (45% vs 35%; *P*=0.035) but not median OS (10.8 vs 8.5 months). Median pain-free survival was similar (*P*=0.06; 10.3 vs 8.5 months) between irinotecan and fluorouracil, as was QOL.
Irinotecan vs BSC Cunningham[98]	279	Primary: OS; secondary: performance status, body weight, tumor-related symptoms, QOL	Compared to best supportive care, OS was improved with irinotecan (13.8% 1-year survival vs 36.2%; *P*=0.0001); survival without deterioration in performance status, weight loss >5%, and pain-free survival were also improved with irinotecan.

(continued)

TABLE 130-9 Comparative Outcomes from Selected Trials in Metastatic Colorectal Cancer (*Continued*)

Trial	Number	Outcome Measures	Results
Cetuximab ± Irinotecan Cunningham[99]	829	Primary: ORR; secondary: TTP, OS	Addition of cetuximab to continuing irinotecan associated with 22.9% ORR compared with 10.9% with cetuximab alone (*P*=0.0074); median survival with cetuximab plus irinotecan similar to cetuximab alone (8.6 vs 6.9 months; *P*=0.48), but TTP was longer with cetuximab plus irinotecan (4.1 vs 1.5 months; HR = 0.54; 95% CI, 0.42-0.71).
Cetuximab ± Irinotecan Sobrero[100]	1,298	Primary: OS; secondary: PFS, RR, QOL	No difference in OS was seen between the cetuximab + irinotecan or irinotecan alone group (10.7 months vs 10.0 months, respectively; HR = 0.975; *P*=0.71). Cetuximab + irinotecan significantly improved PFS (median, 4.0 vs 2.6 months; HR = 0.692; *P*≤0.0001) and QOL.
Irinotecan ± Panitumumab Seymour MT 2013[83]	460	Primary: OS; secondary PFS, RR	Original study design amended to allocate subjects with *KRAS* wild-type tumors to one of 2 treatment groups with panitumumab. Individuals receiving panitumumab did not experience improved OS compared to those receiving irinotecan alone (10.4 vs 10.9 months: *P*=0.91). PFS was improved with the addition of panitumumab to irinotecan (HR = 0.78; *P*=0.015).
Panitumumab vs BSC Van Cutsem[87]	329	Primary: PFS; secondary: ORR, OS, safety	Panitumumab plus BSC prolonged PFS compared to BSC alone, with a median PFS of 8 weeks with panitumumab (HR = 0.54; 95% CI, 0.44-0.66).
FOLFIRI ± Panitumumab Peeters[83]	1,186	Primary: PFS and OS prospectively analyzed by *KRAS* status	In *KRAS* wild-type patients, the addition of panitumumab to chemotherapy demonstrated a significant improvement in PFS (6.7 months for panitumumab + FOLFIRI vs 4.9 months for FOLFIRI; HR = 0.82; *P*=0.023). Median OS was 14.5 months in the panitumumab group, 2 months longer than with FOLFIRI alone (12.5 months; HR = 0.92; *P*=0.37).
FOLFOX4 ± Bevacizumab Giantonio[83]	463	Primary: OS; secondary: PFS, ORR, toxicity	Addition of bevacizumab to FOLFOX4 in patients previously treated with irinotecan and a fluoropyrimidine improved median OS (12.9 vs 10.8 months; HR, 0.75, *P*=0.001), PFS (7.3 vs 4.7 months; HR, 0.75, *P*<0.0001), and ORR (22.7% vs 8.6%, *P*<0.0001) compared with FOLFOX4 alone.
Bevacizumab + chemotherapy continuation after first progression vs chemotherapy alone Bennouna[83]	820	Primary: OS; secondary, PFS, RR	Median OS was 11.2 months for bevacizumab plus chemotherapy and 9.8 months for chemotherapy alone (HR = 0.81; *P*=0.0062). Second-line chemotherapy choice based on what was administered as first-line therapy (patients who received oxaliplatin-based chemotherapy in the first-line received irinotecan-based therapy in the second-line setting and vice versa). PFS and RR improved with bevacizumab.
FOLFIRI ± Aflibercept Van Cutsem[83]	1,226	Primary: OS; secondary: PFS, ORR, adverse effects	Addition of aflibercept to FOLFIRI improved OS compared to FOLFIRI plus placebo (median survival 13.50 vs 12.06 months, respectively; HR = 0.817; *P*=0.0032). Median PFS extended with the addition of aflibercept to 6.90 months vs 4.67 months with placebo.
FOLFIRI ± Ramucirumab Tabernero 2015[101]	1,072	Primary: OS; secondary: PFS, ORR, disease control, adverse events, patient-reported outcomes (QOL)	Ramucirumab treatment median OS was 13.3 months vs 11.7 months with placebo (HR 0.844; *P*=0.0219). PFS significantly longer with ramucirumab compared to placebo, 5.7 months vs 4.5 months, respectively; HR = 0.793; *P*=0.0005.
Refractory Disease			
Panitumumab vs Cetuximab Price 2014[83]	999	Primary: OS, assessed for noninferiority; secondary PFS, RR	Historical HR for cetuximab plus BSC used for primary endpoint analysis. Panitumumab was noninferior to cetuximab with median OS of 10.4 months vs 10.0 months for panitumumab and cetuximab, respectively. Incidence of any grade and moderate to severe toxicities was similar among treatments.
Regorafenib vs Placbo Grothey[83]	753	Primary: OS; secondary PFS	Median OS was 6.4 months for regorafenib and 5.0 months for placebo (HR 0.77; *P*=0.0052). PFS 1.9 for regorafenib vs 1.7 months for best supportive care (HR, 0.49, *P*<0.001).
Trifluridine/tipiracil (TAS-102) vs Placebo Mayer 2015[102]	800	Primary: OS	Median OS was 7.1 months with trifluridine/tipiracil compared to 5.3 months with placebo (HR 0.68; *P*<0.001). Median time to worsening performance status was longer with trifluridine/tipiracil than with placebo (5.7 months vs 4.0 months; HR 0.66; *P*<0.001).

BSC, best supportive care; Capelri, capecitabine plus irinotecan; CapOx: capecitabine plus oxaliplatin; CI: confidence interval; FOLFIRI, fluorouracil plus leucovorin plus irinotecan; FOLFOX, fluorouracil plus leucovorin plus oxaliplatin; FOLFOXIRI, fluorouracil plus leucovorin plus oxaliplatin plus irinotecan; FU/LV, fluorouracil plus leucovorin; HR, hazard ratio; IFL, irinotecan plus fluorouracil plus leucovorin; IROX, irinotecan plus oxaliplatin; ITT, intention to treat; ORR, overall response rate; OS, overall survival; PFS, progression-free survival; QOL, quality-of-life; TTF, time-to-treatment failure; TTP, time-to-tumor progression; XELOX, capecitabine plus oxaliplatin.

and alopecia; diarrhea and neutropenia are dose limiting.[91] Two distinct patterns of diarrhea have been described. Early-onset diarrhea occurs during or within 2 to 6 hours after irinotecan administration and is characterized by lacrimation, diaphoresis, abdominal cramping, flushing, and/or diarrhea. These cholinergic symptoms, thought to be caused by inhibition of acetylcholinesterase, respond to atropine 0.25 to 1 mg given IV or subcutaneously. About 10% of patients experience the acute symptoms during or shortly following the irinotecan. More commonly, late-onset diarrhea occurs 1 to 12 days after irinotecan administration and may last for 3 to 5 days. Late-onset diarrhea may require hospitalization or discontinuation of therapy, and fatalities have been reported. The incidence of late-onset diarrhea can be decreased with aggressive antidiarrheal intervention. Aggressive intervention with high-dose loperamide therapy should consist of 4 mg taken at the first sign of soft or watery stools, followed by 2 mg orally every 2 hours until symptom-free for 12 hours; this regimen can be modified to 4 mg taken orally every 4 hours during the night.

The severity of delayed diarrhea has been correlated with the systemic exposure (ie, area under the concentration-vs-time curve) of irinotecan and SN-38 (irinotecan's active metabolite) and with genetic polymorphisms in the enzyme uridine diphosphate-glucuronosyltransferase (UGT1A1), which is responsible for the glucuronidation of SN-38 to inactive metabolites. Reduced or deficient levels of the UGT1A1 enzyme are observed in Gilbert syndrome, a familial hyperbilirubinemia disorder, and correlate with irinotecan-induced diarrhea and neutropenia.[103] An FDA-approved test for deficiency in this enzyme is available, and clinicians can consider obtaining these results for individual patients prior to initiating irinotecan-based therapy to see if a dose reduction at initiation of therapy is warranted.

Fluorouracil and Leucovorin Plus Oxaliplatin 8 Oxaliplatin, in combination with infusional fluorouracil plus leucovorin, is FDA-approved for use in first-line and salvage regimens for metastatic colorectal cancer (see Table 130-8). Oxaliplatin incorporation into fluorouracil-based regimens as first-line therapy for metastatic colorectal cancer is associated with higher response rates and improved PFS, with variable effects on OS (see Table 131-9).[90] Oxaliplatin is not effective as a single agent in colorectal cancer and is, therefore, only used in combination regimens.

Fluorouracil and Leucovorin plus Oxaliplatin plus Irinotecan 8 To further improve survival rates achieved with FOLFOX and FOLFIRI regimens, a four-drug regimen (FOLFOXIRI) was developed and has been compared with FOLFIRI.[83] FOLFOXIRI improved PFS and OS compared to FOLFIRI, and a higher proportion of patients receiving FOLFOXIRI were able to undergo radical resection of metastases. As expected, FOLFOXIRI causes more neutropenia, neurotoxicity, diarrhea, and alopecia, but may be appropriate for medically fit individuals with diffuse aggressive disease to palliate symptoms and as potential conversion therapy.[58,83,88]

Capecitabine 8 Capecitabine is an oral, tumor-activated, and tumor-selective fluoropyrimidine carbamate. Capecitabine can be administered alone or in combination with oxaliplatin (CapeOx also known as XELOX). When administered alone, it has higher response rates but comparable time-to-tumor-progression and median survival.[92] CapeOx has similar OS and PFS when compared with FOLFOX.[58] Hand–foot syndrome is common with capecitabine, whereas grades 3 or 4 neutropenia and stomatitis are more common with fluorouracil plus leucovorin. The convenience of oral administration and different toxicity profile make capecitabine a useful substitution for infusional fluorouracil in regimens for metastatic disease.

Targeted Therapy 8 Current guidelines and clinical practice recommend the addition of targeted therapy to one of the chemotherapy backbones mentioned earlier.[58]

Bevacizumab 9 Bevacizumab is a recombinant, humanized monoclonal antibody that inhibits vascular endothelial growth factor (VEGF). Bevacizumab, in combination with IV fluorouracil-based chemotherapy, was FDA approved in 2004 for initial treatment of patients with metastatic colorectal cancer. Results from randomized trials show increased PFS and OS benefit as compared with chemotherapy alone.[88] An infusional fluorouracil regimen should be used with the combination of bevacizumab and irinotecan. A randomized phase III trial demonstrated a median OS of 28 months compared with 19.2 months with FOLFIRI and IFL, respectively (HR 1.79; $P = 0.037$) when given in combination with bevacizumab.[93] A third arm of this trial replaced fluorouracil and leucovorin with capecitabine and was found to be inferior to FOLFIRI; during accrual the trial was amended to add bevacizumab to all treatment arms. The capecitabine arm remained inferior to FOLFIRI. Based on these results, capecitabine should not be administered with irinotecan, with or without bevacizumab. In contrast to irinotecan-containing regimens, bevacizumab has also been combined with oxaliplatin in a variety of chemotherapy regimens for the initial treatment of metastatic colon cancer. The method of fluorouracil administration (or substitution with capecitabine) does not appear to significantly affect outcomes.

Hypertension is common with bevacizumab.[58] The hypertension is easily managed with oral antihypertensive agents. Bleeding, thromboembolism, and proteinuria also can occur with bevacizumab. Monitoring for proteinuria is done with urine dipsticks regularly during therapy, and therapy is withheld in patients with 2+ protein or more, confirmed with a 24-hour urine collection. The risk of gastrointestinal perforation is increased by the addition of bevacizumab, and patients complaining of abdominal pain associated with vomiting or constipation should be considered for this rare but potentially fatal complication. Bevacizumab is also associated with a two fold increased risk of arterial thrombotic events, with patients who are older than age 65 or who have a prior history of arterial thrombotic events at greatest risk. Nevertheless, because these individuals derive the same survival benefits with bevacizumab as do other patients, they may be appropriate candidates to receive bevacizumab. Bevacizumab can also interfere with wound healing and it is recommended there be at least a 6 to week interval between the last dose of bevacizumab and elective surgery and wait at least 6-8 weeks to reinitiate bevacizumab after surgery.

EGFR Inhibitors 10 Cetuximab and panitumumab are monoclonal antibodies directed against EGFR. EGFR inhibitors may be used in combination with first-line chemotherapy regimens mFOLFOX4 or FOLFIRI or administered as single agents. The benefit of EGFR inhibitors, however, is limited to patients with wild-type *RAS* tumors and they should not be used in patients with tumor *RAS* mutations.[88] Results of a recent meta-analysis of 14 randomized trials showed that addition of an EGFR inhibitor provides improvement in PFS in patients with *RAS* wild type.[104] See Table 130-9 for information on clinical trials. Tumors harboring *BRAF* mutations are also associated with a poor prognosis and a poor response to EGFR inhibitors in patients with wild-type *RAS*.[57] Therefore, individuals with *BRAF* mutations should not receive EGFR inhibitors.

For reasons that are not well understood, the addition of panitumumab or cetuximab to bevacizumab plus irinotecan- or oxaliplatin-containing chemotherapy reduces PFS and is currently not recommended. The Panitumumab Advanced Colorectal Cancer Evaluation Study trial and the CAIRO2 demonstrated a decrease in PFS of 1.4 months when panitumumab and 1.3 months when cetuximab was added to bevacizumab-containing chemotherapy, respectively.[105,106] Both of these differences were clinically and statistically significant. The results from these trials demonstrate the potential pitfalls of treating patients with multiple targeted agents outside of the setting of a clinical trial and why this practice should be avoided.

Severe infusion reactions, including anaphylaxis, can occur with cetuximab (3%) and panitumumab (1%).[58] Administration of panitumumab seems feasible in those who experienced a reaction with cetuximab based on a small trial.[107] Skin toxicity is also a common side effect with these drugs and is not part of the infusion reaction. The presence of papulopustular skin rash has been shown to correlate with response and survival. It most commonly occurs within 2 to 4 weeks of therapy initiation and preventative therapy with topical corticosteroids with moisturizer, sunscreen and oral doxycycline is recommended unless contraindications exist.[108]

Selection of an Initial Metastatic Regimen Several factors should be considered when selecting first-line therapy for metastatic colorectal cancer when disease palliation is the primary treatment goal. The first factor that should be considered is whether intensive therapy is appropriate for the patient. Those with multiple comorbidities or low performance status would likely better tolerate a less-intensive therapy. The second consideration then is *RAS* status. Those with *RAS* wild type can receive an EGFR inhibitor therapy and those with *RAS* mutation cannot. Once those two factors are known, the selection of the appropriate regimen is based on toxicity profile and convenience of administration for the patient. Based on the comparable results of FOLFIRI versus mFOLFOX6, either of these regimens is considered the reference standard in metastatic colorectal cancer. Most patients will receive first- and second-line regimens and patient preference for either sequence of treatments based on their different toxicity profiles is important. Preexisting neuropathies may lead to FOLFIRI being chosen initially, whereas increased bilirubin or known UGT1A1 deficiency (known risk factors for delayed diarrhea) may lead to mFOLFOX as the initial choice. Alopecia occurs much more frequently with irinotecan compared to oxaliplatin combinations. Because mFOLFOX can cause persistent neuropathy, a rationale for starting with FOLFIRI is based on the observation that time-to progression is longer with first-line treatment than in second line. Therefore, the time to death during which some patients will have to live with neuropathy may be shorter.[88] Capecitabine is an appropriate substitute for IV fluorouracil in oxaliplatin combination regimens. Because of higher response rates and modest survival benefit with FOLFOXIRI, this 4-drug combination may be useful for patients with initially aggressive and symptomatic disease. Select patients who are candidates for FOLFOXIRI may benefit from the addition of bevacizumab, but the incidence of moderate or severe toxicities is increased.[83]

Metastatic Disease: Second-Line and Subsequent Therapy

Systemic chemotherapy represents the mainstay of therapy for patients whose disease progresses following initial treatment for metastatic disease. Table 130-10 lists treatment options for refractory metastatic disease.[58,102] Treatment options are based on the type of and response to prior treatments, the site and extent of disease, and patient factors and treatment preferences.

Systemic Chemotherapy

On disease progression following standard initial therapy, appropriate treatment options depend primarily on the type of prior therapy received (see Table 130-10). Because most patients will have received a combination of a fluoropyrimidine with either irinotecan or oxaliplatin, second-line therapy with the alternate regimen should be considered. Patient survival can exceed 2 years with this approach and it is important for patients to receive all traditional chemotherapy options if possible. Targeted agents can either be added to the aforementioned regimens or used as single agents.

Irinotecan It was initially FDA approved as a second-line treatment for recurrent or progressive disease following fluorouracil. Two phase III trials compared irinotecan to either best supportive care or continuous-infusion fluorouracil in patients who had progressed within 6 months of treatment with fluorouracil.[58] Both trials demonstrated an improvement in OS with irinotecan as compared to the control arms. However, this approach is rarely used since single agent fluorouracil is rarely given as first-line therapy.

TABLE 130-10 Second-line and Salvage Chemotherapy Regimens for Metastatic Colorectal Cancer[58,102]

Disease Progression with First-Line Regimen	Comments
First-Line Therapy: Oxaliplatin-Based Regimen ± Bevacizumab (ie, FOLFOX, CapeOX)	
Second-line options	
1. FOLFIRI ± bevacizumab or ziv-afilbercept or ramucirumab	Bevacizumab is preferred antiangiogenic agent based on toxicity and cost
2. Irinotecan ± bevacizumab or ziv-afilbercept or ramucirumab	Bevacizumab is preferred antiangiogenic agent based on toxicity and cost
3. Single agent cetuximab or panitumumab	Only if *RAS* wild-type; cetuximab improved OS compared to best supportive care
4. FOLFIRI ± cetuximab or panitumumab	Only if *RAS* wild type; increased PFS compared to FOLFIRI alone
First-Line Therapy: Irinotecan-Based Regimen ± Bevacizumab (ie, FOLFIRI)	
Second-line options	
1. FOLFOX or CapOx ± bevacizumab	Bevacizumab FDA-approved to continue with second-line options
2. Irinotecan ± cetuximab or panitumumab	Only if *RAS* wild-type; response rates with combination greater than cetuximab monotherapy
3. Single-agent cetuximab or panitumumab	Only if *RAS* wild type
First-Line Therapy: Fluorouracil-Based Regimen ± Bevacizumab (ie, Fluorouracil/Leucovorin, Capecitabine)	
Second-line options	
1. FOLFOX or CapOx ± bevacizumab or ziv-afilbercept or ramucirumab	Bevacizumab has least toxicity and lower cost of antiangiogenic agents
2. Irinotecan + oxaliplatin (IROX) ± bevacizumab or ziv-afilbercept or ramucirumab	Bevacizumab has least toxicity and lower cost of antiangiogenic agents
3. Irinotecan ± bevacizumab or ziv-afilbercept or ramucirumab	Bevacizumab has least toxicity and lower cost of antiangiogenic agents
4. FOLFIRI ± bevacizumab or ziv-afilbercept or ramucirumab	Bevacizumab has least toxicity and lower cost of antiangiogenic agents
Therapy After Second Progression or Third Progression	
1. Regorafenib	Can be given without regard to *RAS* genotype
2. Irinotecan ± cetuximab or panitumumab	Only if *RAS* wild type; response rates with combination greater than cetuximab monotherapy
3. FOLFOX or CapeOX	Only after second-line irinotecan regimens
4. Cetuximab or panitumumab	Only if *RAS* wild-type and for patients unable to tolerate combination therapy
5. Trifluridine/tipiracil	Only after treatment with fluoropyrmidine-, oxaliplatin-, and irinotecan-based chemotherapy, anti-VEGF biologic product, and anti EGFR-monoclonal antibody if *RAS* wild type
6. Clinical trial	If available and only if patient eligible
7. Best supportive care	Appropriate for patients who do not want to pursue treatment or quality of life is expected to decrease

CapOx, capecitabine plus oxaliplatin; EGFR, endothelial growth factor receptor; FOLFIRI, fluorouracil plus leucovorin plus irinotecan; FOLFOX, fluorouracil plus leucovorin plus oxaliplatin; OS, overall survival; PFS, profession-free survival; VEGF, vascular-endothelial growth factor.

The use of the FOLFIRI regimen after progression with first-line FOLFOX demonstrated an objective response rate of 4% with a median PFS of 2.5 months.[58] These results are consistent with observations that demonstrate improved outcomes in those patients who are able to receive all active cytotoxic agents during the course of their disease.[88]

Based on these results, irinotecan should be considered standard second-line therapy for patients with disease progression with first-line treatment with oxaliplatin-containing regimens. Continuous-infusion fluorouracil (FOLFIRI), with or without targeted therapy, is most commonly given.

Oxaliplatin The oxaliplatin plus fluorouracil and leucovorin should be considered for patients who received primary treatment with irinotecan plus fluorouracil. Despite the low activity of single-agent oxaliplatin against fluorouracil-refractory disease, when oxaliplatin has been administered in a bimonthly regimen with high-dose leucovorin and continuous fluorouracil infusion, a 21% response rate with a median survival in excess of 10 months has been reported.[88] The combination of oxaliplatin plus fluorouracil and leucovorin is also effective as salvage therapy after initial treatment with irinotecan plus fluorouracil and leucovorin, with a similar response rate.[114] Although irinotecan can be used effectively as a single agent in colorectal cancer, it should be noted that oxaliplatin does not have substantial activity alone, and should only be given in combination with a fluoropyrimidine.

Trifluridine/Tipiracil Trifluridine is a thymidine-based nucleoside analog that is incorporated into DNA and inhibits cell proliferation. The addition of tipiracil increases trifluridine exposure by inhibiting its metabolism by thymidine phosphorylase. This combination chemotherapy product has activity in *RAS* wild-type tumors. Trifluridine/tipiracil was FDA approved for treatment of metastatic colorectal cancer patients who have been previously treated with an fluoropyrimidine-, oxaliplatin-, and irinotecan-containing regimens, an anti-VEGF targeted therapy, and an anti-EGFR monoclonal antibody if *RAS* wild type.[102] When compared in a double-blind, placebo-controlled trial of trifluridine/tipiracil and placebo, an improvement in OS was observed (7.1 vs 5.3 months; HR 0.68; $P<0.01$). This chemotherapy product is administered 35 mg/m^2 orally twice daily within 1 hour of completing morning and evening meals on days 1 through 5 and days 8 through 12 of a 28-day cycle. Common adverse effects include myelosuppression, fatigue, diarrhea, nausea/vomiting, abdominal pain, and pyrexia.

Targeted Therapy

10 The addition of targeted therapy to chemotherapy in second and subsequent therapies does improve outcomes, but typically also increases toxicity. EGFR inhibitors may be administered in combination with irinotecan but can be used as single agents in patients who cannot tolerate irinotecan-based chemotherapy. Angiogenesis inhibitors are also used in second-line and subsequent therapy. However, the monoclonal antibodies bevacizumab, ziv-aflibercept, or ramucirumab are not given as single agents.

EGFR Inhibitors 10 Cetuximab is active in chemotherapy-refractory disease as a single agent and in combination with continued irinotecan.[60] As a single agent, cetuximab is associated a 23% improvement in OS compared with best supportive care (HR, 0.77; 95%; P=0.005).[60] The combination of cetuximab and irinotecan has also been evaluated in the second-line setting in patients naïve to irinotecan after oxaliplatin-based failures demonstrating significant improvements in PFS with cetuximab.[100] An important caveat for most initial trials with cetuximab is that *RAS* testing was not initially performed. Retrospective analyses of these studies show that antitumor effects are limited to patients with wild-type *RAS*.[88]

Panitumumab, also administered alone or in combination with irinotecan-containing regimens, may be used as second or subsequent lines of therapy in patients with *RAS* wild type. Results of studies have shown a 46% decrease in the rate of tumor progression with single-agent therapy compared with best supportive care and a 2-month improvement in PFS when compared with FOLFIRI.[83,87]

A randomized, multicenter comparative study of single-agent cetuximab and panitumumab showed noninferiority between agents in terms of OS and similar side effects.[83] Therefore, both monotherapy with panitumumab or cetuximab or combination with chemotherapy regiments such as FOLFIRI or single-agent irinotecan are recommended by current NCCN guidelines as second-line options in patients with wild-type *RAS* who have not had an EGFR as part of initial therapy (see Table 130-10).[58]

Angiogenesis Inhibitors Angiogenesis inhibitors including VEGF inhibitors bevacizumab, ramucircumab, and ziv-alfibrecept and the multikinase inhibitor regorafenib may be used in patients who have progressed on other therapies (see Table 130-10). VEGF inhibitors may be used as second- or subsequent-line therapies, whereas regorafenib is limited to third- or subsequent-line use. The 2016 NCCN guidelines recommend bevacizumab over ramucircumab and ziv-alfibercept based on toxicity and cost. Continuation of bevacizumab as second-line therapy provides a modest improvement in OS based on several clinical trials.[58,83] Bevacizumab may also be added to another second-line therapy in patients who did not receive it as part of their initial therapy, also resulting in a modest improvement in OS (10.8 to 12.1 months [P = 0.001]).[83] Single-agent bevacizumab is not recommended as it has shown inferior efficacy to combination therapy.[58]

Clinical **Controversy...**

Continuation of bevacizumab after disease progression has recently been FDA approved. Originally justified based on retrospective data that demonstrate improved survival, a confirmatory phase III trial demonstrated a small improvement in OS. Benefit of this strategy versus changing the antiangiogenic therapy to a new agent that targets the same pathway or in combination with other targeted agents will need to be determined.

Ziv-aflibercept is a soluble recombinant fusion protein that was designed to block the angiogenic process. The agent was developed by fusing sections of the VEGFR-1 and VEGFR-2 immunoglobulin domains to the F_c portion of human immunoglobulin G1 (IgG1) and blocks VEGF-A, VEGF-B, and placental growth factor (PIGF) by "trapping" the ligands before they get to the native transmembrane receptors. In a phase III randomized trial, FOLFIRI plus ziv-aflibercept was compared to FOLFIRI after progression on an oxaliplatin-based regimen.[83] The trial met its primary end point with an improvement in OS (13.5 months for FOLFIRI/ziv-aflibercept vs 12.06 months for FOLFIRI/placebo; HR, 0.817; P=0.0032). It is dosed at 4 mg/kg as an IV infusion over 1 hour every 2 weeks and is associated with similar adverse effects as bevacizumab. The addition of ziv-aflibercept to oxaliplatin regimens has not been evaluated and therefore is not recommended. Additionally the addition of ziv-aflibercept following failure of a bevacizumab-containing regimen has not been evaluated. Therefore, ziv-aflibercept should only be used in patients naïve to antiangiogenic regimens and only with irinotecan-containing regimens.

Ramucirumab is a human monoclonal antibody that binds directly to the ligand-binding pocket of VEGFR-2 to block binding of VEGF-A, VEGF-C, and VEGF-D. A phase III randomized placebo-controlled trial of patients who had failed an oxaliplatin-based regimen and bevacizumab were randomized to receive FOLFIRI with or without ramuciumab.[101] A modest improvement in OS (13.3 vs 11.7 months; HR, 0.84; *P*=0.02) and PFS (5.7 vs 4.5 months; HR, 0.79; *P*<0.0005) were observed. Ramucirumab is administered as 8 mg/kg IV over 1 hour every 2 weeks and is associated with similar adverse effects as bevacizumab.

Regorafenib, a small-molecule inhibitor of tumor angiogenesis (VEGFR-1, VEGFR-2, and VEGFR-3) and other downstream targets (FGF receptors, PDGF receptors, BRAF, KIT, and RET), is approved for the third- or fourth-line treatment of metastatic colorectal cancer. This oral agent is dosed 160 mg once daily for the first 21 days of each 28-day cycle; although it is common to start at a lower dose (80 or 120 mg) and titrate as tolerated.[58] In a phase III trial of patients with metastatic colorectal cancer and progression during or within 3 months of last chemotherapy, regorafenib demonstrated a 1.4-month improvement in OS when compared to placebo.[83] Patients with mutant or wild-type *RAS* may receive this therapy. Because this is an oral-only regimen, patients must be counseled on its use and potential toxicity. Regorafenib should be taken with a low-fat breakfast and may interact with CYPP450 3A4 inducers and inhibitors. Toxicities include hypertension, hand–foot syndrome, diarrhea, and hepatotoxicity.

Hepatic-Directed Therapies

Patients with unresectable or nonablatable hepatic-predominant metastases or who are unable to undergo surgery may be candidates for chemoembolization, radioembolization, or HAI chemotherapy, as discussed previously.[109] Although various hepatic-directed therapies offer potential disease palliation in select patients with unresectable, yet limited hepatic metastases, no conclusive survival advantage has been demonstrated.

New Strategies and Agents in Development

The number of active cytotoxic agents against cancers of the colon and rectum is limited. These traditional chemotherapy agents, which target rapidly dividing cells, kill both malignant and nonmalignant cells, and new cancer therapies are needed to improve therapeutic outcomes. In particular, targeted therapies aimed at the underlying cancer pathology are increasingly being developed and used in colorectal cancer treatment. A variety of agents targeted toward augmenting the host immune system response have undergone, or are currently undergoing, study for colorectal cancer, including monoclonal antibodies, tumor vaccines, and agents targeting the programmed cell death (PD) receptor or ligand. Additional strategies include regulating tumor growth through the inhibition of various cell proliferation, survival, and death pathways, angiogenesis, and cancer stem cells. Agents that can alter microenvironmental factors that support angiogenesis and tumor metastases may also be of benefit.

PERSONALIZED PHARMACOTHERAPY

Drug therapy for patients diagnosed with colorectal cancers is individualized based on several established tumor and patient pharmacogenetic factors that influence treatment response. In addition, various tumor characteristics, patient genetics, and molecular markers may predict prognosis and/or response to certain therapies and provide the rationale for pharmacogenomic strategies to select appropriate therapies for individual patients. Table 130-11 summarizes potential predictive markers for individualizing colorectal cancer treatment.[15,30,57-60,110-112]

Tumor Genomics

The most important development in biomarkers for colorectal cancer treatment has been validation of *RAS* mutation status as a predictive marker for lack of tumor response to anti-EGFR antibodies.[60,110] Tumors should be genotyped for *RAS* (*KRAS* exon 2 and nonexon 2; *NRAS*) and *BRAF* mutations at diagnosis of stage IV disease; patients with known *KRAS* or *NRAS* mutations should not receive cetuximab or panitumumab.[58] Because fewer than 60% of patients with *KRAS* wild-type tumors respond to cetuximab or panitumumab, additional factors downstream of *RAS* signaling have been explored for their ability to predict response to EGFR inhibitors, including *BRAF* V600E mutation, and mutation or loss of *PTEN* or *PIK3CA*.[30,58] Although the predictive value of *BRAF* mutation status has not been established, retrospective evidence shows its association with a lack of response to anti-EGFR antibodies.[58,110] Also, patients with *BRAF* mutant tumors have a poor prognosis, with shorter survival times.[110] *PIK3CA* mutations are present in up to 30% of tumors; since they are often detected with coexisting *BRAF* or *RAS* mutations, their prognostic and predictive values are difficult to evaluate.[110] However, activation of the PI3K/PTEN/AKT signaling pathway downstream of EGFR, via *PIK3CA* or *PTEN* mutation may contribute to resistance to anti-EGFR antibodies.

Amphiregulin (AREG) and epiregulin (EREG) are EGFR ligands that have undergone study as biomarkers of efficacy of cetuximab. Patients with wild-type *KRAS* tumors and higher levels of ligand expression experienced greater responses to cetuximab monotherapy.[110] Tumor AREG and EREG mRNA expression may help predict cetuximab efficacy and are under investigation.

About 12% to 22% of stage II and III colorectal cancers show high-frequency microsatellite instability (MSI-H), which is associated with an improved prognosis.[60] Findings from pooled analyses of patients with MSI-H tumors who received adjuvant fluorouracil indicate a lack of response to treatment, perhaps due to an improved overall prognosis and/or additional factors. Nevertheless, some practitioners use MSI status to determine which patients with low-risk stage II colorectal cancer should not receive adjuvant fluorouracil. Current NCCN guidelines recommend MSI testing for stage II colon cancers because MSI-H status confers a good prognosis and those patients do not benefit from adjuvant single agent fluoropyrimidine.[58]

Tumors with *P53* mutations demonstrate a high degree of resistance to radiation, fluorouracil, oxaliplatin, and certain other chemotherapeutic agents and are associated with a less-favorable prognosis. However, because of difficulties with adequately sensitive and specific immunohistochemical analysis to identify P53 mutations, widespread testing, and application of this as a marker is unlikely.[57,112]

Chemotherapy Pharmacogenomics

Polymorphisms or epigenetic modifications in genes involved in drug metabolism and transport, DNA repair, and therapeutic targets are potentially predictive of fluoropyrimidine, irinotecan, and oxaliplatin toxicity and/or efficacy.[111] There are currently no clinically useful predictive markers for fluoropyrimidine efficacy, but DPD deficiency is predictive for toxicity. Patients who are deficient in DPD experience severe and potentially life-threatening toxicities with conventional doses of fluorouracil and capecitabine, but determination of DPD activity is relatively time consuming and the techniques are not amenable to routine clinical practice. However, genetic testing for DPYD polymorphisms can identify patients who would require lower fluorouracil doses to avoid severe toxicity and is recognized by the FDA as an approved pharmacogenomic marker to predict toxicities from fluorouracil.[110-112]

Of factors predictive for tumor sensitivity to fluorouracil, TS expression has been most studied. Tumors that overexpress TS, an enzyme that converts deoxyuridine monophosphate to deoxythymidine monophosphate, an essential step for DNA synthesis, are less sensitive to fluorouracil chemotherapy, whereas low TS expression

TABLE 130-11 Potential Predictive Markers for Personalized Pharmacotherapy for Colorectal Cancer

Pathway	Biomarker	Relationship to Response
DNA MMR	MSI (MSI-H)	Improved survival and decreased risk of recurrence following resection; may predict lack of survival benefit (and perhaps detrimental effect) from adjuvant therapy with a fluoropyrimidine alone for stage II disease
DPD	*DPYD* polymorphisms	Absent or reduced DPD associated with risk of severe fluorouracil and capecitabine toxicities; low levels of DPD activity correspond to greater response to fluorouracil-based chemotherapy
EGFR	*KRAS* and *NRAS* mutations (exons 2, 3, and 4)	Predict lack of response to anti-EGFR antibodies
	BRAF exon 15 mutations (including V600E mutation)	Predicts lack of response to anti-EGFR antibodies in *KRAS* wild-type tumors
	PIK3CA mutations (exons 9 and 20)	Predict poor overall response to anti-EGFR inhibitor antibodies May predict patients likely to benefit from adjuvant aspirin or aspirin chemoprevention
	PTEN mutation or reduced PTEN expression	May predict lack of response to anti-EGFR antibodies
	AREG, EREG expression	Higher EGFR ligand mRNA expression may correspond to better anti-EGFR antibody efficacy
	Skin rash with EGFR inhibitor	Development of skin rash with anti-EGFR antibodies may predict response to treatment and improved treatment outcome
Folate	*MTHFR* polymorphisms	Polymorphisms linked to reduced intracellular folate pools associated with fluoropyrimidine toxicity; may influence response to FOLFOX
Glutathione-S-Transferase	*GSTP1* polymorphisms	May help predict oxaliplatin-induced neurotoxicity
Nucleotide Excision Repair	*ERCC1* *ERCC2* *XRCC1*	Polymorphisms and protein expression associated with resistance to platinum-based chemotherapy Decreased ERCC1 protein expression associated with improved survival with FOLFOX
Thymidine phosphorylase	TP expression	Associated with response to capecitabine treatment
Thymidylate synthase	TS expression	Increased TS expression associated with reduced response to fluorouracil; low tumor expression associated with increased sensitivity to fluorouracil; may be prognostic for survival
	TYMS polymorphisms and expression	Gene expression in tumor tissue and certain variants modestly prognostic for treatment outcomes; evaluation of haplotypes may improve predictive value for treatment response
UDP-glucuronosyltransferases	*UGT1A1*28*	Homozygous 7-repeat allele associated with increased risk of severe diarrhea with irinotecan

AREG, amphiregulin; DNA MMR, DNA mismatch repair genes; DPYD, dihydropyrimidine dehydrogenase; EGFR, epidermal growth factor receptor; ERCC1, excision repair cross-complementing group 1; ERCC2, excision repair cross-complementing group 2; EREG, epiregulin; FOLFOX, fluorouracil, leucovorin, and oxaliplatin; MSI, microsatellite instability; MTHFR, methylenetetrahydrofolate reductase; TP, thymidine phosphorylase; TS, thymidylate synthase; *TYMP*, thymidine phosphorylase gene; *TYMS*, thymidylate synthase gene; UGT1A1, uridine diphosphate-glucuronosyltransferase; XRCC1, x-ray repair cross-complementing protein 1.

Data from references 15, 30, 57-60, and 110-112.

contributes to increased chemosensitivity.[57,110,111] Patients whose cancers have higher levels of TS appear to have a significantly worse overall 5-year survival than patients whose cancers have a low level of TS.[112] However, no large cooperative group trial has identified a subgroup of patients who failed to benefit from fluorouracil plus leucovorin therapy based on tumor TS levels, probably due to differential results obtained using different analytic techniques. Also, the importance of TS protein expression is difficult to ascertain given that fluorouracil is generally not administered as a single agent. Therefore, tumor testing for TS overexpression is not routinely used to select fluorouracil treatments.

Tests for polymorphisms in other genes that influence fluoropyrimidine activity with potential to predict treatment toxicity or efficacy have been established but are not routinely used.[111,112] Frequencies of germline polymorphisms in *TYMP* and *MTHFR* vary among ethnic populations; their consequential effects on treatment toxicities and/or efficacy are recognized, but the complexities of testing including haplotype analyses, sample size requirements, and applicable study designs have limited efforts to establish their utility as predictive markers.[112]

Nucleotide excision repair genes (eg, *ERCC1*, *ERCC2*, *ERCC5*, *XRCC1*, and *XRCC3*) have been evaluated as prognostic factors in colorectal cancer and genetic variants in some of these genes confer resistance to anticancer agents, including platinum-based chemotherapy.[57,112] Certain *ERCC1* polymorphisms are associated with decreased ERCC1 protein expression, which may predict for response to and improved survival with FOLFOX chemotherapy.[57] Despite findings from several investigations that certain variants within the DNA repair system may serve useful in optimizing chemotherapy treatments, they are still considered exploratory, as most studies were small, conducted in select populations, and studied a limited number of gene variants.[111]

Patients that are homozygous for a *UGT1A1* 7-repeat allele (*UGT1A1*28*), which is associated with reduced levels of UGT1A1 expression, are at increased risk for severe diarrhea with irinotecan. FDA-approved testing to determine *UGT1A1* genotype is commercially available. Although some individuals advocate testing UGT1A1 genotype prior to starting irinotecan, widespread testing has not been adopted.[57] The prescribing information recommends an initial reduced dose of irinotecan in patients with *UGT1A1*28* genotype.

Therapeutic Drug Monitoring

Because of the wide inter- and intrapatient variability in fluorouracil pharmacokinetics and a narrow therapeutic range, pharmacokinetic optimization of fluorouracil represents a potential strategy to individualize dosing and optimize efficacy and minimize adverse effects.

Published data suggest that only 20% to 30% of patients treated with fluorouracil achieve therapeutic concentrations.[113] A prospective study that compared pharmacokinetically guided fluorouracil dosing with conventional dosing in patients with metastatic colorectal cancer demonstrated that pharmacokinetically guided dose adjustments reduced grade 3/4 toxicities, increased the objective tumor response rate, and provided a higher yet not significantly increased survival rate.[114] Most recently, a pharmacokinetically guided fluorouracil algorithm was used to adjust doses to achieve a target area-under-the-concentration versus time curve in 70 patients with colorectal cancer.[115] This program showed that pharmacokinetically guided fluorouracil dosing resulted in fewer underdosed patients, reduced gastrointestinal toxicities, and is feasible in the community setting. Valid assay methods that facilitate therapeutic drug monitoring are available and are being used in some centers. Algorithms are available for specific treatment protocols that enable practitioners to determine doses based on patient physiological and pathophysiological characteristics. Increased awareness and application of this dosing strategy will be required to determine if it will indeed improve therapeutic outcomes for patients with colorectal cancer.

EVALUATION OF THERAPEUTIC OUTCOMES

The goal of monitoring patients is to either evaluate whether the patient is receiving any benefit from the management of the disease or for those who have completed curative intent therapy, to detect recurrence. During treatment for active disease, patients should undergo monitoring for measurable tumor response, progression, or new metastases; these tests may include chest, abdominal or pelvic CT scans, or radiographs, depending on known sites of disease, and CEA measurements every 3 months if the CEA is or was previously elevated. In addition, a complete blood cell count should be obtained prior to each course of chemotherapy administration to ensure that hematologic indices are adequate. Baseline liver function tests and an assessment of renal function should be evaluated prior to and periodically during therapy. These radiologic tests and other selected laboratories should also be evaluated with the development of any new symptoms or significant change in disease status. Patients should be evaluated during every treatment visit for the presence of anticipated side effects, which generally include loose stools or diarrhea, nausea or vomiting, mouth sores, fatigue, and fever, as well as other side effects such as neuropathy, skin rash, and hepatotoxicity that are typically associated with oxaliplatin, EGFR inhibitors, and regorafenib, respectively. Serum electrolytes, including magnesium, should be monitored for during treatment with EGFR inhibitors. Patients receiving bevacizumab, ziv aflibercept, or regorafenib should be evaluated for hypertension and proteinuria.

Symptoms of recurrence such as pain syndromes, changes in bowel habits, rectal or vaginal bleeding, pelvic masses, anorexia, and weight loss develop in less than 50% of patients. A greater percentage of recurrences are detected in asymptomatic patients because of increased serum CEA levels that lead to further examination. Although the value of CEA monitoring for asymptomatic disease recurrence is questioned by some because of the related expense and emotional stress associated with false-positive elevations, CEA monitoring plays an important role in postoperative follow-up studies for most individuals. A PET scan can be considered to identify localized sites of metastatic disease when a rising CEA level suggests metastatic disease but CT scans and other imaging studies are negative.

Patients who undergo curative surgical resection, with or without adjuvant therapy, require close follow-up based on the premise that early detection and treatment of recurrence could still render them cured. In addition, early treatment for asymptomatic metastatic colorectal cancer appears superior to delayed therapy. Specific practice guidelines for postoperative surveillance examinations following successful treatment for stage II or III disease were developed by NCCN and include: history, physical examination, and CEA test every 3 to 6 months for the first 2 years, then every 6 months for a total of 5 years; annual chest and abdominal and pelvic CT scans for up to 5 years following primary therapy; and colonoscopy at about 1 year after surgery. Repeat colonoscopies are recommended at 3 years, unless findings of polyps warrant closer follow-up. Less intensive surveillance is recommended for patients treated for stage I disease because of low risk of recurrence.[58]

Posttreatment surveillance should also include a survivorship care plan with immunizations for vaccine-preventable diseases, early detection of second primary cancers, and support systems that encourage smoking cessation, establish regular exercise and maintain a healthy BMI, and encourage healthy lifestyle and dietary choices.[58] In addition, if there is a strong family history of colorectal cancer or related malignancies or clinicopathologic findings in an individual consistent with an hereditary syndrome, a consultation with a geneticist is indicated. Recent advances in the treatment for cancer of the colon and rectum now offer the potential to improve patient survival, but for many patients, improved DFS and PFS represent equally important therapeutic outcomes. Although treatment approaches for metastatic colorectal cancer have been historically assessed by their ability to produce a measurable objective tumor response, which is generally believed necessary for any treatment to improve survival, the effects of therapies on survival are clinically more meaningful than their ability to induce a tumor response. However, with the availability of multiple active treatments for metastatic disease, and the likelihood that patients will receive more than one during the course of their treatment, improvements in OS with new therapies will be increasingly difficult to determine.

In the absence of the ability of a specific treatment to demonstrate improved survival, important outcome measures should include the effects of the treatment on patient symptoms, daily activities and performance status, and other quality-of-life indicators, as well as PFS and time-to-treatment failure. Because most metastatic colorectal cancers are incurable, a specific decision regarding an individual patient's care will ultimately be required. This decision should be based on a careful assessment of the balance between risks associated with treatment (or lack thereof) and benefits of treatment. Effort should also be made to ensure that the costs of screening, diagnostic tests, treatments, and procedures for colorectal cancer are consistent with their value in improving patient outcomes.

ABBREVIATIONS

APC	adenomatous polyposis coli (gene)
BMI	body mass index
CapOx	capecitabine plus oxaliplatin
CEA	carcinoembryonic antigen
CIN	chromosomal instability
CIMP	CpG island methylator phenotype
COX	cyclooxygenase
CT	computed tomography
CYP	cytochrome P450 isoenzyme
DCBE	double-contrast barium enema
DFMO	difluoromethylornithine
DFS	disease-free survival
DPD	dihydropyrimidine dehydrogenase
EGFR	epidermal growth factor receptor
ERCC1	excision repair cross-complementing group 1
ERCC2	excision repair cross-complementing group 2

ERCC5	excision repair cross-complementing group 5
FAP	familial adenomatous polyposis
FDA	Food and Drug Administration
FIT	fecal immunochemical test
FLOX	fluorouracil, leucovorin, oxaliplatin
FOBT	fecal occult blood test
FOLFIRI	fluorouracil, leucovorin, and irinotecan
FOLFOX	fluorouracil, leucovorin, and oxaliplatin
FOLFOXIRI	fluorouracil and leucovorin, oxaliplatin, irinotecan
FSIG	flexible sigmoidoscopy
gFOBT	guaiac-based fecal occult blood test
HAI	hepatic artery infusion
HbA_{1c}	glycosylated hemoglobin
HNPCC	hereditary nonpolyposis colorectal cancer
HR	hazard ratio
IFL	irinotecan, fluorouracil, and leucovorin
iFOBT	immunochemical fecal occult blood test
IGF-1	insulin-like growth factor-1
IgG1	immunoglobulin G1
IROX	irinotecan and oxaliplatin
LOH	loss of heterozygosity
MAPK	mitogen-activated protein kinase
MMR	mismatch-repair
MOSAIC	Multicenter International Study of Oxaliplatin/5-Fluorouracil/Leucovorin in the Adjuvant Treatment of Colon Cancer
MRI	magnetic resonance imaging
MTHFR	methylenetetrahydrofolate reductase
MSI	microsatellite instability
NCCN	National Comprehensive Cancer Network
NSAID	nonsteroidal antiinflammatory drug
OS	overall survival
PET	positron emission tomography
PFS	progression-free survival
15-PGDH	15-prostaglandin dehydrogenase
PIGF	placental growth factor
PI3K	phosphatidylinositol 3-kinase
PPE	palmar–plantar erythrodysesthesia
RR	relative risk
RT-PCR	reverse-transcription polymerase chain reaction
sDNA	stool DNA
TGF-β	transforming growth factor-β
TP	thymidine phosphorylase
TS	thymidylate synthase
UGT1A1	uridine diphosphate-glucuronosyltransferase
USPSTF	United States Preventive Services Task Force
VEGF	vascular endothelial growth factor
VEGFR	vascular endothelial growth factor receptor
XRCC1	x-ray cross-complementing group 1
XRCC3	x-ray cross-complementing group 2
XRT	radiation therapy

REFERENCES

1. American Cancer Society. *Cancer Facts & Figures 2016*. Atlanta: American Cancer Society; 2016.
2. American Cancer Society. *Global Cancer Facts & Figures,* 3rd *edition*. Atlanta: American Cancer Society; 2015.
3. American Cancer Society. *Colorectal Cancer Facts & Figures 2014-2016*. Atlanta: American Cancer Society, 2014.
4. Howlader N, Noone AM, Krapcho M, et al (eds). SEER Cancer Statistics Review, 1975-2012, National Cancer Institute. Bethesda, MD, http://seer.cancer.gov/csr/1975_2012/, based on November 2014 SEER data submission, posted to the SEER web site, April 2015, http://seer.cancer.gov/csr/1975_2012/.
5. Lieberman DA, Rex DK, Winawer SJ, et al. Guidelines for colonoscopy surveillance after screening and polypectomy: a consensus update by the US Multi-Society Task Force on Colorectal Cancer. Gastroenterology 2012;143:844-857.
6. Kim E, Change DK. Colorectal cancer in inflammatory bowel disease: the risk, pathogenesis, prevention and diagnosis. *World J Gasteroenterol* 2014;20:9872-9881.
7. Chan AT, Giovannucci EL. Primary prevention of colorectal cancer. *Gastroenterol* 2010;138:2020-2043.
8. Lou W, Cao Y, Liao C, Gao F. Diabetes mellitus and the incidence and mortality of colorectal cancer: a meta-analysis of 24 cohort studies. *Colorectal Dis* 2011;14:1307-1312.
9. Dehal AN, Newton CC, Jacobs EJ, et al. Impact of diabetes mellitus and insulin use on survival after colorectal cancer diagnosis: The Cancer Prevention Study-II Nutrition Cohort. *J Clin Oncol* 2011;30:53-59.
10. Samadder NJ, Japerson K, Burt RW. Hereditary and common familial colorectal cancer evidence for colorectal screening. *Dig Dis Sci* 2015;60:734-747.
11. Rassol S, Rasool V, Naqvi T, Ganai BA, Shah BA. Genetic unraveling of colorectal cancer. *Tumor Biol* 2014;35:5067-5082.
12. Teixeria MC, Braghiroli MI, Sabbaga J, Hoff PM. Primary prevention of colorectal cancer myth or reality. *World J Gastoenterol* 2014;20:15060-15069.
13. Thun MJ, Jacobs EJ, Patrono C. The role of aspirin in cancer prevention. *Nat Rev Clin Oncol* 2012;9:259-267.
14. Rothwell PM. Aspirin in prevention of sporadic colorectal cancer: current clinical evidence and overall balance of risks and benefits. *Recent Results Cancer Res* 2013;191:121-142.
15. Liao X, Lochhead P, Nishihara R, et al. Aspirin use, tumor *PIK3CA* mutation, and colorectal-cancer survival. *N Engl J Med* 2012;367:1596-1606.
16. Rennert G, Rennert HS, Pinchey M, et al. Use of hormone replacement therapy and the risk of colorectal cancer. *J Clin Oncol* 2009;27:4542-4547.
17. Haggar FA, Boushey RP. Colorectal cancer epidemiology: incidence, mortality, survival, and risk factors. *Clin Colon Rectal Surg* 2009;22:191-197.
18. Ma Y, Yang Y, Wang F, et al. Obesity and risk of colorectal cancer risk: a systemic review of prospective studies. *PLoS One* 2013;8:e53916.
19. Campbell PT, Jacobs ET, Ulrich CM, et al. Case-control study of overweight, obesity, and colorectal cancer, overall and by tumor microsatellite instability status. *J Natl Cancer Inst* 2010;102:391-400.
20. Tarraga-Lopez PJ, Albero JS, Rodriguez-Montes JA. Primary and secondary prevention of colorectal cancer. *Clin Med Insights Gastroenterol* 2014;7:33-46.
21. Gong J, Hutter C, Baron JA, et al. A pooled analysis of smoking and colorectal cancer: timing of exposure and interactions with environmental factors. *Cancer Epidemol Biomarkers Prev* 2012;21:1974-1985.
22. McCleary NJ, Niedzwiecki D, Hollis D, et al. Impact of smoking on patients with stage II colon cancer. *Cancer* 2010;116:956-966.
23. Vargas AJ, Thompson PA. Diet and nutrient factors in colorectal cancer risk. *Nutr Clin Pract* 2012;27:612-623.
24. Aune D, Chan DSM, Lau R, et al. Dietary fibre, whole grains, and risk of colorectal cancer: systematic review and dose-response meta-analysis of prospective studies. *BMJ* 2011;343:d6617.
25. Ma Y, Zhang P, Wang F, et al. Association between vitamin D and risk of colorectal cancer: a systematic review of prospective studies. *J Clin Oncol* 2011;29:3775-3782.
26. Hubner RA, Houlston RS. Folate and colorectal cancer prevention. *Br J Cancer* 2009;100:233-239.

27. Heine-Broring RC, Winkels RM, Renkema JMS, et al. Dietary supplement use and colorectal cancer risk: a systematic review and meta-analysis of prospective cohort studies. *Int J Cancer* 2015;136:2388-2401.
28. Gala M, Chung DC. Hereditary colon cancer syndromes. *Semin Oncol* 2011;38:490-499.
29. Markowitz SD, Bertagnolli MM. Molecular basis of colorectal cancer. *N Engl J Med* 2009;361:2449-2460.
30. Fearon ER. Molecular genetics of colorectal cancer. *Annu Rev Pathol* 2011;6:479-507.
31. Al-Sohaily S, Biankin A, Leong R. et al. Molecular pathways in colorectal cancer. *J Gastroenterol Hepatol* 2012;27:1423-1431.
32. Yarom N, Jonker DJ. The role of the epidermal growth factor receptor in the mechanism and treatment of colorectal cancer. *Discov Med* 2011;11:95-105.
33. Lanza G, Messerini L, Gafà R, Risio M. Gruppo Italiano Patologi Apparato Digerente (GIPAD); Società Italiana di Anatomia Patologica e Citopatologia Diagnostica/International Academy of Pathology, Italian division (SIAPEC/IAP). Colorectal tumors: the histology report. *Dig Liver Dis* 2011; (43 suppl 4):S344-S355.
34. Cooper K, Squires H, Carroll C, et al. Chemoprevention of colorectal cancer: systematic review and economic evaluation. *Health Technol Assess* 2010;14:1-206.
35. Zhou P, Cheng SW, Yang R, et al. Combination chemoprevention: future direction of colorectal cancer prevention. *Eur J Cancer Prev* 2012;21:231-240.
36. Uccello M, Malaguarnera G, Basile F, et al. Potential role of probiotics on colorectal cancer prevention. *BMC Surg* 2012;12(suppl 1):S35, doi:10.1186/1471-2482-12-S1-S35. http://www.biomedcentral.com/1471-2482/12/S1/S35.
37. Cuzick J, Otto F, Baron JA, et al. Aspirin and non-steroidal anti-inflammatory drugs for cancer prevention: an international consensus statement. *Lancet Oncol* 2009;10:501-507.
38. U.S. Preventive Services Task Force. Final Recommendation Statement. Aspirin use to prevent cardiovascular disease and colorectal cancer: preventive medication. http://www.uspreventiveservicestaskforce.org/Page/Document/RecommendationStatementFinal/aspirin-to-prevent-cardiovascular-disease-and-cancer. Last accessed August 16, 2016.
39. Chan AT, Arber N, Burn J, et al. Aspirin in the chemoprevention of colorectal neoplasia: An overview. *Cancer Prev Res (Phila)* 2012;5:164-178.
40. Farjardo AM, Piazza GA. Chemoprevention in gastrointestinal physiology and disease. Anti-inflammatory approaches for colorectal cancer chemoprevention. *Am J Physiol Gastrointest Liver Physiol* 2015;309:G59-G70.
41. Nan H, Huytter CM, Lin Y, et al. Association of aspirin and NSAID use with risk of colorectal cancer according to genetic variants. *JAMA* 2015;313:1133-1142.
42. Baron JA, Barry EL, Mott LA. A trial of calcium and vitamin D for the prevention of colorectal adneomas. *N Engl J Med* 2015;373:1519-1530.
43. NCCN Clinical Practice Guidelines In Oncology—Genetic/Familial High-Risk Assessment: Colorectal v1.2016. 2016, http://www.nccn.org/professionals/physician_gls/pdf/genetics_colon.pdf.
44. Qaseem A, Denberg TD, Hopkins RH, et al. Screening for colorectal cancer: a guidance statement from the American College of Physicians. *Ann Intern Med* 2012;156:378-386.
45. Levin B, Lieberman DA, McFarland B, et al. Screening and surveillance for the early detection of colorectal cancer and adenomatous polyps, 2008; a joint guideline from the American Cancer Society, the US Multi-Society on Colorectal Cancer, and the American College of Radiology. *CA Cancer J Clin* 2008;58:138-160.
46. Smith RA, Manassaram-Baptiste D, Brooks D, et al. Cancer screening in the United States, 2015: a review of the current American Cancer Society Guidelines and current issues in cancer screening. *CA Cancer J Clin* 2015;65:30-54.
47. Rex DK, Johnson DA, Anderson JC, et al. American College of Gastroenterology Guidelines for Colorectal Cancer Screening 2008. *Am J Gastroenterol* 2009;104:739-750.
48. U.S. Preventive Services Task Force. Screening for colorectal cancer: U.S. Preventive Services Task Force recommendation statement. *Ann Intern Med* 2008;149:627-637.
49. NCCN Clinical Practice Guidelines In Oncology—Colorectal Cancer Screening v.1.2016. 2016, http://www.nccn.org/professionals/physician_gls/pdf/colorectal_screening.pdf.
50. Paschos A, Bird N. Current diagnostic and therapeutic approaches for colorectal cancer liver metastases. *Hipplkratia* 2008;3:132-138.
51. Locker GY, Hamilton S, Harris J, et al. ASCO 2006 update of recommendations for the use of tumor markers in gastrointestinal cancer. *J Clin Oncol* 2006;24:5313-5327.
52. Gunderson LL, Jessup JM, Sargent DJ, Greene FL, Stewart AK. Revised TN categorization for colon cancer based on national survival outcomes data. *J Clin Oncol* 2010;28:264-271.
53. Gunderson LL, Jessup JM, Sargent DJ, Greene FL, Stewart AK. Revised tumor and node categorization for rectal cancer based on surveillance, epidemiology, and end results and rectal pooled analysis outcomes. *J Clin Oncol* 2010;28:256-263.
54. Colon and rectum. In: Edge SB, Byrd DR, Compton CC, et al. (eds.), American Joint Committee on Cancer. AJCC Cancer Staging Manual, 7th ed. New York: Springer, 2010:143-159.
55. Libutti KS, Saltz LB, Willett CG. Cancers of the gastrointestinal tract: Cancer of the colon. In: DeVita VT, Lawrence TS, Rosenberg SA, eds. Cancer: Principles and Practice of Oncology, 9th ed. Philadelphia: Lippincott Williams & Wilkins, 2011:1084-1126.
56. Zlobec I, Lugli A. Prognostic and predictive factors in colorectal cancer. *J Clin Pathol* 2008;61:561-569.
57. Ross JS, Torres-Mora J, Wagle N, et al. Biomarker-based prediction of response to therapy for colorectal cancer. *Am J Clin Pathol* 2010;134:478-490.
58. NCCN Clinical Practice Guidelines In Oncology—Colon Cancer v.2.2016. 2015, http://www.nccn.org/professionals/physician_gls/pdf/colon.pdf.
59. Kelley RK, Venook AP. Prognostic and predictive markers in stage II colon cancer: Is there a role for gene expression profiling? *Clin Colorectal Cancer* 2011;10:73-80.
60. Cunningham D, Atkin W, Lenz HJ, et al. Colorectal cancer. *Lancet* 2010;375:1030-1047.
61. Phillips JG, Hong TS, Ryan DP. Multidisciplinary management of early-stage rectal cancer. *J Natl Compr Canc Netw* 2012;10:1577-1585.
62. Giantonio BJ, Catalano PJ, Meropol NJ, et al. Bevacizumab in combination with oxaliplatin, fluorouracil, and leucovorin (FOLFOX4) for previously treated metastatic colorectal cancer: results from the Eastern Cooperative Oncology Group Study E3200. *J Clin Oncol* 2007;25:1539-1544.
63. Andre T, Boni C, Navarro M, et al. Improved overall survival with oxaliplatin, fluorouracil, and leucovorin as adjuvant treatment in stage II or III colon cancer in the MOSAIC trial. *J Clin Oncol* 2009;27:3109-3116.
64. Yothers G, O'Connell MJ, Allegra CJ, et al. Oxaliplatin as adjuvant therapy for colon cancer: updated results of NSABP C-07 trial, including survival and subset analyses. *J Clin Oncol* 2011;29:3768-3774.
65. Twelves C, Scheithauer W, McKendrick J, et al. Capecitabine versus 5-fluorouracil/folinic acid as adjuvant therapy for stage III colon cancer: final results from the X-ACT trial with analysis by age and preliminary evidence of a pharmacodynamic marker of efficacy. *Ann Oncol* 2012;23:1190-1197.
66. Haller DG, Tabernero J, Maroun J, et al. Capecitabine plus oxaliplatin compared with fluorouracil and folinic acid as adjuvant therapy for stage III colon cancer. *J Clin Oncol* 2011;29:1465-1471.
67. Wolmark N, Rockette H, Fisher B, et al. The benefit of leucovorin-modulated fluorouracil as postoperative adjuvant therapy for primary colon cancer: results from National Surgical Adjuvant Breast and Bowel Project protocol C-03. *J Clin Oncol* 1993;11:1879-1887.
68. O'Connell MJ, Mailliard JA, Kahn MJ, et al. Controlled trial of fluorouracil and low-dose leucovorin given for 6 months as postoperative adjuvant therapy for colon cancer. *J Clin Oncol* 1997;15:246-250.
69. Van Cutsem E, Labianca R, Bodoky G, et al. Randomized phase III trial comparing biweekly infusional fluorouracil/leucovorin alone or with irinotecan in the adjuvant treatment of stage III colon cancer: PETACC-3. *J Clin Oncol* 2009;27:3117-3125.
70. Chuang VTG, Suno M. Levoleucovorin as replacement for leucovorin in cancer treatment. *Ann Pharmacother* 2012;46:1349-1357.
71. Meta-Analysis Group in Cancer. Toxicity of fluorouracil in patients with advanced colorectal cancer: effect of administration schedule and prognostic factors. *J Clin Oncol* 1998;16:3537-3541.
72. Weikhardt A, Wells K, Messersmith. Oxaliplatin-induced neuropathy in colorectal cancer. *J Oncol* 2011; doi:10.1155/2011/201593.
73. NCCN Clinical Practice Guidelines In Oncology—Rectal Cancer v.1.2016. 2015, http://www.nccn.org/professionals/physician_gls/pdf/rectal.pdf.

74. Cai GX, Cai SJ. Multi-modality treatment of colorectal liver metastases. *World J Gastroenterol* 2012;18:16-24.
75. Chua TC, Morris DL. Therapeutic potential of surgery for metastatic colorectal cancer. *Scand J Gastroenterol* 2012;47:258-268.
76. Cleary JM, Tanabe KT, Lauwers GY, Zhu AX. Hepatic toxicities associated with the use of preoperative systemic therapy in patients with metastatic colorectal adenocarcinoma to the liver. *Oncologist* 2009;14:1095-1105.
77. Schwarz RE, Berlin JD, Lenz HJ. Systemic cytotoxic and biological therapies of colorectal liver metastases: expert consensus statement. *HPB (Oxford)* 2013;15:106-115.
78. Hochster HS, Hart LL, Ramanathan RK, et al. Safety and efficacy of oxaliplatin and fluoropyrimidine regimens with or without bevacizumab as first-line treatment of metastatic colorectal cancer: results of the TREE study. *J Clin Oncol* 2008;26:3523-3529.
79. Stintzing S, Fischer von Weikersthal L, Decker T, et al. FOLFIRI plus cetuximab versus FOLFIRI plus bevacizumab as first-line treatment for patients with metastatic colorectal cancer-subgroup analysis of patients with KRAS: mutated tumours in the randomised German AIO study KRK-0306. *Ann Oncol* 2012;23:1693-1699.
80. Ducreux M, Malka D, Mendiboure J, et al. Sequential versus combination chemotherapy for the treatment of advanced colorectal cancer (FFCD 2000-05): an open-label, randomised, phase 3 trial. *Lancet Oncol* 2011;12:1032-1044.
81. Kabbinavar FF, Hambleton J, Mass RD, et al. Combined analysis of efficacy: the addition of bevacizumab to fluorouracil/leucovorin improves survival for patients with metastatic colorectal cancer. *J Clin Oncol* 2005;23:3706-3712.
82. Feliu J, Safont MJ, Salud A, et al. Capecitabine and bevacizumab as first-line treatment in elderly patients with metastatic colorectal cancer. *Br J Cancer* 2010;102:1468-1473.
83. Fakih MG. Metastatic colorectal cancer: current state and future directions. *J Clin Oncol* 2015;33:1809-1824.
84. Douillard JY, Siena S, Cassidy J, et al. Final results from PRIME: randomized phase III study of panitumumab with FOLFOX4 for first-line treatment of metastatic colorectal cancer. *Ann Oncol* 2014;25(7):1346-1355.
85. Hurwitz HI, Fehrenbacher L, Hainsworth JD, et al. Bevacizumab in combination with fluorouracil and leucovorin: an active regimen for first- line metastatic colorectal cancer. *J Clin Oncol* 2005;23:3502-3508.
86. Martín-Martorell P, Roselló S, Rodríguez-Braun E, et al. Biweekly cetuximab and irinotecan in advanced colorectal cancer patients progressing after at least one previous line of chemotherapy: results of a phase II single institution trial. *Br J Cancer* 2008;99:455-458.
87. Van Cutsem E, Peeters M, Siena S, et al. Open-label phase III trial of panitumumab plus best supportive care compared with best supportive care alone in patients with chemotherapy-refractory metastatic colorectal cancer. *J Clin Oncol* 2007;25:1658-1664.
88. Glimelius B, Cavalli-Björkman N. Metastatic colorectal cancer: current treatment and future options for improved survival. *Scand J Gastroenterol* 2012;47:296-314.
89. Goldberg RM, Sargent DJ, Morton RF, et al. A randomized controlled trial of fluorouracil plus leucovorin, irinotecan, and oxaliplatin combinations in patients with previously untreated metastatic colorectal cancer. *J Clin Oncol* 2004;22:23-30.
90. de Gramont A, Figer A, Seymour M, et al. Leucovorin and fluorouracil with or without oxaliplatin as first-line treatment in advanced colorectal cancer. *J Clin Oncol* 2000;18:2938-2947.
91. Douillard J, Cunningham D, Roth A, et al. Irinotecan combined with fluorouracil compared with fluorouracil alone as first-line treatment for metastatic colorectal cancer: a multicentre randomised trial. *Lancet* 2000;355:1041-1047.
92. Twelves C. Capecitabine as first-line treatment in colorectal cancer. *Eur J Cancer* 2002;38:15-20.
93. Fuchs CS, Marshall J, Barrueco J. Randomized, controlled trial of irinotecan plus infusional, bolus, or oral fluoropyrimidines in first-line treatment of metastatic colorectal cancer: Updated results from the BICC-C study. *J Clin Oncol* 2008;26:689-690.
94. Tournigand C, Andre T, Achille E, et al. FOLFIRI followed by FOLFOX6 or the reverse sequence in advanced colorectal cancer: a randomized GERCOR study. *J Clin Oncol* 2004;22:229-237.
95. Bokemeyer C, Bondarenko I, Makhson A, et al. Fluorouracil, leucovorin, and oxaliplatin with and without cetuximab in the first-line treatment of metastatic colorectal cancer. *J Clin Oncol* 2009;27:663-667.
96. Van Cutsem E, Kohne C-H, Hitre E, et al. Cetuximab plus irinotecan, fluorouracil, and leucovorin as first-line treatment for metastatic colorectal cancer: updated analysis of overall survival according to tumor *KRAS* and *BRAF* mutation status. *J Clin Oncol* 2011;29(15):2011-2019.
97. Rougier P, Van Cutsem E, Bajetta E, et al. Randomised trial of irinotecan versus fluorouracil by continuous infusion after fluorouracil failure in patients with metastatic colorectal cancer. *Lancet* 1998;352:1407-1412.
98. Cunningham D, Pyrhönen S, James R, et al. Randomised trial of irinotecan plus supportive care versus supportive care alone after fluorouracil failure for patients with metastatic colorectal cancer. *Lancet* 1998;352:1413-1418.
99. Cunningham D, Humblet Y, Siena S, et al. Cetuximab monotherapy and cetuximab plus irinotecan in irinotecan-refractory metastatic colorectal cancer. *N Engl J Med* 2004;351:337-345.
100. Sobrero AF, Maurel J, Fehrenbacher L, et al. EPIC: phase III trial of cetuximab plus irinotecan after fluoropyrimidine and oxaliplatin failure in patients with metastatic colorectal cancer. *J Clin Oncol* 2008;26:2311-2319.
101. Tabernero J, Yoshino T, Cohn AL, et al. Ramucirumab versus placebo in combination with second-line FOLFIRI in patients with metastatic colorectal carcinoma that progressed during or after first-line therapy with bevacizumab, oxaliplatin, and a fluoropyrimidine (RAISE): a randomised, double-blind, multicentre, phase 3 study. *Lancet Oncol* 2015;16(5):499-508.
102. Mayer RJ, Van Cutsem E., Falcone A, et al. Randomized trial of TAS-102 for refractory metastatic colorectal cancer. *N Engl J Med* 2015;372(2):1909-1919.
103. Benhaim L, Labonte MJ, Lenz HJ. Pharmacogenomics and metastatic colorectal cancer: Current knowledge and perspectives. *Scand J Gastroenterol* 2012;47:325-339.
104. Vale CL, Tierney JF, Fisher D, et al. Does anti-EGFR therapy improve outcome in advanced colorectal cancer? A systematic review and meta-analysis. *Cancer Treat Rev* 2012;38:618-625.
105. Hecht JR, Mitchell E, Chidiac T, et al. A randomized phase IIIB trial of chemotherapy, bevacizumab, and panitumumab compared with chemotherapy and bevacizumab alone for metastatic colorectal cancer. *J Clin Oncol* 2009;27:672-680.
106. Tol J, Koopman M, Cats A, et al. Chemotherapy, bevacizumab, and cetuximab in metastatic colorectal cancer. *N Engl J Med* 2009;360:563-572.
107. Resch G, Schaberl-Moser R, Kier P, et al. Infusion reactions to the chimeric EGFR inhibitor cetuximab--change to the fully human anti-EGFR monoclonal antibody panitumumab is safe. *Ann Oncol* 2011;22:486-487.
108. Lacotoure ME, Anadkat MJ, Bensadoun RJ, et al. Clinical practice guidelines for the prevention and treatment of EGFR inhibitor-associated dermatologic toxicities. *Support Care Cancer* 2011;19:1079-1095.
109. Mahnken AH, Pereira PL, de Baère T. Interventional oncologic approaches to liver metastases. *Radiology* 2013;266:407-430.
110. Stintzing S, Stremitzer S, Sebio A, Lenz HJ. Predictive and prognostic markers in the treatment of metastatic colorectal cancer (mCRC): personalized medicine at work. *Hematol Oncol Clin North Am* 2015;29(1):43-60.
111. Mattia ED, Cecchin E, Toffoli G. Pharmacogenomics of intrinsic and acquired pharmacoresistance in colorectal cancer: toward targeted personalized therapy. *Drug Resist Updat* 2015;20:39-70.
112. Panczyk M. Pharmacogenetics research on chemotherapy resistance in colorectal cancer over the last 20 years. *World J Gastroenterol* 2014;20(29):9775-9827.
113. Saif MW, Choma A, Salamone SJ, Chu E. Pharmacokinetically guided dose adjustment of 5-fluorouracil: a rational approach to improving therapeutic outcomes. *J Natl Cancer Inst* 2009;101:1543-1552.
114. Gamelin E, Delva R, Jacob J, et al. Individual fluorouracil dose adjustment based on pharmacokinetic follow-up compared with conventional dosage: results of a multicenter randomized trial of patients with metastatic colorectal cancer. *J Clin Oncol* 2008;26:2099-3105.
115. Patel JN, O'Neil BH, Deal AM, et al. A community-based multicenter trial of pharmacokinetically guided 5-fluorouracil dosing for personalized colorectal cancer therapy. *Oncologist* 2014;19:959-965.

131

Prostate Cancer

LeAnn B. Norris and Jill M. Kolesar

KEY CONCEPTS

1 Prostate cancer is the most frequent cancer in men in the United States. African American ancestry, family history, and increased age are the primary risk factors for prostate cancer.

2 Prostate-specific antigen can be used to detect prostate cancer at early stages, predict outcome for localized disease, define disease-free status, and monitor response to androgen-deprivation therapy (ADT) or chemotherapy for advanced-stage disease.

3 The prognosis for prostate cancer patients depends on the histologic grade, the tumor size, and the disease stage. More than 85% of patients with stage A_1 disease but less than 1% of those with stage D_2 can be cured.

4 ADT with a luteinizing hormone-releasing hormone (LHRH) agonist plus an antiandrogen should be used prior to radiation therapy for patients with locally advanced prostate cancer to improve outcomes over radiation therapy alone.

5 ADT, with either orchiectomy, an LHRH agonist alone or an LHRH agonist plus an antiandrogen (combined hormonal blockade), can be used to provide palliation for patients with advanced (stage D_2) prostate cancer. The effects of androgen deprivation are most pronounced in patients with minimal disease at diagnosis.

6 Antiandrogen withdrawal, for patients having progressive disease while receiving combined hormonal blockade with an LHRH agonist plus an antiandrogen, can provide additional symptomatic relief. Mutations in the androgen receptor can cause antiandrogen compounds to act like receptor agonists.

7 Chemotherapy, with docetaxel and prednisone improves survival in patients with castrate-refractory prostate cancer and is considered a first-line therapy option for these patients. Other effective agents include enzalutamide and abiraterone.

Prostate cancer is the most commonly diagnosed cancer in American men.[1] For most men, prostate cancer has an indolent course, and treatment options for early disease include expectant management, surgery, or radiation. With expectant management, patients are monitored for disease progression or development of symptoms. Localized prostate cancer can be cured by surgery or radiation therapy, but advanced prostate cancer is not yet curable. Treatment for advanced prostate cancer can provide significant disease palliation for many patients for several years after diagnosis. The endocrine dependence of this tumor is well documented, and hormonal manipulation to decrease circulating androgens remains the basis for the treatment of advanced disease.

EPIDEMIOLOGY

1 Prostate cancer is the most frequent cancer among American men and represents the second leading cause of cancer-related deaths in males.[1] In the United States alone, it is estimated that 180,890 new cases of prostate carcinoma will be diagnosed and more than 26,120 men will die from this disease in 2016.[1] Although the incidence of prostate cancer increased during the late 1980s and early 1990s related to widespread prostate-specific antigen (PSA) screening, deaths from prostate cancer have been declining since 1995.[1]

ETIOLOGY

Table 131-1 summarizes the possible factors associated with prostate cancer.[2,3] The widely accepted risk factors for prostate cancer are age, race-ethnicity, and family history of prostate cancer.[2,3] The disease is rare in those younger than 40 years, but the incidence sharply increases with each subsequent decade, most likely because the individual has had a lifetime exposure to testosterone, a known growth signal for the prostate.[2,3]

Race and Ethnicity

The incidence of clinical prostate cancer varies across geographic regions. Scandinavian countries and the United States report the highest incidence of prostate cancer, while the disease is relatively rare in Japan and other Asian countries.[4] African American men have the highest rate of prostate cancer in the world, and prostate cancer mortality in African Americans is more than twice that seen in white populations in the United States.[1] Hormonal, dietary, and genetic differences, and differences in access to healthcare may contribute to the altered susceptibility to prostate cancer in these populations.[2,3] Testosterone, commonly implicated in the pathogenesis of prostate cancer, is about 15% higher in African American men compared with white males. Activity of 5-α-reductase, the enzyme that converts testosterone to its more active form, dihydrotestosterone (DHT), in the prostate, is decreased in Japanese men compared with African Americans and whites.[2,3]

In addition, genetic variations in the androgen receptor exist. Activation of the androgen receptor is inversely correlated with CAG repeat length. Shorter CAG repeat sequences have been found in African Americans, and a recent meta-analysis demonstrated that carriers of a short CAG repeat were at increased risk of prostate cancer (odds ratio 1.21, 95% confidence interval [CI] 1.10-1.51) when compared to individuals with long CAG repeats.[3] Therefore the combination of increased testosterone and increased androgen receptor activation may account for the increased risk of prostate cancer for African American men.[2,3] The Asian diet is generally considered to be low in fat and high in fiber with a high concentration of phytoestrogens, potentially explaining their decreased risk.[4]

TABLE 131-1 Risk Factors Associated with Prostate Cancer

Factor	Possible Relationship
Probable Risk Factors	
Age	More than 70% of cases are diagnosed in men older than 65 years old
Race	African Americans have higher incidence and death rate
Genetic	Familial prostate cancer inherited in an autosomal dominant manner
	Mutations *BRCA1*, *BRCA2*, *MSH2*, and *HOXB13* are associated with an increased risk of prostate cancer
Possible Risk Factors	
Environmental	Clinical carcinoma incidence varies worldwide
	Latent carcinoma similar between regions
	Nationalized males adopt intermediate incidence rates between those of the United States and their native country
Occupational	Increased risk associated with cadmium exposure
Diet	Mediterranean diet associated with reduced risk Increased risk associated with high-meat and high-fat diets
	Decreased intake of 25-dihydroxyvitamin D, lycopene, and β-carotene increases risk
Hormonal	Does not occur in castrated men
	Low incidence in cirrhotic patients
	Up to 80% are hormonally dependent; African Americans have 15% increased testosterone
	Japanese have decreased 5-α-reductase activities
	Polymorphic expression of the androgen receptor

Family History

Men with a brother or father with prostate cancer have twice the risk for prostate cancer as compared with the rest of the population and 5% to 10% of prostate cancers are thought to be inherited.[5] Familial clustering of a prostate cancer syndrome has been reported, and genome-wide scans have identified potential prostate cancer susceptibility candidate genes. Male carriers of germline mutations of *BRCA1* mutations have about 4-fold increased risk of prostate cancer and an absolute risk of about 10% by age 65 while those with *BRCA2* mutations have a 2.5- to 8.6-fold increase in prostate cancer risk and a 15% absolute risk by age 65.[5] Other genes implicated in hereditary prostate cancer are *MSH2* and *HOXB13*.[5] Common exposure to environmental and other risk factors may also contribute to increased risk among patients with first-degree relatives with prostate cancer.[4]

Diet

The overall dietary factor associated with the lowest risk of developing prostate cancer appears to be adherence with a Mediterranean diet.[6] The typical Mediterranean diet is high in fruits, vegetables, legumes, fish, olive oil and red wine, with low to moderate amounts of red meat, poultry and dairy. In a meta-analysis including about 1.5 million individuals, adherence to a Mediterranean diet was associated with a small, but significantly reduced risk of prostate cancer (relative risk [RR] 0.96, 95% CI: 0.92-0.99).[6]

Many individual dietary factors have been assessed to ascertain their role in the development or prevention of prostate cancer.[7] Green tea and lycopene are currently considered the most useful, and at least not harmful. Green tea consumption was associated with a reduced risk of prostate cancer in a small case-control study. Lycopene, obtained primarily from tomatoes, was shown to decrease the risk of prostate cancer in small cohort studies, although a meta-analysis failed to show a benefit for high tomato consumption.

Consistent with the beneficial effects of the Mediterranean diet, red meat and high milk intake have been clearly and consistently associated with an increased risk of prostate cancer in epidemiological studies.[7]

Other Factors

Benign prostatic hyperplasia (BPH) is a common problem among elderly men, affecting more than 40% of men older than 70 years (see Chapter 84). BPH results in the urinary symptoms of hesitancy and frequency. Because prostate cancer affects a similar age group and often has similar presenting symptoms, the presence of BPH often complicates the diagnosis of prostate cancer, although it does not appear to increase the risk of developing prostate cancer.[2]

Smoking has not been associated with an increased risk of prostate cancer, but smokers with prostate cancer have an increased mortality resulting from the disease when compared with nonsmokers with prostate cancer (RR 1.5-2).[2] In addition, the results of an observational study showed that alcohol consumption was not associated with the development of prostate cancer.

CHEMOPREVENTION

The use of 5-α-reductase inhibitors, finasteride, and dutasteride to prevent prostate cancer has been debated for more than a decade.[8-11] These drugs inhibit 5-α-reductase, an enzyme that converts testosterone to its more active form, DHT, which is involved in prostate epithelial proliferation. 5-α-reductase exists as two types, type I and type II, and both are implicated in the development of prostate cancer. Finasteride selectively inhibits the 5-α-reductase type II isoenzyme, while dutasteride inhibits both isoenzymes.[9] Both finasteride and dutasteride can falsely lower the PSA by about 50% in patients, and this must be considered when one interprets PSA in patients on these medications.[12]

The efficacy of 5-α-reductase inhibitors in reducing the risk of prostate cancer was evaluated in a Cochrane review.[8] Eight randomized studies involving 41,638 men were included, including the Reduction by Dutasteride of Prostate Cancer Events (REDUCE) study, which compared dutasteride to placebo in more than 8,000 subjects, and the Prostate Cancer Prevention Trial (PCPT) study, which compared finasteride to placebo in more than 18,000 subjects. Compared with placebo, 5-α-reductase inhibitors reduced the risk of prostate cancers detected by 25% (RR 0.75, 95% CI: 0.67-0.83; absolute risk reduction 1.4%, [3.5% vs 4.9%]). Although the incidence of prostate cancers was reduced in both the PCPT[9] and REDUCE[10] trials, the prostate tumors that were diagnosed were significantly more aggressive grades (Gleason 7-10) than those diagnosed in the placebo arm. The studies were not designed to evaluate prostate cancer mortality and 5-α-reductase inhibitors did not reduce mortality in the combined analysis. Adverse effects, including gynecomastia, decreased libido, and erectile dysfunction, were more common in patients treated with 5-α-reductase inhibitors than in placebo.[8]

Based on the concern for development of more aggressive tumors, lack of survival benefit and increased risk of adverse effects, neither finasteride nor dutasteride are approved for preventing prostate cancer.[11] The American Society of Clinical Oncology and the American Urological Association published a joint practice guideline for prostate cancer chemoprevention.[13] The guideline recommends that asymptomatic men with a PSA less than or equal to 3.0 ng/mL (mcg/L) who are regularly screened with PSA for early detection of prostate cancer may benefit from a discussion of both the benefits and the potential risks of dutasteride or finasteride for 7 years for the prevention of prostate cancer.[13] Notably, the guideline does not recommend either chemoprevention or prostate cancer screening. The data from PCPT and REDUCE have been criticized for both selection bias and altered differential sensitivity in diagnosis.[11,12]

Additional post-hoc analyses that account for these potential biases have generally reported that the inherent biases in the trials were most likely responsible for the increased risk of high grade prostate cancer observed in the treatment arms. However, in the current environment where overdiagnosis and overtreatment of prostate cancer are of concern, these analyses have not generated sufficient interest in 5-α-reductase inhibitors as chemoprevention agents. Current research focuses on the ability of the 5-α-reductase inhibitors to reduce the risk of progression in patients with low grade prostate cancers and in those who fail initial therapy.

Selenium and vitamin E alone or in combination were evaluated as possible chemopreventive agents in the *Sel*enium and Vitamin *E* Cancer Prevention *T*rial (SELECT), a clinical trial investigating in healthy men. The data and safety monitoring committee found that, after 5 years, selenium or vitamin E taken alone or together did not prevent prostate cancer. Based on these data and safety concerns, the trial was halted. With longer follow-up of that trial, dietary supplementation with vitamin E significantly increased the risk of prostate cancer by 17% (P=0.008).[14] Other agents, including lycopene, green tea, nonsteroidal anti-inflammatory agents, isoflavones, and statins, are under investigation for prostate cancer and show some promise, but none are currently recommended for routine use outside of a clinical trial.[15]

SCREENING

2 PSA can be used for detecting prostate cancer at early stages, predicting outcome for localized disease, defining disease-free status, and monitoring response to androgen-deprivation therapy (ADT) or chemotherapy for advanced-stage disease. If prostate cancer screening is performed, PSA is the method of choice, although low specificity is a major limitation.[16,17] PSA may be elevated in men with acute urinary retention, acute prostatitis, and prostatic ischemia or infarction, as well as BPH, a nearly universal condition in men at risk for prostate cancer. PSA elevations between 4.1 and 10 ng/mL (mcg/L) cannot distinguish between BPH and prostate cancer, limiting the utility of PSA alone for the early detection of prostate cancer. Additionally, many men with clinically significant prostate cancer do not have a serum PSA outside the reference range.[18]

Early detection of potentially curable prostate cancers is the goal of prostate cancer screening. For cancer screening to be beneficial, it must reliably detect cancer at an early stage, when intervention would decrease mortality. Whether prostate cancer screening fits these criteria is debatable.[17,19-22] The European Randomized Study of Screening for Prostate Cancer (ERSPC) evaluated the effect of PSA screening on prostate cancer mortality.[23] More than 182,000 men from seven different European countries were randomized between being offered screening with PSA to no screening. The frequency of screening and PSA threshold for a biopsy varied by country. Most centers used a PSA cutoff of 3 ng/mL (mcg/L), but Belgium allowed up to 10 ng/mL (mcg/L). Most centers screened every 4 years, although Sweden screened every 2 years. Most (82%) of the men in the screening group had at least one PSA performed. With a median follow-up of 11 years, the cumulative incidence of prostate cancer was 9.6% in the screening group and 6.0% in the control group.[23] The rate ratio for death from prostate cancer in the screening group, compared with the control group, was 0.79 (95% CI: 0.68-0.91, adjusted P=0.001), which corresponds to about one death from prostate cancer per 1,000 men (at a median follow-up of 11 years) prevented in the screened group compared with the unscreened group. Of the 136,689 PSA tests performed, 16.6% of the tests were positive; biopsies were performed for 86% of men with elevated PSAs. Overall mortality was similar in the two study groups (rate ratio 0.99, 95% CI: 0.97-1.01).[23]

In the United States, the Prostate, Lung, Colon and Ovarian Screening (PLCO) study randomized 76,693 men to receive either annual screening (38,343 subjects) or usual care as the control (38,350 subjects).[24] In the screening group, men were offered annual PSA testing for 6 years and DRE for 4 years. Compliance with screening was 85%. Men in the usual care group were able to receive screening, with the rate of PSA testing ranging from 40% to 52% and DRE from 41% to 46%. After 13 years of follow-up, the incidence of death per 10,000 person-years was not significantly different between the two groups with 3.7 (158 deaths total) in the screening group and 3.4 (145 deaths total) in the control group (RR 1.09; 95% CI: 0.87-1.36).[24]

The ERSPC demonstrated that PSA testing every 4 years was better than no PSA testing, decreasing prostate cancer deaths in the screened group by about 1 per 1,000 men screened compared with the unscreened group, but the false-positive rate was 76%, resulting in more than 13,000 unnecessary biopsies.[23] The PLCO screening study showed no reduction in prostate cancer death between the annual (PSA and DRE) screening group and the usual care group, which is not surprising given the small reduction in death expected and that about one-half of the patients in the usual screening groups had PSA and/or DRE screening performed.[24] Both studies demonstrated that screening identifies more prostate cancers than not screening.[23,24] PSA measurements can identify small, subclinical prostate cancers, where no intervention may be required. Detecting prostate cancer in those not needing therapy not only increases the cost of care through unnecessary screening and workups, but also increases harm by subjecting some patients to unnecessary therapy. Based on this evidence, the United States Preventive Services Task Force (USPSTF) recommended against screening for prostate cancer (grade D recommendation) in 2012, based on moderate or high certainty that screening has no net benefit or that the harms outweigh the benefits.[21] The American Urologic Association (AUA) does not recommend routine screening in men between the ages of 40 and 54 years of average risk. In men aged 55 to 69 years, the AUA recommends that the risks and benefits of prostate cancer screening are discussed.[17] For men who elect to be screened, the frequency should be no more than 2 years, and a recent study suggests that screening every 5 years may be adequate. The American Cancer Society recommends that asymptomatic men who have at least a 10-year life expectancy have an opportunity to make an informed decision about prostate cancer screening, including discussion of the uncertainties, risks, and potential benefits associated with screening.[20]

In the United States, PSA screening data from the National Health Interview Survey showed a decline in the prevalence of prostate cancer screening, decreasing from 36% of men undergoing annual PSA screening in 2010 to 31% of men in 2013. The authors suggest that changes in screening patterns were associated with USPSTF guidelines recommending against PSA screening.[22]

Clinical **Controversy...**

Prostate cancer screening with prostate-specific antigen (PSA) tests is controversial. The USPSTF recommends no PSA screening, while the AUA recommends shared decision making with a discussion of risk and benefits for men aged 55 to 69 years. An additional trial of PSA screening (CAP/ProtecT trial) is expected to report initial results in 2016 and may help resolve these issues.

Based on the available evidence, Gulati et al recently evaluated the comparative effectiveness of alternative PSA screening strategies.[25] Examples of alternative screening strategies include the use of higher PSA thresholds for biopsy referral or longer screening intervals. Several of the screening scenarios were predicted to produce similar reductions in prostate cancer mortality and reduce harms.

PATHOPHYSIOLOGY

The prostate gland is a solid, rounded, heart-shaped organ positioned between the neck of the bladder and the urogenital diaphragm (Fig. 131-1). The normal prostate is composed of acinar secretory cells arranged in a radial shape and surrounded by a foundation of supporting tissue. The size, shape, or presence of acini is almost always altered in the gland that has been invaded by prostatic carcinoma. Adenocarcinoma, the major pathologic cell type, accounts for more than 95% of prostate cancer cases.[26,27] Much rarer tumor types include small cell neuroendocrine cancers, sarcomas, and transitional cell carcinomas.

Prostate cancer can be graded systematically according to the histologic appearance of the malignant cell and then grouped into well, moderately, or poorly differentiated grades.[27,28] Gland architecture is examined and then rated on a scale of 1 (well differentiated) to 5 (poorly differentiated). Two different specimens are examined, and the score for each specimen is added. Groupings for total Gleason score are 2 to 4 for well differentiated, 5 or 6 for moderately differentiated, and 7 to 10 for poorly differentiated tumors. Poorly differentiated tumors grow rapidly (poor prognosis), while well-differentiated tumors grow slowly (better prognosis).

Metastatic spread can occur by local extension, lymphatic drainage, or hematogenous dissemination.[28,29] Lymph node metastases are more common in patients with large, undifferentiated tumors that invade the seminal vesicles. The pelvic and abdominal lymph node groups are the most common sites of lymph node involvement (see Fig. 131-1). Skeletal metastases from hematogenous spread are the most common sites of distant spread. Typically, the bone lesions are osteoblastic or a combination of osteoblastic and osteolytic. The most common site of bone involvement is the lumbar spine. Other sites of bone involvement include the proximal femur pelvis, thoracic spine, ribs, sternum, skull, and humerus. The lung, liver, brain, and adrenal glands are the most common sites of visceral involvement, although these organs are not usually initially involved. About 25% to 35% of patients will have evidence of lymphangitic or nodular pulmonary infiltrates at autopsy. The prostate is rarely a site for metastatic involvement from other solid tumors.

Normal growth and differentiation of the prostate depend on the presence of androgens, specifically DHT.[29,30] The testes and the adrenal glands are the major sources of circulating androgens. Hormonal regulation of androgen synthesis is mediated through a series of biochemical interactions between the hypothalamus, pituitary, adrenal glands, and testes (Fig. 131-2). Luteinizing hormone-releasing hormone (LHRH) released from the hypothalamus stimulates the release of luteinizing hormone (LH) and follicle-stimulating hormone (FSH) from the anterior pituitary gland. LH complexes with receptors on the Leydig cell testicular membrane and stimulates the production of testosterone and small amounts of estrogen. FSH acts on the Sertoli cells within the testes to promote the maturation of LH receptors and to produce an androgen-binding protein. Circulating testosterone and estradiol influence the synthesis of LHRH, LH, and FSH by a negative feedback loop operating at the hypothalamic and pituitary level.[31] Prolactin, growth hormone, and estradiol appear to be important accessory regulators for prostatic tissue permeability, receptor binding, and testosterone synthesis.

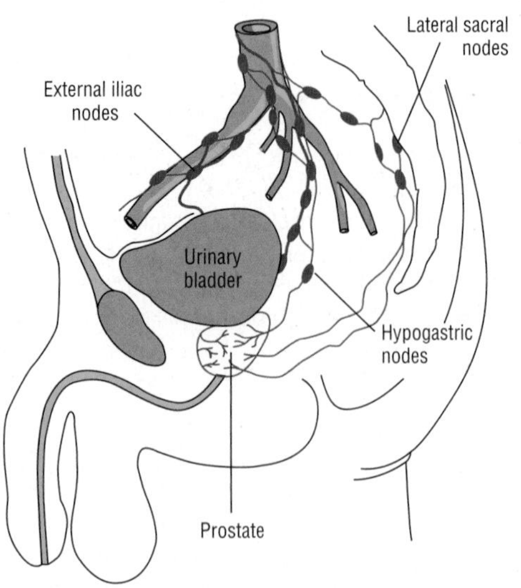

FIGURE 131-1 The prostate gland.

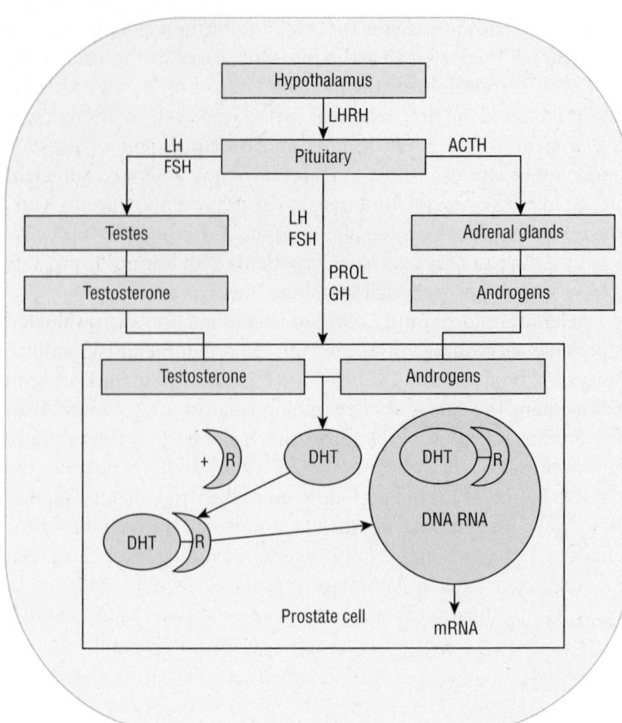

FIGURE 131-2 Hormonal regulation of the prostate gland. (ACTH, adrenocorticotropic hormone; DHT, dihydrotestosterone; FSH, follicle-stimulating hormone; GH, growth hormone; LH, luteinizing hormone; LHRH, luteinizing hormone-releasing hormone; PROL, prolactin; R, receptor.)

Testosterone, the major androgenic hormone, accounts for 95% of the androgen concentration. The primary source of testosterone is the testes, but 3% to 5% of the testosterone concentration is derived from direct adrenal cortical secretion of testosterone or C19 steroids such as androstenedione.[28-30]

In early-stage prostate cancers, aberrant tumor cell proliferation is promoted by the presence of androgens. For these tumors, blockade of androgens induces tumor regression in most patients. Hormonal manipulations to ablate or reduce circulating androgens can occur through several mechanisms[29,30] (Table 131-2). The organs responsible for androgen production can be removed surgically (orchiectomy, hypophysectomy, or adrenalectomy). Hormonal pathways that modulate prostatic growth can be interrupted at several steps (see Fig. 131-2). Interference with LHRH or LH can reduce testosterone secretion by the testes (estrogens, LHRH agonists, progestogens, and cyproterone acetate). Estrogen administration reduces androgens by directly inhibiting LH release, by acting directly on the prostate cell, or by decreasing free androgens by increasing steroid-binding globulin levels.[28-30]

Isolation of the naturally occurring hypothalamic decapeptide hormone, LHRH has provided another group of effective agents for advanced prostate cancer treatment. The physiologic response to LHRH depends on both the dose and the mode of administration.

TABLE 131-2 Hormonal Manipulations in Prostate Cancer

Androgen source ablation	Antiandrogens
Orchiectomy	Flutamide
Adrenalectomy	Bicalutamide
Hypophysectomy	Enzalutamide
LHRH or LH inhibition	Nilutamide
Estrogens	Cyproterone acetate[b]
LHRH agonists	Progesterones
Progesterones[a]	5-α-Reductase inhibition
Cyproterone acetate[b]	Finasteride[b]
Androgen synthesis inhibition	Dutasteride
Aminoglutethimide	
Ketoconazole	
Abiraterone Acetate	
Progesterones[a]	

LH, luteinizing hormone; LHRH, luteinizing hormone-releasing hormone.

[a]Minor mechanisms of action.

[b]Investigational compounds or use.

TABLE 131-3 Diagnostic and Staging Workup for Prostate Cancer

Initial tests	DRE
	PSA TRUS if either DRE is positive or PSA is elevated
	Biopsy
Staging tests	Gleason score on biopsy specimen
	Bone scan
	Complete blood count
	Liver function tests
	Serum phosphatases (acid/alkaline)
	Excretory urogram
	Chest x-ray
Additional staging tests (depends on tumor classification, PSA, and Gleason score)	Skeletal films
	Lymph node evaluation
	Pelvic computed tomography
	^{111}In-labeled capromab pendetide scan
	Bipedal lymphangiogram
	Transrectal magnetic resonance imaging

DRE, Digital rectal examination; PS, Prostate-specific antigen; TRUS, transrectal ultrasonography.

Intermittent pulsed LHRH administration, which mimics the endogenous release pattern, causes sustained release of both LH and FSH, whereas high-dose or continuous IV administration of LHRH inhibits gonadotropin release due to receptor downregulation.[23] Structural modification of the naturally occurring LHRH and innovative delivery have produced a series of LHRH agonists that cause a similar downregulation of pituitary receptors and a decrease in testosterone production.[31]

Androgen synthesis can also be inhibited in the testes or in the adrenal gland. Aminoglutethimide inhibits the desmolase-enzyme complex in the adrenal gland, thereby preventing the conversion of cholesterol to pregnenolone. Pregnenolone is the precursor substrate for all adrenal-derived steroids, including androgens, glucocorticoids, and mineralocorticoids. Ketoconazole, an imidazole antifungal agent, causes a dose-related reversible reduction in serum cortisol and testosterone concentration by inhibiting both adrenal and testicular steroidogenesis.[31] Megestrol is a synthetic derivative of progesterone that exhibits a secondary mechanism of action by inhibiting androgen synthesis. This inhibition appears to occur at the adrenal level, but circulating levels of testosterone are also reduced, suggesting that inhibition at the testicular level may also occur.[31]

Antiandrogens inhibit the formation of the DHT-receptor complex and therefore interfere with androgen activity at the cellular level.[31] The conversion of testosterone to DHT may be inhibited by 5-α-reductase inhibitors.[7]

In advanced stages of disease, prostate cancer cells may be able to survive and proliferate without the signals normally provided by circulating androgens.[31] When this occurs, the tumor is no longer sensitive to therapies that depend on androgen blockade. These tumors are often referred to as hormone refractory or androgen independent.

Prior to the implementation of routine screening, prostate cancers were frequently identified on the investigation of symptoms, including urinary hesitancy, retention, painful urination, hematuria, and erectile dysfunction. With the introduction of screening techniques, most prostate cancers are now identified prior to the development of symptoms, although this may change as routine screening is no longer the norm.

The information obtained from the diagnostic tests is used to stage the patient (Table 131-3). There are two commonly recognized staging classification systems (Table 131-4). The formal international classification system (tumor, node, metastases [TNM]), adopted by the International Union Against Cancer in 1974, was last updated in 2010. The AUS classification is the most commonly used staging system in the United States. Patients are assigned to stages A through D and corresponding subcategories based on size of the tumor (T), local or regional extension, presence of involved lymph node groups (N), and presence of metastases (M). Based on men diagnosed with prostate cancer at Walter Reed Army Medical Center from 1988 to 1998, including more than 2,042 prostate cancer diagnoses, localized prostate cancer (stage T_1 and T_2) was diagnosed more frequently (89% vs 68%), and advanced disease (stages T_3, T_4, and D) was diagnosed less frequently (11% vs 32%) in 1998 as compared to 1988.

3 The prognosis for patients with prostate cancer depends on the histologic grade, the tumor size, and the local extent of the primary tumor.[27] The most important prognostic criterion appears to be the histologic grade, because the degree of differentiation ultimately determines the stage of disease. Poorly differentiated tumors are highly associated with both regional lymph node involvement and distant metastases.[27]

CLINICAL PRESENTATION Prostate Cancer

Localized Disease

- Asymptomatic

Locally Invasive Disease

- Ureteral dysfunction, frequency, hesitancy, and dribbling
- Impotence

Advanced Disease

- Back pain
- Cord compression
- Lower extremity edema
- Pathologic fractures
- Anemia
- Weight loss

TABLE 131-4 Staging and Classification Systems for Prostate Cancer

AUS[a] Stage (A–D)	AJCC-UICC[b] Classification (TNM)
A (occult, nonpalpable)	$T_xN_xM_x$ (cannot be assessed)
A_1: Focal	$T_0N_0M_0$ (nonpalpable)
A_2: Diffuse	T_0: Focal or diffuse
B (confined to prostate)	$T_1N_0M_0$, $T_2N_0M_0$
B_1: Single nodule in one lobe, < 1.5 cm	T_1 (Clinically inapparent tumor not palpable or visible by imaging)
	T_{1a}: Tumor incidental histologic finding in 5% or less of tissue resected
	T_{1b}: Tumor incidental histologic finding in 5% or more of tissue resected
	T_{1c}: Tumor identified by needle biopsy (eg, because of elevated PSA)
B_2: Diffuse involvement of whole gland, > 1.5 cm	T_2: (Tumor confined within the prostate[c]) T_{2a}: Tumor involves half of a lobe or less T_{2b}: Tumor involves more than half a lobe, but not both lobes
	T_{2c}: Tumor involves both lobes
C (localized to periprostatic area)	$T_3N_0M_0$, $T_4N_0M_0$
C_1: No seminal vesicle involvement, < 70 g	T_3: (Tumor extends through the prostatic capsule[d])
	T_{3a}: Unilateral extracapsular extension
	T_{3b}: Bilateral extracapsular extension
	T_{3c}: Tumor invades the seminal vesicle(s)
C_2: Seminal vesicle involvement, > 70 g	T_4: (Tumor is fixed or invades adjacent structures other than the seminal vesicles)
	T_{4a}: Tumor invades any of bladder neck, external sphincter, or rectum
	T_{4b}: Tumor invades levator muscles and/or is fixed to the pelvic wall
D (metastatic disease)	Any T, N_{1-4}, M_0, or N_{0-4}, M_1
D_1: Pelvic lymph nodes or ureteral obstruction	N_1: Metastasis in a single lymph node, 2 cm or less in greatest dimension
D_2: Bone, distant lymph node, organ, or soft tissue metastases	N_2: Metastasis in single lymph node more than 2 cm but not more than 5 cm in greatest dimension; or multiple lymph node metastases, none more than 5 cm in greatest dimension
	N_3: Metastasis in lymph node more than 5 cm in greatest dimension
	M_{1a}: Nonregional lymph node(s)
	M_{1b}: Bone(s)
	M_{1c}: Other site(s)

PSA, prostate-specific antigen.

[a]American Urologic System.

[b]American Joint Committee on Cancer–International Union Against Cancer.

[c]Note: Tumor found in one or both lobes by needle biopsy, but not palpable or visible by imaging, is classified as T_{1c}.

[d]Note: Invasion into the prostatic apex or into (but not beyond) the prostatic capsule is not classified as T_3 but as T_2.

From 1999 to 2005, 5-year overall survival rates were estimated at 100% for whites and 97% for African Americans.[1] For almost the same period, the survival rates for localized or regional disease (100%), and distant disease (30%) in white males were about the same as the survival rates for localized or regional disease (100%), and distant disease (29%) in African American males.[1] A 4.1% decline in age-adjusted mortality has been observed for the period 1994 to 2006. Ten-year cancer-specific survival is estimated as 95% for stage A_1, 80% for stages A_2 to B_2, 60% for stage C, 40% for stage D_1, and 10% for stage D_2. It is estimated that more than 85% of patients with stage A_1 can be cured, while less than 1% of patients with stage D_2 will be cured.

TREATMENT

Desired Outcomes

The desired outcome in early-stage prostate cancer is to minimize morbidity and mortality caused by prostate cancer.[32,33] The most appropriate therapy of early-stage prostate cancer is controversial. Early-stage disease may be treated with surgery, radiation, or expectant management. While surgery and radiation are curative, they are associated with significant morbidity and mortality. Because the overall goal is to minimize morbidity and mortality associated with the disease, watchful waiting is appropriate in selected individuals. Advanced prostate cancer (stage D) is not currently curable, and treatment should provide symptom relief and maintain quality of life. The mainstay of treatment for advanced prostate cancer is ADT, with a goal of reducing testosterone to castrate levels, with either an orchiectomy or an LHRH agonist.

General Approach to Treatment

The initial treatment for prostate cancer depends primarily on the disease stage, the Gleason score, the presence of symptoms, and the life expectancy of the patient.[32] Prostate cancer is usually initially diagnosed by PSA and DRE and confirmed by a biopsy, where the Gleason score is assigned. Asymptomatic patients with a low risk of recurrence, those with a T_1 or T_{2a}, with a Gleason score of 2 through 6, and a PSA of less than 10 ng/mL (mcg/L) may be managed by observation, radiation, or radical prostatectomy (Table 131-5). As patients with asymptomatic early-stage disease generally have an excellent 10-year survival, immediate morbidities of treatment must be balanced with the lower likelihood of dying from prostate cancer. More aggressive treatment of early-stage prostate cancer is generally reserved for younger men, although patient preference is a major consideration in all treatment decisions. In a patient with a normal life expectancy of less than 10 years, observation or radiation therapy may be offered. In those with a normal life expectancy of equal to or greater than 10 years, either observation, radiation (external beam or brachytherapy), or radical prostatectomy with a pelvic lymph node dissection may be offered. Radiation and radical prostatectomy therapy are generally considered therapeutically equivalent for localized prostate cancer, although neither has been proven to be better than observation alone.[34]

Wilt and colleagues conducted a systematic review of 18 randomized trials and 473 observational studies to compare the effectiveness and potential complications from treatment options from prostate cancer. This study showed that the effectiveness of radiation, radical prostatectomy, and ADT could not be compared because of the paucity of high-quality evidence available for analysis. Adverse effect profiles were similar, although severity varied among the treatments.[35] Complications from radical prostatectomy include blood loss, stricture formation, incontinence, lymphocele, fistula formation, anesthetic risk, and impotence. Nerve-sparing radical prostatectomy can be performed in many patients; 50% to 80% regain sexual potency within the first year. However, a recently published prospective study showed that even in patients with good preoperative sexual health, many do not return to baseline after surgery even with the assistance of erectile dysfunction treatments.[36] Acute complications from radiation therapy include cystitis, proctitis, hematuria, urinary retention, penoscrotal edema, and impotence (30% incidence).[27] Chronic complications include proctitis, diarrhea, cystitis, enteritis, impotence, urethral stricture, and incontinence.[27] In addition, ADT can cause cognitive impairment, mood disturbances,

TABLE 131-5 Initial Management of Prostate Cancer Based on Expected Survival and Recurrence Risk

Recurrence Risk	Expected Survival (Years)	Initial Therapy
Very Low		
T_{1c}	< 20	Observation
T_{1c}	20 or more	Observation or Radical prostatectomy with or without pelvic lymph node dissection or Radiation therapy
Low		
T_1–T_{2a} and Gleason 2-6 and PSA less than 10 ng/mL (mcg/L) and < 5% tumor in specimen	10 or more	Observation or Radical prostatectomy with or without pelvic lymph node dissection or radiation therapy
	<10	Observation
Intermediate		
T_{2b}–T_{2c} or Gleason 7 or PSA 10-20 ng/mL (mcg/L)	10 or less	Observation or Radical prostatectomy with pelvic lymph node dissection or Radiation therapy with or without 4-6 months of neoadjuvant androgen deprivation therapy with or without brachytherapy
T_{2b}–T_{2c} or Gleason 7 or PSA 10-20 ng/mL (mcg/L)	10 or more	Radical prostatectomy with pelvic lymph node dissection or Radiation therapy with or without 4-6 months of neoadjuvant androgen deprivation therapy with or without brachytherapy
High		
T_{3a}, Gleason 8-10, PSA > 20 ng/mL (mcg/L)		Radiation therapy and ADT[a] (2-3 years) with or without brachytherapy or Radical prostatectomy and pelvic lymph node dissection
Very High		
T_{3b}-T_4		Radiation therapy and ADT (2-3 years) with or without brachytherapy or Radical prostatectomy and pelvic lymph node dissection or ADT
Very High		
Any T, N_1		ADT (2-3 years) or Radiation therapy and ADT (2-3 years)
Any T, Any N, M_1		ADT with orchiectomy or LHRH agonist[b] + 7 days antiandrogen therapy or LHRH agonist + antiandrogen or LHRH agonist

ADT, androgen-deprivation therapy; LHRH, luteinizing hormone-releasing hormone; PSA, prostate-specific antigen.

[a]Androgen deprivation therapy to achieve serum testosterone levels < 50 ng/dL (1.7 nmol/L).

[b]LHRH agonist, medical castration, or surgical castration are equivalent.

and lack of initiative.[35] Because radiation and prostatectomy have significant and immediate mortality when compared with expectant management alone, many patients may elect to postpone therapy until symptoms develop.

Individuals with T_{2b} and T_{2c} disease or a Gleason score of 7 or a PSA ranging from 10 to 20 ng/mL (mcg/L) are considered at intermediate risk for prostate cancer recurrence.[32] Individuals with less than a 10-year expected survival may be offered observation or radical prostatectomy with pelvic lymph node dissection or radiation therapy with or without 4 to 6 months of neoadjuvant ADT with or without brachytherapy, and those with a greater than or equal to 10-year life expectancy may be offered either radical prostatectomy with or without a pelvic lymph node dissection or radiation therapy with or without 4 to 6 months of neoadjuvant ADT with or without brachytherapy (see Table 131-5).

The treatment of patients at high risk of recurrence (stage T_3, a Gleason score ranging from 8 to 10, or a PSA value greater than 20 ng/mL [mcg/L]) should be treated with androgen ablation for 2 to 3 years combined with radiation therapy with or without brachytherapy (Table 131-5). Selected individuals with a low tumor volume may receive a radical prostatectomy with or without a pelvic lymph node dissection.

Patients with T_{3b} and T_4 disease have a very high risk of recurrence and are usually not candidates for radical prostatectomy because of extensive local spread of disease, although it may be possible for some individuals.[32] (4) ADT with a LHRH agonist plus an antiandrogen should be used prior to radiation therapy for patients with locally advanced prostate cancer to improve outcomes over radiation therapy alone. Recent evidence suggests that androgen ablation should be instituted at diagnosis rather than waiting for symptomatic disease or progression to occur. In a randomized clinical trial of 500 men with locally advanced prostate cancer who were randomized to either immediate initiation of androgen ablation (either orchiectomy or androgen ablation) or deferred hormonal therapy, patients who received immediate therapy had a median actuarial cause-specific survival duration of 7.5 years for immediate treatment as compared with 5.8 years for deferred treatment.[37]

(5) ADT, with orchiectomy, an LHRH agonist alone, an LHRH agonist plus an antiandrogen (combined androgen blockade), or an LHRH with docetaxel without prednisone for six cycles (for patients with visceral metastases and/or four or more bone metastases sites beyond the pelvis or sacrum) can be used to provide palliation for patients with advanced (stage D_2) prostate cancer.

Patients who develop metastatic disease often have tumor progression and develop castration-resistant prostate cancer.[32] This may be described clinically by a rising PSA while on optimal ADT, or the development of symptoms, typically related to bone metastases, including bone pain and fractures. Patients with metastatic disease may be continued on ADT and denosumab ([RANK] ligand inhibitor) or an IV bisphosphonate is added in patients with bone metastases. Importantly, further therapy is determined by the presence of symptomatic disease or whether the metastatic progression is manifested as only a rising PSA.

For clinically asymptomatic patients with a rising PSA, sipuleucel-T is recommended as first-line treatment. Prior to the introduction of sipuleucel-T, standard therapy was a secondary hormonal manipulation, including the addition or withdrawal of antiandrogen therapy.

For those with symptomatic or disease involving internal organs, such as the liver, treatment with docetaxel is recommended as first-line therapy. For patients with symptomatic visceral disease who have a rising PSA enzalutamide or abiraterone acetate are also recommended. Other first-line treatment options following docetaxel chemotherapy include cabazitaxel, a microtubule inhibitor, in combination with prednisone, docetaxel rechallenge, a clinical trial, or mitoxantrone[32] (Fig. 131-3).

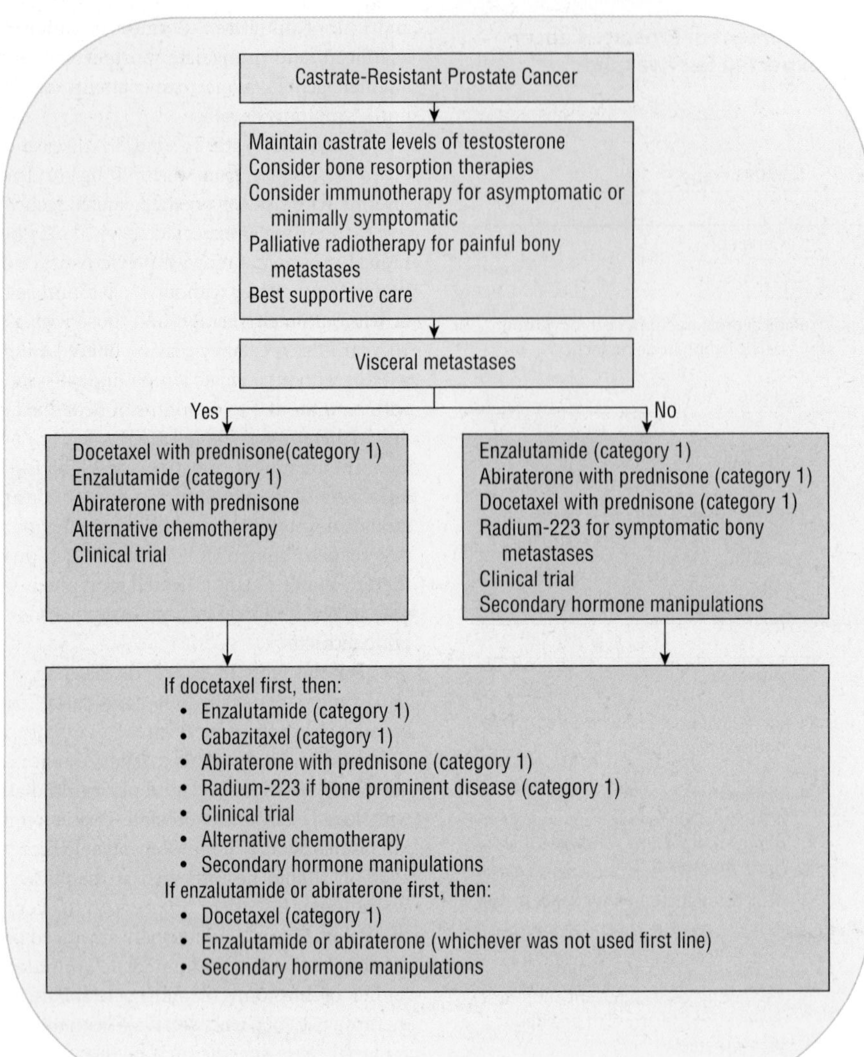

FIGURE 131-3 Treatment of castrate-resistant prostate cancer.

Nonpharmacologic Therapy

Observation

Observation is often referred to as expectant management, active surveillance or watchful waiting. Observation involves monitoring the course of disease and initiating treatment if the cancer progresses. It is estimated that only about 10% of men who are eligible for observation choose this option.[34] A PSA and DRE are performed every 6 months, with a repeat biopsy at any sign of disease progression. The advantages of observation are avoiding the adverse effects associated with definitive therapies such as radiation and radical prostatectomy, and minimizing the risk of unnecessary therapies. The major disadvantage of observation is the risk that the cancer progresses and requires a more intensive therapy.

Orchiectomy

Bilateral orchiectomy, or removal of the testes, is a form of ADT that rapidly reduces circulating androgens to castrate levels (less than 50 ng/dL [1.7 nmol/L]).[22] However, many patients are not surgical candidates because of advanced age, and other patients find this procedure psychologically unacceptable.[26] Orchiectomy is the preferred initial treatment in patients with impending spinal cord compression or ureteral obstruction.

Radiation

The two commonly used methods for radiation therapy are external beam radiotherapy and brachytherapy.[32] In external beam radiotherapy, doses of 70 to 75 Gy (7,000-7,500 rad) are delivered in 35 to 41 fractions in patients with low-grade prostate cancer and 75 to 80 Gy (7,500-8,000 rad) for those with intermediate- or high-grade prostate cancer. Brachytherapy involves the permanent implantation of radioactive beads of 145 Gy (14,500 rad) ^{125}iodine or 124 Gy (12,400 rad) of ^{103}palladium and is generally reserved for individuals with low-risk cancers. Radiation therapy may also be given after surgery in patients with localized disease. Acute complications from radiation therapy include cystitis, proctitis, hematuria, urinary retention, penoscrotal edema, and impotence.[16] Chronic complications include proctitis, diarrhea, cystitis, enteritis, impotence, urethral stricture, and incontinence.[26] Because radiation and prostatectomy have significant and immediate mortality when compared with observation alone, many patients elect to postpone therapy until symptoms develop.

Radical Prostatectomy

Complications from radical prostatectomy include blood loss, stricture formation, incontinence, lymphocele, fistula formation, anesthetic risk, and impotence. Nerve-sparing radical prostatectomy can be performed in many patients; 50% to 80% regain sexual potency within the first year.

Pharmacologic Therapy

Drug Treatments of First Choice

Luteinizing Hormone-Releasing Hormone Agonists LHRH agonists are a reversible method of androgen ablation and are as effective as orchiectomy in treating prostate cancer.[38] Currently available LHRH agonists include leuprolide, leuprolide depot, leuprolide implant, triptorelin depot, triptorelin implant, and goserelin acetate implant. Leuprolide acetate is administered once daily, while leuprolide depot and goserelin acetate implant can be administered either once monthly, once every 12 weeks, or once every 16 weeks (leuprolide depot, every 4 months) (Table 131-6). The leuprolide depot formulation contains leuprolide acetate in coated pellets. The dose is administered intramuscularly, and the coating dissolves at different rates to allow sustained leuprolide levels throughout the dosing interval. Goserelin acetate implant contains goserelin acetate dispersed in a plastic matrix of D, L-lactic, and glycolic acid copolymer and is administered subcutaneously. Hydrolysis of the copolymer material provides continuous release of goserelin over the dosing period. A leuprolide implant is a mini-osmotic pump that delivers 120 mcg of leuprolide daily for 12 months. After 12 months the implant is removed, and a different implant can be placed. Triptorelin LA is administered as an intramuscular injection of 11.25 mg every 84 days. Triptorelin depot is 3.75 mg once every 28 days.

Several randomized trials have demonstrated that leuprolide, goserelin, and triptorelin are effective agents when used alone in patients with advanced prostate cancer.[30] Response rates around 80% have been reported, with a lower incidence of adverse effects as compared with estrogens.[30] The currently available LHRH agonists or the dosage formulations have not been directly compared in clinical trials, but a meta-analysis showed no significant differences in efficacy or toxicity between leuprolide, goserelin, and orchiectomy.[39] Triptorelin is a more recent addition that is generally considered to be equally effective. Therefore the choice between the three agents is usually made based on cost and patient and physician preference for a dosing schedule.

The most common adverse effects reported with LHRH agonist therapy include a disease flare during the first week of therapy, hot flashes, erectile impotence, decreased libido, and injection-site reactions.[30] The disease flare is caused by an initial induction of LH and FSH by the LHRH agonist leading to an initial phase of increased testosterone production, and manifests clinically as either increased bone pain or increased urinary symptoms.[30] This flare reaction usually resolves after 2 weeks and has a similar onset and duration pattern for the depot LHRH products.[40,41] Tumor flare can be minimized by initiating an antiandrogen prior to the administration of the LHRH agonist and continuing for 2 to 4 weeks.[31]

LHRH agonist monotherapy can be used as initial therapy, with response rates similar to those for orchiectomy. The incidence of cardiovascular-related adverse effects is lower with LHRH therapy than with estrogen administration. Patients should be counseled to expect worsening symptoms during the first week of therapy. Appropriate pain and symptom management is required during this period, and a short course of concomitant antiandrogen therapy may need to be considered prior to initiating the LHRH agonist. Caution should be exercised if initiating LHRH agonist therapy in patients with widely metastatic disease involving the spinal cord or having the potential for ureteral obstruction because irreversible complications may occur.

Another potentially serious complication of ADT is a decrease in bone mineral density leading to an increased risk for osteoporosis, osteopenia, and skeletal fractures. During initial therapy, bone mineral density of the hip and spine decreases by 2% to 3%.[42] Additionally, ADT has been associated with a 21% to 45% relative increase in fracture risk.[43-45] Therefore, most clinicians recommend that men starting long-term ADT should have a baseline bone mineral density and be initiated on a calcium and vitamin D supplement.[31,32]

In addition, an antiresorptive agent, either zoledronic acid or denosumab should be considered. A meta-analysis combined data from three identically designed double-blind randomized controlled trials that compared the efficacy and safety of denosumab at a dose of 120 mg with that of zoledronic acid at a dose of 4 mg administered IV.[46] Almost 6,000 patients with breast and prostate cancer and multiple myeloma were included in the meta-analysis. Denosumab reduced the risk of first skeletal-related event (SRE) by 17% (hazard ratio 0.83, 95% CI: 0.76-0.90, $P < 0.001$ for both noninferiority and superiority tests) as compared with zoledronic acid and the median time to first SRE was 27.66 (24.21 to not estimable) months for denosumab versus 19.45 (18.53-21.42) months for zoledronic acid. The benefits were consistent across tumor types evaluated and the incidence of adverse effects was not significantly different between the denosumab and zoledronic acid groups.

ADT has also been associated with a higher incidence of metabolic effects. In a landmark population-based trial, patients treated with an ADT and a gonadotropin-releasing hormone (GnRH) agonist had a greater risk of new-onset diabetes, coronary artery disease, and myocardial infarctions.[47] However, it is not clear whether ADT increases the risk of cardiovascular death. A published meta-analysis of eight trials with 4,141 patients treated with ADT evaluated prostate cancer specific mortality and all-cause mortality.[48] The trials included patients with nonmetastatic disease who were treated with immediate predominantly GnRH-agonist–based ADT versus no immediate ADT (control group). The incidence of cardiovascular deaths was 11.0% (95% CI: 8.3%-14.5%) in the ADT group versus 11.2% (95% CI: 8.3%-15.0%) in the control group. The risk of cardiovascular death for ADT versus control was not significantly different (RR 0.93, 95% CI: 0.79-1.10, P=0.41) and these results suggest that ADT does not lead to increased cardiovascular mortality.[32] Patients receiving ADT should be screened for cardiovascular disease and diabetes and appropriate interventions to prevent and treat these complications should be initiated.[32]

Gonadotropin-Releasing Hormone Antagonists An alternative to LHRH agonists is the approved GnRH antagonist, degarelix. Degarelix works by binding reversibly to GnRH receptors in the pituitary gland, reducing the production of testosterone to castrate levels. The major advantage of degarelix over LHRH agonists is the rapidity at which it reduces testosterone levels. Castration levels are achieved in 7 days or less with degarelix, as compared with 28 days with leuprolide. Tumor flare does not occur and antiandrogens are not required.

In a trial of 610 men with advanced prostate cancer, degarelix was shown to be equivalent to leuprolide in lowering testosterone levels for up to 1 year. Degarelix is available as a 40 mg/mL and a 20 mg/mL vial for subcutaneous injection, and the starting dose is 240 mg followed by 80 mg every 28 days. The starting dose should be divided into two 120 mg injections.[49] Degarelix has not been studied in combination with antiandrogens, and routine use of the combination is not recommended.

The most frequently reported adverse reactions were injection site reactions, including pain (28%), erythema (17%), swelling (6%), induration (4%), and nodules (3%). Most were transient and mild to moderate, leading to discontinuation in less than 1% of study subjects. Other adverse effects included elevations in liver function tests, which occurred in about 10% of study subjects. Osteoporosis may develop, and calcium and vitamin D supplementation should be considered.[49]

Antiandrogens Four antiandrogens, flutamide, bicalutamide, nilutamide, and enzalutamide, are currently available (Table 131-6).[53-64] Cyproterone is another agent with antiandrogen activity, but it is not

TABLE 131-6 Hormonal Therapies for Prostate Cancer[53–64]

Drug (Brand Name)	Usual Dose	Toxicities	Hepatic/Renal Adjustments	Monitoring Parameters	Drug Interactions	Administration
Antiandrogens						
Flutamide (Eulexin)	750 mg/day	Gynecomastia Hot flashes Gastrointestinal disturbances (diarrhea) Loss of libido LFT abnormalities Breast tenderness Methemoglobinemia	Contraindicated in patients with hepatic impairment No dosage adjustment necessary in chronic renal impairment	Serum transaminases should be monitored prior to start of therapy and monthly for first 4 months, then periodically thereafter Monitor for tumor reduction, testosterone/estrogen, and phosphatase serum levels	Substrate of CYP1A2 and CYP3A4	Administered orally in three divided doses; capsule may be opened into applesauce, pudding, or other soft foods
Bicalutamide (Casodex)	50 mg/day (up to 150 mg/day—unlabeled use)	Gynecomastia Hot flashes Gastrointestinal disturbances (diarrhea) Decrease libido LFT abnormalities Breast tenderness	Discontinue if ALT >2 times upper limit of normal or patient develops jaundice	Serum transaminases should be monitored prior to start of therapy and monthly for first 4 months, then periodically thereafter Periodic monitoring of CBC, EKG, echocardiograms, serum testosterone, luteinizing hormone, and PSA	Inhibits CYP3A4 May increase concentration of vitamin K antagonists	May be taken with or without food
Nilutamide (Nilandron)	300 mg/day for first month then 150 mg/day	Gynecomastia Hot flashes Gastrointestinal Disturbances (constipation) LFT abnormalities Breast tenderness Visual disturbances (impaired dark adaptation) Alcohol intolerance Interstitial pneumonitis	Contraindicated in patients with hepatic impairment Discontinue if ALT >2 times upper limit of normal or patient develops jaundice	Serum transaminases should be monitored prior to start of therapy and monthly for first 4 months, then periodically thereafter Chest x-ray at baseline and consideration of pulmonary function testing (at baseline)	Substrate of CYP2C19 and weak inhibitor of CYP2C19	May be taken with or without food
Enzalutamide (Xtandi)	160 mg/day	Gastrointestinal disturbances (diarrhea) Musculoskeletal disorders (back pain, arthralgias, muscle pain, weakness) Asthenia Peripheral edema CNS (headache, dizziness) Seizures LFT abnormalities	No adjustment necessary for renal or hepatic impairment	Complete blood counts baseline and periodically LFTs baseline and periodically	Strong CYP3A4 and moderate CYP2C9 and CYP2C19 inducer; avoid CYP3A4, CYP2C9 and CYP2C19 sensitive substrates. CYP2C8 substrate, avoid strong inducers and inhibitors of CYP2C8 If vitamin K antagonists necessary, conduct additional INR monitoring	May be taken with or without food
Androgen Synthesis Inhibitor						
Abiraterone acetate (Zytiga)	1,000 mg/day + prednisone 5 mg BID	Gastrointestinal disturbances (diarrhea) Edema Hypokalemia Hypophosphatemia LFT abnormalities Hypertriglyceridemia	250 mg daily for Child Pugh Class B; avoid use in Child Pugh Class C Withhold treatment if LFTs >5 times the ULN or bilirubin >3 ULN	Serum transaminases should be monitored prior to start of therapy, every 2 weeks for 3 months, then monthly thereafter Monitor for signs and symptoms of adrenocorticoid insufficiency; monthly for hypertension, hypokalemia, and fluid retention	Substrate of CYP3A4. Use with caution with CYP3A4 inhibitors and inducers. Inhibits CYP1A2, CYP2C19, CYP2C8, CYP2C9, CYP2D6, CYP3A4, and P-glycoprotein Use sensitive substrates with caution	Administer on an empty stomach, at least 1 hour before and 2 hours after food

Luteinizing-Hormone Agonists						
Leuprolide (Lupron)	7.5 mg IM every month 22.5 mg IM every 3 months 30 mg IM every 4 months 45 mg IM every 6 months	Hot flashes Decreased libido Gynecomastia Osteoporosis Fatigue Weight gain	No adjustment necessary for renal or hepatic impairment	Serum testosterone ~4 weeks after initiation, PSA, blood glucose, and $HgbA_{1c}$ prior to initiation and periodically thereafter	May diminish the effects of antidiabetic agents	Vary injection site
Goserelin (Zoladex)	3.6 mg SQ implant every month 10.8 mg SQ implant every 3 months	Hot flashes Decreased libido Gynecomastia Osteoporosis Fatigue Weight gain	No adjustment necessary for renal or hepatic impairment	Monitor bone mineral density, serum calcium, and cholesterol/lipids	May diminish the effects of antidiabetic agents	Vary injection site
Triptorelin (Trelstar)	3.75 mg IM every month 11.25 mg IM every 3 months 22.5 mg IM every 6 months	Hot flashes Decreased libido Gynecomastia Osteoporosis Fatigue Weight gain	No adjustment necessary for renal or hepatic impairment	Monitor serum testosterone levels and prostate specific antigen	May diminish the effects of antidiabetic agents	Vary injection site
Gonadotropin-Releasing Hormone Antagonists						
Degarelix (Firmagon)	240 mg SQ loading dose 80 mg SQ every 28 days (following 28 days after loading dose)	Hot flashes Decreased libido Gynecomastia Osteoporosis Fatigue Weight gain	Use with caution with CL_{cr} <50 mL/min (<0.83 mL/s) Do not use in patients with severe hepatic impairment	Prostate-specific antigen periodically, serum testosterone monthly until castration achieved then every other month, LFTs at baseline in addition to serum electrolytes and bone mineral density	Use with caution with agents that may increase QTC interval	Vary injection site

ALT, alanine aminotransferase; BID, twice daily; CBC, complete blood count; CL_{cr}, creatinine clearance; CNS, central nervous system; CYP, cytochrome P450; EKG, electrocardiogram; $HgbA_{1c}$, hemoglobin A1c; IM, intramuscular injection; INR, international normalized ratio; LFT, liver function test; PSA, prostate-specific antigen; SQ, subcutaneous injection; ULN, upper limit of normal.

available in the United States. Antiandrogens have been used as monotherapy in previously untreated patients, but a recent meta-analysis showed that monotherapy with antiandrogens is less effective than LHRH agonists.[41] Therefore, for advanced prostate cancer, flutamide, bicalutamide, and nilutamide are indicated only in combination with androgen-ablation therapy. Flutamide and bicalutamide are indicated in combination with an LHRH agonist, and nilutamide is indicated in combination with orchiectomy.[50] Antiandrogens can reduce the symptoms from the flare phenomenon associated with LHRH agonist therapy.[31] The Food and Drug Administration (FDA) recently approved the newest androgen-receptor inhibitor, enzalutamide. Enzalutamide, also known as MDV3100, is currently approved as a single agent for patients with metastatic castrate-resistant prostate cancer.[51] As with the other antiandrogens, enzalutamide does not lower androgen levels but inhibits androgen-receptor signaling by competitively inhibiting the binding of androgens without stimulation of the androgen receptor. Enzalutamide may have an advantage over the currently available antiandrogen agents in that it inhibits nuclear translocation of the androgen receptor, DNA binding, and coactivator recruitment. It also has a greater affinity for the androgen receptor and has shown activity in patients resistant to other antiandrogens. Initially approved in docetaxel failure only, the PREVAIL study demonstrated enzalutamide may be used in the first line setting to delay the initiation of chemotherapy.[52]

The most common antiandrogen-related adverse effects are listed in Table 131-7. In the only randomized comparison of bicalutamide plus an LHRH agonist versus flutamide plus an LHRH agonist, diarrhea was more common in flutamide-treated patients. The adverse effects of enzalutamide are similar to those of the other antiandrogens, but enzalutamide does have an increased risk of seizures.

Combined Androgen Blockade Although up to 80% of patients with advanced prostate cancer will respond to initial hormonal manipulation, almost all patients will progress within 2 to 4 years after initiating therapy.[26] Two mechanisms have been proposed to explain this tumor resistance. The tumor could be heterogeneously composed of cells that are hormone-dependent and hormone-independent, or the tumor could be stimulated by extratesticular androgens that are converted intracellularly to DHT. The rationale for combination hormonal therapy is to interfere with multiple hormonal pathways to completely eliminate androgen action. In clinical trials, combination hormonal therapy, sometimes also referred to as maximal androgen deprivation or total androgen blockade, or *combined androgen blockade* (CAB), has been used. The combination of LHRH agonists or orchiectomy with antiandrogens is the most extensively studied CAB approach.

A systematic review of six meta-analyses concluded that the best evidence for CAB came from the largest meta-analysis, conducted by the Prostate Cancer Trialists Collaborative Group including 8,725 patients from 27 trials.[65] That analysis found no difference in overall survival between CAB and castration alone at 2 or 5 years, but a subgroup analysis showed that CAB with nonsteroidal antiandrogens, including flutamide, bicalutamide or nilutamide was associated with a statistically significant improvement in 5-year survival over castration alone (27.6% vs 24.7%, P=0.005). As expected, antiandrogens increased toxicity over placebo.

Although some clinicians consider CAB to be the initial hormonal therapy of choice for newly diagnosed patients, the clinician must weigh the costs of combined therapy against the modest survival benefit.[65] It is appropriate to use either LHRH agonist monotherapy or CAB as initial therapy for metastatic prostate cancer. CAB may be most beneficial in patients with minimal disease and prevents tumor flare, particularly in those with advanced metastatic disease. All other patients may be started on LHRH monotherapy, and an antiandrogen may be added after several months if androgen ablation is incomplete.

It is not clear when to start hormonal-deprivation therapy in patients with advanced prostate cancer.[30] The original recommendation to start therapy when symptoms appeared was based on the Veterans Administration Cooperative Urologic Research Group (VACURG) trials, in which no overall survival difference was demonstrated in patients who either started diethylstilbestrol (DES) initially or crossed over to active treatment when symptoms appeared; the excess mortality was attributed to estrogen administration.[66] Because LHRH agonists and antiandrogens are viable therapies with less cardiovascular toxicity, it is not clear whether delaying therapy is justified with these agents. Reanalysis of the original VACURG data[67] and recent combined ADT trials[66] demonstrate a survival advantage for young, good-performance-status, minimal-disease patients treated initially with hormonal therapy, suggesting that early intervention before symptoms appear may be appropriate.[67]

Alternative Drug Treatments

Secondary or salvage therapies for patients who progress after their initial therapy depend on what was used for initial management.[32] For patients initially diagnosed with localized prostate cancer, radiotherapy can be used in the case of failed radical prostatectomy. Alternatively, androgen ablation can be used in patients who progress after either radiation therapy or radical prostatectomy.

Secondary Hormonal Manipulations In patients treated initially with one hormonal modality, secondary hormonal manipulations may be attempted. This may include adding an antiandrogen to a patient with incomplete suppression of testosterone secretion with an LHRH agonist. In patients that have progression while receiving CAB, withdrawing antiandrogens, or using agents that inhibit androgen synthesis may be attempted. For patients who initially received an LHRH agonist alone, castration testosterone levels should be documented. Patients with inadequate testosterone suppression (greater than 20 ng/dL [0.7 nmol/L]) can be treated by adding an antiandrogen or performing an orchiectomy. If castration testosterone levels have been achieved, the patient is considered to have androgen-independent disease, and palliative androgen-independent salvage therapy can be used.

6 Antiandrogen withdrawal, for patients having progressive disease while receiving CAB with an LHRH agonist plus an antiandrogen, can provide additional symptomatic relief. Mutations in the androgen receptor have been documented that cause antiandrogens to act like receptor agonists.

If the patient initially received CAB with an LHRH agonist and an antiandrogen, then androgen withdrawal is the first salvage manipulation.[32] Objective and subjective responses have been noted following the discontinuation of flutamide,[68] bicalutamide,[69] or nilutamide[70] in patients receiving these agents as part of combined androgen ablation with an LHRH agonist. Mutations in the androgen receptor have been demonstrated that allow antiandrogens such as flutamide, bicalutamide, and nilutamide (or their metabolites) to become agonists and activate the androgen receptor.[71] Patient responses to androgen withdrawal manifest as significant PSA reductions and improved clinical symptoms. Androgen withdrawal responses lasting 3 to 14 months have been observed in up to 35% of patients, and responses appear to be most closely related to longer androgen exposure times. Incomplete cross-resistance has been noted in some patients who received bicalutamide after they had progressed while receiving flutamide.[72] The addition of an agent that blocks adrenal androgen synthesis, such as aminoglutethimide, at the time that androgens are withdrawn may produce a better response than androgen withdrawal alone.[71] Because of the potential for response immediately after antiandrogen withdrawal, a sufficient observation and assessment period (usually 4-6 weeks) is usually

TABLE 131-7 Chemotherapy and Immunotherapy for Prostate Cancer[62-64]

Drug (Brand Name)	Usual Dose	Toxicities	Hepatic/Renal Adjustments	Monitoring Parameters	Drug Interactions	Administration
Antimicrotubule Agents						
Docetaxel (Taxotere)	75 mg/m² IV every 3 weeks	Fluid retention, alopecia, mucositis, myelosuppression, hypersensitivity	Aspartate transaminase/alanine transaminase >1.5 times the upper limit of normal and alkaline phosphatase >2.5 times the upper limit of normal do not administer	CBC with differential, LFTs, bilirubin, alkaline phosphatase, renal function Monitor for hypersensitivity reactions	Avoid concomitant use of CYP3A4 inhibitors	Administer IV infusion over 1 hour. Premedication with corticosteroids for 3 days beginning the day before
Cabazitaxel (Jevtana)	25 mg/m² IV every 3 weeks	Fluid retention, constipation, mucositis, myelosuppression, hypersensitivity	Discontinue if ALT >2 times upper limit of normal or patient develops jaundice	CBC weekly during first cycle, then prior to each treatment. Monitor for hypersensitivity	Avoid concomitant use of CYP3A4 inducers and inhibitors	Administer IV infusion over 1 hour
Immunotherapy						
Sipuleucel-T (Provenge)	Each injection contains >50 million autologous CD54+ cells (obtained through leukapheresis) activated with PAP-GM-CSF. Dose is given ~ every 2 weeks for 3 total doses	Hypersensitivity, chills, fatigue, fever, headache, myalgias	No dosage adjustment necessary for renal or hepatic dysfunction	No specific laboratory monitoring recommended	Immunosuppressants may decrease the therapeutic effects of sipuleucel-T	Administer IV infusion over 1 hour. Observe patient for 30 minutes after the completion of the infusion. Premedicate with acetaminophen and an antihistamine 30 minutes prior to administration

ALT, alanine aminotransferase; CBC, complete blood count; CYP, cytochrome P450; LFT, liver function test; PAP-GM-CSF, prostatic acid phosphatase granulocyte-macrophage colony-stimulating factor.

required before a patient can be enrolled on a clinical trial evaluating a new agent or therapy for advanced prostate cancer.

Androgen synthesis inhibitors, such as aminoglutethimide or ketoconazole, can provide symptomatic relief for a short time in about 50% of patients with progressive disease despite previous androgen-ablation therapy.[32] Adverse effects during aminoglutethimide therapy occur in about 50% of patients.[32] Central nervous system effects that include lethargy, ataxia, and dizziness are the major adverse reactions. A generalized morbilliform, pruritic rash has been reported in up to 30% of patients treated. The rash is usually self-limiting and resolves within 5 to 8 days with continued therapy. Adverse effects from ketoconazole include gastrointestinal intolerance, transient rises in liver and renal function tests, and hypoadrenalism. Ketoconazole is combined with replacement doses of hydrocortisone to prevent symptomatic hypoadrenalism.[32]

Abiraterone is the newest androgen synthesis inhibitor that targets cytochrome P450 (CYP)17A1, which results in a decrease in circulating levels of testosterone.[73] Abiraterone is indicated in patients with metastatic castration-resistant prostate cancer, either before or after docetaxel-based chemotherapy. The initial approval was based on the results of a phase III study of patients previously treated with a docetaxel-containing regimen. The combination of abiraterone and prednisone increased median overall survival by 3.9 months in comparison to placebo. Hypertension, hypokalemia, and edema may occur due to hypoadrenalism. Abiraterone is available as the prodrug, abiraterone acetate, and should be taken on an empty stomach as food increases bioavailability by up to 10-fold. Monitoring of liver function tests is recommended at baseline, every 2 weeks for the first 3 months, and then monthly thereafter. Since abiraterone is an inhibitor of CYP2D6, medication profiles should be reviewed for potential drug interactions prior to initiation of abiraterone therapy.[73]

7 **Chemotherapy** Chemotherapy with docetaxel and prednisone improves survival in patients with castrate-refractory prostate cancer and is considered first-line therapy for these patients. Docetaxel 75 mg/m^2 every 3 weeks combined with prednisone 5 mg twice a day improves survival in hormone-refractory metastatic prostate cancer.[74] The most common adverse events with this regimen are nausea, alopecia, and bone marrow suppression. Other adverse effects of docetaxel include fluid retention and peripheral neuropathy. Docetaxel is metabolized in the liver; patients with hepatic impairment may not be eligible for treatment with docetaxel because of an increased risk for toxicity (see Table 131-7).

Cabazitaxel is a taxane with demonstrated activity in docetaxel resistant cell lines and animal models of human cancer.[75] Cabazitaxel has lower affinity for P-glycoprotein multidrug resistance transporter than docetaxel, which may explain why cabazitaxel is active in the setting of docetaxel resistance. In patients previously treated with docetaxel and prednisone, treatment with cabazitaxel 25 mg/m^2 every 3 weeks with prednisone 10 mg daily significantly improved progression-free survival and overall survival as compared to mitoxantrone and prednisone. Neutropenia, febrile neutropenia, neuropathy, and diarrhea are the most significant toxicities. Hypersensitivity reactions may occur and premedication with an antihistamine, a corticosteroid, and an H_2 antagonist is recommended. Cabazitaxel is extensively metabolized in the liver and should be avoided in patients with hepatic dysfunction (see Table 131-7). Mitoxantrone plus prednisone has not demonstrated a survival improvement after failure of docetaxel, but remains a palliative therapeutic option, specifically in men who are not candidates for cabazitaxel or radium-223 therapy.[32]

Immunotherapy Sipuleucel-T is a novel autologous cellular immunotherapy that was FDA-approved in April 2010 for the treatment of asymptomatic or minimally symptomatic metastatic hormone-refractory prostate cancer.[76] Alternative treatment options for this patient population are secondary hormonal therapy, including antiandrogen therapy, withdrawal of antiandrogen therapy, ketoconazole, abiraterone acetate, enzalutamide, steroids, estrogen, or enrollment on a clinical trial, although none of these options has been shown to improve overall survival. No clinical trials have compared sipuleucel-T to secondary hormonal therapies. Patients treated with sipuleucel-T undergo leukapheresis on day 1 to collect peripheral blood mononuclear cells, the cellular fraction that includes immune effector cells. These cells are incubated with a prostatic acid phosphatase (PAP)–granulocyte-macrophage colony-stimulating factor (GM-CSF) fusion protein; PAP is the specific tumor antigen, and GM-CSF is the immune cell activator. The cellular product is then infused IV into the patient on day 3 or 4, providing an autologous infusion of activated cells. Each course of sipuleucel-T consists of three infusions of activated cells, given every 2 weeks. In the pivotal trial, sipuleucel-T prolonged median survival by 4.1 months and reduced the risk of death by 22% (HR 0.78, 95% CI: 0.61-0.98, P=0.03).[76] Adverse effects related to sipuleucel-T were generally mild and nearly all patients were able to receive the entire course (ie, 3 infusions). A course of sipuleucel-T costs about $93,000, and some insurers have questioned the value of the therapy.

Clinical **Controversy...**

The use of sipuleucel-T is controversial. The treatment is indicated for minimally symptomatic prostate cancer and has not been compared to standard second-line hormonal interventions.

Nuclear Medicine Radium-223, an alpha emitter, can be administered to target specific bone metastases with alpha particles in patients with metastatic, castrate-resistant prostate cancer. Radium-223 administered every 4 weeks improved overall survival by 2.8 months in patients who had received, were not eligible for, or had declined docetaxel therapy. Improvements in skeletal pain, pain-related outcomes, and quality of life were also significant. Opioid needs were decreased in patients who received radium-223 (36% vs 50%). The most common side effects of radium-223 include nausea, diarrhea, vomiting, peripheral edema, and bone marrow suppression .[77] Radium-223 is a category 1 recommendation and may be used in first-, second-, or third-line therapy in patients with metastatic castrate resistant prostate cancer with symptomatic primary bone metastases. Radium-223 has not been approved for use with concomitant chemotherapy.

PERSONALIZED PHARMACOTHERAPY

Prevention strategies for prostate cancer, specifically whether to undergo PSA screening for early detection or whether to start chemoprevention with finasteride or dutasteride in an effort to prevent prostate cancer, are highly personalized decisions and depend on an individual patient weighing the risks and benefits of either strategy. This is a major change from previous recommendations, which uniformly recommended screening regardless of age, health status or patient preference.

Prostate cancer therapy is personalized based on clinical factors, including stage of cancer, life expectancy of the patient, and a patient's fitness for surgical interventions (see Table 131-5). Agents used in the treatment of prostate cancer are often personalized with dose adjustments for organ dysfunction of other clinical characteristics (see Table 131-7). Although there are no current selection strategies where individuals with a specific mutation receive a specific therapy, this remains an important area of research.

EVALUATION OF THERAPEUTIC OUTCOMES

Monitoring of prostate cancer depends on the stage of the cancer.[32] When definitive, curative therapy is attempted, objective parameters to assess tumor response include assessment of the primary tumor size, evaluation of involved lymph nodes, and the response of tumor markers such as PSA to treatment. Following definitive therapy, the PSA level is checked every 6 months for the first 5 years, then annually. Local recurrence in the absence of a rising PSA may occur, so a DRE is also performed. In the metastatic setting, chemotherapy and novel hormonal manipulations have been shown to prolong overall survival. In addition, clinical benefit responses can be documented by evaluating performance status changes, weight changes, quality of life, and analgesic requirements, in addition to the PSA or DRE at 3-month intervals.

ABBREVIATIONS

ADT	androgen-deprivation therapy
AUA	American Urologic Association
BPH	benign prostatic hyperplasia
CAB	combined androgen blockade
CI	confidence interval
CYP	cytochrome P450
DES	diethylstilbestrol
DHT	dihydrotestosterone
DRE	digital rectal examination
ERSPC	European Randomized Study of Screening for Prostate Cancer
FDA	Food and Drug Administration
FSH	follicle-stimulating hormone
GM-CSF	granulocyte-macrophage colony-stimulating factor
GnRH	gonadotropin-releasing hormone
LH	luteinizing hormone
LHRH	luteinizing hormone–releasing hormone
PAP	prostatic acid phosphatase
PCPT	Prostate Cancer Prevention Trial
PLCO	Prostate, Lung, Colon, and Ovarian Screening (study)
PSA	prostate-specific antigen
RANK	receptor activator of nuclear factor k B
REDUCE	Reduction by Dutasteride of Prostate Cancer Events
RR	Relative risk
SELECT	Selenium and Vitamin E Cancer Prevention Trial
SRE	skeletal-related event
TNM	tumor, node, metastases
USPSTF	United States Preventative Services Task Force
VACURG	Veterans Administration Cooperative Urologic Research Group

REFERENCES

1. Siegel RL, Miller KD, Jemal A. Cancer statistics, 2016. *CA Cancer J Clin* 2016;66:7-30.
2. Hsieh K, Albertsen PC. Populations at high risk for prostate cancer. *Urol Clin North Am* 2003;30:669-676.
3. Sun JH, Lee SA. Association between CAG repeat polymorphisms and the risk of prostate cancer: a meta-analysis by race, study design and the number of (CAG)n repeat polymorphisms. *Int J Mol Med* 2013;32:1195-1203.
4. Crawford ED. Epidemiology of prostate cancer. *Urology* 2003;62(6 Suppl 1): 3-12.
5. Maia S, Cardoso M, Paulo P, et al. The role of germline mutations in the BRCA1/2 and mismatch repair genes in men ascertained for early-onset and/or familial prostate cancer. *Fam Cancer* 2015. [Epub ahead of print]
6. Schwingshackl L, Hoffmann G. Adherence to Mediterranean diet and risk of cancer: A systematic review and meta-analysis of observational studies. *Int J Cancer* 2014;135:1884-1897.
7. Mandair D, Rossi RE, Pericleous M, Whyand T, Caplin ME. Prostate cancer and the influence of dietary factors and supplements: A systematic review. *Nutr Metab (Lond)* 2014;11:30.
8. Wilt TJ, Macdonald R, Hagerty K, et al. 5-alpha-Reductase inhibitors for prostate cancer chemoprevention: an updated Cochrane systematic review. *BJU Int* 2010;106:1444-1451.
9. Thompson IM, Goodman PJ, Tangen CM, et al. The influence of finasteride on the development of prostate cancer. *N Engl J Med* 2003;349:215-224.
10. Andriole GL, Bostwick DG, Brawley OW, et al. Effect of dutasteride on the risk of prostate cancer. *N Engl J Med* 2010;362:1192-1202.
11. Lacy JM, Kyprianou N. A tale of two trials: The impact of 5α-reductase inhibition on prostate cancer. *Oncol Lett* 2014;8:1391-1396.
12. Redman MW, Tangen CM, Goodman PJ, Lucia MS, Coltman CA Jr, Thompson IM. Finasteride does not increase the risk of high-grade prostate cancer: A bias-adjusted modeling approach. *Cancer Prev Res (Phila)* 2008;1:174-181.
13. Kramer BS, Hagerty KL, Justman S, et al. Use of 5 alpha-reductase inhibitors for prostate cancer chemoprevention: American Society of Clinical Oncology/American Urological Association 2008 Clinical Practice Guideline. *J Urol* 2009;181:1642-1657.
14. Klein EA, Thompson IM Jr, Tangen CM, et al. Vitamin E and the risk of prostate cancer: the Selenium and Vitamin E Cancer Prevention Trial (SELECT). *JAMA* 2011;306:1549-1556.
15. Thompson IM, Tangen CM, Goodman PJ, Lucia MS, Klein EA. Chemoprevention of prostate cancer. *J Urol* 2009;182:499-507.
16. Cuzick J, Thorat MA, Andriole G, et al. Prevention and early detection of prostate cancer. *Lancet Oncol* 2014;15:e484-e492.
17. Carter HB, Albertsen PC, Barry MJ, et al. Early detection of prostate cancer: AUA Guideline. *J Urol* 2013;190(2):419-426.
18. Thompson IM, Pauler DK, Goodman PJ, et al. Prevalence of prostate cancer among men with a prostate-specific antigen level < or =4.0 ng per milliliter. *N Engl J Med* 2004;350:2239-2246.
19. Shteynshlyuger A, Andriole GL. Prostate cancer: to screen or not to screen? *Urol Clin North Am* 2010;37:1-9.
20. Wolf AM, Wender RC, Etzioni RB, et al. American Cancer Society guideline for the early detection of prostate cancer: update 2010. *CA Cancer J Clin* 2010;60:70-98.
21. Moyer VA. Screening for prostate cancer: U.S. Preventive Services Task Force recommendation statement. *Ann Intern Med* 2012;157:120-134.
22. Sammon JD, Abdollah F, Choueiri TK, et al. Prostate-Specific Antigen Screening After 2012 US Preventive Services Task Force Recommendations. *JAMA* 2015 Nov 17;314:2077-2079.
23. Schroder FH, Hugosson J, Roobol MJ, et al. Prostate-cancer mortality at 11 years of follow-up. *N Engl J Med* 2012;366:981-990.
24. Andriole GL, Crawford ED, Grubb RL 3rd, et al. Prostate cancer screening in the randomized Prostate, Lung, Colorectal, and Ovarian Cancer Screening Trial: mortality results after 13 years of follow-up. *J Natl Cancer Inst* 2012;104:125-132.
25. Gulati R, Gore JL, Etzioni R. Comparative effectiveness of alternative prostate-specific antigen--based prostate cancer screening strategies: Model estimates of potential benefits and harms. *Ann Intern Med* 2013;158:145-153.
26. Khauli RB. Prostate cancer: diagnostic and therapeutic strategies with emphasis on the role of PSA. *J Med Liban* 2005;53:95-102.
27. Iczkowski KA. Current prostate biopsy interpretation: criteria for cancer, atypical small acinar proliferation, high-grade prostatic intraepithelial neoplasia, and use of immunostains. *Arch Pathol Lab Med* 2006;130:835-843.
28. De Marzo AM, Meeker AK, Zha S, et al. Human prostate cancer precursors and pathobiology. *Urology* 2003;62(5 Suppl 1):55-62.
29. Culig Z. Role of the androgen receptor axis in prostate cancer. *Urology* 2003;62(5 Suppl 1):21-26.
30. Marks LS. Luteinizing hormone-releasing hormone agonists in the treatment of men with prostate cancer: timing, alternatives, and the 1-year implant. *Urology* 2003;62(6 Suppl 1):36-42.
31. Sharifi N, Gulley JL, Dahut WL. Androgen deprivation therapy for prostate cancer. *JAMA* 2005;294:238-244.
32. National Comprehensive Cancer Network. National Comprehensive Cancer Network guidelines for the management of prostate cancer. 2015; Available at: http://www.nccn.org/professionals/physician_gls/pdf/prostate.pdf v1.2016.
33. Scher HI. Prostate carcinoma: defining therapeutic objectives and improving overall outcomes. *Cancer* 2003;97(3 Suppl): 758-771.

34. Ganz PA, Barry JM, Burke W, et al. National Institutes of Health State-of-the-Science Conference: Role of active surveillance in the management of men with localized prostate cancer. *Ann Intern Med* 2012;156:591-595.
35. Wilt TJ, MacDonald R, Rutks I, Shamliyan TA, Taylor BC, Kane RL. Systematic review: comparative effectiveness and harms of treatments for clinically localized prostate cancer. *Ann Intern Med* 2008;148:435-448.
36. Dalkin BL, Christopher BA. Potent men undergoing radical prostatectomy: a prospective study measuring sexual health outcomes and the impact of erectile dysfunction treatments. *Urol Oncol* 2008;26(3):281-285.
37. Immediate versus deferred treatment for advanced prostatic cancer: Initial results of the Medical Research Council Trial. The Medical Research Council Prostate Cancer Working Party Investigators Group. *Br J Urol* 1997;79:235-246.
38. Novara G, Galfano A, Secco S, Ficarra V, Artibani W. Impact of surgical and medical castration on serum testosterone level in prostate cancer patients. *Urol Int* 2009;82:249-255.
39. Seidenfeld J, Samson DJ, Aronson N, et al. Relative effectiveness and cost-effectiveness of methods of androgen suppression in the treatment of advanced prostate cancer. *Evid Rep Technol Assess (Summ)* 1999(4): i-x, 1-246, I241-236, passim.
40. Hedlund PO, Henriksson P. Parenteral estrogen versus total androgen ablation in the treatment of advanced prostate carcinoma: effects on overall survival and cardiovascular mortality. The Scandinavian Prostatic Cancer Group (SPCG)-5 Trial Study. *Urology* 2000;55:328-333.
41. Seidenfeld J, Samson DJ, Hasselblad V, et al. Single-therapy androgen suppression in men with advanced prostate cancer: A systematic review and meta-analysis. *Ann Intern Med* 2000;132:566-577.
42. Smith MR, Finkelstein JS, McGovern FJ, et al. Changes in body composition during androgen deprivation therapy for prostate cancer. *J Clin Endocrinol Metab* 2002;87:599-603.
43. Shahinian VB, Kuo YF, Freeman JL, Goodwin JS. Risk of fracture after androgen deprivation for prostate cancer. *N Engl J Med* 2005;352:154-164.
44. Smith MR, Boyce SP, Moyneur E, Duh MS, Raut MK, Brandman J. Risk of clinical fractures after gonadotropin-releasing hormone agonist therapy for prostate cancer. *J Urol* 2006;175:136-139.
45. Smith MR, Lee WC, Brandman J, Wang Q, Botteman M, Pashos CL. Gonadotropin-releasing hormone agonists and fracture risk: a claims-based cohort study of men with nonmetastatic prostate cancer. *J Clin Oncol* 2005;23:7897-7903.
46. Lipton A, Fizazi K, Stopeck AT, et al. Superiority of denosumab to zoledronic acid for prevention of skeletal-related events: A combined analysis of 3 pivotal, randomised, phase 3 trials. *Eur J Cancer* 2012;48:3082-3092.
47. Keating NL, O'Malley AJ, Smith MR. Diabetes and cardiovascular disease during androgen deprivation therapy for prostate cancer. *J Clin Oncol* 2006;24:4448-4456.
48. Nguyen PL, Je Y, Schutz FA, et al. Association of androgen deprivation therapy with cardiovascular death in patients with prostate cancer: A meta-analysis of randomized trials. *JAMA* 2011;306:2359-2366.
49. Klotz L, Boccon-Gibod L, Shore ND, et al. The efficacy and safety of degarelix: A 12-month, comparative, randomized, open-label, parallel-group phase III study in patients with prostate cancer. *BJU In.* 2008;102:1531-1538.
50. Akaza H. Combined androgen blockade for prostate cancer: Review of efficacy, safety and cost-effectiveness. *Cancer Sci* 2011;102:51-56.
51. Scher HI, Fizazi K, Saad F, et al. Increased survival with enzalutamide in prostate cancer after chemotherapy. *N Engl J Med* 2012;367:1187-1197.
52. Beer TM, Armstrong AJ, Rahkopf DE, et al. Enzalutamide in Metastatic Prostate Cancer before Chemotherapy. *NEJM* 2014;371:424-433.
53. Flutamide [package insert]. Kenilworth, NJ: Schering Corporation, 2000.
54. Bicalutamide [package insert]. Wilmington, DE: AstraZeneca Pharmaceuticals LP, 2000.
55. Nilutamide [package insert]. Bridgewater, NJ: Sanofi-Aventis, 2006.
56. Enzalutamide [package insert]. Northbrook, IL: Astellas Pharma, 2015.
57. Abiraterone [package insert]. Horsham, PA: Janssen Biotech, 2015.
58. Leuprolide [package insert]. Irvine, CA: SICOR Pharmaceuticals, 2005.
59. Goserelin [package insert]. Wilmington, DE: AstraZeneca Pharmaceuticals LP, 2012.
60. Triptorelin [package insert]. Kalamazoo, MI: Pharmacia & Upjohn Company, 2001.
61. Degarelix [package insert]. Parsippany, NJ: Ferring Pharmaceuticals, 2012.
62. Docetaxel [package insert]. Bridgewater, NJ: Sanofi-Aventis, 2011.
63. Cabazitaxel [package insert]. Bridgewater, NJ: Sanofi-Aventis, 2012.
64. Sipuleucel-T [package insert]. Seattle, WA: Dendreon Corporation, 2011.
65. Lukka H, Waldron T, Klotz L, Winquist E, Trachtenberg J. Maximal androgen blockade for the treatment of metastatic prostate cancer–a systematic review. *Curr Oncol* 2006;13:81-93.
66. Carcinoma of the prostate: treatment comparisons. *J Urol* 1967;98:516-522.
67. Ryan CJ, Small EJ. Early versus delayed androgen deprivation for prostate cancer: New fuel for an old debate. *J Clin Oncol* 2005;23:8225-8231.
68. Scher HI, Kelly WK. Flutamide withdrawal syndrome: Its impact on clinical trials in hormone-refractory prostate cancer. *J Clin Oncol* 1993;11:1566-1572.
69. Small EJ, Srinivas S. The antiandrogen withdrawal syndrome. Experience in a large cohort of unselected patients with advanced prostate cancer. *Cancer* 1995;76:1428-1434.
70. Huan SD, Gerridzen RG, Yau JC, Stewart DJ. Antiandrogen withdrawal syndrome with nilutamide. *Urology* 1997;49:632-634.
71. Sartor O, Cooper M, Weinberger M, et al. Surprising activity of flutamide withdrawal, when combined with aminoglutethimide, in treatment of "hormone-refractory" prostate cancer. *J Natl Cancer Inst* 1994;86:222-227.
72. Scher HI, Liebertz C, Kelly WK, et al. Bicalutamide for advanced prostate cancer: the natural versus treated history of disease. *J Clin Oncol* 1997;15:2928-2938.
73. de Bono JS, Logothetis CJ, Molina A, et al. Abiraterone and increased survival in metastatic prostate cancer. *N Engl J Med* 2011;364:1995-2005.
74. Tannock IF, de Wit R, Berry WR, et al. Docetaxel plus prednisone or mitoxantrone plus prednisone for advanced prostate cancer. *N Engl J Med* 2004;351:1502-1512.
75. de Bono JS, Oudard S, Ozguroglu M, et al. Prednisone plus cabazitaxel or mitoxantrone for metastatic castration-resistant prostate cancer progressing after docetaxel treatment: a randomised open-label trial. *Lancet* 2010;376:1147-1154.
76. Kantoff PW, Higano CS, Shore ND, et al. Sipuleucel-T immunotherapy for castration-resistant prostate cancer. *N Engl J Med* 2010;363:411-422.
77. Parker C, Nilsson S, Heinrich D, et al. Alpha emitter radium-223 and survival in metastatic prostate cancer. *N Engl J Med* 2013;369:213-223.

132

Lymphomas

Alexandre Chan and Jolynn Sessions

KEY CONCEPTS

1 With all stages and risk-groups of Hodgkin lymphoma, restaging PET-CT following about 8 to 12 weeks of chemotherapy will further guide the patient-specific treatment plan.

2 Patients with early stage Hodgkin lymphoma should be treated with combination chemotherapy with or without involved-site radiation.

3 Combination chemotherapy with doxorubicin (Adriamycin®), bleomycin, vinblastine, and dacarbazine (ABVD) is the primary treatment for patients with advanced-stage Hodgkin lymphoma. Patients with advanced unfavorable disease may be treated with more aggressive regimens, but are associated with a higher risk of secondary malignancies.

4 Some patients with Hodgkin lymphoma will be refractory to initial therapy or will have a recurrence following a complete remission. Response to salvage therapy depends on the extent and site of recurrence, previous therapy, and duration of initial remission. High-dose chemotherapy and autologous hematopoietic stem cell transplantation (HSCT) should be considered in patients with refractory or relapsed disease.

5 The current classification system for non-Hodgkin lymphoma (NHL) is the World Health Organization (WHO) classification system, which is based on the principle that NHLs can be classified into specific disease entities, defined by a combination of morphology, immunophenotype, genetic features, and clinical features.

6 As compared with Hodgkin lymphoma, the clinical presentation of NHL is more variable because of disease heterogeneity and more frequent extranodal involvement.

7 The Ann Arbor staging system correlates poorly with prognosis in NHL because the disease does not spread through contiguous lymph nodes and often involves extranodal sites.

8 Several prognostic models have been developed to estimate prognosis in patients with NHL. The International Prognostic Index (IPI) score is a well-established model for patients with aggressive NHL. The Follicular Lymphoma International Prognostic Index (FLIPI) is a similar model used for patients with follicular and other indolent lymphomas.

9 The clinical behavior and degree of aggressiveness can be used to categorize NHL into indolent and aggressive lymphomas. Patients with an indolent lymphoma usually have a relatively long survival, with or without aggressive chemotherapy. Although these lymphomas respond to a wide range of therapeutic approaches, few if any of these patients are cured of their disease. In contrast, aggressive lymphomas are rapidly growing tumors and patients have a short survival if appropriate therapy is not initiated. Most patients with aggressive lymphomas respond to intensive chemotherapy and many are cured of their disease.

10 Patients with localized follicular lymphoma can be cured with radiation therapy alone. Advanced follicular lymphoma is not curable, and many treatment options are available, including watchful waiting, extended-field radiation therapy, single-agent alkylating agents, anthracycline-containing combination chemotherapy, anti-CD20 monoclonal antibodies, fludarabine, lenalidomide, idelalisib, and high-dose chemotherapy with HSCT.

11 Patients with localized aggressive lymphomas can be cured with several cycles of R-CHOP (rituximab, cyclophosphamide, doxorubicin [hydroxydaunorubicin], vincristine [Oncovin®], prednisone) chemotherapy and involved-field irradiation. Patients with bulky stage II, stage III, or stage IV aggressive lymphomas can be cured of their disease with R-CHOP chemotherapy.

12 Conventional-dose salvage therapy can induce responses in patients with aggressive lymphomas who relapse, but long-term survival and cure are uncommon. Some patients with aggressive lymphoma who relapse and respond to salvage therapy can be cured with high-dose chemotherapy and autologous HSCT.

INTRODUCTION

Lymphomas are a heterogeneous group of malignancies that arise from malignant transformation of immune cells that reside predominantly in lymphoid tissues. They most commonly present as a solid tumor, but can sometimes present as circulating tumor cells in peripheral blood. The differing histology of lymphoma cells has led to classification of Hodgkin lymphoma (Reed–Sternberg cells) or non-Hodgkin lymphoma (NHL) (B- or T-cell lymphocyte markers). NHLs are further classified into distinct clinical entities, which are defined by a combination of morphology, immunophenotype, genetic features, and clinical features. Chemotherapy is the mainstay of treatment in patients with lymphoma, especially those with widespread disease. Overall cure rates are high for many subtypes of lymphomas, even when patients present with advanced disease.

HODGKIN LYMPHOMA

Hodgkin lymphoma is one of the most curable forms of cancer. Although initial reports of Hodgkin lymphoma demonstrated the disease to be uniformly fatal, an impressive 80% of patients can be cured today with recommended treatments.[1] Some of the keys to the success of the treatments for Hodgkin lymphoma include: (1) use of multidrug chemotherapy regimens with differing mechanisms of action and toxicities, and (2) treatment with full doses of chemotherapy and on schedule whenever possible. It is also common to use radiation therapy in the treatment schema. However, the success of treatment has not been without cost. The treatment programs are intense, technically demanding, and associated with considerable acute toxicity and long-term complications. The long-term effects, particularly secondary malignancies, account for a higher cumulative mortality than Hodgkin lymphoma 15 to 20 years after treatment. Long-term toxicities with standard chemotherapy regimens have been more fully documented in recent years and are shaping future therapies.[3-5]

Hodgkin lymphoma is named after Thomas Hodgkin, who first described seven cases of a mysterious disease of the lymph system in 1832. Although Hodgkin lymphoma was not the first cancer to be described, it was one of the first cancers to have methodical investigational treatments that ultimately lead to successful outcomes.[5]

Since many factors influence prognosis of patients with Hodgkin lymphoma, treatment plans must be personalized for each patient. The staging for Hodgkin lymphoma differs from other cancers, and uses the Ann Arbor Staging Classification where the "A" refers to the absence of B-symptoms, and "B" refers to the presence of B-symptoms. Beyond the stage of the disease, certain factors have been associated with a poor prognosis (unfavorable risk). Several research groups have defined these unfavorable factors, and the International Prognostic Score (IPS) is used clinically to predict an individual's risk of recurrence.

Epidemiology and Etiology

Hodgkin lymphoma represents less than 1% of all known cancers in the United States. It is estimated that 8,500 new cases of Hodgkin lymphoma will be diagnosed in the United States in 2016, and there will be 1,150 deaths associated with Hodgkin lymphoma during this same period.[6] Hodgkin lymphoma occurs slightly more frequently in males than in females. It exhibits bimodal distribution in industrialized countries; the first peak occurs in young adults and the second smaller peak occurs after age 50.[3,5] The 5-year overall survival for all stages of Hodgkin lymphoma is about 85%.[7] Death as a consequence of recurrent Hodgkin lymphoma is less than those from all other causes 15 years after treatment.[8]

The etiology of Hodgkin lymphoma is currently unknown, but laboratory and epidemiologic evidence support infectious exposure as a potential cause.[3,5] Studies suggest an increased risk of Hodgkin lymphoma in patients who have been infected with the Epstein-Barr's virus (EBV); and many patients experience EBV activation even before the onset of Hodgkin lymphoma. EBV is found in about 40% of all classical Hodgkin lymphoma cases, and it is frequently observed in cases of mixed cellularity and lymphocyte-depleted Hodgkin lymphoma.[9] Reed–Sternberg cells (large, bilobate, multinuclear cells looking like "owl eyes"), the malignant cells in Hodgkin lymphoma, are linked to EBV. Individuals who are immunosuppressed, such as patients with congenital immunosuppression, solid-organ transplant recipients, and human immunodeficiency virus (HIV)-infection, are also at much higher risk to develop Hodgkin lymphoma. Although the risk of developing Hodgkin lymphoma is up to 25-fold greater in patients with HIV, the CD4 level may be very low or within the normal range at diagnosis. Almost all cases of Hodgkin lymphoma (HL) in HIV-infected individuals are EBV positive, and are most commonly the lymphocyte-deplete subtype of HL. Hodgkin lymphoma is not an AIDS-defining illness.

Genetic factors are also associated with an increased risk of Hodgkin lymphoma. The strongest evidence comes from identical twin studies, which show that the unaffected identical twin has almost a 100-fold increase in risk.[10]

Pathophysiology

Hodgkin lymphoma is a clonal malignant lymphoid disease of transformed B-lymphocytes. The malignant cell in Hodgkin lymphoma is known as the Reed–Sternberg cell named after Dorothy Reed and Carl Sternberg, who were credited with the first definitive microscopic description of Hodgkin lymphoma.[2,3] Procedures to isolate and analyze Reed–Sternberg cells remain a challenge to pathologists because of the relatively small percentage (1%-2%) of Reed–Sternberg cells in an inflammatory microenvironment typically found in the Hodgkin lymphoma mass.[9] Fortunately, new laboratory techniques have led to significant progress in identifying the origin of the Reed–Sternberg cell. Single-cell polymerase chain reaction and DNA microarray analyses indicate that nearly all classic Hodgkin lymphoma cases and all nodular lymphocyte-predominant Hodgkin lymphomas (NLPHLs) have immunoglobulin gene rearrangements, which indicates a germinal center or post-germinal center B-cell origin.[9,11] Interestingly, nearly all Reed–Sternberg cells of classical Hodgkin lymphoma fail to express B-cell specific cell surface proteins.

B-cell transcriptional processes are disrupted during malignant transformation, which prevents B-cell surface marker expression and production of immunoglobulin messenger ribonucleic acid. The normal cellular consequence of failure to express immunoglobulin is apoptosis, but because of alterations in the normal apoptotic pathways, cell survival and proliferation are favored. Reed–Sternberg cells overexpress nuclear factor-κ B, which is associated with cell proliferation and antiapoptotic signals. Infections with viral and bacterial pathogens upregulate nuclear factor-κ B and consequently are hypothesized to be involved with the etiology of Hodgkin lymphoma.[3,9,11] This hypothesis is supported by the presence of EBV in many Hodgkin lymphoma tumors, but it is important to note that not all tumors are associated with EBV. Another signaling pathway, Janus kinase–signal transduction and transcription (JAK–STAT), has also been found to be active in Hodgkin lymphoma.[3,9] As molecular techniques continue to improve, our understanding of the pathophysiology of Hodgkin lymphoma will also improve.

The histopathologic classification of Hodgkin lymphoma has undergone numerous changes over the past three decades. The current classification system is the 2016 World Health Organization (WHO) classification (Table 132-1).[12] This classification divides Hodgkin lymphoma into two major groups: classical Hodgkin lymphoma and NLPHL, which constitute about 95% and 5% of cases, respectively. Classic Hodgkin lymphoma is further divided into four subtypes: nodular sclerosis, mixed cellularity, lymphocyte-depleted, and lymphocyte-rich. The subtypes in these classifications are based on characteristics of the Reed–Sternberg cell, the surrounding cells, and the tissue. Nodular sclerosis has features that make it distinct from the other three subtypes, which represent a continuum of background cellularity, with lymphocyte-predominance being the most cellular and lymphocyte-depletion being the least cellular. Typical immunophenotype for classical Hodgkin lymphoma includes $CD15^+$, $CD30^+$, PAX-5^+ (weak), $CD3^-$, $CD20^-$, $CD45^-$, $CD79a^-$. NLPHL is separated because of its distinct immunophenotype: $CD15^-$, $CD20^+$, $CD30^-$, and $CD45^+$ (the opposite of classical Hodgkin lymphoma). With the introduction of extensive staging, sophisticated radiotherapy, and effective combination chemotherapy, the prognostic value of these subtypes is becoming less clear. The true value of understanding these subtypes is likely tied to the pathogenesis of the disease and its potential prevention in the future.

Clinical Presentation

Most patients with Hodgkin lymphoma present with a painless, rubbery, enlarged lymph node in the supradiaphragmatic area and commonly have mediastinal nodal involvement. Lymphadenopathy

TABLE 132-1 WHO Classification of the Mature B-Cell, T-Cell, and NK-Cell Neoplasms (2016)

B Cell	NK cells	Hodgkin Lymphoma
B-cell chronic lymphocytic leukemia/small lymphocytic lymphoma	T-cell prolymphocytic leukemia	Nodular lymphocyte-predominant Hodgkin lymphoma
B-cell prolymphocytic leukemia	T-cell granular lymphocytic leukemia	Classical Hodgkin lymphoma
Lymphoplasmacytic lymphoma	Aggressive NK cell leukemia	Nodular sclerosis classical Hodgkin lymphoma
Splenic marginal zone B-cell lymphoma (± villous lymphocytes)	Adult T-cell leukemia/lymphoma (HTLV-I+)	Lymphocyte-rich classical Hodgkin lymphoma
Hairy cell leukemia	Extranodal NK/T-cell lymphoma, nasal type	Mixed cellularity classical Hodgkin lymphoma
Plasma cell myeloma/plasmacytoma	Enteropathy-associated T-cell lymphoma	Lymphocyte-depleted classical Hodgkin lymphoma
Extranodal marginal zone B-cell lymphoma of MALT type	Hepatosplenic γ δ T-cell lymphoma	
Mantle cell lymphoma	Subcutaneous panniculitis-like T-cell lymphoma	
Follicular lymphoma	**Mycosis fungoides/Sézary syndrome**	
Nodal marginal zone B-cell lymphoma (± monocytoid B cells)	Anaplastic large cell lymphoma, primary cutaneous type	
Diffuse large B-cell lymphoma (DLBCL)	**Peripheral T-cell lymphoma, not otherwise specified (NOS)**	
Germinal center B-cell type	**Angioimmunoblastic T-cell lymphoma**	
Activated B-cell type	**Anaplastic large cell lymphoma, primary systemic type**	
Burkitt's lymphoma		

HTLV, human T-cell lymphotropic virus; MALT, mucosa-associated lymphoid tissue; NK, natural killer; WHO, World Health Organization.

Note: Not all subtypes are listed. **Malignancies in bold occur in at least 1% of patients.**

Adapted from SH Swerdlow et al: WHO Classification of Tumours of Haematopoietic and Lymphoid Tissues, 4th ed. World Health Organization, 2008.

may come and go, but persistence of lymphadenopathy more than 2 months warrants evaluation. Hodgkin lymphoma is occasionally diagnosed in an asymptomatic patient who has a mediastinal mass found with chest radiography or another imaging procedure. Asymptomatic adenopathy of the inguinal and axillary regions may be present at diagnosis but is less common (Fig. 132-1).[3,5] Patients can also present with constitutional symptoms (B symptoms) before the discovery of lymph node enlargement, and these symptoms include fever greater than 38°C (100.4°F), drenching night sweats, and weight loss greater than 10% within 6 months of diagnosis. At diagnosis, these symptoms may appear in about 25% of all patients and up to 50% of patients with advanced disease. Patients may also experience other nonspecific symptoms including pruritus, fatigue, and development of pain after alcohol consumption at sites where nodes are involved.[5] Extranodal manifestations, such as bowel and hepatic involvements, are much less common in Hodgkin lymphoma than NHL.[3]

Diagnosis, Staging, and Prognostic Factors

Diagnostic and staging procedures are based on recommendations made at the Ann Arbor and Cotswolds conferences and new scientific advances, as described in the National Comprehensive Cancer Network (NCCN) guideline.[1] The diagnosis and pathologic classification of Hodgkin lymphoma can only be made by review of a biopsy (preferably an excisional biopsy) of the enlarged node by an expert hematopathologist.

In addition to a careful physical examination, routine laboratory tests including a complete blood count, complete metabolic panel to assess renal and hepatic function, lactate dehydrogenase (LDH), and erythrocyte sedimentation rate (ESR) will be helpful in treatment planning and aid in prognosis. Pregnancy test and HIV status should be assessed. Computed tomography (CT) scans of the chest, abdomen, and pelvis are routinely performed. Furthermore, positron emission tomography (PET) plays an important role in the initial staging of Hodgkin lymphoma, as it has shown high sensitivity and specificity in the staging of the disease.[13] The use of integrated PET-CT has further improved the staging of Hodgkin lymphoma given that it can provide more sensitive and specific imaging as compared with each imaging alone. The NCCN guideline recommends diagnostic CT and integrated PET-CT scan (preferred) for initial staging.[1] Bone marrow biopsy is now only recommended in patients with cytopenias and a negative PET.

Staging can be based on clinical or pathologic findings. The clinical stage is based on all noninvasive procedures (history, physical examination, laboratory tests, and radiologic findings), whereas the pathologic stage is based on the biopsy findings of strategic sites (bone marrow, spleen, and abdominal nodes). Patients with extranodal disease (bone marrow, bone, or Waldeyer ring) contiguous to

CLINICAL PRESENTATION Hodgkin Lymphoma

General

- Most patients with Hodgkin lymphoma have lymph node involvement in the supradiaphragmatic and mediastinal areas.

Symptoms

- About 25% of all patients present with fever, night sweats, and weight loss (ie, B symptoms), and up to 50% of patients with advanced disease.
- Fatigue, malaise, and pruritus.

Signs

- Enlarged lymph node, which may present as painless and rubbery.

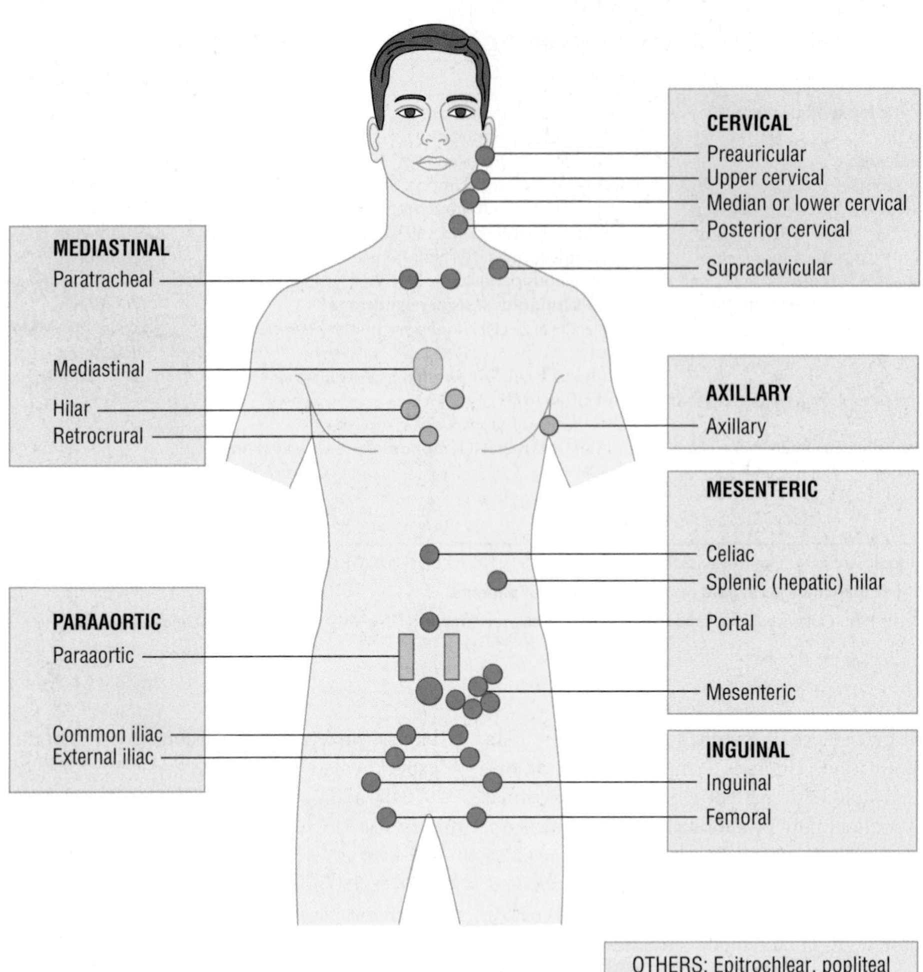

FIGURE 132-1 Areas of lymph nodes used in the staging of Hodgkin and non-Hodgkin lymphoma. Each rectangle corresponds to a nodal area.

involved nodes are classified with the subscript "E" in the Cotswolds staging system.

The Ann Arbor staging classification, which was developed at the 1970 Ann Arbor conference, has proven to be a good schema. At the Cotswolds meeting in 1989, the Ann Arbor classification was modified to incorporate new diagnostic techniques (eg, CT and magnetic resonance imaging), and the understanding that prognosis is associated with the bulk of the disease and the number of involved nodal sites (Table 132-2).[5] After careful staging, about one-half of patients have localized disease (stages I, II, and II_E) and the remainder have advanced disease (stage III or IV). About 10% to 15% present with metastatic disease (stage IV). It is important to note that Hodgkin lymphoma appears to follow a predictable pattern of nodal spread that is not seen with the NHLs.[3,14]

Patient prognosis is predominately driven by age and amount of disease. Patients older than ages 65 to 70 have a lower cure rate than younger patients. The difference in cure rates may be related to the higher incidence of comorbid diseases and decreased organ function in older patients, which impairs their ability to tolerate intensive chemotherapy. Stage is a dominant factor in predicting survival; patients with limited-stage disease (stages I to II) have a 90% to 95% cure rate, while those with advanced disease (stages III to IV) have only a 60% to 80% cure rate.[3,5]

Seven adverse prognostic factors with similar impact on survival (each factor reduced survival by 7%-8% per year) have been identified through an international collaborative effort. These factors can be combined to generate an IPS that can be used to predict progression-free and overall survival (Table 132-3).[15]

TREATMENT

Hodgkin Lymphoma

Desired Outcomes

The current goal in the treatment of Hodgkin lymphoma is to maximize curability while minimizing short- and long-term treatment-related complications. According to the Surveillance, Epidemiology, and End Results (SEER) database, the 5-year age-adjusted relative survival is greater than 80%.[7] Therefore, the initial treatment goal for all stages of Hodgkin lymphoma should be cure.

General Approach to Treatment

Combination chemotherapy is the primary treatment modality for most patients with Hodgkin lymphoma. In general, patients of all stages are initially treated with combination chemotherapy for about 8 to 12 weeks (depending on the regimen), and then restaged with PET-CT. Three combination chemotherapy regimens are primarily used for the initial treatment of classical Hodgkin lymphoma: ABVD, Stanford V, and some version of BEACOPP (bleomycin, etoposide, doxorubicin (Adriamycin®), cyclophosphamide, vincristine (Oncovin®), procarbazine, and prednisone). Depending on the initial radiographic response from the restaging, further chemotherapy with or without radiation is planned. For patients with refractory or recurrent disease, salvage therapy consists of multi-agent chemotherapy with or without high-dose chemotherapy and autologous hematopoietic stem cell transplantation (HSCT).[1,3,5]

TABLE 132-2 The Ann Arbor Staging Classification of Hodgkin Lymphoma

Stage I	Involvement of a single lymph node region or structure (I) or of a single extralymphatic organ or site (I_E)
Stage II	Involvement of two or more lymph node regions on the same side of the diaphragm (II) or localized involvement of an extralymphatic organ or site and of one or more lymph node regions on the same side of the diaphragm (II_E). The number of nodal regions involved should be indicated by a subscript (eg, II_2)
Stage III	Involvement of lymph node regions on both sides of the diaphragm (III), which may also be accompanied by localized involvement of an extralymphatic organ or site (III_E) or by involvement of the spleen (IIIS) or both ($IIIS_E$). III_1: with or without splenic, hilar, celiac, or portal node involvement. III_2: with paraaortic, iliac, or mesenteric node involvement
Stage IV	Diffuse or disseminated involvement of one or more extralymphatic organs or tissues with or without associated lymph node enlargement A—No symptoms B—Fever, night sweats, weight loss (>10%) X—Bulky disease >One-third the width of the mediastinum >10 cm maximal dimension of nodal mass E—Involvement of extralymphatic tissue on one side of the diaphragm by limited direct extension from an adjacent, involved lymph node region S—Involvement of the spleen CS—Clinical stage PS—Pathologic stage

Radiation is often an integral part of the treatment plan. Selected patients with early stage disease (usually nodular lymphocyte-predominant histology) can receive radiation as the only treatment modality, whereas most other patients with early stage disease may receive chemotherapy and radiation depending on the initial bulk of disease and the response to chemotherapy alone. Although radiation is a local therapy, many patients with advanced disease will also receive radiation therapy to residual or bulky disease sites after chemotherapy. Many different radiation techniques targeting different radiation fields have been used over the last few decades, including involved-field radiation (IFRT), extended-field radiation, subtotal nodal irradiation, and total nodal irradiation. The major concern with radiation therapy is its long-term effects, particularly on organs at risk, such as cardiovascular disease and secondary malignancies that commonly occur in the lung, breast, gastrointestinal tract and connective tissue.[16] Involved-site radiation therapy (ISRT) and involved-node radiation therapy are now being used as alternatives to the classic IFRT, and both define a smaller field than IFRT. ISRT targets the nodal sites and extranodal extensions that were involved at diagnosis but is intended to spare adjacent uninvolved organs when lymphadenopathy regresses after chemotherapy and ISRT. Additional techniques help to refine the volume of radiation delivered to the intended sites such as 4D-CT simulation planning, intensity modulated radiation therapy, image-guided RT, and respiratory gating.[17-19]

Although multiple treatment modalities are used to treat Hodgkin lymphoma, surgery has a limited role regardless of stage. Surgery is important for an accurate diagnosis via excisional biopsy, and on certain other occasions, such as placement of a central line. The following sections will review treatment of early stage favorable disease, early stage unfavorable disease, advanced-stage favorable disease, advanced-stage unfavorable disease, and salvage therapy.

TABLE 132-3 The International Prognostic Factors Project Score for Advanced Hodgkin Lymphoma

Risk Factors

Serum albumin (<4 g/dL [<40 g/L])
Hemoglobin (<10.5 g/dL [<105 g/L; 6.52 mmol/L])
Male gender
Stage IV disease
Age (≥45 years)
White blood cell (WBC) count (≥15,000 cells/mm³ [≥15 × 10⁹/L])
Lymphocytopenia (<600 cells/mm³ [<0.6 × 10⁹/L] or <8% of WBC count)

Number of Factors	Freedom from Progression[a]	Overall Survival[a]
0	84 ± 4	89 ± 2
1	77 ± 3	90 ± 2
2	67 ± 2	81 ± 2
3	60 ± 3	78 ± 3
4	51 ± 4	61 ± 4
≥5	42 ± 5	56 ± 5

[a]Percentage of patients at 5 years.

Data from reference 15.

Chemotherapy Regimens

Prior to the 1960s, the outcome for patients with Hodgkin lymphoma was dismal. Treatment with single-agent therapies or broad radiation fields provided excessive toxicities and few durable responses with advanced disease. The mechlorethamine, vincristine, procarbazine, and prednisone (MOPP) regimen was introduced in the early 1960s and was the initial combination chemotherapy regimen shown to cure advanced Hodgkin lymphoma (Table 132-4). This was a tremendous advance in oncology at that time. MOPP chemotherapy was a mainstay of treatment for patients with stages III and IV advanced Hodgkin lymphoma for years to come. However, investigators later learned that MOPP is associated with high rates of sterility and secondary malignancies. The young population of Hodgkin survivors would live long enough to endure these consequences. The research focus was then shifted to maintain the high cure rates obtained with MOPP while decrease the long-term toxicities.

The development of ABVD by Bonnadonna and colleagues at the Milan Cancer Institute about a decade later represents the next important step in the evolution of therapy for Hodgkin lymphoma (see Table 132-4).[20] ABVD was initially shown to be effective in treating MOPP failures and was later compared directly to MOPP in advanced disease, where it produced an 82% complete response rate, as compared to a 67% complete response rate with MOPP. Improved failure-free survival was demonstrated with ABVD, but no significant differences in 5-year overall survival were noted.[21] Because ABVD was less toxic and provided similar or better outcomes than MOPP, it eventually replaced MOPP as the standard regimen for advanced-stage Hodgkin lymphoma.

In the early 1980s, the Goldie–Coldman hypothesis proposed that chemotherapy resistance was related to spontaneous mutation rates and the development of resistant clones. To test that hypothesis, researchers designed several clinical trials to evaluate the efficacy of alternating non–cross-resistant drug combinations in patients with Hodgkin lymphoma.[22] The initial approach adopted by investigators was to alternate or combine the MOPP and ABVD regimens. When MOPP and ABVD (or doxorubicin [Adriamycin®], bleomycin, vinblastine [ABV]) are combined in a monthly cycle, it is referred to as a hybrid regimen. Besides a potential benefit in efficacy, another potential benefit of alternating or hybrid regimens is the decreased risk of long-term toxicities. In the alternating MOPP/ABVD regimen, the cumulative doses of procarbazine and mechlorethamine are reduced by 50%, and the cumulative doxorubicin dose is reduced by 50%. In the hybrid regimen, the cumulative doxorubicin dose

TABLE 132-4 Combination Chemotherapy Regimens for Hodgkin Lymphoma

Drug	Dosage (mg/m²)	Route	Days
MOPP			
Mechlorethamine	6	IV	1, 8
Vincristine	1.4	IV	1, 8
Procarbazine	100	Oral	1-14
Prednisone	40	Oral	1-14
Repeat every 21 days			
ABVD			
Doxorubicin (Adriamycin®)	25	IV	1, 15
Bleomycin	10	IV	1, 15
Vinblastine	6	IV	1, 15
Dacarbazine	375	IV	1, 15
Repeat every 28 days			
MOPP/ABVD			
Alternating months of MOPP and ABVD			
MOPP/ABV hybrid			
Mechlorethamine	6	IV	1
Vincristine	1.4	IV	1
Procarbazine	100	Oral	1-7
Prednisone	40	Oral	1-14
Doxorubicin	35	IV	8
Bleomycin	10	IV	8
Vinblastine	6	IV	8
Repeat every 28 days			
Stanford V			
Doxorubicin	25	IV	Weeks 1, 3, 5, 7, 9, 11
Vinblastine	6	IV	Weeks 1, 3, 5, 7, 9, 11
Mechlorethamine	6	IV	Weeks 1, 5, 9
Etoposide	60	IV	Weeks 3, 7, 11
Vincristine	1.4[a]	IV	Weeks 2, 4, 6, 8, 10, 12
Bleomycin	5	IV	Weeks 2, 4, 6, 8
Prednisone	40	Oral	Every other day for 12 weeks; begin tapering at week 10
One course (12 weeks)			
BEACOPP (standard-dose)			
Bleomycin	10	IV	8
Etoposide	100	IV	1-3
Adriamycin (doxorubicin)	25	IV	1
Cyclophosphamide	650	IV	1
Oncovin® (vincristine)	1.4[a]	IV	8
Procarbazine	100	Oral	1-7
Prednisone	40	Oral	1-14
Repeat every 21 days			
BEACOPP (escalated-dose)			
Bleomycin	10	IV	8
Etoposide	200	IV	1-3
Adriamycin (doxorubicin)	35	IV	1
Cyclophosphamide	1250	IV	1
Oncovin® (vincristine)	1.4[a]	IV	8
Procarbazine	100	Oral	1-7
Prednisone	40	Oral	1-14
Granulocyte colony-stimulating factor		Subcutaneously	8+
Repeat every 21 days			

[a]Vincristine dose capped at 2 mg.

is reduced by 33%, and the cumulative bleomycin dose is reduced by 50%.

Several clinical trials have been performed to evaluate the efficacy of alternating or hybrid MOPP/ABVD regimens. The results of these trials show that alternating and hybrid regimens are superior to MOPP but not to ABVD.[22,23] Another approach evaluated by researchers was the administration of sequential cycles of MOPP and ABVD (MOPP/ABVD). Results of an intergroup trial showed sequential MOPP and ABVD to be inferior to the MOPP/ABV hybrid regimen in terms of response and survival.[23] In yet another randomized comparison trial of the MOPP/ABV hybrid regimen and ABVD, the complete remission rate, failure-free survival, and overall survival were similar between the two regimens.[24] The latter trial was closed prematurely because of an increased number of treatment-related deaths and secondary malignancies in the patients who received the MOPP/ABV hybrid regimen.

More aggressive regimens, such as Stanford V and BEACOPP, have been evaluated as alternatives to MOPP or ABVD. It is important to note that radiation therapy is an integral part of the Stanford V regimen for all patients. The Stanford V regimen generated considerable interest based on the results of phase II trials.[25] Stanford V, ABVD, and an MOPP/ABV hybrid-like regimen (mechlorethamine, vincristine, procarbazine, prednisone, epidoxorubicin, bleomycin, vinblastine, lomustine, doxorubicin, and vindesine [MOPPEB-VCAD]) were then compared in a randomized trial to determine the best regimen to support a reduced radiotherapy program.[26] Five-year failure-free and progression-free survival were significantly worse for the Stanford V regimen as compared to the other two regimens. However, no significant differences in overall response rate or 5-year overall or failure-free survival were observed between Stanford V and ABVD in a published randomized trial of patients with advanced Hodgkin lymphoma (E2496).[29] Investigators have speculated that differences in the application of radiotherapy may explain the divergent results in the randomized trials. More pulmonary toxicity occurred in the ABVD group, but other toxicities occurred more frequently in the Stanford V group.

The German Hodgkin Study Group (GHSG) developed the BEACOPP regimens based on the principles of dose density, dose intensity, and mathematical modeling. BEACOPP uses similar drugs as in the cyclophosphamide, vincristine, procarbazine, and prednisone (COPP)/ABVD regimen, but rearranges the drugs in a shorter 3-week cycle. Several different versions of BEACOPP have been developed: standard-dose BEACOPP, escalated-dose BEACOPP, and dose-dense BEACOPP (BEACOPP-14). Granulocyte colony-stimulating factor support is required for the escalated-dose BEACOPP and BEACOPP-14 regimens.

It is important to note that the initial evidence for these regimens focused on patients with advanced or metastatic disease as described in this section, but subsequent trials have focused on the use of these regimens in early stage disease.

Restaging during Therapy and Risk-adaptive Therapy

1 With all stages and risk-groups of Hodgkin lymphoma, it is current practice to treat with chemotherapy for 8 to 12 weeks and then obtain a restaging PET-CT.[1] This scan is assessed on a PET 5-point scale, also known as Deauville Criteria. Score 1 indicates no uptake, and can be called a complete response, or no measurable disease (Table 132-5).[30] For all stages of Hodgkin lymphoma, further treatment is based on the restaging PET/CT results such that residual uptake at the end of chemotherapy would likely indicate the need for ISRT. If a Deauville score of 5 exists after completion of chemotherapy, then a biopsy of the involved area is indicated. Based on these current guidelines, every patient's treatment plan is personalized based on the response to treatment.

Classical Hodgkin Lymphoma

Hodgkin lymphoma can initially be divided into two broad classifications: classical Hodgkin lymphoma and NLPHL. Although classical Hodgkin lymphoma can be further divided into pathologic subtypes, the treatments are based on risk factors and presence of bulky disease regardless of the subtype of classical Hodgkin lymphoma.

Treatment of Early Stage Favorable Disease

Patients with early stage favorable disease have stage IA or IIA disease and no adverse risk factors (B-symptoms, extranodal disease, bulky disease, three or more sites of nodal involvement, or an ESR of >50 mm/h [>13.9 μm/s]). Extended-field radiation was previously considered to be the treatment of choice for stages IA and IIA disease. Although most patients were cured of their disease, the radiation is associated with long-term toxicities due to large radiation fields such as heart disease, pulmonary dysfunction, and secondary malignancies.[5,16]

Combined modality therapy (chemotherapy and radiation therapy) has replaced radiation therapy alone in patients with early stage favorable disease. With combined modality therapy, both a shorter duration of chemotherapy and newer, more focused radiation techniques (ISRT, others) are used in an attempt to decrease the long-term toxicities of both.

Clinical trials comparing radiation alone to radiation plus chemotherapy show lower relapse rates in patients treated with combined modality therapy (radiation and chemotherapy), but no change in overall survival because of the availability of effective salvage therapy. Ongoing trials focus on questions such as the optimal number of chemotherapy cycles, the volume of radiation that must be used to obtain optimal patient outcomes, and the role of PET scanning to individualize therapy. Long-term results of clinical trials also suggest that as few as two cycles of Stanford V or ABVD chemotherapy followed by IFRT is sufficient in favorable, early stage disease patients.[27,28] Different combination chemotherapy regimens have been used in these studies, and no one regimen is clearly superior to another.

Clinical trials have also investigated the use of chemotherapy alone to treat low-risk early stage Hodgkin lymphoma. Long-term results of clinical trials show a lower rate of disease control versus combined modality therapy. Selected patients can be treated with chemotherapy alone if they achieve a complete response following two cycles of chemotherapy, with a total treatment of four cycles of chemotherapy.

TABLE 132-5 PET 5-Point Scale or Deauville Criteria

Score	PET/CT Scan Result
1	No uptake
2	Uptake ≤ mediastinum
3	Uptake > mediastinum but ≤ liver
4	Uptake moderately higher than liver
5	Uptake markedly higher than liver and/or new lesions
X	New areas of uptake unlikely to be related to lymphoma

Data from Barrington SF, Mikhaeel NG, Kostakoglu L, et al. Role of imaging in the staging and response assessment of lymphoma: consensus of the International Conference on Malignant Lymphomas Imaging Working Group. J Clin Oncol 2014;32:3048-3058.

Clinical **Controversy...**

Some clinicians believe that radiation therapy can and should be excluded altogether for some patients, especially young patients who are at higher risk of reproductive and secondary malignancy concerns.

The current NCCN guideline recommends that patients with early stage favorable disease be treated with two cycles of ABVD plus ISRT or two to four cycles of the Stanford V regimen (doxorubicin, vinblastine, mechlorethamine, etoposide, vincristine, bleomycin, and prednisone), followed by a restaging PET-CT scan. Depending on the response to the initial chemotherapy, consolidative ISRT is recommended if anything less than a complete response is achieved.[1] With this approach, 5-year progression-free and overall survival rates of more than 90% can be achieved in early stage favorable disease.

Treatment of Early Stage Unfavorable Disease

Patients with early stage disease who have certain features associated with a poor prognosis (B symptoms, extranodal disease, bulky disease, three or more sites of nodal involvement, or an ESR >50 mm/h [>13.9 μm/s]) are defined as having unfavorable disease. Different research groups or clinical trials have different definitions for unfavorable disease (Table 132-6). Current guidelines recommend combined modality therapy (combination chemotherapy and ISRT) to reduce the relapse rate and avoid the toxicity associated with extended-field radiation.[1]

Randomized trials show that combined modality therapy reduces the relapse rate in patients with early stage unfavorable disease. Different chemotherapy regimens and number of chemotherapy cycles have been compared in clinical trials. In most studies involving early-stage unfavorable disease, ABVD is the comparator arm. ABVD plus 30 Gy [3,000 rad] ISRT remains the standard of care for patients with early stage unfavorable disease, but the Stanford

TABLE 132-6 Examples of "Unfavorable Risk Factors" for Early-Stage Hodgkin Lymphoma

Risk Factor	NCCN	GHSG	EORTC	NCIC
Age			≥50	≥40
ESR and B-symptoms	>50 mm/h (>13.9 μm/s) or any B symptoms	>50 mm/h (>13.9 μm/s) if A; >30 mm/h (>8.3 μm/s) if B symptoms	>50 mm/h (>13.9 μm/s) if A; >30 mm/h (>8.3 μm/s) if B symptoms	>50 mm/h (>13.9 μm/s) or any B symptoms
Mediastinal mass	MMR > 0.33 or >10 cm	MMR > 0.33	MTR > 0.35	MMR > 0.33 or >10 cm
Number of Nodal Sites	>3	>2*	>3*	>3
Other		Any extranodal lesion		Histology: mixed cellularity or lymphocyte deplete

EORTC, European Organization for the Research and Treatment of Cancer; GHSG, German Hodgkin Study Group; MMR, mediastinal mass ratio—maximum width of mass/maximum intrathoracic diameter; MTR, Mediastinal thoracic ratio—maximum width of mediastinal mass/intrathoracic diameter at T5-6; NCCN, National Comprehensive Cancer Network, USA; NCIC, National Cancer Institute, Canada.

*Definitions of lymph node regions differ.

V regimen plus radiation or BEACOPP for two cycles followed by ABVD for two cycles are both alternatives in select patients.[1] The Stanford V regimen has been studied in several single arm trials[31,32] and comparative trials versus ABVD[29,33] report overall response rates in the 90% range and 5-year overall survival from 88% to 94%. All of these trials included radiation therapy as part of the treatment schema. The GHSG studied the use of a more aggressive regimen of escalated-dose BEACOPP for two cycles followed by ABVD for two cycles versus ABVD for four cycles. Both treatment arms received 30 Gy [3,000 rad] of IFRT. Patients treated with BEACOPP had longer progression-free survival but similar 5-year overall survival as compared with ABVD.[34] BEACOPP is associated with more toxicities than ABVD in early stage unfavorable Hodgkin lymphoma.[35]

2 In summary, most patients with early stage disease will be treated with two to four cycles of ABVD chemotherapy and involved-site radiation. The number of cycles initially administered is based on the classification of favorable versus unfavorable disease. Restaging with a PET-CT after 4 to 12 weeks of chemotherapy further guides the need for more chemotherapy or radiation (ISRT), but most patients with unfavorable disease will require radiation. Clinical trials have demonstrated the utility of PET scans as biomarkers to individualize therapy and minimize the amount of therapy necessary for cure.[13] Although ABVD is the preferred initial regimen (NCCN category 1 recommendation), evidence supports the use of Stanford V in favorable and unfavorable early stage patients and escalated BEACOPP-ABVD in unfavorable early stage patients.[1] Despite excellent results from treatment with ABVD and radiation, about 5% of patients do not respond to initial treatment and another 15% of patients will relapse following an initial response.

Treatment of Advanced-Stage Disease

Advanced-stage disease consists of stages III and IV disease. In some studies, stage IIB with a large mediastinal mass or extranodal disease is also considered advanced-stage disease (see Table 132-2). By definition, patients with stages III and IV disease have tumors on both sides of the diaphragm, which almost always precludes the use of radiation alone as a therapeutic modality. Intensive combination chemotherapy is the mainstay of treatment, although some patients will benefit from radiation following chemotherapy. The prognosis of advanced-stage disease is excellent with 5-year overall survival rates ranging from 56% to 90%. Most patients obtain a complete response from their initial treatment. Prognostic factors have been identified and standardized to predict an individual's prognosis, according to the IPS (see Table 132-3).[15]

Patients with advanced-stage Hodgkin lymphoma can be classified into two groups based on the number of prognostic factors present from the IPS (see Table 132-3). Advanced-stage patients with three or fewer poor prognostic factors are considered to have favorable disease and have about a 60% likelihood of being failure-free at 5 years with traditional combination chemotherapy. Advanced-stage patients with four or more poor prognostic factors are considered to have unfavorable disease and a less than 50% likelihood of being failure-free at 5 years with traditional combination chemotherapy. Cures are possible in patients with high-risk disease, but long-term disease control is a more realistic goal for most patients.

Combination Chemotherapy in Advanced-Stage Disease

Doxorubicin (Adriamycin®), bleomycin, vinblastine, and dacarbazine for (ABVD) decades has continued to be the standard initial regimens utilized for advanced Hodgkin lymphoma in many cancer programs. As discussed in the **Chemotherapy Regimens** section, many multinational, randomized large trials have demonstrated ABVD's sustained positive outcomes and lower toxicity profile as compared to other regimens.

The activity of the Stanford V regimen with ISRT in advanced Hodgkin lymphoma has been demonstrated in prospective trials. In a phase III intergroup trial (E2496) comparing ABVD to Stanford V with radiation therapy in either arm, no significant differences in the 5-year overall or failure-free survival were observed.[29]

The BEACOPP regimens were designed to provide a more aggressive treatment for advanced disease. Several randomized trials have compared BEACOPP to other regimens.[5,36] The GHSG conducted a large randomized comparison of COPP/ABVD (alternating), BEACOPP, or an escalated-dose BEACOPP regimen (HD9 trial).[36] Escalated-dose BEACOPP was the most active regimen in this study, with 10-year freedom from treatment failure at 82% and overall survival at 86%, but this regimen was also associated with more toxicities including secondary leukemias, and was particularly toxic in the elderly.[37,38] In the HD2000 study, patients with advanced Hodgkin lymphoma were randomized to receive six cycles of ABVD, four cycles of escalated-dose BEACOPP with two cycles of standard-dose BEACOPP, or a third chemotherapy regimen that is not a current standard of care.[39] BEACOPP was superior to ABVD for 5-year failure-free survival (78% vs 65%, $P = 0.036$) and progression-free survival (81% vs 68%, $P = 0.038$), but 5-year overall survival was not significantly different between ABVD and BEACOPP. It appears that BEACOPP may be superior to ABVD in patients with high-risk advanced Hodgkin lymphoma (IPS ≥3). Higher rates of neutropenia and severe infections were observed with BEACOPP as compared with ABVD. The HD2000 trial also demonstrated a higher risk of secondary malignancy in the BEACOPP versus ABVD arm (6.7 vs 0.9, $P = 0.027$) at 10 years.[40] Finally, GHSG has conducted several trials to evaluate the optimal number and intensity of BEACOPP. The HD12 and HD15 trials are two examples of this research.[41,42] The results of these studies suggest that escalated-dose BEACOPP is superior to ABVD in the treatment of advanced Hodgkin lymphoma, but at the cost of more treatment-related toxicity.

National Comprehensive Cancer Network currently recommends that patients with advanced disease be treated with ABVD,

Stanford V or escalated-dose BEACOPP. NCCN further recommends that Stanford V may be considered in patients with IPS less than 3 and escalated-dose BEACOPP may be considered in patients less than 60 years old with an IPS of greater than or equal to 4.[1] As with earlier stage disease, combination chemotherapy should be administered for 4 to 18 weeks, depending on the regimen chosen, followed by a restaging PET scan. Based on the residual Deauville score, additional chemotherapy and/or radiation may be administered.

Summary for Advanced-Stage Hodgkin Lymphoma

3 In summary, there are several approaches to the initial treatment of stages III and IV Hodgkin lymphoma. A standard treatment of advanced-stage favorable Hodgkin lymphoma is to administer two cycles of ABVD chemotherapy followed by a restaging PET-CT. If minimal disease is found (Deauville score 1-3), 4 additional courses of ABVD should be given (total of 6 cycles). If residual disease is suspected (Deauville score 4-5), a switch to escalated-BEACOPP for 4 cycles should be considered. If the Stanford V regimen is selected for initial therapy, then the full 12 weeks of planned chemotherapy would be given before the restaging PET-CT. Escalated-dose BEACOPP for 6 cycles should be considered for patients with unfavorable disease. This risk-adapted approach should result in 70% to more than 90% of patients achieving a complete remission and 60% to 80% of patients being cured of their disease. No further treatment is needed for patients who achieve a complete remission (Deauville 1-2) with chemotherapy alone. Patients who achieve a partial remission (Deauville 3-5) should be considered for consolidative radiation to residual sites of disease. As with all stages and risk-groups of HL, if a Deauville score of 5 remains after completion of initial chemotherapy, a biopsy is recommended to determine if refractory disease is present.

Nodular Lymphocyte-Predominant Hodgkin Lymphoma

Nodular lymphocyte-predominant Hodgkin lymphoma has been described as more indolent in nature, and has a better prognosis as compared with classical Hodgkin lymphoma. The use of radiation alone for stages I and II NLPHL patients who choose to omit chemotherapy or who cannot tolerate chemotherapy does not appear to adversely affect survival.[1] The disadvantage of radiation therapy alone as compared with combination chemotherapy plus radiation is the higher relapse rate. Patients who relapse after radiation alone (20%-25%) can be successfully salvaged with chemotherapy. If the decision is made to use radiation alone, ISRT is the preferred method. Patients with advanced-stage disease can be treated with combined chemotherapy and radiation therapy. Historically, MOPP and MOPP/ABVD have been used, but these regimens have fallen out of favor much like classical Hodgkin lymphoma. ABVD is frequently used in these patients due to the available evidence to support its use for classical Hodgkin lymphoma, although other regimens, such as CHOP (cyclophosphamide, doxorubicin, vincristine, and prednisone), and CVP (cyclophosphamide, vincristine, and prednisone), have been studied. No randomized clinical trials of different chemotherapy regimens have been conducted in NLPHL. NLPHL reliably expresses CD20, and therefore rituximab has demonstrated efficacy in both newly diagnosed and progressive NLPHL. Several phase II trials have reported overall response rates of 90% to 100% with single agent rituximab.[43,44] Current NCCN guidelines recommend that patients with stage IA or IIA non-bulky disease preferentially be treated with ISRT alone. In very select patients with stage IA disease that was completely resected with the excisional biopsy, observation may be an option. Patients with IB, IIB, or advanced disease should receive chemotherapy with or without rituximab, with or without ISRT.[1]

Treatment of Refractory or Relapsed Disease

4 Refractory disease is defined as disease that persists following initial therapy, including any response less than a complete response. Relapsed disease suggests tumor recurrence following attainment of a complete response. Patients who experience relapsed disease less than 12 months after the completion of therapy have a poor prognosis. The goal of second-line or salvage therapy is still cure. With the increasing use of chemotherapy with or without radiation, regardless of disease extent, the rate of primary refractory disease is decreasing. Many therapeutic options are available for treatment of refractory or relapsed disease, so each patient's treatment should be personalized. The highest survival and cure rates are reported for patients with chemosensitive disease who are medically able to undergo high-dose therapy and autologous HSCT.[45,46] Since most patients are initially treated with ABVD, doxorubicin should be avoided in salvage chemotherapy regimens if the cumulative dose has reached between 300 and 400 mg/m^2, particularly in those patients who have received mediastinal radiotherapy, because of the higher risk of cardiotoxicity.

The response to salvage therapy depends on the extent and site of recurrence, previous therapy, and duration of initial remission. Patients who relapse after radiation therapy alone have a good chance of being cured with combination chemotherapy, although fewer patients are being treated with radiation alone. High response rates (60%-87%) have been reported with salvage chemotherapy regimens.[3,5] Other patient groups who have a favorable prognosis following salvage therapy include patients who experience a local recurrence in a nonirradiated location and those who relapse more than 1 year after completion of their initial chemotherapy. Patients who experience late relapses can be cured with retreatment with the same chemotherapy regimen, treatment with a different, potentially non–cross-resistant regimen, or high-dose chemotherapy and autologous HSCT.

Patients who have an early relapse (<1 year after treatment) generally respond poorly to standard-dose salvage chemotherapy. High-dose chemotherapy and autologous HSCT is more effective, but also produces a higher risk of treatment-related mortality. Therefore, the choice of salvage treatment should consider the patient's tolerance for a particular set of chemotherapeutic agents and treatment approach (standard-dose chemotherapy vs high-dose chemotherapy and autologous HSCT).[46]

High-dose therapy should be considered in patients who relapse within 12 months of initial remission and in those who are refractory to first-line chemotherapy.[46] Although no single preparative regimen has been shown to be superior to another, most regimens do not include total-body irradiation because of its potential pulmonary toxicity. Most patients are already at higher risk for pulmonary toxicity because of previous exposure to one or more of the following: bleomycin, thoracic radiation, and nitrosoureas.

Brentuximab vedotin is an antibody-drug conjugate (ADC) comprising an anti-CD30 antibody conjugated by a protease cleavable linker to a potent antimicrotubule agent, monomethyl auristatin E (MMAE). After binding of the ADC to CD30 on the cell surface, the ADC-CD30 complex is internalized. This leads to the release of MMAE via proteolytic cleavage in the lysosomal compartment. Tubulin binding by MMAE disrupts the microtubule network, which can lead to apoptotic death of the cancer cells.[47] In a pivotal multicenter phase II study of 102 patients with relapsed or refractory Hodgkin lymphoma after HSCT, objective responses and complete remissions were observed in 75% and 34% of patients treated with brentuximab vedotin, respectively. Brentuximab vedotin has also been evaluated as posttransplant consolidation therapy in a phase III trial in 329 patients undergoing autologous HSCT. All patients had a high risk of relapse, defined as disease refractory to initial therapy or relapsed disease less than 12 months from completion of initial therapy with extranodal disease. Patients randomized to receive 16 cycles of brentuximab had significantly longer median progression-free survival (42.9 vs 24.1 months) as compared with placebo.[48] Common toxicities associated with brentuximab vedotin include neuropathy, neutropenia, nausea, and fatigue.[49] Based on these results, the FDA has approved brentuximab vedotin (Adcetris®) for the treatment of classical Hodgkin lymphoma after failure of autologous HSCT or after failure of at least two prior multi-agent chemotherapy regimens in patients who are not candidates for autologous HSCT, and also for patients with classical Hodgkin lymphoma at high risk of relapse or progression as consolidation therapy after autologous HSCT.

Many single-agent and combination regimens can be used as salvage therapy. In this setting, the goal of therapy is disease control, and cures are unlikely. Gemcitabine, vinorelbine, and pegylated liposomal doxorubicin (GVD), ifosfamide, carboplatin, and etoposide (ICE) and ifosfamide, gemcitabine and vinorelbine are examples of chemotherapy regimens that include drugs with different mechanisms of action and toxicity profiles than regimens used earlier in therapy. Bendamustine, lenalidomide, and everolimus have all shown activity in patients with refractory or relapsed Hodgkin lymphoma.

Checkpoint inhibitors, specifically PD1 inhibitors (programmed death 1 pathway) are being studied in refractory Hodgkin lymphoma. Promising results are emerging from phase II trails that involve patients that are heavily pretreated. One trial with single-agent nivolumab reports an objective response rate of 87% with 17% being complete responses. The rate of progression-free survival at 24 weeks is cited at 86%.[49a]

Long-Term Complications

A variety of acute and chronic toxicities may occur as a result of treatment for Hodgkin lymphoma. Long-term complications of radiation therapy, chemotherapy, and combined modality therapy have become more evident as the curability and long-term survival of Hodgkin lymphoma patients has improved.[1,3,5,16] Gonadal dysfunction (including sterility and hypothyroidism), secondary malignancies, and cardiopulmonary diseases have become important considerations in the treatment of this malignancy. Almost all men and up to 50% of premenopausal women treated with six cycles of regimens containing alkylating agents become sterile. This appears to be a dose-related phenomenon. For men, even a single dose of nitrogen mustard or chlorambucil can cause sterility, so if fertility is a major concern, ABVD is the best alternative.[50]

The risk of secondary malignancies is increased about threefold in long-term survivors of Hodgkin lymphoma. The risk of developing leukemia carries the highest increase in risk and is seen with radiotherapy, chemotherapy, and chemoradiotherapy. Solid tumors, including breast cancers, gastrointestinal cancers, and lung cancers, are also likely to develop more than 10 years after the completion of treatment. A recently published British cohort study suggested that unlike radiotherapy, which may increase the occurrence of cancer at almost all anatomic sites, chemotherapy is associated with an increased risk of leukemia, NHL, and lung cancer.[51] However, studies that evaluate the risk of secondary malignancies (and other complications) must be interpreted cautiously because many factors probably contribute to the development of secondary malignancies. In addition, much of the long-term complication data are derived from patients who were treated with older regimens and extensive field radiotherapy, which are no longer commonly used in clinical practice. As the field of cancer survivorship continues to grow, more specific recommendations for long-term follow-up are developed. Regular mammograms and breast MRI are recommended starting 10 years following the completion of therapy or at age 40 (whichever is earlier) for females. Patients are at increased risk of lung cancer if they have a smoking history, chest irradiation, and/or alkylating agent exposure. These patients should be considered for low-dose screening chest CT. For cardiovascular monitoring, annual blood pressure monitoring and aggressive management of cardiovascular risk factors are strongly encouraged. Hypothyroidism is reported in about 50% of long-term survivors who received irradiation to this area. Thyroid function tests should be performed annually. Monitoring and follow-up should be personalized and patient-specific, after assessing a patient's risks for long-term complications.[1]

NON-HODGKIN LYMPHOMA

The NHLs are a heterogeneous group of lymphoproliferative disorders that affect individuals from early childhood to late adulthood. Advances in molecular biology techniques and our understanding of the human immune system have led to major progress in understanding the pathogenesis and treatment of the lymphomas. NHLs are classified into distinct clinical entities that are defined by a combination of morphology, immunophenotype, genetic features, and clinical features. These differences influence the natural history, and approach and response to treatment. The use of extensive combination chemotherapeutic regimens shows dramatic improvement in survival and cure in patients with a disease that was once considered incurable. The 5-year survival rate for patients with NHL has increased from 48% to 71% over the past 25 years, and the mortality rate actually *declined* from 1997 to 2004.[6,7] Further improvement in survival is anticipated with the continued expansion of our therapeutic armamentarium, including high-dose chemotherapy and biologic therapy.

Epidemiology and Etiology

Non-Hodgkin lymphoma is the fifth most common cause of newly diagnosed cancer in the United States and accounts for about 4% of all cancers. An estimated 72,580 new cases will be diagnosed in 2016, and it is estimated that 19,020 people will die from NHL during this same period.[6] Although the average age of patients at the time of diagnosis is about 67 years, NHL can occur at any age. The incidence rate generally increases with age, and is higher in men than in women and in whites than in blacks.[5] The age-adjusted incidence rate of NHL increased by more than 80% in the United States since the early 1970s, from about 11 cases per 100,000 in 1975 to about 20 cases per 100,000 in 2011 and 2012.[7] The incidence of NHL increased by 3% to 4% from 1975 to 1991, but appears to have stabilized since reaching its peak in 1994. The increased incidence of NHL over the past three decades is second only to melanoma and has been referred to as an epidemic of NHL. Although the increase has been noted particularly among the elderly and patients with acquired immune deficiency syndrome (AIDS), much of it cannot be explained by known risk factors.

The etiology of NHL is unknown, although several genetic diseases, environmental agents, and infectious agents are associated with the development of NHL.[52,53] An increased incidence of NHL is seen in many congenital and acquired immunodeficiency states, supporting the role of immune dysregulation in the etiology of NHL.[53] Patients with congenital immunodeficiency disorders such as Wiskott-Aldrich's syndrome and ataxia telangiectasia, acquired immunodeficiency disorders such as AIDS, and those receiving chronic pharmacologic immunosuppression in the setting of solid-organ transplantation are predisposed to the development of NHL. Autoimmune diseases (Hashimoto's thyroiditis and Sjögren's syndrome) cause chronic inflammation in the mucosa-associated lymphoid tissue (MALT), which predisposes patients to subsequent lymphoid malignancies. Other autoimmune diseases, such as systemic lupus erythematosus and rheumatoid arthritis, are also associated with the development of NHL, but the use of immunosuppressive agents in these diseases makes the pathologic cause less clear.

Certain infections are associated with the development of lymphoma.[52] EBV was discovered in cell lines from tumors of patients with African (endemic) Burkitt lymphoma, and EBV DNA is associated with nearly all cases of endemic Burkitt lymphoma.

However, EBV is associated with sporadic Burkitt lymphoma in 15% to 85% of cases. EBV is also associated with posttransplant lymphoproliferative disorders and some lymphomas in patients with AIDS or congenital immunodeficiencies. The human T-cell lymphotropic virus type 1 was the first human retrovirus associated with a malignancy. Infection with human T-cell lymphotropic virus type 1, especially in early childhood, is strongly associated with an aggressive form of T-cell lymphoma, known as adult T-cell leukemia/lymphoma. Human T-cell lymphotropic virus type 1 is endemic in parts of southern Japan, Africa, South America, and the Caribbean. In endemic areas, more than 50% of all NHL cases are adult T-cell leukemia/lymphoma. A third virus associated with NHL is human herpes virus 8 (also referred as Kaposi sarcoma–associated herpesvirus [KSHV]). This virus was originally isolated from Kaposi sarcoma lesions in AIDS patients. Gastric infection with *Helicobacter pylori*, a gram-negative bacteria that leads to chronic gastritis, is associated with gastric MALT lymphomas. Finally, hepatitis C virus has been associated with splenic and nodal marginal zone lymphomas.

A number of physical agents are also associated with the development of NHL.[53] Exposure to herbicides, particularly phenoxyl herbicides, is associated with the development of NHL. These observations may explain why certain occupations, such as farmers, forestry workers, and agricultural workers, are associated with a higher risk of NHL. Exposure to lawn-care pesticides is also increasing in the general population. A higher risk of NHL is also associated with exposure to other chemical solvents and dyes, exposure to radiation from nuclear explosions, and high intake of meats and dietary fats. Smoking or alcohol consumption is not strongly associated with an increased risk of NHL.

Molecular Abnormalities

Chromosomal translocations have become a hallmark of many lymphoid malignancies.[54,55] The presence of these specific translocations can be helpful in the diagnosis and classification of lymphoid malignancies. The mechanisms leading to the translocations are unknown, but they usually involve the antigen receptor loci. In contrast to most myeloid and some lymphoid leukemias, NHLs usually place a structurally intact cellular protooncogene under the regulatory influence of highly expressed immunoglobulin or T-cell receptor genes, leading to effects on cell growth, cellular differentiation, or apoptosis. The most common chromosomal translocations involve t(8;14), t(14;18), and t(11;14); each translocation involves the immunoglobulin heavy-chain gene locus on chromosome 14 at 14q32. The translocation t(8;14) that involves c-*MYC*, a well-characterized oncogene clearly associated with malignancy, is implicated in nearly all cases of Burkitt lymphoma. The translocation t(14;18) that involves *BCL*-2, one of several putative B-cell lymphoma-associated oncogenes, is found in about 90% of cases of follicular B-cell lymphomas. The translocation t(11;14) that involves *BCL*-1 is found in about 70% of patients with mantle cell lymphoma (MCL). Another putative B-cell lymphoma-associated oncogene, *BCL*-6, is found in about one-third of diffuse large B-cell lymphomas (DLBCLs).

Although mutations in the *p53* tumor suppressor gene have been recognized in many human neoplasms, such mutations have not been consistently found in patients with lymphoma, which suggests that it may occur late in malignant evolution.

Because of their role in the pathogenesis of lymphoma, oncogenes are attractive molecular targets for the development of new and novel therapies.[56]

Pathology and Classification

Non-Hodgkin lymphomas are neoplasms derived from the monoclonal proliferation of malignant B or T lymphocytes and their precursors. About 85% to 90% of NHLs in the United States are of B-cell origin.[53] Proliferation of malignant cells results in the replacement of the normal cells and architecture of lymph nodes or bone marrow with a relatively uniform population of lymphoid cells. The classification of NHLs has evolved over the past five decades, as advances in immunology and genetics have allowed scientists to recognize a number of previously unrecognized subtypes of NHLs (Table 132-7).[57,58] The current classification schemes characterize the NHLs according to the cell of origin (B cell vs T cell), clinical features, and morphologic features. Additional immunohistochemical markers, cytogenetic features, and genotypic characteristics may help to further classify NHL into subtypes.

TABLE 132-7 Evolution in the Classification of Non-Hodgkin Lymphomas

Time	Classification System	Basis for Classification
1950s–1960s	Rappaport	Morphology
1970s–1980s	Luke–Collins	Morphology and immunophenotype
1970s–1980s	Kiel	Morphology and immunophenotype
1980s–1990s	International Working Formulation	Morphology and clinical behavior
1990s	REAL	Disease entities
2001	WHO	Disease entities

REAL, revised European–American Classification of Lymphoid Neoplasms developed by the International Lymphoma Study Group; WHO, World Health Organization.

Morphology

The macroscopic and microscopic appearance of the involved tissue remains one of the most important factors in the diagnosis and classification of NHLs.[57,58] In the 1950s, Rappaport et al. proposed a morphologic classification of malignant lymphomas based on two features: that the malignant cell would disrupt the nodal architecture in a *nodular* or *diffuse* manner, and that lymphomas of histiocytic origin existed. The Rappaport classification gained rapid acceptance in the United States because of its precision, simplicity, and prognostic significance. Application of the system divided NHLs into those with large (ie, incorrectly called "histiocytes") or small cells, with or without a nodular (ie, follicular) growth pattern.

Immunology

In the 1970s, it became apparent that NHLs were tumors of the immune system and were derived from B or T lymphocytes. With the availability of techniques using antibodies to antigens on the surface of lymphoid cells (ie, immunophenotype) and cytochemical assays, expert pathologists independently developed new classification schemes for NHL in the 1970s and 1980s.[57,58] The Kiel classification was based primarily on the work of Lennert in Germany and became widely used in Europe. In North America, the Lukes and Collins classification scheme was used briefly, but was soon superseded by the Working Formulation. Like the Rappaport classification, divisions within the Working Formulation were based largely on cell size (large [histiocytic] vs small [lymphocytic]), cell shape (round vs not round), and growth pattern (follicular [nodular] vs diffuse). Both the Kiel and Working Formulation classification schemes considered the histologic grade of the tumor, but only the Working Formulation considered actual survival curves of patients with the various subtypes of NHL. *Low-grade* indicated longer median survival (ie, indolent) whereas *intermediate-grade* and *high-grade* indicated shorter median survival (ie, aggressive). In the 1980s and early 1990s, the Working Formulation became the most widely used classification scheme in North America. It was based on the premise that NHL was a single disease with a range of histologic grades and clinical aggressiveness.

Disease Entities

In the 1980s and early 1990s, rapid advances in immunology and genetics allowed scientists to recognize a number of previously unrecognized subtypes of NHLs. Cytogenetic and molecular genetic analyses identified the presence of many chromosomal translocations, oncogenes, and their gene products in patients with NHL (see Molecular Abnormalities earlier in this Chapter). In addition, diseases that would have been lumped together as low-grade or intermediate/high grade in the Working Formulation showed marked differences in survival, which prompted scientists to reevaluate lymphoma classification schemes.

Information from these studies allowed scientists to further classify B-cell lymphomas as malignant expansions of cells from the germinal center, mantle zone, or marginal zone of normal lymph nodes.[57,59] Germinal centers are complex structures that form in the spleen and lymph nodes in response to antigenic challenge. In addition to B cells, germinal centers contain antigen-presenting cells and helper T cells that cooperate in mediating the B-cell changes that result in a more potent secondary immune response. Malignant transformation often occurs or is initiated in germinal center B cells. Follicular, Burkitt, and most large cell lymphomas are believed to be tumors of germinal center B cells. Three histologically distinct microenvironments have been described within the germinal center: a mantle zone surrounding interior, dark, and light zones. The mantle zone contains small resting B cells that have not been exposed to antigens (naïve). Tumors of cells from the mantle zone are usually clinically indolent and histologically low grade. Antigen-triggered activation of the densely packed B cells of the dark zone causes cells to proliferate and subjects genomic DNA to somatic hypermutation. Surviving clones from within the dark zone then enter the light zone where proliferation slows and affinity selection occurs. During affinity selection, only cells with surface immunoglobulin receptors with high affinity for the antigen survive. Antigen-specific B cells generated in the germinal center reaction leave the follicle and reappear in the outer mantle zone, to form a marginal zone. Marginal zones are particularly prominent in mesenteric lymph nodes, Peyer's patches, and the spleen. These post-germinal center B cells include memory B cells of the marginal zone and plasma cells. Marginal cell B-cell lymphomas tend to be indolent and may be either extranodal or nodal; extranodal marginal cell B-cell lymphomas are also referred to as MALT lymphomas.

T-cell lymphomas can be classified on the basis of antigen expression as either precursor (thymic) or mature (peripheral) in origin. These classifications clinically translate to precursor lymphoblastic lymphomas or to a heterogeneous group of peripheral T-cell lymphomas. Tumors of natural killer or natural killer-like T cells are uncommon.

The International Lymphoma Study Group, an informal group of 19 hematopathologists from the United States, Europe, and Asia, adopted a new approach to lymphoma classification in 1993. Because it represented a revision of current or prior European and American lymphoma classifications, it was called the Revised European-American Classification of Lymphoid Neoplasms (REAL). The REAL classification system is based on the principle that a classification is a list of "real" disease entities, which are defined by a combination of morphology, immunophenotype, genetic features, and clinical features.[57,58] The relative importance of each of these criteria for both definition and diagnosis differs among different diseases. Morphology is always important, and some diseases are primarily defined by morphology alone (eg, follicular lymphoma), although immunophenotype can be helpful in difficult cases. Some diseases have a specific immunophenotype (eg, MCL, small lymphocytic lymphoma) that is virtually diagnostic of that disease. A specific genetic abnormality is important in some lymphomas—t(11;14) in MCL, t(8;14) in Burkitt lymphoma, and t(14;18) in follicular lymphoma—whereas other lymphomas lack specific genetic abnormalities (eg, MALT lymphoma, DLBCL). Finally, other lymphomas consider clinical features (eg, extranodal vs nodal presentation in marginal zone lymphoma and peripheral T-cell lymphoma).

Since 1995, members of the European and American Hematopathology societies have worked to develop a new WHO classification of hematologic malignancies. The final classification was published in 2001, and revised in 2008 and 2016.[12,57,58] The WHO classification uses an updated version of the REAL classification and expands the principles of the REAL classification to the classification of myeloid and lymphoid malignancies.

5 The 2016 WHO classification categorizes lymphoid malignancies into two major categories: B-cell lymphomas and T-cell (and natural killer cell) lymphomas (see Table 132-1).[12,57,58] B-cell lymphomas represent about 85% to 90% of all NHLs. Lymphomas within each category can be divided into malignancies of precursor or mature cells. Hodgkin lymphoma and multiple myeloma are now recognized as mature B-cell neoplasms. The WHO classification uses the term *grade* to refer to histologic parameters such as cell and nuclear size, density of chromatin, and proliferation fraction, and the term *aggressiveness* to denote clinical behavior of a tumor. This classification scheme includes both lymphomas and lymphoid leukemias because there is no distinction between the solid and circulating forms of these diseases. The WHO classification includes several previously unrecognized types of lymphomas, and new entities not specifically recognized in the Working Formulation account for about 20% to 25% of the cases.

The WHO classification has broad clinical implications. The WHO Clinical Advisory Committee has agreed that clinical groupings of lymphoid neoplasms into prognostic categories are neither necessary nor desirable because such arbitrary groupings are of no practical value and may be misleading.[60]

Clinical Presentation

6 Patients with NHL present with a wide variety of symptoms, depending on the site of involvement and whether tumor involvement is nodal or extranodal. Sites of involvement and dissemination of the malignant cells can sometimes be predicted based on the cell of origin and the tendency of tumors to frequently disseminate to areas where the normal counterparts of the lymphoma cells are located. For example, B-cell lymphomas involve areas of the lymphoid system normally populated by B-lymphocytes such as lymph nodes, spleen, and bone marrow. T-cell lymphomas commonly disseminate to various extranodal sites such as the skin and lungs.[55]

Most patients present with peripheral lymphadenopathy. The lymphadenopathy may be either localized or generalized, and the involved nodes are often painless, rubbery, and discrete, and usually located in the cervical and supraclavicular regions as in Hodgkin lymphoma (see Fig. 132-1). Rapid and progressive lymphadenopathy is more characteristic of aggressive lymphomas. Waxing and waning of lymph nodes, including their complete disappearance and reappearance, is more characteristic of indolent lymphomas. Massive lymphadenopathy can sometimes lead to organ dysfunction. For example, patients with NHL may present with acute renal failure from retroperitoneal adenopathy causing ureteral obstruction or from metabolic abnormalities such as hyperuricemia with uric acid nephropathy.

About 40% of patients with NHL present with fever (temperature >38°C [100.4°F]), weight loss (unexplained weight loss of 10% of body weight over the past 6 months), or night sweats (drenching night sweats). If one or more of these symptoms is present, the patient is noted to have B symptoms, and a B is added to the stage of disease (discussed in the Diagnosis, Staging, and Prognostic Factors section under Hodgkin Lymphoma earlier in this Chapter). B symptoms are more commonly observed in patients with aggressive NHLs.

CLINICAL PRESENTATION Non-Hodgkin Lymphoma

General

- Patients with NHL present with a wide variety of symptoms, depending on the site of involvement and whether tumor involvement is nodal or extranodal.

Symptoms

- About 40% of patients present with fever, night sweats, and weight loss (ie, B symptoms).
- Fatigue, malaise, and pruritus.

Signs

- More than two-thirds of patients present with peripheral lymphadenopathy.

Laboratory Tests

- A complete blood count, tests of renal and liver function, and serum electrolytes should be obtained.
- Serum β_2-microglobulin and LDH levels may be useful as prognostic factors and for monitoring response to therapy.

Other Diagnostic Tests

- Varies depending on sites of involvement.

Patients with Hodgkin lymphoma rarely present with extranodal (ie, extralymphatic) disease, but 10% to 35% of patients with NHL have primary extranodal disease at the time of diagnosis. The frequency of extranodal presentation varies dramatically among different subtypes. The most common extranodal sites are the gastrointestinal tract followed by the skin. The liver or spleen may be enlarged in patients with generalized adenopathy. Patients with mesenteric or gastrointestinal involvement may present with signs and symptoms of nausea, vomiting, obstruction, abdominal pain, a palpable abdominal mass, or gastrointestinal bleeding. Patients with bone marrow involvement may have symptoms related to anemia, neutropenia, or thrombocytopenia. Other sites of extranodal disease include the testes and bone. The incidence of solitary brain lymphoma is increasing, especially in patients with AIDS.

Diagnosis, Staging, and Prognostic Factors

As with Hodgkin lymphoma, the diagnosis of NHL must be established by pathologic review of tissue obtained by biopsy.[55,61] The preferred procedure is an excisional biopsy, where the entire involved lymph node is removed for review by an experienced hematopathologist. This procedure should be done carefully to prevent distortional artifact of the architecture, which could lead to an inaccurate diagnosis. Needle biopsy of the node can sometimes provide adequate tissue for pathologic diagnosis, if an excisional biopsy cannot be performed. When adenopathy is not present, diagnosis may be established by biopsy of cutaneous lesions, bone marrow biopsy and aspiration in patients with unexplained myelosuppression, liver biopsy in patients with hepatomegaly or elevated liver function tests, or biopsy of involved extranodal organs such as bone, Waldeyer's ring, lung, and testis.

After the diagnosis is established, further work-up is required to determine the extent of involvement.[55,61] Clinical staging always begins with a thorough history and physical examination. Patients should be questioned about the presence or absence and extent of fever, night sweats, and weight loss. A detailed history of lymphadenopathy should also be obtained, including when and where the lymph nodes were first noted, and their rate of growth. A complete physical examination is performed to assess the extent of disease involvement, with special attention given to all nodal areas (see Fig. 132-1). All patients should have a complete blood count, serum chemistries including liver and renal profiles, a chest radiograph, and bone marrow aspiration and biopsy. The likelihood of bone marrow involvement varies among the different histologic types of lymphoma (Table 132-8). Lumbar puncture to evaluate the cerebrospinal fluid is recommended in patients who have histologic types of lymphoma that often spread to the CNS.

Imaging studies are usually important in the staging work-up. CT scanning can identify both nodal and extranodal sites of disease, and has largely replaced lymphangiography for the evaluation of retroperitoneal lymphadenopathy. The abdominal and pelvic CT scan can identify mesenteric and retrocrural node involvement. CT scans can also detect tumor involvement of organs, including the kidneys, ovary, spleen, and liver. PET is currently not used routinely for staging of NHL.[61,62] Magnetic resonance imaging is of limited usefulness in the staging of NHL. Gallium scans are sometimes used as part of the staging work-up. Other tests, such as liver-spleen scan, bone scan, upper gastrointestinal series, and IV pyelogram, are sometimes useful in patients with organ symptomatology or serum chemistry abnormalities.

Although staging laparotomy was widely used in the late 1960s and 1970s as part of the staging work-up in patients with lymphoma, it is rarely used today because of technical improvements in imaging studies and the morbidity and potential mortality associated with the procedure.

The Ann Arbor staging classification developed for the clinical staging of Hodgkin lymphoma is also used to stage patients with NHL (see Table 132-2). After completion of the staging work-up, most patients will be found to have advanced disease (stages III and IV). The frequency of localized disease at the time of diagnosis varies depending on the histologic type of lymphoma (see Table 132-8). Stage is a more important prognostic factor in Hodgkin lymphoma than in NHL.

7 The Ann Arbor system emphasizes the distribution of nodal disease sites because Hodgkin lymphoma usually spreads through contiguous lymph nodes and does not involve extranodal sites. But NHL is a disease with tremendous heterogeneity that does not spread through contiguous lymph nodes and that often involves extranodal sites. As a result of these clinical differences between Hodgkin lymphoma and NHL, Ann Arbor stage correlates poorly with prognosis.

8 This lack of accuracy with the Ann Arbor staging system in NHL has led to several international projects to develop prognostic models for the most common types of NHLs—DLBCLs and follicular lymphomas. The International Non-Hodgkin Lymphoma Prognostic Factors Project was based on more than 2,000 patients with diffuse aggressive lymphomas treated with an anthracycline-containing combination chemotherapy regimen in the United States, Europe, and Canada.[63] The Project identified five risk factors that correlated with low complete response rate to chemotherapy and

TABLE 132-8 Clinical Characteristics of Patients with Common Types of Non-Hodgkin Lymphomas

Disease	Median Age (Years)	Frequency in Children	% Male	Stage I/II vs III/IV (%)	B Symptoms (%)	BM Involvement (%)	GI Tract Involvement (%)	% Surviving 5 years
B-cell chronic lymphocytic leukemia/small lymphocytic lymphoma	65	Rare	53	9 vs 91	33	72	3	51
Mantle cell lymphoma	63	Rare	74	20 vs 80	28	64	9	27
Extranodal marginal zone B-cell lymphoma of MALT type	60	Rare	48	67 vs 33	19	14	50	74
Follicular lymphoma	59	Rare	42	33 vs 67	28	42	4	72
Diffuse large B-cell lymphoma	64	≈25% of childhood NHL	55	54 vs 46	33	16	18	46
Burkitt lymphoma	31	≈30% of childhood NHL	89	62 vs 38	22	33	11	45
Precursor T-cell lymphoblastic lymphoma	28	≈40% of childhood NHL	64	11 vs 89	21	50	4	26
Anaplastic large T-/null cell lymphoma	34	Common	69	51 vs 49	53	13	9	77
Peripheral T-cell non-Hodgkin lymphoma	61	≈5% of childhood NHL	55	20 vs 80	50	36	15	25

BM, bone marrow; GI, gastrointestinal; MALT, mucosa-associated lymphoid tissue; NHL, non-Hodgkin lymphoma.

Reproduced with permission from Longo DL. Malignancies of Lymphoid Cells. In: Kasper D, Fauci A, Hauser S, Longo D, Jameson J, Loscalzo J. eds. Harrison's Principles of Internal Medicine, 19e. New York, NY: McGraw-Hill; 2015.

poor survival: age older than 60 years, reduced performance status more than or equal to 2, abnormal serum LDH levels, two or more extranodal sites of disease, and advanced tumor stage (Ann Arbor stage III or IV) (Table 132-9). In patients older than or equal to 60 years old, three risk factors correlated with low complete response rate to chemotherapy and poor survival: reduced performance status, abnormal serum LDH levels, and Ann Arbor stage. It is unclear whether the effect of serum LDH level is related to a tumor or a host event. LDH likely measures cellular catabolism (the enzyme is released from injured cells), or the product of tumor burden and proliferation. Because each of the factors has about the same impact (eg, relative risk) on prognosis, the number of adverse risk factors is summed to provide the IPI. Patients could, therefore, have a score of 0 to 5. For patients older than or equal to 60 years old, a simplified IPI score can be developed based on Ann Arbor stage, serum LDH level, and performance status.

As prognosis improves as a result of more effective therapy, it is important to reevaluate prognostic factors. The IPI was based on patients treated from 1982 to 1987 with anthracycline-based combination chemotherapy; none of the patients received rituximab. In a reexamination of the IPI in a cohort of patients treated with rituximab-containing chemotherapy, Sehn et al. found that the IPI remained predictive, but it only identified two, rather than four, risk groups.[64] When the number of risk factors is redistributed, three risk groups are identified that correlate with prognosis. This revised IPI score may more accurately predict prognosis in patients treated with rituximab-containing combination chemotherapy, but needs to be validated in a larger group of patients.

Although the IPI is often used to predict prognosis in patients with other NHL subtypes, the IPI has several shortcomings when applied to patients with indolent lymphomas. Because only patients with diffuse aggressive lymphomas were used to develop the IPI system, some important prognostic factors may have been missed. Furthermore, the IPI system has limited discriminating power in follicular lymphoma because only about 10% of patients are categorized as high-risk in the IPI system. To address these concerns, an international cooperative study was designed to develop a prognostic model similar to the IPI in patients with follicular lymphoma. The results of that study, which was based on more than 4,000 patients with follicular lymphoma diagnosed between 1985 and 1992, were recently published.[65] Five factors were identified that correlated with poor survival: age older than 60 years, advanced tumor stage (Ann Arbor stage III or IV), low hemoglobin level (<12 g/dL [<120 g/L; <7.45 mmol/L]), five or more nodal sites of disease (see Fig. 132-1), and an abnormal serum LDH level. Analogous to the IPI, the number of adverse risk factors is summed to provide the Follicular Lymphoma International Prognostic Index (FLIPI). Three prognostic groups were identified: low-risk (0-1 factors), intermediate-risk (2 factors), and high-risk (≥3 factors). FLIPI appeared to have higher discriminating power among groups as compared with the IPI system. Table 132-10 shows the correlation between the FLIPI score and overall survival. The survival data from FLIPI, however, may

TABLE 132-9 Risk Factors and Survival According to the International Non-Hodgkin Lymphoma Prognostic Factors Project

All Patients	Patients ≤60 Years of Age
Age >60 years	Abnormal LDH level
Abnormal LDH level	Performance status ≥2
Performance status ≥2	Ann Arbor stage III or IV
Ann Arbor stage III or IV	
Extranodal involvement ≥2 sites	

LDH, lactic dehydrogenase.

Data from reference 67.

TABLE 132-10 Risk Factors and Survival According to the Follicular Lymphoma International Prognostic Index

All Patients	
Age >60 years Ann Arbor stage III or IV Number of nodal sites ≥5 Abnormal lactate dehydrogenase level Hemoglobin <12 g/dL (<120 g/L; <7.45 mmol/L)	
Risk Group (% of Patients)	**Number of Risk Factors**
Low (36)	0–1
Intermediate (37)	2
High (27)	≥3

not reflect current treatment results because none of the patients in the cohort used to derive the FLIPI were treated with rituximab. In an updated prognostic model (FLIPI-2) derived from patients with newly diagnosed follicular lymphoma treated with rituximab-containing chemoimmunotherapy regimens, age older than 60 years, low hemoglobin level (<12 g/dL [<120 g/L; <7.45 mmol/L]), longest diameter of the largest lymph node more than 6 cm, abnormal β_2-microglobulin levels and bone marrow involvement were identified as adverse risk factors. FLIPI-2 was highly predictive of treatment outcomes and separated patients into three distinct risk groups: low-risk (0 factors), intermediate-risk (1 or 2 factors), and high-risk (≥3 factors). Three-year progression-free survival was 91%, 69%, and 51% and overall survival was 99%, 96%, and 84% in low-, intermediate-, and high-risk patients, respectively.[66]

Although IPI and FLIPI are clinically useful tools to estimate prognosis, the factors used to calculate these scores probably represent clinical surrogates for the biologic heterogeneity among NHLs and many researchers are interested in determining the prognostic importance of certain phenotypic and molecular characteristics of NHLs. For example, molecular markers of apoptosis, cell-cycle regulation, cell lineage, and cell proliferation are being evaluated as potentially clinically useful prognostic factors.[67]

Gene expression profiling with microarrays may also correlate with survival. Using gene expression profiling, investigators identified at least two molecularly distinct forms of DLBCLs based on gene expression patterns indicative of different stages of B-cell differentiation: germinal center B-cell–like (GCB) and activated B-cell–like (ABC).[67,68] The GCB subtype of DLBCL probably arises from normal germinal center B-cells while the ABC subtype may arise from post-germinal center B-cells. Many oncogenic pathways are different for the GCB and ABC subtypes, and these differences may lead to the development of targeted therapies for each subtype.[59,67] Patients with the germinal center B-cell profile had significantly better overall survival independent of IPI score after treatment with cyclophosphamide, doxorubicin [hydroxydaunorubicin], vincristine (Oncovin®), prednisone (CHOP) or CHOP-like chemotherapy. In a recently published study of patients with DLBCL treated with either CHOP or rituximab and CHOP (R-CHOP), Lenz et al. identified several gene expressions signatures that predicted survival in both CHOP and R-CHOP cohorts: GCB, stromal-1, and stromal-2.[69] The GCB and stromal-1 signatures were associated with a favorable prognosis while the stromal-2 signature was associated with an unfavorable prognosis. The stromal-1 signature reflects extracellular matrix deposition and histiocytic infiltration whereas the stromal-2 signature reflects tumor blood vessel density. It is speculated that DLBCLs that express the stromal-2 signature may respond to antiangiogenic agents.

Another recently identified molecular subtype is double-hit DLBCL, defined as the existence of both MYC gene arrangement and t(14;18) BCL2 translocation.[70] In one pathologic study that used immunohistochemical scoring, patients with high expression of both BCL2 and MYC protein had the worst prognosis. Double-hit NHL is associated with significantly lower complete response rate, shorter overall survival and shorter progression-free survival.[71] The NCCN guideline suggests that patients with double-hit lymphoma usually have a very poor prognosis, with a median overall survival that is 4 to 6 months even with highly aggressive chemotherapy. Some lymphoma experts suggest that patients with double-hit NHL should be treated with regimens that are more dose-intensive.[67]

Two molecularly distinct profiles of follicular lymphoma also have been identified; the first included genes encoding for T-cell markers and genes highly expressed in macrophages, and the second included genes that are preferentially expressed in macrophages, dendritic cells, or both.[72] Patients with the first molecular signature had a more favorable outcome than those with the second signature. These results suggest that molecular classification of tumors on the basis of gene expression may allow identification of clinically significant subtypes of cancer.

TREATMENT
Non-Hodgkin Lymphoma

Desired Outcomes

The primary goals in the treatment of NHL are to relieve symptoms, cure the patient of the disease whenever possible, and minimize the risk of serious toxicities. The treatment strategy depends on many factors, including the patient's age, concomitant disease, disease type, stage of disease, site of disease, and patient preference.

General Approach

9 Historically, both the clinical behavior and degree of aggressiveness are often used to describe NHLs. Indolent lymphomas, which make up about 25% to 40% of all NHLs, are characterized by their slow-growth behavior. Patients with an indolent lymphoma usually have a relatively long survival (measured in years), with or without aggressive chemotherapy. Although these lymphomas respond to a wide range of therapeutic approaches, there is no convincing evidence of a survival plateau, which indicates that patients are rarely cured of their disease. In contrast, aggressive lymphomas, which make up about 60% to 75% of all NHLs, are characterized by rapid growth rate and short survival (measured in weeks to months), if appropriate therapy is not initiated. Despite their more aggressive nature, many patients with aggressive lymphomas who respond to chemotherapy can experience prolonged disease-free survival and some are cured of their disease. Therefore, the terminology for the NHLs represents a paradox, where "indolent" is bad and "aggressive" is good in terms of the likelihood for cure.

Therapeutic approaches to NHL include radiation therapy, chemotherapy, and biologic agents. The role of radiation therapy in the treatment of NHL differs from its role in the treatment of Hodgkin lymphoma. Although the disease responds to radiation therapy, only a small percentage of patients with NHL present with truly localized disease that can be treated with local or regional radiation therapy. Radiation therapy is used more commonly in advanced disease, primarily as a palliative measure to control local bulky disease.

Effective chemotherapy for NHL ranges from single-agent therapy in indolent lymphomas to aggressive, complex chemotherapy regimens in aggressive lymphomas. The most active agents used in the treatment of NHL include the alkylating agents (eg, cyclophosphamide, chlorambucil), bleomycin, doxorubicin, purine analogs, etoposide, methotrexate, vincristine, and corticosteroids (eg, prednisone, dexamethasone). The most aggressive chemotherapy approaches are dose-dense chemotherapy or high-dose chemotherapy followed by autologous or allogeneic HSCT.

B-cell lymphomas have served as a model for immunotherapy with monoclonal antibodies for more than 20 years, beginning with the successful use of custom-made monoclonal antibodies targeted against the idiotype present on the patient's cancer cells.[73,74] These encouraging results lead to the development of monoclonal antibodies against a more generic target, a molecule on the surface of B cells that would be present on tumor cells. One potential target, the CD20 molecule, is present only on cells in the B-lymphocyte lineage. It is expressed on the surface of both normal and malignant B cells, but not on other normal tissues. Rituximab (Rituxan®) is a chimeric monoclonal antibody directed at the CD20 molecule. Its antitumor activity is mediated through complement-dependent cytotoxicity, antibody-dependent cytotoxicity, and induction of apoptosis.[74] With the availability of monoclonal antibodies and radioimmunoconjugates for the therapy of lymphoma, nearly all patients with NHL will receive one or more biologic agents during the course of their disease.

Objective response to therapy for NHL should be defined according to the International Workshop to Standardize Response Criteria for Non-Hodgkin Lymphoma, which was recently updated to incorporate the results of newer tests to monitor response such as PET, immunohistochemistry, and flow cytometry.[62] The revised guidelines describe criteria for response (eg, complete response, partial response, and stable disease) and survival (eg, overall, disease-free, event-free, and progression-free).

Appropriate therapy for NHL depends on the patient's age, histologic type, stage of disease, site of disease, and presence of adverse prognostic factors (as measured by IPI or FLIPI score), and patient preferences. In general, treatment of lymphoma can be divided into limited disease and advanced disease. Limited disease includes those patients with localized disease (Ann Arbor stages I and II). Advanced disease is defined as all Ann Arbor stage III or IV patients, and also frequently includes Ann Arbor stage II patients with poor prognostic features (see Tables 132-6 and 132-7).[63,65]

The following section discusses the clinical characteristics and therapy of the most common disease entities.

Follicular Lymphomas

The combined group of follicular lymphomas makes up the second most common histologic type of NHL in the United States, comprising about 20% of all NHLs worldwide and up to 70% of indolent lymphomas reported in American and European clinical trials.[75] The WHO classification includes criteria for grading follicular lymphoma based on the number of centroblasts per high-power field: grade 1 to 2 (0-15 centroblasts/high-power field) and grade 3 (>15 centroblasts/high-power field).[12] The clinical behavior and treatment outcome of grades 1 and 2 follicular lymphoma are similar, and they are usually treated as indolent lymphomas. In contrast, grade 3 follicular lymphoma is synonymous with what is often referred to as follicular large cell lymphoma and is usually treated as an aggressive lymphoma.

Follicular lymphomas tend to occur in older adults, with a slight female predominance (see Table 132-6). Most patients have advanced disease at diagnosis, but about 25% to 33% of patients have localized disease (clinical stage I or II) at diagnosis.[76] Extranodal disease, bulky disease, and B symptoms are uncommon features at diagnosis. Most patients with follicular lymphoma have the chromosomal translocation t(14;18) at the time of diagnosis.

The clinical course is generally indolent, with median survivals of 8 to 10 years. But the natural history of follicular lymphoma can be unpredictable. Spontaneous regression of objective disease has been noted in as many as 20% to 30% of patients.[77] There is also a high conversion rate of follicular lymphoma to a more aggressive histology over time that steadily increases after diagnosis and reaches about 30% at 10 years.[78] At autopsy, most patients with follicular lymphoma have some evidence of DLBCL. Patients with transformed indolent lymphoma should be treated in the same way as patients with an aggressive lymphoma.

Most patients have dramatic responses to initial therapy, and their disease course is characterized by multiple relapses, with responses to salvage therapy becoming progressively shorter after every relapse, eventually leading to death from disease-related causes. This pattern of constant relapses over time without evidence of a survival plateau and the failure of randomized controlled trials to show a survival benefit with aggressive chemotherapy led to the conclusion that therapy does not prolong overall survival and patients are not cured of their disease. However, several recently published studies suggest that the use of biologic agents, particularly rituximab, has changed the natural history of the follicular lymphoma. In a study of patients enrolled in Southwest Oncology Group (SWOG) trials over a period of more than 20 years, patients treated with CHOP and a monoclonal antibody had a significantly longer 4-year overall survival than those treated with CHOP alone (91% vs 69%).[79] Similar results were reported in patients treated over a 30-year period at the M.D. Anderson Cancer Center.[80] That study also showed an apparent plateau in the failure-free survival curve.

Certain subsets of patients with follicular lymphoma have a much better or worse prognosis. Some studies suggest that the natural history of follicular large cell lymphoma (ie, grade 3 follicular lymphoma) is similar to that of other aggressive lymphomas and that treatment with intensive combination chemotherapy regimens may result in long-term disease-free survival, including a possible plateau in the survival curve.[75] The recent development of the FLIPI prognostic model should help clinicians to identify patients in different prognostic groups based on disease characteristics at the time of diagnosis.[65] Patients who are predicted to have a poor prognosis (ie, high-risk) could then be offered aggressive or experimental therapy, while those who are predicted to have a good prognosis (ie, low-risk) would be treated with standard therapy, avoiding unnecessary toxicity.

Treatment of Localized Disease (Stages I and II)

Radiation therapy is the standard treatment for early stage follicular lymphoma. Involved-field, extended-field, and total nodal irradiation have been used. Carefully staged patients with either stage I or contiguous stage II disease treated with radiation therapy alone can achieve disease-free survival rates of 40% to 50% and overall survival rates of 60% to 70% at 10 years.[75] Late relapses are uncommon; only 10% of patients who reached 10 years without relapse subsequently experienced a recurrence.

Chemotherapy is not usually given in most patients with localized follicular lymphoma, but it may be helpful in some patients with high-risk stage II disease (eg, multiple sites of involvement or bulky disease).[81]

10 About 40% to 60% of patients with clinical stage I or II follicular lymphoma are cured of their disease with radiation therapy alone.[61] Most centers use radiation at a dose of 30 to 40 Gy (3,000-4,000 rad) to either involved (ie, local) or regional fields, which would consist of irradiation to the involved nodal region plus one additional uninvolved region on each side of the involved nodes. Extended-field irradiation is not usually used because of the absence of a survival benefit and possible increased risk of secondary malignancies. In addition, previous use of extended-field irradiation compromises the ability of that patient to receive subsequent chemotherapy. The current NCCN guideline states that locoregional radiation therapy is preferred for most patients with early stage follicular lymphoma.[61] Immunotherapy (ie, rituximab) with or without chemotherapy is also listed as an option.

Treatment of Advanced Disease (Stages II Bulky, III, and IV)

The management of stages II Bulky, III, and IV indolent lymphomas remains controversial because until recently, no therapeutic approaches had been shown to prolong overall survival despite the high complete remission rates to initial therapy. However, the results of recently published studies suggest that the initial use of biologic therapy such as rituximab is associated with longer overall survival.[79,80] More than 80% of patients with stage III or IV follicular lymphoma are alive at 5 years, and the median survival ranges between 7 and 10 years.

Therapeutic options for these patients are diverse and include watchful waiting, radiation therapy, single-agent chemotherapy, combination chemotherapy, biologic therapy, radioimmunotherapy, and combined-modality therapy.[61] Although complete remission can be achieved in 50% to 80% of patients with various treatments, the median time to relapse is usually only 18 to 36 months. About 20% of patients who have a complete response remain in remission for longer than 10 years. After relapse, patients are retreated, and high remission rates can be achieved. Unfortunately, response rates and duration of response both decrease with each retreatment.

Several different approaches can be used to treat follicular lymphoma. Carefully selected patients may receive no initial therapy followed by single-agent chemotherapy, rituximab, or radiation therapy when treatment is needed. Candidates for the conservative approach are usually older, asymptomatic, and have minimal tumor burden. Patients with symptoms, extensive extranodal involvement, bulky disease, cytopenia due to bone marrow involvement, or impaired end-organ function at the time of diagnosis are not candidates for conservative treatment. Alternatively, patients can be treated aggressively with combination chemotherapy, with or without rituximab early in the disease course. Both conservative and aggressive approaches are listed as possible options in the current NCCN guideline, but the guideline recommends that initial therapy should include rituximab unless contraindicated.[61] Patients who respond to induction therapy may receive maintenance therapy with single-agent rituximab.

At the time of relapse, many of the same treatment options are available, and the following factors must be considered: age, symptomatic status of the patient, tumor burden, rate of regrowth (based on previous assessment of active disease sites), presence or absence of characteristics suggesting transformation or biologic progression, prior therapy, degree and duration of response to prior therapy, availability of clinical trials, and patient preferences.[61]

Watch-and-Wait Because there are no convincing data that standard treatment approaches have improved survival, some clinicians have adopted a "watch-and-wait" approach for asymptomatic patients where therapy is delayed until the patient experiences systemic symptoms or disease progression such as rapidly progressive or bulky adenopathy, anemia, thrombocytopenia, or disease in threatening sites such as the orbit or spinal cord.[81,82] The median time until treatment is required is 3 to 5 years, and about 20% of patients do not require therapy for up to 10 years. The 10-year survival is 73%, which is not significantly different from patients who received therapy at the time of diagnosis. In a randomized study of asymptomatic patients with indolent lymphomas (mostly follicular), patients who underwent watchful waiting had similar cause-specific and overall survival as compared with those who received immediate chlorambucil.[82] With a median length of follow-up of 16 years, about 17% of patients who were randomized to the watchful waiting group died of other causes without receiving chemotherapy and an additional 9% are alive and have not yet had chemotherapy. Due to the frequent use of rituximab in current clinical practice, a recent study has evaluated whether the use of the "watch-and-wait" approach is more effective than the use of rituximab to delay the need for chemotherapy or radiotherapy in patients with advanced-stage, low-tumor-burden follicular lymphoma. Immediate treatment with rituximab significantly delays disease progression and the time until chemotherapy or radiotherapy compared with a watchful waiting approach.[83] However, an overall survival advantage has not been demonstrated with this approach.

As described above, patients with follicular lymphoma who are followed without therapy sometimes have spontaneous regressions that can be complete while the disease in other patients can convert to a more aggressive histology. If the watchful waiting approach is chosen, the patient should be evaluated at least every 3 to 6 months for 5 years and then annually, so that intervention can occur before serious problems occur.[61]

Clinical **Controversy...**

Watch-and-wait is a common approach for managing asymptomatic, indolent follicular lymphomas. Although it is demonstrated that early initiation of induction and maintenance rituximab in this group of patients improves quality of life, it has not been demonstrated to improve overall survival. Some experts suggest that future studies should evaluate whether early induction with rituximab would have an impact on second line therapy.

Chemotherapy Oral alkylating agents, given either alone or combined with prednisone, have been the mainstay of treatment for follicular lymphoma. More intensive chemotherapy has not been shown to improve patient outcome. In a randomized trial of oral chlorambucil, oral cyclophosphamide, or CVP in patients with indolent lymphoma, no significant difference in overall survival or freedom-from-relapse between the three groups was observed.[77] The dosage of single-agent chlorambucil or cyclophosphamide is usually adjusted to maintain a platelet count above 100,000 cells/mm^3 (100×10^9/L) and a white blood cell count above 3,000 cells/mm^3 (3×10^9/L). Although single-agent alkylating agents have a high initial complete remission rate, the time required to achieve a complete response is slow (median time is 9-12 months). Complete responses occur more rapidly with combination chemotherapy, particularly with doxorubicin-containing regimens. Many clinicians will therefore give CHOP or CHOP-like chemotherapy when a rapid response is necessary. The development of the CHOP regimen is described in more detail in the Aggressive Lymphomas section later in this chapter. Table 132-11 shows the CHOP regimen that is widely used in the treatment of NHL. In those who achieve a complete response, the duration of response is relatively short (about 2.5 years). Maintenance therapy with chemotherapy provides no additional benefit. After the "best" response is achieved, many experts will discontinue therapy and observe.

Both single-agent alkylating agents and CVP are well tolerated by most patients. The advantages of oral chlorambucil are no hair

TABLE 132-11 CHOP Regimen

Drug	Dose	Route	Treatment Days
Cyclophosphamide	750 mg/m^2	IV	1
Doxorubicin	50 mg/m^2	IV	1
Vincristine	1.4 mg/m^2	IV	1
Prednisone	100 mg	Oral	1–5
One cycle is 21 days			

Another name for doxorubicin is hydroxydaunorubicin.

[a]Vincristine dose is typically capped at 2 mg.

loss, little or no nausea, and minimal myelosuppression. Because of its mild side effects profile, oral chlorambucil is usually recommended for older patients who are minimally symptomatic or who have other comorbidities. There are some concerns with the risk of secondary acute leukemia in patients receiving continuous exposure to alkylating agents.

Anti-CD20 Monoclonal Antibodies The approval of rituximab is arguably the most important recent development in the treatment of NHL. Its initial approval in 1997 was based on an open-label multicenter study that enrolled 166 patients with relapsed or recurrent indolent lymphoma.[84] Rituximab, given IV at a dose of 375 mg/m^2 weekly for 4 weeks, resulted in an overall response of 48% (complete response: 6%, partial response: 42%). Median time to progression for responders was 13.2 months and median duration of response was 11.6 months. Other studies of single-agent rituximab in patients with relapsed or refractory indolent NHL have reported overall response rates of 40% to 60% and complete response rates of 5% to 10%.[85]

Based on the activity of rituximab in relapsed or refractory patients, it is currently being used as first-line therapy, either alone or in combination with chemotherapy.[73,85,86] When given as a single agent to patients with previously untreated indolent NHL, the overall response rate is 60% to 70% and the complete response rate is 20% to 30%. It is interesting to note that many of these patients remain in molecular remission (ie, polymerase chain reaction–negative) at 12 months. Single-agent rituximab is listed as an acceptable option for first-line therapy of follicular lymphoma, particularly for patients who cannot tolerate more intensive chemotherapy regimens.[61]

The rationale for the use of rituximab in combination with conventional agents is based on clinical activity of both agents/regimens, non–cross-resistant mechanisms of action, nonoverlapping toxicities, and synergistic antitumor activity in vitro. Many clinical trials have evaluated the use of rituximab in combination with other chemotherapy agents. In a phase II trial of six courses of R-CHOP, the overall and complete response rate in 40 patients with previously untreated or relapsed indolent lymphoma was 95% and 55%, respectively.[87] More than 70% of patients were progression-free after 4 years of follow-up. In an updated analysis, median time-to-progression was reached at 82 months.[88] Based on these encouraging results, several randomized controlled trials have evaluated rituximab in combination with various chemotherapy regimens in first-line therapy for follicular or other indolent lymphomas.[73] In the R-CHOP versus CHOP trial, patients who were randomized to receive R-CHOP as initial therapy had significantly higher overall response rates (96% vs 90%), reduced risk for treatment failure (relative risk 0.4), and longer time-to-treatment failure and overall survival.[89] In another randomized trial of R-CHOP versus CHOP in relapsed or resistant follicular lymphoma, patients treated with R-CHOP had higher overall and complete response rates (85% vs 72% and 30% vs 16%, respectively) and lower risk of treatment failure (hazard ratio [HR] 0.65), but no significant difference in overall survival was observed.[90] Similar results were reported when rituximab was added to other combination regimens.[73,74] In a meta-analysis of all randomized controlled trials, patients with indolent lymphoma treated with rituximab and chemotherapy had a significantly higher overall response rate and reduced risk of treatment failure (HR 0.62) and death (HR 0.65).[91] Rituximab is FDA-approved for first-line therapy for follicular lymphoma in combination with CVP chemotherapy. R-CHOP is listed as an acceptable option for first-line therapy of follicular lymphoma (category 1).[61]

Rituximab and CHOP chemotherapy can be combined in many different ways. In the R-CHOP regimen developed by Czuczman et al., two doses of rituximab are given before the start of CHOP therapy; two more doses are given in the middle of the six cycles of CHOP; and two additional doses are given at the end of CHOP therapy.[87] However, in most NHL protocols and in clinical practice, rituximab is given on day 1 of CHOP chemotherapy. In some protocols, rituximab is given on the day before chemotherapy (ie, day 0) or rituximab is given on day 1 and the other drugs are given on day 3.

In patients who respond to rituximab, either alone or combined with chemotherapy, maintenance therapy with single-agent rituximab is often given to prolong the duration of remission. Rituximab is FDA approved as single-agent maintenance therapy in patients achieving a complete or partial response following induction chemotherapy. The FDA approval was based on a randomized controlled trial in previously untreated patients with advanced-stage follicular lymphoma treated with maintenance rituximab after CVP chemotherapy.[92] Three-year progression-free survival was significantly longer in the maintenance rituximab group as compared with the observation group (65% vs 22%).[83] In another recently published randomized controlled trial, patients responding to first-line chemotherapy in combination with rituximab (such as R-CVP, R-CHOP or rituximab, fludarabine, cyclophosphamide, and mitoxantrone [R-FCM]) were randomized to receive rituximab maintenance (12 infusions of 375 mg/m^2 given IV, once every 8 weeks) or no maintenance.[93] After a median follow-up of 24 months, rituximab maintenance significantly improved progression-free survival compared to observation (75% vs 58%). Interestingly, induction therapy with R-CHOP or R-FCM was associated with improved progression-free survival, which suggests that R-CVP was not beneficial in this study. Longer follow-up is needed to evaluate the effect of rituximab maintenance on overall survival.

Although the use of maintenance rituximab improves progression-free survival, no overall survival benefit has been observed in randomized controlled trials. Similar findings were observed in a prospective observational study of more than 2,700 patients with newly diagnosed follicular lymphoma treated in the United States from 2004 to 2007, patients who have received maintenance rituximab after induction chemotherapy were found to have significantly longer progression-free survival and time to next treatment after 5 years of follow-up.[94] And maintenance rituximab is expensive and may be associated with adverse effects, including an increased risk of grades 3 or 4 infections. The NCCN guideline lists maintenance therapy with rituximab (one dose every 8 weeks for up to 2 years) as an option following first-line therapy for patients initially presenting with high tumor burden.[61]

Rituximab maintenance following second-line therapy has also been evaluated in patients with relapsed or refractory disease. Two randomized trials have demonstrated a progression-free survival advantage with rituximab maintenance over observation for patients treated with induction chemotherapy.[95,96] In a recently published trial of patients with relapsed or resistant follicular lymphoma responding to CHOP or R-CHOP induction, maintenance rituximab significantly improved median progression-free survival as compared with observation alone (3.7 years vs 1.3 years). The 5-year overall survival, however, was not significantly different between the study arms (74% vs 64%).[96] It is also important to note that patients who develop progression of disease during or within 6 months of first-line maintenance rituximab will likely experience little, if any, benefit from maintenance therapy in the second-line setting. The NCCN guideline recommends optional maintenance therapy with rituximab (one dose every 12 weeks for 2 years) for patients who are in remission after second-line therapy.[61]

Most of the adverse effects of rituximab are infusion-related, particularly after the first infusion, and consist of fever, chills, respiratory symptoms, fatigue, headache, pruritus, and angioedema. Premedication with oral acetaminophen 650 mg and diphenhydramine 50 mg is usually given 30 minutes before rituximab infusion. The package insert recommends a step-up infusion rate of rituximab to decrease the risk of infusion-related infusion. Duration of infusions, however, may take up to 5 hours. Studies have demonstrated that rapid infusion of rituximab (infused over 90 minutes) is feasible in patients who tolerate their first cycle of rituximab without increasing the risk of infusion-related reactions.[97,98] The FDA has approved rapid infusions of rituximab, but they are not recommended in patients with clinically significant cardiovascular disease and high circulating lymphocyte counts (>5,000 cells/mm^3 [5 × 10^9/L]). Reactivation of hepatitis B has been reported in patients receiving chemotherapy, either alone or combined with rituximab.[99] Hepatitis B testing is recommended in patients who are considering rituximab therapy.[61]

In addition to rituximab, other anti-CD20 antibodies are currently under research development.[74] Ofatumumab, a fully human antibody against CD20, is currently approved for treatment of refractory chronic lymphocytic leukemia. It binds to two sites on the CD20 molecule, which brings the antibody closer to the cell membrane and increases complement-dependent cytotoxicity.[100] Ofatumumab is being evaluated in randomized controlled trials against rituximab-based regimens for treatment of both indolent and aggressive lymphomas.

Bendamustine Bendamustine is an alkylating agent with structural similarities to both alkylating agents and purine analogs. The mechanism of action of bendamustine appears to be different from other alkylating agents and it does not show cross-resistance to other alkylating agents. When used as a single agent, bendamustine shows antitumor activity in relapsed or refractory indolent lymphomas. Overall and complete response rates of 70% to 80% and 30% to 35% have been reported, respectively, in phase II trials.[101] Two randomized, non-inferiority studies have demonstrated that bendamustine and rituximab (BR) is noninferior to R-CHOP for indolent lymphomas. In a Phase III randomized non-inferiority study enrolling Stages 3 and 4 indolent lymphoma (with slightly over half follicular lymphoma patients), patients received either BR or R-CHOP. At a median follow-up of 45 months, median progression-free survival was longer in the BR group than in the R-CHOP group. In the subgroup analysis of patients with follicular lymphoma subtype, a significant benefit for progression-free survival was observed with BR versus R-CHOP.[102] In another study, BR was demonstrated to be noninferior to standard therapies (R-CHOP or R-CVP) for both overall (97% vs 91%) and complete response (31% vs 25%).[103] Both studies also reported that BR was associated with fewer infectious episodes and fewer hematological toxicities such as grade 3 to 4 leukopenia and neutropenia. BR was also associated with less peripheral neuropathy and alopecia.[102,103] However, dermatological toxicities, drug-related hypersensitivities and vomiting were more common with BR. Based on these results, BR, R-CHOP, and R-CVP are all listed as first-line therapy of follicular lymphoma (category 1).[61]

Clinical **Controversy...**

Bendamustine and rituximab is associated with fewer serious adverse events as compared to R-CHOP as first-line therapy for follicular lymphoma. With the increased use of bendamustine-based treatment as first-line therapy for follicular lymphoma in the rituximab era, it is unknown whether maintenance rituximab as consolidation would confer any clinical benefit in this group of patients.

Fludarabine Fludarabine phosphate shows encouraging results in previously untreated and relapsed advanced follicular lymphoma. The mechanism of action is not well understood, but it is accumulated in lymphocytes and are resistant to adenosine deaminase. In patients with relapsed or refractory indolent lymphoma, single-agent fludarabine has an overall response rate of almost 50% and a complete response rate of 10% to 15%. Response rates are higher in previously untreated patients, with overall and complete response rates of 70% and almost 40%, respectively. The median time to progression is less than 6 months for relapsed disease and more than 12 months for previously untreated patients. Combination regimens with fludarabine have also being investigated. Fludarabine, mitoxantrone, and dexamethasone (FND), given with or without rituximab, are examples of fludarabine-containing regimens that show encouraging results in patients with indolent lymphoma.[104]

Fludarabine does not usually cause nausea and vomiting or hair loss, but it is associated with cumulative and prolonged myelosuppression and profound immunosuppression, which increases the risk of opportunistic infections, such as fungal infections, *Pneumocystis jiroveci* pneumonia, and viral infections. Because the use of fludarabine-based regimens may impair stem cell mobilization and collection, some experts avoid fludarabine-based regimens for patients who are potential candidates for autologous HSCT.

Radioimmunotherapy ^{90}Y-ibritumomab tiuxetan (Zevalin®) is an anti-CD20 radioimmunoconjugate which is currently available for patients with indolent NHLs.[105] It is a mouse antibody linked to yttrium-90 $^{(90Y)}$, a radioisotope. Another anti-CD20 radioimmunoconjugate, ^{131}I-tositumomab (Bexxar®), was recently discontinued by the manufacturer because of limited use. Indolent lymphomas are known to be responsive to radiation therapy (ie, radiosensitive), and the rationale of radioimmunotherapy is that the antibody will act as a guided missile to deliver its payload (ie, radiation) to its target (ie, lymphoma cells that express the CD20 antigen). The specificity of the monoclonal antibody allows delivery of the radiation selectively to the tumor (and adjacent normal tissues).

^{90}Y-ibritumomab tiuxetan has shown activity in relapsed and refractory patients with indolent or transformed lymphomas.[105] In patients who respond to radioimmunotherapy, the duration of remission can be more than several years. Although radioimmunotherapy is usually reserved for second-line therapy of follicular lymphoma, some clinicians consider radioimmunotherapy earlier in the disease course. In a phase II study, patients with previously untreated follicular lymphoma were treated with six cycles of CHOP chemotherapy followed 4 to 8 weeks later by ^{131}I-tositumomab.[106] The overall response rate to the entire treatment regimen was 91%, including 69% complete remissions, and the 5-year progression-free survival is estimated to be 67%. Similar results were reported in a phase II trial of ^{131}I-tositumomab given without induction CHOP chemotherapy in previously untreated patients with advanced-stage follicular lymphoma.[107] Durable responses have also been reported with ^{131}I-tositumomab and CVP.[108]

Radioimmunotherapy is generally well-tolerated. The major acute toxicities with both radioimmunoconjugates are infusion-related reactions and myelosuppression.[131] The primary concern with radioimmunotherapy is the development of treatment-related myelodysplastic syndrome or acute myelogenous leukemia.[109]

The decision to use radioimmunotherapy must be made carefully because of the complexity, risks, and costs of the treatment regimen. Because of safety concerns related to delivery of radiation to bone marrow, candidates for radioimmunotherapy usually have limited bone marrow involvement and adequate absolute neutrophil and platelet counts. Although medical oncologists usually select patients for therapy, the radioimmunotherapy regimen must be administered at a radiation oncology or nuclear medicine facility.

Lenalidomide Lenalidomide is an immunomodulating agent which is currently indicated for the treatment of multiple myeloma and myelodysplastic syndromes. There is emerging data suggesting that it has activity in indolent NHL. In a phase II study of lenalidomide and rituximab in previously untreated follicular lymphoma patients, the overall response rate was 98% and the 2-year progression-free survival was 89%.[110] The combination has also been evaluated in the treatment of both patients with previously untreated and relapsed/refractory indolent lymphomas. In another phase II trial of patients with relapsed/refractory indolent NHL, single-agent lenalidomide induced an overall response rate of 27% within the subgroup of patients with follicular lymphoma, with a median progression-free survival for all patients of 4.4 months.[111] Toxicities that are commonly observed with lenalidomide include neutropenia, fatigue and thrombosis. A number of studies are currently evaluating its role as frontline therapy for indolent lymphoma.

Idelalisib Idelalisib is an oral inhibitor of phosphatidylinositol 3-kinase-delta (PI3K delta) which was approved for the treatment of relapsed and refractory FL. PI3K delta mediates B-cell receptor signaling and microenvironmental support signals that promote the growth and survival of malignant B lymphocytes. In a phase II study, patients with relapsed or refractory indolent NHL were given idelalisib 150 mg twice daily until disease progression. The overall response rate was 57%, with a median duration of response of 12.5 months. Common side effects of idelalisib include neutropenia, transaminitis, diarrhea, and pneumonia.[112] The current NCCN guideline lists idelalisib as an option for second-line therapy for patients with relapsed or refractory follicular lymphoma.[61]

Hematopoietic Stem Cell Transplantation High-dose chemotherapy, followed by autologous or allogeneic HSCT, is another option for patients with relapsed follicular lymphoma.[113,114] In patients who are transplanted at the time of initial treatment failure, 5-year event-free survival is about 40% to 50%. Although the rate of recurrence is lower after allogeneic HSCT as compared with autologous HSCT, that benefit is offset by increased treatment-related mortality after allogeneic HSCT. The presence of a survival plateau after allogeneic HSCT suggests that some patients may be cured of their disease.

A recent study has evaluated the role of HSCT in relapsed/refractory follicular lymphoma following disease relapse after prior rituximab-based therapy. Allogeneic HSCT was associated with increased risk of death on analysis. Autologous HSCT, on the other hand, was associated with a 3-year overall survival rates at 87%.[115] The current NCCN guideline lists the use of autologous HSCT as an appropriate consolidative therapy for patients achieving second or third remission.[61]

Diffuse Large B-Cell Lymphoma

Diffuse large B-cell lymphomas are the most common lymphoma in the International NHL Classification Project, accounting for about 30% of all NHLs.[116] DLBCLs are characterized by the presence of large cells, which are similar in size to or larger than tissue macrophages and usually more than twice the size of normal lymphocytes. The median age at the time of diagnosis is in the seventh decade, but DLBCL can affect individuals of all ages, from children to the elderly. Patients often present with a rapidly enlarging symptomatic mass, with B symptoms in about 30% to 40% of cases.[116] About 30% to 40% of patients with DLBCL present with extranodal disease; common sites include the head and neck, gastrointestinal tract, skin, bone, testis, and CNS. DLBCL is the most common type of diffuse aggressive lymphomas, which are characterized by an aggressive clinical behavior that leads to death within weeks to months if the tumor is not treated. Diffuse aggressive lymphomas are also sensitive to many chemotherapeutic agents, and some patients treated with chemotherapy can be cured of their disease.

Several factors have been shown to correlate with response to chemotherapy and survival in patients with aggressive lymphoma. Because the IPI was originally developed based on patients with aggressive lymphoma, IPI score correlates with prognosis (see Table 132-9).[63] As described above, the revised IPI score may more accurately predict prognosis in patients receiving rituximab-containing combination chemotherapy.[64]

Therapy of DLBCL is based on the Ann Arbor stage, IPI (or revised IPI) score, and other prognostic factors.[116] About one-half of patients present with localized (stage I or II) disease. However, many patients present with large bulky masses (ie, larger than 10 cm), and patients with bulky stage II disease are treated with the same approach used for patients with advanced disease (stage III or IV).

Treatment of Localized Disease (Stages I and II)

Before 1980, radiation therapy was the primary treatment for patients with localized DLBCL. Five-year disease-free survival with radiation therapy alone was about 50% and 20% in patients with stage I and stage II disease, respectively.[116] Randomized trials in the 1980s showed that radiation therapy followed by chemotherapy resulted in significantly longer disease-free and overall survival as compared with radiation therapy alone. Other studies reported excellent results with a short course of chemotherapy (three cycles) followed by involved-field radiotherapy or six to eight cycles of CHOP chemotherapy, with or without consolidation radiotherapy. With either of these approaches, 5-year progression-free survival was more than 90% for patients with stage I disease and about 70% for patients with stage II disease.[116]

Because the most effective approach was not clear, the SWOG performed a randomized trial that compared three cycles of CHOP and involved-field radiotherapy or six cycles of CHOP in patients with stage I and nonbulky stage II aggressive lymphoma.[61] Patients treated with three cycles of CHOP plus radiotherapy had significantly better 5-year progression-free (77% vs 64%) and overall (82% vs 72%) survival than did patients treated with CHOP alone. The incidence of life-threatening toxicity was higher in patients who received CHOP alone. But with longer follow-up, more patients who received abbreviated chemotherapy experienced late relapses and the differences in progression-free or overall survival were no longer significant between the two arms. Further subgroup analysis of that trial identified several prognostic factors that led to the development of the stage-modified IPI score. Four adverse risk factors comprise the score: nonbulky stage II disease (bulky stage II disease is considered advanced disease), age older than 60 years, elevated LDH levels, or performance status more than or equal to 2.

The stage-modified IPI score is often used to identify patients with localized aggressive NHL who may have a poor prognosis. Based on the results of this trial, the current standard for therapy of most patients with localized nonbulky aggressive lymphoma without any adverse risk factors is three to four cycles of R-CHOP followed by locoregional radiation therapy (30-40 Gy [3,000-4,000 rad]).[116] Five-year median survival in this favorable group of patients exceeds 90%.

Five-year median survival is reduced to about 70% in patients with at least one adverse risk factor in the stage-modified IPI score. Patients in this high-risk subgroup may benefit from more aggressive chemotherapy (six cycles of R-CHOP) followed by locoregional radiation therapy.[61]

Treatment of Advanced Disease (Bulky Stage II, Stages III and IV)

It has been known since the late 1970s that intensive combination chemotherapy can cure some patients with disseminated DLBCL.[116] Initial studies with cyclophosphamide, vincristine (Oncovin®), and prednisone or prednisolone (COP; same as CVP) produced a plateau on the survival curve of just 10%, with a median survival of less than 1 year. Based on the activity of single-agent doxorubicin, McKelvey et al. developed the CHOP regimen (see Table 132-9).[117] A few years later, a SWOG study showed that CHOP was more active than COP, and CHOP chemotherapy rapidly became the treatment of choice for patients with aggressive lymphomas.[118] Studies in larger numbers of patients showed that about 50% of patients had a complete remission to CHOP chemotherapy, and 50% to 75% of the patients who had a complete response (about one-third of all patients) experienced long-term disease-free survival and cure of their disease.

In an effort to improve these results, many investigators used several general approaches to develop second- and third-generation regimens in the 1980s.[116] Results of phase II trials suggested that these second- and third-generation regimens were more active than CHOP, with slightly higher complete response rates and improved disease-free survival rates. However, they were also more difficult to administer, more toxic, and more expensive. Based on these results, many oncologists adopted one of these second- or third-generation combination regimens as their standard regimen for patients with advanced aggressive lymphomas.

Many randomized studies have compared different combination regimens in patients with aggressive lymphoma. Although the results of these studies show that no one regimen is clearly superior to another, they demonstrate the superiority of anthracycline-containing regimens over those that do not contain an anthracycline. In the largest and most widely quoted study, the SWOG initiated a randomized trial in 1986 that compared CHOP to three of the most commonly used third-generation regimens in nearly 900 patients with bulky stage II, stage III, or stage IV aggressive NHL. At the time of the initial publication (median follow-up: 35 months), no differences in disease-free and overall survival were observed between the four groups.[119] Furthermore, no significant differences in disease-free or overall survival were observed in any subgroup of patients. But the risk of treatment-related mortality was higher in patients receiving one of the third-generation regimens. Extended follow-up of that trial shows that about 35% of patients who participated in that trial are probably cured of their disease, regardless of the initial combination chemotherapy regimen. Interestingly, the overall survival is about 10% higher than the disease-free survival, which probably reflects the effectiveness of salvage high-dose chemotherapy with autologous HSCT (see the Treatment of Refractory or Relapsed Disease section later in this chapter).

Based on the lack of survival benefit with the newer combination chemotherapy regimens, the less complicated and less expensive CHOP regimen was considered as the treatment of choice for most patients with DLBCL and other aggressive NHLs for many years. Even with CHOP chemotherapy, however, less than 50% of patients with DLBCL were cured of their disease and most patients who relapse after an initial response do so in the first 2 years. New treatment approaches were clearly needed.

Several studies attempted to improve treatment results by increasing chemotherapy dose (ie, dose-intensity), shortening the interval between chemotherapy cycles (ie, dose-density), or both. Because of the increased risk of severe neutropenia, these approaches require growth factor support. Although results of these studies have not consistently shown improved survival, encouraging results from several recently published studies suggest that these approaches be evaluated in future randomized trials.[120]

Based on the encouraging results of R-CHOP in indolent lymphomas, several studies evaluated this combination in aggressive lymphomas. The first randomized controlled trial that established the efficacy of R-CHOP in advanced-stage DLBCL showed that R-CHOP significantly increased complete response rates and overall survival in elderly (≥60 years old) patients as compared with CHOP alone (discussed in the Treatment of Elderly Patients with Advanced Disease section later in this chapter).[121,122] Although the results of that study established R-CHOP as standard therapy in older patients, the role of R-CHOP in the treatment of younger patients was not clear. That issue was recently addressed in the MabThera International Trial, which enrolled younger (18-60 years old) patients with good-prognosis DLBCL.[123] Patients randomized to receive rituximab plus CHOP-like chemotherapy had significantly higher complete response rates (86% vs 68%) and longer 3-year event-free and overall survival (79% vs 59% [HR 0.44] and 93% vs 84% [HR 0.40], respectively). Furthermore, in a population-based study conducted in British Columbia, institution of a policy recommending R-CHOP for all patients with newly diagnosed advanced-stage DLBCL resulted in significant improvements in progression-free and overall survival.[124] Based on these trial results, rituximab received FDA approval for first-line treatment in combination with CHOP or CHOP-like chemotherapy and R-CHOP is recommended for all patients with advanced-stage DLBCL in the current NCCN guideline.[61]

Treatment outcomes for high-risk patients according to the IPI (or revised IPI) score are unsatisfactory. High-risk groups generally include all patients older than 60 years and those with an IPI score of 3 or more (or an age-adjusted IPI score of ≥2). Because progression-free survival is only about 50% in these high-risk patients treated with R-CHOP,[64,125] other more aggressive treatments, preferably as part of a clinical trial, should be considered in these patients. Examples of more aggressive approaches include dose-intense or dose-dense chemotherapy with growth factor support, usually combined with rituximab, or high-dose chemotherapy with autologous HSCT.[116,126]

One approach is to give high-dose chemotherapy with autologous HSCT as intensive consolidation in high-risk patients with DLBCL who achieve a remission with standard chemotherapy.[121] A recent published study suggested that this approach improves progression-free survival among patients with high-intermediate-risk or high-risk disease who had a response to CHOP-based chemotherapy.[126]

11 In summary, all patients with bulky stage II, stage III, or stage IV disease should be treated with R-CHOP or rituximab and CHOP-like chemotherapy until a complete response is achieved (usually four cycles).[65] Clinicians are encouraged to adopt the revised response criteria proposed by the International Working Group.[66] In patients who have a positive pretreatment PET scan, PET scanning can be useful in response assessment. A rapid response to chemotherapy (ie, a complete response achieved in the first three treatment cycles) is associated with a more durable remission compared with patients requiring longer treatment cycles. Two or more cycles of chemotherapy should be given following attainment of a complete response (total of six to eight cycles). The use of long-term maintenance therapy following a complete response has not been shown to improve survival. Treatment outcomes for high-risk patients according to the IPI (or revised IPI) score are unsatisfactory and alternative treatment approaches, preferably as part of a clinical trial, should be considered in these patients. High-dose chemotherapy with autologous HSCT should be considered in high-risk patients who respond to standard chemotherapy and are candidates for autologous HSCT.[65]

Treatment of Elderly Patients with Advanced Disease

More than one-half of patients with NHL are older than 60 years of age at diagnosis, and about one-third are older than age 70 years. The International Non-Hodgkin Lymphoma Prognostic Factors Project showed that patients older than 60 years of age had a significantly lower complete response rate and overall survival.[63] The reasons for the poorer outcome in elderly patients are not clear. Older patients do not tolerate intensive chemotherapy as well as younger patients, and some studies report that older patients have a higher risk of treatment-related mortality. As a result, many clinicians treat elderly patients with reduced dose or less-aggressive chemotherapy regimens. In general, these less-intensive regimens have used anthracyclines with less cardiotoxicity than doxorubicin, have substituted mitoxantrone for doxorubicin, or have used short-duration weekly therapy.[116]

Over the past few years, several nonrandomized and randomized trials have evaluated different treatment approaches in older patients with aggressive NHL.[116] The results of these studies suggest that carefully selected elderly patients with good performance status and without significant comorbidities can tolerate aggressive anthracycline-containing regimens as well as younger patients. These patients should be treated initially with full-dose R-CHOP or similar regimens; dosages can be reduced later if severe toxicity occurs. Hematopoietic growth factors may allow elderly patients to maintain dose intensity.

The combination therapy, R-CHOP, has replaced CHOP as standard treatment for elderly patients with aggressive lymphoma, based on the results of the Groupe d'Etude des Lymphomes de l'Adulte (GELA) study.[121,122] In that study of 399 elderly patients with DLBCL, patients who were randomized to receive R-CHOP had a significantly higher complete response rate (76% vs 63%) and longer event-free and overall survival as compared with those who received CHOP. After 10 years of follow-up, progression-free survival was significantly longer among those who received R-CHOP than CHOP (36.5% vs 20.1%).[122] A higher risk of death or development of secondary cancer was not observed with the addition of rituximab to CHOP after 10 years of follow-up. In another randomized controlled trial conducted primarily in the United States (Eastern Cooperative Oncology Group 4494), elderly (≥60 years old) patients who received rituximab, either as induction or maintenance with CHOP chemotherapy, had significantly longer failure-free survival as compared with those not given rituximab during their treatment course.[126] Maintenance therapy with single-agent rituximab did not provide any additional benefit in patients who received R-CHOP as induction therapy. It is important to note that rituximab is given differently in the two studies. In the GELA study, rituximab is given on day 1 (the same day that cyclophosphamide, doxorubicin, and vincristine are administered) with each cycle of CHOP chemotherapy.[121,122] In the Eastern Cooperative Oncology Group 4494 study,[127] R-CHOP was modeled after the regimen developed by Czuczman et al.: two doses of rituximab are given before cycle 1, and one dose is given before cycles 3, 5, and 7 (if administered).[87] In most NHL protocols and in clinical practice, rituximab is given on day 1 of CHOP chemotherapy.

Dose-dense chemotherapy, where the interval between cycles is shortened from 3 to 2 weeks, has been evaluated. Before the rituximab era, patients who were randomized to receive biweekly CHOP (CHOP-14) had significantly longer 5-year event-free and overall survival than patients who received standard CHOP every 21 days (CHOP-21).[128] All patients in the CHOP-14 group received prophylactic growth factors starting from day 4. Toxicity was similar between the two groups. In the next study, the same group of investigators evaluated the addition of rituximab (CHOP-14 vs R-CHOP-14) and the number of treatment cycles (six vs eight cycles).[129] Patients who received rituximab did better than those who did not, but eight cycles were not better than six cycles. The addition of rituximab to the CHOP-14 regimen resulted in significantly longer 3-year event-free and overall survival (67% vs 47% and 78% vs 68%, respectively). In the rituximab era, however, data suggested that R-CHOP-21 remains the standard treatment regimen when compared to R-CHOP-14 for treatment of DLBCL. Two recently published randomized studies confirmed that R-CHOP-14 is not superior to R-CHOP-21 for previously untreated DLBCL patients.[130,131] The NCCN guideline does not recommend dose-dense R-CHOP (R-CHOP-14) as first-line therapy for DLBCL.[61]

Treatment of Refractory or Relapsed Disease

12 Although many patients with aggressive NHL experience long-term survival and cure with intensive chemotherapy, about 10% to 20% of patients fail to achieve a complete remission and about 20% to 30% of patients who do achieve a complete remission will subsequently relapse. Therefore, about 30% to 40% of all patients with aggressive NHL will require salvage therapy at some point during their disease course. Response to salvage therapy depends on the initial responsiveness of the tumor to chemotherapy. Patients who achieve an initial complete remission and then relapse generally have a better response to salvage therapy than those who are primarily or partially resistant to chemotherapy.

Many conventional-dose salvage chemotherapy regimens have been used in patients with relapsed or refractory NHL. Many patients who respond to salvage therapy (ie, chemosensitive relapse) will then receive high-dose chemotherapy with autologous HSCT. In an effort to avoid cross-resistance, most salvage regimens incorporate drugs not used in the initial therapy. Some of the more commonly used salvage regimens include ICE, dexamethasone, cytarabine, cisplatin (DHAP), etoposide, methylprednisolone, cytarabine, cisplatin (ESHAP), and mesna, ifosfamide, mitoxantrone, etoposide (MINE), gemcitabine, dexamethasone, cisplatin (GDP) and no one regimen appears to be clearly superior to any other regimen.[116,132] With these salvage regimens, about 30% to 50% of patients achieve a complete response, with a median duration of remission of 1 to 2 years. Only about 5% to 10% of patients will have long-term disease-free survival.

Rituximab is sometimes added to these salvage regimens. It is recommended, however, to exclude rituximab in second-line therapy if patient's disease is refractory or if the duration of remission is less than 6 months. One study (CORAL study) has compared two salvage regimens (R-ICE and R-DHAP) that are used for treatment of patients with relapsed or refractory DLBCL, followed by autologous HSCT.[133] No significant difference in 3-year event-free survival or overall survival was observed between R-ICE and R-DHAP. However, patients who had received prior rituximab treatment and experienced early relapse (defined as less than 12 months after diagnosis) had a poor prognosis. This suggests that new treatment strategies are needed in order to improve the response rates of salvage regimens.

To improve the cure rate, many studies have evaluated high-dose chemotherapy with autologous HSCT as intensive consolidation therapy in patients who respond to salvage therapy. In the PARMA study, 215 patients with relapsed aggressive NHL who had a response to DHAP salvage therapy were randomized to receive either high-dose chemotherapy or continued DHAP therapy.[134] Patients who received high-dose chemotherapy had significantly longer 5-year disease-free survival (46% vs 12%) and overall survival (53% vs 32%) than those treated with conventional salvage therapy. Further analysis of that study showed that patients who relapsed within 12 months of their initial diagnosis were less likely to benefit from high-dose chemotherapy than patients who relapsed after 12 months. Based on a review of the available evidence, including the PARMA study, high-dose chemotherapy with autologous HSCT is considered to be the treatment of choice in younger patients with chemotherapy-sensitive relapse.[61] High-dose chemotherapy with autologous HSCT is not recommended in patients with untested or chemotherapy-refractory relapse.

Other Aggressive Lymphomas

Mantle cell lymphoma is found in 6% of cases in the International Lymphoma Classification Project.[76] The chromosomal translocation t(11;14) occurs in most cases of MCL. MCL usually occurs in older adults, particularly in men, and most patients have advanced disease at the time of diagnosis (see Table 132-6). Extranodal involvement is found in about 90% of cases. The course of the disease is moderately aggressive; the median overall survival is about 3 years, with no evidence of a survival plateau.

Both aggressive and less-aggressive chemotherapy regimens have been evaluated in patients with disseminated MCL. One widely used aggressive combination regimen is cyclophosphamide, vincristine, doxorubicin, dexamethasone alternating with methotrexate and cytarabine (hyperCVAD) with or without rituximab. Overall response rates to these regimens is about 90%, with about two-thirds of patients achieving a complete response.[61] Because MCL usually expresses CD20, rituximab, either alone or combined with CHOP and bendamustine, has been used with some success in patients with newly diagnosed and relapsed MCL.[91,102] In a phase III study, BR was compared to R-CHOP for first-line therapy in patients with advanced follicular, indolent and MCL. In the MCL subgroup, progression-free survival was higher with BR compared to R-CHOP, and it is associated with less hematological toxicities.[102]

Despite the high response rates, MCL is not considered curable with standard chemotherapy. Consequently, younger patients who have an initial response to chemotherapy often undergo autologous or allogeneic HSCT as consolidation therapy. The NCCN guideline recommends that patients with advanced-stage MCL be treated initially with rituximab and combination chemotherapy, followed by autologous HSCT as first-line consolidation therapy.[61] Unfortunately, most patients with MCL eventually relapse and are treated with salvage therapy or enrolled in trials of investigational agents, some of which are aimed at molecular targets.

Bortezomib (Velcade®) is currently approved for treatment of patients with MCL that has relapsed after at least one prior therapy based on the results of a phase II study that showed a 33% response rate.[135] In a recently published phase III randomized study, patients with newly diagnosed mantle-cell lymphoma who were ineligible or not considered for HSCT received R-CHOP intravenously on day 1 (with prednisone administered orally on days 1-5) or VR-CAP (R-CHOP regimen, but replacing vincristine with bortezomib). After a median follow-up of 40 months, median progression-free survival was longer in the VR-CAP arm compared to R-CHOP (24.7 vs 14.4 months; $P < 0.001$). Rates of neutropenia and thrombocytopenia were higher in the VR-CAP group.[136]

Ibrutinib is an oral Bruton tyrosine kinase (BTK) inhibitor approved for treatment of relapsed or refractory MCL. In a Phase II study, ibrutinib had demonstrated a high response rate of 67% with a median duration of response of 17.5 months. Most of the patients had received three or more prior therapies.[137] The most common side effects of ibrutinib include diarrhea and fatigue. Bleeding can rarely occur, particularly during the first 6 months of ibrutinib therapy.

Non-Hodgkin Lymphoma in Acquired Immune Deficiency Syndrome

The risk of NHL for patients with AIDS is increased more than 100-fold as compared with the general population.[138,139] AIDS-related lymphoma arises as a consequence of long-term stimulation and proliferation of B lymphocytes from HIV and the reactivation of prior EBV infection as a consequence of HIV-induced immunosuppression. AIDS-related lymphoma usually occurs late in the course of HIV infection and is the cause of death in about 15% of HIV-infected individuals. Although HIV infects T cells, more than 95% of AIDS-related lymphomas are B-cell neoplasms. Most cases of AIDS-related lymphomas are classified as Burkitt or DLBCL.

The clinical presentation is similar to that observed in other immunocompromised states. Most patients with AIDS-related lymphoma present with B symptoms and have advanced-stage (III or IV) disease at the time of diagnosis.[138] Involvement of extranodal sites is common. The clinical course of AIDS-related lymphoma is usually aggressive and has improved with the availability of highly active antiretroviral therapy (HAART). Improved survival has been observed, primarily in patients with DLBCL. Patients with AIDS-related lymphoma treated with intensive therapy have a median survival that is similar to the survival of patients with HIV-negative NHLs.[139] In the post-HAART era, many of the prognostic factors have also changed and only lymphoma-related factors such as the IPI remain as independent predictors of prognosis.

The treatment of patients with AIDS-associated lymphomas is difficult because the immunocompromised state of these patients increases their risk of significant toxicity as a consequence of myelosuppressive therapy. Except for primary CNS lymphoma, AIDS-related lymphoma is never considered truly localized and systemic chemotherapy is indicated. For patients with adequate immune function and without a history of an opportunistic infection, chemotherapy regimens similar to that used for aggressive lymphomas may be used.[61] However, many patients with AIDS-related lymphoma were previously treated with less-intensive regimens because of the increased risk of treatment-related toxicity. In the post-HAART era, however, most clinicians believe that standard doses of chemotherapy can be safely administered to patients who achieve a virologic response to HAART.

The results of treatment with standard chemotherapy regimens have been disappointing, particularly in patients with Burkitt lymphoma. In patients with DLBCL, the complete response rate with combination chemotherapy is about 40% to 50%, with 5-year overall survival rates of about 20% to 30%. Newer approaches, such as the dose-adjusted etoposide, prednisone, vincristine, cyclophosphamide, and doxorubicin (EPOCH) regimen developed at the National Cancer Institute, appear promising. In a recently published pooled analysis that included patients with HIV-associated NHL treated in the R-CHOP or R-EPOCH, patients receiving R-EPOCH achieved an improvement of response and survival when compared against R-CHOP.[140] Treatment-associated deaths were more prominent among patients with very low $CD4^+$ counts.

The role of rituximab in the treatment of AIDS-related DLBCL is not clear. In a randomized trial of CHOP versus R-CHOP, no significant differences in progression-free and overall survival were observed.[141] However, 14% of patients treated with R-CHOP died of treatment-related infection as compared with only 2% of those in the CHOP group. NCCN guidelines suggest omission of rituximab in patients at high risk for serious infectious complications (eg, patients on HAART with persistently low $CD4^+$ count).[61]

The optimal timing for HAART is not clear in patients with AIDS-related lymphoma.[138,139] Current NCCN guidelines recommend the use of HAART and growth factor support along with full-dose chemotherapy regimen.[61] If HAART is given concurrently with chemotherapy, patients should be monitored closely for possible pharmacokinetic interactions between HAART and chemotherapy. Prophylactic antibiotics should be continued during chemotherapy and intrathecal chemotherapy should be administered to prevent CNS relapses.

PERSONALIZED PHARMACOTHERAPY

Molecular testing of the lymphoma cells at the time of diagnosis is an essential part of the diagnostic work-up. Molecular subtypes have been identified that predict for survival. For example, two molecular subtypes of DLBCL have been identified, and the ABC subtype appears to be less responsive to chemotherapy than the GCB subtype. Another molecular subtype associated with poor response is double-hit DLBCL, defined as the existence of both MYC gene arrangement and t(14;18) BCL2 translocation.

In addition to disease stage, several prognostic indices such as IPS, IPI, and FLIPI are used clinically to predict response to therapy and survival in individual patients. The results of these evaluations form the basis for risk-adapted therapy, where the intensity of the recommended therapy is tailored to the risk category of the patient. More intensive therapy is generally recommended for higher risk patients, particularly when long-term survival or cure is the treatment goal.

Age or comorbidities often limit the use of chemotherapy regimens. Patients with poor cardiac function may not be able to receive doxorubicin, an important component of combination regimens used to treat both Hodgkin lymphoma and NHL. Patients with preexisting diabetic neuropathy or who develop peripheral neuropathy during chemotherapy may not be able to receive all of their planned doses of vinca alkaloids, particularly vincristine. Most patients with NHL are elderly and these patients may not tolerate the toxicities of intensive chemotherapy regimens. Dosage adjustments or treatment delays may be required.

Interim PET scans are currently being investigated as a biomarker of early response in patients with advanced-stage Hodgkin lymphoma. If validated, PET scans may allow clinicians to decide which patients should receive treatment intensification and which patients should have their treatment discontinued.

EVALUATION OF THERAPEUTIC OUTCOMES

Hodgkin and NHLs tend to respond well to radiation, chemotherapy, and biologic therapy. The goal of therapy for patients with Hodgkin lymphoma and aggressive NHL is long-term survival and cure. The therapeutic goal in patients with indolent NHLs is less clear because of the indolent nature of the disease and the lack of convincing evidence showing that therapy prolongs survival. Therapeutic responses should be evaluated based on physical examination, radiologic evidence, PET/CT scanning, and other positive findings at baseline. Patients with Hodgkin lymphoma and aggressive NHLs are usually evaluated for response at the end of four cycles of therapy or at the end of treatment if fewer than four cycles of therapy are planned. If patients are treated with chemotherapy alone, two additional cycles of chemotherapy are given after the patient has achieved a complete remission. Recent studies have also shown that early interim PET scans may possess prognostic value in patients with advanced Hodgkin lymphoma. The rapidity of response to therapy in patients with indolent NHL depends on the choice of therapy. Responses occur slowly with therapy with oral alkylating agents, but occur much more rapidly with aggressive therapies such as combination chemotherapy with or without rituximab. If radiation alone is used, then a therapeutic evaluation should occur at the end of treatment.

ABBREVIATIONS

ABC	activated B-cell–like
ABV	doxorubicin (Adriamycin®), bleomycin, vinblastine
ABVD	doxorubicin (Adriamycin®), bleomycin, vinblastine, and dacarbazine
ADC	antibody-drug conjugate
AIDS	acquired immune deficiency syndrome
BEACOPP	bleomycin, etoposide, doxorubicin (Adriamycin®), cyclophosphamide, vincristine (Oncovin®), procarbazine, and prednisone
BR	bendamustine and rituximab
BTK	Bruton tyrosine kinase
BVR	bendamustine, rituximab, and bortezomib
CEC	cyclophosphamide, lomustine, vindesine, melphalan, prednisone, epirubicin, vincristine, procarbazine, vinblastine, bleomycin
CHOP	cyclophosphamide, doxorubicin, vincristine (Oncovin®), prednisone
CNS	central nervous system
COP	cyclophosphamide, vincristine (Oncovin®), and prednisone or prednisolone
COPP	cyclophosphamide, vincristine, procarbazine, and prednisone
CT	computed tomography
CVP	cyclophosphamide, vincristine, and prednisone
DHAP	dexamethasone, cytarabine, cisplatin
DLBCL	diffuse large B-cell lymphoma
EBV	Epstein-Barr's virus
EPOCH	etoposide, prednisone, vincristine, cyclophosphamide, and doxorubicin
ESHAP	etoposide, methylprednisolone, cytarabine, cisplatin
ESR	erythrocyte sedimentation rate
FDA	Food and Drug Administration
FLIPI	Follicular Lymphoma International Prognostic Index
FN	fludarabine and mitoxantrone
FND	fludarabine, mitoxantrone, and dexamethasone
GCB	germinal center B-cell–like
GDP	gemcitabine, dexamethasone, cisplatin
GELA	Groupe d'Etude des Lymphomes de l'Adulte
GHSG	German Hodgkin Study Group
GVD	gemcitabine, vinorelbine, and pegylated liposomal doxorubicin
HAART	highly active antiretroviral therapy
HIV	human immunodeficiency virus
HLA	human leukocyte antigen
HR	hazard ratio
HSCT	hematopoietic stem cell transplantation
hyperCVAD	cyclophosphamide, vincristine, doxorubicin, dexamethasone alternating with methotrexate and cytarabine
ICE	ifosfamide, carboplatin, and etoposide
IFRT	involved-field radiation
IPI	International Prognostic Index
IPS	International Prognostic Score
ISRT	involved-site radiation therapy
JAK–STAT	Janus kinase–signal transduction and transcription
KSHV	Kaposi sarcoma–associated herpesvirus
LDH	lactate dehydrogenase
MALT	mucosa-associated lymphoid tissue
MCL	mantle cell lymphoma
MINE	mesna, ifosfamide, mitoxantrone, etoposide
MMAE	monomethyl auristatin E
MOPP	mechlorethamine, vincristine, procarbazine, and prednisone
MOPPEBVCAD	mechlorethamine, vincristine, procarbazine, prednisone, epidoxorubicin, bleomycin, vinblastine, lomustine, doxorubicin, and vindesine
NCCN	National Comprehensive Cancer Network
NHL	non-Hodgkin lymphoma
NLPHL	nodular lymphocyte-predominant Hodgkin lymphoma
PET	positron emission tomography
R-CHOP	rituximab, cyclophosphamide, doxorubicin, vincristine (Oncovin®), prednisone
R-FCM	rituximab, fludarabine, cyclophosphamide, and mitoxantrone
REAL	revised European-American Classification of Lymphoid Neoplasms
RICE	rituximab, ifosfamide, carboplatin, and etoposide
SEER	surveillance, epidemiology, and end results
SWOG	Southwest Oncology Group
WHO	World Health Organization

REFERENCES

1. NCCN Clinical practice Guidelines in Oncology. Hodgkin Lymphoma. V2.2015. Available at: http://www.nccn.org
2. Hodgkin's Disease—Historical Timeline. Available at: http://www.lymphomainfo.net/hodgkins/timeline.html. (Last Accessed on: 10/05/2015)
3. Engert A, Eichenauer DA, Harris NL, et.al. Hodgkin lymphoma. In: DeVita VT, Jr., Hellman S, Rosenberg SA, eds. *Cancer: Principles & Practice of Oncology*. 9th ed. Philadelphia, PA: Lippincott Williams & Wilkins; 2011:1819-1854.
4. Townsend W, Linch D. Hodgkin's lymphoma in adults. *Lancet* 2012;380:836-847.
5. Bartlett NL, Foyil KV. Hodgkin's lymphoma. In: Niederhuber JE, Armitage JO, Dorowhow JH, et. al., eds. *Abeloff's Clinical Oncology*. 5th ed. New York, NY: Churchill Livingstone; 2014:2018-2032.
6. Siegel RL, Miller KD, Jemal A. Cancer statistics 2016. *CA Cancer J Clin* 2016;66:7-30.
7. Howlader N, Noone AM, Krapcho M, et al. SEER Cancer Statistics Review, 1975–2012. 2015. Available at: http://seer.cancer.gov/csr/1975_2012/.
8. Ng AK, Bernardo MP, Weller E, et al. Long-term survival and competing causes of death in patients with early-stage Hodgkin's disease treated at age 50 or younger. *J Clin Oncol* 2002;20: 2101-2108.
9. Kìppers R. New insights in the biology of Hodgkin lymphoma. *Hematology Am Soc Hematol Educ Program* 2012;2012:328-334.
10. Mack TM, Cozen W, Shibata DK, et al. Concordance for Hodgkin's disease in identical twins suggesting genetic susceptibility to the young-adult form of the disease. *N Engl J Med* 1995;332:413-418.
11. Papadaki T, Stamatopoulos K. Hodgkin disease immunopathogenesis: Long-standing questions, recent answers, further directions. *Trends Immunol* 2003;24:508-511.
12. Swerdlow SH, Campo E, Pileri SA, et al. The 2016 revision of the World Health Organization classification of lymphoid neoplasms. *Blood* 2016; 127: 2375-90.
13. Barrington SF, Mikhaeel NG, Kostakoglu L, et al. Role of imaging in the staging and response assessment of lymphoma: Consensus of the International Conference on malignant lymphomas imaging work group. *J Clin Oncol* 2014;32:3048-3058.
14. Mauch PM, Kalish LA, Kadin M, Coleman CN, Osteen R, Hellman S. Patterns of presentation of Hodgkin disease. Implications for etiology and pathogenesis. *Cancer* 1993;71:2062-2071.
15. Hasenclever D, Diehl V. A prognostic score for advanced Hodgkin's disease. International Prognostic Factors Project on Advanced Hodgkin's Disease. *N Engl J Med* 1998;339:1506-1514.
16. Hodgson DC. Late effects in the era of modern therapy for Hodgkin lymphoma. *Hematology Am Soc Hematol Educ Program* 2011;2011:323-329.
17. Hoppe BS, Flampouri S, Su Z, et al. Effective dose reduction to cardiac structures using protons compared to 3DCRT and IMRT in mediastinal Hodgkin lymphoma. *Int J Radiat Oncol Biol Phys* 2012;84:449-455.
18. Paumier A, Ghalibafian M, Gilmore J, et al. Dosimetric benefits of intensity-modulated radiotherapy combined with the deep-inspiration breath-hold technique in patients with mediastinal Hodgkin's lymphoma. *Int J Radiat Oncol Biol Phys* 2012;82: 1522-1527.
19. Filippi AR, Ragona R, Fusella M, et al. Changes in breast cancer risk associated with different volumes, doses, and techniques in female Hodgkin lymphoma patients treated with supra-diaphragmatic radation therapy. *Pract Radiat Oncol* 2013;3:216-222.
20. Bonnadonna G, Zucali R, Monfardini S, De Lena M, Uslenghi C. Combination therapy of Hodgkin's disease with Adriamycin, bleomycin, vinblastine, and imidazole carboxamide versus MOPP. *Cancer* 1975;36:252-259.
21. Canellos GP, Anderson JR, Propert KJ, et al. Chemotherapy of advanced Hodgkin's disease with MOPP, ABVD, or MOPP alternating with ABVD. *N Engl J Med* 1992;327:1478-1484.
22. Goldie JH, Coldman AJ, Gudauskas GA. Rationale for the use of alternating non-cross-resistant chemotherapy. *Cancer Treat Rep* 1982;66:439-449.
23. Glick JH, Young ML, Harrington D, et al. MOPP/ABV hybrid chemotherapy for advanced Hodgkin's disease significantly improves failure-free and overall survival: The 8-year results of the intergroup trial. *J Clin Oncol* 1998;16:19-26.
24. Duggan DB, Petroni GR, Johnson JL, et al. Randomized comparison of ABVD and MOPP/ABV hybrid for the treatment of advanced Hodgkin's disease: Report of an intergroup trial. *J Clin Oncol* 2003;21: 607-614.
25. Horning SJ, Hoppe RT, Breslin S, Bartlett NL, Brown BW, Rosenberg SA. Stanford V and radiotherapy for locally extensive and advanced Hodgkin's disease: Mature results of a prospective clinical trial. *J Clin Oncol* 2002;20:630-637.
26. Gobbi PG, Levis A, Chisesi T, et al. ABVD versus modified Stanford V versus MOPPEBVCAD with optional and limited radiotherapy in intermediate- and advanced-stage Hodgkin's lymphoma: Final results of a multicenter randomized trial by the Intergruppo Italiano Linfomi. *J Clin Oncol* 2005;23:9198-9207.
27. Advani RH, Hoppe RT, Baer D, et al. Efficacy of abbreviated Stanford V chemotherapy and involved-field radiotherapy in early-stage Hodgkin lymphoma: Mature results of the G4 trial. *Ann Oncol* 2013; 24:1044-1048.
28. Engert A, Plutschow A, Eich HT, et al. Reduced treatment intensity in patients with early-stage Hodgkin's lymphoma. *N Engl J Med* 2010;363:640-652.
29. Gordon LI, Hong F, Fisher RI, et al. Randomized phase III trial of ABVD versus Stanford V with or without radiation therapy in locally extensive and advanced-stage Hodgkin lymphoma: An intergroup study coordinated by the Eastern Cooperative Oncology Group (E2496). *J Clin Oncol* 2013;31:684-691.
30. Barrington SF, Mikhaeel NG, Kostakoglu L, et al. Role of imaging in the staging and response assessment of lymphoma: Consensus of the International Conference on Malignant Lymphomas Imaging Working Group. *J Clin Oncol* 2014;32:3048-3058.
31. Horning SJ, Hoppe RT, Breslin S, et al. Stanford V and radiotherapy for locally extensive and advanced Hodgkin's disease: Mature results of a prospective clinical trial. *J Clin Oncol* 2002;20:630-637.
32. Edwards-Bennett SM, Jacks LM, Moskowitz CH, et al. Stanford V program for locally extensive and advanced Hodgkin lymphoma: The Memorial Sloan-Kettering Cancer Center experience. *Ann Oncol* 2010;21:574-581.
33. Hoskin PJ, Lowry L, Horwich A, et al. Randomized comparison of the Stanford V regimen and ABVD in the treatment of advanced Hodgkin's lymphoma: United Kingdom National Cancer Research Institute Lymphoma Group Study ISRCTN 64141244. *J Clin Oncol* 2009;27:5390-5396.
34. von Tresckow B, Plutschow A, Fuchs M, et al. Dose-intensification in early unfavorable Hodgkin's lymphoma: Final analysis of the German Hodgkin Study Group HD14 trial. *J Clin Oncol* 2012;30:907-913.
35. Eich HT, Diehl V, Gorgen H, et al. Intensified chemotherapy and dose-reduced involved-filed radiotherapy in patients with early unfavorable Hodgkin's lymphoma: Final analysis of the German Hodgkin Study Group HD11 trial. *J Clin Oncol* 2010;28:4199-4206.
36. Diehl V, Franklin J, Pfreundschuh M, et al. Standard and increased-dose BEACOPP chemotherapy compared with COPP-ABVD for advanced Hodgkin's disease. *N Engl J Med* 2003;348:2386-2395.
37. Engert A, Diehl V, Franklin J, Lohri A, Dorken B. Escalated-dose BEACOPP in the treatment of patients with advanced-stage Hodgkin's lymphoma: 10 Years of follow-up of the GHSG HD9 study. *J Clin Oncol* 2009;27:4548-4554.
38. Ballova V, Ruffer JU, Haverkamp H, et al. A prospectively randomized trial carried out by the German Hodgkin Study Group (GHSG) for elderly patients with advanced Hodgkin's disease comparing BEACOPP baseline and COPP-ABVD (study HD9 elderly). *Ann Oncol* 2005;16:124-131.
39. Federico M, Luminari S, Iannitto E, et al. ABVD compared with BEACOPP compared with CEC for the initial treatment of patients with advanced Hodgkin's lymphoma: Results from the HD2000 Gruppo Italiano per lo Studio dei Linfomi Trial. *J Clin Oncol* 2009;27:805-811.
40. Merli F, Luminari S, Mammi C, et al. Long-term follow-up analysis of HD2000 trial comparing ABVD versus BEACOPP versus COPP/EBV/CAD in patients with newly diagnosed advanced-stage Hodgkin's lymphoma: A study from the Fondazione Italiana Linfomi. *Blood* 2014;124:Abstract 499.
41. Borchmann P, Haverkamp H, Diehl V, et al. Eight cycles of escalated-dose BEACOPP compared with four cycles of escalated-dose BEACOPP followed by four cycles of baseline-dose BEACOPP with or without radiotherapy in patients with advanced-stage Hodgkin's lymphoma: Final analysis of the HD12 trial of the German Hodgkin Study Group. *J Clin Oncol* 2011;29:4234-4242.
42. Engert A, Haverkamp H, Kobe C, et al. Reduced-intensity chemotherapy and PET-guided radiotherapy in patients with advanced stage Hodgkin's lymphoma (HD15 trial): A randomised, open-label, phase 3 non-inferiority trial. *Lancet* 2012;379:1791-1799.

43. Schulz H, Rehwald U, Morschhauser F, et al. Rituximab in relapsed lymphocyte-predominant Hodgkin lymphoma: Long-term results of a phase 2 trial by the German Hodgkin Lymphoma Study Group (GHSG). *Blood* 2008;111:109-111.
44. Advani RH, Horning SJ, Hoppe RT, et al. Mature results of a phase II study of rituximab therapy for nodular lymphocyte-predominant Hodgkin Lymphoma. *J Clin Oncol* 2014;32:912-918.
45. Majhail NS, Weisdorf DJ, Defor TE, et al. Long-term results of autologous stem cell transplantation for primary refractory or relapsed Hodgkin's lymphoma. *Biol Blood Marrow Transplant* 2006;12:1065-1072.
46. Brice P. Managing relapsed and refractory Hodgkin lymphoma. *Br J Haematol* 2008;141:3-13.
47. de Claro RA, McGinn KM, Kwitkowski VE, et al. U.S. Food and Drug Administration approval summary: Brentuximab vedotin for the treatment of relapsed Hodgkin lymphoma or relapsed systemic anaplastic large cell lymphoma. *Clin Cancer Res* 2012;18:5855-5859.
48. Moskowitz CH, Nademanee A, Masszi T, et al. Brentuximab vedotin as consolidation therapy after autologous stem-cell transplantation in patients with Hodgkin's lymphoma at risk of relapse or progression (AETHERA): A randomized, double-blind, placebo-controlled, phase 3 trial. *Lancet* 2015;385:1853-1862.
49. Younes A, Gopal AK, Smith SE, et al. Results of a pivotal phase II study of brentuximab vedotin for patients with relapsed or refractory Hodgkin's lymphoma. *J Clin Oncol* 2012;30:2183-2189.
49a. Ansell SM, Lesokhin AM, Borrello, et al. PD-1 blockade with nivolumab in relapsed or refractory Hodgkin's lymphoma. *NEJM* 2015;372(4)311-9.
50. Kulkarni SS, Sastry PS, Saikia TK, et al. Gonadal function following ABVD therapy for Hodgkin's disease. *Am J Clin Oncol* 1997;20:354-357.
51. Swerdlow AJ, Higgins CD, Smith P, et al. Second cancer risk after chemotherapy for Hodgkin's lymphoma: A collaborative British cohort study. *J Clin Oncol* 2011;29:4096-4104.
52. Ambinder RF. Infectious etiology of lymphoma. In: Armitage JO, Mauch PM, Harris NL, Coiffier B, Dalla-Favera R, eds. *Non-Hodgkin Lymphoma*. 2nd ed Philadelphia, PA: Lippincott Williams & Wilkins; 2010:83-101.
53. Wang SS, Hartge P. Epidemiology. In: Armitage JO, Mauch PM, Harris NL, Coiffier B, Dalla-Favera R, eds. *Non-Hodgkin Lymphoma*. 2nd ed. Philadelphia, PA: Lippincott Williams & Wilkins; 2010:64-82.
54. Dalla-Favera R, Pasqualucci L. Molecular genetics of lymphoma. In: Armitage JO, Mauch PM, Harris NL, Coiffier B, Dalla-Favera R, eds. *Non-Hodgkin Lymphoma*. 2nd ed. Philadelphia, PA: Lippincott Williams & Wilkins; 2010:115-130.
55. Wilson WH, Armitage JO. Non-Hodgkin's lymphoma. In: Abeloff MD, Armitage JO, Niederhuber JE, Kastan MB, McKenna WG, eds. *Abeloff's Clinical Oncology*. 4th ed. New York, NY: Churchill Livingstone; 2008:2371-2404.
56. Reeder CB, Ansell SM. Novel therapeutic agents for B-cell lymphoma: Developing rational combinations. *Blood* 2011;117: 1453-1462.
57. Swerdlow S, Campo E, Harris NL, et al., eds. *World Health Organization Classification of Tumours of Haematopoietic and Lymphoid tissues*. Lyon: IARC Press; 2008.
58. Harris NL. History and classification of lymphoid malignancies. In: Armitage JO, Mauch PM, Harris NL, Coiffier B, Dalla-Favera R, eds. *Non-Hodgkin Lymphoma*. Philadelphia, PA: Lippincott Williams & Wilkins; 2010:xv-xxix.
59. Lenz G, Staudt LM. Aggressive lymphomas. *N Engl J Med* 2010;362: 1417-1429.
60. Harris NL, Jaffe ES, Diebold J, et al. World Health Organization Classification of neoplastic diseases of the hematopoietic and lymphoid tissues: Report of the Clinical Advisory Committee meeting—Airlie House, Virginia, November 1997. *J Clin Oncol* 1999;17:3835-3849.
61. Oncology NCPGi. Non-Hodgkin's Lymphoma, version 2.2015. 2015. Available at: http://www.nccn.org.
62. Cheson BD, Pfistner B, Juweid ME, et al. Revised response criteria for malignant lymphoma. *J Clin Oncol* 2007;25:579-586.
63. The International Non-Hodgkin's Lymphoma Prognostic Factors Project. A predictive model for aggressive non-Hodgkin's lymphoma. *N Engl J Med* 1993;329:987-994.
64. Sehn LH, Berry B, Chhanabhai M, et al. The revised International Prognostic Index (R-IPI) is a better predictor of outcome than the standard IPI for patients with diffuse large B-cell lymphoma treated with R-CHOP. *Blood* 2007;109:1857-1861.
65. Solal-Celigny P, Roy P, Colombat P, et al. Follicular lymphoma international prognostic index. *Blood* 2004;104:1258-1265.
66. Federico M, Bellei M, Marcheselli L, et al. Follicular lymphoma international prognostic index 2: A new prognostic index for follicular lymphoma developed by the international follicular lymphoma prognostic factor project. *J Clin Oncol* 2009;27:4555-4562.
67. Nowakowski GS, Czuczman MS. ABC, GCB, and Double-Hit Diffuse Large B-Cell Lymphoma: Does subtype make a difference in therapy selection? *Hematology Am Soc Hematol Educ Program* 2015;35:e449-457.
68. Rosenwald A, Wright G, Chan WC, et al. The use of molecular profiling to predict survival after chemotherapy for diffuse large-B-cell lymphoma. *N Engl J Med* 2002;346:1937-1947.
69. Lenz G, Wright G, Dave SS, et al. Stromal gene signatures in large-B-cell lymphomas. *N Engl J Med* 2008;359:2313-2323.
70. Aukema SM, Siebert R, Schuuring E, et al. Double-hit B-cell lymphomas. *Blood* 2011;117:2319-2331.
71. Green TM, Young KH, Visco C, et al. Immunohistochemical double-hit score is a strong predictor of outcome in patients with diffuse large b-cell lymphoma treated with rituximab plus cyclophosphamide, doxorubicin, vincristine, and prednisone. *J Clin Oncol* 2012;30:3460-3467.
72. Dave SS, Wright G, Tan B, et al. Prediction of survival in follicular lymphoma based on molecular features of tumor-infiltrating immune cells. *N Engl J Med* 2004;351:2159-2169.
73. Cheson BD, Leonard JP. Monoclonal antibody therapy for B-cell non-Hodgkin's lymphoma. *N Engl J Med* 2008;359:613-626.
74. Maloney DG. Anti-CD20 antibody therapy for B-cell lymphomas. *N Engl J Med* 2012;366:2008-2016.
75. Freedman AS, Friedberg JW, Mauch PM, Dalla-Favera R, Harris NL. Follicular lymphoma. In: Armitage JO, Mauch PM, Harris NL, Coiffier B, Dalla-Favera R, eds. *Non-Hodgkin's Lymphoma*. 2nd ed. Philadelphia, PA: Lippincott Williams & Wilkins; 2010:266-283.
76. The Non-Hodgkin's Lymphoma Classification Project. A clinical evaluation of the International Lymphoma Study Group classification of non-Hodgkin's lymphoma. *Blood* 1997;89:3909-3918.
77. Horning SJ. Natural history of and therapy for the indolent non-Hodgkin's lymphomas. *Semin Oncol* 1993;20(Suppl 5):75-88.
78. Bernstein SH, Burack WR. The incidence, natural history, biology, and treatment of transformed lymphoma. *Hematology Am Soc Hematol Educ Program* 2009:532-541.
79. Fisher RI, LeBlanc M, Press OW, et al. New treatment options have changed the survival of patients with follicular lymphomas. *J Clin Oncol* 2005;23:8477-8452.
80. Liu Q, Fayad L, Cabanillas F, et al. Improvement of overall and failure-free survival in stage IV follicular lymphoma: 25 Years of treatment experience at the University of Texas M.D. Anderson Cancer Center. *J Clin Oncol* 2006;24:1582-1589.
81. Gribben JG. How I treat indolent lymphoma. *Blood* 2007;109: 4617-4626.
82. Ardeshna KM, Smith P, Norton A, et al. Long-term effect of a watch and wait policy versus immediate systemic treatment for asymptomatic advanced-stage non-Hodgkin's lymphoma: A randomised controlled trial. *Lancet* 2003;362:516-522.
83. Ardeshna KM, Qian W, Smith P, et al. Rituximab versus a watch-and-wait approach in patients with advanced-stage, asymptomatic, non-bulky follicular lymphoma: An open-label randomised phase 3 trial. *The Lancet Oncology* 2014;15:424-435.
84. McLaughlin P, Grillo-Lopez AJ, Link BK, et al. Rituxumab chimeric anti-CD20 monoclonal antibody therapy for relapsed indolent lymphoma: Half of patients respond to a four-dose treatment program. *J Clin Oncol* 1998;16:2825-2833.
85. Cohen Y, Solal-Celigny P, Polliack A. Rituximab therapy for follicular lymphoma: A comprehensive review of its efficacy as primary treatment, treatment for relapsed disease, re-treatment and maintenance. *Haematologica* 2003;88:811-823.
86. Friedberg JW, Taylor MD, Cerhan JR, et al. Follicular lymphoma in the United States: First report of the National LymphoCare Study. *J Clin Oncol* 2009;27:1202-1208.
87. Czuczman MS, Grillo-Lopez AJ, White CA, et al. Treatment of patients with low-grade B-cell lymphoma with the combination of chimeric anti-CD20 monoclonal antibody and CHOP chemotherapy. *J Clin Oncol* 1999;17:268-276.
88. Czuczman MS, Weaver R, Alkuzweny B, Berlfein J, Grillo-Lopez AJ. Prolonged clinical and molecular remission in patients with low-grade or follicular non-Hodgkin's lymphoma treated with rituximab plus CHOP chemotherapy: 9-year follow-up. *J Clin Oncol* 2004;22:4711-4716.
89. Hiddemann W, Kneba M, Dreyling M, et al. Frontline therapy with rituximab added to the combination of cyclophosphamide, doxorubicin, vincristine, and prednisone (CHOP) significantly improves the outcome for patients with advanced-stage follicular

lymphoma compared with therapy with CHOP alone: Results of a prospective randomized study of the German Low-Grade Lymphoma Study Group. *Blood* 2005;106:3725-3732.

90. van Oers MHJ, Klasa R, Marcus RE, et al. Rituximab maintenance improves clinical outcome of relapsed/resistant follicular lymphoma non-Hodgkin's lymphoma in patients both with and without rituximab during induction: Results of a prospective randomized phase 3 intergroup trial. *Blood* 2006;108:3295-3301.
91. Schulz H, Bohlius JF, Trelle S, et al. Immunochemotherapy with rituximab and overall survival in patients with indolent or mantle cell lymphoma: A systematic review and meta-analysis. *J Natl Cancer Inst* 2007;99:706-714.
92. Hochster H, Weller E, Gascoyne RD, et al. Maintenance rituximab after cyclophosphamide, vincristine, and prednisone prolongs progression-free survival in advanced indolent lymphoma: Results of the randomized phase III ECOG1496 study. *J Clin Oncol* 2009;27:1607-1614.
93. Salles G, Seymour JF, Offner F, et al. Rituximab maintenance for 2 years in patients with high tumour burden follicular lymphoma responding to rituximab plus chemotherapy (PRIMA): A phase 3, randomised controlled trial. *Lancet* 2011;377:42-51.
94. Nastoupil LJ, Sinha R, Byrtek M, et al. The use and effectiveness of rituximab maintenance in patients with follicular lymphoma diagnosed between 2004 and 2007 in the United States. *Cancer* 2014;120:1830-1837.
95. Forstpointner R, Unterhalt M, Dreyling M, et al. Maintenance therapy with rituximab leads to a significant prolongation of response duration after salvage therapy with a combination of rituximab, fludarabine, cyclophosphamide, and mitoxantrone (R-FCM) in patients with recurring and refractory follicular and mantle cell lymphomas: Results of a prospective randomized study of the German Low Grade Lymphoma Study Group (GLSG). *Blood* 2006;108:4003-4008.
96. van Oers MH, Van Glabbeke M, Giurgea L, et al. Rituximab maintenance treatment of relapsed/resistant follicular non-Hodgkin's lymphoma: Long-term outcome of the EORTC 20981 phase III randomized intergroup study. *J Clin Oncol* 2010;28:2853-2858.
97. Al Zahrani A, Ibrahim N, Al Eid A. Rapid infusion rituximab changing practice for patient care. *J Oncol Pharm Pract* 2009;15:183-186.
98. Chiang J, Chan A, Shih V, Hee SW, Tao M, Lim ST. A prospective study to evaluate the feasibility and economic benefits of rapid infusion rituximab at an Asian cancer center. *Int J Hematol* 2010;91:826-830.
99. Yeo W, Chan TC, Leung NWY, et al. Hepatitis B virus reactivation in lymphoma patients with prior resolved hepatitis B undergoing anticancer therapy with or without rituximab. *J Clin Oncol* 2009;27:605-611.
100. Beers SA, Chan CH, French RR, et al. CD20 as a target for therapeutic type I and II monoclonal antibodies. *Semin Hematol* 2010;47:107-114.
101. Rummel MJ, Gregory SA. Bendamustine's emerging role in the management of lymphoid malignancies. *Semin Hematol* 2011;48:S24-S36.
102. Rummel MJ, Niederle N, Maschmeyer G, et al. Bendamustine plus rituximab versus CHOP plus rituximab as first-line treatment for patients with indolent and mantle-cell lymphomas: An open-label, multicentre, randomised, phase 3 non-inferiority trial. *Lancet* 2013;381:1203-1210.
103. Flinn IW, van der Jagt R, Kahl BS, et al. Randomized trial of bendamustine-rituximab or R-CHOP/R-CVP in first-line treatment of indolent NHL or MCL: The BRIGHT study. *Blood* 2014;123:2944-2952.
104. McLaughlin P, Hagemeister FB, Rodriguez MA, et al. Safety of fludarabine, mitoxantrone, and dexamethasone combined with rituximab in the treatment of stage IV indolent lymphoma. *Semin Oncol* 2000;27:37-41.
105. Goldsmith SJ. Radioimmunotherapy of lymphoma: Bexxar and Zevalin. *Semin Nucl Med* 2010;40:122-135.
106. Press OW, Unger JM, Braziel RM, et al. Phase II trial of CHOP chemotherapy followed by tositumomab/iodine I-131 tositumomab for previously untreated follicular non-Hodgkin's lymphoma: Five-year follow-up of Southwest Oncology Group Protocol S9911. *J Clin Oncol* 2006;24:4143-4149.
107. Kaminski MS, Tuck M, Estes J, et al. ^{131}I-tositumomab therapy as initial treatment for follicular lymphoma. *N Engl J Med* 2005;352:441-449.
108. Link BK, Martin P, Kaminski MS, Goldsmith SJ, Coleman M, Leonard JP. Cyclophosphamide, vincristine, and prednisone followed by tositumomab and iodine-131-tositumomab in patients with untreated low-grade follicular lymphoma: Eight-year follow-up of a multicenter phase II study. *J Clin Oncol* 2010;28:3035-3041.
109. Armitage JO, Carbone PP, Connors JM, Levine AM, Bennett JM, Kroll S. Treatment-related myelodysplasia and acute leukemia in non-Hodgkin's lymphoma patients. *J Clin Oncol* 2003;21:897-906.
110. Martin P, Jung S-H, Johnson JL, et al. CALGB 50803 (Alliance): A phase II trial of lenalidomide plus rituximab in patients with previously untreated follicular lymphoma. *J Clin Oncol* 2014;32: Abstract 8521.
111. Witzig TE, Wiernik PH, Moore T, et al. Lenalidomide oral monotherapy produces durable responses in relapsed or refractory indolent non-Hodgkin's Lymphoma. *J Clin Oncol* 2009;27:5404-5409.
112. Gopal AK, Kahl BS, de Vos S, et al. PI3Kδ inhibition by idelalisib in patients with relapsed indolent lymphoma. *N Engl J Med* 2014;370:1008-1018.
113. van Besien KW. Allogeneic stem cell transplantation in follicular lymphoma: Recent progress and controversy. *Hematology Am Soc Hematol Educ Program* 2009:610-618.
114. Oliansky DM, Gordon LI, King J, et al. The role of cytotoxic therapy with hematopoietic stem cell transplantation in the treatment of follicular lymphoma: An evidence-based review. *Biol Blood Marrow Transplant* 2010;16:443-468.
115. Evens AM, Vanderplas A, LaCasce AS, et al. Stem cell transplantation for follicular lymphoma relapsed/refractory after prior rituximab: A comprehensive analysis from the NCCN lymphoma outcomes project. *Cancer* 2013;119:3662-3671.
116. Armitage JO, Mauch PM, Harris NL, Dalla-Favera R, Bierman PJ. Diffuse large B-cell lymphoma. In: Armitage JO, Mauch PM, Harris NL, Coiffier B, Dalla-Favera R, eds. *Non-Hodgkin Lymphoma*. 2nd ed. Philadelphia, PA: Lippincott Williams & Wilkins; 2010: 304-326.
117. McKelvey EM, Gottleib JA, Wilson HE, et al. Hydroxydaunomycin (Adriamycin) combination chemotherapy in malignant lymphoma. *Cancer* 1976;38:1484-1493.
118. Jones SE, Grozea PN, Metz EN, et al. Superiority of adriamycin containing combination chemotherapy in the treatment of diffuse lymphoma: A Southwest Oncology Group study. *Cancer* 1979;43:417-425.
119. Fisher RI, Gaynor ER, Dahlberg S, et al. Comparison of a standard regimen (CHOP) with three intensive chemotherapy regimens for advanced non-Hodgkin's lymphoma. *N Engl J Med* 1993;328:1002-1006.
120. Blayney DW, LeBlanc ML, Grogan T, et al. Dose-intense chemotherapy every 2 weeks with dose-intense cyclophosphamide, doxorubicin, vincristine, and prednisone may improve survival in intermediate- and high-grade lymphoma: A phase II study of the Southwest Oncology Group (SWOG 9349). *J Clin Oncol* 2003;21: 2466-2473.
121. Coiffier B, Lepage E, Briere J, et al. CHOP chemotherapy plus rituximab compared with CHOP alone in elderly patients with diffuse large-B-cell lymphoma. *N Engl J Med* 2002;346:235-242.
122. Coiffier B, Thieblemont C, Van Den Neste E, et al. Long-term outcome of patients in the LNH-98.5 trial, the first randomized study comparing rituximab-CHOP to standard CHOP chemotherapy in DLBCL patients: A study by the Groupe d'Etudes des Lymphomes de l'Adulte. *Blood* 2010;116:2040-2045.
123. Pfreundschuh M, Trumper L, Osterborg A, et al. CHOP-like chemotherapy plus rituximab versus CHOP-like chemotherapy alone in young patients with good-prognosis diffuse large B-cell lymphoma: A randomised controlled trial by the MabThera International Trial (MInT) Group. *Lancet Oncol* 2006;7:379-391.
124. Sehn LH, Donaldson J, Chhanabhai M, et al. Introduction of combined CHOP plus rituximab therapy dramatically improved outcome of diffuse large B-cell lymphoma in British Columbia. *J Clin Oncol* 2005;23:5027-5033.
125. Feugier P, Van Hoof A, Sebban C, et al. Long-term results of the R-CHOP study in the treatment of elderly patients with diffuse large B-cell lymphoma: A study by the Groupe d'Etude des Lymphomes de l'Adulte. *J Clin Oncol* 2005;23:4117-4126.
126. Stiff PJ, Unger JM, Cook JR, et al. Autologous transplantation as consolidation for aggressive non-Hodgkin's lymphoma. *N Engl J Med* 2013;369:1681-1690.
127. Habermann TM, Weller EA, Morrison VA, et al. Rituximab-CHOP versus CHOP alone or with maintenance rituximab in older patients with diffuse large B-cell lymphoma. *J Clin Oncol* 2006;24:3121-3127.

128. Pfreundschuh M, Trumper L, Kloess M, et al. Two-weekly or 3-weekly CHOP chemotherapy with or without etoposide for the treatment of elderly patients with aggressive lymphomas: Results of the NHL-B2 trial of the DSHNHL. *Blood* 2004;104:634-641.
129. Pfreundschuh M, Schubert J, Ziepert M, et al. Six versus eight cycles of bi-weekly CHOP-14 with or without rituximab in elderly patients with aggressive CD20$^+$ B-cell lymphomas: A randomised controlled trial (RICOVER-60). *Lancet Oncol* 2008;9:105-116.
130. Cunningham D, Hawkes EA, Jack A, et al. Rituximab plus cyclophosphamide, doxorubicin, vincristine, and prednisolone in patients with newly diagnosed diffuse large B-cell non-Hodgkin lymphoma: A phase 3 comparison of dose intensification with 14-day versus 21-day cycles. *Lancet* 2013;381:1817-1826.
131. Delarue R, Tilly H, Mounier N, et al. Dose-dense rituximab-CHOP compared with standard rituximab-CHOP in elderly patients with diffuse large B-cell lymphoma (the LNH03-6B study): A randomised phase 3 trial. *Lancet Oncol* 2013;14:525-533.
132. Crump M, Kuruvilla J, Couban S, et al. Randomized comparison of gemcitabine, dexamethasone, and cisplatin versus dexamethasone, cytarabine, and cisplatin chemotherapy before autologous stem-cell transplantation for relapsed and refractory aggressive lymphomas: NCIC-CTG LY.12. *J Clin Oncol* 2014;32:3490-3496.
133. Gisselbrecht C, Glass B, Mounier N, et al. Salvage regimens with autologous transplantation for relapsed large B-cell lymphoma in the rituximab era. *J Clin Oncol* 2010;28:4184-4190.
134. Philip T, Guglielmi C, Hagenbeek A, et al. Autologous bone marrow transplantation as compared with salvage chemotherapy in relapses of chemotherapy-sensitive non-Hodgkin's lymphoma. *N Engl J Med* 1995;333:1540-1545.
135. Fisher RI, Bernstein SH, Kahl BS, et al. Multicenter phase II study of bortezomib in patients with relapsed or refractory mantle cell lymphoma. *J Clin Oncol* 2006;24:4867-4874.
136. Robak T, Huang H, Jin J, et al. Bortezomib-based therapy for newly diagnosed mantle-cell lymphoma. *N Engl J Med* 2015;372:944-953.
137. Wang ML, Blum KA, Martin P, et al. Long-term follow-up of MCL patients treated with single-agent ibrutinib: Updated safety and efficacy results. *Blood* 2015;126:739-745.
138. Levine AM, Said JW. Management of acquired immunodeficiency syndrome-related lymphoma. In: Armitage JO, Mauch PM, Harris NL, Coiffier B, Dalla-Favera R, eds. *Non-Hodgkin Lymphoma*. 2nd ed. Philadelphia, PA: Lippincott Williams & Wilkins; 2010:507-526.
139. Mounier N, Spina M, Gisselbrecht C. Modern management of non-Hodgkin's lymphoma in HIV-infected patients. *Br J Haematol* 2007;136:685-698.
140. Barta SK, Lee JY, Kaplan LD, et al. Pooled analysis of AIDS malignancy consortium trials evaluating rituximab plus CHOP or infusional EPOCH chemotherapy in HIV-associated non-Hodgkin lymphoma. *Cancer* 2012;118:3977-3983.
141. Kaplan LD, Lee JY, Ambinder RF, et al. Rituximab does not improve clinical outcome in a randomized phase III trial of CHOP with or without rituximab in patients with HIV associated non-Hodgkin's lymphoma: AIDS Malignancy Consortium trial 010. *Blood* 2005; 106:1538-1543.

133

Ovarian Cancer

Judith A. Smith and Elizabeth K. Nugent

KEY CONCEPTS

1. Ovarian cancer is denoted "the silent killer" because of the nonspecific signs and symptoms that contribute to the delay in diagnosis. The few patients who present with disease still confined to the ovary will have a 5-year survival rate greater than 90%, but most patients present with advanced disease and have a 5-year survival rate of 10% to 30%.
2. Ovarian cancer is a sporadic disease with less than 10% of cases of ovarian cancer attributed to heredity. However, a history of two or more first-degree relatives with ovarian cancer increases a woman's risk of developing ovarian cancer by greater than 50%.
3. Considerable education efforts have been made to identify patients with the persistence, greater than 2 weeks, of nonspecific presenting symptoms of ovarian cancer including: abdominal pressure/pain, difficulty eating or feeling full quickly, urinary urgency/frequency, change in bowel habits, or unexplained vaginal bleeding.
4. CA-125 is a nonspecific antigen used as a tumor marker for diagnosis and monitoring epithelial ovarian carcinoma. If CA-125 is positive at the time of diagnosis, changes in CA-125 levels correlate with disease response and progression.
5. Although most patients will achieve a complete response to initial treatment, more than 50% of patients will have recurrence within the first 2 years. If recurrence occurs less than 6 months after completion of chemotherapy, the tumor is defined to be platinum-resistant. The antitumor activity of second-line chemotherapy regimens is similar, and the choice of treatment for recurrent platinum-resistant ovarian cancer depends on residual toxicities, physician preference, and patient convenience. Participation in a clinical trial is also a reasonable option for these patients.
6. Ovarian cancer is staged surgically with the International Federation of Gynecology and Obstetrics (FIGO) staging algorithm. Tumor debulking and total abdominal hysterectomy–bilateral oophorectomy surgery are the primary surgical interventions for ovarian cancer. After the completion of the staging and primary surgical treatment, the current standard of care is six cycles of a taxane/platinum-containing chemotherapy regimen.
7. The interperitoneal (IP) route of chemotherapy administration has significantly improved progression-free and overall survival, but patients must be carefully selected.
8. A platinum-containing doublet chemotherapy regimen is the standard of care for the first recurrence of platinum-sensitive ovarian cancer.
9. Despite recent advances, enrollment in an investigational study is still the primary treatment recommendation for patients with recurrent platinum-resistant ovarian cancer.
10. The activity of the new class of the poly(adenosine diphosphate [ADP]-ribose) polymerase (PARP) inhibitors depends on BCRA status or "BRCAness" of the tumor.

Ovarian cancer is a gynecologic cancer that usually arises from disruption or mutations in the epithelium of the ovary. It is associated with the highest mortality among the gynecologic cancers, primarily because most patients present with advanced disease. (1) Ovarian cancer is denoted "the silent killer" because of the nonspecific signs and symptoms that often lead to a delay in diagnosis. Ovarian cancers often metastasize via the lymphatic and blood systems to the liver and/or lungs. Common complications of advanced and progressive ovarian cancer include ascites and small bowel obstruction. The few patients who present with disease still confined to the ovary will have a 5-year survival rate greater than 90%, but most patients present with advanced disease and have a 5-year survival rate of 10% to 30%. Primary treatment includes tumor-debulking surgery followed by six cycles of a taxane-platinum chemotherapy regimen. Although 70% of patients achieve an initial complete response to chemotherapy, more than 50% of these patients will have recurrence within the first 2 years from diagnosis.[1]

EPIDEMIOLOGY

It is estimated that 22,280 new cases of ovarian cancer were diagnosed, and 14,240 women died of the disease in 2016 giving an overall mortality rate of 63.9%.[2] Unfortunately, despite clinical advances over the past two decades, the overall mortality rate for ovarian cancer has not changed (Fig. 133-1). Ovarian cancer is still associated with the highest mortality rate among the gynecologic cancers and is the fifth leading cause of cancer-related deaths in women. The high mortality rate is related to the insidious onset of nonspecific symptoms and the lack of adequate screening tools, which allows the disease to go undiagnosed until it has progressed beyond the pelvic cavity.

ETIOLOGY

As with many other cancers, the risk of ovarian cancer increases with increasing age. A woman's risk increases from 15.7 to 54 per 100,000 as her age advances from 40 to 79 years, and the median age at diagnosis is 59.[2] Most cases of ovarian cancer are diagnosed during the peri- and postmenopausal phase of women's reproductive life span.

(2) Heredity accounts for less than 10% of all ovarian cancer cases. Family history is an important risk factor in the development of ovarian cancer. If one family member has a diagnosis of ovarian cancer, the associated lifetime risk is 9%, but this risk increases to greater than 50% if there are two or more first-degree relatives (eg, her mother and sister) with a diagnosis of ovarian cancer or multiple cases of ovarian and breast cancer within the same family.[1]

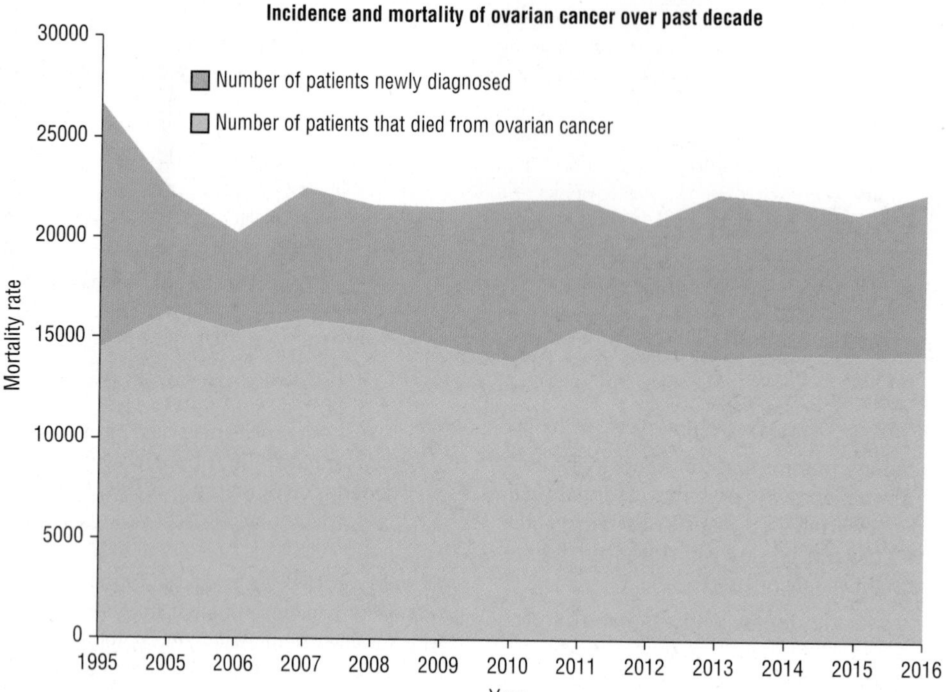

FIGURE 133-1 Incidence and mortality of ovarian cancer over past decade.

BRCA1 and *BRCA2* are the tumor suppressor genes thought to be involved in one or more pathways of DNA damage recognition and repair. The *BRCA1* gene is located on chromosome 17q12–21, and the *BRCA2* gene is located on chromosome 13q12–13. Both *BRCA1* and *BRCA2* mutations are associated with ovarian cancer. However, *BRCA1* is more prevalent, being associated with 90% of inherited and 10% of sporadic cases of ovarian cancer.[3] Patients with *BRCA1*-associated ovarian cancer are usually considerably younger than patients with *BRCA2* mutations, with a mean age of 54 years.[3] Patients usually present with advanced stage at diagnosis, and the *BRCA1*-linked ovarian cancers are more aggressive tumors that typically are serous histology, moderate to high grade. As *BRCA1* and *BRCA2* are thought to be involved in DNA damage or repair, their inactivation/mutations may be associated with an increased resistance of ovarian cancer cells to cytotoxic agents.

Hereditary breast and ovarian cancer syndrome is one of the two different forms of hereditary ovarian cancer that are associated with germline mutations in *BRCA1* and *BRCA2*.[3] The hereditary nonpolyposis colorectal cancer or Lynch syndrome is a familial syndrome with germline mutations causing defects in enzymes involved in DNA mismatch repair, which is associated with up to 12% of hereditary ovarian cancer cases.[3] This syndrome is associated with mutations in DNA mismatch repair genes such as *MSH2, MLH1, PMS1*, and *PMS2* and leads to microsatellite instability.

Hormone exposure, specifically estrogen, and reproductive history are also associated with the risk of developing ovarian cancer. Conditions that increase the total number of ovulations in women's reproductive history, such as nulliparity, early menarche, or late menopause, are associated with an increased risk for epithelial ovarian cancers.[4] Conversely those conditions that limit ovulations are associated with a protective effect. Each time ovulation occurs, the ovarian epithelium is broken, followed by cellular repair. According to the *incessant ovulation hypothesis*, the risk of mutations and, ultimately, cancer increases each time the ovarian epithelium undergoes cell repair.

Finally, ovarian cancer is associated with certain dietary and environmental factors. A diet that is high in galactose, animal fat, and meat may increase the risk of ovarian cancer, whereas a vegetable-rich diet may decrease the risk of ovarian cancer.[5] Although controversial, exogenous factors such as asbestos and talcum powder use in the perineal area are also associated with an increased risk of ovarian cancer.[5]

PATHPHYSIOLOGY

Ovarian carcinomas can be separated into three major entities: epithelial carcinomas, germ cell tumors, and stromal carcinomas. Most ovarian tumors (85%-90%) are derived from the epithelial surface of the ovary.[6] The classification of common epithelial tumors has been developed by the World Health Organization and FIGO.[6] The nomenclature considers cell type, location of the tumor, and the degree of the malignancy, which ranges from benign tumors to tumors of low malignancy to invasive carcinomas. Epithelial tumors classified as low malignancy ("borderline malignancy") are characterized by epithelial papillae with atypical cell clusters, cellular stratification, nuclear atypia, and increased mitotic activity, and have a much better prognosis than those classified as invasive carcinomas. Malignant tumors are characterized by an infiltrative destructive growth pattern with malignant cells growing in a disorganized manner and dissection into stromal planes.

Invasive epithelial adenocarcinomas are characterized by histologic subtype and grade, which measures the degree of cellular differentiation. Although the histologic type of the tumor is not a significant prognostic factor, with the exception of clear cell, the histopathologic grade is an important prognostic factor. Undifferentiated tumors are associated with a poorer prognosis than those lesions that are considered to be well or moderately differentiated. A universal grading system for ovarian cancer was developed that combines mitotic score, nuclear atypia score, and architectural score based on the histologic pattern.[7]

The histologic subtypes of adenocarcinomas include papillary serous, mucinous, endometrioid, clear cell, mixed epithelial, transition-cell, and undifferentiated adenocarcinomas.[1,8] Papillary serous adenocarcinoma is the most common type of epithelial ovarian cancer and accounts for about 46% of cases. The peak age of diagnosis ranges from 45 to 65 years with 63 years as the median age of diagnosis.[6] Serous carcinomas typically display complex papillary and solid patterns and qualify as high-grade carcinomas. Endometrioid carcinomas are seen in women 40 to 50 years of age and comprise about 8% of ovarian carcinomas, of which about 6% are surface epithelial neoplasms.[8] Endometrioid tumors are usually diagnosed as stage I disease and have a better prognosis than tumors with serous histology. Mucinous carcinomas occur in women between 40 and 70 years of age and account for about 36% of all ovarian cancers. The overall prognosis for mucinous carcinoma is better than for serous carcinoma because most patients present with stage I disease. Clear cell carcinoma comprises about 3% of ovarian carcinomas in women, with a mean age of 57 years. Although clear cell carcinoma is the least common ovarian neoplasm, it is most commonly associated with paraneoplastic-related hypercalcemia.[8]

Germ cell tumors of the ovary, including malignant teratoma and dysgerminomas, are rare, comprising about 2% to 3% of all ovarian cancers in Western countries with an increased incidence in black and Asian women.[6] These tumors are highly curable and affect primarily young women. In contrast to epithelial tumors, about 60% to 70% of germ cell tumors are stage I at diagnosis, which is related to earlier detection and response to symptoms in this younger patient population.[6] Serum markers (human β-chorionic gonadotropin and α-fetoprotein) are helpful to confirm the diagnosis and monitor response to treatment.

Finally, ovarian sex cord-stromal tumors account for 7% of all ovarian cancers and tend to be diagnosed at an early stage.[6] Sex cord-stromal tumors are associated with hormonal effects, such as precocious puberty, amenorrhea, and postmenopausal bleeding. Because these tumors are rare, the optimal treatment of ovarian sex cord-stromal tumors is not clear. The current recommended standard of care is surgery followed by treatment with a platinum-based chemotherapy regimen.

Ovarian cancer is usually confined to the abdominal cavity, but spread can occur to the lung, liver, and, less commonly, the bone or brain. Disease is spread by direct extension, peritoneal seeding, lymphatic dissemination, or bloodborne metastasis. Lymphatic seeding is the most common pathway and frequently causes ascites.

SCREENING AND PREVENTION

Screening

Ovarian cancer is an uncommon disease with no known preinvasive component, which has made it difficult to screen patients to detect early disease. In addition, the risk factors for developing ovarian cancer are not well understood, which also makes it difficult to identify a high-risk group of individuals. At the present time, there are no effective screening tools for early detection of ovarian cancer. 3 However, considerable education efforts have been made to help identify patients with the persistence (ie, >2 weeks) of nonspecific presenting symptoms of ovarian cancer including: abdominal pressure/pain, difficulty eating or feeling full quickly, urinary urgency/frequency, change in bowel habits, or unexplained vaginal bleeding.

Pelvic examinations are noninvasive and well accepted and can detect large tumors with a sensitivity of 67% for detecting all tumors.[9] However, because pelvic examinations cannot detect minimal or microscopic disease, they do not usually detect ovarian cancer until it is in an advanced stage. As a result of these limitations, routine pelvic examinations are not an effective screening tool and do not decrease overall mortality.[9]

Transvaginal ultrasound (TVUS) creates an image of the ovary by releasing sound waves. It can be used to evaluate the size and shape and to detect the presence of cystic or solid masses or abdominal fluid. Transvaginal ultrasound can also evaluate blood flow within an ovarian mass. Normal ovarian size cutoff parameters range from 1.25 cm^2 for women 55 to 59 years of age to 1.0 cm^2 for women older than age 65 to 69 years.[17,18] Transvaginal ultrasound is sensitive in identifying ovarian lesions and abnormalities, but its use as a routine screening test is limited by a lack of specificity and an inability to detect peritoneal cancer or cancer in normal-size ovaries.[9]

Serum cancer antigen-125 (CA-125) is a nonspecific inflammatory antigen that can be elevated in numerous conditions associated with inflammation in the abdominal cavity. CA-125 has been extensively studied as a potential tumor marker for ovarian cancer based on the observation that CA-125 levels in a woman without ovarian cancer tend to stay the same or decrease over time, whereas levels associated with malignancy tend to gradually increase over time.[9] However, CA-125 is a nonspecific test that can be elevated in a number of benign conditions, including other gynecologic conditions, such as endometriosis, and many nongynecologic conditions, such as diverticulitis and peptic ulcer disease. Because of these limitations, CA-125 levels are not recommended as a routine screening test for detection of ovarian cancer. Numerous other serologic markers such as carcinoembryonic antigen and lipid-associated sialic acid have been evaluated but cannot be recommended for routine screening for ovarian cancer.

The United States Preventive Services Task Force found fair evidence to support screening with CA-125 or TVUS and concluded that earlier detection would likely have a small effect, at best, on mortality from ovarian cancer.[10] Unfortunately, because of the low prevalence of ovarian cancer and the invasive nature of diagnostic testing after a positive screening test, the United States Preventive Services Task Force also found fair evidence that screening could likely lead to important harms. The United States Preventive Services Task Force concluded that the potential harms outweigh the potential benefits and recommended against any form of routine screening with CA-125 or TVUS for ovarian cancer.

In high-risk women, as defined by family history, most clinicians use a multimodality approach for ovarian cancer screening that includes an annual TVUS in combination with a CA-125 blood test every 6 months. Changes in CA-125 are monitored over time, and changes such as a persistent elevation or consistent increases in CA-125 levels in conjunction with TVUS abnormalities are evaluated further.

Prevention

It is difficult to make recommendations for prevention for the general population because ovarian cancer is a sporadic disease with no established risk factors. Noninvasive measures, such as chemoprevention, have demonstrated some benefit in decreasing the risk of developing ovarian cancer. Ovulation itself is considered a potential insult to the ovarian epithelium, increasing its susceptibility to damage and, ultimately, to cancer. Interventions or reproductive conditions associated with decreasing the number of ovulations, including multiparity, may have a protective effect for the prevention of ovarian cancer. However, the more invasive prevention interventions, such as prophylactic surgery and genetic screening, should be reserved for those women identified to be at high risk based on their heredity for developing ovarian cancer.

Chemoprevention

Although a number of agents have been investigated as chemoprevention of ovarian cancer, including oral contraceptives, aspirin, nonsteroidal anti-inflammatory agents, and retinoids, none of these agents is currently accepted as standard treatment for the prevention of ovarian cancer. Oral contraceptives inhibit ovulation, which reduces the opportunity for potential for damage to the ovarian epithelium. When taken for longer than 10 years, oral contraceptives decrease the relative risk to less than 0.4.[11] Because oral contraceptive use is associated with an increased risk of breast cancer, women with a family history of breast cancer are not candidates for this use of oral contraceptives as chemoprevention of ovarian cancer.[11]

Nonsteroidal anti-inflammatory drugs, aspirin, and acetaminophen also have been suggested for use in the chemoprevention of different cancers, especially hereditary nonpolyposis colon cancer.[12] Although the results of observational studies show that the use of nonsteroidal anti-inflammatory drugs, aspirin, and acetaminophen reduces the risk of ovarian cancer, these findings have not been confirmed in prospective clinical studies. The proposed mechanism of these agents is the anti-inflammatory effect on normal ovulation and inhibition of ovulation.[12]

Prophylactic Surgery

Prophylactic surgical interventions for the prevention of ovarian cancer are reserved for patients with a significant family history or known genetic mutations such as *BRCA1* and should be postponed until after childbearing is completed. The goal is to remove healthy, at-risk organs before any carcinogenic activity is initiated, ultimately reducing the risk of developing cancer. These surgeries include prophylactic oophorectomy or bilateral salpingo-oophorectomy and tubal ligation. These procedures will cause surgical menopause, which can be associated with severe hot flashes, vaginal dryness, sexual dysfunction, and increased risk for development of osteoporosis and heart disease in these women. Because of the potential impact on quality of life and increased health risks, prophylactic surgery is not recommended as a general prevention intervention for the general population.

Although prophylactic surgical interventions are associated with significant reduction in risk of developing ovarian cancer, patients who choose to have a prophylactic oophorectomy/bilateral salpingo-oophorectomy completed need to be informed that complete protection is not guaranteed.[11,13] Although a 67% risk reduction has been shown, a potential 2% to 5% risk of primary peritoneal cancer remains.[13] Primary peritoneal cancers have identical histology of ovarian tumors with diffuse involvement of peritoneal surfaces. Primary peritoneal cancers can often result from "seeding" during the prophylactic surgery. It is recommended for peritoneal washings to be completed during the prophylactic surgery to check for presence of peritoneal surfaces. If positive, then prophylactic surgery would change to staging and treatment surgery to determine extent of disease and remove any other possible lesions.

Tubal ligation is another procedure that can potentially reduce the risk for developing ovarian cancer. In a case-control study, Narod et al. reported that tubal ligation in *BRCA*-positive women was associated with a 63% reduction in risk of developing ovarian cancer.[14] However, it is not recommended as a sole procedure in prophylaxis. The mechanism for its protective effect is not clear, but it has been proposed that tubal ligation may limit exposure of the ovary to environmental carcinogens.

Genetic Screening

Genetic screening should be considered for those women with a significant family history of ovarian cancer. Patients should be evaluated for the presence of genes such as *BRCA1*, *BRCA2*, or other genes such as those associated with hereditary nonpolyposis colorectal cancer or the hereditary breast ovarian cancer (hereditary breast and ovarian cancer syndrome) syndrome.[14] Prior to genetic screening, appropriate patient/family counseling and genetic counseling should be available to help women prepare and deal with the health and psychosocial implications of the genetic screening results.

CLINICAL PRESENTATION

Patients with early ovarian cancer are often asymptomatic and the ovarian mass is often detected incidentally during their annual pelvic examinations. Patients with ovarian cancer often present with nonspecific, vague symptoms such as abdominal bloating, pressure or pain, indigestion, or change in bowel movements.[1] These symptoms can easily be confused with symptoms of common benign gastrointestinal disorders. Patients will often not seek medical attention until these symptoms become unrelenting and bothersome, which allows the disease to progress undetected. Patients with advanced disease may report symptoms such as pain, abdominal distension, and ascites.[1]

Several groups have partnered together to educate women about early signs and symptoms of ovarian cancer. Goff et al. recently developed a symptom index, based on a comparison of symptoms experienced in patients with ovarian cancer and a matched control group.[15] Symptoms that were correlated with ovarian cancer were persistent or recurrent bloating, pelvic or abdominal pain, difficulty eating or feeling full quickly, and urinary symptoms (either urgency or frequency). The Gynecologic Cancer Foundation, Society of Gynecologic Oncologists, and American Cancer Society recommend that women who have any of those problems nearly every day for more than 2 weeks should see a gynecologist, especially if the symptoms are new and quite different from her usual state of health. Furthermore, healthcare professionals should keep ovarian cancer in the differential for women presenting with these persistent symptoms.

CLINICAL PRESENTATION

General

- Ovarian cancer is sometimes referred to as "the silent killer" because of the vague nonspecific signs and symptoms that contribute to the delay in diagnosis.

Symptoms

- The patient may complain of abdominal discomfort, nausea, dyspepsia, flatulence, bloating, fullness, early satiety, urinary frequency, change in bowel function (diarrhea or constipation), weight change, and digestive disturbances.

Signs

- Abdominal or pelvic mass may be palpable.
- Lymphadenopathy may be present.
- Vaginal bleeding may be irregular.
- Patient may have signs of ascites (abdominal distension, shifting, and dullness to percussion—may present like "pregnant abdomen").

Laboratory Tests

- CA-125 may be elevated (normal level is <35 units/mL [kU/L]).
- Abnormalities in liver function tests may suggest hepatic involvement.
- Abnormalities in renal function tests may suggest compression of the renal system by the tumor.

DIAGNOSIS

The diagnostic workup for suspected ovarian cancer includes a careful physical examination including a Papanicolaou (Pap) smear and a pelvic and rectovaginal examination.[3] The presence of a pelvic mass that is unilateral or bilateral, solid, irregular, fixed, or nodular is highly suggestive of ovarian cancer. Unfortunately, by the time a pelvic mass can be palpitated on physical exam, the disease is already advanced beyond the pelvic cavity. A detailed family history should be taken, especially noting the number and pattern of first-degree relatives with malignancies.

A complete blood count, chemistry profile (including liver and renal function tests), and CA-125, carcinoembryonic antigen, and CA19–9 levels should be performed. 4 Although CA-125 is a nonspecific antigen, it is the best current tumor marker for epithelial ovarian carcinoma. A normal CA-125 value is less than 35 units/mL (kU/L). If the CA-125 is elevated at the time of diagnosis, changes in CA-125 levels correlate with tumor burden. Rising CA-125 levels are often associated with disease progression, but CA-125 can be elevated in various other conditions such as different phases of the menstrual cycle, diverticulitis, endometriosis, as well as other nongynecologic cancers. When a patient presents with an abdominal mass, it is important to rule out other cancers in the abdominal cavity. Carcinoembryonic antigen and CA19–9 are markers for other gastrointestinal cancers and may be helpful in the differential diagnosis.

Other diagnostic tests should include a transvaginal or abdominal ultrasonography, chest radiography, computed tomography, magnetic resonance imaging, or positron emission tomography scan. An upper GI series, IV pyelogram, cystoscopy, proctoscopy, or barium enema is sometimes indicated to confirm diagnosis and extent of disease.

TREATMENT
Ovarian Cancer

Desired Outcomes

The goals of treatment of ovarian cancer depend upon the FIGO stage at diagnosis. While ideally "treatment for cure" is desired, it is important to set realistic expectations for the patient. 5 Most patients will achieve a complete response to the initial multimodality treatment, but over 50% of these patients will present with recurrent disease within the first 2 years after completion of treatment. Although overall survival has not significantly changed for ovarian cancer patients, the progression-free survival has improved, which translates to less time on chemotherapy and overall improvement in quality of life for these patients.

In patients who present with metastatic disease or are not surgical candidates, the goal of treatment is to alleviate symptoms and prolong survival as long as quality of life is acceptable. In the setting of recurrent platinum-resistant ovarian cancer, the treatment goal is also to alleviate symptoms and prolong survival as long as quality of life is acceptable.

General Approach

5 A multimodality approach that includes comprehensive surgery and chemotherapy is used for the initial treatment of ovarian cancer with curative intent. Although most patients will initially achieve a complete response, more than 50% will recur within the first 2 years.[1,16] A clinical complete response to treatment is defined as no evidence of disease by physical examination or diagnostic tests and a normal CA-125 level.

Chemotherapy regimens for ovarian cancer have evolved over the past several decades. Treatment regimens began with single-agent melphalan followed by single-agent cyclophosphamide. Shortly after cisplatin was introduced into clinical practice, it was added to cyclophosphamide, and this combination was the "standard of care" for more than a decade until the introduction of paclitaxel in the 1980s. Paclitaxel soon replaced cyclophosphamide, and paclitaxel plus cisplatin became the standard of care. Carboplatin was then substituted for cisplatin because of its improved toxicity profile, and paclitaxel plus carboplatin was adopted. During this same period, many researchers have conducted numerous clinical trials of IP chemotherapy. In 2006, Armstrong and colleagues published the first clinical trial to demonstrate a survival advantage of IP therapy over the standard IV regimen.[17] Long-term follow-up of that trial suggests IP therapy significantly improves overall survival.[18] However, these advances in chemotherapy for the treatment of ovarian cancer have not yet translated into major changes in overall 5-year survival for women diagnosed with advanced ovarian cancer, which remains less than 20%.

Certain subgroups of patients have a better or worse response to chemotherapy. The histologic subtype of the tumor is a prognostic factor; clear cell histology is more likely to be poorly differentiated, faster growing, and have intrinsic drug resistance.[1,6] However, the extent of residual disease, size larger than 1 cm, and tumor grade are better predictors of response to chemotherapy and overall survival.[1]

In general, younger patients have a better performance status and tolerate chemotherapy better than elderly patients. For unknown reasons, white women tend to have a worse prognosis and response to therapy as compared with women of other ethnic backgrounds.[1]

In patients with recurrent ovarian cancer, the goals of treatment are to relieve symptoms such as pain or discomfort from ascites, slow disease progression, and prevent serious complications such as small bowel obstructions.

Surgery

Surgery is the primary treatment intervention for ovarian cancer.[19-21] Surgery may be curative for selected patients with limited stage IA disease. Primary surgical treatment includes a total abdominal hysterectomy with bilateral salpingo-oophorectomy (TAH/BSO), omentectomy, and lymph node dissection (Fig. 133-2).[19-21] The primary objective of the surgery is to optimally debulk the tumor to less than 1 cm of residual disease.[42] Long-term follow-up studies confirm that residual disease smaller than 1 cm correlates with higher complete response rates to chemotherapy and longer overall survival as compared to patients with bulky residual disease (>1 cm).[21]

A comprehensive exploratory laparotomy is vital for the accurate confirmation of diagnosis and staging of ovarian cancer.[19,20] 6 Unlike other cancers that are typically diagnosed by biopsy or laboratory results and clinically staged by results from imaging tests, gynecologic cancers, such as ovarian cancer, are surgically diagnosed and then staged according to the FIGO staging algorithm (Fig. 133-3). The FIGO staging system requires a fairly extensive surgery by an experienced gynecologic oncologist. The skill of the surgeon has a significant effect on prognosis, with definitive benefit of a trained gynecologic oncologist performing surgery as compared with a gynecologist or general surgeon.[22] The reasons for this approach include (a) pelvic tumors cannot be readily biopsied without risk of "tumor seeding," which can increase the risk of recurrence, and (b) surgical staging takes into account the presence of microscopic disease in samples obtained by pelvic washing and lymph node dissection and read by a pathologist during the surgical procedure. It is recommended that the initial surgical staging and tumor-debulking surgery be completed by a trained gynecologic oncology surgeon when ovarian cancer is suspected to prevent understaging and to optimize overall outcome.[23]

Secondary cytoreduction or interval debulking is when surgery is performed after completion of some or all chemotherapy to remove residual disease. Some protocols include additional cycles of

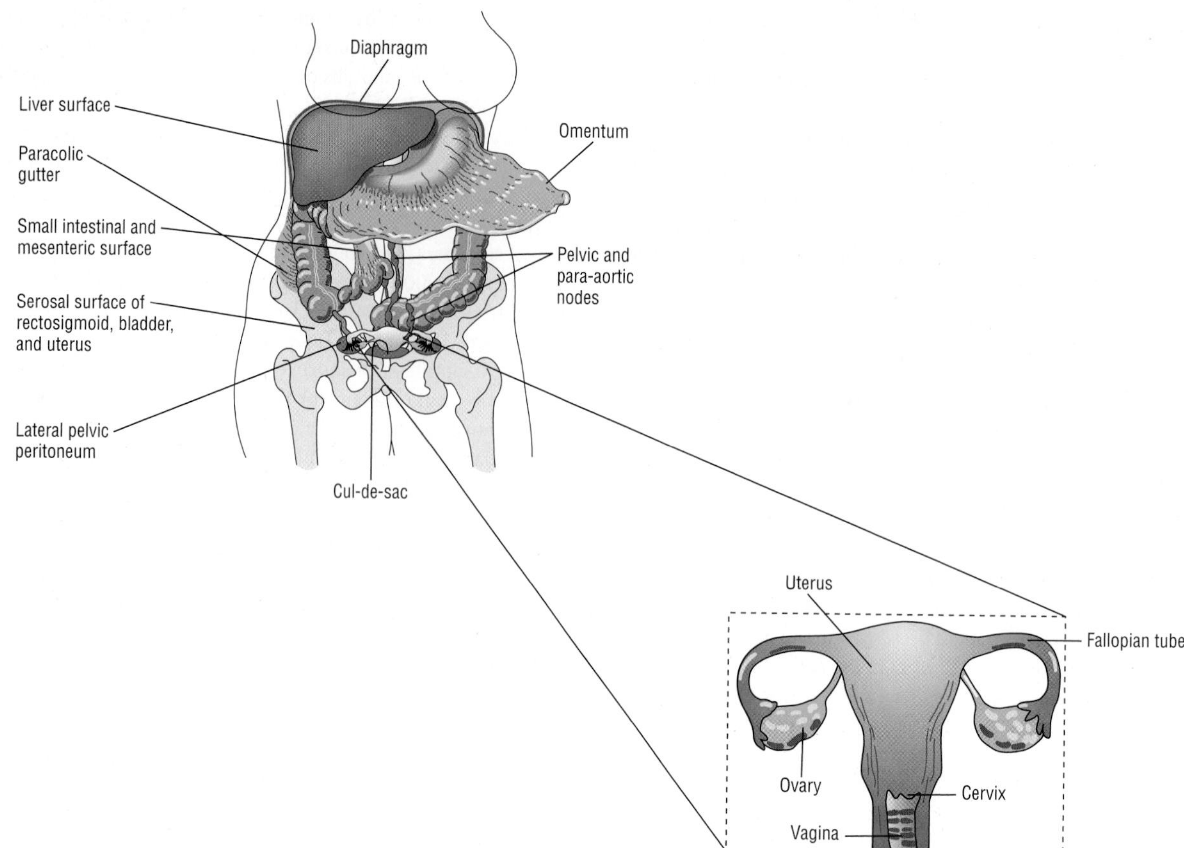

FIGURE 133-2 Staging laparotomy for ovarian cancer with diagram of female reproductive tract (uterus, fallopian tubes, ovaries, and vagina). *Dashed line box* outlines what is removed during the total abdominal hysterectomy with bilateral salpingo-oophorectomy.

chemotherapy after the surgical procedure. The importance of cytoreduction before, during, or after chemotherapy is still controversial, but it has been recommended to facilitate response to chemotherapy and improve overall survival. Randomized trials of secondary surgical cytoreduction have reported conflicting results. In a recently published study of 550 women with stage III or IV disease treated with primary cytoreductive surgery and three cycles of paclitaxel and cisplatin, patients randomized to receive secondary cytoreductive surgery followed by three more cycles of chemotherapy had similar progression-free survival and overall survival as compared with those randomized to receive three more cycles of chemotherapy alone.[24]

The overall effect of interval debulking is influenced by several factors, including initial response to chemotherapy, the amount of residual disease before and after second-look surgery, and the presence of microscopic residual disease. The results of recent trials suggest that secondary surgical cytoreduction does not prolong survival in patients who are treated with maximal primary cytoreductive surgery followed by appropriate postoperative chemotherapy.

"Second-look surgery" is an elective surgical procedure performed in patients who achieve a clinical complete response after primary chemotherapy to determine if any visible or microscopic disease is present in the peritoneal cavity. The benefit of "second-look laparotomy" to evaluate residual disease after completing chemotherapy remains controversial because it has been difficult to establish any impact on overall survival. It has questionable benefit because about 50% of those with a negative second look still relapsed.[24] If visible or microscopic disease is detected during second look, then the clinician may decide to give additional chemotherapy. But if no visible or microscopic disease is detected during second look, the clinician may decide to observe and monitor the patient. Use of laparoscopic surgical techniques is controversial for initial surgery but is sometimes considered in debulking of recurrent or advanced disease when the intent is palliative rather than curative.[21] In patients with recurrent disease, the goal of debulking surgery is to relieve symptoms associated with complications such as small bowel obstructions and to help improve the patient's quality of life.

Radiation

Radiation has a limited role in the management of ovarian cancer. Use of radiation for treatment of early stage disease has had no benefit or impact on overall survival.[25] Radiation therapy is most beneficial for palliation of symptoms in patients with recurrent pelvic disease, often associated with small bowel obstructions. The two forms of radiation therapy used in ovarian cancer are external beam whole-abdominal irradiation and intraperitoneal isotopes such as phosphorus-32 (^{32}P). Alleviation of symptoms with external beam whole-abdominal irradiation is associated with a significant improvement in the patient's quality of life. The recommended dose ranges from 35 to 45 Gy (3500-4500 rad), depending on the treatment history and ability to tolerate radiation treatments.

First-Line Chemotherapy

The mainstay of ovarian cancer treatment is chemotherapy. It is used as a component of first-line treatment after completion of surgery and is the primary modality of treatment for recurrent ovarian cancer. Systemic chemotherapy with a taxane and platinum regimen following optimal surgical debulking is the standard of care for treatment of epithelial ovarian cancer (Fig. 133-4). Table 133-1 summarizes the chemotherapeutic regimens used as the initial treatment of newly diagnosed epithelial ovarian cancer. More than 60 randomized, controlled clinical trials have evaluated combination chemotherapy regimens for the treatment of advanced ovarian cancer, and a meta-analysis of these trials confirmed the efficacy of platinum and taxane regimens over other regimens.[26]

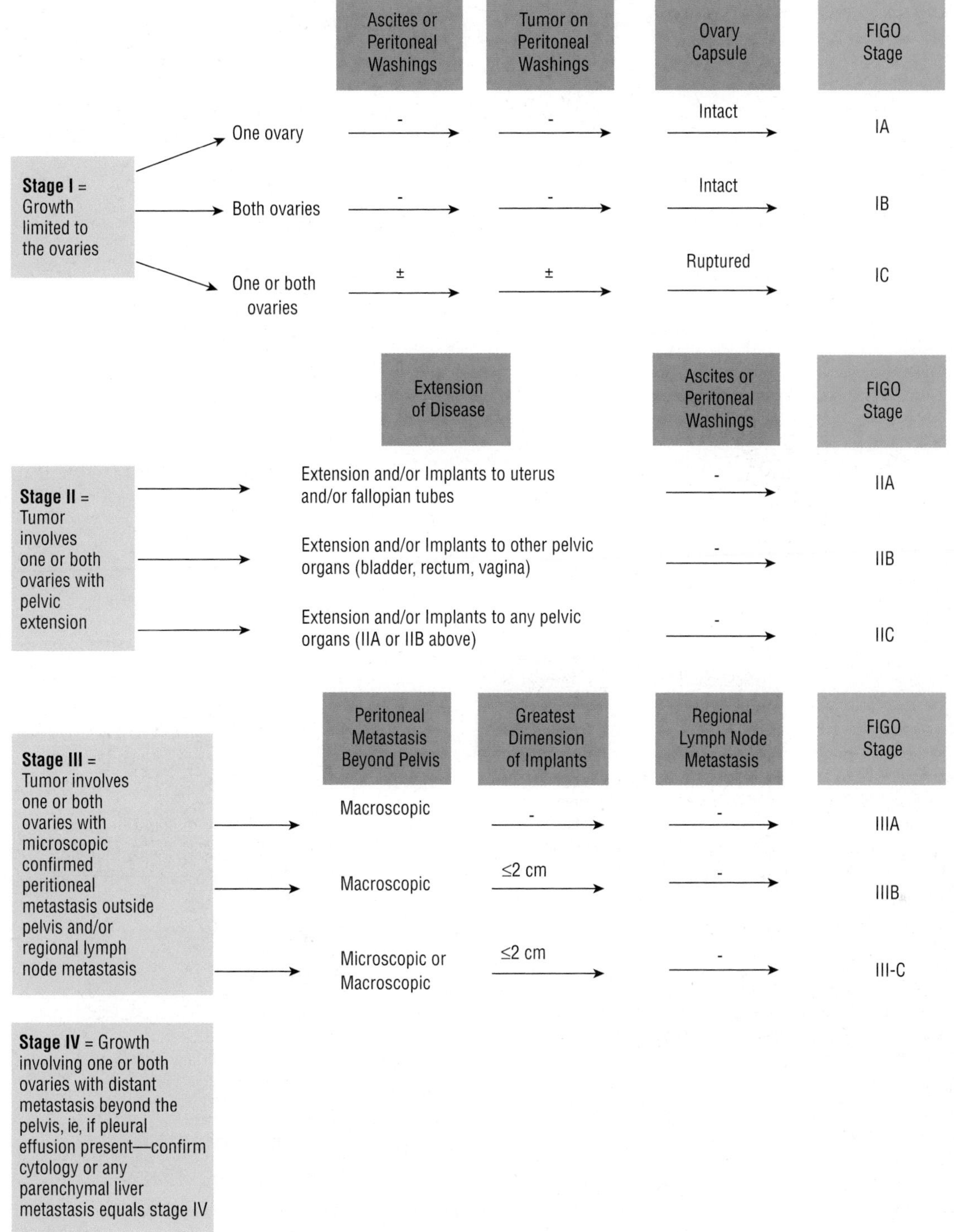

FIGURE 133-3 International Federation of Gynecology and Obstetrics (FIGO) staging algorithm.

Historically, single-agent alkylating agents such as melphalan, and later cyclophosphamide, were used for the treatment of advanced ovarian cancer until the introduction of cisplatin in the 1970s. Combination chemotherapy regimens containing cisplatin and cyclophosphamide achieved higher response rates and overall survival than regimens without cisplatin in patients with advanced ovarian cancer.[16] Based on the results of these trials, the combination of cisplatin plus cyclophosphamide remained the standard of care for the treatment of ovarian cancer until the early 1990s.

The next major advance in the therapy of advanced ovarian cancer occurred with the introduction of paclitaxel into chemotherapy regimens. McGuire et al. reported the results of a Gynecologic Oncology Group (GOG)-111 study that found the combination of paclitaxel 135 mg/m^2 over 24 hours and cisplatin 75 mg/m^2 achieved higher response rates and longer survival than did cyclophosphamide 750 mg/m^2 and cisplatin 75 mg/m^2 in patients with newly diagnosed, suboptimally debulked, stages III and IV ovarian cancer.[27] Survival improved significantly in the paclitaxel arm, with an increase in median progression-free survival (18 vs 13 months) and overall survival (38 vs 24 months). Neutropenia, alopecia, and peripheral neuropathy were more severe in the paclitaxel plus cisplatin group. Similar results were reported in a large European-Canadian Intergroup Phase III randomized trial study (OV10) that also confirmed superior response rates with the paclitaxel 135 mg/m^2 over 24 hours with cisplatin 75 mg/m^2 regimen as compared with cyclophosphamide 750 mg/m^2 with cisplatin 75 mg/m^2 regimen.[28] Based on the results of these studies, paclitaxel plus cisplatin was widely adopted and became the accepted standard of care.

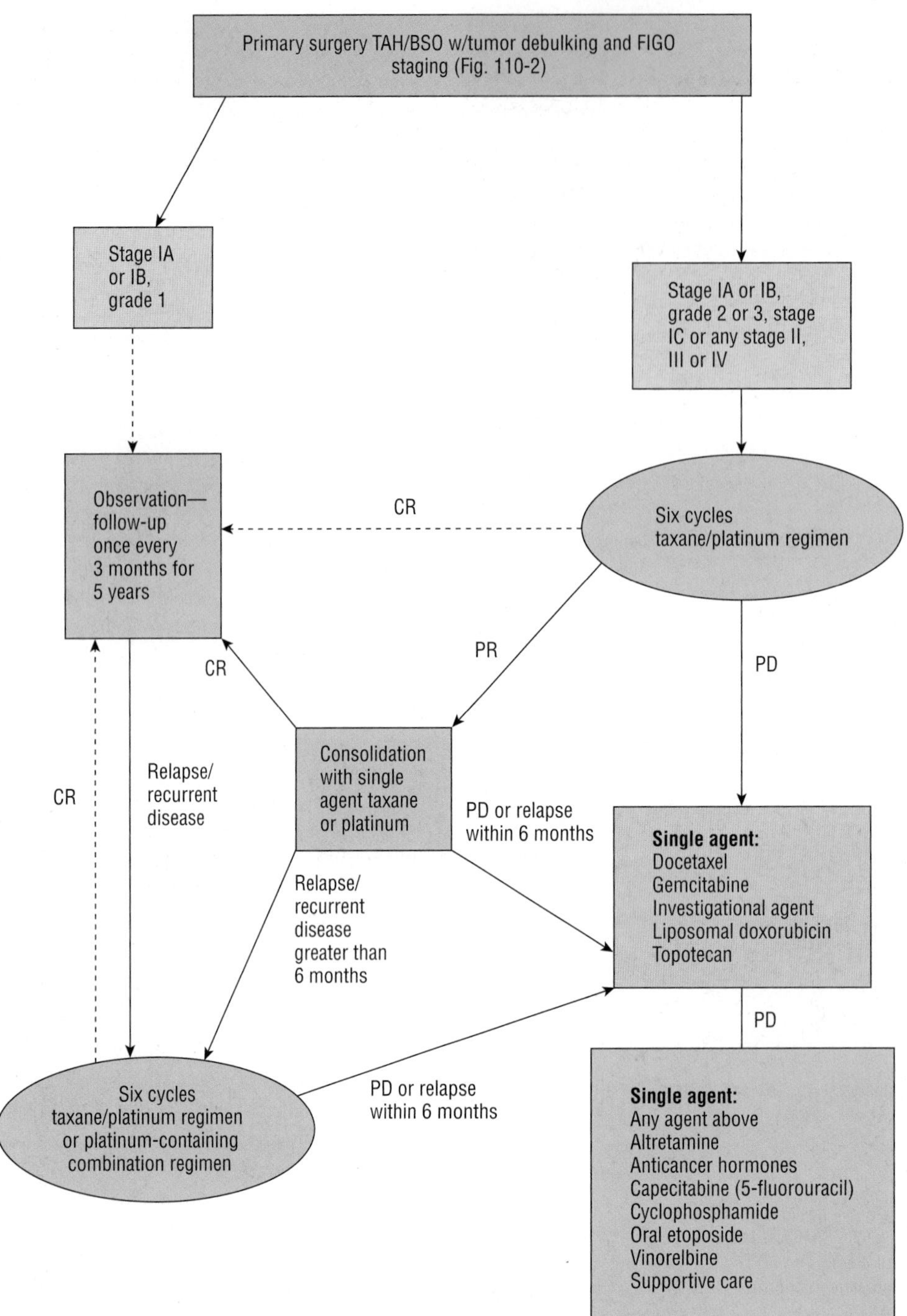

FIGURE 133-4 Management of newly diagnosed, refractory, and progressive epithelial ovarian cancer. All recommendations are category 2A unless otherwise indicated. (CR, complete response; PD, progression of disease; PR, partial response; TAH/BSO, total abdominal hysterectomy/bilateral salpingo-oophorectomy; USO, unilateral salpingo-oophorectomy.)

TABLE 133-1 Initial Chemotherapeutic Regimens of Epithelial Ovarian Cancer

Drug(s)	Brand Name	Initial Dose(s)/Usual Range	Cycle Frequency
Paclitaxel + carboplatin	Taxol/Paraplatin	175 mg/m^2 IV (3-hours infusion) day 1 Dosed to AUC 5-7.5 IV day 1	Every 21 days
Paclitaxel + cisplatin (IV)	Taxol/Platinol	135 mg/m^2 IV (24-h infusion) day 1 75 mg/m^2 IV day 1	Every 21 days
Paclitaxel + cisplatin (IP)	Taxol/Platinol	Day 1: Paclitaxel 135 mg/m^2 IV infused over 24 hours Day 2: Cisplatin 100 mg/m^2 IP infused over 1 hour Day 8: Paclitaxel 60 mg/m^2 IP infused over 1 hour.	Every 21 days
Cisplatin + cyclophosphamide	Platinol/Cytoxan	50-100 mg/m^2 IV day 1 500-1,000 mg/m^2 IV day 1	Every 21-28 days
Docetaxel + carboplatin	Taxotere/Paraplatin	75 mg/m^2 IV day 1	Every 21 days

AUC, area under the curve; IP, interperitoneal.

The availability of carboplatin led to clinical trials to evaluate whether carboplatin could be substituted for cisplatin, which would spare patients from the significant neurotoxicity and nephrotoxicity associated with cisplatin. Several prospective randomized comparisons of carboplatin plus paclitaxel versus cisplatin plus paclitaxel in patients with advanced ovarian cancer have been conducted.[29-32] The results of these trials show that carboplatin plus paclitaxel is equally efficacious and better tolerated than cisplatin and paclitaxel. In the GOG-158 study, 840 previously untreated patients with optimally resected stage III disease (no residual tumor nodule >1 cm) were randomized to carboplatin (area under the curve [AUC] = 7.5) plus paclitaxel 175 mg/m^2 over 3 hours, or cisplatin 75 mg/m^2 plus paclitaxel 135 mg/m^2 over 24 hours administered every 21 days for six cycles.[29,31] The results of that trial showed no difference in progression-free survival between the two treatment arms with a median time-to-progression of 19.4 months in the paclitaxel plus cisplatin arm versus 20.7 months in the paclitaxel plus carboplatin arm. As expected, the incidence of leukopenia, fever, gastrointestinal toxicity, and metabolic toxicity was higher in patients in the cisplatin arm, while patients in the carboplatin arm experienced more thrombocytopenia and pain. Although the incidence of neurotoxicity was similar in the two treatment arms, it was more severe in the paclitaxel plus cisplatin arm. The results of this study showed that the substitution of carboplatin for cisplatin in the regimen does not compromise efficacy and improves tolerability. These findings were confirmed in two other large randomized, controlled studies.[31,32] Based on these results, paclitaxel plus carboplatin became the accepted standard of care.

Other clinical trials have evaluated the use of docetaxel as a substitute for paclitaxel. In the Scottish Randomized Trial in Ovarian Cancer (SCOTROC), Vasey et al. compared carboplatin (AUC = 5) combined with either docetaxel (75 mg/m^2 over 1 hour) or paclitaxel (175 mg/m^2 over 3 hours) administered every 21 days for six cycles as first-line chemotherapy for stages I to IV epithelial ovarian cancer.[33] The results of this study showed that the substitution of docetaxel for paclitaxel does not compromise efficacy and improves tolerability, particularly neurotoxicity. These findings were not confirmed in another randomized, controlled trial. However, based on the results of this study the combination of docetaxel plus carboplatin is considered a reasonable treatment option for patients with advanced ovarian cancer. Six cycles of paclitaxel plus carboplatin following tumor debulking surgery remain the current standard of care for treatment of advanced ovarian cancer.

Although the choice of taxane or platinum agent does not appear to have a major effect on antitumor activity, weekly paclitaxel administration ("dose density") may be superior to administration every 3 weeks.[34-36] In a phase III trial conducted in Japan, Katsumata et al. reported that patients randomized to six cycles of dose-dense weekly paclitaxel plus carboplatin every 3 weeks had longer progression-free survival as compared to the standard paclitaxel plus carboplatin every 3 weeks.[36] Overall survival at 3 years was also significantly longer in patients who received the dose-dense regimen (72% vs 65%, $P = 0.03$). However, over 42% of the patients who received the dose-dense regimen dropped out of the study before completing six cycles because of treatment-related toxicities. A confirmatory GOG phase III trial is ongoing to confirm these results and address concerns regarding the feasibility of the dose-dense regimen in a larger group of patients as well as the elderly population.

IP chemotherapy was initially employed as palliative care in the management of ascites and uncontrolled intraabdominal tumors. In the late 1970s, IP chemotherapy administration as a primary treatment intervention was initiated based on the rationale that exposure of the tumor to high drug concentrations would increase tumor drug uptake by passive diffusion and ultimately cancer cell death.[37] The increase in AUC exposure in the peritoneal cavity was demonstrated, but the correlative increase in drug uptake in tumor tissue has yet to be validated in any preclinical or clinical study.

7 IP chemotherapy has demonstrated a benefit in the first-line treatment of patients with optimally debulked advanced-stage ovarian cancer.[38-40] In a landmark trial, Armstrong et al. reported the results of the GOG-172 study, which evaluated 415 patients randomized to receive either the combination regimen of paclitaxel 135 mg/m^2 over 24 hours and cisplatin 75 mg/m^2 or a new combination regimen that included paclitaxel 135 mg/m^2 IV infused over 24 hours followed by cisplatin 100 mg/m^2 IP infused over 1 hour on day 2, and then paclitaxel 60 mg/m^2 IP infused over 1 hour on day 8.[17] Both treatment regimens were given once every 21 days for a total of six cycles. Patients randomized to the IP chemotherapy arm had a 5.5-month increase in median progression-free survival and a 15.9-month increase in overall survival.[17] A secondary analysis by Tewari et al. of patients from GOG-172 and GOG-114 IP therapy studies reported a 10.4-month improvement in the median overall survival and 23% decreased risk of death in those patients that had received IP chemotherapy compared to IV chemotherapy.[18] Contributing factors that negatively impacted survival included gross residual disease, clear cell or mucinous histology, and not completing all six cycles of IP chemotherapy.

A potential limitation of IP therapy is significantly more toxicity, including pain, fatigue, myelosuppression, gastrointestinal, metabolic, and neurotoxicity.[17,39,41,42] Despite the potential benefit to improve survival, there has been slow adoption of IP therapy into routine clinical use. Burger et al. completed a cohort study of 823 women with advanced ovarian cancer from six National Comprehensive Cancer Network institutions and found that less than 50% of eligible patients had received IP chemotherapy as part of their primary treatment.[43] The significant increase in systemic toxicity, primarily neurotoxicity, has led to the question of whether IP carboplatin could be substituted for IP cisplatin. Although these platinum agents have demonstrated equal efficacy when administered IV to ovarian cancer patients, it is difficult to extrapolate the IP activity of cisplatin to carboplatin because of the difference in molecular size of cisplatin versus carboplatin and the importance of passive diffusion of drug into the tumor.

Clinical **Controversy...**

The use of IP chemotherapy as first-line treatment of advanced ovarian cancer has been recommended by the National Comprehensive Cancer Network (NCCN) guidelines. Most clinical trials have used platinum agents given IP until the Gynecologic Oncology Group (GOG)-172 trial that incorporated IP paclitaxel. Many clinicians are concerned about how to manage hypersensitivity reactions to either platinum or taxane agents when administered IP.

The 2015 NCCN guidelines recommend that IP chemotherapy be considered and offered to appropriate patients as first-line treatment of optimally debulked, ≥1 cm residual disease, ovarian cancer.[42] 7 Because of the significant toxicities associated with IP therapy, only carefully selected patients should receive IP therapy. Ideal candidates for IP therapy are younger patients with good performance status, minimal comorbidities, adequate renal and liver function, and optimally debulked disease without significant bowel resection.[38,41]

In patients who are poor surgical candidates because of comorbidities or bulky tumors, neoadjuvant chemotherapy can be given prior to any surgical interventions.[44] In patients with bulky disease, the goal of neoadjuvant chemotherapy is to reduce tumor burden to make surgery more feasible and optimal tumor debulking more likely. The typical regimen used in neoadjuvant chemotherapy is three cycles of a taxane combined with a platinum agent followed by surgery. After surgery, patients usually receive another three to six cycles, depending on their response to chemotherapy. In patients who are poor candidates for surgery because of comorbidities, the primary intent of neoadjuvant chemotherapy is to relieve symptoms and slow disease progression. In this setting, palliative chemotherapy alone has not been curative for patients with advanced ovarian cancer.[44] If tolerated, these patients will receive the standard taxane plus platinum chemotherapy regimen once every 3 to 4 weeks. Another option for palliative neoadjuvant chemotherapy, especially in elderly patients, is single-agent carboplatin once every 4 weeks.

Neoadjuvant Chemotherapy

Neoadjuvant chemotherapy is first-line treatment for patients who are poor surgical candidates or patients with bulky or significant tumor burden.[44] The neoadjuvant chemotherapy regimen typically includes a combination of taxane with platinum agent and is administered every 21 to 28 days as tolerated with intent to reduce tumor burden to point where it potentially could be surgically resected and ideally optimally debulking during surgery.[44] After surgery, patient will receive another three to six cycles depending on response to chemotherapy. The role of neoadjuvant chemotherapy for all patients presenting with advance ovarian cancer is being revisited in ongoing GOG clinical trials.

Consolidation Therapy

If patients do not achieve a clinical complete response after completion of six cycles of taxane-platinum regimen, then consolidation chemotherapy should be considered in an attempt to achieve a complete response (Fig. 133-3). If the patient has a partial response to first-line chemotherapy, as measured by a greater than 50% decline in CA-125 (as compared with the pre-surgery level) or tumor regression, the cancer is still considered sensitive to the regimen. The typical regimens for consolidation chemotherapy are the taxane plus platinum regimen or single-agent therapy with either a taxane or platinum agent.[16] If the patient had a poor response to taxane and platinum, then alternative second-line agents can be considered.[42] Additional cycles of chemotherapy are given until complete response is achieved. Another alternative in the setting of no or minimal measurable disease after completion of primary chemotherapy is to just observe the patient and provide supportive care as indicated until disease progresses, then reinitiate chemotherapy at that time.[42]

Because the initial clinical complete response observed in first-line treatment has not been durable, optimization of first-line therapy is under investigation. Numerous options have been evaluated, including the use of additional cycles or maintenance chemotherapy and dose intensity.

Maintenance Chemotherapy

Maintenance chemotherapy is similar to consolidation chemotherapy except maintenance chemotherapy is given to those patients who have achieved a clinica complete response. The primary differences between consolidation and maintenance chemotherapy are the types of agents used and duration of therapy. Consolidation therapy usually consists of more aggressive combination regimens, whereas maintenance chemotherapy usually consists of single agents given less frequently (ie, once monthly) to minimize adverse effects. The goal of maintenance chemotherapy is to eliminate any residual microscopic disease that may be present to extend progression-free and overall survival.

Maintenance chemotherapy has gained popularity after the publication of the results of the collaborative Southwest Oncology Group (SWOG) and GOG 178 study that compared single-agent paclitaxel 175 mg/m^2 over 3 hours once every 21 days for three additional cycles versus an additional 12 cycles.[45] Eligible patients had to have been in complete clinical remission after at least five to six cycles of a taxane-platinum regimen. This study was closed after the interim analysis by the SWOG Safety Monitoring Committee because patients receiving the additional 12 cycles had longer progression-free survival than those receiving three cycles of single-agent paclitaxel (28 vs 21 months). After the results were reported, many patients randomized to the three-cycle arm chose to receive nine additional cycles of paclitaxel, which reduced the ability of the trial to show a difference in overall survival.[46] Because this study was closed early and did not demonstrate an overall survival benefit, another randomized, controlled trial through the GOG was initiated to confirm the improvement in progression-free survival and to attempt to determine the impact on overall survival. Until these confirmatory trials are completed, the role of maintenance chemotherapy is controversial in the management of advanced ovarian cancer patients. Maintenance chemotherapy is listed as an option in the 2015 NCCN guidelines (2B recommendation).[42]

Treatment of Recurrent Disease

Although most patients will achieve a complete response to initial treatment, most patients will eventually have recurrence of their disease within the first 2 years. When a patient relapses, the prognostic factors are similar to the factors after initial surgery except that the disease-free interval—defined as the length of time that has lapsed since the completion of chemotherapy—should be considered to determine if the tumor is likely to be drug resistant to agents used in first-line treatment, which included platinum and taxanes. If recurrence occurs less than 6 months after completion of chemotherapy, or if the patient progresses during platinum-based chemotherapy, the tumor is defined as platinum-resistant. Patients with platinum-sensitive disease generally have a better prognosis than platinum-resistant patients.

If the patient has a clinical complete response to first-line chemotherapy and the recurrence occurs more than 6 months after chemotherapy is completed, the tumor is considered platinum-sensitive. 8 In patients with platinum-sensitive ovarian cancer, the standard of care is to treat the first recurrence with a doublet, platinum-containing chemotherapy regimen. Table 133-2 summarizes some of the chemotherapeutic regimens used in the treatment of recurrent or refractory ovarian cancer. Because the chemotherapy agents used for second-line treatment of recurrent or refractory platinum-resistant disease have similar response rates that average less than 30%, the selection of the agent depends on multiple factors including the toxicity profile of the agent, physician preference, patient performance status, residual toxicities, and patient convenience (Fig. 133-3). In this setting, the intent of treatment is to prolong survival and alleviate symptoms, not necessarily to achieve another "complete response" to chemotherapy. 9 Because of poor response rates of the available agents, participation in a clinical trial of an investigational agent is often recommended for patients with recurrent platinum-resistant ovarian cancer.

Platinum-Sensitive Disease

9 Retreatment with a platinum-containing regimen should be considered in patients with platinum-sensitive disease. The International Collaborative Ovarian Neoplasm 4 and Arbeitsgemeinschaft Gynaekologische randomized 802 patients with recurrent platinum-sensitive ovarian cancer to either single-agent platinum, a non–taxane-platinum combination, or a taxane plus platinum combination.[47] Patients treated with the paclitaxel plus platinum regimen had

TABLE 133-2 Single-Agent Chemotherapeutic Regimens for Recurrent or Refractory Ovarian Cancer

Drug(s)	Brand Name(s)	Initial Dose(s)/Usual Range	Cycle Frequency
Docetaxel	Taxotere	75 mg/m² IV day 1	Every 21 days
Pegylated-liposomal doxorubicin	Doxil	40 mg/m² IV day 1	Every 28 days
Gemcitabine	Gemzar	800-1,000 mg/m² IV days 1, 8, and 15	Every 28 days
Paclitaxel	Taxol	60-80 mg/m² IV (1-h infusion) day 1	Every week
Paclitaxel	Taxol	135-175 mg/m² IV day 1	Every 21 days
Carboplatin	Paraplatin	AUC 5 IV day 1	Every 21-28 days
Cisplatin	Platinol	75 mg/m² IV day 1	Every 21-28 days
Topotecan	Hycamtin	1.3-1.5 mg/m² IV once daily for 5 days	Every 21 days
Topotecan	Hycamtin	4 mg/m² IV once a week × 3 weeks, then 1 week off	Every 21 days
Etoposide	Vepesid	50 mg/m² orally once daily days 1-10 repeat every 21 days	Every 28 days
Capecitabine	Xeloda	1,800-2,000 mg/m² in divided dose twice a day for 2 weeks on, 1 week off	Every 21 days
Altretamine	Hexalen	260 mg/m² orally (total daily dose divided in four doses) for 14-21 days	Every 28 days
Tamoxifen	Nolvadex	20 mg orally twice a day	Continuous
Letrozole	Femara	2.5 mg orally once daily	Continuous

AUC, area under the curve.

significantly longer progression-free (29 vs 24 months) and overall survival (hazard ratio 0.82 [95% CI 0.69- 0.97]) as compared with the other two treatment arms.[47,48] Although the taxane-platinum combination was clearly superior in this European study, it is difficult to extrapolate these results to patients treated in the United States because of differences in first-line treatment. At the time that International Collaborative Ovarian Neoplasm 4 (ICON4) was conducted, the standard of care in Europe for first-line treatment was single-agent carboplatin, so most patients enrolled in this study had no prior exposure to a taxane agent.[47] However, the standard of care in the United States has been a taxane-platinum combination since the early 1990s. Confirmatory data are needed to evaluate whether combination regimens would also be more beneficial in these patients for treatment of recurrent ovarian cancer.

Clinical **Controversy...**

In patients with recurrent ovarian cancer that is platinum sensitive, some clinicians will recommend retreatment with a chemotherapy regimen including a platinum agent. Other clinicians suggest that the platinum-free interval for these patients should be extended and will recommend that recurrent disease first be treated with a non-platinum regimen (ie, liposomal doxorubicin) and reserve the platinum agent until the next relapse.

The 2015 NCCN guidelines recommend the combination of platinum agent with gemcitabine, liposomal doxorubicin, or paclitaxel for treatment of platinum-sensitive recurrent ovarian cancer (Table 133-3).[42] In addition, the combination of gemcitabine plus cisplatin has demonstrated improvement in progression-free survival.[48] Carboplatin alone or any of the second-line agents is recommended for patients with platinum-sensitive disease who are unable to tolerate additional combination chemotherapy regimens because of residual toxicity or poor performance status.[42]

Platinum-Resistant Disease

Frequently patients present with recurrent drug-resistant disease after initial platinum-based therapy and cytoreductive surgery.[16] Patients who progress on a platinum agent or have no response are considered "platinum-refractory," whereas those patients who have recurrence within 6 months of completing a platinum-containing regimen are considered "platinum-resistant."[42] The 2015 NCCN guidelines list many possible treatment options for recurrent platinum-resistant or refractory ovarian carcinoma.[42] The optimal chemotherapeutic agent or regimen in the treatment of platinum-resistant disease is currently unclear. Ideally, the agent should be active in ovarian cancer and non–cross-resistant with taxanes or platinum agents. Unfortunately, the response rate is low for all of the agents in platinum-refractory or resistant ovarian cancer.[16] Patients should typically be evaluated for response after treatment with at least three cycles of the chemotherapy agent or regimen. Because partial responses are rare, stable disease with relief of symptoms is considered a treatment success.

TABLE 133-3 Combination Chemotherapy Regimens for Platinum-Sensitive Recurrent Ovarian Cancer

Drug(s)	Brand Name	Initial Dose(s)/Usual Range	Cycle Frequency
Gemcitabine + carboplatin	Gemzar/Paraplatin	800 mg/m² IV day 1 & 8	Every 21 days
Gemcitabine + cisplatin	Gemzar/Platinol	Dosed to AUC 5 IV day 1	Every 21 days
Liposomal doxorubicin + carboplatin	Doxil/Paraplatin	Day 1 & day 8: gemcitabine 800 mg/m² & cisplatin 40 mg/m²	Every 28 days
Cyclophosphamide + bevacizumab	Cytoxan/Avastin	30 mg/m² IV over 1-3 h & carboplatin AUC 5 50 mg PO once daily + bevacizumab 15 mg/kg q 3 weeks	Every 28 days

AUC, area under the curve; PO, by mouth.

If no response is observed, then an alternative chemotherapy regimen may be selected. Because all the potential agents have similar efficacy, the selection of agents and sequence used for treatment as the patient progresses will vary based on residual toxicity, dosing schedule, patient convenience, and physician preference.

Topotecan, an analog of the plant alkaloid 20(S)-camptothecin, is active in patients with metastatic ovarian cancer and is non–cross-resistant with platinum-based chemotherapy.[16] Preclinical studies suggest that protracted schedules of administration with low doses achieve the greatest antitumor response.[16] Topotecan has demonstrated activity in phase II trials as second-line and salvage therapy in patients who have relapsed after, or progressed during, platinum-based therapy.[49] A randomized phase III trial compared topotecan and paclitaxel in patients with advanced ovarian cancer who had failed one platinum-based regimen.[50] Patients were randomized to receive topotecan 1.5 mg/m^2 per day as a 30-minute infusion for 5 days repeated every 21 days or paclitaxel 175 mg/m^2 as a 3-hour infusion every 21 days. The overall response rate was 21% and 13% for the topotecan- and paclitaxel-treated groups, respectively. The median time-to-progression for topotecan-treated patients (32 weeks) was not significantly different from that for paclitaxel-treated patients (20 weeks). Median survival was 61 weeks in the topotecan-treated group and 43 weeks in the paclitaxel-treated group. Topotecan was well tolerated with minimal nonhematologic toxicities.[49,50]

Pegylated liposomal doxorubicin is one of the primary agents used for second-line therapy of recurrent ovarian cancer.[51-53] The drug tends to be better tolerated than topotecan, which is important for heavily pretreated patients with advanced disease. A large, randomized phase III study compared pegylated liposomal doxorubicin 50 mg/m^2 every 4 weeks to topotecan 1.5 mg/m^2 per day for 5 days repeated every 21 days in patients who failed first-line platinum therapy.[53] A total of 474 patients were randomized, 239 to pegylated liposomal doxorubicin and 235 to topotecan. The overall response rates for the pegylated liposomal doxorubicin and topotecan groups were 20% and 17%, respectively. Overall survival tended to favor pegylated liposomal doxorubicin, with a median of 108 weeks versus 71 weeks for topotecan. Differences in toxicity were observed between the arms, with more hematologic toxicity occurring in the topotecan arm and more palmar–plantar erythrodysesthesia (PPE) in the pegylated liposomal doxorubicin arm. However, the incidence of PPE has decreased in current clinical practice because the standard dose of pegylated liposomal doxorubicin used currently, 40 mg/m^2, is less than the dose that was used in the initial clinical trials and approved by the FDA.[54,55]

Gemcitabine, a novel pyrimidine antimetabolite, is also widely used in the treatment of recurrent platinum-resistant ovarian cancer. Although the overall response rate is only about 13% to 22% with single-agent gemcitabine in patients with platinum-refractory recurrent ovarian cancer, an additional 16% to 50% of patients have stable disease for a median of 7 months.[56] The main toxicities include myelosuppression, fatigue, myalgia, and skin rash. Because of its non-cross-resistant activity and in vivo synergy with platinum agents, gemcitabine is being evaluated in doublet regimens in patients with refractory disease and with carboplatin/taxane regimens in previously untreated patients.[56] The combination of gemcitabine with taxanes has demonstrated response rates from 36% to 90%, which if confirmed, are extremely encouraging.[16]

Other agents that have shown an overall response rate of 10% to 25% in patients with recurrent ovarian cancer include altretamine, etoposide, capecitabine, tamoxifen, letrozole, vinorelbine, and oxaliplatin.[16] Response rates tend to be higher in the platinum-sensitive subgroups. Most of these agents are available in oral formulations, which allows for outpatient administration in the palliative care setting.

Although there are no therapeutic guidelines for the selection of agents for the treatment of recurrent platinum-resistant ovarian cancer, the three most commonly used agents in clinical practice include pegylated liposomal doxorubicin, gemcitabine, and topotecan. These agents have demonstrated efficacy when used as a single agent and in combination with other agents. A phase II GOG study is ongoing to help define the optimal chemotherapy combination for treatment of recurrent or refractory platinum-resistant ovarian cancer. Selection of chemotherapy for treatment of recurrent disease is ultimately based on the patient's residual toxicities, scheduling and convenience, and physician preference.

Additional research continues to identify new agents and new targets for the treatment of ovarian cancer. Because platinum agents and taxanes have been identified as the most active classes of agents for treatment of ovarian cancer, drug development has focused on new platinum derivatives, taxanes and taxane analogs, and agents that exert cytotoxic activity by interacting with DNA directly. Specifically, new cytotoxic agents such as trabectedin, pemetrexed, and epothilones are currently being evaluated in clinical trials.

Biologic and Targeted Agents

Monoclonal antibodies such as bevacizumab and cetuximab and small-molecule tyrosine kinase inhibitors such as sunitinib, gefitinib, or sorafenib, are being evaluated to be incorporated into first line and recurrent treatment regimens for ovarian cancer.[16] Although the biologic agents as single agents have not demonstrated significant activity, the results of several clinical trials show that the addition of agents such as bevacizumab into first line and maintenance regimens improves progression-free survival. However, the impact on overall survival is controversial.

Bevacizumab

Bevacizumab is a recombinant humanized monoclonal antibody that targets vascular endothelial growth factor (VEGF), a key mediator of angiogenesis. In the setting of recurrent disease, single-agent bevacizumab produces a response rate similar to other therapies of 16% to 21%.[57,58] Response rates with combinations of bevacizumab range from 15% to 80%.[57-61] However, these phase II trials have also reported a higher risk of bowel perforation in patients treated with bevacizumab-containing regimens.[57,58] Bevacizumab should therefore not be given to patients who have had recent bowel surgery or a history of significant bowel resections. In an open label phase III study (AURELIA Study) that evaluated the combination of bevacizumab in combination with chemotherapy (pegylated liposomal doxorubicin, weekly paclitaxel, or topotecan), the addition of bevacizumab to chemotherapy had no significant impact on overall survival but did improve median progression-free survival (6.4 vs 3.7 months).[62] Based on this study, bevacizumab was approved for use in combination with pegylated liposomal doxorubicin, weekly paclitaxel, or topotecan for treatment of recurrent ovarian cancer.

Recent efforts have focused on the use of bevacizumab in first-line treatment regimens. Perren et al. conducted an international multi-institutional phase III randomized study (ICON-7) that demonstrated a 7.8-month improvement in overall survival in women who had bevacizumab added to first-line treatment.[63] Based on these encouraging preliminary results, the GOG initiated a confirmatory phase III (GOG-218) study comparing six cycles of standard paclitaxel plus carboplatin to six cycles of the same regimen with bevacizumab to determine whether bevacizumab improves the efficacy of paclitaxel plus carboplatin.[64] A third arm evaluated the benefit of maintenance bevacizumab for an additional 10 months. At the conclusion of the study, no difference in overall survival was observed between the three study arms. However, a four month increase in median progression-free survival was observed in the group that received an additional 10 months of maintenance bevacizumab. Cohn et al. completed a cost utility analysis that incorporated quality of life scores to estimate the cost effectiveness of bevacizumab with paclitaxel/carboplatin for first-line treatment of advanced ovarian cancer.[65] In that analysis, the incremental cost effectiveness ratio of the addition of bevacizumab 15 mg/kg once every three weeks to paclitaxel/carboplatin regimen was $632,571 per progression-free year and $792,380 per quality-adjusted progression-free year. Incorporation of quality of life scores resulted in a less favorable incremental cost effectiveness ratio.

Clinical **Controversy...**

Although bevacizumab has demonstrated some progression-free survival advantages when used in combination, its effect on overall survival is not clear. Therefore, it is not clear that the benefits justify the high cost of bevacizumab. As a result, health insurance companies do not consistently reimburse providers for bevacizumab when used for the treatment of ovarian cancer.

Poly(Adenosine Diphosphate [ADP]-Ribose) Polymerase Inhibitors

Poly(adenosine diphosphate [ADP]-ribose) polymerase (PARP) has a critical role in the repair of single strand DNA breaks via the base-excision repair pathway. Specifically PARP keeps the low-fidelity nonhomologous-end-joining DNA repair machinery functioning. PARP inhibition results in double stranded DNA breaks that cannot be repaired in cancer cells with homologous recombinant deficiency such as those with BRCA1/2 mutations. (10) The activity of the new class of the PARP inhibitors depends on BCRA status or "BRCA-ness" of the tumor.

In 2015, olaparib, the first PARP inhibitor was approved for treatment of recurrent, platinum sensitive BRCA1/2 positive ovarian cancer after failure of at least two prior treatments.[66] The recommended dose for olaparib is 400 mg twice a day with patient monitoring once a month. The common adverse effects associated with olaparib include nausea and vomiting and significant anemia with associated fatigue. Patients often require antiemetics and some require transfusion support. Three other PARP inhibitors, veliparib, rucaparib, and niraparib, are currently in phase II and III trials for treatment of BRCA1/2 positive platinum-sensitive ovarian cancer.[66-68] The challenge of combining PARP inhibitors with chemotherapy has been the significant hematological toxicity, primarily anemia, thrombocytopenia and neutropenia.

Other Targeted Agents

Tyrosine kinase inhibitors such as sorafenib, sunitinib, pazopanib, and cediranib inhibit angiogenesis by specifically targeting the VEGF receptor (VEGFR). When given as single agents, tyrosine kinase inhibitors have demonstrated some antitumor activity in ovarian cancer.[69,70] Ongoing trials have focused on combination regimens with cytotoxic agents for first-line treatment and also treatment of recurrent ovarian cancer. Another interesting targeted agent is VEGF Trap (aflibercept), a fusion protein that targets VEGF-A. Aflibercept has been beneficial in the treatment of malignant ascites and is currently being incorporated into first-line regimens. Epidermal growth factor receptor (EGFR) inhibitors such as erlotinib have not demonstrated activity either alone or combined with chemotherapy or bevacizumab for the treatment of ovarian cancer.[71] Newer classes of targeted therapies such as platelet-derived growth factor (PDGF) inhibitors are being investigated in ongoing clinical trials.[72]

PERSONALIZED PHARMACOTHERAPY

Current research efforts are focused on identifying biomarkers which are predictive of response in ovarian cancer. The primary focus has been on response to first-line treatment agents, paclitaxel and platinum and the multidrug resistance (MDR) pathway, specifically ABC-transport protein p-glycoprotein (Pgp).[73]

Epigenetics is a potential source of drug resistance. Epigenetic changes are heritable changes outside of the "traditional" DNA coding sequence. Aberrant DNA methylation and histone acetylation are epigenetic events which can silence tumor suppression genes required for apoptosis or DNA repair and therefore lead to resistance. The acetylation of histones is required for active genes and deacetylation occurs in silenced genes. Histone acetyltransferases (HATs) add acetyl groups and histone deacetylases (HDACs) remove acetyl groups.[74]

Ovarian cancers upregulate a variety of factors involved in DNA repair, angiogenesis, proliferation, and migration; they also downregulate mismatch-repair (MMR), cell adhesion, and apoptotic genes.[74] Tumorigenesis can induce hypermethylation or hypomethylation, which leads to chromosomal instability.[75] Hypermethylation or deacetylation has been shown to silence specific genes such as *hMLH1*, which leads to tumor formation and progression in the ovaries. Deacetylation of p21, a cell cycle regulator, can occur in ovarian carcinomas. Epigenetics may downregulate Apaf-1 and p16 while potentially upregulating MDR1. Finally, resistance to a platinum and taxane regimen may be associated with *hMLH1* methylation.[74]

Genomic information is being gathered to help overcome resistance such as finding amplified or deleted sequences or determining whether single nucleotide polymorphisms (SNPs) are the cause of resistance. Proteomics can also be used to identify mechanisms of resistance by finding over- or underexpressed proteins. These methods could lead to personalized pharmacotherapy if any of these biomarkers are predictive of drug response or resistance.[75]

While most chemotherapy drugs used to treat ovarian cancer are dosed according to body surface area (BSA), carboplatin dosing is personalized based on each individual's renal function with the Calvert formula: carboplatin dose = AUC × (glomerular filtration rate [GFR] + 25).[76] When it was originally developed and validated, measured GFR was used in the Calvert equation. However, the estimated creatinine clearance (CL_{CR}) is now used in clinical practice in place of measured GFR. Despite more than 30 years of clinical use, it is still not clear which equation to use to estimate CL_{CR} and the best method to estimate CL_{CR} in certain patient subgroups. The use of personalized carboplatin dose has reduced potential toxicity such as thrombocytopenia, neuropathy, and nephrotoxicity.[76] Personalized dosing of carboplatin is one of the reasons why it is often the preferred platinum agent over cisplatin for primary treatment for ovarian cancer.[32]

EVALUATION OF THERAPEUTIC OUTCOMES

During chemotherapy patients may experience numerous side effects such as nausea and vomiting, myelosuppression, neuropathy, and changes in organ function. Patients receiving a taxane or platinum chemotherapy regimen should be monitored for signs of hypersensitivity or infusion-related reactions. Patients treated with paclitaxel often experience infusion-related reactions, which have been attributed to the polyethoxylated castor oil (Cremophor) diluent. Premedications including an H_1-blocker, H_2-blocker, and steroid should be administered prior to each chemotherapy administration to prevent hypersensitivity reactions. If a patient has a reaction, increasing the duration of the infusion from 3 to 6 hours may help with infusion-related reactions. For patients with a true taxane allergy, paclitaxel desensitization can be attempted with 24 hours of premedications (H_1-blocker, H_2-blocker, and steroids) followed by paclitaxel given as a titrated infusion (1:1000 → 1:100 → 1:10 → full dose) over 8 hours. With repeated exposure (ie, seven cycles or more) to carboplatin, patients can develop a delayed hypersensitivity reaction. A similar protocol can be used for carboplatin desensitization.

Ovarian cancer patients receive multiple courses of chemotherapy that can have varying effects on kidney and liver function, often with a delayed onset. Appropriate laboratory tests should be ordered to assess organ function so that chemotherapy doses can be adjusted as indicated. Patients on platinum-containing regimens can often experience electrolyte wasting, so patients should be monitored for electrolyte replacement, IV or oral, as indicated. The use of myeloid growth factors should be considered to prevent treatment delays or dose reductions. Prevention of nausea and vomiting, both acute and delayed, is critical for patients receiving emetogenic chemotherapy regimens.

During initial taxane plus platinum chemotherapy, a CA-125 level should be obtained with each cycle and monitored for at least a 50% reduction in CA-125 after completion of four cycles, which is related to an improved prognosis. Patients who achieve a complete response after completion of first-line treatment should have follow-up once every 3 months, including CA-125, physical examination, pelvic examination, and appropriate diagnostic scans (ie, computed tomography, magnetic resonance imaging, or positron emission tomography), which should be evaluated for presence of disease. In addition to routine follow-up examinations, clinicians should monitor for resolution of any residual chemotherapy-related side effects, including neuropathies, nephrotoxicity, ototoxicity, myelosuppression, and nausea and vomiting.

In the progressive disease or recurrent setting, CA-125 levels can still be used to monitor for response and should be checked with each cycle, although no change in therapy is recommended until after completion of at least three cycles of the second-line chemotherapy. In addition to laboratory monitoring, appropriate diagnostic scans (ie, computed tomography, magnetic resonance imaging, or positron emission tomography) should be done once every three cycles. Patients need to be monitored with each cycle of chemotherapy to evaluate for new or persistent toxicities such as neuropathies, fluid retention, PPE, myelosuppression, and nausea and vomiting. Another precaution to keep in mind for patients with significant ascites, the "dry weight" or an adjusted body weight should be used for dosing chemotherapy.

Most patients with ovarian cancer will eventually progress through all chemotherapy regimens and investigational treatment options, after which the best supportive care measures should be provided to maintain patient comfort and quality of life. A plan to treat common complications of progressive ovarian cancer, including thrombosis, ascites, uncontrollable pain, and small bowel obstruction should be developed. This plan should include an opioid-based pain regimen with both long-acting agents and short-acting opioids for breakthrough or progressive pain; it should also include a bowel regimen to prevent opioid-induced constipation. Nausea can be a problem in women with advanced ovarian cancer when disease progression causes ascites or partial/complete bowel obstruction. Both antiemetic medications and non-pharmacotherapy interventions with nutrition and hydration can be helpful. Management of partial or complete small bowel obstruction focuses on controlling symptoms of pain and nausea. Bowel rest with best supportive care may lead to spontaneous resolution of the small bowel obstruction but most often it is a complication associated with rapidly progressive disease.[77] Palliative surgery may be considered in selected patients to relieve symptoms.

ABBREVIATIONS

AUC	area under the curve
BRCA1	breast cancer activator gene 1
BRCA2	breast cancer activator gene 2
BSA	body surface area
CA-125	cancer antigen 125
CI	confidence index
CL_{cr}	creatinine clearance
EGFR	epidermal growth factor receptor
FDA	Food and Drug Administration
FIGO	International Federation of Gynecology and Obstetrics
GFR	glomerular filtration rate
GI	gastrointestinal
GOG	Gynecologic Oncology Group
HAT	histone acetyltransferase
HDAC	histone deacetylase
HSCT	hematopoietic stem cell transplantation
ICON4	International Collaborative Ovarian Neoplasm 4
IP	intraperitoneal
MDR	multidrug resistance
MMR	mismatch-repair
NCCN	National Comprehensive Cancer Network
^{32}P	phosphorus-32
Pap	Papanicolaou
PARP	poly-ADP-ribose polymerase
PDGF	platelet-derived growth factor
Pgp	p-glycoprotein
PPE	palmar–plantar erythrodysesthesia
QOL	quality of life
SBO	small bowel obstruction
SCOTROC	Scottish Randomized Trial in Ovarian Cancer
SNP	single nucleotide polymorphism
SWOG	Southwest Oncology Group
TAH/BSO	total abdominal hysterectomy/bilateral salpingo oophorectomy
TVUS	transvaginal ultrasound
VEGF	vascular endothelial growth factor
VEGFR	vascular endothelial growth factor receptor

REFERENCES

1. Heintz APM, Odicino F, Maisonneuve P, et al. Carcinoma of the ovary. FIGO 6th annual report on the results of treatment in gynecological cancer. *Int J Gynaecol Obstet* 2006;95(Suppl):S161-S192.
2. Siegel R, Miller KD, Jemal A. Cancer statistics, 2016. *CA Cancer J Clin* 2016;66:7-30.
3. Bai H, Cao D, Yang J, et al. Genetic and epigenetic heterogeneity of epithelial ovarian cancer and the clinical implications for molecular targeted therapy. *J Cell Mol Med* 2016. DOI:10.1111/jcmm.12771.
4. RimMertens-Waler I, Baxter RC, Marsh DJ. Gonadotropin signaling in epithelial ovarian cancer. *Cancer Lett* 2012;324:152-159.
5. Permuth-Wey J, Sellers TA. Epidemiology of ovarian cancer. *Methods Mol Biol* 2009;472:413-437.
6. Sundar S, Neal RD, Kehoe S. Diagnosis of Ovarian Cancer. *BMJ* 2015;351:h4443.
7. Silverberg SG. Histopathologic grading of ovarian carcinoma: A review and proposal. *Int J Gynecol Pathol* 2000;19:7-15.
8. Longuespee R, Boyon C, Desmons A, et al. Ovarian cancer molecular pathology. *Cancer Metastat Rev* 2012;31:713-732.
9. Buys SS, Partridge E, Black A, et al. Effect of screening on ovarian cancer mortality: The prostate, lung, colorectal, and ovarian (PLCO) cancer screening randomized controlled trial. *JAMA* 2011;305: 2295-2303.
10. Moyer VA. U.S. Preventive Services Task Force. Screening for ovarian cancer: Recommendation statement. *Ann Intern Med* 2012;157:900-904.
11. Dann JL, Zorn KK. Strategies for ovarian cancer prevention. *Obstet Gynecol Clin North Am* 2007;34:667-686.
12. Harris RE, Beebe-Donk J, Doss H, et al. Aspirin, ibuprofen, and other non-steroidal anti-inflammatory drugs in cancer prevention: A critical review of non-selective COX-2 blockade. *Oncol Rep* 2005;13:559-583.
13. Hartmann LC, Lindo NM. The role of risk-reducing surgery in hereditary breast and ovarian cancer. *N Engl J Med* 2016;374(5): 454-468.
14. Narod SA, Sun P, Ghadirian P, et al. Tubal ligation and risk of ovarian cancer in carriers of *BRCA1* and *BRCA2* mutations: A case control study. *Lancet* 2001;357:1467-1470.

15. Goff BA, Mandel LS, Drescher CW, et al. Development of an ovarian cancer symptom index. *Cancer* 2007;109:221-227.
16. Syrios J, Banerjee S, Kaye SB. Advanced epithelial ovarian cancer: From standard chemotherapy to promising molecular pathway targets—where are we now? *Anticancer Res* 2014;34:2069-2078.
17. Armstrong DK, Bundy B, Wenzel L, et al. Intraperitoneal cisplatin and paclitaxel in ovarian cancer. *N Engl J Med* 2006;354:34-43.
18. Tewari D, Java JJ, Salani R, et al. Long-term survival advantage and prognostic factors associated with intraperitoneal chemotherapy treatment in advanced ovarian cancer: A gynecology oncology group study. *J Clin Oncol.* 2015 May 1;33(13):1460-6. doi: 10.1200/JCO. 2014.55.9898. Epub 2015 Mar 23.
19. Chang SJ, Bristow RE, Chi DS, Cliby WA. Role of aggressive surgical cytoreduction in advance ovarian cancer. *J Gynecol Oncol* 2015;26(4): 336-342.
20. Schorge JO, McCann C, Del Carmen M. Surgical debulking of ovarian cancer: What difference does it make? *Rev Obstet Gynecol* 2010;3:111-117.
21. Ibeanu OA, Bristow RW. Predicting the outcome of cytoreductive surgery for advanced ovarian cancer: A review. *Int J Gynecol Cancer* 2010;20(Suppl 1):S1-S11.
22. Mayer AR, Chambers SK, Graves E, et al. Ovarian cancer staging: Does it require a gynecologic oncologist? *Gynecol Oncol* 1992;47:223-227.
23. Nguyen HN, Averette HE, Hoskins W, et al. National survey of ovarian carcinoma, V: The impact of physician's specialty on patients' survival. *Cancer* 1993;72:3663-3670.
24. Martinek IE, Kehoe S. When should surgical cytoreduction in advanced ovarian cancer take place? *J Oncol* 2010;2010:8520-8528.
25. Lorusso D, Mancini M, Di Rocco R, Fontanelli R, Raspagliesi F. The role of secondary surgery in recurrent ovarian cancer. *Int J Surg Oncol* 2012;2012. DOI: 10.1155/2012/613980.
26. Bohra U. Recent advances in management of epithelial ovarian cancer. *Apollo Med* 2012;9:212-218.
27. McGuire WP, Hoskins WJ, Brady MF, et al. Cyclophosphamide and cisplatin compared with paclitaxel and cisplatin in patients with stage III and stage IV ovarian cancer. *N Engl J Med* 1996;334:1-6.
28. Piccart MJ, Bertelsen K, Stuart G, et al. Long-term follow-up confirms a survival advantage of the paclitaxel-cisplatin regimen over the cyclophosphamide-cisplatin combination in advanced ovarian cancer. *Int J Gynecol Cancer* 2003;13(Suppl 2):144-148.
29. Bookman MA, Greer BE, Ozols RF. Optimal therapy of advanced ovarian cancer: Carboplatin and paclitaxel vs. cisplatin and paclitaxel (GOG 158) and an update on GOG0 182-ICON5. *Int J Gynecol Cancer* 2003;136:735-740.
30. Ozols RF, Bundy BN, Green BE, et al. Phase III trial of carboplatin and paclitaxel compared with cisplatin and paclitaxel in patients with optimally resected stage III ovarian cancer: A Gynecologic Oncology Group Study. *J Clin Oncol* 2003;21:3194-3200.
31. du Bois A, Luck HJ, Meier W, et al. A randomized clinical trial of cisplatin/paclitaxel versus carboplatin/paclitaxel as first-line treatment of ovarian cancer. *J Natl Cancer Inst* 2003;95:1320-1329.
32. Neijt JP, Engelholm SA, Tuxen MK, et al. Exploratory phase III study of paclitaxel and cisplatin versus paclitaxel and carboplatin in advanced ovarian cancer. *J Clin Oncol* 2000;18:3084-3092.
33. Vasey PA, Jayson GC, Gordon A, et al. Phase III randomized trial of docetaxel-carboplatin versus paclitaxel-carboplatin as first-line chemotherapy for ovarian carcinoma. *J Natl Cancer Inst* 2004;96: 1682-1691.
34. Fennelly D, Aghajanian C, Shapiro F, et al. Phase I and pharmacologic study of paclitaxel administered weekly in patients with relapsed ovarian cancer. *J Clin Oncol* 1997;15:187-192.
35. Markman M, Blessing J, Rubin SC, et al. Phase II trial of weekly paclitaxel (80 mg/m^2) in platinum and paclitaxel-resistant ovarian and primary peritoneal cancers: A Gynecologic Group Study. *Gynecol Oncol* 2006;101:436-440.
36. Katsumata N, Yasuda M, Takahashi F, et al. Dose-dense paclitaxel once a week in combination with carboplatin every 3 weeks for advanced ovarian cancer: A phase 3, open-label, randomized controlled trial. *Lancet* 2009;374:1331-1338.
37. Fujiwara K, Armstrong D, Morgan M, Markman M. Principles and practice of intraperitoneal chemotherapy for ovarian cancer. *Int J Gynecol Cancer* 2007;17:1-20.
38. Jaaback K, Johnson N. Intraperitoneal chemotherapy for the initial management of primary epithelial ovarian cancer. *Cochrane Database Syst Rev* 2006;3:1-28.
39. Markman M, Bundy BN, Alberts DS, et al. Phase III trial of standard-dose intravenous cisplatin in small-volume stage III ovarian carcinoma: An intergroup study of the gynecologic oncology group, southwestern oncology group, and eastern cooperative oncology group. *J Clin Oncol* 2001;19:1001-1007.
40. Alberts DS, Liu PY, Hannigan EV, et al. Intraperitoneal cisplatin plus intravenous cyclophosphamide versus intravenous cisplatin plus intravenous cyclophosphamide for stage III ovarian cancer. *N Engl J Med* 1996;335:1950-1955.
41. Walker JL, Armstrong DK, Huang HQ, et al. Intraperitoneal catheter outcomes in a phase III trial of intravenous versus intraperitoneal chemotherapy in optimal stage III ovarian and primary peritoneal cancer: A Gynecologic Oncology Group Study. *Gynecol Oncol* 2006;100: 27-32.
42. National Comprehensive Cancer Network (NCCN) Practice Guidelines in Oncology—Ovarian Cancer, V2. 2015. Available at: http://www.nccn.org. Date accessed 1/9/2016.
43. Wright AA, Cronin A, Milne DE, et al. Use and effectiveness of intraperitoneal chemotherapy for treatment of ovarian cancer. *J Clin Oncol* 2015;33. 2015;33(26):2841-2847.
44. Seward SM, Winer I. Primary debulking surgery and neoadjuvant chemotherapy in the treatment of advanced epithelial ovarian carcinoma. *Cancer Metastasis Rev* 2015;34:5-10.
45. Markman M, Liu PY, Wilczynski S, et al. Phase III randomized trial of 12 versus 3 months of maintenance paclitaxel in patients with advanced ovarian cancer who attained a clinically-defined complete response to platinum/paclitaxel-based chemotherapy: A Southwest Oncology Group and Gynecology Oncology Group trial. *J Clin Oncol* 2003;21:2460-2465.
46. Markman M. Unresolved issues in the chemotherapeutic management of gynecologic malignancies. *Semin Oncol* 2006;33(Suppl 6):S33-S38.
47. ICON and AGO Collaborators. Paclitaxel plus platinum-based chemotherapy versus conventional platinum-based chemotherapy in women with relapsed ovarian cancer: The ICON4/AGO-OVAR-2.2 trial. *Lancet* 2003;361:2099-2106.
48. Bozas G, Bamias A, Koutsoukou, et al. Biweekly gemcitabine and cisplatin in platinum resistant/refractory, paclitaxel pre-treated, ovarian and peritoneal carcinoma. *Gynecol Oncol* 2007;104:580-585.
49. ten Bokkel Huinink W, Gore M, Carmichael J, et al. Topotecan versus paclitaxel for the treatment of recurrent epithelial ovarian cancer. *J Clin Oncol* 1997;15:2183-2193.
50. Creemers GJ, Bolis G, Gore M, et al. Topotecan, an active drug in the second-line treatment of epithelial ovarian cancer: Results of a large European phase II study. *J Clin Oncol* 1996;14:3056-3061.
51. Muggia FM, Hainsworth JD, Jeffers S, et al. Phase II study of liposomal doxorubicin in refractory ovarian cancer: Antitumor activity and toxicity modification by liposomal encapsulation. *J Clin Oncol* 1997;15: 987-993.
52. Gordon AN, Cranai CO, Rose PG, et al. Phase II study of liposomal doxorubicin in platinum- and paclitaxel refractory epithelial ovarian cancer. *J Clin Oncol* 2000;18:3093-3100.
53. Gordon AN, Fleagle JT, Guthrie D, et al. Recurrent epithelial ovarian carcinoma: A randomized phase III trial of pegylated liposomal doxorubicin versus topotecan. *J Clin Oncol* 2001;19:3312-3322.
54. Wilailk S, Linasmita V. A study of pegylated liposomal doxorubicin in platinum-refractory epithelial ovarian cancer. *Oncology* 2004;67: 183-186.
55. Drake RD, Lin WM, King M, et al. Oral dexamethasone attenuates Doxil-induced palmer-plantar erythrodysesthesias in patients with recurrent gynecologic malignancies. *Gynecol Oncol* 2004;94: 320-324.
56. Lund B, Hansen P, Theilade K, et al. Phase II study of gemcitabine (2′,2′-difluorodeoxycytidine) in previously treated ovarian cancer patients. *J Natl Cancer Inst* 1994;6:1530-1533.
57. Cannistra SA, Matulonis UA, Penson RT, et al. Phase II study of bevacizumab in patients with platinum-resistant ovarian cancer or peritoneal serous cancer. *J Clin Oncol* 2007;25:5180-5186.
58. Burger RA, Sill MW, Monk BJ, Greer BE, Sorvosky JI. Phase II trial of bevacizumab in persistent or recurrent epithelial ovarian cancer or primary peritoneal cancer: A gynecologic oncology group study. *J Clin Oncol* 2007;25:5165-5171.
59. Garcia AA, Hirte H, Fleming G, et al. Phase II clinical trial of bevacizumab and low-dose metronomic oral cyclophosphamide in recurrent ovarian cancer: A trial of the California, Chicago, and Princess Margaret Hospital phase II consortia. *J Clin Oncol* 2008;26: 76-82.
60. McGonigle KF, Muntz HG, Vuky J, et al. Combined weekly topotecan and biweekly bevacizumab in women with platinum-resistant ovarian, peritoneal, or fallopian tube cancer: Results of a phase 2 study. *Cancer* 2011;117:3731-3740.
61. Penson RT, Dizon DS, Cannistra SA, et al. Phase II study of carboplatin, paclitaxel, and bevacizumab with maintenance bevacizumab as first-line chemotherapy for advanced müllerian tumors. *J Clin Oncol* 2009;28:154-159.

62. Pujade-Lauraine E, Hilpert F, Weber F. Bevacizumab combined with chemotherapy for platinum resistant recurrent ovarian cancer: The AUREILIA open label randomized phase III trial. *J Clin Oncol* 2014;32.
63. Perren TJ, Swart AM, Pfisterer J. A phase 2 trial of bevacizumab in ovarian cancer. *N Engl J Med* 2011;365:2482-2496.
64. Burger RA, Brady MF, Bookman MA, et al. Incorporation of bevacizumab in the primary treatment of ovarian cancer. *N Engl J Med* 2011;365:2473-2483.
65. Cohn DE, Barnett JC, Wenzel L. A cost-utility analysis of NRG Oncology/Gynecologic Oncology Group Protocol 218: Incorporating prospectively collected quality-of-life scores in an economic model of treatment of ovarian cancer. *Gynecol Oncol* 2015;136:293-299.
66. Kaufman B, Shapirea R, Schmutzler RK, et al. Olaparib monotherapy in patients with advanced cancer and germline BRCA 1/2 mutation. *J Clin Oncol* 2014:244-250.
67. Matulonis UA. PARP Inhibitors: The first potential treatment of hereditary ovarian cancers. The ASCO Post 2015 Vol 6(9). Available at: http://www.ascopost.com/issues/may-25,-2015/parp-inhibitors-the-first-potential-treament-of-hereditary-ovarian-cancers.aspx accessed 12/10/2015.
68. Coleman RL, Sill MW, Bell-McGuinn K, et al. A phase II evaluation of the potent, highly selective PARP inhibitor veliparib in the treatment of persistent or recurrent epithelial ovarian cancer, fallopian tube, or primary peritoneal cancer in patients who carry a germline BRCA1 or BRCA2 mutation: An NRG Oncology/Gynecologic Oncology Group Study. *Gyencol Oncol* 2015;137:386-391.
69. Matulonis UA, Berlin S, Ivy P, et al. Cediranib, an inhibitor of vascular endothelial growth factor receptor kinases, in an active drug in recurrent epithelial ovarian, fallopian tube and peritoneal cancer. *J Clin Oncol* 2009;27:5601-5606.
70. Biagi JJ, Oza AM, Chalchal HI, et al. A phase II study of sunitinib in patients with recurrent epithelial ovarian and primary peritoneal carcinoma: An NCIC Clinical Trials Group Study. *Ann Oncol* 2011;22: 335-340.
71. Banerjee S, Kaye S. The role of targeted therapy in ovarian cancer. *Eur J Cancer* 2011;47(Suppl 3):S116-S130.
72. Marsh S, Paul J, King CR, Gifford G, McLeod H, Brown R. Pharmacogenetic assessment of toxicity and outcome after platinum plus taxane chemotherapy in ovarian cancer: The Scottish Randomized Trial in Ovarian Cancer. *J Clin Oncol* 2007;25:4528-4535.
73. Glasspool RM, Teodoridis JM, Brown R. Epigenetics as a mechanism driving polygenic clinical drug resistance. *Br J Cancer* 2006;94: 1087-1092.
74. Kanai Y. Alterations of DNA methylation and clinicopathological diversity of human cancers. *Pathol Int* 2008;58:544-558.
75. Schiavone MB, Bashir S, Herzog TJ. Biologic therapies and personalized medicine in gynecologic malignancies. *Obstet Gynecol Clin North Am* 2012;39:131-144.
76. Calvert AH, Newell DR, Gumbrell LA, et al. Carboplatin dosage: Prospective evaluation of a simple formula based on renal function. *J Clin Oncol* 1989;7:1748-1756.
77. Tuca A, Guell E, Martinez-Losada, Cordorniu N. Malignant bowel obstruction in advanced cancer patients: Epidemiology, management, and factors influencing spontaneous resolution. *Cancer Manag Res* 2012;4:159-169.

134

Acute Leukemias

Amy Hatfield Seung and Alix Dabb

KEY CONCEPTS

1. Acute leukemias are the most common malignancies in children and the leading cause of cancer-related death in patients younger than age 20 years.
2. Several risk factors correlate with prognosis for acute lymphoblastic leukemia (ALL). Poor prognostic factors include high white blood cell (WBC) count at presentation, very young or very old age at diagnosis, delayed remission induction and presence of certain cytogenetic abnormalities (eg, Philadelphia chromosome positive [Ph^+]).
3. For children with ALL, remission induction therapy includes vincristine, a corticosteroid, and asparaginase, with or without an anthracycline. For adults with ALL, vincristine, prednisone, and an anthracycline are given, and asparaginase is sometimes added.
4. All patients with ALL require prophylactic therapy to prevent CNS disease because of the high risk of central nervous system (CNS) relapse. The choice for therapy includes a combination of the following: cranial irradiation, intrathecal chemotherapy, or high-dose systemic chemotherapy with drugs that cross the blood-brain barrier.
5. Long-term maintenance therapy for 2 to 3 years is essential to eradicate residual leukemia cells and prolong the duration of remission. Maintenance therapy consists of oral methotrexate and mercaptopurine, with or without monthly pulses of vincristine and a corticosteroid.
6. Disease-free survival is lower in adults with ALL and has been attributed to greater drug resistance, poor side effect tolerance with subsequent nonadherence, and possibly less-effective therapy. This population is also more likely to have Ph^+ ALL, which is associated with a worse outcome, but the use of tyrosine kinase inhibitors has improved treatment results.
7. There are several poor prognostic factors for adult acute myeloid leukemia (AML): older age, organ impairment, presence of extramedullary disease, and presence of certain cytogenetic and molecular abnormalities.
8. Therapy of AML usually includes induction therapy with an anthracycline and cytarabine. Postremission therapy is required in all patients and can include either consolidation chemotherapy with or without maintenance therapy, or hematopoietic stem cell transplantation (HSCT).
9. Treatment of acute promyelocytic leukemia (APL) consists of induction therapy, followed by consolidation and maintenance therapy. Induction includes tretinoin and an anthracycline; consolidation therapy consists of two to three cycles of anthracycline-based therapy; maintenance consists of pulse doses of tretinoin, mercaptopurine, and methotrexate for 2 years.
10. Hematopoietic growth factors can be safely and effectively used with myelosuppressive chemotherapy for acute leukemias. The benefits may include reduced incidence of serious infections, reduced hospital stays, and fewer treatment delays, but do not include prolonged disease-free survival or overall survival (OS).

The leukemias are heterogeneous hematologic malignancies characterized by unregulated proliferation of the blood-forming cells in the bone marrow. These immature proliferating leukemia cells (blasts) physically "crowd out" or inhibit normal cellular maturation in bone marrow, resulting in anemia, granulocytopenia, including neutropenia, and thrombocytopenia. Leukemic blasts may also infiltrate a variety of tissues such as lymph nodes, skin, liver, spleen, kidney, testes, and the central nervous system (CNS).

Historically, leukemia has been classified based on the cell of origin and cell line maturation, and as acute or chronic based on differences in clinical presentation, rapidity of progression of the untreated disease, and response to therapy. The four major leukemias are acute lymphoblastic (or lymphocytic) leukemia (ALL), acute myeloid (or myelogenous) leukemia (AML), chronic lymphocytic leukemia, and chronic myeloid leukemia. Undifferentiated immature cells that proliferate autonomously characterize acute leukemias. Chronic leukemias also proliferate autonomously, but the cells are more differentiated and mature. Untreated, acute leukemia is fatal within weeks to months.

EPIDEMIOLOGY

It is estimated that 26,540 new cases of acute leukemia—19,950 cases of AML and 6,590 cases of ALL will be diagnosed in the United States in 2016, accounting for 1.57% of the total cancer incidence.[1] The incidence has been relatively stable for two decades. An estimated 11,860 deaths per year, representing about 2% of all cancer deaths, are caused by acute leukemias.[1]

1 Leukemia is the leading cause of cancer-related deaths in persons younger than age 20 years.[2] For males ages 20 to 39, it is now the leading cause of cancer death, but continues to be an uncommon cause of cancer-related death for both genders after age 40 years.[1] Among adults, acute and chronic leukemias occur at equal rates. More than 90% of the cases of acute and chronic leukemia occur in adults. AML accounts for most cases of acute leukemia in adults, and occurs with increasing frequency in elderly patients. There are about 4.5 cases of AML and 1.5 cases of ALL per 100,000 individuals.[2] The median age at diagnosis of patients with AML is about 67 years, while the peak age for ALL patients is 1 to 4 years.[2] The incidence of AML increases with age from 1.8 per 100,000 in individuals younger than age 65 years to 18.3 per 100,000 in those 65 years or older.[2] Acute leukemia is about 30% more common in males than in females. In the United States, acute leukemia is more common

among whites than among blacks, American Indians, and Hispanic ethnicities.[2]

Despite the low incidence, the acute leukemias are the most common malignancy in persons younger than 20 years of age, accounting for 27% of all childhood malignancies.[2] About 80% of children with leukemia have ALL and 15% AML.[2] Conversely, AML represents about 80% of acute leukemias in adults while only 20% of cases are ALL.[1] Childhood ALL is about 30% more common in males than in females, peaks at 1 to 4 years of age, and is almost twice as likely to affect white children as black children.[2] The incidence of childhood AML is highest in the Hispanic population and occurs throughout childhood without any peak age period. Acute leukemia during the first year of life (infant leukemia) slightly favors ALL over AML.[2] Antineoplastic agents including chemotherapy and targeted therapies have dramatically improved the outlook of patients with acute leukemia. More than 85% of children and young adults with acute leukemia achieve an initial complete remission (CR) of their disease. In comparison, 60% to 85% of adults who are 60 years of age or younger, and only 40% to 60% of patients who are older than 60 years of age achieve an initial CR.[3] For persons younger than 19 years of age, the 5-year survival rate is 90% for ALL and about 65% for AML.[2,4] The prognosis of adult acute leukemia is generally worse than that of childhood leukemia, with only 35% to 40% of patients who are 60 years of age or younger and 5% to 15% of patients who are older than 60 years of age becoming long-term survivors.[5]

ETIOLOGY

The exact cause of the acute leukemias is unknown. A multifactorial process involving genetics, environmental and socioeconomic factors, toxins, immunologic status, and viral exposures is likely. Table 134-1 summarizes the major factors that have been linked to acute leukemias. Infectious and genetic factors have the strongest associations to date.[6-8] In pediatric ALL, a number of environmental factors are inconsistently linked to the disease: exposure to ionizing radiation, toxic chemicals, herbicides and pesticides; maternal use of contraceptives, diethylstilbestrol, or cigarettes; parental exposure to drugs (amphetamines, diet pills, and mind-altering medications), diagnostic radiographs, alcohol consumption, coffee and cola consumption, or chemicals before and during pregnancy; and chemical contamination of groundwater.[9,10] A growing body of evidence indicates that high birthweight is a risk for ALL.[6,11] Ionizing radiation and benzene exposure are the only environmental risk factors strongly associated with ALL or AML.[7-9] A few studies have reported a possible link between electromagnetic fields of high-voltage power lines and the development of leukemia, but larger studies could not confirm this association. In most patients who develop leukemia, a cause cannot be identified.

Childhood AML is associated with Hispanic ethnicity, prior exposure to alkylating agents or epipodophyllotoxins, and in utero exposure to ionizing radiation.[9] Maternal alcohol consumption, maternal coffee and cola consumption, parental and child organophosphate pesticide exposure, and parental benzene exposure are also associated with childhood AML.[10] AML has been associated with both low and high birthweight.[11] Adult AML has been associated with prior anthracycline exposure in addition to prior exposure to alkylating agents or epipodophyllotoxins.[7]

TABLE 134-1 Factors Associated with the Development of Acute Leukemia

Drugs	**Chemicals**
Alkylating agents	Benzene
Anthracyclines	Pesticides
Epipodophyllotoxins	Pyrethroid-based shampoo
Genetic conditions	**Radiation**
Amegakaryocytic thrombocytopenia	Ionizing radiation
Ataxia telangiectasia	**Viruses**
Bloom syndrome	Epstein-Barr virus
Diamond-Blackfan anemia	Human T-lymphocyte virus (HTLV-1 and HTLV-2)
Down syndrome	
Dyskeratosis congenita	**Social habits**
Familial monosomy 7	Cigarette smoking
Fanconi anemia	Maternal marijuana use
Klinefelter syndrome	Maternal ethanol use
Kostmann syndrome	Maternal caffeine consumption
Langerhans cell histiocytosis	
Li Fraumeni syndrome	
Neurofibromatosis type 1	
Noonan syndrome	
Shwachman syndrome	
Severe combined immunodeficiency syndrome	
Wiskott-Aldrich syndrome	

PATHOPHYSIOLOGY

A basic understanding of normal hematopoiesis is needed before one can understand the pathogenesis of leukemia. Chapter e86 has a detailed discussion of hematopoiesis. Normal hematopoiesis consists of multiple well-orchestrated steps of cellular development. A pool of pluripotent stem cells undergoes differentiation, proliferation, and maturation, to form the mature blood cells seen in the peripheral circulation. These pluripotent stem cells initially differentiate to form two distinct stem cell pools. The myeloid stem cell gives rise to six types of blood cells (erythrocytes, platelets, monocytes, basophils, neutrophils, and eosinophils). Lymphoid stem cells differentiate to form natural killer cells, B lymphocytes, and T lymphocytes. Leukemia may develop at any stage and within any cell line.

Two features are common to both AML and ALL. First, both arise from a single leukemic cell that expands and acquires additional mutations, culminating in a monoclonal population of leukemia cells. Second, there is a failure to maintain a relative balance between proliferation and differentiation, so that the cells do not differentiate past a particular stage of hematopoiesis. Cells (lymphoblasts or myeloblasts) then proliferate uncontrollably. Proliferation, differentiation, and apoptosis are under genetic control, and leukemia can occur when the balance between these processes is altered.

Acute myeloid leukemia likely arises from a defect in the pluripotent stem cell or a more committed myeloid precursor, resulting in partial differentiation and proliferation of immature precursors of the myeloid blood-forming cells. In older patients, trilineage leukemia occurs suggesting that the cell of origin is probably a stem or very early progenitor cell. In younger patients, a more differentiated progenitor becomes malignant, allowing maturation of some granulocytic and erythroid populations. These two forms of AML exhibit different patterns of resistance to chemotherapy, with resistance more evident in the older adults with AML. ALL is a disease characterized by proliferation of immature lymphoblasts. In this type of acute leukemia, the defect is probably at the level of the lymphopoietic stem cell or a very early lymphoid precursor.

Leukemic cells have growth and/or survival advantages over normal cells, leading to a "crowding out" phenomenon in the bone marrow. This growth advantage is not caused by more rapid proliferation as compared with normal cells. Some studies suggest that it is caused by factors produced by leukemic cells that either inhibit normal cellular proliferation and differentiation, or reduce apoptosis as compared with normal blood cells.

The types of genetic alterations that lead to leukemia have only recently become evident. The genetic defects may include

(a) activation of a normally suppressed gene (protooncogene) to create an oncogene that produces a protein product that signals increased proliferation; (b) loss of signals for the blood cell to differentiate; (c) loss of tumor suppressor genes that control normal proliferation; and (d) loss of signals for apoptosis. Most normal cells are programmed to die eventually through apoptosis, but the appropriate programmed signal is often interrupted in cancer cells, leading to continued survival, replication, and drug resistance. Signal transduction, RNA transcription, cell-cycle control factors, cell differentiation, and programmed cell death may all be affected.

LEUKEMIA CLASSIFICATION

The World Health Organization (WHO), in collaboration with the Society for Hematopathology and the European Association of Haematopathology, published the current classification system for myeloid neoplasms in 2008 (Table 134-2).[12] This classification system incorporates not only morphologic findings, but also genetic, immunophenotypic, cytochemical, and clinical features. About 40% to 50% of adult patients with AML have no detectable chromosomal abnormality on standard cytogenetic analysis, but the percent increases with age.[13] The WHO classification attempts to formally incorporate the relationship between AML and myelodysplastic syndrome (MDS), and is being used routinely for children and adults.[12] The WHO classification defines acute leukemias as more than 19% blasts in the marrow or blood. A revision of the WHO classification for myeloid neoplasms is currently ongoing.[3]

Lymphoblast analysis is used to classify ALL. Immunophenotype is determined by flow cytometry that analyzes specific antigens, known as clusters of differentiation (often abbreviated "CD"), present on the surface of hematopoietic cells. Although no leukemia-specific antigens have been identified, the pattern of cell-surface antigen expression reliably distinguishes between lymphoid and myeloid leukemia. The immunophenotype defines the cell of origin. The major phenotypes are mature B-cell, precursor B-cell, and T-cell disease, but the WHO classifies ALL as either B lymphoblastic or T lymphoblastic. About 80% of childhood ALL derives from precursor B cells and about 15% from T cells; the remainder is either mixed lineage or from mature B cells. T-cell ALL is more common in teenage males. In adults, about 75% of ALL is B-cell lineage and 25% of cases are T-cell lineage ALL.

Leukemias may also be described by cytogenetic abnormalities. Chromosome alterations include numerical (hyperdiploidy and hypodiploidy), and structural abnormalities due to exchanges of genetic information within (inversion) or between (translocation) chromosomes. Unique translocations can identify specific subtypes of acute leukemia. Twenty-five percent of children with precursor B-cell ALL have the *ETV6-RUNX1* (formerly *TEL-AML1*) fusion gene generated by the t(12;21)(p13;q22) chromosomal translocation.[6,14] This translocation appears to endow the preleukemia cell with altered self-renewal and survival properties. The most common translocation in adult ALL, occurring in 25% of patients, is the t(9;22) or Philadelphia chromosome positive (Ph^+), which causes fusion of the BCR signaling protein to the ABL nonreceptor tyrosine kinase, resulting in constitutive tyrosine kinase activity. More than 50% of childhood T-cell ALL have activating mutations of the *NOTCH1* gene that encodes for a transmembrane receptor implicated in regulation of T-cell development.[6,14] Acute promyelocytic leukemia (APL) is characterized by a specific translocation between chromosomes 15 and 17: t(15;17). Molecular tests may be used to identify products of specific translocations, such as promyelocytic leukemia (PML) retinoic acid receptor-α (RARα) in APL and *AML1-ETO* and *CBFβ/MYH 11* in other subtypes of AML.

A number of factors may affect the cytogenetics of AML in adults. First, in about 5% of patients, simultaneous blood and marrow samples demonstrate normal cytogenetics versus abnormal cytogenetics, respectively.[15] Second, central cytogenetic analysis is done in multicenter trials because of variability in specimen examination. A small number of patients may have a normal karyotype on standard review, but carry fusion genes, which are identical to those of translocations or inversions. These insertions of very small chromosome segments do not alter chromosome morphology but may affect outcome.

TABLE 134-2 World Health Organization Classification of Acute Myeloid Leukemia

Acute myeloid leukemia (AML) with recurrent genetic abnormalities
AML with t(8;21)(q22;q22), (AML1/ETO)
AML with abnormal bone marrow eosinophils and inv(16)(p13;q22) or t(16;16)(p13;q22), (CBFβ/MYH11)
Acute promyelocytic leukemia with t(15;17)(q22;q12), (PML/RARα) and variants
AML with 11q23 (MLL) abnormalities
Acute myeloid leukemia with multilineage dysplasia
Following MDS or MDS/MPD disorder
Without antecedent MDS or MDS/MPD, but with dysplasia in at least 50% of cells or two or more lineages
Acute myeloid leukemia and MDS, therapy-related
Alkylating agent/radiation-related type
Topoisomerase II inhibitor-related type (some may be lymphoid)
Others
Acute myeloid leukemia, not otherwise categorized, classify as
Acute myeloid leukemia, minimally differentiated
Acute myeloid leukemia without maturation
Acute myeloid leukemia with maturation
Acute myelomonocytic leukemia
Acute monoblastic/acute monocytic leukemia
Acute erythroid leukemia (erythroid/myeloid and pure erythroleukemia)
Acute megakaryocytic leukemia
Acute basophilic leukemia
Acute panmyelosis with myelofibrosis
Myeloid sarcoma

MDS, myelodysplastic syndrome; MLL, mixed lineage leukemia; MPD, myeloproliferative disease; PML, promyelocytic leukemia; RARα, retinoic acid receptor-α.

CLINICAL PRESENTATION AND DIAGNOSIS

Common signs and symptoms at presentation result from malignant cells that replace and suppress normal hematopoietic progenitor cells and infiltrate into extramedullary spaces. Many of the signs and symptoms result from low blood cells. Thrombocytopenia can result in bruising, petechiae, and bleeding; low red blood cells can result in fatigue and loss of energy; and low white blood cells (WBCs) can result in signs and symptoms of infection such as fever, chills, and rigors. Patients with ALL may rarely present with small blue-green collections of leukemia cells under the skin called *chloromas*.

In addition to clinical presentation, laboratory and pathology evaluations are required for a definitive diagnosis of leukemia. An abnormal complete blood count is usually the diagnostic test that initiates a leukemia workup. Although leukemic blast cells may be present on the peripheral blood smear, they are not diagnostic of leukemia because there are other causes in which immature blast cells may be present in peripheral blood. The most important diagnostic test is a bone marrow biopsy and aspirate, which is submitted to hematopathology for numerous evaluations, including flow cytometry, cytogenetics, and immunophenotyping. A lumbar puncture is performed to determine if there are blasts in the CNS. A chest radiograph or computed tomography is performed to screen for a mediastinal mass (most common in T-cell disease). The results of these evaluations help to determine the patient's prognosis and therapeutic plan.

CLINICAL PRESENTATION

General

- Recent history of vague symptoms such as tiredness, lack of exercise tolerance, weight loss, and "feeling unwell," but in no obvious distress.

Signs and Symptoms

- Common: Patients with anemia present with pallor, malaise, palpitations, and fatigue. Patients with low platelet counts present with bruising, ecchymoses, and petechiae. Temperature is often elevated and may be caused by disease or infection. Patients may have bone pain from a hyperactive bone marrow.
- Other possible symptoms include epistaxis, dyspnea on exertion, seizures, or headache. Splenomegaly, hepatomegaly, and/or lymphadenopathy are common in patients presenting with ALL, but may also have painless testicular enlargement and rarely, small, blue-green collections of leukemia cells under the skin (chloromas). Patients with AML may present with gum hypertrophy and bleeding.

Laboratory Tests

- Complete blood count with differential. Anemia (43% <7 g/dL [<70 g/L; <4.34 mmol/L]) is normochromic and normocytic (without a compensatory increase in reticulocytes). Thrombocytopenia (severe, <20,000 cells/mm^3 [$<20 \times 10^9$/L]) is present in 28% of ALL and 50% of AML cases. Patients can present with leukopenia or leukocytosis; about 20% of patients will present with a WBC count ≥50,000 cells/mm^3 ($\geq 50 \times 10^9$/L) and 53% of ALL and 20% of AML cases with a WBC <10,000 cells/mm^3 ($<10 \times 10^9$/L). Even patients with elevated counts can be considered functionally neutropenic.
- Uric acid may be elevated because of rapid cellular turnover and is more common in patients presenting with elevated WBC count and with ALL.
- Electrolytes: potassium and phosphate may be elevated with a compensatory decrease in calcium, more common with ALL.
- Coagulation (more common with AML): elevated prothrombin time, partial thromboplastin time, D-dimers; hypofibrinogenemia.

Other Diagnostic Tests

- Bone marrow aspirate and biopsy: send for morphologic examination, cytochemical staining, immunophenotyping, and cytogenetic (chromosome) analysis. Molecular testing for FMS-like tyrosine kinase 3 (FLT3), nucleophosmin (NPM1), and CCAAT/enhancer binding-protein *α* (CEBPA), mutations is warranted for suspected AML.
- All children and adults with ALL should have a screening lumbar puncture performed to assess CNS involvement. Screening in patients with AML is not routine and depends on multiple factors at presentation including symptoms, WBC count, and morphology that includes monocytic disease.

ACUTE LYMPHOBLASTIC LEUKEMIA

Risk Classification

Many clinical and biologic features at diagnosis are associated with response to treatment, as measured by the CR rate, duration of remission, and long-term survival. The patient's response to initial therapy is also strongly associated with response to treatment. Identification of these risk factors allows the clinician to better understand the disease and to tailor treatment according to risk of disease recurrence (ie, risk-adapted therapy). For example, if a patient has many clinical and laboratory features that are associated with a favorable response to antineoplastic therapy ("standard risk"), then the clinician may choose to give less-intensive therapy to reduce the risk of long-term adverse effects. Conversely, if a patient is unlikely to respond well to standard therapy (high-risk or very-high-risk disease), then the clinician may choose to give more intensive antineoplastic therapy. The factors can be grouped as follows: patient characteristics at diagnosis, leukemic cell features at diagnosis, and patient response to initial therapy.

Patient Characteristics

2 The National Cancer Institute (NCI) developed an ALL risk stratification to create a standard for comparison in children.[16] Induction therapy is initially selected based on this classification, which divides children into standard- or high-risk categories based on age and initial WBC count (Table 134-3a). Age remains an independent predictor of outcome with children aged 1 to 9 years having the best event-free survival (EFS). This is partly explained by the more frequent occurrence of favorable cytogenetics in this age group.[17] The presence of CNS disease at diagnosis is associated with a higher relapse rate. About 2% of males have testicular disease at diagnosis, but not all cooperative groups classify it as an adverse prognostic factor. Patients with Down syndrome tend to have lower EFS, but this is mostly attributed to higher treatment-related morbidity and mortality.[18]

Race is controversial, with older studies indicating worse outcomes for minorities. Male race and obesity have been associated with worse outcome in cooperative group studies, but not in single-institution studies.[6] Hepatosplenomegaly and mediastinal mass are both associated with worse outcomes.

Leukemic Cell Characteristics

With current therapy, the cell of origin no longer has prognostic significance as therapy has improved. Several chromosomal (cytogenetic) abnormalities are associated with prognosis. Children with ALL have an average of six DNA copy number alterations.[14] Favorable

TABLE 134-3a National Cancer Institute (NCI) Risk Classification for Pediatric Acute Lymphoblastic Leukemia

Risk Group	Standard Risk	High Risk
Age (years)	1- <10	<1 or ≥10
WBC count ($\times 10^3$ cells/mm^3 or $\times 10^9$/L)	<50	≥50
Karyotype	No t(9;22) or t(4;11)	t(9;22) or t(4;11)

WBC, white blood cell.

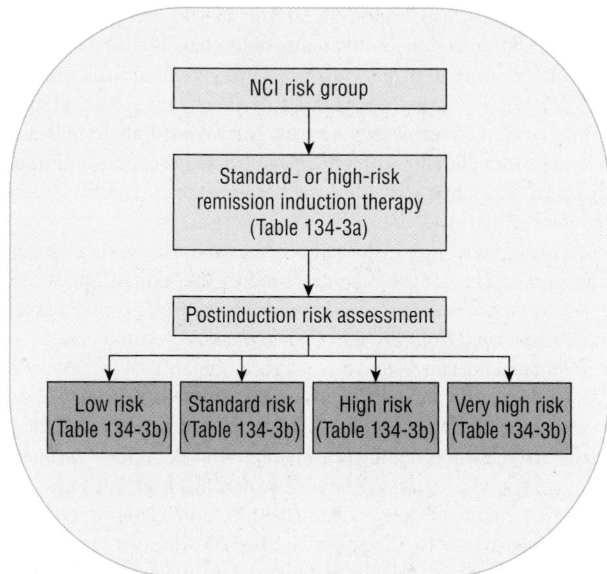

FIGURE 134-1 Pediatric precursor B-cell acute lymphoblastic leukemia risk classification. (NCI, National Cancer Institute.)

outcomes are associated with three copies of chromosomes 4 and 10, high hyperdiploidy (51-65 chromosomes), and the *ETV6-RUNX1* cryptic translocation, t(12;21).[14] *NOTCH1* and *FBXW7* mutations confer a favorable prognosis for patients with T-cell disease.[14] The Philadelphia chromosome is present in 3% to 5% of children and 25% of adults and is historically associated with a poor prognosis.[19] The mixed lineage leukemia (*MLL*) gene rearrangement (11q23), intrachromosomal amplification of chromosome 21 ($iAMP_{21}$), and hypodiploidy (less than 44 chromosomes) are associated with a poorer prognosis.[20]

Initial Response to Therapy

The strongest prognostic factor for outcome for ALL is response to therapy.[21] Both the rapidity of response and the level of residual disease at the end of induction therapy are associated with long-term outcome. Children with a reduction of bone marrow lymphoblasts within 14 days of initiating antineoplastic therapy (rapid early responders) have a more favorable prognosis. Molecular measurement of subclinical minimal residual disease (MRD) by either flow cytometry or polymerase chain reaction has enabled detection of leukemic cells not visible on morphologic examination to assess treatment response and detect relapse in children and adults.[22] This technique allows detection of 1 leukemia cell in 10,000 normal cells, which is about 100-fold more sensitive than morphologic examination.[22] If MRD is detected at the end of induction therapy, the clinician may decide to give more intensive therapy to decrease the risk of relapse.

The Children's Oncology Group uses a risk- and response-based classification of childhood ALL (Fig. 134-1).[23] This classification system uses the NCI risk assignment to initially categorize patients into standard- or high-risk groups (see Table 134-3a). Following induction therapy, risk is reclassified based on the rapidity and completeness of response to therapy, the presence or absence of cytogenetic abnormalities, and CNS involvement (Table 134-3b). Patients are then reclassified as low risk, standard risk, high risk, or very-high risk (see Fig. 134-1). Patients who are initially high risk do not have therapy reduced, but may have it intensified to very-high risk as discussed here.

Children are classified as low risk and will have therapy reduced if they have trisomy 4 and 10 or the *ETV6-RUNX1* cryptic translocation with less than 0.01% MRD on day 8 peripheral blood and day 29 bone marrow samples. Children with testicular disease, more than 5% blasts in the bone marrow by day 15, MRD greater than or equal to 0.01% at day 29, or who received steroids prior to diagnosis have postinduction therapy intensified and are classified as high risk. Childhood precursor B-ALL with more than five WBCs and blasts present in the cerebrospinal fluid (CSF), Ph^+ disease, hypodiploidy, $iAMP_{21}$, induction failure, or *MLL* gene rearrangement have therapy intensified and are considered very-high risk. Infant ALL, trisomy 21, or childhood T-cell ALL have unique risk classification schemas. Children with T-cell leukemia historically have an inferior response to standard-risk therapy and are automatically categorized as high risk to receive augmented therapy and T-cell targeted therapy. T-cell and mature B-cell disease are favorable phenotypes in adults.[6] Age is inversely associated with prognosis in patients with Ph^+ ALL.[6]

TREATMENT

Acute Lymphoblastic Leukemia

Desired Outcomes

The short-term goal for ALL treatment is to rapidly achieve a complete clinical and hematologic remission. A CR is defined as the disappearance of all physical and bone marrow evidence (normal cellularity with less than 5% blasts) of leukemia, with restoration of normal hematopoiesis. After a CR is achieved, the goal is to maintain the patient in continuous CR. In general, a child is considered "cured" after being in continuous CR for 5 years.

Successful treatment of ALL was first developed in children. Cure rates in children have risen from less than 10% with treatments used in the 1960s to current rates of about 90.[21] The reason for this improvement lies largely in improved scheduling of existing drugs, as relatively few new drugs have come to the market since the 1960s. Current regimens result in clinical remission in 96% to 99% of children with ALL at the end of induction.[6] MRD is a strong predictor of relapse in ALL. Children with MRD in the bone marrow at the end of induction have a 5-year EFS of 59% versus 88% in children without MRD.[24] Children with low-risk disease have a 5-year EFS of more than 95%.[25] The 5-year EFS for average-risk disease is 90% to 95%.[25] The 5-year EFS is nearly 90% for high-risk childhood

TABLE 134-3b Pediatric Precursor B-Cell Acute Lymphoblastic Leukemia Risk Classification

	Low	Standard			High		Very High			
NCI Risk[a]	SR	SR	SR	SR	SR	HR (age <13 y)	SR	HR	HR (age >13 y)	Any
Favorable Genetics	Yes	Yes	No	Yes	No	Any	No	Any	Any	Any
Unfavorable Characteristics	None	None	None	None	None	None	None	None	None	Yes
Day 8 PB MRD	<0.01%	≥0.01%	<1%	Any	≥1%	Any	Any	Any	Any	Any
Day 29 Marrow MRD	<0.01%	<0.01%	<0.01%	>0.01%	<0.01%	<0.01%	>0.01%	>0.01%	<0.01%	Any

HR, high-risk; MRD, minimal residual disease; NCI, National Cancer Institute; PB, peripheral blood; SR, standard-risk.

[a]See Table 134-3a for criteria used to categorize patients into risk categories.

B-precursor and T-cell ALL including rapid and slow responders. Children with very-high-risk disease have a 5-year EFS of less than 80%.[25] Response to treatment is determined by intrinsic drug sensitivity and the patient's pharmacogenomics and pharmacodynamics, treatment received, and treatment adherence.

Although treatment results with adult ALL are worse than those with childhood ALL, recent use of aggressive chemotherapy in adult ALL has increased the initial CR rate after induction therapy from 60% to 85%. Long-term EFS in this population, however, remains low (between 30% and 40%) because a higher proportion of adults present with poor-risk disease. CR rates and EFS vary according to a number of poor prognostic factors and certain types of ALL are associated with a very poor outcome.

Treatment Phases

Therapy for childhood ALL is divided into five phases: (a) induction, (b) consolidation therapy, (c) delayed intensification, (d) interim maintenance, and (e) maintenance therapy (Fig. 134-2). CNS prophylaxis is a mandatory component of ALL treatment regimens and is administered longitudinally during all phases of treatment. The total duration of treatment is 2 to 3 years.

Induction

3 The goal of induction is to rapidly induce a complete clinical and hematologic remission. The CR rate is about 98% for standard-risk children treated with vincristine, a glucocorticoid (dexamethasone or prednisone), and pegaspargase.[21] Many treatment protocols include daunorubicin in induction (four-drug induction) for high-risk or very-high-risk ALL. Most children achieve a CR in 4 weeks, which classifies them as rapid early responders. Those who have an M2 (5%-25% blasts) or M3 (more than 25% blasts) marrow on day 15 of induction or have positive MRD at day 29 are classified as slow early responders and receive intensified therapy. Only 2% to 3% of children fail induction therapy and have a 10-year survival rate of 32%.[26]

Prednisone has historically been the primary glucocorticoid used in pediatric ALL regimens.[27] Dexamethasone is now being used in most standard-risk protocols because of its longer duration of action and higher CSF penetration compared to prednisone.[27] When dexamethasone is used in place of prednisone, absolute EFS improves by 5% to 9% and the risk of CNS relapse decreases by 2% to 4%.[27,28] However, dexamethasone increases the risk of side effects such as osteonecrosis, mood alteration, steroid myopathy, hyperglycemia, and infections.[27-29] Patients older than 10 years of age are particularly prone to osteonecrosis and receive prednisone instead of dexamethasone to minimize this side effect. Low serum albumin prolongs dexamethasone exposure and may contribute to increased toxicity.[27] Since patients with Down syndrome have increased infections and mortality with dexamethasone, these patients receive prednisone.[18]

Asparaginase has historically been available in three forms. Asparaginase (no longer manufactured in the United States) and pegaspargase are isolated from *Escherichia coli* while *Erwinia* asparaginase is isolated from *Erwinia chrysanthemi*. A recombinant *E. coli* asparaginase and a pegylated form of recombinant *Erwinia* asparaginase are currently in clinical trials. Pegaspargase is pegylated *E. coli* asparaginase; pegylation prolongs its duration of activity and allows it to be given less frequently. Pegaspargase is used in most protocols and is preferred over asparaginase because of fewer intramuscular injections, decreased antibody formation, and superior response rates. Pegaspargase is also approved for IV administration.[30] The use of prolonged intensive asparaginase treatment compared with shorter treatment increases absolute EFS by 4% to 17%.[31]

Asparaginase products are the antineoplastic agents used in ALL which are most likely to cause hypersensitivity reactions. Depending on the type of asparaginase used and the presence of a coadministered steroid, 8% to 42% of patients may develop hypersensitivity reactions to asparaginase.[32,33] Reactions usually occur during postinduction phases of therapy when asparaginase has not been given for a prolonged period of time.[31] Hypersensitivity reactions to pegaspargase may be delayed in onset (when administered intramuscularly) and prolonged in duration, sometimes requiring hospitalization.[34] *Erwinia* asparaginase is currently only used for patients who are allergic to pegaspargase. Because *Erwinia* asparginase has a short half-life, administration must occur more frequently. A single dose of pegaspargase is replaced by six doses of *Erwinia* asparaginase, given three times per week.[33]

Patients may develop silent inactivation, also known as subclinical hypersensitivity, in which they develop neutralizing antibodies that can rapidly inactivate asparaginase, but without developing a clinical hypersensitivity reaction. Silent inactivation can be detected by therapeutic monitoring of asparaginase activity. If inadequate asparaginase activity is detected, a therapeutic switch from pegaspargase to *Erwinia* asparaginase can be made to optimize activity and outcomes.[35,36] The use of therapeutic drug monitoring to optimize the dosing of asparaginase has also been demonstrated in clinical trials.[37]

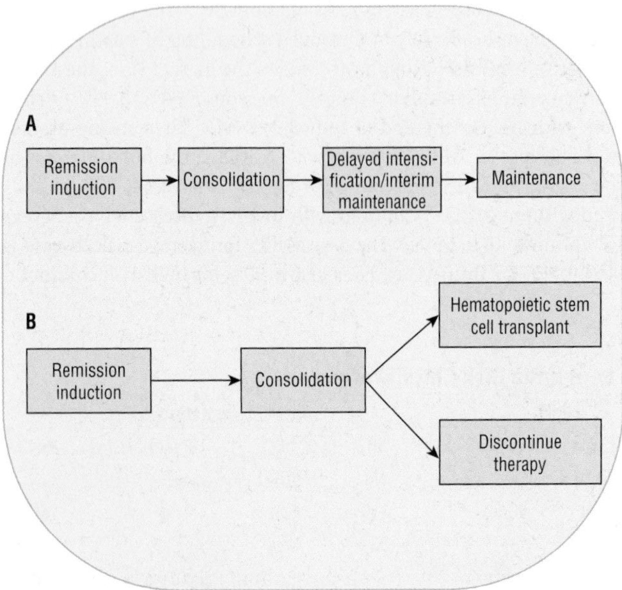

FIGURE 134-2 Treatment algorithm for (*A*) acute lymphoblastic leukemia and (*B*) acute myeloid leukemia.

Clinical **Controversy...**

Should therapeutic drug monitoring of asparaginase products be used routinely? With the recent addition of a commercially available asparaginase activity assay, clinicians have the opportunity to use this tool to monitor and optimize asparaginase therapy. Although published data support the use of therapeutic drug monitoring of asparaginase products to optimize pharmacokinetic differences in preparations and detect suboptimal activity levels, this approach is not routinely used. Clinical trials are needed to determine the role for routine therapeutic drug monitoring of asparaginase and any potential impact that this has on outcomes.

Central Nervous System Prophylaxis

Central nervous system prophylaxis is incorporated throughout all phases of therapy. The rationale for CNS prophylaxis is based on two observations. First, many antineoplastic agents do not readily cross the blood-brain barrier. Second, results from early clinical trials of ALL showed that the majority of patients with ALL experienced a CNS relapse.[21] These observations indicate that the CNS is a potential sanctuary for leukemic cells and undetectable leukemic cells are present in the CNS in many patients at the time of diagnosis, while only 3% of children have detectable CNS involvement at diagnosis.[17]

The goal of CNS prophylaxis is to eradicate undetectable leukemic cells from the CNS while minimizing neurotoxicity and late effects. Once CNS relapse has occurred, patients are at increased risk of bone marrow relapse and death from refractory leukemia. Initial trials of childhood ALL in the 1960s established craniospinal irradiation as the standard for prevention of CNS relapse. However, this approach is associated with long-term sequelae including neuropsychological deficits, precocious puberty, osteoporosis, decreased intellect, thyroid dysfunction, brain tumors, short stature, and obesity. Subsequent trials have demonstrated that irradiation may be replaced by frequent administration of intrathecal chemotherapy in children with ALL.[38] Some centers may treat children with CNS disease at diagnosis or very-high-risk disease with cranial radiation.[21]

4 The CNS prophylaxis regimen is selected based on efficacy, toxicity, and risk of CNS disease. Intrathecal chemotherapy, cranial irradiation, dexamethasone, and high-dose IV methotrexate or cytarabine can be used to treat or prevent CNS disease. Current treatment approaches have reduced isolated CNS relapses to less than 5% among children.[39] Risk factors for CNS relapse include male sex, hepatomegaly, T-cell phenotype, CNS2 disease (the presence of leukemic blasts in a CSF sample that contains less than 5 WBC/mm^3 [less than 5×10^6/L]), age younger than 2 years or older than 6 years, and a bloody diagnostic lumbar puncture.[6,39] Intrathecal therapy consists of methotrexate and cytarabine, given either alone or in combination. When given together, hydrocortisone is commonly added (triple intrathecal therapy) to decrease the incidence of arachnoiditis. Triple intrathecal therapy is typically reserved for children with refractory CNS disease. For standard-risk ALL, triple intrathecal therapy decreased CNS relapse rates by 30% in comparison to intrathecal methotrexate but had no effect on EFS and worsened overall survival (OS).[39] The doses of intrathecal chemotherapy used for childhood ALL are age-based because of differences in the volume of CSF at various ages. For example, intrathecal methotrexate is dosed as 8 mg if less than 2 years, 10 mg for 2 to 2.99 years, 12 mg for 3 to 8.99 years, and 15 mg for more than or equal to 9 years. Liposomal cytarabine given intrathecally induces CNS remission in 57% of relapsed patients, but is associated with a high incidence of arachnoiditis and other CNS-related adverse effects.[40] Currently its use is limited to refractory or relapsed CNS disease in children.

Patients with T-cell leukemia have an increased incidence of CNS disease and usually receive systemic therapy that penetrates the CNS such as high-dose methotrexate. A WBC count greater than 100,000 cells/mm^3 (100×10^9/L) is associated with an increased risk of CNS relapse.[6] Patients with T-cell disease have lower methotrexate polyglutamate accumulation in leukemic blasts and therefore require higher doses of infusional methotrexate (5 g/m^2 compared to 1 g/m^2).[41] Patients with T-cell leukemia may require prophylactic or therapeutic CNS irradiation.[38]

Consolidation Therapy

Consolidation therapy in ALL is started after a CR has been achieved, and refers to continued intensive antineoplastic therapy in an attempt to eradicate clinically undetectable disease in order to secure (consolidate) the remission. Regimens usually incorporate either non–cross-resistant drugs that are different from the induction regimen, or more dose-intensive use of the same drugs.

Randomized trials show that consolidation therapy clearly improves patient outcome in children, but its benefit in adults is less clear.[42] The relative benefit of individual components of treatment regimens is difficult to demonstrate because of the overall complexity of therapy in ALL. Standard consolidation lasts 4 weeks and usually consists of vincristine, mercaptopurine, and intrathecal methotrexate. In children, the intensity of consolidation therapy is based on the child's initial risk classification and response to induction therapy. Children who are slow early responders during induction or have high-risk disease benefit from intensified consolidation that includes the addition of pegaspargase, cyclophosphamide, and low-dose cytarabine to standard therapy.[43] Children with testicular disease usually receive radiation during this phase of therapy if a complete clinical response in the testes is not achieved by the end of induction. Patients with T-cell leukemia also receive nelarabine, a prodrug of ara-G that preferentially accumulates in T lymphoblasts as ara-guanosine triphosphate (GTP), during consolidation and throughout the remainder of their treatment course given the improved EFS when it is added to an intensified therapeutic backbone.[44]

Reinduction (Delayed Intensification and Interim Maintenance)

One or two delayed intensification phases separated by low-intensity interim maintenance cycles can be added to maintain remission and to decrease cumulative toxicity. Delayed intensification usually consists of drugs used during induction and consolidation or agents that lack cross-resistance with those already received such as cyclophosphamide, methotrexate, and limited amounts of doxorubicin. The methotrexate dose is variable; standard-risk children usually receive 1 to 2 g/m^2 while those with T-cell disease usually receive a higher dosage (5 g/m^2). Interim maintenance usually consists of dexamethasone, vincristine, weekly methotrexate, mercaptopurine, and intrathecal methotrexate. Delayed intensification improves EFS for standard-risk children.[41,43] Delayed intensification with dose intensification improved EFS and decreased late relapses for high-risk childhood ALL, but there was no additional benefit for two delayed intensification cycles.[43] Children on the intensified arms of the study received significantly more antimicrobial drugs, blood products, and parenteral nutrition but had no increase in treatment-related mortality.[43] The antimetabolite-based regimens may have a reduced risk of late toxicities, but the more intensive regimens appear to result in better survival for some patients, especially those with higher risk disease.

Maintenance Therapy

5 Maintenance therapy allows long-term drug exposure to slowly dividing cells, allows the immune system time to eradicate leukemia cells, and promotes apoptosis (programmed cell death). The goal of maintenance therapy is to further eradicate residual leukemic cells and prolong remission duration. Although maintenance therapy is clearly beneficial in childhood ALL, the benefit in adults has only recently been demonstrated.

Maintenance therapy usually consists of daily mercaptopurine and weekly methotrexate for 12-week courses, at doses that produce relatively little myelosuppression, with monthly "pulses" of vincristine and a steroid.[45,46] Based on the results of studies that show a trend toward an increase in late relapse (excluding isolated testicular relapse) among male children treated for 2 years versus 3 years, some centers treat female children for 2 years while males receive maintenance for a total of 3 years of therapy.[17]

Interpatient variability in the pharmacokinetics of oral methotrexate and mercaptopurine may also be an important determinant of the effectiveness and toxicity of maintenance therapy. It is recommended that mercaptopurine be administered in the evening rather than in morning based on data demonstrating improved outcomes.[47]

Mercaptopurine cannot be given with milk or milk products because of the presence of xanthine oxidase. Children with an adherence rate less than 95% with mercaptopurine have a 2.7-fold higher risk of suffering a relapse.[48] Factors associated with nonadherence include single-parent household, adolescence, lower socioeconomic status, and Hispanic ethnicity.[49] To account for the interpatient variability, most clinicians will titrate the dose of these agents to achieve adequate myelosuppression.[17] Some protocols overcome bioavailability and poor adherence issues by administering methotrexate IV or intramuscularly. The importance of these pharmacokinetic issues in adults is not well defined.

Philadelphia Chromosome Positive Acute Lymphoblastic Leukemia

Ph⁺ ALL has historically been treated as very-high-risk disease.[19] This includes the use of a four-drug induction regimen with the addition of continuous imatinib mesylate, a signal transduction inhibitor that inhibits *BCR-ABL* kinase, throughout all phases of treatment. This targeted therapeutic approach has resulted in a 3-year EFS of 80% in comparison to 35% for historical controls.[50] The results for patients receiving chemotherapy with imatinib were equivalent to those receiving hematopoietic stem cell transplantation (HSCT). Imatinib is currently incorporated into childhood treatment trials for Ph⁺ ALL in Europe and the United States. Trials are ongoing with the more potent second generation tyrosine kinase inhibitors, nilotinib and dasatinib, and with ponatinib, which is effective in imatinib-resistant leukemia.[51]

Acute Lymphoblastic Leukemia in Infants

Acute lymphoblastic leukemia and AML in infants younger than 1 year of age account for less than 5% of the reported acute leukemias in childhood, but they are associated with poor outcomes. About 70% to 80% of infants with acute leukemia have t(4;11) involving the *MLL* gene, which is associated with worse outcomes.[52] Infants with ALL are more likely to present with a high WBC count, hepatosplenomegaly, and CNS disease. Age younger than 6 months at diagnosis and poor response to prednisone alone given prior to starting other agents are poor prognostic indicators. Infants with *MLL* gene rearrangements are more likely to overexpress FLT3, a tyrosine kinase implicated in leukemogenesis that is associated with a poor prognosis. Current trials are testing the efficacy of FLT3 inhibitors in infants with *MLL* gene rearrangements.[52] Lack of pharmacokinetic data for antineoplastic agents in infants has contributed to toxicity from potential inaccurate dosing of doxorubicin and vincristine. The use of allogeneic HSCT for infants with ALL remains controversial because of a lack of donors, concerns over the long-term toxicity of total body irradiation, excessive mortality in some series, and differing outcomes.[53,54]

Acute Lymphoblastic Leukemia in Down Syndrome

Children with Down syndrome have a markedly increased risk of developing ALL.[55] The clinical presentation of ALL in Down syndrome patients is similar to patients without Down syndrome but there is a lower incidence of high-risk features including T-cell disease, CNS involvement, hepatosplenomegaly, and cytogenetic abnormalities.[18] Therapy for ALL in Down syndrome patients is similar to that of non-Down syndrome patients, with the caveat that anthracycline exposure is limited and methotrexate dosing is reduced and supported with aggressive leucovorin rescue.[18] Children with Down syndrome and ALL have an increased risk of relapse and treatment-related mortality resulting in a decreased OS rate when compared to non-Down syndrome patients with ALL.[56]

Acute Lymphoblastic Leukemia in Adolescents and Young Adults

Although ALL is relatively uncommon in adolescents and young adults (AYA) (15-39 years old), the outcomes are generally worse than for childhood ALL.[57] ALL in AYA has a higher frequency of T-cell immunophenotype and a lower frequency of the t(12;21)(p13;q22) cryptic translocation responsible for hyperdiploidy and the *ETV6-RUNX1* fusion gene; about 5% to 7% of ALL in AYA have Ph⁺ disease (higher than children, but lower than older adults).[14,58] A retrospective comparison of 16- to 20-year-old patients treated on pediatric versus adult protocols in the United States resulted in identical CR rates, but the 7-year EFS favored the patients treated on pediatric regimens (64% vs 34%).[58] Patients treated on the pediatric regimens also had a 10% lower CNS relapse rate. The adult regimens studied were more myelosuppressive due to the use of anthracyclines, cyclophosphamide, and cytarabine, while the pediatric regimens intensified steroids, vincristine, and asparaginase and included aggressive CNS-directed therapy and maintenance therapy. The adult regimens had a higher risk of late effects due to higher doses of daunorubicin and use of cyclophosphamide. A current adult intergroup study is using a pediatric regimen for AYA patients and will be able to evaluate some of the other potential reasons for the outcome disparity, such as adherence and psychosocial differences. AYA patients may receive treatment based on an adult or pediatric regimen depending on institutional preferences, but the trend is shifting toward pediatric regimens.

Acute Lymphoblastic Leukemia in Adults

6 Treatment risk stratification for adult patients differs depending on age and Philadelphia chromosome status. The National Comprehensive Cancer Network (NCCN) guidelines recommend different strategies for AYA, adults 40 to 65, and adults older than 65 years with or without poor performance status.[59] While CR is achieved in 70% to 90% of adults with a four-drug induction regimen containing daunorubicin or doxorubicin, vincristine, an asparaginase formulation, and prednisone, long-term EFS is considerably lower and achieved in only 20% to 40% of patients.[60] Poorer outcomes in adults have been attributed to differences in cytogenetic abnormalities, greater drug resistance, higher risk of treatment-related adverse effects with subsequent nonadherence, and possibly less effective therapy. The value of adding more agents to the basic four-drug induction regimen or higher doses of drugs in the remission induction regimen is not clear. Several different regimens are considered appropriate to use as first-line therapies in adults including the Cancer and Leukemia Group B (CALGB) 8,811 (Larson regimen), Eastern Cooperative Oncology Group (ECOG) 2,993, or Linker regimen.[61] Some studies suggest that high-dose methotrexate and cytarabine alternating with fractionated cyclophosphamide plus vincristine, doxorubicin, and dexamethasone (hyperCVAD) may improve response and survival in adults with ALL.[61] A considerable number of ALL cases occur in patients older than age 65 years, and treatment of this group of patients is an even greater challenge. The response to therapy and durability of response is less than in all other populations. Treatment-related mortality rates during remission induction therapy are also higher in this population.

While the overall incidence of Ph⁺ positive disease is 25% in adults, the incidence rises with increasing age to over 40% in adults older than the age of 50 years.[62] Traditionally, treatment outcomes for patients with Ph⁺ ALL has been extremely poor with reported OS rates of less than 20% and a 2-year OS of 40% to 50% for those continuing to allogeneic HSCT. As compared with historical control patients treated with standard chemotherapy alone, the addition of *BCR-ABL* tyrosine kinase therapy to chemotherapy is associated with an increased CR and OS.[63,64] No randomized trials have compared imatinib or dasatinib and conventional chemotherapy versus conventional chemotherapy alone. The CR rates seen with tyrosine kinase inhibitors appear to be more durable and allow more patients with Ph+ disease to proceed to allogeneic HSCT. This approach also appears to be tolerated in elderly patients.[65] For patients older than 65 years of age or for those with a poor performance status, induction regimens may include concurrent chemotherapy with a tyrosine kinase inhibitor, either alone or combined with corticosteroids. Based on these data, the combination of imatinib or dasatinib with concurrent chemotherapy is currently considered as the standard of care for first-line therapy.

Other *BCR-ABL* tyrosine kinase inhibitors, nilotinib, bosutinib, and ponatinib, have also been evaluated in patients with imatinib-resistant Ph+ leukemias.[61] Responses may be achieved, and they are treatment options in patients with relapsed or refractory Ph+ ALL. A primary concern with the *BCR-ABL* tyrosine kinase inhibitors is the emergence of resistance, specifically T315I mutations. Ponatinib is the only *BCR-ABL* tyrosine kinase inhibitor available in the United States with known activity against T315I mutations.[66] A patient's specific mutation analysis should be considered in the selection of a specific tyrosine kinase inhibitor in the relapsed or refractory setting.

In adults with B-cell ALL, about 50% have leukemic cells that express CD20. CD20 expression has been associated with decreased CR rates, higher risk of relapse, and shorter OS.[67,68] A phase II study has evaluated hyperCVAD and rituximab versus hyperCVAD alone and reported a higher CR rate (70% vs 38%) and longer OS (75% vs 47%) in patients treated with hyperCVAD and rituximab.[69] These results support the use of rituximab in patients who have cells that express CD20.

Hematopoietic stem cell transplantation plays an important role in the treatment of adult patients with ALL. For patients with Ph+ ALL or Ph− ALL who have a CR after induction therapy, consolidation with allogeneic HSCT should be considered if a human leukocyte antigen (HLA)-matched sibling or matched unrelated donor is available. After HSCT, patients with Ph+ ALL should continue with standard maintenance therapy that includes a tyrosine kinase inhibitor. For patients with Philadelphia chromosome negative (Ph−) disease who have MRD after induction therapy an allogeneic HSCT should be considered if a matched donor is available. Allogenic HSCT is preferred over autologous HSCT because of lower disease relapse rates.[70]

Relapsed Acute Lymphoblastic Leukemia

About 20% of children with ALL will relapse, but about 40% will experience long-term OS following relapsed treatment regimens.[21] The most common site for relapse is isolated to the bone marrow, although isolated relapses can occur in the CNS or testicles, in addition to combined sites of involvement.[17] Because marrow relapse usually follows isolated CNS or testicular relapses, patients with isolated extramedullary relapses are treated with localized radiation (cranial or testicular) and aggressive systemic chemotherapy similar to that given to patients with a marrow relapse.[71]

Patients who have completed treatment and remained in remission for longer periods are more likely to achieve remission again. The second CR rate is 78% in children who were in continuous CR for less than 18 months, 78% if the duration of remission was 18 to 36 months, and 93% if the duration of remission was more than 36 months.[72] Three-year OS following bone marrow (28%), CNS (60%), and testicular (60%) relapse is not optimal.[71] Overall, 5-year disease-free survival rates are 27% for second complete remission (CR2) and 15% for third complete remission (CR3).[72]

Clofarabine, a purine antimetabolite, is an option for patients with second or later relapses, but the duration of response is less than 6 months. Nelarabine is an option for relapsed T-cell ALL, especially if the patient had not previously received nelarabine as part of their initial therapy. Other antineoplastic agents that have antileukemic activity in relapsed ALL include liposomal vincristine, moxetumomab pasudotox, inotuzumab ozogamicin, and bortezomib.[73,74]

Blinatumomab received FDA approval in 2014 for relapsed or refractory Ph− B-cell precursor ALL. As a bi-specific T-cell engager (BiTE), blinatumomab binds to both CD19, an antigen that is present throughout B cell development, and CD3, a T-cell receptor. By linking CD19 and CD3, blinatumomab enables a cascade of events resulting in lysis of CD19 cells.[75] Blintumomab has induced a CR and achieved MRD negativity in adult and pediatric patients with relapsed or refractory ALL. Phase III trials of single-agent blinatumomab are ongoing, as are trials combining blinatumomab with conventional antineoplastic agents. Since blinatumomab has a very short half-life, it must be administered as a continuous infusion for 28 days of a 6-week cycle. Adverse reactions occur in most patients, ranging from mild, reversible symptoms such as fever and rigors to more severe toxicities including neurotoxicity, infections, and cytokine release syndrome.[76]

Chimeric antigen receptor (CAR) T-cell therapy is a promising therapeutic option for ALL patients without other curative options. This new therapeutic modality involves genetically engineered T cells designed to express CARs directed against CD19, resulting in T cells targeting leukemic cells that express CD19. Clinical trials have reported a CR rate ranging from 70% to 90% in pediatric and adult patients with relapsed or refractory ALL.[77-79] Significant adverse effects arising after CAR T-cell therapy include hypogammaglobulinemia, encephalopathy, seizures, and cytokine release syndrome, ranging from mild, flu-like symptoms to multiorgan system failure.

Allogeneic HSCT has traditionally been the treatment of choice for early bone marrow relapse (continuous CR less than 36 months) while children who relapse more than 36 months after completion of initial therapy have traditionally received chemotherapy alone.[42] More recent analyses have shown HSCT to be an advantage to all relapsed children, while some have not shown a benefit.[72] Therefore, the question of who would benefit from HSCT continues to be investigated.

Most patients with relapsed or refractory disease are considered for an allogeneic HSCT with a matched sibling or unrelated donor if they achieve a CR2 following salvage chemotherapy. Most elderly patients are not candidates for standard allogeneic HSCT but are candidates for nonmyeloablative transplant (NMT). Patients who undergo an NMT receive a reduced intensity conditioning regimen. An NMT may produce similar outcomes with less treatment-related morbidity and mortality. The National Marrow Donor Program and the American Society for Blood and Marrow Transplantation have developed guidelines for transplant consultation based on current clinical practice and evidence.[70,80]

Late Effects of Treatment

Certain late effects associated with cranial or craniospinal irradiation and corticosteroids were discussed earlier. The Childhood Cancer Survivor Study tracks the health status of adults treated for childhood cancer between 1970 and 1986 and has yielded invaluable information on how to monitor adult survivors.[81] Leukemia survivors are 3.7 times more likely to develop a severe or life-threatening chronic health condition as compared with healthy siblings, and 2.8 times more likely to report multiple chronic conditions.[81]

Older ALL regimens that incorporated intensive use of topoisomerase II inhibitors (etoposide and teniposide) are associated with unacceptably high risks of development of secondary leukemia.[42] High cumulative doses of anthracyclines used in high-risk or relapsed patients can cause cardiomyopathy. Cranial irradiation is also associated with learning deficits, especially in patients younger than 5 years of age at the time of treatment. Patients who received cranial radiation as children also have higher unemployment rates and lower marital rates among females two decades after diagnosis.[81] The Children's Oncology Group has developed long-term follow-up guidelines for survivors of childhood, adolescent, and young adult cancers.[82]

ACUTE MYELOID LEUKEMIA

Risk Classification

Many clinical and laboratory features at diagnosis are associated with response to treatment, as measured by the CR rate, duration of remission, and long-term survival. Identification of these risk factors may allow the clinician to better understand the disease and to tailor treatment according to risk of disease recurrence. For example, if a patient has many clinical and laboratory features that are associated with a favorable response to chemotherapy ("favorable risk"), then the clinician may choose to give less intensive therapy to reduce the risk of long-term toxic effects. Conversely, if a patient is unlikely to respond well to therapy ("high risk"), then the clinician may choose to give more intensive chemotherapy that may include HSCT.

7 Several prognostic factors have been identified for adults with AML. The most important patient factor is age, with younger patients more likely to achieve a CR than patients older than age 60 years.[3] The lower CR rate in older patients results from an increased frequency of fatal infection and bleeding complications and resistance to conventional chemotherapy. The duration of remission is also shorter in older patients as compared to younger patients. Other patient-specific prognostic factors include concurrent infection and any major organ impairment.[13] Patients with extramedullary disease, CNS involvement, or underlying MDS have a worse prognosis. Other unfavorable prognostic factors in adult AML include: age older than 60 years, multidrug-resistance gene expression, WBC greater than 100,000 cells/mm^3 (>100 × 10^9/L), and therapy-related AML.[13] Age must be evaluated as a continuous variable when looking at prognostic factors. The clinical difference between a patient 61 years old and one 71 years old, is much greater than a 59-year-old and a 61-year-old. Certain cytogenetic abnormalities are also known to worsen the response rate and survival of patients with AML (Table 134-4).[13] Chromosome 16 or translocations between chromosome 8 and 21 alter core-binding factor. Core-binding factor is associated with sensitivity to cytarabine.[3,13] In addition, patients who develop a "secondary" leukemia after treatment of another malignancy usually have a very poor response to antileukemic chemotherapy (ie, therapy-related AML). Another factor that needs consideration for any cancer treatment is performance status. A bed-ridden patient with a new diagnosis of AML would not be a good candidate for treatment because of high treatment-related morbidity and mortality. Patients with poor performance status may be offered supportive care.

Cytogenetics may be the most important prognostic factor for a patient newly diagnosed with AML.[3,13] Molecular testing for FLT3-ITD, CEBPA, C-KIT, and *NPM1* is becoming more common in commercial laboratories and referral centers, and should be considered for all newly diagnosed AML patients.[3,13] Patients with core-binding factor with t(8;21)(q22;q22) or inv(16)(p13;q22)/t(16;16)(p13;q22) treated with a cytarabine-based regimen have a relatively favorable prognosis. Adults and children with chromosomal deletions such as 3q[abn(3q)] or 5q[del(5q)], monosomies of chromosome 5 and/or 7(-5/-7) have a poor prognosis with standard chemotherapy for AML, and may benefit from experimental treatments. About 40% of cases have a normal karyotype. Molecular mutations, such as FLT3, *NPM1* (nucleophosmin), C-KIT, and CEBPA (CCAAT/enhancer-binding protein α), can identify subsets of patients with differing outcome who have normal karyotypes. FLT3 is a receptor tyrosine kinase that is mutated in about one-third of patients with AML, including those with normal karyotype, and is associated with higher presenting WBC, decreased duration of CR, and a poorer prognosis. *NPM1* is present in about 30% of patients with AML, even in patients with normal karyotype, and commonly coexists with FLT3, and is associated with a higher CR and reduced relapse risk compared to patients without the mutation.[3,13] C-KIT mutations have been observed in about 20% of patients with core-binding factor AML and are associated with decreased duration of CR and OS.[83] CEBPA is present in about 10% of patients with AML, and is associated with a favorable outcome. The area of cytogenetic and molecular abnormalities is complex and still evolving.

Prognostic factors associated with pediatric AML include response to the first course of remission induction therapy, cytogenetics, and molecular genetics. Poor prognostic factors include monosomy 7, age older than 10 years, black race, internal tandem duplications of FLT3, *MLL* gene rearrangements, and a diagnosis of AML secondary to prior chemotherapy or radiation therapy.[4,84] Conversely, inversion of chromosome 16, trisomy 21, CBF-AML, *PML-RARA*, *NPM1*, biallelic CEBPA, and *RUNX1-RUNX1T1* fusion transcript t(8;21) are associated with a favorable outcome.[4,84]

Acute myeloid leukemia treatment in the future may be based primarily on cytogenetic and molecular classification. Treatment algorithms based on these newer classifications have been proposed, but they are not currently incorporated into the initial remission induction therapy. These tests do provide prognostic information that may be incorporated into subsequent treatment decisions for postremission therapy or relapsed/refractory disease.[15]

TABLE 134-4 Risk Category According to Cytogenetic and Molecular Abnormalities Present

	Risk Category		
Disease	**Good-Risk**	**Intermediate-Risk**	**High-Risk**
AML	t(8;21)(q22;q22); inv(16); t(15;17); t(9;11) trisomy 21 Mutated NPM1 without FLT3-ITD Mutated CEBPA	Normal karyotype; trisomy 8; 11q23; del(7q); del(9q); trisomy 22; t(9;11)	Complex karyotype; −5; −7; del(5q); inv(3p) FLT3 ITD

AML, acute myeloid leukemia; CEBPA, CCAAT/enhancer binding-protein α; FLT3-ITD, Fms-like tyrosine kinase 3 internal tandem duplication; NPM1, nucleophosmin.

TREATMENT

Acute Myeloid Leukemia

Desired Outcomes

The short-term goal of treatment for AML is to rapidly achieve a complete clinical and hematologic remission. In the absence of a CR, a rapid and fatal outcome is inevitable. CR is defined as the disappearance of all clinical and bone marrow evidence (normal cellularity more than 20% with less than 5% blasts) of leukemia, with restoration of normal hematopoiesis (neutrophils more than or equal to 1,000 cells/mm^3 [more than 1 × 10^9/L] and platelets more than 100,000 cells/mm^3 [more than 100 × 10^9/L]).[85] Partial remission is a significant response to treatment (a decrease of at least 50% of blasts), but evidence of residual disease in the bone marrow remains (5%-25% blasts) and is considered a treatment failure requiring additional therapy. The definition of CR has several categories including not only CR (morphologic CR with restoration of normal hematopoiesis), but also CR with complete remission with incomplete hematological recovery (CRi), cytogenetic CR ([CRc] patient with normal cytogenetics in which cytogenetics were previously abnormal), and molecular CR ([CRm] molecular studies negative).[85] If there is a question of residual leukemia on bone marrow biopsy in adults, a bone marrow aspirate/biopsy should be repeated in 1 week.

After a CR is achieved, the goal is to maintain the patient in continuous CR. The occurrence of leukemic relapse in the bone marrow significantly reduces the likelihood of cure. Most patients who will die from acute leukemia die within the first 6 years; the survival curve (percentage alive vs time) beyond the sixth year after therapy does not continue to decline as rapidly ("survival plateau"), and at this time patients can be considered "cured."

With recent advances in antineoplastic therapy and supportive care, 60% to 80% of all patients with AML achieve a CR, and 20% to 40% become long-term survivors.[3] Overall, the median duration of remission is 1 to 2 years. In patients 60 years of age or older, the CR rate averages around 50%, and the median duration of remission is shorter than 1 year.[3] In contrast to ALL, effective therapies used in AML cause severe and often prolonged myelosuppression. As a result, patients with AML, particularly patients older than 60 years of age, are at greater risk for treatment-related fatal infectious and bleeding complications.

Treatment Phases

Remission Induction

As with ALL, the goal of remission induction for AML is to rapidly induce a CR with associated restoration of normal hematopoiesis. Compared to ALL, however, fewer patients with AML achieve CR. Because the CR rate in AML is related to the intensity of the remission induction regimen, the drugs used in AML are given at doses that uniformly cause severe myelosuppression (except tretinoin). One reason for the lower CR rate in AML as compared to ALL is the inability to give optimal doses of chemotherapy because of marrow toxicity. With continued improvement of supportive care for patients undergoing chemotherapy, more intensive treatment regimens are being given in an effort to reduce the high rate of leukemic relapse and increase the proportion of long-term survivors. Most patients achieve a CR after 1 or 2 courses of chemotherapy. Patients who require additional chemotherapy to achieve a CR have been reported to have a poor prognosis, even if remission is ultimately achieved.

8 The most active single agents in AML are the anthracycline antibiotics (daunorubicin, doxorubicin, and idarubicin), mitoxantrone, and the antimetabolite cytarabine. The standard therapy for the treatment of adult AML has not changed in several decades. The most common regimen ("7+3") combines daunorubicin administered as a short infusion of 45 to 60 mg/m^2 per day on days 1 to 3, along with cytarabine administered as a continuous 24-hour infusion of 100 to 200 mg/m^2 per day on days 1 to 7.[3,86] The CR rate with the 7+3 regimen is 65% to 75% in patients 18 to 60 years old. Several trials have attempted to improve on conventional 7+3 therapy, but have shown no improvement by (a) increasing cytarabine to 10 days, (b) shortening cytarabine to 5 days, (c) substituting doxorubicin, idarubicin, or mitoxantrone for daunorubicin, (d) adding other agents such as etoposide, thioguanine, or topotecan, or (e) increasing cytarabine to higher doses (2 g/m^2 every 12 hours for 8-12 doses).[3] The most recent change to the standard 7+3 regimen is to increase the daunorubicin dose. Adults younger than 60 years old with AML who were randomized to receive higher daunorubicin dosages (90 mg/m^2 per day on days 1-3) in combination with 7 days of standard-dose cytarabine (100 mg/m^2 per day) had a significantly higher CR rate (71% vs 57%) and longer median OS (23.7 vs 15.7 months) as compared with those who received the standard 7+3 regimen of daunorubicin (45 mg/m^2 per day on days 1-3) and cytarabine.[87]

Idarubicin and mitoxantrone have been evaluated as alternatives to daunorubicin in combination with standard-dose continuous infusion cytarabine. Trials in younger patients reported improved CR rates with these newer anthracyclines (idarubicin) or anthracenediones (mitoxantrone), and one trial reported prolonged survival. Among older adults, the CR rate and OS do not appear to be different among the different anthracyclines or anthracenediones.[3,86] Therefore, the anthracycline of choice for the standard 7+3 regimen is daunorubicin or idarubicin with many centers adopting idarubicin or higher doses of daunorubicin into the induction regimen in younger AML patients.

Based on experimental tumor models that showed a steep dose-response curve for cytarabine, higher cytarabine doses have been evaluated as a means to increase the antileukemic activity of induction therapy. The decision to give high-dose cytarabine in induction may depend on the treatment plan for postremission or consolidation therapy. The Southwest Oncology has evaluated the impact of adding high-dose cytarabine to induction therapy. This strategy does not improve the CR rate or OS, but does improve EFS.[88] A study specifically in younger patients compared conventional dose cytarabine to high-dose cytarabine demonstrated improved OS in patients aged 15 through 45 years of age.[89] A retrospective study conducted by the European Group for Blood and Marrow Transplantation demonstrated that the cytarabine dose administered during induction and/or consolidation did not influence the outcome in patients who ultimately went on to receive allogeneic or autologous HSCT.[90] These data suggest that high doses of cytarabine during induction may not be needed in patients who receive HSCT as postremission therapy. No data are available using more than daunorubicin 60 mg/m^2 or idarubicin 12 mg/m^2. In summary, the role of high-dose cytarabine during induction remains controversial. If used during induction, high-dose cytarabine is more appropriate in younger patients than in elderly patients because of poor tolerance by elderly patients. Additionally, it may be an option in patients unable to tolerate anthracyclines.

Clinical **Controversy...**

Some studies have reported improved treatment outcomes with high-dose cytarabine (2 g/m^2 every 12 hours for 8-12 doses) given in combination with an anthracycline during induction therapy. Should high-dose be given for induction therapy? If so, should it be given only to younger patients or those with high-risk AML?

The National Comprehensive Cancer Network (NCCN) has published guidelines for the treatment of AML.[91] The classic 7+3 regimen may be inadequate in adults younger than 60 years of age because the duration of remission is less than that reported in some studies that employed high-dose cytarabine in induction. The NCCN guideline recommends that adults younger than 60 years of age without an antecedent hematologic disorder (ie, no preexisting hematologic malignancy such as MDS) be treated with either the 7+3 regimen or more aggressive chemotherapy including high-dose cytarabine with an anthracycline or anthracenedione. In patients 60 years of age or older with good performance status, the conventional 7+3 regimen should be used or the patient should be enrolled in a clinical trial. The approach in patients with an antecedent hematologic disorder differs, and younger patients (less than 60 years) should be offered available clinical trials or proceed to allogeneic HSCT (provided a suitable donor is available).

Older patients (more than or equal to 60 years) with an antecedent hematologic disorder or those with significant comorbidities unrelated to leukemia should be offered a low-intensity therapy with low-dose subcutaneous cytarabine, a hypomethylating agent such as azacitidine or decitabine, a clinical trial or best supportive care because of the dismal outcomes and toxicity risks associated with conventional chemotherapy. Azacitidine and decitabine are pyrimidine nucleoside analogs of cytidine that inhibit DNA methylation. While each agent has shown promising results versus conventional chemotherapy and best supportive care, the agents have not been compared to each other in trials.[92,93] Azacitidine is usually given

75 mg/m^2/dose IV or subcutaneously for 7 days while decitabine is given 20 mg/m^2/dose IV for 5 days. Cycles are repeated about every 28 days. A minimum of 4 to 6 cycles of therapy must be given before evaluation of response. Azacitidine has resulted in OS rates of 50% as compared to 16% in those treated with usual care (chemotherapy, low-dose cytarabine, or best supportive care).[93] These agents are generally well-tolerated with the most significant adverse effect being myelosuppression. Best supportive care includes use of blood product transfusion support.

All adult patients who present with CNS symptoms or asymptomatic monocytic disease should have a diagnostic lumbar puncture, and, if it is positive, should be treated for disease. Methotrexate or cytarabine should be administered intrathecally twice a week until clearance of leukemic blasts from the CSF, and then weekly for 4 to 6 weeks. Continued secondary prophylaxis is recommended following treatment for CNS disease.[91]

Intensive Postremission Therapy

Although most adults with AML achieve a CR, the duration of remission is short (6-9 months) if no further treatment is given. Relapse is presumably a consequence of the presence of residual, but clinically undetectable, leukemic cells after remission induction therapy. The goal of intensive postremission therapy is to eradicate these residual leukemic cells and to prevent the emergence of drug-resistant disease. The need for postremission therapy is based on postmortem analysis and cell kinetic data suggesting that nearly 10^9 residual leukemic cells remain after effective remission induction therapy. Strategies evaluated as postremission therapy include (a) low-dose, prolonged maintenance therapy, (b) short-course intensive chemotherapy-alone regimens, and (c) high-dose chemotherapy with or without radiation therapy followed by allogeneic or autologous HSCT.

Chemotherapy In the treatment of AML, intensive postremission therapy is often referred to as *consolidation therapy*. Results of randomized controlled trials in adults clearly show that intensive postremission therapy following remission induction therapy prolongs survival versus no therapy, although the exact duration of postremission therapy is controversial.[3,5,91]

The intensity of postremission therapy is important. In a large CALGB trial, all patients who achieved a CR after standard 7+3 induction were randomized to receive one of three cytarabine-based consolidation regimens: 100 mg/m^2 per day or 400 mg/m^2 per day as a continuous 24-hour infusion, or 3,000 mg/m^2 every 12 hours on days 1, 3, and 5.[94] For adults younger than age 60 years, the probability of remaining in CR after 4 years was significantly higher in patients who received high-dose cytarabine (25% vs 29% vs 44%, respectively).[94] Elderly patients had lower response rates in all arms and did not benefit from the administration of higher cytarabine doses, probably because they were unable to tolerate the high-dose regimen. Dose-limiting neurotoxicity in the high-dose arm was more common in elderly patients and those patients with impaired kidney function.[94]

It is not clear whether the same agents (cytarabine and an anthracycline) given for remission induction should be used for postremission therapy in higher doses, or whether different agents should be given. If leukemic relapse is caused by a resistant cell line, then the use of different agents that are non–cross-resistant with drugs used in induction might be beneficial.

High-dose cytarabine appears to be an important component of postremission therapy, particularly if it is not used in induction therapy. However, many questions remain, such as the optimal dose (g/m^2), number of doses per cycle, and number of cycles of high-dose cytarabine. Among patients with core-binding factor AML, defined as the presence of either t(8;21) or inv(16), it is clear that multiple cycles are beneficial, generally 3 to 4 cycles. The NCCN guideline recommends 3 to 4 cycles of high-dose cytarabine for adults younger than 60 years of age and with favorable cytogenetics.[91] Patients with intermediate-risk cytogenetics should receive 3 to 4 cycles of high-dose cytarabine, or proceed directly to a matched allogeneic HSCT, while those patients with treatment-related or poor risk disease should continue directly to a matched allogenic HSCT.[91] If a patient is 60 years of age or older, standard-dose cytarabine with or without anthracycline for one to two cycles, a reduced-dose high-dose cytarabine regimen (1-1.5 g/m^2 per day for 4-6 doses) for one to two cycles, continuation of low-intensity therapy such as azacitidine or decitabine, or enrollment in a clinical trial is recommended. Patients with high-risk cytogenetics, underlying MDS, or secondary AML should either be enrolled in a clinical trial or be referred for either a matched sibling or alternative donor allogeneic HSCT.[91]

Allogeneic Hematopoietic Stem Cell Transplantation Allogeneic HSCT represents the most aggressive postremission therapy in the management of AML. Much controversy surrounds this treatment approach, specifically the appropriateness, timing, treatment design, and donor selection.

The antileukemic activity of allogeneic HSCT is based on the administration of pretransplant high-dose chemotherapy (or chemoradiotherapy) and the development of a post-transplant immune-based antileukemic response. The immune-based response, referred to as a graft-versus-leukemia (GVL) effect, often accompanies the graft-versus-host disease (GVHD) reaction. The immune-based benefit of allogeneic HSCT has been demonstrated through the observation of consistently lower relapse rates with allogeneic HSCT as compared to autologous or syngeneic HSCT. This potential benefit of allogeneic HSCT can be offset by the risk of post-transplant complications such as GVHD, sinusoidal obstruction syndrome, graft failure, and infections.

Allogeneic HSCT was first evaluated as a treatment modality for AML in refractory patients, but because of initial success in small numbers of patients, it has also been evaluated as intensive postremission therapy in AML patients in first or subsequent remission. Nonrandomized trials of HLA-identical sibling allogeneic HSCT performed in AML patients in first complete remission (CR1) reported 5-year survival rates of 45% to 60% with relapse rates of 10% to 20%.[3,5,86] Transplant-related mortality following HLA-matched sibling allogeneic HSCT ranges from 15% to 25% in most series.[5,86] As clinicians have gained more experience in this intensive form of therapy and been provided with more effective immunosuppressive and antibiotic regimens, transplant-related mortality rates have decreased and survival rates have increased. Bone marrow registry data indicate that long-term survival rates in AML patients who receive a matched sibling allogeneic HSCT while in first remission have increased from about 45% in the early 1980s to about 60% in the mid-1990s.

Allogeneic HSCT from an HLA-matched sibling donor for AML patients in CR1 results in long-term EFS in 43% to 55% of patients. Although the results vary, some of the studies show longer EFS and lower relapse rates with allogeneic HSCT in AML in CR1 as compared to chemotherapy-alone postremission regimens. Overall, single center prospective trials have not shown an OS advantage for allogeneic HSCT in all patients with AML CR1. Meta-analyses of clinical trials evaluating allogeneic HSCT versus other consolidation strategies in CR1 shows that allogeneic HSCT does provide an OS advantage for patients with intermediate- and high-risk AML.[5]

Myeloablative allogeneic HSCT is generally restricted to patients younger than 60 years of age, which limits the number of patients eligible for treatment of a disease that primarily affects older adults. NMT uses reduced intensity preparative regimens and is now being used in AML patients, particularly in older patients and those with comorbid illnesses that would limit their eligibility for conventional allogeneic HSCT. NMT is designed to provide enough immunosuppression in the preparative regimen to allow for engraftment of donor cells, and depends heavily on the development of a GVL effect as a means to treat and prevent relapse of AML. The procedure is well tolerated in a wide age range of patients is associated with low rates of regimen-related toxicity. A larger trial evaluating 264 patients who had received an NMT from matched related and unrelated donors demonstrated a 5-year OS of 33% and disease-free survival of 32%.[95] Because only 30% of patients have an HLA-matched sibling donor, allogeneic HSCT is further restricted as a treatment alternative for AML patients.[5] Matched unrelated donor HSCT with a phenotypically HLA-matched donor identified from bone marrow registries is also a treatment option in young adults and pediatric AML patients. This approach is associated with long-term EFS rates of 30% to 40%, which are slightly lower than in AML patients undergoing HLA-matched sibling allogeneic HSCT because of a higher risk of treatment-related mortality with the procedure.

The decision to transplant a patient depends a great deal on which prognostic risk group the patient belongs. Among patients with favorable-risk AML, allogeneic HSCT does not result in better outcomes as compared to high-dose cytarabine-based therapy. All patients with high-risk AML, including those with an antecedent hematologic disorder, treatment-related MDS, or induction failure, should undergo evaluation for HSCT. Similarly, patients in CR1 with high-risk cytogenetics and patients in CR2 and beyond should undergo evaluation for allogeneic HSCT.[5,86,91]

Autologous Hematopoietic Stem Cell Transplantation

Compared to allogeneic HSCT, autologous HSCT has the advantage of a lower risk of posttransplant complications because of lack of immunosuppression and GVHD, and more broad applicability because of a lack of donor limitations and fewer age restrictions. Although the preparative regimen still provides antileukemic activity, autologous HSCT is associated with a higher risk of relapse because of a lack of a GVL effect and potential tumor contamination with autologous stem cells. EFS following autologous HSCT for adult AML in CR1 ranges from 40% to 60%, with treatment-related mortality of 5% to 15% and relapse rates of 30% to 50%.[96] Controversies in autologous HSCT include the optimal timing of therapy, the amount of consolidation therapy needed prior to HSCT, the dose of stem cells needed, and the impact of post-transplant therapy.[96]

Clinical **Controversy...**

Intensive postremission therapy may include an HSCT, but there are many questions concerning the use of HSCT in the treatment of AML. When should a patient receive an HSCT during their postremission therapy? Should a patient receive HSCT during CR1 or later after relapse has occurred? For eligible patients with a matched related (sibling) or unrelated donor, what type of HSCT (allogeneic vs autologous) is preferred?

Comparison of Postremission Therapy Options Several randomized trials in AML patients in CR1 have compared outcomes following allogeneic HSCT, autologous HSCT, and/or intensive consolidation chemotherapy. In most trials, eligible patients based on age and donor availability received an allogeneic HSCT and the remaining patients were randomized between autologous HSCT and chemotherapy alone. The effect of stem cell source on EFS and OS is controversial. Several comparative trials of bone marrow versus peripheral blood have been completed in patients with hematologic malignancies, and a meta-analysis of nine randomized trials showed a lower relapse rate for those patients receiving peripheral blood stem cells.[97]

Most transplant centers base their decision to transplant on cytogenetic risk category.[3] Patients with high-risk cytogenetics do poorly with conventional chemotherapy or autologous HSCT (EFS <15%), making allogeneic HSCT the treatment of choice in this population. Patients with favorable-risk cytogenetics should not proceed to transplant in CR1, as neither autologous nor allogeneic HSCT is superior to conventional chemotherapy. The optimal treatment of choice in patients with intermediate-risk cytogenetics is not clear and is based on availability of matched related donor and clinician preference. Many centers consider a relapse probability of 40% to 50% sufficiently high so as to justify the risk of transplant-related mortality. The decision to proceed with HSCT in this group may depend on the results of molecular testing. According to the NCCN guidelines, the decision to proceed to HSCT depends on prognostic risk features including cytogenetics.[91] If the patient has a favorable-risk cytogenetic profile and is younger than age 60 years, then high-dose cytarabine for four cycles or one cycle of high-dose cytarabine-based therapy followed by autologous HSCT is preferred over allogeneic HSCT. If the patient has an unfavorable-risk cytogenetic profile and is younger than 60 years of age, then allogeneic HSCT should be considered early after remission induction. Patients with intermediate-risk cytogenetics should be entered into a clinical trial, but if a clinical trial is not available, either a matched allogeneic HSCT or high-dose cytarabine should be considered. For patients 60 years and older, the NCCN guidelines do not favor a myeloablative HSCT, but NMT is being used more frequently.[5,95] For the AML patient who relapses early after induction therapy, if a sibling or matched unrelated donor is available, then allogeneic HSCT is the primary reinduction therapy because conventional chemotherapy offers little benefit. If the relapse occurs late, then HSCT may be used as postremission consolidation after reinduction therapy.[91]

Acute Myeloid Leukemia in Children

Overall survival rates for pediatric AML are about 60%, which is lower than that for pediatric ALL.[98] About 73% of children with AML are classified as low-risk, based on the presence of certain favorable risk factors, including t(8;21), MRD negativity at the end of induction, or inversion 16, and have an OS of 80%.[99] Children with disease or treatment factors associated with high-risk ALL, such as monosomy 7, 5q deletion, high FLT3-ITD to wild-type allelic ratio, or MRD at the end of induction, have an OS of 35%.[99] Therapy for AML in children includes one to two cycles of induction therapy followed by two to three cycles of consolidation therapy. The number of cycles varies by protocol.[84] Maintenance therapy has no role in pediatric AML (see Fig. 134-2).[4] Induction therapy with cytarabine and an anthracycline is standard. Etoposide is often included in induction but the contribution of this agent to efficacy has been debated.[84] Consolidation therapy relies on the use of high-dose cytarabine in conjunction with an anthracycline and etoposide.[4] The use of intrathecal chemotherapy for CNS prophylaxis is routinely accepted, but the optimal regimen is not known and varies by protocol.[84] Cranial radiation is only used for patients with refractory CNS disease.

Certain patients may be eligible to receive an HSCT as consolidation therapy, instead of continuing chemotherapy. The use of HSCT in CR1 rather than waiting until relapse/CR2 is controversial. Most trials recommend consolidation with chemotherapy for favorable risk patients; the role of HSCT in unfavorable AML may be considered on an individual basis carefully weighing the risks and benefits.

While children younger than 2 years of age at diagnosis are considered high risk, the therapy they receive is not different than older pediatric AML patients. However, infants with AML generally receive therapy dosed on body weight (per kilogram) rather than body surface area. Children with Down syndrome and AML do not need the same intensive therapy that is given to AML patients without Down syndrome. Recent trials have provided dose reductions and shortened duration of overall therapy to AML patient with Down syndrome without any significant change in outcome.[100]

Relapsed or Refractory Acute Myeloid Leukemia

The most common cause of treatment failure in AML patients receiving chemotherapy alone or undergoing HSCT is relapse. In addition, many patients, particularly elderly patients, have refractory disease as defined by the inability to achieve a CR after two courses of induction therapy. In most cases, the preferred method of treatment for relapsed or refractory disease is HSCT if patients are able to tolerate it. Prolonged EFS is observed in 30% to 40% of patients receiving allogeneic or autologous HSCT in first relapse or CR2. Unfortunately, only a small percentage of relapsed or refractory adult patients will be eligible for HSCT, particularly allogeneic HSCT, because of age and donor restrictions. The role of NMT is also being evaluated in this setting.

The timing of HSCT to treat relapse is controversial. Some studies suggest that outcomes of HLA-matched, related allogeneic HSCT are similar regardless of whether the transplant is performed at the time of early first relapse or in CR2. The difficulty with this approach is identifying a patient in "early relapse," as often the patient will present in a florid relapse. While performing the allogeneic HSCT in first relapse eliminates the need for and toxicity of salvage chemotherapy, the feasibility of this approach is limited by the lead time required to activate a donor search. Patients who relapse following allogeneic HSCT have a poor outcome, with a median survival of about 3 to 4 months. In this setting, treatment options depend on performance status, clinical condition, and the time since allogeneic HSCT. Patients relapsing less than 100 days following allogeneic HSCT are unlikely to respond to current therapies, and salvage attempts are often associated with a high treatment-related mortality. For selected patients relapsing more than 1 year after allogeneic HSCT, a second allogeneic HSCT may be an alternative, but the likelihood of prolonged survival is generally less than 10% with a second transplant. Other strategies being investigated for the treatment of relapse after allogeneic HSCT include immune manipulation to stimulate a GVL effect through donor lymphocyte infusions, and premature discontinuation of calcineurin inhibitors and other immunosuppressants.

If patients with relapsed or refractory disease are not candidates for HSCT, the primary mode of treatment is salvage chemotherapy. The ability to achieve a CR2 with salvage chemotherapy is related to the duration of the first remission. About 50% to 60% of patients who relapse longer than 2 years after induction therapy will achieve a CR2, often with the same induction regimen.[3,86] If a patient relapses 1 to 2 years after induction therapy, the CR2 rate decreases to 40%, and only 10% to 20% of patients who relapse within 6 to 12 months following induction are able to achieve a CR2 with alternate salvage chemotherapy regimens. Long-term survival at 3 years ranges from zero in patients who relapse early to 20% to 25% in those who experience a prolonged duration of initial remission. Based on these data, a risk-adapted approach should be taken when considering treatment options.

Treatment strategies for patients who have relapsed are also categorized according to age and ability to tolerate intensive therapy. Cytarabine has been administered alone or in combination with various agents, including etoposide, fludarabine, topotecan, clofarabine, and an anthracycline, as treatment of relapsed or refractory AML. Response rates to such salvage regimens range from 30% to 50%, but are often short-lived. Patients who received high-dose cytarabine during remission induction may be less likely to benefit from such a regimen for treatment of relapse, and thus require alternate salvage strategies. Regimens containing purine analogs such as fludarabine or clofarabine are another option.[91] Clofarabine may be given alone or in combination with agents such as cytarabine. While studies have shown CR rates of about 50%, median OS is less than 12 months.[101] Less intensive therapies for relapsed disease include use of low-dose cytarabine or one of the hypomethylating agents, azacitidine or decitabine.

Several classes of agents are being investigated as alternate treatment approaches for relapsed or refractory AML, including multiple targeted approaches for FLT3, NPM1, and C-KIT.[102] Additionally, histone deacetylase inhibitors (panobinostat and vorinostat), farnesyltransferase inhibitors (tipifarnib), monoclonal antibodies, and cell cycle inhibitors (volasertib and rigosertib) are several other classes actively being studied for this challenging indication.[103]

In children with AML, about 5% have refractory disease and 30% experience a relapse.[4] About one-half the children relapse within 1 year of initial diagnosis and have a poor prognosis.[4] Therapy for relapse should include an anthracycline and antimetabolite followed by allogeneic HSCT if a CR2 is achieved. Several new agents are being investigated for use in the relapsed refractory setting including clofarabine, bortezomib, sorafenib, and gemtuzumab ozogamicin.[4,104]

Late Effects of Therapy

Because of the intense therapy received by children with AML, they are at risk for a variety of long-term sequelae. A recent study reported that more than 50% of survivors have growth abnormalities.[105] Other findings include neurocognitive deficits, transfusion-associated hepatitis, endocrine disorders, cataracts, and cardiomyopathy (median cumulative anthracycline dose 335 mg/m^2). The 20-year cumulative risk for a second malignancy is estimated to be 1.8%.

TREATMENT
Acute Promyelocytic Leukemia

Acute promyelocytic leukemia is a subclass of AML that accounts for about 10% of all cases. APL is the most curable of the AML subtypes, but its clinical presentation is associated with a high early death rate secondary to coagulopathy.[106] Most patients are diagnosed between the ages of 15 and 60 years, and the average age is 44 years.[91] Multiple large cooperative group trials have shown that induction regimens produce CR rates exceeding 90%.[107] Five-year EFS rates of 70% to 80% are reported with APL.[107] APL is clinically unique from the other subclasses because of the common occurrence of severe coagulopathy (characterized by disseminated intravascular coagulation) at diagnosis and during induction therapy, which frequently resulted in intracerebral hemorrhage. In APL, differentiation and maturation arrest are caused by alterations in the retinoic acid receptor (RAR) because of the translocation of chromosomes 15 and 17. The discovery of t(15;17) provides a cytogenetic marker of the disease and is predictive of response to differentiation therapy with tretinoin (commonly referred to as all-*trans* retinoic acid or ATRA). This translocation leads to a fusion protein of the *PML* gene on chromosome 15 and the RARα on chromosome 17.

Prior to the availability of tretinoin in the late 1980s, treatment of APL consisted of the same combination chemotherapy regimens used in the treatment of other subclasses of AML. Such standard regimens produced CR rates of 50% to 60%, but were associated with a high treatment-related mortality rate caused by hemorrhagic complications. The introduction of molecularly targeted therapy with tretinoin allows for high CR rates with a significant reduction in life-threatening bleeding complications. Arsenic trioxide targets the PML moiety, resulting in apoptosis, and appears to be synergistic with tretinoin.

The WBC count at initial presentation is the most important prognostic factor in patients with APL. Risk stratification of patients at diagnosis based on WBC count has improved outcomes. Abnormal creatinine, increased peripheral blast count, and presence of coagulopathy are prognostic factors that predict for early death due to hemorrhage.[107]

Treatment Phases

Induction

Tretinoin, an oral vitamin A analog, is given orally in a dose of 45 mg/m^2 per day, as a single dose or divided into two doses, after a meal. Tretinoin-based regimens achieve CR rates as high as 95% in APL patients within 1 to 3 months. Because tretinoin does not cross the blood-brain barrier, leukemic meningitis should be treated with conventional intrathecal chemotherapy.

Although it is not myelosuppressive, tretinoin therapy is associated with headache, skin and mucous membrane reactions, bone pain, nausea, and the retinoic acid syndrome. When tretinoin is started, rapid onset of differentiation of promyelocytes occurs, which can lead to leukocytosis and retinoic acid syndrome. The retinoic acid syndrome (fever, respiratory distress, interstitial pulmonary infiltrates, pleural effusions, and weight gain) is now referred to as the APL differentiation syndrome or APL hyperleukocytosis syndrome, because it is associated with other treatment modalities in the management of APL. The syndrome is fatal in 5% to 29% of cases. A combination of chemotherapy with tretinoin induction decreases the risk of APL differentiation syndrome, and rapid initiation of dexamethasone 10 mg (0.2 mg/kg per dose in children) twice daily on development of symptoms decreases associated mortality.[108]

A number of clinical trials have evaluated treatment regimens for APL since the discovery of tretinoin.[91,107] These trials show that tretinoin induction therapy, followed by consolidation chemotherapy, produces similar CR rates but decreased relapse and increased EFS and OS as compared to chemotherapy alone for remission induction and consolidation. However, a significant proportion of patients receiving tretinoin in that study relapsed by 4 years, and 25% of patients experienced the APL differentiation syndrome. In an effort to extend the duration of remission and decrease tretinoin-associated toxicity, other trials have evaluated the sequential and concurrent administration of tretinoin with chemotherapy during induction and consolidation therapy. Additionally, the stratification of therapies based on WBC at diagnosis has been used in trials. A combined analysis of the Programa para el Estudio de la Terapeutica en Hemopatıa Maligna (PETHEMA) 99 and the French APL 2000 trial showed that in patients with WBC less than 10,000/mm^3 (less than 10×10^9/L), the regimen containing tretinoin with idarubicin for induction and tretinoin in consolidation produced similar CR rates with decrease relapse rates, whereas for patients with WBC more than 10,000/mm^3 (more than 10×10^9/L), the induction regimen containing cytarabine resulted in higher CR rates and improved OS rates.[109]

9 Based on these data, the current NCCN guideline for induction therapy for newly diagnosed APL patients includes selection of a regimen based on the WBC count at presentation and ability to tolerate anthracyclines. All of these regimens include tretinoin 45 mg/m^2 per day until a CR is achieved, in combination with an anthracycline (either daunorubicin 50-60 mg/m^2 per dose for 3 or 4 days, or idarubicin 6-12 mg/m^2 per dose every other day for four doses) or tretinoin plus arsenic trioxide for patients unable to tolerate anthracycline therapy.[91] Several of the induction regimens also contain cytarabine 200 mg/m^2 per dose for 7 days; similar CR rates are observed with daunorubicin or idarubicin. APL cells appear to be more sensitive to anthracyclines, possibly because of decreased P-glycoprotein expression. The NCCN guidelines also emphasize the use of one published regimen consistently throughout induction, consolidation, and maintenance phases.[91] Children should also be treated with tretinoin, an anthracycline, and cytarabine with results similar to those achieved in adults.

Another difference in the treatment of APL is the timing of bone marrow biopsy. Assessment of response to treatment of APL is completed at the time of count recovery after induction therapy. A day 10 to 14 day bone marrow biopsy, which is completed for monitoring the effect of induction chemotherapy for other types of AML, is not a long enough time from initiation of therapy because leukemic promyelocytes need more time for differentiation. Assessment of molecular remission should be made after consolidation.

Arsenic trioxide is a compound with demonstrated efficacy in relapsed APL. It has been evaluated as part of remission induction therapy in several studies. The concept of a "chemotherapy-free" regimen in this disease is attractive especially for patients unable to tolerate anthracyclines. A combination of tretinoin with arsenic trioxide for induction therapy resulted in CR of 100% of low/intermediate risk patients.[91]

Consolidation Therapy

Consolidation chemotherapy should be administered to patients with APL because of the high relapse rate. Consolidation therapy usually consists of an idarubicin or daunorubicin-based regimen in combination with tretinoin. Arsenic trioxide has also been evaluated in consolidation therapy.

Postconsolidation Therapy

Unlike other subtypes of AML, maintenance therapy is an important but controversial component of therapy for APL. Before the advent of tretinoin, nonrandomized trials suggested a benefit of continuous low-dose methotrexate and mercaptopurine in prevention of relapse of APL. Larger prospective randomized trials have demonstrated decreased relapse rates in patients who received maintenance therapy (either tretinoin or combination chemotherapy) and some trials have demonstrated increased EFS and OS.[107] However, other trials have shown little benefit. In a meta-analysis of nine randomized controlled trials of maintenance therapy versus observation in APL in CR1, no statistically significant improvement in OS with maintenance treatment was observed regardless of tretinoin inclusion or maintenance with other therapies. Disease-free survival was improved with maintenance compared to observation, although the difference was not statistically significant. Current recommendations for maintenance therapy in adult APL patients include tretinoin 45 mg/m^2 per day for 15 days every 3 months, in addition to mercaptopurine 100 mg/m^2 orally daily and methotrexate 10 mg/m^2 per week, for 2 years in patients at high risk. The benefit of maintenance therapy may depend on the induction and consolidation regimens given, and thus the NCCN guidelines recommends following the recommendations for maintenance therapy that are used in conjunction with the induction treatment regimen selected.[91]

Relapsed Acute Promyelocytic Leukemia

The incidence of relapsed APL is 10% to 15% overall with rates as high as 20% to 30% in high-risk disease. Most relapses occur in the first 3 years following induction therapy. Arsenic trioxide is the agent of choice for relapsed APL, and this agent serves as a backbone for treatment regimens. Multiple studies have shown CR rates of about 85%.[91,107]

Arsenic trioxide has induced clinical remissions in relapsed APL through its induction of apoptosis and differentiation.[107] The recommended dose is 0.15 mg/kg per day IV until bone marrow remission, not to exceed 60 doses, followed by consolidation beginning 3 to 6 weeks after completion of induction at the same dose for a total of 25 doses over a period up to 5 weeks. Arsenic trioxide therapy is associated with two specific toxicities. First, it can cause the APL differentiation syndrome, similar to that seen with tretinoin. Management is similar: corticosteroids at first signs of pulmonary distress or a rapidly rising WBC count. The second toxicity is a prolongation of the QT_c interval. Consequently, it is important to obtain a baseline 12-lead electrocardiogram prior to starting therapy with arsenic trioxide, and correct any electrolyte abnormalities, including potassium, calcium, and magnesium. Other medications known to prolong the QT_c interval should be avoided, if possible, during arsenic trioxide therapy. The QT_c interval should not exceed 500 milliseconds at baseline, and if it increases to more than 500 milliseconds during therapy, the patient should be reevaluated. Arsenic trioxide should not be restarted until the QT_c is less than 460 milliseconds. Following induction of a CR2 with arsenic trioxide in relapsed patients, postremission therapy with combination arsenic trioxide and chemotherapy can result in molecular remissions and improved EFS, as compared to chemotherapy or arsenic trioxide alone following remission.[107]

It is recommended for patients to proceed to autologous HSCT following hematologic and molecular remission after arsenic therapy. Outcomes with autologous HSCT depend on the disease status of the patient at the time of transplant. Autologous HSCT in CR2 (vs CR1) is associated with a lower OS, leukemia-free survival, and increased treatment-related mortality. Autologous HSCT have shown increased disease-free survival and OS compared to allogenic HSCT.[91,110]

Patient Monitoring

In comparison to non-APL AML, molecular and cytogenetic testing at the end of remission induction therapy in APL has no prognostic value. Clinicians should not make decisions based on the presence or absence of any genetic abnormalities at this time. Because terminal differentiation of blasts in APL requires more than 40 days, results of a bone marrow biopsy obtained at the end of remission induction can be misleading because insufficient time has elapsed to determine response. Molecular and cytogenetic response assessment should occur after the completion of consolidation treatment.

Detection of residual PML/RARα transcripts in the bone marrow at the end of consolidation therapy is strongly associated with subsequent hematologic relapse. Achievement of PML/RARα-negative status is associated with a higher probability of cure. The use of this molecular technique allows the clinician to assess response to therapy and also detect relapse earlier, which might prevent the development of overt disease recurrence and is associated with improved outcome compared with delaying treatment until overt morphologic relapse.[107] Most experts recommend that APL patients should be routinely evaluated for continuous remission status. Suggested follow-up includes polymerase chain reaction for PML/RARα every 3 to 6 months for 2 years, and then every 6 months for 2 years.[91,107]

ROLE OF HEMATOPOIETIC GROWTH FACTORS IN ACUTE MYELOID LEUKEMIA

10 Hematopoietic growth factors have been evaluated in AML patients to enhance chemotherapy cytotoxicity, shorten the duration of neutropenia, and reduce the incidence and severity of infection following induction and consolidation chemotherapy. Most studies show limited benefit with the use of colony-stimulating factors as "priming" agents administered during remission induction therapy in an effort to recruit leukemia cells into the cycle to enhance susceptibility to cell-cycle–specific chemotherapy agents, leading to increased cell kill. Use of hematopoietic growth factors concurrently during chemotherapy administration is discouraged outside the setting of a clinical trial and is not recommended in the American Society of Clinical Oncology guidelines.[111]

Both filgrastim and sargramostim are FDA approved to prevent neutropenic complications in adult AML patients receiving intensive chemotherapy. Myeloid blast cells have receptors for granulocyte colony-stimulating factor and granulocyte-macrophage colony-stimulating factor, and there was initial concern that the use of these factors would stimulate regrowth of the myeloid leukemia. Although subsequent studies have addressed these concerns, many clinicians do not initiate filgrastim until an initial remission is achieved.

A number of randomized trials, primarily in elderly patients, consistently demonstrate that filgrastim or sargramostim reduces the duration of neutropenia following AML induction chemotherapy.[111] While neutropenia can be reduced from 2 to 12 days depending on the trial, results vary in terms of improvements in infectious morbidity and mortality, resource use, and disease response rates. The American Society of Clinical Oncology Guidelines for the Use of White Blood Cell Growth Factors considers the use of hematopoietic growth factors after initial induction therapy reasonable, with the understanding that the effects on length of hospitalization and incidence of severe infection are modest.[111] Patients older than age 55 years appear to derive the greatest benefit, and use is appropriate in this population where more rapid marrow recovery might decrease the duration of hospitalization.[111] A recent review of 19 trials including a total of 5,256 patients showed no difference in the incidence of bacteremias or invasive fungal infections with the use of hematopoietic growth factors.[112] It also concluded that the use of hematopoietic growth factors after consolidation did not affect CR duration, relapse rates or OS. Further pharmacoeconomic data are required in this setting, but the body of evidence supports their use following consolidation therapy in adults. Other controversial issues surrounding hematopoietic growth factor use in AML include which growth factor to use, what dose, which day to start after chemotherapy, how long to continue, and should the marrow be examined for leukemia prior to starting a colony-stimulating factor. All hematopoietic growth factors have been evaluated in patients with AML, including sargramostim, filgrastim, and pegfilgrastim. Although pegfilgrastim is not FDA approved for this indication, research supports its use in this setting. The use of hematopoietic growth factors can also interfere with the interpretation of the day 14 bone marrow examination. Hematopoietic growth factors should be discontinued at least 7 days prior to a bone marrow aspirate and biopsy to avoid interfering with the interpretation of the results (ie, may see immature myeloid forms that would suggest residual disease).

SUPPORTIVE CARE

The most common and significant toxic effect of antileukemic agents is marrow suppression. With the exception of corticosteroids, tretinoin, asparaginase/pegaspargase, and vincristine, antineoplastic agents used to treat acute leukemia cause myelosuppression. During AML remission and postremission therapy, daily monitoring of the complete blood count and the absolute neutrophil count is necessary to determine when red cell and platelet transfusions are needed and when neutropenia is achieved. Less frequent monitoring may be sufficient during ALL induction. Marrow hypoplasia from the myelosuppressive regimens usually reaches its lowest point (nadir) after 1 to 2 weeks of therapy and lasts for another 1 to 2 weeks. During this period of hypoplasia, infectious and bleeding complications are major causes of death in leukemic patients.

As typical signs and symptoms of infection may be absent in the neutropenic host, frequent monitoring of vital signs (especially fever) and daily physical examination are important.[113] Infection control strategies often include routine hand washing;

dietary restrictions; reverse isolation and laminar-air flow rooms; fungal, *Pneumocystis*, and bacterial prophylaxis; and the empiric use of broad-spectrum antibiotics when fever occurs (see Chapter 122).[113] *Pneumocystis jiroveci* prophylaxis, usually trimethoprim-sulfamethoxazole, is begun in all adults and children with ALL by the end of induction and continues until 6 months after therapy is discontinued. In contrast to the practice at many institutions, the NCCN guidelines do not recommend prophylactic antimicrobials or gut decontamination during induction or consolidation, and leave the choice to the discretion of the treating facility based on local infection patterns and concerns.[114] Several groups have analyzed the evidence supporting the use of prophylactic antibacterials. In general, prophylactic antibacterials should be reserved for patients who are expected to have prolonged (more than 7 days) and profound (absolute neutrophil count less than 100 cells/mm^3 [less than 0.100 $\times$ 10^9/L]) neutropenia. Based on these criteria, prophylaxis following induction chemotherapy is warranted and postconsolidation therapy is warranted on a case-by-case basis.

In children, prophylactic antibiotics have not proven useful and have resulted in increased resistance. Pediatric ALL patients on standard induction regimens, which generally are minimally myelosuppressive, often have recovered blood counts earlier and do not require very aggressive measures. However, they do require close monitoring of vital signs and blood counts until their counts recover. Pediatric AML patients are usually admitted during periods of neutropenia for close observation and rapid initiation of broad spectrum antimicrobials, but the effectiveness of this non-pharmacologic approach to preventing infections is controversial. Infectious complications, especially fungal, are a major cause of morbidity and mortality, therefore antifungal prophylaxis is strongly recommended.[115] The incidence of viridans streptococci has increased with the intensity of therapy and is most associated with high-dose cytarabine. These infections can lead to meningitis or delayed acute respiratory distress syndrome.

Acute leukemia patients, particularly those patients with an initial elevated WBC count, are at risk for tumor lysis syndrome. Preventive measures include allopurinol or rasburicase, and adequate hydration prior to and during chemotherapy to prevent the development of urate nephropathy from rapid destruction of WBCs. Rasburicase, a recombinant urate-oxidase enzyme produced by genetic modification of *Saccharomyces cerevisiae*, catalyzes the enzymatic oxidation of uric acid into the inactive soluble metabolite, allantoin. In children, rasburicase more rapidly reduces uric acid levels in patients with aggressive malignancies compared to allopurinol, and reduces the need for dialysis.[116] Rasburicase has been evaluated in adults, and some studies in adults show that fixed dosing produces equivalent outcomes to a weight-based, mg/kg dosing strategy. Because of its cost, rasburicase is usually limited to patients with ALL who have a high WBC count or bulky extramedullary disease, aggressive lymphoma, or patients with AML with a high presenting WBC. Most institutions also include an elevated uric acid as part of the criteria for use. Rasburicase has a rapid onset of action and long duration of action; so many institutions also limit its use to a single dose and allow repeat doses as needed. Rasburicase is contraindicated in patients with glucose-6-phosphate dehydrogenase deficiency. Tumor lysis syndrome may lead not only to hyperuricemia, but also to hyperkalemia, hyperphosphatemia, hypocalcemia and subsequent renal insufficiency.[116]

Hematologic support consists primarily of platelet and packed red blood cell transfusions. Platelet transfusions are often given for peripheral counts below 10,000 cells/mm^3 (10 $\times$ 10^9/L) or clinical signs of bleeding. Transfusions of packed red cells may also be indicated for a hemoglobin less than 8 g/dL (80 g/L; 4.96 mmol/L), profound fatigue, shortness of breath, tachycardia, or chest pain. APL can release procoagulants that can cause disseminated intravascular coagulation, necessitating close monitoring and replacement of coagulation factors with cryoprecipitate. Because of the gastrointestinal toxic effects of chemotherapy, parenteral nutrition may be required. Patients are frequently receiving infusions of antibiotics, fluids, hyperalimentation, opioids, and blood products simultaneously. To provide the total support needed for these patients, a multiple-lumen central venous access device should be considered at the start of therapy.

PERSONALIZED PHARMACOTHERAPY

Treatment of acute leukemia is highly personalized. A risk-adapted approach is used in the treatment of ALL and AML. In ALL, patients are placed into risk categories based on age and disease characteristics. The initial risk category is sometimes changed based on the rapidity and completeness of response to remission induction therapy. The same risk-adapted approach is used in the treatment of AML, but age and cytogenetics are the most important factors in determining the risk category. Molecular mutations are becoming more important in both ALL and AML.

Genetic polymorphisms may affect drug metabolism, receptor expression, drug transportation, drug disposition, and pharmacologic response. These alterations may contribute to acute and chronic toxicity from ALL therapy and to treatment outcome.[6] The most studied polymorphism involves thiopurine metabolism. Cellular thiopurine *S*-methyltransferase (TPMT) inactivates thiopurines such as mercaptopurine and thioguanine. About 10% of the population has intermediate TPMT activity as a result of heterozygous polymorphisms in the gene encoding for TPMT, and 1 in 300 has extremely low activity as a result of homozygous presence of this TPMT polymorphism. Deficiency of TPMT activity can result in excessive myelosuppression from standard doses of thiopurines. Patients with low activity (homozygous mutant TPMT genotype) require 85% to 90% dose reductions.[117] About 50% of the heterozygous patients will require dose reductions. TPMT status can now be determined directly by DNA-based testing, which may become a standard of care in the near future.

EVALUATION OF THERAPEUTIC OUTCOMES

Appropriate development of a pharmaceutical care plan for the acute leukemia patient begins with establishing the diagnosis and prognosis for the patient. Long-term therapeutic goals for the patient may include long-term EFS, although palliative care is a possibility in some patients. The desired short-term outcome is the establishment of remission. The return of hematologic values to normal and a repeat bone marrow biopsy that demonstrates no evidence of disease serve as documentation that remission has been achieved. Monitoring guidelines for induction or consolidation are similar (Table 134-5). After the appropriate postremission therapy has been completed, the patient may return monthly for 1 year, and then every 3 months, to check hematologic values. If no evidence of disease exists after 5 years from the diagnosis and the patient has been in continuous CR, the patient is considered cured.

Frequent monitoring of fevers, hematologic and chemistry laboratory values, microbiology reports, and the patient's physical condition are necessary to identify infection, risk of bleeding, and tumor lysis syndrome early. A coagulation screening panel will identify patients with ongoing disseminated intravascular coagulation, a particular risk with APL.

During therapy, the pharmacist and other healthcare professionals are important providers of patient and caregiver education. Patients should receive information regarding acute and chronic toxicities of the chemotherapy being administered, as well as possible treatments for those toxicities. Healthcare professionals should

TABLE 134-5 Acute Myeloid Leukemia Assessment and Monitoring

Baseline Workup	Monitoring During Therapy	Postremission Monitoring
History and physical examination CBC with differential, platelets Serum chemistries (creatinine, bilirubin, AST, ALT to assess organ function) Coagulation (PT, PTT, D-dimers, fibrinogen) Bone marrow biopsy and aspirate with cytogenetics Immunophenotyping and cytochemistry Human leukocyte antigen (HLA) typing Cardiac workup (MUGA or echocardiogram; ECG) Intravascular access Lumbar puncture (if symptomatic or monocytic disease) Chest radiography Height and weight Molecular testing for genetic aberrations (FLT3, NPM1, CEBPA)	Daily physical examination CBC with differential, platelets Serum chemistries (including uric acid, K^+, Ca^{+2}, PO_4, SCr during tumor lysis syndrome risk period[a]) Coagulation (PT, PTT, D-dimers, fibrinogen [if APL]) Bone marrow biopsy and aspirate 7-10 days after end of chemotherapy. Repeat bone marrow biopsy and aspirate upon hematologic recovery to document complete response (with cytogenetics if initially abnormal) Temperature curve (initiate antibiotics when febrile) Lumbar puncture (with intrathecal chemotherapy) if initial lumbar puncture was positive for leukemia	Routine physical examination at clinic visit CBC with differential, platelets Bone marrow biopsy and aspirate at set intervals to evaluate ongoing remission and if peripheral blood counts are abnormal or if they fail to recover within 5 weeks of treatment PML/RARα monitoring [if APL]

ALT, alanine aminotransferase; APL, acute promyelocytic leukemia; AST, aspartate aminotransferase; CBC, complete blood cell count; ECG, electrocardiogram; FLT3, FMS-related tyrosine kinase 3; MUGA, multiple-gated acquisition (blood pool scan); NMP1, nucleophosmin; PML/RARα, promyelocytic-leukemia retinoic acid receptor-α; PT, prothrombin time; PTT, partial thromboplastin time; S_{cr}, serum creatinine.

[a]Risk for tumor lysis syndrome during induction therapy only.

follow patients throughout therapy for dosing adjustments and toxicities due to antineoplastic therapy. For example, the health-care team should make sure the patient is receiving corticosteroid and saline eye drops four times daily while the patient is receiving high-dose cytarabine to prevent the ocular toxicity of cytarabine. The pharmacist is an important resource for information regarding antibiotics, antiemetics, nutritional support, hematopoietic growth factors, and other supportive care issues.

Pharmacists should be involved in assessing drug doses and any dose modifications for organ dysfunction or prior toxicity. Pharmacists are often in the best position to recognize the potential risk for medication errors and drug interactions and to help avoid them. Similarly, pharmacists are often able to assess adherence and identify the possibility that patient problems are secondary to drug treatments.

Numerous late sequelae from leukemia therapy have been recognized and should be included in the monitoring plan after therapy is completed. Chapter 140 discusses the long-term consequences of HSCT. Additionally, the Children's Oncology Group Long-Term Follow-Up guidelines provide an additional resource for assessment and monitoring.[82]

ABBREVIATIONS

ALL	acute lymphoblastic leukemia
AML	acute myeloid leukemia
APL	acute promyelocytic leukemia
ATRA	all-*trans* retinoic acid
AYA	adolescents and young adults
BMI	body mass index
CALGB	Cancer and Leukemia Group B
CAR	chimeric antigen receptor
CEBPA	CCAAT/enhancer binding-protein α
CNS	central nervous system
COG	Children's Oncology Group
CR	complete remission
CR1	first complete remission
CR2	second complete remission
CR3	third complete remission
CRi	complete remission with incomplete hematological recovery
CRc	cytogenetic complete remission
CRm	molecular complete remission
CSF	cerebrospinal fluid
ECOG	Eastern Cooperative Oncology Group
EFS	event-free survival
FDA	Food and Drug Administration
GTP	guanosine triphosphate
GVHD	graft-versus-host disease
GVL	graft-versus-leukemia
HLA	human leukocyte antigen
HSCT	hematopoietic stem cell transplantation
hyperCVAD	high-dose methotrexate and cytarabine alternating with fractionated cyclophosphamide plus vincristine, doxorubicin, and dexamethasone
$iAMLP_{21}$	intrachromosomal amplification of chromosome 21
MDS	myelodysplastic syndrome
MLL	mixed lineage leukemia
MRD	minimal residual disease
NCCN	National Comprehensive Cancer Network
NCI	National Cancer Institute
NMT	nonmyeloablative transplant
NPM1	nucleophosmin
OS	overall survival
PETHEMA	Programa para el Estudio de la Terapeutica en Hemopatıa Maligna
Ph^+	Philadelphia chromosome positive
PML	promyelocytic leukemia
RARα	retinoic acid receptor-α
TPMT	thiopurine *S*-methyltransferase
WBC	white blood cell
WHO	World Health Organization

REFERENCES

1. Siegel RL, Miller KD, Jemal A. Cancer statistics, 2016. *CA Cancer J Clin* 2016;66:7-30.
2. Howlader N NA, Krapcho M, et al. (eds). *SEER Cancer Statistics Review*, 1975-2012. Bethesda, MD: National Cancer Institute. Available at: http://seer.cancer.gov/csr/1975_2012/ (based on November 2014 SEER data submission, posted to the SEER web site, April 2015).
3. Dohner H, Weisdorf DJ, Bloomfield CD. Acute Myeloid Leukemia. *N Engl J Med* 2015;373:1136-1152.

4. Creutzig U, van den Heuvel-Eibrink MM, Gibson B, et al. Diagnosis and management of acute myeloid leukemia in children and adolescents: Recommendations from an international expert panel. *Blood* 2012;120:3187-3205.
5. Dohner H, Estey EH, Amadori S, et al. Diagnosis and management of acute myeloid leukemia in adults: Recommendations from an international expert panel, on behalf of the European LeukemiaNet. *Blood* 2010;115:453-474.
6. Pui CH, Robison LL, Look AT. Acute lymphoblastic leukaemia. *Lancet* 2008;371:1030-1043.
7. Deschler B, Lubbert M. Acute myeloid leukemia: Epidemiology and etiology. *Cancer* 2006;107:2099-2107.
8. Inaba H, Greaves M, Mullighan CG. Acute lymphoblastic leukaemia. *Lancet* 2013;381:1943-1955.
9. Belson M, Kingsley B, Holmes A. Risk factors for acute leukemia in children: A review. *Environ Health Perspect* 2007;115:138-145.
10. Thomopoulos TP, Ntouvelis E, Diamantaras AA, et al. Maternal and childhood consumption of coffee, tea and cola beverages in association with childhood leukemia: A meta-analysis. *Cancer Epidemiol* 2015;39:1047-1059.
11. Caughey RW, Michels KB. Birth weight and childhood leukemia: A meta-analysis and review of the current evidence. *Int J Cancer* 2009;124:2658-2670.
12. Vardiman JW, Thiele J, Arber DA, et al. The 2008 revision of the World Health Organization (WHO) classification of myeloid neoplasms and acute leukemia: Rationale and important changes. *Blood* 2009;114:937-951.
13. Estey EH. Acute myeloid leukemia: 2013 update on risk-stratification and management. *Am J Hematol* 2013;88:318-327.
14. Pui CH, Pei D, Campana D, et al. Improved prognosis for older adolescents with acute lymphoblastic leukemia. *J Clin Oncol* 2011;29:386-391.
15. Marcucci G, Haferlach T, Dohner H. Molecular genetics of adult acute myeloid leukemia: Prognostic and therapeutic implications. *J Clin Oncol* 2011;29:475-486.
16. Smith M, Arthur D, Camitta B, et al. Uniform approach to risk classification and treatment assignment for children with acute lymphoblastic leukemia. *J Clin Oncol* 1996;14:18-24.
17. Cooper SL, Brown PA. Treatment of pediatric acute lymphoblastic leukemia. *Ped Clin North Am* 2015;62:61-73.
18. Izraeli S, Vora A, Zwaan CM, Whitlock J. How I treat ALL in Down's syndrome: Pathobiology and management. *Blood* 2014;123:35-40.
19. Arico M, Schrappe M, Hunger SP, et al. Clinical outcome of children with newly diagnosed Philadelphia chromosome-positive acute lymphoblastic leukemia treated between 1995 and 2005. *J Clin Oncol* 2010;28:4755-4761.
20. Moorman AV, Ensor HM, Richards SM, et al. Prognostic effect of chromosomal abnormalities in childhood B-cell precursor acute lymphoblastic leukaemia: Results from the UK Medical Research Council ALL97/99 randomised trial. *Lancet Oncol* 2010;11:429-438.
21. Hunger SP, Mullighan CG. Acute Lymphoblastic Leukemia in Children. *N Engl J Med* 2015;373:1541-1552.
22. Campana D. Minimal residual disease in acute lymphoblastic leukemia. *Semin Hematol* 2009;46:100-106.
23. Schultz KR, Pullen DJ, Sather HN, et al. Risk- and response-based classification of childhood B-precursor acute lymphoblastic leukemia: A combined analysis of prognostic markers from the Pediatric Oncology Group (POG) and Children's Cancer Group (CCG). *Blood* 2007;109:926-935.
24. Borowitz MJ, Devidas M, Hunger SP, et al. Clinical significance of minimal residual disease in childhood acute lymphoblastic leukemia and its relationship to other prognostic factors: A Children's Oncology Group Study. *Blood* 2008;111:5477-5485.
25. Hunger SP, Loh ML, Whitlock JA, et al. Children's Oncology Group's 2013 blueprint for research: Acute lymphoblastic leukemia. *Ped Blood Cancer* 2013;60:957-963.
26. Schrappe M, Hunger SP, Pui CH, et al. Outcomes after induction failure in childhood acute lymphoblastic leukemia. *N Engl J Med* 2012;366:1371-1381.
27. Inaba H, Pui CH. Glucocorticoid use in acute lymphoblastic leukaemia. *Lancet Oncol* 2010;11:1096-1106.
28. Mitchell CD, Richards SM, Kinsey SE, Lilleyman J, Vora A, Eden TO. Benefit of dexamethasone compared with prednisolone for childhood acute lymphoblastic leukaemia: Results of the UK Medical Research Council ALL97 randomized trial. *Br J Haematol* 2005;129:734-745.
29. Kawedia JD, Kaste SC, Pei D, et al. Pharmacokinetic, pharmacodynamic, and pharmacogenetic determinants of osteonecrosis in children with acute lymphoblastic leukemia. *Blood* 2011;117:2340-2347.
30. Silverman LB, Supko JG, Stevenson KE, et al. Intravenous PEG-asparaginase during remission induction in children and adolescents with newly diagnosed acute lymphoblastic leukemia. *Blood* 2010;115:1351-1353.
31. Pieters R, Hunger SP, Boos J, et al. L-asparaginase treatment in acute lymphoblastic leukemia: A focus on Erwinia asparaginase. *Cancer* 2011;117:238-249.
32. Raetz EA, Salzer WL. Tolerability and efficacy of L-asparaginase therapy in pediatric patients with acute lymphoblastic leukemia. *J Pediatr Hematol Oncol* 2010;32:554-563.
33. Salzer WL, Asselin B, Supko JG, et al. Erwinia asparaginase achieves therapeutic activity after pegaspargase allergy: A report from the Children's Oncology Group. *Blood* 2013;122:507-514.
34. Petersen WC Jr., Clark D, Senn SL, et al. Comparison of allergic reactions to intravenous and intramuscular pegaspargase in children with acute lymphoblastic leukemia. *Ped Hematol Oncol* 2014;31:311-317.
35. Asselin B, Rizzari C. Asparaginase pharmacokinetics and implications of therapeutic drug monitoring. *Leuk Lymphoma* 2015:56(8):2273-2280.
36. Bleyer A, Asselin BL, Koontz SE, Hunger SP. Clinical application of asparaginase activity levels following treatment with pegaspargase. *Ped Blood Cancer* 2015;62:1102-1105.
37. Vrooman LM, Kirov II, Dreyer ZE, et al. Activity and toxicity of intravenous Erwinia asparaginase following allergy to *E. coli*-derived asparaginase in children and adolescents with acute lymphoblastic leukemia. *Ped Blood Cancer* 2016;63:228-233.
38. Pui CH, Campana D, Pei D, et al. Treating childhood acute lymphoblastic leukemia without cranial irradiation. *N Engl J Med* 2009;360:2730-2741.
39. Matloub Y, Lindemulder S, Gaynon PS, et al. Intrathecal triple therapy decreases central nervous system relapse but fails to improve event-free survival when compared with intrathecal methotrexate: results of the Children's Cancer Group (CCG) 1952 study for standard-risk acute lymphoblastic leukemia, reported by the Children's Oncology Group. *Blood* 2006;108:1165-1173.
40. Bomgaars L, Geyer JR, Franklin J, et al. Phase I trial of intrathecal liposomal cytarabine in children with neoplastic meningitis. *J Clin Oncol* 2004;22:3916-3921.
41. Seibel NL. Treatment of acute lymphoblastic leukemia in children and adolescents: Peaks and pitfalls. *Hematology/the Education Program of the American Society of Hematology. American Society of Hematology. Education Program*. 2008:374-380.
42. Pui CH, Evans WE. Treatment of acute lymphoblastic leukemia. *N Engl J Med* 2006;354:166-178.
43. Seibel NL, Steinherz PG, Sather HN, et al. Early postinduction intensification therapy improves survival for children and adolescents with high-risk acute lymphoblastic leukemia: A report from the Children's Oncology Group. *Blood* 2008;111:2548-2555.
44. Winter SS, Dunsmore KP, Devidas M, et al. Safe integration of nelarabine into intensive chemotherapy in newly diagnosed T-cell acute lymphoblastic leukemia: Children's Oncology Group Study AALL0434. *Ped Blood Cancer* 2015;62:1176-1183.
45. De Moerloose B, Suciu S, Bertrand Y, et al. Improved outcome with pulses of vincristine and corticosteroids in continuation therapy of children with average risk acute lymphoblastic leukemia (ALL) and lymphoblastic non-Hodgkin lymphoma (NHL): Report of the EORTC randomized phase 3 trial 58951. *Blood* 2010;116:36-44.
46. Conter V, Valsecchi MG, Silvestri D, et al. Pulses of vincristine and dexamethasone in addition to intensive chemotherapy for children with intermediate-risk acute lymphoblastic leukaemia: A multicentre randomised trial. *Lancet* 2007;369:123-131.
47. Schmiegelow K, Glomstein A, Kristinsson J, Salmi T, Schroder H, Bjork O. Impact of morning versus evening schedule for oral methotrexate and 6-mercaptopurine on relapse risk for children with acute lymphoblastic leukemia. Nordic Society for Pediatric Hematology and Oncology (NOPHO). *J Ped Hematol Oncol* 1997;19:102-109.
48. Bhatia S, Landier W, Hageman L, et al. Systemic exposure to thiopurines and risk of relapse in children with acute lymphoblastic leukemia: A Children's Oncology Group Study. *JAMA Oncol* 2015;1:287-295.
49. Bhatia S, Landier W, Shangguan M, et al. Nonadherence to oral mercaptopurine and risk of relapse in Hispanic and non-Hispanic white children with acute lymphoblastic leukemia: A report from the Children's Oncology Group. *J Clin Oncol* 2012;30:2094-2101.

50. Schultz KR, Bowman WP, Aledo A, et al. Improved early event-free survival with imatinib in Philadelphia chromosome-positive acute lymphoblastic leukemia: A Children's Oncology Group Study. *J Clin Oncol* 2009;27:5175-5181.
51. Bernt KM, Hunger SP. Current concepts in pediatric Philadelphia chromosome-positive acute lymphoblastic leukemia. *Front Oncol* 2014;4:54.
52. Brown P. Treatment of infant leukemias: Challenge and promise. *Hematology/the Education Program of the American Society of Hematology. American Society of Hematology. Education Program.* 2013;2013:596-600.
53. Mann G, Attarbaschi A, Schrappe M, et al. Improved outcome with hematopoietic stem cell transplantation in a poor prognostic subgroup of infants with mixed-lineage-leukemia (MLL)-rearranged acute lymphoblastic leukemia: results from the Interfant-99 Study. *Blood* 2010;116:2644-2650.
54. Dreyer ZE, Dinndorf PA, Camitta B, et al. Analysis of the role of hematopoietic stem-cell transplantation in infants with acute lymphoblastic leukemia in first remission and MLL gene rearrangements: A report from the Children's Oncology Group. *J Clin Oncol* 2011;29:214-222.
55. Maloney KW, Taub JW, Ravindranath Y, Roberts I, Vyas P. Down syndrome preleukemia and leukemia. *Ped Clin North Am* 2015;62:121-137.
56. Buitenkamp TD, Izraeli S, Zimmermann M, et al. Acute lymphoblastic leukemia in children with Down syndrome: A retrospective analysis from the Ponte di Legno study group. *Blood* 2014;123:70-77.
57. Curran E, Stock W. How I treat acute lymphoblastic leukemia in older adolescents and young adults. *Blood* 2015;125:3702-3710.
58. Stock W, La M, Sanford B, et al. What determines the outcomes for adolescents and young adults with acute lymphoblastic leukemia treated on cooperative group protocols? A comparison of Children's Cancer Group and Cancer and Leukemia Group B studies. *Blood* 2008;112:1646-1654.
59. National Comprehensive Cancer Network Clinical Practice Guidelines in Oncology. Adolescent and Young Adult (AYA) Oncology. Version 1.2016. September 3.
60. Jabbour E, O'Brien S, Konopleva M, Kantarjian H. New insights into the pathophysiology and therapy of adult acute lymphoblastic leukemia. *Cancer* 2015;121:2517-2528.
61. National Comprehensive Cancer Network Clinical Practice Guidelines in Oncology. Acute Lymphoblastic Leukemia. Version 2.2015. September 22.
62. Burmeister T, Schwartz S, Bartram CR, Gokbuget N, Hoelzer D, Thiel E. Patients' age and BCR-ABL frequency in adult B-precursor ALL: A retrospective analysis from the GMALL study group. *Blood* 2008;112:918-919.
63. Bassan R, Rossi G, Pogliani EM, et al. Chemotherapy-phased imatinib pulses improve long-term outcome of adult patients with Philadelphia chromosome-positive acute lymphoblastic leukemia: Northern Italy Leukemia Group protocol 09/00. *J Clin Oncol* 2010;28:3644-3652.
64. Ravandi F, O'Brien SM, Cortes JE, et al. Long-term follow-up of a phase 2 study of chemotherapy plus dasatinib for the initial treatment of patients with Philadelphia chromosome-positive acute lymphoblastic leukemia. *Cancer* 2015;121:4158-4164.
65. Ottmann OG, Wassmann B, Pfeifer H, et al. Imatinib compared with chemotherapy as front-line treatment of elderly patients with Philadelphia chromosome-positive acute lymphoblastic leukemia (Ph+ALL). *Cancer* 2007;109:2068-2076.
66. Cortes JE, Kim DW, Pinilla-Ibarz J, et al. A phase 2 trial of ponatinib in Philadelphia chromosome-positive leukemias. *N Engl J Med* 2013;369:1783-1796.
67. Thomas DA, O'Brien S, Jorgensen JL, et al. Prognostic significance of CD20 expression in adults with de novo precursor B-lineage acute lymphoblastic leukemia. *Blood* 2009;113:6330-6337.
68. Maury S, Huguet F, Leguay T, et al. Adverse prognostic significance of CD20 expression in adults with Philadelphia chromosome-negative B-cell precursor acute lymphoblastic leukemia. *Haematologica* 2010;95:324-328.
69. Thomas DA, O'Brien S, Faderl S, et al. Chemoimmunotherapy with a modified hyper-CVAD and rituximab regimen improves outcome in de novo Philadelphia chromosome-negative precursor B-lineage acute lymphoblastic leukemia. *J Clin Oncol* 2010;28:3880-3889.
70. Oliansky DM, Larson RA, Weisdorf D, et al. The role of cytotoxic therapy with hematopoietic stem cell transplantation in the treatment of adult acute lymphoblastic leukemia: Update of the 2006 evidence-based review. *Biol Blood Marrow Transplant* 2012;18:16-17.
71. Gaynon PS. Childhood acute lymphoblastic leukaemia and relapse. *Br J Haematol* 2005;131:579-587.
72. Ko RH, Ji L, Barnette P, et al. Outcome of patients treated for relapsed or refractory acute lymphoblastic leukemia: A Therapeutic Advances in Childhood Leukemia Consortium Study. *J Clin Oncol* 2010;28:648-654.
73. Annesley CE, Brown P. Novel agents for the treatment of childhood acute leukemia. *Ther Adv Hematol* 2015;6:61-79.
74. Parikh SA, Litzow MR. Philadelphia chromosome-negative acute lymphoblastic leukemia: Therapies under development. *Future Oncol* 2014;10:2201-2212.
75. Buie LW, Pecoraro JJ, Horvat TZ, Daley RJ. Blinatumomab: A first-in-class bispecific T-cell engager for precursor B-cell acute lymphoblastic leukemia. *Ann Pharmacother* 2015;49:1057-1067.
76. Teachey DT, Rheingold SR, Maude SL, et al. Cytokine release syndrome after blinatumomab treatment related to abnormal macrophage activation and ameliorated with cytokine-directed therapy. *Blood* 2013;121:5154-5157.
77. Davila ML, Riviere I, Wang X, et al. Efficacy and toxicity management of 19-28z CAR T cell therapy in B cell acute lymphoblastic leukemia. *Sci TranslMed* 2014;6:224ra225.
78. Lee DW, Kochenderfer JN, Stetler-Stevenson M, et al. T cells expressing CD19 chimeric antigen receptors for acute lymphoblastic leukaemia in children and young adults: A phase 1 dose-escalation trial. *Lancet* 2015;385:517-528.
79. Maude SL, Frey N, Shaw PA, et al. Chimeric antigen receptor T cells for sustained remissions in leukemia. *N Engl J Med* 2014;371:1507-1517.
80. National Marrow Donor Program. National Marrow Donor Program. Available at: https://bethematch.org. (Accessed September 20, 2015.)
81. Mody R, Li S, Dover DC, et al. Twenty-five-year follow-up among survivors of childhood acute lymphoblastic leukemia: A report from the Childhood Cancer Survivor Study. *Blood* 2008;111:5515-5523.
82. Children's Oncology Group. Long-Term Follow-Up Guidelines. V 4.0-October 2013. Available at: http://www.survivorshipguidelines.org.
83. Paschka P, Marcucci G, Ruppert AS, et al. Adverse prognostic significance of KIT mutations in adult acute myeloid leukemia with inv(16) and t(8;21): A Cancer and Leukemia Group B Study. *J Clin Oncol* 2006;24:3904-3911.
84. Zwaan CM, Kolb EA, Reinhardt D, et al. Collaborative Efforts Driving Progress in Pediatric Acute Myeloid Leukemia. *J Clin Oncol* 2015;33:2949-2962.
85. Cheson BD, Bennett JM, Kopecky KJ, et al. Revised recommendations of the International Working Group for Diagnosis, Standardization of Response Criteria, Treatment Outcomes, and Reporting Standards for Therapeutic Trials in Acute Myeloid Leukemia. *J Clin Oncol* 2003;21:4642-4649.
86. Ferrara F, Schiffer CA. Acute myeloid leukaemia in adults. *Lancet* 2013;381:484-495.
87. Fernandez HF, Sun Z, Yao X, et al. Anthracycline dose intensification in acute myeloid leukemia. *N Engl J Med* 2009;361:1249-1259.
88. Weick JK, Kopecky KJ, Appelbaum FR, et al. A randomized investigation of high-dose versus standard-dose cytosine arabinoside with daunorubicin in patients with previously untreated acute myeloid leukemia: A Southwest Oncology Group Study. *Blood* 1996;88:2841-2851.
89. Willemze R, Suciu S, Meloni G, et al. High-dose cytarabine in induction treatment improves the outcome of adult patients younger than age 46 years with acute myeloid leukemia: Results of the EORTC-GIMEMA AML-12 trial. *J Clin Oncol* 2014;32:219-228.
90. Cahn JY, Labopin M, Sierra J, et al. No impact of high-dose cytarabine on the outcome of patients transplanted for acute myeloblastic leukaemia in first remission. Acute Leukaemia Working Party of the European Group for Blood and Marrow Transplantation (EBMT). *Br J Haematol* 2000;110:308-314.
91. National Comprehensive Cancer Network Clinical Practice Guidelines in Oncology. Acute Myeloid Leukemia. Version 1.2015. December 3.
92. Kantarjian HM, Thomas XG, Dmoszynska A, et al. Multicenter, randomized, open-label, phase III trial of decitabine versus patient choice, with physician advice, of either supportive care or low-dose cytarabine for the treatment of older patients with newly diagnosed acute myeloid leukemia. *J Clin Oncol* 2012;30:2670-2677.
93. Fenaux P, Mufti GJ, Hellstrom-Lindberg E, et al. Azacitidine prolongs overall survival compared with conventional care regimens in elderly patients with low bone marrow blast count acute myeloid leukemia. *J Clin Oncol* 2010;28:562-569.

94. Mayer RJ, Davis RB, Schiffer CA, et al. Intensive postremission chemotherapy in adults with acute myeloid leukemia. Cancer and Leukemia Group B. *N Engl J Med* 1994;331:896-903.
95. Gyurkocza B, Storb R, Storer BE, et al. Nonmyeloablative allogeneic hematopoietic cell transplantation in patients with acute myeloid leukemia. *J Clin Oncol* 2010;28:2859-2867.
96. Breems DA, Lowenberg B. Acute myeloid leukemia and the position of autologous stem cell transplantation. *Semin Hematol* 2007;44:259-266.
97. Allogeneic peripheral blood stem-cell compared with bone marrow transplantation in the management of hematologic malignancies: An individual patient data meta-analysis of nine randomized trials. *J Clin Oncol* 2005;23:5074-5087.
98. Tarlock K, Meshinchi S. Pediatric acute myeloid leukemia: Biology and therapeutic implications of genomic variants. *Ped Clin North Am* 2015;62:75-93.
99. Pui CH, Carroll WL, Meshinchi S, Arceci RJ. Biology, risk stratification, and therapy of pediatric acute leukemias: An update. *J Clin Oncol* 2011;29:551-565.
100. Caldwell JT, Ge Y, Taub JW. Prognosis and management of acute myeloid leukemia in patients with Down syndrome. *Expert Rev Hematol* 2014;7:831-840.
101. Faderl S, Ravandi F, Huang X, et al. A randomized study of clofarabine versus clofarabine plus low-dose cytarabine as front-line therapy for patients aged 60 years and older with acute myeloid leukemia and high-risk myelodysplastic syndrome. *Blood* 2008;112:1638-1645.
102. Grunwald MR, Levis MJ. FLT3 Tyrosine Kinase Inhibition as a Paradigm for Targeted Drug Development in Acute Myeloid Leukemia. *Semin Hematol* 2015;52:193-199.
103. Montalban-Bravo G, Garcia-Manero G. Novel drugs for older patients with acute myeloid leukemia. *Leukemia* 2015;29:760-769.
104. Moore AS, Kearns PR, Knapper S, Pearson AD, Zwaan CM. Novel therapies for children with acute myeloid leukaemia. *Leukemia* 2013;27:1451-1460.
105. Leung W, Hudson MM, Strickland DK, et al. Late effects of treatment in survivors of childhood acute myeloid leukemia. *J Clin Oncol* 2000;18:3273-3279.
106. Park JH, Qiao B, Panageas KS, et al. Early death rate in acute promyelocytic leukemia remains high despite all-trans retinoic acid. *Blood* 2011;118:1248-1254.
107. Coombs CC, Tavakkoli M, Tallman MS. Acute promyelocytic leukemia: Where did we start, where are we now, and the future. *Blood Cancer J* 2015;5:e304.
108. Cardinale L, Asteggiano F, Moretti F, et al. Pathophysiology, clinical features and radiological findings of differentiation syndrome/all-trans-retinoic acid syndrome. *World J Radiol* 2014;6:583-588.
109. Ades L, Guerci A, Raffoux E, et al. Very long-term outcome of acute promyelocytic leukemia after treatment with all-trans retinoic acid and chemotherapy: The European APL Group experience. *Blood* 2010;115:1690-1696.
110. Holter Chakrabarty JL, Rubinger M, Le-Rademacher J, et al. Autologous is superior to allogeneic hematopoietic cell transplantation for acute promyelocytic leukemia in second complete remission. *Biol Blood Marrow Transplant* 2014;20:1021-1025.
111. Smith TJ, Bohlke K, Lyman GH, et al. Recommendations for the Use of WBC Growth Factors: American Society of Clinical Oncology Clinical Practice Guideline Update. *J Clin Oncol* 2015;33:3199-3212.
112. Gurion R, Belnik-Plitman Y, Gafter-Gvili A, et al. Colony-stimulating factors for prevention and treatment of infectious complications in patients with acute myelogenous leukemia. *The Cochrane Database of Systematic Reviews.* 2012;6:Cd008238.
113. Freifeld AG, Bow EJ, Sepkowitz KA, et al. Clinical practice guideline for the use of antimicrobial agents in neutropenic patients with cancer: 2010 Update by the Infectious Diseases Society of America. *Clin Infect Dis* 2011;52:427-431.
114. National Comprehensive Cancer Network Clinical Practice Guidelines in Oncology. Prevention and Treatment of Cancer-Related Infections. Version 2.2015. April 16.
115. Lehrnbecher T, Sung L. Anti-infective prophylaxis in pediatric patients with acute myeloid leukemia. *Expert Rev Hematol* 2014;7:819-830.
116. Coiffier B, Altman A, Pui CH, Younes A, Cairo MS. Guidelines for the management of pediatric and adult tumor lysis syndrome: An evidence-based review. *J Clin Oncol* 2008;26:2767-2778.
117. Relling MV, Gardner EE, Sandborn WJ, et al. Clinical Pharmacogenetics Implementation Consortium guidelines for thiopurine methyltransferase genotype and thiopurine dosing. *Clin Pharmacol Ther* 2011;89:387-391.

135

Chronic Leukemias

Patrick J. Kiel and Christopher A. Fausel

KEY CONCEPTS

1. Chronic myelogenous leukemia (CML) is defined by the presence of the Philadelphia chromosome (Ph), a translocation between chromosomes 9 and 22. The resulting abnormal fusion protein, p210 *BCR-ABL*, phosphorylates tyrosine kinase residues and is constitutively active, resulting in uncontrolled hematopoietic cell proliferation.
2. Without treatment, the disease course of CML is characterized by a progressive increase in white blood cells over a period of years that ultimately transforms to an acute leukemia.
3. The commercially available tyrosine kinase inhibitors, imatinib, dasatinib, nilotinib, bosutinib, and ponatinib have demonstrated efficacy in treatment of newly diagnosed CML patients and in patients with either accelerated phase or blast crisis.
4. CML monitoring requires assessment of milestones throughout the therapy such as hematologic, cytogenetic, and molecular responses, the ideal of which is a molecular response.
5. Allogeneic hematopoietic stem cell transplant (HSCT) is the only known curative treatment option for CML and is reserved for patients with a suitable donor and progression after treatment with tyrosine kinase-based therapy.
6. The management of chronic lymphocytic leukemia (CLL) is highly individualized and includes observation in patients with early-stage disease and treatment with targeted therapy, chemotherapy, biologic therapy, or both in patients with more advanced disease.
7. Alemtuzumab, ofatumumab, obinutuzumab, and rituximab are monoclonal antibodies that are indicated for the treatment of CLL.
8. Regimens such as fludarabine, cyclophosphamide, and rituximab are considered as first-line therapy for patients with CLL who are younger or have more aggressive disease.
9. Novel agents such as ibrutinib and idelalisib provide an oral option for the treatment of CLL. Ibrutinib is approved for treatment of patients with 17p-deletion and for patients with relapsed disease who have received at least one prior therapy. Idelalisib may be used in combination with rituximab as first line therapy when concomitant medical conditions preclude the use of systemic chemotherapy.

The chronic leukemias include chronic myeloid leukemia (CML), chronic lymphocytic leukemia (CLL), hairy cell leukemia, and prolymphocytic leukemia. The typical clinical presentation of the chronic leukemias is an indolent course in contrast to patients with acute leukemia who will die of their disease within weeks to months if not treated. This chapter focuses on the two most common types of chronic leukemia, CML, and CLL.

CHRONIC MYELOGENOUS LEUKEMIA

Chronic myelogenous leukemia is a myeloproliferative disease that results from malignant transformation of a subpopulation of pluripotent hematopoietic stem cells. Bone marrow hyperplasia and accumulation of differentiated myeloid cells in the peripheral blood are the initial presenting features of the disease. The terminal stage of CML is characterized by rapid accumulation of blast cells in the bone marrow and suppression of normal hematopoiesis that ultimately leads to death. CML was the first malignant disease identified with a consistent cytogenetic abnormality, namely the Ph that contains the BCR-ABL oncogene. This dominant cytogenetic abnormality has allowed CML to become the template for development of molecular targeted drug therapies.

Epidemiology and Etiology

It is estimated that 8,220 new cases of CML will be diagnosed in the United States in 2016.[1] The median age of diagnosis is 64. The development of CML is not associated with hereditary, familial, geographic, ethnic, or economic status. An increased risk of CML has been noted with ionizing radiation exposure and in atomic bomb survivors from Hiroshima and Nagasaki.[2,3]

Pathophysiology

Chronic myelogenous leukemia was first described in 1845, but extensive research into the genetic and molecular characteristics of the disease began with the discovery of the Ph in 1960 by Nowell and Hungerford.[4] Research in the 1980s identified the molecular changes that occur as a result of the Ph when an oncogenic protein was identified and implicated in the pathophysiology of CML.[4,5]

Ph is the first karyotypic abnormality specifically implicated in the pathogenesis of cancer, and its discovery has resulted in extensive research into the molecular biology of CML.[6] This chromosomal abnormality is characteristic of CML and is present in about 95% of patients with the disease.[4-6]

(1) Ph, identified as a shortened long arm of chromosome 22, is found in granulocyte and erythrocyte progenitors, macrophages, megakaryocytes, and lymphocytes. The Ph is the consequence of breaks in chromosomes 9 and 22 resulting in a transposition that relocates the 3′ end of *ABL* (Abelson proto-oncogene) from its normal site on chromosome 9 at band 34 to the 5′ end of *BCR* (breakpoint cluster region) on chromosome 22 at band 11 (symbolized as *t*[9;22][q34;q11]).[6,7] This results in the formation of the hybrid *BCR-ABL* fusion gene (Fig. 135-1). Through this chromosomal translocation, the *ABL* protooncogene is able to escape the normal genetic controls on its senescence and is activated into a functional oncogene, directing the transcription of an 8.5-kilobase messenger ribonucleic acid (mRNA) molecule. The mRNA is translated into a 210-kDa protein—p210 *BCR-ABL*—that is constitutively (ie, constantly) activated compared to the 145-kDa protein translated by the normal *ABL* gene.[5-7] Although p210 *BCR-ABL* is the most common tyrosine kinase found

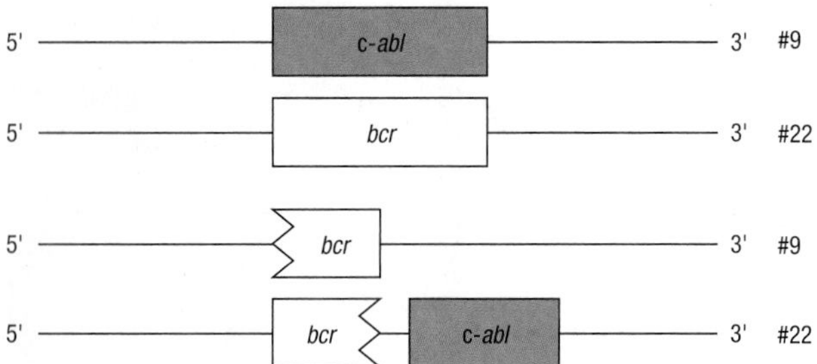

FIGURE 135-1 Diagram of the chromosomal translocation that results in the Philadelphia chromosome. *(Reprinted with permission from Fishleder AJ. Oncogenes and cancer: Clinical applications. Cleve Clin J Med 1990;57:721-726. Copyright © 1990 Cleveland Clinic. All rights reserved.)*

in CML, variations in the breakpoints in the *ABL* gene encode different size proteins. For example, a smaller protein, p190 *BCR-ABL*, is involved in two-thirds of adults with Ph-positive acute lymphoblastic leukemia (ALL), but is rarely found in patients with CML.[6]

Because CML begins with the malignant transformation of a single cell, it is considered a clonal disease. The progeny from this transformed primitive hematopoietic stem cell results in a proliferative advantage over normal hematopoietic cells that displaces normal hematopoiesis. The Ph is found in both myeloid and lymphoid cells, which suggests that the transformed cell of CML is a pluripotent stem cell.[7] This alteration gives the transformed progenitor cell an inheritable growth advantage, leading to the proliferation of a neoplastic, monoclonal population of cells.[8] Disrupted maturation leads to additional divisions by CML progenitor cells before reaching a nonproliferative stage; the resulting number of circulating granulocytes may be many times higher than normal. In the advanced stages of CML, cytopenias may occur in association with fibrotic changes in the bone marrow.

The *BCR-ABL* fusion gene encodes for a constitutively active tyrosine kinase that is involved in both the increased proliferation of the CML clone and the reduction in Fas-mediated apoptosis. Characterization of the adenosine triphosphate binding site on the *BCR-ABL* tyrosine kinase has provided a target for inhibition of tyrosine kinase activity. The first FDA-approved tyrosine kinase inhibitor (TKI), imatinib mesylate (Gleevec®), was indicated for patients in chronic phase who had failed interferon alfa (IFN-α) or for those

TABLE 135-1 Criteria for Different Phases of Chronic Myelogenous Leukemia

Chronic Phase	Accelerated Phase	Blast Crisis
• <10% blasts in peripheral blood or bone marrow	• 10%-19% blasts in peripheral blood or bone marrow • Platelets <100,000 cells/mm^3 (<100 × 10^9/L) or >1,000,000 cells/mm^3 (>1,000 × 10^9/L) Additional findings • Cytogenetic evolution • Progressive splenomegaly	• >20% blasts in peripheral blood or bone marrow • Large clusters of blasts on bone marrow biopsy • Presence of extramedullary infiltrates Additional findings • Fever • Malaise • Splenomegaly

Data from Cortes JE, Talpaz M, O'Brien S, et al. Staging of chronic myeloid leukemia in the imatinib era. Cancer 2006;106:1306-1315.

with advanced disease. Imatinib received additional FDA approval in 2002 for first-line treatment in newly diagnosed CML. Second-generation TKIs with a higher binding affinity and selectivity for *ABL* kinase are approved as both frontline agents and salvage for patients with resistance or intolerance to imatinib.

Clinical Presentation

2 The three clinical phases of CML are: chronic phase (CP), accelerated phase (AP), and blast crisis (BC) (Table 135-1). Nearly 90% of patients present with CP at the time of diagnosis. Often the diagnosis of CML is found incidentally during routine examination or if a complete blood count is obtained for unrelated reasons because patients are often asymptomatic upon presentation. Signs and symptoms include fatigue, sweating, bone pain, weight loss, abdominal discomfort, and early satiety secondary to splenomegaly. Leukocytosis is the hallmark of CP and the white blood cell count can be as high as 1,000,000 cells/mm^3 (1,000 × 10^9/L), placing patients at risk for complications of leukostasis. Symptoms secondary to leukostasis include acute abdominal pain resulting from splenic infarctions, priapism, retinal hemorrhage, cerebrovascular accidents, confusion, hyperuricemia, and gouty arthritis.[6] Patients can survive several years in CP without treatment.

CLINICAL PRESENTATION Chronic Myelogenous Leukemia[1,6]

General

- 90% of patients are diagnosed in CP
- 50% are asymptomatic in CP and often diagnosed following abnormal complete blood count

Signs and Symptoms

- Fatigue
- Left upper quadrant pain
- Abdominal pain or distension
- Weight loss
- Night sweats

Physical Examination

- Splenomegaly
- Hepatomegaly

Laboratory Tests

- Peripheral blood
  - Leukocytosis
  - Thrombocytosis
  - Basophilia
  - Low or undetectable leukocyte alkaline phosphatase
  - Elevated uric acid and lactate dehydrogenase
- Molecular testing
  - Presence of *BCR-ABL* by reverse-transcription polymerase chain reaction (RT-PCR)
- Bone marrow
  - Hypercellular
  - Fully mature myeloid cells
  - Increased megakaryocytes
  - <10% blasts in CP
- Cytogenetics
  - Presence of Ph
  - Additional abnormalities

Initial laboratory workup includes complete blood count with differential, complete metabolic panel, and serum uric acid. A bone marrow aspiration and biopsy is required to confirm the diagnosis of CML. The differential diagnosis of CML includes infection, myeloproliferative disorders (ie, polycythemia vera, essential thrombocythemia, myelofibrosis), and chronic myelomonocytic leukemia. Bone marrow is markedly hypercellular (75%-90%) with increased granulocyte/erythroid ratio increased (10-30:1), erythropoiesis increased megakaryocytes normal. Karyotyping (cytogenetic analysis) is required for a diagnosis. The bone marrow aspiration is analyzed with fluorescence in situ hybridization (FISH) to determine the presence of the Ph chromosome. Quantitative RT-PCR is also performed to assess the baseline *BCR-ABL* transcript levels.

AP is characterized by progressive myeloid maturation arrest and loss of efficacy of drug therapy directed to attenuate the increase in white blood cells. Clinical findings of AP include anemia, increasing peripheral blood and bone marrow blasts and basophils, clonal cytogenetic evolution, extramedullary disease sites (bone, breast, CNS, mucosal tissue, lymph nodes, and skin), exacerbation of splenomegaly, and either thrombocytosis or thrombocytopenia. Nonspecific findings such as bone pain, fever, night sweats, and weight loss may occur. The most commonly observed cytogenetic changes with disease progression are an additional Ph chromosome, trisomy 8, and isochromosome 17q. Survival typically will not exceed several months. The World Health Organization (WHO) classification[6] defines AP CML as one or more of the following changes: 10% to 19% of blasts in the peripheral blood or bone marrow, persistent thrombocytopenia less than 100,000 cells/mm^3 (100×10^9/L) (not related to drug therapy), thrombocytosis greater than 1,000,000 cells/mm^3 ($1{,}000 \times 10^9$/L) despite drug therapy, peripheral basophilia >20%, increasing spleen size and white blood cell count despite drug therapy, bone marrow evidence of progression of the leukemic clone or new cytogenetic abnormalities.

Blast crisis is the terminal stage of disease and clinically resembles acute leukemia where the leukemic clone overwhelmingly dominates the bone marrow at the expense of normal hematopoiesis. The WHO classification defines BC CML as the presence of one or more of the following: greater than 20% blasts in the peripheral blood or bone marrow, extramedullary disease, or large clusters of blasts in the bone marrow.[6] Patients can present occasionally with BC without an apparent AP. One-third of patients present with BC of lymphoid lineage, while two-thirds present with BC of myeloid lineage or undifferentiated like phenotype. The increased proliferative rate in BC CML is the consequence of a number of factors in addition to *BCR-ABL*, such as the activation of the oncogene signaling pathways and loss of tumor suppressors such as p53. Duration of BC is typically days to weeks before death.

Prognosis

Several models have been proposed for estimating prognosis in patients with CML, but the one proposed by Sokal et al. has become the most widely used.[8] The Sokal algorithm uses spleen size, percentage of circulating blasts, platelet count, and age as prognostic factors for patients in CP. However, this scoring system was developed prior to the advent of TKI therapy and may have limited predictive value in the era of imatinib. The median overall survival for patients diagnosed with CP, AP, and BC CML was reported to be 47 months, 12 to 24 months, and 3 to 6 months, respectively, in the era prior to the introduction of TKIs.[9,10]

TREATMENT

Chronic Myelogenous Leukemia

Desired Outcomes

Without effective treatment, CML disease progression leads inexorably to a fatal outcome within 5 years. The overriding treatment goals for CML include the eradication of the leukemic clone from the bone marrow and maintenance of CP with minimal toxicity from treatment. The only proven therapy to eradicate the malignant clone from the bone marrow is allogeneic hematopoietic stem cell transplantation (HSCT). Both immunotherapy with IFN-α and TKI-based therapies have demonstrated the ability to extend CP beyond the expected period of several years. The introduction of TKI therapy has dramatically changed the clinical course of CML where patients can now expect to maintain disease control for many years.[10] The current standard of practice is to initiate TKI therapy for newly diagnosed CML patients. Long-term follow-up from phase III trials have documented a response in excess of 85% of patients that receive imatinib as primary treatment.[11-13] Table 135-2 shows the effect of various treatment modalities on survival in CP CML.

TABLE 135-2 Effect of Therapy on Survival in Patients with Chronic-Phase Chronic Myelogenous Leukemia

Therapy	5-Year Survival (%)	Median Survival (Months)
Busulfan	30-40	40-50
Hydroxyurea	40-50	50-60
IFN-α	50-70	60-80
IFN-α + ara-C	60-80	NR
Allogeneic transplantation		
Matched sibling	60-80	NR
Matched unrelated	40-70	NR
Imatinib	89	NR
Dasatinib	85	NR
Nilotinib	NR	NR
Bosutinib	NR	NR
Omacetaxine	NR	NR
Ponatinib	NR	NR

IFN, interferon; NR, not yet reached.

Clinical response in CML is measured by hematologic, cytogenetic, and molecular indices, all of which have standardized criteria.[6,13] *Hematologic response* is defined as the normalization of peripheral blood counts and is the earliest type of response observed in CML patients. *Cytogenetic responses* are based on the percentage of cells positive for Ph in a bone marrow biopsy. *Complete cytogenetic response* is defined as the elimination of Ph from all cells in the marrow sample whereas *major cytogenetic response* is defined as fewer than 35% Ph-positive cells. Patients who have a major or complete cytogenetic response have an improved survival compared to those who fail to achieve a cytogenetic response.[13]

Because most patients on imatinib achieve a complete cytogenetic response, more sensitive tests to monitor disease status are now used. *Molecular responses* are determined by RT-PCR, which are several logs more sensitive than methods used to measure cytogenetic responses. A *complete molecular response* is the absence of *BCR-ABL* transcripts by RT-PCR. RT-PCR assays should be interpreted carefully because they have varying sensitivities and may show a complete molecular remission even when low levels of *BCR-ABL* transcripts are present.[17] A major molecular response is a greater than 3-log reduction in *BCR-ABL* transcripts by RT-PCR assay. Quantitative RT-PCR should be performed on every patient prior to initiating therapy and throughout therapy to monitor residual disease. Because bone marrow and peripheral blood *BCR-ABL* mRNA levels are correlated, peripheral blood can often be used for this analysis.[12,13]

Conventional Chemotherapy

Conventional cytotoxic chemotherapy is used in CP CML to reduce and temporarily control high peripheral white blood cell (WBC) counts.

Historically, the two agents used for leukoreduction are busulfan (Myleran) and hydroxyurea (Hydrea). Busulfan is no longer used because randomized trials have shown that hydroxyurea treatment provides a modest survival advantage, and busulfan has a risk of potentially life-threatening pulmonary fibrosis.[14]

Hydroxyurea rapidly lowers high circulating WBCs in CP CML by inhibiting ribonucleotide reductase, which inhibits DNA synthesis, eliminating cells in the S phase of the cell cycle, and synchronizing cells in the G_1 or pre-DNA synthesis phase. Hydroxyurea is initiated at 40 to 50 mg/kg/day in divided doses until the WBC count falls to about 10,000 cells/mm^3 (10×10^9/L). Hydroxyurea may be discontinued once adequate control of the WBC count is achieved and a TKI has been initiated. Hydroxyurea is not specifically active against Ph and will not change the natural progression of the disease to BC.

Interferon α

The interferons are a family of glycoproteins involved in many of the functional aspects of the hematopoietic system. Prior to the introduction of imatinib, IFN-*α* was the preferred agent in the treatment of CML. The role of IFN-*α* has since been relegated to patients who fail TKIs and are not candidates for allogeneic HSCT.

3 Use of IFN-*α* in the treatment of CP CML was based on reports that 20% to 50% of patients achieve a major cytogenetic response, which led to prolonged survival.[5,9] In the 10% to 15% of patients achieving a complete cytogenetic response, the median survival was more than 10 years. Patients enrolled on the IFN-*α* arm in the International Randomized Interferon vs STI571 (IRIS) trial had a complete cytogenetic response of 14%, as compared with 76% of patients treated with imatinib.[11] The 2016 National Comprehensive Cancer Network (NCCN) guidelines recommend IFN-*α* only for posttransplant relapse.[12]

IFN-*α* use is also limited by its toxicity profile because it is associated with both short-term constitutional toxicities and potentially dose-limiting long-term toxicities. In the IRIS trial, 26% of patients discontinued IFN-*α* as a result of intolerable side effects.[15] The most predictable early toxicity is a flu-like syndrome characterized by fever, chills, myalgia, headache, and anorexia. These dose-dependent effects may be a result of IFN-*α*–induced leukocytosis and release of inflammatory cytokines. Cardiovascular toxicities (tachycardia, hypotension) are seen in about 15% of patients in the first few weeks. Long-term adverse effects include weight loss, alopecia, neurologic effects (paresthesia, cognitive impairment, and depression), and immune-mediated complications (hemolysis, thrombocytopenia, nephrotic syndrome, systemic lupus erythematosus, and hypothyroidism), which occur in about 5% to 20% of patients.

Despite falling out of clinical favor, IFN-*α* still remains a disease-modifying agent and ongoing clinical trials are investigating the use of imatinib and IFN-*α* in combination for the treatment of CML. Imatinib has been combined with pegylated IFN-α_{2A} in newly diagnosed CP CML yielding improved major molecular response rate at 12 months compared with imatinib 400 mg daily alone (57% vs 38%), but the 12-month complete cytogenetic response rate was similar (66% vs 58%).[15]

Imatinib Mesylate (Gleevec®)

A transformative discovery in cancer therapeutics was the characterization of the adenosine triphosphate binding site on the *BCR-ABL* tyrosine kinase. This specific receptor established a novel drug discovery platform for molecular targeted therapy in CML. Numerous TKIs were in development in the 1990s and STI571 (STI stands for *signal transduction inhibitor*), subsequently named imatinib (Gleevec®), emerged as the drug with the best oral bioavailability and high binding affinity for the *BCR-ABL* tyrosine kinase.[16,17] In 2001, imatinib mesylate received FDA approval for patients in CP CML who had failed IFN-*α* treatment and in patients with AP or BC CML based on phase II studies. In 2002, it received FDA approval for first-line treatment in newly diagnosed CML on the basis of the 2-year follow-up in the IRIS phase III trial.[18]

TABLE 135-3 Cytogenetic and Molecular Response Associated with Tyrosine Kinase Inhibitor Therapy in Chronic Myelogenous Leukemia

Drug (Disease Status)	Daily Dose (mg)	CCyR (%)	MMR	Median Follow-up
Imatinib (CP)	400	82	57%	70 months
	800	90	NR	30 months
Imatinib (AP)	600	43	NR	12 months
	400	11	NR	
Imatinib (BC)	400-800	7.40	NR	—
Dasatinib (CP)	100	83	76%	60 months
Dasatinib (AP)	140	32	NR	15 months
Nilotinib (CP)	600	87	77%	36 months
Nilotinib (AP)	800	16	NR	24 months
Bosutinib (CP–3rd line)	500	24	15%	28.5 months
Bosutinib (CP–1st line)	500	79	59%	12 months
Omacetaxine (CP–2nd line, T315I mutation)	2.5	16	NR	19.1 months
Ponatinib (CP-resistant/ intolerant disease)	45	37	NR	10 months
Ponatinib (CP-T315I mutation)	45	66	NR	10 months

AP, accelerated phase; BC, blast crisis; CCyR, complete cytogenetic response; CP, chronic phase; MCyR, major cytogenetic response; MMR, major molecular response; NR, no response.

Imatinib inhibits several other tyrosine kinases including *BCR-ABL*, C-Kit, and platelet-derived growth factor receptor (PDGFR). Imatinib competitively binds to the adenosine triphosphate (ATP)-binding site on *BCR-ABL*, which inhibits the phosphorylation of proteins involved with CML clone proliferation.[16-18] Table 135-3 summarizes the clinical results of imatinib in CML patients in CP, AP, and BC CML. Table 135-4 summarizes the dosing, food–drug interactions, and drug–drug interactions of TKIs. Early phase I and phase II studies of imatinib, designed to determine maximum tolerated dose and safety, showed higher than expected response rates in all stages of CML.[19]

Chronic Phase

The IRIS study compared imatinib 400 mg orally daily to IFN-*α* plus low-dose subcutaneous cytarabine in 1,106 patients with newly diagnosed CP CML.[18] After a median follow-up of 19 months, patients who received imatinib achieved a complete hematologic response of 96%, major cytogenetic response of 85%, and complete cytogenetic response of 69%. Six percent of patients had progressed to AP or BC and only 4% discontinued imatinib because of an adverse event. The study was designed to allow crossover to the opposite treatment arm for lack of response or intolerance. After 5 years of follow-up, only 3% of patients randomized initially to receive IFN-*α* remained on their initial regimen compared with 69% of patients in the imatinib arm. The 5-year follow-up data from the IRIS trial was published in December 2006 and 8-year follow-up data was presented in December 2009.[11,20] Estimated 5-year and 8-year overall survival of the 553 patients who were originally randomized to receive imatinib is 89% and 85%, respectively. At 8 years, estimated event-free survival (EFS) was 81% and freedom-from-progression to AP or BC

TABLE 135-4 Dosing of Tyrosine Kinase Inhibitors in Chronic Myelogenous Leukemia

Drug	Brand Name	Dose Range	Food–Drug Interactions	Drug–Drug Interactions
Imatinib	Gleevec	400 mg/day (CP) 600 mg/day (AP/BC) 400 mg/day (moderate hepatic impairment) 300 mg/day (severe hepatic impairment)	Take with food and a large glass of water	CYP3A4 inducers may decrease C_{max} and AUC. CYP3A4 inhibitors may increase C_{max} and AUC. Imatinib inhibits CYP3A4 and 2D6. Package labeling recommendations against using warfarin concurrently.
Dasatinib	Sprycel	100 mg/day (CP) 140 mg/day (AP/BC)	With or without meals; do not crush tablets	CYP3A4 inhibitors may increase dasatinib drug levels. CYP3A4 inducers may decrease dasatinib drug levels. H_2 antagonists/PPIs decrease dasatinib drug levels.
Nilotinib	Tasigna	300 mg BID (CP) 400 mg BID (AP/BC)	Take with water; avoid food 2 hours prior to a dose or 1 hour after	Avoid drugs concurrently known to prolong QT interval. CYP inducers may decrease nilotinib serum concentrations. CYP inhibitors may increase nilotinib serum concentrations. Nilotinib is an inhibitor of CYP3A4, CYP2C8, CYP2C9, and CYP2D6. Nilotinib is an inducer of CYP2B6, CYP2C8, and CYP2C9.
Bosutinib	Bosulif	500 mg/day; may increase to 600 mg/day in patients who do not clinically respond by weeks 8-12	Take with food; PPIs may decrease absorption	Concurrent use with CYP3A or Pgp inhibitors increase bosutinib plasma concentrations. Concurrent use with CYP3A inducers reduces bosutinib plasma concentrations.
Ponatinib	Iclusig	45 mg/day (lower dosing may be required as optimal dose is not defined)	With or without food	Concurrent use with CYP3A or Pgp inhibitors increase ponatinib plasma concentrations. Concurrent use with CYP3A inducers reduces ponatinib plasma concentrations.

AP, accelerated phase; AUC, area under the curve; BC, blast crisis; BID, twice daily; C_{max}, maximum concentration; CP, chronic phase; CYP, cytochrome P450; Pgp, P-glycoprotein; PPI, proton pump inhibitor.

was 92% and annual rates of progression to AP or BC in years 4 through 8 were 0.9%, 0.5%, 0%, 0%, and 0.4%. Only 55% of patients remained on imatinib therapy at the 8-year time point.[20]

Cytogenetic and molecular responses secondary to imatinib are associated with EFS and risk of progression to AP or BC. Patients who do not achieve a hematologic response by 3 months, cytogenetic response by 6 months, or a major cytogenetic response by 12 months fare significantly worse compared to responders. In addition, patients with a complete cytogenetic response and at least a 3-log reduction in *BCR-ABL* levels via RT-PCR correlated with a 100% survival without disease progression at 18 months. The risk of disease progression according to the Sokal scoring system predicted the rates of disease progression to be 3%, 8%, and 17% in low-risk, intermediate-risk, and high-risk patients, respectively. However, the Sokal score was not associated with disease progression in patients who achieved a complete cytogenetic response.[11]

4 Although most patients attain a complete cytogenetic response on imatinib, very few patients achieve a complete molecular response. In a study of patients enrolled in the IRIS study, Hughes et al. reported that less than 5% of patients on imatinib have undetectable levels of *BCR-ABL* when analyzed by RT-PCR.[21] Recent data suggest that the level of residual disease is predictive of progression-free survival. A 3-log decline in *BCR-ABL* mRNA within 3 months after achieving a complete cytogenetic response is reported to be a predictor of longer progression-free survival.[22] Careful monitoring of *BCR-ABL* levels by RT-PCR is necessary to guide clinician decision making for therapy modification. The 2016 NCCN guidelines recommend imatinib 400 mg orally daily as one of several options for patients in CP CML (see Table 135-3).[12]

Higher imatinib doses have been evaluated in clinical trials. The European Leukemia Net conducted a randomized phase II trial in high-risk patients defined by the Sokal scoring system to imatinib 400 mg versus 800 mg daily and evaluated the proportion of patients achieving a complete cytogenetic response at 12 months.[23] Patients receiving the higher dose of imatinib achieved a 64% complete cytogenetic response compared to 58% of patients receiving standard dose with a median follow-up period of 12 months (p=0.435). These study results do not justify the routine use of imatinib 800 mg daily as frontline therapy in high-risk patients with CP CML. A phase II trial evaluated imatinib 400 mg daily for 2 weeks, then titrated to 400 mg twice daily in patients with an intermediate-risk Sokal score appeared to have benefit with 88% and 91% of patients achieving a complete cytogenetic response at 12 and 24 months.[24] These data require validation with a phase III clinical trial before a widespread use of a higher dose can become standard of care in CP CML.

Accelerated Phase/Blast Crisis

Response rates for patients with AP or BC CML are lower compared with those in CP CML. A phase II study evaluating imatinib 600 mg daily in patients with AP CML reported complete hematologic and complete cytogenetic response rates of 71% and 19%, respectively.[25] Prior to protocol amendments, patients were able to receive imatinib 400 mg daily, but the rates of hematologic response, cytogenetic response, disease progression, and overall survival were inferior to imatinib 600 mg. The toxicity profile between imatinib 400 mg and 600 mg daily was similar.

Traditional therapy for BC CML has focused on administering cytotoxic chemotherapy in treatment programs similar to acute leukemia induction. Etoposide (VP-16), cytarabine (Ara-C), and carboplatin (VAC-regimen) has demonstrated efficacy in patients with BC CML with a median overall survival of 7 months.[26] Imatinib has demonstrated modest benefit in BC CML. An open-label, nonrandomized trial evaluated imatinib 400 mg daily with dose escalation to 600 mg daily and 400 mg twice daily (for patients not achieving a hematologic response after one month).[27] The primary objectives were to assess hematologic response, complete cytogenetic response, and the return to CP CML. Fifteen percent developed a complete hematologic response, 7.4% achieved a complete cytogenetic response, and 18% achieved a second CP. Imatinib 600 mg was associated with sustained hematologic response. The median overall survival was 6.9 months.

Imatinib Resistance

Despite having high cytogenetic response rates, some patients treated with imatinib will not respond to therapy or will relapse after an initial response.[28] The most prominent mechanism of imatinib resistance is the presence of point mutations in one or more areas on the ABL kinase. More than 100 different mutations have been discovered thus far. Many of these mutations can cause a conformational change in the ATP binding site, which greatly decreases the ability of imatinib to bind and inhibit kinase activity.[13,28] Imatinib binds to *BCR-ABL* by establishing a series of hydrogen bonds with side chains of amino acids within the kinase domain. Mutations which alter this surface can decrease the affinity of imatinib for *BCR-ABL*, potentially preventing binding entirely. The kinase domain of *BCR-ABL*, which encompasses amino acids 225 to 400, can be subdivided into ATP and imatinib binding site (P loop), the catalytic site where the phosphate from ATP is transferred to the substrate protein, and the activation domain that determines the state of the kinase (open or closed). The imatinib binding site is located in the region of amino acids 300 to 325. Resistance is caused by point mutations in one or more areas on the ABL kinase. The T315I mutation occurs directly within the imatinib binding site and completely disrupts imatinib binding.[13,28] This mutation is important because it confers resistance not only to imatinib but also to second-generation *BCR-ABL* kinase inhibitors.

The other known clinically relevant mechanism of resistance is *BCR-ABL* gene amplification. The *BCR-ABL* gene is overexpressed to such an extent that the typical 400 mg daily dose of imatinib is insufficient to inhibit the activity of the kinase. Reports of clinically significant resistance have been published owing to *BCR-ABL* gene amplification, multiple copies of Ph, or both. The largest series published this far included 66 patients, in whom only 2 patients had confirmed *BCR-ABL* genomic amplification.[28] Other proposed mechanisms of resistance to imatinib include differential binding to α_1-acid glycoprotein in serum, overexpression of P-glycoprotein-induced drug efflux, and clonal evolution to acquisition of additional cytogenetic abnormalities.[12,13,28]

Imatinib Monitoring

Imatinib therapy should be frequently monitored to assess response or disease progression. Recommendations for monitoring include baseline molecular and cytogenetic assessment. Patients with CP CML who have an optimal response have a complete hematologic response within 3 months, partial cytogenetic response within 6 months, complete cytogenetic response within 12 months and major molecular response within 18 months of starting imatinib. *BCR-ABL* transcripts should be evaluated by RT-PCR every 3 months and bone marrow cytogenetics performed at 3 months if RT-PCR is unavailable or 12 months if neither complete cytogenetic response nor major molecular response is achieved. Bone marrow cytogenetics are repeated at 18 months if the patient is not in major molecular response or did not have a complete cytogenetic response at 12 months.[12,13] The loss of hematologic or cytogenetic responses or clonal evolution at any time should be considered a treatment failure warranting a change in therapy. *BCR-ABL* kinase domain mutation analysis is performed for patients who have an inadequate initial response at 3, 12, or 18 months, have any sign of loss of response, or demonstrate disease progression to AP or BC.[12,13]

Adverse Effects and Drug Interactions

Tables 135-4 and 135-5 summarize drug–drug interactions, adverse drug reactions, and monitoring of imatinib. Imatinib-induced myelosuppression is one of the most common adverse events. Moderate-to-severe myelosuppression occurs in about 5% to 10% of patients with CP CML and in 50% to 60% of patients in AP or BC.[11-13] The myelosuppression typically occurs within the first 4 weeks of therapy and is more common in patients with advanced disease (ie, high blastic involvement of the bone marrow) and those with a low hemoglobin. Hematopoiesis in patients with CML depends on the amount of Ph-positive progenitors, although some degree of myelosuppression should be expected when the malignant clone is suppressed. However, imatinib also suppresses normal hematopoiesis, which suggests that myelosuppression associated with imatinib is probably related to effects on the Ph clone and normal hematopoietic cells. When imatinib is initiated, patients should have complete blood counts drawn every 1 to 2 weeks to assess for myelosuppression until they have stabilized.[12] Appropriate initial management of myelosuppression is to interrupt imatinib treatment, not dose reduce, as dose reductions below 300 mg daily do not fully inhibit *BCR-ABL* and may lead to the emergence of imatinib resistance.[12]

Nonhematologic toxicities associated with imatinib include gastrointestinal complications, fluid retention, myalgias and arthralgias, rash, and hepatotoxicity. Drug rash frequently occurs but is usually mild and can be managed with antihistamines or topical steroids. Severe rash, while uncommon, has been reported as an important cause for discontinuation of therapy. Algorithms for desensitization for patients that have experienced serious imatinib-associated rash have been published.[29] Hepatotoxicity can occur with imatinib, and the drug should be withheld if liver function tests exceed five times the upper limits of normal. After the liver function tests normalize, imatinib can be restarted at a reduced dose of not less than 300 mg/day. Imatinib is then dose escalated to the initial dose if liver function tests do not rise during 6 to 12 weeks of treatment. Death as a consequence of liver failure has been reported in a patient receiving large doses of acetaminophen concomitantly with imatinib. It is recommended that patients on imatinib limit their use of acetaminophen to 1,300 mg daily.[12] Other medications that are known to be hepatotoxic should be used with caution while patients are treated with imatinib.

Advanced-Generation Tyrosine Kinase Inhibitors

Dasatinib (Sprycel®) and nilotinib (Tasigna®) are approved second-generation TKIs used for the treatment of CML in patients who are resistant or intolerant to imatinib therapy; both drugs are also approved for first-line treatment of CP CML. Dasatinib is an oral *BCR-ABL* TKI that was FDA approved in 2006 for the treatment of imatinib-resistant CML. Dasatinib is an oral TKI of *BCR-ABL*, the SRC family, C-KIT, EPHA2, and PDGFR. Preclinical data show that dasatinib is 300 times more potent than imatinib and inhibits the growth of imatinib-resistant clones, with the exception of the T315I.[30] Dasatinib received accelerated approval based on hematologic and cytogenetic responses seen in imatinib-resistant or imatinib-intolerant patients.

Dasatinib has been evaluated in patients with imatinib-resistant or intolerant CP, AP, and BC CML. In a phase II trial of 186 patients in CP CML receiving dasatinib 70 mg orally twice daily a hematologic response and major cytogenetic response were noted in 90% and 52% of patients, respectively.[31] Kantarjian et al. evaluated imatinib 400 mg twice daily compared to dasatinib 70 mg twice daily in patients who developed resistance or were intolerant to imatinib 400 mg daily dosing. At 2 years follow-up, patients receiving dasatinib were more likely to achieve a complete hematologic response (93% vs 82%; P=0.034), major cytogenetic response (53% vs 33%; P = 0.023), and an increased estimated progression-free survival at 2 years, which suggests that dasatinib is superior to imatinib dose escalation in disease progression.[32] A trial evaluating different dosing strategies of dasatinib showed that 100 mg once daily was as efficacious as dasatinib 70 mg twice daily, 50 mg twice daily or 140 mg once daily but with decreased adverse events such as pleural effusions.[33] The standard dose of dasatinib for patients with CP CML is now accepted to be 100 mg daily.

Dasatinib induces responses in patients who are resistant or intolerant to imatinib with advanced disease CML. In a phase II trial of dasatinib 70 mg twice daily in patients with AP CML, 45% achieved a complete hematologic response and 39% achieved a complete cytogenetic response. At 12 months, 66% had progression-free survival and 82% were alive.[34] A phase III trial comparing dasatinib 70 mg twice daily to 140 mg once daily reported similar efficacy at 15 months

TABLE 135-5 Monitoring of Tyrosine Kinase Inhibitors in Chronic Myelogenous Leukemia

Drug	Adverse Reactions	Monitoring Parameters	Comments
Imatinib	Common: • Myelosuppression • Fluid retention (pleural/pericardial effusion, ascites, periorbital, and peripheral edema) • Nausea/vomiting • Rash • Fatigue • Hepatotoxicity • Hypothyroidism • Myalgias Rare but serious: • Congestive heart failure/left ventricular dysfunction • Hemorrhage • Bullous dermatologic reactions	• CBC for myelosuppression • CMP for hepatotoxicity • Consider baseline echocardiogram if preexisting cardiac dysfunction or risk factors for cardiac dysfunction, repeat if experiencing symptoms of cardiac dysfunction • Thyroid-stimulating hormone	Nausea and vomiting improved when drug is administered with food
Dasatinib	Common: • Myelosuppression • Myalgia • Fluid retention • Cardiotoxicity • Rash • Gastrointestinal toxicity • Hypophosphatemia • Hepatotoxicity Rare but serious: • Pleural effusion • QT prolongation • Congestive heart failure/left ventricular dysfunction • Pulmonary arterial hypertension • Hemorrhage	• CBC for myelosuppression • CMP for hypophosphatemia and hepatotoxicity • ECG if risk factors for QTc prolongation • Chest radiograph for signs and symptoms of pleural effusion • Evaluate for signs/symptoms of underlying cardiopulmonary disease for pulmonary arterial hypertension	Gastrointestinal hemorrhage reported to be fatal; severe pleural effusions requiring thoracentesis; fatal myocardial infarction are reported
Nilotinib	Common: • Myelosuppression • Rash • Gastrointestinal toxicity • Peripheral edema • Liver function abnormalities • Elevated serum lipase/amylase • Electrolyte abnormalities (hypophosphatemia, hypokalemia, hypocalcemia, and hyponatremia) Rare but serious: • Tumor lysis syndrome • Cardiotoxicity (QTc prolongation/sudden cardiac death/left ventricular dysfunction)	• CBC for myelosuppression • CMP for hypophosphatemia and hepatotoxicity • Serum amylase/lipase • ECG if risk factors for QTc prolongation at baseline, 7 days thereafter and then as clinically indicated	Sudden deaths reported with nilotinib; ventricular repolarization abnormalities may have been contributory
Bosutinib	Common: • Myelosuppression • Gastrointestinal toxicity • Fluid retention • Hepatotoxicity • Hypophosphatemia • Rash Rare but serious: • Embryofetal toxicity	• CBC for myelosuppression • CMP for hypophosphatemia and hepatotoxicity • Serum amylase/lipase • ECG if risk factors for QTc prolongation at baseline, 7 days thereafter and then as clinically indicated	Potential for additive risk of hepatotoxicity when given concurrently with letrozole
Ponatinib	Common: • Myelosuppression • Arthralgia • Headache • Fatigue • Fever • Pancreatitis • Elevated lipase • Hypertension • Gastrointestinal toxicity • Dermatologic toxicity • Electrolyte abnormalities • Fluid retention Rare but serious: • Arterial thrombosis • Hepatotoxicity • Cardiotoxicity (arrhythmia/congestive heart failure) • Embryofetal toxicity • Hemorrhage • Tumor lysis syndrome • Impaired wound healing/GI perforation	• CBC for myelosuppression • Serum lipase • CMP for hepatotoxicity, at baseline for tumor lysis syndrome • Blood pressure as clinically indicated	Deaths reported from hepatotoxicity, thrombosis including myocardial infarction and hemorrhage

CBC, complete blood count; CMP, comprehensive metabolic panel; ECG, electrocardiogram; GI, gastrointestinal.

follow-up, but an improved safety profile that established dasatinib 140 mg once daily as the preferred dosing in AP CML.[35] In patients with BC CML, dasatinib induced a hematologic response in 35% and a major cytogenetic response in 33% of patients. Median overall survival for patients receiving dasatinib in BC CML is 11.8 months.[36]

Dasatinib has been evaluated as first-line therapy in a phase III trial of 519 patients with CP CML.[37] Patients were randomized to dasatinib 100 mg once daily or imatinib 400 mg once daily. The rate of complete cytogenetic response at 5 years was higher with dasatinib as compared with imatinib (83% vs 78%, *P*=0.187). The rate of major molecular response was significantly higher in the dasatinib group (76% vs 64%, *P*<0.002). At the time of analysis, 61% of dasatinib and 63% of imatinib patients remained on study with transformation to AP/BC occurring in 4.6% of dasatinib versus 7.3% of imatinib patients. Five-year overall survival was similar in the two groups (91% dasatinib, 90% imatinib). Adverse effects were similar between the two treatment groups, with the exception that 29% of dasatinib-treated patients developed grade 1 or 2 pleural effusions.

Nilotinib has 20 to 30 times the inhibitory activity of the *BCR-ABL* tyrosine kinase than imatinib, with activity against C-KIT and PDGFR (but not SRC kinases) due to a modification of the methylpiperazinyl structure of imatinib. Nilotinib has inhibitory activity against imatinib-resistant mutants with the exception of T315I. In a phase II trial of 280 patients with imatinib-resistant or intolerant CP CML, 59% of patients treated with nilotinib 400 mg twice daily achieved a major cytogenetic response, with an estimated 4-year progression-free and overall survival of 57% and 78%, respectively.[38] In patients with AP CML treated with nilotinib 400 or 600 mg twice daily, 26% achieved a complete hematologic response and 29% achieved a major cytogenetic response.[39] For first-line treatment of CML, results of a randomized trial in 846 patients comparing nilotinib at two doses (300 or 400 mg twice daily) to imatinib 400 mg once daily have been published.[40] The primary end point of the trial was major molecular response. At 5 years, both nilotinib arms had a significantly higher major molecular response rate at 12 months (77% for nilotinib 300 and 400 mg twice daily) as compared to imatinib (60%, *P*<0.0001 for both comparisons). The nilotinib arms also had a significant improvement in the time-to-progression to the AP or BC, as compared to the imatinib arm. The number of patients discontinued from treatment was similar in all three treatment arms. Nilotinib provides an alternative to dasatinib in patients with imatinib-resistant or intolerant CP or AP CML and is one of several options in initial treatment of CP CML.[12] The phase III trial results for both dasatinib and nilotinib have made them viable alternatives to imatinib for first-line treatment for newly diagnosed CP CML.

Two other TKIs were approved for treatment of CML in 2012, bosutinib and ponatinib. Bosutinib has 15 to 100 times the inhibitory activity of the *BCR-ABL* tyrosine kinase as imatinib with activity against SRC kinases with minimal activity against C-KIT and PDGFR. Among 288 patients previously treated with imatinib, 34% achieved a major cytogenetic response at 24 weeks. Among patients previously treated with imatinib followed by dasatinib or nilotinib, 27% achieved a major cytogenetic response at 24 weeks. Grade 3 or 4 nonhematologic adverse events included diarrhea (9%), rash (9%), and vomiting (3%). Based on this study, the bosutinib dose that was recommended for phase II trials was 500 mg daily. A major cytogenetic response was observed in 32% of patients and a complete cytogenetic response was observed in 24% of patients in the phase II trials.[42]

Bosutinib 500 mg daily was compared to imatinib 400 mg daily in a phase III randomized trial of 502 patients in newly diagnosed CP CML.[43] Although the primary end point of complete cytogenetic response rate at 12 months (70% with bosutinib vs 68% with imatinib) was not significantly different observed, the rate of major molecular response was significantly higher in the bosutinib group (41% vs 27%, *P*<0.001). The incidence of adverse events was similar between the groups with the exception that bosutinib had a higher incidence of diarrhea (68% vs 21%) and imatinib had a higher incidence of edema (38% vs 11%).

Ponatinib is considered a third-generation TKI that contains a novel triple-bond linkage in its chemical structure that avoids the steric hindrance caused by the bulky isoleucine residue at position 315 in T315I *BCR-ABL* binding site cleft, providing clinical activity against this resistance phenotype.[44] In the combined phase I and II trials, 147 patients had a T315I mutated *BCR-ABL* CML in either CP, AP, BC or Ph positive ALL, the maximum tolerated dose of ponatinib was 45 mg with dose-limiting toxicities identified as pancreatitis and myelosuppression.[44,45] Of the 76 patients with CP CML, 72% achieved a complete cytogenetic response and 61% a major molecular response. Of the 45 patients with AP or BC CML, the rate of major hematologic response was 58% and 27%, respectively.[44,45] Hepatotoxicity including reports of liver failure, vascular occlusion, heart failure, and death are also included in the black box warning, several of which occurred within 1 week of starting therapy. The manufacturer recommends specific dose modifications for myelosuppression, hepatotoxicity, and elevated lipase. Due to these toxicities, the FDA requires a Risk Evaluation and Mitigation Strategy (REMS) prescribing program in patients with CML and a T315I mutation or in patients in whom no other TKI therapy is indicated.[46]

Tables 135-4 and 135-5 summarize dosing, drug interactions, adverse drug reactions, and monitoring of advanced-generation TKIs. Edema and plural effusions can be managed by dasatinib drug holiday, diuretics, or short courses of steroids. Nilotinib can be associated with indirect bilirubin elevations in 10% to 15% of patients.[38,39] Nilotinib may prolong the QTc interval (black box warning) and patients should have an electrocardiogram at baseline, at 7 days following initiation of therapy, and periodically thereafter. Based on early clinical trial data, bosutinib appears to have similar rates of adverse events of diarrhea, nausea and vomiting, rash, and abdominal discomfort.[41] Like imatinib, advanced-generation TKIs are metabolized by cytochrome P450 (CYP) 3A4. Clinicians need to be aware of possible drug interactions with inducers and inhibitors of the CYP3A4 pathway such as phenytoin, azole antifungals, or macrolide antibiotics.

Clinical **Controversy...**

The controversy of whether to use imatinib or a second-generation TKI therapy as first-line treatment for patients is ongoing. In the first-line setting, a higher proportion of patients treated with nilotinib or dasatinib achieved a major cytogenetic response and *BCR-ABL* transcripts of less than 10% at 3 and 6 months than those on imatinb. The achievement of a major molecular response, especially early in therapy, is associated with long-term disease control. However, the five-year progression-free and overall survival are not significantly different between imatinib and second-generation tyrosine kinase therapy. A generic formulation of imatinib is available that may provide cost savings for payers and patients. The NCCN guidelines currently support that either imatinib, nilotinib, or dasatinib may be used in the first line setting.[12]

Omacetaxine

Omacetaxine was approved by the FDA in October 2012 for treatment of CP or AP CML with resistance or intolerance to two or more TKIs. Omacetaxine is a first-in-class cephalotaxine ester that inhibits protein synthesis independent of direct *BCR-ABL* binding. The putative mechanism is the reduction of *BCR-ABL* oncoproteins and Mcl-1, an anti-apoptotic Bcl-2 family member, via binding to A-site cleft in the peptidyl-transferase center of the large ribosomal subunits. Efficacy with omacetaxine has been demonstrated in two patients groups: CP or AP CML resistant to two or more TKIs and patients previously treated with imatinib harboring the T315I mutation. The former group was evaluated in a combined analysis of two phase II studies for CP and AP CML. Omacetaxine was administered at 1.25 mg/m^2 subcutaneously twice daily for 14 consecutive days every 28 days then for 7 days every 28 days as maintenance.[47] Of the 122 patients enrolled, 81 had CP CML of which 20% achieved a major cytogenetic response, 10% achieved a complete cytogenetic response, with a median overall survival of 34 months.

A phase II trial of omacetaxine was conducted in 62 CP CML patients with a history of the T315I mutation.[48] Patients were treated with the induction regimen as above and transitioned to maintenance when the patient achieved a hematologic response. Hematologic response was achieved in 77%, complete cytogenetic response in 16%, and major cytogenetic response in 23% of patients. The median duration of complete hematologic response was 9.1 months, and major cytogenetic response was 6.6 months. The majority of grade 3/4 toxicities reported in these trials were myelosuppression with occasional reports of myalgias and arthralgias and gastrointestinal toxicity.

Hematopoietic Stem Cell Transplantation

5 Allogeneic HSCT remains the only therapy proven to cure patients with CML, with many patients alive and disease-free decades after transplant. Patients undergoing allogeneic HSCT from a human leukocyte antigen (HLA)-matched sibling donor have 5-year survival rates ranging from 60% to 80% and long-term survival of about 50%.[49,50] In most long-term survivors, the *BCR-ABL* translocation is absent in all diagnostic tests including RT-PCR. Prognostic risk factors associated with survival outcomes include age, phase of disease, and disease duration. Increasing age is associated with poorer prognosis, with higher transplant-related mortality in patients older than age 50 years. Patients with CP who receive allogeneic HSCT have better outcomes than those in AP or BC. The time from diagnosis to transplantation also affects outcomes. Patients who undergo matched-sibling allogeneic HSCT within the first year of diagnosis have a better 5-year survival rate than those who undergo transplantation more than 1 year after their diagnosis (70%-80% vs 50%-60%).[49,50] These data were reported prior to the use of imatinib as first-line therapy for CML.

The major limitation for broad application of HSCT is that fewer than 30% of patients who are transplant-eligible will have an HLA-matched sibling donor. The most practical approach is to use an HLA-matched unrelated donor, if available. Matched unrelated donor HSCT has an overall 5-year survival reported to be 40% to 70%, which approaches overall survival data results reported for matched-sibling donor HSCT.[7,12,49,50] The advent of TKI therapy has resulted in fewer transplants for CML. Data collected to date appear to show that imatinib use prior to transplantation does not negatively affect transplant-related mortality.[51]

Treatment options in patients who relapse after HSCT are limited. Graft-versus-leukemia (GVL) effect, TKIs, omacetaxine, IFN-α, or a clinical trial are reasonable options. The infusion of donor lymphocytes functions as a form of adoptive immunotherapy that can induce a GVL effect. In relapsed CML, donor lymphocytes induce durable responses and these responses strongly correlate with the development of graft-versus-host disease (GVHD).[52] Tumor burden also predicts the likelihood of response to donor lymphocyte infusion in relapsed CML. The optimal method of administering donor lymphocytes remains unclear, but these data suggest it may be possible to partially separate the GVL effect from GVHD.

Imatinib has been used in patients who have residual disease after allogeneic HSCT. Most patients respond to imatinib with complete molecular response of 70%.[53] Use of imatinib or other TKI therapies require further study to determine the magnitude of benefit when applied in the post-HSCT setting.[54] The role of nonmyeloablative transplants in CML is evolving, but preliminary results suggest comparable outcomes to myeloablative transplants. Data from a German registry suggest that 17% of all transplants for CML use a reduced-intensity conditioning regimen.[55]

Personalized Pharmacotherapy

Personalized treatment of CML is mostly directed following initiation of second-line therapy. Mutational analysis of binding sites that confer resistance to TKIs should be evaluated if initial response is inadequate, or the milestones of complete cytogenetic response or major molecular response are lost, or if any signs of disease progression in the form of AP or BC are noted.[12,13] The results of this analysis will guide selection of the appropriate TKI as second-line therapy.[12,13,56] In addition, with the advent of omacetaxine and ponatinib, two agents are now available that are active against the T315I mutation that confers resistance to the rest of the TKIs.

Preliminary data support the role of therapeutic drug monitoring of TKIs in CML. Trough imatinib levels of ≥1 μmol/L have been associated in patients with a higher response than those with <1 μmol/L.[57] Data on nilotinib and dasatinib are more limited. The clinical applicability of therapeutic drug monitoring is still to be determined because the drug assays are not yet commercially available.

Evaluation of Therapeutic Outcomes

Current standard of care is for patients with newly diagnosed CP CML to receive imatinib or one of the second-generation TKIs. The goal of disease monitoring in CML is to differentiate patients who have optimally responded to an initial course of TKI therapy from those at high risk for treatment failure. With imatinib, nilotinib, and dasatinib as appropriate options for frontline therapy for newly diagnosed CP CML, and bosutinib, ponatinib, and omacetaxine approved for salvage therapy, clinicians have a large number of treatment options to consider before allogeneic HSCT. Future research opportunities will focus on how to select second-, third-, and fourth-line therapies and whether combination therapy provides additional long-term benefit.

CHRONIC LYMPHOCYTIC LEUKEMIA

Epidemiology and Etiology

Chronic lymphocytic leukemia is a lymphoproliferative disorder characterized by accumulation of functionally incompetent clonal B lymphocytes.[58] Chronic lymphocytic leukemia is the most common form of leukemia in the United States, but is rare in other countries, such as Japan and China. It is estimated that 18,960 new cases of CLL will be diagnosed in the United States in 2016.[1] Occasional family clusters have been recognized, and first-degree relatives of patients with CLL are at three times the risk of developing a lymphoid malignancy as compared with the general population. Chronic lymphocytic leukemia is a disease of the elderly, with a median age of 71 years, although 20% to 30% of CLL occurs in patients who are younger than 55 years of age. Male sex, white race, family history, and advanced age are known risk factors for the disease.

Pathophysiology

Chronic lymphocytic leukemia cells are comprised of a neoplastic clone of CD5$^+$ cells, which express low levels of surface-membrane immunoglobulin M (IgM) and immunoglobulin D (IgD) compared to normal peripheral blood B cells. Normal CD5$^+$ B lymphocytes are present in the lymph nodes and in the blood. Neoplastic CD5$^+$ cells accumulate in the lymph nodes and spleen because of the loss of apoptosis by either the overexpression of an oncogene, such as *bcl-1* or *2*, or loss of a tumor suppressor gene, such as *RB1*.[58] The bcl-2 protein is a major regulator of apoptosis or programmed cell death.

Evidence is emerging that antigenic stimulation and cytokines drive the proliferation of the CLL cells.

Although CLL lacks a common genetic target as observed in CML, B-cell-receptor signaling has emerged as a driving factor for CLL tumor survival. Bruton's tyrosine kinase (BTK), a member of the Tec family of kinases, is essential for the activation of several constitutively active pathways for CLL cell survival. Bruton's tyrosine kinase leads to activation of the Akt, extracellular signal-regulated kinase (ERK), and nuclear factor kappa light-chain enhancer of active B-cells (NF-κβ) pathways.[59] Additionally, BTK is required for B-cell chemokine-mediated homing and adhesion. Phosphatidylinosital 3-Kinase (PI3K) is a lipid kinas that has a catalytic subunit with four different isoforms: α, β, γ, and δ. When PI3K is activated, it generates phospholipid messengers on the cell membrane that recruit and activate various intracellular enzymes that regulate cell motility, survival, and proliferation.[60] The δ isoform plays a critical role in normal B-cell development, function, and transducing signals from receptors. The PI3Kδ signaling pathway is hyperactive in CLL and other B-cell cancers.

A monoclonal population of B cells with a similar surface antigen phenotype as CLL cells has been recently identified in patients up to several years prior to diagnosis of the disease.[61] This phenomenon, termed monoclonal B-cell lymphocytosis (MBL) appears to predict whether a patient is at risk for developing CLL over time. In a cohort of 77,000 patients enrolled in a cancer screening trial, 45 patients were diagnosed with CLL throughout the duration of the study. Baseline blood samples collected on enrollment of the screening trial were analyzed for the patients who developed CLL. MBL was present in 44 of 45 of the patients by either flow cytometric or molecular analysis (ie, RT-PCR assay) and confirmed in 41 of 45 of these patients by both methods. Samples predated the diagnosis of CLL in a time period ranging from 6 months to 6.4 years. This finding could lead to potentially earlier diagnosis and intervention for CLL.

Cytogenetic abnormalities correlate with disease progression in CLL. About 80% of patients with CLL have a karyotypic abnormality. The chromosomes that are most frequently involved include chromosomes 11, 12, 13, and 17.[62] Additional cytogenetic abnormalities may be acquired during therapy, particularly with deletions of chromosome 17, which have an adverse effect on survival.[63] Somatic point mutations have been identified in a cohort of 91 patients yielding nine mutated genes: *TP53*, *ATM*, *MYD88*, *NOTCH1*, *SF3B1*, *ZMYM3*, *MAPK1*, *FBXW7*, and *DDX3X*.[64] These mutations were associated with cell-cycle and DNA repair pathways, intracellular signaling, inflammatory pathways, and RNA splicing and processing. A correlation was identified with *SF3B1* and chromosome 11 deletions providing insight into how these mutations may impact clinical outcomes.

About 4% of patients with CLL will undergo transformation of their disease to an aggressive non-Hodgkin lymphoma (diffuse large B cell), which is termed as *Richter's syndrome*. Richter's syndrome may be triggered by accumulation of additional cytogenetic abnormalities in the malignant clone of lymphocytes or by viral infections, such as Epstein-Barr's virus.[65]

CLINICAL PRESENTATION Chronic Lymphocytic Leukemia

Constitutional Symptoms

- Fever, fatigue, weight loss

Physical Examination

- Lymphadenopathy (87%)
- Splenomegaly (54%)
- Hepatomegaly (14%)

Laboratory Tests

- Peripheral blood
  - Lymphocytosis
  - Coombs-positive autoimmune hemolytic anemia
  - Hyper- or hypogammaglobulinemia
  - Monoclonal gammopathy
  - Anemia
  - Thrombocytopenia
- Bone marrow
  - Hypercellular
  - Increased mature lymphocytes
  - Increased megakaryocytes
- Molecular markers
  - Cytogenetics (17p-)
  - ZAP-70 mutations

Staging and Prognosis

Survival times for patients with CLL are widely variable, with some patients succumbing to disease within 3 years and others living into a second decade from the time of diagnosis. The Rai and the Binet staging systems are commonly used in CLL with the Rai being favored in the United States and the Binet in Europe. The Rai staging system has been combined into a risk classification scheme: low risk (stage 0), intermediate risk (stages I and II), and high risk (stages III and IV) with median survivals of greater than 10 years, 7 years, and 2 to 4 years, respectively.[58,66]

The disease course for CLL varies within each stage such that one patient may have an indolent course with long survival time, while another patient may have more aggressive disease and a relatively short survival time. The Rai and Binet staging systems incompletely predict for individual patients who may experience more rapid disease progression. Patients with Richter's syndrome will have a rapidly advancing disease course that mimics diffuse large B-cell non-Hodgkin lymphoma. However, successful treatment of the diffuse large B-cell non-Hodgkin lymphoma with combination chemotherapy will not eradicate the underlying clone of CLL cells and patients will ultimately relapse.[65]

Biomarkers, such as CD38 expression and ζ-associated protein 70 (ZAP-70) expression, have been explored as prognostic factors for CLL. CD38 is a cell-surface antigen that is associated with early progression, significantly shorter overall survival, and a poor response to fludarabine.[58,67,68] ZAP-70 is an intracellular protein with tyrosine kinase activity. Once considered as simply a surrogate marker for the unmutated variable region of the immunoglobulin heavy chain gene (IGHV), elevated ZAP-70 expression appears to predict for rapid CLL disease progression and independently correlates with prognosis.[66,68]

Cytogenetic changes such as deletion of the short arm of chromosome 17 (17p-), which corresponds to p53 silencing, can be biomarkers of poor response to therapy. A prospective study showed that newly diagnosed patients with 17p- had a median time-to-progression following first-line therapy with either fludarabine or fludarabine and cyclophosphamide of 10 to 12 months.[63] Patients with chromosomal abnormalities of 11, 12, 13, and 17 have reported median survivals of 133 months, 114 months, 79 months, and 32 months, respectively.[62]

TREATMENT
Chronic Lymphocytic Leukemia

Desired Outcomes

6 The primary goals of treatment for CLL are to achieve and maintain remission duration with minimal treatment-related toxicity. The management of patients with CLL is highly individualized with some patients receiving therapy on diagnosis, while other patients with early-stage disease are managed expectantly. Indications for starting treatment include disease-related symptoms (fatigue, night sweats, weight loss, and fever), threatened end-organ function, bulky disease, doubling of lymphocyte doubling time in less than 6 months, progressive anemia, and platelet count less than 100,000/mm^3 (100 × 10^9/L).[70,71] Consideration of initial treatment options is based on several factors including patient age, disease stage, and high-risk prognostic factors, such as deletion 17p- or 11q.

Most stage 0 patients do not require treatment and can be managed with observation. In patients with stage I disease, treatment is controversial. A consistent survival benefit from early therapy has not been reported in asymptomatic patients.[70,71] Cytotoxic chemotherapy in early stage CLL is usually reserved for patients who have disease characteristics consistent with a more aggressive course, such as short lymphocyte doubling times and presence of biologic markers such as ZAP-70 or high-risk cytogenetics. In stages II through IV disease, treatment is required, with the goal of achieving a partial or complete remission. Table 135-6 shows the regimens used to treat newly diagnosed and previously treated CLL.[69-71]

TABLE 135-6 Treatment for Newly Diagnosed and Previously Treated Chronic Lymphocytic Leukemia

Treatment	Overall Response (%)	Complete Response (%)
Chlorambucil		
Untreated	37	4
Fludarabine alone		
Untreated	60-80	20-30
Previously treated	13-59	3-37
Fludarabine + cyclophosphamide		
Untreated	80-90	25-40
Previously treated	60-70	10-15
Rituximab alone		
Untreated	50-60	10-20
Previously treated	80-90	20-40
Fludarabine + rituximab		
Untreated	80-100	30-50
Previously treated	80-90	20-40
Fludarabine + cyclophosphamide + rituximab		
Untreated	95	70
Previously treated	73	25
Alemtuzumab alone		
Untreated	80-90	20-30
Previously treated	30-50	0-20
Alemtuzumab + fludarabine		
Previously treated	83	17-30
Bendamustine + rituximab		
Untreated	97	38
Previously treated	60	9
Ofatumumab + chlorambucil		
Untreated	82	12
Obinutuzumab		
Previously treated	30-62	0-5
Obinutuzumab + chlorambucil		
Untreated	78	20
Ibrutinib		
Previously treated	71	5
Idelalisib + rituximab		
Previously treated	81	0

Cytotoxic Chemotherapy

Orally administered alkylating agents such as chlorambucil and cyclophosphamide, given either alone or with corticosteroids, historically have been used as primary treatment for CLL. Results from a meta-analysis involving 2,048 patients from six randomized controlled studies evaluated low-dose alkylating agents in CLL.[72] That analysis showed that delayed treatment with alkylating agents in asymptomatic patients did not adversely affect 10-year survival. More importantly, if only deaths caused by CLL were considered, significantly longer survival was observed when treatment was deferred. Chlorambucil continues to be used in elderly, symptomatic patients as initial treatment for CLL, but its use is based on a small number of studies with no demonstrable survival advantage.[71,72] Commonly used dosing schedules for chlorambucil are intermittent pulse dosing of 15 to 40 mg/m^2 orally every 28 days or daily doses of 4 to 8 mg/m^2/day.[71] The dose of chlorambucil is often titrated to circumvent myelosuppression.

Cyclophosphamide produces a similar response rate as chlorambucil (overall response rate: 40%-60%; complete response: 4%) and can be used in patients who cannot tolerate chlorambucil or in whom response is not optimal. Some patients who do not respond to chlorambucil will respond to single-agent cyclophosphamide. Cyclophosphamide is typically given orally at a daily dose of 1 to 3 mg/kg. Oral cyclophosphamide is less commonly used than chlorambucil because of the risk of hemorrhagic cystitis and bladder cancer with prolonged treatment.

Fludarabine-based therapy is a common initial treatment in CLL. It is particularly useful in younger patients and in those patients who can tolerate immunosuppressive chemotherapy. Fludarabine, along with the other purine analogs, 2-chlorodeoxyadenosine (cladribine) and 2-deoxycoformycin (pentostatin), are highly active in CLL, with fludarabine being the most widely studied agent in the class in the treatment of CLL.[70-73] Most patients receive fludarabine 25 to 30 mg/m^2 IV daily for 5 days when used as a single agent. Cladribine and pentostatin have similar activity, although head-to-head trials comparing these three nucleosides have not been conducted.[73-75]

Fludarabine was initially studied in CLL patients who were refractory to chlorambucil. Several trials reported overall response rates to fludarabine in previously treated patients ranging from 13% to 59% and complete response rates of 3% to 37%.[74-77] Fludarabine has higher overall response and complete remission rates than alkylating-based therapies in the frontline setting. In one of the randomized studies that compared fludarabine to chlorambucil in chemotherapy-naïve patients, fludarabine-treated patients had a higher complete remission rate as compared with chlorambucil (20% vs 5%).[75] However, the higher complete remission rate did not translate into a significant difference in overall survival and patients treated with fludarabine had a higher rate of severe neutropenia and infection. The study allowed chlorambucil failures to cross over to fludarabine, which may have hampered the ability to show a survival advantage in the fludarabine arm. A recent review of younger patients enrolled in a large phase III trial showed that 33% of patients receiving fludarabine or fludarabine-based therapy had infectious complications.[76] An increase in *Pneumocystis* infections was not observed, but a 6% increase in herpes and varicella zoster infection was documented. Dose reductions occurred frequently as a result of the infectious episodes. Based on the increased risk of infectious complications, some practitioners recommend antiviral and antibacterial prophylaxis with treatment.[72,76,77]

Bendamustine is an alkylating agent that contains a purine-derivative benzimidazole ring in its chemical structure that yields a compound that is non–cross-resistant with other alkylating agents. Bendamustine induces cell death via single and double-stranded cross-links.[78] The efficacy of bendamustine was established as first-line agent in Binet stage B or C CLL in a phase III trial that randomized 319 patients to bendamustine or chlorambucil.[79,80] Complete response rates of 31% versus 2% and an overall response rate for 68% versus 31% were observed for bendamustine and chlorambucil, respectively. The median progression-free survival was 21.2 versus 8.8 months favoring bendamustine ($P<0.0001$). The median overall survival was not reached in the bendamustine group and was 78.8 months in the chlorambucil group. Adverse events reported for bendamustine include hematologic toxicity in about 25% of patients, and gastrointestinal and cutaneous toxicity.

Biologic Therapy

Monoclonal antibodies, such as rituximab and alemtuzumab, are increasingly being used in the treatment of CLL. Rituximab is a chimeric monoclonal antibody that targets the CD20 antigen expressed on B lymphocytes. Rituximab was initially approved for patients with indolent non-Hodgkin lymphoma and later for aggressive non-Hodgkin lymphoma. Rituximab received FDA approval for the treatment of CD20-positive CLL in 2010. CLL cells have less prominent CD20 expression on their surface as compared to non-Hodgkin lymphoma, which may explain the lower clinical response. Efficacy with rituximab as a single agent in CLL is moderate with a 58% overall response rate reported with 9% complete responses.[70,71] Subsequent studies have used higher rituximab doses (up to 500 mg/m^2 per cycle) when given in combination with other agents.

7 Alemtuzumab is a monoclonal antibody that targets the CD52 antigen found on both B and T lymphocytes (Fig. 135-2). This agent was initially FDA approved in 2001 for the treatment of patients with CLL who had been treated with alkylating agents and had failed fludarabine therapy and is now approved as a single agent for both frontline and salvage treatment of CLL. Alemtuzumab is titrated to a maintenance dose of 30 mg IV or subcutaneously given 3 times a week for 12 weeks. As a single agent, alemtuzumab has produced response rates from 33% to 53% in patients with refractory disease, but complete responses are infrequent.[81-83]

Results from a randomized phase III trial comparing alemtuzumab to chlorambucil in chemotherapy-naïve patients with symptomatic CLL showed higher complete response rates with alemtuzumab than with chlorambucil, 24% versus 2%, respectively.[81] These differences in response rate translated into a significant difference in progression-free survival (hazard ratio, 0.58; 95% confidence interval, 0.43-0.77, $P<0.0001$).

Infusion-related reactions are one of the most frequently reported toxicities with alemtuzumab. The reactions experienced with IV administration include fever, rigors, and hypotension.[82] Alemtuzumab is associated with serious, potentially life-threatening toxicities, including pancytopenia, infusion reactions, and opportunistic infections. Because of alemtuzumab's profound immunosuppression, the 2015 NCCN guidelines recommend antibacterial and antiviral prophylaxis to prevent *Cytomegalovirus* reactivation and *Pneumocystis* infections.[71] Prophylaxis with trimethoprim-sulfamethoxazole and famciclovir or valacyclovir is recommended with the use of alemtuzumab.[71,82] Alemtuzumab is FDA-approved for IV administration, although the use of subcutaneous alemtuzumab has been evaluated to reduce the frequency of these reactions. In a study by Lundin et al. 41 patients received 30 mg of subcutaneous alemtuzumab three times a week for 12 weeks, which yielded a response rate of 87%.[83] Major adverse event were grades 1 and 2 skin reactions in 90% of patients; fever, rigors, and hypotension were infrequent. About 10% of patients had reactivation of *Cytomegalovirus* and required ganciclovir treatment. Similar to IV administration, antiviral and antibacterial prophylaxis is warranted when alemtuzumab is given via the subcutaneous route.[83]

Ofatumumab is a fully human monoclonal antibody to CD20 that was approved as single-agent therapy in 2009 for patients with CLL that is refractory to fludarabine and alemtuzumab. Ofatumumab is administered as an IV infusion with an initial dose of 300 mg then four weekly doses followed by four monthly doses of 2,000 mg. An overall response rate of 58% in patients with fludarabine and alemtuzumab refractory disease and 47% in bulky fludarabine refractory disease was reported.[84] Median time-to-progression was 5.7 and 5.9 months and median overall survival 13.7 and 15.4 months in the fludarabine, alemtuzumab refractory patients and bulky fludarabine

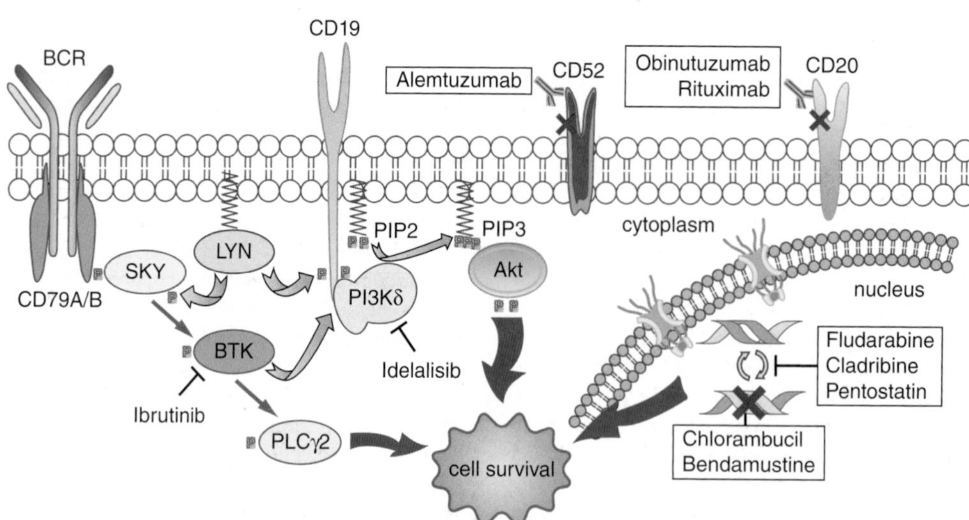

FIGURE 135-2 Current treatments and their molecular targets in chronic lymphocytic leukemia *(Reprinted with permission from Manman W, Wang X, Song Z, et al. Targeting PI3Kδ: Emerging Therapy for Chronic Lymphocytic Leukemia and Beyond. Med Res Rev 2015;35:720-752. Copyright © 2015 John Wiley and Sons. All rights reserved.)*

refractory disease patients, respectively. Adverse events reported in greater than 10% of patients included infection and neutropenia. Infusion-related events were reported in about 60% of patients, 40% during the first infusion, and 25% with the second infusion. Serious toxicities such as fatal infections, progressive multifocal leukoencephalopathy, and hepatitis B reactivation have been reported.

The efficacy of first-line ofatumumab was studied in a phase III trial of 447 patients with previously untreated CLL.[85] Median progression-free survival was significantly longer in the ofatumumab and chlorambucil group versus the chlorambucil alone group (22.4 vs 13.1 months). Grade III toxicity including neutropenia and infusion-related events were reported more frequently in the combination arm although the overall infection rate was similar in both treatment arms. These results led to the approval of ofatumumab in combination with chlorambucil in previously untreated CLL for whom fludarabine-based therapy is considered inappropriate.

Combination Therapy

The single-agent activity of fludarabine has led to incorporation of fludarabine in combination regimens in patients with CLL. The most widely studied combination is fludarabine with cyclophosphamide, which produces complete response rates between 25% and 40% in treatment-naïve patients as compared with 20% to 30% for single-agent fludarabine.[70-75] Although improved response rates and progression-free survival have been reported with fludarabine and cyclophosphamide combinations compared with fludarabine alone, no benefit in overall survival has been observed.

8 The combination of fludarabine and rituximab has promising activity. In vitro studies suggest that rituximab is synergistic with fludarabine and cyclophosphamide and has led investigators to evaluate this combination in clinical trials. Results from an uncontrolled trial of fludarabine, cyclophosphamide, and rituximab (FCR) reported a complete remission rate of 70% in previously untreated CLL patients.[86] FCR has documented a complete remission rate of 25% in previous treated patients. Results of two phase III trials comparing FCR with fludarabine and cyclophosphamide documented a progression-free survival benefit (30 vs 20 months) in patients treated with FCR in patients with refractory disease and an overall survival benefit (87.2% vs 82.5%) in patients with newly diagnosed disease.[87,88] The results of these phase III trials led to FDA approval of rituximab with fludarabine and cyclophosphamide in CLL.

Bendamustine and rituximab (BR) have been combined in two phase II studies in patients with CLL, in the frontline and relapsed setting.[89,90] In the frontline setting, 117 patients were treated with bendamustine 90 mg/m^2 days 1 and 2 and rituximab 375 mg/m^2 IV on day 0 for cycle 1 and then 500 mg/m^2 IV on day 1 for subsequent cycles.[89] Overall, 88% of patients had a clinical response with 23% being complete responses. The median EFS was 34 months with 90% of patients reported being alive at the median follow-up time point of 27 months. Patients with 17p- responded less well, with a 37.5% overall response rate. Grade 3/4 myelosuppression was observed in about 20% of patients. BR is currently being compared to FCR in previously untreated fit patients with CLL. An interim analysis showed overall response rates of 97.8% for both regimens, but the FCR group had a higher complete response rate (47.4% vs 38.1%, P=0.031) and 2-year progression-free survival (85% vs 78.2%, P=0.041).[90] The advantages of FCR need to be balanced by a higher risk of severe adverse events, in particular neutropenia (81.7% vs 56.8%; P<0.001) and infections (39% vs 25.4%; P<0.001) associated with FCR. Based on these results no firm recommendations of FCR or BR can be made in the first-line setting. The risks and benefits of FCR and BR should be discussed with the patient because no overall survival advantage has been reported.

In the relapsed setting, BR was administered as above with the exception of a lower bendamustine dose of 70 mg/m^2 in 78 patients who had received a median of two prior treatments.[91] The overall response rate was 59%, with 9% of patients having a complete response. With a median follow-up of 24 months, the EFS was 14.7 months with a median overall survival of 34 months. About 25% of patients experienced grade 3/4 myelosuppression with three treatment-related deaths related to infection.

Obinutuzumab is a glycoengineered type II anti-CD20 monoclonal antibody that does not induce translocation of CD20 monoclonal antibody complexes or complement-dependent cytotoxicity, but rather stimulates direct cell death via actin reorganization and homotypic adehesion.[91] Obinutuzumab was FDA approved in 2013 in combination with chorlambucil in patients with previously untreated CLL. A Phase III trial randomized 781 patients to one of three groups: 1) chlorambucil 0.5 mg/kg on days 1 to 15; 2) obinutuzumab 1,000 mg on days 1, 8, 15, of cycle 1 and day 1 on cycles 2 through 6 plus chlorambucil; 3) rituximab 375 mg/m^2 on day 1 of cycle 1 then 500 mg/m^2 on day 1 of cycles 2 through 6 plus chlorambucil. Progression-free survival was increased with obinutuzumab and chlorambucil (26.7 months) compared to rituximab and chlorambucil (16.3 months) or chlorambucil (11.1 months).[92] Overall survival favored obinutuzumab and chlorambucil compared to chlorambucil monotherapy (hazard ratio 0.41; 95% CI 0.23-0.74; P=0.002). Treatment with obinutuzumab and chlorambucil versus rituximab and chlorambucil resulted in longer progression-free survival (hazard ratio 0.39; 95% CI 0.31-0.49; P<0.001) and higher rates of complete response (70% vs 20.7%). Infusion-related reactions and neutropenia were more common with the obinutuzumab group than rituximab, but the risk of infection was similar.

9 Targeted Therapy

Ibrutinib is an orally administered compound that covalently binds to the cysteine-481 amino acid of the BTK enzyme and inhibits signaling of ERK, NF-κB, and cytosine phosphate-guanine mediated tumor cell proliferation and migration.[59] Ibrutinib was FDA approved in 2014 for the treatment of CLL. In the phase Ib/II trial, 85 patients with relapsed or refractory CLL received ibrutinib at 420 mg or 840 mg by mouth daily.[59] The overall response rate was 71% for both groups with a partial response observed in 20% and 15%, respectively. In a phase III trial, ibrutinib was compared to ofatumumab in patients with relapsed or refractory CLL with a primary endpoint of progression-free survival.[93] Median progression-free survival in the ibrutinib groups was not reached as compared to 8.1 months in the ofatumumab group (hazard ratio 0.22, 95% CI 0.15-0.32; P<0.001). The overall response rate was significantly higher in the ibrutinib group at 42.6% versus 4.1% with ofatumumab (P<0.001). Overall survival at 12 months also favored ibrutinib, 90% versus 81%. The response rate among patients with a 17p-deletion was 68%, including one complete response, highlighting the ability of ibruitnib to overcome resistance associated with purine analogues and alkylating agents. The most frequent nonhematologic adverse events were diarrhea, fatigue, fever, and nausea. A toxicity unique to ibrutinib is lymphocytosis (69%) secondary to tumor cell mobilization to the peripheral blood. This lymphocytosis is not an indicator of disease progression and ibrutinib should be continued at the standard dose.

Idelalisib is a small-molecule inhibitor of PI3Kδ and interferes with the PI3Kδ-AKT signaling pathway leading to increased apoptosis.[60] Idelalisib 150 mg taken orally twice a day plus rituximab was compared to rituximab plus placebo in a randomized phase III trial in patients with relapsed CLL who had comorbidities that precluded them from being treated with standard chemotherapy.[60] Patients may not have been eligible for systemic chemotherapy for the following reasons: severe neutropenia or thrombocytopenia, an estimated glomular filtration rate of less than 60 mL/min/1.73 m^2, or a score of 6 or more on the Cumulative Illness Rating Scale. The primary endpoint of progression-free survival was not reached in the idelalisib group compared to 5.5 months in the rituximab monotherapy group ($P<0.001$). The overall response rate also favored the idelalisib group, 81% versus 13% ($P<0.001$) as did the 12 months overall survival, 92% versus 80% ($P=0.02$). Black box warnings include hepatic dysfunction, severe diarrhea, colitis, intestinal perforation, and pneumonitis. Patients should have complete blood counts and hepatic function monitored prior to initiation and throughout treatment.

It should be noted that both ibrutinib and idelalisib are metabolized by cytochrome P450 (CYP) 3A4. Therefore, clinicians need to be aware of possible drug interactions with inducers and inhibitors of the CYP3A4 pathway such as phenytoin, azole antifungals, or macrolide antibiotics.

Clinical **Controversy...**

Certain molecular and cellular markers have been identified that may predict CLL disease progression. ZAP-70 expression, CD38 expression, IGHV mutations, and 17p- are associated with a more aggressive clinical course of CLL. Controversy surrounds whether or not treatment should be based on these biologic markers alone. 17p- is the most consistent poor prognostic marker and results in a loss of the tumor suppressor gene, p53. Consensus guidelines delineate treatment options for patients based on the presence of 17p-. If a patient has 17p- more aggressive regimens that contain immunotherapy and purine analogs (eg, fludarabine, cyclophosphamide, and rituximab) are potential first-line treatments. Given that ibrutinib is active against CLL with 17p- it is also a potential first line treatment option. Head-to-head comparisons of ibrutinib versus chemoimmunotherpay in the first line setting are lacking and require further evaluation.[71]

Hematopoietic Stem Cell Transplantation

The experience with the use of HSCT in CLL is limited. Patients treated with allogeneic HSCT achieve higher remission rates and appear to have a longer disease-free survival, but is associated with high treatment-related mortality, which approaches 40%. Contrary to the high mortality reported in most studies, a randomized phase II study of high-risk CLL patients comparing allogeneic and autologous HSCT reported 100-day mortality of 4% in both arms. After 6 years of follow-up, no difference in overall survival (58% autologous and 55% allogeneic) was observed.[93] This low early mortality must be interpreted carefully, given that only 25 carefully selected patients received allogeneic HSCT as compared with 137 who received autologous HSCT. T-cell depletion was performed on the allogeneic grafts, which may reduce 100-day mortality at the cost of increased relapse, infectious complications, or posttransplant lymphoproliferative disorders as a consequence of reduced GVL effect.[94]

Although allogeneic HSCT may offer the potential of cure in CLL, the advanced age of most patients, limited donor availability, and the high treatment-related mortality precludes the routine application in the management of this disease. Allogeneic HSCT is a more viable option for younger patients with aggressive disease. Older patients who are not candidates for full-intensity allogeneic HSCT may be candidates for nonmyeloablative allogeneic HSCT.

Immunotherapy

The use of immunotherapy in CLL had been considered as a potential treatment strategy because of the presence of tumor specific antigens such as CD19. The modification of autologous T cells expressing an anti-CD19 chimeric antigen receptor (CART19) has been explored in patients with refractory CLL.[95] Autologous T cells are collected via leukapheresis and treated with a self-inactivating lentiviral vector to express the CD19 specific chimeric antigen receptor concurrently with the costimulatory CD137 signaling domain. Modified cells are kept for about two weeks for expansion and then harvested for infusion. Patients receive a preparative regimen of standard CLL-directed chemotherapy with the goal of lymphodepleting the patients and enhancing the proliferation of the infused T-cells. A cell dose of about 3×10^8 autologous transduced-T cells is administered within several days of completion of chemotherapy.

In the largest single-center experience, 45 highly refractory CLL patients have been treated with this approach.[95] Overall response rate was reported to be 45% with small numbers of patients having documented persistence of the genetically-modified T-cell population lasting beyond 3 years. Toxicity with the procedure is notable for the expected toxicities of the chemotherapy preparative treatment, cytokine release syndrome, hypogammaglobinemia and B-cell aplasia. Cytokine release syndrome is believed to be an interleukin-6 mediated event characterized by escalating fevers (>40°C), myalgias, nausea, vomiting and diarrhea. Severe cases of cytokine release syndrome can progress to hypotension, capillary leak, and hypoxia requiring critical care level support.

Personalized Pharmacotherapy

Molecular biomarkers are important as predictors for disease time to progression, decision making for initiation of treatment, and prognosis. The most important are cytogenetic abnormalities such as deletion 17p- and 11q, which are associated with more aggressive disease that is less responsive to treatment. Unmutated status of the immunoglobulin heavy chain variable gene locus and overexpression of ZAP-70 and CD38 expression are also predictive of poor prognosis.

The 2015 NCCN guidelines recommend treatment options based on the presence of deletion 17p- or 11q, age older or younger than 70 years, and first- and second-line regimens.[71] Preferred first-line therapy options for patients younger than 70 years without poor-risk cytogenetics or significant comorbidities are aggressive chemoimmunotherapy regimens such as bendamustine, rituximab; fludarabine, cyclophosphamide, rituximab; fludarabine, rituximab; and pentostatin, cyclophosphamide, and rituximab. In patients who are older than 70 years without poor-risk cytogenetics preferred chemotherapy options include: obinutuzumab, chlorambucil; ofatumumab, chlorambucil; rituximab, chlorambucil; or bendamustine, rituximab. In frail patients or those with significant comorbidities and unable to tolerate purine analogs preference of first line therapy may include: obinutuzumab, chlorambucil; ofatumumab, chlorambucil; or rituximab, chlorambucil. The current standard of care for relapsed or refractory CLL is ibrutinib monotherapy and idelalisib plus rituximab.[70,71] For patients who have poor-risk cytogenetics such as 17p- deletion, first-line therapy options consist primarily of more aggressive chemoimmunotherapy treatment options (FCR; fludarabine and rituximab; high-dose methylprednisolone and rituximab) or targeted therapy with ibrutinib. Preferred second-line regimens include ibrutinib or idelalisib plus rituximab regardless of age or comorbidities.[70,71]

Evaluation of Therapeutic Outcomes

Chronic lymphocytic leukemia is an incurable disease and the goal of therapy is to optimize remission duration while minimizing the burden of treatment-related adverse effects. Supportive care for patients undergoing active treatment for CLL is crucial for ensuring a successful outcome. Patients may become hypogammaglobinemic as a consequence of disease progression or treatment will need routine monitoring of serum IgG. If the serum IgG falls below 500 mg/dL (5 g/L), then monthly replacement doses of 300 to 500 mg/kg of IV immune globulin is warranted. Antibiotic prophylaxis for patients receiving fludarabine-based regimens or chemoimmunotherapy should be considered for herpes virus and *Pneumocystis*. Patients who are treated with alemtuzumab will require monitoring for cytomegalovirus (CMV) antigen every 1 to 2 weeks while on therapy and for 2 months after or be given prophylaxis with valganciclovir.

ABBREVIATIONS

ABL	Abelson proto-oncogene
ALL	acute lymphoblastic leukemia
AP	accelerated phase
ATP	adenosine triphosphate
BC	blast crisis
BCR	breakpoint cluster region
BTK	Bruton's tyrosine kinase
CHOP	cyclophosphamide, hydroxydaunorubicin, vincristine, prednisone
CLL	chronic lymphocytic leukemia
CML	chronic myelogenous leukemia
CMV	cytomegalovirus
CNS	central nervous system
CP	chronic phase
CYP	cytochrome P450
EFS	event-free survival
ERK	extracellular signal-regulated kinase
FCR	fludarabine, cyclophosphamide, rituximab
FDA	Food and Drug Administration
FISH	fluorescence in situ hybridization
GVHD	graft-versus-host disease
GVL	graft-versus-leukemia (effect)
HLA	human leukocyte antigen
HSCT	hematopoietic stem cell transplantation
Ig	immunoglobulin M
IGHV	immunoglobulin heavy chain gene
IFN-α	interferon alpha
IRIS	International Randomized study of Interferon vs STI571 trial
MBL	monoclonal B-cell lymphocytosis
mRNA	messenger ribonucleic acid
NCCN	National Comprehensive Cancer Network
PDGFR	platelet-derived growth factor receptor
Ph	Philadelphia chromosome
PI3K	phosphatidylinosital 3-kinase
REMS	Risk Evaluation and Mitigation Strategy
RT-PCR	reverse-transcription polymerase chain reaction
STI	signal transduction inhibitor
TKI	tyrosine kinase inhibitor
WBC	white blood cell
WHO	World Health Organization
ZAP-70	ζ-associated protein 70

REFERENCES

1. Siegel RL, Miller KD, Jemal A. Cancer statistics, 2016. CA Cancer *J Clin* 2016;66:7-30.
2. Corso A, Lazzarino M, Morra E, et al. Chronic myelogenous leukemia and exposure to ionizing radiation—a retrospective study of 443 patients. *Ann Hematol* 1995;70:79-82.
3. Ichimaru M, Ishimaru T, Belsky JL. Incidence of leukemia in atomic bomb survivors belonging to a fixed cohort in Hiroshima and Nagasaki, 1950-71. Radiation dose, years after exposure, age at exposure, and type of leukemia. *J Radiat Res* 1978;19:262-282.
4. Borgaonkar DS. Philadelphia-chromosome translocation and chronic myeloid leukaemia. *Lancet* 1973;1:1250.
5. Stam K, Heisterkamp N, Grosveld G, et al. Evidence of a new chimeric bcr/c-abl mRNA in patients with chronic myelocytic leukemia and the Philadelphia chromosome. *N Engl J Med* 1985;313:1429-1433.
6. Vardiman JW, Harris NL, Brunning RD. The World Health Organization (WHO) classification of myeloid neoplasms. *Blood* 2002;100:2292-2302.
7. Fialkow PJ, Jacobson RJ, Papayannopoulou T. Chronic myelocytic leukemia: Clonal origin in a stem cell common to the granulocyte, erythrocyte, platelet, and monocyte/macrophage. *Am J Med* 1977;63: 125-130.
8. Sokal JE, Cox EB, Baccarani M, et al. Prognostic discrimination in "good-risk" chronic granulocytic leukemia. *Blood* 1984;63:789-799.
9. Cortes JE, Kantargian HM. How I treat newly diagnosed chronic phase CML. *Blood* 2012;120:1390-1397.
10. Jabbour E, Kantarjian H. Chronic myeloid leukemia: 2012 Update on diagnosis, monitoring and management. *Am J Hematol* 2012;87: 1038-1045.
11. Druker BJ, Guilhot F, O'Brien S, et al. Five-year follow-up of patients receiving imatinib for chronic myelogenous leukemia. *N Engl J Med* 2006;355:2408-2417.
12. National Comprehensive Cancer Network. The NCCN Chronic Myelogenous Leukemia Clinical Practice Guideline (Version 1.2016). 2015. http://www.nccn.org. Accessed June 20, 2016.
13. Mathisen MS, Kantarjian HM, Cortes J, et al. Practical issues surrounding the explosion of tyrosine kinase inhibitors for the management of chronic myeloid leukemia. *Blood Rev* 2014;28:179-187.
14. Hehlmann R, Heimpel H, Hasford J, et al. Randomized comparison of busulfan and hydroxyurea in chronic myelogenous leukemia: Prolongation of survival by hydroxyurea. The German CML Study Group. *Blood* 1993;82:398-407.
15. Preudhamme C, Guillhot J, Nicolini FE, et al. Imatinib plus peginterferon alfa-2a in chronic myeloid leukemia. *N Engl J Med* 2010;363:2511-2521.
16. Deininger MWN, Druker BJ. Specific targeted therapy at chronic myelogenous leukemia with imatinib. *Pharmacol Rev* 2003;55: 401-423.
17. Deininger M, Buchdunger E, Druker BJ. The development of imatinib as a therapeutic agent for chronic myeloid leukemia. *Blood* 2005;105: 2640-2653.
18. O'Brien SG, Guilhot F, Larson RA, et al. Imatinib compared with interferon and low-dose cytarabine for newly diagnosed chronic-phase chronic myeloid leukemia. *N Engl J Med* 2003;348:994-1004.
19. Druker BJ, Talpaz M, Resta DJ, et al. Efficacy and safety of a specific inhibitor of the *BCR-ABL* tyrosine kinase in chronic myeloid leukemia. *N Engl J Med* 2001;344:1031-1037.
20. Deininger M, O'Brien SG, Guilhot F, et al. International Randomized Study of Interferon vs. STI-571 (IRIS) 8 year follow-up: Sustained survival and low risk for progression or events in patients with newly diagnosed chronic myeloid leukemia in chronic phase treated with imatinib. *Blood* 2009;116:Abstract e1126.
21. Hughes TP, Kaeda J, Branford S, et al. Frequency of major molecular responses to imatinib or interferon alfa plus cytarabine in newly diagnosed chronic myeloid leukemia. *N Engl J Med* 2003;349: 1423-1432.
22. Press RD, Love Z, Tronnes AA, et al. *BCR-ABL* mRNA levels at and after the time of a complete cytogenetic response (CCR) predict the duration of CCR in imatinib mesylate-treated patients with CML. *Blood* 2006;107:4250-4256.
23. Baccarani M, Rosti G, Castagnetti F, et al. Comparison of imatinib 400 mg and 800 mg daily in the front-line treatment of high-risk, Philadelphia-positive chronic myeloid leukemia: A European Leukemia Net study. *Blood* 2009;113:4497-4504.
24. Castagnetti F, Palandri F, Amabile M, et al. Results of high-dose imatinib mesylate in intermediate Sokal risk chronic myeloid leukemia in early chronic phase: A phase 2 trial of the GIMEMA CML Working Party. *Blood* 2009;113:3428-3434.
25. Talpaz M, Silver RT, Druker BJ, et al. Imatinib induces durable hematologic and cytogenetic responses in patients with accelerated phase chronic myeloid leukemia: Results of a phase 2 study. *Blood* 2002;99:1928-1937.
26. Amadori S, Picardi A, Fazi P, et al. A phase II study of VP-16, intermediate-dose Ara-C and carboplatin (VAC) in advanced acute myelogenous leukemia and blastic chronic myelogenous leukemia. *Leukemia* 1996;10:766-768.
27. Sawyers CL, Hochhaus A, Feldman E, et al. Imatinib induces hematologic and cytogenetic responses in patients with chronic myelogenous leukemia in myeloid blast crisis: Results of a phase II study. *Blood* 2002;99:3530-3539.
28. Milojkovic D, Apperly J. Mechanisms of resistance to imatinib and second-generation tyrosine kinase inhibitors in chronic myeloid leukemia. *Clin Cancer Res* 2009;15:7519-7527.

29. Nelson RP, Cornetta K, Ward KE, Ramanaju S, Fausel C, Cripe L. Desensitization to imatinib in patients with leukemia. *Ann Allergy Asthma Immunol* 2006;97:216-222.
30. Talpaz M, Shah NP, Kantarjian H, et al. Dasatinib in imatinib-resistant Philadelphia chromosome-positive leukemias. *N Engl J Med* 2006;354:2531-2541.
31. Hochhaus A, Kantarjian HM, Baccarani M, et al. Dasatinib induces notable hematologic and cytogenetic responses in chronic-phase chronic myeloid leukemia after failure of imatinib therapy. *Blood* 2007;109:2303-2309.
32. Kantarjian HM, Pasquini R, Levy V, et al. Dasatinib or high-dose imatinib for chronic-phase chronic myeloid leukemia resistant to imatinib at a dose of 400 to 600 milligrams daily. *Cancer* 2009;115:4136-4147.
33. Shah NP, Kantarjian HM, Kim DW, et al. Intermittent target inhibition with dasatinib 100 mg once daily preserves efficacy and improves tolerability in imatinib-resistant and -intolerant chronic-phase chronic myeloid leukemia. *J Clin Oncol* 2008;26:3204-3212.
34. Apperley JF, Cortes JE, Kim DW, et al. Dasatinib in the treatment of chronic myeloid leukemia in accelerated phase after imatinib failure: The START A trial. *J Clin Oncol* 2009;24:3472-3479.
35. Kantarjian HM, Cortes J, Kim DW, et al. Phase 3 study of dasatinib 140 mg once daily versus 70 mg twice daily in patients with chronic myeloid leukemia in accelerated phase resistant or intolerant to imatinib: 15-month median follow-up. *Blood* 2009;113:6322-6329.
36. Cortes J, Kim DW, Martinelli G, et al. Efficacy and safety of dasatinib in imatinib-resistant or -intolerant patients with chronic myeloid leukemia in blast phase. *Leukemia* 2008;22:2176-2183.
37. Cortes J, Saglio G, Baccarani M, et al. Final study results of the phase 3 dasatinib versus imatinib in newly diagnosed chronic myeloid leukemia in chronic phase (CML-CP) trial (DASISION, CA180-056). *Blood* 2014;124:Abstract e152.
38. Giles FJ, le Coutre PD, Pinilla-Ibarz J, et al. Nilotinib in imatinib-resistant or imatinib-intolerant patients with chronic myeloid leukemia in chronic phase: 48-month follow-up results of a phase II study. *Leukemia* 2013;27:107-112.
39. Le Coutre P, Ottmann OG, Giles F, et al. Nilotinib (formerly AMN107), a highly selective BCR-ABL tyrosine kinase inhibitor, is active in patients with imatinib-resistant or -intolerant accelerated phase chronic myelogenous leukemia. *Blood* 2008;111:1834-1839.
40. Larson RA, Kim DW, Issaragrilsil S, et al. Efficacy and safety of nilotinib (NIL) vs imatinib (IM) in patients with newly diagnosed chronic myeloid leukemia in chronic phase (CML-CP): Long term follow-up of ENESTnd. *Blood* 2014;124:Abstract e4541.
41. Gambacorti-Passerini C, Kantarjian HM, Kim DW, et al. Long-term efficacy and safety of bosutinib in patients with advanced leukemia following resistance/intolerance to imatinib and other tyrosine kinase inhibitors. *Am J Hematol* 2015;90:755-768.
42. Khoury HJ, Cortes JE, Kantarjian HG, et al. Bosutinib is active in chronic phase chronic myeloid leukemia after imatinib and dasatinib therapy failure. *Blood* 2012;119:3403-3412.
43. Cortes JE, Kim DW, Kantarjian HM, et al. Bosutinib versus imatinib in newly diagnosed chronic phase chronic myeloid leukemia: Results from the BELA trial. *J Clin Oncol* 2012;30:3486-3492.
44. Cortes JE, Kantarjian H, Shah NP, et al. Ponatinib in refractory Philadelphia chromosome-positive leukemias. *N Engl J Med* 2012;367: 2075-2088.
45. Cortes JE, Kim DW, Pinilla-Ibarz J, et al. A phase 2 trial of ponatinib in Philadelphia chromosome-positive leukemias. *N Engl J Med* 2013;369:1783-1796.
46. Ponatinib (Iclusig) prescribing information. 2016. http://iclusig.com/pi/. Accessed June 20, 2016.
47. Cortes JE, Nicolini FE, Wetzler M, et al. Subcutaneous omacetaxine mepesuccinate in patients with chronic-phase chronic myeloid leukemia previously treated with 2 or more tyrosine kinase inhibitors including imatinib. *Clin Lymphoma Myeloma Leuk* 2013;13:584-591.
48. Cortes J, Lipton JH, Rea D, et al. Phase II study of subcutaneous omacetaxine mepesuccinate after tyrosine kinase inhibitor failure in patients with chronic phase chronic myeloid leukemia with the T315I mutation. *Blood* 2012;120:2573-2580.
49. Gratwohl A, Brand R, Apperly J, et al. Allogeneic hematopoietic stem cell transplantation for chronic myeloid leukemia in Europe 2006: Transplant activity, long-term data and current results. An analysis by the Chronic Leukemia Working Party of the European Group for the Blood and Marrow Transplantation (EBMT). *Haematologica* 2006;91:513-521.
50. van Rhee F, Szydlo RM, Hermans J, et al. Long-term results after allogenic bone marrow transplantation for chronic myelogenous leukemia in chronic phase: A report from the Chronic Leukemia Working Party of the European Group for Blood and Marrow Transplantation. *Bone Marrow Transplant* 1997;20:553-560.
51. Deininger M, Schleuning M, Greinix H, et al. The effect of prior exposure to imatinib on transplant-related mortality. *Haematologica* 2006;91:452-459.
52. Porter D, Levine JE. Graft-versus host disease and graft-versus leukemia after donor leukocyte infusion. *Semin Hematol* 2006;43:53-61.
53. Hess G, Bunjes D, Siegert W, et al. Sustained complete molecular remissions after treatment with imatinib mesylate in patients with failure after allogeneic stem cell transplantation for chronic myelogenous leukemia: Results of a prospective phase II open label multicenter study. *J Clin Oncol* 2005;23:7583-7593.
54. Klyuchnikov E, Kroger N, Brummendorf TH, et al. Current status and perspectives of tyrosine kinase inhibitor treatment in the post-transplant period in patients with chronic myeloid leukemia. *Biol Blood Marrow Transplant* 2010;16:301-310.
55. Bacher U, Klyuchnikov E, Zabelina T, et al. The changing scene of allogeneic stem cell transplantation for chronic myeloid leukemia: A report from the German Registry covering the period from 1998-2004. *Ann Hematol* 2009;88:1237-1247.
56. Soverini S, Hochhaus A, Nicolini FE, et al. BCR-ABL kinase domain mutation analysis in chronic myeloid leukemia patients treated with tyrosine kinase inhibitors: Recommendations from an expert panel on behalf of the European Leukemia. *Blood* 2011;118:1208-1215.
57. Gao B, Yeap S, Clements A, et al. Evidence for therapeutic drug monitoring of targeted anticancer therapies. *J Clin Oncol* 2012;30: 4017-4025.
58. Hallek M. Chronic lymphocytic leukemia: 2015 update on diagnosis, risk stratification, and treatment. *Am J Hematol* 2015;90:446-460.
59. Byrd JC, Furman RR, Coutre SE, et al. Targeting BTK with ibrutinib in relapsed chronic lymphocytic leukemia. *N Eng J Med* 2013;369:32-42.
60. Furman RR, Sharman JP, Coutre SE, et al. Idelalisib and rituximab in relapsed chronic lymphocytic leukemia. *N Eng J Med* 2014;370: 997-1007.
61. Landgren O, Albitar M, Ma W, et al. B-cell clones as early markers for chronic lymphocytic leukemia. *N Engl J Med* 2009;360:659-667.
62. Dohner H, Stilgenbauer S, Benner A, et al. Genetic aberrations and survival in chronic lymphocytic leukemia. *N Engl J Med* 2000;343: 1910-1916.
63. Tam CS, Shanafelt TD, Wierda WG, et al. De novo deletion of 17p13.1 chronic lymphocytic leukemia shows significant clinical heterogeneity: The MD Anderson and Mayo Clinic experience. *Blood* 2009;114:957-964.
64. Wang, L, Lawrence MS, Wan Y, et al. SF3B1 and other novel cancer genes in chronic lymphocytic leukemia. *N Engl J Med* 2011;365: 2497-2506.
65. Tsimberidou AS, O'Brien S, Khouri I, et al. Clinical outcomes and prognostic factors in patients with Richter's syndrome treated with chemotherapy or chemoimmunotherapy with or without stem cell transplantation. *J Clin Oncol* 2006;24:2343-2351.
66. Eisele L, Haddad T, Sellmann L, Durhsen U, Durig J. Expression of CD38 on leukemic B-cells but not on non-leukemic T-cells are comparably stable over time and predict the course of disease in chronic lymphocytic leukemia. *Leuk Res* 2009;33:775-778.
67. Vroblova V, Smolej L, Vrbacky F, et al. Biological prognostic markers in chronic lymphocytic leukemia. *Acta Medica* 2009;52:3-8.
68. Rassenti LZ, Huynh L, Toy TL, et al. ZAP-70 compared with immunoglobulin heavy-chain gene mutation status as a predictor of disease progression in chronic lymphocytic leukemia. *N Engl J Med* 2004;351:893-901.
69. Zenz T, Mertens D, Kuppers R, Dohner H, Stilgenbauer S. From pathogenesis to treatment of chronic lymphocytic leukemia. *Nat Rev Cancer* 2010;10:37-50.
70. Byrd JC, Jones, JJ, Woyach JA, et al. Entering the era of targeted therapy for chronic lymphocytic leukemia: Impact on the practicing clinician. *J Clin Oncol* 2014;32:3039-3047.
71. National Comprehensive Cancer Network. The NCCN Non-Hodgkin's Lymphoma Clinical Practice Guideline (Version 1.2016). 2015. http://www.nccn.org. Accessed June 20, 2016.
72. CLL Trialists' Collaborative Group. Chemotherapeutic options in chronic lymphocytic leukemia: A meta-analysis of the randomized trials. *J Natl Cancer Inst* 1999;91:861-868.
73. Robak T, Blonski JZ, Kasznicki M, et al. Cladribine with or without prednisone in the treatment of previously treated and untreated B-cell chronic lymphocytic leukaemia—updated results of the multicentre study of 378 patients. *Br J Haematol* 2000;108:357-368.
74. Sorensen JM, Vena DA, Fallavollita A, et al. Treatment of refractory chronic lymphocytic leukemia with fludarabine phosphate via the

group C protocol mechanism of the National Cancer Institute: Five-year follow-up report. *J Clin Oncol* 1997;15:458-465.

75. Rai KR, Peterson BL, Appelbaum FR, et al. Fludarabine compared with chlorambucil as primary therapy for chronic lymphocytic leukemia. *N Engl J Med* 2000;343:1750-1757.
76. Eichhorst BF, Busch R, Schweighofer C, et al. Due to the low infection rates no routine anti-infective prophylaxis is required in younger patients with chronic lymphocytic leukemia during fludarabine-based first line therapy. *Br J Haematol* 2007;136:63-72.
77. Keating MJ, O'Brien S, Kontoyiannis D, et al. Results of first salvage therapy for patients refractory to a fludarabine regimen in chronic lymphocytic leukemia. *Leuk Lymphoma* 2002;43:1755-1762.
78. Cheson BD, Rummel MJ. Bendamustine: Rebirth of an old drug. *J Clin Oncol* 2009;27:1492-1501.
79. Knauf WU, Lissichkov T, Aldaoud A, et al. Phase III randomized study of bendamustine compared with chlorambucil in previously untreated patients with chronic lymphocytic leukemia. *J Clin Oncol* 2009;27:4378-4384.
80. Hainsworth JD, Litchey S, Barton JH. Bendamustine compared with chlorambucil in previously untreated patients with chronic lymphocytic leukaemia: Updated results of a randomized phase III trial. *Br J Haematol* 2012;159:67-77.
81. Hillmen P, Skotnicki AB, Robak T, et al. Alemtuzumab compared with chlorambucil as first-line therapy for chronic lymphocytic leukemia. *J Clin Oncol* 2007;35:5616-5623.
82. Osterborg A, Karlsson C, Lundin J, Kimby E, Mellstedt H. Strategies in the management of alemtuzumab-related side effects. *Semin Oncol* 2006;33(Suppl 5):S29-S35.
83. Lundin J, Kimby E, Bjorkholm M, et al. Phase II trial of subcutaneous anti-CD52 monoclonal antibody alemtuzumab (Campath-1H) as first-line treatment for patients with B-cell chronic lymphocytic leukemia (B-CLL). *Blood* 2002;100:768-773.
84. Weirda WG, Kipps TJ, Mayer J, et al. Ofatumumab as a single agent CD20 immunotherapy in fludarabine refractory chronic lymphocytic leukemia: A phase I/II study. *J Clin Oncol* 2010;28:1749-1755.
85. Hillmen P, Robak T, Janssens A, et al. Chlorambucil plus ofatumumab versus chlorambucil alone in previously untreated patients with chronic lymphocytic leukemia (COMPLEMENT-1): A randomized, multicenter, open-label phase 3 trial. *Lancet* 2015;385:1873-1883.
86. Keating MJ, O'Brien S, Albitar M, et al. Early results of a chemoimmunotherapy regimen of fludarabine, cyclophosphamide, and rituximab as initial therapy for chronic lymphocytic leukemia. *J Clin Oncol* 2005;23:4079-4088.
87. Robak T, Dmoszynska A, Solal-Céligny P, et al. Rituximab plus fludarabine and cyclophosphamide prolongs progression-free survival compared with fludarabine and cyclophosphamide alone in previously treated chronic lymphocytic leukemia. *J Clin Oncol* 2010;28:1756-1765.
88. Halleck M, Fischer K, Fingerle-Rowson G, et al. Addition of rituximab to fludarabine and cyclophosphamide in patients with chronic lymphocytic leukaemia: a randomized, open-labeled, phase 3 trial. *Lancet* 2010;376;1164-1174.
89. Fischer K, Cramer P, Busche R, et al. Bendamustine in combination with rituximab for previously untreated patients with chronic lymphocytic leukemia. A multicenter phase II trial of the German Chronic Lymphocytic Leukemia Study Group. *J Clin Oncol* 2012;30:3209-3216.
90. Eichhorst B, Fink AM, Busch R, et al. Frontline chemoimmunotherapy with fludarabine (F), cyclophosphamide (C), and rituximab (R) (FCR) shows superior efficacy in comparison to bendamustine (B) and rituximab (R) in previously untreated and physically fit patients with advanced chronic lymphocytic leukemia(CLL): Final analysis of an international, randomized study of the German CLL Study Group (GCLLSG) (CLL10 Study). *Blood* 2014;124:Abstract e19.
91. Fischer K, Cramer P, Busche R, et al. Bendamustine combined with rituximab in patients with relapsed and/or refractory chronic lymphocytic leukemia. A multicenter phase II trial of the German Chronic Lymphocytic Leukemia Study Group. *J Clin Oncol* 2011;29:3559-3566.
92. Cartron G, deGuibert S, Dilhuydy MS, et al. Obinutuzumab (GA101) in relapsed/refractory chronic lymphocytic leukemia: Final data from the phase 1/2 GAUGUIN study. *Blood* 2014;124:2196-2202.
93. Byrd JC, Brown JR, O'Brien S; RESONATE Investigators. Ibrutinib versus ofatumumab in previously treated chronic lymphocytic leukemia. *N Eng J Med* 2014;371:213-223.
94. Delgado J, Milligan DW, Dreger P. Allogeneic hematopoietic cell transplantation for chronic lymphocytic leukemia: Ready for prime time? *Blood* 2009;114:2581-2588.
95. Mato A, Porter DL. A drive through cellular therapy for CLL in 2015: Allogeneic cell transplantation and CARs. *Blood* 2015;126:478-485.

Multiple Myeloma

Kamakshi V. Rao and Amy M. Pick

136

KEY CONCEPTS

1. Multiple myeloma (MM) is a cancer that develops in plasma cells, leading to excessive production of a monoclonal immunoglobulin.
2. Most patients have skeletal involvement at the time of diagnosis with associated bone pain and fractures. Anemia, hypercalcemia, and renal failure may also be present. A bone marrow biopsy with 10% or more plasma cells and a M-protein spike on plasma or urine electrophoresis confirms the diagnosis.
3. Cytogenetics may play an important role when selecting the appropriate initial therapy for patients with a new MM diagnosis and tools such as the Mayo Stratification for Myeloma and Risk-adapted Therapy (mSMART) approach are available.
4. Induction treatment is based on patients' eligibility for autologous stem cell transplantation. Novel agents such as thalidomide, lenalidomide, pomalidomide, bortezomib, and carfilzomib have gained popularity over traditional chemotherapy because of higher response rates and survival. The increased response rate is at the expense of significant grade 3 and 4 toxicity, which can include myelosuppression, venous thromboembolism (VTE), and neuropathy depending on the regimen used.
5. Thalidomide, lenalidomide, and pomalidomide are immunomodulatory agents that have antiangiogenic and anti-inflammatory activity. Thalidomide's dose limiting toxicity is neuropathy. Lenalidomide is less neurotoxic, but can cause significant myelosuppression. Pomalidomide, the newest of this class, is currently only used in relapsed/refractory MM.
6. The proteasome inhibitors, bortezomib and carfilzomib, are highly active in the treatment of MM, particularly those with high-risk cytogenetics.
7. Autologous hematopoietic stem cell transplantation (HSCT) is used after induction in patients with reasonably good performance status to maximize complete remissions and prolong survival. Combining autologous HSCT with allogeneic HSCT is investigational and should be performed within a clinical trial.
8. Maintenance therapies may be used in both transplant-eligible and ineligible patients. Current regimens typically include lenalidomide or bortezomib with the intent of increasing response rates and progression-free survival.
9. Bisphosphonates are used to treat bone disease associated with MM, which results in decreased pain and skeletal-related events and improved quality of life.
10. Salvage therapy for patients with relapsed or refractory MM can include any of the prior listed therapies and depends on patient's performance status, risk category, and prior treatments used for induction.

INTRODUCTION

1 Multiple myeloma (MM) is a malignancy of plasma cells or immunoglobulin-producing B lymphocytes.[1,2] The cancer is characterized by clonal proliferation and accumulation of a monoclonal immunoglobulin secreted from the plasma cell that can be measured in the plasma or urine. Patients with MM often have osteolytic bone lesions at the time of diagnosis, which is probably related to various bone-mobilizing cytokines secreted from the MM clone and bone marrow stromal cells. Other clinical manifestations include end-organ damage such as renal insufficiency, hypercalcemia, and anemia. The treatment of MM often consists of two or three drug combinations incorporating a proteasome inhibitor and immunomodulator. These regimens have improved response rates and outcomes compared to conventional chemotherapeutic agents. Although therapy is not currently curative, MM continues to be a remarkable example of bench-to-bedside translation in new drug development.

EPIDEMIOLOGY AND ETIOLOGY

In the United States, it was estimated that 30,330 cases of MM were diagnosed in 2016, with 12,650 deaths.[3] It is a disease that affects older adults with a median age of 69 years at diagnosis.[4] MM occurs more frequently in men and African Americans. Familial clusters of MM have been reported with emerging evidence suggesting a genetic predisposition toward the disease.[5]

Certain environmental factors have been implicated with MM. Radiation exposure has been historically linked to the development of MM with atomic bomb survivors having a five times higher risk of MM than nonexposed controls. Data suggest that low levels of radiation may also be a risk factor. MM has been associated with exposure to various chemicals including pesticides, aromatic hydrocarbons, and petroleum products used in farming, cleaning works, mining, and other occupational groups working with these chemicals. Alcohol and tobacco use have not been strongly associated with an increased risk of MM and the association of MM with an infectious etiology has been inconclusive.[6]

Although the pathogenesis of MM has not been fully elucidated, multiple genetic mutations have been identified and our understanding of these cellular events has improved. Decades of research and improved scientific techniques have enabled closer examination of the changes that occur during the development of normal and abnormal B cells.

PATHOPHYSIOLOGY

MM is a genetically heterogeneous disease that is characterized by abnormal clonal plasma cell infiltration in the bone marrow. Monoclonal gammopathy of undetermined significance (MGUS) and smoldering MM may precede active MM. MGUS is associated with monoclonal immunoglobulin in the blood (≤ 3 g/dL [≤ 30 g/L]) without clinical manifestations of the complications of MM (eg, end-organ damage).[7,8] The conversion rate of MGUS to MM is about 1% per year. The molecular changes associated with the conversion of MGUS to MM are not clear, but genome-wide studies have identified several candidate genes associated with disease progression.[2,8,9] Smoldering MM is an advanced premalignant stage that is clinically distinct from MGUS with criteria including high monoclonal immunoglobulin in the blood (≥ 3 g/dL [≥ 30 g/L]) without clinical manifestations of the complications of MM. Although patients with smoldering MM have asymptomatic disease, the risk of progression to MM is about 10% per year for the first 5 years after diagnosis, about 3% per year for the next 5 years, and about 1% per year for the next 10 years.[10,11] Certain cytogenetic characteristics appear to be associated with a higher risk of transformation to active MM including a translocation of 4 and 14.[10] Multiple genetic changes may occur over time leading to more symptomatic disease. Numerous genetic mutations are associated with transformation, with one report of four patients who transformed from smoldering MM to MM acquiring an average of 433 mutations.[9] The molecular mechanisms leading to these mutations remain to be fully elucidated.

MM is characterized by the accumulation of malignant plasma cells in the bone marrow. Both MM and normal plasma cells are produced from differentiated B cells after antigen stimulation. Normal plasma cells will die within days to weeks after differentiation, whereas MM plasma cells are immortalized.[1,6] The malignant plasma cell is involved in the unregulated production of a monoclonal antibody referred to as *M protein*. MM cells are seldom seen in large quantities in the peripheral blood because of their close interaction with bone marrow stromal cells. MM cells are supported by a nurturing bone marrow microenvironment which promotes the further expansion of myeloma clones. Molecules such as interleukin-6 (IL-6), vascular endothelial growth factor (VEGF), insulin-like growth factor 1 (IGF-1), and the transcriptional regulator nuclear factor kappa B (NF-*κB*) are part of the microenvironment and stimulate clonal growth, disease progression, and promote resistance to therapy.[9] The disruption of the microenvironment is an important strategy for therapy.[12] Figure 136-1 shows several of the factors involved in disease pathogenesis and progression and potential mechanisms of action of thalidomide, lenalidomide, pomalidomide, bortezomib, and carfilzomib.

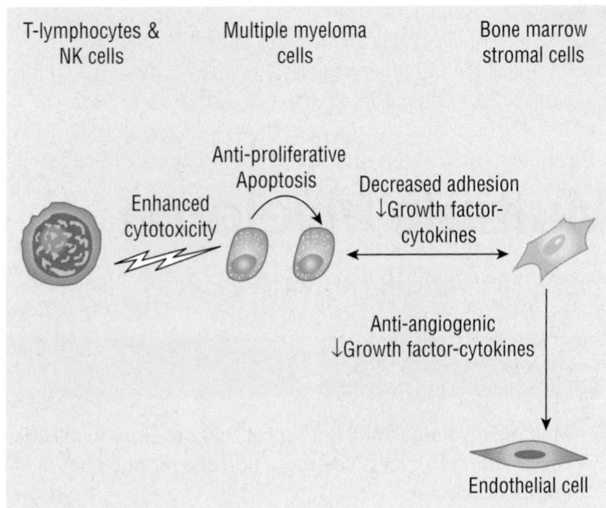

FIGURE 136-1 Proposed mechanisms of action of immunomodulatory drugs.

CLINICAL PRESENTATION

The clinical manifestations are related to the effects of the myeloma cell on the bone microenvironment and the unregulated production of the M protein. (2) Most patients with MM present with complaints of bone pain and fatigue at diagnosis.[6] Initial laboratory evaluation often reveals hypercalcemia, renal insufficiency, anemia, and other abnormalities including β_2-microglobulin that measures tumor burden. Skeletal evaluation shows gross abnormalities in most patients. Bone scans show abnormalities that often include lytic lesions, osteoporosis, and fractures. This group of findings (hyper**c**alcemia, **r**enal insufficiency, **a**nemia, and **b**one lesions) is often referred by the acronym *CRAB* and suggests end-organ damage.[6,7] A confirmed diagnosis is defined by a bone marrow biopsy with 10% or more plasma cells and an M-protein spike on plasma or urine electrophoresis.[7,13] Both the National Comprehensive Cancer Network (NCCN) and International Myeloma Working Group (IMWG) have described criteria to diagnose MM.[13,14]

Following the diagnosis of MM, further workup involves analyzing the isotype of M protein. Serum protein electrophoresis and serum and urine immunofixation identify the M-protein isotype being secreted. In a minority of patients, M protein may not be detected in

CLINICAL PRESENTATION Multiple Myeloma

General Criteria

- 80% of patients present with symptomatic disease

Signs and Symptoms

- Bone pain (fractures, lytic lesions)
- Fatigue (anemia)
- Infection (reduced polyclonal response)
- Neurologic symptoms (nerve compression)
- Polyuria (hypercalcemia)
- Nausea and vomiting (hypercalcemia)

Laboratory Parameters

- Elevated M protein
  - Plasma electrophoresis
  - Urine electrophoresis
  - Immunofixation
- Elevated serum creatinine
- Hypercalcemia
- Low hemoglobin
- Low albumin
- Elevated β_2-microglobulin
- Elevated C-reactive protein

Bone Marrow

- More than or equal to 10% plasma cells

Cytogenetics

- Chromosome 13 deletion
- Translocations of t(4;14), t(11;14) and t(14;16)
- Del (17p)
- Chromosome 1 amplification

the plasma but found in the urine, requiring the urine to be examined as part of a complete diagnostic workup. About 60% of patients have intact monoclonal immunoglobulin G (IgG), 20% have monoclonal IgA, and the remaining 20% secrete only monoclonal light chains. Antibodies are composed of two light chains where antigen binds and two heavy chains. Light-chain immunoglobulins, called Bence Jones proteins, can be secreted by the MM clone and excreted in the urine due to their low molecular weight. Bence Jones proteins are primarily responsible for MM-associated renal failure.[1,6] Serum-free light chains (SFC) may also be measured and these results may provide valuable information on the likelihood of disease progression.[15]

Most patients have bone involvement at the time of diagnosis.[6,7] The effects of MM on the bone result from the abnormal production of cytokines, including IL-1, IL-6, tumor necrosis factor-α (TNF-α), and the receptor for activation of NF-κB ligand (RANK-L). Bone involvement is the net effect of the activation of osteoclasts and inhibition of osteoblastogenesis.[16] This leads to bone destruction and resorption predisposing one to pathologic fractures and lytic lesions. Patients with MM are frequently anemic due to infiltration of the bone marrow with the MM clone and poor erythropoietin response. Patients can have clinically important hypercalcemia, which results from calcium mobilization due to bone resorption. Renal failure can occur as a result of high protein load from the monoclonal protein secretion as well as dehydration.

STAGING AND PROGNOSTIC FACTORS

Two clinical staging systems for MM have been developed. The newer International Staging System (ISS) uses serum β_2-microglobulin and albumin concentrations to stage patients.[17] These two routine laboratory tests predict survival in patients treated with either conventional treatment or autologous hematopoietic stem cell transplantation (HSCT). It does not consider cytogenetics or molecular markers. An older staging system, Durie-Salmon, may also be used. It uses hemoglobin, serum calcium, bone involvement, and M protein to categorize patients into one of three stages.[13] The Durie-Salmon system has variable accuracy in patients undergoing HSCT and with newer novel therapies.[6] Table 136-1 describes the ISS and median survival times for each stage.

3 Certain cytogenetic abnormalities have been identified as important prognostic factors. Shortened overall survival has been demonstrated in patients with chromosomal 13 deletion (del 13), translocation of 4 and 14 (t(4;14)), and deletion of 17p (del (17p)).[6,13] Recent data suggest that the translocation of 11 and 14 may be associated with increased survival. The Mayo Clinic developed a risk-adapted approach, known as the mSMART (Mayo Stratification for Myeloma and Risk-adapted Therapy), that categorizes patients into three risk groups based on cytogenetics and gene expression profiling: high, intermediate, and standard risk.[18] Therapeutic options and treatment length is then provided for each risk group. Additional prognostic factors generally represent the underlying pathologic changes associated with MM, including proinflammatory biomarkers (elevated C-reactive protein), tumor load (increased β_2-microglobulin), and dysregulated cellular growth (labeling index and marrow microvessel density).

TABLE 136-1 The International Staging System for Multiple Myeloma

Stage	Characteristics	Median Survival (mo)
I	Serum β_2-microglobulin <3.5 mcg/mL (mg/L)	62
	Serum albumin ≥3.5 g/dL (≥35 g/L)	
II	Not stage I or stage III	44
III	Serum β_2-microglobulin ≥5.5 mcg/mL (mg/L)	29

Used with permission by the American Society of Clinical Oncology. Greipp PR, Miguel JS, Durie BG, et al. International staging system for multiple myeloma. J Clin Oncol 2005;23:3412-3420.

TREATMENT

Desired Outcomes

The primary goal in the treatment of MM is to prolong the patient's survival and improve quality of life. The different phases of treatment also have specific goals. The goal of induction therapy in newly diagnosed MM patients is to obtain at least a major response.[6,7] Induction therapy is followed by various treatment phases including transplant, consolidation, and maintenance therapy. The goals of these subsequent phases are to further improve response rates. With the integration of novel agents into therapy, progression-free survival and overall survival have steadily improved, and responses have increased in frequency, depth, and duration. Unfortunately, there is no convincing evidence that patients are cured of their disease.

General Approach

The decision to initiate treatment depends on whether the patient is experiencing symptoms of the disease. Watchful waiting is the most common practice for patients with smoldering MM and is currently recommended by the NCCN guidelines.[13] However, this treatment paradigm is evolving with the availability of novel agents. Several small published studies suggest that early treatment with novel agents in patients with high-risk smoldering MM may improve overall survival and delay time to progression.[9] The challenge remains identifying patients with high-risk smoldering MM and developing criteria to assess a treatment response.[9]

4 Initial management of symptomatic MM (refer to "Clinical Presentation") depends on whether patients are candidates for autologous HSCT (Fig. 136-2). Transplant consideration factors include patient age, renal function, performance status, and comorbidities. The determination of transplant eligibility guides further treatment decisions. All patients with symptomatic MM are treated with initial induction therapy, with the selected regimen based on transplant eligibility. Therapies that may compromise stem cell reserve are avoided in transplant-eligible patients and the selected regimen will often be composed of various novel agents. Doublet or triplet combination regimens such as dexamethasone combined with bortezomib and lenalidomide or thalidomide have become common.

Induction therapy is usually continued until the desired response is achieved. Patients who are candidates for autologous HSCT will often receive two to four cycles of therapy and then will proceed to hematopoietic stem cell collection. Most patients undergo autologous HSCT immediately following collection, but some patients may decide to delay the transplant until first relapse. Patients who are not candidates for autologous HSCT usually receive several cycles of consolidation therapy, although the optimal duration of therapy after desired response is achieved is unknown. Single-agent maintenance therapy may be given in both transplant-eligible and ineligible patients. The use of guidelines may assist the clinician with drug therapy selection. Clinicians may be guided by the NCCN and IMWG Guidelines and mSMART treatment recommendations, which are discussed later in the "Initial Therapy" section.

The IMWG has developed uniform response criteria for MM.[19] Clinical response to therapy is generally defined by a reduction in M protein in the blood and urine. Numerous response types have been defined and the depth-of-response correlates with improved outcomes. A complete response (CR) is defined as elimination of the M protein as measured by immunofixation and plasma cells (≤5%) in the bone marrow. A CR is desirable because it is associated with improved overall survival.[20] A stringent complete response (sCR) is a CR with normal free light chain and absence of clonal cells in bone marrow. Lesser responses include partial response (PR), near complete response (nCR), and very good partial response (VGPR). These lesser responses are important because they may also correlate with

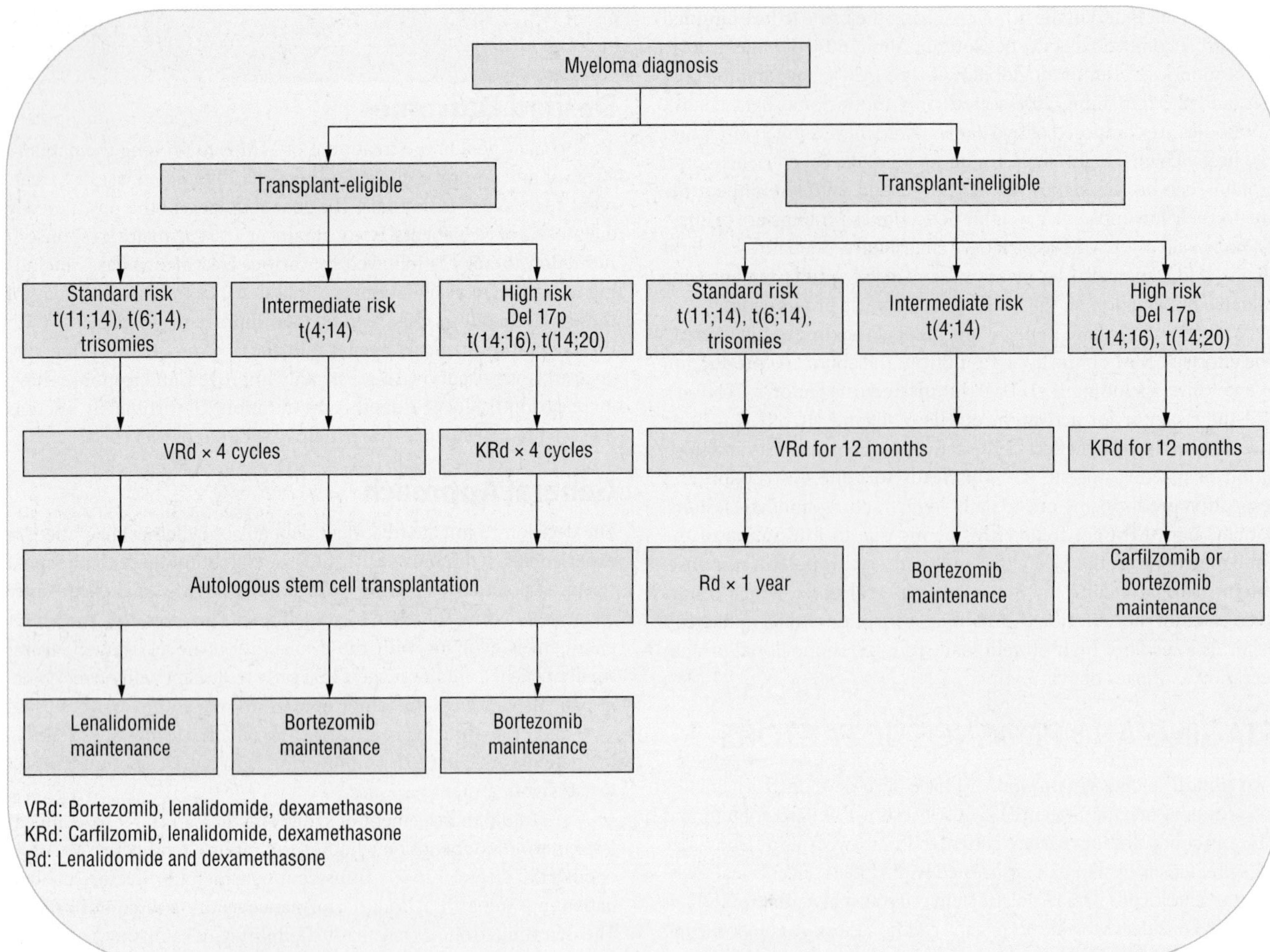

FIGURE 136-2 **Risk adapted treatment of multiple myeloma based on eligibility for hematopoietic stem cell transplantation.** *Adapted from Mayo Clinic mSMART classification.*

improved survival. Table 136-2 describes the most common types of responses that are used clinically.[13]

Pharmacotherapy of Multiple Myeloma

The current treatment of MM is based on novel agents from two classes of drugs, the immunomodulators and proteasome inhibitors. A three-drug regimen is commonly used in the treatment of MM and often incorporates dexamethasone and a drug from each class.

TABLE 136-2 Definition of Clinical Response in Multiple Myeloma

Type of Response	Definition[a]
PR	• ≥50% decrease in serum M protein • Reduction in 24-hour urine light chain by ≥90%
VGPR	• Serum and urine M protein detected on immunofixation but not electrophoresis
CR	• Negative immunofixation on serum and urine • No soft tissue plasmacytomas
sCR	• <5% plasma cells in the bone marrow • CR definition • Normal free light chain ratio • Absence of clonal cells in the bone marrow

CR, complete remission; PR, partial response; sCR, stringent complete response; VGPR, very good partial remission.

[a]Maintained for a minimum of 6 weeks.

Adapted from Mayo Clinic mSMART classification. Mayo Stratification for Myeloma and Risk-adapted Therapy: Newly Diagnosed Myeloma.

The optimal regimen is not clear because of the lack of head-to-head comparative trials.[6,7] Several highly active combination regimens are available. These regimens have improved response rates and survival with acceptable but different toxicity profiles compared to conventional regimens previously used in MM. Tables 136-3 and 136-4 show dosing and monitoring parameters for the newer agents used in the treatment of MM. Dose reductions in elderly patients and in patients with adverse events are often required.[13,20]

Conventional Chemotherapy

Conventional chemotherapy incorporating a corticosteroid was once the mainstay for the treatment of MM. Today, these conventional drugs may be combined with a novel agent to improve overall survival. Two of the common conventional chemotherapy regimens used historically to treat MM were melphalan plus prednisone (MP) and vincristine, doxorubicin, and dexamethasone (VAD).[6,21] The two drug regimen MP is no longer preferred because of inferior overall survival compared with newer regimens and is now often combined with a novel agent.[6,7,20] Melphalan is only recommended in the transplant-ineligible patients because of the adverse effects it has on stem cell mobilization and subsequent autologous HSCT.[6] Melphalan has also been associated with the development of myelodysplastic syndromes which is why the use of VAD chemotherapy as initial treatment became more common.[22] VAD has also been replaced with novel therapies.[13]

Corticosteroids are the cornerstone in MM therapy. Dexamethasone has been used alone as initial therapy and is believed to account for most of the antimyeloma activity of VAD (Table 136-5).

TABLE 136-3 Dosing of Novel Agents in Multiple Myeloma

Drug (Brand Name)	Initial Dose	Usual Dose	Special Population
Thalidomide (Thalidomide®)	50-100 mg/day	200 mg/day	Start low in elderly adults; increase dose every 1-3 weeks
Lenalidomide (Revlimid®)	10-25 mg/day Days 1-21 (28-day cycle) Days 1-28 (35 day cycle)	25 mg/day	Adjust dose in renal impairment: 30-60 mL/min (0.5-1.0 mL/s) (10 mg every 24 h) <30 mL/min (<0.5 mL/s) (15 mg every 48 h) <30 mL/min (<0.5 mL/s) (dialysis) (5 mg every 24 h)
Bortezomib (Velcade®)	1.3 mg/m² Days 1, 4, 8, and 11 Every 21 days		Reduce initial dose in hepatic impairment (serum bilirubin >1.5 × ULN) to 0.7 mg/m²
Carfilzomib (Kyprolis®)	20/m² given on days 1, 2, 8, 9, 15, and 16 of a 28-day cycle	27 mg/m²	
Pomalidomide (Pomalyst®)	4 mg/day for 21 days (28-day cycle)		

ULN, upper limit of the normal range.

TABLE 136-5 Initial Therapies for Multiple Myeloma

Regimen	Type of Response (%) OR	CR	CR/nCR/ VgPR
Melphalan + prednisone	40-50		5-10
Dexamethasone	40-50		
Thalidomide	34-40		
Thalidomide + dexamethasone	50-70	5-10	20-30
Melphalan, prednisone, and thalidomide	50-80	5-25	20-50
VAD chemotherapy	50-60		
Doxorubicin combinations + thalidomide	70-90		40-50
Single autoHSCT	80-90		40-50
Tandem autoHSCT	80-90		30-50
AutoHSCT followed by RI-alloHSCT	80-90		60
Bortezomib	40-50		12
Bortezomib + dexamethasone	80-90		20-30
Bortezomib + chemotherapy	80-98	10–30	43
Bortezomib + thalidomide + dexamethasone	85-95	20–35	50-60
Bortezomib + lenalidomide + dexamethasone	100		50-74
Lenalidomide + LD dexamethasone	70		40
Lenalidomide + high-dose dexamethasone	80		50
Clarithromycin + lenalidomide + dexamethasone	93	43	68
Lenalidomide + chemotherapy	80	15-25	
Carfilzomib + Lenalidomide + LD dexamethasone	98	42 (sCR)	81

alloHSCT, allogeneic hematopoietic stem cell transplantation; autoHSCT, autologous hematopoietic stem cell transplantation; CR, complete response; LD, low dose; OR, overall response (at least partial response); RI, reduced intensity; sCR, stringent complete response; VAD, vincristine, doxorubicin, and dexamethasone.

High-dose dexamethasone is associated with a higher rate of infection and central nervous system toxicity compared to MP which led investigators to conclude that high-dose dexamethasone should be used with caution as initial therapy, particularly in older patients.[23] In current regimens, newer agents (thalidomide, bortezomib, lenalidomide, carfilzomib) are combined with dexamethasone or the MP backbone to maximize initial response rates.[6,7,24] Doxorubicin or liposomal doxorubicin are also combined with various novel agents to improve response rates.

Immunomodulatory Drugs (IMiD)

Thalidomide (Thalomid®) Thalidomide was first used clinically in Europe in the late 1950s as a sedative and antiemetic but its use was largely abandoned when teratogenicity was reported. Its immunomodulatory effects became evident in the treatment of Hansen disease (leprosy), and it continues to be used for this rare indication. These clinical benefits are thought to be related to the anti-TNF activity of thalidomide. Recognizing that TNF may be involved in the pathophysiology of MM led researchers to study thalidomide as a treatment for refractory MM in 1999. The observation that thalidomide had activity against myeloma rejuvenated it as an important therapeutic agent.[6]

TABLE 136-4 Adverse Reactions and Monitoring Parameters for Novel Agents in Multiple Myeloma

Drug	Adverse Drug Reactions	Monitoring Parameters	Comments
Thalidomide	Neuropathy, sedations, constipation, VTE, rash, neutropenia, teratogenicity	Neurologic examination, active bowel sounds, CBC, STEPS Program	Evening dose to ↓ sedation Laxatives VTE prophylaxis
Lenalidomide	Myelosuppression, rash	CBC, renal function, REMS	Adjust dose in renal impairment VTE prophylaxis
Pomalidomide	Myelosuppression, rash, VTE, teratogenicity	CBC, REMS	
Bortezomib	Myelosuppression, neuropathy, infection gastrointestinal	CBC, neurologic examination	VZV prophylaxis
Carfilzomib	Myelosuppression, infection	CBC, fluid status, serum chemistries	Hydration to reduce risk of renal toxicity and TLS Dexamethasone premedication for infusion reactions VZV prophylaxis

CBC, complete blood count; STEPS, System for Thalidomide Education and Prescribing Safety; REMS, Risk Evaluation and Mitigation Strategy; TLS, tumor lysis syndrome; VTE, venous thromboembolism; VZV, varicella zoster.

5 Thalidomide and other IMiDs have complex immune effects and appear to block several pathways that are involved in disease progression in MM.[6,7,25] While not fully understood, IMiDs have anti-angiogenic and anti-inflammatory properties which may directly or indirectly affect the myeloma cell. IMiDs decrease the production of cytokines and growth factors such as IL-6, TNF-α, and VEGF which are believed to have a role in the pathogenesis of the disease. IMiDs may also inhibit nuclear factor-κB (NF-κB) activation, either directly or indirectly via TNF, which results in increased apoptosis of the MM clone.[6] Further discussion of NF-κB can be found in the proteasome inhibitors treatment section. Thalidomide and other IMiDs induce IL-2 mediated T-cell proliferation including natural killer cell activity. Figure 136-1 shows the proposed effects of thalidomide on the myeloma cell.

Thalidomide activity has been demonstrated in numerous trials. Initially, single-agent thalidomide was evaluated in refractory MM and produced overall response rates (including minor responses) in about 30% of patients.[26] Although minor and partial responses were the most common types of responses, these end points were associated with improved survival.[27]

With the activity of thalidomide in refractory MM established, subsequent studies evaluated its activity in newly diagnosed transplant-eligible and -ineligible patients. These studies evaluated thalidomide in combination with other therapies, including dexamethasone, bortezomib, and chemotherapy. PR rates with thalidomide monotherapy in untreated patients were about 30% to 40%.[6] When dexamethasone was added to thalidomide in untreated patients, response rates (≥ PR) increased to about 70% to 80%.[28] In vitro results suggest there may be synergism and reversal of resistance when used in combination.[6] The higher response rate with the combination of thalidomide plus dexamethasone has made this an attractive combination for initial therapy. The addition of bortezomib to the combination of thalidomide and dexamethasone (VTD) has been investigated in transplant-eligible patients. The triple drug regimen was associated with higher overall response rates (CR, vCR, and VGPR) compared to the combination of thalidomide and dexamethasone (TD) following first and second HSCT.[13,29] For this reason, the combination of thalidomide, bortezomib, and dexamethasone is a first-line option for transplant-eligible patients. Clinicians should recognize the higher rate of venous thromboembolism (VTE) with this combination (15%-20%) and consider VTE prophylaxis when used in patients with MM.[6,13]

The addition of thalidomide to chemotherapy also increases response rates (Table 136-5). Three randomized controlled trials evaluated the addition of thalidomide to MP in newly diagnosed MM.[30-32] Two of the three trials showed improvement in progression-free survival and overall survival with melphalan, prednisone, and thalidomide (MPT) compared with MP. The other trial demonstrated only an improvement in progression-free survival but not overall survival. Based on these results, MPT is an option for transplant-ineligible patients including older patients with MM.[13] Clinicians should be aware that the increased response rate of MPT is at the expense of higher rates of grades 3 and 4 toxicity, particularly VTE, peripheral neuropathy, and infection.[31,32]

Thalidomide dose correlates with response and toxicity. When thalidomide is combined with chemotherapy, thalidomide doses of 100 mg/day are associated with high CR rates.[30] Neuropathy is one of the important dose-limiting toxicities and may correlate with cumulative thalidomide doses. Thalidomide-induced neuropathy is usually, but not always, reversible and is associated with demyelinating changes in peripheral neurons. About 10% to 20% of patients are unable to tolerate thalidomide with neuropathy being the toxicity most often associated with discontinuation of therapy.[6,32]

Other common toxicities associated with thalidomide include constipation, sedation, fatigue, and rash. Although these toxicities can be problematic, they rarely require discontinuation of thalidomide treatment and can be therapeutically managed. Stimulant laxatives can be used to prevent severe constipation. The severity of constipation and sedation declines over time in many patients.[33]

The rate of VTE with single-agent thalidomide is relatively low (< 5%) and may not exceed the baseline incidence for MM patients. For this reason, VTE prophylaxis is not recommended in patients receiving single-agent thalidomide.[33] When thalidomide is combined with dexamethasone or chemotherapy, the risk of thrombosis is elevated, with rates reported between 10% and 30%.[30-32] The underlying mechanism for thrombosis in these patients is unknown, however, appears to be multifactorial. The American Society of Clinical Oncology (ASCO) and the IMWG have guidelines for VTE prevention. The ASCO guidelines suggest that patients should receive prophylactic aspirin or low molecular weight heparin (LMWH), depending on VTE risk.[34] The IMWG guidelines include therapeutic doses of warfarin, fixed-dose warfarin, LMWH, or aspirin depending on the patient's risk for VTE.[35] A randomized trial has compared the use of fixed-dose warfarin (1.25 mg/day), aspirin (100 mg/day), or LMWH (enoxaparin 40 mg/day) in MM patients receiving thalidomide combinations. Fixed-dose warfarin and aspirin showed similar efficacy to LMWH based on a composite measure of VTE and cardiac events. However, when only grade 3 to 4 VTEs were evaluated, aspirin prophylaxis was similar to LMWH, but fixed-dose warfarin was inferior.[36] The evidence suggests low-dose aspirin is effective prophylaxis, but should be reserved for patients in whom LMWH is not feasible and in whom there is a low-to-moderate risk of developing VTE.[36]

Lenalidomide (Revlimid®) 5 Lenalidomide is a potent thalidomide analog and shares a similar mechanism of action to other IMiDs by targeting the microenvironment. Lenalidomide is commonly used, due to an improved toxicity profile compared with thalidomide. In phase I studies, patients with relapsed, refractory MM were found to have a maximum tolerated dose of lenalidomide of 25 mg/day, with this dose being the most commonly used dose in subsequent phase II and III studies.[37] Lenalidomide is typically used in combination with low-dose dexamethasone or MP in the treatment of MM. The drug may be used in transplant-eligible or -ineligible patients, but clinicians should be aware that multiple cycles of lenalidomide therapy may impair stem cells, possibly affecting stem cell collection.[13]

Lenalidomide was FDA approved in 2006 for the treatment of relapsed or refractory MM based on the results of two randomized controlled trials. In both trials, patients were randomized to receive a combination of either lenalidomide (25 mg/day on days 1- 21 of a 28-day cycle) and high-dose dexamethasone or an identical lenalidomide placebo and high-dose dexamethasone. In one trial, patients receiving lenalidomide and dexamethasone group had overall response and CR rates of 61% and 14%, respectively, compared with 20% and 0.6% in the dexamethasone alone group (P<0.001).[38] These improved response rates translated into longer median overall survival time in the lenalidomide and dexamethasone group (29.6 vs 20.5 months). Similar results were reported in the second trial (Table 136-5).[39] Lenalidomide subsequently received FDA approval for the treatment of newly diagnosed patient with MM. In this setting, the doublet of lenalidomide and dexamethasone was compared with dexamethasone alone. The trial was halted when a planned interim analysis showed the combination to be more active than dexamethasone alone, with increased progression-free survival and overall response rate in the combination arm.[13]

The most appropriate dosing of dexamethasone with lenalidomide has also been evaluated. An open-label noninferiority phase III trial addressed this question in untreated patients with MM.[40] Patients were randomized to lenalidomide plus high-dose dexamethasone (40 mg on days 1-4, 9-12, and 17-20 of each 28 day cycle) compared with lenalidomide plus low-dose dexamethasone (40 mg/week). The trial reported a superior 2-year overall survival rate in the lenalidomide plus low-dose dexamethasone group (87% vs 75%) and found that lenalidomide with low-dose dexamethasone was associated with higher overall survival and less toxicity than lenalidomide with high-dose dexamethasone. This trial was halted after a second interim analysis and patients were allowed to cross-over to the low-dose arm.[40] Results showed that the lenalidomide plus high-dose dexamethasone arm had a 26% incidence of VTE compared to a 12% rate in those randomized to the lenalidomide plus low-dose dexamethasone arm.[40] The improved survival in the low-dose dexamethasone arm is likely related to lower mortality from adverse events, particularly VTE. Deaths in the high-dose dexamethasone group usually occurred in the first 4 months and in elderly patients. The low risk of VTE in the lenalidomide plus low-dose dexamethasone arm may allow for VTE prophylaxis with low-dose aspirin, LWMH, or warfarin as needed.[40] Lenalidomide plus dexamethasone is considered a category 1 NCCN recommendation for the initial treatment of MM patients regardless of transplant eligibility (see Fig. 136-2).[13]

Lenalidomide is also commonly added to bortezomib-based regimens and chemotherapy. The triplet of bortezomib, lenalidomide, and dexamethasone has demonstrated activity in newly diagnosed and refractory or relapsed MM. It is an option for transplant-eligible MM patients, with ongoing studies to determine its role in this setting (see Fig. 136-2).[13] The triplet regimen of melphalan, prednisone, and lenalidomide (MPL) has been studied in transplant-ineligible patients. In a recent study, MPL was compared to MPT in newly diagnosed patients with MM. No differences in survival and response rates were observed, but MPT was associated with more grade 3 or higher overall toxicity (73% vs 58%; P=0.007).[41] Along with MPT, MPL is recognized by the NCCN as a first-line option for transplant-ineligible patients.[13]

Lenalidomide is considered less toxic than thalidomide. Lenalidomide causes less neurotoxicity, somnolence, and constipation but more myelosuppression than thalidomide.[6] When used as part of combination therapy, the risk of VTE with lenalidomide is similar to that observed with thalidomide, and VTE prophylaxis is recommended.[3,34] Multiple cycles of lenalidomide impair stem cell mobilization.[13,24] IMWG recommends that transplant-eligible patients receiving lenalidomide have stem cells collected within the first four cycles of therapy.[13]

Pomalidomide (Pomalyst®) 5 Pomalidomide is the newest IMiD used in the treatment of myeloma. It is FDA approved in relapsed MM in patients who have received at least two prior therapies including lenalidomide and bortezomib. A phase II trial showed that the combination of pomalidomide with dexamethasone produced a good overall response rate (35%) in heavily pretreated relapsed and refractory MM.[13] The toxicity profile was reasonable and consisted mainly of manageable myelosuppression. Pomalidomide has also been evaluated in phase III trials. An open-label phase III trial compared pomalidomide and low-dose dexamethasone to pomalidomide and high-dose dexamethasone in relapsed or refractory MM. The primary endpoint of progression-free survival was longer in the low-dose dexamethasone arm compared with the high-dose dexamethasone combination (4 vs 1.9 months).[42] Thus, the combination of pomalidomide and dexamethasone is an option for relapsed and refractory MM.

Proteasome Inhibitors

Bortezomib (Velcade®) Bortezomib was the first drug in the class of proteasome inhibitors. It is approved in newly diagnosed and relapsed or refractory MM. The mechanism of action is complex and involves inhibiting the proteasome and NF-*κB* activation. The proteasome is a protease complex responsible for degrading cytosolic proteins that are conjugated to ubiquitin. Ubiquitin is an 8.5-kD polypeptide that tags various proteins for destruction.[43] By reversibly binding to the chymotrypsin site in the catalytic core of the 26S proteasome, bortezomib inhibits the degradation of these targeted proteins.

As discussed earlier, NF-*κB* activity is increased in MM. In the cytosol, NF-*κB* is bound to and is inhibited by I*κB*. The proteasome degrades I*κB*. When the proteasome is inhibited with bortezomib, cytosolic concentrations of I*κB* remain high, and NF-*κB* is retained in the cytosol as an inactive complex. The resulting inhibition of the NF-*κB* signal leads to a reduction in cytokine production and growth inhibition of the MM clone. Other proteins involved in cell-cycle regulation and apoptotic signaling that may be affected by bortezomib include p53, JNK proteins, and caspase 3.[6,43]

Bortezomib was initially approved in 2003 under the FDA's accelerated approval process for relapsed or refractory MM in patients who had failed at least two prior therapies. The approval was based on a phase II trial in which refractory MM received 1.3 mg/m^2 of bortezomib twice weekly for 2 weeks followed by 1 week of rest. Patients received up to 8 cycles. The overall response rate was 35% (includes minor responses) with seven (3.6%) patients achieving a CR.[44] Subsequently, a large phase III study (Assessment of Proteasome Inhibition for Extending Remissions [APEX] trial) demonstrated that bortezomib had superior activity compared with high-dose dexamethasone in relapsed MM.[45] Bortezomib-treated patients had higher complete and partial response rates (38% vs 18%), longer median time-to-progression (6.2 vs 3.5 months), and improved 1-year overall survival (80% vs 66%) compared with patients receiving dexamethasone. The differences in each of these end points were statistically significant.[45] The results from this study led to expanded FDA approval in 2005 to include patients who had relapsed after one therapy.

Combination therapy with bortezomib has shown promising results in relapsed MM. The combination of bortezomib and corticosteroids has reported CR and nCR rates ranging between 5% and 15%.[46] 6 Bortezomib is often part of a three-drug combination and, in addition to dexamethasone, may include doxorubicin, melphalan, thalidomide, or lenalidomide. These regimens have reported CR and nCR rates of 10% to 50% in relapsed MM.[6,13,46]

Numerous studies have investigated bortezomib in newly diagnosed patients in both transplant-eligible and -ineligible patients (Table 136-5). The inclusion of bortezomib in three- or four-drug combinations produces CR and nCR rates of about 19% to 52% in newly diagnosed MM.[6] Commonly used regimens in the treatment of transplant-eligible patients include bortezomib-cyclophosphamide-dexamethasone, bortezomib-thalidomide-dexamethasone, and bortezomib-lenalidomide-dexamethasone.[13] Bortezomib is also part of a regimen known as MPB (melphalan, prednisone, and bortezomib) used in the treatment of transplant-ineligible patients. The most pivotal trial leading to FDA approval as front-line therapy was the VISTA (Velcade as Initial Standard Therapy in multiple myeloma) trial in which MPB was compared with MP. The overall response and CR rates, time-to-progression, and overall survival were significantly better in the MPB group.[13] An update of this study reported a continued survival benefit after 5 years of follow-up.[47] The NCCN guidelines recognize MPB as an option for transplant-ineligible patients.[13] A meta-analysis of phase III trials suggests that MPB may achieve better response rates, including higher CR and more rapid response than MPT. However, no overall survival and progression-free survival differences were demonstrated.[13] Bortezomib-based therapies may also be preferred in patients with higher risk disease. For example, bortezomib may be able to overcome certain cytogenetic abnormalities, including the t(4;14) translocation.[48]

Bortezomib can cause significant toxicity. The most common adverse effects are mild-to-moderate fatigue and gastrointestinal toxicities. Neuropathy occurs frequently and is the most common cause of discontinuation of therapy. Other important toxicities include thrombocytopenia, fever, neutropenia, and infection. An increased risk of shingles has been reported in bortezomib-treated patients, and the NCCN guidelines recommend that herpes zoster prophylaxis be considered.[13] Bortezomib-based therapy is an attractive option for those patients with renal dysfunction since renal dose modifications are not required. Unlike melphalan and lenalidomide, bortezomib does not affect stem cell mobilization.

Neurotoxicity is a concern with bortezomib. The neurotoxicity may be decreased with modifying the route of administration and dosing schedule of bortezomib. In a phase III trial in relapsed MM, therapeutic equivalence was found between intravenous and subcutaneous routes of administration.[49] In addition, subcutaneous administration offers the potential advantage of administration in patients without IV access, convenience and improved safety profile, particularly less peripheral neuropathy. Dose schedules have also been modified to decrease toxicity-related treatment delays. Once-weekly bortezomib has been compared with twice-weekly dosing with similar overall response rates demonstrated (93% vs 88%), respectively.[13] The once-weekly schedule was associated with a reduced incidence of serious neuropathy and fewer dose reductions.[50]

Carfilzomib (Kyprolis®) Carfilzomib is a second-generation, irreversible proteasome inhibitor approved for patients with relapsed and refractory disease. Its mechanism, higher selectivity for the chymotryptic site of the 20S proteasome, and toxicity profile are distinct compared to bortezomib.[51] The dosing schedule is also different than bortezomib. Carfilzomib is more potent, yet tolerable, with two consecutive daily doses. Collectively, clinical trials have generally adopted the administration schedule of days 1, 2, 8, 9, 15, and 16 of a 28-day cycles with carfilzomib, starting at 20 mg/m^2 IV over 2 to 10 minutes on the first cycle/week and increasing to 27 mg/m^2 or more afterward depending on tolerability.[13,51]

Carfilzomib may be used as a single-agent as well as in combination therapy. The single-agent activity of carfilzomib is based on an open-label phase II study of 266 patients with relapsed and refractory MM who had received a median of five previous therapies.[52] Patients received carfilzomib 20 mg/m^2 IV over 2 to 10 minutes twice weekly on 2 consecutive days with dexamethasone premedication for 3 of 4 weeks in cycle 1 and then 27 mg/m^2 in subsequent cycles until disease progression, unacceptable toxicity, or completion of a maximum of 12 cycles. The primary endpoint of overall response rate (≥PR) was 23.7%, and the median duration of response was 7.8 months (95% confidence interval [CI] 5.6-9.2 months). In patients who were refractory or intolerant to both bortezomib and lenalidomide, 37% obtained clinical benefit. In patients refractory to both bortezomib and lenalidomide, the overall response rate (≥PR) was 15.4%. Moreover, unfavorable cytogenetic characteristics did not appear to adversely impact response rates. The median overall survival was 15.6 months compared with the median of 9 months typically seen in this setting.[52]

The activity of carfilzomib in combination regimens as first-line treatment is impressive. Two phase II trials have evaluated carfilzomib in combination with lenalidomide and low-dose dexamethasone and an additional trial has examined carfilzomib with cyclophosphamide and dexamethasone. The overall response rate (VGPR or higher) reported in these trials ranges from 74% to 88%.[13,53] The responses were rapid and increased in depth with additional cycles of therapy. The three-drug regimen containing lenalidomide did not adversely affect stem cell collection, but was associated with peripheral neuropathy, which was predominately grade 1 or 2 and observed in 23% of patients.[53] More data are required before carfilzomib-containing regimens are recommended for first-line therapy. The Endurance trial is currently comparing bortezomib-lenalidomide-dexamethasone versus carfilzomib-lenalidomide-dexamethasone.

Numerous trials of carfilzomib in relapsed myeloma are ongoing. The results from a recent interim analysis showed that the addition of carfilzomib to a lenalidomide-dexamethasone backbone improved progression-free survival (26.3 vs 17.6 months) and health-related qualify of life without any change in adverse effects.[51] Additional trials are examining the role of carfilzomib monotherapy compared with other regimens.

The most mature safety data for carfilzomib come from the compiled results of four phase II studies.[54] The most frequently reported adverse events included fatigue (55%), anemia (47%), nausea (45%), thrombocytopenia (36%), dyspnea (35%), diarrhea (33%), and pyrexia (30%). The most common grade 3 or greater adverse events were thrombocytopenia (23%), anemia (22%), lymphopenia (18%), pneumonia (11%), and neutropenia (10%). Most of these events were manageable. Peripheral neuropathy appears to be minimal with grade 3 or higher neuropathy reported in less than 1% in clinical trials.

Ixazomib (Ninlaro®) Ixazomib is the first oral proteasome inhibitor approved for the treatment of MM. It is a once-weekly medication that may be used as second-line therapy in combination with lenalidomide and dexamethasone. The approval is based on the TOURMALINE-MM1 trial which showed the addition of ixazomib to lenalidomide and dexamethasone extended progression-free survival in patients with relapsed or refractory MM compared with lenalidomide and dexamethasone alone (20.6 vs 14.7 months; HR 0.742; *P*=0.012). The safety profile was similar to the individual agents and included neutropenia, anemia, thrombocytopenia, pneumonia, diarrhea, cutaneous rash, and peripheral neuropathy. The approval of ixazomib is exciting because it allows for an orally administered triple-drug combination in the management of MM. Current studies are examining the role of ixazomib in other MM settings including induction and maintenance therapy.[55]

Monoclonal Antibodies

Two monoclonal antibodies have been recently FDA approved for the treatment of relapsed and refractory MM. Daratumumab (Darzalex®) is an IgG1-κ fully human monoclonal antibody that targets CD38, a glycoprotein highly expressed on MM cells. Accelerated FDA approval was granted after two open-label phase II trials of daratumumab showed single-agent activity (overall response rates of 29% and 36%).[57] Elotuzumab (Empliciti®) is another monoclonal antibody that is directed against signaling lymphocyte activation molecule family 7 (SLAMF7). Elotuzumab was evaluated in a phase III trial in combination with lenalidomide and dexamethasone.[57] The elotuzumab combination demonstrated improved progression-free survival and a higher overall response rate compared to lenalidomide.

Panobinostat (Farydak®)

Inhibitors of histone deacetylase enzymes such as panobinostat and vorinostat have shown activity in MM.[13] Panobinostat was evaluated in a recent phase III trial. Patients with refractory or relapsed MM who had received prior therapy with an IMiD and bortezomib were randomized to receive bortezomib, dexamethasone, and panobinostat or bortezomib, dexamethasone, and placebo.[56] The trial enrolled 768 patients and the primary endpoint of progression-free survival was statistically improved by 3.91 months (11.99 vs 8.08 months). No overall survival data were reported. There were serious adverse effects noted including thrombocytopenia, diarrhea, fatigue, and peripheral neuropathy. This trial led to the FDA approval of panobinostat in combination with bortezomib and dexamethasone in patients with refractory or relapsed MM.

Drugs in Development

There are numerous drugs in development for MM that target the MM microenvironment. Combination therapy incorporating traditional chemotherapeutic agents such as bendamustine are currently in clinical trials.[13] In addition, therapies that activate the immune system are also being explored. ImMucin is a 21-mer cancer vaccine that has demonstrated activity in a phase I/II trial.[58] The vaccine targets the mucin 1, cell surface associated (MUC1) glycoprotein domain, which increases the bodies T cells and antibody response. The trial administered ImMucin along with human granulocyte-macrophage colony-stimulating factor to 15 MUC-1 positive patients with MM and found the vaccine to be well tolerated with 11 patients having stable disease or improvement. For this reason, ImMucin was granted orphan drug designation by the FDA for the treatment of MM.

Initial Therapy

Initial therapy is guided by the NCCN, IMWG, and mSMART recommendations.[13,18,35] These recommendations are based on transplant eligibility (see Fig. 136-2). In patients ineligible for autologous HSCT, thalidomide, lenalidomide, or bortezomib is often added to MP.[13,18,20,21,50] Bortezomib-containing regimens (ie, MPB) may be particularly useful in MM patients with high-risk cytogenetics (t(4;14), 17p-). Lenalidomide plus low-dose dexamethasonse is also an option. The preferred combination is currently unclear and will require randomized controlled comparisons of these combinations. Carfilzomib-based therapy has an important role in heavily pretreated refractory MM and is being evaluated in ongoing phase III trials as induction therapy for newly diagnosed MM patients.

If autologous HSCT is planned after induction therapy, melphalan should be avoided, and thalidomide, bortezomib, or lenalidomide can be added to dexamethasone or VAD-like chemotherapy.[13,20,21,50] The NCCN guidelines list several induction therapy options (see Fig. 136-2). Because there is no standard induction regimen, clinicians can select from a wide range of possible induction regimens.[13] Many clinicians recommend lenalidomide or bortezomib and dexamethasone as two-drug induction regimens or bortezomib, dexamethasone, and either cyclophosphamide, doxorubicin, or lenalidomide as three-drug regimens for patients who are autologous HSCT candidates.[20,21,50]

Some clinicians may choose therapies based on risk using the mSMART model.[18] Bortezomib-containing induction regimens are often utilized in patients with high-risk cytogenetics which is reflected in the mSMART model (see Fig. 136-2).[18] In this approach, high-risk patients receive the combination of bortezomib, lenalidomide, and dexamethasone as induction therapy. Intermediate- and standard-risk patients receive the combination of bortezomib, cyclophosphamide, and dexamethasone or lenalidomide and low-dose dexamethasone. These regimens are continued in transplant-eligible patients for four cycles then followed by transplant, but transplant can be delayed depending on patient preference. Transplant-ineligible patients will receive therapy for about 1 year and then possibly maintenance therapy.[18]

Clinical **Controversy...**

Novel agents, such as thalidomide, bortezomib, and lenalidomide, are routinely used in combination with dexamethasone or chemotherapy as induction therapy. There is no standard induction therapy, and decisions are made based on physician preference and individual characteristics of the patient. Some experts recommend a risk-adapted approach that tailors the treatment based on cytogenetics and gene expression profiling.

Autologous Hematopoietic Stem Cell Transplantation

Although MM is a chemosensitive tumor with significant response rates after treatment with conventional chemotherapy, response durations have been short. In an attempt to improve outcomes with chemotherapy, high-dose chemotherapy regimens with autologous stem cell support have been used after initial induction therapy. The intent of the induction therapy before transplant is to reduce tumor burden. With newer treatment regimens being used for induction, higher rates of quality responses (CR, VGPR, nCR) can be obtained. Recent data suggest that obtaining quality responses during induction improves the outcomes associated with autologous HSCT.[59]

7 Two pivotal, randomized, controlled trials have evaluated the role of high-dose chemotherapy followed by autologous HSCT. In these trials, previously untreated patients were randomized to induction therapy alone versus the same induction therapy followed by high-dose chemotherapy and autologous HSCT. In 1996, the Intergroupe Francophone du Myelome (IFM) reported results of a trial demonstrating a survival advantage for high-dose chemotherapy with autologous HSCT compared with conventional chemotherapy.[60] Since then, six other trials have compared autologous HSCT to conventional chemotherapy.[61-64] Four of the six trials showed improved progression-free survival, while three showed an increase in overall survival associated with the autologous transplant arms. It is worth noting that only one of these trials used newer myeloma induction regimens. The other trials used induction regimens that are rarely used in the modern era of therapy. Palumbo et al. evaluated an induction regimen of lenalidomide and dexamethasone followed by either chemotherapy (melphalan/prednisone/lenalidomide) or tandem melphalan-based autologous transplants.[64] Results of this trial showed a progression-free survival and overall survival benefit for the autologous transplant arm. Based on all available data, guidelines from the American Society of Blood and Marrow Transplantation (ASBMT) support high-dose chemotherapy and autologous HSCT as a level A recommendation.[65]

Induction regimens containing at least one of the novel agents may make a significant difference in response and survival outcomes after autologous HSCT.[66] A randomized phase III trial performed by the French group compared the combination of bortezomib and dexamethasone to VAD as induction before autologous HSCT.[67] Patients were randomized to one of four treatment arms, which included either bortezomib plus dexamethasone or VAD as induction therapy. All arms underwent autologous HSCT with melphalan preparation (200 mg/m^2). Postinduction CR and nCR rates were 15% in the bortezomib-containing arms compared to 6% in those receiving VAD. Progression-free survival was superior in the patients in whom autologous HSCT was preceded by bortezomib plus dexamethasone induction. Two other studies that used bortezomib-based induction before autologous HSCT showed similar benefit.[66]

The optimal timing of autologous HSCT (early vs late) in MM was investigated in three trials. In a landmark trial, patients were randomized to early (within 12 months of diagnosis, $n = 91$) or late transplantation (>12 months after diagnosis, $n = 94$), and no significant difference in 5-year overall survival was observed between the groups.[68] Event-free survival, however, was significantly longer in the early transplantation group (39 months vs 13 months). In an analysis that factors in the time without symptoms, treatment, or treatment toxicity (TWisTT), patients receiving early transplantation had a longer time in a state associated with a good quality of life (27.8 vs 22.3 months). The results of this study supported early autologous HSCT because of its effects on event-free survival and quality of life. Since then, two retrospective studies comparing early versus delayed autologous HSCT have been published.[69,70] These studies included MM patients who received either lenalidomide or thalidomide-based induction regimen, or another novel-therapy based induction regimens. Both trials demonstrated similar time-to-progression and overall survival in the early (within 12 months) and delayed transplant groups. The results of these two retrospective evaluations may support the idea that, in the setting of novel therapy, delaying transplant may be feasible, but the lack of rigorous, prospective, randomized data prevents the uniform recommendation to delay transplant. Enrollment in clinical trials is highly recommended for most patients when evaluating the appropriate timing of stem cell transplantation in MM.[13]

A specialized form of autologous HSCT, tandem transplantation, involves the use of two separate autologous HSCT procedures separated by a rest period of several months. It was theorized that this more intensive approach would lead to improvements in therapeutic outcomes. Since the initial evaluation showing a benefit to the tandem transplant approach, a number of trials have investigated this approach to therapy. Two large meta-analyses evaluated single versus tandem autologous HSCT in the setting of MM.[71,72] Combined, these meta-analyses included nine individual trials in their evaluations. Both analyses concluded that the use of tandem autologous HSCT was associated with an improvement in response rate but did not result in improvements in event-free survival or overall survival. Further, it was noted that the improvement in response rates may have come at the expense of a significant increase in transplant-associated mortality with the use of tandem transplantation.

The primary conclusion from the current data on autologous HSCT as consolidation therapy in MM is that it should be used in younger patients with good performance status. Before transplant, all patients should receive induction therapy to reduce tumor burden. Because of higher transplant-related mortality, a second autologous HSCT is not currently recommended for patients with a diagnosis of MM. There is controversy surrounding the potential value of upfront autologous HSCT in an era of novel induction therapy. Some experts recommend a risk-adapted approach to treatment that included autologous HSCT in the algorithm. For example, the Mayo Clinic offers autologous HSCT to transplant-eligible intermediate- and high-risk patients after bortezomib-based induction therapy. Standard-risk patients are given the option of autologous HSCT followed by maintenance therapy or induction followed by maintenance therapy.[18]

Maintenance Therapy

8 Even with the advances in induction therapy and autologous HSCT, most patients eventually progress within 3 to 5 years, suggesting that effective maintenance therapy is needed to control or delay disease progression. The International Myeloma Working Group has published a consensus document on maintenance therapy in MM.[73]

Historically, variable efficacy and high toxicities have been reported with interferon-α (IFN-α) and dexamethasone maintenance, and neither drug can be recommended outside of a clinical trial.[23] IFN-α at one time was considered to be the maintenance drug of choice after autologous HSCT based on data from a randomized trial showing superior progression-free survival and overall survival following autologous HSCT.[74] A meta-analysis supports the benefit of IFN-α maintenance, but the benefit is limited by high toxicity and intolerance.[75] A randomized trial conducted by the Southwest Oncology Group evaluated the benefit of prednisone maintenance therapy in 125 patients.[76] Patients who received high-dose steroids had significantly longer progression-free survival and overall survival at the expense of high toxicity. Although IFN-α or corticosteroid maintenance has not been widely adopted because of toxicity profile, these therapies served as proof of principle for maintenance therapy and led to trials evaluating thalidomide, lenalidomide, and bortezomib in this setting.

Thalidomide has been studied as maintenance after autologous HSCT. Six trials have evaluated the role of thalidomide maintenance therapy.[21] In all six trials, treatment with thalidomide was associated with improvements in overall response rate, progression-free survival, and event-free survival. Overall survival was improved in three of the six trials.[21] Toxicity assessments showed that patients receiving thalidomide experienced significantly higher rates of clinically significant toxicities, leading to discontinuation of maintenance therapy in a large number of patients. Of note, three of these studies found that in patients who relapsed after transplant, survival after relapse was shorter if they had received prior thalidomide therapy. Additionally, follow up from the MRC Myeloma IX trial demonstrated that in patients with adverse-risk cytogenetics, use of maintenance thalidomide resulted in shorter overall survival.[77]

Overall, the evidence demonstrates that thalidomide maintenance significantly reduces disease progression and prolongs event-free survival, but the effect on overall survival is unclear. The toxicities associated with thalidomide also make it a less than optimal choice in the maintenance setting.

Lenalidomide has largely replaced thalidomide as maintenance therapy because of its more favorable toxicity profile. Two pivotal, randomized phase III trials have investigated the use of lenalidomide maintenance after autologous HSCT.[78] In the CALGB 100104 study, 460 patients with myeloma underwent autologous HSCT, after which subjects were randomized to receive placebo or lenalidomide maintenance. Interim analysis of the data showed significant improvement in time-to-progression in the lenalidomide arm, which led to the study being unblinded. Upon unblinding, 86 of 128 patients receiving placebo crossed over to active treatment with lenalidomide. Despite this large crossover, time-to-progression and overall survival were still improved in the lenalidomide group. In the IFM-2005 trial, patients after autologous HSCT received two cycles of lenalidomide consolidation, followed by randomization to either further lenalidomide maintenance or placebo. In this trial, lenalidomide treatment was associated with an improvement in progression-free survival, but overall survival was similar between groups.[79,80] One unique adverse effect noted in these trials was second primary malignancy, including solid tumors, hematologic malignancies, and non-melanoma skin cancers, associated with lenalidomide treatment. In both trials, these second malignancies occurred at significantly higher rate compared to placebo or control arms. Based on the data, the FDA issued a safety announcement to be added to the warning section of the lenalidomide drug labeling, detailing this increased risk. Given the risk, some practitioners have advocated limiting the use of maintenance lenalidomide to 2 years after transplant in order to minimize risk.[78]

Bortezomib maintenance after autologous HSCT has been evaluated in three separate studies.[20,21] Unfortunately, there is significant variability in the regimens used in these studies, and most included bortezomib in both the induction and maintenance setting, making it difficult to clearly define the clinical benefit of bortezomib in the maintenance setting. In the largest of these trials, 827 patients with newly diagnosed myeloma were randomized to receive induction therapy with vincristine/doxorubicin/dexamethasone (VAD) or bortezomib/doxorubicin/dexamethasone (PAD) followed by autologous HSCT.[81] Maintenance for the VAD group consisted of thalidomide, while maintenance for the PAD group consisted of bortezomib. After 2 years of maintenance, CR rates and progression-free survival were improved in the PAD group. Twelve months after randomization, progression-free survival and overall survival were improved for the PAD arm. Although data supports the activity of bortezomib, the exact role, dose, schedule, and duration of therapy remains unclear.

Given the available data, NCCN and ASBMT do not recommend the use of dexamethasone or IFN-α in the maintenance setting.[13,65] Both thalidomide and lenalidomide are recommended maintenance agents by both NCCN and ASBMT (category 1, grade A). ASBMT guidelines note that in most cases, lenalidomide is the preferred agent. Bortezomib is also a feasible maintenance option, though data are limited. NCCN lists bortezomib as a maintenance option with a category 2A recommendation. ASBMT guidelines identify bortezomib as a grade D recommendation for maintenance therapy, with potential utility in those with cytogenetic high risk disease. The decision to use any of these agents in the maintenance setting must include careful consideration of the benefits and risks.

Allogeneic Hematopoietic Stem Cell Transplantation

Allogeneic HSCT uses a stem cell source other than the patient and is therefore a transplant across immunologic barriers. Unlike autologous HSCT, which is simply a method of increasing the dose intensity of chemotherapy, allogeneic HSCT is a form of immune therapy. The interest in allogeneic transplantation for MM exists from the notion of using a disease-free stem cell source which may potentially offer longer disease control and possible cure. The major post-transplant complications associated with allogeneic transplant are acute and chronic graft-versus-host disease (GVHD). GVHD may be accompanied by graft-versus-myeloma effect. The graft-versus-myeloma effect, which is mediated by antitumor effector cells from the GVHD reaction, reduces relapse risk and may offer the patient the best chance for long-term disease-free survival.[82]

Myeloablative allogeneic HSCT has traditionally been associated with a high rate of morbidity and mortality, between 20 and 50%.[83] Historically, allogeneic transplant has been used after patients have received and progressed after an autologous HSCT. Several trials have compared tandem autologous transplants to autologous followed by allogeneic stem cell transplant, although there is wide variability in trial design patient selection, and protocols for the prevention and treatment of GVHD).[65] In all trials to date, there have been no consistent findings of improvements in overall survival or progression-free survival. Meta-analyses have shown that the use of allogeneic HSCT may confer a higher CR rate, but this comes at the cost of a higher rate of transplant-related mortality.[84,85]

Allogeneic HSCT may have a role in the management of patients with high risk disease. Ongoing clinical trials are evaluating the role of allogeneic HSCT in patients with MM who have high risk cytogenetic characteristics, who are likely to either respond poorly to upfront therapy or who relapse quickly after upfront therapy or autologous HSCT. There is increasing interest in the use of reduced intensity conditioning regimens. With the current available data, upfront myeloablative allogeneic HSCT is not routinely recommended.

Supportive Care

Bone-Modifying Agents

9 Along with anti-MM therapy, supportive care measures are aggressively used to stabilize skeletal abnormalities. Patients with MM have a high rate of bone involvement of their disease. The mechanism of MM-associated bone disease is thought to be mediated through a number of pathways, including IL-6, IL-1, and TNF-α, but the most targeted pathway is that involving receptor activator factor kappa B ligand (RANK-L) and osteoprotegerin (OPG).[16] In normal bone, RANK-L and OPG are both produced by osteoblasts. RANK-L binds to RANK receptors on osteoclasts, to stimulate bone resorption, and to OPG, a "decoy receptor," to inhibit bone resorption and stimulate bone formation. A balance between RANK-L and OPG is the basis for normal bone remodeling. In MM, an imbalance in normal bone homeostasis leads to increased osteoclast activity and the formation of osteolytic bone lesions which can lead to clinically significant skeletal-related events, including fracture, hypercalcemia, and bone pain.

Bone-modifying agents are frequently used in the treatment of bone-related complications associated with MM. Bisphosphonates are the most studied and used of these agents. Bisphosphonates bind to crystalline calcium in the bone, and are then phagocytized by osteoclasts, leading to osteoclast apoptosis.[86,87] In addition to osteoclast inhibition, bisphosphonates may also promote apoptosis in MM cells. This effect may result from the inhibition of the mevalonic acid pathway, which produces several molecules required for growth of the MM clone.[88] In addition, other potential antimyeloma effects of bisphosphonates may include modifying the cytokine microenvironment, inhibiting the adhesion of MM cells to bone marrow matrix cells, and inhibiting angiogenesis.[89] Although it is possible that bisphosphonates have an antimyeloma effect, there is little direct clinical evidence to support this activity.

The use of bisphosphonates in MM is based on the results of several large, randomized, controlled trials. In the first published study of pamidronate in myeloma, the drug was compared with placebo in a group of MM patients undergoing their first or second course of chemotherapy.[90] Several clinical end points were found to be positively impacted by pamidronate therapy. The investigators reported that patients in the pamidronate group had a lower risk of skeletal-related events, lower pain scores, and improved quality of life. Importantly, a survival advantage was observed in the pamidronate-treated patients who had already received one or more courses of antimyeloma chemotherapy. This finding of improved survival in subgroup analysis is part of the circumstantial evidence to propose an antimyeloma effect for the bisphosphonates.

In 2003, the long-term follow-up results of a trial comparing zoledronic acid to pamidronate were published.[91] This trial included a total of 1,648 patients, although only 194 of these patients had a diagnosis of MM. Patients were randomized to receive zoledronic acid 8 mg (reduced to 4 mg), zoledronic acid 4 mg, or pamidronate 90 mg every 4 weeks for 24 months. With 25 months of follow-up, results showed that zoledronic acid reduced the proportion of patients overall with skeletal-related events, and decreased skeletal morbidity. These findings were less pronounced in the MM subgroup, where time to first skeletal-related event was similar amongst the groups.

Other randomized, controlled trials have been conducted, and the results of these trials were pooled in a recent systematic review.[92] Twenty randomized trials were included, which accounted for 6,692 MM patients. The risk of vertebral fractures and pain was significantly lower in the bisphosphonate-treated patients, and there was no difference between zoledronic acid or pamidronate. Given that the aggregate data in the systematic review agreed with the large controlled studies described earlier, the effect on vertebral fractures and pain are well-supported benefits of bisphosphonate therapy. An overall survival benefit associated with bisphosphonate use in MM patients remains unclear, but this meta-analysis reported that zoledronic acid improved overall survival compared with placebo.

Of interest, a study sponsored by the Myeloma Research Council was published in 2010, comparing zoledronic acid to clodronate in 1,960 patients with newly diagnosed MM. The results of this trial demonstrated a 16% reduction in mortality associated with zoledronic acid. Median overall survival was also significantly extended in the zoledronic acid arm. These results have provided further interest in the potential that bisphosphonate therapy may have some direct anti-myeloma activity, although the mechanism of this activity is largely unknown.[93]

Pamidronate and zoledronic acid, the two most commonly used bisphosphonates in MM, are usually well tolerated. Flu-like symptoms can occur after the administration of bisphosphonates. Acute renal impairment can occur with both agents and is related to both infusion time and dose. For zoledronic acid, the risk of acute renal impairment is higher with the 8 mg dose (vs 4 mg) and when the duration of infusion is 5 minutes (vs 15 minutes). Patients with moderate renal impairment (creatinine clearance: 30-60 mL/min [0.5-1.0 mL/s]) should have their dose of zoledronic acid adjusted downward by 25% (3 mg). This recommendation is included in the zoledronic acid package insert and is based on a greater renal toxicity in patients with preexisting renal impairment.[94] Randomized studies suggest that renal effects are similar between pamidronate and zoledronic acid, and patients on bisphosphonate therapy should have serum creatinine measured at baseline and then periodically thereafter.[95]

Osteonecrosis of the jaw (ONJ) is characterized by an area of exposed necrotic bone and often affects the mandible and the maxilla, but it can also affect the soft palate. Treatment of ONJ involves surgical debridement and antimicrobial therapy and is often suboptimal.[96] The development of ONJ may be related to dental disease and tooth extraction and appears to be more common with IV bisphosphonates compared with oral, and more common with zoledronic acid than with pamidronate. The incidence of ONJ is unknown but may be as high as 10% in MM patients receiving zoledronic acid for extended periods of time. A strong recommendation on a preferred bisphosphonate based on ONJ incidence is likely not warranted. A recent meta-analysis found no difference between the bisphosphonate used and the risk of ONJ.[92]

Recommendations for the treatment of MM-related bone disease were published by the International Myeloma Working Group in 2013.[97] These guidelines recommend that bisphosphonate therapy be initiated in patients with or without bone lesions at diagnosis, and should continue for 1 to 2 years. After 2 years, patients who have achieved a CR or VGPR may consider discontinuing therapy because of the increased risk of ONJ. In addition to recommendations regarding bisphosphonate therapy, this publication also provides guidance for nonpharmacologic interventions to optimize bone health, including radiation, surgery, and kyphoplasty or vertebroplasty.

More recently, a new class of bone-modifying agents has emerged. Denosumab is a first-in class monoclonal antibody directed towards RANK-L. By binding to RANK-L, denosumab prevents binding of RANK-L to RANK, reducing osteoclast activity and allowing bone formation and osteoblast function to predominate. A phase III trial evaluated the efficacy and safety of denosumab compared to zoledronic acid in patients with MM and other cancers.[98] Initial results from this study showed denosumab to be noninferior to zoledronic acid in delaying time to first skeletal-related event. Rates of overall survival, disease progression, and ONJ were similar between groups. Of note, renal adverse effects occurred at a higher rate with zoledronic acid. Denosumab does not require dose adjustments for those with impaired renal function. In a subset analysis of patients with MM, the hazard ratio for death was 2.26 for patients receiving zoledronic acid. While the exact reason for this increase in mortality associated with denosumab is unknown, it is not recommended to routinely use denosumab in place of a bisphosphonate for patients with MM.

Clinical **Controversy...**

Although bisphosphonates are indicated in MM patients with bone disease, controversies surrounding the selection of the best agent and duration of therapy remain. Because of the risk of ONJ in MM patients, a cautious approach on bisphosphonate use is prudent. Some experts recommend that the duration of bisphosphonate therapy should be limited to 2 years. The preference of pamidronate over zoledronic acid is also controversial given that ONJ has also been reported with pamidronate, and the higher risk of ONJ with zoledronic acid is based on observational studies rather than head-to-head randomized comparisons.

Relapsed or Refractory Disease

10 A variety of factors must be considered when determining the most appropriate therapy for an individual who suffers relapses, including the type and duration of previous therapies, whether the patient received a transplant, presence or absence of adverse prognostic factors, toxicity of prior therapies (eg, peripheral neuropathy), organ dysfunction (eg, renal impairment), and how much time has elapsed from initial response to relapse.[13,20,21] The same drugs used to treat MM initially can also be used as salvage therapy in patients who have relapsed. Patients who suffer relapse more than 6 months after initial induction therapy may have same induction therapy repeated.[13] The treatment of patients with relapsed or refractory MM can be with active agents in combination or single agents used sequentially. With the growing number of highly active agents, combination salvage therapy has become predominant. The NCCN has five category 1 recommendations and lists many other additional regimens.[13] Bortezomib is widely used in relapsed and refractory MM. One reason is that bortezomib has activity in patients with high-risk cytogenetics and high-risk patients are more likely to suffer relapse and require salvage therapy. Bortezomib may be used as a single agent or in combination therapy. The addition of dexamethasone, liposomal doxorubicin, panobinostat, lenalidomide, or thalidomide to patients who progress on single-agent bortezomib has been shown to improved response.[50] Interestingly, prior use of IMiDs or high-dose chemotherapy does not appear to affect bortezomib activity in relapsed MM. A phase III trial reported that bortezomib with or without dexamethasone had activity in relapsed or refractory disease despite prior thalidomide therapy or autologous HSCT.[99] Several IMiD combination regimens may also be used in relapsed and refractory MM. Lenalidomide is the IMiD most commonly utilized and has received a category 1 recommendation in relapsed or refractory patients when combined with dexamethasone alone or in combination with carfilzomib and dexamethasone.[13,50]

Treatment decisions for individual patients with relapsed disease may potentially be improved by taking into account patient-specific information such as the type of previous therapies, adverse cytogenetics, and end-organ dysfunction. For example, in patients with relapsed MM, combined bortezomib and liposomal doxorubicin has shown improved time-to-progression compared with bortezomib alone, including in patients who had received prior anthracyclines, lenalidomide, and thalidomide.[50] In contrast, treatment with lenalidomide and dexamethasone resulted in a significantly shorter time-to-progression in patients who had previously been treated with thalidomide compared with thalidomide-naïve patients.[38,39] Despite clear progress, most salvage therapies produce less than a 50% response rate, and new drugs and drug combinations are needed.

Questions remain on the optimal timing for autologous HSCT. For patients who are eligible for autologous HSCT and did not receive transplant as part of initial therapy, it is appropriate to offer autologous HSCT at first relapse. It is important to emphasize that although higher quality of life was realized when autologous HSCT was used as consolidation therapy, there was no difference in overall survival based on timing of transplant. The use of salvage autologous HSCT in patients who received a prior autologous HSCT seemed to be most beneficial in patients who had a response of greater than 24 months after initial autologous HSCT.[100] In patients with relapsed or refractory MM, autologous HSCT followed by nonmyeloablative allogeneic HSCT has potential benefit but at the expense of increased transplant-related mortality requiring treatment only be performed as part of a clinical protocol.

PERSONALIZED PHARMACOTHERAPY

Therapy for MM is personalized based on staging (eg, ISS), cytogenetics, gene expression profiling, performance status of the patient, age of the patient, and preexisting risk for drug toxicity. Personalized therapy has been driven by the explosion of new treatment options in MM and a better understanding of the MM biology and therapeutic targets. As described previously, the Mayo Clinic recommends a risk-adapted approach that tailors therapy based on risk category (eg, high, intermediate, or standard).

The use of a risk-adapted approach is reasonable in newly diagnosed patients (see Fig. 136-2). MM is currently not curable, and the disease will evolve as the disease progresses, which will require evaluation of biomarkers at times of relapse and progression to tailor therapy in each stage of the disease.

In addition to molecular characteristics of the tumor, a number of patient-related factors guide personalized treatment. For example, older patients with poor performance status would not be candidates for autologous HSCT. Patients with preexisting severe peripheral neuropathy would be less likely to receive thalidomide or bortezomib because of neurotoxicity. Patients with risk factors for VTE would be more likely to receive bortezomib-containing combinations because the risk of VTE is lower compared with thalidomide or lenalidomide combinations. Patients with preexisting renal failure may be less likely to receive lenalidomide because it requires dose adjustment based on renal function. With personalized therapy, patients will have the opportunity to benefit from the use of novel agents.

EVALUATION OF THERAPEUTIC OUTCOMES

As MM is currently an incurable disease, the goals of therapy are to prolong survival and to improve quality of life. Patients with asymptomatic MM are usually followed and not treated. Asymptomatic patients are assessed every 3 to 6 months for disease progression, which would then warrant therapy. Assessment involves measurement of M protein in blood and urine and laboratory tests that include complete blood count, serum creatinine, and calcium. Patients are treated as the disease produces symptoms. Disease response is defined by a decline in M protein. After completion of the initial course of therapy and once a response is obtained, patients should be monitored every 3 months. Bone surveys are performed yearly or as required because of changes in symptoms. Various other tests, including bone marrow biopsy, magnetic resonance imaging, and positron emission tomography, or computed tomography scan, are performed on an as-needed basis to evaluate disease status.

ABBREVIATIONS

ASBMT	American Society of Bone Marrow Transplant
ASCO	American Society of Clinical Oncology
CI	confidence interval
CR	complete remission
I*κB*	inhibitory factor kappa B
IFN	interferon
IGF-1	insulin-like growth factor
IL	interleukin
IL-6	interleukin-6
IMiD	immunomodulatory drug
HSCT	hematopoietic stem cell transplantation
IFM	Intergroupe Francophone du Myelome
IgG	intact monoclonal immunoglobulin
ImiD	immunomodulatory drug
IMWG	International Myeloma Working Group
ISS	International Staging System
LMWH	low-molecular-weight heparin
MGUS	monoclonal gammopathy of undetermined significance
MM	multiple myeloma
MP	melphalan plus prednisone
MPB	melphalan, prednisone, and bortezomib
MPL	melphalan, prednisone, and lenalidomide
MPT	melphalan, prednisone, and thalidomide
mSMART	Mayo Stratification for Myeloma and Risk-adapted therapy
MUC-1	mucin-1
NCCN	National Comprehensive Cancer Network
NF-*κB*	nuclear factor kappa B
nCR	near complete response
ONJ	osteonecrosis of the jaw
OPG	osteoprotegerin
PAD	bortezomib/doxorubicin/dexamethasone
PR	partial response
RANK	receptor activator of nuclear factor-κB
RANK-L	receptor for activation of NF-*κB* ligand
SFC	Serum free light chains
TNF-*α*	tumor necrosis factor-*α*
VAD	vincristine, doxorubicin, and dexamethasone
VEGF	vascular endothelial growth factor
VGPR	very good partial response
VTE	venous thromboembolism

REFERENCES

1. Mahindra A, Hideshima T, Anderson KC. Multiple Myeloma: Biology of the disease. *Blood Reviews* 2010;S5-S11.
2. Morgan GJ, Walker BA, Davies FE. The genetic architecture of multiple myeloma. *Nature Reviews* 2012;12:335-348.
3. Siegel R, Miller KD, Jemal A. Cancer statistics, 2016. CA *Cancer J Clin* 2016;66:7-30.
4. Surveillance, Epidemiology, and End Results (SEER) Program. SEER Stat Facts Sheets: Myeloma. Available at: http://seer.cancer.gov/statfacts/html/mulmy.html. Last accessed October 1, 2015.
5. Landgren O, Kristinsson SY, Goldin LR, et al. Risk of plasma cell and lymphoproliferative disorders among 14,621 first-degree relatives of 4,458 patients with monoclonal gammopathy of undetermined significance in Sweden. *Blood* 2009;114(4):791-795.
6. Munshi NC, Anderson KC. Plasma cell neoplasms. In: Devita VT, Hellman S, Rosenberg SA, eds. *Cancer Principles and Practice of Oncology*, 9th ed. Philadelphia, PA: Lippincott Williams & Wilkins; 2011:2305-2342.
7. Palumbo A, Anderson K. Multiple myeloma. *N Engl J Med* 2011;364:1046-1060.
8. Kyle RA, Therneau TM, Rajkumar SV, et al. Prevalence of monoclonal gammopathy of undetermined significance. *N Engl J Med* 2006;354:1362-1369.
9. Ahn IE, Mailankody S, Korde N, Landgren O. Dilemmas in treating smoldering multiple myeloma. *J Clin Oncol* 2015;33:115-123.
10. Rajikumar SV, Gupta V, Fonseca R, et al. Impact of primary molecular cytogenetic abnormalities and risk of progression in smoldering multiple myeloma. *Leukemia* 2013;27(8):1738-1744.
11. Landgren O. Monoclonal gammopathy of undetermined significance and smoldering multiple myeloma: biological insights and early treatment strategies. *Hematology* 2013;478-487.
12. Mahindra A, Laubach J, Raje N, et al. Latest advances and current challenges in the treatment of multiple myeloma. *Nat Rev Clin Oncol* 2012;9:135-143.
13. National Comprehensive Cancer Network. The NCCN Multiple Myeloma Clinical Practice Guidelines in Oncology (Version 2.2016). 2015. Available at: http://www.NCCN.org. Last accessed October 1, 2015.
14. Rajkumar SV, Dimopoulus MA, Palumbo A, et al. International Myeloma Working Group updated criteria for the diagnosis of multiple myeloma. *Lancet Oncology* 2014;15(12):e538-548.
15. Dispenzieri A, Kyle R, Merlini G, et al. International myeloma working group guidelines for serum light chain analysis in multiple myeloma and related disorders. *Leukemia* 2009;23:215-224.
16. Roodman GD. Pathogenesis of myeloma bone disease. *Leukemia* 2009;23:435-441.
17. Greipp PR, Miguel JS, Durie BG, et al. International staging system for multiple myeloma. *J Clin Oncol* 2005;23:3412-3420.
18. Mikhael JR, Dingli D, Roy V, et al. Management of Newly Diagnosed Symptomatic Multiple Myeloma: Updated Mayo Stratification of Myeloma and Risk-Adapted Therapy (mSMART) Consensus Guidelines 2013. *Mayo Clin Proc* 2013;88:360-376.

19. Rajkumar SV, Harousseau JL, Durie, et al. Consensus recommendations for the uniform reporting of clinical trials: report of the International Myeloma Workshop Consensus Panel 1. *Blood* 2011;117:4691-4695.
20. Mateos MV, San Miguel JF. How should we treat newly diagnosed multiple myeloma patients? *Hematology Am Soc Hematol Educ Program* 2013.2013:488-495.
21. Moreau P, Attal M, Facon T. Frontline therapy of multiple myeloma. *Blood* 2015;125(20):3076-3084.
22. Thomas A, Mailankody S, Korde N, et al. Second malignancies after multiple myeloma: From 1960s to 2010s. *Blood* 2012;119:2731-2737.
23. Facon T, Mary JY, Pegourie B, et al. Dexamethasone-based regimens versus melphalan prednisone for elderly multiple myeloma patients ineligible for high dose therapy. *Blood* 2006;107:1292-1298.
24. Rajkumar SV. Doublets, triplets, or quadruplets of novel agents in newly diagnosed myeloma? *Hematology Am Soc Hematol Educ Program* 2012;2012:354-361.
25. Kotla V, Gold S, Nischal S, et al. Mechanism of action of lenalidomide in hematological malignancies. *J Hematol Oncol* 2009;2:36.
26. Reece DE, Leitch HA, Atkins H, et al. Treatment of relapsed and refractory myeloma. *Leuk Lymphoma* 2008;49:1470-1485.
27. Barlogie B, Desikan R, Eddlemon P, et al. Extended survival in advanced and refractory multiple myeloma after single-agent thalidomide: Identification of prognostic factors in a phase 2 study of 169 patients. *Blood* 2001;98:492-494.
28. Larocca A, Palumbo A. Evolving paradigms in treatment of newly diagnosed multiple myeloma. *J NCCN* 2011;9:1186-1196.
29. Cavo M, Tacchetti P, Patriarca F, et al. Bortezomib with thalidomide plus dexamethasone compared with thalidomide plus dexamethasone as induction therapy before, and consolidation therapy after, double autologous stem-cell transplantation in newly diagnosed multiple myeloma: a randomized phase 3 study. *Lancet* 2010;116:3143-3151.
30. Palumbo A, Bringhen S, Liberati AM, et al. Oral melphalan with prednisone and thalidomide in elderly patients with multiple myeloma: Updated results of a randomized controlled trial. *Blood* 2008;112:3107-3114.
31. Facon T, Mary JY, Hulin C, et al. Melphalan and prednisone plus thalidomide versus melphalan and prednisone alone or reduced-intensity autologous stem cell transplantation in elderly patients with multiple myeloma (IFM 99–06): A randomised trial. *Lancet* 2007;370:1209-1218.
32. Hulin C, Facon T, Rodon P, et al. Efficacy of melphalan and prednisone plus thalidomide in patients older than 75 years with newly diagnosed multiple myeloma: IFM 01/01 Trial. *J Clin Oncol* 2009;27:3664-3670.
33. Gleason C, Nooka A, Lonial S. Supportive therapies in multiple myeloma. *J Natl Compr Canc Netw* 2009;7:971-979.
34. Lyman GH, Khorana AA, Kuderer NM, et al. Venous thromboembolism prophylaxis and treatment in patients with cancer: American Society of Clinical Oncology Clinical Practice Guideline Update. *J Clin Oncol* 2013;31(17):2189-2204.
35. Palumbo A, Rajkumar SV, San Miguel JF, et al. International Myeloma Working Group consensus statement for the management, treatment, and supportive care of patients with myeloma not eligible for standard autologous stem-cell transplantation. *J Clin Oncol* 2014;32(6):587-600.
36. Palumbo A, Cavo M, Bringhen S, et al. Aspirin, warfarin, or enoxaparin thromboprophylaxis in patients with multiple myeloma treated with thalidomide: A phase III open label randomized trial. *J Clin Oncol* 2011;29:986-993.
37. Armoiry X, Auglagner G, Facon T. Lenalidomide in the treatment of multiple myeloma: A review. *J Clin Pharm Ther* 2008;33:219-226.
38. Weber DM, Chen C, Niesvizky R, et al. Lenalidomide plus dexamethasone for relapsed multiple myeloma in North America. *N Engl J Med* 2007;357:2133-2142.
39. Dimopoulous M, Spencer A, Attal M, et al. Lenalidomide plus dexamethasone for relapsed or refractory multiple myeloma. *N Engl J Med* 2007;357:2123-2132.
40. Rajkumar SV, Jacobus S, Callander NS, et al. Lenalidomide plus high-dose dexamethasone versus lenalidomide plus low-dose dexamethasone as initial therapy for newly diagnosed multiple myeloma: an open-labeled randomized control trial. *Lancet Oncol* 2010;11:29-37.
41. Steward AK, Jacobus S, Fonseca R, et al. Melphalan, prednisone, and thalidomide vs melphalan, prednisone, and lenalidomide (ECOG E1A06) in untreated multiple myeloma. *Blood* 2015;126(11):1294-1301.
42. San Miguel J, Weisel K, Moreau P, et al. Pomalidomide plus low-dose dexamethasone versus high-dose dexamethasone alone for patients with relapsed and refractory multiple myeloma (MM-003): A randomized, open-label, phase 3 trial. *Lancet Oncol* 2013;14:1055-1066.
43. Shah JJ, Orlowski RZ. Proteasome inhibitors in the treatment of multiple myeloma. *Leukemia* 2009;23:1964-1979.
44. Richardson P, Barlogie B, Berenson J, et al. A phase II study of bortezomib in relapsed, refractory myeloma. *N Engl J Med* 2003;348:2609-2617.
45. Richardson PG, Sonneveld P, Schuster MW, et al. Bortezomib or high dose dexamethasone in relapsed multiple myeloma. *N Engl J Med* 2005;352:2487-2498.
46. Richardson PG, Mitsiades C, Ghobrial I, Anderson K. Beyond single agent bortezomib: Combination regimens in relapsed multiple myeloma. *Curr Opin Oncol* 2006;18:598-608.
47. San Miguel JF, Schlag R, Khuageva NK, et al. Persistent overall survival benefit and no increased risk of secondary malignancies with bortezomib-melphalan-prednisone versus melphalan-prednisone in patients with previously untreated multiple myeloma. *J Clin Oncol* 2013;31:448-455.
48. Avet-Loiseua H, Leleu X, Roussel M, et al. Bortezomib plus dexamethasone induction improves outcomes of patients with t(4;14) myeloma but not outcomes of patients with del(17p). *J Clin Oncol* 2010;28(30):4630-4634.
49. Arnulf B, Pylypenko H, Grosicki S, et al. Updated survival analysis of a randomized Phase III study of subcutaneous verus intravenous bortezomib in patients with relapsed multiple myeloma. *Hematologica* 2012;97:1925-1928.
50. Rakjumar SV. Multiple myeloma: 2014 update on diagnosis, risk-stratification and management. *Am J Hematol* 2014;89(10): 998-1009.
51. Stewart AK, Rajkumar S, Dimopoulos MA, et al. Carfilzomib, lenalidomide and dexamethasone for replased multiple myeloma. *N Engl J Med* 2015;372(2):42-152.
52. Siegel DS, Martin T, Wang M, et al. A phase 2 study of single agent carfilzomib (PX-171-003-A1) in patients with relapsed and refractory multiple myeloma. *Blood* 2012;120:2817-2825.
53. Jakubowiak AJ, Dytfeld D, Griffith KA, et al. A phase 1/2 study of carfilzomib in combination with lenalidomide and low-dose dexamethasone as a frontline treatment for multiple myeloma. *Blood* 2012;120:1801-1809.
54. Siegel D, Martin T, Nooka A, et al. Integrated safety profile of single-agent carfilzomib: Experience from 527 patients enrolled in 4 phase II clinical studies. *Haematologica* 2013;98(11):1753-1761.
55. Ixazomib, an Investigational Oral Proteasome Inhibitor (PI), in Combination with Lenalidomide and Dexamethasone (IRd), Significantly Extends Progression-Free Survival (PFS) for Patients (Pts) with Relapsed and/or Refractory Multiple Myeloma (RRMM): The Phase 3 Tourmaline-MM1 Study. American Society of Hematology 2015 Annual Meeting (Abstract #727).
56. San-Miguel JF, Hungria VT, Yoon SS, et al. Panobinostat plus bortezomib and dexamethasone versus placebo plus bortezomib and dexamethasone in patients with relapsed or relapsed and refractory multiple myeloma: A multicenter, randomized, double-blind phase 3 trial. *Lancet Oncol* 2014;14:1195-1206.
57. Afifi S, Michael A, Lesokhin A. Immunotherapy: a new approach to treating multiple myeloma with daratumumab and elotuzumab. *Ann Pharmacother* 2016;50:555-568.
58. Carmon L, Aviv I, Kovjazin R, et al. Phase I/II study exploring ImMucin, a pan-major histocompatibility complex, anti-MUC1 signal peptide vaccine, in multiple myeloma patients. *British Journal of Haematology* 2015;169:44-56.
59. Rosinol L, Oriol A, Teruel AI, et al. Superiority of bortezomib, thalidomide, and dexamethasone (VTD) as induction pre-transplantation in multiple myeloma: A randomized Phase 3 PETHEMA/GEM study. *Blood* 2012;120:1589-1596.
60. Attal M, Harousseau JL, Stoppa AM, et al. A prospective, randomized trial of autologous bone marrow transplantation and chemotherapy in multiple myeloma. *N Engl J Med* 1996;335:91-97.
61. Child JA, Morgan GJ, Davies FE et al. High-dose chemotherapy with hematopoietic stem cell rescue for multiple myeloma. *N Engl J Med* 2003;348:1875-1883.
62. Blade J, Rosinol L, Sureda A, et al. High dose therapy intensification compared with continued standard chemotherapy in multiple myeloma patients responding to the initial chemotherapy: long term results from a prospective randomized trial from the Spanish cooperative group PETHEMA. *Blood* 2005;106:3755-3759, #85.

63. Palumbo A, Bringhen S, Petrucci MT, et al. Intermediate-dose melphalan improves survival of myeloma patients aged 50 to 70: Results of a randomized controlled trial. *Blood* 2004;104:3052-3057, #84.
64. Palumbo A, Cavallo F, Gay F, et al. Autologous transplantation and maintenance therapy in multiple myeloma. *N Engl J Med* 2014;371: 895-905.
65. Shah N, Callander N, Ganguly S, et al. Hematopoietic Stem Cell Transplantation for Multiple Myeloma: Guidelines from the American Society for Blood and Marrow Transplantation. *Biol Blood Marrow Transplant* 2015;21(7):1155-1166.
66. Giralt S. Stem cell transplantation for multiple myeloma: Current and future status. *Hematology Am Soc Hematol Educ Program* 2012;2012:191-196.
67. Harousseau JL, Avet-Loiseau H, Attal M, et al. Bortezomib plus dexamethasone is superior to VAD as induction treatment prior to ASCT in newly diagnosed multiple myeloma: Results of the IFM 2005-01 Phase III trial. *J Clin Oncol* 2010;28:4621-4629.
68. Fermand JP, Ravaud P, Chevaer S, et al. High dose therapy and autologous peripheral blood stem cell transplantation in multiple myeloma: Up-front or rescue treatment? Results of a multicenter sequential randomized clinical trial. *Blood* 1998;92:3131-3136.
69. Kumar SK, Lacy MQ, Dispenzieri A, et al. Early versus delayed autologous transplantation after immunomodulatory agents based induction therapy in patients with newly diagnosed multiple myeloma. *Cancer* 2012;118:1585-1592.
70. Dunavin NC, Wei L, Elder P, et al. Early versus delayed autologous stem cell transplant in patients receiving novel therapies for multiple myeloma. *Leuk Lymphoma* 2013;54:1658-1664.
71. Kumar A, Kharfan-Dabaja MA, Glasmacher A, Djulbegovic B. Tandem versus single autologous hematopoietic cell transplantation for treatment of multiple myeloma: A systematic review and meta-analysis. *J Natl Cancer Instit* 2009;101:100-106.
72. Neumann-Winter F, Greb A, Borchmann P, et al. First-line tandem high-dose chemotherapy and autologous stem cell transplant versus single high-dose chemotherapy and autologous stem cell transplant in multiple myeloma, A systematic review of controlled studies. *Cochrane Database Syst Rev* 2012;10:CD004626.
73. Ludwig H, Durie BG, McCarthy P, et al. IMWG consensus on maintenance therapy in multiple myeloma. *Blood* 2012;119: 3003-3015.
74. Mandelli F, Avvisati G, Amadori S, et al. Maintenance treatment with recombinant interferon-alpha 2b in patients with multiple myeloma responding to conventional induction chemotherapy. *N Engl J Med* 1990;322:1430-1434.
75. Fritz E, Ludwig H. Interferon-alpha treatment in multiple myeloma: Meta-analysis of 30 randomized trials among 3948 patients. *Ann Oncol* 2000;11:1427-1436.
76. Berenson JR, Crowley JJ, Grogan TM, et al. Maintenance therapy with alternate-day prednisone improves survival in multiple myeloma patients. *Blood* 2002;99:3163-3168.
77. Morgan GJ, Gregory WM, Davies FE, et al. The role of maintenance thalidomide therapy in multiple myeloma: MRC Myeloma IX results and meta-analysis. *Blood* 2012;119:7-15.
78. Rajkumar SV. Lenalidomide maintenance – perils of a premature denouement. *Nature Reviews* 2012;9:372-373.
79. Attal M, Lauwers-Cances V, Marit G, et al. Lenalidomide maintenance after stem cell transplant for multiple myeloma. *N Engl J Med* 2012;366:1782-1791.
80. McCarthy PL, Owzar K, Hofmeister CC, et al. Lenalidomide after stem cell transplantation for multiple myeloma. *N Engl J Med* 2012;366:1770-1781.
81. Sonneveld P, Schmidt-Wolf I, van der Holt B, et al. Bortezomib induction and maintenance treatment in patients with newly diagnosed multiple myeloma: Results of the randomized Phase III Hovon-65/GMMG-HD4 trial. *J Clin Oncol* 2012;30:2946-2955.
82. Laterveer L, Verdonck LF, Peeters T, et al. Graft-versus-myeloma may overcome the unfavorable effect of deletion of chromosome 13 in multiple myeloma. *Blood* 2003;101:1201-1202.
83. Bruno B, Giaccone L, Sorasio R, Boccadoro M. Role of allogeneic stem cell transplantation in multiple myeloma. *Semin Hematol* 2009;46:158-165.
84. Armeson KE, Hill EG, Costa LJ. Tandem autologous vs autologous plus reduced intensity allogeneic transplantation in the upfront management of multiple myeloma: meta-analysis of trials with biological assignment. *Bone Marrow Transplant* 2013;48:562-567.
85. Kharfan-Dabaja MA, Hanadani M, Reljic T, et al. Comparative efficacy of tandem autologous versus autologous followed by allogeneic hematopoietic cell transplantation in patients with newly diagnosed multiple myeloma: a systematic review and meta-anlysis of randomized controlled trials. *J Hematol Oncol* 2013;6:2.
86. Russell RG. Bisphosphonates: From bench to bedside. *Ann N Y Acad Sci* 2006;1068:367-401.
87. Papapoulos SE. Bisphosphonate actions: Physical chemistry revisited. *Bone* 2006;38:613-616.
88. Baulch-Brown C, Molloy TJ, Yeh SL, et al. Inhibitor of the mevalonate pathway as potential therapeutic agents in multiple myeloma. *Leuk Res* 2007;31:341-352.
89. Neville-Webbe HL, Holen I, Coleman RE. The anti-tumor activity of bisphosphonates. *Cancer Treat Rev* 2002;28:305-319.
90. Berenson JR, Lichtenstein A, Porter L, et al. Long-term pamidronate treatment of advanced multiple myeloma patients reduces skeletal events. Myeloma Aredia Study Group. *J Clin Oncol* 1998;16:593-602.
91. Rosen LS, Gordon D, Kaminski M, et al. Long-term efficacy and safety of zoledronic acid compared with pamidronate disodium in the treatment of skeletal complications in patients with advanced multiple myeloma or breast carcinoma. *Cancer* 2003;98(8):1735-1744.
92. Mhaskar R, Redzepovic J, Wheatley K, et al. Bisphosphonates in multiple myeloma: A network meta-analysis. *Cochrane Database Syst Rev* 2012;5:CD003188.
93. Morgan GJ, Davies FE, Gregory WM, et al. First-line treatment with zoledronic acid as compared with clodronic acid in multiple myeloma: A randomized control trial. *Lancet* 2010;376:1989-1999.
94. Zometa®[package insert]. East Hanover, New Jersey: Novartis Pharmaceuticals Corporation. Last accessed October 1, 2015.
95. Pozzi S, Raje N. The role of bisphosphonates in multiple myeloma: Mechanisms, side-effects, and future. *Oncologist* 2011;16:651-662.
96. Reid IR, Cornish J. Epidemiology and pathogenesis of osteonecrosis of the jaw. *J Nat Rev Rheumatol* 2012;8:90-96.
97. Terpos E, Morgan G, Dimopoulos MA, et al. International Myeloma Working Group Recommendations for the Treatment of Multiple Myeloma-Related Bone Disease. *J Clin Oncol* 2013;31:2347-2357.
98. Henry DH, Costa L, Goldwasser F, et al. Randomized, Double-Blind Study of Denosumab versus Zoledronic Acid in the Treatment of Bone Metastases in Patients with Advanced Cancer (Excluding Breast and Prostate Cancer) or Multiple Myeloma. *J Clin Oncol* 2011;29:1125-1132.
99. Mikhael JR, Belch AR, Prince HM, et al. High response rates to bortezomib with or without dexamethasone in patients with relapsed or refractory multiple myeloma: Results of a global phase IIIb expanded access programs. *Br J Hematol* 2009;144:169-175.
100. Lemieux E, Hulin C, Caillot D, et al. Autologous stem cell transplant: An effective salvage therapy in multiple myeloma. *Biol Blood Marrow Transplant* 2013;19(3):445-449.

Myelodysplastic Syndromes

e137

Kristen B. McCullough and Julianna A. Merten

KEY CONCEPTS

1. Myelodysplastic syndromes (MDS) primarily affect elderly adults, with median age at diagnosis of 76 years.
2. MDS are associated with environmental, occupational, and therapeutic exposures to chemicals or radiation.
3. The clonal population of cells manifested as MDS results from enhanced self-renewal of a hematopoietic stem cell or acquisition of self-renewal in a progenitor cell, increased proliferative capacity in the abnormal clone, impaired cell differentiation, evasion of immune regulation, and antiapoptotic mechanisms in the disease-sustaining cell.
4. Most patients with MDS present with fatigue and lethargy or symptoms related to anemia-induced tissue hypoxia.
5. The prognosis of patients with MDS is variable. Overall survival time ranges from a few months to several years and is most accurately estimated with the International Prognostic Scoring System—Revised (IPSS-R).
6. The primary goal of therapy is hematologic improvement for lower-risk patients and alteration in the natural course of the disease for higher-risk patients. Palliation of symptoms and improvement in quality of life are goals of therapy for all patients.
7. Current guidelines recommend erythropoietin (EPO) or darbepoetin with or without filgrastim for management of anemia in patients with lower-risk MDS.
8. Hypomethylating agents are appropriate for patients with lower-risk MDS with clinically significant neutropenia or thrombocytopenia, patients with anemia who are unlikely to respond to or have not responded to a trial of EPO or immunosuppressive therapy.
9. Antithymocyte globulin is appropriate treatment for patients with lower risk, HLA DR15 positive expressing MDS who have symptomatic anemia that is unlikely to respond to erythropoietic agents.
10. Lenalidomide is recommended for initial treatment of lower-risk 5q- syndrome accompanied by symptomatic anemia.
11. Allogeneic hematopoietic stem cell transplantation offers potentially curative therapy to patients with MDS who have a donor and are healthy enough for the procedure.

INTRODUCTION

Myelodysplastic syndromes (MDS) are myeloid clonal, heterogeneous, stem cell disorders characterized by predominantly hypercellular bone marrows, anemia, thrombocytopenia, leukopenia, and an inherent predisposition toward evolution to acute myeloid leukemia (AML).[1,2] The diagnostic hallmark for MDS is the presence of bone marrow dysplasia in at least 10% of cells of a single myeloid lineage.[1] The clinical course of patients with MDS varies from a slowly progressing indolent disease to more aggressive disease characterized by excess bone marrow blasts and rapid progression to AML in up to 30% of cases.[3,4]

Our understanding of the molecular genetics behind MDS has advanced in recent years, but few targeted treatments have been approved in MDS. Aberrations in epigenetic regulator genes, spliceosome component pathways, DNA damage response genes, and genes regulating transcription factors have redefined the molecular landscape in MDS and several additional chromosomal abnormalities have been incorporated into prognostic models predicting survival and leukemic transformation.[5,6] Between 2004 and 2006, three medications (azacitidine, decitabine, and lenalidomide) were approved by the FDA for the treatment of MDS with both azacitidine and lenalidomide improving survival in MDS.[7,8] Despite progress in disease classification, identification of over 40 recurrently mutated genes, improvement in risk stratification, and development of new treatment options in the past two decades, the ability to provide patient specific, targeted therapy remains elusive.

EPIDEMIOLOGY

1 MDS primarily affect elderly adults, with a median age at diagnosis of 76 years and a slight male predominance, with an estimated male-to-female ratio of about 1.75 to 1.[9,10] An estimated 3 to 12 cases of MDS are diagnosed per 100,000 persons per year. The risk of MDS increases with age; in patients older than 65 to 70 years, an estimated 27 to 75 new cases occur per 100,000 persons per year.[10-12] The Surveillance, Epidemiology and End Results (SEER) Program estimates about 19,600 new cases of MDS are diagnosed in the United States each year.[10] Recent reports suggest that the incidence of MDS has been grossly underestimated, with analyses of Medicare claims databases indicating it could be as high as 45,000 per year.[12,13] Many experts predict that the incidence of MDS will increase as the population of the United States ages and clinicians become more aware of MDS.[9]

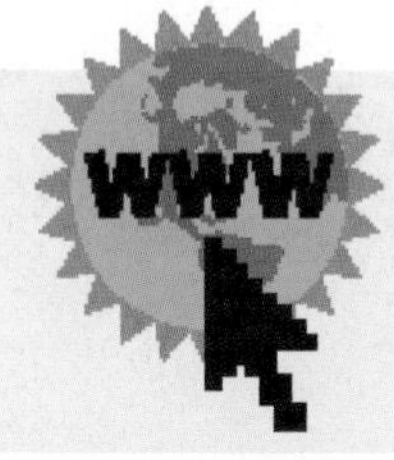

The complete chapter, learning objectives, and other resources can be found at **www.pharmacotherapyonline.com.**

Renal Cell Carcinoma

Christine M. Walko and Daniel J. Crona

e138

KEY CONCEPTS

1. Renal cell carcinoma (RCC) predominantly occurs later in life, with about 70% of all cases diagnosed between the ages of 55 and 84 years.
2. Established risk factors for RCC include smoking, obesity, hypertension, and inherited susceptibility.
3. Inactivation of the von Hippel-Lindau tumor suppressor gene is the hallmark of the most common type of RCC, the clear cell histologic subtype.
4. More than 50% of RCC cases are diagnosed by incidental findings on routine imaging for unrelated reasons.
5. The Memorial Sloan-Kettering Cancer Center Prognostic Factors Model for Survival classifies patients into low-, intermediate-, and high-risk groups based on five clinical factors and can predict survival among both untreated patients and those treated with immunotherapy and/or targeted agents.
6. Surgical excision of the primary tumor, either by radical or partial nephrectomy, is the preferred treatment modality for patients with stage I-III RCC, but some patients with stage IV disease may also benefit from surgery.
7. Historically, immunotherapy (interleukin [IL]-2 and interferon [IFN]-*α*) was considered the preferred first-line therapy for metastatic RCC (mRCC) but has largely been replaced by targeted agents because of their improved efficacy and tolerability. Nivolumab is a new immunotherapy option for mRCC patients who have received prior targeted therapy.
8. Sunitinib, pazopanib, and axitinib are oral small molecule inhibitors of vascular endothelial growth factor (VEGF) and platelet-derived growth factor and are treatment options as first-line therapy for mRCC. Bevacizumab and IFN-α is also a first-line option.
9. The multikinase inhibitors sorafenib and cabozantinib, and the mammalian target of rapamycin (mTOR) inhibitor everolimus, are the oral agents used as second-line therapy options for mRCC patients who progress on a targeted therapy or cytokine-based therapy first-line regimen.
10. Temsirolimus is an IV administered mTOR inhibitor indicated for first-line therapy in patients with high-risk mRCC.

INTRODUCTION

Renal cell carcinoma (RCC) represents about 2% of all adult malignancies and is the most common type of malignancy of the kidney and renal pelvis. Until a decade ago, there were few treatment options, and those that were available had modest activity and were poorly tolerated by patients. However, treatment for the disease has been revolutionized by targeted agents that were developed based on an increased understanding of RCC pathophysiology. Clear cell is the predominant subtype of RCC (up to 75% of all cases), and is the result of inactivation of the von Hippel-Lindau (*VHL*) tumor suppressor gene located on chromosome 3p25. *VHL* inactivation leads to increased production of growth factors, such as vascular endothelial growth factor (VEGF), transforming growth factor (TGF), platelet-derived growth factor (PDGF), and others responsible for angiogenesis and cell growth.[1] Prior to 2005, the primary therapeutic option for patients with advanced or metastatic RCC (mRCC) after nephrectomy was immunotherapy, which induced few durable responses and caused high rates of severe toxicities. However, nine new drugs have been approved as first- or second-line therapy for RCC: sorafenib, sunitinib, temsirolimus, bevacizumab (in combination with interferon-*α* [IFN-*α*]), everolimus, pazopanib, axitinib, nivolumab, and cabozantinib.[2-9] Each drug is an example of targeted therapy against growth factors important in the pathophysiology of RCC and has yielded much needed progress in a disease with few therapeutic options. RCC serves as an example of rational development of targeted agents based on knowledge of tumor biology and molecular signaling pathways for the treatment of other malignancies.

EPIDEMIOLOGY

About 62,000 new cases of kidney and renal pelvis cancer are diagnosed each year in the United States, with two-thirds of these cases occurring in men. More than 13,000 people in the United States will die of kidney cancer each year. Kidney cancer is the seventh most common cancer in men, and the number of new cases diagnosed each year is similar to non-Hodgkin lymphoma and melanoma. In women, kidney cancer is the eighth most common cancer, occurring at a rate similar to the rates for ovarian and pancreatic cancers.[10] The incidence of RCC has increased over the past three decades. The rate has increased more rapidly in blacks than whites and in women than men. In the United States, between 2002 and 2006, the age-adjusted incidence rate in black men was 21.3, white men 19.2, black women 10.3, and white women 9.9 per 100,000 person years.[11] This increase may be related to improved imaging techniques and greater use of these imaging modalities, although the higher prevalence of some risk factors may also explain the increased incidence.

1 Kidney cancer is most commonly diagnosed between the ages of 40 and 70 years, with a peak in the sixth and seventh decades of life. Nearly 70% of all cases of kidney cancer are diagnosed in people between the ages of 55 and 84 years, with less than 3% of all cases diagnosed in patients younger than 34 years.[11]

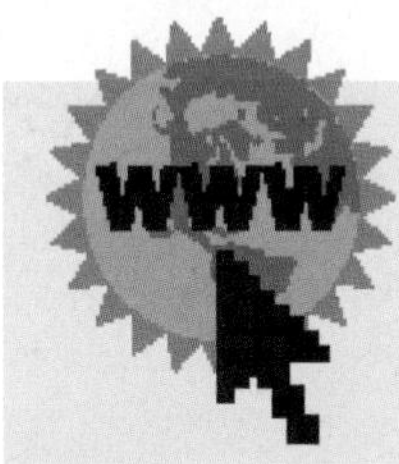

The complete chapter, learning objectives, and other resources can be found at **www.pharmacotherapyonline.com.**

139

Melanoma

Cindy L. O'Bryant and Jamie C. Poust

KEY CONCEPTS

1. Cutaneous melanoma is an increasingly common malignancy, but it is a cancer that can be cured if detected early. Public education about screening and early detection is one strategy to control the increase in incidence and the mortality associated with cutaneous melanoma.
2. Surgical resection can cure patients with early-stage melanoma.
3. Adjuvant therapy should be considered in patients with locally advanced disease; recommended options include IFN-α_{2b}, ipilimumab or participation in a clinical trial.
4. Single agent chemotherapy offers limited benefit in metastatic melanoma. Combination chemotherapy has not been shown to be superior to single-agent therapy.
5. Advances in immunotherapy with ipilimumab, pembrolizumab, and nivolumab have led to long durable responses in some patients with metastatic melanoma and have significantly impacted overall survival.
6. The immune-related toxicities associated with immunotherapy can be severe and life-threatening. Consequently, the use of these agents warrants appropriate patient selection, close monitoring and toxicity management by an experienced healthcare team.
7. As the biology of melanoma has been further delineated, a growing number of potential targets for drug therapy have been identified. BRAF mutations appear in up to 70% of melanoma patients. The use of BRAF inhibitors with or without MEK inhibitors has been shown to improve overall survival in patients with this mutation.
8. Treatment of melanoma is determined by many factors. As the number of treatment options for patients with metastatic melanoma grows, it will be important to consider disease- and patient-related aspects when determining appropriate therapy.

INTRODUCTION

Skin cancer is the most common malignancy worldwide and is associated with chronic ultraviolet (UV) exposure. The two types of skin cancer are nonmelanoma skin cancers (NMSCs) and melanoma. Although NMSCs are the most common malignancy of the skin, cutaneous melanoma accounts for up to 75% of all skin cancer-related deaths. Melanoma cases are increasing globally with the highest rates found in Australia, New Zealand, North America, and Northern Europe. Melanoma is the sixth most common cancer in the United States. The incidence of melanoma has steadily increased in the United States since the 1970s, and for the last decade, has raised an average of 1.4% each year.[1] When detected early, patients generally have a good prognosis. With the rise in the number of melanoma skin cancers and the associated mortality, it is essential to consider issues of care beyond that of disease treatment. Skin cancer prevention and screening have a major impact on public health, and on the success of treatment, for those individuals diagnosed with both NMSC and melanoma. Skin cancers tend to occur more frequently in older individuals with a median age of diagnosis 63 years old.[1] Therefore, as the population continues to age, effective strategies to prevent, detect, and treat individuals with these cancers are necessary. An understanding of the biology of melanoma has led to the development of targeted therapies toward somatic mutations and immunotherapies, which have shown improved outcomes in patients with advanced melanoma.

EPIDEMIOLOGY

In the United States, about one in every 50 individuals will be diagnosed with melanoma in their lifetime. The lifetime risk is greater in men than women, but rates are higher in women before the age of 50. Risk also varies with ethnicity, with the majority of melanoma occurring in non-Hispanic whites.[2,3] In 2016, it is estimated that 76,380 new cases of melanoma would be diagnosed in the United States.[3] Unfortunately, this estimate may not be accurate as many superficial, and in situ melanomas, are managed in facilities that do not routinely report their cases to cancer registries. Childhood and adolescent melanoma account for only 1% of new melanoma cases each year, but is the most common skin cancer in individuals younger than 20 years old. The incidence in this age group is increasing by 2% per year. Adolescents between the age of 15 and 19 years have the highest rates of melanoma (18%) compared to younger children, with the incidence in girls being higher than boys in all age ranges.[4]

The estimated number of individuals expected to die of melanoma in 2016 in the United States is 10,130.[3] Survival rates have gradually increased over the past four decades. The 5- and 10-year relative survival rates are 91% and 89%, respectively, but survival declines to 16% with more advanced disease.[1] Although the overall mortality rate has remained stable, those younger than 50 years of age had a 2.6% decrease from 2007 to 2011 while those over 50 years of age had a 0.6% increase.[3]

A number of patient-specific factors and environmental factors have been identified (Table 139-1), and it is likely these factors alone, or in combination, increase the risk of cutaneous melanomas.

Individual physical characteristics can determine responses to UV radiation. Caucasians with fair-colored hair (red or blond), light-colored eyes (blue or green), high degrees of freckling, and those who have a tendency to burn, and rarely tan with exposure to sunlight, appear to be especially at risk. Both UVB and UVA are known carcinogens and are related to the development of melanoma. Clinical and epidemiologic research shows a higher rate of

TABLE 139-1 Risk Factors for Melanoma

Patient-Specific Risk Factors
Adulthood (age older than 15 years)
History of cutaneous melanoma
Dysplastic nevi
High density of common nevi and atypical nevi
Cutaneous melanoma in first-degree relative
Immunodeficiency or immunosuppression
High degree of freckling
Sunburns easily or tans rarely
Blonde or red hair
Blue, green, or gray eyes
Socioeconomic status (higher > lower)
Race (Caucasians > Hispanics > African Americans)
External Risk Factors
Intense intermittent sun exposures
History of sunburn
More than four painful sunburns before age 15 years
Recreational sun exposure

melanoma in those who have extensive or repeated intense UV and sun exposure.[5] Intermittent intense sun exposure, blistering sunburns, the use of tanning beds, and the time of life when exposed to the sun are critical factors for development of cutaneous melanoma. Individuals with a history of these factors are at highest risk. The risk is lower in individuals who have had chronic sun exposure, without a history of burning, and those with occupational exposure. The risk with sunlight and UV radiation seems to be greatest during childhood and adolescence and is more hazardous than exposure during adult life.

An important risk factor for melanoma is the number and size of melanocytic nevi (pigmented lesions or moles) on the body. The formation of these nevi has been shown to be directly related to cumulative sun exposure. The relative risk of developing melanoma increases with the number of typical nevi an individual has. A second risk factor is the presence of atypical melanocytic nevi. Atypical nevi may progress from a normal nevus or be dysplastic from the onset. Up to 20% of melanomas develop from atypical nevi. Congenital melanocytic nevi may be present at birth or within the first few months after birth, and the associated risk of melanoma increases with size.

Immunocompromised patients are at an increased risk for development of cutaneous melanoma and these cases have been shown to have a poor prognosis.[6] Immunodeficiency includes individuals with chronic lymphocytic leukemia, Hodgkin lymphoma, and immunosuppression after organ transplant. Acquired immunodeficiency syndrome (AIDS) has been shown to increase the risk of developing cutaneous melanoma and the disease often is more aggressive. A personal history of NMSC or melanoma skin cancers is a risk factor for subsequent melanoma and may be associated with a poor prognosis. Xeroderma pigmentosum is a rare skin disorder associated with an increased risk for melanoma.

A number of genes have been implicated in melanoma development and progression, and molecular profiling studies have identified several distinct molecular subclasses of melanoma. Familial atypical multiple mole syndrome (FAMMS) or dysplastic nevus syndrome is a hereditary disease characterized by a predisposition to develop dysplastic nevi and cutaneous melanoma. It is estimated that up to 12% of cases of melanoma are associated with a family history or hereditary dysplastic nevus syndrome. FAMMS is associated with mutations in the *CDKN2A* gene located at chromosome 9p21. *CDKN2A* encodes two distinct proteins: inhibitor of cyclin-dependent kinase 4 (INK4A or $p16^{INK4a}$) and ARF (alternative reading frame; p14ARF). INK4A regulates cell cycle progression at the G_1/S checkpoint by inhibiting the G_1 cyclin-dependent kinases that phosphorylate and inactivate the retinoblastoma protein. ARF inhibits p53 degradation and loss of ARF inactivates p53. The frequencies of *CDKN2A* mutations vary in melanoma, but are more commonly found in individuals with familial inheritance patterns and are associated with multiple cases of melanoma in a family, young age at diagnosis, multiple primary melanomas among family members, and pancreatic cancer.[7]

ETIOLOGY

Melanoma arises from the melanocytes in the basal layer of the epidermis. DNA damage, most commonly a result of UV radiation, causes cellular mutations which transform the cell, allow uncontrolled proliferation, and lead to the formation of tumors. The identification of these genetic alterations has led to the recognition of molecular subgroups of melanoma, and more focused drug development for treatment. The first insights to the role of genetics were seen with the relationship of *CDKN2A* mutations and FAMMS.

One of the major signaling pathways found to be associated with the development of melanoma is the mitogen-activated protein kinase pathway (MAPK), which mediates receptor tyrosine kinases, resulting in activation of RAS and downstream BRAF. Activating *BRAF* mutations are the most common somatic genetic event in human melanoma, occurring in 25% to 70% of melanoma patients and primarily noted by a single point mutation (V600E). In the V600E mutation, a valine is substituted for glutamic acid at codon 600. *BRAF* is a somatic mutation and its high prevalence appears to be an epidemiologic link between UV radiation and melanoma. *BRAF* mutations are common in melanomas arising from skin with intermittent sun exposure.[8]

Upstream of BRAF, mutations in *NRAS* and c-*Kit* have also been found as molecular drivers in the development of melanoma. Mutations in *NRAS* are found in 15% to 20% of patients. These tumors are associated with more advanced disease at diagnosis, high growth rates, and shorter survival times than those with *BRAF* mutations.[8] c-*Kit* is a transmembrane receptor tyrosine kinase which, when activated, signals the MAPK andphosphatidyl-inosital-3-OH kinase (PI3K) pathways, resulting in transcription and cell proliferation. Mutations in c-*Kit* are commonly found in acral and mucosal melanomas.[8]

Other genetic alterations involved with the development of melanoma include *MITF* (microphthalmia-associated transcription factor), which is a gene important to the survival of melanocytes. When mutated, *MITF* acts as an oncogene.[9] The melanocortin 1 receptor gene (*MC1R*), is prevalent in individuals with melanoma and signals through the MITF pathway. It is involved in melanin synthesis and is associated with the red hair and fair skin phenotype. Variants in *MCIR* lead to a shift in the production from eumelanin (brown/black pigment) to pheomelanin (red/yellow pigment).[10]

PREVENTION AND DETECTION

1 Skin cancer is recognized as a major health problem in the United States. As a result, in 2014 the US Surgeon General released Call to Action to Prevent Skin Cancer. The Call to Action addresses the following goals to support skin cancer prevention: increase opportunities for sun protection in outdoor settings; provide individuals with the information they need to make informed, healthy choices about UV radiation exposure; promote policies to advance the national goal of preventing skin cancer; reduce harms from indoor tanning; and strengthen research, surveillance, monitoring, and evaluation related to skin cancer prevention.[11] As such, the mainstay of melanoma prevention remains strategies to protect individuals from the harmful effects of the sun (Table 139-2). There are three different strategies for melanoma chemoprevention: primary chemoprevention in healthy individuals; secondary chemoprevention to prevent

TABLE 139-2 Options for Sun Protection Sunscreens

Behavioral	Sunscreens	
	Physical Blockers (Reflectants)	Chemical Absorbers
Protective clothing and accessories	Zinc oxide	Ultraviolet B absorbers
Seek shade (avoid peak sun hours)	Talc	Salicylates
Avoid tanning equipment	Titanium dioxide	Cinnamates
	Red petrolatum	Camphor derivatives
		Aminobenzoates
		Ultraviolet A absorbers
		Benzopehnone-6
		Dibenzoylmethanes

premalignant melanoma precursors from becoming melanoma; and tertiary chemoprevention to prevent melanoma recurrence.

UV exposure plays a major role in melanoma development and is the most preventable cause of melanoma. For most people, the sun is the most common source of UV exposure and an important environmental factor in the pathogenesis of melanoma. The incidence of melanoma has been associated with latitude and the intensity of solar exposure among susceptible populations. Radiation in the UVB range (280-320 nm) is historically considered to be the critical factor linking sunlight and melanoma, although prolonged exposure to UVA radiation (320-400 nm) is also important.

Education, and reeducation, about the importance of sun protection have the potential to decrease the rising incidence of this disease. Strategies such as sun avoidance, especially during peak hours of sun intensity (10 AM-4 PM), and staying in the shade when outdoors, are important education concepts for individuals who are in the sun for prolonged periods or who are at high risk for burning. Skiers and winter sports enthusiasts should be cautioned about exposure to UV radiation because the reflection off snow and high altitude contribute to increased UV exposure. The use of protective clothing to minimize damage to the skin for individuals who spend time in the sun is also an option. Clothing and hats designed to protect an individual from sun exposure, but allow for physical activities, such as water sports and hiking, are widely available. In addition, the use of sunglasses, with both UVA and UVB protection, is important. The use of tanning beds has also been associated with development of melanoma. A recent meta-analysis reported that about 6,000 cases of melanoma may be related to indoor tanning in the United States each year.[12] In 2009, the World Health Organization International Agency for Research on Cancer declared UV light emitted from tanning beds was a human carcinogen.[13] To aid in the prevention of skin cancers here in the United States, the Food and Drug Administration (FDA) reclassified UV tanning devices to class II (moderate-to-high risk) devices.[14] Furthermore, regulations have been put in place to restrict minors' access to indoor tanning in 44 states, including 13 which prohibit the use of indoor tanning for anyone younger than 18 years of age.[11]

The use of sunscreens is another strategy to decrease UV exposure. Historically, people have been educated that the risk of skin cancer can be limited by the use of sunscreens with a sun protection factor (SPF) of 15 or greater. In 2011, the FDA mandated new testing and labeling regulations for sunscreen products. Under these regulations, sunscreens labeled as broad spectrum must protect against both UVA and UVB radiation. A product labeled as broad spectrum with a SPF of 15 or higher when used regularly, as directed, and with other sun protective measure, will help prevent sunburn and reduce the risk of skin cancer. Additionally, the regulations limit the SPF value on sunscreen labels to 50+ because of the lack of evidence to show that products with SPF values greater than 50 provide greater protection.[15]

It is important to counsel patients about the appropriate use of sunscreens to optimize benefits from these products. Sunscreens should be applied 30 minutes before going into the sun and should be reapplied every 2 hours, after swimming, and after perspiring heavily. About 1 oz (30 mL) of sunscreen (a "palmful") should be used to cover the arms, legs, neck, and face of the average adult. Sun protection must be used regularly and not merely limited to times of recreation or anticipated "prolonged" exposure. Times of season changes, when the potential for sun exposure can be perceived as erratic, are possible times for the "first-of-the-season sunburn."

Thickness and stage of the disease are inversely related to melanoma survival. Early detection can play a large part in the secondary and tertiary prevention of melanoma. Many healthcare organizations, and skin cancer groups, recommend monthly self-skin examination (SSE) to serve as a mechanism for recognizing moles or marks on the skin that may be melanoma. Patients with a strong family history should have additional clinical examinations, and in some cases, screening photography to document the size, shape, and location of moles. Both patients and clinicians need to be properly educated in the clinical features of the disease to ensure more appropriate diagnosis. Currently, there are no consistent recommendations for the screening and early detection of melanoma.

PATHOPHYSIOLOGY

Melanomas most often arise within epidermal melanocytes of the skin, although they can also arise from noncutaneous melanocytes. During fetal development, melanocytes migrate over a predictable route to a variety of sites within the body including the skin, uveal tract, meninges, and ectodermal mucosa. Primary melanoma can arise in any area of the body with melanocytes. The skin is the most frequent site of melanoma; cutaneous melanoma constitutes 90% of all melanomas. Primary melanoma can arise in the eye (ocular melanoma), the mucosa, and in some cases, as metastatic disease with unknown primary site.[16]

Melanocytes synthesize melanin to protect various tissues, such as the skin, from UV damage and reach the keratinocytes in the upper layers of the epidermis via dendrites. Tyrosinase is an essential enzyme within melanosomes that synthesizes melanin. They are resistant to severe UV radiation, unlike keratinocytes, and their survival leads to the proliferation of mutated genes.

The pathogenesis of human melanoma involves a series of morphologic stages: melanocytic atypia, atypical melanocytic hyperplasia, radial growth phase in which limited growth and radial expansion of the nevi may occur without metastatic competence, primary melanoma in the vertical growth phase with or without in-transit metastasis, regional lymph node metastatic melanoma, and distant metastatic melanoma. Primary melanoma is characterized by radial growth and limited vertical thickness (less than 0.75 mm). Primary melanoma demonstrates little tendency to metastasize. Melanoma has a potential for metastasis formation with the onset of a vertical growth phase. Therefore, the thickness of a primary melanoma is an important prognostic factor and is used in the staging classification of cutaneous melanoma. Of note, melanomas can skip steps in this development pathway.

Melanoma cells secrete a variety of growth autocrine and paracrine factors which may facilitate proliferation. As disease progresses, melanoma cells increase production of certain growth factors and cytokines which, in turn, activate cellular growth and survival pathways. Understanding the biology of melanoma has provided potential targets for drug therapy. Pathways, such as MAPK and PI3K/AKT, have been targeted by RAF and MEK inhibitors and mammalian target of rapamycin (mTOR) inhibitors, respectively. As new pathways are identified and as agents that inhibit these pathways are developed, there is growing excitement about the opportunities to impact treatment of melanoma in new and effective ways.

The immune response appears to be more involved in the progression of melanoma than other solid tumors. Spontaneous cancer regressions are rare but are a well-documented phenomenon seen in melanoma and appear to be associated with host immunity.[17] Recombinant cytokines including interleukin-2 (IL-2) and interferons (IFNs) have been used in the treatment of melanoma to stimulate the immune system through T cell activation. Immune checkpoint receptors, such as cytotoxic T lymphocyte antigen 4 (CTLA-4) and programmed death-1 (PD-1), both found on the surface of activated T cells, appear to have an inhibitory effect on the cells. Blocking these receptors is an effective strategy for increasing the T-cell antitumor response. Vaccines against melanoma-associated antigens and the use of adoptive T cell therapy (ACT) and chimeric antigen receptors (CARs) T cell therapy are other immunotherapeutic approaches currently under investigation.[17,18]

HISTOLOGIC SUBTYPES

Cutaneous melanomas are categorized by growth patterns. Four major histologic subtypes, or growth patterns of primary cutaneous melanoma, have been identified: superficial spreading melanoma (SSM), nodular melanoma, lentigo maligna melanoma (LMM), and acral lentiginous melanoma (ALM). Clinical outcomes of the four major melanoma subtypes are similar if the comparison controls for depth of penetration or tumor thickness. Any of the four subtypes can present as an amelanotic variant. Amelanotic melanomas appear to be devoid of clinically apparent pigmentation. Desmoplastic melanoma is a less common subtype found in about 1% of cases. It is frequently seen in older individuals, and its clinical presentation is similar to that seen in NMSCs. If a biopsy of the lesion is not obtained, the disease may be mismanaged.

SSM is the most common morphologic type of cutaneous melanoma, accounting for about 75% of all melanomas and is associated with intense, intermittent sun exposure. Early in lesion development, SSM is flat, growing radially before vertically. SSM evolves slowly, typically over 1 to 5 years. As the lesion progresses it may become raised or ulcerated. The borders are often irregular and asymmetrical as the lesion progresses and may vary in color (blue, black, brown, pink, or other colors). SSMs may occur at any anatomic site on the body, but are more commonly seen on the back in men, and on the legs in women.[19] The average age of a diagnosis of SSM is 50 years old. These lesions can be linked to mutations in *BRAF*.

LMM represents 10% to 20% of melanomas and is commonly found on the head and neck. It is unique from other histologic subtypes; because of prolonged radial growth phase, it does not have the same propensity to metastasize. LMM arises on chronically sun-exposed sites in older individuals and presents as a freckle-like lesion. LMMs are generally large flat, tan-colored lesions with shades of brown and black. The lesions gradually grow, develop, and begin to change in color.[19] Evolution into invasive melanoma is characterized by nodular development within the flat lesion. Median age at diagnosis is 65 years old. These lesions can be linked to mutations in *KIT*.

Nodular melanoma is the second most common growth pattern of melanoma, occurring in 15% to 30% of patients. Since nodular melanoma is a pure vertical growth phase disease, it is more aggressive and develops more rapidly than other subtypes.[19] Nodular melanomas are dark blue–black and often uniform in color with a shiny surface, although a small percentage of nodular melanomas are amelanotic and have a fleshy appearance. Nodular melanomas are raised and often symmetric. Although they can occur at any age, they typically occur around 50 years of age, and are most common on the trunk, head, and neck. Nodular melanomas are more common in men.

ALM makes up about 5% of melanomas and is not related to UV exposure. It presents as three distinct clinical subtypes: melanoma on the palms of the hands or soles of the feet, subungual melanoma, and mucosal melanoma.[6] Most ALMs are located on the soles of the feet and appear as a large tan or brown stain. The lesions often have irregular convoluted borders and may be masked by thick skin on the feet. Suspicious lesions on the palms or soles of the feet should be evaluated. Subungual melanoma arises in the nail matrix or nail bed. The most common presentation is a brown or black line in the great toe or the thumbnail. Mucosal melanoma is rare but can occur on any mucosal surface. Mucosal melanoma occurs most commonly in the oropharyngeal mucosa followed by the anal and rectal, genital, and urinary mucosa. Unfortunately, mucosal melanoma often does not become clinically apparent until the mass is large or the lesion bleeds. ALM is the most common type of melanoma reported in individuals with a dark complexion (eg, African Americans, Asians, and Hispanics).[19] Similar to LMMs, this subtype is characterized by a protracted radial growth phase and are associated with mutations in *c-KIT*.

Uveal melanoma is currently considered a separate disease from cutaneous melanoma. It is the most common primary intraocular malignancy seen in adults but is an uncommon tumor. Unlike cutaneous melanoma, the frequency and mortality rates of uveal melanoma have remained steady. This melanoma arises from the pigmented epithelium of the choroid. Iris melanoma is a subset of uveal melanoma and tends to have a more benign course. The risk of metastasis varies with the histologic type and size of the tumor as well as the location in the eye and most frequently metastasizes to the liver but can spread to a variety of tissues.[20]

CLINICAL SUBTYPES

With the understanding of the role of genetic alterations in the treatment and outcomes of patients with melanoma, four distinctive clinical subtypes have emerged based on UV exposure and anatomic site. The four subtypes are divided into 1) nonchronic sun damage (non-CSD): melanomas on skin without chronic sun-induced damage; 2) CSD: melanomas on skin with chronic sun-induced damage characterized by the presence of solar elastosis; 3) acral; and 4) mucosal. A genomic analysis revealed differences in the activation of the MAPK and PI3K between the different clinical subtypes. The data showed *BRAF* mutations predominantly occur in non-CSD and less commonly in the other groups. About 10% to 20% of all the subtypes contain *NRAS* mutations and these mutations occur independent of BRAF.[21,22] Further studies showed *c-KIT* mutations are found in almost 40% of acral and mucosal subtypes, in almost a third of CSD melanomas and not at all in non-CSD melanomas.[21,22] This data further emphasizes the need for continued refinement of tumor classifications in melanoma based on genetic and biological features with the hope this will ultimately lead to more personalized treatment options and improved outcomes for patients.

CLINICAL PRESENTATION

Benign nevi often occur in sun-exposed areas and are typically 4 to 6 mm in diameter (about the size of a pencil eraser), raised or flat, uniform in color and round in shape. Dysplastic nevi, an intermediate between benign nevi and melanoma, tend to be larger than common nevi (greater than 5 mm), appear as flat macules with asymmetry, have a fuzzy or ill-defined shape, and vary in color.

The initial clinical presentation of melanoma is often a cutaneous lesion and depends on the histologic subtype and the stage of development of the lesion. The cardinal clinical feature of a cutaneous melanoma is a pigmented skin lesion which changes over a period of time. Any changes in the skin surrounding a nevus, including redness or swelling, are important clinical signs. Uncommonly, the lesion may become itchy or tender and painful. Friability of the

CLINICAL PRESENTATION

General

- Any lesion that changes in appearance over time

Local Signs and Symptoms

- The clinical features used to describe questionable lesions are highlighted with the mnemonic "ABCDE"
  - (A) Asymmetry: Melanoma lesions are often asymmetric
  - (B) Border: Melanoma lesions have irregular borders
  - (C) Color: Color is often variegated in a melanoma ranging from tan, blue-black, red, purple, or white
  - (D) Diameter: Melanoma lesions are frequently greater than 6 mm
  - (E) Enlargement or evolution: A sudden enlargement or change in lesion is concerning for melanoma
- Other signs of melanoma include a lesion that swells, bleeds, or oozes

Systemic Signs and Symptoms

- Palpable lymph nodes
- Depending on the site of metastasis, shortness of breath, abdominal pain, bone pain, headache, and mental status changes

Laboratory Tests

- In addition to a comprehensive metabolic panel, LDH should be evaluated

Other Diagnostic Tests

- Biopsy and pathology review for staging with molecular testing for BRAF and *c-Kit*
- When applicable, SLNB
- Systemic staging should include chest, abdomen, and pelvic CT scan or CT/PET bone scan, and brain MRI

CT, computed tomography; LDH, lactate dehydrogenase; MRI, magnetic resonance imaging; PET, positron emission tomography; SLNB, sentinel lymph node biopsy.

lesion, resulting in bleeding or oozing, is a danger sign. Perhaps, the most important warning sign of danger is the evolution in any characteristic of a lesion. A biopsy of the lesion is critical to establish diagnosis of melanoma. Subsequent pathologic interpretation of the biopsy will help provide information on prognosis and treatment options. An excisional biopsy, with a 1- to 2-mm margin of normal-appearing skin, is recommended for a suspicious lesion and should include a portion of underlying subcutaneous fat for microstaging. For larger lesions, an incisional or punch biopsy can be performed, and should include a core of full-thickness skin and subcutaneous tissue. When excisional biopsies are not appropriate, as with the face or palmar surface of the hands, a full-thickness incisional or punch biopsy is preferred. A shave biopsy is never appropriate because it can underestimate the thickness of the lesion and may not fully remove the lesion. Additionally, scarring may mask the remaining tumor.

Evaluation of any individual with a suspected melanoma includes a complete history and total-body skin examination. The focus of the patient history is identifying potential risk factors including family history of melanoma, personal history of skin cancer or nevus excisions, sun exposure, and phenotype. A total dermatologic examination is necessary to determine melanoma risk factors (eg, mole pattern, mole type, or freckling) and for staging. Melanoma commonly spreads to the lymph nodes; therefore, individuals suspicious for advanced disease should be examined for lymphadenopathy. Lactate dehydrogenase (LDH) should be measured as elevated serum levels are an independent predictor of decreased survival.[23] In addition, any other signs or symptoms suggestive of metastatic disease should be completely evaluated.

1 Improved survival rates for melanoma have been attributed to the identification and treatment of disease at an early stage when the disease is limited and has not yet metastasized. It follows that one strategy to improve survival rates would be to increase efforts to identify early-stage melanoma. The cost-effectiveness of massive screening for all adults by a physician has never been demonstrated. However, routine examination of the skin by physicians is recommended for individuals, adults, and children who are at high risk. The entire cutaneous surface, including the scalp, should be examined.

It has been estimated that about 50% of the initial melanoma lesions found are discovered by self-examination. Therefore, one of the most direct strategies to improve early detection would be a method to increase effective SSE by the individual, the individual's partner, or a caregiver. Identification of early melanoma allows the opportunity to treat lesions when they are early stage and curable, thus lowering the mortality rate of the disease. Healthcare professionals who routinely work with the public, such as community pharmacists, have an opportunity to increase public awareness concerning the benefits and appropriate methods for SSE. Educational pamphlets describing SSE (Table 139-3) for the public are widely available through the American Cancer Society, American Academy of Dermatology, and Skin Cancer Foundation. If a newly discovered pigmented lesion is identified, or if a preexisting pigmented lesion changes, the individual should be evaluated by a physician immediately.

SSE is of special interest in elderly adults. As the population of older adults (greater than or equal to 65 years of age) increases, it is expected that the mortality rate from melanoma also will increase. Barriers to successful SSE in elderly adults, such as failing eyesight, lack of partners, and poor memory, impact older adults in detecting new or changing lesions. These barriers, coupled with the higher

TABLE 139-3 Self-Examination of Suspicious Moles

1. Examine your body front and back in the mirror and then the right and left sides with the arms raised
2. Bend the elbows and look carefully at the forearms and upper arms and palms
3. Look at the backs of the legs and feet. Look specifically in the spaces between toes and at the soles of the feet
4. Examine the back of the neck and scalp with the help of a hand-held mirror; part the hair (or use a blow dryer) to lift the hair and give yourself a closer look
5. Check the back and buttocks with a handheld mirror

Derived from publications of the American Academy of Dermatology.

incidence of melanoma in men, present challenges and opportunities for healthcare professionals to target education to this growing segment of our population.

STAGING AND PROGNOSTIC FACTORS

The size of a primary melanoma lesion is associated with the likelihood of metastasis. The Breslow tumor thickness of the primary melanoma lesion is commonly used as prognostic factor to determine predicted outcomes.[24] Tumor thickness is quantified to the nearest tenth of a millimeter with an ocular micrometer, measuring from the top of the granular layer of the overlying epidermis to the deepest contiguous invasive melanoma cell. The correlation between tumor thickness and probability of tumor metastasis is strong but does not include aspects such as tumor satellites, defined rather arbitrarily, as skin involvement within 2 cm of the primary lesion, and vascular invasion. Patients with satellitosis have a worse prognosis than patients with thick primary lesions (tumor thickness greater than 4 mm), and prognosis is more similar to that of patients with nodal metastasis. Mitotic rate, defined as the number of mitosis per square millimeter, is another important prognostic factor for developing metastatic disease. Increasing mitotic rate represents a more aggressive lesion and is associated with a poorer survival rate despite tumor size. The American Joint Committee on Cancer (AJCC) developed a staging system for melanoma which divides patients with localized melanoma into four stages according to microstaging criteria of Breslow, but data from large patient databases demonstrated that the different cut off values for primary thickness may better predict overall survival. Additionally, ulceration of the melanoma and satellite lesions of the primary tumor should be considered when making decisions about therapy. As a result, the AJCC revised the staging system for cutaneous melanoma which was updated in 2009.[23] It is important to carefully examine older clinical trials to determine which staging system was used to determine patient inclusion and exclusion criteria, as results may differ based on these patient criteria. Clinical staging includes microstaging of the primary melanoma with clinical, laboratory and radiologic evaluation. It is used after complete excision of the primary melanoma along with clinical assessment to determine regional and distant metastasis. Pathologic staging includes microstaging of the primary melanoma and pathologic information about the regional nodes after partial or complete lymphadenectomy. At this time, it appears that patients with very limited disease (in situ or stage 0) do not require pathologic evaluation of lymph nodes (Tables 139-4 and 139-5).[22]

As with other solid tumors, the presence of regional lymph node involvement is a powerful predictor of tumor burden and patient outcome. Sentinel lymph node biopsy (SLNB) is a minimally invasive procedure which determines if a patient is a candidate for a complete lymph node dissection. The rationale for lymphatic mapping and subsequent SLNB is based on the observation that regions of the skin have patterns of lymphatic drainage to specific lymph nodes in the regional lymphatic basin. The sentinel lymph node is believed to be the first node in the lymphatic basin into which the primary melanoma drains. Unlike other solid tumors, melanoma appears to progress in an orderly nodal distribution. SLNB allows for detection of micrometastases as a result of more thorough examination of a single sentinel node than is possible when examining multiple lymph nodes with a lymph node dissection, and may be most useful for melanomas located in ambiguous drainage sites such as the head and neck areas. SLNB is associated with low false-negative rates and low complication rates.[25] Detection of clinically undetectable disease in a lymph node basin not directly adjacent to the primary lesion, may allow for upstaging of patients who initially are believed to have node-negative disease. The American Society of Clinical Oncology and Society of Surgical Oncology joint clinical practice guidelines recommend SLNB for patient with any intermediate-thickness melanoma.[25]

TABLE 139-4 Melanoma Tumor (T), Node (N), Metastasis (M) Classification

T Classification	Thickness	Ulcerative Status
T_X	Primary tumor cannot be addressed (eg, shave biopsy)	
T_0	No evidence of primary tumor	
T_{is}	Melanoma in situ	
T_1	≤1 mm	A: No ulceration and mitosis <1/mm^2 B: With ulceration or mitosis ≥1/mm^2
T_2	1.01-2 mm	A: No ulceration B: With ulceration
T_3	2.01-4 mm	A: No ulceration B: With ulceration
T_4	>4 mm	A: No ulceration B: With ulceration
N Classification	**No. of Metastatic Nodes**	**Nodal Metastatic Mass**[a]
N_X	Regional lymph nodes cannot be assessed	
N_0	No regional lymph nodes	
N_1	1 node	A: Micrometastasis B: Macrometastasis
N_2	2-3 nodes	A: Micrometastasis B: Macrometastasis C: In-transit metastases or satellite(s) without metastatic nodes
N_3	≥4 metastatic lymph nodes or matted nodes or in-transit metastases or satellite(s) with metastatic node(s)	
M Classification	**Site**	**Serum Lactate Dehydrogenase**
M_X	Distant metastases cannot be assessed	
M_0	No detectable distant metastasis	
M_{1a}	Distant skin, subcutaneous tissue, or nodal metastatic disease	Normal
M_{1b}	Lung metastases	Normal
M_{1c}	All other visceral metastases Any distant metastasis	Normal Elevated

M, metastasis; N, node; T, tumor.

[a]Micrometastases are diagnosed after sentinel or elective lymphadenectomy. Macrometastases are defined as clinically detectable lymph node metastases confirmed by therapeutic lymphadenectomy or when any lymph node metastasis exhibits extracapsular extension.

Data from Balch CM, Gershenwald JE, Soong SJ, et al. Final version of 2009 AJCC melanoma staging and classification. J Clin Oncol 2009;27:6199-6206.

The stage of melanoma, based on tumor thickness, level of tumor invasion, and ulceration, at the time of diagnosis, is one of the primary indicators of the natural history of the disease and contributes to prognosis. Other factors such as tumor growth pattern, or histological subtype, mitotic rate, density of tumor infiltrating lymphocytes (TILs) in the tumor tissue, elevated LDH level, satellite lesions, angiolymphatic invasion, gender, and age also have been reported to influence survival (Table 139-6). The location of the primary tumor on the skin is also important as tumors of the extremities have an increased survival compared with those with axial, neck, head, and trunk tumors. In addition, a number of additional prognostic factors

TABLE 139-5 American Joint Committee on Cancer Tumor (T), Node (N), Metastasis (M) Stage Grouping for Cutaneous Melanoma

Pathologic Stage	T	N	M
0	T_{is}	N_0	M_0
IA	T_{1a}	N_0	M_0
IB	T_{1b}	N_0	M_0
	T_{2a}	N_0	M_0
IIA	T_{2b}	N_0	M_0
	T_{3a}	N_0	M_0
IIB	T_{3b}	N_0	M_0
	T_{4a}	N_0	M_0
IIC	T_{4b}	N_0	M_0
IIIA	$T_{1\text{-}4a}$	N_{1a}	M_0
	$T_{1\text{-}4a}$	N_{2a}	M_0
IIIB	$T_{1\text{-}4b}$	N_{1a}	M_0
	$T_{1\text{-}4b}$	N_{2a}	M_0
	$T_{1\text{-}4a}$	N_{1b}	M_0
	$T_{1\text{-}4a}$	N_{2b}	M_0
	$T_{1\text{-}4a}$	N_{2c}	M_0
IIIC	$T_{1\text{-}4b}$	N_{1b}	M_0
	$T_{1\text{-}4b}$	N_{2b}	M_0
	$T_{1\text{-}4b}$	N_{2c}	M_0
	Any T	N_3	M_0
IV	Any T	Any N	M_1

Clinical Stage	T	N	M
0	T_{is}	N_0	M_0
IA	T_{1a}	N_0	M_0
IB	T_{1b}	N_0	M_0
	T_{2a}	N_0	M_0
IIA	T_{2b}	N_0	M_0
	T_{3a}	N_0	M_0
IIB	T_{3b}	N_0	M_0
	T_{4a}	N_0	M_0
IIC	T_{4b}	N_0	M_0
III	Any	N_1	M_0
IV	Any T	Any N	M_1

have been identified in patients with advanced disease. The number of metastatic sites, disease involvement of the gastrointestinal tract, liver, pleura, or lung, Eastern Cooperative Oncology Group (ECOG) performance status of 1 or greater, male sex, and prior immunotherapy have been associated with poor prognosis.[26]

TREATMENT

Desired Outcomes

Treatment of cutaneous melanoma depends on the stage of disease. Local disease is managed, and often cured, with surgical ablation. Regional disease is treated with surgical resection of the primary lesion and, depending on the risk of recurrence, adjuvant therapy in an effort to eradicate any residual disease and cure the patient. The role of interferon-α (IFN-α) as adjuvant therapy after surgical resection remains controversial. Until recently, metastatic melanoma has been a difficult disease to treat. The treatment goals for metastatic disease are to slow tumor progression, prolong life, relieve acute symptoms, and improve quality of life. With the advent of new immunotherapy and molecular targeted therapy, the management of metastatic melanoma has drastically changed. After more than a decade of ineffective drug development, several new treatment options now exist for the treatment of metastatic melanoma such as CTLA-4 inhibitors, BRAF inhibitors, MEK inhibitors, and PD-1 inhibitors. Molecular targeted agents offer rapid and high response rates with prolonged time to disease progression, while immunotherapy can induce durable responses. These new treatment options have increased survival expectations to an all-time high in the history of melanoma treatment.

TABLE 139-6 Prognostic Factors for Cutaneous Melanoma

Tumor-Related Factors
Tumor thickness
Level of tumor invasion
Ulceration
Histologic subtype
Anatomic site of primary tumor
Mitotic rate
Lymphangitic invasion
Occurrence of microsatellites
Presence of tumor-infiltrating lymphocytes
Patient-Related Factors
Age
Gender

Surgery

Patients who present with a suspicious pigmented lesion should undergo a full-thickness excisional biopsy, if possible. A full-thickness incisional or punch biopsy is preferred, in cases where an excisional biopsy not possible, to provide microstaging and ultimately determine therapy.

2 Localized cutaneous melanoma can often be cured with surgical excision. The cure rates for melanomas smaller than 1 mm are as high as 98%. The extent of the excision margin is important in preventing local recurrence and ultimate survival. For melanoma in situ, excision of the visible lesion or biopsy site with a 0.5 to 1 cm border of clinically normal skin, and a layer of subcutaneous tissue with confirmation of histologically negative peripheral margins, is recommended. The recommended clinical margin for invasive melanoma depends on tumor thickness. Excision with a 1 cm margin of clinically normal skin, and underlying subcutaneous tissue, is recommended for invasive melanomas 1 mm thick or smaller. Current guidelines recommend a 1 to 2 cm margin for melanoma with tumor thickness of 1.01 to 2 mm.[22] Lesions which are 2 to 4 mm thick should be excised with a 2 cm margin. Primary tumors more than 4 mm thick require at least a 2 cm margin, whether a larger margin is beneficial is unclear. Surgical management of lentigo maligna melanoma is problematic as subclinical extension of atypical junctional melanocytic hyperplasia

may extend beyond the visible margins. Complete excision of these lesions is important.

When isolated regional lymph nodes are detected via physical examination, in the absence of distant disease, therapeutic lymphadenectomy is recommended. The extent of therapeutic lymph node dissection often is modified according to the anatomic area of the lymphadenopathy. Selective regional lymphadenectomy performed after scintigraphic and dye lymphographic identification of the affected sentinel draining lymph node(s), is the standard of care for melanomas more than 1 mm thick. If the sentinel node is found to have micrometastatic melanoma, regional dissection of the involved nodal basin is performed. If the lesion is 0.75 to 1 mm in thickness with ulceration or is Clark level IV or V, lymphatic mapping with SLNB may be considered based on patient characteristics, such as ulceration of the tumor.[27] The likelihood of detecting metastatic disease in the sentinel lymph node is about 1% in tumors which are smaller than 0.8 mm, but increases to more than 30% in tumors 4 mm thick.[27] Final results, with 10 years of follow-up, from the Multicenter Selective Lymphadenectomy Trial I showed no difference in disease-specific survival when SLNB was compared to the watch and wait approach (remove nodes once palpable).[28] These results support current clinical practice to remove microscopic metastasis before they become problematic. The Multicenter Selective Lymphadenectomy Trial II is currently enrolling patients to assess whether or not a complete lymph node dissection after a positive SLNB improves overall survival. SLNB results are important for accurate staging, therapeutic lymphadenectomy, and to aid in the decision to offer adjuvant treatment.[27]

One of the most important aspects of surgical management of cutaneous melanoma is the role of patient follow-up.[22] Postsurgical follow-up of patients who have had a melanoma excised is essential to monitor for undetected metastatic disease and the development of a second primary cutaneous melanoma or nonmelanoma primary malignancy. Scheduled screening, in addition to routine surgical follow-up, is required for any patient with a melanoma; the recommended frequency and duration depend on the stage of melanoma. The optimal duration of follow-up remains controversial. Most patients who develop recurrent disease do so in the first 5 years after treatment, but late recurrences, more than 10 years after surgery, have been observed. The increased lifetime risk of developing a second primary melanoma supports lifetime dermatologic surveillance for all patients.

A patient with stage III melanoma commonly has lymph node involvement and in-transit metastases may also occur. In-transit metastasis is the clinical manifestation of tumor which develops in lymphatics between the primary melanoma and the regional lymph node basin.[5] In-transit metastases are more than 2 cm from the original lesion. In-transit metastases are more common in individuals with thick, ulcerated lesions. Surgery is used for management of in-transit lesions, with the goal of complete resection. Unfortunately, subsequent recurrence in the same extremity often occurs after initial resection of in-transit metastasis.

The role of surgery beyond that of cure is less clear, although surgery may offer palliation for patients with isolated metastasis.[27] In these cases, surgery may extend survival time in select patients with metastatic disease. Patients whose metastasis can be completely resected may experience improved quality of life, improved overall survival, and occasionally long-term disease control.[27]

Brain metastasis is a frequent complication of advanced melanoma. About 20% to 50% of patients with stage IV disease develop clinically apparent central nervous system (CNS) involvement. Surgical resection, with or without radiation, has been used in select individuals. More recently, high control rates of brain metastasis have been achieved with focal radiation therapy such as linear accelerator-based stereotactic radiosurgery or gamma-knife technologies.[29] Melanoma in the gastrointestinal tract can lead to bowel obstruction. Appropriate resection or bypass may provide significant relief of symptoms. Despite the lack of controlled clinical trials, the impact on palliative surgery should be evaluated in the context of a patient's comfort and quality of life. The risk of relapse and death after resection of a local, or regional cutaneous melanoma, is the primary determinant for use of adjuvant therapy after primary resection. Adjuvant trials have focused on patients at intermediate or high risk for recurrence.

Adjuvant Therapy

3 Melanoma is considered one of the most immunogenic solid tumors, and it appears to interact with, and respond to, the immune system of the host in which it arises. Spontaneous regressions of melanoma suggest the importance of the immune system in disease modulation. Lymphoid infiltration into the primary melanoma also suggests that immunomodulation may impact the biology of melanoma. Early work has shown that nonspecific immunomodulators, such as levamisole and Bacillus Calmette-Guérin (BCG) for treatment of melanoma, were associated with some regression of the tumor, although many of these responses were limited and short-lived. Because melanoma is generally resistant to traditional treatment modalities such as radiation and chemotherapy, immunotherapy offers an avenue of treatment. In early trials, patients who showed the highest response to immunotherapy had minimal disease burden. The use of adjuvant immunotherapy to treat these patients has been investigated to prevent distant recurrence and improve long term survival.

Interferon

One of the oldest, and most controversial, immunotherapy approaches for the treatment of melanoma is the use of IFNs. The IFNs are a group of proteins with diverse immunomodulatory and antiangiogenic properties. A number of studies evaluated various doses and schedules of recombinant IFN for treatment of metastatic melanoma. Response rates in metastatic melanoma range from 10% to 30%, and overall response rates are about 15% for IFN-α. In clinical trials of IFN therapy for patients with metastatic melanoma, response rates were highest in patients with limited disease. Responses were seen at all sites of disease, but were most frequent in subcutaneous, lymph node, and pulmonary metastasis. The activity of IFN in patients with minimal disease encouraged investigators to evaluate the role of adjuvant IFN. A large, multicenter cooperative group trial (E1684) of adjuvant IFN-α_{2b} versus observation was designed for 287 patients with high-risk (stages IIB and III disease based on the 1997 AJCC staging criteria) melanoma after curative surgical resection. IFN-α_{2b} was given IV as an induction therapy at maximum tolerated doses of 20 million IU/m^2 per dose 5 days per week for 4 weeks; treatment was continued for 48 weeks with subcutaneous IFN-α_{2b} 10 million IU/m^2 per dose 3 times per week. This therapy now is often referred to as *high-dose interferon* (HDI). With a median follow-up period of 6.9 years, patients treated with HDI had significantly longer relapse-free and overall survival compared with patients who were observed after surgical resection (1.72 vs 0.98 years and 3.8 vs 2.8 years, respectively).[30] Both the 5-year relapse-free and overall survival rates were higher with HDI. This data led to the 1995 FDA approval of HDI as standard of care. With longer follow-up (median, 12.6 years), however, the difference in overall survival was no longer significant.[31] Further analysis showed that the greatest reduction in melanoma recurrence occurred during the first few months of treatment. Subgroup analysis of this study indicated that patients with large primary tumors and node-negative disease did not receive the same benefit from therapy, but the small number of patients in this group made it difficult to draw definite conclusions about the role of IFN for adjuvant therapy in this setting.

Pegylated IFN-α_{2b} has also been evaluated in the adjuvant setting with the hope for a better efficicy and toxicity profile. The European

Organization for Research and Treatment of Cancer (EORTC) 18991 trial evaluated 1,256 patients with resected stage III melanoma. Patients were randomized to observation or pegylated IFN. Pegylated IFN was given less frequently compared with nonpegylated IFN. Updated results demonstrated an improvement in relapse-free survival, but no difference in overall survival or distant metastasis-free survival.[32] Based on this data, the FDA approved pegylated IFN-α_{2b} as an option for adjuvant treatment.

HDI treatment is associated with multiple toxicities, including flu-like syndrome. Toxicities of IFN therapy in the adjuvant HDI trials were common and severe. About one-third of patients will need a dose modification during induction and only half of the patients are able to complete the year of therapy in an outpatient setting. One strategy for reducing toxicities associated with IFN is to modify the dose and duration. A subsequent ECOG trial (E1690) of low-dose IFN (3 million IU per dose given subcutaneously three times weekly *low-dose interferon* [LDI]) for 24 months compared with the HDI regimen described earlier versus observation did not demonstrate an overall survival advantage of HDI versus observation.[33] At a median follow-up period of 52 months, the 5-year estimated relapse-free survival rates for HDI, LDI, and observation were 44%, 40%, and 35%, respectively. With longer follow-up, however, the difference in relapse-free survival was no longer significant.[33] A significant overall survival benefit was not seen for HDI or LDI compared with observation, although the investigators speculated that this analysis of survival was affected by the number of patients in the observation arm who received IFN therapy after disease progression.[33]

The use of IFN in the adjuvant setting remains controversial. Although the HDI regimen is used in the United States, the LDI strategy remains standard in many European countries. In a pooled analysis of 713 patients who participated in two randomized controlled trials (E1684 and E1690), HDI was associated with a significant reduction in relapse-free survival compared with observation ($P<0.006$).[31] No benefit in overall survival was observed in the pooled analysis. The results of nine randomized clinical trials of adjuvant HDI or LDI versus observation in melanoma were included in a systematic review. The systematic review observed a trend toward reduced risk of recurrence of melanoma and of death among the IFN-treated patients in nearly all studies.[34] Because of differences in dose, frequency, and duration of IFN-α treatment in the various trials, the review was not able to compare LDI versus HDI. Furthermore, the wide variability in number of patients enrolled, end points, patient selection, quality, type of therapy, duration of treatment, and follow-up precluded statistical analysis of the pooled results. Although the differences in overall survival have not always been statistically significant, HDI remains the only adjuvant treatment shown to prolong survival in prospective randomized trials. IFN-α_{2b} is approved by the FDA for treatment of patients with primary melanomas larger than 4 mm (stages IIB and IIC) and in patients with melanoma involving regional lymph nodes who are disease-free after lymph node dissection (stage III).

For patients who receive IFN, it is important to effectively prevent and manage treatment-related toxicities. A common syndrome seen with IFN-α therapy is a diverse group of side effects referred to as *constitutional symptoms*, which can include acute symptoms such as fever, chills, myalgia, and fatigue, and can encompass some of the more chronic toxicities such as fatigue, anorexia, and depression.[35] Acetaminophen can be used to prevent or minimize acute dose-related symptoms such as fever, myalgia, and chills. Opiates, such as meperidine, are often required when patients experience severe chills or rigors, most commonly during the initial month of the HDI induction phase. Nonsteroidal anti-inflammatory drugs (NSAIDs) have been used to manage IFN-related myalgia, but may have overlapping side effects with IFN, such as a decrease in renal blood flow. NSAIDs and acetaminophen may mask fevers which occur in patients who experience neutropenia while undergoing therapy. Additionally, NSAIDs may increase the risk of bleeding in the setting of thrombocytopenia caused by IFN. Fatigue is one of the most frequently observed dose-limiting toxicities seen with IFN therapy, occurring in 70% to 100% of patients.[35] IFN-induced fatigue appears to be dose related and may worsen with continued therapy. Pharmacologic (eg, methylphenidate) and nonpharmacologic (eg, exercise, psychosocial techniques, distraction, energy management, and dietary modifications) may improve IFN-related fatiguein patients. Depression is common and should be fully evaluated. Contributing factors such as IFN-induced hypothyroidism or concomitant IFN symptoms (eg, nausea and fatigue) should be evaluated concurrently with depression symptoms to optimize treatment decisions. Antidepressants, such as selective serotonin reuptake inhibitors, have been studied in IFN-induced depression with notable benefit.[35] Anorexia is reported in about 70% of patients receiving adjuvant IFN therapy for melanoma and is thought to be mediated through direct effects on hypothalamic neurons, modification of normal hypothalamic neurotransmitters or neuropeptides, or effects from stimulation of other cytokines.[35] Taste alterations may contribute to anorexia. Glucocorticoids should not be used for appetite stimulation or as part of an antiemetic therapy as they may adversely impact the immunomodulatory effects of IFN. Other toxicities, such as hematologic or hepatic toxicities, require monitoring and appropriate dose modification.

CTLA-4 Checkpoint Inhibitor

One of the major advances in the treatment of metastatic melanoma has come through targeting specific immune checkpoints. T-cells play a role in cell-mediated immunity and cancer immunotherapy. T-cells are activated when the T-cell receptor (TCR) interacts with its antigen followed by the interaction of CD28 on the T-cell with the co-stimulatory molecule, B7 on antigen presenting cells. To prevent over activation of T-cells receptors, such as CTLA-4, function as a co-inhibitory receptor for the co-stimulatory molecule B7. Crosslinking of CTLA-4 by B7 inhibits T-cell activation, transcription, translation, and transduction. CTLA-4 blockade overcomes this inhibition and results in activation and proliferation of Tcells.[17] Ipilimumab, a monoclonal antibody to CTLA-4, has demonstrated efficacy in the metastatic melanoma setting. More recently, the EORTC 18071 trial evaluated 475 patients treated with high-dose ipilimumab 10 mg/kg IV every 3 weeks × 4 doses, then every 3 months for up to 3 years, compared to placebo in the adjuvant setting. Recurrence-free survival was 26.1 months in patients treated with high-dose ipilimumab compared to 17.1 months in patients treated with a placebo ($P=0.0013$).[36] The effect on overall survival remains to be determined.

CTLA-4 antibodies produce several immune-related adverse effects (irAEs) that are distinct and different than adverse events associated with conventional cancer treatments. CTLA-4 antibodies cause autoimmune-irAEs by promoting the activation of self-reactive T cells. The incidence of irAEs is as high as 60%, and up to 20% of patients experience Grade 3 or 4 irAEs.[37] The most common serious irAEs include dermatitis, enterocolitis, hepatitis, and endocrinopathies.[17] These adverse reactions are dose-related and follow a predictable pattern: skin related toxicities occur first after the first dose; colitis follows after the second dose; and hepatitis and endocrinopathies occur last, after third or fourth dose.[38] Most irAEs are reversible with treatment and resolve after 6 to 8 weeks, with the exception of endocrinopathies which may require lifelong hormonal treatment. Close monitoring for irAEs and participation in a risk evaluation and mitigation strategy (REMS) program while on therapy is necessary.[22] It is recommended that patients obtain a comprehensive metabolic panel (with liver function tests), complete blood count, and thyroid function tests at baseline, throughout treatment and for up to 6 months after treatment.[38] Ipilimumab therapy should be held for moderate-to-severe irAEs. High-dose systemic corticosteroids should be initiated for patients who do not improve from withholding therapy or for grade 3 immune-related events. Ipilimumab can be restarted when adverse events improve to grade 0 or 1 and systemic corticosteroid doses have been minimized. In early studies, corticosteroids were discouraged for concern they would blunt the desired immune response. But studies show that the efficacy of ipilimumab is not compromised with steroid use.[39] For patients who are steroid refractory, defined as no response to high dose IV steroids within 48 to 72 hours of initiation, other immunosuppressive agents have been utilized. Agents such as infliximab and mycophenolate can be used for patients who develop steroid refractory colitis and hepatitis, respectively.[38] Due to its own hepatotoxicity potential, infliximab should be used with caution. Published guidelines for the treatment of irAEs are available.[38] In cases of severe or life-threatening irAEs, permanent discontinuation of therapy is recommended. In clinical studies reported to date, patients who experienced grade 3 or 4 autoimmune toxicities were also the most likely to exhibit tumor regression and increased time-to-relapse in the metastatic setting.[37] The most common adverse effects observed in the EORTC 18071 adjuvant trial were autoimmune colitis and autoimmune hepatitis, consistent with known adverse effects. Autoimmune endocrinopathies occurred at a higher frequency than in the metastatic disease trials. irAE led to the discontinuation of treatment in 52% of patients who were treated with ipilimumab. Of concern, five deaths were attributed to drug-related adverse effects.[36]

Although IFN is approved for the adjuvant setting, many experts continue to question its use given the considerable treatment toxicities and the uncertain overall survival advantage. High-dose ipilimumab provides a new treatment option for patients with high risk disease. Further evaluation is needed to determine its effect on overall survival. Given the significant toxicities associated with high-dose ipilimumab, the decision to treat a patient should be based on careful evaluation of the risk versus benefit. Patients who receive ipilimumab must be carefully monitored for irAEs. The National Comprehensive Cancer Network (NCCN) guidelines for melanoma list IFN-α and ipilimumab as treatment options in the adjuvant setting. Other options include observation, and most importantly, clinical trials.[22]

Clinical **Controversy...**

The role of ipilimumab in the adjuvant setting for high-risk patients after surgical resection of melanoma needs further investigation. In the adjuvant trial, ipilimumab was dosed at 10 mg/kg while the FDA approved dose in the metastatic setting remains 3 mg/kg. The optimal dose to balance efficacy and toxicity remains unknown.

Treatment of Metastatic Melanoma

Chemotherapy and Biochemotherapy

4 Although many drugs show in vitro activity against melanoma, only a few drugs have consistently shown a response rate greater than 10% in individuals with metastatic melanoma. Most clinical trials of new agents in melanoma measure antitumor activity in terms of response rates, which does not always correlate with survival, and do not evaluate benefit to the patient. Complete responses can be durable in a small number of patients.

Dacarbazine, a cytotoxic drug thought to exert its antitumor effect through alkylation, currently is the most effective chemotherapeutic agent for treatment of melanoma. Dacarbazine remains the only FDA-approved chemotherapeutic agent for treatment of metastatic melanoma in the United States. Prospective controlled clinical trials have observed response rates of 10% to 25%, with an average duration of response of 5 to 7 months.[40] Complete responses are uncommon, with fewer than 5% of patients treated with single-agent dacarbazine sustaining long-term complete responses. The optimum dose schedule of dacarbazine has never been determined; doses of 250 mg/m^2/day for 5 days or 800 to 1,000 mg/m^2 every 3 weeks are seen in practice. Common adverse effects of dacarbazine therapy include myelosuppression, severe nausea and vomiting, and flu-like symptoms after high doses. Nausea and vomiting can be prevented and managed with available antiemetics and are not a major complication.

Temozolomide is an oral prodrug of the active metabolite of dacarbazine and is less emetogenic than dacarbazine. Temozolomide appears to cross into the CNS and was initially thought to have benefit for patients with CNS metastasis. In a phase III trial of chemotherapy-naïve individuals with metastatic melanoma, temozolomide showed efficacy at least equivalent to that of dacarbazine in terms of objective response rates, time-to-progression, and overall and disease-free survival but appeared to be associated with improvement in some aspects of quality of life.[40]

Other chemotherapeutic agents such as *platinum analogues*, *taxanes*, and *nitrosureas* have been evaluated as single agents in the treatment of metastatic melanoma and have been found to exhibit minimal benefit. Of note, a phase III trial comparing *albumin-bound paclitaxel* with dacarbazine in chemotherapy-naïve melanoma patients reported an increase in progression-free survival and a trend in overall survival in patients receiving albumin-bound paclitaxel. Neuropathy and neutropenia were more common in the albumin-bound paclitaxel arm.[41] At this time, these agents are not routinely used as single-agent therapy for melanoma, but are being incorporated into multidrug strategies against metastatic melanoma.

In an attempt to improve the limited responses seen with single-agent chemotherapy, a variety of combination chemotherapy regimens have been evaluated in both small and large clinical trials. The combination of dacarbazine with other chemotherapy, most commonly cisplatin, increased response rates with minimal survival benefit. The initial reports with the cisplatin, vinblastine, and dacarbazine (CVD) regimen were exciting, with reported response rates greater than 50%, a 4% complete response rate, a median response duration of 9 months, and acceptable toxicities.[42] Subsequent reports showed no difference in response rates or survival.

The Dartmouth regimen is a combination which includes carmustine, dacarbazine, cisplatin, and tamoxifen. Initial reports with this regimen demonstrated high response rates of 20% to 50%, but few patients achieve long-term survival. A controlled clinical trial from the National Cancer Institute of Canada demonstrated no benefit in response or survival from tamoxifen in this combination.[43] Further trials showed no benefit of the Dartmouth regimen compared with single-agent dacarbazine.[40] Of concern, toxicities were higher with the combination study and included bone marrow suppression, nausea, vomiting, and fatigue.

Low overall response rates and toxicity have limited the routine use of chemotherapy alone in the management of metastatic disease. The strategy of a combination of chemotherapy (dacarbazine, platinum agents, or vinca alkaloids) and cytokines (aldesleukin or IFN) often termed *biochemotherapy*, has been a focus of investigation in the management of metastatic melanoma. The primary rationale for this combination is to increase overall activity and perhaps response rates based on preclinical trials which suggest potential synergistic interactions between cytokines and some chemotherapy agents. As with other treatment strategies in melanoma, results from initial trials suggested higher response rate with biochemotherapy than with either chemotherapy or biotherapy alone. Despite encouraging results with combination chemotherapy and combination biotherapy, the results of clinical studies have not demonstrated a clear advantage with biochemotherapy compared with chemotherapy alone. A meta-analysis of 18 randomized trials of chemotherapy versus biochemotherapy showed that biochemotherapy was associated with a significantly higher response rate in treatment of metastatic melanoma but the higher response rate did not translate into a significant difference in overall survival.[44] Toxicities can be severe and are consistent with the individual agents in the regimen.

Biochemotherapy has also been evaluated in the adjuvant setting. Early published data was encouraging. Recently, results from larger phase III studies comparing biochemotherapy with IFN, as adjuvant therapy in high-risk stage III disease, were published. This trial demonstrated that biochemotherapy significantly improved relapse-free survival, but no difference in overall survival was observed.[45]

The role of chemotherapy and biochemotherapy in metastatic melanoma is limited because of low response rates and a lack of survival benefit. NCCN currently recommends these treatment approaches as second-line or subsequent treatment options for patients with metastatic melanoma.[22]

Immunotherapy

Significant attention has been given to immunotherapy as a treatment modality in metastatic melanoma due to its general resistance to traditional treatment modalities. Although complete response rates seen with biotherapy are relatively low, the responses can be durable. Over the past few years, advances in immunotherapy for the treatment of melanoma have significantly impacted survival in patients with metastatic melanoma.

Interleukin-2 Interleukin-2 is a glycoprotein produced by activated lymphocytes. IL-2 was first identified as a T-cell growth factor, but IL-2 is also a growth factor for a variety of cells, including lymphocytes and natural killer (NK) cells. IL-2 also may be immunosuppressive.

The precise mechanism of cytotoxicity of IL-2 is unknown. In vitro and in vivo, IL-2 stimulates the production and release of many secondary monocyte-derived and T-cell–derived cytokines, including IL-4, IL-5, IL-6, IL-8, tumor necrosis factor (TNF)-α, granulocyte-macrophage colony-stimulating factor, and IFN-γ, which may have direct or indirect antitumor activity. In addition, IL-2 stimulates the cytotoxic activities of NK cells, monocytes, lymphokine-activated killer (LAK) cells, and cytotoxic T lymphocytes (CTLs). IL-2 also appears to activate endothelial cells, which results in increased expression of adhesion molecules.[46]

High-dose aldesleukin was evaluated is a series of trials with objective response rates around 16%. Of significance, 6% of those patients produced a complete response which were durable (median response, 70 months).[46] Responses were seen at a number of metastatic sites such as the lung, liver, bone, lymph nodes, and subcutaneous tissue. The FDA approved high-dose aldesleukin regimen used for treatment of metastatic melanoma is 600,000 IU/kg per dose every 8 hours for 14 doses maximum in a 5-day period given for two cycles, with a 10- to 14-day rest period between cycles. At these doses, cytokine-induced capillary leak syndrome is a common problem and often is accompanied by significant hypotension, visceral edema, dyspnea, tachycardia, and arrhythmias. Increased permeability of capillary walls allows for a fluid shift from the intravascular space into tissue. As the patient becomes intravascularly dehydrated, hypotension may occur, resulting in reflex tachycardia and arrhythmias. In addition, the decrease in blood volume may result in decreased renal blood flow and urine output, manifesting as increases in blood urea nitrogen, serum creatinine, edema, and weight gain and a decrease in urine output (input greater than output). Visceral edema may result in pulmonary congestion, pleural effusions, and edema. The management of patients receiving high-dose aldesleukin requires extensive supportive care medications, careful monitoring, and staff trained in aspects of critical care such as hypotension management. Constitutional symptoms are a frequent complication of aldesleukin therapy and become more intense as therapy progresses. Additional side effects seen with aldesleukin include pruritus, eosinophilia, bone marrow suppression, increased liver function tests, neurologic disturbances, diarrhea, and nausea

Careful patient selection for aldesleukin therapy is important. Pretreatment factors such as performance status, site of metastasis, and LDH may predict who will respond. Based on reports of long-term responses (greater than 10 years) experienced by some patients, the benefit certainly exceeds the risk for those individuals. Unfortunately, at this time, it is difficult to determine which individuals will respond to aldesleukin therapy because no biologic or immunologic biomarkers have been found to correlate with response. The decision to treat an individual with high-dose aldesleukin should be based on an analysis of an individual patient's risk versus potential benefit. With newer agents now available on the market, and complexity of administration, the role of aldesleukin has diminished.

5 **CTLA-4 Checkpoint Inhibitors** CTLA-4 was the first immune checkpoint inhibitor identified as a target for anticancer therapies and ipilimumab was the first drug in this class of drugs to demonstrate efficacy in metastatic melanoma. Results from phase I and II trials with ipilimumab demonstrate up to 20% response rates in advanced disease.[47] In a phase III trial of 676 HLA-A*0201-positive patients with refractory metastatic melanoma, ipilimumab (3 mg/kg) plus a glycoprotein 100(gp100) peptide vaccine was compared with ipilimumab (3 mg/kg) alone or gp100 alone.[48] The median overall survival time was significantly longer in patients treated with ipilimumab, alone or combined with gp100, as compared with patients treated with gp100 alone (10.0 or 10.1 vs 6.4 months, hazard ratio [HR] 0.66, $P = 0.003$). Another phase III trial compared a higher dose of ipilimumab (10 mg/kg) plus dacarbazine with dacarbazine alone in patients previously untreated for metastatic melanoma.[49] Ipilimumab plus dacarbazine demonstrated significantly longer overall survival (11.2 vs 9.1 months, HR 0.72, $P < 0.001$) and higher survival rates at 1 year (47.3% vs 36.3%), 2 years (28.5% vs 17.9%), and 3 years (20.8% vs 12.2%) than dacarbazine alone. In 2011, ipilimumab, dosed at 3 mg/kg IV every 3 weeks × 4 doses, became the first FDA approved drug for the treatment of unresectable or metastatic melanoma with a survival benefit. With longer follow-up data, the survival benefit is maintained for patients who had an initial response to ipilimumab. Five-year follow-up data from clinical trials demonstrates survival rates of 13% to 23% with survival durations of 13 to 16 months.[50] It is also important to note that the 3-year survival mark is noteworthy for patients treated with ipilimumab. Up to 85% of the patients who were alive at 3 years were alive at 4 years, suggesting that the 3-year survival mark may be a useful surrogate endpoint.[51] After a period of time, it is felt that the balance between immune response and tumor growth can shift leading to disease relapse after an extended duration of response. Re-treatment can be an option for patients who had an initial clinical benefit and has been shown to re-induce a response; no additional toxicities have been observed with re-induction.[52]

One of the greatest lessons learned from early clinical trials with ipilimumab was the differing kinetics of response and how to evaluate response to treatment. Patients appeared to have no regression of disease for many weeks after treatment initiation. Even more alarming was around 10% of patients initially experienced a significant increase in tumor burden which suggested disease progression. This was then followed by a delayed response to the drug after 12 weeks of therapy; some patients continued to have a steady reduction in tumor burden over time which eventually produced a durable clinical benefit.[53] It is hypothesized that the delayed response is related to the time needed to stimulate the immune system.[50] Due to this phenomenon, the Response Evaluation Criteria in Solid Tumors (RECIST) developed immune-related response criteria (irRC) to evaluate immunotherapies. The most significant additions were the allowance of up to 25% increase in tumor volume and deferral of assessing response until 12 weeks from the start of therapy.[50]

TABLE 139-7 Management of Immune-Related Adverse Effects

Organ Toxicity	Signs/Symptoms	Management	Comments
Skin and Mucosa	Pruritus, rash, desquamation, mucositis	Grade 1 or 2 Topical corticosteroids (betamethasone 0.1%) Urea based creams Oral antipruritic as needed (diphenhydramine or hydroxyzine) Grade 3 or 4 Prednisone 1-2 mg/kg/day or equivalent	Rare cases of toxic epidermal necrosis and Stevens-Johnson syndrome have been reported with ipilimumab
Gastrointestinal	Diarrhea, hematochezia, abdominal cramping, nausea and vomiting	Grade 1 Oral hydration Electrolyte repletion Loperamide Grade 2 Diphenoxylate hydrochloride and atropine Budesonide 9 mg daily Grade 3 or 4 Methylprednisolone 125 mg IV once followed by prednisone 1-2 mg/kg/day or equivalent	Infliximab 5mg/kg IV every 2 weeks may be given if symptoms do not improve with 48-72 hours of high dose steroids. Bowel perforation and obstruction may occur in cases of severe colitis
Hepatic	Transaminitis, jaundice, sclera icterus	Grade 1 or 2 Hold therapy Grade 3 or 4 Prednisone 1-2 mg/kg/day or equivalent	Mycophenylate mofetil 500 mg IV/PO Q12 hours can be used in patients who do not respond to steroids within 48 hours
Neurologic	Muscle weakness, motor neuropathies, sensory neuropathies	Grade 1 Monitor Grade 2 Consider holding therapy Grade 3 or 4 Prednisone 1-2 mg/kg/day or equivalent	Rare case reports of Guillian-Barre' syndrome and myasthenia gravis have been reported with ipilimumab
Endocrine	Headache, weakness, visual changes, behavioral changes, electrolyte imbalances	Grade 1 or 2 Appropriate hormone replacement therapy Grade 3 or 4 Methylprednisolone 1-2 mg/kg IV then 1-2 mg/kg/day of oral prednisone or equivalent	Potential endocrinopathies include Addison's disease, pan-hypopituitarism, adrenal crisis and hypophysitis. These effects may be permanent
Ocular	Photophobia, eye dryness, blurred vision	Grade 1 or 2 Prednisolone acetate 1% topical Grade 3 or 4 Prednisone 1-2 mg/kg/day or equivalent	Rare cases of episcleritis and uveitis have been reported
Pulmonary	Dyspnea, new or worsened cough, chest pain, hemoptysis	Grade 2 Prednisone 1-2 mg/kg/day or equivalent Grade 3 or 4 Methylprednisolone 1-2 mg/kg IV then 1-2 mg/kg/day of oral prednisone or equivalent	Pneumonitis is more common with pembrolizumab and nivolumab than ipilimumab

[a]Hold immunotherapy for grade 3 or 4 irAEs. Data from references 53 and 56.

(6) The greatest challenge with the use of ipilimumab is management of irAEs. Patients must be thoroughly educated on signs and symptoms of irAEs and when to seek medical attention. Providers should be familiar with the differing type, timing and appropriate management of irAEs (Table 139-7). As previously discussed, management of irAEs should follow established treatment guidelines.[38]

(5) PD-1 and PD-L1 Checkpoint Inhibitors PD1 protein is an immune checkpoint upregulated on activated T-cells in response to inflammation. Antibodies directed against PD-1 block the binding of program death-ligand 1 (PD-L1) and 2 (PD-L2) to the receptor on tumor cells, thus allowing Tcells to remain stimulated and the immune response to continue.[8] Pembrolizumab (formerly known as lambrolizumab) and nivolumab are two monoclonal antibodies directed against PD-1. These agents have demonstrated response rates of 30% with long term clinical benefit in early phase I trials.[54] Most notably from these trials, PD-1 inhibitors had a more favorable safety profile with significantly fewer irAEs compared to ipilimumab. Additionally, benefits were seen in patients who had been previously treated with ipilimumab with no difference in response rates. The KEYNOTE-001 trial evaluated the efficacy of pembrolizumab in patients who were previously treated with ipilimumab. The trial reported that overall response rate was 26%, progression-free survival at 24 weeks was 45%, and 1-year overall survival was 58%.[55] Treatment was well tolerated with grade 3 or 4 adverse effects only occurring in 12% of patients. In the randomized controlled trial of patients previously treated with ipilimumab, nivolumab produced higher response rates (32% vs 11%) with fewer irAEs when compared to chemotherapy.[56] An important observation from these studies is the lack of cross resistance between ipilimumab and PD-1 inhibitors. As with ipilimumab, if patients are able to achieve a response to these agents, that response can be maintained for an extended duration. In 2014, the FDA approved both pembrolizumab at 2 mg/kg IV every 3 weeks and nivolumab 3 mg/kg IV every 2 weeks for the treatment of patients with advanced or unresectable melanoma who progressed on previous ipilimumab therapy and, if applicable, a BRAF inhibitor.

(6) Like ipilimumab, the response to PD-1 inhibitors is delayed. One notable difference is response to the PD-1 inhibitors may be slightly faster than with ipilimumab. The most common adverse effects of pembrolizumab and nivolumab are fatigue, cough, nausea, pruritis, rash, decreased appetite, constipation, arthralgias and diarrhea.[55,56] The risk of grade 3 or 4 irAEs is significantly lower compared to ipilimumab. The incidence of grade 3 or 4 diarrhea/colitis with PD-1 inhibitors is dramatically lower and occurs in only1% to 2% of patients. A higher incidence of autoimmune pneumonitis (1%-2%) is seen with nivolumab and pembrolizumab compared to ipilimumab.[38] Patients should be counseled to notify a provider if they notice new or worsening cough,

chest pain or shortness of breath. Treatment of irAEs follows the same established treatment algorithms as ipilimumab (Table 139-7).

First line therapy with PD-1 inhibitors has been evaluated for the treatment of unresectable or metastatic melanoma. In the KEYNOTE-006 trial, pembrolizumab was compared directly to ipilimumab for first line treatment. In this trial, 834 patients with unresectable or metastatic melanoma were randomized to receive 10 mg/kg every 2 weeks or every 3 weeks or ipilimumab 3 mg/kg every 3 weeks for 4 doses. One-year overall survival rates were 75% for the pembrolizumab every 2 weeks (HR 0.63, $P=0.005$), 68.4% for the pembrolizumab every 3 weeks (HR 0.69, $P=0.0036$) and 58.2% for ipilimumab.[57] Treatment-related grade 3 or 4 adverse effects were lower in both the pembrolizumab arms. With better efficacy and less toxicity compared to ipilimumab, the FDA has approved pembrolizumab 2 mg/kg IV every 3 weeks as a first line treatment option for metastatic melanoma. Similarly, in a randomized controlled trial, nivolumab produced significantly better 1-year overall survival rates (73% vs 42%, HR 0.42, $P<0.001$), median progression-free survival (5.1 vs 2.2 months, HR 0.43, $P<0.001$), and overall response rates (40% vs 14%) when compared to dacarbazine in the first line treatment of *BRAF* wild-type metastatic melanoma.[58] The NCCN Guidelines recommend both pembrolizumab and nivolumab as first-line treatment options for patients with unresectable or metastatic disease.

5 **Combination CTLA-4 and PD-1 Checkpoint Inhibitors** The mechanism of inhibition of CTLA-4 and PD-1 is complementary. A combination of a CTLA-4 inhibitor, which exerts its immune inhibition at the central level in the priming phase of activated T cells, and a PD-1 inhibitor, which acts in the peripheral phase within the tumor microenvironment, can result in synergistic activity. Impressive survival rates of 90% at 1-year and greater than 80% at 2-years are unprecedented in the treatment of metastatic melanoma in early trials.[37] This combination was studied in 945 previously untreated patients with unresectable stage III or IV melanoma. Patients were randomized to nivolumab alone, nivolumab plus ipilimumab, or ipilimumab alone. The median progression-free survival was 11.5 months with nivolumab plus ipilimumab, compared with 2.9 months with ipilimumab (HR 0.42, $P<0.001$).[59] 6 One of the most significant concerns of combining two immune checkpoint inhibitors is the safety profile. Grade 3 and 4 treatment-related adverse effects are significantly higher with the combination arm-compared to the ipilimumab arm (55% vs 27.3%). The risk of hepatotoxicity was higher in the combination arm. A second trial, CheckMate-069 trial confirmed the benefits of this combination. In this double-blind trial, 142 untreated melanoma patients were randomized to receive ipilimumab 3 mg/kg and nivolumab 1 mg/kg or the same dose of ipilimumab with placebo once every 3 weeks for 4 doses. Ipilimumab was then discontinued and patients received nivolumab or placebo at the same dose every 2 weeks until disease progression or unacceptable toxicity.[60] Objective response rate was 61% for patients receiving the combination versus 11% for patients receiving ipilimumab alone ($P<0.001$). Complete responses were seen in 22% of the combination arm and none in the ipilimumab arm. Responses were seen regardless of BRAF mutational status. Median progression-free survival was significantly longer in the combination arm (HR 0.40, $P<0.001$). As with previous studies, the responses appeared to be durable, with 82% of responding patients in the combination arm maintaining their response. The higher response rate with combinations of immune checkpoint inhibitors comes at the cost of greater toxicity. The risk of grade 3 or 4 drug-related adverse reactions was higher in the combination arm (54% vs 24%). As a result of data from these two trials, the FDA granted approval of combination therapy with nivolumab and ipilimumab inpatients with *BRAF* V600 wild-type unresectable or metastatic melanoma. While this combination offers higher response rates, some of which can be durable, judicious monitoring and aggressive management of toxicities are important.

Clinical **Controversy...**

The combination of ipilimumab and nivolumab leads to higher response rates compared to ipilimumab alone. Autoimmune toxicities with the combination are significantly higher and must be aggressively managed. Future trials are needed to evaluate if ipilimumab and nivolumab produce higher responses compared to nivolumab alone.

With the rapid advances in immunotherapy, the treatment of melanoma with these new therapies offers new hope to patients. Improved survival has been seen with both CTLA-4 and PD-1 inhibition. While pembrolizumab and nivolumab have better efficacy with less toxicity, ipilimumab is still effective and irAEs can be managed. The combination of ipilimumab and nivolumab has significantly higher responses compared to ipilimumab alone, but the risk of irAEs is also significantly higher. The NCCN guidelines list all of these regimens as potential treatment options for metastatic melanoma.

Despite advances in the treatment of melanoma, several questions still surround the use of immunotherapy. First, who is the best treatment candidate for immunotherapy? Some clinicians are hesitant to treat elderly patients with ipilimumab because of concern for toxicity. Similarly, patients with existing autoimmune conditions have been excluded from treatment with ipilimumab. These unique patient populations require further investigation. Second, what are the biomarkers of response to immunotherapy? Immunologic markers as well as biomarkers have been investigated without success to help identify patients who respond to ipilimumab.[37] Tumors that express PD-L1, regardless of the cancer, have demonstrated higher responses to PD-1/PD-L1 blockade. However, patients with tumors that do not express PD-1/PD-L1 do benefit and should not be excluded from this treatment option. Additionally, it remains unclear as to the best approach for assessing PD-L1 expression, definition of positivity in the assay, and clinical application.[54] Lastly, what is the optimal sequencing of immunotherapeutic agents and with immunotherapy and other therapeutic options? Studies are ongoing looking at sequencing of CTLA-4 inhibitors, PD-L/PD-L1 inhibitors, BRAF/MEK inhibitors, chemotherapy and other investigational agents.

Clinical **Controversy...**

Treatment with immunotherapy is expensive. The projected cost of combination therapy with ipilimumab and nivolumab is $250,000 the first year of therapy and $150,000 per year thereafter. Further analysis is needed to assess the cost-effectiveness of these therapies and the economic burden on patients and society.

Other Immunotherapy Approaches *Vaccine therapy* has been investigated for over a decade in metastatic melanoma. The rationale for vaccination is that antigens expressed on the surface of tumor cells differ from normal cells and vaccines have the ability to induce effective tumor-specific immune responses with less toxicity than conventional chemotherapy or other immunotherapies.

A variety of melanoma vaccines, based on whole tumor cells, peptides, and proteins have been evaluated for treatment of patients with metastatic disease and for intermediate- and high-risk patients after surgical resection of disease and to date none have shown a survival advantage.[17] Occasional clinical responses have been observed in clinical trials of melanoma vaccines, which demonstrate their potential. Vaccines in combination with other biologic therapies have

TABLE 139-8 Dosing of Oral Targeted Therapies

Drug	Brand Name	Dose	Food–Drug Interactions	Drug–Drug Interactions
Trametinib	Mekinist	2 mg Daily Store in the refrigerator (36-46°F)	Administration with a high-fat, high-calorie meal may decrease AUC Take 1 hour before or 2 hours after a meal	Trametinib may enhance the adverse effect of dabrafenib
Cobimetinib	Cotellic	60 mg daily on days 1-21 of 28	Take with or without meal Avoid grapefruit and grapefruit juice	CYP3A4 inducers may decrease cobimetinib drug levels CPY3A4 inhibitors may increase cobimetinib drug levels
Vemurafenib	Zelboraf	960 mg twice daily A missed dose may be take up to 4 hours prior to the next dose	Take with or without meal Avoid grapefruit and grapefruit juice	Vemurafenib may increased drug levels of CYP1A2 and Pg-P substrates CYP3A4 inhibitors may increase vemurafenib drug levels CYP3A4 inducers may decrease vemurafenib drug levels Monitor closely if vemurafenib is use concurrently with other drugs known the prolong QT interval
Dabrafenib	Tafinlar	150 mg twice daily A missed dose may be take up to 6 hours prior to the next dose	Take 1 hour before or 2 hours after a meal High-fat meals decrease Cmax and AUC Avoid grapefruit and grapefruit juice	Dabrafenib may decrease drug levels of CYP2B6, CYP2C19, CYP2C8, CYP2C9, and CYP3A4 substrates CYP2C8 and CYP3A4 inhibitors may increase dabrafenib drug levels CYP2C8 and CYP3A4 inducers may decrease dabrafenib drug levels Concurrent use with antacids, H2-Antagonists and proton pump inhibitors may decrease dabrafenib concentrations

AUC, area-under-the-curve; CYP, cytochrome P450.

been evaluated. Although tumor responses with some of these combination approaches have been observed in phase I and II trials, none of the vaccine responses or improvement in survival have been confirmed in phase III trials.[17] Clinical trials looking at way to incorporate vaccines into currently approved immunotherapeutic treatments are ongoing.

Oncolytic immunotherapy is currently being investigated for the treatment of metastatic melanoma. Talimogene laherparepvec (T-VEC) is a genetically modified oncolytic immunotherapy derived from herpes simplex-1. T-VEC works by two distinct mechanisms: 1) modification of attenuated HSV-1 to selectively replicate within the tumor environment causing death while sparing other cells and 2) secretion of GM-CSF to attract dendritic cells to the site to start the process of antigen presentation and T cells activation. Activated T cells can then target the cancer cells systemically. In a phase III study, T-VEC demonstrated better response rates (including complete responses) and a trend toward improved survival compared to GM-CSF alone.[61] It was well tolerated with fatigue, chills, and fever being the most common adverse effect with few severe adverse effects reported. T-VEC was recently FDA approved for the local treatment of unresectable cutaneous, subcutaneous, and nodal lesions in patients with recurrent melanoma after initial surgery. T-VEC is administered intratumorally (injected directly into the tumor) and as such patients with internal visceral disease are not appropriate candidates for treatment. With its favorable toxicity profile, ongoing studies are evaluating T-VEC in combination with other immune-directed treatments.

Targeted Therapy

7 Protein kinase inhibitors have emerged as standard therapy for malignancies such as renal cell carcinoma, chronic myelogenous leukemia, subsets of lung cancer and gastrointestinal stromal tumors. As our understanding of the biology of melanoma grows, there is increasing interest in targeted therapies against molecular targets involved in the development and progression of melanoma. Several orally administered targeted therapies are FDA approved for treatment of melanoma (Tables 139-8 and 139-9).

The MAPK and PI3K/AKT pathways are involved in tumor cell growth and differentiation and are activated in melanoma. BRAF is downstream in the MAPK pathway. *BRAF* mutations have been described in melanoma cell lines, and it appears that up to 70% of melanomas exhibit BRAF alteration.[8] In a phase I/II trial, vemurafenib, an orally available inhibitor of mutated BRAF, showed activity in patients with melanoma that had *BRAF* with the V600E mutation. In a phase III trial comparing vemurafenib with dacarbazine in patients with unresectable, previously untreated stage IIIC or IV melanoma with a *BRAF* V600E mutation, vemurafenib significantly improved response rate (48% vs 5%) and overall survival.[62] Patients treated with vemurafenib had longer median progression-free survival (5.3 vs 1.6 months) and a higher overall survival rate at 6 months (84% vs 64%). The median time-to-response was also shorter with vemurafenib than dacarbazine (1.45 vs 2.7 months). Dabrafenib, another oral selective BRAF inhibitor, demonstrated similar activity to vemurafenib in early stage clinical trials in patients with previously untreated *BRAF* V600E mutated melanoma. In a phase III study, dabrafenib 150 mg orally twice daily was compared to dacarbazine in patients with untreated stage IV or unresectable stage III melanoma. Patients in the dabrafenib arm had longer median progression-free survival (5.1 vs 2.7 months, HR 0.30, $P < 0.0001$).[63] A follow-up analysis showed that overall survival at 12 months was 70% with dabrafenib as compared to 63% with dacarbazine.[63] Both vemurafenib and dabrafenib have been studied in melanoma patients with CNS metastasis with some activity. Other drugs targeted toward mutated *BRAF*, such as sorafenib, have not reported encouraging results.

BRAF inhibitors are generally well tolerated (Table 139-9). Skin complications comprising of cutaneous squamous cell carcinoma or keratoacanthoma and photosensitivity reactions, are a major

TABLE 139-9 Monitoring of Oral Targeted Therapies

Drug	Adverse Reaction	Monitoring Parameters	Comments
Trametinib	Common: • Hypertension • Skin toxicity (most commonly puritis, acneiform rash, erythema, skin rash) • Hypoalbuminermia • Diarrhea • Stomatitis • Anemia • Lymphedema • Hyperglycemia • Increased liver function tests • Fever Rare but serious: • Cardiomyopathy • Hemorrhage • Rhabdomyolysis • Interstitial lung disease • Serious febrile events • Retinal detachment • Retinal vein occlusion • Basal cell carcinoma, squamous cell carcinoma or primary melanoma	• CBC at baseline and periodically for myelosuppression • CMP at baseline and periodically for hepatotoxicity and hyperglycemia • LVEF at baseline, 1 month after therapy initiation, then at 2- to 3-month intervals for cardiomyopathy • Ophthalmological evaluation periodically especially if patients report visual disturbances • Evaluate for signs/symptoms of pulmonary toxicity (eg, cough, dyspnea, hypoxia, pleural effusions, infiltrates) • Blood pressure • Signs and symptoms of bleeding concerning for hemorrhage • Dermatologic exams when used with dabrafenib at baseline, every 2 months during treatment, then 6 months after discontinuation for secondary skin malignancies	• Hospitalization may be required for severe skin toxicities • Intracranial hemorrhage reported to be fatal • The risk of adverse effects increases when trametinib is used in combination with dabrafenib
Cobimetinib	Common: • Nausea/vomiting/diarrhea • Hypertension • Photosensitivity • Electrolyte disturbances • Hypoalbuminemia • Lymphocytopenia • Anemia • Increased liver function tests • Increased CPK • Increase in serum creatinine • Fever Rare but serious: • Cardiomyopathy • Hemorrhage (GI and cerebral) • Secondary skin malignancies (cutaneous squamous cell carcinoma or keratoacathoma, basal cell carcinoma or secondary primary melanoma) • Retinal vein occlusion/Retinopathy • Hepatotoxicity • Rhabdomyolysis	• CMP at baseline and monthly during treatment for hepatotoxicity, renal dysfunction and electrolyte replacement • CPK at baseline and periodically during treatment for rhabdomyolysis • LVEF at baseline, 1 month after initiation of therapy, and every 3 months for cardiomyopathy • Dermatologic exams at baseline, every 2 months during treatment, then 6 months after discontinuationfor secondary skin malignancies • Ophthalmological evaluation periodically especially if patients reports visual disturbances • Signs and symptoms of hemorrhage and rhabdomyolysis	
Vemurafenib	Common • Nausea/vomiting/diarrhea • Skin toxicity (most commonly rash, photosensitivity, pruritus) • Headache • Alopecia • Peripheral edema • Arthralgias/myalgias • Hyperkeratosis • Fever • Decreased appetite Rare but serious: • Renal failure • Prolonged QT interval • SJS/TEN • Hepatotoxicity • Secondary skin malignancies (squamous cell carcinoma, basal cell carcinoma or keratocanthoma) • Hypersensitivity • Uveitis	• CMP at baseline and monthly or as clinically indicated for hepatotoxicity and renal failure • LVEF at baseline, 1 month after initiation of therapy, and every 3months for cardiomyopathy • Dermatologic exams at baseline, every 2 months during treatment, then 6 months after discontinuation for secondary skin malignancies • Eye pain, photophobia or vision changes	• Off label indication for *BRAF* V600K mutation

(*continued*)

TABLE 139-9 Monitoring of Oral Targeted Therapies (*Continued*)

Drug	Adverse Reaction	Monitoring Parameters	Comments
Dabrafenib	Common • Nausea/vomiting/diarrhea • Skin rash pruritus • Hyperkeratosis • Fever • Hypophosphatemia • Peripheral edema • Headache • Alopecia • Palmar-plantar erythrodysesthesia • Increased liver function tests • Hyperglycemia • Hemolytic anemia • Arthralgias Rare but serious: • Interstitial nephritis • Pancreatitis • Secondary skin malignancies (squamous cell carcinoma, basal cell carcinoma or keratocanthoma) • Uveitis • Hypersensitivity • Hemorrhage • Serious febrile event	• CMP with electrolytes for hypophosphatemia, hyperglycemia, and hepatotoxicity • CBC for myelosuppression • Dermatologic exams at baseline, every 2 months during treatment, then 6 months after discontinuation for secondary skin malignancies • Eye pain, photophobia or vision changes for uvetitis	• The risk of secondary skin malignancies decreases when used in combination with a MEK inhibitor • Assess LEVF when used in combination with a MEK inhibitor • Patients with G6PD deficiency are at risk for hemolytic anemia

CBC, complete blood count; CMP, comprehensive metabolic panel; CPK, creatine phosphokinase; DVT, deep vein thrombosis; LFT's, liver function tests; LEVF, left ventricular function; PE, pulmonary embolism.

concern with the use of these agents. In clinical trials, the incidence of cutaneous squamous cell carcinoma or keratoacanthoma with vemurafenib is 18% and 6% with dabrafenib.[22] The development of these lesions is thought to result from activation of the MAPK pathway in healthy skin cells lacking *BRAF* alterations. As a result, patients receiving a BRAF inhibitor should have dermatologic evaluations prior to starting therapy, every 2 months while on therapy and for up to 6 months following discontinuation of therapy. Cutaneous complications can be effectively managed by surgical resection, and treatment with the BRAF inhibitor can continue without dose adjustment.[64]

Unfortunately, patients develop resistance to BRAF inhibitors, typically after 5 to 6 months of therapy. Resistance is potentially caused by mutations in *MEK*, dependency on MEK/ERK antiapoptotic signaling, PI3K/AKT pathway involvement, *NRAS* mutation, or MAPK pathway reactivation. The use of MEK inhibitors in combination BRAF inhibitors has been found to delay the development of acquired resistance.[62,64]

7 MEK inhibitors have been studied in the treatment of metastatic melanoma and have shown modest activity as monotherapy. Trametinib is an inhibitor of MEK1/2. Compared with chemotherapy (dacarbazine or paclitaxel) in *BRAF*-mutated patients in a phase II trial, patients treated with trametinib had improved progression-free survival, overall survival, and response rates. These results were confirmed in a phase III trial that compared trametinib to chemotherapy (dacarbazine or paclitaxel). In this trial, median progression-free survival was 4.8 months versus 1.5 months in the trametinib and chemotherapy arms respectively (HR 0.45, $P<0.001$). Overall survival at 6 months was 81% for trametinib and 67% for chemotherapy (HR 0.54, $P=0.01$), even with crossover at progression. Common adverse events seen with trametinib were rash, diarrhea, and peripheral edema. Interestingly, secondary skin neoplasms were not observed in this trial.[65]

In addition to delaying drug resistance, the combination of a MEK inhibitor and a BRAF inhibitor has shown efficacy in the treatment of melanoma. The combination of trametinib 2 mg orally once daily and dabrafenib 150 mg orally twice daily received accelerated approval for the treatment in patients with unresectable or metastatic melanoma with *BRAF* mutations based on higher objective response rates compared to either agent alone. Additional trials with this combination compared to a BRAF inhibitors in the same patient population confirmed early findings and led to a full FDA approval. In a clinical trial that compared the combination to dabrafenib alone, patients randomized to the combination had longer median progression-free survival (9.3 vs 8.8 months, HR 0.75, $P=0.03$), overall survival at 6 months (93% vs 85%, HR 0.63, $P=0.02$) and higher overall response rates (66% vs 51%) as compared with dabrafenib alone.[66] In another phase III trial, the combination of dabrafenib and trametinib showed significantly longer median overall survival (not reached vs 17.2 months, HR 0.69, $P=0.005$) and higher overall survival at 12 months (72% vs 65%). Median progression-free survival was also significantly longer (11.4 vs 7.3 months, HR 0.56, $P<0.001$) and overall response rate was higher (64% vs 51%, $P<0.001$) in patients treated with the combination.[67] The safety profile with the combination was similar to that observed with either drug given alone, with the notable exception of deceased incidence of skin complications in the combination arms.

Cobimetinib is another inhibitor of MEK1/2 which was recently FDA approved for the treatment of patients with unresectable or metastatic melanoma with a *BRAF* mutation in combination with vemurafenib. The recommended dosing with this regimen is vemurafenib 960 mg orally twice daily on days 1 to 28 and cobimetinib 60 mg orally once daily on days 1 to 21 of a 28 day cycle. In a phase III trial, median progression-free survival was significantly improved with the combined regimen of cobimetinib and vemurafenib versus vemurafenib alone (9.9 vs 6.2 months, HR 0.51, $P<0.001$). Longer follow-up is needed to evaluate overall survival. Overall response rates were 68% and 45% for the combination and single agent arms, respectively. Adverse events were similar across the two groups and similar to the other MEK and BRAF combination, the number of secondary cutaneous cancer was decreased.[68]

Another agent of interest is imatinib mesylate, an oral agent that inhibits *c-KIT* and platelet-derived growth factor receptor. *c-KIT* is expressed primarily on acral and mucosal melanomas. Imatinib suppressed melanoma cell growth in preclinical studies. In clinical trials with unselected patients, imatinib is not active in metastatic melanoma despite downregulation of phosphorylated *c-KIT*.[22] However, a phase II trial of imatinib in patients with *c-KIT* mutations reported that 23% had a partial response, 30% had stable disease, and progression-free survival was 3.5 months.[8] Reponses in these patients were short similar to what is seen with BRAF inhibitors.

Other important potential molecular targets in the treatment of melanoma include vascular endothelial growth factor (VEGF) and cyclin-dependent kinases. Studies with drugs that inhibit these pathways are currently ongoing. With the success of immunotherapy, combining targeted agents with immunotherapeutic agents is another area of research interest. Reports from a phase I trial combining vemurafenib and ipilimumab showed significant hepatotoxicity, which shows the importance of patient selection to identify the best candidates for combined modality therapy.[69]

Other Approaches

Radiation The role of radiation in the adjuvant treatment of melanoma is being investigated based on retrospective data that suggests patients treated with therapeutic lymphadenectomy for lymph node field relapse benefit from postoperative radiation to the nodal basins. Overall, these data demonstrate improvement in locoregional control with reasonable toxicity, but with no impact on overall survival. Results of a phase III trial indicated adjuvant radiotherapy reduced the risk of lymph node field relapse in patients who had undergone therapeutic lymphadenectomy for metastatic melanoma in regional lymph nodes.[70] No difference in relapse-free survival was observed. Radiation can be used patients with in-transit metastasis or for extranodal tumor extension. For patients with metastatic melanoma, radiation is palliative to symptomatic areas of disease progression. Adjuvant whole brain radiation after resection of brain lesions is controversial and is currently being investigated.[71]

Limb Perfusion and Limb Infusion Isolated limb perfusion is a surgical procedure involving regional intravascular delivery of chemotherapy or biotherapy (or both) into an extremity with cutaneous melanoma.[72] When in-transit metastasis occur in extremities, local therapy with isolated limb perfusion or isolated limb infusion has been used. Isolated limb perfusion is a method for escalating the dose of chemotherapeutic drugs to a specific region of the body while limiting the systemic toxicities of the agent. Most perfusions can be performed with drug exposures of less than 2%. The most significant side effect of isolated limb perfusion are regional toxicity because the skin, subcutaneous tissue, and tissue of the extremity receives the same dose and is subjected to the same perfusion conditions as the tumor located within the extremity. After regional perfusions, objective response rates greater than 50% in treated limbs have been reported, with overall response rates possibly as high as 80%. The role of hyperthermia (38.9°C-40°C [102°F-104°F]) with regional isolated perfusion is not clearly defined. Although most clinical trials have used melphalan, it is not known whether the combination of melphalan with other agents may improve results.[73] Agents that have been combined with melphalan include actinomycin D, nitrogen mustard, thiotepa, and cisplatin. Work with biologic response modifiers, such as TNF-α, has been encouraging.[74] A simplified form of isolated limb perfusion, called isolated limb infusion, is a low-flow isolated limb perfusion performed under hypoxic conditions via small-caliber arterial and venous catheters. It has been proposed that the hypoxia that develops during isolated limb infusion may be beneficial with certain cytotoxic agents such as melphalan.

PERSONALIZED PHARMACOTHERAPY

Treatment of cutaneous melanoma is determined by both disease-related and patient-related issues. Treatment recommendations are based on stage of disease. Treatment of localized disease is surgical excision, with the extent of excision based on the tumor size. Wide excision is recommended for in situ melanoma and wide excision with SLNB for stage IA, IB, and II disease.

The role of adjuvant therapy in the management of individuals at high risk for recurrence remains controversial. One controversy is to identify which patients are appropriate candidates for treatment after resection of the primary tumor. Another controversy with adjuvant therapy is the choice of therapy. HDI has the most evidence supporting its use and is FDA approved for this indication. The challenges with this therapy have been discussed and its use has limited worldwide acceptance. Based on positive clinical trial results, ipilimumab is now an acceptable option in the adjuvant setting. Patient selection must be carefully considered given the irAEs. New therapies and combinations must be evaluated to answer the remaining questions about adjuvant therapy in melanoma. The most appropriate option at this time is a clinical trial, if available.

8 Due to the rapid influx of effective therapies, the management of metastatic melanoma has become complex. The NCCN guidelines list a variety of preferred systemic therapies for advanced or metastatic melanoma, including ipilimumab, pembrolizumab, nivolumab, dabrafenib with or without trametinib, vemurafenib with or without cobimetinib, high-dose aldesleukin, and clinical trial. Dacarbazine, temozolomide, combination chemotherapy, or biochemotherapy are also included as treatment options.[22] The choice of drug therapy should be based on *BRAF* mutational status, the aggressiveness of the disease, and disease-related symptoms. Patients with a more indolent clinical picture may respond better to immunotherapy. Pembrolizumab or nivolumab are now recommended as first line treatment in *BRAF* wild-type melanoma over ipilimumab. Patients with a documented *BRAF* mutation are candidates for treatment with a BRAF inhibitor with or without a MEK inhibitor. These agents may be particularly beneficial in patients with *BRAF* mutations who are symptomatic from their disease because of the rapid response rates that are seen with their use. In patients who harbor the *c-KIT* mutation, imatinib can be offered as first-line therapy.[22] Combination chemotherapy or biochemotherapy should be reserved for patients who do not respond to immunotherapy or targeted therapy upfront. These modalities may be beneficial in stabilizing disease in patients who are *BRAF* wild-type with rapid disease progression. Best supportive care is also an option in some individuals. Data suggest that surgical treatment of metastatic melanoma should be considered in select individuals based on the extent and location of disease and performance status.

In patients who develop brain metastasis, treatment of CNS disease is independent of systemic therapy. Depending on the size and location of metastasis, surgical resection can be offered as the first-line treatment modality in patients with a favorable prognosis. Stereotactic radiosurgery is an acceptable alternative for patients who are unable to undergo resection. Whole-brain radiotherapy is generally reserved for patients with a large volume of metastasis because of the concern of cognitive decline.[75] In many cases, after brain metastasis have been treated, patients can continue with their systemic treatment. The role of targeted treatments and immunotherapy in patients with brain metastasis is ongoing. Early trials with ipilimumab excluded patients with active brain metastasis. Recently, several case reports have described activity in this patient population.[76] An important consideration for treatment of melanoma is the clinical presentation of the disease. As discussed, treatment of melanoma isolated to the limb may be most appropriately treated with regional therapy. Treatment options for metastatic uveal melanoma include strategies for managing hepatic metastasis.

EVALUATION OF THERAPEUTIC OUTCOMES

The outcome of patients treated with melanoma depends on the stage of disease at presentation. The prognosis of patients with thin tumors (less than 1 mm in thickness) and localized disease is good with long-term survival in more than 90% of patients. The risk of regional nodal involvement rises with increasing tumor thickness and survival rates decrease in patients with nodal involvement. Long-term survival in patients with distant metastasis is even lower. Therefore, early diagnosis and appropriate treatment of early disease are essential. Patients with suspicious pigmented lesions should be evaluated and the lesion excised whenever possible. Treatment is determined by patient factors and stage of disease.

Clinical practice guidelines published by the NCCN and European Society of Clinical Oncology (ESMO) provide guidance for treatment and follow-up of patients with melanoma.[22,77] Intensive surveillance has the benefit of early detection of recurrent disease, which may lead to better options of surgical resection. Emphasis on evaluation of locoregional areas is important. For patients with in situ melanoma, periodic skin examinations for life are recommended, with frequency determined based on patient risk factors. Local recurrence is associated with aggressive tumor biology and frequently is a manifestation of an aggressive primary tumor. If a local recurrence occurs after inadequate primary disease management, the patient should undergo a workup based on the lesion thickness of the original melanoma. Patients with nodal recurrence should be evaluated for lymph node metastasis. Patients with systemic recurrence should be evaluated and treated in a fashion similar to patients presenting with systemic disease.

ABBREVIATIONS

AJCC	American Joint Committee on Cancer
ALM	acral lentiginous melanoma
ARF	alternative reading frame
bFGF	basic fibroblast growth factor
CTL	cytotoxic T lymphocyte
CTLA-4	cytotoxic T lymphocyte antigen 4
ECOG	Eastern Cooperative Oncology Group
EORTC	The European Organization for Research and Treatment of Cancer
ESMO	European Society of Clinical Oncology
FDA	Food and Drug Administration
HR	hazard ratio
HDI	high-dose interferon
HLA	human leukocyte antigen
IFN	interferon
IL-2	interleukin-2
irAEs	immune related adverse effects
INK4A	inhibitor of cyclin-dependent kinase 4
LAK	lymphokine-activated killer
LDH	lactate dehydrogenase
LDI	low-dose interferon
LMM	lentigo maligna melanoma
MAPK	mitogen-activated protein kinase pathway
mTOR	mammalian target of rapamycin
NCCN	National Comprehensive Cancer Network
NK	natural killer
NMSC	nonmelanoma skin cancer
NSAID	nonsteroidal antiinflammatory drug
PD-1	programed death receptor 1
PET	positron emission tomography
PI3K	phosphatidyl-inosital-3-OH kinase
SLNB	sentinel lymph node biopsy
SPF	sun protection factor
SSE	skin self-examination
SSM	superficial spreading melanoma
TNF	tumor necrosis factor
TIL	tumor-infiltrating lymphocyte
UV	ultraviolet
UVA	ultraviolet A
UVB	ultraviolet B
VEGF	vascular endothelial growth factor

REFERENCES

1. SEER Cancer Statistics Factsheets: Melanoma of the Skin. National Cancer Institute. Bethesda, MD. *http://seer.cancer.ogv/statfacts/html/melan/html*. Last accessed December 20, 2015.
2. Rigel DS. Trends in dermatology: Melanoma incidence. *Arch Dermatol* 2010;146:318.
3. American Cancer Society. Cancer Facts & Figures 2016. Atlanta. *American Cancer Society* 2016.
4. Wong JR, Harris JK, Rodriguez-Galindo C, Johnson KJ. Incidence of childhood and adolescent melanoma in the United States: 1973-2009. *Pediatrics* 2013;131:846-854.
5. Lin SW, Wheeler DC, Park Y, et al. Prospective study of ultraviolet radiation exposure and risk of cancer in the United States. *Int J Cancer* 2012;131:E1015-E1023.
6. Kubica AW, Brewer JD. Melanoma in immunosuppressed patients. *Mayo Clin Proc* 2012;87: 991-1003.
7. Eckerle Mize D, Bishop M, Resse E, et al. Familial Atypical Multiple Mole Melanoma Syndrome. In: Riegert-Johnson DL, Boardman LA, Hefferon T, et al., eds. Cancer Syndromes [electronic version]. Bethesda (MD): *National Center for Biotechnology Information (US)*; 2009-. *http://www.ncbi.nlm.nih.gov/books/NBK7030/*.Last accessed December 20, 2015.
8. Amaria RN, Gonzalez R. Updated approach to the patient with metastatic melanoma. *Emerg Cancer Ther* 2012;3:583-602.
9. Garraway LA, Widlund HR, Rubin MA, et al. Integrative genomic analyses identify MITF as a lineage survival oncogene amplified in malignant melanoma. *Nature* 2005;436:117-122.
10. Kanetsky PA, Rebbeck TR, Hummer AJ, et al. Population-based study of natural variation in the melanocortin-1 receptor gene and melanoma. *Cancer Res* 2006;66:9330-9337.
11. U.S. Department of Health and Human Services. The Surgeon General's Call to Action to Prevent Skin Cancer. Washington, DC: U.S. Dept of Health and Human Services, Office of the Surgeon General 2014.
12. Wehner MR, Chren M, Nameth D, et al. International prevalence of indoor tanning: A systematic review and meta-analysis. *JAMA Dermatol* 2014;150:390-400.
13. El Ghissassi F, Baan R, Straif K, et al. A review of human carcinogens-part D: Radiation. *Lancet Oncol* 2009;10:751-752.
14. Ogden N. General and plastic surgery devices: Reclassification of ultraviolet lamps for tanning, henceforth to be known as sunlamp products and ultraviolet lamps intended for use in sunlamp products. *https://www.federalregister.gov/articles/2014/06/02/2014-12546/general-and-plastic-surgery-devices-reclassification-of-ultraviolet-lamps-for-tanning-henceforth-to*. Last accessed December 20, 2015.
15. Department of Health and Human Services, Food and Drug Administration 21 CFR Parts 201 and 310, Labeling and Effectiveness Testing; Sunscreen Drug Products for Over-the- Counter Human Use. *https://www.gpo.gov/fdsys/pkg/FR-2011-06-17/pdf/2011-14766.pdf*. Last accessed December 20, 2015.
16. Gangadhar TC, Fecher LA, Miller CJ, et al. Melanoma. In: Neiderhuber JE, Armitage JO, Doroshow JH, et al., eds. *Ableoff's Clinical Oncology*. 5th ed. Philadelphia, PA: Churchill Livingstone; 2014:1071-1091.
17. Zhu Z, Liu W, Gotlieb V. The rapidly evolving therapies for advanced melanoma: Towards immunotherapy, molecular targeted therapy, and beyond. *Crit Rev Oncol Hematol* 2015 Dec 10. pii: S1040-8428(15)30091-3.
18. Rotte A, Bhandaru M, Zhou Y, McElwee KJ. Immunotherapy of melanoma: Present options and future promises. *Cancer Metastasis Rev* 2015;34:115-128.
19. Linares MA, Zakaria A, Nizran P. Skin Cancers. Primary Care: *Clinics in Office Practice* 2015;42;645-659.
20. Goh AY, Layton CJ. Evolving systemic targeted therapy strategies in uveal melanoma and implications for ophthalmic management: A review. *Clin Experiment Ophthalmol* 2015 Nov 25.
21. Curtin JA, Busam K, Pinkel D, et al. Somatic activation of KIT in distinct subtypes of melanoma. *J Clin Oncol* 2006;24:4340-4346.
22. National Comprehensive Cancer Network. NCCN Melanoma Clinical Practice Guidelines in Oncology, version 2. *http://www.nccn.org*. Last accessed Dec 20, 2015.

23. Balch CM, Gershenwald JE, Soong SJ, et al. Final version of 2009 AJCC melanoma staging and classification. *J Clin Oncol* 2009;27:6199-6206.
24. Breslow A. Thickness, cross-sectional areas and depth of invasion in the prognosis of cutaneous melanoma. *Ann Surg* 1970;172:1902-1908.
25. Wong SL, Balch CM, Hurley P, et al. Sentinel lymph node biopsy for melanoma: American Society of Clinical Oncology and Society of Surgical Oncology Joint Clinical Practice Guideline. *J Clin Oncol* 2012;30:2912-2918.
26. Wisco OJ, Sober AJ. Prognostic factors for melanoma. *Dermatol Clin* 2012;30:496-485.
27. Wargo JA, Tanabe K. Surgical management of melanoma. *Hematol Oncol Clin North Am* 2009;23:565-581.
28. Morton DL, Thompson JF, Cochran AJ, et al. Final trial report of sentinel-node biopsy versus nodal observation in melanoma. *N Engl J Med* 2014;370:599-609.
29. Bernard ME, Wegner RE, Reineman K, et al. Linear accelerator based stereotactic radiosurgery for melanoma brain metastasis. *J Cancer Res Ther* 2012;8:215-221.
30. Kirkwood JM, Straderman MH, Ernstoff MS, et al. Interferon alfa-2b adjuvant therapy of high-risk resected cutaneous melanoma: The Eastern Cooperative Oncology Group Trial. *J Clin Oncol* 1996;14:7-17.
31. Kirkwood JM, Manola J, Ibrahim J, et al. A pooled analysis of Eastern Cooperative Oncology Group and Intergroup trials of adjuvant high-dose interferon for melanoma. *Clin Cancer Res* 2004;10:1670-1677.
32. Eggermont AM, Suciu S, Testori A, et al. Long-term results of the randomized phase III trial EORTC 18991 of adjuvant pegylated interferon alfa-2b versus observation in resected stage III melanoma. *J Clin Oncol* 2012;30:3810-3818.
33. Kirkwood JM, Ibrahim JG, Sondak VK, et al. High- and low-dose interferon alfa-2b in high risk melanoma: First analysis of intergroup trial E1690/S9111/C9190. *J Clin Oncol* 2000;18:2444-2458.
34. Lens MB, Dawes M. Interferon alfa therapy for malignant melanoma: A systematic review of randomized controlled trials. *J Clin Oncol* 2002;20:1818-1825.
35. Hauschild A, Gogas H, Tarhini A, et al. Practical guidelines for the management of interferon-alpha-2b side effects in patients receiving adjuvant treatment for melanoma. *Cancer* 2008;112:982-994.
36. Eggermont AMM, Chiarion-Sileni V, Grob JJ, et al. Adjuvant ipilimumab versus placebo after complete resection of high-risk stage III melanoma (EORTC 18071): A randomised, double-blind, phase 3 trial. *Lancet Oncol* 2015;16:522-530.
37. Eggermont AMM, Maio M, Robert C. Immune checkpoint inhibitors in melanoma provide the cornerstones for curative therapies. *Semin Oncol* 2015;42:429-435.
38. Weber JS, Yang JC, Atkins MB, Disis ML. Toxicities of immunotherapy for the practitioner. *J Clin Oncol* 2015:2092-2099.
39. Horvat TZ, Adell NG, Dang TO, et al. Immune-related adverse events, need for systemic immunosuppression, and effects on survival and time to treatment failure in patients with melanoma treated with ipilimumab at Memorial Sloan Kettering Cancer Center. *J Clin Oncol* 2015;33;3193-3198.
40. Yang AS, Chapman PB. The history and future of chemotherapy for melanoma. *Hematol Oncol Clin North Am* 2009;23:583-597.
41. Hersh E, DelVecchio M, Brown M, et al. Phase 3, randomized, open-label, multicenter trial of nab-paclitaxel vs dacarbazine in previously untreated patients with metastatic malignant melanoma. Society for Melanoma Research 2012 Congress. *Pigment Cell Melanoma Res* 2012;25:836-903.
42. Legha SS, Ring S, Papadopoulos N, et al. A prospective evaluation of a triple-drug regimen containing cisplatin, vinblastine and DTIC (CVD) for metastatic melanoma. *Cancer* 1989;64:2024-2029.
43. Rusthoven JJ, Quirt IC, Iscoe NA, et al. Randomized, double-blind, placebo-controlled trial comparing the response rates of carmustine, dacarbazine, and cisplatin with and without tamoxifen in patients with metastatic melanoma. National Cancer Institute of Canada clinical trials group. *J Clin Oncol* 1996;14:2083-2090.
44. Ives NJ, Stowe RL, Lorigan P, Whearley K. Chemotherapy compared with biochemotherapy for the treatment of metastatic melanoma. A meta-analysis of 18 trials involving 2,621 patients. *J Clin Oncol* 2007;25:5426-5434.
45. Flaherty LE, Moon J, Atkins MB, et al. Phase III trial of high-dose interferon alpha-2b versus cisplatin, vinblastine, DTIC plus IL-2 and interferon in patients with high risk melanoma (SWOG S0008): An intergroup study of CALGB, COG, ECOG and SWOG [abstract]. *J Clin Oncol* 2012;30:541s.
46. Sim GC, Radvanyi L. The IL-2 cytokine family in cancer immunotherapy. *Cytokine GrowthFactor Rev* 2014;25:377-390.
47. Sarnaik AA, Weber JS. Recent advances using anti-CTLA-4 for the treatment of melanoma. *Cancer J* 2009;15:169-173.
48. Hodi FS, O'Day SJ, McDermott DF, et al. Improved survival with ipilimumab in patients with metastatic melanoma. *N Engl J Med* 2010;363:711-723.
49. Robert C, Thomas L, Bondarenko I, et al. Ipilimumab plus dacarbazine for previously untreated metastatic melanoma. *N Engl J Med* 2011;364:2517-2526.
50. Delyon J, Maio M, Lebbé C. The ipilimumab lesson in melanoma: Achieving long-term survival. *Semin Oncol* 2015;42:387-401.
51. McDermott D, Lebbe C, Hodi FS, et al. Durable benefit and the potential for long-term survival with immunotherapy in advanced melanoma. *Can Treat Review* 2014;40:1056-1064.
52. Chiarion-Sileni V, Pigozzo J, Ascietro PA, et al. Ipilimumab retreatment in patients with pretreated advanced melanoma: the expanded access programme in Italy. *Br J Can* 2014;110:1721-1726.
53. Weber JS, Kahler KC, Hauschild A. Management of immune-related adverse events and kinetics of response with ipilimumab. *J Clin Oncol* 2012;30:2691-2697.
54. Postow MA, Callahan MK, Wolchok JD. Immune checkpoint blockade in cancer. *J Clin Oncol* 2015;33:1974-1982.
55. Ribas A, Hodi FS, Kefford R, et al. Efficacy and safety of the anti-PD-1 monoclonal antibody MK-3475 in 411 patients with melanoma. *J Clin Oncol* 2014;32:5s.
56. Weber JS, D'Angelo SP, Minor D, et al. Nivolumab versus chemotherapy in patients with advanced melanoma who progressed after anti-CTLA-4 treatment (CheckMate 037): A randomised controlled, open-label, phase 3trial. *Lancet Oncol* 2015;16:375-384.
57. Robert C, Schachter J, Long GV, et al. Pembrolizumab versus ipilimumab in advanced melanoma. *N Engl J Med* 2015;372:2521-2532.
58. Roberts C, Long GV, Brady B, et al. Nivolumab in previously untreated melanoma without *BRAF* mutation. *N Engl J Med* 2015;372:320-330.
59. Larkin J, Chiarion-Sileni V, Gonzalez R, et al. Combined nivolumab and ipilimumab or monotherapy in untreated melanoma. *N Engl J Med* 2015;373:23-34.
60. Postow MA, Chesney J, Pavlick AC, et al. Nivolumab and ipilimumab versus ipilimumab in untreated melanoma. *N Engl J Med* 2015;372:2006-2017.
61. Andtbacka RHI, Collichio FA, Amatruda T, et al. OPTiM: A randomized phase III trial of talimogene laherparepvec (T-VEC) versus subcutaneous (SC) granulocyte-macrophage colony-stimulating factor (GM-CSF) for the treatment of unresected stage IIIB/C and IV melanoma. *J Clin Oncol* 2015;58:3377.
62. Chapman PB, Hauschild A, Robert C, et al. Improved survival with vemurafenib in melnoma with BRAF V600E mutation. *N Engl J Med* 2011;364:2507-2516.
63. Hauschild A, Grob JJ, Demidov LV, et al. Dabrafenib in BRAF-mutated melanoma: Amuticentre, open-label, phase 3 randomised controlled trial. *Lancet* 2102;380:358-365.
64. Muñoz-Couselo E, García JS, Pérez-García JM, et al. Recent advances in the treatment of melanoma with BRAF and MEK inhibitors. *Ann Transl Med* 2015;3:207.
65. Flaherty KT, Robert C, Hersey P, et al. Improved survival with MEK inhibition in BRAF-mutated melanoma. *N Engl J Med* 2012;367:107-114.
66. Long GV, Stroyakovskiy D, Gogas H, et al. Combined BRAF and MEK inhibition versus BRAF inhibition alone in melanoma. *N Engl J Med* 2014;371:1877-1888.
67. Robert C, Karaszewska B, Schachter J, et al. Improved overall survival in melanoma with combined dabrafenib and trametinib. *N Engl J Med* 2015;372:30-39.
68. Larkin J, Ascierto B, Dreno V, et al. Combined vemurafenib and cobimetinib in BRAF-mutated melanoma. *N Engl J Med* 2014;371:1867-1876.
69. Ribas A, Hodi FS, Callahan M, et al. Hepatotoxicity with combination of vemurafenib and ipilimumab. *N Eng J Med* 2013;368:1365-1366.
70. Burmeister BH, Henderson MA, Ainslie J, et al. Adjuvant radiotherapy versus observation alone for patients at risk of lymph-node field relapse after therapeutic lymphadenectomy for melanoma: A randomised trial. *Lancet Oncol* 2012;13:589-597.
71. Fogarty G, Morton RL, Vardy J, et al. Whole brain radiotherapy after local treatment of brain metastasis in melanoma patients: A randomised phase III trial. *BMC Cancer* 2011;11:142.

72. Coleman A, Augustine CK, Beasely G, et al. Optimizing regional infusion treatment strategies for melanoma extremities. *Expert Rev Anticancer Ther* 2009;9:1599-1609.
73. Sanki A, Kam PCA, Thompson JF. Long-term results of hyperthermic isolated limb perfusion for melanoma. *Ann Surg* 2007;245:591-596.
74. Lejeune FJ, Eggermont AMM. Hyperthermic isolated limb perfusion with tumor necrosis factor is a useful therapy for advanced melanoma of the limbs. *J Clin Oncol* 2007;25:1449-1450.
75. Gibney GT, Forsyth PA, Sondak VK. Melanoma of the brain: Biology and therapeutic options. *Melanoma Res* 2012;22:144-183.
76. Di Giacomo AM, Margolin K. Immune checkpoint blockade in patients with melanoma metastatic to the brain. *Semin Oncol* 2015; 42:459-465.
77. Dummer R, Hauschild A, Lindenblatt N, Pentheroudakis G, Keilholz U. Cutaneous malignant melanoma: ESMO Clinical Practice Guidelines. *Ann Oncol* 2015;25:v126-v132.

Hematopoietic Stem Cell Transplantation

140

Susanne Liewer and Janelle Perkins

KEY CONCEPTS

1. Hematopoietic stem cell transplantation (HSCT) is a process that involves intravenous infusion of hematopoietic stem cells from a donor into a recipient, after the administration of chemotherapy with or without radiation. The rationale is to increase tumor cell kill by increasing the dose of chemotherapy. Immune-mediated effects also contribute to the tumor cell kill observed after allogeneic HSCT.
2. Hematopoietic stem cells used for transplantation can come from the recipient (autologous) or from a related or unrelated donor (allogeneic). If the related donor is a twin, the transplant is referred to as a syngeneic transplant.
3. Human leukocyte antigen (HLA) mismatching of allogeneic donor–recipient pairs at either class I or class II loci increases the risk of graft failure, graft-versus-host disease (GVHD), and worsens survival. The ideal donor is one that is matched at HLA-A,B,C, DRB1, and DQ.
4. Hematopoietic stem cells are found in the bone marrow, peripheral blood, and umbilical cord blood. Because of the rarity and similarity to other cells, hematopoietic stem cells are difficult to isolate and measure. These stem cells express the CD34 antigen, and measurement of the number of $CD34^+$ cells is a clinically useful measure of the number of hematopoietic stem cells.
5. Because of clinical and economic advantages, peripheral blood has replaced bone marrow as the source of hematopoietic stem cells in the autologous and adult allogeneic HSCT setting.
6. The purpose of the preparative (or conditioning) regimen in traditional myeloablative transplants is twofold: (a) maximal tumor cell kill and (b) immunosuppression of the recipient to reduce the risk of graft rejection (allogeneic HSCT only).
7. Reduced-intensity conditioning regimens (including those that are nonmyeloablative) have been developed in order to reduce early posttransplant morbidity and mortality while maximizing the graft-versus-malignancy (GVM) effect. The advantage to this approach is that patients who would otherwise not be eligible for allogeneic HSCT can now be offered a potentially curative therapy.
8. Transplant-related mortality associated with allogeneic HSCT ranges from 10% to 80% depending mostly on age, donor, and disease status. Major causes of death include infection, organ toxicity, and GVHD. The most common cause of death after autologous HSCT is disease relapse; transplant-related mortality is usually less than 5%, depending on the conditioning regimen, age, and disease status.
9. Patients undergoing allogeneic HSCT are given prophylactic immunosuppressive therapy, which inhibits T-cell activation, proliferation, or both. The most commonly used GVHD prophylaxis regimens are cyclosporine or tacrolimus and methotrexate. Sirolimus or mycophenolate mofetil are often substituted for methotrexate.
10. Initial treatment of both acute and chronic GVHD consists of prednisone, either alone or combined with cyclosporine or tacrolimus. Treatment of patients with steroid-refractory GVHD is unsatisfactory.

INTRODUCTION

1 Hematopoietic stem cell transplantation (HSCT) is a process that involves intravenous infusion of hematopoietic stem cells from a compatible donor into a recipient, usually after administration of high-dose chemotherapy with or without radiation (called conditioning or preparative regimens). The original rationale for HSCT for treatment of malignant disease is based on studies showing that most anticancer drugs have a steep dose–response relationship and that myelosuppression limits the chemotherapy dosage that can be safely administered. Although standard-dose chemotherapy can prolong survival in many cancer patients, most patients are not cured of their disease with this strategy alone. Infusion of hematopoietic stem cells allows administration of very high doses of chemotherapy (as much as 10-fold higher) by reestablishing hematopoiesis. If tumor cells that are resistant to standard doses are sensitive to higher doses of chemotherapy, then tumor cell kill will be greatly increased, and the likelihood of cure would be higher with HSCT compared with standard dose chemotherapy. However, the chemotherapy dose cannot be escalated indefinitely because of the risk for death caused by nonhematologic toxicity (**Fig. 140-1**).

HSCT is an important modality for treatment of a variety of malignant and nonmalignant diseases. More than 18,000 transplants were performed in the United States in 2012, primarily for malignant diseases.[1] The most common malignancies treated with HSCT are multiple myeloma, lymphomas, and leukemias. The number of transplants has grown steadily over the past decade because of an increase in the number of patients receiving alternative donor transplants and an increase in the number of patients older than 60 years undergoing transplantation.

Although HSCT is most commonly used for treatment of malignant diseases, many nonmalignant hematologic disorders, including aplastic anemia, thalassemia, and sickle cell anemia; immunodeficiency disorders; and other genetic disorders are also potentially curable with allogeneic HSCT. Transplantation is also being investigated as a treatment modality for patients with life-threatening autoimmune diseases, such as rheumatoid arthritis, systemic and multiple sclerosis, and systemic lupus erythematosus.

This chapter summarizes the procedures involved in HSCT and the common complications associated with HSCT. More detailed information on HSCT can be found in published reviews and books.[2-5] Information on HSCT also can be found on several

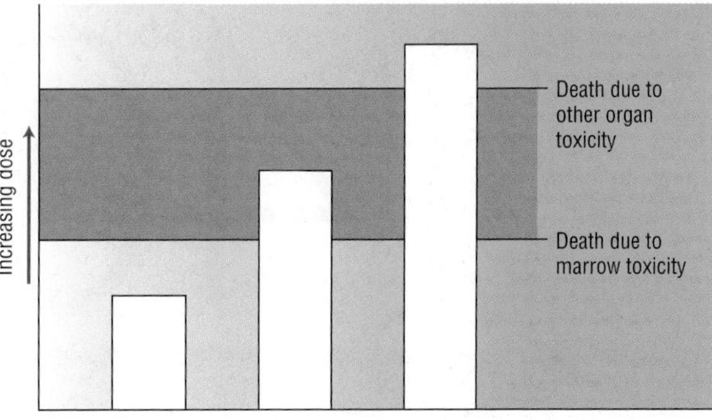

FIGURE 140-1 Patients represented by the middle column are the best candidates for hematopoietic stem cell transplantation because the technique allows for administration of chemotherapy or radiation in doses that otherwise would be intolerable because of severe myelosuppression.

websites, including *http://www.cibmtr.org* (Center for International Blood and Marrow Transplant Research [CIBMTR]) and *https://bethematch.org/* (National Marrow Donor Program [NMDP]).

HISTOCOMPATIBILITY TESTING AND DONOR SELECTION

2 Different types of donors are used in HSCT. The choice of donor depends on the diagnosis and disease status of the recipient as well as his or her age and comorbidities. The role and indications for HSCT are discussed in detail within individual disease chapters of this text. In *autologous* transplants, patients receive their own hematopoietic stem cells, which were collected and stored before administration of the transplant conditioning regimen. In *syngeneic* transplants, an identical twin serves as the donor. In *allogeneic* transplants, the donor is genetically not identical to the recipient but shares some common cell surface antigens called human leukocyte antigens (HLAs). These antigens are encoded by the major histocompatibility complex (MHC), a cluster of genes located on the sixth chromosome.[6] The MHC contains three distinct regions designated as class I, class II, and class III. Class I and class II genes encode for HLA; products of class III genes have other important roles in the immune system. Class I and class II HLA antigens differ in their tissue distribution, structure, and function. Their primary function is to aid the immune system in recognizing cells or tissues as "self" or "nonself." The genes (and the corresponding antigens they encode for) important in HSCT are the class I antigens, HLA-A, HLA-B, and HLA-C and the class II antigen, HLA-DRB1. Because of the polymorphism of the HLA system, there are many different HLA antigens within each different class of HLA. To reduce the chance of graft rejection and graft-versus-host disease (GVHD), a donor is chosen based on how many of these HLA antigens are the same as those of the recipient. Thus, an ideally matched donor would be a "8/8" match, matching at each of the HLA loci mentioned above.

To identify a suitable allogeneic donor, both the recipient and potential donors are HLA typed (ie, specific HLA antigens are identified); the potential donor who is most closely matched is generally chosen to be the transplant donor. HLA typing is accomplished by DNA-based techniques that use polymerase chain reaction (PCR) amplification of specific HLA genes from genomic DNA. DNA typing methods are categorized by the level of discrimination they provide in defining the sequence of an HLA gene.[6] Low-resolution methods provide limited sequence information about a particular HLA gene and are typically used to identify sibling donors. However, low-resolution techniques cannot distinguish the extremely polymorphic nature of many of the HLA antigens. HLA antigens are characterized by thousands of genetic variations (alleles), and each allele may correspond to a unique HLA molecule. Different alleles can be distinguished only by high-resolution typing techniques; high-resolution methods are used to identify suitable unrelated donors.

3 The degree of HLA mismatching correlates with the risk of graft rejection, GVHD, and survival.[6] Mismatches at HLA-A, HLA-B, HLA-C, and HLA-DRB1 are similarly associated with increased risk of GVHD and mortality.[7] HLA-DQ mismatching is less predictive of negative outcomes suggesting an 8/8 match is as beneficial as a 10/10 match. As the number of mismatches increase, the risk of GVHD and transplant-related mortality also increases. In the search for an allogeneic donor, the patient's siblings are typed first. The odds that any one full sibling will match a patient are one in four. About 30% of Americans have an HLA-identical sibling. In an effort to offer allogeneic HSCT to patients who lack an HLA-identical sibling donor, alternative donors are being used. The most common type of alternative donor is an individual unrelated to the recipient who is fully or closely HLA matched. To facilitate identification of these donors, the NMDP (https://bethematch.org) was started in 1986 with initial funding from a US Navy contract. To date, the NMDP has registered more than 16 million donors in the United States and has facilitated more than 60,000 unrelated donor transplants. Donors outside the United States can also be accessed by the NMDP through agreements with international cooperative registries. About one-third of the allogeneic HSCTs performed worldwide are from unrelated donors.[1] The NMDP currently requires that the recipient be typed by high-resolution methodology at HLA-A,B,C, and DRB1. Although it is the transplant center's responsibility to select the donor, the NMDP recommends that selected donor and recipient be matched at HLA-A,B,C, and DRB1 by high-resolution typing when possible for bone marrow or peripheral blood HSCT.[8] If more than one suitable HLA-matched unrelated donor is identified, other factors can be used to select the donor, such as younger age, being male or a nulliparous female, and negative cytomegalovirus (CMV) serostatus.

The likelihood of a recipient finding an HLA-matched unrelated donor ranges from one in 100 to one in 1,000,000 depending on the prevalence of the recipient's HLA type, race, and ethnic background. With the current size and racial make-up of the NMDP registry, the matching likelihood is higher for whites than for patients from other racial or ethnic groups. Agreements between NMDP and international registries may improve the likelihood of finding donors for these patients and NMDP has launched a major effort to promote participation among nonwhite volunteers. Another limitation is the time needed to search for a potential donor. While searches are generally done in an expeditious manner, some donor searches may take up to 3 to 4 months, and patients with acute leukemia can relapse while waiting for completion of the search. With improved HLA typing techniques and better supportive care, most reported outcomes with matched unrelated donors are no longer significantly different than those reported with related sibling donors.[9]

Unfortunately, not every patient who could benefit from an allogeneic donor transplant will have a matched related or unrelated donor available. This has sparked interest in evaluating the use of alternative donor options such as umbilical cord blood (discussed in the next section), mismatched unrelated donors or related haploidentical donors.[10] Potentially useful HLA-mismatched unrelated donors are those who are mismatched at one or, at most, two HLA loci. By allowing for minimal mismatching, the chance of finding an unrelated donor increases significantly. Although mismatched unrelated donor transplants are inferior with respect to GVHD, transplant-related mortality and overall survival when compared to matched unrelated donors, these transplants do offer a curative therapeutic option in select populations.[11] Research is being focused on evaluating the relative effect of mismatches at specific loci to determine if some are less detrimental (permissive) than others in order to improve outcomes. In addition, NMDP recommends testing the recipient for donor-specific HLA antibodies as graft failure is more common when the antibodies are present.[6]

Related haploidentical donors are those that are a complete half mismatch to the recipient; the donor and recipient are matched at 3 of 6 or 4 of 8 HLA loci. Donors can be parents, children or siblings of the recipients. Historically, haploidentical allogeneic transplants (Haplo-HSCT) generated poor outcomes related to high rates of graft failure and GVHD. Strategies to reduce the incidence of graft failure and GVHD have included various methods of T-cell depletion including administration of anti-thymocyte globulin (ATG), alemtuzumab, or posttransplant cyclophosphamide.[11,12] The use of high dose posttransplant cyclophosphamide (PTCy) on days 3 and 4 after infusion of stem cells has provided encouraging results. Three observational studies have compared outcomes after Haplo-HSCT and PTCy to traditional matched related and unrelated donor transplants and have shown that GVHD and survival outcomes were similar.[12] Two parallel prospective studies with identical objectives, eligibility criteria and clinical endpoints were conducted with reduced-intensity conditioning regimens in either Haplo-HSCT with PTCy or umbilical cord blood transplant (UCBT).[13] While the trials were not designed for results to be compared directly, patients receiving Haplo-HSCT had higher rates of engraftment, lower incidence of acute and chronic GVHD and less nonrelapse mortality than reported in the UCBT trial. However, relapse rates were lower after UCBT leading to similar progression-free and overall survival between the two studies. These trials reproduce promising single-center results with Haplo-HSCT or UCBT and suggest that survival rates with these alternative donor sources are comparable to those observed after matched unrelated donors. Based on these results, a phase III study comparing the two alternative stem cell sources is currently underway (BMT-CTN 1101, NCT01597778). Until the results of that trial and other randomized controlled trials are available, choosing an alternative donor in the absence of a HLA-matched sibling or unrelated donor will remain controversial and depends on patient characteristics, physician preference and center experience.

HEMATOPOIETIC STEM CELLS

Hematopoietic stem cells serve as "mother" cells for all blood cells, including erythrocytes, leukocytes, and platelets (see Chapter e86). Stem cells have varying degrees of "stemness." True pluripotent stem cells are capable of replicating indefinitely and can give rise to stem and progenitor cells of all tissues. Multipotent stem cells, such as hematopoietic stem cells, have the capacity for self-renewal and can differentiate into more than one cell type in a particular tissue lineage. Because of their capacity for self-renewal, hematopoietic stem cells are capable of repopulating the recipient's marrow, which has been "emptied" by administration of high-dose chemotherapy, either alone or combined with radiation.

4 Hematopoietic stem cells are rare cells, comprising less than 0.01% of all bone marrow cells. Isolation and quantitative measurement of hematopoietic stem cells are extremely difficult because of their rarity and their similar appearance to other cells. For these reasons, surrogate markers are used to measure the number of stem cells. CD34 is an antigen expressed on hematopoietic stem cells and other early progenitor cells. Determination of the number of cells expressing the CD34 antigen ($CD34^+$ cells), as determined by flow cytometry, has become the standard method of measuring hematopoietic stem cell content.

Hematopoietic stem cells are found in the bone marrow, peripheral blood, and umbilical cord blood (UCB). Hematopoietic stem cells from the bone marrow are obtained by multiple aspirations from the anterior and posterior iliac crests while the donor is under general anesthesia. The procedure takes about 1 hour and yields 200 to 1,500 mL, depending on the size of the donor. In allogeneic bone marrow transplantation (BMT), the marrow stem cells are given to the recipient 12 to 24 hours after harvest. In autologous BMT, the marrow is frozen and stored until needed. After intravenous infusion, the marrow stem cells enter the systemic circulation and find their way to the bone marrow cavity, where they reseed and grow in the bone marrow microenvironment. Although the donor experiences local soreness for a few days, the procedure usually is well tolerated, with no delayed complications resulting from the marrow aspiration. The major risk of serving as a marrow donor is the risk of undergoing general anesthesia.

Hematopoietic stem cells in peripheral blood (peripheral blood stem cells [PBSCs]) are found in the mononuclear fraction of white blood cells (lymphocytes and monocytes) and are collected by a procedure called leukapheresis (or apheresis). This is an outpatient procedure that involves withdrawal of blood from a vein (through a specialized IV catheter), selective removal of mononuclear cells (containing the hematopoietic stem cells) by an apheresis machine, and reinfusion of the unneeded blood components back to the patient. During this process, about 10 to 15 L of blood is processed over several hours during each daily apheresis session. Most of the blood cells are returned to the donor, and each apheresis yields about 200 mL of cells. Leukapheresis is continued daily until a target number of $CD34^+$ cells (which include hematopoietic stem cells) are collected.

The number of hematopoietic stem cells that circulate in peripheral blood normally is too low for apheresis to be technically feasible. Without mobilization techniques, at least six aphereses are usually required to collect a sufficient number of PBSCs. Several methods have been used clinically to "mobilize" hematopoietic stem cells from the bone marrow into peripheral blood for use in autologous transplantation. Figure 140-2 shows representative schemas for mobilization and collection of PBSCs. The most commonly used mobilization method in both donor populations (healthy donors and autologous donors) is administration of a recombinant hematopoietic growth factor such as granulocyte colony-stimulating factor (G-CSF [filgrastim]) or granulocyte-macrophage colony-stimulating factor (GM-CSF [sargramostim]). Both agents are approved by the Food and Drug Administration (FDA) for this indication, but filgrastim is more commonly used. Head-to-head comparisons report superior outcomes with filgrastim in terms of number of stem cells collected, and posttransplant patient outcomes such as hematopoietic recovery, transfusion and antibiotic support.[14] Chemotherapy followed by a hematopoietic growth factor in the autologous transplant population increases the number of PBSCs to a greater extent than growth factor alone. This approach is more expensive and is

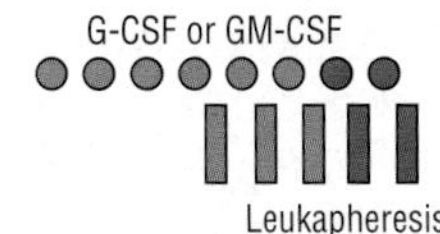

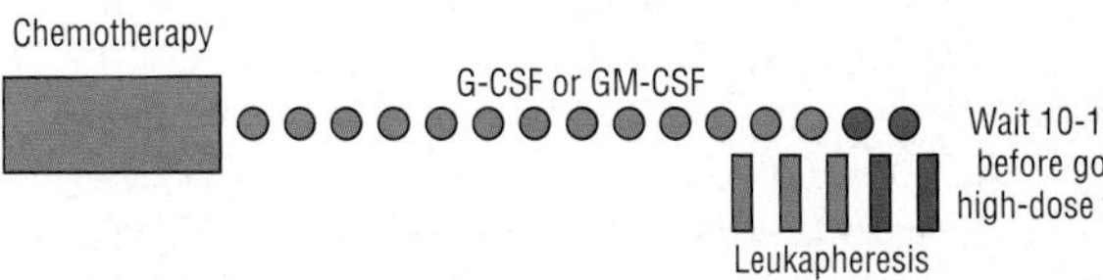

FIGURE 140-2 Schema for collection of peripheral blood progenitor cells after hematopoietic growth factor administration (top) or after chemotherapy and hematopoietic growth factor administration (bottom). Symbols with darker shading represent procedures performed only if adequate numbers of $CD34^+$ cells have not been collected. (G-CSF, granulocyte colony-stimulating factor; GM-CSF, granulocyte-macrophage colony-stimulating factor.)

associated with more adverse effects, but the number of aphereses is reduced, and the additional chemotherapy may further reduce the tumor burden before transplant. However, these benefits have not translated into improved transplant outcomes so this approach is generally not used.[14] Pegfilgrastim (pegylated filgrastim) has also been evaluated in the mobilization setting, either alone or after chemotherapy (6 and 12 mg doses). Its prolonged half-life of 33 hours allows for single-dose administration, increasing patient convenience. Studies of single agent pegfilgrastim are limited by small numbers and report varying degrees of success.[14] The combination of pegfilgrastim and chemotherapy mobilization has resulted in similar CD34$^+$ cell collections and transplant-related outcomes to chemotherapy and filgrastim mobilization.[14]

An ongoing area of controversy is the use of biosimilar filgrastim agents during stem cell mobilization. Most of the data to support the use of biosimilars is in the setting of chemotherapy-induced neutropenia. A meta-analysis summarized the results in over 900 subjects that included healthy donors and patients with hematologic malignancies who used biosimilar agents to collect PBSCs. Mobilization with biosimilars resulted in expected CD34$^+$ stem cell yields with similar posttransplant engraftment and side effects to filgrastim, which suggests that biosimilars may be an acceptable option in mobilization.[15] The European Bone Marrow Transplantation Association (EBMT), World Marrow Donor Association (WMDA), as well as American Society for Blood and Marrow Transplantation (ASBMT) recommend that filgrastim biosimilars only be used within the context of a clinical trial until further information is available.[16,17]

Plerixafor is a novel inhibitor of the CXCR4 chemokine receptor that is FDA approved as a mobilizing agent in combination with filgrastim in autologous transplant candidates. Two phase III trials of plerixafor combined with filgrastim reported the combination was associated with higher CD34$^+$ cell yields, fewer apheresis sessions, increased likelihood of achieving CD34$^+$ target yields, and lower graft failure rates compared to single-agent filgrastim.[18,19] Based on the results of these trials, plerixafor is being routinely used to mobilize stem cells in autologous HSCT patients. However, because most patients are able to mobilize efficiently with filgrastim alone and plerixafor is expensive, transplant centers generally use a risk-adapted or preemptive approach to identify which patients are appropriate candidates for plerixafor. One approach is to give plerixafor to patients with certain characteristics that have been associated with a high risk of poor mobilization (ie, risk-adapted approach). These characteristics include older age, diagnosis of non-Hodgkin lymphoma (NHL), extensive chemotherapy history, previous radiation therapy, previous exposure to lenalidomide or purine analogs, previous mobilization failure and low preapheresis circulating peripheral blood CD34$^+$(PBCD34$^+$) cell counts.[14] However, these characteristics lack sensitivity and specificity in predicting poor mobilization outcomes and thus patients may be either over or under treated.[20] Another approach is often referred to as a preemptive strategy, which identifies poor mobilizers based on PB ("PBCD") CD34$^+$ cell counts on day 4 or 5 of filgrastim administration or on the first apheresis collection. Low numbers of CD34$^+$ cells after filgrastim administration have been associated with mobilization failure. Patients who do not have a minimal number of CD34$^+$ cells receive plerixafor.[14] Many transplant centers use these preemptive approaches to guide their mobilization strategies thereby limiting plerixafor use to patients at high risk for not obtaining the target CD34$^+$ yield. These algorithms have been reported to improve initial mobilization rates while efficiently managing resources.[14]

In about 20% to 30% of autologous transplant candidates, an optimal number of CD34$^+$ cells will not be obtained after the first attempt with standard mobilization regimens.[14] Several strategies for overcoming the obstacle of poor mobilization have been evaluated, including remobilization with the same or higher doses of the same hematopoietic growth factor, a combination of hematopoietic growth factors (ie, filgrastim and sargramostim), or a combination of chemotherapy and a hematopoietic growth factor. Each of these remobilization strategies has been used with varying success. Unfortunately these strategies are associated with failure rates that exceed 70%.[14] Bone marrow harvest is also an option if other strategies fail.

Current consensus guidelines suggest that plerixafor be used in remobilization regimens for patients failing primary mobilization attempts, regardless of whether it was used in the primary mobilization.[14] When combined with filgrastim, plerixafor is associated with failure rates of less than 30%, which compares favorably with other secondary mobilization strategies but is also more costly, especially if multiple doses of plerixafor are required.[21] The use of plerixafor combined with chemotherapy and filgrastim may a promising strategy, but further data are needed to better understand the appropriate timing and use of this regimen. The selection of a secondary mobilization regimen should be based on patient-specific factors and clinician judgment.

Several studies show that the number of CD34$^+$ cells infused correlates significantly with the rate of neutrophil and platelet recovery after high-dose chemotherapy.[14] Rapid neutrophil recovery usually is observed in patients who receive at least 2×10^6 CD34$^+$ cells/kg (body weight of recipient). More rapid platelet recovery is observed when at least 5×10^6 CD34$^+$ cells/kg is transplanted compared with lower cell doses. As a result, consensus guidelines recommend 2×10^6 CD34$^+$ cells/kg as a minimum number to collect for autologous transplant, with an optimal target of 5×10^6 CD34$^+$ cells/kg.[14] The decision to use a collection yield of less than 2×10^6 CD34$^+$ cells/kg should be limited to those cases in which the potential benefit of a HSCT outweighs the risks of infusing a suboptimal CD34$^+$ cell dose. For patients with multiple myeloma undergoing tandem transplants, cells for both transplants are collected before the first transplant. A minimum of 4×10^6 CD34$^+$ cells/kg is required, and generally the entire cell dose collected is divided into two equal aliquots, one for each transplant.

5 Use of peripheral blood instead of bone marrow as a source of hematopoietic stem cells offers several clinical and economic advantages. For autologous transplant patients the most clinically important advantage is that patients who receive mobilized PBSCs experience more rapid hematopoietic engraftment. Although engraftment of all lineages is more rapid when PBSCs are used, the most significant effect is observed with platelet recovery. Patients who receive mobilized PBSCs experience platelet recovery as much as 2 to 3 weeks earlier and require fewer platelet transfusions than those who receive bone marrow stem cells. As a result, patients usually are discharged earlier from the hospital, so the overall cost of autologous HSCT is reduced with the use of PBSCs. PBSCs may be less likely to be contaminated with malignant cells compared with marrow stem cells. Finally, because PBSCs are collected from the mononuclear cell fraction, a fraction that also contains immunocompetent cells (eg, natural killer [NK] cells and T lymphocytes), some investigators believe that infusion of PBSCs represents a form of "adoptive immunotherapy." In this model, NK cells and lymphocytes targeted against tumor cells help to kill residual tumor cells. As a result of these clinical and economic advantages, peripheral blood has replaced bone marrow as the source of stem cells in the autologous setting.

Peripheral blood has also become the predominant source of hematopoietic stem cells in adult allogeneic HSCT.[22] About two-thirds of allogeneic HSCTs performed in adults currently come from PBSCs harvested from normal donors receiving filgrastim mobilization. Filgrastim is generally well tolerated in the normal donor population. Short-term effects are similar to those seen in cancer patients receiving filgrastim (eg, bone pain, headache, fever, arthralgias, malaise). Although there are concerns about increased risk of acute myelogenous leukemia (AML) in healthy subjects given filgrastim, no higher risk has been observed thus far.[23] Because of the long latent period of drug-related AML and the very low incidence of AML in the general population, longer follow-up of thousands of healthy donors will be required to definitively rule out an association between filgrastim and AML.

Randomized controlled trials and meta-analyses have shown that the stem cell source can influence posttransplant outcomes in allogeneic HSCT. Traditionally, matched related PBSCT have been associated with a more rapid hematopoietic recovery and required fewer transfusions compared with patients receiving bone marrow.[24] The difference in the rate of engraftment may be related to the threefold higher numbers of CD34$^+$ cells infused in recipients of PBSC transplants. Although increased risk of acute GVHD or transplant-related mortality in patients receiving allogeneic PBSC transplants has not been reported, a higher risk of chronic GVHD has been observed in many retrospective studies and meta-analyses.[24] The Blood and Marrow Transplant Clinical Trials Network (CTN) reported results from a trial that randomized 551 patients to allogeneic PBSC or bone marrow from matched unrelated donors.[25] Two years after transplant, there were no differences in overall survival, relapse, acute GVHD or mortality not related to relapse. However, a higher incidence of chronic GVHD was reported in patients who received PBSC transplants. Two-year survival is an early outcome, and further follow-up will need to be done to determine if these results are maintained over time. The published reports describing the impact of stem cell source on transplant related outcomes has focused primarily on transplants using myeloablative conditioning (discussed below). The CIBMTR reported retrospective data of patients with hematologic malignancies who received reduced intensity unrelated donor transplant with either PBSCs or bone marrow. Time-to-engraftment, risks of acute or chronic GVHD, relapse, non-relapse morality and overall survival were not significantly different between the two groups. Subgroup analysis suggests that GVHD prophylaxis may impact survival in this patient population and warrants further evaluation.[26] Selection of the optimal source of hematopoietic stem cells for an individual patient should be based on the risk of relapse, chronic GVHD, graft failure, and donor preference.

Hematopoietic stem cells found in UCB are an attractive source for several reasons.[27] Because the stem cells are collected from placental blood, there is a very low risk of transmissible infectious diseases, no risk to the mother or the baby, and the cells are immediately available. UCB initially was obtained from siblings, but now recipients of transplants from unrelated donors account for almost all patients who receive UCB transplants. More than 600,000 UCB grafts are available in more than 100 UCB banks, and more than 30,000 unrelated UCB transplants have been performed worldwide.[27]

Recipients of UCB transplants usually receive a CD34$^+$ cell dose more than 1 log lower than that given to recipients of BMT, and this difference in CD34$^+$ cell dose may explain the delayed engraftment in recipients of UCB transplants. The number of infused total nucleated and CD34$^+$ cells correlates with outcomes after UCB transplantation. The CIBMTR compared outcomes for adults with acute leukemia who were transplanted with unrelated bone marrow or PBSC versus UCB. Overall and leukemia-free survival were similar in all transplant groups. The risk of acute and chronic GVHD was lower in UCB recipients compared with PBSC, and the risk of chronic GVHD was lower in UCB compared with bone marrow. However, transplant-related mortality was higher after UCB as compared with other stem cell sources. These data support the use of UBCs as a source of stem cells when matched PBSCs or bone marrow are not immediately available.[28]

A major limitation of UCB transplants is the small volume of blood collected, usually 60 to 150 mL with resultant low numbers of CD34$^+$ cells. The relatively low numbers of hematopoietic cells may limit its use for larger recipients. This has led to "pooling" 2 or more units of UCB for one recipient (referred to as double cord transplant). The Seattle and Minnesota groups published their experience in more than 500 patients older than 10 years of age who received a matched related donor, matched unrelated donor, mismatched unrelated donor, or double cord transplant. Leukemia-free survival was similar in all groups, but the double cord transplant recipients had a higher risk of transplant-related mortality.[11] The Blood and Marrow Transplant CTN conducted a phase II trial in which a reduced-intensity conditioning regimen was administered with subsequent unrelated double cord transplant.[13] At 1 year posttransplant, the nonrelapse mortality remained high compared to alternative donor sources. Although the role of double cord transplantation has not yet been fully defined, these results suggest that pooled UCB units may provide an option for patients in which no other appropriate donors are available.

Initially, Haplo-HSCT generated poor outcomes related to high rates of graft failure and GVHD.[12] The use of PTCy on days 3 and 4 after infusion of stem cells has provided some encouraging results. Three observational studies have compared outcomes between Haplo-HSCT with PTCy to traditional matched related and unrelated donors and reported similar transplant outcomes. Two parallel prospective studies of reduced intensity conditioning regimens in Haplo-HSCT with PTCy or UCBT reported higher rates of engraftment and lower rates of acute and chronic GVHD and nonrelapse mortality in the Haplo-HSCT group. However, relapse rates were lower after UCBT leading to similar progression-free survival and overall survival between the two studies.[13] Based on these results, a phase III study comparing the two alternative stem cell sources is currently underway.

Clinical **Controversy...**

For patients that do not have a fully matched related or unrelated donor, the optimal alternative stem cell source, such as umbilical cord blood, mismatched unrelated, or HLA-haploidentical donors, is not clear. An ongoing phase III trial will directly compare two of these stem cell sources and may provide more definitive recommendations.

APPROACHES TO ERADICATE MALIGNANT CELLS

Conditioning Regimens

6 The purpose of the pretransplant conditioning regimen (also called the preparative regimen) depends on the type of transplant and the indication for its use. In the autologous setting, conditioning is used to eradicate malignant cells.[29] This is also the case in allogeneic HSCT for malignant diseases, but the conditioning regimen also serves a dual purpose to suppress the recipient's immune system to allow for donor cell engraftment. Two types of conditioning regimens are used, myeloablative and reduced intensity. Myeloablative conditioning (MAC) regimens contain very high doses of chemotherapy with or without radiation that would lead to life-threatening or fatal myelosuppression if hematopoietic stem cells were not infused.[30] Patients undergoing autologous HSCT receive only MAC regimens. Reduced-intensity conditioning (RIC) regimens are only used in allogeneic HSCT and consist of lower doses or different types of chemotherapy or lower doses of radiation than used in MAC regimens. RIC regimens were developed after the observation was made that some of the antitumor effect of the allogeneic transplant was mediated by a reaction between the donor's immune system and the recipient's cancer cells. This meant that very high doses of chemotherapy, radiation, or both may not be needed. Because RIC regimens use lower doses of chemotherapy or radiation or less toxic

TABLE 140-1 Dose-Limiting Nonhematologic Toxicities for Selected Chemotherapeutic Agents Included in Myeloablative Conditioning Regimens in Hematopoietic Stem Cell Transplantation

Drug	Conventional Dose[a] (mg/m²)	HSCT Dose (mg/m²)	Dose-Limiting Toxicity
Busulfan (oral)	2	450	Hepatic
Carboplatin	400	2,000	Hepatic, renal
Carmustine	200	1,200	Pulmonary, hepatic
Cisplatin	100	200	Renal, peripheral neuropathy
Cyclophosphamide	1,000	7,500	Cardiomyopathy
Etoposide	300-600	2,400	Mucositis
Ifosfamide	5,000	18,000	Renal
Melphalan	40	225	Mucositis
Thiotepa	20-50	1,125	Mucositis, central nervous system

HSCT, hematopoietic stem cell transplantation.

[a]Doses are approximate and are for drugs used as single agents. When combinations are used, doses may need to be decreased.

Eder JP, Elias A, Shea TC, et al. A phase I–II study of cyclophosphamide, thiotepa, and carboplatin with autologous bone marrow transplantation in solid tumor patients. J Clin Oncol 1990;8:1242. Reprinted with permission. © 1990 American Society of Clinical Oncology. All right reserved.

drugs, older patients and those with comorbidities are now able to undergo allogeneic transplant. Both types of regimens are discussed in detail below.

Myeloablative Conditioning Regimens

MAC regimens usually include at least one anticancer drug with a relatively steep dose-response curve and myelosuppression as their dose-limiting toxicity, such as alkylating agents. Cyclophosphamide, melphalan, busulfan, and carmustine are examples of chemotherapy agents commonly used in MAC regimens. Other agents are usually added that have additive or synergistic effects with these alkylating agents in specific types of cancers; other alkylating agents have also been used. Table 140-1 lists chemotherapeutic agents that are frequently used in MAC regimens as well as the doses used and their dose-limiting toxicity in the transplant setting.

Total-body irradiation (TBI) is also used in some pretransplant conditioning regimens. In patients with malignant disease, the rationale of TBI is to eradicate malignant cells located in areas inaccessible to the systemic circulation and thus to the chemotherapeutic agents (eg, CNS and testicles). TBI also has significant immunosuppressive activity. TBI doses for MAC regimens range from 10 to 15 Gy (1,000-1,500 rads or cGy), which is more than twice the lethal myelosuppressive dose of radiation for a normal person. TBI in these doses is typically fractionated (split over several days, once or twice a day) rather than given as a single-dose. Fractionated TBI has an improved therapeutic ratio compared with single-dose administration, that is, destruction of more leukemic cells and marrow stem cells while sparing other normal tissues. The acute toxicities of TBI consist of fever, nausea, vomiting, diarrhea, mucositis, and tender swelling of the parotid gland. Long-term complications of TBI-containing regimens include cataract formation, growth retardation, carcinogenesis, permanent reproductive sterility, and secondary malignancies.

Based on its immunomodulatory and antineoplastic effects, cyclophosphamide (60 mg/kg/day for 2 days) is commonly combined with TBI (CyTBI). Other chemotherapy agents have been used with TBI but there is no evidence to suggest that any of these combinations are more effective than CyTBI.[31] Due to the toxicities seen with high dose TBI, chemotherapy only regimens also have been developed. Many of these regimens contain busulfan due to its activity against a variety of malignancies. Busulfan can either be given IV or orally. The use of IV busulfan-containing regimens has been associated with improved survival compared to TBI containing regimens in patients with myeloid malignancies.[32] At some transplant centers, plasma busulfan concentrations are monitored and doses adjusted as systemic exposure has been shown to correlate with both efficacy and toxicity and use of a preparative regimen with targeted busulfan may improve patient outcomes.[31,33] Busulfan was originally combined with cyclophosphamide (BuCy) but more recently has been combined with fludarabine (BuFlu) to increase regimen tolerability when used in the allogeneic transplant setting.

Several studies, both prospective and retrospective, have been done evaluating differences between allogeneic transplant MAC regimens.[31,32] In general, there is no definitive data showing the superiority of one regimen over another, such that the choice of regimens before allogeneic HSCT generally is based on the experience of the transplant center, patient characteristics, diagnosis, and disease status.

Conditioning regimens used in autologous HSCT are exclusively myeloablative and generally include at least one alkylating agent with other agents added that may have specific activity against the tumor type being treated.[29,31] TBI usually is not commonly used and is not included in the conditioning regimen in patients who have received prior radiotherapy. MAC regimens used in patients with lymphoma generally include different combinations of cyclophosphamide, carmustine, etoposide, and cytarabine. Rituximab is commonly added in patients with CD20-positive lymphomas, although randomized controlled studies supporting the use of rituximab in this setting are lacking.[29] The Blood and Marrow Transplant CTN conducted a prospective comparative trial randomizing patients with diffuse large B cell lymphoma to receive high-dose chemotherapy with rituximab or iodine-131 tositumomab followed by autologous HSCT.[29] Progression-free survival and overall survival were not significantly different between the two groups, and thus anti-CD20 radiolabeled monoclonal antibodies are not used routinely as part of conditioning for patients with NHL undergoing autologous HSCT. Single-agent melphalan (200 mg/m²) is the standard conditioning regimen for patients undergoing autologous HSCT for myeloma. The addition of other agents to melphalan has not been proven to be superior to melphalan alone.[29]

Reduced-Intensity Conditioning Regimens

7 Donor T cells contribute to the tumor cell kill and prevention of relapse observed after allogeneic HSCT, an effect referred to as the graft-versus-malignancy (GVM) effect. Evidence for the GVM effect is based on retrospective studies showing that patients who developed GVHD had a lower risk of leukemic relapse than those who did not develop GVHD. However, the overall survival rate was not different because of the increased nonrelapse mortality associated with GVHD. Other anecdotal evidence supporting a T cell-mediated GVM effect includes the increased risk of relapse found with T cell-depleted

transplants compared with unmodified transplants and the efficacy of donor lymphocyte infusions (DLIs) in producing responses in patients who have relapsed after allogeneic HSCT.[31]

RIC regimens containing lower doses of chemotherapy or radiation or less toxic agents were developed to take advantage of the GVM effect but with a lower incidence of regimen-related toxicity than that of MAC regimens. Animal data demonstrated that MAC was not required for engraftment of donor cells (the other important role of conditioning in allogeneic HSCT), thus paving the way for the evaluation of RIC in humans.[31] The major advantage of RIC is that potentially curative transplants can be offered to patients who typically would not be considered for allogeneic HSCT because of their unacceptably high risk of transplant-related complications due to increased age or moderately compromised organ function. Use of RIC regimens has steadily increased in patients aged 50 and older.[1] In addition, because of the lower rate of toxicity, allogeneic HSCT with RIC can be offered to patients who have relapsed after traditional myeloablative autologous or allogeneic transplants, provided they are healthy enough to tolerate a second transplant. Because RIC regimens may not be completely myeloablative, host hematopoiesis can persist and lead to mixed chimerism (blood cells from both donor and recipient are present) (Fig. 140-3).[34] Several studies have reported significant correlations between donor T-cell chimerism levels and the risk of graft rejection, GVHD, and relapse. For example, a low percentage of donor T and NK cells present on day 14 has been associated with graft rejection, but high T-cell donor chimerism on day 28 has been associated with acute GVHD. Achievement of full donor chimerism was associated with better GVM effect and longer progression-free survival. These data suggest that monitoring donor chimerism after transplant may allow early interventions to prevent graft rejection or relapse.[34]

A number of RIC regimens that vary in their cytotoxic, myelosuppressive, and immunosuppressive activity have been developed.[31] Most regimens include fludarabine (125-240 mg/m^2) because of its potent immunosuppressive activity, combined with either low-dose TBI (at doses up to 8 Gy [800 rad]) or an alkylating agent, such as cyclophosphamide (2-3.6 g/m^2 or 120-200 mg/kg), busulfan (up to 10 mg/kg), or melphalan (up to 180 mg/m^2). ATG or alemtuzumab is sometimes given for additional immunosuppression, and other purine analogs (eg, pentostatin or clofarabine) are sometimes used instead of fludarabine. Rituximab has also been included in patients with CD20-positive lymphoid malignancies. Many of these regimens are myeloablative but are defined as RIC because of the reduced doses of chemotherapy.[30]

Some RIC regimens are considered nonmyeloablative because they result in little to no myelosuppression and do not require hematopoietic cell support for recovery of hematopoiesis. Nonmyeloablative regimens are associated with very little regimen-related toxicity but, similar to other RIC regimens, are immunosuppressive enough to result in full engraftment of important donor immune effector cells.[30] Two of the most common nonmyeloablative regimens are fludarabine (25 mg/m^2/day for 3-5 days) combined with cyclophosphamide (60 mg/kg/day × 2 days) or with TBI (less than or equal to 2 Gy [less than or equal to 200 rad]). Although these regimens are clearly nonmyeloablative, the distinction may be more difficult with other regimens as definitions remain somewhat arbitrary.

Progression-free and overall survival varies depending on the specific RIC regimen, disease type and status at the time of transplant, donor type, and patient age and comorbidities. Patients with indolent lymphoid malignancies generally have the lowest relapse rate after RIC transplants; those with advanced myeloid and lymphoid malignancies have higher relapse rates.[35] Several large retrospective registry-based studies have reported the results of RIC regimens.[35] In general, regimen-related toxicity and nonrelapse mortality have been reported to be lower than that of historical or concurrent control participants receiving MAC regimens in nonrandomized comparisons. This is remarkable considering the older age and higher incidence of comorbidities in patients receiving RIC transplants. Of concern, however, has been an increased rate of relapse in patients receiving RIC regimens, resulting in similar overall survival. One randomized trial has been published to date comparing RIC (FluTBI) versus MAC (CyTBI) regimens in patients 18 to 60 years of age with AML in first complete remission.[36] The two groups were well matched for age, cytogenetic abnormalities and donor type. The trial was stopped early due to slow accrual. Overall and progression-free survival were similar between the groups but, because the study was closed early, it likely lacked power to show a difference in the primary endpoints. The Blood and Marrow Transplant CTN performed a large randomized trial comparing RIC versus MAC in patients with AML or MDS. Eligibility criteria included age less than or equal to 65, disease in complete remission and

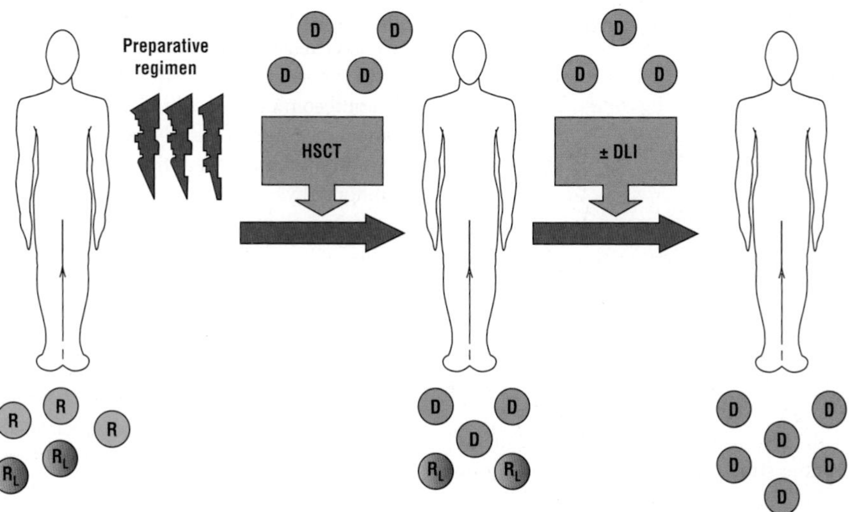

FIGURE 140-3 Schema for nonmyeloablative transplantation for hematologic malignancy. Recipients (R) receive a reduced-intensity conditioning regimen and an allogeneic hematopoietic stem cell transplant (HSCT). Initially, mixed chimerism is present with the coexistence of donor (D) cells and recipient-derived normal and leukemia/lymphoma (R_L) cells. Donor-derived T cells mediate a graft-versus-host hematopoietic effect that eradicates residual recipient-derived normal and malignant hematopoietic cells. Donor lymphocyte infusions (DLIs) can be administered to enhance graft-versus-malignancy effects.

minimal comorbidities. This trial was halted prematurely because a benefit in the MAC arm of the study was observed. The results, when published in a peer-reviewed journal, will assist clinicians in selecting the appropriate choice of regimen for the population represented in the study.[31] For other populations, clinicians will consider patient and disease characteristics as well as donor type when choosing an appropriate conditioning regimen until more evidence is available.

Clinical **Controversy...**

Although RIC regimens reduce transplant-related mortality, whether this approach results in improved survival compared with MAC regimens is not clear. Direct comparison of the results of RIC versus MAC transplants is difficult because patients undergoing RIC transplants tend to be older and have more comorbidities. Randomized controlled trials addressing these questions are ongoing, and the results of these studies should better define the role of RIC transplants.

Posttransplant Therapy

Relapse of primary disease remains the most common cause of death for both allogeneic and autologous HSCT patients. As a result, much research has been directed at both preventing and treating posttransplant relapse or progression of disease.[37-40] The use of therapy posttransplant can be categorized either as "maintenance (or consolidation) therapy" or "salvage therapy." Maintenance/consolidation therapy is used to prevent relapse whereas salvage therapy is given to treat active relapse. Methods of identifying relapsed disease for many transplantable malignant diseases have become quite sensitive, and often disease can be detected at the molecular level (ie, minimal residual disease) and used to direct posttransplant therapy. Several posttransplant therapies have been evaluated both in the maintenance and salvage settings, including immunotherapy, conventional chemotherapy, and targeted therapy. Relapse after autologous transplant can often be treated with standard doses of chemotherapy, a second autologous transplant, or even an allogeneic transplant, depending on the diagnosis, disease status, side effects, response, and duration of response to the first transplant. Treatment options for most patients who relapse after allogeneic HSCT are more limited, and prognosis is generally poor. Disease-specific chemotherapy and immunotherapy can be considered for some patients. A second allogeneic HSCT may be considered but is associated with a mortality rate of up to 45%.[38]

Immunotherapy

The rationale for posttransplant immunotherapy after allogeneic HSCT is based on the GVM effect. To take advantage of the GVM effect in patients who relapse after allogeneic HSCT, immunosuppressive therapy being used for GVHD is withdrawn as quickly as possible without inducing a serious GVHD flare. In rare cases, this is enough to reinduce a remission, but further therapy is usually required. In addition, this is not a viable option in patients with active GVHD. Induction of the GVM effect has been investigated with several immunostimulatory drugs including interleukin-2, cyclosporine, interferon-gamma, and interleukin-1. None of the randomized trials done with these agents showed survival benefit.[40] Other posttransplant immune strategies include DLI and monoclonal antibodies.

Donor Lymphocyte Infusion Perhaps the most commonly used form of posttransplant immunotherapy is DLI.[41,42] Lymphocytes are collected from the same donor who provided hematopoietic stem cells for the original allogeneic transplant, thus limiting this option to patients with available donors. Response to DLI is disease specific. More than 80% of patients with CML who are in cytogenetic or molecular relapse respond to DLI. The response rate of patients in more advanced phases is about 15% to 30%. Although the time to response is delayed (median, 3-4 months), patients often have a durable molecular remission to DLI. Response rates to DLI of patients with other myeloid malignancies, such as AML and myelodysplasia, are generally lower (25%-30%) than the rates of patients with CML. This may be related to the rapid proliferation of acute leukemia within the often prolonged time to response after DLI. Patients with relapsed AML after HSCT are more likely to achieve a complete response to DLI if they had a longer remission period after transplant and have some GVHD after the DLI; low tumor burden, remission at the time of DLI, and good-risk cytogenetics have also been shown to be favorable characteristics. Administration of induction chemotherapy or therapeutic agents with novel mechanisms of action (eg, 5-azacitidine, lenalidomide, and bortezomib) before DLI administration may improve the antitumor activity of DLI in patients with AML or other rapidly proliferating malignancies, but this method has not been tested in a randomized study.[38] DLI has been shown to have limited benefit in patients with relapsed acute lymphocytic leukemia (ALL) after transplant.

DLI appears to be effective in patients with multiple myeloma who relapse after allogeneic HSCT, with reported response rates of 40% to 50%. Chemotherapy followed by DLI may induce a GVM effect in patients with relapsed lymphoma. The highest response rates were reported in patients with indolent NHL while more aggressive malignancies had lower response rates.

The most serious complications of DLI are pancytopenia and GVHD, and DLI is not usually given to patients with active GVHD. The cytopenias generally are transient and can be treated with hematopoietic growth factors. Some patients may have a more prolonged course of aplasia with associated risk of infection, bleeding, and anemia and these patients may benefit from another infusion of donor hematopoietic stem cells.

New strategies being evaluated to improve outcomes with DLI include priming the donor with filgrastim, infusion of selected subsets of T-lymphocytes to promote GVM, preemptive use of DLI based on the presence of minimal residual disease or evidence of molecular/cytogenetic relapse, or prophylactic DLI in patients who are at high risk of relapse.[41]

Monoclonal Antibodies Although earlier studies showed potential benefit of rituximab as maintenance therapy for certain types of NHL patients after autologous HSCT, more recent randomized controlled trials with mature follow up have not consistently demonstrated benefit.[29,40] Therefore, routine use of rituximab maintenance is not recommended. Rituximab may be useful in combination with other active agents for salvage therapy of posttransplant relapse.

Brentuximab vedotin (anti-CD30 antibody conjugated to monomethyl auristatin E, a microtubule-disrupting agent) was evaluated as maintenance therapy in a randomized placebo-controlled study in patients with Hodgkin lymphoma after autologous HSCT.[43] Progression-free survival was significantly improved in patients randomized to brentuximab (hazard ratio 0.57, 95% confidence interval 0.4-0.81). Consistent benefit was seen across all subgroups that were analyzed. The most frequent adverse events in the brentuximab group were peripheral sensory neuropathy and neutropenia. No difference in overall survival was seen, likely because patients receiving placebo were allowed to crossover to brentuximab treatment at the time of progression. These results are encouraging given the generally poor prognosis of patients with relapsed/refractory Hodgkin lymphoma.

Chemotherapy or Targeted Therapy

Tyrosine kinase inhibitors (TKIs), such as imatinib, dasatinib, and nilotinib have been shown to be effective in the prevention and treatment of relapse after allogeneic HSCT in patients with CML and Philadelphia chromosome–positive (Ph+) ALL.[44] In patients with CML who experience hematologic relapse (presence of leukemic blasts in blood or bone marrow) after allogeneic HSCT, imatinib has been reported to induce complete hematologic responses (disappearance of leukemic blasts) and complete cytogenetic responses (disappearance of cytogenetic markers of disease) in a majority of these patients. Outcomes in patients with Ph+ ALL have also been encouraging. TKIs are also given soon after transplant to prevent relapse.[44,45] Patients with Ph+ ALL and CML without evidence of disease after transplant who are treated with TKIs to prevent relapse appear to have sustained cytogenetic remissions (without evidence of cytogenetic markers of disease). In a study of patients with Ph+ ALL, 50% of patients who had minimal residual disease detected after stem cell transplant had a complete response to TKI therapy.[45] TKIs are generally well tolerated after transplant. Commonly reported side effects include neutropenia, thrombocytopenia, liver function abnormalities, edema, and muscle pain, which may require dosage reductions or discontinuation. Larger comparative studies will be required to clearly define the benefit of TKIs after transplant, as well as the optimal dosing, timing, and duration of therapy.

Based on its activity in AML and MDS, 5-azacitidine is being evaluated in the posttransplant setting to prevent or treat relapse in patients with these diagnoses. Investigators at the MD Anderson Cancer Center performed a dose and schedule finding study with 5-azacitidine maintenance therapy in patients who were in a complete remission after HSCT. The dose-limiting toxicity was thrombocytopenia, and the optimal dose was 32 mg/m^2 given subcutaneously for 5 days for 4 cycles. This study demonstrated that low-dose 5-azacitidine may be administered in this population safely, and it may prolong event-free survival and overall survival, justifying further studies to confirm these preliminary findings.[40,46] 5-azacitidine maintenance therapy has also been associated with a reduction in GVHD and increasing donor chimerism which delayed disease relapse.[39] Retrospective analyses of 5-azacitidine used to treat posttransplant relapse of AML have reported a response rate of 50% to 75% but overall survival remains poor (15%-20% at 2 years) and toxicity is substantial.[47] Improved results have been seen when DLI is given after 5-azacitidine.[39] Other therapies being investigated as maintenance therapy after allogeneic HSCT include panobinostat (deacetylase inhibitor) and the FLT3 tyrosine kinase inhibitors (sorafinib, quizartinib, and midostaurin).[39] Posttransplant therapy is also being evaluated in patients with multiple myeloma. Previous studies showed a potential benefit of thalidomide to prevent relapse after autologous transplant, but its use is limited by neurotoxicity and other bothersome adverse effects. When given after autologous transplant in patients with nonprogressing disease, lenalidomide has been shown to prolong progression-free survival compared with patients receiving placebo.[40] However, a small but significant increased incidence of second primary cancers was reported in the lenalidomide-treated patients. Further study is needed to better define the risk of second malignancies. Patients should be aware of this potential safety issue when discussing treatment with lenalidomide after autologous HSCT. Bortezomib maintenance therapy after autologous HSCT has also been associated with prolonged progression-free survival.[40]

TRANSPLANT-RELATED COMPLICATIONS

8 Although many patients with cancer who are treated with high-dose chemotherapy and autologous or allogeneic HSCT experience long-term survival and cure of their disease, this modality is associated with many serious and potentially life-threatening complications.[29,32] In spite of the availability of improved broad-spectrum anti-infective agents, immunosuppressive drugs, and hematopoietic growth factors which has improved survival over the last four decades, the transplant-related mortality rate after allogeneic HSCT with HLA-matched sibling and unrelated donors is 20% to 30%. The mortality rate is generally lower with the use of RIC regimens but higher when alternative donors are used. Causes of nonrelapse-related death are a result of transplant-related organ toxicity, GVHD, or immunosuppression. The risk of transplant-related mortality after autologous HSCT generally is less than 5%, depending on patient population and conditioning regimen.[29] The mortality rate is lower with autologous transplants because of the lack of GVHD and associated complications of immunosuppression. Transplant-related mortality in autologous HSCT usually is caused by regimen-related toxicity or infection.

Table 140-1 lists the dose-limiting nonhematologic toxicities for several drugs that are commonly included in MAC regimens. These toxicities may be uncommon or rare with administration of conventional doses of specific drugs. When these agents are given in high doses, the toxicities seen with conventional doses (eg, mucositis, enteritis, nausea, vomiting, and hematuria) can be more frequent or severe. Several unusual and severe manifestations of regimen-related toxicities are discussed in this section.

Sinusoidal Obstruction Syndrome

Sinusoidal obstruction syndrome (SOS), formerly known as hepatic venoocclusive disease (VOD), occurs as a result of chemotherapy-induced damage to the sinusoidal endothelial cells of the liver, which leads to release of proinflammatory cytokines and further damage to the endothelium. Gaps develop between the endothelial cells allowing cellular debris to accumulate, causing the sinusoids to narrow and eventually become occluded. In addition, injury to the endothelial cells produces fibrin deposition and clot formation, further narrowing the sinusoids.[48] These histologic changes can lead to obstruction of sinusoidal flow, reduced hepatic venous outflow, portal hypertension, and hepatic failure. Clinical signs of SOS include fluid retention (resulting in sudden weight gain and ascites), hepatomegaly (sometimes painful), and hyperbilirubinemia or jaundice. SOS usually occurs within the first 4 weeks after transplant, and the incidence of SOS ranges from 5% to 20% in most published series. Severe SOS is fatal in 50% to 75% of cases. Factors that have been reported to increase the risk of SOS include use of TBI-containing conditioning regimens (dose dependent), use of sirolimus for the prevention of GVHD, increased systemic exposure to busulfan, oral administration of busulfan, individual variability in cyclophosphamide metabolism, chronic viral hepatitis, and elevated liver function test results before transplant. Pretransplant exposure to gemtuzumab ozogamicin (Mylotarg®) has been implicated in the development of SOS in patients undergoing allogeneic HSCT, especially when given within a few months of transplant.[48]

Prostaglandin E_1, unfractionated low-molecular-weight heparin, and ursodiol have all been studied in prevention of SOS.[32,48] Ursodiol has been found to not only reduce the risk of SOS in patients undergoing MAC allogeneic transplants but has also been associated with reduced transplant-related mortality and GVHD. Defibrotide, a polydisperse oligonucleotide with fibrinolytic properties, is another agent that has been used successfully in the prophylaxis of SOS. It is being routinely used in some European transplant centers in patients at high risk for SOS.[48]

Treatment of SOS is generally supportive, including fluid and electrolyte management. Hepato- and nephrotoxic drugs should be avoided. Mild-to-moderate disease generally resolves without specific therapy. Recombinant tissue plasminogen activator has been given to patients with severe SOS because of the possible role of the coagulation cascade in the pathogenesis of SOS. Responses have been reported, but patients also experienced a higher risk of bleeding.[48] Mounting evidence supports the use of defibrotide in the treatment of patients with severe SOS, demonstrating improved response rates and lower mortality compared with historical control participants.[48] Defibrotide (Defitelio®) was recently approved by the FDA in 2016 and its role in the treatment of SOS is still being defined.

Pulmonary Complications

Pulmonary complications after HSCT can be categorized as infectious and noninfectious (infectious complications are discussed in Chapter 122). Noninfectious complications can be caused by direct damage to the pulmonary tissue by chemotherapy or radiation used in the conditioning regimen, immune effects of the graft, or other causes not clearly understood. Early complications include diffuse alveolar hemorrhage, periengraftment respiratory distress syndrome, and idiopathic interstitial pneumonitis.[49] Diffuse alveolar hemorrhage is characterized by dyspnea, hypoxia, dry cough, and fever; chest radiography usually shows diffuse infiltrates in an alveolar pattern. Diffuse alveolar hemorrhage is diagnosed by examination of bronchoalveolar lavage fluid via bronchoscopy, which reveals progressively bloodier fluid with each instilled aliquot and negative findings on microbiologic analysis. Although the condition can be life-threatening or fatal, prompt treatment with high doses of corticosteroids is sometimes beneficial.[49]

Periengraftment respiratory distress syndrome is characterized by fever, erythrodermatous skin rash, and noncardiogenic pulmonary edema can occur during neutrophil recovery after HSCT.[49] The incidence of engraftment syndrome is not known because of the lack of uniform diagnostic criteria, although some series report that about 10% of patients who receive autologous HSCT develop the syndrome. This syndrome can progress to life-threatening respiratory failure with or without multiple organ failure. Corticosteroids are effective in some patients.

Idiopathic interstitial pneumonitis (also called idiopathic pneumonia syndrome) is defined as widespread alveolar injury in the absence of active lower respiratory tract infection after HSCT.[50] Patients with idiopathic interstitial pneumonitis are clinically indistinguishable from patients with interstitial pneumonitis related to infection. Idiopathic interstitial pneumonitis is postulated to have a multifactorial etiology, including toxic effects of MAC, immunologic cell-mediated injury, inflammatory cytokine-induced lung damage, and occult pulmonary infections. The risk is similar in recipients of autologous or allogeneic HSCT but appears to be higher in patients who are conditioned with a TBI-containing regimen or who have acute GVHD. A mortality rate as high as 70% has been reported, and treatment consists of supportive care only as the efficacy of corticosteroids is not well described. Etanercept may be beneficial in some patients with idiopathic interstitial pneumonitis.[51]

Late pulmonary complications cover a wide spectrum of disorders and include both obstructive and restrictive lung diseases.[49,52] The best described of these disorders is bronchiolitis obliterans with or without organizing pneumonia. Although bronchiolitis obliterans is thought to be a result of chronic GVHD affecting the lungs, its pathogenesis has not been completely elucidated. Therapy consists of corticosteroids, which are about 50% effective. Patients with mild-to-moderate airflow impairment appear to have the best response. The survival rate at 5 years from diagnosis of bronchiolitis obliterans is less than 20%.

Graft Failure

Initial engraftment of hematopoietic cells after high-dose chemotherapy conditioning regimens usually occurs in the first 2 to 4 weeks after transplant. Engraftment is evidenced by rising peripheral blood counts and the presence of hematopoietic precursor cells in the marrow. In allogeneic HSCT, the presence of donor cells (ie, chimerism) is confirmed by PCR-based analysis of polymorphic DNA sequences of cells from the bone marrow and peripheral T cells. Full chimerism is defined as greater than 95% of cells of donor origin. In most patients, engraftment is sustained with complete recovery of hematopoiesis.

However, graft failure (loss of bone marrow function with resultant loss in peripheral blood counts) can occur after both allogeneic and autologous HSCT. It can be the result of heavy pretreatment with chemotherapy or radiation therapy (or both); infusion of insufficient numbers of hematopoietic stem cells; viral infection; recurrence of primary hematologic malignancy; drug reaction (eg, to ganciclovir); development of a secondary myelodysplasia; or in the allogeneic setting, an immunologic reaction between the donor and recipient caused by inadequate immunosuppression of the recipient (ie, graft rejection). Two syndromes have been observed. Whereas early graft failure occurs when the rate of hematopoietic recovery is delayed or does not occur at all (primary graft failure or delayed engraftment), late graft failure is characterized by a decline in peripheral blood counts after initial engraftment (secondary graft failure). With widespread use of PBSCs and posttransplant growth factors, primary graft failure is rare after autologous and HLA-matched allogeneic HSCT but is not uncommon after UCBT. Graft failure that occurs after allogeneic HSCT, characterized by regrowth of immunocompetent recipient cells and a simultaneous loss of donor cells, is referred to as *graft rejection*. Graft rejection occurs rarely after HLA-matched allogeneic HSCT. An increased risk of graft rejection has been observed in recipients of hematopoietic stem cells from HLA-mismatched donors, recipients of T cell-depleted marrow, and patients with severe aplastic anemia. In a large retrospective analysis of over 20,000 patients undergoing myeloablative allogeneic HSCT the incidence of primary graft failure was reported was 5.5%.[53] In this analysis, risk factors for primary graft failure included bone marrow (vs peripheral blood) grafts, diagnosis of a myeloproliferative disorder, HLA mismatched transplants, ABO incompatibility, and BuCy conditioning. The long-term prognosis of patients with graft failure is poor. Despite supportive care and treatment with hematopoietic growth factors, death may result from infection or bleeding. In some patients with an allogeneic donor, a second infusion of stem cells can be attempted.[32]

Hematopoietic growth factors usually are given after transplant to patients who receive autologous HSCT, based on several benefits associated with their use including fewer antibiotic days and decreased length of stay. Decreasing resource utilization after transplant (total antibiotic days and length of stay) can help justify the cost of growth factors in this patient population. Growth factors can be initiated the day of, the day after, or as late as 7 days after the infusion of stem cells and are continued until neutrophil recovery to greater than an arbitrary number of neutrophils (500-1,000 cells/mm^3 [$0.5\text{-}1.0 \times 10^9$/L]). Pegfilgrastim appears to be equally efficacious to filgrastim in this setting.

Hematopoietic growth factors also accelerate the rate of neutrophil recovery in patients undergoing allogeneic HSCT. However, filgrastim does not reduce infection rates, antibiotic days or length of stay. The decision to whether or not to use filgrastim must be made by each institution and may be reserved for use in patients who are at risk for a prolonged rate of neutrophil recovery (eg, UCB transplants).

Results of studies with platelet growth factors, such as thrombopoietin and interleukin-11 (IL-11), given posttransplant have been disappointing. Platelet transfusions remain the standard of care in patients with thrombocytopenia below a given threshold (eg, 10,000 cells/mm^3 [10×10^9/L]) and in patients with significant bleeding.

Anemia may be problematic in the posttransplant setting, especially in patients receiving allogeneic HSCT. The etiology is unclear and most likely is multifactorial. Although erythropoietin administration may be useful in reducing the need for red blood cell transfusions, its use in cancer patients is associated with an increased risk of adverse events and is limited by FDA warnings and restrictions.

Graft-Versus-Host Disease

GVHD is caused by immunocompetent allogeneic donor T cells reacting against recipient/host antigens on the surface of antigen-presenting cells (APCs). In that setting, donor T cells recognize unmatched major or minor histocompatibility antigens of the host as genetically foreign, become activated, proliferate, and attack recipient tissue, thereby producing the clinical syndrome of GVHD.

Two different clinical syndromes of GVHD (acute and chronic) are recognized, each with two subcategories. Classic acute GVHD occurs within 100 days after transplant or DLI while persistent, recurrent or late-onset acute GVHD occurs beyond 100 days after transplant, withdrawal of immunosuppression or DLI.[54] Both subcategories of acute GVHD occur in the absence of chronic GVHD. Classic chronic GVHD usually occurs after day 100, with only clinical manifestations that can be attributed to chronic GVHD. Chronic GVHD may occur after resolution of acute GVHD or de novo (no prior acute GVHD). Acute and chronic overlap syndrome is a newly defined entity in which features of both acute are chronic GVHD appear together. Chronic GVHD usually develops before resolution of acute GVHD (also called progressive onset). The clinical manifestations of GVHD are distinct. Whereas acute GVHD usually is limited to the gastrointestinal tract, skin, and liver, signs and symptoms of chronic GVHD resemble an autoimmune disorder and can affect many organ systems.

A "hyperacute" form of GVHD may occur in patients with multiple HLA mismatches and in patients who receive T cell–replete transplants without adequate GVHD prophylaxis, especially after MAC regimens.[55] Descriptions of hyperacute GVHD vary but usually include fever, generalized erythroderma, desquamation, and edema. More severe forms with accompanying organ failure have been seen in haploidentical donors. Hyperacute GVHD typically occurs about 1 week after transplant before engraftment of neutrophils. The response rate to first-line therapy appears to be lower in patients with hyperacute GVHD compared with patients who develop GVHD later after transplant, but no difference in survival has been observed.

Acute Graft-Versus-Host Disease

The pathophysiology of acute GVHD has been described as a three-step process.[56] In step 1, the conditioning regimen causes damage to the intestinal mucosa, leading to release of lipopolysaccharides into the systemic circulation. This stimulates secretion of inflammatory cytokines such as IL-1 and tumor necrosis factor-α (TNF-α). These cytokines upregulate MHC gene products and host APCs such as dendritic cells, which play a critical role in this immune response. In step 2, donor T cells are activated, and secretion of other cytokines (IL-2 and interferon-γ) by activated T cells results in recruitment of macrophages and alteration of target cells in the gastrointestinal tract and skin so that they are more susceptible to damage. In step 3, multiple cytotoxic effector cells (T cells and macrophages) are generated and contribute to target tissue injury by secreting more inflammatory cytokines that cause target cell apoptosis. The term "cytokine storm" is sometimes used to describe the critical role of inflammatory cytokines in this process. Three general approaches have been used to prevent GVHD in humans. The first is to reduce host tissue damage with the use of RIC regimens. The second and most widely used approach is to modulate donor T cells by reducing T-cell numbers (T-cell depletion), activation (most immunosuppressive agents), or proliferation (antiproliferative agents). The third approach is to block inflammatory stimulation and effectors (eg, TNF-α inhibition, IL-1 receptor blockade).

The principal target organs in acute GVHD are the skin, liver, and gastrointestinal tract.[56] Acute GVHD is classified into four grades, depending on the number of organs involved and the degree of involvement of each organ (Table 140-2). Grade I disease involves only the skin. Grades II through IV involve the skin and the liver, gastrointestinal tract, or both. Acute skin GVHD usually is manifested as a generalized maculopapular rash that initially involves the face, ears, palms, soles, and upper trunk. The skin rash can spread to the rest of the body and, if untreated or refractory to treatment, will progress to bullae formation and desquamation similar to a burn injury. Gastrointestinal GVHD presents as a secretory diarrhea but may progress to abdominal pain or cramping and ileus; hemorrhage may also occur. GVHD of the upper intestinal tract appears as persistent nausea, vomiting, anorexia, and dyspepsia. The diagnosis of gastrointestinal GVHD should be made by biopsy of the intestinal

TABLE 140-2 Consensus Grading of Acute Graft-versus-Host Disease

Organ/Extent of Involvement			
	Skin	**Liver**	**Intestinal Tract**
Stage			
1	Rash on <25% of skin[a]	Bilirubin 2-3 mg/dL (34.2-51.3 μmol/L)[b]	Diarrhea >500 mL/day[c] or persistent nausea[d]
2	Rash on 25%-50% of skin	Bilirubin 3-6 mg/dL (51.3-102.6 μmol/L)	Diarrhea >1,000 mL/day
3	Rash on >50% of skin	Bilirubin 6-15 mg/dL (102.6-256.5 μmol/L)	Diarrhea >1,500 mL/day
4	Generalized erythroderma with bulla formation	Bilirubin >15 mg/dL (>256.5 μmol/L)	Severe abdominal pain with or without ileus
Grade			
0	None	None	None
I	Stage 1-2	None	None
II	Stage 3	or Stage 1	or Stage 1
III	—	Stage 2-3	or Stage 2-4
IV[e]	Stage 4	or Stage 4	—

[a]Use the "rule of nines" to determine body surface area involvement.

[b]Range given as total bilirubin. Downgrade one stage if an additional cause of elevated bilirubin has been documented.

[c]Volume of diarrhea applies to adults. For pediatric patients, the volume of diarrhea should be based on body surface area.

[d]Persistent nausea with histologic evidence of graft-versus-host disease in the stomach or duodenum.

[e]Grade IV may include lesser organ involvement but with extreme decrease in performance status.

tract (stomach, duodenum, or rectum). Hepatic GVHD usually is asymptomatic, consisting of hyperbilirubinemia and elevated alkaline phosphatase levels; increases in serum transaminases occur less consistently. The diagnosis can be made by biopsy, if possible.

The overall incidence of moderate-to-severe (grades II-IV) acute GVHD ranges from 20% to more than 80%.[57] Mortality directly attributable to acute GVHD or its treatment occurs in about 20% of patients. The incidence of GVHD is related to the degree of histocompatibility, number of T cells in the graft, donor and recipient age and gender, intensity of the conditioning regimen, source of hematopoietic cells (bone marrow vs peripheral blood), and prophylactic regimen. The most severe acute GVHD is observed in allogeneic HSCT with non-HLA-identical donors. In this setting, the incidence of grades II to IV acute GVHD can exceed 50% despite aggressive GVHD prophylaxis. Severe acute GVHD is a major cause of mortality with the risk of death increasing as the grade of GVHD increases. This risk is further increased if initial therapy is not effective.

Multiorgan acute GVHD and the drugs given to prevent or treat the disease are associated with delayed immunologic recovery and increased susceptibility to infections. Infection is often the primary cause of death in patients with GVHD. Patients with GVHD treated with an immunosuppressive regimen should receive prophylactic antiviral, antibacterial, and antifungal therapy and be monitored routinely for the occurrence of these infections.

Prevention of Acute Graft-Versus-Host Disease 9 Because treatment of established acute GVHD often is unsatisfactory, aggressive preventive measures usually are taken. The most common strategy used to prevent acute GVHD is to block the activation of T cells by administration of immunosuppressive agents.[56,57] Several immunosuppressive agents have been used, including methotrexate (MTX), cyclosporine (CSA), tacrolimus (TAC), sirolimus, mycophenolate mofetil, ATG, corticosteroids, and monoclonal antibodies directed at T cells. Table 140-3 shows the doses, toxicities, and monitoring of immunosuppressive agents used to prevent or treat GVHD. Most GVHD prophylaxis regimens combine immunosuppressive agents that affect different stages of T-cell activation. The most commonly used GVHD prophylaxis regimens are CSA or TAC and MTX. Another strategy is removing or depleting most T cells from donor bone marrow ex vivo before transplant by physical separation or by treatment with monoclonal antibodies directed at T cells.

Initially, acute GVHD prophylaxis was single agent MTX administered on days 1, 3, 6, and 11 after transplant and then weekly. However, when a short course of MTX was combined with CSA, the two agents showed synergy and a survival benefit. The addition of a third agent, such as prednisone, to the CSA/MTX combination failed to improve overall outcomes. TAC, another calcineurin inhibitor, was shown to have similar results to CSA when combined with a short course of MTX. The combination of a calcineurin inhibitor with MTX remains a standard immunosuppressive regimen used today. Intravenous CSA or TAC is usually started a few days before or on the day of transplant. Patients are converted to oral formulations when they can be tolerated. CSA or TAC typically are given at full doses until days 50 to 100, gradually tapered in the absence of GVHD, and discontinued by day 180. MTX is still given IV on days 1, 3, 6, and 11 after transplant. About 70% of patients are able to receive all four doses of MTX. Elimination of one or more MTX doses may be associated with an increased risk of GVHD. However, toxicities such as severe mucositis, hepatotoxicity or the development of conditions that may prolong MTX systemic exposure (eg, renal failure or third spacing) are common reasons to omit the day 11 dose of MTX. For patients who experience significant toxicity from MTX, monitoring of MTX levels with leucovorin rescue may be warranted.

Despite standard prophylaxis with CSA or TAC and MTX, grade II to IV acute GVHD still occurs in 30% to 50% in matched related donor transplants and 40% to 70% in matched unrelated donor transplants. Because of the gastrointestinal and hematologic toxicities of MTX, and in an effort to improve prevention, other prophylactic regimens have been evaluated. Sirolimus, an mTOR inhibitor, has been successfully used for the prevention of rejection in solid organ transplant patients and has theoretical advantages when used as GVHD prophylaxis. This agent has been reported to promote immune tolerance through generation of regulatory T cells, has antiviral properties (CMV and Epstein-Barr virus), and has antitumor activity against some hematologic malignancies.[58] Several studies have shown encouraging results with sirolimus when combined with a calcineurin inhibitor (TAC or CSA) in the prevention of GVHD, and many clinicians believe that the combination of TAC and sirolimus is less toxic and more efficacious than CSA and sirolimus. A phase III randomized trial was conducted by the Blood and Marrow CTN that compared TAC and sirolimus with TAC and MTX as GVHD prophylaxis.[59] The primary endpoint, grade II to IV acute GVHD-free survival at day 114, and the incidence of grade II to IV GVHD were similar between the two groups (67% vs 62%, P=0.38; 26% vs 34%, P=0.48). Neutrophil and platelet engraftment were more rapid in the TAC and sirolimus group by two and three days, respectively. Toxicities were similar between the two groups, except that oropharyngeal mucositis was less severe in the TAC and sirolimus arm. Chronic GVHD, disease relapse and overall survival at 2 years from transplantation were not different between groups. Based on similar long-term outcomes and shorter time-to-engraftment, TAC and sirolimus can be considered as an alternative to TAC and MTX.

Other MTX-sparing strategies have been evaluated for GVHD prophylaxis. Mycophenolate mofetil through its metabolite, mycophenolic acid, inhibits proliferation of lymphocytes and is synergistic with calcineurin inhibitors. Mycophenolate mofetil with TAC was compared with TAC and MTX in recipients of matched related and unrelated donors. The results of two small randomized trials have shown less toxicity with mycophenolate mofetil with similar rates of acute GVHD or overall survival.[60,61]

Single-agent PTCy is another GVHD prophylaxis strategy which does not include a calcineurin inhibitor. Its immunosuppressive activity is related to its antiproliferative effects on rapidly dividing alloreactive T cells. Hematopoietic stem cells have high levels of aldehyde dehydrogenase, thus sparing them from the antiproliferative activity of Cy. In patients receiving MAC with single-agent Cy posttransplant prophylaxis, 43% developed grade II to IV GVHD, and 10% had grade III to IV GVHD. The incidence of chronic GVHD was 10% at 26 months.[62] The use of posttransplant Cy combined with other immunosuppressive agents such as mycophenolate mofetil and a calcineurin inhibitor has shown to be effective immunosuppression for Haplo-HSCT patients.

Other novel agents, such are bortezomib, and pentostatin have shown activity in preventing GVHD. The addition of bortezomib, given on days 1, 4, and 7 after transplant, to standard TAC and MTX in RIC mismatched unrelated donor transplants showed an incidence of grade II to IV GVHD that was comparable to patients who received HLA-matched transplants.[63] Pentostatin 1.5 mg/m^2 weekly for 4 weeks combined with a calcineurin inhibitor and MTX increased the proportion of patients alive without GVHD at day 100 compared with control participants.[64] Although the addition of these novel agents is intriguing, the role of these agents in GVHD prophylaxis is not clear. The Blood and Marrow CTN is conducting a phase II trial evaluating the activity of several novel three-drug GVHD prophylaxis regimens: bortezomib or maraviroc added to TAC and MTX; and PTCy added to TAC and mycophenolate mofetil (BMT-CTN 1203, NCT02208037).

TABLE 140-3 Immunosuppression for the Prevention and Treatment of GVHD

Agent	Dose	Drug Monitoring
Prevention		
Tacrolimus[54]	0.02-0.03 mg/kg/day IV beginning 1-3 days before transplant; change to PO when able to tolerate	Check serum levels ~72 hours after start and then 2-3 times/wk until stable (trough serum levels, 5-15 mcg/L [6.2-18.6 nmol/L]); serum creatinine for renal toxicity, CBC for hematologic toxicity, blood pressure for hypertension, and BMP for electrolyte abnormalities
Cyclosporine[54]	3-5 mg/kg/day IV beginning 1-3 days before transplant; change to PO when able to tolerate	Check blood levels ~72 hours after start and then 2-3 times/wk until stable (trough blood levels, 150-450 mcg/L [125-374 nmol/L]); serum creatinine for renal toxicity, CBC for hematologic toxicity, blood pressure for hypertension, and BMP for electrolyte abnormalities
Sirolimus[58]	Loading dose 12 mg PO on day +1 followed by 4 mg PO daily starting on day +2	Check serum levels ~24 hours after start and then 2-3 times/wk until stable (trough serum levels, 3-12 mcg/L [3-13 nmol/L]); serum creatinine for renal toxicity and CBC for hematologic toxicity
Methotrexate[54]	15 mg/m² IV on day +1 followed by 10 mg/m² IV on days +3, 6, and 11 *or* 5 mg/m² IV on days +1, 3, 6, and 11	Monitor for toxicity: mucositis, LFTs for hepatic dysfunction, serum creatinine for renal impairment, fluid retention, and CBC for hematologic toxicity; methotrexate levels are not routinely monitored unless the patient develops renal dysfunction or third spacing; doses may be omitted if severe mucositis or hepatotoxicity develops
Mycophenolate[60]	15 mg/kg/dose IV twice daily beginning on day 0; change to PO when able to tolerate	Monitor for toxicity: CBC for neutropenia and severe GI symptoms
Pentostatin[64]	1.5 mg/m² IV weekly × 4 doses beginning day +8	Monitor for toxicity: BMP for renal impairment and CBC for thrombotic thrombocytopenic purpura
Cyclophosphamide[12]	50 mg/kg/day IV on days +3 and +4	Monitor for toxicity: BMP for renal impairment, LFTs for hepatic toxicity (including SOS), urinalysis for hemorrhagic cystitis, vital signs and possible cardiac workup for pericarditis (only for symptomatic patients)
Rabbit anti-thymocyte globulin (ATG)[67]	2.5-5 mg/kg/day IV beginning 3 days before transplant	Monitor for toxicity: frequent vital signs during infusion for fever, rash, cardiovascular and GI dysfunction, anaphylaxis and serum sickness
Alemtuzumab[65]	10-20 mg/day IV daily beginning 4-5 days before transplant	Monitor for toxicity: fever, chills, infection, and anaphylaxis
Treatment		
Methylprednisolone[a] *or* Prednisone[a,57]	1-2 mg/kg/day	Monitor for toxicity: glucose for hyperglycemia, blood pressure for hypertension, labile mood, bone osteopenia, avascular bone necrosis, impaired wound healing, and adrenal insufficiency
Mycophenolate[57]	1.5-2 g PO daily in divided doses	As above
Sirolimus[57]	1-2 mg/day; then adjust based on levels	As above
Denileukin diftitox[57]	9 mcg/kg on days 1, 3, 5, 15, 17, and 19	Monitor for toxicity: LFTs for hepatic toxicity
Infliximab[57]	10 mg/kg/wk for at least 4 doses	Monitor for toxicity: anaphylaxis (rare)
Etanercept[57]	0.4 mg/kg/dose (maximum dose, 25 mg) SC twice weekly for 8 weeks	Monitor for toxicity; generally well tolerated
Rabbit ATG[57]	0.5 mg/kg for first dose followed by 1-1.5 mg/kg for subsequent doses	As above
Pentostatin[57]	1.5 mg/m² IV on days 1-3 and 15-17	As above

BMP, basic metabolic panel; CBC, complete blood count; GI, gastrointestinal; LFT, liver function test; PO, orally; SC, subcutaneous; SOS, sinusoidal obstruction syndrome.

[a]Considered 1st line therapy.

Another strategy to reduce the risk of acute GVHD is to reduce the number of donor T cells in the stem cell donation. In vivo T-cell depletion may be incorporated into conditioning regimens with agents such as ATG or alemtuzumab.[65] Uncontrolled trials of ATG with MAC regimens suggested that ATG could prevent GVHD, but may increase the risk of relapse and graft failure. A Cochrane review of six trials reported that ATG given with MAC regimens did decrease the risk of grade II to IV acute GVHD, but did not significantly improve overall survival, disease relapse or nonrelapse mortality.[66] The role of ATG with RIC transplantation has not been evaluated in a randomized controlled trial. The CIBMTR has reported that ATG recipients were more likely to have disease relapse, shorter overall and disease-free survival.[67] However, another observational study of European patients receiving RIC regimens reported reduced incidences of acute and chronic GVHD with similar relapse risk, nonrelapse mortality and survival.[68] Results from that study also suggested a dose effect with ATG doses of less than 6 mg/kg associated with improved outcomes. Based on these conflicting data, the use of ATG in RIC transplants should be reserved for clinical trials.

The role of ex vivo T-cell depletion is controversial.[56] Earlier reports of this technique were associated with an increased risk of graft failure, delayed immune reconstitution, leukemic relapse, CMV reactivation, and Epstein-Barr virus–related lymphoproliferative disorders. Most of these studies occurred when bone marrow was the preferred stem cell source. In a comparative analysis of patients who received ex vivo T-cell depletion or the standard calcineurin inhibitor and MTX prophylaxis, T cell–depleted stem cells had lower rates of chronic GVHD. No differences in rates of graft rejection, leukemia relapse, treatment-related mortality, or overall survival rates were reported.[69]

It is difficult to predict which patients will develop acute GVHD. Risk factors are unable to accurately identify patients who will go onto develop GVHD. Biomarkers that could predict the development of GVHD could direct treatment before the patient develops severe disease. An ideal biomarker would be predictive of both disease onset and prognosis, inexpensive, and readily available in order to facilitate real-time clinical decision making. Many biomarkers have been studied including IL-2 receptor alpha, IL-8, peptidase inhibitor-3, regenerating islet-derived 3α (REG 3α), hepatocyte growth factor, serum albumin and microRNAs.[70] Although several biomarkers appear promising, they should not be used outside of a clinical trial.

Treatment of Acute Graft-Versus-Host Disease 10 Patients with mild skin-only acute GVHD (grade I) can be treated with topical corticosteroid preparations and counseled on the appropriate use of sunscreen. If a patient develops grades II to IV GVHD, prophylactic agents are continued, and high-dose corticosteroids in the form of IV methylprednisolone or oral prednisone are given.[56] The usual dosage is 1 to 2 mg/kg/day given in two divided doses; higher dosages have not been shown to be more efficacious. About 25% to 40% of patients with established acute GVHD respond to high-dose corticosteroids. If the patient responds, the corticosteroid dose is tapered gradually over several weeks to months, depending on response. In patients who experience a flare in GVHD during the taper phase, therapy consists of increasing the corticosteroid dose and then tapering more slowly. Oral beclomethasone dipropionate, a topically active corticosteroid, has been shown to reduce the frequency of gastrointestinal GVHD relapses when continued after prednisone taper.[71] Administration of beclomethasone has been associated with a better survival at 200 days and 1 year after transplant. Budesonide, another nonabsorbable corticosteroid, has also been evaluated in uncontrolled studies and may also reduce the need for sustained use of high-dose systemic corticosteroid administration.[71]

GVHD-associated mortality is strongly correlated to response to initial treatment and ranges from about 25% in patients who had a complete response to about 80% in patients who had no response or progressive disease. Several randomized trials have evaluated other agents combined with methylprednisolone in an effort to improve response to initial therapy for acute GVHD.[56] In a randomized phase II trial, 180 patients were treated with methylprednisolone 2 mg/kg/day combined with etanercept, mycophenolate mofetil, denileukin diftitox, or pentostatin.[72] After 28 days of treatment, efficacy and toxicity data suggested that the use of mycophenolate mofetil plus corticosteroids was the most promising regimen to compare with corticosteroids alone in a definitive phase III trial. This trial was halted early when a futility rule was met at a planned interim analysis. GVHD-free survival 56 days after randomization was not different between the groups. Based on the current published data, the use of glucocorticoid treatment with an additional agent for initial therapy of acute GVHD should only be done within the confines of a clinical trial.[57]

The mortality rate of patients with steroid-refractory GVHD is high. Criteria and indications for initiating secondary therapy for steroid-refractory acute GVHD have not been well defined in the literature. Although different centers may have varying criteria, in general, if the manifestations of acute GVHD in any organ worsen over 3 days of corticosteroid treatment or symptoms do not improve by 5 days, the patient likely will not respond to corticosteroids, and secondary therapy should be considered.[57] There is no standard treatment of patients with steroid-refractory acute GVHD because very few prospective comparative studies have been conducted to assess the efficacy of individual agents. Second-line therapy has consisted of continuation of corticosteroids with the addition of one or more of the following: ATG, mycophenolate mofetil, sirolimus, infliximab, etanercept, denileukin diftitox, alemtuzumab, or pentostatin.[57,73] One approach that has shown benefit as corticosteroid-sparing therapy is extracorporeal photopheresis. During this procedure, the patient's blood is exposed extracorporeally to 8-methoxypsoralen followed by ultraviolet A radiation and then returned to the patient. This process is thought to result in suppression of T-cell reactivity and induction of regulatory T cells. Clinical results have been positive, especially in patients with skin GVHD.[74] The choice of a second-line regimen for acute GVHD should be based on the risk of potential toxicities, interactions with other agents, convenience, and cost.

Clinical **Controversy...**

Optimal treatment of steroid-refractory GVHD is unclear. Comparative trials are needed to determine a standard approach to this difficult clinical condition.

Chronic Graft-Versus-Host Disease

Chronic GVHD is the major determinant of late transplant-related morbidity and mortality. The pathophysiology of chronic GVHD is poorly understood and likely involves inflammation, cell mediated immunity as well as humoral immunity and fibrosis.[75] The presentation of chronic GVHD is diverse and resembles a variety of autoimmune disorders. The incidence of chronic GVHD is 30% to 70%, and while its clinical manifestations usually present during the first year, it can also develop many years after transplant. Both HLA mismatching and transplantation from unrelated donor transplants help explain the growing incidence of chronic GVHD. The diagnosis of chronic GVHD is often based on clinical presentation, but biopsies of affected organs can help differentiate acute from chronic GVHD. More recently, the use of biomarkers has been studied in order to facilitate diagnosis and predict treatment response.[75] The risk of chronic GVHD increases with a previous history of acute GVHD, increasing donor and recipient age, patients who receive transplants from HLA-nonidentical donors and in patients who receive PBSC transplants (especially with higher $CD34^+$ cell doses). Unlike acute GVHD, prophylactic immunosuppression does not appear to reduce the incidence or severity of chronic GVHD.

Chronic GVHD resembles autoimmune diseases and can affect any organ or tissue of the body. The most common sites involved are the skin, mouth, liver, and eye, but other sites include the gastrointestinal tract, joints, muscles, and lungs. The National Institutes of Health (NIH) Consensus Development Project developed standardized criteria for the diagnosis of chronic GVHD and proposed a clinical scoring system for the evaluation of patients with chronic GVHD based on the extent of organ damage and degree of functional impairment.[75] The Working Group recommends that the diagnosis of chronic GVHD be made with the presence of at least one diagnostic clinical sign of chronic GVHD (eg, poikiloderma or esophageal web) or a distinctive manifestation (eg, keratoconjunctivitis sicca) confirmed by biopsy or other test (eg, Schirmer test). For patients with overlap syndrome, the NIH Working Group now recommends documenting all specific manifestations (acute and chronic) when establishing a diagnosis.

The clinical scoring system categorizes chronic GVHD into mild, moderate, and severe.[75] Mild chronic GVHD involves only one or two organs or sites (except the lung) with no clinically significant functional impairment. Moderate chronic GVHD involves at least one organ or site with clinically significant but no major disability, three or more organs or sites with no clinically significant functional impairment, or mild lung involvement. Severe chronic GVHD indicates major disability caused by chronic GVHD or at least moderate lung involvement.

Patients with mild skin-only chronic GVHD can be treated with a variety of topical preparations, such as clobetasol, TAC, and pimecrolimus.[76] Other organs such as mouth, eyes and genital tract may also be treated with aggressive local therapy. Initial treatment of patients with more severe or systemic involvement of chronic GVHD consists of prednisone 0.5 to 1 mg/kg/day followed by taper with or without a calcineurin inhibitor. Although calcineurin inhibitors do not conclusively improve outcomes, they are often used to reduce toxicities of prolonged steroid therapy, especially in patients who may be at high risk for prednisone-related complications.[77] Treatment is continued until signs and symptoms of the disease have resolved and then are tapered gradually over an extended period of time. Patients with chronic GVHD may require prolonged immunosuppressive treatment for an average of 2 to 3 years from the initial diagnosis.

In addition to treatment specifically for chronic GVHD, ancillary therapies and supportive care should be recommended to lessen the symptoms of chronic GVHD.[77] Patients should be educated on the use of sunscreens (and avoidance of sun exposure) to reduce skin injury and exacerbation of GVHD skin lesions. Nonsclerotic skin lesions without erosions or ulcerations may respond well to emollients in addition to topical corticosteroids. Patients should be advised to maintain good oral hygiene with routine dental care. Saliva substitutes can be given for dry mouth symptoms, and topical corticosteroid gels can be used for localized and symptomatic oral lesions. Artificial tears or, if necessary for more severe symptoms, CSA or corticosteroid eye drops are useful for patients with chronic GVHD manifesting as dry eyes or conjunctivitis. Physical therapy is recommended to reduce functional loss as a result of steroid myopathy, joint contractures, and deconditioning.

Patients who do not respond to initial therapy have a very poor prognosis. Indications for secondary treatment include worsening symptoms, involvement of new organs, no improvement of symptoms after 1 month of therapy, inability to decrease steroid dose or significant treatment-related toxicity. Uncontrolled trials have investigated several therapies with varying degrees of success. To date, no consensus has been reached regarding the optimal choice for salvage therapy. When choosing initial salvage therapy, clinicians should consider agents with documented activity and an adequate safety profile as well as agents that are steroid sparing. Agents with reported activity in refractory chronic GVHD include thalidomide, extracorporeal photophoresis, TAC, sirolimus, pentostatin, mycophenolate mofetil, hydroxychloroquine, rituximab, imatinib, and others.[77,78]

Monitoring for long-term drug toxicities and infectious complications is critical during long-term immunosuppression. Infection is the primary cause of death in patients with chronic GVHD, and antimicrobial prophylaxis is an important component of the care of patients being treated for chronic GVHD.[77,78] Patients should receive oral trimethoprim–sulfamethoxazole, penicillin, an antifungal azole agent, and acyclovir to prevent infections commonly seen in immunocompromised patients. Routine monitoring for CMV reactivation should be performed. Some HSCT centers also administer IV immunoglobulin to patients with low serum immunoglobulin G levels. Patients who remain on long-term steroids should be monitored for steroid-induced osteoporosis and diabetes mellitus. Other potential long-term complications of chronic GVHD therapies include hyperlipidemia, cataracts, myelosuppression, elevated blood pressure, and renal dysfunction.

Infection

Patients undergoing high-dose chemotherapy with autologous or allogeneic HSCT are severely immunocompromised and therefore are at high risk for bacterial, fungal, and viral infections.[29,32] Management of these infections is discussed in detail in Chapters 121 and 122.

Late Complications

With the success of HSCT, the number of long-term survivors has grown. Many survivors experience delayed complications of transplantation and treatments used to prevent or treat those complications, including restrictive and obstructive pulmonary disease, bone and joint disease (including osteoporosis and avascular necrosis), cataract formation, endocrine dysfunction (including sterility and thyroid dysfunction), impaired growth and development, infections, cardiovascular disease, chronic renal and hepatic dysfunction, and secondary malignancies.[29,32,79] These effects are more frequent after allogeneic compared with autologous HSCT and among allogeneic HSCT patients, those with chronic GVHD tend to have a higher prevalence of multiple health conditions than those without chronic GVHD.[29,79] Physical recovery tends to occur earlier than psychological or work recovery. Full recovery usually takes several years, and about two-thirds of patients are without major limitations by 5 years. Both allogeneic and autologous transplants are associated with a several-fold increase in risk of premature death; relative mortality decreased with time but remained significantly elevated even 10 years after transplant. The leading cause of death is relapse of primary disease in both allogeneic and autologous HSCT patients, but allogeneic HSCT patients also continue to die from complications of chronic GVHD, while autologous HSCT patients more frequently succumbed to secondary malignancies.[29,79] Long-term monitoring of HSCT patients is required, both by transplant clinicians and primary care providers who are knowledgeable in the care of these patients, to screen for, prevent and treat late complications when such interventions are available. In 2012, the CIBMTR (in partnership with leading transplant organizations) published posttransplant care recommendations for adult and pediatric autologous and allogeneic HSCT recipients (www.cibmtr.org/posttransplant).

ABBREVIATIONS

ALL	acute lymphocytic leukemia
AML	acute myelogenous leukemia
APC	antigen-presenting cell
ASBMT	American Society of Blood and Marrow Transplantation
ATG	anti-thymocyte globulin
BMT	bone marrow transplantation
CIBMTR	Center for International Blood and Marrow Transplant Research
CML	chronic myeloid leukemia
CMV	cytomegalovirus
CSA	cyclosporine
CTN	Clinical Trials Network
DLI	donor lymphocyte infusion
EBMT	The European Bone Marrow Transplantation Association
G-CSF	granulocyte colony-stimulating factor; filgrastim
GM-CSF	granulocyte-macrophage colony-stimulating factor; sargramostim
GVHD	graft-versus-host disease
GVM	graft-versus-malignancy (effect)
Haplo-HSCT	haploidentical allogeneic transplant
HLA	human leukocyte antigen
HSCT	hematopoietic stem cell transplantation
MAC	myeloablative conditioning
MDS	myelodysplastic syndrome
MHC	major histocompatibility complex
MTX	methotrexate
NHL	non-Hodgkin lymphoma
NK	natural killer (cells)

NMDP	National Marrow Donor Program
PCR	polymerase chain reaction
Ph+	Philadelphia chromosome–positive
PBSC	peripheral blood stem cell
PTCy	post-transplant cyclophosphamide
RIC	reduced-intensity conditioning
SOS	sinusoidal obstruction syndrome
TAC	tacrolimus
TBI	total-body irradiation
TKI	tyrosine kinase inhibitor
TNF-α	tumor necrosis factor-α
TKI	tyrosine kinase inhibitor
UCB	umbilical cord blood
UCBT	umbilical cord blood transplant
VOD	venoocclusive disease

REFERENCES

1. Pasquini MC ZX. *Current uses and outcomes of hematopoietic stem cell transplantation: 2014 CIBMTR Summary Slides*. http://www.cibmtr.org. Last accessed, February 12, 2016.
2. Wingard J, Gastineau D, Leather H, Synder E, Szczepiorkowski Z, eds. *Hematopoietic Stem Cell Transplantation: A Handbook for Clinicians*, 2nd ed. Bethesda, MD: AABB; 2015.
3. Forman SJ, Negrin RS, Antin JA, Appelbaum FR., eds. *Thomas' Hematopoietic Cell Transplantation*. 5th ed. Oxford, UK: Wiley-Blackwell; 2015.
4. Gyurkocza B, Rezvani A, Storb RF. Allogeneic hematopoietic cell transplantation: The state of the art. *Expert Rev Hematol* 2010;3:285-299.
5. Copelan EA. Hematopoietic stem-cell transplantation. *N Engl J Med* 2006;354:1813-1826.
6. Fung MK, Benson K. Using HLA typing to support patients with cancer. *Cancer Control* 2015;22:79-86.
7. Petersdorf EW. Optimal HLA matching in hematopoietic cell transplantation. *Curr Opin Immunol* 2008;20:588-593.
8. Spellman SR, Eapen M, Logan BR, et al. A perspective on the selection of unrelated donors and cord blood units for transplantation. *Blood* 2012;120:259-265.
9. Majhail NS, Chitphakdithai P, Logan B, et al. Significant improvement in survival after unrelated donor hematopoietic cell transplantation in the recent era. *Biol Blood Marrow Transplant* 2015;21:142-150.
10. Eapen M, O'Donnell P, Brunstein CG, et al. Mismatched related and unrelated donors for allogeneic hematopoietic cell transplantation for adults with hematologic malignancies. *Biol Blood Marrow Transplant* 2014;20:1485-1492.
11. Ballen KK, Koreth J, Chen YB, et al. Selection of optimal alternative graft source: Mismatched unrelated donor, umbilical cord blood, or haploidentical transplant. *Blood* 2012;119:1972-1980.
12. Kanakry CG, de Lima MJ, Luznik L. Alternative donor allogeneic hematopoietic cell transplantation for acute myeloid leukemia. *Semin Hematol* 2015;52:232-242.
13. Brunstein CG, Fuchs EJ, Carter SL, et al. Alternative donor transplantation after reduced intensity conditioning: Results of parallel phase 2 trials using partially HLA-mismatched related bone marrow or unrelated double umbilical cord blood grafts. *Blood* 2011;118:282-288.
14. Giralt S, Costa L, Schriber J, et al. Optimizing autologous stem cell mobilization strategies to improve patient outcomes: Consensus guidelines and recommendations. *Biol Blood Marrow Transplant* 2014;20:295-308.
15. Schmitt M, Publicover A, Orchard KH, et al. Biosimilar G-CSF based mobilization of peripheral blood hematopoietic stem cells for autologous and allogeneic stem cell transplantation. *Theranostics* 2014;4:280-289.
16. Duong HK, Savani BN, Copelan E, et al. Peripheral blood progenitor cell mobilization for autologous and allogeneic hematopoietic cell transplantation: Guidelines from the American Society for Blood and Marrow Transplantation. *Biol Blood Marrow Transplant* 2014;20:1262-1273.
17. Shaw BE, Confer DL, Hwang WY, et al. Concerns about the use of biosimilar granulocyte colony-stimulating factors for the mobilization of stem cells in normal donors: Position of the world marrow donor association. *Haematologica* 2011;96:942-947.
18. DiPersio JF, Stadtmauer EA, Nademanee A, et al. Plerixafor and G-CSF versus placebo and G-CSF to mobilize hematopoietic stem cells for autologous stem cell transplantation in patients with multiple myeloma. *Blood* 2009;113:5720-5726.
19. DiPersio JF, Micallef IN, Stiff PJ, et al. Phase III prospective randomized double-blind placebo-controlled trial of plerixafor plus granulocyte colony-stimulating factor compared with placebo plus granulocyte colony-stimulating factor for autologous stem-cell mobilization and transplantation for patients with non-Hodgkin's lymphoma. *J Clin Oncol* 2009;27:4767-4773.
20. Costa LJ, Nista EJ, Buadi FK, et al. Prediction of poor mobilization of autologous CD34+ cells with growth factor in multiple myeloma patients: Implications for risk-stratification. *Biol Blood Marrow Transplant* 2014;20:222-228.
21. Perkins JB, Shapiro JF, Bookout RN, et al. Retrospective comparison of filgrastim plus plerixafor to other regimens for remobilization after primary mobilization failure: Clinical and economic outcomes. *Am J Hematol* 2012;87:673-677.
22. Korbling M, Freireich EJ. Twenty-five years of peripheral blood stem cell transplantation. *Blood* 2011;117:6411-6416.
23. Moalic V. Mobilization and collection of peripheral blood stem cells in healthy donors: Risks, adverse events and follow-up. *Pathol Biol (Paris)* 2013;61:70-74.
24. Holtick U, Albrecht M, Chemnitz JM, et al. Comparison of bone marrow versus peripheral blood allogeneic hematopoietic stem cell transplantation for hematological malignancies in adults-a systematic review and meta-analysis. *Crit Rev Oncol Hematol* 2015;94:179-188.
25. Anasetti C, Logan BR, Lee SJ, et al. Blood and Marrow Transplant Clinical Trials Network. Peripheral-blood stem cells versus bone marrow from unrelated donors. *N Engl J Med* 2012;367:1487-1496.
26. Eapen M, Logan BR, Horowitz MM, et al. Bone marrow or peripheral blood for reduced-intensity conditioning unrelated donor transplantation. *J Clin Oncol* 2015;33:364-369.
27. Ballen KK, Gluckman E, Broxmeyer HE. Umbilical cord blood transplantation: The first 25 years and beyond. *Blood* 2013;122:491-498.
28. Eapen M, Rocha V, Sanz G, et al. Effect of graft source on unrelated donor haemopoietic stem-cell transplantation in adults with acute leukaemia: A retrospective analysis. *Lancet Oncol* 2010;11:653-660.
29. Hamadani M. Autologous hematopoietic cell transplantation: An update for clinicians. *Ann Med* 2014;46:619-632.
30. Bacigalupo A, Ballen K, Rizzo D, et al. Defining the intensity of conditioning regimens: Working definitions. *Biol Blood Marrow Transplant* 2009;15:1628-1633.
31. Gyurkocza B, Sandmaier BM. Conditioning regimens for hematopoietic cell transplantation: One size does not fit all. *Blood* 2014;124:344-353.
32. Arnaout K, Patel N, Jain M, et al. Complications of allogeneic hematopoietic stem cell transplantation. *Cancer Invest* 2014;32:349-362.
33. Ciurea SO, Andersson BS. Busulfan in hematopoietic stem cell transplantation. *Biol Blood Marrow Transplant* 2009;15:523-36.
34. Mickelson DM, Sproat L, Dean R, et al. Comparison of donor chimerism following myeloablative and nonmyeloablative allogeneic hematopoietic SCT. *Bone Marrow Transplant* 2011;46:84-89.
35. Pingali SR, Champlin RE. Pushing the envelope-nonmyeloablative and reduced intensity preparative regimens for allogeneic hematopoietic transplantation. *Bone Marrow Transplant* 2015;50:1157-1167.
36. Bornhauser M, Kienast J, Trenschel R, et al. Reduced-intensity conditioning versus standard conditioning before allogeneic haemopoietic cell transplantation in patients with acute myeloid leukaemia in first complete remission: A prospective, open-label randomised phase 3 trial. *Lancet Oncol* 2012;13:1035-1044.
37. Avigan D, Hari P, Battiwalla M, et al. Proceedings from the national cancer institute's second international workshop on the biology, prevention, and treatment of relapse after hematopoietic stem cell transplantation: Part II. Autologous transplantation-novel agents and immunomodulatory strategies. *Biol Blood Marrow Transplant* 2013;19:1661-1669.
38. de Lima M, Porter DL, Battiwalla M, et al. Proceedings from the national cancer institute's second international workshop on the

biology, prevention, and treatment of relapse after hematopoietic stem cell transplantation: Part III. Prevention and treatment of relapse after allogeneic transplantation. *Biol Blood Marrow Transplant* 2014;20:4-13.

39. Oran B. Is there a role for therapy after transplant? *Best Pract Res Clin Haematol* 2015;28:124-132.
40. Hourigan CS, McCarthy P, de Lima M. Back to the future! The evolving role of maintenance therapy after hematopoietic stem cell transplantation. *Biol Blood Marrow Transplant* 2014;20:154-163.
41. Chang YJ, Huang XJ. Donor lymphocyte infusions for relapse after allogeneic transplantation: When, if and for whom? *Blood Rev* 2013;27:55-62.
42. Deol A, Lum LG. Role of donor lymphocyte infusions in relapsed hematological malignancies after stem cell transplantation revisited. *Cancer Treat Rev* 2010;36:528-538.
43. Moskowitz CH, Nademanee A, Masszi T, et al. AETHERA Study Group. Brentuximab vedotin as consolidation therapy after autologous stem-cell transplantation in patients with hodgkin's lymphoma at risk of relapse or progression (AETHERA): A randomised, double-blind, placebo-controlled, phase 3 trial. *Lancet* 2015;385:1853-1862.
44. Klyuchnikov E, Kroger N, Brummendorf TH, et al. Current status and perspectives of tyrosine kinase inhibitor treatment in the posttransplant period in patients with chronic myelogenous leukemia (CML). *Biol Blood Marrow Transplant* 2010;16:301-310.
45. Lee HJ, Thompson JE, Wang ES, Wetzler M. Philadelphia chromosome-positive acute lymphoblastic leukemia: Current treatment and future perspectives. *Cancer* 2011;117:1583-1594.
46. de Lima M, Giralt S, Thall PF, et al. Maintenance therapy with low-dose azacitidine after allogeneic hematopoietic stem cell transplantation for recurrent acute myelogenous leukemia or myelodysplastic syndrome: A dose and schedule finding study. *Cancer* 2010;116:5420-5431.
47. Tessoulin B, Delaunay J, Chevallier P, et al. Azacitidine salvage therapy for relapse of myeloid malignancies following allogeneic hematopoietic SCT. *Bone Marrow Transplant* 2014;49:567-571.
48. Carreras E. How I manage sinusoidal obstruction syndrome after haematopoietic cell transplantation. *Br J Haematol* 2015;168:481-491.
49. Chi AK, Soubani AO, White AC, Miller KB. An update on pulmonary complications of hematopoietic stem cell transplantation. *Chest* 2013;144:1913-1922.
50. Panoskaltsis-Mortari A, Griese M, Madtes DK, et al. American Thoracic Society Committee on Idiopathic Pneumonia Syndrome. An official american thoracic society research statement: Noninfectious lung injury after hematopoietic stem cell transplantation: Idiopathic pneumonia syndrome. *Am J Respir Crit Care Med* 2011;183:1262-1279.
51. Yanik GA, Horowitz MM, Weisdorf DJ, et al. Randomized, double-blind, placebo-controlled trial of soluble tumor necrosis factor receptor: Enbrel (etanercept) for the treatment of idiopathic pneumonia syndrome after allogeneic stem cell transplantation: Blood and marrow transplant clinical trials network protocol. *Biol Blood Marrow Transplant* 2014;20:858-864.
52. Bacigalupo A, Chien J, Barisione G, Pavletic S. Late pulmonary complications after allogeneic hematopoietic stem cell transplantation: Diagnosis, monitoring, prevention, and treatment. *Semin Hematol* 2012;49:15-24.
53. Olsson RF, Logan BR, Chaudhury S, et al. Primary graft failure after myeloablative allogeneic hematopoietic cell transplantation for hematologic malignancies. *Leukemia* 2015;29:1754-1762.
54. Pavletic SZ, Fowler DH. Are we making progress in GVHD prophylaxis and treatment? *Hematology Am Soc Hematol Educ Program* 2012;2012:251-264.
55. Saliba RM, de Lima M, Giralt S, et al. Hyperacute GVHD: Risk factors, outcomes, and clinical implications. *Blood* 2007;109:2751-2758.
56. Holtan SG, Pasquini M, Weisdorf DJ. Acute graft-versus-host disease: A bench-to-bedside update. *Blood* 2014;124:363-373.
57. Martin PJ, Rizzo JD, Wingard JR, et al. First- and second-line systemic treatment of acute graft-versus-host disease: Recommendations of the american society of blood and marrow transplantation. *Biol Blood Marrow Transplant* 2012;18:1150-1163.
58. Abouelnasr A, Roy J, Cohen S, et al. Defining the role of sirolimus in the management of graft-versus-host disease: From prophylaxis to treatment. *Biol Blood Marrow Transplant* 2013;19:12-21.
59. Cutler C, Logan B, Nakamura R, et al. Tacrolimus/sirolimus vs tacrolimus/methotrexate as GVHD prophylaxis after matched, related donor allogeneic HCT. *Blood* 2014;124:1372-1377.
60. Perkins J, Field T, Kim J, et al. A randomized phase II trial comparing tacrolimus and mycophenolate mofetil to tacrolimus and methotrexate for acute graft-versus-host disease prophylaxis. *Biol Blood Marrow Transplant* 2010;16:937-947.
61. Bolwell B, Sobecks R, Pohlman B, et al. A prospective randomized trial comparing cyclosporine and short course methotrexate with cyclosporine and mycophenolate mofetil for GVHD prophylaxis in myeloablative allogeneic bone marrow transplantation. *Bone Marrow Transplant* 2004;34:621-625.
62. Luznik L, Bolanos-Meade J, Zahurak M, et al. High-dose cyclophosphamide as single-agent, short-course prophylaxis of graft-versus-host disease. *Blood* 2010;115:3224-3230.
63. Koreth J, Stevenson KE, Kim HT, et al. Bortezomib-based graft-versus-host disease prophylaxis in HLA-mismatched unrelated donor transplantation. *J Clin Oncol* 2012;30:3202-3208.
64. Parmar S, Andersson BS, Couriel D, et al. Prophylaxis of graft-versus-host disease in unrelated donor transplantation with pentostatin, tacrolimus, and mini-methotrexate: A phase I/II controlled, adaptively randomized study. *J Clin Oncol* 2011;29:294-302.
65. Poire X, van Besien K. Alemtuzumab in allogeneic hematopoetic stem cell transplantation. *Expert Opin Biol Ther* 2011;11:1099-1111.
66. Theurich S, Fischmann H, Shimabukuro-Vornhagen A, et al. Polyclonal anti-thymocyte globulins for the prophylaxis of graft-versus-host disease after allogeneic stem cell or bone marrow transplantation in adults. *Cochrane Database Syst Rev* 2012;9:CD009159.
67. Soiffer RJ, Lerademacher J, Ho V, et al. Impact of immune modulation with anti-T-cell antibodies on the outcome of reduced-intensity allogeneic hematopoietic stem cell transplantation for hematologic malignancies. *Blood* 2011;117:6963-6970.
68. Baron F, Labopin M, Blaise D, et al. Impact of in vivo T-cell depletion on outcome of AML patients in first CR given peripheral blood stem cells and reduced-intensity conditioning allo-SCT from a HLA-identical sibling donor: A report from the acute leukemia working party of the European Group for Blood and Marrow Transplantation. *Bone Marrow Transplant* 2014;49:389-396.
69. Pasquini MC, Devine S, Mendizabal A, et al. Comparative outcomes of donor graft CD34+ selection and immune suppressive therapy as graft-versus-host disease prophylaxis for patients with acute myeloid leukemia in complete remission undergoing HLA-matched sibling allogeneic hematopoietic cell transplantation. *J Clin Oncol* 2012;30:3194-3201.
70. Tomuleasa C, Fuji S, Cucuianu A, et al. MicroRNAs as biomarkers for graft-versus-host disease following allogeneic stem cell transplantation. *Ann Hematol* 2015;94:1081-1092.
71. Hockenbery DM, Cruickshank S, Rodell TC, et al. A randomized, placebo-controlled trial of oral beclomethasone dipropionate as a prednisone-sparing therapy for gastrointestinal graft-versus-host disease. *Blood* 2007;109:4557-4563.
72. Alousi AM, Weisdorf DJ, Logan BR, et al. Etanercept, mycophenolate, denileukin, or pentostatin plus corticosteroids for acute graft-versus-host disease: A randomized phase 2 trial from the blood and marrow transplant clinical trials network. *Blood* 2009;114:511-517.
73. Pidala J, Anasetti C. Glucocorticoid-refractory acute graft-versus-host disease. *Biol Blood Marrow Transplant* 2010;16:1504-1518.
74. Abu-Dalle I, Reljic T, Nishihori T, et al. Extracorporeal photopheresis in steroid-refractory acute or chronic graft-versus-host disease: Results of a systematic review of prospective studies. *Biol Blood Marrow Transplant* 2014;20:1677-1686.
75. Jagasia MH, Greinix HT, Arora M, et al. National institutes of health consensus development project on criteria for clinical trials in chronic graft-versus-host disease: I. the 2014 diagnosis and staging working group report. *Biol Blood Marrow Transplant* 2015;21:389-401.e1.
76. Wolff D, Gerbitz A, Ayuk F, et al. Consensus conference on clinical practice in chronic graft-versus-host disease (GVHD): First-line and topical treatment of chronic GVHD. *Biol Blood Marrow Transplant* 2010;16:1611-1628.
77. Flowers ME, Martin PJ. How we treat chronic graft-versus-host disease. *Blood* 2015;125:606-615.
78. Socie G, Ritz J. Current issues in chronic graft-versus-host disease. *Blood* 2014;124:374-384.
79. Mosesso K. CE: Adverse late and long-term treatment effects in adult allogeneic hematopoietic stem cell transplant survivors. *Am J Nurs* 2015;115:22-34.

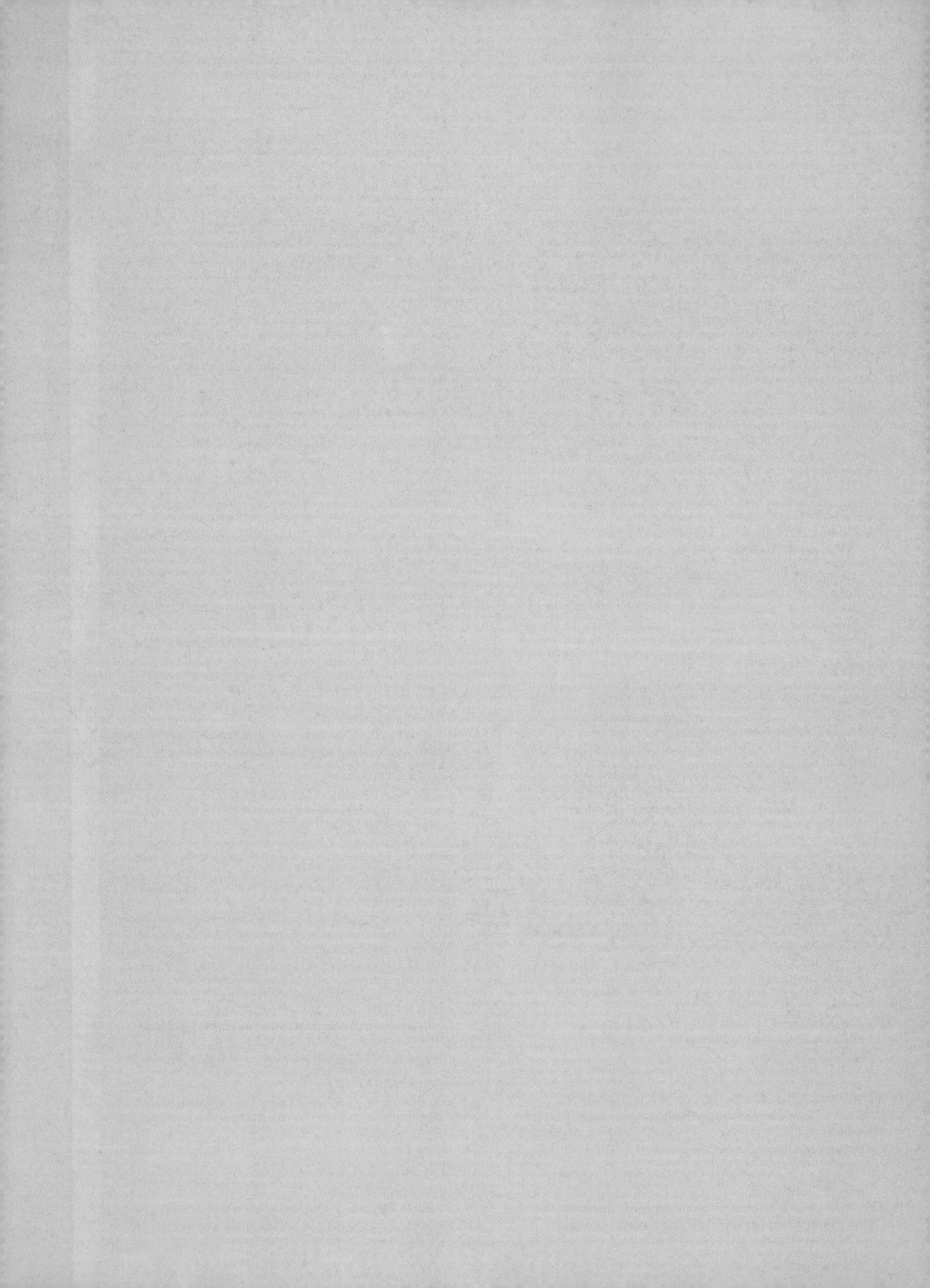

Assessment of Nutrition Status and Nutrition Requirements

141

Katherine Hammond Chessman and Vanessa J. Kumpf

KEY CONCEPTS

1. Malnutrition encompasses both overnutrition (obesity) and undernutrition.
2. Nutrition screening is distinct from assessment; it should be designed to quickly and consistently identify those with preexisting malnutrition or those at risk for malnutrition.
3. A comprehensive nutrition assessment is required to formulate a nutrition care plan for an individual found to be nutritionally-at-risk for nutrition-related poor outcomes.
4. A nutrition-focused physical examination and medical, surgical, and dietary history are essential components of a comprehensive nutrition assessment.
5. Evaluation of anthropometric measurements (weight, height, and head circumference) should be based on published standards.
6. Laboratory assessment of visceral proteins and other nutrition-related parameters must be interpreted in the context of physical findings, medical and surgical history, including acute and chronic inflammation, and clinical status.
7. Micronutrient or macronutrient deficiencies or toxicities or risk factors for these deficiencies or toxicities can be identified by a comprehensive nutrition assessment.
8. Evidence-based patient-specific goals should be established considering the patient's clinical condition and the need for maintenance or repletion in adults or continued growth and development in children.
9. Validated predictive equations are most often used to determine energy requirements; however, if available, indirect calorimetry is the most accurate bedside method to determine energy requirements.
10. Drug–nutrient interactions can affect nutrition status and the response to and adverse effects seen with drug therapy.

Nutrition care is a vital component of quality patient care and nutrition screening and assessment are integral parts of the nutrition care process. No single clinical or laboratory parameter is an absolute indicator of nutrition status, so information from a number of them must be collected and analyzed. This chapter reviews the tools most commonly used for accurate, relevant, and cost-effective nutrition screening and assessment, including various methods used to determine patient-specific macro- and micronutrient requirements and potential drug–nutrient interactions.

CLASSIFICATION OF NUTRITION DISEASE

1 Malnutrition is a consequence of nutrient imbalance. In general, deficiency states can be categorized as those involving protein and calories or single nutrients such as individual vitamins or trace elements. Starvation-associated malnutrition, marasmus, results from prolonged inadequate intake, absorption, or utilization of protein and energy. It occurs in patients with an inadequate food supply, anorexia nervosa, major depression, and malabsorption syndromes (Fig. 141-1). Somatic protein (skeletal muscle) and adipose tissue (subcutaneous fat) wasting occurs, but visceral protein (albumin [ALB] and transferrin [TFN]) production is usually preserved. Weight loss may exceed 10% of usual body weight (UBW; typical weight). Patients with starvation-associated malnutrition commonly have a prototypical wasted appearance.[1,2] Kwashiorkor, a form of starvation-associated malnutrition develops as a consequence of inadequate protein intake and is usually seen in areas where there is famine or limited food supply. In the United States, kwashiorkor has been seen in children and elderly individuals who are abused or neglected. Patients with kwashiorkor may not appear malnourished because of relative adipose tissue sparing, especially with mild undernutrition, but visceral (and to some degree somatic) protein stores are depleted, resulting in severe hypoalbuminemia and edema in more advanced cases. In patients with starvation-related malnutrition, enhancing nutritional intake or bypassing impaired absorption with specialized nutrition support can reverse the condition.[1,2]

Malnutrition can also develop as the result of an acute or chronic disease, especially those associated with mild-to-severe inflammation (see Fig. 141-1).[3,4] Patients with severe acute disease or injury (major infections, burns, trauma, and traumatic brain injury) or with chronic inflammatory diseases, organ failure, or cancer can develop disease-related malnutrition because of increased metabolic demands despite seemingly adequate nutrition intake. Individuals with starvation-related malnutrition can develop marked malnutrition when a severe injury or inflammatory process occurs simultaneously. In patients with disease-related, acute or chronic, malnutrition, simply providing nutrients in usual or even increased amounts may not be sufficient to reverse the nutrient imbalance. Regardless of the cause, undernutrition can result in changes in subcellular, cellular, or organ function that increase the individual's risks of morbidity and mortality.

Nutrition assessment can also be used to identify overnutrition: overweight and obese individuals and those at risk of becoming overweight or obese. Obesity is a major global healthcare concern: during 2011 to 2014, approximately 69% of U.S. adults were overweight (defined as a body mass index [BMI] greater than or equal to 25 kg/m^2)[5], and about 36.5% (82 million) were obese

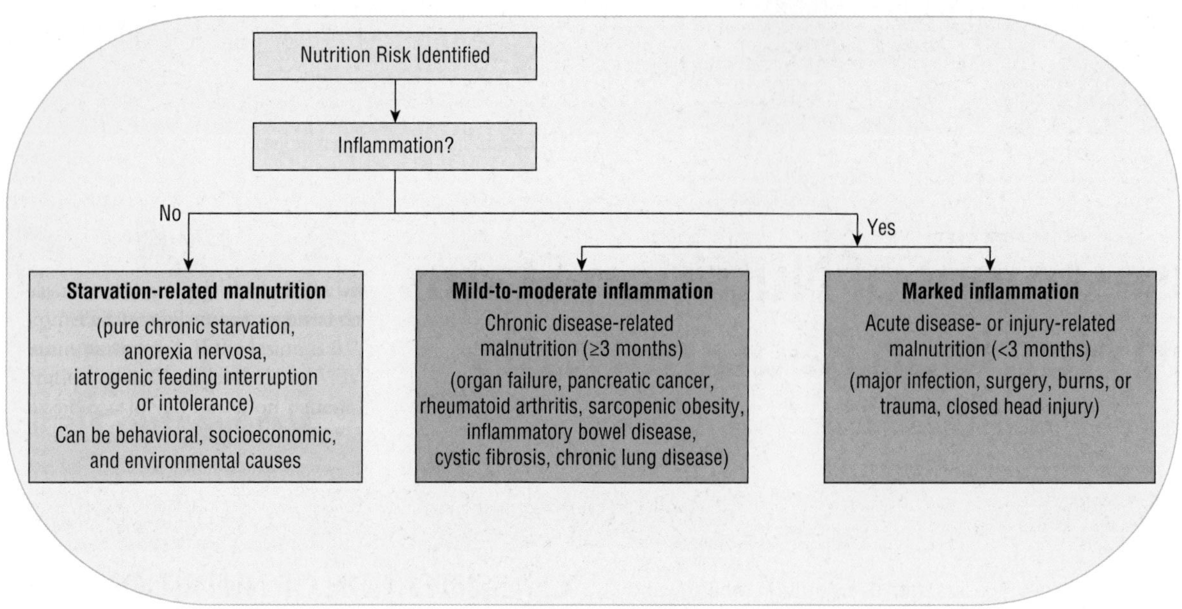

FIGURE 141-1 Etiologic basis for malnutrition diagnosis. (*Adapted from references 4 and 35.*)

(BMI greater than or equal to 30 kg/m^2).[6] Obesity prevalence in 2014 ranged from 21% in Colorado to about 36% in West Virginia, Arkansas, and Mississippi.[7] Additionally, 17% (12.7 million) of all U.S. children and adolescents (age 2-19 years) were obese (BMI greater than or equal to 95th percentile for age on the gender-appropriate BMI-for-age Centers for Disease Control and Prevention's [CDC] 2000 growth chart).[5,6,8] Many more children (approximately 32%) were overweight (BMI greater than or equal to 85th percentile for age).[5] Interestingly, there was no change in obesity prevalence among U.S. adults or children from 2011 to 2014 compared with 2003 to 2004.[6] After a steady increase in obesity prevalence since 1999, this leveling trend is encouraging. The consequences of obesity are numerous and include type 2 diabetes mellitus, cardiovascular disease, hypertension, and stroke (see Chapter 144).

Malnutrition is associated with higher morbidity and mortality rates in many settings. An effective nutrition screening program will consistently identify patients at nutrition-related risk alerting trained clinicians to perform a comprehensive nutrition assessment to accurately characterize baseline nutrition status, estimate nutrition needs, and develop a patient-specific nutrition care plan. Diligent monitoring of ongoing nutrition status can ensure that nutrition-related goals are being met and improve patient outcomes.

NUTRITION SCREENING

2 Nutrition screening is distinct from nutrition assessment.[9] It is not practical, cost-effective, or clinically warranted to conduct a comprehensive nutrition assessment on every individual; thus, nutrition screening provides a reliable, systematic method to identify persons for whom a detailed nutrition assessment is needed. A nutrition screen can be used to detect those who are overweight, obese, malnourished, or at risk for malnutrition; predict their health outcomes as a result of nutrition-related factors; and identify those who would benefit from nutritional intervention.

The ideal nutrition screening tool is quick, simple, and noninvasive and can be done by lay and healthcare providers in homes, long-term care facilities, ambulatory care clinics, and hospitals. Since 1995, the Joint Commission has included nutrition screening and assessment in its performance standards for accredited healthcare institutions.[10] Each entity must have a written nutrition screening process and criteria that determine when a more in-depth assessment will be performed. In hospitals, a nutrition screen must be completed within 24 hours of admission on all patients unless the institution's policy excludes certain patient populations. In hospitals, most screens are done by nurses.[11] For patients who are determined to be '*nutritionally-at-risk*' by the screening criteria, a comprehensive nutrition assessment must be completed within 48 to 72 hours. Periodic rescreening should occur at regular intervals determined by the institution and the patient population, usually every 3 to 7 days. Most nutrition assessments are completed by dietitians but may be completed by others including pharmacists with training in nutrition support.[11] For outpatients, nutrition screening should occur ideally at the first visit with a new provider and thereafter as warranted by the patient's condition.

Risk factor identification is the foundation of appropriate nutrition screening. Risk factors for undernutrition include recent unintended weight loss, presence and severity of acute and chronic disease states, drug and or other treatments, and socioeconomic factors that may result in a decreased nutrient intake or altered nutrient absorption, metabolism, or utilization. Risk factors for obesity include a family history of obesity, certain medical diagnoses (eg, polycystic ovary syndrome, Prader-Willi syndrome, and Cushing's syndrome), poor dietary habits, inadequate exercise, and some drug therapies. Various rating and classification systems have been proposed to screen for nutrition risk and guide subsequent interventions.[2,9,12–17] The Malnutrition Screening Tool (MST)[16] and the Subjective Global Assessment (SGA) are among the most frequently utilized.[17,18] In general, checklists of varying complexity are used to quantify a person's food and alcohol consumption habits; ability to buy, prepare, and eat food; weight history; diagnoses; medical and surgical procedures; drug therapies; and, history of specialized nutrition support (enteral or parenteral nutrition). Nutrition screening for children is based on the evaluation of growth parameters against the CDC or World Health Organization (WHO) growth charts[8,19] and the presence of medical conditions known to increase nutrition risk. Current estimates of the prevalence of in-hospital malnutrition for pediatric and adult patients, range from 13% to 88% depending on the patient population, disease severity, and the criteria used to identify its occurrence.[11] In any setting, patients determined to be nutritionally-at-risk should receive a timely comprehensive nutrition assessment to verify nutrition-related risk and to formulate a nutrition care plan with monitoring parameters to ensure that desired outcomes are met.

ASSESSMENT OF NUTRITION STATUS

3 A comprehensive nutrition assessment is the first step in formulating a patient-specific nutrition care plan. Goals of nutrition assessment include identification of the risk factors associated with malnutrition, including disorders resulting from macro- or micronutrient deficiencies (undernutrition), obesity (overnutrition), or impaired nutrient absorption, metabolism or utilization; determination of the risk of nutrition-related complications; estimation of nutrition needs; and establishment of baseline nutrition parameters against which to measure nutrition therapy outcomes. Nutrition assessment should include a nutrition-focused medical, surgical, and dietary history; a nutrition-focused physical examination, including anthropometrics; and laboratory measurements.

Nutrition-Focused History and Physical Examination

4 The nutrition-focused medical, surgical, and dietary history serves to identify factors that predispose to malnutrition (eg, prematurity, chronic diseases, gastrointestinal [GI] dysfunction, alcohol abuse, and acute or chronic inflammation [cancer, surgery, and trauma]), and overnutrition (eg, poor dietary habits, limited exercise, chronic disease, and family history). The clinician should determine any history of weight gain or loss (intended or unintended), anorexia, vomiting, diarrhea, decreased or restrictive food intake, including enteral or parenteral nutrition (Table 141-1).

The nutrition-focused physical examination should assess each body system for physical findings associated with nutrition-related problems, such as muscle wasting, edema, or loss of subcutaneous fat.[20,21] The presence of findings commonly associated with malnutrition such as alopecia, dermatitis, glossitis, cheilosis, or jaundice should be noted (Table 141-2). Additionally, nonspecific indicators of ongoing inflammation or stress (eg, fever and tachycardia) should be documented (Table 141-3).

The SGA is a representative example of a relatively simple, reproducible, cost-effective, bedside approach to nutrition assessment.[17,18] This screening tool assesses five aspects of the medical and dietary history: weight change in the previous 6 months, dietary changes, GI symptoms, functional capacity of the patient, and disease states known to affect nutrition status. Weight loss of less than 5% of UBW is considered a "small" loss, 5% to 10% loss is "potentially significant," and more than a 10% loss is "definitely significant."

TABLE 141-1 Pertinent Data from a Nutrition-Focused Medical, Surgical, and Dietary History

Nutrition intake and dietary habits
Anorexia
Unusual or absent taste
Dietary intake, including vegetarianism
Specialized diets, including enteral or parenteral nutrition
Supplemental vitamin, mineral, or herbal intake
Food allergies or intolerance
Underlying pathology with nutritional effects
Chronic infections or inflammatory states
Neoplastic diseases
Endocrine disorders
Chronic illness, including pulmonary disease, liver cirrhosis, and kidney failure
Hypermetabolic states, such as trauma, burns, and sepsis
Digestive or absorptive disease, nausea, vomiting, diarrhea, and constipation
Hyperlipidemia
End-organ effects
Weight changes
Skin or hair changes
Exercise intolerance or fatigue
Gastrointestinal tract symptoms such as diarrhea, vomiting, and constipation
Gastrointestinal surgery
Bariatric surgery
Small bowel or colon resection or diversion
Gastrectomy
Miscellaneous
Catabolic medications or therapies, including corticosteroids, immunosuppressive agents, radiation, or chemotherapy
Other medications, including diuretics, laxatives, antipsychotics, or anabolic steroids
Genetic background, including body habitus of parents, siblings, and family
Alcohol or drug abuse

Data from references 1, 2, 9, 12, and 15-18.

TABLE 141-2 Physical Examination Findings Suggestive of Malnutrition

General
Edema (especially ankle and sacral)
Cachexia or obesity
Ascites
Signs and symptoms of dehydration, including poor skin turgor, sunken eyes, orthostasis, or dry mucous membranes
Muscle wasting or loss of subcutaneous fat
Fever
Tachycardia
Alopecia/dry brittle hair
Skin and mucous membranes
Thin, shiny, dry, or scaly skin
Decubitus ulcers
Ecchymoses or perifollicular petechiae
Poor healing of surgical or traumatic wounds
Pallor or redness of gums or fissures at mouth edge
Glossitis, stomatitis, or cheilosis
Musculoskeletal
Retarded growth or short stature
Bone pain or tenderness or epiphyseal swelling
Muscle mass less than expected for habitus, exercise level
Neurologic
Ataxia, positive Romberg test result,[a] or decreased vibratory or position sense
Nystagmus
Seizures or paralysis
Encephalopathy
Failure to meet age-appropriate developmental milestones
Hepatic
Jaundice
Hepatomegaly

[a]The Romberg test is a neurologic test used to detect problems with balance.
Data from references 2, 9, 12, 13, and 15-22.

TABLE 141-3 Assessment of Inflammation

Laboratory Assessment	Clinical Findings	Acute/Chronic Disease States
Decreased	Fever	Cancer
Albumin	Hypothermia	Celiac disease
Transferrin	Infection	Cystic fibrosis
Prealbumin	Urinary tract	Inflammatory bowel disease
Nitrogen balance	Pneumonia	Organ failure
Elevated	Bacteremia	Pancreatitis
CRP	Wound/incision	Rheumatologic disorders
Glucose	Abscess	Rheumatoid arthritis
% neutrophils	Trauma	Systemic lupus erythematosus
Decreased or increased	Burns	
WBC		
Platelets		

CRP, C-reactive protein; WBC, white blood cell count.
Data from reference 4.

Dietary intake is characterized as normal or abnormal, and the duration and degree of abnormal intake are noted. The presence of daily GI symptoms (anorexia, nausea, vomiting, and diarrhea) for longer than 2 weeks is significant. Functional capacity assesses the patient's energy level and whether the patient is active or bedridden. Finally, disease state impact on metabolic demands (no, low, moderate, or high stress) is documented. Four physical examination findings are rated as normal, mild, moderate, or severe: loss of subcutaneous fat (triceps and chest), muscle wasting (quadriceps and deltoids), edema (ankle and sacral), and ascites. The patient's nutrition status is then rated as adequately nourished, moderately malnourished or suspected of being malnourished, or severely malnourished. Critics of the SGA find it time-consuming and complex.[2] Another example of a simple screening tool, the Mini Nutritional Assessment, has been used extensively in geriatric patients and found to be useful in several care settings.[2,22]

Anthropometric Measurements

5 Anthropometric measurements, which are physical measurements of the size, weight, and proportions of the human body, are important parameters used to assess nutrition status. Common measurements are weight, stature (standing height or recumbent length), head circumference (for children younger than 3 years of age), and waist circumference. Measurements of limb size, such as skinfold thickness, midarm muscle circumference, and wrist circumference, may be useful in selected individuals. Bioelectrical impedance analysis (BIA) is also an anthropometric assessment tool. An individual's body measurements can be compared with normative population standards to identify clinical concerns and may be repeated at various intervals to monitor response to a nutrition care plan. In adults, nutrition-related changes in anthropometric measurements tend to occur slowly; several weeks or more may be required before detectable changes are noted. In infants and young children, changes occur more quickly. Significant acute changes in weight and skinfold thickness usually reflect changes in hydration, which must be considered when interpreting these parameters.

Weight, Stature, and Head Circumference

Body weight is a nonspecific measure of body cell mass, representing skeletal mass, body fat, and the energy-using component lean body mass (LBM). Fat-free mass includes skeletal muscle, bone, connective tissue, organs, and water while fat mass includes the subcutaneous fat beneath the skin and the visceral (internal) fat. Change in weight over time, particularly in the absence of edema, ascites, or voluntary losses, is an important indicator of altered LBM. Actual body weight (ABW) interpretation should include consideration of ideal weight-for-height, referred to as ideal body weight (IBW), UBW (typical weight), fluid status, and age (Table 141-4). Patients

TABLE 141-4 Evaluation of Body Weight and Waist Circumference

Parameter	Interpretation	NHLBI Obesity Classification	Waist Circumference	
ABW compared with IBW				
ABW <69% IBW	Severe malnutrition			
ABW 70%-79% IBW	Moderate malnutrition			
ABW 80%-89% IBW	Mild malnutrition			
ABW 90%-120% IBW	Normal			
ABW >120% IBW	Overweight			
ABW ≥150% IBW	Obese			
ABW ≥200% IBW	Morbidly obese			
ABW compared with UBW				
ABW 85%-95% UBW	Mild malnutrition			
ABW 75%-84% UBW	Moderate malnutrition			
ABW <75% UBW	Severe malnutrition			
BMI (kg/m²)				
Adults				
<16	Severe malnutrition			
16-16.9	Moderate malnutrition			
17-18.9	Mild malnutrition			
19-24.9	Healthy		Disease risk above BMI-related risk[a]—Waist Circumference	
Older Adults 22-30	Healthy		Women ≤89 cm (35 in) Men ≤102 cm (40 in)	Women >89 cm (35 in) Men >102 cm (40 in)
25-29.9	Overweight		Increased	High
30-40	Moderate obesity			
30-34.9		I	High	Very high
35-39.9		II	Very high	Very high
>40	Severe or morbid obesity	III	Extremely high	Extremely high
Children				
BMI for age <5th percentile	Underweight			
BMI for age 5th-84th percentile	Healthy			
BMI for age 85th-94th percentile	Overweight			
BMI for age ≥95th percentile	Obese			

[a]Increased risk for Type 2 diabetes mellitus, hypertension, and cardiovascular disease.

ABW, actual body weight; BMI, body mass index; IBW, ideal body weight; NHLBI, National Heart, Lung, and Blood Institute; UBW, usual body weight.

Data from references 8, 13, 36, and 38-41.

who are dehydrated will have a decreased ABW but not a loss of LBM. Once rehydrated, these patients must be reweighed to establish a baseline weight for nutrition evaluation. Edema and ascites increase total body water (TBW), thus increasing ABW but not LBM. Because the ABW of patients with severe edema and ascites should not be used for nutrition assessment; practitioners often use an estimated "*dry weight*" to account for this increase in TBW. Both acute and chronic changes in fluid status can affect the ABW; these changes often can be detected by monitoring the patient's daily fluid intake and output. Accurate weight measurement can be difficult in critically ill patients because of their clinical condition and stress-related water retention.

The IBW is a population reference standard against which the ABW can be compared. IBW-for-height reference tables are available, and IBW can be calculated using mathematical equations based on gender and height. Using the Hamwi method, IBW is calculated as (48 kg [106 lb] + 2.7 kg [6 lb] × [inches over 5 feet]) for adult men and for adult women as (45 kg [100 lb] + 2.3 [5 lb] × [inches over 5 feet]).[23] Using the Devine equations, IBW is calculated as 50 kg + (2.3 × inches over 60 feet) for adult men and 45.5 kg + (2.3 × inches over 6 feet) for adult women.[24] For both equations, a range of ± 4.5 kg for large or small frame size is used for interpretation purposes. For obese adults, use of an adjusted ABW has been recommended for nutrition-related calculations, where adjusted ABW = ([ABW − IBW] × 0.25-0.5) + IBW.[25-27] The use of this adjusted ABW is not evidence-based because most of the metabolic rate equations were formulated using ABW in a mix of obese and non-obese individuals.[25,27,28] The IBW of a child can be calculated as ([height in cm]^2 × 1.65)/1,000. Alternatively, IBW-for-height can be determined by identifying the body weight corresponding to the same growth channel as the child's measured stature on the appropriate CDC or WHO growth chart. Comparison with the 50th percentile weight-for-age has been suggested but can be misleading if the child's height is not also at the 50th percentile.

Change in weight over time can be calculated as a percentage of UBW (see Table 141-4). Use of UBW as a reference point may provide a more accurate reflection of clinically significant weight changes over time. However, unless documented in the medical record, determining UBW depends on patient or family recall, which may be inaccurate. The use of UBW avoids the inherent problems with normative tables and documents comparative changes in body weight. All weight changes should be interpreted relative to time. Unintentional weight loss, especially rapid weight loss (5% of UBW in 1 month or 10% of UBW in 6 months), increases the risk of nutrition-related poor clinical outcomes.[13,14]

Adult stature is determined by both genetics and nutrition. In infants, recumbent length is measured; in older children and adults, a standing height is preferred. If a standing height cannot be measured, the measurement of demispan can be used to estimate height. Demispan is determined in a seated patient by measuring the distance from the sternal notch to the web between the middle and ring fingers along a horizontally outstretched arm with the wrist in neutral rotation and zero extension or flexion. Demispan may more accurately assess stature in elderly adults, especially those with kyphosis or vertebral collapse. After the demispan is measured, height is estimated using the following equations: women: height (cm) = (1.35 × demispan [cm]) + 60.1; men: height (cm) = (1.4 × demispan [cm]) + 57.8.[29] Knee height may also be used to estimate stature and is especially helpful in patients with limb contractures, such as patients with cerebral palsy.[29-31] Knee height is measured from just under the heel to the anterior surface of the thigh just proximal to the patella. Using the average of two measurements rounded to the nearest 0.1 cm, height can be estimated using the following equations: women: height (cm) = 84.88 (0.24 × age [years]) + (1.83 × knee height [cm]); men: height (cm) = 64.19 (0.04 × age [years]) + (2.02 × knee height [cm]).[31]

Appropriate growth is the best indicator of adequate nutrition in a child. At each medical encounter, weight, stature, head circumference (until 3 years), and BMI (after 2 years) should be plotted on the WHO (younger than 2 years) or CDC gender- and age-specific growth curves.[8,19] The CDC charts were revised in 2000 from U.S. data only and indicate how U.S. children grow. The WHO charts developed in 2006 are preferred in those younger than 2 years because they include data from infants from six industrialized countries including the United States who were predominantly breastfed for the first 4 months of life and who were receiving some breast milk at 12 months, conditions felt to ensure optimal growth.[19] Specialized charts are also available for assessment of short- and long-term growth of premature infants.[32,33] For premature infants with corrected postnatal age of 40 weeks or more, the WHO growth charts can be used; however, weight-for-age, length-for-age, and head circumference-for-age should be plotted according to corrected postnatal age until 2 years, 3.5 years, and 3 years of age, respectively.

Recommended intervals between measurements in young children are weight, 7 days; length, 4 weeks; height, 8 weeks; and head circumference, 7 days in infants and 4 weeks in children until 3 years of age. Growth velocity can be used to assess growth at intervals too close to plot accurately on a growth chart (Table 141-5). In newborns, average weight gain is 10 to 20 g/kg/day (24-35 g/day in term infants; 10-25 g/day in preterm infants). The rate of weight gain declines considerably after 3 months of age; children 6 to 10 years of age gain about 2 to 3 kg/yr. The adolescent 'growth spurt' typically begins at 9 to 10 years in girls and 11 to 12 years in boys. During the 11 to 13 year-old-interval of maximum growth in height, girls will gain about 10 kg (22 lb) while boys gain 15.5 kg (33 lb). Length increases rapidly in infancy (see Table 141-5). In children 6 to 10 years of age, height increases by 2 to 3 in/yr (approximately 5-7.5 cm/yr) and continues until about 16 to 18 years of age in girls and 18 to 20 years of age in boys. Head growth (measured by head circumference), usually 0.5 cm/wk (0.2 in/wk) during the first year of life, can be compromised during periods of critical illness or malnutrition. Rapid head growth, especially at a rate faster than expected, suggests hydrocephalus and should be further evaluated.

Failure to thrive (growth failure) in children has commonly been defined as weight-for-age, length-for-age, BMI-for-age, or weight velocity below the 5th percentile or a weight deceleration crossing two or more major percentiles (major percentiles are defined as 97th, 95th, 90th, 75th, 50th, 25th, 10th, 5th, and 3rd).[34] In children, a significant weight loss is defined as: greater than 2% in 1 week; greater than 5% in 1 month; greater than 7.5% in 3 months; and, greater than 10% in 6 months. Malnutrition can be defined by using z-scores for weight-for-length, BMI-for-age, or length- or

TABLE 141-5 Expected Growth Velocities in Term Infants and Children

Age	Weight (g/day)	Height (cm/mo)[a]
0-3 mo	24-35	2.8-3.4
4-6 mo	15-21	1.7-2.4
7-12 mo	10-13	1.3-1.6
1-3 yr	5-9	0.6-1
4-6 yr	5-6	0.5-0.6
7-10 yr	7-11	0.4-0.5

Example of growth assessment

Age: 2 mo; weight: 3.2 kg; weight at 1 mo of age, 3.1 kg; time since last weight was obtained: 30 days.

Growth velocity = ([3.2 kg−3.1 kg] × 1,000 g/kg)/30 days = 3.3 g/day.

Interpretation: suboptimal growth; comprehensive nutrition assessment needed.

[a]Growth velocity of 1 cm/mo is equivalent to 0.4 in/mo.

Data from references 8 and 19.

height-for age: -1, mild malnutrition -2, moderate malnutrition; and, -3, severe malnutrition.[35] Weight-for-height evaluation is age independent and helps differentiate a stunted child (chronic malnutrition) from a wasted child (acute malnutrition). Short stature can be associated with chronic undernutrition, but short stature in the absence of poor weight gain suggests another etiology, such as growth hormone deficiency or constitutional growth delay.

Body Mass Index

Body mass index can be calculated as either body weight in kilograms divided by height in meters squared (kg/m^2) or body weight in pounds multiplied by 703 divided by height in inches squared (lb/in^2). The 2013 AHA/ACC/TOS joint guideline for management of obesity in adults endorses using BMI as the first step but not the sole criterion, to judge potential health risk.[36] A BMI of 25 kg/m^2 or higher is considered a risk factor for premature death and disability. Health risks increase as the BMI increases; however, individual variation, especially in very muscular persons, can lead to erroneous classification of nutrition status when BMI alone is used. Thus, BMI should be interpreted based on characteristics such as sex, frame size, race/ethnicity, and age. For example, at the same BMI, a woman tends to have more body fat than a man, and an older adult would have more body fat than a younger one. Also, Asians may have more body fat than whites, especially at lower BMIs, and thus health risks may be associated with lower BMIs in individuals of Asian descent.[37]

In general, a BMI between 18.5 and 24.9 kg/m^2 is indicative of a healthy weight, between 25 kg/m^2 and 29.9 kg/m^2 signifies being overweight, and 30 kg/m^2 or higher indicates obesity (see Table 141-4).[13,36,38] These BMI classifications may not be appropriate for those older than 60 years, where a BMI between 25 kg/m^2 and 30 kg/m^2 is not associated with the same increased nutrition-related risks seen in younger individuals.[39,40] BMI has also been used to assess undernutrition (less than 18.5 kg/m^2 indicates undernutrition), but this relationship is not as well established.[13,38] Children 2 years of age and older are considered overweight if their BMI is at or above the 85th percentile on the age- and gender-specific CDC BMI chart and obese if the BMI is at or above the 95th percentile.[8] Use of these charts at each medical encounter helps to heighten awareness of children whose BMI and family history put them at risk for adult obesity and its associated complications.

Waist Circumference

Waist circumference is a simple measurement used to assess abdominal (visceral) fat. Extra weight around the waist rather than peripheral (subcutaneous) fat confers a greater health risk than extra weight around the hips and thighs. The larger the waist, the greater the risk of obesity-related complications, especially diabetes mellitus, cardiovascular disease, and all-cause mortality.[36,41] Waist circumference is determined by measuring the distance around the smallest area below the rib cage and the top of the iliac crest. Men are at increased risk (beyond the BMI-related risk) if the waist circumference is greater than 40 inches (102 cm); women are at increased risk if the waist circumference is greater than 35 inches (89 cm) (see Table 141-4); and children are at risk if the waist circumference is at the 75th percentile or greater (16-17-year-old girls) or 90th percentile (all others) according to CDC age- and gender-specific standards.[42]

Waist-to-Hip and Waist-to-Height Ratios

The waist-to-hip ratio is determined by dividing the waist circumference by the hip circumference (maximal posterior extension of the buttocks). In adults, a waist-to-hip ratio of greater than 0.9 in men and 0.85 in women is considered an independent risk factor for adverse health consequences.[41] Waist-to-height ratio (both measured in centimeters) has been used to evaluate children at risk for the metabolic syndrome because, unlike waist circumference, it is independent of age and gender. A child with a waist-to-height ratio of more than 0.5 is considered at risk for developing the metabolic syndrome.[43]

Skinfold Thickness and Mid-Arm Muscle Circumference

More than 50% of the body's fat is subcutaneous; thus, changes in subcutaneous fat reflect changes in total body fat. Skinfold thickness measurement provides an estimate of subcutaneous fat, and mid-arm muscle circumference, which is calculated using the skinfold thickness and mid-arm circumference, estimates skeletal muscle mass. Although simple and noninvasive, these anthropometric measurements are used most commonly in population analysis and long-term monitoring of individuals. Triceps skinfold thickness is used most often, but reference standards also exist for subscapular and suprailiac measurements.[44] Consistent technique in the use of pressure-regulated calipers is essential for reproducibility and reliability in measuring triceps skinfold thickness.[45] Standards do not account for variation in bone size, muscle mass, hydration, or skin compressibility, and they do not consider obesity, ethnicity, illness, and increased age. Results should be interpreted cautiously as these parameters change slowly in adults, often requiring weeks before significant alterations from baseline can be detected. They will change more rapidly in young children.

Bioelectrical Impedance

Bioelectrical impedance is a simple, quick (less than 15 minutes), noninvasive, portable, and relatively inexpensive technique used to measure body composition.[46,47] When a weak, alternating electric current is applied to two appendages (wrist and ankle or both feet), impedance (resistance) to flow is measured as it passes through the body. Current is well conducted by water and electrolyte-rich tissues such as blood and muscle and poorly conducted by fat, bone, and air-filled spaces. Assessment of LBM, TBW, and water distribution can be determined with BIA. Increased TBW decreases impedance; thus, it is important to evaluate hydration along with BIA. Other potential limitations of BIA include variability with electrolyte imbalance and interference by large fat masses, environment, ethnicity, menstrual cycle phase, and underlying medical conditions.[47] Although BIA equations have high validity when used in the population in which they were developed (mostly young healthy adults), BIA calculations are subject to considerable errors if applied to other populations and if conditions are not identical (eg, electrode placement must be identical).[47] The lack of reference standards that reflect variations in individual body size and clinical condition also limits BIA use in clinical practice.[46]

OTHER NUTRITION ASSESSMENT TOOLS

Functional status assessment has been recommended as part of nutrition assessment, but the specific components of this assessment are not well defined. Muscle function is an end-organ response; thus diminished skeletal muscle function can be a useful indicator of malnutrition. Muscle function also recovers more rapidly in response to adequate nutrition support than anthropometric measurements. Simple assessments of functional status include ability to perform activities of daily living, participate in physical and occupational therapy, and wean from the ventilator. Hand-grip strength (forearm muscle dynamometry), respiratory muscle strength, and muscle response to electrical stimulation also have been used. Measuring hand-grip strength is a relatively simple, noninvasive, and inexpensive procedure that correlates well with patient outcome.[48,49] Normative standards supplied by the manufacturer of the dynamometer can be used. Hand grip strength is a proxy for LBM making it a good parameter for assessment of undernutrition. However, conditions that limit hand grip strength include rheumatoid arthritis, stroke, neuromuscular disease, dementia, and heavy sedation. Ulnar nerve stimulation causes measurable muscle contraction and can be used in most intensive care units to monitor neuromuscular blockade. In malnourished patients, increased fatigue and a slowed muscle relaxation rate are noted; these indices return to normal with refeeding.

Other methods have been used to determine body composition in the research setting, including bioimpedance spectroscopy, dual energy x-ray absorptiometry (DXA), quantitative CT, air displacement plethysmography (BodPod®), three-dimensional photonic scanning, MRI, quantitative MRI, ultrasonography, and positron emission tomography.[47,50,51] These methods are complex and expensive to perform. DXA, best known for its use in measuring bone density, is a promising method for routine clinical practice because it can quantify mineral, fat, and LBM compartments and is available in most hospitals and many outpatient facilities. A central body DXA scanner requires a fair amount of space, and the cost depends on the scanner's complexity. Portable (or peripheral) DXA devices can be used to measure bone density in peripheral bones, such as the wrist, fingers, or heel, and have also been used to assess subcutaneous fat. Portable DXA scanners are much less expensive (about $10,000 compared to $80,000 for a central scanner) and can be used in community screenings. Further research is needed to determine how DXA can be used clinically in nutrition assessment. MRI and CT can measure subcutaneous, intra-abdominal, and regional fat distribution and thus also have the potential to be useful clinically.

Laboratory Assessment

6 Biochemically, LBM can be assessed by measuring the serum concentrations of the visceral proteins, ALB, TFN, and prealbumin (also known as transthyretin). C-reactive protein (CRP) can be useful as a marker of inflammation. Creatinine-height index has historically been calculated to assess LBM but is seldom used now because of the lack of evidence to support its value.

Visceral Proteins

Visceral proteins synthesized by the liver with the greatest relevance for nutrition assessments are serum ALB, TFN, and prealbumin. It is assumed that in undernutrition states, a low serum protein concentration reflects diminished hepatic protein synthetic mass and indirectly reflects the functional protein mass of other organs (heart, lung, kidney, and intestines). Many factors other than nutrition can affect serum concentrations of these proteins including age; abnormal kidney (nephrotic syndrome), GI tract (protein-losing enteropathy) or skin (burns) losses; hydration (dehydration results in hemoconcentration, overhydration in hemodilution); liver function (synthesis); and metabolic stress and inflammation (sepsis, trauma, surgery, and infection). Thus, visceral protein concentrations must be interpreted relative to the individual's overall clinical condition (Table 141-6). The significant influence of inflammation on visceral protein concentrations is now well established; thus these negative acute phase proteins may be considered to reflect the presence of inflammation more than the presence of malnutrition in many circumstances (see Table 141-3). Visceral protein concentrations for nutrition assessment are of greatest value in the presence of uncomplicated starvation and recovery. During severe acute stress (trauma, burns, and sepsis), these proteins are relatively poor markers of nutrition status because the resultant increased vascular permeability can lead to dramatic fluid shifts and the reprioritizing of liver protein synthesis increases the production of acute-phase reactants such as CRP, ferritin, fibrinogen, and haptoglobin.[52] CRP can be used in these cases to assess the degree of inflammation present: if CRP is elevated, then inflammation is a likely major contributing factor to decreased visceral protein concentrations. Assessing individual patient trends is most useful in these cases.

Albumin, the most abundant serum protein, is involved in maintenance of colloid oncotic pressure and binding and transport of numerous hormones, anions, drugs, and fatty acids. Although it has been widely used as a marker of chronic malnutrition, it is a relatively insensitive index of protein malnutrition because there is a large amount normally in the body (4-5 g/kg of body weight), it is extensively distributed in the extravascular compartment (60%), and it has a long half-life (18-20 days). However, chronic protein deficiency in the setting of adequate non-protein calorie intake leads to marked hypoalbuminemia because of a net ALB loss from the intravascular and extravascular compartments. Serum ALB concentrations also are affected by moderate-to-severe calorie deficiency and liver, kidney, and GI disease. ALB is a negative acute-phase reactant, and serum concentrations decrease with inflammation, infection, trauma, stress, and burns. Serum ALB concentrations less than 2.5 g/dL (25 g/L) can be expected to exacerbate ascites and peripheral, pulmonary, and GI mucosal edema as a result of decreased colloid oncotic pressure. Hypoalbuminemia also affects the interpretation of serum concentrations of calcium and highly protein bound drugs (eg, phenytoin and valproic acid).

Transferrin is a glycoprotein that binds and transports ferric iron to the liver and reticuloendothelial system for storage. Because it has a shorter half-life (8-9 days) and there is less of it in the body (less than 100 mg/kg of body weight), TFN will decrease in response to protein and energy depletion before the serum ALB concentration decreases. If a direct measure of serum TFN is not available, TFN concentration can be estimated indirectly from measurement of total iron-binding capacity, where TFN (in mg/dL) = (total iron-binding capacity [mcg/dL] × 0.8) – 43. Alternatively, TFN (mg/dL) = 0.7 × total iron-binding capacity (mcg/dL) and TFN (g/L) = 0.039 × total iron-binding capacity (μmol/L). TFN is also a negative acute-phase reactant, and its concentration is decreased in the presence of critical illness and inflammation. Iron stores also affect serum TFN concentrations: in iron deficiency, hepatic TFN synthesis is increased, resulting in increased serum TFN concentrations.

TABLE 141-6 Visceral Proteins Used for Assessment of Lean Body Mass

Serum Protein	Half-Life (Days)	Function	Factors Resulting in Increased Values	Factors Resulting in Decreased Values
Albumin	18-20	Maintains plasma oncotic pressure; transports small molecules	Dehydration, anabolic steroids, insulin, infection	Fluid overload; edema; kidney dysfunction; nephrotic syndrome; poor dietary intake; impaired digestion; burns; heart failure; cirrhosis; thyroid, adrenal, or pituitary hormones; trauma; sepsis
Transferrin	8-9	Binds Fe in plasma; transports Fe to bone	Fe deficiency, pregnancy, hypoxia, chronic blood loss, estrogens	Chronic infection, cirrhosis, burns, enteropathies, nephrotic syndrome, cortisone, testosterone
Prealbumin	2-3	Binds T_3 and, to a lesser extent, T_4; retinol-binding protein carrier	Kidney dysfunction	Cirrhosis, hepatitis, stress, surgery, inflammation, hyperthyroidism, cystic fibrosis, burns, zinc deficiency

T_3, triiodothyronine; T_4, thyroxine.

Prealbumin (transthyretin) is the transport protein for thyroxine and a carrier for retinol-binding protein. Prealbumin stores are low (10 mg/kg of body weight), and it has a very short half-life (2-3 days); thus, the serum prealbumin concentration may be reduced quickly after a significant reduction in calorie and protein intake (NPO status) or in patients with severe metabolic stress (trauma, burns). Prealbumin is most useful in monitoring the short-term, acute effects of nutrition support or deficits, as it responds very quickly in both situations. As with ALB and TFN, prealbumin synthesis is decreased in liver disease. Increased prealbumin concentrations may be seen in patients with kidney disease because of impaired excretion.

Clinical **Controversy...**

Serum visceral proteins (ALB, TFN, and prealbumin) have been used for many years as markers of nutrition status. With the growing recognition of the role that inflammation plays in the development of both acute and chronic malnutrition, the use of these visceral proteins as markers of malnutrition has been challenged. Assessing CRP concomitantly with these traditional visceral protein markers can assist the clinician in assessing their usefulness. However, the role of CRP in nutrition assessment requires further investigation.

Immune Function Tests

Nutrition status affects immune function either directly, via actions on the lymphoid system, or indirectly by altering cellular metabolism or organs that are involved with immune system regulation. Immune function tests most often used in nutrition assessment are the total lymphocyte count and delayed cutaneous hypersensitivity (DCH) reactions. Both tests are simple, readily available, and inexpensive. A lack of specificity, however, limits the usefulness of these tests as nutrition status markers.

Total lymphocyte count reflects the number of circulating T and B lymphocytes. Tissues that generate T cells are very sensitive to malnutrition, undergoing involution resulting in decreased T-cell production and eventually lymphocytopenia. A total lymphocyte count less than 1,500 cells/mm^3 (1.5 × 10^9 cells/L) has been associated with nutrition depletion.[2] Total lymphocyte count is reduced in the presence of infection (eg, human immunodeficiency virus [HIV], other viruses, and tuberculosis), immunosuppressive drugs (eg, corticosteroids, cyclosporine, tacrolimus, sirolimus, chemotherapy, and antilymphocyte globulin), leukemia, and lymphoma.

Delayed cutaneous hypersensitivity is commonly assessed using recall antigens to which the patient was likely previously sensitized, such as mumps and *Candida albicans*. Anergy is associated with severe malnutrition, and response is restored with nutrition repletion. Other immune function tests used in research include lymphocyte surface antigens (CD4, CD8, and the CD4:CD8 ratio), T-lymphocyte responsiveness, and various serum interleukin concentrations. A number of factors affect DCH, including fever, viral illness, recent live-virus vaccination, critical illness, irradiation, immunosuppressive drugs, diabetes mellitus, HIV, cancer, and surgery. Nutrients such as arginine, omega-3 fatty acids, and nucleic acids given in pharmacologic doses may improve immune function (see Chapter 143). Monitoring efficacy of a nutrition care plan that includes these potentially immune-modulating nutrients may include immune function assessment.

SPECIFIC NUTRIENT DEFICIENCIES AND TOXICITIES

7 A comprehensive nutrition assessment should include an evaluation for possible trace element, vitamin, and essential fatty acid deficiencies (EFAD) or toxicities. Because of their key role in metabolic processes (coenzymes and cofactors), a deficiency of any of these nutrients may result in altered metabolism and cell dysfunction. An accurate history to identify symptoms and risk factors for a specific nutrient deficiency or toxicity is critical. A nutrition-focused physical examination and biochemical assessment to confirm a suspected deficiency or toxicity should be done in all nutritionally-at-risk patients. Ideally, biochemical assessment would be based on the nutrient's function (eg, metalloenzyme activity) rather than simply measuring the serum concentration. Unfortunately, few practical methods to assess micronutrient function are available; thus, the nutrient's serum concentration is most often measured (Table 141-7).

Trace Elements

The trace elements that are essential in humans (at least one important role and a range of intakes within which homeostasis is maintained) are zinc, copper, manganese, selenium, chromium, iodine, molybdenum, and iron.[53-58] Each trace element is involved in a variety of biologic functions and is necessary for normal metabolism, serving as a coenzyme or playing a role in hormonal metabolism or erythropoiesis. Toxicities can occur with excess intake of some trace elements. With the current interest in complementary medicine, clinicians must ask patients about their use of all dietary supplements (see Table 141-7).

Iron is the most abundant trace element and is an important component of hemoglobin, myoglobin, and cytochrome enzymes; it is also involved in oxygen transport and cellular energy production. Patients with iron-deficiency anemia generally present with fatigue, weakness, and pallor, but they may have other symptoms (see Chapter 100). Inadequate iron intake, malabsorption, and blood loss are the principal causes of iron-deficiency anemia. Iron toxicity (overload) with possible organ damage can occur when chronic iron intake exceeds requirements, such as in patients receiving multiple blood transfusions over an extended period of time (1 unit of packed red blood cells provides 200 mg elemental iron). Iron deficiency or overload is confirmed by assessment of body iron stores, as reflected indirectly by measurement of hemoglobin, serum iron, total iron-binding capacity, and serum ferritin or directly by bone marrow staining or liver biopsy. Direct methods are the most accurate but are invasive and rarely necessary. Because indirect parameters may be altered by acute or chronic illness independent of iron stores, concomitant illness must be considered in their interpretation.[54,56]

Zinc, the second-most abundant trace element, is a cofactor in many enzymatic reactions involved in protein, fat, and carbohydrate metabolism and is involved in the regulation of gene expression, wound healing, and liver regeneration.[54,56,59] Most of the body's zinc (85%) is found in muscle and bone; less than 1% is found in the serum. Excess zinc intake is usually eliminated by the kidneys and GI tract; thus, zinc toxicity is uncommon except in overdoses. Patients at risk for zinc deficiency include those with anorexia, alcohol dependence, excessive bile, intestinal, or urine losses, increased metabolic demands (burns) or after bariatric surgery.[59] Zinc deficiency can develop in 14 days to 3 months with insufficient intake and is characterized by skin lesions (acrodermatitis enteropathica), a moist eczematous dermatitis that is most apparent in the nasolabial folds and around orifices, and other symptoms (see Table 141-7). Recovery is rapid with oral zinc supplementation; severe dermatitis can remit in as little as 4 to 5 days.[58] Zinc deficiency can be documented by the presence of low serum zinc concentrations.[53,59] However, serum zinc concentrations decrease during acute stress states (trauma, burns, and infection) and generally remain depressed until the stress resolves. Hair zinc analysis and urinary zinc excretion can also be used as biomarkers of zinc status.

Copper is a cofactor in oxidative enzymes vital to the function of hematopoietic, vascular, and skeletal tissue, as well as structure and function of the nervous system.[60-62] It is a component of ceruloplasmin and key metalloenzymes involved in iron metabolism

TABLE 141-7 Assessment of Trace Element Status

Trace Element	Signs of Deficiency	Signs of Toxicity	Factors Associated with Altered Plasma Concentrations	Monitoring
Chromium	Impaired glucose/protein utilization, peripheral neuropathy, low RQ, weight loss, increased LDL-C, increased free fatty acid concentrations	Industrial exposure: skin or nasal septum lesions, allergic dermatitis, increased incidence of lung cancer	**Decreased**: long-term inadequate intake **Increased**: kidney failure	Serum glucose, plasma chromium (unreliable)
Copper	Menkes' syndrome: progressive mental deterioration, vomiting, diarrhea, protein-losing enteropathy, hypopigmentation, bone and hair changes Deficiency: neutropenia, hypochromic anemia, pallor, dermatitis, neurological dysfunction, osteoporosis, myopathy, thrombocytopenia, decreased bone mineralization (children)	Wilson's disease: cirrhosis, Kayser-Fleischer rings,[a] kidney dysfunction, neurologic or psychiatric symptoms (tremors, slow speech, inappropriate behavior, personality changes) Mild chronic toxicity: fatigue, anemia, thrombocytopenia Acute toxicity: nausea, vomiting, diarrhea	**Decreased**: high zinc, iron, or vitamin C intake; corticosteroid use **Increased**: infection, rheumatoid arthritis, pregnancy, oral contraceptives, decreased biliary excretion	Serum copper and ceruloplasmin with CRP[b], CBC
Iodine	Hypothyroid goiter, neuromuscular impairment, deaf-mutism, increased embryonic and postnatal mortality, cognitive impairment, impaired fertility, congenital hypothyroidism (severe cases)	Thyrotoxicosis: nodular goiter, weight loss, tachycardia, muscle weakness, warm skin	**Decreased**: long-term inadequate intake	Serum T3,T4,TSH
Iron	Microcytic, hypochromic anemia (weakness, pallor, fatigue), glossitis, headache, dysphasia, nail changes, gastric atrophy, paresthesia, decreased cognitive function	Cirrhosis, cardiomyopathy, pancreatic damage, skin pigmentation changes	**Increased**: blood transfusion **Decreased**: blood loss; long-term iron-free PN	Serum ferritin[c], iron, percent iron saturation, iron binding capacity; CBC
Manganese	Nausea; vomiting; dermatitis; hair color changes; hypocholesterolemia; growth retardation; defective carbohydrate, lipid, and protein metabolism	Parkinsonian-like symptoms, hyperirritability, hallucinations, libido disturbances, ataxia, mental confusion, lack of attention, memory loss, weakness, seizures, facial nerve abnormalities, headache, dizziness, dystonia, peripheral neuropathy	**Increased**: decreased biliary excretion, high iron or vitamin C intake	Whole blood manganese, brain MRI
Molybdenum	Tachycardia, tachypnea, altered mental status, visual changes, headache, nausea, vomiting	Gout-like syndrome, increased urinary copper	**Decreased**: low birth weight, excessive GI losses	Urinary hypoxanthine, xanthine, and sulfite oxidase
Selenium	Muscle weakness or pain, cardiomyopathy, skin and hair pigmentation changes, macrocytosis, alopecia and growth retardation in infants	Nausea, vomiting, hair or nail loss, tooth decay, skin lesions, irritability, fatigue, peripheral neuropathy	**Decreased**: malignancy, liver failure, pregnancy, stress, infection **Increased**: reticuloendothelial-neoplasia	Plasma, serum, or whole blood selenium, RBC glutathione peroxidase; CBC
Zinc	Dermatitis (scaly, hyperpigmented skin lesions), stomatitis, glossitis, perioral and periungual ulceration, altered taste and smell, alopecia, diarrhea, apathy, depression, growth retardation, impaired wound healing, anorexia, confusion, immunosuppression, delayed sexual maturation, hypogonadism (decreased sperm count and function)	Acute: diarrhea, vomiting, nausea, dizziness, garlic-smelling breath; death with large IV doses Chronic: immunosuppression, decreased HDL-C, copper deficiency	**Decreased**: infection, burns, stress, hypoalbuminemia, corticosteroids, pregnancy, inflammation **Increased**: tissue injury, hemolysis, contaminated collection tube	Plasma or serum zinc with albumin and CRP, stool or ostomy output

CBC, complete blood count; CRP, C-reactive protein; GI, gastrointestinal; HDL-C, high-density-lipoprotein cholesterol; LDL-C, low-density-lipoprotein cholesterol; MRI, magnetic resonance imaging; PN, parenteral nutrition; RBC, red blood cell; RQ, respiratory quotient; TSH, thyroid stimulating hormone.

[a]Kayser-Fleischer rings are dark rings that appear to encircle the iris of the eye.

[b]If CRP > 4 mg/dL (> 40 mg/L), serum copper concentration will be falsely elevated. Ceruloplasmin increased with inflammation, pregnancy, liver disease, malignancy, and myocardial infarction.

[c] If ferritin low, iron deficiency; if high, inflammation.

Data from references 13, 20, 53, 54, 56-58, and 61.

(ceruloplasmin), electron transport and energy metabolism (cytochrome oxidase), connective tissue and collagen cross-linking (lysyl oxidase, elastase, and monoamine oxidase), and free radical scavenging (superoxide dismutase), among other functions. Copper is absorbed in the duodenum and excreted through the bile bound to bile salts. Most copper (67%) is found in bone and muscle, and 60% to 95% of serum copper is bound to ceruloplasmin.[62] Signs and symptoms of copper deficiency are listed in Table 141-7 and include anemia, neutropenia, and thrombocytopenia, and neurologic dysfunction. In severe cases, such as in Menkes' syndrome, copper deficiency is further manifested as hypothermia, hair and skin depigmentation, progressive mental deterioration, and growth retardation. Factors predisposing to copper deficiency include generalized malabsorption, protein-losing enteropathy, nephrotic syndrome, and copper-free parenteral nutrition.[60,62] Patients undergoing bariatric surgery are also at risk for developing copper deficiency as early as 2 months after surgery. Resolution typically occurs within 1 to 3 weeks after initiation of copper supplementation (1 mg/day). Copper deficiency is assessed using serum copper concentrations along with CRP and ceruloplasmin, which appear to reflect changes in copper status in both copper-depleted and copper-replete individuals.[61] While they are reliable indicators of severe copper deficiency, serum copper and ceruloplasmin concentrations may not detect marginal copper deficiency because serum concentrations may be altered by a variety of conditions including inflammation (see Table 141-7). Copper concentrations should be monitored routinely in patients receiving long-term parenteral nutrition. While long-term parenteral nutrition supplemented with copper increases the risk of copper toxicity, copper deficiency has been reported as a result of copper-free parenteral nutrition most often because of concern for accumulation with cholestasis and the resulting decrease in biliary elimination.[62] The chronic ingestion of excessive copper or inadequate elimination can result in cirrhosis as seen in Wilson's disease, an autosomal-recessive genetic disorder. Copper concentrations should be monitored every 2 to 6 months in patients receiving long-term parenteral nutrition.

Trivalent chromium is needed for insulin function and maintenance of normal blood glucose concentrations. A low-molecular-weight chromium binding substance, "*the glucose tolerance factor*", may enhance insulin receptor response to insulin.[63] Chromium is stored in the liver, spleen, soft tissues, and bones and excreted by the kidney. Chromium deficiency is characterized by glucose intolerance, increased insulin requirements, and impaired protein utilization. Patients with chromium deficiency also may have increased free fatty acid concentrations and a low respiratory quotient (RQ) (see Table 141-7). Chromium deficiency has only been identified in patients receiving long-term chromium-free parenteral nutrition. Serum chromium concentrations do not accurately reflect total body chromium status, presumably because the biologically active form of chromium is the low-molecular-weight chromium binding substance. Toxicity from trivalent chromium is not a common clinical concern; toxicity has been reported only with contaminated drinking water or industrial exposure. Chromium supplementation as an adjunct to aerobic exercise for weight loss has not been proven effective[64] (see Chapter 142).

Manganese is needed for the proper function of metalloenzymes, including arginase (amino acid metabolism via the urea cycle), pyruvate carboxylase and phosphoenolpyruvate carboxykinase (carbohydrate and cholesterol metabolism), superoxide dismutase (mitochondrial antioxidant), glycosyltransferases (bone formation via proteoglycans), and prolidase (wound healing).[54,56] Excess manganese is eliminated mainly in bile. Manganese deficiency has only been reported in association with the ingestion of chemically defined manganese-deficient oral diets. Table 141-7 lists common symptoms associated with manganese deficiency. Manganese toxicity is more concerning and has been described in industrial exposures via inhaled manganese and in patients receiving long-term manganese-supplemented parenteral nutrition in the setting of chronic cholestasis.[65-68] Manganese can accumulate in brain tissue and the newborn brain may be more susceptible to the effects of manganese toxicity.[66] Increased signal intensity on T1-weighted MRI of the globus pallidus has been found in patients with manganese toxicity. Whole-blood manganese concentrations are used to assess manganese status; serum concentrations do not correlate with either whole blood concentrations or MRI.[67] Clinical toxicity is evidenced primarily by extrapyramidal symptoms mimicking Parkinson's disease, such as headache, dizziness, tremors, ataxia, facial muscle spasms, and other symptoms.[54,65] These symptoms may be preceded by psychiatric symptoms, including irritability, aggressiveness, and hallucinations. In most reported cases, removing manganese from the parenteral nutrition solution resulted in resolution of neurologic symptoms within 6 months with partial or total normalization of the MRI after 1 to 2 years.

Selenium is incorporated into at least 25 enzymes known as selenoproteins, about half of which have a defined metabolic function. Important selenoproteins include selenoprotein P (antioxidant activity), glutathione peroxidase (antioxidant activity), iodothyronine deiodinase (thyroid hormone regulation), thioredoxin reductase (vitamin C), selenoprotein V (spermatogenesis), and selenoprotein S (inflammation and immune response).[54,56,69] Selenoprotein P is the major (60%) circulating form of selenium in serum. A key metabolic function of selenium is its role in the enzymatic cofactor selenocysteine, the 21st amino acid.[56] Prematurity, critical illness, chronic GI losses, and long-term selenium-free parenteral nutrition are associated with low serum selenium concentrations and decreased glutathione peroxidase activity.[54,56,69] The clinical significance of reduced serum selenium concentrations is unclear, but low selenium concentrations may increase susceptibility to physiologic stressors. Although critically ill patients require higher selenium intakes than normal, the optimal intake is unknown. Current recommendations range from 20 to 1,000 mcg/day.[70] Low serum selenium concentrations in critically ill patients correlate with low triiodothyronine (T_3) concentrations.[70] Serum selenium concentrations reflect acute distribution between tissues rather than selenium stores. Selenium deficiency is associated with muscle pain, wasting, and weakness (see Table 141-7), but severe biochemical deficiency is not always accompanied by these symptoms. Fatal cardiomyopathy has been reported in several cases.

Serum, erythrocyte, and whole-blood selenium, serum selenoprotein P, and serum, platelet, and whole-blood glutathione peroxidase activity respond to changes in selenium intake, but the response is heterogeneous.[69] Decreased serum selenium concentrations may indicate selenium deficiency, but reductions have also been observed in patients with malignancies, liver failure, pregnancy, alcoholism, and HIV; in patients receiving statins or corticosteroids; and in smokers. Selenium toxicity (selenosis) generally occurs only in those with long-term exposure to foods grown in selenium-rich soil (eg, U.S. Great Plains area) and may occur when intake exceeds 400 mcg/day for prolonged periods; although, the lowest reported adverse event intake is 850 mcg/day. Selenium toxicity results in hair and nail brittleness and loss, GI disturbance, skin rash, garlic breath odor, fatigue, irritability, and nervous system abnormalities.

Molybdenum is a cofactor for enzymes involved in catabolism of sulfur-containing amino acids, purines, and pyrimidines (xanthine, aldehyde, and sulfite oxidases).[54,56,71] Molybdenum deficiency is uncommon, but a rare genetic defect that prevents sulfite oxidase synthesis resulting in molybdenum deficiency has been identified. One case of molybdenum deficiency has been reported in a patient receiving long-term molybdenum-free parenteral nutrition who presented with symptoms that included tachycardia, tachypnea, headache, night blindness, nausea, vomiting, central scotomas, lethargy, disorientation, and ultimately coma (see Table 141-7). Symptoms were reversed when molybdenum was added to the parenteral nutrition solution.[72] Factors predisposing to molybdenum deficiency appear to be low birth weight,[73] excessive GI losses, and long-term inadequate intake. Biochemical abnormalities expected in molybdenum deficiency include very low serum and urine uric acid concentrations (low xanthine oxidase activity) and low urine inorganic sulfate concentrations with high urine inorganic sulfite concentrations (low sulfate oxidase activity).[71] Molybdenum toxicity has not been described.

Iodine is found primarily in the thyroid gland (70%-80%). Iodine deficiency may result in goiter formation (see Chapter 75). However, not everyone with an iodine-deficient diet will develop a goiter. Measurement of thyroxine (T_4), T_3, and TSH (thyroid stimulating hormone) can be used to assess iodine status (see Table 141-7). Intravenous iodine supplementation is not necessary except during long-term parenteral nutrition with minimal enteral intake. Iodine needs may be met by consumption of iodized salt or cutaneous iodine absorption from povidone–iodine, a topical antiseptic, used in catheter care. Use of povidone–iodine for this indication has virtually been eliminated with increased chlorhexidine use for catheter care, putting long-term parenteral nutrition patients at higher risk. Iodine excess is rarely a clinical concern when thyroid and kidney functions are normal except in overdoses.

Vitamins

Vitamins act as both catalysts (cofactors) and substrates in essential metabolic reactions. A comprehensive nutrition-focused history and physical examination is the most valuable means of assessing patients for vitamin deficiency or toxicity (**Table 141-8**). A thorough review of vitamins and their complex effects on nutrition and metabolism is beyond the scope of this chapter.[56,57,74,75] Generalized malnutrition is often associated with multiple vitamin deficiencies or increased needs; however, single vitamin deficiencies do occur. Thiamine (B_1) deficiency can result in early symptoms (dry or wet beriberi and GI symptoms) or advanced symptoms (lactic acidosis, Wernicke's encephalopathy, polyneuropathy, ataxia, and mental confusion) due to impaired oxidative and energy metabolism often leading to serious and potentially irreversible neurological damage or death.[56,76] Macrocytic anemia, peripheral neuropathy, and neuropsychiatric sequelae are also caused by vitamin B_{12} (cyanocobalamin) deficiency which can occur after gastric or ileal resection. Vitamin B_{12} deficiency has been reported with increasing frequency in adults, especially with prolonged gastric acid suppression.[77] There is a high prevalence of subclinical vitamin K deficiency in patients with chronic kidney disease, including those on hemodialysis or peritoneal dialysis. Vitamin K deficiency is a modifiable risk factor for cardiovascular disease and bone fracture in this patient population.[78]

The increasing prevalence of vitamin D deficiency is a worldwide concern, including all ages, genders, and racial/ethnic groups, especially children, elderly adults, individuals with dark skin, invalids and shut-ins, patients on long-term parenteral nutrition, and those living in temperate and higher latitudes.[79,80] Laboratory assessment can confirm the clinical suspicion of a deficiency state. Vitamins D2 (ergocalciferol) and D3 (cholecalciferol) are quickly converted to 25-OH-vitamin D via hydroxylation in the liver. The best marker for vitamin D deficiency is the serum concentration of 25-OH-vitamin D. Reference ranges for U.S. laboratories are typically 20 to 100 ng/mL (50-250 nmol/L) but the optimal range is likely above 30 ng/mL (75 nmol/L) based on the concentration associated with parathyroid hormone (PTH) stimulation and calcium absorption efficiency.[79] The first indication of a deficiency is usually a decrease in circulating serum concentrations of 25-OH-vitamin D. Subsequently, there is a decrease in urinary excretion of vitamin D, which is followed by diminished tissue concentrations. Because 1,25-$(OH)_2$-vitamin D is produced only when needed, not stored, and dependent on kidney function, intact PTH concentration, and calcium and phosphorus supply, it is not a useful marker of vitamin D deficiency (see Table 141-8; see Chapter 44)

Vitamin toxicity can occur, especially with fat-soluble vitamins (A, D, E, and K), which are stored in the body. Excessive dietary vitamin A intake (hypervitaminosis A) is linked to an increased risk of hip fractures in both men and women.[81,82] Vitamin D toxicity can cause significant hypercalcemia. With the exception of cyanocobalamin, which is stored in the liver, water-soluble vitamins are not stored in the body; consequently, the toxicity risk is minimal unless ingested in very high doses. Recent evidence, however, suggests that even water-soluble vitamins may be associated with adverse events when taken chronically in high doses. Although folic acid administration is definitively associated with a reduction in neural tube defects, its effect on some cardiac outcomes (as a result of its effect on homocysteine concentrations) is not established.[83] The administration of folic acid, vitamin B_6 (pyridoxine), and vitamin B_{12} after coronary artery stenting has been associated with an increased risk of stent restenosis.[84] With Americans' current use of nutrition supplements, clinicians should be alert for signs of hypervitaminosis (see Table 141-8) and inappropriate vitamin use and discuss rational supplement use with all patients.

Essential Fatty Acids

The human body can synthesize all fatty acids except the essential fatty acids, linoleic acid (an omega-6 fatty acid) and α-linolenic acid (an omega-3 fatty acid). Essential fatty acid deficiency (EFAD) can be prevented if approximately 5% of total calories are ingested as these fatty acids.[85,86] EFAD is rare in adults and children but can occur with prolonged use of lipid-free parenteral nutrition, severe fat malabsorption, very low-fat enteral feeding formulations or diets, high medium chain triglyceride-containing diets, and severe malnutrition, especially in stressed patients. Although the time course to develop EFAD is variable, overt EFAD has been shown to occur after 4 weeks of lipid-free parenteral nutrition, and biochemical evidence can occur within 1 week.[86] Because newborns, especially those born prematurely, have limited fat stores, they may develop EFAD more rapidly than adults. Biochemical evidence of EFAD has been noted within 72 hours after birth in preterm infants receiving fat-free intravenous solutions.[87] Symptoms of EFAD include dermatitis (dry, cracked, and scaly skin), alopecia, impaired wound healing, growth failure, thrombocytopenia, and anemia.

Linoleic acid is converted to arachidonic acid (20:4ω-6; a tetraene fatty acid). When linoleic acid is unavailable, oleic acid (18:1ω-9) is the preferred substrate, resulting in production of eicosatrienoic acid (20:3ω-9; a triene fatty acid). Thus, EFAD is associated with decreased tetraene and increased triene production. The usual ratio of trienes to tetraenes is less than 0.4; a ratio of greater than 0.2 indicates subclinical EFAD, but clinical symptoms of EFAD are generally only seen when the ratio is greater than 0.4.[88] EFAD diagnosis is generally made based on risk assessment and clinical findings with confirmation by measuring serum fatty acid concentrations.

Carnitine

Carnitine is a quaternary amine required for transport of long-chain fatty acids into the mitochondria for β-oxidation and energy production. Additionally, acyl compounds that are trapped within cells due to cell membrane impermeability to them can be esterified with carnitine and transported out of the cell, aiding in their elimination (detoxification), especially when the acyl compounds accumulate to inhibitory or toxic concentrations. Carnitine is available from a wide variety of dietary sources (especially meats) and can be synthesized by the liver and kidneys from lysine and methionine. Hepatic synthesis is decreased in premature infants, and low serum carnitine concentrations and overt carnitine deficiency have been documented in premature infants receiving carnitine-free parenteral nutrition or diets, as well as in those with inborn errors of carnitine metabolism.[89] Other predisposing factors for carnitine deficiency include chronic kidney[90] or liver disease,[89] chronic valproic acid[89] and zidovudine use,[91] and a vegetarian diet. The clinical presentation of carnitine deficiency includes generalized skeletal muscle weakness, hypotonia, failure-to-thrive, fasting hypoglycemia, encephalopathy, and coma.[89]

Although tissue concentrations, especially muscle, are higher than serum concentrations, in clinical practice, carnitine status is most often assessed by measurement of serum total and free

TABLE 141-8 Assessment of Vitamin Status

Vitamin	Signs of Deficiency	Laboratory Assay	Comments
Water-Soluble Vitamins			
Thiamine (B_1)	Early: anorexia, fatigue, depression, impaired memory or concentration Late: paresthesia, nystagmus, GI beriberi (nausea, vomiting, abdominal pain, lactic acidosis), beriberi (heart failure, edema), Wernicke's encephalopathy, Korsakoff's psychosis, peripheral neuropathy	Whole blood or erythrocyte transketolase activation test Blood thiamine pyrophosphate Erythrocyte glutathione reductase activity coefficient	Increased need with hemo- and peritoneal dialysis, alcoholism, malabsorption, hypermetabolism
Riboflavin (B_2)	Mucositis, dermatitis, cheilosis, glossitis, photophobia, corneal vascularization, lacrimation, decreased vision, impaired wound healing and growth, normocytic anemia	Urine riboflavin	
Pantothenic acid	Fatigue, malaise, headache, insomnia, vomiting, abdominal cramps	Serum pantothenic acid	
Niacin	Pellagra: dermatitis, dementia, glossitis, diarrhea, memory loss, headaches	Urine niacin and N_1-methylnicotinamide Erythrocyte NAD and NADP concentrations to determine "niacin number"	Flushing, nausea, and vomiting seen with hyperlipidemia treatment; increased need with hemo- and peritoneal dialysis
Pyridoxine (B_6)	Pellagra, dermatitis, glossitis, cheilosis, distal limb numbness or paresthesia, convulsions, microcytic anemia	Plasma pyridoxal 5-phosphate Urine 4-pyridoxic acid	Sensory neuropathy and seizures with very high doses (>2 g/day)
Folic acid	Macrocytic anemia, diarrhea, glossitis, cheilosis, angular stomatitis, fatigue, difficulty concentrating, irritability, headache, palpitations, shortness of breath, heart failure, tachycardia, postural hypotension, lactic acidosis, neural tube defects, impaired cellular immunity, paranoid behavior	Serum or plasma folate (acute) Red blood cell folate (chronic) Serum homocysteine	Decreased with increased cellular/tissue turnover (pregnancy, malignancy, hemolytic anemia); masks diagnosis of vitamin B_{12} deficiency; decreases risks of neural tube defects
Cyanocobalamin (B_{12})	Pernicious (megaloblastic) anemia, glossitis, spinal cord degeneration, peripheral neuropathy, paresthesias, pancytopenia, personality changes, dementia, depression, psychosis	Serum cobalamin Plasma homocysteine Urine or plasma methylmalonic acid[a] CBC	Decreased absorption in the elderly, distal ileal resection, loss of gastric intrinsic factor due to gastrectomy or long-term gastric acid suppression
Biotin	Dermatitis, depression, lassitude, somnolence	Urine biotin	
Ascorbic acid (C)	Enlargement or keratosis of hair follicles, impaired wound healing, anemia, lethargy, depression, bleeding, ecchymosis, scurvy	Plasma ascorbic acid Leukocyte ascorbate	GI disturbances, hyperoxaluria and kidney stones, excess iron absorption with excess intake; smokers need 35 mg/day more than nonsmokers; rebound scurvy with abrupt discontinuation after long-term high doses
Fat-Soluble Vitamins			
Vitamin A (includes retinol, retinal, retinoic acid, and retinyl esters)	Dermatitis, night blindness, xerophthalmia, Bitot spots,[b] pruritus, follicular hyperkeratosis, excessive deposition of periosteal bone, hair changes, poor growth and wound healing, impaired resistance to infection Irreversible: punctate keratopathy, keratomalacia, corneal perforation	Serum retinol Serum retinol-binding protein Serum retinyl esters (toxicity)	Teratogenic, liver toxicity with excessive intake; alcohol intake, liver disease, hyperlipidemia, and severe protein malnutrition increase susceptibility to adverse effects of high intake; β-carotene supplements recommended only for those at risk of deficiency (fat malabsorption); may reverse corticosteroid-induced poor wound healing
D	Rickets, osteomalacia, osteoporosis, muscle weakness, poor growth, hypocalcemia, immune dysfunction, cardiomyopathy	Serum 25-hydroxy-vitamin D	Elevated intake causes hypercalcemia, nephrocalcinosis, azotemia, poor growth; decreased in uremia, elderly (especially in winter), fat malabsorption
α-Tocopherol (E)	Hemolysis	Serum α-tocopherol Ratios of serum α-tocopherol to total lipids	Excess intake: hemorrhagic toxicity; increased risk of bleeding with anticoagulants; impaired leukocyte function
K	Bleeding (ecchymosis, petechiae, hematomas)	Prothrombin time INR	Anticoagulant therapy can be affected by supplements or diet

CBC, complete blood count; GI, gastrointestinal; INR, international normalized ratio; NAD, nicotinamide adenine dinucleotide; NADP, nicotinamide adenine dinucleotide phosphate.

[a]Plasma methylmalonic acid concentrations increase with vitamin B_{12} deficiency.

[b]Bitot spots are spots which are oval, triangular, or irregular in shape and located superficially in the conjunctiva.

Data from references 13, 20, 21, 56, 57, and 75.

carnitine concentrations and acylcarnitine. Serum and urine carnitine concentrations are most helpful in primary carnitine deficiency (an inborn error of metabolism); acylcarnitine concentrations are more helpful in secondary causes of carnitine deficiency. When only total and free concentrations are available, the free is subtracted from the total to give the acylcarnitine concentration.[89]

NUTRIENT REQUIREMENTS

8 Individual nutrient requirements vary with age, gender, size, disease state, and clinical condition. Nutrition status, physical activity, and the need for continued maintenance of adequate nutrition or repletion in those with ongoing metabolic stress or malnutrition dictate the nutrient requirements for an individual. For obese patients, usual nutrition requirements may be altered because of desired weight loss or after bariatric surgery. In children, there is the added consideration of sustaining or reestablishing normal growth and development. Organ function (intestine, kidney, liver, and pancreas) may affect nutrient utilization. Nutrient requirements can be estimated using various methods interpreted in the context of patient-specific factors.

Recommended Dietary Allowances

The recommended daily allowances (RDAs) were first established in 1941, and in 1997, the Food and Nutrition Board introduced a new designation for nutrition reference values: the dietary reference intakes (DRIs).[92] The four DRI categories are estimated average requirements (EARs), RDAs, adequate intakes (AIs), and tolerable upper intake levels (ULs). The nutrient intake that meets the needs of half of the healthy persons in a group (EAR) can be used for planning nutrient intakes for groups. The RDA, the nutrient intake that meets the needs of almost all persons in a designated group, is approximately 2 standard deviations above the EAR for nutrients for which the requirement is well defined and 1.2 times the EAR for other nutrients. To evaluate an individual's daily intake, the RDA is the most appropriate comparator. AI, defined as the average intake for the designated group that appears to sustain a particular nutrition state, growth, or other functional indicator of health, is reserved for nutrients for which no EAR or RDA has been determined. Finally, the UL is the maximum nutrient intake unlikely to pose adverse effects in almost all persons in a designated group.[92]

Dietary reference intakes have been established for six nutrient groups: calcium, phosphorus, magnesium, vitamin D, and fluoride; folate and other B vitamins; antioxidants (eg, selenium and vitamins C and E); trace elements; macronutrients (eg, protein, fat, carbohydrates, and fiber); and electrolytes and water. Because of the increased prevalence of vitamin D deficiency, calcium and vitamin D recommendations were revised in 2010.[93] The U.S. Department of Agriculture's website includes an Interactive DRI for Healthcare Professionals, which calculates a generally healthy individual's DRI-based nutrition needs.[94]

According to the DRIs, adults and children older than 1 year of age should consume 45% to 65% of their total calories as carbohydrates. Recommended fat intakes vary by age: 1 to 3 years, 30% to 40%; 4 to 18 years, 25% to 35%; and, adults, 20% to 35% of total calories. Infants, especially premature infants, require a higher proportion of calories from fat (approximately 40%-50% of total calories) to ensure normal neurological development. Protein recommendations also vary by age: 1 to 3 years, 5% to 20%; 4 to 18 years, 10% to 30%; and, adults, 10% to 35% of total calories.[85]

Energy

9 Energy requirements of individuals can be estimated using published, validated equations or can be measured directly. The most appropriate method is determined by a variety of factors, including severity of illness and resource availability.

Estimating Energy Expenditure

Daily energy expenditure consists of the basal energy expenditure (BEE), diet-induced thermogenesis (10%), and energy used for physical activity. In sick or injured patients, the BEE is increased because of stress-related hypermetabolism, but the physical activity and the energy needed for metabolism are usually reduced. For example, continuous infusion enteral feeding, often used in critically ill patients, results in minimal diet-induced thermogenesis (5%) when overfeeding is not present.[28] Failure to account for these changes can result in overfeeding.

More than 200 methods for determining an individual's daily energy requirement have been published.[2,28,95-97] These methods use population estimates of calories per kilogram of body weight (kcal/kg), equations that estimate energy expenditure (kcal/day or kJ/day; 1 kcal is equivalent to 4.184 kJ), or indirect calorimetry. The simplest method to determine energy requirements is to use population estimates of calories required per kilogram of body weight. This method assumes standard values for health or the energy requirements associated with various disease states or clinical conditions, as well as the additional requirements for repletion of a malnourished individual. Most do not take into consideration age- or gender-related differences in energy needs. No stress or activity modifiers are used with these equations because the effect of the clinical condition (hypermetabolism) has been captured in the calculation. Daily adult requirements by this method can be estimated as shown below:[95-97]

1. Healthy, normal nutrition status, minimal illness severity: 20 to 25 kcal ABW/kg/day (84-105 kJ ABW/kg/day).
2. Illness, metabolic stress (BMI less than 30 kg/m^2): 25 to 30 kcal ABW/kg/day (105-126 kJ ABW/kg/day).
3. Illness, metabolic stress (BMI greater than or equal to 30 kg/m^2): 11 to 14 kcal ABW/kg/day (46-59 kJ ABW/kg/day) or 22 to 25 kcal IBW/kg/day (92-105 kJ ABW/kg/day).
4. Major burn injury (greater than or equal to 50% total body surface area) or repletion: greater than or equal to 30 kcal ABW/kg/day (greater than or equal to 126 kJ ABW/kg/day).[98]

When using the ranges in 3 above, as the BMI increases, the number derived using ABW compared to IBW becomes quite disparate. Accuracy is improved by using the ABW recommendation for patients with BMI 30-50 kg/m^2 and the IBW recommendation when the BMI is greater than 50 kg/m^2. When these recommendations are used for patients with a BMI of 30 kg/m^2 or more, the calories provided allow for permissive underfeeding (provision of approximately 80% of estimated or measured energy needs), which decreases infection rates and hospital length of stay.[28] Table 141-9 shows suggested calorie intakes (kcal/kg) for maintenance and normal growth of healthy infants and children.[85] These maintenance energy requirements are approximately 150% of the basal metabolic rate, with the additional calories provided to support usual activity and growth. For all ages, energy requirements increase with fever, sepsis, major surgery, trauma, burns, and long-term growth failure and in the presence of chronic conditions such as bronchopulmonary dysplasia, congenital heart disease, and cystic fibrosis. Energy needs may decrease with obesity and neurologic disability (eg, cerebral palsy).

Numerous equations are available to estimate energy expenditure in adults and children (Tables 141-10 and 141-11, respectively).[2,28,95-97] The Harris-Benedict equations, derived in 1919 from a study of 239 individuals, are still used by some clinicians for assessing energy requirements in adults. They have the advantage of incorporating the patient's age, height, weight, gender, and clinical condition into the estimation. These equations were derived from oxygen consumption measurements made in normally nourished healthy individuals who were in a fasting and resting state. Although they are commonly referred to as the "BEE equations," they actually estimate resting energy expenditure (REE), the amount of energy

TABLE 141-9 Dietary Reference Intakes for Energy and Protein in Healthy Children

Age (Reference age/weight)	Estimated Energy Requirement (kcal/day)[a]		Protein RDA (g/kg/day)[b]
	Boys	Girls	
0-6 mo (3 mo/6 kg)	570	520	1.52[c]
7-12 months (9 mo/9 kg)	743	676	1.5
1-2 yr (24 mo/12 kg)	1,046	992	
1-3 yr (24 mo/12 kg)			1.1
3-8 yr (6 yr/20 kg)	1,742	1,642	
4-8 yr (6 yr/20 kg)			0.95
9-13 yr (11 yr/M: 36 kg; F: 37 kg)	2,279	2,071	0.95
14-18 yr (16 yr/M: 61 kg; F: 54 kg)	3,152	2,368	0.85

F, female; M, male; RDA, recommended dietary allowance.

[a]1 kcal is equal to approximately 4.18 kJ.

[b]Protein requirements in children with moderate to severe stress increase by 50% or more.

[c]Adequate intake.

Data from reference 85.

expended at rest by a fasting, awake individual in a temperature-controlled environment performing only basal functions such as breathing, circulation, and metabolic processes.

Because these equations approximate REE, the results have been historically modified by a factor that adjusts for the individual's clinical condition. For example, an individual who is confined to bed may require a calorie intake that is only 20% to 30% above the REE, while a person who has sustained a severe burn injury may require 150% to 200% of the calculated REE. Some clinicians multiply the calculated REE by both a stress factor and an activity factor.

TABLE 141-10 Estimates of Energy Expenditure in Adults[a]

Healthy Adults
Harris-Benedict[b] Equations (kcal/day)
Men: BEE = 66 + (13.75W + 5H [cm]) – (6.8A)
Women: BEE = 655 + (9.6W + 1.8H [cm]) – (4.7A)
DRI Equations (kcal/day)[c]
Men: EER = 662 – 9.53A + (PA × 15.91W) + 539.6H (m)
Women: EER = 354 – 6.91A + (PA × 9.36W) + 726H (m)
PA = 1 if sedentary; 1.12 if low active; 1.27 if active; and 1.45 if very active
Mifflin-St. Jeor Equations (kcal/day)
Men: 10W + 6.25H (cm) – 5A + 5
Women: 10W + 6.25H (cm) – 5A – 161
Critically Ill Adults
Penn State Equations (kcal/day)
Age ≥60 years with BMI ≥30 kg/m^2: Mifflin(0.71) + T_{max}(85) + Ve(64) – 3085
All others: Mifflin(0.96) + T_{max}(167) + Ve(31) – 6212

A, age in years; BEE, basal energy expenditure; BMI, body mass index; DRI, dietary reference intakes; EER, estimated energy requirement; H, height in centimeters or meters, as indicated; PA, physical activity factor; T_{max}, maximum body temperature in the previous 24 hours in degrees centigrade; Ve, minute ventilation in L/min; W, actual body weight in kilograms.

[a]No real consensus exists as to which formula is best in all situations. Many clinicians use more than one equation and calculate a range of acceptable intakes.

[b]The common practice of using an adjusted body weight for obesity in these calculations is not supported by the original data that used actual body weight in all cases up to a BMI of 56 kg/m^2 in men and 40 kg/m^2 in women.

[c]1 kcal is equal to approximately 4.18 kJ.

Data from references 2, 28, 95, and 96.

TABLE 141-11 Equations to Estimate Energy Expenditure in Children[a,b]

FAO/WHO/UNU 2001 (kcal/day)[b]
0-12 Months
Breastfed
TEE (kcal/day) = –152 + 92.8W
TEE (MJ[c]/day) = –0.635 + 0.388W
Formula fed
TEE (kcal/day) = –29 + 82.6W
TEE (MJ[c]/day) = –0.122 + 0.346W
Boys 1-17 Years
TEE (kcal/day) = 310.2 + 63.3W – 0.263W^2
TEE (MJ[c]/day) = 1,298 + 0.265W – 0.0011W^2
Girls 1-17 Years
TEE (kcal/day) = 263.4 + 65.3W – 0.454W^2
TEE (MJ[c]/day) = 1,102 + 0.273W – 0.0019W^2
DRI Equations (kcal/day)
Birth through 2 years of age
EER = (89W – 100) + GF
GF = 175 kcal if 0-3 months; 56 kcal if 4-6 months; 22 kcal if 7-12 months; 20 kcal if 13-35 months
3-18 years of age
Boys: EER = 88.5 – (61.9A) + PA (26.7W + 903H) + GF
Girls: EER = 135.3 – (30.8A) + PA (10W + 934H) + GF
GF = 20 kcal if 3-8 years; 25 kcal if 9-18 years
PA = 1 if sedentary; 1.13-1.16 if low activity; 1.26-1.31 if normal activity; and 1.42-1.56 if very active

A, age in years; DRI, dietary reference intakes; EER, estimated energy requirement; FAO/WHO/UNU, Food and Agriculture Organization/World Health Organization/United Nations University; GF, growth factor; H, height in meters; PA, physical activity factor; TEE, total energy expenditure; W, actual body weight in kilograms.

[a]No real consensus exists as to which formula is best in all situations. Many clinicians use more than one equation and calculate a range of acceptable intakes.

[b]Additional daily calories are needed for growth; about 2 kcal/g of weight gain desired.

[c]1 kcal is equivalent to approximately 4.18 kJ; 1 MJ = 1,000 kJ.

Data from references 85, 101, and 102.

Because validation studies have shown that these equations overestimate REE by 6% to 15%, the calculated REE should be multiplied by either a stress factor or an activity factor to avoid further overestimation of the individual's energy needs.[2] It should also be noted that ABW (up to a BMI of 56 kg/m^2 in men and 40 kg/m^2 in women), not IBW or adjusted body weight, was used to generate the original data with these equations and thus should be used for these calculations.[96] Overestimation of energy needs with the Harris-Benedict equations is well documented.[28,96] When compared to indirect calorimetry, the accuracy has been shown to be about 34%.[99] The Mifflin-St. Jeor equations tend to be more accurate in healthy adults than the Harris-Benedict equations (see Table 141-10): the accuracy rate is 80% in patients who are not obese (BMI less than or equal to 30 kg/m^2) and 70% in obese patients (BMI greater than 30 kg/m^2).[28,99]

There is no individual method proven to accurately determine the energy needs of all critically ill patients.[95] The Penn State equations are the most accurate in critically ill adults receiving mechanical ventilation[28] (see Table 141-10), but the accuracy is only about 67% when compared to indirect calorimetry measurements.[99] The Penn State modified appears to be more accurate in older obese patients, with an accuracy of approximately 74% when compared to indirect calorimetry measurements in the same individuals.[99] There is no consensus as to the best equation for critically ill adults who are not mechanically ventilated. The metabolic response to stress in children appears to be different than in critically ill adults; thus, "stress factors" used in adults, shown in Table 141-12, are not appropriate for use in estimating energy use in children.[100-102]

TABLE 141-12 Stress Factors for Use in Adults

Condition	Factor
No Stress	
Confined to bed	1.2
Out of bed: normal activity	1.3
Catch-up growth	1.5
Mild Stress[a]	
Postoperative recovery: uncomplicated surgery	1-1.15
Trauma: mild (eg, long-bone fracture)	1.2
Moderate Stress[a]	
Sepsis (moderate)	1.2-1.4
Trauma: CNS (sedated)	1.3
Trauma: moderate to severe	Children: 1.5
	Adults: 1.3-1.4
Severe Stress[a]	
Sepsis (severe)	Children: 1.6
	Adults: 1.3
Trauma: CNS (severe)	Children: up to 2.0
	Adults: up to 1.3
Burns (proportionate to burned area)[b]	Up to 2.0

CNS, central nervous system.

[a]Assumes decreased activity during periods of stress.

[b]Formulas specifically for estimating energy needs in burned children and adults have been published and are likely to be more accurate. See reference 98.

Data from reference 2.

Clinical **Controversy...**

Many equations have been published for estimating energy requirements of patients in a variety of settings. Indirect calorimetry is becoming more widely available for use in many patient settings. Whether estimating energy needs using an appropriate validated equation is cost-effective and/or improves outcomes versus measuring the energy requirements using indirect calorimetry is not yet established.

Measuring Energy Expenditure

The most accurate method to determine energy expenditure in clinical practice is to measure it using indirect calorimetry (metabolic gas monitoring), but capital and operational costs limit its availability. Handheld calorimeters have been shown to produce similar results to metabolic carts and may be a viable alternative to the more expensive equipment in both the inpatient and outpatient setting.[103]

Indirect calorimetry methodology is based on pulmonary gas exchange: when a substrate (carbohydrate, fat, or protein) is oxidized, heat is produced, oxygen is consumed, and carbon dioxide is expired in a constant amount depending on the substrate being oxidized. More carbon dioxide is produced when a gram of glucose is metabolized than either a gram of protein or a gram of fat. Indirect calorimetry is a noninvasive procedure in which oxygen consumption (VO_2, mL/min) and carbon dioxide production (VCO_2, mL/min) are measured, and the measured resting energy expenditure (MREE; kcal/day) is calculated using the abbreviated Weir equation as MREE $= ([3.94\ VO_2 + 1.11\ VCO_2] + [2.17\ uN_2]) \times 1.44$.[99,104,105] The urinary nitrogen component (uN_2) is often omitted when calculating energy expenditure because it accounts for less than 4% of the energy expenditure in critically ill patients, and its omission results in only a 1% to 2% calculation error.[28,105] Excluding the nitrogen component obviates the need for a 24-hour urine collection, which can be difficult in many patients and delay the measurement in others.

The MREE represents the total energy expended during the time period over which the measurements were taken extrapolated to a 24-hour period to approximate daily energy requirements. MREE reflects changes in energy requirements resulting from diseases or clinical conditions, but it does not include energy required for repletion of a malnourished individual or growth in a child. The energy intake required for these functions is accounted for by multiplying MREE by a metabolic or activity factor: mechanically ventilated, critically ill, 1; critically ill, no mechanical ventilation, 1 to 1.1; adult acute, not critically ill, 1.1 to 1.4, depending on activity; adult needing repletion or a child, 1.3 to 2; adult outpatient, 1.1 to 2, depending on activity; and adult depletion (weight loss), less than 1.[104,105]

Indirect calorimetry also can be used to determine the patient's RQ, calculated as VCO_2/VO_2, which reflects substrate oxidation and characterizes substrate utilization. RQ values for nutrient substrates are fat, 0.7; carbohydrate, 1; protein, 0.8; and mixed substrate (fat, carbohydrate, and protein), 0.85. RQ values greater than 1 represent either lipogenesis or hyperventilation; less than 0.7 may indicate a ketogenic diet, fat gluconeogenesis, or ethanol oxidation. Values outside the physiologic range of 0.67 to 1.3 suggest an invalid test. Clinically, the RQ is used to determine if a patient is being overfed, which is likely if the RQ value is greater than 1.

Indirect calorimetry is a respiratory measurement that does not reflect metabolism in all clinical situations. Indirect calorimetry overestimates REE for patients with hyperventilation, metabolic acidosis, overfeeding, and if there are air leaks anywhere in the ventilator circuit. Underestimation of REE is likely with hypoventilation, metabolic alkalosis, underfeeding, and gluconeogenesis. Mechanically ventilated patients are technically easier to study because the indirect calorimeter can be integrated into the ventilator circuit. However, the patient must be at complete rest for 1 hour, must not receive bolus feedings either by feeding tube or orally for 4 hours, should have no changes in substrate delivery for 12 hours, and must be on a fraction of inspired O_2 of less than 0.6 with a positive end-expiratory pressure less than 5 cm H_2O (approximately 0.5 kPa) to ensure an accurate steady-state reading. Unfortunately, many of the patients in whom indirect calorimetry would be most useful will not meet these requirements. Indirect calorimetry should be considered in any patient in whom uncertainty in estimating energy requirements needs to be minimized, such as adults and children who are severely malnourished (BMI less than 18.5 kg/m^2) or obese (BMI greater than 30 kg/m^2), who have unexplained high partial arterial pressure of carbon dioxide ($PaCO_2$) concentrations or minute ventilation, spinal cord injuries, who experience weight loss despite apparently receiving adequate protein and energy intakes, critically ill surgery patients receiving parenteral nutrition, and patients unable to be weaned from the ventilator.[28,104,105]

Protein

Daily protein requirements are based on age, gender, nutrition status, disease state, and clinical condition. Table 141-9 lists the RDAs for protein for children; for individuals older than 18 years of age, the RDA is 0.8 g/kg/day, which is significantly less than most Americans typically consume.[85] In adults older than 60 years of age, protein needs are increased to 1.5 g/kg/day to reduce the loss of LBM that occurs with aging, and 1.5 to 2 g/kg/day or more may be needed in states of metabolic stress (infection, trauma, and surgery).[85,97,106] Protein requirements are also higher in pregnant and lactating women (1.1 g/kg/day or 6-10 g protein per day above the usual RDA).[85]

Protein metabolism depends on both kidney and liver function. Critical illness results in a hypercatabolic state in which there is both increased protein synthesis and degradation. The goal of protein administration is to minimize catabolism by maximizing protein synthesis. Consequently, protein requirements are increased to 1.2 to 2 g/kg/day in critically ill patients. For obese critically ill patients, protein needs are 2 g/kg IBW or more if the BMI is between 30 and 40 kg/m^2 and 2.5 g/kg IBW or more if the BMI is greater than 40 kg/m^2.[95] Adults with significant total body surface area burns have protein requirements as high as 2.5 to 3 g/kg ABW/day. In children with significant burns, between 20% and 25% of their total calorie needs should be provided as protein.[98] Soft tissue defects and large stool or ileostomy losses also increase protein requirements. Liver failure typically results in the need for protein restriction (0.5 g/kg/day) unless a hypercatabolic state is also present, which will increase requirements to 1.5 g/kg/day. Protein needs in patients with kidney failure are variable and affected by the various renal replacement therapies available. The application of these protein intake guidelines requires both clinical judgment and frequent monitoring of kidney and liver function, serum chemistries, clinical condition, and nutrition outcomes.

Nitrogen is found only in protein and at a relatively constant ratio of 1 g nitrogen per 6.25 g of protein. This ratio may vary somewhat for enteral and parenteral feeding formulations, depending on the biologic value of the protein source. The adequacy of protein intake can be assessed clinically by a nitrogen balance study—measuring urinary nitrogen excretion and comparing it with nitrogen intake. Nitrogen balance indirectly reflects protein use or the protein catabolic rate, which increases with hypercatabolism. As the stress level increases, a concomitant increase in protein catabolism results in an increase in urinary nitrogen excretion. The amount of urine urea nitrogen (UUN) measured in a 24-hour urine collection in healthy individuals, accounts for 80% to 90% of the total urine nitrogen (TUN) excreted. Nitrogen output (g/day) can be approximated as 24-hour UUN + 4, where 4 is a factor representing usual skin, fecal, and respiratory nitrogen losses. At higher UUN values (30 g nitrogen or more), then the use of a factor of + 6 may yield a more accurate measure of nitrogen output.[107] Alternatively, if available, TUN can be measured and may be more accurate, especially in critically ill patients who excrete more nitrogen-containing substances such as 3-methylhistidine. If TUN is used, then the best estimate of nitrogen output is TUN + 1.05.[107] In patients with kidney failure, in which case neither UUN nor TUN accurately represents net protein degradation, nitrogen balance can be approximated only with equations based on urea nitrogen appearance.[108]

Fat

The daily AI for men and women for α-linolenic acid is 1.6 and 1.1 g, respectively; for linoleic acid, it is 14 to 17 g/day for men and 11 to 12 g/day for women.[85] Overall, for adults, fat should represent no more than 10% to 35% of total calories, with the recommendation that saturated fatty acids, *trans* fatty acids, and dietary cholesterol intake be kept as low as possible while a nutritionally adequate diet is consumed. Fat should constitute 30% to 40% of energy in children 1 to 3 years of age and 25% to 35% of energy in children 4 to 18 years of age.[85] Fat intake in children younger than 3 years of age is critical for proper central nervous system growth and development; generally, fat-restricted diets (skim milk) should not be imposed until after the age of 2 to 3 years except under medical supervision. A lower limit of 15% of total energy intake has been suggested as the minimum fat intake in children when fat restriction is warranted.[109]

Fiber

Reduced risk of coronary heart disease and maintenance of normal laxation have been attributed to dietary fiber intake.[110] Fiber intake may also have a role in colon cancer prevention and may promote weight control through its effect on satiety. Men and women 50 years of age and younger should ingest 38 g/day and 25 to 26 g/day, respectively, of total fiber. For men and women older than 50 years of age, the recommended intakes are 30 g/day and 21 g/day, respectively.[85] The AI for fiber has not been set for children younger than 1 year of age. Breast milk and infant formulas are essentially fiber-free. For older children, the recommended fiber intake is 19 g/day for children 1 to 3 years of age, 24 g/day for children 4 to 8 years of age, and 26 to 31 g/day for children 9 to 13 years of age.[85]

TABLE 141-13 Factors That Alter Fluid Requirements

Increased Requirements	Decreased Requirements
Fever	Fluid overload
Radiant warmers	Heart failure
Diuretics	Decreased urine output
Vomiting	Heat shields
Nasogastric suction	Relatively high humidity
Ostomy or fistula drainage	Humidified air via endotracheal tube
Diarrhea	Kidney failure
Glycosuria	Hypoalbuminemia with starvation
Phototherapy	Syndrome of inappropriate secretion of antidiuretic hormone (SIADH)
Diabetes insipidus	
Increased ambient temperatures	
Hyperventilation	
Prematurity	
Excessive sweating	
Increased metabolism (eg, hyperthyroidism)	

Fluid

The daily fluid requirement for an adult depends on many factors but is generally estimated to be 30 to 35 mL/kg, 1 mL for each kcal (or 4.18 kJ) ingested, or 1,500 mL/m^2. Fluid requirements per kilogram of body weight are higher for children and even higher for preterm infants because of their higher percentage of TBW and basal energy needs. Additionally, premature neonates have increased fluid requirements because of greater insensible losses and the kidneys' inefficiency in concentrating urine. The Holliday-Segar method is a commonly used, quick, and simple method for estimating minimum daily fluid needs of children and adults. Children weighing less than 10 kg should receive at least 100 mL/kg/day. An additional 50 mL/kg/day should be provided for each kilogram of body weight between 11 kg and 20 kg and 20 mL/kg/day for each kilogram above 20 kg. Thus, the minimum fluid required for a child weighing 8 kg would be 800 mL/day, a 17-kg child would need 1,350 mL/day; and a 50-kg individual would need 2,000 mL/day.

Table 141-13 lists factors that alter fluid needs for both adults and children. All sources of fluid intake should be considered (eg, fluid vehicles for intravenous medications and intravenous or feeding tube flushes) when determining fluid requirements. Urine output and specific gravity as well as serum electrolytes and weight changes can be used to assess fluid status. A urine output of at least 1 mL/kg/h (in children) and approximately 40 to 50 mL/h (in adults) is considered adequate to ensure tissue perfusion. Urine output should be higher if large fluid volumes or high renal solute loads (eg, parenteral nutrition or concentrated enteral feeding formulations) are being administered. Urine specific gravity depends on the kidney's concentrating and diluting capabilities. Concomitant diuretic therapy, resulting in increased solute excretion, limits the usefulness of urine specific gravity as an assessment of fluid status.

Micronutrients

Requirements for micronutrients (electrolytes, minerals, trace elements, and vitamins) vary with age, gender, and the route by which the nutrient is ingested (Table 141-14; see Chapters 49 to 51).[53-58,74,92,111] Oral and parenteral requirements vary as a result of bioavailability considerations. Micronutrients poorly absorbed via the GI tract usually are required in greater amounts when given by the enteral than parenteral route. However, many water-soluble micronutrients are excreted more rapidly via the kidneys when administered intravenously. In these situations, the intravenous dose is

TABLE 141-14 Recommended Daily Electrolyte, Trace Element, and Vitamin Intake[a]

	Adult (≥19 yr of age)		Pediatric	
Nutrient	**Enteral**	**Parenteral**	**Enteral**	**Parenteral**
Electrolytes and Minerals				
Acetate[b]	—	—	—	—
Calcium	1,000-1,200 mg	0-15 mEq (0-7.5 mmol)	0-12 mo: 210-270 mg 1-3 yr: 700 mg 4-8 yr: 1,000 mg 9-18 yr: 1,300 mg	Premature: 2-4 mEq/kg (1-2 mmol/kg) Other: 1-2.5 mEq/kg (0.5-1.25 mmol/kg)
Chloride[b]		—	—	2-6 mEq/kg (2-6 mmol/kg)
Magnesium	M: 400-420 mg W: 310-320 mg	10-20 mEq (5-10 mmol)	0-6 mo: 30 mg 7-12 mo: 75 mg 1-3 yr: 80 mg 4-8 yr: 130 mg 9-18 yr: 240-410 mg	0.25-1 mEq/kg (0.12-0.5 mmol/kg)
Phosphorus	700 mg	20-45 mmol	0-6 mo: 100 mg 7-12 mo: 275 mg 1-8 yr: 460-500 mg 9-18 yr: 1,250 mg	Premature: 1-2 mmol/kg Others: 0.5-1 mmol/kg
Potassium[c,d]	4,700 mg	60-100 mEq (60-100 mmol) (1-2 mEq/kg [1-2 mmol/kg])	0-6 mo: 400 mg 7-12 mo: 700 mg 1-8 yr: 3,000-3,800 mg 9-18 yr: 4,500-4,700 mg	2-5 mEq/kg (2-5 mmol/kg)
Sodium[c,d]	1,200-1,500 mg	60-100 mEq (60-100 mmol) (1-2 mEq/kg [1-2 mmol/kg])	0-6 mo: 120 mg 7-12 mo: 370 mg 1-8 yr: 1,000-1,200 mg 9-18 yr: 1,500 mg	2-6 mEq/kg (2-6 mmol/kg)
Trace Elements				
Chromium[e] (mcg)	20-45 (varies with age and sex)	10-15	0-6 mo: 0.2 7-12 mo: 5.5 1-8 yr: 11-15 9-18 yr: 21-35	0.14-0.2 mcg/kg (maximum, 5 mcg)
Copper[f] (mcg)	900 1,000 (pregnancy) 1,300 (lactation)	0.3-1.5 (increased with GI loss)	0-12 mo: 200-220 1-8 yr: 340-440 9-18 yr: 700-890	20 mcg/kg (maximum, 300 mcg)
Fluoride (mg)	M: 4 W: 3	1	0-6 mo: 0.01 mg 7-12 mo: 0.5 mg 1-8 yr: 0.7-1 mg 9-18 yr: 2-3 mg	—
Iodine[g] (mcg)	150 220 (pregnancy) 290 (lactation)	70-140 (not well defined)	0-12 mo: 110-130 1-8 yr: 90 9-18 yr: 120-150	1 mcg/kg
Iron (mg)	M: 8 W (≤50 yr): 18 27 (pregnancy) 9 (lactation) W (>50 yr): 8	1 1.5 (blood loss)	0-6 mo: 0.27 7 mo-8 yr: 7-11 M (9-18 yr): 8-11 F (9-13 yr): 8 F (14-18 yr): 15	Varies
Manganese[f] (mg)	W: 1.8 2 (pregnancy) 2.6 (lactation) M: 2.3	0.15-1	0-6 mo: 0.003 7-12 mo: 0.6 1-8 yr: 1.2-1.5 9-18 yr: 1.6-2.2	1 mcg/kg (maximum, 50 mcg)
Molybdenum (mcg)	45 50 (pregnancy, lactation)	100-200	0-12 mo: 2-3 1-8 yr: 17-22 9-18 yr: 34-43	0.25 mcg/kg (maximum, 5 mcg)
Selenium (mcg)	55 60 (pregnancy) 70 (lactation)	20-60[h] 100+ with deficiency	0-12 mo: 15-20 1-8 yr: 20-30 9-18 yr: 40-55	1.5-3 mcg/kg (maximum, 30 mcg)
Zinc[i] (mg)	W: 8 M, pregnancy: 11 Lactation: 12	2.5-5[h] (increased with GI loss)	0-12 mo: 2-3 1-8 yr: 3-5 9-18 yr: 8-11	Premature: 300-400 mcg/kg Other: 50-250 mcg/kg

(*continued*)

TABLE 141-14 Recommended Daily Electrolyte, Trace Element, and Vitamin Intake[a] (*Continued*)

	Adult (≥19 yr of age)		Pediatric	
Nutrient	**Enteral**	**Parenteral**	**Enteral**	**Parenteral**
vitamins				
Ascorbic acid (mg) (vitamin C)	75-90	100	0-12 mo: 40-50 1-8 yr: 15-25 9-18 yr: 45-75	80
Biotin (mcg)	30	60	0-12 mo: 5-6 1-8 yr: 8-12 9-18 yr: 20-25	20
Cobalamin (mcg) (vitamin B_{12})	2.4	5	0-12 mo: 0.4-0.5 1-8 yr: 0.9-1.2 9-18 yr: 1.8-2.4	1
Folic acid (mcg)	400	400	0-12 mo: 65-80 1-8 yr: 150-200 9-18 yr: 300-400	140
Niacin (mg NE)	14-16	40	0-12 mo: 2-4 1-8 yr: 6-8 9-18 yr: 12-16	17
Pantothenic acid (mg)	5	15	0-12 mo: 1.7-1.8 1-8 yr: 2-3 9-18 yr: 4-5	5
Pyridoxine (mg) (vitamin B_6)	1.3-1.7	4	0-12 mo: 0.1-0.3 1-8 yr: 0.5-0.6 9-18 yr: 1-1.3	1
Riboflavin (mg)	1.1-1.3	3.6	0-12 mo: 0.3-0.4 1-8 yr: 0.5-0.6 9-18 yr: 0.9-1.3	1.4
Thiamine (mg)	1.1-1.2	3	0-12 mo: 0.2-0.3 1-8 yr: 0.5-0.6 9-18 yr: 0.9-1.2	1.2
Vitamin A (mcg RE) (retinol)	700-900	600-1,000 (3,300-5,500 international units)	0-12 mo: 400-500 1-8 yr: 300-400 9-18 yr: 600-900	700 (2,300 international units)
Vitamin D (mcg)	≤70 yr: 15 (600 international units) >70 yr: 20 (800 international units)	5 (200 international units)[h]	All ages: 15 (600 international units)	5-10 (200-400 international units)[h]
Vitamin E (mg TE) (α-tocopherol)	15 (15 international units)	10 (10 international units)	0-12 mo: 4-5 (4-5 international units) 1-8 yr: 6-7 9-18 yr: 11-15	7 (7 international units)
Vitamin K (mcg)	90-120	0.7-2.5 mg	0-12 mo: 2-2.5 1-8 yr: 30-55 9-18 yr: 60-75	200

M, men; NE, niacin equivalents; RE, retinol equivalents; TE, tocopherol equivalent; W, women.

[a]Data represent either the recommended dietary allowance (RDA) or the adequate intake (AI) for each nutrient where established.

[b]Not established; as needed to maintain acid–base balance.

[c]Newborns and low-birth-weight or very-low-birth-weight infants or with concomitant disease (eg, necrotizing enterocolitis) may have higher requirements. Intake in nonhealthy children must be individualized.

[d]No RDA or AI has been established.

[e]An additional 20 mcg/day is recommended in patients with significant intestinal losses.

[f]May accumulate in cholestasis.

[g]Long-term parenteral nutrition only if no topical preparations containing iodide or iodized table salt are used.

[h]Higher doses may be required in patients with short bowel syndrome receiving long-term parenteral nutrition.

[i]Additional intake needed with small bowel losses, which can be 12 mg zinc/L or 17 mg zinc/kg of stool or ileostomy output; an additional 2 mg/day needed for acute catabolic stress.

Data from references 53-58, 74, 75, and 93.

greater than the oral dose. Other factors that affect micronutrient requirements include GI losses through diarrhea, vomiting, or high-output fistula or ostomies; wound healing; and hypermetabolism or hypercatabolism. Cutaneous micronutrient losses (eg, zinc, copper, and selenium) also may be significant after major burn injury. Sodium, potassium, magnesium, and phosphorus excretion are particularly dependent on kidney function, and in the settings of acute kidney injury or chronic kidney disease, intake will likely need to be restricted. Calcium needs, on the other hand, may be increased in these patients (see Chapters 44 and 45). Patients who are severely malnourished will have increased electrolyte requirements during early refeeding owing to preexisting deficiencies and rapid intracellular uptake with anabolism. Failure to provide adequate electrolyte replacement, especially phosphorus, and vitamin supplementation (thiamine) before delivery of full calories during refeeding has resulted in death from the refeeding syndrome.[112,113]

DRUG–NUTRIENT INTERACTIONS

10 Drug-induced nutrient deficiency, poor therapeutic response, enhanced drug toxicity, and failure to achieve desired nutrition outcomes can occur if either nutrition support or drug therapy is stopped as a consequence of adverse effects. Patient outcomes may be enhanced when an effective screening method to identify significant drug–nutrient interactions is coupled with a patient counseling program. An important part of the screening process is to recognize risk factors that influence drug–nutrient interactions. The potential for drug–nutrient interactions is greatest in pediatric and elderly individuals, those with poor nutrition status (obesity and marasmus), and those receiving multiple drug therapies or tube feedings.[114-120]

Mineral and electrolyte serum concentrations may change because of drug therapy. For example, with loop diuretics, urine sodium, potassium, calcium, and magnesium wasting may occur, causing a reduction in their respective serum concentrations. Alternatively, calcium excretion is reduced with thiazide diuretics (see Chapter 49). Serum electrolyte concentrations also may increase as a direct result of the drug's mechanism (potassium-sparing diuretics) or because of the drug's salt form (sodium piperacillin/tazobactam). Corticosteroids and cyclosporine are known to cause hyperglycemia; other drugs are prescribed to pharmacologically lower blood glucose concentrations (eg, insulin and oral hypoglycemics; see Chapter 74).

Vitamin and trace element status also may be affected by drugs (Table 141-15). For example, sulfasalazine therapy causes a decrease in folic acid, isoniazid therapy causes pyridoxine deficiency, and furosemide therapy may result in decreased thiamine concentrations. Drug therapy outcomes also may be affected by vitamin intake. For instance, the ingestion of high folic acid doses may decrease methotrexate's therapeutic effect, and changes in an individual's usual vitamin K or vitamin E intake may cause variability in warfarin's anticoagulant effects.

Drug-delivery vehicles also may contain nutrients. Most intravenous therapies (maintenance intravenous fluids, drugs, and electrolyte replacements) are delivered using solutions of either dextrose (dextrose 5% or 10% in water) or sodium (0.9% NaCl). Lipid emulsion (10%) is used as the vehicle for the anesthetic agent propofol and the intravenous calcium channel blocker clevidipine and contributes fat calories (1.1 kcal/mL or 4.6 kJ/mL) when continuous infusions are used. In these instances, nutrition support regimens must be adjusted to accommodate calories and other nutrients delivered through these therapies to avoid overfeeding and other complications.

TABLE 141-15 Drug and Nutrient Interactions

Drug	Effect
Antacids	Thiamine deficiency
Antibiotics	Vitamin K deficiency
Aspirin	Folic acid deficiency; increased vitamin C excretion
Cathartics	Increased requirements for vitamins D, C, and B_6
Cholestyramine	Vitamins A, D, E, and K and β-carotene malabsorption
Colestipol	Vitamins A, D, E, and K and β-carotene malabsorption
Corticosteroids	Decreased vitamins A, D, and C
Diuretics (loop)	Thiamine deficiency
Efavirenz	Vitamin D deficiency caused by increased metabolism of 25(OH)-vitamin D and 1,25-$(OH)_2$-vitamin D
Histamine$_2$ antagonists	Vitamin B_{12} malabsorption (reduced acid results in impaired release of B_{12} from food)
Isoniazid	Vitamin B_6 and niacin deficiency
Isotretinoin	Vitamin A increases toxicity
Mercaptopurine	Niacin deficiency
Methotrexate	Folic acid inhibits effect
Orlistat	Vitamins A, D, E, and K malabsorption caused by fat malabsorption
Pentamidine	Folic acid deficiency
Phenobarbital	Increased vitamin D metabolism
Phenytoin	Increased vitamin D metabolism, decreased folic acid concentrations
Primidone	Folic acid deficiency
Protease inhibitors	Vitamin D deficiency (impaired renal hydroxylation)
Proton pump inhibitors	Vitamin B_{12} malabsorption (reduced acid results in impaired release of B_{12} from food)
Sulfasalazine	Folic acid malabsorption
Trimethoprim	Folic acid depletion
Warfarin	Vitamin K inhibits effect; vitamins A, C, and E may affect prothrombin time
Valproic acid	Zinc
Zidovudine	Folic acid and B_{12} deficiencies increase myelosuppression

Data from references 114-120.

PRACTICAL GUIDELINES FOR NUTRITION ASSESSMENT

The value of any marker used for nutrition screening is only as good as its ability to accurately identify the patient with malnutrition and to correlate with nutrition-related complications. The response of the various nutrition status markers to nutrition therapy and the correlation between improvement in these markers and decreased morbidity and mortality support their validity. However, when applied to an individual, most of these markers lack specificity and sensitivity, which makes the development of a clinically useful, cost-effective approach to nutrition screening challenging.

The importance of the nutrition-focused history and physical examination in both nutrition screening and nutrition assessment cannot be overemphasized. The minimum amount of objective data that can further substantiate the clinical impression and provide a baseline for subsequent monitoring is weight and serum ALB concentration. The cost effectiveness of the addition of other biochemical parameters is unknown. The assessment of other anthropometric measures is most useful in the setting of anticipated long-term nutrition support in which these measurements will serve as a longitudinal marker of response to the nutrition care plan.

Initially, nutrition requirements are determined on the basis of assumptions made about the patient's clinical condition and the nutrition needs associated with repletion or growth, if needed. After a nutrition intervention has been initiated, periodic reassessment of nutrition status is critical to determine the accuracy of the initial estimate of nutrition requirements. Nutrition requirements are dynamic in the setting of acute or critical illness—as the patient's clinical status changes, so will protein and energy requirements, further emphasizing the need for continued reassessment.

Better markers of nutrition status and methods for determining patient-specific nutrition requirements are needed to allow further refinement of estimates of an individual's nutrition needs.

Functional tests and simple, noninvasive tests for body composition analysis hold promise for the future. However, until better methods of assessment become available clinically and are demonstrated to be cost effective, the currently available battery of tests will continue to be the mainstay of nutrition assessment.

ABBREVIATIONS

ABW	actual body weight
AI	adequate intake
ALB	albumin
BEE	basal energy expenditure
BIA	bioelectrical impedance analysis
BMI	body mass index
CDC	Centers for Disease Control and Prevention
CRP	C-reactive protein
DCH	delayed cutaneous hypersensitivity
DRI	dietary reference intake
DXA	dual-energy x-ray absorptiometry
EAR	estimated average requirement
EFAD	essential fatty acid deficiency
GI	gastrointestinal
HIV	human immunodeficiency virus
IBW	ideal body weight
LBM	lean body mass
MREE	measured resting energy expenditure
MRI	magnetic resonance imaging
MST	Malnutrition Screening Tool
RDA	recommended dietary allowance
REE	resting energy expenditure
RQ	respiratory quotient
SGA	Subjective Global Assessment
TBW	total body water
TFN	transferrin
TUN	total urine nitrogen
UBW	usual body weight
UL	tolerable upper intake level
UUN	urine urea nitrogen
VCO_2	carbon dioxide production
VO_2	oxygen consumption
WHO	World Health Organization

REFERENCES

1. Jensen GL, Hsiao PY, Wheeler D. Adult nutrition assessment tutorial. *J Parenter Enteral Nutr* 2012;36:267-274.
2. DeLegge MH, Drake LM. Nutritional assessment. *Gastroenterol Clin North Am* 2007;36:1-22.
3. White JV, Guenter P, Jensen GL, et al. Consensus statement: Academy of Nutrition and Dietetics and the American Society for Parenteral and Enteral Nutrition: Characteristics recommended for the identification and documentation of adult malnutrition (undernutrition). *J Parenter Enteral Nutr* 2012;36:275-283.
4. Malone A, Hamilton C. The Academy of Nutrition and Dietetics/The American Society for Parenteral and Enteral Nutrition Consensus Malnutrition Characteristics: Application in practice. *Nutr Clin Pract* 2013;28:639-649.
5. Ogden CL, Carroll MD, Kit BK, Flegal K. Prevalence of childhood and adult obesity in the United States, 2011-2012. *JAMA* 2014;311:806-814.
6. Ogden CL, Carroll MD, Fryar CD, Flegal KM. Prevalence of obesity among adults and youth: United States, 2011-2014. *NCHS Data Brief* 2015;219:1-8.
7. Centers for Disease Control and Prevention. Overweight and Obesity: Adult Obesity Facts. 2013. Available at: http://www.cdc.gov/obesity/data/adult.html. (Accessed December 15, 2015)
8. Centers for Disease Control and Prevention. Growth Charts. Available at: http://www.cdc.gov/growthcharts/. (Accessed December 15, 2015)
9. Charney P. Nutrition screening vs nutrition assessment: How do they differ? *Nutr Clin Pract* 2008;23:366-372.
10. Joint Commission on Accreditation of Healthcare Organizations. *2015 Hospital Accreditation Standards*. Oakbrook Terrace, IL: Joint Commission Resources. Available at: http://www.jointcommission.org. (Accessed December 15, 2015)
11. Patel V, Romano M, Corkins MR, et al., the American Society for Parenteral and Enteral Nutrition. Nutrition screening and assessment in hospitalized patients: A survey of current practice in the United States. *Nutr Clin Pract* 2014:29:483-490.
12. Kondrup J, Allison SP, Elia M, et al. ESPEN guidelines for nutrition screening 2002. *Clin Nutr* 2003;22:415-421.
13. Jensen GL, Hsiao PY, Wheeler D. Nutrition screening and assessment. In: Mueller C, ed. *The A.S.P.E.N. Adult Nutrition Support Core Curriculum*. 2nd ed. Silver Spring, MD: American Society for Parenteral and Enteral Nutrition; 2012:155-169.
14. Skipper A, Ferguson M, Thompson K, et al. Nutrition screening tools: An analysis of the evidence. *J Parenteral Enteral Nutr* 2012;36:292-298.
15. Anthony PS. Nutrition screening tools for hospitalized patients. *Nutr Clin Pract* 2008;23:373-382.
16. Ferguson M, Capra S, Bauer J, Banks M. Development of a valid and reliable malnutrition screening tool for adult acute hospital patients. *Nutrition* 1999;15:458-464.
17. Makhija S, Baker J. The subjective global assessment: A review of its use in clinical practice. *Nutr Clin Pract* 2008;23:405-409.
18. Keith J. Bedside nutrition assessment past, present, and future: A review of the subjective global assessment. *Nutr Clin Pract* 2008;23:410-416.
19. Centers for Disease Control and Prevention. Use of World Health Organization and CDC growth charts for children aged 0-59 months in the United States. *Morb Mortal Wkly Rep* 2010;59(RR-9):1-16.
20. Esper DH. Utilization of nutrition-focused physical assessment in identifying micronutrient deficiencies. *Nutr Clin Pract* 2015;30:194-202.
21. Corkins KG. Nutrition-focused physical examination in pediatric patients. *Nutr Clin Pract* 2015;30:203-209.
22. Bauer JM, Kaiser MJ, Anthony P, et al. The Mini Nutritional Assessment®: Its history, today's practice, and future perspectives. *Nutr Clin Pract* 2008;23:388-396.
23. Hamwi GJ. Changing dietary concepts. In: Danowski TS, ed. *Diabetes Mellitus: Diagnosis and Treatment*. Vol. 1. New York: American Diabetes Association, Inc.; 1964:73-78.
24. Devine BJ. Gentamicin therapy. *Drug Intell Clin Pharm* 1974;8:650-655.
25. Barak N, Wall-Alsonso E, Sitrin MD. Evaluation of stress factors and body weight adjustments currently used to estimate energy expenditure in hospitalized patients. *J Parenter Enteral Nutr* 2002;26:231-238.
26. Krenitsky J. Adjusted body weight, Pro: Evidence to support the use of adjusted body weight in calculating calorie requirements. *Nutr Clin Pract* 2005;20:468-473.
27. Ireton-Jones C. Adjusted body weight, Con: Why adjust body weight in energy-expenditure calculations? *Nutr Clin Pract* 2005:20:474-479.
28. Frankenfield DC, Ashcraft CM. Estimating energy needs in nutrition support patients. *J Parenter Enteral Nutr* 2011;35:563-570.
29. Hickson M, Frost G. A comparison of three methods for estimating height in the acutely ill elderly population. *J Hum Nutr Diet* 2003;16:13-20.
30. Bell KL, Davies PS. Prediction of height from knee height in children with cerebral palsy and non-disabled children. *Ann Hum Biol* 2006;33:493-499.
31. Chumlea WC, Guo SS, Steinbaugh ML. Prediction of stature from knee height for black and white adults and children with application to mobility-impaired or handicapped persons. *J Am Diet Assoc* 1994;94:1385-1388.
32. Fenton TR. A new growth chart for preterm babies: Babson and Benda's chart updated with recent data and a new format. *BMC Pediatr* 2003;3:13.
33. Rao SC, Tompkins J, World Health Organization. Growth curves for preterm infants. *Early Hum Dev* 2007;83:643-651.
34. Cole SZ, Lanham JS. Failure to thrive: an update. *Am Fam Physician* 2011;83:829-834.
35. Mehta NM, Corkins MR, Lyman B, et al. Defining pediatric malnutrition: A paradigm shift toward etiology-related definitions. *J Parenter Enter Nutr* 2013;37:460-481.
36. Jensen MD, Ryan DH, Apovian CM, et al. 2013 AHA/ACC/TOS guideline for the management of overweight and obesity in adults:

A report of the American College of Cardiology/American Heart Association Task Force on Practice Guidelines and The Obesity Society. *J Am Coll Cardiol* 2014;63(25 Pt B):2985-3023. Erratum in *J Am Coll Cardiol* 2014;63(25 PT B):3029-3030.

37. Deurenberg P, Deurenberg S-Yap M, Guricci S. Asians are different from Caucasians and from each other in the body mass index/body fat per cent relationship. *Obes Rev* 2002;3:141-146.
38. Centers for Disease Control and Prevention. Body Mass Index (BMI). Available at: http://www.cdc.gov/healthyweight/assessing/bmi. (Accessed December 15, 2015)
39. Cook Z, Kirk S, Lawrenson S, Sandford S. Use of BMI in the assessment of undernutrition in older subjects: Reflecting on practice. *Proc Nutr Soc* 2005;64:313-317.
40. DiMaria-Ghalili RA. Integrating nutrition assessment in the comprehensive geriatric assessment. *Nutr Clin Pract* 2014;29:420-427.
41. Ness-Abramof R, Apovian CM. Waist circumference measurement in clinical practice. *Nutr Clin Pract* 2008;23:397-404.
42. Fernández JR, Redden DT, Pietrobelli A, Allison DB. Waist circumference percentiles in nationally representative samples of African-American, European-American, and Mexican-American children and adolescents. *J Pediatr* 2004;145:439-444.
43. Maffeis C, Banzato C, Talamini G, on behalf of the Obesity Study Group of the Italian Society of Pediatric Endocrinology and Diabetology. Waist-to-height ratio, a useful index to identify high metabolic risk in overweight children. *J Pediatr* 2008;152:207-213.
44. Frisancho AR. *Anthropometric Standards for the Assessment of Growth and Nutritional Status*. Ann Arbor: The University of Michigan Press; 1990.
45. NHANES III Anthropometrics Procedures Video. Available at: http://www.cdc.gov/nchs/nhanes/nhanes3/anthropometric_videos.htm. (Accessed December 15, 2015)
46. Mulasi U, Kuchnia AJ, Cole AJ, Earthman CP. Bioimpedance at the bedside: Current applications, limitations, and opportunities. *Nutr Clin Pract* 2015;30:180-193.
47. Earthman CP. Body composition tools for assessment of adult malnutrition at the bedside: A tutorial on research considerations and clinical applications. *J Parenter Enteral Nutr* 2015;39:787-822.
48. Schlüssel MM, dos Anjos LA, de Vasconcellos MTL, et al. Reference values of handgrip dynamometry of healthy adults: A population-based study. *Clin Nutr* 2008;27:601-607.
49. Kerr A, Syddall HE, Cooper C, et al. Does admission grip strength predict length of stay in hospitalized older patients? *Age Ageing* 2006;35:82-84.
50. Fields DA, Gunatilake R, Kalaitzoglou E. Air displacement plethysmography: Cradle to grave. *Nutr Clin Pract* 2015;30:219-226.
51. Baracos V, Caserotti P, Earthman CP, et al. Advances in the science and application of body composition measurement. *J Parenter Enteral Nutr* 2012;36:96-107.
52. Crook MA. Hypoalbuminemia: The importance of correct interpretation. *Nutrition* 2009;25:1004-1005.
53. Hardy G, Menendez AM, Manzanes W. Trace element supplementation in parenteral nutrition: Pharmacy, posology, and monitoring guidance. *Nutrition* 2009;25:1073-1084.
54. Fessler TA. Trace elements in parenteral nutrition: A practical guide for dosage and monitoring for adult patients. *Nutr Clin Pract* 2013;28:722-729.
55. Food and Nutrition Board, Institute of Medicine, National Academy of Sciences. Dietary Reference Intakes: Elements. 2009. Available at: http://www.iom.edu/Home/Global/News%20Announcements/~/media/48FAAA2FD9E74D95BBDA2236E7387B49.ashx. (Accessed December 15, 2015)
56. Clark SF. Vitamins and trace elements. In: Mueller C, ed. *The A.S.P.E.N. Adult Nutrition Support Core Curriculum*. Silver Spring, MD: American Society for Parenteral and Enteral Nutrition; 2012:121-154.
57. Sriram K, Lonchyna VA. Micronutrient supplementation in adult nutrition therapy: Practical considerations. *J Parenter Enteral Nutr* 2009;33:548-562.
58. Kleinman RE, ed. Trace elements. In: *Pediatric Nutrition Handbook*. 6th ed. Elk Grove Village, IL: American Academy of Pediatrics; 2009:423-451.
59. Livingstone C. Zinc: Physiology, deficiency, and parenteral nutrition. *Nutr Clin Pract* 2015;30:371-382.
60. Hurwitz M, Garcia MG, Poole RL, Kerner JA. Copper deficiency during parenteral nutrition: A report of four pediatric cases. *Nutr Clin Pract* 2004;19:305-308.
61. Harvey LJ, Ashton K, Hooper L, et al. Methods of assessment of copper status in humans: A systematic review. *Am J Clin Nutr* 2009;89(Suppl):2009S-2024S.
62. MacKay M, Mulroy CW, Street J. Assessing copper status in pediatric patients receiving parenteral nutrition. *Nutr Clin Pract* 2015;30:117-121.
63. Vincent JB. Quest for the molecular mechanism of chromium action and its relationship to diabetes. *Nutr Rev* 2000;58:67-72.
64. Tian H, Guo X, Wang X, et al. Chromium picolinate supplementation for overweight and obese adults. *Cochrane Database Syst Rev* 2013;11:CD010063.
65. Dickerson RN. Manganese intoxication and parenteral nutrition. *Nutrition* 2001;17:689-693.
66. Erikson KM, Thompson K, Aschner J, Aschner M. Manganese neurotoxicity: A focus on the neonate. *Pharmacol Ther* 2007;113:369-377.
67. Iinuma Y, Kubota M, Uchiyama M, et al. Whole-blood manganese levels and brain manganese accumulation in children receiving long-term home parenteral nutrition. *Pediatr Surg Int* 2003;19:268-272.
68. Takagi Y, Okada A, Sando K, et al. Evaluation of indexes of in vivo manganese status and the optimal intravenous dose for adult patients undergoing home parenteral nutrition. *Am J Clin Nutr* 2002;75:112-118.
69. Ashton K, Hooper L, Harvey LJ, et al. Methods of assessment of selenium status in humans: A systematic review. *Am J Clin Nutr* 2009;89(Suppl):2025S-2039S.
70. Manzanares W, Langlois PL, Heyland DK. Pharmaconutrition with selenium in critically ill patients: What do we know? *Nutr Clin Pract* 2015;30:34-43.
71. Sardesai VM. Molybdenum: An essential trace element. *Nutr Clin Pract* 1993;8:277-281.
72. Abumrad NN, Schneider AJ, Steet D, et al. Amino acid intolerance during prolonged total parenteral nutrition reversed by molybdenum therapy. *Am J Clin Nutr* 1981;34:2551-2559.
73. Friel JK, MacDonald AC, Mercer CN, et al. Molybdenum requirements in low-birth-weight infants receiving parenteral and enteral nutrition. *J Parenter Enteral Nutr* 1999;23:155-159.
74. Food and Nutrition Board, Institute of Medicine, National Academy of Sciences. Dietary Reference Intakes: Vitamins. 2009. Available at: http://www.iom.edu/Home/Global/News%20Announcements/~/media/48FAAA2FD9E74D95BBDA2236E7387B49.ashx. (Accessed December 15, 2015)
75. Kleinman RE, ed. Vitamins. In: *Pediatric Nutrition Handbook*. 6th ed. Elk Grove Village, IL: American Academy of Pediatrics; 2009:453-495.
76. Frank LL. Thiamin in clinical practice. *J Parenter Enteral Nutr* 2015;39:503-520.
77. Lam JR, Schneider JL, Zhao W, Corley DA. Proton pump inhibitor and histamine 2 receptor antagonist use and vitamin B_{12} deficiency. *JAMA* 2013;310:2435-2442.
78. McCabe KM, Adams MA, Holden RM. Vitamin K status in chronic kidney disease. *Nutrients* 2013;5:4390-4398.
79. Lappe JM. The role of vitamin D in human health: A paradigm shift. *J Evid-Based Comp Alt Med* 2011;16:58-72.
80. Bharadwaj S, Gohel RD, Deen OJ, et al. Prevalence and predictors of vitamin D deficiency and response to oral supplementation in patients receiving long-term home parenteral nutrition. *Nutr Clin Pract* 2014;29:681-685.
81. Peskanich D, Singh V, Willett WC, Colditz GA. Vitamin A intake and hip fractures among postmenopausal women. *JAMA* 2002;287:47-54.
82. Michaëlsson K, Lithell H, Vessby B, Melhus H. Serum retinol levels and the risk of fracture. *N Engl J Med* 2003;348:287-294.
83. The Heart Outcomes Prevention Evaluation (HOPE) 2 Investigators. Homocysteine lowering with folic acid and B vitamins in vascular disease. *N Engl J Med* 2006;354:1567-1577.
84. Lange H, Suryapranata H, De Luca G, et al. Folate therapy and in-stent restenosis after coronary stenting. *N Engl J Med* 2004;350:2673-2681.
85. Food and Nutrition Board, Institute of Medicine, National Academy of Sciences. Dietary Reference Intakes for Energy, Carbohydrate, Fiber, Fat, Fatty Acids, Cholesterol, Protein, and Amino Acids. 2005. Available at: http://www.nap.edu/books/0309085373/html/R2.html. (Accessed December 15, 2015)
86. Hise M, Brown JC. Lipids. In: Mueller C, ed. *The A.S.P.E.N. Adult Nutrition Support Core Curriculum*. Silver Spring, MD: American Society for Parenteral and Enteral Nutrition; 2012:63-82.
87. Foote KD, MacKinnon MJ, Innis SM. Effect of early introduction of formula versus fat-free parenteral nutrition on essential fatty acid status of preterm infants. *Am J Clin Nutr* 1991;54:93-97.
88. Gramlich L, Meddings L, Alberda C, et al. Essential fatty acid deficiency in 2015: The impact of novel intravenous lipid emulsions. *J Parenter Enter Nutr* 2015;39(Suppl 1):61S-66S.

89. Crill CM, Helms RA. The use of carnitine in pediatric nutrition. *Nutr Clin Pract* 2007;22:204-213.
90. Schreiber B. Levocarnitine and dialysis: A review. *Nutr Clin Pract* 2005;20:218-243.
91. Scruggs ER, Dirks Naylor AJ. Mechanisms of zidovudine-induced mitochondrial toxicity and myopathy. *Pharmacology* 2008;82:83-88.
92. Food and Nutrition Board, Institute of Medicine, National Academy of Sciences. Dietary Reference Intakes (DRIs): The Development of DRIS 1994-2004: Lessons Learned and New Challenges. 2008. Available at: http://books.nap.edu/openbook.php?record_id=12086&page=R1. (Accessed December 15, 2015)
93. Food and Nutrition Board. Committee to Review Dietary Reference Intakes for Vitamin D and Calcium. Dietary Reference Intakes for Calcium and Vitamin D. Report brief. November 2010. Available at: http://www.iom.edu/vitamind. (Accessed December 15, 2015)
94. United States Department of Agriculture, National Agriculture Library. Interactive DRI for Healthcare Professionals, 2015. Available at: http://fnic.nal.usda.gov/fnic/interactiveDRI/. (Accessed December 15, 2015)
95. McClave SA, Taylor BE, Martindale RG, et al. Guidelines for the provision and assessment of nutrition support therapy in the adult patient: Society of Critical Care Medicine (SCCM) and American Society for Parenteral and Enteral Nutriiton (A.S.P.E.N.). *J Parenter Enter Nutr* 2006;40:159-211.
96. Wooley JA, Frankenfield D. Energy. In: Mueller C, ed. *The A.S.P.E.N. Adult Nutrition Support Core Curriculum.* Silver Spring, MD: American Society for Parenteral and Enteral Nutrition; 2012:22-35.
97. FAO/WHO/UNU Expert Consultation. Food and Nutrition Technical Report Series. Human Energy Requirements. October 2001;1-103. ftp://ftp.fao.org/docrep/fao/007/y5686e/y5686e00.pdf. (Accessed December 15, 2015)
98. Chan MM, Chan GM. Nutrition therapy for burns in children and adults. *Nutrition* 2009;25:261-269.
99. Cooney RN, Frankenfield DC. Determining energy needs in critically ill patients: Equations or indirect calorimetry. *Curr Opin Crit Care* 2012;18:174-177.
100. McClave SA, Martindale RG, Kiraly L. The use of indirect calorimetry in the intensive care unit. *Curr Opin Clin Nutr Metab Care* 2013;16:202-208.
101. Meyer R, Kulinskaya E, Briassoulis G, et al. The challenge of developing a new predictive formula to estimate energy requirements in ventilated critically ill children. *Nutr Clin Pract* 2012;27:669-676.
102. Mehta NM, Compher C, A.S.P.E.N. Board of Directors. A.S.P.E.N. clinical guidelines: Nutrition support of the critically ill child. *J Parenter Enteral Nutr* 2009;33:260-276.
103. Hipskind P, Glass C, Charlton D, Nowak D, Dasarathy S. Do handheld calorimeters have a role in assessment of nutrition needs in hospitalized patients? A systematic review of literature. *Nutr Clin Pract* 2011;26:426-433.
104. Haugen HA, Chan L-N, Li F. Indirect calorimetry: A practical guide for clinicians. *Nutr Clin Pract* 2007;22:377-388.
105. Moreira de Rocha EE, Alves VGF, da Fonseca RBV. Indirect calorimetry: Methodology, instruments and clinical application. *Curr Opin Clin Nutr Metab Care* 2006;9:247-256.
106. Wolfe RR, Miller SL, Miller KB. Optimal protein intake in the elderly. *Clin Nutr* 2008;27:675-684.
107. Velasco N, Long CL, Otto DA, et al. Comparison of three methods for the estimation of total nitrogen losses in hospitalized patients. *J Parenter Enteral Nutr* 1990;14:517-522.
108. Wolk R, Foulks C. Renal disease. In: Mueller C, ed. *The A.S.P.E.N. Adult Nutrition Support Core Curriculum.* Silver Spring, MD: American Society for Parenteral and Enteral Nutrition; 2012:491-510.
109. Kleinman RE, ed. Fats and fatty acids. In: *Pediatric Nutrition Handbook*, 6th ed. Elk Grove Village, IL: American Academy of Pediatrics; 2009:357-386.
110. American Dietetic Association. Position of the American Dietetic Association: Health implications of dietary fiber. *J Am Diet Assoc* 2008;108:1716-1731.
111. Greene HL, Hambidge KM, Schanler R, Tsang RC. Guidelines for the use of vitamins, trace elements, calcium, magnesium, and phosphorus in infants and children receiving total parenteral nutrition: Report of the Subcommittee on Pediatric Parenteral Nutrient Requirements from the Committee on Clinical Practice Issues of the American Society for Clinical Nutrition. *Am J Clin Nutr* 1988;48:1324-1342.
112. Kraft MD, Btaiche IF, Sacks GS. Review of the refeeding syndrome. *Nutr Clin Pract* 2005;20:625-633.
113. Skipper A. Refeeding syndrome or refeeding hypophosphatemia: A systematic review of cases. *Nutr Clin Pract* 2012;27:34-40.
114. Jefferson JW. Drug and diet interactions: Avoiding therapeutic paralysis. *J Clin Psychiatry* 1998;59:31-39.
115. Saito M, Hirata-Koizumi M, Matsumoto M, et al. Undesirable effects of citrus juice on the pharmacokinetics of drugs: Focus on recent studies. *Drug Saf* 2005;28:677-694.
116. Santos CA, Boullata JI. An approach to evaluating drug–nutrient interactions. *Pharmacotherapy* 2005;25:1789-1800.
117. McCabe BJ. Prevention of food–drug interactions with special emphasis on older adults. *Curr Opin Clin Nutr Metab Care* 2004;7:21-26.
118. Hester EK. HIV medications: An update and review of metabolic complications. *Nutr Clin Pract* 2012;27:51-64.
119. Yilmaz Y, Tasdemir HA, Paksu MS. The influence of valproic acid treatment on hair and serum zinc levels and serum biotinidase activity. *Eur J Paediatr Neuro* 2009;13:439-443.
120. Robien K, Oppeneer SJ, Kelly JA, Hamilton-Reeves JM. Drug–vitamin D interactions: A systematic review of the literature. *Nutr Clin Pract* 2013;28:194-208.

Parenteral Nutrition

142

Todd W. Mattox and Catherine M. Crill

KEY CONCEPTS

1. Development and implementation of an appropriate, individualized nutrition care plan requires definition of nutrition goals, determination of nutrition requirements and appropriate route of nutrient delivery, and design of a monitoring plan to evaluate suitability of the nutrition regimen as a patient's clinical condition changes.
2. The appropriate route of nutrition support depends on the functional condition of the patient's gastrointestinal (GI) tract, risk of aspiration, expected duration of nutrition therapy, and clinical condition.
3. Suitable candidates for parenteral nutrition (PN) therapy can be identified on the basis of their age, nutrition status, expected duration of GI dysfunction, and potential risks of PN therapy.
4. PN formulations include injectable amino acids, dextrose, fat, water, electrolytes, vitamins, trace elements, and other additives.
5. PN solutions may be appropriately formulated for administration by peripheral or central venous access.
6. PN formulations are available as standardized commercial premixed products or they may be compounded with an automated compounding device (ACD).
7. PN solutions may be infused continuously or intermittently.
8. Biochemical and clinical measurements for effective monitoring of patients receiving PN include serum chemistries, vital signs, body weight, total daily fluid intake and losses, and nutritional intake.
9. Non–catheter-related complications of PN therapy can be minimized by using age-appropriate nutrient dosing guidelines, frequent monitoring, and implementing rational adjustments to the PN regimen when metabolic abnormalities occur.
10. Individualized PN therapy should be based on nutrition therapy goals determined from a patient-specific nutrition assessment, type of available IV access, and macronutrient and micronutrient requirements.
11. A patient's nutrient requirements are affected by age, degree of metabolic demand, organ function, drug therapy, exogenous losses, acid–base status, and enteral intake in patients with recovering GI function.

INTRODUCTION

Maintenance of adequate nutrition status during illness has been recognized for more than 50 years as an integral part of the treatment plan for patients who are unable to attain and sustain oral nourishment. Successful techniques for providing IV nutrition support were introduced to clinical practice in adults and subsequently, infants in the late 1960s.[1] Use of central venous access was investigated to reduce risk of metabolic complications associated with IV fluid overload and electrolyte imbalances. The use of large central vessels permitted infusion of concentrated formulas, which decreased the fluid volume required and avoided the phlebitis that commonly occurred when hypertonic infusions were given peripherally.

Clinical experience and research fostered development of protocols that promoted better patient care and resulted in a decline in complications and costs associated with parenteral nutrition (PN) therapy.[2] The scope of practice for nutrition support clinicians has broadened as a result of increasing knowledge regarding the metabolic consequences associated with acute injury and chronic disease states. The pharmacist's role in providing safe and effective nutrition-support care requires knowledge of the principles of patient selection, initial therapy design, outcome monitoring, and strategies for providing therapy during PN product shortages.[3,4] In addition, the pharmacist is uniquely prepared to take on the responsibility for PN order verification as well as compounding and dispensing of the PN admixture. The PN order must be verified by a pharmacist to ensure the order is clear, complete, and correctly transcribed. A clinical review should be performed to confirm appropriate indication, nutrient dosing, and non-nutrient medication dosing. A pharmaceutical review should be performed to confirm compatibility of ordered nutrients and any non-nutrient medications in addition to the expected stability of the formulation.[4,5] Other responsibilities of the nutrition support pharmacist may include development of policy and procedures as well as quality improvement activities for patient care and operational processes associated with providing parenteral and enteral nutrition.[4-7] The clinical role of other healthcare professionals may be similar because of the evolving interprofessional approach to nutritional support.[8-10] This chapter reviews indications for PN, components of PN formulations, routes of IV administration, practical aspects of regimen design, solution admixture, outcome monitoring, and management of complications for both adult and pediatric (neonates, infants, and children) patients.

DESIRED OUTCOMES

1 The primary objective of nutrition support therapy is to promote positive clinical outcomes of an illness and improve a patient's quality of life. Four fundamental steps are key to providing optimal care for patients who require nutrition support. They are establishing patient-specific nutrition goals, determining nutrient requirements to achieve the nutrition goals, assuring delivery of the required nutrients, and subsequently assessing the nutrition regimen.[5-7]

A patient's nutrition goals can be established after a thorough nutritional assessment (see Chapter 141). Nutrient requirements and an appropriate route for delivery of the required nutrients can then be determined. Nutrition support goals include correction of the patient's caloric and nitrogen imbalances and any fluid, electrolyte, vitamin, or trace element abnormalities. An additional goal is to lessen the metabolic response to injury by minimizing oxidant stress and favorably modulating immune response. These interventions should not cause or worsen other metabolic complications.

2 The gastrointestinal (GI) tract is the optimal route for providing nutrients unless obstruction or other GI complications are present (see Chapter 143).[11,12] Two other considerations that may impact selection of the optimal route for delivery of nutrition support include expected duration of nutrition therapy and risk of aspiration. Patients who have nonfunctional GI tracts or are otherwise not candidates for enteral nutrition may benefit from PN.

INDICATIONS FOR PARENTERAL NUTRITION SUPPORT

The association between malnutrition and development of complications and mortality is well documented for adult and pediatric patients.[12,13] Although improvement in various clinical nutrition markers has been reported for patients who received PN, the impact on clinical outcome has been difficult to demonstrate in many adult populations. Several investigations have reported a positive effect of PN on complications and mortality, but others have failed to confirm these findings.[11,14,15] Early studies have been criticized for defective study design, such as small sample sizes, inappropriate randomization, and inconsistent baseline nutrition status among the study and control groups, which hindered demonstration of the effectiveness of PN therapy. The impact of PN on clinical outcome has been more consistently demonstrated for critically ill infants and children, particularly those with acquired or congenital GI tract anomalies.[16] Consensus guidelines for PN use for adults (Table 142-1) and pediatric (Table 142-2) patients are based on clinical experience and investigations in specific patient populations.[11,12,14,16-20] Unfortunately, conflicting data have resulted in a lack of consistency in published guidelines from different sources, which complicates identification of the patient who is most likely to benefit from PN. However, these published reports may serve as resources for development of institution-specific standards.

3 The decision to initiate PN is based on the findings of an assessment performed after a patient demonstrates an inability to meet nutritional needs enterally for an extended time period. This assessment must include an evaluation of the patient's nutrition status, clinical status, age, and potential risks of initiating therapy (eg, infection and other metabolic abnormalities). The appropriate length of time to wait before starting PN therapy depends on patient age and clinical status.[11,12,14,16-20] Adult PN therapy is not an emergent intervention and should not be initiated until the patient is hemodynamically stable.[11] In general, previously well-nourished, clinically stable adults who are not candidates for enteral nutrition, should be considered candidates for PN after 7 to 14 days of suboptimal nutritional intake.[11,14,20] PN should be initiated as soon as possible in severely malnourished critically ill patients in whom EN is not feasible. Supplemental PN should be considered after 7-10 days in critically ill patients in whom greater than 60% of energy and protein requirements cannot be met by the enteral route alone.[11] The most appropriate time to initiate therapy for infants and children varies with age and nutritional status. Because early PN results in enhanced protein accretion and improved growth in extremely low-birth-weight infants, initiation of PN within the first 24 hours of life in preterm neonates has been recommended.[18,21,22] Withholding PN for 2 to 3 days after birth, coupled with slow advancement of nutrient substrate, only appears to deplete limited energy reserves and contribute to growth failure for many neonates.[21] PN should be initiated within 5 to 7 days for other pediatric patients who are unable to meet their nutrient requirements with via the enteral route.[16] Earlier intervention should be considered for term infants (within 2-3 days), critically ill pediatric patients (within 3-5 days), and those with preexisting malnutrition.

TABLE 142-1 Indications for Adult PN

1. Inability to absorb nutrients via the GI tract because of one or more of the following:
   a. Massive small bowel resection: Usually patients with less than 100 cm of small bowel distal to the ligament of Treitz without a colon or less than 50 cm of small bowel with an intact colon
   b. Intractable vomiting when adequate EN is not expected for 7–14 days.
   c. Severe diarrhea
   d. Bowel obstruction
   e. GI fistulae: PN is indicated in patients with prolonged inadequate nutritional intake longer than 5–7 days who are not candidates for EN
2. Cancer: Antineoplastic therapy, radiation therapy, or HSCT
   a. PN may be used in moderately to severely malnourished patients receiving active anticancer treatment who are not candidates for EN.
   b. PN is not routinely indicated for well-nourished or mildly malnourished patients undergoing surgery, chemotherapy, or radiation therapy.
   c. PN is unlikely to benefit patients with advanced cancer whose malignancy is unresponsive to treatment. However, use may be appropriate for carefully selected patients who have failed trials of less invasive medical therapies and have good performance status, an estimated life expectancy of longer than 40–60 days, and strong social and financial support.
   d. PN is appropriate in patients undergoing HSCT who are malnourished and who are anticipated to be unable to ingest or absorb adequate nutrients for 7–14 days. PN should be discontinued as soon as toxicities have resolved after stem cell engraftment.
3. Pancreatitis: PN may be used in patients with severe pancreatitis with prolonged inadequate nutritional intake longer than 5–7 days who are not candidates for EN. PN should be used when EN exacerbates abdominal pain, ascites, or fistula output.
4. Critical care
   a. PN should be used in malnourished patients in whom EN is contraindicated or is unlikely to provide adequate nutritional requirements as soon as possible after ICU admission and adequate resuscitation.
   b. PN should be reserved and initiated only after the first 7 days of hospitalization for previously well-nourished patients.
   c. Organ failure (liver, renal, or respiratory): PN should be used in patients with moderate to severe catabolism when EN is contraindicated.
   d. Burns: PN should be used in those patients in whom EN is contraindicated or is unlikely to provide adequate nutritional requirements within 4–5 days.
5. Perioperative PN
   a. Preoperative: For 5–7 days for patients with moderate to severe malnutrition who are undergoing major GI surgery if the operation can be safely postponed
   b. Postoperative: PN should be used in patients in whom EN is contraindicated or is unlikely to provide adequate nutritional requirements within 7–14 days after surgery.
6. Hyperemesis gravidarum: when EN is not tolerated
7. Eating disorders: PN should be considered for patients with anorexia nervosa and severe malnutrition who are unable or unwilling to ingest adequate nutrition.

EN, enteral nutrition; GI, gastrointestinal; HSCT, hematopoietic stem cell transplantation; ICU, intensive care unit; PN, parenteral nutrition; SBS, short-bowel syndrome.

Data from references 11, 14, 15, 19, and 20.

Clinical **Controversy...**

Early enteral nutrition (within 24-48 hours of admission to an intensive care unit) is recommended as the preferred route for nutrition support in critically ill patients. Many clinicians maintain PN should be withheld unless enteral nutrition cannot be achieved within 7 days because of data that associate early PN with negative clinical outcomes. Conversely other clinicians may recommend early supplemental PN to prevent the protein–energy deficit that has been associated with worsening clinical outcomes in some studies.

TABLE 142-2 Indications for Pediatric PN

1. When enteral nutrition is unlikely to provide adequate nutritional requirements
   a. Premature infant within 24–48 hours
   b. Other pediatric patients within 5–7 days
2. When the GI tract is not functional or cannot be assessed
   a. Massive small bowel resection resulting in short-bowel syndrome
   b. Neonatal necrotizing enterocolitis
   c. Congenital anomalies of the GI tract
   d. Severe inflammatory bowel disease
   e. Intractable diarrhea or vomiting
   f. Graft vs host disease
   g. After chemotherapy
3. Infants and children requiring extracorporeal membrane oxygenation
4. Organ failure (liver, renal, pulmonary, pancreas) or congenital heart disease when enteral nutrition is contraindicated and the child is catabolic

GI, gastrointestinal; PN, parenteral nutrition.

Data references, 12, 16 to 18, 21, and 22.

COMPONENTS OF PARENTERAL NUTRITION

4 PN formulations include IV sources of protein, dextrose, fat, water, electrolytes, vitamins, trace elements, and other additives. PN solutions should provide the optimal combination of macro- and micronutrients to provide a patient's specific nutritional requirements. Macronutrients include water, protein, dextrose, and fat (Table 142-3). Micronutrients include vitamins, trace elements, and electrolytes. Both macronutrients and micronutrients are necessary for maintenance of normal metabolism. In general, macronutrients are used for energy (dextrose and fat) and as structural substrates (protein and fat). Micronutrients on the other hand support a variety of metabolic activities necessary for cellular homeostasis such as enzymatic reactions, fluid balance, and regulation of electrophysiologic processes.

Over the past 5 to 7 years, shortages of all PN components have been reported.[3,23] The unavailability of these products has resulted in delays in PN therapy initiation, restricted or limited nutrient dosing, and negative effects on all steps of the PN process that have compromised patient health and safety. Providing safe therapy during PN product shortages can be challenging for PN patients and practitioners.[5] Conservation recommendations and alternative therapy measures may need to be employed to optimize quality of care and avoid patient harm.[3]

Amino Acids

Protein in PN solutions is provided in the form of crystalline amino acids (CAAs), which when oxidized for energy yield 4 cal or approximately 17 J per gram of protein. However, including the caloric contribution from protein when calculating calories provided by the PN regimen is controversial.[24] While sufficient energy substrate should be provided to allow utilization of amino acids for protein synthesis rather than an energy source, oxidation of amino acids for energy has been demonstrated in critically ill patients and is thought to occur because of metabolic derangements seen during severe metabolic stress. Hence, some practice settings may differ in expressing calories provided by a PN regimen as total calories (protein, carbohydrate, and fat calories) or non-protein calories (carbohydrate and fat calories).

Commercially available CAA solutions may be categorized as standard amino acid solutions or modified amino acid solutions. Standard CAA solutions are designed for patients with "normal" organ function and nutritional requirements (see Table 142-3). Although standard CAA solutions differ in the proportion of specific amino acids, they contain a balanced profile of essential, semi-essential, and nonessential L-amino acids. Despite these differences,

TABLE 142-3 Macronutrient Components of PN Solutions

Nutritional Substrate	IV Source	Description
Fluid	Sterile water for injection USP	
Nitrogen	Crystalline amino acids Standard solutions	Contain a balanced profile of essential, semi-essential, and nonessential L-amino acids
	Disease-specific solutions	
	Hepatic encephalopathy	Amino acid profile includes higher BCAA concentrations and lower AAA and methionine concentrations
	Renal failure	Amino acid profile includes higher EAA and histidine concentrations
	Metabolic stress or trauma	Amino acid profile provides standard essential, semi-essential, and nonessential amino acids with higher BCAA concentrations
	Pediatrics	Amino acid profile includes standard essential, semi-essential, and nonessential amino acids with lower methionine, phenylalanine, and glycine concentrations; these solutions also contain taurine, glutamate, and aspartate
Energy		
Carbohydrate	Dextrose	
	Glycerol	Used in ProcalAmine (B. Braun Medical, Inc.)
Fat	IV fat emulsion LCT emulsions Mixed fat emulsions Alternative fat emulsions (investigational)	Fatty acid source Soybean Soybean-Olive Oil SMOF (soybean oil, MCT, olive, and fish oils) Olive oil Fish oil Mixed fat emulsions: MCT-LCT MSF (MCT, soybean, and fish oils)

AAA, aromatic amino acids (includes phenylalanine and tyrosine); BCAA, branched-chain amino acids (leucine, isoleucine, and valine); EAA, essential amino acids (leucine, isoleucine, valine, phenylalanine, tryptophan, methionine, threonine, and lysine); LCT, long-chain triglycerides; MCT, medium-chain triglycerides; MSF, MCT, soybean, and fish oils; PN, parenteral nutrition; SMOF, soybean oil, MCT, olive, and fish oils; USP, United States Pharmacopeia.

similar effects on markers of protein use have been reported.[25] The protein concentration, total nitrogen, and electrolyte content may also differ among products. Because the nitrogen concentration of dietary protein is approximately 16%, 6.25 (100 g protein/16 g nitrogen) is commonly accepted as the conversion figure for calculating the nitrogen amount provided by CAA protein. Differences in nitrogen content per gram of amino acids among CAA products may affect calculation of nitrogen amounts infused when determining nitrogen balance.[25,26] The clinical significance of these differences in determining nitrogen balance for routine clinical use is unknown.[26]

Electrolyte composition of standard CAA solutions varies from small, obligatory amounts to the provision of maintenance requirements of most electrolytes for an adult. Electrolytes provided by CAA solutions must be considered when determining a patient's individual requirements. CAAs are available in several different concentrations, which facilitates compounding of patient-specific PN regimens. Use of highly concentrated products (15%-20% amino acids) is attractive for critically ill patients who typically require fluid restriction but have large protein needs. Modified amino acid solutions are designed for patients who have altered protein requirements, such as those with hepatic encephalopathy, renal failure, and metabolic stress or trauma, as well as for neonates and pediatric patients (see Table 142-3). These solutions tend to be more expensive than standard CAA solutions. The rationale for and clinical efficacy of modified amino acids in disease-specific PN regimens is also controversial because of inconsistency in clinical outcomes reported in multiple clinical trials.[11,15,19,27]

Several commercially available CAA solutions are designed to provide conditionally essential amino acids, which are considered nonessential during health because they are produced from other amino acids. However, under certain physiologic conditions, such as prematurity or sepsis, these amino acids cannot be synthesized in sufficient quantities.[25] CAA solutions specifically designed for neonates and pediatric patients contain increased amounts of taurine, aspartic acid, and glutamic acid. Other conditionally essential amino acids, such as cysteine, carnitine, and glutamine, are not available in commercial CAA solutions in pharmacologic amounts because they are relatively unstable or poorly soluble.[25]

Clinical **Controversy...**

Exclusive use of standardized, commercially prepared premixed IV products has been advocated to improve medication safety. However, the American Society for Parenteral and Enteral Nutrition (A.S.P.E.N.) has reported that patient safety data do not support the general use of standardized PN formulations across healthcare organizations.

Consequently, PN solutions may need to be modified to provide the desired amount of supplemental conditionally essential amino acids. For example, cysteine is a conditionally essential amino acid for preterm and term infants because of their enzymatic immaturity of the trans-sulfuration pathway. Cysteine may be added to PN solutions at the time of compounding as a supplement to CAA solutions and to enhance calcium and phosphate solubility by decreasing solution pH.[28] Carnitine is a quaternary amine required for long-chain fatty acid transport into the mitochondria for β-oxidation and energy production. Newborns are at risk for carnitine deficiency because of their immature biosynthetic capacity. Decreased plasma carnitine concentrations have been reported in infants and children receiving PN without carnitine.[18] Supplemental carnitine may be added to the PN solution at the time of compounding. Although the benefit of carnitine supplementation in PN has not been clearly identified, positive effects on nutritional markers, including improved fatty acid oxidation, weight gain, and nitrogen balance, have been documented. In general, carnitine supplementation is reserved for neonates expected to receive PN support for 7 days or longer.[18]

Glutamine is the most abundant free amino acid in the body and is an important intermediate for many metabolic processes. Glutamine is reported to have an important role in maintaining intestinal integrity, immune function, and protein synthesis during conditions of metabolic stress.[29] Investigations in humans and animals have reported positive effects on nutritional markers such as nitrogen balance, but others have reported significant improvement in other outcome markers, such as decreased length of hospitalization, incidence of infections, and GI toxicities associated with chemotherapy or radiation.[29] Unfortunately, the best candidate for response to glutamine therapy has not been clearly identified.[29] Use of both intravenous and enteral glutamine in combination with a variety of antioxidant supplements in critically ill adult patients has been associated with increased mortality.[30] Although an association between increased brain volume and head circumference has been reported in school-aged children, who were premature at birth and received glutamine during the first year of life,[31] the clinical usefulness of glutamine in neonates and infants is not clear.[29,32,33] Plasma glutamine concentrations increase with supplementation, but no beneficial effect on sepsis incidence or outcome, enteral feeding tolerance, necrotizing enterocolitis, growth, or mortality has been reported.[29,32,33] The clinical use of glutamine is further complicated because there is no parenteral glutamine formulation commercially available in the United States. Currently available CAA solutions do not contain glutamine because of poor solubility and instability. Use of parenteral glutamine requires special manufacturing techniques not readily available in many institutional pharmacies.[29] However, parenteral glutamine has been made available from several licensed pharmacies that extemporaneously compound glutamine crystalline powder under sterile conditions either as a separate parenteral solution or as a part of a CAA solution. Recent Food and Drug Administration (FDA) mandated changes in conditions under which a human drug product that has no applicable United States Pharmacopeia (USP) or National Formulary (NF) monograph or is not a component of an FDA-approved drug can be used to compound a prescription medication may create further obstacles to obtaining extemporaneously compounded glutamine-containing PN formulations. The FDA's Pharmacy Compounding Advisory Committee, which provides advice on scientific, technical, and medical issues concerning drug compounding, has recommended to not allow the use of alanyl-L-glutamine in compounding due to insufficient information to fully assess safety related to impurities of the product.[34,35]

Dextrose

The primary energy source in PN solutions is carbohydrate, usually in the form of dextrose monohydrate, hereafter referred to as dextrose which is available in concentrations ranging from 5% to 70%. When oxidized, each gram of dextrose provides 3.4 kcal (14.2 kJ). The appropriate IV dextrose dose depends on the patient's age, estimated caloric requirements, and clinical condition. For example, minimum dextrose requirements for neonates are estimated to be approximately 6 to 8 mg/kg/min and infusion rates should not exceed 14 to 18 mg/kg/min for infants or 4 to 7 mg/kg/min for adults.[18,21,36] The recommended dextrose dose for routine clinical care rarely exceeds 5 mg/kg/min for adolescents and adults.[18,36] Maintaining an age-appropriate dextrose infusion rate is necessary to minimize risk of adverse effects. If the dextrose infusion rate exceeds the glucose oxidation rate, metabolically expensive pathways, such as glycogen repletion and lipid synthesis, are favored, resulting in increased energy expenditure, increased oxygen consumption, and increased carbon dioxide production. Excessive dextrose infusion rates also may contribute to the development of hyperglycemia and an increase in the concentration of biochemical markers indicative of fatty infiltration of the liver.[36,37]

Carbohydrate sources that are not insulin-dependent have been investigated as an alternative to dextrose to improve glycemic control for patients with impaired insulin secretion or activity who require PN. Glycerol, a sugar alcohol, that provides 4.3 kcal/g (18 kJ/g), is the only dextrose alternative commercially available. It is available as an isotonic, 3% solution in combination with 3% amino acids and supplemental electrolytes (ProcalAmine, B. Braun Medical, Irvine, CA). Although the solution may be peripherally infused, a major disadvantage of this product is the dilute amino acid and carbohydrate concentrations. Most adult patients require up to 3 to 4 L/day of ProcalAmine solution together with IVFE as a caloric source to meet minimum energy requirements.[38] IV glycerol use for catabolic adults is safe and effective, but similar data are not available for infants and children.[39]

Intravenous Fat Emulsion

Intravenous fate emulsion (IVFE) is used as a concentrated source of calories and essential fatty acids. Although commercially available IVFE products have traditionally contained soybean oil (SO) or a combination of SO and safflower oil, IVFE products containing safflower oil are no longer commercially available. However, a new IVFE product containing a mixture of SO and olive oil (OO) was recently approved for use in adults.[40] SO-based IVFE products have been marketed in 10%, 20%, and 30% concentrations while the SO-OO product is only marketed as a 20% emulsion. The 10% SO IVFE products are currently unavailable because of discontinued production or a prolonged manufacturer's stock shortage.[18] Both types of IVFE contain egg phospholipids as an emulsifying agent and glycerol to make the emulsion isotonic. Although the caloric contribution of fat is 9 kcal/g (38 kJ/g), the caloric content of 10% IVFE is 1.1 kcal/mL (4.6 kJ/mL), 2 kcal/mL (8.4 kJ/mL) for the 20% emulsion, and 3 kcal/mL (12.6 kJ/mL) for the 30% emulsion because of the caloric contribution of the egg phospholipid and glycerol.[18] The fatty acid composition of SO IVFEs varies between approximately 44% to 62% linoleic acid and 4% to 11% linolenic acid.[41] While the fatty acid composition of the SO-OO product is approximately 14% to 22% linoleic acid, 0.5% to 4% linolenic acid, 44% to 80% oleic acid, 8% to 19% palmitic acid, and 0.7% to 5% stearic acid.[40] Linolenic acid, an omega-3 fatty acid, and linoleic acid, an omega-6 fatty acid, are both polyunsaturated long-chain triglycerides (LCTs).[41] Palmitic and stearic acids are saturated LCTs while oleic acid is an unsaturated LCT.[41] The concentrated SO IVFEs (20% and 30%) have a lower phospholipid-to-triglyceride ratio compared with 10% SO IVFE.[18,42] Because higher amounts of circulating phospholipids are associated with impaired triglyceride clearance in neonates and infants, 20% SO IVFE is the preferred product for this population. The more concentrated 30% IVFE would be an attractive alternative as well but its use is approved only for the preparation of total nutrient admixture (TNA) formulations which are not recommended for use in neonates and infants.[5,18,42]

SO–based IVFE is effective for treatment or prevention of essential fatty acid deficiency (EFAD) in both adult and pediatric patients. EFAD is the result of a biochemical deficiency of linoleic acid and arachidonic acid, which are considered essential for humans.[43] Linoleic and linolenic acids are important for a variety of functions such as cellular integrity, platelet function, postnatal brain development, and wound healing.[43] Normally, linoleic acid is converted to the tetraene arachidonic acid. When linoleic acid is not present in sufficient amounts, oleic acid is converted to the triene 5,8,11-eicosatrienoic acid, a fatty acid of lesser physiologic integrity, and as a result EFAD develops. EFAD may be prevented by providing 2% to 4% of total calories as linoleic acid and 0.25% to 0.5% of total calories as linolenic acid.[44] This may be achieved for most adult patients by giving approximately 100 g SO IVFE weekly.[36,44] Neonates and infants require a minimum of 0.5 to 1 g/kg daily.[18,45] The SO-OO product is currently not approved for use in pediatric patients because of its lower linoleic and linolenic acid content and lack of clinical data demonstrating provision of adequate essential fatty acids to prevent or treat EFAD when used in recommended doses.[40]

Plasma IVFE clearance is directly related to gestational age of infants and appears to be influenced by the infusion rate and the patient's clinical status.[18,42,45] The risk of developing hypertriglyceridemia decreases with longer infusion times.[42,44,45] Rapid IVFE infusions are reported to contribute to decreased oxygenation for neonates.[45,46] Adverse pulmonary effects are thought to be caused by polyunsaturated fatty acid (PUFA)–driven prostaglandin production, which results in altered vascular tone. Although the association between IVFE and pulmonary dysfunction is not clear, a boxed warning appears in the FDA product labeling for both SO and SO-OO IVFE that acknowledges deaths in preterm infants associated with pulmonary fat accumulation thought to be related to IVFE infusions.[18,40,47] In addition, data for animals and humans also suggest that rapid infusion of long-chain fatty acid formulations may have a negative impact on immunocompetence by saturating the reticuloendothelial system.[36,48]

As a caloric source, IVFE use may facilitate provision of adequate calories and minimize complications of nutrition therapy such as hyperglycemia, hepatotoxicity, or increased carbon dioxide production.[36] Although the frequency of acute adverse effects is reported to be less than 1% with current formulations, patients receiving their first IVFE dose should be monitored for dyspnea, chest tightness, palpitations, and chills. Headache, nausea, and fever also have been reported and might be associated with a rapid infusion rate. In general, IVFE use is contraindicated for patients with an impaired ability to clear fat emulsion, such as patients with pathologic hyperlipidemia, lipoid nephrosis, and hypertriglyceridemia associated with pancreatitis.[47] Finally patients with an egg allergy should be evaluated carefully for the nature and severity of the reaction before deciding to initiate a fat-based PN regimen.

Commercially available 10% and 20% IVFE products may be administered by either the central or the peripheral route. They may be added directly to the PN solution as a TNA, also referred to as a three-in-one system (lipids, protein, glucose, and additives), or they may be co-infused with the CAA-dextrose solution, commonly referred to as a two-in-one admixture.[44,47] The more concentrated 30% IVFE is only approved for use in the preparation of TNA and is not intended for direct IV administration.

IVFEs with SO as the lipid source have negative effects on immune function as the result of omega-6 PUFA influence on proinflammatory eicosanoid production. These negative effects on immune function have stimulated a search for alternative IVFE sources that provide adequate essential fatty acids but lower amounts of omega-6 FA such as the SO-OO emulsion.[41,48] The SO-OO IVFEs provide essential fatty acids, are a rich source of vitamin E, and appear to have a neutral effect on immune function because of the decreased amount of omega-6 PUFA linoleic acid.[41] Medium-chain triglycerides (MCTs) may offer several advantages, especially for critically ill patients. MCTs are hydrolyzed and cleared more rapidly than LCTs, and they do not accumulate in the liver. In addition, MCTs do not require carnitine for entrance into mitochondria for oxidation. However, MCTs are not a source of essential fatty acids. Subsequent studies of IV MCT-LCT mixtures in a number of patients demonstrate safety and efficacy comparable with standard LCT emulsions.[41,48]

Several alternative IVFE products are not currently available in the United States. However, one mixed IVFE product available in Europe that includes soybean oil, MCT, olive oil and fish oil was recently FDA-approved for use in adults. Other IVFE that are available outside the United States include a fish oil-based emulsion, and a soybean, MCT, and fish oil combination (Table 142-3).[41,48] (see Table 142-3). Fish oil–based IVFE contain predominantly omega-3 PUFAs, which are metabolized to cytokine mediators that may be less inflammatory and immunosuppressive than those derived from omega-6 PUFAs. The clinical effect of IVFE administration on immune function, as well as on patient morbidity and mortality, is not clear.[41,48] However, investigations of enteral solutions with a higher concentration of omega-3 PUFAs have reported decreased infections and improvement of in vitro immunologic indices in critically ill patients.[43,49] Recent evidence suggests that SO–based IVFE, which contains phytosterols and predominantly omega-6 PUFAs, may play a greater role in the development of PN-associated liver disease (PNALD).[50] Investigations of fish oil–based IVFE have reported improvement in or reversal of PNALD.[41,50] The SO-OO emulsion contains phytosterols as well, but the effect on development of PNALD is not known.

Clinical **Controversy...**

The association between SO IVFE and PNALD has stimulated modifications to standard clinical practice, including SO IVFE dose restriction and / or the replacement of SO IVFE with fish oil–based IVFE. The risk for developing EFAD as a result of decreased LCT when reducing or eliminating SO IVFE from the parenteral diet is controversial.

Although IVFE products remain the most common source of parenteral fat, a number of drugs have been introduced that contain lipid either as a vehicle for delivery or as a portion of the drug formulation. Propofol, an IV anesthetic, is delivered in a SO-in-water emulsion that has essentially the same composition and caloric concentration as 10% IVFE. This agent is used commonly for continuous sedation of mechanically ventilated patients and should be considered a potentially significant source of calories that may require adjustment of a patient's nutrition regimen.[51] Clevidipine is an injectable calcium channel blocker that contains 20% IVFE as a vehicle that may be a potentially clinically significant source of IV fat when used as a continuous infusion for multiple days of therapy.[52] The antifungal amphotericin B is available in several lipid-containing combinations such as liposomal and lipid complex formulations. The caloric contribution from these products when used in standard doses generally is small and is not clinically relevant.

Vitamins

The Nutrition Advisory Group of the American Medical Association (NAG-AMA) recommended in 1975 the daily parenteral supplementation of 13 essential (four fat-soluble and nine water-soluble) vitamins for pediatric and adult patients based on requirements for healthy people.[53]

Since these original recommendations, the NAG-AMA has revised the guidelines for children to primarily reflect changes for preterm infants requiring PN.[53] The FDA also mandated in 2000 changes in adult parenteral vitamin formulations (inclusion of vitamin K and higher doses of vitamins B_1, B_6, and C).[53]

The amount of vitamin K supplementation in parenteral multivitamin formulations has been debated. The NAG-AMA recommendation for vitamin K for adults is 2 to 4 mg weekly, while other practitioners recommend larger doses of 0.5 to 1 mg/day or 5 to 10 mg weekly.[44] Vitamin K was not included in early multivitamin formulations due to the potential for drug-nutrient interactions in patients receiving anticoagulants, and the amount mandated to be included in 2000 (150 mcg/day) was considerably lower than other recommended requirements. However, an investigation of patients receiving long-term IVFE-containing PN with vitamin K–free parenteral multivitamins at home suggested that supplemental vitamin K may not be necessary to maintain normal prothrombin times and plasma vitamin K concentrations.[54] SO used in IVFEs is a natural source of phylloquinone (vitamin K_1). However, the vitamin K concentration is dependent on the SO concentration in the IVFE.[54-56] Mean concentrations of 30.9 and 67.5 mcg/100 mL were reported for 10% and 20% Intralipid (Baxter Healthcare Corporation, Deerfield, IL), a SO–based IVFE. The bioavailability of vitamin K from IVFEs is unknown. Although hospitalized patients who received no additional vitamin K supplementation during short-term PN that included a low vitamin K-containing IVFE experienced minimal effects on international normalized ratio, supplemental vitamin K may be given intramuscularly or subcutaneously or added to the PN solution if needed.[55] Current recommendations suggest supplemental vitamin K is unnecessary when a vitamin K-containing multiple-vitamin product is used.[44]

The 2012 A.S.P.E.N. recommendations advocate for the continued availability of multivitamin products with and without vitamin K so that clinicians have the ability to withhold vitamin K supplementation in patients receiving warfarin therapy. Most adult parenteral multiple-vitamin products which are available commercially contain vitamin K. MVI-12, multivitamin infusion without vitamin K is available from Hospira, Inc. Lake Forest, IL. Two parenteral multiple-vitamin products are commercially available for use for pediatric patients. MVI-Pediatric (Hospira Inc.) and Infuvite Pediatric (Baxter Healthcare Corporation) are formulated to meet the revised NAG-AMA guidelines for infants weighing less than 1 kg (2.2 lb) and children up to 11 years. However, there are no commercially available injectable multivitamin products designed to specifically meet the unique requirements of premature infants, including higher vitamin A and lower doses of vitamins B_1, B_2, B_6, and B_{12}.

Vitamin requirements may be altered in malnutrition and other specific disease states or with certain drug therapies. Individual and combination products are available to provide additional or tailored supplementation, which may be necessary to prevent development of vitamin toxicities or deficiencies caused by altered metabolism or drug therapy.

The 2012 A.S.P.E.N. recommendations question whether the vitamin D content of parenteral multivitamins is adequate to meet current Recommended Dietary Allowances (RDA) and advocate for the addition of a parenteral vitamin D product for PN-dependent patients who are unresponsive to additional enteral vitamin D supplementation.[53] In addition, the recommendations support the continued production of adult injectable multivitamin products with and without vitamin K and for the supplementation of carnitine (2-5 mg/kg/day) in neonatal PN and choline in all patients receiving PN.[53]

Trace Elements

Many trace elements are an important part of metalloenzymes and function as cofactors in a variety of regulatory metabolic pathways.[57] Although 17 trace elements have demonstrated biologic importance, clear deficiency syndromes in humans have been described only for cobalt (as vitamin B_{12}), copper, iodine, iron, and zinc.[57-59] In 1979, the NAG-AMA recommended chromium, copper, manganese, and zinc supplementation for patients receiving PN.[53,57] Recommendations followed in 1984 to also supplement with selenium.[53,57] Although a clear deficiency syndrome for manganese has not been reported in humans, the NAG-AMA considered manganese essential based on case reports of patients receiving PN with metabolic complications that corrected after manganese supplementation. Reports of deficiency syndromes associated with selenium and molybdenum suggest that they also may be essential.[57,58] Although iodine deficiency has not been reported for patients receiving short-term PN, it has been observed in patients receiving long-term PN and may be related to the use of chlorhexidine for central-line care instead of povidone–iodine.[60]

Injectable trace elements are available as single-trace element solutions and as multiple-trace element combinations. The use of single-entity injectable products allows for individualization of trace mineral supplementation of chromium, copper, iodine, manganese, selenium, and zinc. Recent shortages have threatened the supply of both the combination and single-entity products.[3] Most combination products for adults provide the daily requirements for the trace elements considered essential by the NAG-AMA (ie, chromium, copper, manganese, selenium, and zinc).[18] While combination products approved for use in the United States for neonates and pediatric patients have contained only chromium, copper, manganese, and zinc, additional options are now available.[18] (Table 142-4) In response to widespread injectable trace element product shortages, the FDA implemented in 2013 a temporary enforcement discretion to allow the importation of alternative injectable trace element products.[61] A combination product for adults provides fluoride, iodine, molybdenum, and iron, in addition to the standard five trace elements included in US adult products

TABLE 142-4 Imported Sterile Injectable Parenteral Nutrition Products[61-63]

Imported Product (Manufacturer)	Content
Sodium Glycerophosphate Injection Glycophos™ (Fresenius Kabi, USA LLC)	- Contains 1 mmol phosphate and 2 mEq Na per mL compared to US products which contain 3 mmol phosphate and 4 mEq Na per mL.
Adult Trace Elements Addamel™ N (Fresenius Kabi, USA LLC)	- Copper contains 9 trace elements: zinc chloride chloride, manganese chloride, chromic chloride, sodium selenite, ferric chloride, sodium molybdate, potassium iodide, and sodium fluoride.
Pediatric Trace Elements Peditrace™ (Fresenius Kabi, USA LLC)	- Contains 6 trace elements: zinc chloride, copper chloride, manganese chloride, sodium selenite, potassium iodide, and sodium fluoride.
Zinc Injectable Zinc gluconate trihydrate (Aguettant)	- Active substance is equivalent to 1 mg of elemental zinc per mL.

(chromium, copper, manganese, selenium, zinc).[61] The pediatric combination product content differs from the US products in that it lacks chromium and includes selenium, fluoride, and iodine.[61] A single-entity injectable zinc product has also recently been made available.[62] Clinicians should be cautious when transitioning between products to ensure correct doses are being ordered, compounded, and administered to patients because the United States and imported products vary not only by trace element content but also by salt form and trace element doses per unit.[61] In addition, potential interactions resulting in stability or compatibility problems should be considered because frequently information for use of imported injectable products with US products is limited.

Requirements for trace elements also vary on the basis of the patient's clinical condition. For example, higher doses of supplemental zinc likely are necessary for patients with high-output ostomies or diarrhea because the GI tract is the predominant excretion route for zinc. Whereas manganese and copper are excreted through the biliary tract, chromium, molybdenum, and selenium are excreted renally. Hence, these trace elements should be restricted or withheld from PN solutions for patients with cholestatic liver disease and renal failure, respectively.

A.S.P.E.N. recommended formulation changes to the available injectable multiple-trace element preparations for PN patients.[53] The recommendations support overall decreased contamination of trace elements in large- and small-volume PN products.[53] The recommendations advocate for decreased copper and manganese, no (or decreased) chromium, and inclusion and increased dose of selenium in all injectable adult multiple-trace products.[53] The recommendations also support products with no chromium, decreased manganese, and the inclusion of selenium in all injectable pediatric multiple-trace products.[53]

Electrolytes

Electrolytes such as sodium, potassium, calcium, magnesium, phosphorus, chloride, and acetate are necessary PN components for the maintenance of many cellular functions. Electrolytes may be given to maintain normal serum concentrations or to correct deficits. Patients who have "normal" organ function and relatively normal serum concentrations of any electrolyte should receive "normal" maintenance electrolyte doses when PN is initiated and daily thereafter. Specific electrolyte requirements vary according to the patient's age, disease state, organ function, previous and current drug therapy, nutrition status, and extrarenal losses. Electrolytes are available commercially as single- and multiple-nutrient solutions. Multiple-electrolyte solutions are useful for stable patients with normal organ function who are receiving PN. Concentrated multiple-electrolyte solutions designed for addition to PN solutions generally contain only sodium, potassium, calcium, and magnesium. Phosphorus must be added as a separate additive. In response to a severe injectable phosphorus shortage, the FDA implemented a temporary enforcement discretion to allow importation of sodium glycerophosphate injection.[63] (see Table 142-4) This injectable organic phosphorus product has been reported to be more soluble with calcium chloride and calcium gluconate in PN solutions. However, widely used published calcium-phosphorus solubility data is only available for inorganic sodium phosphate with PN products available in the United States which makes use difficult with ACDs and compounding software. Further information regarding metabolism and requirements of vitamins, trace elements, and electrolytes is given elsewhere.[44,64]

DESIGNING A PARENTERAL NUTRITION REGIMEN

5 Several factors, including the patient's venous access, fluid status, and macronutrient and micronutrient requirements, are important considerations when designing the PN regimen. A patient's venous access and fluid status determines the maximum PN osmolar concentration which will impact the nutrient amount that may be provided. PN solutions may be administered by central or peripheral venous access. The patient's clinical condition determines which route is most appropriate.

Parenteral nutrition formulations may be provided as a two-in-one admixture that contains dextrose, CAA, and other necessary micronutrients or as a three-in-one admixture or TNA that contains dextrose, CAA, and IVFE, as well as other necessary micronutrients. Use of TNA solutions offers several potential advantages, including reduced inventory (infusion pumps, tubing, and other related supplies), decreased time for compounding and administration, a potential decrease in manipulations of the infusion line (which should correspond with a decreased risk of catheter contamination), and ease of delivery and storage for patients receiving home PN.[65] Potential disadvantages include increased risk of infections and stability and compatibility concerns. For example, the stability of TNA admixtures is less predictable than that of two-in-one admixtures, which makes their use less desirable in some patient populations such as neonates and infants.[44,66]

Routes of Parenteral Nutrition Administration

Peripheral Route

Peripheral parenteral nutrition (PPN) is an option for mild to moderately stressed patients for whom central access is unavailable or undesirable and function of their GI tract is expected to return within 10 to 14 days.[20,67] Potential PPN candidates should not be fluid-restricted or require large nutrient amounts. Lower concentrations of amino acids (3%-5% final concentration), dextrose (5%-10% final concentration), and micronutrients compared with central parenteral nutrition (CPN) must be used for peripheral administration. Because PPN solutions are relatively dilute, larger volumes are usually necessary to provide nutrient requirements. Additionally, many patients who receive PPN likely will require IVFE to achieve the desired caloric intake at levels consistent with CPN regimens. The primary advantages of PPN include a lower risk of infectious, metabolic, and technical complications.[67] Patients who have poor venous access as the result of multiple courses of chemotherapy, malnutrition, and illness of long duration which has required multiple venous accesses for fluid and medication administration as well as premature infants and the elderly are likely to be poor candidates for PPN.

TABLE 142-5 Osmolarities of Selected Parenteral Nutrients

Nutrient	Osmolarity
Amino acid	100 mOsm/%
Dextrose	50 mOsm/%
Lipid emulsion (20%)	1.3–1.5 mOsm/g
Sodium (acetate, chloride)	2 mOsm/mEq
Sodium phosphate	3 mOsm/mEq sodium
Potassium (acetate, chloride)	2 mOsm/mEq
Potassium phosphate	1.7–2.7 mOsm/mEq potassium
Magnesium sulfate	1 mOsm/mEq
Calcium gluconate	1.4 mOsm/mEq

PPN use is also limited by relatively poor peripheral vein tolerance to hypertonic solutions. Thrombophlebitis is a commonly reported complication for patients receiving PPN.[66] Although the risk of phlebitis is greater with solution osmolarities greater than 600 to 900 mOsm/L, peripherally administered TNA with much higher osmolarities to adults has been associated with low infusion-site complications in some centers.[66,67] Efforts to minimize development of phlebitis or infiltration sequelae for patients receiving PPN include addition of IVFE as a possible venous lumen protectant, subtherapeutic heparin doses (0.5-1 unit/mL) to prevent thrombus formation, or small doses of hydrocortisone (5 mg/L) to minimize access site inflammation.[66,67] However, the coinfusion of IVFE with PPN (ie, not provided as a TNA) has not been shown to reduce phlebitis. In addition, heparin has not been shown to reduce catheter-related thrombosis and is not compatible for use in TNAs.[66] Midline catheter use may offer some advantage and has been associated with a reduced risk of thrombophlebitis.[68] Although these catheters are not central venous access devices, they are longer and infuse into larger venous vessels that may dilute the PPN solution to a more tolerable osmolarity. The osmolarity of a PN solution may be estimated by using the guidelines for osmolarities of selected PN components in Table 142-5.

Central Route

CPN is the preferred route for PN delivery and is used predominantly for patients who require PN for periods of more than 7 to 14 days during hospitalization or indefinitely at home.[20,44,69] These patients may have large nutrient requirements; poor peripheral venous access; or fluctuating fluid requirements, such as metabolically stressed patients with extensive surgery, trauma, sepsis, multiple-organ failure, or malignancy. CPN solutions are highly concentrated hypertonic solutions that must be administered through a large central vein. Unlike peripheral veins, central veins have a higher blood flow, which quickly dilutes the hypertonic solutions. Disadvantages of CPN include risks associated with catheter insertion, routine catheter use, and care of the access site. Relative to peripheral venous access, central venous catheter (CVC) access is associated with a greater potential for infection. In addition, the risk of more serious catheter-induced trauma and related sequelae and other serious technical or mechanical problems is are greater than that with peripheral access.

The choice of central venous access site depends on a number of factors, including the patient's age and anatomy. CVCs vary in composition, lumen size, number of injection ports, and other features that affect ease or convenience of care and maintenance. CVCs for short-term use for adults are commonly inserted percutaneously into the subclavian vein and advanced so that the tip is at the superior vena cava.[68] If this approach is not possible, the internal jugular vein can be used. Frequently, short-term central venous access is obtained for critically ill neonates via a catheter placed in the umbilical vein. Other sites for central venous access in infants and older children are similar to those in adults. When therapy is expected to last longer than 4 weeks, the catheter usually is tunneled subcutaneously before entering the central vessel, secured initially with retaining sutures, and anchored in place with a felt cuff that promotes subcutaneous fibrotic tissue growth around the catheter. The injection port may remain external or may be concealed entirely beneath the skin. Implanted CVCs have a larger port or reservoir that is surgically placed beneath the skin surface and anchored in the chest wall muscle. Peripherally inserted central catheters (PICCs) are venous access devices that are inserted into a peripheral vein (basilic, cephalic, or brachial) and advanced so that the tip is at the superior vena cava.[65] PICCs are increasingly used for both short- and long-term central venous access in acute or home care settings because of ease and economy of bedside placement.[44,69]

Constructing a Parenteral Nutrition Regimen

After the route of delivery is chosen, the components of the PN regimen are determined based on the patient's nutritional assessment. Although not recommended due to increased potential for errors, some healthcare systems may require the entire PN order to be written in individual components and additives on traditional paper order forms without the use of a standard order form. Standardized electronic PN orders suitable for computerized prescriber order entry (CPOE) have been recommended for all patients to minimize risk of errors associated with the ordering process.[5,44] Standardized order forms or clinical decision support within electronic PN ordering systems promote education of practitioners by providing brief guidelines for initiating PN and foster cost-efficient nutrition support by minimizing errors in ordering, compounding, and administration.[5,44,66] Standardized order forms also may include options for ordering certain related procedures, laboratory tests, protocols for patient management, or consultations with other medical services related to the patient's nutrition support.

Adult Parenteral Nutrition Solutions

6 In general, there are two methods for ordering adult PN. The "standard formula approach" offers a variety of admixtures with a fixed nonprotein-calorie-to-nitrogen ratio. This method usually includes different formulas for mild to moderately stressed patients, and those who have kidney or liver failure or are fluid-restricted. Because the nonprotein-calorie-to-nitrogen ratio is fixed, the daily amount of nutrient delivered depends solely on the volume infused. Standard institutional PN formulations may be compounded; however, standardized commercial PN products or "premixed" solutions are available from several manufacturers.[70] A standard institutional formula may promote clinician prescribing of a complete, balanced formulation and promote consistent provision of stable and compatible admixtures. However, efficiencies associated with use of the standard formula approach may be hindered if there is a frequent need to modify the PN formulation. Finally, standard PN formulations may be difficult to use in complicated patients, such as neonatal or pediatric patients, and those with severe malnutrition, organ failure, glucose intolerance, large GI losses, or critical illness.[70]

The "individualized formula approach" permits compounding of patient-specific admixtures. Compounding of the PN admixture is limited only by the concentrations of stock solutions and stability of the additives. The nutrient amount delivered depends on the daily volume of the PN solution infused and the nutrient amounts in the PN solution. The total daily amount of PN solution may be prepared in multiple bags or more cost-effectively in a single container.[44]

Traditionally, adult PN formulations have been ordered by expressing the final concentrations of each component in the solution. For example, CAA and dextrose are ordered commonly in final percentage, electrolytes in milliequivalents in milliequivalents (or millimoles) per liter, and per liter, and other additives in amount (milliliters or units) per day. This inconsistency may promote confusion and misinterpretation of PN admixture contents that may result in harm, especially when patients are transferred between health system environments. To ensure that PN labels in all health system environments clearly and accurately reflect the PN admixture contents, guidelines for standardized adult PN labeling have been recommended.[5,44] In addition to including a variety of other information on the label such as dosing weight and administration route, the guidelines recommend expressing PN ingredients in amounts per daily volume, which minimizes the need for pharmaceutical calculations to determine the nutrient value of the admixture. Commercially available computer software for calculating PN formulations include the recommended A.S.P.E.N. labeling guidelines (Baxter Healthcare, Deerfield, Il.; B. Braun Medical Inc., Bethlehem, PA)[5,44] Pharmaceutical calculations of a an adult TNA PN regimen are briefly reviewed (Fig. 142-1).

Several guidelines are available to help simplify calculation of a PN regimen after a patient's nutritional requirements have been decided. For example, adult patients receiving only PN therapy may need larger volumes of fluid to provide maintenance requirements and replace extrarenal losses. However, patients requiring other IV drug therapy may receive adequate fluid from an additional IV maintenance solution (eg, 0.45% NaCl in 5% dextrose) or co-infused medications (or both). Depending on individual institutional

Calculation of an Adult PN Regimen

Patient case: A patient's daily nutritional requirements have been estimated to be 105 g protein and 2,200 total kcal. The patient has central venous access and reports no history of diabetes, hyperlipidemia, or egg allergy. The patient is not fluid-restricted. The PN formulation will be compounded as an individualized regimen using a single-bag, 24-hour infusion of a TNA. Determine the total PN volume and administration rate by calculating the macronutrient solution volumes required to provide the desired daily nutrients. The PN products used for this regimen are 10% CAA, 70% dextrose, and 30% IVFE.

1. Determine the daily IVFE calories and volume.
   - 2,200 kcal/day × 30%–40% of total calories as fat = 660 – 880 kcal/day
   - Choose 660 kcal to minimize IVFE calories; calculate 30% IVFE volume

     660 kcal ÷ 3 cal/mL 30% IVFE = X mL — X = 220 mL 30% IVFE

   - Calculate IVFE gram amount
     30 g/100 mL = X g/220 mL 30% IVFE — X = 66 g IVFE

2. Determine the appropriate volume of 70% dextrose to deliver the desired dextrose calories

   - Dextrose calories = Total kcal – IVFE kcal – Protein kcal
     = 2,200 kcal – 660 kcal IVFE – (4 kcal × 105 g CAA) = 1,120 kcal

   - Calculate required dextrose (grams):

     1,120 kcal ÷ 3.4 kcal/g dextrose = 329 g dextrose

   - Determine 70% dextrose volume
     70 g/100 mL = 329 g/X mL 70% dextrose; — X = 470 mL 70% dextrose

2. Determine the appropriate volume of 10% CAA
   10 g/100 mL = 105 g/X mL 10% CAA — X = 1,050 mL 10% CAA

3. Determine the TNA PN volume and administration rate
   - Calculate CAA/dextrose/IVFE volume:
     470 mL 70% dextrose + 1,050 mL 10% CAA + 220 mL 30% IVFE = 1,740 mL
   - Add 100-200 mL for additives:
     Total TNA volume = approximately 1,840-1,940 mL/day
   - Calculate the administration rate:
     1,840 to 1,940 mL/day ÷ 24 h = 77 to 81 mL/h; round up to 80 to 85 mL/h

4. Choose final TNA regimen and determine final concentrations of CAA, dextrose, and IVFE
   - Final TNA regimen
     105 g CAA/329 g dextrose/66 g IVFE in 1,920 mL/d to infuse at 80 mL/h

   - Calculate final concentrations of CAA, dextrose, and IVFE

     - 105 g CAA/1,920 mL = X g/100 mL — X = 5.5% CAA
     - 329 g dextrose/1,920 mL = X g/100 mL — X = 17.1% dextrose
     - 66 g IVFE/1,920 mL = X g/100 mL — X = 3.4% IVFE

FIGURE 142-1 Calculation of an adult PN regimen. To convert to energy units of kilojoules (kJ) multiply values with kilocalories as the numerator (kcal, kcal/mL, kcal/kg, kcal/g) by 4.18 to give the corresponding value in kilojoules (kJ, kJ/mL, kJ/kg, kJ/g). (CAA, crystalline amino acids; IVFE, intravenous fat emulsion; PN, parenteral nutrition; TNA, total nutrient admixture.)

practices, maximally concentrating the PN admixture and using an inexpensive maintenance fluid to manage hydration may provide a cost-effective regimen that requires fewer adjustments. Another guideline that may be helpful in designing a PN regimen is to allow a volume of approximately 100 to 150 mL/L of base solution (approximately 200-300 mL/day) for electrolytes and other additives. PN regimens for patients who require very small amounts of additives, such as patients with kidney failure, may need further concentration.

Pediatric Parenteral Nutrition Solutions

Pediatric PN admixtures are typically ordered using an individualized approach because current safe clinical practice guidelines recommend nutrient intakes based on the patient's weight.[5,44] To simplify pediatric PN ordering, many institutions use a pediatric-specific PN order form that expresses daily nutrient amount based on weight. For example, protein and fat are ordered as grams per kilogram per day, dextrose as milligrams per kilogram per minute, and electrolytes as milliequivalents per kilogram per day. However, some institutions may order macronutrients by expressing the final concentration of each component in the solution. Current safe practice guidelines recommend ordering all PN ingredients based on weight as "amount per kilogram per day."[5,44] The PN bag label should accurately reflect the weight-based order as well. Calculations for determining a pediatric PN admixture are reviewed to illustrate fundamental concepts for ordering pediatric PN formulations (Fig. 142-2). Additional features of the pediatric PN label include the dosing weight, administration date and time, expiration date, infusion rate, and duration of infusion. Because infants and children generally receive daily maintenance fluid from the PN regimen, supplemental IV solutions are rarely needed. Pediatric PN may be provided as a two-in-one admixture or TNA. However, the TNA system is not recommended for compounding neonatal and infant PN because of IVFE instability with the often needed higher calcium and phosphorus concentrations.[44,66] The IVFE labeling guidelines for pediatric PN are similar to adult IVFE labeling recommendations.

Administration Techniques

PN admixtures should be administered with an infusion pump. The IV administration line for CAA-dextrose solutions should include a 0.22-micron inline filter to remove particulate matter, air, and any microorganisms that may be present in the solution. IVFE's may be administered separately from the CAA-dextrose solution by co-infusion into the PN line. A port beyond the inline filter must be used because the average size of IVFE particles is approximately 0.5 microns.[5,44] However, co-infused IVFE should also be filtered with a 1.2 micron filter.[47] The FDA recommends use of a 1.2-micron filter with TNA solutions, which may be effective in preventing catheter occlusion caused by precipitates or lipid aggregates.[5,44] This filter size is also reported to remove *Candida albicans.*

INITIATING AND ADVANCING THE PARENTERAL NUTRITION INFUSION

Adult Parenteral Nutrition

The patient's nutrition status, current clinical status, history of glucose tolerance, and dextrose concentration in the formula will dictate the infusion rate at which the adult PN solution should be initiated. Stable patients with normal organ function and stable baseline serum glucose concentrations have demonstrated minimal effect on serum glucose concentrations when PN is abruptly initiated or discontinued.[5,71] However, another approach is to begin the PN infusion and increase the rate gradually over 12 to 24 hours to the desired rate. The infusion rate may likewise be reduced in a stepwise fashion, such as decreasing the rate by 50% for 1 hour before discontinuation.[5,71] This approach should prevent development of hyperglycemia and rebound hypoglycemia, respectively. Alternatively, the PN regimen may be initiated at the goal infusion rate but with a hypocaloric dextrose dose. The dextrose dose can be increased daily to the goal based on patient response. Tapered initiation and cessation should be considered for patients receiving intermittent subcutaneous regular insulin; patients with severe kidney or liver disease; and patients with other disease states that have an increased risk for development of hyperglycemia or hypoglycemia, such as severe diabetes or pancreatic malignancy.

Although the IVFE dose should not exceed 2.5 g/kg per day or 60% of total daily calories, lower doses of 1 g/kg per day not to exceed 30% of calories have been recommended to minimize negative effects associated with long-chain fatty acids.[44] Manufacturer's information recommends IVFE infusion over 4 to 8 hours for adults.[47] However, co-infusion over 12 hours as a separate infusion with 2-in-1 admixtures and infusion over no longer than 24 hours in a TNA formulation appears to be the best clinical strategy to promote IVFE clearance and minimize risk of negative effects on infection control and pulmonary and immune function.[5,44]

The manufacturer's guidelines recommend initiating IVFE for adults with a test dose of 0.5 to 1 mL/min for the first 15 to 30 minutes because of the potential for an immediate hypersensitivity reaction.[47] For most patients, this is probably not necessary because of the relatively low incidence and benign nature of acute adverse reactions. In addition, infusion over 12 to 24 hours eliminates the need for a test dose because the infusion rate is within the range of the recommended test dose rates. Appropriate electrolytes should be provided to patients with normal organ function based on standard nutrient ranges.[44] Adjustments may be necessary depending on the patient's clinical condition. Adults and children older than 11 years should receive daily amounts of trace elements and an adult vitamin formulation.

Pediatric Parenteral Nutrition

Pediatric PN solutions are typically initiated with a volume calculated to provide the patient's daily maintenance fluid requirements on the first day of therapy. Individual nutrient substrates are then advanced daily as tolerated with the goal PN regimen generally being achieved by day 3 of therapy. However, the PN formulation should be initiated with the goal of achieving the desired protein dose on day one. The initial dextrose dose for older infants and children is based on their previous glucose tolerance. Although practices may vary, one approach is to start with 10% dextrose and advance the concentration in 5% increments daily, as tolerated, to goals of 10 to 14 mg/kg/min in infants, 8 to 10 mg/kg/min in children, or 5 to 6 mg/kg/min in adolescents.[18] Initial dextrose doses for premature infants should approximate fetal nutrient delivery rates of 5 to 6 mg/kg/min. Frequently, this results in a final PN dextrose concentration of 5% to 10%. The dextrose concentration for the neonatal PN should be advanced daily by 1% to 2.5% or by 2 to 4 mg/kg/min increments to a goal of 10 to 14 mg/kg/min (maximum, 14-18 mg/kg/min).[18] IVFE is usually initiated at 0.5 g/kg/day for neonates and 0.5 to 1 g/kg/day for infants and children and increased daily by 0.5 to 1 g/kg/day. Incremental increases of IVFE dose allow daily serum triglyceride evaluation and early detection of those with impaired fat clearance. The IVFE dose should not exceed 60% of total daily calories for neonates and 30% of total calories for children, and the maximum IVFE dose should not exceed 3 g/kg/day (approximately 30 kcal/kg/day [126 kJ/kg/day]) for infants and 2.5 g/kg/day for children.[18] The best clinical strategy for minimizing the risk of adverse effects associated with IVFE administration and promoting IVFE clearance is to infuse IVFE over 20 to 24 hours or at a rate of no more than 0.15 g/kg/h.[18,45,66]

IV electrolytes, vitamins, and trace elements should be initiated on the first day of therapy and continued as a daily component of

Calculation of a Pediatric PN Regimen

The nutrition requirements for a 2-week-old preterm neonate (28 weeks gestation; weight 1.2 kg) have been estimated to be 3.5 g/kg/day protein, 3 g/kg/day IVFE, 100 nonprotein kcal/kg/day, and 150 mL/kg/day fluid. The neonate has central access and no prior history of hyperlipidemia or egg allergy. The PN regimen will be compounded as an individualized regimen using a single-bag, 24-hour infusion of a 2-in-1 solution with 20% IVFE co-infused into the PN infusion line. Determine the macronutrient calculations to deliver this neonate's nutrition goals; 10% pediatric CAA and 70% dextrose stock solutions will be used to compound the solution.

1. Determine the goal daily IVFE amount, volume, and administration rate
   - 3 g/kg/day IVFE × 1.2 kg = 3.6 g
   - Calculate 20% IVFE volume
     - 20 g/100 mL = 3.6 g/X mL
     - X = 18 mL/day of 20% IVFE (15 mL/kg/day)
   - Calculate the IVFE administration rate:
     - 18 mL 20% IVFE ÷ 24 hours = 0.75 mL/h (rate may need to be rounded up to 0.8 mL/h or down to 0.7 mL/h depending on precision capability of infusion pump)
2. Determine the goal 2-in-1 PN volume and administration rate
   - Total volume based on maintenance fluid requirements
     - 150 mL/kg/day (estimated fluid goal) – 15 mL/kg/day (20% IVFE) = 135 mL/kg/day for PN volume
     - 135 mL/kg/day × 1.2 kg = 162 mL/day
   - PN infusion rate is 162 mL/day ÷ 24 hours = 6.75 mL/h (rate may need to be rounded up to 6.8 mL/h or down to 6.7 mL/h depending on precision capability of infusion pump)
3. Determine the daily protein amount and the corresponding 10% CAA volume
   - Calculate the goal protein amount
     - 3.5 g/kg/day × 1.2 kg = 4.2 g/day
   - Calculate the 10% pediatric CAA stock solution volume
     - 10 g/100 mL = 4.2 g/X mL 10% pediatric CAA
     - X = 42 mL 10% pediatric CAA
4. Determine the daily dextrose amount, corresponding 70% dextrose volume, and final dextrose concentration in the 2-in-1 PN solution
   - Goal is to provide approximately 14 mg/kg/min dextrose
     - 14 mg x 1.2 kg × 1,440 minutes/day ÷ 1,000 mg/g = 24.2 g dextrose
   - Calculate the 70% dextrose volume
     - 70 g/100 mL = 24.2 g/X mL 70% dextrose
     - X = 34.6 mL 70% dextrose
   - Calculate the final dextrose concentration of the PN solution
     - 24.2 g dextrose/162 mL = X g/100 mL
     - X = 14.9% dextrose (round up to 15% dextrose final concentration)
     - 162 mL × 15% dextrose = 162 × 15 g/100 mL = 24.3 g dextrose
5. Determine the available volume for additives
   - 162 mL – 42 mL (10% pediatric CAA) – 34.6 mL (70% dextrose) = 85.4 mL
   - Depending on volume needed for additives, sterile water may be necessary to add to formulation to make final total volume of 162 mL
6. Determine the final PN regimen and provided nutrient amounts
   - Final PN regimen
     - 3.5 g/kg/day pediatric CAA and 15% dextrose to infuse at 6.75 mL/h
     - 3 g/kg/day (or 18 mL) 20% IVFE to infuse at 0.75 mL/h
   - Macronutrient calories

Dextrose:	24.3 g × 3.4 kcal/g	=	82.6 kcal
Protein:	4.2 g × 4 kcal/g	=	16.8 kcal
20% IVFE	18 mL × 2 kcal/mL	=	36 kcal
Total kcal (kcal/kg):			135.4 kcal (113 kcal/kg)
Nonprotein kcal (kcal/kg):			118.6 kcal (99 kcal/kg)

FIGURE 142-2 Calculation of a pediatric PN regimen. To convert to energy units of kilojoules, multiply values with kilocalories as the numerator (kcal, kcal/mL, kcal/kg, kcal/g) by 4.18 to give the corresponding value in kilojoules (kJ, kJ/mL, kJ/kg, kJ/g). (CAA, crystalline amino acids; IVFE, intravenous fat emulsion.)

the PN solution.[44] Children younger than 11 years should receive a vitamin product formulated for pediatric patients. Two multivitamin dosing schemas have been suggested for infants and children.[44] One method recommends 2 mL/kg/day for infants weighing less than 2.5 kg (less than 5.5 lb) and 5 mL/day for infants and children weighing 2.5 kg (5.5 lb) or greater. The other suggests 30% of a vial (1.5 mL/day) for infants weighing less than 1 kg (less than 2.2 lb), 65% of a vial (3.25 mL/day) for infants weighing 1 to 3 kg (2.2-6.6 lb), and 100% of the vial (5 mL/day) for children weighing more than 3 kg (6.6 lb) (up to 11 years of age). Adult injectable vitamin products should not be used for infants because of potential neurotoxicity from accumulation of polysorbate and propylene glycol preservatives. Weight-based dosage recommendations for pediatric multiple trace element products are 0.3 mL/kg for children weighing less than 3 kg (less than 6.6 lb) and 0.2 mL/kg for children weighing 3 kg (6.6 lb) or greater (maximum, 5 mL/day). Children weighing more than 25 kg (55 lb) should receive an adult trace element product. The weight-based dosage recommendation for the imported pediatric multiple trace element product is different than that for the US products (1 mL/kg up to a maximum of 15 mL per day).[61] Weight-based doses of the multiple trace element products do not provide the recommended daily intake for all trace elements, so additional supplementation or individual dosing with single-entity products may be necessary. Individualized dosing allows for dose adjustment based on serum trace element assessment, individual patient characteristics (eg, cholestasis, stool losses, wounds), and the need to minimize administration of trace elements that accumulate in patients receiving chronic PN such as chromium and manganese. Pediatric patients receiving PN commonly transition from PN support to enteral nutrition gradually, over a period of days to weeks, by decreasing the PN infusion rate while increasing the enteral intake. The PN infusion rate should be reduced for 1 to 2 hours before stopping the infusion for neonates and infants because of their immature counter-regulatory mechanisms that contribute to an increased risk for developing rebound hypoglycemia.[16] Blood glucose concentrations should be measured within 15 to 60 minutes after the PN infusion ends.

Continuous versus Cyclic Infusions

7 Continuous infusions are attractive for patients with unstable fluid balance or glucose homeostasis. The intermittent or cyclic infusion of PN over less than 24 hours, usually for 12 to 18 hours each day, is useful for hospitalized patients with limited venous access in whom administration of multiple other medications requires interruption of the PN infusion.[71] Cyclic PN also may minimize the incidence or reverse the liver injury associated with continuous PN therapy. In addition, this delivery mode allows patients receiving PN at home the ability to resume a relatively normal lifestyle.[69,71] Various protocols have been reported that suggest incremental increases to the maximum infusion rate for a desired period of time followed by a gradual taper to discontinue the solution have been sugested.[16,71] However, metabolically stable adults and children older than 2 years receiving IVFE–based PN regimens are likely candidates for abrupt initiation and discontinuation of their intermittent PN regimen.[5,16,71,72] Cyclic PN should be used with caution for those with severe glucose intolerance, diabetes, or unstable fluid balance.

EVALUATION OF THERAPEUTIC OUTCOMES

8 Thorough and consistent monitoring of patients who are receiving PN is necessary to ensure that the desired nutritional outcomes are achieved and to prevent the occurrence of adverse effects or complications. Routine evaluation should include the assessment of the patient's clinical condition with a focus on nutritional and metabolic effects of the PN regimen. Serial documentation of a patient's response to their PN regimen is a helpful guide for determining appropriate adjustments in fluid, electrolyte, and nutrient therapies.

Serum concentrations of electrolytes, hematologic indices, and biochemical markers for kidney and liver function, and nutrition status should be measured before PN initiation and periodically thereafter depending on the patient's age, nutrition status, and clinical condition. The frequency of blood laboratory measurements for neonates and infants tends to be more conservative because of their smaller blood volumes and, in some cases, lack of central vascular access. Other important clinical measurements include vital signs, weight, total fluid intake and output, and nutritional intakes. Weekly measurements of height, length, and head circumference are helpful for monitoring nutritional changes in neonates. Monitoring parameters considered important for patients receiving PN and the suggested frequency of measurement for each are outlined in Fig. 142-3. Appropriate assessment and evaluation of patient data can identify potential complications that may be avoided or treated early. Monitoring protocols should be developed and tailored for the patient population, medical practices, and resources of individual practice settings.

COMPOUNDING, STORAGE, AND INFECTION CONTROL

The USP Chapter 797 details the procedures and requirements for compounding sterile preparations, including PN admixtures.[73] These standards apply to all healthcare settings in which sterile preparations are compounded and are used by boards of pharmacy, the FDA, and accreditation organizations such as The Joint Commission. Compounded sterile preparations are defined by risk level (immediate use, low, low with 12-hour beyond-use date, medium, and high) based on the probability of microbial, chemical, or physical contamination. PN solutions are classified as a medium-risk compounded sterile preparation. In general, PN solutions should be prepared using aseptic technique in a device or room that meets International Organization for Standardization (ISO) class 5 standards that is located in an ISO class 7 buffer area with an ISO class 8 ante area.[73] Preparation of PN formulations should be supervised by a pharmacist experienced in compounding IV solutions and knowledgeable about the stability, compatibility, and storage of PN admixtures. Quality assurance procedures should be developed to maintain safe and accurate admixture preparation. A standardized process for PN ordering, labeling, determining nutrient requirements, screening of the PN order, PN administration, and monitoring has been recommended to minimize risk of potentially life-threatening compounding errors.[5,44,70] The potential risk of infectious complications associated with PN solution contamination can be decreased greatly when pharmacy-based admixture programs follow specific guidelines developed to ensure proper compounding of PN solutions.[5,73]

In general, the type of solution being prepared dictates the compounding, storage, and infusion methods. Currently, the two most commonly used types of PN solutions are two-in-one admixtures with or without IVFE co-infused into the PN line and TNAs. Methods for compounding PN admixtures vary based on a healthcare system's patient population and medical practices and the number of PN admixtures that need to be prepared. PN base admixtures may be prepared by using gravity-driven transfer of CAA stock solutions to partially filled bags of concentrated dextrose stock solutions.[44,74] Other practice settings may use standardized commercial PN products with CAA and dextrose, and more recently, IVFE separated within a single bag that must be mixed before use.[44,70] Advances in compounding technology have facilitated the use of ACDs for preparing PN solutions. These devices are computer-based systems that perform the calculations necessary to determine volumes of nutrient-stock solutions for PN admixtures. In addition, most ACD systems include software that communicates the determined calculations directly to a transfer pump device that delivers fluid from the source container to the final container by either a volumetric or gravimetric fluid pumping system.[74] Advantages of ACDs include reduced personnel time and compounding materials and improved compounding accuracy. Disadvantages include the potential for equipment failure. Because of their acidic pH and hypertonicity, two-in-one PN admixtures are poor media for microbial growth.[44] However, several characteristics of IVFE, such as isoosmotic tonicity, near neutral to alkaline pH, glycerol content, and preservative-free

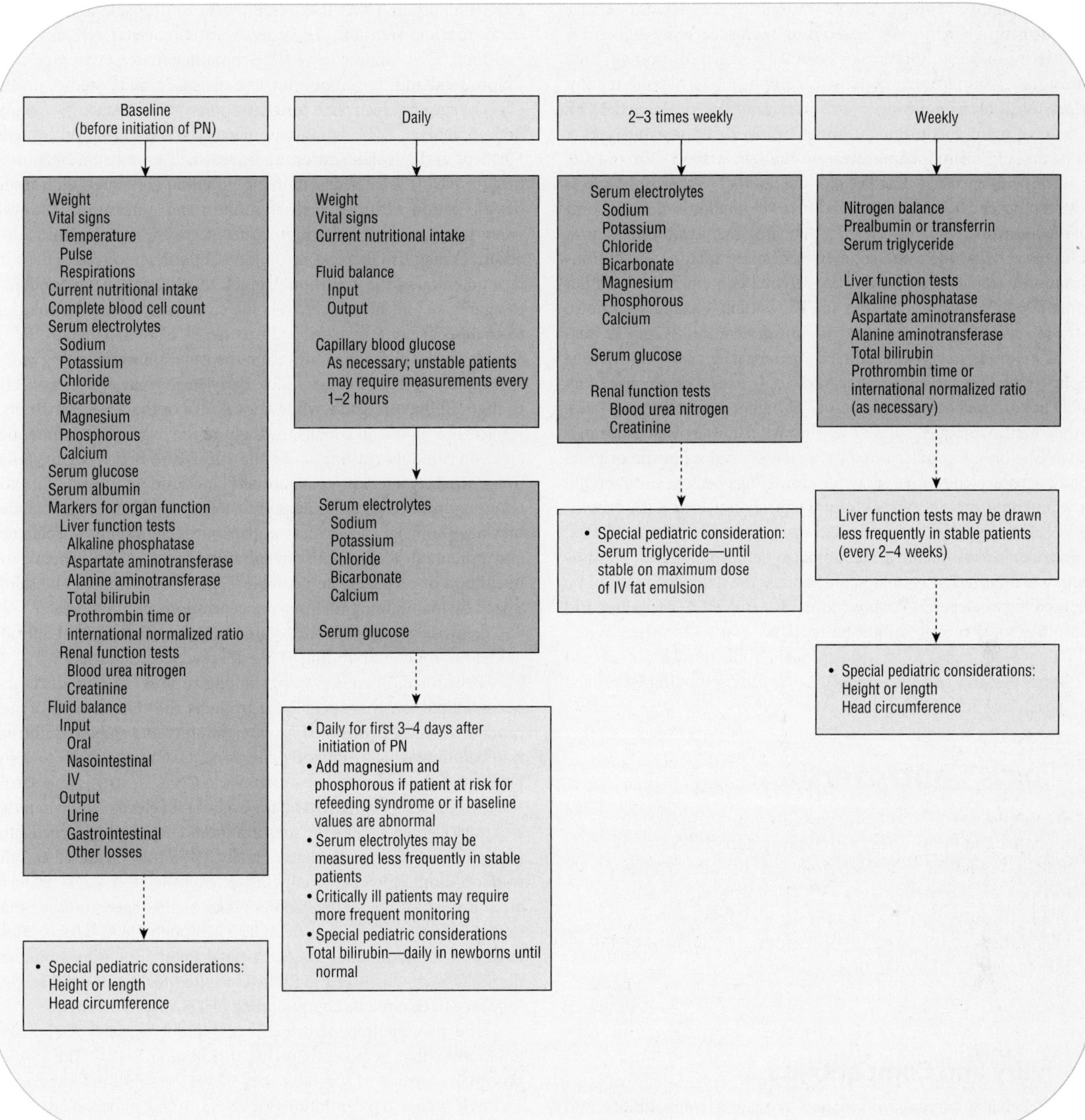

FIGURE 142-3 Monitoring strategy for patients receiving parenteral nutrition (PN).

formulations favor microbial growth, particularly at room temperature.[44] Other factors contributing to the potential for compromised IVFE stability or sterility include the container material, length of IVFE co-infusion with PN, length of time between administration set change, effect of infusion from the source container such as the original container, and infusion of IVFE transferred to a secondary container. When IVFEs are added to dextrose-CAA solutions to make TNAs, the growth potential is decreased, presumably because of the protective effects of the hypertonic dextrose-CAA solution and decreased pH.[66]

Because of the risk for microbial contamination, manufacturers recommend storage of PN solutions for as little time as possible after preparation. The USP 797 standards recommend storage times of not more than 30 hours at controlled room temperature (20°C to 25°C [68°F to 77°F]) and not more than 9 days at refrigerated temperatures (2°C to 8°C [36°F to 46°F]) for all medium-risk compounded sterile preparations, including PN admixtures.[73]

When co-infusing IVFE with PN (ie, not as a TNA), the appropriate IVFE dosage form (original packaging or re-packaged doses) and administration time to minimize risk of contamination is controversial. Unfortunately, The Centers for Disease Control and Prevention (CDC) guidelines offer no guidance for administration times.[68] Instead, the guidelines recommend administration tubing replacement every 24 hours for both IVFE infused separately or when given as part of a TNA. The guidelines also recommend administration tubing replacement no more frequently than at 96-hour intervals but at least every 7 days for tubing used continuously for infusion of IV solutions other than blood, blood products, or IVFE. More conservative recommendations have been presented.[5,44,66] The A.S.P.E.N. 2013 PN Safety Consensus suggests a 24-hour infusion time and administration tubing replacement every 24 hours for TNAs and 2-in-1 PN formulations and a 12-hour infusion time and administration tubing replacement every 12 hours for IVFE co-infused separately.[5]

Compliance with A.S.P.E.N. recommendations in pediatric patients is problematic. For example, an infant receiving 3 g/kg/day IVFE at an maximum infusion rate of 0.15 g/kg/h to promote lipid clearance and minimize metabolic complications, would require at least a 20-hour infusion.[18,45] To accommodate prolonged IVFE infusions, many institutions routinely infuse IVFE separately over 24 hours and change administration tubing for the IVFE and PN solution with each new bag because the use of TNA formulations is not recommended in neonates and infants. In addition, since commercially available IVFE products are not manufactured in unit volumes suitable for safe use in neonates and infants, institutions commonly transfer IVFE from the original container into another container to accommodate the smaller patient-specific volume to decrease risk of adverse events from infusion-related errors. A variety of methods have been utilized for repackaging IVFE. Syringe repackaging and aseptic transfer into sterile bags with the use of an ACD are not recommended because of higher contamination rates. Other methodologies, such as aseptic withdrawal of an appropriate IVFE volume resulting in a patient-specific dose in the original manufacturer's container (drawing-down) has been recommended as a potential option.[66] These multifactorial concerns with providing IVFE to pediatric patients have been addressed by the A.S.P.E.N. Safety Consensus Recommendations.[5] When prolonged IVFE infusions are required in neonates and infants, the daily dose should be divided in two separate 12-hour infusions. The IVFE container and administration tubing should be replaced every 12 hours.[5] When utilizing repackaged IVFE, the infusion time should not exceed 12 hours per unit and the administration tubing should be changed with each new infusion.[5,66]

Clinical **Controversy...**

The safety of repackaging IVFE before administration to neonates and infants has been heavily debated. Some clinicians maintain that the benefits of cost effectiveness and increased patient safety with administering smaller IVFE units outweigh the risks of microbial contamination, while others continue to advocate for the delivery of IVFE direct from the manufacturer's container to decrease infection risk.

Stability and Compatibility

Comprehensive current information regarding compatibility and stability of PN solutions can be found in several reference sources such as *Handbook on Injectable Drugs*[75] and *King Guide to Parenteral Admixtures*.[76] In many cases, the answer to a compatibility question may not be readily available, and a review of the primary literature may be necessary. When information is not available, clinical judgment and experience must be used to resolve the situation.

The stability of a PN formulation is determined by the rate or degree of component degradation and any resulting changes in chemical integrity or pharmacologic activity that may render the formulation unsuitable for safe administration. In general, the sterile combination of PN components accelerates the rate of physicochemical destabilization of all of the components in the formulation; certain amino acids, vitamins, and IVFE are the most susceptible nutrients.[44] When compounded and stored appropriately, the degree of degradation is usually not clinically relevant for most patients receiving short-term PN because many patients have sufficient stores of those susceptible nutrients to support any short-term periods of suboptimal intake. However, nutrient degradation that is more extensive may be problematic for patients with marginal nutrient stores who receive long-term PN. TNAs present additional stability challenges because of the presence of IVFE in the solution. IVFE stability in TNAs is affected by the amino acid and dextrose concentration, solution pH, order of mixing, electrolyte amounts, and final TNA volume as well as container material, storage conditions, and addition of nonnutrient drugs. Stability studies on the effect of specific electrolyte concentrations on TNA stability are limited. In general, IVFE stability is affected by the PN cation content. Divalent and trivalent cation additives such as calcium and magnesium have a greater destabilizing potential compared with monovalent cation additives such as sodium and potassium. However, when given in sufficiently high concentrations, monovalent cation additives may also increase instability. Cations act to reduce the surface potential of the emulsion droplet, thereby enhancing tendency to aggregate and ultimately, in some cases, destabilize the solution to coalescence or a "cracked" admixture.[5,28,44] When a cracked IVFE occurs, the oil phase separates from the water phase, resulting in the appearance of free oil fat globules. Early stages may appear as subtle changes in the uniformly white appearance of the TNA, which may progress to yellow oil streaks throughout the bag or development of an amber oil layer at the top of the admixture bag. TNA formulations with any visible free oil should be considered unsafe for parenteral administration because infusion of circulating fat globules may be of sufficient size to accumulate in the pulmonary vasculature and potentially compromise respiratory function. In general, the likelihood of preparing an unstable TNA formulation can be minimized by maintaining the final concentrations of CAA greater than 4%, dextrose greater than 10%, and IVFE greater than 2%.[5] Specific guidelines for compounding TNAs are reviewed elsewhere.[28,65]

Because of differences in pH among various CAA products and phospholipid content among IVFE products, the manufacturer of each product should be consulted for compatibility and stability information before routinely admixing components. One approach to compounding TNAs manually is to combine CAA, dextrose, and sterile water (if necessary) followed by the addition of electrolytes, vitamins, and trace elements. Then the solution should be visually inspected for precipitate or other particulates. Finally, IVFE may be added and the solution should then be visually inspected again to ensure a uniform emulsion exists.[28,44] Mixing components in this specific order may not be possible with the use of ACDs. Although CAA, dextrose, and IVFE may be simultaneously transferred to an admixture container, the ACDs manufacturer should be consulted for the optimal mixing sequence to ensure safe compounding of TNA formulations.

The precipitation of calcium and phosphorus is a common interaction that is potentially life-threatening.[18,28,44,77] The risk of precipitate formation is greater with increased solution temperature and pH, higher concentrations of calcium and phosphorus, lower concentrations of amino acids and dextrose, use of the chloride salt of calcium, improper mixing sequence when adding calcium and phosphorus salts, and the presence of other additives (including IVFEs).[18,28,44,77] In general, steps to minimize risk of calcium and phosphate precipitation in PN admixtures include the use of calcium gluconate instead of calcium chloride because it is less reactive, adding phosphate salts early in the mixing sequence, adding calcium last or nearly last, and agitating the mixture throughout the admixture process to achieve homogeneity. PN admixtures with a lower final pH should be used when clinically appropriate. Higher final concentrations of dextrose and CAA and lower final concentrations of IVFE favor a lower admixture pH. CAA product-specific solubility curves that are available from the manufacturer or primary literature should be consulted to project calcium and phosphorous solubility. The calculation of a sum or product of calcium and phosphate concentrations should not be used as the sole criterion for determining solubility because the product of calcium and phosphate concentrations vary inconsistently as calcium concentration decreases and phosphate concentration increases.[77]

Electrolyte stability in TNA solutions is difficult to assess because of poor visualization of a precipitate if one occurs.

PN solutions for neonates and infants tend to contain larger amounts of calcium and phosphorus, as well as other divalent cations, that limit the use of TNAs. Because of the limited amount of published stability information, the use of a two-in-one admixture with separate administration of IVFEs is recommended for neonates and infants.[44] In general, alternative methods of delivering electrolytes or medications should be pursued in any clinical situation in which TNA compatibility information is lacking. Because the addition of bicarbonate to acidic PN admixtures may result in the formation of carbon dioxide gas and insoluble calcium and magnesium carbonates, sodium bicarbonate use in PN admixtures is not recommended.[44] Use of a bicarbonate precursor salt such as acetate usually is preferred.

Vitamins may be affected adversely by changes in solution pH, presence of other additives, storage time, solution temperature, and exposure to light.[28] Because of variable stabilities of individual vitamins, IV vitamin solutions should be added to the PN solution as near to the time of administration as is clinically feasible and should not be in the PN solution longer than 24 hours.

Increased peroxide concentrations have been reported in IVFE and dextrose–amino acid solutions after addition of injectable multivitamins or exposure to air or light.[78] Multiple in vitro experiments have reported negative effects of peroxides and associated metabolites on organ and immune function. Peroxides are associated with neonatal hypoxic–ischemic encephalopathy, intraventricular hemorrhage, periventricular leukomalacia, chronic lung disease, retinopathy of prematurity, and necrotizing enterocolitis.[78] Neonates and infants are at increased risk for harmful effects of peroxides because they receive a higher daily peroxide load from PN solutions compared to adults and they have lower endogenous antioxidant levels. Protecting PN and IVFE solutions from light is therefore recommended to minimize peroxide formation.[78]

Many patients receiving PN also receive other IV medications. The compatibility of these medications with the PN solution is an important consideration for safe and effective drug delivery. Although some medications may be added directly to the PN solution and administered at the same rate as the PN infusion, most are administered as a separate admixture co-infused in the PN line. Several criteria should be considered before medications are added directly to the PN solution because of the potential for ineffective drug therapy or other complications associated with physiochemical incompatibility and stability of the PN solution.[44] First, the drug should be stable for at least 24 hours and should have pharmacokinetic properties appropriate for continuous infusion. Second, the chemical and physical compatibility of the medication with PN admixture components and other medications that may be co-infused concomitantly into the PN line should be verified. Advantages of using PN admixtures as drug vehicles include consolidation of dosage units, improved pharmacodynamics for certain drugs, conservation of fluid in volume-restricted patients, fewer venous catheter violations, and decreased compounding and administration times. However, a major disadvantage to the use of PN solutions as drug-delivery vehicles is the lack of compatibility and stability data. Medications frequently added to PN solutions include regular insulin and histamine-2 receptor antagonists.[41,75,76]

COMPLICATIONS OF PARENTERAL NUTRITION

Mechanical and Technical Complications

Mechanical and technical complications include malfunctions in the system used for IV delivery of the solution, such as infusion pump failure, problems with administration sets or tubing, or the CVC. Although problems associated with infusion pumps and administration sets can be decreased by appropriate equipment selection and routine care and monitoring, CVC-related complications are potentially life-threatening. Pneumothorax, catheter misdirection or migration into the wrong vein or improper positioning within the cardiac chambers, arterial puncture, bleeding, and hematoma formation may occur during surgical placement of the catheter. Many of these complications, in addition to venous thrombosis and air embolism, can occur after insertion. CVCs occasionally occlude or break during use and if these problems cannot be rectified easily, the catheter may need to be surgically replaced.

Infectious Complications

Infectious complications can be a major hazard for patients receiving CPN because of the increased risk associated with the presence of an indwelling CVC. The source of a CVC infection may be skin organisms from the catheter insertion site, contamination of the catheter hub, or hematogenous seeding of the catheter from a distant site. In addition, patients receiving PN therapy are often predisposed to infection because of compromised immunity or concomitant infection. Frequent use of broad-spectrum antibiotic therapy and malnutrition are also predisposing factors for development of infection. The risk of catheter infection is increased for those who require multiple manipulations of the line used for PN administration as well as those who experience failure of in-line bacterial filter, poor catheter placement technique, and poor CVC and insertion site care.[68]

Infection rarely develops secondary to solution contamination.[68,79] Strict adherence to protocols for preparation of PN admixtures should minimize this occurrence.[44,73] Catheter-related bloodstream infections (CRBSIs), defined as the presence of clinical manifestations of infection (eg, fever, chills, hypotension) associated with bacteremia or fungemia resulting from no apparent source other than the catheter, are common sources of systemic infection.[79] Before this diagnosis can be made, there should be evidence of more than one positive blood culture result obtained from the peripheral vein with growth of the same organism from a blood culture obtained from the catheter or catheter segment. When a CRBSI is suspected or confirmed, appropriate antimicrobial therapy should be initiated. Retention or removal of the central catheter depends on the patient's severity of illness, the suspected or identified pathogen, and the type of catheter involved. The catheter may be removed and replaced in the same site, the catheter may be removed and replaced at a different anatomic location, or it may not be replaced.[79] Filling the catheter with antimicrobials such as vancomycin or antiseptics such as 70% alcohol and allowing the solution to dwell for a period of time while the catheter is not in use is referred to as a catheter lock.[68] Antimicrobial catheter locks have been used to prevent and treat CRBSI in patients with long-term catheters such as those receiving home PN.[68,69] Specific guidelines for treatment of CRSBI have been recently reviewed.[79]

Clinical **Controversy...**

Ethanol catheter lock therapy has offered promise for the prevention and treatment of CRBSI. The best method for ethanol removal from the CVC after ethanol catheter lock is not known. If the ethanol is withdrawn from the CVC, blood is introduced into the CVC, which may increase the risk of biofilm formation. Alternatively, clearing the catheter by flushing the ethanol into the patient is concerning because there is no known safe amount of ethanol to routinely infuse into patients, particularly neonates and infants.

Metabolic and Nutritional Complications

9 Metabolic and nutritional complications associated with PN therapy are numerous; frequently multifactorial in origin; and if left untreated, potentially fatal. Metabolic abnormalities related

to substrate intolerance, fluid and electrolyte disorders, and acid-base disorders are summarized in multiple recent review articles and their management is briefly summarized in the following sections.[36,37,43,44,64,71]

Liver Disease

Parenteral nutrition–associated liver disease presents as elevations in total bilirubin, aspartate aminotransferase, alanine aminotransferase, and alkaline phosphatase. Both adult and pediatric patients who receive PN are at risk for developing PNALD; it is reported to occur in approximately 50% to 60% of children who receive long-term PN, with a higher incidence in premature infants.[37,80] No single etiology has been identified, although several risk factors have been reported, such as, degree of prematurity, sepsis, hypoxia, lack of enteral nutrition, small bowel bacterial overgrowth, GI conditions requiring surgical intervention, duration of PN therapy, and long-term administration of excessive calories.[37,80] PNALD in infants is characterized clinically by a serum direct bilirubin concentration greater than 2 mg/dL (more than 34.2 μmol/L).[37] Taurine deficiency has been proposed as an etiology of cholestasis for preterm infants and neonates.[37] Taurine is a conditionally essential amino acid that is not present in standard CAA solutions but is important for neonatal and infant bile metabolism. However, the preventative or therapeutic benefit of PN regimens with CAA solutions containing supplemental taurine is unclear. Recent studies have focused on the potential relationship between IVFE and the development of PNALD.[50] SO-based IVFEs contain large concentrations of plant sterols or phytosterols, which are inefficiently metabolized to bile acids by the liver. Experimental data suggest parenteral phytosterols may impair bile flow. Improvement or reversal of PNALD has been reported for patients who received a fish oil–based IVFE that is not currently commercially available in the United States.[50] Other PNALD treatments that have been investigated include providing reduced doses of SO–based IVFE and use of enteral fish oil in patients with limited oral intake.[50,81]

Risk factors for PNALD in adults include preexisting liver disease, sepsis, preexisting malnutrition, extensive bowel resection, prolonged duration of PN therapy, lack of enteral intake, nutrient deficiencies such as choline deficiency, and long-term administration of excessive calories.[37,80] PNALD in adults typically presents as steatosis and steatohepatitis on biopsy. Clinically, PNALD is characterized by mild elevations in serum liver enzymes, usually less than three times the upper limit of normal, with peak enzyme levels usually occurring between 1 and 4 weeks after initiating PN. In many cases, the liver abnormalities improve or resolve with manipulation of substrate intake or discontinuation of PN therapy. However, in severe cases, liver dysfunction may progress to overt failure and death despite use of traditional therapies such as using cyclic PN, ursodiol, and oral antibiotics for bacterial overgrowth; maximizing enteral feeding; and avoiding sepsis and parenteral overfeeding.[37,80] Intestinal transplant with or without liver transplantation has become a treatment option for PN-dependent patients who have progressive PNALD.

Hypertriglyceridemia

Hypertriglyceridemia, defined as serum triglyceride concentrations greater than 400 mg/dL (4.52 mmol/L) for adults and 150 mg/dL (1.70 mmol/L) to 200 mg/dL (2.26 mmol/L) for preterm infants, neonates, and older pediatric patients, may occur in patients receiving IVFE–based PN. Risk factors include preexisting liver or pancreatic dysfunction, sepsis, multiple-organ failure, degree of prematurity, IVFE infusion rate, and dose.[44,45]

IVFE–associated hypertriglyceridemia is generally thought to be caused by defective lipid clearance or an excessive rate of IVFE administration.[42,44] Premature infants and neonates have relatively slower lipid clearance than do adults because of immature metabolic pathways, including decreased lipoprotein lipase activity.[42,45] Reducing the IVFE infusion rate or dose or withholding IVFE therapy should be considered when patients present with hypertriglyceridemia or lipemic serum.[42,44] Use of low-dose heparin (1 unit/mL of two-in-one PN formulation) to stimulate lipoprotein lipase activity has been suggested as a potential therapeutic intervention to treat IVFE–associated hypertriglyceridemia in neonates.[16,42] However, others have suggested that the risk associated with heparin delivery via PN outweighs the clinical benefits because of the potential for compounding errors associated with confusion between heparin and insulin doses.[82] The role of carnitine for treatment of IVFE–associated hypertriglyceridemia is not clear.[16,42]

Hyperglycemia

Hyperglycemia is one of the most common complications of PN administration and is associated with a history of diabetes, metabolic stress, adverse effects of medications such as glucocorticoids, and excessive carbohydrate administration. In the pediatric population, additional risks for hyperglycemia include prematurity and surgery. The optimal blood glucose concentration for acutely ill hospitalized patients receiving PN is not known. However, a target range of 140 to 180 mg/dL (7.8-10 mmol/L) has been suggested for adults, and less than 150 mg/dL (8.3 mmol/L) has been suggested for neonates.[83,84] Clinical management of PN patients with hyperglycemia has not been well studied and is largely empiric. Blood glucose concentrations can be controlled with regular insulin, which may be given subcutaneously or added to the PN formulation. One approach for adult PN patients requiring insulin or oral hypoglycemic agents before starting PN therapy is to initiate PN with approximately 100 to 200 g of dextrose and add 0.05 to 0.1 units of regular insulin per gram of dextrose in the PN solution for those patients with mild hyperglycemia (130-150 mg/dL [7.2-8.3 mmol/L]). The insulin dose may be increased to 0.15 to 0.2 units per gram of dextrose for patients with moderate hyperglycemia (151-200 mg/dL [8.4-11.1 mmol/L]).[44,85] Blood glucose concentrations should be monitored every 4 to 6 hours. Blood glucose measurements above the goal range should be treated with regular insulin administered subcutaneously according to an appropriate sliding scale (see Chapter 74). The insulin dose is modified daily by adding 60% to 100% of the sliding-scale insulin given over the previous 24 hours to the PN formulation daily until blood glucose concentrations are stable and within the target range. When blood glucose measurements are stable, the dextrose dose may be advanced to achieve the therapeutic goal and the frequency of monitoring blood glucose concentrations may be decreased after blood glucose concentrations are stable within the target range at the goal dextrose dose. Use of a separate IV insulin infusion is most commonly used for pediatric patients, but it may also provide better and safer glycemic control for patients with very large insulin requirements or those with unstable marked fluctuations in their blood glucose concentrations.

Refeeding Syndrome

Severe and rapid declines in serum phosphate, potassium, and magnesium concentrations; fluid retention; and other micronutrient deficiencies are common features of the refeeding syndrome.[86,87] Individuals at greatest risk for refeeding syndrome are severely malnourished patients with significant weight loss who receive aggressive nutritional supplementation. In addition, those who are unfed for 7 to 10 days with evidence of stress or nutritional depletion; those with chronic diseases causing undernutrition such as cancer, cardiac cachexia, chronic obstructive pulmonary disease, or cirrhosis; and individuals who were previously morbidly obese and have experienced massive weight loss are at heightened risk for this syndrome.[87] Electrolyte abnormalities appear to be related to acute provision of macronutrient substrates that promote anabolism in an environment of depleted total body stores of phosphorus, potassium, and magnesium. Recommendations for initiating PN in adults at risk for refeeding syndrome include providing 25% to 50% of the calculated nonprotein caloric requirements initially. The dextrose dose should be initiated at approximately 100 to 200 g/day. Calories should be advanced over 3 to 4 days to the desired goal. Because the metabolic abnormalities described with refeeding syndrome appear to be related primarily to acute provision of large amounts of dextrose, the goal protein dose may be provided with the initial PN infusion. Pediatric PN regimens are usually advanced over several days as a general practice for all pediatric patients. Additional recommendations for minimizing the risk of refeeding syndrome for pediatric patients include provision of additional phosphorus and potassium above standard nutrient requirements at the time PN is initiated.[88]

Complications Associated with Long-Term Parenteral Nutrition

Other nutritional complications of PN therapy may develop over a prolonged course of therapy (weeks to months) as a result of inappropriate intake of a particular nutrient. Certain conditions, such as metabolic stress in a previously malnourished patient, may elicit symptoms of deficiency much earlier if a nutrient is not appropriately provided. For example, lactic acidosis and other life-threatening complications associated with severe thiamine deficiency have been reported in patients who received PN solutions without multivitamin supplementation.[53] Maintenance doses of vitamins, trace elements, and essential fatty acids should be provided to all patients with normal age-related organ function receiving PN.

Essential Fatty Acid Deficiency

Patients receiving PN regimens without IVFEs for weeks to months are at risk for development of EFAD. Clinical signs of EFAD include hair loss, desquamative dermatitis, thrombocytopenia, malabsorption, and diarrhea resulting from changes in intestinal mucosa.[43,44] EFAD also may be diagnosed by evaluating plasma fatty acid profiles. Although this assessment is not routinely available, it can be provided by several larger regional laboratories. Historically, a triene-to-tetraene ratio more than 0.4 has been considered biochemical evidence for EFAD, however, individual laboratory reference ranges should be used when evaluating patients for EFAD.[18] Although the time in which EFAD may develop depends on the patient's nutrition status, disease state, and age, these manifestations may occur 2 to 4 weeks after initiation of fat-free PN in adults and within 48 hours in newborn infants.[43,45]

Metabolic Bone Disease

Metabolic bone disease has been reported for adults and children receiving long-term home PN.[37] This disorder in adults is characterized by osteomalacia with or without osteoporosis that may present without associated clinical, radiologic, or biochemical abnormalities. The diagnosis may not be made for premature infants until after the development of bone fractures or overt rickets. The etiology is poorly understood and likely multifactorial. Treatment options include pharmacologic intervention, calcium and vitamin D supplementation, and exercise. Because excessive vitamin D has also been implicated in the development of metabolic bone disease, others have recommended removal of vitamin D from the PN for patients with a normal 25-hydroxyvitamin D concentration and low serum parathyroid hormone and 1,25-hydroxyvitamin D concentrations.[16,37]

Trace Element and Vitamin Complications

Clinical symptoms of trace element deficiencies, although rare, have been reported for patients receiving long-term PN. More commonly, decreased serum trace element concentrations have been reported in a variety of patient populations. However, the clinical significance of abnormally low concentrations of many trace elements is not known because serum concentrations often do not correlate with total body stores.[53] Occasionally, patients may develop clinical toxicities from elevated vitamin or trace element concentrations as the result of increased intake or decreased metabolism. These abnormalities are frequently associated with an underlying disease state such as severe kidney or hepatic failure and may necessitate reduction in vitamin and trace element intake.

Many trace elements are present in PN components as contaminants.[53] Some investigations of patients with normal organ function who were receiving PN supplemented with commercially available parenteral multiple trace element solutions have reported concern with elevated serum concentrations of trace elements such as chromium and manganese.[53] Aluminum is a common contaminant of many sterile IV solutions, including those used for compounding PN. Calcium and phosphorus solutions are among those components with the highest levels of aluminum contamination.[89,90] Aluminum accumulation may occur during long-term PN therapy, especially for patients with reduced kidney function, and is associated with abnormal neurologic and hematologic function and metabolic bone disease in adults and premature infants.[37,89,90] Preterm infants are at higher risk of aluminum toxicities because they receive larger doses (micrograms per kilogram) from PN solutions than adults.[90] Preterm infants are also more likely to retain aluminum because of immature renal kidney function. Although the maximum safe level of IV aluminum intake is unknown, the FDA has reported that parenteral doses of 4 to 5 mcg/kg/day were associated with central nervous system and bone toxicity.[91] Even smaller amounts may result in tissue accumulation but no documented toxicity.

The FDA implemented a mandate in 2004 to restrict aluminum content in large-volume PN stock solutions (CAA, dextrose, sterile water for injection, IVFE) to a maximum of 25 mcg/L and for manufacturers to indicate the maximum aluminum concentration at expiration for both large- and small-volume parenteral products used for PN.[91] Investigations have determined actual aluminum concentrations in parenteral products to be lower than the amounts reported on the manufacturer's label, however, aluminum amounts in PN solutions still exceed FDA guidelines.[89,90] In addition, the aluminum content of parenteral products appears to vary considerably during the shelf life of the products and increases with time because of leaching from glass containers. The amount of aluminum contamination delivered to patients receiving long-term parenteral therapy such as chronic PN patients or dialysis patients, can be substantially reduced if newer stock solutions are used to prepare their PN.[89,90]

The amount of aluminum present in alternative imported trace element products is unknown because their initial approval was not based on FDA criteria.[61]

HOME PARENTERAL NUTRITION

Advances in technology for the delivery of IV solutions have allowed medically stable patients who require extended PN therapy to be maintained indefinitely on IV nutrition. An increasing concern for cost containment of healthcare services has fostered use of sophisticated infusion devices to provide PN at home. Numerous programs are now available outside the traditional healthcare setting to support patients who require long-term or permanent PN. Standards have been developed to promote safe and effective care.[69] Home PN services may be coordinated and administered through a hospital or by a commercial home care company.[69]

Many factors are considered in selecting candidates for home PN therapy. Significant benefit must be expected from the therapy. Examples of patients who have been maintained successfully with home PN include those with severe GI dysfunction secondary to Change from Crohn disease to Crohn's disease, ischemic bowel disease, severe GI motility disorders, extensive intestinal obstruction, and congenital bowel dysfunction.[69] The patient and the patient's caregiver must be willing to complete training and assume numerous responsibilities for managing the new daily routine. Other logistics such as funding, procurement of solutions and supplies, and clinical management and follow-up must be individualized for each patient in order to achieve the desired outcomes.[69]

Patients commonly receive PN solutions from their home care provider. IV vitamins or other additives may be added daily by the patient or caregiver, depending on the arrangement with the home care provider. The solution generally is administered through the night by infusion pump over 8 to 20 hours.[69,71] A cycled regimen allows the patient time away from the pump during daylight hours and provides many patients with the freedom to have a reasonably normal daily routine. Clinical management and follow up are performed periodically according to the needs of the patient and the protocol of the home care provider or the managing healthcare team. A coordinated effort among several healthcare professionals, including physicians, pharmacists, nurses, dietitians, social workers, and the patient and the patient's caregiver, as well as the suppliers, is paramount to providing safe and effective management. Home PN affords some patients the potential for an ambulatory lifestyle while maintaining an IV feeding regimen that was previously only available in the hospital setting. For others, home PN may contribute to a better quality of life in the comfort of their homes.[69]

PHARMACOECONOMIC CONSIDERATIONS

Determining the true cost of PN support is difficult because numerous variables affect the provision of PN and the clinical response to therapy. PN therapy cost variables include the underlying indication for treatment, the administration setting (home or acute care), timing of PN initiation, therapy associated complications, and the type of PN formulation provided (compounded or standardized commercial PN product).[69,92-97] Expenses associated with PN therapy may be categorized as direct and indirect costs.[95] Direct costs may be further categorized as fixed or variable costs. Fixed costs do not depend on the volume of patients receiving therapy. For example, an ACD and the tubing sets required to transfer volumes of stock solutions to the administration bag would be considered fixed costs in many practice settings. These costs per patient tend to be highest in low-volume environments. Variable costs such as PN administration bags or standard commercial PN products depend directly on the number of patients receiving PN. Other direct costs include ancillary services required by patients receiving PN and costs related to the management of PN associated complications.

Clinical benefits and other clinical effects of PN (ie, reduction in hospital length of stay and frequency of complications) in specific patient populations have been evaluated but few investigations have reported a comprehensive economic assessment of PN therapy. Attempting to measure the cost or cost savings associated with reported benefits of PN therapy and other clinical effects based on results of controlled clinical trials is difficult.[93,94] Clinical outcome measurements and hence economic outcomes are influenced by multiple factors, including experimental design, sample size, and specific health system practices.[93,95,96,98,99] More recent cost analyses for PN therapy have focused on timing of initiating therapy in critically ill patients and choice of PN formulation (compounded or standard commercial PN product). In general, although individual investigations have reported cost savings with supplemental PN in critically ill patients unable to meet nutritional goals within 24 to 48 hours of intensive care unit (ICU) admission, others have reported no cost advantage with early PN intervention.[96] Similarly, while cost savings have been reported with use of standard commercial PN products compared to PNs compounded with an ACD, others have reported increased costs with other supportive care usually provided with compounded PN when standard commercial PN products were used.[98,100]

Although the results of economic analyses of PN remain controversial, similarities among several reports provide a basis for minimizing the costs of PN therapy:

1. Use PN only for the most appropriate patients as described by institution-specific criteria based on current consensus statements. Enteral nutrition should be used whenever feasible because the associated costs and complications are demonstrated to be less than those associated with PN.[97,101]
2. Reassess the need for routine laboratory monitoring measurements used for PN therapy. In general, the level of laboratory monitoring should decrease as a patient's clinical condition stabilizes.
3. Minimize the direct cost of PN by using efficient purchasing practices for PN solutions and compounding supplies through contract purchasing, streamlined compounding procedures, standardized administration times, single-bag PN solutions, and optimized monitoring plans. Some institutions may realize direct cost savings with use of standardized, commercial PN products depending on the usual daily PN census and patient population.[99] Others may reduce direct costs by outsourcing PN compounding to a third-party compounding pharmacy facility.

PERSONALIZED PHARMACOTHERAPY

10 11 Considerations for individualizing a patient's PN regimen include: goals determination based on a patient-specific nutrition assessment, selection of the optimal type of available vascular access, and macronutrient and micronutrient requirements. In general, both macronutrient and micronutrient doses are age and weights based but are also affected by the patient's degree of metabolic demand, organ function, other drug therapy, exogenous losses, and acid–base status. Nutrient amounts provided by the PN may also require adjustment based on enteral intake either orally or by feeding tube in patients with recovering GI tract function.

Patient-specific caloric goals include (a) adequate energy intake to promote normal growth and development in neonates, infants, and children; (b) energy equilibrium and preservation of fat calorie stores in well-nourished adults; and (c) positive energy balance in malnourished patients with depleted endogenous fat stores. Overweight patients with a body mass index above 30 kg/m^2 may require less caloric support than nonobese patients with the same clinical condition.[11] Critically ill adults may also benefit from a hypocaloric regimen.[11] Specific nitrogen goals are positive nitrogen balance or nitrogen equilibrium and improvement in the serum concentration of visceral protein markers such as transferrin or prealbumin in patients without systemic inflammation. Routine monitoring is necessary to ensure that the nutrition regimen is suitable for a given patient as the patient's clinical condition changes and to minimize or treat complications. The PN component doses usually require individualized adjustments as the patient's clinical condition affects further changes in metabolic stress, organ function, fluid and electrolyte balance, and acid–base status.

Appropriate patient selection, assessment, and monitoring are key to successful PN therapy and the prevention of unnecessary complications. Because pharmacists are actively involved in the provision of PN at many levels, including order verification, PN compounding and dispensing, direct patient care, education, and research, nutrition support is recognized as a pharmacy practice specialty.[102] In addition, as the interprofessional team based approach to specialized nutrition support has evolved, standards of practice have been defined for pharmacists as well as for other healthcare professionals.[4,8-10] Standardized order forms and monitoring protocols are useful tools to ensure safe administration and monitoring of PN therapy. The future of PN therapy and the role of nutrition-support clinicians will be affected primarily by new insights from clinical research and economic challenges in the evolving healthcare environment.

ABBREVIATIONS

AAP	American Academy of Pediatrics
A.S.P.E.N.	American Society for Parenteral and Enteral Nutrition
CAA	crystalline amino acid
CDC	Centers for Disease Control and Prevention
CPN	central parenteral nutrition
CRBSI	catheter related bloodstream infection
CVC	central venous catheter
EFAD	essential fatty acid deficiency
FDA	Food and Drug Administration
GI	gastrointestinal
ICU	intensive care unit
IVFE	IV fat emulsion
LCT	long-chain triglyceride
MCT	medium-chain triglyceride
NAG-AMA	Nutrition Advisory Group of the American Medical Association
NF	National Formulary
OO	olive oil
PICC	peripherally inserted central catheter
PN	parenteral nutrition
PNALD	parenteral nutrition–associated liver disease
PPN	peripheral parenteral nutrition
PUFA	polyunsaturated fatty acid
SO	soybean oil
TNA	total nutrient admixture
USP	United States Pharmacopeia

REFERENCES

1. Dudrick SJ, Palesty JA. Historical highlights of the development of total parenteral nutrition. *Surg Clin N Am* 2011;693-717.
2. Delegge MH, Kelley AT. State of nutrition support teams. *Nutr Clin Pract* 2013;28:691-697.
3. Mirtallo JM, Holcombe B, Kochevar M. Parenteral nutrition product shortages: The A.S.P.E.N. strategy. *JPEN J Parenter Enteral Nutr* 2012;27:385-391.
4. Tucker A, Ybarra J, Bingham A, et al. American Society for Parenteral and Enteral Nutrition (A.S.P.E.N.) Standards of Practice for Nutrition Support Pharmacists. *Nutr Clin Pract* 2015;30:139-146.
5. Ayers P, Adams S, Boullata J, et al. A.S.P.E.N. Parenteral Nutrition Safety Consensus Recommendations. *JPEN J Parenter Enteral Nutr* 2014;38:296-333.
6. Ukleja A, Freeman KL, Gilbert K, et al; Task Force on Standards for Nutrition Support: Adult Hospitalized Patients, and the American Society for Parenteral and Enteral Nutrition Board of Directors. Standards for nutrition support: Adult hospitalized patients. *Nutr Clin Pract* 2010;25:403-414.
7. Corkins MR, Griggs KC, Groh-Wargo S, et al. Standards for nutrition support: Pediatric hospitalized patients. *Nutr Clin Pract* 2013; 263-276.
8. Brantley SL, Russell MK, Mogensen KM, et al. American society for parenteral and enteral nutrition and academy of nutrition and dietetics revised 2014 standards of practice and standards of professional performance for registered dietitian nutritionists (competent, proficient, and expert) in nutrition support. *Nutr Clin Pract* 2014;29:792-828.
9. American Society for Parenteral and Enteral Nutrition (A.S.P.E.N.) Board of Directors and Nurses Standards Revision Task Force, DiMaria-Ghalili RA, Bankhead R, Fisher AA, et al. Standards of practice for nutrition support nurses. *Nutr Clin Pract* 2007;22: 458-465.
10. Mascarenhas MR, August DA, DeLegge MH, et al; Task Force on Standards for Nutrition Support Physicians; American Society for Parenteral and Enteral Nutrition Board of Directors; American Society for Parenteral and Enteral Nutrition. Standards of practice for nutrition support physicians. *Nutr Clin Pract* 2012;27: 295-299.
11. McClave SA, Taylor BE, Martindale RG, et al. Guidelines for the provision and assessment of nutrition support therapy in the adult critically ill patient: Society of Critical Care Medicine (SCCM) and American Society for Parenteral and Enteral Nutrition (A.S.P.E.N.). *JPEN J Parenter Enteral Nutr* 2016;40:159-211.
12. Mehta NM, Compher C, and A.S.P.E.N. Board of Directors. A.S.P.E.N. Clinical guidelines: Nutrition support of the critically ill child. *JPEN J Parenter Enteral Nutr* 2009;33;260-276.
13. White JV, Guenter P, Jensen G, et al; Academy of Nutrition and Dietetics Malnutrition Workgroup, A.S.P.E.N. Malnutrition Task Force, A.S.P.E.N. Board of Directors. Consensus statement: Academy of Nutrition and the American Society for Parenteral and Enteral Nutrition: Characteristics recommended for the identification and documentation of adult malnutrition (undernutrition). *JPEN J Parenter Enteral Nutr* 2012;36:275-283.
14. August DA, Huhmann MB; American Society for Parenteral and Enteral Nutrition (A.S.P.E.N.) Board of Directors. A.S.P.E.N. clinical guidelines: Nutrition support therapy during adult anticancer treatment and in hematopoietic cell transplantation. *JPEN J Parenter Enteral Nutr* 2009;33:472-500.
15. Koretz RL, Avenell A, Lipman TO. Nutritional support for liver disease (Review). *Cochrane Database Syst Rev* 2012 (May 16);5: CD008344.
16. A.S.P.E.N. Board of Directors and the Clinical Guidelines Taskforce. Administration of specialized nutrition support—Issues unique to pediatrics. *JPEN J Parenter Enteral Nutr* 2002;26(Suppl A): 97SA-110SA.
17. A.S.P.E.N. Board of Directors and the Clinical Guidelines Taskforce. Specific guidelines for disease—Pediatrics. *JPEN J Parenter Enteral Nutr* 2002;26(Suppl A):111SA-138SA.
18. Crill CM, Gura KM. Parenteral nutrition support: In: Corkins MR, ed. The A.S.P.E.N. *Pediatric Nutrition Support Core Curriculum,* 2nd ed. Silver Spring, MD: American Society for Parenteral and Enteral Nutrition (A.S.P.E.N.); 2015:593-614.
19. Brown RO, Compher C; American Society for Parenteral and Enteral Nutrition Board of Directors. A.S.P.E.N. clinical guidelines: Nutrition support in adult acute and chronic renal failure. *JPEN J Parenter Enteral Nutr* 2010;34:366-377.
20. Mirtallo J, Patel M. Overview of Parenteral Nutrition. In: Mueller CM, ed. The A.S.P.E.N. *Adult Nutrition Support Core Curriculum,* 2nd ed. Silver Spring, MD: American Society for Parenteral and Enteral Nutrition (A.S.P.E.N.); 2012;234-244.
21. Ehrenkranz RA. Early, aggressive nutritional management for very low birth weight infants: What is the evidence? *Semin Perinatol* 2007;31:48-55.
22. Moyses HE, Johnson MJ, Leaf AA, Cornelius VR. Early parenteral nutrition and growth outcomes in preterm infants: As systematic review and meta-analysis. *Am J Clin Nutr* 2013;97:816-826.
23. FDA Drug Shortages-Current and Resolved Drug Shortages and Discontinuations Reported to FDA. 3 Oct. 2014. Available at: www.accessdata.fda.gov/scripts/drugshortages/default.cfm. Accessed July 10, 2015.
24. Van Way CW. Editorial: Total calories vs nonprotein calories. *Nutr Clin Pract* 2001;16:271-272.
25. Furst P, Stehle P. Are intravenous amino acid solutions unbalanced? *New Horizons* 1994;2:215-223.
26. Dickerson RN. Using nitrogen balance in clinical practice. *Hosp Pharm* 2005;40:1081-1085.
27. Yarandia SS, Zhaob VM., Gautam Hebbara, and Thomas R. Ziegler TR, Amino acid composition in parenteral nutrition: What is the evidence? *Curr Opin Clin Nutr Metab Care.* 2011;14:75-82.
28. Trissel LA. Amino Acids. In: Trissel LA, ed. *Handbook on Injectable Drugs,* 17th ed. Bethesda, MD: American Society of Health-System Pharmacists; 2013:38-70.
29. Vanek VW, Matarese LE, Robinson M, et al; Novel Nutrient Task Force, Parenteral Glutamine Workgroup; American Society for Parenteral and Enteral Nutrition (A.S.P.E.N.) Board of Directors. A.S.P.E.N. position paper: Parenteral nutrition glutamine supplementation. *Nutr Clin Pract* 2011;26:479-494.
30. Heyland D, Muscedere J, Wischmeyer PE, et al. A Randomized Trial of Glutamine and Antioxidants in Critically Ill Patients. *N Engl J Med* 2013; 368:1489-1497.
31. de Kieviet JF, Vuijk PJ, van den Berg A, et al. Glutamine effects on brain growth in very preterm children in the first year of life. *Clin Nutr* 2014;33:69-74.

32. Moe-Byrne T, Wagner JV, McGuire W. Glutamine supplementation to prevent morbidity and mortality in preterm infants. *Cochrane Database Syst Rev* 2012;(3):CD001457.
33. Brown JV, Moe-Byrne T, McGuire W. Glutamine supplementation for young infants with severe gastrointestinal disease. *Cochrane Database Syst Rev* 2014;(12):CD005947.
34. fda.gov/downloads/AdvisoryCommittees/CommitteesMeetingMaterials/Drugs/PharmacyCompoundingAdvisoryCommittee/UCM466379.pdf. Accessed October 28, 2015.
35. fda.gov/Drugs/GuidanceComplianceRegulatoryInformation/PharmacyCompounding/ucm375804.htm. Accessed October 28, 2015.
36. Btaiche IF, Khalidi N. Metabolic complications of parenteral nutrition in adults, part 1. *Am J Health Syst Pharm* 2004;61:1938-1949.
37. Btaiche IF, Khalidi N. Metabolic complications of parenteral nutrition in adults, part 2. *Am J Health Syst Pharm* 2004;61:2050-2057.
38. Waxman K, Day AT, Stellin GP, et al. Safety and efficacy of glycerol and amino acids in combination with lipid emulsion for peripheral parenteral nutrition support. *JPEN J Parenter Enteral Nutr* 1992;16:374-378.
39. ProcalAmine. Product information. Irvine, CA: B. Braun Medical, 2015.
40. Clinolipid. Product information. Deerfield, IL: Baxter Healthcare, 2013.
41. Vanek VW, Seidner DL, Allen P, et al; Novel Nutrient Task Force, Intravenous Fat Emulsions Workgroup; American Society for Parenteral and Enteral Nutrition (A.S.P.E.N.) Board of Directors. A.S.P.E.N. position paper: Clinical role for alternative intravenous fat emulsions. *Nutr Clin Pract* 2012;27:150-192.
42. Parenteral Nutrition. In: Kleinman RE, ed. American Academy of Pediatrics Committee on Nutrition. *Pediatric Nutrition Handbook*, 6th ed. Elk Grove, IL: American Academy of Pediatrics; 2009:519-540.
43. Bistrian BR. Clinical aspects of essential fatty acid metabolism: Johnathon Rhoads Lecture. *JPEN J Parenter Enteral Nutr* 2003;27:168-175.
44. Task Force for the Revision of Safe Practices for Parenteral Nutrition. Safe practices for parenteral nutrition. *JPEN J Parenter Enteral Nutr* 2004;28:539-570.
45. Kerner JA Jr, Poole RL. The use of IV fat in neonates. *Nutr Clin Pract* 2006;21:374-380.
46. Hicks RW, Becker SC, Chuo J. A summary of NICU fat emulsion medication errors and nursing services. Data from MEDMARX. *Adv Neonatal Care* 2007;7:299-310.
47. Intralipid. Product information. Deerfield, IL: Baxter Healthcare Corporation, 2014.
48. Waitzberg DL, Torrinhas RS. Fish oil based lipid emulsions and immune response: What clinicians need to know. *Nutr Clin Pract* 2009;24:487-499.
49. Marik PE, Zaloga GP. Immunonutrition in critically ill patients: A systematic review and analysis of the literature. *Intensive Care Med* 2008;11:1980-1990.
50. Nandivada P, Carlson SJ, Chang MI, et al. Treatment of parenteral nutrition-associated liver disease: The role of lipid emulsions. *Adv Nutr* 2013;4:711-717.
51. Diprivan. Product information. Schaumburg, IL: APP Pharmaceuticals, LLC, 2009.
52. Cleviprex (clevidipine) injectable emulsion. Product information. Graz, Austria: Fresenius Kabi Austria GmbH, 2008.
53. Vanek VW, Borum P, Buchman A, et al; Novel Nutrient Task Force, Parenteral Multi-Vitamin and Multi–Trace Element Working Group; American Society for Parenteral and Enteral Nutrition (A.S.P.E.N.) Board of Directors. A.S.P.E.N. Position paper: Recommendations for changes in commercially available parenteral multivitamin and multi-trace element products. *Nutr Clin Pract* 2012;27:440-491.
54. Chambrier C, Lellerq M, Saudin F, et al. Is vitamin K_1 supplementation necessary in long-term parenteral nutrition? *JPEN J Parenter Enteral Nutr* 1998;22:87-90.
55. Helphingstine CJ, Bistrian BR. New food and drug administration requirements for inclusion of vitamin K in adult parenteral multivitamins. *JPEN J Parenter Enteral Nutr* 2003;27:220-224.
56. Lennon C, Davidson KW, Sandowski JA, Mason JB. The vitamin K content of intravenous lipid emulsion. *JPEN J Parenter Enteral Nutr* 1993;17:142-144.
57. Greene HL, Hambidge KM, Schanler R, Tsang RC. Guidelines for the use of vitamins, trace elements, calcium, magnesium, and phosphorus in infants and children receiving total parenteral nutrition: Report of the Subcommittee on Pediatric Parenteral Nutrient Requirements from the Committee on Clinical Practice Issues of the American Society for Clinical Nutrition. *Am J Clin Nutr* 1988;48:1324-1342.
58. Misra S, Kirby DF. Micronutrient and trace element monitoring in adult nutrition support. *Nutr Clin Pract* 2000;15:120-126.
59. Aggett PJ. Trace elements of the micropremie. *Clin Perinatol* 2000;27:119-129.
60. Zimmermann MB, Crill CM. Iodine in enteral and parenteral nutrition. *Best Pract Res Clin Endocrinol Metab* 2010;24:143-158.
61. Current Drug Shortage Bulletins: Trace Elements Injection. Available at: ashp.org/menu/DrugShortages/CurrentShortages/Bulletin.aspx?id=785. Accessed October 31, 2015.
62. Laboratoire Aguettant (Lyon, France). Dear Healthcare Professional Letter. Zinc Injection Availability. July 24, 2013. Accessed August 10, 2015.
63. Current Drug Shortage Bulletins: Sodium Phosphate Injection. ashp.org/menu/DrugShortages/CurrentShortages/Bulletin.aspx?id=770. Accessed October 31, 2015.
64. Kraft MD, Btaiche IF, Sacks GS, Kudsk KA. Treatment of electrolyte disorders in adult patients in the intensive care unit. *Am J Health Syst Pharm* 2005;62:1663-1682.
65. Gervasio J. Total nutrient admixtures (3-in-1): Pros vs cons for adults. *Nutr Clin Pract* 2015;30:331-335.
66. Boullata JI, Gilbert K, Sacks G, et al. A.S.P.E.N. Clinical Guidelines: Parenteral Nutrition Ordering, Order Review, Compounding, Labeling, and Dispensing. *JPEN J Parenter Enteral Nutr.* 2014;38:334-377.
67. Anderson ADG, Palmer D, MacFie J. Peripheral parenteral nutrition. *Br J Surg* 2003;90:1048-1054.
68. O'Grady NP, Alexander M, Burns LA, et al; Healthcare Infection Control Practices Advisory Committee. Guidelines for the prevention of intravascular catheter-related infections. *Am J Infect Control* 2011;39(Suppl):S1-S34.
69. Kirby DF, Corrigan ML, Speerhas RA, Emery DM. Home parenteral nutrition tutorial. *JPEN J Parenter Enteral Nutr.* 2012;36:632-644.
70. A.S.P.E.N. Board of Directors and Task Force on Parenteral Nutrition Standardization, Kochevar M, Guenter P, Holcombe B, et al. A.S.P.E.N. Statement on Parenteral Nutrition Standardization. *JPEN J Parenter Enteral Nutr* 2007;31:441-448.
71. Speerhas R, Wang J, Seidner D, Steiger E. Maintaining normal blood glucose concentrations with total parenteral nutrition: Is it necessary to taper total parenteral nutrition? *Nutr Clin Pract* 2003;18:414-416.
72. Stout ST, Cober MP. Metabolic effects of cyclic parenteral nutrition infusion in adults and children. *Nutr Clin Pract* 2010;25:277-281.
73. USP <797> Guidebook to Pharmaceutical Compounding—Sterile Preparations. Rockville, MD: United States Pharmacopeia Convention, 2008.
74. American Society for Health-System Pharmacists. ASHP guidelines on the safe use of automated compounding devices for the preparation of parenteral nutrition admixtures. *Am J Health Syst Pharm* 2000;57:1343-1348.
75. *Handbook on Injectable Drugs,* 18th ed. Bethesda, MD: American Society of Health-System Pharmacists, 2014.
76. King JC, Catania PN, ed. *King Guide to Parenteral Admixtures,* Napa, CA: King Guide Publications, 2012.
77. Newton DW, Driscoll DF. Calcium and phosphate compatibility: Revisited again. *Am J Health-Syst Pharm* 2008;65:73-80.
78. Hoff DS, Michaelson AS. Effects of light exposure on total parenteral nutrition and its implications in the neonatal population. *J Pediatr Pharmacol Ther* 2009;14:132-143.
79. Mermel LA, Allon M, Bouza E, et al. Clinical practice guidelines for the diagnosis and management of intravascular catheter-related infection: 2009 Update by the Infectious Diseases Society of America. *Clin Infect Dis* 2009;49:1-45.
80. Tillman EM. Review and clinical update on parenteral nutrition-associated liver disease. *Nutr Clin Pract* 2013;28:30-39.
81. Tillman EM, Helms RA. Omega-3 long chain polyunsaturated Fatty acids for treatment of parenteral nutrition-associated liver disease: A review of the literature. *J Pediatr Pharmacol Ther* 2011;16:31-38.
82. ISMP Medication Safety Alert!® Acute Care. Action needed to prevent dangerous heparin-insulin confusion. May 3, 2007. Available at: www.ismp.org/Newsletters/acutecare/articles/20070503.asp. Access on August 29, 2016.
83. McMahon MM, Nystrom E, Braunschweig C, et al; American Society for Parenteral and Enteral Nutrition (A.S.P.E.N.) Board of Directors.

A.S.P.E.N. Clinical guidelines: Nutrition support of adult patients with hyperglycemia. *JPEN J Parenter Enteral Nutr* 2012;37(1):23-36.

84. Arsenault D, Brenn M, Kim S, et al; American Society for Parenteral and Enteral Nutrition Board of Directors, Puder M. A.S.P.E.N. Clinical Guidelines: Hyperglycemia and hypoglycemia in the neonate receiving parenteral nutrition. *JPEN J Parenter Enteral Nutr* 2012;36:81-95.
85. Newton L, Garvey WT. Nutritional and medical management of diabetes mellitus in hospitalized patients. In: Mueller C, ed. The A.S.P.E.N. *Adult Nutrition Support Core Curriculum,* 2nd ed. Silver Spring, MD: American Society for Parenteral and Enteral Nutrition (A.S.P.E.N.); 2012;580-602.
86. Mehanna HM, Moledina J, Travis J. Refeeding syndrome: What it is, and how to prevent and treat it. *BMJ* 2008;336;1495-1498.
87. Kraft MD, Btaiche IF, Sacks G. Review of the refeeding syndrome. *Nutr Clin Pract* 2005;20:625-633.
88. Schmidt GL. Fluid and electrolytes. In: Corkins MR, ed. *The A.S.P.E.N. Pediatric Nutrition Support Core Curriculum*. Silver Spring, MD: American Society for Parenteral and Enteral Nutrition (A.S.P.E.N.); 2010:87-102.
89. Gura KM. Aluminum contamination in products used in parenteral nutrition: Has anything changed? *Nutrition* 2010;26:585-594.
90. Gura KM. Aluminum contamination in parenteral products. *Curr Opin Clin Nutr Metab Care* 2014;17:551-557.
91. Food and Drug Administration. Aluminum in large and small volume parenterals used in total parenteral nutrition. *Fed Regist* 2000;65:4103-4111.
92. Howard L. Home parenteral nutrition: Survival, cost, and quality of life. *Gastroenterology* 2006;130:S52-S59.
93. Lipman TO. The cost of TPN: Is the price right? *JPEN J Parenter Enteral Nutr* 1993;17:199-200.
94. Eisenberg JM, Glick HA, Buzby GP, et al. Does perioperative total parenteral nutrition reduce medical care costs? *JPEN J Parenter Enteral Nutr* 1993;17:201-209.
95. Eisenberg JM, Glick H, Hillman AL, et al. Measuring the economic impact of perioperative total parenteral nutrition: Principles and design. *Am J Clin Nutr* 1988;47:382-391.
96. Bost RBC, Tjan DHT, Van Zanten ARH. Timing of (supplemental) parenteral nutrition in critically ill patients: A systematic review. *Ann Intensive Care* 2014;4:31.
97. DeLegge MH, Base MD, Bannister C, Budak AR. Parenteral nutrition (PN) use for adult hospitalized patients: A study of usage in a tertiary medical center. *Nutr Clin Pract* 2007;22:246-249.
98. Busch RA, Curtis CS, Leverson GA, Kudsk KA. Use of piggyback electrolytes for patients receiving individually prescribed vs premixed parenteral nutrition. *JPEN J Parenter Enteral Nutr* 2015; 39:586-590.
99. Bozat E, Korubuk G, Abbasoglu O. Cost analysis of premixed multichamber bags versus compounded parenteral nutrition: Breakeven point. *Hosp Pharm* 2014;49:170-176.
100. Turpin RS, Canada T, Liu FX, et al. Nutrition therapy cost analysis in the US. Pre-mixed multi-chamber bag vs compounded parenteral nutrition. *Appl Health Econ Health Policy* 2011;9:281-292.
101. Zaloga GP. Parenteral nutrition in adult inpatients with functioning gastrointestinal tracts: Assessment of outcomes. *Lancet* 2006;367:1101-1111.
102. Mirtallo JM. Advancement of nutrition support in clinical pharmacy. *Ann Pharmacother* 2007;41:869-872.

143

Enteral Nutrition

Vanessa J. Kumpf and Katherine H. Chessman

KEY CONCEPTS

1. The gastrointestinal (GI) tract defends the host from toxins and antigens by both immunologic and nonimmunologic mechanisms, collectively referred to as the gut barrier function. Whenever possible, enteral nutrition (EN) is preferred over parenteral nutrition (PN) because it is associated with a lower risk of metabolic and infectious complications and is less expensive and invasive.
2. Candidates for EN are those with a sufficiently functioning GI tract to allow adequate nutrient absorption who cannot or will not eat and in whom enteral access can be safely obtained.
3. The most common route for both short- and long-term EN access is directly into the stomach. The method of delivery may be continuously via an infusion pump, intermittently via a pump or gravity drip, or bolus administration via gravity or syringe.
4. Patients unable to tolerate tube feeding into the stomach because of impaired gastric motility may benefit from feeding tube placement into the duodenum or jejunum. When feeding into the small bowel, the continuous method of delivery via an infusion pump is required to enhance tolerance.
5. Selection of the enteral feeding formulation depends on nutritional requirements, the patient's primary disease state and related complications, and nutrient digestibility and absorption. A standard polymeric formulation will be appropriate for the majority of adults and children.
6. Measurement of gastric residual volumes (GRVs) is often used to monitor GI tolerance in patients receiving gastric feeding. Although the practice has not been consistently reported to decrease aspiration risk, a high GRV may provide an early sign of GI dysfunction and alert the clinician to the need for intervention.
7. Management of diarrhea in patients receiving EN should focus on identification and correction of the most likely cause(s). Tube feeding-related causes include too rapid delivery or advancement, intolerance to the formula composition, and occasionally formula contamination.
8. Medication administration through a feeding tube requires selection of an appropriate dosage form and verification of appropriate enteral access. Medications that should not be crushed and administered through a tube include enteric-coated or sustained-release capsules or tablets and sublingual or buccal tablets.
9. The coadministration of medications with EN can result in alterations in bioavailability and/or changes in the desired pharmacologic effects. Medications known to interact with EN include phenytoin, warfarin, select antibiotics, antacids, and proton-pump inhibitors.

INTRODUCTION

Enteral nutrition (EN) is defined as the delivery of nutrients by tube or by mouth into the gastrointestinal (GI) tract. This chapter focuses on nutrient delivery through a feeding tube rather than oral food ingestion. The terms *enteral nutrition* and *tube feeding* are thus used interchangeably in this context. The goal of EN is to provide calories, macronutrients, and micronutrients to those patients who are unable to achieve these requirements from an oral diet. Increased recognition of malnutrition, along with improvements in enteral access techniques, feeding formulations, and methods to prevent and manage complications, have resulted in an increased use of EN across all healthcare settings. In this chapter, principles and practices related to the safe and successful use of EN therapy are described.

GASTROINTESTINAL TRACT PHYSIOLOGY

The GI tract plays a key role in the processing of ingested foods. Many of the processes involved in digestion, absorption, and utilization of nutrients are modifiable by the presence of acute and chronic illnesses.

Digestion and Absorption

Digestion and absorption are GI processes that generate the body's usable fuels.[1,2] Ingested nutrients are primarily large polymers that cannot be absorbed across the intestinal cell membrane unless they are transformed into an absorbable molecular form. Digestion consists of the stepwise conversion of a complex chemical and physical nutrient into a molecular form that is absorbable by the intestinal mucosa. Absorption from the GI tract is a multistep process that includes the transfer of a nutrient across the intestinal cell membrane. The nutrient ultimately reaches the systemic circulation through the portal venous or splanchnic lymphatic systems, provided that the GI or biliary tract does not excrete it. In addition, a coordinated interplay of GI motility and neurohormonal secretion is required to facilitate adequate digestion and absorption.

Nutrient digestion involves the complex coordination of multiple mechanical, enzymatic, and physiochemical processes.[1,2] Mechanical dissolution of food occurs by chewing, then mixing and grinding the stomach contents. Food stimulates secretion of numerous hormones and enzymes from the salivary glands, stomach, liver and biliary system, pancreas, and intestines (Table 143-1). As food traverses the gut lumen, these hormones modulate GI motility and the secretions from other organs of the digestive system. Nutrient absorption occurs within the gut lumen and is a specific function of the intestinal cell membrane, which is comprised of fingerlike projections called villi. Each individual villus is made up of epithelial cells called enterocytes. The enterocyte surface contains special luminal projections called microvilli, which provide an increased surface area that is referred to as the brush-border membrane.

TABLE 143-1 Gastrointestinal Enzymes and Hormones

Enzyme/Hormone	Site of Secretion	Main Actions
Amylase	Salivary glands, pancreas	Converts carbohydrates, starch, and glycogen to simple disaccharides
Cholecystokinin	Duodenum, jejunum	Stimulates pancreatic enzyme secretion and gallbladder contraction
Chymotrypsinogen	Pancreas	Breaks down proteins into peptides
Enteroglucagon	Duodenum, small intestine	Inhibits pancreatic enzyme secretion and bowel motility
Gastric inhibitory peptide	Small intestine	Decreases gastric motility and stimulates insulin secretion
Gastrin	Stomach, duodenum	Stimulates gastric acid secretion and mucosal growth
Glucagon	Pancreas	Stimulates hepatic glycogenolysis and inhibits motility
Lipase	Pancreas	Hydrolyzes dietary fat to release fatty acids
Pancreatic polypeptide	Pancreas	Inhibits gallbladder contraction and pancreatic and biliary secretion
Pepsinogen	Stomach	Converts large proteins into polypeptides
Secretin	Small intestine	Stimulates hepatic and pancreatic water and bicarbonate release
Trypsinogen	Pancreas	Breaks down proteins into peptides
Vasoactive inhibitory peptide	Small intestine, pancreas	Vasodilator; stimulates water and bicarbonate secretion, insulin and glucagon release, and small bowel secretions

The digestion and absorption of carbohydrate, fat, and protein within the small intestine are illustrated in Figure 143-1. Carbohydrates are presented to the small intestine in either a digestible or a nondigestible form. Polysaccharides (starches) and oligosaccharides (sucrose and lactose) undergo enzymatic digestion to simple sugars. The simple sugars are absorbed via active and passive transport mechanisms and are eventually released into the portal vein. Polysaccharides, such as cellulose complexes and other fiber components, pass undigested to the colon, where they are digested by bacteria and enzymes to short-chain fatty acids. Colonic absorption of short-chain fatty acids stimulates sodium and water reabsorption. The short-chain fatty acids serve as a systemic energy source and they provide nourishment for the colonic mucosa cells.

Fat is most often presented to the small intestine as long-chain triglycerides. Fat digestion requires pancreatic lipase release and formation of mixed bile salt micelles, which are then absorbed across the intestinal enterocyte. Within the enterocyte, triglycerides are reesterified and packaged into chylomicrons that are then transported into the lymphatic system. Medium-chain triglycerides (MCTs) can be absorbed intact by the mucosal membrane and are acted on by intracellular lipase within the enterocyte to release free fatty acids that pass directly into the portal vein.[3]

Protein is presented to the small intestine primarily as large polypeptides and to a lesser extent as free amino acids because of protein denaturation in the stomach. Polypeptide digestion generates oligopeptides, which are further hydrolyzed to dipeptides and tripeptides. Peptide absorption occurs via a peptide transport system while free amino acids are absorbed via specific amino acid transporters. These peptide carriers are very efficient, whereas free amino acid absorption appears to less efficient.[2]

Understanding the mechanisms involved in digestion and absorption can greatly enhance the rational use of EN in patients with normal or altered GI anatomy and/or function. Various circumstances may alter the efficacy of nutrient digestion and absorption. For example, the functional immaturity of the neonatal gut may lead to clinical problems associated with inadequate digestion and absorption of EN.

Gut Host Defense Mechanisms

1 Besides digesting and absorbing nutrients to maintain nutritional health, the GI tract is actively involved in defending the host

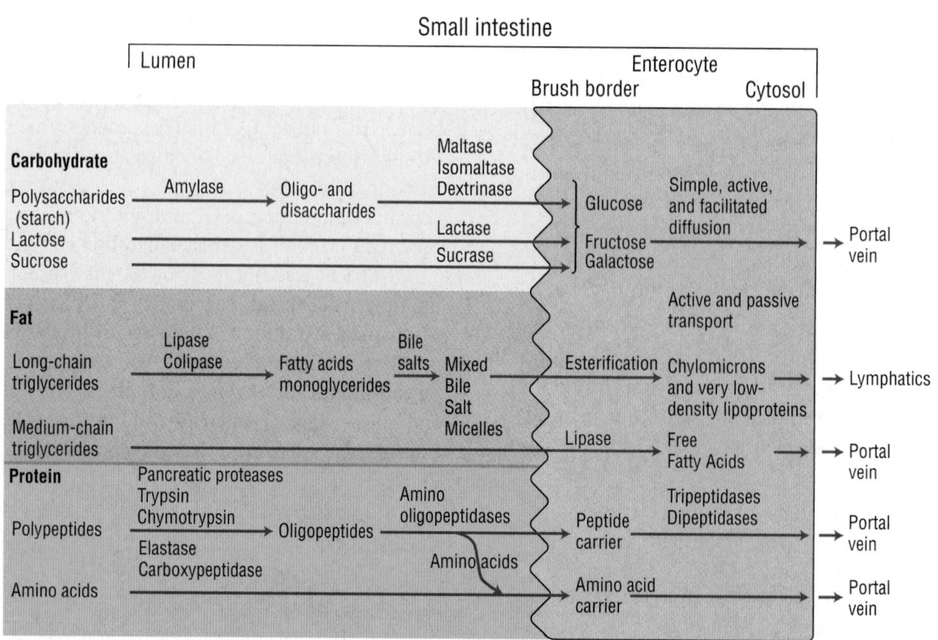

FIGURE 143-1 Schematic of carbohydrate, fat, and protein digestion.

from toxins and antigens by both immunologic and nonimmunologic mechanisms.[4] These gut host defense mechanisms are collectively referred to as the gut barrier function. The gut barrier acts to prevent the systemic spread of intraluminal bacteria and endotoxins to other organs and tissues. Hydrochloric acid secreted by the stomach kills most of the bacteria ingested with food. Under normal circumstances, a mucus layer coats the intestinal epithelium and thereby alters the adherence of bacteria to the cells of the GI tract but provides a favorable environment for anaerobic bacteria. Anaerobic bacteria, which normally colonize the mucus layer, aid in preventing tissue colonization by potential pathogens. Small bowel peristalsis further prevents bacterial stasis and overgrowth. The gut barrier function is also maintained by the intestinal immune system, known as the gut-associated lymphoid tissue (GALT). GALT regulates the local immune response to antigens within the GI tract. Specific immunoglobulins are secreted to kill the remaining organisms and neutralize any toxins they produce. The liver Kupffer cells help to maintain gut barrier function by clearing the portal blood of gut-derived bacteria and endotoxins. Gut barrier integrity may be affected negatively by numerous pathogenic insults, such as physiologic stress and ischemia, and a variety of drugs, including chemotherapeutic agents. The administration of certain probiotics can modify intestinal flora and may have beneficial effects in various disease states and patient populations by positively affecting the maintenance of gut barrier function and intestinal immune function.[5-7]

INDICATIONS FOR ENTERAL NUTRITION

2 The decision to initiate EN is based on a variety of factors. Suitable candidates are those who cannot or will not eat a sufficient amount to meet their nutritional requirements, those who exhibit a sufficient functioning GI tract to allow for nutrient absorption, and those in whom a method of enteral access can be safely initiated.[8-11] Thus, EN may be indicated in a variety of conditions or disease states (Table 143-2). For example, patients who have difficulty swallowing due to stroke, altered mental status, or obstruction in the head, neck, or esophagus due to cancer may benefit from EN. Extreme prematurity necessitates tube feeding because the suck–swallow-and-breath mechanism is not matured sufficiently to allow safe oral intake.[12]

TABLE 143-2 Potential Indications for Enteral Nutrition

Neoplastic disease	**Neurologic impairment**
Chemotherapy	Comatose state
Radiation therapy	Cerebrovascular accident
Upper GI tumors	Demyelinating disease
Cancer cachexia	Severe depression
Organ dysfunction	Cerebral palsy
Liver disease/failure	**Other indications**
Kidney insufficiency/failure	AIDS
Cardiac cachexia	Anorexia nervosa
ARDS/ALI	Complications during pregnancy
Bronchopulmonary dysplasia	Failure-to-thrive
Congenital heart disease	Geriatric patients with multiple chronic diseases
Organ transplantation	Extreme prematurity
Hypermetabolic states	Inborn errors of metabolism
Closed head injury	Cystic fibrosis
Burns	
Trauma	
Postoperative major surgery	
Sepsis	
GI disease	
Inflammatory bowel disease	
Short bowel syndrome	
Esophageal motility disorder	
Pancreatitis	
Fistulas	
Gastroesophageal reflux disease (severe)	
Esophageal or intestinal atresia	

AIDS, acquired immune deficiency syndrome; ALI, acute lung injury; ARDS, acute respiratory distress syndrome.

Critically ill patients who are endotracheally intubated represent a large percentage of hospitalized patients requiring EN. Traditionally, EN in the critically ill population was regarded as supportive care designed to provide nutrients during the period of time the patient was unable to maintain adequate oral dietary intake. Current evidence also supports the use of EN as a tool to modulate the stress response to critical illness and improve patient outcomes. Nutrition guidelines support the initiation of EN in critically ill adults[13-15] and children[16] who are unable to maintain volitional intake. Some of these patients may have reduced gastric emptying caused by sepsis, GI surgery, anesthetic agents, opioid analgesics, and underlying pathology, such as diabetic gastroparesis and burns. However, successful EN can often be achieved by advancing the tip of the feeding tube beyond the pylorus into the duodenum, or preferably into the jejunum. Small bowel feeding may also be appropriate for patients with gastric outlet obstruction, those with pancreatitis, those with moderate to severe gastroesophageal reflux, or those with high aspiration risk.

Contraindications to EN use and/or tube placement are distal mechanical intestinal obstruction, bowel ischemia, active peritonitis, uncorrectable coagulopathy, and necrotizing enterocolitis.[1,17,18] Conditions that my result in significant challenges to EN use include severe diarrhea, protracted vomiting, enteric fistulas, severe GI hemorrhage, hemodynamic instability, and intestinal dysmotility.

BENEFITS OF ENTERAL NUTRITION

The importance of maintaining nutrient delivery through the GI tract in patients without a contraindication to its use is well supported. The beneficial effects of EN, specifically in the critically ill patient, are further enhanced if EN is initiated within 24 to 48 hours of admission to an intensive care unit (ICU).[13-15]

Enteral Versus Parenteral Nutrition

Clinical studies comparing EN and parenteral nutrition (PN) in the critically ill adult patient demonstrate a decrease in infectious complications with the use of EN.[19-21] Infectious complications are thought to be less common with EN in part because EN supports functional gut integrity by stimulating bile flow and the release of endogenous trophic agents, such as cholecystokinin, gastrin, and bile salts. Provision of enteral nutrients appears to help maintain the intestinal mucosal villous height and support the mass of secretory immunoglobulin A (IgA)-producing immunocytes that comprise the GALT. In the setting of critical illness or severe injury, adverse changes in gut permeability and gut barrier function that result in increased risk for systemic infection and multiorgan dysfunction syndrome have been noted. By supporting gut integrity, the enteral feeding route is thought to lower infection risk and minimize organ failure.[13]

The incidence of infectious complications has been documented to be lower in EN patients with abdominal trauma, burns, severe head injury, major surgery, and acute pancreatitis. This reduction in infectious complications is primarily due to the lower incidence of pneumonia and catheter-related bloodstream infections and a decrease in abdominal abscess in trauma patients.[19-21] Unfortunately, interpretation of these studies is often complicated by small sample size and lack of standardization in timing of EN initiation and achievement of nutrition goals. Recently, the CALORIES trial randomized 2,400 adult critically ill patients who were expected to require nutritional support for at least 2 days to either EN or PN and initiated therapy within 36 hours of ICU admission.[22] No significant differences in infectious complications or mortality was noted and these findings challenge EN use as the preferred route for early nutritional support in critically ill patients.. There are no randomized, controlled trials that compare the use of EN and PN in children.[16]

Enteral nutrition is more physiologic than PN in terms of nutrient utilization and therefore is generally associated with fewer metabolic complications, such as glucose intolerance and elevated insulin requirements.[23] Enteral formulations contain both complex and simple carbohydrates, which results in slower carbohydrate absorption compared with the simple carbohydrate, dextrose, used in PN. In addition, enteral formulations that contain fiber and/or a high fat content will further slow carbohydrate absorption and reduce blood sugar elevations by delaying gastric emptying, accounting for better blood glucose control when carbohydrates are given via the enteral route. An additional physiologic benefit of enteral feeding is that it stimulates bile flow through the biliary tract and thus reduces the risk of developing cholestasis, gallbladder sludge, and gallstones, conditions that have been associated with long-term PN and bowel rest.[24] EN avoids the potential infectious and technical complications associated with the placement and use of a central venous access device required for PN. Finally, EN is less costly than PN when all factors associated with the therapy are considered.

Timing of Initiation

The timing of initiation of EN in the critically ill patient is of clinical significance. Initiating EN in the first 24 to 72 hours following admission appears to attenuate the stress response and may reduce disease severity and infectious complications when compared with the initiation of feedings after 72 hours.[13-15] Early EN has also been associated with a decrease in the release of inflammatory cytokines and fewer effects on gut permeability.[25] Clinical studies demonstrating reductions in infectious complications with EN compared with PN have been reported in the critically ill patient when feeding was initiated within 24 to 48 hours of hospital admission.[13-15,26] The benefit of fewer infectious complications was not apparent when the initiation of EN was delayed. A review of available studies comparing early versus delayed EN in critically ill patients revealed a trend toward a reduction in infectious complications with early EN.[13-15] In addition, a trend toward reduction in mortality associated with early EN has been noted.[13-15,26]

In critically ill patients who are hemodynamically unstable, early EN may result in gut ischemia because of poor gut blood flow and increased oxygen demand. Consequently, it is recommended that initiation of EN be delayed until the patient is fluid resuscitated and has an adequate perfusion pressure.[13] Once this goal is achieved, the initiation of EN at a low administration rate is considered appropriate, along with clinical monitoring to ensure GI tolerance and continued hemodynamic stability. Therefore, early EN (within 24-48 hours after hospital admission) is recommended in critically ill adult patients.[13-15] Although no randomized, controlled trials have assessed early EN in critically ill children, initiation of EN within 48 to 72 hours of admission is common.[16]

Early EN initiation is not warranted for previously well nourished, mild to moderately stressed adult patients. When oral intake is inadequate, it is reasonable to delay the initiation of EN for 5 to 7 days in these patients.[8] In the mild to moderately stressed adult patient who is moderately to severely malnourished, most clinicians would initiate EN sooner.

ENTERAL ACCESS

Advances in enteral access techniques have contributed to the expanded use of EN for conditions in which PN had previously been used. In particular, improved methods of achieving jejunal access for feeding have allowed the EN use during the early postoperative and post-injury period when gastric motility is typically impaired. As outlined in Table 143-3, various factors influence the selection of enteral access site and device, including anticipated duration of use and whether to feed into the stomach or small bowel. Figure 143-2 illustrates the predominant enteral access options.

Short-Term Access

3 Short-term enteral access is easier to initiate, less invasive, and less costly than the establishment of long-term access.[27] The most frequently used routes for short-term enteral access are established by inserting a tube through the nose or mouth and passing the tip into the stomach (nasogastric [NG]; orogastric [OG]), or jejunum (nasojejunal [NJ]; orojejunal [OJ]). In general, these tubes are used in the hospitalized patient when the anticipated tube feeding duration is less than 4 to 6 weeks. The orogastric route is generally

TABLE 143-3 Options and Considerations in the Selection of Enteral Access

Access	EN Duration/Patient Characteristics	Tube Placement Options	Advantages	Disadvantages
Nasogastric or orogastric	Short term Intact gag reflex Normal gastric emptying	Manually at bedside	Ease of placement Allows for all methods of administration Inexpensive Multiple commercially available tubes and sizes	Potential tube displacement Potential increased aspiration risk
Nasojejunal or orojejunal	Short term Impaired gastric motility or emptying High risk of GER or aspiration	Manually at bedside Fluoroscopically Endoscopically	Potential reduced aspiration risk Allows for early postinjury or postoperative feeding Multiple commercially available tubes and sizes	Manual transpyloric passage requires greater skill Potential tube displacement or clogging Bolus or intermittent feeding not tolerated
Gastrostomy	Long term Normal gastric emptying	Surgically Endoscopically Radiologically Laparoscopically	Allows for all methods of administration Low-profile buttons available Large-bore tubes less likely to clog Multiple commercially available tubes and sizes	Attendant risks associated with each type of procedure Potential increased aspiration risk Risk of stoma site complications
Jejunostomy	Long term Impaired gastric motility or gastric emptying High risk of GER or aspiration	Surgically Endoscopically Radiologically Laparoscopically	Allows for early postinjury or postoperative feeding Potential reduced aspiration risk Multiple commercially available tubes and sizes Low-profile buttons available	Attendant risks associated with each type of procedure Bolus or intermittent feeding not tolerated Risk of stoma site complications

EN, enteral nutrition; GER, gastroesophageal reflux.

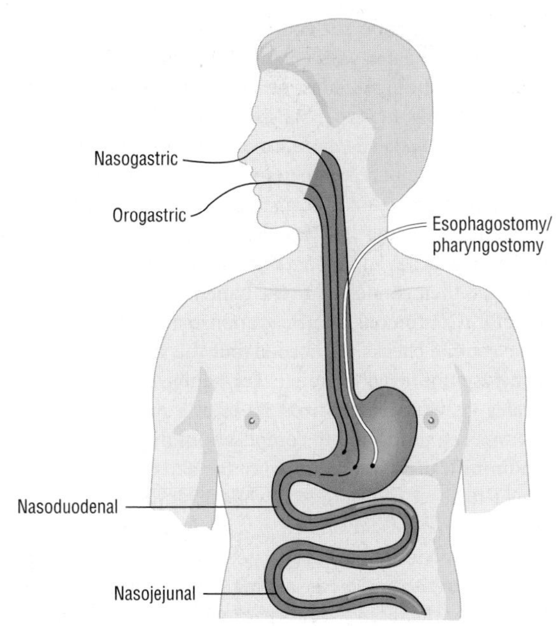

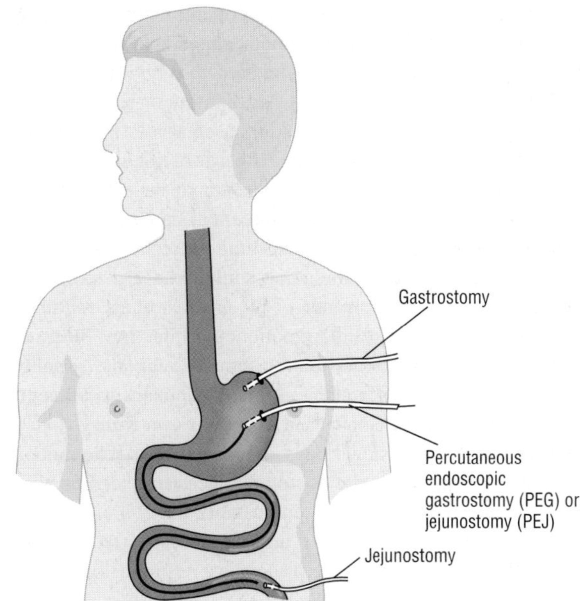

FIGURE 143-2 Access sites for tube feeding.

reserved for patients in whom the nasopharyngeal area is inaccessible or in young infants who are obligate nasal breathers. Because these routes do not require surgical intervention, they are the least invasive. The most common technique for placement is blind passage at the bedside by trained medical personnel. Several techniques have been described in the literature to help facilitate bedside placement and greater skill is required to advance the tip of the feeding tube beyond the pylorus.[17] Metoclopramide, a prokinetic agent, has been used with variable success to aid passage of the tube beyond the pylorus. A bedside electromagnetic tube placement device has also been used to guide tip position into the small bowel by attracting a metal tip on the end of the tube.[28,29] Alternatively, a variety of endoscopic and fluoroscopic techniques have been described to insert tubes into the small bowel.[17,27] Radiographic confirmation of appropriate tip placement should be obtained prior to use for all bedside placed feeding tubes.[9,17]

Nasogastric tubes vary in diameter and stiffness. Large-bore (greater than or equal to 14F) rigid NG tubes are used primarily to decompress the stomach but can also be used for feeding. There is a low incidence of clogging with these tubes, and they provide a reliable way to measure gastric residual volumes (GRVs). The major disadvantage associated with the use of these tubes is patient discomfort. Small-bore nasal tubes designed solely for feeding are available in varying lengths (12-60 inches [30-152 cm]) and diameters (3.5F-12F) to accommodate both pediatric (including neonates) and adult patients. The tip of the tube can be placed into the stomach or into the duodenum or jejunum (also referred to as transpyloric placement). These tubes consist of a lightweight, pliable silicone or polyurethane material that is designed for patient comfort. A disadvantage of small-bore tubes is that they more easily occlude, often as a result of improper medication administration or flushing technique. The feeding tube is frequently held in place only by a piece of tape on the nose or face; therefore, it can be inadvertently dislodged relatively easily. Nasal bridles have been used with variable results to secure the nasoenteric tube in place.[17] A bridle involves passing a piece of thin tubing or suture into one nostril, then around the bony portion of the nose, and out the other nostril, and finally tying the tubing around the feeding tube.

4 In general, gastric feeding is the least expensive and the least labor-intensive method for enteral feeding; however, feeding into the stomach is not always tolerated. Patients with impaired gastric motility may be predisposed to aspiration and pneumonia when fed into the stomach. Many critically ill, injured, and postoperative patients exhibit delayed gastric emptying, which limits their ability to tolerate gastric feeding. In addition, patients with diabetic gastroparesis or patients with severe gastroesophageal reflux disease or intractable vomiting are at a higher risk for aspiration of gastric contents, resulting in pneumonia. In these patients, placing the tip of the tube into the duodenum or jejunum has been suggested as a method to decrease aspiration risk.[17] Transpyloric feeding has been associated with a lower rate of vomiting and ventilator-associated pneumonia when compared to NG feeding.[30] However, the evidence to support the difference in aspiration and aspiration pneumonia risk associated with gastric and small bowel feeding is inconclusive. In general, small bowel feeding may be beneficial in patients who do not tolerate gastric feeding and offers an alternative to PN.[13-16]

Long-Term Access

Feeding tubes used for short-term enteral access are usually not optimal for long-term use because of patient discomfort, complications, and mechanical failures that develop over time. Long-term access should generally be considered when the need for EN is anticipated to be longer than 4 to 6 weeks. Many techniques can be used to establish long-term enteral access, including laparotomy, laparoscopy, endoscopic and image guidance (eg, fluoroscopy and ultrasound).[17] The ability to perform the various techniques will be somewhat dependent on the expertise and facilities available within each institution. Long-term enteral access options include gastrostomy and jejunostomy tubes.

A gastrostomy is the most common type of long-term enteral access. It eliminates the nasal irritation and discomfort associated with nasoenteric feeding tubes and inadvertent removal is uncommon. In addition, because feeding gastrostomies use large-bore tubes, clogging is less of a problem. The most commonly placed is the percutaneous endoscopic gastrostomy (PEG). The technique is minimally invasive and can be performed safely and cost-effectively in an endoscopy suite or at the bedside using conscious sedation and local anesthesia. Young children, however, will usually require general anesthesia for the procedure. Gastrostomy tubes are available in various sizes (12F-28F; 0.8-5 cm shaft lengths), material (eg, silicone and polyurethane), and have different retention mechanisms. Since smaller-diameter tubes are prone to more frequent occlusion and dysfunction, the largest diameter size possible is preferred. For patient convenience, comfort, and cosmetic appearance, a low-profile skin-level gastrostomy device may be used. It is typically placed as an exchange tube for a preexisting gastrostomy or jejunostomy once the tract has matured but can also be used at the time of initial tube placement. This "gastric button" consists of a short, silicone, self-retaining conduit with either a mushroom tip or a balloon at the internal end and a one-way valve and small flange at the skin surface. Because this averts the external tube presence, it tends to be preferred in children or ambulatory adults who are receiving intermittent feedings. The exit site of all gastrostomies requires general stoma care to prevent inflammation and infection. Routine replacement of the gastrostomy tube at defined intervals (usually 3-6 months) is a standard of practice of many clinicians to prevent failure of the retention mechanism that can occur over time.[17]

In patients with a functional bowel but impaired gastric motility, pancreatitis, or who otherwise do not tolerate gastric feeding and require long-term enteral access, a jejunostomy may be an appropriate option.[27] Various endoscopic and fluoroscopic techniques are available for direct jejunostomy placement. A surgically placed jejunostomy may be an option if the patient requires a laparotomy or laparoscopy for other reasons. For patients who require small bowel feeding with simultaneous gastric decompression, a gastrojejunal tube may be placed utilizing various endoscopic, fluoroscopic, and surgical techniques.[15,30] Because jejunostomies use smaller-bore tubes, occlusion occurs more commonly than with gastrostomy tubes. Gastrojejunostomy tubes are often replaced every 3 to 6 months to prevent occlusion.

There are ethical implications regarding determination of appropriate candidates for long-term feeding tube placement.[17,31-35] Because a gastrostomy is relatively easy to place and many patients, families, and clinicians overestimate the benefits of EN, it is prone to inappropriate use. In certain patient populations, such as those with advanced dementia or other near end-of-life conditions, the placement of a gastrostomy is not recommended. Artificial nutrition and hydration (ANH) has not been shown to promote the healing of pressure ulcers, increase patient comfort or functional status, or prolong survival when compared to hand feeding in patients with advanced dementia.[31] From a clinical standpoint, ANH does not increase a patient's comfort or improve nutrition parameters of most terminally ill individuals and can result in medical complications.[32] Studies consistently demonstrate that survival rates are not improved in older patients with advanced dementia who receive tube feedings and it is associated with substantial burden, including agitation, greater use of physical and chemical restraints, recurrent aspiration, and tube-related complications.[33,34] Evaluation by a multidisciplinary team is warranted for all patients near the end of life to establish whether the benefit of EN outweighs the risks of feeding tube placement.[31,33-35]

ADMINISTRATION METHODS

Enteral nutrition may be administered by continuous, cyclic (continuous rate over a portion of the day), intermittent (infused over 20-60 minutes), or bolus (generally given in 5-10 minutes) methods and may be accomplished by syringe, gravity, or pump-controlled techniques. The deliver method depends on the location of the tip of the feeding tube, the patient's clinical condition and intestinal function, and the patient's tolerance to the tube feeding.

Continuous

Pump-assisted continuous administration of EN is generally the method of choice for most hospitalized patients, especially when initiating therapy. They may be candidates for transitioning to intermittent or bolus feeding for long-term use as their medical condition stabilizes, as described below. However, when EN is to be delivered into the small intestine, the continuous method is always preferred because it is associated with enhanced tolerance. The rapid delivery of feeding into the small intestine may contribute to abdominal distension, cramping, hyperperistalsis, and diarrhea (also referred to as *dumping syndrome*). Therefore, conversion to intermittent or bolus administration is not recommended for those with jejunostomies.

The delivery system for continuous administration generally includes a feeding set with attached reservoir bag or spike set that connects to a feeding container. The feeding set is attached to a pump and then connected to the patient's enteral access tube with an adaptor. Continuous administration may increase nursing time because routine checks are needed, but this disadvantage is usually offset by the improved tolerance. For adults, target EN administration rates generally range from 50 to 125 mL/h, although higher rates have been used without complications. In infants and children, goal administration rates vary with age and weight and should be sufficient to meet caloric needs while maintaining good GI tolerance. The primary disadvantage to this method of administration is the cost and inconvenience associated with the pump and administration sets. In the home care setting, battery-operated ambulatory enteral pumps that fit into a backpack with the feeding bag are available to allow the patient greater mobility.

Cyclic

A patient who is not eating well during the day because of complaints of fullness and lack of appetite or who is not able to consume enough calories during the day to meet increased needs (eg, trauma and burns) may benefit from cyclic EN, in which the enteral feeding is administered by pump only at night. In addition, nocturnal EN administration will free the patient from the pump during the day and allow for greater mobility. This increased mobility may be particularly useful for the home patient or patient requiring rehabilitation. This method may be used in patients with either gastric or small bowel access.

Bolus

The bolus administration of EN is commonly used for patients in the home or long-term care setting who have a gastrostomy. This administration technique involves the delivery of the enteral feeding formulation over 5 to 10 minutes. Essentially, the only equipment needed is a syringe to instill the feeding volume into the tube. Depending on the patient's nutritional requirements, a feeding volume of 240 to 500 mL is generally used and repeated four to six times daily. From a convenience standpoint, it is generally preferable to adjust the bolus volume in increments of the feeding formulation container size (usually 240-250 mL). Bolus volumes given to infants and children vary with age and weight (usually 30-240 mL) and should be sufficient to meet the patient's calorie needs. In neonates and young infants, the bolus regimen is usually begun with an every 3-hour schedule; in older infants and children, feedings may be given at a frequency needed to deliver four to five feedings daily.[18] In patients with duodenal or jejunal access, bolus delivery may result in cramping, nausea, vomiting, aspiration, and diarrhea. Bolus administration also should be avoided in patients with delayed gastric emptying and in patients who are at high risk of aspiration.

Intermittent

If a patient is experiencing intolerance to bolus administration over 5 to 10 minutes, it may be helpful to administer the prescribed volume over a longer time period, generally 20 to 60 minutes. For this method, the desired volume of feeding formulation is emptied into a reservoir bag or container with attached tubing and administered by an enteral pump or via gravity drip using a roller clamp. The bolus method of administration is more consistent physiologically with normal eating patterns than the continuous method.

One study in infants demonstrated that normal gallbladder emptying did not occur with continuous feedings but was present in those infants receiving bolus feedings.[36] Thus, those patients who need long-term EN and PN, especially children, may benefit when this approach is used because it may minimize the development of cholestatic liver disease.

INITIATION AND ADVANCEMENT PROTOCOL

Guidelines for the initiation and advancement of enteral feeding formulations vary greatly and are primarily tailored to patient tolerance. The typical recommendation for continuous EN administration for adults is to start at 20 to 50 mL/h and advance by 10 to 25 mL/h every 4 to 8 hours until the desired goal is achieved. For intermittent administration, the typical recommendation is to start with 120 mL every 4 hours and advance by 30 to 60 mL every 8 to 12 hours.[8,9] In children, continuous administration is often initiated at a rate of 1 to 2 mL/kg per hour (no more than 25-30 mL/h) or 2 to 4 mL/kg per bolus (no more than 30-90 mL) with advancement by similar amounts every 4 to 24 hours. In premature infants, feedings may be initiated at lower rates usually 10 to 20 mL/kg per day and advanced by similar rates daily.[11,18] Schedules for progression of tube feeding from initial to target rates are important and may influence tolerance. If the protocol is too conservative, it may take an excessively long period of time to reach nutrient goals. The practice of diluting enteral feeding formulations is not recommended unless necessary to increase fluid intake.[9] The development of an EN protocol within an institution that outlines initiation and advancement criteria is recommended to optimize achievement of nutrient goals.[13,14] Due to frequent interruptions of EN, some institutions have implemented volume-based feeding protocols to improve success in meeting targeted goals. Such a protocol shifts the focus from an hourly rate target goal to a 24-hour volume goal and provides guidance on how to adjust the rate of administration when EN is interrupted for reasons unrelated to GI tolerance.[37,38]

ENTERAL FEEDING FORMULATION SELECTION

Historically, enteral formulas were designed primarily to provide essential nutrients. Over the years, enhancements have been made to meet specific patient needs and improve tolerance. For example, nutrient composition has been enhanced by changing the content of the amino acids (eg, glutamine and arginine), increasing the omega-3 polyunsaturated fatty acid content, and adding RNA to enhance immune function and improve therapeutic outcomes. These specific nutrients have been called nutraceuticals or pharmaconutrients because of the intent to use them to modify disease processes and improve clinical outcomes. Currently, enteral feeding formulations are categorized by the FDA as medical foods.[9] They are considered components of supportive care and are simply regulated to ensure sanitary manufacture. Unfortunately, they are not subject to rules governing health claims, and promotion of medical foods for therapeutic intent is currently not regulated by the FDA.[39]

The macronutrient content of enteral formulas (namely, protein, carbohydrate, and fat) varies in nutrient complexity (Table 143-4). Nutrient complexity refers to the amount of hydrolysis and digestion a substrate requires prior to intestinal absorption. Polymeric or intact substrates are of similar molecular form as the foods we eat. Enteral formulas that contain partially hydrolyzed or elemental substrates are characterized as elemental or defined-formula diets. The caloric contribution of each of the macronutrients is as follows: carbohydrates, 4 kcal/g (17 kJ/g); protein, 4 kcal/g (17 kJ/g); and fat, 9 kcal/g (38 kJ/g).

TABLE 143-4 Enteral Formula Nutrient Complexity

Nutrient	Polymeric or Intact	Partially Hydrolyzed or Elemental
Carbohydrate	Starches Fruit, vegetable, cereal solids Glucose polymers Corn syrup solids Polysaccharides	Oligosaccharides Maltodextrins Disaccharides Maltose, sucrose, lactose Monosaccharides Glucose Galactose
Fat	Long-chain triglycerides Polyunsaturated fatty acids Corn oil Safflower oil Soybean oil Canola oil Marine oils	Medium-chain triglycerides Coconut oil Palm kernel oil Free fatty acids Linoleic
Protein	Whole Egg, milk, wheat, whey Isolates Caseinate salts Lactalbumin	Oligopeptides Dipeptides Tripeptides L-amino acids

Protein Composition

The essential amino acid content of the protein source determines the quality of the protein, and most commercially available enteral feeding formulations contain proteins of high quality. The form of the protein source in enteral formulas will determine the amount of digestion that is required for absorption. Polymeric or intact protein sources require digestion to smaller peptides and free amino acids before absorption. Protein sources, such as meat, milk, eggs, and caseinates, require digestion by hydrochloric acid, specific protein enzymes, and pancreatic proteases. Enteral formulations may also contain protein sources that are partially hydrolyzed to peptides or L-amino acids. As the molecular form of protein is reduced in size, the osmotic load of the enteral formulation is increased. Many commercially available enteral feeding formulations contain combinations of intact and partially hydrolyzed protein sources. Most enteral formulations are gluten-free.

Conditionally Essential Amino Acids

Glutamine and arginine are generally considered nonessential amino acids. However, during periods of high physiologic stress, the need for these nutrients may be increased beyond the body's synthetic ability; consequently, these amino acids are characterized as conditionally essential. Because they are usually present in low amounts in most enteral feeding formulations, formulations targeted for the critically ill may be supplemented with glutamine and/or arginine.

Glutamine serves as a key fuel for rapidly dividing cells, including enterocytes, endothelial cells, lymphocytes, and fibroblasts. The primary site of glutamine production is skeletal muscle. During critical illness, skeletal muscle catabolism provides an increased glutamine supply, but this may not be enough to meet the high rate of glutamine use by cells of the immune system and other cells involved in recovery and repair. Glutamine depletion may develop, particularly during prolonged periods of metabolic stress. Favorable outcomes have been documented in critically ill patients when enteral formulations have been supplemented with glutamine.[13,40] Its use has specifically been recommended in burn and trauma patients.[15] However, high dose glutamine supplementation in critically ill patients with shock and multiorgan failure should be used with caution.[14] This concern is based on a study in over 1,200 critically ill adults that showed no benefit and a trend toward increased mortality when high-dose glutamine was given as a combined parenteral and enteral supplement for 28 days.[41]

Arginine has been added to some immune-modulating enteral formulations in concentrations that range from 4.5 to 14 g/L. However, arginine supplementation remains controversial, especially in patients with sepsis.[40,42] Many of arginine's physiologic effects are mediated by its conversion to nitric oxide, which, in turn, modulates immune function, inflammation, and vasodilation. Some of these effects may be potentially harmful in the patient with sepsis, especially when higher arginine intakes are used.[13]

Carbohydrate Composition

The carbohydrate component of enteral feeding formulations usually provides the major source of calories. Polymeric or intact enteral formulations contain starches and numerous types of glucose polymers, which require digestion to monosaccharides prior to intestinal absorption (see Fig. 143-1). As the extent of hydrolysis of carbohydrates increases within an enteral formulation, the osmolality of the formulation increases. Simple sugars, such as glucose and galactose, contribute significantly to the osmolality of enteral formulations. Consequently, polymeric entities, rather than elemental sugars, are preferred. Glucose polymers provide a useful carbohydrate source that is tolerated by most individuals (see Table 143-4). The polymers are large chains that provide minimal osmotic load, yet are absorbed easily in the intestine. The one shortcoming of glucose polymers and oligosaccharides is that they are not as sweet as simple glucose and thus may decrease the palatability of orally consumed products. Finally, almost all commercially available enteral feeding formulations used in adults and older children are lactose-free because disaccharidase production within the gut lumen is reduced during illness and periods of prolonged bowel rest. Additionally, there is a high incidence of lactose intolerance in those of certain ethnic decent. Infant formulas are available with or without lactose.

Fat and Fatty Acid Composition

Fat is an important constituent in the diet because it provides a concentrated calorie source and serves as a carrier for fat-soluble vitamins. Sufficient linoleic acid is required to prevent essential fatty acid deficiency and should approximate at least 1% to 3% of total daily calories. The most common fat sources in enteral feeding formulations are vegetable oils (soy or corn) that are rich in polyunsaturated fatty acids. The fat concentration varies between less than 2% and 45% of total calories. High dietary fat content is associated with delayed gastric emptying. Enteral feeding formulations can also contain fat in the form of MCTs derived from palm kernel or coconut oils. Because MCTs do not contain linoleic acid, enteral formulations that contain MCTs will also have a source of long-chain triglycerides to provide essential fatty acids. Potential advantages of MCTs compared to long-chain triglycerides are that they are more water soluble, undergo rapid hydrolysis, require no pancreatic lipase or bile salts for absorption, and do not require carnitine for transport into the mitochondria, where they are converted to energy. They also do not require chylomicron formation for small bowel enterocyte absorption and are not transported via the lymphatic system.

The source of long-chain fat within some enteral formulations has been modified from omega-6 to omega-3 fatty acids in an effort to modulate the inflammatory response in patients with acute respiratory distress syndrome (ARDS), acute lung injury (ALI), and sepsis.[43] The omega-6 fatty acids are high in linoleic acid and are derived from vegetable oil, whereas the omega-3 fatty acids, derived from cold-water fish oils, are high in linolenic acid. Omega-6 fatty acids serve as precursors to certain arachidonic acid-derived cytokines that are potent inflammatory mediators and also decrease cell-mediated immune response; whereas omega-3 fatty acids are precursors for eicosapentanoic acid-derived cytokines which are less inflammatory. It has been proposed that if the dietary proportion of omega-3 fatty acids is increased and omega-6 fatty acids is decreased, less inflammation and immunosuppression may occur during metabolic stress.

Docosahexaenoic acid (DHA) and arachidonic acid (ARA) are two fatty acids abundant in human milk, but until recently, they were not contained in commercial infant formulas. Although the role of ARA supplementation is unclear, DHA is important in brain and eye development. In some studies, DHA and ARA supplementation provided benefits to a child's visual function and/or cognitive and behavioral development.[44] The FDA has classified plant-based fatty acid blends of DHA and ARA as generally recognized as safe (GRAS), and most infant formulas, as well as some products for pregnant and lactating women, are supplemented with these fatty acids.

Fiber Content

Fiber, in both soluble and insoluble forms, is added to several adult and pediatric enteral feeding formulations in amounts ranging from 5.9 to 24 g/L. Infant formulas generally do not contain fiber; however, at least one formula intended for use in infants with diarrhea contains soy fiber. Fiber supplementation is common in clinical practice, primarily because fiber-free enteral formulations are implicated as a contributing factor to both diarrhea and constipation. Soluble fiber undergoes bacterial degradation within the colon to produce short-chain fatty acids. Potential benefits of soluble fiber are its trophic effects on the colonic mucosa and promotion of sodium and water absorption within the colon. Insoluble fiber is undigested and may help decrease GI transit time by increasing fecal weight. Fiber supplementation may help to regulate bowel function in both normal individuals and those with altered colonic motility. In addition, the resulting short-chain fatty acids are an excellent energy source. Although beneficial effects of fiber supplementation have not been clearly proven in clinical studies, there is experimental evidence that fiber may play an integral role in normal nutrition, and risk is generally minimal, particularly in non-critically ill patients.[45] Fiber supplementation may be beneficial when long-term EN is required or in patients who experience diarrhea or constipation while receiving a fiber-free enteral formulation. Soluble fiber may also be beneficial in the critically ill patient who is hemodynamically stable and develops diarrhea while receiving EN.[13] Insoluble fiber should be avoided in all critically ill patients due to case reports of bowel obstruction.[13]

Osmolality and Renal Solute Load

The unit of measure of osmolality is milliosmoles per kilogram (mOsm/kg) or millimoles per kilogram (mmol/kg); iso-osmolar is considered to be approximately 300 mOsm/kg (mmol/kg). Osmolality and renal solute load can affect tolerance to enteral feeding formulations. The osmolality of a given enteral formulation is a function of the size and quantity of ionic and molecular particles, primarily related to the protein, carbohydrate, electrolyte, and mineral content within a given volume. Enteral formulations with greater amounts of partially hydrolyzed or elemental substrates have a higher osmolality than formulations containing polymeric or intact substrates. Therefore, formulations that contain sucrose or glucose, dipeptides and tripeptides, and amino acids are generally hyperosmolar. Increased caloric density also increases the osmolality of an enteral formulation. In general, the osmolality of commercially available enteral feeding formulations ranges from 300 to 900 mOsm/kg (mmol/kg). American Academy of Pediatrics guidelines recommend that enteral formulations for use in infants have an osmolality of 450 mOsm/kg (mmol/kg) or less which equates to an osmolality of 400 mOsm/L.[46]

Symptoms of gastric retention, diarrhea, abdominal distension, nausea, and vomiting have been attributed to enteral formulations with a high osmolality based on the assumption that higher osmolality draws water into the gut lumen. However, clinical evidence to support this relationship between osmolality and GI tolerance is lacking. The practice of diluting hyperosmolar formulations has not been shown to enhance tolerance and should be discouraged unless dilution is done to increase fluid intake.[9] Factors, such as concurrent antibiotic therapy, method of enteral feeding administration, and the formulation's composition, are likely to play a greater role in GI tolerance than the osmolality.

The renal solute load is determined by the protein, sodium, potassium, and chloride content of the enteral formulation. Formulations that contain a greater solute load increase the obligatory water loss via the kidney. It is estimated that 40 to 60 mL of water is the minimal amount necessary to excrete 1 g of nitrogen. Those receiving high-protein enteral formulations unable to ingest or tolerate supplemental water may be at risk for developing dehydration.

CLASSIFICATION OF ENTERAL FEEDING FORMULATIONS

5 Most patients' nutritional needs can be met using a standard enteral feeding formulation; however, certain disease states or clinical conditions may warrant the use of a specialty feeding formulation. Development of an evidence-based, enteral formulary should focus on clinically significant characteristics of available formulations and avoid duplication. Categorizing enteral feeding formulations according to therapeutic class is necessary in developing a formulary system for adults (Table 143-5) and children (Table 143-6).

Standard Polymeric

A large number of commercially available enteral feeding formulations fall into the standard polymeric formulation category. These formulations are approximately isotonic (300 mOsm/L [300 mmol/L]), provide 1 to 1.2 kcal/mL (4.2-5 kJ/mL), and are composed of intact nutrients in a nutritionally balanced mix of carbohydrate, fat, and protein. They may contain dietary fiber. The nonprotein calorie-to-nitrogen ratio of these products is approximately 125:1 to 150:1. This ratio is a useful parameter for assessing protein density in relation to calories provided (see Chapter 141). Certain feeding formulations in this category may be promoted as high nitrogen but actually fall within standard protein amounts. To maintain isotonicity, many products within this category are not sweetened, making them unpalatable and generally suited only for tube feeding; however, flavored products are available for oral supplementation. The nutrient requirements of the majority of adults and children older than 1 year receiving EN can generally be met using feeding formulations in this category. Many term and preterm infant formulas will also fall into this category and available in formulations that provide 19 to 24 kcal/oz (2.7-3.5 kJ/mL) or 22 to 30 kcal/oz (3.1-4.2 kJ/mL), respectivly.[46]

High Protein

Enteral feeding formulations with a nonprotein calorie-to-nitrogen ratio less than 125:1 can be categorized as high protein. The lower the ratio, the higher the protein density in relation to calories provided. In patients with high protein requirements, it is generally unacceptable to use a feeding formulation with standard protein amounts because the volume necessary to meet protein requirements will result in excessive calorie intake. Patients who may be candidates for a high-protein feeding formulation are critically ill patients and those with pressure sores, surgical wounds, and high output enterocutaneous fistulas. In general, adult patients with estimated protein requirements exceeding 1.5 g/kg per day may benefit from a high-protein formulation. High-protein formulations may also be beneficial in mechanically ventilated patients who are receiving propofol for sedation. The vehicle for propofol is a soybean fat emulsion that contains 1.1 kcal/mL (4.6 kJ/mL). At therapeutic dosages, propofol intake can significantly contribute to caloric intake, and a high protein formulation may be beneficial in allowing for the provision of protein requirements while minimizing overfeeding.

TABLE 143-5 Adult Enteral Feeding Formulation Classification System

Category	Features	Indications
Standard polymeric	Isotonic 1-1.2 kcal/mL (4.2-5 kJ/mL) NPC:N 125:1-150:1 May contain fiber	Designed to meet the needs of the majority of patients Patients with functional GI tract Not suitable for oral use
High protein	NPC:N <125:1 May contain fiber	Patients with protein requirements >1.5 g/kg/day, such as trauma patients and those with burns, pressure sores, or wounds Patients receiving propofol
High caloric density	1.5-2 kcal/mL (6.3-8.4 kJ/mL) Lower electrolyte content per calorie Hypertonic	Patients requiring fluid and/or electrolyte restriction, such as kidney insufficiency
Elemental	High proportion of free amino acids Low in fat	Patients who require low fat Use has generally been replaced by peptide-based formulations
Peptide-based	Contains dipeptides and tripeptides Contains MCTs	Indications/benefits not clearly established Trial may be warranted in patients who do not tolerate intact protein due to malabsorption
Disease-specific		
Kidney	Caloric dense Protein content varies Low electrolyte content	Alternative to high caloric density formulations, but generally more expensive
Liver	Increased branched-chain and decreased aromatic amino acids	Patients with hepatic encephalopathy
Lung	High fat, low carbohydrate Antiinflammatory lipid profile and antioxidants	Patients with ARDS and severe ALI
Diabetes mellitus	High fat, low carbohydrate	Alternative to standard, fiber-containing formulation in patients with uncontrolled hyperglycemia
Immune-modulating	Supplemented with glutamine, arginine, nucleotides, and/or omega-3 fatty acids	Patients undergoing major elective GI surgery, trauma, burns, head and neck cancer, and critically ill patients on mechanical ventilation Use with caution in patients with sepsis Select nutrients may be beneficial or harmful in subgroups of critically ill patients
Oral supplement	Sweetened for taste Hypertonic	Patients who require supplementation to an oral diet

ALI, acute lung injury; ARDS, acute respiratory distress syndrome; MCT, medium-chain triglyceride; NPC:N, nonprotein calorie-to-nitrogen ratio.

TABLE 143-6 Pediatric Enteral Feeding Formulation Classification System

Formula Type	Features	Indications
Infants		
Cow's milk-based	Standard energy density for feeding: 20-24 kcal/oz (2.8-3.3 kJ/mL); also available in concentrate (40 kcal/oz [5.6 kJ/mL]) and powder forms Standard formulation contains lactose, but also available as lactose-free	Normal, healthy infant
Soy protein-based	Standard energy density for feeding: 20 kcal/oz (2.8 kJ/mL); also available in concentrate (40 kcal/oz [5.6 kJ/mL]) and powder forms Lactose free May contain added soy fiber	Lactase deficiency or lactose intolerance, galactosemia, diarrhea (fiber added)
Prematurity	Standard energy density for feeding: 24 kcal/oz (3.3 kJ/mL); also available in 20 (2.8 kJ/mL) and 30 kcal/oz (4.2 kJ/mL) forms	Preterm infants weighing <2-3 kg (<4.4-6.6 lb)
Transition	Standard energy density for feeding: 22 kcal/oz (3.1 kJ/mL) Provide higher calcium and phosphorus content compared with term infant formulas	Preterm infants weighing <3 kg (<6.6 lb) and ready for discharge
Semi-elemental/ elemental	Standard energy density for feeding: 20 kcal/oz (2.8 kJ/mL) Hydrolyzed protein and free amino acids May contain ARA and DHA Lactose free Typically contain MCTs ranging from 5% to 86% of fat content	Malabsorption, cow's milk protein allergy, chylothorax, cystic fibrosis, biliary atresia, short bowel syndrome, food allergies
Special diets	Low electrolyte/mineral content	Kidney disease
Children Ages 1-10 Years		
Standard	Standard energy density for feeding: 30 or 45 kcal/oz (1 or 1.5 kcal/mL [4.2 or 6.3 kJ/mL]) Intact protein; 30-38 g/L May contain added fiber	Functioning GI tract requiring tube feedings
Semi-elemental/ elemental	Standard energy density for feeding: 20-30 kcal/oz (2.8-4.2 kJ/mL) Hydrolyzed protein and free amino acids Lactose-free MCTs range from 33% to 87% of fat content	Malabsorption, cow's milk protein allergy, chylothorax, cystic fibrosis, biliary atresia, short bowel syndrome, food allergies

ARA, arachidonic acid; DHA, docosahexaenoic acid; MCT, medium-chain triglyceride.

High Caloric Density

High caloric density formulations are concentrated to provide less fluid and electrolyte intake in comparison to a standard polymeric formulation. They provide approximately 2 kcal/mL (8.4 kJ/mL) and similar calorie and protein intake can be achieved as a standard polymeric formulation, using half the volume. High caloric density formulations are often necessary for patients who require fluid and/or electrolyte restriction, such as those with kidney or heart failure. Although specialty enteral formulations targeted for acute kidney injury and chronic kidney disease are available, many patients with kidney failure can be managed using a product in this category.

Elemental/Peptide-Based

Formulations in this category contain protein and/or fat components that are hydrolyzed into smaller, predigested forms. Traditionally, enteral formulations in this category were referred to as elemental and contained a high proportion of protein in the form of free amino acids and a low amount of fat. Many of these formulations have been reformulated to provide a portion of the protein in the form of dipeptides and tripeptides and fewer free amino acids because dipeptides and tripeptides are more readily absorbed than an equivalent intake of free amino acids.[48] These peptide-based formulations may be beneficial in patients with impaired digestion or absorption. Peptide-based formulations are generally higher in fat than the more elemental formulations and use MCTs in varying proportions as the fat source.

Evidence to support the use of elemental or peptide-based formulations is limited, and their routine use is generally not recommended. Patients who do not tolerate standard, intact nutrient formulations as a result of malabsorption or short bowel syndrome might be candidates for a trial of a peptide-based formulation. In addition, elemental or peptide-based products that have higher percentages of MCTs and small amounts of long-chain triglycerides may be beneficial for patients with severe pancreatic insufficiency, such as chronic pancreatitis and cystic fibrosis; severe abnormalities of the intestinal mucosa, such as untreated celiac disease; biliary tract disease, such as biliary atresia or severe cholestasis; or chylothorax or chylous ascites.

Disease Specific

Enteral feeding formulations also have been designed to meet unique nutrient requirements and manage metabolic abnormalities associated with specific disease states. Specialized enteral feeding formulations are marketed for use in adult patients with kidney and liver failure; lung disease, including ARDS; diabetes mellitus; wound healing; and metabolic stress. There are no disease-specific enteral products currently marketed for use in infants or children younger than 10 years of age. Thus, modular supplements may be necessary in these patients (see discussion in Modular Products section).

Specialized enteral formulations designed to modulate the inflammatory response in adult patients with severe metabolic stress have been referred to as immune-modulating formulations or immunonutrition. These formulations are supplemented with nutrients such as glutamine, arginine, antioxidants, nucleotides, and omega-3 polyunsaturated fatty acids, because of their potential role in regulating immune function. There is lack of consensus between the professional nutrition societies guidelines regarding the use of immune-modulating enteral formulations in critically ill patients.[13-15] Positive results have been reported in patients undergoing major elective GI surgery and cancer surgery of the head and neck, those with severe trauma or burns, and critically ill patients on mechanical ventilation. The use of immune-modulating enteral formulations in these select patient populations has resulted in significant reductions in infectious complications, hospital length of stay, and duration of mechanical ventilation.[43,49] In contrast, two recent multicenter trials revealed no improvement in infectious complications or other clinical end points and possible harm with immune-modulating formulations[50] or when enteral immunonutrition was a provided as a twice daily supplement.[51] The heterogeneity of studies and lack of consistency between the various immunonutrition supplementation regimens makes it impossible to recommend their use in critically ill adult patients at this time. Immune-modulating formulations are not currently recommended for use in children because of the lack of evidence to support their use.[16]

Clinical **Controversy...**

The value of adding probiotics to EN in the ICU setting is controversial. The use of probiotics has reduced ventilator-associated pneumonia, antibiotic-associated diarrhea, and overall infections in critically ill patients. However, increased risk of mortality has been shown when probiotics are used concomitant with fiber and jejunal feeding in patients with severe acute pancreatitis. The benefits of probiotics appear to be variable and likely product-specific and dose dependent. Recommendations regarding their use are difficult to provide at this time.

Oral Supplements

In general, oral supplements are not intended for tube feeding but to enhance an oral diet. They are sweetened to improve taste and therefore are hypertonic (approximately 450-700 mOsm/kg [mmol/kg]), but osmolality is rarely a problem in the patient with a functioning GI tract. However, in the tube-fed patient, a sweetened product is unnecessary and may contribute to GI intolerance, particularly diarrhea. Powder supplements that are mixed with milk should be avoided in lactose-intolerant patients. In addition to liquid supplements, puddings, gelatins, bars, and milkshake-like supplements are available.

Modular Products

A module is a powder or liquid form of a nutrient (eg, protein, carbohydrate, fat, and dietary fiber) that is used to supplement nutrition intake when the diet or commercially available enteral formulation does not fully meet a patient's needs.[47] Alternatively, formulations available in powder or concentrate can be mixed with less water than needed for the standard dilution to deliver more nutrients in less volume. Infant formulas can be prepared to provide increased caloric density beyond the standard 19 to 20 kcal/oz (2.7-2.8 kJ/mL); concentrations of 22 to 30 kcal/oz (3.1-4.2 kJ/mL) are routinely used. The mixing process required for modular components increases the potential for bacterial contamination and incorrect preparation. Contamination is a particular concern with the use of blenders and reconstitution of powders.[9,52] A number of methods are used to fortify human milk so that it meets the needs of a premature infant fortify for added calories, protein, and minerals. They have been shown to improve nutritional outcomes in human milk-fed premature infants.[53,54]

Rehydration

Oral rehydration formulations are useful in maintaining hydration or treating dehydration in adult and pediatric patients with high GI output. Such formulations are available commercially in powder or liquid form or can be extemporaneously compounded. They can be administered orally or given via a feeding tube. The glucose content of oral rehydration solutions is important because it stimulates active transport systems, which, in turn, stimulate passive glucose-coupled sodium and water uptake. Therefore, oral or enteral administration of rehydration solutions may decrease fecal water loss and generate a positive fluid and electrolyte balance.[55,56]

FORMULARY AND DELIVERY SYSTEM CONSIDERATIONS

For an institution's enteral formulary, generally no more than one product per category is necessary, and it may be possible to omit certain categories based on the specific patient population cared for within a given institution. Additional selection criteria include container size and type, liquid or powder form, shelf life, ease of use, and cost.

Most enteral products are available as ready-to-use, prepackaged liquids, but a few are available in the powdered state and require reconstitution prior to use. Advantages of ready-to-use liquid formulations are convenience and reduced susceptibility to microbiologic contamination. One disadvantage is that more storage space may be required. The ease or convenience of a ready-to-use liquid is especially important for self-care patients, the disabled, and those who have difficulty reading or following printed instructions. Ready-to-use liquid enteral formulations are generally available in ready-to-hang rigid plastic containers or bags (*closed system*), cans, or bottles. Bolus administration of EN is usually achieved using formulas available in cans or bottles. However, when formula from a can/bottle is used for continuous or cyclic administration, it must first be poured into a feeding bag and attached to an administration set to allow for administration via a pump. This "open system" has a higher risk of microbial contamination than the ready-to-hang containers. The use of a powder formula is also considered an open delivery system.

Contamination of enteral feeding formulations is a potential cause of diarrhea.[8,9] Contamination is caused by a lack of attention to proper handling techniques, inadequate cleaning and disinfection of preparation equipment, and the use of nonsterile or contaminated tube-feeding additives. Unlike liquid formulations, powdered products are not guaranteed by the manufacturer to be sterile because it is not possible to sterilize the powder without destruction of some of its components. Contamination of milk powder and consequently powdered infant formulas with *Enterobacter sakazakii* (*Cronobacter* species) has been reported.[52] Contamination of one infant formula at the manufacturing site with *E. sakazakii* was implicated in the death of an infant in a neonatal ICU, prompting FDA warnings regarding the use of powdered formulations in premature neonates and other immunocompromised infants.[57] Closed-system containers supply a ready-to-hang, prefilled, sterile supply of formula in volumes of 1 to 1.5 L. Most but not all enteral formulations intended for use in adults and some pediatric formulations are available in the closed-administration system. The closed-administration system also offers the advantage of not requiring refrigeration and allowing hang times up to 48 hours, whereas the conventional open-delivery system necessitates hang times of generally 4 to 8 hours.

New enteral connectors are currently being integrated into the EN marketplace to prevent enteral misconnections and improve patient safety. An enteral misconnection occurs when a component of the enteral feeding system is inadvertently connected to a non-enteral site, such as a tracheostomy tube, peritoneal dialysis catheter, or other medical device or IV tubing. Misconnections are commonly attributed to the use of universal connectors that allow for misconnections between incompatible systems.[58] Due to several reports of serious patient harm, including death, an international standard (ISO 80369) has been developed to guide the redesign of all small-bore connectors and the new enteral connectors, referred to as the ENFit™ system.[59] The ENFit™ connector provides a unique connection that is not compatible with any other device and has been specifically designed for all nutrition sources, enteral administration sets, enteral syringes, and all feeding tubes.[59] Filling and administration instructions for syringes used to deliver medications via feeding tubes will differ from oral syringes. Information about these processes and other resources is available at the Global Enteral Device Supplier Association (GEDSA) web site (www.stayconnected.org).[60]

COMPLICATIONS AND MONITORING

The majority of complications associated with EN are metabolic, GI, or mechanical. The early detection and management of potential complications is necessary to allow for the safe and successful use of EN. In addition, measures to avoid complications should be incorporated into the management of all patients receiving EN (Table 143-7).

Metabolic Complications

Metabolic complications associated with EN are similar to those associated with PN, but the incidence tends to be lower.[23] Critically ill patients, especially those with underlying organ dysfunction, are at risk of developing complications related to hydration and electrolyte imbalance and altered glucose control. Patients who present with a history of minimal dietary intake for an extended period of time and have experienced significant weight loss are at risk of developing refeeding syndrome which can be evidenced by hypophosphatemia, hypokalemia, hypomagnesemia, thiamine deficiency, and sodium retention.[61] The frequency of clinical and laboratory assessment to monitor hydration, electrolytes, organ function, and glucose adequately for a patient who is critically ill or at risk of developing refeeding syndrome is greater than for a stable hospitalized patient or patients residing in rehabilitation units or at home (see Table 143-7). Patients receiving long-term EN at home may require laboratory monitoring only every 2 to 3 months, depending on their clinical status. Besides macronutrient content, it is important to evaluate the actual water and micronutrient content provided by the enteral formulation, especially in critically ill patients. Supplemental fluid, electrolytes, and minerals may be required in some patients. Conversely, for patients who have fluid retention or elevated serum electrolytes, the enteral formulation may need to be changed to one that is more concentrated or provides less of a particular nutrient, if available.

TABLE 143-7 Suggested Monitoring for Patients on Enteral Nutrition

Parameter	During Initiation of EN Therapy	During Stable EN Therapy
Vital signs	Every 4-6 hours	As needed with suspected change (ie, fever)
Clinical assessment		
Weight	Daily	Weekly
Length/height (children)	Weekly-monthly	Monthly
Head circumference (<3 years of age)	Weekly-monthly	Monthly
Total intake/output	Daily	As needed with suspected change in intake/output
Tube-feeding intake	Daily	Daily
Enterostomy tube site assessment	Daily	Daily
GI tolerance		
Stool frequency/volume	Daily	Daily
Abdomen assessment	Daily	Daily
Nausea or vomiting	Daily	Daily
Gastric residual volumes	Every 4-8 hours (varies)	As needed when delayed gastric emptying suspected
Tube placement	Prior to starting, then ongoing	Ongoing
Laboratory		
Electrolytes, blood urea nitrogen/serum creatinine, glucose	Daily until stable, then 2-3 times/week	Every 1-3 months
Calcium, magnesium, phosphorus	Daily until stable, then 2-3 times/week	Every 1-3 months
Liver function tests	Weekly	Every 1-3 months
Trace elements, vitamins	If deficiency/toxicity suspected	If deficiency/toxicity suspected

EN, enteral nutrition.

Gastrointestinal Complications

6 The GI complications associated with tube feeding include nausea, vomiting, abdominal distension, cramping, aspiration, diarrhea, and constipation. GRV refers to the volume of contents in the stomach and is measured by using a syringe and aspirating from a large-bore NG or gastrostomy tube. Although it has been recommended as a method to identify patients at risk of vomiting, aspiration and/or ventilator-associated pneumonia, this has not been validated in clinical studies.[8,62-64] However, it remains a widely used tool to help clinicians assess GI tolerance in patients receiving gastric tube feeding via continuous administration. The frequency of measuring GRV generally varies between every 4 and 8 hours, and most institutions follow a protocol that directs the frequency of monitoring and at what volume and for how long to hold feedings.[64] In critically ill patients receiving gastric feeding, GRVs should be measured every 4 hours.[13] Measurement of GRV is not recommended in patients receiving bolus or intermittent feedings.

If high GRVs occur, the response is often to stop or decrease the rate of continuous feedings. However, other signs and symptoms of intolerance should also be considered before stopping feeding because frequent interruptions in EN delivery can adversely affect the attainment of nutrition outcome goals. A trend toward increased GRV is generally more important than one isolated high measurement. Generally, in the absence of other signs of intolerance, EN should not be held when the GRV is less than 500 mL.[13,65] If symptoms are present, and GRVs are elevated, a decrease in the tube feeding rate or discontinuation may be warranted. Measures to reduce aspiration risk should be implemented when GRVs are consistently elevated, including elevating the head of the patient's bed to a 30° to 45° angle and changing to postpyloric continuous feeding. In addition, it may be beneficial to initiate a prokinetic agent such as metoclopramide or erythromycin to improve gastric emptying rate.[13,66] Other potential interventions include minimizing the use of narcotics, sedatives, or other agents that may slow gastric emptying and correcting underlying fluid and electrolyte imbalances that can impair GI motility.[67] Unless GRVs are excessive (greater than 500 mL in adults), they should generally be reinstilled (refed) through the tube to minimize nutrient, fluid, and electrolyte losses.[9,68]

Aspiration pneumonia is considered the most serious complication associated with tube feeding. Although aspiration is a fairly common event for critically ill patients receiving tube feeding, progression to aspiration pneumonia is difficult to predict. Risk factors for aspiration include a previous aspiration episode, decreased consciousness, neuromuscular disease, structural airway or GI tract abnormalities, endotracheal intubation, vomiting, persistently high GRVs, and prolonged supine positioning.[62] Identification of these risk factors, along with close GRV monitoring, is recommended for all critically ill patients receiving tube feeding. Historically, blue food coloring had been added to enteral formulations in an attempt to detect aspiration. However, because of its low sensitivity for detection and association with several serious adverse events, including death, the addition of blue food dye to enteral formulations is not advised.[13,69] There are currently no reliable methods available to detect aspiration in enterally fed patients.[13,70]

Clinical Controversy...

The optimal dose of EN in critically ill adult patients is a subject of debate. The intentional use of "permissive" underfeeding or trophic EN (10-20 mL/h) in critically ill adult patients requiring short ICU lengths of stay may result in improved GI tolerance and similar short-term outcomes when compared to full feeding. However, the strategy of intentional underfeeding may not be appropriate for patients at high nutrition risk as defined by disease severity, preexisting malnutrition, and anticipated prolonged ICU length of stay.

Diarrhea is the most common GI complication in patients receiving EN, but the actual incidence is unclear due to the lack of a standard definition and the large number of contributing factors.[8,23] When monitoring for diarrhea, stool frequency, consistency, and volume should be evaluated, and previous bowel habits should be considered. Diarrhea has been defined as more than three liquid stools daily or a stool volume of more than 250 to 500 mL/day (20-25 mL/kg per day in children) for at least two consecutive days.[23] Therefore, the intermittent occurrence of one or two loose stools does not constitute diarrhea or require intervention.

7 Diarrhea in patients receiving tube feeding may be caused by a number of factors, and management should be directed at identifying and correcting the most likely cause(s).[71] Tube feeding-related factors that may contribute to diarrhea include too rapid delivery or advancement of formula, intolerance to the formula composition, administration of large volumes of feeding into the small bowel, and formula contamination. Thus, measures to prevent or manage diarrhea related directly to the tube feeding should address these potential causes.[23,67,72] If diarrhea occurs when using a fiber-free formulation, a fiber-containing formulation may be considered. If using a high-fat formulation, it may be beneficial to switch to a formulation lower in fat or having a higher proportion of the fat supplied as MCTs; although, a high MCT concentration has also been associated with diarrhea. Finally, it is important to assess the risk of bacterial contamination of the formula and take steps to minimize any potential risk factors. If infectious etiologies have been excluded, severe diarrhea may require pharmacologic treatment with loperamide, diphenoxylate/atropine, or opioids (see chapter 36).

Drug therapy, particularly the use of broad-spectrum antibiotics, is a common cause of diarrhea that is unrelated to tube feeding. Sorbitol, used as a sweetening agent in many liquid formulations to enhance palatability, is an osmotic laxative that can cause diarrhea. In addition, many drugs available in a liquid form are hyperosmolar, which may contribute to diarrhea, especially when these medications are not diluted properly before administration. Because many patients receiving tube feeding also receive medications in a liquid form, all medications should be evaluated for their potential contribution. Infectious causes, such as antibiotic-induced bacterial overgrowth by *Clostridium difficile* or other intestinal flora, need to be considered when diarrhea develops. Malabsorption, secondary to the underlying disease state or condition, may also cause diarrhea.

Mechanical Complications

Mechanical complications of EN are those associated with the feeding tube, including tube occlusion or malposition, and inadvertent nasopulmonary intubation. Feeding tube occlusion usually results from improper medication administration and/or flushing. Kinking of the tube also may cause occlusion. Adult feeding tubes should be flushed with at least 15 to 30 mL of water before and after administering any medication. If more than one medication is scheduled for a given time, each should be administered separately, and the tube should be flushed with 5 to 15 mL of water between drugs.[9,73] Flush volume will be less for children but should be adequate to ensure complete flushing of the medication through the tube.[74] The frequency of flushing should be at least every 8 hours during continuous feeding and before and after each intermittent feeding. If tube occlusion occurs, the tube should be irrigated with warm water. Other fluids such as colas and cranberry juice have been used to irrigate occluded tubes but have not been shown to be any more effective than warm water. Some success in reestablishing patency has been shown with the use of pancreatic enzymes mixed with sodium bicarbonate.[73] Declogging devices that are specifically designed to unclog feeding tubes are available. They have been designed to either mechanically break through or remove the occlusion or provide an applicator and syringe prefilled with pancreatic enzymes and various powders targeted to restore patency.[8,73]

Inadvertent nasoenteric tube removal or displacement has been reported in approximately 40% of patients receiving EN.[75] An agitated or confused patient may pull at the feeding tube and cause its removal or malposition. Measures to decrease agitation and confusion should be attempted. Securing the tube with tape may be helpful, as well as marking the tube with permanent ink at the exit site to assess for position change. A nasal bridle that uses a magnetic retrieval system has proven to be a simple and effective method for securing nasoenteric feeding tubes and preventing accidental removal.[70]

When a feeding tube is inserted nasally or orally, there is a risk that the tube may inadvertently enter the tracheobronchial tree. The risk may be higher in patients who have an impaired cough or gag reflex and when a stylet is used for tube insertion. Proper positioning of the tube should always be confirmed by radiography prior to feeding initiation and routinely reassessed to avoid inadvertent administration of enteral formula into the lung.

Other Complications

Infectious complications of feeding tube placement include sinusitis (with nasoenteric placement), exit site-related infections (eg, cellulitis, subcutaneous abscess, and necrotizing fasciitis), and intraabdominal infections (eg, peritonitis and abscess). Leaking and bleeding around the exit site can also occur.[17] Formation of excessive granulation tissue around the exit site is often the cause of leaking and bleeding and can be managed by applying silver nitrate and topical corticosteroids.

A unique complication of tube feeding use in children, especially in the first year of life, is the development of oral hypersensitivity, poor oral/motor skills, and food aversion when oral feeding is held. In these children, transitioning from tube to oral nutrition can be difficult and protracted. The involvement of an occupational or speech therapist, behavioral psychologist, or other trained individual, as well as perseverance by the family, often is necessary to improve oral intake. Avoidance of a strict nothing by mouth (NPO) status, if possible, and oral stimulation programs for those children who must remain NPO are recommended to avoid this complication.[76]

NUTRITION CARE PLAN

A nutrition care plan that incorporates nutrition assessment and therapy goals should be developed for all EN patients (see Chapter 141). Desired outcomes of EN are to promote an adequate nutritional state in adults and to promote growth and development of infants and children. The EN goals are individualized and based on meeting estimated fluid, calorie, protein, and micronutrient requirements. The desired end point should be included in the care plan. The end point may be resolution of a disease or condition that impairs ability to eat, such as in a critically ill trauma patient who is expected to transition back to an oral diet. EN may be considered a lifelong therapy for those with a permanent impairment that restricts or limits eating, such as gastroparesis.

Assessing the outcome of EN requires monitoring objective measures of body composition, protein and energy balance, and muscle function and wound healing. In addition to optimizing nutrition, the goal of EN is to reduce disease-related morbidity and mortality. Measures of disease-related morbidity include length of hospital stay, infectious complications, and the patient's functional status and sense of well-being. A target weight should be established for each patient and energy content from the EN regimen adjusted as needed to safely achieve or maintain the target weight. In general, in adults, no more than 1 to 2 pound [approximately 0.45-0.9 kg] per week should be gained or lost. Children should be followed using standard growth velocity expectations. EN may be used to supplement an oral diet when oral intake is inadequate and should be modified as needed based on changes in tolerance.

DRUG DELIVERY VIA FEEDING TUBE

Using enteral feeding tubes to deliver drugs is a common practice and offers an alternative for patients unable to take drugs by the oral route. However, in addition to tube occlusion, effects on drug bioavailability and other potential interactions need to be considered when using this route. Medications have been given as a concomitant bolus administration via the feeding tube or admixed with the enteral feeding formulation.

Concomitant Drug Administration

8 Concomitant administration of medications with enteral feedings can be extremely complicated and potentially deleterious. Delivering medications directly into the stomach allows for the normal process of drug dissolution. Medication delivery directly into the small bowel however may result in alterations in drug dissolution because the stomach is bypassed. In addition, therapeutic effects designed to occur within the stomach, such as with antacids and sucralfate, may not be achieved. Because many drugs are best absorbed in the fasting state, they should be administered on an empty stomach whenever possible. Patients on bolus gastric feeding must receive these medications appropriately spaced between feedings, and patients on continuous feeding will require feeding interruptions for drug administration.

Selecting the proper medication dosage form for coadministration with the tube feeding is another important consideration. Medications in sublingual form, sustained-release capsules or tablets, and enteric-coated tablets should not be crushed and therefore should not be administered via enteral feeding tubes.[9,73] Solid dosage forms that are appropriate to crush should be prepared as a very fine powder and mixed with 15 to 30 mL of water or other appropriate solvent before administering through the tube. In addition, many capsules may be opened and the contents administered in the same manner. Pellets contained inside microencapsulated dosage forms should generally not be crushed. It may be acceptable to administer intact pellets through larger bore feeding tubes, provided that the pellets are small enough and drug absorption is not compromised.[77,78] To avoid the need to crush a solid dosage form, liquid dosage forms are commonly preferred for administration through feeding tubes. However, the risk of GI intolerance should be considered because of the hyperosmolality of many liquid formulations and possible sorbitol content.[73,79] Although the use of a liquid dosage preparation may be more convenient than a solid dosage form, it may not be the best choice if GI intolerance is an issue.

Clinical Controversy...

The source of water used to flush the feeding tube and maintain patient hydration via the feeding tube is controversial. Tap water is adequate for the otherwise healthy, immunocompetent patient. However, the acute or chronically ill patient receiving EN may be at higher risk from exposure to nonsterile tap water and may benefit from the use of purified water. Nosocomial infections from contaminated tap water sources have been reported in critically ill patients. The use of purified water for tube-feeding flushes in at-risk patients has been recommended by some clinicians.

Admixture of Drugs with Enteral Feeding

Mixing liquid medications with certain enteral feeding formulations is associated with several types of physical incompatibilities, including granulation, gel formation, separation, and precipitation.[73,77] Not only can these physical incompatibilities inhibit drug absorption, but gel formation may clog small-bore feeding tubes. Physical incompatibility with medications is more common in formulations that contain intact protein than in those with hydrolyzed protein. Also, medication and enteral formula incompatibilities are more common with the use of acidic pharmaceutical syrups. The most prudent recommendation is to avoid the routine admixture whenever possible, especially for nonaqueous preparations and syrups. In the clinical setting, exceptions do exist, such as adding sodium or magnesium to enteral formulas to assist in maintaining or repleting electrolytes.

Drug–Nutrient Interactions

9 The most significant drug–nutrient interactions that can occur during continuous enteral feeding are those in which the drug's bioavailability is reduced, and the desired pharmacologic effect is not achieved (Table 143-8).[80] Unfortunately, limited clinical studies are available to document the extent of this problem with enteral feeding. Most of the observations are anecdotal case reports involving few patients. One of the well-documented interactions is between phenytoin and enteral feeding. Phenytoin serum concentrations may decrease by 50% to 75% when phenytoin is given concomitantly with EN, possibly as a result of the binding of phenytoin to calcium caseinates or protein hydrolysates in the enteral formulation. Patients typically require higher than normal phenytoin doses while receiving EN.[73,77] The patient's clinical response and phenytoin serum concentrations should be monitored to assure that the desired therapeutic effects are achieved.

Decreased bioavailability of certain antibiotics, particularly quinolones, has been documented when coadministered with enteral feeding due to complexation with multivalent cations such as calcium, magnesium, and iron contained in the feeding.[73,77] Although the practice of holding tube feeding for 30 minutes before and 30 minutes after quinolone administration has been recommended, it has not been shown to improve drug absorption. Another option is to increase the quinolone dose when given concurrently with EN. There is evidence to suggest that ciprofloxacin absorption is significantly decreased when given via a jejunostomy tube, so this practice should be avoided, if possible.[73]

Warfarin resistance has been documented during enteral feeding, possibly as a consequence of decreased absorption or the antagonist effects of vitamin K in the feeding formulation. Before 1980, it was thought that the content of vitamin K (up to 1,330 mcg/1,000 kcal [or 317 mcg/1,000 kJ] of enteral feeding formula) was contributing to the pharmacologic interaction with warfarin. Subsequently, the vitamin K content within formulas intended for use in adults was

TABLE 143-8 Medications with Special Considerations for Enteral Feeding Tube Administration

Drug	Interaction	Comments
Phenytoin	Reduced bioavailability in the presence of tube feedings Possible phenytoin binding to calcium caseinates or protein hydrolysates in enteral feeding	To minimize interaction, holding tube feedings 1-2 hours before and after phenytoin has been suggested; this has no proven benefit Adjust tube-feeding rate to account for time held for phenytoin administration Monitor phenytoin serum concentration and clinical response closely Consider switching to IV phenytoin if unable to reach therapeutic serum concentration
Fluoroquinolones Tetracyclines	Potential for reduced bioavailability because of complexation of drug with divalent and trivalent cations found in enteral feeding	Consider holding tube feeding 1 hour before and after administration Avoid jejunal administration of ciprofloxacin Monitor clinical response
Warfarin	Decreased absorption of warfarin because of enteral feeding; therapeutic effect antagonized by vitamin K in enteral formulations	Adjust warfarin dose based on INR Anticipate need to increase warfarin dose when enteral feedings are started and decrease dose when enteral feedings are stopped Consider holding tube feeding 1 hour before and after administration
Omeprazole Lansoprazole	Administration via feeding tube complicated by acid-labile medication within delayed-release, base-labile granules	Granules become sticky when moistened with water and may occlude small-bore tubes Granules should be mixed with acidic liquid when given via a gastric feeding tube An oral liquid suspension can be extemporaneously prepared for administration via a feeding tube

INR, International normalized ratio.

reduced to less than 200 mcg/1,000 kcal (or 48 mcg/1,000 kJ). However, warfarin resistance continues to be reported, and a warfarin dosage increase may be required in patients receiving EN.[73,81] The International Normalized Ratio should be closely monitored in patients receiving both warfarin and enteral feedings. Conversely, when EN is discontinued, a reduction in warfarin dosage may be required.

CLINICAL BOTTOM LINE

Identifying appropriate candidates for EN and designing a personalized EN regimen and monitoring plan is a complex process that is often under-appreciated. The successful use of EN can minimize the need for PN in patients unable to meet nutrient requirements with an oral diet. Ultimately, no disease process can improve with prolonged starvation and malnutrition. A.S.P.E.N. has identified safety issues related to the administration and management of EN and created practice recommendations based on evidence-based research and expert opinion.[9] These guidelines address the provision and assessment of nutrition support therapy, including EN, for adult and pediatric critically ill patients.[13,16] A multidisciplinary team approach, either as a formal nutrition support service or as a team of caregivers within the practice setting, is recommended to optimize patient outcomes.

ABBREVIATIONS

ALI	acute lung injury
ANH	artificial nutrition and hydration
ARA	arachidonic acid
ARDS	acute respiratory distress syndrome
DHA	docosahexaenoic acid
EN	enteral nutrition
GALT	gut-associated lymphoid tissue
GI	gastrointestinal
GRV	gastric residual volume
ICU	intensive care unit
IgA	immunoglobulin A
MCT	medium-chain triglyceride
NG	nasogastric
NJ	nasojejunal
NPO	nothing by mouth
OG	orogastric
OJ	orojejunal
PEG	percutaneous endoscopic gastrostomy
PN	parenteral nutrition

REFERENCES

1. Colaizzo-Anas T. Nutrient intake, digestion, absorption, and excretion. In: Mueller CM, ed. *The A.S.P.E.N. Adult Nutrition Support Core Curriculum*. 2nd ed. Silver Spring, MD: American Society for Parenteral and Enteral Nutrition; 2012:3-21.
2. Abumrad NA, Nassir F, Marcus A. Digestion and absorption of dietary fat, carbohydrate, and protein. In: Feldman M, Friedman LS, Brandt LJ, eds. *Sleisenger & Fordtran's Gastrointestinal and Liver Disease: Pathophysiology/Diagnosis/Management*. 10th ed. Philadelphia, PA: Saunders Elsevier; 2016:1736-1764.
3. Hise ME, Brown JC. Lipids. In: Mueller CM, ed. *The A.S.P.E.N. Adult Nutrition Support Core Curriculum*. 2nd ed. Silver Spring, MD: American Society for Parenteral and Enteral Nutrition; 2012:63-82.
4. Dotan I, Mayer L. Mucosal immunology and inflammation. In: Feldman M, Friedman LS, Brandt LJ, eds. *Sleisenger & Fordtran's Gastrointestinal and Liver Disease: Pathophysiology/Diagnosis/Management*. 10th ed. Philadelphia, PA: Saunders Elsevier; 2016:16-27.
5. Shanahan F, Dinan TG, Ross P, Hill C. Probiotics in transition. *Clin Gastroenterol Hepatol* 2012;10:1220-1224.
6. Wallace B. Clinical use of probiotics in the pediatric population. *Nutr Clin Prac* 2009;24:50-59.
7. Lau CSM, Chamberlain RS. Probiotic administration can prevent necrotizing enterocolitis in preterm infants: A meta-analysis. *J Pediatr Surg* 2015;50:1405-1412.
8. Kozeniecki M, Fritzshall R. Enteral nutrition for adults in the hospital setting. *Nutr Clin Pract* 2015;30:634-651.
9. Bankhead R, Boullata J, Brantley S, et al. A.S.P.E.N. enteral nutrition practice recommendations. *JPEN J Parenter Enteral Nutr* 2009;33:122-167.
10. Brantley SL, Mills ME. Overview of enteral nutrition. In: Mueller CM, ed. *The A.S.P.E.N. Adult Nutrition Support Core Curriculum*. 2nd ed. Silver Spring, MD: American Society for Parenteral and Enteral Nutrition; 2012:170-184.
11. Vermilyea S, Goh VL. Enteral feeding in children: Sorting out tubes, buttons, and formulas. *Nutr Clin Pract* 2016;31(1):59-67.
12. Corkins MR, McKown CG, Gosa MM. Mechanics of nutrient intake. In: Corkins MR, ed *The A.S.P.E.N. Pediatric Nutrition Support Core Curriculum*. 2nd ed. Silver Spring, MD: American Society for Parenteral and Enteral Nutrition; 2015:3-14.
13. McClave SA, Martindale RG, Vanek VW, et al. Guidelines for the provision and assessment of nutrition support therapy in the adult

critically ill patient: Society of Critical Care Medicine (SCCM) and American Society for Parenteral and Enteral Nutrition (A.S.P.E.N.). *JPEN J Parenter Enteral Nutr* 2009;33:277-316.

14. Dhaliwal R, Cahill N, Lemieux M, Heyland DK. The Canadian critical care nutrition guidelines in 2013: An update on current recommendations and implementation strategies. *Nutr Clin Pract* 2014;29:29-43.
15. Kreymann KG, Berger MM, Deutz NEP, et al. ESPEN guidelines on enteral nutrition: Intensive care. *Clin Nutr* 2006;25:210-223.
16. Mehta NM, Compher C, A.S.P.E.N. Board of Directors. A.S.P.E.N. clinical guidelines: Nutrition support of the critically ill child. *JPEN J Parenter Enteral Nutr* 2009;33:260-276.
17. Itkin M, DeLegge MH, Fang JC, et al. Multidisciplinary practical guidelines for gastrointestinal access for enteral nutrition and decompression from the Society of Interventional Radiology and American Gastroenterological Association (AGA) Institute, with endorsement by Canadian Interventional Radiological Association (CIRA) and Cardiovascular and Interventional Radiological Society of Europe (CIRSE). *Gastroenterology* 2011;141:742-765.
18. Monczka J. Enteral nutrition support: Determining the best way to feed. In: Corkins MR, ed. *The A.S.P.E.N. Pediatric Nutrition Support Core Curriculum*. 2nd ed. Silver Spring, MD: American Society for Parenteral and Enteral Nutrition; 2015:641-646.
19. Dhaliwal R, Heyland DK. Nutrition and infection in the intensive care unit: What does the evidence show? *Curr Opin Crit Care* 2005;11:461-467.
20. Simpson F, Doig GS. Parenteral vs. enteral nutrition in the critically ill patient: A meta-analysis of trials using the intention to treat principle. *Intensive Care Med* 2005;31:12-23.
21. Gramlich L, Kichian K, Pinilla J, et al. Does enteral nutrition compared to parenteral nutrition result in better outcomes in critically ill adult patients? A systematic review of the literature. *Nutrition* 2004;20:843-848.
22. Harvey SE, Parrott F, Harrison, DA, et al. Trial of the route of early nutritional support in critically ill adults. *N Engl J Med* 2014;371:1673-1684.
23. Malone A, Seres D, Lord L. Complications of enteral nutrition. In: Mueller CM, ed. *The A.S.P.E.N. Adult Nutrition Support Core Curriculum*. 2nd ed. Silver Spring, MD: American Society for Parenteral and Enteral Nutrition; 2012:218-233.
24. Kumpf VJ. Parenteral nutrition-associated liver disease in adult and pediatric patients. *Nutr Clin Pract* 2006;21:279-290.
25. McClave SA, Heyland DK. The physiologic response and associated clinical benefits from provision of early enteral nutrition. *Nutr Clin Pract* 2009;24:305-315.
26. Doig GS, Heighes PT, Simpson F, et al. Early enteral nutrition, provided within 24 h of injury or intensive care unit admission, significantly reduces mortality in critically ill patients: A meta-analysis of randomized controlled trials. *Intensive Care Med* 2009;35:2018-2027.
27. Fang JC, Bankhead R, Kinikini M. Enteral access devices. In: Mueller CM, ed. *The ASPEN Adult Nutrition Support Core curriculum*. 2nd ed. Silver Spring, MD: American Society for Parenteral and Enteral Nutrition; 2012:206-217.
28. Koopmann MC, Kudsk KA, Szotkowski MJ, Rees SM. A team-based protocol and electromagnetic technology eliminate feeding tube placement complications. *Ann Surg* 2011;253:297-302.
29. Rivera R, Campana J, Hamilton C, Lopez R, Seidner D. Small bowel feeding tube placement using an electromagnetic tube placement device: Accuracy of tip location. *JPEN J Parenter Enteral Nutr* 2011;35(5):636-642.
30. Hsu CW, Sun SF, Lin SL, et al. Duodenal versus gastric feeding in medical intensive care patients: A prospective, randomized, clinical study. *Crit Care Med* 2009;37:1866-1872.
31. Barrocas A, Geppert C, Durfee SM, et al. A.S.P.E.N. ethics position paper. *Nutr Clin Pract* 2010;25:672-679.
32. Dorner B, Posthauer ME, Friedrich EK, Robinson GE. Enteral nutrition in older adults in nursing facilities. *Nutr Clin Pract* 2011;26:261-272.
33. Schwartz DB, Barrocas A, Wesley JR, et al. Gastrostomy tube placement in patients with advanced dementia or near end of life. *Nutr Clin Pract* 2014;29:829-840.
34. American Geriatrics Society Ethics Committee and Clinical Practice and Models of Care Committee. American Geriatrics Society feeding tubes in advanced dementia position statement. *J Am Geriatr Soc* 2014;62:1590-1593.
35. Komatz KC. Ethical issues in providing nutrition. In: Corkins MR, ed *The A.S.P.E.N. Pediatric Nutrition Support Core Curriculum*. 2nd ed. Silver Spring, MD: American Society for Parenteral and Enteral Nutrition; 2015:641-646.
36. Jawaheer G, Shaw NJ, Pierro A. Continuous enteral feeding impairs gallbladder emptying in infants. *J Pediatr* 2001;138:822-825.
37. McClave SA, Saad MA, Esterle M, et al. Volume-based feeding in the critically ill patient. *JPEN J Parenter Enteral Nutr* 2015;39:707-712.
38. Taylor B, Brody R, Denmark R, Southard R, Byham-Gray L. Improving enteral delivery through the adoption of the "Feed early enteral diet adequately for maximum effect (FEED ME)" protocol in a surgical trauma ICU: A quality improvement review. *Nutr Clin Pract* 2014;29:639-648.
39. Cresci G, Lefton J, Esper DH. Enteral formulations. In: Mueller CM, ed. *The A.S.P.E.N. Adult Nutrition Support Core Curriculum*. 2nd ed. Silver Spring, MD: American Society for Parenteral and Enteral Nutrition; 2012:185-205.
40. Chen Y, Peterson SJ. Enteral nutrition formulas: Which formula is right for your adult patient? *Nutr Clin Pract* 2009;24:344-355.
41. Heyland D, Muscedere J, Wischmeyer PE, et al. A randomized trial of glutamine and antioxidants in critically ill patients. *N Engl J Med* 2013;368:1487-1495.
42. Marik PE, Zaloga GP. Immunonutrition in critically ill patients: A systematic review and analysis of the literature. *Intensive Care Med* 2008;34:1980-1990.
43. Singer P, Theilla M, Fisher H, et al. Benefit of an enteral diet enriched with eicosapentaenoic acid and gamma-linolenic acid in ventilated patients with acute lung injury. *Crit Care Med* 2006;34:1033-1038.
44. Koletzko B, Lien E, Agostoni C, et al. The roles of long-chain polyunsaturated fatty acids in pregnancy, lactation and infancy: Review of current knowledge and consensus recommendations. *J Perinat Med* 2008;36:5-14.
45. Zaman MK, Chin K, Rai V, Majid HA. Fiber and prebiotic supplementation in enteral nutrition: A systematic review and meta-analysis. *World J Gastroenterol* 2015;21:5372-5381.
46. Commentary on breast-feeding and infant formulas, including proposed standards for formulas. *Pediatrics* 1976;57:278-285.
47. Corkins KG, Beck A. Infant formulas and complementary feedings. In: Corkins MR, ed. *The A.S.P.E.N. Pediatric Nutrition Support Core Curriculum*. 2nd ed. Silver Spring, MD: American Society for Parenteral and Enteral Nutrition; 2015:169-184.
48. Young LS, Kearns LR, Schoefel SL, Clark NC. Protein. In: Mueller CM, ed. *The A.S.P.E.N. Adult Nutrition Support Core Curriculum*. 2nd ed. Silver Spring, MD: American Society for Parenteral and Enteral Nutrition; 2012:83-97.
49. Doley J, Mallampalli A, Sandberg R. Nutrition management for the patient requiring prolonged mechanical ventilation. *Nutr Clin Pract* 2011;26:232-241.
50. van Zanten AR, Sztark F, Kaisers UX, et al. High-protein enteral nutrition enriched with immune-modulating nutrients vs standard high-protein enteral nutrition and nosocomial infections in the ICU: A randomized clinical trial. *JAMA* 2014;312:514-524.
51. Rice TW, Wheeler AP, Thompson BT, et al. Enteral omega-3 fatty acid, γ-linolenic acid, and antioxidant supplementation in acute lung injury. *JAMA* 2011;306:1574-1581.
52. Chenu JW, Cox JM. Cronobacter (*Enterobacter sakazakii*): Current status and future prospects. *Lett Appl Microbiol* 2009;49:153-159.
53. Groh-Wargo S, Sapsford A. Enteral nutrition support of the preterm infant in the neonatal intensive care unit. *Nutr Clin Prac* 2009;24:363-376.
54. Wessell JJ. Human milk. In: Corkins MR, ed. *The A.S.P.E.N. Pediatric Nutrition Support Core Curriculum*. 2nd ed. Silver Spring, MD: American Society for Parenteral and Enteral Nutrition; 2015:153-168.
55. Atia AN, Buchman AL. Oral rehydration solutions in non-cholera diarrhea: A review. *Am J Gastroenterol* 2009;104:2596-2604.
56. Tarleton S, DiBaise JK. Short bowel syndrome. In: Mueller CM, ed. *The A.S.P.E.N. Adult Nutrition Support Core Curriculum*. 2nd edition. Silver Spring, MD: American Society for Parenteral and Enteral Nutrition; 2012:511-522.
57. Himelright I, Harris E, Lorch V, Anderson M. *Enterobacter sakazakii* infections associated with the use of powdered infant formula—Tennessee, 2001. *J Am Med Assoc* 2002;287:2204-2205.
58. Simmons D, Symes L, Guenter P, Graves K. Tubing misconnections: Normalization of deviance. *Nutr Clin Pract* 2011;26:286-293.
59. Guenter P. New enteral connectors: Raising awareness. *Nutr Clin Pract* 2014;29:612-614.
60. Global Enteral Device Supply Associate (GEDSA). Stay Connected. Available at: www.StayConnected.org. (Accessed November 16, 2015)
61. Skipper A. Refeeding syndrome or refeeding hypophosphatemia: A systematic review of cases. *Nutr Clin Pract* 2012;27:34-40.
62. McClave SA, Lukan JK, Stefater JA, et al. Poor validity of residual volumes as a marker for risk of aspiration in critically ill patients. *Crit Care Med* 2005;33:324-330.

63. Reignier J, Mercier E, Le Gouge A, et al. Effect of not monitoring residual gastric volume on risk of ventilator-associated pneumonia in adults receiving mechanical ventilation and early enteral feeding: A randomized controlled trial. *JAMA* 2013;309:249-256.
64. Elke G, Felbinger TW, Heyland DK. Gastric residual volume in critically ill patients: A dead marker or still alive? *Nutr Clin Pract* 2015;30:59-71.
65. Montejo JC, Minambres E, Bordejé L, et al. Gastric residual volume during enteral nutrition in ICU patients: The REGANE study. *Intensive Care Med* 2010;36:1386-1393.
66. Fraser RJL, Bryant L. Current and future therapeutic prokinetic therapy to improve enteral feed tolerance in the ICU patient. *Nutr Clin Pract* 2010;25:26-31.
67. Btaiche IF, Chan LN, Pleva M, Kraft MD. Critical illness, gastrointestinal complications, and medication therapy during enteral feeding in critically ill adult patients. *Nutr Clin Pract* 2010;25:32-49.
68. Juvé-Udina ME, Valls-Miró C, Carreno-Granero A, et al. To return or to discard? Randomised trial on gastric residual volume management. *Intensive Crit Care Nurs* 2009;25:258-267.
69. Maloney JP, Ryan TA, Brasel KJ, et al. Food dye use in enteral feedings: A review and a call for a moratorium. *Nutr Clin Pract* 2002;17:168-181.
70. Maloney JP, Ryan TA. Detection of aspiration in enterally fed patients: A requiem for bedside monitors of aspiration. *JPEN J Parenter Enteral Nutr* 2002;26(6 Suppl):S34-S42.
71. Jack L, Coyer F, Courtney M, Venkatesh B. Diarrhoea risk factors in enterally tube fed critically ill patients: A retrospective audit. *Intensive Crit Care Nurs* 2010;26:327-334.
72. Whelan K, Schneider S. Mechanisms, prevention, and management of diarrhea in enteral nutrition. *Curr Opin Gastroenterol* 2011;27:152-159.
73. Williams NT. Medication administration through enteral feeding tubes. *Am J Health Syst Pharm* 2008;65:2347-2357.
74. Lyman B, Shah SR. Nutrition access. In: Corkins MR, ed. *The A.S.P.E.N. Pediatric Nutrition Support Core Curriculum*. 2nd ed. Silver Spring, MD: American Society for Parenteral and Enteral Nutrition; 2015: 567-582.
75. Gunn SR, Early BJ, Zenati MS, Ochoa JB. Use of a nasal bridle prevents accidental nasoenteral feeding tube removal. *JPEN J Parenter Enteral Nutr* 2009;33:50-54.
76. Rommel N, DeMeyer AM, Feenstra L, Veereman-Wauters G. The complexity of feeding problems in 700 infants and young children presenting to a tertiary care institution. *J Pediatr Gastroenterol Nutr* 2003;37:75-84.
77. Wohlt PD, Zheng L, Gunderson S, et al. Recommendations for the use of medications with continuous enteral nutrition. *Am J Health Syst Pharm* 2009;66:1458-1467.
78. Magnuson BL, Clifford TM, Hoskins LA, Bernard AC. Enteral nutrition and drug administration, interactions, and complications. *Nutr Clin Pract* 2005;20:618-624.
79. Klang M, McLymont V, Ng N. Osmolality, pH, and compatibility of selected oral liquid medications with an enteral nutrition product. *JPEN J Parenter Enteral Nutr* 2013;37:689-694.
80. Chan LN. Drug-nutrient interactions. *JPEN J Parenter Enteral Nutr* 2013;37:450-459.
81. Dickerson RN, Garmon WM, Kuhl DA, Minard G, Brown RO. Vitamin K-independent warfarin resistance after concurrent administration of warfarin and continuous enteral nutrition. *Pharmacotherapy* 2008;28:308-313.

Obesity

144

Amy Heck Sheehan, Judy T. Chen, Jack A. Yanovski, and Karim Anton Calis

KEY CONCEPTS

1. Two clinical measures of excess body fat, regardless of sex, are the body mass index (BMI) and the waist circumference (WC). BMI and WC provide a better assessment of total body fat than weight alone and are independent predictors of obesity-related disease risk.
2. Excessive central adiposity increases risk for development of type 2 diabetes, hypertension, and dyslipidemia.
3. Weight loss of as little as 5% of total body weight can significantly improve blood pressure, lipid levels, and glucose tolerance in overweight and obese patients. Sustained, large weight losses (eg, after bariatric surgery) are associated with a lower risk of cardiovascular events and death and with long-term improvements in many of the complications associated with obesity.
4. Clinicians should consider the weight-altering effects of medications used to treat comorbid conditions (eg, antidepressants, antipsychotics, antiepileptics, and antidiabetics) and select medications that promote weight loss or are weight-neutral.
5. Bariatric surgery is reserved for patients with extreme obesity having a BMI more than or equal 40 kg/m^2 or BMI more than or equal to 35 kg/m^2 with significant comorbidities.
6. Pharmacotherapy may be considered an adjunctive treatment in patients with a BMI more than or equal to 30 kg/m^2 or BMI of 27 to 30 kg/m^2 with a comorbidity if comprehensive lifestyle modifications (ie, diet, exercise, and behavioral modification) fail to achieve or sustain weight loss.
7. Weight regain occurs with a high probability when pharmacotherapy for obesity is discontinued.
8. Pharmacotherapy should be discontinued if weight loss of at least 5% is not achieved after 12 weeks of maximum-dose therapy with lorcaserin, phentermine-topiramate, or bupropion-naltrexone because significant weight loss is unlikely to be achieved despite continued therapy. Liraglutide should be discontinued if weight loss of at least 4% is not achieved after 16 weeks of therapy.
9. The Food and Drug Administration (FDA) does not regulate labeling of herbal and food supplement diet agents, and content is not guaranteed.

INTRODUCTION

Since 1980, the prevalence of obesity worldwide has more than doubled.[1] It is now estimated that at least two of every three women and three of every four men are overweight or obese in the United States, and the number of obese women outnumbers those who are overweight.[2] While the rise in childhood obesity appears to have reached a plateau, the prevalence remains historically high with one of every three adolescents currently considered overweight or obese.[3] The presence of obesity and overweight is associated with a significantly increased risk for the development of many diseases (Table 144-1),[4-19] poorer outcomes of comorbid disease states, and increased healthcare costs. As of 2008, it was estimated that obesity accounted for 9.1% of total medical expenditures in the United States, and the cost of treating obesity-related illnesses in adults approached national health spending of $147 billion annually.[20] National and global initiatives to stem the obesity epidemic have been established through prevention strategies, consensus guidelines, and best practices.[5,21-24] This chapter reviews the epidemiology, pathophysiology, and therapeutic approaches for the management of obesity. Although nonpharmacologic treatment modalities are discussed, the pharmacotherapy of obesity is highlighted, and the role of pharmacotherapy relative to the other therapeutic options is critically reviewed.

EPIDEMIOLOGY

One of the global health targets set by the World Health Assembly is to halt the rise of diabetes and obesity.[23] Obesity in the United States has increased in prevalence since the 1960s. The National Health and Nutrition Examination Survey (NHANES) II data (1976-1980) estimated the prevalence of obesity among adults in the United States at 15%.[25] During NHANES 1999 to 2000, the prevalence increased twofold to 30.9%, and by 2011 obesity affected 34.9% of the adult population.[2,3] While the trends in obesity appear to have leveled off in recent years, prevention of obesity remains a public health priority due to its high prevalence. Children who are overweight are likely to remain overweight as adults. Furthermore, overweight or obese children and adolescents have a higher risk of premature mortality and morbidity as adults.[26] Therefore, childhood and early adulthood are critical intervention periods for prevention of obesity in the future. The prevalence of obesity varies by sex among racial and ethnic minorities within the United States. The highest prevalence is observed among non-Hispanic black women (56.8% obese) compared with 39.2% for non-Hispanic black men.[2] Non-Hispanic blacks are more likely to have extreme obesity compared to other ethnic groups. This gender disparity is also associated with the level of parental education. Young black women from the lowest educated families are at greater risk of obesity compared with young black men.[27] Obesity is reported in approximately one-third of White men and women, and the prevalence is also high among Hispanic men and women, exceeding 35%.[2] Educational achievement, which is linked to socioeconomic status, is also correlated with the fraction of people who are overweight; the prevalence of overweight is greatest in those with less than a high school education.

ETIOLOGY

Obesity occurs when there is increased energy storage resulting from an imbalance between energy intake and energy expenditure over time. The specific etiology for this imbalance in the vast majority of

TABLE 144-1 Conditions More Prevalent Among Patients with Obesity

Cancer	Genitourinary
Breast cancer (postmenopausal)	Chronic kidney disease
Colorectal cancer	Increased serum urate
Gallbladder cancer	End-stage renal disease
Endometrial cancer	Obesity-related glomerulopathy
Esophageal carcinoma	Urinary stress incontinence
Hepatic cancer	**Metabolic**
Kidney cancer	Diabetes mellitus
Ovarian cancer	Hyperlipidemia
Pancreatic cancer	Hyperinsulinemia
Prostate cancer	Hypertriglyceridemia
Rectal cancer	Low high-density lipoprotein
Cardiovascular	Impaired glucose tolerance
Atrial fibrillation	Metabolic syndrome
Cerebral vascular accidents	**Musculoskeletal**
Congestive heart failure	Degenerative joint disease
Coronary artery disease	Diff use idiopathic skeletal hyperostosis
Cor pulmonale	Disc disease
Hypertension	Gait disturbance
Left ventricular hypertrophy	Gout and hyperuricemia
Myocardial infarction	Fibromyalgia
Peripheral vascular disease	Immobility
Peripheral venous insufficiency	Low back pain/back strain
Pulmonary embolism	Osteoarthritis (knee, hips, ankles, feet)
Thrombophlebitis	Plantar fasciitis
Varicose veins	**Neurologic**
Venous thromboembolism	Carpal tunnel syndrome
Dermatologic	Idiopathic intracranial hypertension
Acanthosis nigricans	Meralgia paresthetica
Cellulitis	Pseudotumor cerebri
Intertrigo, carbuncles	Stroke
Lymphedema	**Oral Health**
Skin tags	Dental caries
Status pigmentation of legs	Loss of teeth
Striae distensae (stretch marks)	Periodontitis
Psoriasis (women)	Xerostomia
Endocrine and Reproductive	**Psychological**
Amenorrhea and other menstrual disorders	Affective disorders
Congenital anomalies	Body image disturbance
Fetal abnormalities	Depression
Hirsutism	Eating disorders
Hypogonadism (male)	Low self-esteem
Infertility	Social stigmatization
Polycystic ovarian syndrome	**Respiratory**
Hyperandrogenism	Asthma
Pregnancy complications	Chronic obstructive pulmonary disease
Sexual dysfunction	Dyspnea
Gastrointestinal	Hypoventilation syndrome
Cholelithiasis	Obstructive sleep apnea
Gastroesophageal reflux disease	Pickwickian syndrome
Hepatic cirrhosis	Pneumonia
Hernias	Pulmonary hypertension
Nonalcoholic fatty liver disease	

Data from references 4 to 19.

individuals is multifactorial, with genetic and environmental factors contributing to various degrees. In a small minority of individuals, excess weight may be attributed to an underlying medical condition or an unintended effect of a medication.

Genetic Influences

Observational studies in humans and experimental studies in animal models have demonstrated the strong role of genetics in determining both obesity and distribution of body fat. In some individuals, genetic factors are the primary determinants of obesity, whereas in others, obesity may be caused primarily by environmental factors. The genetic contribution to the actual variance in body mass index (BMI) and body fat distribution is estimated to be up between 40% and 70%.[28] A number of single-gene mutations producing extreme obesity have been identified, but such mutations are rare and account for a relatively small number of the total cases of obesity.[28] The total number and identity of contributing genes are still being determined, as is the means by which the many potential so-called "obesity" genes interact with each other and with the environment to produce the obese phenotype.

Environmental Factors

Many of the societal changes associated with economic development over the past 40 years have been implicated as potential causes for the increase in the prevalence of obesity.[29] These include an abundant and easily accessible food supply and the material comforts of modern life in Western civilizations, which have contributed to a reduction in physical activity. Advances in technology and automation have resulted in more sedentary lifestyles during both work and leisure time for most individuals. At the same time, there has been a significant increase in the availability and portion size of high-fat foods, which are aggressively marketed and are often more convenient and less expensive than healthier alternatives. This modern environment has been described by some as "obesogenic" because it is likely to result in a state of positive energy balance in many individuals (Fig. 144-1).[30] Obesity has also been reported more frequently among individuals within close social networks (eg, siblings, spouses, and friends), with a person's risk of becoming obese increasing significantly if a friend in his or her social network is obese.[31] Finally, it should be noted that cultural factors, socioeconomic status, and religious beliefs may influence eating habits and body weights.

Medical Conditions

Occasionally, patients present with obesity secondary to an identifiable medical condition. Conditions associated with weight gain include iatrogenic and idiopathic Cushing syndrome, growth hormone deficiency, insulinoma, leptin deficiency, and various psychiatric disorders, such as depression, binge-eating disorder, and schizophrenia. Hypothyroidism is often included in this list, but it mostly causes fluid retention (myxedema) and is generally not a cause of significant obesity. Genetic syndromes that have obesity as a major component are extremely rare and include Prader-Willi, Wilms' tumor, aniridia, genitourinary abnormalities or gonadoblastoma, and mental retardation (WAGR), Simpson-Golabi-Behmel, Cohen, Bardet-Biedl, Carpenter, Börjeson, and Wilson-Turner syndromes. The clinician evaluating a patient for obesity needs to be aware of these potential conditions. The physical examination of obese patients always should include an assessment for secondary causes of obesity, including genetic syndromes.

Medications

An increasing number of medications are associated with unintended weight gain.[32] These include several anticonvulsants (eg, carbamazepine, gabapentin, pregabalin, and valproic acid), antidepressants (eg, mirtazapine and tricyclic antidepressants), atypical antipsychotics (eg, clozapine, olanzapine, quetiapine, and risperidone), conventional antipsychotics (eg, haloperidol), and hormones (eg, corticosteroids, insulin, and medroxyprogesterone). Although the pharmacologic mechanism responsible for weight gain is usually drug-specific, in most cases the precise mechanism is unknown.

PATHOPHYSIOLOGY

The pathophysiology of obesity involves numerous factors that regulate appetite and energy balance.[33-35] Disturbance of these homeostatic functions results in an imbalance between energy intake and energy expenditure.

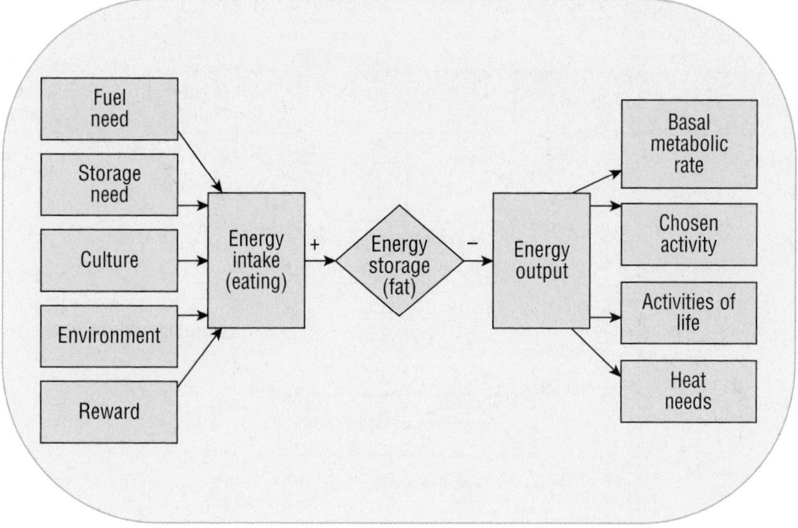

FIGURE 144-1 Net energy stores are determined by various inputs and outputs. Simply stated, obesity occurs when there is an imbalance between energy intake and expenditure.

Appetite

Human appetite is a complex process that is the net result of many inputs within a neural network involving principally the hypothalamus, limbic system, brainstem, hippocampus, and elements of the cortex.[33-35] Within this neural network, many neurotransmitters and neuropeptides have been identified that can stimulate or inhibit the brain's appetite network and thereby affect total caloric intake. The first receptor systems found to alter food intake in animals and humans were the biogenic amines. Serotonin, also known as 5-hydroxytryptamine (5-HT), and cells known to respond to 5-HT are found throughout the central nervous system (CNS) and the periphery. Currently, two major noradrenergic receptor subtypes are recognized (α and β), each with multiple subtypes. Histamine and dopamine also demonstrate multiple receptor subtypes, but their role in the regulation of human eating behaviors and food intake is less well documented. Table 144-2 summarizes the major effects of direct receptor stimulation, inhibition, and changes in synaptic cleft amine concentrations on food intake.

Many neuropeptides also influence appetite within the hypothalamus. Most research has focused on the neural projection between parts of the hypothalamus and the arcuate nucleus with signals to the paraventricular nucleus. The key peptides in this projection are thought to include neuropeptide Y and α-melanocyte–stimulating hormone. Neuropeptide Y is the most potent known stimulator of eating, and α-melanocyte–stimulating hormone action at the melanocortin 3 and 4 receptors is one of the crucial inhibitors of eating.[33] The lateral hypothalamus has been referred to as the "hunger" center within the brain. The most prominent of the lateral hypothalamic peptides, orexin, increases food intake stimuli within the lateral hypothalamus.[33] Another important neuropeptide stimulator of eating that principally originates in the lateral hypothalamus is melanocyte-concentrating hormone. Neurons in the lateral hypothalamus use orexin and melanocyte-concentrating hormone to communicate with other neurons throughout the brain and thereby affect a number of functions beyond appetite.[33] Table 144-2 summarizes the major effects of various neuropeptides on food intake. Although hunger and satiety functions are thought to be primarily regulated by the hypothalamus, humans eat in response to a broad set of stimuli, including reward, pleasure, learning, and memory.

Peripheral appetite signals also dramatically affect food intake.[33,34] Leptin, a hormone that is secreted by adipose cells, acts on the arcuate nucleus of the hypothalamus and elsewhere in the brain to decrease appetite and increase energy expenditure.[33,34] Studies conducted in leptin-deficient mice and humans revealed that exogenous leptin administration produced significant weight loss. However, recombinant leptin replacement therapy in obese humans who are not leptin deficient has not proved successful because obese humans appear to be leptin resistant.[33] Figure 144-2 shows the peripheral link that leptin appears to provide in signaling the CNS about the status of fat cell mass.

Other peripheral signals important to the brain's processing of appetite include several gut hormones, notably those released by the intestine in response to passage of digesting food such as glucagon-like peptide-1 (GLP-1), oxyntomodulin, and peptide YY.[34] Each of these

TABLE 144-2 Effects of Various Neurotransmitters, Receptors, and Peptides on Food Intake[33,34]

Anatomic Region	Increased Eating	Decreased Eating
Arcuate nucleus of hypothalamus	NPY AgRP	α-MSH CART Leptin Insulin GLP-1 PYY
Paraventricular nucleus of hypothalamus	NPY AgRP	α-MSH, melanocortin CRH CCK
Lateral hypothalamus	Orexin MCH	
Hypothalamus	Norepinephrine α_2 Serotonin 5-HT_{1A}	Norepinephrine α_1 and β_2 Serotonin 5-HT_{1B} and 5-HT_{2C} Histamine H_1 and H_3
Nucleus accumbens	Dopamine	
Brainstem (hindbrain)	NPY AgRP Opioids (especially μ)	Leptin α-MSH, melanocortin CCK
Vagus nerve	Ghrelin	Leptin CCK GLP-1 PYY

AgRP, agouti-related protein; CART, cocaine-and-amphetamine-regulated transcript; CCK, cholecystokinin; CRH, corticotropin-releasing hormone; GLP-1, glucagon-like peptide-1; MCH, melanocyte concentration hormone; α-MSH, α-melanocyte-stimulating hormone; NPY, neuropeptide Y; PYY, peptide YY.

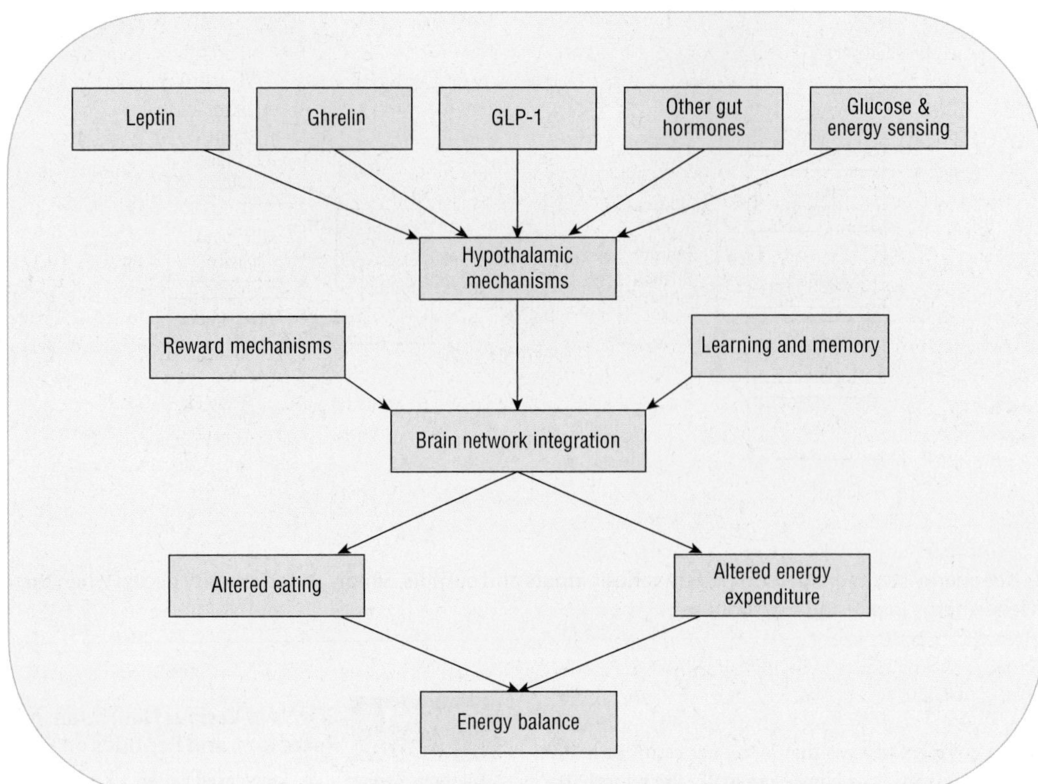

FIGURE 144-2 Intrinsic hypothalamic hunger and satiety mechanisms are modified by input from fat tissue via leptin, and from the gut via ghrelin, glucagon-like peptide-1 (GLP-1), and other hormones. Additional input is derived by direct sensing of prevailing glucose and other energy signals. The hypothalamus generates signals that are integrated within brain networks, which also receive additional signals. The brain network effects change in energy balance by modifying food intake and energy expenditure.

hormonal signals suppresses eating in animals and humans. GLP-1 has other effects, most importantly as an incretin, which facilitates release of insulin by pancreatic β cells in response to meal-related glucose. Ghrelin, another important gut hormone that is released from the distal stomach and duodenum, stimulates appetite. An understanding of the relationships among the brain, its many neurotransmitters and neuropeptides, environmental stimulation of brain activities, and other hormones is still evolving.

Energy Balance

The net balance of energy ingested relative to energy expended by an individual over time determines the degree of obesity (see Fig. 144-1). An individual's metabolic rate is the single largest determinant of energy expenditure. Resting energy expenditure (REE) is defined as the energy expended by a person at rest under conditions of thermal neutrality. Basal metabolic rate (BMR) is defined as the REE measured soon after awakening in the morning at least 12 hours after the last meal. Metabolic rate increases after eating based on the size and composition of the meal. It reaches a maximum approximately 1 hour after the meal is consumed and returns to basal levels 4 hours after the meal. This increase in metabolic rate is known as the *thermogenic effect of food.* The REE measures the energy costs of the wakeful state and may include the residual thermogenic effect of a previous meal. Physical activity is the other major factor that affects total energy expenditure and is the most variable component. With regard to energy storage, there are two major types of adipose tissue, white and brown. The primary function of white adipose tissue is lipid manufacture, storage, and release. Brown adipose tissue, once believed to be found only in infants, is now recognized to exist in most adults.[36] It is more commonly identified in lean than obese individuals, but its importance for human obesity remains unclear. Whereas lipid storage occurs in response to insulin, lipid release is seen during periods of calorie restriction. Brown adipose tissue is notable for its ability to dissipate energy via uncoupled mitochondrial respiration.[36] Both white and brown adipose tissues are highly innervated by the sympathetic nervous system, and adrenergic stimulation via β-adrenergic receptors (β_1, β_2, and β_3) is known to activate lipolysis in fat cells as well as increase energy expenditure in adipose tissue and skeletal muscle.

CLINICAL PRESENTATION

Although obesity is readily apparent, most obese patients seek healthcare only when obesity-associated comorbidities become problematic. The National Institutes of Health (NIH) has established a stratification of weight excess based on associated medical risks.[37] These levels of excess weight are defined on the basis of BMI, a measure of total body weight relative to height. Using metric units, BMI (kg/m^2) is defined as weight in kilograms divided by height in meters squared (kg/m^2). Using pounds and inches, BMI (kg/m^2) is estimated as (weight [lb]/height [inches^2]) × 703. Adults with a BMI of 25 to 29.9 are considered "*overweight*"; the terms *obese*, and *extreme obese* are reserved for those with a BMI of 30 to 39.9, and 40 and over, respectively. While the precise definition of childhood obesity is still lacking, the Endocrine Society clinical practice guideline currently classifies children and adolescents ages 2 to 18 years with a BMI at the 95th percentile or above as obese, and those with a BMI between the 85th and 94th percentiles as overweight.[38] Because BMI may overestimate the degree of excess body fat in some clinical situations (eg, edematous states, extreme muscularity, muscle wasting, and short stature), the assessment of body composition in such cases often requires clinical judgment.

1 BMI is an acceptable measure of obesity and is the practical method of defining obesity in the clinic and epidemiologic studies;

however, it does not always correspond to excess fat. There are well-established differences in the relationship between BMI and obesity-related risks among disparate racial, sex, and ethnic groups. For example, BMI underestimates risks among Asians;[39] whereas Caucasians tend to have higher level of visceral adipose tissue than African American adults at higher levels of BMI and waist circumference.[40] Central obesity reflects high levels of intra-abdominal or visceral fat, and this pattern of obesity is associated with an increased propensity for the development of hypertension, dyslipidemia, type 2 diabetes, and cardiovascular disease (sometimes referred to as the "metabolic syndrome"). Thus, in addition to the absolute excess fat mass, the distribution of this fat regionally in the body has important clinical effects. Intra-abdominal fat is best estimated by imaging techniques such as computed tomography (CT) and magnetic resonance imaging (MRI) but can be approximated through measurement of waist circumference (WC). Clinically, WC is the narrowest circumference measured in the area between the last rib and the top of the iliac crest. The current definition for high-risk WC is greater than 40 inches (102 cm) in men and greater than 35 inches (89 cm) in women.[6] Routine determination of WC should be implemented in those with BMIs between 25 and 34.9 kg/m^2 to assess additional metabolic risk. However, after a patient's BMI reaches 35 kg/m^2, it is not necessary to measure WC because it will likely be elevated and adds little in terms of risk prediction.[5]

2 Although BMI and WC are related, each measure independently predicts disease risk. Both measurements should be assessed and monitored during therapy for obesity.[5,6] The risks for development of type 2 diabetes, hypertension, or cardiovascular disease at various stages of obesity based on BMI or WC are outlined in Table 144-3. Note that increased WC confers increased risk even in normal-weight individuals.

Comorbidities

Obesity and overweight are associated with an increased risk of all-cause mortality. The greater the BMI, the greater the risk of cardiovascular diseases (CVD), type 2 diabetes, and all-cause mortality in both men and women.[5] Substantial reduction in life expectancy has been predicted in adults with BMIs greater than 35 kg/m^2.[41] Excessive body fat affects virtually all organ systems. A plethora of evidence continue to link obesity with numerous disease states and health conditions (see Table 144-1).[4-19] Therefore, it is important for clinicians to assess the presence of these chronic conditions in all overweight and obese individuals.[35] Because obese individuals are also at risk for developing many malignancies, adherence to routine age- and risk- appropriate cancer screening guidelines is recommended.[35] Furthermore, hypertension, hyperlipidemia, coronary heart disease, cerebrovascular accidents, insulin resistance, glucose intolerance, and diabetes are all known cardiac risk factors that tend to cluster in obese individuals. Aggressive management of these comorbid cardiovascular risk factors and other obesity-related medical conditions (eg, sleep apnea, major depression, osteoarthritis, nonalcoholic fatty liver disease) is warranted in an obese individual regardless of an individual's weight loss efforts.[6,35]

TABLE 144-3 Classification of Overweight and Obesity by Body Mass Index, Waist Circumference, and Associated Disease Risk

			Disease Risk[a] (Relative to Normal Weight and Waist Circumference)	
			Men	
			≤40 in (≤102 cm)	>40 in (>102 cm)
			Women	
	BMI (kg/m^2)	Obesity Class	≤35 in (≤89 cm)	>35 in (>89 cm)
Underweight	<18.5		—	—
Normal weight[b]	18.5-24.9		—	High
Overweight	25.0-29.9		Increased	High
Obesity	30.0-34.9 35.0-39.9	I II	High Very high	Very high Very high
Extreme obesity	≥40	III	Extremely high	Extremely high

BMI, body mass index.

[a]Disease risk for type 2 diabetes, hypertension, and cardiovascular disease.

[b]Increased waist circumference can also be a marker for increased risk even in persons of normal weight.

Adapted from Preventing and Managing the Global Epidemic of Obesity. Report of the World Health Organization Consultation on Obesity. Geneva: World Health Organization, 1997. Reprinted with permission from National Institutes of Health, National Heart, Lung and Blood Institute. 1997, http://www.nhlbi.nih.gov/guidelines/obesity/ob_home.htm.

TREATMENT

Available treatment options for the chronic management of obesity include reduced caloric intake, comprehensive lifestyle intervention, pharmacotherapy, implantable medical devices, and bariatric surgery.

Desired Outcomes

Weight management is commonly considered successful when a predefined amount of weight has been lost such that a final goal is achieved. The ultimate goal of treatment must be defined clearly and may be absolute weight loss if obesity is present without other comorbid conditions. If improvement in blood glucose, blood cholesterol, and hypertension are primary goals, then these must be defined appropriately and may include setting target levels for low-density lipoprotein cholesterol, glycosylated hemoglobin, or blood pressure. In 2013, an updated evidence-based guideline on the management of overweight and obesity was published by the Obesity Society (TOS), American Heart Association (AHA), and American College of Cardiology (ACC),[5] which recommended the initial weight loss goal for adults to be approximately 5% to 10% of the baseline weight over a 6-month period. Success may also include end points of decreasing the rate of weight gain or maintaining a weight-neutral status. All too often patients expect to lose weight overnight, only to be disappointed. Thus, it is important to set a time course for the plan. A significant number of web-based resources for supporting both patient and practitioner weight-management activities are available.[6,22,42]

General Approach to Treatment

To achieve meaningful weight loss goals, successful obesity treatment plans require incorporation of comprehensive lifestyle interventions such as healthy diet, adequate physical activity, and behavioral modifications as the cornerstone of weight management.[5] Once the need for weight loss has been determined, the clinician needs to assess a patient's readiness to engage in weight loss efforts and identify any potential barriers to success. They need to initiate a dialogue with each patient who is overweight or obese to ensure they understand the potential health consequences of excess body weight and benefits of appropriate weight management. Specific weight goals should be established that are consistent with medical needs and the patient's personal desire. For most overweight and obese patients, a weight loss goal of 5% to 10% of initial weight is reasonable. Patients should not be allowed to attain an abnormally low body weight (ie, less than their estimated ideal body weight).

3 Patients seeking help for obesity do so for many reasons, including improvement in their quality of life, a reduction in associated morbidity, and increased life expectancy. Because weight stigma is prevalent in the western culture, numerous individuals seek therapy for obesity primarily for cosmetic purposes and often have unrealistic goals and expectations. Aggressive marketing of weight loss programs, therapies, and diets—parallel to the fashion industry's standards of desirable body profiles—has led many individuals to set impossible goals and expectations. In some cases, these individuals will go to extreme measures to achieve weight loss. Consequently, clinicians must be careful to fully discuss the risks of therapies and to clearly define the achievable benefits and magnitude of weight loss. Obese patients should be redirected away from trying to achieve an "ideal weight" to the more realistic goal of modest (eg, loss of 5%-10% of body weight) but sustained, medically relevant weight loss. In practice, goals should be set based on many factors, including initial body weight, patient motivation and desire, presence of comorbid conditions, and age. The Look Action for Health in Diabetes (AHEAD) study found that patients with diabetes who maintained weight loss of at least 7% with intensive lifestyle modifications for a period of almost 10 years did not experience a reduced incidence of cardiovascular events, but they did have a reduced need for diabetes medications and improvement in physical function and other health benefits.[43] Indeed, in overweight and obese patients with diabetes, lifestyle modification with sustained weight loss of greater than 5% have been shown to improve HbA1c level, ameliorate hyperglycemia, hyperlipidemia, and hypertension within a year.[44] For obese individuals with osteoarthritis, significantly more weight reduction may be required to improve symptoms. These data emphasize the importance of defining end points and measures of success in any weight-loss plan.

4 Weight-loss interventions must be founded on lifestyle changes, such as a modification in eating practices; complemented by drug therapy, if indicated; and in some cases, surgery (Fig. 144-3). Before recommending any therapy, the clinician must evaluate the patient for the presence of secondary causes of obesity. If a secondary cause is suspected, then a more complete diagnostic workup and the initiation of appropriate therapy may be warranted. The next step in patient evaluation is to determine the presence and severity of other medical conditions that are either directly associated with obesity (eg, diabetes, cardiovascular diseases, uncontrolled hypertension) or that have an impact on therapeutic decision making (eg, history of pancreatitis, cardiac arrhythmia, seizure disorders, concurrent medications).[35] The Endocrine Society Clinical Practice Guideline for the Pharmacological Management of Obesity emphasizes that clinicians should always consider the potential weight-altering effects of all medications a patient is receiving for the management of comorbid conditions and select medications that are weight-neutral or promote weight loss (strong recommendation with moderate quality evidence).[35] For example, in patients with type 2 diabetes, antidiabetic agents that promote weight loss (eg, metformin, glucagon-like pepetide-1 analogs or sodium-glucose-linked transporter-2

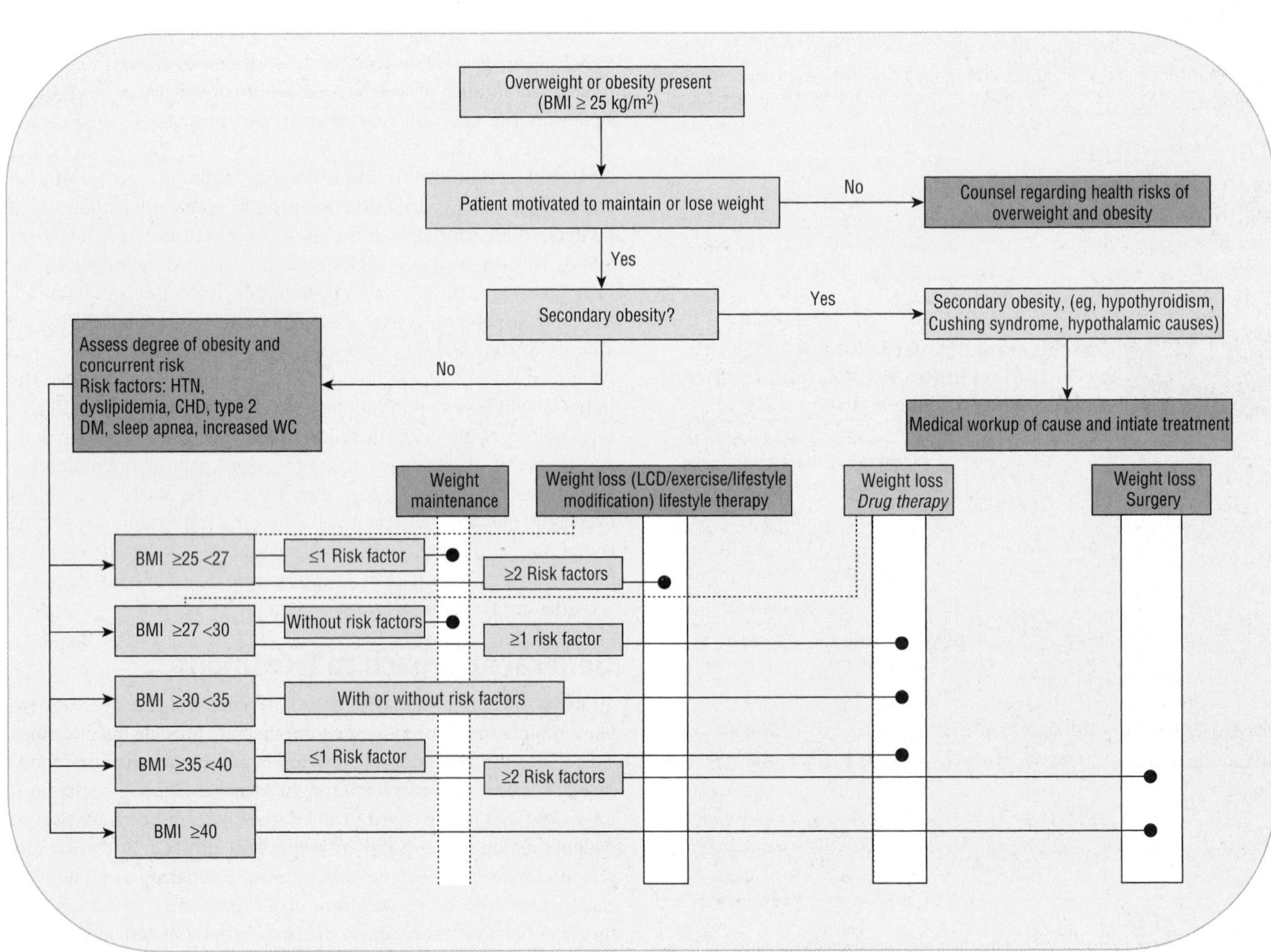

FIGURE 144-3 Treatment algorithm. Candidates for pharmacotherapy are selected on the basis of body mass index and waist circumference criteria along with consideration of concurrent risk factors. Medication therapy is always used as an adjunct to a comprehensive weight-loss program that includes diet, exercise, and behavioral modification.[5,35] CHD, coronary heart disease; DM, diabetes mellitus; HTN, hypertension; LCD, low-calorie diet; WC, waist circumference (more than or equal to 40 inches [more than or equal to 102 cm] for men and more than or equal to 35 inches [more than or equal to 89 cm] for women).

inhibitors) are preferred. Appropriate laboratory tests to exclude or quantify the degree of specific conditions such as diabetes, liver dysfunction, and nephropathy should be performed as indicated by the history and physical examination. Based on the outcome of this medical evaluation, the patient should be counseled on treatment options, benefits, and risks. Ultimately, lifelong therapeutic goals should consist of maintenance of reduced body weight and prevention of weight gain.

Nonpharmacologic Therapy

Nonpharmacologic therapy, including reduced caloric intake, increased physical activity, and behavioral modification is the mainstay of obesity management. This combination is recommended as first-line therapy for all patients with BMI more than or equal to 25 kg/m^2 by The Endocrine Society Clinical Practice Guidelines for the Pharmacological Management of Obesity (graded as strong recommendation with high quality evidence).[35] Although the difference is subtle, it should be noted that the AHA/ACC/TOS Guidelines for the Management of Overweight and Obesity in Adults do not recommend weight loss therapy for patients with BMI between 25 and 29.9, unless the patient has CVD risk factors.[5] Weight loss will require significant effort on the part of the patient to change their lifestyle and comply with the management plan. If the patient is not ready to meet these expectations, then early counseling will reduce the chance of frustration for the patient, clinician, and possibly other family members. Providing basic education can lead to a significant change in motivation and desire to lose weight and improved compliance.

Reduced Caloric Intake

Current adult guidelines recommend reduced caloric intake through adherence to a low-calorie diet (LCD).[5] The LCD should provide a daily caloric deficit of 500 to 750 kcal (2,092-3,138 kJ), which generally correlates to a total intake of 1,200 to 1,500 kcal/day (5,021-6,276 kJ/day) for women and 1,500 to 1,800 kcal/day (6,276-7, 531 kJ/day) for men. Severely obese individuals will require more energy, at least at the start of dietary restriction. Adherence to the LCD has been shown to result in an average weight loss of 8% after 6 months.[6]

Numerous diet and nutrition plans are available to aid patients in their pursuit of weight loss, and current guidelines allow for choice among many potential evidence-based diet plans.[5,6] Popular diets include moderate energy-deficient plans (eg, Weight Watchers, LEARN [Lifestyle, Exercise, Attitude, Relationships, Nutrition], and Jenny Craig), vegetarian-based plans (eg, Ornish), and low carbohydrate plans (eg, Zone and Atkins). Short-term weight loss is significant for almost all diet plans. However, long-term weight loss and maintenance of weight loss are less promising, primarily because of difficulty with adherence. Therefore, the choice of diet plan should be determined based on patient-specific preferences, health status, and ability to consistently adhere to the specific recommendations of the diet.[5] A recent meta-analysis of 48 clinical trials assessing the efficacy of various diets concluded that differences in weight loss among popular named diets are not clinically significant,[45] highlighting the general consensus that macronutrient composition of the diet may not be as important as consistent adherence to reduced energy consumption.

Very-low-calorie diets, providing less than 800 kcal/day (3,349 kJ/day), are generally not recommended.[6] Although very-low-calorie diets can often result in early weight loss, long-term results have been disappointing because it is difficult for individuals to maintain compliance.[44] Additionally, very-low-calorie diets require intensive medical monitoring and should only be used in certain situations under the supervision of an experienced clinician. Regardless of the diet program, it is clear that energy consumption must be less than energy expenditure to achieve weight loss (see Fig. 144-1). The challenge is to develop a diet plan that leads to consistent adherence by the patient and sustained weight loss and maintenance.

Comprehensive Lifestyle Intervention

Comprehensive lifestyle intervention encompasses the combination of reduced caloric intake, increased physical activity, and behavioral modification. Increased physical activity is an important component in achieving the state of greater energy expenditure than energy intake that is necessary to lose weight and maintain weight loss. When increased physical activity is attempted as monotherapy, only modest weight loss has been reported.[46] However, when it is combined with reduced calorie intake and behavior modification, it can augment weight loss and improve obesity-related comorbidities and cardiovascular risk factors.[5,6] Moderate physical activity for at least 30 minutes per day, on most days of the week, is recommended. Greater levels (ie, 200-300 min/wk) may be required to augment weight loss and maintain lost weight. Patients should be advised to start slowly and gradually increase intensity. All obese patients should receive a medical examination before embarking on a physical activity program.

Current adult guidelines recommend initiation of a comprehensive lifestyle program to help overweight and obese patients adhere to the prescribed LDC and increase physical activity per week (NHLBI Grade A; strong recommendation).[5] On-site, individual or group, behavioral counseling sessions offered by a trained clinician on at least 14 occasions during a 6-month time period are preferred. However, electronic or commercial based programs may also be effective. For patients who have successfully lost weight during the first 6 months, long-term participation in a comprehensive lifestyle program is recommended. The primary aim is to help patients choose lifestyles that are conducive to safe and sustained weight loss. Most such programs use self-monitoring of diet and exercise to increase patient awareness of behavior and as a tool for the clinician to determine patient compliance as well as patient motivation. Clinical studies evaluating the efficacy of high-intensity comprehensive lifestyle interventions that include a reduced-calorie diet, increased exercise, and in-person behavioral counseling sessions have reported an average weight loss of 8 kg after 6 months.[5,6]

Implantable Medical Devices

Recently, the FDA approved two new implantable medical devices for weight reduction in obese patients. vBloc® neurometabolic therapy, is indicated for weight loss in adults with a BMI of 40 to 45 kg/m^2, or a BMI of 35 to 39.9 kg/m^2 with at least one comorbidity who have failed a supervised weight management program within the past 5 years.[47,48] The vBloc® neurometabolic therapy, delivered via a pace-maker like device called the Maestro® Rechargeable system, is implanted subcutaneously on the vagal trunk with the electrodes designed to intermittently block the communication with the vagus nerve. The vagus nerve is known to regulate digestion through autonomic communication between the brain and the stomach. Blockage of the vagal communication is believed to alter multiple physiological mechanisms related to food intake and energy metabolism, thus resulting in increased satiety and weight loss. The implanted neuroregulator is controlled by the clinician with an external programming device to deliver at least 12 hours of intermittent vagal nerve block. The ReCharge trial evaluated the effect of vagal nerve block in patients with morbid obesity, the percentage of excess weight loss (defined as weight loss above a BMI of 25 kg/m^2) was significant with 24% excess weight loss (9% of initial body weight) reported in the vagal nerve block treatment group compared to 16% excess weight loss (6% of initial body weight) reported in the sham control group.[47] In obese patients with type 2 diabetes, 25% excessive weight loss was reported along with 1% decrease in A1c for those who received the vBloc® device which was active for 12 to 15 hours daily.[48] Patients with cirrhosis, portal hypertension, esophageal varices, hiatal hernia, planned MRI or diathermy, and patients with a permanently implanted, electrical-powered medical device are contraindicated for the vBloc® therapy. Common adverse events with vBloc® therapy include neuroregulator site pain, nausea, abdominal pain, heartburn or dyspepsia. Although safety and efficacy of this device has only been studied up to 1 year, long-term data continue to be collected from ongoing clinical trials.[47,48] Unfortunately, once the device is turned-off, patients will often regain the weight lost.

The ReShape Dual Balloon device is indicated for weight reduction in patients with BMI of 30 to 40 kg/m^2 with one or more obesity-related comorbidities who have failed previous weight loss attempts with diet and exercise alone.[49] The balloon device is implanted into the stomach through a minimally invasive endoscopic procedure. After placement, the balloon is then inflated with saline and blue dye (methylene blue) to trigger the feelings of fullness by occupying the space in the stomach which helps patients reduce hunger and improve appetite control. While the balloon device does not alter the stomach's nature anatomy like bariatric surgery, the placement is only intended to be temporarily and should be removed 6 month after insertion as the device itself will deflate over time. Patients who failed to have the device removed after 6 months experienced an increased risk of intestinal obstruction due to migration of the deflated balloon and may require surgical removal of the device. In clinical trials, the average weight loss reported with the ReShape Dual Balloon device was 14.3 lbs (6.5 kg; 6.8% of total body weight) compared with 7.2 lbs (3.3 kg; 3.3% of total body weight) reported in the control group.[49] Six months following the removal of the device, patients treated with the balloon device maintained an average reduction of 9.9 pounds (4.5 kg) of the 14.3 pounds (6.5 kg) that was initially lost. Potential adverse effects from this procedure are primarily related to endoscopic sedation. Once the device is placed in the stomach, patients may experience vomiting, nausea, abdominal pain, diarrhea, and feelings of indigestion. Therefore, this balloon device is not indicated in patients with previous gastrointestinal (GI) or bariatric surgery, inflammatory intestinal or bowel disease, large hiatal hernia, symptoms of delayed gastric emptying, severe liver damage, or active *Helicobacter pylori* infection. In addition, patients who are pregnant, breastfeeding or taking anticoagulants, anti-inflammatory, or other gastric irritates daily are not candidates for the device. Finally, patients currently taking selective serotonin reuptake inhibitors (SSRIs), serotonin-norepinephrine reuptake inhibitors (SNRIs), and monoamine oxidase inhibitors (MAOIs) should use this device with caution due to the potential for balloon rupture and release of methylene blue which with these concurrent therapies can increase risk of developing serotonin syndrome.

Clinical **Controversy...**

Current practice guidelines state that bariatric surgery may be considered in patients with a BMI of 40 kg/m^2 or above or BMI of 35 kg/m^2 with significant comorbidities, as an increasing body of literature indicates improvements in comorbidities and prolongation of life after bariatric surgery. Most long-term data are for the Roux-en-Y gastric bypass procedure; the long-term outcomes of other approaches remain somewhat uncertain. Researchers are also beginning to study the effects of bariatric procedures among patients with BMIs below 35 kg/m^2 for remediation of comorbid conditions such as diabetes, but the long-term benefits, risks, and cost-effectiveness of this approach remain unclear.

Bariatric Surgery

5 Consistent with the growing obesity epidemic, the demand for bariatric surgery has increased drastically over the past 2 decades. Surgery currently remains the most effective and durable intervention for the treatment of obesity. Current clinical practice guidelines recommend that surgical intervention be reserved for patients with extreme obesity (BMI ≥ 40 kg/m^2) or BMI greater than 35 kg/m^2 with significant comorbidities such as hypertension, type 2 diabetes, or obstructive sleep apnea (NHLBI Grade A; strong recommendation).[5,50] Surgery may also be offered to patients with BMI between 30 kg/m^2 and 34.9 kg/m^2 with diabetes or metabolic syndrome but the long-term data have yet to demonstrate its overall benefits.[5,50]

Surgical weight loss options should only be considered in patients who have met the eligibility criteria and have failed other recommended methods for weight loss. It is critical for bariatric surgical candidates to fully understand the surgical risks and be able to adhere to the extensive postoperative care plan, follow-ups, and necessary lifelong dietary and lifestyle adjustments to ensure the long-term success of the procedure.

The four common surgical procedures are (1) adjustable gastric banding, (2) sleeve gastrectomy, (3) biliopancreatic diversion with duodenal switch, and (4) conventional Roux-en-Y gastric bypass. The adjustable gastric banding and sleeve gastrectomy are designed to reduce the volume of the stomach and thus restrict the rate of nutrient intake. The biliopancreatic diversion with duodenal switch is primarily malabsorptive in nature, and the length of the diversion determines the extent of nutrient malabsorption. The conventional roux-en-Y gastric bypass is the most common procedure currently performed in the United States and worldwide.[51] This hybrid procedure combines a restrictive approach with a degree of malabsorption induced by reducing the size of the stomach pouch and causing food to bypass parts of the small intestine. Techniques that involve redirection of the flow of nutrients so as to have humoral and malabsorptive effects, generally yield greater and longer lasting weight loss than the purely restrictive methods.[51] Ultimately, reductions in excess body weight of approximately 23.4% (range 14%-52%) can be achieved within the first 1 to 2 years, with a modulation to 16.1% after 10 years as patients often experience weight regain after surgical procedures.[51] The extent of weight loss and the potential for weight regain after bariatric surgery is multifactorial as metabolic, anatomic, and lifestyle changes can all impact the outcome of the procedure. Improvements in the peri- and postoperative care of gastric surgery patients have reduced morbidity and mortality associated with bariatric surgeries. The operative 30-day mortality rates reported range from 0.1% to 1.2%, depending on the type of procedure.[51] Some of the most common early surgical complications are gastric and anastomotic leaks, bleeding, wound infections, and pulmonary emboli. Due to the disruption of the normal gastric anatomy and physiology, postsurgical patients are often at risk for severe micronutrient deficiencies such as vitamin B_{12} and anemia.[52] Therefore, empiric supplementation with daily adult multivitamin plus minerals, elemental calcium, vitamin D, folic acid, thiamine, elemental iron, and vitamin B_{12} is essential to prevent nutritional deficiencies in bariatric patients.[50] All bariatric surgical patients should undergo routine and nutritional monitoring after the procedure. Weight losses resulting from bariatric surgery are often accompanied by dramatic improvements, and sometimes complete resolution, of many obesity-related complications.[51,53] Significant reduction in risks of stroke, myocardial infarction, cardiovascular deaths, as well as the incidence of type 2 diabetes and cancer (in women), have also been documented after bariatric surgery.[53-57] Furthermore, a significant 52% reduction in mortality for patients who underwent bariatric surgery compared with those who did not receive any surgical intervention has been noted.[54]

After experiencing weight loss, many gastric surgery patients are able to discontinue pharmacotherapy for glucose lowering, dyslipidemia, hypertension[50] and reduce medication costs.[55] However, the need for use of proton-pump inhibitors or H_2-receptor antagonists are often increased.[52] It is imperative for clinicians to recognize that bariatric interventions not only alter nutrient absorption but also may impede drug absorption and can cause potential serious consequences.[52,58]

Achlorhydria, reduced surface area for intestinal and gastric absorption, and alterations in drug metabolism via the intestinal metabolic pathways (eg, cytochrome P450 enzymes or efflux transporters) after bariatric surgery can lead to altered dissolution and/or absorption of many medications. Reduced bioavailability has been reported for some antimicrobials, immunosuppressives, anticonvulsants, highly lipophilic tricyclic antidepressants, SSRIs, and levothyroxine.[52] Furthermore, concurrent administration of proton-pump inhibitors may also alter bioavailability of weak basic drugs such as antifungals (eg, ketoconazole), certain antibiotics and some cardiovascular medications (eg, digoxin) as well as hinder the absorption of micronutrients.[52] Therefore, clinicians need to recognize that the standard dosage regimens recommended for presurgical patients may need to be adjusted. Close therapeutic monitoring of all orally administered medications after surgery, particularly those with narrow therapeutic ranges, is highly recommended because dosage form selection, dose conversion, or therapeutic interchange may be necessary to avoid or minimize absorption problems and ensure optimal patient outcomes.

Pharmacologic Therapy

6 and 7 The debate regarding the appropriateness of obesity pharmacotherapy remains heated, fueled by the recognized national need to treat a growing epidemic and the medical and litigious fallout from the adverse effects of medications which were ultimately withdrawn from the US market (ie, fenfluramine [Pondomin], dexfenfluramine [Redux], and sibutramine [Meridia]). Strategies for the pharmacologic management of obesity have historically focused on modulating central or peripheral sites that regulate energy balance. Long-term pharmacotherapy may have a place in the treatment of obesity for patients who have no obvious contraindications to approved drug therapy, as the likelihood of weight regain after treatment discontinuation is quite high.[59] According to current guidelines, pharmacotherapy is an adjunct to comprehensive lifestyle intervention in adults who are motivated to lose weight, have failed to achieve or sustain weight loss with lifestyle changes alone, and have a BMI more than or equal to 30 kg/m^2 or a BMI more than or equal to 27 kg/m^2 with at least one weigh-related comorbidity (Graded as a strong recommendation with high quality evidence).[35] Furthermore, patients who meet the BMI requirements and have a history of failed attempts to lose weight or maintain weight loss with comprehensive lifestyle intervention alone may also be candidates for pharmacotherapy.[35] A pharmacotherapy treatment algorithm based on these treatment guidelines is depicted in Fig. 144-3. Table 144-4 lists the status of the most common classes of agents currently available.

A multidisciplinary team approach to the management of obesity is necessary to ensure long-term success. It is common for patients to use a combination of nonprescription, prescription, and other complementary and alternative therapies to attain the desired weight loss goal. Therefore, clinicians should maintain a high degree of sensitivity toward the potential polypharmacy practices of patients with obesity. Finally, it is prudent to consider specific patient factors and characteristics along with the efficacy and safety profiles of individual therapies when determining if use of a pharmacologic intervention is warranted.

Agents Approved for Long-Term Use

8 There are currently five products approved in the United States for the chronic management of obesity. These include the lipase inhibitor orlistat (Xenical, Genentech USA, South San Francisco, CA; Alli, GlaxoSmithKline, Middlesex, UK), the serotonin 2C receptor agonist lorcaserin (Belviq, Arena Pharmaceuticals GmbH, Zofingen, Switzerland), the combination product phentermine–topiramate extended release (Qsymia, Vivus, Inc, Mountain View, CA), the combination product naltrexone-bupropion extended-release tablets (Contrave, Takeda Pharmaceuticals America Inc, Deerfield, IL), and the GLP-1 receptor agonist liraglutide (Saxenda, Novo Nordisk Inc, Plainsboro, NJ). Pharmacotherapy management guidelines recommend discontinuation of drug therapy in patients who fail to lose sufficient amounts of body weight after 3 months and in patients who experience significant adverse events, with consideration given to potential alternative weight loss agents (strong recommendation with high-quality evidence).[35] Table 144-6 lists clinical and economic considerations for use of the products approved for long-term use.[35,59]

Clinical **Controversy...**

Obesity is considered a chronic disease. None of the FDA-approved agents for obesity has been shown to have cardiovascular benefit, and the optimal treatment duration remains unknown. Because discontinuation of drug treatment tends to result in weight regain, continuation of an effective and well-tolerated drug regimen is common practice.

Lipase Inhibitor: Orlistat Excessive intake of dietary fat is one of the contributing factors in the development of obesity. GI (gastric, pancreatic, and carboxyl ester) lipases are essential in the absorption of the long-chain triglycerides. Additionally, lipase is known to play a role in facilitating gastric emptying and secretion of other pancreaticobiliary substances. Orlistat (Xenical) is a synthetic derivative of lipstatin, a natural lipase inhibitor produced by *Streptomyces toxytricini*. The drug is minimally absorbed and induces weight loss by persistent lowering of dietary fat absorption through selective inhibition of the GI lipase. Furthermore, lower luminal free fatty acid concentrations result in malabsorption of cholesterol. Up to 30% reduction in fat absorption occurred with daily doses of 120 mg three times daily with meals.[59] A nonprescription formulation of orlistat (Alli) is approved in the United States at a reduced daily dose of 60 mg three times daily.[59] The drug must be taken within 1 hour of consuming foods that contain fat in order to exert its effect. If a meal is skipped or contains no fat, the dose of orlistat can be omitted.

Clinical studies using orlistat as an adjunct to diet therapy demonstrate dose-dependent reductions in fat absorption. Overall, results from clinical trials demonstrate that orlistat modestly increases the amount of weight lost and decreases the amount of weight regained during medically supervised weight loss programs.[59,60] The longest trial that evaluated the safety and efficacy of orlistat is XENDOS (XENical in the prevention of Diabetes in Obese Subjects), a 4-year, double-blind, randomized, placebo-controlled prospective study.[61] Although weight regain was observed with continual therapy beyond the first year of orlistat therapy, results from this study show moderate weight loss sustained after 4 years of treatment compared with placebo, 12.8 lb (5.8 kg) and 6.6 lb (3.0 kg), respectively. Weight loss using orlistat also decreased the rate of development of type 2 diabetes by 37.3% in patients with impaired glucose tolerance. Improved glycemic control can be attained in patients with type 2 diabetes by inducing or increasing weight loss with orlistat in addition to diet management.[59,60] In some cases, dosages or the number of antidiabetic medications may be reduced or discontinued.[60] Significant improvements in lipid profile (reduction in total and low-density lipoprotein [LDL] cholesterol), glucose control, and other markers of metabolism are seen when using orlistat in addition to the diet.[59,60] Orlistat is approved for the chronic treatment of obesity in adults and adolescents between ages 12 abd 16 years. The recommended dose is 120 mg three times daily taken within 1 hour of consuming a fat-containing meal.

At least one GI complaint (soft stools, abdominal pain or colic, flatulence, fecal urgency, or incontinence) has been reported in up to

TABLE 144-4 FDA-Approved Pharmacotherapeutic Agents for Weight Loss

Drug	Brand Name	Initial Dose	Usual Range	Special Population Dose	Comment
Gastrointestinal Lipase Inhibitor					
Orlistat	Xenical	120 mg three times daily with each main meal containing fat	120 mg three times daily with each main meal containing fat		Approved for long-term use Take during or up to 1 hour after the meal Omit dose if meal is occasionally missed or contains no fat
Orlistat	Alli[a]	60 mg three times daily with each main meal containing fat	60 mg three times daily with each main meal containing fat		Same as Xenical
Serotonin 2C Receptor Agonist					
Lorcaserin	Belviq	10 mg twice daily	10 mg twice daily	Use with caution in moderate renal impairment and severe hepatic impairment; not recommended in patients with end state renal disease	Approved for long-term use Controlled substance: C–IV
Phentermine–Topiramate Combination					
Phentermine and topiramate extended release	Qsymia	3.75 mg of phentermine and 23 mg of topiramate once daily for 14 days; then increase to 7.5 mg of phentermine and 46 mg of topiramate once daily	7.5 mg of phentermine and 46 mg of topiramate once daily to a maximum dose of phentermine 15 mg and topiramate 92 mg once daily	Maximum dose for patients with moderate or severe renal impairment or patients with moderate hepatic impairment is 7.5 mg of phentermine and 46 mg of topiramate	Approved for long-term use Take dose in the morning to avoid insomnia Controlled substance: C–IV
Naltrexone-Bupropion Combination					
Bupropion and naltrexone extended release	Contrave	8 mg naltrexone/90 mg bupropion (1 tablet) once daily in the morning for 1 week; then 8 mg naltrexone/90 mg bupropion twice daily (morning and evening) for 1 week; then 16 mg naltrexone/180 mg bupropion in the morning and 8 mg naltrexone/ 90 mg bupropion in the evening for 1 week; then 16 mg naltrexone/180 mg bupropion twice daily (morning and evening)	16 mg naltrexone and 180 mg bupropion (2 tablets) twice daily	Maximum dose for patients with moderate or severe renal impairment is 8 mg naltrexone/90 mg bupropion (1 tablet) twice daily Maximum dose for patients with hepatic impairment is 8 mg naltrexone/90 mg bupropion (1 tablet) once daily in the morning	Approved for long-term use Do not take dose with high-fat meal
Glucagon-Like Peptide-1 Antagonist					
Liraglutide	Saxenda	0.6 mg once daily for 1 week 1.2 mg once daily for 1 week 1.8 mg once daily for 1 week 2.4 mg once daily for 1 week 3.0 mg once daily for 1 week * administered by subcutaneous injection	3 mg once daily	Use with caution in mild, moderate, and severe renal and hepatic impairment	Approved for long-term use Inject subcutaneously in the abdomen, thigh, or upper arm Administer at any time of day without regard to the timing of meals
Noradrenergic Agents					
Phendimetrazine	Bontril PDM; Bontril Slow-Release	Conventional tablet: start at 17.5 mg two or three times daily, given 1 hour before meals Extended-release capsule: 105 mg once daily 30-60 minutes before morning meal	70-105 mg/day	Use caution in patients with renal impairment	Approved for short-term monotherapy Controlled substance: C–III Prescriptions should be written for the smallest quantity to minimize possibility of overdose
Phentermine	Adipex-P, Suprenza	Orally disintegrating tablet: 15 or 30 mg once every morning Phentermine hydrochloride: 15-37.5 mg/day given in one or two divided doses; administer before breakfast or 1-2 hours after breakfast	Orally disintegrating tablet: 15 or 30 mg once every morning Phentermine hydrochloride: 15-37.5 mg/day given in one or two divided doses; administer before breakfast or 1-2 hours after breakfast	Use with caution in patients with renal impairment	Approved for short-term monotherapy Controlled substance: C–IV Prescriptions should be written for the smallest quantity to minimize possibility of overdose Individualize to achieve adequate response with lowest effective dose

(continued)

TABLE 144-4 FDA-Approved Pharmacotherapeutic Agents for Weight Loss (*Continued*)

Drug	Brand Name	Initial Dose	Usual Range	Special Population Dose	Comment
Diethylpropion	Tenuate, Tenuate Dospan	Immediate release: 25 mg three times daily administered 1 hour before meals Controlled release: 75 mg once daily administered at midmorning	75 mg/day	Use with caution in patients with renal impairment	Approved for short-term monotherapy Dose should not be administered in the evening or at bedtime Controlled substance: C–IV

[a]Available without a prescription.

80% of individuals using prescription-strength orlistat. These complaints are most common in the first 1 to 2 months of therapy, are mild to moderate in severity, and tend to improve with continued orlistat use. Limiting dietary fat before initiation of orlistat therapy may be beneficial in decreasing initial GI complaints. Severe diarrhea secondary to orlistat use can affect the absorption of orally administered drugs, such as oral contraceptives, fat-soluble vitamins (A, D, E, and K), and β-carotene.[60] Therefore, supplementation with a multivitamin should be considered during therapy. In the presence of severe diarrhea, women receiving oral contraceptives should be advised of the need to use alternative backup methods because absorption of oral contraceptive may be reduced.[60] Although orlistat does not appear to alter the pharmacokinetic profiles of other agents, including digoxin, glyburide, metformin, phenytoin, fluoxetine, amitriptyline, phentermine, losartan, nifedipine, captopril, atenolol, furosemide, alcohol, or atorvastatin, reduced fat absorption can potentially affect the absorption of lipophilic drugs, such as lamotrigine, valproic acid, gabapentin, and amiodarone.[62,63] Decreased vitamin K absorption has also been noted and can alter the patient's warfarin dosage needs. Clinicians should also be aware that orlistat may directly interfere with the absorption of other narrow therapeutic range drugs, such as cyclosporine and levothyroxine.[33] In patients requiring concomitant therapies with orlistat, close monitoring is warranted to ensure an adequate therapeutic response. Separation of the administration times of the medications may minimize these potential drug interactions. Finally, there have been rare postmarketing reports of liver damage with the use of orlistat.[63] Although causality has not been definitively linked to orlistat, patients are advised to notify their healthcare providers if they notice signs and symptoms of liver injury, such as development of itching, yellow eyes or skin, dark urine, loss of appetite, or light-colored stools.

Serotonin Receptor Agonist Lorcaserin (Belviq) is a selective serotonin (5-HT_{2C}) receptor agonist, approved for chronic weight management in patients who are obese (BMI of greater than or equal to 30 kg/m^2) or overweight (BMI of greater than 27 kg/m^2) with at least one weight-related comorbidity.[64] At the recommended dose of 10 mg twice daily, lorcaserin selectively activates central 5-HT_{2C} receptors on hypothalamic anorexigenic pro-opiomelanocortin neurons. Activation of central 5-HT_{2C} receptors results in appetite suppression, leading to reduced energy intake and enhanced satiety.

Clinical trials evaluating the efficacy of loracaserin, used in combination with a LCD and exercise counseling, have reported a modest but significantly greater weight loss compared with placebo.[65,66] The Behavioral Modification and Lorcaserin for Overweight and Obesity Management (BLOOM) trial was a 2-year, randomized, placebo-controlled, double-blind, prospective trial that enrolled more than 3,000 obese and overweight patients.[65] Mean weight loss at 1 year was 5.8 kg (12.8 lb) in the lorcaserin group compared with 2.2 kg (4.8 lb) in the placebo group. Patients in the lorcaserin-treated group also experienced significant improvements in fasting glucose, insulin, total cholesterol, LDL cholesterol, and triglyceride concentrations at the end of the first year. Although weight regain was observed during the second year of the trial, 68% of the

TABLE 144-5 Clinical and Economic Considerations for Long-Term Pharmacotherapy Options

Drug	Brand Name	Weight Loss Above Diet and Exercise Alone (1 year)[35,59,73]	Cost for 30 days of Therapy[a]	Comments[35]
Orlistat	Xenical	2.9-3.4 kg (6.5-7.5 lb)	$512.11	—Use may be limited by GI intolerance —Suggested for patients with cardiovascular disease (The Endocrine Society; weak recommendation with low quality evidence)
Lorcaserin	Belviq	3.6 kg (7.9 lb)	$199.50	—Increased risk of serotonin syndrome if used in combination with other serotonergic and dopaminergic drugs —Suggested for use in patients with cardiovascular disease (The Endocrine Society; weak recommendation with low quality evidence)
Phentermine and topiramate extended release	Qsymia	6.6-8.6 kg (14.5-18.9 lb)	$186.00- 7.5 mg-46 mg $199.50- 15 mg-92 mg	—Limited distribution under FDA Risk Evaluation Mitigation Strategy (REMS)
Bupropion and naltrexone extended release	Contrave	4.9 kg (10.8 lb)	$199.50	—Lowers seizure threshold (bupropion) —Rare reports of hepatotoxicity (naltrexone) —Drug interactions with opioids, CYP2B6 inducers and CYP2D6 substrates
Liraglutide	Saxenda	5.8 kg (12.8 lb)	$1,068.00	—Injectable —Reduces HbA1c and fasting glucose —Risk of medullary thyroid carcinoma and Multiple Endocrine Neoplasia syndrome type 2 —Rare reports of pancreatitis, gall bladder disease, and suicidal ideation

[a]Cost of therapy based on maintenance dose using wholesaler acquisition cost (WAC) as of August 24, 2015.

TABLE 144-6 Drug Monitoring

Drug	Brand Name	Adverse Reactions	Monitoring Parameters	Comments
Gastrointestinal Lipase Inhibitor				
Orlistat	Xenical, Alli[a]	Soft stools, diarrhea, abdominal pain or colic, flatulence, fecal urgency, incontinence, liver damage (rare)	BMI; calorie and fat intake; serum glucose in patients with diabetes; thyroid function in patients with thyroid disease; liver function tests in patients exhibiting symptoms of hepatic dysfunction	Supplement with a multivitamin during therapy to prevent vitamin deficiency
Serotonin 2C Receptor Agonist				
Lorcaserin	Belviq	Headache, dizziness, fatigue, nausea, dry mouth, constipation, hypoglycemia in patients with diabetes, psychiatric disorders, priapism, elevated serum prolactin level	BMI; calorie and fat intake; serum glucose in patients with diabetes; complete blood count, depression or suicidal thoughts; signs or symptoms of serotonin syndrome; signs or symptoms of valvular heart disease	Discontinue if 5% weight loss not achieved by week 12
Phentermine–Topiramate Combination				
Phentermine and topiramate extended release	Qsymia	Constipation, dry mouth, paraesthesia, dysgeusia, insomnia, hypoglycemia in patients with diabetes	BMI; calorie and fat intake; serum glucose in patients with diabetes; pregnancy; depression or suicidal thoughts; mood or sleep disorders; heart rate; serum electrolytes and creatinine at baseline and during treatment	Discontinue or escalate dose if 3% weight loss not achieved by week 12 on phentermine 7.5 mg and topiramate 46 mg Discontinue if 5% weight loss not achieved by week 12 on phentermine 15 mg and topiramate 92 mg Gradually discontinue phentermine 15 mg and topiramate 92 mg to prevent possible seizure
Bupropion-Naltrexone Combination				
Bupropion and naltrexone extended release	Contrave	Nausea, constipation, headache, vomiting, dizziness, insomnia, dry mouth and diarrhea	BMI; calorie and fat intake; serum glucose in patients with diabetes; heart rate and blood pressure; signs and symptoms of hepatotoxicity, neuropsychiatric reactions, and suicidal thoughts or behavior	Discontinue if 5% weight loss not achieved by week 12
Glucagon-Like Peptide-1 Antagonist				
Liraglutide	Saxenda	Nausea, diarrhea, constipation, vomiting, dyspepsia, hypoglycemia, and abdominal pain	BMI; calorie and fat intake; serum glucose in patients with diabetes; signs and symptoms of pancreatitis; heart rate; signs and symptoms of gallbladder disease and suicidal ideation	Discontinue if 4% weight loss not achieved by week 16
Noradrenergic Agents				
Phendimetrazine Phentermine Diethylpropion	Bontril PDM; Bontril Slow-Release Adipex-P, Suprenza Tenuate, Tenuate Dospan	Increased blood pressure, ischemic events, palpitations, tachycardia, valvular disease, urticaria, agitation, dizziness, headache, insomnia, overstimulation, psychosis, restlessness, dry mouth, constipation, thirst, diarrhea	Baseline cardiac evaluation (for preexisting valvular heart disease, pulmonary hypertension); echocardiogram during therapy; weight, waist circumference; blood pressure	Approved as monotherapies only for short-term use (a few weeks). Discontinue if satisfactory weight loss has not occurred within the first 4 weeks of treatment or if tolerance develops Abrupt discontinuation after prolonged high doses may be associated with extreme fatigue and depression

BMI, body mass index.

[a]Available without a prescription.

patients who had previously achieved 5% weight loss during the first year were able to maintain this level of weight loss by the end of the second year. The efficacy of lorcaserin has also been shown in patients with type 2 diabetes, with an average weight loss of 4.5% and significant improvements in HbA_{1c} and fasting glucose after 1 year of treatment.[67] Based on data from clinical trials, the approved label states that lorcaserin therapy should be discontinued if 5% weight loss not is not achieved by week 12 because it is unlikely that a benefit will be seen.[64]

The most common adverse effects associated with the use of lorcaserin in clinical trials were headache, dizziness, constipation, fatigue, and dry mouth.[65] Previous serotonergic agents (eg, dexfenfluramine) used for weight loss have been associated with cardiac valvulopathy.[62,68] The mechanism for this toxicity is thought to be related to stimulation of $5HT_{2B}$ receptors on cardiac cells. At therapeutic doses, lorcaserin is selective for central $5HT_{2C}$ receptors. During clinical trials, the incidence of cardiac valvulopathy was not significantly different between patients who received lorcaserin (2.4%) and those who received placebo (2%).[64] However, patients should be counseled to contact their healthcare providers if they experience signs or symptoms of cardiac valve disease such as dyspnea or edema. Lorcaserin should not be used in combination with other serotonergic and dopaminergic drugs because of the increased risk of serotonin syndrome or neuroleptic malignant syndrome–like reactions. Lorcaserin should be used cautiously in patients with congestive heart failure because these patients may be at an increased risk for cardiac valvulopathy. Additional rare adverse effects that clinicians should be aware of include psychiatric disorders, priapism, and elevated serum prolactin concentrations. Lorcaserin is classified as a controlled substance in class IV due to potential for abuse.

Phentermine–Topiramate Extended Release A combination product containing phentermine and topiramate extended release (Qsymia) is approved for chronic weight management in patients who are obese (BMI of greater than or equal to 30 kg/m^2) or overweight (BMI of greater than 27 kg/m^2) with at least one weight-related comorbidity.[69] Phentermine is structurally similar to amphetamine, but it has less severe CNS stimulation and a lower abuse potential. Its mechanism of action centers on its ability to enhance norepinephrine (NE) and dopamine neurotransmission, resulting in appetite suppressing effects. Topiramate is an antiepileptic drug. Although the exact mechanism for its efficacy in weight management is not known, it may decrease appetite and increase satiety through multiple pathways, including effects on γ-aminobutyrate, voltage-gated ion channels, excitatory glutamate receptors, or carbonic anhydrase.[69] The doses of phentermine (3.75-15 mg) and topiramate (23-92 mg) in this combination are significantly lower than the therapeutic doses of each separate product when used as monotherapy for obesity (37.5 mg) and epilepsy (400 mg), respectively. The recommended dosing strategy for phentermine–topiramate extended release involves gradual titration, staring with 3.75 mg of phentermine and 23 mg of topiramate once daily for 14 days and then increasing the dose to 7.5 mg of phentermine and 46 mg of topiramate once daily.[69] After 12 weeks of therapy, the dose may be increased again to 11.25 mg of phentermine and 69 mg of topiramate for 14 days and then to a maximum dose of 15 mg of phentermine and 92 mg of topiramate daily. Likewise, when discontinuing therapy, the dose should be gradually decreased by taking a dose every other day for at least 1 week to prevent the possible precipitation of seizures.

Clinical trials evaluating the efficacy of phentermine–topiramate, when used as an adjunct to a reduced-calorie diet and lifestyle changes, have reported dose-dependent weight loss and significant reductions in blood pressure, total cholesterol, LDL cholesterol, triglycerides, fasting glucose, and HbA$_{1c}$.[70,71] The CONQUER trial was a randomized, placebo-controlled, double-blind, prospective trial of 2,487 overweight or obese patients with two or more obesity-related comorbidities.[70] After a 4-week dose titration phase, subjects were randomized to receive (a) placebo, (b) 7.5 mg of phentermine with 46 mg of topiramate, or (c) 15 mg of phentermine with 92 mg of topiramate daily. Weight loss at 1 year was significantly greater than placebo in both of the treatment groups, with a mean weight loss of 8.1 kg (17.8 lb) in the 7.5-mg phentermine and 46-mg topiramate group and a mean weight loss of 10.2 kg (22.4 lb) in the 15-mg phentermine and 92-mg topiramate group. The efficacy of phentermine–topiramate has also been documented in patients with class II and class III obesity (mean BMI, 42 kg/m^2), with a reported mean weight loss of 10.9% after 1 year of treatment.[71]

The most common adverse effects associated with the use of phentermine–topiramate in clinical trials were constipation, dry mouth, paraesthesia, dysgeusia, and insomnia.[70,71] Because topiramate is a known teratogen, this drug is contraindicated in pregnancy because fetal exposure in the first trimester increases the risk of cleft lip or cleft palate. To manage the potential risk of teratogenicity, the drug is only available through a limited distribution process under a risk evaluation and mitigation strategy (REMS).[69] All women of childbearing age must have a documented negative pregnancy test result before beginning treatment and then monthly to continue therapy. Topiramate has been associated with acute myopia associated with secondary angle-closure glaucoma, and phentermine can cause mydriasis from adrenergic stimulation. Therefore, this product is also contraindicated in patients with glaucoma. The potential for hypertensive crisis with coadministration of phentermine and MAOIs exists; therefore, patients should have stopped an MAOI for at least 14 days before use of any adrenergic agent. Phentermine–topiramate is also contraindicated in patients with untreated hyperthyroidism.

Monitoring parameters and drug interactions that clinicians should be aware of include known issues related to both components of the formulation. Of note, increases in heart rate greater than 10 beats/min were observed in approximately 50% of patients receiving phentermine–topiramate during clinical trials.[69] In patients receiving the highest dose, 19% experienced increases in heart rate that were greater than 20 beats/min. Therefore, heart rate should be monitored in all patients, particularly those with preexisting CVD. Decreases in serum bicarbonate were also noted in clinical trials, which were generally mild with peak decreases observed after 4 weeks of therapy. Decreases in serum potassium and increases in serum creatinine were also reported. Therefore, monitoring of serum electrolytes and creatinine is recommended at baseline and during therapy. Clinicians should be aware that concomitant use of non–potassium-sparing diuretics may potentiate the risk for hypokalemia. Although pregnancy risk is not expected, use of phentermine–topiramate concomitantly with oral contraceptives may result in breakthrough bleeding because of increased exposure to progestin and decreases exposure to estrogen. Phentermine–topiramate is classified as a controlled substance in schedule IV because of the abuse potential of phentermine. Similarly to lorcaserin, therapy should be discontinued if 5% weight loss is not achieved after 12 weeks.[69]

Naltrexone–Bupropion Extended Release A combination product containing naltrexone and bupropion extended release (Contrave) was approved in 2014 for chronic weight management in patients who are obese (BMI of more than or equal to 30 kg/m^2) or overweight (of more than or equal to 27 kg/m^2) with at least one weight-related comorbidity.[72] Naltrexone and bupropion are both approved separately for treatment of alcohol and opioid dependence, and depression and smoking cessation, respectively.[73] Bupropion is a dopamine and norepinephrine reuptake inhibitor, and naltrexone is an opioid antagonist. Although the exact weight-loss mechanism of action is not known for this drug combination, stimulation of release of α-MSH in hypothalamus by bupropion and inhibition of endogenous opioids by naltrexone are thought to contribute to a decrease in appetite.[73] The recommended dosing strategy for naltrexone-bupropion extended-release involves gradual titration, starting with one tablet (8-mg naltrexone/90-mg bupropion) per day and slowly increasing the dose over a period of 4 weeks to a maintenance dose of two tablets twice daily. Doses greater than 32 mg of naltrexone and 360 mg of bupropion (ie, 4 tablets) per day are not recommended. Patients should be advised to not take their dose with a high-fat meal as this would result in increased systemic exposure to both naltrexone and bupropion.

Four randomized, placebo-controlled, clinical trials evaluating the efficacy of naltrexone/bupropion, when used in combination with a reduced-calorie diet and lifestyle changes, have reported significantly more weight loss with naltrexone/bupropion compared to placebo, as well as improvements in high-density lipoprotein (HDL) cholesterol, triglycerides, glucose, and insulin.[74-77] The average total weight loss reported among the four studies was 7.3 kg (95% CI, 7.0-7.6 kg) following 1 year of treatment,[73] with the greatest amount of weight loss (9.7 kg) reported in nondiabetic subjects who were also receiving intensive behavior modification therapy.[76]

The most common adverse effects associated with the use of naltrexone/bupropion in clinical trials were nausea, constipation, headache, vomiting, dizziness, insomnia, dry mouth, and diarrhea.[72] Approximately 24% of patients who received naltrexone-bupropion in clinical trials discontinued treatment due to adverse events, with nausea being the most frequently cited reason.[72] Statistically significant increases in heart rate (2.1 beats/min) and blood pressure (1.8-2.3 mm Hg systolic and 1.7-2.1 mm Hg diastolic) were observed in patients receiving naltrexone-bupropion compared with those who received placebo during the first 3 months of therapy. Although the clinical significance of these increases is unknown, blood pressure and pulse should be monitored at baseline and at regular intervals following initiation of therapy. Naltrexone-bupropion should not be used in patients with uncontrolled hypertension.[72] Naltrexone monotherapy has been associated with rare reports of hepatotoxicity, and patients receiving naltrexone-bupropion should be advised of the signs and symptoms of acute hepatitis. Bupropion lowers the seizure threshold in a dose-dependent manner, and has been associated with serious neuropsychiatric reactions and an increased risk of suicidal thoughts and behavior when used for smoking cessation and treatment of depression. Bupropion has also been reported to cause activation of mania, serious allergic reaction, and angle-closure glaucoma.

Clinicians should also be aware of potential drug interactions with naltrexone-bupropion. Because of the opioid antagonist effects of naltrexone, naltrexone-bupropion is contraindicated in patients receiving chronic opioid or opiate agonist therapy, and also in patients undergoing abrupt withdrawal of chronic alcohol, benzodiazepine, barbiturate or antiepileptics. Bupropion is metabolized by cytochrome P450 2B6 (CYP2B6) and inhibits cytochrome P450 2D6 (CYP2D6). Therefore, any medication that induces CYP2B6 (ie, rifampin, carbamazepine, etc) could potentially reduce the effects of bupropion, and bupropion could increase the effects of medications that are CYP2D6 substrates (ie, SSRIs, tricyclic antidepressants, antipsychotics, etc). Bupropion is also contraindicated with concomitant use of MAOIs As with other long-term pharmacologic treatments for obesity, weight loss may increase the risk of hypoglycemia in patients with type 2 diabetes receiving antidiabetic medications. Finally, treatment with naltrexone-bupropion should be discontinued if 5% weight loss is not achieved after 12 weeks.

Glucagon-Like Peptide-1 Receptor Agonist Liraglutide Liraglutide (Saxenda), an analog of GLP-1, is the latest medication approved in the United States for chronic weight management in patients who are obese (BMI of more than or equal to 30 kg/m^2) or overweight (BMI of more than 27 kg/m^2) with at least one weight-related comorbidity.[78] Endogenous GLP-1 is released in response to food digestion and stimulates GLP-1 receptors in the brain to reduce appetite. GLP-1 also stimulates insulin secretion and reduces glucagon secretion. For that reason, several GLP-1 receptor agonists, including liraglutide, are currently approved for the treatment of type 2 diabetes at recommended doses of 1.2 mg or 1.8 mg daily far less than the maintenance dose for weight loss of 3 mg daily.[78] Liraglutide is administered subcutaneously and is available in prefilled, multidose pens. When used for weight loss, a 5-week dose escalation schedule is recommended to improve tolerability of GI adverse events. It should be initiated at a dose of 0.6 mg daily, and increased weekly by 0.6-mg increments to a final maintenance dose of 3 mg daily. If the patient cannot tolerate the GI adverse events at any point during the dose escalation phase, a dose increase may be delayed by a week. Patients should be instructed on the proper technique for subcutaneous injection into the abdomen, thigh, or upper arm.

The efficacy of liraglutide for the management of overweight and obesity has been studied in patients with and without diabetes.[78-80] The Satiety and Clinical Adiposity-Liraglutide Evidence in Nondiabetic and Diabetic Individuals (SCALE) Obesity and Prediabetes study was a 56-week, randomized, placebo-controlled, double-blind, prospective trial of approximately 3,700 obese and overweight patients without diabetes.[79] Mean weight loss after 1 year of treatment was 8.4 kg (18.5 lb) in the liraglutide group compared with 2.8 kg (6.1 lb) in the placebo group. As expected, patients in the liraglutide-treated group also experienced significant improvements in HbA_{1c}, fasting glucose and insulin, and had a lower prevalence of prediabetes at the end of the trial. In the SCALE Diabetes trial, 840 overweight or obese subjects with type 2 diabetes were randomized to liraglutide 3 mg daily, liraglutide 1.8 mg daily, or placebo in combination with a LCD and exercise program for 56 weeks.[80] The average weight loss after 1 year of treatment was 6.4 kg (14 lbs) for the liraglutide 3-mg group, 5 kg (11 lbs) for the liraglutide 1.8-mg group, and 2.2 kg (4.8 lbs) in the placebo group. Significant improvements in fasting glucose and the number of subjects achieving HbA_{1c} targets of less than or equal to 7% (≤ 0.07; ≤ 53 mmol/mol Hb) (69.2% vs 27.2%) and less than or equal to 6.5% (≤ 0.065; ≤48 mmol/mol Hb) (56.5% vs 15%) in the liraglutide 3-mg group compared to the placebo group.

The most common adverse effects associated with the use of liraglutide in clinical trials were nausea, diarrhea, constipation, vomiting, dyspepsia, hypoglycemia, and abdominal pain.[78-80] GI complaints are the most common reason for premature discontinuation of therapy, underscoring the importance of the slow dose-escalation schedule with initiation of therapy. Rare cases of acute pancreatitis (0.3%), potentially leading to fatal hemorrhagic or necrotizing pancreatitis, have been reported with the use of liraglutide.[78] Small increases in resting heart rate averaging 2 to 3 beats/min have been reported in clinical trials. However, in some cases increases were as high as 20 beats/min. Although the clinical significance of these increases is unknown, heart rate should be regularly monitored in all patients receiving liraglutide. Cholelithiasis (1.5%), cholecystitis (0.6%), and suicidal ideation (0.2%) have also been observed during clinical trials.[78] Liraglutide carries a boxed-warning about the risk of thyroid C-cell tumors, including medullary thyroid carcinoma (MTC), and is contraindicated in patients with a personal or family history of MTC or multiple endocrine neoplasia syndrome type 2 (MEN2). Hypoglycemia may occur when liraglutide is used in combination with other antidiabetic agents (particularly sulfonylureas and insulin) in patients with type 2 diabetes. Therefore, dose adjustments of antidiabetic medications may be necessary. Because liraglutide increases gastric emptying time, clinicians also should be aware that absorption of concomitantly administered oral medications may be altered. Liraglutide should be discontinued if weight loss of at least 4% is not achieved after 16 weeks of therapy.

Agents Approved for Short-Term Use Several noradrenergic agents are currently approved by the FDA for short-term weight loss. Because short-term therapy is not consistent with current national guidelines for the chronic management of obesity, these agents have limited clinical utility in practice.

Phentermine Phentermine is available in both immediate-release and sustained-release formulations. However, the value of sustained-release formulations is questionable based on the reported phentermine plasma half-life of 12 to 24 hours.[81] Phentermine is an effective adjunct to diet, exercise, and behavior modification for producing weight loss in excess of that seen with placebo.[81,82] Intermittent phentermine therapy appears to elicit comparable weight loss as that seen with continuous use. However, most individuals experience weight regains during therapy and generally always after discontinuing use.[81] A single dose of 30 mg once daily in the morning provides effective appetite suppression throughout the day. Divided doses of 8 mg immediately before meals, however, are common. Doses greater than 30 mg daily do not improve effectiveness.[82] Evening or nighttime dosing should be avoided because of insomnia. Significant increases in blood pressure, palpitations, and arrhythmias can occur with phentermine administration. Use is not advisable in hypertensive patients. Pharmacotherapy management guidelines recommend against the use of sympathomimetic agents in patients with uncontrolled hypertension or a history of CVD (strong recommendation with high-quality evidence).[35]

The potential for hypertensive crisis with coadministration of phentermine and MAOIs is noted in the product labeling of each agent; therefore, patients should be off an MAOI for at least 14 days before use of any adrenergic agent to avoid excessive adrenergic stimulation syndromes.[83] Phentermine use is contraindicated in patients with hyperthyroidism or agitated states and in those who are abusers of substances such as cocaine, phencyclidine, and methamphetamine, again because of the potential for excessive adrenergic stimulation syndromes and abuse potential. Mydriasis from adrenergic stimulation can worsen glaucoma, and patients diagnosed with glaucoma should not receive phentermine. Patients with diabetes may experience altered insulin or oral hypoglycemic dosage requirements soon after beginning therapy and before any substantial weight loss. Phentermine remains the most widely prescribed weight management medication by obesity specialists despite product labeling that indicates short-term (a few weeks), monotherapy use only.[81] This usage pattern deviates from the current national recommendations that promote only long-term drug intervention when obesity pharmacotherapy is appropriate.[35]

Clinical **Controversy...**

Although phentermine is only approved for short-term use, it continues to be the most widely prescribed weight loss drug in the United States. Some clinicians consider use of long-term phentermine to be reasonable in select patients given the low cost and a lack of serious long-term adverse events reported in the literature over the past 20 years. Select patients include those without evidence of CVD, psychiatric disease, or substance abuse; without clinically significant increases in blood pressure or heart rate while receiving phentermine; and documentation of significant weight loss while receiving phentermine.

Diethylpropion Diethylpropion stimulates NE release from presynaptic storage granules. Increased adrenergic neurotransmitter concentrations activate hypothalamic centers, which result in decreased appetite and food intake. This drug undergoes extensive first-pass hepatic metabolism. Active metabolites are eliminated renally and account for about 70% of the administered dose. The elimination half-life of these metabolites is about 8 hours.[82] Less than 10% of the parent compound is recovered in urine. No specific dosing recommendations exist for use in patients with renal or hepatic insufficiency. Diethylpropion can be taken in divided daily doses, generally 25 mg three times daily before meals. An extended-release formulation is also used by some clinicians, usually as 75 mg taken once daily in the morning or midmorning. Both dosing regimens are effective in achieving short-term weight loss in excess of placebo.[84] Complaints of insomnia increase if late afternoon dosing is used. Diethylpropion causes less stimulation of the CNS than mazindol and generally causes less insomnia than phentermine. Patients with severe hypertension or significant CVD should not receive diethylpropion. Patients with diabetes may experience decreased insulin or oral hypoglycemic dosage requirements soon after beginning therapy and before any substantial weight loss. More frequent blood glucose self-monitoring and medical follow-up are warranted when treating diabetic patients with diethylpropion.

Amphetamines Appetite suppressant effects of the amphetamines were well recognized in the 1930s. Amphetamines activate central noradrenergic receptor systems as well as dopaminergic pathways at higher doses by stimulating neurotransmitter release. Increases in blood pressure and mild bronchodilation are attributed to peripheral α- and β-receptor activation. Amphetamines are no longer widely used for the treatment of obesity because of their powerful stimulant effects and addictive potential.

Off-Label Use of Serotonergic Agents Serotonin is an important neurotransmitter involved in many human physiologic systems such as sleep–wake cycles, sensitivity to pain, blood pressure, mood, and eating behaviors. Increasing central serotonin levels disrupts the body's natural development of satiety by decreasing the amount of food consumed and prolongs the time between food intake.[85] Some serotonergic agents increase central serotonin concentrations via stimulating release of presynaptic stores or inhibition of reuptake into storage granules. Additionally, either the parent compound or metabolites of these agents may stimulate postsynaptic 5-HT receptors directly. Peripheral serotonin effects that have an impact on appetite, such as slowing gastric motility, have been described. A major distinction between serotonergic and noradrenergic anorexiants is that serotonergic agents lack the central stimulant effects and thus the abuse potential seen with the noradrenergic compounds.[84] Conversely, decreased wakefulness, altered sleep patterns, and changes in affect can be seen. Some of the serotonergic agents were first studied as antidepressants and when weight loss was noted in some patients, they began to be used as weight management agents. These drugs are not approved by the FDA as weight management agents and are currently not recommended for the treatment of obesity. Nonetheless, some practitioners have prescribed these agents for the treatment of obesity "off label" either alone or in combination with phentermine.

Fluoxetine is a serotonergic agent that has been prescribed as an appetite-suppressing agent. Higher doses of fluoxetine (60 mg) were generally used for weight loss as opposed to the lower doses (20 mg) frequently used for the treatment of depression. A meta-analysis of five fluoxetine trials in patients with diabetes resulted in weight loss of 4.3 kg (9.4 lb) compared with placebo over periods of up to 1 year.[86] Evidence also demonstrates sustained benefits in fasting blood glucose, HbA_{1c}, and triglycerides in patients with poor glycemic control. However, weight regain was noted to occur with discontinuation of medication.

The safety and efficacy of phentermine–serotonin reuptake inhibitor combinations is limited. A case report of adverse experiences (eg, impaired mentation, tremor, hyperreflexia, and GI symptoms) with unintentional concurrent use of phentermine and fluoxetine reinforces the need for caution by prescribers of this unapproved combination therapy.[87] Although cases of pulmonary hypertension have been reported in patients exposed to fluoxetine,[88] serious adverse effects such as cardiac valve abnormalities in excess of baseline prevalence have not been reported in relation to SSRI use for obesity therapy.[89]

Noradrenergic–Serotonergic Agents Until 2010, sibutramine was available as Meridia in the United States for long-term use for weight loss. This agent induced weight loss by decreasing appetite and maintaining or increasing thermogenesis via increasing the synaptic concentration of serotonin, NE, and dopamine through reuptake inhibition. The Sibutramine Cardiovascular OUTcomes (SCOUT) study—the first prospective trial that evaluated the potential benefits of sibutramine on cardiovascular outcomes in obese or overweight individuals with preexisting CVD, type 2 diabetes mellitus, or both, failed to provide any reassurance regarding sibutramine's safety.[90] Although individuals taking sibutramine had modest weight loss, improvement in cardiovascular outcomes was not seen. Conversely, subjects with preexisting CVD actually had an increased risk of nonfatal myocardial infarction and nonfatal stroke. Because of concerns that the effectiveness of sibutramine on weight loss is counterbalanced by increased rather than decreased cardiovascular risk, the drug was voluntarily withdrawn from the US market.

Complementary and Alternative Therapies 9 Many complementary and alternative therapy products are currently promoted for weight loss. A nationwide survey of US consumers reported that about 34% of adults reported that they had used "dietary supplements" specifically for the purposes of weight loss.[91] It is important for clinicians to be aware that the regulation of dietary supplements is less rigorous than that of prescription and over-the-counter drug products. As such, a manufacturer of a dietary supplement does not have to prove the safety or effectiveness of the product before it is marketed. Of concern, some herbal and food supplement diet agents contain pharmacologically active substances that should be used with caution or avoided in obese patients with conditions such as diabetes, hypertension, and significant CVD. In addition, many marketed products have been reported to lack consistency in labeling versus actual product content, and a number of dietary supplements have been found to contain undeclared prescription drugs.[92] Common herbal and natural products that have been used for weight loss include hoodia, green tea, citrus aurantium, fenugreek, caffeine, ephedrine, capsaicin, yohimbine, chitosan, guar gum, hydroxycitric acid, and garcina cambogia.[93,94]

PERSONALIZED PHARMACOTHERAPY

Genetic influences are estimated to contribute between 40% and 70% of the actual variance in body weight and fat distribution.[28] As such, identifying specific genes involved in the development of obesity is an area of extensive research. Several gene variants associated with the development of obesity have been identified through the use of genome-wide association studies (GWAS).[95] However, the use of personalized pharmacotherapy to treat obesity has only been documented in patients with congenital leptin deficiency.[96] This is an extremely rare condition in which administration of recombinant human leptin results in significant improvement in body weight and other associated abnormalities of leptin deficiency. Recommendations regarding how currently available medications can be individualized to maximize patient benefit are not yet available.

EVALUATION OF THERAPEUTIC OUTCOMES

The evaluation and management of a patient with obesity requires careful clinical; biochemical; and, if necessary, psychological evaluation. This evaluation should include an assessment of the patient's current medical condition and medication regimen. A multidisciplinary team including, but not limited to, a physician, nutritionist, psychologist, behavioral expert, and pharmacist should be involved in the care of obese individuals.

Monitoring the Pharmaceutical Care Plan

Assessment of patient progress should be documented frequently.[5] Each encounter should document weight, WC, BMI, blood pressure, medical history, and patient assessment of obesity medication tolerability.[5] Chronic use of obesity medications should be consistent with the approved product labeling. According to current pharmacologic management guidelines, efficacy and tolerability of the medication should be assessed monthly for the first 3 months, followed by visits every 3 months thereafter (weak recommendation with low quality evidence).[35] If the patient has failed to demonstrate weight loss or maintenance of prior weight, medication therapy should be discontinued after 3 months (strong recommendation with high quality evidence).[35] To achieve optimal weight loss, patients should be instructed about the importance of adherence to prescribed medication and lifestyle changes. The Short Form 36 (SF-36) has been used as a quality-of-life evaluation tool for obese patients undergoing programmatic weight loss. Quarterly assessments of well-being and quality of life using validated assessment tools can be helpful in objectively quantifying the effectiveness of therapy.

Patients with diabetes receiving weight loss medication require more intense medical monitoring and self-monitoring of blood glucose. Insulin therapy may need to be adjusted with the start of obesity medication therapy. Some patients with diabetes may require daily telephone contact with a healthcare provider to assist in adjusting their hypoglycemic therapy. Weekly patient visits to a healthcare setting may be necessary for 1 to 2 months until the effects of diet, exercise, and weight loss medication become more predictable. As frequent as quarterly assessment of HbA_{1c} may be appropriate in patients with type 2 diabetes who lose weight to aid in adjustment of hypoglycemic therapy. Lipid profiles can normalize or improve with weight loss. Lipid status should be assessed semi-annually or annually in patients with hyperlipidemia to determine the need for continued hyperlipidemia therapies. Weight loss also can result in normalization of blood pressure in hypertensive obese patients. Assessment of appropriateness of antihypertensive therapy should occur with each follow-up visit.

CONCLUSION

Obesity is a chronic disease with a prevalence that has increased dramatically over the past 30 years. Increased body weight is a consequence of increased energy storage resulting from an imbalance between energy intake and energy expenditure over time, which is influenced by many factors, including genetics and the environment. Nonpharmacologic therapy, including reduced caloric intake, increased physical activity, and behavioral modification, is currently the mainstay of obesity management. Drug therapy may be considered as an adjunct for patients who fail to achieve adequate weight loss with comprehensive lifestyle modifications. Currently, five products—orlistat, lorcaserin, phentermine–topiramate extended release, naltrexone-bupropion extended release, and liraglutide—are approved by the FDA for the long-term treatment of overweight and obesity. Bariatric procedures have evidence for long-term efficacy for weight reduction, but they also introduce surgical comorbidities and, for the most efficacious procedures, may cause significant nutritional deficiencies. Treatment of obesity should be individualized, considering factors such as patient desires, age, degree and duration of obesity, and the presence or absence of medical conditions both directly related to obesity and those that may have an impact on the therapeutic decisions. Regardless of the chosen treatment plan, the management of obesity is a lifelong process requiring patient support and careful monitoring for safety and efficacy.

ACKNOWLEDGMENT

This research was supported in part by the Intramural Research Program of the National Institute of Child Health and Human Development, National Institutes of Health.

ABBREVIATIONS

5-HT	5-hydroxytryptamine (serotonin)
AHEAD	Action for Health in Diabetes
BLOOM	Behavioral Modification and Lorcaserin for Overweight and Obesity Management
BMI	Body mass index
BMR	basal metabolic rate
CNS	central nervous system
CT	computed tomography
CVD	cardiovascular disease
FDA	Food and Drug Administration
GI	gastrointestinal
GLP-1	glucogen-like peptide-1
GWAS	genome-wide association studies
HbA_{1c}	hemoglobin A_{1c}
HDL	high-density lipoprotein
LCD	low-calorie diet

LDL	low-density lipoprotein
MAOI	monoamine oxidase inhibitor
MEN2	multiple endocrine neoplasia syndrome type 2
MRI	magnetic resonance imaging
MTC	medullary thyroid carcinoma
NE	norepinephrine
NHANES	National Health and Nutrition Examination Survey
NIH	National Institutes of Health
REE	resting energy expenditure
REMS	risk evaluation and mitigation strategy
SCALE	Satiety and Clinical Adiposity-Liraglutide Evidence in Nondiabetic and Diabetic Individuals
SCOUT	Sibutramine Cardiovascular OUTcomes
SF-36	Short Form 36
SNRI	serotonin-norepinephrine reuptake inhibitor
SSRI	selective serotonin reuptake inhibitor
WAGR	Wilms' tumor, aniridia, genitourinary abnormalities or gonadoblastoma, and mental retardation
WC	waist circumference
XENDOS	XENical in the prevention of Diabetes in Obese Subjects

REFERENCES

1. World Health Organization. Obesity and overweight. Fact sheet No. 311, January 2015. Available at: http://www.who.int/mediacentre/factsheets/fs311/en/. Last accessed August 18, 2015.
2. Yang L, Colditz GA. Prevalence of Overweight and Obesity in the United States, 2007-2012. *JAMA Intern Med* 2015;175(8):1412-1413.
3. Ogden CL, Carroll MD, Kit BK, Flegal KM. Prevalence of childhood and adult obesity in the United States, 2011-2012. *JAMA* 2014;311(8):806-814.
4. U.S. Department of Health and Human Services. National Heart Lung and Blood Institute. Obesity Initiative Expert Panel on the Identification, Evaluation, and Treatment of Overweight and Obesity in Adults. Washington, DC: U.S. Public Health Service, 1998.
5. Jensen MD, Ryan DH, Apovian CM, et al. 2013 AHA/ACC/TOS Guideline for the Management of overweight and Obesity in adults: a report of the American College of Cardiology/American Heart Association Task Force on Practice Guidelines and The Obesity Society. *Circulation* 2014;129 (Suppl 2):S102-S138.
6. National Heart, Lung, and Blood Institute. Managing Overweight and Obesity in Adults: Systemic Review From the Obesity Expert Panel, 2013. Available at http://www.nhlbi.nih.gov/sites/www.nhlbi.nih.gov/files/obesity-evidence-review.pdf Last accessed August 19, 2015.
7. Lavie CJ, Milani RV, Ventura HO. Obesity and cardiovascular disease: Risk factor, paradox, and impact of weight loss. *J Am Coll Cardiol* 2009;53(21):1925-1932.
8. Anandacoomarasamy A, Caterson I, Sambrook P, Fransen M, March L. The impact of obesity on the musculoskeletal system. *Int J Obes* 2008;32(2):211-222.
9. Kolotkin RL 1, Zunker C, Østbye T. Sexual functioning and obesity: A review. *Obesity (Silver Spring)* 2012 Dec;20(12):2325-2333.
10. Keum N, Greenwood DC, Lee DH, et al. Adult weight gain and adiposity-related cancers: A dose-response meta-analysis of prospective observational studies. *J Natl Cancer Inst* 2015;107(2).
11. Kushner RF, Roth JL. Assessment of the obese patient. *Endocrinol Metab Clin North Am* 2003;32(4):915-933.
12. Ueda H, Yagi T, Amitani H, et al. The roles of salivary secretion, brain-gut peptides, and oral hygiene in obesity. *Obes Res and Clin Prac* 2013;7:e321-e329.
13. Murugan AT, Sharma G. Obesity and respiratory diseases. *Chron Respir Dis* 2008;5(4):233-242.
14. Naguib MT. Kidney disease in the obese patient. *South Med J* 2014 Aug;107(8):481-485.
15. Bhaskaran K, Douglas I, Forbes H, et al. Body-mass index and risk of 22 specific cancers: A population-based cohort study of 5·24 million UK adults. *Lancet* 2014;384(9945):755-765.
16. Tobin AM, Ahern T, Rogers S, Collins P, O'Shea D, Kirby B. The dermatological consequences of obesity. *Int J Dermatol* 2013;52(8):927-932.
17. Stothard KJ, Tennant PW, Bell R, Rankin J. Maternal overweight and obesity and the risk of congenital anomalies: A systematic review and meta-analysis. *JAMA* 2009;301(6):636-650.
18. Segula D. Complications of obesity in adults: a short review of the literature. *Malawi Med J* 2014;26(1):20-24.
19. Reis JP, Macera CA, Araneta MR, Lindsay SP, Marshall SJ, Wingard DL. Comparison of overall obesity and body fat distribution in predicting risk of mortality. *Obesity* 2009;17(6):1232-1239.
20. Trogdon JG, Finkelstein EA, Feagan CW, Cohen JW. State- and payer-specific estimates of annual medical expenditures attributable to obesity. *Obesity* 2012;20(1):214-220.
21. Whitlock EP, O'Connor E, Williams SB, Beil TL, Lutz KW. *Effectiveness of Weight Management in Children and Adolescents*. Rockville, MD: Agency for Healthcare Research and Quality; 2008. AHRQ Publication 08-E014, Evidence Report/Technology Assessment 170. Available at: http://www.ahrq.gov/research/findings/evidence-based-reports/chwght-evidence-report.pdf. Last accessed August 18, 2015.
22. Ryan D, Heaner M. Guidelines (2013) for managing overweight and obesity in adults. Preface to the full report. *Obesity* 2014;22 Suppl 2:S1-3.
23. World Health Organization. Resolutions and decisions. Sixty-sixth World Health Assembly, May 20-27, 2013. WHA66/2013/REC/1. Geneva: World Health Organizations, 2013.
24. Moyer VA. Screening for and management of obesity in adults: US Preventative Services Task Force Recommendation Statement. *Ann Intern Med* 2012;157(5):373-378.
25. Ogden CL, Yanovski SZ, Carroll MD, Flegal KM. The epidemiology of obesity. *Gastroenterology* 2007;132(6):2087-2102.
26. Reilly JJ, Kelly J. Long-term impact of overweight and obesity in childhood and adolescence on morbidity and premature mortality in adulthood: Systematic review. *Int J Obes* 2011;35(7):891-898.
27. Robinson WR, Gordon-Larsen P, Kaufman JS, Suchindran CM, Stevens J. The female-male disparity in obesity prevalence among black American young adults: Contributions of sociodemographic characteristics of the childhood family. *Am J Clin Nutr* 2009;89(4):1204-1212.
28. Waalen J. The genetics of human obesity. *Transl Res* 2014;164:293-301.
29. Huneault L, Mathieu ME, Tremblay A. Globalization and modernization: an obesogenic combination. *Obes Rev* 2011;12(5):64-72.
30. Berthoud HR. The neurobiology of food intake in an obesogenic environment. *Pro Nutr Soc* 2012;71(4):478-487.
31. Christakis NA, Fowler JH. The spread of obesity in a large social network over 32 years. *N Engl J Med* 2007;357(4):370-379.
32. Domecq JP, Prutsky G, Leppin A, et al. Clinical review: drugs commonly associated with weight change: a systematic review and meta-analysis. *J Clin Endocrinol Metab* 2015;100(2):363-370.
33. Schneeberger M, Gomis R, Claret M. Hypothalamic and brainstem neuronal circuits controlling homeostatic energy balance. *J Endocrinol* 2014;220:T25-T46.
34. Camilleri M. Peripheral mechanism in appetite regulation. *Gastroenterology* 2015;148:1219-1233.
35. Apovian CM, Aronne LJ, Bessesen DH, et al. Pharmacological Management of Obesity: An Endocrine Society Clinical Practice Guideline. *J Clin Endocrinol Metab* 2015;100:342-362.
36. Sidossis L, Kajimura S. Brown and beige fat in humans: thermogenic adipocytes that control energy and glucose homeostasis. *J Clin Invest* 2015;125(2):478-486.
37. Clinical guidelines on the identification, evaluation, and treatment of overweight and obesity in adults: The Evidence Report. National Institutes of Health. *Obes Res* 1998;6(Suppl 2):51S-209S.
38. August GP, Caprio S, Fennoy I, et al. Prevention and treatment of pediatric obesity: an endocrine society clinical practice guideline based on expert opinion. *Clin Endocrinol Metab* 2008;93(12):4576-4599.
39. Wulan SN, Westerterp KR, Plasqui G. Ethnic differences in body composition and the associated metabolic profile: a comparative study between Asians and Caucasians. *Maturitas* 2010;65(4):315-319.
40. Conway JM, Yanovski SZ, Avila NA, Hubbard VS. Visceral adipose tissue differences in black and white women. *Am J Clin Nutr* 1995;61:765-771.
41. Finkelstein EA, Brown DS, Wrage LA, Allaire BT, Hoerger TJ. Individual and aggregate years-of-life-lost associated with overweight and obesity. *Obesity* 2010;18(2):333-339.
42. Center for Disease Control and Prevention. Overweight and Obesity: Strategies to take actions for me. Available at: http://www.cdc.gov/obesity/strategies/me.html. Last accessed, August 20, 2015.
43. Look AHEAD Research Group. Cardiovascular effects of intensive lifestyle intervention in type 2 diabetes. *N Engl J Med* 2013;369(2):145-54.

44. Franz MJ, Boucher JL, Rutten-Ramos S, VanWormer JJ. Lifestyle Weight-Loss Intervention Outcomes in Overweight and Obese Adults with Type 2 Diabetes: A Systematic Review and Meta-Analysis of Randomized Clinical Trials. *J Acad Nutr Diet* 2015;S2212-2672(15): 00259-2. doi: 10.1016/j.jand.2015.02.031.
45. Johnston BC, Kanters S, Bandayrel K, et al. Comparison of weight loss among named diet programs in overweight and obese adults: a meta-analysis. *JAMA* 2014;312(9):923-933.
46. Shaw K, Gennat H, O'Rourke P, Del Mar C. Exercise for overweight or obesity. *Cochrane Database Syst Rev* 2006;(4):CD003817.
47. Shikora S, Toouli J, Herrera MF, et al. Vagal blocking improves glycemic control and elevated blood pressure in obese subjects with type 2 diabetes mellitus. *J Obes* 2013;2013:245683.
48. Ikramuddin S, Blackstone RP, Brancatisano A, et al. Effect of reversible intermittent intra-abdominal vagal nerve blockade on morbid obesity. *JAMA* 2014;32:915-922.
49. ReShape™ Medical product labeling. San Clemente, California: Reshape Medical, Inc.; August 2015.
50. Mechanick JI, Youdim A, Jones DB, et al. American Association of Clinical Endocrinologists, the Obesity Society, and American Society for Metabolic and Bariatric Surgery. Clinical practice guidelines for the perioperative nutritional, metabolic, and nonsurgical support of the bariatric surgery patient--2013 update. *Endocr Prac.* 2013;19(2):337-72.
51. Piché MÈ, Auclair A, Harvey J, Marceau S, Poirier P. How to choose and use bariatric surgery in 2015. *Can J Cardiol* 2015;31(2):153-166.
52. Stein J, Stier C, Raab H, Weiner R. Review article: The nutritional and pharmacological consequences of obesity surgery. *Aliment Pharmacol Ther* 2014;40(6):582-609.
53. Svane MS, Madsbad S. Bariatric surgery - Effects on obesity and related co-morbidities. *Curr Diabetes Rev* 2014;10(3):208-214.
54. Kwok CS, Pradhan A, Khan MA, et al. Bariatric surgery and its impact on cardiovascular disease and mortality: A systematic review and meta-analysis. *Int J Cardiol* 2014;173(1):20-28.
55. Courcoulas AP, Yanovski SZ, Bonds D, et al. Long-term outcomes of bariatric surgery: A National Institutes of Health symposium. *JAMA Surg.* 2014;149(12):1323-1329.
56. Sjöström L. Review of the key results from the Swedish Obese Subjects (SOS) trial - a prospective controlled intervention study of bariatric surgery. *J Intern Med.* 2013;273(3):219-234.
57. Halperin F, Ding SA, Simonson DC, et al. Roux-en-Y gastric bypass surgery or lifestyle with intensive medical management in patients with type 2 diabetes: feasibility and 1-year results of a randomized clinical trial. *JAMA Surg* 2014;149(7):716-726.
58. Padwal R, Brocks D, Sharma AM. A systematic review of drug absorption following bariatric surgery and its theoretical implications. *Obes Rev* 2010;11(1):41-50.
59. Yanovski SZ, Yanovski JA. Long-term drug treatment for obesity: A systematic and clinical review. *JAMA* 2014;311(1):74-86.
60. McClendon KS, Riche DM, Uwaifo GI. Orlistat: Current status in clinical therapeutics. *Expert Opin Drug Saf* 2009;8(6):727-744.
61. Torgerson JS, Hauptman J, Boldrin MN, Sjostrom L. XENical in the prevention of diabetes in obese subjects (XENDOS) study: A randomized study of orlistat as an adjunct to lifestyle changes for the prevention of type 2 diabetes in obese patients. *Diabetes Care* 2004;27(1):155-161.
62. Halpern B, Halpern A. Safety assessment of FDA-approved (orlistat and lorcaserin) antiobesity medications. *Expert Opin Drug Saf* 2015;14(2): 185-189.
63. Xenical® [package insert]. South San Francisco, CA: Genetech USA, Inc., 2015.
64. Belviq® [package insert]. Zofingen, Switzerland: Arena Pharmaceuticals, 2014.
65. Smith SR, Weissman NJ, Anderson CM, et al. Multicenter, placebo-controlled trial of lorcaserin for weight management. *N Engl J Med* 2010;363:245-256.
66. Fidler MC, Sanchez M, Raether B, et al. A one-year randomized trial of lorcaserin for weight loss in obese and overweight adults: The BLOSSOM trial. *J Clin Endocrinol Metab* 2011;96(10): 3067-3077.
67. O'Neil PM, Smith SR, Weissman NJ, et al. Randomized placebo-controlled clinical trial of lorcaserin for weight loss in type 2 diabetes mellitus: The BLOOM-DM study. *Obesity* 2012;20(7):1426-1436.
68. Halford JC, Boyland EJ, Lawton CL, et al. Serotonergic anti-obesity agents: Past experience and future prospects. *Drugs* 2011;71(17): 2247-2255.
69. Qsymia™ [package insert]. Mountain View, CA: Vivus Inc, 2014.
70. Gadde KM, Allison DB, Ryan DH, et al. Effects of low-dose, controlled-release, phentermine plus topiramate combination on weight and associated comorbidities in overweight and obese adults (CONQUER): A randomized, placebo-controlled, phase 3 trial. *Lancet* 2011;377:1341-1352.
71. Allison DB, Gadde KM, Garvey WT, et al. Controlled-release phentermine/topiramate in severely obese adults: A randomized controlled trial (EQUIP). *Obesity* 2012;20(2)330-342.
72. Contrave® [package insert]. La Jolla, CA: Orexigen Therapeutics; 2014.
73. Yanovski SZ, Yanovski JA. Naltrexone extended-release plus bupropion extended-release for treatment of obesity. *JAMA* 2015;313(12): 1213-1214.
74. Greenway FL, Fujioka K, Plodkowski RA, et al. Effect of naltrexone plus bupropion on weight loss in overweight and obese adults (COR–I): A multicentre, randomised, double-blind, placebo-controlled, phase 3 trial. *Lancet* 2010;376(9741):595-605.
75. Apovian CM, Aronne L, Rubino D, et al. A randomized, phase 3 trial of naltrexone SR/bupropion SR on weight and obesity-related risk factors (COR-II). *Obesity* 2013;21:935-943.
76. Wadden TA, Foreyt JP, Foster GD, et al. Weight loss with naltrexone SR/bupropion SR combination therapy as an adjunct to behavior modification: The COR–BMOD Trial. *Obesity (Silver Spring)* 2011; 19(1):110-120.
77. Hollander P, Gupta AK, Plodkowski R, et al. Effects of naltrexone sustained-release/bupropion sustained-release combination therapy on body weight and glycemic parameters in overweight and obese patients with type 2 diabetes. *Diabetes Care* 2013;36:4022-4029.
78. Saxenda [package insert]. Plainsboro, NJ: Novo Nordisk Inc; 2014.
79. Pi-Sunyer X, Astrup A, Fujioka K, et al. A randomized, controlled trial of 3.0 mg of liraglutide in weight management. *N Engl J Med* 2015;373:11-22.
80. Davies MJ, Bergenstal R, Bode B, et al. Efficacy of liraglutide for weight loss among patients with type 2 diabetes: The SCALE diabetes trial. *JAMA* 2015;314(7):687-699.
81. Bray GA, Ryan DH. Update on obesity pharmacotherapy. *Ann N Y Acad Sci* 2014;1311:1-13.
82. Silverstone T. Appetite suppressants: A review. *Drugs* 1992;43(6): 820-836.
83. Adipex-P (phentermine hydrochloride) product information. Horsham, PA: Teva Pharmaceuticals, 2015.
84. Li Z, Maglione M, Tu W, et al. Meta-analysis: pharmacologic treatment of obesity. *Ann Intern Med.* 2005;142(7):532-546.
85. Halford JC, Harrold JA, Boyland EJ, Lawton CL, Blundell JE. Serotonergic drugs: Effects on appetite expression and use for the treatment of obesity. *Drugs* 2007;67(1):27-55.
86. Ye Z, Chen L, Yang Z, et al. Metabolic effects of fluoxetine in adults with type 2 diabetes mellitus: A meta-analysis of randomized placebo-controlled trials. *PLoS One* 2011;6(7):e21551.
87. Bostwick JM, Brown TM. A toxic reaction from combining fluoxetine and phentermine. *J Clin Psychopharmacol* 1996;16(2):189-190.
88. Anchors M. Fluoxetine is a safer alternative to fenfluramine in the medical treatment of obesity. *Arch Intern Med* 1997;157(11):1270.
89. Whigham LD, Dhurandhar NV, Rahko PS, Atkinson RL. Comparison of combinations of drugs for treatment of obesity: Body weight and echocardiographic status. *Int J Obes* 2007;31(5):850-857.
90. James WPT, Caterson ID, Coutinho W, et al. Effect of sibutramine on cardiovascular outcomes in overweight and obese subjects. *N Engl J Med* 2010;363(10):905-917.
91. Pillitteri JL, Shiffman S, Rohay JM, et al. Use of dietary supplements for weight loss in the United States: results of a national survey. *Obesity* 2008;16(4):790-796.
92. Cohen PA. American roulette: Contaminated dietary supplements. *N Engl J Med* 2009;361(16):1523-1525.
93. Bhamani M, Eftekhari Z, Saki K, et al. Obesity phytotherapy: Review of native herbs used in traditional medicine for obesity. J Evid Based Complementary Altern Med August 12, 2015;
94. Marquez R, Babio N, Bullo M, Salas-Salvado J. Evaluation of the safety and efficacy of hydroxycitric acid or Garcinia cambogia extracts in humans. *Crit Rev Food Sci Nutr* 2012;52(7)585-594.
95. Yazdi FT, Clee SM, Meyre D. Obesity genetics in mouse and human: back and forth, and back again. *Peer J* 2015; DOI 10.7717/peerj.856.
96. Farooqi IS, Matarese G, Lord GM, et al. Beneficial effects of leptin on obesity, T cell hyporesponsiveness, and neuroendocrine/metabolic dysfunction of human congenital leptin deficiency. *J Clin Invest* 2002; 110(8):1093-1103.

Index

Page numbers followed by *f*, *t*, or *b* indicate figures, tables, or clinical presentation boxes, respectively.

B

E

INDEX

M

INDEX

O

INDEX